D1037410

FOURTH EDITION

GREENFIELD'S SURGERY

SCIENTIFIC PRINCIPLES AND PRACTICE

FOURTH EDITION

GREENFIELD'S SURGERY

SCIENTIFIC PRINCIPLES AND PRACTICE

Editors

Michael W. Mulholland, MD, PhD
Frederick A. Coller Distinguished Professor
Surgeon-in-Chief
Chairman, Department of Surgery
University of Michigan
Ann Arbor, Michigan

Keith D. Lillemoe, MD
Jay L. Grosfeld Professor and Chairman
Department of Surgery
Indiana University School of Medicine
Surgeon-in-Chief
Indiana University Hospital
Indianapolis, Indiana

Gerard M. Doherty, MD
N.W. Thompson Professor of Surgery
Head, Section of General Surgery
Chief, Division of Endocrine Surgery
University of Michigan
Ann Arbor, Michigan

Ronald V. Maier, MD
Jane and Donald Trunkey Professor
and Vice-Chairman of Surgery
University of Washington
Surgeon-in-Chief
Harborview Medical Center
Seattle, Washington

Gilbert R. Upchurch, Jr., MD
Associate Professor of Surgery
Leland Ira Doan Research Professor of
Vascular Surgery
Department of Surgery
University of Michigan
Ann Arbor, Michigan

With 216 contributors

Illustrations by Holly R. Fischer, MFA

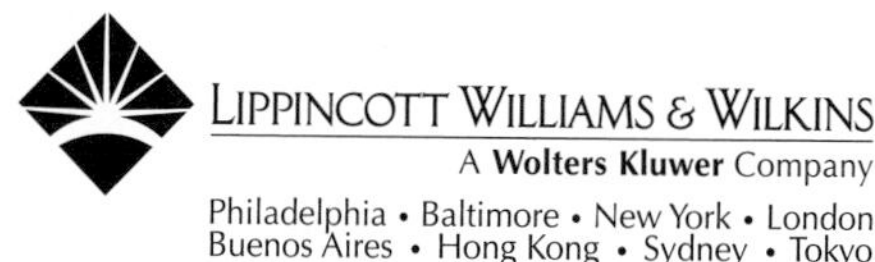

Philadelphia • Baltimore • New York • London
Buenos Aires • Hong Kong • Sydney • Tokyo

Acquisitions Editor: Brian Brown
Managing Editor: Julia Seto
Developmental Editor: Grace Caputo, Dovetail Content Solutions
Production Manager: Bridgett Dougherty
Senior Manufacturing Manager: Benjamin Rivera
Associate Director of Marketing: Adam Glazer
Design Coordinator: Doug Smock
Production Services: Nesbitt Graphics, Inc.
Printer: RR Donnelley

© 2006 by LIPPINCOTT WILLIAMS & WILKINS

530 Walnut Street
Philadelphia, PA 19106 USA
LWW.com

All rights reserved. This book is protected by copyright. No part of this book may be reproduced in any form or by any means, including photocopying, or utilized by any information storage and retrieval system without written permission from the copyright owner, except for brief quotations embodied in critical articles and reviews. Materials appearing in this book prepared by individuals as part of their official duties as U.S. government employees are not covered by the above-mentioned copyright.

Printed in the USA

0-7817-5624-3
Library of Congress Cataloging-in-Publication Data
Available upon request

Care has been taken to confirm the accuracy of the information presented and to describe generally accepted practices. However, the authors, editors, and publisher are not responsible for errors or omissions or for any consequences from application of the information in this book and make no warranty, expressed or implied, with respect to the currency, completeness, or accuracy of the contents of the publication. Application of this information in a particular situation remains the professional responsibility of the practitioner.

The authors, editors, and publisher have exerted every effort to ensure that drug selection and dosage set forth in this text are in accordance with current recommendations and practice at the time of publication. However, in view of ongoing research, changes in government regulations, and the constant flow of information relating to drug therapy and drug reactions, the reader is urged to check the package insert for each drug for any change in indications and dosage and for added warnings and precautions. This is particularly important when the recommended agent is a new or infrequently employed drug.

Some drugs and medical devices presented in this publication have Food and Drug Administration (FDA) clearance for limited use in restricted research settings. It is the responsibility of the health care provider to ascertain the FDA status of each drug or device planned for use in their clinical practice.

To purchase additional copies of this book, call our customer service department at (800) 639 -3030 or fax orders to (301) 824-7390. International customers should call (301) 714-2324.

Visit Lippincott Williams & Wilkins on the Internet: at LWW.com. Lippincott Williams & Wilkins customer service representatives are available from 8:30 am to 6pm, EST.

10 9 8 7 6 5 4 3 2 1

CONTRIBUTING AUTHORS

Keith D. Aaronson, MD
Associate Professor
Department of Internal Medicine
Division of Cardiovascular Medicine
University of Michigan
Ann Arbor, Michigan

N. Scott Adzick, MD
Surgeon in Chief
Department of Surgery
Children's Hospital of Philadelphia
Philadelphia, Pennsylvania

Steven A. Ahrendt, MD
Associate Professor and Director
Section of Gastrointestinal Surgery
Department of Surgery and Pathology
University of Rochester
Rochester, New York

John J. Aiken, MD
Associate Professor of Pediatric Surgery
Medical College of Wisconsin
Milwaukee, Wisconsin

Dana K. Anderson, MD
Professor
Department of Surgery
University of Massachusetts
Worcester, Massachusetts

Saman Arbabi, MD, MPH
Assistant Professor of Surgery
Section of General Surgery
Division of Trauma Burn Critical Care
University of Michigan
Ann Arbor, Michigan

J. Pablo Arnoletti, MD
Assistant Professor of Surgery
University of Alabama at Birmingham
Birmingham, Alabama

Subodh Arora, MD
Associate Professor of Surgery
George Washington University
Washington, DC

Massimo Asolati, MD
Assistant Professor of Surgery
University of Texas Southwestern Medical Center at Dallas
Staff Surgeon, Surgical Service
VA North Texas Health Care Center
Dallas, Texas

Ali Azizzadeh, MD
Assistant Professor
Cardiothoracic and Vascular Surgery
University of Texas at Houston Medical School
Medical Director, Vascular Laboratory, Staff Vascular Surgeon
Memorial Hermann Hospital
Houston, Texas

Ariel L. Barkan, MD
Professor of Medicine and Neurosurgery
University of Michigan
Ann Arbor, Michigan

Barbara L. Bass, MD
Professor
Department of Surgery
Weill Medical College of Cornell University
Ithaca, New York;
Carolyn and John F. Bookout Chair
Department of Surgery
The Methodist Hospital
Houston, Texas

B. Timothy Baxter, MD
Department of Surgery
University of Nebraska Medical Center
Methodist Hospital
Omaha Medical Center
Omaha, Nebraska

Michael Belkin, MD
Associate Professor of Surgery
Harvard Medical School
Chief, Division of Vascular and Endovascular Surgery
Brigham and Women's Hospital
Boston, Massachusetts

Timothy R. Billiar, MD
The George Vance Foster Professor and Chair
Department of Surgery
Presbyterian University Hospital
University of Pittsburgh Medical Center
Pittsburgh, Pennsylvania

John D. Birkmeyer, MD
George D. Zuidema Professor of Surgery
Section of General Surgery
University of Michigan
Ann Arbor, Michigan

C. Richard Boland, MD
Chief, Division of Gastroenterology
Baylor University Medical Center
Dallas, Texas

Steven F. Bolling, MD
Professor of Medicine
Professor of Surgery, Section of Cardiac Surgery
Gayle Halperin Kahn Professor of Integrative Medicine
University of Michigan
Ann Arbor, Michigan

Edward L. Bove, MD
Helen and Marvin Kirsch Professor
Professor and Section Head, Cardiac Surgery
C.S. Mott Children's Hospital
Ann Arbor, Michigan

Scott M. Bradley, MD
Professor of Surgery
Department of Surgery
Chief, Pediatric Cardiac Surgery
Medical University of South Carolina
Charleston, South Carolina

Robert S. Bresalier, MD
Professor of Medicine
Department of Gastrointestinal Medicine and Nutrition
University of Texas, MD Anderson Cancer Center
Houston, Texas

Robert E. Bristow, MD
Associate Professor and Director
Department of Gynecology and Obstetrics
Johns Hopkins Medical Institutions
Baltimore, Maryland

Jonathan S. Bromberg, MD, PhD
Professor, Department of Surgery
Surgical Director, Kidney/Pancreast Transplantation
Recanti/Miller Transplantation Institute
The Mount Sinai Medical Center
New York, New York

David L. Brown, MD, FACS
Assistant Professor of Surgery
Division of Plastic Surgery
University of Michigan
Ann Arbor, Michigan

F. Charles Brunicardi, MD
Professor and Chairman
Michael E. DeBakey Department of Surgery
Baylor College of Medicine
Houston, Texas

Steven R. Buchman, MD
Professor, Plastic Surgery
Chief, Pediatric Plastic Surgery
Director, Craniofacial Anomalies Program
University of Michigan Health Systems
Ann Arbor, Michigan

Eileen M. Bulger, MD
Associate Professor
Department of Surgery
University of Washington School of Medicine;
Associate Director
Emergency Surgical Services
Harborview Medical Center
Seattle, Washington

Arthur L. Burnett, MD
Professor of Urology
The Johns Hopkins Hospital
Baltimore, Maryland

John L. Cameron, MD
Professor of Surgery
The Johns Hopkins University
Baltimore, Maryland

Darrell A. Campbell, Jr., MD
H. King Ransom Professor of Surgery
Chief, Office of Clinical Affairs
Division of Transplantation Surgery
University of Michigan
Ann Arbor, Michigan

Darrell L. Cass, MD
Assistant Professor
Michael E. DeBakey Department of Surgery
and Department of Pediatrics
Baylor College of Medicine
Co-Director, Texas Center for Fetal Surgery
Houston, Texas

Paul S. Cederna, MD
Associate Professor of Surgery
Department of Surgery
University of Michigan
Ann Arbor, Michigan

David Y. Chan, MD
Assistant Professor of Urology and Pathology
Director of Outpatient Urology
Johns Hopkins Medical Institution
Baltimore, Maryland

William F. Chandler, MD
Professor
Department of Neurosurgery
University of Michigan
Ann Arbor, Michigan

Andrew C. Chang, MD
Assistant Professor of Surgery
Section of Thoracic Surgery
University of Michigan
Ann Arbor, Michigan

Alfred E. Chang, MD
Hugh Cabot Professor of Surgery
Chief, Division of Surgical Oncology
University of Michigan
Ann Arbor, Michigan

Jens R. Chapman, MD
Professor of Orthopaedic Surgery
and Sports Medicine
Joint Professor of Neurologic Surgery
HansJoerg Wyss Endowed Chair
University of Washington School of Medicine
Harborview Medical Center
Seattle,Washington

Randall M. Chesnut, MD
Associate Professor, Neurosurgery
Director of Neurotrauma;
Chief, Neurosurgical Spine Service
University of Washington
Harborview Medical Center
Seattle, Washington

Kevin C. Chung, MD, MS
Associate Professor
Plastic and Reconstructive Surgery
University of Michigan
Ann Arbor, Michigan

Robert E. Cilley, MD
Professor of Surgery and Pediatrics
Penn State University College of Medicine
Milton S. Hershey Medical Center
Hershey, Pennsylvania

G. Patrick Clagett, MD
Professor and Chairman, Division of Vascular and Endovascular Surgery
Department of Surgery
Jan and Bob Pickens Distinguished Professorship in Medical Science
Director, Center for Vascular Disease
University of Texas Southwestern Medical Center
Dallas, Texas

Alexander W. Clowes, MD
Professor and Chief
Division of Vascular Surgery
Department of Surgery
University of Washington School of Medicine
Seattle, Washington

Raul Coimbra, MD, PhD
Associate Professor
Department of Surgery
University of California San Diego
Director, Surgical Intensive Care Unit
Associate Director of Trauma
Division of Trauma and Surgical Critical Care
USSD Medical Center
San Diego, California

Geoffrey Cundiff, MD
Associate Professor and Chairman
Department of Gynecology-Obstetrics
Johns Hopkins at Bay View
Baltimore, Maryland

Steven A. Curley, MD
Professor
Department of Surgical Oncology
Chief, Gastrointestinal Tumor Surgery
The University of Texas M.D. Anderson Cancer Center
Houston, Texas

Joseph Cuschieri, MD
Assistant Professor
Department of Surgery
University of Washington School of Medicine
Harborview Medical Center
Seattle, Washington

Michael C. Dalsing, MD
E. Dale and Susan E. Habeggar Professor of Surgery
Director of Vascular Surgery
Indiana University School of Medicine
Indianapolis, Indiana

David C. Dawson, PhD
Professor and Chair
Department of Physiology and Pharmacology
Oregon Health Sciences University
Portland, Oregon

E. Patchen Dellinger, MD
Professor and Vice Chairman, Surgery
Associate Medical Director and Chief of General Surgery
University of Washington School of Medicine
Seattle, Washington

Keith A. Delman, MD
Assistant Professor
Division of Surgical Oncology
Department of Surgery
Emory University School of Medicine
Attending Surgeon
Division of Surgical Oncology
Winship Cancer Institute
Emory University Hopital
Atlanta, Georgia

Eric J. DeMaria, MD
Professor and Chairman, General Surgery Division
Virginia Commonwealth University/MCV Medical Center
Director, Center for Minimally Invasive Surgery
Richmond, Virginia

Thomas R. DeMeester, MD
Professor and Chairman, Department of Surgery
Keck School of Medicine
University of Southern California
Los Angeles, California

Eric J. Devaney, MD
Assistant Professor of Surgery
Section of Cardiac Surgery
University of Michigan
Ann Arbor, Michigan

Peter W. Dillon, MD
Professor of Surgery and Pediatrics
Penn State University College of Medicine
Milton S. Hershey Medical Center
Hershey, Pennsylvania

Verdi J. DiSesa, MD
Staff Surgeon
The Cardiovascular Center at the Chester County Hospital
West Chester, Pennsylvania

Gerard M. Doherty, MD
N.W. Thompson Professor of Surgery
Head, Section of General Surgery
Chief, Division of Endocrine Surgery
University of Michigan
Ann Arbor, Michigan

Matthew J. Eagleton, MD
Assistant Professor, Vascular Surgery
Cleveland Clinic Lerner College of Medicine of Case Western Reserve University
Staff, Vascular Surgery
The Cleveland Clinic Foundation
Cleveland, Ohio

Jean C. Emond, MD
Thomas S. Zimmer Professor of Surgery
Vice Chairman and Chief of Transplantation Services
College of Physicians & Surgeons of Columbia University
New York, New York

Anthony L. Estrera, MD
Assistant Professor and Director, Cardiovascular Intensive Care Unit
Cardiothoracic and Vascular Surgery
University of Texas at Houston
Memorial Hermann Hospital
Houston, Texas

Mary E. Fallat, MD
Professor of Surgery
Department of Surgery, Division of Pediatric Surgery
University of Louisville
Chief of Surgery and Trauma
Kosair Children's Hospital
Louisville, Kentucky

Alessandro Fichera, MD
Assistant Professor of Surgery
University of Chicago
Pritzker School of Medicine
Chicago, Illinois

Neil A. Fine
Associate Professor
Department of Surgery
Northwestern University Feinberg School of Medicine
Chicago, Illinois

Robert J. Fitzgibbons, Jr., MD
Harry E. Stuckenhoff Professor of Surgery and Chief, Division of General Surgery
Department of Surgery
Creighton University Medical Center
Omaha, Nebraska

Yuman Fong, MD
Murray F. Brennan Chair in Surgery
Chief, Gastric and Mixed Tumor Service
Department of Surgery
Memorial Sloan-Kettering Cancer Center
Professor of Surgery
Cornell University Medical College
New York, New York

Douglas L. Fraker, MD
Jonathan E. Rhoads Professor of Surgery
Department of Surgery
University of Pennsylvania
Philadelphia, Pennsylvania

David C. Frankenfield, MS, RD, CNSD
Chief Clinical Dietician
Penn State College of Medicine
M.S. Hershey Medical Center
Hershey, Pennsylvania

Chris E. Freise, MD
Associate Professor of Surgery
Transplant Division
University of California, San Francisco
San Francisco, California

Eric R. Frykberg, MD
Professor of Surgery
University of Florida College of Medicine
Chief, Division of General Surgery
Shands Jacksonville Medical Center
Jacksonville, Florida

Paul G. Gauger, MD
Associate Professor of Surgery and Medical Education
University of Michigan
Ann Arbor, Michigan

Eli V. Gelfand, MD
Clinical Fellow in Medicine
Harvard Medical School
Fellow in Cardiovascular Diseases
Beth Israel Deaconess Medical Center
Boston, Massachusetts

Larry M. Gentilello, MD
Professor of Surgery
University of Texas Southwestern Medical Center
Chairman, Division of Burns, Trauma, Critical Care
Parkland Memorial Hospital
Dallas, Texas

Nicole S. Gibran, MD
Professor of Surgery
University of Washington
Director, University of Washington Burn Center
Harborview Medical Center
Seattle, Washington

Joseph Giglia, MD
Assistant Professor of Surgery
Department of Surgery
University of Cincinnati, College of Medicine;
Cincinnati, Ohio

Amy Kim Gira, MD
Lecturer
Department of Dermatology
University of Michigan
Ann Arbor, Michigan

Robert L. Giuntoli, II, MD
Assistant Professor
Department of Gynecology and Obstetrics
The Johns Hopkins Medical Institutions
Baltimore, Maryland

Thomas G. Gleason, MD
Assistant Professor of Surgery
Division of Cardiothoracic Surgery
Northwestern University
Chicago, Illinois

Toby A. Gordon, ScD
Associate Professor
Departments of Surgery and Health Policy Management
Johns Hopkins University
Baltimore, Maryland

Linda M. Graham, MD
Professor of Surgery
Cleveland Clinic Lerner College of Medicine
Staff, Department of Vascular Surgery
Cleveland Clinic Foundation,
Cleveland, Ohio

Joseph S. Gruss, MD
Professor
University of Washington
Division of Plastic Surgery
Harborview Medical Center
Seattle, Washington

John W. Hallett, Jr., MD
Clinical Professor of Surgery
Medical University of South Carolina
Medical Director
Roper Saint Francis Heart and Vascular Center
Charleston, South Carolina

Maureen Heldmann, MD
Department of Radiology
Louisiana State University Health Sciences Center in Shreveport
Shreveport, Louisiana

Peter K. Henke, MD
Associate Professor of Surgery
Section of Vascular Surgery
University of Michigan
Ann Arbor, Michigan

Jennifer C. Hirsch, MD
Instructor in Surgery
Section of Cardiac Surgery
University of Michigan
Ann Arbor, Michigan

Richard A. Hodin, MD
Associate Professor
Department of Surgery
Harvard Medical School;
Massachusetts General Hospital
Boston, Massachusetts

Julian T. Hoff, MD
Professor
Department of Neurosurgery
University of Michigan
Ann Arbor, Michigan

Richard A. Hopper, MD
Assistant Professor
University of Washington
Division of Plastic Surgery
Harborview Medical Center
Seattle, Washington

David B. Hoyt, MD
Professor
Department of Surgery
University of California, San Diego
Chief, Division of Trauma, Burns, and Surgical Critical Care
Department of Surgery
UCSD Medical Center
San Diego, California

Emina Huang, MD
Assistant Professor of Surgery
Section of General Surgery
Division of Colorectal Surgery
University of Michigan
Ann Arbor, Michigan

Thomas S. Huber, MD, PhD
Associate Professor
Department of Surgery
University of Florida College of Medicine
Staff Surgeon
Shands Hospital at the University of Florida
Gainesville, Florida

Roger D. Hurst, MD
Associate Professor
Department of Surgery
University of Chicago
Pritzker School of Medicine
Chicago, Illinois

Tam T. T. Huynh, MD
Assistant Professor
Cardiothoracic and Vascular Surgery
University of Texas at Houston Medical School
Memorial Hermann Hospital
Houston, Texas

Michael T. Jaklitsch, MD
Assistant Professor of Surgery
Harvard Medical School
Boston, Massachusetts

Marcus D. Jarboe, MD
Resident
Department of Surgery
University of Cincinnati, College of Medicine
Cincinnati, Ohio

Thomas W. Jarrett, MD
Associate Professor of Urology
Co-director, Endourology Fellowship
Chief, Division of Endourology and Laparoscopy
Johns Hopkins Medical Institutions
Baltimore, Maryland

Raymond J. Joehl, MD
Professor of Surgery, Program Director General Surgery Residency
Department of Surgery
Loyola University Medical Center
Maywood, Illinois;
Chief, Surgical Service and Manager, Surgery Service Line
The Charles B. Puestow Surgical Service
Edward Hines, Jr. VA Hospital
Hines, Illinois

Timothy M. Johnson, MD
Professor of Dermatology, Otolaryngology, and Surgery
Chief, Cutaneous Surgery and Oncology Program
University of Michigan
Ann Arbor, Michigan

Gregory J. Jurkovich, MD
Professor
Department of Surgery
University of Washington
Chief, Trauma Service
Harborview Medical Center
Seattle, Washington

Seema Khan
Associate Professor
Department of Surgery
Northwestern University Medical School
Chicago, Illinois

Larry R. Kaiser, MD
John Rhea Barton Professor and Chairman
Department of Surgery
University of Pennsylvania
Chief of Surgery
Hospital of the University of Pennsylvania
Philadelphia, Pennsylvania

Riyad Karmy-Jones, MD
Associate Professor of Surgery
University of Washington
Chief, Cardiothoracic Surgery
Harborview Medical Center
Seattle, Washington

Donald R. Kauder, MD
Associate Professor of Surgery
Vice-chief, Division of Traumatology and Surgical Critical Care
Department of Surgery
University of Pennsylvania Medical Center
Philadelphia, Pennsylvania

Lawrence T. Kim, MD
Associate Professor of Surgery
Director of Surgical Endocrinology
University of Arkansas for Medical Sciences
Chief, Surgical Service
Central Arkansas Veterans Healthcare System
Little Rock, Arkansas

Andrew S. Klein, MD, MBA
Director, Comprehensive Transplant Center
Cedars-Sinai Medical Center
Los Angeles, California

Gary B. Korus, MD
Assistant Professor of Clinical Surgery
University of Pennsylvania Health System
Philadelphia, Pennsylvania

Alexander S. Krupnick, MD
Instructor of Surgery
University of Washington School of Medicine
Seattle, Washington

James K. Kuan, MD
Acting Instructor
Department of Urology
University of Washington
Attending Department of Urology
Harborview Medical Center
Seattle, Washington

John C. Kucharczuk, MD
Assistant Professor of Surgery
University of Pennsylvania
Philadelphia, Pennsylvania

William M. Kuzon, MD
Professor and Section Head, Plastic Surgery
University of Michigan
Ann Arbor, Michigan

John S. Lane, MD
Assistant Professor
Department of Surgery
UCSF Division of Vascular Surgery;
Chief, Vascular Surgery
Department of Surgery
San Francisco General Hospital
San Francisco, California

Michael P. LaQuaglia, MD
Professor and Chief
Pediatric Surgery
Memorial-Sloan Kettering Cancer Center
New York, New York

Martin LeBoutillier, III, MD
Staff Surgeon
The Cardiovascular Center at the Chester County Hospital
West Chester, Pennsylvania

W. Anthony Lee, MD
Assistant Professor, Vascular Surgery
Department of Surgery
University of Florida College of Medicine
Gainesville, Florida

Jean-Christophe Leveque, MD
Clinical Instructor
Department of Neurosurgery
University of Michigan
Ann Arbor, Michigan

Steven K. Libutti, MD
Senior Investigator
Surgery Branch, Center for Cancer Research
National Cancer Institute
Bethesda, Maryland

Keith D. Lillemoe, MD
Jay L. Grosfeld Professor and Chairman
Department of Surgery
Indiana University School of Medicine
Surgeon-in-Chief
Indiana University Hospital
Indianapolis, Indiana

Ricardo V. Lloyd, MD, PhD
Professor of Pathology
Mayo Clinic College of Medicine
Consultant at Mayo Clinic
Rochester, Minnesota

Robert D. Madoff, MD
Professor of Surgery
University of Minnesota
Minneapolis, Minnesota

John C. Magee, MD
Associate Professor of Surgery
Section of General Surgery
Division of Transplantation Surgery
University of Michigan
Ann Arbor, Michigan

David K. Magnuson, MD
Assistant Professor of Surgery and Pediatrics
Case Western Reserve University
Chief, Division of Pediatric Surgery
Rainbow Babies & Children's Hospital
Cleveland, Ohio

Ronald V. Maier, MD
Jane and Donald Trunkey Professor and Vice-Chairman of Surgery
University of Washington
Surgeon-in-Chief
Harborview Medical Center
Seattle, Washington

Jocelyne Martin, MD, MSc, FRCSC
Assistant Professor, Department of Surgery
Université de Montréal
Thoracic Surgeon
Department of Surgery
CHUM–Hôpital Notre–Dame
Montréal, Quebec, Canada

Michael R. Marvin, MD
Assistant Professor of Surgery
Westchester Medical Center
New York Medical College
Hawthorne, New York

Jeffrey B. Matthews, MD
Christian R. Holmes Professor and Chairman
Department of Surgery
University of Cincinnati
Chief of Surgery
Department of Surgery
University Hospital
Cincinnati, Ohio

Matthew T. Menard, MD
Co-Director of Endovascular Surgery
Division of Vascular and Endovascular Surgery
Brigham and Women's Hospital
Instructor in Surgery
Harvard Medical School
Boston, Massachusetts

Robert M. Merion, MD
Professor of Surgery
Department of Surgery
University of Michigan
Attending Surgeon
Division of Transplantation
University of Michigan
Ann Arbor, Michigan

Louis M. Messina, MD
Professor and Chief of Vascular Surgery
University of California, San Francisco
San Francisco, California

Fabrizio Michelassi, MD
Lewis Atterbury Stimson Professor of Surgery
Chairman, Department of Surgery, Weill Medical College of Cornell University
Surgeon-in-Chief, New York Presbyterian Hospital-Weill Cornell Medical Center
New York, New York

Charles C. Miller, III, PhD
Professor
Cardiothoracic and Vascular Surgery
Center for Clinical Research and Evidence-Based Medicine
Center for Biotechnology
University of Texas at Houston Medical School
Houston, Texas

Eugene Minevich, MD
Assistant Professor
Department of Surgery
Division of Pediatric Urology
University of Cincinnati
Pediatric Urologist
Cincinnati Childrens Hospital Medical Center
Cincinnati, Ohio

R. Scott Mitchell, MD
Professor of Cardiovascular Surgery
Stanford School of Medicine
Stanford, California

H. David Moehring, MD
Professor
Department of Orthopaedic Surgery
University of California, Davis School of Medicine
Sacramento, California

Susan D. Moffatt-Bruce, MD, PhD
Cardiothoracic Fellow
Stanford University Medical Center
Stanford, California

Ernesto P. Molmenti, MD, PhD, MBA
Professor and Chief, Section of Abdominal Transplantation
Department of Surgery
University of Arizona College of Medicine
Tucson, Arizona

Arden M. Morris, MD
Assistant Professor of Surgery
Section of General Surgery
Division of Colorectal Surgery
University of Michigan
Ann Arbor, Michigan

Monica Morrow, MD
Chairman
G. Willing Pepper Chair in Cancer Research
Department of Surgery
Fox Chase Cancer Center
Professor of Surgery
Temple University School of Medicine
Philadelphia, Pennsylvania

Ralph S. Mosca, MD
Associate Professor of Surgery
Columbia University College of Physicians and Surgeons
Associate Attending Surgeon
New York-Presbyterian Hospital/Columbia University Medical Center
New York, New York

Jeffrey S. Moyer, MD
Assistant Professor
Department of Otolaryngology–Head and Neck Surgery
University of Michigan
Ann Arbor, Michigan

Michael W. Mulholland, MD, PhD
Frederick A. Coller Distinguished Professor
Surgeon-in-Chief
Chairman, Department of Surgery
University of Michigan
Ann Arbor, Michigan

Joseph T. Murphy, MD
Associate Professor of Surgery
University of Texas Southwestern Medical School
Dallas, Texas

Thomas A. Mustoe, MD
Chief of Plastic Surgery
Department of Surgery
Feinberg School of Medicine
Northwestern University
Chicago, Illinois

Attila Nakeeb, MD
Associate Professor
Department of Surgery
Indiana University
Attending Surgeon
Indiana University Hospital
Indianapolis, Indiana

Avery B. Nathens, MD, PhD, MPH
Associate Professor of Surgery
University of Washington School of Medicine
Director, Surgical Critical Care Service
Division of General Surgery and Trauma
Harborview Medical Center
Seattle, Washington

Santhat Nivatvongs, MD
Professor of Surgery
Mayo Clinic College of Medicine
Rochester, Minnesota

Richard G. Ohye, MD
Assistant Professor, Departments of Surgery and Pediatrics and Communicable Diseases
Surgical Director, Pediatric Cardiac Transplantation
Director, Pediatric Cardiovascular Surgery Fellowship Program
University of Michigan
Ann Arbor, Michigan

Grant E. O'Keefe, MD
Associate Professor of Surgery
Department of Surgery
University of Washington School of Medicine
Surgeon
Harborview Medical Center
Seattle, Washington

Keith T. Oldham, MD
Surgeon in Chief and Marie Z. Uihlein Chair
Department of Pediatric Surgery
Medical College of Wisconsin
Milwaukee, Wisconsin

John A. Olson, Jr., MD, PhD
Associate Professor
Department of Surgery
Duke University
Durham, North Carolina

Mary F. Otterson, MD
Associate Professor of Surgery
Minimally Invasive Gastrointestinal Surgery
Medical College of Wisconsin
Milwaukee, Wisconsin

C. Keith Ozaki, MD
Associate Professor
Vascular Surgery
Department of Surgery
University of Florida College of Medicine
Gainesville, Florida

Francis D. Pagani, MD, PhD
Associate Professor of Surgery
Section of Cardiac Surgery
University of Michigan
Ann Arbor, Michigan

Jeffrey H. Peters, MD
Seymour I. Schwartz Professor and Chairman
Department of Surgery
University of Rochester School of Medicine and Dentistry
Rochester, New York

Robin N. Pierson, III, MD
Associate Professor of Surgery
Department of Surgery
University of Maryland Medical Center
Clinical Director, Heart and Lung Transplantation
Department of Surgery
University of Maryland Medical Center and Baltimore VAMC
Baltimore, Maryland

Henry A. Pitt, MD
Professor and Vice Chairman
Department of Surgery
Indiana University
Indianapolis, Indiana

Eyal E. Porat, MD
Assistant Professor
Cardiothoracic and Vascular Surgery
University of Texas at Houston Medical School
Director, Minimally Invasive Surgery and Robotics Program
Memorial Herman Hospital
Houston, Texas

Jeffrey D. Punch, MD
Associate Professor of Surgery
Section of General Surgery
Chief, Division of Transplantation Surgery
University of Michigan
Ann Arbor, Michigan

Thomas H. Quinn, PhD
Professor of Biomedical Science and Surgery
Creighton University School of Medicine
Omaha, Nebraska

Steven E. Raper, MD
Associate Professor
Department of Surgery
University of Pennsylvania
Surgeon
Department of Surgery
Hospital of the University of Pennsylvania
Philadelphia, Pennsylvania

Todd E. Rasmussen, MD
Assistant Professor of Surgery
Uniformed Services University of Health Sciences
Bethesda, Maryland
Chief of Vascular Surgery
Wilford Hall USAF Medical Center
Lackland Air Force Base, Texas

Daniel J. Reddy, MD
D. Emerick and Eve Szilagyi Chair in Vascular Surgery
Henry Ford Hospital
Detroit, Michigan

Taylor Sohn Riall, MD
Assistant Professor
Department of Surgery
University of Texas Medical Branch
Galveston, Texas

Alan T. Richards, MD
Associate Professor and Attending Surgeon
Creighton University Medical Center
Omaha, Nebraska

Ronald Rodriguez, MD, PhD
Assistant Professor of Urology, Medical Oncology, and Cellular and Molecular Medicine
Johns Hopkins Medical Institutions
Baltimore, Maryland

Matthew R. Rosengart, MD
Assistant Professor
Department of Surgery
University of Pittsburgh School of Medicine
Pittsburgh, Pennsylvania

M. L. Chip Routt, Jr., MD
Professor
Department of Orthopaedic Surgery
University of Washington
Harborview Medical Center
Seattle, Washington

Grace S. Rozycki, MD
Professor and Vice Chair
Department of Surgery
Emory University School of Medicine
Director, Trauma/Surgical Critical Care
Grady Memorial Hospital
Atlanta, Georgia

Valerie W. Rusch, MD
Chief, Thoracic Service
Department of Surgery
Memorial-Sloan Kettering Cancer Center
Professor of Surgery
Cornell University Medical College
New York, New York

Timothy W. Rutter, MD
Associate Professor
Department of Anesthesiology
University of Michigan
Ann Arbor, Michigan

Michael S. Sabel, MD
Assistant Professor of Surgery
Division of Surgical Oncology
University of Michigan
Ann Arbor, Michigan

Hazim J. Safi, MD
Professor and Chairman
Cardiothoracic and Vascular Surgery
The University of Texas at Houston Medical School
UTH Medical Center
Houston, Texas

Sergio X. Salles-Cunha, MD
Jobst Vascular Center
Toledo, Ohio

Isaac Samuel, MD
Assistant Professor of Surgery
Department of Surgery
Roy J. and Lucille A. Carver College of Medicine
University of Iowa
Iowa City, Iowa

George Andrew Sarosi, Jr., MD
Assistant Professor
Department of Surgery
University of Texas Southwestern Medical Center at Dallas
Assistant Chief, Surgical Service
VA North Texas Health Center
Dallas, Texas

Thomas T. Sato, MD
Associate Professor of Pediatric Surgery
Medical College of Wisconsin
Children's Hospital of Wisconsin
Milwaukee, Wisconsin

Mandeep S. Saund, MBBS, MS
Instructor in Surgery
Harvard Medical School
Staff Surgeon
Department of Surgery
Brigham and Women's Hospital
Boston, Massachusetts

David W. Scaff, DO
Instructor of Surgery
Department of Surgery
Division of Traumatology & Surgical Clinical Care
University of Pennsylvania
Philadelphia, Pennsylvania

Richard D. Schulick, MD
Associate Professor of Surgery, Oncology, Gynecology and Obstetrics
Johns Hopkins Medical Institutions
Baltimore, Maryland

C. William Schwab, MD
Professor
Department of Surgery
University of Pennsylvania School of Medicine
Hospital of the University of Pennsylvania
Philadelphia, Pennsylvania

James M. Seeger, MD
Professor and Chief, Vascular Surgery
Associate Chair, Department of Surgery
University of Florida College of Medicine
Gainesville, Florida

Neal E. Seymour, MD
Associate Professor of Surgery
Department of Surgery
Tufts University School of Medicine
Chief, Division of General Surgery
Department of Surgery
Baystate Medical Center
Springfield, Massachusetts

Steven R. Shackford, MD
Professor and Chairman
Department of Surgery
College of Medicine, University of Vermont
Burlington, Vermont

Curtis A. Sheldon, MD
Professor of Surgery
Cincinnati's Children Hospital Medical Center
Cincinnati, Ohio

Alexander D. Shepard, MD
Senior Staff Surgeon
Henry Ford Hospital
Detroit, Michigan

Anton N. Sidawy, MD, MPH
Chief, Surgical Service
VA Medical Center
Professor of Surgery
George Washington and Georgetown Universities
Washington, DC

Diane M. Simeone, MD
Associate Professor of Surgery
Section of General Surgery
University of Michigan
Ann Arbor, Michigan

Niten Singh, MD, MS
Assistant Professor of Surgery
Uniformed Services University of the Health Sciences
Georgetown/Washington Hospital Center
Washington, DC

Michael J. Sise, MD
Medical Director, Trauma
Scripps Mercy Hospital
San Diego, California

J. Stanley Smith, Jr., MD
Professor of Surgery
Department of Surgery
Pennsylvania State University College of Medicine
Professor
Department of Surgery
M.S. Hershey Medical Center
Hershey, Pennsylvania

Wiley W. Souba, MD, DSc, MBA
John A. Waldhausen Professor of Surgery
Pennsylvania State University College of Medicine
Chair, Department of Surgery
M.S. Hershey Medical Center
Hershey, Pennsylvania

David I. Soybel, MD
Associate Professor of Surgery
Harvard Medical School
Staff Surgeon
Department of Surgery
Brigham & Women's Hospital
Boston, Massachusetts

Martinus T. Spoor, MD
Instructor
Section of Cardiac Surgery
University of Michigan
Ann Arbor, Michigan

Sunita D. Srivastava, MD
Assistant Professor
Section of Vascular Surgery, Department of Surgery
Cleveland Clinic Lerner College of Medicine of Case Western University
Staff, Department of Vascular Surgery
The Cleveland Clinic Foundation
Cleveland, Ohio

James C. Stanley, MD
Handleman Professor of Surgery
Section of Vascular Surgery
Department of Surgery
University of Michigan
Ann Arbor, Michigan

Peter Stock, MD
Professor
Department of Surgery
University of California, San Francisco
UCSF Hospital
San Francisco, California

David J. Sugarbaker, MD
Professor of Surgery
Brigham & Women's Hospital
Division of Thoracic Surgery
Boston, Massachusetts

Randall S. Sung, MD
Assistant Professor of Surgery
Department of General Surgery, Transplantation Division
University of Michigan
Ann Arbor, Michigan

John F. Sweeney, MD
Associate Professor of Surgery
Chief, Division of General Surgery
Michael E. DeBakey Department of Surgery
Baylor College of Medicine
Houston, Texas

Theodoros N. Teknos, MD
Associate Professor
Department of Otolaryngology–Head and Neck Surgery
Chief
Division of Head and Neck Surgery
University of Michigan
Ann Arbor, Michigan

Jason Thompson, MD
Clinical Instructor
Department of Orthopaedic Surgery and Sports Medicine
Harborview Medical Center
Seattle, Washington

Kevin K. Tremper, MD
Professor and Chair
Department of Anesthesiology
University of Michigan
Ann Arbor, Michigan

Richard H. Turnage, MD
Professor and Chair
Department of Surgery
Louisana State University Health Science Center
Shreveport, Louisiana

Douglas J. Turner, MD
Assistant Professor
Department of Surgery
University of Maryland
Baltimore, Maryland

Gilbert R. Upchurch, Jr., MD
Associate Professor of Surgery
Leland Ira Doan Research Professor of Vascular Surgery
Department of Surgery
University of Michigan
Ann Arbor, Michigan

Selwyn M. Vickers, MD
Professor and Chairman
Section of Gastrointestinal Surgery
Department of Surgery
University of Alabama at Birmingham
Birmingham, Alabama

Richard B. Wait, MD, PhD, FACS
Clinical Professor of Surgery
Department of Surgery
Tuft's University School of Medicine
Boston, Massachusetts
Chairman of Surgery
Department of Surgery
Baystate Medical Center
Springfield, Massachusetts

Thomas W. Wakefield, MD
S. Martin Lindenauer Professor of Surgery
Department of Surgery, Section of Vascular Surgery
University of Michigan
Ann Arbor, Michigan

Thomas J. Watson, MD
Assistant Professor
University of Rochester
Department of Surgery
Rochester, New York

Sharon Weber, MD
Assistant Professor
Department of Surgery
Section of Surgical Oncology
University of Wisconsin
Chief of Surgery
William S. Middleton Veterans Hospital
Madison, Wisconsin

Hunter Wessells, MD
Professor
Department of Urology
University of Washington
Chief
Department of Urology
Harborview Medical Center
Seattle, Washington

Edward E. Whang, MD
Assistant Professor of Surgery
Dpeartment of Surgery
Brigham and Women's Hospital
Harvard Medical School
Boston, Massachusetts

Edwin G. Wilkins, MD, MS
Associate Professor of Surgery
Section of Plastic Surgery
University of Michigan
Ann Arbor, Michigan

John A. Williams, MD, PhD
Professor and Chair, Department of Physiology
University of Michigan
Ann Arbor, Michigan

David H. Wisner, MD
Vice-Chair and Professor
Department of Surgery
University of California Davis
Sacramento, California

James S. T. Yao, MD, PhD
Professor of Surgery
Division of Vascular Surgery
Feinberg School of Medicine, Northwestern University
Chicago, Illinois

Charles J. Yeo, MD
Professor and Chairman—Department of Surgery
Jefferson Medical College
Chief, Division of General and Gastrointestinal Surgery
Thomas Jefferson University Hospital
Philadelphia, Pennsylvania

Gerald B. Zelenock, MD
Chief of Surgery
Department of Surgery
William Beaumont Hospital
Royal Oak, Michigan

Lambros Zellos, MD
Instructor
Department of Surgery
Brigham and Women's Hospital
Boston, Massachusetts

FOREWORD

It has been fourteen years since Michael Mulholland and I developed our concept of a contemporary textbook of surgery that would cover the broad field of surgery in a manner that attracted the full spectrum of readers from students to residents, teachers, and practitioners. First and foremost, we wanted to integrate the basic sciences and clinical practice. By selecting younger authors who were actively contributing new knowledge to the field, we were assured of a fresh, forward-looking approach to each subject. We recognized the importance of imagery in visualizing concepts, and selected one artistic style for consistency in illustrations. The result was the first edition in 1993 of *Surgery: Scientific Principles and Practice*. The response exceeded our expectations. In two succeeding editions, we continued to add improvements and introduce new authors without deviating from our original vision and mission. Now, for the fourth edition, the same logic that acknowledges the value of change leads us to a seamless transition of editorial responsibilities. In addition to Drs. Mulholland and Lillemoe's new position as Editors-in-Chief, the new editorial team adds Gerard Doherty, Ronald Maier, and Gilbert Upchurch, Jr., who have established themselves as leaders in their fields with a broad view of the discipline of surgery.

We are taught not to judge a book by its appearance, but appearances do count. This edition adds color to the illustrations throughout, and new teaching tools. Particularly helpful will be the inclusion of decision-making algorithms in the practice chapters and summary Key Points for each chapter.

We are also taught that we stand on the shoulders of our predecessors. From my perspective, we predecessors have the advantage as we look up to the next generation of surgeons with admiration and full confidence that the art, knowledge, and craft of surgery will continue to evolve.

Lazar J. Greenfield, MD

PREFACE

The editors are pleased to present the fourth edition of *Greenfield's Surgery: Scientific Principles and Practice*. The past decade has witnessed an explosive growth in the knowledge base of clinical surgery. Surgical practice is being transformed through advancements in physiologic and cellular investigation, integration of new techniques and concepts from molecular biology into patient care, and the emerging field of bioinformation. The rapidly accelerating pace of scientific progress has demanded an adoption of new ideas into surgical therapy and a commitment to lifelong learning. Accordingly, the new edition of Surgery seeks to integrate new scientific knowledge with evolving changes in surgical care.

The fourth edition has been enhanced in every way, with dramatic changes to the book's editorial board, authorship, content, organization, and visual presentation. The first three editions of *Surgery: Scientific Principles and Practice* were guided by Lazar J. Greenfield, MD. His perceptive wisdom helped to create a truly unique book that is the basis of the latest iteration. As his name moves from the list of editors to the book's title, we thank him for his continuing help and welcome three new associate editors—Gerard M. Doherty, MD, Ronald V. Maier, MD, and Gilbert R. Upchurch, Jr., MD. Their energy and new perspectives have invigorated this volume.

We have elicited contributions from well over 200 authors, all chosen because of their scientific sophistication. Each contributor is currently an active practitioner in the field of surgery. Moreover, many have presented seminal articles and developed the new concepts in their disciplines that are featured in the text. An excellent example is the new chapter "Quality Assessment in Surgery." Several more chapters are also debuting in this edition, including "Terrorism," "Fetal Intervention," and "Vascular Diagnostics."

Organizationally, trauma and transplantation are now in the form of separate sections rather than subdivided chapters. The content within each has been presented as individual chapters in appreciation of the significance of each topic. Elsewhere, related topics have been combined into a single chapter (e.g., "Renal Artery Occlusive and Aneurysmal Disease") to avoid duplication of content.

Perhaps the most obvious change is the book's appearance. The design has been overhauled inside and out to create a text that not only looks better but also *works* better. The text has gone from only two colors—blue and black—to a full range of hues, creating both more immediate visual impact and more opportunity to convey information quickly and with greater meaning. As part of our continuing commitment to superb medical art, line drawings—almost all created by a single artist—have been enhanced with full-color highlighting, ensuring a presentation that maximizes teaching effectiveness and clinical utility. In addition, color photographs have been used liberally within the chapters, with special emphasis on pathologic findings. More than 60 individually numbered decision-making algorithms are featured throughout the book to provide diagnostic and management information in a simplified format (these can be easily located using the list that follows the Contents). Many tables now carry classification bars, such as Diagnosis or Results, useful both when scanning the text for information and when accessing the book's contents digitally. To aid review, each chapter ends with a list of the Key Points covered therein, and the most important articles and chapters on the topic are highlighted in the reference list. We believe that even small additions, such as the color-coded tabs in the right margin, will improve the utility and readability of this edition of *Surgery*.

This edition is highly integrated with a new electronic format to provide supplemental educational material. These materials include review questions for reinforcement of concepts and for board examination preparation. Access to supplemental text and journal content produced by Lippincott Williams & Wilkins is an additional advantage of this electronic integration.

In three editions, *Surgery: Scientific Principles and Practice* has become a standard text in the field. We believe that with the many improvements implemented in this fourth edition—color art throughout, user-oriented design, new pedagogical features, increased electronic accessibility, and, most important, updated and improved content—it will soon be the text by which all other surgery texts are judged.

Michael W. Mulholland, M.D., Ph.D.

DEDICATION

We dedicate this book to our mentors, residents, and students, who challenge and inspire us daily, and to our families, our best and truest supporters.

To my family: Patricia, Erin, Kevin, Katie, and Brenna.

—M.W.M.

To my wife, Cheryl, and children, Chris, Shannon, Becky, and Heather, for your love and support.

—K.D.L.

To my wonderful family: Faith, Kevin, and Megan.

—G.M.D.

To Lauren, Michael, and Anna, for all you sacrifice for me.

—R.V.M.

To my wife, Nancy, who provided me with the extra time to work on this book, and to my boys, Rivers, Walker, and Joe, who help me to focus on the thing that is most important in my life—my family. And to my parents, Gilbert R. Upchurch, Sr., and Mary Anne Upchurch, who always encouraged me to pursue medicine and made it possible for me to do so.

—G.R.U.

ACKNOWLEDGMENTS

We gratefully acknowledge our surgical patients, past and future, whom we are privileged to serve.

I express my appreciation for the efforts of the contributing authors, whose scholarship makes this work possible. We have been fortunate to maintain a happy working relationship with our publisher, Lippincott Williams & Wilkins, and I wish to specifically acknowledge the support of Brian Brown as acquisitions editor and Grace Caputo as developmental editor.

—M.W.M.

My gratitude to John Cameron, M.D., who provided me with the opportunity for success in academic surgery, and to The Johns Hopkins Hospital and Indiana University surgical house staff for providing the constant stimulus for greater achievement.

—K.D.L.

I appreciate the efforts of the faculties and residents at the University of Michigan, Washington University, and UCSF with whom I have had the privilege to work.

—G.M.D.

Thanks to the housestaff and students, whose dedication, inquisitiveness, and challenges provide the stimulus and rewards for this effort.

—R.V.M.

I am grateful to the long line of academic surgeons I have been fortunate enough to be trained by and work for. They include George Johnson, Jr., George Sheldon, John Mannick, Anthony D. Whittemore, Mike Belkin, Lazar Greenfield, Michael Mulholland, and James C. Stanley.

—G.R.U.

CONTENTS

PART ONE ■ SCIENTIFIC PRINCIPLES

PART TWO ■ SURGICAL PRACTICE

SECTION A ■ TRAUMA

Background to Trauma Care

Initial Care Phase

Definitive Care Phase

PART TWO ■ SURGICAL PRACTICE

SECTION G ■ PANCREAS

SECTION H ■ HEPATOBILIARY AND PORTAL VENOUS SYSTEM

SECTION I ■ COLON, RECTUM, AND ANUS

PART TWO ■ SURGICAL PRACTICE

LIST OF ALGORITHMS

PART ONE
SCIENTIFIC PRINCIPLES

CHAPTER 1 ■ CELL STRUCTURE AND FUNCTION

JOHN A. WILLIAMS AND DAVID C. DAWSON

Clinical medicine is in the midst of a revolution. The explosive growth in basic biologic science during the past two decades has provided unprecedented insights into normal physiology and disease processes. The bases of human illness are understood increasingly in cellular and molecular terms, and novel approaches to treatment have resulted. The pace of scientific advancement is likely to accelerate. This new knowledge requires that future surgeons learn a new scientific vocabulary. All clinicians must understand the tenets of cellular and molecular biology to appreciate both the power and the limitations of these approaches.

CELL STRUCTURE

The human body, like all living organisms, is composed of cells. Individual cells express widely differing shapes and functions, but all possess common structural and functional elements that allow the cell to use energy, maintain homeostasis, grow, and divide.[1,2] Cells become differentiated for specific functions by expressing particular, specialized elements. For example, all cells possess membrane proteins that act as ion channels and participate in the maintenance of the intracellular ionic milieu, but in nerve cells, these ion channels have diversified and are highly voltage dependent, providing the basis for information transmission in the form of electrical impulses.

In many cases, proteins do not function as individual molecules but within larger structures specialized for specific functions. These structures, when visible by light and electron microscopy, are termed *organelles* (Fig. 1.1). In most cases, organelles compartmentalize the cell; they are surrounded by a biologic membrane based on a lipid bilayer that is structurally similar to the plasma membrane. This section reviews the structure of the major cell organelles as well as that of the cytoskeleton, a collection of structural proteins that form large, supramolecular aggregates.

Membranes and Organelles

Plasma Membrane

The plasma membrane defines the boundary of the cell and serves to contain and concentrate enzymes and the other macromolecular constituents.[3] The plasma membrane is composed of amphipathic molecules, mainly phospholipids, sphingolipids, and proteins, that contain distinct regions that are either insoluble in water (hydrophobic) or soluble in water (hydrophilic). By orienting themselves so that their hydrophobic portions are in contact with each other, phospholipids can spontaneously form closed vesicles and planar lipid bilayers, within which proteins and hydrophobic components such as cholesterol are embedded (Fig. 1.2). Individual lipid molecules are able to diffuse in the bilayer. Embedded proteins can also move, although their movement is slower and often restricted by cytoskeletal attachment. The lateral mobility of lipids and proteins can be quantitated by fluorescence recovery after photobleaching. The plasma membrane forms a continuous barrier between the aqueous extracellular and intracellular fluids. In addition to physically restraining macromolecules within the cell, the hydrophobic core of the lipid bilayer presents a barrier to small, charged molecules such as ions, amino acids, and adenosine triphosphate (ATP). This arrangement allows specialized transport proteins in the membrane, which act as regulated channels or transporters, to maintain an intracellular ionic milieu that is clearly different from extracellular fluid. Transport proteins and receptors are usually transmembrane proteins whose hydrophobic regions in the lipid bilayer are most often present in an α-helical configuration. Other membrane proteins on the inside of the plasma membrane, such as Ras, are attached by fatty acid chains or isoprenyl derivatives, whereas some proteins on the external face are linked to phosphatidylinositol (PI) situated in the outer leaflet of the bilayer. Most plasma membrane proteins extending externally

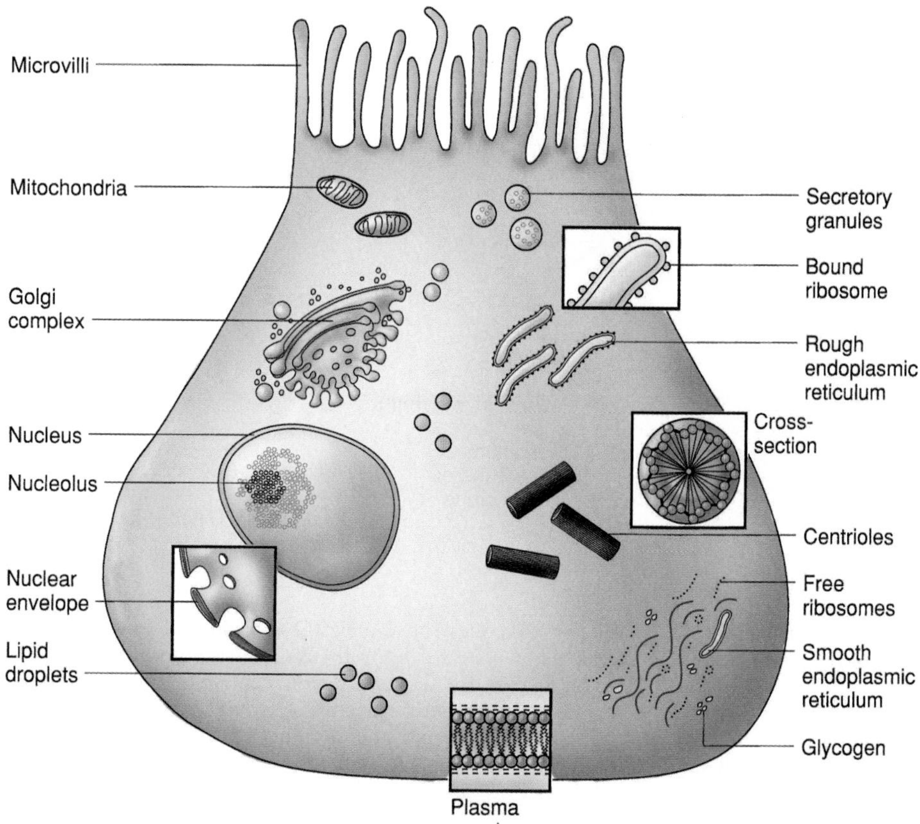

FIGURE 1.1 Schematic diagram of a typical epithelial cell, showing the common internal organelles.

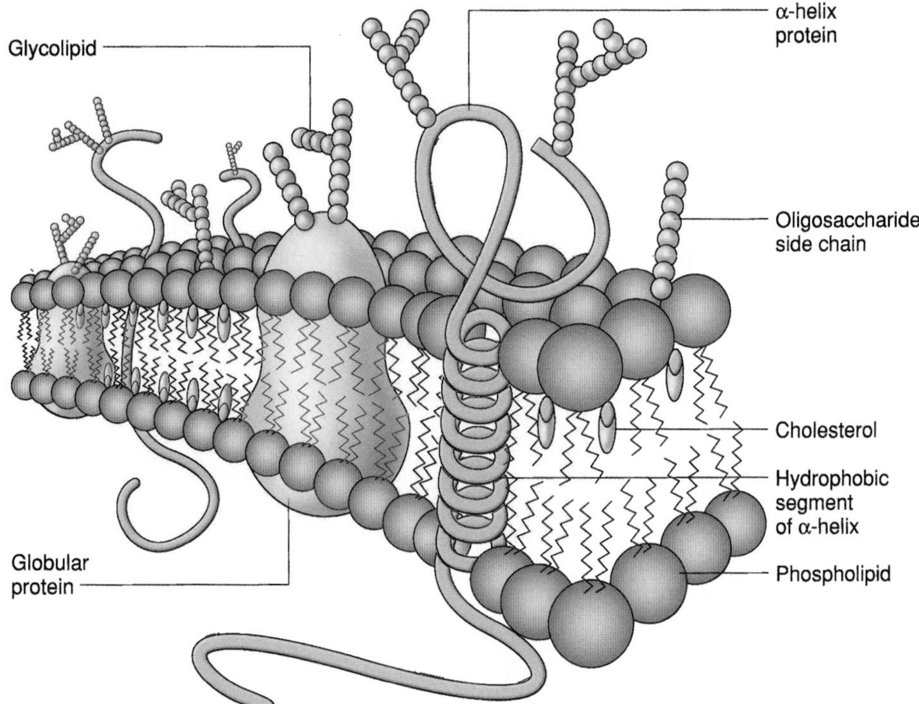

FIGURE 1.2 Structure of the cell membrane as a fluid mosaic consisting of a phospholipid bilayer that contains cholesterol and embedded proteins.

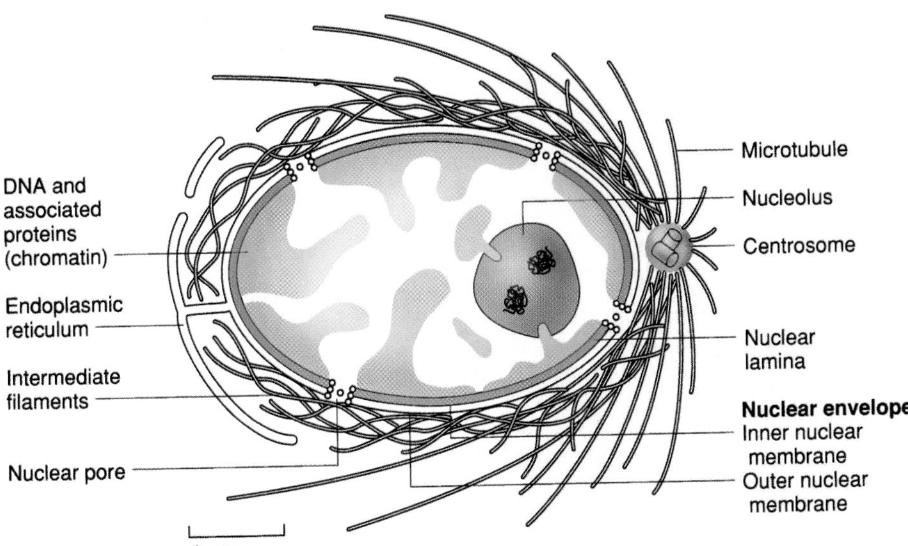

FIGURE 1.3 Detailed structure of the cell nucleus.

bear carbohydrate moieties primarily as oligosaccharide chains, which contribute to the cell coat or glycocalyx. Finally, cells can restrict lipid and protein components to specific membrane domains. This is especially prominent in ion-transporting epithelial cells of gut and kidney, which have distinct apical and basolateral domains, and in cells with specialized secretory regions such as neurons.

Nucleus

The largest of the cellular organelles is the nucleus, usually 3 to 8 tm in diameter. The nucleus is defined by an envelope consisting of two membranes, the inner and outer nuclear membranes (Fig. 1.3). Just inside the inner nuclear membrane is a supporting meshwork of intermediate filaments, the nuclear lamina. The outer membrane is continuous with the rough endoplasmic reticulum (ER) and is studded with ribosomes. All of the chromosomal DNA is contained in the nucleus in association with a specialized class of acidic proteins termed *histones*. Histones and DNA exist together as chromatin fibers. The contents of the nucleus communicate with the cytoplasm by means of openings in the nuclear envelope called *nuclear pores*. These ringlike pores are composed of specialized proteins that function as energy-dependent channels to regulate the movement of material between nucleus and cytoplasm. The nucleus also contains a specialized region, the nucleolus, where ribosomes are assembled.

The remainder of the cell, external to the nucleus and contained by the plasma membrane, is termed *cytoplasm*. Cytoplasm is composed of a nonparticulate "soup," or cytosol, as well as a number of membranous organelles and the filamentous cytoskeleton.

Mitochondria

Mitochondria are sausage-shaped organelles that are 0.2 to 0.5 μm in diameter and up to several micrometers in length. They are defined by a smooth outer membrane and an inner membrane characterized by infoldings, called cristae, which protrude into the central matrix (Fig. 1.4). Mitochondria are the major source of energy production in eukaryotic cells. The enzymes involved with electron transport and oxidative phosphorylation exist in an ordered array of small, stalked particles protruding inward from the inner membrane. Enzymes involved in the final oxidation of sugars and lipids are present in the matrix space, which also contains granules of mitochondrial DNA and a few ribosomes. Mitochondria contain the genetic codes for and synthesize some of their own proteins. They also divide by fission, consistent with the notion that mitochondria originated from captive or symbiotic bacteria. Both mitochondrial membranes have unique characteristics. The outer membrane contains porins, proteins forming large channels that render the membrane permeable to molecules of up to 10 kd. The inner mitochondrial membrane is almost entirely protein, with the lowest lipid content of common biologic membranes. Oxidative phosphorylation at the inner membrane generates an electrochemical proton gradient, and the downhill movement of H^+ through adenosine triphosphatase (ATPase) molecules provides energy to synthesize ATP.

Endoplasmic Reticulum

The ER is a network of interconnected membranes forming closed vesicles, tubules, and saccules. The ER has a number of functions and is primarily involved in the synthesis of protein and lipids. The ER is divided into rough ER, which is studded with ribosomes and involved in the synthesis of exportable proteins (Fig. 1.5), and smooth ER, which lacks ribosomes and is involved in the synthesis of fatty acids and lipids (Fig. 1.6). Rough ER is especially prominent in cells such as pancreatic acinar cells and plasma cells that secrete large amounts of

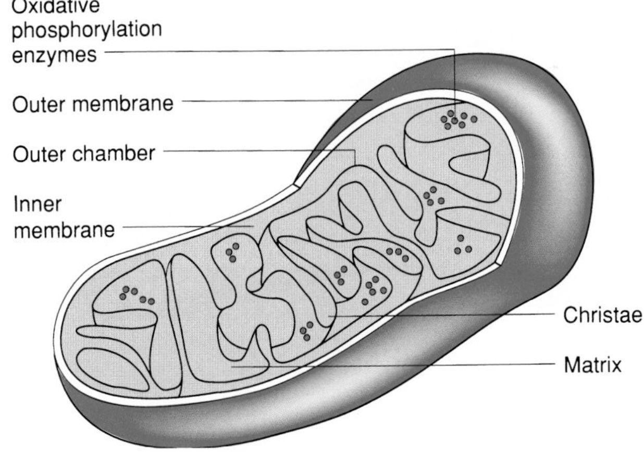

FIGURE 1.4 Schematic structure of a typical mitochondrion.

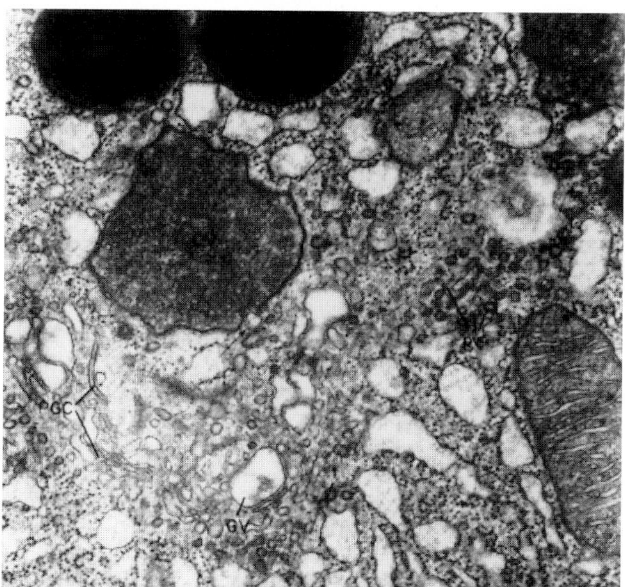

FIGURE 1.5 Electron photomicrograph of a portion of a pancreatic acinar cell showing endoplasmic reticulum, Golgi apparatus, and forming secretory granules. There is an abundance of small transport vesicles, which shuttle secretory proteins between the various membrane-limited organelles. CV, condensing vacuole; PGC, post-Golgi cisternae; PV, peripheral vesicles; GV, Golgi vacuole; t, transition element of the RER. (Courtesy of J. Jamieson, Yale University, New Haven, CT.)

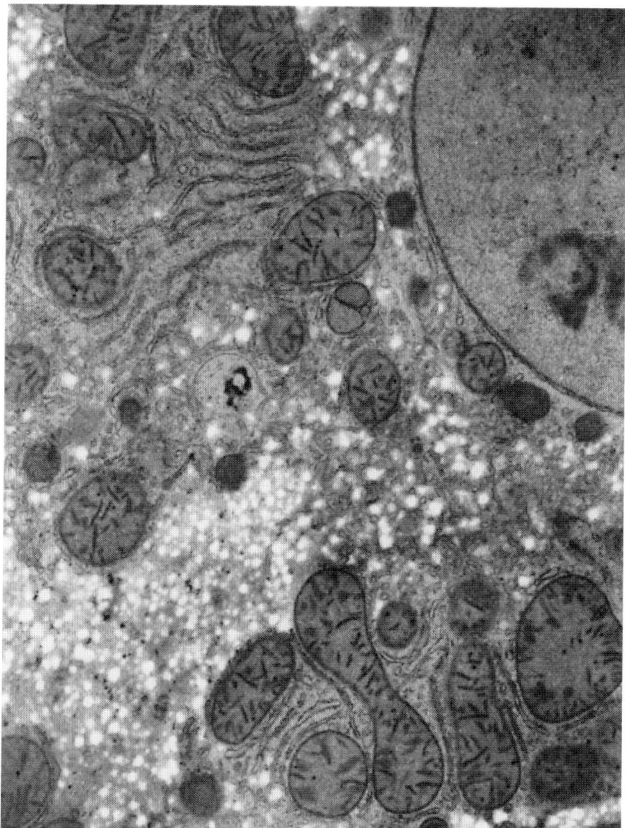

FIGURE 1.6 Electron photomicrograph of a portion of a hepatocyte, showing a nucleus, mitochondria, and smooth and rough endoplasmic reticulum. (Courtesy of A.K. Christensen, University of Michigan, Ann Arbor, MI.)

protein; its functional role in protein synthesis is discussed later. Smooth ER is especially prominent in cells producing lipid derivatives, such as the adrenal cortex, and in the hepatocyte. Smooth ER also contains enzymes that modify or detoxify endogenous metabolites and foreign molecules such as drugs and pesticides.

Golgi Complex

Adjacent to the rough ER and functionally involved in the sorting and packaging of secreted protein is the Golgi complex (see Figs. 1.1, 1.5). Each complex consists of a series of flattened membrane sacs, or cisternae, surrounded by a number of vesicles. These vesicles are transport containers that shuttle proteins destined for secretion from the rough ER to the Golgi complex. During this process, secretory proteins are modified or processed, for example, by addition of sugar residues. The Golgi complex is also the compartment involved in directing secretory proteins into either lysosomes, small vesicles that rapidly move to the periphery of the cell and release their contents, or larger secretory granules, where the contents condense and are stored to await a regulatory signal that initiates fusion with the plasma membrane and secretion (see section on intracellular synthesis, transport, and organization of macromolecules).

Lysosomes and Peroxisomes

Lysosomes are membrane-limited organelles containing acid hydrolytic enzymes that degrade polymers such as proteins, carbohydrates, and nucleic acids.[4] Lysosomal enzymes all work best at an acid pH. The interior of the lysosome is maintained at a pH of approximately 5.0 by an H^+-transporting ATPase located in the lysosomal membrane in conjunction with a Cl^- channel protein. This enzyme uses ATP hydrolysis to pump H^+ into the lysosomal lumen. Lysosomes are frequently classified as primary lysosomes, which are small, spherical structures containing only hydrolytic enzymes, or secondary lysosomes, larger and irregularly shaped, containing membranes or particles that are being digested. Secondary lysosomes result from the fusion of primary lysosomes with engulfed or abnormal organelles or with endocytotic vesicles that are bringing extracellular material into the cell for degradation. The cell is normally protected from lysosomal enzymes by their sequestration in a membrane-limited compartment. In addition, if the lysosome ruptures into the cytoplasmic compartment, the digestive enzymes have little activity because cytoplasmic pH is maintained near 7.0. The lysosomal membrane is permeable to amino acids, monosaccharides, and other similarly sized molecules that are released after hydrolysis. These molecules can be reused by the cell.

Peroxisomes are small (0.2 to 1 μm), membrane-bounded organelles that contain enzymes involved in the oxidation of fatty acids.[5] They are involved in degrading various toxic molecules. Their name is derived from the fact that they generate and degrade large amounts of hydrogen peroxide.

Cytoskeleton

The cytoskeleton is a collection of filamentous protein structures that allows cells (a) to assume and maintain a variety of shapes, (b) to produce directed movement of organelles within the cell, and (c) to effect movement of the entire cell relative to other cells.[6,7] Thus, the cytoskeleton is involved with the movement of organelles in cells, the movement of cells such as leukocytes on a substrate, muscle contraction, and the changes in cell shape that occur during development. These multiple activities depend on three main types of filaments: actin filaments, intermediate filaments, and microtubules. Each type of filament is formed from protein monomers and a variety of accessory proteins that serve to cross-link individual filaments or to attach them to membranes. Additional accessory proteins regulate polymerization, that is, assembly and disassembly of filaments or movement, as in muscle and cilia.

Actin-based Filaments

Actin filaments are threadlike structures, about 8 nm in diameter, composed of a tight helix of actin monomers (Fig. 1.7). Actin filaments are polar structures with two different ends that are in equilibrium with free monomers. In muscle cells, most actin exists in stable filaments (F-actin) made from the globular subunits (G-actin). In nonmuscle cells, about half of the actin is in the free monomer pool, and filaments can form by addition of subunits to the positive end. Disassembly occurs by deletion from the negative end. This equilibrium is also regulated by a number of cytosolic actin-binding proteins, including thymosin and profilin that bind G-actin. Polymerization is also regulated by cell surface receptors acting through heterotrimeric and small guanosine triphosphate (GTP)-binding proteins of the Rho family.[8]

In skeletal muscle, actin forms a regular array of thin filaments, each with the positive end attached to a Z disk. The other major protein of skeletal muscle, myosin II, contains two heavy chains, each of molecular weight 230 kd, which together form two globular heads, a hinge region, and a coiled, rodlike tail (see Fig. 1.7). Also attached to each head are two distinct light chains of approximately 20 kd molecular weight. In skeletal and cardiac muscle, 300 to 400 of these myosin dimers pack together by interaction between their rodlike tails to form a bipolar aggregate, called the *thick filament.* The protruding heads of the thick filament myosin bundles interact with actin in an ATP-dependent manner to create movement by ratcheting the myosin head down the actin filament toward the positive end. This movement causes the thick and thin filaments to overlap and the muscle to shorten. Other proteins, including troponins and tropomyosin, are involved in the regulation of this interaction. One of the troponins (troponin C) binds Ca^{2+}, leading to activation of the myosin ATPase. In smooth muscle and nonmuscle cells, myosin is not as abundant or as well organized,

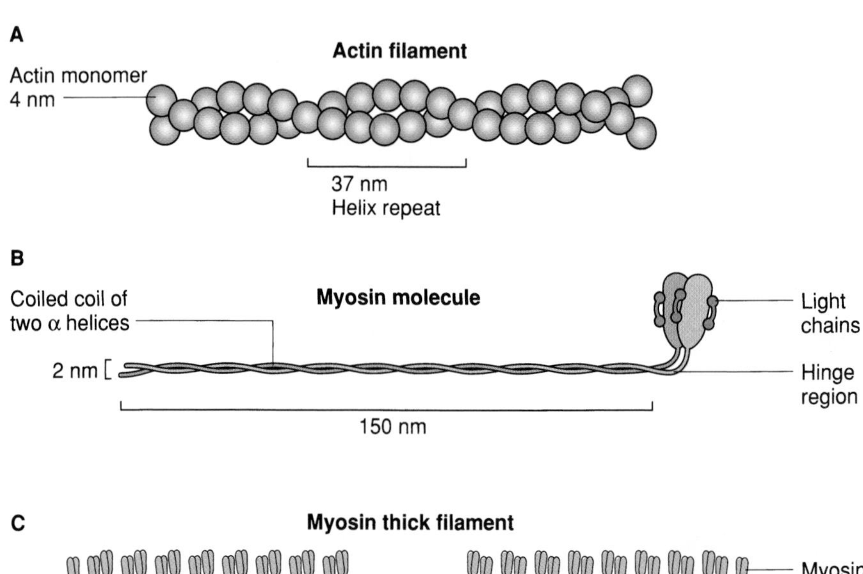

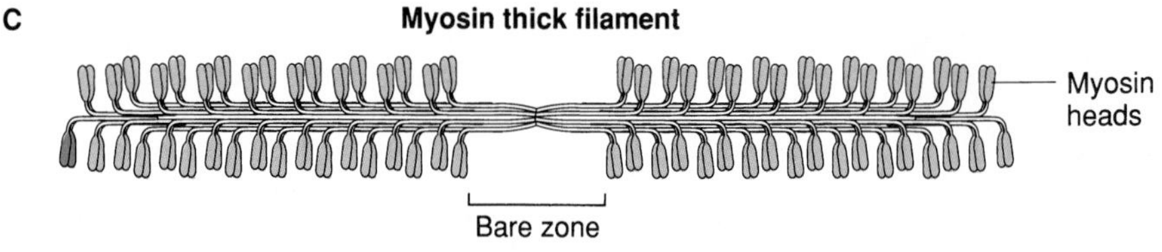

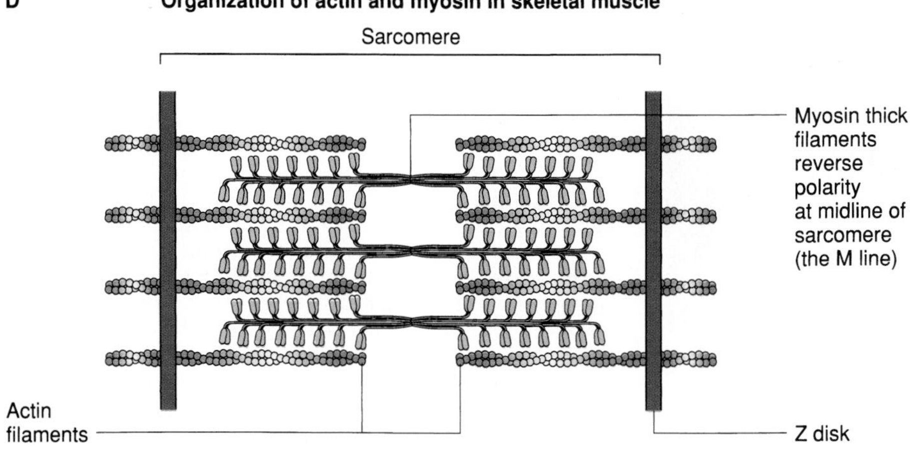

FIGURE 1.7 Structures of actin and myosin, their organization into filaments, and the organization of actin thin filaments and myosin thick filaments in striated muscle.

but bipolar filaments of 15 to 20 myosin molecules exist and can interact with actin to produce movement. In this case, activation is controlled by Ca^{2+} interaction with the calcium-binding protein, calmodulin. Calmodulin activates the enzyme, myosin light-chain kinase, which phosphorylates one of the light chains of myosin and thus promotes the actin–myosin interaction.

Nonmuscle cells also contain a distinct, smaller form of myosin, termed *minimyosin* or *myosin*,[9] which does not form filaments. Rather, its smaller tail is attached to membranes or organelles, whereas its single head, which is similar to that of regular myosin, can interact with and move along an actin filament. When the actin is fixed, this can lead to organelle movement, as in cytoplasmic streaming. Other isoforms of myosin exist but are less well characterized.

Muscle-like bundles of actin and myosin can form transiently in nonmuscle cells and can be involved in specialized functions. An example of such a temporary cellular structure is the contractile ring that leads to the separation of the two daughter cells during cell division. The contractile ring contains actin and myosin, and its formation constricts the middle of a cell. When cell division is complete, the ring disappears. Other, less transitory assemblies of actins and myosin are involved in the folding of epithelial cell sheets and in the maintenance of epithelial polarity. The latter is maintained by a belt of filaments running circumferentially around the apical end of the cell. The filaments attach to junctional complexes that connect adjacent cells.

Actin filaments are also involved in the maintenance of cell shape. An especially dense network of actin, sometimes termed the *cell web,* is present just beneath the plasma membrane. The cell web consists of a three-dimensional network of actin filaments stabilized by cross-linking proteins, one of the most abundant of which is filamen.[10] Filamen exists as a dimer joined head-to-head with each tail possessing an actin-binding site. The loose actin network is also connected to the plasma membranes by other proteins, including spectrin and fodrin. Because the network must disassemble to allow secretion or endocytosis, it is not surprising that actin-severing proteins also exist. When activated by Ca^{2+}, one of these, gelsolin, severs and forms a cap on the new positive end of the actin filament, thereby leading to a local and usually transient disappearance of the network. Another, cofilin, is regulated by reversible phosphorylation. Actin filaments are also stabilized by capping proteins such as CapZ and tropomodulin.

Another example of a specialized structure based on an actin-containing cytoskeleton are the microvilli found on many cells but especially on intestinal enterocytes. In the intestine, microvilli serve to increase absorptive surface area. The core of each microvillus contains a bundle of 20 to 30 parallel actin filaments attached at the tip by the positive end and extending down to anchor in a specialized cortex at the apical pole of the cell. The actin filaments are held together by several small actin-binding proteins, such as fimbrin and villin. Fimbrin contains two actin-binding sites on a single polypeptide chain such that the actin filaments are tied into a compact bundle with regular spacing. The bundle is also connected to the overlying plasma membrane by lateral arms that contain a minimyosin-like molecule.

Intermediate Filaments

Intermediate filaments are a heterogeneous class of tough protein fibers named for their thickness (≈10 nm), which is intermediate between the thin and thick filaments of muscle cells.[11] These structural elements usually form a basket around the nucleus and extend out to the cell periphery. Intermediate filaments are formed from fibrous proteins that associate side to side in overlapping arrays to form long, tough, stable filaments. In contrast to actin filaments and microtubules, which are made up of unique subunits, intermediate filaments are made up of a variety of subunit proteins with homology to one another in the fiber-forming domain of each molecule.

Intermediate filaments are classified on the basis of amino acid structure into four types. Type I are the keratins, found primarily in epithelial cells and sometimes subdivided into acidic and basic. A large number of tissue-specific classes of keratin exist and can be used to distinguish the cell type of origin for certain tumors. Type II intermediate filaments include vimentin, desmin, and glial fibrillary protein. Type III are neurofilaments and are restricted to neurons. Type IV proteins are nuclear lamins that form a two-dimensional sheet just inside the inner nuclear membrane (see Fig. 1.3).

Intermediate filaments are believed to be structural elements designed to resist stress and provide support. As such, they are often associated with other, more dynamic cytoskeletal elements such as microtubules (Fig. 1.8), and with the plasma membrane, where they associate with desmosomes. In some cases, their assembly is controlled by phosphorylation.

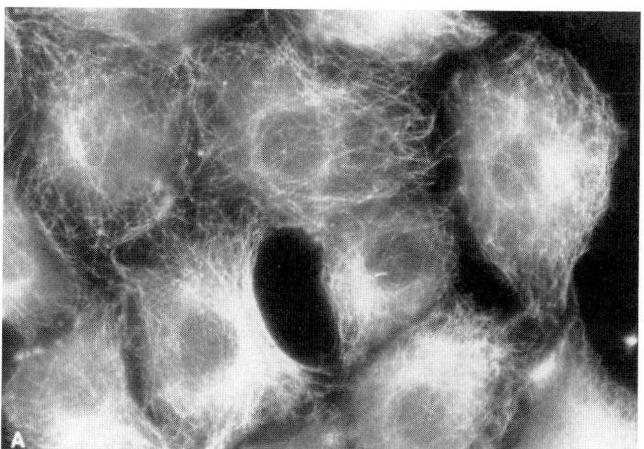

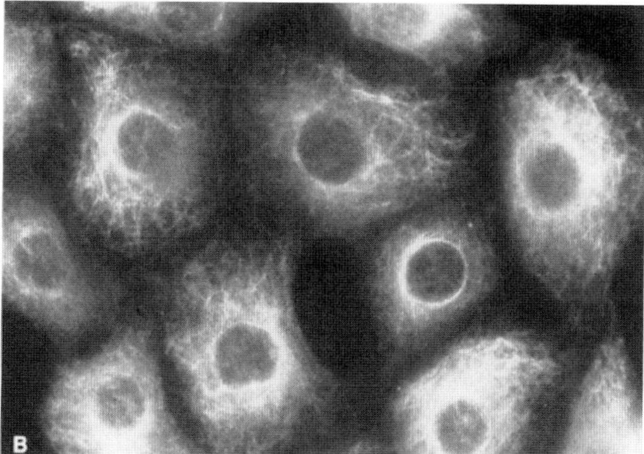

FIGURE 1.8 The distribution of cytoskeletal elements in pulmonary endothelial cells as detected by fluorescence-specific antibodies. Although surrounded by a cytoskeletal network, the nuclei are unstained. (*A*) Antitubulin stain. (*B*) Antivimentin stain. (Courtesy of M.J. Welsh, University of Michigan, Ann Arbor, MI.)

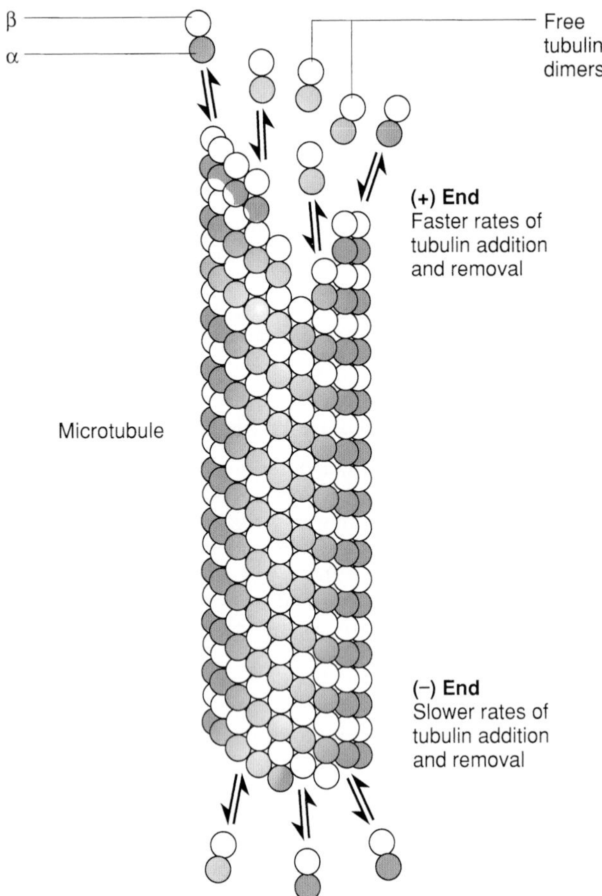

FIGURE 1.9 Diagram of a microtubule composed of longitudinal rows of tubulin dimers. The α- and β-tubulin dimers add to or dissociate from the two ends.

This is especially true for nuclear lamins, which are phosphorylated and disassemble during mitotic division as the nuclear envelope disappears.

Microtubules

Microtubules are found in all cells except erythrocytes. Structurally, they are hollow fibers 24 nm in diameter that vary in length from less than one up to hundreds of micrometers. Their basic structure consists of 13 parallel rows, or protofilaments, each composed of globular subunits (Fig. 1.9). Chemically, microtubules contain two related major proteins, α- and β-tubulin, each with a molecular weight of approximately 50 kd. In the cell, these subunits exist as an ab heterodimer called tubulin. Tubulin dimers arranged αβ-αβ-αβ make up the protofilament. As a result of this organization, microtubules are oriented with a positive and a negative end, and all structures that contain microtubules are polarized. Specialized cellular structures based on microtubules include cilia, neuronal axons, and the mitotic spindle.

Microtubules are frequently associated with a specialized organelle, the centriole (see Fig. 1.1). A centriole is a short, cylindric structure composed of nine groups of triplet microtubules. Centrioles usually exist in pairs oriented at right angles to each other. All cells contain at least one pair of centrioles near the nucleus, surrounded by a cloud of amorphous material, called the *microtubule-organizing center.* The centriole divides during DNA replication. After forming the organizing center for each pole of the mitotic spindle, one centriole remains with each daughter cell. Because microtubules always have their negative pole associated with a centriole or microtubule-organizing center, and because growth occurs faster on the positive end, microtubules can be observed to grow out from the organizing center. Cilia are made up of an ordered array of microtubules, and each is attached to a modified centriole, termed the *basal body.*

Within the cell, microtubules exist in a dynamic state in which they are continually forming and dissociating as tubulin subunits are added to or removed from the ends.[12] This dynamic equilibrium involves the conversion of GTP bound to tubulin to guanosine diphosphate (GDP). Each tubulin molecule possesses a binding site for colchicine, and binding of this drug prevents microtubule formation. Colchicine binding leads to the disappearance of formed microtubules and is the basis of the antimitotic action of this class of compounds. Other antimitotic agents that act on microtubules include vinblastine, which induces formation of paracrystalline aggregates of tubulin, and paclitaxel (Taxol), which stabilizes formed microtubules, preventing their depolymerization. Microtubules also depolymerize at low temperatures. Although microtubules in dividing or motile cells such as leukocytes rapidly disappear in response to colchicine or low temperature, microtubules in organized parenchymal or epithelial cells disappear more slowly, and some microtubules, such as those in cilia, appear resistant. This difference, which is related to the function of the organelle (i.e., whether it needs to be stable or dynamic), is due in large part to other associated proteins, termed *microtubule-associated proteins* (MAPs). The MAPs are responsible for holding microtubules together in permanent arrays, attaching them to other organelles, including membrane vesicles, and generating the force that is involved in microtubule-based movement. Many MAPs are high-molecular-weight proteins or complexes of proteins. One prominent lower-molecular-weight class is termed *tau protein;* it acts to facilitate microtubule polymerization.

The transport of organelles in cytoplasm is usually associated with microtubules. The most specialized case is axonal flow, whereby vesicles move at rates of 3 μm/second (250 mm/day) along the axon. When viewed in the electron microscope, a cross-bridge structure exists, connecting the moving particle to the microtubule. A motor protein, kinesin, has been isolated that mediates movement along microtubules in the negative-to-positive direction and is responsible for antegrade rapid axonal transport.[13] Kinesin is composed of heavy-chain subunits, which bind tubulin and possess ATPase activity, and light chains, which attach to cellular organelles. When ATP is hydrolyzed, the kinesin moves along the microtubule, transporting the bound vesicle (Fig. 1.10). Kinesin is now known to belong to a family of motor proteins that

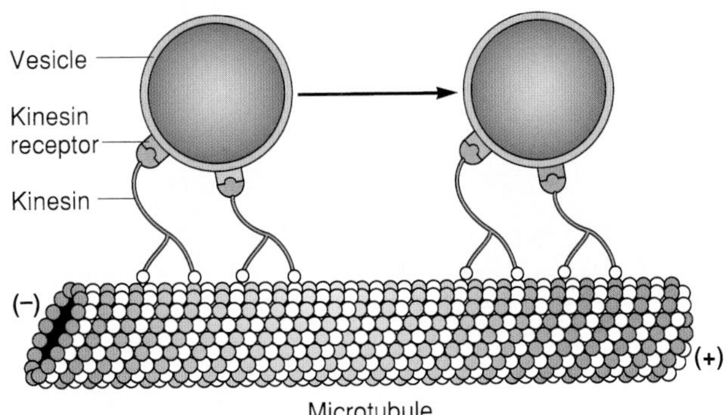

FIGURE 1.10 Model of kinesin-mediated transport of vesicles along a microtubule. The kinesin molecules move along the microtubule by interacting with tubulin in an adenosine triphosphate-requiring manner.

include cytosolic kinesins responsible for vesicle and organelle transport, spindle kinesins that participate in spindle assembly and chromosomal movement during mitosis, and cytosolic dyneins, which are the primary negative end-directed motor proteins.

A specialized form of microtubule-based motility is the beating cilium. Each cilia has a basic structure of nine microtubule doublets surrounding a central microtubule pair. The entire structure, called an *axoneme,* also contains other linker proteins that hold the unit together and a specialized MAP protein, dynein, which makes contact with the adjacent microtubule doublet. Dynein is a large protein (400 kd) with ATPase activity and, like kinesin, generates force on the adjacent microtubule in one direction. Because the microtubules are attached to one another, what would otherwise be a sliding motion is converted into a bending or whiplike motion. Cilia are especially prominent in the respiratory tract, where they generate movement of mucus out of the bronchial system.

CELL–CELL INTERACTION

All cells must interact with their neighbors, and most are arranged in assemblies called *tissues.* The cells in a tissue are in contact with the extracellular matrix, which in cases such as connective tissue may surround the cells. In other cases, epithelial cells are directly attached to each other and the extracellular matrix is reduced to a thin layer, the basal lamina, which underlies the cellular sheet. Although cells such as neurons and endocrine cells influence other cells by specialized secretions, this section considers direct physical interactions mediated by molecules in the cell membrane and by the cytoskeleton.

Cell Junctions

Cell junctions were originally identified and classified by their structure as observed using the electron microscope. Functionally, cell junctions can be classified as occluding, anchoring, or communicating.[2] The major occluding junction is the tight junction or zonula occludens, which connects cells in epithelia and thereby allows epithelia to serve as selective permeability barriers. As discussed later, epithelia are almost always engaged in transcellular transport. Tight junctions make this possible both by preventing backflux between cells of transported molecules and by maintaining distinct apical and basal membrane proteins. Tight junctions are normally located near the apical pole of the cell and form a belt that completely encircles the cell (Fig. 1.11). In transmission electron microscopy, the junction appears as a series of focal contacts between the outer leaflets of adjacent plasma membrane. In freeze-fracture electron microscopy, the junction appears as an anastomosing network of sealing strands. Although all tight junctions are impermeable to macromolecules, the barrier to ions and water is related to the number of sealing strands. The strands are composed of long rows of transmembrane proteins, occludin and claudin.[14] Attached to their cytosolic domains are the proteins ZO-1, ZO-2, and ZO-3, which are also bound to actin.

Anchoring junctions connect the cytoskeleton of the cell to extracellular matrix or neighboring cells.[15] Morphologically,

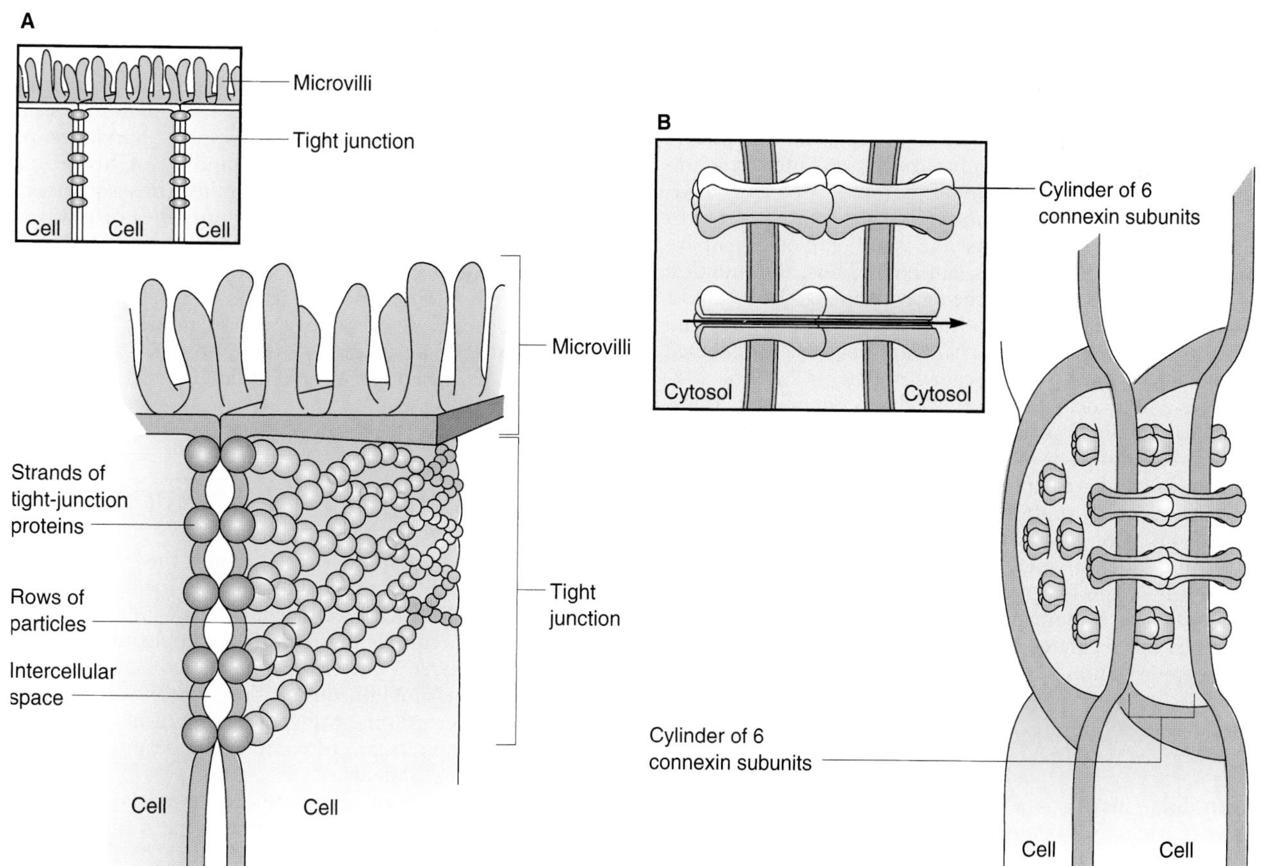

FIGURE 1.11 Schematic view of two intracellular junctions.

these are adherens junctions or desmosomes. Adherens junctions occur in epithelia as a continuous adhesion belt, the zonula adherens, located just below the tight junction. Morphologically, this consists of a long stretch of continuous contact between cell membranes. The membranes are held together by a linker protein, E-cadherin, also called *uvomorulin.* E-cadherin is a single-pass transmembrane glycoprotein with four extracellular Ca^{2+}-binding domains and a terminal domain that binds to the same domain on another cadherin molecule. The properties of this molecule account for the Ca^{2+} dependence of cell adhesion. Within the cell, the adhesion belt is attached by the cytoplasmic end of cadherin molecules to contractile bundles of actin filaments by a set of intracellular linker proteins, including catenins, vinculin, and α-actinin. In nonepithelial cells, adherens junctions are localized as focal contacts or adhesion plaques where bundles of actin filaments terminate and serve primarily as attachment sites to the extracellular matrix. In addition to participating in anchoring junctions in adult cells, the cadherin family of cell-adhesion molecules, along with the structurally distinct nerve-cell adhesion molecule (N-CAM), intercellular adhesion molecule (ICAM), and selectins, play important roles in morphogenesis and in the adhesion of leukocytes to endothelial cells during inflammation.

The other type of anchoring junction is the desmosome. Desmosomes are button-like points of attachment with a prominent intracellular plaque that weld together adjacent cells by serving as anchoring sites for intermediate filaments in the cell. The particular type of intermediate filament depends on the cell type and is keratin in most epithelial cells and desmin in cardiac muscle cells. The transmembrane-linker proteins in desmosomes are cadherins that, as discussed earlier, bind each other by a Ca^{2+}-dependent mechanism. Hemidesmosomes, or half-desmosomes, are morphologically similar to desmosomes but are chemically and functionally distinct and are considered in the next section (cell–matrix adhesion).

The third functional type of cell junction is the gap junction,[16,17] which is specialized for cell communication (see Fig. 1.11B). In conventional electron micrographs, it appears as a patch where adjacent membranes are separated by a uniform narrow gap of approximately 20 nm. This gap, however, is spanned by protein molecules that form an array of channels through which ions and small molecules up to approximately 1,000 daltons can pass. Thus, the junction mediates both electrical and chemical coupling. This is most dramatic in cardiac and smooth muscle but also plays an important role in embryogenesis. Gap junctions are formed from transmembrane proteins called *connexins.* Multiple connexins have been identified, each of which contains four transmembrane domains and a variable cytoplasmic domain; many of these are identified by their apparent mass (i.e., connexin-32, connexin-26) and are expressed in a tissue-specific manner. A ring of six identical connexins forms a *connexon,* with a central aqueous pore. The connexons protrude from the membrane, and, when aligned with a connexon on an adjacent cell, both hold the two membranes at the characteristic distance and form a channel. These channels are not continuously open but regulated by Ca^{2+}, intracellular pH, and protein phosphorylation.

Cell–Matrix Adhesion

Extracellular matrix is a meshwork of negatively charged polysaccharide glycosaminoglycan chains and protein fibers. The protein fibers are mainly structural, such as collagen and elastin, or adhesive, such as fibronectin and laminin. The principal protein molecules in the plasma membrane that serve as receptors for matrix molecules are the integrins.[18] Integrins are so named to indicate that they integrate the extracellular matrix and the cytoskeleton. Evidence is now emerging that integrins are functional as well as structural integrators and that they are involved in bidirectional signaling across the plasma membrane.

Integrins are noncovalently attached heterodimeric glycoproteins composed of α and β subunits. So far, 17 α and 8 β subunits have been identified. Different cell types express and synthesize different $\alpha\beta$ complexes, with the combination of α and β determining the ligand specificity. For example, $\alpha_5\beta_1$ is a fibronectin receptor, whereas $\alpha_6\beta_1$ is a laminin receptor; both are expressed on most cells. By contrast, β_2 chains are primarily expressed on white blood cells and mediate cell–cell interactions (e.g., between white blood cells and vascular endothelium). A significant amount of redundancy occurs; most integrins bind several adhesive glycoproteins, and most adhesive glycoproteins bind to more than one protein.

Each integrin subunit spans the membrane once with a large extracellular domain and a small cytoplasmic domain. Divalent cation-binding motifs are present in both subunits near the presumed ligand-binding site. Most integrins are clustered into focal adhesion plaques and attach to actin through linker proteins, particularly talin and α-actinin.[19] In fibroblasts, these focal adhesions colocalize with the termination of stress fibers. Other proteins in the adhesion plaque include a 125-kd tyrosine kinase termed $p25^{FAK}$ (focal adhesion kinase). By virtue of this connection to the cytoskeleton, cells can orient the matrix macromolecules they secrete, and in turn, matrix macromolecules can organize the cytoskeleton. A special case is the integrin found in hemidesmosomes $\alpha_6\beta_4$, which connects intracellularly to intermediate filaments by distinct linker proteins. Whereas keratin filaments associated with desmosomes have lateral attachments to the desmosome, many filaments associated with hemidesmosomes end in the plaque.

Integrins are components of inside-out signal transduction. Various β_2-integrins on monocytes and neutrophils are stimulated (i.e., show an increased binding affinity) in response to inflammatory mediators. Platelet activation induces its integrins to bind fibrinogen. In other cases, phosphorylation of a β_1-integrin during mitosis inhibits binding of fibronectin, allowing the cell to round up or detach. Integrins also mediate outside-in signaling. The binding of antibodies or glycoproteins to integrins can affect intracellular pH and Ca^{2+} as well as tyrosine phosphorylation and lead to cellular differentiation, activation, or proliferation. An integrin-associated protein appears to function as a Ca^{2+} channel. The protein $p125^{FAK}$ can be activated by both integrins and peptide growth factors, although its role in cell function remains to be determined.

MEMBRANE TRANSPORT

The plasma membrane physically defines the boundaries of the cell and acts as a dynamic interface that mediates all interactions of the cell with the extracellular environment. The survival of the cell requires that cytosolic composition be maintained within narrow limits, despite the constant influx of nutrients and the simultaneous outflow of waste. This section focuses on the membrane transport mechanisms that enable the cell to maintain its unique composition despite the continual turnover of its contents.

A striking feature of living cells is the marked difference between the composition of the cytosol, the fluid within the cell, and the fluid of the extracellular milieu, as illustrated in Fig. 1.12. The most familiar example is the distribution of sodium (Na^+) and potassium (K^+). Cells are typically rich

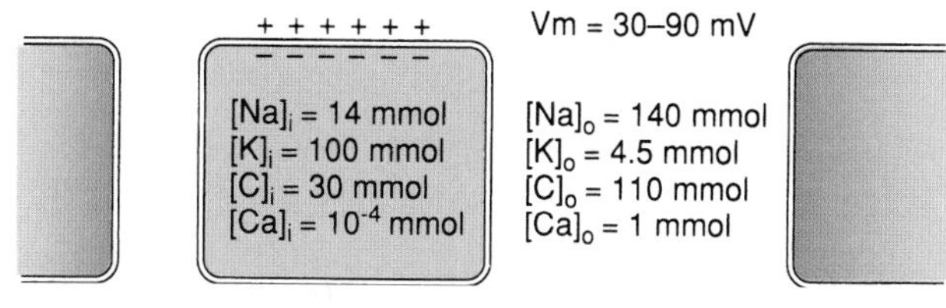

FIGURE 1.12 Intracellular ionic composition differs markedly from that of the surrounding extracellular fluid. Representative values for intracellular and extracellular ion concentrations are shown.

in K^+ and contain relatively little Na^+, despite the fact that they are constantly bathed by a fluid with precisely the opposite composition. Even more impressive is the distribution of ionized (as opposed to bound) Ca^{2+}. The extracellular concentration of this ion is typically of the order of 10^{-3} mol/L (1 mmol/L), whereas that of the cytosol is typically 10^{-7} mol/L (10^{-4} mmol/L), a 10,000-fold gradient. These and many other examples establish the fact that the cell and its environment are not in equilibrium. Such nonequilibrium ion distributions are all the more remarkable in light of the fact that the plasma membrane is, to varying degrees, leaky to ions such as Na^+, K^+, and Ca^{2+}. The key to understanding the ability of the cell to maintain nonequilibrium cellulap composition is found in two fundamental properties of the plasma membrane—selectivity and energy conversion.

Selectivity and Its Modulation

The plasma membrane is leaky to a variety of substances, but it exhibits an astounding ability to discriminate, or select, one substance over another. For example, the plasma membrane of many cells is 10 to 100 times more leaky to K^+ than Na^+. Even more spectacular is the selectivity for some organic compounds: n-glucose is often favored over the L-isomer by 1,000-fold. The molecular basis for this selectivity lies in the properties of membrane-spanning proteins, which exhibit an enzyme-like specificity for particular molecules and can thus catalyze their selective transport across the plasma membrane. Much of the research in the field of membrane transport is devoted to identifying and characterizing the specific membrane proteins that constitute highly selective transport pathways.

The selectivity of biologic membranes can be altered drastically as a result of regulatory or signaling processes that occur in the cell. In nerve and muscle cells, for example, the resting membrane is 10- to 100-fold selective for K^+ over Na^+, but in a matter of milliseconds, at the peak of an action potential, this selectivity can be completely reversed so that the membrane becomes 100-fold selective for Na^+ over K^+. In the appropriate cell types, insulin can cause a 30-fold increase in the leakiness to glucose. This modulated selectivity is the basis for cellular signaling as well as regulatory processes that protect the integrity of individual cells and act as crucial elements in epithelial transport processes.

Energy-converting Transport

The selectivity of the plasma membrane, although impressive, cannot account for the nonequilibrium composition of living cells. A cell can be maintained in a nonequilibrium state only by the continual expenditure of energy. The maintenance of steady-state, nonequilibrium cellular composition is possible because the plasma membrane is the site of energy converters, membrane proteins that function as biologic transport machines using the energy derived from metabolic processes to perform transport work. The archetype for the biologic transport machine is the Na^+-K^+-ATPase, a membrane protein that hydrolyzes cytosolic ATP and couples the resulting free energy to the transport of Na^+ and K^+. The catalytic cycle involves the binding of internal Na and external K in such a way that the hydrolysis of one molecule of ATP is associated with the movement of exactly three Na^+ out of and two K^+ into the cell.

The energy conversion that occurs in the Na^+-K^+-ATPase is often referred to as an example of primary active transport, whereby energy is derived directly from ATP hydrolysis. A second and equally important type of energy-converting transporter is one in which the energy inherent in a transmembrane ion gradient, usually that of Na^+, can be used to drive the transport of a second species (e.g., protons, calcium, amino acids, or glucose). Such secondary active transport processes are extremely important to the cell because they allow energy that has been invested in the transmembrane Na gradient by the Na^+-K^+-ATPase to be used to perform various kinds of transport work (Fig. 1.13).

Cell composition is determined by the interaction of energy converters and selective leak pathways. This can be seen in Fig. 1.14. Two cells are diagrammed, one a symmetric cell and the other a polarized cell, such as is found in an epithelial cell layer. Mechanisms for Na transport are diagrammed for both cells. In either case, a steady-state, intracellular Na concentration is achieved by a balance between the net inflow of Na and the net efflux of Na. In the case of the symmetric cell, Na is shown entering by a variety of mechanisms, Na channels, Na-dependent cotransport, and countertransport. Na leaves the cell through the Na^+-K^+-ATPase. The balance between these opposing processes determines the level of intracellular Na. Similarly, in the polarized cell, net transcellular Na transport is achieved by the serial arrangement of apical Na entry and basolateral Na exit, so that the level of intracellular Na is determined by the balance between these two processes. Despite similarities, these two cellular processes may differ significantly with regard to one important variable, the turnover rate. The symmetric cell is typically designed to maintain static gradients at a minimum rate of turnover; that is, leak rates are low, so pump rates are low. In contrast, the polarized cell is specialized for throughput. Entry and exit rates are elevated to produce significant transcellular Na transport that is important, for example, in the function of the airways, kidney, and gastrointestinal tract.

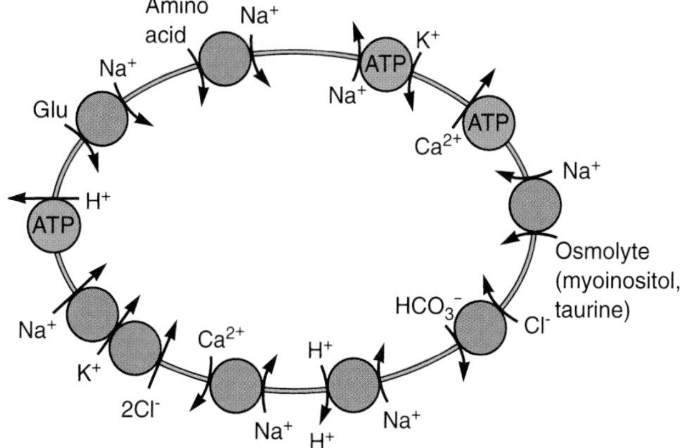

FIGURE 1.13 The plasma membrane contains a variety of energy-converting transporters, which function to maintain intracellular composition away from equilibrium.

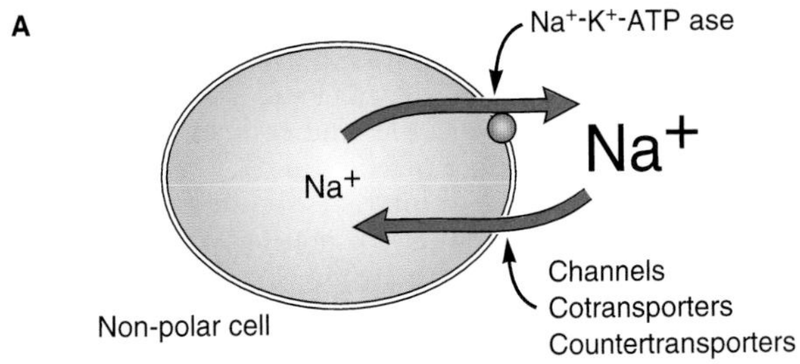

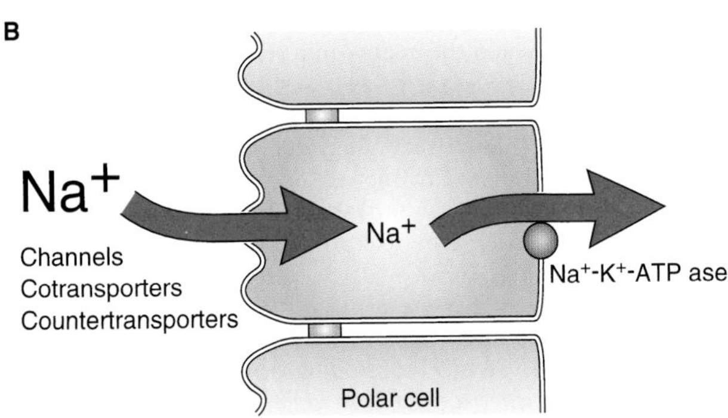

FIGURE 1.14 Cytosolic composition is maintained in a steady state by balancing pumps and leaks. Shown here are mechanisms that maintain low intracellular Na^+ concentration in two cells, one a symmetric cell (*A*) and the other a polar, epithelial cell (*B*). In the symmetric cell, Na^+ efflux by the pump is balanced by the sum of all the Na^+ leaks into the cell. In the polar cell, Na^+ influx at the apical (lumen-facing) side is balanced by active Na^+ efflux at the basolateral (blood-facing) side. The rates of Na^+ transport are typically much greater for the polar cell, which is designed to effect the net transcellular movement of Na^+ that is important for the function of the kidney and gastrointestinal tract.

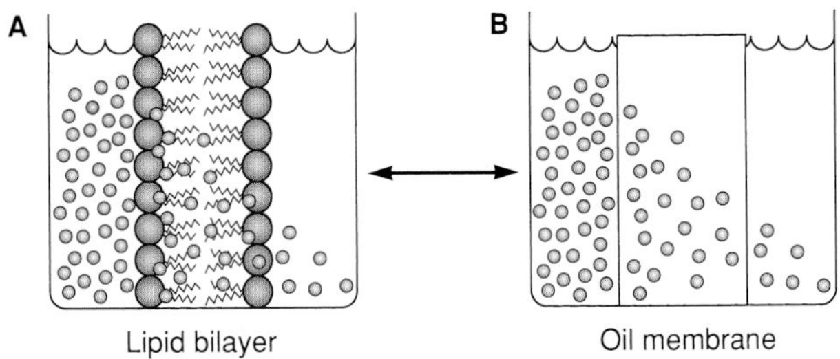

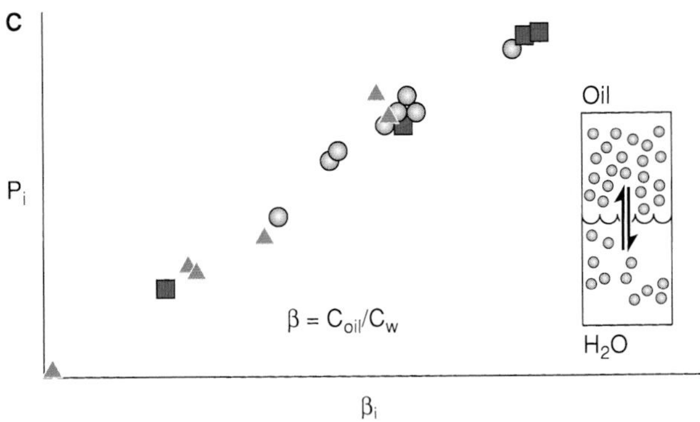

FIGURE 1.15 Lipophilic substances can cross a lipid bilayer by solubility diffusion. The lipid bilayer (*A*) can be approximated by a layer of oil (*B*), and the permeability of the oil membrane to various substances is expected to be proportional to β_i, the oil–water partition coefficient or solubility of the substance in oil (*C*). The *inset* illustrates the determination of β_i as an oil–water partition coefficient.

Membrane Composition: Implications for Selectivity and Energy Conversion

Plasma membranes are mosaic structures, consisting of a matrix of lipid in which are embedded the membrane proteins responsible for the specialized transport properties of the cell interface (see Fig. 1.2). It is instructive to consider some of the general features of the lipid and protein regions of the plasma membrane, as an introduction to the molecular basis for membrane selectivity.

Lipid is a major component of the plasma membrane. Membrane phospholipids, being amphipathic molecules with polar and nonpolar ends, exhibit a strong tendency to organize into a stable, bimolecular layer (Fig. 1.15). The hydrocarbon layer formed by the fatty acid tails of phospholipids exhibits the transport properties that are expected for a layer of oil. Substances can penetrate this layer by a process of solubility–diffusion, that is, dissolving into the hydrocarbon and diffusing across. A model based on the simple notion of dissolving (partitioning) and diffusion predicts the transport properties of a lipid bilayer with amazing accuracy, and the tenet that plasma membranes are in general permeable to lipophilic molecules remains one of the most useful generalizations in cell biology.

The planar nature of the bimolecular lipid layer, combined with the physical properties of the fatty acid hydrocarbon tails of the phospholipids, has led to the concept of the plasma membrane as a "two-dimensional fluid." Experiments with labeled molecules indicate that individual phospholipids can move about relatively freely within the plane of each monolayer, but the polar head groups anchor the molecules so effectively in the aqueous phase that movement from one monolayer to another is relatively rare. Another reflection of the fluidity of the lipid bilayer is that some membrane proteins exhibit lateral mobility; that is, they can move about within the plane of the bilayer. The degree of fluidity exhibited by a lipid bilayer is affected by the type of phospholipid (particularly the degree of unsaturation of the fatty acid side chains) and the cholesterol content. Cholesterol intercalates between phospholipids and decreases membrane fluidity.

Membrane Proteins: Specific Transport Pathways

The movement of substances like glucose and ions across the plasma membrane requires specialized permeation pathways, which are formed by membrane-spanning proteins. In the earlier literature, a variety of transmembrane transport processes were attributed to components referred to as "carriers." The word *carrier* naturally evokes a picture of a mobile membrane component that could bind the transported substance and shuttle it back and forth across the lipid bilayer. Some antibiotic molecules, such as valinomycin, facilitate transmembrane ion movement in precisely this way. There is little doubt, however, that the endogenous mediators of specific transmembrane transport processes are proteins that span the bilayer to provide a path from one side to the other, which is a hospitable environment for non-lipid-soluble (hydrophilic) moieties such as ions, sugars, and amino acids. These transport proteins can be divided into two broad categories: channels and carriers. In the former, the protein forms a pore that can open and close and provides a mechanism for passive flow of solutes or water across membranes. In the latter, the protein is likely to form a porelike structure, but translocation is coupled to specific conformational changes in the protein (see later).

The transport function of membrane-spanning proteins requires that they have a dual nature chemically—they must interact both with the hydrocarbon of the bilayer and the transported substrate. Accordingly, such proteins are amphiphilic, with a hydrophobic portion that permits the protein to pass through the lipid layer and hydrophilic portions that are stable in the aqueous environments of the cytoplasm and the extracellular fluid. The functional, three-dimensional structure of such a protein may require that it cross the membrane as many as 10 or 12 times. Such proteins may consist of alternating hydrophilic and hydrophobic regions (Fig. 1.16). If the amino acid sequence is known, as a result of cloning the cDNA, it is possible to estimate the relative ability of various portions of the protein to interact with the bilayer. Stretches of amino acids that are highly hydrophobic (or hydropathic) are more likely to reside in the bilayer. A plot of the hydropathy index versus the position of the amino acids in the primary sequence (see Fig. 1.16) is used to identify regions of the protein that are likely to be associated with the membrane. This hydropathy plot provides a valuable first guess as to the number of membrane-spanning regions of the protein and points to possible large intracellular or extracellular domains. In the case of transport proteins, one expectation is that the membrane-spanning region is associated with the transport process per se, whereas large cytoplasmic or extracellular regions may be involved in regulatory functions, such as the binding of second messengers or hormones.

A membrane-spanning polypeptide chain usually adopts an α-helical conformation. This conformation is dictated by the fact that, in the absence of water, the polar peptide bonds tend to form hydrogen bonds with each other. The α-helical conformation maximizes the number of such bonds and usually forms in such a way as also to enable nonpolar amino acid side chains to interact with the lipid bilayer matrix. An important tertiary structure thought to be common to ion channel proteins is the juxtaposition of a number of membrane-spanning a helices, arranged like barrel staves, to form a central pore that is highly polar and thus a hospitable environment for ion conduction (see Fig. 1.16B).

Transport: Energetics and Mechanism

All transport mechanisms, regardless of their complexity, can be viewed as consisting of three steps: (a) the entry of the transported substance into the membrane on one side, (b) a translocation event that conveys the substance to the other side, and (c) the exit of the substance from the membrane and

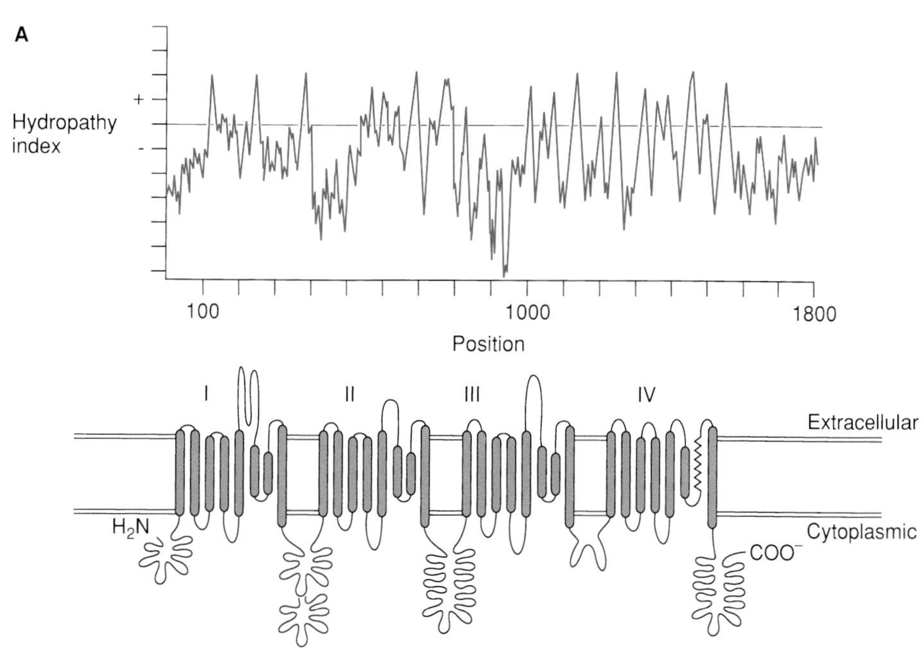

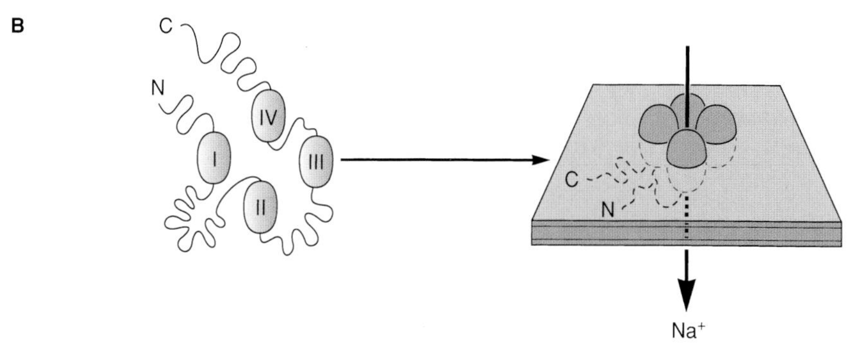

FIGURE 1.16 (*A*) The amino acid sequence of a sodium channel protein derived from the cDNA can be analyzed by plotting the hydropathy index versus the position of the amino acid. (*B*) Regions predicted to be hydrophobic (+) are represented in the diagram as putative membrane-spanning domains. The four repeated motifs are shown as folding around a central pore to form an ion channel. (After Trimmer JS, Agnew WS. Molecular diversity of voltage-sensitive Na channels. *Annu Rev Physiol.* 1989;51:401.)

into the aqueous compartment. Understanding the mechanism for this process means comprehending the physical processes that govern each of these three steps. A complementary approach to understanding transport mechanisms is to inquire about the energetics of the transport process. Is the transporter a passive leak pathway, or does the transport event involve energy conversion?

The basis for energetic analysis of transport processes is the concept of equilibrium.[20,21] If the distribution of any substance, say glucose, Na, or K, is not at equilibrium, then flow of that substance is expected to be in a direction so as to restore equilibrium. If the distribution is maintained away from equilibrium, this means that some process is moving the substance "uphill," and such a process must involve energy conversion. For uncharged substances, the analysis is particularly simple. Consider, for example, the distribution of glucose across a cell membrane (Fig. 1.17). The equilibrium condition is $[\text{glucose}]_{in} = [\text{glucose}]_{out}$. In this condition, there is no net flow of glucose through a simple glucose leak pathway. If $[\text{glucose}]_{in}$ is less than $[\text{glucose}]_{out}$, net passive glucose flow through a leak pathway is into the cell. If $[\text{glucose}]_{in}$ is greater than $[\text{glucose}]_{out}$, glucose leaves the cell through such a transporter. Because this is a leak pathway (non-energy converting), glucose flow can only be "downhill," from a high glucose concentration to a low glucose concentration.

It is useful to analyze equilibrium for such a solute in terms of free energy, rather than concentration. To do this, we define the difference in chemical potential for glucose across the membrane, $\Delta\mu_{glu}$, as follows:

$$\Delta\mu_{glu} \text{ (in J/mol)} = RT \ln \frac{(\text{glucose})_i}{(\text{glucose})_o}$$

where R = the universal gas constant, and T = the absolute temperature.

In terms of free energy, the equilibrium condition is specified by $\Delta\mu_{glu} = 0$. If $\Delta\mu_{glu} \neq 0$, there is a driving force for net flow, and the flow occurs in a direction so as to restore equilibrium.

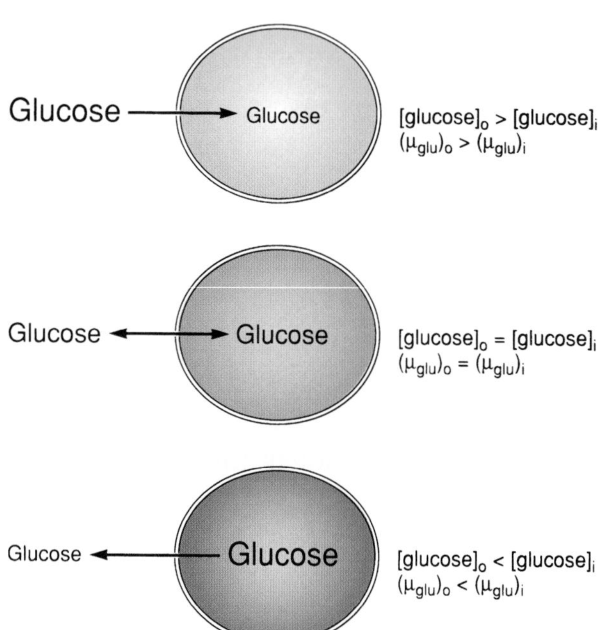

FIGURE 1.17 For a substance that moves by a non–energy-dependent transport mechanism, the direction of the net flow is determined by the passive driving force. In this example, the movement of glucose is determined by the orientation of the concentration gradient (the chemical potential gradient).

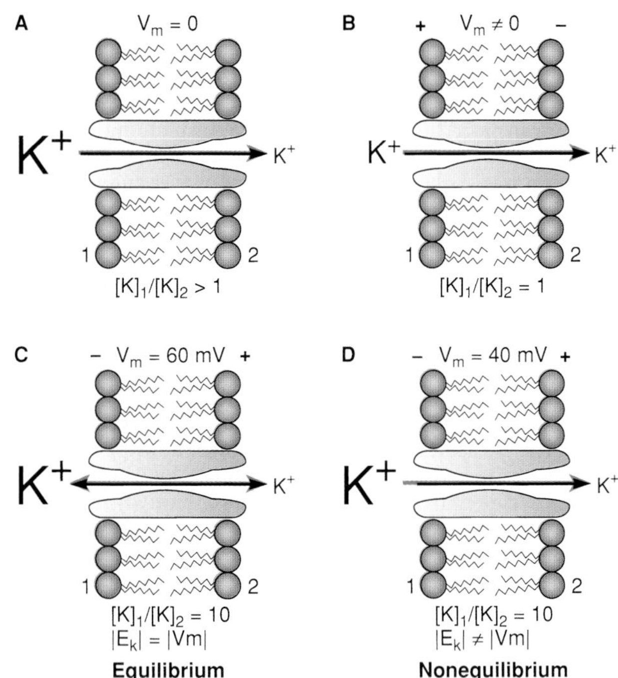

FIGURE 1.18 The direction of passive ion flow is determined by the *electrochemical potential gradient.* The total driving force is the sum of that due to the K concentration gradient (*A*) and that due to the electrical potential difference (*B*). If the driving force due to the concentration gradient is equal in magnitude and opposite in direction to the electrical potential (*C*), the total passive force is zero (i.e., the ion is distributed at equilibrium). (*D*) A net driving force exists because there is an imbalance between E_K and V_m.

Ion flow through a channel can be driven by either an ion concentration gradient or an electrical potential difference (Fig. 1.18). To express both of these driving forces in the same units, the electrochemical potential difference, $\Delta\bar{\mu}_i$ can be defined. For K ions, $\Delta\bar{\mu}_K$ is given by the following equation:

$$\Delta\bar{\mu}_K = RT \ln ([K]_i/[K]_o) + zFV_m$$

where $[K]_i$ and $[K]_o$ = K concentrations; z = the valence; F = the Faraday constant; and V_m = the membrane potential.

If $\Delta\bar{\mu}_K = 0$, the driving force for ion flow is zero and the ion is distributed at equilibrium. If $\Delta\bar{\mu}_K \neq 0$, there is a driving force for ion flow. The total driving force, $\Delta\bar{\mu}_K$, is the sum of two parts—one due to the K concentration gradient $[(RT \ln ([K]_i/[K]_o)]$ and the other due to the electrical potential (zFV_m). The electrochemical potential difference can be regarded as a generalized potential function that encompasses driving forces due to both concentration gradients and electrical potential. $\Delta\bar{\mu}_K$ enables one to express the driving forces due to a concentration gradient and an electrical potential in the same units. This is perhaps most obvious as illustrated in Fig. 1.18, in which all terms are expressed using electrical units (i.e., millivolts), so that the driving force for K^+ flow can be written as follows:

$$\frac{\Delta\bar{\mu}_K}{zF} = V_m - E_K$$

where $E_K = RT/zF \ln ([K]_o/[K]_i)$, a measure of the driving force due to the potassium concentration gradient in electrical units.

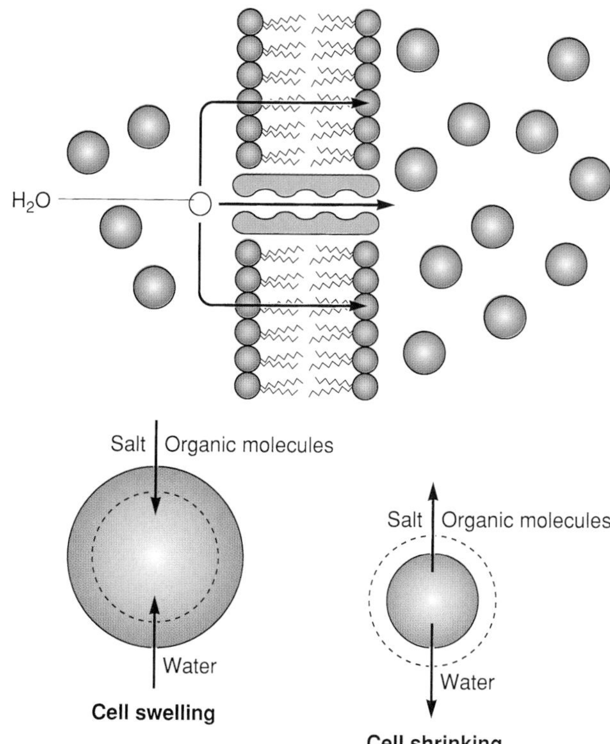

FIGURE 1.19 Water permeates the plasma membrane by means of *solubility-diffusion* through the lipid bilayer and, in some cells, through specialized water channels. Cell volume is normally determined by *solute* distribution because plasma membrane water permeability is high and cells tend to approach osmotic equilibrium.

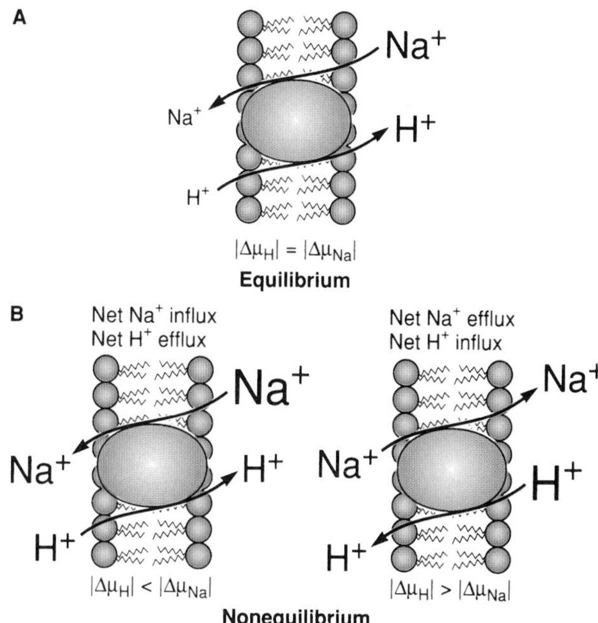

FIGURE 1.20 The Na^+–H^+ exchanger is an example of a *countertransporter,* a mechanism by which energy invested in the Na gradient can be used to drive protons out of the cell. The direction of turnover of the exchange process is determined by the balance of the chemical potential gradients for Na^+ and H^+.

Driving Force for Water Flow

The energetics of water movement across cell membranes is simplified by the fact that water moves only passively owing to gradients of hydrostatic pressure or water concentration. Hydrostatic pressure is an important driving force only for certain specialized cells—the capillary endothelium and the glomerulus of the kidney. For most of the cells in the body, the transmembrane hydrostatic pressure is zero (owing to membrane elasticity), and water moves only in response to water concentration gradients.

Because the concentration of water is determined by the amount of dissolved solute, the difference in water concentration is typically expressed as a function of the difference in solute concentration or, as it is more commonly known, osmotic pressure difference (Fig. 1.19). Because there are no specialized, energy-converting transport mechanisms for water, water is distributed at equilibrium. Water distribution is determined entirely by solute distribution. If a cell gains solute, it swells by gaining water. If a cell loses solute, it shrinks because of the obligatory efflux of water.

Active Transport: Conservation of Energy

Transport processes can be conceptualized in terms of the relation between work available and work done, as suggested by Fig. 1.20, which illustrates an example of a coupled transport process: Na^+–H^+ antiport or Na^+–H^+ exchange. From this perspective, the function of an Na^+–H^+ antiporter is to use the energy available in the transmembrane Na^+ gradient to drive protons out of the cell. This available energy has been invested in the Na^+ gradient by the action of the Na^+-K^+-ATPase. The work done moving protons is given by the electrochemical potential difference for protons multiplied by the number of protons (or moles of protons) moved per cycle. Similarly, the work *available* is given by the electrochemical potential difference for Na^+ times the mole number.

What would happen if we were artificially to *increase* ΔpH by acidifying the solution bathing the cell in Fig. 1.20 so that ΔH^+ exceeds ΔNa^+? Like any chemical reaction, the antiporter would run backward. Protons would enter the cell and drive Na^+ out. The energetics of any coupled transporter is an important experimental test for the coupling process.

Transport Mechanisms

The composition of the lipid bilayer suggests that its transport properties should be those of a layer of oil or, more accurately, a layer of hydrocarbon, formed by the fatty acid side chains of the phospholipids. To penetrate the lipid bilayer, a substance must enter the bilayer by dissolving, or partitioning, into it. Movement across the bilayer occurs by diffusion. The overall process is referred to as *solubility–diffusion* and is the mechanism of membrane transport for moderately lipophilic solutes and water. Cells may also have specialized transport proteins called aquaporins[22] that function as water channels, but for most cells, water movement across the plasma membrane can be accounted for by simple solubility–diffusion of H_2O across the lipid bilayer. The coexistence in some cells of two pathways for water movement is a bit puzzling, but the implied redundancy is highlighted by the observation that congenital absence of aquaporin 1 is not associated with any clinical phenotype.

At equilibrium, the partitioning of a solute between the aqueous and hydrocarbon phases can be described by an

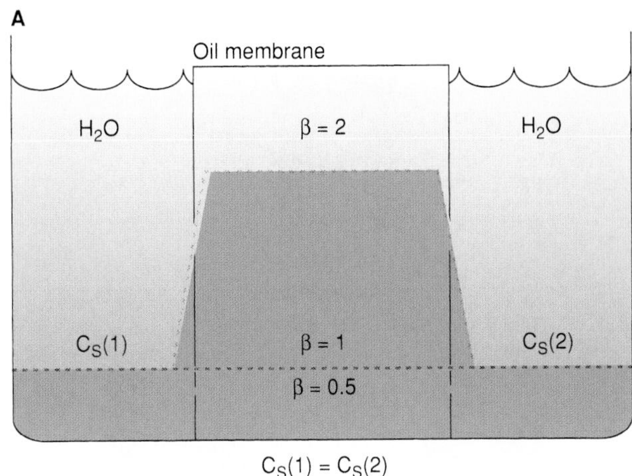

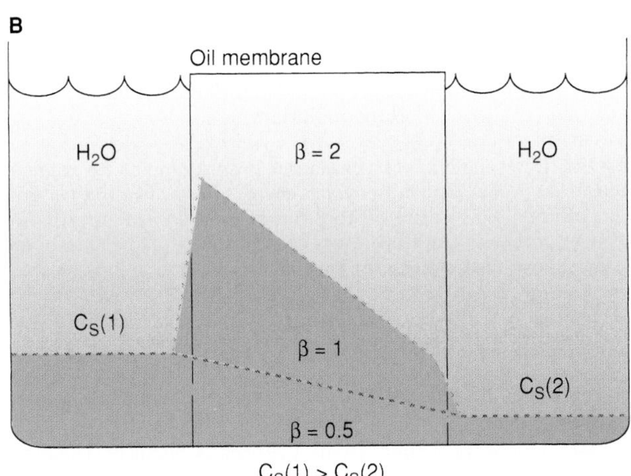

FIGURE 1.21 Moderately lipophilic solutes can cross the plasma membrane by solubility diffusion through the lipid bilayer, modeled here as an oil membrane. Three hypothetical solutes are depicted as having oil–water partition coefficients (β_i) of 0.5, 1, and 2. The concentration profiles in the absence (*A*) and in the presence (*B*) of a concentration gradient are shown. The dominant factor in the determination of permeability is the partition coefficient β_i.

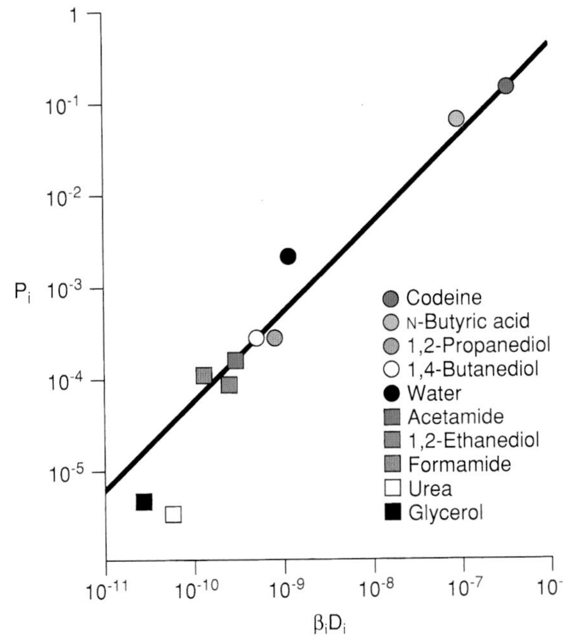

FIGURE 1.22 The permeability of a planar lipid bilayer to a series of lipophilic solutes is highly correlated with the product of the oil–water partition coefficient and the diffusion coefficient (i.e., $\beta_i D_i$).

oil–water partition coefficient, β_{oil}, expressed as C_{oil}/C_{water}, the ratio of the concentration of the substance in oil to that in water. This equilibrium partitioning is illustrated in Fig. 1.21A for a solute that is present at the same concentration on both sides of an oil membrane. The concentration profile is shown as the concentration of the solute in the aqueous and oil phases plotted versus distance along the y-axis. Concentration profiles are illustrated for three hypothetical solutes exhibiting three different partition coefficients, 13 = 0.5, 1, and 2. In this case, because the concentration is identical on both sides of the membrane ($C_1 = C_2$),there is no flow across the membrane. The diffusion of lipophilic nonelectrolytes is a purely passive leak process; if there is no concentration gradient, there is no driving force for net flow. Figure 1.21B shows the concentration profiles in the presence of a concentration gradient ($C_1 > C_2$), illustrating the influence of the partition coefficient on the amount of solute in the membrane. The permeability of lipid membranes to moderately lipophilic solutes is highly correlated with the value of the oil–water partition coefficient. Figure 1.22 illustrates the correlation using data from a planar lipid bilayer. Note the position of water in this plot.

Ion Channels

Ion channels are transmembrane proteins that form pores that can conduct ions across the plasma membrane. The lipid portion of the plasma membrane is virtually impermeable to small ions such as Na^+, K^+, Cl^-, and Ca^{2+}. The inability of ions to cross a hydrophobic layer results from the enormous energy required to move an ion from a highly polar aqueous environment into the relatively nonpolar region formed by the hydrocarbon tails of the phospholipids. Ion channels are formed by membrane-spanning peptides that are arranged so that polar moieties line a central pore, as suggested in Fig. 1.16B. These polar groups take the place of the water of hydration, which stabilizes an ion in an aqueous solution. The polar groups create, in essence, a water-like environment into which the ion can partition and move in the presence of an appropriate driving force. The recent crystal structure obtained for the bacterial K channel showed that when a K^+ ion enters the channel, four of its inner sphere waters of hydration are "replaced" by interactions with a halo of four carbonyl oxygen ligands.[23]

The movement of an ion through a channel implies the movement of charge or current flow and hence is referred to as a *conductive process*. The physical interactions that underlie the conduction process determine both the rate at which ions can traverse the channel and the selectivity of the channel, the degree to which the channel discriminates between ions. The size of the single-channel conductance and the selectivity of the channel provide important criteria for distinguishing one channel from another on the basis of function. For example, most cells contain a variety of channels that are selective for specific ions (e.g., Na^+, K^+, Cl^- Ca^{2+}, HCO_3^-). Selectivity provides a broad classification of channels. Most cells contain several subtypes of selective channels, which are often distinguished on the basis of the size of the single-channel conductance. It is likely that channels differentiated on the basis of function reflect the properties of distinctly different membrane proteins. The existence of channel diversity suggests that different channel proteins may play different roles in the life of the cell.

Gating of Ion Channels

Ion channels are permissive transport elements: ions flow through a channel only in the presence of an appropriate driving force. Records of the current flowing through single channels (Fig. 1.23) show clearly that even in the presence of a driving force, an ion channel does not conduct all of the time. Rather, the form of the single-channel current record suggests that the channel protein undergoes conformational changes between conducting (open) states and nonconducting (closed) states. These conformational changes are collectively referred to as *gating*. Gating of ion channels is crucial to the survival of cells and organisms because gating is the basis for the regulation of ion flow through membrane channels.

The simplest model for the gating process recognizes two states of the ion channel protein—closed (nonconducting) and open (conducting), which can be represented as a reversible chemical reaction:

$$\text{closed} \underset{\alpha}{\overset{\beta}{\rightleftharpoons}} \text{open}$$

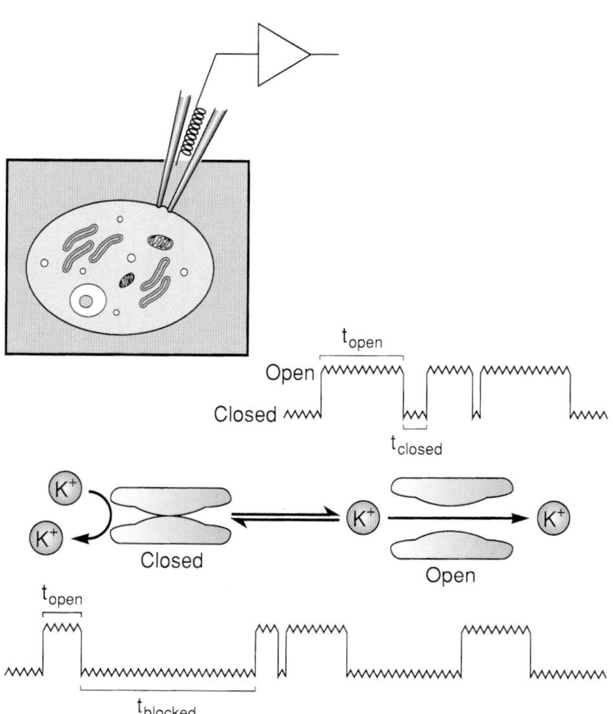

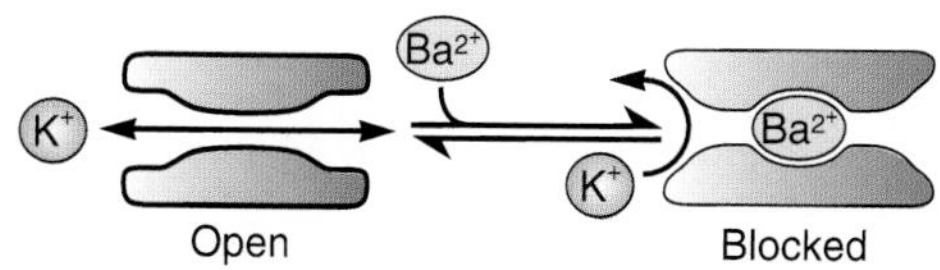

FIGURE 1.23 The patch-clamp method permits the recording of the currents that flow through a single open ion channel. The gating (opening and closing) of the channel is reflected in the changes in the single-channel current between two values—zero and the open-channel value. A channel blocker such as barium can induce long, nonconducting intervals because it binds in the channel and blocks ion flow.

The gating process can be envisioned as being the result of the incessant thermal vibration, or "twitching," of the protein. Occasionally, one such thermal twitch has enough energy to precipitate a change in the conformation of the protein, a change from closed to open, for example. The rate coefficients, α and β, are a measure of the likelihood of these conformational changes. The relative values of α and β determine the fraction of time that the channel spends in one state or another, or, more accurately, the probability of finding the channel in a particular state. For example, if $\alpha = \beta$, then, regardless of the individual values of α and 43, the channel conducts half the time. In general, the probability of finding the channel in the open state would be given by the following equation:

$$P_o = \beta(\alpha + \beta)$$

Channel gating provides the molecular basis for exquisite regulation of the rate of ion flow across a membrane. For example, consider the rate of K flow through a population, or ensemble, of a particular type of K channel. The total conductance due to the population is given by g_K using the formula:

$$g_K = \gamma_K(N_K)_o$$

where γK = conductance of a single K channel, and $(N_K)_o$ = average number of open channels. $(N_K)_o$, however, is given by the formula

$$(N_K)_o = N_K P_o$$

where N_K = *total* number of channels in the cell membrane (counting open *and* closed), and P_o = probability of finding any one channel in the open state.

Combining, this relation is obtained:

$$g_K = \gamma_K N_K P_o$$

This important equation relates the macroscopic conductance, g_K, to the properties of individual channel proteins. Contained within the three parameters γ_K, N_K, and P_o is the basis for the regulation of ion transport. The conductance, or leakiness, of a membrane to a particular ion can be modulated by altering P_o, N_K, or γ_K.

Ion Channel Conduction Can Be Blocked

The conduction process can be blocked by ions or organic compounds that enter the channel, bind there, and occlude the pore. Typically, channel blockade is a reversible binding reaction, so that the efficacy of the blocker is determined by the affinity of the blocker for the binding site; this affinity determines how long the blocking molecule remains in the pore. Figure 1.23 shows the blockage of a K channel by the divalent ion, barium. The recording of the single-channel current allows us to resolve a single blocking event—that is, the interaction of one blocker molecule with a single-channel protein. The blocking events are clearly discernible as long, nonconducting intervals in the record of single-channel current.

Channel blockade is an important mechanism of action for toxins and some therapeutic agents. For example, the deadly toxin of the puffer fish, tetrodotoxin, acts by blocking the Na^+ channels that are responsible for the conduction of the nerve impulse. The diuretic, amiloride, acts by blocking the Na channels that inhabit the apical membrane of the epithelial cells of the distal nephron. Local anesthetics such as lidocaine (Xylocaine) act by blocking ion channels.

Modulation of Ion Channel Gating

Two of the most important mechanisms that operate to gate ion channels are voltage and ligand binding. Voltage-gated ion channels are the molecular basis for excitability in nerve and muscle and the conduction of the nerve impulse (action potential) from the cell body along the axon to the synaptic terminus. Voltage-dependent gating of Na and K channels is the basis of the action potential. Because Na-selective channels open more rapidly than K-selective channels, the initial effect of a depolarizing stimulus is to increase an inward Na current and further depolarize V_m. Subsequently, K channels are opened by the depolarization, and the increased K conductance tends to repolarize V_m. During an action potential, the Na conductance of the axon membrane can increase by 100-fold in less than 1 second. During this change, the number of channels in the membrane does not increase; the increase in Na conductance is due solely to a dramatic increase in the probability that an Na channel is open.

The mechanism of voltage-dependent gating is not completely understood, but data suggest that in voltage-gated channels the conformational change from closed to open is associated with the movement of a charged group on the protein. Depolarization of the membrane reduces the free energy (work) required to open the channel by reducing the work required to move this so-called gating charge. Several voltage-gated channels have been cloned, and a region has been identified that has properties appropriate for a voltage sensor. Interestingly, this region appears to be highly conserved in Na, K, and Ca channels (Fig. 1.24).

The term *ligand-gated channels* refers to a broad class of channels that can be opened (or closed) in response to the binding of some ligand to the channel protein. The ligand can be a neurotransmitter, such as acetylcholine, or an intracellular messenger, such as calcium. The binding of a ligand can increase membrane conductance by favoring the open configuration of the channel (Fig. 1.25).

Water Channels

The plasma membrane of most cells is highly permeable to water because water can cross the lipid bilayer at significant rates by means of solubility–diffusion. A few cells in the body are specialized so that they can exhibit a highly regulated water permeability. These cells include epithelial cells found in the distal tubule of the mammalian kidney. In such cells, the water permeability can be exquisitely regulated by antidiuretic hormone (ADH). ADH is a peptide hormone that binds to receptors located in the basolateral membranes of epithelial cells and, by means of a cyclic adenosine monophosphate (cAMP)-dependent mechanism, leads to the insertion of water-conducting channels in the apical membrane. Regulated water permeability requires that two basic conditions be met: (a) there must be a regulatable pathway for water transport (i.e., water channels); and (b) the background, or non–ADH-dependent water permeability of the membrane, must be relatively low. The apical membranes of ADH-sensitive epithelia are specialized in both of these ways. The resting water permeability (or hydraulic conductivity) of these membranes is relatively low, so that in the absence of ADH, even a substantial osmotic gradient produces little water flow. ADH can effect a dramatic increase in water permeability by inducing the insertion of water-conducting channels into the apical membrane of such cells. The ADH-sensitive water channel has been identified as aquaporin 2, and congenital absence of this protein can contribute to nephrogenic diabetes insipidus.[22] To be an effective instrument for the regulation of body fluid composition, these channels must be selective for water. If water channels exhibited significant ion permeability, for example, the ability of the kidney to regulate body fluid osmolality would be compromised by salt flows.

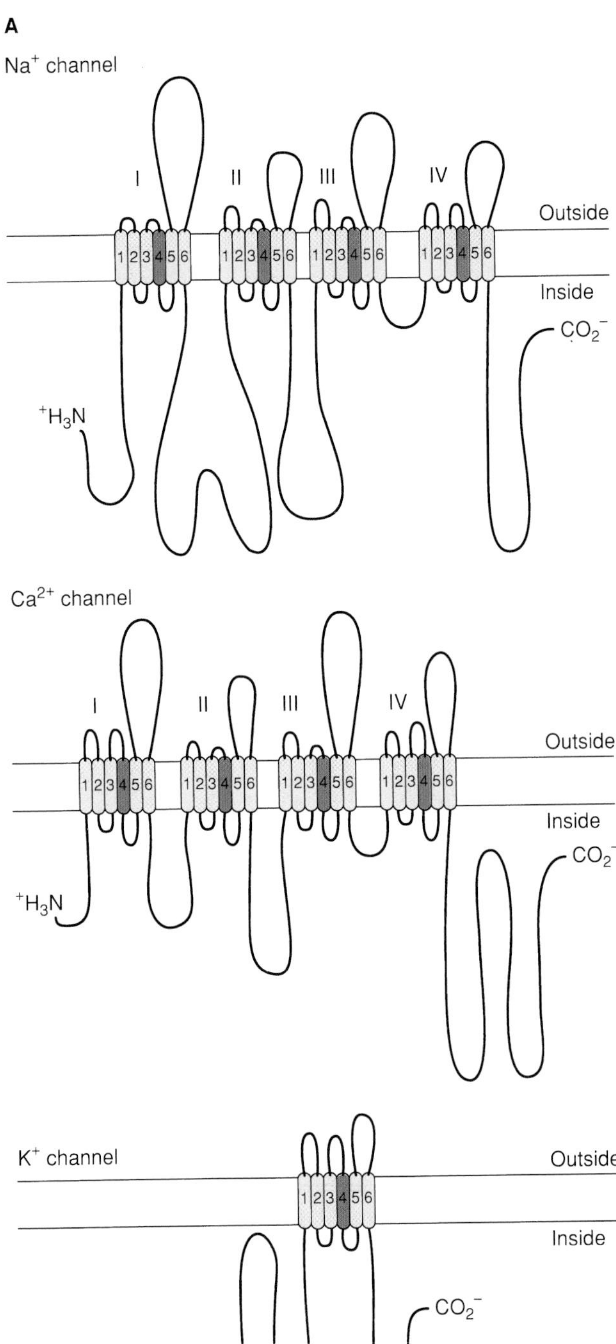

FIGURE 1.24 (*A*) Hydropathic analysis of predicted amino acid sequences for three voltage-dependent ion channels—Na^+, Ca^{2+}, and K^+—yields clues to the configuration of the proteins in the plasma membrane. Na^+ and Ca^{2+} are thought to contain four repeating motifs in one protein, which can fold to make a channel, whereas K^+ channels are tetramers. All three channels contain a highly conserved region, thought to be the voltage sensor. (*B*) Voltage-dependent gating is thought to be effected by charges in the S4 region that cause this segment to undergo a twisting motion in an electric field. (After Catterall WA. Structure and fraction of voltage-sensitive ion channels. *Science* 1988;242:50–61.)

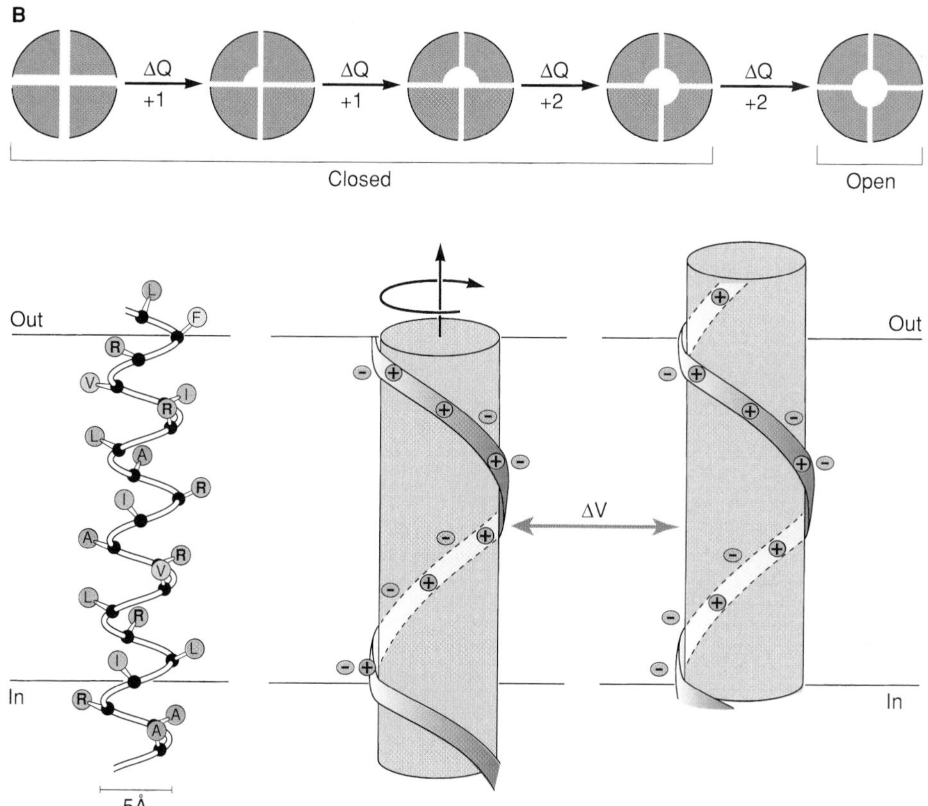

FIGURE 1.24 *(continued)*

Carrier Proteins

Most transport proteins appear to function as carriers rather than as channels. Membrane carriers are a broad class of transmembrane proteins that include simple leaks as well as energy-converting mechanisms such as the ATPases, countertransporters, and cotransporters. For membrane carriers, the mechanism of translocation is probably more complicated than for an open channel. Although the details of the mechanisms are not well understood, important distinctions can be made between carrier-type and channel-type mechanisms on the basis of transport kinetics.

The most important difference between a channel mechanism and a carrier mechanism is the role in the transport event played by conformational changes in the membrane protein. For a channel, the gating process is envisioned as involving a conformational change between conducting and nonconducting states that operates like a gate. Conduction is associated only with the open state of the channel, and the gating process is not coupled to the translocation event. In a carrier mechanism, available information suggests that the translocation event is directly linked to, or caused by, a conformational change in the membrane protein.

Figure 1.26 compares the transport mechanism for a channel and a carrier. The channel (see Fig. 1.26A) is depicted as having two states, closed and open, so that it operates like a switch. In contrast, carrier transport (see Fig. 1.26B) is envisioned as requiring a cycle of conformational changes. In the absence of substrate, the carrier can assume one of two conformations, which are distinguished by location of the substrate binding site, an inward-facing and an outward-facing conformation. Binding of substrate permits or initiates a conformational change that translocates the site, and the bound substrate, from one side to the other. The unoccupied site can then revert to the inward-facing form, and the cycle can be repeated. The transport of one molecule of substrate requires one complete cycle of the carrier. This sort of analysis suggests that carriers can be distinguished from channels based on the accessibility of the binding site. In a channel mechanism, binding sites within the open pore are equally accessible from either side of the membrane, whereas in a carrier mechanism, the binding site is available only on one side of the membrane at any instant.

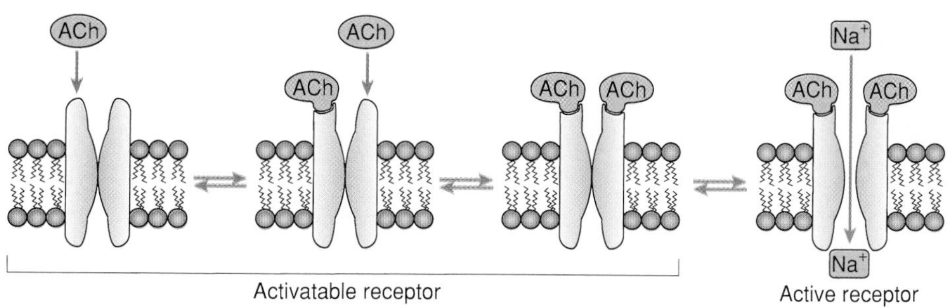

FIGURE 1.25 The acetylcholine receptor is an example of a ligand-gated channel. Two molecules of acetylcholine must bind before the channel can reach the open (conducting) conformation.

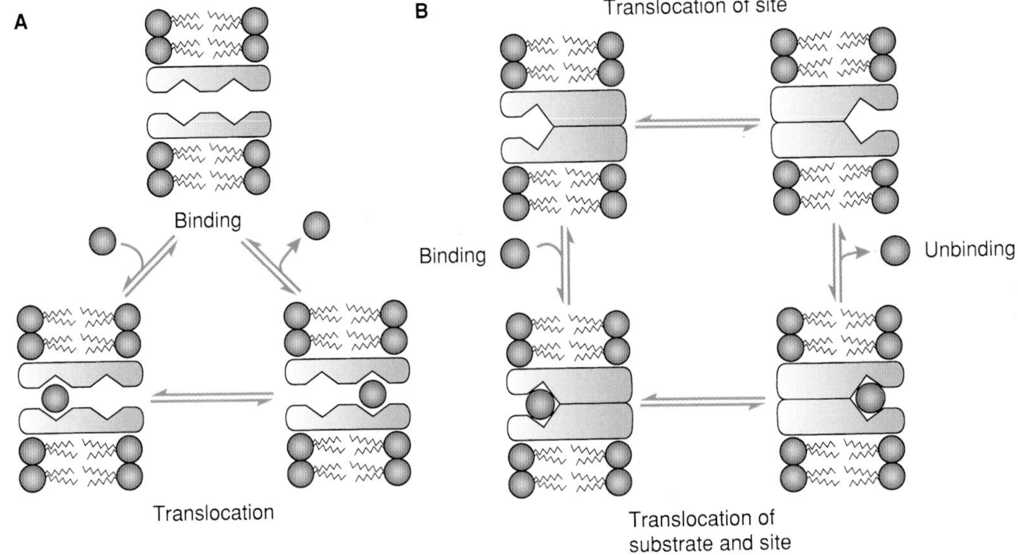

FIGURE 1.26 (*A*) Ion translocation through an open channel can be envisioned as involving a binding step, followed by translocation and unbinding of the ion. (*B*) In contrast, carrier-mediated flow involves binding followed by a conformational change that is coupled to the translocation of the substrate. In this model, the unbound site can translocate.

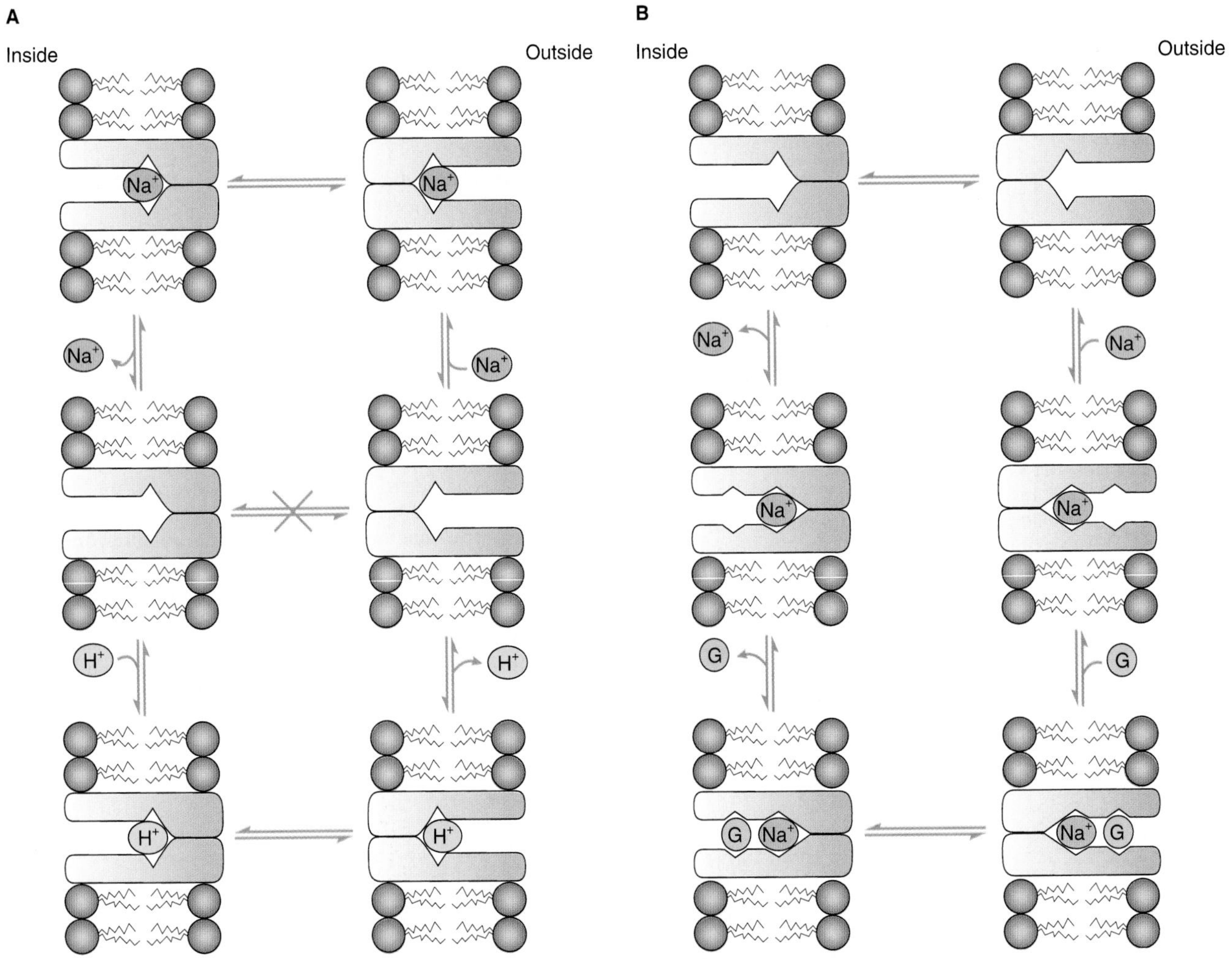

FIGURE 1.27 (*A*) An exchanger, or antiporter, is created by disallowing the translocation of the unbound site. For example, the catalytic cycle diagrammed here leads to the exchange of Na^+ for H^+ (i.e., Na^+–H^+ antiport). (*B*) An obligatory cotransporter is created by permitting only two forms of the protein to undergo translatory conformational changes—the doubly bound and the unbound. Here, the binding of Na^+ facilitates the subsequent binding of glucose, leading to the Na^+-dependent cotransport of Na^+ and glucose.

The cyclic nature of the carrier transport mechanism has several important consequences. First, the linkage of transport to conformational changes renders the process slower than that of a channel by approximately one order of magnitude. A distinguishing feature of channel-mediated ion transport is the high rate of transport, of the order of 10^6 ions/second. A second consequence of the conformational cycling in carriers is that the conformation of the carrier can be strongly influenced by the transmembrane distribution of the transported substrate. This creates a mechanism for the coupling of the flows of two substrates. The intimate link between conformational change and translocation makes it possible to envision a variety of mechanisms for the coupling of the flow of one substrate to that of a second substrate flow or to a chemical reaction (an ATPase). These mechanisms are diagrammed in Fig. 1.27. A cotransporter (e.g., Na^+–glucose) is envisioned as one in which the translocation event requires the binding of both Na and glucose (Fig. 1.26A). In one scheme, the binding of Na to one site would increase the affinity of a second site for glucose. Thus, an Na^+ gradient creates a net flow of glucose by favoring inward glucose flow. The fact that the Na^+ binds with its charge means that the inside negative membrane potential represents another force, which drives the cycle so as to favor inward glucose flow.

If the conformational changes of the unbound site are disallowed, the resulting mechanism is an exchanger or antiporter because the only possible transport event is the obligatory exchange, or swapping, of one substrate molecule for another. This process is presumed to be the basis for the energy-converting countertransport that occurs, for example, in Na^+–H^+ exchange (Fig. 1.26A). Here, the imposition of an Na^+ gradient can drive protons out of the cell. Because of the Na^+ gradient, Na^+ dominates the out-to-in portion of the cycle, whereas H^+ dominates the in-to-out portion of the cycle. There is evidence for an activation site on the cytoplasmic face of the Na^+–H^+ antiporter, which functions to turn on Na^+–H^+ exchange only when cytosolic pH falls below a certain set point. It has been suggested that hormones and growth factors that influence Na^+–H^+ exchange do so in part by modulating the activating site.

The archetype for biologic pumps is the Na^+-K^+-ATPase. For this transporter, the biochemical events in the catalytic cycle have been examined in great detail, although the exact nature of the translocation events still is not well understood. Figure 1.28 illustrates how the inclusion of a phosphorylation event in the catalytic cycle could result in the coupling of the free energy of hydrolysis of ATP to the translocation of ions, in this case, the exchange of Na^+ for K^+ in the ratio of three Na^+ to two K^+ This unequal stoichiometry results in the transfer of net charge during the catalytic cycle, so that the normal pumping mode is associated with an outwardly directed membrane current.

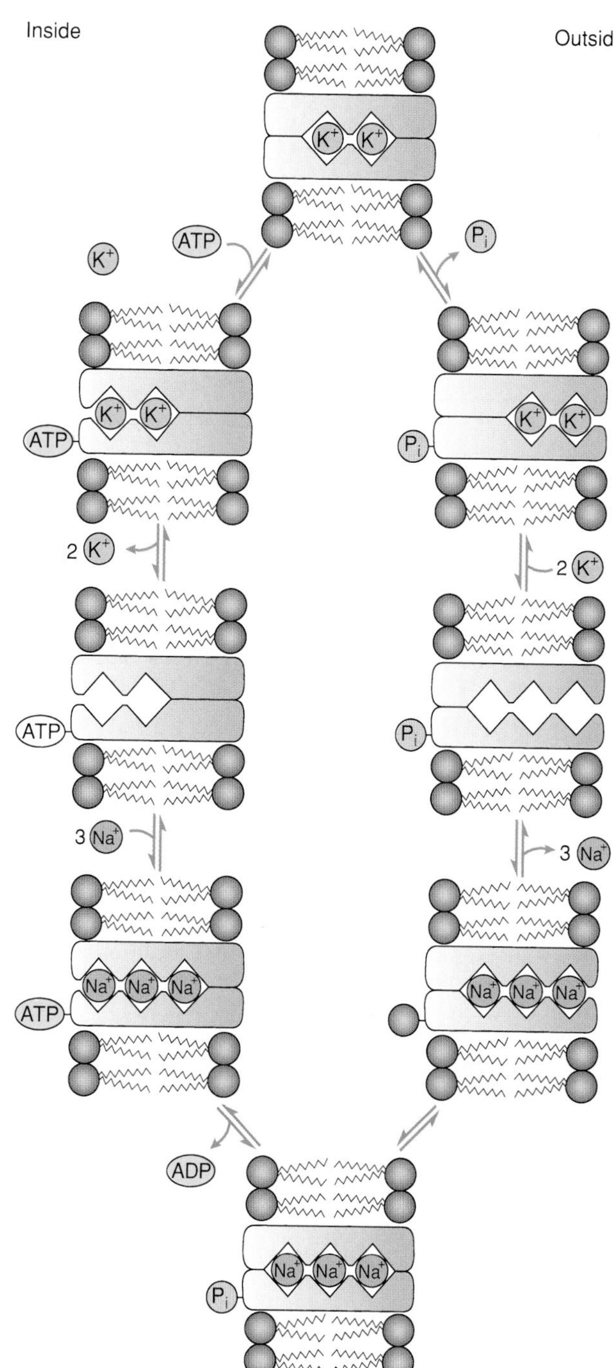

FIGURE 1.28 The Na^+-K^+-adenosine triphosphatase (ATPase) has a complicated catalytic cycle that involves not only the binding and unbinding of Na^+ and K^+ but the binding of ATP, phosphorylation of the protein, and subsequent dephosphorylation, so that one ATP is hydrolyzed per transport cycle.

Volume Regulation

One important function of the solute transport mechanisms that inhabit the plasma membrane is the maintenance and regulation of cell volume. Water distribution, as noted earlier, is determined in most cells entirely by solute distribution. Thus, the volume of a cell is determined by the same mechanisms that maintain the steady-state solute composition of the cell. Many, if not all, cells have the capacity to respond actively to a perturbation in cell volume—that is, they are capable of volume regulation. Volume regulatory responses are based on membrane transporters that enable the cell to undergo a net loss or a net gain of solute and hence lose or gain water. For example, if a cell is swollen by exposure to a hypotonic medium, the permeability of the cell membrane to K^+ and Cl^- is markedly increased, such that a net efflux of salt and water occurs, bringing about a regulatory volume decrease (Fig. 1.29). Similarly, shrinking a cell by exposing it to an impermeant solute activates mechanisms for solute entry, usually NaCl. Another type of volume regulatory mechanism involves the movements of organic solutes such as taurine or myoinositol. These solutes are accumulated by cells through Na-dependent cotransporters and can account for a significant fraction of intracellular osmolality. Cell swelling leads to the opening of channels that mediate rapid efflux of these osmolytes from the cell, thus initiating a regulatory volume decrease.

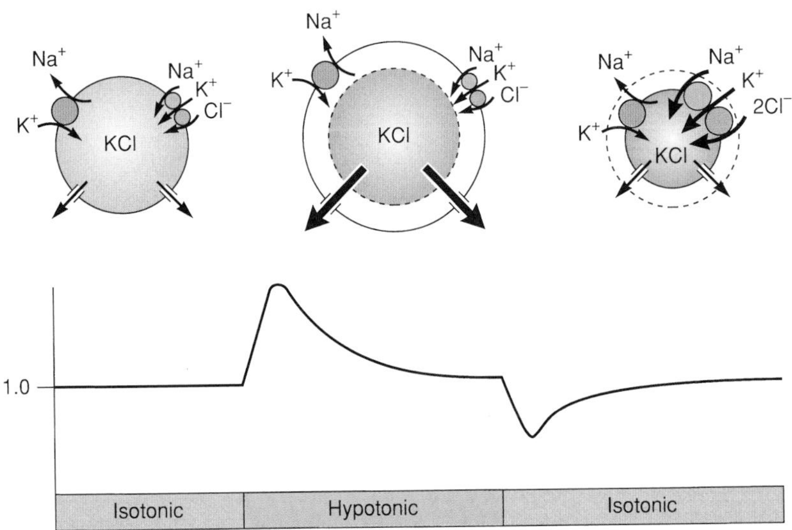

FIGURE 1.29 Many cells actively regulate their volume by turning on and off specific transport pathways. A hypotonic solution is shown here as causing cell swelling and activating channels for K^+ and Cl^- so that salt leaves the cell, promoting shrinkage. A return to isotonic conditions leads to water efflux and cell shrinkage, which activates a coupled, Na^+-K^+-$2Cl^-$ entry process that results in a gain of salt and water and a return to normal volume.

INTRACELLULAR SYNTHESIS, TRANSPORT, AND ORGANIZATION OF MACROMOLECULES

Cell structure and function are ultimately determined by the proteins present in a particular cell type and their spatial arrangement in distinct organelles. It is important to understand how the synthesis of proteins is carried out, how it is regulated, and how the newly synthesized proteins are directed or targeted to a specific cellular location or transported to the cell surface and secreted from the cell. Because protein structure is coded for by DNA, this section initially reviews how genetic information is stored in DNA, transcribed into RNA, and then translated into unique proteins.[1,2,24] After this, the intracellular targeting and transport of proteins are discussed.

DNA, RNA, and Protein Synthesis

The genetic blueprint of an organism is carried in the nucleus of every cell, encoded by the sequence of the four bases—adenine (A), guanine (G), cytosine (C), and thymine (T)—which together make up two long chains bound together by hydrogen bonds to form a DNA double helix. Bases in opposite strands of the double helix are specifically paired by hydrogen bonding. A is paired with T by two hydrogen bonds, and C is paired with G by three hydrogen bonds. This base-pair complementarity is the central principle on which DNA replication, RNA transcription, and protein synthesis are based.

A gene is a segment of DNA that is transcribed into a corresponding RNA molecule that either codes for a protein or forms a structural RNA molecule (Fig. 1.30). Genes are commonly between 10,000 and 100,000 base pairs in length and include, in addition to the coding sequence, flanking regions and intervening sequences, called *introns*. Introns are removed from the primary RNA transcript by a process called *splicing*. Each strand of DNA has polarity, and information is read from the 5′ to the 3′ direction, with the numbers referring to the free hydroxyl group on the deoxyribose moiety. The basic unit of information is the codon, a sequence of three bases or a triplet. The four nucleotide bases arranged as triplets lead to 64 possible codons. Sixty-one of these code for the 20 known amino acids, and 3 are termination signals called *stop codons*. The code is degenerate in that some amino acids are specified by up to six codons.

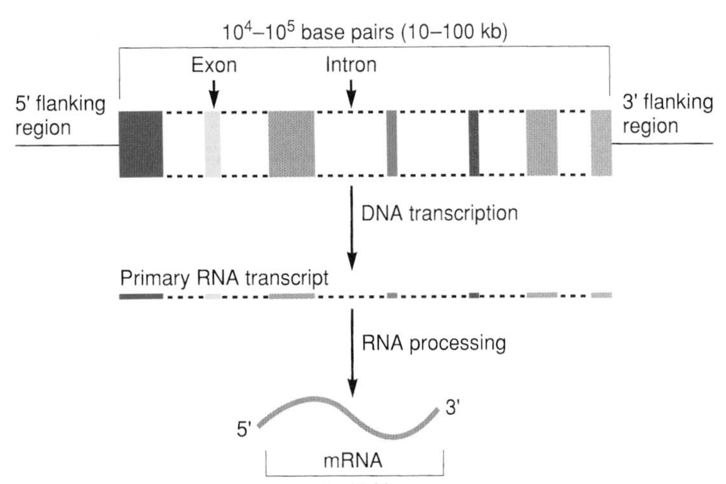

FIGURE 1.30 Structure of a typical gene, its primary RNA transcript, and the resulting mature mRNA. The entire coding region of the gene *is* initially transcribed, and the regions coded for introns are then spliced out during processing. The mature mRNA is then an RNA copy of the exon regions of the gene.

When cells divide, the two DNA chains that constitute the double helix separate, and each serves as a template for synthesis of a complementary strand directed by the enzyme DNA polymerase.[1] One of the new double helices goes to each daughter cell, so that the amount and sequence of DNA in each new cell is the same as that of the parent cell. To direct the synthesis of protein, the DNA sequence has to be transcribed into three types of RNA—messenger RNA (mRNA), transfer RNA (tRNA), and ribosomal RNA (rRNA). RNA contains the nucleoside uridine (U) instead of thymidine and usually exists as a single-stranded, linear polymer. RNA synthesis is directed by an RNA polymerase enzyme that makes an RNA copy of DNA. Eukaryotic cells contain three types of RNA polymerase—termed I, II, and III—each of which catalyzes the formation of a different type of RNA. RNA polymerase II directs the formation of mRNA.

Transcription of a gene begins at an initiation site associated with a specific DNA sequence, called a *promotor region*. Recognition of this region by the polymerase is aided by specific proteins, called *transcription factors,* which bind to the DNA, and by *initiation factors,* which bind to the polymerase. Some transcription factors determine tissue specificity, whereas others, such as steroid hormone receptors, are regulatory and act in various cells to increase or decrease transcription rates of specific genes. After binding to DNA, the RNA polymerase opens up a short region of the double helix to expose the nucleotides. Once the two strands of DNA are separated, the strand containing the promoter acts as a template to which ribonucleoside triphosphates base pair by hydrogen bonds. Nucleotides are then joined together with elongation, proceeding in a 5′ to 3′ direction as the RNA polymerase moves stepwise along the DNA (Fig. 1.31). Behind the polymerase, the DNA double helix reforms, displacing the nascent RNA polymer. When a termination signal is reached, the polymerase releases both the template and the newly made RNA strand and is free to rebind to another promoter region. The average length of the RNA transcript is approximately 8,000 nucleotides, although much longer molecules are common.

The initial products of RNA polymerase II are known as heterogeneous nuclear RNA because of their large size variation. These primary transcripts are then processed to form mRNA. Processing includes addition of a methylguanosine to the 5′ end as a cap, addition of a long sequence of adenosine bases to the 3′ end as a tail, and removal of a number of long nucleotide sequences. As mentioned earlier, these sequences, or introns, are present in the gene but not in mature RNA (see Fig. 1.30). The gene regions represented in mRNA are termed *exons,* for expressed regions. The joining of coding regions on either side of an intron sequence, or splicing, accounts for mature mRNA being much shorter than nuclear RNA. Moreover, alternative splicing can lead to the production of different mRNA molecules and, in some cases, different proteins from the same gene. mRNA is exported from the nucleus only after processing is complete. A typical mammalian cell can contain as few as 1 or 2 or up to 10,000 copies of each mRNA molecule at any one time. Although the number of copies is primarily a function of the rate of transcription (synthesis), mature mRNA is degraded in the cytoplasm, and the rate of degradation of each species also contributes to its relative abundance. mRNA species that need to be rapidly regulated probably carry a sequence that tags them for more rapid destruction.

The synthesis of protein involves conversion from a four-letter nucleotide language to one of 20 chemically distinct amino acids. Accordingly, this process is referred to as *translation.* There is no mechanism for direct chemical recognition between specific nucleic acid bases and specific amino acids. Instead, an adapter molecule, tRNA, is used. tRNAs are small RNA molecules of 70 to 90 nucleotides, traditionally represented as a cloverleaf (Fig. 1.32). The loop on one end contains an anticodon nucleotide triplet that lines up with the complementary sequence of the mRNA, whereas the other end binds the amino acid specified by the mRNA codon. Each tRNA carries only one amino acid and must be recognized by a distinct enzyme, termed an *aminoacyl tRNA synthetase,* which catalyzes the covalent attachment of the carboxyl terminus of the amino acid to the 3′ of the tRNA in a process using ATP. Covalent attachment to the tRNA allows amino acids to be added to a growing protein in the sequence specified by the nucleic acid code. The attachment to tRNA also activates the amino acid by generating a high-energy intermediate. This energy is used to drive the reaction by which the amino acid is added to the nascent protein.

Protein synthesis occurs by the formation of a peptide bond between the carboxyl terminus of the growing polypeptide chain and the free amino group of the activated amino acid tRNA. This event does not occur in free solution but within ribosomes. Ribosomes are protein-synthesizing machines that bring all the necessary components together in the correct sequence and spatial orientation.[25] Each ribosome is a complex of more than 80 proteins and RNA molecules arranged into two subunits, a small and a large, with an

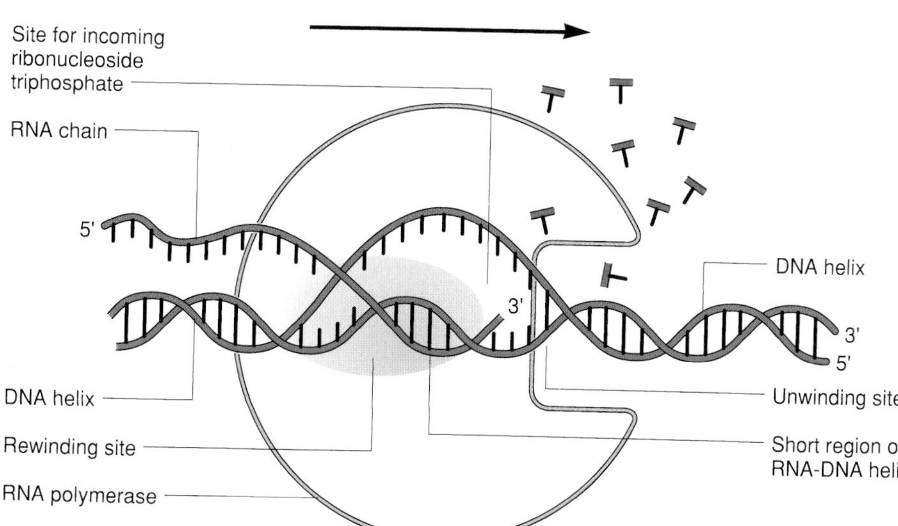

FIGURE 1.31 Transcription of DNA. RNA polymerase acts to unwind the DNA helix, catalyzes the formation of a transient RNA–DNA helix, and then releases the RNA as a single-strand copy while the DNA rewinds. In the process, the polymerase moves along the DNA from a start sequence to a stop sequence.

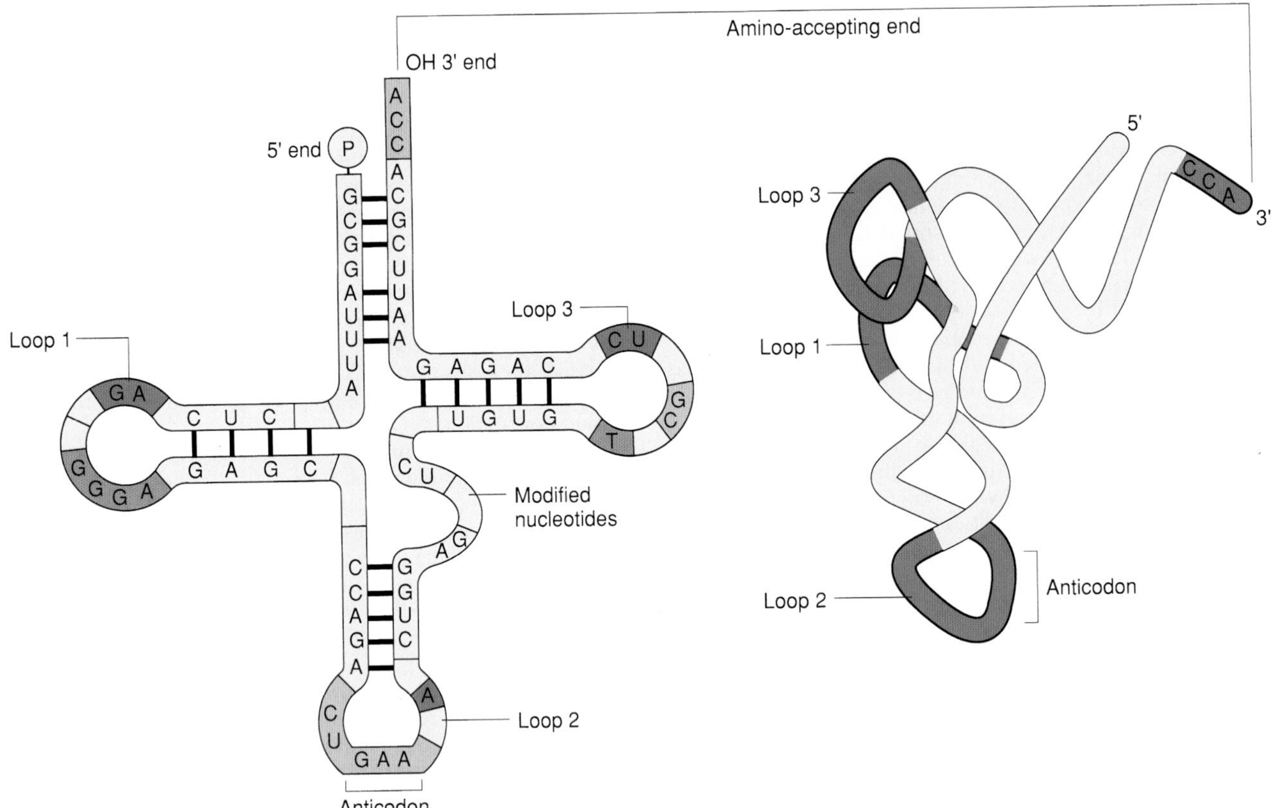

FIGURE 1.32 Structure of a transfer or tRNA molecule. The structure is shown as a stylized cloverleaf (*left*) and as it is believed to exist in three dimensions (*right*). Note the opposite regions for binding an amino acid and the anticodon that forms a base pair with mRNA.

aggregate molecular mass of approximately 4 million. Each ribosome contains three RNA-binding sites, one for mRNA and two for tRNA (Fig. 1.33). One of the latter, termed the *P-site,* holds the tRNA attached to the last amino acid added to the growing polypeptide chain, whereas the other, the A-site, holds the aminoacyl tRNA carrying the next amino acid to be added to the chain. After formation of each new peptide bond, the resulting peptidyl tRNA is transferred from the A-site to the P-site. The free tRNA produced in the P-site is released, and a new aminoacyl tRNA can enter the A-site to begin a new cycle. In the process, the ribosome moves exactly three nucleotides along the mRNA molecule. Protein synthesis consumes a great deal of energy because four high-energy phosphate bonds must be split to make each peptide bond.

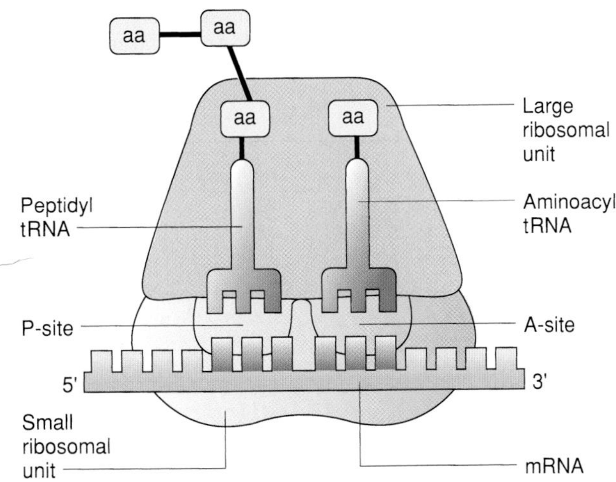

FIGURE 1.33 Schematic view of the elongation phase of protein synthesis on a ribosome. As the ribosome moves along the mRNA, incoming aminoacyl–tRNA complexes bind to the A-site on the ribosome, after which a new peptide bond is formed with the nascent polypeptide chain previously attached to the peptide tRNA. The ribosome then moves, ejecting the now-empty tRNA and opening the A-site for the next aminoacyl–tRNA complex.

Protein synthesis requires identification of the appropriate starting and ending points on the mRNA.[26] The synthesis of all eukaryotic proteins begins with a methionine coded for by an AUG triplet. Only one specific methionine tRNA can initiate synthesis. This initiator tRNA, charged with methionine, forms a complex with the small ribosomal subunit and a protein, eukaryotic initiation factor 2. This complex then binds to an mRNA, which is in most cases identified as such by its 5′ 7-methylguanosine cap, and is then joined by other proteins (initiation factors). The small ribosomal subunit moves along the RNA until its initiating tRNA reaches the start site defined by the AUG sequence. At this time, some of the initiating factors dissociate, and a large ribosomal subunit joins the complex. Chain elongation can then occur by the binding of a free aminoacyl tRNA. Chain termination occurs when the ribosome reaches one of three different stop codons. Termination involves additional proteins, called *release factors,* which catalyze the addition of a water molecule rather than an amino acid to the carboxyl terminus of the polypeptide chain. At this point, there is no longer attachment to a tRNA, and the completed polypeptide is released into the cytoplasm. The ribosome then dissociates into its two subunits and releases the mRNA.

The complete synthesis of a single protein takes 30 seconds to a few minutes, but multiple ribosomes can initiate translation and be moving down the mRNA molecule simultaneously, thus increasing the rate of protein synthesis. This complex of multiple ribosomes on an mRNA molecule is called a *polyribosome*. Protein synthesis can be blocked by a number of antibiotic molecules. Some, such as tetracyclines and streptomycin, selectively block prokaryotic protein synthesis and are therefore therapeutic agents for bacterial infections. Others, such as puromycin and cycloheximide, which act on eukaryotic protein synthesis, are useful as experimental tools. All of these inhibitors block specific steps in the complex sequence of initiation and elongation.

Targeting of Newly Synthesized Protein

After synthesis, a new protein molecule must be directed or targeted to its appropriate location in the cell. Many proteins also undergo posttranslational processing, such as the removal of some amino acids, blockage of the amino or carboxyl terminus, or the addition of carbohydrate, lipid, or phosphate residues. In the process of targeting, all proteins, except those destined to remain cytosolic, must be inserted into or cross a membrane. Posttranslational processing may occur simultaneously with this transmembrane transport or after the new protein resides in a specialized subcellular compartment possessing the necessary enzymes.

Cytosolic proteins fold rapidly and spontaneously into a structure containing most secondary structures such as α helices and β sheets. Further attainment of the final three-dimensional configuration involves helper proteins called *chaperones*.[27] Most chaperones are heat-shock proteins because their synthesis is greatly increased after brief exposure to elevated temperature; they are identified by size in kilodaltons, for example, hsp60 and hsp70. These proteins bind and hydrolyze ATP and, by binding to exposed hydrophobic regions, "massage" the protein into a mature state.

Information specifying intracellular protein targeting resides in the sequence or structure of the protein and interaction with a receptor capable of recognizing that sequence. The targeting information usually resides in a sequence of 15 to 40 amino acids, termed a *signal sequence* or *signal peptide*.[28] The sole function of this sequence is to direct targeting, and the sequence is frequently removed after that function is complete. In other cases, targeting information resides in a signal patch of amino acid residues, which are adjacent after protein folding but are located at different regions in the primary sequence. The definition of signal areas on proteins is evolving, and only some of the better-understood examples are presented.

After protein synthesis, the first "decision" in the targeting process is whether a newly synthesized protein is to enter the secretory pathway or remain in the cell in the cytoplasm or other organelles. The secretory pathway includes proteins to be secreted from the cell as well as those destined to reside in the plasma membrane or lysosomes or destined to remain permanently within the lumen or membranes of the ER or Golgi. Secretory pathway proteins are known to be synthesized on ribosomes bound to the ER, whereas other proteins are synthesized on cytoplasmic free ribosomes. All protein synthesis originates on ribosomes in the cytosol, but proteins destined for the secretory pathway rapidly bind to the ER. The elucidation of the process by which secretory proteins are directed into the ER lumen provided the first understanding of targeting mechanisms.

Secretory Pathway Targeting

Proteins targeted for the secretory pathway most commonly contain an amino-terminal signal sequence (Fig. 1.34). Characteristically, this sequence has a positively charged amino acid near the amino terminus, followed by a stretch of hydrophobic amino acids. When protein synthesis is studied in vitro in the presence of microsomes (fragmented ER), the protein ends up within the lumen, and the signal sequence has been removed. The enzyme responsible for this cleavage is called *signal peptidase* and is located in the ER lumen. If in vitro synthesis is completed without microsomes, the full length, or a "preprotein," results, which usually is incapable of entering subsequently added microsomes.

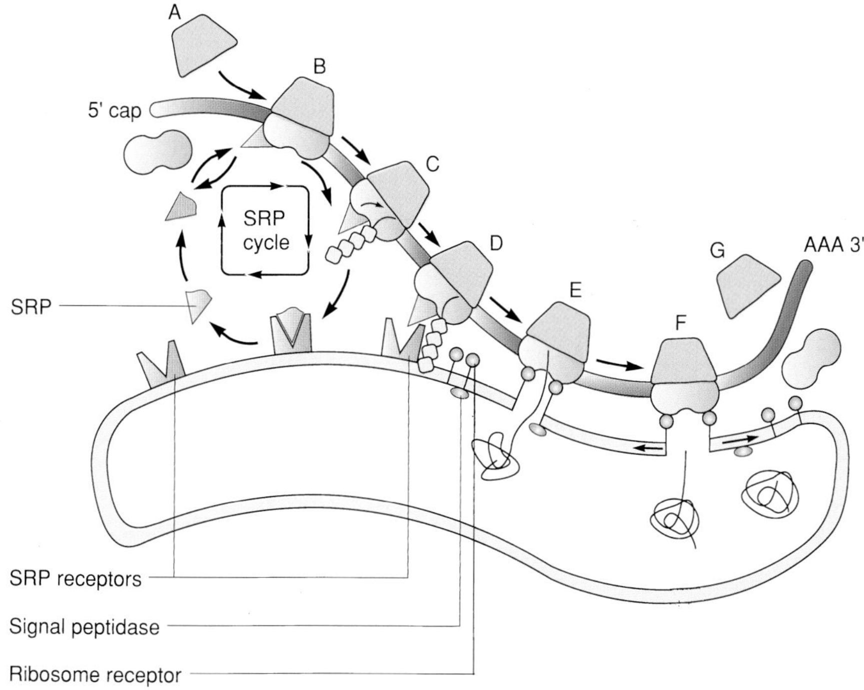

FIGURE 1.34 Synthesis and sequestration of secretory protein. Synthesis begins on the left as ribosomal subunits aggregate (*A*) and begin to translate mRNA (*B*). The signal-recognition particle (SRP) binds to the complex (*C*) and arrests peptide-chain elongation until SRP binds to a receptor in the endoplasmic reticulum membrane (*D*). The nascent polypeptide is then extruded into the lumen (*E* and *F*) with the aid of ribosome receptors, and SRP is released to recycle. The amino-terminal sequence may be cleaved by a signal peptidase. On chain termination, the ribosome dissociates (*G*), and its subunits can recycle.

Insertion into the ER lumen involves a ribonucleoprotein complex, termed the *signal recognition particle* (SRP), and a receptor on the ER, called the *SRP receptor* or *docking protein*.[28] The SRP is a complex of six polypeptide chains and a 300-nucleotide RNA molecule that binds to the nascent signal peptide emerging from the ribosome after the synthesis of approximately 70 amino acids (see Fig. 1.34). After this interaction, translational arrest occurs until the ribosome SRP complex binds to an SRP receptor. The SRP receptor is an integral membrane protein of two polypeptide subunits exposed on the cytosolic surface of the ER membrane. At this point, translation resumes, the ribosome is passed on to bind to a ribosomal receptor protein, and SRP dissociates. Next, the signal peptide binds to another multiprotein complex termed the *translocon,* which makes up a protein-lined channel through which the nascent secretory protein is extruded.[29] In the absence of a ribosome, the translocon is closed at the cytoplasmic end. In the most common case, the secretory protein is completely extruded into the lumen, the signal peptide is cleaved off, and the ribosome dissociates. Insertion of the nascent peptide through the membrane requires the hydrolysis of bound GTP. Energy released by the spontaneous folding of the secretory protein in the ER lumen may also help to pull it across. Translocation and folding are also assisted by the intraluminal binding protein, BiP, which is related to hsp70 proteins.

Lysosomal proteins are similarly inserted into the ER and later sorted into their appropriate organelles. As is the case for many other secretory proteins, lysosomal enzymes are glycosylated on certain asparagine residues as protein synthesis is occurring.[30] This process involves the transfer of a preformed oligosaccharide-containing glucose, mannose, and N-acetylglucosamine from a lipid-linked dolichol phosphate (Fig. 1.35). While still in the ER, the glucose is removed, exposing mannose. The oligosaccharide moiety is then further processed in the Golgi.

Proteins destined to reside in the plasma membrane or in the ER membrane (such as ribosome receptor) have to stop part way through their transmembrane passage[31] (Fig. 1.36). This placement is directed by another amino acid sequence in the nascent protein, termed a *stop transfer* or *membrane anchor sequence.* In the simplest case, the amino terminus of the molecule is extruded through the membrane, the process stops at the anchor sequence, and synthesis of the carboxyl terminus continues in the cytosol. An example of such a protein is the low-density lipoprotein (LDL) receptor. Because the lumen of the ER corresponds topologically to the outside of the cell, after vesicular transport through the Golgi to the surface, the amino terminus of the LDL receptor ends up on the external surface of the plasma membrane. This portion of the molecule may be glycosylated within the ER and Golgi lumina, with the result that the carbohydrate residues are located on the external surface of the plasma membrane. A more complex sequence of events occurs for proteins with an amino terminus that remains in the cytoplasm, such as the asialoglycoprotein and transferrin receptors, or for proteins that have multiple membrane-spanning regions. Both are thought to involve internal signal–anchor sequences. These internal sequences usually form a helices and are thought to insert into the bilayer as a hairpin loop (see Fig. 1.36). In the case of membrane proteins that span the bilayer multiple times, this process must be repeated with a separate insertion for each extracellular loop. Examples of such proteins are heterotrimeric G-protein-coupled receptors that contain seven membrane-spanning segments and many ion channels and transporters.

Nuclear and Mitochondrial Targeting

Nuclear proteins, such as histones, DNA and RNA polymerases, and gene regulatory proteins, are synthesized on cytoplasmic free ribosomes and must then enter the nucleus through the nuclear pores. Studies with fluorescent-labeled proteins have shown free passage through these pores by polypeptides with a size cutoff point of approximately 60 kd, consistent with a water-filled pore approximately 9 nm in

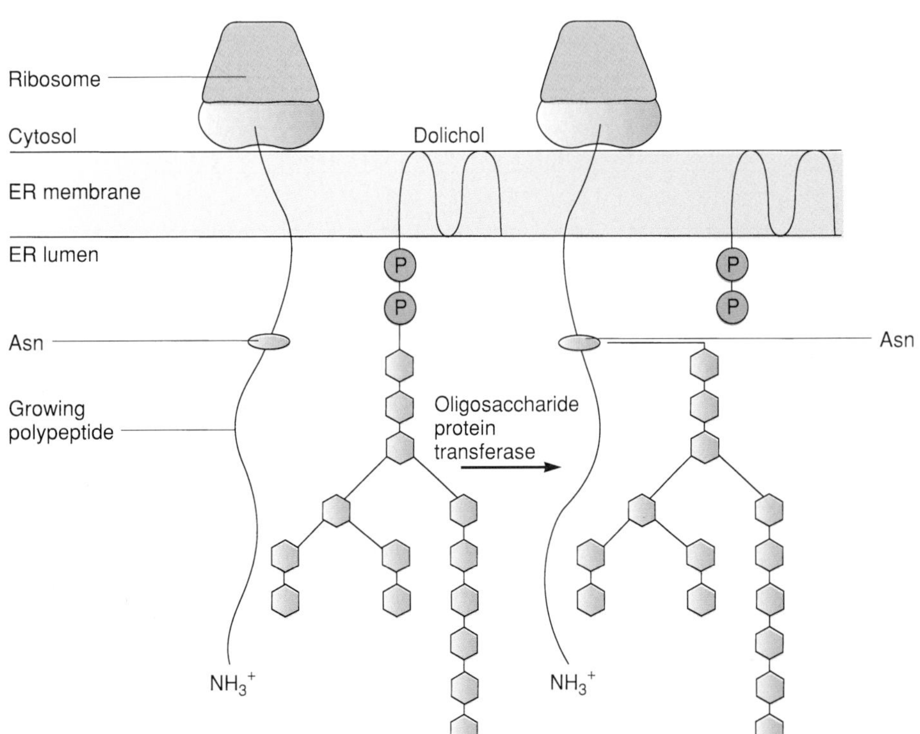

FIGURE 1.35 Biosynthesis of an asparagine-linked glycoprotein in the endoplasmic reticulum (ER) lumen. The sugar core is transferred as a preformed unit from a carrier lipid, dolichol phosphate, to the protein as it is being synthesized.

SCIENTIFIC PRINCIPLES

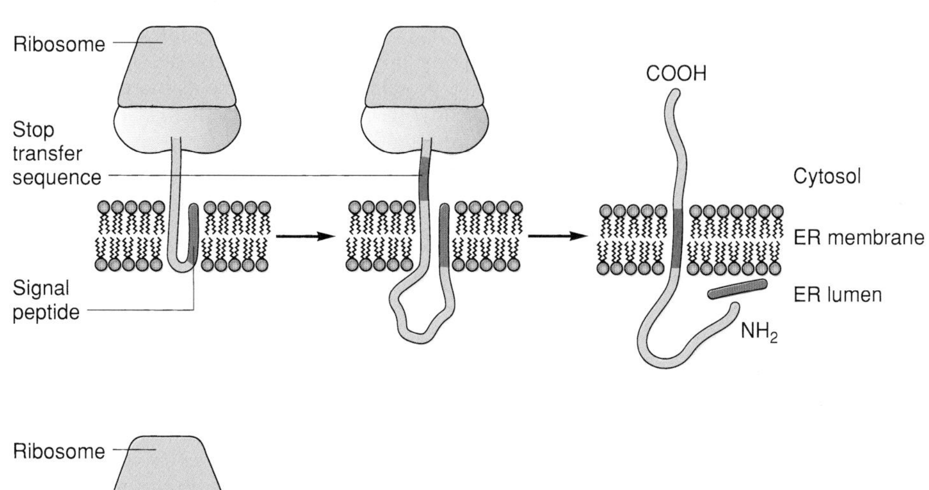

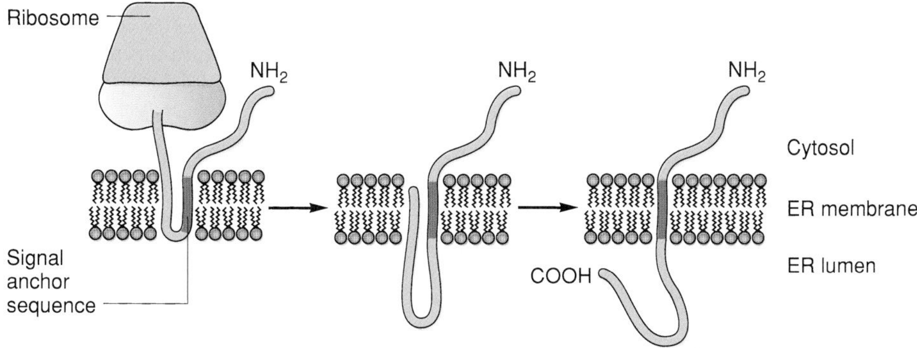

FIGURE 1.36 The topology of membrane proteins is the result of signals in the primary sequence. In this case, the two proteins end up with their opposite ends external. The occurrence of multiple signal anchor sequences can result in multiple transmembrane domains.

diameter. This pore serves to keep cytoplasmic organelles and large proteins out of the nucleus, except those specifically targeted. Entry of large proteins into the nucleus is energy dependent and involves use of ATP and interaction with proteins of the nuclear pore complex. Nuclear targeting is specified by a short amino acid sequence rich in positively charged lysine and arginine residues and usually containing proline. The sequence can occur anywhere in the molecule and is not cleaved after entry. The nuclear localization sequence binds to cytoplasmic proteins termed *importins* and then interacts with the nuclear pore complex. Both nuclear import and export also involve the small GTPase Ran.[32] In contrast to secretory proteins, which are targeted only once, long-lived nuclear proteins may have to be targeted multiple times because the nuclear envelope breaks down and reforms during each mitosis, after which nuclear proteins must reaccumulate. The nuclear pore complex is also involved in regulation of nucleocytoplasmic transport of pre-mRNA.

Mitochondria contain DNA and synthesize some proteins, but most mitochondrial proteins are imported from the cytoplasm (Fig. 1.37). Translocation of matrix proteins must occur across two membranes, the outer and inner mitochondrial

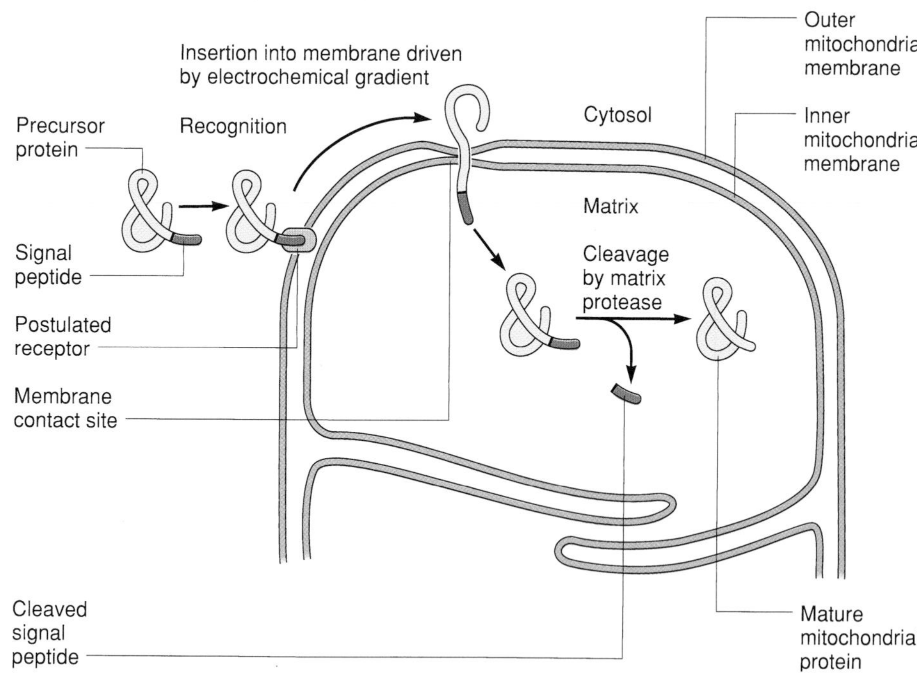

FIGURE 1.37 Insertion of newly synthesized protein into the mitochondrion is specified by a terminal signal peptide that interacts with a postulated receptor. These proteins are originally synthesized on free ribosomes and released into the cytoplasm, from which they insert into the mitochondrion.

membranes, and with the protein in an unfolded state.[33] Cytosolic chaperone proteins of the hsp70 family bind the precursor protein as it is released from the ribosome and prevent it from folding spontaneously before it binds to a receptor protein on the mitochondria. Protein import is believed to occur at points of contact where the two membranes appear to be joined. Mitochondrial proteins have a signal sequence at their amino terminus. Molecular genetic studies have shown that the signal sequence can be as short as 12 amino acids, and, if engineered onto the amino terminus of a cytosolic protein, the sequence causes its insertion into the mitochondria. The signal sequence contains positively charged amino acids every third or fourth residue and forms an amphipathic a helix that is recognized by a specific import receptor. This receptor is part of a multisubunit complex termed Tom (transport across outer membrane) proteins. Some of these proteins appear to form a channel. Once the protein has moved through this channel across the outer membrane, it crosses the inner membrane driven by the mitochondrial membrane potential and ATP hydrolysis through a complex of Tim proteins. Once within the mitochondrial matrix, the signal peptide is cleaved, and the protein folds to assume its mature configuration. This also involves mitochondrial matrix chaperones such as Hsc70 and Hsc60.

Secretory Pathway

Once secretory proteins have been translocated across a lipid bilayer into the lumen of the ER, they must fold properly and form disulfide bonds, with the latter process being aided by the enzyme protein disulfide isomerase[34] and several ER resident chaperones. Then they pass through a number of compartments, including the Golgi, where they are further processed and sorted and end up in a secretory vesicle or lysosome[35,36] (Fig. 1.38). This passage involves movement by a distinct process, that of vesicular transport. In this mechanism, the proteins do not cross membranes but are transferred

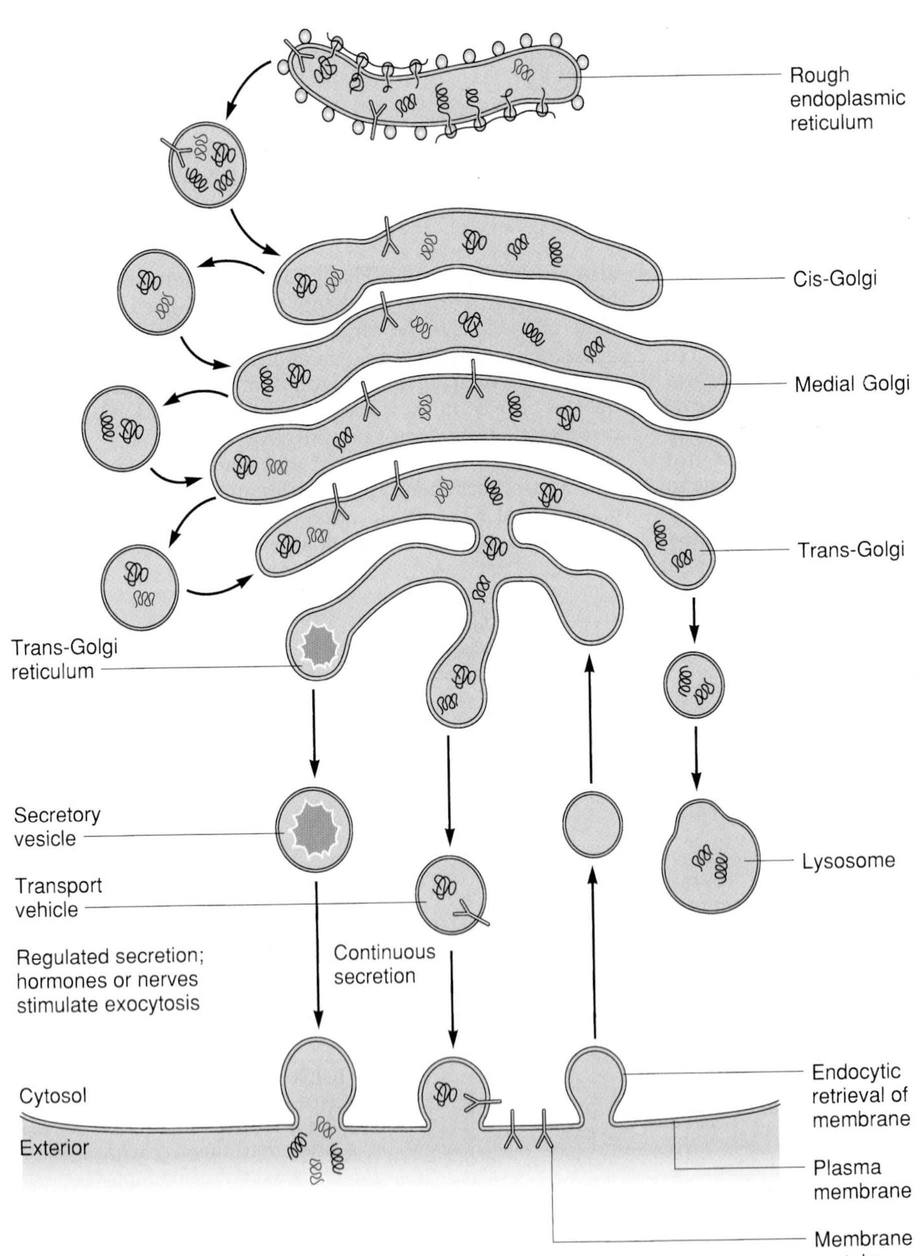

FIGURE 1.38 Intracellular transport and sorting of proteins destined for secretion, insertion into the plasma membrane, or targeting to the lysosome. After insertion into the endoplasmic reticulum lumen, movement from one compartment to another is by vesicular transport, which buds off one compartment and fuses with the next. Sorting signals intrinsic to the newly synthesized proteins specify the pathway to be taken.

between the lumina of compartments. A small vesicle buds off from one compartment such as ER and then fuses with another—in this case, the Golgi. In some cases, vesicular transport is a bulk movement of all luminal contents; in other cases, it is selective, with vesicular receptors binding only certain proteins in the luminal fluid.

The first vesicular transport event in the secretory pathway is movement of newly synthesized protein from ER to Golgi.[37] The Golgi apparatus, which is made up of flattened saccules, can be subdivided into *cis,* medial, and *trans* elements, *cis* being adjacent to the ER. Vesicles approximately 50 urn in diameter bud off from smooth areas of ER, called *transitional elements,* by an ATP-requiring process and fuse with the *cis*-Golgi cisternae. These vesicles are coated, that is, they have a protein visible in electron micrographs that surrounds the vesicle. The coat is composed of coat proteins called *COPS;* these are distinct from the first identified coat protein, clathrin. Low-molecular-weight GTP-binding (LMWG) proteins, which are related to the protooncogene ras, serve as molecular switches in that they are active when binding GTP and inactive when binding GDP. Coat assembly is initiated by the LMWG protein ARF binding to a receptor that initiates COP binding, coat assembly, and budding. Transport vesicles also contain membrane-targeting proteins called *v-SNARES.* After GTP hydrolysis and uncoating, the v-SNARE binds to a docking protein in the target membrane termed the *t-SNARE* (Fig. 1.39), a process that also requires additional cytosolic

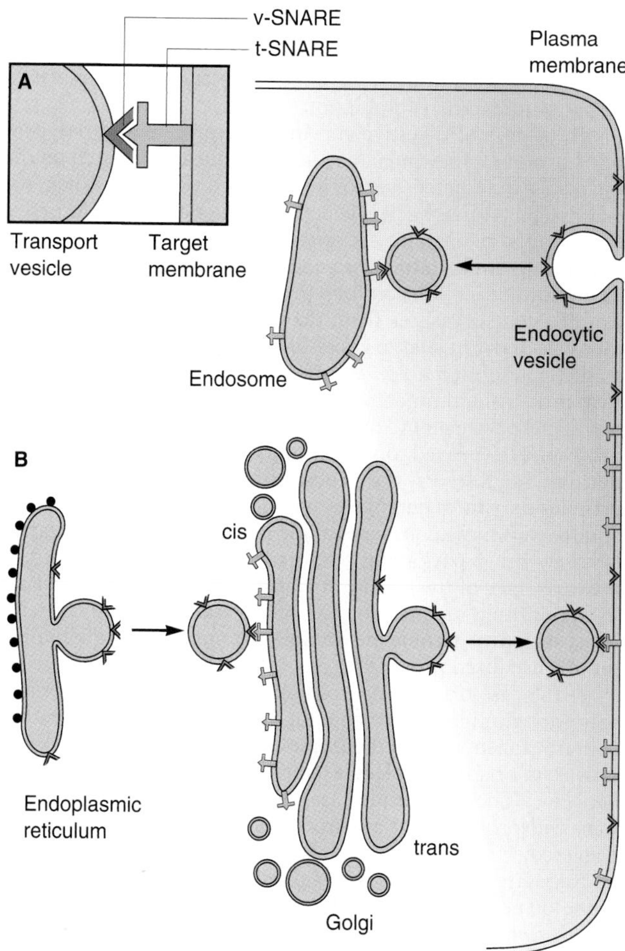

FIGURE 1.39 Vesicular transport is guided by distinct proteins termed *SNARES.* (After Rothman JE. Mechanisms of intracellular protein transport. *Nature* 1994;372:55.)

proteins. Another large family of LMWG proteins, the Rab proteins, also appear to be involved in imposing specificity because different Rab species are associated with different membrane compartments in the cell; for example, Rab1 is associated with ER-to-Golgi transport.[38]

The transport event moves both content and membrane proteins. Proteins destined to reside in the ER lumen, such as protein disulfide isomerase, are not transported but are retained in the ER lumen by virtue of a specific four-amino acid signal sequence, KDEL, in their C-terminus that interacts with a receptor in the ER.

The Golgi apparatus is structurally and functionally divided. Each cisterna constitutes a functional compartment. This compartmentation is demonstrated by the localization of specific enzymes to separate compartments. The functional corollary of Golgi compartmentation is that different processing steps occur in distinct regions. For example, phosphate is added to mannose residues of future lysosomal enzymes in the *cis*-Golgi cisternae. In the processing of secreted glycoproteins, the removal of mannose residues occurs in the medial cisternae, whereas the addition of sialic acid occurs in the *trans*-Golgi cisternae. Such events have been used to develop *in vitro* models demonstrating vesicular transport from one Golgi compartment to another, which occurs similarly to transport from ER to Golgi. Coated vesicles bud from cisternal rims, uncoat, and then fuse selectively with the next compartment. Although all secretory proteins flow unidirectionally from *cis*- to medial to *trans*-Golgi compartments, other vesicles with a distinct coat protein move retrograde and serve to retrieve ER resident proteins that have migrated to the Golgi. From the *trans* cisternae, secretory proteins move directly into a tubular network, called the *trans-Golgi network.* It is here that sorting takes place between secretory proteins and lysosomal enzymes.

The Golgi complex is especially prominent in exocrine cells, such as pancreatic and parotid acinar cells, and in endocrine cells, such as the islets of Langerhans or anterior pituitary. In goblet and other mucus-secreting cells, the Golgi is also prominent and is where proteoglycan synthesis takes place on the nascent protein core. This involves the addition of large glycosaminoglycan polymers to serine residues on the protein core. In a later step in the *trans*-Golgi cisternae, sulfate is added. The same process, albeit to a lesser extent, takes place in many cell types that secrete proteoglycan basement membrane components.

In endocrine cells and neurons, many polypeptide hormones and neuropeptides are synthesized as larger precursors and then cleaved or processed beginning in the *trans*-Golgi and continuing in the secretory granule. In some cases, more than one biologically active peptide results. Although the rationale for this process is not always clear, it allows production of small peptides, such as enkephalins (five amino acids), that otherwise would be too small to be handled by the secretory pathway.

The biosynthesis of lysosomes[36] involves the production of both lysosomal enzymes and specific lysosomal membrane proteins such as the H^+-transporting vacuolar ATPase; these proteins separate from other secretory proteins and proteins destined for the plasma membrane in the *trans*-Golgi network (Fig. 1.40). The sorting signal for lysosomal hydrolases is known to be mannose-6-phosphate (M6P) groups. Phosphate is added in the *cis*-Golgi, where the responsible enzymes must distinguish nascent lysosomal hydrolases from other secretory glycoproteins. Once phosphorylated, the M6P can interact with an M6P receptor protein to concentrate these enzymes in a region of the *trans*-Golgi network. These regions then bud off into vesicles coated with the protein clathrin. The coat is then shed, and the vesicle fuses with a lysosome. Once exposed to acid pH, the lysosomal acid hydrolase rapidly dissociates

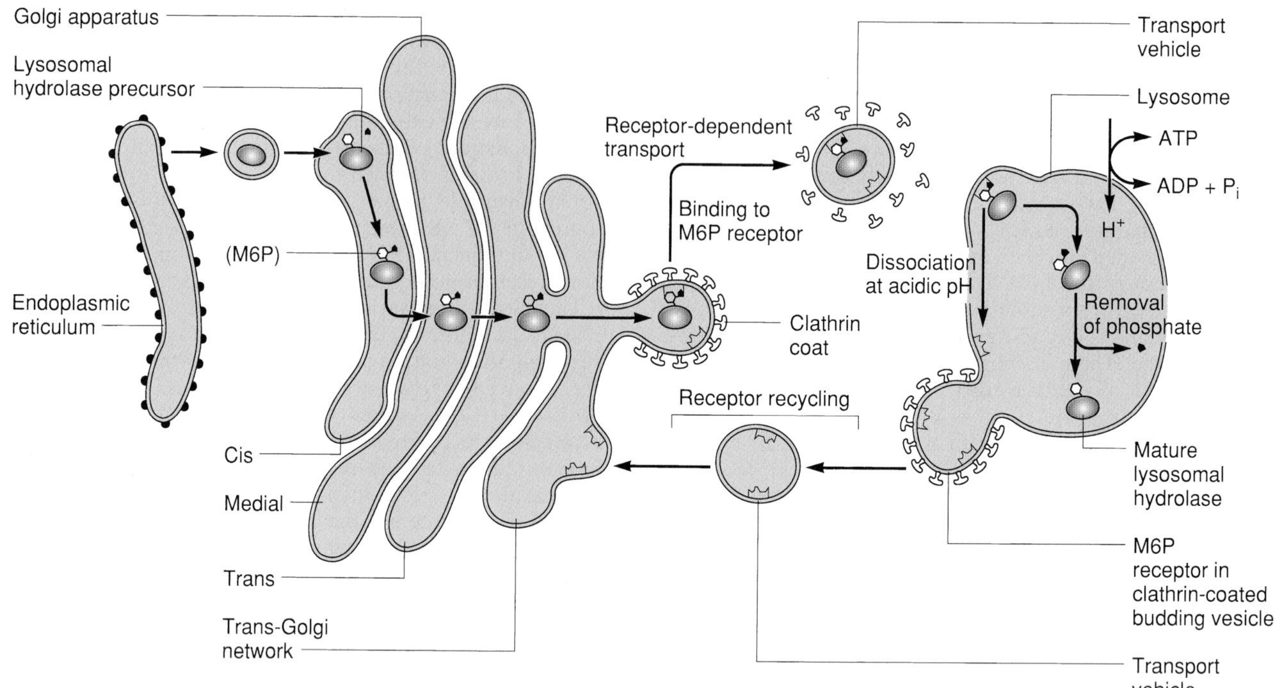

FIGURE 1.40 Biosynthesis of lysosomal proteins. Targeting is specified by phosphorylation of mannose and interaction with a mannose-6-phosphate receptor. The role of clathrin in the budding-off of transport vesicles is also illustrated.

from the M6P receptor, which then cycles back to the *trans*-Golgi network, again by means of coated vesicles. In some cells, M6P receptors are also present on the plasma membrane, where they concentrate any lysosomal enzymes released into the extracellular medium. These receptors are concentrated in coated pits that bud off and return to the *trans*-Golgi network as a scavenger pathway.

Transport to the Cell Surface: Exocytosis

Transport vesicles that bud off from the *trans*-Golgi network carry both material to be secreted from the cell and proteins destined to become components of the plasma membrane (see Fig. 1.38). These vesicles can fuse with the plasma membrane. This process, termed *exocytosis,* results in the release of vesicle content and the incorporation of the vesicle membrane into the plasma membrane with the former internal surface of the vesicle now facing the outside of the cell.

Vesicular transport to the cell surface can be divided into two components—constitutive and regulated secretion.[39] Constitutive secretion involves small, coated vesicles that rapidly move to the plasma membrane and fuse. This mechanism, which occurs in all cells, is probably analogous to vesicular transport from ER to Golgi and that between Golgi cisternae. In the absence of a specific sorting mechanism, secretory and plasma membrane proteins take this route, which can be thought of as a default pathway. This pathway appears to transport basement membrane components that are secreted by all cells and also delivers membrane proteins such as Na^+-K^+-ATPase to the plasma membrane. Liver cells exhibit an active constitutive secretion of serum proteins, such as albumin and clotting factors.

Regulated secretion occurs in cells secreting digestive enzymes, hormones, and other regulatory molecules and neurotransmitters. In regulated secretion, the material to be secreted is sorted into a storage vesicle or granule; fusion with the plasma membrane and exocytosis then takes place in response to external stimulation.

In the case of digestive enzymes and protein and polypeptide hormones, there must be a signal sequence or patch on the molecules that directs it into the regulated pathway. When, for example, a pituitary cell is genetically engineered to synthesize trypsinogen or insulin, the foreign protein is packaged into secretory granules along with endogenous pituitary hormones. The production of secretory granules involves budding of clathrin-coated vesicles from the *trans*-Golgi network, which then fuse to form a large vesicle of dilute content. This vesicle, sometimes termed a *condensing vacuole,* concentrates secretory proteins and, in some cases, completes the processing of the secretory protein. In the case of insulin, its precursor, proinsulin, is cleaved to yield insulin and C peptide in the condensing vacuoles. In the process of condensation, secretory proteins may form complexes with ions such as Ca^{2+} or Zn^{2+} and may even assume a crystalline array. This process is facilitated by other packaging or organizing proteins attached to the inner face of the granule membrane and by an H^+-ATPase in the granule membrane that acidifies the granule content. Most secretory granule membranes contain a relatively limited set of specialized proteins.

In the case of some neurons and mast cells, newly formed secretory granules do not contain secretory material but rather contain transporters and enzymes necessary for the uptake or synthesis of small molecules such as histamine and norepinephrine. These molecules are then condensed with counterions and proteins and are stored until regulated secretion is triggered.

Regulated secretion is triggered in most cases by a hormone or neurotransmitter (Fig. 1.41). The ensuing process is called *stimulus–secretion coupling.* In most cases, the coupling involves an increase in the cytoplasmic concentration of Ca^{2+}, but it may also involve generation of 1,2-diacylglycerol (DAG) or production of cAMP, which activate kinases or phosphatases. Evidence has accumulated invoking a role for Rab

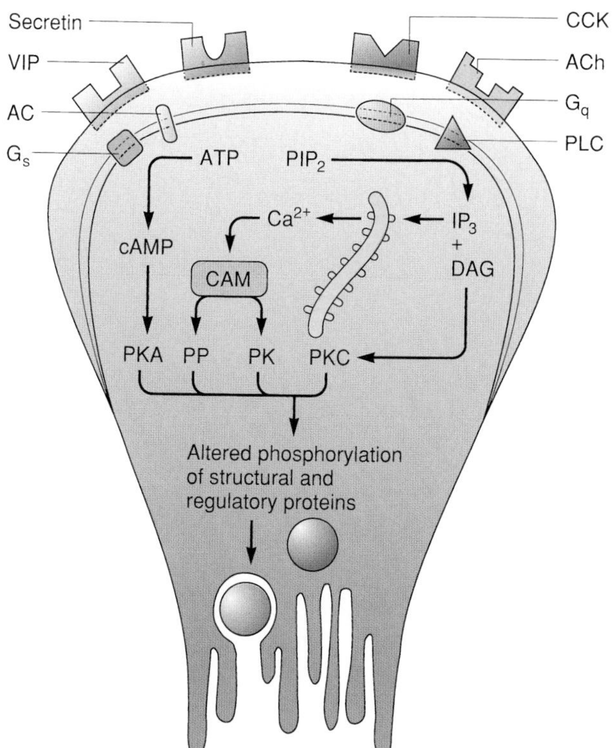

FIGURE 1.41 Scheme for control of regulated secretion for pancreatic acinar cells that secrete digestive enzymes. Vasoactive intestinal peptide (VIP) and secretin activate adenylate cyclase (AC) to promote adenosine monophosphate (AMP) formation, whereas cholecystokinin (CCK) and acetylcholine (ACh) activate phospholipase C (PLC), leading to production of inositol trisphosphate (IP_3) and diacylglycerol (DAG). IP_3 releases intracellular Ca^{2+}, which interacts with calmodulin (CAM). These second messengers (cAMP, Ca^{2+}, DAG) activate a battery of protein kinases (PK) and protein phosphatases (PP), which then induce secretion.

proteins, particularly Rab3 in this process, in a manner analogous to their role in vesicular fusion in intracellular transport. In some secretory cells, such as mast cells and neurons that secrete within seconds, secretory vesicles or granules are prepositioned or "docked" adjacent to the plasma membrane and may need only an increase in Ca^{2+} to fuse. In other cases, granules are dispersed in the cytoplasm and must be continually moved to the membrane over minutes or hours. Such a process, as occurs in pancreatic acinar cells after a meal, involves the cytoskeleton and particularly microtubules. The fusion event itself involves protein–protein interactions between the outside of the granule membrane and the cytosolic face of the plasma membrane. This interaction generates a small fusion pore, which then widens by flow of membrane lipids. At this point, decondensation of secretory granule contents occurs, facilitated by a flow of ions and water across the granule membrane.

The protein machinery involved in mediating docking and fusion[40] is best known for synaptic vesicles and involves proteins functioning as v-SNARES and t-SNARES, which are believed to be synaptobrevin and syntaxin, respectively. Other proteins such as n-Sec1 block the SNARE interaction until triggering. Synaptic vesicle fusion is triggered directly by Ca^{2+} entering the cell through gated channels in the plasma membrane and binding to a Ca^{2+} sensor protein, probably synaptotagmin.

Because fusion of secretory granules with the plasma membrane greatly increases membrane surface area, there may be a transient increase in plasma membrane surface area. This increase is compensated for by an increase in endocytosis, by which coated vesicles bud from the plasma membrane and return to the *trans*-Golgi network. Endocytosis also serves a recycling function because components of the secretory granule membrane can be reused without requiring resynthesis.

Polarized Secretion in Epithelial Cells

Many cells are polarized with two distinct membrane domains. Polarization is especially prominent in epithelial cells, such as those that compose the renal tubule or the intestinal epithelium. Tight junctional complexes form a connecting belt around and between epithelial cells near their apical borders and allow apical and basolateral membranes to maintain distinct protein and even lipid composition. For example, in the small intestinal absorptive cell, the Na^+-coupled glucose transporter and digestive enzymes such as sucrase are localized exclusively in the apical membrane, whereas Na^+-K^+-ATPase is present exclusively in the basolateral membrane. Generation of cell polarity is a complex morphogenetic event, and its maintenance requires the continual resupply of specific membrane components. In polarized secretory cells, such as goblet cells and pancreatic acinar cells, the regulated secretory pathway is usually structurally polarized. The fact that acinar cell granules fuse only with the apical membrane and not with the lateral membrane implies specificity in the proteins controlling fusion. Epithelial cells may need to secrete one set of components apically and another basally. That such sorting can occur is shown by the fact that, after viral infection, some viral proteins move to one membrane, whereas in the same cell, a distinct viral protein may bud from the other side of the cell.

Endocytosis

Opposite in direction to secretion of macromolecules but occurring by similar mechanisms is the process of endocytosis. A portion of the membrane invaginates and pinches off to form an intracellular vesicle containing both membrane proteins and ingested material. As in the secretory pathway, the ingested macromolecules do not mix with the cytoplasm and are transferred within the cell by budding and fusion of vesicles. The process of endocytosis or pinocytosis, which involves the formation of small vesicles, is mechanistically distinct from phagocytosis, by which specialized cells take up larger particles, such as bacteria or erythrocytes (Fig. 1.42).

All cells continually take up portions of their cell membranes in the form of small endocytic or pinocytic vesicles. Pinocytosis, or "cell drinking," refers to the capture of surrounding fluid in the vesicle. The recovery of membrane molecules and any attached ligands is more important functionally. Endocytosis begins at a specialized region, the coated pit, which appears in electron micrographs as a depression of the membrane. The coated pit is further identified by a bristle-like coating on the cytoplasmic surface. This coating is composed of the protein clathrin, whose individual unit is a three-armed structure called a *triskelion*. Triskelions assemble into a basket-like lattice, and this assembly is believed to provide the force resulting in the invagination. The lifetime of a coated pit is short; the pit pinches off within minutes to form a coated vesicle.[41] Dynamin, a large cytosolic GTPase protein, is essential for the pinching-off process, which requires the hydrolysis of bound GTP. After formation, coated vesicles rapidly shed their coats, which can be reused at the membrane. The vesicle moves into the cell, guided by microtubules, to a perinuclear area near the *trans*-Golgi network.

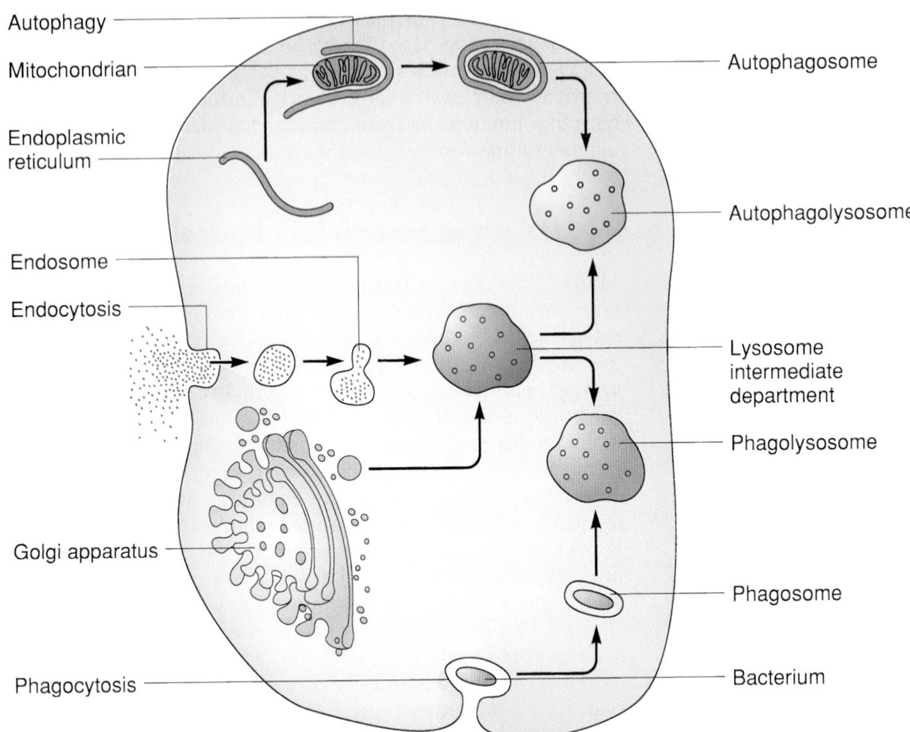

FIGURE 1.42 Formation of lysosomes by combination of transport vesicles from the Golgi-containing lysosomal enzymes with material that has been phagocytosed, endocytosed, or internalized by autophagy.

At this point, the vesicles fuse to form a larger structure, the endosome. Specific LMWG Rab proteins, particularly Rab4 and Rab5, are involved in this process. Unless specifically sorted and removed, the contents of the endosome are passed on to lysosomes, where they are digested.

Many membrane receptor molecules have a cytoplasmic portion that allows them to localize in coated pits (Fig. 1.43). This may occur spontaneously, as with the LDL receptor, or after binding of ligand, as is the case for the epidermal growth factor (EGF) receptor. Concentration of receptors in coated pits allows their selective uptake, a process called *receptor-mediated endocytosis*. In the case of the LDL receptor, this is the major mechanism whereby cells take up cholesterol. A more specialized case is the asialoglycoprotein receptor,

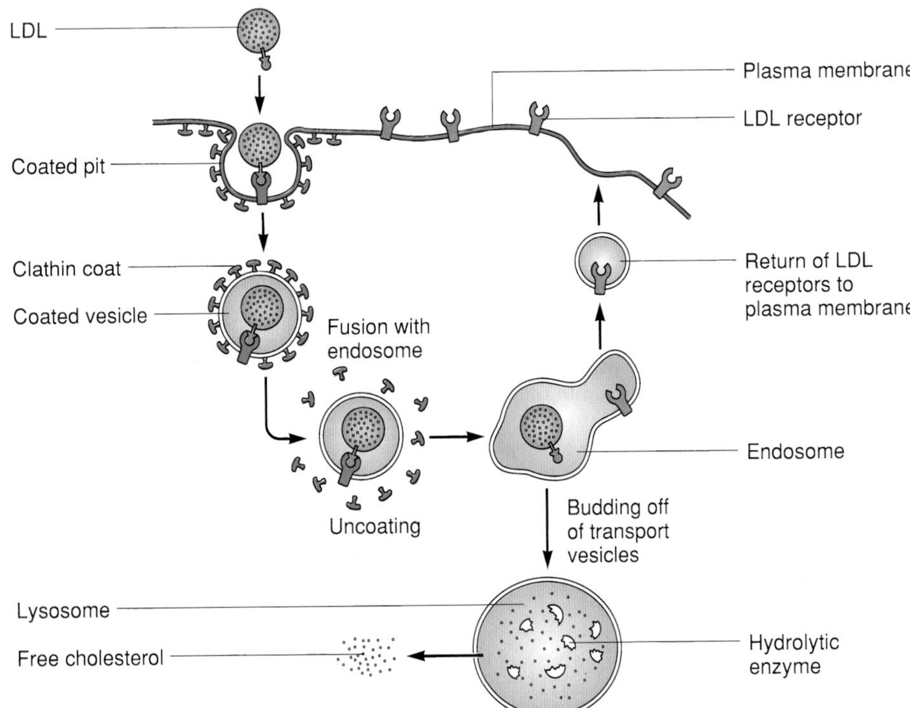

FIGURE 1.43 Receptor-mediated endocytosis of low-density lipoprotein (LDL), with resultant degradation of the endocytosed LDL and recycling of the receptor.

expressed only on hepatocytes, which take up plasma glycoproteins lacking terminal sialic acid residues. Other examples of receptor-mediated endocytosis are the uptake of transferrin with its bound iron and the uptake by absorptive cells of the ileum of vitamin B_{12}.

Ligand–receptor complexes are sorted in the endosome. The contents of the endosome are maintained at an acidic pH of approximately 5.0 as a result of a specific vacuolar H^+-ATPase that transports H^+ into the endosomal lumen. Many ligand–receptor interactions are pH sensitive. The ligands dissociate in the endosome, after which the dissociated ligand is transported to lysosomes and digested. The freed receptor is sorted and buds off as part of a transport vesicle that returns to the cell membrane, where the receptor can undergo another round of endocytosis. This sequence occurs for the LDL and asialoglycoprotein receptors. Some receptors, such as the EGF receptor, do not recycle but are degraded in the lysosome, resulting in a reduced number of cell surface receptors. This process is referred to as *receptor down-regulation.* In the case of transferrin, the low pH of the endosome separates Fe from transferrin, and the binding protein recycles to the cell surface and is released.

Phagocytosis is a specialized form of endocytosis by which large particles are internalized by specialized cells, primarily macrophages and neutrophils (see Fig. 1.42). To be phagocytosed, particles must bind to the surface of the phagocytic cell, usually as a result of specific antibody coating the particle. The phagocytic cell then extends pseudopods to engulf the particle. This event is followed by membrane fusion and a pinching off. This process does not involve clathrin but rather actin. Cytochalasin, a drug that inhibits actin polymerization, inhibits phagocytosis. After internalization, the engulfed particle, called a phagosome, fuses with lysosomes to form a phagolysosome, a type of secondary lysosome. In this terminology, the primary lysosomes are the structures budded off from the *trans*-Golgi network containing lysosomal enzymes or, in the case of neutrophils, specialized storage granules containing lysosomal enzymes. A physiologically relevant site of phagocytosis is the thyroid gland, where thyroid follicular cells phagocytose and digest thyroglobulin from the lumen of the thyroid follicle, thereby releasing the thyroid hormones thyroxine and triiodothyronine.

REGULATION OF CELL FUNCTION

The growth, differentiation, and function of all cells are highly regulated events. Cell regulation can be thought of as the effector side of cell communication. Communication can occur in a number of ways, including direct physical contact or passage of small molecules from cell to cell through gap junction channels (see Fig. 1.11). Most commonly, cell regulation occurs by means of extracellular chemical messengers. Depending on how the extracellular messenger arrives, cell regulation can be classified as paracrine, endocrine, or neurocrine (Fig. 1.44). In paracrine regulation, a chemical messenger or mediator is produced and acts locally. This restricted domain of action is due to the limitations of diffusion and to the fact that the mediators are taken up or inactivated by target cells. Examples of paracrine regulators include histamine released from gastric enterochromaffin-like cells, prostaglandins that are made by cells in all mammalian tissues, nitric oxide (NO), and certain brain–gut peptide regulators such as somatostatin. In endocrine regulation, the extracellular messengers (hormones) are released into the blood and act on target cells anywhere in the body that possess appropriate receptors. In neurocrine regulation, neurons secrete transmitters into a highly localized region, the synaptic cleft, so that regulation depends on a physical connection between the neuron and the target cell and on the presence of a specific receptor.

In almost all cases of cell regulation, the extracellular signal or stimulus is restricted to being an informational molecule. This information is received by a receptor on or in the target cell, which usually has an affinity for the signal molecule such that changes in its concentration result in changes in the fraction of receptors that are occupied. Hormone receptors in general have an affinity (K_d) for the ligand (a generic term for the molecule that binds to the receptor) of the order of 10^{-11} to 10^{-9} mol/L, whereas receptors for neurotransmitters usually display lower affinities, ranging from 10^{-7} to 10^{-4} mol/L. Besides exhibiting high affinity for appropriate ligands, receptors must be selective and discriminate a specific extracellular mediator from all other extracellular molecules.

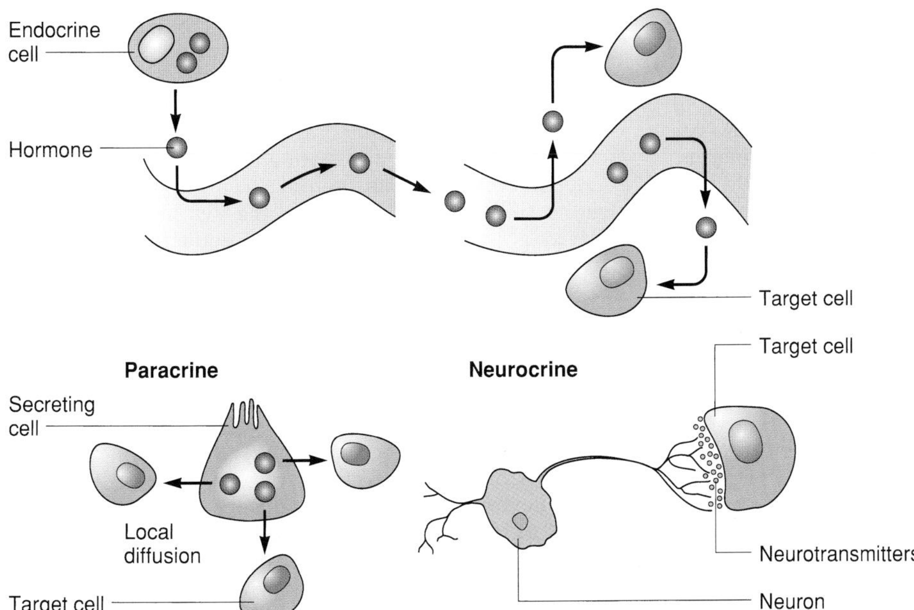

FIGURE 1.44 Endocrine, paracrine, and neurocrine modes of cell-to-cell communication.

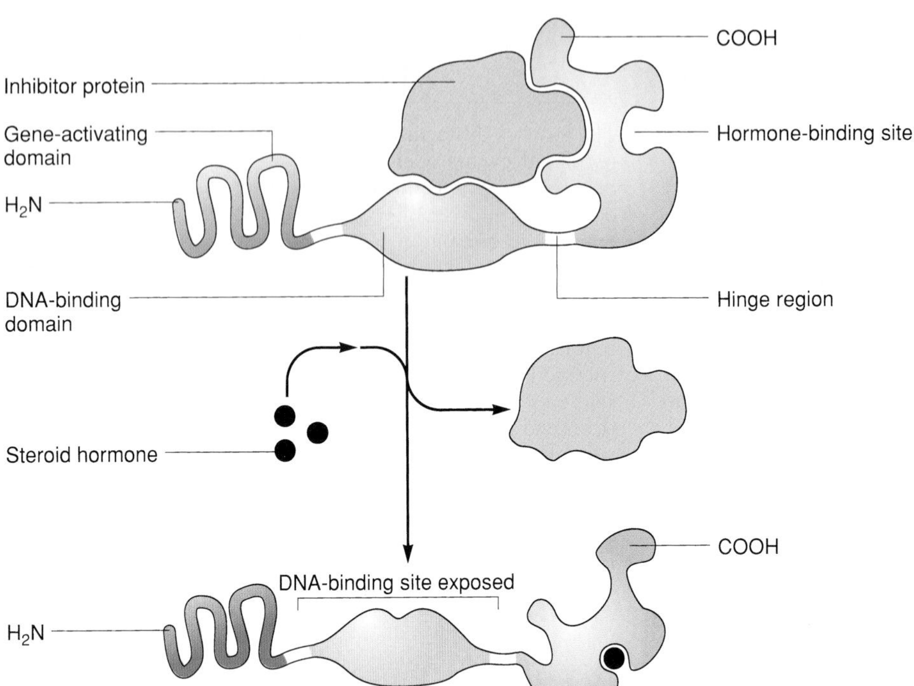

FIGURE 1.45 Schematic diagram of the domain structure of a steroid hormone receptor and its associated inhibitor protein. After steroid binding, the inhibitor dissociates, exposing the DNA-binding site.

Most receptors are protein molecules, existing either in the plasma membrane or intracellularly. Clearly, one important determinant of cell regulation is the nature of the specific complement of receptors and receptor subtypes expressed by a particular cell. Another major determinant of the cell response is its genetic programming. Thus, the same regulator may have different actions on different tissues. For example, adrenal corticosteroids such as cortisol cause cytolysis of lymphocytes but induce the synthesis of enzymes necessary for the production of glucose in the liver.

Most hormones, local mediators, and neurotransmitters are water soluble and cannot readily cross plasma membranes. They vary in size from small amines, such as histamine and norepinephrine, to medium-sized glycoproteins, such as follicle-stimulating hormone and thyroid-stimulating hormone. Receptors for these mediators are localized on the cell membrane and transduce hormone binding into altered levels of intracellular messengers. The ligand itself, particularly polypeptide hormones, may enter the cell by receptor-mediated endocytosis, but intracellular actions of internalized peptides have not been convincingly documented. Another group of regulators, including steroid and thyroid hormones, are lipophilic. These molecules are usually carried in the plasma, bound to specific binding proteins. By virtue of their hydrophobicity, they are able to penetrate readily the lipid portion of the cell membrane. Receptors for these hormones exist intracellularly in the cytoplasm or nucleus and usually act as regulators of gene expression. These hydrophobic signaling molecules exist in plasma bound to protein, so that the concentration of this class of regulators does not fluctuate rapidly in plasma, and their actions are in general slower in onset and more prolonged than those of the water-soluble class.

Intracellular Receptors and the Control of Gene Expression

The primary molecular structure of most intracellular receptors is known from molecular cloning. Receptors for steroid hormones, thyroid hormones, vitamin D, and retinoic acid are homologous and form a superfamily of receptors with similar structure and function.[42,43] All have two properties in common: they bind DNA, and they also bind a particular ligand (hormone). The DNA-binding region in the center of the molecule is highly homologous within the superfamily. The carboxyl-terminal end binds the ligand, and the amino terminus is a variable region believed to be active in regulating gene transcription (Fig. 1.45). Other receptors of unknown function exist, termed *orphan receptors*.

Most cells contain approximately 10,000 receptors for one or more steroid hormones or other, similar receptors. Some types of steroid receptors, particularly for glucocorticoids, are located in the cytosol in the inactive state; others, including thyroid hormone receptors, are located in the nucleus.[42] Once the ligand binds, the receptor undergoes a conformational change, termed *activation*. This allows cytoplasmic receptors to move into the nucleus and bind to DNA. Receptors already in the nucleus increase their affinity for DNA. In the case of glucocorticoid receptors and probably others of this class, the inactive receptor is associated with another protein, the heat-shock protein (molecular weight of 90 kd). Heat-shock proteins block the DNA-binding domain of the receptor. Activation involves the dissociation of the inhibitor protein.

Activated steroid and thyroid receptors bind to specific regions of DNA and influence the synthesis of specific mRNA,[43,44] thereby regulating the production of proteins that mediate the cellular response to the hormone (Fig. 1.46). The specific region of DNA occupied by the receptor can be identified because the bound protein makes this region resistant to cleavage by nucleases. Electrophoretic analysis of a mixture of DNA fragments resulting from a nuclease digestion in the presence of a bound receptor is called *DNA footprinting*. The receptor-binding DNA sequence (called *a response element)* consists of 8 to 10 base pairs. Response elements for glucocorticoids (termed *glucocorticoid response elements*) exhibit homology sufficient that the consensus sequence can be used to identify potential glucocorticoid-regulated genes. Deletion of these sequences abolishes glucocorticoid regulation, and their transfer to another gene confers regulation. Thyroid hormone receptors interact with a different sequence,

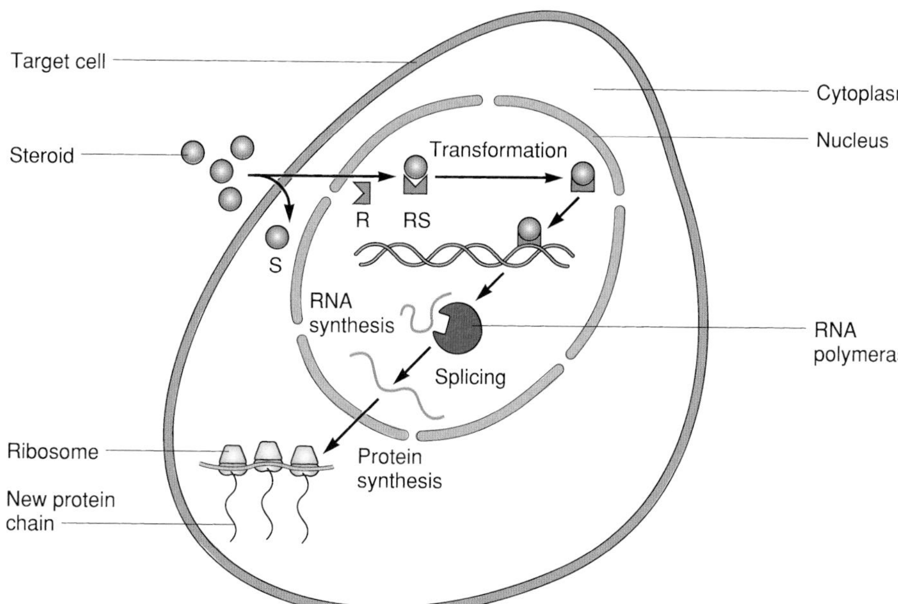

FIGURE 1.46 Schematic diagram of steroid hormone action. Steroids (S) enter the target cell and bind to a receptor (R), which is then transformed and binds to DNA in the nucleus, where it acts as a transcription factor to regulate the binding of RNA polymerase and the synthesis of new mRNA.

termed a *thyroid hormone response element.* The interaction of these receptors with DNA is believed to involve a cysteine-rich region of the receptor that forms loops or fingers coordinated by Zn^{2+}. This so-called *zinc finger structure* is also present in other transcription factors that interact with DNA.

Only a small number of genes are immediately influenced by a particular steroid hormone (primary response). Synthesis of other steroid-regulated proteins occurs later. This observation has led to the concept that some of the primary gene products may in turn activate other genes responsible for the later or secondary response (Fig. 1.47). In addition to stimulating gene expression, steroid hormones may also inhibit transcription of genes. Furthermore, steroids do not induce the same gene in all cells, which indicates that the steroid receptor does not work alone but must interact with other transcription factors termed *coactivators,* some of which are cell-type specific.

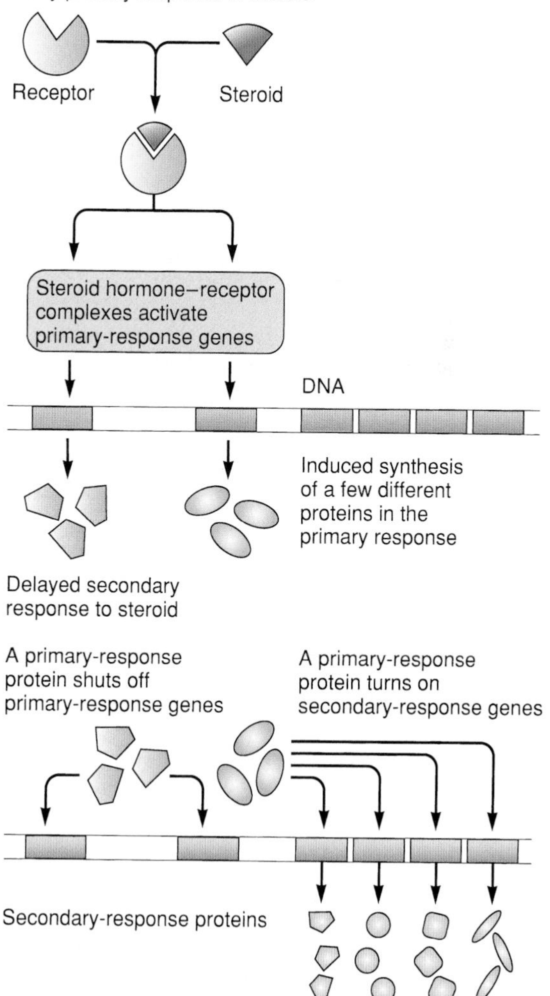

FIGURE 1.47 Pattern of gene expression in response to steroid hormone, whereby a few different primary-response genes are activated, and their products then regulate the expression of secondary-response genes.

Transduction by Cell Surface Receptors

All water-soluble regulatory molecules, including peptide and protein hormones and smaller neurotransmitters, bind to cell surface receptor proteins. Binding of the appropriate ligand evokes an intracellular signal, which usually regulates enzyme activity, membrane transport, or, in some cases, gene expression. The notion that the role of the ligand is to generate a conformational change in the receptor is supported by the observation that antibodies directed against the receptor can sometimes mimic the effect of the normal ligand. This is the case in which autoantibodies against the thyroid-stimulating hormone receptor overactivate thyroid cells and result in the disease state of hyperthyroidism. The number of receptors can vary from a few hundred to 100,000 or more per cell. In polarized cells, receptors may be limited to a specific membrane domain, usually that which is in closest contact with the blood supply.

Most cell surface receptors belong to one of three functional classes. These are ion channel receptors, catalytic receptors, and G-protein-linked receptors (Fig. 1.48A–C). Ion channel receptors, such as the nicotinic cholinergic receptor, are multisubunit assemblies; each subunit has multiple membrane-spanning segments. Together, these subunits

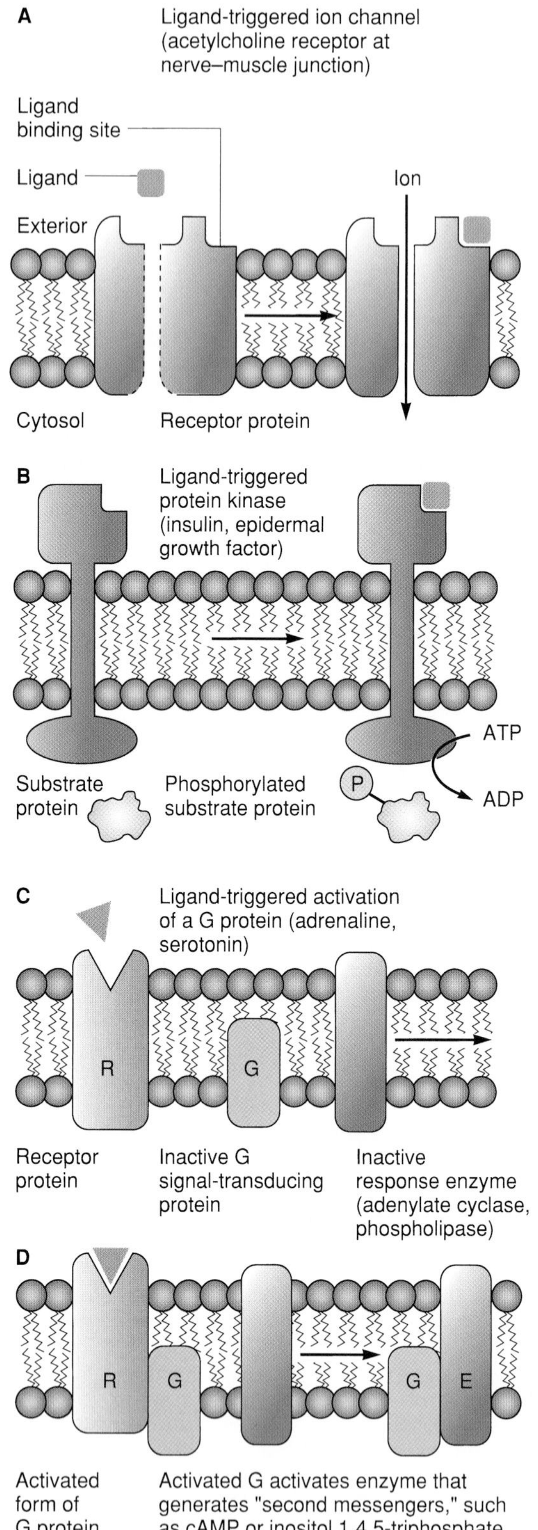

FIGURE 1.48 Types of cell surface receptors. (*A*) Ligand-activated ion channel; binding results in a conformational change, opening or activating the channel. (*B*) Ligand-activated protein kinase; binding activates the kinase domain, which phosphorylates substrate proteins. (*C* and *D*) Ligand activation of a G protein, which then activates an enzyme that generates second, or intracellular, messengers.

form an ion-selective pore that can be gated (i.e., opened or closed) by a change in the transmembrane electrical potential or by the binding of a ligand to one of the subunits. These channels are in general restricted to nerve, muscle, and some endocrine cells and transduce information either by changing the membrane potential or by allowing entry of Ca^{2+}.

Catalytic receptors are membrane proteins that possess enzymatic activity. They usually consist of three regions—an extracellular ligand-binding domain, a membrane-spanning region, and an intracellular catalytic domain. The best understood receptors of this class are tyrosine kinases,[45] which transfer phosphate from ATP to tyrosine residues. Other catalytic receptors possess enzymatic activity as serine kinases, tyrosine phosphatases, and as a form of guanylate cyclase, the enzyme synthesizing cyclic guanosine monophosphate (cGMP) from GTP. Receptors with tyrosine kinase activity include those for EGF, platelet-derived growth factor, and insulin. The insulin receptor contains four disulfide-linked chains, two of which span the membrane and are in proximity. The EGF receptor is a single chain but has been shown to dimerize in the membrane after binding EGF. Interaction between protein subunits may be involved in the signal transduction mechanism by which extracellular ligand binding alters the activity of an intracellular enzyme. In the case of the tyrosine kinase receptors, the kinase initially phosphorylates itself on tyrosine residues (autophosphorylation), a process that may involve the adjacent member of the dimer. Subsequently, the kinase may also phosphorylate tyrosine residues on cytoplasmic proteins such as the insulin-receptor substrate-1 (IRS-1). Multiple signaling pathways are initiated by the binding of intracellular proteins to the phosphotyrosine residues on the receptor or on IRS-1. These proteins include a GTPase-activating protein, phospholipase Cγ, a tyrosine phosphatase, and PI 3-kinase, all of which possess a highly conserved domain called SH2 (for *src* homology), which was first found in the oncogene *src*. A pathway for activation of MAP kinase[46,47] (Fig. 1.49) involves the adaptor protein Grb2, which binds the activated receptor by an SH2 domain and then binds an effector, SOS (named after a gene in *Drosophila*), which promotes the release of GDP from Ras, allowing it to bind GTP and thereby becoming active. Activated Ras binds the protein kinase Raf, causing it to translocate to the plasma membrane, where it is activated. The protein kinase Raf initiates a kinase cascade by phosphorylating a MAP kinase kinase (also called MEK), which phosphorylates and activates a MAP kinase, extracellularly regulated kinase (ERK).

It is now known that mammalian cells possess three parallel kinase cascades, each containing three kinases acting in series and leading to activation of ERKs, JNKs (Jun N-terminal kinase), and p38.[48] All three MAP kinases are activated by dual phosphorylation on threonine and tyrosine residues and, when activated, can phosphorylate structural molecules, enzymes, and transcription factors, as shown for ERKs in Fig. 1.49. Whereas ERKs are key enzymes in cell growth, JNKs and p38 are activated by cell stress and are sometimes called *stress kinases*. The balance of the three kinase cascades along with other cell signaling mechanisms, including NF-kB, can lead to apoptosis (programmed cell death).

Other receptors, such as those for growth hormone, erythropoietin, and various cytokines, are not themselves tyrosine kinases, but when activated by a specific ligand, the cytoplasmic portion of the receptor binds a cytoplasmic tyrosine kinase of the janus family such as JAKs, which then phosphorylates the receptor itself, and intracellular targets including members of the Stat family of transcription factors. This promotes dimerization of the Stat and translocation to the nucleus. This JAK-Stat pathway is another major pathway by which these membrane receptors regulate gene transcription.[49] In an analogous manner, the transforming growth factor-β receptor, which possesses serine kinase activity, phosphorylates another intracellular protein, Smad, which dimerizes and translocates to the nucleus to regulate transcription.

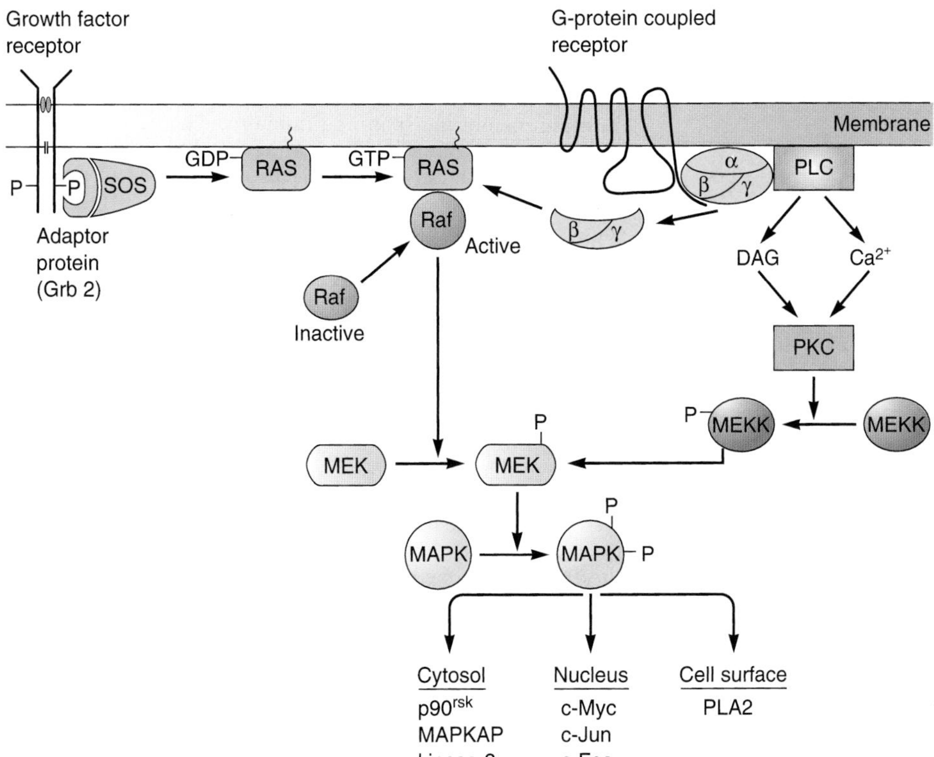

FIGURE 1.49 Schematic diagram for activation of the membrane-associated protein (MAP) kinase cascade, leading to extracellularly regulated kinase (ERK) activation.

The largest family of cell surface receptors is the G-protein-linked receptors. These are homologous structurally in that they possess seven membrane-spanning hydrophobic domains, an extracellular amino terminus, three extracellular connecting loops, three intracellular connecting loops, and a carboxyl tail (Fig. 1.50). They are also functionally homologous in that they all interact with guanine nucleotide–binding proteins (G proteins), which both activate the production of the intracellular message and influence the affinity of the receptor.

The transmembrane segments form a binding pocket for small molecules such as acetylcholine and catecholamines. The external segments are more important in the interaction with peptide hormones. The third cytoplasmic loop between the fifth and sixth transmembrane domains is the largest and most variable and is believed to interact with the appropriate G protein. Phosphorylation of serine, threonine, and tyrosine residues in the carboxyl tail are important in desensitization, whereby continued occupancy of the receptors leads to the loss of the cell response.

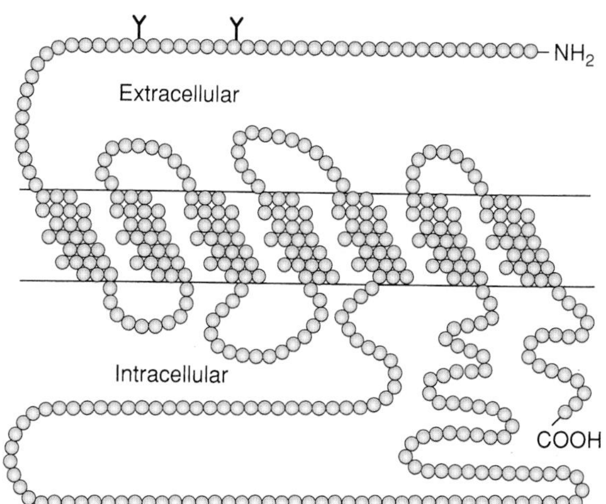

FIGURE 1.50 Schematic view of a G-protein–coupled receptor, showing the typical seven-transmembrane domain structure. Each sphere represents an amino acid. Y indicates N-linked sugar side chain.

The G proteins are a family of proteins that bind and hydrolyze GTP.[50,51] Those in the plasma membrane were originally identified as a component in the activation of adenylate cyclase but are now known also to be involved in the inhibition of adenylate cyclase, the activation of phospholipases C and A_2, the regulation of Ca^{2+} and K^+ channels, and the perception of light and odor. G proteins involved in membrane signal transduction are heterotrimeric proteins with unique a subunits and common or extremely similar β and γ subunits.[51] The α subunits for the G-protein–stimulating adenylate cyclase (α_s) and for the G-protein–inhibiting adenylate cyclase (α_i) have been identified and shown to exist in multiple isoforms. Other homologous a subunits have been identified by purification and molecular cloning, which regulate other membrane effectors. One, termed (α_o) (the G protein is termed G_o is especially abundant in brain and is believed to regulate ion channels. A G-protein–activating phospholipase C, termed G_q, and its a subunit, (α_q), also exist, as do related a subunits α_{11}, α_{14}, and α_{15}. In all cases, it is the α subunit that binds the guanine nucleotide. The $\beta\gamma$ dimer portion of the G protein is involved in anchoring the complex to the membrane but has also been shown to mediate specific biologic effects such as activation of K^+ channels and the MAP kinase cascade.

In a generally accepted model of G-protein function, binding of the ligand to its receptor allows the receptor to interact with the G protein.[52] This interaction leads to the dissociation of the bound GDP from the a subunit, which allows it to be replaced by GTP (Fig. 1.51). The receptor–G-protein complex rapidly dissociates, so that each receptor can interact with multiple G proteins. The GTP-α subunit then dissociates from the $\beta\gamma$ complex and activates or inhibits its effector

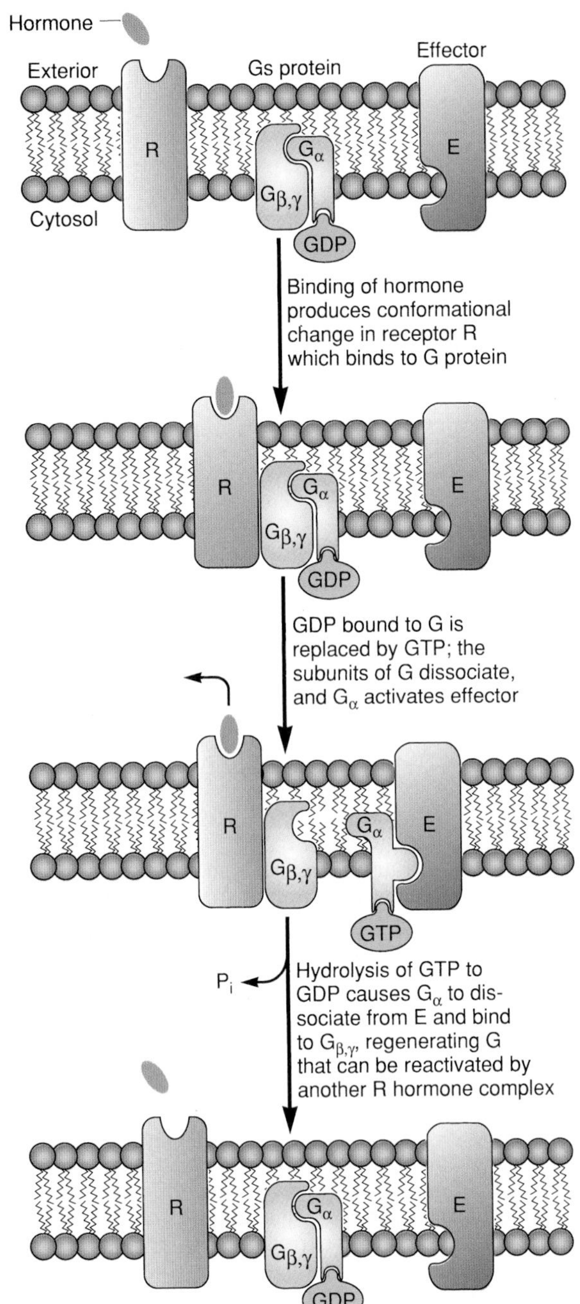

FIGURE 1.51 Activation of a membrane enzyme such as adenylate cyclase by the binding of hormone to its receptor. The G protein is shown here with its constituent α, β, and γ subunits. Blue units are in the activated state.

(i.e., adenylate cyclase, phospholipase C). The system amplifies because the lifetime of the GTP-α complex is much longer than that of the hormone receptor complex. Moreover, it allows multiple receptors to interact with the same or similar G proteins to regulate the same physiologic events. Eventually, GTP is cleaved to GDP by an intrinsic GTPase activity, and the a subunit reassociates with $\beta\gamma$.

The final component in signal transduction by G-protein–linked cell surface receptors is the effector that generates the intracellular messenger. The two best understood effectors are adenylate cyclase, which converts ATP to cAMP, and the polyphosphoinositide-specific phospholipase C, which cleaves PI 4,5-bisphosphate (PIP_2), producing 1,4,5-inositol trisphosphate (IP_3) and DAG. Adenylate cyclase has been cloned, and its primary structure is consistent with an integral membrane protein with a molecular size of 150 kd with multiple membrane-spanning domains. The catalytic site is clearly intracellular. The PI-specific phospholipase C has also been purified and cloned and is known to exist in multiple forms (β, γ, and δ), which are expressed in different tissues.[53] The importance of multiple forms and whether they couple to the same or distinct G proteins remains to be established. The γ isoform, however, can be activated in a different manner, involving tyrosine phosphorylation by the EGF receptor.

Other specific effectors activated by G proteins may include phosphatidylcholine-specific phospholipases C and D, phospholipase A_2, Na^+–H^+ ion exchangers, and various ion channels. Regulation of ion channels is distinct mechanistically from that in which a ligand binds directly to a subunit of the channel. An example of G-protein regulation of ion channels occurs in the heart, where certain types of α_i activate K^+ in response to cholinergic receptor occupancy channels, thereby slowing the heart rate.

Intracellular Messengers Cyclic Nucleotides

The prototypic intracellular messenger cAMP is produced by the action of the enzyme adenylate cyclase in the plasma membrane. In liver cells, cAMP causes glycogenolysis by activation of the enzyme glycogen phosphorylase. To function as a mediator, the concentration of cAMP must change rapidly. In resting cells, cAMP exists at a concentration of 10^{-8} to 10^{-6} mol/L, and is continually being degraded by a specific enzyme, cAMP phosphodiesterase. cAMP levels can increase 10-fold or more within seconds of receptor binding through activation of adenylate cyclase. The rise is reversed on cessation of stimulation by the phosphodiesterase. The cAMP response system can also be modulated in some cases by regulation of phosphodiesterase activity. The increase in cAMP can also be inhibited by regulators activating the inhibitory G protein (Fig. 1.52).

Cyclic adenosine monophosphate acts as an allosteric regulator, and most if not all of its actions are mediated by activation of cAMP-dependent protein kinase A (PKA), which catalyzes the phosphorylation of proteins. In its inactive form, PKA consists of two regulatory subunits that bind cAMP and two catalytic subunits (Fig. 1.53). cAMP binds to the regulatory subunit, causing it to release the active catalytic subunit. In some cases, cAMP action is localized within a cell by a family of anchoring proteins termed AKAPs that bind the regulatory subunit of PKA. The active kinase then catalyzes the phosphorylation of serine and threonine residues of target proteins, thus effecting a change in their activity. For example, phosphorylation of phosphorylase kinase in liver and muscle *activates glycogenolysis. Phosphorylation of hormone-sensi*tive lipase in fat cells activates lipolysis. A great many other structural and enzymatic proteins are known to be phosphorylated in response to various hormones, but the physiologic significance of the phosphorylation is not always understood. In some cases, cAMP is known to activate gene expression. All genes activated by cAMP contain a DNA sequence termed a cAMP-*response element* (CRE), which functions analogously to steroid response elements. When activated, PKA translocates to the nucleus and phosphorylates the transcription factor CREB (CRE binding protein), which, in conjunction with the coactivator protein CBP/300,[54] stimulates transcription.

cAMP also inhibits the dephosphorylation by intracellular phosphatases of proteins phosphorylated by PKA. It does so

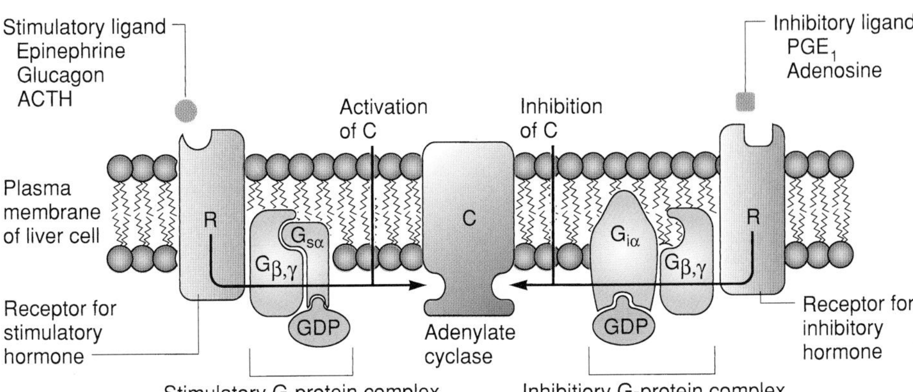

FIGURE 1.52 Stimulatory and inhibitory regulation of adenylate cyclase (C) by different G proteins. The $\beta\gamma$ subunits are the same in both stimulatory and inhibitory G proteins, whereas the a subunits and receptors differ.

by phosphorylating an inhibitor protein, which allows it to bind to and inhibit certain protein phosphatases.

cAMP is not the only cyclic nucleotide that is active as an intracellular messenger. Most animal cells also produce cGMP from GTP, and this cyclic nucleotide is known to activate a specific protein kinase. In most cases, cGMP is produced by a cytoplasmic enzyme, guanylate cyclase, which is activated by NO[55] or oxidative radicals. NO is produced by NO synthase enzymes from arginine and diffuses locally both within and between cells as a gaseous mediator. Membrane-associated forms of guanylate cyclase also exist, and one has been identified as the receptor for atrial natriuretic factor. cGMP also plays a signaling role in rod cells of the retina, although in this situation, the fall in cGMP by a light-induced, G-protein–mediated phosphodiesterase influences Na^+ channels and the receptor potentials of these cells.

Ca^{2+} and Diacylglycerol

Intracellular calcium ions function as second messengers in many cells.[56] The intracellular concentration of Ca^{2+} increases as a result of the enzymatic hydrolysis of PIP_2 by a specific phospholipase C enzyme. PIP_2, which accounts for less than 1% of cellular phospholipid, is produced by the ATP-dependent phosphorylation of PI (Fig. 1.54) and is believed to exist primarily in the inner leaflet of the plasma membrane. PIP_2 is cleaved by a phospholipase C that is activated by receptors coupled through a G protein of the G_q, or in some cases G, family. The cleavage of PIP_2 generates two products—IP_3, which is water soluble and diffuses through the cell, and DAG, which remains in the membrane and activates the enzyme protein kinase C (PKC).[57,58]

IP_3 in the cytoplasm binds to a receptor on the ER, which as a homotetramer forms a gated Ca^{2+} channel[59]; its opening leads to the release of sequestered Ca^{2+}. Normally, cytoplasmic Ca^{2+} [$(Ca^{2+})_i$] is maintained at a concentration of approximately 100 nmol/L by a system of pumps and leaks in the plasma membrane and by a Ca^{2+}-ATPase, which sequesters Ca^{2+} in intracellular organelles. By releasing sequestered Ca^{2+}, an increase in IP_3 can transiently increase $[Ca^{2+}]_i$ to as much as 1 gmol/L, although this level usually falls within a few minutes (Fig. 1.55). Continued maintenance of an elevated $[Ca^{2+}]_i$ requires additional Ca^{2+} influx from extracellular fluid, which may be controlled by a metabolite of IP_3 or by virtue of depletion of the intracellular stores. This latter mechanism, known as the *capacitative model,* implies an unknown mediator that regulates plasma membrane Ca^{2+} channels. After its production, IP_3 is rapidly hydrolyzed to IP_2 and IP by specific phosphatases or phosphorylated to 1,3,4,5-IP_4 and higher phosphate derivatives by IP_3 kinase.[58] 1,3,4,5-IP_4 is hydrolyzed to yield the inactive isomer 1,3,4-IP_3.

When cells are stimulated by submaximal concentrations of agonist, Ca^{2+} is released and taken back up by intracellular stores, leading to repetitive $[Ca^{2+}]_i$ oscillations.[57,60] In some larger cells, such as oocytes or neurons, an increase in $[Ca^{2+}]_i$ can be seen to propagate across the cell. This propagation, along with other evidence, has led to the concept of Ca^{2+}-induced Ca^{2+} release as being important after an initial triggering of Ca^{2+} release by IP_3.

Both Ca^{2+} and DAG exert many of their effects by altering protein phosphorylation. Most of the actions of Ca^{2+} are mediated by binding to proteins that can be thought of as intracellular Ca^{2+} receptors. The most common of these are troponin C in skeletal muscle and calmodulin, which is found in all animal and plant cells. Calmodulin binds four Ca^{2+} ions with an affinity of approximately 1 gmol/L. Calmodulin must bind at least two Ca^{2+} ions before it undergoes a conformational change and is able to activate enzymes. In some cases, calmodulin exists as a permanent regulatory subunit of a multisubunit enzyme, as is the case for phosphorylase kinase; in most cases, the calmodulin exists free, and after binding Ca^{2+} can interact with target proteins, which include cyclic nucleotide phosphodiesterase, some Ca^{2+} transport ATPases, and NO synthase (Fig. 1.56). A variety of Ca^{2+}-calmodulin–activated protein kinases exist, including myosin light-chain kinase, which is specific for myosin, and Ca^{2+}-calmodulin-regulated kinase II, which has a broad substrate specificity. These are all serine- and threonine-specific kinases. Ca^{2+}-calmodulin also activates a specific serine—threonine phosphatase, calcineurin. This phosphatase has been shown to be essential for T-cell activation and is the target for immunosuppressants such as cyclosporine.[61]

The DAG that is produced by PIP_2 hydrolysis has as its primary function the activation of another kinase, PKC,[62] which also requires the presence of Ca^{2+} and acidic phospholipids.

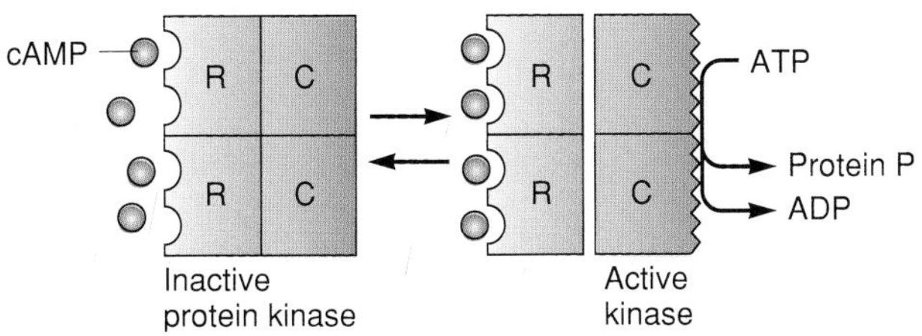

FIGURE 1.53 Activation of adenosine monophosphate (AMP)–dependent protein kinase by cyclic AMP (cAMP). Binding of cAMP to the regulatory (R) subunits induces dissociation and activation of the catalytic (C) subunits. C is enzymatically active only when dissociated.

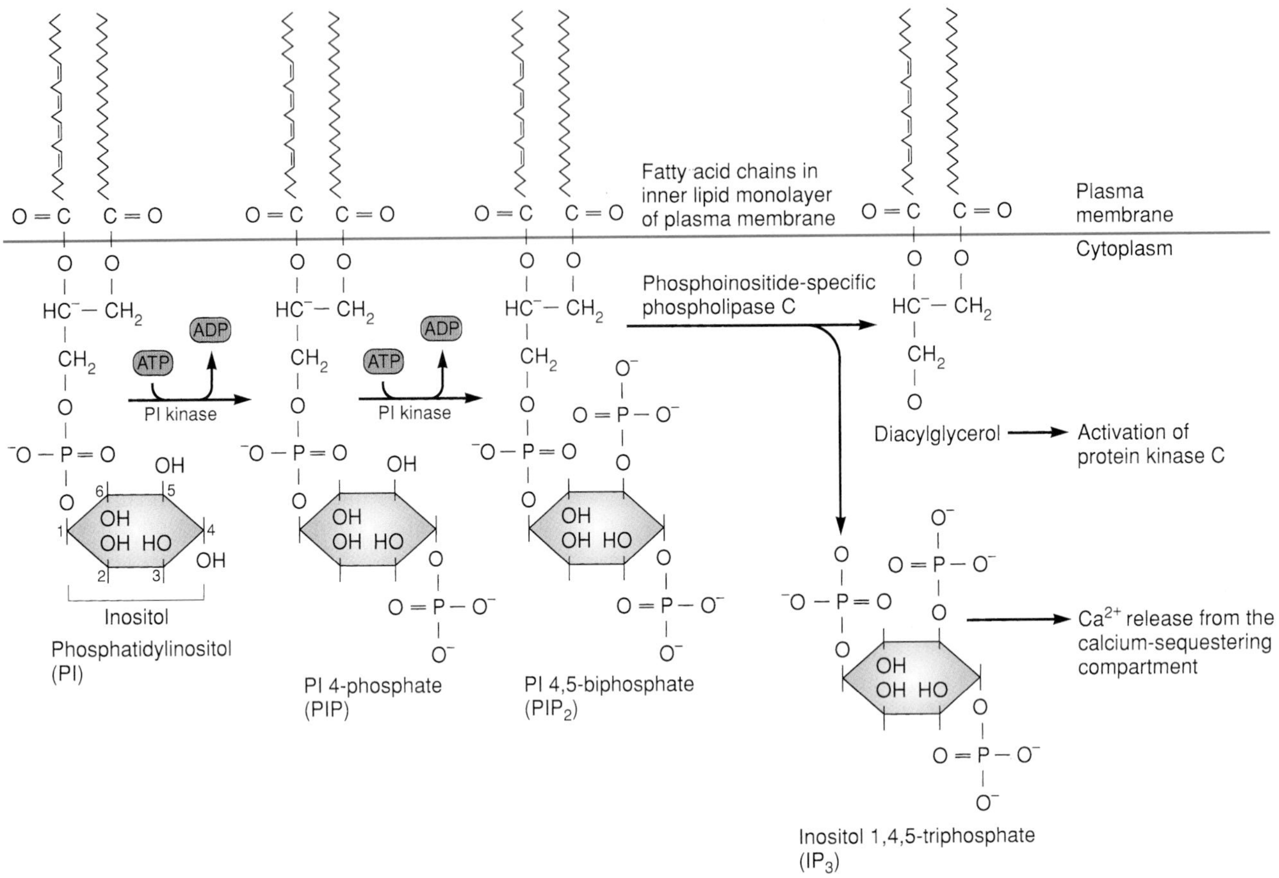

FIGURE 1.54 Synthesis and hydrolysis of inositol phospholipids. Phosphatidylinositol is phosphorylated in the membrane to produce polyphosphoinositides, PIP and PIP_2. PIP_2 is the primary target for phosphoinositide-specific phospholipase; the products of this enzymatic cleavage are inositol trisphosphate (IP_3), which releases intracellular Ca^{2+}, and diacylglycerol, which activates protein kinase C.

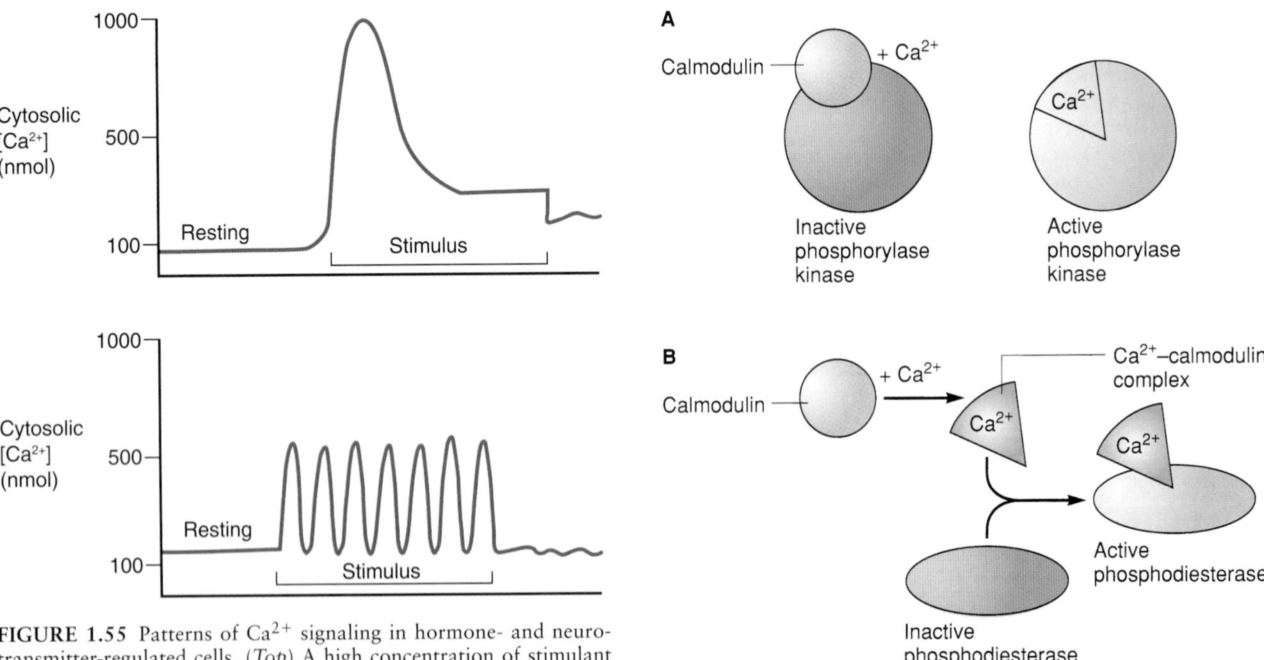

FIGURE 1.55 Patterns of Ca^{2+} signaling in hormone- and neurotransmitter-regulated cells. (*Top*) A high concentration of stimulant induces a large amount of inositol trisphosphate (IP_3), which transiently increases Ca^{2+} to approximately 1 gmol by release of Ca^{2+} from intracellular stores, followed by a much lower sustained increase, which is due to Ca^{2+} influx across the cell membrane. (*Bottom*) Low concentrations of stimulant that induce small increases in IP_3 lead to transient release and reuptake of sequestered intracellular Ca^{2+}, leading to oscillations in intracellular free Ca^{2+}.

FIGURE 1.56 Ca^{2+} binding to the protein calmodulin alters its conformation and thereby activates enzymes. In the case of phosphorylase kinase, calmodulin is an integral subunit of the enzyme, whereas for other enzymes, such as phosphodiesterase, the activated calmodulin binds to the inactive enzyme, thereby activating it.

The action of DAG is to lower the Km for Ca^{2+} such that the enzyme can be activated even at resting $[Ca^{2+}]_i$ concentrations. An increase in $[Ca^{2+}]_i$ probably contributes to activation because Ca^{2+} also promotes binding of the cytoplasmic enzyme to membranes. When activated by DAG and Ca^{2+}, PKC transfers phosphates from ATP to serine and threonine residues on target proteins. PKC can also be activated by phorbol esters, tumor promoters that bind to PKC and are used experimentally to activate this pathway.[63] DAG can be produced not only by PIP_2 hydrolysis but also by hydrolysis of other membrane phospholipids, particularly phosphatidylcholine, which may be cleaved by either a phospholipase C or phospholipase D enzyme. This means that DAG and Ca^{2+} signals, although initially coordinated, may diverge and that some extracellular signals can increase DAG without an increase in Ca^{2+}. It has also been discovered that PKC is actually a family of kinases and that some forms possess lipid binding but lack Ca^{2+}-binding domains.

PRC is believed to phosphorylate a number of important membrane molecules, including the Na^+–H^+ exchanger, ion channels, and certain receptors. Much of the evidence for this is based on the use of phorbol esters to activate PKC artificially. PKC is also able to activate the MAP kinase cascade. In some cases, the activation of PKC increases the transcription of specific genes, which are said to contain a phorbol ester response element. This probably involves activation of a DNA-binding transcription factor after a PKC-mediated phosphorylation.

KEY POINTS

- **The plasma membrane is composed of amphipathic molecules, mainly phospholipids, sphingolipids, and proteins, that contain distinct regions that are either insoluble in water (hydrophobic) or soluble in water (hydrophilic).**
- **Transport proteins and receptors are usually transmembrane proteins whose hydrophobic regions in the lipid bilayer are most often present in an α-helical configuration.**
- **All of the chromosomal DNA is contained in the nucleus in association with a specialized class of acidic proteins, termed *histones*.**
- **Mitochondria are the major source of energy production in eukaryotic cells and contain the genetic codes for and synthesize some of their own proteins.**
- **Endoplasmic reticulum has a number of functions and is primarily involved in the synthesis of protein and lipids.**
- **Lysosomes are membrane-limited organelles containing acid hydrolytic enzymes that degrade polymers such as proteins, carbohydrates, and nucleic acids.**
- **Cell junctions can be classified as occluding, anchoring, or communicating.**
- **Extracellular matrix is a meshwork of negatively charged polysaccharide glycosaminoglycan chains and protein fibers, which bind to receptors in the plasma membrane (integrins).**
- **Ion channels are transmembrane proteins that form pores that can conduct ions across the plasma membrane.**

References

1. Lodish H, Berk A, Zipursky SL, et al. *Molecular cell biology,* 4th ed. New York: WH Freeman; 1999.
2. Aberts B, Bray D, Lewis J, et al. *Molecular biology of the cell,* 3rd ed. New York: Garland; 1994.
3. Bretscher MS. The molecules of the cell membrane. *Sci Am.* 1985;253:100.
4. **Cuervo AM, Dice JF. Lysosomes: a meeting point of proteins, chaperones, and proteases. *J Mol Med.* 1998;76:6-12.**
5. Masters C, Crane D. Recent developments in peroxisome biology. *Endeavor* 1996;20:68.
6. Schliwa M. *The cytoskeleton.* New York: Springer-Verlag; 1986.
7. Bray D. *Cell movements.* New York: Garland; 1992.
8. Hall A. Rho GTPases and the actin cytoskeleton. *Science* 1998;279:509.
9. Coluccio L. Myosin I. *Am J Physiol.* 1997;273:C347.
10. Furukawa R, Fechheimer M. The structure, function, and assembly of actin filament bundles. *Int Rev Cytol.* 1997;175:29.
11. Fuchs E, Cleveland DW. A structural scaffolding of intermediate filaments in health and disease. *Science* 1998;279:514.
12. Maccioni RB, Cambiazo V. Role of microtubule associated proteins in the control of microtubule assembly. *Physiol Rev.* 1995;75:835.
13. Hirokawa N. Kinesin and dynein superfamily proteins and the mechanism of organelle transport. *Science* 1998;279:519.
14. Mitic L, Anderson J. Molecular architecture of tight junctions. *Annu Rev Physiol.* 1998;60:121.
15. Geiger B, Volk T, Volberg T. Molecular heterogeneity of adherins-type junctions. *J Cell Biol.* 1985;101:1523.
16. Bennett MVL. Gap junctions: new tools, new answers, new questions. *Neuron* 1991;6:305.
17. Simon AM, Goodenough DA. Diverse functions of vertebrate gap junctions. *Trends Cell Biol.* 1998;8:477.
18. Hynes RO. Integrins: versatility, modulation, and signaling in cell adhesion. *Cell* 1992;69:11.
19. Yamada KM, Geiger B. Molecular interactions in cell adhesion complexes. *Curr Opin Cell Biol.* 1997;9:76.
20. Finkelstein A, Mauro A. Physical principles and formalisms of electrical excitability. In: Kandel ER, ed. *Handbook of physiology: the nervous system, vol I.* Bethesda, MD: American Physiological Society; 1977:161.
21. **Dawson D. Principles of membrane transport. In: Schultz SG, ed. *Handbook of physiology: the gastrointestinal system.* Bethesda, MD: American Physiological Society; 1991:1.**
22. Deen PMT, van Os CH. Epithelial aquaporins. *Curr Opin Cell Biol.* 1998;10:435.
23. Doyle DA, Morais Cabral J, Pfuetzner RA, et al. The structure of the potassium channel: molecular basis of K^+ conduction and selectivity. *Science* 1998;280:69.
24. Stryer L. *Biochemistry,* 4th ed. New York: WH Freeman; 1995.
25. **Frank J. How the ribosome works. *Am Sci.* 1998;86:428.**
26. Pain VM. Initiation of protein synthesis in eukaryotic cells. *Eur J Biochem.*996;236:747.
27. Georgopoulous C, Welch WJ. Role of the major heat shock proteins as molecular chaperones. *Annu Rev Cell Biol.*993;9: 601.
28. Walter P, Lingoppa VR. Mechanism of protein translocation across the endoplasmic reticulum membrane. *Annu Rev Cell Bio.*1986;2:499.
29. Matlack K, Mothes W, Rappaport TA. Protein translocation: tunnel vision. *Cell* 1998;92:381.
30. Kornfeld R, Kornfeld S. Assembly of asparagine-linked oligosaccharides. *Annu Rev Biochem.* 1985;45:631.
31. Spies M. Heads or tails: what determines the orientation of proteins in the membrane. *FEBS Lett.* 1995;369:76.
32. Melchoir F, Gerace L. Two-way trafficking with Ran. *Trends Cell Biol.* 1998;8:175.
33. Schatz G. The protein import system of mitochondria. *J Biol Chem.* 1996;271:31763.
34. Gilbert H. Protein disulfide isomerase and assisted protein folding. *J Biol Chem.* 1997;272:29399.
35. **Rothman JE. Mechanisms of intracellular protein transport. *Nature* 1994;372:55.**
36. Kornfeld S. Trafficking of lysosomal enzymes. *FASEB J.* 1987;1:462.
37. Farquhar MG, Palade GE. The Golgi apparatus: 100 years of progress and controversy. *Trends Cell Biol.* 1998;8:2.
38. Schimmoller F, Simon I, Pfeffer SR. Rab GTPases, directors of vesicle docking. *J Biol Chem.* 1998;273:22161.
39. Burgess TL, Kelly RB. Constitutive and regulated secretion of proteins. *Annu Rev Cell Biol.* 1987;3:243.
40. Pfeffer SR. Transport-vesicle targeting: tethers before SNAREs. *Nature Cell Biol.* 1999;1:E17.
41. Riezman H, Woodman PG, vanMeer G, et al. Molecular mechanisms of endocytosis. *Cell* 1997;91:731.
42. Evans RM. The steroid and thyroid hormone receptor super-family. *Science* 1988;240:889.
43. Mangelsdorf DJ, Thummel C, Beato M, et al. The nuclear receptor superfamily: the second decade. *Cell* 1995;83:835.
44. Johnson PF, McKnight SL. Eukaryotic transcriptional regulatory proteins. *Annu Rev Biochem.* 1989;58:799.
45. **Fantl WJ, Johnson DE, Williams LT. Signaling by receptor tyrosine kinases. *Annu Rev Biochem.* 1993;62:453.**
46. Blenis J. Signal transduction via the MAP kinases: proceed at your own RSK. *Proc Natl Acad Sci USA.* 1993;90:5889.
47. Seger R, Krebs EG. The MAPK signaling cascade. *FASEB J.* 1995;9:726.
48. Cano E, Mahadevan LC. Parallel signal processing among mammalian MAPKs. *Trends Biochem Sci.* 1995;20:117.
49. Schindler C, Darnell JE. Transcriptional responses to polypeptide ligands: the JAK-STAT pathway. *Annu Rev Biochem.* 1995;64:621.
50. Bourne HR, Saunders DA, McCormick F. The GTPase super-family: conserved structure and molecular mechanism. *Nature* 1991;349:117.
51. Simon MI, Strathman MP, Gautam N. Diversity of G proteins in signal transduction. *Science* 1991;252:802.

52. Bourne HR. How receptors talk to trimeric G proteins. *Curr Opin Cell Biol.* 1997;9:134.
53. Singler WD, Brown HA, Sternweis PC. Regulation of eukaryotic phosphatidylinositol-specific phospholipase C and phospholipase D. *Annu Rev Biochem.* 1997;66:475.
54. Goldman PS, Tran UK, Goodman RH. The multifunctional role of the co-activator CBP in transcriptional regulation. *Recent Prog Hormone Res.* 1997;52:103.
55. Hobbs AJ. Soluble guanylate cyclase: the forgotten sibling. *Trends Pharmacol Sci.* 1997;18:484.
56. Rasmussen H. The cycling of calcium as an intracellular messenger. *Sci Am.* 1989;261:66.
57. **Berridge MJ. Inositol trisphosphate and calcium signaling. *Nature* 1993; 361:315.**
58. Majerus PW. Inositol phosphate biochemistry. *Annu Rev Biochem.* 1992; 61:225.
59. Mikoshiba K. The InsP3 receptor and intracellular Ca^{2+} signaling. *Curr Opin Neurobiol.* 1997;7:339.
60. Berridge MJ. Elementary and global aspects of calcium signaling. *J Physiol (Lond).* 1997;499:291.
61. Bierer BE, Hollander G, Fruman D, et al. Cyclosporin A and FK506: molecular mechanisms of immunosuppression and probes for transplantation biology. *Curr Opin Immunol.* 1993;5:763.
62. Parker PJ, Kour G, Marais RM, et al. Protein kinase C: a family affair. *Mol Cell Endocrinol.* 1989;65:1.
63. Ron D, Kazanietz MG. New insights into the regulation of protein kinase C and novel phorbol ester receptors. *FASEB J.* 1999;13:1658.

CHAPTER 2 ■ SUBSTRATE METABOLISM IN SURGERY

STEVEN E. RAPER

INTERMEDIARY METABOLISM: AN OVERVIEW

Intermediary metabolism may be defined as the fate of dietary carbohydrate, fat, and protein after digestion and absorption. The major intermediary metabolites are glucose, fatty acids, glycerol, and amino acids. Ultimately, these metabolites are processed by a variety of metabolic pathways to acetyl coenzyme A (CoA). Glucose is metabolized to pyruvate and lactate by glycolysis. Aerobic metabolism allows conversion of pyruvate to acetyl CoA. Acetyl CoA enters the citric acid cycle resulting in carbon dioxide, water, and reducing equivalents (a major source of ATP). In the absence of oxygen, glycolysis ends in lactate. Glucose can be stored as or created from glycogen. Glucose can also enter the phosphogluconate pathway where it is converted to reducing equivalents for fatty acid synthesis and ribose five-carbon sugars important in nucleotide formation. Glucose can be converted into glycerol for fat formation and pyruvate for amino acid synthesis. Gluconeogenesis allows synthesis of glucose from lactate, amino acids, and glycerol.

With regard to lipid metabolism, long-chain fatty acids arise from dietary fat or synthesis from acetyl CoA. Fatty acids can be oxidized to acetyl CoA by the process of β-oxidation or converted to acyl glycerols (fat) for storage as the main energy reserve. In addition to the fates noted previously, acetyl CoA can be used as a precursor to cholesterol and other steroids and in the liver can form the ketone bodies acetoacetate and 3-hydroxybutyrate, which are critical sources of energy during periods of starvation.

Proteins are degraded in two major ways: energy independent, usually in lysosomes, and energy requiring, usually through the ubiquitin pathway. Of amino acids generated in protein catabolism, about three fourths are reutilized for protein synthesis, and one fourth are deaminated with the resulting ammonia converted to urea. Amino acids may be divided into nutritionally essential and nonessential. Nonessential amino acids require fewer enzymatic reactions from amphibolic intermediates or essential amino acids. On a daily basis, humans turnover 1% to 2% of total body protein.

CARBOHYDRATE METABOLISM

The products of intestinal carbohydrate digestion are glucose (80%) and fructose and galactose (20%). Fructose and galactose are rapidly converted to glucose, and the body uses glucose as the primary molecule for transport and uptake of carbohydrates by cells throughout the body. Blood glucose levels are tightly regulated by the liver despite wide fluctuations in dietary intake. About 90% of portal venous glucose is removed from the blood by liver cells through carrier-facilitated diffusion. Large numbers of carrier molecules on the sinusoidal domain of the hepatocyte are capable of binding glucose and transferring it to the cytoplasm. The rate of glucose transport is enhanced (up to 10-fold) by insulin. Given the critical role of glucose in survival, complex metabolic pathways have evolved for the storage of glucose in the fed state, the release of glucose from glycogen, and synthesis of new glucose.

Blood glucose is stored, primarily in liver and muscle, as glycogen. Glycogen is a complex polymer of glucose with an average molecular weight of 5 million. On a daily basis, the liver can convert up to 100 g of glucose into glycogen by the process of glycogenesis. The liver can also release glucose into the blood by glycogenolysis, which is the breakdown of glycogen, or by gluconeogenesis, which is the formation of new glucose from substrates such as alanine, lactate, or glycerol. Hormones play a key role in the hepatic regulation of glycogen balance. Insulin, for example, stimulates glycogenesis, and glycolysis; glucagon stimulates glycogenolysis and gluconeogenesis.[1]

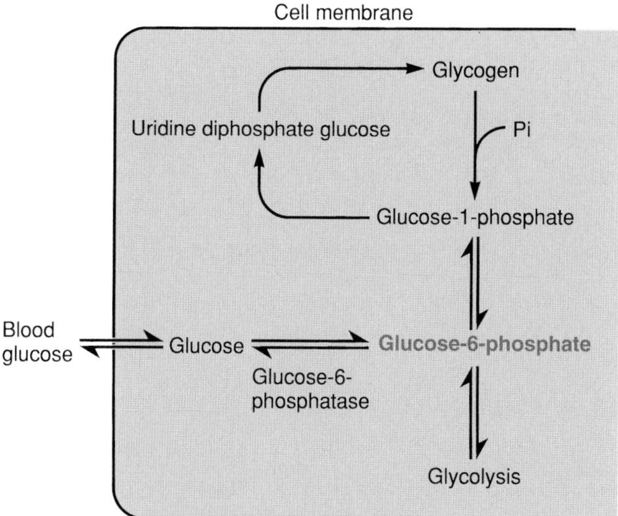

FIGURE 2.1 The chemical reactions of glycogenesis and glycogenolysis. Glucose-6-phosphatase allows hepatic glucose to be transported out of the hepatocyte for use in other tissues. Glucose-6-phosphate, in blue, plays a central role in carbohydrate metabolism.

Glycogenesis and Glycogenolysis

The first step in glycogen storage is the transport of glucose through the plasma membrane. Once in the hepatocyte, glucose and ATP are converted by the enzyme glucokinase to glucose-6-phosphate (G6P), the first intermediate in the synthesis of glycogen (Fig. 2.1). Because complete oxidation of one molecule of G6P generates 37 molecules of ATP, and storage uses only one molecule of ATP, the overall efficiency of glucose storage as glycogen is a remarkable 97%. Glycogenolysis does not occur by simple reversal of glycogenesis. Each succeeding glucose on a glycogen chain is released by glycogen phosphorylase (Fig. 2.2). Eventually, G6P is re-formed. G6P cannot exit from cells and must first be converted back to glucose. The conversion of G6P to glucose is catalyzed by glucose-6-phosphatase, found only in hepatocytes, kidney, and intestinal epithelial cells. Neither brain nor muscle cells, which use glucose as a primary fuel source, contain the phosphatase enzyme. This lack of glucose-6-phosphatase ensures a ready supply of glucose for the energy needs of brain and muscle. Liver does not use glucose primarily for fuel but as a precursor for other molecules.

Glycolysis

Glycolysis is the pathway—found in all mammalian cells—by which glucose is converted to pyruvate or lactate (Fig. 2.3). The glycolytic pathway is interesting in that glucose can be metabolized in the presence (aerobic) or absence (anaerobic) of oxygen. The aerobic conversion of glucose to pyruvate has three effects: (a) a net gain of two ATP molecules, (b) generation of two reducing equivalents of the nicotinamide adenine nucleotide (NADH + H^+), or (c) conversion of pyruvate to acetyl CoA with subsequent degradation of acetyl CoA in the citric acid cycle (see later). The conversion of glucose to pyruvate is regulated by three enzymes: hexokinase (glucokinase), phosphofructokinase, and pyruvate kinase, which are non-equilibrium reactions and as such, functionally irreversible.

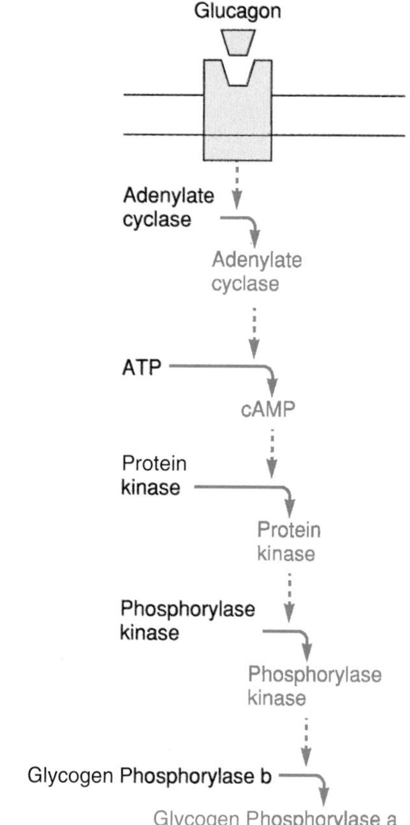

FIGURE 2.2 Glucagon-stimulated enzyme cascade, responsible for the control of glycogen metabolism. Inactive forms are shown in black, active forms in blue.

Under anaerobic conditions, NADH + H^+ cannot be reoxidized by transfer of reducing equivalents through the electron transport chain to oxygen. Instead, pyruvate is reduced by the NADH + H^+ to lactate. Glycolysis takes place in the cytoplasm, in contrast to the citric acid cycle, which is a mitochondrial process. During times of glucose excess, as in the fed state, hepatic glycolysis can generate energy in the form of ATP, but the oxidation of ketoacids is a preferred hepatic energy source.

In erythrocytes, a unique variant of glycolysis enhances oxyhemoglobin dissociation. The first site in glycolysis for generation of ATP is bypassed, leading to the formation of 2,3 bisphosphoglycerate by an additional enzyme called bisphosphoglycerate mutase. Kinetics of the mutase present in erythrocytes allow the presence of high concentrations of 2,3 bisphosphoglycerate to build up. The 2,3 bisphosphoglycerate displaces oxygen from hemoglobin allowing a shift of the oxyhemoglobin dissociation curve to the right.

Gluconeogenesis

There is an absolute minimum requirement for glucose in humans. Below a certain blood glucose concentration, brain dysfunction causes coma and death. When glucose becomes scarce, as in the fasting state, glycogenolysis occurs. Once glycogen stores have been depleted, the liver and kidneys are capable of synthesizing new glucose by the process of gluconeogenesis. Glucagon is produced in response to low blood sugar levels and stimulates gluconeogenesis. Gluconeogenesis is not a simple reversal of the glycolytic

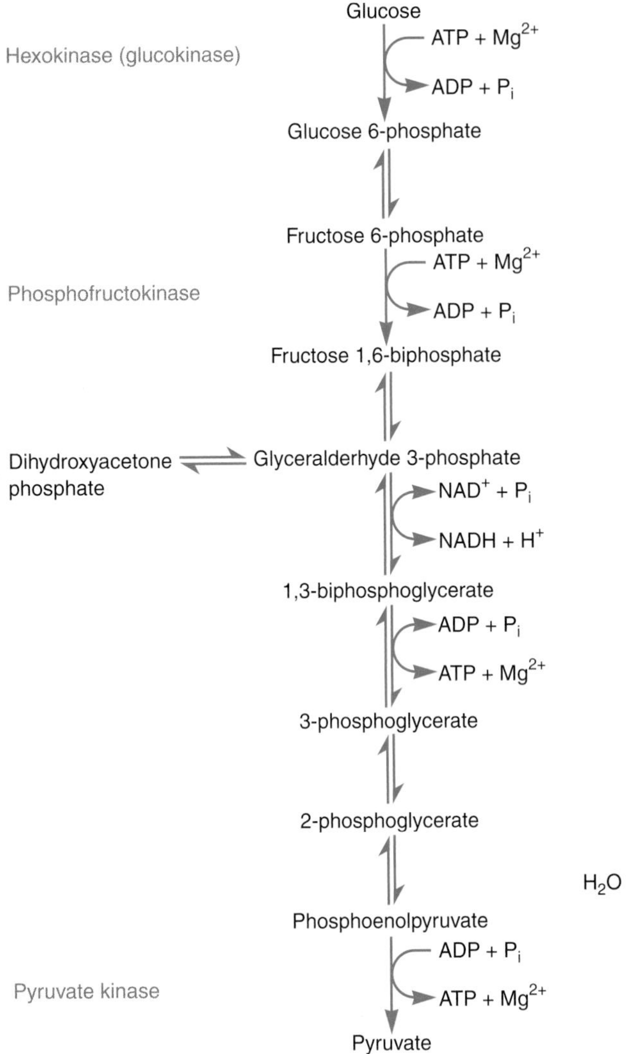

FIGURE 2.3 The glycolytic pathway. There is a net gain of two adenosine triphosphate molecules per glucose molecule. Phosphofructokinase is the key regulatory enzyme in this pathway; however, all the enzymes in red catalyze irreversible reactions. The pathway shown here is active only in the presence of aerobic conditions.

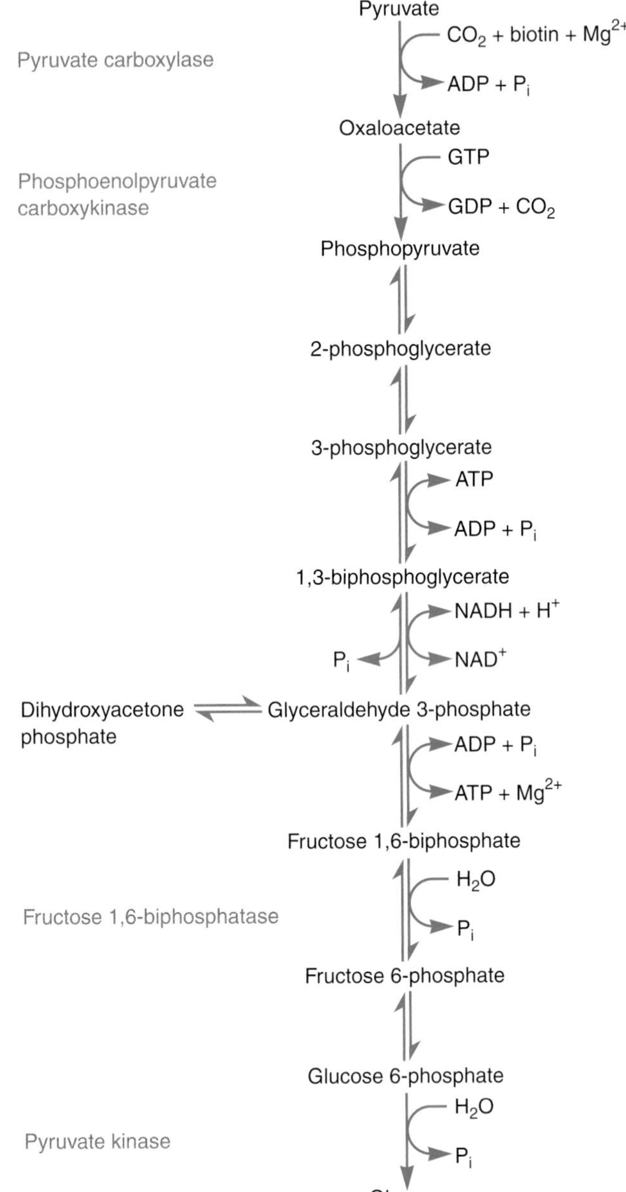

FIGURE 2.4 The gluconeogenesis pathway. The irreversible nature of the glycolytic pathway requires that a different sequence of biosyntheses are required for glucose production. The enzymes in red catalyze irreversible reactions that are different from those in glycolysis. In mammals, glucose cannot be synthesized from acetyl CoA, only from cytosolic pyruvate.

pathway. In glycolysis, as noted previously, the conversion of glucose to pyruvate is a one-way reaction. As a result, four separate, functionally irreversible enzyme reactions are required to convert pyruvate into glucose (Fig. 2.4). These enzymes are pyruvate carboxylase, phosphoenolpyruvate carboxykinase, fructose 1,6-bisphosphatase, and glucose 6-phosphatase. Other enzymes are shared with the glycolytic pathway.

About 60% of the naturally occurring amino acids, glycerol, or lactate can also be used as substrates for glucose production. Alanine is the amino acid most easily converted into glucose. Simple deamination allows conversion to pyruvate, which is subsequently converted to glucose. Other amino acids can be converted into three-, four-, or five-carbon sugars and then enter the phosphogluconate pathway (see later). Gluconeogenesis is enhanced by fasting, critical illness, and periods of anaerobic metabolism. Active skeletal muscle and erythrocytes form large quantities of lactate. In patients with large wounds, lactate also accumulates. The conversion of lactate (through pyruvate) to glucose—a process possible only in the presence of oxygen—is an important means of preventing severe lactic acidosis (Fig. 2.5).

Phosphogluconate Pathway

When glucose enters the liver, glycogen is formed until the hepatic glycogen capacity is reached (about 100 g). If excess glucose is still available, the liver converts it to fat by the phosphogluconate pathway (also known as the pentose phosphate pathway) (Fig. 2.6). The cytosolic phosphogluconate pathway can completely oxidize glucose, generating CO_2 and nicotinamide adenine dinucleotide phosphate

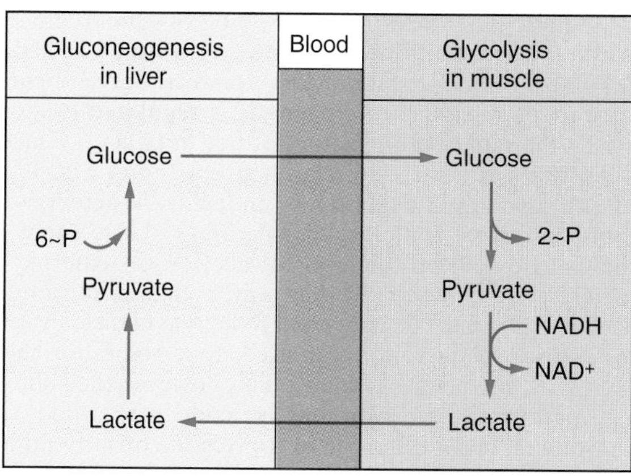

FIGURE 2.5 The Cori cycle, an elegant mechanism for the hepatic conversion of muscle lactate into new glucose. Pyruvate plays a key role in this process.

(NADPH) through what is known as the oxidative phase. Hydrogen atoms released in the phosphogluconate pathway combine with oxidized nicotinamide adenine dinucleotide phosphate ($NADP^+$) to form reduced nicotinamide adenine dinucleotide phosphate ($NADPH + H^+$).[2] The oxidative phase is present only in tissues, such as the adrenal glands and gonads, that require reductive biosyntheses such as steroidogenesis or other forms of lipid synthesis. Essentially, all tissues contain the nonoxidative phase, which is reversible and produces ribose precursors for nucleotide synthesis. In erythrocytes, the phosphogluconate pathway provides reducing equivalents for the production of reduced glutathione by glutathione reductase. Reduced glutathione can remove hydrogen peroxide, which increases the conversion of oxyhemoglobin to methemoglobin and subsequent hemolysis.

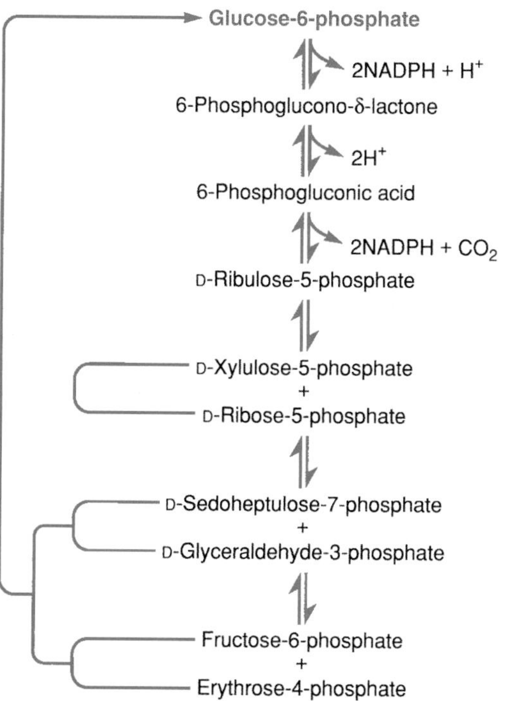

FIGURE 2.6 The phosphogluconate pathway. One of the major purposes of this pathway is to generate reduced nicotinamide adenine dinucleotide, which can serve as an electron donor and allow the liver to perform reductive biosynthesis.

LIPID METABOLISM

Lipid Transport

Lipid transport throughout the body is made complicated by the fact that lipids are insoluble in water. To overcome this physicochemical incompatibility, dietary triglycerides are first split into monoglycerides and fatty acids by the action of intestinal lipases. After absorption into the small intestinal cells, triacylglycerols are re-formed and aggregate into chylomicrons, which then enter the bloodstream by way of the lymph. Chylomicrons are removed from the blood by the liver and adipose tissue. The capillary surface of the liver contains large amounts of lipoprotein lipase, which hydrolyzes triglycerides into fatty acids and glycerol. The fatty acids freely diffuse into the hepatocytes for further metabolism. Similar to chylomicrons, very low-density lipoproteins (VLDLs) are synthesized by the liver and are the main vehicle for transport of triacylglycerols to extrahepatic tissues. The intestines and liver are the only two tissues capable of secreting lipid particles. In addition to chylomicrons and VLDLs, there are two other major groups of plasma lipoproteins: low-density lipoproteins (LDLs), and high-density lipoproteins (HDLs). LDL and HDL contain predominantly cholesterol and phospholipid.

The structure of all classes of lipoproteins is similar. There is a core of nonpolar lipids, either triacylglycerols or cholesteryl esters, depending on the particular lipoprotein. This nonpolar core is coated with a surface layer of amphipathic phospholipid or cholesterol oriented so that the polar ends are in contact with the plasma. A protein component is also present. The A apolipoproteins are found in chylomicrons and HDL. The B apolipoproteins come in two forms: B-100 is the predominant apolipoprotein of LDL, whereas the shorter B-48 is found in chylomicrons. The C apolipoproteins can transfer between VLDL, LDL, and HDL. Apolipoprotein D and E also exist. Apolipoproteins have several functions in lipid transport and storage. Some, such as the B apolipoproteins, are an integral part of the lipoprotein structure. Other apolipoproteins are enzyme cofactors, such as C-II for lipoprotein lipase. Lastly, the apolipoproteins act as ligands for cell surface receptors. As an example, both B-100 and E serve as ligands for the LDL receptor.[3,4]

Fatty Acid Metabolism

Most human fatty acids found in plasma are long-chain acids (C-16 to C-20). Because long-chain fatty acids are not readily absorbed by the intestinal mucosa, they must first be incorporated into chylomicrons. In contrast, short-chain and medium-chain fatty acids are absorbed directly into the portal circulation and are avidly taken up by the liver. Free fatty acids in the circulation are noncovalently bound to albumin and are transferred to the hepatocyte cytosol by way of fatty acid-binding proteins. Fatty acid CoA esters are synthesized in the cytosol after hepatic uptake of fatty acids. These fatty acid CoA esters can be converted into triglyceride, transported into mitochondria for the production of acetyl CoA and reducing equivalents, or stored in the liver as triglycerides. The rate-limiting step in the synthesis of triglyceride is the conversion of acetyl CoA to malonyl CoA. Malonyl CoA in turn inhibits the mitochondrial uptake of fatty acid CoA ester, favoring triglyceride synthesis. The liver also contains dehydrogenases that can unsaturate essential dietary fatty acids. Structural elements of all tissues contain significant amounts of unsaturated fats, and the liver is responsible for the production of these unsaturated fatty acids. As another example, dietary linoleic acid is elongated and dehydrogenated to the prostaglandin precursor arachidonic acid.

Under basal conditions, most free fatty acids are catabolized for energy by cardiac and skeletal muscle. Under conditions of adipocyte lipolysis, the liver can take up and metabolize fatty acids. Although fatty acid synthesis occurs in the cytosol, fatty acid oxidation occurs in the mitochondria. Fatty acid CoA esters bind carnitine, a carrier molecule, and in the absence of cytosolic malonyl CoA, they enter the mitochondria, where they undergo β-oxidation to acetyl CoA and reducing equivalents (Fig. 2.7). Acetyl CoA can then take one of the following routes: (a) enter the tricarboxylic acid cycle and be degraded to carbon dioxide; (b) be converted to citrate for fatty acid synthesis; or (c) be converted into 3-hydroxy-3-methylglutaryl CoA (HMG-CoA), a precursor of cholesterol and ketone bodies. The mitochondrial hydrolysis of fatty acids is a source of large quantities of ATP. The conversion of stearic acid to carbon dioxide and water, for instance, generates 136 molecules of ATP and demonstrates the highly efficient storage of energy as fat. By a process called β-oxidation, acetyl-CoA molecules are cleaved from fatty acids. The acetyl-CoA is then metabolized through the citric acid cycle under normal circumstances.

In times of unrestrained lipolysis, such as starvation, uncontrolled diabetes, or other conditions of triglyceride mobilization from adipocyte stores, ketone bodies—predominantly 3-hydroxybutyrate and acetoacetate—are formed in hepatic mitochondria from free fatty acids and are a source of energy for extrahepatic tissues. Ketogenesis is regulated predominantly by the rate of mobilization of free fatty acids. Once in the liver mitochondria, the relative proportion of acyl-CoA destined to undergo β-oxidation is limited by the activity of an enzyme—carnitine palmitoyltransferase-1. Last, there are mechanisms that keep the levels of acetyl-CoA entering the citric acid cycle constant, so that only at high mitochondrial levels will acetyl-CoA be converted to ketone bodies. Even the brain, in times of starvation, can use ketone bodies for half of its energy requirements. At some point, however, the ability of liver to perform β-oxidation may be inadequate. Under such circumstances, hepatic storage of triglyceride or fatty infiltration of the liver can be significant leading to the development of nonalcoholic steatohepatitis (NASH). Triglyceride storage by itself does not appear to be a cause of hepatic fibrosis, but fatty infiltration may be a marker for the derangement of normal processes by alcohol or drug toxicity, diabetes, or long-term total parenteral nutrition. A specific type of microvesicular fatty accumulation is also seen in a variety of diseases, such as Reye's syndrome, morbid obesity, and acute fatty liver of pregnancy.

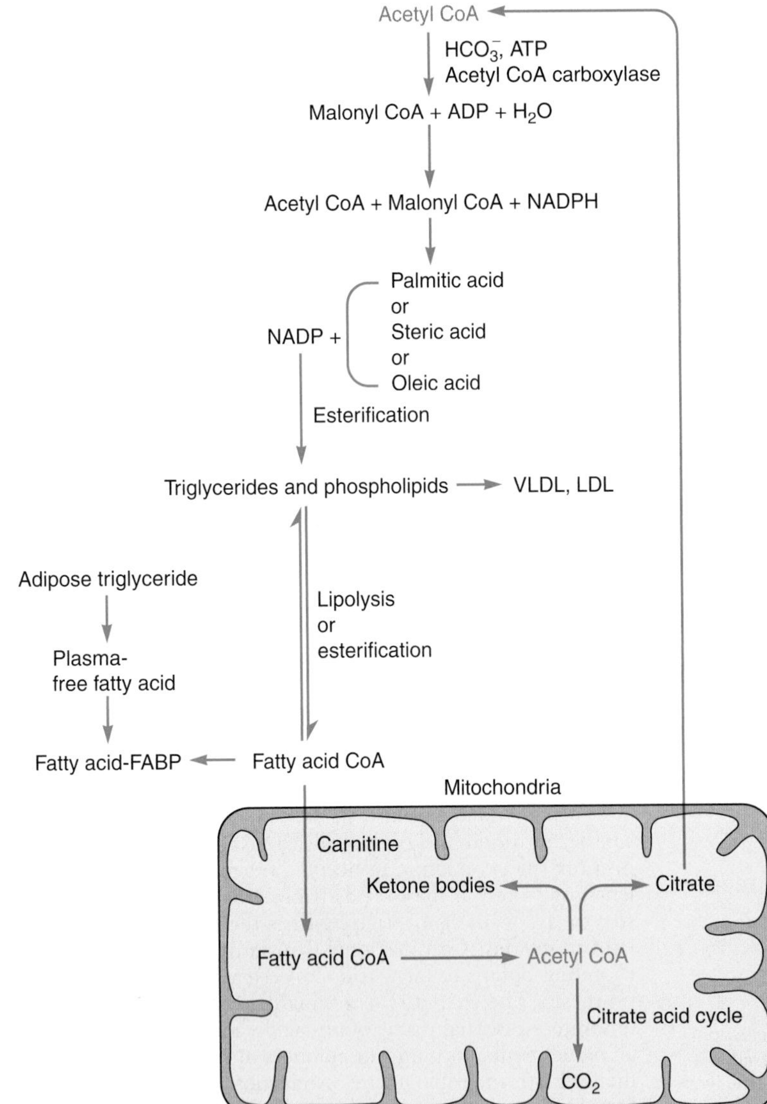

FIGURE 2.7 Diagram of hepatic fatty acid metabolism. Both dietary and newly synthesized fatty acids are esterified and subsequently degraded in the mitochondria for energy, first as reducing equivalents then ATP via the electron transport chain.

Cholesterol Metabolism

Cholesterol is an important regulator of membrane fluidity and is a substrate for bile acid and steroid hormone synthesis. Cholesterol may be available by dietary intake or by de novo synthesis. In mammals, most new cholesterol is synthesized in the liver from its precursor, acetyl CoA. Dietary cholesterol intake can suppress endogenous synthesis by inhibiting the rate-limiting enzyme in the cholesterol biosynthetic pathway, HMG-CoA reductase. A competitive antagonist, lovastatin, can also block HMG-CoA reductase and effectively lower plasma cholesterol by blocking cholesterol synthesis, stimulating LDL receptor synthesis, and allowing an increased hepatic uptake and metabolism of cholesterol-rich LDL lipoproteins. The structure of the LDL receptor is known and serves as a model for the structure and function of other cell membrane receptors (Fig. 2.8).

Cholesterol is lipophilic and hydrophobic, and most plasma cholesterol is found in lipoproteins esterified with oleic or palmitic acid. The liver can process cholesterol esters from all classes of lipoproteins. Hepatocytes can also take up chylomicron remnants containing dietary cholesterol esters. Newly synthesized hepatic cholesterol is used primarily to synthesize bile acids for further intestinal absorption of dietary fats. A large proportion of the bile acids secreted by the liver into bile are returned to the liver via the enterohepatic circulation (Fig. 2.9). Abnormally elevated levels of cholesterol in VLDL or LDL are associated with atherosclerosis, whereas HDL levels are protective.

Phospholipids

The three major classes of phospholipid synthesized by the liver are lecithins, cephalins, and sphingomyelins. Although most cells in the body are capable of some phospholipid synthesis, the liver produces 90%. Phospholipid formation is controlled by the overall rate of fat metabolism and also by the availability of choline and inositol. The main role of phospholipids of all types is to form plasma and organelle membranes. The amphiphilic nature of phospholipids makes them essential for reducing surface tension between membranes and surrounding fluids. Phosphatidylcholine, one of the lecithins, is the major biliary phospholipid and is important in promoting the secretion of free cholesterol into bile. Thromboplastin, one of the cephalins, is needed to initiate the clotting cascade. The sphingomyelins are necessary for the formation of the myelin nerve sheath.

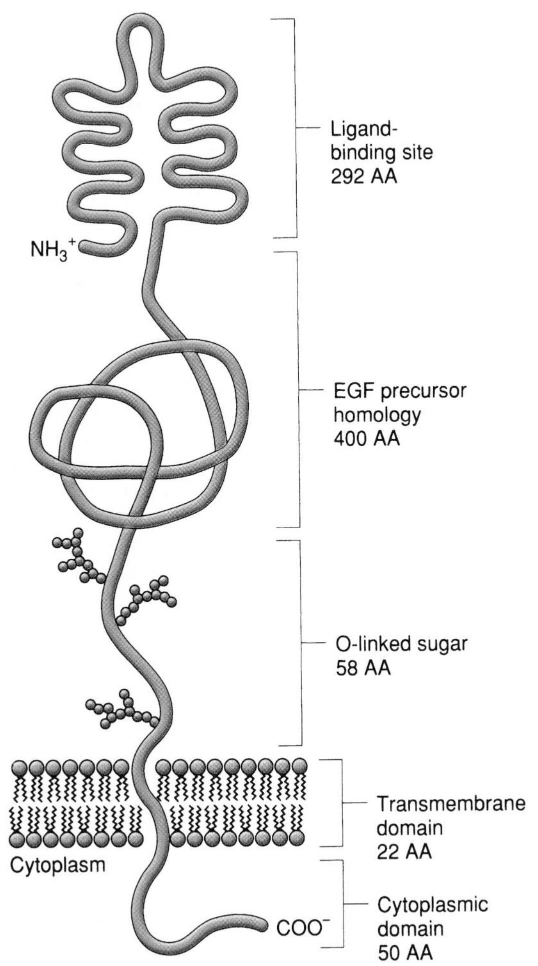

FIGURE 2.8 The low-density lipoprotein (LDL) receptor, an example of a transmembrane receptor that participates in receptor-mediated endocytosis. The LDL receptor specifically binds lipoproteins that contain apolipoprotein B-100 or E. Once internalized, the lipoproteins are degraded. AA, amino acids.

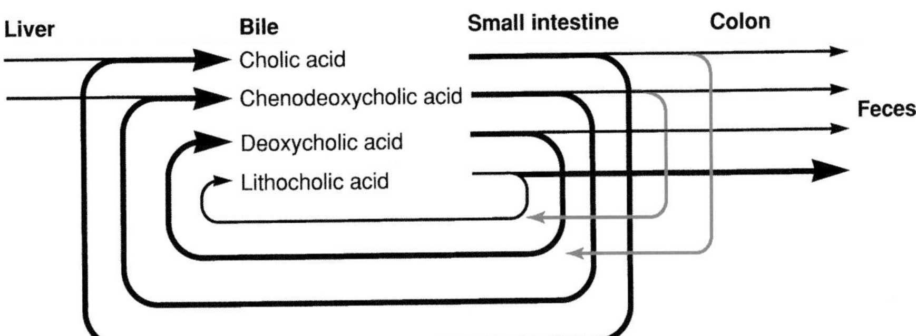

FIGURE 2.9 The enterohepatic circulation of bile acids. The primary bile acids, cholic acid and chenodeoxycholic acid, are synthesized in the liver from cholesterol. Deoxycholic acid and lithocholic acid are formed in the colon (blue lines) during bacterial degradation of the primary bile acids. All four bile acids are conjugated with glycine or taurine in the liver. Most of the lithocholic acid is also sulfated, which decreases reabsorption and increases fecal excretion. Bile acids are absorbed passively in the epithelium of the small and large intestine and actively in the distal ileum.

PROTEIN METABOLISM

Formation and Catabolism of Plasma Proteins

Essentially all albumin, fibrinogen, and apolipoproteins are derived from the liver, which can add up to 50 g of protein to the plasma a day. Of the total hepatic protein synthesized, 75% is destined for export in plasma. Most newly synthesized proteins are not stored in the liver, and the rate of protein synthesis is primarily determined by the intracellular levels of amino acids. The tertiary structure of many proteins undergoes post-translational modification after they have been synthesized in the liver rough endoplasmic reticulum (ER). Glycosylation, or the addition of carbohydrate moieties, occurs in the smooth ER. Sialation, or the addition of sialic acid, occurs in the Golgi. Glycosylation is important in allowing some proteins to bind with specific receptors for subsequent hepatic uptake and processing. Removal of sialic acid residues, or desialation, from the terminal galactose molecules of glycoproteins allows them to bind the asialoglycoprotein (ASGP) receptor in the liver and undergo degradation. Desialation, therefore, is important in the clearance of senescent proteins from the plasma.

Intracellular proteases hydrolyze proteins into peptides, and the peptides are in turn hydrolyzed by peptidases. Ultimately, free amino acids are generated. Unlike carbohydrate and lipids, excess amino acids are degraded if not immediately reincorporated into new proteins. Protein degradation occurs primarily by one of two routes. Asialoglycoproteins are internalized into lysosomes via receptor mediated endocytosis. The lysosomal enzymes do not require ATP and are nonselective in their activities; more than 20 known hydrolytic enzymes are present in lysosomes. A second pathway involves the covalent attachment of ubiquitin, named for the fact that it exists in all mammalian cells, targeting proteins for destruction. This pathway is ATP dependent and generally is used for proteins with shorter half lives.[5]

Amino Acid Synthesis

Essentially all the end products of dietary protein digestion are amino acids, which are absorbed by the enterocytes into the portal circulation in an ionized state. Liver amino acid uptake occurs by one of several active transport mechanisms. Amino acids are not stored in the liver but are rapidly used in the production of plasma proteins, purines, heme proteins, and hormones. Under certain conditions, the amine group is removed from amino acids, and the carbon chain is used for carbohydrate, lipid, or nonessential amino acid synthesis.[6]

Ten nutritionally essential amino acids must be obtained from dietary intake (Table 2.1). However, human tissues contain transferases, which convert the α-keto acids of leucine, valine, and isoleucine so that the corresponding α-keto acids can be used as dietary supplements. The remaining nutritionally nonessential amino acids can be synthesized in one to three enzyme catalyzed reactions. Hydroxyproline and hydroxylysine do not have a corresponding tRNA and arise by post-translational modification of proline or lysine by mixed function oxidases. Glutamate, glutamine, and proline are derived from the citric acid cycle intermediate α-ketoglutarate. Aspartate and asparagine are synthesized from oxaloacetate. Serine and glycine are synthesized from the glycolysis intermediate 3-phosphoglycerate. Cysteine and tyrosine are formed from essential amino acids (methionine and phenylalanine, respectively).[7]

Catabolism of Amino Acid Nitrogen

Ammonia, derived largely from the deamination of amino acids, is toxic to all mammalian cells. The ammonia formed as a result of the deamination of amino acids is detoxified by one of two routes.[8] The most important pathway involves the conversion of ammonia to urea by enzymes of the Krebs-Henseleit, or urea cycle, found only in the liver (Fig. 2.10). A second route of ammonia metabolism involves synthesis of L-glutamine from ammonia and glutamate by renal glutamine synthetase.

TABLE 2.1

AMINO ACIDS REQUIRED BY ADULT HUMANS

	Nutritionally Nonessential	
Nutritionally Essential	**Amino Acid**	**Precursor**
Arginine	Alanine	Pyruvate
Histidine	Asparagine	Oxaloacetate
Isoleucine	Aspartate	Oxaloacetate
Leucine	Cysteine	Methionine
Lysine	Glutamate	α-Ketoglutarate
Methionine	Glutamine	α-Ketoglutarate
Phenylalanine	Glycine	3-Phosphoglycerate
Threonine	Hydroxyproline	α-Ketoglutarate
Tryptophan	Hydroxylysine	Lysine
Valine	Proline	α-Ketoglutarate
	Serine	3-phosphoglycerate
	Tyrosine	Phenylalanine

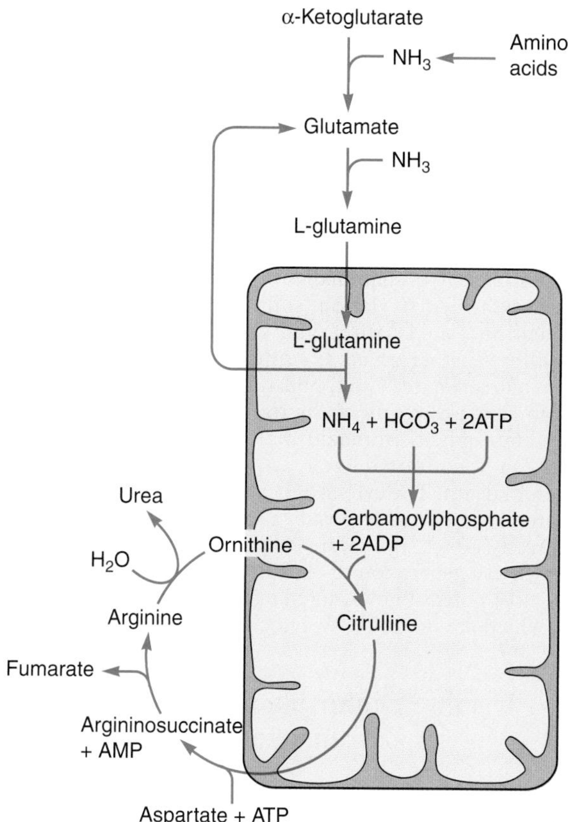

FIGURE 2.10 The urea cycle. Ammonia entering the urea cycle is derived from protein and amino acid degradation in tissues (endogenous) and the colonic lumen (exogenous).

THE CITRIC ACID CYCLE AND INTEGRATION OF METABOLIC PATHWAYS

The major function of the citric acid cycle is to act as a common pathway for the oxidation of carbohydrate, lipid, and protein. Conversely, the citric acid cycle also plays important roles in gluconeogenesis, lipogenesis, and amino acid metabolism. In the fed state, a large proportion of ingested energy from foodstuffs is converted to glycogen or fat. The metabolism of sugars, fats, and proteins, then, allows adequate fuels for all tissue types under conditions from fed to fasting to starvation. The body accomplishes production of fuel substrates for organs and regulates intestinally absorbed nutrients for tissue consumption or storage by integrating three key metabolites—glucose-6-phosphate, pyruvate, and acetyl CoA (Fig. 2.11). Each of these three simple chemical molecules can be extensively modified to allow a large number of metabolites.

The citric acid cycle comprises a series of mitochondrial enzyme reactions. The substrate that drives the citric acid cycle is acetyl CoA.[9] In the mitochondria, acetyl CoA combines with oxaloacetate to form citrate. Through a series of enzymic reactions involving both dehydrogenases and decarboxylases, citrate is catabolized to result in the generation of hydrogen reducing equivalents and carbon dioxide (Fig. 2.12). Each molecule of acetyl CoA catabolized through the citric acid cycle yields three molecules of NADH + H^+ and one molecule of $FADH_2$. These reducing equivalents are transported to the inner mitochondrial membrane and the electron transport chain to generate more ATP. Each molecule of NADH + H^+ is oxidized to yield three molecules of ATP, and each molecule of $FADH_2$ is oxidized to yield two molecules of ATP. One molecule of ATP is generated at the substrate level in the conversion of succinyl-CoA to succinate; thus, the total molecules of ATP generated per molecule of acetyl CoA is 12.

G6P can be stored as glycogen or converted into glucose, pyruvate, or ribose-5-phosphate (a nucleotide precursor). Pyruvate can be converted into lactate, alanine (and other amino acids), and acetyl CoA, or it can enter the tricarboxylic acid cycle by conversion to oxaloacetate. Acetyl CoA is converted to HMG-CoA (a cholesterol and ketone body precursor) or citrate (for fatty acid and triglyceride synthesis), or it is degraded to carbon dioxide and water for energy. In humans, acetyl CoA cannot be converted into pyruvate due to the irreversible reaction of pyruvate dehydrogenase. Thus, lipids cannot be converted into either carbohydrates or glucogenic amino acids.

Regardless of the fed state of the human body, there is a requirement for glucose utilization. The nervous system and erythrocytes have an absolute requirement for glucose. Glucose is a source of glycerol-3-phosphate for adipose tissue, and most other tissues for integrity of the citric acid cycle. To maintain adequate glucose for survival, other fuels can be used depending on environmental conditions. Under conditions of carbohydrate shortage, ketone bodies and free fatty acids are utilized to spare oxidation of glucose in muscle. These alternate fuels increase intracellular citrate, which inhibits both phosphofructokinase and pyruvate dehydrogenase. In starvation, fatty acid oxidation results in the production of glycerol, which along with gluconeogenesis from amino acids is the only source of the required glucose. Ultimately, even the brain can substitute ketone bodies for about half of its energy requirements. The preferred energy substrates for liver are ketoacids derived from amino acid degradation even in well-fed states. This is designed to allow the consumption of glucose by obligate tissues. Glucose produced by the dephosphorylation of G6P rapidly diffuses out of the cell and is taken up by the brain, muscles, and other organs. Hepatic glycolysis is used primarily for the production of intermediates of metabolism and not for energy. Hepatic fatty acid degradation for energy is also inhibited under most circumstances and is seen only during adipocyte lipolysis.

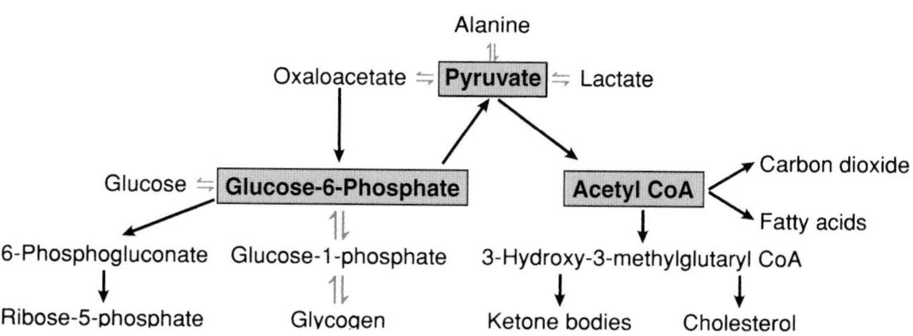

FIGURE 2.11 Summation of the key regulatory molecules used by the liver during diverse metabolic functions. Essentially, any compound found in the body can be synthesized in the liver from glucose-6-phosphate, acetyl coenzyme A, or pyruvate. As a consequence of the inability of mammalian liver to convert acetyl coenzyme A to pyruvate, fats cannot be converted to carbohydrates.

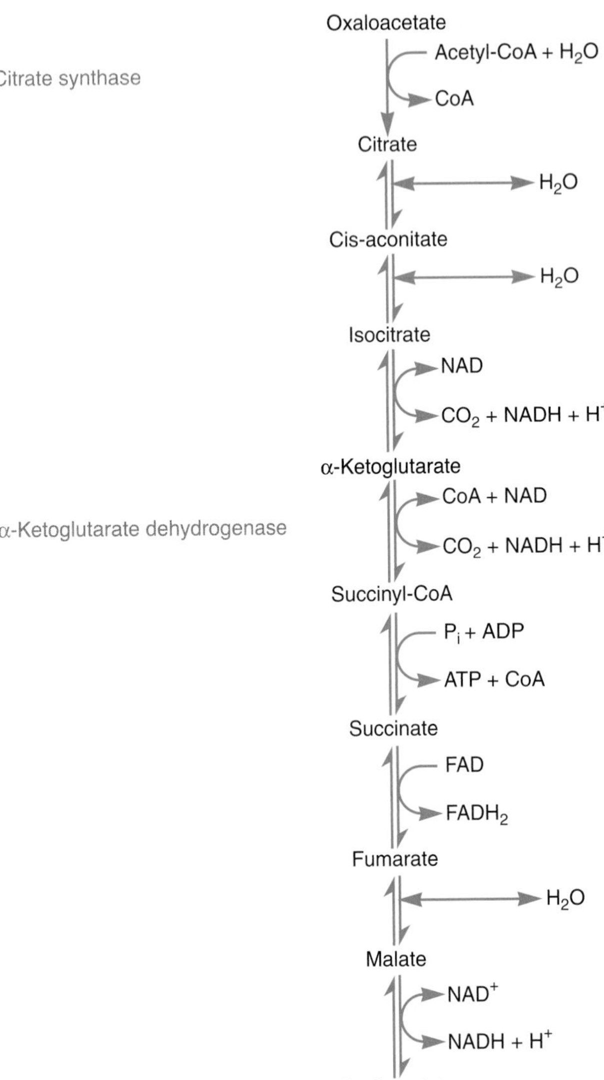

FIGURE 2.12 The citric acid cycle. Reduced nicotinamide adenine dinucleotide and reduced flavin adenine dinucleotide, formed in the citric acid cycle, are subsequently oxidized in mitochondria by means of the electron transport chain to generate adenosine triphosphate. Acetyl coenzyme A plays a key role.

BIOTRANSFORMATION

Biotransformation is defined as the intracellular metabolism of endogenous organic compounds (e.g., heme proteins and steroid hormones) and exogenous compounds (e.g., drugs and environmental compounds). Most biotransformation also occurs chiefly in the liver, which contains enzyme systems that can expose functional groups, such as hydroxyl ions (phase I reactions), or alter the size and solubility of a wide variety of organic and inorganic compounds by conjugation with small polar molecules (phase II reactions). A general strategy is to convert hydrophobic, potentially toxic compounds into hydrophilic conjugates that can then be excreted into bile or urine.

The four general enzyme families responsible for hepatic biotransformation are the cytochromes P-450, the uridine diphosphate-glucuronyl (UDP-glucuronyl) transferases, the glutathione (GSH) S-transferases, and the sulfotransferases. Biotransforming enzymes are not distributed uniformly within the cells of the hepatic lobule. This heterogeneity may account for the ability of some drugs to cause damage preferentially in zone 3 hepatocytes (those nearest the central venule).

Cytochromes P-450

The cytochromes P-450 are named for their ability to absorb light maximally at 450 nm in the presence of carbon monoxide. These enzymes are bound to the ER and collectively catalyze reactions by using NADPH and oxygen. The P-450 isozymes present in mammalian liver catalyze reactions such as oxidation, hydroxylation, sulfoxide formation, oxidative deamination, dealkylation, and dehalogenation. Such reactions allow further phase II conjugation with polar groups such as glucuronate, GSH, and sulfate. The cytochromes P-450 can also create potentially toxic metabolites. Drugs such as acetaminophen, isoniazid, halothane, and the phenothiazines can be converted into reactive forms that cause cellular injury and death. The cytochromes also are responsible for the formation of organic free radicals, reactive metabolites that can directly attack and injure cellular components or act as a hapten in the generation of an autoimmune response. Several of the most potent known carcinogens are aromatic hydrocarbons, which are modified by cytochrome P-450.

Uridine Diphosphate-Glucuronyl Transferases

Glucuronidation is the conjugation of UDP-glucuronic acid to a wide variety of xenobiotics by either ester (acyl) or ether linkages. The transferases catalyzing these reactions reside in the ER. Many common compounds are metabolized in this way, including bilirubin, testosterone, aspirin, indomethacin, acetaminophen, chloramphenicol, and oxazepam. Clinically significant loss of activity can occur with acute ethanol exposure or acetaminophen overdose, when formation of UDP-glucuronic acid from UDP-glucose is outstripped by use. Some acyl linkages lead to the generation of electrophilic centers that can react with other proteins. The covalent linkage of conjugated bilirubin to albumin is believed to occur by this mechanism.

Glutathione S-Transferases

The GSH transferases are more selective in the biotransformations they perform. GSH conjugation occurs only with compounds that have electrophilic and potentially reactive centers. The role of GSH conjugation catalyzed by the GSH S-transferases is best seen with acetaminophen. In this drug, cytochrome P-450 creates an electrophilic center that reacts with protein thiol groups or GSH.[10] The presence of GSH S-transferase allows the preferential detoxification of acetaminophen rather than the potentially injurious binding to thiol groups. A class of GSH S-transferases, known as *ligandins,* appears to facilitate the uptake and intracellular transport of bilirubin, heme, and bile acids from plasma to liver. In addition to the detoxification of potential toxins, GSH is a substrate for GSH peroxidase, an enzyme important in the metabolism of hydrogen peroxide.

Sulfotransferases

The sulfotransferases catalyze the transfer of sulfate groups from 3′-phosphoadenosine-5′-phosphosulfate (PAPS) to compounds such as thyroxine, bile acids, isoproterenol, α-methyldopa, and acetaminophen. They are located primarily in the cytosol. Although many P-450 derivatives can be further conjugated by either the sulfotransferases or the glucuronyl transferases, a

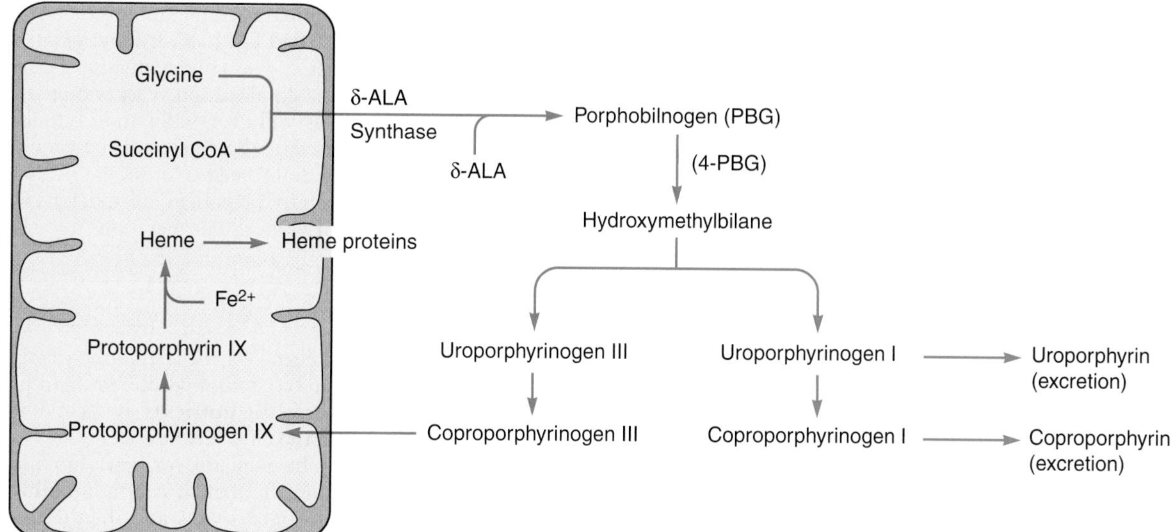

FIGURE 2.13 The heme biosynthetic pathway. Inherited defects of each of the heme biosynthetic enzymes except δ-aminolevulinic acid synthase have been described and lead to the clinical disorders known as the porphyrias.

limited ability of the liver to synthesize PAPS makes glucuronidation the predominant mechanism.

HEME AND PORPHYRIN METABOLISM

Heme is formed from glycine and succinate and is the functional iron-containing center of hemoglobin, myoglobin, cytochromes, catalases, and peroxidases. From glycine and succinate precursors, δ-aminolevulinic acid (δ-ALA) is synthesized by the rate-limiting enzyme ALA synthase. The porphyrinogens are intermediates in the pathway from δ-ALA to heme, and porphyrins are oxidized forms of porphyrinogen (Fig. 2.13). Inherited enzyme defects in the heme synthetic pathway cause the overproduction of various porphyrinogens, which can in turn cause clinical manifestations known as the *porphyrias*.[11] Acquired porphyria can be caused by heavy metal intoxication, estrogens, alcohol, or environmental exposure to chlorinated hydrocarbons.

Bilirubin IXa is the predominant heme degradation product in humans and is derived mostly from hemoglobin. The enzyme heme oxygenase, found in cells of the reticuloendothelial system, is primarily responsible for this conversion. Heme oxygenase is located in the ER and requires NADPH as a cofactor. Hepatic processing of bilirubin is further detailed in the section on bile formation.

METAL METABOLISM

Iron uptake appears to occur by two distinct processes: (a) receptor-mediated endocytosis of iron–transferrin complexes and (b) facilitated diffusion across the plasma membrane. More iron is taken up and stored by the liver than by any other organ, with the exception of the bone marrow. Transferrin is synthesized in the liver and has specific plasma membrane receptors on a number of different tissues. After endocytosis, the transferrin and iron dissociate and the transferrin and transferrin receptor return to the cell surface for recycling. A pathway appears to involve the dissociation of iron and transferrin at the plasma membrane and subsequent internalization by carrier-mediated diffusion. Once internalized, iron is stored and complexed to apoferritin. Each apoferritin molecule is capable of storing several thousand iron molecules. The iron–apoferritin complex, called *ferritin,* is responsible for iron storage under physiologic conditions. Iron storage in a protein-bound form is essential because free iron can catalyze free radical formation, leading to cell injury.[12]

Copper is transported to the liver bound to albumin or histidine and enters the hepatocytes by a process of facilitated diffusion. Once inside the cell, copper can bind to several intracellular proteins for storage or as a necessary enzyme cofactor. Copper-binding proteins include metallothionein, monoamine oxidase, cytochrome *c* oxidase, and superoxide dismutase. *Ceruloplasmin* is a liver-derived protein that binds hepatic copper for transport to other tissues. The low levels of ceruloplasmin seen in patients with Wilson's disease suggest a pathogenetic defect.

Zinc is taken up by and competes for the same binding sites as copper. In hepatocytes, zinc binds predominantly to metallothionein and is excreted into bile, in which it enters the enterohepatic circulation. Other metals, usually found in trace amounts, are lead, cadmium, selenium, mercury, and nickel. These metals are usually bound to metallothionein or GSH, and intoxication is associated with free radical formation and liver injury.

METABOLOMICS—THE EMERGING SCIENCE OF METABOLIC ANALYSIS

The need to understand metabolism—the inter-relation of fundamental intracellular biochemical reactions—is brought into sharp focus by the recent rapid advances in sequencing of the human genome. As every gene contained in the complement of human chromosomes is sequenced and identified, it has become increasingly clear that mere identification of genes is not enough when trying to understand human variation, human development, or the problem of human disease. The need for functional genomics—or the comprehensive analysis of RNA transcripts, proteins, and metabolites—has led to development of transcriptomics, proteomics, and metabolomics, respectively.

Metabolites are the end products of cellular regulatory processes, and their levels can be regarded as the ultimate response of biologic systems to inherited or environmental pressures. The set of metabolites synthesized by a biologic system constitute its "metabolome." These emerging technologies can be expected to identify ways—both expected and unexpected—that genes act in biologic systems. Metabolomic analysis aims at a comprehensive characterization of biologic samples.[13] For metabolomics, gas and liquid chromatography coupled to mass spectrometry have been used to identify and quantitate small-molecular-weight metabolites. Capillary electrophoresis, in conjunction with mass spectroscopy and nuclear magnetic resonance spectroscopy, have also been adapted for metabolomic analysis. Each of these critical technologies has strengths and drawbacks depending on the physicochemical structure of the studied metabolites. Analyses using the technologies noted previously can be performed on large sample numbers and with reasonable measurement times. Thus, metabolomics is emerging as a key technology for systems biology.

Biologically meaningful interpretations are often limited by an incomplete understanding of the metabolites and poor spatiotemporal resolution of acquired data sets. Further, each type of sample preparation may alter the available set of metabolites. The challenges for the future include how reaction pathway structures generate metabolic networks, the need to investigate integrative biochemical networks, and how to develop novel methods of bioinformatics and data visualization. Although metabolomics is still nascent, the identification of gene function; the effects of toxicologic, pharmaceutical, nutritional, and environmental manipulation; and the development of integrated databases of metabolite concentrations across human and research animal populations are all being accomplished.

Currently, there are several anticipated advantages of metabolomics when compared to traditional genetic analysis. Metabolites, like the proteins that synthesize them, are context dependent. The complement of metabolites in a given cell changes depending on the physiologic, developmental, and pathologic state of the cell of interest. In addition, unlike genes and messenger RNA, proteins and metabolites are functional entities. Perhaps most intriguing, however, is the realization that there are far fewer metabolites in cells than genes, message, or proteins. As an example, in the well-studied yeast *Saccharomyces cerevisiae* more than 6,000 genes have been identified, and yet only 600 low-molecular intermediates have been discovered.[14] As a result it is clear that there is no one-to-one correspondence as there is for the classic central dogma of DNA to RNA to protein.

There are several goals for the study of metabolomics: one is a complete computer representation of the chemical species of individual cell types and subsequently, organisms. The use of systems biology approaches will allow computational predictions of the higher-level metabolic complexity of intracellular processes and organ interaction from genomic information. One bioinformatics resource which is being created to perform such computation is named KEGG, for the Kyoto Encyclopedia of Genes and Genomes.[15] Another active area of investigation is the analysis of "silent" genes which do not manifest an overt phenotype in terms of development, growth rate, or other cellular function when deleted from the genome. Current attempts to generate a phenotype that allows the identification and analysis of a gene mutation are limited by gross morphologic abnormalities. Clearly, a variety of subtle changes in phenotype are missed because there is no dramatic change in morphology. Sophisticated analyses are being carried out based on the concept that the lack of a phenotype in silent genes is due to alteration of intracellular metabolites that can compensate for a missing gene function. Concentration changes in a select series of metabolites relative to one selected metabolite caused by the deletion of a silent gene should identify the site of action of the silent gene action. Again, using yeast, a comparative metabolomics approach to functional genomics is called FANCY, or Functional ANalysis by Co-responses in Yeast.[16] The same mathematics, strategies, and computer algorithms developed in yeast and other simpler plant and animal models will eventually and undoubtedly be useful in *Homo sapiens*. For the reasons listed previously, as well as the more immediate need to understand and apply knowledge of metabolism to the patient, all surgeons would do well to keep the principles of cellular metabolism in mind.

KEY POINTS

- **Intermediary metabolism—as the metabolic manipulation and balancing of ingested carbohydrate, fat, and protein—ultimately can process all nutrients to acetyl CoA for energy production in the citric acid cycle.**
- **Glucose must always be available for brain function; if not available directly from the diet, it can be mobilized for a brief period from glycogen stores and then derived from proteins in the liver and kidneys.**
- **Free fatty acids are a direct source of energy catabolized by cardiac and skeletal muscle.**
- **Hepatic protein synthesis, when excess amino acids are available, includes albumin, fibrinogen, and apolipoproteins and can reach 50 g per day.**
- **The citric acid cycle comprises a series of mitochondrial enzymes that transform acetyl CoA into water, carbon dioxide, and hydrogen-reducing equivalents; the hydrogen-reducing equivalents are then transformed into ATP by the electron transport chain. Each molecule of acetyl CoA that enters the citric acid cycle yields 12 molecules of ATP.**
- **Biotransformation of potentially toxic, often hydrophobic, compounds into hydrophilic, excretable compounds occurs mainly in the liver by the cytochromes P-450, the uridine diphosphate-glucuronyl (UDP-glucuronyl) transferases, the glutathione (GSH) S-transferases, and the sulfotransferases.**

References

1. Cellular energetics. In: Lodish H, Berk A, Zipursky LS, et al., eds. *Molecular cell biology*. New York: WH Freeman; 2004:301–350.
2. The Calvin cycle and the pentose phosphate pathway. In: Berg J, Tymoczko J, Stryer L, eds. *Biochemistry*, 5th ed. New York: WH Freeman; 2002:551–576.
3. Havel RJ, Hamilton RL. Hepatocytic lipoprotein receptors and intracellular lipoprotein catabolism. *Hepatology* 1988;8:1869.
4. Mayes PA. Lipid transport and storage. In: Murray RK, Granner DK, Mayes PA, Rodwell VW. *Harper's biochemistry*, 25th ed. New York: McGraw-Hill; 2000:268.
5. Bonifacino JS, Weissman, A. Ubiquitin and the control of protein fate in the secretory and endocytic pathways. *Annu Rev Cell Dev Biol.* 1998;14:19.
6. **Brosnan JT. Interorgan amino acid transport and its regulation. *J Nutr.* 2003;133[6 Suppl 1]:2068S-2072S.**
7. The biosynthesis of amino acids. In: Berg J, Tymoczko J, Stryer L, eds. *Biochemistry*, 5th ed. New York: WH Freeman; 2002:665–692.
8. **Morris SM Jr. Regulation of enzymes of the urea cycle and arginine metabolism. *Annu Rev Nutr.* 2002;22:87.**
9. Kornberg H. Krebs and his trinity of cycles. Nat Rev *Mol Cell Biol.* 2000;1:225.
10. Lee T, Li L, Ballatori N. Hepatic glutathione and glutathione S-conjugate transport mechanisms. *Yale J Biol Med.* 1997;70:287-300.
11. Gross U, Hoffmann GF, Doss MO. Erythropoietic and hepatic porphyrias. *J Inherit Metab Dis.* 2000;23:641.
12. **Hentze MW, Muckenthaler MU, Andrews NC. Balancing acts: molecular control of mammalian iron metabolism. *Cell* 2004;117:285.**
13. Weckwerth W. Metabolomics in systems biology. *Annu Rev Plant Biol.* 2003;54:669.
14. Oliver SG, Winson MK, Kell DB, Baganz F. Systematic functional analysis of the yeast genome. *Trends Biotechnol.* 1998;16:373.
15. **http://www.genome.jp/kegg/pathway.html**
16. **Raamsdonk LM, Teusink B, Broadhurst D, et al. A functional genomics strategy that uses metabolome data to reveal the phenotype of silent mutations. *Nat Biotechnol.* 2001;19:45.**

CHAPTER 3 ■ NUTRITION AND METABOLISM

J. STANLEY SMITH, JR., DAVID C. FRANKENFIELD, AND WILEY W. SOUBA

Nutrition support is indicated in surgical patients if they are significantly malnourished prior to surgery, if they are expected to remain nil per os (NPO) for more than 5 days postoperatively, or if they are critically ill. The main feature of nutrition support in the surgical patient is the presence of the inflammatory response. The inflammatory response is critical to survival from surgical or traumatic injury; however, it poses challenges in the nourishment of these patients. If the response is not present, nutrition support in surgery is similar to that in simple starvation. If the response is present, the nutrition support plan must take into account alterations in carbohydrate, lipid, and protein metabolism, metabolic rate, and catabolism.

The goal of nutrition support is to minimize protein loss and to provide key nutrients to maintain immune and other critical functions during and after surgical or traumatic injury. Often, the disease will be the initiating source for malnutrition, but many patients will lose additional weight during their hospitalization prior to their surgery as a result of fasting for testing or procedures. Critically ill patients are even more at risk because of anorexia, withholding food, and the inflammatory state generated by their illness.

This chapter addresses the areas of nutritional assessment, metabolism, and therapy including the nutritional response to inflammation.

BASIC NUTRITIONAL METABOLIC PRINCIPLES

Body Composition

Total body mass comprises aqueous and nonaqueous components. The nonaqueous portion is made up of bone mineral and the lipid portion of adipose tissue. The aqueous phase is divided between the body cell mass, which is made up of skeletal muscle, organs, skin, the cellular components of blood and adipose tissue, and the extracellular fluids and proteins, such as the interstitial and intravascular volume, serum proteins, tendons, ligaments, and cartilage. The body cell mass is the metabolic engine of the body, whereas the extracellular contents form the supporting structure for the body cell mass. Total body water makes up about 55% to 60% of total body mass. In the prototypical 70-kg male, this is 40 L, with about 22 L intracellular, 14 L interstitial, and 3 to 3.5 L as plasma. Body composition varies as a function of age and sex (Fig. 3.1) and becomes altered following injury or surgery,[1] characterized by a loss of lean body mass, a loss of body fat, and expansion of the extracellular fluid compartment.[2]

Bioelectrical impedance is one way to measure this change in lean body mass, as electrical resistance is proportional to the fluid and electrolyte content of tissue. Because the lean body mass has most of the fluid and electrolyte content, this is a measure of the lean body or "fat free" mass.[3] This works well in both healthy and critically ill patients and can give the practitioner a guide to accurately gauge nutritional and fluid support.

Energy Metabolism

From a simplistic mechanical standpoint, the human body is nothing more than an engine. It burns fuel to generate energy used to perform work. The human body does several kinds of work essential for life including mechanical work (e.g., locomotion, breathing), transport work (e.g., carrier-mediated uptake of nutrients into cells), and synthetic work (biosynthesis of proteins and other complex molecules). The body has the capacity to "oxidize" several types of fuels, among these being glucose (carbohydrates), amino acids (proteins), fatty acids (lipids), ketone bodies, and alcohol. Thus, the body converts energy stored in the chemical bonds of nutrients into internal (i.e., enzymatic catalysis) and external work (i.e., muscular contraction for locomotion). During starvation or following operative procedures when no nutrition is provided, the body oxidizes stored energy sources to generate this work. In humans, this process is relatively inefficient, because about half of this potential energy is lost as heat. Some of the heat generated during this process is used to help maintain body temperature via carefully controlled regulatory mechanisms in the hypothalamus. Excess heat is released primarily through the skin via evaporation, radiation, convection, and conduction. In surgical patients, these central regulatory mechanisms often become "reset" leading to the development of fever. An increase in body temperature results in an increase in enzymatic reactions that are necessary to support the inflammatory process.[4]

The body contains fuel reserves that it can mobilize and utilize during times of starvation or stress (Table 3.1). The greatest energy component is calorically dense fat, providing 9 kilocalories (kcal) per gram. Body protein comprises the next largest source of potential energy, but amino acids yield only about

TABLE 3.1

FUEL RESERVES OF A HEALTHY (70-kg) ADULT MALE

Energy source	Kilograms	kcal value
Fat	14	125,000
PROTEIN		
Skeletal muscle	6	24,000
Other	6	24,000
GLYCOGEN		
Muscle	0.15	600
Liver	0.075	300
Free glucose	0.02	80

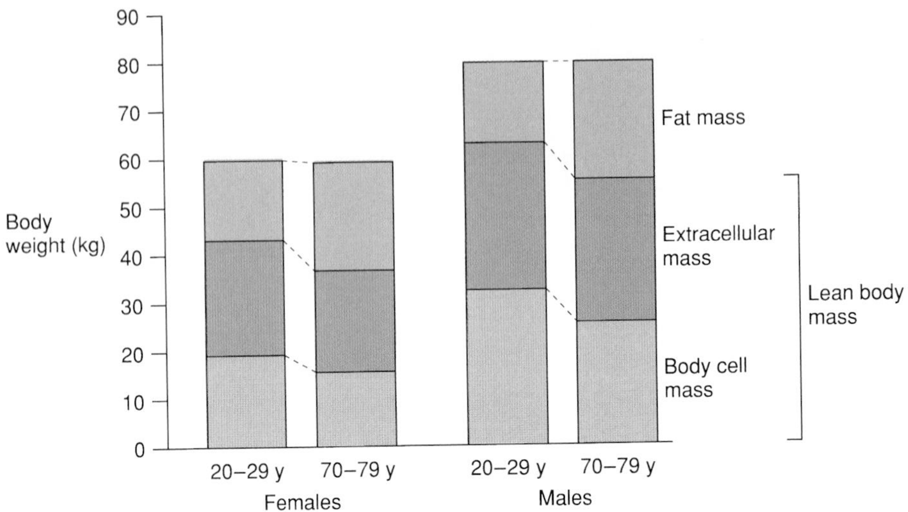

FIGURE 3.1 Body composition as a function of sex and age. (Data from Cohn SH, Vaartsky D, Yasumura S, et al. Compartmental body composition based on total-body nitrogen, potassium, and calcium. *Am J Physiol.* 1980;239:E524–E530).

4 kcal per gram. Unlike fat reserves, body protein is a structural and functional component of the body and its loss can have functional consequences. In undernourished states, proteolysis is accelerated to generate amino acids to support gluconeogenesis and other key synthetic processes. A chronic catabolic state can lead to erosion of body protein stores such that susceptibility to infection is increased, wound healing is impaired, and outcome is unfavorably impacted. Carbohydrate stores are minimal and exist as glucose or liver glycogen, which can be depleted quickly unless replenished from exogenous sources. Thus, carbohydrate and protein metabolism are linked because the body draws on endogenous protein to produce new glucose to meet the demand.

Energy sources are measured in calories. A calorie is the amount of heat required to raise the temperature of 1 g of water from 14.5°C to 15.5°C at a pressure of one standard atmosphere. A kilocalorie (1,000 calories) is the unit of energy measurement used in the United States when referring to body metabolism and nutrition. Basal energy requirements are those used mainly for transport work and synthetic work within cells. A surprisingly small percentage (<5%) of this energy is spent on cardiac output and the work of breathing in normal subjects. Thus, the resting energy expenditure (REE) accounts for the basal energy expenditure plus any extra required by the patient's disease process.[5,6]

Caloric requirements (metabolic rate) are related to oxygen consumption by the formula:

$$\text{Metabolic rate} = 4.83 \times O_2 \text{ consumption}$$

where metabolic rate is expressed in kcal/minute and O_2 consumption (VO_2) is expressed in liters of oxygen consumed per minute. In common usage, metabolic rate is expressed in calories/day, and VO_2 is expressed in mL/minute, so the value of 4.83 heat equivalent of one liter of oxygen is multiplied by 1.44, resulting in the equation, VO_2 (mL/minute) × 7 = calories/day. For example, the average resting postabsorptive 70-kg male consumes about 0.25 L oxygen/minute (360 L/day). This is equal to ~1750 kcal/day (250 mL/min × 7 or 360 L/day × 4.83).

In the majority of non–intensive care unit (ICU) adult surgical patients, energy requirements can be estimated from body weight without the use of more complex equations (Table 3.2).

TABLE 3.2

APPROXIMATE BASAL METABOLIC RATE (BMR) IN ADULTS

Weight (kg)	BMR (kcal/day)
50	1,300
60	1,450
70	1,600
80	1,750
90	1,900
100	2,050

Metabolic rate varies with age and sex, but much of this effect is through modification of body composition. In the more complex situation of critical illness, equations developed for this special population may improve the accuracy of calorie prediction and thus be better guides to calorie replacement.[7]

In critically ill patients, body weight is referenced to height combined with physical appearance.[5]

Ultimately, REE can be measured at the bedside by indirect calorimetry. Patients must be either intubated or able to tolerate a hood placed over their face for exhaled gas capture. Protocols have been developed to measure the REE with just a 5-minute steady state, which saves time yet yields a reliable figure for 24-hour REE.[7] In general, energy needs increase as the severity of the illness increases (Table 3.3). The expenditure of kilocalories is only minimally increased after elective surgery. The largest increase in energy expenditure occurs in patients with severe multiple trauma or major thermal injury. However, the average-sized adult who sustains even a major burn rarely increases energy expenditure to more than 3,000 kcal/day.

Carbohydrate Metabolism

The basic unit of carbohydrate metabolism in humans is glucose. Nearly all dietary carbohydrate is converted to glucose, and glucose is the form of carbohydrate for oxidation.

TABLE 3.3

CALORIC REQUIREMENTS FOR THE AVERAGE ADULT (70-kg) MALE

Disease process	kcal/day
Basal	1,450
Postop (uncomplicated)	1,500–1,700
Sepsis	2,000–2,400
Multiple trauma (ventilator)	2,200–2,600
Major burn	2,500–3,000

The human body has a constant need for glucose oxidation in the central nervous system and blood cells. A glucose supply of approximately 12 hours is available as glycogen, which is sufficient to cover glucose needs between meals. In periods of fasting extending beyond the glycogen supply, the body converts amino acids to glucose, recycles the available glucose, and eventually induces ketone production from fat, which can substitute for some but not all of the body's glucose need. Resumption of glucose intake completely reverses these metabolic adaptations. In surgical nutrition, the stress response accelerates the rate of glucose production from amino acids, minimizes glucose recycling, and limits ketone production, leading to pronounced gluconeogenesis from amino acids for as long as the inflammatory response is present. These metabolic adaptations are much less responsive to dextrose infusion that the system for simple starvation.

Lipid Metabolism

Triglycerides are made up of three fatty acids bound to a glycerol molecule. Naturally occurring fatty acids may be saturated (no double bonds) or unsaturated (one or more double bonds). In most tissues, fatty acids are readily oxidized for energy and are especially important energy sources for the heart, the liver, and skeletal muscle. In adipose tissue, fatty acids may be re-esterified with glycerol and stored as triacylglycerols (triglyceride) in adipocytes. This stored fat is mobilized during starvation and stress, whereas structural lipid is generally preserved. The major lipids in plasma do not circulate in free form. Free fatty acids are bound to albumin whereas cholesterol, triglycerides, and phospholipids are transported as lipoprotein complexes. Lipoproteins are cleared from the circulation by the action of lipoprotein lipase, an enzyme located on the surface of the capillary endothelium.

A second lipase regulating the supply of free fatty acids to tissues is hormone-sensitive lipase. The counter-regulatory stress hormones, epinephrine, norepinephrine, and glucagon rapidly activate hormone-sensitive lipase. Growth hormone (GH) and glucocorticoids also increase the activity of hormone-sensitive lipase, but more slowly. Thus, during stress, the activity of hormone-sensitive lipase increases leading to mobilization of fat. The general rule for the amount of fat administered to patients receiving total parenteral nutrition (TPN) is between 15% and 30% of total nonprotein caloric needs. However, the currently available parenteral fat sources are n-6 polyunsaturated fatty acids, which may be immunosuppressive and counter to the needs of the critically ill patient.

Free fatty acids must be activated in the cytoplasm by condensation with coenzyme A (CoA) before they can be oxidized. The resulting fatty acyl CoA molecules are transported into the mitochondria by means of a shuttle system in which L-carnitine acts as an acyl-carrier. This process may be rate limiting in severe stress states.

Protein and Amino Acid Metabolism

Protein is the building block of life and is a key nutrient for support of surgical patients. About 15% of total body weight is composed of proteins, half of which are intracellular and half extracellular. Extracellular proteins include those that circulate in the bloodstream (i.e., albumin, transferrin, hemoglobin) and those that compose the intercellular matrix such as collagen and other fibrous proteins. Protein is composed of amino acids, 20 of which are dietary essentials.

Absorption of dietary protein involves first the digestion of the protein into amino acids and small peptides by pancreatic and enteric enzymes. Small peptides are absorbed passively, but free amino acids must be carried actively into the enterocyte cytoplasm via functionally and biochemically distinct amino acid transport systems. Many factors, including nutritional status, specifically or nonspecifically alter amino acid transport activities. One example is a reversible hyperplasia of the intestinal mucosa after a prolonged period of oral hyperalimentation, resulting in an increase of epithelial cell numbers and absorptive surface area. This nonspecific hyperplasia can increase amino acid uptake by a factor of five. A second mechanism is a reversible several-fold increase of specific amino acid transport activities. Surgery, infection, and cancer also influence intestinal transport activity.

Absorbed amino acids pass first through the liver, where portions are extracted for synthesis of circulating proteins. The branched-chain amino acids (BCAAs) (leucine, isoleucine, and valine) are untouched by the liver and so are transported to and extracted by muscle. Excess amino acids are degraded and their carbon skeletons are oxidized to produce energy or incorporated into glycogen or free fatty acids. In addition to the metabolism of dietary amino acids, the existing proteins in the cell are continuously recycled, such that total protein turnover in the body is about 300 g/day (Fig. 3.2). Vertebrates cannot reutilize nitrogen with 100% efficiency; therefore, obligatory nitrogen losses occur, mainly in the urine. Urinary nitrogen losses will diminish in individuals fed a protein-free diet but will never become zero because of the body's inability to completely reutilize nitrogen. In stressed patients, this ability to adapt to starvation is compromised such that proteolysis of body proteins continues at a substantial rate (Fig. 3.3). Although it is often assumed that skeletal muscle bears the brunt of this protein wasting, net proteolysis also occurs in organs such as the gut and liver. If protein synthesis is compromised by malnutrition or disease, function is correspondingly impacted. This may manifest as impaired wound healing, immunoincompetence, or breakdown of the gut mucosal barrier.

Stressed surgical patients have increased energy and nitrogen needs. The recommended daily allowance for protein in the United States is 0.8 g/kg/day; this requirement may triple in critically ill patients because of their profound catabolism and inefficient protein economy (Table 3.4). One gram of nitrogen, on the average, is equivalent to 6.25 g of protein.

TABLE 3.4

AMINO ACID REQUIREMENTS FOR THE AVERAGE ADULT (70-kg) MALE

Disease process	Amino acids (kg/day)
Postop (uncomplicated)	1–1.5
Sepsis	1.5–2.0
Multiple trauma (ventilator)	1.5–2.0
Major burn	2.0–3.0

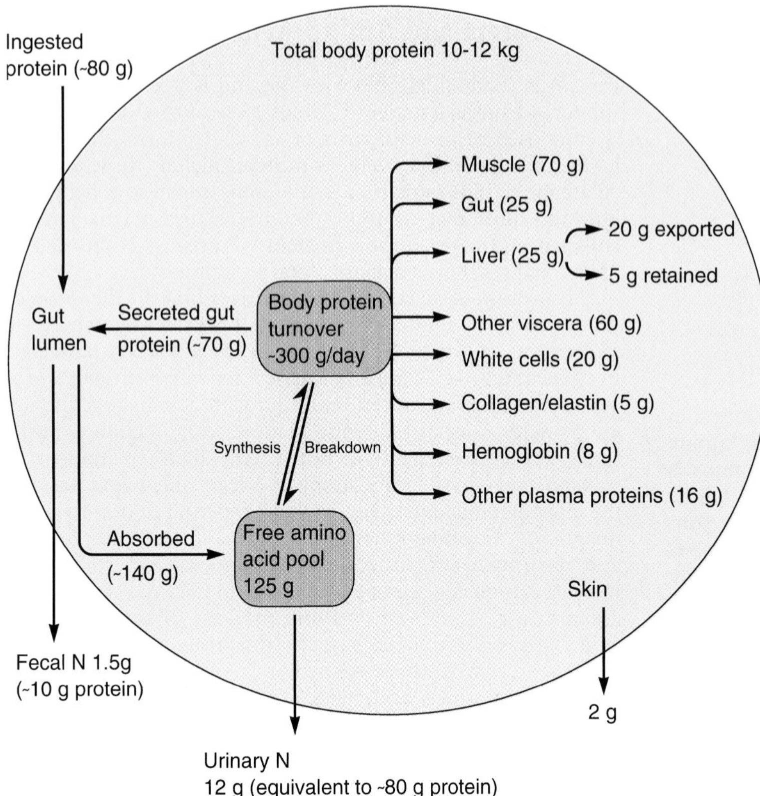

FIGURE 3.2 Whole body protein metabolism in a normal 70-kg man.

Nitrogen (N) balance is an indicator of whether protein intake is keeping up with protein catabolism, and it may be the most important nutritional test in patients receiving nutrition support. Nitrogen balance can be calculated from the difference between the amount of nitrogen taken in by the patient and the amount of nitrogen lost in the urine, stool, skin, wounds, and fistula drainage. Nitrogen balance is measured from the amount of nitrogen given minus the amount excreted in the urine in a 24-hour sample. Nitrogen intake is estimated from protein intake (g protein/6.25). Nitrogen output from skin and stool is usually very small (<2 g/day), difficult to measure, and therefore usually accounted for with a

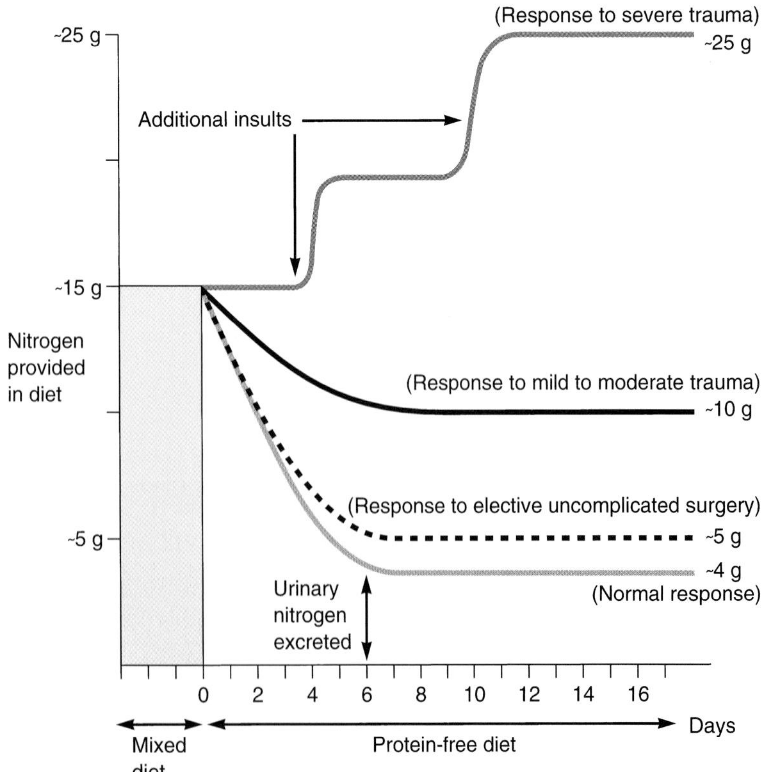

FIGURE 3.3 The response to starvation in normal, postoperative, and septic individuals. The normal person adapts to starvation by conserving body protein, which is manifested by a decrease in nitrogen excretion in the urine. Septic patients do not adapt to starvation by using ketones for energy and therefore urinary nitrogen losses are much greater.

constant of 2 in the balance equation. It is ideal to quantitate total urinary nitrogen (TUN), but many laboratories only measure urea nitrogen. If urea nitrogen (UUN) is measured, an additional 2 to 3 g should be added to the output side of the nitrogen balance equation to account for these unmeasured losses. Over relatively long periods, the healthy adult remains in nitrogen equilibrium (zero nitrogen balance). In contrast, surgical patients are prone to develop negative nitrogen balance because of their underlying disease process and inflammation.

Metabolism of amino acids (from enteral or parenteral feedings) generates ammonia, which is one of the most toxic and reactive compounds in physiologic fluids. However, ammonia levels in blood are generally kept at nontoxic concentrations (20 to 40 μM) due to liver conversion of ammonia to urea, a nontoxic soluble compound. Excretory or transport amino acids, primarily glutamine and alanine, serve as vehicles for transporting ammonia in a nontoxic form from peripheral tissues to the visceral organs. Ammonia is then reformed and either excreted (kidneys) or detoxified to urea (liver). Only the liver has all the enzymes of urea synthesis. These enzymes are located only in periportal hepatocytes; thus, diseases affecting the periportal areas lead to an increased ammonia load in the systemic circulation.

Urea is a highly soluble (2 mol/L), nontoxic molecule with a high nitrogen content (47%), but little chemical energy is required for its biosynthesis. Normal human subjects that ingest a Western diet excrete about 30 g of urea daily (14 g urea nitrogen). This may increase to more than 60 g a day (28 g urea nitrogen) in catabolic surgical patients. Urea accounts for 85% of the total urinary nitrogen with the remaining 15% contributed by ammonia and creatinine.

In the postabsorptive state (after an overnight fast), the gut lumen is empty of ingested proteins. Therefore, absorption of luminal amino acids is relatively low. Circulating amino acid levels are maintained by the release of preformed amino acid pools and the breakdown of cellular proteins. Protein degradation generates amino acids exported directly to the circulation as well as provides amino acid precursors for synthesis of other amino acids subsequently released. In catabolic surgical patients, protein synthesis in skeletal muscle may be increased but the protein breakdown is accelerated to a greater extent, such that net proteolysis and depletion of the amino acid pool is observed (Fig. 3.4). This is manifested clinically as loss of lean body mass and negative nitrogen balance.

Overfeeding

Although the provision of enough calories is beneficial, giving too many calories can "overfeed" the patient. Excess calories, especially in the form of sugars, lead to lipogenesis and hepatic steatosis interfering with hepatic function. To avoid overfeeding, critically ill patients may require indirect calorimetry to accurately measure energy expenditure.

The only significant source of usable energy in mammalian tissues is the carbon-hydrogen bond in carbohydrates, fats, and amino acids. When the bond is broken, energy is liberated, and carbon dioxide and water are formed as well as adenosine triphosphate (ATP). This requires a pool of phosphate to be available to form the ATP from ADP. In chronically malnourished or starved patients, this pool of phosphate may be depleted and become dangerously low as dextrose is reintroduced to the metabolism. This hypophosphatemia can lead to an irreversible cardiac arrest and is known as the "refeeding syndrome." Although uncommon in elective surgical patients, this may manifest in cancer or critically injured patients receiving only borderline nutrition. Serum potassium and magnesium levels may also be affected. Measuring and repleting phosphate, potassium,

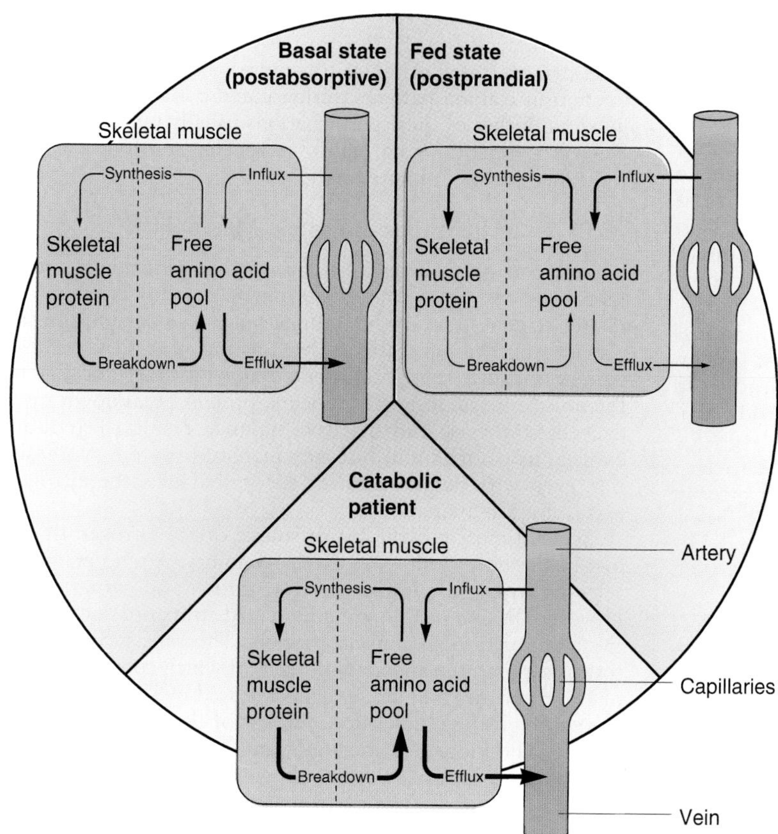

FIGURE 3.4 Relative rates of protein synthesis and breakdown in skeletal muscle in postabsorptive, postprandial, and catabolic states. After an overnight fast, muscle releases net amounts of amino acids to help maintain circulating pool. Breakdown exceeds synthesis, although this may not be measurable using standard techniques. Following a meal, muscle amino uptake is greater than release and protein synthesis is greater than catabolism. In the catabolic surgical patient, protein synthesis may be increased but this rate is exceeded by the rate of breakdown. In the absence of nutritional support, profound muscle wasting can occur.

and magnesium in these patients prior to and during nutrition support is critical.

Substrate Utilization

The mix and total amount of substrate utilized in metabolism is proportional to the steady state volumes of carbon dioxide and oxygen exchanged across the lungs. Indirect calorimetry can be used to assess substrate utilization using the parameter of *respiratory quotient (RQ)*.

RQ is the ratio between the volume of CO_2 produced and the volume of O_2 utilized:

$$RQ = VCO_2/VO_2$$

The RQ for glucose oxidation is six moles of CO_2 to six moles of oxygen, or 1.00.

For the oxidation of fats, less carbon dioxide is produced per mole of oxygen consumed and thus the RQ is less than one. The oxidation of triglyceride is as follows:

$$2\ C_{51}H_{98}O_6 + 145\ O_2 \longrightarrow 102\ CO_2 + 98\ H_2O$$

The RQ is 102/145, which equals 0.7.

The RQ for proteins is more difficult to calculate because the composition of the amino acids varies. However, on average, the RQ for protein is 0.82.

The RQ can rise above 1.0 during excessive overfeeding with carbohydrate resulting in storage of fat in the liver, oxygen consumption, and carbon dioxide production without the generation of ATP. This can increase minute ventilation from the high amounts of carbon dioxide produced.

Thermoregulation

Alterations in the body's central thermostat located in the hypothalamus almost always occur in patients with systemic infection. Core temperature reflects the balance between heat production and heat loss, both of which can be altered in surgical patients. Most of the heat produced in the postabsorptive basal state occurs in the brain and in the abdominal organs. Increase in heat production occurs following an infectious challenge and is due to a re-setting of the hypothalamic setpoint. Such an increase in body temperature is thought to be an adaptive one because rates of cellular reactions increase as a function of temperature. Metabolic rate increases about 10% for each degree (Celsius) increase in body temperature.[4]

Heat loss is regulated by adjustments in skin blood flow and in perspiration. In cooler environments heat loss is via dissipation of skin heat; in warmer environments, heat loss occurs primarily through sweating. During surgery, general anesthesia may reduce the capacity for shivering leading to heat loss and increased evaporation from the open body cavities may lead to hypothermia.

THE BODY'S RESPONSE WHEN STRESSED BY INJURY OR SURGERY

In the 1930s, Cuthbertson[8] described the time course for many of the post-traumatic responses and two distinct periods were identified. The early "ebb" or shock phase was usually brief in duration (12 to 24 hours) and occurred immediately following injury. Blood pressure, cardiac output, body temperature, and oxygen consumption were reduced. These events were often associated with hemorrhage and resulted in hypoperfusion and lactic acidosis. With restoration of blood volume, ebb-phase alterations gave way to more accelerated responses. The flow phase was then characterized by hypermetabolism, increased cardiac output, increased urinary nitrogen losses, altered glucose metabolism, and accelerated tissue catabolism. The flow-phase responses to accidental injury are similar to those seen following elective operation. The response to injury, however, is usually much more intensive and extends over a long period.

Characteristics of the Flow Phase of the Injury Response

Hypermetabolism

Hypermetabolism is defined as an increase in basal metabolic rate (BMR) above that predicted on the basis of age, sex, and body size in a healthy person. The degree of hypermetabolism (increased oxygen consumption) is generally related to the severity of the inflammatory response to the injury with temperature serving as a reasonable indicator of the higher metabolic rate.[4]

Altered Glucose Metabolism

Hyperglycemia commonly occurs following injury, and the elevation of fasting blood sugar levels generally parallels the severity of stress in the ebb phase. During the ebb phase, insulin levels are low and glucose production is only slightly elevated. Later, during the flow phase, insulin concentrations are normal or elevated; however, hyperglycemia persists. Hepatic glucose production is increased and studies show that much of the new glucose generated by the liver arises from three-carbon precursors released from peripheral tissues.

Measurements of substrate exchange across injured and uninjured extremities of severely burned patients indicate that glucose is used in small amounts by the uninjured extremity. In contrast, the injured extremity extracts large amounts of glucose. The wound converts most of the glucose to lactate, which is recycled to the liver in the Cori cycle. Other studies have demonstrated a failure to suppress hepatic glucose production in trauma patients during glucose loading or insulin infusion. Either of these perturbations usually inhibits hepatic glucose production in normal subjects. Thus, profound insulin resistance occurs in injured patients.

Alterations in Protein Metabolism

Extensive urinary nitrogen loss occurs following major injury. Like other responses, the loss of nitrogen following injury is related to the extent of the trauma, but it also depends on the previous nutritional status, as well as the age and sex of the patient, because these factors determine, in part, the size of the muscle mass. In unfed patients, protein breakdown rates exceed synthesis, and negative balance results. Providing exogenous calories and nitrogen increases protein synthesis, but, even with achievement of energy balance, the nitrogen loss is not attenuated.[9]

Skeletal muscle is the major source of the nitrogen that is lost in the urine following extensive injury. Amino acids are released by muscle in increased quantities following injury; however, the composition of amino acid efflux does not reflect the composition of muscle protein. The release is skewed towards glutamine and alanine, each of which comprise about one third of the total amino acids released by skeletal muscle, even though they make up only 5% of the protein mass of muscle. The kidney extracts glutamine, where it contributes ammonium groups for ammonia generation, a process that excretes acid loads. The gastrointestinal (GI) tract also takes up glutamine to serve as an oxidative fuel and substrate for

TABLE 3.5

DIFFERENCES BETWEEN ELECTIVE SURGERY AND ACCIDENTAL INJURY

Insult	Elective operation	Accidental injury (trauma)
Tissue damage	Minimal; tissues are dissected with care and reapproximated	Can be substantial; tissues usually torn or ripped; débridement often necessary
Hypotension	Uncommon: preoperative hydration employed and fluid status is carefully monitored intraoperatively	Fluid resuscitation often not immediate; blood loss can be substantial leading to shock
Pain/fear/anxiety	Generally can be alleviated with preop medication	Generally present
Infectious complications	Uncommon; prophylactic antibiotics often administered	More common due to contamination, hypotension, and tissue devitalization
Overall stress response	Controlled and of lesser magnitude; starvation better tolerated	Uncontrolled; proportional to the magnitude of the injury; malnutrition poorly tolerated

RNA synthesis. The gut enterocytes convert glutamine primarily to ammonia and alanine, and these two substances are released into the portal venous blood. This ammonia is then removed by the liver and is converted to urea, and the alanine may be removed by the liver and serve as a gluconeogenic precursor. Following elective surgical stress, glutamine consumption by the bowel and the kidney is accelerated in a reaction that appears to be regulated by the increased elaboration of the glucocorticoids. Although skeletal muscle releases alanine at an accelerated rate, the GI tract and kidney also release increased amounts of alanine. The alanine is then extracted by the liver to be used in the synthesis of glucose and acute-phase proteins. Hence, glutamine and alanine are important participants in the transfer of nitrogen from skeletal muscle to visceral organs; however, their metabolic pathways favor the production of urea and ammonia, both of which are terminal uses of nitrogen and must be excreted from the body.

Alterations in Fat Metabolism

To support the hypermetabolism, increased gluconeogenesis, and interorgan substrate flux, stored triglyceride is mobilized and oxidized at an accelerated rate. Glucose administration poorly attenuates this lipolysis, which may be the result of continuous stimulation of the sympathetic nervous system. Although mobilization and use of free fatty acids are accelerated in injured subjects, ketosis during brief starvation is blunted, and the accelerated protein catabolism remains unchecked. If unfed, severely injured patients rapidly deplete their fat and protein stores. Such malnutrition increases their susceptibility to added stresses of hemorrhage, surgery, and infection and may contribute to organ system failure, sepsis, and death.

Homeostatic Responses and Adjustments to Stress

Built into the body's defense mechanism is a set of orchestrated responses initiated within moments of injury or insult. These responses are indelible, essential for survival, and are designed to maintain body homeostasis at a time when key physiologic processes are threatened. Later factors reinitiating or perpetuating these responses include invasive infection and starvation. These events are generally related to the severity of injury; that is, the greater the insult, the more pronounced the specific response. The synthesis of key hormones and peptides allows the body to respond to such insults with remarkable resilience.

Whether the body is injured accidentally or within the carefully monitored confines of an operating room, the responses to such trauma are similar. However, such settings are also different in ways that will influence the extent and magnitude of the stress response (Table 3.5). Accidental injury is unplanned and uncontrolled; tissues are torn, ripped, bruised, and contaminated. The associated volume loss may be substantial leading to tissue hypoperfusion, which, if prolonged, will result in cellular deterioration and death in tissues that were not initially traumatized. Pain, excitement, and fear are generally heightened and uncontrolled. As a consequence, the magnitude of the physiologic response to major accidental injury is considerable.

In contrast, the "elective" tissue trauma that is inflicted within the confines of an operating room is calculated, planned, and monitored. Although elective surgery causes pain, often interrupts food intake, and is generally associated with the removal of an organ or tissue, the perioperative management of elective surgical patients is often designed to attenuate such changes. Appropriately selected pharmacologic agents are used to block undesirable cardiovascular responses, and specific techniques such as epidural anesthesia or patient-controlled anesthesia are effective in minimizing postoperative pain. As a consequence, the physiologic responses to elective surgery are generally of a lesser magnitude than those following major accidental injury. Improvements in surgical and anesthetic care now allow us to perform major elective operations with minimal morbidity and mortality. However, in the critically ill, an inflammatory cascade may be launched reaching beyond the limits of the beneficial response.

The Inflammatory Response

The response to operative stresses (elective injury) or accidental injury (trauma) comprises two components: a neurohormonal arm and an inflammatory arm. These pathways work together to determine the magnitude of the response. The inflammatory response is the major metabolic feature of injury and infection and is one of the main reasons why nutrition support in such patients can be a challenge. Recently, the extent to which the inflammatory response underlies the nutritional issues of chronic diseases has been appreciated.[10,11] An inflammatory component exists in the body composition changes of such disparate diseases as congestive heart failure, cancer, chronic obstructive pulmonary disease (COPD), HIV, and rheumatologic disorders.[12–15] Recognition that inflammation drives what has been traditionally thought of as purely nutritionally related effects of disease opens a whole new avenue for the management of the body wasting of disease (cachexia).

The inflammatory response is a primitive, complex, and indispensable part of the nonspecific immune system.[16] Importantly, the changes in body composition caused by inflammation are part of an orchestrated response by the body to the acute challenge to homeostasis. Localized inflammatory responses occur frequently in the body with no systemic consequences.[16] Moderate inflammation is still localized, but its effects are more obvious. For example, the response to a piece of foreign material (e.g., a wood splinter) may include classic signs of inflammation: rubor, tumor, calor, dolor, and functio laesa (redness, swelling, pain, heat, loss of function).[16] Multiple traumatic/surgical injury may cause exuberant inflammation and systemic effects (hypermetabolism, body protein catabolism, insulin resistance, fever, acute phase protein response), initiating severe inflammation. However, dysregulation of this response causes the uncontrolled inflammation of septic multiple organ failure with widespread endothelial damage and organ dysfunction.[16,17] This type of inflammation-driven illness is a major cause of death in the ICU.[16] Severe loss of lean body mass is a feature of patients who survive this, but once convalescence is achieved, the inflammatory metabolism can normalize and the body can be repleted with proper nutrition and exercise.

The inflammatory response can convert from the acute to a chronic condition, in which the systemic manifestations of altered acute phase protein synthesis, impaired intermediary metabolism, and cachexia are present.[18] This form of inflammation is maladaptive and is a feature of many pre-existing chronic disease states in surgical patients, such as renal failure, hepatic failure, congestive heart failure, rheumatoid diseases, and cancer. Thus, although inflammation is an important component of recovery from acute illnesses, in chronic illness it can become pathologic leading to malnutrition.

Despite the costs to the body, the advantages of the inflammatory response are (a) rapid mobilization of fuel and substrates from muscle and adipose tissue to maximize visceral functions leading to recovery (gluconeogenesis, glutamine synthesis, acute phase protein synthesis), (b) initiation of the process of local control and elimination of the offending agent (fever response, neutrophil and macrophage recruitment), (c) presentation of signals to the specific immune system to induce its participation in elimination of the offending agent, and (d) reduction of fluid loss to maintain hydration in the face of interrupted intake. In other words, the inflammatory response can be thought of crudely as a form of internal nutrition support, fluid resuscitation, and antibiotic therapy.

Inflammation is mediated by a host of biochemicals, including hormones, growth factors, enzymes, kinins, complement, cytokines, and eicosanoids. The initial injury stimulates local mast cells to release numerous mediators.[16] Chief among these mediators are the cytokines and eicosanoids. There are pro- and anti-inflammatory forms of each of these. The proinflammatory forms predominate early [tumor necrosis factor (TNF), interleukin (IL)-1, IL-6, prostaglandin-2 series (PGE_2), leukotriene-4 (LT_4)]. TNF and the prostaglandins are expressed early and along with IL-1 elicit the acute phase response (fever, acute phase protein synthesis, insulin resistance). The TNF and IL-1 peak early and then disappear from plasma, but first they stimulate IL-6 release. One of the effects of IL-6 is to reduce the level of insulin-like growth factor (IGF-1), which leads to proteolysis and amino acid release from muscle.

Early in the inflammatory process, there is a marked rise in the elaboration of the counter-regulatory hormones glucagon, glucocorticoids, and epinephrine. During the ebb phase of injury, the sympathoadrenal axis helps maintain the pressure-flow relationships necessary for an intact cardiovascular system to maintain blood flow in a low volume state. With the onset of hypermetabolism, characteristic of the flow phase, these and other hormones exert a variety of metabolic effects. Glucagon along with insulin resistance has potent glycogenolytic and gluconeogenic effects on the liver, which signal the hepatocytes to produce glucose from hepatic glycogen stores and gluconeogenic precursors. Cortisol mobilizes amino acids from skeletal muscle and increases hepatic gluconeogenesis. The catecholamines stimulate hepatic glycolysis and gluconeogenesis and increase lactate production from peripheral tissues (skeletal muscle). Catecholamines also increase metabolic rate and stimulate lipolysis. The level of GH is elevated, but there is resistance to its action (possibly because of suppressed levels of IGF-1) and thyroid hormone levels are reduced to low-normal concentrations. Infusion of counter-regulatory hormones into normal subjects reproduces many of the metabolic alterations that are characteristic of injury.[19] As the inflammatory stimulus is controlled and eliminated, the anti-inflammatory cytokines (IL4, IL-10, IL-13) and eicosanoids (PGE_3, LT_5) begin to predominate and bring the inflammatory response to a conclusion.

The genes that regulate cytokine biosynthesis are highly conserved.[20] Although excess production can be dangerous to the host, cytokines exert a number of beneficial nutritional effects under the majority of circumstances, which appear to outweigh the detrimental effects observed in extreme pathophysiologic states (Fig. 3.5).

Mobilization of Amino Acids and Stimulation of Acute-phase Protein Synthesis. Cytokines act in concert with other mediators to promote mobilization of amino acids from skeletal muscle. This response provides key nutrients to support cellular metabolism at a time when food cannot be acquired.

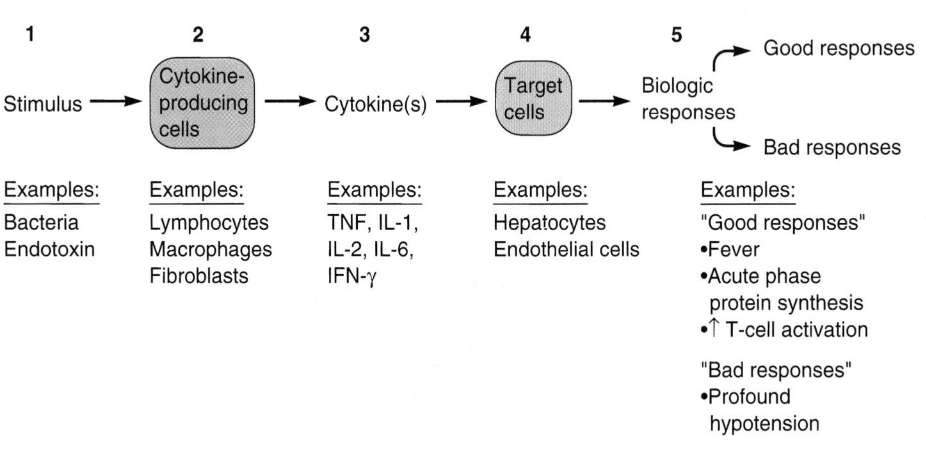

FIGURE 3.5 Cytokines can elicit both beneficial and deleterious responses.

The primary metabolic component of the acute phase response affected by IL-6 is a qualitative alteration in hepatic protein synthesis with a resulting alteration in plasma protein composition. Characteristically, proteins acting as serum transport and binding molecules (albumin, transferrin) are reduced in quantity, and acute phase proteins (fibrinogen, C-reactive protein) are increased. Although the true physiologic role of many of the acute phase proteins remains unclear, many act as antiproteases, opsonins, or coagulation and wound-healing factors, and they likely inhibit the generalized tissue destruction that is associated with the local initiation of inflammation. For example, increases in fibrinogen enhance thrombus formation, whereas antiproteases reduce tissue damage caused by proteases released by dead or dying cells. C-reactive protein has been hypothesized to have a scavenger function and its serum level can be a measure of the inflammatory response.

Hypoferremia and Hypozincemia. Serum iron and zinc levels are reduced in septic patients, an event that is cytokine-mediated. The decrease in serum iron is probably important in protecting the host against various bacteria, by inhibiting the growth rate of microorganisms that have a strict requirement for iron as a growth factor. Both TNF and IL-1 have been shown to mediate hypoferremia, hypozincemia, and other alterations in trace element metabolism. In chronic disease states, the milieu of mediators remains predominantly pro-inflammatory, leading to prolonged tissue damage and systemic effects on immune function, body composition, and metabolism.

Induction of the inflammatory response requires a stimulus. Physical injury and invasion of antigen are the stimuli most often described (trauma, pancreatitis, infection). However, local areas of hypoxia can be an inflammatory stimulus, so that heart failure and COPD may be added to the list of conditions that might cause inflammation. Conversion of self to non-self tissue (e.g., cancer) or faulty recognition of self versus non-self tissue (e.g., inflammatory bowel disease, rheumatologic conditions) can also elicit inflammation.

SPECIFIC STIMULANTS OF THE STRESS RESPONSE

Volume Loss and Tissue Hypoperfusion

Following hemorrhage or plasma loss, the body immediately attempts to compensate to maintain adequate organ perfusion. Pressure receptors in the aortic arch and carotid artery and volume (stretch) receptors in the wall of the left atrium detect the fall in blood volume and immediately respond by signaling the brain. Heart rate and stroke volume increase. Afferent nerve signals are also initiated which stimulate the release of both antidiuretic hormone (ADH) and aldosterone. These mechanisms are only partially effective and, in the absence of adequate resuscitation, severe hemorrhage often leads to a prolonged low-flow state (shock). Under these circumstances, oxygen delivery is inadequate to meet tissue demands and the cell is forced to switch to anaerobic metabolism leading to lactic acidosis.

Tissue Damage, Pain, and Fear

Injury of body tissues appears to be the most important factor initiating the stress response. Hypovolemia and starvation do not initiate a hypermetabolic/hypercatabolic response unless they result in infection or tissue injury. Afferent neural pathways from the wound signal the hypothalamus that injury has occurred; tissue destruction is generally sensed in the conscious patient as pain. Efferent pathways from the brain are immediately triggered and stimulate a number of responses designed to maintain homeostasis. Pain and fear are established components of the stress response. Both lead to excessive production of the catecholamines preparing the body for the "fight or flight" response.

Lack of Nutrient Intake and the Consequences of Malnutrition

The metabolic response to injury and surgery demands increased energy expenditure. In many patients undergoing surgery, nutrient intake is inadequate for a period (1 to 5 days) following operation. If energy intake is minimal (e.g., 5% dextrose infusion), oxidation of body fat stores and erosion of lean body mass occur, with the resultant loss of weight. Body glycogen stores are limited and are depleted within 24 to 36 hours. Consequently, glucose, which is required by the central nervous system and white blood cells, must be synthesized de novo. Amino acids, released principally by skeletal muscle, are the major gluconeogenic precursors. When weight loss exceeds 15% of body weight, the complications of undernutrition interact with the stress process impairing the body's ability to respond appropriately to the injury and may impair responses to added complications such as infection.

A major goal of nutritional support is to match the energy and nitrogen expenditure that occurs following injury to aid host defense. In contrast to injured patients, the catabolic and hypermetabolic responses that occur after elective operations are of a lesser magnitude. Consequently, well-nourished patients undergoing major operations do not require nutritional support after surgery unless it is anticipated that food intake will be precluded for more than seven days.

Invasive Infection

The major complication observed in surgical patients is infection. Most patients, particularly those in ICUs, are exposed to a variety of infectious agents in the hospital. Normal barrier defense mechanisms are disrupted by multiple indwelling foreign materials such as intravenous catheters and nasotracheal and nasogastric tubes. Breakdown of skin and mucous membranes allow portals of entry for bacteria. Infection alone may initiate catabolic responses that are similar to those described following injury in noninfected patients. Both processes cause fever, hyperventilation, tachycardia, accelerated gluconeogenesis, increased proteolysis, and lipolysis, with fat utilized as the principal fuel source. Inflammatory cells release a variety of soluble mediators that aid host resistance and wound repair, but undernutrition may compromise the available host defense mechanisms and thereby increase the likelihood of invasive sepsis, multiple organ system failure, and death.

DETERMINANTS OF HOST RESPONSES TO SURGICAL STRESS

The pattern of physiologic changes elicited in response to surgical stress results from the specific interaction of an individual patient with the stressful stimulus. The host must be capable of transmitting and integrating injury signals, both neural and humoral, and then mounting an appropriate response that requires the interaction of a number of organ systems. The nature, intensity, and duration of the stress are fundamental

TABLE 3.6

METABOLIC DIFFERENCES BETWEEN THE RESPONSE TO SIMPLE STARVATION AND TO INJURY

	Simple starvation	Severe injury
Basal metabolic rate	—	++
Presence of mediators	—	+++
Major fuel oxidized	Fat	Mixed
Ketone body production	+++	±
Hepatic ureagenesis	+	+++
Negative nitrogen balance	+	+++
Gluconeogenesis	+	+++
Muscle proteolysis	+	+++
Hepatic protein synthesis	+	+++

determinants of both the host mediators activated and the physiologic changes observed. The responses that follow a minor elective operation are similar to those observed during a comparable, brief period of fasting and bed rest. Major thermal injury results in a prolonged period of hypermetabolism and a severe drain on the body's energy and protein stores, resolving only with wound closure and resolution of sepsis. Thus, there are profound metabolic differences between the body's response to simple starvation and major stress (Table 3.6).

Body Composition and Gender

Body composition is a major determinant of the metabolic responses observed during surgical illness. Post-traumatic nitrogen excretion is directly related to the size of the body protein mass. The balance of nitrogen intake versus output from the body serves as a marker of protein metabolism. The net loss of nitrogen from the body implies the net breakdown of the corresponding amount of protein. In women, the size of the skeletal muscle mass is about one half that of age-matched men; thus, it is the muscular young man in whom nitrogen losses are most marked after injury.

Nutritional Status

A strong relation between protein depletion and postoperative complications exists in nonseptic, nonimmunocompromised patients undergoing elective major GI surgery. Protein-depleted patients have significantly lower preoperative respiratory muscle strength and vital capacity, an increased incidence of postoperative pneumonia, and longer postoperative hospital stays. Impaired wound healing and decreased respiratory, hepatic, and muscle function in protein-depleted patients awaiting surgery have also been reported.

Age

Many of the changes in the metabolic responses to surgical illness that occur with aging can be attributed to alterations in body composition and to longstanding patterns of physical activity. Although weight remains more or less stable, fat mass tends to increase with age whereas muscle mass tends to decrease. The capacity of muscle to serve as an energy source may be limited during prolonged illness in the elderly patient, and muscle strength may rapidly become inadequate for respiratory and other vital muscle function.

After the limited stress of elective operation, increases in energy expenditure are independent of age. Endocrine responses to elective operation and to trauma appear intact in older patients in terms of plasma cortisol levels and urinary excretion of adrenaline, noradrenaline, and 17-hydroxycorticosteroids.

The prevalence of cardiovascular and pulmonary diseases increases with age. Diminished arterial compliance, impaired vasoconstriction, altered autonomic function and sensitivity to catecholamines, and decreased baroreflex sensitivity may all impair the maintenance of cardiovascular homeostasis during acute surgical illness. Thus, the delivery of oxygen to the tissues may be impaired in the elderly and may be inadequate when oxygen demands are highest.

The Gut Mucosal Barrier Dysfunction as a Mediator of the Stress Response

Under certain circumstances, the gut may become a source of sepsis and serve as the motor of the systemic inflammatory response syndrome. The maintenance of an intact brush border and intercellular tight junctions prevents the movement of toxic substances into the intestinal lymphatics and circulation. Maintenance of a gut mucosal barrier requires normal perfusion, an intact epithelium, and normal mucosal immune mechanisms. Microbial translocation is the process by which microorganisms migrate across the mucosal barrier and invade the host. Translocation can be promoted in three general ways: (a) altered permeability of the intestinal mucosa, (b) decreased host defense, and (c) an increased number of bacteria within the intestine. Hemorrhagic shock, hypoxemia, sepsis, distant injury, or administration of cell toxins lead to altered permeability. Glucocorticoid administration, immunosuppression, or protein depletion decrease host defense. Bacterial overgrowth in association with intestinal stasis may cause translocation. Even if actual migration of whole bacteria does not occur, the gut may absorb endotoxin into the portal venous system. A number of retrospective and epidemiologic studies have associated infection in specific patient populations with bacterial invasion from the gut. These studies have demonstrated an increase in mucosal permeability in both normal volunteers who received endotoxin and infected burn patients. Because many of the factors that facilitate bacterial translocation occur simultaneously in surgical patients and their effects may be additive or cumulative, patients in an ICU may be extremely vulnerable to the invasion of enteric bacteria or to the absorption of their toxins. Methods currently used to support critically ill patients neither facilitate repair of the intestinal mucosa nor maintain gut barrier function. Provision of early enteral feeds and glutamine do the most to prevent translocation.

Elective Operations and Physiologic Responses to Surgery

The physiologic responses to surgical stress are multiple and complex (Fig. 3.6). One of the earliest consequences of a surgical procedure is the rise in levels of circulating cortisol in response to adrenocorticotropic hormone (ACTH) from the anterior pituitary gland. Cortisol has generalized effects on tissue catabolism and mobilizes amino acids from skeletal muscle that provide substrates for wound healing and serve as precursors for the hepatic synthesis of acute phase proteins or new glucose. Associated with the activation of the adrenal cortex is stimulation of the adrenal medulla through the sympathetic nervous system, with elaboration of epinephrine and norepinephrine. These circulating neurotransmitters play an

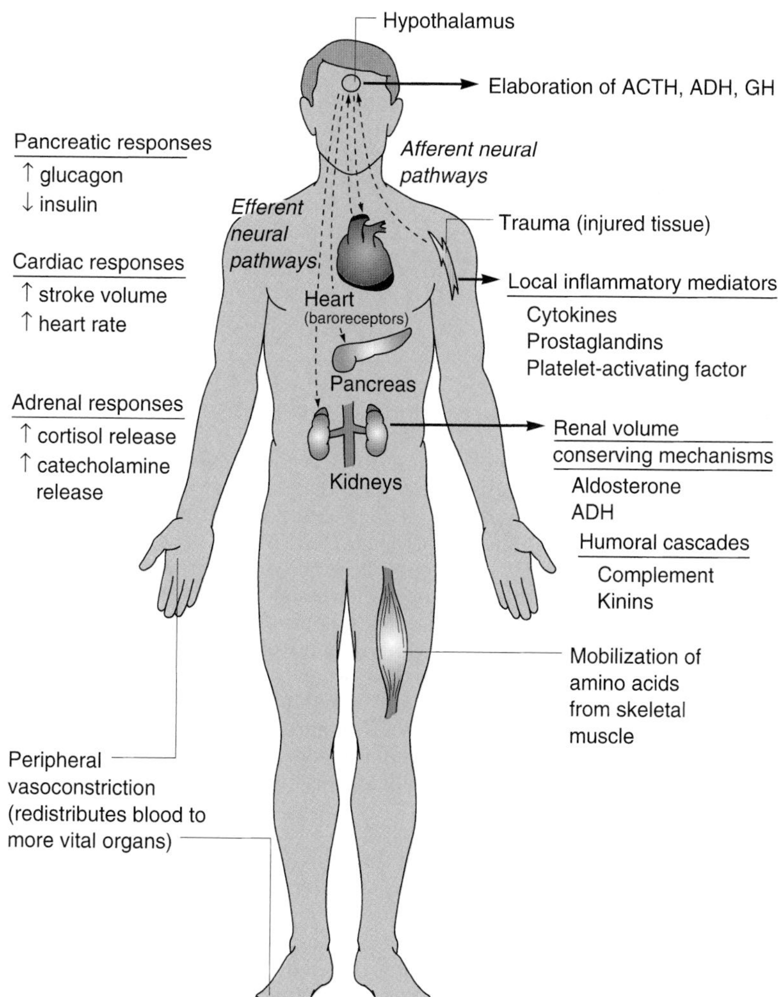

FIGURE 3.6 Homeostatic adjustments initiated after injury.

important role in circulatory adjustment but may also elicit metabolic responses if the augmented secretion rate continues over a prolonged period.

The neuroendocrine responses to operation also modify the various mechanisms that regulate salt and water excretion. Aldosterone is a potent stimulator of renal sodium retention, whereas ADH stimulates renal tubular water reabsorption. Thus, the ability to excrete a water load after elective surgical procedures is restricted and weight gain secondary to salt and water retention is usual following operation. Edema occurs to a varying extent in all surgical wounds, and this accumulation is proportional to the extent of tissue dissection and local trauma. This "third-spaced" fluid eventually returns to the circulation as the wound edema subsides and diuresis commences 2 to 4 days following the operation.

Alterations occur in the response of the endocrine pancreas following elective operation. In general, insulin elaboration is diminished, and glucagon concentrations rise. This response may be related to increased sympathetic activity or to the rise in levels of circulating epinephrine known to suppress insulin release. The rise in glucagon and the corresponding fall in insulin are a potent signal to accelerate hepatic glucose production, and, with the help of other hormones (epinephrine and glucocorticoids), gluconeogenesis is maintained.

The period of catabolism initiated by operation characterized by a combination of inadequate nutrition and alteration of the hormonal environment has been termed the "adrenergic-corticoid phase." This phase generally lasts 1 to 3 days and is followed by the "adrenergic-corticoid withdrawal phase," which lasts 1 to 3 days. This period is followed by the onset of anabolism, which occurs at a variable time in the patient's convalescence. In general, in the absence of postoperative complications, this phase starts 3 to 6 days after an abdominal operation, often concomitant with the commencement of oral feedings. The patient then enters a prolonged period of early anabolism characterized by positive nitrogen balance and weight gain. Protein synthesis is increased as a result of sustained enteral feedings, and this change is related to the return of lean body mass and muscular strength.

NUTRITIONAL SUPPORT OF ELECTIVE SURGICAL PATIENTS

Most patients undergoing elective operations are adequately nourished. Unless the patient has suffered significant preoperative malnutrition, characterized by a weight loss >10% to 15%, or has a major intraoperative or postoperative complication, solutions containing 5% dextrose may be administered for 5 to 7 days before the return of feeding with no detrimental effect on outcome. Therefore, the increased cost of feedings and the potential complications associated with intravenous nutrition cannot be justified. The use of jejunal feedings in the postoperative period may be useful in some patients, especially those undergoing extensive upper GI surgery.

Nutritional Assessment

The two major objectives of nutritional assessment are (1) to determine the patient's nutritional status and (2) to determine energy, protein, and other nutrient requirements. Part of the careful medical history and physical examination should be focused to inquire about associated diseases and history of weight loss and to establish the diagnosis of cachexia, protein-energy malnutrition, or specific nutrient deficiencies.

Immunologic status has been used to evaluate nutritional status. Total lymphocyte count, delayed hypersensitivity, and lymphocyte transformation have all been used as indicators of immunocompetence in the critically ill patient. The depressed immune function often returns to normal with nutritional repletion, but altered immunologic responses are nonspecific and can be observed in patients with advanced malignant disease or in those who have had a severe injury. Serum albumin and transferrin are the most common serum proteins measured, and they correlate well with body protein deficiency in isolated cases of malnutrition. Evidence that the inflammatory state is active can be obtained from serum albumin and C-reactive protein levels. Serum albumin can be depressed for various nutritional and non-nutritional reasons, but C-reactive protein can only be elevated if inflammation is present.

Determining Nutritional Requirements

Total energy requirements are based on several factors: (a) the BMR, (b) the degree of stress imposed by the disease process, and (c) the amount of energy expended with activity. Standard nomograms relate normal metabolic requirements to a person's age, sex, height, and weight. The principal determinants of nitrogen requirement in surgical patients are total energy intake, nitrogen intake, and the metabolic state of the patient. Malnourished patients with intact protein-conserving mechanisms can achieve nitrogen equilibrium when 15% of the total caloric needs are provided as protein. This translates into a calorie-to-nitrogen ratio of approximately 150 kcal: 1 g N_2. Hypermetabolic catabolic patients have a diminished protein economy and require much more protein.

Routes of Feeding

For patients who can eat and who have a functional GI tract, adequate nutrition can best be provided by the regular hospital diet. The enteral route is always the preferred route of feeding and a variety of enteral diets are available for patients with a functional intestinal tract who will not or cannot eat. For patients with a diseased or nonfunctional GI tract, parenteral nutrition may be necessary. Peripheral venous feedings provide dilute nutrients in a large fluid volume and rely on fat emulsions as principal calorie sources. Central venous feedings consist of hypertonic glucose and amino acid solutions infused through a catheter placed in the superior vena cava. Adequate calories can be administered in a small fluid volume, but this method of feeding requires placement and care of a central venous catheter and risks infectious complications.

TRAUMA: NUTRITIONAL SUPPORT OF THE INJURED PATIENT

Consequences of Malnutrition

The metabolic response to injury results in increased energy expenditure. If energy intake is less than expenditure, oxidation of body fat stores and erosion of lean body mass occurs, with resultant loss of weight. When body weight loss exceeds 10% to 15%, the complications of undernutrition interact with the disease process increasing morbidity and mortality rates. Undernutrition may compromise the available host defense mechanisms and may thus increase the likelihood of invasive sepsis, multiple organ system failure, and death. Additional consequences of malnutrition include poor wound healing, decreased mobility and activity, the occurrence of pressure sores and decubitus ulcers, altered GI function, and the occurrence of edema secondary to reduced colloid osmotic pressure.

Goals of Nutritional Support

The majority of injured persons are not malnourished at the time of injury, but the increased metabolic demands following injury will quickly lead to a malnourished state if the patient is not nutritionally supported. The goal of all nutritional support is the maintenance of lean body cell mass and the limitation of weight loss to less than 10% of preinjury weight. The nutritional requirements of the trauma patient can be determined as shown in Table 3.7.

SEPSIS: GENERAL OVERVIEW AND TIME COURSE OF THE METABOLIC RESPONSE TO SEPSIS

The response patterns following major infection are less predictable than those following elective operations and trauma. The invasion of the body by microorganisms initiates many host responses including mobilization of phagocytes, an

TABLE 3.7

DETERMINING THE NUTRITIONAL REQUIREMENTS OF THE TRAUMA PATIENT

1. Determine basal metabolic rate (BMR) for age, sex, and body surface area (BSA) (BMR is expressed in kcal/day).
2. Determine the percentage of increase in metabolic rate due to the injury.
3. If active, add 25% × BMR for hospital activity (walking, physical therapy, sitting, treatment).
4. The sum of steps 1 to 3 is an estimated daily caloric requirement for maintenance of body weight.
5. Divide step 4 by 150 to determine nitrogen requirements (convert to protein = 6.25 × nitrogen).
6. Give approximately 70% of caloric requirement as glucose. Give remaining caloric requirement as fat. Reassess energy and nitrogen needs at least twice weekly.
7. If nutritional support seems inadequate because of progressive weight loss, consider direct measurement of oxygen consumption or measurement of nitrogen balance.

inflammatory response at the local site, fever, tachycardia, and other systemic responses. Systemic events during the hyperdynamic phase of sepsis can be categorized into two general types of responses: (1) those related to the host's immunologic defenses and (2) those related to the body's general metabolic and circulatory adjustments to the infection. The changes in metabolism relate to alterations in glucose, nitrogen, and fat metabolism, as well as the redistribution of trace metals.

Systemic Metabolic Responses

Severe infection is characterized by fever, hypermetabolism, diminished protein economy, altered glucose dynamics, and accelerated lipolysis much like the injured patient. These effects are compounded in the patient with sepsis by multiorgan system failure, which includes the GI tract, liver, heart, and lungs.

Hypermetabolism

Oxygen consumption is usually elevated in the infected patient. The extent of this increase is related to the severity of infection, with peak elevations reaching 50% to 60% above normal. If the patient's metabolic rate is already elevated to a maximal extent because of severe injury, no further increase will be observed. In patients with only slightly accelerated rates of oxygen consumption, the presence of infection causes a rise in metabolic rate that appears additive to the pre-existing state. A portion of the increase in metabolism may be ascribed to the increase in reaction rate associated with fever (Q10 effect). Calculations suggest that the metabolic rate increases 10% to 13% for each elevation of 1°C in central temperature.

Altered Glucose Dynamics

The increase in glucose production in infected patients appears to be additive to the augmented gluconeogenesis following injury. For example, uninfected burn patients have an accelerated glucose production rate approximately 50% above normal; with the onset of bacteremia in similar individuals, hepatic glucose production increases to twice basal levels. Glucose dynamics following infection are complex, and profound hypoglycemia and diminished hepatic glucose production have also been described in both animals and human patients. Deterioration in gluconeogenesis is associated with more progressive stages of infection and may be related to alterations in splanchnic blood flow.

Alterations in Protein Metabolism

Accelerated proteolysis, increased nitrogen excretion, and prolonged negative nitrogen balance occur following infection, and the response pattern is similar to that described for injury. Amino acid efflux from skeletal muscle is accelerated in patients with sepsis, and this flux is matched by accelerated visceral amino acid uptake. In infected burn patients, splanchnic uptake of amino acids is increased 50% above rates in uninfected burn patients with injuries of comparable size. These amino acids serve as glucose precursors and are used for synthesis of acute phase proteins. Studies in animals have demonstrated that an increase in hepatic amino acid uptake during systemic infection is due to an increase in the activities of specific amino acid transporters that reside in the hepatocyte plasma membrane.

Severe infection is often associated with a hypercatabolic state that initiates marked changes in interorgan glutamine metabolism (Fig. 3.7). The cycle may begin with a breakdown

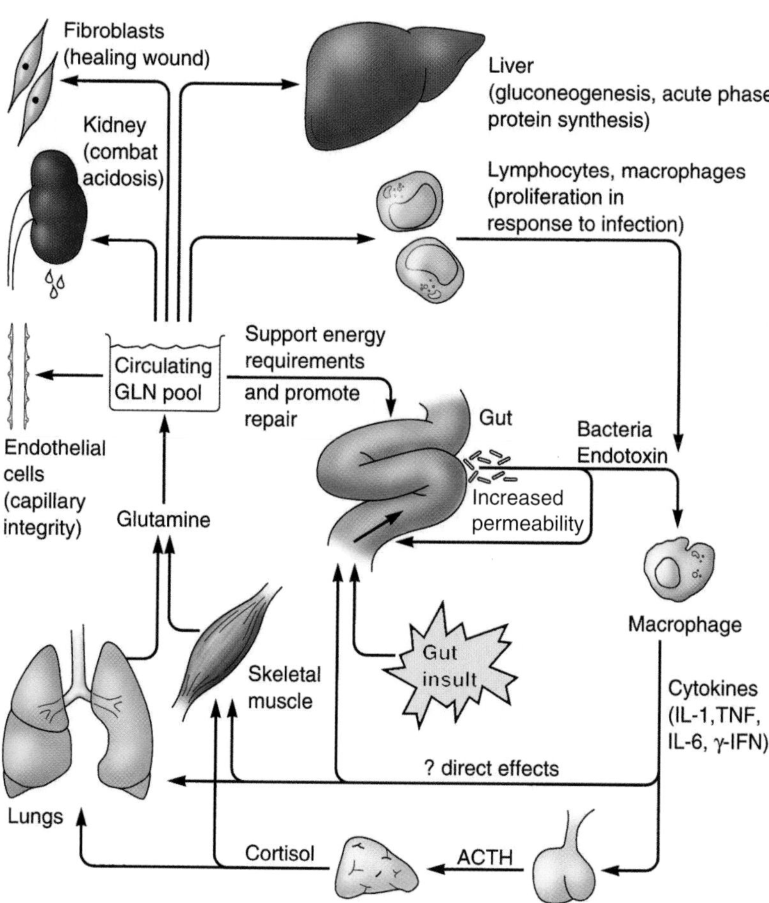

FIGURE 3.7 The *interorgan glutamine cycle* can be initiated by any local and/or systemic catabolic insult that re-directs the flow of glutamine and results in glutamine depletion. In the case illustrated here, the patient develops a breakdown in the gut mucosal barrier, which cause an increase in bowel permeability and bacterial translocation. Bacteria and endotoxins stimulate macrophages to release cytokines [tumor necrosis factor (TNF), interleukin (IL)-1, IL-6], which exert direct effects on glutamine metabolism in various organs and also stimulate release of the counter-regulatory hormones. These mediators work together to mobilize glutamine stores from muscle and to stimulate glutamine production by the lungs. A central goal is to support the increased glutamine requirements in other tissues. It is unclear why organs such as the gut should subserve other tissues, but it is apparent that if the cycle persists, or if the patient is unable to take oral feedings or remains glutamine deficient, a prolonged catabolic state develops.

in the gut mucosal barrier resulting in microbial translocation. Bacteria and their endotoxins stimulate macrophages to release cytokines that activate the pituitary-adrenal axis. The release of cortisol stimulates glutamine synthesis and release by tissues such as the lungs and skeletal muscle. The bulk of the glutamine is taken up by the liver at the expense of the gut. Acidosis frequently occurs in the patient with sepsis, and this stimulus serves as a signal for accelerated glutamine uptake by the kidney. Because the glutamine arises from skeletal muscle proteolysis, this complication of sepsis is yet another stimulus of heightened skeletal muscle breakdown.

Alterations in Fat Metabolism

Fat is a major fuel oxidized in infected patients, and the increased metabolism of lipids from peripheral fat stores is especially prominent during a period of inadequate nutritional support. Lipolysis is most probably mediated by the heightened sympathetic activity that is a potent stimulus for fat mobilization and accelerated oxidation. Marked hypertriglyceridemia has been associated with gram-negative infection on occasion, but plasma triglyceride concentrations are usually normal or low, indicating enhanced clearance by other organs. Infected patients cannot convert fatty acids to ketones efficiently in the liver and hence do not adapt to starvation as fasted, unstressed individuals do. The low ketone levels of infection may be a consequence of the hyperinsulinemia associated with catabolic states.

Changes in Trace Mineral Metabolism

Changes in balance of magnesium, inorganic phosphate, zinc, and potassium generally follow alterations in nitrogen balance. Although the iron-binding capacity of transferrin is usually unchanged in early infection, iron disappears from the plasma, especially during severe pyrogenic infections; similar alterations are observed with serum zinc levels. Both iron and zinc accumulate within the liver, and this accumulation appears to be another host defense mechanism. The administration of iron to the infected host, especially early in the disease, is contraindicated because increased serum iron concentrations may impair resistance. Unlike iron and zinc, copper levels generally rise, and the increased plasma concentrations can be ascribed almost entirely to the increase in ceruloplasmin produced by the liver.

Nutritional Requirements and Special Feeding Problems

As with all patients, the primary objectives of nutritional assessment are to evaluate the patient's present nutritional status and to determine energy, protein, and macro- and micronutrient requirements. Weight gain and anabolism are generally difficult to achieve during the septic process, but they do occur once the disease process has abated. Total energy requirements can be calculated using the stress equation; mild-to-moderate infections increase energy requirements 20% to 30%, and severe infection with fever increases caloric needs ~50% above basal levels. The current treatment of systemic infection consists of (a) removal or drainage of the septic source; (b) use of appropriate antibiotics; (c) supportive therapy of specific organ failure, whether cardiac, pulmonary, hepatic, renal, or GI; and (d) vigorous support of the host through nutritional means.

Respiratory Insufficiency

Patients often require intubation and vigorous ventilatory support, and hypermetabolism is a common feature of septic illness. Hypermetabolism is accompanied by increased oxygen consumption that drives carbon dioxide production as more substrate must be oxidized to support the hypermetabolic response. The composition of the diet (carbohydrate vs. fat) is relatively unimportant in determining the carbon dioxide burden (carbohydrate at RQ 1.0 releasing more CO_2 than fat at RQ 0.7). Avoidance of overfeeding is the primary concern in reducing the nutritional contribution to CO_2 production. The decision to reduce carbohydrate intake and increase lipid intake must be weighed carefully because high fat diets, especially fats high in n-6 fatty acids, may exacerbate lung injury.

Renal Failure

Renal failure significantly compromises the body's ability to clear the byproducts of protein metabolism but does not reduce the catabolic rate or the need for dietary protein. Under such conditions, it is important to avoid overfeeding protein, but it is also important to be aggressive with dialytic therapy so that protein is not restricted to less than the body's requirement. Careful assessment of needs is therefore critical.

Gut Dysfunction

Sepsis causes marked changes in GI function. The most common abnormality is ileus, which can result from intra-abdominal disease or from the effects of bacteria elsewhere. Breakdown of the gut mucosal barrier with translocation of luminal bacteria and their toxins can initiate a prolonged hypermetabolic state.

Hepatic Failure

Hepatic dysfunction is a common manifestation of septicemia. The degree of dysfunction is variable and may appear early as a slight elevation of liver enzymes, or it may cause severe jaundice and hyperbilirubinemia. Hepatic dysfunction generally resolves on resolution of the sepsis, but if the inflammatory process persists, adjustments in the feeding formulation will be necessary. Balanced carbohydrate and fat intake are important. The patient should be observed for the presence of encephalopathy; if this complication occurs and cannot be controlled by lactulose, then the protein load should be reduced. Another indication for limiting protein to <1.5 g/kg body weight is an elevated prothrombin time, as this may indicate impairment of hepatic protein synthetic function. Vitamin K deficiency and anticoagulants must be eliminated as causes of the change.

Cardiac Dysfunction

The myocardial dysfunction that occurs in sepsis may be secondary to the elaboration of cytokines such as TNF or IL-1, which have direct myocardial depressant activity. Alternatively, the heart failure may be secondary to pulmonary insufficiency with an increased pulmonary vascular resistance and right ventricular overload. Malnourished patients with sepsis may be sensitive to volume overload. A concentrated enteral or parenteral feeding solution may be indicated to maximize calories and to minimize volume.

NUTRITIONAL SUPPORT IN CANCER AND ACQUIRED IMMUNODEFICIENCY SYNDROME

Nutrition support of the cancer or AIDS patient is directed at two major areas: providing nutrition when symptoms of the disease or side effects of treatment prevent adequate intake and fighting the inflammatory state created by the tumor.

Cancers of the aerodigestive tract interfere with swallowing and/or digestion precluding adequate caloric or protein intake. Dysgeusia (altered taste perception) may also prevent adequate intake as may mouth sores and irritation of the pharynx and esophagus from chemotherapy, fungal infections, and radiation. Careful attention to a patient's symptoms and provision of zinc and B vitamins may help with taste. Soft foods, slushies, or slurries may help patients get better intake through an irritated or partially obstructed throat or esophagus. Treatment of nausea and constipation allows more interest in food.

Cancer cachexia accompanies many tumors and especially aggressive ones. The later stages of AIDS have a cachexia just like cancer. The cachectic state is a chronic inflammatory state that cannot be reversed even with adequate calories and protein. Proinflammatory cytokines (TNF, IL-1, IL-6) are constantly released in response to the tumor and lead to a chronic state of muscle wasting and fat loss. Only a reversal of the inflammatory response can ameliorate the cachexia. Cancer or AIDS cachexia cannot be cured, but only managed, and so removing the stimulus for inflammation is not possible. Pharmacologic options for interruption of inflammation include several of the nonsteroidal anti-inflammatory drugs (including celecoxib) and anticytokine medications. The nutritional strategies range from regular foods to functional foods to food supplements.

Among the most promising nutritional agents for promoting an anti-inflammatory milieu is the balance of n-6 to n-3 fatty acids in the body.[21] The source of these fatty acids is the diet, and dietary fatty acids are quickly incorporated into cell membranes, influencing the membranes' characteristics and function. These fatty acids are also the raw material for eicosanoid production.[22] The dietary and intravenous n-6 fatty acid is linoleic acid, which is incorporated into cell membranes as arachidonic acid which gives rise to proinflammatory PG_2 and LT_4. The dietary n-3 fatty acids are alpha-linolenic, eicosapentaneoic, and docosahexaenoic acid and are incorporated into cell membranes as the more anti-inflammatory PG_3 and LT_5. These anti-inflammatory eicosanoids interrupt the release of IL-6, thus potentially allowing IGF-1 levels to normalize in the patient with cachexia.[23] The typical modern Western diet is high in the ratio of n-6 to n-3 fatty acids (about 15:1). A more therapeutic ratio would be 2:1 to 4:1. In managing cachexia, the nutritional recommendation is to increase calorie and protein intake by any means possible. This often means dairy foods and protein sources from cold water fish, which will tend to keep the n-3 level high.

In three studies, pancreatic cancer patients consumed 3 g of eicosapenteneoic acid (EPA), a marine source of n-3 fatty acid, in a calorie/protein liquid supplement.[24–26] By doing so, patients gained weight (as fat-free mass, an indicator of anabolism); increased their grip strength; reduced their levels of C-reactive protein, IL-6, and resting metabolic rate (markers of decreased inflammation); and improved their scores on quality of life and functional status questionnaires. In another randomized trial, daily supplementation of 18 g n-3 fatty acid improved survival time in malnourished patients with solid tumors.[27]

Another possible nutritional intervention in cachexia of chronic illness is amino acid supplementation, specifically arginine, glutamine, and/or branched chain amino acids (leucine, isoleucine, valine). Two double-blind, randomized clinical trials of a commercially available amino acid supplement containing 14 g arginine, 14 g glutamine, and 3 g B-hydroxy-B-methylbutyrate (an analog of leucine) has shown that such supplementation can increase the fat-free mass of cachectic cancer patients (stage IV solid tumors) and patients with stage III AIDS.[28,29]

OTHER METHODS OF MODIFYING THE CATABOLIC RESPONSE TO SURGERY AND CRITICAL ILLNESS

In addition to nutritional intervention, other methods to modify the physiologic and biochemical response to operation have been studied in an effort to reduce the magnitude of the stress response and to provide insight into possible mechanisms. Regional anesthetic techniques block afferent signals from the wound and interrupt sympathetic nervous efferent signals to the adrenal gland and possibly the liver, reducing the apparent magnitude of the stress response. Others have studied stress responses in sympathectomized animals by blocking the efferent limb of the neuroendocrine reflex response. These reports indicate that central nervous system blockade interrupts afferent signals stimulated by operative procedures.

More recent studies have documented the safety and efficacy of long-term exogenous recombinant GH administration.[30] GH stimulates protein synthesis during hypocaloric feedings and increases retention of sodium and potassium by the kidney. The potential synergistic effects of specialized nutrition in combination with GH require further study. Cyclooxygenase inhibitors such as aspirin and ibuprofen attenuate the symptoms and endocrine responses that occur with critical illness without altering cytokine elaboration.

Research Findings

One of the difficulties in applying the research on nutritional modulation of the inflammatory response is that research protocols target particular diseases, and so results are often not generalizable. Although novel approaches to the management of the inflammatory response are becoming clinical realities, the current standard of supplemental macro and micronutrients should not be ignored. Akner and Cederholm[10] reviewed the literature and found that in 60% of 36 randomized controlled trials standard supplementation of nutrient intake improved function/morbidity and in 80% of 41 randomized controlled trials standard supplementation improved anthropometric variables. However, this leaves a large percentage of studies in which standard support of calorie, protein, and micronutrient intake did not have a positive effect.

CHOICE OF NUTRITION IN SURGICAL PATIENTS: ENTERAL OR PARENTERAL?

Although the physiologic advantage of enteral nutrition is apparent, preoperative nutritional repletion via the enteral route has not been as extensively studied as preoperative total parenteral nutrition (TPN). Although its use can be associated with the development of nausea, diarrhea, and distention, the use of enteral nutrition (via a feeding tube or as between-meal supplements) in malnourished patients seems preferable if it is feasible. Candidates must have a functional GI tract and must be able to receive adequate amounts of calories and nitrogen. In many critically ill patients, enteral nutrition-related GI complications are high and associated with decreased nutrient intake from the ordered levels.[31,32] Furthermore, forcing the enteral issue in patients who are intolerant of enteral nutrition is more detrimental than properly managed parenteral nutrition.

Nutrition as Primary Therapy

1. Patients with enterocutaneous fistulas (parenteral preferred but enteral could be used with a low output fistula)

Patients with GI-cutaneous fistulas represent the classical indication for TPN. Several comprehensive reviews have concluded that TPN clearly impacts on the treatment and course of disease for patients with GI fistulas. The following conclusions can be drawn from studies evaluating the use of TPN in patients with enterocutaneous fistulas: (a) TPN increases the spontaneous closure rate of enterocutaneous fistulas, but does not markedly decrease the mortality rate in patients with fistulas (improvements in mortality are mainly due to improved surgical and metabolic care); (b) if spontaneous closure of the fistula does not occur, patients are better prepared for operative intervention because of the nutritional support they received; and (c) certain fistulas (radiated bowel) are associated with a higher failure rate of closure than others and should be treated surgically after a defined period of nutritional support (unless closure occurs).

2. Patients with short bowel syndrome (parenteral)

Prospective randomized trials designed specifically to examine the impact of TPN on patients with short bowel syndrome have not been initiated, mainly because such patients have no alternative but to receive TPN. Most of these patients, who would have certainly died prior to the availability of TPN, now survive for long periods on home parenteral nutrition. In selected patients with residual small intestine (at least 18 in), postresectional hyperplasia may develop with time such that they can tolerate enteral feedings. Studies by Wilmore and colleagues[33] have demonstrated that the requirement for TPN could be decreased or even eliminated in patients with short gut syndrome by providing a nutritional regimen consisting of supplemental glutamine; GH; and a modified high carbohydrate, low fat diet. There was a marked improvement in the absorption of nutrients with this combination therapy and a decrease in stool output. In addition, TPN requirements were reduced by 50% as were the costs associated with care of these individuals. Discontinuation of the GH did not increase TPN needs in these patients once they had undergone successful gut rehabilitation.

3. Patients with hepatic failure (enteral formulae preferred)

Individuals with liver disease may be malnourished because of excessive alcohol intake, diminished food intake, or an inflammatory state from viral infection. These individuals are protein depleted yet they are intolerant of protein because of their tendency to become encephalopathic with a high nitrogen intake. Because of liver damage and portasystemic shunting these patients develop derangements in circulating levels of amino acids. The plasma aromatic/BCAA ratio is increased favoring the transport of aromatic amino acids across the blood–brain barrier. These amino acids are precursors of false neurotransmitters that contribute to lethargy and encephalopathy. Treatment of individuals with liver failure with solutions enriched in BCAAs and deficient in aromatic amino acids results in improved tolerance to the administered protein and clinical improvement in the encephalopathic state.

4. Patients with major thermal injury (enteral preferred if possible)

Aggressive nutritional support in patients with major burns seems to be associated with improved survival, particularly when increased amounts of dietary protein are provided.[34] Burned patients often require ventilatory support and/or suffer from ileus, which prevents using the GI tract for feeding. Even if the GI tract is usable, such patients are often unable to eat enough because of frequent trips to the operating room combined with the anorexia of severe injury. Most burn authorities believe that aggressive nutritional support in patients with major thermal injury has influenced outcome in a positive manner.

5. Patients with acute renal failure (also enteral preferred)

TPN with amino acids of high biologic value may decrease the mortality in patients with acute renal failure.[35] The use of solutions containing high-quality amino acids can improve nitrogen balance and diminish urea production. This translates into a decreased frequency of dialysis.

Total Parenteral Nutrition as Secondary Therapy

1. Prolonged ileus after operative procedure

Occasionally, patients will develop a prolonged ileus after an abdominal procedure, which precludes the use of the intestinal tract as a route of feeding. This is generally unpredictable and the cause of the ileus is often not demonstrated. If the patient is unable to eat by the seventh postoperative day, TPN should be started. The ileus may persist for several weeks. Although provision of TPN does not influence the disease process per se, it is beneficial because it prevents further erosion of lean body mass.

2. Acute radiation and chemotherapy enteritis

Malnourished patients who receive abdominal or pelvic radiation or chemotherapy may develop mucositis and enterocolitis that precludes using the GI tract for prolonged periods. TPN should be provided until the enteritis resolves and oral feeding can be resumed.

3. Preoperative TPN in the perioperative setting

In general, one cannot justify the use of perioperative nutrition (particularly parenteral feedings) unless a clear benefit can be demonstrated. The results of prospective randomized trials evaluating the efficacy of preoperative TPN are conflicting because of the variations in the nutritional status of patients studied, the differences in types of diseases in these malnourished patients, the differences in the type and length of nutritional support administered, and the failure to accrue enough patients to avoid type II statistical error.

One of the best studies to date evaluating the efficacy of preoperative TPN was published by the Veterans Affairs Total Parenteral Nutrition Cooperative Study Group.[36] More than 3,500 patients requiring mainly elective abdominal surgery were entered into this prospective randomized trial. They were initially screened for evidence of malnutrition using subjective criteria and/or by determining their Nutritional Risk Index Score, which included objective criteria such as percent weight loss and serum albumin level. The patients were then assigned to one of four groups: well-nourished, borderline malnourished, moderately malnourished, or severely malnourished. Patients in each malnourished category were randomized to receive at least 7 days of preoperative TPN or to proceed with surgery without preoperative TPN. Patients randomized to receive TPN received 1,000 kcal/day in excess of calculated caloric requirements. Lipid was provided on a daily basis. One criticism of this study was that patients were allowed to eat in addition to receiving parenteral feedings.

Analysis of the data from this study indicated that there was no difference in short-term or long-term complications between groups. Infectious complications including pneumonia, abscess, and line sepsis were statistically significantly higher for patients receiving TPN. Noninfectious complications (impaired wound healing) were significantly lower only in those patients receiving TPN who were in the severely malnourished group (>15% weight loss and serum albumin <2.9 mg%). This study strongly suggests that preoperative TPN should be

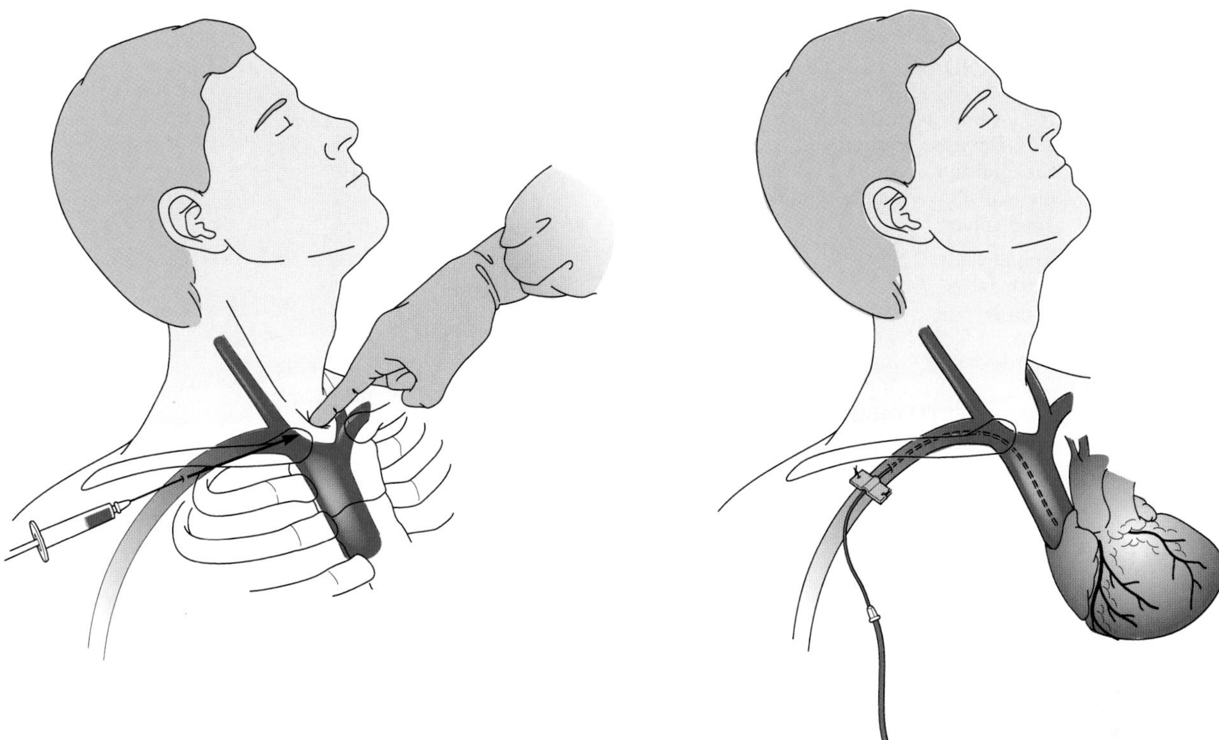

FIGURE 3.8 Technique for insertion of a subclavian catheter (see text for details).

provided only to severely malnourished patients who cannot be nourished by the enteral route. Contraindications to the use of preoperative TPN include patients requiring emergency operation and those who are only mildly or moderately malnourished. In such patients, TPN should be continued postoperatively only if the GI tract cannot be utilized for tube feedings. Nasojejunal or jejunostomy tubes should also be considered in patients undergoing major upper abdominal procedures in whom it is anticipated that oral feedings may not be resumed for 7 to 10 days after surgery.

Composition of TPN Formulations

TPN solutions are administered through a central venous catheter generally inserted into the subclavian vein (Fig. 3.8). The composition of a standard TPN solution is shown in Table 3.8. Because of the hyperosmolarity of such solutions, they must be delivered into a high flow system to prevent venous sclerosis. Patients receiving TPN should be monitored regularly by measuring blood sugar, serum electrolytes, and liver function tests. Elevations in serum glucose are common in surgical patients receiving TPN, especially if the patient is stressed and is relatively glucose intolerant. Hyperglycemia can generally be controlled by adding insulin to the TPN formulation or by decreasing the amount of glucose in the solution. It has been shown that an injured man can maximally oxidize about 4 to 5 mg of glucose/kg/minute. For a 70-kg man this is equal to approximately 400 to 500 g/day (1600 to 2000 kcal/day). Excess glucose calories are converted to fat, deposited in the liver, and result in hyperglycemia and glycosuria. The amounts of the various electrolytes that are provided to patients receiving TPN will vary depending on factors such as previous nutritional and hydration status. Careful monitoring is critical because as new cell mass is built, potassium and phosphate move intracellularly, which can lead to severe hypokalemia or hypophosphatemia. These electrolyte disturbances can develop rapidly and are much more life threatening than hyponatremia. Vitamin (Table 3.9) and trace mineral (Table 3.10) requirements must also be taken into consideration.

The use of lipids in TPN was developed to meet the requirement for essential fatty acids (linoleic acid) and the full caloric needs in hypermetabolic patients. Intravenous fat emulsions are comprised of soy or safflower oils (vegetable fat emulsions), which contain primarily long-chain triglycerides (LCTs) comprised of fatty acids with 16 and 18 carbon chain lengths. The fat provides essential linoleic acid, inhibits lipogenesis from carbohydrates, and lowers the RQ, which may benefit patients with respiratory compromise. However, the high content of n-6 polyunsaturated fatty acids (in particular linoleic acid) in these emulsions may have harmful effects on pulmonary and immune function.[37] Standard intravenous fat emulsions may alter the cell membrane phospholipid composition of cells of the reticuloendothelial system resulting in changes in membrane fluidity such that clearance of bacteria and toxins is impaired. In addition, n-6 polyunsaturated fatty acids may alter the local production of eicosanoids and cytokines such that chemotaxis is negatively impacted. Newer nutritional methods of modifying the catabolic response to injury and infection propose the use of the n-3 fatty acids, which may decrease eicosanoid biosynthesis and thereby diminish the vasoconstriction, platelet aggregation, and immunosuppression that may occur when n-6 derivatives are administered. Omega-3 fatty acids have been added to enteral formulas but are not in parenteral formulae available in the United States.

Fat is an important fuel source for critically ill patients. Septic and injured patients seem to preferentially utilize endogenous fat as an energy source, which appears to be related in part to the effects of counter-regulatory hormones on stimulating fat mobilization. These patients have a relative unresponsiveness to the administration of carbohydrates in that FFA mobilization is only marginally decreased and FFA oxidation is not suppressed as in "pure starvation." Glucose infusion above energy expenditure in a hormonal milieu that favors fat mobilization and oxidation only leads to hepatic steatosis.

TABLE 3.8

COMPOSITION OF A STANDARD CENTRAL VENOUS SOLUTION

Volume	10% Amino acid solution	500 mL
	50% Dextrose solution	500 mL
	Fat emulsion	—
	Electrolytes + vitamins + minerals	~50 mL
	Total volume	~1050 mL
Composition	Amino acids	50 g
	Dextrose	250 g
	Total N	50/6.25 = 8 g
	Dextrose kcal	250 g × 3.4 kcal/g = 840 kcal
	MOsms/L	~2000

ELECTROLYTES ADDED TO TOTAL PARENTERAL NUTRITION SOLUTIONS

Electrolyte	Usual concentration (mEq/L)	Range of concentrations (mEq/L)
Sodium	60	0–150
Potassium	40	0–80
Acetate	50	50–150
Chloride	50	0–150
Phosphate	15	0–30
Calcium[a]	4.5	0–20
Magnesium	5	5–15

[a]Generally added as calcium gluconate or calcium chloride one ampule of calcium gluconate = 1 g of calcium = 4.5 mEq.

Potential Complications of Total Parenteral Nutrition

Advances in technology, monitoring, and catheter care have greatly reduced the incidence of complications associated with the use of TPN. The establishment of a nutrition support team (physician, dietitian, nurse, pharmacist) and the recognition of such a team as an important part of overall patient care has also been a key factor in reducing complications. Complications of TPN occur and can be divided into three types: mechanical, metabolic, and infectious (Table 3.11). The management of the patient who becomes septic while receiving TPN is shown in Algorithm 3.1.

TABLE 3.9

VITAMIN REQUIREMENTS

Vitamin	Unit	Recommended dietary allowance for daily oral intake	Daily requirement of the moderately injured	Daily requirement of the severely injured	Amount provided by one vitamin pill	Daily amount provided by standard intravenous preparations
Vitamin A (retinol)	IU	1,760 (women)–3,300 (men)	5,000	5,000	10,000	3,300 (retinol)
Vitamin D (ergocalciferol)	IU	200	400	400	400	200
Vitamin E (tocopherol)	mg TE	8–10	Unknown	Unknown	15	10[a]
Vitamin K (phylloquinone)	μg	20–40[b]	20	20	0	0[c]
Vitamin C (ascorbic acid)	μg	60	75	300	100	100
Thiamine (vitamin B_1)	μg	1.0–1.5	2	10	10	3.0
Riboflavin (vitamin B_2)	μg	1.2–1.7	2	10	10	3.6
Niacin	mg	13–19	20	100	100	40
Pyridoxine (vitamin B_6)	μg	2.0–2.2	2	40	5	4.0
Pantothenic acid	mg	4–7 (adults)[b]	18	40	20	15
Folic acid	mg	0.4	1.5	2.5	0	0.4
Vitamin B_{12}	mg	3.0	2	4	5	5
Biotin	mg	100–200[b]	Unknown	Unknown	0	60

[a]Equivalent to recommended dietary allowance.
[b]Estimated to be safe and adequate in dietary intakes.
[c]Must be supplemented in peripheral venous solutions.
From Rombeau JL, Rolandelli RH. Nutritional support. In: Wilmore DW, Brennan MF, Harken RH, et al., eds. *Care of the surgical patient: II. Care in the ICU*. New York: Scientific American Medicine; 1989:6.

TABLE 3.10

MINERAL AND TRACE ELEMENT REQUIREMENTS

Mineral	Recommended dietary allowance for daily oral intake (mg)	Suggested daily intravenous intake (mg)	Daily amount provided by a commercially available mixture (mg)
Zinc	15	2.5–5.0[a]	5.0
Copper	2–3[b]	0.5–1.5	1.0
Manganese	2.5–5.0[b]	0.15–0.8	0.5
Chromium	0.05–0.2[b]	0.01–0.015	0.1
Iron	8 (women)–10 (men)	3	0

[a]Burn patients require an additional 2 mg.
[b]Estimated to be safe and adequate in dietary intakes.
From Rombeau JL, Rolandelli RH. Nutritional support. In: Wilmore DW, Brennan MF, Harken RH, et al., eds. *Care of the surgical patient: II. Care in the ICU*. New York: Scientific American Medicine; 1989:6.

TABLE 3.11

COMPLICATIONS ASSOCIATED WITH THE USE OF TPN

Complication	Cause	Treatment
MECHANICAL		
Pneumothorax	Puncture/laceration of lung pleura	Serial CXRs; chest tube if indicated
Subclavian artery injury	Penetration of subclavian artery during needle stick	CXR; Serial monitoring of vital signs
Air embolism	Aspiration of air into the subclavian vein and right heart	Place patient in Trendelenburg and left lateral decubitus; aspirate air
Catheter embolization	Shearing off the tip when withdrawing catheter	Retrieve catheter transvenously under fluoroscopic guidance
Venous thrombosis	Clot formation in great vein secondary to catheter	Heparinization if clinically significant
Catheter malposition	Tip of catheter directed into IJ or opposite subclavian	Reposition under fluoroscopy
METABOLIC		
Hyperglycemia	Excessive glucose calories or glucose intolerance	Decrease glucose calories; administer insulin
Hypoglycemia	Sudden cessation of TPN	Bolus 50% glucose solution monitor blood glucose
Carbon dioxide retention	Infusion of glucose calories in excess of energy needs	Decrease glucose calories and replace with fat
Hyperglycemic, hyperosmolar nonketotic coma (HHNC)	Dehydration from excessive diuresis	Discontinue TPN immediately; give insulin; monitor glucose/electrolytes
Hyperchloremic metabolic acidosis	Excessive chloride administration	Give Na and K as acetate salts
Azotemia	Excessive amino acid administration with inadequate calories	Decrease amino acids; increase glucose calories
Essential fatty acid deficiency	Inadequate essential fatty acid administration	Administer fat solution
Hypertriglyceridemia	Rapid fat infusion of decreased fat clearance	Slow rate of fat infusion
Hypophosphatemia	Inadequate administration of electrolyte in question	Increase administration
Hypocalcemia		
Hypomagnesemia		
Hypokalemia		
Bleeding	Vitamin K deficiency	Administer vitamin K
SEPTIC		
Line sepsis	Catheter tip infected	Remove catheter; antibiotics
Infection at skin site	Bacteria at site of catheter entry into skin	Remove catheter; local wound care

CXR, chest x-ray; IJ, internal jugular; TPN, total parenteral nutrition.

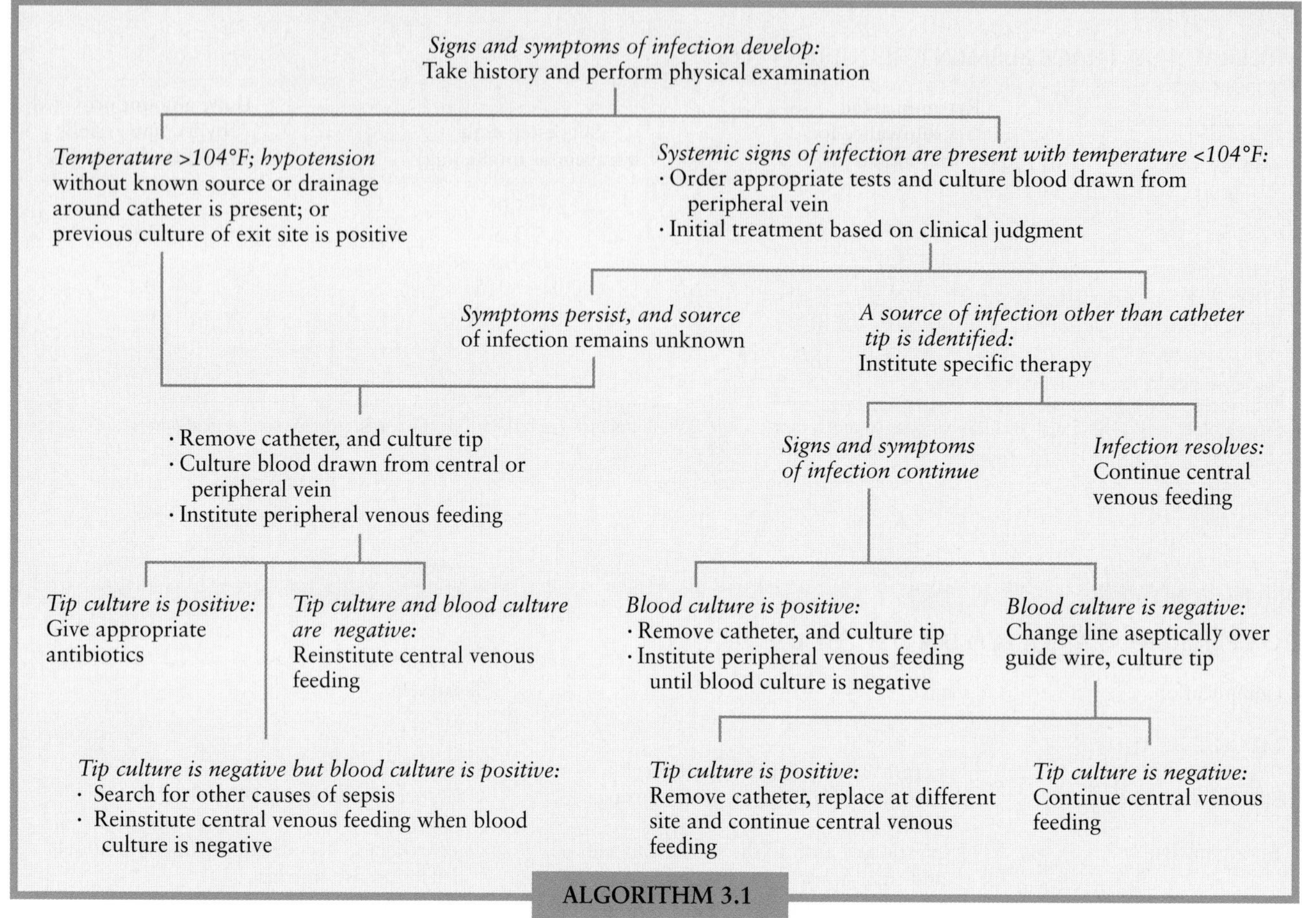

ALGORITHM 3.1 Management of the total parenteral nutrition patient who becomes septic.

The Effects of Total Parenteral Nutrition on the Gastrointestinal Tract

The studies examining the effects of TPN on intestinal function and immunity in animals demonstrate that TPN has a down-side. A unique feature of TPN is that subjects can remain on bowel rest for prolonged periods without concomitant malnutrition. In rats, TPN results in significant disruption of the intestinal microflora and bacterial translocation from the gut lumen to the mesenteric lymph nodes. In addition, when stresses such as burn injury, chemotherapy, or radiation are introduced in these models, animals on TPN have a much higher mortality. This suggests that TPN, under certain circumstances, may predispose patients to an increase in gut-derived infectious complications.[38]

A provocative study in human volunteers demonstrated that individuals receiving TPN had an accentuated systemic response to endotoxin challenge compared to enterally fed volunteers.[31] The study is consistent with an impairment in gut barrier function during parenteral feedings, which may promote the release of bacteria and/or cytokines leading to pronounced systemic responses and possibly multiple organ failure.

Supporting the Gut in Critically Ill Patients

The intestinal tract has long been considered an organ of inactivity following operation or injury. Ileus is generally present, nasogastric decompression is often necessary, and the gut is usually unused in the immediate postoperative period. Disuse of the GI tract, either via starvation or nutritional support by TPN, may lead to numerous physiologic derangements as well as changes in gut microflora, impaired gut immune function, and disruption of the integrity of the mucosal barrier. Thus, maintaining gut function in the perioperative period may be essential to minimize septic complications and organ failure. Treatment strategies designed to support the gut during critical illness are directed to provide appropriate nutrition and to maintain mucosal structure and function.[39]

Nutrition Support: Enteral Feedings

Enteral feedings are probably the single best method of maintaining mucosal structure and function if the bowel is functional. The trophic effects of luminal nutrition are key and the beneficial effects are well-documented even if relatively small amounts of nutrients are provided.

Gut-specific Nutrients. The composition of the diet as well as the route of delivery plays an important role in maintaining gut structure and function. Several gut-specific nutrients have been studied but glutamine has received the most attention. Glutamine has been classified as a nonessential or nutritionally dispensable amino acid. Because this categorization implies that glutamine can be synthesized in adequate quantities from other amino acids and precursors, it has not been considered necessary to include glutamine in nutritional formulas. It has been eliminated from TPN solutions because of its relative instability and short shelf life compared to other amino acids. With few exceptions, glutamine is present in oral and enteral diets only at the low levels of its concentration in most animal and plant proteins (about 7% of total amino acids).

Several recent studies have demonstrated that glutamine may be a conditionally essential amino acid during critical illness, particularly as it relates to supporting the metabolic requirements of the intestinal mucosa.[32,38] In general, these studies demonstrate that dietary glutamine is not required during states of health but appears to be beneficial when glutamine depletion is severe and/or when the intestinal mucosa is damaged by insults such as chemotherapy and radiation therapy. Addition of glutamine to enteral diets reduces the incidence of gut translocation but these improvements are dependent on the amount of supplemental glutamine and the type of insult studied. Glutamine-enriched TPN partially attenuates the villous atrophy that develops during parenteral nutrition. The use of intravenous glutamine in humans appears to be safe and effective and diminishes complications while reducing hospital stay.

In contrast to glutamine, short-chain fatty acids (SCFAs) are the primary energy source for colonocytes. Diets enriched in SCFAs have been shown to increase colonic DNA content and mucosal morphometrics as well as strengthen colonic anastomoses in rats. From diet, SCFAs are obtained from consumption of dietary fiber and fermentation in the colon by bacteria.

Other Factors to Support the Gut Mucosa

Specific growth factors that may promote intestinal mucosal growth have been implicated in a number of physiologic processes including growth, tissue repair, and regeneration. Among these is epidermal growth factor (EGF), a polypeptide secreted by submaxillary glands and by Brunner's glands of the small intestine. The most widespread effect of EGF on the GI mucosa is the overall stimulation of DNA synthesis as evidenced by thymidine incorporation.

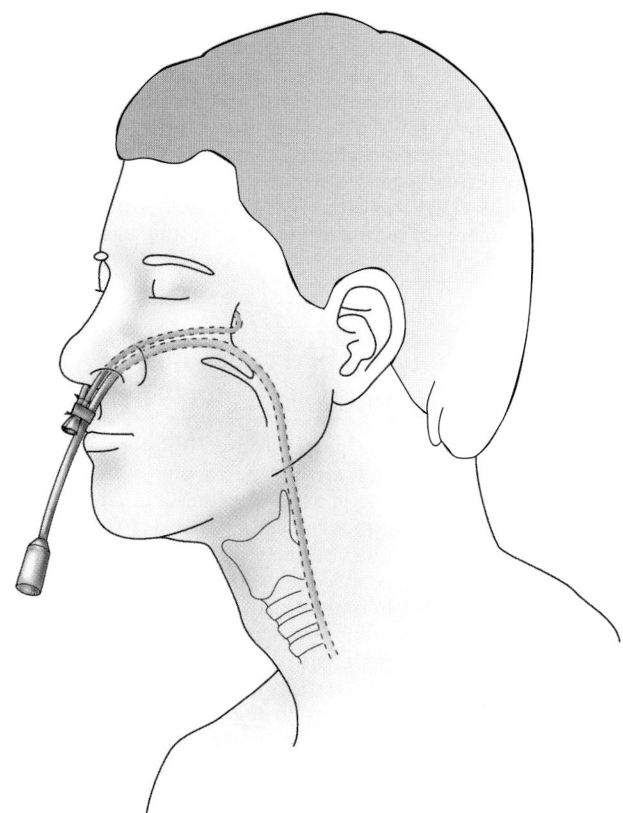

FIGURE 3.9 Use of a feeding tube bridle for patients who are prone to extubate the feeding catheter.

TECHNIQUES OF NUTRITIONAL SUPPORT

Transnasal (Nasogastric and Nasoduodenal) Feeding Catheters

The use of transnasal feeding catheters for intragastric feeding or for duodenal intubation is a popular adjunct for providing nutritional support by the enteral route. Intragastric feedings provide several advantages for the patient. The stomach has the capacity and reservoir for bolus feedings. Feeding into the stomach results in the stimulation of biliary-pancreatic axis, which is probably trophic for the small bowel, and gastric secretions will have a dilutional effect on the osmolarity of the feedings reducing the risk of diarrhea. The major risk of intragastric feeding is the regurgitation of gastric contents resulting in aspiration into the tracheobronchial tree. This risk is highest for patients who have an altered mental status or who are paralyzed.

The placement of the feeding tube through the pylorus into the fourth portion of the duodenum reduces the risk of regurgitation and aspiration of feeding formulas. To place a transnasal intraduodenal feeding catheter, the patient should be in the sitting position with the neck slightly flexed. This will allow for the passage of a lubricated 8-French polyurethane feeding catheter (with a stylette in place) through the patient's nose in a posterior and inferior direction bringing the catheter to the level of the pharynx. The head is brought back to a neutral position and the patient is instructed to swallow while the feeding catheter is passed into the esophageal lumen. The advancement of the catheter is continued for a distance of about 45 to 50 cm. The stylette is removed and the position of the catheter is confirmed radiographically prior to the initiation of feedings. Tubes can be positioned fluoroscopically if necessary. The patient who frequently removes the feeding catheter may be a candidate for feeding tube bridle as shown in Fig. 3.9.

A variety of enteral formulas are commercially available and can be adjusted for calorie, nitrogen, or fiber content.

Technique for Gastrostomy Placement

A feeding gastrostomy should be considered for patients requiring long-term enteral nutrition and in patients with obstruction of the esophagus or locally advanced head and neck cancers, which preclude eating. A temporary Stamm gastrostomy is a popular method for access to the gastric lumen and can be performed at the time of any major abdominal procedure. A square pursestring suture (0 polypropylene) with a 1.0-cm diameter is placed in the body of the anterior wall of the stomach. The ideal location is in the midportion of the stomach closer to the greater curvature in a relatively avascular area. A second hexagonal or octagonal pursestring suture (also 0 polypropylene) is placed outside the first one. The feeding catheter (often a Foley catheter) is then brought through a stab wound in the abdominal wall (left upper quadrant). Using the electrocautery, a puncture is made in the anterior portion of the stomach directly in the center of the concentric pursestring sutures. The feeding catheter is introduced into the gastric lumen and the inner concentric suture is secured in place. The second pursestring is then secured, inverting the gastric mucosa completely. The catheter balloon is inflated and the stomach is drawn upward toward the anterior abdominal wall. Placement of seromuscular silk sutures in all four quadrants around the catheter will secure the stomach to the anterior abdominal wall. The catheter is then secured to the skin by the placement of a bolstering disk at the base of the catheter exit site.

Technique of Percutaneous Endoscopic Gastrostomy

Percutaneous endoscopic gastrostomy (PEG) to provide access for gastric feedings can be performed without the need for a laparotomy or general anesthesia. Using intravenous sedation and topical anesthetic, a gastroscope is passed through the mouth into the esophagus and stomach. The light from the gastroscope is then transilluminated through the anterior abdominal wall in the epigastrium or left subcostal area. The abdomen is prepped and draped and a wheal of local anesthetic is injected right at the area of transillumination. A 1-cm vertical incision is made and an Angiocath or needle is inserted through the abdominal wall into the stomach under the direct vision of the gastroscope. A wire loop is passed through the catheter into the stomach and grasped with a snare passed through the gastroscope. The scope and wire loop are withdrawn through the mouth and the wire is looped through a corresponding wire on the end of the PEG tube. By pulling the wire out through the abdominal wall, the PEG tube is pulled in through the mouth and out the anterior abdomen while followed through the esophagus by the scope. The scope then visualizes the inner part of the PEG tube to ensure that it seats properly against the stomach wall. The tube protruding through the abdominal wall is then bolstered at the exit site to prevent accidental dislodgment. The tube can later be removed with firm traction.

Feeding Catheter Jejunostomy Placement and Witzel Jejunostomy

A feeding catheter jejunostomy should be considered following any major upper abdominal procedure if prolonged enteral nutrition support is anticipated. The simplest method is a needle jejunostomy performed at the end of the definitive operation. A 14- or 16-gauge needle is used to create a tunnel subserosally approximately 30 to 40 cm distal to the ligament of Treitz and then the needle tip is introduced into the jejunal lumen. A feeding catheter is inserted through the needle and advanced 30 to 40 cm distally into the bowel lumen to the desired location, and the needle is withdrawn. The loop of jejunum is then anchored to the parietal peritoneum with permanent sutures. The catheter is then secured to the skin with nylon sutures. A recent prospective trial in major upper GI surgery showed feeding started earlier and progressed more easily with routine placement of a needle catheter jejunostomy.[40]

A feeding jejunostomy can also be performed by utilizing the Witzel technique. A loop of proximal jejunum 20 to 30 cm from the ligament of Treitz is delivered into the wound. A pursestring suture is placed on the antimesenteric border of the bowel and an incision is made with electrocautery in the intestinal wall in the center of the pursestring suture. A red rubber catheter (14 Fr) is inserted into the lumen of the jejunum and advanced distally. The pursestring suture is then secured in place. A serosal tunnel is then constructed with 000 silk sutures from the catheter's exit site extending then 5 to 6 cm proximally. The catheter is then delivered through the abdominal wall through a separate stab incision. This loop of intestine is then anchored to the peritoneum with two 000 silk sutures spread over 2 to 3 cm to prevent twisting of the loop and possible obstruction. The catheter is secured to the skin with a 3-0 nylon suture. Jejunal feeding catheters can be used immediately following the operation.

Peripheral Intravenous Feedings

Peripheral veins may be used for infusion of glucose, amino acid solutions, and fat emulsions. However, these solutions must be nearly isotonic to avoid peripheral vein sclerosis. Ten percent glucose solutions may be used to increase the efficacy of amino acid utilization. Fat emulsions can be administered simultaneously with glucose and amino acid solutions, because they provide an efficient fuel source and are isotonic. The major disadvantage of these peripherally administered mixtures is limited caloric delivery to meet catabolic demands within tolerated fluid volumes. Indications for peripheral vein feeding include the following: (a) as a supplement when enteral feedings can be only partially tolerated because of GI dysfunction, (b) as a method of nutritional support when the GI tract must be kept relatively empty for short periods during diagnostic workup, and (c) as preliminary feedings prior to subclavian catheter insertion in patients requiring TPN.

Technique of Central Venous Catheter Placement

The preferred method of access to the superior vena cava is by percutaneous cannulation of the subclavian vein. Alternate sites include the jugular approach, but with the catheter exiting in the neck region this makes it more difficult to secure the dressing site and maintain sterility.

An individual who is experienced in the technique should perform the placement of a central venous catheter. To reduce the risk of bleeding complications, patients with a platelet count below 50,000/mm^3 should receive fresh platelets prior to catheter insertion. The procedure is performed utilizing aseptic technique; the surgeon should wear a hat, mask, gown, and gloves. The patient is placed in the Trendelenburg position with both arms at the sides and the head turned away from the site of insertion. The chest is shaved, prepped, and draped in a sterile fashion. Local anesthesia is infiltrated near the insertion site and the underlying tissues along the inferior border of the clavicle. The tip of the needle is inserted into the skin and subcutaneous tissues at the midpoint of the clavicle aiming for the suprasternal notch.

The needle is directed parallel to the patient's bed, insinuating beneath the clavicle and at all times with negative pressure applied to the syringe. The prompt inflow of blood into the syringe indicates entrance into the subclavian vein and the needle is advanced a few millimeters to ensure the entire bevel is within the lumen of the vessel. The patient is instructed to perform a Valsalva maneuver to prevent an air embolism, the syringe is disconnected from the needle and the guide wire is passed through the needle lumen, and the needle is then withdrawn over the guidewire. The passage of the wire through the needle should be met with minimal resistance and the needle should be removed only after 15 cm of the wire has been passed into the vessel. A small incision is made at the guide wire exit site and a dilator is passed over the wire. The dilator is then removed over the wire and is replaced by the catheter which is fully advanced. The wire is withdrawn and the catheter is flushed with sterile saline. The catheter is then sutured into position, the insertion site cleaned, and a sterile dressing placed. A portable chest x-ray is done to confirm placement of the catheter and to rule out pneumothorax.

Complications from long-term central venous catheterization include venous thrombosis and catheter-related infections. Thrombosis of the central vessels is a complication that is often overlooked. The clinical suspicion of subclavian vein thrombosis is only about 3%, whereas studies that use phlebography or radionuclide venography indicate that the prevalence is as high as 35%. Febrile episodes are not uncommon in the cancer patient population particularly in the neutropenic individual. If primary catheter sepsis is confirmed, the catheter must be removed immediately and the tip cultured.

Nutrition support of the surgical patient should strive to preserve body composition, provide needed nutrients, and minimize the inflammatory response to promote a decreased risk and better surgical outcome.

KEY POINTS

- **The goal of perioperative or post-traumatic nutritional support is to replete or maintain protein and energy stores as a part of lean body mass, to allow recovery from illness.**
- **Inflammation can increase energy utilization and alter the metabolism of glucose, protein, fat, and trace minerals.**
- **To identify nutritional requirements, estimate basal metabolic rate for age, gender, and body surface area and increase by 25% to 100% based on severity of stress.**
- **Supply 70% of calories as protein, remainder as fat, and calorie/nitrogen ratio of 150:1.**
- **Use the enteral route for feedings when practical.**
- **Assess the adequacy of nutritional support to determine further needs.**

References

1. Frankenfield DC, Cooney RN, Smith JS, Rowe WA. Age-related differences in the metabolic response to injury. *J Trauma* 2000;48:49.
2. Frankenfield DC, Rowe WA, Cooney RN, et al. Limits of body mass index to detect obesity and predict body composition. *Nutrition* 2001;17:26.
3. **Frankenfield DC, Cooney RN, Smith JS, Rowe WA. Bioelectrical impedance plethysmographic analysis of body composition in critically injured and healthy subjects. *Am J Clin Nutr.* 1999;69:426.**
4. Frankenfield DC, Smith JS, Cooney RN, et al. Relative association of fever and injury with hypermetabolism in critically ill patients. *Injury* 1997;28:617.
5. **Frankenfield DC, Rowe WA, Smith JS, Cooney RN. Validation of several established equations for resting metabolic rate in obese and non obese people. *J Am Dietetic Assoc.* 2003;103:1152.**
6. Frankenfield D, Smith JS, Cooney RN. Validation of 2 approaches to predicting resting metabolic rate in critically ill patients. *J Parenter Enteral Nutr.* 2004;28:259.
7. Frankenfield DC, Sarson GY, Blosser SA, et al. Validation of a 5-minute steady state indirect calorimetry protocol for resting energy expenditure in critically ill patients. *J Am Coll Nutr.* 1996;15:397.
8. Cuthbertson DP. Observation of disturbance of metabolism poduced by injury of the limbs. *Q J Med.* 1932;1:233.
9. Frankenfield DC, Smith JS, Cooney RN. Accelerated nitrogen loss after traumatic injury is not attenuated by achievement of energy balance. *JPEN* 1997;21:324.
10. Akner G, Cederholm T. Treatment of protein-energy malnutrition in chronic non-malignant disorders. *Am J Clin Nutr.* 2001;74:6.
11. Kotler DP. Cachexia. *Ann Intern Med.* 2000;133:622.
12. Kaysen G, Eisenrich JP. Characteristics and effects of inflammation in end-stage renal disease. *Semin Dial.* 2003;16:438.
13. Espat NJ, Moldower LL, Copeland EM. Cytokine-mediated alterations in host metabolism prevent nutritional repletion in cachectic cancer patients. *J Surg Oncol.* 1995;58:77.
14. Schulze PC, Gielen S, Adams V, et al. Muscular levels of proinflammatory cytokines correlate with a reduced expression of insulin like growth factor in chronic heart failure. *Basic Res Cardiol.* 2003;98:267.
15. Debigare R, Cote CH, Maltais F. Peripheral muscle wasting in chronic obstructive pulmonary disease. *Am J Resp Crit Care Med.* 2001;164: 1712.
16. Chrousos GP. The hypothalamic-pituitary-adrenal axis and immune-mediated inflammation. *N Engl J Med* 1995;332:1351.
17. Steinborn W, Anker SD. Cardiac cachexia: pathophysiology and clinical implications. *Basic Appl Myol.* 2003;13:191.
18. Anker SD, Coats AJS. Cardiac cachexia. A syndrome with impaired survival and immune and neuroendocrine activation. *Chest* 1999;115:836.
19. Bessey PQ, Watters JM, Aoki TT, Wilmore DW. Combined hormonal infusion simulates the metabolic response to injury. *Ann Surg.* 1984;200:264.
20. Souba WW. Cytokines: key regulators of the nutritional/metabolic response to critical illness. *Curr Prob Surg.* 1994;31:577.
21. Bagga D, Wang L, Farias-Eisner R, et al. Differential effects of prostaglandin derived from n-6 and n-3 polyunsaturated fatty acids on COX-2 and IL-6 secretion. *Proc Natl Acad Sci USA* 2003;100:1751.
22. Scholz H. Prostaglandins. *Am J Physiol Regul Integr Comp Physiol.* 2003;285:R512.
23. Wigmore SJ, Fearon KC, Maingay JP, et al. Down-regulation of the acute-phase response in patients with pancreatic cancer cachexia receiving oral eicosapentaenoic acid is mediated via suppression of interleukin-6. *Clin Sci.* 1997;92:215.
24. Barber MD, McMillan DC, Preston T, et al. The metabolic response to feeding in weight-losing pancreatic cancer patients and its modulation by a fish oil-enriched nutritional supplement. *Clin Sci.* 2000;98:389.
25. Barber MD, Ross JA, Preston T, et al. Fish oil-enriched nutritional supplement attenuates progression of the acute phase response in weight-losing patients with advanced pancreatic cancer. *J Nutr.* 1999;129:1120.
26. Barber MD, Ross JA, Voss AC, et al. The effect of an oral nutritional supplement enriched with fish oil on weight loss in patients with pancreatic cancer. *Br J Cancer* 1999;81:80.
27. Gogos CA, Ginopoulos P, Salsa B, et al. Dietary omega-3 polyunsaturated fatty acids plus vitamin E restore immunodeficiency and prolong survival for severely ill patients with generalized malignancy. *Cancer* 1998;82:395.
28. May PE, Barber A, D'Olympio JT, et al. Reversal of cancer-related wasting using oral supplementation with a combination of B-hydroxy-B-methylbutyrate, arginine, and glutamine. *Am J Surg.* 2002;183:471.
29. Clark RH, Feleke G, Din M, et al. Nutritional treatment for acquired immunodeficiency virus-associated wasting using B-hydroxy-B-methylbutyrate, glutamine, and arginine: a randomized, double-blind, placebo-controlled study. *J Parenter Enteral Nutr.* 2000;24:133.
30. Jiang ZM, He GZ, Zhang SY, et al. Low-dose growth hormone and hypocaloric nutrition attenuates the protein-catabolic response after major operation. *Ann Surg.* 1989;210:514.
31. **Fong Y, Marano MA, Barber A, et al. Total parenteral nutrition and bowel rest modify the metabolic response to endotoxin in humans. *Ann Surg.* 1989;210:449.**
32. Ziegler TR, Young LS, Benfell K, et al. Clinical and metabolic efficacy of glutamine-enriched parenteral nutrition following bone marrow transplantation: a double-blind randomized controlled trial. *Ann Intern Med.* 1992;116:821.
33. Byrne TA, Persinger RL, Young LS, et al. A new treatment for patients with the short bowel syndrome: growth hormone, glutamine, and a modified diet. *Ann Surg.* 1995;222:243.
34. Alexander JW, MacMillan BG, Stinnert JD, et al. Beneficial effects of aggressive protein feeding in severely burned children. *Ann Surg.* 1980;192:505.
35. Abel RM, Beck CH, Abbott WM, et al. Improved survival from acute renal failure following treatment with intravenous essential L-amino acids and glucose: results of a prospective, double-blind study. *N Engl J Med.* 1973;288:695.
36. **Buzby GP and The Veterans Affairs Total Parenteral Nutrition Cooperative Study Group. Perioperative total parenteral nutrition in surgical patients. *N Engl J Med.* 1991;325:525.**
37. **Batistella FD, Widergren JT, Anderson JT, et al. A prospective randomized trial of intravenous fat emulsion administration in trauma victims requiring total parenteral nutrition. *J Trauma* 1997;43;52.**
38. van der Hulst RRWJ, van Kreel BK, von Meyenfeldt MF, et al. Glutamine and the preservation of gut integrity. *Lancet* 1993;341:1363.
39. Scheltinga MR, Young LS, Benfell K, et al. Glutamine-enriched intravenous feedings attenuate extracellular fluid expansion after standard stress. *Ann Surg.* 1991;214:385.
40. **Chin KF, Townsend S, Wong W, Miller GV. A prospective cohort study of feeding needle catheter jejunostomy in an upper gastrointestinal surgical unit. *Clin Nutr.* 2004;23:691.**

CHAPTER 4 ■ WOUND HEALING

NEIL A. FINE AND THOMAS A. MUSTOE

An understanding of wound healing is fundamental to all of surgery and involves a broad range of cellular actions and interactions. Wound healing is a fundamental homeostatic process in response to injury. It involves the activation of basic cellular processes of inflammation, cell proliferation, and growth as well as regulation of these processes once repair is complete. Increased understanding of the cellular and molecular events involving growth factors and cytokines, and the realistic prospects for pharmacologic manipulation, have focused a great deal of research interest from a broad range of disciplines. Although much new knowledge has been gained, there remain many unanswered questions. This chapter outlines a basic set of concepts regarding wound healing, with emphasis on the clinical principles of basic surgical techniques and the care of surgical incisions and open, acute, and chronic wounds.

NORMAL WOUND HEALING

Wound healing is the body's response to injury. Injury can be acute or chronic and involve multiple tissues, but wound healing is most clearly illustrated by examining the response to full-thickness injury (e.g., a cut or an incision) to the epidermis and dermis. This injury sets in motion a sequence of interrelated reparative forces. Although the events overlap in time, it is helpful to consider the process as stages or phases of wound healing; these are presented as separate events. This provides for clear conceptualization of the individual events and conforms to standard conventions. These events, however, do not occur independently, and the degree of temporal overlap is significant (Fig. 4.1).[1]

Every tissue in the body undergoes reparative processes after injury. Bone has the unique ability to heal without scar. Liver has the potential to regenerate parenchyma and is the only organ that has maintained that ability in the adult human. Although liver does regenerate, it often heals with scar (cirrhosis). With these exceptions, all other human tissues heal with scar. This chapter reviews the healing process of human skin with particular emphasis on surgical applications. Delineation of the individual mediators is still evolving, so the emphasis is on the underlying physiologic processes and the patterns of response.

Inflammatory Phase

The inflammatory phase of acute wound healing begins immediately after injury. The initial response to the disruption of blood vessels is bleeding. The homeostatic response to this is clot formation to stop hemorrhage. Platelet plug formation initiates the hemostatic process along with clotting factors activated by collagen and basement membrane proteins exposed by the injury. Fibrin, converted from fibrinogen by the clotting cascade, binds the platelet plug and forms the provisional matrix for the cellular responses that follows. After injury, transient vasoconstriction is mediated by catecholamines, thromboxane, and prostaglandin $F_{2\alpha}$ ($PGF_{2\alpha}$). Platelet degranulation, the emptying of the granules into the extracellular space, provides the contents of α granules and dense granules, most notably platelet-derived growth factor (PDGF) and transforming growth factor β (TGF-β). These substances initiate chemotaxis and proliferation of inflammatory cells, beginning

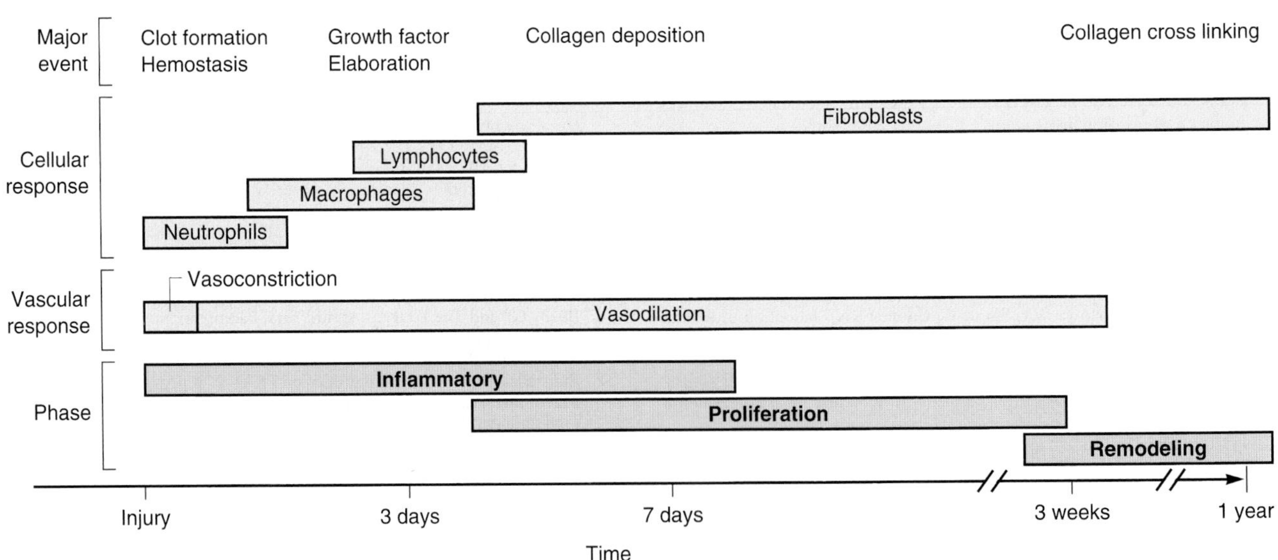

FIGURE 4.1 Time line of phases of wound healing with dominant cell types and major physiologic events.

TABLE 4.1

PLATELET GRANULES AND MEDIATORS OF PLATELET AGGREGATION

PLATELET GRANULES
α Granules: Contain Platelet-specific Proteins
Platelet factor 4
β-Thromboglobulin
Platelet-derived growth factor
Transforming growth factor-β
Dense Granules
Adenosine diphosphate
Serotonin
Calcium
MEDIATORS OF PLATELET AGGREGATION
Thromboxane A_2
Thrombin
Platelet factor 4

the inflammatory response that will ultimately heal the wound (Table 4.1). Transient vasoconstriction is necessary to decrease blood loss at the time of the initial wounding and also to allow clot formation. Vasoconstriction lasts for 5 to 10 minutes. Once a clot has been formed and active bleeding has stopped, vasodilation increases local blood flow to the wounded area, supplying cells and substrate necessary for further wound repair. The vascular endothelial cells also deform, increasing vascular permeability. The vasodilation and increased endothelial permeability are mediated by histamine, prostaglandin E_2 (PGE_2), and prostaglandin I_2 (prostacyclin; PGI_2) as well as vascular endothelial cell growth factor (VEGF). These vasodilatory substances are released by injured endothelial cells and mast cells and enhance the egress of cells and substrate into the wounded tissue (Fig. 4.2).

At this stage, the wound is full of debris from the initial injury. This material consists of a mixture of injured, devitalized tissue (fat, muscle, epithelium), clot (platelets, erythrocytes, fibrin), bacteria (from the skin surface and external environment), extravasated serum proteins (glycoproteins and mucopolysaccharides), and foreign material introduced at the time of injury (suture, dirt). During the next several days, the wound is cleared of bacteria, devitalized tissue, and foreign material by recruited and activated phagocytic cells. Polymorphonuclear leukocytes (PMNs) begin to arrive immediately, attaining large numbers within 24 hours. The process of clearing the wound of debris usually takes several days, but the time varies depending on the amount of material to be cleared. The PMNs are followed temporarily by macrophages, which appear in wounds in significant numbers within 2 or 3 days. The macrophages are mononuclear phagocytic cells derived from circulating monocytes or resident tissue macrophages. They complete the process of removing all material not necessary for the ensuing steps of wound healing.

In the absence of significant bacterial contamination, macrophages promptly replace PMNs as the dominant cell type during the inflammatory phase. The role of the macrophages is not limited to phagocytosis.[2] In addition, macrophages are the sources of more than 30 different growth factors and cytokines. These growth factors induce fibroblast proliferation, endothelial cell proliferation (angiogenesis), and extracellular matrix production, and they recruit and activate additional macrophages. The result is the induction of a wound healing amplification cycle as growth factors recruit macrophages and elicit additional growth factor release. Specific antibodies that destroy PMNs or block certain aspects of amplification function (such as adhesion) have shown that wounds heal normally in the absence of bacteria, but that healing is significantly impaired without functional macrophages (even in the absence of bacteria). These studies confirm the dominant role of the macrophage in the inflammatory phase of wound healing. The amplification process is so powerful that only scattered fibroblasts and endothelial cells are seen in a surgical incision or at the edge of an open wound at day 3, but by day 5 the wound is very cellular with active proliferation. By day 7, the incisional wound is strong enough to allow suture removal, and proliferating fibroblasts and angiogenesis give the wound an appearance similar in many respects to the stroma surrounding tumors.

Lymphocytes also appear in wounds in small numbers during the inflammatory phase. The role of lymphocytes in the wound healing process remains to be clarified, but they are thought to be related more to chronic inflammatory processes than to the initial response to wounding. Because recombinant growth factors are available in sufficient quantities for clinical use, the prospect of using growth factors as pharmacologic agents to stimulate wound healing (and potentially modulate abnormal scarring) has been the focus of much research. Dozens of growth factor studies have been performed in humans, based on animal studies that have demonstrated wound healing activity by about a dozen different growth factors [PDGF, TGF-β1, TGF-β2, TGF-β3, fibroblast growth factor (FGF)2, FGF7, keratinocyte growth factor (KGF), granulocyte-macrophage colony-stimulating factor (GMCSF), insulin-like growth factor (IGF1) plus insulin-like growth factor binding protein (IGFBP1), and epidermal growth factor (EGF) represent a partial list), and to date only PDGF has been approved.[3] After a 7-year process, involving 1,000 patients, PDGF (Regranex) was approved in 1997 by the Food and Drug Administration (FDA) for use in diabetic foot ulcers. The failure of so many clinical trials is a reflection of both the complexity and variability of human wounds, which make it difficult to demonstrate efficacy in all but the largest of studies, and also the multiple factors that result in chronic wounds, which are discussed later.

Another product, an artificial skin equivalent made of a dermis-like matrix covered with cultured epithelium from heterologous human foreskins (Apligraf) was FDA approved in 1998 for use in venous ulcers of more than 1-year duration that had failed other therapies. This product's main effect is most likely due to the delivery of growth factors produced by the neonatal cells. Increased knowledge of the role of growth factors in wound healing has also provoked the evaluation of strategies using other pharmacologic agents to indirectly modulate growth factor levels in wounds.

Proliferative Phase

The proliferative phase begins with the formation of a provisional matrix of fibrin and fibronectin as part of initial clot formation. Initially, the provisional matrix is populated by macrophages; however, by day 3, fibroblasts appear in the fibronectin–fibrin framework and initiate collagen synthesis. Fibroblasts proliferate in response to growth factors to become the dominant cell type during this phase. Growth factors produced by macrophages simultaneously induce angiogenesis, which induces the ingrowth and proliferation of endothelial cells, forming new capillaries. This neovascularity is visible through the epithelium and gives the wound a pink or purple-red appearance. Capillary ingrowth provides the fibroblasts with oxygen and nutrients to sustain cell proliferation and support the production of the permanent wound matrix. This matrix is composed of collagen and proteoglycans or ground substance and replaces the provisional fibronectin–fibrin matrix.

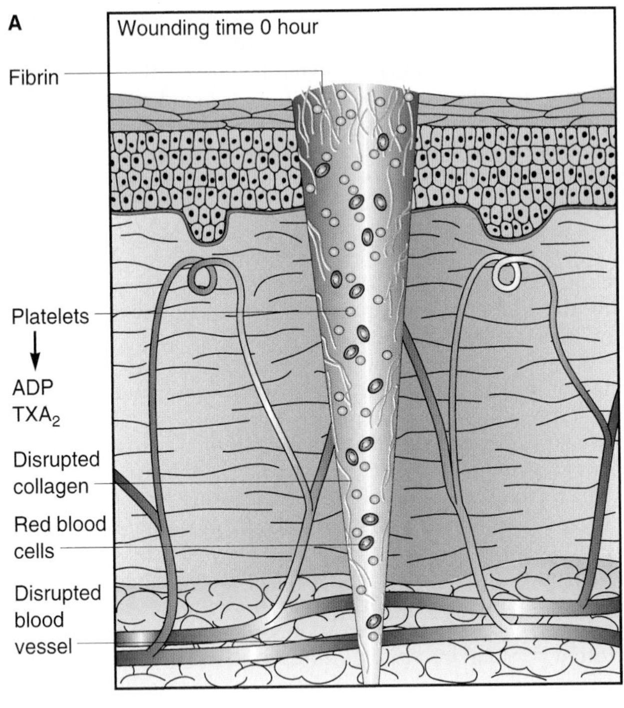

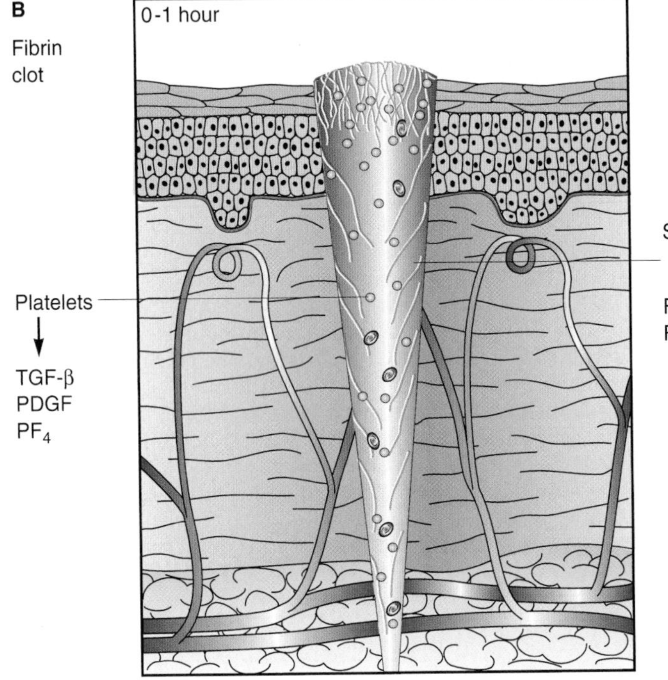

FIGURE 4.2 Schematic representation of wound healing processes. ADP, adenosine diphosphate; TXA_2, thromboxane A_2; TGF, transforming growth factor; PDGF, platelet-derived growth factor; PF_4, platelet factor 4; TNF-α, tumor necrosis factor α; FGF, fibroblast growth factor; PAF, platelet-activating factor; KGF, keratinocyte growth factor.

Collagen is the dominant structural molecule in the wound matrix and in the final scar. This is not surprising because collagen is the principal structural protein in skin, bone, and indeed all human tissue. Collagen is synthesized into an organized cable-like network in a multistep process with both intracellular and extracellular components (Fig. 4.3). The collagen molecule has abundant quantities of two unique amino acids, hydroxyproline and hydroxylysine. The hydroxylation process that forms these amino acids requires ascorbic acid (vitamin C) and is necessary for the subsequent stabilization and cross-linkage of collagen. Procollagen is formed within the fibroblasts as a long linear amino acid segment with regular repeats of hydroxyproline every third amino acid and with terminal extension peptides. Procollagen molecules aggregate in the case of type 1 collagen (the most common) as three α chains to form a triple-helical complex (see Fig. 4.3*A*). The triple helix is maintained by intramolecular disulfide bonds between specific cystine residues. Procollagen is secreted in its triple-helical form; extracellular peptidases cleave the extension peptides at the amino and carboxy termini, leaving the central collagen molecule. Collagen cross-linking (see Fig. 4.3*B*) then occurs in the extracellular space as the collagen molecules aggregate into larger structures. Lysyl oxidase catalyzes the conversion of lysine and hydroxylysine into aldehyde forms. These aldehydes form intermolecular bonds by undergoing spontaneous

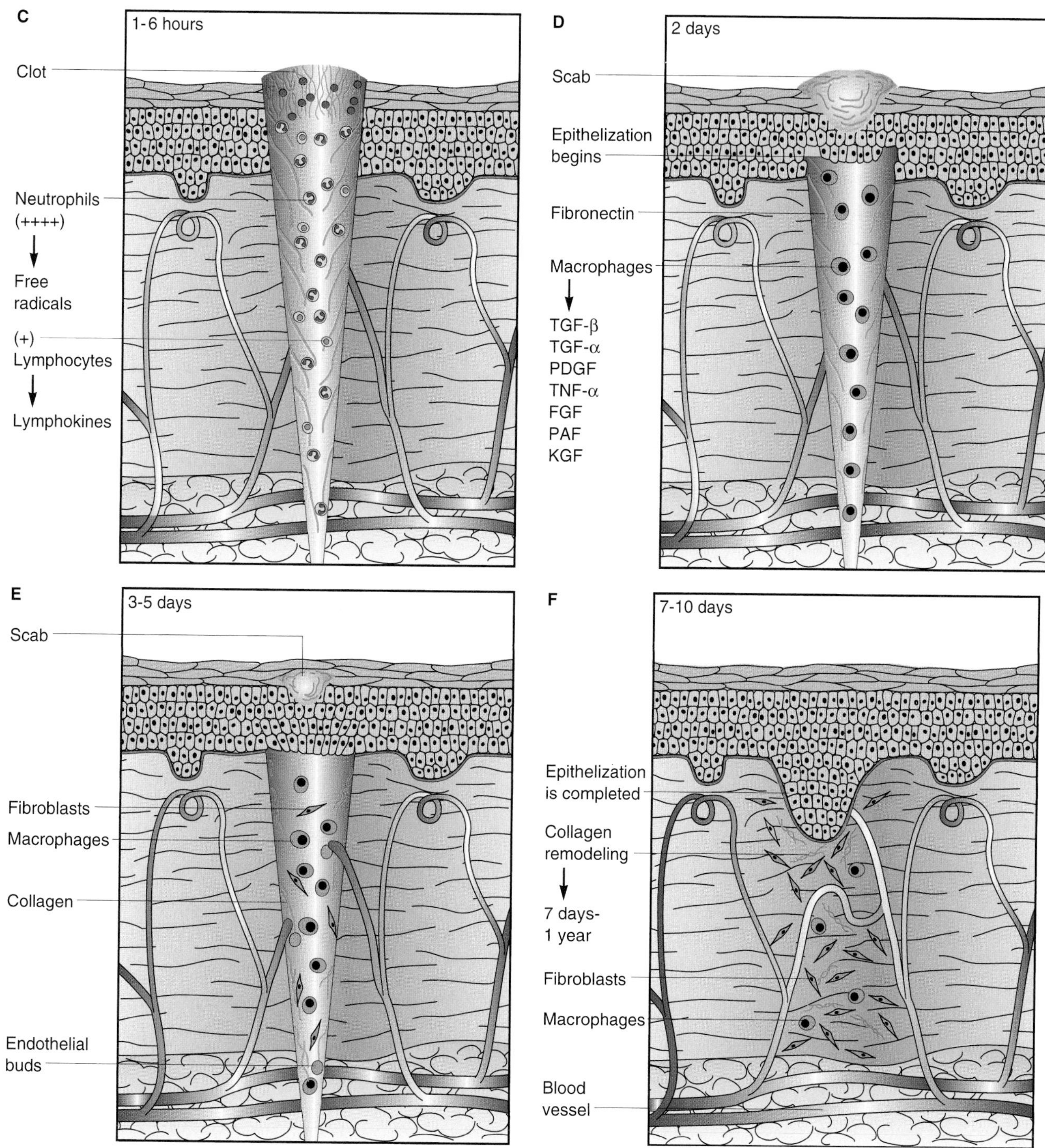

FIGURE 4.2 *(continued)*

condensation. This produces stable, cross-linked collagen fibrils. These intramolecular and intermolecular bonds provide strength and stability. As the wound matures, fibrils cross-link to form large cables of collagen, providing increased tensile strength (see Fig. 4.3C). The wound is now more appropriately considered a scar.

Although there are many types of collagen, type I predominates throughout the body. The principal collagen in scar is type I, with lesser amounts of type III collagen present. Other collagen types make important contributions to the basement membrane, cartilage, and other structures (Table 4.2).

Remodeling Phase: The Formation of Scars

The transition from the proliferative phase to the remodeling phase is defined by reaching collagen equilibrium. Collagen accumulation within the wound reaches a maximum within 2 to 3 weeks after wounding. Although supranormal rates of synthesis and degradation continue throughout remodeling, there is no further change in total collagen content.[4] Tensile strength gradually increases as random collagen fibrils are replaced by organized fibrils with more intermolecular bonds. During the initial phase of wound healing, there is a relative

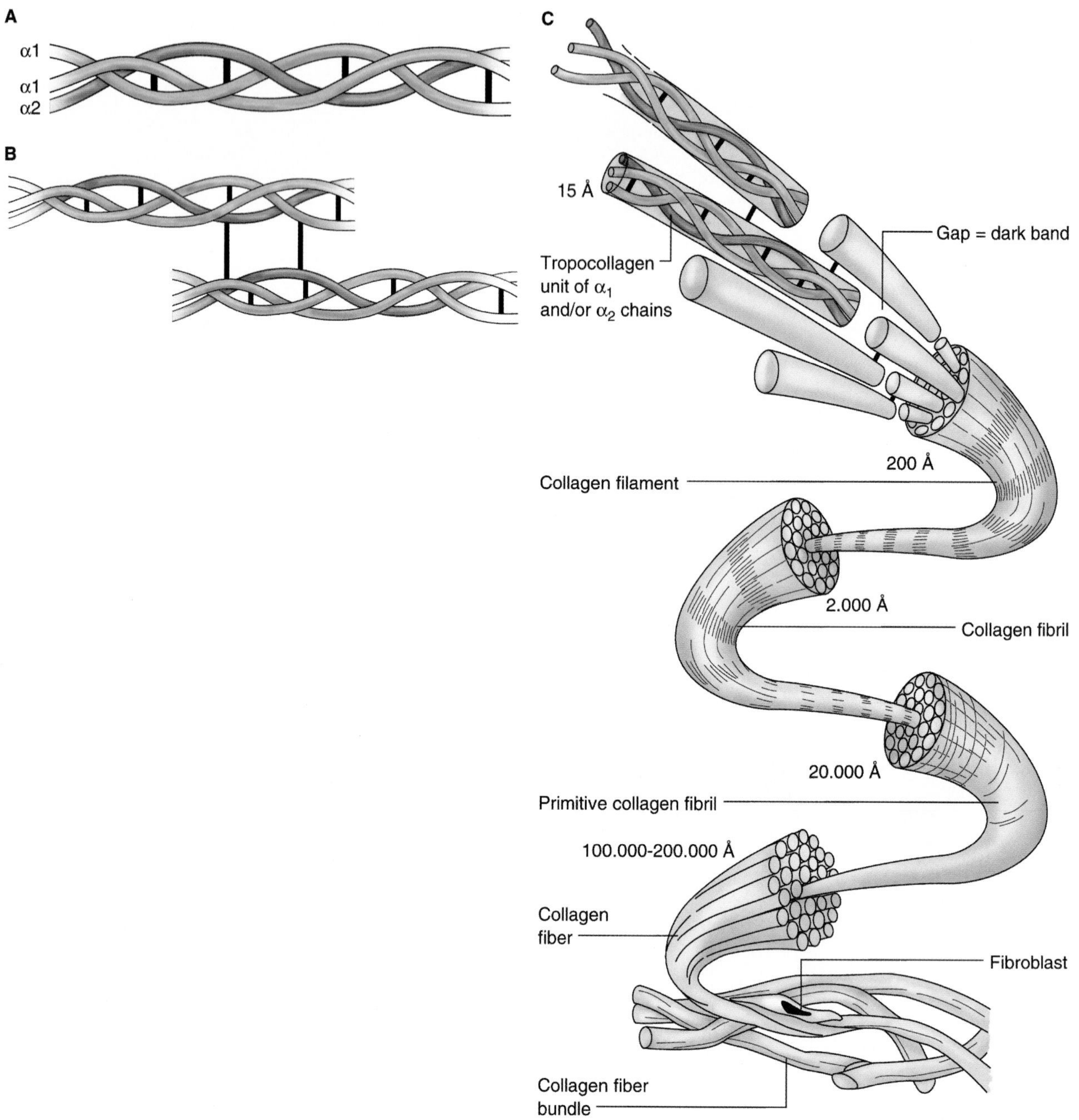

FIGURE 4.3 (*A*) Type I collagen showing triple helix and intramolecular cross-links. (*B*) Intermolecular cross-links provide tensile strength. (*C*) Assembly of collagen fibrils, fibers, and fiber bundles.

abundance of type III collagen in the wound. With remodeling, the normal adult ratio of 4:1 (type I to type III) collagen is restored. Under normal wound healing conditions, the capillary density gradually diminishes, and the number of fibroblasts is reduced. The wound loses its pink or purple vascular color and becomes progressively pale. The collagen undergoes constant remodeling. New collagen is formed, and collagen degradation by specific collagenases is ongoing. Collagenase activity is balanced against new production of collagen to produce a steady state. As equilibrium is achieved, the collagen fibrils align themselves in a longitudinal arrangement as dictated by stress placed on the wound. Scars never achieve the degree of order achieved by collagen in normal skin or tendons, but they do increase in strength for 6 months or longer, eventually reaching 70% of the strength of unwounded skin (Fig. 4.4).

The other important component of the extracellular matrix is the ground substance or proteoglycans. These substances are composed of a protein backbone with long hydrophilic carbohydrate side chains. The hydrophilic nature of these molecules accounts for much of the water content of scars. In the early immature wound, there is a disproportionately large amount of proteoglycans (particularly hyaluronic acid). During the maturation phase, the proteoglycan content returns to a level that closely approximates that of normal skin.

Until recently, the extracellular matrix (predominantly collagen and proteoglycans) was thought to be inert. It is becoming

TABLE 4.2

COLLAGEN TYPES

Type	Property of aggregate unit	Tissue distribution
I	Rigid fibrils	All connective tissue except cartilage
II	Rigid fibrils	Cartilage and vitreous
III	Elastic fibrils	Elastic tissue (e.g., fetal skin, blood vessels, uterus)
IV	Sheet	Basement membrane
V	Fibril	Widespread
VI	Beaded filaments	Widespread
VII	Anchoring fibrils	Interface of basement membrane and underlying stroma
VIII	Sheet	Descemet's membrane
IX	Fibril	Hyaline cartilage
X	Sheet	Hypertrophic cartilage
XI	Fibril	Hyaline cartilage
XII	Fibril	Similar to type I

increasingly clear, however, that extracellular matrix signals certain cells through cell attachment receptors (integrins) and serves as a reservoir for growth factors. Via integrin receptors, the extracellular matrix influences intracellular signal transduction with an impact on cell motility and migration, cellular proliferation, and growth factor production. The role of proteoglycans as signaling molecules is just beginning to be understood. In addition, mechanical forces on tissue are transmitted from the matrix to the cells that are attached to the matrix, and increasing evidence indicates that mechanical forces result in signal transduction, which can result in cellular proliferation, apoptosis, and other signal transduction processes.[5]

Epithelialization

The skin is composed of two layers, the epidermis and the dermis. The outermost layer, the epidermis, is the protective barrier that forms the external interface between the body and the environment. The epidermis protects against water loss, allowing the other cells of the body to live in a liquid environment, as well forming a barrier to bacteria and other environmental factors. Reconstruction of the epithelial barrier (epithelialization) begins within hours of the initial injury. As an initial step, epithelial cells from the basal layer at the wound edge flatten and migrate across the wound, completing wound coverage within 18 to 24 hours in a coapted surgical wound. The cells along the margin are also dividing to re-form the characteristic basilar to apical differentiation of multilayered mature epithelium (see later). Epithelial cells exhibit contact inhibition; that is, they continue to migrate across an appropriate bed until a single continuous layer is formed. Epithelial cell migration occurs by a process in which the epithelial cells send out pseudopods, attaching to the underlying extracellular matrix by integrin receptors. Bacteria, large amounts of protein exudate from leaky capillaries, and necrotic tissue all compromise this process, delaying epithelialization. Delayed epithelialization results in a more profound and prolonged inflammatory process, thereby contributing to unsatisfactory or hypertrophic scarring. There is increasing evidence that reestablishment of a mature epithelium with a multilayered keratin layer (stratum corneum), which completely restores the normal water barrier, is an important component of the scar resolution process. Cell signals from the epithelium have been implicated in the pathogenesis of keloids, and reestablishment of an epithelial barrier

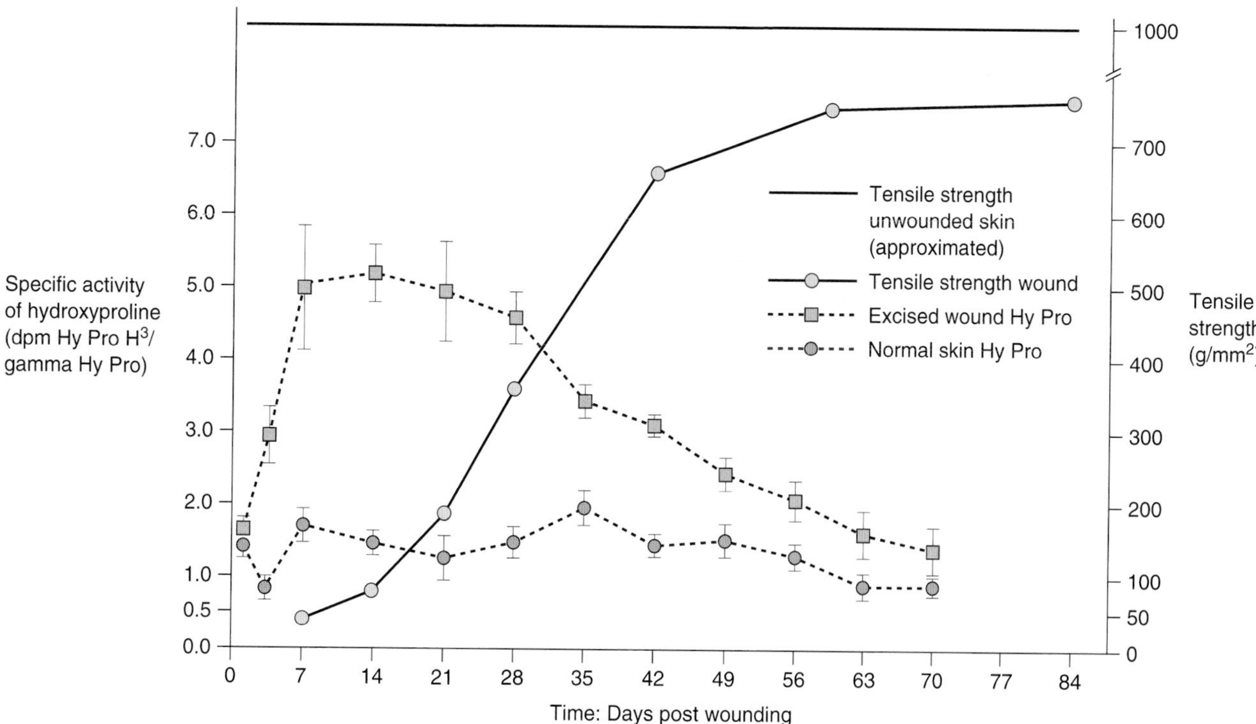

FIGURE 4.4 Relation of the rate of collagen synthesis to the gain of tensile strength of rat skin wounds. (After Madden JW, Peacock EE Jr. Studies on the biology of collagen during wound healing. 1. Rate of collagen synthesis and deposition in cutaneous wounds of the rat. *Surgery* 1968;64:288, with permission.)

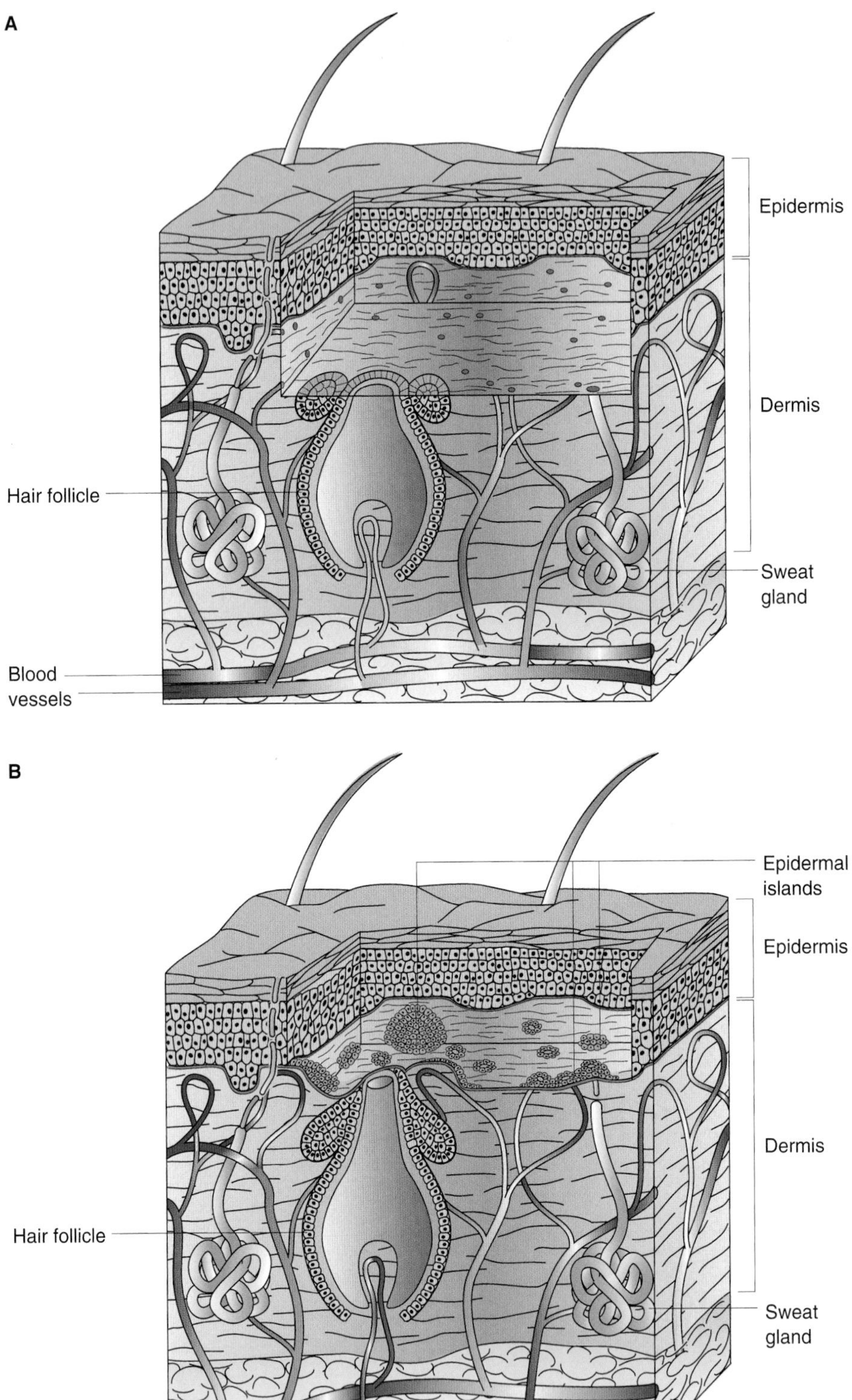

FIGURE 4.5 Reepithelialization of a partial-thickness wound.

by skin graft or flap results in reduction in inflammation and apoptosis of the underlying dermis.[6]

In superficial, partial-thickness wounds, epithelialization results from migration of epithelial cells from remaining dermal appendages, sweat glands, and hair follicles (Fig. 4.5). This is relatively rapid because the distance between hair follicles and sweat glands is short; epithelialization is usually complete within 7 to 10 days. In deeper injuries, however, such as deep second-degree burns, the combination of increased necrosis and fewer remaining dermal appendages can result in delayed epithelialization with prolongation of the inflammatory process.

A partial-thickness burn or abrasion that requires more than 2 weeks to epithelialize has a high incidence of hypertrophic scarring. The increased scarring is presumably

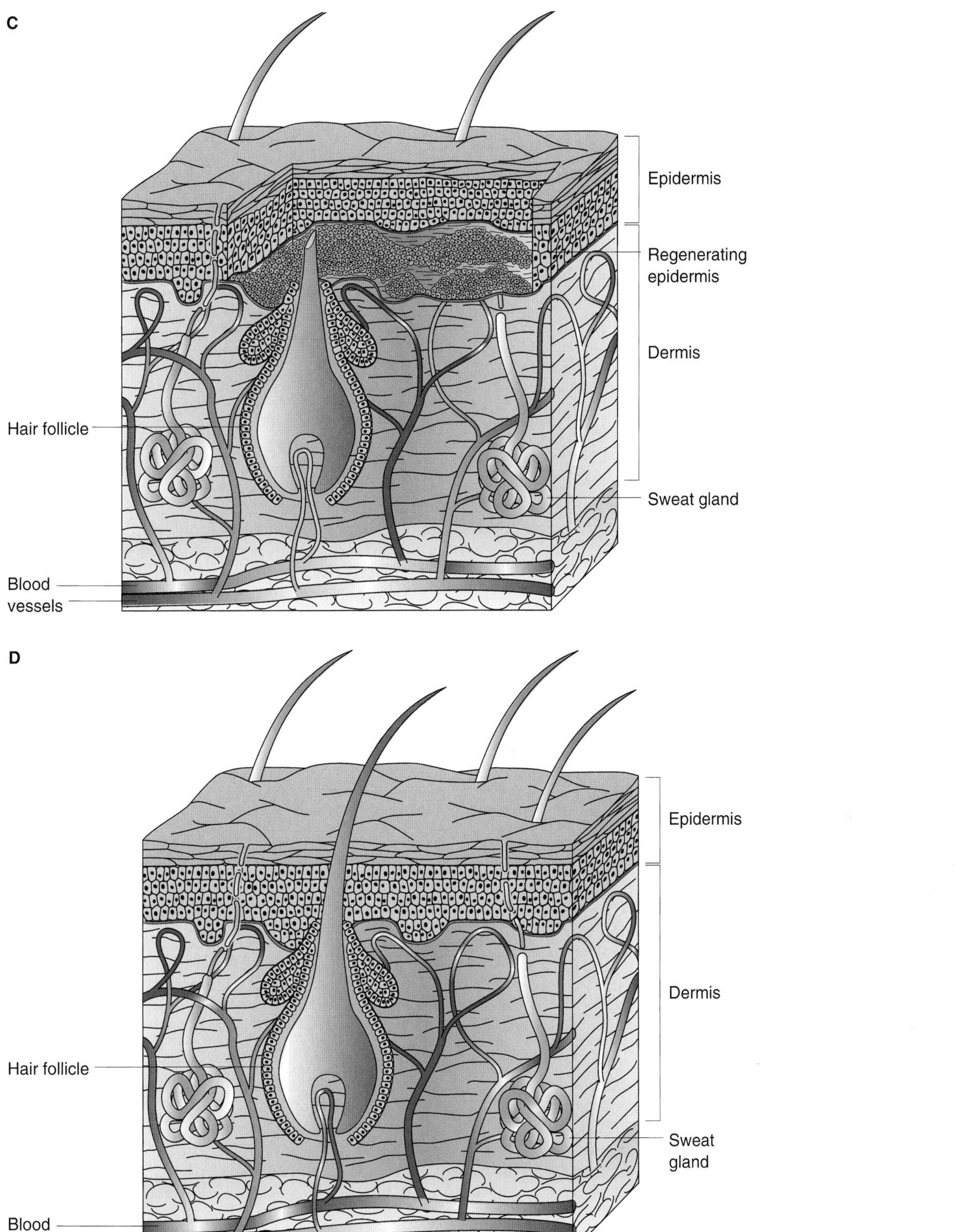

FIGURE 4.5 *(continued)*

secondary to prolonged inflammation. This can be minimized by achieving a closed wound through skin grafting or other techniques. With a partial-thickness wound or abrasion, it is important to achieve rapid epithelialization through maintaining a moist environment and preventing bacterial proliferation by continually removing protein-containing exudates that provide a substrate for bacterial growth.

In full-thickness injury, the entire dermis is destroyed or removed. Epithelialization occurs only from the margins of the wound, at a maximal rate of 1 to 2 mm/day. In practice, adequate coverage of sizable wounds is rarely achieved. Thus, lower leg ulcers rarely heal faster than 1 cm/month; that is, a 2-cm diameter ulcer typically takes 2 months to heal under ideal conditions. In an open wound, the rate of epithelialization is critically dependent on the vascularity and health of the underlying granulation tissue (neodermis) across which it migrates. In addition, cellular migration is dependent on the condition of the matrix. Excess bacterial burden results in secondary PMN influx with protease degradation of the matrix and a hostile environment for cellular attachment and migration. Thus, although chronic wounds are manifested by a failure of epithelial migration, the cause is most often a problem in the underlying wound bed.

The epithelial cells alone provide little strength when not anchored to dermis. They are therefore prone to injury. The basal epidermal cells are attached to the underlying dermis by hemidesmosomes. These structures attach to keratin filaments within the epithelial cells. The hemidesmosomes connect by a series of intermediate proteins to anchoring filaments, long proteins that intertwine with the collagen network of the dermis. Intact epithelium is resistant to sheer forces due to these strong dermal attachments. Without an adequate dermal base, however, epidermis provides unstable wound coverage and is characterized by chronic and recurrent breakdown.

After the first layer of cells restores the epithelial barrier, additional layers develop, restoring the basilar-to-apical order. As the cells mature, they resume keratin formation. This regenerates the stratum corneum of the epidermis and completes the restorative process of epithelialization and provides stable coverage.

Scar

Visible scarring occurs only when the injury extends deeper than the superficial dermis. Superficial abrasions and burns usually heal without scarring even if the superficial dermis is involved, because a thin layer of scar in the superficial dermis is not visible. Whenever the dermis is incised, a scar forms. Scar formation at the molecular level is due to disorganized collagen. In response to injury, dermal integrity is restored by collagen synthesis and deposition. Over the time of scar maturation (6 months to several years), scar remodeling results in progressive collagen linking and increased organization, but the parallel organized collagen layers of normal skin are never completely reconstituted, resulting in visible scar. The prominence of the scar is variable and can be minimized by location and closure technique. If an incision is made, however, a scar is inevitable. The quality of the scar is impacted by a number of factors. The underlying genetic tendency to scar is a significant factor. It is well known that some Africans form keloids from even minor insults, and approximately 5% to 10% of African-Americans are keloid prone. Many Asians (as many as 50% of Chinese, Korean, and Japanese) have some tendency to form hypertrophic scars. Elderly patients heal with less inflammation and rarely form hypertrophic scars. Scars parallel to collagen fibers in relaxed skin tension lines form much better scars than those perpendicular to relaxed skin tension lines. As discussed previously, mechanical forces stimulate cell proliferation and collagen synthesis, so that scars closed under tension after skin excision or in locations subjected to tension such as the sternum or shoulder are prone to scar hypertrophy.[7]

Stretch marks are a unique type of scar. Stretch marks occur when the collagen fibers in the dermis are stretched to the point of disruption, but the epidermis is not disrupted. This results in scar formation in the dermis that is visible through an intact, unscarred epidermis. There is no treatment for stretch marks other than excision of the skin (which of course results in scar from wound closure) or tissue destruction, which can in exceptional circumstances result in wound contraction and some shrinkage of the stretch marks (the rationale for treating stretch marks with laser).

Clinical Implications

Optimal Outcomes from Surgical Closure

This review of normal wound healing has numerous practical implications to the care of wounds and surgical incisions. Meticulous hemostasis reduces the inflammation and phagocytosis necessary to clear the wound of blood. The use of electrocautery should be judicious. Electrocautery results in a band of tissue necrosis that varies in thickness in relation to heat generated. The benefits in hemostasis from cautery must be balanced with the thermal injury that results, to minimize stimuli for inflammation. Atraumatic handling of tissue decreases the load of necrotic or nonviable cells at the wound margin. This is best achieved using fine forceps or skin hooks to retract and assist in coapting the dermis. Crush injury to the epidermis with forceps should be avoided. Deep sutures are best placed only into collagen-laden structures that can hold tension, that is, fascia and dermis. These tissues have the tensile strength to hold sutures under tension. Fat does not contain collagen and does not hold tension. Therefore, fatty tissue should not be sutured as a separate layer. Dead space obliteration and fluid evacuation are best achieved by suction drainage rather than by adding additional foreign material to the wound in the form of suture material. Therefore, in closing a laparotomy incision, even in a morbidly obese patient with a 2-inch panniculus, the closure should be limited to the abdominal fascia, the skin, and rarely the Scarpa's fascia.

Under normal circumstances, epithelialization of an incision is complete within 24 to 48 hours, and there is no reason to protect the incision from water beyond this time. Allowing the patient to wash or shower 1 or 2 days after surgery has significant psychologic benefit and gently débrides the incision and keeps it clean by rinsing away surface bacteria and debris. Blood and protein exudate are an excellent culture media for any skin surface bacteria. Showers reduce the chance of bacterial accumulation in surface crusts along the incision and on the sutures. This decreases inflammation and prevents breakdown of the fragile epithelial layer over the incision, improving the quality of the scar. In addition, there is increasing acceptance of the concept that covering immature epidermis for a period of as long as 2 months with paper tape, silicone gel sheeting, or other materials improves scar outcome, most likely due to restoring the water barrier of mature stratum corneum, as discussed previously.[7]

OPEN WOUNDS (ACUTE)

Open wounds, whether ulcers or open surgical incisions closing by secondary intention, heal with the same sequence of inflammation, matrix deposition, epithelialization, and scar maturation as previously described. However, there are some important differences. In the closed (sutured) incisional wound, the healing process progresses through an orderly temporal sequence. In an open wound, the healing events are spatially separated. In the healing wound, a bed of granulation tissue forms over the exposed subcutaneous tissue. Granulation tissue is composed of new capillaries; proliferating fibroblasts; and an immature matrix of collagen, proteoglycans, substrate adhesion molecules (including fibronectin, laminin, and tenascin), and acute and chronic inflammatory cells. In addition, there are variable amounts of bacteria and protein exudate, depending on the "health" of the wound. At the advancing edge of epithelium, the process of acute inflammation is present. Behind the advancing edge, there is a proliferative area, and further behind, the scar is maturing and remodeling.

An understanding of the biologic principles of wound healing has direct clinical implications in wound care, particularly in the case of chronic wounds (e.g., pressure sores, lower leg ulcers, diabetic foot ulcers).

The most important clinical factor in the healing of surgical incisions is the gain in tensile strength of the wound. This was discussed previously and depends almost entirely on collagen deposition. The rate of collagen synthesis determines the initial wound strength; ultimate wound strength is determined by the degree of collagen organization and cross-linking. The healing of open wounds is defined primarily by epithelialization, and successful healing is related more to the maintenance of epithelial integrity than to the tensile strength of the scar. As discussed earlier, the rate of epithelialization in open wounds is limited by the rate of migration of the proliferating epithelial edge. Factors that regulate epithelial migration are an area of active research. There is clear evidence that the extracellular matrix (collagen, fibronectin, basement membrane proteins, and glycosaminoglycans) is composed of structural elements that are not inert. They function as an essential substrate, with adhesion molecules regulating intercellular communication. The cellular occupants of the matrix express specific receptors that recognize amino acid sequences on the matrix proteins. This allows for cellular attachment at specific sites, cell locomotion, and intracellular signal transduction. Rapid epithelialization is therefore dependent on an optimal matrix, synthesized by the underlying granulation tissue, as well as on optimal delivery of nutrients and oxygen by an adequate blood supply.

Inflammatory cells in open wounds, especially the macrophages, release growth factors. Growth factors enhance migration and proliferation of fibroblasts and endothelial cells in wounds. In an open wound, this leads to the formation of granulation tissue, the cobblestone-like, pink surface of healthy new tissue. The ability of an open wound to form granulation tissue is governed by the blood supply to the tissue and the relative absence of devitalized tissue and bacteria. Therefore, wounds that form granulation should heal or be amenable to surgical closure with flaps or skin grafts. Wounds that do not form granulation tissue are very likely to be recalcitrant to all treatments except those directed at the underlying cause of the failure to form granulation tissue, that is, vascular bypass to restore adequate blood flow to an ischemic extremity wound.

Wound Contraction

Wound contraction is an important event that contrasts the healing of open wounds with closed incisions. When open wounds contract, the surrounding skin is pulled over the wound to reduce its size. This can occur much faster than epithelialization. In addition to increasing the speed of wound closure, another advantage is that the open wound is resurfaced by the normal sensate skin surrounding the wound. Most animals are loose skinned—meaning that the skin (epithelium, dermis, subcutaneous fat) is only loosely attached to the underlying muscle fascia. Some animal wounds heal almost entirely by contraction; for example, a 2-cm ulcer heals to a 3-mm point in a loose-skinned animal. Humans, however, do not have this degree of skin mobility in most sites; the skin is tightly adherent and less elastic, especially in the lower leg. Therefore, although contraction may account for 90% of the reduction in wound size on the perineum, it accounts for at most 30% to 40% of the healing of a lower leg ulcer. This is one important reason why leg ulcers are so slow to heal. All healing wounds generate a strong contractile force.[8] When this contractile force is exerted across a joint, such as the neck, axilla, or elbow, it may result in a scar contracture. A scar contracture is a scar that limits the functional range of motion of a joint.

At the cellular level, the forces that drive wound contraction come from the fibroblasts. Fibroblasts, like muscle cells, contain actin microfilaments. When these filaments increase in number, the cells take on the morphologic appearance of myofibroblasts. Myofibroblasts are seen in increased numbers in contracting wounds, but their role is unclear. It is unknown whether the fibroblasts that attach to the collagen fibrils by means of integrin receptors move collagen fibers together using a locomotor action or whether the contraction comes from intrinsic cellular contraction, but it is likely that contraction is due to a combination of the two. The forces of contraction continue as long as there is inflammation and collagen remodeling.

Unless created and dressed under sterile conditions, all open wounds are contaminated by the bacterial flora on the surrounding skin and from the environment. Even when dressed under sterile conditions, bacterial colonization will occur within about 48 hours from the surrounding skin. Bacterial colonization of the wound is routine and is not deleterious to normal healing. Bacterial infection, however, is deleterious and can delay or prevent healing. Cellulitis or invasive bacterial infection of the surrounding tissues is relatively easy to diagnose with experience. Treatment typically requires systemic antibiotic therapy. Distinguishing wound colonization from excess bacterial load resulting in excess inflammatory cells, protease degradation of matrix, and impaired healing, however, can be difficult. The burn wound experience has demonstrated that bacterial counts of more than 10^5 organisms per gram of tissue on quantitative analysis are associated with failure of surgical wound closure. This is an important technique, because clinical judgment is inadequate. The failure of wound closure in this circumstance is in part due to bacterial and phagocytic proteases that prevent healing. In a similar fashion, if the bacterial count is above this threshold in the wound granulation tissue, the endotoxins and excessive proteases, derived from both bacteria and PMNs, delay epithelialization. Several experimental systems have demonstrated that an excess of PMNs in wound delays healing. Clinical experience with pilonidal wounds, with no other risk factors for impaired healing other than an increased bacterial burden, indicates resolution of that one variable can result in rapid healing of wounds that have remained open for months or even years.

Any nonepithelialized wound leaks plasma. With more inflammation, capillary permeability is further increased. Increased microvascular permeability results from endothelial cell injury or dysfunction. This is mediated by many components of the inflammatory cascade, including histamine, kinins, complement, PGE_2, PGI_2, and others. This exudate of serum proteins and inflammatory cells serves as a rich culture medium, which may continue the cycle of bacterial proliferation and leads to more exudate formation. The net result of this cycle is delayed or absent wound healing. In addition, the edema that results from capillary dysfunction increases the distance for diffusion from oxygen and nutrient sources to their metabolic targets.

Clinical Features

Basic principles of wound care should be tailored to assist the mechanism elaborated earlier, leading to more rapid healing. Although many varieties of wound care are practiced, Winter and Scales[9] first recorded that epithelialization is more rapid under moist conditions than dry conditions. Without dressings, a superficial wound, or one with minimal devitalized tissue, forms a scab or crust. The scab forms when blood and serum coagulate, dry, and form a protective moisture barrier over the open wound (Fig. 4.6). Epithelialization occurs with

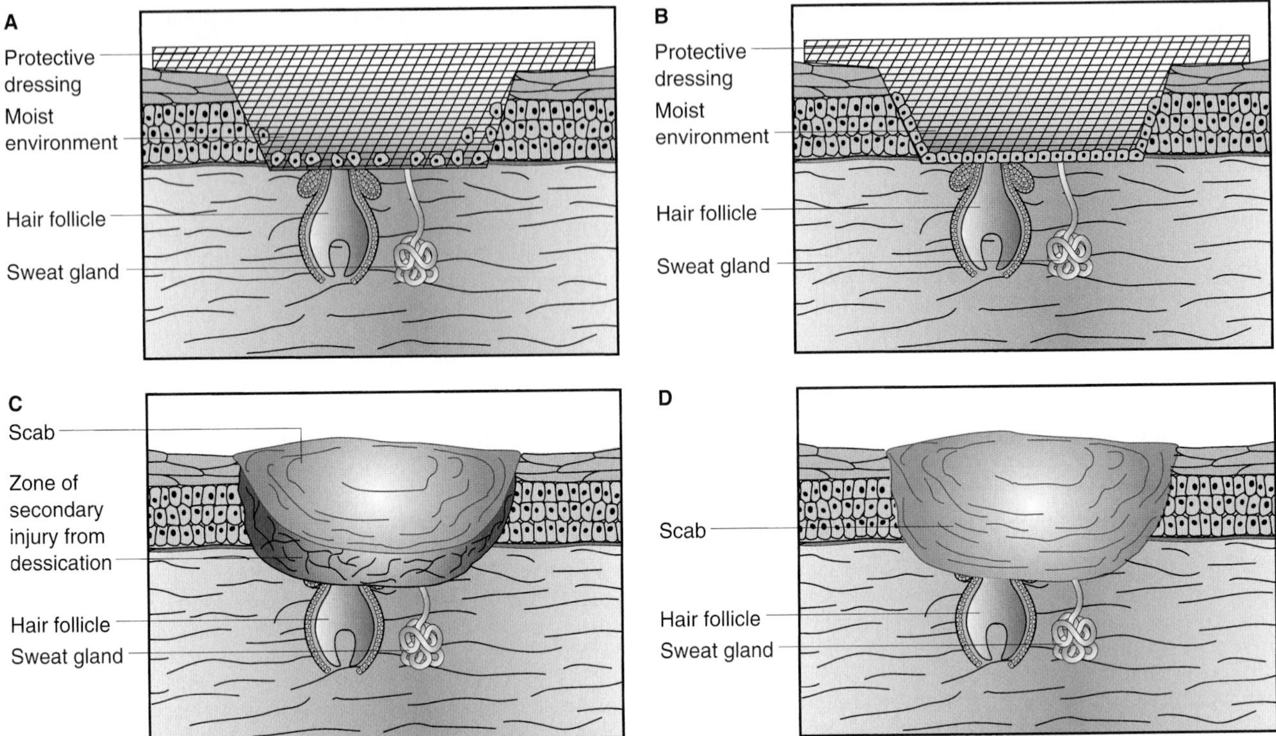

FIGURE 4.6 Rapid epithelialization occurs in a moist environment. Desiccation delays healing by causing tissue necrosis in the exposed wound. The scab ultimately forms a moisture barrier, and epithelialization occurs from the wound edge and any remaining dermal appendages (see Fig. 4.5).

controlled clot proteolysis and migration of the epithelium under the clot. If the wound is kept moist with an occlusive dressing, however, and the exudate does not become infected, then epithelial migration is optimized. A skin graft donor site, for example, epithelializes several days faster under an occlusive dressing than a dry dressing. In addition, the pain of an open wound or skin graft donor site is dramatically reduced under an occlusive dressing.

Moist healing can be achieved by occlusive dressings, occlusive ointments or creams, or continually moistened dressings. The traditional wet to dry dressing, however, if truly left to dry, simply produces desiccation and necrosis of the surface layer of the wound, delaying epithelialization. Although wet to dry dressings can be effective for débridement of wound exudate, they are generally less desirable than a moist healing environment combined with effective cleaning of the wound (i.e., water irrigation).

Role of Oxygen

Oxygen is necessary for normal metabolic cellular function, but in wounds with actively proliferating and metabolically stimulated cells, it is even more critical. PMNs require ambient PO_2 levels of 25 mm Hg to produce superoxide radicals, which serve an essential role in bacterial killing. The enzyme system that generates superoxide and its derivative oxidant products functions optimally at PO_2 levels greater than 50 mm Hg. Collagen synthesis is also highly dependent on an adequate tissue oxygen tension. A fresh wound is initially avascular and is always hypoxic relative to the surrounding tissues. In the center of a new wound, the tissue PO_2 can drop to near zero. After angiogenesis and the delivery of oxygenated blood, the tissue PO_2 quickly rises. Generally, the tissue oxygen tension in a wound is lower than that of surrounding normal tissues. Atherosclerosis of major arteries, small vessel disease from other causes, impaired oxygen delivery, local scarring with fibrosis, and other events may reduce local tissue PO_2 levels from normal (about 40 mm Hg) to less than 25 mm Hg. If so, tissue hypoxia results in significantly impaired wound healing. In the postoperative patient, suboptimal skin perfusion due to even modest hypovolemia, smoking-related arteriopathy, or excess circulating epinephrine can result in a low tissue PO_2. Subcutaneous tissue oxygen levels have been correlated clinically with surgical complication rates. Supplemental oxygen, optimal fluid administration, pain control, and arterial reconstruction all have potential roles in the effort to enhance the tissue PO_2. Oxygen delivery to tissue is the primary determinant of healing; anemia alone is not specifically detrimental to wound healing.[10]

Hyperbaric oxygen therapy (HBO) can achieve high oxygen levels in most wounds for the duration of the treatment, usually 1.5 hours at a time. The patient is placed in the hyperbaric chamber and is exposed to 2 to 2.5 atmospheres of pressure and 100% oxygen. Although oxygen is a necessary component in aerobic metabolism, it may also act as a signaling molecule for growth factor production. There is extensive clinical experience suggesting clinical efficacy of HBO, but conclusive prospective randomized trials have not been conducted. It is clear that HBO can raise the PO_2 in ischemic wounds, but the indications, length of treatment, and number of treatments is still empiric. Based on the success of a number of retrospective studies, the usage of HBO in recent years has become widespread, particularly with diabetic foot ulcers and wounds that have been irradiated.

The role of oxygen is a therapeutic agent has been in part stimulated by an increased understanding of the role of oxygen in intracellular signaling. Previously, oxygen was thought to play an essential role in oxidative metabolism, but oxygen sensors were thought to be limited to the kidney (erythropoietin synthesis), the carotid body, and other specialized organs. However, there has been a great deal of interest, in recent years, on the existence in every cell of signal transduction pathways in response to hypoxia. These pathways are mediated by hypoxia inducible factor that is transported to the nucleus and binds to the promoter region to activate synthesis of many genes including growth factors, VEGF, and TGF-β. Therefore, there is a plausible role for intermittent oxygen therapy to induce signal transduction and improve wound healing. The amount of oxygen necessary to result in a therapeutic effect is unknown, but in the acute surgical situation there are data indicating a beneficial effect from supplemental oxygen in the immediate postoperative period. For the treatment of chronic wounds, placing the wound in an enriched oxygen environment has had some anecdotal interest.[11]

Another approach to increasing local tissue oxygenation is to increase blood flow. A number of studies have suggested that increasing local skin temperature has resulted in improved wound healing.

Role of Edema

In normal tissue, each cell is only a few cell diameters away from the nearest capillary and receives nutrients and oxygen by diffusion. However, with inflammation, venous insufficiency, or any other causes of edema formation, the sequestered extracellular and extravascular fluid increases the diffusion distance for oxygen and results in a lower tissue PO_2. In the case of lower extremity venous insufficiency, the chronic protein leak from the capillaries results in pericapillary deposition. This "cuffing" is a further barrier to oxygen and nutrient diffusion and possibly functions as a site of nonspecific binding of growth factors, making them less available to the wound environment. The importance of edema control is often underestimated. Even in extremities that are not noticeably swollen, elevation and other methods of edema control (elastic wraps, compression stockings, and sequential compression machines) can be of substantial benefit. The most important therapeutic maneuver in the healing of leg ulcers associated with venous insufficiency is edema control with leg elevation, compression stockings or compressive dressings, and, in severe cases, intermittent or sequential compression devices.

Role of Tissue Necrosis and Exudate

Open wounds often contain devitalized tissue as a result of injury and may be aggravated by infection or suboptimal tissue perfusion. If the amount of dead tissue is large, the impairment to healing is obvious, but it is often not fully appreciated that smaller amounts of necrotic tissue or fibrinous exudate also delay healing. In addition, any open wound constantly produces an exudate of serum proteins and dead inflammatory cells, which increases devitalized tissue, if present. The net result is increased exudate, higher bacterial counts, edema, more proteases and other inflammatory mediators, and a deleterious effect on healing. Therefore, devitalized tissue, especially dermis, generally requires surgical excision. If necrotic dermis is left in place, the underlying subcutaneous tissue (fat), which is less vascular, eventually becomes infected. Small amounts of devitalized tissue and exudate can be débrided or removed with dressings, enzyme application, whirlpools, water irrigation, or simple washing. However, the mechanical débriding action must be sufficient and frequent enough to remove the exudate and debris, producing a clean wound before healing is optimal. Because wounds are painful and the dressings or washing insufficient, the exudate is often not removed adequately. This results in delayed healing. The impact of water irrigation in cleaning a wound and reducing tissue bacterial counts has been underappreciated. Whirlpool can gently clean a wound and modestly reduce tissue bacteria counts, but water under pressure (pulse lavage, syringe irrigation with sufficient force, or even a shower stream or dental water pic), can reduce bacterial counts in tissue by several logs.

CHRONIC WOUNDS

A practical definition of a chronic wound is one that has failed to heal within 3 months. Although there are a variety of underlying causes, most can be categorized as pressure sores, diabetic foot ulcers, or leg ulcers. An important question is whether chronic wounds are intrinsically different than acute wounds. For instance, does local tissue senescence make healing a chronic wound impossible? Or, do chronic wounds have the inherent potential to heal, but a combination of factors lead to delayed healing? Research in the past few years has begun to address the question of what is different about the environment in a chronic wound.

Clinicians have long recognized that most chronic wounds do indeed have the potential to heal. Healing usually does not occur because of inadequate attention to the basic principles of open wound care—adequate cleansing, débridement, edema control, avoidance and treatment of ischemia, and achievement of a moist wound healing environment. However, the wound environment in many chronic wounds does differ in important ways from acute wounds. Studies have examined wound fluid and biopsies collected from chronic wounds. These reveal significant increases in tissue levels in proteases and collagenases, which are capable of degrading matrix proteins and growth factors. Degradation of growth factors inhibits their crucial functions of proliferation and chemotaxis. When wound fluid from a chronic wound is compared with fluid from an acute surgical wound, there is indeed a decreased level of growth factors. It is not clear what influence bacteria have in this process, although the direct release of bacterial proteases and the indirect effect of protease release from phagocytic cells are both relevant. It is unknown whether growth factor levels are depressed because of proteolysis, primary inhibition of release, or secondary phenotypic changes in the cells of the chronic wound.

Another important factor in the genesis of chronic wounds is the fact that their occurrence is generally in the aged who have an impaired response to the stress factors of local tissue hypoxia, the increase in reactive oxygen species generated by inflammatory cells, and the existing bacterial burden. As mentioned previously, most chronic wounds are of three types: pressure sores, diabetic foot ulcers, and venous leg ulcers. In all three cases, the inciting injury is an ischemia reperfusion injury. In the first two, pressure exceeding tissue perfusion resulting in a period of ischemia is followed by reperfusion. Repeated cycles of ischemia and reperfusion are much more damaging than an ischemic insult by itself. Experimental evidence in animals supports the notion of an increase in tissue damage in response to an ischemia reperfusion injury.[12]

In chronic wounds, there is some evidence that cells in the periphery of the wound can become senescent after the prolonged stimulus of many months. This is likely a more problematic factor in the elderly and provides a theoretical basis for the efficacy of surgical débridement and excision of the "rind" or callus of a chronic wound, converting it to an acute wound and converting a nonhealing wound to a healing wound.

WOUND MANAGEMENT

Surgical Incisions

It takes at least 3 weeks for collagen to undergo sufficient remodeling and cross-linking to attain moderate strength. Figure 4.4 shows that at 1 to 2 weeks, the time when most sutures are removed, a wound has a small fraction of its eventual strength and may therefore disrupt with even modest stresses. Therefore, deep sutures are placed in collagen-containing structures to hold prolonged tension. Dermis, intestinal submucosa, muscular fascia, tendon, ligament, Scarpa's fascia, and blood vessel wall represent a partial list of tissues with high collagen content. These deep sutures are often absorbable. The most common absorbable material, polygalactic acid (Vicryl, Dexon), retains tensile strength for about 3 weeks. Sutures used for tendon and abdominal fascia are usually permanent or if absorbable should ideally retain their tensile strength for close to 6 weeks. After 6 weeks, wounded tissue has gained about 50% of its eventual strength. To prevent hernia formation, heavy lifting is avoided after major abdominal surgery for 6 weeks. Tendon repairs are splinted and activity restricted to avoid full tension for a similar period.

As discussed in earlier sections, the fibroblasts in a wound respond to mechanical forces, and because skin has elastin fibers and tends to retract in response injury, virtually all wounds are closed under some tension. If the tension forces are relatively large (in excisional wounds, for instance), sutures that effectively splint the wound, preventing the wound fibroblasts from experiencing large mechanical forces, will result in less collagen excess (scar hypertrophy) and less scar stretch. Most absorbable sutures retain their tensile strength for only 3 weeks or so. Studies in humans have demonstrated that this is insufficient to prevent scar widening and results in no better scars than those in which all sutures are removed at 7 days. Therefore, to achieve optimal scars in wounds closed under tension or in areas such as the shoulder, permanent sutures should be left in place for 6 months until collagen remodeling is essentially complete. A continuous intradermal Prolene suture or intradermal interrupted clear nylon sutures with buried knots will achieve that objective.

Open Wound Dressings

There are at least 150 dressing products commercially available at present. These include multiple topical antibiotics, irrigants, and débriding agents. Although PDGF (Regranex) and an artificial skin equivalent made of a dermis-like matrix covered with cultured epithelium from heterologous human foreskins (Apligraf) have been shown to decrease healing times in certain wounds, standard treatment, which adheres to the principles outlined earlier, may be successfully applied to the vast majority of wounds. There are many good alternative treatments, but to avoid confusion they should be judged according to the following criteria:

1. How effectively is the wound cleaned or débrided?
2. Is moist wound healing achieved?
3. Is edema minimized in the peri-wound tissue?
4. Are new pressure (ischemia reperfusion) insults or wound soilage prevented?
5. Is tissue oxygenation (blood flow) adequate?

In some situations, reduction of tissue bacteria is also an important additional need; this is most often addressed by adequate cleaning and débridement. In the absence of large amounts of necrotic tissue, wound débridement does not need to be accomplished surgically. Proteinaceous exudate can be tenacious, however, and simple application of moist dressings may not be adequate to remove it. Water irrigation either in whirlpools or by water from a handheld shower spray or even from dental water cleaning devices can be gentle and yet generate enough power to effectively débride.[13] Frequent moist dressing changes can accomplish this as well, and in some cases, occlusive absorptive dressings can generate enough tissue proteases to effectively degrade proteins that the absorptive dressings remove. This deceptively simple principle is the most frequently overlooked in wound care. The typical open surgical wound often contains deep interstices that packing or other absorptive dressings may not effectively reach. The deeper portions of the wound may then accumulate exudate and bacteria. This is one example in which water irrigation may be particularly useful. Commonly used agents such as hydrogen peroxide are actually harmful to normal tissue and are weak oxidants and thus do a poor job of débriding. These are to be avoided. Enzymatic débriding agents can be effective when properly used.

As discussed, a desiccated wound undergoes delayed healing. Most wounds require an absorptive dressing to remove exudate. This can be gauze, which is inexpensive and effective but which requires frequent dressing changes and is not occlusive so that an ointment or cream must be added. Skin graft donor sites do well with an occlusive polyurethane film dressing. Most of the newer dressing products have been designed to be more absorptive and achieve moist healing without infection from excess exudate. An emphasis has been to decrease the frequency of dressing changes. It must be emphasized that although factors such as convenience, patient acceptance, and cost are good reasons for choosing a product, as long as moist healing is achieved, there is no evidence that one is better than another.

Edema is detrimental to wound healing and is often undertreated, in part because of difficulties in patient education. Edema can be a factor in virtually any ulcer of the lower extremity, although venous insufficiency is the most important. Because patients often have personal habits that are hard to modify, this can be a refractory problem. Patients often object to compression stockings, the most effective method for limiting edema. This leaves intermittent leg elevation, elastic wraps, and elevation of the foot of the bed as alternative measures. The critical factor is getting the patient to realize that leg swelling must be avoided, and so in the course of the day, each patient must modify behavior sufficiently to treat this problem.

Systemic Factors Affecting Wound Healing

Several important systemic factors or conditions influence wound healing. Interestingly, there are no known systemic conditions that lead to more rapid wound healing. The discussion that follows relates to factors that may retard or inhibit wound healing.

Nutrition

Wound healing requires energy and is an anabolic process. Patients who are severely malnourished or who are actively catabolic demonstrate impaired healing. Although there is no single measure of nutritional adequacy, the serum albumin level is the most readily available and clinically useful parameter. A serum albumin greater than 3.5 g/dL suggests adequate protein stores and positive nitrogen balance. However, albumin has a serum half life of 19 days. Therefore, the serum albumin level does not drop early in a catabolic process and is slow to rise when protein stores are repleted and an anabolic state returns. Serum transferrin has a shorter half-life and, therefore, responds more promptly to nutritional fluctuations, but it is not part of a routine chemistry panel and has not gained widespread clinical usage. There is no consensus on nutritional parameters that accurately predict surgical complications. In considering closure of a chronic wound such as a pressure sore, the ability to form granulation tissue and begin wound contraction are clinical indications of acceptable wound healing potential. The presence of a granulating, contracting wound argues strongly that the patient has adequate nutrition to undergo surgery, just as its lack argues strongly against. Certainly an albumin level of less than 3 mg/dL raises concern for potential wound healing problems. Most surgeons avoid trying to close chronic wounds surgically until nutritional levels are considered acceptable.

Vitamins play an important role in wound healing as well. Vitamin A is involved in the stimulation of fibroplasia, collagen cross-linking, and epithelialization. In animal studies, vitamin A reverses the inhibitory effects of glucocorticoids on the inflammatory phase of wound healing.[14] Although there is no conclusive evidence in humans, vitamin A may be useful clinically for steroid-dependent patients who have problematic wounds or who are undergoing an extensive surgical procedure. Vitamin A may be used either topically or systemically, but attention should be paid to the dosage and duration of therapy as vitamin A is fat soluble and has a well-defined toxicity state. An oral dose of 25,000 IU daily or topical application of 200,000 IU ointment three times a day should be sufficient.

Vitamin C is a necessary cofactor in the hydroxylation of lysine and proline in collagen synthesis and cross-linkage. The deficiency state, scurvy, is rarely seen in the Western world today. The utility of vitamin C supplementation in patients who are taking a normal diet is not established.

Vitamin E is applied to wounds and incisions by many patients. The evidence to support this practice is entirely anecdotal, and, in fact, large doses of vitamin E have been found to inhibit wound healing.[15] Only massage, pressure, and silicone sheeting have been shown to flatten and soften scars. Many people perceive a healing benefit from topical creams, but it is very difficult to exclude the two main variables in scar formation: (a) Scars improve with passage of time and (b) natural variability in scar formation, between different individuals and in the same individual in different locations and at different ages.

Essential fatty acids are required for all new cell synthesis. Essential fatty acid deficiency is first noted in areas of high cellular turnover, such as healing wounds, skin, and gastrointestinal mucosa. Early experience with total parenteral nutrition in which essential fatty acids were lacking showed that patients developed difficult wounds and dramatic skin changes. These were rapidly reversed with the addition of fat to the parenteral nutritional program.

Zinc and copper are also important cofactors for many enzyme systems that are important to wound healing. Deficiency states have been seen with parenteral nutrition but are rare and now readily recognized and treated with supplements.

Vitamin and mineral deficiency states clearly show the necessity of these agents for wound healing. However, these deficiency states are extremely rare in the absence of parenteral nutrition or other extreme dietary restrictions. There is no evidence to support the concept that supranormal provision of these factors enhances wound healing in normal patients. Significant complications, especially with excessive fat soluble vitamin supplementation, are reported. However, malnutrition can be a significant problem in the elderly and debilitated patient. These patients require nutritional supplementation and should receive vitamin and mineral supplementation as part of their protein and caloric repletion.

Aging

There are important age-dependent aspects of wound healing. The elderly heal more slowly and with less scarring. There is gradual attenuation of the inflammatory response with age and decreased wound healing is one of the consequences. In vitro studies have documented an age-dependent decrease in the proliferative potential of fibroblasts and epithelial cells. Clinically, these account for the formation of finer scars and improved cosmetic appearance in the elderly. Hypertrophic scars are rarely seen in the elderly. Sutures should be left in place longer to allow for the slower gain in tensile strength in the aged. This may be done without formation of suture marks as slower epithelialization occurs along the sutures. Although the aged usually heal surgical incisions without complications, the combination of age and other adverse factors can result in severe healing deficits and high surgical complication rates (see the previous section on chronic wounds).

Pharmacologic Impairment to Wound Healing

Bone marrow suppression, a common consequence of chemotherapy, is detrimental to wound healing. Quantitative and qualitative lymphocyte and monocyte deficiency impairs cellular proliferation in the inflammatory phase of wound healing. Any chemotherapeutic agent that suppresses the bone marrow will impair healing. Fortunately, this is predictably reversible with cessation of chemotherapy. Glucocorticoids inhibit wound healing based on their anti-inflammatory and immunosuppressive effects. The anti-inflammatory effect of steroids is in part the result of inhibiting arachidonic acid metabolism by impairing macrophage migration and by altering neutrophil function. Glucocorticoids also inhibit synthesis of procollagen by fibroblasts, delaying wound contraction. Steroid-dependent patients have a persistent decrease in wound tensile strength even after healing is complete. Patients who require chronic systemic steroids have attenuation of the dermis and it is therefore susceptible to injury. Even minor shearing forces may produce tearing of the skin and full-thickness wounds due to the decreased tensile strength.

Ischemia

Adequate tissue oxygenation plays a critical role in wound healing.[16] Oxygen is needed for aerobic metabolism and also for proper neutrophil function, especially in bacterial killing. Oxygen is also a requirement for hydroxylation of proline and lysine to form stable collagen fibrils (Table 4.3).

Smoking. Smoking or nicotine patches inhibit oxygen delivery via sympathomimetic vasoconstriction. In addition, smoking elevates carboxyhemoglobin levels in the blood. This effect shifts the oxygen delivery curve to the left due to the high

TABLE 4.3

FACTORS THAT CONTRIBUTE TO WOUND ISCHEMIA

Poor arterial inflow—atherosclerosis
Poor venous flow—venous stasis
Smoking
Radiation
Edema
Diabetes mellitus—accelerates atherosclerosis
Vasculitis
Fibrosis—chronic scarring
Pressure—pressure sores or decubitus ulcer

affinity of carboxyhemoglobin for oxygen, resulting in less available oxygen in the wound. Animal studies demonstrate that even moderate decreases in tissue oxygen tension result in severe impairment of wound healing with substantially increased infection rates. Smoking has been shown to increase wound complication rates when skin flaps are elevated with marginal distal blood supply.

Radiation. Radiation injury leads to arteriolar fibrosis and impaired oxygen delivery. In addition, there is progressive obliteration of blood vessels in the radiated area over time. Radiation also causes intranuclear and cytoplasmic damage to fibroblasts, and this change appears to limit their proliferative potential.

Edema. Edema impairs local oxygen delivery as outlined earlier. In addition, edema is often associated with increased venous pressure. This post capillary obstruction decreases the perfusion pressure in the capillary bed, resulting in ischemia. Increased venous pressure also leads to protein extravasation and pericapillary cuffing. This effect acts as a diffusion barrier to oxygen, further impairing tissue oxygenation and wound healing.

Diabetes. Diabetes mellitus is often associated with decreased healing of open wounds and increased susceptibility to infection. Many factors contribute to poor healing in diabetic patients, and most of these reflect local wound ischemia. However, healing is not impaired in a normally perfused area in a well-controlled diabetic patient. This subject is discussed in detail later.

Neuropathy. There is considerable evidence that neuropeptides promote healing and their absence in the setting of spinal cord injury is a factor in impaired wound healing and may be a factor in the neuropathy of diabetes. This is not a condition that can be treated, although the neuropeptides that impact wound healing are a focus of active research.

Other Local Conditions

Peripheral arterial occlusive disease secondary to atherosclerosis can be a primary cause of impaired healing and may also be a cofactor with other conditions discussed. In addition, conditions such as vasculitis, prolonged pressure, lower leg venous insufficiency, and tissue fibrosis affect wound healing through the mechanism of local tissue ischemia.

Chronic Wound Care

As noted, a chronic wound is commonly defined as an open wound that has failed to respond to standard care and remains open at 3 months. Typically, the wound size is static with an absence of a visible advancing epithelial edge. The etiology of a chronic wound is often multifactorial. One or more factors that impair wound healing, such as advanced age, ischemia, bacterial contamination, edema, and malnutrition or immunosuppression, are often present in patients with chronic wounds. A systematic approach is needed to identify these factors. Once all of the potentially applicable factors have been identified, those amenable to treatment are reversed. Although age is fixed, some impact can be made on most other factors. Wounds should be débrided, and topical as well as systemic antibiotics may be indicated for true bacterial infection. Arterial revascularization can increase oxygenation in the wound and elevation and compression dressings can decrease edema. Skin grafting or other surgical procedures are indicated as long as the underlying processes has been identified and is appropriately treated. The underlying causes of some chronic wounds cannot be corrected. Patients with diabetes or venous insufficiency are among these.

Specific chronic wounds are discussed in the sections that follow.

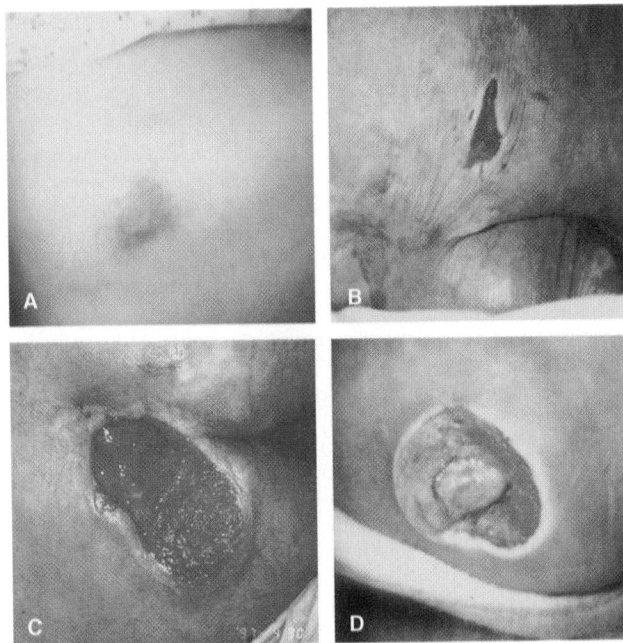

FIGURE 4.7 Pressure ulcer staging. (*A*) Stage I—erythema. (*B*) Stage II—breakdown of the dermis. (*C*) Stage III—full-thickness skin breakdown. (*D*) Stage IV—bone, muscle, and supporting tissue involved. (From Nettina SM. *The Lippincott manual of nursing practice,* 7th ed. Philadelphia: Lippincott Williams & Wilkins, 2001, with permission.)

Pressure Sores

Pressure sores are sometimes mistakenly referred to as bed sores or decubitus ulcers (Fig. 4.7). These sores do not always develop in bed or while lying flat in a decubitus position. All pressure sores, regardless of location, do involve prolonged pressure over a bony prominence followed by reperfusion, which produces much of the injury particularly when there are repeated cycles. The ability of tissue to withstand pressure is defined by the duration of the pressure, the amount of pressure, and related sheer forces. The most frequent locations of pressure sores are overlying the ischium, sacrum, and trochanter. The heel, knee, and ankle are less common locations.

Prolonged pressure produces ischemia in the tissue by occluding the microcirculation. This occurs when the tissue pressure exceeds the capillary filling pressure of 25 mm Hg. Pressure on the tissue overlying the sacrum can reach 80 mm Hg in a recumbent patient, so that tissue necrosis can occur within hours if not relieved by frequent changes in position.

Skin is more resistant to pressure than is the underlying subcutaneous fat (which has less blood supply) or muscle (which, although having an excellent blood supply, is very sensitive to ischemia). This sensitivity accounts for the common finding of a small skin ulceration overlying a large area of subcutaneous necrosis. Efforts to identify and control factors that contribute to impaired wound healing should be made. Nutrition is often a problem as is bacterial overgrowth. If the patient can avoid pressure on the involved area and other contributing factors are controlled, most pressure sores will heal. There is a higher incidence of recurrence if pressure sores are allowed to heal by secondary intention rather than by surgical closure. This difference is explained by the increased scarring that occurs in healing by secondary intention and the fact that this places the scar directly over the pressure point. Because scars are never as strong as intact skin, they are more prone to breakdown than intact skin that has been placed over these pressure points by surgical closure. Patients with significant life expectancy, such as young paraplegics who have a precipitating factor leading to development of a pressure sore, are best treated with surgical flap closure. The recurrence rate can be as high as 90% if chronic issues such as depression are not adequately treated (leading to neglect).

Leg Ulcers

Leg ulcers are perhaps the most common type of chronic ulcer. The underlying disease process is most often local tissue ischemia. The underlying cause of this local tissue ischemia should be identified and appropriate treatment initiated.

About 90% of leg ulcers in the United States are secondary to venous insufficiency (valvular incompetence) (Fig. 4.8). Venous ulcers lead to local tissue ischemia by increased venous pressure, which lowers the transcapillary perfusion pressure, and by leg edema. Initial treatment should be directed to cleansing and débriding the wound of proteinaceous exudate and limiting the edema and protein loss with compression dressings and elevation. A common treatment has been the Unna boot, a paste bandage that is absorptive, limits edema and can be changed weekly. This allows the physician to control treatment with weekly visits. If this dressing is made compressive by adding an elastic wrap, it is highly effective in reducing edema, absorbing exudate, and providing an occlusive wound environment. Its limitations are that it requires weekly visits and precludes normal showering or bathing. Another alternative that has become standard in many venous leg ulcer studies is the four-ply compression garment, in which multiple layers result in effective compression over many days. With effective compression, over 50% of venous ulcers can be healed within a 3- to 4-month period. Compression garments or elastic wraps with frequent dressing changes, thorough cleaning, and an occlusive dressing can be equally effective. Surgical treatment of venous insufficiency is addressed elsewhere and is useful only in isolated instances in which an incompetent perforator can be identified proximal to an ulcer. Valve reconstruction has not achieved widespread acceptance in the United States.

Additional causes of leg ulcers include arterial insufficiency and other vasculitis syndromes. These are treated best by correcting the underlying disease and local wound care. If the underlying problem cannot be treated, there is little hope of securing a stable, healed wound.

Diabetic Foot Ulcers

Diabetic foot ulcers are caused by pressure over bony prominences, usually the metatarsal heads, or calcaneus, in the setting of neuropathy (Fig. 4.9). There is, however, no evidence to support the often-cited concept that these ulcers may result from small vessel disease. This theory originated with a nonblinded study of the microvasculation in amputation specimens by Goldenberg in 1959. Subsequent blinded studies have failed to reveal any architectural differences in small blood vessels of diabetic amputation specimens. The ischemia in diabetic foot ulcers is due to prolonged pressure on insensate toes and feet, with subsequent reperfusion. This pressure ischemia is enhanced by the increase in blood viscosity related to nondeforming erythrocytes, which develop because of nonenzymatic glycosylation of cell membrane proteins. These rigid red blood cells plug capillary beds and decrease microvascular flow. In addition, glycosylated hemoglobin has increased affinity for oxygen, thereby making less oxygen available to the tissues. Diabetic patients also have a predilection for infrapopliteal arterial occlusive disease and may therefore benefit from arterial reconstructive surgery. The requirements for successful treatment of diabetic ulcers include pressure relief with non–weight-bearing strategies and aggressive débridement of callus and marginally vascularized wound edges. Preventive measures with appropriate orthotic shoes are essential once healing is achieved. It should be remembered that it is in clean diabetic forefoot wounds

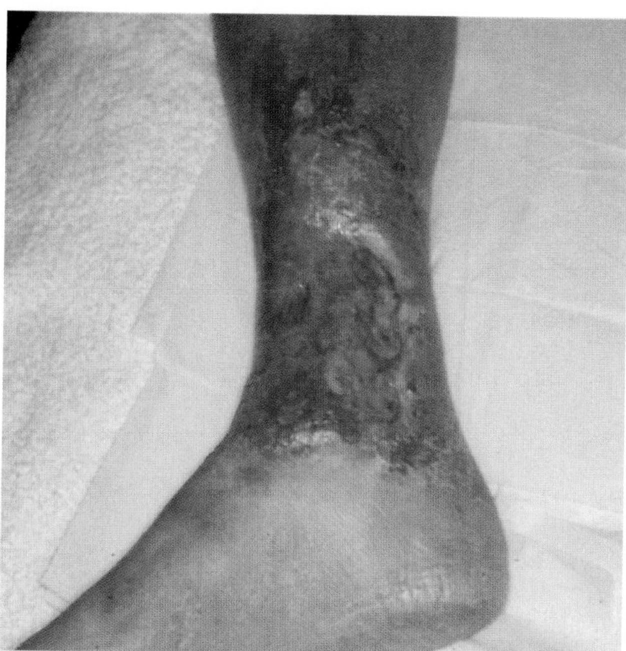

FIGURE 4.8 Venous ulcer. (From Nettina SM. *The Lippincott manual of nursing practice,* 7th ed. Philadelphia: Lippincott Williams & Wilkins, 2001, with permission.)

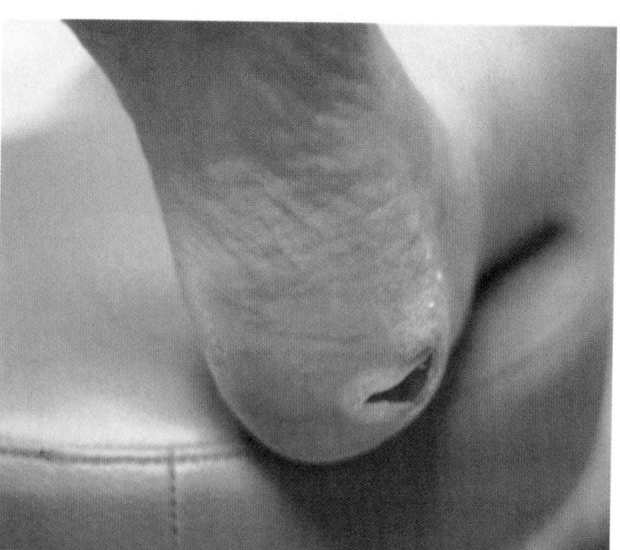

FIGURE 4.9 Diabetic ulcer of the heel. These lesions are noted at sites of pressure, such as the heel in this patient. (From Goodheart HP. *Goodheart's photoguide of common skin disorders,* 2nd ed. Philadelphia: Lippincott Williams & Wilkins, 2003, with permission.)

TABLE 4.4

WOUND DRESSINGS

Classification	Composition	Indications	Functions	Examples
Films	Semiocclusive (semipermeable)—polyurethane or copolyester	Acute partial- or full-thickness wounds with minimal exudate Nondraining primarily closed wounds	Mimics skin performance Is water vapor permeable Is water and bacterial impermeable Is retention dressing for gel Is retention dressing for tubes Provides moist environment	Op-site Bioclusive Tegaderm Blisterfilm Visulin
Hydrocolloids	Contain hydrophilic colloidal particles (quar, karaya, gelatic, carboxymethyl cellulose) in an adhesive mass (usually polysorbutylene)	Acute or chronic partial- or full-thickness wounds Stage I to IV decubitus ulcers	Absorbs fluid Débrides soft necrotic tissue by autolysis Protects wounds Provides good adhesiveness without adherence to wound Encourages granulation Promotes reepithelialization Protects wounds from trauma	Cutinova Hydro Duoderm Comfeel Restore Intrasite Ultec J&J ulcer dressing
Hydrogels	Contain 80%–99% water Cross-linked polymer such as polyethyleneoxide, polyvinyl pyrrolidone, or acrylamide	Acute or chronic partial-thickness wounds with minimal exudate	Creates moist environment Usually requires secondary dressing Has low absorbency Débrides minimally Decreases pain Does not adhere to wound	Vigilon Geliperm Elastogel Intrasite gel
Foams	Either hydrophilic or hydrophobic Nonocclusive Usually polyurethane or gel film-coated High absorbency	Acute or chronic partial-thickness wounds that are highly secreting and require mechanical débriding	Débrides Has high absorbancy Water vapor permeable	Cutinova Plus Lyofoam Allevyn
Impregnates	Fine-mesh gauze impregnated with moisturizing, antibacterial, or bactericidal compounds Nonadherent	Acute or chronic partial-thickness wounds with minimal to moderate exudate	Does not adhere to wound Promotes reepithelialization May contain antibacterial or bactericidal agents Requires secondary dressing	Aquaphor-Gauze Adaptic Biobrane Scarlet Red
Absorptive powders and pastes	Consist of starch, copolymers, or colloidal hydrophilic particles Can absorb up to 100 times their weight in fluid	Chronic full-thickness wounds with large amounts of exudate	Has high absorbancy Débrides necrotic and fibrous material from wound	Spand-Gel Geliperm Envisan paste Bard absorption dressing Duoderm granules Hydrogran Hollister Exudate Absorber

Compiled by M.C. Crossland, RN, Wound Healing Center, Medical College of Virginia, Richmond, VA.

that the clinical effectiveness of becaplermin gel has been demonstrated.

Diabetic foot ulcers are best treated in a multidisciplinary clinic with a combination of surgical and adjunctive measures. If vascular studies indicate significant underlying disease and reduced toe pressures, the leg should be revascularized if possible. Often, diabetics develop altered pressures on their metatarsals and midfeet secondary to neuropathy and loss of functioning intrinsic muscles in the foot. The Achilles tendon can also shorten. In addition to orthotics, surgical procedures to partially correct the altered pressure patterns such as Achilles tendon lengthening can be beneficial. Aggressive surgical débridement to remove callus and convert the chronic wound to a well-vascularized acute wound can be therapeutic. Becaplermin gel has been most efficacious in the setting of aggressive serial débridements.

Agents to Optimize Wound Healing

Dressings

Becaplermin gel has been shown to speed healing in diabetic forefoot wounds and probably has a role in other chronic wounds in which there is a paucity of pharmacologic agents. The biologic dressings Apligraf and Dermagraft have been approved for use in venous ulcers and diabetic ulcers, respectively, and some clinicians feel they play a role in recalcitrant wounds. Many types of dressings are commercially available, and none have been demonstrated to be effective if standard care is ignored. Despite marketing claims, standard wound care, keeping wounds clean, moist, and as free of edema and bacteria as possible, is still the most important factor in wound healing.

The ideal dressing should be simple, inexpensive, highly absorptive, and nonadherent. It should achieve moist healing and have antibacterial properties. Other factors to be considered are less frequent dressing changes, an all-in-one dressing that does not require tape or an overlay, and a gentle adhesive that is effective but not injurious to the skin when removed.[17]

The simplest dressing is gauze and tape—it is inexpensive, is absorptive, and when used with an ointment, can achieve moist healing. The primary disadvantages are the necessity for frequent dressing changes and the potential for tape irritation and wound desiccation. Other products are classified into films, foams, hydrocolloids, hydrogels, and absorptive powders (Table 4.4). Films are semipermeable to water, generally made of polyurethane, and nonabsorptive. These are useful to achieve a moist wound healing environment over minimally exudative wounds, such as a split-thickness skin graft donor site.

Other dressing types have been designed to increase the absorptive capacity of the dressing. This requires fewer dressing changes and maintains an environment for moist healing.

The hydrocolloids deserve special mention because they have achieved widespread use. These contain hydrophilic materials, such as quar, karaya, gelatin, or carboxymethylcellulose, with an adhesive material and are covered by a semipermeable polyurethane film. The material adheres to the skin surrounding a wound, is highly absorptive, and achieves a moist healing environment. Adhesion is maintained until the absorptive capacity is exhausted, and then atraumatic removal is easily done. Similar materials have been extensively used for peristomal care. These are best used for open wounds that have only moderate exudate.

The increased absorptive capacity of these products allows infrequent, minimally traumatic dressing changes. This, along with ease of use and achievement of moist healing, are their principal advantages.

Antibiotics

The role of antibiotics in wound care is controversial. All open wounds are colonized with bacteria. Only when the surrounding tissue is invaded (cellulitis) are systemic antibiotics clearly indicated. Antibiotics may be useful in other situations, such as when the granulation tissue has a high bacterial count or in a case of reduced resistance to bacteria, such as in a diabetic foot ulcer, but these situations are not clearly defined. The routine use of systemic antibiotics for chronic wounds should be avoided to reduce the development of resistant bacterial strains within the wound.

Topical antibiotics are frequently used and can be useful. The ointment vehicle may help keep the wound moist, and the bacteria count in a wound may be lowered as a result. With most antibiotics, however, resistant organisms emerge quickly and development of allergic, hypersensitivity reactions are common. Most topical antibiotic ointments should be limited to 3 weeks of therapy to avoid developing a rash or other signs of inflammation as a result of the antibiotic ointment not bacteria. The expense is substantial, and the benefits are not well demonstrated. Silver sulfadiazine, frequently used for burn care, is also useful for chronic wounds. Its broad spectrum of activity, the lack of relevant drug-resistant plasmids in bacteria, and its low cost make it a good choice.

In recent years, silver impregnated dressings have become available and achieved widespread acceptance. They have the antibacterial activity of silver ions, without the potential for allergy with sulfadiazines, and combine a powerful broad spectrum antibacterial activity without the problems of drug resistance, with the absorptive activities of many dressings.

Débriding Agents

Collagenases have been used to débride wounds for 20 years and can be a highly effective adjunct in the treatment of chronic wounds with necrotic tissue. These agents are used after surgical débridement to help clean a wound and to avoid a painful mechanical débridement. Collagenases that are combined with antibiotic powder have been proposed as a useful treatment for chronic wounds.

Pharmacologic Agents

Growth factors found naturally in wounds have improved healing in both normal and complex animal wounds (Table 4.5). The growth factors with the most evidence for efficacy are PDGF, TGF-β, epidermal growth factor, and members of the FGF family, although IGF1, interleukin (IL)-1, IL-2, granulocyte-macrophage colony-stimulating factor, and VEGF have also shown improved rates of healing in animal models.[18,19] Clinical trials are in progress, and only becaplermin (PDGF) has been approved by the FDA. PDGF has shown efficacy in accelerating healing for patients with clean, well-vascularized diabetic forefoot ulcers. A limiting factor in these clinical trials has been the variability in patients, in terms of both systemic factors that impact healing and the number of variables in the wounds. The clinical studies are therefore difficult to perform and interpret.

Growth hormone deserves brief mention because it has been used successfully in some situations to reverse the catabolic impact of many severe injuries. Wound healing is a fundamentally anabolic event (creating new tissue), and in the setting of a severe burn, growth hormone administration significantly accelerates donor site healing, presumably because of its effects in minimizing catabolism.

TABLE 4.5

SELECTED GROWTH FACTORS RELEVANT TO WOUND HEALING

Factor	Source	Target	Function
TGF-β	All cells	All cells	Fibrosis Proliferation
TGF-α	Platelets Keratinocytes Macrophages	Epithelial cells Fibroblasts Endothelial cells	Proliferation
PDGF	Platelets Macrophages Fibroblasts Endothelial cells Smooth muscle cells	Neutrophils Macrophages Fibroblasts Smooth muscle cells	Chemotaxis Proliferation Collagenase synthesis
FGF	Macrophages Fibroblasts Endothelial cells	Endothelial cells Epithelial cells Fibroblasts Chondroblasts	Proliferation Chemotaxis Angiogenesis
EGF	Platelets Macrophages Keratinocytes	Epithelial cells Endothelial cells Fibroblasts	Proliferation Chemotaxis
IGF-I/Sm-C	Fibroblasts	Fibroblasts Endothelial cells	Cell replication Collagen synthesis
IL-I	Macrophages	Fibroblasts Neutrophils	Proliferation Collagenase synthesis Chemotaxis

TFG-β, transforming growth factor-β; TGF-α, transforming growth factor-α; PDGF, platelet-derived growth factor; FGF, fibroblast growth factor; EGF, epidermal growth factor; IGF-I/Sm-C, insulin-like growth factor I/somatomedin C; IL-I, interleukin-1.

Vacuum Assisted Closure (VAC)

In recent years, VAC therapy has gained increasing acceptance for a wide variety of difficult wounds. This proprietary treatment involves the application of a moderate vacuum to an occlusive dressing with a sponge to allow wicking of the exudates up into the sponge and out of the wound. On theoretical grounds, the VAC is an optimal wound therapy. The negative pressure results in reduction of wound edema and resulting increase in local tissue perfusion. Continual removal of wound exudates removes the media for bacterial growth and results in removal of the bacteria as well, with a resulting reduction in bacterial burden, and the negative pressure accelerates wound contraction. The VAC has found uses in the treatment of chronic wounds and difficult acute wounds; for adherence of skin grafts; and in recent years in the treatment of open sternotomy wounds and exposed joint prostheses, as well as in a variety of other applications. Often, use of the VAC has allowed secondary closure with a skin graft or straightforward secondary closure rather than a complex flap.[20,21]

EXCESSIVE SCARRING

Many factors are involved in the formation of an ideal scar. The most important of these are as follows:

Accurate alignment of sharply incised tissue parallel to the natural lines of resting skin tension

Closure of the wound without tension on the epidermis and without underlying dead space

Primary healing without complications such as infection or dehiscence

The patient's genetic makeup and the location of the wound on the body are also important factors. The more negative factors associated with a particular wound, the more likely it will form a scar that is less than ideal. From an evolutional viewpoint, wound healing has been programmed to be rapid and exuberant to minimize the problems of an open wound. As part of the aging process, the proliferative phase of wound healing becomes less exuberant, and although wound healing is slower, scars are improved (see the remodeling phase section).

The distinctions between an unsightly scar, a hypertrophic scar, and a true keloid can be confusing. An accurate diagnosis of most scars can be made by clinical observation and the history of the lesion.

Keloids

True keloids are uncommon and occur predominantly in dark-skinned people with a genetic predisposition for keloid formation.[7] In most cases, the gene appears to be transmitted in an autosomal dominant pattern. The primary difference between a keloid and a hypertrophic scar is that a keloid extends beyond the boundary of the original tissue injury. It behaves as a benign tumor and extends into or invades the normal surrounding tissue. This creates a scar that is larger than the original wound (Fig. 4.10).

Histologically, keloids contain an overabundance of collagen. The absolute number of fibroblasts is not increased, but the production of collagen continually outpaces the activity of collagenase, resulting in a scar of ever-increasing dimensions. The cause of keloid formation is unknown. Immunoglobulin G levels are increased, which suggests possible autoimmune stimulation resulting in a chronic inflammatory response with continued collagen deposition.

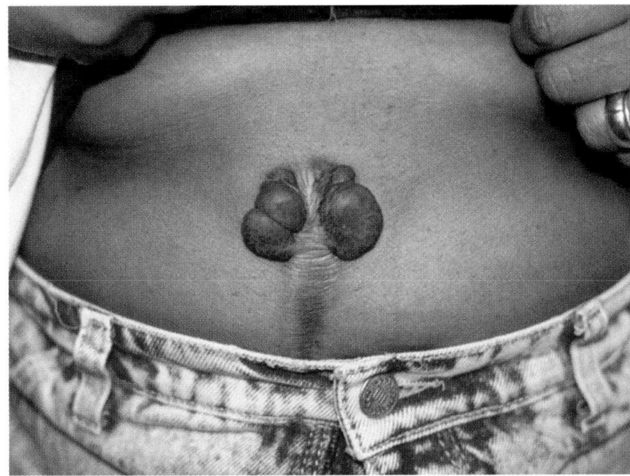

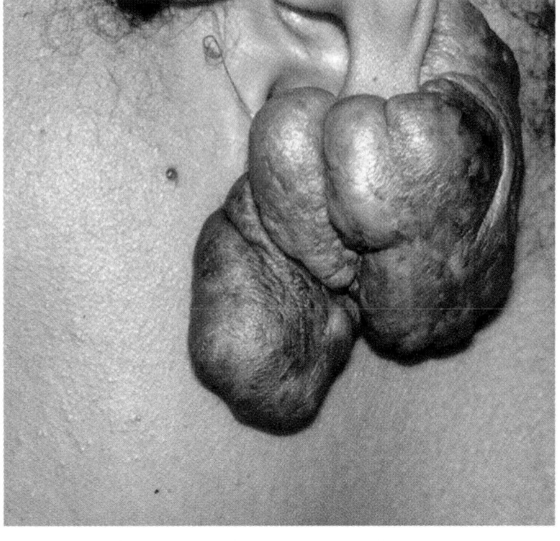

FIGURE 4.10 Keloids. (*A*) This lesion is growing well beyond the border of cesarian section scar. (*B*) The ear lobes are a common location. (From Goodheart HP. *Goodheart's photoguide of common skin disorders,* 2nd ed. Philadelphia: Lippincott Williams & Wilkins, 2003, with permission.)

The treatment of keloids is difficult: The cause is unknown, and the underlying disorder is not resolved by any specific therapy. Some improvement is usually seen with excision followed by intralesional steroid injection.[22] In unresponsive cases, excision followed by a short course of radiotherapy has been successful, but the resulting scar is unpredictable and potentially worse. Keloids typically develop several months after injury and rarely, if ever, subside. Although many therapies have been tried, with anecdotal reports of success, none is ideal.[23]

Hypertrophic Scars

Hypertrophic scars are histologically similar to keloids. They contain an overabundance of dermal collagen. Hypertrophic scars, however, respect the boundaries of the original injury and do not extend into normal unwounded tissue. They have less genetic predisposition, but hypertrophic scars also occur more frequently in Asians and African skin. They are often seen on the upper torso and across flexor surfaces. They usually develop within the first month after wounding and often subside gradually (Fig. 4.11).

Improvement of hypertrophic scars may be obtained with pressure garments, topical silicone gel sheeting applications, or reexcision and closure.[6,24] Reexcision and closure should be considered if conditions of the closure can be improved. This is especially true for wounds that originally healed by secondary intention or were complicated by infection. Simple reexcision and closure is unlikely to improve a scar that was closed with proper alignment and that healed primarily without complications.[25]

Unsightly Scars

A wound that is closed under tension or without adequate or accurate alignment, or a wound that runs across the lines of natural skin tension, is often unsightly. Surgical excision and closure with attention directed to correcting the underlying cause of the unsightly scar usually results in improvement. When reexcising either a hypertrophic scar or unsightly scar from other causes, reclosure with attention to relieving mechanical tension by the use of semipermanent or permanent intradermal sutures and everting wound closure, followed by treatment with taping and/or silicone gel sheeting, and judicious of injected intralesional steroids can result in substantial improvement in the quality of the scar in a high percentage of cases.

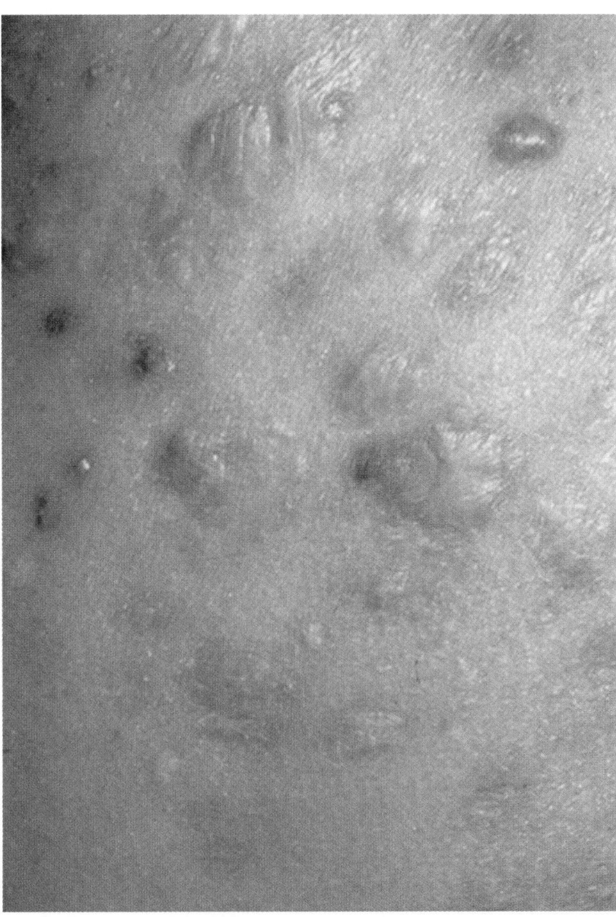

FIGURE 4.11 Hypertrophic scars. These lesions are characteristic of acne scars that occur on the trunk. (From Goodheart HP. *Goodheart's photoguide of common skin disorders,* 2nd ed. Philadelphia: Lippincott Williams & Wilkins, 2003, with permission.)

FETAL WOUND HEALING

Much interest and research have focused on the process of fetal wound healing. It has been demonstrated that humans and several other mammalian species undergo fetal skin healing with little or no scar if the injury occurs early enough during gestation.[26,27]

The physiologic mechanisms involved in scarless fetal healing have been under active investigation. Adult wounds heal with a significant inflammatory response followed by abundant collagen deposition and remodeling into a mature scar. Numerous studies have shown that fetal wounds heal with little or no inflammation and no excess collagen formation. The fetal wound matrix is also higher in hyaluronic acid than the adult wound. This substance is seen only early in adult healing. Amniotic fluid is rich in hyaluronic acid and may provide the hyaluronic acid found in the fetal wound. Experiments that have exposed adult skin to amniotic fluid, however, demonstrate adult-type healing with scar formation. One important factor is that after the second trimester, fetal wounds begin to heal with scar suggesting that the increased cell differentiation that occurs with maturation of the fetus is a critical factor in the scarless versus scarring phenotype.

Clearly, the fetal wound differs from the adult wound in several ways. The scarless healing appears multifactorial. Further research may identify factors (i.e., growth factors) that can be applied to wounds to diminish scar formation. This has potentially important application in virtually all of surgery but has proved to be elusive despite aggressive research interest.

KEY POINTS

- **The inflammatory phase of acute wound healing begins immediately after injury. The initial response to the disruption of blood vessels is bleeding.**
- **The proliferative phase begins with the formation of a provisional matrix of fibrin and fibronectin as part of initial clot formation.**
- **The transition from the proliferative phase to the remodeling phase is defined by reaching collagen equilibrium.**
- **Reconstruction of the epithelial barrier (epithelialization) begins within hours of the initial injury.**
- **Visible scarring occurs only when the injury extends deeper than the superficial dermis.**
- **A practical definition of a chronic wound is one that has failed to heal within 3 months. Although there are a variety of underlying causes, most can be categorized as pressure sores, diabetic foot ulcers, or leg ulcers.**
- **It takes at least 3 weeks for collagen to undergo sufficient remodeling and cross-linking to attain moderate strength.**
- **A chronic wound is commonly defined as an open wound that has failed to respond to standard care and remains open at 3 months.**
- **The primary difference between a keloid and a hypertrophic scar is that a keloid extends beyond the boundary of the original tissue injury.**

References

1. Singer AJ, Clark RA. Cutaneous wound healing. *N Engl J Med.* 1999;341:738.
2. Leibovich SJ, Ross R. The role of the macrophage in wound repair: a study with hydrocortisone and antimacrophage serum. *Am J Pathol.* 1975;78:71.
3. Cross KC, Mustoe TA. Growth factors in wound healing. *Surg Clin North Am.* 2003;83:531–546.
4. Madden JW, Peacock EE. Studies on the biology of collagen during wound healing. I. Rate of collagen synthesis and deposition in cutaneous wounds of the rat. *Surgery* 1968;64:288.
5. Ruoslahti E. Stretching is good for a cell. *Science* 1997;276:1345–1346.
6. Mustoe TA. Editorial: treatment of scars and keloids. *BMJ* 2004;328: 1329–1330.
7. Mustoe TA, Cooter R, Gold M, et al. International clinical guidelines for scar management. *Plast Reconstr Surg.* 2002;110:560–572.
8. Peacock EE Jr. *Wound repair,* 3rd ed. Philadelphia: WB Saunders; 1984.
9. Winter GD, Scales JT. Effect of air drying and dressings on the surface of a wound. *Nature* 1963;197:91.
10. Jonsson K, Jensen JA, Goodson WH, et al. Tissue oxygenation, anemia, and perfusion in relation to wound healing in surgical patients. *Ann Surg.* 1991;214:6.
11. Davidson JD, Mustoe TA. Commentary. Oxygen in wound healing: more than a nutrient. *Wound Repair Regen.* 2001;9:175–177.
12. Mustoe TA. Understanding chronic wounds: a unifying hypothesis on their pathogenesis, and implications for therapy. *Am J Surg.* 2004;187:S65–70.
13. Gross A, Cutright DE, Bhaskar SN. Effectiveness of pulsating water jet lavage in treatment of contaminated crushed wounds. *Am J Surg.* 1972;124:373.
14. Seifter E, Rettura G, Padawer J, et al. Impaired wound healing in streptozotocin diabetes: prevention by supplemental vitamin A. *Ann Surg.* 1981;194:42.
15. Ehrlich P, Tarver H, Hunt TK. Inhibitory effect of vitamin E on collagen synthesis and wound repair. *Ann Surg.* 1972;175:235.
16. LaVan FB, Hunt TK. Oxygen and wound healing. *Clin Plast Surg.* 1990;17:463.
17. Carver N, Leigh IM. Synthetic dressings. *Int J Dermatol.* 1992;31:10.
18. Mustoe TA, Pierce GF, Thomason A, et al. Accelerated healing of incisional wounds in rats induced by transforming growth factor-β. *Science* 1987;237:1333.
19. Brown GL, Nanney LB, Griffen J, et al. Enhancement of wound healing by topical treatment with epidermal growth factor. *N Engl J Med.* 1989;321:76.
20. Argenta LC, Morykwas MJ. Vacuum-assisted closure: A new method for wound control and treatment: Clinical experience. *Ann Plast Surg.* 1997;38:563–577.
21. Moues CM, Vos MC, van den Bemd GJ, et al. Bacterial load in relation to vacuum-assisted closure wound therapy: a prospective randomized trial. *Wound Repair Regen.* 2004;12:11–17.
22. Griffith H. The treatment of keloids with triamcinolone acetonide. *Plast Reconstr Surg.* 1966;38:202.
23. Lawrence WT. In search of the optimal treatment of keloids: report of a series and a review of the literature. *Ann Plast Surg.* 1991;27:164.
24. Ahn ST, Monafo WW, Mustoe TA. Topical silicone gel: a new treatment for hypertrophic scars. *Surgery* 1989;106:781.
25. Khouri RK, Mustoe TA. Trends in the treatment of hypertrophic scars. *Adv Plast Reconstr Surg.* 1991;8.
26. Mast BA, Diegelmann RF, Krummel TM, et al. Scarless wound healing in the mammalian fetus. *Surg Gynecol Obstet.* 1992;174:441.
27. Siebert JW, Burd AR, McCarthy JG, et al. Fetal wound healing: a biochemical study of scarless healing. *Plast Reconstr Surg.* 1990;85:503.

CHAPTER 5 ■ HEMOSTASIS

THOMAS W. WAKEFIELD AND PETER K. HENKE

BASIC CONSIDERATIONS

The coagulation mechanism is a dynamic, interactive network that relies on the interaction between platelets and coagulation complexes for clot formation. Initiating agents for coagulation include collagen and tissue factor (TF). TF, released from injured cells, activates the extrinsic pathway of coagulation. Disruption of the endothelium of blood vessels exposes underlying collagen to platelets, activating them. In the blood, TF complexes with activated factor VII, activating factors IX and X to factors IXa and Xa (activated factors IX and X).[1] The enzyme responsible for the initial activation of factor VII is unknown. However, factors Xa and VIIa catalyze activation of factor VII, so there is amplification for the formation of factor VIIa.[2] At the same time, activated platelets contract, with externalization of negatively charged procoagulant phospholipids, including phosphatidylserine and phosphatidylinositol (termed platelet factor 3).[3] This allows for the coagulation proteins to assemble on the surfaces of platelets, accelerating the coagulation reactions[4] (Fig. 5.1). Platelet membranes contribute critical surfaces for coagulation complex assembly. Activated but not resting platelets express binding sites for coagulation factors. During platelet activation, granules release their contents and membranes are exposed that are rich in receptors for factors Va and VIIIa[5,6] as well as fibrinogen, von Willebrand factor (vWF), and ADP, a potent activator of other platelets. vWF is responsible for platelet adhesion through binding to glycoprotein (Gp) Ib,[7] whereas fibrinogen forms bridges between activated platelets by binding to GpIIb/IIIa on adjacent stimulated platelets.[8] Unstimulated platelets can also attach to immobilized fibrinogen by the same receptor.[9] Platelet activation also leads to the release of arachidonic acid metabolites such as thromboxane A_2, a powerful initiator of platelet aggregation.[10] Contraction of platelets during their activation does lead to a shape change, which then results in the externalization of negatively charged procoagulant phospholipids, including phosphatidylserine and phosphatidylinositol. Platelets also release microparticles, rich in TF and other procoagulant products.

Once the platelet plug has formed, the stage is set for coagulation protein assembly. Activated factor X (Xa), activated factor V (Va), ionized calcium, and factor II (prothrombin) form on the platelet phospholipid surface to initiate the prothrombinase complex, which catalyzes the formation of thrombin faster than can be achieved with factor Xa alone[4]

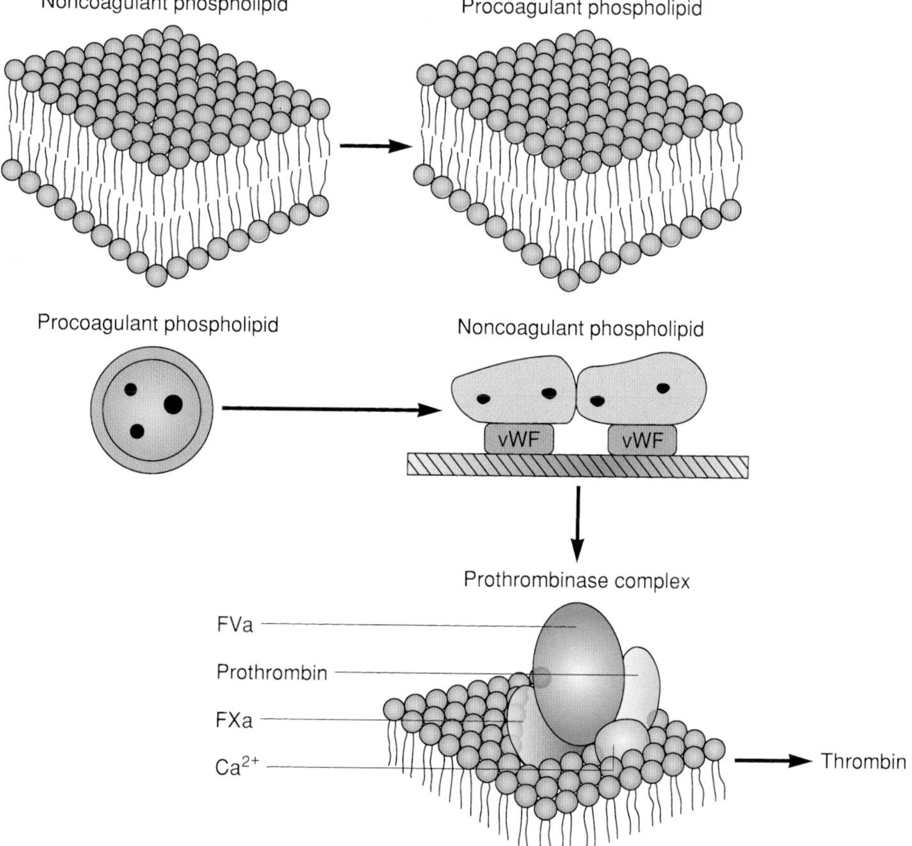

FIGURE 5.1 Formation of coagulation cascade assembly on the platelet phospholipid surface. (After Hassouna HI. Laboratory evaluation of hemostatic disorders. *Hematol Oncol Clin North Am.* 1993;7:1188, with permission.)

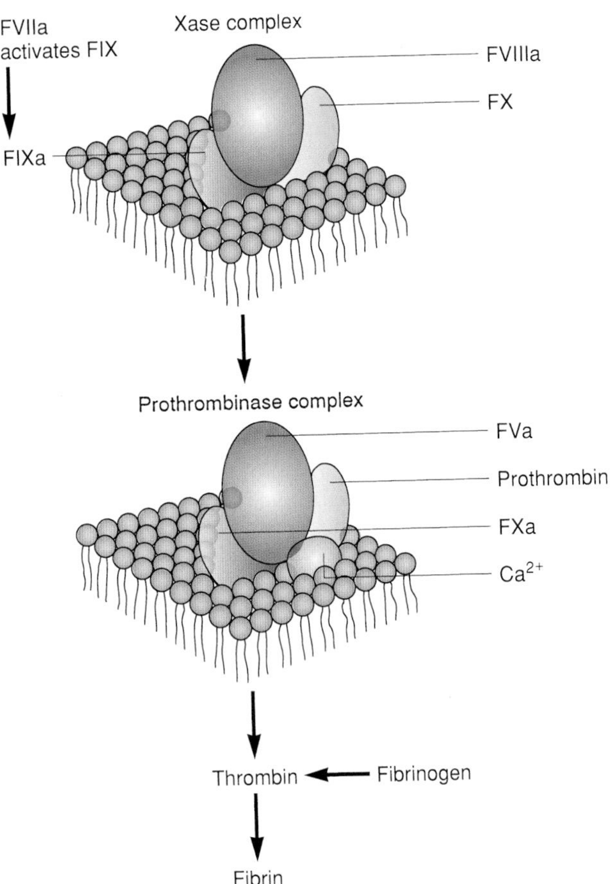

FIGURE 5.2 Formation of the Xase complex and prothrombinase complex with amplification of thrombin and fibrin formation. (After Hassouna HI. Laboratory evaluation of hemostatic disorders. *Hematol Oncol Clin North Am.* 1993; 7:1177, with permission.)

(Fig. 5.2). When the amount of TF is limited, activation of factor IX rather than factor X is favored,[12,13] allowing for coagulation in situations of low TF concentration. The pathway described up to this point corresponds to the classic extrinsic pathway of coagulation. Thrombin is central to all coagulation and acts to cleave fibrinopeptide A (FPA) from the α chain of fibrinogen and fibrinopeptide B (FPB) from the β chain.[14] This leads to the release of fibrinopeptides and the formation of new fibrin monomers, which then cross-link, resulting in fibrin polymerization. Thrombin also activates factor XIII, which catalyzes the cross-linking of fibrin to make the clot firm,[15] activates platelets, and activates factors V and VIII, two nonenzymatic cofactors, to Va and VIIIa.[4] This is important because only activated factors Va and VIIIa are involved in coagulation. Factor XIIIa also cross-links other plasma proteins, such as fibronectin and α_2-antitrypsin, resulting in their incorporation into clot.[16]

The intrinsic pathway of blood coagulation requires activation of factor XI to XIa. This may occur by both the contact activation system through activation of factor XII, plasma prekallikrein, and high-molecular-weight kininogen and, more important, through thrombin with negatively charged surfaces.[17] Factor XIa activates factor XI autocatalytically[17] and also catalyzes the conversion of factor IX to IXa.[18] After activation, factor VIIIa dissociates from vWF and assembles with factors IXa and X. Factor IXa, factor X, ionized calcium, and thrombin-activated factor VIII (VIIIa) then assemble on the platelet surface in a complex called the *Xase complex* to

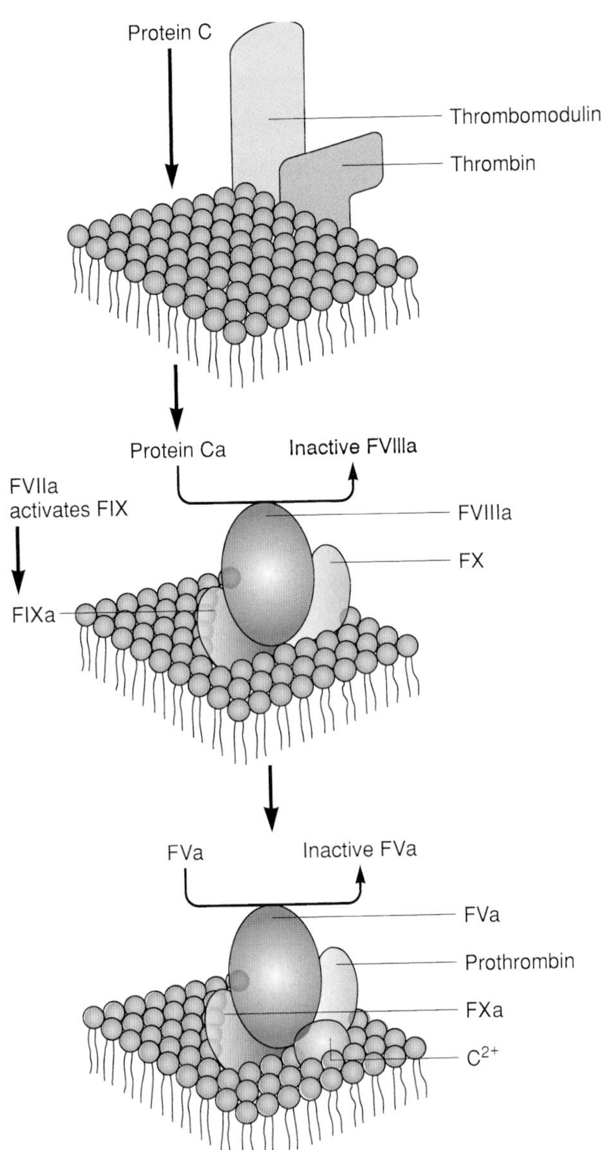

FIGURE 5.3 Activation of protein C by thrombin–thrombomodulin interaction. (After Hassouna HI. Laboratory evaluation of hemostatic disorders. *Hematol Oncol Clin North Am.* 1993;7:1175, with permission.)

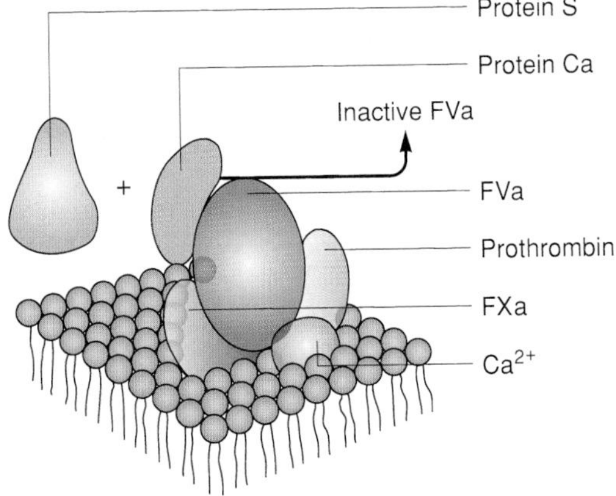

FIGURE 5.4 Actions of protein S. (After Hassouna HI. Laboratory evaluation of hemostatic disorders. *Hematol Oncol Clin North Am.* 1993;7:1176, with permission.)

catalyze the activation of factor X to Xa[4] (see Fig. 5.2). Factor Xa then shunts into the prothrombinase complex for further amplification of thrombin formation. The importance of a mechanism of factor XI activation independent of the contact activation system is apparent because patients deficient in those factors of the contact activation system, including factor XI, bleed, whereas patients deficient in factor XII, prekallikrein, and high-molecular-weight kininogen do not usually bleed.[16] The contact activation system is the most important coagulation process involved in extracorporeal bypass circuits, including cardiopulmonary bypass and extracorporeal membrane oxygenation (ECMO).

NATURAL ANTICOAGULANT MECHANISMS

At the same time that thrombin forms, natural anticoagulant mechanisms oppose further thrombin formation and help to localize thrombin activity to areas of vascular injury. Just as thrombin generation is key to coagulation, antithrombin (AT) is the central anticoagulant protein. This glycoprotein of 70-kd molecular weight binds to thrombin, preventing the removal of FPA and FPB from fibrinogen,[19] preventing the activation of factors V and VIII, and inhibiting the activation and aggregation of platelets. In addition, AT directly inhibits factors IXa,[20] Xa, and XIa.[21] A second natural anticoagulant is activated protein C (APC), which inactivates factors Va[22,23] and VIIIa,[24] thus reducing the Xase and prothrombinase complex acceleration of the rate of thrombin formation. In the circulation, protein C is activated to protein Ca on endothelial cell surfaces by thrombin complexed with one of its receptors, thrombomodulin[25–27] (Fig. 5.3), in a one-to-one complex,[28] highlighting another important role for thrombin. The formation of this thrombin–thrombomodulin complex accelerates the activation of protein C compared with thrombin alone. Thrombin, at the same time, by binding to thrombomodulin, loses its platelet-activating activity[29] as well as its enzymatic activity for fibrinogen and factor V.[30] Protein S is a cofactor for protein Ca[31] (Fig. 5.4). Another innate anticoagulant is tissue factor pathway inhibitor (TFPI). This factor is bound to low-density lipoprotein (LDL) in plasma and is also called lipoprotein-associated coagulation inhibitor. The protein binds to TF-VIIa complex, inhibiting the activation of factor X to Xa and the formation of the prothrombinase complex.[16,32,33] Factor IX activation is not inhibited. A fourth natural anticoagulant is heparin cofactor II.[34] Its concentration in plasma is estimated to be significantly less than that of AT, and its action is implicated primarily in the regulation of thrombin formation in extravascular tissues. Finally, thrombin is inactivated when it becomes incorporated into the clot.

FIBRINOLYSIS

During the process of thrombus formation, there is a constant process of clot lysis, which prevents physiologic thrombus formation from leading to pathologic intravascular thrombosis. Plasminogen, tissue plasminogen activator (tPA), and α_2-antiplasmin (α_2-AP) become incorporated into the fibrin clot as it forms[4] (Fig. 5.5). In fact, thrombin (both α and γ) promotes tPA release from endothelial cells as well as the production of plasminogen activator inhibitor (PAI-1) from endothelial cells.[35,36] tPA converts plasminogen to plasmin, the main fibrinolytic enzyme. This is a serine protease whose main substrates include fibrin, fibrinogen, and other coagulation factors. Plasmin also interferes with platelet adhesion through vWF by proteolysis of GpIb.[37] Fibrin, when digested by plasmin, yields one molecule of fragment E and two molecules of fragment D. In physiologic clot formation, fragment D is

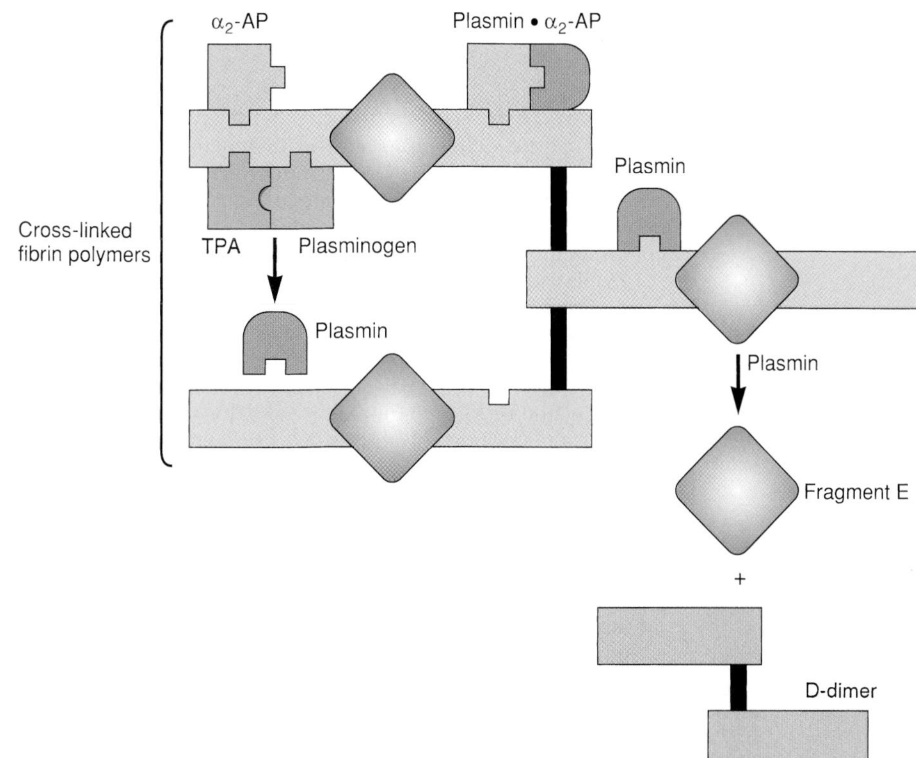

FIGURE 5.5 Incorporation of plasminogen, tissue plasminogen activator (tPA), and α_2-antiplasmin (α_2-AP) into the fibrin clot as it forms with production of D-dimer fragments. (After Hassouna HI. Laboratory evaluation of hemostatic disorders. *Hematol Oncol Clin North Am.* 1993;7:1186, with permission.)

released in dimeric form (D-dimer).[4] The D-dimer fragment is a marker for ongoing thrombosis and fibrinolysis of formed clot (fibrin). The natural inhibitor of excess plasmin, α_2-AP, is also released by endothelial cells. In physiologic fibrinolysis, α_2-AP is bound to fibrin and excess plasmin is readily inactivated. In fibrinolytic states (fibrinogenolysis), however, and during treatment with fibrinolytic agents, circulating fibrinogen, in addition to clot-bound fibrin, is degraded by circulating plasmin, which is not readily inactivated by α_2-AP. Circulating fibrinogen is degraded by removal of FPB and the carboxyl-terminal portion of the α chain, yielding fragment X, which clots slowly.[38] Fragment X is further degraded to one molecule of fragment D and a fragment Y, neither of which clot thrombin; fragment Y is broken down to two molecules of fragment D and one molecule of fragment E[4] (Fig. 5.6). In these fibrinogenolytic states, the D fragments are not cross-linked, and D-dimer is not formed. The Y and D fragments are potent inhibitors of fibrin formation.

The major categories of plasminogen activators include exogenous factors, such as streptokinase; endogenous factors, such as tPA and urokinase; and intrinsic factors.[4] Intrinsic factors include factor XII, prekallikrein, and high-molecular-weight kininogen. These factors of the contact system are more important in clot lysis than thrombus formation. Activated forms of factor XII, kallikrein, and factor XI independently can convert plasminogen to plasmin.[39] These enzymes may also liberate bradykinin from high-molecular-weight kininogen, resulting in an increase in vascular permeability, prostacyclin liberation, and tPA secretion. Finally, APC (factor Ca) has been found to inactivate proteolytically the inhibitor to tPA, thus promoting tPA activity and fibrinolysis.[28]

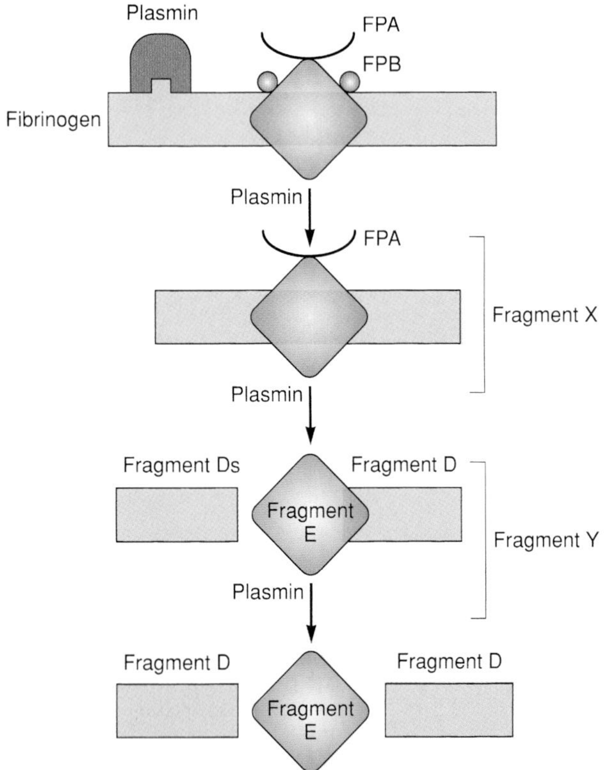

FIGURE 5.6 Process of fibrinogenolysis and formation of non-cross-linked fragment Ds. (After Hassouna HI. Laboratory evaluation of hemostatic disorders. *Hematol Oncol Clin North Am.* 1993;7:1193, with permission.)

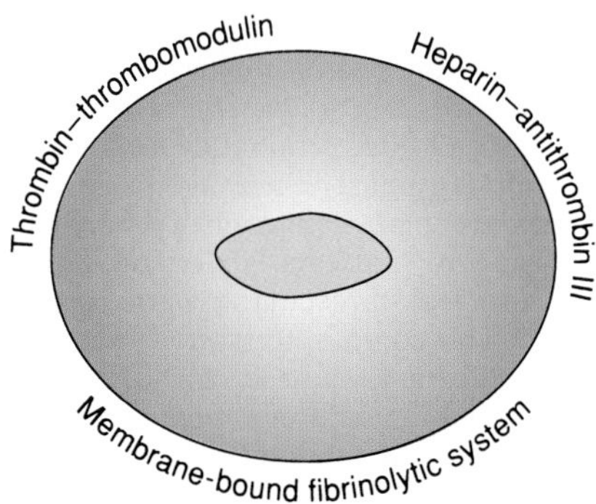

FIGURE 5.7 Vessel wall endothelial cell antithrombotic properties.

The endothelial cell itself appears to be in an excellent position to act as a nonthrombogenic surface (Fig. 5.7). It has three systems for the promotion of a nonthrombotic surface, including thrombin–thrombomodulin interaction, heparin–AT III binding, and a membrane-bound fibrinolytic system. Circulating plasminogen exists in an N-terminal glutamic acid form (Glu-Plg). On the endothelial cell surface, Glu-Plg is converted to its N-terminal lysine form (Lys-Plg) by locally generated plasmin.[40] Local cell concentrations of tPA may be great enough to saturate high-affinity receptors, elaborate small amounts of plasmin, and convert Glu-Plg to Lys-Plg. Lys-Plg is then converted to plasmin with improved catalytic efficiency and the generation of a local fibrinolytic response.

In summary, coagulation is an ongoing process of thrombus formation, inhibition of thrombus formation, and thrombus dissolution. The central mediator is thrombin[4] (Fig. 5.8). Abnormalities in coagulation occur when one process—thrombus formation, thrombus inhibition, or fibrinolysis—overcomes the others and dominates the delicate balance that is hemostasis.

ENDOTHELIUM AND HEMOSTASIS

Through its ability to express procoagulants and anticoagulants, vasoconstrictors and vasodilators, as well as key cell adhesion molecules and cytokines, the endothelial cell is a key regulator of hemostasis. Vascular endothelium sustains a vasodilatory and local fibrinolytic state in which coagulation, platelet adhesion and activation, and leukocyte activation are suppressed. Endothelial products which are vasodilatory include adenosine, nitric oxide (NO), and prostacyclin (PGI_2).[41] A nonthrombogenic endothelial surface is maintained through four main mechanisms, including endothelial production of thrombomodulin and subsequent activation of protein C, endothelial expression of surface heparin- and dermatan-sulfate, constitutive expression of TFPI by endothelium (which is markedly accelerated in response to heparin), and local production of tPA and urokinase plasminogen activator (uPA). Finally, the elaboration of NO_3 and interleukin (IL)-10 by endothelium inhibits leukocyte adhesion and activation.[41]

In contrast, during states of endothelial disturbances, a prothrombotic and proinflammatory state of vasoconstriction is supported by the endothelial surface.[41] Endothelial release of platelet activating factor (PAF) and endothelin-1 promotes vasoconstriction.[42] Endothelial cells increase production of vWF, TF, PAI-1, and factor V to augment thrombosis during times of prothrombotic stimuli.[42] Finally, in response to

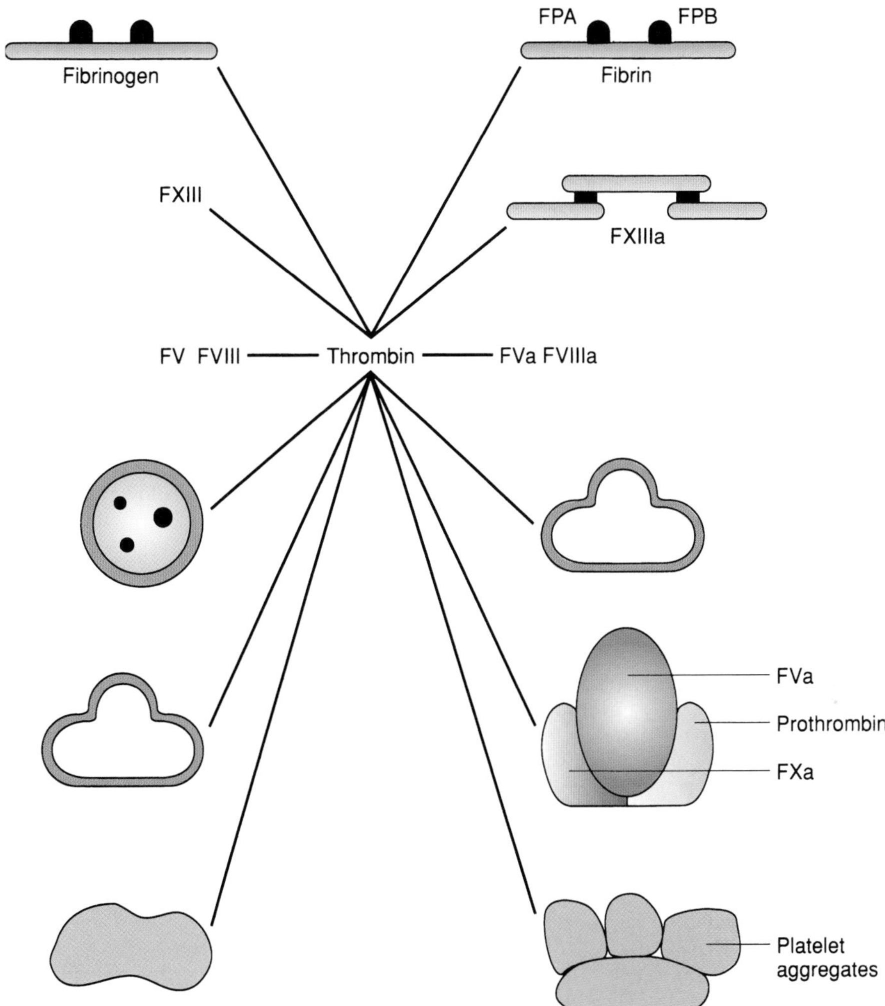

FIGURE 5.8 Thrombin as the central mediator of coagulation. (After Hassouna HI. Laboratory evaluation of hemostatic disorders. *Hematol Oncol Clin North Am.* 1993;7:1177, with permission.)

endothelial injury, endothelial cells are activated resulting in increased surface expression of cell adhesion molecules (such as P- or E-selectin), promoting leukocyte adhesion and activation. This initiates and amplifies inflammation and thrombosis.

THROMBOSIS AND INFLAMMATION

Thrombosis and inflammation are closely linked. Tumor necrosis factor alpha (TNFα), a polypeptide cytokine of stimulated macrophages released in response to inflammation and sepsis, down-regulates thrombomodulin expression through endocytosis and degradation of thrombomodulin.[43] TNFα increases the level of C4b-binding protein, decreasing the amount of free protein S available to function as a cofactor for protein C. In addition, TNF induces TF expression on the surface of endothelial cells. In a study of six normal human volunteers given TNFα, factor X was activated to Xa early after administration, followed by prothrombin activation in a more gradual pattern of increase observed hours after maximal concentrations of factor Xa had been reached.[44] TNFα also inhibits fibrinolysis by suppressing the release of tPA and inducing the expression of tPA inhibitor type I.[45–50] In vivo, TNFa initially increases plasma plasminogen activator activity, followed by an even greater increase in PAI-1 antigen, leading to an overall inhibition of the fibrinolytic system.[51]

In addition, by down-regulating thrombomodulin, TNFα decreases protein C production. Because protein C inhibits PAI-1, a decrease in protein C decreases the fibrinolytic potential of the blood. Along with its effects on coagulation, TNFα facilitates inflammation. TNFα and other cytokines stimulate adherence proteins on endothelial cells[52–55] for leukocytes and induce endothelial and vascular wall smooth muscle cell production of IL-8 gene expression and monocyte chemotactic protein-1 mRNA expression.[56] These cytokines activate neutrophils in vitro and stimulate neutrophil and monocyte movement in vivo. They are also involved in the process of cytokine networking, in which one cytokine activates other cytokines, producing a physiologic response.

A model for the possible interactions between thrombosis and inflammation has been proposed[57] (Fig. 5.9). In this model, vascular injury results in the margination of circulating platelets along the vessel wall, probably mediated by vWF binding to GpIb on the platelet surface. The platelets then activate and aggregate in an interaction mediated by fibrinogen, resulting in platelet plug formation. Blood clotting is stimulated by the expression of TF, and the clotting complexes are propagated on the phospholipid surfaces of activated platelets, resulting in the formation of a fibrin clot. Circulating neutrophils and monocytes then interact with the platelets through P-selectin and with the endothelial cells through P-selectin and E-selectin, events that result in the stable interaction between leukocytes and platelets at the thrombus–wall interface. Neutrophils and monocytes participate in this local

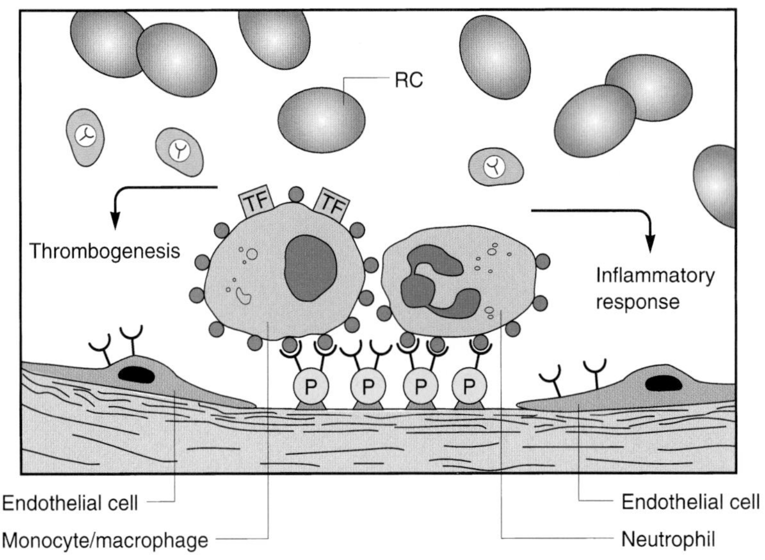

FIGURE 5.9 Cellular basis for blood coagulation, including platelets (P), neutrophils, monocytes, P-selectin (Y), and red blood cells (RC). (After Furie B, Furie BC. Molecular and cellular biology of blood coagulation. *N Engl J Med.* 1992; 326:803, with permission.)

inflammatory response, and monocytes may specifically contribute to clot formation by further TF expression on their surface. This has been suggested in a study involving fibrin formation under the influence of a monoclonal antibody to P-selectin in a primate arteriovenous fistula model.[58]

In the venous circulation, a series of steps linking thrombosis and inflammation has been suggested.[59] In step 1, thrombus formation involving platelets, neutrophils, and monocytes is initiated at venous confluences, saccules, and valve pockets. In step 2, adherent neutrophils and platelets become activated, releasing substances such as adenosine diphosphate (ADP) (in platelets) and neutrophil-activating peptide-2 (NAP-2) (in platelets and neutrophils), activating and attracting more platelets and neutrophils. Cathepsin G, secreted from activated neutrophils, converts β-thromboglobulin (secreted from platelets) into NAP-2 by proteolytic cleavage.[60] This NAP-2 stimulates more cathepsin G secretion, which in turn stimulates more platelet secretion,[61,62] providing more substrate for NAP-2 and causing feedback activation for the recruitment of more platelets and neutrophils. In step 3, coagulation is initiated and promoted on the phospholipid surface of the platelets. Finally, in step 4, new layers of neutrophils and platelets form on the surface of fibrin, activate, and begin another round of the clotting process.

Leukocytes extravasate into the vein wall by a chemotactic gradient that develops in the wall in response to the venous thrombosis. In a baboon model of stasis deep vein thrombosis (DVT), the presence of a venous catheter for a short time, and the administration of the thrombogenic reagents TNFα and antibody to protein C, we have observed by enzyme-linked immunosorbent assay (ELISA) protein measurements and immunohistochemical tissue staining the presence of inflammatory cytokines in the vein wall directly beneath the luminal thrombus, including IL-8, IL-6, monocyte chemotactic protein-1 (MCP-1), epithelial neutrophil-activating protein-78 (ENA-78), and macrophage inflammatory protein-1α (MIP-1α).[63] We have similarly observed in a pure stasis model of inferior venal caval thrombosis in both primates and rats a similar occurrence in the vein wall, with the early influx of neutrophils followed by the later extravasation of monocytes and lymphocytes in a typical inflammatory progression. This suggests that the sequence may lead to a complete inflammatory response in the vein wall. Further research to block the inflammatory response and the subsequent effect this interference may have on the detrimental interactions between the thrombus and the vein wall and valves may have significant implications for treatment of venous thrombosis. Approaches to interfere with the inflammatory response include blocking initial leukocyte adhesion, leukocyte activation, or both.

ARTERIAL VERSUS VENOUS THROMBOSIS

The elements required for the initiation of thrombosis were described by Virchow as stasis, endothelial injury, and hypercoagulability of the blood. In the arterial circulation, endothelial injury (whether acute or chronic) is key to thrombosis. This is most clearly demonstrated by the typical atherosclerotic plaque. In advanced lesions, the lipid core of the plaque is rich in inflammatory cells, cholesterol crystals, and TF (generated by activated macrophages within the plaque). Plaque ulceration exposes highly thrombogenic lipid to the bloodstream, activating coagulation, platelet aggregation, and activation, and leads to the deposition of clot.[64] Platelet deposition occurs at the apex of stenoses, the point of maximal shear force. In contrast, venous blood stasis and changes in its composition (leading to hypercoagulability) incite the formation of thrombus from local procoagulant events, including small endothelial disruptions at venous confluences, saccules, and valve pockets. Neutrophils and platelets then become activated, generating inflammatory and procoagulant mediators that amplify thrombosis further.[59] Additionally, microparticles are elaborated by inflammatory cells, platelets, and endothelial cells. These microparticles are procoagulant by virtue of TF on their surface or the presence of certain phospholipids on their surface and they accumulate in the thrombus, leading to its amplification. With progression, leukocytes (initially neutrophils and subsequently monocytes) extravasate into the vein wall in response to the chemokine gradient generated by the initial thrombotic event, resulting in transmural venous inflammation. The ultimate vein wall response is determined by a balance between pro-inflammatory and anti-inflammatory cytokines and chemokines.

The earliest elevated glycoprotein on endothelial cells and platelets is P-selectin. This glycoprotein plays an important

TABLE 5.1

FREQUENCY OF VTE DUE TO HYPERCOAGULABLE STATES

Hypercoagulable state	Frequency (%)
Factor V Leiden	20–60
Hyperhomocysteinemia	10
PT G20210A	4–6
Protein C deficiency	3–5
Protein S deficiency	2–3
Dysfibrinogenemia	1–3
Antithrombin	1–2
Dysplasminogenemia	<1

VTE, venous thromboembolism.

role in venous thrombogenesis. In models of venous thrombosis, P-selectin inhibition given prophylactically decreases thrombosis in a dose-dependent fashion. Additionally, P-selectin inhibitors (both antibodies to P-selectin and antagonists to the P-selectin receptor) can treat established venous thrombosis as effectively as heparin without anticoagulation.[65,66] It is hypothesized that selectins, expressed after a thrombogenic stimulus, facilitate these proposed interactions between leukocytes and endothelial cells, leukocytes and leukocytes, and leukocytes and platelets. Additionally, microparticles are released with the interaction of P-selectin with its receptor.

PROCOAGULANT STATES

Refer to Tables 5.1 to 5.3 and Algorithm 5.1.

TABLE 5.2

SEVERITY OF VTE DUE TO HYPERCOAGULABLE STATES

High risk for thrombosis
- AT deficiency
- Protein C deficiency
- Protein S deficiency
- HIT/HITTS
- Antiphospholipid antibody syndrome

Lower risk for thrombosis
- Factor V Leiden
- Hyperhomocysteinemia
- PT G20210A
- Dysfibrinogenemia
- Dysplasminogenemia
- Elevated factors VIII, IX, and XI

AT, antithrombin; HIT, heparin-induced thrombocytopenia; HITTS, heparin-induced thrombocytopenia and thrombosis syndrome; VTE, venous thromboembolism.

TABLE 5.3

ANATOMIC LOCATION OF VTE DUE TO HYPERCOAGULABLE STATES

Arterial
- Elevated fibrinogen
- Abnormal platelet aggregation
- Atherosclerosis
- Lipoprotein(a)

Both arterial and venous
- Hyperhomocysteinemia
- HITTS
- Antiphospholipid antibody
- Elevated PAI-1

Venous
- AT
- Protein C
- Protein S
- Factor V Leiden
- PT G20210A
- Dysfibrinogenemia
- Elevated factors XI, IX, and VIII

AT, antithrombin; HITTS, heparin-induced thrombocytopenia and thrombosis syndrome; PAI-1, plasminogen activator inhibitor; VTE, venous thromboembolism.

Defects with High Risk for Thrombosis

Antithrombin Deficiency

Venous is much more common than arterial.

AT is a serine protease inhibitor (SERPIN) of thrombin, kallikrein, and factors Xa, IXa, VIIa, XIIa, and XIa. It is synthesized in the liver and has a half-life of 2.8 days. AT deficiency, accounts for approximately 1% to 2% of episodes of venous thromboembolism (VTE) and may occur at unusual sites such as mesenteric or cerebral veins. Arterial and graft thrombosis have also been described in AT deficiency.[67,68] Most cases become apparent by 50 years of age.[69] As heparin works to potentiate the anticoagulant effects of AT,[70] AT deficiency is suspected with an inability or failure for heparin to produce anticoagulation or failure of heparin to prevent thrombosis. Homozygous patients usually die *in utero*, whereas heterozygous patients usually demonstrate AT levels <70% of normal. Acquired AT deficiency results from liver disease, malignancy, sepsis,[71] disseminated intravascular coagulation (DIC), malnutrition, and renal disease.[72] Less frequent causes of AT deficiency include defective AT activity with normal quantitative levels (an abnormal protein) and AT deficiency with an abnormal interaction between heparin and AT.[73]

The diagnosis of AT deficiency is suspected in a patient who cannot be adequately anticoagulated with heparin or who develops thrombosis while on heparin and is made by measuring AT antigen and activity levels. However, patients should not have been exposed to heparin or related compounds for at least 2 weeks to have accurate values. Heparin decreases AT levels 30%, and this effect can be seen up to 10 days after stopping intravenous heparin therapy.[74] Conversely, warfarin increases AT levels.

For a patient with AT deficiency, anticoagulation with heparin requires the administration of fresh frozen plasma to provide AT, two units every 8 hours, decreasing to one unit every 12 hours, followed by oral anticoagulation. AT concentrates are also available.[75] A reasonable alternative includes anticoagulation with direct thrombin inhibitors such as

SCIENTIFIC PRINCIPLES

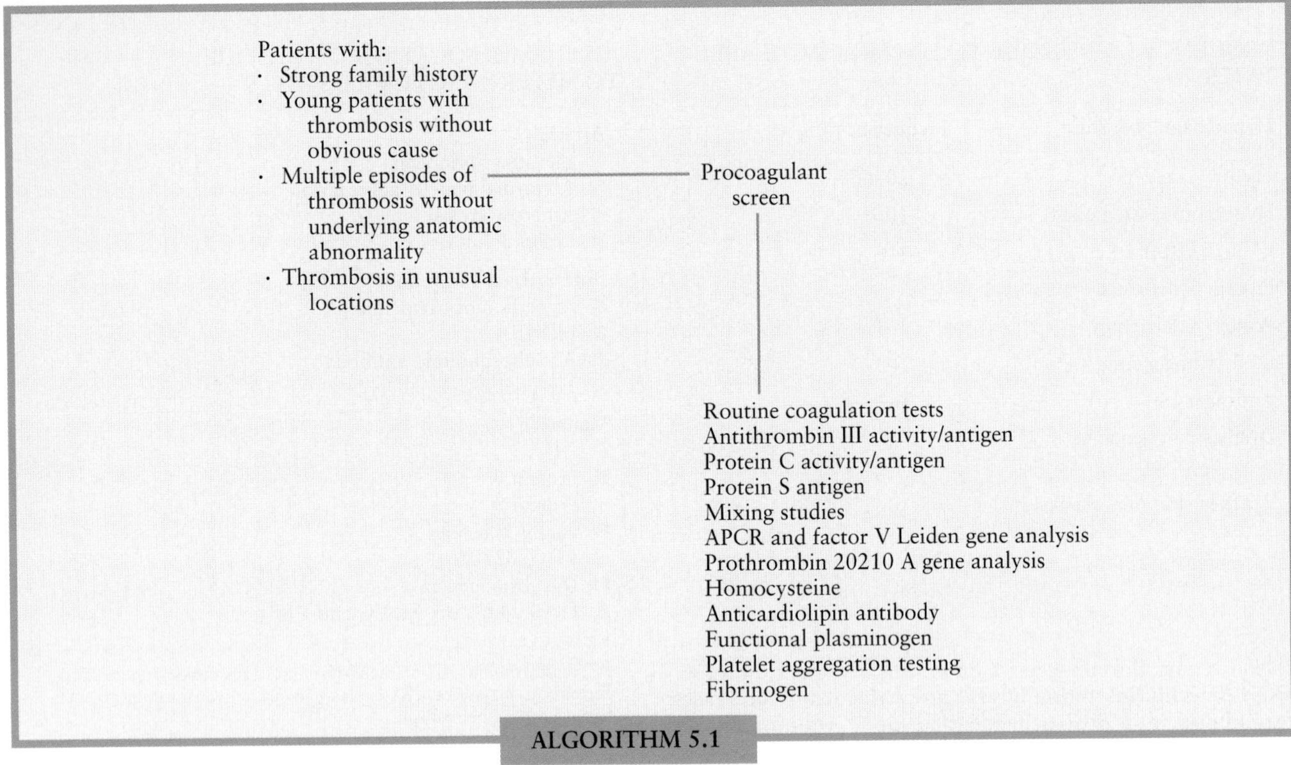

ALGORITHM 5.1 Coagulation analysis.

hirudin, argatroban, or bivalirudin.[76] Aggressive prophylaxis against VTE is recommended during the perioperative period, and lifelong anticoagulation therapy is required after a first episode of VTE.[77]

Protein C and S Deficiencies

Venous is much more common than arterial.

Protein C and its cofactor protein S are both vitamin K-dependent factors synthesized in the liver with half-lives of 4 to 6 hours and 12 to 14 hours, respectively. The majority of cases of protein C or protein S deficiency are inherited as autosomal dominant (Fig. 5.10). Patients present with VTE, often between the ages of 15 and 30 years.[77,78] Protein C and S deficiency states are responsible for approximately 2% to 5% of patients with VTE. However, cases of arterial thrombosis have also been reported.[79] If present as a homozygous state at birth, infants usually die from unrestricted clotting and fibrinolysis, a condition of extreme DIC termed *purpura fulminans*. Patients heterozygous for protein C deficiency usually have antigenic protein C levels less than 60% of normal.[74,80] Acquired protein C deficiency occur with liver failure, DIC, and nephrotic syndrome.

Protein S is a cofactor to protein C and is regulated by complement C4b binding protein. Free protein S is functionally active as an anticoagulant. The deficiency of protein S results in a clinical state identical to protein C deficiency. Nephrotic syndrome can lead to a reduction in free protein S and acquired hypercoagulable state,[81] whereas inflammatory states such as systemic lupus erythematosus (SLE) can result in an elevation of C4b binding protein, reducing free protein S.

The diagnosis of protein C or S deficiency is made by measuring plasma protein C and S levels.[4,82] For protein C, both antigen and activity are measured, whereas for protein S, only antigen is measured. A condition also exists in which there is an abnormality in the function of protein C itself, resulting in a decrease in protein C activity without a decline in antigenic protein C.[78]

Treatment consists of anticoagulation, initially with heparin, followed by lifelong oral anticoagulation. However, not all patients with low levels develop VTE. Many heterozygous family members of homozygous protein C–deficient infants also are unaffected.[83] Thus, the institution of anticoagulation therapy in patients should occur only following an episode of thrombosis. However, aggressive anticoagulant prophylaxis during perioperative periods or high-risk environmental situations is necessary for asymptomatic heterozygote carriers.

With the initiation of oral anticoagulation, blood may become transiently hypercoagulable as the vitamin K–dependent factors with short half-lives are inhibited (factor VII, protein C) before the other vitamin K–dependent factors (factors II, IX, and X).[84] In someone already partially deficient in protein C or S, the levels of these anticoagulant factors will diminish even further with the initiation of warfarin. This results in temporary hypercoagulability, resulting in thrombosis in the microcirculation and warfarin-induced skin necrosis.[85] This leads to full-thickness skin loss, especially over fatty areas such as the breasts, buttocks, and abdomen. This complication can be prevented by initiating warfarin therapy under the protection of systemic heparin anticoagulation or a direct thrombin inhibitor (in patients with VTE).

Heparin-Induced Thrombocytopenia and Thrombosis Syndrome (HITTS)

Venous is more common than arterial.

Heparin-induced thrombocytopenia (HIT) occurs in 0.6% to 30% of patients in whom heparin is given, although severe

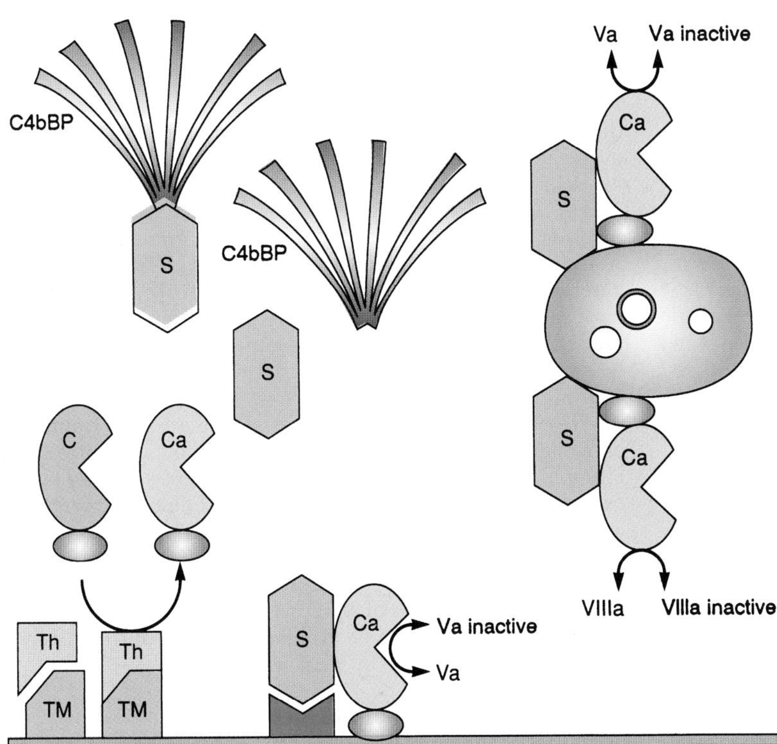

FIGURE 5.10 Role of proteins C and S. Th, thrombin; TM, thrombomodulin; C4bBP, C4b binding protein. (After Esmon CT. The regulation of natural anticoagulant pathways. *Science* 1987;235:1348, with permission.)

thrombocytopenia associated with thrombosis (HITTS) is seen much less frequently.[86,87] Approximately one half of HIT patients have thrombosis that is noted clinically or by duplex imaging. In an analysis of 11 prospective studies, the incidence was reported to be 3%, with thrombosis in 0.9%.[88] Although earlier morbidity and mortality rates of 61% and 23% had been reported,[89] with early diagnosis and appropriate treatment, these rates have declined to 6% and 0%, respectively.[90] HIT is caused by a heparin-dependent immunoglobulin G (IgG) antibody that, when bound to platelet factor 4 (PF_4), induces platelet aggregation.[91,92] The antibody may not be heparin specific, as the degree of sulfonation of the heparin-like compound has been suggested to be critical for this aggregation.[93] Both porcine and bovine standard unfractionated heparins as well as low-molecular-weight heparins (LMWHs) have been found with HIT.[94] The syndrome usually begins 3 to 14 days after heparin is begun. Both arterial and venous thromboses have been reported, and even small exposures to heparin (heparin coating on catheters) can cause the syndrome.[86,95,96]

The diagnosis should be suspected when a patient experiences a 50% or greater decline in platelet count, when there is a fall in platelet count below 100,000/mL during heparin therapy or in any patient who experiences thrombosis during heparin administration.[86,96–98] The syndrome may be difficult to diagnose as many hospitalized patients have multiple reasons for low platelet counts.

The laboratory diagnosis of HIT/HITTS is made by a number of assays. The serotonin release assay (SRA) was the "gold standard." An ELISA test detecting the antiheparin antibody in the patient's plasma directed against the heparin-PF_4 complex is commonly used today.[86,99] This assay is less specific but easier to perform and interpret than the serotonin assay.

When the diagnosis is made, cessation of heparin is mandatory. This includes removing heparin from intravenous catheters and flushes.[95] Patients demonstrate circulating platelet microparticles, which lead to an ongoing prothrombotic state. Warfarin should not be administered until an adequate alternative anticoagulant has been started to prevent venous limb gangrene development.[100] LMWHs have high rates of cross-reactivity with the HIT antibody and therefore should not be merely substituted for standard heparin in patients with HIT.[101]

A number of new anticoagulants are now available to substitute for patients with this diagnosis. The direct thrombin inhibitors hirudin (Lepirudin/Refludan) and argatroban are the treatments of choice.[86,102–104] These agents show no cross-reactivity to heparin antibodies. Antiplatelet agents have not become standard agents for this condition.

Lupus Anticoagulant/Antiphospholipid Syndrome (Antiphospholipid Antibody)

Venous is more common than arterial.

This condition, despite its name, is a prothrombotic state. The antiphospholipid antibody syndrome consists of an elevated antiphospholipid antibody titer in association with thrombosis, recurrent fetal loss, thrombocytopenia, and livedo reticularis.[105,106] Strokes, myocardial infarction, visceral infarction, and extremity gangrene may also occur. Although the lupus anticoagulant has been noted often in patients with SLE, it does occur in patients without SLE. It may also be induced in patients by medications, cancer, and certain infections.[107]

This syndrome is associated with antiphospholipid antibodies that are most commonly IgG. Antiphospholipid antibody syndrome is a particularly virulent hypercoagulable state that results in arterial and venous thrombosis at 5- to 16-fold greater risk.[107–109] A number of possible thrombotic mechanisms have been suggested, including inhibition of prostacyclin synthesis or release from endothelial cells,[110] inhibition of protein C activation by thrombin/thrombomodulin,[111] elevated PAI-1 levels,[112] platelet activation,[113] endothelial cell activation,[114] and interference with the endothelial cell-associated annexin V anticoagulant activity.[115] Increased TF expression on monocytes and low free protein S plasma levels have also been found with the antiphospholipid syndrome and a history of thrombosis.[116]

Thrombosis can also involve both venous and arterial circulations, especially peripheral vessels of the extremities.[117] At least one third of patients with lupus anticoagulants have a history of one or more thrombotic events, 70% or more VTE.[118] Graft thrombosis has been observed in 27% to 50% of patients positive for antiphospholipid antibody.[119,120] Although the incidence of antiphospholipid antibodies was elevated in a group of young white men with chronic lower leg ischemia,[121] a prospective comparison of elective infrainguinal bypass grafting revealed that there was minimal difference in primary or assisted patency rates, limb salvage, or survival between patients positive and negative for antiphospholipid antibodies.[122]

The diagnosis should be suspected in someone with a prolonged activated partial thromboplastin time (aPTT) with other standard coagulation tests normal, along with the presence of an increased antiphospholipid or anticardiolipin antibody titer and elevation of α_2 glycoprotein I.[4,123] The prolongation in the aPTT is strictly a laboratory phenomenon. The antiphospholipid antibody interacts with the anionic phospholipids in the aPTT assay, prolonging the aPTT. The dilute Russell viper venom time confirms the presence of a lupus anticoagulant.

There is imperfect agreement between diagnostic tests for this abnormality. Approximately 80% of patients with a prolonged aPTT will have a positive antiphospholipid antibody, but only 10% to 50% of patients with a positive antiphospholipid antibody will have a prolonged aPTT.[124] Patients with both tests positive are reported to have the same thrombotic risk as those with either test alone.

Heparin followed by warfarin [international normalized ratio (INR) >3.0] has been recommended for the treatment of the antiphospholipid syndrome.[118,125] For recurrent fetal loss, heparin or LMWH use through pregnancy is recommended. In patients with lupus anticoagulants, heparin is monitored by antifactor Xa levels.

Defects with Lower Risk for Thrombosis

Resistance to Activated Protein C (Factor V Leiden)

Venous is much more common than arterial.

Resistance to APC has been reported to be present in 20% to 60% of cases of idiopathic VTE and is the most common underlying abnormality associated with VTE. This disorder is present in 1% to 2% of the general population.[126–128] It confers a relatively low risk for thrombosis, however. It is more common in whites than in nonwhite Americans.[126] As a result of the substitution of a single amino acid, glutamine for arginine, at position 506 in the protein for factor V (termed factor V Leiden) caused by a nucleotide substitution of guanine for adenine at 1691 in Factor V gene, hypercoagulability is conferred by resistance to inactivation of factor Va by APC.[129–131] Additionally, less VIIIa is interfered with, compounding the hypercoagulability. Thrombotic manifestations are noted in those individuals both homozygous and heterozygous for this mutation. The relative risk for VTE in patients heterozygous for factor V Leiden is sevenfold, whereas the relative risk is 80-fold for those homozygous for factor V Leiden.[132] In contrast to factor deficiency states, persons homozygous for this mutation usually do not die in infancy. Additionally, thrombosis is potentiated in the presence of additional acquired risk factors, such as women using oral contraceptives, pregnancy, and coexistent hyperhomocysteinemia.[130,133,134]

Combined defects with other hypercoagulable states, such as protein C and S deficiency or prothrombin G20210A, increase the thrombotic risk.[135,136] In addition to cases of VTE, recurrent VTE is also more common in patients with this entity, with a relative risk 2.4-fold.[137] Although VTE predominates in patients with this syndrome, arterial thrombosis has also been reported.[138]

The diagnosis of APC resistance is made by a clot-based functional assay with the addition of APC (modified APTT). Additionally, genetic analysis should be performed to confirm heterozygosity versus homozygosity, as treatment decisions may be different between the two states. If the patient has a known lupus anticoagulant syndrome, this entity may interfere with the clot-based APC resistance assay[139] and genetic analysis is more accurate.

Treatment options for APC resistance after VTE include anticoagulation, initially heparin, followed by oral anticoagulation. The long-term use of warfarin is controversial. No data exist to suggest that long-term warfarin should be given after a first episode of VTE in a patient heterozygous for the mutation.[140] The fact that APC resistance is a relatively low risk for recurrent thrombosis (2.4-fold) suggests that not all patients after their first episode of VTE need long-term anticoagulant treatment. Patients must be evaluated in light of their overall risk for thrombosis.[141]

Hyperhomocystinemia

Venous is approximately equal to arterial.

Hyperhomocystinemia has been a known risk factor for atherosclerosis and vascular disease for more than 25 years, though a direct cause and effect relationship has not been established.[142–144] However, a recent meta analysis suggests the risk of VTE to be 2.5-fold with elevated homocysteine levels,[145] and hyperhomocystinemia is responsible for up to 10% of VTE. Two enzyme deficiencies, N^5, N^{10}, methylene tetrahydrofolate reductase (MTHFR) or cystathionine beta synthase, are responsible for elevated homocysteine levels.[146] Deficiencies in vitamins B_6 and B_{12} and folate also contribute to elevations in homocysteine. Although mutations in these enzymes are not infrequent, the common polymorphism in MTHFR alone is not a factor in either the elevation of plasma homocysteine or thrombosis.[147] Hyperhomocystinemia also has been found to be a risk factor for VTE in those younger than 40 years,[148] in women[142] and for recurrent venous thrombosis in patients between 20 and 70 years of age.[143] The combination of hyperhomocystinemia and factor V Leiden results in an increased risk of venous and arterial thromboses.[149] Elevated plasma homocysteine results in abnormal endothelial function.[150–154] Additionally, elevated homocysteine increases lipid peroxidation, impairing NO synthetase and degrading NO[155,156] and increasing thromboxane B_2 while decreasing prostacyclin levels.[157] The sum is that homocysteine elevation injures endothelial cells.

Fasting homocysteine levels are determined from serum, usually on two occasions. The test may also be performed after a methionine oral loading regimen.[158,159]

Homocysteine elevation is treated with folate supplements. Although the association between hyperhomocystinemia and VTE has been established, treatment to lower homocysteine levels and the long-term effects of such treatment on procoagulant activity have yet to be validated.[142]

Prothrombin G20210 Polymorphism

Venous is much more common than arterial.

Prothrombin (factor II), a vitamin K-dependent factor synthesized in the liver, becomes thrombin when activated. A recently recognized genetic polymorphism in the distal 3′ untranslated region of the gene for prothrombin has been described in patients with VTE. This results in a normal prothrombin but at increased levels.[133,160,161] This polymorphism, called G20210A, confers an increased risk for VTE by two- to sevenfold. It is associated with 4% to 6 % of patients with VTE.[141,162,163] This thrombosis risk is increased in pregnant women,[164] in women with early myocardial infarctions[165] and in synergy with factor V Leiden.[133] Most patients are heterozygous for this mutation, which affects whites more often. It rarely affects patients of Asian or African descent.[165] Genetic analysis for the 20210 (G to A) mutation is the marker for this abnormality.[166]

Patients who present with VTE should be treated according to current standards and akin to the treatment for heterozygous factor V Leiden. Individuals with prothrombin G20210A who have recurrent episodes of VTE should undergo lifelong anticoagulation, as should those patients with both prothrombin G20210A and factor V Leiden.[133]

Other Disorders Associated with Thrombosis

Defective Fibrinolysis/Dysfibrinogenemia/Lipoprotein(a)

Venous is approximately equal to arterial.

Abnormal plasminogens (dysplasminogenemias), although rare (<1%), have been described in cases of spontaneous arterial or VTE.[167] Other defects in fibrinolysis may affect up to 10% of the normal population.[168] Abnormal fibrinogens may account for 1% to 3% of patients with venous thrombosis and those presenting with digital ischemia.[169] Numerous molecular defects have been classified. Defective thrombin binding or resistance to plasmin-mediated breakdown has been described.[170] Although not clearly documented, defects in plasminogen activators, tPA, or uPA may incite thrombotic events.[171] Moreover, elevated PAI-1 has been associated with DVT and myocardial infarction.[167] Although the relationship between VTE and abnormal fibrinolysis is debated, it is clear that in the postoperative period there is a connection between fibrinolysis and VTE.[167,172,173] Additionally, PAI-1 is up-regulated by thrombin, endotoxin, and IL-1, explaining the elevated circulating levels of PAI-1 during infections.[174] Lipoprotein(a), associated with LDL, has both atherogenic and prothrombotic properties.[175–177] It prevents plasminogen from binding to cells or fibrin and inhibits fibrinolysis.[178] Elevated levels of lipoprotein(a) have been associated with VTE in childhood; it is a weak thrombotic risk factor in adults.[179]

A confirmatory test for dysfibrinogenemia includes a fibrinogen clotting activity-to-antigen ratio. It may also be detected by a prolonged thrombin clotting time (TCT) or reptilase time.[180] Abnormal plasminogens are detected by the presence of reduced activity to antigen ratios. PAI-1 levels have to be measured directed by activity or antigen assay. Lipoprotein(a) levels are measured in serum.

When an individual with thrombosis presents with one of the previously mentioned abnormalities, standard anticoagulation is necessary.[181,182]

Abnormal Platelet Aggregation

Arterial is more common than venous.

It has been recognized for some time that there are patients who have thrombosis and may have hyperactive/hyperresponsive platelets; this entity is poorly defined. Diabetes mellitus, which is known to be associated with hyperactive platelets and hyperlipidemic states, may be a contributing factor. Two clinical settings in which abnormal platelet aggregation has been associated with thrombosis include advanced malignancy of the lung and uterus and after carotid endarterectomy. Hyperactive platelets have also been noted during graft thrombosis in peripheral vascular reconstructions.[183] Although platelet aggregation assays may be helpful in making the diagnosis, these assays are not commonly performed or standardized and, thus, the incidence and importance of platelets to thrombosis are not well known. Bleeding time measurements are not specific and not recommended for making this diagnosis.

Standard anticoagulant treatment is recommended for this condition. Aspirin and the thienopyridine derivatives such as clopidogrel may be useful, but their utility is unknown.[184]

Elevated Procoagulant Factors: VIII, IX, and XI

Venous is more common than arterial.

Elevated prothrombotic factors have only recently been associated with primary and recurrent VTE.[141,185] A dose-response effect has been observed and elevated factor VIII has been best studied.[185–187] Factor VIII:C above the 90th percentile is associated with a five times increased risk of VTE.[187,188] Factor VIII:C elevation is also affected by blood type and race. Elevation of factor XI above the 90th percentile is associated with a two times increase in VTE, independent of other hypercoagulability factors.[189] Similar increases in VTE risk have been observed with elevated factor IX.[190] Acquired and environmental factors precipitate VTE in patients with elevation of these factors, as opposed to inherited deficiencies of AT, protein C, and protein S that confer higher VTE risk.[191]

The diagnosis is made by the direct measurement of these factors with activity assays. If VTE occurs with one of these factor elevated, the standard of care of anticoagulant management should be undertaken.[182]

Disseminated Intravascular Coagulation

DIC is the primary form of acute thrombosis. Causes of DIC include abruptio placentae, gram-positive and gram-negative sepsis, endotoxemia, malignant tumors, pelvic operations, certain snake bites, hematologic malignancies, and hepatic failure.[4] Coagulation is activated by the release into the circulation of TF, which activates factor VII to VIIa, leading to massive thrombin production and fibrin generation. Fibrinolysis then becomes activated, leading to bleeding in the later stages of the syndrome because of the consumption of clotting factors, depletion of fibrinogen, and unchecked plasmin activity. Laboratory values in DIC reveal a decline in platelet count and fibrinogen level with a concomitant elevation in fibrin split products and the presence of a positive D-dimer test. A more chronic form of DIC has been reported, with the release of small amounts of TF into the circulation in conditions such as tumors of the prostate, diabetes mellitus, use of factor IX concentrates, total hip replacement, and abdominal aortic aneurysm.[4] In a prospective study of 76 patients with extensive aortic aneurysms, 4% of patients (especially those with thoracoabdominal involvement) exhibited clinically overt DIC before surgery.[192] In this more chronic form of DIC, fibrinogen tends to remain within the normal range.

Summary of Hypercoagulable States

A number of conditions can lead to a procoagulant state. A procoagulant screen should include routine coagulation tests such as the aPTT and platelet count, AT III activity and antigen assay, protein C antigen and activity levels, protein

S antigen level, and mixing studies to identify a lupus anticoagulant (if indicated); APC resistance assay and factor V Leiden gene analysis; prothrombin 20210 genetic analysis; homocysteine level; an antiphospholipid antibody screen that includes anticardiolipin antibody; fibrinogen level; functional plasminogen assay; and platelet aggregation testing, if possible. Although conditions exist that lead to these hypercoagulable states, only 10% to 15% of patients with venous thrombosis have one of the conditions listed here, with the most frequent condition involving abnormalities in factor V Leiden. The incidence increases with the concentration of patients at high risk in specialized coagulation centers[193] and may be even higher with the measurement of new parameters such as resistance to protein C in which the incidence may be as high as 20% to 40%.[194–196] Thus, not every patient with a thrombotic event should be screened. However, patients with strong positive family histories, young patients with arterial and venous thromboses without obvious cause, and patients with multiple episodes of thrombosis without an underlying anatomic abnormality should be investigated and screened.

BLEEDING DISORDERS

Although the surgeon deals more often with procoagulant states than bleeding disorders, it is important to recognize these disorders when they occur.

Coagulation Factor Deficiency

Coagulation factor deficiency states are important causes of bleeding. Factor VIII and IX deficiency states are involved in hemophilia A and B and type I von Willebrand disease (VWD). Hemophilia A (Fig. 5.11) is inherited as a sex-linked recessive deficiency of factor VIII, with fewer cases secondary to spontaneous mutation. The incidence of this abnormality is approximately 1 in 10,000 births. Clinical findings range from bleeding into joints and muscles, epistaxis, hematuria, and bleeding after minor trauma, to prolonged postoperative bleeding, retroperitoneal bleeding, and intramural bowel hemorrhage. Laboratory screening tests usually reveal a prolongation of the aPTT along with decreased factor VIII levels; other test results are normal. The minimum level of factor VIII required for hemostasis is 30%, and spontaneous bleeding is uncommon with factor VIII levels greater than 5% to 10% of normal.[197] Levels less than 2% constitute severe, 2% to 5% moderate, and greater than 5% mild deficiency.[198] Severe deficiency with levels less than 1% poses the risk for spontaneous bleeding episodes. Although the half-life of factor VIII is 2.9 days in normal subjects, the half-life of factor VIII concentrates is only 9 to 18 hours.[4] Levels between 80% to 100% of normal should be attained for surgical bleeding or life-threatening hemorrhage. Acquired deficiency has been reported to occur with the development of antibodies to factor VIII after therapy. Inhibitor antibodies develop in approximately 10% to 15% of patients with hemophilia A, although the incidence of antibody formation may be much higher in previously untreated patients and in those with severe hemophilia A. A new recombinant factor VIII preparation has been developed and tested in children and infants. Despite the development of low levels of inhibitors in 20% of children at a mean 9 days after first administration, these inhibitors either disappeared or remained at low levels.[199] Because this recombinant preparation is virus free, the benefits outweigh the risks of low levels of inhibitor development for the treatment of hemophilia A (especially because in 1992, almost 30% of the entire hemophilic population in the United States had reported AIDS and more than 22% had died of AIDS).[200]

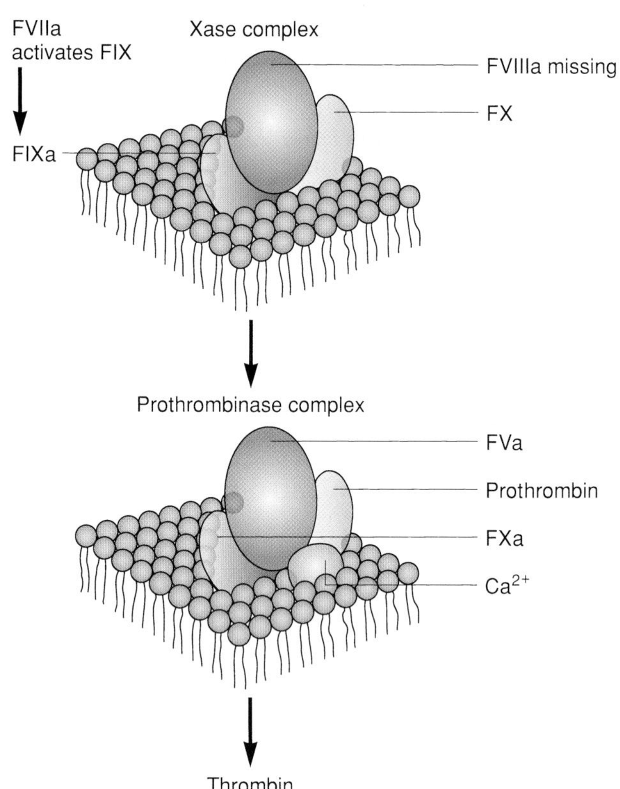

FIGURE 5.11 Hemophilia A involves a deficiency of factor VIII. (After Hassouna HI. Laboratory evaluation of hemostatic disorders. *Hematol Oncol Clin North Am.* 1993;7:1187, with permission.)

Factor IX deficiency (Christmas factor), known as hemophilia B (Fig. 5.12), is transmitted as an X-linked recessive trait. It also may be acquired because of enhanced factor IX clearance in states such as the nephrotic syndrome, abnormal protein production in vitamin K deficiency, and acquired specific inhibitors to factor IX in various autoimmune diseases, such as SLE. It is clinically indistinguishable from hemophilia A, and laboratory screening tests reveal a prolonged aPTT, with other test results normal, although a greater proportion of patients have only mild or moderate deficiency.[201] Severe deficiency (approximately 30% of cases) is defined as a level of activity less than 4% of normal, whereas moderate deficiency is reported with activity levels between 20% and 40%.[4] Treatment consists of plasma or factor IX concentrates and vitamin K. It has been recommended that levels greater than 30% be achieved for hemostasis.[197]

vWF causes platelet adhesion to collagen, initiating platelet plug formation. It also forms a complex with factor VIII in the blood. Produced in endothelial cells and megakaryocytes (compared with the liver for factor VIII), it has a circulating half-life of 6 to 20 hours.[4] VWD, a deficiency of vWF, is the most common of the inherited coagulation disorder. A number of different subtypes have been identified for its deficiency state (Fig. 5.13), and the syndrome is transmitted as both autosomal dominant (heterozygous) and autosomal recessive (homozygous) forms. Variants include types I and III (quantitative decreases in normal-appearing vWF) and type II (qualitative abnormalities in structure and function of vWF).[202] vWF deficiency is probably as common as hemophilia A, although the true incidence may surpass what is generally appreciated because many mild cases probably remain undiagnosed. The classic syndrome is caused by a reduction of factor VIII activity (although not as great as

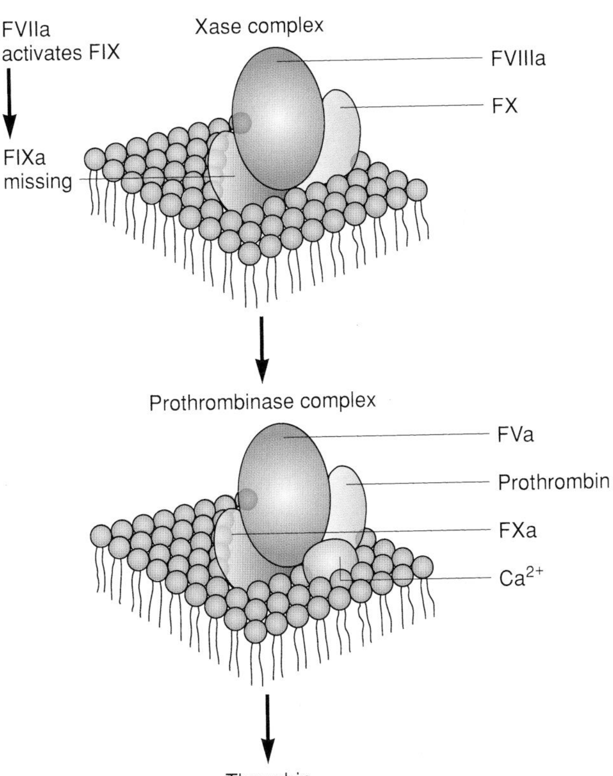

FIGURE 5.12 Hemophila B involves a deficiency of factor IX. (After Hassouna HI. Laboratory evaluation of hemostatic disorders. *Hematol Oncol Clin North Am.* 1993;7:1190, with permission.)

in hemophilia A) and vWF (vWF–factor VIII complex). Clinical manifestations include easy bruisability, mild to moderate epistaxis, gingival bleeding, menorrhagia, rare joint or muscle bleeding, prolonged bleeding following surgery, and subcutaneous bleeding.[4] Spontaneous bleeding is not as common as in

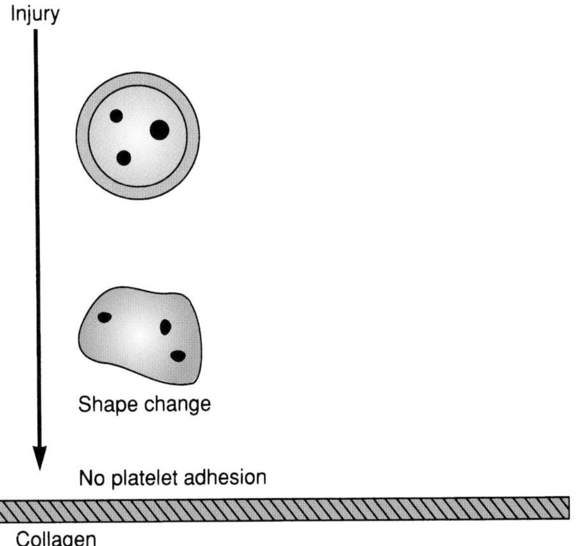

FIGURE 5.13 von Willebrand's disease involves an absence of platelet adhesion to collagen. (After Hassouna HI. Laboratory evaluation of hemostatic disorders. *Hematol Oncol Clin North Am.* 1993;7:1187, with permission.)

hemophilia A. Screening laboratory tests include prolonged aPTT, with other coagulation test results normal; a prolonged bleeding time; a decreased level of factor VIII activity; decreased immunoreactive levels of the vWF; and abnormal platelet aggregation response to ristocetin.[4] The most reliable source of vWF is cryoprecipitate, although many concentrates of factor VIII have vWF present and show promise. Desmopressin acetate (DDAVP) is available for the treatment of mild cases; serum levels of 25% to 50% are needed for hemostasis.[197] Recently, recombinant factor VIII/vWF concentrates that avoid the infectious risks of transfusion have become available.

Other specific factor deficiencies are much less common and receive only a brief mention here. Factor XI (plasma thromboplastin antecedent), complexed to high-molecular-weight kininogen in the plasma, has a half-life of 40 to 80 hours.[4] Deficiency of this factor carries an autosomal recessive inheritance. Homozygous patients have levels up to 20% of normal, whereas heterozygous patients typically show levels between 30% and 65% of normal.[4] This syndrome is particularly frequent in certain ethnic groups such as Ashkenazi Jews. Screening tests include a prolonged aPTT and whole-blood clotting time, with other coagulation test results normal.[4] A factor XI assay is the definitive test for the diagnosis. Treatment includes administration of fresh frozen plasma, and hemostasis requires at least 25% of normal factor XI activity.[197]

Factor V (proaccelerin) deficiency is rare. This factor produced in the liver has a half-life of 12 to 36 hours, and its deficiency is inherited as autosomal recessive.[4] Severe deficiency (called *parahemophilia*) occurs with 1% plasma activity, whereas moderate deficiency is characterized by 25% plasma activity.[4] Deficiency of factor V becomes important in the coagulopathy associated with early liver transplantation. Dysfunctional factor V syndrome has also been described. An acquired syndrome has been seen in patients with acute and chronic liver disease.[4] Screening tests include prolonged aPTT, prothrombin time (PT), and whole-blood clotting times; levels of factor V may be measured. Treatment consists of fresh frozen plasma; levels at least 15% of normal are needed for hemostasis.[197]

Factor VII (proconvertin) deficiency is inherited as an autosomal recessive trait. Homozygous deficiency is found with levels of 10% of normal, whereas heterozygous patients have levels 40% to 60% of normal.[4] A dysfunctional syndrome has also been described with normal levels of factor VII and decreased enzymatic activity. Again, this deficiency state can also be acquired in the presence of liver disease and vitamin K deficiency. Heterozygous patients do not have symptoms, but homozygous patients often display bleeding. Screening tests include a prolonged PT, with other coagulation test results normal.[4] A factor VII assay confirms the diagnosis, and treatment involves the administration of fresh frozen plasma. Levels as low as 10% of normal allow for hemostasis.[197]

Factor X (Stuart-Power factor) deficiency is transmitted as an autosomal recessive, heterogeneous, incomplete recessive trait. Homozygous patients (severe deficiency) have less than 1% of normal plasma activity, whereas those with moderate deficiency demonstrate levels between 10% and 20% of normal plasma activity.[4] Acquired deficiency states have been described. Screening tests include a prolonged aPTT, PT, and whole-blood clotting time with a normal TCT; a specific factor X assay exists. Clinical findings include minor or major bleeding episodes, and treatment involves the use of fresh frozen plasma. Plasma levels should be maintained above 10% of normal to prevent bleeding.[197]

The rarest of the inherited disorders of bleeding is factor II deficiency. This deficiency, transmitted as an autosomal recessive trait, can also be related to liver disease, oral anticoagulation, and the newborn period. Screening tests include a prolonged aPTT and PT, with normal TCT and platelet function.[4] Factor II has a half-life of 2 to 5 days, and treatment involves the use of fresh frozen plasma and prothrombin concentrates; levels of 40% are needed for hemostasis.[197]

Deficiencies of fibrinogen can also lead to bleeding disorders. This is the only factor deficiency state in which the TCT is prolonged. It is generally believed that a fibrinogen level of 100 mg/mL should be achieved to stop bleeding related to fibrinogen abnormalities. Fibrinogen deficiency may also occur from consumption during DIC and from primary fibrinolytic states.

Platelet Disorders

Platelet disorders are another important cause of bleeding. Platelets have three major roles in coagulation: (a) initial adhesion to areas of endothelial denudation; (b) externalization of a phospholipid surface for coagulation complex assembly, accelerating the speed of coagulation; and (c) aggregation for platelet plug formation. Platelet function can be related to three distinct zones. The outer zone contains the glycoprotein receptors responsible for platelet adhesion (GpIb) and platelet aggregation (GpIIb/IIIa); receptors for fibrinogen, vWF, and fibronectin (GpIIb/IIIa); and the receptor for thrombospondin (GpIIIb).[4] The second zone, the sol-gel zone, contains elements that allow platelet contraction; the third zone, the organelle zone, contains electron-dense bodies that store calcium, serotonin, ADP and adenosine triphosphate, and the nondense α granules that store markers for platelet activation.[4] Bleeding associated with platelets includes mucosal bleeding (e.g., epistaxis), easy bruisability, petechiae, purpura, and menorrhagia.

Extracorporeal bypass circuits, such as cardiopulmonary bypass and ECMO, activate platelets regardless of the type of oxygenator used and can produce bleeding. During cardiopulmonary bypass, after fibrinogen and IgG become adsorbed onto the bypass circuit, platelets are immediately activated. These activated platelets change their shape, aggregate, and adhere to the fibrinogen surface through multiple interactions between the GpIIb/IIIa receptor and the exposed binding sites on the carboxyl terminus of the g chain of fibrinogen and the Fc regions of IgG antibodies. Fibrinogen also can induce both platelet activation and aggregation. Platelets release granule contents, such as PF_4, β-thromboglobulin, serotonin, adenine nucleotides, and thromboxane, and their sensitivity to various platelet agonists decreases. Some adherent platelets break away and leave membrane fragments on the surface of the extracorporeal circuit. Platelet aggregates form; new, larger platelets arrive from the bone marrow; and a heterogeneous mixture of platelet fragments, degranulated platelets, resealed platelets with damaged membranes, reversibly activated platelets, and new platelets results.[203] Thus, bleeding time increases are usually recorded. In addition, cardiopulmonary bypass activates factor XII and complement (the contact activation system), leading to neutrophil activation, release of lysosomal enzymes, generation of oxygen free radicals, and the harmful "inflammatory" response noted with extracorporeal circuits along with the direct activation of the fibrinolytic system by plasmin activation. Prosthetic vascular grafts likewise activate platelets and platelet uptake on both Dacron (Fig. 5.14) and expanded polytetrafluoroethylene grafts has been found in a number of animal models and in patients for up to 6 months to 10 years after graft implantation.[204] This platelet uptake appears to be mostly a phenomenon of recruitment with

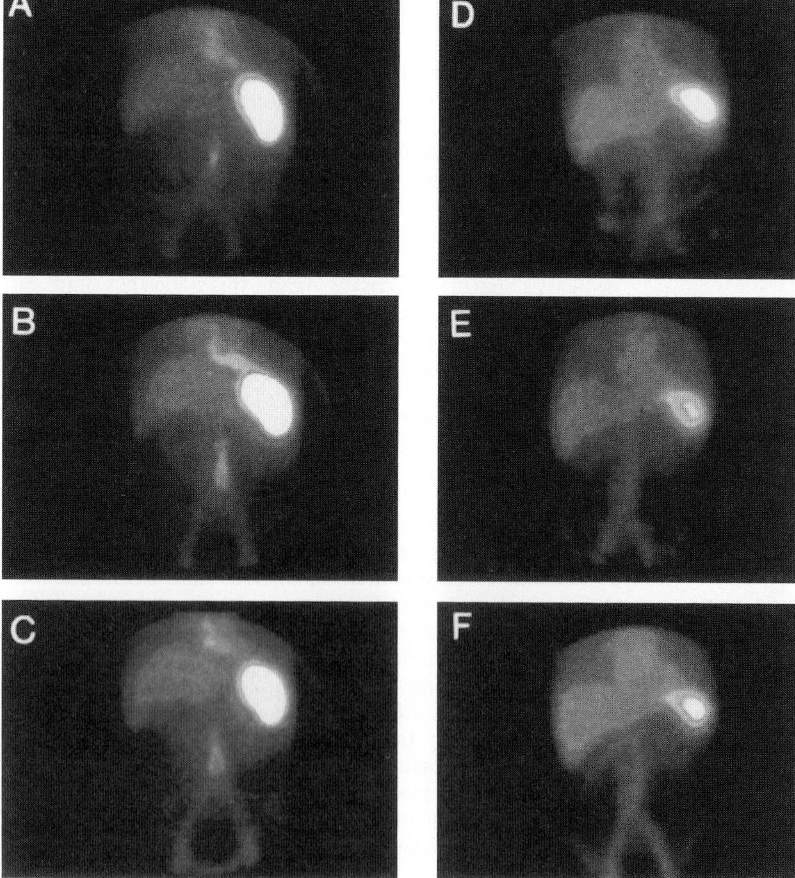

FIGURE 5.14 Human Dacron aortic graft platelet activity at 1 week (*A*), 3 months (*B*), and 6 months (*C*), versus absence of human expanded polytetrafluoroethylene (ePTFE) aortic graft platelet activity at 1 week (*D*), 3 months (*E*), and 6 months (*F*). (After Wakefield TW, Shulkin BL, Fellows EP, et al. Platelet reactivity in human aortic grafts: a prospective, randomized mid-term study of platelet adherence and release products in Dacron and ePTFE grafts. *J Vasc Surg.* 1989;9:238, with permission.)

three different mechanisms: the release of ADP from activated platelets, the production of thromboxane from activated platelets, and the generation of thrombin.

Inherited defects of platelet receptors include defects of GpIIb/IIIa (Glanzmann's thrombasthenia), characterized by impaired platelet binding to vWF, fibrinogen, and fibronectin. In patients with defects in GpIb (Bernard-Soulier syndrome), the absolute number of platelets is decreased, the platelets are larger, and platelet aggregation and adhesion are abnormal.[4] Acquired deficits occur in uremia, both GpIb and GpIIb/IIIa receptors are defective, resulting in impaired adhesion and aggregation. Acquired deficits also occur in patients who previously received platelet transfusions and then acquire immune-mediated anti-platelet antibodies. Patients with Glanzmann's thrombasthenia also show abnormalities in the sol-gel zone, and their platelets lack the ability to contract and retract. A number of platelet disorders associated with abnormalities of the organelle zone have also been described.

Abnormalities in Fibrinolysis

Abnormalities in fibrinolysis may play a role in abnormal bleeding disorders. Genetic or acquired deficiencies in α_2-AP may be associated with bleeding, whereas deficiencies in factor XIII (fibrin stabilizing factor) may lead to highly lysable clot. α_2-AP deficiency is treated with e-aminocaproic acid or tranexamic acid. Homozygous patients with factor XIII deficiency and less than 1% of normal plasma activity often show bleeding from the umbilical cord at birth, bleeding after trauma or surgery, and delayed bleeding 24 to 36 hours later.[4] Intracranial bleeding also has been noted. Screening test results include a shortened euglobulin lysis time.[4] A specific assay for factor XIII activity exists. Treatment consists of fresh frozen plasma, cryoprecipitate, and factor XIII concentrates. Finally, a deficiency of PAI-1 has been described that may lead to bleeding.

PHARMACOLOGIC AND NONPHARMACOLOGIC INTERVENTIONS

Heparin

Heparin, discovered by Jay McLean in 1916, is a heterogeneous mixture of sulfated polysaccharide molecules of varying molecular weights, ranging from 2 to 40 kd. Heparin is obtained from beef lung or porcine intestine. Heparin accelerates the reaction between thrombin and antithrombin III, accelerating the inhibition of thrombin and other serine proteases by AT III. Heparin also directly binds and inhibits coagulation proteases and is important for the selective inhibitor of thrombin, heparin cofactor II. After bolus injection, heparin's half-life is approximately 90 to 120 minutes, although the half-life depends on the amount injected—the more injected, the longer the half-life. Activated factor X and activated factor II are most sensitive to the heparin–AT III complex. Heparin is cleared through the reticuloendothelial system and does not cross the placental barrier. Clinical use of heparin in venous thrombosis and pulmonary embolism (PE) and as a prophylactic agent has been established.[205] A lower frequency of bleeding complications has been found with continuous infusion rather than bolus injections. In addition, a lesser degree of thrombin accumulation has been found with continuous administration. In monitoring heparin, an aPTT 1.5 times control or a TCT two times control reflects adequate anticoagulation. Activated clotting times (ACTs) in a range of 150 to 200 seconds also suggest adequate anticoagulation. In many situations, direct measurements of heparin levels do not correlate with the level of anticoagulation as measured by aPTT. Heparin decreases platelet aggregability while enhancing the generation of thromboxane from platelets.[206] Noncoagulant high-molecular-weight heparin fragments may also potentiate platelet aggregation, and heparin-associated thrombocytopenia from an immune mechanism is a potential complication of heparin use. Monitoring of platelet counts should begin on the fourth day of heparin therapy (earlier if the patient has previously been on heparin) and repeated approximately on days 7, 10, and 14. The most common complication of heparin therapy is bleeding. The risk of hemorrhage is increased in the elderly; in postmenopausal women; and in patients with preexisting abnormalities of coagulation, thrombocytopenia, and uremia. Long-term therapy may be associated with alopecia and osteoporosis; osteoporosis has been found in patients receiving large doses of heparin for longer than 6 months.

The use of low-dose heparin therapy has been endorsed for a number of applications by a consensus statement on venous thrombosis prophylaxis.[207,208] In a meta-analysis of 70 randomized trials in 16,000 patients comparing low-dose heparin with standard therapy for venous thrombosis prophylaxis, the odds of development of DVT with low-dose heparin decreased 67% ± 4%, whereas for PE (both fatal and nonfatal), the odds decreased 47% ± 10%.[209] For fatal PE, the odds reduction was even greater (64% ± 15%). No increase in mortality from other causes was found in patients treated with low-dose heparin. Importantly, these reductions were seen in urologic, elective orthopedic, and traumatic orthopedic procedures. This is somewhat at variance concerning urologic and orthopedic patients, in whom low-dose heparin is not thought to be efficacious, but it may reflect previous errors in interpretation of studies with small numbers of patients (type II error). Bleeding complications were more frequent in the heparin-treated patients, with no difference between 5,000 units twice a day and 5,000 units three times a day. Low-dose heparin prophylaxis appears to be a good means of preventing venous thromboembolic events during many surgical procedures but should be confined to those patients known to be at high risk owing to the potential for increased bleeding complications.[208]

Because of the bleeding complications related to low-dose heparin, there is considerable interest in LMWH for venous thrombosis prophylaxis. Standard heparin is a mixture of polysaccharide molecules that vary in size from 2 to 40 kd. The anticoagulant effect is primarily centered over the lower end of the molecular weight spectrum. Standard unfractionated heparin is able to inhibit thrombin because it is large enough to make a ternary complex between itself, thrombin, and AT III. LMWHs are not large enough to make this complex because the minimum chain length necessary for formation of such a ternary complex is 18 saccharide units. Thus, LMWHs demonstrate less AT activity. However, for inhibition of factor Xa, such a ternary complex is not necessary. Thus, LMWHs are able to inhibit factor Xa. Each LMWH preparation has its own antifactor Xa–to–antifactor IIa (thrombin) ratio, depending on its size and molecular weight. Most commercially available LMWHs have ratios between 4:1 and 2:1, whereas standard unfractionated heparin has a 1:1 ratio. Because the bleeding potential of heparin is related largely to its AT activity, LMWHs should have a lower bleeding potential. In addition, LMWHs have less antiplatelet activity and less risk for HIT.

The LMWHs have other advantages over standard unfractionated heparin. These include an improved pharmacokinetic profile due to reduced nonspecific binding to plasma proteins, less lipolysis, a half-life that is not dose dependent, more constant antifactor Xa inhibition, less interference with protein C activation, less complement activation and interference with appropriate platelet aggregation, less risk for osteoporosis, and a lower level of fibrin monomer production.[210] High and sustained plasma antifactor Xa levels exist for greater than 16 hours after LMWH administration in therapeutic doses, and its excretion is primarily renal. There is no available agent effective for complete LMWH reversal as measured by antifactor Xa levels.[211]

The LMWHs were first used in DVT prophylaxis, and they have become the prophylactic agent of choice in orthopedic hip and knee surgery and in high-risk general surgery patients.[209] More recently, they have been used in the full treatment of DVT and PE. A number of level 1 studies and meta-analyses have compared LMWH with standard unfractionated heparin in the treatment of DVT.[212,213] Together, these studies demonstrate a lower risk of major bleeding, a lower risk of recurrent thromboembolic events, and a lower risk of death than with standard unfractionated heparin. Even for PE, LMWH appears at least equivalent if not superior to standard unfractionated heparin but much more convenient.[214] It is not necessary to monitor LMWH with coagulation testing except in specific situations such as renal failure, and most dosage schemes use either fixed-dose or weight-adjusted dosing given subcutaneously. Because there is no need for coagulation testing, outpatient treatment has become a reality. However, a number of different services need to be coordinated for such outpatient treatment to be successful, including home nursing, pharmacy, coagulation (for warfarin monitoring), and physician.

LMWH has also been studied in unstable angina.[210] LMWH has been found superior to placebo and equivalent or superior to standard unfractionated heparin when evaluating the outcomes death or myocardial infarction, without any increase in major bleeding. The question remains whether one preparation of LMWH will be found superior to another, or whether all preparations are equivalent and share the same advantages for the treatment of DVT, PE, and unstable angina.

Reversal of heparin anticoagulation with protamine sulfate may be associated with adverse hemodynamic and hematologic side effects, including hypotension, bradycardia, pulmonary artery hypertension or hypotension, declines in oxygen consumption, leukopenia, and thrombocytopenia.[215,216] Although the pulmonary changes have been observed in up to 3% to 4% of cases, hypotension is more frequent. In addition, deaths have been reported after the use of protamine, with noncardiogenic pulmonary edema and right heart failure accompanying the most severe reactions. In a survey sent to members of the Society for Vascular Surgery and the European Society for Vascular Surgery, the incidence of noteworthy protamine-related side effects was significant at 4% to 5%, as reported by approximately 650 surgeons. The most likely cause of the hypotension appears to involve the elaboration of a vasodilator factor, such as NO, as well as a direct depression of myocardial function, including the development of bradycardia.[217,218] Pulmonary artery hypertension, on the contrary, is thought to result from thromboxane release from nonplatelet sources in the pulmonary circulation.[219] Finally, thrombocytopenia and leukopenia are most likely the result of a direct effect of protamine on phospholipid membranes of these blood elements.[220] Immunologic reactions also may occur in patients with prior exposure to protamine, especially in diabetic patients taking NPH insulin that contains protamine (to allow for more prolonged absorption) or those previously exposed to protamine. Unfortunately, no other effective and safe agent for heparin neutralization exists, and in those situations when heparin must be reversed, such as at the completion of major aortic reconstructions and cardiopulmonary bypass, protamine must be given. Although it has been suggested that the rate of administration is the most crucial factor in protamine-related reactions, declines in hemodynamic parameters and oxygen consumption still occur with slow administration.[216] Work from our laboratory has demonstrated that total cationic charge appears to be an important determinant for both anticoagulation reversal efficacy and hemodynamic toxicity.[221]

Warfarin

Warfarin oral anticoagulant therapy is recommended for chronic treatment of venous thromboembolism. Warfarin interferes with the vitamin K–dependent clotting factors II, VII, IX, and X; protein C; and protein S. In the liver, these factors are γ-carboxylated in a reaction catalyzed by the reduced form of vitamin K. During this reaction, 10 to 12 glutamic acid residues are converted to γ-carboxyglutamic acid residues (Fig. 5.15). When these factors are released from the liver, they are secreted as active proteins.[4] The carboxyglutamic acid residues are responsible for these proteins binding to phospholipid membranes and the formation of the Xase and prothrombinase complexes on activated platelet surfaces. Warfarin prevents the reduction of vitamin K once it has functioned as a cofactor for the γ-carboxylation (Fig. 5.16). The level of anticoagulation is monitored with the PT. At levels higher than a one-stage PT of 1.4 times control, there is nearly a fivefold increase in the frequency of bleeding complications.[222] Because of variations in the thromboplastins used for the PT determinations in various countries, the INR system, in which the sensitivity of thromboplastins has been standardized, was developed.[223] Using this system, the proper range for treatment of venous thrombosis by warfarin is an INR of 2 to 3.

Major complications of sodium warfarin therapy include recurrent thrombosis, bleeding, and skin necrosis. It is recommended that warfarin be continued 3 to 6 months after an initial episode of DVT. Between 10 weeks and 4 months after DVT, the recurrent thrombosis rate is 8.3 episodes per 1,000 patient months. Between 4 months and 3 years, this incidence falls to four episodes per 1,000 patient months. At approximately 4 months, the risk of bleeding matches and exceeds the benefit from anticoagulant therapy. With recurrent DVT, the thrombotic risk is greater, and sustained anticoagulation is appropriate. Further, repeat venous thrombosis has been found in up to 20% of patients with recurrent venous thrombosis who are treated with only a short, 6-month course of warfarin.[224] In addition, for idiopathic DVT, a prolonged course greater than 3 months may be appropriate.[225] A recent multicenter trial suggested that for idiopathic DVT, low-dose warfarin (INR 1.5 to 2.0) was superior to placebo over a 4-year follow-up.[226] However, a second study suggested that full-dose warfarin (INR 2.0 to 3.0) was superior to low-dose warfarin in these same patients without a difference in bleeding, suggesting that idiopathic DVT requires long-term oral anticoagulation of some still to be defined duration.[227]

Patients at highest risk for bleeding on warfarin include the elderly, patients with gynecologic or urologic disorders, women after childbirth, and patients given large warfarin loading doses. A final important complication of warfarin is skin necrosis, which occurs more frequently in patients with protein C deficiency. This usually involves full-thickness skin sloughing over fatty areas such as the breasts and buttocks but can also be seen in other anatomic distributions such as the extremities and digits.

Antiplatelet Agents

Antiplatelet agents are used to prevent cardiovascular events such as coronary thrombosis and neointimal hyperplasia. Platelet aggregation is mediated by receptors that are part of

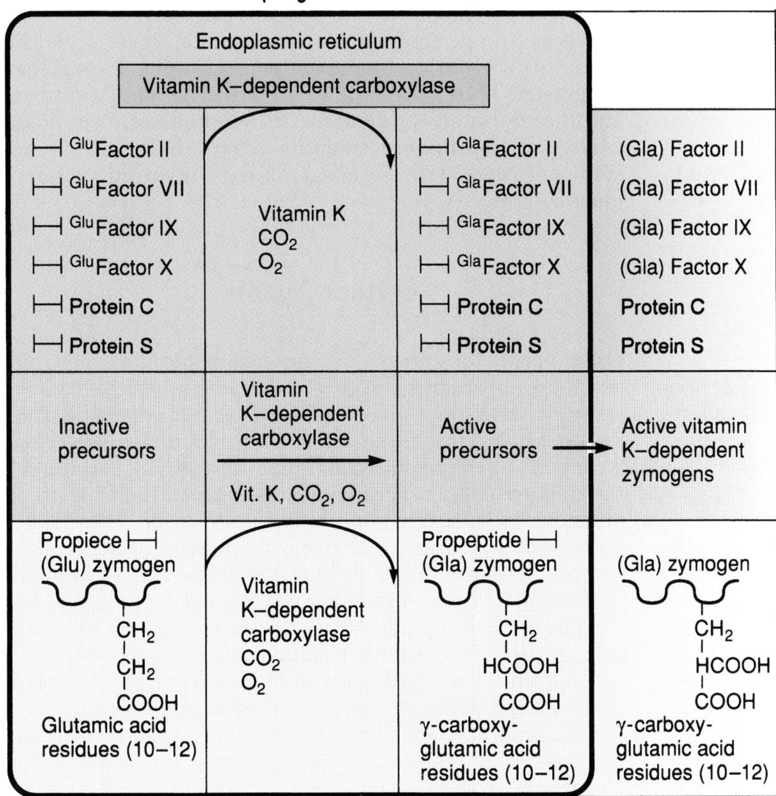

FIGURE 5.15 Conversion of glutamic acid residue to γ-carboxyglutamic acid residues by vitamin K-dependent carboxylase for factors II, VII, IX, and X, protein C, and protein S. (After Hassouna HI. Laboratory evaluation of hemostatic disorders. *Hematol Oncol Clin North Am.* 1993;7:1219, with permission.)

the mammalian integrin family. This family includes the β_1 family, mediating platelet interaction with cells, collagen, fibronectin, and laminin; the β_2 family (LeuCAM), present on leukocytes mediating interactions between leukocytes and other cells important in inflammation; and the β_3 family (cytoadhesion), including the megakaryocyte-specific GpIIb/IIIa receptor and the vitronectin receptor present on platelets and other cells.[228] Platelet aggregation is mediated by GpIIb/IIIa, which binds fibrinogen, vWF, fibronectin, vitronectin, and thrombospondin to activated platelets. These high-density receptors are hidden on unactivated platelets; they become exposed on the surface of activated platelets. Evidence suggests that fibrinogen on the surface of biomaterials can also bind these receptors and itself activate platelets. Fibrinogen's dimeric structure allows for platelet–platelet interactions and platelet aggregation. At high shear rates on biomaterials, however, vWF may mediate platelet aggregation. The GpIIb/IIIa receptor contains a binding site for the tripeptide sequence arginine–glycine–aspartic acid (RGD), which is common to many of the receptor proteins. Agonists for platelets expose

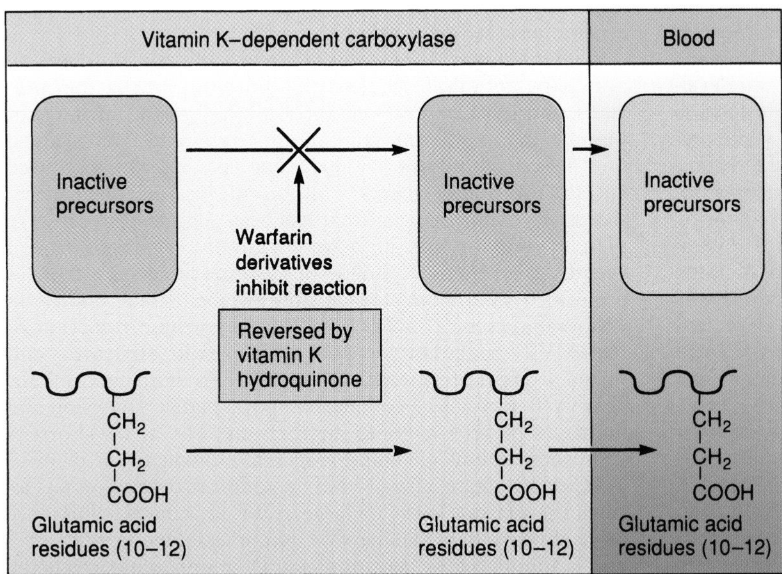

FIGURE 5.16 Secretion of inactive vitamin K-dependent precursor factors from the liver into the blood after warfarin administration. (After Hassouna HI. Laboratory evaluation of hemostatic disorders. *Hematol Oncol Clin North Am.* 1993;7:1220, with permission.)

this receptor, cause aggregation, and initiate the release of arachidonic acid, leading to thromboxane A_2 release and further platelet aggregation. Arachidonic acid release is not necessary for aggregation, however, because most agonists can directly expose GpIIb/IIIa. In addition, initial platelet adhesion is a stimulus for platelet aggregation and receptor exposure.

Platelet aggregation can be inhibited by the following methods:

1. Blocking cyclooxygenase, the first step converting arachidonic acid to thromboxane and prostacyclin
2. Blocking thromboxane synthase, the enzyme leading to thromboxane A_2
3. Blocking the thromboxane A_2 receptor
4. Increasing intraplatelet levels of cyclic adenosine monophosphate (cAMP) or guanosine monophosphate (GMP), which inhibit the exposure of the platelet GpIIb/IIIa receptor
5. Directly blocking the platelet receptor GpIIb/IIIa

Aspirin and indomethacin inhibit cyclooxygenase. Although aspirin inhibits thromboxane, it also inhibits prostacyclin. In clinical situations, the use of lower doses of aspirin in an attempt to inhibit thromboxane generation but preserve prostacyclin generation has not proven successful. Methylxanthines, such as dipyridamole (Persantine; Boehringer Ingelheim, Ridgefield, CT), inhibit phosphodiesterase, the enzyme that normally degrades cAMP, leading to higher levels of cAMP. Endothelium-derived relaxing factor (nitric acid), nitroglycerin, and nitroprusside inhibit platelet aggregation through modulation of cyclic GMP. In addition, monoclonal antibodies to GpIIb/IIIa itself or synthetic peptide blockers of this receptor containing the RGD sequence or the fibrinogen γ-chain carboxyl-terminal sequence directly inhibit the function of this receptor. Receptor blockage is the most specific way to inhibit aggregation; when the GpIIb/IIIa receptor is blocked, even high concentrations of agonists cannot stimulate platelets. In models of prosthetic vascular graft–platelet interactions, thromboxane synthase inhibitors appear less effective than aspirin, suggesting that endoperoxide intermediates are proaggregatory and can interact at the platelet thromboxane receptor, thus subverting any potential antiaggregatory effect of thromboxane reduction. Thromboxane receptor antagonists thus should rectify this situation and exhibit a synergistic effect with thromboxane synthase inhibitors. Thromboxane synthase inhibitors, not thromboxane receptor antagonists, are associated with a decreased urinary excretion of thromboxane metabolites and a marked increase in prostacyclin generation. Combined compounds with both thromboxane synthase inhibition and receptor antagonism have been developed with the intent of enhancing prostacyclin production from endoperoxide intermediates (antiaggregatory) while preventing these intermediates from combining with the thromboxane receptor and augmenting platelet aggregation. Ticlopidine inhibits the exposure of the GpIIb/IIIa receptor by unknown mechanisms. This agent, however, takes several days to become effective. Because of ticlopidine-associated neutropenia, an analogue of ticlopidine, clopidogrel, was developed. This thienopyridine compound is not associated with the same degree of neutropenia and has been shown to reduce the composite end points of stroke, myocardial infarction, and death in patients with vascular disease.[3]

Direct inhibitors of the GpIIb/IIIa receptor were first developed as murine-derived monoclonal antibodies. The compound C7E3Fab (ReoPro; Eli Lilly, Indianapolis, IN), a human chimeric monoclonal antibody directed at GpIIb/IIIa, is the first agent of this class to become clinically available.[3] Its receptor binding is nonspecific and it binds to other cell surface integrins. Other agents include RGD mimics that are competitive antagonists to the GpIIb/IIIa receptor, including the cyclic peptide eptifibatide (Integrilin; Key Pharmaceutical, Kenilworth, NJ), the parenteral nonpetide mimetics tirofiban (Aggrastet; Merck & Co., West Point, PA), and lamifiban; and the oral nonpeptide mimetics xemilofiban, orbofiban, roxifiban, sibrafiban, lefradafiban, and SB 214857.[229] All studies to date with these agents have involved coronary interventions.

Other Agents

Other agents for anticoagulation include hirudin, aprotinin, desmopressin acetate, and ancrod. Hirudin, obtained from the saliva of leeches, is a single-chain polypeptide composed of 65 amino acids, with three disulfide bonds and a molecular weight of 8,000 to 9,000 daltons. It is highly specific for thrombin inhibition. Hirudin has a short half-life of 15 to 30 minutes and is excreted unchanged in the urine. Hirudin has no natural inhibitors, compared with heparin, which has the natural inhibitors PF_4 and fibrin II monomer. As an inhibitor of thrombin, hirudin prevents conversion of fibrinogen to fibrin; thrombin-catalyzed activation of factors V, VIII, and XIII; and, importantly, thrombin-induced platelet aggregation.[230] In addition to its small size and high potency for thrombin, hirudin has a dominant antiplatelet effect, even with platelet-rich thrombi. Hirudin has been found to be more effective than heparin in reducing platelet deposition and mural thrombus at similar aPTT levels.[231] aPTT levels two to three times control (0.7 to 1.0 mg/kg hirudin) are effective in limiting arterial thrombosis and platelet deposition. Hirudin prevents thrombus growth at both high and low shear rates of blood flow and has even been found to stop thrombus growth in severe stenoses. Unlike heparin, which can inhibit only free, circulating, unbound thrombin, hirudin and other thrombin inhibitors act against both circulating and clot-bound thrombin. The high incidence of bleeding from hirudin, however, limits its usefulness clinically.[230] The gene for hirudin was cloned in 1986, leading to the recombinant production of analogues such as Hirulog (The Medicines Co., Cambridge, MA) and lepirudin (Reflodan; Aventis Pharmaceuticals). Hirulog is less potent than hirudin but also demonstrates an apparent lack of toxicity and immunogenicity.[230] Argatroban (a synthetic organic AT) has been found useful for the treatment of patients with HIT, and lepirudin has now been approved by the FDA for use in this syndrome, with an acceptable bleeding profile.

The inhibition of prekallikrein and kallikrein produces an anticoagulant state, whereas the inhibition of plasmin prevents fibrinolysis. However, aprotinin has greater affinity for plasmin than kallikrein, and an anticoagulant effect is noted only at very high doses.[232] This agent has successfully reduced transfusion requirements and blood loss in open heart surgery.[233] Another agent that has been suggested to preserve platelet function and improve coagulation is desmopressin acetate, a synthetic analogue of vasopressin, which releases preformed vWF from storage sites (Weibel-Palade bodies) in endothelial cells.[234] vWF then stimulates the production of factor VIII coagulant protein, stabilizes its structure, and forms a circulating noncovalent complex with factor VIII. This vWF–factor VIII complex supports platelet adhesion and improves platelet–platelet interactions. The aPTT shortens and prothrombin consumption increases owing to the increase in factor VIII coagulant protein. In addition, desmopressin elevates the plasma levels of larger vWF multimers, which are more effective than smaller vWF multimers. Finally, tPA secretion is stimulated by desmopressin. Desmopressin corrects the hemorrhagic tendency in mild hemophilia A and VWD and has been found to reduce blood loss and the need for transfusion by 30% to 40% in complex cardiac operations. Qualitative platelet defects found in uremia and cirrhosis of the liver may be corrected transiently,[235] and the platelet lesion caused by small doses of aspirin also may be corrected by desmopressin acetate. Despite the effectiveness of desmopressin acetate, it has not been shown to increase the risk of thrombosis.

Another anticoagulant that has been used in place of heparin is ancrod, a thrombin-like enzyme derived from the Malayan pit viper.[236] This enzyme produces a controlled decrease in fibrinogen levels by depleting FPA from fibrinogen but not FPB. The fibrin monomers that result stimulate the local production of tPA. Both of these actions lead to a state of anticoagulation. The amount of fibrinogen depletion must be carefully titrated to prevent bleeding. Other agents under development but not discussed include factor X inhibitors, TFPI, and APC.

Two new therapeutic classes of agents have demonstrated the promise of greater efficacy with less bleeding for both VTE prophylaxis and treatment. These include direct thrombin inhibitors and specific factor Xa inhibitors. The direct thrombin inhibitor, Ximelagatran/Melagatran, (Exanta, AstraZeneca), can be taken orally. It is an alternative to warfarin and does not need the same level of monitoring as warfarin. Oral ximelagatran is metabolized to the active Melagatran. It has a half-life of 4 to 5 hours, and approximately 80% of its excretion is renal. There is no increase in bleeding with this agent. In a large prospective study comparing oral Ximelagatran to placebo for 18 additional months after 6 months of standard anticoagulant treatment for DVT in 1,223 patients, the recurrent DVT/PE rate was reduced significantly from 12.6% to 2.8%[237] Major and minor bleeding events were equal at 23.9% and 21.0%. This agent has been found effective in DVT prophylaxis in orthopedic surgery patients. A concerning abnormality with the drug is an increase in liver function tests in approximately 6% of patients. However, this elevation appears to normalize on its own over time. This agent has been approved in Germany for DVT prophylaxis in elective hip/knee replacement but has not been approved by the U.S. Food and Drug Administration.

The specific factor Xa inhibitor pentasaccharide [Fondaparinux (Arixtra; Sanofi-Synthelab)] potentiates approximately 300-fold factor Xa neutralization by AT. It has a half-life of 17 hours and does not bind to plasma proteins. It is primarily excreted through the kidneys. Large prospective randomized studies for both DVT and PE treatment have been conducted.[238,239] For DVT, with 2,205 patients (>30% outpatients), the recurrent DVT/major hemorrhage rate for pentasaccharide (3.9%/1.1%) was equivalent to LMWH (4.1%/1.2%). For PE, with 2,213 patients (with >15% outpatients), recurrent PE/major hemorrhage rate for pentasaccharide (3.8%/1.3%) was equivalent to standard unfractionated heparin (5%/1.1%). Mortality rates were equal between pentasaccharide and conventional treated patients. In orthopedic surgery, this agent has also shown superiority to the best currently available DVT prophylaxis using LMWH. In fact, in hip fracture and knee reconstruction surgery, this agent has decreased the incidence of DVT by greater than 50%. In a meta-analysis of more than 7,000 patients, pentasaccharide decreased the odds 55% of VTE as compared to enoxaparin with no difference in critical bleeding, although major bleeding was slightly greater.[240–242] It has also shown a significant decrease in DVT in prolonged prophylaxis in hip fracture patients after 7 days of in-hospital DVT prophylaxis.[243] There is no good reversal drug for this agent, and this has been one of the factors that has prevented its wider adoption into the medical and surgical communities. Other new alternative agents are in various stages of development, such as oral heparins, oral LMWHs, P-selectin inhibitors, factor VIIa inhibitors, TFPIs, PAI-1 inhibitors, and APC. These agents, available now and in the future, will likely revolutionize the whole field of VTE prophylaxis and treatment.

Fibrinolytic Agents

Fibrinolytic agents are direct or indirect activators of plasminogen, the inactive proteolytic enzyme of plasma that binds to fibrin during the formation of thrombus. Fibrin-bound plasminogen is more susceptible to activation than is free plasminogen in plasma. Streptokinase isolated from group C β-hemolytic streptococci and acylated plasminogen–streptokinase (APSAC) act through a streptokinase–plasmin complex; urokinase, single-chain urokinase-type plasminogen activator (SCU-PA), and recombinant tPA act directly on plasmin without an intermediate drug–plasmin complex[244] (Fig. 5.17). tPA (originally isolated from a melanoma cell line and now produced through recombinant DNA technology), APSAC, and SCU-PA are termed *fibrin selective* because of their high ratio of activity for fibrin-bound plasminogen compared with circulating plasminogen.

Acylation of the streptokinase–plasminogen complex on the active serine moiety on the light chain stabilizes the catalytic serine site, making this complex inert to circulating plasminogen. Binding to fibrin occurs through the heavy-chain lysine–plasminogen portions; over time, the acetyl group leaves the complex, resulting in a fibrin-specific thrombolytic effect. Urokinase, a double-chain polypeptide, is formed by the cleavage of SCU-PA by plasmin to single-chain urokinase (a proenzyme-like substance); this cleavage is fibrin specific and occurs through a mechanism whereby SCU-PA activates plasminogen at the fibrin surface, converting it to plasmin. This activation is 10-fold more active at a fibrin surface than in circulating blood. Thus, only the fibrin-bound plasminogen is converted to plasmin for thrombolysis at the fibrin clot surface. tPA occurs in either a single- or double-polypeptide chain form. tPA has a fibrin-binding site and a catalytic site that are widely separated from each other. This separation allows tPA to be activated to its fibrin target, thus establishing its fibrin-specific nature. The level of the lytic state is greatest with streptokinase and APSAC, intermediate with urokinase, less with SCU-PA, and least with single-chain tPA[244] (Table 5.4). Half-lives also vary among different agents, from 5 minutes for single-chain recombinant tPA to 90 minutes for APSAC.[245] Streptokinase and APSAC, produced by group C β-hemolytic streptococci, are antigenic; urokinase and SCU-PA, produced from human fetal kidney cells in tissue culture, are nonantigenic. Because of its antigenicity, allergic reactions to streptokinase have been reported in 2% to 20% of cases. In addition, serum sickness has been reported with streptokinase.

Bleeding complications associated with fibrinolytic agents (reported in up to half of patients receiving systemic fibrinolytic agents for venous thrombosis) are related to the invasive procedures associated with drug therapy. Factors involved in bleeding include hypo-fibrinogenemia and fibrin degradation products. The latter inhibit fibrin polymerization and, in combination with a decrease in the clotting factors V and VIII (from excess plasmin not neutralized by α_2-AP), inhibit the ability of blood to clot. Although coagulation tests in general do not correlate well with bleeding, a fibrinogen level less than 100 mg/dL is associated with an increased risk and severity of bleeding. In addition, newly formed thrombi are easily lysed as they form. Platelets are both inhibited and stimulated by fibrinolytic agents. Because fibrinogen is a necessary cofactor for ADP-induced platelet aggregation, low fibrinogen levels aggravate a platelet defect. At the same time, plasminogen

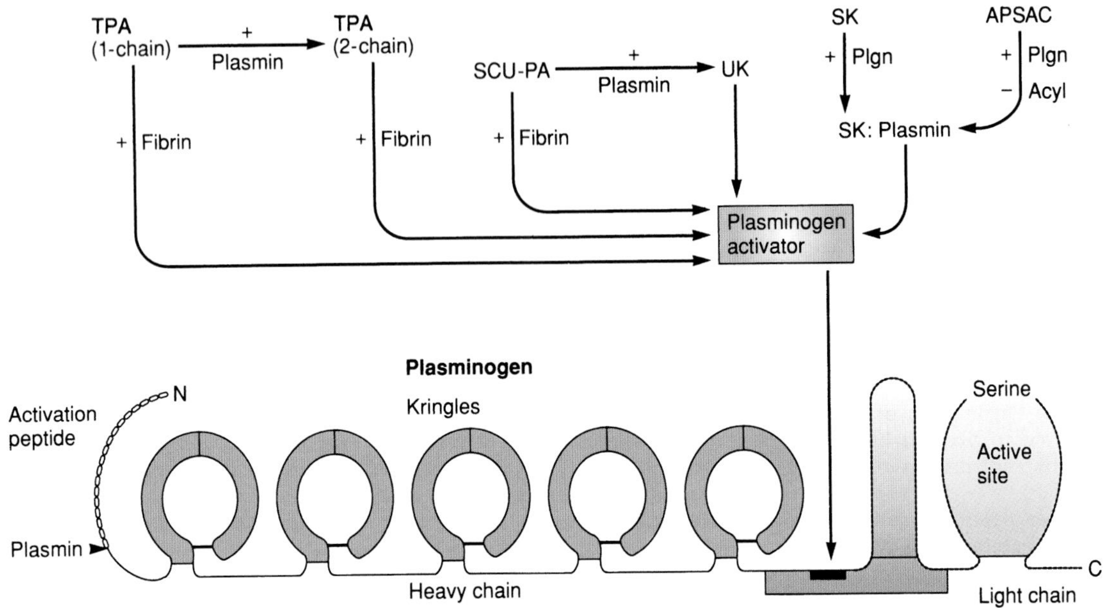

FIGURE 5.17 Sites of action of plasminogen activators on plasminogen. TPA, tissue plasminogen activator; SCU-PA, single-chain urokinase plasminogen activator; UK, urokinase; SK, streptokinase; Plgn, plasminogen; APSAC, acylated plasminogen–streptokinase. (After Marder VJ, Sherry S. Thrombolytic therapy: current status. *N Engl J Med.* 1988;318:1513, with permission.)

bound to platelets leads to impaired adhesion and a decrease in their ability to aggregate. Plasmin-induced cleavage of adhesive proteins, such as thrombospondin, fibronectin, and fibrin, also disrupts the bonds that hold platelet aggregates together. In addition, plasmin formed on the endothelial cell surface impairs platelet adhesion to areas of vascular injury during therapy with fibrinolytic agents. Despite these mechanisms that decrease the clotting ability of blood during fibrinolytic therapy, it has been found that these agents promote reocclusion in up to 30% of cases early after thrombolysis through platelet activation, suggesting that platelet activation occurs early after lysis and platelet inhibition occurs later.[228] In addition, increased synthesis of endothelial cell PAI-1 has been demonstrated experimentally after treatment with tPA,

TABLE 5.4

CHARACTERISTICS OF FIBRINOLYTIC AGENTS[a]

	SK	APSAC	UK	SCU-PA	rTP[a] 2-Chain	rTP[a] 1-Chain
Half-life (min)	23	90	16	7	8	5
Fibrin enhancement	1+	1+	2+	4+	4+	3+
Plasma proteolytic state	4+	4+	3+	2+	2+	1+
Duration of infusion	60 min	2–5 min	5–15 min	Several hours	Several hours	Several hours
Thrombus specificity (vs. hemostatic plug)	0	0	0	0	0	0
Incidence of reperfusion (% within 3 h)	60–70	60–70	60–70	60–70	60–70	60–70
Speed of reperfusion (min)	45	45	45	45	45	45
Frequency of reocclusion (estimated %)	15	10	10	NA	20	20
Simultaneous administration of heparin	No	No	No	Yes	Yes	Yes
Bleeding complications	4+	4+	4+	4+	4+	4+
Allergic side effects	Yes	Yes	No	No	No	No
Antigenicity	Yes	Yes	No	NK	NK	NK
Expense	1+	2+	3+	4+	4+	4+

[a]The clinical data were derived mostly from reported experience with current intravenous dosages in the treatment of acute myocardial infarction. SK, streptokinase; APSAC, acylated plasminogen–streptokinase activator complex; UK, urokinase; SCU-PA, recombinant single-chain urokinase plasminogen activator; rTPA, recombinant tissue-type plasminogen activator; NA, data not available; NK, not known; 0, none; 4+, highest. From Marder VJ, Sherry S. Thrombolytic therapy: current status. *N Engl J Med.* 1988;318:1514.

another mechanism that could potentially contribute to early thrombotic reocclusion.[245]

Indications for thrombolytic therapy remain controversial. Clearly, in DVT, fibrinolytic agents allow for greater clot lysis than heparin and help preserve valve function to a greater degree, but at the risk of a higher rate of bleeding complications.[246] Thirteen studies of thrombolytic therapy for acute DVT have been compiled from the literature.[247] In these studies, patients were assessed with venography. Of those patients treated with anticoagulants, only 4% had complete lysis and 14% revealed partial lysis. In contrast, 45% of patients treated with thrombolytic agents showed significant or complete clot lysis and an additional 18% revealed partial lysis. Two studies evaluated the long-term success of thrombolytic therapy compared with anticoagulation for DVT. In 39 patients with follow-up of 1.6 to 5 years, 21% of patients treated with heparin had no evidence of postthrombotic symptoms, and 64% of patients treated with streptokinase did not have symptoms.[248,249] Similarly, significant functional benefit was reported 5 to 10 years after therapy in patients with significant clot lysis as measured by photoplethysmography (PPG) times and foot volumetric studies, although PPG did not completely normalize in the lysis group. In addition, in a large prospective study in patients followed after DVT with either heparin or streptokinase, no major improvement in deep venous valvular competence was found with lytic agents at 2-year follow-up, and venous functional preservation appeared the same whether clot lysis was complete or incomplete.[250] Approximately half of patients who present with their first episode of DVT and who begin lytic therapy within 72 hours of the onset of symptoms achieve significant dissolution of their thrombus. Only approximately 15% of patients who present acutely with lower extremity DVT, however, fit into this category because most patients who have leg swelling or leg pain for the first time do not immediately seek medical attention.[251] The use of thrombolytic therapy for DVT thus remains controversial.

The main questions about the use of lytic therapy for DVT are which agent, what dose, and for how long? In a study comparing streptokinase to urokinase in DVT,[252] little cost difference was found after considering the longer infusion time and greater bleeding complications associated with streptokinase versus urokinase. Another study[253] compared tPA, 0.5 mg per kilogram twice over 4 hours or 8 hours, with heparin versus placebo plus heparin for proximal venous thrombosis. Over 50% total clot lysis was found in 58% of a group of patients treated over 4 hours, 23% in a group treated for 8 hours, and only 7% complete clot lysis in the placebo-treated group. Follow-up of patients who achieved greater than 50% clot lysis revealed evidence of chronic venous insufficiency in only 25%, compared with 56% of those with less than 50% clot lysis, a difference that was close to but not statistically significant ($p = .07$). This study suggests that further investigation into the use of the fibrin-specific agents for proximal DVT may be enlightening.

Fibrinolytic therapy has been suggested for use in upper extremity effort venous thrombosis, catheter-induced venous thrombosis, Paget-Schroetter syndrome, and superior vena caval thrombosis. An interesting approach combining thrombolytic therapy and thoracic outlet decompression has been proposed.[254] Thrombolytic therapy is initiated locally with urokinase (250,000 IU bolus, then 1,000 to 4,000 IU per minute) by a small catheter positioned from a basilic vein approach. After clot lysis, anticoagulation is continued for 3 months, with heparin followed by sodium warfarin to allow for thrombophlebitis (the inflammatory response in the vein that occurs due to the thrombus) to resolve. In approximately 3 months, thoracic outlet decompression is performed. Percutaneous transluminal angioplasty is not successful in the presence of an anatomic defect. Long-term results have been reported to be excellent and correlate well with the initial ability to clear the thrombus. A recent trend to more immediate thoracic outlet decompression has been advocated, avoiding the 3-month wait interval.

Thrombolytic therapy in PE has been extensively studied. Two carefully designed studies have evaluated the use of either urokinase or streptokinase. Although both agents rapidly lysed clot and improved pulmonary hemodynamics, there was no difference in patient mortality rate or recurrence rate of PE compared with heparin alone.[255,256] Urokinase dissolved pulmonary arterial clot within 24 hours of treatment and, in certain instances, reversed shock. By 7 days, both the thrombolytic- and heparin-treated patients revealed equal improvement in pulmonary hemodynamics, and there was no difference in lung scan resolution. In addition, no difference was seen between urokinase and streptokinase. Bleeding complications were more frequent in the thrombolytic-treated patients. Patients who received urokinase responded better if they were younger, if the embolus was less than 48 hours old, or if the embolus was large.

tPA, 0.6 mg per kilogram over 2 minutes, plus heparin, versus placebo plus heparin for patients with PE has also been reported, with use of lung scans at 24 hours and 7 days to document treatment efficacy.[253] No increase in bleeding complications was noted and lysis was significantly improved at 24 hours in the tPA group (34.4%) versus the placebo group (12%, $p = .026$). However, again, the advantage for tPA had disappeared by 7 days (59% lysis compared with 56% lysis). As a general guide, thrombolytic therapy for PE should be considered when there is angiographically documented lobar or greater PE causing acute pulmonary hypertension and right ventricular failure; lesser degrees of PE should be treated with standard heparin or LMWH anticoagulation.

Thrombolytic therapy for peripheral arterial applications is becoming more frequently used, especially when the agents are given intra-arterially. The method of McNamara and Fischer[257] has gained the most recognition, involving passage of a guidewire through the thrombus and then infusion of a large dose of urokinase at 4,000 IU per minute for 1 to 2 hours, directly into the clot. If progress is made, further thrombolytic therapy is given at 1,000 to 2,000 IU per minute for 6 to 12 hours or until complete clot lysis has occurred. Using this method, the mean infusion time was found to be 18 hours, and the incidence of bleeding was significantly lessened. McNamara and Fischer[257] compared these results with those of streptokinase from the literature and found a 13% incidence of severe bleeding with streptokinase versus only a 4% incidence with high-dose intraarterial urokinase therapy. McNamara and Bomberger[258] reported on their first 100 cases of selective intra-arterial infusion of urokinase and found complete clot lysis in 77%, with native arterial occlusions responding better than arterial graft occlusions (71% vs. 41% success) at 6-month follow-up. After thrombolytic therapy has reopened an occluded vessel or graft, however, radiologic or surgical correction of the lesion responsible for the thrombosis must be addressed for long-term success. A 1-year graft patency rate of 89% in those grafts in which an underlying lesion was successfully repaired, compared with 23% in grafts without a correctable lesion, has been reported.[259] At 2 years, this difference was even greater (79% compared with 10%). Complications associated with thrombolytic therapy for arterial thrombosis include bleeding, rethrombosis, embolization treated with further thrombolytic therapy, and sepsis from prolonged catheter placement. The most recent innovation in intra-arterial thrombolytic therapy involves lacing the entire length of the thrombus with high-dose urokinase before continuous infusion and then using pulse-spray techniques. The application of tPA to peripheral vascular cases has been reported; although promising results were described, 17% of patients still responded with a decrease in systemic fibrinogen levels to less than 100 mg/dL.[260] In addition, three patients had groin hematomas, and one had a stroke soon after therapy had been completed. Although fibrin specific, tPA can still cause systemic thrombolytic effects.

The use of intraoperative thrombolytic therapy has been advocated for situations in which complete clot evacuation cannot be accomplished (as may be seen in up to 40% of patients undergoing balloon embolectomy with an embolectomy catheter for acute arterial occlusion) or when the distal vasculature is occluded and precludes appropriate inflow patency.[246] One method involves urokinase administration distal to an occluding clamp, infused at 250,000 IU combined with 1,000 IU of heparin in 250 mL saline, and allowed to remain for 30 minutes. If necessary, another 125,000 IU is infused for 30 minutes. Using this technique, 70% of limbs with critical ischemia at the completion of successful balloon embolectomy were spared amputation, with only one bleeding complication.[261] For patients with multivessel occlusions or for whom any degree of systemic fibrinolysis would be risky, a new, high-dose isolated limb perfusion technique has been described. This technique involves anticoagulation, limb exsanguination with an Esmarch bandage, application of a proximal tourniquet, and direct arterial infusion of 1,000,000 IU or more of urokinase for 45 to 60 minutes, with direct drainage of the venous effluent below the tourniquet.

Contraindications to thrombolytic therapy, whether regional or systemic, are well defined and consist of active internal bleeding, recent surgery or trauma (usually within 10 days of infusion), recent cerebrovascular accident (within 2 months), or documented left heart thrombus (Table 5.5).

TABLE 5.5 INDICATIONS/CONTRAINDICATIONS

CONTRAINDICATIONS TO THROMBOLYTIC THERAPY

ABSOLUTE
- Active internal bleeding
- Recent (<2 mo) cerebrovascular accident
- Intracranial disease

RELATIVE

Major
- Recent (<10 d) major surgery, obstetric delivery, or organ biopsy
- Left heart thrombus
- Active peptic ulcer or gastrointestinal abnormality
- Recent major trauma
- Uncontrolled hypertension

Minor
- Minor surgery or trauma
- Recent cardiopulmonary resuscitation
- Atrial fibrillation with mitral valve disease
- Bacterial endocarditis
- Hemostatic defects (i.e., renal or liver disease)
- Diabetic hemorrhagic retinopathy
- Pregnancy

CONTRAINDICATIONS TO STREPTOKINASE
- Known allergy
- Recent streptococcal infection
- Previous therapy within 6 mo

Data from NIH Consensus Development Conference. Thrombolytic therapy in treatment. *Ann Intern Med* 1980;93:141, with permission.

Relative contraindications include recent surgery, gastrointestinal bleeding or trauma, severe hypertension, mitral valve disease, endocarditis, a history of a defect in hemostasis, or pregnancy. Finally, the recent withdrawal of urokinase from the market needs to be kept in mind when considerations turn to the use of thrombolytic agents.

Dextran

Dextran is a high-molecular-weight polysaccharide produced from sucrose by *Leuconostoc mesenteroides*. Fractionation and hydrolysis produce a product with an average molecular weight of either 40 kd [dextran-40 (Rheomacrodex; Medisan, Parsippany, NJ)] or 70 kd (Dextran-70). Dextran-40 has been studied in detail for its ability to augment patency of difficult lower extremity bypass grafts in the early postoperative period. Dextran-40 acts as a volume expander, causing hemodilution, decreasing blood viscosity, decreasing platelet adhesiveness, reducing factor VIII activity, and increasing the lysability of clots.[262] In addition, dextran has been found to coat endothelial cell surfaces, decreasing their electronegativity.

Mechanical Measures

Mechanical measures are used for the prevention of DVT during operative procedures or in patients who cannot be given pharmacologic prophylaxis. These measures include early ambulation, elastic stockings, electrical calf muscle stimulation, and external pneumatic compression, with either uniform-pressure stockings or graded-pressure stockings. In many well controlled studies of venous prophylaxis, intermittent pneumatic compression has been found as effective as low-dose heparin therapy. In addition to augmentation of venous return with these devices, local and systemic fibrinolysis appears to be stimulated, even in areas remote from the application of the compression. The length of time that intermittent pneumatic compression should be used has not been adequately determined, but most data suggest that at least 5 days or longer in the face of prolonged immobilization may be optimal.

LABORATORY MONITORING OF COAGULATION AND ANTICOAGULATION

Tests of Platelet Function

Platelet tests include peripheral platelet counts, bleeding times, and platelet aggregation. Usually, a platelet count of 50,000/mL or more ensures adequate hemostasis, whereas counts less than 10,000/mL are dangerous and may lead to spontaneous bleeding. Thrombocytosis is considered to exist when the platelet count exceeds 500,000/mL, although in some cases (especially those involving myeloproliferative disorders or following splenectomy), counts may be greater than 1,000,000/mL.[4] Bleeding time assays assess the ability of platelets to form hemostatic plugs and are usually shorter than 8 minutes. A bleeding time between 8 and 15 minutes most often reflects a low plasma level of vWF, the use of antiplatelet drugs, the presence of lupus-like antibodies, or a factor XI deficiency.[4] A bleeding time greater than 15 minutes is clearly prolonged and indicates severe platelet functional impairment, very low levels of vWF, or afibrinogenemia and severe factor V deficiency. Platelet aggregation testing involves the use of a number of different agonists, such as

ADP, collagen, epinephrine, arachidonic acid, calcium ionophores, platelet-activating factor, thromboxane, and thrombin.

Coagulation Tests

Coagulation tests include PT (intrinsic and extrinsic pathways and fibrinogen), PTT and aPTT (contact and intrinsic pathway), TCT (fibrinogen conversion to fibrin), and ACT (whole blood and platelets). The only abnormality that causes an isolated elevation in PT with all of the other test results normal is factor VII deficiency, the factor that is activated by TF and then stimulates generation of the extrinsic pathway of coagulation. In addition, the PT is sensitive to small decreases in factor V levels. The PT is the most common manner of measuring the level of oral anticoagulant therapy. The aPTT identifies abnormalities of the contact and intrinsic phases of coagulation. The aPTT evolved from the PTT, first described in 1953 and 1954. The PTT uses a phospholipid derived from either brain or lung tissue to mimic the function of platelets in the scheme of coagulation. The aPTT standardizes the activation of factor XII by agents such as cephaloplastin. Because the blood specimen, activator, and phospholipid must be incubated for a period, the blood specimen must be anticoagulated during the activation step; this is usually accomplished with sodium citrate. After incubation, the specimen is recalcified to begin the test. Conditions that cause a prolonged aPTT include the presence of heparin; deficiencies in factors VIII, IX, and XII; and the presence of lupus-like anticoagulants.[4] aPTT values have variably been shown to correlate with heparin dosages and serum heparin levels. Heparin levels of 0.2 IU/mL or greater usually correlate with an aPTT of 1.5 times normal or greater. TCT is a measurement of the time it takes for exogenously added thrombin to turn plasma fibrinogen into fibrin clot. As such, it is extremely sensitive to levels of heparin and is an excellent means of measuring the level of heparin-induced anticoagulation. The beauty of the TCT is that it is not specific for any disease condition; thus, it may be used to differentiate factor deficiencies from the presence of heparin or to separate lupus anticoagulant from abnormalities in fibrinogen levels.[4] The ACT is a measurement of the ability of whole blood to clot and as such is an available technique for monitoring intraoperative heparin levels. The ACT responds linearly to increasing heparin dosage and correlates well with observed clinical anticoagulation (thrombus-free surface on cardiopulmonary bypass devices).[263] Adequate anticoagulation for extracorporeal circulation is defined as an ACT of 480 seconds or more, but most cardiovascular surgeons would agree that any value between 300 and 600 seconds is acceptable. For peripheral vascular applications, values of 250 seconds or greater are considered appropriate levels representative of full intraoperative anticoagulation. The ACT may be affected by hemodilution, cardioplegia solutions, hypothermia, platelet dysfunction, hypofibrinogenemia, and other coagulopathies, as well as by certain medications and excess protamine administration.

Tests of Fibrinolysis

Tests of fibrinolysis are less well characterized. The euglobulin lysis test time is a crude screening test for problems with fibrinolysis.[4] Patients with accelerated fibrinolysis are often found to have a deficiency of α_2-AP (of which the total amount normally is only half of the total plasmin that can be generated) or the fibrin clot-stabilizing factor XIII.[4] A deficiency of PAI-1 also may lead to accelerated fibrinolysis. During normal clot formation and breakdown, the D-dimer fragment of fibrinogen is a marker for ongoing thrombosis and physiologic fibrinolysis, whereas for fibrinogenolysis, the two D fragments that are produced are not cross-linked into the D-dimer form.[4]

KEY POINTS

- **At the same time that thrombin forms, natural anticoagulant mechanisms oppose further thrombin formation and help to localize thrombin activity to areas of vascular injury. Just as thrombin generation is key to coagulation, antithrombin is the central anticoagulant protein.**
- **The endothelial cell acts as a nonthrombogenic surface.**
- **Thrombosis and inflammation are closely linked.**
- **The elements required for the initiation of thrombosis include stasis, endothelial injury, and hypercoagulability of blood.**
- **Heparin-induced thrombocytopenia (HIT) occurs in 0.6% to 30% of patients in whom heparin is given; severe thrombocytopenia associated with thrombosis (HITTS) is much less frequent.**
- **Disseminated intravascular coagulation (DIC) is the primary form of acute thrombosis. Laboratory values in DIC reveal a decline in platelet count and fibrinogen level with an elevation in fibrin split products (D-dimer).**
- **Factor VIII and IX deficiency states are involved in hemophilia A and B and von Willebrand's disease.**

References

1. Zur M, Radcliffe RD, Oberdick J, et al. The dual role of factor VII in blood coagulation: initiation and inhibition of a proteolytic system by a zymogen. *J Biol Chem.* 1982;257:5623.
2. Radcliffe R, Nemerson Y. Mechanism of activation of bovine factor VII: products of cleavage by factor Xa. *J Biol Chem.* 1976;251:4749.
3. Ferguson JJ, Waly HM, Wilson JM. Fundamentals of coagulation and glycoprotein IIb/IIIa receptor inhibition. *Eur Heart J.* 1998;19[Suppl D]:D3.
4. Hassouna HI. Laboratory evaluation of hemostatic disorders. *Hematol Oncol Clin North Am.* 1993;7:1161.
5. Sims PJ, Faioni EM, Wiedmer T, et al. Complement proteins C5b-9 cause release of membrane vesicles from the platelet surface that are enriched in the membrane receptor for coagulation factor Va and express prothrombinase activity. *J Biol Chem.* 1988;263:18205.
6. Gilbert GE, Sims PJ, Wiedmer T, et al. Platelet-derived microparticles express high affinity receptors for factor VIII. *J Biol Chem.* 1991; 266:17261.
7. Hickey MJ, Williams SA, Roth GA. Human platelet glycoprotein IX: an adhesive prototype of leucine-rich glycoproteins with flank-center-flank structures. *Proc Natl Acad Sci U S A.* 1989;86:6773.
8. Bennett JS, Vilaire G, Cines DB. Identification of the fibrinogen receptor on human platelets by photoaffinity labeling. *J Biol Chem.* 1982; 257:8049.
9. Savage B, Ruggeri ZM. Selective recognition of adhesive sites in surface-bound fibrinogen by glycoprotein IIb/IIIa on nonactivated platelets. *J Biol Chem.* 1991;266:11277.
10. Shapiro AD. Platelet function disorders. *Haemophilia* 2000;6[Suppl 1]: 120–127.
11. Ferguson JJ, Waly HM, Wilson JM. Fundamentals of coagulation and glycoprotein IIb/III receptor inhibition. *Eur Heart J.* 1998; 19[Suppl D]:D3.
12. Osterud B, Rapaport SI. Activation of factor IX by the reaction product of tissue factor and factor VIII: additional pathway for initiating blood coagulation. *Proc Natl Acad Sci U S A.* 1977;74:5260.
13. Bauer KA, Kass BL, ten Care H, et al. Factor IX is activated in vivo by the tissue factor mechanism. *Blood* 1990;76:731.
14. Blomback, B, Blomback M. The molecular structure of fibrinogen. *Ann N Y Acad Sci.* 1972;202:77.
15. Folk JE, Finlayson JS. The epsilon-(gamma-glutamyl) lysine crosslink and the catalytic role of transglutamines. *Adv Protein Chem.* 1977;31:1.
16. Davie EW, Fujikawa K, Kisiel W. The coagulation cascade: initiation, maintenance, and regulation. *Biochemistry* 1991;30:10363.
17. Naito K, Fujikawa K. Activation of human blood coagulation factor XI independent of factor XII: factor XI is activated by thrombin and factor XIa in the presence of negatively charged surfaces. *J Biol Chem.* 1991;266:7353.
18. DiScipio RG, Kurachi K, Davie EW. Activation of human factor IX (Christmas factor). *J Clin Invest.* 1978;61:1528.
19. Rosenberg RD, Damus PS. The purification and mechanism of action of human antithrombin-heparin cofactor. *J Biol Chem.* 1973;248:6490.

20. Kurachi K, Fujikawa K, Schmer G, et al. Inhibition of bovine factor IXa and factor Xab by antithrombin III. *Biochemistry* 1976;15:373.
21. Kurachi K, Davie EW. Activation of human factor XI (plasma thromboplastin antecedent) by factor XIIa (activated Hageman factor). *Biochemistry* 1977;16:5831.
22. Kisiel W, Canfield WM, Ericsson LH, et al. Anticoagulant properties of bovine plasma protein C following activation by thrombin. *Biochemistry* 1977;16:5824.
23. Marlar RA, Kleiss AJ, Griffin JH. Mechanism of action of human activated protein C, a thrombin dependent anticoagulant enzyme. *Blood* 1982;59:1067.
24. Vehar GA, Davie EW. Preparation and properties of bovine factor VIII (antihemophilic factor). *Biochemistry* 1980;19:401.
25. Esmon CT, Owen WG. Identification of an endothelial cell cofactor for thrombin-catalyzed activation of protein C. *Proc Natl Acad Sci U S A.* 1981;78:2249.
26. Owen WG, Esmon CT. Functional properties of an endothelial cell cofactor for thrombin-catalyzed activation of protein C. *J Biol* Chem. 1981;256:5532.
27. Esmon NL, Owen WG, Esmon CT. Isolation of a membrane-bound cofactor for thrombin-catalyzed activation of protein C. *J Biol Chem.* 1982;257:859.
28. Esmon CT. The regulation of natural anticoagulant pathways. *Science* 1987;235:1348.
29. Esmon NL, Carroll RC, Esmon CT. Thrombomodulin blocks the ability of thrombin to activate platelets. *J Biol Chem.* 1983;258:12238.
30. Esmon CT, Esmon NL, Harris KW. Complex formation between thrombin and thrombomodulin inhibits both thrombin-catalyzed fibrin formation and factor V activation. *J Biol Chem.* 1982;257:7944.
31. Walker FJ. Regulation of activated protein C by a new protein: a possible function for bovine protein S. *J Biol Chem.* 1980;255:5521.
32. Tollefsen DM, Majerus PW, Blank MK. Heparin cofactor II: purification and properties of a heparin-dependent inhibitor of thrombin in human plasma. *J Biol Chem.* 1982;257:2162.
33. Broze GJ, Girard TJ, Novotny WF. Regulation of coagulation by a multivalent Kunitz-type inhibitor. *Biochemistry* 1990;29:7539.
34. Rapaport SI. Inhibition of factor VIIa/tissue factor-induced blood coagulation: with particular emphasis upon a factor Xa-dependent inhibitory mechanism. *Blood* 1989;73:359.
35. Gelehrter TD, Sznycer-Laszuk R. Thrombin induction of plasminogen activator inhibitor in cultured human endothelial cells. *J Clin Invest.* 1986;77:165.
36. Dichek D, Quertermous T. Thrombin regulation of mRNA levels of tissue plasminogen activator and plasminogen activator inhibitor-1 in cultured human umbilical vein endothelial cells. *Blood* 1989;74:222.
37. Adelman B, Michelson AD, Loscalzo J, et al. Plasmin effect on platelet glycoprotein Ib–von Willebrand factor interactions. *Blood* 1985;65:32.
38. Schmaier AH. Disseminated intravascular coagulation: pathogenesis and management. *J Intensive Care Med.* 1991;6:209.
39. Hajjar KA, Nachman RL. Endothelial cell–mediated conversion of Glu-plasminogen to Lys-plasminogen: further evidence for assembly of the fibrinolytic system on the endothelial cell surface. *J Clin Invest.* 1988; 82:1769.
40. Coleman RW. Activation of plasminogen by human plasma kallikrein. *Biochem Biophys Res Commun.* 1969;35:273.
41. Becker BF, Heindl B, Kupatt C, et al. Endothelial function and hemostasis. *Z Kardiol.* 2000;89:160–167.
42. Gross PL, Aird WC. The endothelium and thrombosis. *Semin Thromb Hemost.* 2000;26:463–478.
43. Esmon NL, Esmon CT. Protein C and the endothelium. *Semin Thromb Hemost.* 1988;14:210.
44. Van der Poll T, Buller HR, ten Cate H, et al. Activation of coagulation after administration of tumor necrosis factor to normal subjects. *N Engl J Med.* 1990;322:1622.
45. Nawroth PP, Stern DM. Modulation of endothelial cell hemostatic properties by tumor necrosis factor. *J Exp Med.* 1986;163:740.
46. Bevilacqua MP, Pober JS, Majeau GR, et al. Recombinant tumor necrosis factor induces procoagulant activity in cultured human vascular endothelium: characterization and comparison with the actions of interleukin-1. *Proc Natl Acad Sci U S A.* 1986;83:4533.
47. Conway EM, Bach R, Rosenberg RD, et al. Tumor necrosis factor enhances expression of tissue factor mRNA in endothelial cells. *Thromb Res.* 1989;53:231.
48. Schleef RR, Bevilacqua MP, Sawdey M, et al. Cytokine activation of vascular endothelium: effects on tissue-type plasminogen activator and type I plasminogen inhibitor. *J Biol Chem.* 1988;263:5797.
49. Van Hinsbergh VW, Kooistra T, van den Berg EA, et al. Tumor necrosis factor increases production of plasminogen activator inhibitor in human endothelial cells in vitro and rats in vivo. *Blood* 1988;72:1467.
50. Medina R, Schocher SH, Han JH. Interleukin-1, endotoxin, or tumor necrosis factor/cachectin enhance the level of plasminogen activator messenger RNA in bovine aortic endothelial cells. *Thromb Res.* 1989;54:41.
51. Van der Poll T, Levi M, Buller HR, et al. Fibrinolytic response to tumor necrosis factor in healthy subjects. *J Exp Med.* 1991;174:729.
52. Pohlman TH, Stanness KA, Beatty PG, et al. An endothelial cell surface factor(s) induced in vitro by lipopolysaccharide, interleukin-1, and tumor necrosis factor-alpha increases neutrophil adherence by CD18 dependent mechanism. *J Immunol.* 1986;136:4548.
53. Schleimer RP, Rutledge BK. Cultured human endothelial cells acquire adhesiveness for neutrophils after stimulation with interleukin-1, endotoxin, and tumor-promoting phorbol diesters. *J Immunol.* 1986;136:649.
54. Rothlein R, Dustin ML, Marlin SD, et al. A human intercellular adhesion molecule (ICAM-1) distinct from LFA-1. *J Immunol.* 1986;137:1270.
55. Bevilacqua MP, Stengelin S, Gimbrone MA, et al. Endothelial leukocyte adhesion molecule 1: an inducible receptor for neutrophils related to complement regulatory proteins and lectins. *Science* 1989;243:1160.
56. Kunkel SL, Standiford T, Metinko AP, et al. Endothelial cell-derived novel chemotactic cytokines. In: Lefant C, ed. *Lung vascular injury: molecular and cellular response.* New York: Marcel Dekker; 1991:213–226.
57. **Furie B, Furie BC. Molecular and cell biology of blood coagulation. *N Engl J Med.* 1992;326:800.**
58. Palabrica T, Lobb R, Furie BC. Leukocyte accumulation promoting fibrin deposition is mediated in vivo by P-selectin on adherent platelets. *Nature* 1992;359:848.
59. Stewart GJ. Neutrophils and deep venous thrombosis. *Haemo-stasis* 1993;23:127.
60. Holt JC, Yan Z, Lu W, et al. Isolation, characterization, and immunological detection of neutrophil-activating peptide 2: a proteolytic degradation product of platelet basic protein. *Proc Soc Exp Biol Med.* 1992;199:171.
61. Ferrer-Lopez P, Renesto P, Schattner M, et al. Activation of human platelets by C5a-stimulated neutrophils: a role for cathepsin G. *Am J Physiol.* 1990;258:C1100.
62. Evangelista V, Rajtar G, de Gaetano G, et al. Platelet activation by fMLP-stimulated polymorphonuclear leukocytes: the activity of cathepsin G is not prevented by antiproteases. *Blood* 1991;77:2379.
63. Wakefield TW, Greenfield LJ, Rolfe MW, et al. Inflammatory and procoagulant mediator interactions in an experimental baboon model of venous thrombosis. *Thromb Haemost.* 1993;69:164.
64. Rauch U, Osende JI, Fuster V, et al. Thrombus formation on atherosclerotic plaques: pathogenesis and clinical consequences. *Ann Intern Med.* 2001;134:224–238.
65. Myers DD Jr, Schaub R. Wrobleski SK, et al. P-Selectin antagonism causes dose-dependent venous thrombosis inhibition. *Thromb Haemost.* 2001; 85:423–429.
66. Myers D, Wrobleski S, Londy F, et al. New and effective treatment of experimentally induced venous thrombosis with anti-inflammatory rPSGL-Ig. *Thromb Haemost.* 2002; 87:374–382.
67. Flinn WR, McDaniel MD, Yao JS, et al. Antithrombin III deficiency as a reflection of dynamic protein metabolism in patients undergoing vascular reconstruction. *J Vasc Surg.* 1984;1:888.
68. Towne JB, Bernhard VM, Hussey C, et al. Antithrombin deficiency—a cause of unexplained thrombosis in vascular surgery. *Surgery* 1981; 89:735.
69. Pabinger I, Schneider B. Thrombotic risk in hereditary antithrombin III, protein C, or protein S deficiency. *Arterioscler Thromb Vasc Biol.* 1996; 16:742–774.
70. **Hirsh J, Raschke R, Warkentin TE, et al. Heparin: mechanism of action, pharmacokinetics, dosing considerations, monitoring, efficacy, and safety. *Chest* 1995;108:258S.**
71. Perry DJ. Review: acquired antithrombin deficiency in sepsis. *Br J Haematol.* 2001;112:26–31.
72. Flinn WR, McDaniel MD, Yao JS, et al. Antithrombin III deficiency as a reflection of dynamic protein metabolism in patients undergoing vascular reconstruction. *J Vasc Surg.* 1984;1:888.
73. Eby CS. A review of the hypercoaguable state. Coagulation disorders: Part II. *Hematol Oncol Clin North Am.* 1993;7:1.
74. **de Moerloose P, Bounameaux HR, Mannucci PM. Screening tests for thrombophilic patients: which tests, for which patient, by whom, when, and why? *Semin Thromb Hemost.* 1998;24(4):321–327.**
75. Menache D: Antithrombin III concentrates. Coagulation disorders: Part I. *Hematol Oncol Clin North Am.* 1992;6:1115.
76. Lubenow N, Greinacher A. Hirudin in heparin-induced thrombocytopenia. *Semin Thromb Hemost.* 2002;28:431–438.
77. **Seligsohn U, Lubetsky A. Genetic susceptibility to venous thrombosis. *N Engl J Med.* 2001;344:1222–1231.**
78. Bick RL. Prothrombin G20210A mutation, antithrombin, heparin cofactor II, protein C, and protein S defects. *Hematol Oncol Clin North Am* 2003;17(1):9–36.
79. Donaldson MC, Belkin M, Whittemore AD, et al. Impact of activated protein C resistance on general vascular surgical patients. *J Vasc Surg.* 1997;25:1054.
80. Franco RF, Reitsma PH. Genetic risk factors of venous thrombosis. *Hum Genet.* 2001;109:369–384.
81. Siddiqi FA, Tepler J, Fantini GA. Acquired protein S and antithrombin III deficiency caused by nephrotic syndrome: an unusual cause of graft thrombosis. *J Vasc Surg.* 1997;25:576.
82. Jennings I, Cooper P. Screening for thrombophilia: a laboratory perspective. *Br J Biomed Sci.* 2003;60:39–51.
83. Esmon CT. The regulation of natural anticoagulant pathways. *Science* 1987;235:1348.
84. Dahlbäck B: Blood coagulation. *Lancet* 2000;355:1627.
85. Cole MS, Minifee PK, Wolma FJ. Coumadin necrosis: a review of the literature. *Surgery* 1988;103:271.

86. Alving B. How I treat heparin-induced thrombocytopenia and thrombosis. *Blood* 2001;101(1).
87. Ansell JE, Price JM, Shah S, et al. Heparin-induced thrombocytopenia: what is its real frequency? *Chest* 1985;88:878.
88. Cancio LC, Cohen DJ. Heparin-induced thrombocytopenia and thrombosis. *J Am Coll Surg.* 1998;186:76.
89. Comp PC, DeBault LE, Esmon NL, Esmon CT. Human thrombomodulin is inhibited by IgG from two patients with non-specific anticoagulants. *Blood* 1983;62[Suppl 1]:299a(abst).
90. Almeida J, Coats R, Liem TK, Silver D. Reduced morbidity and mortality rates of the heparin-induced thrombocytopenia syndrome. *J Vasc Surg.* 1998;27:309.
91. Kelton JG, Smith JW, Warkentin TE, et al. Immunoglobulin G from patients with heparin-induced thrombocytopenia binds to a complex of heparin and platelet factor 5. *Blood* 1994;83:3232–3239.
92. Walenga JM, Jeske WP, Messmore HL. Mechanisms of venous and arterial thrombosis in heparin-induced thrombocytopenia. *J Thromb Thrombolysis* 2000;10:S13–S20.
93. Greinacher A, Michels I, Mueller-Eckhardt C. Heparin-associated thrombocytopenia: the antibody is not heparin specific. *Thromb Haemost.* 1992;67:545.
94. Warkentin TE, Levine MN, Hirsch J, et al. Heparin-induced thrombocytopenia in patients treated with low-molecular-weight heparin or unfractionated heparin. *N Engl J Med.* 1995;332:1330–1335.
95. Laster J, Silver D. Heparin-coated catheters and heparin-induced thrombocytopenia. *J Vasc Surg.* 1988;7:667.
96. George JN, Alving B, Ballem P. Platelets. In: McArthur JR, Benz EJ, eds. *Hematology—1994: the educational program of the American Society of Hematology.* Washington, DC: American Society of Hematology; 1994:66.
97. Jackson MR, Krishnamurti C, Aylesworth CA, et al. Diagnosis of heparin-induced thrombocytopenia in the vascular surgery patient. *Surgery* 1997;121:419.
98. Warkentin TE. Heparin-induced thrombocytopenia: a clinicopathologic syndrome. *Thromb Haemost.* 1999;82:439–447.
99. Greinacher A, Michels I, Kiefel V, et al. A rapid and sensitive test for diagnosing heparin-associated thrombocytopenia. *Thromb Haemost.* 1991; 66:734.
100. Warkentin TE, Elavathil LJ, Hayward CP, et al. The pathogenesis of venous limb gangrene associated with heparin-induced thrombocytopenia. *Ann Intern Med.* 1997;127:804.
101. Slocum MM, Adams JG Jr, Teel R, et al. Use of enoxaparin in patients with heparin-induced thrombocytopenia syndrome. *J Vasc Surg.* 1996; 23:839.
102. Greinacher A, Volpel H, Janssens U, et al. Recombinant hirudin (Lepirudin) provides safe and effective anticoagulation in patients with heparin-induced thrombocytopenia. *Circulation* 1999;99:73–80.
103. Lewis BE, Iaffaldano R, McKiernan TL, et al. Report of successful use of argatroban as an alternative anticoagulant during coronary stent implantation in a patient with heparin-induced thrombocytopenia and thrombosis syndrome. *Cathet Cardiovasc Diagn.* 1996;38:206.
104. Lubenow N, Greinacher A. Hirudin in heparin-induced thrombocytopenia. *Semin Thromb Hemost.* 2002;28:431–438.
105. Lockshin MD. Antiphospholipid antibody syndrome. *JAMA.* 1992; 268:1451.
106. Lockshin MD. Antiphospholipid antibody: babies, blood clots, biology. *JAMA.* 1997;277:1549.
107. Khamashta MA, Cuadrado MJ, Mujic F, et al. The management of thrombosis in the antiphospholipid-antibody syndrome. *N Engl J Med.* 1995;332:993.
108. Eldrup-Jorgensen J, Flanigan DP, Brace L, et al. Hypercoagulable states and lower limb ischemia in young adults. *J Vasc Surg.* 1989;9:334.
109. Galli M, Luciani D, Bertolini G, et al. Lupus anticoagulants are stronger risk factors for thrombosis than anticardiolipin antibodies in the antiphospholipid syndrome: a systematic review of the literature. *Blood* 2003;101:1827–1832.
110. Carreras LO, Defreyn G, Machin SJ, et al. Arterial thrombosis, intrauterine death, and "lupus" anticoagulant: detection of immunoglobulin interfering with prostacyclin formation. *Lancet* 1981;1:244.
111. Comp PC, DeBault LE, Esmon NL, Esmon CT. Human thrombomodulin is inhibited by IgG from two patients with non-specific anticoagulants. *Blood* 1983;62[Suppl 1]:299a(abst).
112. Eldrup-Jorgensen J, Flanigan DP, Brace L, et al. Hypercoagulable states and lower limb ischemia in young adults. *J Vasc Surg.* 1989;9:334.
113. Vermylen J, Blockmans D, Spitz B, et al. Thrombosis and immune disorders. *Clin Haematol.* 1986;15:393.
114. Ferro D, Pittoni V, Quintarelli C, et al. Coexistence of anti-phospholipid antibodies and endothelial perturbation in systemic lupus erythematosus patients with ongoing prothrombotic state. *Circulation* 1997;95:1425.
115. Rand JH, Wu XX, Andree HA, et al. Pregnancy loss in the antiphospholipid-antibody syndrome—a possible thrombogenic mechanism. *N Engl J Med.* 1997;337:154.
116. Reverter JC, Tassies D, Font J, et al. Hypercoagulable state in patients with antiphospholipid syndrome is related to high induced tissue factor expression on monocytes and to low free protein S. *Arterioscler Thromb Vasc Biol.* 1996;16:1319.
117. Williams FM, Hunt BJ. The antiphospholipid syndrome and vascular surgery. *Cardiovasc Surg.* 1998;6:10.
118. Greenfield LJ. Lupus-like anticoagulants and thrombosis. *J Vasc Surg.* 1988;7:818.
119. Ahn SS, Kalunian K, Rosove M, et al. Postoperative thrombotic complications in patients with the lupus anticoagulant: Increased risk after vascular procedures. *J Vasc Surg.* 1988;7:749.
120. Nielsen TG, Nordestgaard BG, von Jessen F, et al. Antibodies to cardiolipin may increase the risk of failure of peripheral vein bypasses. *Eur J Vasc Endovasc Surg.* 1997;14:177.
121. Valentine RJ, Kaplan HS, Green R, et al. Lipoprotein (a), homocysteine, and hypercoaguable states in young men with premature peripheral atherosclerosis: a prospective, controlled analysis. *J Vasc Surg.* 1996;23:53.
122. Lee RW, Taylor LM Jr, Landry GJ, et al. Prospective comparisons of infrainguinal bypass grafting in patients with and without antiphospholipid antibodies. *J Vasc Surg.* 1996;24:524.
123. de Moerloose P, Bounameaux HR, Mannucci PM. Screening tests for thrombophilic patients: which tests, for which patient, by whom, when, and why? *Semin Thromb Hemost.* 1998;24(4).
124. Lynch A, Marlar R, Murphy J, et al. Antiphospholipid antibodies in predicting adverse pregnancy outcome: A prospective study. *Ann Intern Med.* 1994;120:470.
125. Khamashta MA, Cuadrado MJ, Mujic F, et al. The management of thrombosis in the antiphospholipid-antibody syndrome. *N Engl J Med.* 1995;332:993.
126. Ridker PM, Miletich JP, Hennekens CH, et al. Ethnic distribution of factor V Leiden in 4047 men and women: Implications for venous thromboembolism screening. *JAMA.* 1997;277:1305.
127. Rosendaal FR, Koster T, Vandenbroucke JP, et al. High risk of thrombosis in patients homozygous for factor V Leiden (activated protein C resistance). *Blood* 1995;85:1504.
128. Svensson PJ, Dahlback B. Resistance to activated protein C as a basis for venous thrombosis. *N Engl J Med.* 1994;330:517.
129. Kalafatis M, Mann KG. Factor V Leiden and thrombophilia. *Arterioscler Thromb Vasc Biol.* 1997;17:620.
130. Mann KG, Kalafatis M. Factor V: a combination of Dr. Jekyll and Mr. Hyde. *Blood* 2003;101:20–30.
131. Simioni P, Prandoni P, Lensing AW, et al. The risk of recurrent venous thromboembolism in patients with an Arg^{506} to Gln mutation in the gene for factor V (factor V Leiden). *N Engl J Med.* 1997;336:399.
132. Carreras LO, Defreyn G, Machin SJ, et al. Arterial thrombosis, intrauterine death, and "lupus" anticoagulant: detection of immunoglobulin interfering with prostacyclin formation. *Lancet* 1981;1:244–246.
133. de Stefano V, Martinelli I, Mannucci PM, et al. The risk of recurrent deep venous thrombosis among heterozygous carriers of both Factor V Leiden and the G20210A prothrombin mutation. *N Engl J of Med.* 1999; 341:801.
134. Gerhardt A, Scharf RE, Beckmann MW, et al. Prothrombin and Factor V mutations in women with a history of thrombosis during pregnancy and the puerperium. *N Engl J Med.* 2000;342:374.
135. Koeleman BP, Reitsma PH, Allaart CF, et al. Activated protein C resistance as a additional risk factor for thrombosis in protein C-deficient families. *Blood* 1994;84:1031.
136. Koeleman BP, van Rumpt D, Hamulyak K, et al. Factor V Leiden: an additional risk factor for thrombosis in protein S deficient families? *Thromb Haemost.* 1995;74:580.
137. Svensson PJ, Dahlback B. Resistance to activated protein C as a basis for venous thrombosis. *N Engl J Med.* 1994;330:517.
138. Ouriel K, Green RM, DeWeese JA, et al. Activated protein C resistance: prevalence and implications in peripheral vascular disease. *J Vasc Surg.* 1996;23:46.
139. Van Cott EM, Soderberg BL, Laposata M. Activated protein C resistance, the Factor V Leiden mutation, and a laboratory testing algorithm. *Arch Pathol Lab Med.* 2002;126:577–582.
140. Hooper WC, Evatt BL. The role of activated protein C resistance in the pathogenesis of venous thrombosis. *Am J Med Scientific* 1998; 316(2):120–128.
141. Seligsohn U, Lubetsky A. Genetic susceptibility to venous thrombosis. *N Engl J Med.* 2001;344:1222–1231.
142. de Stefano V, Casorelli I, Rossi E, et al. Interaction between hyperhomocysteinemia and inherited thrombophilic factors in venous thromboembolism. *Semin Thromb Hemost.* 2000;26(3):305–311.
143. den Heijer M, Blom HJ, Gerrits WB, et al. Is hyperhomocysteinaemia a risk factor for recurrent venous thrombosis? *Lancet* 1995;345:882.
144. den Heijer M, Koster T, Blom HJ, et al. Hyperhomocysteinemia as a risk factor for deep-vein thrombosis. *N Engl J Med.* 1996;334:759.
145. den Heijer M, Keijzer M. Hyperhomocysteinemia as a risk factor for venous thrombosis. *Clin Chem Lab Med.* 2001;39:710–713.
146. Legnani C, Palareti G, Grauso F, et al, Hyperhomocysteinemia and a common methylenetetrahydrofolate reductase mutation (Ala^{223} Val MTHFR) in patients with inherited thrombophilic coagulation defects (Abstract). *Arterioscler Thromb Vasc Biol,* 1997;17:2924.
147. Kottke-Marchant K. Genetic polymorphisms associated with venous and arterial thrombosis. *Arch Pathol Lab Med.* 2002;126:295–304.
148. Falcon CR, Cattaneo M, Panzeri D, et al. High prevalence of hyperhomocyst(e)inemia in patients with juvenile venous thrombosis. *Arterioscler Thromb.* 1994;14:1080.

149. Mandel H, Brenner B, Berant M, et al. Coexistence of hereditary homocystinuria and factor V Leiden—effect on thrombosis. *N Engl J Med.* 1996;334:763.
150. Hayashi T, Honda G, Suzucki K. An atherogenic stimulus homocysteine inhibits cofactor activity of thrombomodulin and enhances thrombomodulin expression in human umbilical vein endothelial cells. *Blood* 1992; 79:2930.
151. Loscalzo J. The oxidant stress of hyperhomocyst(e)inemia. *J Clin Invest.* 1996;98:5.
152. Rodgers GM, Conn MT. Homocysteine, an atherogenic stimulus, reduces protein C activation by arterial and venous endothelial cells. *Blood* 1990;75:895.
153. Tawakol A, Omland T, Gerhard M, et al. Hyperhomocyst(e)inemia is associated with impaired endothelium-dependent vasodilation in humans. *Circulation* 1997;95:1119.
154. Upchurch GR, Welch GN, Randev N, et al. The effect of homocysteine on endothelial nitric oxide production. *FASEB J.* 1995;9:A876(abst).
155. Blom HJ, Kleinveld HA, Boers GH, et al. Lipid peroxidation and susceptibility of low-density lipoprotein to in vitro oxidation in hyperhomocysteinemia. *Eur J Clin Invest.* 1995;25:149.
156. Rees MM, Rodgers GM. Homocystinemia: association of a metabolic disorder with vascular disease and thrombosis. *Thromb Res.* 1993;71:337.
157. Graeber JE, Slott JH, Ulane RE, et al. Effect of homocysteine and homocystine platelet and vascular arachidonic acid metabolism. *Pediatr Res.* 1982;16:490.
158. George JN, Alving B, Ballem P. Platelets. In: McArthur JR, Benz EJ, eds. *Hematology 1994: the educational program of the American Society of Hematology.* Washington, DC: American Society of Hematology; 1994:66.
159. Ueland PM, Refsum H, Brattstrom L. Plasma homocysteine and cardiovascular disease. In: Francis RB Jr, ed. *Atherosclerotic cardiovascular disease, hemostasis, and endothelial function.* New York: Marcel Dekker; 1993:183.
160. Bick RL. Prothrombin G20210A mutation, antithrombin, heparin cofactor II, protein C, and protein S defects. *Hematol Oncol Clin North Am.* 2003;17(1):9–36.
161. Vicente V, González-Conejero R, et al. The prothrombin gene variant 20210A in venous and arterial thromboembolism. *Haematologica* 1999;84:356–362.
162. Cumming AM, Keeney S, Salden A, et al. The prothrombin gene G20210A variant: prevalence in a U.K. anticoagulant clinic population. *Br J Haematol.* 1997;98:353.
163. Martinelli I, Sacchi E, Landi G, et al. High risk of cerebral vein thrombosis in carrier of a prothrombin gene mutation and in users of oral contraceptives. *N Engl J Med.* 1998;338:1793–1797.
164. Gerhardt A, Scharf RE, Beckmann MW, et al. Prothrombin and factor V mutations in women with a history of thrombosis during pregnancy and the puerperium. *N Engl J Med.* 2000;342:374.
165. Ridker PM, Hennekens CH, Miletich JP. G20210A mutation in prothrombin gene and risk of myocardial infarction, stroke, and venous thrombosis in a large cohort of US men. *Circulation* 1999;99:999–1004.
166. McGlennen RC, Key NS. Clinical and laboratory management of the prothrombin G20210A mutation. *Arch Pathol Lab Med.* 2002; 126:1319–1325.
167. Reiner AP, Siscovick DS, Rosendaal FR. Hemostatic risk factors and arterial thrombotic disease. *Thromb Haemost.* 2001;85:584–595.
168. Towne JB, Bandyk DF, Hussey CV, et al. Abnormal plasminogen: a genetically determined cause of hypercoagulability. *J Vasc Surg.* 1984;1:896.
169. Kwaan HC, Levin M, Sakurai S, et al. Digital ischemia and gangrene due to red blood cell aggregation induced by acquired dysfibrinogenemia. *J Vasc Surg.* 1997;26:1061.
170. Roberts HR. Review of the dysfibrinogenemias. *Br J Haematol.* 2001;114:249–257.
171. Nilsson IM, Ljungner H, Tengborn L. Two different mechanisms in patients with venous thrombosis and defective fibrinolysis: low concentrations of plasminogen activator or increased concentration of plasminogen activator inhibitor. *Br Med J Clin Res Ed.* 1985;290:1453.
172. Prins MH, Hirsh J. A clinical review of the evidence supporting a relationship between impaired fibrinolytic activity and venous thromboembolism. *Arch Intern Med.* 1991;151:1721.
173. van Tilburg NH, RosendaalFR, Bertina RM. Thrombin activatable fibrinolysis inhibitor and the risk for deep venous thrombosis. *Blood* 2000; 95:2855–2859.
174. Paramo JA, Perez JL, Serrano M, et al. Types 1 and 2 plasminogen activator inhibitor and tumor necrosis factor alpha in patients with sepsis. *Thromb Haemost.* 1990;64:3.
175. Ishibashi S. Lipoprotein(a) and atherosclerosis. *Arterioscler Thromb Vasc Biol.* 2001;21:1–2.
176. Liao JK, Shin WS, Lee WY, et al. Oxidized low-density lipoprotein decreases the expression of endothelial nitric oxide synthase. *J Biol Chem.* 1995;270:319.
177. Valentine RJ, Kaplan HS, Green R, et al. Lipoprotein (a), homocysteine, and hypercoaguable states in young men with premature peripheral atherosclerosis: a prospective, controlled analysis. *J Vasc Surg.* 1996;23:53.
178. Griffin JH, Fernández JA, Deguchi H. Plasma lipoproteins, hemostasis, and thrombosis. *Thromb Haemost.* 2001;86:386–394.
179. Nowak-Göttl U, Junker R, Hartmeier M, et al. Increased lipoprotein(a) is an important risk factors for venous thromboembolism in childhood. *Circulation* 1999;100:743–748.
180. Cunningham MT, Brandt JT. Laboratory diagnosis of dysfibrinogenemia. *Arch Pathol Lab Med.* 2002;126:499–505.
181. Mosesson MW. Dysfibrinogenemia and thrombosis. *Semin Thromb Hemost.* 1999;25: 311–319.
182. Rosendaal FR. Venous thrombosis: a multicausal disease. *Lancet* 1993; 353:1167–1173.
183. Eldrup-Jorgensen J, Flanigan DP, Brace L, et al. Hypercoaguable states and lower limb ischemia in young adults. *J Vasc Surg.* 1989;9:334.
184. Harker LA. Platelets in thrombotic disorder: quantitative and qualitative platelet disorders predisposing to arterial thrombosis. *Semin Hematol.* 1998;35:241–251.
185. Kamphuisen PW, Lensen R, Houwing-Duistermaat JJ, et al. Heritability of elevated factor VIII antigen levels in factor V Leiden families with thrombophilia. *Br J Haematol.* 2000;109:519–522.
186. Koster T, Blann AD, Briët E, et al. Role of clotting factor VIII in effect of von Willebrand factor on occurrence of deep venous thrombosis. *Lancet* 1995;345:152–155.
187. O'Donnell J, Mumford AD, Manning RA, et al. Elevation of FVIII:C in venous thromboembolism is persistent and independent of the acute phase response. *Thromb Haemost.* 2000;83:10–13.
188. Mansvelt EPG, Laffan M, McVey JH, et al. Analysis of the F8 gene in individuals with high plasma factor VIII:C levels and associated venous thrombosis. *Thromb Haemost.* 1998;80:561–565.
189. Meijers JC, Tekelenburg WL, Bouma BN, et al. High levels of coagulation factor XI as a risk factor for venous thrombosis. *N Engl J Med.* 2000; 342:696–701.
190. van Hylckama V, Van der Linden IK, Bertina RM, et al. High levels of factor IX increase the risk of venous thrombosis. *Blood* 2000;95:3678–3682.
191. Lane DA, Grant PJ. Role of hemostatic gene polymorphisms in venous and arterial thrombotic disease. *Blood* 2000;95:1517–1532.
192. Fisher DF Jr, Yawn DH, Crawford ES. Preoperative disseminated intravascular coagulation associated with aortic aneurysms: a prospective study of 76 cases. *Arch Surg.* 1983;118:1252.
193. Eby CS. A review of the hypercoagulable state. *Hematol Oncol Clin North Am.* 1993;7:1121.
194. Nielsen TG, Nordestgaard BG, von Jessen F, et al. Antibodies to cardiolipin may increase the risk of failure of peripheral vein bypasses. *Eur J Vasc Endovasc Surg.* 1997;14:177.
195. Nilsson IM, Ljungner H, Tengborn L. Two different mechanisms in patients with venous thrombosis and defective fibrinolysis: low concentrations of plasminogen activator or increased concentration of plasminogen activator inhibitor. *Br Med J Clin Res Ed.* 1985;290:1453.
196. Nordström J, Lindblad B, Anderson H. Deep venous thrombosis and occult malignancy: an epidemiological study. *BMJ* 1994;308:891–894.
197. Collins JA. Blood transfusion and disorders of surgical bleeding. In: Sabiston DC, ed. *Textbook of surgery,* 14th ed. Philadelphia: WB Saunders, 1991:85.
198. Lusher JM, Warrier I. Hemophila A. *Hematol Oncol Clin North Am.* 1993;7:1021.
199. Lusher JM, Arkin S, Abildgaard CF, et al. Recombinant factor VIII for the treatment of previously untreated patients with hemophilia A: safety, efficacy, and development of inhibitors. *N Engl J Med.* 1993;328:453.
200. Telfer MC. Clinical spectrum of viral infections in hemophilic patients. *Hematol Oncol Clin North Am.* 1993;7:1047.
201. Larson PJ, High KA. Biology of inherited coagulopathies: factor IX. *Hematol Oncol Clin North Am.* 1993;7:999.
202. Ginsburg D. Biology of inherited coagulopathies: von Willebrand factor. *Hematol Oncol Clin North Am.* 1993;7:1011.
203. Edmunds LH. Blood contact activation during cardiopulmonary bypass. *J Vasc Surg.* 1990;12:213.
204. Wakefield TW, Shulkin BL, Fellows EP, et al. Platelet reactivity in human aortic grafts: a prospective randomized midterm study of platelet adherence and release products in Dacron and ePTFE grafts. *J Vasc Surg.* 1989;9:234.
205. Hirsh J. Heparin. *N Engl J Med.* 1991;324:1565.
206. Saba HI, Saba SR, Morelli GA. Effect of heparin on platelet aggregation. *Am J Hematol.* 1984;17:295.
207. Kakkar VV. The current status of low-dose heparin in the prophylaxis of thrombophlebitis and pulmonary embolism. *World J Surg.* 1978;2:3.
208. Clagett GP, Anderson FA Jr, Geerts W, et al. Prevention of venous thromboembolism. *Chest* 1998;114:531S.
209. Collins R, Scrigmeour A, Yusuf S, et al. Reduction in fatal pulmonary embolism and venous thrombosis by perioperative administration of subcutaneous heparin: overview of results of randomized trials in general, orthopedic, and urologic surgery. *N Engl J Med.* 1988;318:1162.
210. Hirsh J. Low–molecular-weight heparin. *Circulation* 1998;98:1575.
211. Salzman EW. Low–molecular-weight heparin: is small beautiful? [Editorial]. *N Engl J Med.* 1986;315:957.
212. Leizorovicz A. Comparison of the efficacy and safety of low molecular weight heparins and unfractionated heparin in the initial treatment of deep venous thrombosis: an updated meta-analysis. *Drugs* 1996;52[Suppl 7]:30.
213. Siragusa S, Cosmi B, Piovella F, et al. Low–molecular-weight heparins and unfractionated heparin in the treatment of patients with acute venous thromboembolism: results of a meta-analysis. *Am J Med.* 1996;100:269.

214. **Simonneau G, Sers H, Charbonnier B, et al. A comparison of low-molecular-weight heparin with unfractionated heparin for acute pulmonary embolism. *N Engl J Med.* 1997;337:663.**
215. Horrow JC. Protamine: a review of its toxicity. *Anesth Analg.* 1985; 64:348.
216. Wakefield TW, Ucros I, Kresowik TF, et al. Decreased oxygen consumption as a toxic manifestation of protamine sulfate reversal of heparin anticoagulation. *J Vasc Surg.* 1989;9:772.
217. Pearson PJ, Evora RR, Ayrancioglu K, et al. Protamine releases endothelium-derived relaxing factor from systemic arteries: a possible mechanism of hypotension during heparin neutralization. *Circulation* 1992;86:289.
218. Wakefield TW, Bies LE, Wrobleski SK, et al. Impaired myocardial function and oxygen utilization due to protamine sulfate in a isolated rabbit heart preparation. *Ann Surg.* 1990;212:387.
219. Morel DR, Zapol WM, Thomas SJ, et al. C5a and thromboxane generation associated with pulmonary vaso- and broncho-constriction during protamine reversal of heparin. *Anesthesiology* 1987;66:597.
220. Eika C. On the mechanism of platelet aggregation induced by heparin, protamine, and polybrene. *Scand J Haematol.* 1972;9:248.
221. DeLucia A, Wakefield TW, Andrews PC, et al. Efficacy and toxicity of differently charged polycationic protamine-like peptides for heparin anticoagulation reversal. *J Vasc Surg.* 1993;18:49.
222. Coon WW. Anticoagulant therapy. *Am J Surg.* 1985;150:45.
223. Hirsh J. Oral anticoagulant drugs. *N Engl J Med.* 1991;324:1865.
224. Hull R, Carter C, Jay R, et al. The diagnosis of acute, recurrent, deep-vein thrombosis: a diagnostic challenge. *Circulation* 1983;67:901.
225. **Kearon C, Gent M, Hirsh J, et al. A comparison of three months of anticoagulation with extended anticoagulation for a first episode of idiopathic venous thromboembolism. *N Engl J Med.* 1999;340:901.**
226. **Ridker PM, Goldhaber SZ, Danielson E, et al. Long-term, low-intensity warfarin therapy for the prevention of recurrent venous thromboembolism. *N Engl J Med.* 2003;348:1425.**
227. **Kearon C, Ginsberg JS, Kovacs MJ, et al. Comparison of low-intensity warfarin therapy with conventional-intensity warfarin therapy for long-term prevention of recurrent venous thromboembolism. *N Engl J Med.* 2003;349:631.**
228. Coller BS. Platelets and thrombolytic therapy. *N Engl J Med.* 1990; 322:33.
229. Madan M, Berkowitz SD, Tcheng JE. Glycoprotein IIb/IIIa integrin blockade. *Circulation* 1998;98:2629.
230. Fenton JW, Ofosu FA, Brezniak DV, et al. Thrombin and antithrombotics. *Semin Thromb Haemost.* 1998;24:87.
231. Jang IK, Gold HK, Ziskind AA, et al. Prevention of platelet-rich arterial thrombosis by selective thrombin inhibition. *Circulation* 1990;81:219.
232. Quereshi A, Lamont J, Burke P, et al. Aprotinin: the ideal anti-coagulant? *Eur J Vasc Surg.* 1992;6:317.
233. Royston D, Bidstrup BP, Taylor KM, et al. Effect of aprotinin on need for blood transfusion after repeat open heart surgery. *Lancet* 1987;2:1289.
234. Salzman EW, Weinstein MJ, Reilly D, et al. Adventures in hemostasis. Desmopressin in cardiac surgery. *Arch Surg.* 1993;128:212.
235. Mannucci PM. Desmopressin: a nontransfusional form of treatment for congenital and acquired bleeding disorders. *Blood* 1988;72:1449.
236. Cole CW, Bormanis J, Luna GK, et al. Ancrod versus heparin for anticoagulation during vascular surgical procedures. *J Vasc Surg.* 1993;17:288.
237. Schulman S, Wahlander K, Lundstrom T, et al. Secondary prevention of venous thromboembolism with the oral direct thrombin inhibitor ximelagatran. *N Engl J Med.* 2003;349:1713–1721.
238. Matisse Investigators. The Matisse-DVT and PE trials. *J Thromb Haemost.* 2003;1[Suppl 1]:abstracts OC331, OC332.
239. Bueller HR, Davidson BL, Decousus H, et al. Subcutaneous fondaparinux versus intravenous unfractionated heparin in the initial treatment of pulmonary embolism. *N Engl J Med.* 2003;349:1695–1702.
240. Eriksson BI, Bauer KA, Lassen MR, et al. Fondaparinux compared with enoxaparin for the prevention of venous thromboembolism after hip-fracture surgery. *N Engl J Med.* 2001;345:1298–1304.
241. Bauer KA, Eriksson BI, Lassen MR, et al. Fondaparinux compared with enoxaparin for the prevention of venous thromboembolism after elective major knee surgery. *N Engl J Med.* 2001;345:1305–1310.
242. Turpie AG, Bauer KA, Eriksson BI, et al. Fondaparinux vs enoxaparin for the prevention of venous thromboembolism in major orthopedic surgery. *Arch Intern Med.* 2002;162:1833–1840.
243. Eriksson BI, Lassen MR, for the PENTasaccharide in hip-fracture surgery plus (PENTHIFRA Plus) Investigators. *Arch Intern Med.* 2003;613:1337–1342.
244. Marder VJ, Sherry S. Thrombolytic therapy: current status (first of two parts). *N Engl J Med.* 1988;318:1512.
245. Fuji S, Sawa H, Saffitz JE, et al. Induction of endothelial cell expression of the plasminogen activator inhibitor type I gene by thrombosis in vivo. *Circulation* 1992;86:2000.
246. Quinones-Baldrich WJ. Principles of thrombolytic therapy. In: Rutherford RB, ed. *Vascular surgery,* 4th ed. Philadelphia: WB Saunders; 1995:334.
247. Comerota AJ, Aldridge SC. Thrombolytic therapy for acute deep vein thrombosis. *Semin Vasc Surg.* 1992;5:76.
248. Elliot MS, Immelman EJ, Jeffrey P, et al. A comparative randomized trial of heparin versus streptokinase in the treatment of acute proximal venous thrombosis: an interim report of a prospective trial. *Br J Surg.* 1979; 66:838.
249. Arnsen H, Hoiseth A, Ly B. Streptokinase or heparin in the treatment of deep vein thrombosis: follow-up results of a prospective study. *Acta Med Scand.* 1982;211:65.
250. Kakkar VV, Lawrence D. Hemodynamic and clinical assessment after therapy for acute deep vein thrombosis: a prospective study. *Am J Surg.* 1985;150:54.
251. Porter JM, Taylor LM. Current status of thrombolytic therapy. *J Vasc Surg.* 1985;2:239.
252. Graor RA, Young JR, Risius B. Comparison of cost effectiveness of streptokinase and urokinase in the treatment of deep vein thrombosis. *Ann Vasc Surg.* 1987;1:524.
253. Turpie AGG. Thrombolytic agents in venous thrombosis. *J Vasc Surg.* 1990;12:196.
254. Machleder HI. Evaluation of a new treatment strategy for Paget-Schroetter syndrome: spontaneous thrombosis of the axillary-subclavian vein. *J Vasc Surg.* 1993;17:305.
255. National Heart and Lung Institute Cooperative Study Group. Urokinase pulmonary embolism trial: phase 1 results. *JAMA.* 1970;214:2163.
256. National Heart and Lung Institute Cooperative Study Group. Urokinase-streptokinase embolism trial: phase 2 results. *JAMA.* 1974;229:1606.
257. McNamara TO, Fischer JR. Thrombolysis of peripheral arterial and graft occlusions: improved results using high-dose urokinase. *AJR Am J Roentgenol.* 1985;144:769.
258. McNamara TO, Bomberger RA. Factors affecting initial and 6 months patency rates after intraarterial thrombolysis with high-dose urokinase. *Am J Surg.* 1986;152:709.
259. Gardiner GA, Sullivan KL. Catheter directed thrombolysis for the failed lower extremity bypass graft. *Semin Vasc Surg.* 1992;5:99.
260. Graor RA, Risius B, Young JR, et al. Peripheral artery and bypass graft thrombolysis with recombinant tissue-type plasminogen activator. *J Vasc Surg.* 1986;3:115.
261. Comerota AJ, White JV. Intraoperative, intra-arterial thrombolytic therapy as an adjunct to revascularization in patients with residual and distal arterial thrombus. *Semin Vasc Surg.* 1992;5:110.
262. Rutherford RB, Jones DN. The role of Dextran-40 in preventing early graft thrombosis. In: Bergqvist D, Lindblad B, eds. *Pharmacological intervention to increase patency after arterial reconstructions.* Malmo, Sweden: ICM AB; 1989:44.
263. Stenbjerg S, Berg E, Albrechtsen OK. Heparin levels and activated clotting times (ACT) during open heart surgery. *Scand J Haematol.* 1981;26:281.

CHAPTER 6 ■ INFLAMMATION

MATTHEW R. ROSENGART AND TIMOTHY R. BILLIAR

The concept of inflammation has undergone considerable revision since the initial description of the four cardinal signs and symptoms by Celsus in the first century AD: "rubor et tumor cum calor et dolore," redness and swelling with heat and pain.[1] Centuries later John Hunter postulated that inflammation provides a survival mechanism to preserve the host. Ironically, he commented that an exuberant inflammatory response could be deleterious; the pathologic sequelae of excessive inflammation [i.e., acute respiratory distress syndrome (ARDS), multiple-organ dysfunction syndrome (MODS)] are encountered more frequently as technology affords survival of the initial insult.[1] The 19th century witnessed milestone contributions to our understanding of this process. Rudolph Virchow detailed the cellular pathology of inflammation, Julius Cohnheim provided microscopic details of the acute phases of inflammation (vasodilatation, edema formation, and leukocyte emigration), and Elie Metchnikoff described the events of phagocytosis.[1–3] The evidence culminated into a cellular and humoral concept of inflammation, both of which were deemed critical in host defense against foreign pathogens.

In the 20th century, technologic advancements in molecular biology and biochemistry facilitated more detailed investigation and enabled the rapid expansion of knowledge of the many interwoven facets of the inflammation process. Evidence began to accumulate that the ramifications of these processes extend beyond the confines of the insult. Many humoral mediators, in addition to local effects, influenced distant targets, such as the liver and neurohormonal centers. Recently, it has become clear that the immune system, endocrine system, and nervous system comprise an integrated network sharing similar mediators and their receptors. Such an integrative view, introduced by J. Edwin Blalock, when combined with Hans Selye's concept of stress led to the contemporary understanding of sickness behavior, defined by Robert Dantzer as a highly organized strategy of the organism to fight infections and to respond to other environmental stressors. Hence, what originated nearly 2 millennia ago as a simple concept founded on a constellation of signs and symptoms, now is considered an intense, coordinated interplay of the nervous, vascular, endocrine, and immune systems to any injurious insult. It is the culmination of millions of years of evolution. Without it, life would be an arduous, painful, and brief existence, at best.

This chapter attempts to summarize this enormous quantity of information. An initial description of the elements involved in inflammation provides the foundation on which to discuss the sequence of events and interactions that constitute the inflammatory cascade.

INNATE VERSUS ADAPTIVE IMMUNITY

The initial security against microbes is the responsibility of our innate immunity, a system comprising both cellular and humoral components, already poised to respond prior to any stimulus.[4] Phylogenetically it is ancient and conserved, notably providing the primary mechanism of invertebrate host defense. The response it provides is uniform and consistent with each successive infection. Subsequent reinforcement is provided by the more specific and targeted efforts of the adaptive immune system. In contrast to innate immunity, subsequent exposure to the inciting agent during adaptive immunity elicits responses of increased magnitude and defensive capabilities.[4] This exquisite specificity for individual microbes, the capacity to "learn," "remember," and modify subsequent responses to repeated exposures, has provided the impetus for the name.

Both arms of immunity comprise cellular and serum components. In the adaptive immune response this has been divided into humoral immunity, which is mediated primarily by antibodies, and cell-mediated immunity. These are not distinct systems and form an integrated system of host defense.

CELLULAR COMPONENTS

Neutrophils

Neutrophils are integral to immunity, providing the initial defense against invading viral, bacterial, and parasitic pathogens. This importance is underscored by the fact that 55% to 60% of the hematopoietic output of bone marrow is dedicated to the production of neutrophils.[5] On exiting the marrow they circulate for 7 to 10 hours before taking up residence in the tissues for 1 to 2 days (Table 6.1).[6,7] They are uniquely sensitive to minute concentration gradients of microbial products and inflammatory mediators and rapidly accumulate at sites of infection where they ingest and dispose of a wide array of pathogens with their vast microbicidal armamentarium. This pathogenicity, however, carries with it an implicit capacity for host injury, and accordingly, neutrophil function must be tightly regulated.

Recruitment

Neutrophil recruitment may be viewed as a sequence of events progressing from initial adhesion to activated endothelium, to subsequent extravasation and emigration toward inflammatory foci, to the ultimate elimination of foreign microorganisms through phagocytosis, generation of reactive oxygen species (ROS), and the release of microbial substances.[4] These processes function in a similar context in other inflammatory cells that migrate to foci of infection or inflammation.

After injury, local and regional vasodilation induces hyperemia and facilitates the delivery of leukocytes. Extravasation of plasma creates edema and, in combination with the release of vasoactive substances, leads to hemoconcentration, which promotes the peripheral margination of leukocytes.[8,9]

Circulating neutrophils transiently interact with the endothelial cell surface molecules during "rolling," a process that involves a series of loose and reversible attachments (Fig. 6.1). These interactions are prerequisite for subsequent tighter interactions. The family of selectin receptors binds

TABLE 6.1

LEUKOCYTE SUBSETS

Cell	Neutrophil	Monocyte	Lymphocyte	Eosinophil	Basophil
Size (μm)	13	16–20	9–16	12–16	15
Differential (%)	40–75	2–6	20–45	1–6	<1
Life span	6 h to 7 d	1 d to years	Months to years	8 to 12 d	1 year
Activators	G-CSF, IL-8	M-CSF, GM-CSF, IFNγ, TNF α	IL-2, IL-12(T_H1), IL-4(T_H2)	G-CSF, IL-5	G-CSF, IL-3

G-CSF, granulocyte colony-stimulating factor; M-CSF, monocyte colony-stimulating factor; IL, interleukin, T_H, helper T cell; IFNγ, interferon gamma; TNF, tumor necrosis factor.
Modified from Burkitt G, Young B, Heath JW, eds. *Wheater's functional histology: a text and colour atlas*, 3rd ed. Edinburgh, New York: Churchill Livingstone, 1993.

with their counterligands, the sialyl Lewis family, and other fucosylated and sulfated structures that mediate this process. E-selectin and P-selectin are present on endothelium and L-selectin is found on leukocytes.[4]

Consequent to stimulation with inflammatory mediators [thrombin; histamine; complement fragments; oxygen species; lipopolysaccharide (LPS); and cytokines such as interleukin (IL)-1, tumor necrosis factor alpha (TNFα), and interferon gamma (IFNγ)], vascular endothelial cells express P- and E-selectin, which may engage the neutrophil surface glycoprotein P-selectin glycoprotein ligand 1 (PSGL-1) or sialyl Lewis. P-selectin is stored intracellularly and can be rapidly mobilized for expression within minutes of cellular activation. They also translocate ligands for neutrophil L-selectin and release mediators such as platelet activating factor (PAF) and IL-8. Cytokines such as TNFα, granulocyte-macrophage colony stimulating factor (GM-CSF), and granulocyte colony stimulating factor (G-CSF) increase the affinity of leukocyte L-selectin for its counter-receptor. In addition to mechanical anchorage, these selectins induce signal transduction pathways that influence cellular function. P-selectin facilitates neutrophil degranulation and superoxide production, and cross-linking L-selectin primes the neutrophil for increased superoxide production.[10–12]

After rolling, L-selectin is rapidly shed in preparation for leukocyte diapedesis and emigration. Subsequent exposure to chemoattractant gradients results in conversion of the neutrophil to a state of tight stationary adhesion (see Fig. 6.1). The receptors mediating this interaction are members of the β_2 integrin family, most importantly leukocyte function antigen 1 (LFA-1, CD11a/CD18) and Mac-1 (CD11b/CD18), and their expression is enhanced in response to selectin binding. Secretory vesicles are a major reservoir for these receptors. Both integrin receptors engage the intercellular adhesion molecule (ICAM)-1 and ICAM-2 in mediating adhesion; yet, each provides additional important functions. Leukocyte emigration is primarily an LFA-1 dependent process, as mice deficient in this receptor show reduced neutrophil attachment to ICAM-1 and endothelial cells. By contrast, mice lacking Mac-1 demonstrate impaired degranulation, superoxide production, and phagocytosis. Mac-1 also binds fibrinogen, heparin, and factor X and is implicated in neutrophil

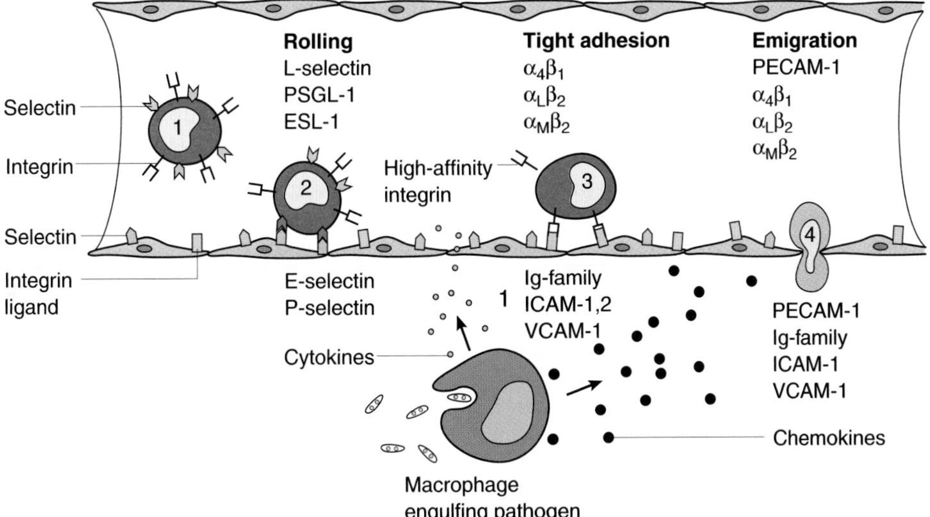

FIGURE 6.1 Leukocyte recruitment. (1) Circulating leukocytes express integrins in a low-affinity conformation. (2) Exposure to activated endothelium leads to rolling, which is mediated by L-selectin and P-selectin on the neutrophil and E-selectin on endothelium. (3) Leukocyte exposure to cytokines released by macrophages phagocytosing pathogens induces a high-affinity integrin conformation. Tight leukocyte-endothelial adhesion involves integrin engagement with counterligand expressed on the endothelium. (4) Subsequent exposure to chemokines leads to diapedesis, which is further mediated by the family of β_1 and β_2 integrins. (After Abbas AK, Lichtman AH. *Cellular and molecular immunology*, 5th ed. Philadelphia: Elsevier; 2003.)

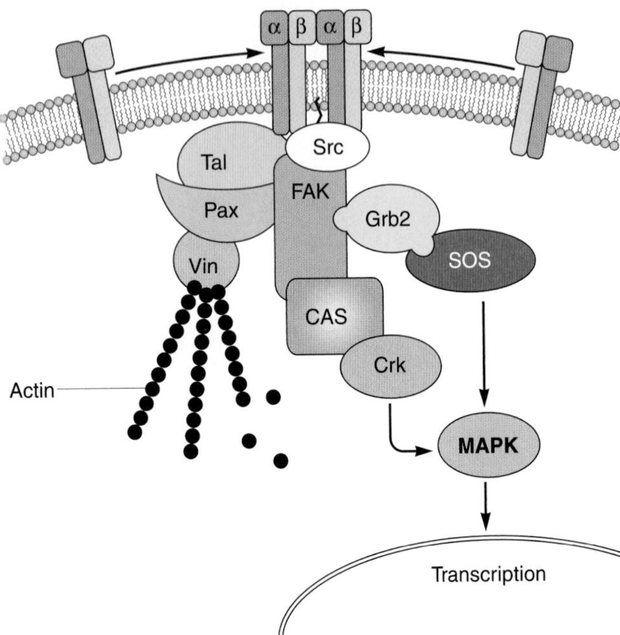

FIGURE 6.2 Integrin signaling. Integrins comprise a large family of cell surface receptors that are composed of two subunits, α and β, and are activated by dimerization. The cytoplasmic tails are devoid of enzymatic activity, and hence, signal transduction is effected by adapter proteins that connect the receptor to the cytoskeleton, cytoplasmic kinases, and transmembrane growth factor receptors. As integrins bind the extracellular matrix they become clustered and associated with the cytoskeletal proteins talin, paxillin, and vinculin and signaling complexes. Actin stress fibers form, which increase integrin clustering. Ultimately, focal adhesion kinase (FAK) is recruited via interactions with talin and paxillin or with the β integrin subunit. Subsequent autophosphorylation on tyrosine 397 provides a binding site for the Src homology 2 (SH2) domain of Src. The Src kinase phosphorylates a number of focal adhesion components including paxillin and tensin and p130CAS, a docking protein that recruits Crk, which can subsequently activate proximal elements in the JNK cascade of the mitogen-activated protein kinase (MAPK) family. FAK may also be phosphorylated by Src on tyrosine 925, creating a binding site for the complex of the adapter Grb2 and Ras guanosine 5′-triphosphate exchange factor mSOS. These interactions also lead to activation of MAPK cascades, and ultimately the induction of a variety of genes. (After Giancotti F, Ruoslahti E. Integrin signaling. *Science* 1999;285:1028–1032.)

phagocytosis-induced apoptosis, a process essential for resolution of the inflammatory process (vida infra). The very late antigen 4 (VLA-4) binds vascular cellular adhesion molecule 1 (VCAM-1) and may provide an additional mechanism for tight adhesion. In addition to providing mechanical anchorage, these receptors interact with the cytoskeleton and other structural proteins and signaling cascades and are thought to represent a biochemical link between the external environment and intracellular signal transduction cascades that induce a cellular phenotype more appropriate for the inflammatory environment (Fig. 6.2).[13–15]

Once tightly adhered, neutrophils must diapedese between endothelial cells and across the basement membrane to arrive at the focus of inflammation. Platelet-endothelial cell adhesion molecule 1 (PECAM-1) and integrin-associated protein are integral during transmigration (see Fig. 6.1).[13,14,16,17] PECAM-1 is concentrated along the intercellular junctions of endothelial cells, and both leukocyte and endothelial PECAM-1 appear to be essential for neutrophil and monocyte diapedesis. Other candidate receptors include the β_1 integrins, or VLAs, which possess affinity for many constituents of the extracellular matrix, including laminin, fibronectin, and collagens, and the β_3 family of integrins including the glycoprotein (gp) IIβIIIα and the vitronectin receptor.[4] Further "directions" for migration to the focus of inflammation are delivered by the concentration gradients of chemotactic factors, including complement C5a, IL-8, LTB_4, and the bacterial product formyl-methionyl-leucyl-phenylalanine (fMLP).[18–20]

The clinical significance of even minor derangements in any aspect of this process is evident in the disease leukocyte adhesion deficiency, characterized by complete absence of CD18 and therefore all β_2 integrins. Patients usually succumb to recurrent skin and mucosal infections within the initial 10 years of life.[4]

Phagocytosis

Microbial elimination commences when the neutrophil first encounters foreign pathogen. It is facilitated by opsonization, a process whereby microbes are coated by immune globulins and/or complement, which subsequently bind to their respective cell-surface receptors, FcγRs and Mac-1.[21–23] Neutrophils constitutively express low-affinity immune globulin receptors FcγRII and FcγRIII and can be induced to express high affinity FcγRI by incubation with IFNγ or cross-linking β_2 integrins.[5,24] Complement-dependent phagocytosis is mediated by interactions between the leukocyte Mac-1 receptor and the complement opsonin iC3b.

Once engaged, FcγRs are phosphorylated on tyrosine residues within an immunoreceptor tyrosine activation motif (ITAM) by the Src-family kinases.[24] These phosphorylated sites serve as docking regions for a variety of proteins, in particular Syk. The importance of Syk is underscored by the observation that mice deficient in Syk are incapable of ingesting IgG-opsonized particles. A series of enzymes are subsequently activated including phosphoinositol 3-kinase, phospholipase C, and protein kinase C. Ultimately, the actin cytoskeleton undergoes rearrangement and the local plasmalemma is remodeled in the formation and sealing of the phagosome.[4,24]

This immature phagosome undergoes a series of maturation steps, whereby it acquires the machinery necessary for the killing and disposal of internalized microorganisms. Alterations in cytosolic calcium concentration induce the fusion of secretory vesicles and granules containing the microbicidal armamentarium with the immature phagosome.[24] Proteins effected by calcium concentration and that may govern phagosomal maturation include synaptotogamins, actin, calmodulin, and the Src family of kinases.[24] The soluble N-ethylmaleimide-sensitive-fusion-protein attachment protein receptor (SNARE) proteins are thought to assist in fusion by engaging cognate receptors on the target membrane and approximating the two membranes. Antibodies to the SNARE 5, syntaxin 6 and SNAP-23, inhibited exocytosis of azurophilic and specific granules, respectively.[24]

Neutrophil Granules and Secretory Vesicles

There are two arms to the microbicidal capacity of the neutrophil: an oxygen-dependent pathway, or "respiratory burst," that generates toxic oxygen derivatives and an oxygen-independent pathway that utilizes toxic proteinases.[25] These two components are compartmentalized into four distinct granules or vesicles that also contain adhesion molecules and important inflammatory mediators (Table 6.2).[26] They are mobilized in a hierarchical fashion in response to gradual elevations in the intracellular calcium level, which parallels their respective contents and the current needs of the cell.[27]

Primary, or azurophil (affinity for the dye azure A), granules target the destruction of phagocytosed organisms (see Table 6.2). The myeloperoxidase (MPO) within these granules

TABLE 6.2

NEUTROPHIL GRANULES AND SECRETORY VESICLES

Azurophil granules	Specific granules	Gelatinase granules or vesicles	Secretory vesicles
MEMBRANE			
Myeloperoxidase (MPO)	Lysozyme	Gelatinase	Plasma proteins
Lysozyme	Phospholipase A_2	Lysozyme	
Cathepsins	Gelatinase	β_2-Microglobulin	
Elastase	Collagenase	Acetyltransferase	
Proteinase 3	Lactoferrin		
Azurocidin	TNF		
BPI	β_2-microglobulin		
Defensins	Histaminase		
iNOS	Heparinase		
α1-Antitrypsin	uPA		
α-Mannosidase			
sialidase			
Acid mucopolysaccharide			
β-Glycerophosphatase			
Elastase			
CYTOSOL			
CD63	Mac-1	Mac-1	Mac-1
CD68	SNAP proteins	SNAP proteins	SNAP proteins
	CD15	Cytochrome b558	Cytochrome b558
	CD66	fMLP R	CR1
	CD67	DAG-deacylating enzyme	CD14
	Cytochrome b558	uPA R	CD45
	Fibronectin R		fMLP R
	Laminin R		uPA R
	Vitronectin R		C1q R
	Thrombospondin R		
	fMLP R		
	uPA R		

BPI, bactericidal/permeability-increasing protein; CD, cluster of differentiation; CR1, complement component C3b; fMLP, N-formylmethionl-leucyl-phenylalanine; iNOS, inducible nitric oxide synthase; SNAP, synaptosomal-associated protein; R, receptor; TNF, tumor necrosis factor; uPA, urokinase-type plasminogen activator.
Modified from Faurschou M, Borregaard N. Neutrophil granules and secretory vesicles in inflammation. *Microbes Infect.* 2003;5:1317–1327.

generates hypochlorous acid from products generated by reduced nicotinamide adenine dinucleotide phosphate (NADPH) oxidase and also imparts the characteristic greenish color of pus.[9,27] Other major constituents include α-defensins, cytotoxic proteins that scaffold into transmembrane pores within the microbial cell wall and perturb the maintenance of vital transmembrane gradients, and bactericidal/permeability-increasing protein (BPI), which binds to gram-negative organisms and induces rearrangement of membrane lipids and inhibits growth.[27–30] Elastase cleaves constituents of the extracellular matrix, including proteoglycans, collagen (types I, III, IV), and fibronectin, and, of course, elastin.[31] Azurocidin is chemotactic for monocytes and stimulates LPS-induced release of IL-6 and TNFα from monocytes.[4,27]

The contents of specific granules, which are rich in antimicrobial substances, are released extracellularly (see Table 6.2).[26] Lactoferrin, by sequestering iron, retards bacterial growth and can bind bacterial cell membranes and induce irreversible membrane damage and lysis.[27] Phospholipase A_2 (PLA_2) participates in the degradation of bacterial membrane phospholipids. Lysozyme, present in all granules, is a cationic antimicrobial peptide that cleaves peptidoglycan polymers of bacterial cell walls. Other extracellular matrix degrading enzymes include gelatinase and collagenase.[27] These granules also possess receptors for a variety of extracellular matrix proteins and cell surface ligands, such as the β_2 integrin Mac-1 that mediates firm adhesion to the endothelium. In addition to the mechanical function of cellular anchorage, engagement of these receptors with their respective counterligands induces phenotypic alterations such as degranulation and enhanced ROS production.[4,27]

Gelatinase granules contain an eclectic array of mediators that contribute to many aspects of inflammation (see Table 6.2). They contain matrix metalloproteases, zymogens that on proteolytic activation degrade the interstitial matrix including collagens, fibronectin, proteoglycans, and laminin; this may facilitate neutrophil extravasation and migration. They are a source of cell surface adhesion molecules.[4,27,30]

Secretory vesicles contain many of the cell surface adhesion molecules operant during and essential for leukocyte recruitment. Their membranes are dense with the β_2 integrins LFA and Mac-1, the complement receptor CR1, the LPS receptor CD14, and the FcγRIII. Through fusion with the plasmalemma, the cell surface is enriched with these receptors, which facilitates firm neutrophil-endothelial engagement and the capacity to respond to a variety of stimuli.[4,27] Not surprisingly, because of the essential nature of leukocyte recruitment, secretory vesicles possess the lowest threshold for release, followed by gelatinase, specific, and azurophil granules (see Table 6.2).[27]

TABLE 6.3

MAJOR ROS AND THEIR METABOLISM

ROS molecule	Main sources	Enzymatic defense systems	Products
Superoxide ($O_2^{\bullet-}$)	Leakage from electron transport chain Activated phagocytes Xanthine oxidase Flavoenzymes	Superoxide dismutase Superoxide reductase	$H_2O_2 + O_2$ H_2O_2
Hydrogen peroxide (H_2O_2)	From $O_2^{\bullet-}$ via superoxide dismutase NADPH oxidase Glucose oxidase Xanthine oxidase	Glutathione peroxidase Catalase Peroxiredoxins	H_2O + GSSG $H_2O + O_2$ H_2O
Hydroxyl radical ($O_2^{\bullet-}$)	From ($O_2^{\bullet-}$) and H_2O_2 via transition metals		
Nitric oxide (NO)	Nitric oxide synthases	Glutathione/TrxR	GSNO

NADPH, nicotinamide adenine dinucleotide phosphate; ROS, reactive oxygen species; TrxR, thioredoxin.
Modified from Nordberg J, Arner E. Reactive oxygen species, antioxidants, and the mammalian thioredoxin system. *Free Radical Biol Med.* 2001;31:1287–1312.

Oxidative Burst and Oxidant Metabolites

The generation of toxic oxygen metabolites or ROS is the cardinal characteristic of the neutrophil but may also be produced by the monocyte/macrophage. Their essential antimicrobial properties are equally destructive to host tissues and implicated in the pathophysiology of many inflammatory disorders (Table 6.3).

A free radical is any species possessing one or more unpaired electrons; the valence is irrelevant. They are categorized under the broader term ROS, which encompasses all molecules capable of radical formation. Despite a very brief existence (10^{-11} to 10^{-6} seconds) extensive damage may occur through the induction of free radical chain reactions. Species operant during both physiologic and pathophysiologic inflammation includes the following: the superoxide anion ($O_2^{\bullet-}$), the hydroxyl radical (·OH), hydrogen peroxide (H_2O_2), and singlet oxygen, as well as the reactive nitrogen intermediates nitric oxide (NO) and peroxynitrite ($ONOO^-$) (see Table 6.3). In addition to their antimicrobial properties, ROS may modulate the immune response by activating inflammatory cells and inducing proinflammatory cytokine secretion.[32,33]

Implicit with the capacity for pathogen elimination, however, is the potential for destruction of host tissues. Hence, numerous regulatory mechanisms provide temporal and spatial control of the ROS production. The NADPH oxidase complex itself exists in a disassembled state, and only on cell activation and the need for ROS production are the subunits approximated and enzymatic function restored.[34] In addition, high plasma and tissue concentrations of antioxidants provide continuous surveillance and systemic control. However, such regulation is incomplete as evidenced by such diseases as rheumatoid arthritis, chronic obstructive pulmonary disease, and autoimmune vasculitis, which are the consequence of damage due to neutrophil-derived ROS.[34]

NADPH oxidase is a heteromeric complex composed of six subunits: flavocytochrome b558, the electron transporting apparatus, which is subdivided into gp91(phox) and p22(phox); the cytosoloic complex p40(phox), p47(phox), and p67(phox); and the oxidase factor rac-2 (Fig. 6.3).[34] Microorganisms or high concentrations of chemoattractants bind to cell surface receptors and initiate oxidase activation, heralded by phosphorylation of p47(phox). Cytochrome b558 (gp91 and p22), which exists within the plasmallema and the membranes of specific granules and secretory vesicles, is recruited by phagocytosis and granule fusion. Phosphorylation of p47(phox) induces a conformation change that enables its incorporation within the membrane, wherein it facilitates the translocation of rac2 and p67(phox) and stabilizes the association of this cytosolic complex with cytochrome b558, thereby rendering the complex functional.[34]

At the redox center of the oxidase, an electron is transferred from NADPH to oxygen, thereby generating superoxide:[35]

$$O_2 + e^- = O_2^{\bullet-}$$

Other mechanisms of superoxide production include uncoupling of the xanthine dehydrogenase system, uncoupling

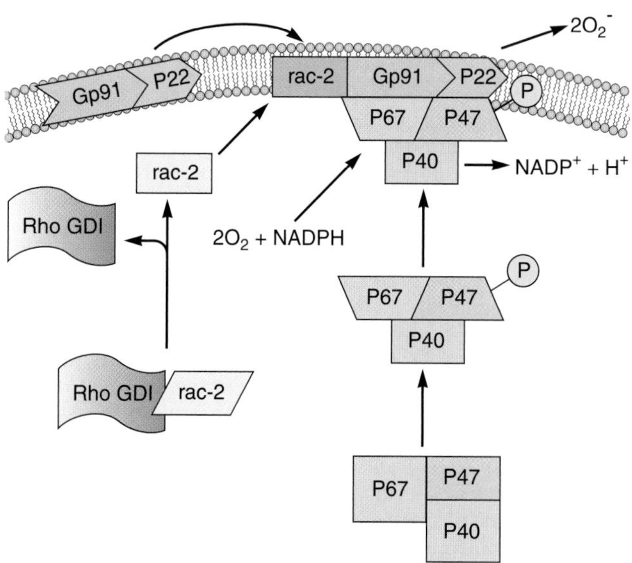

FIGURE 6.3 Reduced nicotinamide adenine dinucleotide phosphate (NADPH) oxidase assembly. In the resting neutrophil, the cytochrome subunits gp91 and p22 are tightly bound in the membrane. P47(phox), p67(phox) and rac-s complex are in the cytosol. On activation, GDI releases rac-2, and p47(phox) becomes phosphorylated. This causes translocation of rac-2, p47(phox), and p67(phox) to the membrane and complex formation with the cytochrome components, thereby completing the assembly of the active oxidase. (After Burg ND, Pillinger MH. *Clin Immunol.* 2001;1:7–17.)

of mitochondrial and endoplasmic reticulum electron transport chains, and nonenzymatic reactions such as autooxidation of hemoglobin.[36,37]

Superoxide is relatively weak and of low bactericidal potency. However, its membrane permeability and role as a reactant in reactions yielding highly toxic products confers on it high potential for cellular and tissue damage.[35]

Superoxide can spontaneously or enzymatically (superoxide dismutase) dismutate into hydrogen peroxide:[34,35]

$$2H^+ + O_2^{\bullet-} \Leftrightarrow H_2O_2 + O_2$$

It can also be converted to the more potent hydroxyl radical through the metal-catalyzed Haber-Weiss reaction:[34,35]

$$H_2O_2 + O_2^{\bullet-} + Fe^{3+} \Leftrightarrow O_2 + OH^- + \cdot OH + Fe^{2+}$$

or through the Fenton equation[34,35]

$$H_2O_2 + Fe^{2+} \Leftrightarrow Fe^{3+} + OH^- + \cdot OH + Hb\text{—}Fe^{2+} + H_2O_2 \Leftrightarrow Hb\text{—}Fe^{3+} + OH^- + \cdot OH$$

Under physiologic conditions, lactoferrin found in neutrophil specific granules provides the iron catalyst for the Haber-Weiss reaction. In the Fenton reaction, superoxide or other biologic reducing agents such as lactate or ascorbate donate electrons to generate the ferrous ions required to react with hydrogen peroxide to produce the hydroxyl radical.[34,35,38]

The hydroxyl anion is highly reactive and induces DNA strand breaks and base hydroxylations leading to adenosine triphosphate (ATP) depletion and gene mutations. It can attack lipid side chains of membrane phospholipids to form hydrogen peroxide and lipid hydroperoxides in a process called lipid peroxidation. These products can disrupt membrane function, serve as substrates for the production of cytotoxic aldehydes, or uncouple calcium-ATPase and increase cytosolic calcium concentration, thereby activating calcium-dependent proteases and phospholipases that propagate cellular damage.[38]

Superoxide can react with NO to produce peroxynitrite ($ONOO^-$) and hydroxyl radical:[35,39]

$$NO^\bullet + O_2^{\bullet-} \Leftrightarrow ONOO^- + H^+ \Leftrightarrow ONOOH \Leftrightarrow \cdot OH + NO_2^\bullet$$

The hemoprotein MPO yields the potently bactericidal hypochlorous acid (HOCl) from the reactants chloride and H_2O_2. HOCl oxidizes amino acids, nucleotides, and hemoproteins; can activate neutrophil collagenases and permit unabated elastase injury by inhibiting α1-antitrypsin; and contribute to hydroxyl radical and singlet oxygen production.[32,38,40] Though short-lived, subsequent reactions with secondary amines generate secondary chloramines, which are equally toxic but much more stable. These metabolites can oxidize similar cellular components. They can combine with halide anions to generate toxic free halides or with taurine chloramines that induces membrane attack complex (MAC) complement formation.[32,38,40]

In light of the pivotal role of MPO during inflammation and pathogen elimination, it is surprising that MPO deficiency is both common and relatively benign. Though MPO-deficient neutrophils show early depressed bacterial killing, bactericidal function normalizes within 60 minutes.[41] It is hypothesized that, although bacterial killing is impaired, postphagocytosis-oxidase-dependent neutrophil apoptosis is normal, resulting in appropriate regulation of the inflammatory response.[41]

Singlet oxygen, a highly reactive and extremely short-lived species, is formed by an input of energy to O_2 that reverses the spin direction of one of the outermost unpaired electrons away from a parallel spin. It is produced during reactions of the MPO-H_2O_2-halide system and is a potential product of superoxide dismutation and the Haber-Weiss reaction. It is highly electrophilic, reacting with compounds containing electron-rich double bonds and may react with membrane lipids to produce peroxides.[38]

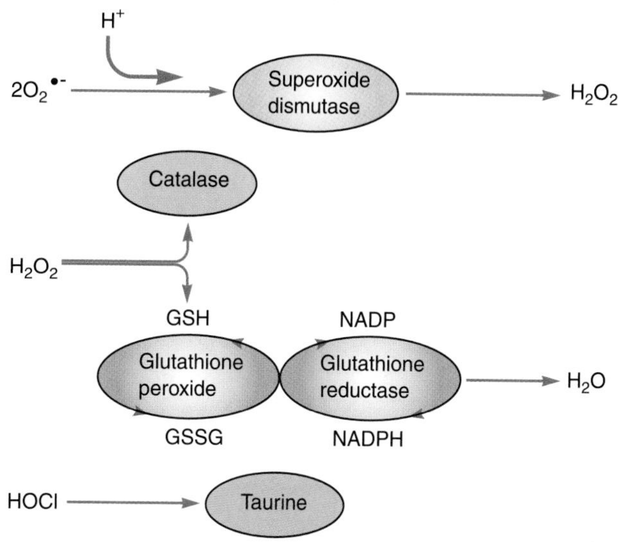

FIGURE 6.4 Scavengers of reactive oxygen species (ROS). (After Klebanoff SJ. In: Gallin JI, Snyderman R, eds. *Inflammation: basic principles and clinical correlates,* 3rd ed. Philadelphia: Lippincott Williams & Wilkins; 1999:723.)

The destructive potential of these ROS for both host and pathogen necessitates a mechanism of continuous tight spatial and temporal regulation. The oxidase complex itself exists spatially disaggregated; only on cellular activation are its constituents assembled and enzymatic function restored (see Fig. 6.3).[34,41] As elegant as is the mechanism to control ROS production, so too are the measures employed to eliminate these products when they are no longer needed. Superoxide, the proximal reactant necessary for many of the ROS generating reactions, is removed by both spontaneous and enzymatic (superoxide dismutase) dismutation to H_2O_2 (Fig. 6.4). H_2O_2 is subsequently reduced to oxygen and water by catalase.[35,38] In the extracellular environment, this function is performed by glutathione (GSH) peroxidase, a selenium-dependent enzyme that reduces H_2O_2 while oxidizing reduced GSH to its oxidized form. There is evidence that increasing GSH concentrations in monocytes and macrophages blocks ROS-mediated activation of NFκB and subsequent proinflammatory cytokine production.[38] Mechanisms of preventing hydroxyl radical-induced tissue damage include the binding of transition metal ions by albumin, ceruloplasmin, haptoglobin, lactoferrin, and transferrin.[32,35,38] Taurine is a scavenger for HOCl. Other antioxidants that may assist in controlling the reaction, include vitamins E (tocopherol) and C. Vitamin C has many antioxidant properties, including the ability to regenerate α-tocopherol. It can prevent activation of neutrophil-derived collagenase and is a powerful scavenger of HOCl, superoxide, singlet oxygen, and hydroxyl radicals. Carotenoids have long double bonds to attract and sequester free radicals. Uric acid is a powerful scavenger of water-soluble radicals such as HOCl and singlet oxygen. It can also bind copper and iron ions to suppress hydroxyl radical formation. Stress proteins or heat-shock proteins are induced by oxygen radicals and ischemia and may play a role in defense. Furthermore, heme oxygenase-1 (HO-1) catalyzes the cleavage of heme to

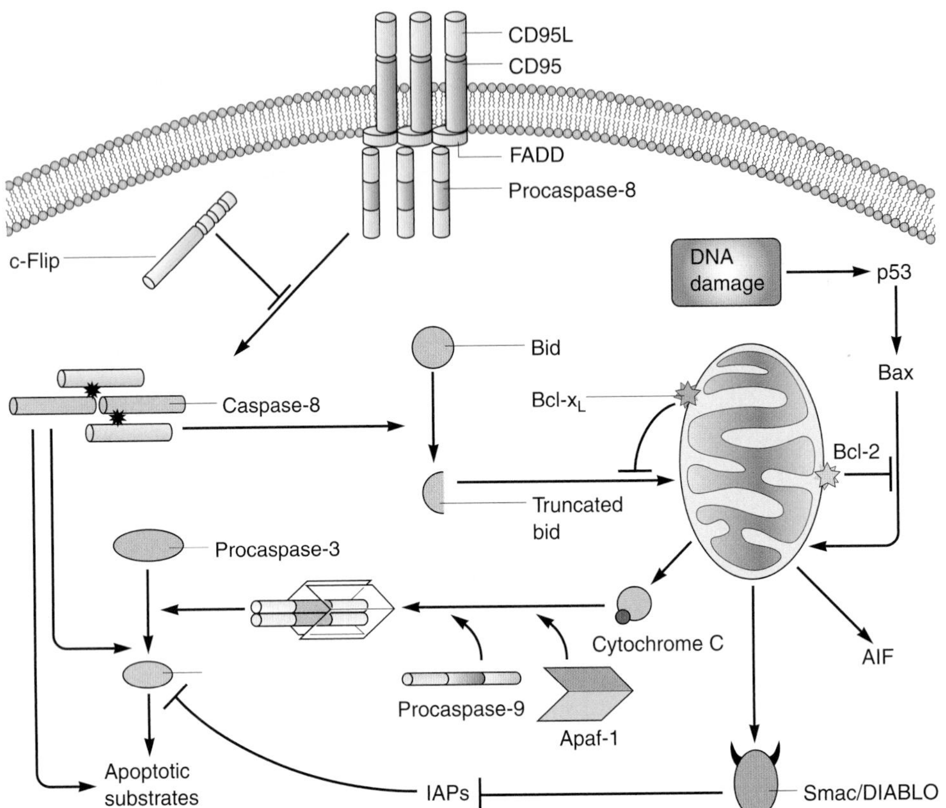

FIGURE 6.5 Apoptosis. CD95L binds CD95, induces receptor clustering and the formation of a death-inducing signaling complex. This complex recruits, through the adapter molecule Fas-associated death domain (FADD) protein, procaspase-8, resulting in caspase-8 activation; this event can be blocked by the caspase homologue c-FLIP. These diverse response pathways converge on mitochondria, often through the activation of a proapoptotic member of the Bcl-2 family. Unlike Bcl-2, which is primarily membrane-associated, Bax, Bad, Bim, and Bid, can shuttle between the cytosol and organelles. Proapoptotic signals redirect these proteins to the mitochondria. Proapoptotic and antiapoptotic Bcl-2 family members converge on the mitochondrium to compete to regulate cytochrome c exit. If the proapoptotic camp wins, an array of molecules is released from the mitochondrial compartment. Principal among these is cytochrome c, which associates with Apaf-1 and then procaspase-9 to form the apoptosome. The death receptor and mitochondrial pathways converge at the level of caspase-3 activation. Caspase-3 activity is antagonized by the IAP proteins, which themselves are antagonized by the Smac/DIABLO protein. Integration between the death receptor and mitochondrial pathways is provided by Bid, a proapoptotic Bcl-2 family member. Caspase-8-mediated cleavage of Bid greatly increases its pro-death activity and results in its translocation to mitochondria, where it promotes cytochrome c exit. (After Hengartner MO. *Nature* 2000;407:700–707.)

biliverdin, which is subsequently converted to bilirubin, an efficient free radical scavenger.[32,35,38]

All of the aforementioned participants of the NADPH oxidase are vital for health, as evidenced by those who suffer from chronic granulomatous disease.[34,41] These patients have deficient superoxide production and experience ineffective inflammatory reactions to infection. They commonly suffer from repeated bacterial infections (pneumonia, cutaneous abscesses and hepatic and perihepatic abscess, and osteomyelitis) by organisms that are catalase positive (*Staphylococcus aureus*). Organisms that produce large amounts of peroxide are less of a threat as the neutrophils can utilize bacterial peroxide to produce toxic metabolites. The use of prophylactic antibiotics and IFNγ has reduced the frequency of serious infections in this patient population.[34,41]

Regulation of Inflammation

In addition to the previously described mechanisms for controlling the inflammatory response of neutrophils, there is substantial evidence supporting the role of apoptosis in resolving the inflammatory response (Fig. 6.5; Appendix A at the end of this chapter).[42] The timely execution of a controlled cell death program in human polymorphonuclear leukocytes (PMNs) is essential for preventing damage to healthy tissues and for the resolution of inflammation. Within 90 minutes of phagocytosis, more than 250 genes are induced, of which more than 30 encode proteins integral to at least three distinct apoptotic pathways.[42] These observations suggest that the mechanism inducing apoptosis is initiated quite proximal in the inflammatory cascade and, in fact, just subsequent to phagocytosis. During some processes such as sepsis or trauma, neutrophil apoptosis appears to be delayed, which might contribute to a failure to resolve inflammation.

The inflammatory capacity of neutrophils is also transcriptionally regulated. Genes encoding proinflammatory mediators or signal transduction molecules such as receptors for IL-8, IL-10, IL-13 are down-regulated early after activation and decrease rapidly after the initiation of apoptosis.[42] In addition, regulating oxidative stress and ROS achieve high priority as the genes involved in GSH and thioredoxin metabolism and heme catabolism are up-regulated as is the production of reduced GSH.[42] Hence, activation-induced apoptosis in neutrophils stimulates self-directed regulation and facilitates removal of neutrophils by macrophages.

Mononuclear Phagocytes

Monocytes circulate for about 1 to 2 days; then they constitutively hone to a particular tissue to differentiate into macrophages possessing a phenotype specific to the resident tissue [e.g., dendritic cells (DCs), Kupffer cells] (see Table 6.1).[4,43,44] Resident macrophages are typically found at interfaces with blood (liver and spleen) and with lymph, where they can readily detect, ingest, and destroy invading organisms.[38] Mononuclear cells function as antigen presenting cells in T-cell-mediated adaptive immune responses, presenting antigen in the appropriate context to effector T cells. Their function is integral to both innate and adaptive immune responses.

Recruitment

Monocytes are recruited and emigrate to foci of inflammation utilizing similar mechanisms of adhesion and diapedesis as described for neutrophils (see Fig. 6.1). PAF, C5a, the CC chemokines, regulated on activation, normally T-cell expressed and secreted (RANTES), macrophage inflammatory protein (MIP)-1α, and chemokines of the membrane cofactor protein (MCP) family are potent monocyte-macrophage chemotaxins (Table 6.4).[45,46] The selectin family of adhesion receptors mediates the initial tethering of monocytes to endothelial cells.[18] Firm adhesion to the endothelium involves the interactions β_1 and β_2 integrins on monocytes with the endothelial adhesion molecules ICAM-1 and VCAM-1.[18]

TABLE 6.4

MONOCYTE/MACROPHAGE PRODUCTS

Product	Functions
Enzymes	Antimicrobial
Lysozyme	Plasminogen activation and fibrinolysis
Collagenase	Connective tissue degradation
Urokinase	Vasopressor
ACE	
Cytokines	
IL-1	Multiple
TNFα	Multiple
Interferon α/β	Antiviral, immune modulation
IL-6	Acute-phase response
IL-10	Antiinflammatory
IL-12, IL-18	Stimulate IFN γ production
IL-8	Neutrophil chemoattraction
FGF	Fibroblast growth
GM-CSF	Granulocyte, macrophage differentiation
MIP-1 α/β	Chemoattractant
MCP-1	Monocyte recruitment
RANTES	Monocyte/T_H cell recruitment
Complement proteins	Opsonization, complement activation
Coagulation factors	Coagulation
Adhesion, matrix molecules	Localization, migration
Fibronectin, proteoglycan	
Transport proteins	
Transferring	Iron transport
B_{12}-binding protein	Vitamin transport
Bioactive lipids	
Cyclooxygenase	Inflammation
Lipoxygenase	Inflammation
PAF	Platelet activation
Reactive oxygen intermediates	
Superoxide, hydrogen peroxide oxygen singlet	Antimicrobial
Reactive nitrogen intermediates	Antimicrobial
NO, nitrates, nitrites	
Defensins	Antibacterial

ACE, angiotensin-converting enzyme; FGF, fibroblast growth factor; GM-CSF, granulocyte/macrophage colony-stimulating factor; IFN, interferon; IL, interleukin; MCP, membrane cofactor protein; MIP, macrophage inflammatory protein; NK, natural killer, NO, nitric oxide; PAF, platelet activating factor; RANTES, regulated on activation, normally T-cell expressed and secreted; TNF, tumor necrosis factor. Modified from Gordon S. Development and distribution of mononuclear phagocytes: relevance to inflammation. In: Gallin JI, Snyderman R, eds. *Inflammation: basic principles and clinical correlates,* 3rd ed. Philadelphia: Lippincott Williams & Wilkins, 1999.

Phagocytosis

Phagocytosis involves both the IgG receptor (FcγR) and the receptor for the complement factor C3b. Terminal sugar patterns on microbial surfaces also allow recognition by macrophages for nonspecific phagocytosis.[22] However, phagosomal maturation differs from that which occurs in the neutrophil in that monocytes and macrophages have an endocytic pathway targeting the phagosome to a lysosome.[24] After endocytosis of a receptor-ligand complex, the contents of a vesicle are targeted to an early endosome, the ligand and receptor dissociate, and the receptor is recycled to the cell surface.[24] This early endosome undergoes a series of maturation steps in which it is acidified (pH 5.5 to 6.0). Ultimately, the endosome fuses with a lysosome, which is characterized by its extreme acidity (pH <5.0) and elevated concentration of proteases.[24] Lysosomes are the terminal destination of phagocytosed material to be degraded.

This acidification is requisite for optimal protease and hydrolase activity involved in pathogen killing. It may also be integral for phagosome maturation as titrating the acidity inhibits phagosome-lysosome fusion.[24]

After fusion, MPO released into phagosomes can react with hydrogen and halides to yield toxic hypohalous acids, superoxide anion, hydrogen peroxide, and hydroxyl radical (see Table 6.3). Macrophages may also use peroxidase generated by adjacent neutrophils, eosinophils, and monocytes and acquired through endocytosis to generate these ROS. In addition to supporting the inflammatory response, macrophages also play an important immunoregulatory role in inflammation by scavenging apoptotic neutrophils at sites of inflammation.[38]

Activation

IFNγ derived primarily from T cells is the primary activator of macrophages.[4,44,47] Optimal macrophage activation requires both IFNγ and a sensitizing agent, both of which can be provided by activated T lymphocytes. CD40 ligand on T cells can bind CD40 on macrophages to sensitize the cell. Alternatively, membrane-associated TNFα or lymphotoxin from lymphocytes can activate macrophage TNFα synthesis and thereby sensitize the macrophage to IFNγ.[38] IL-10 promotes monocyte maturation and macrophage differentiation.[48] Other activators include GM-CSF, IL-1, and LPS.

Activated monocytes and macrophages can produce approximately 100 different inflammatory products, including GM-CSF, M-CSF, G-CSF, IL-1, TNFα, and NO.[38,49] Mononuclear phagocytes are important sources of chemoattractants such as IL-8, PAF, and leukotriene B_4 (LTB_4) that recruit other neutrophils and leukocytes. The respiratory burst and subsequent production of toxic ROS mirrors that of neutrophils.

Antigen Presentation

T cells recognize only those antigens associated with surface major histocompatibility complex (MHC) molecules. MHC class I molecules are expressed on all nucleated cells, whereas MHC class II molecules are restricted to antigen-presenting cells (APCs). After phagocytosing pathogen, mononuclear cells process and display antigen to T cells and, in doing so, initiate the development of the adaptive response. There is evidence that the heat shock protein receptor CD91 may also participate in this process (vide infra). This processed antigen is presented in the context of MHC molecules on the APC surface that are specifically recognized by T-cell receptors and essential for T-cell activation. $CD4^+$ T cells, or helper T cells (T_H), recognize antigen coexpressed with MCH class II molecules and induce B-cell differentiation into either memory or antigen-specific antibody-producing plasma cells. These T_H cells can also induce macrophage production of NO, ROS, and other inflammatory mediators. $CD8^+$ cytotoxic T lymphocytes (CTLs) recognize antigen in the context of MHC class I molecules and induce target cell lysis; they destroy host cells infected with intracellular pathogens or cells of malignant potential.[50] Activated mononuclear phagocytes release IL-12, a potent stimulus for T_H cells and the production of inflammatory cytokines, and elaborate IL-15 that functions similar to IL-2.[51,52]

The three professional APCs are DCs, macrophages, and B cells. Dendritic cells are a specialized APCs, which process and present antigen to naïve T cells. Monocytes stimulated with GM-CSF and IL-4 or IL-13 differentiate toward DC. Maturation of the DC requires TNFα or LPS stimulation.[38] Epidermal Langerhans cells, once encountering antigen, migrate through the lymphoid organs and differentiate into mature DCs and acquire the capacity to provide the costimulatory signal. DCs are particularly effective at presenting viral antigen. They present antigen in the context of both MHC I and MHC II and thereby induce both a T_H1 and T_H2 response, respectively. DCs can also present antigens derived from apoptotic cells in the context of MHC class I.[53–55]

Macrophages present antigenic peptides from ingested pathogens that persist in the phagosomes. These peptides, usually of bacterial origin, are expressed in conjunction with MHC class II molecules. B cells, by contrast, bind specific soluble molecules (insect toxins, venom, and allergens) via immunoglobulin. This is endocytosed, processed, and presented with surface MHC II.[38,55–57]

Lymphocytes

B, T, and natural killer (NK) cells constitute this lineage of inflammatory cells (see Table 6.1). B and T cells are central to the adaptive immune response, whereas NK cells lack antigen specificity and primarily function during innate immune response. NK cells are the first line of defense against many viral infections; the loss of surface expression of MHC class I molecules on virus-infected cells serves as a target for NK cells.[38,58] Alternatively, NK cells bind cell-bound antibody and participate in antibody-dependent cell cytotoxicity. Cells targeted by either mechanism are induced to undergo cell death.

B Lymphocytes

B cells are of bone marrow origin, yet attain full maturation within extramedullary sites such as lymph nodes, the spleen, and the mucosal lymph nodules of tonsils and Peyer patches. With activation, B cells differentiate into antibody-producing plasma cells, which through the elaboration of antibody, aid the neutralization of viruses and bacterial toxins and facilitate opsonization for phagocytosis and complement activation.[4] Activation requires antigen binding to cell surface receptors and stimulation by T_H cell-derived cytokines; they do not need the assistance of APCs. Polyclonal B-cell activation can occur in a T-cell independent mechanism if the antigen has a large repeating polymeric sequence.[38,59]

T Lymphocytes

Development of T lymphocytes begins within the marrow and is completed in the thymus. The final population profile is determined by apoptotic processes of both positive and negative selection.[60] Any protein or antigen of host origin is presented by APCs, and thymocytes reactive to these self-proteins are deleted.[61] Alternatively, expansion of cell lines recognizing foreign, or rather non-self, antigen occurs through positive selection. IL-7 provides the stimulation for proliferation and differentiation of developing T cells. Ultimately, two lines of mature cells, $CD4^+$ and $CD8^+$, will develop.[62]

Lymphocytes, the smallest of the leukocytes, constitute approximately 20% of circulating leukocytes.[4] Most circulating lymphocytes are T cells, and 60% of those are $CD4^+$, a marker of a T_H phenotype. The other 40% are $CD8^+$, called cytotoxic T cells (T_C). The normal ratio of $CD4^+/CD8^+$ is 2:1.[4] Lymphocytes continuously recirculate through lymph nodes, spleen, lymphatics, lymph nodules, and blood, providing continuous surveillance. Encounter with a particular antigen initiates activation toward an effector T cell. Activation of a T cell requires specific antigen binding plus a costimulatory signal provided by the interaction between costimulatory molecules on the APC and their cognate receptors on the T cell.[38]

Naïve T cells circulate continuously between blood and lymphoid organs, making contact with many APCs and the epitopes of the antigens they express.[63] Initially, lymphocytes enter the cortical region of lymph nodes by migrating across the high endothelial venules, a process mediated by the selectin family of receptors. L-selectin, which is found constitutively on all lymphocytes, binds sialyl Lewis carbohydrate on the endothelium.[38] For example, L-selectin on lymphocytes binds GlyCAM-1 on the high endothelial venules in lymph nodes. In mucosal tissues, endothelial MAdCAM-1 guides L selectin-mediated emigration. Migration across the endothelium requires integrins, in particular LFA-1.[64] Binding of LFA-1 to ICAM-1 and ICAM-2 on endothelial cells facilitates migration. Most lymphocytes are carried back to the blood by the efferent lymphatics. If a T lymphocyte recognizes its specific antigen on the surface of an APC, it can remain for several days and then return to the blood as an armed effector T cell.[38]

Adhesion molecules mediate many of the transient interactions between T cells and APCs required for the T cell to sample each antigen it encounters. Lymphocyte LFA-1 can bind the APC in a loose, reversible fashion by any of the ICAM molecules on APCs. If a match between T cell and antigen is found, conformational changes in LFA-1 greatly increase its affinity for ICAM-1 and ICAM-2 to stabilize the interaction. The T cell can then proliferate and differentiate into an effector cell. Effector T cells lose surface expression of L-selectin and no longer circulate through lymphoid tissue. Instead they express VLA-4, an integrin, which binds vascular endothelium at sites of infection. Effector T cells also have increased LFA-1 and CD2 adhesion molecule expression that facilitate tight binding to target cells.[65,66]

Antigen binding in the appropriate context provides the signal for clonal expansion and differentiation of T cells into effector and memory lymphocytes. The appropriate contact comprises antigen complexed with MHC class II molecules on APCs, costimulators, and cytokines produced by the APCs and by the T cells themselves. This first encounter of naïve T cells with antigen is the primary immune response, which serves to induce the formation of effector and memory T cells. These activated T cells hone to peripheral tissues where, on reexposure to the antigen for which they are specific, they activate macrophages to eliminate phagocytosed microbes and induce B-cell differentiation and antigen-specific secretion. The $CD8^+$ CTLs kill infected host cells and tumor cells that display class I MHC associated antigen. Naïve T cells require activation by DCs, whereas effector T cells can respond to antigens presented by a wider variety of APCs, such as macrophages and B lymphocytes. Not surprisingly, differentiated effector and memory T cells possess lower thresholds for costimulation and require lower antigen concentration for activation than naïve T cells.

In general, antigen presented on MHC II molecules is the prototypical stimulus for $CD4^+$ T-cell activation and the subsequent production of a variety of cytokine mediators, including IL-2, which stimulate further expansion and activation. However, the circumstances under which this activation occurs may dictate disparate paths of differentiation, producing T-cell subsets with distinct cytokine profiles and effector functions. These differing phenotypes have been utilized to characterize two distinct subsets: T_H1 and T_H2.[51,52,67] IL-12 derived from phagocytes infected with intracellular pathogen provides the necessary signal for T_H1 differentiation.[38] IL-12 also stimulates production of IFNγ, the principle macrophage activator, by NK cells and $CD4^+$ lymphocytes. Interferons stimulate T_H1 development by augmenting phagocytic IL-12 production and by maintaining IL-12 receptor expression on $CD4^+$ T cells. The principal effector action of T_H1 cells is the activation of macrophages through the production of IFNγ, GM-CSF, TNFα, CD40L, and FasL.[38,51,52,67] They regulate production of opsonizing and complement fixing antibodies and are effectors of phagocyte-dependent responses. This inflammatory response is also referred to as cell mediated immunity or delayed-type hypersensitivity, provides one major arm of the adaptive immune response, and is mediated by $CD4^+$ and $CD8^+$ lymphocytes and macrophages.

The principal stimulus for T_H2 differentiation is IL-4, which is derived from T cells, mast cells, and basophils.[51,52,67] These cells are the cellular effectors of humoral immunity and provide the other major arm of the adaptive immune response, which is mediated by T_H2 $CD4^+$ cells, B cells, plasma cells, and antibodies. They produce IL-4, IL-5, and CD40L, thereby inducing B-cell activation and antibody production, and a host of other proinflammatory and antiinflammatory cytokines.[38] Activation of mast cells and eosinophils by extracellular pathogens is associated with activation of T_H2 cells. T_H2 cells quell the inflammatory response by inhibiting macrophage functions and T_H1 responses; they are considered the antiinflammatory arm of cell-mediated inflammation. Helper T cells that express both T_H1 and T_H2 patterns of cytokine expression have been called T_H0 cells and further studies will certainly discern other subsets of T cells.[4,67]

T-cell activation, differentiation, and expansion are orchestrated by the T cell itself. The responding T cell, in an autocrine fashion, serves as both source and target of a variety of mediators stimulating growth. The principal autocrine growth factor is IL-2. IL-15 stimulates the proliferation of $CD8^+$ T cells, especially memory cells of the $CD8^+$ subset. After antigen exposure, the numbers of T cells specific for that antigen may increase to about 1 in 10 for $CD8^+$ and 1 in 1,000 to 10,000 for $CD4^+$ cells.[4]

After activation, some proliferating cells will differentiate into effector cells that eliminate antigens and may activate other immune cells. Mature $CD4^+$ cells induce the activation of mononuclear phagocytes and B cells. $CD8^+$ cells differentiate into CTLs that recognize viral and other intracellular pathogen antigens that are presented in the context of MHC class I molecules and induce target cell death by releasing the cytotoxins perforin and granzymes from cytoplasmic granules. Granzymes are serine proteases that trigger DNA fragmentation and apoptosis. Perforin stimulates cell membrane pore formation that facilitates granzyme entrance into cells. Apoptosis can also be induced by the binding of Fas ligand on a CTL to fas on the target cell. CTLs also release the cytokines IFNγ, TNFα, and CC chemokines. IFNγ and certain CC chemokines have antiviral properties, and both are potent activators of macrophage function. IL-2 produced by CTL and local helper $CD4^+$ lymphocytes expands the CTL, and IL-12 released by the APC stimulates CTL activity. As with $CD4^+$ cells, early evidence suggests that the population $CD8^+$ may be divided into T_C1 and T_C2 cells based on their cytokine profiles and effector functions.[38,50–52]

Other T cells will mature into long-lived functionally quiescent memory cells. A cell surface rich in adhesion molecules such as integrins and CD44 facilitates rapid and efficient migration to peripheral sites of infection and inflammation upon antigen reexposure.[4] These cells accumulate over time and in the adult human comprise more than half of the circulating T cells.

As aforementioned, mere antigen exposure is insufficient for activation of naïve T cells; proliferation and differentiation require costimulatory signals provided by molecules on APCs. The best characterized costimulator pathway involves the T cell surface molecule CD28 and its counterligand B7-1 and B7-2 expressed on activated APCs.[4,38] CD28 delivers signals that enhance T-cell survival, by increasing expression of the anti-apoptotic protein Bcl-X, the production of cytokines such as IL-2 and the IL-2 receptor, and the differentiation of immature T cells. *In vitro*, purified populations of $CD4^+$ cells challenged with antigen by APCs that express B7 proliferate and secrete cytokines but not if B7 is absent. The costimulatory signal must come from the same APC that provides the initial signal. DCs are the most potent APC because they express both classes of MHC molecules and the B7 molecules. Macrophages and B cells must be activated to express the costimulatory molecules. This expression of costimulators is regulated so as to ensure that T-cell activation is temporally and spatially appropriate. For instance, during T-cell activation, engagement of CD40 ligand with CD40 induces up-regulation of B7 costimulators on the APCs. In addition it increases the secretion of cytokines such as IL-12 that promote T-cell differentiation and activation. A protein called CTLA-4 is homologous to CD28, binds B7-1 and B7-2, and is expressed on activated T cells. Unlike CD28, CTLA-4 functions to terminate T-cell responses and plays a role in self-tolerance. On the basis of many experimental studies of costimulators, antagonists against B7 molecules and CD40L are in clinical trials to prevent the rejection of organ allografts.[4,38]

The differentiation of naïve $CD8^+$ T cells to CTLs requires a stronger costimulatory signal. This can be provided by either DCs, as they have the greatest intrinsic costimulatory activity, or by a $CD4^+$ helper T lymphocyte. Naïve helper T cells attached to the same APC as the $CD8^+$ T cell can be activated to elaborate IL-2. Attached effector helper T cells can stimulate the APC to express more costimulatory molecules. In the case of virulent viruses, cytotoxicity substitutes for CD28 costimulation, and so the typical costimulatory signal is not required for activation. For less virulent viruses, costimulation is necessary for CTL induction.[38,68]

The absence of costimulation results in an unresponsive or anergic T cell. Anergic T cells do not produce IL-2 and therefore cannot proliferate and differentiate into effector cells even when presented with antigen at a later time.[38]

The affinity of most TCRs for peptide-MHC complexes is low, with dissociation constants on the order of 10^{-5} to 10^{-7} and an estimated TCR-antigen interaction of less than 10 seconds. Furthermore, on any APC, fewer than 1000 of the 10^5 available MHC molecules are likely to be displaying any one peptide at any particular time. Therefore, one APC can engage a small fraction of the 10^4 to 10^5 antigen receptors on a single T cell.[4] Activation of an individual T cell may require multiple sequential engagements of that cell's antigen receptors by peptide-MHC complexes on APCs. With engagement, there is clustering of membrane receptors, tyrosine phosphorylation of several proteins, and recruitment and activation of adaptor proteins. TCRs are devoid of enzymatic activity and must utilize other signal transducing proteins.[4]

After TCR-MHC engagement, several membrane surface proteins and intracellular signaling proteins are rapidly recruited, including the TCR complex, CD4 or CD8, receptors for costimulators such as CD28, and enzymes and adaptor proteins.[4] After TCR clustering, activated tyrosine kinases that are associated with the cytoplasmic domains of CD3 phosphorylate tyrosine residues on both CD3 and TCR (Fig. 6.6). These phosphorylation sites provide docking sites for other tyrosine and protein kinases, such as Lck, a Src family tyrosine kinase, and ZAP-70, a tyrosine kinase. These kinases become activated with phosphorylation. Activated ZAP-70 phosphorylates several adaptor proteins that subsequently induce a variety of signal transduction cascades. Adaptor proteins contain structural domains that bind other proteins and thereby facilitate the correct spatial orientation to promote the activation of signal transduction pathways. The ras pathway is also activated, which is an early step in the activation of the mitogen-activated protein kinases (MAPKs) that can activate a variety of transcription factors. Ras is a member of a family of guanine nucleotide-binding proteins (GDP/GTP) that is involved in diverse activation responses in different cell types. This pathway is an amplification process by which few upstream kinases

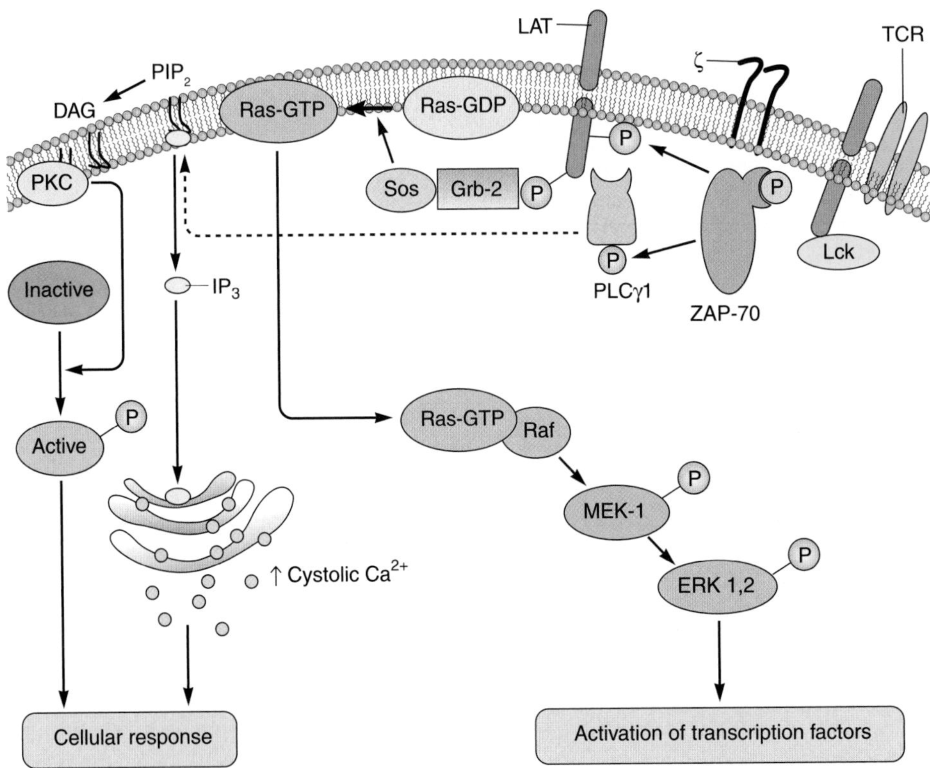

FIGURE 6.6 T-cell signaling and activation. (After Abbas AK, Lichtman AH. *Cellular and molecular immunology.* Philadelphia: Elsevier; 2003.)

TABLE 6.5

TRANSCRIPTION FACTORS

Transcription factor	Stimuli	Effector genes
AP-1	TNFα, IL-1, UV light, H_2O_2, LPS, stress, ROS, hypoxia	TNFα, IL-1, IL-2, IL-5, IFN-γ, ICAM-1, E-selectin, GM-CSF, MMPs, COX-2
NFκB	TNFα, IL-1, UV light, H_2O_2, LPS, ROS	IL-1, IL-2, IL-6, IL-8, IL-12, TNFα, E-selectin, VCAM-1, ICAM-1, MIP-1, MCP-1, RANTES, iNOS, eotaxin, PLA_2, G-CSF, GM-CSF, IFN-β
STAT	IFNs, CSFs, GFs, IL-1 to IL-15	FOS, E-selectin, Myc, ICAM-1, Fc γRI
NFAT	TCR, BCR, FcεR, FcγR, histamine and thrombin receptors	IL-2, IL-3, IL-4, IL-5, IL-8, IL-13, TNFα, GM-CSF, IFN-γ, CD40L, FASL

AP, activator protein; CSF, colony-stimulating factor; COX, cyclooxygenase; GF, growth factor; ICAM, intercellular adhesion molecule; IFN, interferon; IL, interleukin; iNOS, inducible nitric oxide synthase; LPS, lipopolysaccharide; MMP, matrix metalloproteinase; MPO, myeloperoxidase; NFAT, nuclear factor of activated T cells; NFκB, nuclear factor kappa-B; PLA_2, phospholipase A_2; ROS, reactive oxygen species; STAT, signal transducer and activator or transcription; TNF, tumor necrosis factor; UV, ultraviolet; VCAM, vascular cell adhesion molecule.
Modified from Gallin JI, Snyderman R, eds. *Inflammation: basic principles and clinical correlates,* 3rd ed. Philadelphia: Lippincott Williams & Wilkins, 1999.

lead to the activation of several downstream kinases. Ultimately activation of the terminal extracellular regulated kinase (ERK 1/2) leads to the phosphorylation of the protein ELK, which stimulates the transcription of fos, a component of the activation protein 1 (AP-1) transcription factor (Table 6.5; Appendix B). Concomitantly, c-Jun N-terminal kinase (JNK) is activated, which phosphorylates c-Jun, the second component of AP-1. The third member of the MAPK family, p38, is also activated. The activities of the MAPKs are terminated by specific protein tyrosine/threonine phosphatases that are regulated by the MAPKs themselves. Hence, the entire system is self-regulated by a negative feedback system.[4]

Activation of TCR also leads to the induction of phospholipase C (PLC), in particular PLCγ1 (see Fig. 6.6). Phosphorylated PLCγ1 catalyzes the hydrolysis of phosphatidylinositol 4,5-bisphosphate (PIP_2) into inositol 1,4,5-triphosphate (IP_3) and diacylglycerol (DAG) and activates enzymes that generate additional active transcription factors. IP_3 increases cytosolic free calcium that leads to a large increase in cytoplasmic calcium from both intracellular and extracellular sources with subsequent activation of calcium and calmodulin-dependent proteins. DAG activates protein kinase C (PKC), which activates additional transcription factors. The role of PKC and calcium in T-cell function is made evident by studies in which pharmacologic activation of PKC and or elevation of intracellular calcium concentration stimulates T-cell cytokine secretion and proliferation.[4]

Regulation of kinases operant in T-cell signaling involves protein tyrosine phosphatases. Through dephosphorylation they modulate TCR signaling. Two phosphatases induced with TCR clustering are SHP-1 and SHP-2. In contrast, calcineurin, a calcium/calmodulin-dependent phosphatase, is integral in T-cell activation through modulation of the transcription factors, nuclear factor of activated T cells (NFAT), and NF-κB (see Table 6.5).[4]

The ultimate goal of all these signaling transduction pathways is to activate nuclear transcription factors that bind to gene promoter regions and enhance transcription. Three transcription factors that are activated in T cells and appear critical for most T-cell responses are NFAT, AP-1, and NFκB (see Table 6.5).

A third mechanism of T-cell activation involves lipid antigens such as cell wall components from intracellular bacteria. These antigens bind CD1, a MHC-related cell surface molecule that presents these antigens to certain subtypes of T cells. Last, a superantigen is an unprocessed bacterial or retroviral product that binds the MHC molecule and the T-cell receptor outside the usual antigen-binding sites. This engagement leads to a polyclonal and nonspecific stimulation of a large proportion of the T-cell population. An overwhelming activation of all arms of the immune system ensues and underlies much of the pathophysiology of toxic shock syndrome. Intravenous gamma globulin, by binding and blocking this antigen, is thought to be of therapeutic benefit.

Eosinophils

Eosinophils are marrow-derived granulocytes that share some properties of neutrophils and are involved in the eradication of helminthic infections and allergen reaction (see Table 6.1). IL-3, GM-CSF, and IL-5 promote eosinophil differentiation, the induction of effector functions, and survival by inhibiting apoptosis.[69] They emigrate through inflamed endothelium and on exiting release inflammatory mediators and toxic agents from cytoplasmic granules. They generate superoxide anion and hydrogen peroxide, though less efficiently than neutrophils. Eosinophils act in conjunction with basophils and mast cells as primary effectors in allergy and inflammation. They express IgE receptors and stimulate histamine release from basophils and mast cells through major basic protein (MBP). They can also regulate basophil and mast cell function by releasing enzymes that inactivate histamine and slow-reacting substance of anaphylaxis (SRS-a). On exiting the marrow, their intravascular half-life is but a few hours, whereafter they enter the mucosa of the lung, gastrointestinal, and genitourinary tracts.[38,69]

Recruitment and Activation

Eosinophils are primarily recruited to sites of parasitic infection and allergen challenge. Mast cells and macrophages responding to either allergen or parasite secrete cytokines (IL-5, PAF, LTB-4) that up-regulate expression of endothelial adhesion molecules. Eosinophils themselves are more responsive to CC chemokines (MIP-1 α, RANTES, and MCP-3) and the cytokines produced with T_H2 activation. Engagement of the β_1 integrin VLA_4 of eosinophil with VCAM-1 and fibronectin on the endothelium initiates the process of emigration. IL-4 from T_H2 can activate both the binding and the up-regulation of endothelial cell VCAM-1. Diapedesis and tissue infiltration also involves members of the β_2 integrin family (Mac-1 and LFA) similar to that employed during neutrophil recruitment.[38,70]

Eosinophils are activated by IL-3, GM-CSF, IL-5, PAF, CC chemokines, and C3a and C5a of complement. IL-5 is a potent activating agent and enhances the ability of eosinophils to release granule contents on FcR cross-linking. A positive feedback cycle ultimately is established, in which recruited eosinophils produce cytokines and chemokines that recruit more eosinophils and other leukocytes.

Granules

Eosinophils possess a compartmentalized armamentarium of toxic substances to assist in the elimination of organisms, in particular helminths. Their specific granules contain GM-CSF and MBP, the latter of which is cytotoxic to parasites and normal cells and a stimulus for histamine release from mast cells and basophils.[71] The granule matrix contains eosinophil peroxidase (EPO), eosinophil-derived neurotoxin, lysosomal enzymes, catalase, TNFα, transforming growth factor β (TGF-β), and eosinophilic cationic proteins that stimulate formation of transmembrane pores to increase target cellular permeability.[72] EPO is released extracellularly on target cell surfaces where it generates hydrogen peroxide and hydrogen halides. Approximately 30% of oxygen consumed by stimulated eosinophils is utilized in the formation of halogenated species. Thiocyanate may be the major halide for the EPO-H_2O_2 system.[73] If ingested by a neighboring phagocyte, EPO can combine with H_2O_2 and halides to form hypohalous acids. EPO also stimulates neutrophil aggregation and adhesion to endothelial cells. Although they express Fc receptors for IgG, IgA, and IgE, they are relatively insensitive to activation by antigen-mediated cross-linking of these receptors. However, they can kill microorganisms by antibody-dependent cell-mediated cytotoxicity (ADCC).[4,38]

The primary targets of eosinophils are extracellular parasites. The size of these pathogens prohibits phagocytosis, and their integument is relatively resistant to the microbicidal products of neutrophils and macrophages; however, they can be killed by MBP, which is released after cross-linking of Fc bound IgE coating the parasite. The T_H2 response to parasitic invasion produces IL-4, IL-5, and IL-13. IL-4 stimulates the production of specific IgE antibodies, which opsonize helminths. IL-5 activates eosinophils, which bind to the IgE-coated helminths via Fc receptors. Activated eosinophils then release their granule contents and generate ROS and hypohalous acids. EPO also stimulates neutrophil aggregation and adhesion to endothelial cells. The sparse uncompartmental granules contain Charcot-Leyden crystals and have lysophospholipase activity. Finally, eosinophils produce and release lipid mediators such as PAF, prostaglandins, and leukotrienes, which contribute to the process of allergic diseases.[4,74,75]

Basophils and Mast Cells

Basophils and mast cells are central to the development of allergic inflammation and produce cytokines, lipid mediators, vasoactive amines, and proteases that participate in nonallergic inflammatory responses (see Table 6.1). Both cells share a common progenitor cell, which diverges early during differentiation. The primary growth factors for basophil development are IL-3 and GM-CSF, whereas stem cell factor is the primary stimulus for mast cell maturation.[76] Although basophils and mast cells are distinct cell types, they are often grouped together because of their similarity in granule content, activating stimuli, and effector functions.[38]

Mature basophils constitute only 0.5% to 1% of the circulating leukocytes, and mast cells primarily reside fixed in connective tissue. Engagement of IgE-bound antigen with the high-affinity IgE antibody receptor, FceR, provides the primary stimulus for basophil and mast cell activation and degranulation. In addition, diverse agents such as contrast media, opiates, anaphylatoxins, chemokines, and neuropeptides may serve as activators. Basophils and mast cells elaborate both preformed and newly synthesized inflammatory mediators. The main basophil proteoglycan is chondroitin sulfate A, whereas mast cells contain heparin, chondroitin sulfate, and chondroitin sulfate E and also store neutral proteases.[77] The lipid mediators LTB_4, LTC_4, and PGD_2 are synthesized de novo in response to stimulation. The leukotrienes are powerful vasoconstrictors, bronchoconstrictors, and chemoattractants for neutrophils and eosinophils. PGD_2 inhibits platelet aggregation and is chemotactic for neutrophils. Both basophils and mast cells synthesize and secrete histamine. Histamine, or 2-(4-imidazolyl)-ethylamine, is formed by the carboxylation of histidine. It is stored in preformed granules at acid pH as a complex with proteins and proteoglycans. Mast cells carry greater quantities of histamine than do basophils. The classic vasoactive properties of arteriolar dilatation, increased vascular permeability, and bronchoconstriction are mediated by the histamine H_1 receptors. H_2 receptors are involved in modulation of the immune response and stimulating gastric output and mucus secretion. H_3 receptors participate in neuroconduction.[38,77,78]

Platelets

Though classically considered in the context of hemostasis, platelets are integral to both normal and pathologic inflammation and link the processes of hemostasis, inflammation, and tissue repair. They are activated in a variety of inflammatory conditions, such as rheumatoid arthritis and inflammatory bowel disease, a testimony to their role in inflammation.[79] On activation, they release factors that enhance vascular permeability, chemokines, microbicidal proteins, and mitogens for endothelial cells, smooth muscle cells, and fibroblasts. They assist leukocytes in promoting the inflammatory reaction and killing microbes by providing an adhesive surface to facilitate emigration, by stimulating adhered leukocytes, and by further modulating chemokine synthesis (Table 6.6).[79,80]

Humans possess about 150 to 400 $\times$ 10^9 platelets per liter of blood.[79] Thrombopoiesis is regulated by thrombopoietin (TPO) as well as a variety of other peptides (IL-3, IL-4, IL-6, IL-7, and IL-11). In fact, human IL-11 is clinically used to stimulate thrombopoiesis in patients undergoing chemotherapy.[81] After release from the marrow, they circulate with a half-life of approximately 12 days. Interferon α is inhibitory for megakaryocyte growth, and the elevated levels induced with some viral and inflammatory conditions may explain the relative thrombocytopenia observed in these conditions.[79,82]

Recruitment and Activation

Platelets are activated and aggregate by exposure to thrombin or activated endothelium. Clot formation triggers the release of vasoactive agents [PGE_2, PGI_2, $PGF_{2\alpha}$, and platelet-derived growth factor (PDGF)] and inflammatory mediators. Serotonin, PGE_2, and PAF increase vascular permeability. The adhesion molecule PECAM-1 and the β_3 integrins mediate platelet plug formation, endothelial cell adhesion, and leukocyte emigration. The integrin IIb/IIIa and P-selectin facilitate platelet interactions with other inflammatory cells. The α granules are rich in membrane-bound P-selectin; on fusion with the cell surface membrane they markedly enhance the cell surface density of this receptor. On stimulation, both receptors are expressed on the platelet surface in an activated state. IIb/IIIa binds various adhesive proteins containing the RGD sequence (i.e., fibrinogen), which serve as a mechanical link to other platelets, leukocytes, and the endothelium. Possibly the

TABLE 6.6

PLATELET-DERIVED MEDIATORS

Chemoattractants
- C5a
- 12-HETE
- PAF
- α-granule proteins
- PDGF
- PF_4
- RANTES

Growth factors
- Transforming growth factors α and β
- Fibroblast growth factor
- PDGF

Antimicrobial activity
- Cationic bactericidal protein
- IgE-mediated oxidant production by platelets directed at schistosomes

Vascular reactions
- Prostaglandin E_2
- Prostaglandin I_2
- Prostaglandin $F_{2\alpha}$
- Serotonin
- PDGF
- Serotonin
- PAF
- Cationic proteins
- Vascular endothelial growth factor

HETE, hydroxyeicosatetraenoic acid; PAF, platelet activating factor; PDGF, platelet-derived growth factor; PF_4, platelet factor 4; RANTES, regulated on activation, normal T cell expressed and secreted. Klinger MHF, Jelkmann W. Role of blood platelet in infection and inflammation. *J Interferon Cytokine Res.* 2002;22:913–922.

immobilization on the vessel wall of activated platelets with induced P-selectin biochemically and functionally promotes the adhesion of neutrophils to endothelial cells.[79,82]

Platelets are a primary source of chemoattractants for neutrophils. Neutral proteinases released from stimulated platelets cleave complement factor C5, liberating the chemoattractant C5a. PDGF binds strongly to the extracellular matrix, providing a long-acting source of chemoattractant. Platelet factor 4 (PF_4) is a cationic protein that penetrates the vascular wall and is a chemoattractant. Activated platelets also bind monocytes via P-selectin and PSGL-1 and induce the expression and secretion of monocyte chemotactic protein-1 (MCP-1) and IL-8. Thrombospondin released from activated platelets mediates monocyte binding to platelets. Together these substances promote leukocyte margination, activation, and recruitment to the sites of injury.[38]

Granules

The vasoactive substances and inflammatory mediators of platelets are either stored in cytoplasmic granules or synthesized de novo. A platelet contains about 35 α granules and 5 dense bodies. The dense granules contain adenosine diphosphate (ADP), ATP, serotonin, and calcium, mediators operant during the initial phase of inflammation. ADP is the principal platelet agonist during platelet aggregation and augments the oxidative burst of neutrophils. Serotonin increases vascular permeability and enhances the superoxide production by macrophages.[79]

The more abundant α granules contain fibrinogen, RANTES, MIP-1α, thrombospondin, P-selectin, PF_4, PDGF, TGF-β, β-thromboglobulin, high-molecular-weight kininogen (HMWK), and many other biologically active proteins. PF_4 and β-thromboglobulin initiate leukocyte recruitment and activation. PF_4 induces neutrophil adherence to unstimulated endothelium and the release of secondary granules, whereas it inhibits monocyte apoptosis and promotes macrophage differentiation. PF_4 can also stimulate histamine release from basophils. RANTES is deposited on the endothelium and recruits monocytes from the circulation. MIP-1α is chemotactic for $CD8^+$ T lymphocytes. PAF induces platelet aggregation, increases vascular permeability, and enhances phagocyte free radical formation and the adhesion of platelets to neutrophils. Platelet activation appears to occur in allergic asthma and may precede the delayed accumulation of eosinophils in the lung after allergen exposure. The α granules also carry several important growth factors, including vascular endothelial growth factor (VEGF), PDGF, and TGF-β. VEGF promotes extravasation and aids recruitment of leukocytes. PDGF is chemotactic for neutrophils and monocytes. TGF-β is chemotactic for and activates neutrophils and monocytes early during inflammation but displays immunosuppressive effects during later stages of inflammation.[79]

Platelets are an important source of eicosanoids, including thromboxane and $PGF_{2\alpha}$ and PGE_2. Thromboxane synthetase in platelets is responsible for the production of TXA_2, a potent vasoconstrictor that also increases vascular permeability and stimulates platelet aggregation. Aspirin and other nonsteroidal antiinflammatory drugs (NSAIDs) inhibit platelet function by inhibiting TXA_2 production. As this effect is irreversible, new platelets must be produced (7 to 10 days) to restore normal clot formation. $PGF_{2\alpha}$ causes vasoconstriction, whereas PGE_2 vasodilates and modulates pain.[83,84]

Platelets participate in transcellular lipoxygenase (LO) metabolism, which refers to the production of eicosanoids through interactions with neighboring inflammatory cells. Endothelial cells utilize platelet-derived endoperoxides to synthesize PGI_2. Platelets interact with neutrophils in several pathways, providing a direct link between thrombosis and inflammation. 12-hydroxyeicosatetraenoic acid (HETE) released from activated platelets can be used by unstimulated neutrophils to produce the chemoattractant 12,20-HETE. 12-HETE and 5-HETE from activated platelets and neutrophils, respectively, can combine in either cell type to form 5,12 diHETE, an antiinflammatory compound, which diverts production away from the proinflammatory leukotrienes. 12-LO from platelets and LTA_4 formed by neutrophils can produce the intermediate 5(6)-epoxytetraene. This intermediate produces lipoxins A_4 and B_4 that have primarily counterinflammatory functions.[38,80,83,85]

In addition to modulating inflammation, platelets possess some direct microbicidal activity. Platelets are activated and degranulate when exposed to certain bacteria. Electron microscopic studies have shown that activated platelets internalize bacteria and viruses. The α granules contain antibacterial proteins called thrombocytins (TCs) in humans that support the killing of adherent bacteria. The two antibacterial proteins isolated from human platelets (TC-1, TC-2) are bactericidal for *Escherichia coli* and *S. aureus*.[79]

NONCELLULAR COMPONENTS

Cytokines

Cytokines are soluble protein mediators secreted by the cells of the innate and adaptive immunity in response to microbes and other antigens and mediate many of the functions of these cells (Table 6.7). They influence the host response to both acute and

TABLE 6.7

CYTOKINES

Cytokine	Receptor	Signal transduction	Cellular source	Targets	Effects
INNATE/EARLY CYTOKINES					
TNFα	TNF R	TRAFS Death domains	Mo/Mϕ, MC, Ba, Eo, NK, B, T, F, Ep	EC PMN Many cells	↑ inflammation, coagulation, adhesion molecules ↑ activation ↑ apoptosis ↑ fever, APP, catabolism
IL-1	Ig family	IRAK	Mo/Mϕ, B, EC, Ep, F	EC PMN Mo	↑ inflammation, coagulation, adhesion molecules ↑ activation and emigration ↑ activation and emigration ↑ shock, fever, APP production
Chemokines/ IL-8	7 transmembrane	G protein	Mo/Mϕ, T, PMN, F, EC, Ep	PMN T Mo/Mϕ EC Ba	↑ activation, adherence, and migration ↑ emigration ↑ emigration ↑ adhesion molecules ↑ histamine release
IL-12	Type I	JAK/STAT	Mϕ	T NK	T_H1 differentiation, interferon γ synthesis, ↑ cytolytic activity
Interferons (Type I)	Type II	JAK/STAT	All	All	Antiviral, antitumor, increases MHC I Activates T, Mϕ, NK cells
IL-10	Type II	JAK/STAT	Mo/Mϕ, T, B, MC	Mo/Mϕ T B, NK, MC	↓ IL-12, costimulators, MHC II ↓ T_H1 differentiation
IL-6	Type I	JAK/STAT	Mo/Mϕ, B, F, EC, Ep	T B Mo/Mϕ E	Differentiation ↑ antibody-producing cells APP synthesis
IL-15	Type I	JAK/STAT	Mϕ	NK T	Proliferation Proliferation
IL-18	Ig family	IRAK	Mϕ	T, NK	↑ interferon γ
ADAPTIVE/LATE CYTOKINES					
IL-2	Type I	JAK/STAT	T	T B NK	T activation and proliferation, Fas apoptosis ↑ proliferation, antibody synthesis ↑ proliferation and activation Mo/Mϕ activation
IL-4	Type I	JAK/STAT	T, Ba, MC	T B Mo/Mϕ	T_H2 differentiation and proliferation, ↓ Th1 Isotype switching to IgE ↓ interferon-γ–mediated function
IL-5	Type I	JAK/STAT			
Interferon γ	Type II	JAK/STAT	T, NK	Mϕ T B	Mϕ activation T_H1 differentiation IgG secretion ↑ MHC I and II ↑ antiviral ↑ fever, anorexia, shock, capillary leak ↑ APP synthesis, inflammatory cytokine induction
TGF-β			All	T Mϕ B	↓ T proliferation and effector functions ↓ Mϕ function ↓ proliferation ↑ matrix protein synthesis
Lymphotoxin	TNF R	TRAFS Death domains	T	PMN	Recruitment and activation
IL-13	Type I	JAK/STAT	T	Mo/Mϕ B EC	↓ Mϕ function, switching to isotype IgE ↑ adhesion molecules and CC chemokines

APP, acute-phase proteins; B, B cell; Ba, basophils; EC, endothelial cell; Ep, epithelial cell; F, fibroblast; IL, interleukin; IRAK, IL-1R-associated kinase; JAK/STAT, janus kinase/signal transducer and activator of transcription; MC, mast cells; MHC, major histocompatability complex; Mo, monocyte; Mϕ, macrophage; NK, natural killer; PMN, polymorphonuclear leukocyte; T, T cell; TNF, tumor necrosis factor; TRAF, tumor necrosis factor receptor-associated factor.
Modified from Abbas AK, Lichtman AH. *Cellular and molecular immunology,* 5th ed. Philadelphia: Elsevier; 2003:79, 181–182.

chronic bacterial, viral, fungal, and parasitic infections; trauma; burns; allograft rejection; ischemia/reperfusion injury; and autoimmune disease. They govern lymphocyte differentiation during adaptive immunity and activate effector cells of both arms of inflammation to eliminate microbes. Cytokines play important roles in tumor biology as well as in angiogenesis. Though essential for a normal immune response, excessive cytokine release underlies a variety of pathophysiologic inflammatory states such as ARDS and MODS.[86–89]

Cytokine secretion is brief and, because cytokines typically are not stored preformed, necessitates transcription and de novo synthesis, which is also transient as the messenger RNA is unstable. Their functions are pleiotropic and redundant, which has been interpreted as a teleologic safety mechanism. However, such protective characteristics greatly limit the therapeutic utility of either cytokine administration or blockade, respectively. Cytokines often influence the synthesis and actions of other cytokines, such as IL-1-induced T-cell IL-2 production; this interaction may be synergistic (additive or multiplicative) or antagonistic. They may function in an autocrine, paracrine, or even endocrine function, although the inability to correlate plasma cytokine concentrations with the extent of tissue damage suggests that they are designed for local rather than systemic inflammation.[4,38,86]

Their actions are mediated by specific membrane receptors on target cells to which they bind with high affinity (Kd α 10^{-10} to 10^{-12}); hence, only minute quantities are necessary to elicit a response. Such efficiency is accompanied by a narrow therapeutic index and potential for unwanted global effects (i.e., MODS) with even small systemic concentrations. The receptors and the cells expressing them are regulated by external stimuli, which provides some degree of specificity to the response even though the cytokines themselves are not antigen-specific. Receptor binding alters cellular gene transcription (induction or suppression) that may result in proliferation, differentiation, and the acquisition of new or suppression/enhancement of preexisting functions.[4]

All cytokine receptors consist of at least one transmembrane protein with an extracellular portion for ligand binding and an intracellular domain mediating signal transaction. Current receptor classification is based on structural homologies among the extracellular cytokine binding domains. Type I cytokine receptors contain a domain with two conserved pairs of cysteine residues and a membrane proximal sequence of tryptophan-serine-X-tryptophan-serine where X is any amino acid (WSXWS). Type II resemble type I receptors, however the WSXWS motif is absent. The Ig superfamily consists of receptors with extracellular Ig domains. TNF receptors belong to a family of receptors with conserved cysteine-rich extracellular domains. Finally seven-transmembrane α-helical receptors mediate the functions of cytokines called chemokines through GTP-binding (G) proteins.[4]

Translating ligand engagement to the signaling events that alter cellular phenotype involves a variety of signaling cascades dependent on the structure of the cytoplasmic tail of the particular receptor (see Table 6.7). This is another method by which to classify cytokine receptors. These individual signaling cascades are discussed in the context of the various cytokines and respective receptors employing them.

Early Cytokines/Innate Immunity

Tumor Necrosis Factor Alpha. TNFα is the principal mediator of the inflammatory response to gram-negative bacteria and other infectious pathogens. It is an important early mediator of inflammation and is essential for the normal initiation, maintenance, and repair of tissue injury. However, aberrant production may underlie the pathologic sequelae of many inflammatory and infectious states (i.e., MODS). Mononuclear phagocytes are the principle source of TNFα, usually in response to the potent prototypical stimulus LPS.[90,91] LPS-induced TNFα production may be augmented by concomitant stimulation with IFNγ, IL-4, and IL-10, whereas, corticosteroids are suppressive.[92] Secondary sources include mast cells, NK cells, and T and B lymphocytes, and stimuli include complement C5a, GM-CSF, hypoxia, IL-1, NO, ROS, and TNFα itself.[38]

Shedding of extracellular domains of the two TNFα receptors by metalloproteinases can further alter the biologic activity of TNFα by decreasing the number of cell signaling sites on target tissues and increasing the amount of circulating receptors acting as inhibitors. Unlike other members of the TNF family that are primarily involved in regulation of cell proliferation, TNFα has both proinflammatory and apoptosis-inducing properties.[86,93]

TNFα is expressed on the cell membrane as a bioactive protein and is cleaved into its soluble form by a specific TNFα converting enzyme. There are two distinct TNF receptors present on virtually all cell types (Fig. 6.7).[94] Ligand binding to TNF-RII leads to recruitment of TNF receptor-associated factors (TRAFs) that ultimately activate the transcription factors NFK B and AP-1 and thereby influence gene expression and cellular phenotype.[4] Alternatively, binding to TNF-RI activates caspases and triggers apoptosis, in addition to signaling transcription factors. The manner by which either a proinflammatory or an apoptotic path is chosen is unknown, although the net effect of TNFα binding is probably the culmination of differential adaptor protein expression and downstream signal transduction cascades. TNF-R1 appears to be more important in host defense as knockout TNF-RII mice show a greater degree of impairment in host defense than mice lacking TNF-RI.[4]

The principal function of TNFα is to recruit neutrophils and monocytes to foci of infection and to activate these cells to eradicate microbes. TNFα activates the endothelium to up-regulate the expression of the adhesion molecules E- and P- selectin, ICAM-1, PECAM-1, and VCAM-1 and stimulates these cells and macrophages to secret chemokines (IL-8, MIP-1α, and Gro-α) that enhance the affinity of leukocyte integrins for their ligands and induce leukocyte chemotaxis and recruitment.[95] TNFα induces a state of hypercoagulability by stimulating the release of tissue factor, PAF, von Willebrand factor, and thromboplastin. By inhibiting tissue-type plasminogen activator and thrombomodulin, it suppresses fibrinolysis, decreases protein C and S activation, and increases thrombin formation. However, TNFα also induces the release of a variety of anticoagulants (prostacyclin), fibrinolytics (urokinase-type plasminogen activator), and vasodilators (NO, PGE_2), which may balance the tendency toward a procoagulant state. Most likely, the ultimate effect of TNFα depends on the location and quantity in which it is produced and the vascular bed with which it interacts.[4,86]

In severe infections, exuberant production and aberrant release of TNFα enables it to function as an endocrine hormone and cause a plethora of pathologic sequelae. These systemic effects include fever, acute-phase protein production by the liver, cachexia (due to inhibition of hunger and increased lipoprotein lipase activity), inhibition of myocardial contractility and vascular tonus, and intravascular thrombosis due to loss of normal anticoagulant properties of the endothelium and the production of tissue factor. TNFα is central to the pathogenesis of systemic inflammatory response syndrome (SIRS) and septic shock, and either state can be reproduced by administration of LPS or TNFα.[96–98] The organ dysfunction characteristic of either state may result from the hypercoagulability and subsequent tissue ischemia induced by this cytokine. Antagonists of TNFα can prevent mortality in experimental models, but clinical trials with anti-TNFα antibodies or with soluble TNFα receptors have been to no avail.[4,96]

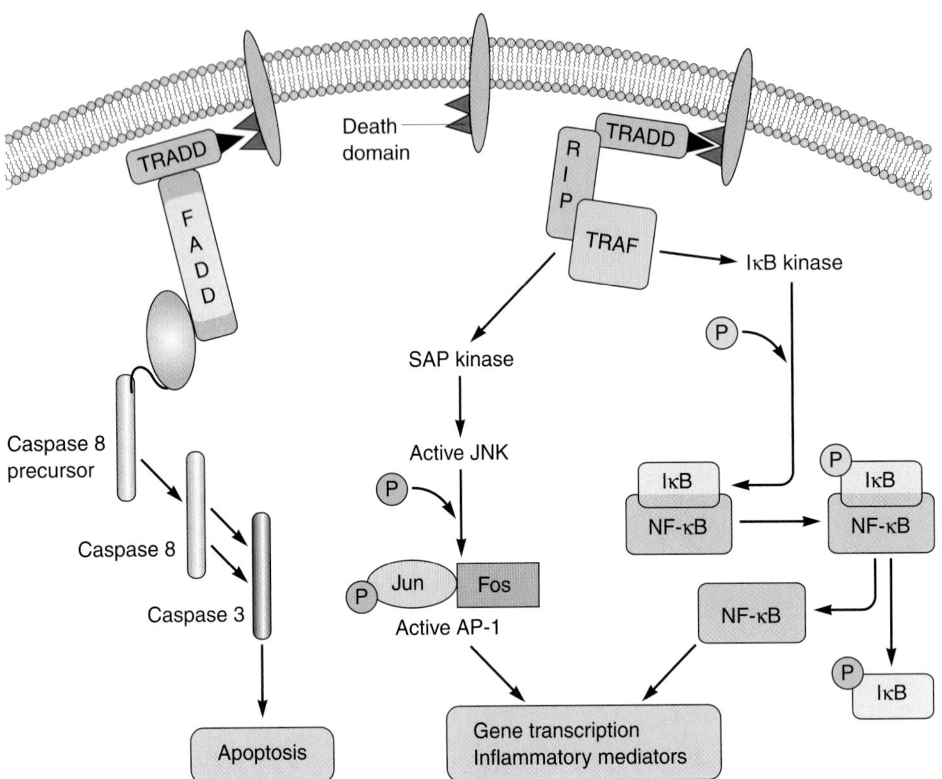

FIGURE 6.7 Tumor necrosis factor (TNF) receptor signaling pathway. (After Abbas AK, Lichtman AH. *Cellular and molecular immunology.* Philadelphia: Elsevier; 2003.)

Soluble TNF receptors formed by proteolytic processing of both types of receptors bind and neutralize TNFα and serve as an endogenous regulator of cytokine activity.[38] Also, TNFα directly induces the expression and release of TNFα inhibitors, including IL-10, corticosteroids, and prostanoids, which in a negative feedback loop suppress TNFα production and processing.[86] Hence, TNFα serves as its own regulator.

Interleukin 1. Interleukin 1 functions similarly to TNFα in mediating a proinflammatory host response to insult and is frequently released concomitantly with TNFα (see Table 6.7).[99] The major source of IL-1 is the mononuclear phagocyte. Synthesis and release are induced by LPS, cytokines (TNFα, IL-2, TGF-β, all the interferons), antigen-antibody complexes, C5, and hypoxia.[86] IL-1 is also produced by neutrophils, B cells, helper T cells, epithelial cells, fibroblast, renal mesangial cells, and endothelial cells.

There are two forms of IL-1, IL-1a and IL-1β. Both forms are active, bind to the same receptors, and mediate the same effects. Most IL-1 found in circulation is IL-1β.[4]

The two IL-1 receptors (IL-1R) are members of the Ig superfamily. IL-1RI is universally expressed and transduces the majority of IL-1 responses.[100,101] IL-1RII expression is restricted to B cells but may be induced on other cells. There is little evidence that this latter receptor serves any function and, in fact, may serve as a decoy.[102] The cytoplasmic portion of IL-1RI is homologous to a domain of Toll-like receptors (TLR), which mediate the cellular response to endotoxin (Fig. 6.8). Engagement of IL-1 with IL-1RI induces the activation of the IL-1 receptor-associated kinase (IRAK) and the subsequent induction of the transcription factors NF-κB and AP-1.[4,101]

The functions of IL-1 mirror those of TNFα, and synergy between the two cytokines is evident.[99] IL-1 activates endothelial cells to increase cell surface expression of adhesion molecules and the production of prostaglandins, PAF, and a variety of colony-stimulating factors (CSFs). In doing so, it facilitates the recruitment and activation of appropriate leukocyte populations for specific localized immune responses. IL-1 also induces a procoagulant state by suppressing fibrinolysis through enhanced plasminogen activator inhibitor-1 and decreased tissue-type plasminogen activator activity and increasing thrombosis by stimulating tissue-factor-like procoagulant and thromboplastin production and suppressing thrombomodulin release. It induces the synthesis of PAF, a potent vasoconstrictor and stimulus for platelet and leukocyte activation. However, similar to TNFα, it also stimulates the production of prostacyclin and urokinase-type plasminogen activator, which promotes an antithrombotic state.[103] At larger concentrations, its effects become systemic causing fever (hence the name endogenous pyrogen) by stimulating the production of PGE_2 by the hypothalamus, the synthesis of acute-phase proteins, cachexia, myalgia, somnolence, and hypotension. It stimulates arachidonic acid and prostaglandin metabolism and the release of pituitary stress hormones. It stimulates collagenase release and is a potent mitogen for neutrophils. Though similar in effect to TNFα, probably by activating similar signaling cascades and transcription factors, IL-1 does not induce apoptosis, and even at high concentrations does not cause the physiologic derangements of septic shock.[38,99]

Mononuclear cells produce the natural inhibitor of IL-1, IL-1ra. This IL-1 structural homologue is an inactive competitive inhibitor and may function as an endogenous regulator of IL-1. As with TNFα, attempts to inhibit IL-1 have not been of clinical benefit in human trials of sepsis.[38]

Chemokines. This is a large family of cytokines that primarily govern leukocyte chemotaxis, hence the name[104–108] (see Table 6.7). Those bound on the endothelial surface induce leukocyte integrins to express a high affinity state for their ligands, which is critical for tight leukocyte adherence and subsequent migration into the extravascular space. However, they are also constitutively produced and assist in orchestrating the migration of immune cells into lymphoid organs. Unlike other chemoattractants, members of this family possess

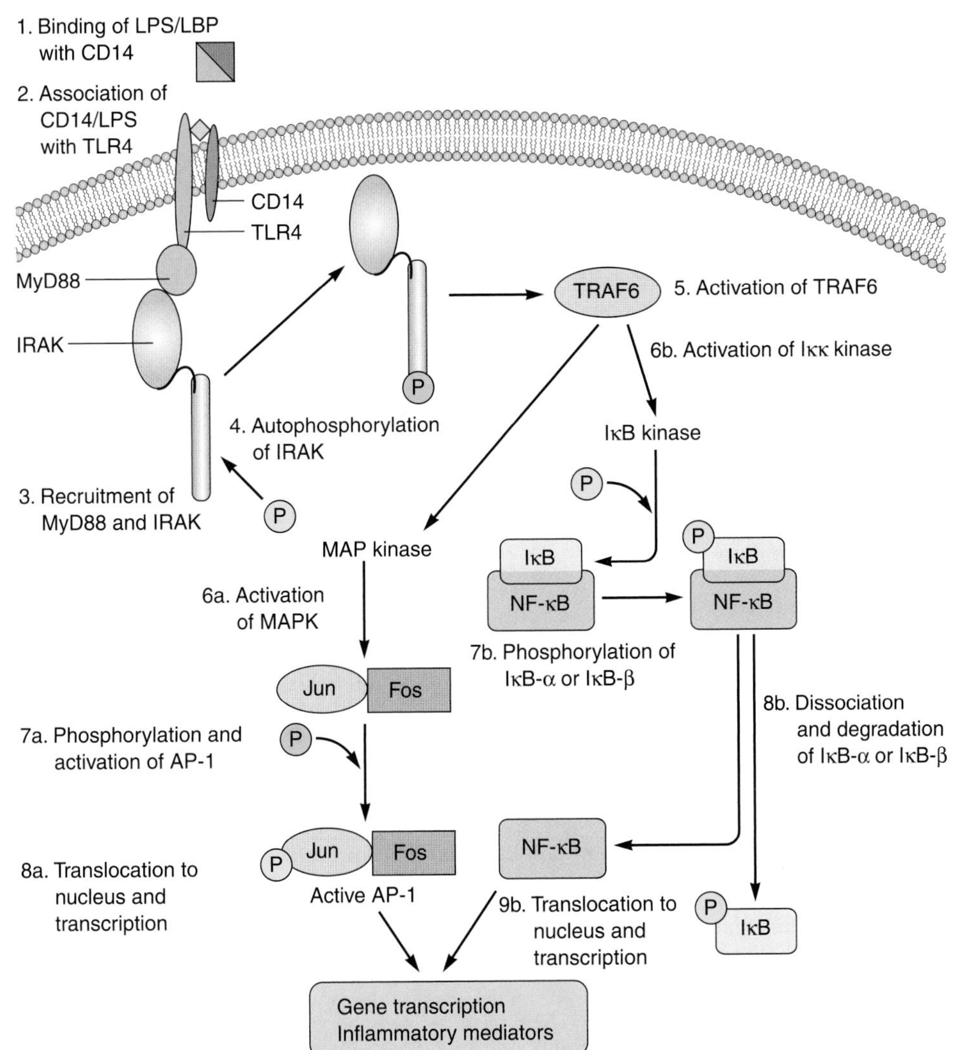

FIGURE 6.8 Toll-like receptor (TLR) signaling pathway. (After Abbas AK, Lichtman AH. *Cellular and molecular immunology*. Philadelphia: Elsevier; 2003.)

a degree of specificity, influencing the recruitment of discrete subsets of leukocytes. They mediate their effects both directly as well as indirectly through the induction of other mediators such as histamine and ROS. Though some chemokines, in particular those regulating cell traffic through tissues, are constitutively produced (MIP-3β and RANTES), most necessitate cellular stimulation for synthesis and release, in particular those involved in inflammatory reactions. They are typically produced by macrophages; leukocytes; endothelial cells; fibroblasts; and many other cell types stimulated by LPS, phagocytosis, and inflammatory cytokines such as IL-1, TNFα, IL-6, and IFNγ.[38]

Chemokines can be classified into four families based on the number and location of N-terminal cysteine residues. The two major families are the CC chemokines, in which the cysteine residues are adjacent, and the CXC chemokines, in which one amino acid is interposed between these cysteine residues. This amino acid sequence appears to account for the disparate influence, either promotion or inhibition, on neutrophil chemotaxis. The three amino acids that immediately precede the first cysteine are critical in defining receptor binding and neutrophil activation.[109,110] This area has been designated the ELR motif. The other two chemokine families are represented by lymphotactin (C chemokine) and fractalkine (CX3C chemokine).[38]

Chemokine receptors are seven transmembrane receptors that signal by G proteins and the formation of the second messengers, IP_3 and DAG (see Fig. 6.6). Currently 6 CXC chemokine receptors, 11 CC, and 1 receptor each for the last two subfamilies have been identified and defined. The pattern of cellular expression of the receptors determines the specificity of the cellular response to binding.[4,110]

CXC chemokines primarily govern the chemoattraction and activation of neutrophils and, to a lesser degree, lymphocytes, in particular T cells. At least 12 different chemokines have been identified. They are clustered on chromosome 4 and demonstrate 20% to 50% homology at the amino acid level. IL-8 is the prototypical CXC chemokine.[89] It is produced by an array of immune and nonimmune cells including monocytes, alveolar macrophages, neutrophils, keratinocytes, mesangial cells, epithelial cells, fibroblasts, and endothelial cells. TNFα and IL-1 are key molecules for inducing IL-8. It is chemotactic for all granulocytes and influences nearly every aspect of neutrophil function. It stimulates neutrophil degranulation, phagocytosis, transendothelial migration and shedding of L-selectin, up-regulation of β_2 integrins, and augments superoxide production. It is also a potent angiogenic factor. It binds to both the CXCR1 and CXCR2, receptors that also engage the chemokines GCP-2, GRO-α, and ENA-78. ENA-78 is a potent neutrophil chemotaxin produced by the endothelium in response to TNFα or IL-1, neutrophils, or monocytes. Studies have demonstrated that ELR-containing CXC chemokines are angiogenic, whereas those lacking this motif are angiostatic.[38,86,109–111]

The interferon-influenced chemokines IP-10 and Mig do not target neutrophils, and the ELR motif is absent. They induce IFNγ production and may play a more prominent role in mediating the inflammatory response to viral infections and autoimmune disorders. Mig is chemotactic for tumor-infiltrating lymphocytes, activated T cells, and monocytes and promotes CTL activity. IP-10 is chemotactic for monocytes, T cells, and NK cells and augments T-cell adhesion. Both chemokines bind the CXCR3 receptor found on IL-2-activated T cells. IFNγ attenuates the expression of both IL-8 and ENA-78 and hence may serve as an important mechanism to the control and regulate inflammation.[38,86] Stromal cell derived factor-1 (SDF-1) is the only known ligand for the CXCR4 receptor and in the presence of IL-7 stimulates proliferation of pre-B-cell clones and growth of bone marrow B progenitor cells. The receptor has gained much interest since it was identified as a coreceptor for HIV-1. PF_4 and neutrophil-activating protein-2 are CXC chemokines of platelet origin. PF-4 has angiostatic properties and inhibits the growth of various cancer cell lines in a manner that appears to be related to its angiostatic properties. It binds heparin with high affinity to stimulate coagulation.[38]

The CC chemokines recruit monocytes, granulocytes, T cells, NK cells, and DCs. RANTES is produced by stimulated T cells, platelets, and endothelials cells and is constitutively produced in resting T cells, which implies a homeostatic function. MIP-1α and β are produced by activated T cells and are chemotactic for neutrophils, monocytes, eosinophils, basophils, and T lymphocytes. They are also mitogenic for hematopoietic progenitor cells and up-regulate TNFα, IL-1, and IL-6. The MCP family of chemokines influences the recruitment of monocytes and T cells. Their influence upon the function of these target cells is dictated by the cell's specific profile of receptor expression. MCP-1 is produced by nonlymphocytic cells (endothelial cells, epithelial cells, fibroblasts, smooth muscle cells, macrophages, and mast cells). Binding to CCR1 enhances chemotaxis, whereas activation of CCR2 increases the release of intracellular substances such as histamine and leukotrienes from basophils.[38]

Lymphotactin is the only member of the C chemokine family and is produced by $CD8^+$ lymphocytes, thymocytes, and NK cells and, to a lesser degree, by DCs and activated mast cells. It selectively recruits lymphoid cells.[38]

Fractalkine is the sole CX3C chemokine and is produced by endothelium. In its membrane-bound form it may act as a solid-phase adhesion molecule, but on cleavage serves as a soluble chemoattractant for lymphoid cells and monocytes.[38]

Interleukin 12 (NK Cell Stimulatory Factor, Cytotoxic Lymphocyte Maturation Factor). IL-12 is integral in the innate immune response (see Table 6.7). It is produced early during innate immune reactions against intracellular microbes and stimulates subsequent adaptive responses that confer further host protection against these pathogens; hence, it is an important link between innate and adaptive immune responses. IL-12 is critical for initiating a sequence of responses involving macrophages, NK cells, and T lymphocytes that results in the eradication of intracellular microbes. It is primarily derived from activated mononuclear phagocytes and DCs and most importantly stimulates IFNγ from T cells and NK cells. There are two pathways leading to IL-12 production: a T-cell dependent and an independent pathway. During innate immunity, LPS, infection by intracellular bacteria, and viral infections may induce IL-12 production. In addition, interactions between CD40 ligand and CD40 on activated lymphocytes and APCs, respectively, induce the release of APC IL-12.[112,113] Thus, IL-12 is produced during the induction of and the effector phases of cell-mediated immune response when APCs present antigens to T cells.[4,38]

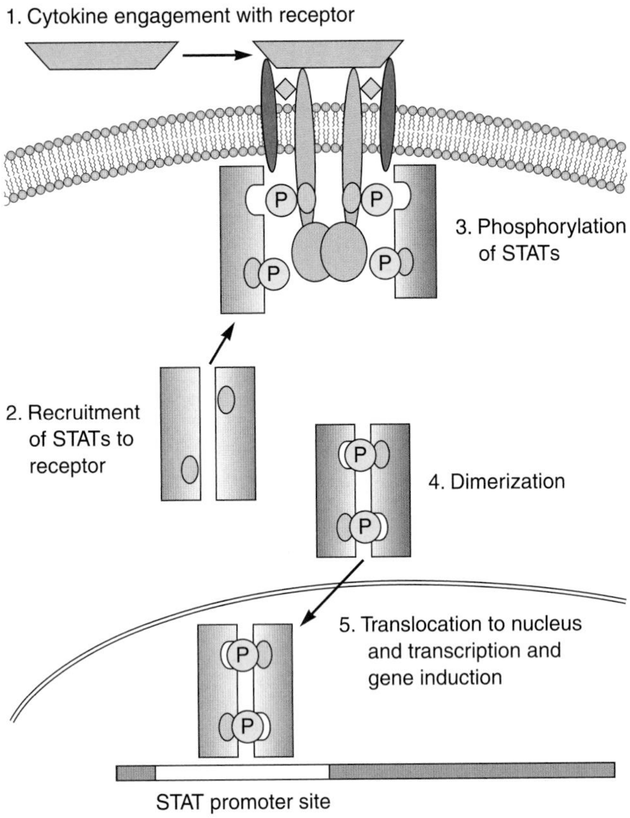

FIGURE 6.9 JAK/STAT signaling pathway. Janus kinase (JAK) components are associated in an inactive form with the cytoplasmic portion of cytokine receptors. Cytokine binding leads to receptor aggregation. Adjacent JAK proteins become activated and phosphorylate each other and tyrosine residues. Through the Src homology domain, signal transduction and activator of transcription (STAT) proteins bind phosphotyrosine residues on the cytoplasmic portion of cytokine receptors. Bound STAT proteins are phosphorylated by bound JAK proteins and subsequently dissociate. Phosphorylated STAT proteins dimerize and then move to the nucleus where they induce transcription by binding to STAT binding regions within the promoter. (After Abbas AK, Lichtman AH. *Cellular and molecular immunology.* Philadelphia: Elsevier; 2003.)

The IL-12 receptor is a heterodimer composed of $\beta1$ and $\beta2$ subunits, the latter of which is involved in signaling, although both are required for engaging ligand. The receptor signals through the JAK/STAT pathway (Fig. 6.9).[4] This signal transduction pathway is employed by numerous cytokines including interferons, IL-6, IL-12, IL-2, IL-7, IL-9, IL-4, and IL-10. A characteristic of this cytokine is the generation of a positive amplification loop, which heightens the inflammatory response. Expression of the IL-12 receptor is induced by IFNγ. Activated NK cells and T_H1 cells produce IFNγ that potentiates macrophage IL-12 production. IL-12 stimulates further production of IFNγ by NK cells and T lymphocytes, which continues to fuel the reaction in a positive feedback mechanism. Ultimately, IFNγ activates macrophages to kill and degrade phagocytosed microbes. IL-12 potentiates bacterial LPS-induced macrophage TNFα production. IL-12 antagonists reduce mortality in experimental models of LPS-induced septic shock; however, there is no evidence of their efficacy in human clinical trials.[4]

$CD4^+$ helper T lymphocytes, under the influence of IL-12, differentiate into T_H1 cells, which subsequently activate phagocytes in cell-mediated immunity. It enhances the cytolytic functions of activated NK cells and $CD8^+$ CTLs and suppresses T_H2 cell differentiation and effector activity.

TABLE 6.8

ACUTE-PHASE PROTEINS

Acute-phase protein	Function
INCREASE	
C-reactive protein	Opsonin
Serum amyloid A	Apolipoprotein
α_1-acid glycoprotein	Platelet inhibitor
Fibrinogen	Coagulation, tissue repair
α_2-,macroglobulin	Antiprotease
α_1-protease inhibitor	Antiprotease
α_1-antichymotrypsin	Antiprotease
Haptoglobin	Antioxidant
Hemopexin	Antioxidant
Ceruloplasmin	Antioxidant
C3	Complement
Factor b	Complement
C1 inhibitor	Complement
C4b-binding protein	Complement
Mannose-binding lectin	Complement
DECREASE	
Albumin	Transport
Prealbumin	Transport
Transferrin	Transport

The inhibition of T_H2 and IL-4 activity confers antiallergic properties to IL-12. IL-12 knockout mice demonstrate diminished IFNγ production and defective T_H1 cell development and cell-mediated immunity against intracellular organisms.[4,38]

Interleukin 6. IL-6 regulates the acute-phase response to inflammation, characterized by altered thermoregulation (i.e., fever), perturbation in nitrogen balance (i.e., cachexia and catabolism), and the generation of the acute-phase reactants of innate immunity by the liver (Tables 6.7 and 6.8).[86,114] It functions in both innate and adaptive immunity to enable the host to recover. Despite *in vitro* data demonstrating that a variety of cells can produce IL-6, the most prominent *in vivo* sources of IL-6 are monocytes and macrophages stimulated with LPS or IL-1 or TNFα stimulated fibroblasts and endothelial cells.[115] Steroids inhibit the induction of IL-6. The receptor for IL-6 consists of cytokine-binding protein and a signal-transducing subunit, which belong to the type I cytokine receptor family. It signals through the JAK-STAT pathway (see Fig. 6.9).[4]

In conjunction with IL-1 and TNFα, IL-6 regulates the systemic manifestations of the acute-phase response.[114] It potentiates the immune response by inducing B-cell differentiation and activating T cells. It interacts with TNFα to enhance T-cell proliferation and promotes neutrophil activation and accumulation. In adaptive immunity, IL-6 stimulates the growth of B lymphocytes that have differentiated into antibody producing plasma cells. IL-6 antagonizes LPS-induced TNFα production and TNFα-induced IL-1 production.[116,117]

High Mobility Group 1 Protein (HMGB1). HMGB1 was initially identified as an architectural chromatin-binding factor that bends DNA and directs protein assembly on specific DNA targets. It is abundant, ubiquitous, and evolutionarily conserved as evident by the 99% amino acid homology between rat and human proteins.[118] Thirty years after the original discovery of HMGB1, Tracy and colleagues demonstrated that it acts as a late mediator of mortality in murine endotoxemia and sepsis. HMGB1 appeared 8 hours poststimulation and plateaued at 16 to 32 hours, very distinct from the acute rise and fall of early mediators (TNFα, IL-1β) of severe sepsis and septic shock.[118]

HMGB1 is released by activated macrophages via an active process that necessitates shuttling the protein from nucleus to cytoplasm. HMGB1 has many of the intercellular signaling activities characteristic of cytokines and therefore is often classified as a proinflammatory cytokine and potent regulator of the inflammatory response. Signaling is thought to occur by binding to the receptor for end-glycation products (RAGE) with subsequent activation of p21ras, MEK, the MAPK kinases, and NFκB.[119,120] This receptor is expressed on mononuclear phagocytes, vascular smooth muscle cells, and neurons. Blocking antibodies to RAGE fail to completely prevent cellular activation suggesting the presence of an alternate receptor. Recent studies suggest that both TLR2 and TLR4 may mediate HMGB1-induced activation of NFκB in macrophages and neutrophils. This observation is very important as it demonstrates that a receptor classically considered specific for microbial danger signals may interact with an endogenous molecule.[118–120]

HMGB1-RAGE interactions induce numerous proinflammatory events. Endothelial cells increase the expression of adhesion molecules and also secrete TNFα and IL-8.[121] In neutrophils, HMGB1 activated the MAPKs and enhanced the expression of proinflammatory cytokines in a NFκB-dependent manner. In addition, it is chemotactic for neutrophils, monocytes, and macrophages in models of acute lung injury.[120] In vivo studies are corroborative. Intratracheal administration of HMGB1 to LPS-resistant mice stimulated lung neutrophil accumulation and the local production of proinflammatory cytokines.[120] However, intravenous administration of HMGB1 does not cause shock as does TNFα. Systemic levels are markedly elevated in patients that die of sepsis. Recombinant HMGB1 mimics the lethality of high-dose LPS and induces the release of TNFα by macrophages. In a series of elegant studies, anti-HMGB1 antibodies conferred a dose-dependent protection in animal models of endotoxemia, even when the first dose of anti-HMGB1 antibodies was delayed for 2 hours. This occurs without changes in TNFα, IL-1β, or MIP-2 concentrations. Even more striking are the in vivo CLP models, in which anti-HMGB1 administration up to 24 hours after CLP significantly increased survival, 72% versus 28%. This wider therapeutic window may enable the development of inhibitors of HMGB1 for treat of sepsis.[120,122–124]

Such observations have stimulated the search for other inhibitors of HMGB1. Ethyl pyruvate, a nontoxic food additive, dose-dependently inhibits HMGB1 release and confers significant protection against the lethality of sepsis, even when the first dose is administered 24 hours after the onset of sepsis. In addition, it inhibits the translocation of NFκB and p38 MAPK signaling.[120,122,125,126]

HMGB1 may also serve as a danger signal for other perturbations in homeostasis, as it can also be released passively by necrotic or injured cells but not by apoptotic cells.[124,127–129] Hypoacetylation of chromatin on the induction of apoptosis enhances HMGB1 binding, thereby preventing release during apoptotic processes. Thus, HMGB1 binding to chromatic depends on the viability of the cell and clearly distinguishes necrotic from apoptotic cells. This enables the innate immune response to respond to injury and further induce inflammation.[124,127–129]

HMGB1 is also elevated during hemorrhage shock. In a clinical case, serum HMGB1 levels increased significantly within 24 hours of hemorrhagic shock and returned toward basal levels as the clinical condition improved. High levels have also been found in other conditions of sterile inflammation such as rheumatoid arthritis. Hence, HMGB1 may serve as a signal of danger from endogenous threats or perturbations.

Interleukin 15. IL-15 is produced by various cells in response to LPS and other stimuli, though the principal cellular source is mononuclear phagocytes (see Table 6.7). It is structurally homologous to IL-2 as is its receptor and the IL-2R. IL-15 stimulates the proliferation of NK cells similarly to the manner by which IL-2 functions later in the adaptive immune response. It also acts as a T-cell growth and survival factor especially for long-lived memory $CD8^+$ T cells.[4]

Interleukin 18. IL-18 is structurally homologous to IL-1 and utilizes a similar IRAK signaling pathway (see Table 6.7). Macrophages responding to microbial challenge or exposure to LPS are the principal source. Its primary function is to stimulate the production of IFNγ by NK cells and T cells, and in synergizing with IL-12, it augments cell-mediated immunity. Knockout mice lacking IL-18 are deficient in IFNγ production, and concomitant IL-12 deficiency eliminates all IFNγ production and any T_H1 response.[4]

Interferons (Type I). Type I interferons possess potent antiviral and antitumor properties (see Table 6.7). It is from this ability to interfere with viral infection that the name is derived. They are subcategorized into α and β interferons. Mononuclear phagocytes are the major source of interferon α, whereas many cell types produce interferon β. The most potent stimulus inducing the synthesis and release of either is viral infection, particularly double-stranded RNA produced during viral replication. Other inducers include IL-1, TNFα, LPS, and antigen-activated T cells. Both groups bind to the same cell surface receptor and induce similar responses by signaling through the JAK/STAT pathway (see Fig. 6.9).

These cytokines provide the first line of defense against viral infection and promote cell-mediated immunity against intracellular pathogen. They are secreted from virally infected cells to protect neighboring uninfected ones by inducing the synthesis of a number of enzymes that interfere with viral RNA or DNA transcription and viral replication. Through enhanced expression of class I MHC molecules, the type 1 interferons facilitate recognition of class I-associated viral antigens on infected cells by CTLs and increase the efficiency of CTL-mediated killing. Type I interferon stimulates the development of T_H1 cells by promoting these cells to express IL-12 receptor. They can also stimulate B-cell development, proliferation, and immunoglobulin heavy chain switching from IgM to IgG.[130–132] Knockout mice lacking the receptor for these cytokines are susceptible to viral infections. Interferons are currently in clinical use for hepatitis B and C infection, multiple sclerosis, chronic myelocytic leukemia (CML), and Kaposi's sarcoma.[130–132]

Interleukin 10 (Cytokine Synthesis Inhibiting Factor). IL-10 inhibits activated macrophages and APCs and functions in a counter-regulatory mechanism to suppress innate immune reactions (see Table 6.6). It is produced mainly by macrophages and hence functions by negative feedback. T lymphocytes, particularly the T_H2 subset; B cells; and some other nonlymphoid cells produce IL-10, in response to a variety of stimuli including LPS, TNFα, IL-2, IL-4, and IL-13.

IL-10 binds to a type II (interferon) receptor. Though the manner by which it effects curtailment of the inflammatory response is unknown, its presence inhibits NK-κB activation and the generation of inflammatory mediators perhaps by inhibiting in some manner the activation of signal transduction cascades and gene activation in proinflammatory pathways.[4,133]

IL-10 terminates many of the functions of activated macrophages and participates in reestablishing homeostasis as the infection resolves. It down-regulates proinflammatory cytokine (TNFα, IL-1, IL-6, and IL-8) production, suppresses the production of IL-12 production, and inhibits IFNγ production and the innate and cell-mediated immune responses.[4,51,86] It represses the expression of costimulators and class II MHC molecules on APCs, thereby terminating T-cell activation and inhibiting cell-mediated immunity.[4] In neutrophils it inhibits cytokine release, superoxide generation, migration, and even survival.[134] In combination with IL-4, it inhibits IFNγ release and IL-12 production to limit differentiation and function of T_H1 cells, favoring a T_H2 profile.[51]

IL-10 knockout develop inflammatory bowel disease, which is hypothesized to result from unregulated macrophage reaction to enteric microbes.[135] In observational studies of ARDS or MODS, serum IL-10 levels were often elevated, and those patients with the highest systemic concentrations died.[133] It is unclear whether this is actually a pathologic response or merely a marker of disease severity. Contemporary belief is that IL-10 is not a mediator of immunosuppression but, rather, important for immunoregulation.

Late Cytokines/Adaptive Immunity

Interleukin 2 (T-Cell Growth Factor). IL-2 stimulates the growth and proliferation of T lymphocytes and is responsible for T-cell clonal expansion after antigen recognition (see Table 6.7).[136] IL-2 is produced by $CD4^+$ T cells and to a lesser extent by $CD8^+$ T cells. The receptor is heterotrimeric, consisting of three noncovalently associated proteins, α, β, and γ. The α and β chains are involved in cytokine binding, and the β and γ chains mediate signal transduction.[4] Antigen recognition enhances the expression of functional IL-2 receptors, which confers a degree of specificity, as those T cells recognizing antigen are preferentially induced to proliferate in response to IL-2. Though the α chain appears on T-cell activation and binds IL-2, signal generation necessitates the β and γ chains. Cells expressing the complete α, β, and γ complex bind IL-2 with higher affinity (Kd of 10^{-11} M), and growth stimulation of such cells occurs at a low IL-2 concentration.[4] On antigen receptor-mediated T-cell activation, IL-2R α is rapidly up-regulated, which reduces the concentration of IL-2 needed to stimulate growth. Therefore, antigen-stimulated T cells are more responsive to IL-2 than naïve T cells. This receptor signals through numerous signal transduction pathways including the JAK/STAT and MAPK pathways (see Figs. 6.5 and 6.8).

IL-2 functions in an autocrine and paracrine fashion to induce the proliferation of the antigen-specific cells. After exposure to IL-1, there is a rise in cyclins and activation of cyclin-dependent kinases that stimulates the progression from the G1 to the S phase of the cell cycle. A reduction in p27, an inhibitor of cyclin-kinase complexes, facilitates this progression, and the induction of Bcl-2, an anti-apoptotic protein, facilitates survival. It also stimulates the production of other cytokines such as IFNγ and IL-4.[4]

IL-2 promotes the proliferation and differentiation of many immune cells. NK cells are stimulated to grow and transform into lymphokine-activated killer (LAK) cells. In combination with IFNγ and IL-12, IL-2 can trigger a positive feedback cycle of NK activation. IL-2 stimulates B-cell growth and antibody synthesis. Repeated activation of $CD4^+$ T cells in the presence of IL-2 sensitizes these cells to apoptosis by fas-fas-ligand. IL-2 may also stimulate the development of regulatory T cells, and IL-2 knockout mice develop autoimmunity. Knockout mice lacking the γ chain develop X-linked severe combined immunodeficiency syndrome. This is probably due to an inability of immature T cells to respond to IL-7. IL-2 has been used in the management of cancer, in particular renal cell carcinoma.[137]

Interleukin 4. IL-4 is the major stimulus for the production of IgE antibodies and for the development of T_H2 cells from naïve $CD4^+$ T cells (see Table 6.7). The principle cellular sources are $CD4^+$ T cells, mast cells, and basophils. The IL-4 receptor belongs to the type I cytokine receptor family and signals through the JAK/STAT pathway[138] (see Fig. 6.8). IgE is integral in orchestrating the defense against parasitic infections. It stimulates IgE production and mast cell/eosinophil-mediated reactions and induces B-cell Ig heavy chain class switching to the IgE isotype. However, IL-4 also serves a counter-regulatory role by inducing T_H2 cell differentiation and growth. IL-4 antagonizes the macrophage-activating effects of IFNγ and thus inhibits cell-mediated immunity.

Interleukin 5. IL-5 is produced by T_H2 cells and activated mast cells and activates eosinophils (see Table 6.7). It signals through the type I cytokine receptor and the JAK/STAT pathway (see Fig. 6.8). IL-5 is an inducer of eosinophil growth, differentiation, and activation and also participates the eradication of helminthic infection. IL-5 also stimulates the proliferation of B cells and the production of IgA antibodies.[4]

Interleukin 13. IL-13 is produced by T_H2 cells and some epithelial cells and is structurally homologous and functionally similar to IL-4 (see Table 6.7). The receptor is found mainly on nonlymphoid cells and can be activated by either IL-13 or IL-4. IL-13 down-regulates the expression of Fcγ on monocytes and macrophages, thereby decreasing antibody-dependent cellular cytotoxicity. It increases 15S-HETE and lipoxin A_4, both of which antagonize proinflammatory leukotrienes. However, they can increase the expression of MHC class II and costimulatory molecules on monocytes and thereby serve an immunostimulatory function. The major action is to inhibit the activation of macrophages and to antagonize IFNγ.[139]

Interferon γ (IFNγ). IFNγ is produced by NK cells, T_H1 cells, and $CD8^+$ cells and, as the principal stimulus for macrophage activation, provides necessary functions during both innate and adaptive immune responses (see Table 6.7). It modulates cellular differentiation, cytotoxicity, cytokine production, cellular adhesion, and oxidative metabolism. During innate immunity, NK cells secrete it on exposure to pathogen or IL-12. $CD8^+$ T cells and the T_H1 subset of $CD4^+$ T cells produce it in response to MHC-bound peptide antigen with a costimulatory signal. The IFNγ receptor is composed of two homologous proteins belonging to the type II cytokine receptor family and functions through the JAK/STAT pathway (see Fig. 6.9).[4]

The antiviral and antitumor properties of IFNγ are redundant with those of type I interferons. In concert with TNFα and IL-12 it forms one arm of a positive feedback loop fueling the activation of both NK cells and macrophages. Stimulated macrophages activate NK cells by releasing TNFα and IL-12. These NK cells produce IFNγ, which further stimulates macrophages to secrete more TNFα and IL-12.[140,141]

IFNγ induces the genes encoding the enzymatic machinery required for generating ROS generation and provides the principle stimulus for macrophages to kill phagocytosed microbes. It regulates the expression of MHC molecules class I and class II molecules and costimulators of APCs and induces the transcription of enzymes regulating antigen processing.[140,141]

IFNγ synergizes with TNFα to activate the endothelium and up-regulate adhesion molecule expression; in doing so, it facilitates lymphocyte and leukocyte recruitment. Interferon promotes the differentiation of naïve $CD4^+$ cells into T_H1 cells and inhibits the proliferation of T_H2 cells, in part by inducing IL-12, the major T_H1 inducing cytokine, from activated mononuclear phagocytes. It promotes B-cell switching to certain IgG subclasses, notably IgG2a, and inhibits the switching to IL-4 dependent isotypes such as IgE and IgG1. These IgG subclasses bind the Fcγ receptors on phagocytes and activate complement, thereby promoting phagocytosis of opsonized microbes. It activates PMNs and stimulates the cytolytic activity of NK cells. The net effect is to promote macrophage-rich inflammatory reactions while inhibiting IgE-dependent eosinophil-rich reactions. IL-10, by suppressing macrophage release of TNFα and IL-12, negatively regulates IFNγ production.

IFNγ also demonstrates counter-regulatory properties. It selectively inhibits LPS-induced expression of CXC chemokines. It up-regulates macrophage production of IP-10, MIG, and ELR-negative chemokines that inhibit neutrophil chemotaxis and activation and decreases macrophage release of ELR-positive CXC chemokines (IL-8), which are chemotactic for additional neutrophils.[4]

Transforming Growth Factor β. TGF-β is a homodimer synthesized and secreted by activated T cells, macrophages, and many other cells (see Table 6.7). It is primarily immunosuppressive and inhibits the proliferation and activation of lymphocytes and other leukocytes. It promotes wound healing by increasing extracellular matrix protein synthesis and stimulating mononuclear cell and fibroblast influx.[142–144] Though the family consists of three closely related isoforms, most cells utilize TGF-β. Its effects are mediated through two high affinity TGF receptors (type I and II) that signal through a serine/threonine kinase domain that phosphorylates transcription factors called SMADS.[4]

TGF-β inhibits the proliferation and differentiation of T cells and the activation of macrophages. It favors differentiation of $CD4^+$ cells to the T_H2 subset and inhibits MHC class II surface expression. By suppressing the expression of MHC class II antigen, it abrogates the adaptive immune response. Macrophages demonstrate diminished ROS production and TNFα and NO release. It directly counteracts the influence of proinflammatory cytokines on PMNs and endothelial cells and, in combination with IL-4, IL-13, and IL-10 can antagonize the production or effects of these proinflammatory mediators. Knockout mice deficient in TGF-β develop uncontrolled inflammatory lesions.[4,38]

Cytokines that Stimulate Hematopoiesis

Cytokines are necessary for normal hematopoiesis. Several of the cytokines stimulated during both innate and adaptive immune responses are mitogenic for and induce differentiation of bone marrow progenitor cells.

CSFs are cytokines made by activated T cells, macrophages, endothelial cells, and bone marrow stromal cells that stimulate increased production of inflammatory leukocytes by bone marrow progenitors. Receptors for GM-CSF and G-CSF are of the class I family of cytokine receptors. GM-CSF is expressed by T and B cells, macrophages, mast cells, fibroblasts, and endothelium in response to stimuli such as IL-1, IL-2, LPS, and TNFα. It stimulates neutrophils, monocytes, macrophages, and DCs and is a powerful inducer of hematopoiesis. It enhances cytokine release, degranulation, and phagocytosis of opsonized particles in neutrophils. In monocytes and macrophages, it enhances cytotoxicity and cytokine release. It promotes the activity of APCs and the maturation of bone marrow cells into DCs and monocytes.[145] G-CSF is produced by macrophages, endothelial cells, fibroblasts, and bone marrow stromal cells. It functions as an endocrine hormone to mobilize neutrophils and induces subsequent leukocyte proliferation and maturation. In 1991, the Food and Drug Administration (FDA) approved the use of G-CSF for use in patients with neutropenia.[146,147]

Stem cell factor or c-Kit ligand is synthesized by marrow stromal cells and binds to a cell surface tyrosine kinase receptor on pluripotent stem cells that is the protein product of the cellular proto-oncogene c-kit. Its effects appear permissive as it is corequisite for stem cell responsiveness to other CSFs;

SCIENTIFIC PRINCIPLES

however, in isolation it does not stimulate colony formation. It may also play a role in sustaining the viability and proliferative capacity of immature T cells in the thymus.[4]

IL-3 is a product of CD4$^+$ T cells that promotes the differentiation of immature marrow progenitors into all known mature cell types. It also promotes the growth and development of mast cells. Surprisingly, despite these important functions, murine knockouts do not manifest noticeable impairment of hematopoiesis.[4]

IL-7 is secreted by bone marrow stromal cells and promotes the growth and survival of immature precursors committed to the B and T lymphocyte lineages. Knockout mice, deficient in IL-7 or its receptor, are lymphopenic with diminished populations of B and T cells.[4]

The Complement System

The complement system is integral to both innate and adaptive immunity. It has the capacity to independently eliminate organisms and to facilitate host defense by marking foreign particles for phagocytosis through opsonization. Many pathophysiologic inflammatory diseases, immune complex diseases, ischemia/reperfusion injury, and ARDS are considered, in part, consequences of aberrant function of this system.[148–151]

The system consists of three pathways comprising approximately 30 serum and cell surface proteins that interact with one another and with other molecules of the immune system in a highly coordinated fashion. These cascades involve the sequential proteolytic activation of zymogens to generate enzymes with proteolytic activity. This mechanism for activation amplifies the response because each individual enzyme activated can cleave numerous zymogens in the next step and generate multiple activated enzyme molecules. Ultimately, the products of complement activation adhere to microbial cell surfaces or to antibody-bound microbes and other antigens to directly or indirectly eliminate these pathogens. Temporal and spatial regulation to the focus of infection is ensured both by the transience of activation of these enzymes in the absence of microbes or antigens and by several circulating proteins that provide surveillance.[148,150]

The complement cascade is divided into three distinct pathways: the classical pathway (humoral immunity), which is activated by antibody bound to antigen; the alternative pathway (innate immunity), in which complement is activated by components of microbial cell surfaces; and the mannose/lectin pathway (innate immunity), which is activated by a plasma lectin that binds to mannose residues on microbes. Despite differences in which the cascade is activated, all three complement pathways ultimately result in the cleavage of C3 and share the same subsequent late cascade.[148,150]

The alternative pathway functions in the absence of antibody and is phylogenetically the oldest pathway (Fig. 6.10). Bacteria, viruses, fungi, and parasites all function as stimuli. Initial activation begins with the cleavage of C3 and the stable attachment of its product C3b to the microbial surface. Bound C3b finds Factor B, which is subsequently cleaved by a plasma serine protease called Factor D to generate Bb. The C3bBb complex is called the alternative pathway C3 convertase and functions to cleave more C3. In doing so, the convertase serves as an amplification step in both the classical and alternative pathways. Properdin prolongs the half-life of C3 convertase by delaying the release of Bb from C3bBb. C3b is the recognition component of the alternate pathway and is responsible for the opsonization of bacteria. C3a in conjunction with C5a and C4a induces acute inflammation by activating mast cells and neutrophils. These inflammatory mediators play a significant role in increasing blood vessel permeability, vasodilatation, edema formation, neutrophil adhesion and activation, chemotaxis, and the release of toxic oxygen species and lysosomal enzymes from phagocytic cells. The binding of another C3b to this complex generates the alternative pathway C5 convertase, C3bBb3b.[4,148,150]

Activation of the alternative pathway is restricted to the cell surface of microbes, as mammalian cells possess several regulatory proteins to rapidly degrade any C3bBb. Excessive amplification is regulated by β1H globulin factor H and factor I. Factor H accelerates the decay and delays the formation of C3bBb. It also acts as a cofactor for I to degrade C3 into iC3b, which is unable to bind B to generate C3 convertase. Decay acceleration factor (DAF) hinders C3 convertase assembly and mediates its dissociation in all three pathways. Also, the protein properdin, which stabilizes this alternative pathway C3 convertase, has a higher affinity for microbial than mammalian cell surfaces.[4,148,150]

The classical pathway is the primary mediator of adaptive humoral immunity and is initiated by binding of the complement protein C1 to IgG or IgM molecules engaged with antigen

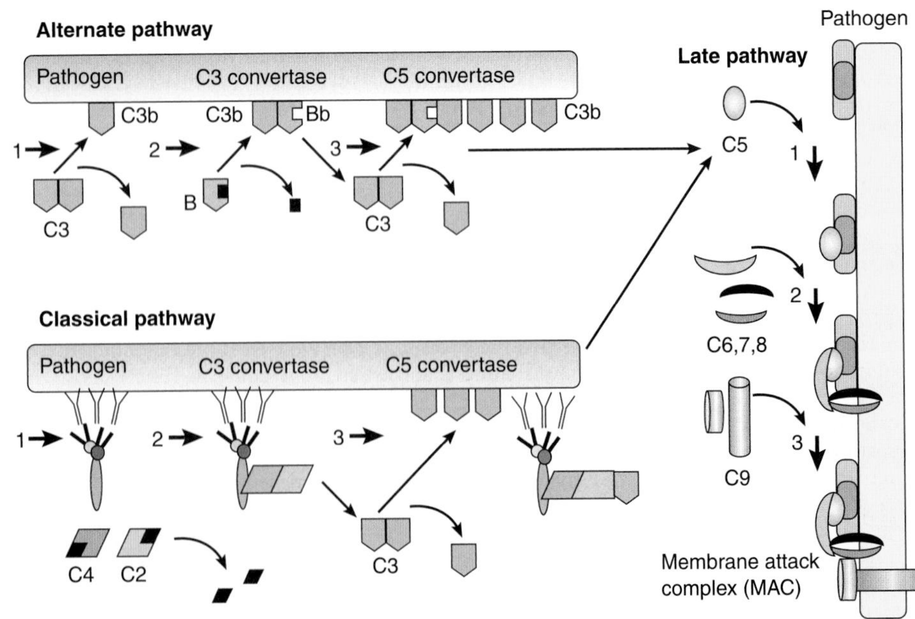

FIGURE 6.10 Complement pathways. Alternate pathway: (1) C3 is cleaved to C3b. (2) C3b binds and cleaves B to Bb to form C3 convertase (C3bBb). (3) Another C3b binds C3 convertase to form C5 convertase (C3bBbC3b). Classical pathway: (1) C1 binds immunoglobulin. (2) C1 binds and cleaves C4 and C2 to C4b and C2a to form C3 convertase (C4b2a). (3) C4b2a binds another C3b to generate C5 convertase (C4b2aC3b). Late pathway: (1) C5 convertase cleaves C5 to form C5b, which integrates into the plasmalemma. (2) C6-8 are recruited, forming the C5b-8 complex. 3. C5b-8 recruits numerous C9 subunits, which form a pore in the pathogen cell wall. (After Abbas AK, Lichtman AH. *Cellular and molecular immunology*. Philadelphia: Elsevier; 2003.)

(see Fig. 6.9). Other substances such as lipid A in endotoxin and mitochondrial membranes may activate this pathway independent of antigen-antibody complexes in vitro.[148,152]

C1 is a calcium-dependent trimeric protein consisting of C1q, which recognizes and binds the Fc region of the immunoglobulin, and C1r and C1s, which are proteases. C1q engages the Fc portion of the immunoglobulin μ and γ heavy chains. Each Fc region has a single C1q binding site, yet for activation, each C1q molecule must bind to two Ig heavy chains. Hence, multiple antibodies must be approximated for activation, which restricts activation to foci of immunoglobulin engagement. IgM exists as a pentamer enabling it to bind to two C1q molecules, and hence it is more efficient at complement activation.[4,148,152]

Interaction between C1q and the immunoglobulin Fc region induces a conformational change in C1q that activates C1r, which subsequently cleaves and activates C1s. C1s cleaves C4 to generate C4b and C4a. The C4a anaphylatoxin possesses properties similar to those described for C3a. C4b localizes to immune complexes on the cell surface. C2, after complexing with C4b, is cleaved by C1s, thereby generating the classical C3 convertase C4b2a complex, which has the ability to cleave C3. The C3b generated can bind Bb, producing more C3 convertase and amplifying the signal. The key early steps of the alternative and classical pathways are analogous: C3 and factor B of the alternative pathway are homologous to C4 and C2 in the classical pathway. C3b can also combine with the classical C3 convertase to generate C4b2a3b, the classical C5 convertase.[4]

Numerous regulatory mechanisms exist to restrict activation to sites of inflammation. Excessive classical C3 convertase activity is prevented by the rapid decay of C2a from the complex, which renders the complex unstable. C1 inhibitor covalently binds C1s, reducing the half-life of activated C1 to only 13 seconds. C4 binding protein enhances spontaneous dissociation of C4b2a and also acts as a cofactor for C3b/C4b inactivator, which degrades C4b.[38]

The mannose-binding lectin (MBL) pathway is activated by the binding of microbial polysaccharides to circulating lectins; MBL serves as the recognition unit of the MBL pathway. This pathway recognizes polysaccharides with high mannose content and other oligosaccharides with characteristic linkages found exclusively on pathogens and not on normal host components. Binding is calcium-dependent and results in the activation of mannose-binding lectin-associated serine proteases (MASP-1 and MASP-2). Activated MASP-2 cleaves and activates C4 and C2 in the same fashion as the classical complement pathway. Subsequent steps of complement activation of the MBL pathway mirror those of the classical complement pathway.[148,153,154]

The C5 convertases generated during either the classical or alternative pathway initiates a cascade of events that culminates in the formation of the cytocidal MAC. Specifically, C5 convertase cleaves C5, yielding C5a and C5b. C6 and C7 bind to generate the C5b67 complex. This hydrophobic moiety penetrates deeply into the lipid bilayer as a high affinity receptor for C8. Binding of C8 forms the complex C5b-8 that recruits numerous C9 subunits, which polymerize to form pores in the plasma membrane. The pores structurally resemble the membrane pores formed by perforin, the cytolytic granule protein found in CTLs and NK cells. Their diameter may span 100 angstroms, which prevents the maintenance of vital ionic gradients and induces osmotic lysis and ultimately the death of target cells or pathogens. Patients with deficiencies in the terminal components of C5, C6, C7, and C8 are susceptible to meningococcal and gonococcal infections.[4,155]

The effects of complement are in part mediated through several complement receptors. Opsonization and phagocytosis are important mechanisms for pathogen destruction, and phagocytic cells express receptors for complement factor C3 components. Complement receptor type I (CR1), the receptor for C3b and C4b, mediates engagement of and facilitates phagocytosis of complement bound microbes and the clearance of immune complexes from the circulation. It is expressed on a variety of cells including red blood cells (RBCs), neutrophils, monocytes, eosinophils, and T and B cells. RBCs facilitate elimination by transporting these opsonized particles to the liver and spleen where the immune complexes are removed by phagocytes. CR2 stimulates humoral immune response by enhancing B-cell activation by antigen and by promoting the trapping of antigen-antibody complexes in germinal centers. In humans, this receptor is the receptor for Epstein-Barr virus (EBV). CR3 and CR4 are β_2 integrins that bind the iC3b-processed fragment of C3 and promote macrophage and neutrophil phagocytosis of iC3b-opsonized antigen.[4,38]

This entire cascade is under strict regulation to ensure that any activation is restricted to sites of inflammation and infection. Several circulating proteins function to do this. This regulation is needed as low level activation is always occurring and, if not quelled, would certainly damage normal tissues. Even when locally activated, byproducts may damage nearby cells and tissues.

C1r and C1s are inhibited by C1 inhibitor, a serine protease inhibitor that mimics C1r and C1s. C1 inhibitor targets activated C1qrs, and after attachment, C1r-C1s dissociate and activation of classical complement ceases. This inhibition prevents the accumulation of active C1r-C1s, thereby limiting the duration during which active C1r-C1s can initiate the cascade.[4] C1 inhibitor also inhibits other circulating inflammatory serine proteases including kallikrein and factor XII, both of which can activate the formation of bradykinin.[4] Hereditary angioneurotic edema is an inherited deficiency of C1 inhibitor and manifests as acute intermittent edema of the skin and mucosa causing abdominal pain, vomiting, diarrhea, and airway obstruction.

MCP, CR1, and DAF are regulatory proteins that bind to C3b and C4b deposited on cell surfaces and competitively inhibit the binding of other components of the C3 and C5 convertases, such as Bb and C2a, and thereby block further progression of the cascade. These proteins are only produced by mammalian cells. Deficiency of an enzyme required to form the linkages necessary to express DAF underlies paroxysmal nocturnal hemoglobinuria, a disease characterized by recurrent intravascular hemolysis due unregulated complement activation on the surface of erythrocytes. Cell-associated C3b is proteolytically degraded by a plasma serine protease called factor I that is active only in the presence of regulatory proteins such as MCP, factor H, C4BP, and CR1. MAC formation is inhibited by CD59, a membrane protein that incorporates itself into growing MACs and inhibits the incorporation of C9. It is not present in microbes. The function of these regulatory proteins may be overcome by increasing amounts of complement activation.[4]

Lipid Mediators

Eicosanoids

Eicosanoids are 20-carbon lipid inflammatory mediators derived from membrane arachidonic acid that are involved in numerous homeostatic processes and inflammation. These lipid mediators are not stored in tissues but are synthesized de novo within seconds in response to a variety of stimuli, including mechanical trauma, or specific cytokines, growth factors, and other mediators (Fig. 6.11). Although most cells are capable of producing eicosanoids, neutrophils and macrophages are

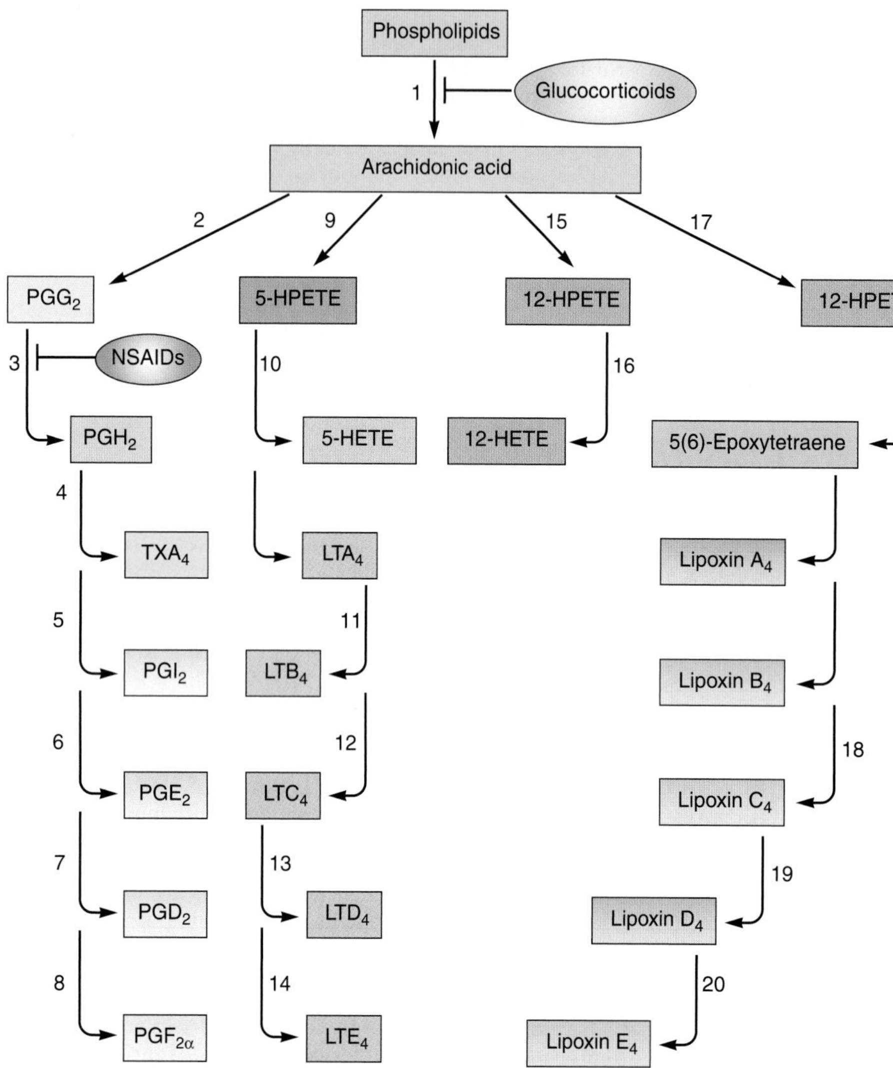

FIGURE 6.11 Eicosanoid production. (1) Phospholipases; (2) cyclooxygenase; (3) hydroperoxidase; (4) thromboxane synthetase; (5) prostacyclin synthetase; (6) E-isomerase; (7) D-isomerase; (8) F-reductase; (9) 5-lipoxygenase; (10) glutathione peroxidase; (11) hydrolase; (12) glutathione S-transferase; (13) γ-glutamyl transpeptidase; (14) cysteinyl glycanase; (15) 12-lipoxygenase; (16) peroxidase; (17) 15-lipoxygenase; (18) GSH-cis-11-trans lipoxin A_4; (19) α-glutamyl transferase; and (20) dipeptidase.

the predominant source during inflammation. They are rapidly degraded in the circulation, which limits their role primarily to that of autocrine and paracrine mediators of local inflammatory changes.[156–158]

The liberation of the precursor molecule, arachidonic acid, is the major rate-limiting step. The family of phospholipases A_2 (PLA_2), in particular type IV cytosolic PLA_2, is responsible for eicosanoid production; cells lacking type IV PLA_2 are devoid of eicosanoid synthesis.[159] Many molecules of the PLA_2 family are transcriptionally regulated by IL-1 and TNFα, whereas others are regulated by the MAPK pathway and by calcium-dependent translocation to membranes. Once formed, arachidonic acid metabolism proceeds along one of two pathways.[156–158]

Cyclooxygenase Pathway (Prostaglandins)

Cyclooxygenase catalyzes the initial step of a series of reactions that converts arachidonic acid to prostanoids (see Fig. 6.11). There are two isoforms, COX1 and COX2; the former is constitutively expressed, whereas COX2 is inducible. COX2 is considered more important during inflammatory processes such as fever, hyperalgesia, and edema formation. Either enzyme catalyzes the conversion of arachidonic acid to the endoperoxidase PGG_2, which is subsequently converted to PGH_2. PGH_2 serves as the precursor to numerous specific prostaglandins. All of these products possess very short half-lives and are rapidly inactivated.[159,160]

Prostaglandins mediate their effects through G protein signaling (Table 6.9). Prostacyclin (PGI_2) is produced by the endothelium as a potent vasodilator and inhibitor of platelet aggregation and adhesion, characteristics that enhance tissue perfusion. PGI_2 inhibits neutrophil chemotaxis and activation and interacts synergistically with PGE_2 to increase vascular permeability through the bradykinin pathway. PGE_2 is the predominant antiinflammatory prostaglandin and is produced by nearly all inflammatory cells. It is produced in response to IL-1 and mediates the hypothalamic fever response and synergizes with bradykinin and histamine to mediate pain. It is a bronchodilator, inhibits both IL-1 production and T-cell responsiveness to IL-1, and at low concentrations suppresses TNFα production. It also inhibits neutrophil chemotaxis and activation and T_H1 lymphocyte proliferation.[159,160] There is some suggestion from animal studies that PGE_2, PGE_1, and PGI_2 may be beneficial in response to sepsis through their endogenous counter-regulatory properties. Administration of each of these has been shown to improve survival in several animal models of hypovolemic and traumatic shock.[160] PGD_2 is a potent bronchodilator that inhibits neutrophil chemotaxis and activation. TXA_2, PGG_2, and PGH_2 oppose the actions of

TABLE 6.9

PROSTANOID EFFECTS

Effect	PGG_2	PGH_2	PGI_2	PGE_2	TXA_2
Chemotaxis	↑	↑	↓	↓	↑
Bronchial resistance	↑	↑	↓	↓	↑
Platelet aggregation	↑	↑	↓	↓	↑
Systemic vascular resistance			↓	↓	↑
Pulmonary vascular resistance	↑	↑	↓	↓	↑

prostacyclin by promoting platelet aggregation and inducing bronchoconstriction. TXA_2 produced by platelets and macrophages is a powerful vasoconstrictor that induces neutrophil accumulation and increases vascular permeability.[156–158,161] There is substantial evidence that TXA_2 plays a significant role in early acute-phase organ injury.[160]

Lipoxygenase Pathway (Leukotrienes and Lipoxins)

Leukotrienes and lipoxins are leukocyte-derived molecules synthesized by the oxidation of arachidonic acid by one of three LO enzymes: 5-LO, 12-LO, and 15-LO (see Fig. 6.11). 5-LO associates with the perinuclear membrane protein 5-LO-activating protein (FLAP) to catalyze the formation of 5-hydroperoxyeicosatetraenoic acid (5-HPETE). 5-HPETE is subsequently converted to LTA_4 by the combined efforts of a dehydrase and 5-LO. LTA_4 serves as the precursor for either LTB_4 or LTC_4. LTC_4 can in turn be successively hydrolyzed to the dipeptide derivative LTD_4 and LTE_4. Additional LO activity results in the production of 12-HPETE, 12-HETE, and 15-HPETE. These compounds exhibit biologic activity, although they are not as potent as the leukotrienes or prostaglandins. The leukotrienes are inactivated by oxidation followed by dehydration.[157–159,161,162]

The major LO product of neutrophils is LTB_4, though macrophages may also synthesize this compound. This compound is potently chemotactic for both neutrophils and eosinophils and by up-regulating endothelial cell surface adhesion molecules promotes leukocyte recruitment. It increases vascular permeability, either directly or through interaction with neutrophils and endothelial cells. LTB_4 has also been shown to induce hyperalgesia.[85,159]

LTC_4, LTD_4, and LTE_4 compose the family of slow-reacting substances of anaphylaxis (SRSA), compounds synthesized by mast cells during anaphylactic reactions. LTC_4 is the major eicosanoid product of eosinophils and the only product of LO. These three leukotrienes are potent vasoconstrictors and the most powerful bronchoconstrictors in humans, being three orders of magnitude more potent than histamine. They also increase vascular permeability and are vasodilatory in skin.[41,159]

Lipoxins are biosynthesized by several routes in a tissue-specific manner. Current evidence implicates the eosinophil. A 5(6)-epoxytetraene intermediate can be formed by 5-LO activity on 15-HPETE. This reaction when carried out in blood vessels requires the interaction between platelets and neutrophils. On mucosal surfaces, 12-LO and 5-LO activity on LTA_4 can result in formation of this lipoxin intermediate through leukocyte-epithelial interactions. The 5(6)-epoxytetraene intermediate is then converted to lipoxin A_4, lipoxin B_4, or lipoxin C_4, the last of which serves as the precursor for lipoxins D_4 and E_4.[83,163,164]

Though many of the functions of lipoxins have yet to be elucidated, they appear to counter-regulate the actions of leukotrienes. They inhibit leukotriene production by down-regulating 5-LO as 15-LO is up-regulated. The antiinflammatory cytokines IL-4 and IL-13 further contribute to suppression of inflammatory responses by enhancing 15-LO activity. In addition to inhibiting synthesis, lipoxins inhibit the actions of LTB_4 and LTD_4. Lipoxins A_4 and B_4 are potent vasoactive compounds, though this effect is tissue-specific for lipoxin B_4, as it induces vasoconstriction in selective tissue beds. Lipoxins influence smooth muscle and vascular tonus by increasing NO and prostacyclin production, increasing arachidonate release, and reversing endothelin-induced vasoconstriction. Counterinflammatory functions of lipoxin A_4 include inhibition of leukotrienes, fMLP, and other chemoattractants. Lipoxin A_4 also down-regulates LTB_4-mediated delayed-type hypersensitivity reactions.[83,163–165]

A large number of antiinflammatory drugs, many of which are in clinical use, act by interfering with eicosanoid synthesis. The antiinflammatory properties of corticosteroids are mediated at least in part by the inhibition of PLA_2 through the induction of lipocortin. NSAIDs block the synthesis of both prostaglandins and thromboxanes by inhibiting COX activity. Newer NSAIDs have been developed to selectively inhibit COX2 activation without affecting COX1. In contrast to the other NSAIDs, aspirin inhibits COX in an irreversible manner, and restoration of platelet function necessitates the administration of platelets. Recently, aspirin, by either acetylating COX2 or by inducing the oxidation of arachidonic acid by cytochrome P-450 or 5-LO, has been shown to stimulate the formation of 15R-HETE in endothelial or epithelial cells. These 15-epilipoxins exhibit higher potency in suppressing inflammation because of their prolonged half-lives. A potential complication of NSAID use and COX inhibition is the shunting of arachidonate through the 5-LO pathway and subsequent greater production of proinflammatory leukotrienes (asthma); such consequences minimize any benefit achieved from reducing other eicosanoid levels. In addition, most NSAIDs act systematically in a nonselective manner, so that inhibition of prostaglandin synthesis can result in dangerous side effects in locations where prostaglandins normally exert cytoprotective effects (e.g., gastric mucosa).[160,164,166]

Platelet Activating Factor

PAF is a heterogeneous mixture of 1-0-alkyl-2-acetyl-sn-glycero-3-phosphocholines that plays a prominent role in both physiologic and pathologic inflammatory states. It does not exist preformed but is rapidly produced by activated cells. Synthesis involves either the remodeling of membrane phospholipids by PLA_2, usually more important under inflammatory conditions, or by de novo synthesis as occurs in resting cells. De novo synthesis is regulated by substrate availability and involves a constitutively active enzyme that produces PAF in small basal amounts.[167] The membrane phospholipid precursor is present in high amounts in neutrophils. Other cells that can synthesize PAF include platelets, basophils, monocytes, eosinophils, mast cells, and vascular endothelial cells. Similar to eicosanoid production, the synthesis of PAF is initiated by calcium-dependent activation of PLA_2, which yields 1-0-alkyl-sn-glycerophosphocholine (lyso-PAF); subsequent acetylation generates PAF. PAF may be released from the cell, or it may be converted back to lyso-PAF by an acetylhydrolase and to the precursor ether-phosphatidylcholine.[167]

The actions of PAF are mediated by G-protein activation. As the name implies, PAF induces platelet aggregation and degranulation, yet also possesses many other critical functions for inflammation. Its vasoactive properties include vasodilation and increased permeability, and it is an equally potent bronchoconstrictor. PAF enhances arachidonic acid metabolism, leading to increased leukocyte motility, degranulation, and free radical formation. PAF plays an integral role in promoting activation and adherence of inflammatory cells to the endothelium.[168] During the early inflammatory response, activated endothelial cells synthesize and express PAF on the cell surface. Leukocytes tethered by selectins to the endothelium are activated by endothelial PAF, which results in the induction of tight integrin-dependent adhesion and subsequent emigration and chemotaxis toward the inflammatory focus. Acyl-PAF, the major acetylated lipid from mast cells, basophils, and endothelial cells, is a less potent derivative of PAF that likely plays a similar role in the regulation of neutrophil recruitment. PAF also promotes platelet and neutrophil aggregation, thereby contributing to the prothrombotic state of acute inflammation. In circumstances of persistent pathologic stimuli, PAF may be liberated systemically, thereby causing the sequelae of an excessive inflammatory response. As a mediator of sepsis, PAF augments endotoxin-induced hypotension and neutrophil and platelet accumulation in the lungs. There is evidence that the NO-induced hypotension in experimental models of endotoxemia is mediated by PAF.[169] PAF infusion leads to a shock state that is similar to septic shock in that there is tissue hypoperfusion despite adequate fluid resuscitation. In animal studies, PAF has been shown to contribute many manifestations of sepsis including coronary vasoconstriction, reduced cardiac contractility, reduced preload, peripheral vasodilation, pulmonary vasoconstriction, increased microvascular permeability, gastrointestinal hemorrhage, and thrombocytopenia.[160] Two prospective randomized, placebo-controlled trials of PAF inhibition in sepsis have suggested a benefit.[160]

PAF acetylhydrolase, an enzyme regulated by dexamethasone, estrogen, and PAF itself, is the enzyme responsible for degradation of PAF.

Kinins

Kinins (i.e., bradykinin and lysyl bradykinin) are small vasoactive peptides generated during the inflammatory response (Fig. 6.12). Three mechanisms of kinin formation are operant during inflammation: plasma proteins, tissue proteins, and cellular proteinases.[170–173]

Production of Bradykinin

Biosynthesis commences with the activation of Hageman factor (HF), or factor XII of the coagulation cascade (see Fig. 6.12). HF is activated by exposure to anionic surfaces such as the basement membrane of injured endothelium, heparin, or lipid A of endotoxin. It can also be proteolytically cleaved and activated by kallikrein. Prekallikrein circulates complexed with HMWK, a nonenzymatic protein. Kininogen enhances the binding of prekallikrein to negatively charged surfaces. Activated HF converts prekallikrein to kallikrein, which in turn activates more HF in a positive feedback cycle. HFf, a cleavage product of activated HF, is also capable of activating prekallikrein. Kallikrein in plasma, tissues, and secretions specifically cleaves HMWK to release the nonapeptide bradykinin. In addition to bradykinin production, kallikrein participates in the activation of plasminogen and C1q of the complement system, yet another link between inflammation and the coagulation system. The only major plasma inhibitor of activated HF is C1 inhibitor. The primary inhibitors of kallikrein in plasma are C1 inhibitor and α_1 macroglobulin.[38,170]

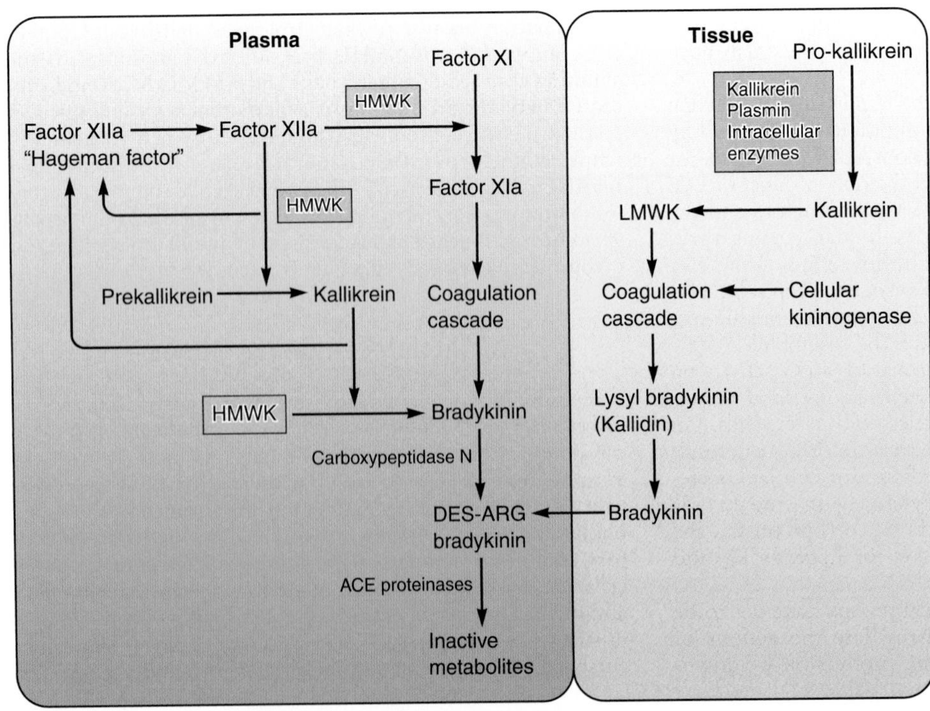

FIGURE 6.12 Kinin pathway. (Modified from Proud D, Kaplan AP. Kinin formation: mechanisms and role in inflammatory disorders. *Annu Rev Immunol.* 1988;6:49.)

Kinin Production in Tissue

Lysyl-bradykinin (kallidin) is the cleavage product of either HMWK or low-molecular-weight kininogen (LMWK) by tissue kallikreins, which are proteins distinct from their plasma counterparts. LMWK is present in higher concentrations intracellularly compared with HMWK. Whereas both HMWK and LMWK can be converted to lysyl-bradykinin by tissue kallikrein, only HMWK is cleaved by plasma kallikrein. Kallidin itself can be converted to bradykinin by a plasma aminopeptidase. Both kallidin and bradykinin use the same receptors and perform similar functions, but kallidin is approximately 85% as potent as bradykinin. Tissue kallikrein is synthesized from a preproenzyme and is converted intracellularly to tissue prokallikrein by enzymes that are not yet well characterized. The secreted prokallikrein is then converted to tissue kallikrein extracellularly by plasmin or plasma kallikrein. The only significant inhibitor of tissue kallikreins is α_1-proteinase inhibitor.[38,170]

Cellular Kininogenase Activity

Neutrophils, mast cells, and basophils are sources of kininogenase activity. Neutrophils produce leukokinins by way of cathepsin D. Their role in inflammation is unclear. Bradykinin is metabolized sequentially to the partially active eight amino acid peptide, des-Arg-bradykinin, by carboxypeptidase N, and then to inactive five-amino acid and three-amino acid fragments by the angiotensin-converting enzyme (ACE). ACE is the predominant enzyme to inactivate bradykinin in the pulmonary vasculature. Arginine released as a byproduct of the carboxypeptidase N reaction may contribute further to the modulation of inflammation by acting as a substrate for the formation of NO.[38,170,174]

There are three kinin receptors, of which two are well characterized.[170,172] B1 receptors are expressed primarily on the vasculature under pathologic conditions such as tissue injury. They bind des-Arg-bradykinin and des-Arg-kallidin and may mediate the hypotension characteristic of sepsis as well as pain.[170,175] Both B1 and the more widely distributed B2 receptors are G-protein coupled receptors. Activation of B2 receptors stimulates PLC, resulting in the accumulation of the second messengers IP_3, DAG, and calcium. The B2 receptors are more important in mediating the effects of inflammatory kinins, such as bradykinin and lysyl-bradykinin. These kinins induce arteriolar dilatation and mediate pain. Similar to histamine, bradykinin increases the gaps between postcapillary venule endothelial cells to increase in vascular permeability. It is a potent constrictor of bronchial, uterine, and gastrointestinal smooth muscle, as well as the coronary and pulmonary vasculature.[172] Activation of endothelial B2 receptors stimulates production of NO to further enhance vasodilatation. Kinins have been implicated in mediating the antihypertensive and cardioprotective effects of ACE inhibitors.[176] ACE, in addition to catalyzing the formation of angiotensin II from angiotensin I, promotes the hydrolysis of bradykinin to inactive metabolites. In addition, bradykinin can modulate platelet function by stimulating endothelial cell secretion of PGI_2 and thromboxane through activation of PLA_2.[170]

Neuropeptides

Neuropeptides may provide the neuroendocrine link between psychological stress and inflammatory diseases such as psoriasis and inflammatory bowel disease. Like cytokines, their actions are pleiotropic and redundant. Neuropeptides execute their inflammatory and immunomodulatory effect by binding to specific G-protein-coupled receptors on the surfaces of target cells, and the resultant effect may be proinflammatory, antiinflammatory, or both. For example, substance P mediates the hypothalamic fever response to PGE_2 induced by IL-1 and TNFα, whereas adrenocorticotropic hormone (ACTH), arginine vasopressin (AVP), and α-melanocyte stimulating hormone (α-MSH) suppress it. The pituitary peptides prolactin, corticotropin-releasing hormone (CRH), and AVP have been shown to augment immune responses by enhancing T_H1 activity.[38,177,178]

Tachykinins are important proinflammatory neuropeptides that mediate pain and vasodilatation and promote the classic inflammatory signs of erythema and edema. Substance P stimulates monocyte and neutrophil influx and neutrophil phagocytosis. Its inflammatory effects appear to be mediated by the proinflammatory cytokines TNFα and IL-1 from mast cells, monocytes, macrophages, bone marrow, and endothelial cells. During allergic inflammation, substance P stimulates histamine release from mast cells. As an effector of immune function, substance P promotes T-cell proliferation and antibody production. Substance P released locally by nerve terminals is important in mediating the perception of pain.[38,170]

CRH induces the release of IL-1, IL-6, and superoxide anion from macrophages and regulates its own proinflammatory effects through cortisol release. Cortisol down-regulates production of proinflammatory cytokines such as IL-1, TNFα, and IL-2; metalloproteinases; and inducible nitric oxide synthase (iNOS), and through this negative feedback loop, it inhibits the production of CRH as well as ACTH and AVP. AVP, growth hormone, and prolactin are other important proinflammatory neuropeptides.[38,177,178]

Vasoactive intestinal peptide (VIP) and its homologues display both proinflammatory and antiinflammatory effects. VIP is widely distributed throughout the central and peripheral nervous systems and serves as a chemoattractant for macrophages, neutrophils, and T cells and may play an important role in granulomatous reactions. VIP stimulates the release of histamine and IL-5 and is a potent vasodilator. It inhibits IL-6, TNFα, and IL-12 release and iNOS expression in activated macrophages. VIP has also been shown to stimulate the production of the antiinflammatory cytokine IL-10 by macrophages and inhibit T-lymphocyte proliferation and the production IL-2 and IFN-γ production.[179]

Somatostatin and α-MSH are primarily antiinflammatory in action. Somatostatin, which colocalizes with substance P in sensory nerves, inhibits IgE formation and NK cell activity. α-MSH inhibits leukocyte chemotaxis and IFN-γ production and down-regulates T_H1 activity. ACTH, calcitonin, and β endorphin are other neuropeptides with predominantly antiinflammatory properties.[38]

Calcitonin gene-related peptide (CGRP) is an immunomodulator that inhibits the activity of T cells and macrophages, in part through the induction of IL-10. It also is an inhibitor of antigen presentation. CGRP promotes vasodilatation and neutrophil influx and synergizes with bradykinin and histamine to promote edema formation.

Nitric Oxide

The endogenous synthesis of NO was first identified in 1987, and NO was the first gaseous molecule shown to be synthesized for the purpose of cell signaling.[180] NO is a weakly reactive radical that diffuses short distances from cell to cell independent of membrane channels or receptors. Its half-life is short because of its rapid inactivation by hemoglobin and other endogenous substances; thus, it functions primarily in a paracrine and autocrine fashion. The enzyme nitric oxide synthase (NOS) catalyzes the formation of NO and citrulline from the substrates L-arginine and oxygen.[47,181–183]

NOS contains prosthetic groups for flavin-adenine dinucleotide, flavin mononucleotide, tetrahydrobiopterin, iron protoporphyrin IX, and zinc. Three isoforms of NOS have been identified. The calcium-dependent constitutive isoforms, neuronal NOS (nNOS) and endothelial NOS (eNOS) generate the small amounts of NO necessary for those processes maintaining physiologic homeostasis, such as neurotransmission and endothelial regulation of vascular tone. The expression of iNOS, however, requires stimulation and produces larger, sustained amounts of NO with both cytoprotective and cytotoxic properties. This distinction is not absolute, as certain cell populations express low basal levels of iNOS, and constitutive NOS transcripts can be enhanced by certain stimuli such as shear and hypoxia.[47,181–183]

Many of the physiologic effects of NO are mediated by the activation of soluble guanylate cyclase. Increased levels of intracellular cyclic guanosine monophosphate trigger a reduction in calcium concentration and promote vascular smooth muscle relaxation and the inhibition of platelet aggregation and adhesion. The cellular response to NO also likely involves multiple signal transduction mechanisms including the MAPK pathway.

Inflammation secondary to endotoxemia, hemorrhagic shock, and ischemia/reperfusion are associated with increased NO production by iNOS. iNOS, first described in macrophages can be expressed in essentially any cell type in response to immunologic stimuli and, unlike nNOS and eNOS, does not depend on elevations in intracellular calcium levels for its activity.[47,181–183] Important activators of iNOS up-regulation include LPS, IL-1, TNFα, and IFN-γ. Expression is primarily transcriptionally regulated, although stabilization of iNOS mRNA also appears to play a role. IFN-γ stabilizes iNOS mRNA, whereas TGF-β can destabilize it. Transcription of the iNOS gene is controlled by NFκB, IFN-γ-responsive element, and TNF-responsive element. Induction of iNOS can be inhibited by glucocorticoids, thrombin, macrophage deactivation factor, PDGF, IL-4, IL-8, IL-10, and IL-13.[47,181–183] Dexamethasone may inhibit iNOS induction by impairing the DNA binding capacity of NFκB and by increasing levels of IκB.[184,185]

The endothelial dysfunction and vascular hyporeactivity characteristic of septic shock is mediated in part by iNOS production of NO.[186] NO has been shown to be the effective mediator of the negative myocardial inotropy of TNFα, IL-6, and IL-2 and the TNFα-induced vasodilatation in the systemic and microcirculations.[187] NO may indirectly increase prostaglandin production by increasing the catalytic activity of cyclooxygenase and decrease leukotriene production by inhibiting 5-LO.[188] NO plays an autoregulatory role in the T_H1 subset of T_H cells by limiting their own proliferation.[189]

NO can mediate tissue injury in inflammation by modulating organ perfusion, mediating interactions with neutrophils, contributing to proinflammatory signaling, and regulating apoptosis.[190] Whereas eNOS primarily regulates perfusion during homeostasis, both eNOS and iNOS modulate organ flow in pathophysiologic states. Basal NO production from eNOS prevents the adherence of neutrophils to the endothelium and inhibits chemotaxis under physiologic conditions. Animal studies in endotoxemia implicate an anti-adhesive role for iNOS.[190] Conversely, similar experiments have demonstrated that pharmacologic inhibition of iNOS or genetic deletion of iNOS attenuates neutrophil accumulation in organs after ischemia/reperfusion injury, suggesting that the effect of induced NO on neutrophil accumulation is insult specific.[191] Activated neutrophils can be stimulated by fMLP, PAF, and LTB_4 to produce NO. NO produced by neutrophils at sites of inflammation can combine with superoxide to form peroxynitrite as another means of effecting toxicity.[38,192]

The reaction of NO with superoxide is the only reaction that outcompetes the reaction of superoxide with superoxide dismutase. Although small amounts of peroxynitrite are produced under basal conditions from constitutively produced NO and superoxide from mitochondria and other cellular sources, endogenous antioxidants such as GSH, vitamin E and C, and superoxide dismutase likely limit its toxicity. A low concentration of peroxynitrite has been shown to inhibit neutrophil adhesion. Higher concentrations of peroxynitrite can initiate a wide range of toxic oxidative reactions through a peroxynitrous acid intermediate. These include the initiation of tyrosine nitration, lipid peroxidation, and direct inhibition of mitochondrial respiratory enzymes. The balance between superoxide and NO determines the reactivity of peroxynitrite; excess NO reduces the oxidation elicited by peroxynitrite. In addition, peroxynitrite may contribute to cytotoxicity by a more indirect pathway. Peroxynitrite-induced single strand breaks in DNA activate the nuclear enzyme poly (ADP-ribose) synthetase, leading eventually to irreversible energy depletion of the cells and necrotic-type cell death.[38,39]

Inducible NOS plays a key role in host defense, with NO or peroxynitrite exhibiting potent antimicrobial activity against a number of pathogens including viruses, fungi, and bacteria. Although microbicidal susceptibility to NO-mediated killing can vary considerable between species, essential roles have been identified in tuberculosis and bacterial peritonitis.[193] Induced NO has been shown to be essential for the up-regulation of the inflammatory response in hemorrhage shock and is likely to be so in other inflammatory processes. NO produced by iNOS leads to the activation of NFkB.[194] This is followed by the induction of proinflammatory cytokines and increased leukocyte recruitment and activation.

NO has demonstrated both proapoptotic and antiapoptotic effects depending on the circumstances. NO derived from eNOS may inhibit apoptosis.[195] Pro-apoptotic effects appear to be associated with pathophysiologic conditions in which iNOS is up-regulated. Low concentrations of peroxynitrite have also been shown to induce apoptosis, whereas higher concentrations promote cell necrosis in vitro. The role of NO-mediated apoptosis in the regulation of the inflammatory response is yet to be more clearly defined.

In summary, NO mediates tissue injury both directly through the formation of peroxynitrite and indirectly through the amplification of the inflammatory process. Like many mediators, however, NO has dual regulatory functions and is therefore difficult to characterize as either proinflammatory or antiinflammatory. In general, basal levels of NO produced by constitutive NOS may confer antiinflammatory effects, whereas induced NO may tend to promote the up-regulation of the inflammatory response. It is likely that an optimal level of NO is necessary in host defense; too little NO may be as harmful as too much.

Heme Oxygenase

Heme oxygenase (HO) catalyzes the breakdown of heme to iron, biliverdin, and carbon monoxide (CO). Three isoforms of HO have been identified. HO-2 is constitutively expressed in many tissues, whereas HO-3 expression appears to be limited to the brain. HO-1 is not expressed constitutively but is rapidly up-regulated during hypoxia, following redox stress, and during inflammation. NO is a potent inducer of HO-1 expression. HO-1 has profound antiapoptotic and antiinflammatory effects mediated through the antioxidant properties of biliverdin. Bilirubin is converted to biliverdin by biliverdin reductase and both molecules have antioxidant properties. Carbon monoxide alone can mimic many of the actions of HO-1 and has been shown to protect in models of sepsis, hemorrhagic shock, and ischemia/reperfusion when administered as an inhaled gas.

RECOGNITION AND ACTIVATION PROCESSES

Exogenous and Endogenous Danger Recognition

The previous discourse illuminates the complexities and intricacies of the many mediators and activation cascades operant during inflammation. The current velocity with which science is unraveling these processes is increasing on an exponential scale; at the present, we understand a fraction of what occurs. Recent literature has begun to elucidate the manner by which these cascades are set into motion. Many of the receptors for infectious insults have been previously described. However, an inflammatory reaction can also be triggered in a noninfectious environment, indicating that damaged cells can themselves produce and release molecules functioning as danger signals. It is becoming apparent that specific receptors exist by which to recognize and distinguish either extrinsic threat (pathogen) and intrinsic altered self (cytokines, oxidized mitochondrial DNA, heat-shock proteins, and uric acid).

Receptors for Danger Recognition

CD14/TLR. The prototypical receptor identifying external infectious threat is CD14. CD14 was identified as the LPS receptor when transfection of CD14-negative CHO cells with CD14 conferred responsiveness to LPS.[196] It has been identified on cells of the myeloid lineage, B cells, liver parenchymal cells, and fibroblasts. Differential expression is observed, ranging from high levels on peritoneal and pleural macrophages to lower levels on Kupffer cells, alveolar macrophages, monocytes, and PMN. Expression may be modified as human PMN express low levels of CD14 that is up-regulated by TNFα, G-CSF, GM-CSF, and fMLP. It currently is believed that CD14 binds LPS bound to LPS-binding protein (LBP) and presents it to TLR4. It is also important in TLR2 signaling, whereby it presents bacterial products other than LPS.

However, CD14 is a glycosylphosphatidylinositol-linked receptor devoid of any transmembrane domain. This in combination with the identification of a soluble form of CD14, necessitated identifying the manner by which LPS induced activation.[197] In 1996 the *Drosophila* protein Toll was shown to be required for an effective immune response to the fungus *Aspergillus fumigatus.* In 1998, TLR4 was identified as the LPS receptor and shown to be essential for murine defense against gram-negative bacteria. These findings revealed that the proximal innate immune sensing apparatus of insects and mammals are related by descent and suggested a central role for TLRs in the primary recognition of infectious pathogens by mammals.[196]

Thirteen mammalian TLR receptors have been identified of which each recognizes a specific set of conserved microbial molecules, so that collectively they can detect most microbes. Despite significant conservation within the binding regions, different TLRs can recognize several structurally unrelated ligands. The subcellular localization of different TLRs correlates to some extent with the molecular patterns of their ligands.[198] TLR1, TLR2, and TLR4 are located on the cell surface and are recruited to phagosomes after activation by their respective ligands. By contrast, TLR3, TLR7, and TLR9, all of which are involved in the recognition of nucleic-acid like structures, are not expressed on the cell surface.

TLR4 is required for the innate response to gram-negative LPS. Individuals with the D299G polymorphism demonstrate increased risk of gram-negative infections, and other studies have linked this with an increased incidence of SIRS. In addition, this polymorphism has been associated with alterations in the susceptibility to other inflammatory and potentially infectious processes (carotid artery atherosclerosis, coronary artery disease). HSP60 of chlamydial origin has been found in atherosclerotic plaques and can bind TLR4. Perhaps recognition of HSP60 by human TLR4 might exacerbate the inflammatory component of atherosclerosis, whereas people with the D299G polymorphism might be at least partly protected from this exacerbation.[199]

TLR2 is the major mammalian receptor for lipoproteins derived from the cell wall of bacteria such as *Treponema pallidum* and *Mycoplasma fermentans.* The R753Q polymorphism in the TLR2 is associated with decreased response to these bacteria and may increase susceptibility to staphylococcal infections or tuberculosis.[199]

Four adaptor proteins, MyD88 (myeloid differentiation factor 88), MAL/TIRAP (MyD88-adaptor-like/TIR-associated protein), TRIF (Toll-receptor-associated activator of interferon), and TRAM (Toll-receptor-associated molecule), transduce signals from all of the TIR [Toll-interleukin-1 receptor (IL-1R) homologous region] domains, activating protein kinases and then transcription factors that cause inflammatory effects.[196,198–200]

Most of this research has occurred in the realm of sepsis and provided insight into the manner by which organisms identify infectious threats and activate the inflammatory pathway to preserve the host. However, several circumstances of sterile inflammation suggest a role of the TLRs in mediating inflammation in response to endogenous danger signals (uric acid, mitochondrial DNA, HMGB1).[196]

RAGE. RAGE is an immunoglobulin superfamily molecule that belongs to the multiligand receptors that recognize families of ligands rather than a single polypeptide.[88,201,202] It has a single transmembrane spanning domain and a highly charged cytoplasmic tail that, although lacking known signaling motifs, is critical for cellular activation. It is thought that signaling necessitates clustering into a particular orientation, which facilitates binding of cytosolic signaling complexes.[88,201] Its ligands include products of nonenzymatic glycoxidation [e.g., advanced glycation end-products (AGEs)], the amyloid-β precursor protein, the S100/calgranulin family of proinflammatory cytokine-like mediators, and the high mobility group 1 DNA binding proteins (HMGB-1), and its expression is up-regulated at sites of diverse pathologies including atherosclerosis and Alzheimer's disease. In fact RAGE-mediated cellular stimulation is thought to increase expression of the receptor itself, thereby generating a positive feedback mechanism and perpetuating the proinflammatory state.[88,201,202]

Recent studies demonstrate the activation of multiple signal transduction cascades subsequent to ligand binding, including the MAPK family (p38, ERK1/2, and JNK) and rho gtpases (cdc42 and rac).[202] It is currently hypothesized that RAGE-ligand interaction induces a new heightened basal state of activation. With a superimposed stimulus, cellular perturbation is magnified. Rather than returning to homeostasis, cellular signal transduction mechanisms favor augmented dysfunction.[88,201]

Studies have implicated RAGE to be an important receptor during various acute and chronic inflammatory processes as well as tumor biology. RAGE expression and function directly correlated with tumor growth in RAGE-transfected C6 glioma cells. In a murine tumor model, mice treated with soluble RAGE, which functions as a decoy, demonstrated a reduction in lung metastases, cellular invasion, and expression of matrix metalloproteinases.[202]

RAGE has also been identified as a receptor for S100A12, a member of the S100/calgranulin family of proinflammatory mediators. Endothelial cells cultured with S100A12 displayed RAGE-dependent expression of VCAM-1 and tissue factor. Mononuclear phagocytes displayed S100A12-RAGE chemotaxis, expression of tissue factor, and elaborated IL-1 and TNFα. In vivo studies of delayed type hypersensitivity demonstrated reduced inflammatory response when mice were treated with anti-RAGE F(ab')$_2$, anti-S100 F(ab')$_2$, or soluble RAGE. Treated animals also displayed reduced NFκB activation and IL-1 and TNF expression.[202]

The angiopathy of diabetes is thought to be consequent to inflammatory processes generated by elevated glucose concentrations. Hyperglycemia has been demonstrated to activate numerous signaling cascades. One process that might mediate these effects is through the nonenzymatic formation of AGEs.[88,201,202] AGE-RAGE interactions on endothelium lead to the expression of procoagulant tissue factor and VCAM-1 and macrophage released tissue factor. Animals treated with soluble RAGE showed decreases in atherosclerotic lesion area and number and a marked reduction in lesion complexity. Also, treated animals had reduced expression of adhesion molecules, tissue factor, MCP-1, and matrix metalloproteinases.[88,201,202]

CD91. The immunologic properties of heat shock proteins (HSP) were discovered by their ability to elicit antitumor immunity. It was later discovered that this antigenic specificity was determined by the peptides they chaperoned. APCs can bind and internalize HSP-peptide complexes derived from virus-infected cells or tumors and represent them on major histocompatibility MHC class I molecules. In addition, APC engagement of HSP-peptide complexes induces maturation, the expression of costimulatory molecules, and the induction and release of cytokines (TNFα, IL-1, IL-12, IL-6, GM-CSF, MIP-1, RANTES, and NO).[203,204]

CD91 had been identified as a receptor for the serum protein α_2 macroglobulin, a natural protease inhibitor that like HSPs is found across many species. In fact α_2 macroglobulin is the evolutionary precursor of the C3 complement component. It is thought that by binding pathogen proteases utilized during invasion and shuttling them for endocytosis, α_2 macroglobulin hindered pathogen invasion.[203,205]

However, such a method of host defense would be ineffective for intracellular pathogens that gain access by alternative means, such as mimicking host proteins and developing ligands for host receptors. Hence, another method of signaling danger is necessary. It is currently thought that on cell death, HSPs contained within the cell transfer information regarding the infected intracellular environment to CD91. This large cell surface receptor, complexed with the HSPs, is internalized and delivers antigen into the classical MHC class I pathway. The MHCs bind and present them to CD8$^+$ T cells. On recognizing nonself, T cells are induced to proliferate and mediate killing. This mechanism could be generalized to implicate CD91 and HSP interactions in the recognition of all cellular stress that culminates in injury and death.[205]

CD91 was first identified by Binder et al.[204,207] as the receptor for gp96 and then by Basu as a common receptor for other HSPs (HSP70, HSP90, and calreticulin). This large multidomain 600-kD protein possesses multiple binding sites for at least 32 ligands. The binding of this receptor to many members of the HSP family has been corroborated by several independent functional and structural studies.[205]

Several in vivo studies suggest a physiologic relevance for HSP-CD91 interaction. Mice immunized with tumor-derived gp96-peptide complexes reject a subsequent tumor challenge. If CD91 antiserum is mixed with the HSP-peptide inoculum, the mice fail to reject the tumors. Binder et al.[204,206] noted that blocking of CD91 completely inhibits the phenomenon of representation of peptides that are carried or chaperoned by HSPs, suggesting that not only is CD91 a receptor for HSPs but also it may be the sole receptor involved in antigen representing.

HSPs have been shown to chaperone antigenic peptides (tumor, viral, minor histocompatibility antigens) from all cellular compartments. The HSPs thus appear to be a universal mechanism for antigen capture, and they permit a high-efficiency antigen uptake through a receptor-mediated mechanism.

Evidence that HSP-peptide-CD91 interactions serve to signal cellular stress is beginning to culminate. Basu et al.[207] demonstrate that hsp70, hsp90, gp96, and calreticulin are released from cells as a result of necrotic cell death but not apoptotic cell death. Similarly, Melcher et al.[208] reported that tumor cells undergoing necrotic death are highly immunogenic as compared to those undergoing apoptotic death. Actual necrosis may be unnecessary as stressed cells and cancer cells have been reported to express cell surface HSP molecules, which may activate APCs. Zheng et al.[209] observed that physical contact of tumor cells artificially engineered to express cell surface HSPs with immature DCs elicits a powerful maturation of DCs.

Other HSP Receptors. CD40 was reported as a receptor for hsp70 when anti-CD40 antibodies were observed to inhibit macrophage chemokine secretion in response to mycobacterial hsp70. Subsequently, Becker noted the association of recombinant GST-tagged CD40 with murine hsp70.[210,211] They further demonstrated enhanced binding after the APCs were stimulated with LPS. As LPS induces expression of a number of cell surface molecules, the authors concluded that CD40 mediates recognition and binding of hsp70.[212]

CD36 has been implicated as a receptor for gp96. Transfection of CD36 into CD36-negative cells has been shown to enhance gp96 binding. In addition, CD36-/ macrophages have a 52% reduction in gp96 binding compared with wild-type controls, suggesting that some role for CD36 as a hsp receptor.[212]

LOX-1, a member of the same scavenger superfamily as CD91 and CD36, has been postulated to be an additional receptor for endocytic uptake of hsp70 and chaperoned peptides by human DCs. Anti-LOX-1 antibodies and LOX-1 ligand-acetylated albumin competed with hsp70 for binding to DCs.[103]

Both TLRs and CD14 have been implicated as receptors for HSPs, such as hsp70.[213] hsp70 stimulates macrophage IL-12p40 production that is partially abrogated by inhibiting downstream TLR signaling cascades. In addition, human hsp60 activated NFκB and TNFα production by 293T cells transfected with either TLR-2 or TLR-4 and MD-2.[214] hsp60 also activated JNK kinase and IKK kinase signaling and TNFα production by macrophages, an effect that was partially eliminated by knocking out MyD88 or TRAF6. Similar functional studies have proposed that CD14 might serve as an hsp70 receptor in APCs. All of these studies heavily suggest a role of TLRs or CD14 in HSP binding, although several investigators call into question the potential for contamination with LPS to be mediating much of these effects.[212]

The Stress Response

The stress response is the cellular reaction to any external perturbation or disruption in equilibrium and serves to restore homeostasis. It is often referred to as the heat-shock response after the identification in the 1960s of a group of genes expressed after exposure to heat, the heat-shock proteins (supra vida).[215] However, subsequent investigations delineated additional cellular proteins that were expressed in response to a wide variety of insults. Inducers of the stress response include physical stresses (burns, radiation, trauma), chemical agents and mediators (toxin, heavy metals, cytokines, ROS), infectious agents (bacteria, viruses, parasites), and allergens. Clinically, expression of HSP has been observed under conditions in which oxygen delivery is compromised, as in hemorrhage or ischemia.[216]

Activation of the stress response is characterized by both morphologic and metabolic cellular alterations. Morphologic alterations include the accumulation of unprocessed forms of mRNA in the nucleolus and increased numbers of actin microfilaments in the cytoplasm. Changes in cellular metabolism include a rapid reduction in intracellular ATP levels, most likely correlated with alterations in the integrity of mitochondria. The stress response is characterized by transient down-regulation of most cellular products and by the up-regulation of stress proteins.[217] It is the induction of stress proteins that confers the primary adaptive and protective effects of the stress response. After expression of stress genes, cells become resistant to subsequent stresses. Members of the stress protein family include heme oxygenase (supra vida); the multiple-drug resistance gene product or P-glycoprotein, ubiquitin, involved in targeting proteins for degradation; scavengers such as superoxide dismutase, ferritin, and metallothioneins; and the glycolytic enzymes enolase and glyceraldehyde 3-phosphate dehydrogenase. The most extensively characterized are the HSPs.[38]

Heat-shock proteins are molecular chaperones that may either be constitutively expressed or induced upon cellular stress.[218] Classification is based on their molecular mass and degree of homology. The most extensively studied is the hsp70 family, members of which possess a mean molecular mass of 70 kd and greater than 70% homology. Members of the Hsp70 family bind ATP, and under conditions of energy depletion the stress response is induced. Hsp70 is integral in cellular adaptation to and survival during environmental stresses. Both Hsp72 and Hsp 73 are present in the cytosol and nucleus; the former is constitutively expressed, whereas, expression of Hsp 72 is exclusively induced after stress. In most studies Hsp72 is used as a marker of HSP induction.[38,216,219,220]

The Hsp60 family members are also referred to as chaperonins. The glucose-regulated protein group of HSP is induced with glucose starvation, inhibitors of N-glycosylation, and calcium ionophores. The decrease in glucose content may affect the pool of sugar donors during protein glycosylation. The low-molecular-weight HSP (molecular masses of 20 to 30 kd) may be important regulatory components of the actin-based cytoskeleton.[216]

Transcription is mediated by the activation of heat-shock elements in the gene promoters. Two heat-shock transcriptional factors (HSF) have been identified, HSF1 and HSF2. HSF1 activates transcription of the Hsp72 gene in response to heat, heavy metals, and other inducers of the stress response. With stimulation, unbound HSF1 oligomerizes, translocates to the nucleus, and binds to the HSP promoter to activate the transcription of the gene. HSF2 is not activated by the classic inducers of heat shock genes but may be important in controlling the activities of HSP gene expression in the normal or unstressed cell.[38,216,219,220]

HSP can play multiple roles in modulating the inflammatory response. A number of inflammatory states such as rheumatoid arthritis, ARDS, and asthma have been shown to benefit experimentally from increased HSP expression.[215–217,220] Functions of HSP during inflammation include enhancement of immune responses, thermotolerance, regulation of apoptosis, hemostasis, and cytoprotection against ROS and other inflammatory mediators. HSP-CD91 interaction are integral to the processing and representation of antigen by APCs. HSP may shift the balance between T_H1 and T_H2 toward an increase in more antiinflammatoryantiinflammatory T_H2 cells. ROS, including H_2O_2, hydroxyl radical, and peroxynitrite, activate HSP synthesis. In the presence of iron, ROS also induce the oxidation-specific stress protein heme oxygenase or ferritin, proteins contributing protection against oxidative stress by binding iron and preventing it from participating in the Fenton reaction. Mechanisms of HSP-mediated cytoprotection from the toxic effects of ROS include the maintenance of cellular GSH levels (Hsp27) and mitochondrial protection (Hsp70). Hence, ROS induce a cytoprotective response that counteracts their own toxicity. Other inflammatory mediators such as NO have also been shown to induce expression of HSP.[38]

HSP may participate in intracellular signaling pathways that modulate the production or function of inflammatory mediators. For example, Hsp90 has been shown to facilitate signaling that leads to NO formation by eNOS.[221] Hsp70 has been reported to prevent apoptosis, which may promote propagation rather than resolution of inflammation. In addition, the body's immune response to bacterial and parasitic stress proteins likely protects the host from infection. The bacterial homologue of Hsp60, GroEL, is a major target of the mammalian humoral response to bacterial infections. Many activators of HSF1 are potent inhibitors of the proinflammatory transcription factor NFκB. Aspirin and other NSAIDs activate HSF while inhibiting NFκB. Therefore, the antiinflammatory effects associated with the stress response might be related more to the inhibition of NFκB activation.[216,222]

The Acute-Phase Response

The acute-phase response consequent to trauma or cellular injury is characterized by alterations in hepatic metabolism; activation of the central nervous system, leading to fever and adaptive behaviors; altered hematopoiesis; activation of complement and the fibrinolytic and coagulation cascades; and the release of neuropeptides, kinins, and hormones. It is a rapid, nonspecific response that accompanies both acute and chronic inflammatory disorders. Many of the processes induced during the acute-phase response are mediated by cytokines; IL-6, IL-1, and TNFα play particularly central roles.[223,224] Though considered a defense mechanism promoting host survival, aberrant or unregulated production of many of these inflammatory mediators can be lethal.

Acute-Phase Proteins

An acute-phase protein is defined as a protein whose concentration increases by at least 25% during inflammation (see Table 6.8).[224,225] These changes are primarily due to altered hepatic synthesis, typically occur within approximately 6 hours of the inciting stimulus, and function to restore homeostasis. These functions include hemostatic functions (fibrinogen), microbicidal and phagocytic functions (complement components, C-reactive protein), antithrombotic properties (plasminogen, protein S), antioxidant properties (haptoglobin), and antiproteolytic actions (α_2 macroglobulin, α_1 protease, α_1 chymotrypsin). The negative acute-phase proteins albumin, prealbumin, transferrin, and retinol-binding protein decrease by at least 25%. Levels of the negative acute-phase proteins albumin and transferrin drop almost immediately after operation and remain depressed for several days. The rapid initial loss of these proteins is likely due to increased vascular permeability and loss to the extravascular space. The magnitude of the response is proportional to the severity of the stress and is specific to the genetic composition of the patient. Whereas trauma and burns lead to significant increases in acute-phase reactants, exercise and psychiatric illness induce more moderate responses.

The two major acute-phase proteins in humans are C-reactive protein (CRP) and serum amyloid A (SAA). CRP, named because of its reaction with pneumococcal C-polysaccharide, displays both proinflammatory and antiinflammatory effects. It has been shown to activate complement, recognize foreign pathogens, bind phagocytic cells, and enhance activation of tissue factor, the main initiator of coagulation. CRP can also inhibit superoxide production by neutrophils and inhibit neutrophil adhesion by decreasing surface expression of L-selectin. Changes in plasma or serum CRP, although nonspecific, may reflect the magnitude of an inflammatory process and may aid the differentiation of inflammatory from noninflammatory conditions. Measurement of CRP is more precise than the erythrocyte sedimentation rate, which largely depends on plasma fibrinogen levels and is influenced by a variety of other, unrelated factors in the circulation. SAA may affect cholesterol metabolism and promote chemotaxis and adhesion of phagocytes during inflammation.[38]

C1 inhibitor is of special interest as an acute-phase protein because of its effects outside of the complement cascade. This antiprotease inhibits the activity of HF, limiting kinin production and factor XI production. Thus, enhanced expression of a complement inhibitor protein during the acute phase influences such diverse processes as the coagulation, fibrinolysis, and kinin pathways.

Systemic Manifestations

Systemic manifestations include neuroendocrine changes, shifts in the hematologic profile, and metabolic and chemical alterations. The classic neuroendocrine manifestation is fever. IL-1, IL-6, and TNFα mediate the fever response by resetting the hypothalamic temperature setpoint through the synthesis of PGE_2. The secretion of neuropeptides such as CRH and AVP and of hormones such as glucagon, insulin, thyroxine, and aldosterone is also characteristic of the acute-phase response. CRH and AVP released by the hypothalamus increase ACTH and cortisol levels. The rise in plasma cortisol levels occurs rapidly and may function to inhibit the fever response and cytokine gene expression, thereby serving a potential regulatory function in the acute-phase response. Glucocorticoids also stimulate macrocortin synthesis, which by inhibiting synthesis of PLA_2, limits the availability of arachidonic acid for prostaglandin synthesis. Glucocorticoids increase the rate of synthesis of certain acute-phase proteins involved in connective tissue repair and clotting, as well as antioxidants and antiproteinases. They also may function to counteract the hypoglycemic response to insulin overproduction during infection or stress.

Other alterations include a prominent leukocytosis, thrombocytosis, and the anemia of chronic disease. Metabolic changes include altered lipid metabolism and negative nitrogen balance. Changes in the chemical and enzymatic profile include increased hepatic production of metallothionein, iNOS, heme oxygenase, manganese superoxide dismutase, and GSH. Plasma levels of zinc and iron are noted to drop, whereas copper levels increase slightly. This persists for the duration of inflammation and is likely due to sequestration induced by IL-6, glucocorticoids, and catecholamines. Low levels of iron and zinc may confer protective antimicrobial effects because they are essential for microbial growth.[38]

Mediators

Bacterial products such as LPS are probably the most potent activators of tissue macrophages, the initiators of the acute-phase response. LPS, through its interactions with LPS-binding protein, CD14, and Toll-like receptors, induces macrophage synthesis of ROS, including NO; lipid derivatives such as PGE_2, thromboxane A_2, and PAF; and acute-phase cytokines. The primary signals inducing synthesis of acute-phase cytokines in the absence of bacterial infection may be free radicals, prostaglandins, or modified proteins acting like foreign materials.[38]

Acute-phase cytokines can be proinflammatory (IL-1, TNFα, IFNγ, IL-8) or antiinflammatory (IL-10, IL-4, IL-13, TGF-β). However, it is IL-6 and IL-6-type cytokines that are most critical in the acute-phase response. IL-6 is the major inducer of acute-phase proteins synthesis and, together with IL-1 and TNFα, is responsible for the systemic features classically associated with the acute-phase response (fever, anorexia, leukocytosis, and hormonal changes).[38]

In addition to the aforementioned cytokines, IFNγ is a potent inducer of complement components. The antiinflammatory cytokine TGF-β stimulates synthesis of antiproteases, urokinase, and negative acute-phase proteins. IL-4 is inhibitory to some acute-phase proteins. Growth factors, including hepatocyte growth factor and TGF-β are also able to modulate the synthesis of acute-phase proteins. Glucocorticoids augment the response to cytokines, and insulin attenuates the cytokine-induced rise in acute-phase proteins.[38]

Effects of the cytokines are influenced by cytokine receptors, receptor antagonists, and hormones. IL-1RA competes with IL-1 and attenuates the acute-phase response in vivo. Soluble receptors for IL-1 and TNFα act as antagonists. In contrast, soluble receptors for IL-6 act as agonists.

Regulation of Acute-Phase Cytokines and Proteins

Several major families of transcription factors participate in the up-regulation of acute-phase cytokines and proteins, the most important being NF-IL-6, AP-1, and NFκB.[226] NF-IL6 participates in the induced expression of the cytokines IL-1, TNFα, IL-6, and IL-8, among others. Activation of cytokine gene expression by NFκB is probably the most important pathway. The triggering of IL-6 in monocytes in vitro by IFNγ involves a change in the amount of the phosphorylated transcription factor Sp1, together with the induction and activation of IFN-regulatory factor.

All known acute-phase proteins are regulated primarily at the transcriptional level. Activation of TNFα and IL-1 receptors triggers signaling pathways that activate transcription factors AP-1 and NFκB. Many type I acute-phase proteins genes contain response elements for NFκB, NF-IL6, and AP-1. Acute-phase protein responses to IL-6 are mediated through the JAK-STAT signal transduction pathway. In addition, both IL-1 and IL-6 signal transduction mechanisms activate the MAPK pathway that activates transcription factors NF-IL6, linking the IL-1 and IL-6 pathways.

Reperfusion Injury

Prolonged tissue ischemia produces irreversible injury and cell death. Timely restoration of perfusion may salvage some tissue, though paradoxically can induce injury as well. Reperfusion injury is the damage caused by the restoration of blood flow in previously ischemic tissue (i.e., myocardial ischemia, transplantation, vascular surgery). Injury is the direct consequence of activation of the inflammatory response, especially complement activation and neutrophil recruitment. Components of the complement cascade promote tissue damage through the generation of anaphylatoxins and by the formation of the MAC. Invading neutrophils injure tissue through the generation of ROS and the release of proteolytic enzymes.

Alterations in the microvascular endothelium are central to the pathophysiologic process of reperfusion injury. Early loss of constitutive NO production facilitates neutrophil adherence and the up-regulation of cell adhesion molecules such as P-selectin and inhibits vasorelaxation and perfusion.[227] Low oxygen tension induces the conversion of xanthine dehydrogenase to xanthine oxidase. Reperfusion and reoxygenation yields the formation of superoxide anion and H_2O_2 and induce oxidant injury. Neutrophils and other cellular effectors are progressively recruited and activated, releasing ROS, cytokines, and NO, further contributing to increased vascular permeability and tissue injury. PAF released by neutrophils activates circulating platelets and promotes vascular plugging. Platelets also release factors that enhance platelet-neutrophil adhesion. Both cell types also release vasoconstricting agents that can further exacerbate no-reflow. Capillary plugging by neutrophils and platelets can impair local blood flow and cause the "no-reflow phenomenon."[38]

Neutrophils mediate direct toxicity to the surrounding tissue through the elaboration of ROS and granule contents. Peroxynitrite formed by the reaction of NO and superoxide can contribute directly to tissue injury during reperfusion. Neutrophil granule proteases such as elastase, collagenase, and gelatinase alter the vascular permeability and are highly destructive to local tissue. The significance of the neutrophil in mediating these effects are apparent in neutrophil depletion studies demonstrating attenuated tissue injury compared with subjects with normal numbers of neutrophils.[228] Animal studies using blocking monoclonal antibodies to selectins and β_2 integrins show improved organ function following ischemia/reperfusion.[229]

The mechanism by which complement is activated with reperfusion is not completely understood. Ischemia may alter the cell's plasma membrane or through the exposure of basement membrane or subcellular organelle components, creating a complement-activating surface. Alternatively, binding of natural antibody may lead to induction of these cascades.[151] Complement activation has been shown to occur in the setting of therapeutic thrombolysis. The generation of plasmin-dependent fibrinolytic agents and plasmin after tissue plasminogen activator administration has been associated with complement activation.[230]

Anaphylatoxins are important effectors of complement-mediated injury. They alter vascular permeability and induce smooth muscle cell contraction and the release of histamine from mast cells and basophils. C3a and C5a are potent chemoattractants especially for neutrophils. C5 can be activated by oxygen free radicals, which are abundant. The subsequent generation of the MAC perturbs the maintenance of vital ion gradients, induces cell lysis, and facilitates neutrophil recruitment. In addition it can induce the expression of numerous inflammatory mediators, including cytokines (TNFα, IL-1, IL-8), ROS, prostaglandins, leukotrienes, and cell surface adhesion molecules.[231]

Systemic Inflammatory Response Syndrome

The inability of host defenses to control a localized inflammatory process or an unchecked systemic inflammatory response can result in SIRS. A recent consensus conference defined SIRS as the presence of any two of the following physiologic parameters: (a) a temperature greater than 38°C or less than 36°C; (b) leukocytosis (>12,000/mm^3), leukopenia (<4,000/mm^3), or more than 10% bands; (c) pulse greater than 90 beats per minute; (d) tachypnea (respiratory rate greater than 20 or PaCO2 <32 mm Hg).[232] Infection underlies only a significant minority of cases as a third of patients with SIRS will have a documented infection and meet the criteria for sepsis. There is a continuum from the development of SIRS to sepsis, to severe sepsis, septic shock, and MODS.[233] The outcome depends on the balance between SIRS and host compensatory mechanisms. In one prospective study, 26% of patients with SIRS developed sepsis and 7% died.[234]

SIRS may be initiated by infectious or noninfectious causes, such as trauma, autoimmune reactions, or pancreatitis. Gram-negative organisms, rich in LPS, induce a potent inflammatory response mediated through the CD14/TLR4/MyD88 pathway previously described and account for the majority of infectious SIRS cases. Gram-positive organisms can generate a similarly impressive degree of inflammation either through TLR2 or alternative mechanisms; streptococcal superantigen may induce a global and nonspecific activation of T cells that culminates in massive systemic elaboration of cytokines and cardiovascular collapse termed toxic shock syndrome. Trauma, either through tissue injury (HMGB1-RAGE, HSP-CD91) or the ischemia/reperfusion consequent to hemorrhage, can culminate in inflammatory pathophysiology indistinguishable from that accompanying these other inflammatory states. As evidence continues to grow, we are replacing the former concept that these stimuli possess individual receptor-signaling mechanisms with one that emphasizes the similarities and integration. Though there are clearly mechanisms by which host distinguishes normal self from endogenous (trauma) and exogenous (infection) dangers, there is considerable overlap in the receptors utilized and all stimuli appear to converge on similar signaling mechanisms in the attaining the goal of preserving the host.

The development of SIRS has been described as progressing through three stages: Stage I—local cytokine production recruits inflammatory cells to the injured site; Stage II—an acute-phase response is initiated and small quantities of cytokines are released into the circulation to enhance the local response; and Stage III—homeostasis cannot be reestablished.[235] Enhanced levels of CRP, the major acute-phase protein in humans, are seen in SIRS/sepsis, and clinical resolution is preceded by a drop in CRP levels.

The elaboration of proinflammatory cytokines (IL-1, TNFα, and IL-6) is central to the pathogenesis of SIRS regardless of the initiating stimulus. Their elaboration triggers increased expression of adhesion molecules, leukocyte recruitment, and the production of secondary proinflammatory mediators, such as chemokines. Endotoxin, or LPS, is one of the most powerful triggers of SIRS. LPS activates the complement and coagulation cascades, induces endothelial cell activation, and increases TNFα and IL-1 synthesis and late release of HMGB1. However, noninfectious tissues injury induces a similar inflammatory response. LPS, TNFα, and IL-1 also induce increased production of NO by iNOS in macrophages and other inflammatory cells. PGI_2 along with other metabolites of arachidonic acid together with NO contribute to decreased systemic vascular resistance and hypotension. Autocrine and paracrine NO production also results in myocardial depression. Increased vascular permeability promotes extravasation of fluid and edema formation. Activated endothelial cells express tissue factor, PECAM, and TXA_2, which promote a procoagulant local environment that predisposes to microthrombi formation. Adherent leukocytes further exacerbate organ injury by mechanically impeding microvascular blood flow and by damaging the endothelial cells and surrounding connective tissue. The results are end-organ hypoperfusion, inadequate oxygen delivery, initiation of anaerobic metabolism, and end-organ failure. The metabolic and nutritional sequelae of this activated cytokine milieu includes fever, catabolism, cachexia, and altered fat, glucose, and trace mineral metabolism.

SIRS is counteracted by the concomitant induction of an antiinflammatory response termed the compensatory antiinflammatory response syndrome (CARS).[235] Many of the proinflammatory mediators that participate in SIRS modulate the immune function of lymphocytes and mononuclear cells. Proinflammatory mediators can inhibit their own synthesis or enhance the synthesis of natural antagonists by negative feedback mechanisms. Thus, at any given time, the clinical manifestation is SIRS; CARS; or, more likely, an intermediate, mixed inflammatory response syndrome. The spectrum of features that characterize these syndromes has been termed CHAOS (cardiovascular shock, homeostasis, apoptosis, organ dysfunction, and immune suppression). Studies employing a variety of specific anticytokine agents have failed to observe an improvement in the outcome of patients with SIRS or sepsis. However, two studies of immunomodulation have noted significant effects in septic populations. The PROWESS study of activated protein C underscores the importance of the coagulation cascade during inflammation. This randomized controlled trial noted a 19.6% relative reduction and 6.1% absolute reduction in mortality for those patients with severe sepsis who received activated protein C.[236] Another study used a combination of corticosteroid and mineralocorticoid replacement for those patients with sepsis and who had relative adrenal insufficiency as defined by a less than 10-unit increase in cortisol after a Cortrosyn stimulation test. They documented a 33% relative reduction and 10% absolute reduction in the risk of death for those patients who received steroids.[237]

Chronic Inflammation

There are no clear boundaries between an acute and a chronic inflammatory response. In general, if the source of an acute inflammatory process is incompletely eliminated, a state of chronic inflammation eventually ensues. Chronicity is usually not characterized by the signs classically associated with acute responses, such as swelling, heat, or redness. Pain is minimal if not absent. Microscopically, a mononuclear cell infiltrate predominates (lymphocytes, monocytes, plasma cells) with proliferation of fibroblasts and vascular elements.

Any agent may create a state of chronic inflammation, including persistent infectious agents, remnants of dead organisms, foreign bodies, and metabolic byproducts. Ultimately, chronicity of inflammation is a result of the immune response to a persistent antigen. Furthermore, a chronic inflammatory response can develop in the absence of a preceding acute response, such as infections with agents of low toxicity such as *Mycobacterium* and *Treponema*. $CD4^+$ T cells and macrophages are the primary cellular orchestrators of chronic inflammatory response.[238] T_H1 cell-mediated immunity (CMI) responses are protective against most microbes and usually result in the elimination of the pathogen. If the microbe persists, the ongoing T_H1 response results in inflammatory tissue injury. Cytokines and growth factors released by T lymphocytes and macrophages stimulate proliferative responses. Neutrophils and eosinophils contribute to the release of proteolytic enzymes and oxygen derivatives. Eosinophilia is seen with chronic parasitic infections and hypersensitivity conditions. Fibroblasts are actively recruited by chemoattractants such as fibrin, collagens, and cytokines. Local IL-1 stimulates fibroblast proliferation and collagen production. Irreversible tissue damage can occur through the replacement of normal parenchyma with fibrous connective tissue. Fibroblasts can release metalloproteinases that degrade normal tissue, further contributing to tissue destruction. Mast cells are elevated in chronic conditions and may play a part in cell-mediated immune responses. Inflammatory cyst formation may occur as a result of epithelial hyperplasia.

APPENDIX A. APOPTOSIS

Apoptosis is an integral component in the regulatory mechanisms that limit and resolve inflammation. Unlike cell necrosis, which is characterized by loss of membrane integrity, cellular edema and lysis, and release of intracellular products that incite an inflammatory reaction, apoptosis is a physiologic process of programmed cell death, characterized by DNA fragmentation and plasma membrane blebbing, with the compartmentalization of cytoplasmic and membrane particles into apoptotic bodies consisting of cytoplasmic and membrane fragments. Cytoplasmic contents are not released and, consequently, an inflammatory response is not induced. Neutrophils are programmed to undergo apoptosis constitutively, and the signal transduction pathways culminating in apoptosis are activated early in acute inflammation (see Fig. 6.5). Subsequent neutrophil apoptotic particles are phagocytosed by resident macrophages, which causes a suppression in macrophage activation. This is the preferred mechanisms for clearing neutrophils from inflammatory foci and has also been implicated in the clearance of eosinophils, monocytes, and lymphocytes.

Apoptosis plays a prominent role in the immune system. Most developing T cells undergo apoptosis during the selection process in the thymus. Termination of the cellular immune response also involves cytokine-induced apoptosis. Apoptosis can be used by lymphocytes as a means of effecting death in other cells. CTLs kill target cells by inducing apoptosis via a Fas-induced pathway and a perforin- and granzyme-mediated pathway. Increased apoptosis has been observed in lymphoid tissues of patients dying of sepsis, suggesting that excessive lymphocyte apoptosis may contribute to fatal sepsis.

Inducers of apoptosis include oxidant stress, radiation, viral infection, trauma, and cytokines. Many of these pathologic agents that induce apoptosis at low concentrations can cause necrosis at higher concentrations. Apoptogenic stimuli activate the apoptotic pathway through both receptor-dependent and independent pathways. The sphingomyelin breakdown product ceramide is implicated as a transducer of apoptosis. DNA damage secondary to radiation or oxygen radical formation results in the accumulation of the tumor suppressor gene *p53*. *p53* promotes non-receptor-mediated modulation of apoptosis.

Receptor-mediated pathways involve the "death receptors" that belong to the TNF receptor superfamily. Ligands shown to induce apoptosis include FasL, TNF, TNF-related apoptosis-inducing ligand (TRAIL), nerve growth factor, and CD40L. The best-characterized death receptors are Fas-bound FasL and TNFRI-bound TNF and lymphotoxin α. Although primarily produced by macrophages, TNF is produced by many cell types, whereas FasL is restricted to the surfaces of CTLs, macrophages, and neutrophils. TNF and FasL also differ in that FasL directly activates a cell death pathway, whereas TNF does so indirectly and concurrently stimulates pathways that inhibit apoptosis. Independent and divergent proinflammatory signaling pathways by TNF lead to the induction of NFκB, an inhibitor of apoptosis. The mechanism by which several cytokines, including IL-1, IL-6, and GM-CSF, inhibit apoptosis is through induction of NFκB and apoptosis is one of many factors that ultimately determine the cell's fate.

Ligation of death receptors recruits "death domain" containing adaptor proteins that interact with the receptor's intracellular death domain. This interaction initiates the enzyme cascade responsible for apoptosis effector mechanisms, the caspases. All signaling pathways converge on the activation of cysteine proteases related to IL-1β converting enzyme called caspases. Caspases propagate apoptotic signaling by cleaving/activating other caspases and eventually execute terminal events in apoptosis by cleaving specific target proteins. Caspases 8 and 10 activate apoptosis signaling by linking Fas-associated death domain protein (FADD) with the caspase cascades. Caspases 3 and 7 are the executor molecules in the nucleus that cleave death substrates, including nuclear structural proteins, protein kinases, and proteins involved in cell cycle regulation or DNA fragmentation. Cytochrome C release from mitochondria is a key component in the activation of caspases. Cytochrome C release, and therefore apoptosis, is inhibited by Bcl-2, the primary death protection protein that belongs to the Bcl family of proapoptotic and antiapoptotic proteins involved in the regulation of apoptosis.

APPENDIX B. TRANSCRIPTION FACTORS

The inflammatory response requires the rapid induction of genes that encode effector proteins. This transcription is regulated by specific DNA-binding transcription factors that bind regulatory elements in gene promoters. Engagement of cell surface receptors triggers intracellular signal transduction pathways, transcription factor activation, and transcription, thereby linking the extracellular environment with the nucleus. Stimuli such as redox stress and ROS operate through similar pathways in a receptor independent manner. Transcription factors of particular importance during inflammation include NFκB, activator protein-1 (AP-1), signal transduction and activator of transcription (STAT) proteins, nuclear factor of activated T cells (NFAT), and nuclear factor IL-6 (NF-IL6).

Activation of NFκB is critical for maximal expression of many proinflammatory cytokines (TNF, IL-1, IL-6, and IL-8). NFκB binding sites have been identified within the promoters of genes encoding growth factors, adhesion molecules and acute-phase proteins, as well as COX-2 and iNOS. This prototype NF is a heterodimeric protein composed of DNA-binding subunits p50 and p65. However, it can be composed of dimers of any combination of Rel DNA binding proteins. A group of IκB inhibitor proteins sequester NFκB in the cytoplasm of immune and inflammatory effector cells. Cellular activation by ROS, cytokines, NO, hypoxia, redox stress, and bacterial metabolites induces IκB phosphorylation and subsequent ubiquitination, which leads to IκB degradation and NFκB release. Free NFκB translocates to the nucleus, where it binds to regulatory elements in target gene promoters to induce gene expression and ultimately protein synthesis (see Table 6.5).

Many of the stress stimuli that trigger NFκB also activate AP-1. AP-1 consists of homodimers or heterodimers of members of c-Jun and c-Fos families of proto-oncogenes. These proteins are exclusively nuclear proteins. The signal for AP-1 activation arises from a group of serine/threonine kinases, the MAPKs. Small G proteins such as Ras activated by cell surface receptor binding trigger a series of phosphorylation sequences that activates the final MAPK. MAPKs can be grouped into three major classes: extracellular-regulated kinase (ERK1/2), c-Jun N-terminal kinases (JNK), and p38. ERK 1/2 is primarily involved in cell cycle regulation and differentiation, whereas JNK and p38 transduce signals from proinflammatory cytokines and sources of cellular stress (heat shock, ROS, ultraviolet light, radiation, osmotic stress). Not surprisingly, there is evidence of cooperative interactions between AP-1 and NFκB activation pathways that can result in functional synergy (see Table 6.5).

The STAT proteins mediate the cellular effects of most cytokines. There are seven STAT proteins identified to date. Janus Kinase (JAK) proteins that associate with cell surface cytokine receptors activate these proteins. On cytokine binding the JAKs dimerize and transphosphorylate each other. STAT proteins associate with the phosphorylated JAKs and are themselves phosphorylated. The activated STAT proteins dimerize and translocate to the nucleus, where they bind to recognition sequences in the promoter regions of genes to induce transcription (see Table 6.5).

Nuclear factor of activated T cells (NFAT) is primarily involved in regulating the production of effector proteins of the immune responses. Although first identified in the IL-2 promoter of T cells, it is expressed in a host of cell types, including mast cells, mononuclear phagocytes, eosinophils, and endothelial cells and is required for the expression of IL-2, IL-4, and TNFα. It is activated by stimulation of receptors coupled to calcium mobilization. Examples of such receptors are antigen receptors on T and B lymphocytes, the FcεR on mast cells and basophils, the Fcγ receptor on macrophages, and G-protein-coupled receptors. Receptor binding activates PLC, leading to increased calcium concentrations. Calcineurin, a calcium/calmodulin-dependent phosphatase activated by elevated levels of intracellular calcium, activates NFAT. NFAT participates in multiple cooperative interactions with AP-1.

KEY POINTS

- **Inflammation is caused by the host immune response, which comprises complex, interactive, redundant systems involving both innate and adaptive immunity.**
- **The initial host defense against infection is innate immunity, comprising both cellular and humoral components.**
- **Each cellular and humoral component of the host immunoinflammatory response has evolved as a "double-edged sword" with both beneficial and, when deficient or excessive, potential significant deleterious impact on the host.**
- **The major etiology of multiple organ dysfunction in the critically ill patient derives from immune dysregulation with primarily an excessive, nondiscriminant immunoinflammatory response.**
- **Therapeutic interventions focused on isolated components of the innate or adaptive immune response are unlikely to improve patient outcomes due to the redundancy and complexity of the immune response.**

References

1. Cotran RS. Inflammation: historical perspectives. In: Gallin J, SR, eds. *Inflammation: basic principles and clinical correlates,* 3rd ed. Philadelphia: Lippincott Williams & Wilkins; 1999.
2. Heifets L. Centennial of Metchnikoff's discovery. *J Reticuloendothel Soc.* 1982;31:381–391.
3. Cotran RS, Kumar V, Robbins T. *Robbins pathologic basis of disease,* 6th ed. Philadelphia: WB Sanders; 1999.
4. Abbas AK, Lichtman AH. *Cellular and molecular immunology,* 5th ed. Philadelphia: WB Saunders; 2003.
5. Wheeler JG, Abramson JS. *The neutrophil.* Oxford, England: IRL Press at Oxford University Press; 1993.
6. Bainton D. The cells of inflammation: a general view. In: Weisserman G, ed. *The cell biology of inflammation,* Vol. 2. New York: Elsevier/North-Holland; 1980.
7. Dancey JT, et al. Neutrophil kinetics in man. *J Clin Invest.* 1976;58:705–715.
8. Omann GM, Hinshaw DB. Inflammation. In: Greenfield LJ, Mulholland MW, Oldham KT, et al., eds. *Surgery: scientific principles and practice,* 2nd ed. 1997, Philadelphia: Lippincott-Raven; 1997:130–159.
9. Trowbridge H, Emling R. Inflammation: a review of the process. In: T. HO and E. RC, eds. Chicago: Quintessence; 1997.
10. Dustin ML, Springer TA. Role of lymphocyte adhesion receptors in transient interactions and cell locomotion. *Annu Rev Immunol.* 1991;9:27–66.
11. Kansas GS. Selectins and their ligands: current concepts and controversies. *Blood* 1996;88:3259–3287.

12. Tedder TF, et al. The selectins: vascular adhesion molecules. *FASEB J.* 1995;9:866–873.
13. Frenette PS, Wagner DD. Adhesion molecules—Part II: Blood vessels and blood cells. *N Engl J Med.* 1996;335:43–45.
14. Frenette PS, Wagner DD. Adhesion molecules—Part 1. *N Engl J Med.* 1996;334:1526–1529.
15. Hynes RO. Integrins: versatility, modulation, and signaling in cell adhesion. *Cell* 1992;69:11–25.
16. **Muller WA. Leukocyte-endothelial-cell interactions in leukocyte transmigration and the inflammatory response. *Trends Immunol.* 2003;24:327–334.**
17. Vaporciyan AA, et al. Involvement of platelet-endothelial cell adhesion molecule-1 in neutrophil recruitment in vivo. *Science* 1993;262: 1580–1582.
18. Thornhill M, Haskard D. Leukocyte adhesion to endothelium. In: Horton M, ed. *Blood cell biochemistry, vol 5: Macrophages and related cells.* New York: Plenum Press; 1993.
19. Rot A. The role of leukocyte chemotaxis in inflammation. In: Whicker J, Evans S, eds. *Biochemistry and inflammation.* Boston: Kluwer Academic; 1992.
20. Wagner JG, Roth RA. Neutrophil migration during endotoxemia. *J Leukoc Biol.* 1999;66:10–24.
21. Indik ZK, et al. Structure/function relationships of Fc gamma receptors in phagocytosis. *Semin Immunol.* 1995;7:45–54.
22. Ezekowitz R. The mannose receptor and phagocytosis. In: Furth RV, ed. *Mononuclear phagocytes: biology of monocytes and macrophages.* Boston: Kluwer Academic; 1992.
23. Ezekowitz RA, et al. Local opsonization by secreted macrophage complement components. Role of receptors for complement in uptake of zymosan. *J Exp Med.* 1984;159:244–260.
24. Lee WL, Harrison RE, Grinstein S. Phagocytosis by neutrophils. *Microbes Infect.* 2003;5:1299–1306.
25. Zychlinsky A, Weinrauch Y, Weiss J. Introduction: forum in immunology on neutrophils. *Microbes Infect.* 2003;5:1289–1291.
26. Borregaard N, Cowland JB. Granules of the human neutrophilic polymorphonuclear leukocyte. *Blood* 1997;89:3503–3521.
27. Faurschou M, Borregaard N. Neutrophil granules and secretory vesicles in inflammation. *Microbes Infect.* 2003;5:1317–1327.
28. Lehrer RI, Ganz T, Selsted ME. Defensins: endogenous antibiotic peptides of animal cells. *Cell* 1991;64:229–230.
29. Elsbach P. The bactericidal/permeability-increasing protein (BPI) in antibacterial host defense. *J Leukoc Biol.* 1998;64:14–18.
30. Beamer LJ, Carroll SF, Eisenberg D. The BPI/LBP family of proteins: a structural analysis of conserved regions. *Protein Sci.* 1998;7:906–914.
31. Gabay JE, et al. Antibiotic proteins of human polymorphonuclear leukocytes. *Proc Natl Acad Sci U S A.* 1989;86:5610–5614.
32. Chapple IL. Reactive oxygen species and antioxidants in inflammatory diseases. *J Clin Periodontol.* 1997;24:287–296.
33. Kasahara Y, et al. Involvement of reactive oxygen intermediates in spontaneous and CD95 (Fas/APO-1)-mediated apoptosis of neutrophils. *Blood* 1997;89:1748–1753.
34. Roos D, van Bruggen R, Meischl C. Oxidative killing of microbes by neutrophils. *Microbes Infect.* 2003;5:1307–1315.
35. Nordberg J, Arner ES. Reactive oxygen species, antioxidants, and the mammalian thioredoxin system. *Free Radic Biol Med.* 2001;31:1287–1312.
36. Winyard PG, et al. The role of toxic oxygen species in inflammation with special reference to DNA damage. In: Whicker JT, Evans SW, eds. *Biochemistry of inflammation.* Boston: Kluwer Academic; 1992.
37. Nohl H. Generation of superoxide radicals as byproduct of cellular respiration. *Ann Biol Clin (Paris)* 1994;52(3):199–204.
38. Schuchert RD, Billiar TR. Inflammation. In: Greenfield LJ, ed. *Surgery: scientific principles and practice,* 3rd ed. Philadelphia: Lippincott Williams & Wilkins; 2001:134–178.
39. Szabo C. The pathophysiological role of peroxynitrite in shock, inflammation, and ischemia-reperfusion injury. *Shock* 1996;6(2):79–88.
40. Warren J, Ward P, Johnson K. Oxygen radicals as mediators of inflammation. In: Henson PM and Murphy RC, eds. *Handbook of inflammation,* Vol. 6. New York: Elsevier Science Publishers BV; 1989.
41. Burg ND, Pillinger MH. The neutrophil: function and regulation in innate and humoral immunity. *Clin Immunol.* 2001;99:7–17.
42. Kobayashi SD, Voyich JM, DeLeo FR. Regulation of the neutrophil-mediated inflammatory response to infection. *Microbes Infect.* 2003;5: 1337–1344.
43. Burkitt HG, Young B, Heath JW. *Wheater's functional histology: a text and colour atlas,* 3rd ed. Edinburgh: Churchill Livingston; 1993.
44. **Ma J, et al. Regulation of macrophage activation. *Cell Mol Life Sci.* 2003;60:2334–2346.**
45. Ben-Baruch A, Michiel DF, Oppenheim JJ. Signals and receptors involved in recruitment of inflammatory cells. *J Biol Chem.* 1995;270:11703–11706.
46. Kuijpers T, et al. Membrane surface antigen expression on human monocytes: changes during purification, in vitro activation and transmigration across monolayers of endothelial cells. In: Furth RV, ed. *Mononuclear phagocytes: biology of monocytes and macrophages.* Boston: Kluwer Academic; 1992.
47. Nathan C, Xie QW. Nitric oxide synthases: roles, tolls, and controls. *Cell* 1994;78:915–918.
48. de Waal Malefyt R, et al. Interleukin-10. *Curr Opin Immunol.* 1992;4:314–320.
49. MacMicking J, Xie QW, Nathan C. Nitric oxide and macrophage function. *Annu Rev Immunol.* 1997;15:323–350.
50. Griffiths GM. The cell biology of CTL killing. *Curr Opin Immunol.* 1995;7:343–348.
51. Romagnani S. Understanding the role of Th1/Th2 cells in infection. *Trends Microbiol.* 1996;4:470–473.
52. Mosmann TR, Coffman RL. TH1 and TH2 cells: different patterns of lymphokine secretion lead to different functional properties. *Annu Rev Immunol.* 1989;7:145–173.
53. Lane PJ, Brocker T. Developmental regulation of dendritic cell function. *Curr Opin Immunol.* 1999;11:308–313.
54. Banchereau J, Steinman RM. Dendritic cells and the control of immunity. *Nature* 1998;392:245–252.
55. Braciale TJ, et al. Antigen presentation pathways to class I and class II MHC-restricted T lymphocytes. *Immunol Rev.* 1987;98:95–114.
56. Razi-Wolf Z, et al. Expression and function of the murine B7 antigen, the major costimulatory molecule expressed by peritoneal exudate cells. *Proc Natl Acad Sci U S A.* 1992;89:4210–4214.
57. Lanzavecchia A. Receptor-mediated antigen uptake and its effect on antigen presentation to class II-restricted T lymphocytes. *Annu Rev Immunol.* 1990;8:773–793.
58. Gumperz JE, Parham P. The enigma of the natural killer cell. *Nature* 1995;378:245–248.
59. **Janeway C, Travers P, eds. *Immunobiology: the immune system in health and disease,* 3rd ed. London: Garland Publishers; 1997.**
60. Surh CD, Sprent J. T-cell apoptosis detected in situ during positive and negative selection in the thymus. *Nature* 1994;372:100–103.
61. von Schacky C. Mechanisms of tolerance induction in major histocompatibility complex class II-restricted T cells specific for a blood-borne self-antigen. *J Exp Med.* 1994;180:2089–2099.
62. Zal T, Volkmann A, Stockinger B. Mechanisms of tolerance induction in major histocompatibility complex class II-restricted T cells specific for a blood-borne self-antigen. *J Exp Med.* 1994;180:2089–2099.
63. Picker LJ. Control of lymphocyte homing. *Curr Opin Immunol.* 1994;6:394–406.
64. Dustin ML, Springer TA. T-cell receptor cross-linking transiently stimulates adhesiveness through LFA-1. *Nature* 1989;341:619–624.
65. Springer TA. Traffic signals for lymphocyte recirculation and leukocyte emigration: the multistep paradigm. *Cell* 1994;76:301–314.
66. Janeway Jr CA, Bottomly K. Signals and signs for lymphocyte responses. *Cell* 1994;76:275–285.
67. Mosmann TR, Sad S. The expanding universe of T-cell subsets: Th1, Th2 and more. *Immunol Today* 1996;17(3):138–46.
68. Lee KP, Harlan DM, June CH. Role of co-stimulation in the host response to infection. In: Gallin JI, Snyderman R, eds. *Inflammation: basic principles and clinical correlates,* 3rd ed. Philadelphia: Lippincott Williams & Wilkins; 1999.
69. Broide DH, Hoffman H, Sriramarao P. Genes that regulate eosinophilic inflammation. *Am J Hum Genet.* 1999;65:302–307.
70. Elsner J, Kapp A. Regulation and modulation of eosinophil effector functions. *Allergy* 1999;54:15–26.
71. Weller PF, Bach DS, Austen KF. Biochemical characterization of human eosinophil Charcot-Leyden crystal protein (lysophospholipase). *J Biol Chem.* 1984;259:15100–15105.
72. Giembycz MA, Lindsay MA. Pharmacology of the eosinophil. *Pharmacol Rev.* 1999;51:213–340.
73. Slungaard A, Mahoney Jr JR. Thiocyanate is the major substrate for eosinophil peroxidase in physiologic fluids. Implications for cytotoxicity. *J Biol Chem.* 1991;266:4903–4910.
74. Wardlaw AJ, Moqbel R, Kay AB. Eosinophils: biology and role in disease. *Adv Immunol.* 1995;60:151–266.
75. Wedi B, et al. Delayed eosinophil programmed cell death in vitro: a common feature of inhalant allergy and extrinsic and intrinsic atopic dermatitis. *J Allergy Clin Immunol.* 1997;100:536–543.
76. Valent P, et al. Interleukin-3 is a differentiation factor for human basophils. *Blood* 1989;73:1763–1769.
77. Nilsson G, Cost J, Metcalfke D. Mast cells an basophils. In: G. JI and S. R, eds. *Inflammation: basic principles and clinical correlates,* 3rd ed. Philadelphia: Lippincott Williams & Wilkins; 1999.
78. Metcalfe DD, Baram D, Mekri YA. Mast cells. *Physiol Rev.* 1997;77:1033–1079.
79. Klinger MH, Jelkmann W. Role of blood platelets in infection and inflammation. *J Interferon Cytokine Res.* 2002;22:913–922.
80. Marcus A. Platelets: their role in hemostasis, thrombosis, and inflammation. In: Gallin J, Synderman R, eds. *Inflammation: basic principles and clinical correlates,* 3rd ed. Philadelphia: Lippincott Williams & Wilkins; 1999.
81. Du X, Williams DA. Interleukin-11: review of molecular, cell biology, and clinical use. *Blood* 1997;89:3897–3908.
82. **Weyrich AS, Lindemann S, Zimmerman GA. The evolving role of platelets in inflammation. *J Thromb Haemost.* 2003;1:1897–1905.**
83. Serhan CN. Lipoxins and novel aspirin-triggered 15-epi-lipoxins (ATL): a jungle of cell-cell interactions or a therapeutic opportunity? *Prostaglandins* 1997;53(2):107–137.

84. Marcus AJ, et al. Platelet-neutrophil interactions. (12S)-hydroxyeicosatetraen-1,20-dioic acid: a new eicosanoid synthesized by unstimulated neutrophils from (12S)-20-dihydroxyeicosatetraenoic acid. *J Biol Chem.* 1988;263:2223–2229.
85. Serhan CN, Haeggstrom JZ, Leslie CC. Lipid mediator networks in cell signaling: update and impact of cytokines. *FASEB J.* 1996;10:1147–1158.
86. Colletti LM. Cytokines. In: Greenfield LJ, ed. *Surgery: scientific principles and practice,* 3rd ed. Philadelphia: Lippincott Williams & Wilkins; 2001.
87. Thomson A, ed. *The cytokine handbook,* 3rd ed. New York: Academic Press; 1998.
88. Schmidt AM, et al. The biology of the receptor for advanced glycation end products and its ligands. *Biochim Biophys Acta.* 2000;1498(2–3):99–111.
89. Strieter RM, et al. Host responses in mediating sepsis and adult respiratory distress syndrome. *Semin Respir Infect.* 1990;5:233–247.
90. Cerami A. Inflammatory cytokines. *Clin Immunol Immunopathol.* 1992;62(1 Pt 2):S3–10.
91. Bauss F, Droge W, Mannel DN. Tumor necrosis factor mediates endotoxic effects in mice. *Infect Immun.* 1987;55:1622–1625.
92. Philip R, Epstein LB. Tumour necrosis factor as immunomodulator and mediator of monocyte cytotoxicity induced by itself, gamma-interferon and interleukin-1. *Nature* 1986;323:86–89.
93. Tartaglia LA, et al. A novel domain within the 55 kd TNF receptor signals cell death. *Cell* 1993;74:845–853.
94. Adam-Klages S, et al. Distinct adapter proteins mediate acid versus neutral sphingomyelinase activation through the p55 receptor for tumor necrosis factor. *J Leukoc Biol.* 1998;63:678–682.
95. Meager A. Cytokine regulation of cellular adhesion molecule expression in inflammation. *Cytokine Growth Factor Rev.* 1999;10(1):27–39.
96. Tracey KJ, et al. Anti-cachectin/TNF monoclonal antibodies prevent septic shock during lethal bacteraemia. *Nature* 1987;330:662–664.
97. Tracey KJ, Lowry SF, Cerami A. Cachetin/TNF-alpha in septic shock and septic adult respiratory distress syndrome. *Am Rev Respir Dis.* 1988;138:1377–1379.
98. Tracey KJ, Lowry SF, Cerami A. Cachectin/TNF mediates the pathophysiological effects of bacterial endotoxin/lipopolysaccharide (LPS). *Prog Clin Biol Res.* 1988;272:77–88.
99. Le J, Vilcek J. Tumor necrosis factor and interleukin 1: cytokines with multiple overlapping biological activities. *Lab Invest.* 1987;56:234–248.
100. Sims JE, et al. cDNA expression cloning of the IL-1 receptor, a member of the immunoglobulin superfamily. *Science* 1988;241:585–589.
101. Kuno K, Matsushima K. The IL-1 receptor signaling pathway. *J Leukoc Biol.* 1994;56:542–547.
102. Colotta F, et al. The type II 'decoy' receptor: a novel regulatory pathway for interleukin 1. *Immunol Today* 1994;15:562–566.
103. Bevilacqua MP, et al. Regulation of the fibrinolytic system of cultured human vascular endothelium by interleukin 1. *J Clin Invest.* 1986;78:587–591.
104. Baggiolini M, Dewald B, Moser B. Human chemokines: an update. *Annu Rev Immunol.* 1997;15:675–705.
105. Bacon K, et al. Chemokine/chemokine receptor nomenclature. *J Interferon Cytokine Res.* 2002;22:1067–1068.
106. Bacon KB, et al. The expanding universe of C, CX3C, and CC chemokines. In: Thomson A, ed. *The cytokine handbook,* 3rd ed. New York: Academic Press; 1998.
107. Rollins BJ. Chemokines. *Blood* 1997;90:909–928.
108. Schall TJ, Bacon KB. Chemokines, leukocyte trafficking, and inflammation. *Curr Opin Immunol.* 1994;6:865–873.
109. Hebert CA, Vitangcol RV, Baker JB. Scanning mutagenesis of interleukin-8 identifies a cluster of residues required for receptor binding. *J Biol Chem.* 1991;266:18989–18994.
110. Clark-Lewis I, et al. Platelet factor 4 binds to interleukin 8 receptors and activates neutrophils when its N terminus is modified with Glu-Leu-Arg. *Proc Natl Acad Sci U S A.* 1993;90:3574–3577.
111. Clark-Lewis I, et al. Structure-activity relationships of chemokines. *J Leukoc Biol.* 1995;57:703–711.
112. D'Andrea A, et al. Production of natural killer cell stimulatory factor (interleukin 12) by peripheral blood mononuclear cells. *J Exp Med.* 1992;176:1387–1398.
113. Shu U, et al. Activated T cells induce interleukin-12 production by monocytes via CD40-CD40 ligand interaction. *Eur J Immunol.* 1995;25:1125–1128.
114. Gauldie J, et al. Interferon beta 2/B-cell stimulatory factor type 2 shares identity with monocyte-derived hepatocyte-stimulating factor and regulates the major acute phase protein response in liver cells. *Proc Natl Acad Sci U S A.* 1987;84:7251–7255.
115. Van Snick J. Interleukin-6: an overview. *Annu Rev Immunol.* 1990;8:253–278.
116. LeMay LG, et al. In vivo evidence that the rise in plasma IL 6 following injection of a fever-inducing dose of LPS is mediated by IL 1 beta. *Cytokine* 1990;2(3):199–204.
117. Tilg H, et al. Interleukin-6 (IL-6) as an anti-inflammatory cytokine: induction of circulating IL-1 receptor antagonist and soluble tumor necrosis factor receptor p55. *Blood* 1994;83:113–118.
118. Wang H, Yang H, Tracey KJ. Extracellular role of HMGB1 in inflammation and sepsis. *J Intern Med.* 2004;255:320–331.
119. Chen G, et al. Bacterial endotoxin stimulates macrophages to release HMGB1 partly through CD14- and TNF-dependent mechanisms. *J Leukoc Biol.* 2004;76:994–1001.
120. Chen G, et al. Extracellular HMGB1 as a proinflammatory cytokine. *J Interferon Cytokine Res.* 2004;24:329–333.
121. Fiuza C, et al. Inflammation-promoting activity of HMGB1 on human microvascular endothelial cells. *Blood* 2003;101:2652–2660.
122. Andersson U, Tracey KJ. HMGB1 in sepsis. *Scand J Infect Dis.* 2003;35:577–584.
123. Andersson U, et al. High mobility group 1 protein (HMG-1) stimulates proinflammatory cytokine synthesis in human monocytes. *J Exp Med.* 2000;192:565–570.
124. Andersson UG , Tracey KJ. HMGB1, a pro-inflammatory cytokine of clinical interest: introduction. *J Intern Med.* 2004;255:318–319.
125. Riedemann NC, Guo RF, Ward PA. Novel strategies for the treatment of sepsis. *Nat Med.* 2003;9:517–524.
126. Sama AE, et al. Bench to bedside: HMGB1-a novel proinflammatory cytokine and potential therapeutic target for septic patients in the emergency department. *Acad Emerg Med.* 2004;11:867–873.
127. Erlandsson Harris H, Andersson U. Mini-review: the nuclear protein HMGB1 as a proinflammatory mediator. *Eur J Immunol.* 2004;34:1503–1512.
128. Rovere-Querini P, et al. HMGB1 is an endogenous immune adjuvant released by necrotic cells. *EMBO Rep.* 2004;5:825–830.
129. Scaffidi P, Misteli T, Bianchi ME. Release of chromatin protein HMGB1 by necrotic cells triggers inflammation. *Nature* 2002;418:191–195.
130. Bogdan C. The function of type I interferons in antimicrobial immunity. *Curr Opin Immunol.* 2000;12:419–424.
131. De Maeyer E, De Maeyer-Guignard J. Type I interferons. *Int Rev Immunol.* 1998;17(1–4):53–73.
132. Uze G, Lutfalla G, Mogensen KE. Alpha and beta interferons and their receptor and their friends and relations. *J Interferon Cytokine Res.* 1995;15(1):3–26.
133. Selzman CH, et al. Therapeutic implications of interleukin-10 in surgical disease. *Shock* 1998;10:309–318.
134. Cassatella MA, et al. Interleukin 10 (IL-10) inhibits the release of proinflammatory cytokines from human polymorphonuclear leukocytes. Evidence for an autocrine role of tumor necrosis factor and IL-1 beta in mediating the production of IL-8 triggered by lipopolysaccharide. *J Exp Med.* 1993;178:2207–2211.
135. Neurath MF, Meyer zum Buschenfelde KH. Protective and pathogenic roles of cytokines in inflammatory bowel diseases. *J Investig Med.* 1996;44:516–521.
136. Smith KA. Interleukin-2: inception, impact, and implications. *Science* 1988;240:1169–1176.
137. Smith KA. Lowest dose interleukin-2 immunotherapy. *Blood* 1993;81:1414–1423.
138. Zurawski SM, et al. Receptors for interleukin-13 and interleukin-4 are complex and share a novel component that functions in signal transduction. *Embo J.* 1993;12:2663–2670.
139. de Waal Malefyt R, et al. Effects of IL-13 on phenotype, cytokine production, and cytotoxic function of human monocytes. Comparison with IL-4 and modulation by IFN-gamma or IL-10. *J Immunol.* 1993;151:6370–6381.
140. Billiau A, et al. Immunomodulatory properties of interferon-gamma. An update. *Ann N Y Acad Sci.* 1998;856:22–32.
141. Boehm U, et al. Cellular responses to interferon-gamma. *Annu Rev Immunol.* 1997;15:749–795.
142. Lawrence DA. Transforming growth factor-beta: an overview. *Kidney Int Suppl.* 1995;49:S19–23.
143. Lawrence DA. Transforming growth factor-beta: a general review. *Eur Cytokine Netw.* 1996;7:363–374.
144. Wahl SM, et al. Transforming growth factor type beta induces monocyte chemotaxis and growth factor production. *Proc Natl Acad Sci U S A.* 1987;84:5788–5792.
145. Romani N, et al. Proliferating dendritic cell progenitors in human blood. *J Exp Med.* 1994;180:83–93.
146. Crawford J, et al. Reduction by granulocyte colony-stimulating factor of fever and neutropenia induced by chemotherapy in patients with small-cell lung cancer. *N Engl J Med.* 1991;325:164–170.
147. Metcalf D, Nicola NA. Proliferative effects of purified granulocyte colony-stimulating factor (G-CSF) on normal mouse hemopoietic cells. *J Cell Physiol.* 1983;116:198–206.
148. Cooper NR. Biology of the complement system. In: Gallin JI, Snyderman R, eds. *Inflammation: basic principles and clinical correlates,* 3rd ed. Philadelphia: Lippincott Williams & Wilkins; 1999.
149. Frank MM, Fries LF. The role of complement in inflammation and phagocytosis. *Immunol Today* 1991;12:322–326.
150. Roitt I, Brostoff J, Male D. Complement. 3rd ed. In: Roitt I, Brostoff J, Male D, eds. *Immunobiology,* 3rd ed. St. Louis: Mosby; 1993.
151. Weiser MR, et al. Reperfusion injury of ischemic skeletal muscle is mediated by natural antibody and complement. *J Exp Med.* 1996;183:2343–2348.
152. Cooper NR. The classical complement pathway: activation and regulation of the first complement component. *Adv Immunol.* 1985;37:151–216.

153. Matsushita M, Fujita T. Activation of the classical complement pathway by mannose-binding protein in association with a novel C1s-like serine protease. *J Exp Med.* 1992;176:1497–1502.
154. Sim RB, Malhotra R. Interactions of carbohydrates and lectins with complement. *Biochem Soc Trans.* 1994;22(1):106–111.
155. Muller-Eberhard HJ. The membrane attack complex of complement. *Annu Rev Immunol.* 1986;4:503–528.
156. Marnett LJ, et al. Arachidonic acid oxygenation by COX-1 and COX-2. Mechanisms of catalysis and inhibition. *J Biol Chem.* 1999;274: 22903–22906.
157. Seeds MC, Bass DA. Regulation and metabolism of arachidonic acid. *Clin Rev Allergy Immunol.* 1999;17(1–2):5–26.
158. Smith WL, Garavito RM, DeWitt DL. Prostaglandin endoperoxide H synthases (cyclooxygenases)-1 and -2. *J Biol Chem.* 1996;271:33157–33160.
159. Funk CD. Prostaglandins and leukotrienes: advances in eicosanoid biology. *Science* 2001;294:1871–1875.
160. Bulger EM, Maier RV. Lipid mediators in the pathophysiology of critical illness. *Crit Care Med.* 2000;28[Suppl]:N27–36.
161. Gerritsen ME. Physiological and pathophysiological roles of eicosanoids in the microcirculation. *Cardiovasc Res.* 1996;32:720–732.
162. Serhan CN. Inflammation. Signalling the fat controller. *Nature* 1996;384:23–24.
163. Leff JA. Leukotriene modifiers as novel therapeutics in asthma. *Clin Exp Allergy* 1998;28[Suppl 5]:147–153; discussion 171–173.
164. McMahon B, Godson C. Lipoxins: endogenous regulators of inflammation. *Am J Physiol Renal Physiol.* 2004;286(2):F189–201.
165. Marcus AJ. Transcellular metabolism of eicosanoids. *Prog Hemost Thromb.* 1986;8:127–142.
166. De Caterina R, et al. Macrophage-specific eicosanoid synthesis inhibition and lipocortin-1 induction by glucocorticoids. *J Appl Physiol.* 1993;75:2368–2375.
167. Snyder F, Fitzgerald V, Blank ML. Biosynthesis of platelet-activating factor and enzyme inhibitors. *Adv Exp Med Biol.* 1996;416:5–10.
168. Snyder F. Metabolic processing of PAF. *Clin Rev Allergy* 1994;12:309–327.
169. Noguchi K, et al. Involvement of nitric oxide and eicosanoids in platelet-activating factor-induced haemodynamic and haematological effects in dogs. *Br J Pharmacol.* 1996;118:941–950.
170. Blais Jr C, et al. The kallikrein-kininogen-kinin system: lessons from the quantification of endogenous kinins. *Peptides* 2000;21:1903–1940.
171. Erdos EG. Kinins, the long march—a personal view. *Cardiovasc Res.* 2002;54:485–491.
172. Hall JM. Bradykinin receptors: pharmacological properties and biological roles. *Pharmacol Ther.* 1992;56(2):131–190.
173. Schreiber AD. Plasma inhibitors of the Hageman factor dependent pathways. *Semin Thromb Hemost.* 1976;3:32–51.
174. Volpe AR, et al. Biosynthesis of endothelium-derived nitric oxide by bradykinin as endogenous precursor. *Immunopharmacology* 1996; 33(1–3):287–290.
175. Dell'Italia LJ, Oparil S. Bradykinin in the heart: friend or foe? *Circulation* 1999;100:2305–2307.
176. Tschope C. et al. Antihypertensive and cardioprotective effects after angiotensin-converting enzyme inhibition: role of kinins. *J Card Fail.* 1997;3(2):133–148.
177. Chikanza IC, Grossman AB. Neuroendocrine immune responses to inflammation: the concept of the neuroendocrine immune loop. *Baillieres Clin Rheumatol.* 1996;10:199–225.
178. Whicker JT, Evans SW. A role for neuropeptides in inflammation. In: Whicker JT, Evans SW, eds. *Biochemistry of inflammation.* Boston: Kluwer Academic; 1992.
179. Delgado M, et al. Vasoactive intestinal peptide and pituitary adenylate cyclase-activating polypeptide enhance IL-10 production by murine macrophages: in vitro and in vivo studies. *J Immunol.* 1999;162:1707–1716.
180. Palmer RM, Ferrige AG, Moncada S. Nitric oxide release accounts for the biological activity of endothelium-derived relaxing factor. *Nature* 1987;327:524–526.
181. Moncada S, Palmer RM, Higgs EA. Nitric oxide: physiology, pathophysiology, and pharmacology. *Pharmacol Rev.* 1991;43(2):109–142.
182. Alderton WK, Cooper CE, Knowles RG. Nitric oxide synthases: structure, function and inhibition. *Biochem J.* 2001;357(Pt 3):593–615.
183. Geller DA, Billiar TR. Molecular biology of nitric oxide synthases. *Cancer Metastasis Rev.* 1998;17(1):7–23.
184. De Vera ME, et al. Dexamethasone suppresses iNOS gene expression by upregulating I-kappa B alpha and inhibiting NF-kappa B. *Am J Physiol.* 1997;273(6 Pt 1):G1290–1296.
185. Kleinert H, et al. Glucocorticoids inhibit the induction of nitric oxide synthase II by down-regulating cytokine-induced activity of transcription factor nuclear factor-kappa B. *Mol Pharmacol.* 1996;49(1):15–21.
186. Titheradge MA. Nitric oxide in septic shock. *Biochim Biophys Acta* 1999;1411:437–455.
187. Finkel MS, et al. Negative inotropic effects of cytokines on the heart mediated by nitric oxide. *Science* 1992;257:387–389.
188. Goodwin DC, Landino LM, Marnett LJ. Effects of nitric oxide and nitric oxide-derived species on prostaglandin endoperoxide synthase and prostaglandin biosynthesis. *FASEB J.* 1999;13:1121–1136.
189. Allione A, et al. Nitric oxide suppresses human T lymphocyte proliferation through IFN-gamma-dependent and IFN-gamma-independent induction of apoptosis. *J Immunol.* 1999;163:4182–4191.
190. Ou J, et al. Differential effects of nonselective nitric oxide synthase (NOS) and selective inducible NOS inhibition on hepatic necrosis, apoptosis, ICAM-1 expression, and neutrophil accumulation during endotoxemia. *Nitric Oxide* 1997;1:404–416.
191. Isobe M, et al. Beneficial effects of inducible nitric oxide synthase inhibitor on reperfusion injury in the pig liver. *Transplantation* 1999;68:803–813.
192. Xia Y, Zweier JL. Superoxide and peroxynitrite generation from inducible nitric oxide synthase in macrophages. *Proc Natl Acad Sci USA.* 1997;94:6954–6958.
193. Szabo C, Billiar TR. Novel roles of nitric oxide in hemorrhagic shock. *Shock* 1999;12(1):1–9.
194. Hierholzer C, et al. Essential role of induced nitric oxide in the initiation of the inflammatory response after hemorrhagic shock. *J Exp Med.* 1998;187:917–928.
195. Tzeng E, et al. Adenoviral transfer of the inducible nitric oxide synthase gene blocks endothelial cell apoptosis. *Surgery* 1997;122:255–263.
196. Beutler B. Inferences, questions and possibilities in Toll-like receptor signalling. *Nature* 2004;430:257–263.
197. Triantafilou M, Triantafilou K. Lipopolysaccharide recognition: CD14, TLRs and the LPS-activation cluster. *Trends Immunol.* 2002;23:301–304.
198. Akira S, Takeda K. Toll-like receptor signalling. *Nat Rev Immunol.* 2004;4:499–511.
199. Cook DN, Pisetsky DS, Schwartz DA. Toll-like receptors in the pathogenesis of human disease. *Nat Immunol.* 2004;5:975–979.
200. Palsson-McDermott EM, O'Neill LA. Signal transduction by the lipopolysaccharide receptor, Toll-like receptor-4. *Immunology* 2004;113(2):153–162.
201. Schmidt AM, et al. The multiligand receptor RAGE as a progression factor amplifying immune and inflammatory responses. *J Clin Invest.* 2001;108:949–955.
202. Stern D, et al. Receptor for advanced glycation endproducts: a multiligand receptor magnifying cell stress in diverse pathologic settings. *Adv Drug Deliv Rev.* 2002;54:1615–1625.
203. Stebbing J, et al. The common heat shock protein receptor CD91 is up-regulated on monocytes of advanced melanoma slow progressors. *Clin Exp Immunol.* 2004;138:312–316.
204. Binder RJ, Han DK, Srivastava PK. CD91: a receptor for heat shock protein gp96. *Nat Immunol.* 2000;1(2):151–155.
205. Srivastava P. Interaction of heat shock proteins with peptides and antigen presenting cells: chaperoning of the innate and adaptive immune responses. *Annu Rev Immunol.* 2002;20:395–425.
206. Binder RJ, Srivastava PK. Essential role of CD91 in re-presentation of gp96-chaperoned peptides. *Proc Natl Acad Sci USA.* 2004; 101: 6128–6133.
207. Basu S, et al. Necrotic but not apoptotic cell death releases heat shock proteins, which deliver a partial maturation signal to dendritic cells and activate the NF-kappa B pathway. *Int Immunol.* 2000;12:1539–1546.
208. Melcher A, et al. Tumor immunogenicity is determined by the mechanism of cell death via induction of heat shock protein expression. *Nat Med.* 1998;4:581–587.
209. Zheng H, et al. Cell surface targeting of heat shock protein gp96 induces dendritic cell maturation and antitumor immunity. *J Immunol.* 2001;167:6731–6735.
210. Heilmann HP, et al. [Results of radiotherapy of bronchial carcinoma (author's transl)]. *Dtsch Med Wochenschr.* 1976;101:1557–1562.
211. Becker T, Hartl FU, Wieland F. CD40, an extracellular receptor for binding and uptake of Hsp70-peptide complexes. *J Cell Biol.* 2002;158:1277–1285.
212. Binder RJ, Vatner R, Srivastava P. The heat-shock protein receptors: some answers and more questions. *Tissue Antigens* 2004;64:442–451.
213. Asea A, et al. HSP70 stimulates cytokine production through a CD14-dependant pathway, demonstrating its dual role as a chaperone and cytokine. *Nat Med.* 2000;6:435–442.
214. Vabulas RM, et al. Endocytosed HSP60s use toll-like receptor 2 (TLR2) and TLR4 to activate the toll/interleukin-1 receptor signaling pathway in innate immune cells. *J Biol Chem.* 2001;276:31332–31339.
215. Polla BS, et al. Heat shock proteins in inflammation and asthma: Dr Jekyll or Mr Hyde? *Clin Exp Allergy* 1998;28:527–529.
216. Polla BS, et al. Stress proteins in inflammation. *Ann N Y Acad Sci.* 1998;851:75–85.
217. Multhoff G, Botzler C. Heat-shock proteins and the immune response. *Ann N Y Acad Sci.* 1998;851:86–93.
218. Perdrizet GA. Heat shock and tissue protection. *New Horiz.* 1995;3:312–320.
219. Mathew A, Morimoto RI. Role of the heat-shock response in the life and death of proteins. *Ann NY Acad Sci.* 1998;851:99–111.
220. Ribeiro SP, Villar J, Slutsky AS. Induction of the stress response to prevent organ injury. *New Horiz.* 1995;3:301–311.
221. Garcia-Cardena G, et al. Dynamic activation of endothelial nitric oxide synthase by Hsp90. *Nature* 1998;392:821–824.
222. Wong HR, Ryan M, Wispe JR. Stress response decreases NF-kappaB nuclear translocation and increases I-kappaBalpha expression in A549 cells. *J Clin Invest.* 1997;99:2423–2428.

223. Moshage H. Cytokines and the hepatic acute phase response. *J Pathol.* 1997;181:257–266.
224. Pepys MB, ed. *Acute phase proteins in the acute phase response.* New York: Springer-Verlag; 1989.
225. **Gabay C, Kushner I. Acute-phase proteins and other systemic responses to inflammation. *N Engl J Med.* 1999;340:448–454.**
226. Koj A. Initiation of acute phase response and synthesis of cytokines. *Biochim Biophys Acta* 1996;1317(2):84–94.
227. Giraldez RR, et al. Decreased nitric-oxide synthase activity causes impaired endothelium-dependent relaxation in the postischemic heart. *J Biol Chem.* 1997;272:21420–21426.
228. Romson JL, et al. Reduction of the extent of ischemic myocardial injury by neutrophil depletion in the dog. *Circulation* 1983;67:1016–1023.
229. Vedder NB, et al. A monoclonal antibody to the adherence-promoting leukocyte glycoprotein, CD18, reduces organ injury and improves survival from hemorrhagic shock and resuscitation in rabbits. *J Clin Invest.* 1988;81:939–944.
230. Agostoni A, et al. Activation of complement and kinin systems after thrombolytic therapy in patients with acute myocardial infarction. A comparison between streptokinase and recombinant tissue-type plasminogen activator. *Circulation* 1994;90:2666–2670.
231. Morgan BP. Complement membrane attack on nucleated cells: resistance, recovery and non-lethal effects. *Biochem J.* 1989;264:1–14.
232. Muckart DJ, Bhagwanjee S. American College of Chest Physicians/Society of Critical Care Medicine Consensus Conference definitions of the systemic inflammatory response syndrome and allied disorders in relation to critically injured patients. *Crit Care Med.* 1997;25:1789–1795.
233. **Bone RC. Sepsis, sepsis syndrome, and the systemic inflammatory response syndrome (SIRS). Gulliver in Laputa. *JAMA.* 1995;273: 155–156.**
234. Rangel-Frausto MS, et al. The natural history of the systemic inflammatory response syndrome (SIRS). A prospective study. *JAMA.* 1995;273:117–123.
235. Davies MG, Hagen PO. Systemic inflammatory response syndrome. *Br J Surg.* 1997;84:920–935.
236. Bernard GR, et al. Efficacy and safety of recombinant human activated protein C for severe sepsis. *N Engl J Med.* 2001;344:699–709.
237. Annane D, et al. Effect of treatment with low doses of hydrocortisone and fludrocortisone on mortality in patients with septic shock. *JAMA.* 2002;288:862–871.
238. Dvorak HF, Galli SJ, Dvorak AM. Cellular and vascular manifestations of cell-mediated immunity. *Hum Pathol.* 1986;17:122–137.

CHAPTER 7 ■ SURGICAL INFECTIONS

E. PATCHEN DELLINGER

Although there is no official definition of a surgical infection, it is commonly understood as an infection that will not resolve with antimicrobial therapy alone but also requires surgical intervention. Surgical intervention may be as significant as a major laparotomy or thoracotomy or as simple as removing sutures from an infected surgical incision or draining a superficial abscess. It also includes interventions by radiologists or other specialists such as computed tomography (CT)-guided percutaneous drainage of an intra-abdominal abscess or placement of a stent through a biliary stricture in a patient with cholangitis. A unifying characteristic of all surgical infections is an anatomic manipulation, such as draining a closed space, closing a perforated viscus, or removing dead tissue or foreign body, that must be performed to achieve resolution of the infection. Many "medical" infections involve single pathogens that are able to establish themselves and grow through intrinsic pathogenic mechanisms despite intact skin or mucosa. Examples include pneumococcal pneumonia, streptococcal pharyngitis, meningococcal meningitis, and salmonella enteritis. Surgical infections typically occur after a mechanical breach of normal epithelial barriers and often involve multiple organisms, typically endogenous to the area of epithelial injury. Examples include peritonitis after perforated appendicitis or diverticulitis and surgical site infections (SSIs) caused by skin flora after clean operations. An exception to this principle for surgical infections is the occurrence of necrotizing soft tissue infections secondary to Group A beta-hemolytic streptococci (hemolytic streptococcal gangrene), which can occur following trivial injuries or no known prior injury. In this chapter we also discuss nonsurgical infections that typically occur in hospitalized surgical patients. These include catheter-related bloodstream infections, pneumonia, and urinary tract infections (UTIs).

In approaching the topic of surgical infections each area is approached in the following order: prevention, diagnosis, treatment. The first element of prevention is the natural host defense mechanisms of the patient. The most important of these for surgical infections is the epithelial covering that separates the sterile portions of the body from those with normal endogenous flora. Thus the skin on the outside of the body and the gastrointestinal (GI) mucosa lining the alimentary tract are the sites of complex microbiologic flora and serve to bar those flora from the tissues in most cases. Once these mechanical barriers are breached, by trauma, medical or surgical procedures, neoplasm, inflammation, or ischemia, cellular and humoral defenses become important.

The array of host defenses is large and complex, and our understanding of these processes is continually advancing. Initial, nonspecific defenses begin with fixed tissue macrophages and circulating polymorphonuclear leukocytes (PNMs), which engulf and kill small numbers of invading microorganisms. The macrophages and dendritic cells also have the ability to ingest pathogens and to process their antigens for presentation to T lymphocytes for the subsequent development of specific antibodies by B lymphocytes. The first presentation of an antigen leads to the formation of IgM class antibodies that are produced over the next 1 to 2 weeks. Subsequent exposure to the same antigen leads to much more rapid production of IgG antibodies. Antibodies bound to microorganisms promote more efficient phagocytosis and killing and also serve to activate complement proteins, another element in the humoral defense system. The complement system exists in a quiescent form, which when activated leads to a cascade of activated complement proteins and fractions that enhance phagocytosis, increase vascular permeability, stimulate inflammation, and lead to direct lysis of some pathogens.

There are many interactions between the cellular and humoral aspects of host defense. Host defense cells manufacture the humoral components, and when activated, the humoral components stimulate the cells. In addition, there is extensive cross talk among the cellular elements of host defenses involving a large number of cytokines including tumor necrosis factor (TNF) and many interleukins, signified by IL-n, with the number n increasing as new cytokines are discovered and characterized. The successful interaction of these elements is essential to normal host defenses, but when the mechanisms of control fail and cytokines spread beyond their intended local actions, these host defense mechanisms can turn against the host, resulting in a spectrum of conditions variously called the systemic inflammatory response syndrome (SIRS) and multiple organ dysfunction syndrome (MODS). Many attempts to modify this process through the development of specific antagonists to various elements of this system have so far failed to produce clinically useful products although research continues.

When injury occurs and blood vessels are opened, the coagulation cascade, similar in some ways to the complement cascade, is also initiated. In recent years it has been recognized that a number of elements in the coagulation response and the inflammatory response are shared, and local thrombosis and fibrinogen deposition is a prominent component of acute inflammation. Inflammation stimulates a procoagulant state and can also promote distant thromboembolic events. More recently, a clinical trial of activated protein C, a component of the coagulation cascade that has antithrombotic, antiinflammatory, and profibrinolytic properties, has proved beneficial for some patients with combined SIRS, infection, and organ failure.[1]

PREVENTION

Despite the success of intrinsic host defenses, in many circumstances infections do occur, especially after surgical interventions, both elective and urgent. It is incumbent on the surgical team to understand and to apply what is known regarding elements of patient care and delivery of surgical procedures that reduce the risk of subsequent infection as much as possible. In general terms, these preventive measures can fall into three broad categories. The patient should come to an operative procedure with host defenses in the best possible condition. The procedure should be conducted in a manner that reduces to the minimum introduction of pathogens into the sterile compartments of the body. The perioperative management of the patient should be conducted in a manner that optimally supports and maintains the patient's host defenses. In actual practice, many items of patient care will relate to more than one of these goals. These items are discussed in more detail in the section dealing with SSIs.

DIAGNOSIS

Although details specific to the diagnosis of specific surgical infections and other infections in surgical patients are covered in those individual sections, some items of diagnosis are common to all. Some relatively straightforward infections such as superficial SSIs or subcutaneous abscesses are properly treated by simply opening the wound or draining the abscess without the use of antimicrobial agents and do not require routine culture. However, most surgical infections require at least the initial use of antimicrobial agents that are most effective if active against the primary pathogens involved. If initial treatment is clearly successful, then knowledge of the specific pathogens and their susceptibilities are not critical for the treatment of that patient. However, when the patient does not respond as expected, then knowledge of the pathogens and their susceptibilities can be extremely useful, and this information will not be available unless the appropriate cultures were obtained prior to initiating antibiotic therapy.

Material sent to the microbiology laboratory from the operating room or the interventional radiology suite is preferable. Surface swabs taken from open or draining wounds or material from drains that have been in place for days have a high probability of returning information about contaminating or colonizing organisms that are not responsible for the infection needing treatment. Samples of tissue or fluid are always preferable to swabs from the operating room. Blood cultures are helpful when positive but are positive in less than one third of surgical infections in most reported series. An early source of information from such specimens is the Gram stain, which should be available to the physician in less than an hour after obtaining the specimen. The initial choice of antimicrobial agents for a serious infection will be quite different if the Gram stain shows gram-positive cocci than if the stain shows predominantly gram-negative rods. Microbial growth and preliminary identification will usually be available within 24 hours for most surgical pathogens, but susceptibility information will not be reported for one or more additional days. Thus, knowledge of the susceptibility patterns in the hospital, or even more specifically, in a specific intensive care unit (ICU), can be invaluable in directing initial empiric antimicrobial choices for a critically ill patient.[2] This is another reason to culture severe infections. The body of information about pathogens and their susceptibilities locally helps to direct therapy for patients in the future, and these patterns can change over time. Thus current culture information is always helpful. Although antimicrobial susceptibility data currently take 2 days or more in most cases, advances in the modern microbiology laboratory may someday provide this information more rapidly. Detection of specific nucleic acid sequences has the potential to identify certain common and well-characterized resistance genes such as the *mecA* gene that codes for methicillin resistance in *Staphylococcus aureus.* Other diagnostic advances that are making their way to the clinical microbiology laboratory include antigen and antibody detection systems and polymerase chain reaction (PCR) for amplifying small amounts of nucleic acids.

Diagnosis of infection always involves history and physical examination, but these are more efficiently discussed in relation to specific infections. Fever and leukocytosis are frequent accompaniments of infection but are not specific and are variously sensitive depending on the specific infection. They may drive further diagnostic efforts including physical and radiologic examination but are not sufficient reason to initiate antimicrobial treatment in isolation from other data. Radiologic examinations can be very helpful in some specific circumstances but should not substitute for or precede history and physical examination and clinical judgment.

TREATMENT

Treatment of surgical infections, as discussed initially in the definition of surgical infections always involves a procedure and often involves the use of one or more antimicrobial agents. The generic term for a procedure directed at the resolution of a surgical infection is *source control.* Source control refers to the mechanical or anatomic procedure that is used to drain an abscess, relieve an obstruction, repair a perforation, or resect dead, ischemic, or inflamed tissue or a foreign body to promote the resolution of a surgical infection. In recent years there has been growing recognition that the literature regarding surgical infections is incomplete when it does not adequately describe and evaluate the effectiveness of source control.[3] This is particularly true for publications comparing different antimicrobial treatments of surgical infections. When the differences between two regimens are small, a difference in the delivery of source control to patients in the comparative regimens can skew the results.[4] The appropriate use of antimicrobial agents is also important in many situations and is addressed in the sections regarding specific infections. Although the choice of specific agents, and to a lesser extent dosing, have been addressed, there is very little relevant data regarding the appropriate duration of antimicrobial treatment for most surgical infections. Trends in recent years have been to decrease this duration in many cases. Only in the area of prophylaxis are good data available.

SURGICAL SITE INFECTIONS

Infections that occur in a surgical incision were previously called wound infections. In recent years, a consensus conference involving surgical and medical societies and the Centers for Disease Control (CDC) developed the concept of SSI.[5,6] This includes any infection that occurs in an operative site. An infection of the subcutaneous tissue only (the vast majority of "wound infections") is termed a superficial SSI. One that involves the muscular and fascial layers and includes a partial or complete fascial dehiscence is a deep SSI. An infection that occurs within the organ or deep space of the wound such as peritonitis, an intra-abdominal abscess, an empyema, or a joint space infection is called an organ/space SSI. Data from the National Nosocomial Infection Surveillance (NNIS) system of the CDC shows that of all SSIs, 47% are superficial, 23% are deep, and 30% are organ/space.[7] Only 46% of these SSIs are diagnosed during the original hospitalization, whereas 16% after discharge as outpatients and 38% on readmission to the hospital. Although 58% of all organ/space SSIs are diagnosed during the original hospitalization, 59% of other SSIs are diagnosed only after discharge.[7]

Surgeons have traditionally divided wounds into the classes of clean, clean-contaminated, contaminated, and dirty (Table 7.1)[8] based on the probability that the wound would be contaminated by bacteria during the operative procedure. These classes roughly divide wounds into different risks for the development of SSI. More recently, examination of data bases that include many thousands of wounds have led to the development of newer risk classification systems that provide a more accurate estimate of risk. The NNIS index[9] assigns up to one risk point for each of (a) contaminated or dirty wound, (b) American Society of Anesthesiologists (ASA) class 3 or higher, and (c) duration of operation exceeding the 75th percentile for that operation.[9] Thus, an operation may fall into one of four classes between 0 and 3. Table 7.2[9] demonstrates the increased precision of this system compared with the older system that refers only to wound class. This system can be used to roughly compare the performance of a hospital or surgical department against the NNIS data base by comparing expected with observed infection rates.[10] Of course, much more precise risk data can be developed for single operative procedures through analysis of large data bases in which the heterogeneity imposed by multiple different procedures is eliminated.[11,12]

TABLE 7.1 CLASSIFICATION

WOUND CLASSIFICATION

Class	Definition
Clean	An uninfected operative wound in which no inflammation is encountered and the respiratory, alimentary, genital, or infected urinary tract is not entered. In addition, clean wounds are closed primarily and, if necessary, drained with closed drainage.
Clean-contaminated	An operative wound in which the respiratory, alimentary, genital, or urinary tracts are entered under controlled conditions and without unusual contamination.
Contaminated	Open, fresh, accidental wounds. Operations with major breaks in sterile technique or gross spillage from the gastrointestinal tract, and incisions in which acute, nonpurulent inflammation is encountered.
Dirty	Old traumatic wounds with retained devitalized tissue and those that involve existing clinical infection or perforated viscera.

TABLE 7.2

COMPARISION OF WOUND CLASSIFICATION AND NNIS SYSTEM FOR EVALUATING RISK OF SURGICAL SITE INFECTION

	NNIS Risk Index				
Wound class	0	1	2	3	All
Clean	1.0	2.3	5.4	—	2.1
Clean-contaminated	2.1	4.0	9.5	—	3.3
Contaminated	—	3.4	6.8	13.2	6.4
Dirty	—	3.1	8.1	12.8	7.1
All	1.5	2.9	6.8	13.0	2.8
Maximum ratio[a]	2.1	1.7	1.8	1.0	

NNIS, National Nosocomial Infection Surveillance System.
[a]Ratio of lowest to highest infection rate in wound class or in risk index.
Adapted from Dellinger EP, Ehrenkranz NJ. Surgical infections. In: Bennett JV, Brachman PS, eds. *Hospital infections*. Philadelphia: Lippincott-Raven; 1998:571–585, with permission.

Many other factors that influence the risk of SSI have been proposed, and a relatively complete summary of these factors is provided in a publication by the Hospital Infection Control Practices Advisory Committee (HICPAC) of the CDC.[6] Some of these are summarized in Table 7.3, which lists the category 1 recommendations that are readily influenced by the surgeon. It is likely that the majority of these are important in most operative procedures, although most have been generated through analysis of single procedures or limited classes of procedures and have not been reproduced in all cases. Many, such as the patient's weight and smoking status or the presence of an infection at a distant site, are modifiable prior to scheduled operation. Others such as age or underlying immune disorders cannot be improved. Some, such as diabetes, cannot be eliminated, but recent information suggests that tight control of perioperative glucose levels can greatly reduce the risk associated with this diagnosis.[13,14]

Prevention

Preventing SSIs is clearly a prime responsibility of any operating surgeon. Although many surgeons think first of prophylactic antibiotics for prevention, and these are clearly important, antibiotics are most effective when they complement maximal efforts for prevention by other means. Two classic papers in surgical prophylaxis, each of which demonstrated the superiority of prophylactic antibiotics to placebo in randomized prospective trials, also demonstrated an increased infection rate in the face of prophylaxis when hemostasis was not ideal[15] or when gross contamination was observed during the operative procedure.[16] Each patient should be brought to the operating

TABLE 7.3

CATEGORY 1 RECOMMENDATIONS FROM THE HOSPITAL INFECTION CONTROL PRACTICES ADVISORY COMMITTEE FOR THE PREVENTION OF SURGICAL SITE INFECTIONS

■ Do not operate on patients with active infections	■ Use sterile instruments
■ Do not shave patient in advance	■ Avoid flash sterilization
■ Control glucose in diabetic patients	■ Wear a mask[a]
■ Stop tobacco use in patient	■ Cover all hair[a]
■ Have patient shower with antiseptic soap	■ Wear sterile gloves[a]
■ Prepare skin with appropriate agent	■ Use gowns and drapes that resist fluid penetration
■ Surgeon's nails should be short	■ Gentle tissue handling
■ Surgeons scrub hands	■ Closed suction drains (when used)
■ Exclude infected surgeons	■ Delayed primary closure for heavily contaminated wounds
■ Give prophylactic antibiotics when indicated	■ Sterile dressing for 24–48 hr
■ Maintain prophylactic antibiotic levels during operation	■ Use CDC definitions for SSI
■ Keep O.R. doors closed	■ SSI surveillance with feedback to surgeons

[a]These items are required by OSHA regulations and are not actually supported by class 1 data.
From Mangram AJ, et al. Guideline for prevention of surgical site infection, 1999. Hospital Infection Control Practices Advisory Committee. *Infect Control Hosp Epidemiol.* 1999;20:250–278, with permission.

room only after the correctable items noted in Table 7.3 have been corrected to the degree possible. In addition, in recent years several elements of the immediate perioperative management of surgical patients have been demonstrated to have a significant effect on the risk for SSI. Beyond these issues most surgeons believe that the technical conduct of the operation, including the handling of tissues, number of ties and other foreign material and devitalized tissue, and the length of operation all influence the risk of SSI. Unfortunately no validated method for assessing these issues exists. In addition, although data clearly demonstrate that the risk for SSI increases with increasing duration of operation and increasing transfusion, it is not clear that operations that take longer or require more transfusion are the same as shorter procedures that do not require transfusion. Thus the precise role of these issues is not clear. Certainly no surgeon should take longer than he or she thinks necessary for a procedure, nor should he or she transfuse a patient when it is not considered important.

Inspired Oxygen Tension

Multiple animal models of infection demonstrate that oxygen tension within the surgical wound correlates with risk for SSI. Low oxygen tensions increase risk, whereas higher tensions decrease it.[17] Another report examined the subcutaneous oxygen tension in 130 surgical patients in the postanesthesia recovery room.[18] The same relationship was found between oxygen tension and risk for SSI. Recently, a prospective trial comparing inspired oxygen concentrations of 30% to 80% in patient having colectomy demonstrated a significant decrease in infection rates in the high inspired oxygen group.[19] Subsequently, a paper from a different group of investigators reported a much smaller number of patients having mixed GI procedures with an opposite conclusion, a higher infection rate in the patients receiving 80% oxygen compared with 35%.[20] Until more data are available, we must consider the ideal inspired oxygen concentration for reducing risk of SSI in surgical patients to be unsettled.

Temperature Control

The temperature of a patient in the operating room is known to influence skin and subcutaneous blood flow and oxygen tension.[21] Animal models have demonstrated increased infection risk when body temperature is lowered. Recently, two prospective controlled trials have demonstrated a reduction in SSI in patients who were actively warmed. One trial in patients submitted to colectomy compared active warming in the operating room to no efforts at warming.[22]A threefold reduction in infection rate was found in the warmed patients. In another study of minor procedures (hernia repair, varicose vein operation, or breast procedure with incision >3 cm) active prewarming, either of the whole patient or of the operative site, also significantly reduced the incidence of SSI and of postoperative antibiotic use by physicians blind to the treatment group.[23] It is increasingly the standard to maintain normal body temperature for operative patients, but without specific protocols to achieve this in all patients, it frequently is not achieved.[24]

Glucose Control

It has long been known that diabetics have a higher risk for SSI than nondiabetic patients. It has been assumed that this related to underlying defects in host defense associated with the diagnosis. Recently, analysis of a large series of patients, both diabetic and nondiabetic, having an open heart procedure demonstrated that the risk for SSI was most strongly correlated with the occurrence of hyperglycemia (glucose >200 mg%) during the first 48 hours after operation.[13] When this occurred, the risk for SSI was doubled regardless of whether the patient was diabetic or not. Forty-seven percent of the patients with hyperglycemia in this study were not diabetic. This relation has also been shown for a group of mixed GI and cardiovascular operations in diabetic patients.[25] Another cardiac surgery group has shown the same relationship between glucose levels and infection risk and has also demonstrated that improved perioperative glucose control with intravenous insulin infusions has reduced both the incidence of SSI and mortality in their diabetic patients.[14,26] Although the strongest evidence exists for diabetic cardiac surgical patients, it is likely that all hyperglycemic surgical patients will benefit from perioperative glucose control.

Antibiotic Prophylaxis

Antibiotic prophylaxis for surgical procedures began shortly after the initial introduction of penicillin with the hope that antibiotics would reduce the risk of surgical wound infections. Prior to 1960, prophylactic antibiotics commonly were started after surgery; a technique that we now know is ineffective. Furthermore, antibiotics were given most often to patients at special risk of infection. Consequently, patients given antibiotics were more likely to develop infections than untreated patients.[27]

TABLE 7.4

TYPICAL INFECTION RATES AND REDUCTION WITH PROPHYLAXIS

	Prophylaxis (%)	Placebo (%)	NNT[a]
Colon	4–12	24–48	3–5
Other (mixed) GI	4–6	15–29	4–9
Vascular	1–4	7–17	10–17
Cardiac	3–9	44–49	2–3
Hysterectomy	1–16	18–38	3–6
Craniotomy	0.5–3	4–12	9–29
Total joint replacement	0.5–1	2–9	12–100
Breast and hernia operations	3.5	5.2	58

GI, gastrointestinal.
[a]Approximate number needed-to-treat (NNT) to avoid one surgical site infection.

Subsequent animal experiments and human trials demonstrated that giving antibiotics before wound contamination occurred (i.e., preoperatively) significantly reduces SSI.[28] Subsequent study has shown that the ideal time for antibiotic administration is just before the incision because this regimen produces better tissue antibiotic concentrations at both the beginning and end of the operation than other administration times.[29]

Prophylactic antibiotics are indicated for all GI (including appendectomy), obstetrical, gynecologic, oropharyngeal, vascular (abdominal and leg), and open-heart procedures. Typical reductions in SSI rate in early placebo-controlled trials of prophylactic antibiotics are given in Table 7.4. The use of prophylactic antibiotics for clean operations remains controversial. Although prophylactic antibiotics reduce the infection rate even in clean procedures, the baseline infection rate is low in these cases.[30,31] Consequently, the number-needed-to-treat for each infection prevented is so large that the reduction in infection risk may not justify the cost and complications associated with antibiotic administration. Nonetheless, prophylactic antibiotic treatment is used routinely for clean procedures such as open-heart operations, joint replacement, vascular prostheses, and craniotomy in which the consequences of SSI are especially severe.[32]

Antibiotics should be dosed to maintain adequate tissue concentrations throughout the period of potential contamination. For example, doses should be increased in larger patients.[33] Similarly, doses should be repeated after one or two half-lives have elapsed.[34,35] Numerous trials comparing shorter and longer durations of prophylactic antibiotics failed to show any benefit of extending antibiotic administration beyond the operating room.[36,37] Furthermore, prolonged prophylaxis is associated with recovery of resistant bacteria.[38] An expert panel assembled by the Center for Medicare and Medicaid Services (CMS) thus recommended that prophylactic antibiotics be initiated within the hour before starting an operation and stopped within 24 hours of completion.[39]

Naturally, the antibiotic(s) must be active against the relevant pathogens. This is most clearly illustrated by the requirement that the agent used have activity against enteric anaerobes for procedures involving the lower GI tract. Although yet to be studied in a systematic manner, there is general agreement that antibiotic agents used for prophylaxis should be different from agents usually chosen as first-line choices for treatment of established infections. Thus, although imipenem/cilastatin or piperacillin/tazobactam would undoubtedly be efficacious as prophylactic agents for colon operations, they are not recommended for this purpose. Table 7.5 gives the spectrum of antibiotic recommendations that have been published by different professional societies and organizations. In general, one can choose a first-generation cephalosporin for operations not expected to encounter anaerobes and a second-generation cephalosporin with anaerobic activity for procedures in which anaerobic contamination is likely.

Beta-lactam allergies are often cited as a problem for surgical antibiotic prophylaxis. However, many patients reported as allergic do not have true allergy and instead have experienced minor adverse reactions such as *Candida* overgrowth or GI upset. Before choosing an alternate prophylactic agent, one should confirm the nature of the previous reaction. Patients who have had immediate, anaphylactic type reactions should not receive a cephalosporin, but most others can safely receive one or two doses in the perioperative period. For patients with true beta-lactam allergies, vancomycin is the most common prophylactic choice when the primary risk of infection is from skin organisms, and clindamycin is another appropriate alternative. There are no controlled trials of prophylaxis in colon operations using agents appropriate for beta-lactam allergic patients. Logic suggests that the combination of clindamycin or metronidazole with either an aminoglycoside or a fluoroquinolone or the combination of clindamycin with aztreonam should be effective. Although vancomycin has been recommended for routine prophylactic use in hospitals with high rates of methicillin-resistant *Staphylococcus aureus* (MRSA), infection rates were not reduced in the only relevant prospective trial and the number of infections due to sensitive staphylococci was increased in the vancomycin arm.[40] Vancomycin prophylaxis appears to be most appropriate in patients proved by preoperative nasal culture to be MRSA carriers.

Shaving

Removing hair at the operative site remains routine in many settings, although there is no evidence that it reduces infection rate. In contrast, studies show that avoiding hair removal or using depilatories rather than shaving reduces infection rates after clean operations.[41,42] For example, infection rates are reduced when hair is clipped rather than shaved, even when performed on the day of operation. It may be helpful to warn patients not to shave their operative sites before surgery as some do in an effort to be helpful. If hair removal at the incision site is considered necessary, it should be performed with clippers during the immediate preoperative period.

TABLE 7.5

SUMMARY OF PUBLISHED GUIDELINES ON ANTIMICROBIAL PROPHYLAXIS FOR OPERATIONS TARGETED FOR SURVEILLANCE IN THE NATIONAL SURGICAL INFECTION PREVENTION PROJECT

Operations	Prophylactic antibiotic recommendation	Comments
Cardiothoracic surgery	Cefazolin Cefuroxime Cefamandole If β-lactam allergy: Vancomycin Clindamycin	Most of the guidelines agree that duration of prophylaxis for cardiac surgery should not exceed 24 hours. The American Society of Health-System Pharmacists (ASHP) suggests continuation of prophylaxis for cardiothoracic surgery for up to 72 hours; however, the authors suggest that prophylaxis for 24 hours or less may be appropriate. Cefamandole is not available in the United States.
Vascular surgery	Cefazolin Cefuroxime If β-lactam allergy: Vancomycin Vancomycin with or without gentamicin Clindamycin	
Colon surgery	Oral: Neomycin plus erythromycin base Neomycin plus metronidazole Parenteral: Cefoxitin or cefotetan Cefazolin plus metronidazole	Currently, none of the guidelines address antimicrobial prophylaxis for those patients with documented β-lactam allergy. Patients with a documented β-lactam allergy undergoing colon surgery are currently excluded from the denominator of the antibiotic selection performance measure for the National Surgical Infection Prevention Project. Cefmetazole is not available in the United States. Although a recent study indicates that the combination of oral prophylaxis with parenteral antimicrobial prophylaxis may result in lower wound infection rates, this is not specified in any of the published guidelines.
Hip or knee arthroplasty	Cefazolin If β-lactam allergy: Vancomycin Clindamycin	Although not addressed in any of the published guidelines, the Workgroup recommends that the prophylactic antimicrobial be completely infused prior to the inflation of a tourniquet.
Vaginal or abdominal hysterectomy	Cefazolin Cefotetan Cefoxitin Cefuroxime	Metronidazole monotherapy is recommended in the ACOG Practice Bulletin as an alternative to cephalosporin prophylaxis for patients undergoing hysterectomy. Patients with a documented β-lactam allergy undergoing hysterectomy are currently excluded from the denominator of the antimicrobial selection performance measure for the National Surgical Infection Prevention Project. Trovafloxacin, although still available in the United States, is recommended on a limited basis only.

Adapted from Bratzler DW, Houck PM. Antimicrobial prophylaxis for surgery: an advisory statement from the national surgical infection prevention project. *Clin Infect Dis.* 2004;38:1706–1715, with permission.

Delayed Primary Closure

A classic technique to avoid SSI has been to leave the wound open at the original procedure and then to attempt delayed primary closure a few days later or to leave the wound open for closure by secondary intention. This practice was widely used by the military during World War II, and although there have been many series recommending this practice, it has rarely been subject to controlled trial. A recent prospective trial randomized patients undergoing an operative procedure with dirty wounds either to have primary closure of the incision or to have it left open with delayed primary closure.[43] Although the authors concluded that there were fewer SSIs in the group with wounds left open, it is instructive that there were very few differences in overall patient course, and more patients went home with open wounds requiring dressing changes when the wounds were left open than when they were closed primarily in the operating room. There were no differences in overall hospital stay or in charges.

Diagnosis of Surgical Site Infection

One can easily diagnosis an SSI when the wound opens and discharges pus. However, it is preferable to make the diagnosis earlier and to initiate prompt intervention. Most SSIs are not clinically evident before the fourth or fifth postoperative day. The rare exceptions to this are infections caused by beta-hemolytic streptococci and by histotoxic *Clostridium* sp. and, even more rarely, wound toxic shock. These can be evident within 1 day and, although rare, can be very severe. If a patient manifests severe systemic signs of infection during the first few days after an operation, the incision should be inspected for signs of infection (Algorithm 7.1). Streptococcal infections usually have local signs of inflammation with marked erythema and pain and wound fluid containing white blood cells (WBCs) and gram-positive cocci. Wounds infected by clostridia usually lack signs of inflammation but cause severe pain out of proportion to other findings and drain a thin, brackish wound fluid lacking leukocytes due to the action of the exotoxins on leukocytes causing lysis. In these cases, gram-positive rods without spores are evident on Gram smear. Wound blisters or desquamation of skin associated with SSI are late findings and predictive of significant morbidity.

Thirteen cases of wound toxic shock were confirmed by the CDC during an 18-month period, representing less than 1% of all cases of toxic shock reported during that period. More than half of these presented within 48 hours of an operation.[44] The earliest signs were fever, diarrhea, and vomiting.

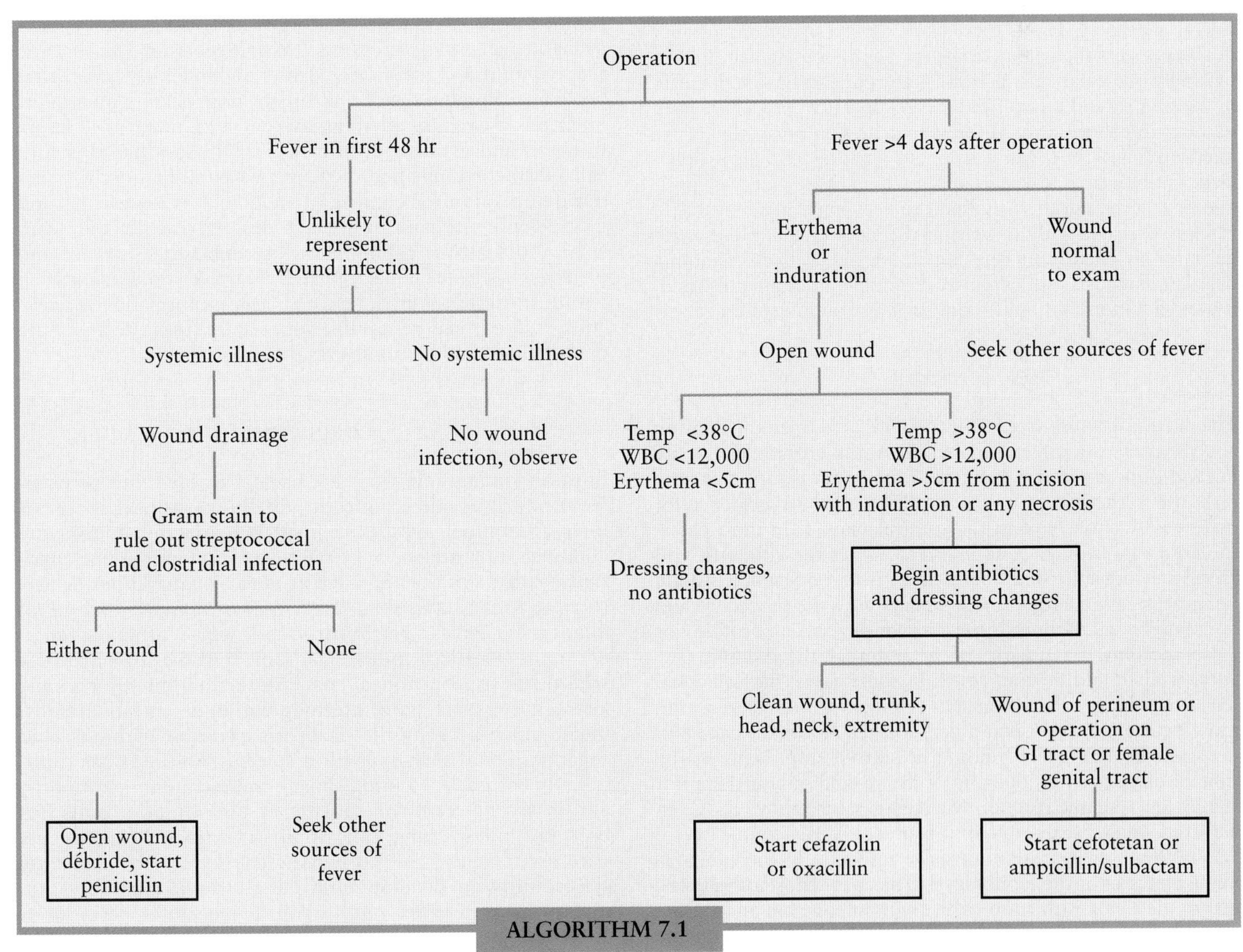

ALGORITHM 7.1 Managing potential surgical site infections. (Adapted from Dellinger EP. Post-operative wound infections. In: Schlossberg D, ed. Current therapy of infectious diseases, 2nd ed. Philadelphia: Mosby Year Book; 2001:409–412, with permission.)

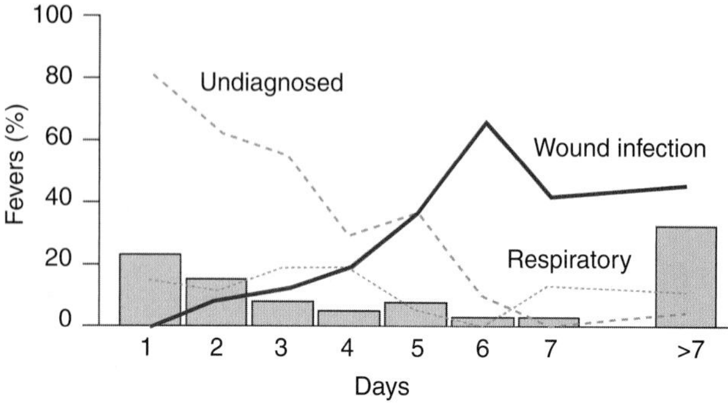

FIGURE 7.1 Percentage of all postoperative fevers occurring on the indicated day following an operative procedure. Lines indicate the percent of fevers occurring on each day attributable to the cause indicated. (After Dellinger EP. Approach to the patient with postoperative fever. In: Gorbach S, Bartlett J, Blacklow N, eds. *Infectious diseases.* Philadelphia: Lippincott Williams & Wilkins; 2004.)

Erythroderma and hypotension were also present. Often, local signs of wound infection were initially absent. Drainage and irrigation of the wound in combination with a systemic anti-staphylococcal antibiotic is recommended.

Although most wound infections are diagnosed within 2 weeks after the procedure, diagnosis may occasionally be considerably delayed. This is more likely when a significant amount of tissue covers the operative site such as abdominal incisions in morbidly obese patients. Because many patients have some fever in the first several days after a major operative procedure even without infection, fever is not a specific sign of postoperative infection (Fig. 7.1).[45] Many surgeons want to continue prophylactic antibiotics or to restart antibiotics in cases with early postoperative fever, but this is unlikely to be helpful. In addition, SSI cannot be treated without opening the incision. If antibiotics are given for an SSI without opening the wound, this can result in a delay in diagnosis and definitive treatment, additional morbidity, and additional complications such as wound dehiscence.

Therapy

The most important treatment for a SSI is to open the incision and evacuate the infected material. Antimicrobial agents are needed only when a patient exhibits a significant systemic response to the infection or when there is clinical evidence for invasive infection beyond the surgical wound. In most cases, the entire incision will be involved under the skin and will have to be opened. When an incision is first opened, it should be inspected by a surgeon who understands the procedure and the underlying anatomy. If the procedure was a laparotomy or a thoracotomy, the integrity of the closure of the abdominal or chest wall should be confirmed. In some cases, the incisional SSI is not the primary event but is a sign of more severe and more extensive infection at a deeper level, an organ/space SSI.

Antimicrobial agents should be started empirically at the time of diagnosis and opening of the wound only if there is a significant systemic reaction with temperature above 38°C, an elevated pulse rate, or an absolute WBC count above 12,000/mm^3 or if there is invasive infection in the subcutaneous space or at the fascial level. The agent chosen should be determined by Gram stain of the wound contents and by the prior procedure. SSI after an operation that did not enter the alimentary tract and was not on the perineum or axilla are often caused by *S. aureus* or less commonly streptococcal species. If Gram stain confirms gram-positive cocci, one can use an initial dose of cefazolin or oxacillin. Antimicrobial treatment should be continued only as long as systemic signs of infection or local cellulitis continues to be present, usually 3 days or less.

For SSI that follow operations in the axilla, gram-negative bacilli are found more often, and after operations on the perineum or involving the alimentary or genital tract, both facultative and obligate anaerobes are common. In these cases, if antimicrobial therapy is necessary, treatment can be started with cefotetan, cefoxitin, or ampicillin-sulbactam. Patients allergic to penicillin and cephalosporins can receive ciprofloxacin or levofloxacin combined with either clindamycin or metronidazole. Again, the treatment should usually be 3 days or less.

INTRA-ABDOMINAL INFECTIONS

Prevention

Most intra-abdominal infections are the result of spontaneous disease including such conditions as appendicitis, diverticulitis, obstructed or perforated carcinomas, or inflammatory bowel disease. Here, prevention depends on early diagnosis and treatment of the underlying condition. However, an increasing proportion of intra-abdominal infections from series published in the past few decades have been postoperative, reflecting the increasing number of operative procedures performed and the increasing risk status of the patients and the complexity of the operations performed. In the case of postoperative intra-abdominal infections, there are few data available regarding prevention. It is safe to assume that factors that reduce risk of incisional SSI after abdominal operations are probably helpful in the case of organ/space or intra-abdominal infections as well. In addition, avoidance of unintended injury to bowel and optimal performance of GI anastomoses is critical. When contamination of the peritoneum does occur, either during operation or because of spontaneous disease, natural host defense mechanisms actually deal very successfully with small inocula by a combination of lymphatic clearance and phagocytosis by local macrophages. However, if contamination with a small inoculum is repeated, abscess formation is likely. And, if continued contamination occurs, local defenses are overwhelmed and peritonitis results.

Diagnosis

Intra-abdominal infections are usually divided into peritonitis, a poorly localized infection of the peritoneal space, or intra-abdominal abscess, a localized infection within the abdomen. Peritonitis can be relatively local within one quadrant or region of the abdomen as in early gangrenous or perforated appendicitis or diffuse in two or more abdominal quadrants. Diffuse peritonitis has a worse prognosis than peritonitis localized to one quadrant.[46] Abscesses may occur within the free peritoneal space in the subphrenic regions, lateral gutters, pelvis, or interloop within the intestinal folds, or they may occur in the retroperitoneum or within a solid organ (visceral) such as liver or spleen. Peritonitis has traditionally been divided into primary and secondary peritonitis, and in recent years the concept of tertiary peritonitis has been proposed. Primary peritonitis describes those patients with ascites due either to hepatic cirrhosis or to nephrotic syndrome who develop infected ascites presumably secondary to bacteremia and without evidence for perforation or underlying GI tract pathology. If the diagnosis of primary peritonitis can be made, these patients are best treated with antimicrobial agents alone and without operation. Because of their severe underlying disease, they are at high risk for poor outcome.

Secondary peritonitis refers to peritoneal infection that occurs secondary to another underlying disease such as bowel perforation. Tertiary peritonitis is a condition first recognized toward the end of the last century and describes patients who continue to have evidence for poorly localized intra-abdominal infection after initial operative and antimicrobial treatment of secondary infection. At subsequent interventions, these patients tend to have evidence for diffuse inflammation without bowel perforation, and cultures return a variety of bacteria that are not common pathogens in the peritoneum such as coagulase-negative staphylococci, *Candida* species, enterococcus, and *Pseudomonas* species.[47] The categorization of secondary intra-abdominal infection can also be divided into spontaneous infection, those cases arising from underlying disease, and postoperative infection, occurring after operative intervention or other procedures or trauma. Recent series show that approximately 66% of intra-abdominal infections are spontaneous and 34% are postoperative.[46]

The diagnosis of intra-abdominal infection is almost always first suggested by abdominal pain. This supplemented with a directed history and an exam demonstrating abdominal tenderness strengthens the case. Fever and elevated WBC count are often present, but early cases of appendicitis and diverticulitis will sometimes present with normal temperature and/or WBC count. In patients with diffuse peritonitis such as follows freely perforated bowel or ulcer, the diagnosis is usually made by clinical examination and this can be followed by resuscitation and operative management without additional sophisticated studies. With abscess, however, the clinical picture is often less straightforward and the addition of cross-sectional imaging techniques, particularly CT scan, can be very helpful, whereas radionuclide scans have limited usefulness in the diagnosis of intra-abdominal abscess.

Treatment—Source Control

The treatment of intra-abdominal infection always involves the combination of both source control and antimicrobial agents. Diffuse peritonitis involves inflammation and fluid production throughout the peritoneal surface, an area comparable to total body surface area. This is a major hemodynamic challenge and inflammatory stress to the host organism and must be addressed by attention to circulating blood volume, respiratory status, and other systemic parameters just as in any other critical systemic illness. The fluid requirements of diffuse peritonitis approximate those of a 50% body surface area burn. These fluid shifts accompanied by the cytokine response to peritonitis can easily lead to respiratory and renal failure initially followed by MODS if not treated early and aggressively. Attention to airway, breathing, and circulation must occur simultaneously with antimicrobial management. The systemic disturbance associated with intra-abdominal infection is most readily measured by critical care scores such as Acute Physiology and Chronic Health Evaluation (APACHE) II score, which has been demonstrated to correlate with mortality and inversely with successful initial treatment of intra-abdominal infection.[48]

Diffuse peritonitis essentially always implies an uncontrolled leak from the GI tract and always mandates operative exploration for source control. If intra-abdominal abscess is diagnosed or suspected, drainage is required, but this can often be accomplished by drains placed percutaneously using the radiologic guidance of fluoroscopy, CT, or ultrasound. Although no prospective trials have been performed comparing open drainage with percutaneous drainage, comparative series suggest that resolution of abscess and mortality are essentially equal between the techniques.[49] Open drainage of intra-abdominal abscess is usually reserved for those cases in which percutaneous access to the abscess is prevented by overlying viscera. Regardless of the approach to source control, review of multiple series suggests that in approximately one fourth of cases a second effort at source control will be necessary to resolve the infection. This may be another open operation or another percutaneous drain or conversion from one approach to the other. A subsequent intervention is indicated when the patient fails to improve or worsens following the primary intervention. Ideally, the initial effort at source control should be successful. When the operating surgeon is asked to rate the initial source control procedure, outcome is greatly inferior when he or she is not satisfied with this procedure.[46,50]

Treatment—Antimicrobial Therapy

The initial antimicrobial treatment of intra-abdominal infection is always empiric. The diagnosis is made clinically, and antimicrobial therapy is started when the diagnosis is made and while the patient is being prepared for the source control procedure. Cultures should be taken in the operating room or radiology suite, but bacterial identification will not be available for at least a day for aerobic and facultative species and for at least 2 days or more for anaerobes. Susceptibility data will not be available for an equivalent amount of time after that. Accordingly, the first 2 to 5 days of treatment are empiric and will be completed without specific susceptibility data. The potential bacterial flora of peritonitis is complex. At least 400 different bacterial species can be identified in the human colon.[51] Despite this clinical microbiology laboratories usually recover only 3 to 5 different pathogens from intra-abdominal infections and fewer than 15 species account for 80% to 90% of the isolates in reported series.[52–55] The clinical findings represent a major simplification of the flora that is the usual contaminating source.

Modern concepts regarding antimicrobial agent choice for intra-abdominal infection come from clinical trials comparing antimicrobial agents and from classical animal experiments demonstrating the basic principles in this field. A mouse peritonitis model with defined bacterial inocula showed that an early bacteremic phase was caused by facultative Enterobacteriaceae, primarily *Escherichia coli,* and a late abscess phase was dependent on anaerobes, especially *Bacteroides fragilis.*[56,57] Antimicrobial agents active against Enterobacteriaceae prevented early mortality, and agents active against the anaerobes prevented late abscess formation. Clinical trials in humans have demonstrated that when antimicrobial regimens are compared, most demonstrate equivalence when both regimens have good activity against both anaerobes and Enterobacteriaceae. A smaller number of trials have demonstrated a clinically and statistically significant difference between antimicrobial regimens and have confirmed that in humans it is important to have coverage against Enterobacteriaceae and against anaerobes.

A number of observational studies have found a strong correlation between the presence of one or more organisms resistant to the antimicrobial agents being used and clinical failure.[53,58–60] One pathogen that has frequently been correlated with failure is the enterococcus, a common enteric organism.[61] However, no prospective trial has demonstrated a superior result for a regimen that has activity against enterococci when compared with one that does not. In addition, patients who have been hospitalized before the onset of intra-abdominal infection or who develop postoperative intra-abdominal infection have an increased risk of resistant organisms. Despite this, no prospective trial has demonstrated an advantage for a more comprehensive, or "broad-spectrum" regimen for such patients.[58,62] For these reasons, a consensus has developed that an empiric antimicrobial regimen for the treatment of peritonitis should have broad activity against aerobic and facultative gram-negative bacilli and against enteric anaerobes. The regimen should not be completely inactive against staphylococcus and streptococcus species. Single and

TABLE 7.6

ANTIMICROBIAL AGENTS FOR INTRA-ABDOMINAL INFECTION

Single Agents
- Cefoxitin
- Cefotetan
- Ampicillin/sulbactam
- Ticarcillin/clavulanic acid
- Piperacillin/tazobactam
- Imipenem/cilastatin
- Meropenem

Combination Regimens
- Cefuroxime plus metronidazole
- Third-/fourth-generation cephalosporin (cefotaxime, ceftriaxone, ceftizoxime, ceftazidime, cefepime) plus an antianaerobe
- Aztreonam plus clindamycin
- Ciprofloxacin plus metronidazole
- Aminoglycoside (gentamicin, tobramycin, netilmicin, amikacin) plus an antianaerobe (clindamycin or metronidazole)

Adapted from Mazuski JE et al. The Surgical Infection Society guidelines on antimicrobial therapy for intra-abdominal infections: an executive summary. *Surg Infect (Larchmt).* 2002;3(3):161–173, with permission.

combination antimicrobial regimens that have these characteristics and have been tested in prospective trials are listed in Table 7.6.[63,64] For some patients it may be helpful for the regimen to have activity against *Pseudomonas aeruginosa* and against enterococcus species, but accurate criteria for choosing such patients are lacking. A Surgical Infection Society committee has concluded that it is reasonable, based on retrospective series and expert opinion, to provide an agent with activity against enterococcus for patients at high risk of failure with enterococcus.[63]

NECROTIZING SOFT TISSUE INFECTIONS

Necrotizing soft tissue infection refers to a spectrum of surgical infections that involve tissue necrosis but are not localized or walled off as abscesses are. These include clostridial infections, which are rare, and nonclostridial infections. Historically, a great variety of labels have been applied to the nonclostridial infections, and in some cases attempts are made to distinguish one from another (Table 7.7).[65] However, these conditions have more in common than the small differences recorded. All present with external signs at the skin level that are far less extensive than the underlying infection and thus the potential for late diagnosis and treatment. And, all possess the potential for major tissue loss, significant morbidity, and high mortality. Differences that have been stressed include the pathogen (beta-hemolytic streptococcus vs. mixed infection), the location (perineum vs. other location), and depth of involvement (involving only superficial tissues vs. muscle also involved). The most common term applied is necrotizing fasciitis, but in most cases the involvement is limited to skin and subcutaneous tissue, and the deeper muscular aponeurosis is not involved. Deeper tissues tend to be involved when the original injury (or operation) breached those areas (e.g., intramuscular hematoma). Necrotizing infection of the abdominal wall can occur after abdominal operations involving bowel entry or treatment of intra-abdominal infection, and the risk is increased when the

TABLE 7.7

TERMS APPLIED TO SIMILAR NECROTIZING SOFT TISSUE INFECTIONS

- Gangrenous erysipelas
- Necrotizing erysipelas
- Hemolytic streptococcal gangrene
- Nonclostridial crepitant cellulitis
- Nonclostridial gas gangrene
- Synergistic necrotizing cellulitis
- Bacterial synergistic gangrene
- Necrotizing fasciitis
- Necrotizing cellulitis
- Fournier's gangrene

Adapted from Dellinger EP. Necrotizing soft-tissue infections. In: Davis JM, Shires GT, eds. *Principles and management of surgical infections.* Philadelphia: Lippincott; 1991:23–39.

patient is hemodynamically unstable or when the abdominal wall is closed under tension, causing ischemia in the wound.

Histotoxic clostridial infections or myonecrosis, commonly called "gas gangrene," are less common than the nonclostridial infections, which are less likely to but still frequently contain gas due to microbial metabolism. Toxins, produced when clostridia grow in anaerobic conditions kill muscle and inhibit neutrophil chemotaxis, thus facilitating the spread of infection and systemic toxicity.[66,67] The most common clostridial organism is *Clostridium perfringens*, followed by *Clostridium novyi*, *Clostridium septicum*, and *Clostridium sordelli.* Although nearly all cases of myonecrosis originate in a traumatic wound, *C. septicum* is capable of causing spontaneous myonecrosis if it gains access to the body through compromised bowel mucosa, which can occur with GI malignancies, such as colon cancer, or during chemotherapy for other malignancies.[65]

Diagnosis

The most important aspect for effective treatment of necrotizing soft tissue infections is early diagnosis. Delay in diagnosis affects outcome adversely. The following physical signs are strongly suggestive of necrotizing infection and merit exploration of the wound in the operating room: any skin necrosis, crepitus, gas in tissue detected by radiologic examination, bullae, or ecchymosis. Other suggestive criteria include marked, or "woody," edema beyond the area of inflammation or progression of the infection despite apparently appropriate antimicrobial therapy. Although necrotizing soft tissue infections have a reputation for progressing very rapidly, and many do, leading to potential early death, they can also be more indolent and simply persist until diagnosed and débrided.[68]

The diagnostic significance of infection-associated gas is worth an explanation. When aerobic and facultative bacteria are able to use oxidative metabolic pathways, they produce CO_2 as do mammals. CO_2 is highly soluble and is readily carried away by blood flow in perfused tissue. However, when facultative and anaerobic bacteria are forced to use nonoxidative metabolic pathways, they rely on fermentation, denitrification, or deamination. These processes produce nitrogen and hydrogen, which are relatively insoluble and accumulate in the surrounding tissue. Thus, the presence of gas in tissue with infection implies anaerobic metabolism, which is incompatible with living host tissue. This implies that the infection is in nonperfused, dead tissue and requires débridement or drainage.

The persistent difficulty of diagnosis using signs and symptoms has led clinicians to search for other aids to diagnosis. Multiple reports examining the role of ultrasound, CT scans, and magnetic resonance imaging suggest that these techniques have increased sensitivity for detecting abnormalities in affected tissues but are not specific and frequently are unhelpful in distinguishing between soft tissue infections that require operative intervention from those that do not.[68] In addition, biopsy and frozen section examination of affected tissues has been suggested.[69] However, if enough suspicion exists to do a biopsy, most experienced surgeons can recognize the extent of the process and need for débridement visually when the incision is made.[68]

Treatment

Operative management of these infections requires exposure of all affected tissue. This usually necessitates incision through uninvolved skin for a significant distance. Necrotic tissue should be débrided, and involved areas must be exposed, but this does not necessarily require excision of overlying tissues unless they are rendered ischemic by the incisions. Careful planning of incisions should be able to avoid this in most cases. On an extremity, amputation may be required for a clostridial infection, and, although this is uncommon for nonclostridial soft tissue infections, amputation may still be lifesaving and not delayed if indicated. Intraoperatively, lack of muscular contraction in response to electrical stimulation, using cautery, is frequently used to identify dying or dead muscle requiring more extensive débridement. All patients who require operative intervention for a necrotizing soft tissue infection should be scheduled for a second look in the operating room during the next 24 to 48 hours. Decision regarding further operative intervention can be made at that time. Large wounds are common, and secondary closure or skin grafts may be required after the infection is completely resolved.

Antimicrobial treatment is initially empiric and must be directed against a presumed mixed flora or aerobic and anaerobic pathogens. The choice of agents is essentially the same as for intra-abdominal infection. Initially, high-dose penicillin, gentamicin, and clindamycin are frequently implemented. There is suggestive evidence from animal experiments that high-dose clindamycin, by binding to RNA in the bacteria, may reduce toxin formation by clostridial species and by toxin producing streptococci and staphylococci.[70] As with other severe infections, patients with necrotizing soft tissue infections have a marked systemic response and require attention to fluid resuscitation, gas exchange, and renal function.

SEPSIS, SHOCK, AND MULTIPLE ORGAN DYSFUNCTION

A severe systemic response to infection including hemodynamic instability and progression to multiple organ dysfunction can occur after either medical or surgical infections. They can occur after either gram-positive or gram-negative infections but appear to be more common with gram-negative infections and are often triggered by a complex systemic host response to lipopolysaccharide (LPS). Within the context of surgical infections, the best outcome for a patient consists of prompt diagnosis and treatment of infections to prevent the onset of sepsis. A number of studies show that early, aggressive correction of physiologic abnormalities seen in early sepsis[71] along with prompt aggressive treatment of the infection itself, both with antimicrobial agents and source control,[72,73] results in the best outcome. Currently, the only additional medical treatment with demonstrated benefit is the administration of activated protein C (drotrecogin alpha) to patients who fit the entry criteria for this trial with sepsis and concomitant organ dysfunction in more than one organ.[1] The risk of increased bleeding complications must be balanced against potential benefits, particularly following recent surgical procedures.

OTHER NOSOCOMIAL INFECTIONS IN SURGICAL PATIENTS

Surgical patients are also susceptible to a number of nonsurgical nosocomial infections during hospitalization. The appropriate care of these patients demands an understanding of the prevention and treatment of these infections as well.

Catheter-Related Bloodstream Infections

Although both peripheral venous and arterial catheters and central venous catheters can be infected, diagnosis is often easier with peripheral catheters, and serious bloodstream infections are more common with central catheters. One of the first principles in preventing these infections is to restrict the use of catheters and to ask each day whether the patient actually needs the catheters that are in place. Another important element of prevention is the insertion technique, especially for central catheters. Although full barrier precautions with wide draping and use of glove, gown, hat, and mask by the inserting physician results in lower infection rates,[74] this is not always followed. An institutional education program to emphasize the importance of insertion technique has been shown to lower infection rates.[75] Skin preparation with a chlorhexidine solution results in lower infection rates than preparation with povidone-iodine solutions.[76] All intravascular devices are susceptible to infection, and the risk increases the longer the catheter is in place. However, changing central lines on a particular schedule does not decrease infection risk.[77,78] The final risk is related to the number of days that any catheter is in place. Subclavian central venous catheters have a lower risk of infection than internal jugular catheters. Recommendations for the use of antimicrobial-coated catheters are not well established because one must balance the risk of line infection against the risk of additional antimicrobial exposure to the patient and to the environment. When the local rate of infection is high, they are probably justified.[77]

The diagnosis of catheter-related bloodstream infection is made by isolating the same organism from the bloodstream and from a semiquantitative culture of the catheter tip. When the diagnosis is made, the catheter should be removed. Bacteremia should be treated by a specific antimicrobial agent and, for *S. aureus*, gram-negative rods, or fungi, should be continued for 10 to 14 days.[79] For coagulase-negative staphylococci, the most common pathogen, duration of treatment can be limited to the period of systemic response after removal of the catheter.

Pneumonia

Pneumonia is less common than SSI and UTI on surgical services but when it occurs is a major source of morbidity and mortality. Prevention of postoperative pneumonia is best accomplished by policies and procedures that emphasize the early extubation of ventilated patients, the use of noninvasive positive pressure ventilation when feasible, and elevation of the head of the bed for ventilated patients. Diagnosis can be made by physical examination and chest radiograph in the spontaneously breathing postoperative patient. The diagnosis can be much more challenging in the ventilated ICU patient. These patients often have abnormal chest films and physical findings as well as fever and leukocytosis in the absence of pneumonia. In addition, all patients with an endotracheal tube for more than a few days are likely to have bacteria in tracheal aspirates independent of infection. Overtreatment of suspected infection is common, and restriction of treatment for patients without demonstrated pneumonia improves outcome.[80] On the other hand, delayed, specific treatment of true infection increases mortality.[81,82] For this reason, procedures that produce more specific diagnosis of pneumonia and that help to rule out the diagnosis when pneumonia is not present, such as bronchoalveolar lavage and protected specimen brush cultures, have an important role in the care of ventilated ICU patients.[83–86] Culture of expectorated sputum or of simple endotracheal aspirates are very nonspecific and of little use in diagnosing pneumonia.

Urinary Tract Infection

The most common etiologic agent of UTI in hospitalized patients is the indwelling bladder catheter. Many surgical patients have urinary catheters placed in the operating room. A primary preventive measure for UTI is to use urinary catheters only when actually necessary due to the location of the operative procedure or the length and complexity of the operation. When a catheter is required it should be removed as soon as possible, often at the end of the operative procedure or on the first postoperative day. When a catheter must be left in place, a closed system should always be used. The risk of UTI doubles on any day when the integrity of a close system is violated.

In a patient without a catheter, the diagnosis of UTI is traditionally made when a quantitative culture shows greater than 10^5 organisms per milliliter of urine. In patients with catheters much lower colony counts may represent true infection. Attempts to clear bacteriuria when the catheter is in place usually fail. If the patient is symptomatic, specific antimicrobial treatment should be followed by a catheter change. If the patient is not symptomatic, specific antimicrobial treatment should be given after the catheter has been removed.

PATHOGENS

As noted in the introduction, most surgical infections are caused by endogenous microorganisms that gain access to the body after violation of an epithelial barrier. Specific pathogens are identified through culture in the microbiology laboratory, but earlier information can be obtained through examination of a Gram-stained smear of material taken from the infected site. Gram-positive cocci are very commonly found in soft tissue infections and can represent *Staphylococcus* species, either *S. aureus* or coagulase-negative staphylococci, or streptococcal species. Coagulase-negative staphylococci are the most common pathogens found in catheter-related bloodstream infections but cause serious infections in other locations rarely. *S. aureus* possess virulence characteristics that enable them to invade healthy tissues and form abscesses and are usually significant when recovered. Extensive use of beta-lactam antibiotics has led to the emergence of MRSA in many areas, and recently some strains of vancomycin intermediate *Staphylococcus aureus* (VISA) and vancomycin resistant *Staphylococcus aureus* (VRSA) strains have emerged.

Beta hemolytic streptococci, especially from group A have significant virulence properties that allow them to invade uninjured or minimally injured tissues to cause severe soft tissue infections as previously discussed in the section on necrotizing soft tissue infections. They are uncommon surgical pathogens otherwise. Group D streptococci, or enterococci, are frequently recovered from intra-abdominal infections, but studies fail to demonstrate superior outcomes when antimicrobial regimens are directed toward enterococci. However, this species can clearly cause severe disease in immune compromised patients, especially liver transplant patients. In this setting the occurrence of vancomycin-resistant enterococci (VRE) in recent years has presented a very difficult treatment challenge.

Facultative gram-negative rods, which can grow either in aerobic or anaerobic environments are commonly associated with surgical infections, especially those arising from intra-abdominal sources. These include the familiar genera *Escherichia, Proteus, Klebsiella, Enterobacter, Morganella, Providencia,* and *Serratia.* These pathogens are most commonly treated with advanced generation cephalosporins, expanded-spectrum penicillins, carbapenems, or fluoroquinolones. In recent years, a number of these pathogens have developed expanded-spectrum beta-lactam enzymes capable of inactivating even third-generation cephalosporins. Obligate aerobic gram-negative rods encountered in surgical patients include *Pseudomonas* species and *Acinetobacter* species. These are most commonly found in the respiratory tract but can also occur in the abdomen. These pathogens often exhibit an even higher degree of antimicrobial resistance than the facultative gram-negative rods.

Anaerobic bacteria are the most common inhabitants of the GI tract in humans and cause significant disease in intra-abdominal infections, but they are not represented in infections proportional to their density in the bowel. The most common isolates are members of the *Bacteroides* genus, especially *B. fragilis* and *B. thetaiotaomicron.* The most effective antibiotics against these organisms are metronidazole, clindamycin, the carbapenems, and advanced generation penicillins combined with a beta-lactam inhibitor. The anaerobic cocci are also susceptible to the same antibiotics. *Clostridium* species, as noted in the section on necrotizing soft tissue infections, are most important in that setting. When anaerobes are recovered from a surgical infection or from the bloodstream, this means that bacteria are growing in the body in an anaerobic environment. These are always surgical infections and require source control in addition to antimicrobial treatment.

Fungi, most commonly *Candida* species, are rarely primary causative agents in surgical infections. However, they are often secondary pathogens, overgrowing on skin and the gut under the influence of broad-spectrum antibacterial therapy. In this setting they become important opportunistic invaders. The most common strain found is *Candida albicans.* Most *Candida* infections are currently treated with fluconazole, but increasing use of this agent tends to provide pressure to increase the presence of resistant strains such as *Candida glabrata* or *Candida krusei.* In these cases, treatment with voriconazole, caspofungin, or amphotericin may be required.

Viruses do not cause surgical infections. Surgical patients are most susceptible to viral infection as a result of blood transfusion, which may transmit hepatitis B, hepatitis C, or the human immunodeficiency virus (HIV). Recent advances in nucleic acid detection technology have rendered the blood supply in the United States increasingly safe so that the current risk for transmission of any of these agents by transfusion is less than one in two million.[87] Transplant patients are susceptible to a number of viral infections due to their immune compromised state, especially cytomegalovirus.

ANTIMICROBIAL AGENTS

Antimicrobial agents are used in combination with source control and other treatment modalities to prevent or resolve surgical infections. The goal should be to use these agents when they are required and to withhold them when they are not. Overuse of antimicrobial agents contributes to bacterial resistance and limits their effectiveness when they are needed. They should be used in a manner that ensures therapeutic levels at the site of infection for the appropriate duration. Recent data have demonstrated that the pharmacodynamic principles of antibiotic use differ for different classes of drugs. The factors that go into an antibiotic's effectiveness include its minimal inhibitory concentration (MIC) for a particular pathogen, its half-life and mode of elimination from the body, and its mechanism of action.[88,89] Beta-lactam antibiotics such as penicillins and cephalosporins bind to penicillin-binding proteins (PBP) in the bacterial cell wall and inhibit bacterial cell wall synthesis. Once drug levels are achieved that are well above MIC, the rate of bacterial killing does not increase with higher drug levels. Their effectiveness depends on the percent of time during therapy that the drug levels exceed the MIC at the site of infection. Thus, a dose and time of administration that achieves levels above MIC for more than 50% of the time between doses will provide optimal therapy. This favors drugs with long half-lives or continuous administration of drugs with shorter half-lives. Alternatively, aminoglycosides kill by inhibiting microbial protein synthesis, and higher levels of drug above the MIC kill bacteria more rapidly. In addition, these drugs exhibit a "postantibiotic effect" in which bacteria do not begin to grow again for a time after the drug levels have fallen below the MIC. This has led to the once daily administration of aminoglycoside antibiotics, which achieve very high serum levels shortly after administration and take advantage of the postantibiotic effect after serum levels have fallen. In addition, renal toxicity of the drugs is equal or less with once-daily administration compared with three times daily administration, which was the former practice. For quinolones, the best results correlate with the ratio between the area under the curve (AUC) when time is graphed against serum concentration in mg/L. A ratio of AUC/MIC >125 correlates with clinical success.

When antimicrobial agents are used to treat an infection, response to treatment should be evaluated in a regular and ongoing schedule. If improvement is not evident within 2 to 3 days of treatment, the situation should be assessed and an explanation sought. These questions should be asked: Was the original source control adequate? Has a complication of the source control procedure occurred? Has a superinfection developed? Is enough of the proper drug being given in an appropriate manner? The wrong antibiotic is not the most common cause of failure in treating a surgical infection.

Once the patient is improving, we need to decide how long to continue antimicrobial agents. For most surgical infections, these agents can be stopped when the patient has demonstrated a return to normal temperature and WBC count with improvement in general condition as long as the source control was adequate. There is an absence of objective, prospective data demonstrating the necessary duration of drug treatment. Prolonged antimicrobial agent administration predisposes the patient to superinfections, to colonization with resistant bacteria, and to development of drug adverse reactions and organ damage.

This chapter does not provide a detailed discussion of each antimicrobial drug available. The list is very large and frequently changes. Detailed discussions of indications and doses for individual drugs are available in several reference sources, which are updated on a yearly basis. Table 7.8 lists the classes and individual drugs that are most commonly used by surgeons, grouped by class and antimicrobial activity.

TABLE 7.8

ANTIBIOTICS

PENICILLIN CLASS	**CARBAPENEMS**
The original	Imipenem/cilastatin
Penicillin G	Meropenem
Antistaphylococcal	Ertapenem
Methicillin	
Nafcillin	**FLUOROQUINOLONES**
Oxacillin	Ciprofloxacin
Limited gram-negative activity	Levofloxacin
Ampicillin	Gatifloxacin
Amoxicillin	Moxifloxacin
Broader gram-negative activity	
Carbenicillin	**AMINOGLYCOSIDES**
Ticarcillin	Gentamicin
Piperacillin	Tobramycin
Beta-lactamase inhibitor combinations	Amikacin
Ampicillin/sulbactam	Netilmicin
Amoxicillin/clavulanate	
Ticarcillin/clavulanate	**VARIOUS ANTIANAEROBIC DRUGS**
Piperacillin/tazobactam	Chloramphenicol
	Clindamycin
CEPHALOSPORIN CLASS	Metronidazole
First generation	
Cephalothin	**ANTIMICROBIALS WITH ACTIVIY AGAINST MRSA**
Cefazolin	Vancomycin
Cephalexin	Quinupristin/dalfopristin
Cephradine	Linezolid
Second generation	Daptomycin
Cefuroxime	
Cefoxitin	**ANTIFUNGAL DRUGS**
Cefmetazole	Amphotericin
Cefotetan	Fluconazole
Third generation	Voriconazole
Cefotaxime	Caspofungin
Ceftizoxime	
Ceftriaxone	
Cefoperazone	
Ceftazidime	
Cefepime	

MRSA, methicillin-resistant *Staphylococcus aureus*.

KEY POINTS

- **Surgical infections require surgical intervention, that is, "source control," which refers to a mechanical or anatomic procedure to drain an abscess, relieve an obstruction, repair a perforation, or resect dead, ischemic, or inflamed tissue or foreign body to promote resolution.**
- **Source control is combined with empiric antibiotic therapy that is later modified based on microbiologic susceptibility patterns.**
- **Empiric antibiotic therapy requires knowledge of the current patterns of pathogens involved and antibiotic susceptibility within the institution and, even, specific units, such as the ICU.**
- **Surgical site infections (SSI) are dependent on numerous factors, including extent of contamination, hemostasis, tissue handling, length of operation, tissue hypoxia, patient temperature, and glucose control, in addition to minimizing comorbidities.**
- **Antibiotic prophylaxis should be dosed to maintain adequate tissue concentrations during the period of potential contamination, starting approximately 1 hour prior to surgery, repeated after one to two half-lives, increased in large patients, and stopped within 24 hours postoperatively. Choose a first-generation cephalosporin if no anaerobes are expected and second generation if anaerobic activity is likely.**
- **With peritonitis, antibiotics active against aerobic gram-negative organisms prevent early mortality and those active against anaerobic organisms prevent abscesses. Thus, broad-spectrum antibiotics are needed.**
- **Necrotizing soft tissue infections are hard to diagnose, present with external skin changes under-representing the extent of underlying disease, and have potential for major tissue loss and high morbidity and mortality.**

References

1. Bernard GR, Vincent JL, Laterre PF, et al. Efficacy and safety of recombinant human activated protein C for severe sepsis. *N Engl J Med.* 2001;344:699–709.
2. Namias N, Harvill S, Ball S, et al. Empiric therapy of sepsis in the surgical intensive care unit with broad-spectrum antibiotics for 72 hours does not lead to the emergence of resistant bacteria. *J Trauma* 1998;45:887–891.
3. **Marshall JC, Schein M. *Source control: a guide to the management of surgical infections.* Berlin: Springer; 2002.**
4. Solomkin JS, Yellin AE, Rotstein OD, et al. Ertapenem versus piperacillin/tazobactam in the treatment of complicated intraabdominal infections: results of a double-blind, randomized comparative phase III trial. *Ann Surg.* 2003;237:235–245.
5. Horan TC, Gaynes RP, Martone WJ, et al. CDC definitions of nosocomial surgical site infections, 1992: a modification of CDC definitions of surgical wound infections. *Am J Infect Control* 1992;20:271–274.
6. Mangram AJ, Horan TC, Pearson ML, et al. Guideline for prevention of surgical site infection, 1999. Hospital Infection Control Practices Advisory Committee. *Infect Control Hosp Epidemiol.* 1999;20:250–278; quiz 279–280.
7. Gaynes RP, Culver DH, Horan TC, et al. Surgical site infection (SSI) rates in the United States, 1992-1998: the National Nosocomial Infections Surveillance System basic SSI risk index. *Clin Infect Dis.* 2001;33[Suppl 2]:S69–77.
8. Howard JM, Barker WF, Culbertson W, et al. Postoperative wound infections: the influence of ultraviolet irradiation on the operating room and of various other factors. *Ann Surg.* 1964;160[Suppl 2]:1–196.
9. Culver D, Horan T, Gaynes R. Comparing surgical site infection (SSI) rates using the NNIS SSI index and the standardized infection ratio. *Am J Infect Control* 1994;22:102.
10. Nosocomial infection rates for interhospital comparison: limitations and possible solutions. A Report from the National Nosocomial Infections Surveillance (NNIS) System. *Infect Control Hosp Epidemiol.* 1991;12:609–621.
11. Roy MC, Herwaldt LA, Embrey R, et al. Does the Centers for Disease Control's NNIS system risk index stratify patients undergoing cardiothoracic operations by their risk of surgical-site infection? *Infect Control Hosp Epidemiol.* 2000;21:186–190.
12. Minnema B, Vearncombe M, Augustin A, et al. Risk factors for surgical-site infection following primary total knee arthroplasty. *Infect Control Hosp Epidemiol.* 2004;25:477–480.
13. Latham R, Lancaster AD, Covington JF, et al. The association of diabetes and glucose control with surgical-site infections among cardiothoracic surgery patients. *Infect Control Hosp Epidemiol.* 2001;22:607–612.
14. Furnary AP, Zerr KJ, Grunkemeier GL, et al. Continuous intravenous insulin infusion reduces the incidence of deep sternal wound infection in diabetic patients after cardiac surgical procedures [see comments]. *Ann Thorac Surg.* 1999;67:352–360; discussion 360–362.
15. Polk HC Jr, Lopez-Mayor JF. Postoperative wound infection: a prospective study of determinant factors and prevention. *Surgery* 1969;66:97–103.
16. Hojer H, Wetterfors J. Systemic prophylaxis with doxycycline in surgery of the colon and rectum. *Ann Surg.* 1978;187:362–368.
17. Hunt TK, Linsey M, Grislis H, et al. The effect of differing ambient oxygen tensions on wound infection. *Ann Surg.* 1975;181:35–39.
18. Hopf HW, Hunt TK, West JM, et al. Wound tissue oxygen tension predicts the risk of wound infection in surgical patients. *Arch Surg.* 1997;132:997–1004; discussion 1005.
19. Greif R, Akca O, Horn EP, et al. Supplemental perioperative oxygen to reduce the incidence of surgical-wound infection. Outcomes Research Group [see comments]. *N Engl J Med.* 2000;342:161–167.
20. Pryor KO, Fahey 3rd TJ, Lien CA, et al. Surgical site infection and the routine use of perioperative hyperoxia in a general surgical population: a randomized controlled trial. *JAMA.* 2004;291:79–87.
21. Rabkin JM, Hunt TK. Local heat increases blood flow and oxygen tension in wounds. *Arch Surg.* 1987;122:221–225.
22. **Kurz A, Sessler DI, Lenhardt R. Perioperative normothermia to reduce the incidence of surgical-wound infection and shorten hospitalization. Study of Wound Infection and Temperature Group [see comments]. *N Engl J Med.* 1996;334:1209–1215.**
23. Melling AC, Ali B, Scott EM, et al. Effects of preoperative warming on the incidence of wound infection after clean surgery: a randomised controlled trial. *Lancet* 2001;358:876–880.
24. Sessler DI. Perioperative heat balance. *Anesthesiology* 2000;92:578–596.
25. Pomposelli JJ, Baxter 3rd JK, Babineau TJ, et al. Early postoperative glucose control predicts nosocomial infection rate in diabetic patients. *JPEN J Parenter Enteral Nutr.* 1998;22(2):77–81.
26. **Furnary AP, Gao G, Grunkemeier GL, et al. Continuous insulin infusion reduces mortality in patients with diabetes undergoing coronary artery bypass grafting. *J Thorac Cardiovasc Surg.* 2003;125:1007–1021.**
27. McKittrick LS, Wheelock Jr FC. The routine use of antibiotics in elective abdominal surgery. *Surg Gynecol Obstet.* 1954;99:376–377.
28. Burke J. The effective period of preventive antibiotic action in experimental incisions and dermal lesions. *Surgery* 1961;50:161–168.
29. Classen DC, Evans RS, Pestotnik SL, et al. The timing of prophylactic administration of antibiotics and the risk of surgical-wound infection [see comments]. *N Engl J Med.* 1992;326:281–286.
30. Platt R, Zaleznik DF, Hopkins CC, et al. Perioperative antibiotic prophylaxis for herniorrhaphy and breast surgery. *N Engl J Med.* 1990;322:153–160.
31. Platt R. Antibiotic prophylaxis in clean surgery: does it work? Should it be used if it does? *New Horiz.* 1998;6[2 Suppl]:S53–57.
32. Dellinger EP, Gross PA, Barrett TL, et al. Quality standard for antimicrobial prophylaxis in surgical procedures. Infectious Diseases Society of America. *Clin Infect Dis.* 1994;18:422–427.
33. Forse RA, Karam B, MacLean LD, et al. Antibiotic prophylaxis for surgery in morbidly obese patients. *Surgery* 1989;106:750–756.
34. Scher KS. Studies on the duration of antibiotic administration for surgical prophylaxis. *Am Surg.* 1997;63:59–62.
35. Zanetti G, Giardina R, Platt R. Intraoperative redosing of cefazolin and risk for surgical site infection in cardiac surgery. *Emerg Infect Dis.* 2001;7:828–831.
36. Kriaras I, Michalopoulos A, Turina M, et al. Evolution of antimicrobial prophylaxis in cardiovascular surgery. *Eur J Cardiothorac Surg.* 2000;18:440–446.
37. McDonald M, Grabsch E, Marshall C, et al. Single- versus multiple-dose antimicrobial prophylaxis for major surgery: a systematic review [see comments]. *Aust N Z J Surg.* 1998;68:388–396.
38. Harbarth S, Samore MH, Lichtenberg D, et al. Prolonged antibiotic prophylaxis after cardiovascular surgery and its effect on surgical site infections and antimicrobial resistance. *Circulation* 2000;101:2916–2921.
39. **Bratzler DW, Houck PM. Antimicrobial prophylaxis for surgery: an advisory statement from the national surgical infection prevention project. *Clin Infect Dis.* 2004;38:1706–1715.**
40. Finkelstein R, Rabino G, Mashiah T, et al. Vancomycin versus cefazolin prophylaxis for cardiac surgery in the setting of a high prevalence of methicillin-resistant staphylococcal infections. *J Thorac Cardiovasc Surg.* 2002;123:326–332.
41. Alexander JW, Fischer JE, Boyajian M, et al. The influence of hair-removal methods on wound infections. *Arch Surg.* 1983;118:347–352.
42. Ko W, Lazenby WD, Zelano JA, et al. Effects of shaving methods and intraoperative irrigation on suppurative mediastinitis after bypass operations. *Ann Thorac Surg.* 1992;53:301–305.
43. Cohn SM, Giannotti G, Ong AW, et al. Prospective randomized trial of two wound management strategies for dirty abdominal wounds. *Ann Surg.* 2001;233:409–413.
44. **Bartlett P, Reingold AL, Graham DR, et al. Toxic shock syndrome associated with surgical wound infections. *JAMA.* 1982;247:1448–1450.**

45. Dellinger EP. Approach to the patient with postoperative fever. In: Gorbach S, Bartlett J, Blacklow N, eds. *Infectious diseases.* Philadelphia: Lippincott Williams & Wilkins; 2004:817–823.
46. Seiler CA, Brugger L, Forssmann U, et al. Conservative surgical treatment of diffuse peritonitis. *Surgery* 2000;127:178–184.
47. Nathens AB, Rotstein OD, Marshall JC. Tertiary peritonitis: clinical features of a complex nosocomial infection. *World J Surg.* 1998;22:158–163.
48. **Christou NV, Barie PS, Dellinger EP, et al. Surgical Infection Society intra-abdominal infection study. Prospective evaluation of management techniques and outcome. *Arch Surg.* 1993;128:193–198; discussion 198–199.**
49. Levison MA. Percutaneous versus open operative drainage of intra-abdominal abscesses. *Infect Dis Clin North Am.* 1992;6:525–544.
50. Ohmann C, Yang Q, Hau T, et al. Prognostic modeling in peritonitis. Peritonitis Study Group of the Surgical Infection Society Europe. *Eur J Surg.* 1997;163:53–60.
51. Finegold SM, Sutter VL, Mathisen GE. Normal indigenous intestinal flora. In: Hentges DJ, ed. *Human intestinal microflora in health and disease.* New York: Academic Press; 1983:3–31.
52. Solomkin JS, Dellinger EP, Christou NV, et al. Results of a multicenter trial comparing imipenem/cilastatin to tobramycin/clindamycin for intra-abdominal infections. *Ann Surg.* 1990;212:581–591.
53. Mosdell DM, Morris DM, Voltura A, et al. Antibiotic treatment for surgical peritonitis. *Ann Surg.* 1991;214:543–552.
54. Barie PS, Vogel SB, Dellinger EP, et al. A randomized, double-blind clinical trial comparing cefepime plus metronidazole with imipenem-cilastatin in the treatment of complicated intra-abdominal infections. Cefepime Intra-abdominal Infection Study Group. *Arch Surg.* 1997;132:1294–1302.
55. Solomkin JS, Reinhart HH, Dellinger EP, et al. Results of a randomized trial comparing sequential intravenous/oral treatment with ciprofloxacin plus metronidazole to imipenem/cilastatin for intra-abdominal infections. The Intra-Abdominal Infection Study Group. *Ann Surg.* 1996;223: 303–315.
56. Bartlett JG, Onderdonk AB, Louie T, et al. A review. Lessons from an animal model of intra-abdominal sepsis. *Arch Surg.* 1978;113:853–857.
57. Weinstein WM, Onderdonk AB, Bartlett JG, et al. Antimicrobial therapy of experimental intraabdominal sepsis. *J Infect Dis.* 1975;132:282–286.
58. Christou NV, Turgeon P, Wassef R, et al. Management of intra-abdominal infections. The case for intraoperative cultures and comprehensive broad-spectrum antibiotic coverage. The Canadian Intra-abdominal Infection Study Group. *Arch Surg.* 1996;131:1193–1201.
59. Hopkins JA, Lee JC, Wilson SE. Susceptibility of intra-abdominal isolates at operation: a predictor of postoperative infection. *Am Surg.* 1993;59:791–796.
60. Montravers P, Gauzit R, Muller C, et al. Emergence of antibiotic-resistant bacteria in cases of peritonitis after intraabdominal surgery affects the efficacy of empirical antimicrobial therapy. *Clin Infect Dis.* 1996;23:486–494.
61. Burnett RJ, Haverstock DC, Dellinger EP, et al. Definition of the role of enterococcus in intraabdominal infection: analysis of a prospective randomized trial. *Surgery* 1995;118:716–721.
62. Dupont H, Carbon C, Carlet J. Monotherapy with a broad-spectrum beta-lactam is as effective as its combination with an aminoglycoside in treatment of severe generalized peritonitis: a multicenter randomized controlled trial. The Severe Generalized Peritonitis Study Group. *Antimicrob Agents Chemother.* 2000;44:2028–2033.
63. **Mazuski JE, Sawyer RG, Nathens AB, et al. The Surgical Infection Society guidelines on antimicrobial therapy for intra-abdominal infections: an executive summary. *Surg Infect (Larchmt).* 2002;3:161–173.**
64. Mazuski JE, Sawyer RG, Nathens AB, et al. The Surgical Infection Society guidelines on antimicrobial therapy for intra-abdominal infections: evidence for the recommendations. *Surg Infect (Larchmt).* 2002;3:175–233.
65. Dellinger EP. Necrotizing soft-tissue infections. In: Davis JM, Shires GT, eds. *Principles and management of surgical infections.* Philadelphia: Lippincott; 1991:23–39.
66. Stevens DL, Tweten RK, Awad MM, et al. Clostridial gas gangrene: evidence that alpha and theta toxins differentially modulate the immune response and induce acute tissue necrosis. *J Infect Dis.* 1997;176:189–195.
67. Stevens DL, Mitten J, Henry C. Effects of alpha and theta toxins from Clostridium perfringens on human polymorphonuclear leukocytes. *J Infect Dis.* 1987;156:324–333.
68. **Marshall JC, Maier RV, Jimenez M, et al. Source control in the management of severe sepsis and septic shock: an evidence-based review. *Crit Care Med.* 2004;32:S513–526.**
69. Stamenkovic I, Lew PD. Early recognition of potentially fatal necrotizing fasciitis. The use of frozen-section biopsy. *N Engl J Med.* 1984;310: 1689–1693.
70. Stevens DL, Bryant AE, Hackett SP. Antibiotic effects on bacterial viability, toxin production, and host response. *Clin Infect Dis.* 1995;2:S154–157.
71. Rivers E, Nguyen B, Havstad S, et al. Early goal-directed therapy in the treatment of severe sepsis and septic shock. *N Engl J Med.* 2001;345: 1368–1377.
72. Kumar A, Wood K, Gurka D, et al. Duration of hypotension prior to antimicrobial administration is a critical determinant of outcome in human septic shock. In: *Interscience Conference on Antimicrobial Agents and Chemotherapy.* Washington, DC: American Society for Microbiology, 2004.
73. Kumar A, Wood K, Gurka D, et al. Outcome of septic shock correlates with duration of hypotension prior to source control implementation. In: *Interscience Conference on Antimicrobial Agents and Chemotherapy.* Washington, DC: American Society for Microbiology, 2004.
74. Raad II DC, Hohn BJ, Gilbreath, et al. Prevention of central venous catheter-related infections by using maximal sterile barrier precautions during insertion. *Infect Control Hosp Epidemiol.* 1994;15[4 Pt 1]: 231–238.
75. Sherertz RJ, Ely EW, Westbrook DM, et al. Education of physicians-in-training can decrease the risk for vascular catheter infection. *Ann Intern Med.* 2000;132:641–648.
76. Maki DG, Ringer M, Alvarado CJ. Prospective randomised trial of povidone-iodine, alcohol, and chlorhexidine for prevention of infection associated with central venous and arterial catheters. *Lancet* 1991;338: 339–343.
77. **O'Grady NP, Alexander M, Dellinger EP, et al. Guidelines for the prevention of intravascular catheter-related infections. Centers for Disease Control and Prevention. *MMWR Recomm Rep.* 2002;51(RR-10):1–29.**
78. Cook D, Randolph A, Kernerman P, et al. Central venous catheter replacement strategies: a systematic review of the literature. *Crit Care Med.* 1997;25:1417–1424.
79. Mermel LA, Farr BM, Sherertz RJ, et al. Guidelines for the management of intravascular catheter-related infections. *Clin Infect Dis.* 2001;32: 1249–1272.
80. Singh N, Rogers P, Atwood CW, et al. Short-course empiric antibiotic therapy for patients with pulmonary infiltrates in the intensive care unit. A proposed solution for indiscriminate antibiotic prescription. *Am J Respir Crit Care Med.* 2000;162[2 Pt 1]:505–511.
81. Kollef MH, Sherman G, Ward S, et al. Inadequate antimicrobial treatment of infections: a risk factor for hospital mortality among critically ill patients. *Chest* 1999;115:462–474.
82. Mathevon T, Souweine B, Traore O, et al. ICU-acquired nosocomial infection: impact of delay of adequate antibiotic treatment. *Scand J Infect Dis.* 2002;34:831–835.
83. Chastre J. Prospective evaluation of the protected specimen brush for the diagnosis of pulmonary infections. *Am Rev Respir Dis.* 1984;130: 924–929.
84. Croce MA, Fabian TC, Schurr MJ, et al. Using bronchoalveolar lavage to distinguish nosocomial pneumonia from systemic inflammatory response syndrome: a prospective analysis. *J Trauma* 1995;39:1134–1139; discussion 1139–1140.
85. Pugin J, Auckenthaler R, Mili N, et al. Diagnosis of ventilator-associated pneumonia by bacteriologic analysis of bronchoscopic and nonbronchoscopic "blind" bronchoalveolar lavage fluid. *Am Rev Respir Dis.* 1991;143[5 Pt 1]:1121–1129.
86. Pereira Gomes JC, Pedreira Jr WL, Araujo EM, et al. Impact of BAL in the management of pneumonia with treatment failure: positivity of BAL culture under antibiotic therapy. *Chest* 2000;118:1739–1746.
87. Dodd RY, Notari EPT, Stramer SL. Current prevalence and incidence of infectious disease markers and estimated window-period risk in the American Red Cross blood donor population. *Transfusion* 2002;42: 975–979.
88. **Ebert SC, Craig WA. Pharmacodynamic properties of antibiotics: application to drug monitoring and dosage regimen design. *Infect Control Hosp Epidemiol.* 1990;11:319–326.**
89. Leggett JE, Ebert S, Fantin B, et al. Comparative dose-effect relations at several dosing intervals for beta-lactam, aminoglycoside and quinolone antibiotics against gram-negative bacilli in murine thigh-infection and pneumonitis models. *Scand J Infect Dis Suppl.* 1990;74:179–184.

CHAPTER 8 ■ SHOCK

JOSEPH T. MURPHY AND LARRY M. GENTILELLO

The history of shock is interesting because for many years the nature and purpose of the heart and circulatory system was either unknown or misunderstood. Galen was perhaps the first physician to investigate the heart's purpose. He proposed that the arteries carry blood, not air, as was previously thought. However, he also believed that blood dissolved in the body after it left the heart but was rapidly remanufactured by the liver. Because much of his dissection work was carried out on frogs he concluded that the heart had only two chambers and blood passed from the right to left chamber through invisible pores in the septum.[1]

These conclusions remained unchallenged for nearly 1,500 years until Vesalius, in the 17th century, described dissection of the human body. He demonstrated that blood did not flow directly from the right to left ventricle. Although he provided elaborate drawings of the body's network of blood vessels, he did not anticipate that blood circulated through the body and could not discern the heart's purpose. Shortly thereafter, Harvey moved beyond anatomy to the study of physiology, discovered the closed nature of the circulation, and concluded that the heart was its pumping mechanism. Although the microscope had not yet been invented, he proposed the existence of capillaries that connect the arterial and venous system.[1]

In the following century, military surgeons such as Henri le Dran (1740) noted that injured soldiers left unattended for several hours suddenly deteriorated as if there had been a *secousse* (jolt) to the system, which probably led to use of the word "shock."[1] Surgeons began to notice that even when a wounded extremity was amputated the physiologic effects of the injury often continued, and shock was increasingly recognized as a distinct systemic syndrome apart from the wound itself.[1]

In the early 20th century, Blalock concluded that shock was due to blood loss into tissues. Subsequently, third-spaced fluid loss was recognized to be much greater in quantity than the amount of blood loss. Therapy began to focus not only on restoring intravascular volume but also on replacing interstitial fluid with a balanced salt solution. Investigators then became increasingly intrigued by the fact that, at some point, shock becomes irreversible and is no longer responsive to further volume resuscitation. As stated more than 50 years ago by Wiggers, "at a certain stage an adequate circulation cannot be restored by merely filling the system, as one does an automobile radiator."[2] At some point the wound, infection, cardiac dysfunction, or other initiating event is no longer the primary threat. Other factors sustain the shock state, blood pressure cannot be restored, improvements are only transient, and death occurs shortly thereafter.

The modern approach to shock acknowledges that uncorrected hypovolemia and critical oxygen delivery deficits lead to irreversible shock but recognizes that future therapies must move beyond fluid resuscitation and indices of tissue oxygenation and target the internal machinery of the cell itself. Thus, investigators are increasingly looking to gain an understanding of the chain of events that occur that lead to organ damage and irreversibility. This chapter provides an overview of these events, discusses the therapeutic approaches utilized in current management, and offers a brief perspective on what may lie in the future.

TYPES OF SHOCK

Hypovolemic Shock

Hypovolemic shock is the form of shock most commonly encountered in surgical practice (Table 8.1). The essential feature is a reduction in intravascular volume to a level that prevents the heart from being able to pump sufficient blood to vital organ systems. Substantial blood (>20% circulating volume) or plasma (via soft tissue or enteric sequestration or gastrointestinal, urinary, or insensible losses) losses are required to produce this syndrome.

Hypovolemic shock secondary to hemorrhage has been classified based on the volume of blood loss and the associated systemic response.[3] Class I hemorrhage (500 to 700 mL, or 10%–15% of blood volume in a 70-kg individual) is well tolerated in otherwise healthy individuals, with minimal tachycardia and no significant change in blood pressure. With Class II hemorrhagic shock (750 to 1,500 mL, or 20%–30% blood volume), physical findings become more prominent, including tachycardia, narrow pulse pressure, poor capillary refill, and increasing anxiety. Class III shock (1,500–2,000 mL, or 30%–40% of blood volume) is the first level that is consistently characterized by hypotension and the classic findings of tachycardia, oliguria, pallor, diaphoresis, and confusion. Class IV shock (>2,000 mL or >40% blood loss) results in profound hemodynamic instability and clear evidence of inadequate perfusion to critical organs (kidneys, brain) and is a preterminal event.

In practice, individual susceptibility to blood loss varies greatly and is affected by age, pre-existing disease, prescription and nonprescription medications, adequacy of compensatory mechanisms, and other factors that are poorly characterized.

Hypovolemia due to plasma losses may also lead to hypovolemic shock. The clinical findings of hemorrhagic shock are typically present, but significant differences do exist. Hemoconcentration, elevated blood urea nitrogen (BUN) and creatinine, and hypernatremia are typical of acute plasma and/or free water losses and are not necessarily present in other forms of shock.

Septic Shock

Septic shock is defined as a systemic inflammatory response to infection in conjunction with arterial hypotension, despite adequate fluid resuscitation. It occurs when bacterial products interact with cells of the immune system, leading to elaboration

TABLE 8.1

CLASSIFICATION SYSTEM AND CAUSES OF SHOCK

Classification	Etiology	Specific causes
Hypovolemic	Hemorrhagic	Obvious bleeding Occult bleeding
	Nonhemorrhagic	Absolute fluid loss (renal, gastrointestinal) Relative fluid loss (redistribution secondary to injury, drugs)
Cardiac		
Intrinsic	Myocardial failure	Ischemia, infarction Cardiomyopathy Drug effect Metabolic (hypophosphatemia, hypocalcemia, acidosis) Excess afterload Myocardial rupture Myocardial injury (e.g., contusion)
	Valve failure	Infection Proximal aortic dissection Injury Ruptured papillary muscle Obstruction from thrombus, myxoma Stenosis
	Conduction	Tachyarrhythmia, bradyarrhythmia
Compressive	Pericardial tamponade compromise, outflow blockage	Acute (injury) Chronic (uremia, infection, neoplasm)
	Increased intrathoracic pressure	Tension pneumothorax Excess positive end-expiratory pressure
	IVC obstruction	Gravid uterus on IVC
	Pulmonary embolism	Tumor, thrombus
Septic	Infection	Invasive infection with systemic response
	Noninfectious systemic inflammatory	Burn, pancreatitis, other causes response syndrome
	Acute adrenal insufficiency	
	Anaphylaxis, drug reactions	
Neurogenic	Anatomic	Spinal trauma, tumor
	Induced	Spinal or epidural anesthetic
Miscellaneous	Toxins	Carbon monoxide, cyanide poisoning
	Metabolic	Myxedema coma
Mixed	Combinations	

IVC, inferior vena cava.

of mediators that cause circulatory disturbances and direct and indirect cell damage.[4] Hemodynamic changes are defined as early (warm or hyperdynamic) or late (cold or hypodynamic). These stages are primarily characterized by the degree of ventricular contractility and peripheral vasomotor impairment present. Early septic shock is distinguished by peripheral vasodilation, flushed and warm extremities, and a compensatory elevation in cardiac output. Although an increase in venous capacitance diminishes venous return to the heart, cardiac output is maintained via tachycardia and the decrease in afterload.

Late septic shock is characterized by impaired myocardial contractility, worsening peripheral perfusion, vasoconstriction, extremity mottling, oliguria, and hypotension. Peripheral oxygen utilization may be severely impaired by bacterial toxins, such as lipopolysaccharide (LPS) and the inflammatory products of the host's own immune response, resulting in metabolic dysfunction and acidosis despite a high systemic oxygen delivery (Fig. 8.1). Hypoperfusion and the altered tissue metabolism create a vicious cycle that propagates the inflammatory response initiated in reaction to the initial infectious challenge.

In addition to source control, immediate treatment of septic shock should address cardiac function and microvascular hypoperfusion. Unresolved perfusion deficits contribute significantly to multiple organ failure and high mortality. The volume of fluid needed may exceed that required for treatment of other forms of shock, as microvascular endothelial capillary leak precipitates a profound loss of intravascular fluids into the interstitial tissues.

Traumatic Shock

Traumatic shock results from direct tissue or bony injury, resulting in a combination of hypovolemia caused by fluid and blood loss and an immunologic and neuroendocrine response to tissue destruction and devitalization. This combined insult complicates what might otherwise be straightforward hemorrhagic shock by inducing a systemic response that utilizes many of the inflammatory mediators present in septic shock (see Fig. 8.1).[5] These mediators propagate and intensify the effects of the initial hypovolemia and make subsequent multiple organ failure far more likely than occurs with hypovolemic shock alone.

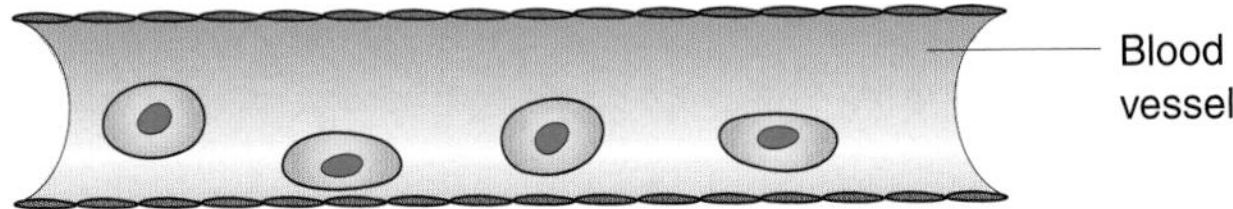

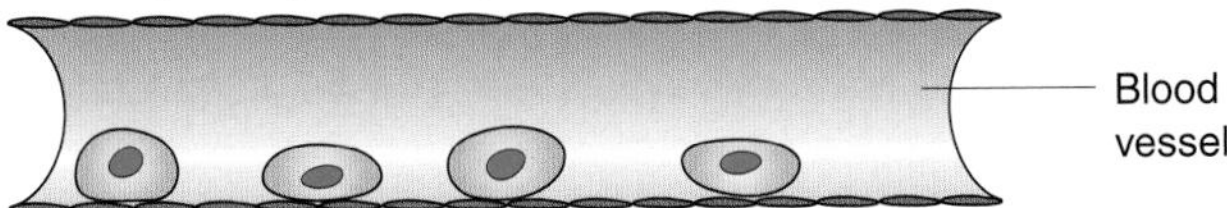

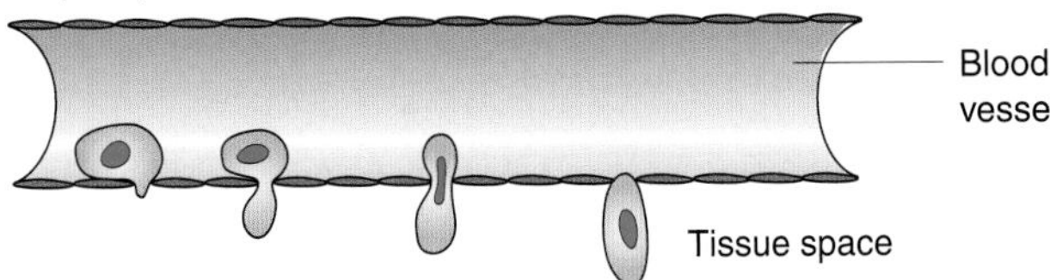

FIGURE 8.1 Activated polymorphonuclear leukocyte (PMN) microvascular transmigration at injury site. (After Bernhard GR, Vincent J-L, Laterre P-F, et al. Efficacy and safety of recombinant human activated protein C for severe sepsis. *N Engl J Med.* 2001;344:699.)

Cardiogenic Shock

The clinical definition of cardiogenic shock is decreased cardiac output with tissue hypoperfusion, despite presence of adequate intravascular volume. It is caused by a primary problem with the cardiac muscle, electrical conduction system, or valves. The most common cause is anterior wall myocardial infarction, although in surgical patients it is often precipitated by pulmonary embolus, myocardial contusion, or pulmonary hypertension.

Distinguishing cardiogenic shock from other shock etiologies is occasionally difficult. It is not uncommon to see combined cardiogenic and traumatic shock in the elderly patient, with one often being the precipitating event for the other. The hallmarks of the hemodynamic and neuroendocrine response to systemic hypoperfusion from other causes are also typical of cardiogenic shock. Eliciting a history of pre-existing cardiac disease, and physical findings such as pulmonary rales, cardiac murmurs, an S3 gallop, and jugular venous distension may be helpful. An electrocardiogram may detect significant ischemia or other pathology. A chest radiograph may reveal bilateral pulmonary infiltrates typical of cardiogenic edema, and cardio-specific serum tests [(troponin I, creatine phosphokinase (CPK)] may indicate myocardial damage.

Like other forms of shock, cardiogenic shock tends to be self-perpetuating. Myocardial perfusion depends on the pressure gradient between the coronary artery and the left ventricle and the duration of diastole. Both are compromised by the hypotension and tachycardia that characterizes this condition. High-volume fluid resuscitation, sometimes necessary for treatment of other forms of shock, is poorly tolerated and likely to be detrimental to an individual with the compromised myocardial function of cardiogenic shock.

A subset of patients with cardiogenic shock do not have intrinsic cardiac disease but have pump failure due to extrinsic compression that limits diastolic filling and cardiac output. Cardiac tamponade, tension pneumothorax, diaphragmatic herniation of abdominal viscera, mediastinal hematoma, and, occasionally, positive pressure mechanical ventilation may all precipitate cardiogenic shock by exerting pressure on the myocardium. The key to diagnosis and appropriate therapy is the physical examination, supplemented by use of appropriate diagnostic modalities.

The classical physical findings of cardiac tamponade, Beck's triad, comprise hypotension, muffled heart sounds, and jugular venous distention. Unfortunately, these nonspecific clinical findings are seldom present together. Elevated jugular venous pressure, noted by either physical examination of measurement of central venous pressure (CVP), although not specific for cardiac compression, is usually present. Pulsus paradoxus can be useful for the diagnosis of cardiac tamponade. Although it may be caused by other conditions, it is virtually always present in patients with tamponade.

Neurogenic Shock

Neurogenic shock is defined as failure of the nervous system to provide effective peripheral vascular resistance, resulting in inadequate end-organ perfusion. Warm, flushed, flaccid extremities; paraplegia; confusion; oliguria; and hypotension are the classic clinical findings. Injury to the proximal spinal cord, with interruption of the autonomic sympathetic vasomotor pathways, disrupts basal vasoconstrictor tone to peripheral veins and arterioles. Profound vasodilation of all microvascular beds below the level of cord injury diminishes venous return to the heart, reduces cardiac output, and precipitates hypotension. Injuries at or above the fourth thoracic vertebrae disrupt sympathetic enervation to the heart, resulting in significant bradycardia and severe decompensation.

Similar to the initial therapy for shock resulting from hypovolemia, treatment of the relative hypovolemia due to vasodilation of neurogenic shock requires intravenous volume resuscitation. Restoration of the pathologically expanded intravascular space improves preload and cardiac output and may reverse hypotension. However, maintenance of adequate hemodynamics often requires vasopressor support in an effort to avoid the administration of excessive fluids. CVP monitoring to assess cardiac preload should be considered as a means of determining adequate and nonexcessive filling pressures, as loss of vasomotor capacity within the pulmonary circulation predisposes these patients to pulmonary edema. As spinal cord injury is often associated with other traumatic injuries, diagnosis of isolated neurogenic shock must be a process of exclusion.

Hypoadrenal Shock

The role of adrenocortical hormones in providing resistance to shock is well recognized. The reduction in effective blood volume and changes in blood chemistry that occur after adrenalectomy are similar to those of shock and hemorrhage. Adrenalectomized animals have markedly diminished tolerance to both trauma and hypovolemia. Adrenal cortical hormones also play a key role in maintaining normal capillary tone and permeability. In recent years, the concept of functional or relative adrenal insufficiency has received increasing attention as a cause of unrecognized shock and hypoperfusion. Most critically ill patients have elevated cortisol levels, but some have low concentrations in relation to the degree of stress imposed by their disease. Administration of physiologic doses of steroids to correct this insufficiency may result in stabilization of hemodynamics and possible survival benefits.

Diagnosis of hypoadrenal shock is difficult, as classic signs of Addison's disease are absent. The only clinical clues may be unexplained hypotension and refractory response to high-dose vasopressors. An isolated serum cortisol level is difficult to interpret because the range of values observed in critically ill patients varies considerably. A cortisol level below 15 μg/dL suggests a high likelihood of adrenal insufficiency, whereas a value above 35 μg/dL suggests adequate renal function.[6] The adrenocorticotropic hormone (ACTH) stimulation test may be used to identify hypoadrenal patients when the diagnosis is unclear. Although hypoadrenal shock may complicate various types of shock, there is evidence to support the use of supplemental corticosteroids in patients with septic shock if there is biochemical evidence of hypoadrenalism.

ORGAN-SPECIFIC RESPONSE TO SHOCK

Cardiac and Microvascular Response

Cardiovascular physiology is profoundly affected by shock (Table 8.2). Reduced stroke volume is caused by an absolute or relative loss of preload. Intrinsic neuroendocrine and renal compensatory responses, along with additional intravenous fluid, are needed to increase ventricular end-diastolic volume. Restoration of adequate preload alone is often sufficient to return cardiac output to levels required to overcome peripheral perfusion deficits. However, some cases are complicated by acquired myocardial contractility derangements. Contractile function under these conditions is less a function of preload and more related to intrinsic myocardial dysfunction.

A defining characteristic of shock is compromise of microvascular perfusion (see Table 8.2). Far from being a passive conduit, the microvasculature actively participates in the response to shock. Arteriolar vessels are innervated by sympathetic nerves, as are small veins and venules. The vasoconstriction of hypovolemic shock and the vasodilation of septic and neurogenic shock are a result of these autonomic responses. The majority of the circulating blood volume resides in the venous system, and normal physiologic compensation mechanisms rely on this venous blood pool as an autotransfusion reservoir. Collapse of underperfused veins passively propels

TABLE 8.2

HEMODYNAMIC CHANGES WITH SHOCK

Type of Shock	CVP / PCWP	Cardiac output	SVR	SvO_2
Hypovolemic	↓	↓	↑	↓
Cardiogenic	↑	↓	↑	↓
Septic				
Hyperdynamic	↑↓	↑	↓	↑
Hypodynamic	↑↓	↓	↑	↑↓
Traumatic	↓	↑↓	↑↓	↓
Neurogenic	↓	↓	↓	↓
Hypoadrenal	↓↑	↓	↓	↓

CVP, central venous pressure; PCWP, pulmonary capillary wedge pressure; SVR, systemic vascular resistance, SvO_2, mixed venous oxygen saturation.

blood toward the heart, while α-adrenergic venoconstriction actively mobilizes the venous pool. Profound peripheral vasoconstriction via α-adrenergic, vasopressin, angiotensin II, and endothelin-1 stimulation of arteriolar and precapillary smooth muscle sphincters selectively diminishes perfusion to dermal, renal, muscle, and splanchnic vascular beds to preserve perfusion of critical central organs, primarily the central nervous system (CNS) and myocardium.[7]

The capillary endothelial monolayer maintains a semipermeable barrier between the intra- and extraluminal spaces and is compromised by shock.[8] Circulating inflammatory mediators and byproducts of infection [LPS, thrombin, tumor necrosis factor alpha (TNFα), interleukin (IL)-1, nitric oxide, and endothelin-1] generated in response to traumatic or septic shock have been shown to induce and sustain endothelial capillary leak (see Fig. 8.1). Although the exact mechanisms of endothelial monolayer dysfunction are unclear, the only available therapies to reverse microvascular decompensation are timely restoration of peripheral perfusion, rapid elimination of infectious and necrotic tissue, and pharmacologic and mechanical support of cardiopulmonary function.

Neuroendocrine Response

The neuroendocrine reaction to shock comprise involuntary responses by the hypothalamus, autonomic nervous system, and secretory endocrine glands and is directed toward restoration of tissue perfusion and a redirected utilization of metabolic substrates. The autonomic response is initially triggered by hypoxia, hypotension, or hypovolemia detected by aortic and carotid baro- and chemoreceptors. Subsequently, sympathetic vasoconstriction of specific vascular beds, induced by direct synaptic release of norepinephrine, results in redistribution of circulating blood volume from tissue of low metabolic activity to more metabolically demanding organs. Cardiac output, diminished by loss of preload, is augmented by inhibition of cardiac vagal activity and a resulting reflex tachycardia.

Circulating epinephrine and norepinephrine alter several aspects of glucose utilization, availability, and metabolism. The hyperglycemia of stress results from catecholamine induced glycogenolysis, gluconeogenesis, and decreased pancreatic insulin release. Simultaneously, hypothalamic stimulation of the anterior pituitary induces release of ACTH, which in turn prompts cortisol and aldosterone release by the adrenal cortex. Elevated serum cortisol contributes to postinjury hyperglycemia by increasing gluconeogenesis, enhancing lipolysis, and diminishing peripheral utilization of glucose and amino acids. The pancreatic response is characterized by a decrease in insulin release and an increase in glucagon secretion, which further stimulates hepatic gluconeogenesis. The combined actions of catecholamines, cortisol, and glucagon are synergistic and create a shock-related hyperglycemia that is often refractory to insulin treatment.

Renal juxtaglomerular secretion of renin in response to adrenergic stimulation and renal hypoperfusion triggers the formation of angiotensin I in the liver, which is subsequently converted to angiotensin II by the lungs. Angiotensin II, a potent vasoconstrictor, augments shock-induced catecholamine-mediated peripheral and splanchnic vasoconstriction and stimulates aldosterone release from the adrenal cortex. Renal tubular resorption of sodium in response to elevated circulating aldosterone creates highly concentrated, low-volume urine. Vasopressin secretion by the posterior pituitary similarly contributes to compensatory restoration and maintenance of intravascular volume by promoting water reabsorption by the renal distal tubules and by causing peripheral and splanchnic vasoconstriction. A major result is a prolonged severe hypoperfusion of the splanchnic vascular bed, further augmenting the deleterious host response.

Immunoinflammatory Response

Many shock-inducing events, particularly those associated with septic or traumatic shock, simultaneously trigger a massive systemic inflammatory response. Although inflammatory mediators (TNF-α, ILs, chemokines, etc.) play an integral role in the recovery of local tissue to trauma and infection, an uncontrolled systemic inflammatory response contributes to organ failure. Immunologically active cells involved in the systemic inflammatory response include nucleated blood cells (monocytes, polymorphonuclear leukocytes) and platelets, microvascular endothelial cells, and tissue macrophages. These cells generate and secrete scores of signal-amplifying inflammatory mediators ranging in complexity from individual molecules (nitric oxide) to large multisubunit, extensively modified proteins (TNF-α, IL-1, etc.). Even transient systemic elevation of any of these mediators has profound physiologic consequences.

Local tissue destruction, microbial contamination, and infection similarly activate the coagulation cascade and induce platelet aggregation and release of numerous platelet, endothelial, and clot-derived vasoactive mediators. Persistent, profound, and recurring microvascular hypoperfusion of the splanchnic and other organs likewise causes local tissue ischemia, parenchymal cell injury, microvascular coagulation, activation of inflammatory cells, and release of inflammatory mediators. Circulating monocyte, lymphocyte, and PMN adherence to activated endothelium results in extraluminal transmigration of these inflammatory cells into tissues remote from the area of injury (Fig. 8.2). This hyperdynamic immunologic response, with continued generation of proinflammatory mediators, is responsible for the progression of systemic inflammatory response syndrome (SIRS) toward multiple organ failure syndrome (MOFS)[9] (see Fig. 8.1).

Regulation of the systemic inflammatory response has been an active area of shock research for several decades. Elimination of particular inflammatory mediators from the systemic circulation, or inhibition of particular cell–cell interactions in experimental animal systems, has been shown to improve outcomes after shock resuscitation. However, to date, all efforts to regulate the SIRS response with therapeutic elimination or supplementation of specific proinflammatory and antiinflammatory mediators have proven ineffective or even harmful in humans. This lack of efficacy may relate to inadequacy of current animal models of shock, sepsis, and organ failure or to inadequate understanding of key elements that regulate this syndrome. Unfortunately, the network of inflammatory mediators and affected cells are so complex and redundant that no single agent is likely to be effective at interrupting this response. As a result, there is probably no single common pathway likely to respond to a "silver bullet" approach.

Pulmonary Response

The lung is the organ system most sensitive to systemic insult and injury and is frequently the first organ to fail in the progression to MOFS. Adult respiratory deficiency syndrome (ARDS) represents a high-mortality form of pulmonary insufficiency that is often precipitated by sepsis or traumatic shock (see Fig. 8.1). It is triggered and perpetuated by the numerous

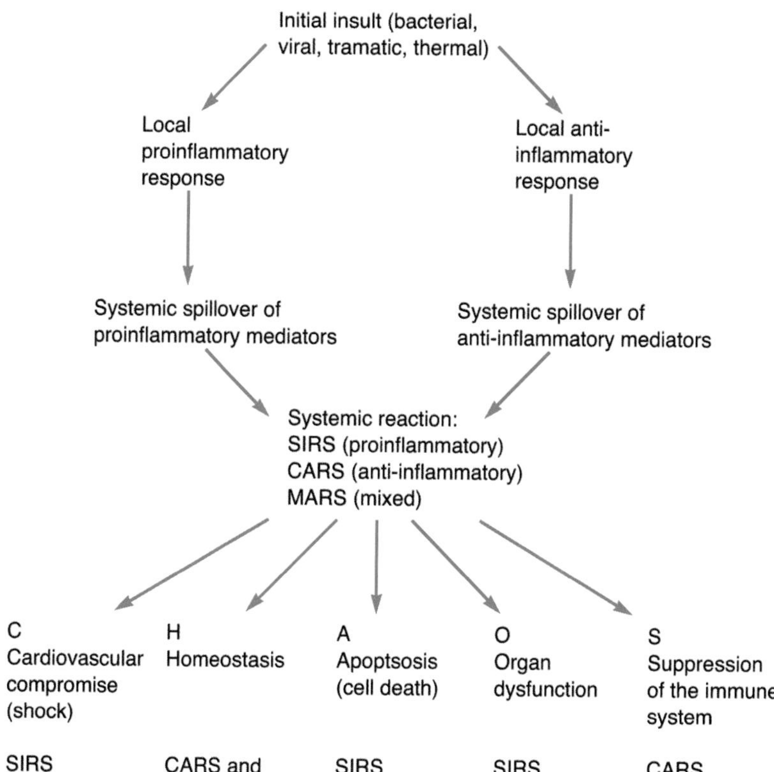

FIGURE 8.2 Clinical sequelae of the systemic inflammatory response syndrome (SIRS) and the compensatory anti-inflammatory response syndrome (CARS). (After Bone RC. Sir Isaac Newton, sepsis, SIRS, and CARS. *Crit Care Med.* 1996;24:1125–1128.)

inflammatory mediators created in the hypoperfused microvasculature elsewhere in the body.[10]

Interstitial edema and subsequent reduced compliance results in diminished tidal volume and tachypnea, compromising gas exchange. Surfactant abnormalities contribute to alveolar collapse, resulting in loss of functional residual capacity (FRC) and the onset of pulmonary insufficiency. The pulmonary microvascular response mirrors the systemic response, with angiotensin and α-adrenergic-induced vasoconstriction creating significant elevations of pulmonary vascular resistance, further straining the heart. Pulmonary parenchymal injury may be propagated by excessive positive pressure ventilation and alveolar overdistension in particular, further contributing to alveolar damage.

Renal Response

Direct sympathetically induced renal vasoconstriction increases afferent arteriole resistance in response to shock. This effect is reinforced by elevated circulating angiotensin II and catecholamines. The resulting decrease in renal blood flow and glomerular filtration rate (GFR), along with elevated circulating aldosterone and vasopressin (ADH), produce oliguria and prerenal azotemia. Acute tubular necrosis (ATN) may result from prolonged decreases in renal cortical blood flow, as well as from toxins generated during sepsis. Oliguric renal failure, like the pulmonary insufficiency of ARDS, is a common component of MOFS.

Distinguishing low urine output due to oliguric renal failure from the oliguria of decreased renal perfusion pressure can be aided by analyzing urine sodium and osmolality. Renal hypoperfusion usually results in a urine sodium of less than 20 mEq/L with an osmolality of >400 mosmol/kg, and acute tubular injury impairs sodium reabsorption and is associated with a low urinary osmolality. Fractional excretion of sodium of less than 2% may also help determine whether the cause is renal or prerenal.

Early detection of abnormal kidney function is critical to prevent progression to renal injury. Abnormal renal function can be detected as a decline in creatinine clearance. The correlation between a creatinine clearance based on a 24-hour collection and a sample collected over a shorter interval is poor. However, the 24-hour value represents an average value over that time. A sample obtained over a shorter period may reflect the time in question and allow timely recognition and treatment of renal dysfunction.

Genetic Regulation of the Response to Shock

Individuals vary considerably in their susceptibility to shock and in their ability to recover from its consequences. Recently, unique host-specific responses have been identified as important determinants of the outcome of sepsis and septic shock. Genetic predispositions in an individual's immunoinflammatory response may dictate whether infection is adequately or inadequately countered. These differences in response may be partially explained by single nucleotide polymorphisms (SNPs) in the genetic sequences for various inflammatory mediators.

These subtle nucleotide variations may affect the transcription or translation of associated genes, or the secretion or function of the corresponding proteins.

The recognition that genetic background may regulate the response to severe sepsis and septic shock has led to the identification of an array of genetic markers associated with enhanced risk of septic mortality. These SNPs are in genes encoding proteins involved in pathogen recognition (Toll-like receptors 2, 4, and 5, CD14, and mannose binding lectin), cytokine expression (TNF-α, IL-1, IL-6, and IL-10), and several other genes involved in mediating and controlling the innate immune response and the inflammatory cascade.[11]

Investigation into genetic polymorphisms should provide important insights into the pathophysiology of shock. SNP identification leading to early diagnosis of individuals at risk of developing or dying from the complications of shock may allow therapies to become more preemptive and effective.

COMPLICATIONS OF SHOCK

Ischemia-Reperfusion Injury

Inadequate microvasculature flow results in activation of leukocytes and converts local endothelial cells to a proinflammatory, prothrombotic phenotype. On reperfusion, the re-introduction of oxygen prompts these cells to generate superoxide anion, hydroxyl radicals, and hydrogen peroxide, further injuring local tissue. Microvascular endothelial adherence, monolayer transmigration, and local oxidative burst by activated neutrophils, along with the profound loss of endothelial monolayer integrity (i.e., microvascular capillary leak), contribute to massive interstitial edema after reperfusion (see Fig. 8.2). Although all tissues are sensitive to varying degrees, ischemia-reperfusion injury appears to be most detrimental to the pulmonary vasculature and the splanchnic circulations. Pulmonary interstitial edema and alveolar fluid accumulation are associated with the development of ARDS, whereas extensive visceral edema may contribute to development of abdominal compartment syndrome.

Second-Hit Phenomena

Patients who have been successfully resuscitated from shock are at risk for what is referred to as the second-hit phenomena. A single episode of severe or prolonged shock may precipitate organ failure, but, more commonly, the initial insult "primes" the inflammatory response, resulting in an augmented response to a subsequent insult such as an infection, a second episode of blood loss, or major surgery.[12] For example, after the primary event, circulating neutrophils demonstrate enhanced superoxide anion production, increased endothelial cell adherence, augmented cytokine response, and increased cytotoxicity. Due to preferential vasoconstriction during shock, the ischemic gut is thought to serve as a bed for priming circulating neutrophils and may play a pivotal role in producing the second hit.

Multiple Organ Failure Syndrome

MOFS rarely develops as a result of isolated cardiogenic or neurogenic shock but is most often precipitated by septic and traumatic shock complicated by second-hit events such as repeated episodes of hypovolemia, subsequent infection, or repeated blood transfusions. Similarly, the presence of an unresolved inflammatory focus (such as devitalized necrotic tissue), undrained bodily fluids, or unresolved regional perfusion deficits, are the primary causes for the persistence of SIRS and the transition to MOFS.

There is also a compensatory antiinflammatory phase of the SIRS response that is evolutionarily designed to counter the locally generated hyperimmune response and check systemic spread of proinflammatory mediators. If the compensatory antiinflammatory response syndrome (CARS) results in excessive immunosuppression, it may contribute to susceptibility to primary and secondary infections that can then lead to organ failure.[13]

Unfortunately, few therapeutic agents designed to counter immune dysfunction have had significant impact on the prevention and treatment of MOFS. Numerous clinical trials utilizing proinflammatory and antiinflammatory mediators as therapeutic interventions have been conducted. With the exception of activated protein C, all have failed to sufficiently and appropriately stimulate or suppress the SIRS response and improve outcomes.[14]

Abdominal Compartment Syndrome

Splanchnic ischemia and reperfusion result in extensive visceral capillary leak and interstitial edema of the bowel. Grossly edematous viscera within the closed space of the abdomen dramatically increases intra-abdominal pressure, which compromises intra-abdominal organ function, increases renovascular resistance, limits diaphragmatic excursion, and may decrease cardiac output and elevate intra-cranial pressure. The clinical hallmarks of abdominal compartment syndrome are a distended and tense abdomen, diminished tidal volume, pulmonary edema, decreased cardiac output, oliguria, and elevated urinary bladder pressure. Presence of all or part of this syndrome should prompt consideration of an operative procedure to decompress the abdomen.

Hypothermia

Human beings produce heat as a result of oxygen consumption (combustion). Because shock can be defined as a reduction in oxygen delivery to a level that decreases oxygen consumption, all patients in shock have diminished heat production. Hypothermia ($<35°C$) is associated with cardiac contractile dysfunction, impaired oxygen dissociation from hemoglobin, inhibition of platelet aggregation, slowing of the enzymatic reactions of the coagulation cascade, and an increase in blood and fluid resuscitation requirements.[15] Hypothermia contributes significantly to a refractory shock state and is associated with high mortality.

Under certain conditions, hypothermia decreases tissue metabolic rate and oxygen requirements. Successful application after circulatory arrest due to primary cardiac events has extended interest in this technique for use in treatment of profound hemorrhagic shock due to injuries that would otherwise be survivable after repair during induced hypothermic circulatory arrest. Clinical trials will require development of new devices to rapidly cool the brain and body, as well as perfusate fluids that will work synergistically with hypothermia to stabilize cellular energy stores.

TREATMENT

Fluid Therapy

Early investigators of hemorrhagic shock noted that decreased CVP and a reduction in total body oxygen delivery (DO_2) were key early findings. If the decrease in oxygen delivery was severe or prolonged, a reduction in total body oxygen consumption ensued. After adequate fluid resuscitation, oxygen delivery and consumption increased above the baseline value for several hours, as if the body was paying back an "oxygen debt." Failure to display this hyperdynamic response to resuscitation was almost always fatal. Because early death from shock appeared to be explained by the dynamics of oxygen delivery and utilization, therapy focused on restoring hemodynamics and oxygen transport with fluid and inotropes.

The provision of additional fluid beyond the amount of blood loss was associated with improved survival in both clinical and experimental studies of hemorrhagic shock, leading to widespread acceptance of aggressive fluid infusion. However, some researchers have recently described a significant increase in mortality associated with crystalloid over-resuscitation and have postulated that excessive fluid administration increases the clinical risk of ARDS.[16] Because massive volumes of fluid are only provided to patients with severe shock, it is unclear if it is the excessive fluid or the associated underlying shock that increases the risk of ARDS, organ failure, or death after massive fluid resuscitation.

Edema and fluid shifts are unavoidable after shock. Edema occurs when capillary hydrostatic pressure exceeds capillary oncotic pressure (25–28 mm Hg). Shock often results in a protein leak that abolishes the gradient between intravascular and interstitial colloid oncotic pressure. In such cases, hydrostatic forces favoring fluid movement out of the vascular space are unopposed, and lung, intestinal, cerebral, and total body interstitial fluid accumulates at normal or even low capillary pressure.[17] Thus, Starling forces governing fluid movement across the capillary membrane indicate that increases in capillary pressure play a major role in causing and perpetuating fluid shifts during capillary leak syndromes and are, at least to some extent, dependent on the volume of resuscitation fluids.[18]

A balanced salt solution such as 0.9% normal saline contains 9 g of sodium per liter, far more than the 2 to 4 gram per day limitation often recommended to elderly patients with cardiac disease and a predisposition to edema formation. Volume overload may be particularly severe when the inflammatory response activates salt- and water-conserving mechanisms. The type of fluid administered for resuscitation may also have significant consequences. Lactated Ringer's solution increases expression of adhesion molecules, promotes release of proinflammatory cytokines, and is associated with cellular apoptosis and endothelial cell dysfunction.[19] It is poorly retained in the intravascular space, and large volumes are often required.

Hypertonic saline solutions stabilize arterial blood pressure and cardiac output with small-volume infusion and have been shown to have beneficial effects on immune function. However, no benefit was demonstrated when used for initial resuscitation of hypotensive patients with traumatic brain injury, and an adverse effect was reported in burn patients, with no reduction in ultimate cumulative fluid load.[20,21]

Colloids have been of interest since the demonstration that infusion of 1 L of lactated Ringer's solution in patients with shock expanded the plasma volume by only 194 mL, with most fluid moving to the interstitial space, whereas 100 mL of a 25% albumin solution expanded plasma volume by 465 mL.[22] However, at least one large, multicenter randomized trial failed to demonstrate a benefit in intensive care unit (ICU) patients, and two meta-analyses of colloid use also failed to demonstrate a beneficial effect.[23]

Aggressive fluid resuscitation is clearly a lifesaving modality, and a key strategy in the treatment of shock and prevention of secondary consequences (Algorithm 8.1). However, indiscriminate fluid loading causes problematic edema in the lungs, gut, brain, and other organs. The amount of fluid used for resuscitation should be titrated to carefully selected hemodynamic and oxygen transport endpoints. Solutions currently in development ("artificial blood") with oxygen transport

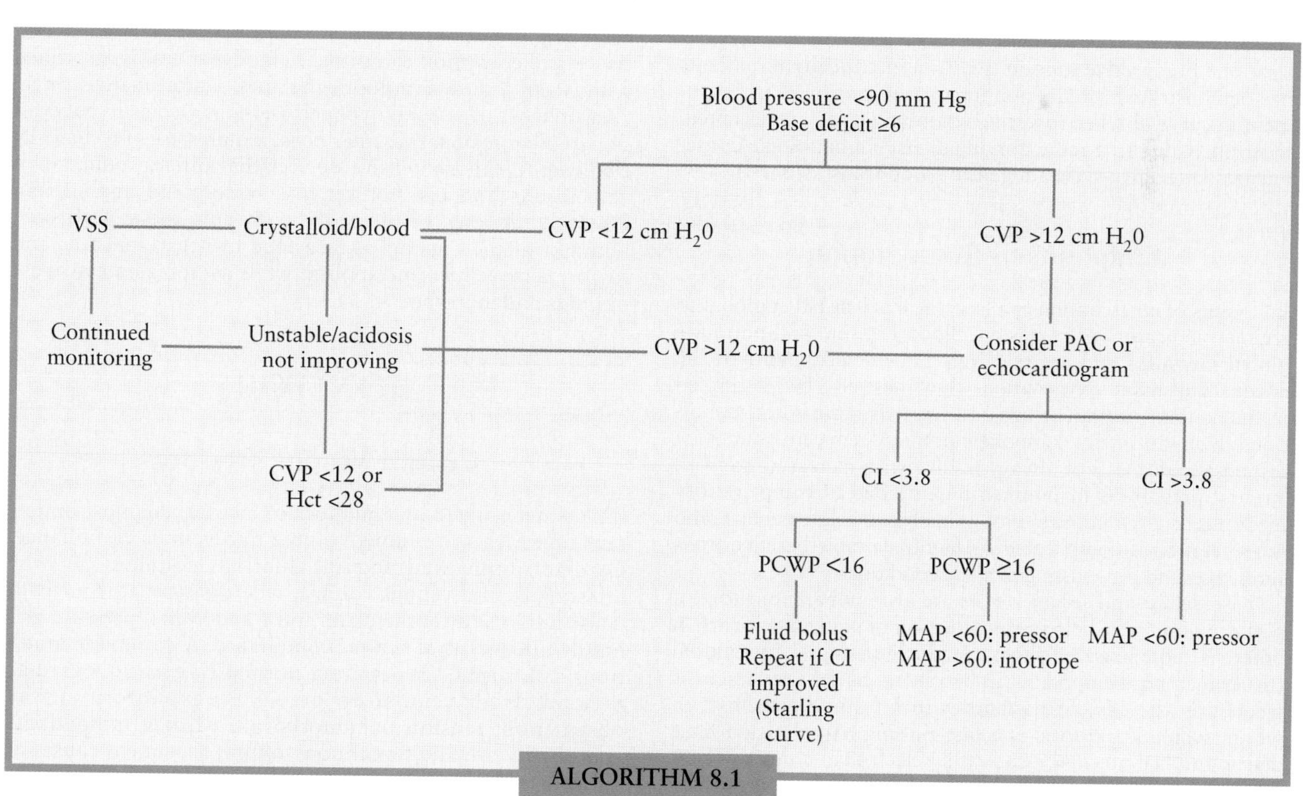

ALGORITHM 8.1 Shock resuscitation algorithm.

capabilities may hold the potential of restoring oxygen transport while minimizing the need for large volumes.

Permissive Hypotension

Elevation of systemic arterial pressure in patients with disruption of the arterial system or major solid organ injury, especially after penetrating trauma, may cause acceleration of hemorrhage, disrupt natural clotting mechanisms, and cause dilution of clotting factors. Laboratory and clinical evidence support judicious use of intravenous fluids until hemorrhage is controlled by surgery, angiography, or direct pressure.[24] Fluid resuscitation for patients with multisystem blunt trauma, especially with concomitant traumatic brain injury, represents a more complicated decision process, as maintaining cerebral perfusion pressure is a competing priority. Avoidance of both excessive fluid administration and prolonged hypoperfusion is best achieved in all patients not by maintenance of a marginal blood pressure but by rapid surgical or angiographic intervention to control bleeding.

Transfusion

Anemia prompts clinical concerns because it may signify blood loss or hematologic disease, but it rarely causes tissue ischemia. The hemoglobin level that causes concern should depend on the adequacy of other mechanisms involved in oxygen delivery such as arterial oxygen saturation and cardiac output, the specific clinical situation, and the organ systems most at risk, balanced against the risk of transfusion. Clinical evidence suggests that hemoglobin values above 7 mg/dL are adequate in most patients, with the exception of those with coronary ischemic syndromes or traumatic brain injury, in whom local factors may restrict blood flow even though oxygen delivery may be adequate to other parts of the body. At least one prospective randomized trial in critically ill patients has demonstrated a reduction in complications and improvement in survival when lower hemoglobin values are accepted, most likely due to a reduction in adverse immunologic consequences associated with allogeneic blood transfusion.[25]

Endpoints of Resuscitation

Endpoints of resuscitation can be categorized as either global or regional indicators of perfusion. Blood pressure and pulse are global measures and are relatively poor determinants of the adequacy of tissue oxygenation. They must also be interpreted in the context of patient age and pre-existing medical conditions. Tachycardia is a component of the systemic inflammatory response and does not always resolve with increased preload. Arterial pressure is maintained by a myriad of compensatory mechanisms, even in the face of a significant volume deficit, and interpretation is complicated by highly variable baseline pressures, age, and pre-existing medical conditions.

Base deficit and serum lactate are also global indicators of perfusion and may help in the detection of patients who are in otherwise compensated shock. Acidosis arising from regional tissues may not be apparent in peripheral blood samples, as is frequently the case in patients with intestinal ischemia, in whom systemic acidosis is a late finding. An elevated base deficit and lactate can be caused by electrolyte abnormalities, accelerated glycolysis or pyruvate production, and decreased clearance by the liver. They may also reflect a period of hypoperfusion that has already resolved and does not need further treatment. A positive response toward correction, however, is indicative of appropriate resuscitation.

A pulmonary artery catheter (PAC) has obvious appeal as a monitor because ensuring adequate oxygen delivery is paramount in the treatment of shock (see Algorithm 8.1). A progressive decline in systemic oxygen delivery (DO_2) results in an increase in oxygen extraction ratio, evident as a reduction in pulmonary mixed venous oxygen saturation. When DO_2 is reduced below the level needed to maintain normal tissue metabolic activity, anaerobic metabolism occurs. This is evident as a decrease in total body oxygen consumption (VO_2). Adequate resuscitation requires eliminating any pathologic decrease in VO_2 by restoring oxygen delivery to an adequate level. In clinical practice, however, there is no precise level of VO_2 that can be used as an endpoint, as tissue oxygen needs vary according to the patient's condition, level of sedation, body temperature, and other factors, and are affected by endogenous and exogenously administered catecholamines.

Oxygen consumption may be especially difficult to interpret in patients with late stage sepsis because acquired defects in mitochondrial respiration may prevent utilization of oxygen, resulting in decreased consumption and progressive acidosis despite normal or high DO_2.

The adequacy of resuscitation can also be assessed by measurement of end-organ function and perfusion, in addition to global measures. Blood flow to the most vital organs (brain and heart) is preserved during shock at the expense of flow to the skin, muscles, gut, and, ultimately, the kidneys. Detection of ischemia in less vital organs could theoretically identify patients in compensated shock who have otherwise normal global indicators.

Low urine output (0.5–1.0 mL/kg/hour) is an indicator of inadequate end-organ perfusion, but urine output may initially be maintained by peripheral venoconstriction and maintenance of cardiac output due to tachycardia. The use of gastric tonometry to measure intramucosal pH has highlighted the uneven recovery from shock by visceral organs. Persistent visceral hypoperfusion, as demonstrated by intramucosal acidosis despite correction to normal hemodynamics, is associated with organ failure and poor outcomes. Unfortunately, direct measurement of visceral hypoperfusion, as well as hypoperfusion in other regional vascular beds, requires use of technically challenging, labor-intensive devices that often produce variable results and has not yet had widespread application. Presently, the goal of therapy is to restore tissue perfusion, both global and regional as measured by organ function, and to normalize cellular metabolism while avoiding excessive use of fluids and inotropes.

MONITORS

Central Venous Pressure

CVP is determined by a number of factors, the most important of which are venous volume and venous compliance. Cardiac output and arterial dilation modulate CVP by affecting central venous volume, whereas sympathetic venoconstriction and thoracic and intra-abdominal pressure primarily affect central venous compliance. A variety of conditions can raise CVP despite a normal or even low cardiac preload. High ventilatory pressures, expiratory airway obstruction, tension pneumothorax, cardiac tamponade, and obesity are additional non-volume-dependent causes of an elevated CVP.

Circulating catecholamines cause vasoconstriction, with maintenance of venous pressure despite reduced circulating volume. In such cases, fluid therapy may reduce the intensity of vasoconstriction by reducing tone, with no net change in

CVP. Following the change in CVP in response to a fluid challenge may be the only way to accurately estimate preload in some patients. Although an elevated CVP does not guarantee adequate preload, a low CVP is a reliable indicator of hypovolemia. Inspiratory stridor is the only condition that can falsely reduce CVP and mimic hypovolemia by reducing pleural pressure.

Pulmonary Artery Catheter

Hemodynamic monitoring utilizing a flow-directed PAC has been a standard in the treatment of shock for decades and has been considered to be essential for optimal management of certain forms of shock (see Table 8.2). However, as a result of a multicenter study that reported that use of a PAC was associated with increased mortality, the indications for PAC use have recently been questioned.[26] PAC patients were retrospectively compared to matched control patients that were selected using a scoring system. This scoring system has not been validated, which raises the possibility that physicians inserted a PAC in the more critically ill patients.

ICU staffing practices may have also been a factor explaining these surprising results. The study was conducted in "open" ICUs, where any physician on the medical staff could admit a patient to the unit and insert a PAC. Clinicians may not always interpret PAC data appropriately. In a multicenter study of physicians' knowledge and interpretation of PAC data, nearly half (47%) were unable to appropriately determine the wedge pressure from a clear tracing, and a similar percentage (44%) could not identify the determinants of oxygen delivery.[27] Studies have demonstrated improved outcome when patients are managed in ICUs staffed by specialists in critical care, despite their more frequent use of PACs.[28]

An additional consideration regarding the controversy over the utility of PACs is that currently used endpoints for PAC-guided resuscitation may be inappropriate. For example, efforts to augment systemic oxygen delivery have not convincingly demonstrated any benefits to this approach, whereas treatments used to alter the variables ascertained with the catheter may themselves cause harm (fluid overload, excessive inotropes, blood transfusions). Finally, PACs are associated with specific complications, including the risk of central venous catheter insertion, endocarditis, and pulmonary artery injury, which may outweigh any potential benefits. As the safety and utility of the PAC have not yet been evaluated with prospective clinical trials in specific shock states, its usefulness in the management of shock remains to be determined.

Newer versions of the PAC have been developed that provide additional hemodynamic information, including continuous determination of cardiac output, ejection fraction, and calculated right ventricular end-diastolic volume. The pulmonary artery wedge pressure is a proxy for preload. However, the amount of precontractile stretch achieved with any given wedge or chamber pressure is modulated by the compliance of the ventricle. Therefore, cardiac chamber pressure may not be an accurate indicator of ventricular end-diastolic volume, just as end-diastolic volume may not be an accurate indicator of pulmonary wedge pressure and risk of pulmonary edema. The combination of both wedge pressure and end-diastolic volume may be used to maximize preload while avoiding excessive pulmonary capillary pressure.

A comparison of the pH and pCO_2 of mixed venous blood with a matched arterial blood sample can provide evidence of shock with tissue hypoxia. Hypoxic cells generate a hydrogen ion that is buffered by bicarbonate, resulting in increased production of H_2O and CO_2. An increase in venous pCO_2 results in an abnormal gap between mixed venous and arterial pCO_2 and pH and is a sign of anaerobic metabolism. With cessation of hydrogen ion production, this abnormal gap is quickly eliminated, whereas base deficit and hyperlactatemia may persist for several hours.

PHARMACEUTICAL SUPPORT

Inotropic augmentation of cardiac output may be required when restoration of venous preload fails to provide sufficient cardiac output to satisfy tissue oxygen demands. The effect of inotropic agents depends on the specific adrenergic receptor affinity, chronotropic effects. and demands placed on myocardial oxygen consumption of the individual agents (Table 8.3). Vasodilators reduce demands on the myocardium and augment cardiac function via reduction in systemic vascular resistance (SVR) or afterload or by dilating the venous system and reducing cardiac preload. Afterload reduction may preserve stroke volume in face of a failing myocardium, whereas venodilation reduces pulmonary capillary wedge pressure and pressure-driven pulmonary edema. Agents that increase afterload may be needed when blood pressure falls below the autoregulatory range of the coronary, cerebral, and renal vascular beds.

Inotropes and Vasopressors

Dopamine

Dopamine is an endogenous sympathetic amine with effects that change with increasing doses. The highest affinity receptors are occupied at low serum concentrations (infusions $<$2–3 μg/kg/minute) and consist of dopaminergic receptors in the renal and splanchnic beds that serve to augment regional blood flow, increase urine output, and cause natriuresis. However, multiple studies, including prospective randomized trials, have failed to demonstrate that low-dose dopamine prevents acute renal failure or decreases the need for dialysis in critically ill patients. At modest concentrations (3–5 μg/kg/minute) dopamine occupies cardiac β_1-adrenergic receptors and increases myocardial contractility and heart rate. Higher doses ($>$5 μg/kg/minute) cause an increase in heart rate and blood pressure. Alpha-adrenergic receptors are stimulated at higher dose ranges ($>$10 μg/kg/minute), resulting in elevation of blood pressure and peripheral vascular resistance. Dopamine is therefore an effective agent for increasing blood pressure in hypotensive patients after appropriate fluid resuscitation. Because the relationship among a specific dose, receptor affinity, and clinical effect is unique to each patient, individual titration is required to achieve the desired effect.

Dobutamine

Dobutamine, a synthetic catecholamine, has a predominant affinity for β-adrenergic receptors. At clinically relevant doses (5–20 μg/kg/minute), dobutamine enhances myocardial contractility with mild to moderate changes in heart rate. It also induces peripheral vasodilation, which limits its utility in patients with hypotension. It is an appropriate agent when cardiac output augmentation, not blood pressure support, is required and when a drop in peripheral resistance and preload is clinically tolerable or beneficial. Treatment of cardiogenic shock following myocardial infarction typically requires support of myocardial contractility and reduction of peripheral resistance, which makes dobutamine an excellent choice in this setting.

TABLE 8.3

PHARMACODYNAMICS OF INOTROPIC/VASOCONSTRICTOR AGENTS

		Sites of action				Hemodynamic response			
Drug	Metabolism	Heart β1	Heart β2	Vessels α	Vessels β2	Renal perfusion	CO	SVR	BP
Isoproterenol 1 mg/250 mL 1–2 μg/min initially	Renal	+++	+++	0	+++	+/−		−	+/−
Dobutamine 250 mg/250 mL 3 μg/kg/min initially	Hepatic	+++	0/+	0/+	0/+			−	0/+
Dopamine 200 mg/250 mL 2–5 μg/kg/min low dose 20–50 μg/kg/min High dose	Hepatic	+++	+	0	Low dose High dose	−	Low dose High dose	0/+ −	
Epinephrine 2 mg/250 mL 2 μg/min initially	Renal	+++	+++	+++	++	−		−	
Norepinephrine 4 mg/250 mL 4 μg/min initially	Renal	++	++	+++	0	−	+/−		
Phenylephrine	Renal	0	0	+++	0	−	−		

α (alpha) vasoconstrict peripheral arterioles; β1 (beta-1) myocardial inotropy, chronotropy, enhance AV conduction; β2 (beta-2) chronotropy, vasodilate mesenteric/skeletal bed, bronchodilation; dopaminergic vasodilate mesenteric/renal bed.
BP, blood pressure; CO, cardiac output; SVR, systemic vascular resistance.

Epinephrine

When epinephrine is administered as a pharmacologic agent (0.01–0.05 μg/kg/minute), β_1–adrenergic effects predominate, causing increased stroke volume, heart rate, and contractility, along with modest β_2-receptor stimulation. At higher infusion rates, α-adrenergic receptors are stimulated, which overcomes β_2-mediated peripheral vasodilation, resulting in an increase in blood pressure and SVR. Renal and splanchnic vasoconstriction, cardiac dysrhythmias, and increased myocardial oxygen demands limit the prolonged use of high-dose epinephrine. Transient increases in serum lactate have also been noted, possibly due to impaired regional blood flow. Epinephrine should be considered as a potential short-term agent for use in patients with impaired cardiac function not responsive to other agents such as dobutamine.

Norepinephrine

Norepinephrine also has concentration dependent cardiovascular effects. It should be considered as a drug with predominantly α-constrictor effects and less pronounced β-stimulation and is therefore appropriate for use in patients who remain hypotensive despite dopamine administration or as a dopamine alternative. Combined α and β stimulation typically results in an increase in afterload and renal glomerular perfusion pressure, with preservation of cardiac output. Despite the potential for renal vasoconstriction, as a result of its effects on mean arterial pressure, norepinephrine is associated with an increase in urine output and creatinine clearance in hypotensive, septic patients.[29]

Phenylephrine

Phenylephrine is a pure α-agonist and is an effective agent for increasing peripheral vascular resistance and arterial blood pressure. Although it has no direct effect on the myocardium, the increase in afterload increases left ventricular work and oxygen demand and may cause a decrease in stroke volume and cardiac output. It is often used as a first-line agent in patients with neurogenic shock, but its use is otherwise generally restricted to patients who remain hypotensive when the dosage of agents such as dopamine or norepinephrine cannot be increased due to excessive tachycardia.

Vasopressin

Vasopressin acts directly on V_1 receptor in vascular smooth muscle to cause vasoconstriction and increases the reactivity of vascular smooth muscle to catecholamines. Release of endogenous vasopressin is a normal physiologic response to shock. After septic or prolonged hemorrhagic shock circulating vasopressin levels are decreased, possibly due to depletion of hypophyseal secretory stores. This relative deficiency may play a role in causing refractory hypotension. Vasopressin has minimal effects on normotensive patients, but in patients with septic shock it is effective in increasing SVR and mean arterial pressure. Vasopressin does not have inotropic properties and is a potent splanchnic and coronary vasoconstrictor. It has been associated with decreased cardiac output due to myocardial ischemia and increased afterload and may worsen metabolic acidosis in patients in shock by causing splanchnic ischemia.

Amrinone and Milrinone

Amrinone and milrinone are inotropes with cardiovascular effects similar to dobutamine, but with minimal chronotropic activity. As steroid-like phosphodiesterase antagonists, they increase smooth muscle cyclic adenosine monophosphate (cAMP) and alter calcium metabolism. Cardiac contractility, stroke volume, heart rate, and cardiac output are increased, while a concomitant reduction in afterload offsets cardiac workload. The increase in cardiac performance with minimal demands on myocardial oxygen consumption offers some utility in the treatment of cardiogenic shock or as a potential alternatives to dobutamine infusion. Both agents have a relatively long half-life of nearly 3 hours and should therefore be used with caution in patients at risk of developing hypotension.

Vasodilators

Nitroprusside and Nitroglycerin

Nitroprusside is a potent arterial and venous smooth muscle vasodilator. It causes a reduction in afterload that increases cardiac output and has a less prominent venodilatory effect that reduces pulmonary venous pressure and preload. Hypotension may limit its use, particularly in the presence of contractility deficits or inadequate preload. Infusions (>3 μg/kg/minute) continued for greater than 48 hours require monitoring of serum thiocyanate levels and arterial pH to detect complications of cyanide toxicity.

Nitroglycerin is primarily a venous smooth muscle vasodilator, with less significant arterial vasodilation effects than nitroprusside. Thus, although nitroprusside predominantly decreases afterload, nitroglycerin predominantly increases venous capacitance. It is an effective treatment for acute myocardial ischemia because it reduces excessive preload and ventricular end-diastolic pressure, thereby diminishing myocardial oxygen demand.

Miscellaneous Therapeutics

Corticosteroids

In septic shock, ACTH resistance may diminish the normal cortisol response. Also, peripheral tissue resistance to corticosteroids may develop through down-regulation of normal corticosteroid receptors. Initial clinical trials showed no reduction in mortality when short courses of high-dose corticosteroids were used as adjuncts in the treatment of septic shock. However, recent studies utilizing low or physiologic doses (<300 mg/day) of hydrocortisone for a longer duration (>5 days) of treatment have demonstrated a beneficial impact on mortality in septic patients.[30] Evaluation of refractory septic shock should include performance of a cosyntropin challenge test to evaluate the ability of the adrenal glands to secrete cortisol. Low basal cortisol levels, or cortisol levels that fail to augment after infusion of ACTH analogue, suggest adrenal insufficiency, and administration of hydrocortisone should be implemented.

Activated Protein C

Decades of cellular and humoral inflammation research have failed to produce an effective immunologic intervention in humans with septic shock and organ failure. However, coagulation pathway dysfunction, the mediators of which are also part of the innate host response to infection, has recently been shown to correlate with disease severity and mortality. Specifically, septic shock is associated with rapid depletion of protein C and blunted endogenous protein C activation. The protein C pathway serves to regulate thrombosis and may play a role in limiting the inflammatory response and diminishing endothelial cell injury in response to inflammatory cytokines (Fig. 8.3).

A recent phase III trial of recombinant activated protein C (APC) in severe sepsis demonstrated a 6.1% absolute reduction in 28-day mortality compared with placebo. Although the short- and long-term survival rates associated with APC were better in patients at high risk of death, treatment with APC was also associated with a slightly increased risk of serious bleeding compared with placebo, particularly during infusion (3.5% vs. 2.0%), and must be considered in the patient in the early postoperative period.[31]

Metabolites and Electrolytes

Severe shock is frequently associated with hypocalcemia. Severe hypocalcemia that causes cardiac dysfunction or electrical instability should be rapidly treated. Calcium chloride rapidly corrects calcium deficits, whereas calcium gluconate must be degraded in the liver to release calcium ion, resulting in slower

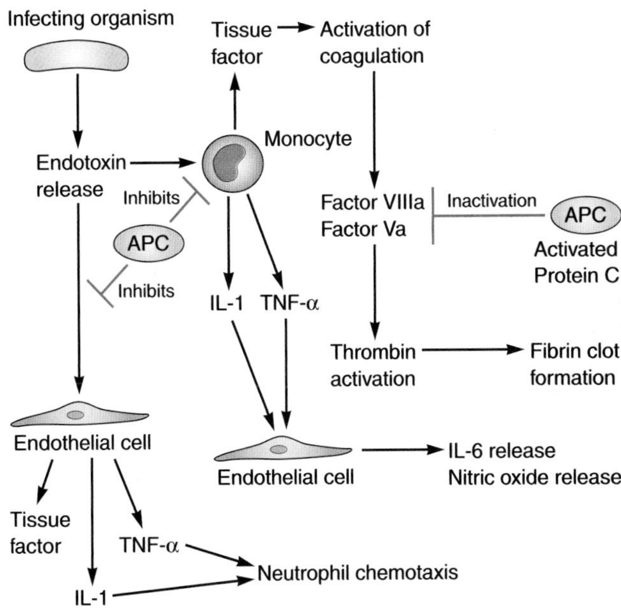

FIGURE 8.3 Events associated with the cytokine cascade in shock. Endotoxin and other antigenic components of infecting organism stimulate monocytes and local endothelial cells, resulting in elaboration of interleukin (IL)-1, tumor necrosis factor (TNF)-α, and tissue factor (primary stimulant for the coagulation cascade). Activated protein C (APC) is shown to inhibit several areas of pathway. (After Fitch SJ, Gossage JR. Optimal management of septic shock: rapid recognition and institution of therapy are crucial. *Postgrad Med.* 2002;111:53–66.)

correction of deficits but less risk of tissue reaction. In the absence of evidence of cardiac dysfunction, attempts to restore plasma calcium to normal during shock are not warranted. Ischemia results in decreased cell membrane ATP and failure of the membrane calcium pump. Increased cytosolic calcium causes release of lysosomal enzymes and activation of phospholipases, protein kinases, and proteases that cause membrane damage and cytoskeletal destruction. Reduced serum calcium levels during severe shock are probably due to movement of ionized calcium into the cells. Administration of exogenous calcium may worsen uncontrolled calcium influx, whereas effective resuscitation will usually restore circulating calcium levels to normal.

Many shock resuscitation protocols emphasize correction of metabolic acidosis with fluids and inotropes until the pH begins to normalize. When interpreting an acid-base disorder, the presence of an anion gap is supportive evidence of lactic acidosis. However, a non-anion gap acidosis with worsening base deficit frequently occurs when normal saline is administered in large volumes. Efforts to correct a non-anion gap acidosis with additional fluids that may no longer be needed may increase the risk of fluid overload.

Future Therapies

When initiating therapy for shock the clinician does not know if therapy has been started early when salvage is still possible or late, after irreversible changes have occurred within the cell and death is inevitable. Failure to respond to fluids, inotropes, and vasopressors with restoration of normal oxygen consumption and aerobic metabolism probably represents a defect in cellular and subcellular function in critical organ systems. There are many active areas of investigation that reflect the progression of our understanding of shock that have been outlined in this chapter and that have begun to move the field beyond the basics of fluid resuscitation and hemodynamic monitoring.

Efforts to control ischemia-reperfusion injury include controlled reperfusion with carbon monoxide or other compounds to reduce oxidative stress. Induced hypothermia may interrupt generation of harmful byproducts of ischemia and enable restoration of circulation and repair of structural injuries in a cellular environment where hypoxia is no longer critical. New biosensors using near-infrared light may enable transcutaneous identification of critical limitations of blood flow and enable clinicians to more accurately target areas of regional hypoperfusion.[32] A search for agents that optimize circulation in the microvascular by preventing activation of the endothelium may enable resuscitative efforts to restore oxygen to cells as needed to maintain normal respiration and provide critical nutrients. Further understanding of functional genomics may enable clinicians to target transcription and translational events triggered by shock and thus alter outcome.

KEY POINTS

- **Shock is the clinical syndrome that results from inadequate tissue perfusion from numerous causes, including hypovolemic, septic, traumatic, cardiogenic, neurogenic, and hypoadrenal shock.**
- **Hypovolemic shock due to ongoing blood and/or plasma loss leads to progressive cardiovascular deterioration ultimate hypotension, oliguria, confusion, irreversible cell injury, and death.**
- **Septic and traumatic shock are systemic inflammatory responses to infection or tissue injury with cellular breakdown, producing hypotension requiring massive volume resuscitation and high risk of multiple organ failure and death.**
- **Cardiogenic shock is decreased tissue perfusion due to intrinsic or extrinsic (tamponade, tension pneumothorax, etc.) pump failure.**
- **Complications of an episode of shock include ischemia-reperfusion injury from oxidant stress; potential secondary immunosuppression with enhanced nosocomial infection risk; hypothermia and coagulopathy; and multiple organ failure syndrome, including abdominal compartment syndrome.**
- **Treatment of shock involves aggressive volume resuscitation with control of the underlying etiology and careful monitoring of adequacy of end-organ perfusion to avoid over-resuscitation.**

References

1. Bogolioubov A, Keefe DL, Groeger JS. Circulatory shock. *Crit Care Clin.* 2001;17:697–719.
2. Wiggers C. The present status of the shock problem. *Physiol Rev.* 1942;22:74–123.
3. American College of Surgeons Committee on Trauma: *Advanced trauma life support course: instructor manual.* Chicago: American College of Surgeons; 2004:83–89.
4. Levy MM, Fink MP, Marshall JC, et al. 2001 SCCM/ESICM/ACCP/ATS/SIS International Sepsis Definitions Conference. *Crit Care Med.* 2003;31: 1250–1256.
5. **Goris RJ. Pathophysiology of shock in trauma. [Review] [106 refs]. *Eur J Surg.* 2000;166:100–111.**
6. Coursin DB, Wood KE. Corticosteroid supplementation for adrenal insufficiency. *JAMA.* 2002;287:236–240.
7. **Parker MM. Pathophysiology of cardiovascular dysfunction in septic shock. *New Horiz.* 1998;6:130–138.**
8. Peters J, Mack GW, Lister G. The importance of the peripheral circulation in critical illnesses. *Intensive Care Med.* 2001;27:1446–1458.
9. Gabay C, Kushner I. Acute-phase proteins and other systemic responses to inflammation. *N Engl J Med.* 1999;340:448–454.
10. **Khadaroo RG, Marshall JC. ARDS and the multiple organ dysfunction syndrome. Common mechanisms of a common systemic process. *Crit Care Clin.* 2002;18:127–141.**
11. Texereau J, Pene F, Chiche JD, et al. Importance of hemostatic gene polymorphisms for susceptibility to and outcome of severe sepsis. *Crit Care Med.* 2004;32:S313–S319.
12. **Rotstein OD. Modeling the two-hit hypothesis for evaluating strategies to prevent organ injury after shock/resuscitation. *J Trauma* 2003;54[Suppl 6].**
13. **Sharma S, Kumar A. Septic shock, multiple organ failure, and acute respiratory distress syndrome. *Curr Opin Pulmon Med.* 2003;9:199–209.**
14. Bernard GR, Vincent JL, Laterre PF, et al. Efficacy and safety of recombinant human activated protein C for severe sepsis. *N Engl J Med.* 2001;344:699–709
15. Gentilello LM. Practical approaches to hypothermia. In: Maull KI, ed. *Advances in trauma and critical care,* vol. 9. St. Louis: Mosby-Year Book; 1994:39–79.
16. Lyons W. Perioperative ARDS. *Pan Am Med Assoc J.* 1996;73:42–44.
17. Orlinsky M, Shoemaker W, Reis ED, et al. Current controversies in shock and resuscitation. *Surg Clin North Am.* 2001;81:1217–1262.
18. Zarins CK, Rice CL, Peters RM, et al. Lymph and pulmonary response to isobaric reduction in plasma oncotic pressure in baboons. *Circ Res.* 1978;43:925–930.
19. Pope A, French G, Longnecker DE. *Fluid resuscitation: state of the science for treating combat casualties and civilian injuries.* Committee on Fluid Resuscitation for Combat Casualties, Institute Of Medicine. Washington, DC: National Academy Press; 1999.
20. **Cooper DJ, Myles PS, McDermott FT, et al. Prehospital hypertonic saline resuscitation of patients with hypotension and severe traumatic brain injury: a randomized controlled trial. *JAMA.* 2004;291:1350–1357.**
21. Huang PP, Stucky FS, Dimick AR. Hypertonic sodium resuscitation is associated with renal failure and death. *Ann Surg.* 1995;221:543–554.
22. Hauser CJ, Shoemaker WC, Turpin I, et al. Oxygen transport responses to colloids and crystalloids in critically ill surgical patients. *Surg Gynecol Obstet.* 1980;150:811–816.
23. **The SAFE Study Investigators. A comparison of albumin and saline for fluid resuscitation in the intensive care unit. *N Engl J Med.* 2004;350: 2247–2256.**
24. Bickell WH, Wall Jr MJ, Pepe PE, et al. Immediate versus delayed fluid resuscitation for hypotensive patients with penetrating torso injuries. *N Engl J Med.* 1994;331:1105–1109.
25. Hebert PC, Wells G, Blajchman MA, et al. A multicenter, randomized, controlled clinical trial of transfusion requirements in critical care. Transfusion Requirements in Critical Care Investigators, Canadian Critical Care Trials Group. *N Engl J Med.* 1999;340:409–417.

26. Connors Jr AF, Speroff T, Dawson NV, et al. The effectiveness of right heart catheterization in the initial care of critically ill patients. SUPPORT Investigators. *JAMA.* 1996;276:889–897.
27. Iberti TJ, Fischer EP, Leibowitz AB, et al. A multicenter study of physicians' knowledge of the pulmonary artery catheter. Pulmonary Artery Catheter Study Group. *JAMA.* 1990;264:2928–2932.
28. Reynolds HN, Haupt MT, Thill-Baharozian MC, et al. Impact of critical care physician staffing on patients with septic shock in a university hospital medical intensive care unit. *JAMA.* 1988;260:3446–3450.
29. Albanese J, Leone M, Garnier F, et al. Renal effects of norepinephrine in septic and nonseptic patients. *Chest* 2004;126:534–539.
30. Annane D, Bellissant E, Bollaert PE, et al. Corticosteroids for treating severe sepsis and septic shock. *Cochrane Database Syst Rev.* 2004:CD002243.
31. Dhainaut JF, Yan SB, Claessens YE. Protein C/activated protein C pathway: overview of clinical trial results in severe sepsis. *Crit Care Med.* 2004;32:S194–201.
32. Hopf HW. Molecular diagnostics of injury and repair responses in critical illness: what is the future of "monitoring" in the intensive care unit? *Crit Care Med.* 2003;31[Suppl 23].

CHAPTER 9 ■ CRITICAL CARE

AVERY B. NATHENS AND RONALD V. MAIER

ORGANIZATIONAL STRUCTURE OF THE INTENSIVE CARE UNIT

A significant proportion of patients under the care of surgeons receive some form of critical care during their hospital stay. The exposure to the intensive care unit (ICU) may take one of several forms, ranging from routine postoperative monitoring in the high-risk surgical patient to the management of life-threatening postoperative complications. Additionally, many patients experience significant physiologic derangements due to their surgical illness (e.g., trauma, peritonitis) such that they require ICU care.

The ICU environment is conducive to the support of acute life-threatening organ dysfunction through the provision of mechanical ventilation and invasive cardiac monitoring. These services require specific equipment and nursing expertise not found in or available throughout the hospital setting. As a result of these requirements, the ICU is typically spatially separated from the acute care beds in most hospitals. This spatial separation leads to one of two possibilities for the provision of medical care by physicians. The surgeon responsible for the care of the patient's underlying disease may assume primary responsibility for the provision of critical care services. This approach is in keeping with the ethical standards of the American College of Surgeons under which surgeons are responsible for the postoperative care of their patients. In this context, the ICU is simply a location where advanced monitoring and organ support are available. The surgeon continues with clinical responsibilities outside the ICU while also caring for critically ill patients. This organizational approach is typically referred to as an "open" ICU.[1] Alternatively, the surgeon may relinquish care of the patient to an intensivist who may be specifically trained in the care of the critically ill patient and certified by one of several medical specialty boards including internal medicine, anesthesiology, or surgery. In this context, the intensivist has no other responsibilities outside the ICU that would limit his or her immediate accessibility and is primarily available to the critically ill patient. This organizational approach is often referred to as a "closed" ICU or an intensivist-model ICU.[1]

The argument for maintaining the involvement of the surgeon as the primary physician responsible for the direction of critical care services is to ensure that there is continuity of care. Putatively, this continuity of care results in a well-defined, cohesive management plan that is necessary to ensure optimal outcomes. However, in a retrospective analysis of the effect of conversion from an open to a closed surgical ICU in a tertiary-care academic center, complications and mortality were lower and the use of consultants was less frequent when patients were primarily cared for by surgeons or anesthesiologists who were board-certified in critical care.[2] In another report in a similar surgical ICU setting, two different concurrent care models were compared. One group was managed exclusively by the critical care attending service and the other by the general surgery faculty and house staff. Despite increased severity of illness, the critical care cohort had a shorter ICU length of stay, fewer days of mechanical ventilation, fewer consultations, fewer complications, and lower hospital charges.[3] Last, in a large observational study, Pronovost et al.[4] evaluated outcomes following abdominal aortic surgery in the state of Maryland. This cohort of patients was well chosen because these individuals are at high risk of postoperative complications both related to the operative intervention and from significant comorbidity. These investigators demonstrated that daily rounds by a dedicated intensivist were associated with a significant reduction in the risk of postoperative complications and death.

Taken together, these data and a recent systematic review suggest that critically ill patients are best cared for by intensivists.[5] For surgical patients, this argues for the continued training and involvement of surgeons in the field of critical care. In the absence of a surgical intensivist, the most recent recommendations from the American College of Critical Care Medicine are that the intensivist and the surgeon proactively collaborate in the ongoing care of the patients.[6]

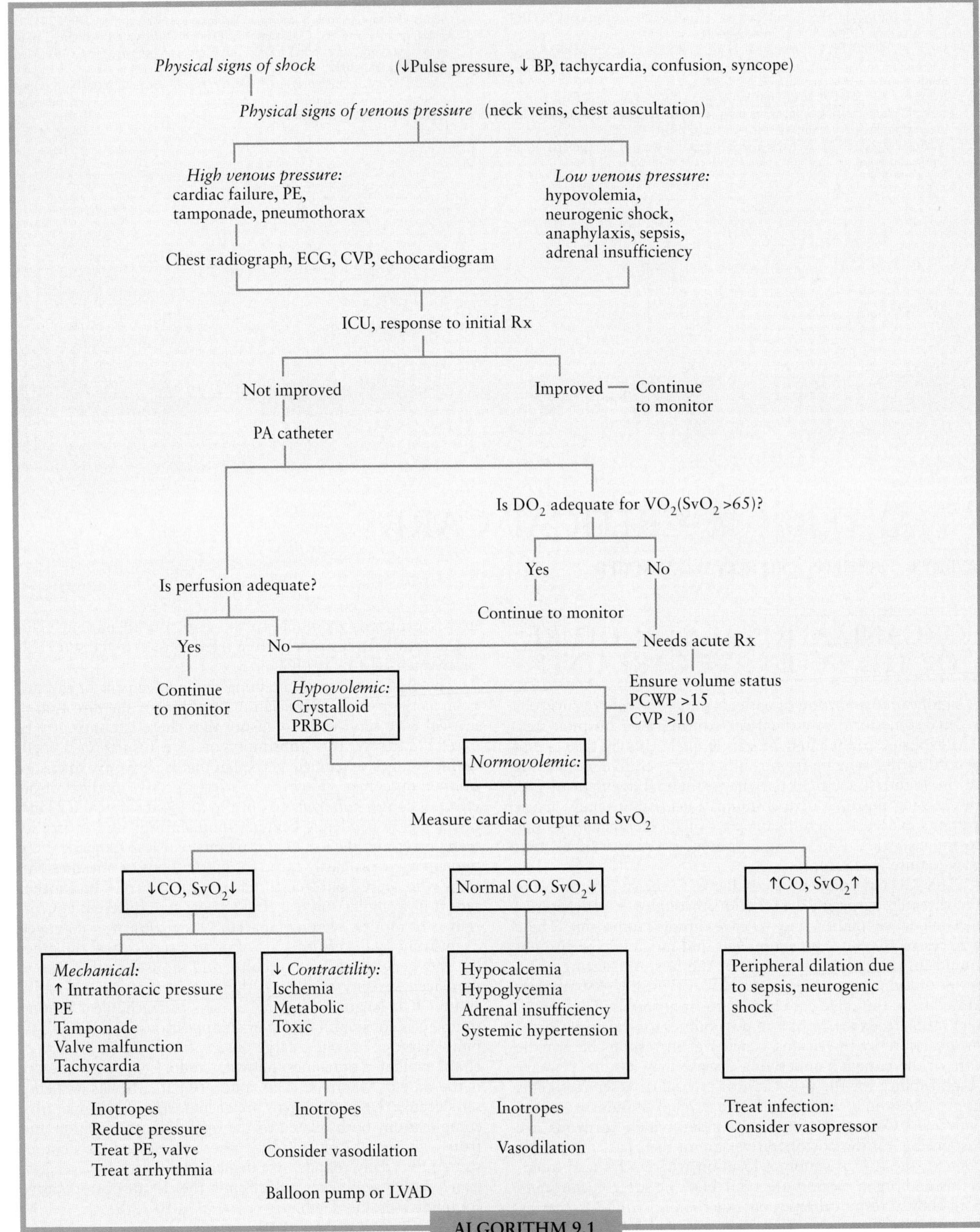

ALGORITHM 9.1 Management of hemodynamic problems. (Modified from Bartlett RH. *University of Michigan critical care handbook*. Boston: Little, Brown; 1996.)

PURPOSES OF THE INTENSIVE CARE UNIT

The ICU serves several purposes. First, the availability of both electronic physiologic monitors and a high nurse-to-patient ratio (typically 1:1 or 1:2) provides an opportunity for very early detection of a critical change in status of the patient. This change might relate to postoperative bleeding, the development of a neurologic deficit after craniotomy or spinal surgery (or injury to the brain or spinal cord), or changes in the patients' cardiorespiratory status. Common to all of these scenarios is a high likelihood of a need for urgent intervention. In this context, the ICU serves the purpose of monitoring to identify and prevent adverse consequences in a patient at great risk.

The more familiar role of the ICU is an environment with all the resources to support an acute deterioration of vital organ function. To ensure optimal outcomes, it is critical that the physician understands the physiology of organ dysfunction, the tools he or she has available for their monitoring and support, and their limitations. Without this understanding, the physicians with the resources availed in the ICU have the potential to inflict great harm. The most frequent challenges in the critical care environment are the support of the failing cardiovascular system, lungs, and kidneys. During this period of support, the patient must receive adequate nutritional support until the acute physiologic derangements have normalized. The focus of this chapter is these aspects of critical care, followed by a discussion of prognostic scoring systems and ethics in the ICU.

ASSESSMENT AND MANAGEMENT OF THE FAILING CARDIOVASCULAR SYSTEM

Support of the failing cardiovascular system is geared toward achieving adequate tissue oxygen delivery (Algorithm 9.1). To achieve this end, it is important to understand the relationship between oxygen delivery and consumption. Oxygen consumed in the process of metabolism is expressed as the volume of oxygen per minute ($\dot{V}O_2$). $\dot{V}O_2$ is normally 100 to 120 mL/m^2/minute, or 200 mL/minute for a typical adult. $\dot{V}O_2$ decreases under conditions of hypothermia, paralysis, and hypothyroidism. $\dot{V}O_2$ increases during exercise or other muscular activity, hyperthermia, profound hypothalamic injury, and hyperthyroidism. Most pertinent to the critically ill surgical patient in the ICU is the profound increase in $\dot{V}O_2$ induced by high circulating levels of catecholamines and inflammatory mediators. Inadequate levels of tissue oxygen delivery in the face of either normal or increased levels of $\dot{V}O_2$ result in anaerobic tissue metabolism and are reflected clinically as a state of shock (i.e., cellular dysfunction). We have little control over tissue oxygen consumption, save for avoiding or treating hyperthermia and pharmacologic paralysis.

Oxygen Delivery

In contrast to $\dot{V}O_2$, many interventions in the ICU focus on manipulating tissue oxygen delivery ($\dot{D}O_2$) to meet either normal or elevated levels of tissue $\dot{V}O_2$. The amount of O_2 that is delivered to peripheral tissues is the product of the O_2 content in arterial blood (CaO_2) and the cardiac output. Normally, CaO_2 is about 20 mL/dL and the normal cardiac index (CI) is 3.2 L/m^2/minute, or 5 L/minute for a typical adult. Therefore, the normal systemic delivery of O_2 ($\dot{D}O_2$) is 20 mL/dL $\times$ 50 dL/minute, or 1,000 mL/minute. Although the O_2 content is the most important measure of O_2 in blood, the partial pressure of oxygen (PO_2) and the oxyhemoglobin saturation are more commonly measured in the ICU; hence, it is necessary to convert these measurements. Each gram of hemoglobin (Hgb) can bind 1.36 mL of O_2. If the Hgb level of the blood is normal (15 g/dL) and the Hgb is 98% saturated, the amount of O_2 bound to Hgb is 19.9 mL/dL. In addition, a small amount of O_2 is physically dissolved in the water that makes up plasma and red blood cells. The solubility coefficient for O_2 is 0.0031 mL/mm Hg per deciliter; therefore, the amount of O_2 dissolved in 1 dL of blood at a PaO_2 of 100 mm Hg is 0.3 mL, so that the O_2 content of normal arterial blood 19.9 + 0.3 or 20.2 mL/dL, conveniently rounded off to 20 mL/dL. Through the same arithmetic, the O_2 content of venous blood (CvO_2), which is 80% saturated, is 16 mL/dL; hence, the normal arteriovenous difference in O_2 content (avO_2 difference) is 4 mL/dL. Expressed mathematically:

$$\dot{D}O_2 = CI \times CaO_2$$

where: $CaO_2 = 1.36 \times Hgb + 0.0031 \times PaO_2$ and CI = stroke volume $\times$ heart rate and, therefore, $\dot{V}O_2 = CI \times (CaO_2 - CvO_2)$

The relation among PO_2, saturation, and O_2 content for different concentrations of Hgb is shown in Figure 9.1. Note that the arterial partial pressure of oxygen (PaO_2) and saturations are the same as for normal arterial and venous blood due to an increase in CI, even though the O_2 content is severely decreased in anemia.

Relationship Between Oxygen Supply and Demand

When a change in $\dot{V}O_2$ occurs, a proportional change in $\dot{D}O_2$ occurs almost immediately, mediated completely by a change in

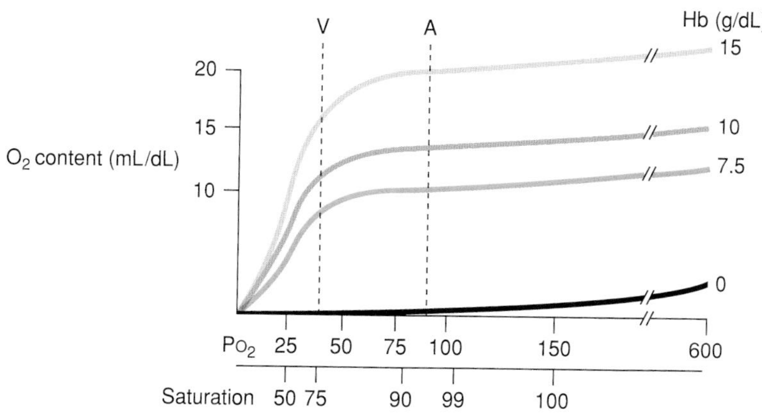

FIGURE 9.1 The relation of O_2 content, saturation, and PO_2. Typical normal levels in arterial and venous blood are defined at various levels of hemoglobin. (After Bartlett RH. *University of Michigan critical care handbook*. Boston: Little, Brown; 1996, with permission.)

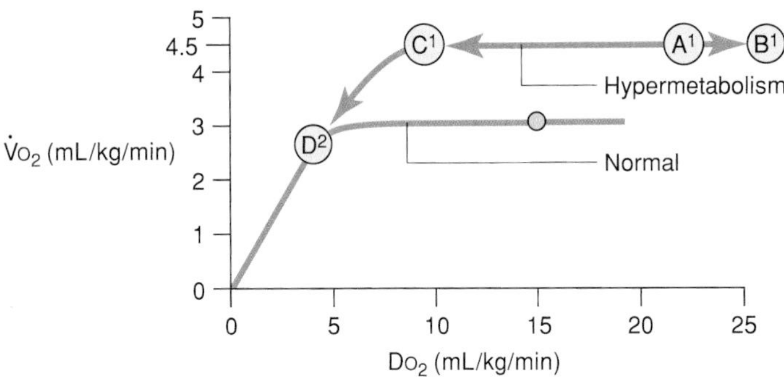

FIGURE 9.2 The relation of O_2 consumption to a wide range of changes in O_2 delivery. Examples are shown for normal metabolism (*circle*) and hypermetabolic status (A^1). (After Bartlett RH, Anderson HL. Multiorgan failure. In: Zelenock GB, D'Alecy LG, Fantone JC, et al., eds. *Clinical ischemic syndromes: mechanisms and consequences of tissue injury*. St. Louis: Mosby; 1989:565, with permission.)

cardiac output. For example, if a person goes from rest to mild exercise, an increase in $\dot{V}O_2$ occurs, followed promptly by an increase of cardiac output (A to A^1 in Fig. 9.2). The mechanism that mediates this change in cardiac output is not fully understood but is probably related to a chemoreceptor on the venous side of the circulation. This autoregulation occurs whether the change in $\dot{V}O_2$ is an increase or a decrease and whether it is caused by exercise, sepsis, catecholamines, or other mediators.

Shock states are characterized by limitations in $\dot{D}O_2$ leading to a mismatch of supply and demand. For example, hemorrhagic shock leads to a reduction in preload (thus affecting stroke volume and CI) and a reduction in DO_2, which is further decreased by the drop in CaO_2 due to loss of Hgb. The end result of this limitation in DO_2 is tissue hypoxia which is thought to play a causal role in the development of multiple organ failure. When DO_2 falls below the level of $\dot{V}O_2$, $\dot{V}O_2$ becomes supply-dependent and a state of anaerobic metabolism occurs (Fig. 9.3).

The relation between DO_2 and $\dot{V}O_2$ is reflected in the amount of O_2 in venous blood. Under normal conditions, DO_2 is 1,000 mL/min and $\dot{V}O_2$ is 200 mL/min. The amount of O_2 extracted is 20% of that delivered, with 80% of the O_2 still present in venous blood returning to the heart. This latter parameter, referred to as mixed venous blood saturation (SvO_2), must be obtained from either blood in the right ventricle or pulmonary artery to allow mixing of superior vena caval, inferior vena caval and coronary sinus blood as the relative rates of extraction in organs served by these circulations differ. In the critical care setting, SvO_2 is typically obtained from a pulmonary artery catheter (PAC) and can be monitored continuously using oximetric probes at the tip of the catheter. As mentioned above, the normal SvO_2 is in the range of 70% to 80%. Reductions in SvO_2 are indicative of a mismatch between supply and demand. If VO_2 increases with no further increase in delivery, then the percent of oxygen extraction must increase resulting in a drop in SvO_2. More frequently, SvO_2 is affected by changes in DO_2. Relatively small reductions in CI, SaO_2, or Hgb concentrations can result in significant increases in oxygen extraction, manifested as a drop in SvO_2. In the context of a very dynamic clinical situation with multiple perturbations occurring concurrently, continuous measurement of SvO_2 provides a good estimate of the net effect of any intervention on the balance between oxygen supply and demand.

In critically ill patients, $\dot{V}O_2$ may be elevated or depressed, but a slight to moderate elevation in $\dot{V}O_2$ is the most common abnormality in critically ill patients. $\dot{V}O_2$ is elevated in proportion to the degree of inflammation (either bacterial or sterile, as in burns and pancreatitis). A febrile patient with significant signs of sepsis typically has a $\dot{V}O_2$ that is 1.5 to 2 times normal. It is unusual for the $\dot{V}O_2$ of a critically ill patient to be more than twice normal. This occurs only in situations of severe muscular activity, as in seizures or tetanus. $\dot{V}O_2$ is decreased in critically ill patients who are hypothermic.

During hypermetabolism, a change in $\dot{V}O_2$ is followed promptly by a proportional change in DO_2; thus, it is normal for a hypermetabolic patient to have a high cardiac output and pulse rate, that is, to be hyperdynamic. Rarely, the hyperdynamic response exceeds the increase in $\dot{V}O_2$; this situation, reflected in a ratio of DO_2 to VO_2 higher than 5:1 and a venous saturation above 80%, can occur when a large arteriovenous fistula is present, caused either by direct vascular communication or by hyperperfusion of tissues, as in portal hypertension with excessive perfusion of the splanchnic viscera. More commonly, patients cannot mount an increased DO_2 in response to an increased $\dot{V}O_2$ because of any combination of hypoxia, anemia, and myocardial dysfunction. If this occurs, the amount of O_2 extracted from each deciliter of blood increases. This increase in oxygen extraction is reflected by a lower SvO_2.

Invasive Hemodynamic Monitoring

Given the importance of adequate oxygen delivery, it is evident that a tremendous amount of effort among intensivists is

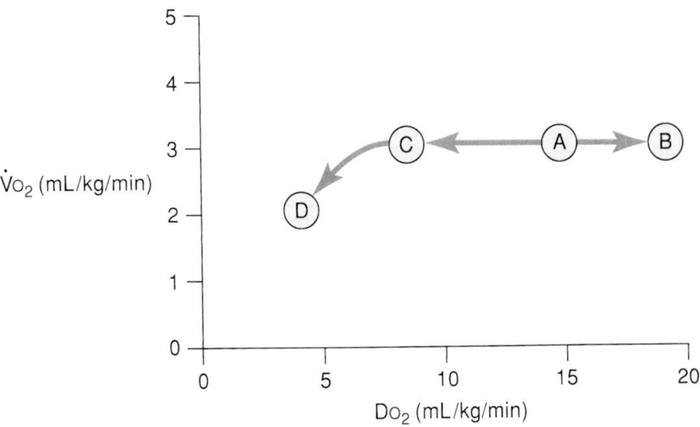

FIGURE 9.3 Normally (A), systemic O_2 delivery is about 15 mL/kg per minute and O_2 consumption is 3 mL/kg per minute. Consumption becomes supply-dependent when delivery is very low (C to D). Delivery increases in response to increased metabolism (A to B). (After Bartlett RH, Anderson HL. Multiorgan failure. In: Zelenock GB, D'Alecy LG, Fantone JC, et al., eds. *Clinical ischemic syndromes: mechanisms and consequences of tissue injury*. St. Louis: Mosby; 1989:565, with permission.)

geared toward optimizing delivery. There are three important parameters that can be modified to affect systemic oxygen delivery: CI, Hgb, and hemoglobin saturation (SaO_2). The principal tool to measure and manipulate DO_2 and that which has generated the greatest controversy is the PAC. The balloon-tip flow-directed pulmonary artery (or Swan-Ganz) catheter is inserted into the central venous system where it is enters the right heart and rests in the pulmonary artery where it provides continuous monitoring of pulmonary artery pressures. The catheter has more proximal ports such that central venous pressure is also monitored. Using the thermal dilution method, the catheter provides information regarding CI. More recent modifications of the PAC have resulted in the capability of continuous measurement of cardiac output, mixed venous oxygen saturation (SvO_2), and right ventricular end-diastolic volume. When the balloon is inflated, the catheter advances slightly and wedges into a small pulmonary artery branch. This pulmonary capillary wedge pressure (PCWP) provides an estimate of left ventricular end-diastolic pressure (LVEDP). The assumption is that a static, nonflowing column of blood that extends from the catheter's lumen to the pulmonary arterioles, capillaries, and veins of that lung segment provides a measure of the pressure downstream from the catheter tip ending in the left ventricle. Barring circumstances described later, LVEDP tracks left ventricular end-diastolic volume (LVEDV). LVEDV represents the volume of the left ventricle (i.e., myocardial stretch, or preload) that we aim to effect through increases in intravascular volume.

The parameters made available through placement of a PAC, when used in concert with simultaneously measured SaO_2 (and SvO_2) and Hgb concentration, provide information regarding DO_2. DO_2 can be manipulated through alterations in Hgb or SaO_2; however, the perceived greatest value of the PAC is information obtained regarding intravascular volume status (PCWP) and CI, which guide fluid resuscitation and the use of inotropic support. However, when the PCWP is used to guide administration of fluids, it is important to understand that several of the assumptions whereby PCWP tracks LVEDV might be violated. The ability to derive information regarding a volume (LVEDV) from a pressure (PCWP) first assumes that the myocardial compliance is normal. However, myocardial compliance is often affected by ischemia, massive volume resuscitation, high intra-abdominal or intrathoracic [e.g., high levels of positive end-expiratory pressure (PEEP)] pressures, or longstanding hypertension. Focusing on the PCWP to guide therapy in these circumstances will lead to an overestimate of preload. Mitral stenosis will also increase the PCWP while LVEDV might be low. Not realizing the importance of these assumptions and how they might be violated often leads to incorrect treatment strategies.

Many have advocated the use of the right ventricular end-diastolic volume index (RVEDVI), a measure of right ventricular filling, as a better measure to assess for adequate preload and to estimate preload-recruitable CI.[7] Specifically, if the RVEDVI is low, fluid administration will increase the cardiac output. Not infrequently, the RVEDVI and PCWP are discordant—typically the RVEDVI is low while the PCWP is high. This scenario might occur in the presence of a very noncompliant myocardium. Alternatively, if the PAC is wedged in a segment of the lung where the alveolar pressure exceeds the pulmonary capillary pressure then a similar combination of findings will occur. In this scenario, the assumption of a static intact column of blood from the catheter tip to the pulmonary veins is violated. In these circumstances, fluid administration will increase the cardiac output; however, the cost of doing so might be an excessive increase in hydrostatic forces and development of pulmonary edema.

The PAC is merely a monitoring device; thus, any benefit derived from its use will depend on the therapeutic strategies implemented following collection of various hemodynamic

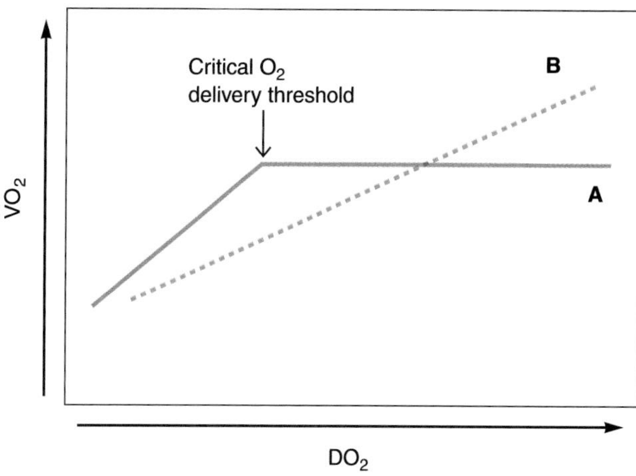

FIGURE 9.4 Normal supply dependency of oxygen consumption (VO_2) on oxygen delivery (DO_2) implies the presence of a critical oxygen delivery threshold at which the tissues receive all the oxygen that can be consumed (*A*). Beyond this point there is no further consumption with increasing delivery. In this context, there is no point in pushing oxygen delivery beyond the inflection point. Pathologic supply dependency suggests that consumption continues to increase with increasing delivery (*B*). The lack of a discrete inflection point and plateau suggests that resuscitation should be geared toward specific empirically derived elevated endpoints.

parameters. In this regard, two approaches have been used. In the first, referred to as a goal-directed strategy, CI is increased to achieve a specific level of DO_2. In several retrospective studies, patients, in whom the CI exceeds 4.5 L/minute/m^2 or DO_2 exceeds 600 mL/minute, had improved outcomes compared to those not reaching these endpoints. Attempting to achieve these "supranormal" goals was derived from the concept that there exists a pathologic supply dependency of VO_2 on DO_2 (Fig. 9.4), a hypothesis that has since been refuted.[8,9] Despite the benefit identified in retrospective studies, three prospective, randomized trials in which subjects were randomized to a supranormal goal-oriented approach (i.e., interventions were directed to achieving these endpoints) demonstrate either no benefit or worse outcomes compared to those in whom specific goals were not targeted.[10–12] As a result, there is general consensus that this approach, at least in patients with sepsis, is not beneficial and might in fact be harmful.[13] An alternative approach is to consider that the relationship between DO_2 and VO_2 is unique for each patient. Using this strategy, the purpose of hemodynamic optimization would be to increase DO_2 until VO_2 consumption no longer increases, or SvO_2 exceeds 75% to 80%, suggesting that delivery has met the metabolic demands of the tissues.

Despite the conceptual appeal of invasive hemodynamic monitoring and the information it provides, there are no data suggesting that the use of a PAC offers benefit. In fact, the opposite is true. In a large retrospective analysis, resource utilization and rates of death were higher in patients with sepsis undergoing right heart catheterization.[14] In one trial of 201 patients with shock or acute respiratory failure, patients with a PAC had more fluid administration, a higher incidence of renal failure, and a greater incidence of thrombocytopenia.[15] In another such study involving almost 700 patients with shock and/or the acute respiratory distress syndrome (ARDS), patients receiving a PAC had equivalent outcomes to those without.[16] In a randomized trial of PAC use in high-risk surgical patients, those randomized to the PAC arm had a higher rate of pulmonary embolism and no evidence of benefit. Other retrospective studies have confirmed a lack of benefit and potential higher risk of congestive heart failure and renal failure, two complications that one would think a PAC would help prevent. Given these data, it is important to realize that the PAC offers no clear benefit in the resuscitation of patients. If there are specific subgroups that benefit, they have not yet been identified in either retrospective or prospective studies.

Recent attention has focused on the use of a central venous catheter with an oximetric probe that rests in the superior vena cava. In addition to providing information regarding central venous pressure (and thus intravascular volume status), this catheter provides information regarding superior vena caval oxygen saturation ($SvcO_2$, normally ~5% to 10% greater than SvO_2). In a randomized controlled trial, early use of this catheter, along with a directed protocol to normalize the central venous pressure and $SvcO_2$ has been shown to reduce mortality in patients with severe sepsis.[17] These data speak to the importance of early intervention to achieve relatively normal (rather than supranormal) physiologic endpoints. The value of normalizing $SvcO_2$ in other clinical settings (e.g., hemorrhagic shock, trauma) is untested.

New Modalities for Cardiac Output Measurement

The difficulties in using the PAC along with the questions regarding their safety has been the impetus for the development of several less invasive means of monitoring cardiac output. Esophageal probes, placed in a similar fashion to a nasogastric tube, measure blood flow velocity in the descending aorta by means of a Doppler transducer. The measured parameter is the aortic velocity waveform, which is converted to stroke volume using a standardized algorithm. An accurate velocity measurement requires good alignment between the Doppler beam and blood flow. In general, the agreement between cardiac output obtained by means of the thermodilution technique and that obtained through measurement of the aortic velocity waveform appears to be acceptable.[18]

Pulse contour analysis has also been investigated as a means to continuously monitor cardiac output. Pulse contour methods use the pressure waveform as an input for a model of the systemic circulation to predict instantaneous flow. The pressure waveform is obtained from peripheral artery (radial or femoral), which requires assumptions regarding the changes in pulse shape between these different locations. The values attributed to model parameters (e.g., arterial resistance and compliance) are initially estimated according to the patient's sex and age and from the pressure waveform. They are then refined following a calibration of mean cardiac output using an indicator technique (e.g., transpulmonary thermodilution or lithium chloride dilution). Several reports indicate that there is fair agreement between cardiac output measured by thermodilution and pulse contour analysis.[19]

Which of the previously mentioned techniques, if any, will be widely adopted is unknown. They both appear to be safer than the PAC, but whether they will change management and, more importantly, improve outcome remains to be seen.

SUPPORT OF THE FAILING RESPIRATORY SYSTEM

Impending or established respiratory failure is a common reason for admission of surgical patients to the ICU. However, it is important to recognize that not all patients requiring an airway (endotracheal or nasotracheal intubation) and mechanical ventilatory support have respiratory failure. There are a large proportion of patients who have airway instability requiring endotracheal intubation (postoperative patients, traumatic brain injury, intoxication) but whose need for mechanical ventilatory support is relatively limited. By contrast, patients with respiratory failure due to ARDS, trauma, cardiogenic pulmonary edema, exacerbation of chronic obstructive pulmonary edema, or other less common etiologies require a mechanical ventilator to support gas exchange.

Pulmonary Gas Exchange

By gas exchange, we mean the process by which oxygen is taken up by the pulmonary capillaries from the alveolus and CO_2 ultimately excreted in each expired breath. These two processes—oxygen uptake and CO_2 excretion are regulated by different mechanisms and have to be managed with these differences in mind.

Oxygen Uptake

Gas transfer in the lung and the causes of hypoxemia are demonstrated in Figure 9.5. Under normal conditions, red blood cells in the pulmonary capillaries become fully

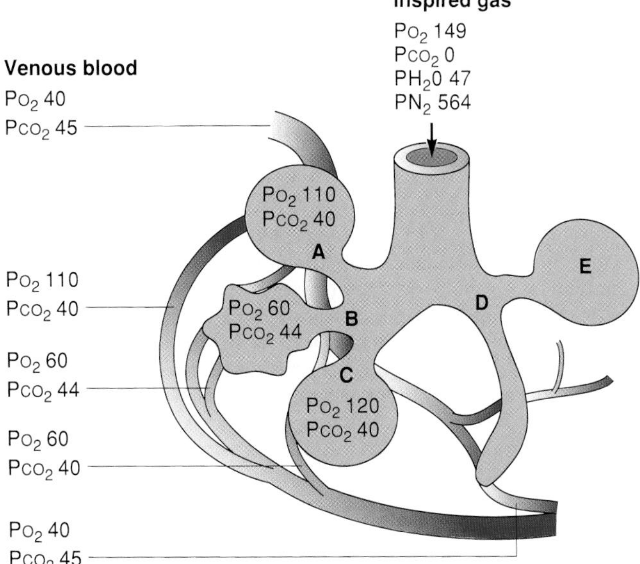

FIGURE 9.5 Variables affecting pulmonary gas exchange while air is breathed. In alveolus *A*, blood flow and ventilation are equal and normal. The values in the alveolus and the exiting blood represent the end of a normal resting exhalation. Alveolus *B* represents hypoventilation. Alveolus *C* represents diffusion block. Alveolus *D* represents collapse or transpulmonary shunt. Alveolus *E* is ventilated without blood flow. (After Bartlett RH. Posttraumatic pulmonary insufficiency. In: Cooper P, Nyhus L, eds. *Surgery annual, 1971*. New York: Appleton-Century-Crofts; 1971, with permission.)

saturated and O_2 dissolves in the plasma; the result is a blood PO_2 of 100 mm Hg (when equilibrium is reached at the end of a resting expiration) and a saturation of 100% (alveolus *A* in Fig. 9.5). This equilibration may be disturbed by hypoventilation in relation to perfusion, or $\dot{V}/\dot{Q}$ mismatch (alveolus *B* in Fig. 9.5); diffusion block caused by interstitial fibrosis or edema (alveolus C in Fig. 9.5); or perfusion of nonventilated alveoli (shunt), which is simply the extreme of hypoventilation (alveolus *D* in Fig. 9.5). Diffusion block and $\dot{V}/\dot{Q}$ mismatch can usually be overcome by breathing 100% O_2; thus, persistent hypoxemia during exposure to high alveolar PO_2 is caused by total $\dot{V}/\dot{Q}$ mismatch, called *transpulmonary shunting* or *venous admixture*. Under normal conditions, about 5% of the blood entering the left atrium has been shunted away from the pulmonary capillaries and oxygenation, either as a result of bronchial nutritive blood flow or through thebesian veins opening directly into the left side of the heart. This phenomenon, combined with the normal minor $\dot{V}/\dot{Q}$ mismatch associated with shallow breathing at rest and positional effects on pulmonary blood flow, results in a normal arterial PO_2 of 90 to 100 mm Hg and a normal arterial blood oxygen saturation (SaO_2) of 98%. The extent to which various degrees of transpulmonary shunting affect arterial oxygenation is shown in Figure 9.6. The shunt fraction is actually calculated by assuming that the blood in capillaries in those alveolar units that are functioning normally is fully saturated and oxygenated. In addition, it is assumed that the blood passing through areas of transpulmonary shunt is identical to venous blood. With these assumptions, the fraction of blood passing through the shunt can be calculated as the O_2 content of blood leaving the capillaries of normal alveoli minus the O_2 content of arterial blood divided by the O_2 content of blood leaving normal alveoli minus the O_2 content of venous blood.

Obviously, the effect of the O_2 content of venous blood in the shunt calculation is considerable; when O_2 delivery is decreased because of low cardiac output or a low Hgb concentration, the venous saturation falls and the shunt fraction is increased. It is not generally appreciated that the reductions in mixed venous oxygen saturation as a result of inadequate cardiac output or severe anemia might lead to profound hypoxemia refractory to increases in fraction of inspired oxygen (FIO_2). This effect occurs only in the presence of some

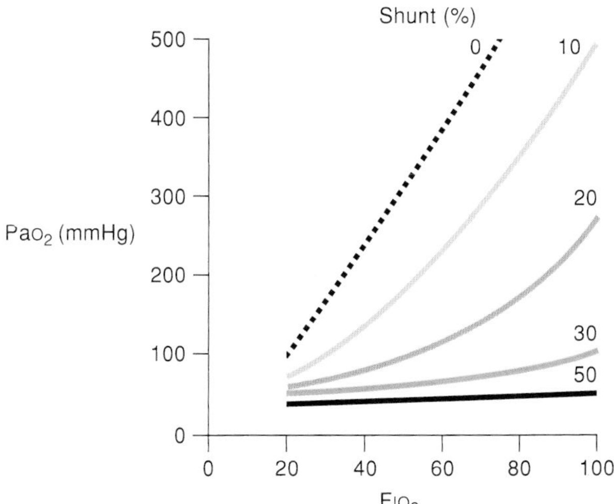

FIGURE 9.6 The PaO_2 values achieved at variable levels of FIO_2 and variable levels of shunt. These calculations assume normal hemoglobin and a venous saturation of 75%. (After Bartlett RH. *University of Michigan critical care handbook*. Boston; Little, Brown; 1996, with permission.)

degree of intrapulmonary shunting and is not evident in patients with normal lungs. For example, if one assumes there is some degree of shunt due to atelectasis, blood perfusing the atelectatic lung mixes with blood perfusing the more normal lung, so that overall pulmonary venous oxygen content is significantly lowered. Increasing the inspired O_2 to 100% may result in a large increase in PO_2 in the blood leaving the normal lung but little increase in arterial oxygen saturation because the pulmonary venous blood from normal alveoli was already maximally saturated. The large increase in PO_2 is associated with a small increase in O_2 *content* because the O_2 that raises the PO_2 (e.g., from 100 to 500 mm Hg) does increase the small amount dissolved in plasma. However, the oxygenation of the arterial blood is an average of the O_2 content of blood from the two areas of lung, not an average of the PO_2. Therefore, systemic hypoxia persists regardless of the FIO_2. This physiology should be kept in mind—at times improvements in arterial oxygen saturation may only be gained through increasing O_2 by improving CI or Hgb concentration, both of which would serve to increase the mixed venous oxygen saturation.

The shunt fraction can be calculated for any FIO_2, but such a calculation will also include components of diffusion block and $\dot{V}/\dot{Q}$ mismatch when the FIO_2 is less than 1. The level of lung dysfunction can be similarly estimated by calculating the alveolar–arterial (Aa) gradient for O_2 or the PaO_2 divided by the FIO_2. The Aa gradient is calculated as follows:

$$AaO_2 \text{ gradient} = (P_B - P_{H_2O}) \times FIO_2 - PaCO_2/R - PaO_2$$

where: P_B = barometric pressure (~ >60 mm Hg at sea level), P_{H_2O} = 47 mm Hg at 37°C, and R = respiratory quotient (usually 0.8) and the alveolar PCO_2 is identical to the arterial PCO_2.

With these assumptions, the normal Aa gradient is about 10 mm Hg, and an Aa gradient above 500 mm Hg corresponds to about 30% transpulmonary shunt. Dividing the PaO_2 by the FIO_2 is simply a shortened method to characterize the Aa gradient without all the calculations. The normal value is 500, and a value of 100 corresponds to a 30% shunt.

Finally, interruption of the blood flow to alveoli has no effect on oxygenation, except for the diversion of blood flow to all the other areas of lung (alveolus *E* in Fig. 9.5). If the remainder of the lung is basically normal, then occlusion of the pulmonary arteries should have no effect on oxygenation. Patients with pulmonary embolism can become hypoxic, however, because (a) blood flow must increase through areas of $\dot{V}/\dot{Q}$ mismatch and shunting, (b) right atrial pressure increases to the point at which right-to-left shunting occurs through a patent foramen ovale, or (c) the residence time of red blood cells in pulmonary capillaries becomes so short that the time for oxygenation is inadequate. Of these causes, the latter can be largely corrected with supplemental O_2, which raises the gradient for O_2 diffusion in the pulmonary capillaries.

Excretion of CO_2

The rate of alveolar ventilation is the principal parameter affecting the excretion of carbon dioxide (CO_2). This differs from oxygen uptake because CO_2 is much more diffusible than O_2 and because a large amount of CO_2 is excreted during a short period of hyperventilation.

The total amount of CO_2 produced by systemic metabolism is roughly equivalent to the amount of O_2 consumed (100 to 120 mL/m^2/minute, or 200 mL/minute in a typical adult). The ratio between CO_2 produced and O_2 consumed is referred to as the *respiratory quotient* (RQ) and varies slightly depending on whether carbohydrate or fat is being metabolized, with a normal value being 0.8. An RQ of 1 or greater

TABLE 9.1

CALORIC VALUE OF METABOLIC SUBSTRATES

	kcal/g	kcal/L O_2	RQ
Carbohydrate	4.0	5.0	1.0
Fat	9.5	4.7	0.7
Protein	4.8	4.5	0.8

RQ, respiratory quotient.

suggests that the principal nutrient being metabolized is carbohydrate, whereas an RQ of 0.7 indicates that primarily lipids are being utilized (Table 9.1).

The production of CO_2 is increased or decreased by each of the factors that cause an increase or decrease in $\dot{V}O_2$. Most of the CO_2 in blood is present as bicarbonate ion, the amount of which cannot change quickly (somewhat analogous to the total blood Hgb or red cell mass in relation to O_2). The metabolically produced CO_2, however, is mostly present as dissolved CO_2, added to the blood in the peripheral tissues and excreted in the lung. In a steady state, the amount of CO_2 excreted through the lung is exactly equal to the amount of CO_2 produced in peripheral tissues. Because the amount excreted is so easily influenced by minor changes in ventilation, however, the assurance of a steady state is particularly important when $\dot{V}CO_2$ is measured at the airway. The amount of CO_2 excreted is a function of ventilation of perfused alveoli (i.e., alveolar ventilation per minute, or minute ventilation). The relation between alveolar ventilation and CO_2 excretion is shown in Figure 9.7.

As excretion of CO_2 is directly related to alveolar ventilation, even if 70% to 80% of the alveoli are not inflated, hyperventilation of the remaining 25% can maintain normocarbia in arterial blood, whereas profound hypoxemia results from 70% to 80% shunt regardless of the level of FIO_2 or ventilation of the remaining alveoli. These relations are shown in Figure 9.8, which again illustrates that oxygenation is a function of matching blood flow to alveolar inflation, whereas CO_2 excretion is a function of ventilation or hyperventilation of alveoli with some blood flow. Normally, the end-tidal CO_2 represents mixed alveolar gas that is in equilibrium with pulmonary capillary blood and hence with arterial blood. Therefore, the end-tidal CO_2 and the partial pressure of arterial carbon dioxide ($PaCO_2$) should be almost identical. The respiratory center is very sensitive to the $PaCO_2$, so that

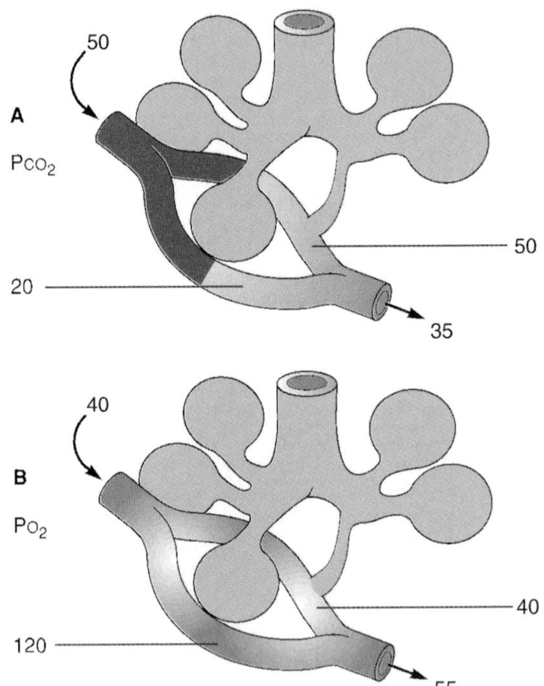

FIGURE 9.8 The effects of collapsed alveoli (transpulmonary shunt) on the exchange of O_2 and CO_2 in the lung. (*A*) Exchange of CO_2 is limited by ventilation of perfused lung. (*B*) Exchange of O_2 is limited by blood uptake of O_2 in ventilated lung. (After Bartlett RH. Pulmonary pathophysiology in surgical patients. *Surg Clin North Am.* 1980;60:1323, with permission.)

the automatic rate and depth of breathing are regulated to maintain the $PaCO_2$ at 40 mm Hg. The end-tidal CO_2 should be the same or just slightly less. There is no way that the $PaCO_2$ can be lower than the end-tidal CO_2. If some of the end-tidal gas has not been in equilibrium with pulmonary capillary blood, the gas does not contain CO_2 and the CO_2 is diluted in end-tidal measurements, so that the end-tidal CO_2 is lower than the $PaCO_2$. This situation occurs whenever a significant amount of lung is ventilated but not perfused (i.e., dead space) or is overventilated and minimally perfused or when some of the end-tidal gas represents inflation gas that is simply compressed and released, never having reached the alveoli. The latter situation inevitably occurs under any positive-pressure ventilation circumstance but creates a significant end-tidal $PaCO_2$ gradient only when peak airway pressures

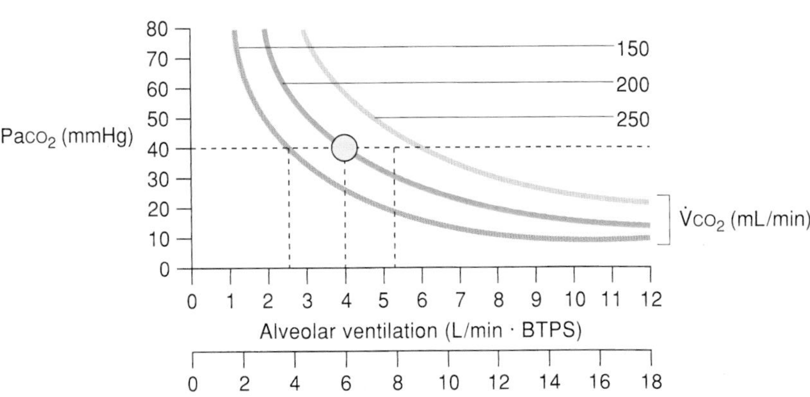

FIGURE 9.7 Alveolar ventilation required to excrete different levels of metabolically produced CO_2. (Adapted from Nunn JF. *Applied respiratory physiology.* London: Butterworth-Heineman; 1969;2:9, with permission.)

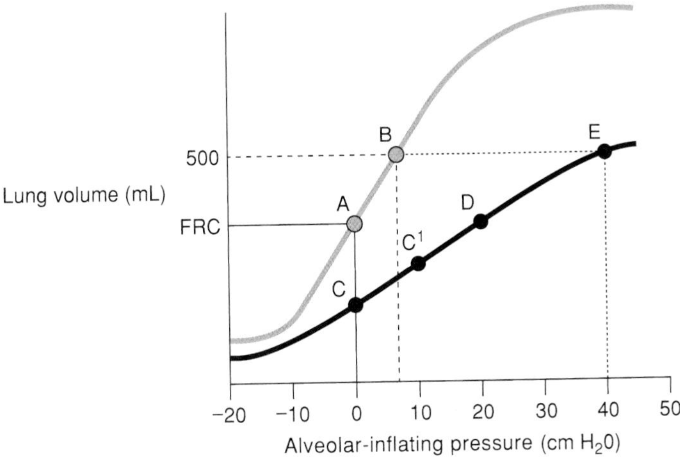

FIGURE 9.9 Volume–pressure (compliance) curves representing a normal lung (*A* and *B*) and an atelectatic or edematous lung (*C* through *E*). The functional reserve capacity is decreased (*A* to *C*), and more pressure is required for inflation (*C* to *D* to *E*). (After Bartlett RH. Use of mechanical ventilation. In: Holcroft J, ed. *Care of the surgical patient,* vol 1. *Critical care.* New York: Scientific American Medicine; 1989;2:9, with permission.)

are very high and when the compression volume is a significant component of each exhaled breath. However, the end-tidal CO_2 measurement becomes a useful continuous monitor of $PaCO_2$ when the lung is nearly normal, as in ventilator weaning. In addition, the gradient between end-tidal and arterial CO_2, when it is large, serves as an indirect measure of nonperfused alveoli (dead space) or compression volume, or both.

Pulmonary Mechanics

The interrelations of gas volumes and pressures in ventilation are referred to as *pulmonary mechanics.* How these volumes and pressures relate depend on pulmonary compliance. The standard compliance or volume–pressure curve, shown in Figure 9.9, is drawn by measuring volume and pressure at stages of lung *deflation* after total inflation. Volume–pressure curves for normal lungs in three different patients are shown in Figure 9.10. Notice that the curve for a normal 35-kg child is the same as that for an adult with major atelectasis. (It would be similar after pneumonectomy in an adult.) This emphasizes the point that the functional lung in acute respiratory failure is smaller, but not necessarily "stiffer." Computed tomographic studies of patients with ARDS support this concept. The lung injury in ARDS is heterogeneous such that, in the presence of normal tidal volumes, the relatively few alveoli that remain ventilated might very well be overdistended.[20] These findings have significant implications for ventilatory strategies in these patients.

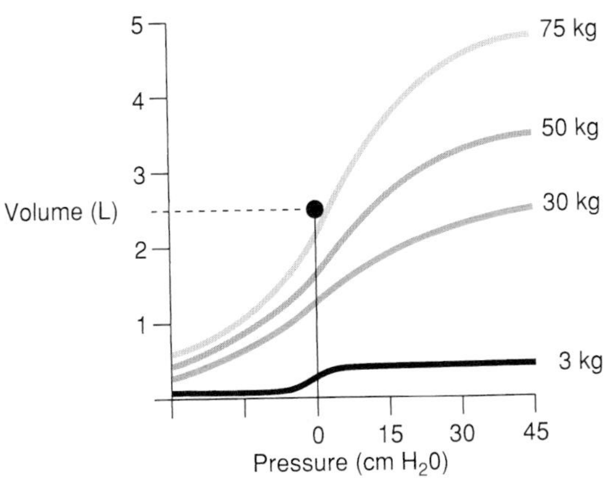

FIGURE 9.10 Lung volume and pressure in patients of different sizes (or lung volumes of different sizes in an adult patient). The decreased compliance in acute respiratory distress syndrome occurs because the lung is smaller not because it is stiffer.

In the example shown in Figure 9.9, inflation of the normal lung with 500 mL of gas requires a pressure of 8 cm H_2O and moves the patient from point *A* to point *B*. When the pressure is released, exhalation occurs passively, and lung volume returns to point *A*. Periodic inflation to 25 or 30 cm H_2O would achieve near-total alveolar inflation without causing over distention. In acute respiratory failure, the cause of decreased compliance is almost always associated with a decrease in the functional residual capacity (FRC) (see Fig. 9.9). The decreased FRC represents lost alveoli, which are either collapsed or filled with fluid but still perfused with blood. Because the lung is smaller, the compliance curve is shifted to the right, and much higher pressures are required to achieve the same level of inflation. To inflate the lung to point *E*, for example, a pressure of 40 cm H_2O would be necessary. One way of managing ventilation in this circumstance is to maintain PEEP at 10 cm H_2O (C^1 in Fig. 9.9) and ventilate to point *D* with tidal breathing. The PEEP is set at this level to maintain the inflation of alveoli that might close at lower end-expiratory pressures. The elevated inspiratory pressures may also be helpful in recruiting closed alveoli. When that happens, the functional lung is bigger, and the entire compliance curve shifts back toward the left.

PEEP has beneficial effects on gas exchange and lung compliance; however, if used without understanding the potential downsides, it might cause harm. For example, high levels of PEEP in relatively compliant lungs might increase intrathoracic pressure sufficiently to inhibit venous flow and reduce preload and cardiac output. High intrathoracic pressures might have dramatic effects on patients with elevated intracranial pressure due to increased impedance to cerebral venous return. Caution must also be exercised in patients with a unilateral lung process (e.g., aspiration, pulmonary contusion, alveolar hemorrhage), as the increased pressures might harm the uninjured normal lung through overdistention.

Several measurements must be taken to determine whether positive airway pressure is recruiting collapsed alveoli or simply distending normal alveoli (Fig. 9.11). As the most normal areas of lung have the best compliance, they are the most vulnerable to overdistention, and this vulnerability contributes to

Positive pressure
Distention
↓ Vol/P
↑ V_D/V_T
↓ CO
Shunt →
↑ Air leak
Recruitment
↑ Vol/P
↓ V_D/V_T
CO →
↓↓ Shunt
Air leak →

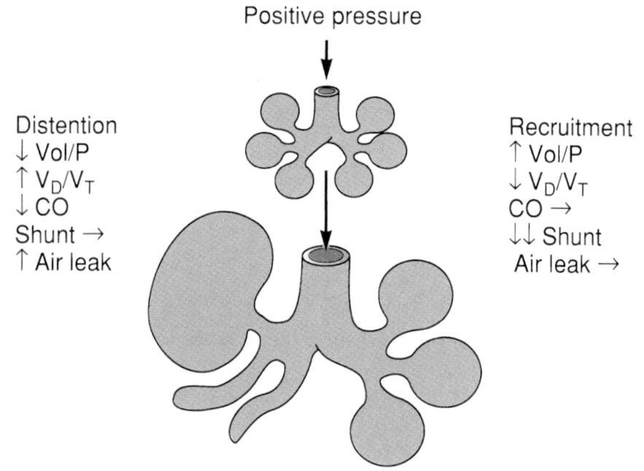

FIGURE 9.11 During mechanical ventilation, the gas volume may inflate alveoli equally (recruitment) or overdistend selected alveoli (distention). (After Bartlett RH. Pulmonary pathophysiology in surgical patients. *Surg Clin North Am* 1980;60:1323, with permission.)

the steady progression of lung dysfunction in patients ventilated at either excessive pressures or tidal volumes. As collapsed alveoli are reinflated, compliance improves, dead space ventilation decreases, and oxygenation increases at the same ventilator settings as shunt decreases. These principles and measurements must be kept in mind during the treatment of the patient on a mechanical ventilator.

Management of Respiratory Failure

When confronted with a patient in acute respiratory failure, the first priority is to identify and treat easily remediable causes. Examples include a pneumothorax requiring a chest tube, acute pulmonary edema requiring diuresis, or an acute asthma exacerbation that may respond to bronchodilator therapy. In the absence of a readily reversible cause, most patients will require mechanical ventilatory support (Algorithm 9.2). Setting up the ventilator can be intimidating because the terminology is complex and continues to evolve with advances

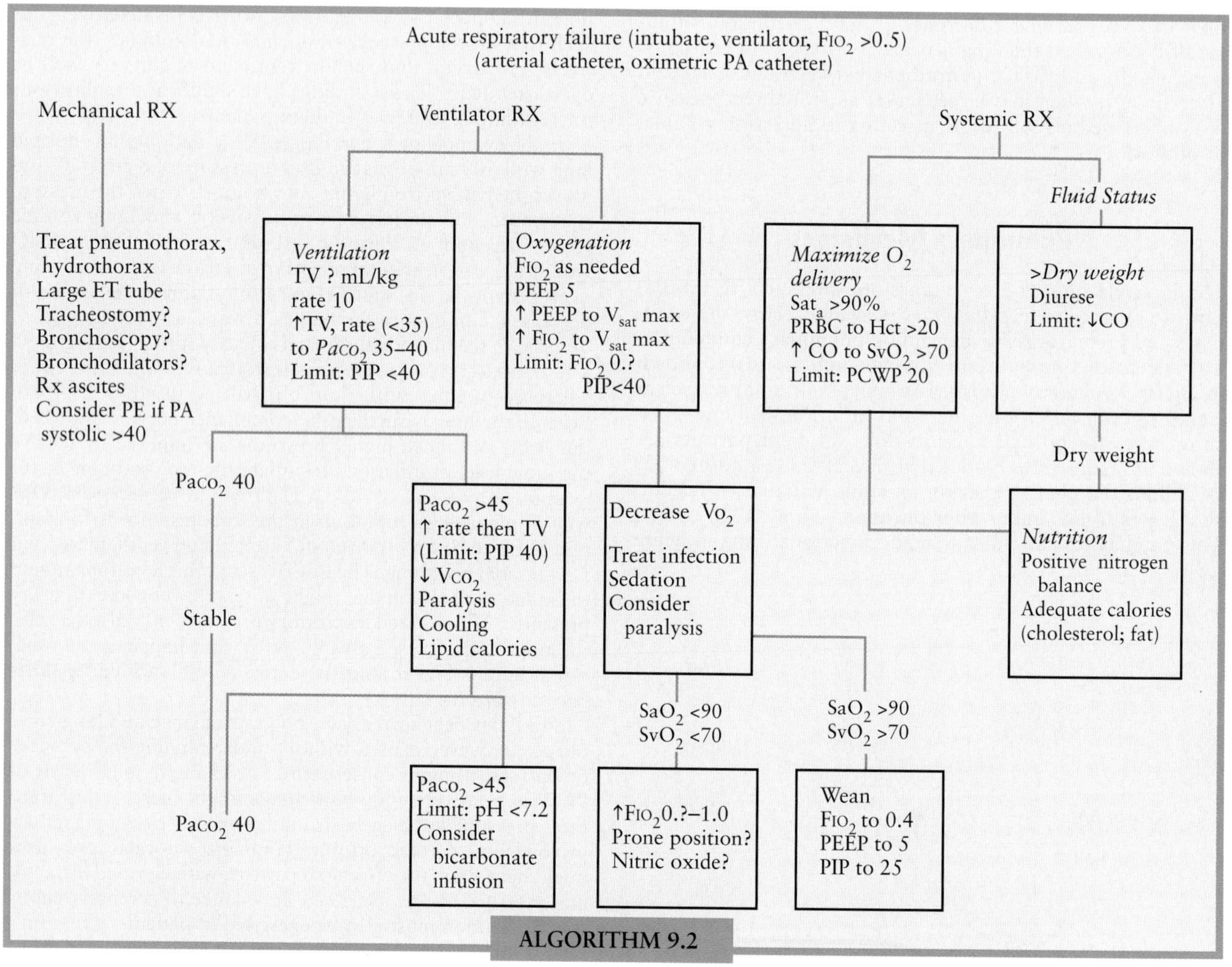

Acute respiratory failure (intubate, ventilator, FIO_2 >0.5)
(arterial catheter, oximetric PA catheter)
Mechanical RX
Ventilator RX
Systemic RX
Treat pneumothorax, hydrothorax
Large ET tube
Tracheostomy?
Bronchoscopy?
Bronchodilators?
Rx ascites
Consider PE if PA systolic >40
Ventilation
TV ? mL/kg
rate 10
↑TV, rate (<35) to $Paco_2$ 35–40
Limit: PIP <40
Oxygenation
FIO_2 as needed
PEEP 5
↑ PEEP to V_{sat} max
↑ FIO_2 to V_{sat} max
Limit: FIO_2 0.?
PIP<40
Maximize O_2 delivery
Sat_a >90%
PRBC to Hct >20
↑ CO to SvO_2 >70
Limit: PCWP 20
Fluid Status
>Dry weight
Diurese
Limit: ↓CO
Dry weight
Nutrition
Positive nitrogen balance
Adequate calories (cholesterol; fat)
$Paco_2$ 40
Stable
$Paco_2$ >45
↑ rate then TV
(Limit: PIP 40)
↓ Vco_2
Paralysis
Cooling
Lipid calories
Decrease Vo_2
Treat infection
Sedation
Consider paralysis
SaO_2 <90
SvO_2 <70
SaO_2 >90
SvO_2 >70
$Paco_2$ 40
$Paco_2$ >45
Limit: pH <7.2
Consider bicarbonate infusion
↑$FIO_2$0.?–1.0
Prone position?
Nitric oxide?
Wean
FIO_2 to 0.4
PEEP to 5
PIP to 25
ALGORITHM 9.2

ALGORITHM 9.2 Management of respiratory failure. ET, endotracheal; PE, pulmonary embolism; PA, pulmonary artery; PEEP, positive end-expiratory pressure; TV, tidal volume; PRBC, packed red blood cells; PCWP, pulmonary capillary wedge pressure. (Modified from Bartlett RH. *University of Michigan critical care handbook*. Boston: Little, Brown; 1996.)

in technology. Only the most commonly used modes are discussed next.

In principle, three parameters determine the mode of ventilation: *trigger, limit,* and *cycle.* Trigger refers to the signal to initiate the inspiratory phase and is set according to whether or not the patient has spontaneous respiratory effort. Mandatory modes such as continuous mandatory ventilation (CMV) use a time trigger, whereas spontaneous modes such as pressure support use a flow or pressure change initiated by the patient. Mandatory modes of ventilation are required if the patient has inadequate or no spontaneous respiratory effort.

The limit variable refers to the flow or pressure that is set during inspiration and cannot be exceeded. By convention, if the limit variable is flow, then the mode is labeled volume control (VC) ventilation (volume = flow × time). Alternatively, if the limit variable is pressure, then the mode is termed pressure control (PC) or pressure support ventilation (PSV). Although both are pressure-limited modes, PSV requires spontaneous inspiratory effort, whereas PC can be used as either a mandatory or spontaneous mode.

Cycle is the variable that terminates the inspiratory cycle, which might be time, flow, pressure, or volume. In general, setting the cycle variable is equivalent to setting the inspiratory time and is manipulated based on pulmonary mechanics and the desired ratio of inspiratory to expiratory time. Intermittent mandatory ventilation (IMV) and assist control (A/C) modes both represent forms of volume control ventilation in which breaths are delivered at a set tidal volume with a set frequency. In A/C mode, if the patient initiates a breath, the tidal volume delivered will be the set volume, whereas in IMV mode, the tidal volume of spontaneous breaths is determined by the patient. However, when the ventilator is triggered (machine or patient), a fixed flow of gas is generated for a specific time providing a preset inspiratory volume (volume = flow × time). Volume-limited ventilation is generally easier to regulate but may be less comfortable for the awake patient as the flow curve is a square wave and markedly different from the normal inspiratory flow pattern in a nonventilated patient. The major advantage of volume-controlled modes of ventilation is the assurance that the patient will receive a guaranteed minimum minute ventilation.

PSV is the most frequently used form of pressure-limited ventilation. In this mode, the patient triggers a breath and a variable flow is delivered to meet a set pressure. Cycling in this mode is determined by the decrease in flow rate and causes the ventilator to stop the inspiratory phase. As the lung inflates, compliance decreases and flow decreases to maintain a constant inspiratory pressure. When flow reaches a percentage of the maximal flow rate (typically around 80% of maximum, depending on the ventilator model) inspiratory flow ceases, and the patient exhales passively. Tidal volumes will be determined by lung compliance—the more compliant the lung, the larger the tidal volume at a set pressure. PSV is often used as a partial mode of ventilatory support in alert patients who may not tolerate more controlled forms of mechanical ventilation.

Pressure control ventilation (PCV) is related to pressure support in that the flow is descending in amplitude during the inspiratory cycle. In contrast to PSV, with PCV the inspiratory time is set by the ventilator, not the patient. PCV is generally used in the A/C, which allows full support of patient-initiated breaths in addition to those initiated by the ventilator (mandatory, or time triggered). The purported advantages of PCV relate to the decelerating flow curve, which is thought to allow more time for alveolar inflation and gas exchange. It is important to recognize that the tidal volume (and therefore minute ventilation) might change quite rapidly with changes in lung compliance. Thus, without continued reassessment of tidal volumes, there is a possibility that the patient might be significantly hypo- or hyperventilated. Pressure-regulated volume control (PRVC) is a mode similar to PCV in which the pressure is autoregulated (within a specified range) to ensure tidal volumes are maintained despite changes in lung compliance.

Ventilator Strategies

Endotracheal intubation and mechanical ventilation provide vital support yet are associated with disadvantages, including a greater risk of pneumonia and aggravation of alveolar injury, respectively. Additionally, there is increasing evidence that the manner by which patients are ventilated and weaned might have significant effects on outcome. For example, in a large randomized controlled trial, patients with ARDS or acute lung injury (a form of hypoxemic respiratory failure, Table 9.2[21]) ventilated with lower tidal volumes (6 mL/kg) had a significantly lower mortality than those ventilated at higher tidal volumes (12 mL/kg).[22] Clinical and experimental studies suggest that higher tidal volumes lead to ventilator-induced lung injury (by means of over distending alveoli), which incites a greater local and systemic inflammatory response. Patients ventilated with lower tidal volumes also had significantly lower ventilatory pressures (plateau pressures <30 cm H_2O), thus it is unclear which offered benefit—the lower tidal volumes or the

TABLE 9.2

RECOMMENDED CRITERIA FOR ACUTE LUNG INJURY AND ACUTE RESPIRATORY DISTRESS SYNDROME[a]

	Timing	Oxygenation	Chest radiograph	Pulmonary artery wedge pressure
Acute lung injury (ALI)	Acute onset	$PaO_2/FiO_2 \leq 300$ regardless of PEEP level	Bilateral infiltrates on frontal chest radiograph	≤18 when measured or no clinical evidence of left atrial hypertension
Acute respiratory distress syndrome (ARDS)	Acute onset	$PaO_2/FiO_2 \leq 200$ regardless of PEEP level	Bilateral infiltrates on frontal chest radiograph	≤18 when measured or no clinical evidence of left atrial hypertension

[a]In setting of known risk factors of either direct lung injury (aspiration, diffuse pulmonary infection, near drowning, toxic inhalation, pulmonary contusion) or indirect lung injury (sepsis, severe nonthoracic trauma, massive transfusion, cardiopulmonary bypass or ischemia/reperfusion insult). Adapted from Bernard GR, Artigas A, Brigham KL, et al. The American-European Consensus Conference on ARDS. Definitions, mechanisms, relevant outcomes, and clinical trial coordination. *Am J Respir Crit Care Med.* 1994;149:818–824.

lower plateau pressures. Many centers have since adopted this lung protective ventilatory strategy.

A frequent point of controversy in managing the hypoxemic patient are the relative merits of using high levels of PEEP and lower levels of FIO_2 or using lower levels of PEEP with a correspondingly higher FIO_2. By convention, many intensivists use higher levels of PEEP to maintain the FIO_2 <0.6, believing that higher levels of oxygen might induce hyperoxic lung injury. However, results from a randomized controlled trial comparing a high PEEP strategy with a high FIO_2 strategy demonstrated similar outcomes.[23] Given these data, the risks and benefits of using PEEP should be assessed for each patient depending on the nature of their underlying lung disease and associated conditions (e.g., low cardiac output state, high intracranial pressure, unilateral lung disease).

The process of weaning from the ventilator has changed significantly with evidence that the most rapid means of liberating a patient from the ventilator is through daily trials (30 to 90 minutes) of spontaneous breathing with low levels of continuous positive airway pressure (CPAP). This approach is superior to the gradual withdrawal of ventilation using pressure support or IMV.[24–27] If the patient tolerates the trial of spontaneous breathing, it is likely that he or she can be extubated with a low risk of requiring reintubation, providing he or she can protect the airway. Patients who fail a trial of spontaneous breathing should be rested for at least 24 hours using a stable, nonfatiguing form of ventilatory support. A partial support mode of ventilation (e.g., pressure support) probably offers benefit in terms of patient comfort while allowing a period of rest, as the patient can determine the respiratory rate, the flow rate, inspiratory time, and the tidal volume.

TRANSFUSION THERAPY IN THE INTENSIVE CARE UNIT

Virtually half of patients admitted to an ICU will receive a transfusion during the course of their ICU stay.[28] In those staying in the ICU for at least 1 week, 85% will require an average of nine units over the course of their ICU stay.[29] The causes are multifactorial and include blood loss from the underlying disease(s), repeated blood draws for laboratory tests, and suppression of erythropoietin release. In the past, transfusions were provided liberally to maintain Hgb in the range of 10 g/dL with the belief that allogeneic transfusions were not harmful and would improve oxygen delivery. However, in a study in nonbleeding euvolemic patients with low oxygen delivery, the relative increase in oxygen delivery at the tissue level achieved with transfusion was far below that obtained through measures to increase cardiac output.[30] An increase in the rigidity of red blood cell membranes associated with prolonged storage might impair the ability of these cells to navigate the microvasculature, resulting in sludging.[31] Additionally, the transfusion of allogeneic red blood cells has been associated with an increased risk of nosocomial infection in a variety of clinical settings.

A large clinical trial in which nonbleeding, euvolemic critically ill patients were randomized to either a liberal transfusion strategy (Hgb of 10 g/dL) or a restrictive strategy (Hgb of 7 g/dL) demonstrated that patients in the liberal group fared no better than those in the restrictive group who received far fewer transfusions.[32] In fact, younger patients (<55 years) and those with Acute Physiology and Chronic Health Evaluation (APACHE) II scores of less than 20 had lower mortality and lower rates of organ dysfunction. In a subset of patients requiring prolonged ventilator support, the rate of liberation from mechanical ventilation was higher in patients randomized to the restrictive arm, suggesting there is no benefit to transfusing patients for the purposes of improving their ability to wean off the ventilator.[33] It appears that the risk of adverse outcomes related to a strict transfusion strategy is higher only in patients with unstable cardiovascular disease (unstable angina, acute myocardial infarction).[34]

Several approaches may be used to reduce transfusion requirements in the critically ill patient. Blood sampling should be reduced to only that is required to alter patient care. Pulse oximetry should be used rather than arterial blood gases when there are changes in PEEP or FIO_2, and end-tidal CO_2 monitoring can guide changes in minute ventilation. Weekly recombinant human erythropoietin (rHuEPO) administration has been evaluated in patients with an anticipated prolonged ICU stay. In one randomized controlled trial, erythropoietin reduced transfusion requirements by approximately 20% and reduced the need for any transfusion by 17%, without affecting length of stay, rates of organ dysfunction, or mortality.[35] Given these findings, it is not clear whether the benefits associated with a more restrictive transfusion policy are due to a lower Hgb concentration or fewer transfusions.

METABOLISM AND NUTRITION

Metabolic and nutritional support are vital if the critically ill patient is to survive the ICU stay. Depletion of energy and protein reserves leads to an inability to wean off the ventilator, immunologic failure, and a high probability of death due to overwhelming infection. Thus, in the ICU a tremendous amount of effort is geared toward assessing and maintaining adequate nutritional support.

Energy Sources

The major sources of energy are carbohydrates (including ketones and alcohols) and fats. Protein can be oxidized through gluconeogenesis and is often a significant source of energy in critically ill patients. The goal of nutritional support is to supply energy from sources other than protein, so that endogenous and exogenous protein can be used for anabolism rather than catabolism. In normal volunteers and surgical patients, the breakdown of protein is decreased by giving the subject exogenous fuel, typically in the form of carbohydrate or fat. This is referred to as the *protein-sparing effect.* Small amounts of glucose (400 cal/day) provide some degree of protein sparing, but full caloric support is required for maximal effect.

Carbohydrate is the major source of energy during the normal, nonstarving state. The brain and red cells are obligate users of glucose. They require glucose as the primary energy source under normal conditions. Other organs also use glucose preferentially as a source of energy. The brain and red blood cells can develop the capacity to use ketones as an energy source, a process called *starvation adaptation.* When fully oxidized, carbohydrate produces 4 cal of energy per gram of substrate metabolized, 5 cal of energy per liter of O_2 consumed and one molecule of CO_2 for each molecule of O_2 consumed. The latter ratio is the RQ, discussed previously in the context of CO_2 production (see Table 9.1).

Fat is the most efficient source of energy. Fat produces 9 cal of energy per gram of substrate metabolized and 4.7 cal of energy per liter of O_2 consumed in this oxidation; its RQ is 0.7. Fat is stored as triglyceride, and for every three molecules of fatty acid oxidized to produce energy, one molecule of glycerol is also oxidized. Endogenous fat is the major source of energy during starvation. The glycogen stores are virtually depleted after a day of fasting, following which fat becomes the major source of energy, with protein breakdown supplying glucose through the process of gluconeogenesis.

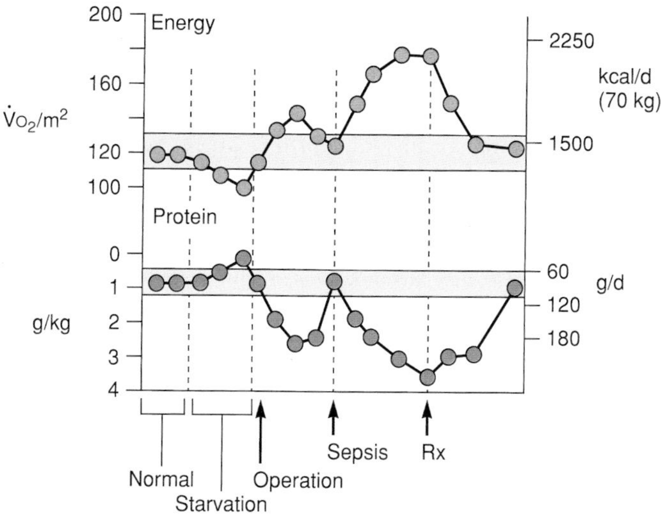

FIGURE 9.12 Energy and protein metabolism in normal, starving, operative, and septic states. (After Bartlett RH. Nutritional support. In: Dantzker DR, ed. *Cardiopulmonary critical care.* Orlando, FL: Grune & Stratton; 1986:263, with permission.)

TABLE 9.3

PREDICTED INCREASE IN CALORIC REQUIREMENTS AS A FUNCITON OF STRESSOR

Physiologic stress	Stress factor
Operation	1.1
Peritonitis, major infection, or long bone fracture	1.25
Severe injury/infection or multiple organ failure	1.5
Thermal injury	
10% BSA	1.25
20–30% BSA	1.5
40% BSA	1.75
>50% BSA	2.0

BSA, body surface area.

Metabolic Requirements

The typical expenditures of energy and protein in normal subjects and critically ill patients are shown in Figure 9.12. Protein and energy requirements are continuous. These are met by endogenous sources during fasting or through exogenous treatment (nutrition). Energy expenditure is referred to as the *basal metabolic rate,* or the *basal energy expenditure.* The term basal metabolic rate describes the energy required to maintain cell integrity in the resting state and at thermoneutrality. The latter term means an ambient temperature, usually close to 80°F (28°C) at which the heat loss and the need for increased heat production to maintain the body temperature are minimal. The basal energy expenditure (BEE) decreases with advancing age and varies with sex and body size. It is a function of cellular metabolism and hence of the body cell mass. The basal energy expenditure (in kilocalories) is usually estimated from the Harris-Benedict equation, which incorporates age, sex, and body size:

Women:

$$\text{BEE} = 655 + (9.6 \times \text{weight in kilos}) + (1.8 \times \text{height in cm}) - (4.7 \times \text{age in years}).$$

Men:

$$\text{BEE} = 66 + (13.7 \times \text{weight in kilos}) + (5 \times \text{height in cm}) - (6.8 \times \text{age in years}).$$

Requirements are most often expressed as kcal/kg/day. Basal requirements are typically in the range of 25 kcal/kg/day.

Estimating and Measuring Energy Requirements

The actual metabolic rate of any given patient can be estimated by modifying the predicted basal rate according to the clinical condition. For example, the metabolic rate is decreased by 10% in a starving person and increased by 10% with minor activity. This further estimation of metabolic activity in the resting (as opposed to basal) state is referred to as the *resting energy expenditure.* Trauma, stress, sepsis, and surgical operations are all known to increase the metabolic rate. As a result, the BEE is usually multiplied by a stress factor to better approximate caloric requirements (Table 9.3). In general, the critically ill patient requires approximately 35 kcal/kg/day.

Although most of the studies on nutrition in critical illness have been based on estimated energy expenditure, actual measurement is much more accurate and is an important aspect of critical care. The most commonly used method of measurement is indirect calorimetry. In the ICU, indirect calorimetry is the only accurate and clinically feasible method of measuring energy expenditure. It is called indirect because the caloric burn rate is calculated from a measurement of oxygen uptake. Direct calorimetry implies a measurement of heat released by the body, which is technically difficult and clinically impractical. Indirect calorimetry relies on the fact that burning 1 kilocalorie requires approximately 200 mL of oxygen. Because of this very direct relationship between caloric burn and oxygen consumed, measurements of oxygen uptake (VO_2) and caloric burn rate are virtually interchangeable.

Indirect calorimetry can be carried out at the patient's bedside and requires the measurement of the differences in oxygen and carbon dioxide concentrations between a known volume of inspired and expired gas. Assuming the patient is in a steady state, oxygen consumption and carbon dioxide production can be quantitated. With measurement of O_2 consumption and CO_2 production, the RQ (VCO_2/VO_2) can be calculated, thus providing an assessment of the relative oxidation of carbohydrates and fat (see Table 9.1). Thus, indirect calorimetry provides some indication of which substrates are being utilized to fulfill energy requirements. Usually the RQ is approximately 0.8; very infrequently the RQ might be in excess of 1 and as high as 2.5, indicative of lipogenesis (synthesis of fat from carbohydrates) and indicative of excess availability of carbohydrates.

Measurement of the RQ is helpful as an internal check on the accuracy of the calorimetry measurements and as a guideline to patient management. For example, if a patient has been receiving only 500 cal/day and has a metabolic rate of 2,500 cal/day one would expect that the use of fat would be maximal, and the RQ should be 0.7 or less. If such a patient is treated with parenteral nutrition and glucose used as the major source of energy, the RQ should be 1 when the caloric replacement matches caloric losses. If the RQ exceeds 1, then some of the excess infused carbohydrate is being converted to fat and excess CO_2 is produced, which leads to a need for a higher minute ventilation. Thus, hypercaloric feeding with glucose can cause respiratory failure that requires mechanical ventilation simply by increasing the load of CO_2.

Protein Metabolism

Estimating and Measuring Protein Requirements

In normal protein metabolism, a continuous excretion of nitrogen (mostly as urea) equivalent to about 50 g of protein each day is matched by a protein intake of 50 g/day. The rate of protein synthesis and breakdown is about 300 g/day, with most endogenous amino acids being recycled into new protein. In starvation, protein catabolism continues (although at a slower rate) without a corresponding protein intake, leaving the patient in a negative protein balance. This protein flux is most conveniently measured as nitrogen flux; consequently, the condition is commonly referred to as *negative nitrogen balance.* During critical illness, the rate of protein catabolism generally increases while intake stops, so that a significant negative nitrogen balance results. It is convenient to think of this protein breakdown as necessary to produce critically required glucose through gluconeogenesis when other carbohydrate stores have been exhausted.

Protein Sources

The fact that the nitrogen balance is negative does not mean that protein synthesis stops or slows down. On the contrary, the synthesis of new cells, inflammatory cells, collagen, coagulation factors, antibodies, and scores of other proteins occurs at an accelerated rate during critical illness. Amino acids derived from muscle tissue or other somatic and visceral proteins become the building blocks for protein in healing tissue and host defenses. The site of a traumatic or surgical wound or an area of acute inflammation diverts protein from other body tissues. Proteins that would otherwise strengthen the diaphragm or myocardium or participate in host defense processes are no longer available, thus significantly compromising the patient. A large part of the goal of nutritional management is to provide sources of energy so that endogenous proteins are not required for energy (i.e., protein sparing) and to supply exogenous proteins so that all the needs of protein synthesis can be met without a breakdown of endogenous sources. Although oversimplified, a convenient number to remember for the basal protein requirement is 0.8 g/kg per day. The average critically ill surgical patients might require 1.5 g/kg per day, whereas patients with severe thermal injury and head injuries might have requirements in excess of 2 g/kg per day.

Nitrogen Balance

Protein balance is most frequently determined through assessment of nitrogen balance. Nitrogen balance can be determined by measuring the amount of nitrogen excreted. This is most conveniently done by measuring the amount of urea excreted in the urine if one assumes that urea constitutes 85% of the total nitrogen excretion. It is better to measure the total nitrogen in urine and other lost fluids because the percentage contained in urea can vary considerably. Each gram of nitrogen represents 6.25 g of protein, thus total protein intake can be compared with protein loss through an estimate of daily urea excretion.

Indirect assessments of protein reserves are based on the single measurement of body substances that are maintained at normal levels by rapid protein synthesis. A variety of visceral proteins that have relatively short half-lives have been assessed for their relationship to protein status. Prealbumin ($t_{1/2}$ = 2 days), retinol-binding protein ($t_{1/2}$ = 10 hours), and transferrin ($t_{1/2}$ = 8 days) have all been used in the evaluation of nitrogen balance. Albumin has limited utility given its relatively long half-life ($t_{1/2}$ = 21 days). Some advocate insulin-like growth factor-1 as another short-lived serum visceral protein, with the major benefit being its relative independence to the inflammatory state of the patient. For example, prealbumin is a negative acute phase reactant and serum levels will decrease in the presence of ongoing, acute inflammation. As a result, increasing levels of prealbumin might be consistent with the deposition of new protein or an abating inflammatory response, whereas a decrease might suggest a negative nitrogen balance or a new focus of inflammation or infection. For these reasons, these rapid-turnover visceral proteins should be used as only one measure of protein status.

Fat Metabolism

In a normal 80-kg man, about 1,000 cal are readily available as glycogen and other stored carbohydrates, 24,000 cal available as protein, and approximately 140,000 cal are stored as fat. A 10,000 cal deficit accrued over 5 to 6 days of semistarvation in a critically ill patient is considered a severe, acute energy deficit. This seems paradoxical given the large amount of calories stored as fat. However, the problem of a 10,000 cal deficit is not the loss of a few kilograms of fat but rather the protein catabolism commonly associated with an energy deficit of this size.

With the exception of essential fatty acids, the critically ill patient has little need for the administration of exogenous lipid. If the entire nonprotein caloric requirement were administered solely as carbohydrate, glycemic control and CO_2 retention (or a need for a higher minute ventilation) would be the only potential adverse effects. Thus, lipid is provided to prevent essential fatty acid deficiency and as a source of nonprotein calories.

There is significant debate regarding the value of administering intravenous fat emulsions in patients requiring parenteral nutritional support. Selected studies report an increased risk of infection and other complications, including potential lung toxicity from released fatty acids, compared to patients not receiving lipid emulsions.[36] It is entirely possible that the improved outcomes in the patients not receiving lipids were related to withholding the fat infusions or due to the hypocaloric nutritional regimen (underfeeding) these patients received, which might simplify glycemic control with all of its inherent benefits (see later).

Vitamins and Minerals

A hypermetabolic patient catabolizes vitamins more rapidly than is normal and can reach a deficiency state sooner. Additionally, the oxidative stress associated with reperfusion injury and a systemic inflammatory response leads to depletion of vitamins E and C. In this regard, there is evidence to suggest that high doses of vitamins E and C might improve outcome and lower the risk of multiple organ failure in critically ill surgical patients.[36] Adequate levels of other vitamins are readily available in commercially prepared formulations used for enteral or parenteral administration.

Mineral and trace metals must be managed more carefully than vitamins because a deficiency can occur sooner and overdose can be deleterious. Calcium, phosphorus, and magnesium are lost continuously through the urine, stool, gastric juices, and other drainage. Although large body stores (particularly of calcium and phosphorous) are available, deficiency can develop rapidly. Enteral and parenteral feeding must include these elements. Serum levels of calcium, phosphorus, and magnesium should be measured at regular intervals. Zinc, copper, chromium, selenium, and manganese must be supplied to patients who are supported with enteral or parenteral feeding for more than 2 weeks.

Nutritional Support

Nutritional status should be assessed at the time of admission to the ICU with a view to determining whether the patient is malnourished and the likelihood of return to normal oral intake. Patients who are malnourished at the time of admission should receive nutritional support as soon as possible, typically once the acute resuscitation phase is over. In a systematic review of randomized controlled trials, early enteral nutrition (initiation within 36 hours of admission) was associated with a significantly lower risk of infections and a shorter hospital length of stay.[38] A reasonable goal for nutritional support is to meet the caloric and protein requirements within 5 days of ICU admission in adequately nourished patients in whom a return to oral intake is not imminent (Algorithm 9.3).

The critically ill patient is best provided energy and protein using the gastrointestinal tract whenever possible. This route has fewer risks of complications and is less costly than the parenteral route. Enteral feeding can be accomplished through a tube passed directly into the duodenum or jejunum at surgery or through a soft, small-bore feeding tube passed into the stomach through the nose or mouth. It is generally possible to accomplish tube feeding with gastric infusion. There appears to be no specific benefit to postpyloric enteral feeding with respect to rates of pneumonia due to aspiration.[39] However, in the case of intolerance, postpyloric feeding should be considered. Intolerance of gastric feeding usually manifests as large volumes (>300 mL) of residual feeds in the stomach on aspiration from the feeding tube. In this scenario, the feeding tube should be advanced beyond the pylorus using endoscopy or fluoroscopy. Alternatively prokinetic agents like metoclopramide or erythromycin may be effective.

Feedings should be given by continuous infusion rather than as large boluses. The patient should be positioned in a semirecumbent or sitting position (at a minimum of a 30-degree angle) to prevent regurgitation and aspiration.

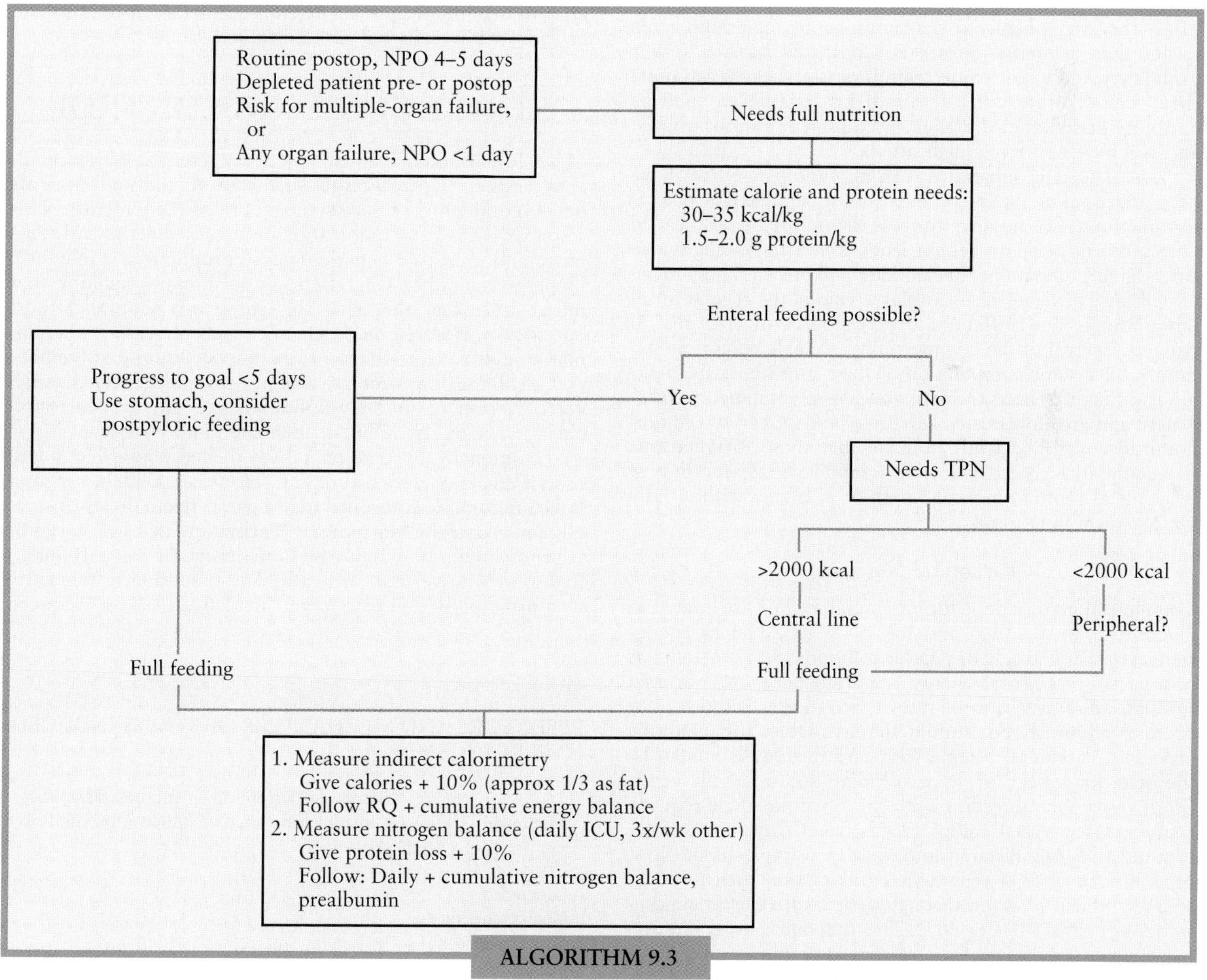

ALGORITHM 9.3 Nutritional management. TPN, total parenteral nutrition; RQ, respiratory quotient. (Modified from Bartlett RH. *University of Michigan critical care handbook*. Boston: Little, Brown; 1996.)

SCIENTIFIC PRINCIPLES

Gastric residuals should be checked if the patient feels uncomfortable or appears distended, but it is not necessary to check the residual more than once a day under most circumstances. With continuous tube feeding, a residual of 200 to 300 mL is normal.

It is better to start with a small amount of full-strength formula rather than a large amount of diluted formula. The rate can be advanced and gradually increased until the desired volume is reached. Hypernatremia can occur in patients who receive high protein formulas or concentrated formulas or in those patients with significant free water losses. Hypernatremia should be managed by administering free water via the feeding tube. A serious problem with tube feeding is complete cessation of feedings because of diarrhea or a large gastric residual. If the tube feeding needs to be curtailed for any reason, it should be reinstituted the next hour at a smaller volume and gradually increased until the prescribed caloric load is reached.

Enteral Formulations

Commercially available formulae for enteral feeding generally contain 1 to 2 cal/mL and include 16% to 25% of calories as protein. Most of the calories are supplied as maltodextrins, hydrolyzed corn syrup, corn syrup solids, and sucrose. Those that are considered elemental, supplying amino acids rather than proteins, or are concentrated have a higher osmolarity and might cause cramps or diarrhea. When diarrhea occurs, other causes should be considered such as antibiotic-associated diarrhea, pseudomembranous colitis, and sorbitol-containing medications.

Several specific substrates with immunologic effects have been added, alone or in combination, to a variety of enteral formulations. The number of these key nutrients, also called nutraceuticals or pharmaconutrients, is now increasing but to date arginine, glutamine, nucleotides, and omega-3 polyunsaturated fatty acids all seem to play a role in the regulation of immunologic and inflammatory responses in critically ill patients. Several of the commercially available enteral preparations have some combination of these nutraceuticals, making it difficult to assess which alone or in combination offer benefit and are more costly. Several systematic reviews of randomized controlled trials indicate that these formulations reduce the incidence of infectious complications, duration of mechanical ventilation, and length of ICU stay without any improvement in mortality.[38,40,41]

Parenteral Nutrition

Commercial preparations for parenteral feeding are limited to glucose (20% to 70%) and fat (10% to 20%) as energy sources and amino acid or peptide solutions (5.5% to 15%) as protein sources. Total energy requirements should be met through administration of fat, carbohydrate, or both. Any protein administered should be available for anabolic processes. Parenteral feeding with carbohydrate is limited by the sclerotic effect of hyperosmolar solutions on veins. Effective parenteral feeding with carbohydrate alone requires solutions of at least 1 cal/mL (25% sugar). This type of solution must be administered into an area of rapid blood flow, generally the superior vena cava. Fat is a more efficient energy source and can be given through peripheral veins in concentrations of either 10% or 20%. The total daily energy requirement can be given as fat, or a major portion can be given as fat with the rest as carbohydrate. Both fat and carbohydrate are equally effective sources of energy. The ratio between fat and carbohydrate energy sources and the ratio between total energy sources and grams of protein vary depending on the clinical state. For example, a patient with cardiac failure may require a solution that is low in volume and low in sodium but high in calories and protein. A patient with multiple intestinal fistulae may require large volumes, which allow fewer calories and grams of protein per milliliter. As a rule of thumb, half of the calories can be provided by carbohydrate, 30% as fat, and the remainder as protein.

The standard solution can be modified for individual patients by raising or lowering the concentration of glucose and amino acids and by varying the electrolyte and trace metal composition. Vitamins and trace minerals are added to the solution at regular intervals. The standard solution must be supplemented with intravenous fat to provide at least 100 g of fat emulsion each week to preclude fatty acid deficiency. Fat emulsion may be administered through a peripheral vein or through a central catheter at the same time as the hypertonic glucose solution.

The most common complication of total parenteral nutrition is infection on or around the intravascular catheter. Of course, infection can occur with any indwelling vascular catheter, but it is more likely in the presence of hypertonic glucose and protein solutions. If catheter infection is suspected, the catheter must be removed and a new catheter placed. Hyperglycemia is common and should be aggressively managed with an insulin infusion. A sudden increase in blood glucose levels in a patient receiving parenteral nutrition is often an early sign of infection. When this occurs, the patient should be thoroughly evaluated with this in mind.

STRICT GLYCEMIC CONTROL

The cytokine and hormonal milieu characteristic of critical illness leads to hyperglycemia such that virtually all patients have blood glucose levels in excess of 120 mg/dL. This response is due to a combination of increased peripheral resistance and increased hepatic glucose production (Table 9.4). Hyperglycemia has several effects on immune function that might increase the risk of infectious complications. Specifically, elevated blood glucose levels increase proinflammatory cytokine production from monocytes; impair lymphocyte proliferation; decrease serum opsonic activity through glycosylation of immunoglobulins; and impair neutrophil chemotaxis, oxidative burst, adherence, and phagocytosis.

Traditionally, hyperglycemia was treated only if blood glucose levels exceeded 200 mg/dL. However, evidence from a large randomized controlled trial suggests that a policy of strict glycemic control is warranted.[42] Patients treated with a protocol to maintain blood glucose in the range of 80 to 100 g/dL had a 44% lower risk of death. The reduction in mortality was principally due to a lower incidence of sepsis-induced

TABLE 9.4

EFFECTORS AND MECHANISMS OF STRESS-INDUCED HYPERGLYCEMIA

Mediator	Increased peripheral insulin resistance	Increased hepatic glucose production
Cortisol	X	
Glucagon		X
Growth hormone	X	
Norepinephrine		X
Epinephrine		X
TNF-α	X	
IL-1	X	

IL-1, interleukin 1; TNF-α, tumor necrosis factor alpha.

multiple organ failure. These and other supporting data argue for the routine implementation of protocols to maintain strict glycemic control in all critically ill patients. Ideally, these protocols should be based on continuous intravenous infusions of insulin, rather than intermittent boluses or subcutaneous administration. Erratic absorption from subcutaneous sites in edematous patients in whom skin perfusion is variably impaired increases the risk of both hyper- and hypoglycemia.

ACUTE RENAL FAILURE

Acute renal failure (ARF), by definition, is an abrupt decrease in kidney function that results in the accumulation of nitrogenous solutes. ARF may be oliguric (urine output <400 mL/day) or nonoliguric (urine output is normal or increased while solute clearance is markedly decreased) (Table 9.5). The mortality of ARF in the surgical ICU is high (50% to 90%) because ARF is usually just one component of severe multiple-organ failure. The mortality from nonoliguric ARF is significantly less than that from oliguric ARF, although many patients progress to oliguria with its poor outcome. Regardless of urine output, the sequelae of ARF result from the retention of metabolic wastes indicated by a progressive rise in blood urea nitrogen (BUN) and serum creatinine concentrations. Hypervolemia and electrolyte imbalances further complicate the management of oliguric ARF.

The pathogenesis of ARF is commonly classified as prerenal, postrenal, or intrinsic parenchymal disease. This discussion is limited to parenchymal disease. Parenchymal abnormalities include acute tubular necrosis, pigment nephropathy (secondary to circulating myoglobin and Hgb), and those caused by nephrotoxic agents (various drugs and contrast material). Other causes of parenchymal renal disease, such as acute glomerular nephritis and vasculitis, are not typically responsible for ARF in the surgical patient and are not discussed in this chapter.

Acute Tubular Necrosis

Acute tubular necrosis results from ischemia in the renal parenchyma and is the most common pathologic etiology of ARF. Under conditions of diminishing renal blood flow, perfusion of the kidneys is first maintained by vasomotor responses, which dilate the afferent arteriole and constrict the efferent arteriole. As continued hypotension is detected by the juxtaglomerular apparatus, the renin–angiotensin system is activated in concert with the sympathetic release of other vasoactive hormones. These substances produce vasoconstriction systemically, including the afferent arteriole and further exacerbate cortical hypoperfusion. Casts of cellular debris obstruct the lumen, and cellular edema occurs. As tubular cells become necrotic and slough off, the leakage of glomerular ultrafiltrate back across the proximal tubular membrane into the interstitium causes edema. Acute tubular necrosis comprises a spectrum of effects of cortical ischemia, ranging from polyuria with tubular dysfunction to temporary anuria to renal cortical necrosis with chronic anuria.

TABLE 9.5

STANDARD MEASUREMENTS IN THE DIAGNOSIS OF RENAL FAILURE

Test	Prerenal	Parenchymal
Urine osmolarity (mOsm)	>500	250–350
U/P osmolality	>1.5	<1.1
U/P creatinine	>20	<10
Urine sodium	<20	>40
FE_{Na}	<1%	>3%

FE_{Na}, fraction of excreted sodium; U/P, urine-to-plasma ratio.

Pigment Nephropathy

Pigment nephropathy is a common cause of ARF and may occur after trauma, burns, operation, or hemodynamic catastrophe. In surgical patients, pigment nephropathy is most often due to myoglobin; however, hemoglobinemia due to massive intravascular hemolysis might also give rise to ARF. During ischemia or after blunt injury to large muscle masses, myoglobin is released into the circulation. This syndrome, referred to as rhabdomyolysis leads to ARF in up to one third of patients. In the context of rhabdomyolysis, there are three main mechanisms leading to the development of renal failure: decreased renal perfusion related to hypovolemia and renal vasoconstriction in response to myoglobin, cast formation with tubular obstruction, and the direct toxic effects of myoglobin on the renal tubules. Although myoglobin is not a direct nephrotoxin, in the presence of aciduria, myoglobin is converted to ferrihemate, which is toxic to renal cells. Rhabdomyolysis should be suspected in patients with burns, trauma, seizures, alcohol or drug intoxication, prolonged ischemia in muscle groups, and extended coma.

The presence of myoglobin in the urine can be first suspected by the presence of dark, tea-colored urine and then confirmed with a positive urine dipstick, which reacts with the heme groups of both myoglobin and Hgb. The absence of red cells on microscopy confirms that the discolored urine is caused by myoglobin. High serum levels of creatinine phosphokinase (CPK) or myoglobin, in combination with evidence of urine myoglobin, confirm the diagnosis. Hyperkalemia and elevated serum creatinine are also consistent with injury to muscle masses.

Patients with either CPK >20,000 IU/L or serum myoglobin >10,000 ng/mL are at highest risk for pigment nephropathy. Measures should be instituted to prevent pigment nephropathy and lower the likelihood of requiring renal replacement therapy (RRT). The most important measure is volume expansion with or without administration of diuretics to achieve a urine output of 200 mL/hour. Mannitol is an ideal diuretic in this sense as it induces an osmotic diuresis and as an oxidant scavenger might reduce iron-mediated oxidative injury to the renal tubules. Many intensivists also attempt to alkalinize the urine (pH ≥7) through the administration of sodium bicarbonate solutions, although evidence supporting this approach is marginal. Forced diuresis should continue until the urine is clear of myoglobin.

Nephrotoxic Agents

Drug-induced ARF is responsible for about 5% of all cases of ARF. Its pathophysiology differs according to the offending agent. Through normal reabsorption and secretion, the kidney is exposed to high concentrations of drugs and solutes, which may be toxic. This problem is compounded by hypovolemia, which causes an increased reabsorption of water and solutes and exposes the lumen to even higher concentrations of toxins. Although the damage to tubular function can be significant, much drug-induced ARF remains nonoliguric because of the sparing of glomerular function.

Radiographic contrast dye has been documented to cause ARF. The incidence of contrast nephropathy is about 1% to 10% and may be predicted according to a number of risk factors. These include contrast load, age, preexisting renal insufficiency, and diabetes, although some of these factors are disputed. The incidence in patients with normal renal function is a significantly lower, at 1% to 2%. Contrast nephropathy is usually experienced as an asymptomatic, transient rise in creatinine but may progress to oliguric renal failure that requires hemodialysis (HD). Volume expansion (500 mL of normal saline) before contrast injection may decrease the incidence and severity of ARF in high-risk patients. Potentially beneficial adjunctive prophylactic measures include administration of sodium bicarbonate or N-acetylcysteine.

Management of Acute Renal Failure

In surgical patients, ARF rarely occurs in isolation. Rather, ARF is only one component of a syndrome of multiple-organ failure that is often accompanied by infection. The treatment of these patients, therefore, should be focused on managing the underlying disease processes. The development of ARF complicates the care of surgical patients by introducing difficulties in fluid, electrolyte, and nutritional management. The adverse effects of renal replacement therapies further compound these problems. A favorable outcome can be achieved only through aggressive intervention. This includes surgical drainage of infectious foci, excision of necrotic tissue, early implementation of effective RRT, and full nutritional support (Algorithm 9.4).

General Care

With nonoliguric ARF, the treatment may differ little from that required for identical patients with normal renal function. The management of fluids, solutes, and nutrition is usually unaffected by nonoliguric ARF, although the BUN may be elevated. The extent of renal dysfunction is limited and almost always reversible. The use of renal replacement therapies (and their inherent complications) is rarely necessary.

Oliguria and anuria pose several management difficulties. In the absence of normal urine output, problems of fluid overload

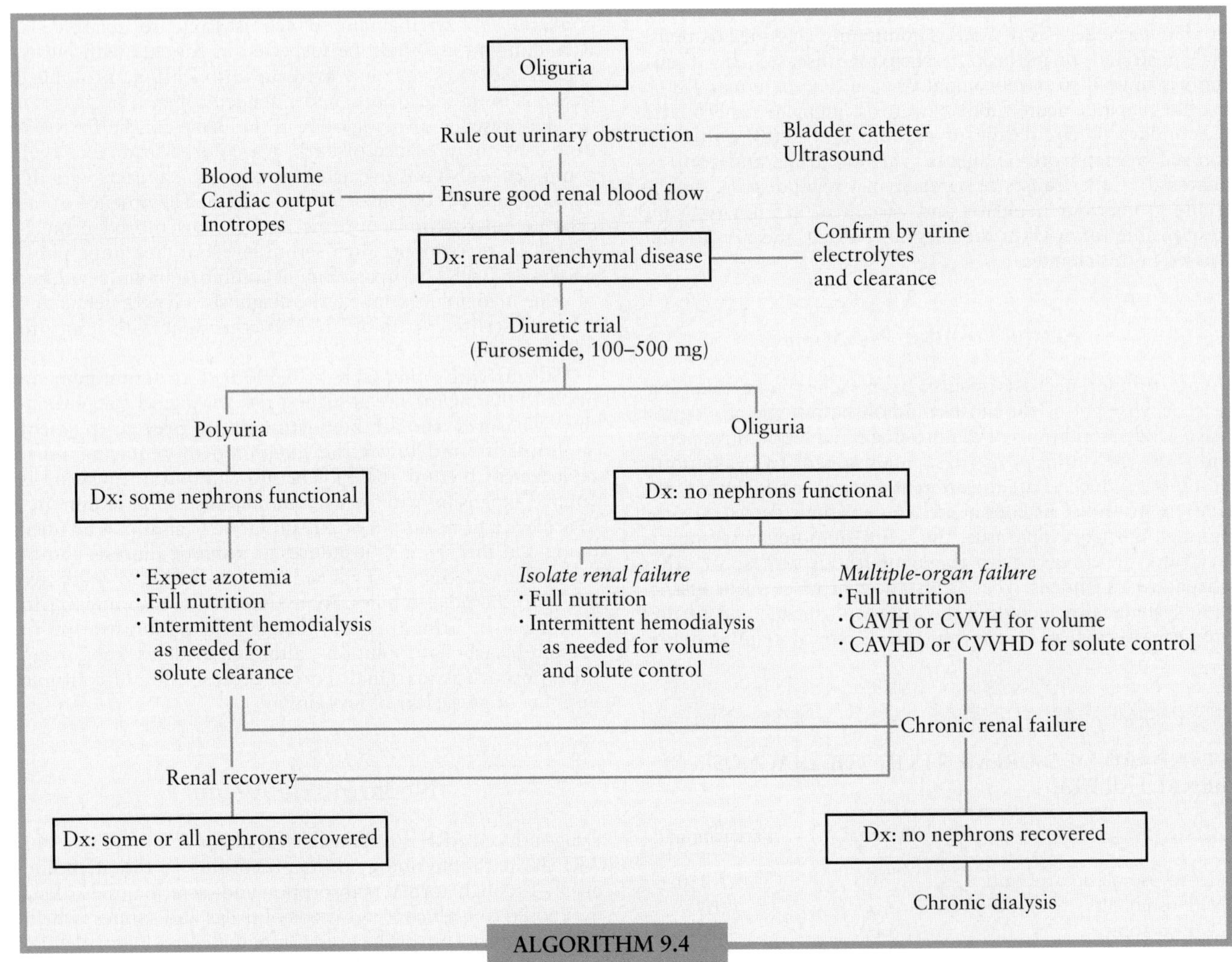

ALGORITHM 9.4 Management of acute renal failure. PD, peritoneal dialysis; CAVH, continuous arteriovenous hemofiltration; CAVHD, continuous arteriovenous hemodialysis.

can lead to anasarca, pulmonary edema, and congestive heart failure. The pharmacokinetics of drugs becomes difficult to predict as a result of decreased elimination and increased volume of distribution. In light of these risks, the volume status of patients with ARF must be carefully monitored. Fluid intake and output must be precisely tabulated, and the body weight should be measured daily. Pulmonary artery catheterization may be necessary to monitor the fluid status of these patients more closely. Treatment options for hypervolemia consist of fluid restriction or fluid removal with some form of RRT. Fluid restriction, however, limits the administration of intravenous medications and may preclude adequate nutrition.

ARF can create severe derangements in electrolyte and acid–base physiology. Serum electrolytes should be measured daily. Of all the electrolyte abnormalities that can occur with ARF, hyperkalemia is the most serious. Under the conditions of hypercatabolism and tissue necrosis that characterize these patients, large amounts of potassium may be generated and accumulate during a short period of time. Acute hyperkalemia causes a decrease in cardiac excitability, which can ultimately result in asystole. The removal of potassium must be accomplished with RRT or ion-exchange resins. Other electrolyte abnormalities, such as hyponatremia, hyperphosphatemia, hypocalcemia, and metabolic acidosis, are common in ARF and must be monitored closely. Treatment consists of appropriate additions or restrictions of intravenous solutions and effective use of the RRT.

Platelet dysfunction and coagulopathy are often associated with ARF. A reproducible platelet defect can be demonstrated experimentally with a BUN of 100 mg/dL. This defect can be transiently reversed with administration of desmopressin (DDAVP). Platelet transfusion in this clinical setting will be ineffective because the transfused platelets will rapidly acquire the same dysfunction at the patient's platelets. Anemia also accompanies ARF in surgical patients. In addition to the loss of blood during hemorrhage or operation, the production of erythropoietin has been shown to decrease in direct proportion to the decrease in renal function.

Nutritional Support in Acute Renal Failure

The goal of nutritional support in ARF is to provide optimal amounts of calorie and protein substrates to minimize autocatabolism and allow tissue anabolism, wound healing, and sustained immune function. In any discussion of nutrition and renal failure, it is necessary to point out the distinction between acute and chronic renal failure. Patients with chronic renal failure are generally healthy, and their energy requirements differ little from those of persons without chronic renal failure. Protein intake is required only for metabolic turnover and is restricted to minimize the generation of urea and other products of protein metabolism.

By contrast, the metabolic requirements of a patient with ARF are those of a critically ill, hospitalized patient. Actual measurement of resting energy expenditure has shown that the caloric requirements of patients with multiple-organ failure and ARF are often 50% above those of normal, healthy subjects. Measured protein requirements may be increased to as much as 2.5 g/kg to provide for anabolic wound healing and sustained immune function. For these patients, protein restriction is counterproductive and potentially detrimental. Urea generation is best minimized by providing enough energy substrates (carbohydrates and lipids) to prevent the cannibalization of endogenous protein as an energy source.

A positive energy balance may also make the management of uremia and hyperkalemia less difficult. When a patient receives fewer calories than those expended, the difference must be made up from endogenous stores. In a well-nourished person, carbohydrate stores rarely exceed 2,500 kcal. After these stores have been depleted, lipid and protein stores are mobilized. In the diseased state, endogenous protein has been shown to be catabolized preferentially as an energy substrate in the absence of readily available glucose. With the catabolism of protein, urea is generated. In addition, catabolic wasting of tissues and cells liberates excess potassium. Maintaining a positive energy balance with glucose and lipids should reduce protein catabolism, urea generation, and hyperkalemia.

Renal Replacement Therapy

Indications for the use of RRT include fluid overload (pulmonary edema, congestive heart failure), hyperkalemia, metabolic acidosis, uremic encephalopathy, coagulopathy, and acute poisoning[43] (Table 9.6). The optimal timing of initiation of therapy has not been definitively established, but it is preferable to begin renal replacement before complications occur. In one randomized controlled trial, there was no improvement in mortality or renal recovery in patients in whom RRT was initiated within 12 hours of developing ARF compared to initiation once conventional indications for dialysis were met.[44]

Three modalities of RRT are available for the treatment of ARF: intermittent HD, continuous RRT, and peritoneal dialysis. Peritoneal dialysis is performed by infusing several liters of a sterile electrolyte solution with hypertonic glucose into the abdominal space. With the peritoneal membrane used as a selective barrier, the dialysate solution creates an osmotic pressure gradient that extracts extracellular fluid and solutes out of the mesenteric circulation and into the peritoneal cavity, which is then drained after an equilibration period of 1 to 2 hours. Complications of peritoneal dialysis include hyperglycemia, respiratory distress secondary to reduced diaphragmatic compliance resulting from increased intra-abdominal pressure, and significant daily protein losses. For these reasons, peritoneal dialysis is typically not used in critically ill patients with ARF.

TABLE 9.6

PROPOSED CRITERIA FOR INITIATION OF RENAL REPLACEMENT THERAPY IN CRITICALLY ILL PATIENTS WITH ACUTE RENAL FAILURE

Pulmonary edema
Unable to meet nutritional requirements due to volume load (pulmonary edema)
Oliguria: urine output <200 mL in 12 h
Anuria: urine output <50 mL in 12 h
Hyperkalaemia: potassium concentration >6.5 mmol/L
Severe acidemia: pH <7.0
Azotaemia: urea concentration >30 mmol/L
Uremic encephalopathy
Uremic neuropathy/myopathy
Uremic pericarditis
Plasma sodium abnormalities: concentration >155 mmol/L or <120 mmol/L
Hyperthermia
Drug overdose with dialyzable toxin

Adapted from Lameire N, Van Biesen W, Vanholder R. Acute renal failure. *Lancet* 2005;365:417–430.

SCIENTIFIC PRINCIPLES

Intermittent Hemodialysis

In intermittent HD, blood is circulated through a porous, hollow-fiber membrane that is permeable to solutes of less than 2,000 d. An isotonic solution surrounding the membrane provides a concentration gradient for the selective removal of solutes such as potassium, urea, and creatinine, whereas plasma concentrations of sodium, chloride, and bicarbonate are unchanged. A roller pump is used to maintain an extracorporeal blood flow of about 300 mL/minute through an arteriovenous shunt or a double-lumen venovenous access. The transmembrane pressure gradient created by the pump affects the desired amount of fluid removal. Full systemic anticoagulation is required for this procedure, although less heparin may be used in patients with a baseline coagulopathy. Solute and volume removal with HD is considered very efficient relative to removal with the other methods of renal replacement. This efficiency is reflected in the clearance of water-soluble drugs such as aminoglycosides, cephalosporins, and penicillins. Plasma concentrations may be decreased by as much as 50% per treatment; accordingly, these drugs should be administered after treatments with close monitoring of serum concentrations. HD is also the method of choice for the rapid removal of life-threatening toxins and poisons.

Although the incidence of complications of HD is insignificant in the treatment of patients with chronic renal failure, frequent and often profound complications may occur when it is used to treat critically ill patients with ARF. In the acute setting, HD has been shown to cause hypotension, hypoxemia, and hemolysis and to precipitate cardiac arrhythmia. These events limit the application of HD in patients who are hemodynamically unstable.

Continuous Renal Replacement Therapy

Continuous renal replacement techniques offer the advantage of improved hemodynamic stability with continuous clearance of toxic metabolites and fluid removal. Continuous venovenohemodialysis (CVVHD) is the most commonly used method in the ICU. In this technique, venous access is obtained by means of a temporary double-lumen central venous dialysis catheter, which is placed percutaneously in the subclavian, internal jugular, or femoral vein. Blood is pumped by a peristaltic pump through a filter against the flow of dialysate, which is pumped into the nonblood portion of the filter in the opposite direction. Rates of fluid removal are adjusted as necessary to maintain hemodynamic stability while the concentrations of solutes in the dialysate are adjusted to ensure adequate clearance of potassium, acid and other products of uremia. Continuous arteriovenous hemodiafiltration (CAVHD) is similar to CVVHD but requires large-bore arterial access in addition to venous access. The pressure gradient between the arterial and venous limbs of the circuit, rather than a pump, drives the flow of blood in the circuit. Continuous RRT allows for slow but continuous removal of fluid and clearance of toxic wastes. Compared with intermittent HD, continuous RRT provides better hemodynamic stability, maintenance of cerebral perfusion, and control of fluid balance. It is therefore indicated in patients with renal failure and critical illness and may be the treatment of choice for ARF in this patient population.

There are no good prospective data supporting the use of continuous versus intermittent techniques in critically ill patients with ARF; thus, the choice should be dependent on local resource availability and patient-specific factors (Table 9.7). Regardless of which modality is selected, there is good evidence to suggest that "higher dose" dialysis offers benefit. In a randomized controlled trial comparing daily HD for 4 hours versus 4 hours every other day, patients in the more frequent dialysis group had a lower mortality rate and a faster recovery from ARF, which seemed most likely related to a much lower incidence of episodes of intradialytic hypotension.[45] In addition, daily HD was associated with a lower incidence of oliguria after initiation of dialysis and the development of clinical complications, such as respiratory failure, delirium, and gastrointestinal bleeding. In a study in which patients receiving CVVHD were randomized to one of

TABLE 9.7

ADVANTAGES OF INTERMITTENT HEMODIALYSIS AND CONTINUOUS RENAL REPLACEMENT THERAPY

Intermittent hemodialysis	Continuous renal replacement therapy
ADVANTAGES	
Lower risk of systemic bleeding	Better hemodynamic stability
Facilitates transport for other interventions	Fewer cardiac arrhythmias
More suitable for severe hyperkalemia	Improved nutritional support
Lower cost	Better pulmonary gas exchange
	Better fluid control
DISADVANTAGES	
Availability of dialysis staff	Greater vascular access problems
More difficult hemodynamic control	Higher risk of systemic bleeding
Inadequate dialysis dose (frequency)	Long-term immobilization of patient
Inadequate fluid control	More filter problems (rupture, clotting)
Inadequate nutritional support	Greater cost
Not suitable for patients with intracranial hypertension	
No removal of cytokines (theoretical)	
Potential complement activation by non-biocompatible membranes	

Adapted from Lameire N, Van Biesen W, Vanholder R. Acute renal failure. *Lancet* 2005;365:417–430.

three doses of hemofiltration (20 mL/kg/day, 35 mL/kg/day, and 45mL/kg/day adjusted by changes in pump blood flow rate), patients randomized to the low hemofiltration group had a significantly higher mortality than the other two groups after adjustment for severity of illness.[46]

Prognosis in Acute Renal Failure

The survival of patients with ARF depends on the successful treatment of the primary disease causing renal failure. The anephric patient supported with RRT survives until disease of some other organ system supervenes. In a study of patients with "pure" acute tubular necrosis after renal transplantation, Mentzer et al. reported the mortality rate of ischemic acute tubular necrosis without other organ failure to be 6%. In contrast, the mortality rate of multiple-organ failure complicated by ARF ranges from 50% to 90%.

For patients who survive the acute phase of illness, the recovery of renal function after ARF depends on the type and extent of injury to the renal parenchyma. RRT may be required for several weeks until urine output and solute excretion return to acceptable levels. If renal function has not returned after 6 weeks, recovery is unlikely, and provisions should be made for long-term renal substitution therapy.

PROGNOSTICATION AND INTENSIVE CARE UNIT OUTCOME

The critical care environment is filled with an abundance of data. Data are collected at the time of admission and almost daily, allowing repeated assessment of physiologic status over time. This data-rich environment has led to the development of scoring systems that provide information regarding the likelihood of survival based on information available early during the course of the ICU stay. Many systems that have been developed focus not on prognosticating survival but rather on the assessment of outcome, typically in the degree of organ dysfunction. The differences in these two approaches are highlighted in Table 9.8.

Prognostic Scoring Systems

Prognostic scores were developed to maximize their predictive capacity. The APACHE, the simplified acute physiology score (SAPS II), and the mortality prediction model (MPM) systems constitute the three most widely used prognostic models. Each model assumes that mortality will be influenced by extreme physiologic derangement that occurs early in the course of the illness and before optimal resuscitation. Each uses data that are available early in the ICU admission to construct a composite severity of illness measure.

The most frequently utilized prognostic score is the APACHE II system, comprising data derived from 12 physiologic variables, age, and chronic health status, yielding a score of 0 to 71. Major limitations of this system include the fact that risk predictions are based on outcomes of treatment from 1979–1982; the system was not designed to predict outcome for individual patients; and there is lead time bias—unless all admissions were entered at the same time in the course of the patient's illness, there will be errors in prediction. APACHE III is a more recent model and is derived from information on 17 variables. APACHE III is proprietary and has not been widely adopted.

SAPS II is composed of 17 variables, which include 12 physiologic variables, age, type of admission (medical, surgical, scheduled surgical, unscheduled surgical), and variables that are related to specific underlying diseases. The MPM is less based on physiology than APACHE II or SAPS and was designed to measure mortality risk at 24 and 48 hours after ICU admission. This longer time interval provides a revised risk based on patient response to resuscitation and early treatment. There are minor differences across these prognostic measures in terms of their predictive capacity, but there are no data to support that one offers significant improvement over another. Pertinent to the discussion on futility (see later), these severity of illness systems provide only estimates of mortality. For example, a mortality estimate of 75% means that approximately 75 of 100 patients with this probability would be expected to die, but it is not possible to ascertain whether any specific, individual patient will be 1 of the 75 patients that dies or 1 of the 25 that lives.

TABLE 9.8

SCORING SYSTEMS IN THE ICU

	Prognostic scales: severity of illness	Outcome measures: organ dysfunction scales
Uses	Prognostication; risk stratification	Outcome prediction; evaluation of clinical course over time
Timing of ascertainment	Early during ICU stay	Following resuscitation; at any time during ICU stay
Selection of variables	Physiologic measures	Measures of physiology or therapeutic response
	Worst values	Stable, representative values
	Selected to maximize predictive capacity	Selected to reflect clinical construct
Calibration	Maximize prediction	Maximize description

ICU, intensive care unit.
From Marshall JC. Risk prediction and outcome description in critical surgical illness. In: Norton JA, Bollinger RR, eds. *Surgery basic science and clinical evidence*. New York: Springer Verlag; 2001:306.

TABLE 9.9

ORGAN DYSFUNCTION SCORING: THE MARSHALL MULTIPLE ORGAN DYSFUNCTION SCORE

Organ system	0	1	2	3	4
Respiratory (PaO_2/FIO_2)	>300	226–300	151–225	76–150	≤75
Renal (serum creatinine, mg/dL)	≤1.1	1.2–2.3	2.4–3.9	4.0–5.6	>5.7
Hepatic (serum bilirubin, mg/dL)	≤1.1	1.2–3.5	3.6–7.1	7.2–14.1	>14.2
Cardiovascular (PAR*)	≤10.0	10.1–15.0	15.1–20.0	20.1–30.0	>30.0
Hematologic (platelet count × 10^{-3})	>120	81–120	51–80	21–50	≤20
Neurologic (Glasgow coma score)	15	13–14	10–12	7–9	≤6

*

Adapted from Marshall JC, Cook DJ, Christou NV, et al. Multiple organ dysfunction score: a reliable descriptor of a complex clinical outcome. *Crit Care Med.* 1995;23:1638.

Outcome Measures

Organ failure is a relatively frequent occurrence in critically ill patients and has resulted in attempts to describe and quantify organ dysfunction. This is a difficult process because organ failure is dynamic and represents a broad spectrum of disease. Which organ systems to include and which measures one should use to quantitate organ dysfunction remain controversial. Most scores focus on six organ systems: respiratory, cardiovascular, hematologic, central nervous system, renal, and hepatic. These outcome measures have conceptual appeal for several reasons. First, they provide an estimate of baseline severity for entry into clinical trials, whereas serial evaluation might provide information on mortality risk. With these organ dysfunction measures, the burden of disease experienced by the patient throughout the course of ICU stay is captured. By contrast, with prognostic scoring systems there is but an early snapshot of the patient's physiologic status, whereas information regarding the remainder of the patient's course is lost.

The most commonly used outcome measures include the Sequential Organ Failure Assessment (SOFA) Score and the Multiple Organ Dysfunction (MOD) Score or Marshall Score, both of which capture data on the six aforementioned systems (Table 9.9). A Marshall score of ≥4 (≥6 in select studies) is used to indicate MOD. By contrast, post-traumatic multiple organ failure is often assessed using a discrete scoring system limited to only four organ systems (also known as the Denver Score).[47] Hematologic dysfunction and neurologic dysfunction are not captured, likely due to the frequency of coagulopathy and traumatic brain injury, which relate to the initial injury rather than the development of organ dysfunction. A Denver score of ≥4 is indicative of MOD. Like the prognostic scoring systems, no single measure of organ dysfunction is superior.

ETHICS IN THE INTENSIVE CARE UNIT

The availability of advanced technologies to prolong life in the ICU has resulted in a number of controversies centered on their appropriate use. The controversies have developed under the guise of the technologic imperative, implying that the availability of technology requires that this technology be used. To counter the technologic imperative, physicians have often invoked the concept of futility to limit its inappropriate use, resulting in confusion and, at times, conflict when caring for critically ill patients.

In the strictest sense, true medical futility occurs rarely and signifies interventions that simply should not be offered. For example, we do not offer ongoing medical care to a patient who meets criteria for brain death. The majority of therapies that physicians judge to be futile are not truly futile. They should more accurately be considered inadvisable or inappropriate because the chances of achieving the intended goal are exceedingly low, their benefits are controversial, or their costs are excessively great. Implicit in this definition is a clear understanding of the real or perceived therapeutic endpoint, that is, it is meaningless to say an intervention is futile without specifying the goal of the intended therapy. Conflicts arise when there are disagreements about the intended goal, whether the desired goal is appropriate, and whether the probability of success is sufficiently great. In this sense, there are both qualitative (value-driven) and quantitative (probabilistic) aspects to the understanding and application of futility in the ICU.

Quantitative futility describes a clinical situation in which the application of an intervention has a very low probability of producing a satisfactory outcome—usually survival. There have been a large number of prognostic scoring systems developed to compare outcomes in large groups of patients. Although these scoring systems were not devised to predict outcome in individual patients, there has been some effort on the part of physicians to adapt these measures for this purpose. In effect, if the probability of survival is below a certain threshold, the intervention might be considered futile or inadvisable and not instituted. Physicians are not very capable at assigning an estimated probability of outcome for an individual patient. Further, this threshold varies across physicians and patients, making decisions based on quantitative futility difficult.

Qualitative futility describes the clinical situation in which the outcome is survival but with an unsatisfactory quality of life. Excellent examples of qualitative futility include patients in a persistent vegetative state or patients dependent on intensive medical care. Conflict arises when what is defined as unsatisfactory for one party might be acceptable for the other. For example, the family of a critically ill, severely debilitated elderly stroke patient might consider the maintenance of life of greatest importance, whereas the physicians believe that given the expected quality of life, further care would be futile.

Inappropriate declarations of futility are common; we rarely can predict with absolute certainty whether a patient will survive their ICU stay. In effect, we offer opinions colored by our own values not objective data. The tendencies to frame value judgments as medical decisions based on such data are inappropriate. Therapeutic interventions should be directed not toward eliciting a desired physiologic effect but toward an agreed on goal that is consistent with the wishes of the patient while maintaining professional integrity. Failure to reach the prespecified goal renders the treatment futile. Intensivists should consider the use of ethics consultations when the goals cannot be agreed on or when confusion exists. Consultation with an ethicist is not to decide the answer but to receive input from an impartial individual who often brings a fresh approach to a difficult situation. In one randomized controlled trial, the use of ethics consultations shortened the duration of ICU stay and reduced the use of life-sustaining treatments without altering overall mortality.[48] In this study, the majority of physicians, nurses, and patients/surrogates agreed that ethics consultations in the ICU were helpful in addressing treatment conflicts.

KEY POINTS

- **Critical care units provide monitoring to identify and guide intervention prior to life-threatening physiologic deterioration and utilize advanced technology to support failing organs until treatment and recovery can occur.**
- **Oxygen delivery to tissues must match cellular metabolic needs. To prevent cellular failure, adequate tissue oxygenation relies on oxygen-carrying capacity of blood (hemoglobin), loading of oxygen (gas exchange), and cardiac output (heart function).**
- **Respiratory dysfunction involves inadequate gas exchange, ventilation, or both. Oxygenation requires matching pulmonary perfusion to alveolar ventilation, whereas CO_2 excretion relies primarily only on ventilation. Ventilator support should be tailored to individual needs.**
- **Excessive transfusion (hematocrit >21 mL/dL) and hyperglycemia (blood glucose >110 mg/dL) have each been shown to correlate with increased complications and mortality.**
- **Full nutritional support (enteral route preferred) based on estimated needs should be provided as soon as possible. Carbohydrates should match metabolic needs to protect against excess nitrogen losses from protein breakdown. Essential fatty acids, vitamins, and mineral intake should recognize excessive losses in the critically ill.**
- **Acute renal failure rarely occurs as an isolated organ failure. Dialysis is indicated for fluid overload, acidosis, electrolyte abnormalities, or coagulopathy. Replacement therapy should preferably be continuous arteriovenous or venovenous dialysis.**
- **Multiple scores of critical illness have been developed to produce both an objective prognosis in the critically ill and an assessment of outcome by utilizing multiple organ failure severity.**

References

1. Brilli RJ, Spevetz A, Branson RD, et al. Critical care delivery in the intensive care unit: defining clinical roles and the best practice model. *Crit Care Med.* 2001;29:2007–2019.
2. Ghorra S, Reinert SE, Cioffi W, et al. Analysis of the effect of conversion from open to closed surgical intensive care unit. *Ann Surg.* 1999;229:163–171.
3. Hanson III CW, Deutschman CS, Anderson III HL, et al. Effects of an organized critical care service on outcomes and resource utilization: a cohort study. *Crit Care Med.* 1999;27:270–274.
4. Pronovost PJ, Jenckes MW, Dorman T, et al. Organizational characteristics of intensive care units related to outcomes of abdominal aortic surgery. *JAMA.* 1999;281:1310–1317.
5. Pronovost PJ, Angus DC, Dorman T, et al. Physician staffing patterns and clinical outcomes in critically ill patients: a systematic review. *JAMA.* 2002;288:2151–2162.
6. Haupt MT, Bekes CE, Brilli RJ, et al. Guidelines on critical care services and personnel: recommendations based on a system of categorization of three levels of care. *Crit Care Med.* 2003;31:2677–2683.
7. Cheatham ML, Nelson LD, Chang MC, Safcsak K. Right ventricular end-diastolic volume index as a predictor of preload status in patients on positive end-expiratory pressure. *Crit Care Med.* 1998;26:1801–1806.
8. Phang PT, Cunningham KF, Ronco JJ, et al. Mathematical coupling explains dependence of oxygen consumption on oxygen delivery in ARDS. *Am J Respir Crit Care Med.* 1994;150:318–323.
9. Ronco JJ, Fenwick JC, Tweeddale MG, et al. Identification of the critical oxygen delivery for anaerobic metabolism in critically ill septic and nonseptic humans. *JAMA.* 1993;270:1724–1730.
10. Gattinoni L, Brazzi L, Pelosi P, et al. A trial of goal-oriented hemodynamic therapy in critically ill patients. *N Engl J Med.* 1995;19:1025–1032.
11. Hayes MA, Timmins AC, Yau EHS, et al. Elevation of systemic oxygen delivery in the treatment of critically ill patients. *N Engl J Med.* 1994;330:1717–1722.
12. Velmahos GC, Demetriades D, Shoemaker WC, et al. Endpoints of resuscitation of critically injured patients: normal or supranormal? A prospective randomized trial. *Ann Surg.* 2000;232:409–418.
13. Dellinger RP, Carlet JM, Masur H, et al. Surviving sepsis campaign guidelines for management of severe sepsis and septic shock. *Crit Care Med.* 2004;32:858–873.
14. Connors AF, Speroff T, Dawson NV, et al. The effectiveness of right heart catheterization in the initial care of critically ill patients. *JAMA.* 1996;276:889–897.
15. Hodes A, Cusack RJ, Newman PJ, et al. A randomised, controlled trial of the pulmonary artery catheter in critically ill patients. *Intensive Care Med.* 2002;28:256–264.
16. Richard C, Warszawski J, Anguel N, et al. Early use of the pulmonary artery catheter and outcomes in patients with shock and acute respiratory distress syndrome: a randomized controlled trial. *JAMA* 2003;290:2713–20.
17. Rivers E, Nguyen B, Havstad S, et al. Early Goal-Directed Therapy Collaborative Group. Early goal-directed therapy in the treatment of severe sepsis and septic shock. *N Engl J Med.* 2001;345:1368–1377.
18. Valtier B, Cholley BP, Belot JP, et al. Noninvasive monitoring of cardiac output in critically ill patients using transesophageal Doppler. *Am J Respir Crit Care Med.* 1998;158:77–83.
19. Berton C, Cholley B. Equipment review: new techniques for cardiac output measurement—oesophageal Doppler, Fick principle using carbon dioxide, and pulse contour analysis. *Crit Care* 2002;6:216–221.
20. Gattinoni L, Caironi P, Pelosi P, Goodman LR. What has computed tomography taught us about the acute respiratory distress syndrome? *Am J Respir Crit Care Med.* 2001;164:1701–1711.
21. Bernard GR, Artigas A, Brigham KL, et al. The American–European Consensus Conference on ARDS. Definitions, mechanisms, relevant outcomes, and clinical trial coordination. *Am J Respir Crit Care Med.* 1994;149:818–824.
22. Ventilation with lower tidal volumes as compared with traditional tidal volumes for acute lung injury and the acute respiratory distress syndrome. The Acute Respiratory Distress Syndrome Network. *N Engl J Med.* 2000;342:1301–1308.
23. Brower RG, Lanken PN, MacIntyre N, et al. Higher versus lower positive end-expiratory pressures in patients with the acute respiratory distress syndrome. *N Engl J Med.* 2004;351:327–336.
24. Ely EW, Baker AM, Dunagan DP, et al. Effect on the duration of mechanical ventilation of identifying patients capable of breathing spontaneously. *N Engl J Med.* 1996;335:1864–1869.
25. Esteban A, Frutos F, Tobin MJ, et al. A comparison of four methods of weaning patients from mechanical ventilation. Spanish Lung Failure Collaborative Group. *N Engl J Med.* 1995;332:345–350.
26. Esteban A, Alia I, Tobin MJ, et al. Effect of spontaneous breathing trial duration on outcome of attempts to discontinue mechanical ventilation. Spanish Lung Failure Collaborative Group. *Am J Respir Crit Care Med.* 1999;159:512–518.
27. MacIntyre NR, Cook DJ, Ely EW Jr, et al. Evidence-based guidelines for weaning and discontinuing ventilatory support: a collective task force facilitated by the American College of Chest Physicians; the American Association for Respiratory Care; and the American College of Critical Care Medicine. *Chest* 2001;120[6 Suppl]:375S–395S.
28. Corwin HL, Gettinger A, Pearl RG, et al. The CRIT Study: anemia and blood transfusion in the critically ill—current clinical practice in the United States. *Crit Care Med.* 2004;32:39–52.
29. Corwin HL, Parsonnet KC, Gettinger A. RBC transfusion in the ICU. Is there a reason? *Chest* 1995;108:767–771.
30. Silverman HJ, Tuma P. Gastric tonometry in patients with sepsis. Effects of dobutamine infusions and packed red blood cell transfusions. *Chest* 1992;102:184–188.
31. Marik PE, Sibbald WJ. Effect of stored-blood transfusion on oxygen delivery in patients with sepsis. *JAMA.* 1993;269:3024–3029.
32. Hebert PC, Wells G, Blajchman MA, et al. A multicenter, randomized controlled clinical trial of transfusion requirements in critical care. *N Engl J Med.* 1999;340:409–417.
33. Hebert PC, Blajchman MA, Cook DJ, et al. Do blood transfusions improve outcomes related to mechanical ventilation? *Chest* 2001;119:1850–1857.
34. Hebert PC, Yetisir E, Martin C, et al. Is a low transfusion threshold safe in critically ill patients with cardiovascular diseases? *Crit Care Med.* 2001;29:227–234.
35. Corwin HL, Gettinger A, Pearl RG, et al. Efficacy of recombinant human erythropoietin in critically ill patients: a randomized controlled trial. *JAMA.* 2002;288:2827–2835.
36. Battistella FD, Widergren JT, Anderson JT, et al. A prospective, randomized trial of intravenous fat emulsion administration in trauma victims requiring total parenteral nutrition. *J Trauma* 1997;43:52–58.
37. Nathens AB, Neff MJ, Jurkovich GJ, et al. Randomized, prospective trial of antioxidant supplementation in critically ill surgical patients. *Ann Surg.* 2002;236:814–822.

38. Marik PE, Zaloga GP. Early enteral nutrition in acutely ill patients: a systematic review. *Crit Care Med.* 2001;29:2264–2270.
39. Montejo JC, Grau T, Acosta J, et al. Multicenter, prospective, randomized, single-blind study comparing the efficacy and gastrointestinal complications of early jejunal feeding with early gastric feeding in critically ill patients. *Crit Care Med.* 2002;30:796–800.
40. Heyland DK, Novak F, Drover JW, et al. Should immunonutrition become routine in critically ill patients? A systematic review of the evidence. *JAMA.* 2001;286:944–953.
41. Montejo JC, Zarazaga A, Lopez-Martinez J, et al. Immunonutrition in the intensive care unit. A systematic review and consensus statement. *Clin Nutr.* 2003;22:221–233.
42. Van den BG, Wouters P, Weekers F, et al. Intensive insulin therapy in the critically ill patients. *N Engl J Med.* 2001;345:1359–1367.
43. Lameire N, Van Biesen W, Vanholder R. Acute renal failure. *Lancet* 2005;365:417–430.
44. Bouman CS, Oudemans-Van Straaten HM, Tijssen JG, et al. Effects of early high-volume continuous venovenous hemofiltration on survival and recovery of renal function in intensive care patients with acute renal failure: a prospective, randomized trial. *Crit Care Med.* 2002;30: 2205–2211.
45. Schiffl H, Lang SM, Fischer R. Daily hemodialysis and the outcome of acute renal failure. *N Engl J Med.* 2002;346:305–310.
46. Ronco C, Belomo R, Homel P, et al. Effects of different doses in continuous veno-venous haemofiltration on outcomes of acute renal failure: a prospective randomised trial. *EDTNA ERCA J.* 2002;[Suppl 2]:7–12.
47. Sauaia A, Moore FA, Moore EE, et al. Early predictors of postinjury multiple organ failure. *Arch Surg.* 1994;129:39–45.
48. Schneiderman LJ, Gilmer T, Teetzel HD, et al. Effect of ethics consultations on nonbeneficial life-sustaining treatments in the intensive care setting: a randomized controlled trial. *JAMA.* 2003;290:1166–1172.

CHAPTER 10 ■ FLUIDS, ELECTROLYTES, AND ACID–BASE BALANCE

RICHARD B. WAIT AND NEAL E. SEYMOUR

A thorough understanding of fluid and electrolyte composition and management is essential to the effective care of surgical and critically ill patients. Disease- and injury-related alterations in fluid volume and electrolyte physiology are complex and cannot be fully understood without first understanding normal physiologic mechanisms of fluid and electrolyte homeostasis, inclusive of acid–base balance considerations. In this chapter, these mechanisms are reviewed and used as a starting point for presentation of fluid and electrolyte pathophysiology and management of specific clinical situations. Newer fluid administration options are also discussed.

BODY FLUIDS

Total Body Water and Body Fluid Compartments

Traditionally, most scientists used a two-compartment model of tissues within the body: the fat compartment and the fat-free or lean tissue compartment. Over the past 20 years, technology has added significantly to our knowledge of body composition, and more complex models have been developed, the simplest of which is the four-compartment model. In this model, the fat-free mass is actually composed of three separate compartments: water, protein, and bone ash. The remaining compartment is fat, which is considered to be triglycerides, because adipose tissue, a more general descriptor, also contains small amounts of water. *Total body water* (TBW) is defined as the total volume of water within the body. TBW has traditionally been measured using indicator dilution techniques in which radioactive tracers such as deuterium oxide (D_2O) were given to subjects and a steady state allowed to develop before measurements of the D_2O in the plasma were made. More recently, other techniques have added greatly to our ability to measure TBW content as well as the content of all of the elements within the body. Perhaps the most sophisticated method of measurement of body composition, involves *neutron activation analysis,* techniques in which the body is exposed to a source of thermal neutrons. These neutrons enter the atomic nuclei, resulting in the transformation of that nucleus to a more activated energy state. This activated state is transient and later returns to the baseline, resulting in energy release from the nucleus in the form of gamma radiation, which can then be measured using whole-body shielded gamma detectors.[1] Using these techniques, total body oxygen, carbon, hydrogen, nitrogen, calcium, phosphorus, sulfur, potassium, sodium, and chlorine can be measured. These measurements, in turn, can be used to calculate steady state body composition using standard formulas. For example, total body protein can be calculated as total body nitrogen × 0.625, because 99% of the body's nitrogen is found within protein. More complex mathematical models are needed when calculating the composition of components using elements that are distributed among more than one component of the body (e.g., TBW and fat).

The relationship between TBW and body weight varies according to percentage of body fat. Differences in percent TBW between individuals can generally be accounted for by differences in relative body fat content. Average TBW is 60% of body weight in adult men and 50% in adult women. In infants, water makes up approximately 80% of body weight. This figure decreases to approximately 65% by 1 year of age and continues to decrease slowly throughout life, primarily related to decreases in lean body mass. Estimates of TBW can be empirically adjusted for the obese and thin body habitus. In obesity, estimates of TBW can be decreased by 10% to 20%. In very thin individuals, estimates can be increased by up to 10%.

TBW is distributed into specific compartments in dynamic equilibrium with one another. The principal of these are the intracellular and extracellular compartments (Table 10.1). Intracellular fluid (ICF) makes up approximately two thirds of the TBW, and the remaining one third is composed of

TABLE 10.1

BODY FLUID COMPARTMENTS

	Body weight (%)	Total body water (%)
Total	60	100
Intracellular	40	67
Extracellular	20	33
Intravascular	5	8
Interstitial	15	25
Transcellular	2	4

extracellular fluid (ECF). The ECF compartment has traditionally been measured using *inulin,* which distributes itself primarily within the ECF. More recently, ECF estimates have been made by measuring the volume of distribution of either bromide or sulfate isotopes, both of which are distributed primarily within the ECF. Using these techniques, ECF volume estimates range from 30% to 33% of TBW, or approximately 20% of body weight.

ICF cannot be measured directly, however, because the majority of potassium within the body resides within the intracellular space; measurements of total body potassium (TBK) can be used to estimate intracellular water. This is accomplished using a technique similar to neutron activation analysis. Normally, potassium within the body exists in two states, nonradioactive ^{39}K and radioactive ^{40}K. Because ^{40}K represents a stable proportion of total K within the body (0.0118%), measurement of the gamma radiation of the ^{40}K radioisotope using the sensing equipment similar to that used in neutron activation analysis can be accomplished. The TBK can then be calculated as TBK (mmol) = $^{40}K/0.000118$.[2] If one knows the size of the ECF compartment and multiplies this by the known quantity of ^{40}K measured in a serum sample, the ICF can then be calculated by subtracting this total from the TBK.

The ECF compartment is subdivided into the intravascular, and interstitial spaces. The intravascular space accounts for 25% of the ECF and contains the plasma volume, which is approximately 8% of the TBW or 5% of body weight. Interstitial water volume is calculated as ECF—intravascular space volume and constitutes approximately 25% of TBW, or 15% of body weight. The interstitial space extends from the blood vessels to the cells themselves and includes the complex ground substance making up the acellular tissue matrix. The water in this space exists in free and bound phases. The free phase contains water that is freely exchangeable with intravascular, lymphatic, and intracellular water and that is in a constant state of flux. The bound or *gel* phase is much less freely exchangeable and is composed of water that hydrates matrix materials such as glycosaminoglycans and mucopolysaccharides. The transcellular space, a third and smaller component of ECF, consists of water that is separated from other compartments by endothelial and epithelial barriers, including cerebrospinal, ocular, and synovial fluids, as well as fluid in the gastrointestinal (GI) tract. Under normal circumstances, fluid in the transcellular space is not easily exchangeable with that in other compartments.

Composition of Body Fluids

Sodium and potassium are the dominant cations in the body. Sodium is restricted primarily to the ECF and potassium to the ICF. Sodium content in the average adult is approximately 60 mEq/kg. Approximately 25% is confined to bone and is nonexchangeable. Of the exchangeable fraction, approximately 85% is in the ECF. Potassium, calcium, and magnesium make up the remainder of the cations present in the ECF. As mentioned, potassium is the dominant cation in the ICF. TBK is normally approximately 42 mEq/kg, and most of this potassium is intracellular and freely exchangeable. Magnesium and sodium ions also contribute to the cationic component of the ICF. These cations are balanced by phosphate and sulfate anions as well as bicarbonate and intracellular proteins (Table 10.2).

Similarly, ECF cations are in electrochemical balance with chloride, bicarbonate, phosphate, and sulfate anions, although chloride is the major contributor to this balance. In addition, anionic proteins contribute to ion balance in plasma but not in interstitial fluid, which is essentially an ultrafiltrate of plasma that normally contains little protein. As a result, the content of

TABLE 10.2

ELECTROLYTE CONCENTRATIONS OF INTRACELLULAR AND EXTRACELLULAR FLUID COMPARTMENTS

	Extracellular fluid (mEq/L)		
	Plasma	Interstitial	Intracellular fluid (mEq/L)
Cations			
Na^+	140	146	12
K^+	4	4	150
Ca^{2+}	5	3	10^{-7}
Mg^{2+}	2	1	7
Anions			
Cl^-	103	114	3
HCO_3^-	24	27	10
SO_4^{2-}	1	1	—
HPO_4^{3-}	2	2	116
Protein	16	5	40
Organic anions	5	5	—

both cations and anions in interstitial fluid are slightly higher than in plasma (see Table 10.2).

The Donnan equilibrium describes the relationship between solutions of permeable and impermeable complex anions when these anions are unevenly distributed across a semipermeable membrane. This special type of equilibrium exists between the ICF and ECF because of the high concentration of protein and nondiffusible phosphates in the cell. Interstitial fluid, by comparison, contains little protein. These impermeable intracellular negative charges tend to favor diffusion of permeant anions into the ECF. The Donnan equilibrium also exists across the capillary endothelial membrane because the concentration of protein is higher on the blood side of the capillary than on the interstitial fluid side. Thus, the concentrations of diffusible ions are not necessarily equal across these membranes because of the presence of these complex anions.

Concentration of Body Fluids

Despite the difference in composition between the ECF and ICF, the overall concentration of solutes in water in these fluids is identical. Transient concentration differences may develop; however, because water freely equilibrates between compartments, these quickly disappear. The concentration of solutes in the fluid compartments depends on the osmotic activity generated by the ion species contained in each compartment.

Osmotic Activity of Body Fluids

When two solutions are separated by a semipermeable membrane, water moves across the membrane to equalize the concentration of osmotically active particles to which the membrane is impermeable. The maintenance of osmotic equilibrium across a semipermeable membrane is based primarily on the number of solute particles rather than on the molar concentration of the solution on each side of the membrane. The correct measurement to reflect osmotic activity is made by multiplying the molar concentration of the substance by the number of particles into which it can freely dissociate in water. The unit of measurement of osmotically active particles is the osmole (Osm) or milliosmole (mOsm) rather than the conventional units of solute concentration such as milliequivalents per liter (mEq/L). When one mol of NaCl dissociates in water to Na^+ and Cl^-, it produces two osm. The same relationship holds true of dissociating salts of multivalent ions such as calcium and magnesium. One mol of a nondissociating molecule, such as glucose, produces one osm (1,000 mOsm). Osmolarity (mOsm/L) and osmolality (mOsm/kg water) define the osmotic activity of particles in solution. The measured osmolality of a solution may not equal the calculated osmolality if the ions do not totally dissociate. The osmotic coefficient of a solution describes the degree to which dissociation of the ions in solution occurs, and can be calculated as follows:

Osmotic coefficient = observed (measured) osmolality/calculated osmolality

Body fluids are aqueous solutions composed of water and various solutes within the different body fluid compartments. Because cells are bounded by a semipermeable membrane, adding free water to the fluid surrounding a cell causes water to move across the cell membrane to equalize the osmolality differential between the intracellular and extracellular compartments. On a larger scale, adding free water to the ECF of the body causes an immediate expansion of the extracellular space, followed by a redistribution of water into the intracellular compartment (Fig. 10.1A).

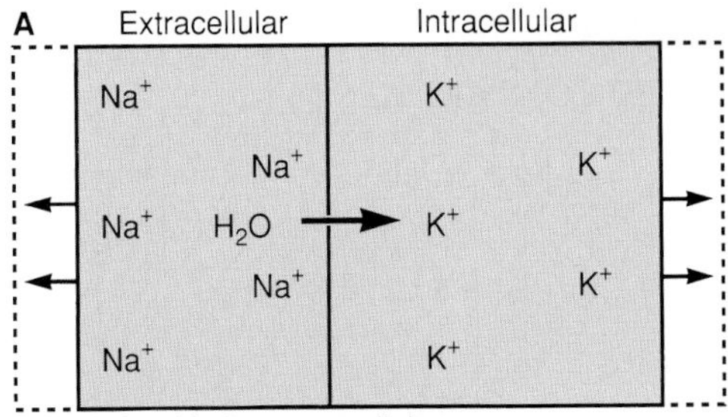

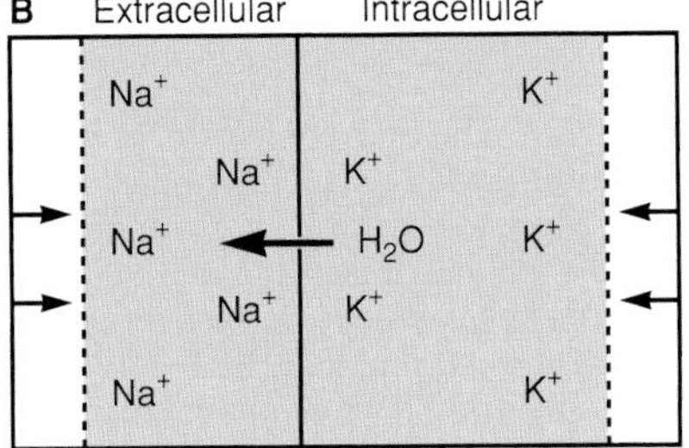

FIGURE 10.1 (*A*) The equilibration of water from the extracellular to the intracellular space after the addition of free water to the extracellular fluid compartment. Osmolality transiently decreases in the extracellular compartment, causing water to move across the cell membranes into the intracellular space. (*B*) Similar shifts after free water loss from the extracellular compartment. Water moves from the intracellular space to the extracellular space in response to the osmolal gradient that is established.

Conversely, loss of free water from the extracellular space ultimately leads to a shift of water from the intracellular to the extracellular space (see Fig. 10.1B). An osmotic gradient of just 1 mOsm generates a pressure gradient of 19.3 mm Hg.

Whereas *osmolality* defines the concentration of osmotically active particles in solution, *tonicity* refers to the effect of the particles on cell volume. Permeant solutes can freely cross cell membranes, whereas impermeant solutes cannot. Although permeant solutes contribute to the osmolality of a solution, they have no effect on tonicity because they contribute neither to oncotic gradients across cell membranes nor to alterations in cell volume. Sodium is an example of an impermeant solute that affects both osmolality and tonicity. Urea and ethanol are permeant solutes that contribute to osmolality but have little effect on tonicity because they distribute equally across membranes.

Both impermeant and permeant solutes can contribute to *hyperosmolar* and *hypoosmolar* states. However, hypoosmolar states are always accompanied by hypotonicity, whereas hyperosmolar states are not always associated with hypertonicity. There may be marked hyperosmolality without hypertonicity with elevation of blood urea nitrogen (BUN) levels because urea is a freely permeable molecule. In contrast, elevated levels of plasma glucose in diabetic patients is associated with hyperosmolarity and associated hypertonicity. Insulin increases the transport of glucose across cell membranes, rendering these osmoles *ineffective* and reducing hypertonicity. Plasma hyperglycemia is associated with the movement of intracellular water to the extracellular space. This causes expansion of ECF and plasma volume and a consequent decrease in the concentration of plasma sodium. For every 100 mg/dL elevation in blood glucose, measured serum sodium falls 1.5 mEq/L, without an actual alteration of body sodium content. This fluid shift and apparent hyponatremia, termed *pseudohyponatremia,* are corrected with insulin administration, as glucose moves into the cells water follows and, thus, no longer contributes to the hypertonic state.

Plasma osmolality (P_{osm}) is an excellent measure of total body osmolality. Osmolality differentials between fluid compartments are only transient because fluid shifts maintain isosmotic conditions. Sodium is the predominant extracellular cation; thus, estimates of P_{osm} can be made by simply doubling the serum sodium concentration (serum [Na^+]):

$$P_{osm}\ (\text{mOsm/L}) = 2 \times \text{serum}\ [Na^+]$$

Because glucose and BUN may make significant contributions to P_{osm} in certain disease states, this formula is modified for glucose and for BUN:

$$P_{osm}\ (\text{mOsm/L}) = 2 \times \text{serum}\ [Na^+] + \text{glucose}/18 + \text{BUN}/2.8$$

Discrepancies of greater than 15 mOsm/L between calculated P_{osm} and P_{osm} measured in the clinical laboratory may be the result of the presence of other osmotically active particles, such as mannitol, ethanol, or ethylene glycol, or of a reduced fraction of plasma water secondary to high levels of myeloma proteins or hypertriglyceridemia.

Colloid Oncotic Pressure (Colloid Osmotic Pressure)

Plasma proteins are confined primarily to the intravascular space and contribute to the osmotic pressure developed between the plasma and the interstitial fluid. Normal plasma protein levels of 7 g/dL contribute approximately 0.8 mOsm/L. The van't Hoff equation is used to convert osmolality to osmotic pressure:

$$p = CRT$$

where p = osmotic pressure, C = osmolal solute concentration, R = gas constant, and T = absolute temperature. At body temperature, each milliosmole develops a 19.3 mm Hg pressure gradient; thus, normal plasma protein concentrations generate a colloid oncotic pressure of 15.4 mm Hg (19.3 mm Hg × 0.8 mOsm/L). When measured directly, plasma oncotic pressure equals approximately 24 mm Hg. The difference between the calculated and measured pressures is due to the shift in solute particles caused by the pressure of protein anions on one side of a semipermeable membrane as explained by the Donnan equilibrium.

Osmoregulation

Osmolality of body fluids stays fairly constant at approximately 289 mOsm/L as the result of tightly regulated water balance. Osmoreceptor cells in the paraventricular and supraoptic nuclei of the hypothalamus exert central control over the thirst mechanism and antidiuretic hormone (ADH) secretion from the posterior pituitary. In the presence of excess free water, ECF osmolality falls toward 280 mOsm/kg H_2O, thirst is inhibited, and ADH levels decline. In the absence of ADH, the permeability of renal collecting tubules to water is decreased causing free water reabsorption to decrease and excretion to increase. Urine osmolality (U_{osm}) can decline to 100 mOsm/kg H_2O (Fig. 10.2). As excess free water is eliminated, P_{osm} begins to rise. Conversely, free water depletion causes an increase in P_{osm}. As P_{osm} approaches 295 mOsm/kg H_2O, thirst is stimulated as is ADH secretion. As ADH levels rise to approximately 5 pg/mL, the renal collecting tubules become maximally permeable to water. Water is reabsorbed from the collecting ducts in response to the concentration gradient developed in the renal medullary interstitium. Thus, the final concentration of urine depends on both the permeability of the collecting ducts (controlled by ADH secretion) and the concentration of the medullary interstitium. Maximal U_{osm} may approach 1200 mOsm/kg H_2O. The net effect of these mechanisms is to promptly return high or low P_{osm} to normal. The high sensitivity of the osmoreceptors, and the responsiveness of the ADH feedback system, ensures that even small changes in P_{osm} result in marked alterations in urine concentration. This relation can be expressed as follows:

$$\text{Urine osmolality} = 95 \times \text{plasma osmolality}$$

Thus a 1 mOsm change in P_{osm} results in a 95-fold change in U_{osm}.

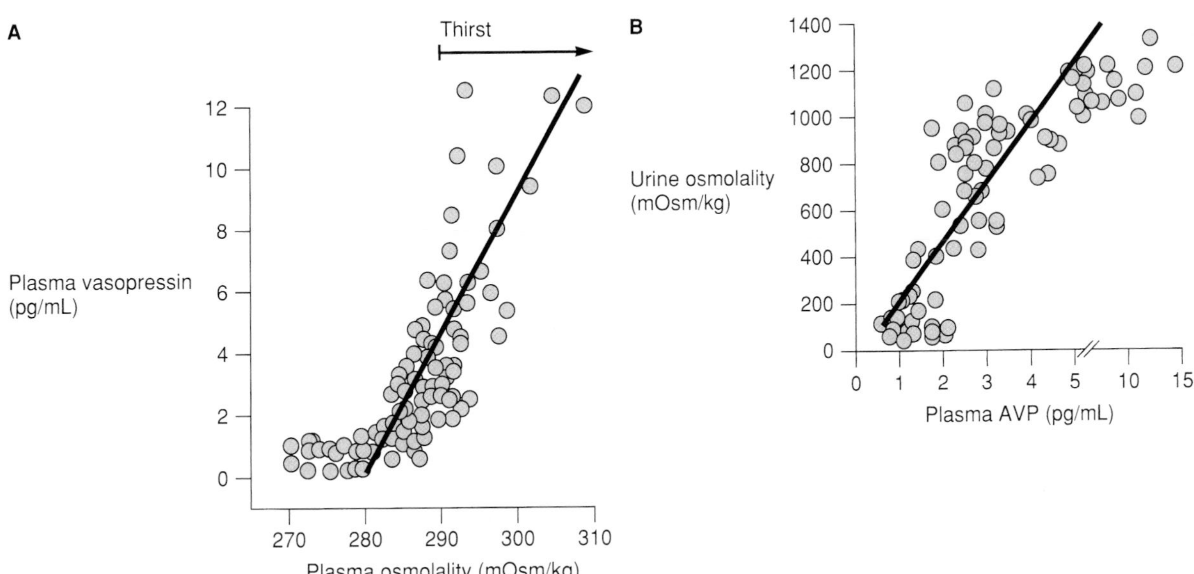

FIGURE 10.2 The relation of plasma antidiuretic hormone (arginine vasopressin or AVP) secretion to plasma (*A*) and urine (*B*) osmolality in healthy adults in varying states of water balance. (From Robertson GL, Berl T. Water metabolism. In: Brenner BM, Rector FC Jr, eds. *The kidney.* Philadelphia: WB Saunders; 1986:392, with permission.)

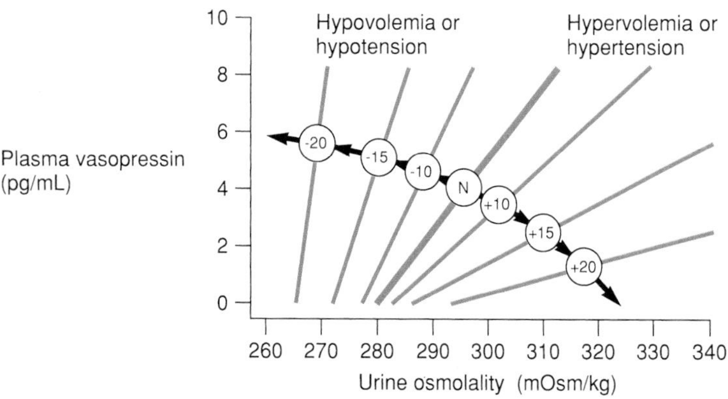

FIGURE 10.3 Effect of acute changes in blood volume or pressure on the osmoregulation of antidiuretic hormone (ADH; vasopressin). The heavy oblique line in the center represents the relation between plasma ADH and osmolality under normovolemic, normotensive conditions. The lines to the left and right show the shift in the relation when blood volume or blood pressure is acutely decreased or increased by the percentage indicated in the circles. [From Robertson GL. Physiology of ADH secretion. *Kidney Int.* 1987;32 (Suppl 21):520, with permission.]

Angiotensin II and neural input from medullary baroreceptors can also influence ADH secretion and thirst, thus tying water balance to hemodynamic alterations. Relatively small changes in pressure have little effect on ADH secretion, but large decreases in pressure can cause tremendous increases in ADH release. Although changes in osmolality tend to have a much greater effect on ADH secretion than do hemodynamic changes, ADH responses to high or low P_{osm} can be profoundly affected by large changes in blood pressure (Fig. 10.3).

FLUID BALANCE

Sodium Concentration and Water Balance

Changes in TBW content are reflected by changes in the extracellular solute concentration. Because sodium is the primary extracellular cation and potassium is the predominant intracellular cation, the serum [Na^+] approximates the sum of the exchangeable total body sodium (Na_e^+) and exchangeable TBK (K_e^+) divided by TBW:

$$\text{Serum }[Na^+] = Na_e^+ + K_e^+/\text{TBW}$$

Because total body solute content ($Na_e^+ + K_e^+$) remains relatively stable over time, changes in TBW content result in inversely proportional changes in serum Na^+ (Fig. 10.4).

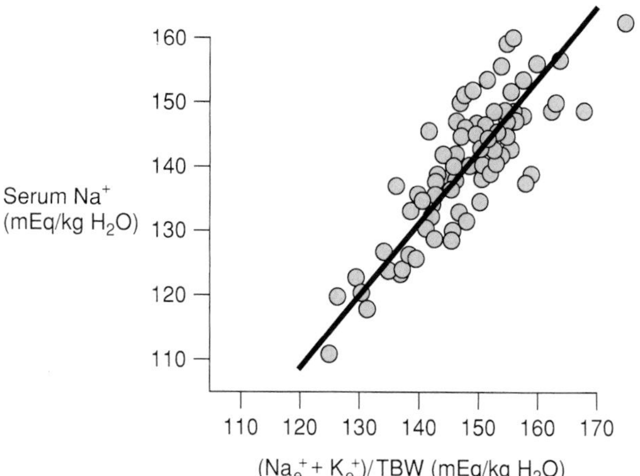

FIGURE 10.4 Relation between serum [Na^+] and the ratio of (Na_e^+ + K_e^+) to total body water (TBW). (From Edelman IS, Liebman J, O'Meara MP, et al. Interrelationships between serum sodium concentration, serum osmolarity and total exchangeable sodium, total exchangeable potassium and total body water. *J Clin Invest.* 1958;37:1236, with permission.)

Thus, abnormalities in serum sodium are usually an indication of abnormal TBW content.

Volume Control

Changes in volume are detected both by osmoreceptors, which detect changes in P_{osm}, and baroreceptors, which are sensitive to changes in pressure. The osmoreceptors are responsible for the day-to-day fine-tuning of volume, whereas the baroreceptors contribute relatively little to the control of fluid balance under normal conditions.[3] As mentioned previously, large changes in circulating volume (10% to 20% blood volume loss) can modify the osmoregulation of ADH secretion. Cardiac atrial baroreceptors control volume by means of sympathetic and parasympathetic neural mechanisms, whereas atrial natriuretic peptide (ANP) released by atrial myocytes in response to atrial wall distention may influence sodium-linked volume control by inhibition of renal sodium reabsorption.

Baroreceptor Modulation of Volume Control

Effective circulating volume describes that portion of the extracellular volume that perfuses the organs of the body and affects the baroreceptors. The effective circulating volume normally corresponds to the intravascular volume. However, in disease states such as congestive heart failure and arteriovenous fistula, where a smaller percentage of intravascular volume than normal is available for organ perfusion, effective circulating volume is reduced.

Changes in the effective circulating volume are sensed by volume receptors in the intrathoracic capacitance vessels and atria, pressure receptors of the aortic arch and carotid arteries, intrarenal baroreceptors, and hepatic and cerebrospinal volume receptors. These stretch receptors respond to changes in pressure and circulating volume and, through a complex system of neural and hormonal actions, alter sodium and water balance in the kidneys. Hormonal effects are mediated by the renin-angiotensin system, aldosterone, ANP, dopamine, and the renal prostaglandins.

Baroreceptor Function

The low-pressure baroreceptors of the intrathoracic vena cava and atria are located in vessels that are distensible and not affected by sympathetic stimulation; thus, they are ideally situated to detect changes in venous volume.[4] These receptors send continuous signals through vagal afferent nerves to the cardiovascular control centers of the medulla and hypothalamus, which, in turn, send signals through parasympathetic and sympathetic fibers to the heart and kidneys. Changes in stretch of these vessels result in changes in the frequency of signal output from these receptors. Increases in atrial distention cause decreased nerve signal traffic, which ultimately causes increased sympathetic tone to the heart, which results in tachycardia and inhibition of sympathetic tone to the kidney. This leads to increased renal blood flow and decreased tubular sodium reabsorption. Conversely, low volume in the intrathoracic vessels results in increased sympathetic tone to the kidneys, decreased renal blood flow, and increased sodium reabsorption.

Experimental evidence indicates that stimulation of the sympathetic innervation of renal arterioles and tubules results in decreased renal blood flow and increased tubular sodium reabsorption. The effects of sympathetic activity on renal sodium reabsorption are probably mediated both by direct tubular innervation and by β-adrenergic stimulation of renin production. Whether this effect is crucial to fine regulation of sodium balance under normal physiologic conditions is unclear. Renal denervation in conscious, unstressed animals results in minimal alteration of either blood flow or sodium reabsorption. The effects of renal denervation become much more marked with anesthesia administration or hypotension, suggesting that sympathetic effects on renal function may be important during periods of physiologic stress.

Arterial baroreceptors are located in the aortic arch and carotid arteries. They respond to changes in heart rate, arterial pressure, and the rate of rise in the arterial pressure. Arterial baroreceptors are important during periods in which there are extremes in the changes in arterial pressure characteristics, as occur during hemorrhage. They are probably not involved in controlling subtle volume or pressure changes. In addition to large-vessel baroreceptors, there are arterial baroreceptors in the afferent arterioles of the kidneys. These baroreceptors modulate renin secretion. Increases in transmural pressure cause suppression of renin release, and decreases in transmural pressure stimulate renin release.

Hormonal Mediators of Volume Control

Renin-Angiotensin System. Renin is a 40-kd proteolytic enzyme that is released from the juxtaglomerular cells of afferent arterioles in the kidney in response to several stimuli. These include changes in arterial pressure, changes in sodium delivery to the macula densa of the distal convoluted tubule, increases in β-adrenergic activity, and increases in cellular cyclic adenosine monophosphate.

Renin cleaves the decapeptide angiotensin I from circulating angiotensinogen, an α_2-globulin produced by the liver. Angiotensin I is cleaved to the octapeptide angiotensin II by angiotensin-converting enzyme (ACE), which is produced by vascular endothelial cells. One pass through the pulmonary microvasculature converts most angiotensin I to angiotensin II. Angiotensin II acts both locally and systemically to increase vascular tone. It also stimulates catecholamine release from the adrenal medulla, increases sympathetic tone through central effects, and stimulates catecholamine release from sympathetic nerve terminals. Angiotensin II affects sodium reabsorption by decreasing renal blood flow and glomerular filtration. This results in altered tubuloglomerular feedback, the mechanism by which changes in distal tubular NaCl delivery alter glomerular blood flow. Finally, angiotensin II increases sodium reabsorption by direct tubular action as well as by stimulation of aldosterone release from the adrenal cortex. The multiplicity of actions of angiotensin are depicted in Figure 10.5.

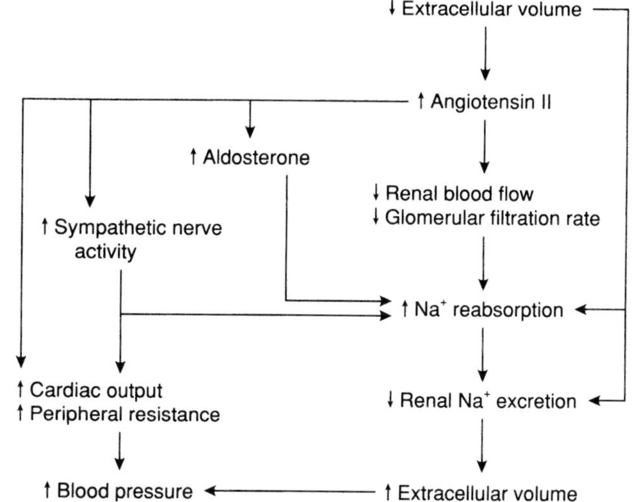

FIGURE 10.5 Multiple effects of increased angiotensin II release in response to the stimulus of decreased extracellular volume.

Aldosterone. Aldosterone is a mineralocorticoid produced in the zona glomerulosa of the adrenal cortex. Aldosterone increases renal tubular reabsorption of sodium. Aldosterone acts directly on the distal tubule cells by modifying gene expression and stabilizing the epithelial Na^+ channel in the open state and by increasing the number of channels in the apical membrane of these cells.[5] By increasing protein production in these tubular cells, aldosterone induces an influx of sodium, which causes an increase in cellular Na^+-K^+-adenosine triphosphatase activity. The net result is increased sodium reabsorption and increased potassium excretion. Although the primary regulator of aldosterone secretion is angiotensin II, aldosterone release is also stimulated by increased potassium levels, adrenocorticotropic hormone, endothelins, and prostaglandins.

Atrial and Renal Natriuretic Peptides. ANP is synthesized and released by atrial myocytes in response to atrial wall distention. As mentioned previously, small changes in right atrial pressure produce large increases in plasma levels of ANP.[6] There is evidence that ANP has a direct inhibitory effect on renal sodium reabsorption, which is probably maximal at the level of the medullary collecting tubules. Although pharmacologic doses of ANP can cause changes in both renal blood flow and glomerular filtration rate, physiologic levels do not appear to have any major effect on these parameters. Other active fragments of the ANP prohormone have been found to have natriuretic activity. The best described is urodilatin, also known as *renal natriuretic* peptide. Urodilatin is a peptide with ANP-like activity that was first isolated from human urine. It is synthesized and luminally secreted by cortical collecting tubule cells. Like ANP, it is released in the kidney tubules in response to atrial distention and saline loading. It is at least twice as potent as ANP, acting in the distal nephron to cause a rise in intracellular cyclic guanosine monophosphate, leading to sodium, chloride, and water diuresis. ANP and other peptides may play an important role in controlling intravascular volume and water and electrolyte secretion.[7]

Renal Prostaglandins. Renal prostaglandins appear to play a role in volume control, although under normal physiologic conditions, this role may be minimal. Disease states such as sepsis and jaundice, or the induction of anesthesia, may make the contribution of the prostaglandins more pronounced.

Prostaglandin E_2 (PGE_2) and prostaglandin I_2 (PGI_2) appear to be the predominant prostaglandins produced in the kidney. PGE_2 is produced primarily by the interstitial cells of the renal medulla. The release of PGE_2 has been shown to depend on increases in interstitial pressure, which can be induced by changes in renal perfusion, ureteral obstruction, or alterations in oncotic pressure. Under these conditions, PGE_2 increases sodium excretion in the absence of changes in glomerular filtration rate. PGE_2 antagonizes the action of vasopressin (ADH) and inhibits ADH-induced sodium reabsorption along the medullary collecting duct and thick ascending limb. PGI_2 is produced by the glomeruli and endothelial cells of the kidney and is present in the greatest concentrations in the renal cortex. PGI_2 is a vasodilator, and its effects on renal vascular resistance increase both renal blood flow and glomerular filtration rate. PGI_2 production is augmented by increases in angiotensin, catecholamines, and sympathetic tone and may act to counterbalance their vasoconstricting effects. Although under normal physiologic conditions, inhibition of prostaglandin production has little effect on renal function, administration of nonsteroidal antiinflammatory agents, which inhibit cyclooxygenase, to patients with conditions known to cause renal dysfunction (e.g., cirrhosis) can precipitate renal failure, presumably because of loss of the protective effects of the renal prostaglandins.[8]

Endothelins. Endothelins are peptide vasoconstrictors that are involved in volume and pressure regulation. Endothelin is produced and released by endothelial and other cells act on adjacent smooth muscle cells. In addition to increasing peripheral resistance, endothelin infusion has a direct inotropic effect on the myocardium. In contrast to its vasoconstrictive effects, endothelin stimulates the release of other vasoactive mediators, particularly endogenous vasodilators like nitric oxide, which act to limit its intense vasoconstrictor effect.

Endothelin exerts a complex influence on sodium and water exchange through varied interactions with many other hormones that govern fluid and electrolyte balance. One net effect of endothelin is a decrease in the filtered load of sodium in the kidney. This results in inhibition of water reabsorption and decreased sodium excretion. Endothelin increases ANP secretion, activates ACE, and inhibits renin release by the juxtaglomerular apparatus. At low doses, endothelin-1 produces a dose-dependent natriuresis and diuresis. Endothelin also modulates the biosynthesis of aldosterone, thereby inhibiting water reabsorption through aldosterone-controlled mechanisms. Vasopressin-mediated water reabsorption is also inhibited. Endothelin appears to have complex interactions with other regulators of renal perfusion and handling of water and electrolytes, which has stimulated research to evaluate the contribution of endothelin to the pathophysiology of various renal diseases.[7,9]

Nitric Oxide. Nitric oxide is a short-lived free radical produced from L-arginine by nitric oxide synthases. Although this substance has numerous biologic functions that are beyond the scope of this chapter, including regulation of vascular tone and tissue blood flow,[7,10] its effects in the kidney as they relate to fluid and electrolyte homeostasis deserve mention. Nitric oxide is produced in renal smooth muscle cells, mesangial cells, tubules, and endothelial cells and participates in the regulation of renal hemodynamics and renal handling of water and electrolytes. Nitric oxide and PGI_2 each independently cause renal vasodilation in response to a variety of stimuli. Nitric oxide is important in the regulation of medullary (vasa recta) blood flow. Pressure-dependent sodium excretion is ablated by inhibitors like L-NG-monomethyl-arginine and restored with L-arginine. Nitric oxide also contributes to tubuloglomerular feedback, which modulates the delivery and reabsorption of sodium and chloride in the renal tubules. Nitric oxide synthase in macula densa cells is activated by tubular solute reabsorption to release nitric oxide as a vasodilating component of the tubuloglomerular feedback response. Nitric oxide also participates in regulating renin release by the juxtaglomerular apparatus. Finally, nitric oxide produced in the proximal tubule may mediate the effects of angiotensin on tubular reabsorption.[11]

Normal Water and Electrolyte Exchange

The body's normal homeostatic mechanisms control both the volume and composition of the fluid compartments such that a remarkably stable internal milieu is maintained. Surgical patients are prone to fluid and electrolyte abnormalities, not only because of disease but because perioperative fluid replacement may sidestep some of these homeostatic mechanisms. Although it is important to recognize and correct disease, trauma, and stress-related abnormalities, it is equally important to understand normal fluid and electrolyte balance and to avoid iatrogenic perturbations of these systems.

Normal Water Exchange

Water losses are both sensible (measurable) and insensible (unmeasurable). Sensible losses include losses through urine, stool, and sweat. Table 10.3 summarizes the normal sensible and insensible losses encountered in a 24-hour period. The volumes of these losses may vary considerably. Urinary loss usually varies in proportion to intake plus other losses. The minimal amount of water needed to excrete normal metabolic waste products is approximately 300 mL/day.

Water loss in stool is usually small, on the order of 150 mL/day but may increase markedly in disease conditions. The GI tract has a net secretory action down to the level of the jejunum, and the reabsorptive capacity of the remainder of the small and large intestines keeps water loss by this route to a minimum. Bowel obstruction, severe diarrhea, and enterocutaneous fistulas are examples of conditions that may increase GI losses of water and electrolytes.

Sweat does not usually account for much of the daily water loss. Sweating is an active process involving the secretion of a hypotonic mixture of electrolytes and water, and it should be differentiated from the insensible water loss of evaporation from the skin.

Insensible water loss is the evaporatory loss of water from both the skin and the respiratory tract (see Table 10.3). Evaporatory skin losses are determined by the body surface area and temperature of the patient, as well as by the relative humidity of the environment. Evaporation through the skin functions as a mechanism for heat loss and is proportional to calories expended. Approximately 30 mL of water is lost for every 100 kcal expended. Respiratory exchange depends on the ambient temperature and the relative humidity as well as on the rate of air exchange. Respiratory water loss is also energy dependent; thus, at normal respiratory rates, 13 mL of water is lost for every 100 kcal expended. Overall, normal insensible water losses average approximately 8 to 12 mL/ kg/day. Insensible water loss increases 10% for each degree of body temperature above

TABLE 10.3

WATER LOSSES IN A 60- TO 80-KG MAN

	Average daily volume (mL)	Minimal daily volume (mL)
Sensible losses		
Urinary	800–1,500	300
Intestinal	0–250	0
Sweat	0	0
Insensible losses		
Lungs and skin	600–900	600–900

Adapted from Shires GT, Canizaro PC. Fluid and electrolyte management of the surgical patient. In: Sabiston DC, ed. *Textbook of surgery.* Philadelphia: WB Saunders; 1986:77, with permission.

37.2°C (99°F). In addition, patients with tracheostomies who breathe unhumidified air lose additional free water. Conversely, patients who are on respirators or who breathe air that is 100% humidified have no respiratory losses and may gain free water.

A person normally consumes approximately 2,000 mL/day of water, although this quantity is highly variable. Approximately one third of this amount comes from water bound to food, and the remainder originates from free water intake. In addition, water may be gained when carbohydrates and proteins, which are kept in solution by water in the cell, are metabolized. Although this gain is usually minimal, catabolic states may increase the amount of oxidative free water gain to approximately 500 mL/day. To maintain proper fluid volumes, intake and excretion are well balanced through thirst mechanisms and the changes in renal excretion described earlier.

Normal Salt Exchange

In industrialized nations, daily sodium intake averages 100 to 250 mEq/day. This intake is balanced by losses through sweat, stool, and urine. Fine control of sodium balance is achieved by renal sodium excretion. In cases of hyponatremia, the kidney is capable of reducing urinary losses of sodium to less than 1 mEq/day. Conversely, urinary excretion can be increased to rates up to 5,000 mEq/day if necessary to achieve sodium balance. The normal sodium requirement is in the range of 1 to 2 mEq/kg/day.

Potassium balance in the body is also finely controlled. Because most potassium remains in the intracellular compartment, potassium homeostasis is maintained by a balance between intake and GI and renal losses and by a balance between extracellular and intracellular potassium. With a normal diet, approximately 40 to 120 mEq of potassium is ingested daily. Of this potassium, 10% to 15% is excreted in the feces, and the remainder is excreted in the urine. Normal daily potassium requirements are approximately 0.5 to 1 mEq/kg/day. Abnormal renal function markedly changes this figure; consequently, potassium intake must be minimized in patients with renal failure.

FLUID AND ELECTROLYTE THERAPY

Parenteral Solutions

Crystalloids

Solutions of electrolytes and water are collectively referred to as *crystalloids* and are the most widely used fluids for parenteral administration. Crystalloids are inexpensive, are highly effective for fluid maintenance and replacement, and have outstanding safety profiles. Crystalloid-induced hypercoagulability, possibly related to reduction in antithrombin III,[12] has been reported.[13,14] However, it is not clear that this represents a significant clinical problem.

A number of electrolyte solutions are available for parenteral administration (Table 10.4). Selection of the appropriate fluid requires assessment of the patient's maintenance fluid requirements, existing fluid deficits, and anticipated ongoing fluid losses. When a single solution does not accurately replace the electrolyte components of the losses or deficits, more than one type of solution may be administered. Ions such as potassium, magnesium, or calcium may be necessary and can be added to parenteral solutions to suit the patient's requirements.

Lactated Ringer's solution is commonly used to replace losses of fluid with the ionic composition of plasma, such as blood loss, edema fluid, and small bowel losses. It is ideal for the replacement of existing fluid deficits when serum electrolyte concentrations are normal. Although sodium content (130 mEq/L) is low compared with plasma, normal renal function usually ensures that the extra free water in this solution (150 mL/L) is excreted. Hyponatremia can occur with extended use of lactated Ringer's solution or with use in patients who have impaired renal function, especially dilutional abnormalities such as those secondary to increased ADH secretion. Because the lactate anions in lactated Ringer's solution are readily metabolized to bicarbonate in the liver, this solution does not appear to contribute to acidosis if tissue perfusion has been maintained or restored. Recent work comparing the DL racemic mixture of lactate in lactated Ringer's solution with its L-isomer have implicated the D-isomer in leukocyte activation, although at present there are no compelling data to suggest that resuscitation with this solution increases the inflammatory response.[15] Utilization of only the L-isomer in resuscitation solutions eliminates this theoretical problem.

Isotonic saline (0.9% or normal saline) contains 154 mEq of both sodium and chloride. Although this solution can be useful in patients with hyponatremia or hypochloremia, the excess of both sodium and chloride can lead to electrolyte and acid–base disturbances. Infusion of large volumes of 0.9% saline can lead to total body sodium overload and hyperchloremia. The added chloride load can result in a hyperchloremic metabolic acidosis or can aggravate preexisting acidosis. In addition, the pH of this solution and of the related solutions (0.45%, 0.33%, and 0.2% saline) is 4.0 to 5.0.

Following correction of deficits, less-concentrated saline solutions are more appropriate to replace ongoing fluid losses (i.e., nasogastric tube losses) and for maintenance fluid therapy. Although the practical differences between 0.45%,

TABLE 10.4

ELECTROLYTE CONTENT OF COMMONLY USED INTRAVENOUS CRYSTALLOID SOLUTIONS

	Electrolyte (mEq/L)					
Solution	Na^+	K^+	Ca^{2+}	Mg^{2+}	Cl^-	HCO_3^-
0.9% NaCl	154	—	—	—	154	—
0.45% NaCl	77	—	—	—	77	—
0.33% NaCl	56	—	—	—	56	—
0.2% NaCl	34	—	—	—	34	—
Lactated Ringer's	130	4	4	—	109	28
3.0% NaCl	513	—	—	—	513	—
5.0% NaCl	855	—	—	—	855	—

0.33%, and 0.2% saline solutions are not large, the specific fluid product selection is best determined by calculated requirements. These fluids are hypoosmotic and hypotonic with respect to plasma. In theory, rapid infusion of very hypotonic solutions can result in red blood cell lysis. For this reason, 5% dextrose (50 g of dextrose per liter) is added to these solutions to increase tonicity. In addition, 5% dextrose represents 200 kcal in each liter of solution.

Hypertonic saline solutions (3% NaCl and 5% NaCl) are generally used to replace sodium deficits in patients with symptomatic hyponatremia. However, these and even more concentrated (7.5% NaCl) solutions have also been used for resuscitation of hemorrhagic shock, head trauma, and burn patients.[16] Hypertonic saline appears to increase intravascular volume in these patients more quickly than isotonic solutions, and the total resuscitation volume requirement may be decreased. Advantages of hypertonic solutions used for resuscitative purposes have not been clearly demonstrated, except potentially in patients with head trauma in whom these solutions may more rapidly increase cerebral perfusion and reduce cerebral edem.[17] Patients resuscitated with hypertonic solutions require close monitoring of serum electrolytes to prevent hypernatremia and hyperosmolar coma. Although hypertonic saline resuscitation may have some utility in unique circumstances, other resuscitative fluids are safer in general.

Colloids

Colloid plasma volume expander solutions offer the potential benefits of promoting retention of fluid in the intravascular space and of reducing excess interstitial fluid (edema). Worldwide, albumin and artificial colloids are relied on to varying degrees in fluid management of the surgical patient. In the United States, concerns regarding the effectiveness and potential complications of colloid administration have limited their use to specific clinical situations.

Albumin

Albumin (69-kDa) derived from human plasma and heat-treated to reduce infection risk, is available in 5% and 25% solutions. These act by increasing plasma oncotic pressures and theoretically retarding or even reversing movement of water into the interstitial space. However, many of the conditions associated with edema are also associated with abnormalities in microvascular permeability. Examples include the pulmonary circulation in the adult respiratory distress syndrome, regional circulatory beds in burns or infections, and the systemic circulation in sepsis. Exogenously administered protein in colloid solutions can extravasate into the interstitial space and intensify, rather than decrease interstitial edema. Numerous studies have failed to show any consistent benefit in the use of albumin as compared to crystalloid in the fluid management of critically ill patients. In contrast with artificial colloid solutions, the safety profile of albumin is quite good, although it is a very expensive product.

Hetastarch

Hydroxyethyl starches (HES) are synthetic plasma expanders derived from hydrolyzed amylopectin, with variable degrees of substitution (DS) of hydroxyl groups for carbon groups on glucose molecules. HES is available commercially in the United States as a 6% solution of high molecular weight (450,000), highly hydroxyethyl substituted (DS 0.7) HES (Hetastarch) in 0.9% saline. Hetastarch has been used as a resuscitative solution in a variety of clinical settings with variable results. Coagulopathy and bleeding complications have been widely reported after administration of highly substituted, high molecular weight HES.[18,19] This appears to be associated with reduced factor VIII and von Willebrand factor levels, a prolonged partial thromboplastin time, and impaired platelet function.[20] Because of its long half-life, coagulopathy does not quickly reverse after cessation of HES administration. Reports of renal insufficiency or renal failure after HES 450/0.7, HES 250/0.45 (Pentaspan), and HES 200/0.62 administration add to the concerns regarding overuse of these volume expanders, particularly in patients with preexisting renal impairment.

Hextend, a balanced 6% hetastarch (MW 720,000) in lactated Ringer's solution, has been forwarded as a much-improved alternate resuscitation product as compared to 6% Hetastarch in saline. In a phase III trial of Hextend and 6% Hetastarch in saline, Hextend was found to be as effective for resuscitation but without adversely affecting the coagulation profile.[21] Although the safely profile of this alternative colloid resuscitative fluid appears to be better than that of 6% Hetastarch in saline, the data regarding its safety in situations of massive resuscitation are not clear. In a recent study using an experimental model of traumatic brain injury, Hextend was found to reduce fluid requirement, eliminate the need for mannitol, and improve neurologic outcome as compared to crystalloid and mannitol resuscitation. Furthermore, it had no adverse effect on coagulation.[22] In another recent experimental report, Hextend was found to have no significant platelet-inhibitory effects.[23]

Low molecular weight, low-substituted (MW 130 kDa; DS 0.4) HES (Voluven) has recently been introduced and demonstrated to have a far smaller effect on coagulation than other HES solutions.[24] In addition, there is evidence that renal impairment does not occur after administration of HES 130/0.4, in contrast to the high-molecular-weight, highly substituted HES solutions.[25] Although numerous reports now suggest that this type of alternative HES is a very good option when plasma volume expansion is indicated, the safety of wide use of large-volume Voluven administration remains to be demonstrated.

Dextrans

Dextrans are glucose polymers synthesized by *Leuconostoc mesenteroides* bacteria grown on sucrose media. These are available as synthetic plasma expanders in 40,000 MW (Dextran 40; Rheomacrodex) and 70,000 MW (Dextran 70; Macrodex) solutions. Although neither are used frequently for volume expansion, Dextran 70 has been preferred because of its significantly longer half life and better retention in plasma. The most accepted current use of dextran solutions is to lower blood viscosity. Both should be avoided in patients with known renal dysfunction, but Dextran 40 has been shown to represent a particular risk for renal injury.[26] Anaphylactoid reactions can occur with either Dextran 40 or 70.

Gelatins

Gelatin solutions produced from bovine collagen are effective as plasma volume expanders, and are available outside the United States in urea-linked (Gelofusin) and succinate-linked (Haemaccel) formulations. Gelofusin has been used in similar clinical settings to HES, with similar clinical results, although one randomized trial comparing the two colloids in trauma patients suggested that HES (MW 250; DS 4.5) was more effective in reducing capillary leak.[27] Coagulopathy does not appear to be an issue with gelatins, although renal impairment has been reported with these colloids as well. Allergic reactions ranging in severity from pruritus to anaphylaxis can occur with both gelatin formulations.[28]

Artificial Oxygen Carriers

Although the subject of transfusion is beyond the scope of this chapter, new developments in the area of oxygen-carrying synthetic volume expanders deserve brief mention. Early difficulties with perfluorocarbon-based solutions have increased the intensity of investigation to develop hemoglobin-based oxygen-carrying (HBOC) solutions, and the results of recent clinical trials with these substances have been encouraging.[29,30] In the future, these solutions may prove beneficial when volume expansion in conjunction with increased oxygen-carrying capacity is required and will avoid the immunologic consequences of allogenic blood transfusions.

Goals of Fluid and Electrolyte Therapy

The goals of fluid therapy are to normalize hemodynamic parameters and body fluid electrolyte concentrations. This is accomplished by correction of both volume and electrolyte abnormalities, as well as by replacement of both normal daily losses and additional ongoing losses associated with disease states and surgical treatments.

CORRECTION OF VOLUME ABNORMALITIES

Volume Deficits

Hypovolemia is common among surgical and trauma patients. Its occurrence may be related to direct loss of blood or other fluids but frequently occurs in the absence of external fluid loss. In critically ill patients, this can be due to vasodilation or diffuse capillary leak. Large volumes of fluid can be sequestered in extravascular spaces (third-space losses) as a consequence of inflammation, sepsis, or shock-related endothelial injury, and increased endothelial permeability.[31] This situation is characterized by a movement of proteins and fluid from the intravascular to the interstitial compartment. Examples of disorders that cause third-space loss include bowel obstruction with edema of the bowel wall and transudation of fluid into the bowel lumen and pancreatitis with often massive retroperitoneal fluid extravasation. Third-space fluid in the interstitial space is poorly exchangeable with the intravascular compartment while the disease process persists. With the resolution of pathologic conditions and normalization of microvascular permeability, these fluid losses stop and sequestered fluid is returned to the intravascular space at variable rates.

Volume deficits can be either acute or chronic. Chronic volume deficits may manifest as decreased skin turgor, weight loss, sunken eyes, hypothermia, oliguria, orthostatic hypotension, and tachycardia. In addition, serum BUN and creatinine may be elevated, with a high BUN/creatinine ratio (above 15:1), and the hematocrit may be elevated as well. Assuming no change in red cell mass, the hematocrit can be expected to increase 6 to 8 percentage points for each liter deficit in intravascular volume. In this situation, urine concentration is usually high, and urine sodium excretion is low (<20 mEq/L Na^+). Unlike urine sodium levels, plasma sodium is not an indicator of intravascular volume. Plasma sodium concentration remains normal when fluid loss is isotonic, despite the volume of fluid lost.

Acute volume losses are usually manifested by changes in vital signs. If organ perfusion is compromised, urine output may be low. Attempts to quantify volume deficits are usually of little value. The volume of fluid required to restore blood pressure, heart rate, and urine output is the best estimate of what the volume deficit has been. Fluid resuscitation for hypovolemia is initiated with an isotonic solution such as lactated Ringer's solution. Urine flow in critically ill patients is monitored with an indwelling Foley catheter with a goal of at least 0.5 mL/kg/hour output. After fluid resuscitation has been initiated, a thorough history and physical examination may help to determine the origins of the volume deficits, and the underlying causes can be appropriately addressed. Invasive monitoring with a central venous or pulmonary artery catheter should be considered in elderly patients or patients with cardiac disease.

Volume Excess

Clinical manifestations of volume excess may occur with excessive parenteral volume administration, particularly in at-risk patients such as the elderly and those with cardiac disease. Volume overload can occur if appropriate adjustments to fluid therapy are not made. Possible manifestations of volume overload are weight gain, elevated central venous pressure (CVP), pulmonary congestion or edema, and peripheral edema. Intravascular volume excess is treated by volume restriction and use of loop diuretics.

MAINTENANCE FLUID THERAPY

Calculation of maintenance fluid replacement does not include replacement of either preexisting deficits or ongoing additional losses. Basal requirements for water and electrolytes are determined by sensible and insensible losses. Insensible water loss averages 8 to 12 ml/kg/day and increases 10% for every degree of body temperature above 37.2°C. Urinary and fecal losses must be added to this figure. Maintenance fluid volume requirements can be calculated based on body weight taking into account a larger per kilogram volume requirement of smaller body weight individuals (Table 10.5). A10-kg child requires 100 mL kg/day or 1,000 mL/day. A 70-kg man requires 1,000 mL/day for the first 10 kg (100 mL/kg × 10 kg), plus 500 mL/day for the second 10 kg (50 mL/kg × 10 kg), plus 1,000 mL/day for the last 50 kg (20 mL/kg × 50 kg) for a total daily water requirement of 2,500 mL/day. In patients who may be intolerant of hypervolemia (i.e., cardiac disease, elderly patients) the requirement per kilogram over 20 kg is decreased to 15 mL/kg/day.

One to 2 mEq/kg/day of sodium is required for maintenance therapy, with any administered excess managed by urinary sodium excretion. Potassium requirements are approximately 0.5 to 1 mEq/kg/day. If sodium is replaced at 2 mEq/kg/day and potassium is replaced at 1 mEq/kg/day,

TABLE 10.5

CALCULATION OF MAINTENANCE FLUID REQUIREMENTS

Body weight	Fluid requirement[a]	
For 0–10 kg	Give 100 mL/kg/d	A
For the next 10–20 kg	Give an additional 50 mL/kg/d	B
For weight >20 kg[b]	Give 20 mL/kg/d	C

[a]Maintenance fluid requirements = sum of A + B + C.
[b]For elderly patients or patients with cardiac disease, this amount should be reduced to 15 mL/kg/d.

a 70-kg patient requires 2,500 mL of water containing 140 mEq of sodium and 70 mEq of potassium. Each liter of parenteral solution would contain 56 mEq of sodium and 28 mEq of potassium. 0.33% saline solution (56 mEq/L Na^+) is the solution that best fits this patient's daily maintenance requirements. Potassium chloride can be added to each liter of solution (20 to 30 mEq/L), with appropriate adjustments for the patient's electrolyte and renal functional status.

Short-term maintenance therapy generally does not require addition of calcium, phosphate, or magnesium. However, patients who require long-term parenteral fluid therapy should receive these electrolytes by the most practical route. If the enteral route is unavailable, these are administered in parenteral nutrition solutions along with trace elements, vitamins, and appropriate caloric sources.

REPLACEMENT OF ONGOING FLUID LOSSES

Once volume deficits have been replaced and maintenance fluids have been calculated and given, the overall fluid balance of the patient can be maintained by replacement of fluid losses beyond those considered to be maintenance. Ongoing losses from nasogastric tubes, stomas, fistulae, and other measurable sources are recorded during the course of care and can be replaced in fairly straightforward fashion. The electrolyte contents of these fluids can be estimated or measured and used to guide the choice of replacement fluid type (Table 10.6).

Intraoperative Fluid Therapy

Anesthesia interrupts normal baroreceptor reflexes, so the patient with volume depletion that was compensated preoperatively by increased vascular resistance and heart rate may become acutely hypotensive on induction of anesthesia. For this reason, adequate resuscitation before surgery is mandatory. During operative procedures fluid losses result from blood loss, third-space sequestration, and evaporative losses from open wounds. Operative blood loss can often be measured. Evaporative losses and shifts of intravascular fluid to the extravascular space (third-space) cannot be measured but should be anticipated. Intraoperative replacement with isotonic solutions is usually accomplished at rates of 500 to 1,000 mL/hour. Close monitoring of blood pressure and urine output, as well as judicious use of invasive monitoring techniques, aids the surgeon and anesthesiologist in avoiding problems associated with intraoperative volume depletion.

Postoperative Fluid Therapy and Monitoring

Fluid therapy during the postoperative period is adjusted to the patient's volume status at the completion of the operative procedure, as well as to anticipated ongoing fluid losses. Isotonic solutions should be used for volume resuscitation during the early postoperative period. It is best not to give potassium supplements during this period, unless they are specifically required as indicated by serum electrolyte measurements, until adequate renal function is confirmed.

Routine monitoring of postoperative fluid status consists of serial vital signs and urine output measurements. Fluid intake and output data are recorded in the patient's medical record and used to plan ongoing fluid therapy. Weight should also be recorded daily. In the postsurgical patient, rapid fluctuations in weight are generally related to changes in TBW. Adequate fluid is given to maintain a urine output of >0.5 mL/kg/hour. Urine specific gravity can also be measured and serves as an indicator of both volume status and renal ability to concentrate and dilute the urine. Urine specific gravity of greater than 1.010 to 1.012 indicates that the urine is being concentrated (relative to plasma), and a urine specific gravity of less than 1.010 indicates that dilute urine is being produced. Both volume depletion and cardiac failure are accompanied by increased urine concentration and low urine outputs. Urine specific gravity in the range of plasma (1.010 to 1.012) may indicate either adequate hydration or the inability of the kidneys either to dilute or concentrate the urine.

Renal failure in the postoperative period may be accompanied by low urine volumes (oliguric renal failure, <500 mL/day), or normal or high urine volumes (nonoliguric or high-output renal failure). Measurement of urine electrolytes and creatinine clearance can help clarify questions regarding volume status and renal function. CVP measurement can be used to more accurately assess volume status and guide fluid administration. Normal CVP may range from 5 to 12 mm Hg. Higher pressures usually indicate volume overload or cardiac failure, whereas pressures below this range indicate intravascular volume depletion. There are significant limitations to CVP measurement as a reflection of circulating volume, particularly in critically ill patients. Abnormalities of cardiac performance and vascular tone may confound interpretation of CVP measurements, and pulmonary artery catheterization may be required to resolve volume status questions.

TABLE 10.6

ELECTROLYTE CONCENTRATIONS IN GASTROINTESTINAL SECRETIONS

	Electrolyte (mEq/L)					
Secretion	Na^+	K^+	Cl^-	HCO_3^-	H^+	Rate (mL/d)
Salivary	50	20	40	30	—	100–1,000
Gastric						
Basal	100	10	140	—	30	1,000
Stimulated	30	10	140	—	100	4,200
Bile	140	5	100	—	—	500–1,000
Pancreatic	140	5	75	—	—	1,000
Duodenum	140	5	80	—	—	100–2,000
Ileum	140	5	70	—	—	100–2,000
Colon	60	70	15	—	—	—

ELECTROLYTES

Concentration Changes in Body Fluids

Volume excess or deficits are often isotonic but may be accompanied by changes in extracellular sodium concentration and osmolality. The mechanisms controlling normal osmoregulation may be affected by the same processes responsible for controlling volume. Volume depletion is the most common disorder of volume status encountered in surgical and trauma patients. These patients usually present with isotonic dehydration (Fig. 10.6A). In this condition, the volume lost is isotonic with plasma. Examples of isotonic volume deficits include blood loss, third-space losses, and GI losses. Volume depletion may also be accompanied by hypoosmolar conditions (hypotonic dehydration; see Fig. 10.6B), which is often iatrogenic and the result of incomplete volume resuscitation with hypotonic solutions. Dehydration associated with hyperosmolar states (hypertonic dehydration; see Fig. 10.6C) is infrequent and usually indicates impaired consciousness and thirst mechanisms or a patient's inability to drink or obtain water. As mentioned previously, volume excesses often occur some time after hospitalization rather than at presentation. The most frequent concentration defect associated with volume excess is hyponatremia.

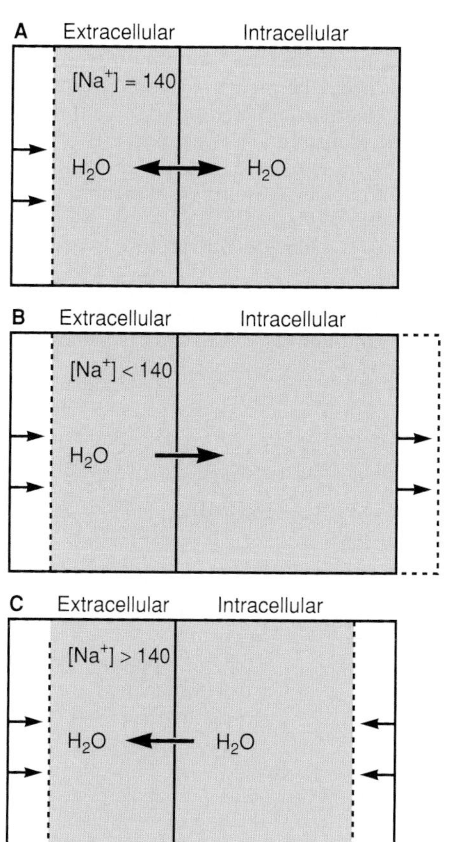

FIGURE 10.6 (*A*) Isotonic dehydration. Extracellular fluid is lost, but sodium concentration and osmolality remain unchanged. There is no change in intracellular volume. (*B*) Hypotonic dehydration caused by an extracellular fluid deficit with hyponatremia. Water moves into the intracellular space, causing further extracellular depletion and intracellular fluid (ICF) expansion. (*C*) Hypertonic dehydration caused by loss of extracellular free water, resulting in hypernatremia. Water from the ICF shifts to the extracellular space, resulting in contraction of both ICF and extracellular fluid compartments.

Hyponatremia

Causes. Hyponatremia may result from direct sodium loss, or from dilution of sodium by excessive free water under hypovolemic, euvolemic, or hypervolemic conditions. Hyponatremia is frequently seen in the postoperative or postinjury period when ADH is elevated as a component of the normal stress response to injury. Inflammatory and stress cytokines such as C-reactive protein, interleukin-6, interleukin-1, and tumor necrosis factor all increase ADH levels. Volume expansion due to increased ADH-stimulated free water reabsorption may stimulate natriuresis and exacerbate hyponatremia. Because volume expansion and hyponatremia diminish the effects of ADH on the collecting tubules, hyponatremia is usually self-limited under these circumstances, with serum sodium concentration rarely falling below 130 mEq/L unless exacerbated by exogenous free water administration.

The *syndrome of inappropriate ADH secretion* (SIADH) occurs as the result of ADH release under circumstances that are inappropriate to the patient's volume status. The diagnosis can be made when hyponatremia occurs in the presence of euvolemia (or hypervolemia) and normal renal and adrenal function. SIADH can be encountered in wide range of clinical problems (Table 10.7). The diagnosis requires that the patient have a low plasma osmolality with a high urine osmolality secondary to high urinary sodium excretion in a low volume of urine. SIADH is usually treated with a combination of an osmotic diuretic (mannitol), a loop diuretic (furosemide), and water restriction of approximately 50% maintenance fluid volume. Nonpeptide vasopressin (V_2) antagonists can also be used, which work by competitively blocking the binding of ADH (arginine vasopressin) to V_2 receptors.

Hyponatremia can also be associated with low effective circulating volume. This most commonly occurs in edematous states or cirrhosis with ascites, but it can also result from dehydration with concomitant volume replacement with hypotonic solutions. Because of the low intravascular volume, renal plasma flow and glomerular filtration rate are low, resulting in increased sodium reabsorption by the kidneys. This renal compensation may not be sufficient to correct the abnormality.

Although hyponatremia most often results from excess free water, it can occur in the presence of excess solute, as previously described, with increased P_{osm} in hyperglycemic conditions (pseudohyponatremia). Other types of solute may contribute to hyperosmolality and water shifts from the intracellular to the extracellular space, with consequent hyponatremia. These include exogenously administered or

TABLE 10.7

CAUSES OF THE SYNDROME OF INAPPROPRIATE ADH SECRETION

Tumor hypersecretion of ADH	Lung Pancreas Bladder Prostate
CNS disorders	Head trauma Neurosurgical interventions Brain tumors Alcohol withdrawal Stroke
Other	Infection Medication-induced

ADH, antidiuretic hormone; CNS, central nervous system.

TABLE 10.8

SYMPTOMS OF HYPONATREMIA

Central nervous system	Headaches Confusion Delirium Coma Seizures
Gastrointestinal	Anorexia Nausea Vomiting
Musculoskeletal	Weakness Fatigue Muscle cramps

ingested mannitol, ethanol, methanol, or ethylene glycol. In addition to shifts in water, cellular exchange of potassium for sodium as a compensatory mechanism for potassium loss may result in hyponatremia. In both hyperosmolar and hypokalemic conditions, total body sodium remains normal.

Finally, hyperproteinemia and hyperlipidemia can cause falsely low sodium values. This pattern of *pseudohyponatremia* is due to an anomaly of laboratory measurement of sodium and is not accompanied by any symptoms attributable to hyponatremia.

Clinical Features. Chronic hyponatremia is often asymptomatic until serum [Na^+] falls below 110 to 120 mEq/L. A more acute drop in serum [Na^+] to the 120 to 130 mEq/L range may result in central nervous system (CNS), musculoskeletal, or GI symptoms (Table 10.8). Symptoms related to the CNS result largely from cellular water intoxication, and permanent CNS injury can occur if hyponatremia is left untreated.

Diagnosis. Differentiating the causes of hyponatremia may be difficult. Once hyperosmolar hyponatremia (caused by hyperglycemia, mannitol administration, or radiologic contrast medium) has been excluded and pseudohyponatremia has been eliminated from the differential diagnosis, the clinician must determine whether the effective circulating volume is low (hyponatremic dehydration) or normal.

Hyponatremic dehydration may be caused by renal or extrarenal sodium losses. Renal sodium losses are usually the result of diuretic use, chronic renal failure, adrenal insufficiency, or a defect in aldosterone secretion. The hallmark of these disorders is a urine sodium level above 20 mEq/L in the face of hyponatremia. This is in contradistinction to extrarenal sodium loss such as that caused by vomiting; diarrhea; or fluid loss through nasogastric tubes, fistulas, or drains. The dehydration resulting from these conditions causes increased renal sodium reabsorption and urine sodium levels below 20 mEq/L. Normal or high effective circulating volume in combination with hyponatremia is almost always caused by SIADH or by increased sensitivity of the renal collecting tubules to the action of normal levels of ADH.

Treatment. Hypovolemic patients with hyponatremia can frequently be treated by rehydration with isotonic saline or lactated Ringer's solution because symptoms in this situation are often caused by dehydration rather than hyponatremia. Overly rapid normalization of volume may lead to hypernatremia, and serum [Na^+] must be serially monitored during volume replacement. Most surgical patients with hyponatremia are euvolemic or hypervolemic. Asymptomatic patients in this category are best treated by free water restriction.

Patients who have significant symptoms require aggressive treatment with a clear recognition that overzealous therapy may lead to CNS injury. Rapid infusion of hypertonic saline may result in central pontine myelinolysis and the quadriplegia, dysarthria, and dysphasia of the "locked-in" syndrome. This risk is greatest in patients who have been hyponatremic for longer than 48 hours. In these patients, 5% or 3% saline solution is given relatively slowly to increase serum [Na^+] at a rate not exceeding 0.5 mEq/L/hour. The amount of sodium needed to increase the serum [Na^+] to a desired level can be calculated as follows:

$$Na^+ \text{ required (in mEq)} = (\text{desired } [Na^+]_s - \text{actual } [Na^+]_s) \times \text{TBW}$$

where $[Na^+]_s$ = serum sodium concentration. For example, a 70-kg patient has been hyponatremic for more than 48 hours and has a serum sodium level of 120 mEq. Correction of hyponatremia during the first 24 hours is limited to 0.5 mEq/L/hour × 24 hours = 12 mEq/L. Assuming TBW 60% of body weight:

$$Na^+ \text{ required} = (132 - 120) \times (0.6[70]) = 504 \text{ mEq}$$

Because 5% saline contains 850 mEq/L of sodium, the volume of 5% saline required to provide 504 mEq of sodium in the first 24 hours of treatment is as follows:

$$504 \text{ mEq}/850 \text{ mEq} = 0.593 \text{ L } 5\% \text{ saline}$$

For more acute symptomatic hyponatremia (<48 hours duration), more rapid treatment may be used. Five percent or 3% hypertonic saline may be administered at a rate of 1 to 2 mEq/L/hour. Hyperacute hyponatremia, which may result from inadvertent infusion of large volumes of water or from dialysis accidents, can be treated at rates of 5 mEq/L/hour. The treatment goal is to achieve a serum sodium level above 125 mEq/L or to achieve resolution of symptoms.

Hypernatremia

Hypernatremia is a less common problem in surgical patients than hyponatremia but can occur due to a number of causes (Table 10.9). Although hypernatremia is usually the result of excessive free water loss associated with hypovolemia, it can

TABLE 10.9

CAUSES OF HYPERNATREMIA

Volume status	Cause
Low	Free water loss Insensible -skin, respiratory Gastrointestinal loss Excessive hyperosmotic peritoneal dialysis Renal -diuretics, diabetes insipidus, nonoliguric renal failure
Normal	Same as "Low" volume status but with improper correction
High	Free water loss Increased mineralocorticoids -hyperaldosteronism, hypercortisolism Iatrogenic Excessive sodium administration

also occur in euvolemic and hypervolemic states. Euvolemic hypernatremia tends to occur for the same reasons as in hypovolemic situations, with the added factor of improper correction of free water loss (i.e., with sodium-containing fluids). Water loss may be due to nonrenal or renal causes. Nonrenal free water losses can be characterized as insensible as in respiratory losses in patients with tracheostomies who breathe unhumidified air or skin losses in patients with high fevers. Large volumes of free water can also be lost when hypertonic glucose solutions are used for peritoneal dialysis. *Diabetes insipidus,* seen most frequently in head trauma or neurosurgical patients, is due to depressed secretion of ADH. The free water diuresis in this condition can at times be massive.

Hypernatremia can also be caused by increased total body content of sodium, which is usually related to exogenous administration of sodium. Infusion of excessive amounts of sodium bicarbonate during acute resuscitation from cardiopulmonary arrest is frequently associated with subsequent hypernatremia. Administration of solutions containing large amounts of sodium for replacement of free water deficits may also lead to hypernatremia.

Clinical Features. Moderate degrees of hypernatremia are tolerated well, and symptoms rarely develop unless serum $[Na^+]$ levels exceed 160 mEq/L or serum osmolality exceeds 320 to 330 mOsm/kg. Rapid onset of hypernatremia is associated with earlier onset of symptoms. The symptoms of hypernatremia are related to the hyperosmolar state. Cellular dehydration occurs as water passes into the extracellular space. CNS effects predominate. The most common symptoms are restlessness, irritability, ataxia, fever, tonic spasms, and seizures. Subarachnoid hemorrhage may also occur.

Treatment. Once hypernatremia becomes symptomatic, it is associated with significant morbidity and mortality if prompt treatment is not instituted. Rapid correction carries a significant risk of cerebral edema and brain stem herniation. In chronic hypernatremia, the cells in the brain gradually adapt by increasing intracellular osmotic solute content, thereby regaining cellular volume. These cellular changes are not readily reversed. A sudden decrease in extracellular sodium concentration, and therefore osmolality, results in cell swelling. Because chronic hypernatremia is relatively well tolerated, there are few advantages to correcting the free water deficit rapidly. Free water is administered to correct serum $[Na^+]$ at a rate not exceeding 0.7 mEq/L/hour. The amount of water required to correct a hypernatremic state depends on the free water deficit, the insensible free water losses, and the urinary free water excretion rate. The water requirement to replace the free water deficit can be calculated using the following formula:

$$\text{water requirement} = \frac{\text{desired change in } [Na^+]_s \times \text{TBW}}{\text{desired } [Na^+]_s}$$

For example, a 70-kg patient with a TBW of 42 L (TBW 60% of body weight) has a serum sodium of 170 mEq/L. The maximum desired change in serum sodium over 1 day would be approximately 16 mEq (0.7 mEq/L/hour). Therefore, water requirement = 16 × 42/154 = 4.3 L.

The desired level of serum sodium would not be achieved unless insensible losses (approximately 8 mL/kg/day) and urinary free water losses were also replaced. Urinary losses of free water can be determined by calculating free water clearance:

$$CH_2O = V - C_{osm}V - \frac{U_{osm} \times V}{P_{osm}}$$

where CH_2O = free water clearance rate, C_{osm} = osmolar clearance rate, V = urine flow rate, and U_{osm} and P_{osm} = urine and plasma osmolalities, respectively.

The U_{osm} and P_{osm} can be estimated by the total sodium and potassium concentrations. Therefore,

$$CH_2O = V - \frac{(U_{Na} + U_K) \times V}{[Na^+]_s}$$

where U_{Na} and U_K = urinary sodium and potassium concentrations, respectively. A positive number signifies net free water loss and adds to the water requirement, whereas a negative number indicates free water absorption and is subtracted from the water requirement. Thus, the total water requirement to achieve the desired decrease in serum $[Na^+]$ is the sum of the calculated water deficit plus the calculated insensible water loss plus the urinary free water clearance.

Compositional Changes in Body Fluids

Potassium

Potassium is the major intracellular cation and is the major determinant of intracellular osmolality. Normally, intracellular potassium concentration is approximately 150 mEq/L, whereas extracellular potassium levels range from 3.5 to 5 mEq/L. Because of the large difference between intracellular and extracellular potassium concentrations, a transmembrane potential is generated. Alterations in the potassium concentration gradient have profound effects on transmembrane potential and consequently on cellular function. This is especially true for cardiac, skeletal, and smooth muscle. The membrane potential (E_m) developed in cells is described by the Nernst equation:

$$E_m = -\log 60\ [K_I]/[K_E]$$

where $[K_I]$ and $[K_E]$ = intracellular and extracellular potassium concentrations, respectively.

Normally, the membrane potential of cells is approximately −90 mV as produced by a $[K_I]/[K_E]$ ratio of 30:1. Intracellular potassium levels are relatively stable, but extracellular potassium levels are often altered in pathologic situations. Overall potassium balance is determined by potassium intake and by renal and extrarenal excretion.

Approximately 90% of ingested potassium is excreted in the urine, and the remainder (5 to 10 mEq/day) primarily in feces. Most potassium filtered by the glomerulus is reabsorbed in the proximal tubule, so that net excretion is determined by the amount of potassium secreted by the distal tubule and collecting duct of the nephron. In these nephron segments, movement of potassium into the tubular lumen is determined by the difference between intracellular and luminal fluid K^+ concentrations, the permeability of the luminal cell membranes to K^+, and the electrical potential gradient across the luminal cell membrane. Potassium secretion is stimulated by increased urine flow in the distal nephron segments, increased sodium delivery to these segments, high plasma potassium concentrations, and alkalosis. In addition, humoral factors, including aldosterone, vasopressin, and β-adrenergic agonists, stimulate renal excretion of K^+. Because of the central role of the kidneys in potassium excretion, renal failure can lead to hyperkalemia. Nonrenal losses may increase greatly in hyperkalemic states or in renal failure.

Extracellular potassium levels can be greatly influenced by the acute shifts of potassium into or out of the cells. Insulin causes potassium to move into the cell, inducing a change in membrane potential and stimulating glycolysis. Alkalosis causes K^+ to shift into cells in exchange for H^+. Conversely, acidemia induces the cellular exchange of intracellular K^+ for extracellular H^+. A redistribution of K^+ into the ECF can also occur in hyperosmolar conditions because the movement of water into the extracellular compartment causes "solvent drag" which may increase the flux of potassium.

Hyperkalemia

Causes. Hyperkalemia rarely develops from excessive potassium intake given the high capacity for renal potassium excretion. In the surgical patient, diminished renal function is probably the most common problem leading to hyperkalemia. Both chronic and acute renal failure result in a defect in potassium excretion. Nonoliguric renal failure may lead to hyperkalemia despite apparently adequate urine output. Serum potassium levels may increase by 0.3 to 0.5 mEq/L/day in noncatabolic patients with acute renal failure, but this level can increase to 0.7 mEq/L/day or more in catabolic patients or those with other sources of potassium intake. Hospitalized patients may also receive excess potassium in intravenous fluids and total parenteral nutrition formulas. Less obvious sources include medications that are bound to potassium (i.e., β-lactam antibiotics).

In patients with chronic renal disease, potassium balance is normalized by increased colonic potassium excretion, as well as increased potassium excretion per functional nephron. Infusion of cationic amino acid solutions, such as arginine and lysine, can be associated with hyperkalemia because these amino acids are taken up by cells in exchange for potassium. Patients with impaired renal function or diabetes are also at risk for developing hyperkalemia when given ACE inhibitors and/or angiotensin or aldosterone receptor inhibitors.[32]

Cellular disruption with release of potassium may result in hyperkalemia. The classic example of this is hyperkalemia associated with crush injuries. Reperfusion of ischemic limbs can lead to substantial elevations in potassium when reflow of blood washes out the byproducts of ischemia-induced cell lysis. Hyperkalemia may also occur when potassium is released from lysed erythrocytes in large hematomas or after massive blood transfusion. Similarly, potassium release from tumor lysis may result in increased serum potassium. Hyperkalemia can also be associated with the depolarizing muscle relaxants (e.g., succinylcholine). Although unusual, hyperkalemia can also result from absorption of potassium after the use of solutions containing high potassium levels, such as cardioplegia solutions or organ preservation solutions.

Clinical features. The clinical manifestations of hyperkalemia are primarily related to membrane depolarization caused by a decrease in the $[K_I]/[K_E]$ ratio. The most life-threatening manifestations are related to the cardiac effects of membrane depolarization. Mild hyperkalemia results in peaked T waves on the electrocardiogram (ECG) and can cause paresthesias and/or weakness. More severe forms of hyperkalemia cause flattened P waves, prolongation of the QRS complex, and deep S waves on the ECG. Ventricular fibrillation and cardiac arrest can follow. Neuromuscular manifestations of severe hyperkalemia include weakness progressing to flaccid paralysis.

Treatment. The treatment of hyperkalemia is dictated by the serum level and by ECG changes or symptoms. Severe hyperkalemia with ECG abnormalities requires urgent treatment. The effects of hyperkalemia on membrane potentials can be reduced by increasing calcium levels. Rapid infusion of 10% to 20% calcium gluconate may be lifesaving. The effects are transient and usually last approximately 30 minutes. Administration of sodium bicarbonate is another temporary measure. The increase in serum sodium antagonizes the effects of hyperkalemia on the membrane potential, whereas the increase in extracellular pH shifts potassium into the cells. Movement of potassium into the intracellular compartment can also be achieved by giving 10 to 20 units of regular insulin. Twenty-five to 50 g of glucose (50 to 100 mL of 50% glucose solution) is administered concurrently to avoid insulin-induced hypoglycemia.

Definitive therapy of hyperkalemia requires increasing potassium excretion. This may be accomplished by the administration of K^+/Na^+ exchange resins such as sodium polystyrene sulfonate (Kayexalate). The usual oral dose is 40 g dissolved in 20 to 100 mL of sorbitol. Each gram removes approximately 1 mEq of potassium. Kayexalate can also be given as a retention enema in a dose of 50 to 100 g in 200 mL of water. Retention of the enema may be facilitated by inflating the balloon of a Foley catheter in the rectum. Each gram removes approximately 0.5 mEq of potassium. Peritoneal dialysis or hemodialysis is indicated for severe hyperkalemia and for patients with renal failure.

Hypokalemia

Causes. Hypokalemia can be caused by TBK depletion secondary to decreased potassium intake, increased extrarenal potassium losses, or increased renal potassium losses. Normally, hypokalemia is not secondary to diminished potassium intake, although intravenous fluid replacement with potassium-free solutions for prolonged periods can result in hypokalemia, especially in patients with ongoing potassium losses.

Decreased serum potassium levels may also be caused by redistribution of potassium into the intracellular space. Acute increases in blood pH secondary to bicarbonate administration during resuscitation can cause acute hypokalemia, as can administration of insulin to hyperglycemic diabetic patients. Causes of hypokalemia are listed in Table 10.10.

Clinical features. Symptoms of hypokalemia, like those of hyperkalemia, are manifestations of disturbances in the $[K_I]/[K_E]$ ratio with resultant alterations in membrane potentials. As potassium levels fall below 2.5 mEq/L, muscle weakness is common. Severe hypokalemia can cause paralysis involving the muscles of respiration. Intestinal peristalsis can be impaired and result in intestinal ileus. Cardiac muscle abnormalities are reflected by the predisposition to digitalis intoxication; the development of cardiac arrhythmias, including ventricular fibrillation; and sensitization to epinephrine. ECG abnormalities include flattened T waves, depressed ST segments, prominent U waves, and prolongation of the QT interval. Renal changes include decreased renal blood flow and glomerular filtration rate. These effects may be relatively minor, and they may be accompanied by polyuria, polydipsia, metabolic alkalosis, and sodium retention. Decreased peripheral vascular resistance with ensuing hypotension may be due to a decrease in vascular sensitivity to angiotensin II.

TABLE 10.10

CAUSES OF HYPOKALEMIA

- Shift of potassium to the intracellular space
- Acute alkalosis
- Administration of glucose and insulin
- Catecholamines
- Increased gastrointestinal loss
- Diarrhea
- Mucus-secreting colon tumors (villous adenoma)
- Excessive renal loss
- Metabolic alkalosis
- Magnesium deficiency
- Hyperaldosteronism (adrenal adenoma or hyperplasia)

Treatment. The primary treatment of hypokalemia is potassium replacement, although the patient's acid–base balance should be considered before initiating therapy. The route and rate of potassium replacement depends on the presence and severity of symptoms. A reduction in serum potassium of 1 mEq/L represents a TBK deficiency of approximately 100 to 200 mEq. Potassium should be administered intravenously if the symptoms are severe, if the serum concentration is below 2 mEq/L, or if the patient is unable to take oral potassium. Intravenous potassium can be administered at a rate of approximately 10 mEq/hour, and the concentration of potassium should be 40 mEq/L or less. If less fluid is desired, up to 20 mEq in 100 mL of intravenous solution can be given, although no more than 40 mEq should be administered per hour. Potassium should be given orally if possible. Oral formulations include potassium salts such as potassium chloride, potassium phosphate, and potassium bicarbonate.

Calcium

Calcium is a divalent cation found in abundance in the human body. Approximately 99% of total body calcium is located in bone in the form of hydroxyapatite crystals. Although the bulk of this calcium is not readily exchangeable, the calcium on the surface of bones can be exchanged and serves as the major store of calcium for maintenance of calcium balance. Calcium homeostasis depends on exchange of calcium between bone and ECF, renal excretion, and intestinal absorption. These three processes are controlled to a great extent by parathyroid hormone (PTH).

The total plasma calcium concentration is approximately 10 mg/dL. In ECF, calcium exists in three forms: ionized, nonionized, and protein-bound. Ionized calcium, which makes up approximately 45% of total calcium, is responsible for most physiologic actions of calcium in the body, and its level is tightly controlled by regulatory mechanisms. Normal serum concentration of ionized calcium is approximately 4.5 mg/dL. Some nonionized calcium is complexed with nonprotein anions, including phosphate and citrate, and does not easily dissociate. These molecular forms make up only 15% of the total calcium present in plasma. Approximately 40% of extracellular nonionized calcium is bound to proteins. Most is bound to albumin, with the remainder bound to α- and β-globulins.

Changes in either plasma protein levels or pH can alter the proportion of calcium in the ionized state. The protein binding of calcium is pH dependent because of competition by H^+ for protein-binding sites. Prompt correction of changes in ionized calcium by various homeostatic mechanisms usually prevents symptoms from occurring, but rapid changes in pH can result in symptoms. The change in ionized calcium can be predicted if the changes in pH and protein concentrations are known. A 0.1 change in pH alters protein-bound calcium by 0.17 mg/dL in the same direction as the pH change. Thus, acidosis decreases protein-bound calcium levels and increases ionized calcium levels. Similarly, a change in albumin concentration of 1 g/dL changes protein-bound calcium by 0.8 mg/dL in the same direction. Because little of the calcium is bound to globulins, changes in globulin concentration of 1 g/dL change protein-bound calcium by only 0.16 mg/dL.

Despite a 10,000-fold concentration gradient with the ECF, intracellular calcium concentration is normally maintained at extremely low levels, 10^{-7} mol/L. This is accomplished by active transport of calcium out of the cell and by sequestration of calcium in mitochondria and the endoplasmic reticulum. Calcium influx occurs through calcium channels, and cytosolic calcium is often bound to specific calcium-binding proteins such as calmodulin. These control mechanisms are key to the central role of calcium as a second messenger in multiple cellular functions such as neural transmission, muscle contraction, and enzyme regulation.

Calcium Homeostasis. Calcium homeostasis is maintained through a balance of bone exchange, renal excretion, and intestinal absorption. All of these functions are controlled to a great degree by PTH. Of these three homeostatic mechanisms, calcium exchange with bone is the most important. Decreased levels of ionized calcium lead to increases in PTH and increases in 1,25-dihydroxyvitamin D_3, both of which stimulate bone absorption by increasing osteoclastic activity. Increased levels of ionized calcium result in decreased PTH and 1,25-dihydroxyvitamin D_3, which decreases bone absorption. In addition, an elevated ionized calcium concentration results in increased calcitonin and 24,25-dihydroxyvitamin D, which increases osteoblastic activity.

Intestinal absorption of calcium depends primarily on 1,25-dihydroxy vitamin D_3, which stimulates calcium absorption from all parts of the small intestine. Renal excretion of calcium is regulated by PTH and vitamin D, which increase distal tubular reabsorption of calcium, and by calcitonin which inhibits calcium reabsorption. Both metabolic and respiratory alkalosis can increase calcium excretion. Acidosis has the opposite effect. The fundamentals of the regulation of calcium homeostasis are depicted in Fig. 10.7.

Hypercalcemia

Causes. The most common causes of hypercalcemia are hyperparathyroidism and malignancy. Hyperparathyroidism is termed primary when one or more parathyroid glands produce inappropriately elevated amounts of PTH in relation to the serum calcium level. This is the result of a parathyroid adenoma in approximately 80% to 90% of cases. Chief cell hyperplasia accounts for an additional 15% of cases, whereas parathyroid cancer is responsible for less than 1% of cases. In secondary hyperparathyroidism, elevated PTH secretion occurs because of an abnormality of an organ system other than the parathyroid glands. Usually this is the result of renal failure, although Paget's disease, osteogenesis imperfecta, and multiple myeloma are other known etiologies. Renal failure can contribute to hypocalcemia in several ways: (a) poor renal excretion of phosphate produces rises in serum phosphate levels that result in decreased serum calcium levels, (b) gut absorption of calcium is decreased because of a deficiency in renal vitamin D metabolism, and (c) diseased kidneys are not capable of clearing the breakdown products of PTH. Tertiary hyperparathyroidism is the development of parathyroid hyperplasia with autonomous PTH production. As a result, up to 30% of patients with prerenal transplantation hyperparathyroidism have persistent elevations in the PTH and calcium after renal transplantation despite the fact that renal function has returned toward normal.

Hypercalcemia can be caused by malignant disease, either because of bony destruction from metastases, or from autonomous tumor secretion of PTH-like substances that alter calcium homeostasis. Common causes of hypercalcemia associated with bone destruction include multiple myeloma, lymphoma, or metastatic breast carcinoma. Interleukin-1, colony-stimulating factor, and tumor necrosis factor have been implicated as local mediators of the osteolytic activity associated with tumor metastases. Tumors that elaborate humoral factors resulting in hypercalcemia are primarily squamous cell carcinomas of the head and neck, esophagus, lung, kidney, and genitourinary tract. Secretion of PTH-like peptides, prostaglandins, transforming growth factor, and vitamin D metabolites has been reported. Humorally mediated hypercalcemia may also occur with metastatic tumors, especially breast carcinoma.

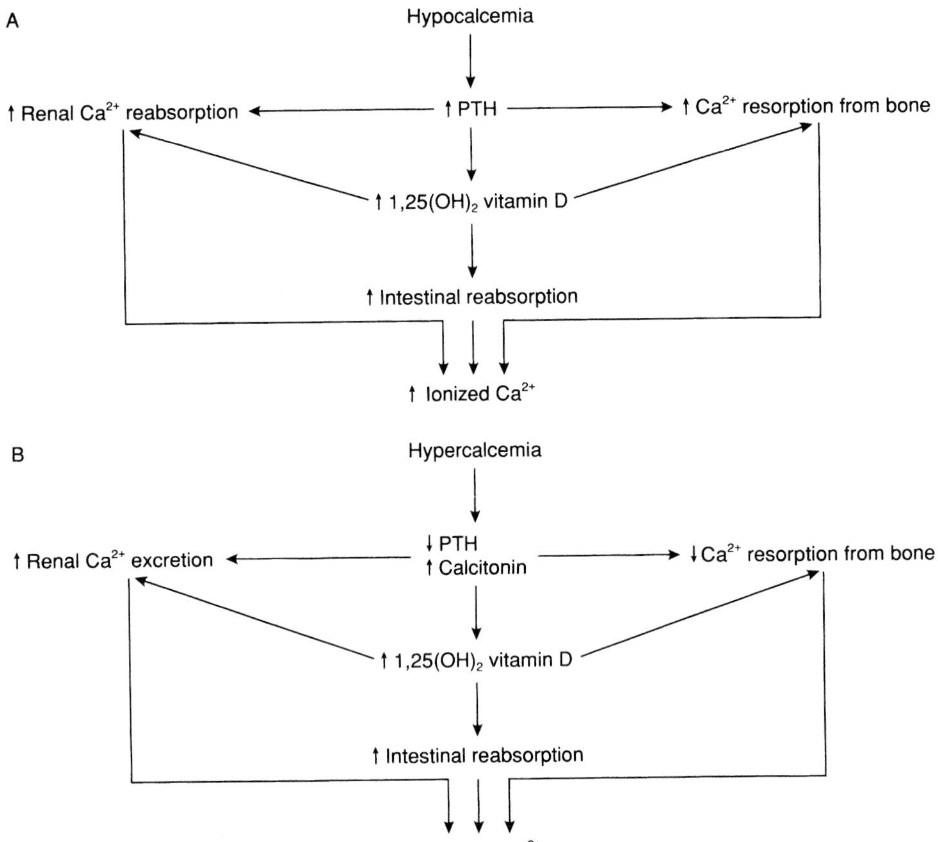

FIGURE 10.7 Effects of hypocalcemia (*A*) and hypercalcemia (*B*) on the mediators of calcium homeostasis. PTH, parathyroid hormone.

Other causes of hypercalcemia include the use of thiazide diuretics, acute adrenal insufficiency, granulomatous disease, milk-alkali syndrome, hyperthyroidism, and prolonged immobilization in otherwise young and healthy patients.

Clinical features. The clinical manifestations of hypercalcemia depend on both the severity and duration of the abnormality. Neuromuscular effects may be the earliest manifestations and include muscle fatigue, weakness, personality disorders, psychoses, confusion, depression, and coma. Cardiovascular effects are less prominent, with hypertension being the most frequent problem encountered. ECG changes include shortening of the QT interval. GI side effects, such as nausea, vomiting, and abdominal pain, are not uncommon. Pancreatitis and increased gastric acid secretion with ulcer formation have also been reported.

The renal side effects of chronic hypercalcemia are numerous and can be severe. The combination of increased renal calcium excretion and decreased intestinal calcium reabsorption in response to hypercalcemia results in a new state of equilibrium at a higher serum concentration of calcium. A decrease in glomerular filtration rate, which may be a direct effect of hypercalcemia or secondary to dehydration from vomiting, can exacerbate the hypercalcemia by increasing calcium reabsorption by the kidney. In addition, nephrocalcinosis can occur, ultimately leading to chronic renal failure. Nephrolithiasis, interstitial nephropathy, renal tubular acidosis (RTA), and nephrogenic diabetes insipidus may also accompany prolonged hypercalcemia.

Treatment. Elevation of serum calcium concentrations to greater than 14 mg/dL requires prompt treatment to prevent potentially lethal complications of hypercalcemia. This is even more urgent for hypercalcemia associated with hyperphosphatemia because of the risk of metastatic calcification. Immediate measures are directed toward maximizing renal excretion of calcium. Because these patients are often dehydrated, 0.9% or 0.45% saline solution with 20 to 30 mEq/L of potassium is administered intravenously. Hydration should proceed at rates of 200 to 300 mL/h to promote diuresis. Once adequate hydration is achieved, furo-semide may be given to enhance calcium excretion.

Long-term treatment depends on the underlying cause of the hypercalcemia. Primary hyperparathyroidism is treated by parathyroidectomy. Secondary or tertiary hyperparathyroidism may be treated by either subtotal parathyroidectomy or total parathyroidectomy with autonomous parathyroid transplantation. Hypercalcemia secondary to tumor secretion of hormonal mediators may be controlled by extirpation of the tumor. In the presence of metastatic bone disease, inhibition of bone resorption with mithramycin or calcitonin may yield good results. In addition, hypercalcemia due to metastatic breast carcinoma or hematologic malignancies may respond to steroid therapy. Intravenous administration of bisphosphonates have been shown to be extremely effective and safe for treatment of patients with hypercalcemia associated with cancer.[33] Patients with renal failure benefit from dialysis using a low-calcium dialysate.

Hypocalcemia

Causes. Hypocalcemia secondary to hypoparathyroidism can complicate thyroid or parathyroid surgery by either inadvertent total parathyroidectomy or loss of parathyroid function due to devascularization. This has been reported to occur in as many as 2% to 3% of patients undergoing total thyroidectomy, although this figure appears to be declining. After resection of a parathyroid adenoma, hypocalcemia can occur because of atrophy of the remaining glands. Calcium replacement therapy may be required until the remaining glands resume normal function.

Hypocalcemia can also complicate acute pancreatitis owing to calcium precipitation into the peripancreatic tissues. In addition, pancreatic and small bowel fistulae may result in loss of calcium-rich fluid. Long-standing vitamin D deficiency secondary to malnutrition, malabsorption, or lack of exposure to sunlight can lead to hypocalcemia. Renal failure can lead to a deficiency in 1,25-dihydroxyvitamin D_3 and result in diminished intestinal absorption of calcium. Severe magnesium deficiency can also lead to hypocalcemia because of suppression of PTH levels.

Clinical features. Serum calcium levels below 8 mg/dL may be associated with symptoms and signs that are primarily manifestations of neuromuscular abnormalities. These include muscle cramps, perioral tingling, paresthesia, laryngeal stridor, tetany, seizures, and psychotic behavior. Classic signs of hypocalcemia include hyperactive deep tendon reflexes. Two well-described physical findings occur when a patient becomes hypocalcemic. One of these is Chvostek's sign, which consists of facial muscle spasm when the trunk of the facial nerve is tapped. The other finding is Trousseau's sign, carpal spasms when a blood pressure cuff is inflated to occlude the brachial artery for 3 minutes. This finding indicates latent tetany. ECG changes include a prolonged QT interval caused by prolongation of the ST segment.

Treatment. Asymptomatic hypocalcemia, which may be secondary to low protein or albumin levels with normal ionized calcium levels, need not be treated. Symptomatic hypocalcemia is best treated with intravenous infusion of calcium in the form of calcium gluconate or calcium chloride. Calcium chloride dissociates primarily to the ionized form and is therefore more efficacious in raising ionized calcium levels. Calcium should be administered at a rate not exceeding 50 mg/minute (2.5 mEq/minute). Prolonged calcium replacement is given orally in the form of calcium lactate, calcium citrate, or calcium carbonate. Vitamin D_3, also known as calcitriol, increases the rate of intestinal absorption and decreases the oral calcium dose requirement.

Magnesium

Total body content of magnesium in the average adult is 2,000 mEq, half of which is confined to bone. Most of the remaining magnesium is distributed in the intracellular space. Less than 1% of total body magnesium is located in the extracellular space, at concentrations of 1.4 to 2 mEq/L (or 1.7 to 2.3 mg/dL). Sixty percent of this magnesium exists in the ionized form, 25% is in the protein-bound state, and the remainder is complexed with nonprotein anionic species.

Approximately 25 mEq per day of magnesium is consumed in the diet, a variable amount of which is absorbed by the small intestine. Magnesium absorption may be influenced by the levels of 1,25-dihydroxyvitamin D_3. Bone stores constitute the other major source of available magnesium, although regulation of magnesium exchange with bone is poorly understood.

Magnesium is excreted primarily by the kidneys. Approximately 40% of the filtered magnesium is reabsorbed in the proximal tubule, predominantly in the ascending limb of Henle. Thus, loop diuretics cause a marked increase in magnesium excretion. Magnesium excretion is also increased by hypermagnesemia, hypercalcemia, metabolic acidosis, and phosphate depletion. Conversely, magnesium excretion is decreased by metabolic alkalosis.

Hypermagnesemia

Causes. Because of the ability of the kidneys to excrete large magnesium loads, hypermagnesemia rarely occurs if renal function is normal. In chronic or acute renal failure, administration of magnesium-containing antacids or laxatives is frequently the cause of hypermagnesemia. Severe burns, crush injuries, and other causes of rhabdomyolysis may lead to high magnesium levels due to the release of magnesium from injured tissues. Severe metabolic acidosis, extracellular volume depletion, and renal insufficiency with creatinine clearances below 30 mL/minute may also cause hypermagnesemia.

Clinical features. Neuromuscular function is depressed by hypermagnesemia because of the inhibition of synaptic acetylcholine release. Loss of deep tendon reflexes can occur with magnesium levels above 8 mg/dL. Paralysis and eventually coma can develop if levels exceed 12 to 18 mg/dL. Hypotension or even cardiac arrest can occur if levels exceed 18 mg/dL.

Treatment. Magnesium-containing medications must be avoided in patients with hypermagnesemia. Calcium antagonizes the effects of magnesium, and infusion of 5 to 10 mEq of calcium by slow intravenous injection may serve as adequate emergency treatment. Volume expansion, correction of acid–base disturbances, administration of loop diuretics, and hemodialysis may also be used to decrease magnesium levels.

Hypomagnesemia

Causes. Because the kidneys are able to conserve magnesium well in states of magnesium depletion, hypomagnesemia rarely occurs from poor intake alone, although malnutrition is a common cause of hypomagnesemia. Malabsorptive states, especially steatorrhea, can result in significant losses of magnesium. The combination of diminished intake and increased GI losses can lead to hypomagnesemia. Other causes of hypomagnesemia include prolonged periods of intravenous fluid replacement without magnesium replacement and chronic use of loop diuretics. Drugs, such as cyclosporine, aminoglycosides, cisplatin, and insulin, can also produce magnesium depletion. Burns, acute pancreatitis, treatment of diabetic ketoacidosis (DKA), and the diuretic phase of acute renal failure have been associated with the development of hypomagnesemia.

Clinical features. Magnesium plays an integral role as a cofactor in many enzyme systems and also affects neuromuscular function. Deficiencies in magnesium may present symptoms and signs similar to hypocalcemia. Muscle fasciculations and weakness, tetany, carpopedal spasm, nausea, vomiting, and personality changes may occur. Electrolyte disturbances may also be caused by hypomagnesemia. Hypocalcemia caused by impaired PTH secretion and PTH resistance may develop. Hypokalemia caused by renal potassium wasting may also occur.

Treatment. Magnesium may be administered orally in mild cases of hypomagnesemia, but large oral doses frequently lead to diarrhea. Correction of major deficits is therefore managed by intravenous administration of magnesium sulfate at a dose of 50 to 100 mEq/day. Treatment of patients who have severe symptoms with up to 3 g of magnesium sulfate may be accomplished by bolus intravenous injection followed by an infusion of 1 to 2 mEq/kg/day.

ACID–BASE BALANCE

Definitions

An acid is defined as a chemical that can donate a hydrogen ion (H^+), for example, HCl and H_2CO_3, and a base is a chemical that can accept a H^+, for example, OH^- and HCO_3^-.

Ampholytes are both acids and bases; an example is $H_2PO_4^-$, which can donate a H^+ to become HPO_4^{2-} but can also accept H^+ to become H_3PO_4. Because HCl is a strong acid that almost completely dissociates, Cl^- is not considered a base. Bases are commonly anions, but neutral substances can also function as bases (e.g., ammonia and creatinine). Some chemicals do not fit the classic definition of an acid, although they retain acidic properties when dissociated in water. For example, when $CaCl_2$ is dissolved in water, the Ca^{2+} accepts OH^- to form $Ca(OH)_2$. Because $[H^+] \times [OH^-]$ in water remains constant at 10 to 14, the consumption of OH^- by Ca^{2+} results in increased dissociation of water. Consequently, the concentration of hydrogen ions increases, and $CaCl_2$ dissolved in water is an acidic solution.

The concentration of hydrogen ions $[H^+]$ determines the acidity of a solution. The pH is the negative logarithm of $[H^+]$ expressed in moles per liter (mol/L). The concentration of H^+ in biologic systems is in the range of nanomoles (10^{-9} mol) per liter (nmol/L). When

$$[H^+] = 40 \text{ nmol/L} = 4 \times 10^{-10} \text{ mol/L}$$

then

$$pH = -\log [H^+] = -(-7.4) = 7.4$$

When

$$[H^+] = 80 \text{ nmol/L} = 8 \times 10^{-10} \text{ mol/L}$$

then

$$pH = -\log [H^+] = -(-7.1) = 7.1$$

The degree to which an acid dissociates determines its strength. If an acid, HA, dissociates to H^+ and A^-, then

$$[H^+] \times [A^-]/[HA] = K$$

where K = dissociation constant. The greater the value of K, the greater the ability to dissociate and therefore the greater the strength of the acid. Because most acids have a K value considerably below 1.0

$$pK = -\log K$$

Rearranging

$$[H^+] = K \times [HA]/[A^-]$$

$$-\log [H^+] = -\log K \times -\log [HA]/[A^-]$$

$$pH = pK \times \log [A^-]/[HA]$$

This is the derivation for the Henderson-Hasselbalch equation.

Buffer Systems

Buffers are chemicals in solution that tend to minimize changes in pH that would otherwise occur after the addition of acid or alkali. If a strong acid is added to the salt of a weak acid and a strong base, the reaction produces another salt and a weak acid:

$$HCl + NaHCO_3 \longrightarrow NaCl + H_2CO_3$$

Thus, the decrease in pH that would have occurred in the absence of $NaHCO_3$ is minimized. Conversely, if a strong base is added to a weak acid, the base is neutralized:

$$NaOH + H_2CO_3 \longrightarrow NaHCO_3 + H_2O$$

The elevation in pH after the addition of NaOH is prevented.

One type of buffer is a mixture of a weak acid and its salt, which forms an amount of weak acid or base equivalent to the amount of strong acid or base added to the system. The presence of such buffer systems in the body is crucial in minimizing changes in pH secondary to the daily production of the 70 mEq of acid generated from dietary precursors. There is a relatively narrow range of pH for optimal function of the chemical reactions necessary for cell function.

The principal intracellular buffers are organic phosphates, bicarbonate, and peptides. In addition, hemoglobin functions as a significant buffer in red blood cells. The major extracellular buffer is bicarbonate. An approximation of the total body buffer capacity is 15 mEq/kg. More than half of the total body alkaline buffer content is located outside the ECF and may in large part reside in bone.[34] The buffer pair carbonic acid/bicarbonate (H_2CO_3/HCO_3^-) is the focus of the ensuing discussion because it is the primary buffer system of the body and the components of this buffer system are easily measured. Because all body buffer systems are in equilibrium, the state of the H_2CO_3/HCO_3^- system essentially reflects the state of all the body buffers.

From a chemical point of view, the ideal buffer should have a pK that approximates the pH to be preserved. The H_2CO_3/HCO_3^- buffer system has a pK of only 6.1, but this buffer system is efficient because of the presence of large amounts of bicarbonate, the conversion of its acid H_2CO_3 to CO_2 that is rapidly excreted through the lungs, and an inexhaustible supply of CO_2, although at low concentrations.

The H_2CO_3/HCO_3^- buffer system is defined by the Henderson-Hasselbalch equation:

$$pH = pK + \log [HCO_3^-]/[H_2CO_3]$$

In the clinical use of this equation, $[H_2CO_3]$ is replaced by $[CO_2]$ because measurement of the low concentrations of $[H_2CO_3]$ present in body fluids is difficult, whereas $[CO_2]$, which is in equilibrium with $[H_2CO_3]$ in a fixed ratio, can be readily measured. Making this substitution, the equation becomes

$$pH = pK + \log [HCO_3^-]/[CO_2]$$

Because the pK for this buffer system is 6.1

$$pH = 6.1 + \log [HCO_3^-]/[CO_2]$$

Using normal values for $[HCO_3^-]$ (24 mEq/L) and $[CO_2]$ (1.2 mmol/L)

$$\begin{aligned} pH &= 6.1 + \log 24/1.2 \\ &= 6.1 + \log 20 = 7.4 \end{aligned}$$

A pH of 7.4 is maintained as long as the ratio of $[HCO_3^-]$ to $[CO_2]$ remains 20:1. The amount of $[CO_2]$ in solution is estimated from PCO_2 and its solubility coefficient (0.03 in plasma). Making these substitutions

$$pH = 6.1 + \log [HCO_3^-]/(P\text{CO}_2 \times 0.03)$$

Anion Gap

The anion gap is defined as follows:

$$\text{Anion gap} = [Na^+] - ([Cl^-] + [HCO_3^-])$$

Normally, the difference between the serum $[Na^+]$ and the sum of the chloride and bicarbonate anion concentrations is a reflection of the sum of the serum proteins, sulfate anions, inorganic phosphates, and organic acids present in low concentrations. The anion gap is usually 12 ± 2 mEq/L. Variances from the normal may be caused by a change in unmeasured anions or cations. Calculation of the anion gap may help define both simple and mixed forms of acid–base disturbances. Acidosis associated with a high anion gap is usually secondary to increases in endogenously produced acids (e.g., lactic acidosis or ketoacidosis), decreases in renal excretion of acid, or ingestion of toxins.

TABLE 10.11

HCO_3^- AND PCO_2 DERANGEMENTS IN PRIMARY AND SECONDARY ACID–BASE DISTURBANCES

		Primary		Secondary	
Disorder	pH	HCO_3^-	PCO_2	HCO_3^-	PCO_2
Metabolic acidosis	↓	↓			↓
Metabolic alkalosis	↑	↑			↑
Respiratory acidosis	↓		↑	↑	
Respiratory alkalosis	↑		↓	↓	

Acid–Base Disturbances

There are four primary acid–base disturbances, each of which are related to changes in either [HCO_3^-] or PCO_2. Metabolic acidosis is a decrease in pH as a result of a primary decrease in [HCO_3^-], whereas metabolic alkalosis is an increase in pH caused by a primary increase in [HCO_3^-]. Respiratory acidosis is a decrease in pH secondary to a primary increase in PCO_2, and respiratory alkalosis is an increase in pH caused by a primary decrease in PCO_2. In each of these disorders, compensatory changes occur to minimize changes in the relative ratio of [HCO_3^-] to PCO_2 and thereby blunt the effect of the primary disturbance on pH (Table 10.11).

Metabolic Acidosis

Three mechanisms result in a decrease in extracellular bicarbonate concentration and metabolic acidosis:

1. Dilutional acidosis. Rapid infusion of an alkali-free solution results in dilution of the bicarbonate concentration.
2. Cellular retention of K^+ in exchange for Na^+ and H^+. Buffering of the H^+ may result in a transient decrease in extracellular bicarbonate concentration.
3. Decreased body bicarbonate content. This occurs when net loss of bicarbonate exceeds bicarbonate generation.

The first two mechanisms are relatively infrequent and usually produce only mild, self-limiting metabolic acidosis; however, aggressive "overresuscitation" of surgical or trauma patients with normal saline solution may result in a dilutional acidosis. Most clinically significant metabolic acidosis is related to net loss of bicarbonate, which occurs when consumption due to either loss or titration is greater than bicarbonate generation. Under normal circumstances of ingestion of the average amount of protein in the American diet, approximately 70 mEq of acid is generated daily. The major source of acid production is sulfuric acid from the metabolism of sulfur-containing amino acids. In addition, normal physiologic processes result in the generation of organic acids, the titration of which consumes bicarbonate. Although the resulting organic anions are further metabolized with regeneration of bicarbonate, urinary excretion of some organic anions occurs and results in net loss of bicarbonate.

These sources of acid gain are partially offset by net GI absorption of metabolizable anions, such as citrate, which are metabolized to yield bicarbonate. The remainder of the excess acid is balanced by renal excretion of acid with simultaneous generation of bicarbonate. A decrease in body bicarbonate content may therefore be the result of a primary increase in net acid generation, termed *extrarenal acidosis*, or a primary reduction in renal acid excretion, termed *renal acidosis*.

In extrarenal acidosis, the normal compensatory mechanism is increased renal excretion of acid, usually as ammonia, with generation of bicarbonate. This mechanism is sensitive to decreases in bicarbonate concentration and has the capacity to generate large amounts of bicarbonate.

In contrast, renal acidosis is not as readily compensated because the renal abnormality is the primary mechanism. The level to which serum bicarbonate concentration decreases depends on several factors, including the magnitude of the disparity in acid production and acid excretion as well as its duration. In general, the development of renal acidosis is slow but progressive, whereas the development of extrarenal acidosis is rapid but usually self-limiting. Despite persistent net loss of bicarbonate, extracellular bicarbonate concentration may stabilize at a subnormal level rather than continue to decrease. This may be due to bone buffering, which has the capacity to buffer as much as 28 to 37 mEq/day of acid.

Mechanisms Resulting in Decreased Body Bicarbonate Content

Increased production of organic acids. Increased protein intake and tissue catabolism resulting in greater metabolism of sulfur-containing amino acids can lead to generation of increased amounts of sulfuric acid. With normal kidney function, any decline in serum bicarbonate concentration stimulates renal acid excretion, which can compensate nearly completely for the increase in acid production.

Administration of exogenous acid. Ingestion of a sufficient quantity of exogenous acid can exceed renal compensatory capacity and result in metabolic acidosis. Examples of acids that may be ingested include ammonium chloride, calcium chloride, nitric acid, sulfuric acid, and hydrochloric acid.

Nonrenal loss of bicarbonate. Diarrhea, intestinal or pancreatic fistulas, and burns can cause metabolic acidosis secondary to loss of bicarbonate. Urinary diversion with segments of GI tract (ureterosigmoidostomy and ureteroileostomy) can result in loss of bicarbonate with reabsorption of NH_4Cl from the urine. The potential for fistulas to result in metabolic acidosis depends on the concentration of bicarbonate in the fluid and the rate of external drainage. Thus, metabolic acidosis is less common with biliary fistulae than pancreatic fistulas because bicarbonate concentration in bile is usually less than 50 to 60 mEq/L, and the amount of drainage tends to be modest. Bicarbonate concentration in pancreatic juice approaches 150 mEq/L, and the drainage can be profuse.

Organic acidosis. Organic acidosis describes conditions of acidosis brought about by abnormal endogenous production of specific acid compounds. The two most common types of organic acidosis are *ketoacidosis* and *lactic acidosis*.

Ketoacidosis. Normally, free fatty acids generated from breakdown of triglycerides in adipose tissue are either used as an energy source by tissues such as muscle or carried to the liver, where they are reesterified to triglycerides. Ketoacids are produced by mitochondrial metabolism of free fatty acids to acetyl-CoA, with subsequent formation of acetoacetate and b-hydroxybutyrate (redox forms of the same compound). Under normal conditions, a small amount of ketoacidosis is produced. During prolonged starvation, production of ketoacids increases to modest levels, providing an important source of energy to nonhepatic tissues, particularly the brain.

In DKA, the ketoacid production is excessive because of insulin deficiency, which drives ketoacid production by increasing free fatty acid release from adipose tissue, increasing transport of free fatty acids into hepatic mitochondria, promoting conversion of acetyl-CoA to ketoacids, and impairing extrahepatic use of ketoacids.[35] Insulin deficiency also contributes to hyperglycemia by decreasing the metabolism of glucose by extrahepatic tissues and increasing hepatic production of glucose. The resulting osmotic glucose diuresis causes increased renal excretion of sodium and water. Additional losses of sodium and potassium occur as the result of renal excretion of the excess ketoacid anions. Potassium excretion is further enhanced by hyperaldosteronism due to the increased delivery of sodium to the distal tubule that occurs in association with the osmotic diuresis. Despite TBK depletion, serum potassium concentration is often increased in DKA secondary to metabolic acidosis, renal insufficiency, insulin deficiency, and hyperosmolality. These pathophysiologic changes result in the typical clinical presentation, which includes dehydration, polyuria, polydipsia, hyperglycemia, hyperventilation, and metabolic acidosis with an increased anion gap. Spontaneous decarboxylation of acetoacetate to acetone occurs with excretion of acetone through the lungs, resulting in the characteristic odor described in DKA. Patients may demonstrate impaired mental status or coma in severe cases.

In hyperosmolar, hyperglycemic, and nonketotic coma, moderate acidosis may be observed. The mechanism of the acidosis is not clear. In contrast to the moderate hyperglycemia, averaging 600 mg/dL, seen in DKA, the marked hyperglycemia, averaging 1,200 mg/dL, that occurs in hyperosmolar nonketotic hyperglycemia is not associated with ketoacidosis.

Lactic acidosis. Lactic acidosis can be characterized as type A (caused by tissue hypoxia), and type B (other causes). Hypoxia impairs the mitochondrial oxidation of the reduced form of nicotinamide-adenine dinucleotide (NADH) to NAD, which is necessary for glycolysis. Under these conditions, NADH is oxidized by the reduction of pyruvate, the end product of glucose metabolism in the Embden-Meyerhof pathway, to lactic acid. Thus, generation of lactic acid is the final step of anaerobic glycolysis. Lactic acid is normally produced by muscle, blood elements, intestine, and skin and is used by the liver and kidney. Normal serum lactate concentration is below 2 mEq/L. Lactic acidosis secondary to hypoxia is usually due to increased production of lactate as well as decreased use, and serum lactate concentration is greater than 6 mEq/L.

The most common cause of type B lactic acidosis is ethanol intoxication. Lactic acidosis is caused by increased generation of NADH by the metabolism of alcohol, which interferes with hepatic gluconeogenesis and, therefore, lactate use.

In lactic acidosis, the L-isomer is usually elevated because of the specificity of mammalian lactate dehydrogenase. Various bacteria found in colonic flora are capable of generating large amounts of D-lactic acid. D-Lactic acidosis has been reported in humans only in the presence of short-gut syndrome because the small bowel normally absorbs the dietary substrate for bacterial D-lactic acid production. In addition, the colon must be selectively colonized by bacteria that possess D-lactate dehydrogenase. Typically, the patient has short-gut syndrome, and the acidosis is preceded by food ingestion and is accompanied by characteristic neurologic findings, including mental confusion, slurred speech, staggering gait, and nystagmus. These neurologic manifestations are secondary to bacterial neurotoxins. The acidosis is accompanied by an increased anion gap, but L-lactate and ketone levels are normal. Treatment includes oral antibiotics, recolonization of the colon with non-D-lactate dehydrogenase-forming bacteria, and a low-carbohydrate diet.

Metabolic Acidosis Caused by Drugs and Toxins. Acetylsalicylic acid (aspirin) is rapidly metabolized to salicylic acid and then more slowly to other metabolites that are excreted by the kidney. Ingestion of more than 4 to 6 g/day results in salicylate intoxication with an anion gap metabolic acidosis, as well as renal excretion of unmetabolized salicylic acid. Acidosis increases the toxicity of salicylate by increasing the concentration of its nonionized form, which can achieve high intracellular concentrations. A respiratory alkalosis occurs due to direct stimulation of the respiratory center. Manifestations of salicylate overdose include tinnitus, asterixis, noncardiogenic pulmonary edema, hypotension, vascular collapse, vomiting, seizures, and coma. Treatment consists of alkalinization of the urine to prevent reabsorption of salicylate and hemodialysis in patients with severe neurologic symptoms.

Ethylene glycol, the principal component of antifreeze, is converted by alcohol dehydrogenase to glycoaldehyde, then to glycolic acid with production of one NADH at each step. The acidosis produced by ingestion of ethylene glycol is secondary to accumulation of glycolic acid, although lactate also accumulates because of the production of NADH. Bicarbonate is not regenerated when the glycolate is further metabolized, so exogenous alkali is required to replace what was titrated. In addition, 3% to 10% of ethylene glycol is converted to oxalic acid, which may result in hypocalcemia and contribute to acute renal failure. Three stages of toxicity are described. CNS dysfunction characterizes the first stage. This is followed by cardiopulmonary failure and finally by oliguric acute renal failure. Treatment includes the administration of ethanol, which has greater affinity for alcohol dehydrogenase and delays the metabolism of ethylene glycol to its toxic metabolites. Treatment also includes hemodialysis or peritoneal dialysis to remove ethylene glycol and glycolate.

Metabolism of methanol by alcohol dehydrogenase results in the formation of formaldehyde and formic acid, both of which are severely toxic. The acidosis is associated with an increase in anion gap secondary to the accumulation of formate. The clinical presentation includes blurred vision or blindness associated with the funduscopic findings of hyperemic discs and retinal edema, malaise, headache, abdominal pain, vomiting, convulsions, and coma. Treatment includes ethanol infusion to delay the metabolism of methanol by alcohol dehydrogenase, hemodialysis, bicarbonate administration, and intravenous folate to enhance metabolism of formate.

Renal Acidosis: Decreased Net Acid Excretion. The impaired ability of the kidney to excrete acid may be secondary to a decrease in the number of functioning nephrons and is termed *uremic acidosis* or *renal tubular acidosis*. Uremic acidosis, which can occur in both acute and chronic renal failure, is primarily caused by a reduction in ammonia excretion secondary to a reduction in the number of functioning proximal tubular cells. In addition, decreased proximal tubular bicarbonate reabsorption contributes to the development of acidosis. Although the onset of uremic acidosis may be related to declining renal function, its appearance can also be influenced by diet-dependent protein and organic anion ingestion, use of diuretic therapy that stimulates acid excretion, and the extent of tubular versus glomerular injury.

RTA can be classified as distal (type I) or proximal (type II), depending on the primary site of the renal tubular defect leading to acidosis. Distal RTA is characterized by a defect in urinary acidification. It is associated with either hypokalemia or hyperkalemia, depending on the underlying pathophysiologic mechanisms. Proposed mechanisms of distal RTA with hypokalemia include reduced H^+ pump activity and increased tubular permeability with back-leak of secreted H^+ into the tubular cell. In RTA with hyperkalemia, the mechanism is decreased luminal negativity secondary to impaired sodium reabsorption. The major defect in proximal RTA is proximal tubular dysfunction resulting in diminished reabsorption of filtered bicarbonate. Urinary excretion greater than 15% of the filtered load of bicarbonate at normal serum bicarbonate levels is pathognomonic for proximal RTA. Other indicators of proximal tubular dysfunction include glycosuria, aminoaciduria, uricosuria, and phosphaturia.

Clinical Features of Acute Metabolic Acidosis. The major cardiovascular effects of acute metabolic acidosis are peripheral arteriolar dilatation, decreased cardiac contractility, and central venous constriction. These can lead to cardiovascular collapse and pulmonary edema. Catecholamine secretion is stimulated by metabolic acidosis, and in mild cases (pH >7.1), heart rate may be increased. In more severe metabolic acidosis (pH <7.1), the direct effects of acidosis override the catecholamine effects and result in bradycardia and decreased contractility. These depressive effects are magnified by beta blockers. In addition to these cardiovascular effects, metabolic acidosis can increase oxygen delivery by shifting the oxygen–hemoglobin dissociation curve to the right. In more prolonged metabolic acidosis, this may be partially offset by decreased production of 2,3-diphosphoglycerate in red blood cells because of a slower rate of glycolysis. Metabolic acidosis can also cause gastric distention, abdominal pain, nausea, and vomiting.

Compensatory Mechanisms

Renal compensation. The kidney is extremely sensitive to changes in serum bicarbonate concentration and responds by increasing net acid excretion primarily by increasing ammonia excretion. Maximal renal compensation requires 2 to 4 days. In addition, the maximal amount of ammonia excreted during acidosis depends on factors that include the rate of glutamine delivery, effects on glomerular filtration rate by associated conditions such as dehydration, and the type of anion that accompanies the acid because renal acid secretion is stimulated to varying degrees by different anions. Although renal compensation is effective in achieving normal net acid excretion with extrarenal causes of metabolic acid, variable results are seen with renal acidosis. Compensation at times is complete for proximal RTA, whereas compensation usually is incomplete for distal RTA.

Respiratory compensation. Delay in achieving maximal renal response to an increased acid load causes blood pH to decline, which stimulates hyperventilation. Although effective in promptly raising blood pH, early ventilatory compensation is only partial. Full respiratory compensation can occur in 12 to 24 hours. The magnitude of the decrease in P_{CO_2} in response to a given degree of metabolic acidosis can be used to determine whether the metabolic acidosis is complicated by coexisting respiratory acidosis or respiratory alkalosis. Although a number of sophisticated mathematic models relating P_{CO_2} to serum bicarbonate, serum hydrogen ion, and pH have been described, the following is a simple equation that is readily applicable to the clinical situation:

$$dP_{CO_2} = 1.2 \times d[HCO_3^-] \pm 2.0$$

where dP_{CO_2} = expected decrease in P_{CO_2} given the measured decrease in serum bicarbonate concentration. For example, if serum bicarbonate is 18, $d[HCO_3^-]$ is 6 (24 − 18). The expected dP_{CO_2} is 7.2 ± 2, or P_{CO_2} = 32.8 (40 − 7.2) ± 2 mm Hg. This equation is applicable in mild to moderate metabolic acidosis because pulmonary edema complicating severe metabolic acidosis interferes with maximal ventilatory compensation.

Treatment

Acute metabolic acidosis. In surgical and trauma patients, metabolic acidosis is often the result of inadequate tissue perfusion and consequent lactic acidosis. Volume resuscitation alone may be enough to correct this acidosis. Attempts to correct acidosis with exogenous bicarbonate without addressing inadequate tissue perfusion will be unsuccessful. Bicarbonate is best reserved for patients with metabolic acidosis that is either not easily reversible or is so severe that the patient is in danger of cardiovascular collapse. Older patients and those with cardiovascular disease have decreased tolerance for acidosis, and it may be appropriate to administer bicarbonate in these groups before the pH has fallen to critically low levels. The amount of bicarbonate required to increase its serum concentration to any given level cannot be calculated. The goal is to increase the pH to 7.2 to 7.3 by administering one or two ampules of bicarbonate (44.5 to 50 mEq/amp) initially, basing the need for additional bicarbonate on repeated arterial blood gas results. Rapid correction to achieve normal serum bicarbonate concentration may be harmful because organic anions are precursors of bicarbonate, and their eventual metabolism combined with administered bicarbonate may result in metabolic alkalosis. This may be further complicated by persistent hyperventilation in the face of rapidly normalized serum bicarbonate concentration, resulting in the superimposition of a respiratory alkalosis. In addition, rapid correction of serum bicarbonate concentration may not allow reversal of 2,3-diphosphoglycerate depletion in red blood cells. The resulting leftward shift of the oxygen–hemoglobin dissociation curve may result in tissue hypoxia.

Chronic acidosis. Distal RTA may be treated with daily doses of alkali to correct acidosis and prevent nephrocalcinosis and nephrolithiasis, and potassium supplementation if hypokalemia as also present. Mild proximal RTA in adults does not require specific therapy. Severe cases ($[HCO_3^-]$ <18) are treated with thiazide diuretics and a low-salt diet aimed to achieve modest volume depletion, which reduces bicarbonate requirement. Children are particularly susceptible to the growth-retarding effects of even mild acidosis, and the threshold for treatment should be low.

Diabetic ketoacidosis. The correction of both acidosis and hyperglycemia is best achieved by administration of insulin. Metabolism of the anions of the ketoacids begins promptly with insulin therapy and results in the generation of bicarbonate. In addition, insulin inhibits ketone formation and gluconeogenesis and stimulates peripheral uptake of ketones and glucose. An intravenous (IV) dose of 20 IU of regular insulin may be given to initiate therapy, followed by a continuous intravenous infusion of 5 to 10 IU/h. Insulin administration should continue until acidosis resolves. Volume resuscitation requirements in DKA averages 4 to 5 L in the first 24 hours. By alternating liters of normal and half-normal saline risk of cerebral edema is minimized. Potassium should be administered even in the face of normal or high serum potassium, because hypokalemia develops as acidosis and hyperglycemia are corrected. Unrecognized hypokalemia is a major cause of death from DKA.

Hyperosmolar nonketotic acidosis. The key to successful treatment is to seek, recognize, and treat any underlying cause for the hyperosmolar nonketotic hyperglycemia, such as gram-negative sepsis. Hyperglycemia is corrected by the administration of insulin, as described previously. Volume depletion can be more severe than that seen with DKA. Potassium supplementation must be given as well.

Metabolic Alkalosis

Causes. Sustained metabolic alkalosis occurs only if extracellular bicarbonate concentration is increased and renal excretion of excess bicarbonate is inhibited. Extracellular bicarbonate concentration increases can occur through several mechanisms. In surgical patients, loss of HCl is a frequent cause of metabolic alkalosis, most commonly due to vomiting or nasogastric drainage in the face of gastric outlet obstruction. External loss of gastric acid results in a net gain in bicarbonate (generated by equimolar gastric secretion of HCl), which causes the alkalosis. Although the kidney can excrete excess bicarbonate, this must be accompanied by excretion of sodium. Renal excretion of sodium is limited in the face of the volume depletion which also occurs with external losses of gastric secretion. As volume depletion progresses, sodium is conserved in exchange for hydrogen, and urine will become acidic, even in the presence of severe metabolic alkalosis. This phenomenon is referred to as *paradoxic aciduria.*

Increased extracellular bicarbonate concentration can occur with administration of either bicarbonate or precursors of bicarbonate, such as lactate, citrate, or calcium carbonate, or as a result of increased renal production of bicarbonate. Conditions in which acid excretion exceeds endogenous acid production and in which the renal threshold for bicarbonate reabsorption is increased can result in metabolic alkalosis. Such conditions include moderate potassium depletion, excess mineralocorticoids, and high P_{CO_2}.

Hypokalemia and cellular exchange of potassium for hydrogen can also lead to metabolic alkalosis. Hypokalemia results in enhanced proximal tubular bicarbonate reabsorption and distal tubular acid excretion. When potassium leaves the cell, it is exchanged for either sodium or hydrogen to maintain electrical neutrality. Loss of potassium from the body then results in a net gain in bicarbonate in the ECF.

Maintenance of elevated extracellular bicarbonate concentration can occur by a number of mechanisms. Volume contraction leads to decreases in renal blood flow and glomerular filtration rate that reduce the filtered load of bicarbonate. This, in addition to increased proximal tubular reabsorption of bicarbonate, maintains high extracellular concentrations of bicarbonate. High P_{CO_2} causes an increase in renal threshold for bicarbonate secondary to decreased intracellular pH of the renal tubular cell. The net result is increased bicarbonate reabsorption.

Hypercalcemia and low PTH levels both result in increased proximal tubular reabsorption of bicarbonate, which may be enhanced by a decrease in glomerular filtration rate. Renal failure also leads to an inability of the kidney to excrete excess bicarbonate. Diuretics can cause or exacerbate metabolic alkalosis by both causing rapid contraction of intravascular volume and increasing renal excretion of acid. Chloride deficiency is another common factor that maintains an alkalotic state. In some instances of metabolic alkalosis, urinary excretion of chloride is markedly reduced. Reversal of metabolic alkalosis in these cases can be readily achieved by administration of chloride-containing solutions. Although chloride deficiency per se can result in an increased renal threshold for bicarbonate and in increased renal reabsorption of bicarbonate, this apparent association may also be related to volume contraction. Metabolic alkalosis can be divided into chloride-responsive and chloride-resistant types.

Respiratory Compensation. The major compensatory mechanism in metabolic alkalosis is respiratory because the presence of the metabolic alkalosis implicates renal dysfunction in either generating or failing to excrete increased amounts of bicarbonate. Hypoventilation is limited by the development of hypoxemia, which stimulates ventilation, and P_{CO_2} rarely exceeds 60 mm Hg (Table 10.12). Among the four major types of acid–base disorders, this compensatory mechanism is the least effective. For a given degree of metabolic alkalosis, the following equation can be used to predict the compensatory increase in P_{CO_2}:

$$dP_{CO_2} = 0.7 \times d[HCO_3^-] \pm 5$$

where dP_{CO_2} = expected increase in P_{CO_2} given the measured increase in serum bicarbonate concentration.

Clinical Features. Clinical signs of metabolic alkalosis may not be prominent because the condition usually develops relatively slowly. If acute, CNS manifestations of confusion, obtundation, stupor, and coma may be present as well as tetany and neuromuscular irritability.

Treatment. Correction of the underlying cause is the mainstay of treatment in this disorder. In general, correction of potassium depletion and volume depletion corrects the

TABLE 10.12

CALCULATIONS FOR ESTIMATING THE COMPENSATORY RESPONSES TO PRIMARY ACID–BASE DISTURBANCES

Type of disorder	Compensation requirement	Time
Metabolic acidosis	$dP_{CO_2} = d[HCO_3^-] \times 1.2 \pm 2$	12–24 h
Metabolic alkalosis	$dP_{CO_2} = d[HCO_3^-] \times 0.7 \pm 5$	12–24 h
Acute respiratory acidosis	$d[HCO_3^-] = dP_{CO_2} \times 0.07 \pm 1.5$	Minutes
Chronic respiratory acidosis	$d[HCO_3^-] = dP_{CO_2} \times 0.4 \pm 3$	3–5 d
Acute respiratory alkalosis	$d[HCO_3^-] = dP_{CO_2} \times 0.2 \pm 2.5$	Minutes
Chronic respiratory alkalosis	$d[HCO_3^-] = dP_{CO_2} \times 0.5 \pm 2.5$	2–3 d

metabolic alkalosis. Renal excretion of bicarbonate cannot occur in the face of persistent volume depletion. Volume depletion should be corrected with chloride-containing solutions. In patients without intravascular volume deficits, renal excretion of bicarbonate can be enhanced by administration of the carbonic acid anhydrase inhibitor diuretic acetazolamide. If renal excretion of bicarbonate cannot be increased because of underlying renal insufficiency or if the metabolic alkalosis is severe, acid may be administered to titrate directly the excess extracellular bicarbonate. Acids that can be used include ammonium chloride, arginine hydrochloride, lysine hydrochloride, or dilute hydrochloric acid (0.1 N). Partial correction of the alkalosis is the initial goal. A general guide is that 2.2 mEq/kg of acid decreases serum bicarbonate by approximately 5 mEq/L. In the face of renal failure, dialysis may be necessary to remove excess bicarbonate.

Respiratory Alkalosis

Respiratory alkalosis is defined as increased extracellular pH secondary to decreased P_{CO_2} with hyperventilation. Hyperventilation and the ensuing fall in P_{CO_2} may be secondary to hypoxia, reflex stimulation from decreased pulmonary compliance, drugs, mechanical ventilation, and other causes.

Hypoxia stimulates ventilation through peripheral chemoreceptors in the carotid and aortic body. Decrease in arterial P_{O_2}, rather than in oxygen content, is the main stimulus. Acute drops in arterial P_{O_2} result in sustained hyperventilation only when the P_{CO_2} decreases below 60 mm Hg. Although hyperventilation occurs with even slight degrees of hypoxia, the resulting increase in brain pH suppresses the stimulus for hyperventilation unless severe hypoxia is present. In contrast, chronic hypoxia results in hyperventilation even with mildly decreased P_{CO_2} because brain pH is lowered by metabolic compensation. The two most common causes of hypoxia resulting in respiratory alkalosis are pulmonary disease and exposure to high altitudes.

Compensatory Mechanisms. Tissue buffering is the initial response to a decrease in P_{CO_2}. Red blood cells provide one third of the buffering. Consumption of bicarbonate results from cellular liberation of H^+. Although immediate, the magnitude of tissue buffering is slight and can be predicted by the following formula:

$$d[HCO_3^-] = dP_{CO_2} \times 0.2 \pm 2.5$$

Renal compensation is achieved not by increasing excretion of bicarbonate but by decreasing net acid excretion, primarily through reductions in ammonia excretion and increases in organic anion excretion. These organic anions are excreted as sodium and potassium salts. As a result, potassium excretion is increased, resulting in hypokalemia. Complete renal compensation requires 2 or 3 days.

Clinical Features. Chronic respiratory alkalosis is usually asymptomatic because compensatory mechanisms are successful in maintaining pH close to normal. Acute respiratory alkalosis may cause sensations of breathlessness, dizziness, and nervousness and can result in circumoral and extremity paresthesias, altered levels of consciousness, and tetany. These signs are related to decreased cerebral blood flow secondary to decreased P_{CO_2} and decreased ionized calcium concentration secondary to the increased blood pH.

Treatment. The underlying stimulus for the hyperventilation should be addressed. The cause of hypoxemia should be determined and corrected. In acute symptomatic respiratory alkalosis, rebreathing or breathing 5% CO_2 temporarily relieves the symptoms. If the condition is secondary to mechanical ventilation, adjustment of tidal volume or respiratory rate should result in resolution of the respiratory alkalosis.

Respiratory Acidosis

Respiratory acidosis, the decrease in extracellular pH from a primary increase in P_{CO_2}, is due to inadequate ventilation. Causes of hypoventilation include the various causes of CNS depression, as well as impaired thoracic ventilatory mechanics, airway obstruction, and chronic obstructive pulmonary disease. In addition, inappropriate ventilator settings may result in respiratory acidosis in patients on mechanical ventilation.

Compensatory Mechanisms. Increased P_{CO_2} results in increased H_2CO_3, which dissociates into H^+ and HCO_3^-. Cellular exchange of Na^+ and K^+ for H^+ allows the reaction to continue in this direction with increased extracellular bicarbonate. This tissue buffering is accomplished within minutes. Persistently elevated P_{CO_2} also stimulates increased renal acid excretion, primarily the chloride salt of ammonia, and results in increased renal generation of HCO_3^-. Full renal compensation occurs over 3 to 5 days. The following formula describes chronic respiratory acidosis:

$$d[HCO_3^-] = dP_{CO_2} \times 0.4 \pm 3$$

Clinical Features. The magnitude of clinical manifestations depends on the chronicity and rate of development of respiratory acidosis. Acute increases in P_{CO_2} result in cerebral acidosis, manifested by drowsiness, restlessness, tremor, as well as stupor or coma in more severe cases. Cerebral vasculature dilation occurs in response to acidosis, resulting in increased cerebral blood flow. This may, in turn, result in increased intracranial blood pressure, headache, and papilledema. Systemic acidosis results in peripheral vasodilatation, depressed cardiac contractility, and insensitivity to catecholamines.

Treatment. Treatment should be directed to the underlying cause of hypoventilation. Endotracheal intubation to achieve adequate ventilation is key to the treatment of acute respiratory acidosis of any cause. The treatment of chronic, compensated respiratory acidosis may be complicated by the accompanying hypoxemia. In chronic hypercapnia, the central chemoreceptors may be insensitive, and the accompanying hypoxemia may supply the main respiratory drive through stimulation of peripheral chemoreceptors. In such patients, complete correction of the hypoxemia may further suppress respiration and worsen the respiratory acidosis. In addition, P_{CO_2} should not be normalized rapidly. Reequilibration of cerebral bicarbonate concentration lags behind systemic changes. Thus, even if P_{CO_2} is normal, cellular and cerebral metabolic alkalosis may develop.

Mixed Acid–Base Disorders

Combinations of two or more of the four primary acid–base disorders may occur and should be suspected when blood pH approaches normal despite abnormal P_{CO_2} and $[HCO_3^-]$, or when compensatory changes appear to be either excessive or inadequate (Fig. 10.8). Familiarity with the acid–base disorders associated with various clinical situations and the expectation of mixed abnormalities allows appropriate interpretation of arterial blood gases and serum electrolyte determinations. A summary of the calculations for estimating the compensatory responses and timing of these responses is presented in Table 10.12.[36]

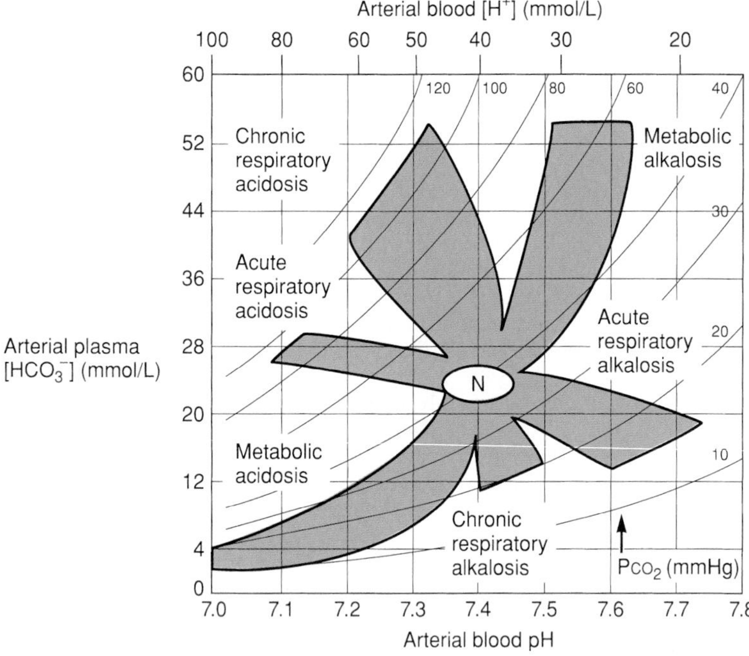

FIGURE 10.8 Acid–base nomogram. Shown are the 95% confidence limits of the normal respiratory and metabolic compensations for primary acid–base disturbances. (From Cogan MG, Rector FC Jr. Acid–base disturbances. In: Brenner BM, Rector FC Jr, eds. *The kidney.* Philadelphia: WB Saunders; 1986:473, with permission.)

KEY POINTS

- The human body is conceptualized as composed of at least four compartments: water, protein, fat, and bone ash.
- Sodium (ECF) and potassium (ICF) are the dominant cations and, whereas composition varies between ECF and ICF, overall concentration of solutes in these fluids is identical.
- Osmolality is kept constant by tight regulation of water balance by osmoreceptor-induced control of ADH and thirst.
- Effective circulating volume is sensed by volume receptors (capacitance vessels, atria, hepatic, and CNS) and pressure receptors (aortic arch, carotid, and intrarenal) that alter sodium and water balance mediated by renin-angiotensin, aldosterone, ANP, dopamine, and renal prostaglandins.
- Water losses involve both sensible (measurable) via urine, stool, and sweat and insensible (unmeasurable) via evaporative loss from both skin and respiratory tract.
- Goals of fluid therapy are to normalize hemodynamic parameters and body fluid electrolyte concentrations and can be achieved with crystalloids (preferable) or colloids, both correcting deficits and matching ongoing or expected losses.
- The major cations (Na^+, K^+, Ca^{2+}, and Mg^{2+}) should be monitored and replaced, recognizing unique distributions and impact of various diseases.
- Acid–base balance is carefully buffered within very narrow limits. Acid–base disturbance and compensation are frequently mixed, involving respiratory and metabolic-renal responses.

References

1. Kehayias JJ, Valtuena, S. Neutron activation analysis determination of body composition. *Clin Nutr Metab Care.* 1999;2:453–463.
2. Pietrobeloi A, Wang Z, Heymsfield SB. Techniques used in measuring human body composition. *Clin Nutr Metab Care* 1998;1:439–448.
3. Briggs JP, Sawaya BE, Schnerman J. Disorders of salt balance. In: Kokko JP, Tannen RL, eds. *Fluid and electrolytes.* Philadelphia: WB Saunders; 1990:70.
4. Thompson CA, Tatro DL, Ludwig DA, et al. Baroreflex responses to acute changes in blood volume in humans. *Am J Physiol.* 1990;259:R792–798.
5. Stockand JD. New ideas about aldosterone signaling in epithelia. *Am J Physiol Renal Physiol.* 2002;51:F559-F576.
6. Boland DG, Abraham WT. Natriuretic peptides in heart failure. *Congestive Heart Failure* 1998;4:23–33.
7. Schrier R, Abraham W. Mechanisms of disease: hormones and hemodynamics in heart failure. *N Engl J Med.* 1999;341:577–585.
8. Wait RB, Kahng KU. Renal failure complicating obstructive jaundice. *Am J Surg.* 1989;157:256.
9. Reuzzi G, Benigni A. Endothelins in the control of cardiovascular and renal function. *Nature* 1993;342:589.
10. Rodeberg DA, Chaet MS, Bass RC, et al. Nitric oxide: an overview. *Am J Surg.* 1995;170:292.
11. Bachman S, Mundel P. Nitric oxide and the kidney: synthesis, localization, and function. *Am J Kidney Dis.* 1994;24:112.
12. Ruttmann TG, James MFM, Lombard EM. Haemodilution induced enhancement of coagulation is attenuated in vitro by restoring antithrombin III to predilution concentrations. *Anaesth Intensive Care* 2001;29:489.
13. Ng KFJ, Lam CCK, Chan LC. In vivo effect of haemodilution with saline on coagulation: a randomized controlled trial. *Br J Anaesth.* 2002;88:475.
14. Ruttmann TG, James MFM, Finlayson J. Effects on coagulation of intravenous crystalloid or colloid in patients undergoing peripheral vascular surgery. *Br J Anaesth.* 2002;89:226.
15. Koustova E, Standon K, Gushchin V, et al. Effects of lactated Ringer's solution on human leukocytes. *J Trauma* 2002;53:872–878.
16. Wade CE, Kramer GC, Grady JJ, et al. Efficacy of 7.5% saline and 6% dextran-70 in treating trauma. A meta-analysis of controlled clinical studies. *Surgery* 1997;122:609.
17. Shackford SR, Bourguignon PR, Wald SL, et al. Hypertonic saline resuscitation of patients with head injury: a prospective, randomized clinical trial. *J Trauma Injury Infect Crit Care* 1998;44(1):50–58.
18. Cope JT, Banks D, Mauney MC, et al. Intraoperative hetastarch infusion impairs hemostasis after cardiac operations. *Ann Thorac Surg.* 1997;63:78.
19. Martin G, Bennett-Guerrero E, Wakeling H, et al. A prospective, randomized comparison of thrombelastographic coagulation profile in patients receiving lactated Ringer's solution, 6% hetastarch in a balanced-saline vehicle, or 6% hydroxyethyl starch in saline during major surgery. *J Cardiothorac Vasc Anesth.* 2002;16:441.
20. Omar MN, Shouk TA, Khaleq MA. Activity of blood coagulation and fibrinolysis during and after hydroxyethyl starch (HES) colloidal volume replacement. *Clin Biochem.* 1999;32:269.
21. Gan TJ, Bennett-Guerrero E, Phillips-Bute B, et al. Hextend, a physiologically balanced plasma expander for large volume use in major surgery: a randomized phase III clinical trial. Hextend Study Group. *Anesth Analg.* 1999;88:992.
22. King DR, Cohn SM, Proctor KG. Changes in intracranial pressure, coagulation, and neurologic outcome after resuscitation from experimental traumatic brain injury with hetastarch. *Surgery* 2004;136:355.
23. Deusch E, Thaler U, Kozek-Langenecker SA. The effects of high molecular weight hydroxyethyl starch solutions on platelets. *Anesth Analg.* 2004;99:665.

24. Franz A, Bräunlich P, Gamsjäger T, et al. The effects of hydroxyethyl starches of varying molecular weights on platelet function. *Anesth Analg.* 2001;92:1402–1407.
25. Jungheinrich C, Scharpf R, Wargenau M, et al. The pharmacokinetics and tolerability of an intravenous infusion of the new hydroxyethyl starch 130/0.4 (6%, 500 mL) in mild-to-severe renal impairment. *Anesth Analg.* 2002;95:544.
26. Biesenbach G, Kaiser W, Zazgornik J. Incidence of acute oligoanuric renal failure in dextran 40 treated patients with acute ischemic stroke stage III or IV. *Ren Failure* 1997;19:69.
27. Allison KP, Gosling P, Jones S, et al. Randomized trial of hydroxyethyl starch versus gelatine for trauma resuscitation. *J Trauma* 1999;47 :1114.
28. Russell WJ, Fenwick DG. Anaphylaxis to Haemaccel and cross reactivity to Gelofusin. *Anaesth Intensive Care* 2002;30:481.
29. Sprung J, Kindscher JD, Wahr JA, et al. The use of bovine hemoglobin glutamer-250 (Hemopure) in surgical patients: results of a multicenter, randomized, single-blinded trial. *Anesth Analg.* 2002;94:799.
30. Levy JH, Goodnough LT, Greilich PE, et al. Polymerized bovine hemoglobin solution as a replacement for allogeneic red blood cell transfusion after cardiac surgery: results of a randomized, double blind trial. *J Thorac Cardiovasc Surg.* 2002;124:35.
31. Fleck A, Raines G, Hawker F, et al. Increased vascular permeability: a major cause of hypoalbuminaemia in disease and injury. *Lancet* 1985; 1:781.
32. Palmer BF. Managing hyperkalemia caused by inhibitors of the renin-angiotensin-aldosterone system. *N Engl J Med.* 2004, 351:585–592.
33. Stewart AF. Hypercalcemia associated with cancer. *N Engl J Med.* 2005;352:373–379.
34. Lemann JJR, Lennon EJ. Role of diet, gastrointestinal tract, and bone in acid–base homeostasis. *Kidney Int.* 1972;1:275.
35. Hood VL, Tannen RL. Mechanisms of disease: protection of acid-base balance by pH regulation of acid production. *N Engl J Med.* 1998;339:819–826.
36. Carroll HJ, Oh MS. Water, electrolyte and acid–base metabolism. Philadelphia: JB Lippincott; 1989:206.

CHAPTER 11 ■ BURNS

NICOLE S. GIBRAN

Comprehensive care of the patient with thermal injuries involves sophisticated surgical decision making, critical care management, rehabilitation, and psychosocial interventions. With early excision and grafting and better critical care management, survival rates have improved markedly since the mid 1970s. Therefore, in the 21st century, clinical goals must focus on optimizing outcomes and returning patients to their premorbid level of function. This chapter presents a management philosophy that correlates optimal clinical management of patients with thermal injuries with increasing understanding of burn pathophysiology and promotes a systematic multidisciplinary approach.

MANAGEMENT PHILOSOPHY

Whereas the coordinated care of a burn center may primarily benefit patients with complicated life-threatening large burn injuries, poor management of smaller burns bears long-term negative impact on patient outcome—both aesthetic and functional. The focused approach of an organized burn center allows for early surgical excision and closure of the burn wounds, critical care support, patient and family psychosocial support, patient and family education, continuous long-term rehabilitation, reentry into society, and reconstructive surgical needs. Therefore, all patients with burns that meet American Burn Association criteria (Table 11.1) for transfer to a burn center soon after initial assessment are likely to benefit from a multidisciplinary specialized burn care plan. (Guidelines for the Operations of Burn Units, pp. 55–62, Resources for Optimal Care of the Injured Patient: 1999, Committee on Trauma, American College of Surgeons.)

With modern burn care, survival with an excellent quality of life can be expected for most patients with severe burns. There remains no reliable formula for predicting burn survival despite the easily remembered "Age + % total body surface area burn = mortality" formula. Predicting mortality is difficult in burned patients. In one statistical evaluation, age older than 60 years, full-thickness burn size over 40% of the total body surface area (TBSA), and the presence of inhalation injury were found to be important prognostic factors. Experienced burn surgeons report that they may limit resuscitation based on burn size, availability of donor sites, patient age, comorbidity, and inhalation injury; however, this approach to providing comfort care for devastating injuries must be carefully and thoroughly discussed by knowledgeable burn care providers with consideration for patient values and interests.

Successful burn patient outcomes require a well-organized care plan. Deciding whether outpatient management is appropriate for a patient with small burns (1% to 5% of TBSA) that do not involve joints or vital structures and when to discharge a patient with a large burn depends on clear communication with the patient and family. Outpatient management often fails because insufficient teaching in a busy emergency room leads to inadequate pain control, wound infection, and limited movement. Indications for burn patient hospitalization include wound care needs, physical therapy, and pain management. A short hospital stay immediately after the injury allows the patient to learn how to properly clean and dress the burn, especially extremity burns before swelling, infection, or functional limitations hinder long-term recovery. A burn specialty therapist can educate the patient about expected range of motion exercises and activity programs. Pain including background pain (pain experienced with ordinary daily activities), procedural pain (pain experienced during wound care), and anxiety should be carefully assessed, and analgesic and antianxiolytic medication should be titrated to the individual pain levels. Inadequate pain management frequently leads to hospital readmission. Pain levels may increase as epithelial buds emerge in a healing partial-thickness burn, and new stinging pain may indicate a superficial wound infection. This change in symptoms indicates that the burn should be evaluated for signs of infection, including erythema or breakdown of a previously healed wound; an infected burn may have no cellulitis.

TABLE 11.1

ABA CRITERIA FOR PATIENT TRANSFER TO A BURN CENTER

1	Partial-thickness burns greater than 10% total body surface area (TBSA)
2	Burns that involve the face, hands, feet, genitalia, perineum, or major joints
3	Third-degree burns in any age group
4	Electrical burns, including lightning injury
5	Chemical burns
6	Inhalation injury
7	Burn injury in patients with preexisting medical disorders that could complicate management, prolong recovery, or affect mortality
8	Any patients with burns and concomitant trauma (such as fractures) in which the burn injury poses the greatest risk of morbidity or mortality. If the trauma poses the greater immediate risk, the patient may be initially stabilized in a trauma center before being transferred to a burn center. Physician judgment will be necessary in such situations and should be in concert with the regional medical control plan and triage protocols.
9	Burned children in hospitals without qualified personnel or equipment for the care of children
10	Burn injury in patients who will require special social, emotional, or long-term rehabilitative intervention

Simple wound care is a key to successful transition to outpatient management. For all but major burns >20% TBSA, once-daily dressing changes are adequate. Burns are effectively washed during a daily shower or bath with tap water and nonperfumed soap. Using a soapy washcloth to wipe the topical ointment and bacteria that have accumulated over the past day from the wound provides adequate wound care; there is no need to scrub the wound to débride superficial exudates. Intact blisters provide a useful protective biologic wound dressing unless they limit mobility, in which case blisters should be incised, débrided, and covered with a topical antimicrobial dressing that allows full range of motion.

A common misconception is that joint immobilization promotes burn wound healing. In reality, extremity immobilization leads to swelling, which worsens tissue injury, exacerbates pain, and increases the risk of wound infection. Patients with hand burns must learn exercises to maintain range of motion, and patients with foot burns must ambulate without assistive devices so that muscle contraction can facilitate lymphatic drainage of the lower extremity. Patients must elevate burned extremities when they are not actively exercising to reduce swelling. Many burn patients underestimate the time and commitment they must dedicate to physical therapy for optimal functional recovery.

EPIDEMIOLOGY

Because burns are an unreported disease, the annual incidence of thermal injuries is unknown. However, extrapolation from 2003 Centers for Disease Control (CDC) data (http://www.cdc.gov/ncipc/) on fire-related injuries suggests that approximately 1 million burn injuries occur annually in the United States. Fire-related deaths in the United States in 2003 are estimated to be 3,700 (1.3 deaths per 100,000); this compares to 322,000 (5.2 deaths per 100,000) worldwide deaths (http://www.who.int/violence_injury_prevention).

TABLE 11.2

RISK FACTORS FOR BURN INJURIES

Alcohol or drug use
Age (very young/very old)
Smoking
Low socioeconomic status
Occupation
Violence
Epilepsy

In general, burn injuries affect vulnerable populations (Table 11.2): the very young and old, the impaired, and those in lower socioeconomic groups. Workplace injuries comprise a significant component of burn injuries among young adults. Structural fires historically were associated with large numbers of patients with large burns. However, introduction of smoke detectors has dramatically reduced the numbers of these burns except in cases where the alarms are tampered or when the inhabitants are cognitively or physically impaired. As with other trauma, alcohol and drugs are often implicated in epidemiology of burn injuries. Suggestion of a nonaccidental injury or potential neglect mandates admission for full evaluation of the home situation; if the history and the burn distribution are consistent with abuse, the patient must be referred to protective services. Likewise, suggestion of a self-induced burn injury should trigger admission for psychological evaluation; the presence of multiple small cigarette burns in various phases of healing is an absolute indication for admission to the hospital for psychological evaluation, even though the burns themselves may be easily cared for at home with bandages. Patients with language barriers may also benefit from a brief hospital admission to be sure they understand the treatment plan. Underinsured and homeless patients may not have the resources to care for a wound outside the hospital and should be admitted for initial wound care and comprehensive discharge planning.

Despite regulations established after mass burn casualties such as the Cocoanut Grove Fire in Boston in 1942, the risk of burn mass casualties in public places continues to be a public concern as evidenced by the 2002 Rhode Island night club fire that killed 100 people and injured approximately 200 others. Extensive legislative efforts and public outreach programs have decreased the incidence of many nonaccidental burn injuries. Examples include state mandates that hot water heaters in multidwelling facilities be set at 120°F have led to a decreased incidence of nonaccidental hot water injuries. Inconsistent application across states of these laws remains a problem. Smoke detectors and annual drives to change the battery have decreased serious injuries in house fires. Federal requirements that children's sleepwear be fire-retardant, implemented in 1972, represented a transiently successful national burn-prevention program that died in 1996 when Congress reversed regulations. Abuse and neglect continue to impact pediatric patients and require ongoing public awareness campaigns. One recent legislative lobbying effort is the implementation of laws requiring that cigarettes have reduced propensity to ignite furniture or mattresses by using less dense tobacco, less porous paper, a smaller diameter, filter tip, and no added citrates to the paper. Thus far, New York State has passed a state law requiring that cigarettes sold in that state meet these fire-safe requirements.

BIOLOGY OF SKIN

Two distinct layers—the epidermis and the dermis—comprise the skin. The outer epidermis acts as the barrier against the environment and protects against infection, toxin absorption, ultraviolet light exposure, fluid evaporation, and thermal regulation. It has five progressively differentiated layers of keratinocytes, leading to the outermost nonviable and relatively impermeable stratum corneum, which provides the barrier mechanism that protects the underlying tissues. In contrast, the dermis comprises a more complicated cellular and extracellular layer that contributes cutaneous durability and elasticity. The fibroblast, the principal cell of the dermis, synthesizes and degrades mesenchymal proteins. The epidermis and dermis both harbor bone marrow-derived inflammatory cells that contribute to cutaneous inflammatory responses. Dermal connective tissue projections, known as dermal papillae, interdigitate with epidermal projections, known as rete ridges, to create the dermal-epidermal junction (DEJ). Here, the basement membrane, a complex extracellular matrix layer made up of structural proteins that anchor the basal keratinocytes to the papillary dermis separate the two cutaneous layers.

BURN PATHOPHYSIOLOGY

Jackson's 1953 classification of burn wound depth remains a basis for our understanding of the pathophysiology of cutaneous thermal injury. He described three zones of tissue injury following burn injury (Fig. 11.1A and B). The central, most severely damaged area is the zone of coagulation because the tissue is coagulated or necrotic and irreparably injured; this region represents a full-thickness burn (or third degree) (see Fig. 11.1C) that will not heal and must be débrided and grafted. Surrounding the zone of coagulation is a zone of stasis, characterized by vasoconstriction and ischemia. With careful wound management, this partial-thickness burn (or second degree) (see Fig. 11.1D) can convert to a shallower wound; however, edema, infection, or poor perfusion increase the risk that the injured tissue will convert to a deeper burn that will require excision and grafting. The outermost area of a burn is the zone of hyperemia or superficial partial-thickness burn (see Fig. 11.1D), which usually heals quickly without scarring. Superficial burns such as sunburns are often referred to as first-degree burns and are not included in burn size calculations.

Tissue repair represents a continuum that begins immediately following injury. An initial hemostatic response involves coagulation and microvasculature constriction. The extrinsic and intrinsic coagulation pathways also provide provisional matrix scaffolding for subsequent cellular migration into the wound bed. Tissue factor activation of the coagulation cascade leads to cleavage of fibrinogen to fibrin, which serves as both clot matrix and wound bed matrix. Wound inflammatory cells generate plasmin for clot resolution, a process tightly regulated by plasminogen activator inhibitors to ensure that the clot does not resolve too rapidly. Interestingly, animal studies suggest that exogenous tissue plasminogen activator promotes conversion of the zone of stasis in an acute burn wound to a zone of hyperemia.

The well-recognized vasodilatation and capillary leak associated with the resuscitative phase of a burn injury follow the early transient vascular constriction. Vascular permeability contributes to inflammatory cell migration into the wound bed but also causes extravascular leak, which complicates overall patient outcome by causing pulmonary edema, compartment syndrome, and conversion of burns to a deeper injury. Many inflammatory cytokines contribute to this response. In addition to the many interleukins and prostaglandins, sensory nerve-derived neuropeptides induce histamine release by mast cells, cytokine and adhesion molecule up-regulation by keratinocytes and endothelial cells, inflammatory cell chemotaxis, and fibroblast proliferation. Serotonin, histamine, bradykinin, and the arachidonic acid metabolites prolong vasodilatation and capillary permeability.

Resident cutaneous cells may be the most important contributors to cutaneous inflammation. Skin-associated lymphoid tissue includes bone marrow-derived cells, such as Langerhans' cells and dermal dendrocytes, and also keratinocytes and microvascular endothelial cells. Keratinocytes and dermal microvascular cells synthesize cytokines, including interleukins,[13–17] monocyte chemoattractant protein-1, and tumor necrosis factor.[19,20] Before margination into the wound bed, neutrophils adhere to endothelial cell adhesion molecules and plug the capillaries, thereby inducing further cytokine release and potential tissue ischemia. In burn wounds, the zone of stasis represents ischemic tissue that may convert to a zone of coagulation with neutrophil-mediated reperfusion injury. Whereas inhibition of the neutrophil-endothelial adherence in deep dermal rabbit contact burns speeds healing, these studies have not been verified in human burn patients.

Granulation tissue, with its capillary arcades, is well-recognized clinical evidence that a wound is healthy and is ready for closure. However, normal excisional wound closure occurs with angioinhibition[22,23] suggesting that secondary wound repair may not require angiogenesis. In contrast, skin grafts and tissue flaps do require angiogenesis for engraftment. Whereas delivery of oxygen and nutrients to a skin graft by imbibition—or diffusion—suffices for a few days, skin graft take requires neovascularization, which occurs by inosculation, the linkage between existent capillaries in the graft and in the wound bed. Excessive wound granulation actually hinders burn wound healing as it prevents migration of the epithelial tongue; many burn surgeons débride the granulation tissue in a healing burn before applying a skin graft to eliminate the associated bacterial contamination and exuberant inflammatory response to maximize graft take. In addition, excessive granulation tissue has been associated with increased hypertrophic scar formation in the healed wound.[24,25]

An epithelialized burn equals a healed burn. Full-thickness wounds heal from the wound edges (Fig. 11.2A) but an advancing epithelial tongue can migrate for approximately 1 cm before it stops migrating and heaps up at the wound edge. In contrast, partial-thickness wounds heal from epidermal appendages (i.e., hair follicles, sweat glands, and sebaceous glands) in the wound bed (see Fig. 11.2B). Whereas completion of this process by no means represents the end of burn wound healing, epithelialization restores the three protective barrier functions of the outer layer of the skin: fluid maintenance, temperature regulation, and prevention of microbial or toxin invasion. Epithelialization may also represent an essential transition in the wound inflammatory state. Growing evidence suggests that epidermal–dermal interactions regulate cutaneous morphogenetic processes such as fetal skin development and wound repair. Just as the epidermis responds to mesenchyme-derived mediators, activated keratinocytes in the advancing epidermal tongue may secrete cytokines and growth factors to promote dermal inflammation.[28,29] Once cell–cell contact is achieved with complete wound epithelialization, release of the inflammatory mediators may stop. Evidence for epidermal influence on dermal inflammatory responses includes clinical observations that partial-thickness wound coverage with viable allograft eliminates granulation tissue formation and promotes healing. Because it takes time for a mature basement membrane to develop, epithelialized wounds undergo epidermolysis (blistering) until the anchoring structures mature.

A

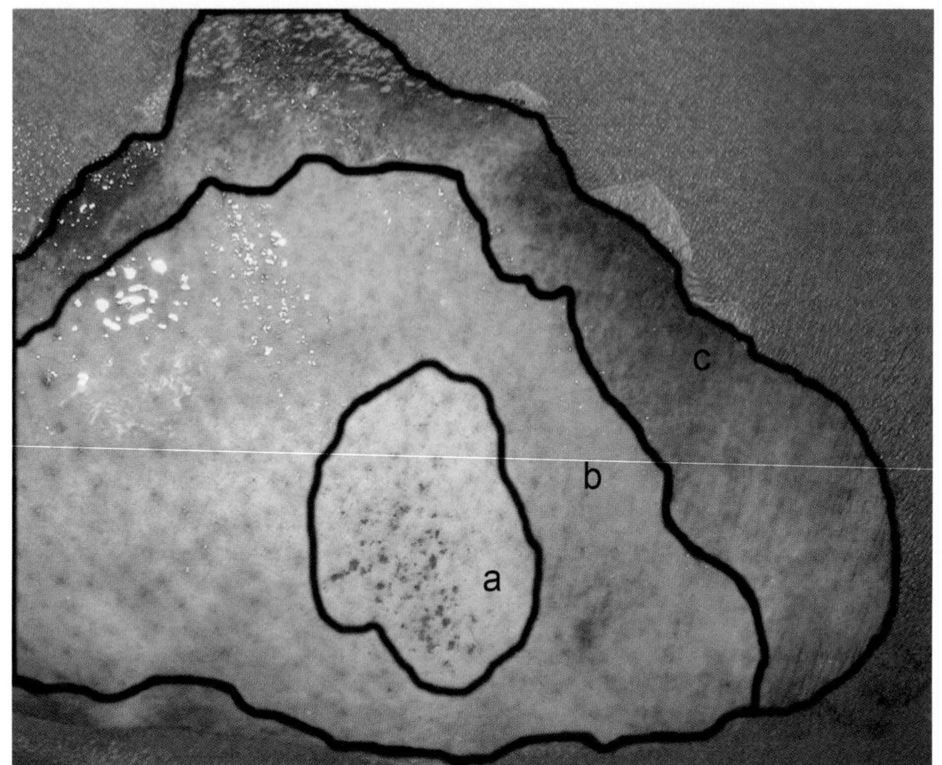

B

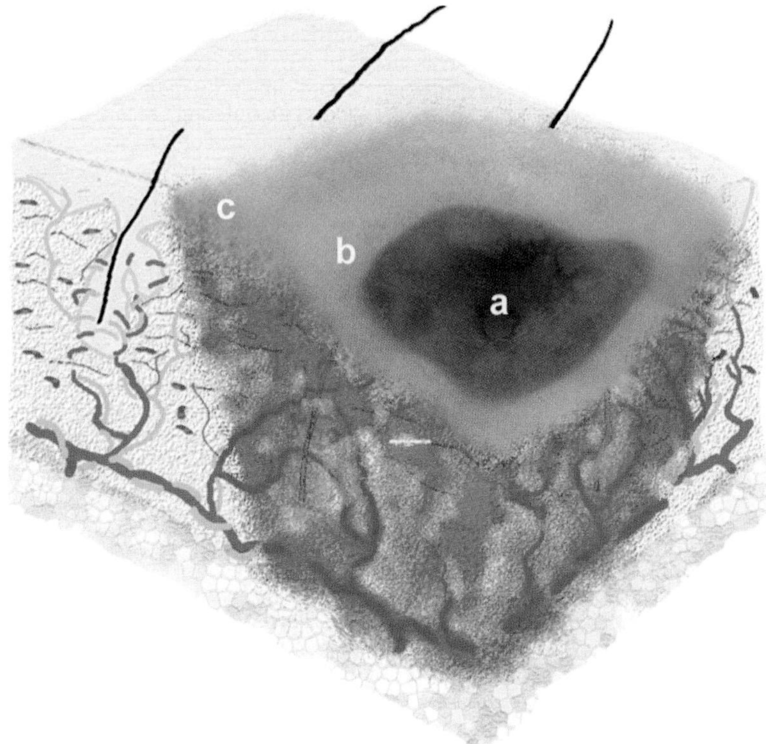

FIGURE 11.1 Zone of injury correlates with burn depth. In (*A*) and (*B*), the central zone of coagulation (*a*) represents a full-thickness burn (as shown in C); the surrounding zone of stasis (*b*) represents a partial-thickness burn (as shown in *D*) that may extend into the reticular dermis (deep partial thickness) or the papillary dermis (superficial partial thickness). The peripheral zone of hyperemia correlates with a superficial or first-degree burn and might be similar to a sunburn.

Whereas clinicians consider an epithelialized wound to be healed, long-term dermal and subcutaneous fibrogenesis may be the most critical determinants of long-term wound appearance and cutaneous tensile strength. Deposition of fibrin, thrombin, fibronectin, and vitronectin into the site of injury promotes cellular migration and proliferation for angiogenesis and fibrogenesis. As fibroblasts migrate into the wound from the margins, they synthesize collagen. The result is deposition of collagen III and subsequently collagen I in a dense mat that is characteristic of dermal scar. As collagen I fibrils are cross-linked into cables, dermal breaking strength increases but never meets that of uninjured skin. Matrix remodeling begins

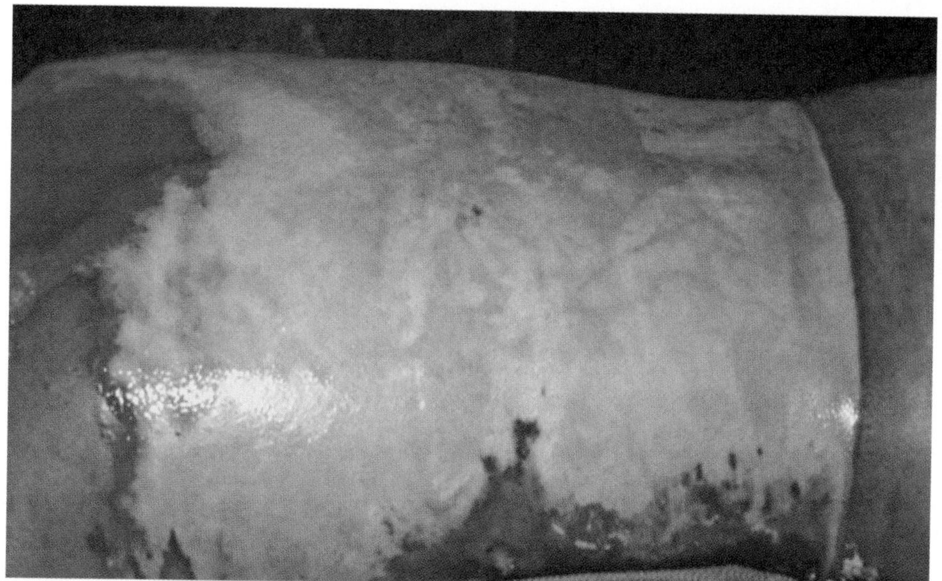

C

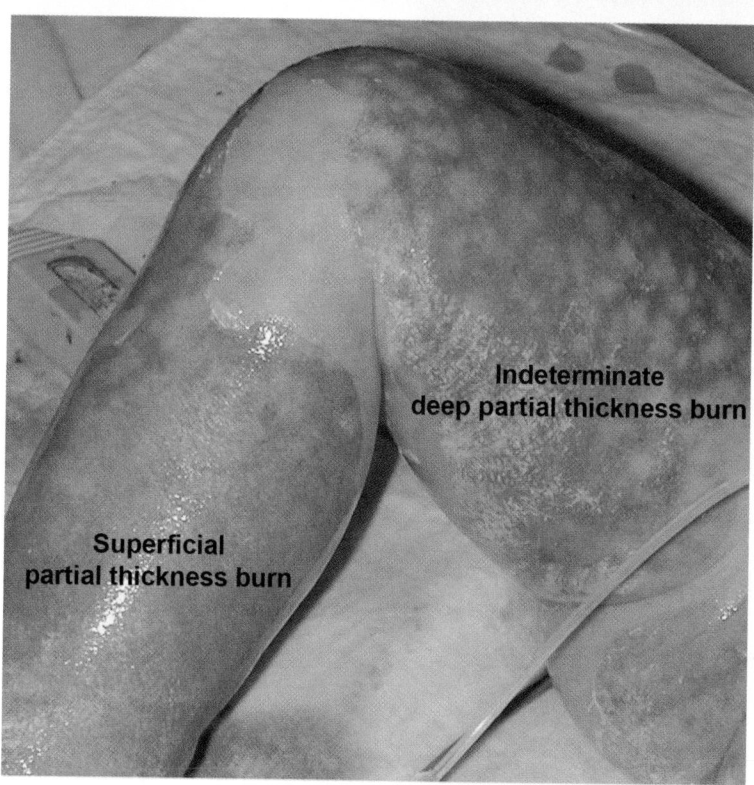

D

FIGURE 11.1 *(continued)*

with fibrin clot dissolution and ends with a mature wound 12 to 24 months later. Matrix metalloproteinases (MMPs) have been implicated in keratinocyte migration, angiogenesis, and dermal matrix remodeling.[33,34] Expression levels of MMPs appear to be decreased in hypertrophic scars.

Contraction, resulting from centrifugal forces in the center of the wound, constitutes an important wound closure mechanism. Myofibroblasts, specialized fibroblasts characterized by intracellular smooth muscle actin filaments, may contribute to this means of closure. A pathologic extension of wound contraction over joints is contracture—a debilitating scarring process that compromises return to function in many patients with large burns. Constant attention to stretching, exercising, and splinting can minimize contracture development, but surgical release of the tight bands may be necessary to restore normal function of extremities, the neck, or mouth.

Just as the dermis undergoes changes, the epidermis also evolves after injury. Melanocytes migrate from the wound edge and from epidermal appendages soon after the epithelial cells (see Fig. 11.2C). Patients must be informed that pigmentation in healed burn wounds can be unpredictable and may result in either increased or decreased melanin. Most clinicians advise patients that exposure to ultraviolet rays exacerbates pigmentation changes in the wound. Use of topical bleaching agents should also be discouraged. Patients with healing partial-thickness wounds complain of pruritus. Hypertrophic scars, which are classically very pruritic, have increased numbers of sensory nerves compared to normal scars and uninjured skin.[36,37]

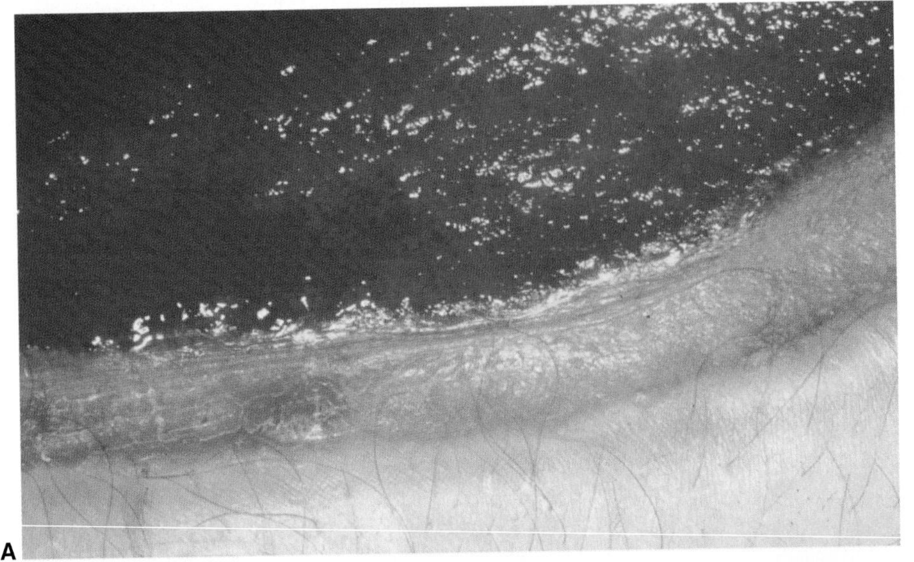

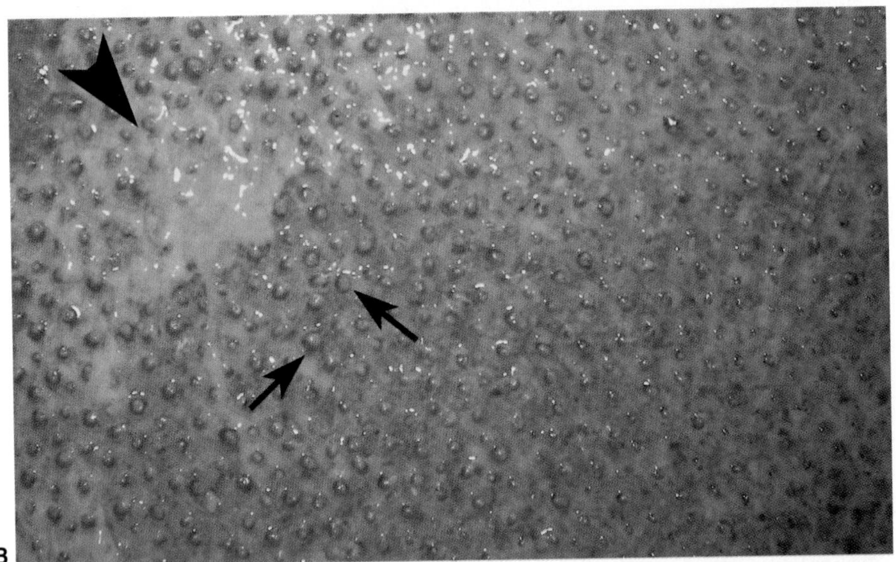

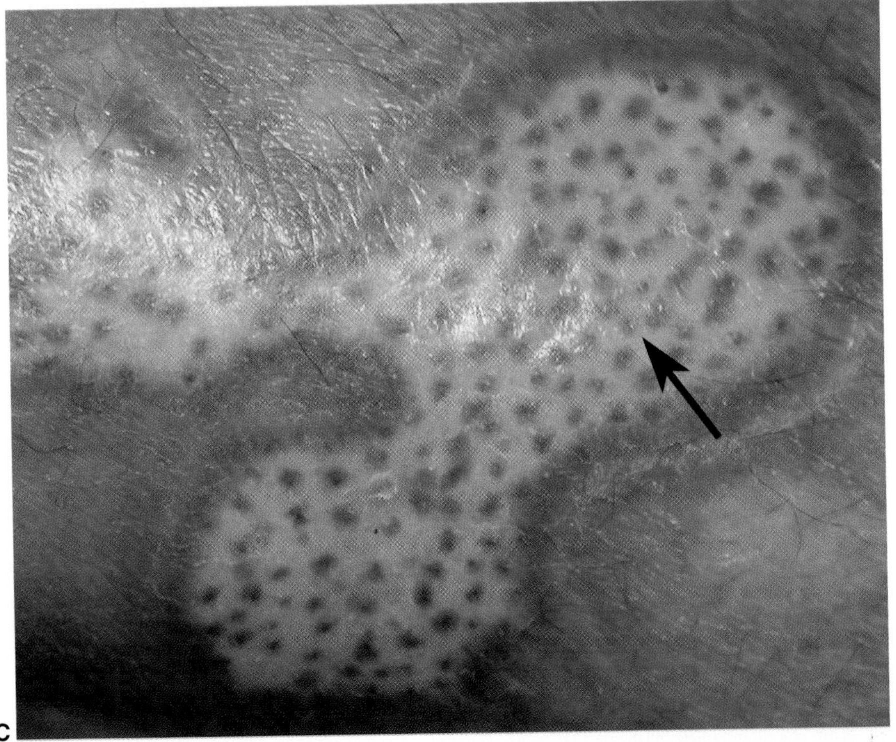

FIGURE 11.2 (*A*) Epithelialization of a full-thickness wound occurs from the wound edge. (*B*) Partial-thickness wounds heal from the epidermal appendages throughout the wound bed; the arrow depicts "buds" of epithelium at each of the appendages. The arrowhead shows the silver sulfadiazine that should be gently washed daily from the wound surface. (*C*) Repigmentation of healed wounds occurs as melanocytes migrate from the epidermal appendages across the wound bed. Skin color in a healed wound is difficult to predict. Exposure to ultraviolet radiation can permanently increase the pigmentation. Bleaching agents are discouraged because of the risk of further tissue damage.

Systemic Response to Burn Injury

Cutaneous inflammatory cells from the injured tissue release mediators that drive the systemic response to cutaneous thermal injury leading to accelerated intravascular volume depletion, inadequate tissue perfusion, and ultimately risk of multiorgan dysfunction. Therefore, patients with large burns require continuous intravenous (IV) replacement to compensate for the capillary leak. The leak associated with a burn larger than 30% TBSA (or smaller if there is concomitant inhalation injury) can cause clinically significant interstitial edema in soft tissues including muscle compartments, lungs, and abdomen. The potential morbidity from the edema includes compartment syndrome in injured and noninjured extremities, abdominal compartment syndrome, and pulmonary edema leading to development of respiratory distress syndrome. Careful attention to fluid status of the acutely injured burn patient is critical to avoid resuscitation failures including both inadequate and excessive resuscitation.

INITIAL EVALUATION

A burn patient is a trauma patient and should be addressed with the same organized approach as for any seriously injured patient that begins with the primary survey to assess airway, breathing, and circulation. A systematic early comprehensive secondary survey is also mandatory, especially for burn patients with associated trauma such as seen in motor vehicle collisions. Evidence suggests that even a small burn injury significantly worsens prognosis in patients with multiple injuries and high injury severity scores (unpublished UW Burn Center data). Therefore, close coordination between the trauma and burn teams is indicated, especially during the resuscitative phase of response to injury.

Because workup of a trauma patient is covered extensively, this section focuses on elements of the workup relevant to evaluation of the burn component of the injuries. Expeditious transfer of a critically burned patient to a burn intensive care unit is essential to avoid hypothermia and resuscitation complications; this mandates minimal evaluation in the emergency department. If the patient is not taken to a burn center initially, a rapid evaluation and initiation of resuscitation should be started and immediate transfer arranged. Table 11.3 is an example of a transfer protocol that outlines initial management of the burn patient prior to transfer to a burn center.

A crucial part of the initial evaluation of the extent of injury in a burn patient is estimation of the size and depth of the burn. This is the basis for subsequent fluid resuscitation and care plans. Because the zones of injury in a burn wound evolve for up to 72 hours (see previous discussion on the zones of injury), burn depth determination at the initial examination can be erroneous. Although numerous burn depth indicators have been investigated including laser Doppler flow meters, IV fluorescein, burn wound biopsy, thermography, light reflectance, magnetic resonance imaging, and IV dyes,[38–40] no technology has been proven more accurate than an experienced burn surgeon. Therefore, many indeterminate burns must be placed in a "wait and watch" plan to determine whether the burn will heal within 3 weeks or whether excision and grafting will be necessary to close the wound.

On the other hand, to estimate burn size, two simple formulas exist. The rule of nines (Fig. 11.3) provides an anatomic estimate in which each arm is considered to be 9% TBSA, each leg 18%, the anterior trunk 18%, the posterior trunk 18%, and the head 9%; this method underestimates head size in children. Another easy method involves using the patient's full palm, including digits, to represent 1% TBSA. First-degree burns should not be included in the calculation of burned areas. Soot should be gently cleaned from the patient because this often misleads an unfamiliar evaluator and erroneously increases the estimated burn size.

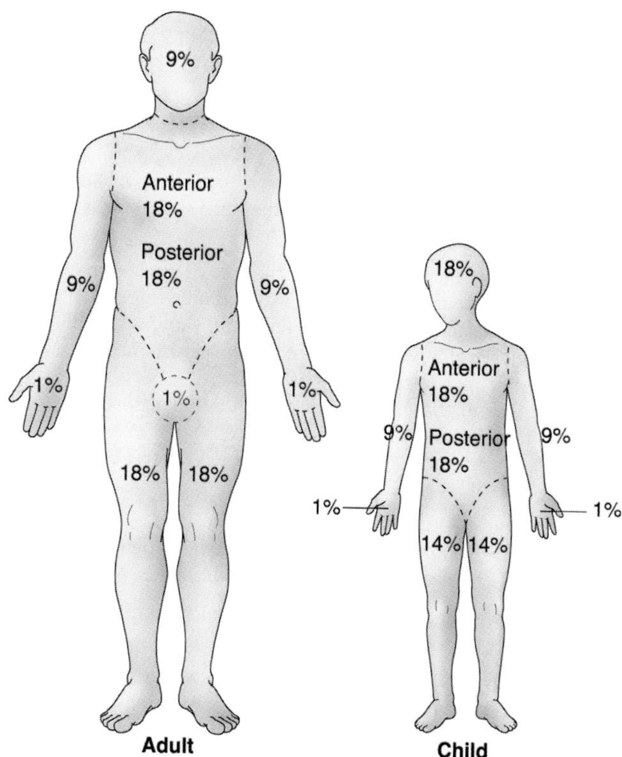

FIGURE 11.3 Estimating burn size accurately is essential for care of the burn patient. The rule of nines provides a simple algorithm for calculating the burned surface area.

Initial assessment of the burn patient requires few laboratory or radiologic studies. Patients with a history of exposure to noxious fumes should have arterial PaO_2, $PaCO_2$, pH, and carboxyhemoglobin percentage determined. Patients with isolated burns and no other injuries rarely need blood products during the resuscitative phase of their care, but a routine blood sample can be sent to the blood bank as a type and screen. Routine hematology and chemistry profiles have limited use, but baseline electrolyte levels and renal function [blood urea nitrogen (BUN), creatinine] and hematocrit, white blood cell count, and platelet count should be established. The efficacy of following laboratory values such as base deficits and lactic acid levels has not been established in burn patients. Urinalysis may be helpful to diagnose myoglobinuria in patients with electrical injuries or deep thermal burns, but if the urine appears clear, treatment is not warranted. Need for radiographical assessments must be based on mechanism of injury, but a baseline chest radiograph is sufficient for an isolated burn without other evidence of trauma.

AIRWAY ASSESSMENT AND MANAGEMENT

Airway assessment and management in the burn patient must include diagnosis of an inhalation injury because this significantly increases morbidity and mortality of patients with thermal injuries. Diagnosis of an inhalation injury should be

TABLE 11.3 MANAGEMENT

UW BURN CENTER TRANSFER STABILIZATION PROTOCOL

Remove source of heat.
Remove clothing that is burned, covered with chemicals or constrictive.

Intubate patients for loss of consciousness, increasing stridor or hoarseness, evidence of posterior pharyngeal burns or if the burn size exceeds 60% total body surface area (TBSA).

Initiate fluid resuscitation.
- Estimate the burn size based on the rule of nines or based on patient palm size (1% TBSA) to calculate the resuscitation fluid volume (Fig. 11.3).
- Administer lactated Ringer's solution at 3 mL/kg/%TBSA burn.
- For children that weigh <20 kg administer maintenance D51/2NS crystalloid at maintenance intravenous (IV) rate.
- Except for maintenance fluids in children, dextrose solutions cause osmotic diuresis and confuse assessment of resuscitation.
- Unless mean arterial blood pressure is less than 60 mm Hg, IV fluid boluses are not necessary for burn resuscitation.

Insert nasogastric tube in intubated patients and patients with burns larger than 20% TBSA.
Enteral tube feedings should be started if the patient will not be transported to a burn center within 12 hours; if feeding is contraindicated, a proton pump inhibitor should be started.

Insert Foley catheter in patients with burns >20 percent TBSA to assess urine output as a measure of resuscitation.

Adequate urine output is 30 mL/hr in adults and 1.5 mL/kg/hr in a child less than 20 kg.
- Observe urine for burgundy color (seen with massive injuries or electrical burns). The high incidence of renal failure associated with myoglobinemia from these injuries warrants prompt and aggressive intervention.
- If the urine is red or brown, consult burn center staff for further fluid management.

Escharotomy
- If transfer will occur within 12 hours of injury, escharotomies are rarely needed.
- Burned extremities should be elevated.

Medications
- A tetanus shot should be given on admission to the emergency department.
- Antibiotics are NOT indicated for acute burn management.
- Short-acting pain medication may be titrated in small doses.

Wound care
- Débridement and application of topical antimicrobials is usually unnecessary.
- Transport patient in dry sheets and blankets, keeping patient warm.
- Avoid hypothermia.

Special considerations for chemical burns
- Remove ALL clothing.
- Brush powered chemicals off wound: then flush burns for a minimum of 30 minutes with running water. Be careful to protect yourself.
- Irrigate burned eyes with a gentle stream of saline. Follow with an ophthalmology consult if transport is not imminent.

Special considerations for electrical injuries
- Elevate burned extremities above the level of the heart on pillows.
- Monitor distal pulses and neurologic examination.
- Maintain UOP >100mL/hr if myoglobinuria present.

considered for any patient involved in a closed space fire, but inhalation injury may also occur in a patient who is injured outdoors; a patient that throws gasoline onto a bonfire can inhale the petroleum fumes or liquid and sustain a significant chemical pneumonitis. Clues in physical examination include singed nasal hairs and facial burns, but these do not in themselves indicate the presence of an inhalation injury. The decision to intubate should be based on respiratory and mental status; hoarseness, wheezing, or stridor suggest pharyngeal swelling and indicate a potential need for intubation. In patients with these signs and symptoms, direct laryngoscopy should be performed to confirm posterior pharyngeal mucosal sloughing or carbonaceous sputum coming up through the vocal cords. Patients with large burns who will receive massive IV resuscitation volumes should be intubated for airway protection as swelling progresses. With swelling or with face burns, securing the endotracheal tube can be a challenge and requires that an umbilical tie be used rather than adhesive surgical tape. Nasotracheal intubation should be avoided if possible because of the risks of sinusitis and erosion of the nasal columella, especially if the nose is burned. Intubated patients with inhalation injuries should have the head of their bed elevated to at least 45 degrees to reduce swelling and to prevent aspiration.

TABLE 11.4

CARBOXYHEMOGLOBIN LEVEL CORRELATIONS WITH PATIENT SYMPTOMS

Carboxyhemoglobin level (%)	Symptoms
<10	None
15–25	Nausea, headache
30–40	Confusion, stupor, weakness
40–60	Coma
>60	Death

Inhalation Injury

Inhalation injury complicates approximately one third of all major burns. Whereas isolated inhalation injuries do not result in high mortality, they significantly increase mortality in patients with cutaneous burns.[41–46] Presumably, the combined injuries lead to recurrent or persistent bacteremia from the burn wound that potentiates the pulmonary injury.

Carbon Monoxide Poisoning

Carbon monoxide (CO) toxicity is the most commonly diagnosed form of inhalation injury because clinical signs and symptoms correlate with arterial carboxyhemoglobin levels (Table 11.4). CO toxicity is easily treated with 100% inhaled oxygen, which rapidly accelerates CO dissociation from hemoglobin (Table 11.5).

Hyperbaric oxygen (HBO) treatment has been proposed as an expeditious way to reduce carboxyhemoglobin levels but data are controversial.[47–49] Hyperbaric treatment may be appropriate in the patient who has isolated CO toxicity with impaired neurologic status and a markedly elevated carboxyhemoglobin level (≥25%). However, the risks for a burn patient (≥10% TBSA) undergoing resuscitation in an isolated hyperbaric chamber may be too significant; reported life-threatening complications in burn patients undergoing hyperbaric therapy include aspirations, inadequate resuscitation with hypovolemia and metabolic acidosis, inadequate ventilation with respiratory acidosis, electrolyte abnormalities with associated cardiac dysrhythmias, hypothermia, and barotrauma. Inhalation injury complicated by cardiac arrest is uniformly fatal regardless of aggressive therapy, including HBO. Hydrogen cyanide toxicity, which may occur in structural fires, disrupts cellular oxidation and causes lactic acidosis, which resolves with ventilation in most patients without need for sodium thiosulfate treatment.

TABLE 11.5

CARBON MONOXIDE-HEMOGLOBIN HALF-LIFE WITH OXYGEN TREATMENT

Carboxyhemoglobin half-life	Treatment modality
4 hours	Room air
45–60 minutes	100% oxygen
20 minutes	100% oxygen at 2 atm [hyperbaric oxygen (HBO)]

Upper Airway Thermal Injury

Upper airway burns occur due to hot air or chemical toxins and can be diagnosed by direct visualization of the posterior pharynx at the time of intubation. The heat absorptive capacity of the oropharynx is sufficiently efficient that thermal burns to the lower airway are rare; however, steam can cause a lower airway thermal burn. Upper airway thermal injury constitutes an important indication for prophylactic intubation, because it is mandatory to control the airway before airway edema develops during resuscitation.

The diagnosis of upper airway thermal injury is achieved with direct laryngoscopic visualization of the posterior oropharyngeal cavity. The decision to intubate should be based on visual evidence of posterior pharyngeal swelling, mucosal sloughing, or carbonaceous sputum coming from below the level of the vocal cords.

Treatment for upper airway injuries includes hospital admission for observation and provision of humidified oxygen, pulmonary toilet, bronchodilators as needed, and endotracheal intubation as indicated. Upper airway thermal burns usually manifest within 48 hours of injury, and airway swelling usually is maximal 12 to 24 hours after the injury. A patient with an upper airway burn may require airway protection for 72 hours. In a patient with a small burn (<15%), a short course of systemic or inhaled steroids may facilitate earlier resolution of airway edema, but steroids are contraindicated in patients with large burns due to the risk of infection and failure to heal. The patient can be extubated based on pulmonary weaning parameters and the presence of an air leak around the endotracheal tube. Once it is safe to extubate, removing the endotracheal tube should be expedited because of the potential nosocomial complication of ventilator-associated pneumonia.

Lower Airway Burn Injury

Burn injury to the tracheobronchial tree and the lung parenchyma results from combustion products in smoke (Table 11.6) and—under unique conditions—inhaled steam. Numerous irritants in smoke or the vaporized chemical reagents in steam can cause direct mucosal injury, leading to mucosal slough and bronchial edema, bronchoconstriction, and bronchial obstruction. Tracheobronchial mucosal damage and loss of ciliary clearance of the debris induces parenchymal inflammation, which leads to exudate formation and microvascular permeability and ultimately may progress to pulmonary edema, pneumonia, or acute respiratory distress syndrome (ARDS). Significant inhalation of aerosolized toxins can reduce myocardial contractility and cause resuscitation failure. A diagnosis of lower airway inhalation injury can be confirmed by bronchoscopy or ^{133}xenon ventilation-perfusion scan, but these modalities often underdiagnose the extent of injury and do not change therapeutic choices or clinical outcome. Therefore, these technologies are not crucial to management of the burn patient early after injury. Given the high rate (up to 50%) of pneumonia in patients with lower airway inhalation injuries, successful treatment requires aggressive pulmonary toilet and frequent chest physiotherapy.

Acute Respiratory Distress Syndrome

ARDS is an independent risk factor for death in burn patients.[55,56] Understanding of ARDS pathophysiology and management has improved since its initial description in the late 1960s, but 40% to 70% of patients with ARDS still die. ARDS is defined by the clinical findings of pulmonary edema, hypoxemia, diffuse pulmonary infiltrates, and reduced lung

TABLE 11.6

PRODUCTS OF COMBUSTION THAT CAN BE PREDICTED TO CAUSE SIGNIFICANT PULMONARY PARENCHYMAL INJURY

Source	Product of combustion
Organic matter	Carbon monoxide Carbon dioxide
Petroleum products (gasoline, kerosene, propane, plastics)	Carbon monoxide, nitrogen oxide, benzene
Wood, paper, anhydrous ammonia	Nitrogen oxides (NO, NO_2)
Polyvinyl chloride (plastics)	Hydrogen chloride
Wool, silk, polyurethane (nylon)	Hydrogen cyanide
Wood, cotton, paper	Aldehydes
Polyurethane (nylon)	Ammonia

compliance; radiographic findings usually are nonspecific. Histologically, ARDS has diffuse alveolar epithelial damage, microvascular permeability and subsequent inflammatory cell infiltration into the lung parenchyma, interstitial and alveolar edema, hyaline membrane formation, and ultimately fibrosis.

The development of ARDS is often presaged by high fluid resuscitation requirements reflecting increased microvascular permeability and leading to increased pulmonary edema. ARDS commonly develops within 7 days after injury. Burn patients with inhalation injury have as high as a 73% incidence of respiratory failure (defined by hypoxemia, pulmonary infections, or prolonged ventilator support) and a 20% incidence of ARDS, compared to burn patients without inhalation injury who have a 5% incidence of respiratory failure and a 2% incidence of ARDS. Advanced age may also be a risk factor for development of ARDS. Acute pulmonary failure rarely develops in patients with inhalation injury but without cutaneous burns.[46,60]

FLUID RESUSCITATION

Vascular access should be obtained early during the evaluation before swelling obscures venous markings. Two large-bore peripheral IV lines should provide adequate prehospital venous access; because the early burn is not contaminated with bacteria, these IV lines can be placed through eschar but care should be taken to secure them well. For children, intraosseous cannulae can provide temporary life-saving resuscitation, but IV access should be obtained as soon as possible.

Multiple organ failure due to inadequate resuscitation and decreased tissue perfusion was a common cause of death in burn patients before fluid formulas were developed to estimate fluid needs. Several proposed fluid resuscitation formulas estimate fluid requirements in the patient with large burns, suggesting that no one formula satisfactorily estimates fluid requirements for all patients. It is essential to remember that each of these formulas estimate fluid needs, but fluid volumes should be constantly adjusted based on patient physiologic responses during resuscitation (urine output, alert sensorium, pulse, and blood pressure). Patients may require more or less fluid depending on size and depth of burn (deeper burns often are associated with a greater inflammatory response and more fluid needs), presence of inhalation injury, associated injuries, or comorbidities.

One of the commonly used resuscitation formulas has been the Baxter (or Parkland) formula, which calls for 3 to 4 mL of crystalloid per percentage of TBSA burned over 24 hours. Half of this volume is delivered during the first 8 hours after injury; the other half is delivered over the subsequent 16 hours. If a patient receives all of the 24-hour estimated volume during the first 2 hours after injury, that fluid has likely leaked into the interstitial extracellular tissues and the patient still must receive the estimated crystalloid volumes to maintain intravascular volumes. The reliability of the Parkland formula directly depends on an accurate initial assessment of burn depth and size as described above (see Fig. 11.3).

Reliable clinical resuscitation endpoints include maintaining a mean arterial blood pressure greater than 60 mm Hg and urine output of 30 mL per hour for adults. Pediatric fluid requirements often exceed estimated formula estimates likely due to less well developed renal concentrating abilities. Therefore, the urinary output goal for infants and very young children (<20 kg) should be 1.5 mL/kg/hour. Large-volume crystalloid boluses should be restricted to hypotensive episodes and should be accompanied by an increase in the hourly volume by 10%. Decreased urine output for 1 or 2 hours does not require a large-volume crystalloid bolus and can be managed by increasing the hourly resuscitation fluid rate by 10%. Stabilization of the flux of mediators and closure of capillary leaks occurs gradually 12 to 48 hours after the burn injury. As capillary leak resolves, the amount of fluids needed to maintain these endpoints should progressively decrease and the IV rate generally can be slowly weaned by 10% per hour. Most burn patients do not require pulmonary artery catheter (PAC) monitoring during resuscitation and will be overresuscitated if IV fluid administration is based on pulmonary artery wedge pressures. A PAC may be useful in patients with underlying cardiac comorbidity at risk for cardiac shock and congestive heart failure.

Patients with extremely deep burns, electrical burns, or compartment syndrome may develop rhabdomyolysis with myoglobinuria (Fig. 11.4) and subsequent acute tubular necrosis. In these patients, maintaining a brisk urine output of 100 mL/hour is indicated. Alkalinization of the urine with IV sodium bicarbonate (0.12 to 0.5 mEq/kg/hour) theoretically increases myoglobin solubility and decreases precipitation in the renal tubules but requires careful serum pH monitoring and is not routinely implemented. Rarely, osmotic diuresis with mannitol is required to maintain urine output but this treatment should be carefully considered because osmotic diuresis reduces urine output reliability as an endpoint for determining intravascular volume status.

Colloid administration (albumin or fresh frozen plasma) after the capillary leak has closed (12 to 48 hours postinjury) may restore intravascular volume in patients with persistent low urine output and hypotension despite adequate crystalloid

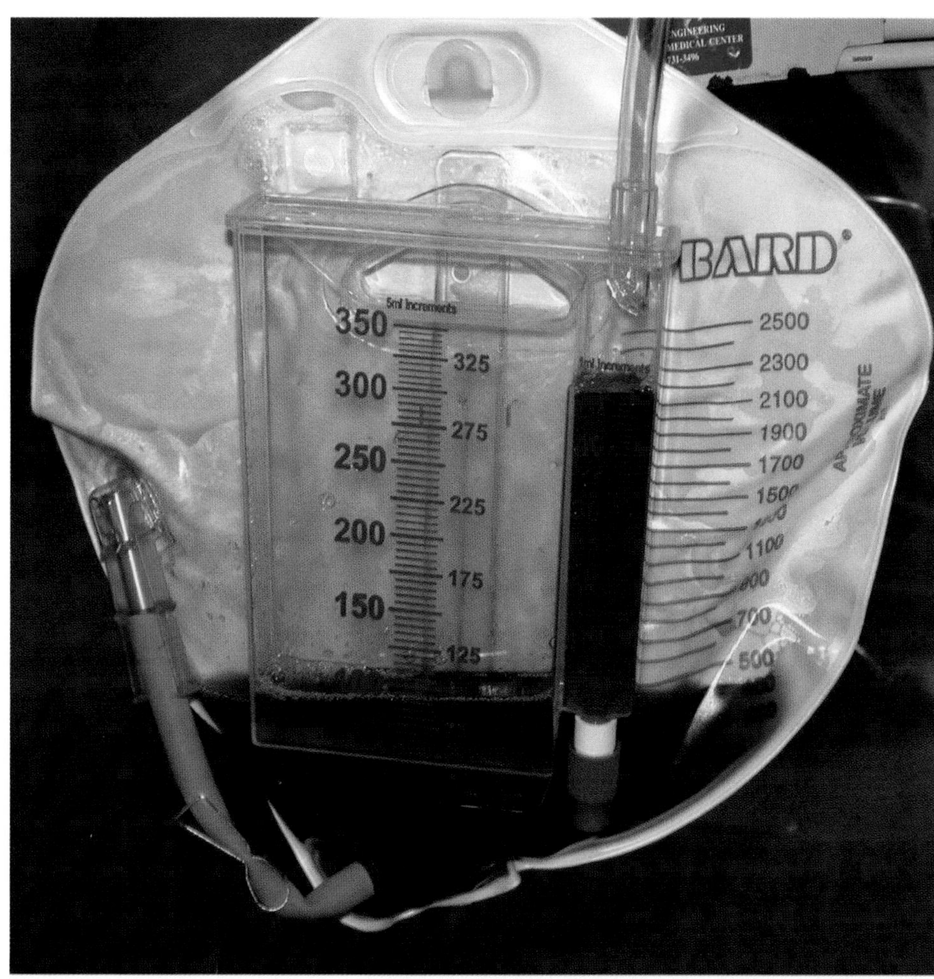

FIGURE 11.4 Myoglobinuria with dark pigment in the urine.

administration. In such cases, 5% albumin (0.3 to 0.5 ml/kg/% TBSA burn) can be administered over 24 hours. Plasmapheresis also reduces IV fluid requirements in patients who do respond to standard crystalloid resuscitation. Indications for plasmapheresis include a sustained MAP of less than 60 mm Hg and UOP less than 30 mL/hour in a patient whose ongoing fluid needs are more than twice fluid volume estimates. Early plasmapheresis (12 to 24 hours postinjury) appears to decrease the incidence of complications from administration of excessive fluid such as extremity compartment syndromes, abdominal compartment syndrome, and pulmonary edema. The mechanism by which plasmapheresis works is unknown, but theoretically the plasma exchange removes circulating cytokines that drive the systemic inflammatory response and cause ongoing vasodilatation and capillary leak.

Once resuscitation is complete (24 to 48 hours postinjury), insensible losses and hyperthermia associated with a hyperdynamic state may require increased ongoing maintenance IV or enteral fluid administration. Reliable daily weights are often useful for determining insensible fluid losses or fluid retention.

Fluid Resuscitation Complications

Overresuscitation causes complications such as poor tissue perfusion, abdominal or extremity compartment syndrome, pulmonary edema, and pleural effusion. Because of the risk for compartment syndrome in patients undergoing large-volume resuscitation, burned extremities should be elevated and hourly neurovascular examinations should be performed; tight bands of eschar are often evident before vascular inflow is compromised and indicate need for escharotomies. Decreased chest compliance with circumferential burns can also improve with thoracic escharotomies, especially in children. An effective thoracic escharotomy must extend along each anterior axillary line and connect at the infraclavicular and subcostal lines (Fig. 11.5A). Extremity escharotomies should extend through the skin only and should not violate the fascia; the arm must be in anatomic position when medial and lateral incisions are made extending across the wrist (see Fig. 11.5B). Eschar on the dorsal hand must often be released to restore vascular signals in the palmar arch (see Fig. 11.5C); there is no benefit to digital escharotomies and risk of injury to the digital arteries and nerves is significant.

Increased abdominal pressure decreases lung compliance and impedes lung expansion, resulting in elevated airway pressures and hypoventilation Abdominal compartment syndrome also classically has decreased venous return, oliguria, and intraabdominal pressures exceeding 25 mm Hg. Bedside decompressive laparotomy through burn wounds, if necessary (Fig. 11.6), can alleviate abdominal compartment syndrome, in patients with hemodynamic instability, hypoventilation with hypoxemia, and elevated abdominal pressures.

Composition of the resuscitation fluid is important to prevent electrolyte imbalance and acidosis. Typically, lactated Ringer's solution is the primary resuscitative fluid

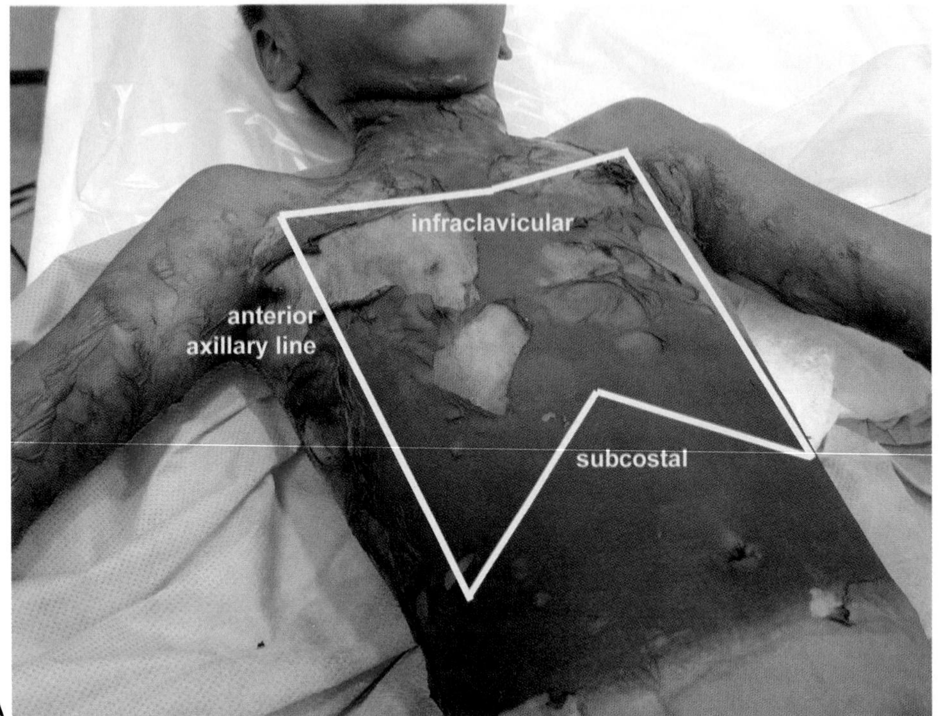

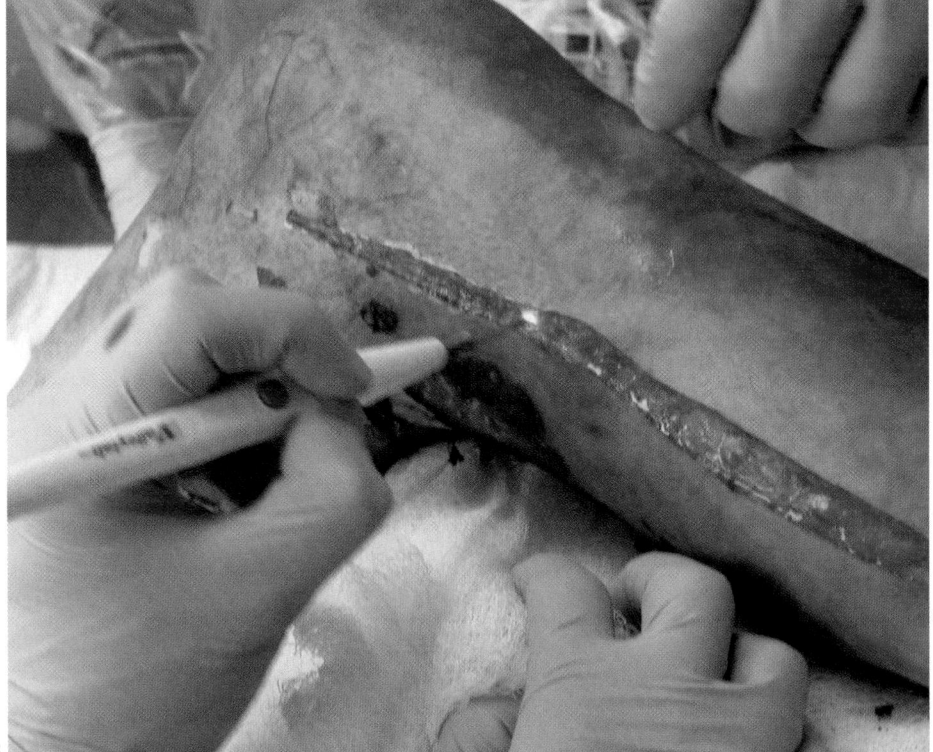

FIGURE 11.5 Escharotomies can be useful for improving chest wall compliance, and relieving extremity compartment syndromes but are very unaesthetic unless a fascial excision will be necessary. (*A*) For the torso escharotomies, incisions across the infraclavicular and subcostal chest that connect the anterior axillary incisions facilitate ventilation, especially in children. (*B*) Extremity escharotomies are performed with the limb in its anatomic position along the medial and lateral axes. (*C*) Hand escharotomies should be placed in the spaces between the metacarpals.

because of the risk for metabolic hyperchloremic acidosis and hypernatremia in patients who receive large volumes of 0.9% normal saline solution. The resuscitative fluid solution should not contain glucose because hyperglycemia and osmotic diuresis may confound resuscitation. However, pediatric patients who weigh less than 20 kg do not have large glycogen stores in their liver and should receive 0.45% half normal saline with 5% dextrose at a maintenance rate (3 to 4 mL/kg/hour).

WOUND MANAGEMENT

Topical Antimicrobials

Prophylactic systemic antibiotics do not have a role in the management of the patient with acute burn injuries. Because eschar is devitalized and avascular, systemic antibiotics cannot

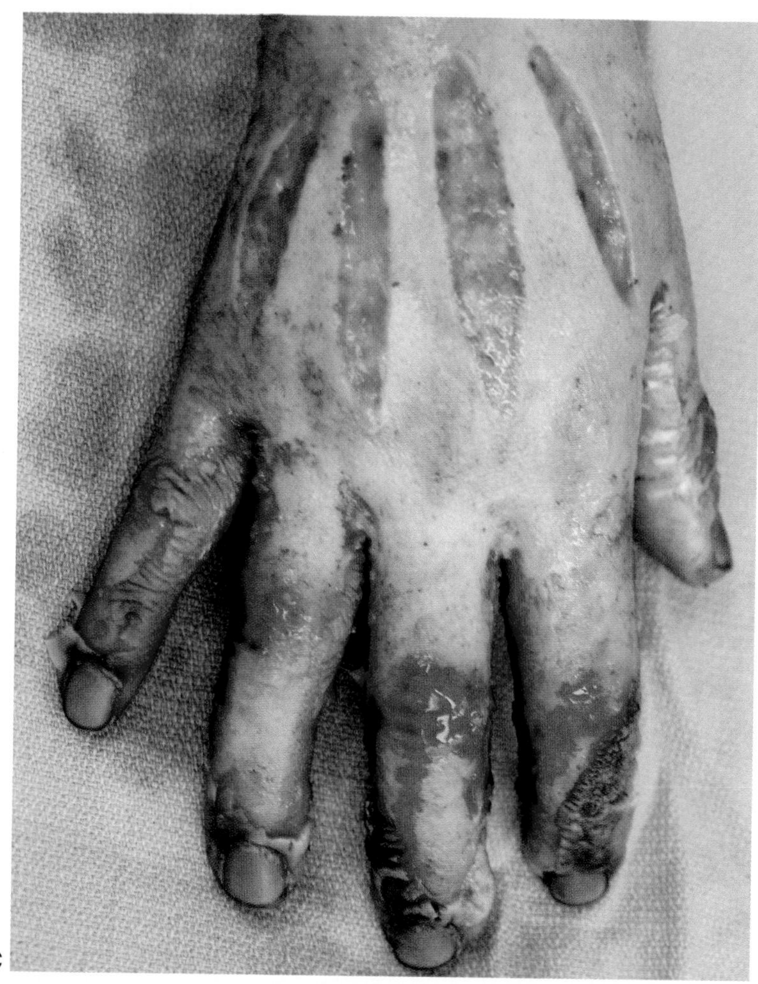

FIGURE 11.5 *(continued)*

reach the eschar surface where the bacterial colonization occurs. Topical antimicrobial agents delay wound colonization and infection but they in themselves have not changed mortality in the way that early excision and grafting has. All agents commonly used in the United States have benefits and side effects (Table 11.7).

Silver sulfadiazine is the most commonly used antimicrobial agent for burns because it has a broad spectrum of antimicrobial activity, is soothing, and has no significant metabolic or electrolyte implications. Because silver sulfadiazine does not penetrate eschar, it is ineffective against already established burn wound infections. Silver sulfadiazine has been

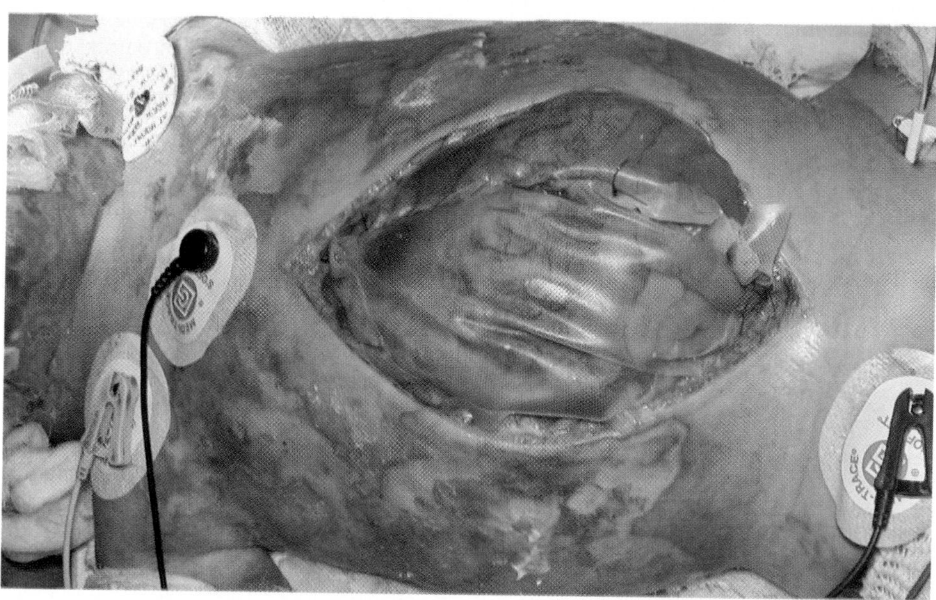

FIGURE 11.6 Decompressive laparotomy can be safely performed through a burn but significantly increases morbidity and should be avoided by closely monitoring fluid resuscitation.

TABLE 11.7

ADVANTAGES AND DISADVANTAGES OF ANTIMICROBIAL TOPICAL AGENTS

Antimicrobial agent	Coverage	Advantages	Disadvantages
Silver sulfadiazine	Broad spectrum, especially *Pseudomonas*	Soothing	Poor eschar penetration May impede epithelial cell migration
Mafenide acetate	Broad spectrum including *Clostridium*	Good eschar penetration Excellent for both treatment and prophylaxis	Carbonic anhydrase inhibition with secondary metabolic acidosis Painful
Silver nitrate	Broad spectrum	Excellent prophylaxis	Poor eschar penetration Hyponatremia Methemoglobinemia
Bacitracin	Gram-positive bacteria	Good for shallow facial burns	Expensive Often delivered in combination with neomycin and polymyxin B, which are nephrotoxic
Mupirocin	Methicillin-resistant *Staphylococcus*	Excellent for methicillin-resistant *Staphylococcus*	Very expensive
Acticoat	Broad coverage	Good for shallow burns, grafts, and donor sites	Hides wound Can cause discomfort when dried Nonadhesive and slips from wound

associated with early post burn neutropenia, but this is more likely related margination of neutrophils due to the overall inflammatory response to injury rather than to the topical agent. The neutropenia is typically self-limited and rarely requires change in antimicrobial therapy. Patients with sulfa allergies typically do not have adverse reactions to silver sulfadiazine; a test patch in a small area of the burn will cause pain or a rash in the unusual case of an allergy.

Mafenide acetate is unique because it penetrates eschar, making it effective in both treating and preventing burn wound infections. This attribute has lead to its frequent use on ears to protect against suppurative chondritis; however, silver sulfadiazine appears to be equally effective. Mafenide provides excellent coverage against gram-negative organisms. Mafenide is available as either a cream or a solution, which is a useful topical agent for skin grafts when the wound bed is considered likely to benefit from postoperative antimicrobial treatment. The major disadvantage is that mafenide inhibits carbonic anhydrase and causes metabolic acidosis that may complicate ventilator management. Topical mafenide can be painful especially on application to partial-thickness burns.

Silver nitrate provides broad-spectrum antimicrobial coverage, including good activity against staphylococci and gram-negative organisms, but it does not penetrate eschar well. Dressings must be irrigated with the aqueous 0.5% solution every 4 hours to keep the dressing moist and prevent precipitation of the silver nitrate onto the wound surface. Because concentrated silver nitrate causes a chemical burn, the bacteriostatic solution used for burn wounds is very hypotonic (it is reconstituted in water rather than saline to avoid silver chloride precipitation) and causes osmotic dilution in the tissues leading to hyponatremia and hypochloremia. These can become severe enough to warrant treatment with oral salt tablets. Use of silver nitrate solution can also rarely lead to methemoglobinemia, which can be successfully treated with IV methylene blue; treatment should also include discontinuation of the silver nitrate. A secondary disadvantage of silver nitrate solution is that it stains everything black.

Bacitracin, neomycin, and polymyxin B used for coverage of superficial wounds in conjunction with petrolatum gauze promote epithelialization and minimize bacterial colonization. These ointments are commonly used for superficial face burns. All three should be limited to relatively small burns because of potential nephrotoxicity. Mupirocin has the advantage of being effective against methicillin-resistant *Staphylococcus aureus* (MRSA) and its use should be restricted for this indication.

Acticoat (Smith & Nephew, London, England) is one of several recently introduced dressings that are impregnated with elemental silver, which has unique antimicrobial properties and works by disrupting bacterial cellular respiration. Acticoat can be used for superficial partial-thickness burns, donor sites, and meshed skin grafts. The advantage of the Acticoat dressing is its decreased need for dressing changes because it can stay in place until a shallow burn or donor site heals. The reduced frequency of dressing changes simplifies burn care but can hinder evaluation of evolving partial-thickness burns, so its use should be limited to wounds that are likely to heal or do not need frequent evaluations. Because Acticoat is nonadherent, an adhesive tape such as Hypafix (Smith & Nephew) must be used to secure the dressing to the wound bed. After 7 days, the tape can be removed and the Acticoat can be washed and towel-dried daily until it peels off the epithelialized wound.

Burn Excision and Grafting

The beneficial impact of early excision and grafting on outcomes following thermal injuries has been remarkable. Because of this change in therapy from a nonoperative to an operative approach,[68–71] mortality in burn patients has dramatically dropped and functional outcomes have improved over the past 30 years. Other advantages include shortened

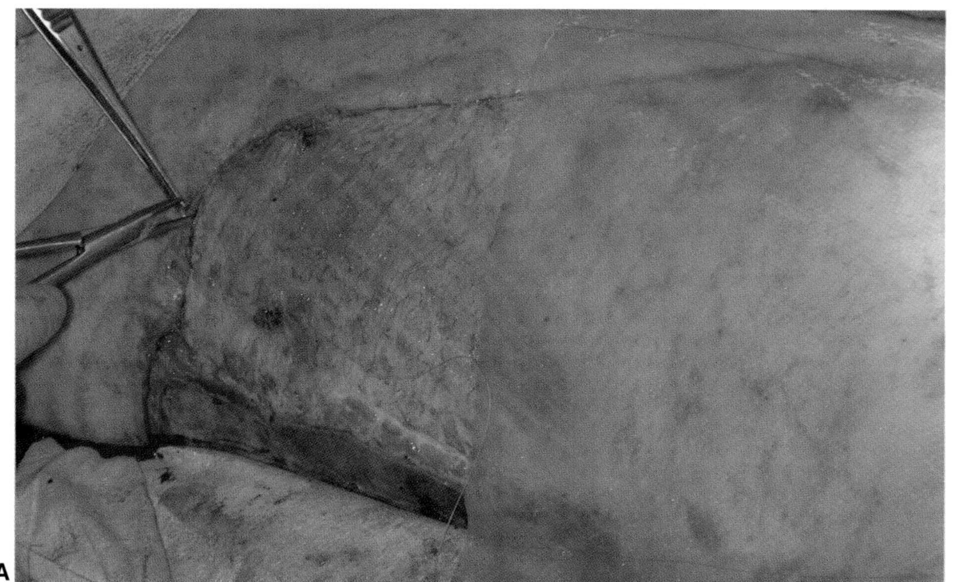

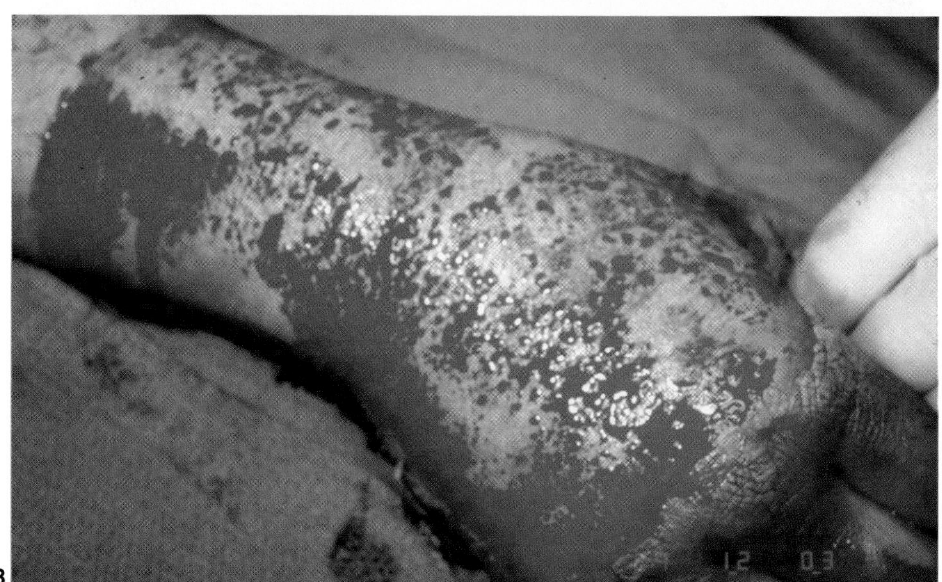

FIGURE 11.7 (*A*) Fascial excision limits bleeding but results in suboptimal aesthetic outcomes and should be avoided if possible. If necessary because of burn depth, care can be taken to tack down the edges to minimize the ledge that interferes with function. (*B*) Tangential excision requires serial tissue removal until the wound bed has diffuse punctate bleeding; ideally this allows a thin pearly white dermal layer to remain in the wound bed.

length of hospital stay, lower costs, and fewer reconstructive surgeries. The timing for initial excision of deep burn wounds should occur as soon after the resuscitative phase of recovery as feasible. Excising large burns during the first 24 hours complicates fluid resuscitation with the risk of hypothermia and bleeding and is not recommended. By 3 to 4 days after injury, burn excision and wound coverage should be a safe option depending on the patient's hemodynamic and pulmonary status, comorbidities, and associated injuries. A patient with large, deep, partial-thickness or full-thickness burns should undergo the initial excision within 7 days of injury. Staged excisions can be performed every 2 to 3 days until the entire burn wound is excised. However, many burns are not homogeneous with both shallow and deep areas. Such indeterminate depth burns can be safely treated with topical antimicrobial ointment for 7 to 10 days until the deeper portion that requires grafting becomes evident; this situation is common in patients with scald or grease burns. By 72 hours after injury, an experienced burn care provider can often differentiate burns that will heal with topical antimicrobial treatment within 3 weeks from deeper injuries that will require excision.

Surgical excision of the burn wound involves one of two technical approaches: fascial excision or tangential excision. Fascial excision involves excising the burned tissue and the underlying subcutaneous tissue down to the muscle fascia using electrocautery, which limits surgical bleeding (Fig. 11.7A). Advantages of a fascial excision include an easily defined, well-vascularized plane that can readily accept a graft. A major disadvantage to this approach is the inevitable removal of healthy, viable subcutaneous tissue, which leads to unaesthetic contour deformities; without the cushioning of the subcutaneous tissue, the grafts on the fascia are often fragile for years after the injury.

Tangential excision involves sequential excision of eschar until the wound bed displays diffuse punctate bleeding indicative of viable tissue that can support a skin graft (see Fig. 11.7B). Tangential excision can be performed with a handheld knife (Weck or Watson), adjusting the guard to control depth of excision. A disadvantage of tangential excision includes diffuse bleeding from the wound bed.

As surgeons have become more comfortable with early excision and grafting, they have developed strategies to minimize surgical blood loss. Topical epinephrine solution (1:10,000),

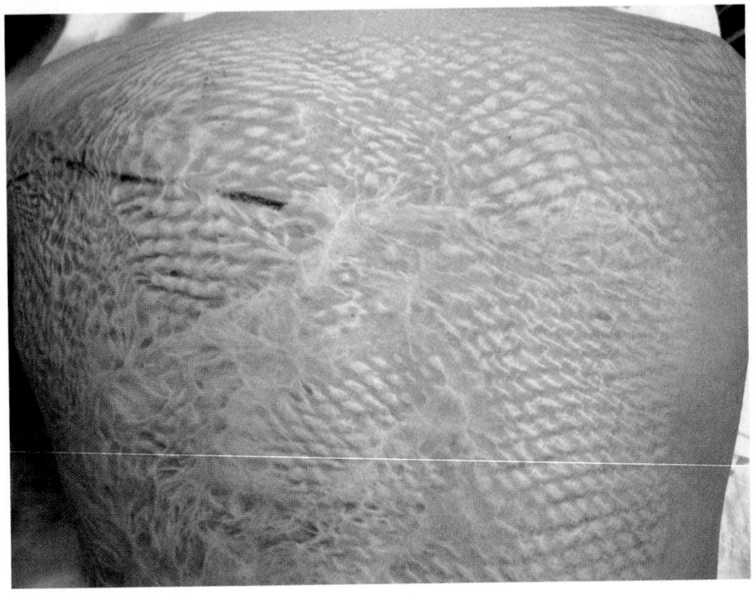

FIGURE 11.8 Traditional widely meshed skin grafts leave hypertrophic interstices long after the wounds are mature.

electrocautery, and compression were recognized early on to minimize blood loss. With experience, other methods evolved including using pneumatic tourniquets for extremity burns and using subeschar injection of dilute epinephrine solution to vasoconstrict the capillaries before excision. Both of these techniques require substantial experience to assess tissue viability because there will be no diffuse bleeding in the wound bed. A commercially available fibrinogen and thrombin spray system (Tisseel Fibrin Sealant; Baxter, Deerfield, Illinois) improves hemostasis and promotes graft adherence to the wound bed with fewer and smaller underlying postoperative fluid collections.

Wound Closure Alternatives

Once the eschar is excised to viable tissue, the wound should be closed as soon as possible, ideally with immediate autografting. Whereas, the best cutaneous replacement would be full-thickness skin grafts, this is not possible for most patients, especially those with large burns and limited donor sites. Traditionally, wounds that could not be autografted immediately were covered with a biologic dressing while donor sites healed. Human allograft is one temporary biologic dressing that is meshed 1:1 to allow wound drainage and applied to excised wound beds. Allograft vascularizes and engrafts and provides physiologic wound closure for 2 to 4 weeks when it typically is rejected and must be replaced with either new allograft or preferably autograft from reharvested donor sites. Porcine xenograft can also be used as a cheaper alternative, but it will not vascularize and will not engraft. When widely meshed skin grafts are necessary, overlaid sheets of allograft can be used on top of the autografts to protect the wound bed as the meshed interstices epithelialize. This minimizes wound bed desiccation and reduces pain. The disadvantage of this technique was the long time till definitive wound closure, the need to recrop donor sites and the potential for significant hypertrophic scar formation in the interstices of the widely meshed grafts (Fig. 11.8A) and in the reharvested donor sites.

Alternative approaches using skin substitutes have improved patient long-term functional and aesthetic outcomes. Two types of skin substitutes exist: epidermal and dermal. Both technologies have advantages and disadvantages (Table 11.8.)

Epidermal skin substitutes consisting of cultured autologous keratinocytes with or without a subjacent layer of autologous fibroblasts suggested great promise for scarless wound closure in the late 1980s. Whereas future advances in burn wound management will depend on improvements in cultured epithelial cell technology,[78,79] current available products have not significantly evolved burn wound management.

TABLE 11.8

ADVANTAGES AND DISADVANTAGES OF SKIN SUBSTITUTES

	Dermal substitutes	Epidermal substitutes
Pros	Useful with limited donor sites Replaces mesenchyme Thin donor sites Decreases scar formation	Useful with limited donor sites Replaces epidermis Fewer donor sites
Cons	Expensive Prone to infection Requires completely viable wound bed Requires fastidious post-operative wound care	Expensive Prone to infection Prone to sheering Prolonged immobilization with delayed rehabilitation Prolonged LOS

Dermal substitutes have been more successful in early clinical use.[80,81] Integra dermal template (Integra Lifesciences, Plainsboro, NJ) is one commercially available product, designed to be combined with ultrathin autograft or cultured epithelium. Its advantage is that it is a bilaminate product comprised of a temporary outer silastic layer and an inner matrix layer of type 1 collagen and chondroitin sulfate.[83,84] The silastic layer provides early wound closure following eschar excision and the inner layer serves as a template that autologous fibroblasts, endothelial cells, and other mesenchymal cells populate. Once the product is vascularized (2 to 3 weeks), an ultrathin autograft can be placed on the neodermis. Histologic evaluation suggests that the Integra neodermis architecture is more comparable to uninjured dermis than regular scar (Fig. 11.9A).

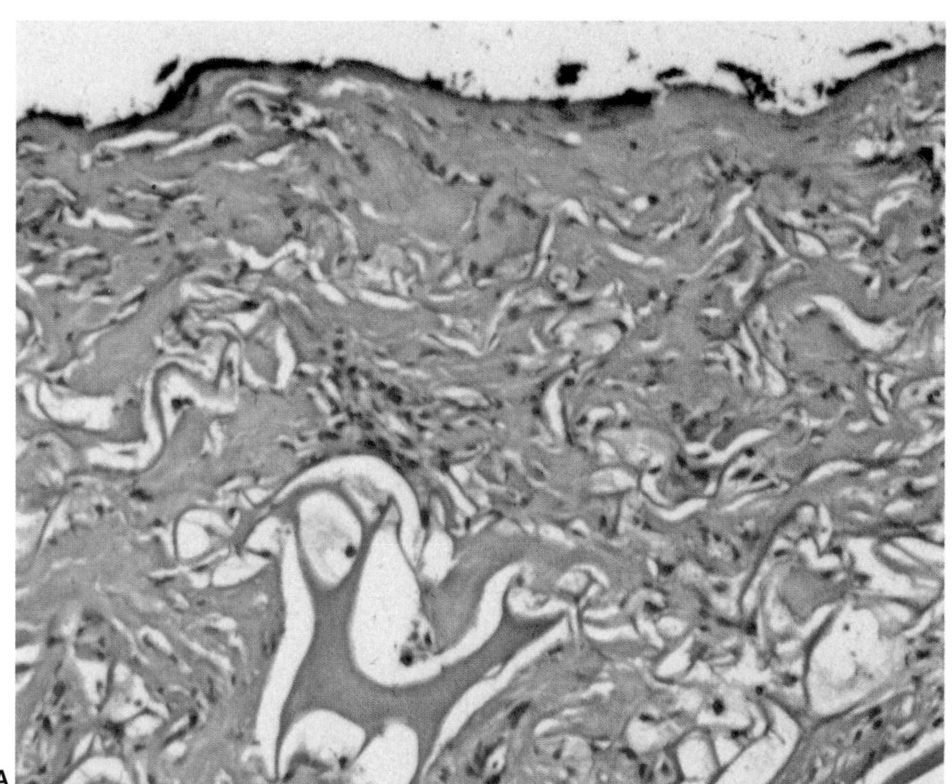

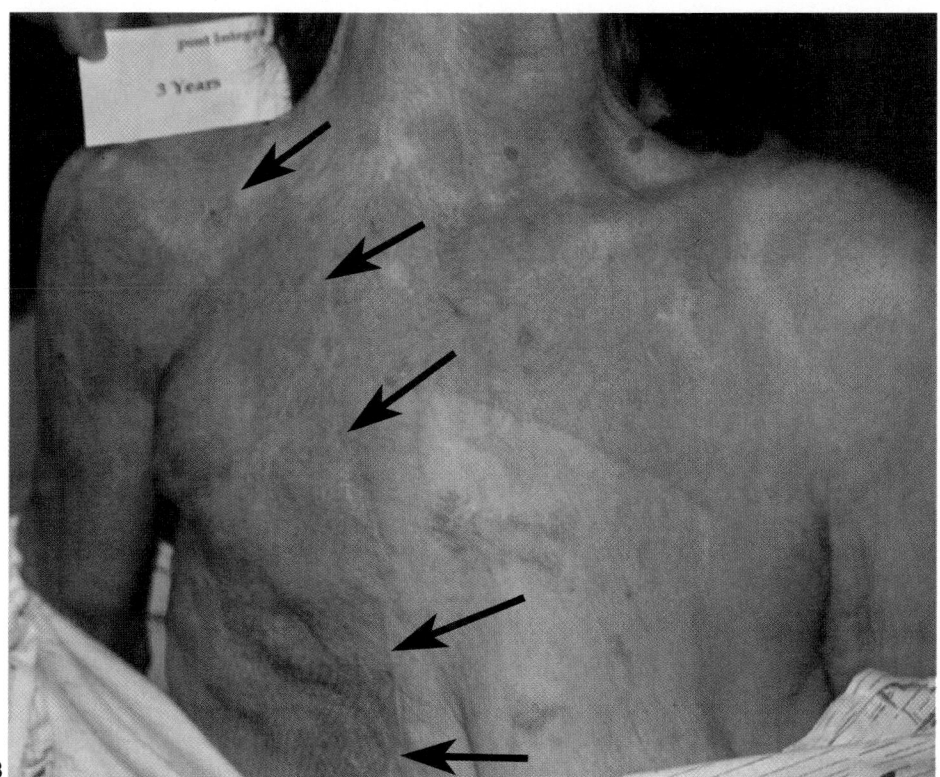

FIGURE 11.9 (*A*) Histology of Integra neodermis appears more like uninjured dermis than regular scar. (*B*) Integra covered with ultrathin skin grafts (arrows) is softer and more elastic than the traditional wide meshed grafts. (*C*) Donor sites for the ultrathin grafts heal quickly without the long-term scars typical of standard depth donor sites.

C 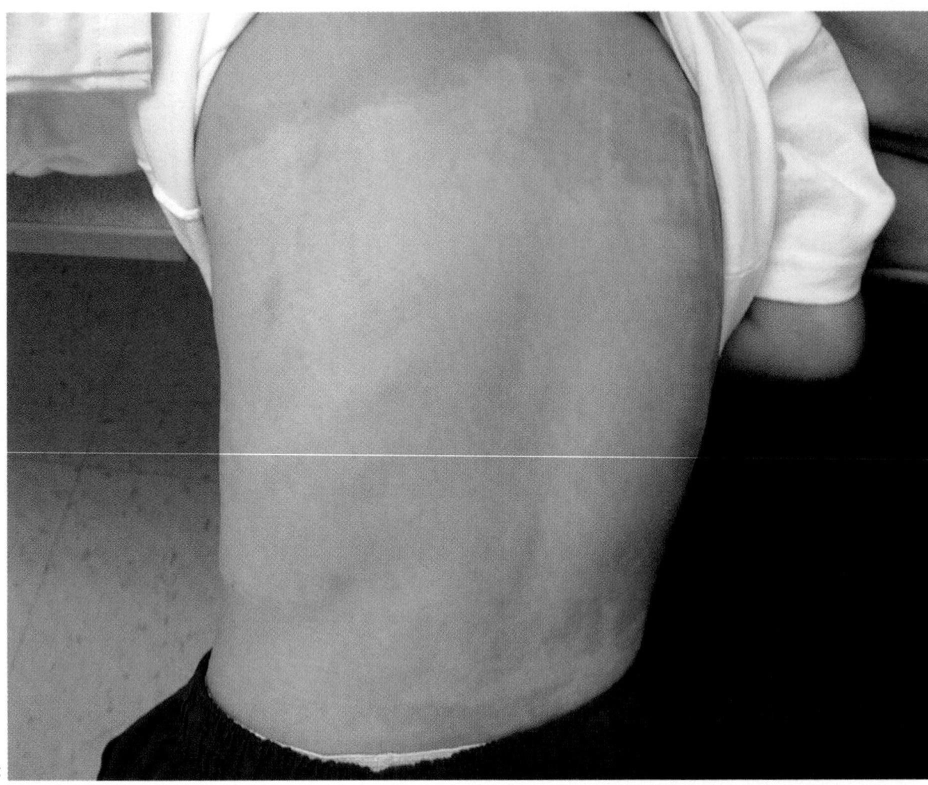

FIGURE 11.9 *(continued)*

Integra use has been reported to have improved long-term aesthetic and functional results (see Fig. 11.9B) but requires meticulous surgical excision and postoperative care to minimize infection; success is improved if a topical antimicrobial agent is used postoperatively. A significant advantage is the rapid healing and minimal scarring in ultrathin donor sites (see Fig. 11.9C).

Another promising dermal substitute is AlloDerm (LifeCell, The Woodlands, TX), a cryopreserved human dermal allograft. The advantage of this product is the native mesenchymal structure without the allogenic cellular components that cause allograft rejection. This dermal substitute requires immediate autografting because there is no outer barrier.

METABOLIC AND NUTRITIONAL SUPPORT

Patients with major thermal injury develop a hypermetabolic state characterized by increased basal metabolic rate, increased oxygen consumption, negative nitrogen balance, and weight loss. As a consequence, these patients have increased caloric requirements to prevent delayed wound healing, decreased immune competence, and cellular dysfunction.

Protein catabolism in a 60-kg patient with a large burn may result in loss of 150 to 200 g of nitrogen per day. Nitrogen excreted in the urine can be measured, but large amounts of nitrogen lost from wounds are insensible. Therefore, measured 24-hour total urea nitrogen levels underestimate nitrogen losses in burn patients (Table 11.9).

The catabolic state continues until the wounds are closed. Once a patient becomes anabolic, preburn muscle mass takes three times as long to regain as it did to lose.[89,90] Several equations can be used to estimate calorie needs. The Harris-Benedict equation estimates basal energy expenditure according to gender, age, height, and weight; the basal energy expenditure is multiplied by an activity factor that reflects the severity of injury or the degree of illness; for burns, this multiplier is 2, the maximal factor for this formula. The Harris-Benedict equation overestimates caloric needs for patients with a moderate burn size. The Curreri formula based on patient weight and burn size overestimates caloric needs for patients with large burns and is best used for patients with small- or moderate-sized burns (<40% TBSA).[92,93]

TABLE 11.9

NUTRITIONAL ASSESSMENT OF BURN PATIENTS

	Wound size (% TBSA)	Nitrogen loss from wounds (g/kg/day)	Protein loss from wounds in a 60-kg adult (g/day)	Nutritional needs
Small burn	<10	0.02	~8	Oral intake only
Moderate burn	11–30	0.05	~19	Supplemental enteral feeding if oral intake is insufficient
Large burn	>31	0.12	~45	Enteral feeding to meet nutritional goals with oral intake as tolerated

Infection, ARDS, or creation of donor sites increase catabolism and alter caloric needs. Healing and skin grafting close wounds and decrease the catabolic state. Hence, repeated evaluation of the metabolic state of a burn patient is necessary to account for changes in wound size and clinical condition. As discussed previously, 24-hour total urea nitrogen levels in the urine must be augmented to estimate nitrogen losses from the wound. Serum albumin levels are not sensitive markers of adequate nutrition; they are typically low in patients with burns larger than 20% TBSA. Transthyretin or prealbumin levels correlate more closely with catabolic status and a trend over several weeks may correlate with patient caloric needs. C-reactive protein levels provide an indication of the patient's general inflammatory state and may correlate with catabolic status. Indirect calorimetry may be useful for measuring caloric needs in intubated burn patients by quantifying oxygen consumption and carbon dioxide expiration and calculating nutritional requirements based on the formula: kcal/day = $(3.9 \times VO_2 + 1.1 \times VCO_2) \times 1.44$. Pulmonary artery catheters can also indirectly provide this information by using the Fick equation: kcal/day = cardiac output $\times$ (arterial pO_2 − venous pO_2) $\times 10 \times 6.96$.

Enteral Nutrition

Prolonged ileus and gastric stress ulcers in burn patients have been largely eliminated by early feeding. Multiple studies have shown that patients with major thermal injury can receive adequate calories soon after injury. At the University of Washington Burn Center, tube feeding is started a median of 5 hours after admission (unpublished quality improvement data).

Benefits of gastric feeding versus duodenal feeding continue to be debated. Although feeding distal to the pylorus theoretically should cause less aspiration risk, enteral formula can be found in pulmonary secretions of 7% of patients receiving gastric feeds compared with 13% of patients receiving transpyloric feeding.[100] Hence, for burn patients with high caloric needs, the delay in feeding for confirmation of tube placement may not be worth the effort.

Continuation of tube feeds during surgery in intubated burn patients who require multiple operations maximizes caloric intake and decreases wound infection[101]; however, intraoperative positioning may necessitate stopping feeds preoperatively—especially if the patient will be prone. Critically ill burn patients that have undergone decompressive laparotomy for abdominal compartment syndrome also tolerate continuous tube feedings.[102]

Glucose Management

Hyperglycemia negatively impacts wound healing and increases morbidity and mortality in critically ill patients—even in those without underlying diabetes mellitus.[103] Increased risk of infection, reduced skin graft take, and higher mortality[104] underscore the importance of maintaining blood sugars between 80 to 120 mg/dL.[105]

Albumin

Hypoalbuminemia typically persists in burn patients until the wounds are healed. Patients with large burns typically have serum albumin levels of 1.7 g/dL and rarely exceed 2.5 g/dL. Administration of exogenous albumin to attain serum levels above 1.5 g/dL does not appear to impact length of stay, complication rate, or mortality.[106]

Nutritional Supplementation

Studies to determine benefits of specialized nutritional supplements such as arginine, glutamine, and omega-3 fatty acids in burn patients are contradictory.[107–109] However, there are reports that anabolism can be promoted in burn patients with metabolically active agents such as insulin, recombinant human growth factor, the anabolic steroid oxandrolone, and propranolol.[109] Oxandrolone in particular has been reported to improve weight gain and functional recovery in burn survivors.[110] Early administration of the antioxidants alpha-tocopherol and ascorbic acid reduces the incidence of organ failure and shortens intensive care unit (ICU) length of stay in critically ill trauma patients.[111] Whether a multicenter study will be necessary to repeat this trial in burn patients is unclear, but the potential benefit and the low cost makes antioxidant supplementation an attractive low-risk intervention for burn patients at risk for multiple organ dysfunction.

INFECTION

We have determined that as many as 80% of patients with large burns develop an infection from one or more sources during the hospital stay (unpublished data). Nevertheless, judicious antibiotic use must be employed in treating infections to limit development of opportunistic infections in individual patients and to establish responsible epidemiologic infection control in the burn unit. Therefore, targeted systemic antibiotics should be used for diagnosed infections based on clinical judgment and supportive laboratory and radiologic findings. Prophylaxis against gram-positive organisms leads to development of gram-negative bacterial infections or fungal and mold infections and are therefore contraindicated in patients with burns. Tetanus prophylaxis continues to be recommended because the disease is so devastating and vaccination has theoretically minor risk. However, modern medical literature has few reports of tetanus developing in patients who have been immunized during childhood.[112]

DEEP VEIN THROMBOSIS

The incidence of deep vein thrombosis (DVT) has been reported to be as high as 25% in hospitalized burn patients.[113] It has also been reported to be responsible for only 0.14% of deaths in burn patients; hence a standard of care for DVT prophylaxis in burn patients has never been defined.[114] At the University of Washington Burn Center, patients with burns larger than 20% TBSA developed clinically evident thromboembolic disease in 9% of those who received prophylaxis with unfractionated heparin and in 18% of those who received low-molecular-weight heparin (unpublished data). On the basis of these data, patients with burns larger than 20% TBSA receive prophylaxis with subcutaneous unfractionated heparin, 5,000 U twice a day. A dropping platelet count suggests heparin-induced thrombocytopenia (HIT), which causes generalized microvascular thrombosis and can be associated with thromboembolic disease.

ANEMIA

Acute blood loss soon after injury is uncommon in a patient with an isolated burn injury; therefore, a dropping hematocrit during resuscitation may be a sign that a patient has associated injuries or a bleeding diathesis. Procedures such as central venous line placement or escharotomies should not be associated with significant blood loss.

Patient age, overall condition, and comorbidity should contribute to the determination for the need for a transfusion.

The risks of viral transmission, transfusion reaction, and cost must also be considered. For a healthy patient who does not need surgery, a hematocrit as low as 20% may be well tolerated. However, inhalation injury, severe infection, or unstable cardiac ischemia may require a higher hematocrit to maximize oxygen-carrying capacity. Patients with large burns and anticipated blood loss should receive iron supplements. Erythropoietin is an expensive recombinant supplement that has not been shown to prevent anemia or decrease transfusion requirements in acutely burned patients.[115]

PAIN MANAGEMENT

Pain management for patients with burn injuries works best with simple pharmaceutical approaches. Use of several narcotics with varying half-lives will confuse health-care providers, the patient, and the family. However, burn patients experience three different classes of pain—background, breakthrough, and procedural pain, which require different approaches.

Burn patients experience background pain 24 hours per day until their wounds are healed; long-acting pain relievers are well suited for this type of discomfort. A hospitalized patient with large burns can be easily treated with methadone or controlled-release morphine sulfate. An outpatient with a small burn often does well with a nonsteroidal antiinflammatory drug (NSAID); NSAIDs should be stopped at least 7 days before any surgery.

Breakthrough pain occurs when exercise or other activities of daily living exacerbate background burn wound discomfort. Short-acting narcotics or acetaminophen can alleviate occasional breakthrough pain. Persistent breakthrough pain suggests that the long-acting medication dosage should be increased.

Procedural pain occurs during wound care and dressing changes and usually requires treatment with a short-acting narcotic. For inpatients with larger burns, oral narcotics or transmucosal fentanyl citrate[116,117] work well for wound care; IV morphine or fentanyl can be used for uncontrolled pain. For outpatients, oxycodone (5 to 15 mg) usually suffices for daily wound care. Anxiety about wound care or therapy is often misconstrued as pain, especially in children. Therefore, patients with large burns requiring daily wound care should be evaluated for potential benefit from a short-acting anxiolytic agent for procedures. Complications of excessive narcotic use, such as prolonged sedation, delirium, and, more urgently, loss of airway control, must be avoided in young children and elderly patients, who may have decreased narcotic tolerance.[118]

Nonpharmacologic approaches can augment pain management in burn patients. Hypnosis can be administered either by trained health-care providers or by patients themselves to reduce narcotic use.[119] Virtual reality has also shown promise as a distraction modality to enhance patient comfort during wound care and intense physical therapy.

Discomfort in the healed wound due to paresthesias and itching may persist for months after injury but generally do not respond to narcotics; exercise and deep massage are effective modalities that patients should be encouraged to use. Diphenhydramine, cyproheptadine, or cetirizine may relieve itching. Use of doxepin ointment may also abrogate itching in healed wounds.[120] Keeping the wound moist with a topical salve or lotion may be as effective as other pharmacologic approaches.

SPECIALIZED BURN AREAS

Burns of the Face, Ocular Adnexa, and Ears

The structures in the midface can be difficult to excise and reconstruct. Therefore, the face is commonly treated nonoperatively with topical antimicrobial agents for 10 days.[121,122] Areas that remain unhealed at that time should be excised and grafted with thick sheet autograft. The nasal tip and alar rims are especially difficult to reconstruct and excision should be sparing. Periocular burns can lead to acute and late sequelae. Early after injury, edema can cause conjunctival desiccation with eventual keratitis and corneal ulceration. Lubrication with ophthalmologic antibiotics is mandatory but tarsorrhaphy may be necessary. If the lid burns are deep, earlier excision and skin grafting may be indicated. Ear burns can lead to suppurative chondritis if infection develops. Many texts suggest that all ear burns must be treated with mafenide cream,[123] but studies have verified that silver sulfadiazine has comparable results. More importantly, pressure on the burned auricle from objects such as pillows and tight dressings or ties should be avoided by using a foam egg crate for a pillow and very loose dressings.

Burns of the Hands and Feet

Optimal functional outcome of hand burns is facilitated by an organized, multidisciplinary approach to the injuries with emphasis on the therapist. The initial evaluation of the burned hand must include evaluation of capillary refill, temperature, and Doppler signals in the palmar arch. It is not enough simply to demonstrate that there is blood flow in the radial or ulnar arteries. If the arm or upper arm are circumferentially burned, escharotomies of the proximal upper extremity and dorsal hand may be indicated (see Fig. 11.5C). Digital escharotomies are never indicated because the potential injury to the digital vessels and nerves outweighs the benefit. For high-voltage electrical injury or deep fourth- or fifth-degree thermal burns, fasciotomy may be required for forearm compartment syndrome or progressive neurovascular impairment. In equivocal cases, it is most prudent to proceed to decompression promptly rather than wait until ischemia has advanced.

Extremity elevation benefits all hand burns by limiting edema and subsequently allowing range of motion and limiting risk of infection. Active range of motion should be the goal for all hand burns; this will decrease edema and maintain manual function. If the patient is unable to cooperate, passive range of motion should be performed at least twice per day. Splinting the hand in a functional position, with the metacarpophalangeal joints at 70 to 90 degrees, the interphalangeal joints in extension, the thumb in neutral position with the first web space open, and the wrist in 20 to 30 degrees of extension, may be indicated for a critically injured patient. Deep partial-thickness and full-thickness burns should be excised and sheet grafted as soon as practical (Fig. 11.10). Hands are immobilized in a functional position for 5 days after surgery to prevent shearing of the graft before range of motion exercises are resumed. Deeper hand burns that involve the extensor mechanisms, joint capsules, or bone, are difficult clinical problems. They also often require temporary or long-term axial Kirschner wire fixation of open and unstable interphalangeal or metacarpophalangeal joints. These burns may require groin or abdominal flap coverage[124] to achieve a tissue bed that can be grafted. With these approaches, patients with deep hand burns should be able to function independently.

Palm burns are especially common in the toddler age group as they begin to explore and touch hot surfaces such as ovens or gas-fireplace glass. Because palmar skin is thick, many burns do not require resurfacing. Therefore, a nonoperative approach facilitates preservation of the specialized attachment of the palmar skin to the underlying fascia and regeneration of the unique Pacinian mechanoreceptors in the palmar skin. If necessary, full-thickness injuries that do not heal in 3 to 4 weeks or show signs of healing by contraction should be grafted with full-thickness or thick split-thickness sheet grafts and splinted in extension to maintain the palm in an open

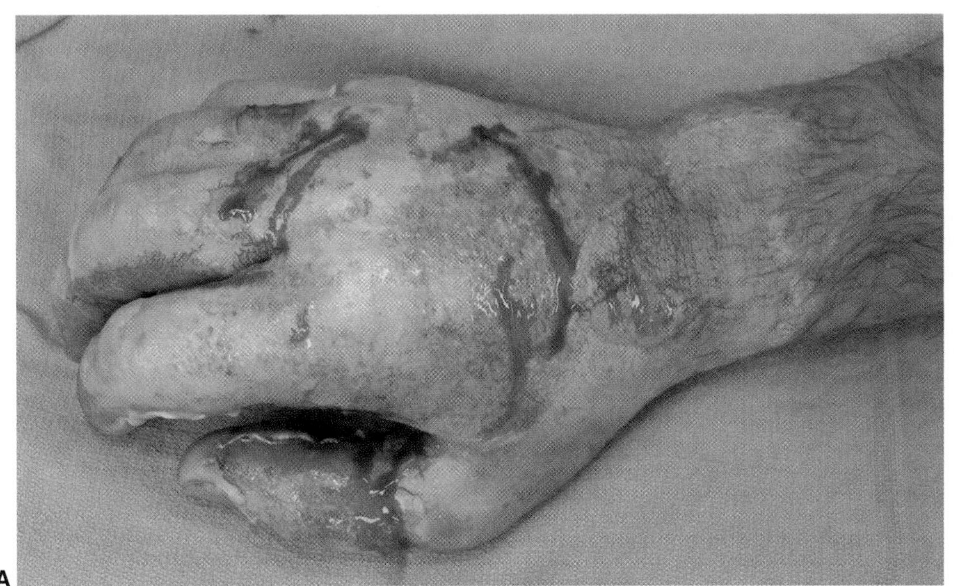

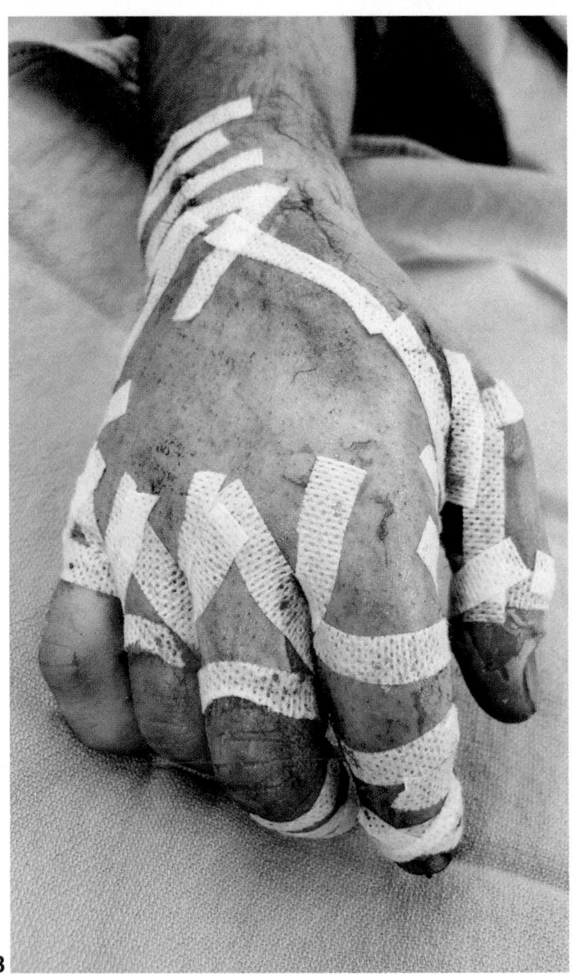

FIGURE 11.10 (*A*) A deep grease/flame burn to hand can be grafted as soon after injury as feasible to expedite return to function. (*B*) Sheet grafts for the hands provide the optimal functional and aesthetic outcomes.

position. Likewise, burns of the plantar surface of the feet should be grafted with full- or thick split-thickness sheet grafts if they fail to heal within 3 weeks.

Genital Burns

Genital burns should initiate an investigation of abuse or neglect. A burned foreskin must be reduced to a normal position so edema does not cause paraphimosis. Penile and scrotal burns often heal well without excision and grafting. Urethral stenting and bladder catheter drainage are not required for genital burn management and increase the risk of urinary tract infection. Bladder catheters should be removed when close monitoring of the urine output is no longer required. Likewise, with aggressive wound care, diversion of the intestinal tract is not required in the management of perineal burns.

MISCELLANEOUS BURN INJURIES

Electrical Injuries

Electrical injuries can be grouped into three categories: high voltage, involving contact with more than 1,000 volts; low voltage, caused by contact with less than 1,000 volts; and those caused by lightning. Electrical flash burns occur when a high-voltage current arcing (jumping) from a high-tension wire toward a human being generates heat and produces a flash skin burn; this does not involve electrical current and should not be confused with an electrical injury. Low-voltage injuries may cause locally destructive injuries but rarely cause systemic sequelae. High-voltage injuries can cause local destruction at the contact wounds; a deep-tissue injury secondary to the passage of current, deep wounds where the current arcs across joints; flash burns or deep flame burns if clothing ignites; axial spine fractures due to tetanic contraction of paravertebral muscles; and other blunt injuries related to a fall. Hence, patients with high-voltage electrical burns require a complete trauma evaluation including radiographic skeletal series, cardiac monitoring, bladder catheterization to evaluate the urine for presence of myoglobinuria, and serial neurovascular examinations in extremities at risk for compartment syndrome; because many electrical injuries involve the hand, carpal tunnel syndrome and impaired median nerve function deserve special immediate attention. Increased compartment pressures due to edema of the injured muscle leads to additional ischemic injury and rhabdomyolysis and warrant immediate fasciotomy; likewise, progressive loss of median nerve function suggests that a carpal tunnel release may be indicated. Surveys of trauma and burn surgeons suggest that practices vary with regard to cardiac monitoring and musculoskeletal workup. Given the paucity of evidence-based data on outcomes following electrical injuries, establishing standards of care for treating this injury is challenging.

A low-voltage electrical injury especially unique to children occurs when a child puts an electrical extension cord connector into its mouth to pull the two plugs apart. The classic finding is a full-thickness tissue injury to the lateral mouth (Fig. 11.11) with delayed bleeding from the facial artery when the eschar falls off. Maintaining the oral opening is essential to prevent contracture.

Late sequelae of high-voltage electrical injuries include progressive demyelinating sensory and/or motor neurologic loss and early cataract formation; these can develop within weeks to months of the injury. All patients admitted for evaluation and treatment of a high-voltage electrical injury should undergo a comprehensive neurologic and ophthalmologic examination to establish baseline status.

Chemical Injuries

Regardless of whether a chemical burn is alkali or acid, the initial treatment should be copious irrigation with tap water for 30 minutes. Cement and concrete powder or powdered lye should be brushed dry from the patient because contact with water activates the aluminum hydroxide. For eye burns,

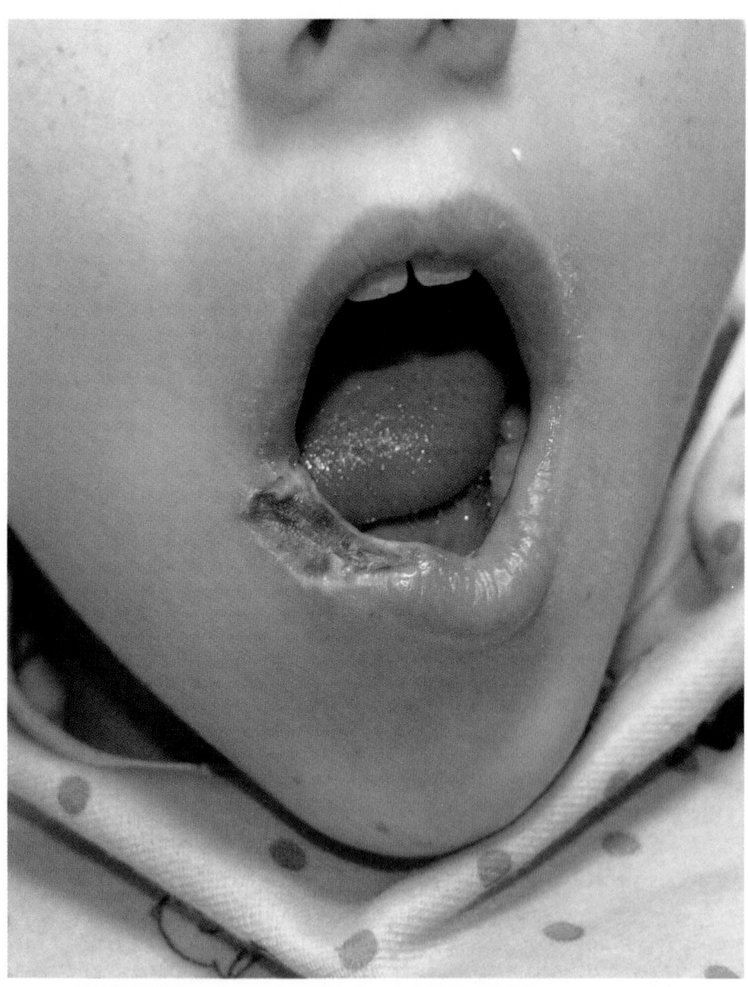

FIGURE 11.11 Full-thickness tissue destruction due to an electrical burn to the commissure of the mouth in young children can lead to oral contractures. The importance of range of motion exercises must be emphasized to the parents.

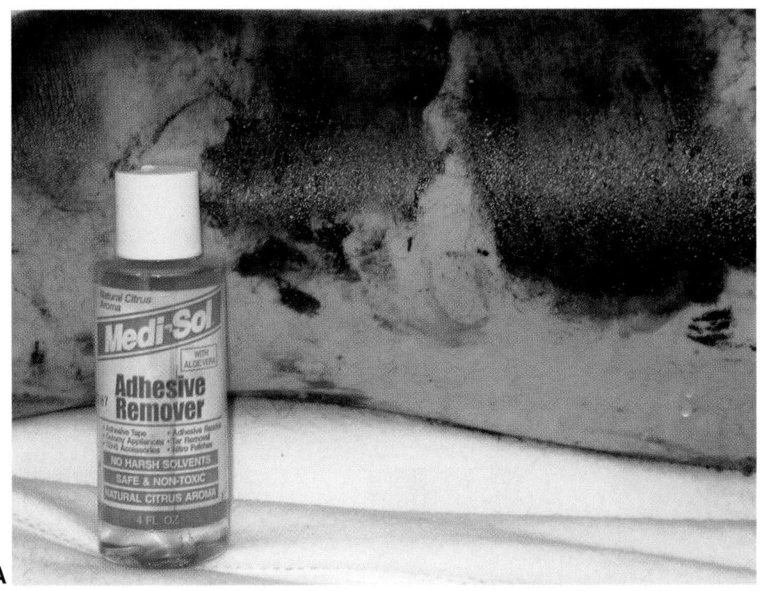

A

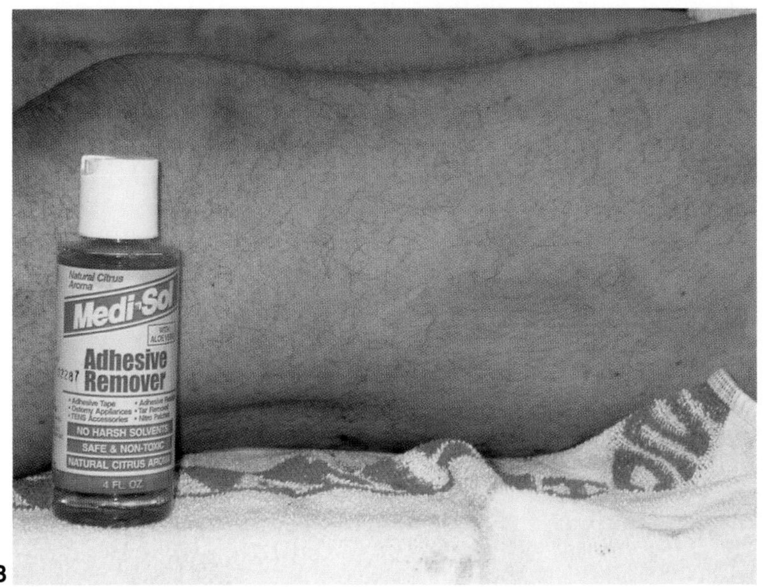

B

FIGURE 11.12 A: Congealed tar should be removed with a lipophilic solvent to determine whether there is a burn underneath. **B:** Cleaning wounds thoroughly with Medi-Sol is safe and essential for correctly determining an accurate burn size.

topical ophthalmic anesthetics can facilitate relief of the conjunctivitis and blepharospasm that limits affective irrigation; ophthalmologic antibiotics should be used if a fluorescent examination confirms presence of a corneal abrasion.

Hydrofluoric acid is one chemical that does have a specific antidote because exposure can induce life-threatening hypocalcemia as the fluoride binds calcium in the tissue.[125] In addition to irrigation with water, topical calcium gluconate gel can be soothing[126] but is inefficient. These burns are often located on the hands of manual workers and can be treated with calcium gluconate intraarterial infusion over 4 hours.[127] This approach requires cardiac monitoring in an ICU. If the burn involves a large area and hypocalcemia persists, emergency burn wound excision is indicated.

Tar Injuries

Tar is often heated to more than 300°F and commonly causes a deep burn, especially if the source is the "mother pot." Adherent tar can be initially cooled by tap water irrigation to limit the progression of the injury. It can be easily removed from the skin (Fig. 11.12) with a lipophilic solvent such as Medi-sol (The Orange-sol Group of Companies, Gilbert, Arizona). Once the wound is exposed, it can be treated like other thermal injuries with topical antimicrobial ointments until the need for surgery is determined.

NONACCIDENTAL BURN INJURIES

Neglect and abuse affect enough children that providers should consider these diagnoses in any child that has burns. If there is any question that either contributed to the injury, the child should be admitted to the hospital for further assessment. If expert opinion suggests that the injuries are suspicious, they should be filed with the appropriate local agency. Radiographic evaluation of the head, ribs, and long bones should be obtained for further documentation of other types of abuse; ophthalmologic evaluation should also be performed to rule out retinal detachment—often a sign of shaken baby syndrome. Too often abuse in other vulnerable populations is overlooked; learning disabled and the elderly[128] are also at-risk groups and suspicious injuries should be reported to adult protective services.[129] Finally, self-mutilation should be treated cautiously. Even patients with multiple small burns such as cigarette burns should be admitted for psychological evaluation.[130]

NONBURN CONDITIONS COMMONLY CARED FOR IN BURN CENTERS

Wound care and critical care services in burn centers[131,132] lend themselves to management of other conditions with large cutaneous deficits such as purpura fulminans, toxic epidermal necrolysis (TEN), staphylococcal scalded skin syndrome, or major soft tissue avulsions.

TEN (Fig. 11.13A), scalded skin syndrome (see Fig. 11.13B), and graft versus host disease (see Fig. 11.13C) are similar blistering disorders with vastly different etiologies. TEN, a variant of erythema multiforme major, involves epidermal slough at the dermal–epidermal junction. Common associations include prior use of sulfa drugs, anticonvulsants, and NSAIDs, but nonspecific viral syndromes may be the only prodromic event leading to the skin loss. This condition is characterized by sloughing of all of stratified squamous epithelial cell surfaces including the oral mucosa and anus. Typically, the skin between the blisters can be sheered with minimal digital pressure in a test known as a Nikolski sign.

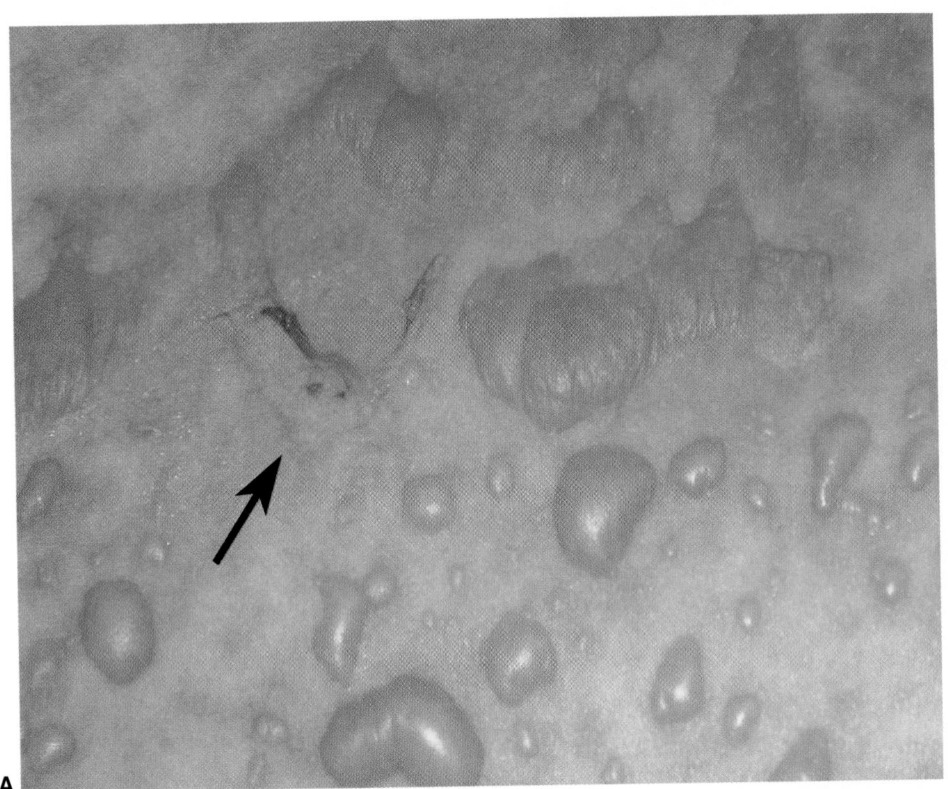

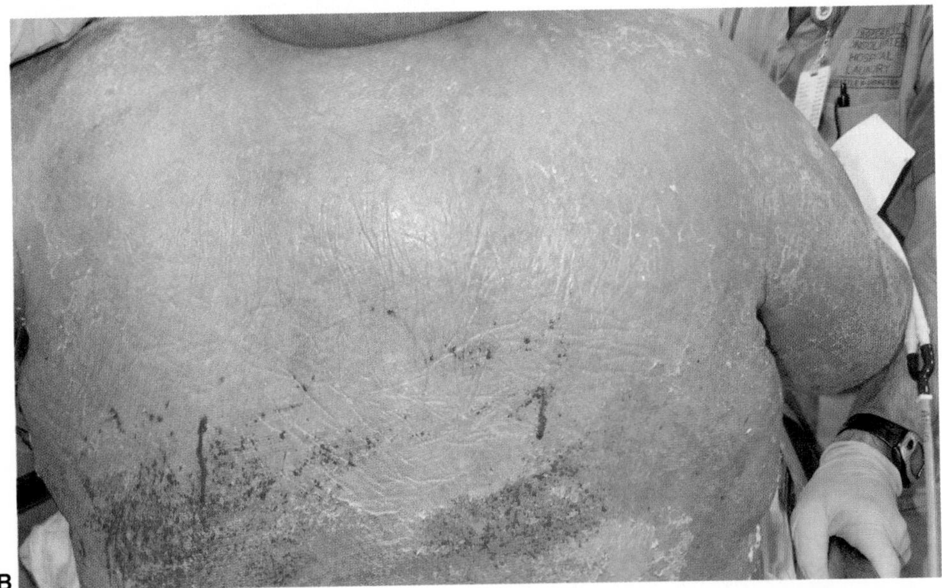

FIGURE 11.13 (*A*) Toxic epidermal necrolysis (TEN), a severe variant of erythema multiforme major, causes distinct blisters and a characteristic Nikolski sign (arrow) of normal appearing skin sloughing between the bullae. (*B*) Scalded skin with diffuse erythema appears more diffuse and when the skin sloughs, the underlying epidermis is often healed. (*C*) Graft versus host disease can be confused in appearance with TEN, but history of a recent transplant (solid or hematologic) is pathognomonic. (*D*) Removal of the sloughed skin and protection of the underlying viable wound bed by applying a biologic dressing such as xenograft improves survival in patients with TEN.

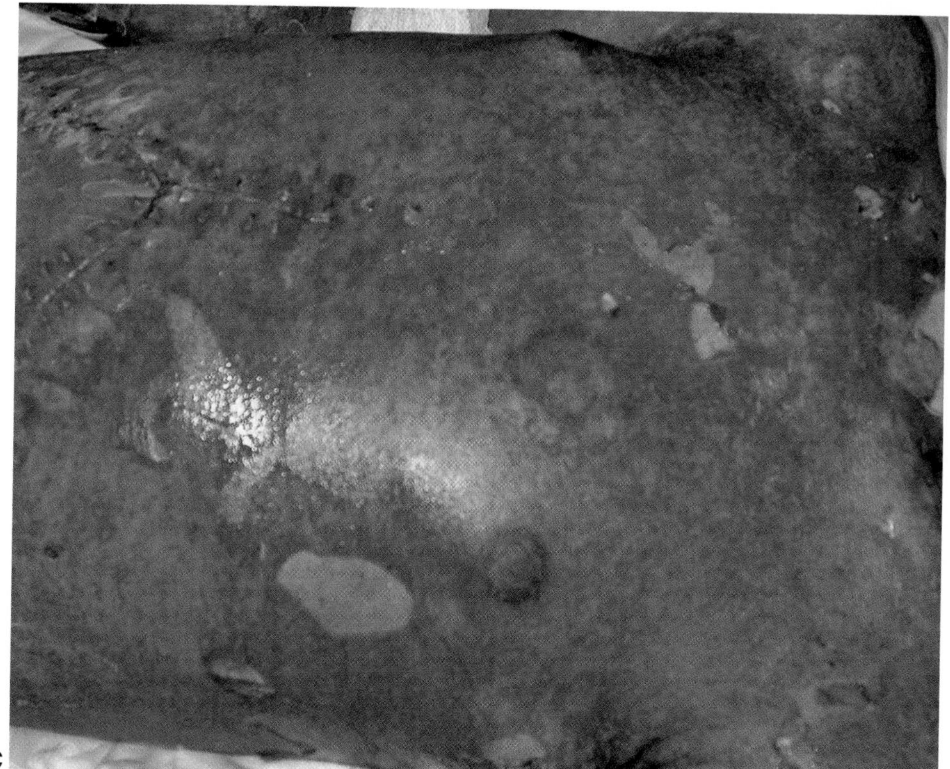

C

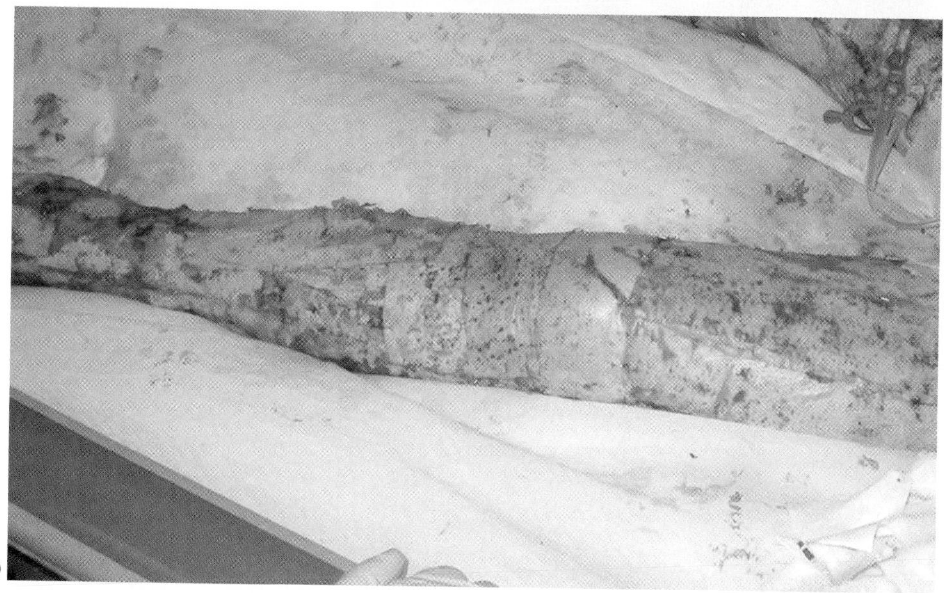

D

FIGURE 11.13 *(continued)*

Treatment depends on extent of skin sough. Small scattered areas can be treated with Acticoat or greasy gauze. When epidermal sloughing involves more than 25% TBSA, gentle débridement of the confluent areas of sloughed skin and placement of a biologic dressing such as xenograft[133] is indicated to prevent skin desiccation and superinfection (see Fig. 11.13D). Systemic steroid treatment is associated with a poorer prognosis as are topical treatment with silver nitrate solution and total peripheral nutrition.[134] Recent suggestions that the process can be effectively limited with intravenous immunoglobulin (IVIG) treatment[135] have not been definitively demonstrated in clinical trials. Prophylactic antibiotics are associated with increased mortality. Patients with severe oropharyngeal involvement may require intubation for airway protection and early enteral tube feeding while the oral lesions heal. Daily ophthalmologic evaluation is essential to prevent synechiae forming. Likewise, daily separation of the external genitalia and vaginal lubrication is indicated to prevent painful mucosal scarring.

Differentiation between TEN and staphylococcal scalded skin syndrome can be difficult on clinical grounds and, if there is a question, warrants a skin biopsy for histologic confirmation. Patients with scalded skin syndrome typically do not present with positive blood cultures because the staphylococcal exotoxin is responsible for the epidermal separation at the granular layer. These wounds are more superficial than TEN and usually heal quickly. Mucous membrane and conjunctiva involvement are not typical and may provide a useful differentiation between staphylococcal scalded skin syndrome and TEN.

Empiric antistaphylococcal antibiotics should be administered but a detailed physical examination should be performed to identify a source of infection.

Purpura fulminans is typically a complication of meningococcal or streptococcal sepsis.[136] Many patients with this condition have multiorgan failure due to the underlying septic shock coupled with the significant vasopressive agents required for cardiovascular support; ischemia affects end organs including patchy cutaneous necrosis (Fig. 11.14A) especially digits (see Fig. 11.14B). Treatment of the wounds is supportive until the patient is stable enough to undergo excision and grafting; excision or amputation may be indicated earlier if the necrotic wounds become secondarily infected. Amputations are common in survivors.

Necrotizing Soft Tissue Infection

Necrotizing fasciitis should be considered in any patient with cellulitis and a history of IV drug abuse, diabetes, obesity, vascular insufficiency, or immunosuppression. Signs and symptoms that help to differentiate a necrotizing infection (Fig. 11.15A) from uncomplicated cellulitis reflect the severity of illness and are summarized in Table 11.10. Delayed diagnosis and surgical treatment are associated with significantly increased mortality. If a necrotizing soft tissue infection is suspected, wide surgical débridement should be performed emergently (see Fig. 11.15B). A central venous catheter should be placed for fluid resuscitation and preoperative antibiotics: penicillin (4 million units), gentamicin (7 mg/kg), and clindamycin (1,200 to 1,600 mg) should be administered. During wide débridement of necrotic tissue, an immediate Gram stain and culture swab should be obtained and reviewed. One should assume clostridial infection if there are gram-positive rods with a paucity of white blood cells (WBCs) and assume beta-hemolytic streptococcal infection if there are abundant gram-positive cocci. Plans should be made to reexplore the wound within 24 hours of the original operation; this may be sooner if the patient undergoes clinical deterioration or if the WBC count increases. Broad-spectrum antibiotics should be continued until the microbiology results are final to direct focused therapy. For patients in septic shock, perioperative IVIG may be indicated to bind the toxin. Anecdotal

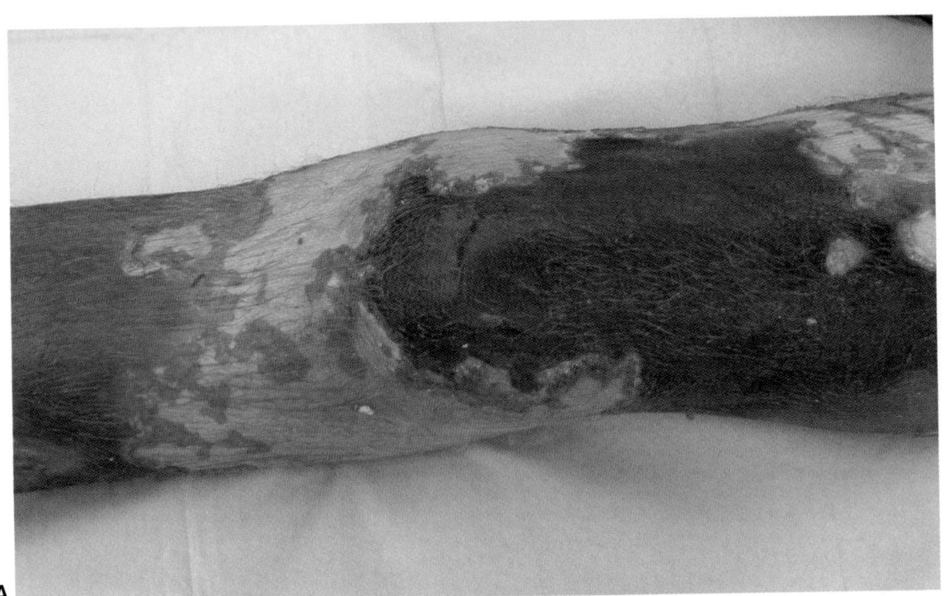

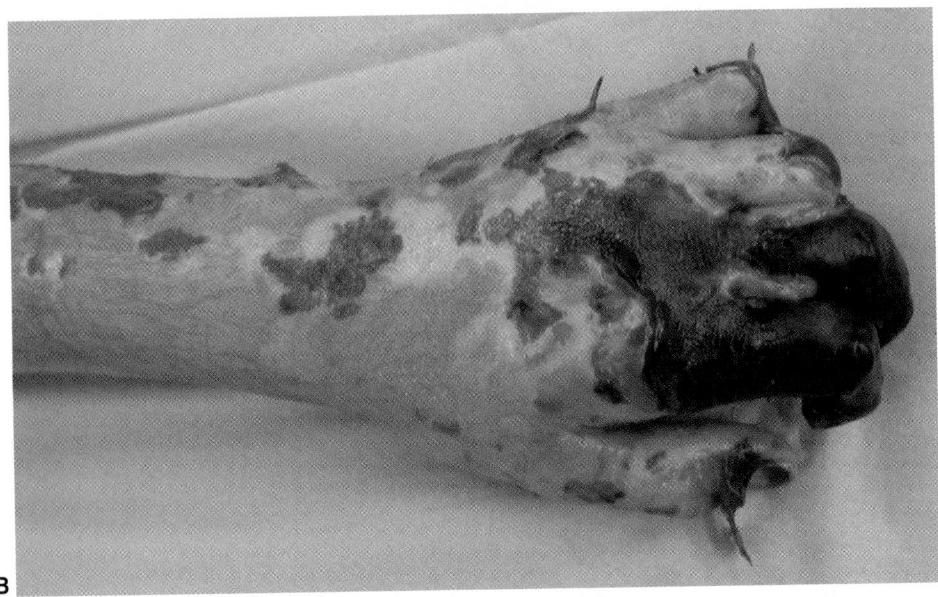

FIGURE 11.14 Purpura fulminans resulting from meningococcemia or streptococcemia causes patchy cutaneous necrosis on many body surfaces (**A**) but especially the digits (**B**).

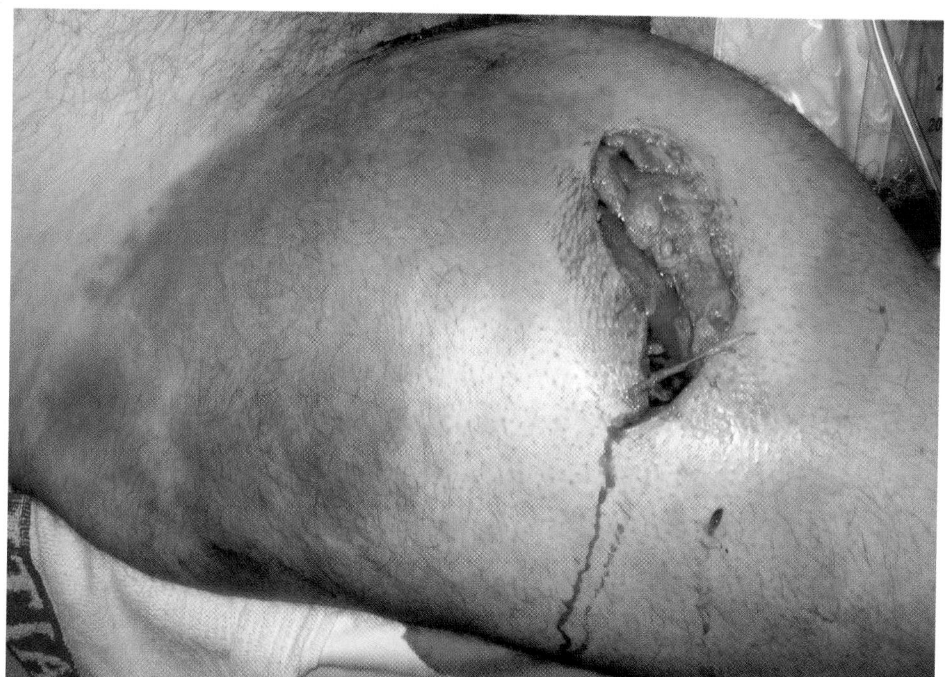

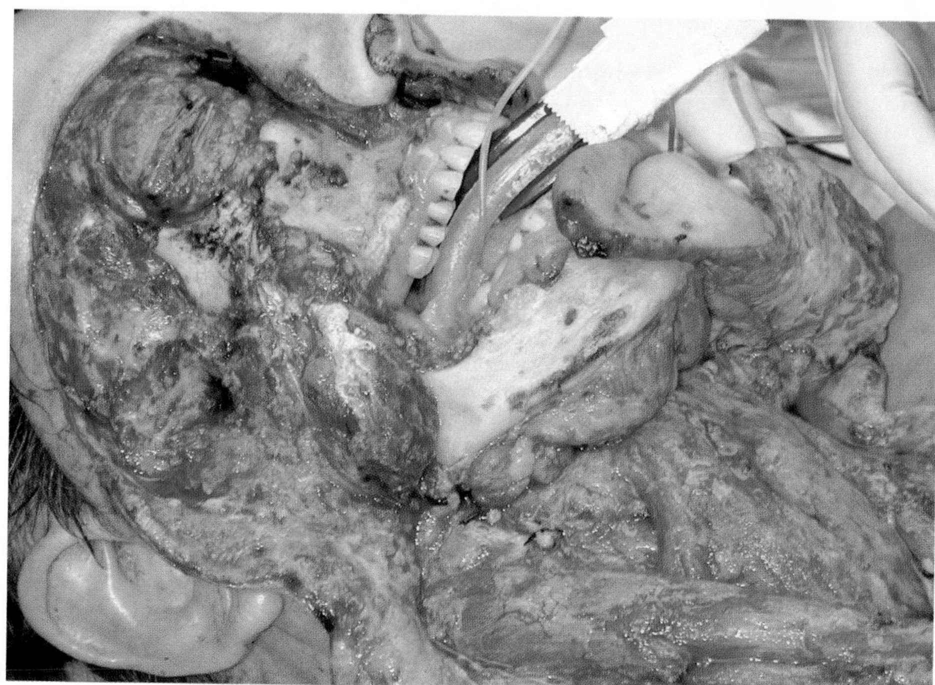

FIGURE 11.15 (*A*) Necrotizing soft tissue infections must be differentiated from cellulitis based on systemic physiology. (*B*) Wide surgical débridement of all involved tissues is the mainstay of treatment for this life-threatening tissue infection, even if it exposes vital structures.

evidence also indicates that plasmapheresis may improve outcome in septic patients.

HYPERTROPHIC SCARRING AND RECONSTRUCTIVE SURGERY

Hypertrophic scar formation is a devastating complication of burns and partial-thickness wounds (Fig. 11.16). The scars are raised, hyperemic, warm, and very pruritic reflecting the histologic findings of increased microvessels and nerves.[36,37] We know from clinical experience that hypertrophic scars form in wounds that take longer to heal, suggesting that either wound depth or complications in healing are important. We also know that they occur in anatomic locations such as the presternal chest and central face more frequently than sites such as the forehead, scalp, and palms or soles. Hypertrophic scars are more prevalent in patients with pigmented skin, especially Asians and Hispanics. The decreased incidence in elderly patients with atrophic skin and senescent cellular responses suggests that high cellular activity may contribute to scar formation. Despite the misery associated with hypertrophic scar formation, our understanding of the pathophysiology is very limited; this basic lack of knowledge is aggravated by the absence of an animal model of scar hypertrophy.

TABLE 11.10 DIAGNOSIS

SIGNS AND SYMPTOMS OF NECROTIZING SOFT TISSUE INFECTION

White blood cell count 20,000/mm^3 Thin, gray drainage Marked induration Edema of entire limb Hyponatremia (Na <135 mEq/L) Skin blistering/sloughing Skin necrosis Crepitus/soft tissue gas on x-ray Pain out of proportion to skin findings Sepsis (tachycardia, hypotension, high fluid requirements)
If patient meets any of these criteria, consider early surgical consultation.

However, recent studies suggest that the female red Duroc pig generates a cutaneous scar[137] that parallels many clinical, histologic, and biochemical findings in human hypertrophic scar tissues.

The ability to regulate development of hypertrophic scars is limited as is treatment for the symptoms. Custom fit compression garments are worn within 2 weeks of wound healing and often continue until the wounds mature at 1 or 2 years after injury. Topical silicone anecdotally improves hypertrophic scar size and symptoms, but the mechanism is not clear and use can be accompanied by skin irritation and rashes. Intradermal steroid injection has also been described but is very painful and unreliable in the management of hypertrophic scarring; furthermore, the wound size that can be treated is limited by the risk of systemic steroid effects. Patients with persistent symptomatic hypertrophic scarring that limit function or activities of daily living often require excision and primary wound closure or wound closure with sheet autografts or tissue flaps. Patients who have survived large burns may require several sequential reconstructive procedures during the first few years after injury to attain the optimal cosmetic and functional results.

REHABILITATION AND RECONSTRUCTION

As survival following major burns has improved, more emphasis has been placed on functional recovery, societal reintegration, and return to school or work. In the early 1990s, The National Institute of Disability and Rehabilitation Research (NIDRR; http://www.ed.gov/offices/osers/nidrr), whose mission is to generate, disseminate, and promote new knowledge to improve independent living options for disabled persons, recognized that burn survivors would likely benefit from organized rehabilitation model systems that had been established for survivors of traumatic brain injuries. Since then NIDRR has continuously funded projects to advance knowledge in burn rehabilitation by providing multicenter grants to four centers of excellence.

Physical function requires continual participation of burn occupational and physical therapists from the time of the acute injury until long after discharge from the hospital. Initially, therapists are involved with twice daily passive or active range-of-motion exercises of all joints and positioning and splinting of hands, extremities, or the neck. In patients with small burns or in those with almost healed large injuries, therapy involves strengthening, ambulation, active and passive range of motion, performance of activities of daily living, and, in older adolescents and adults, development of work-related skills and if necessary development of adaptive skills with modified utensils or prosthetic devices. Therapists often provide the essential human bridge between inpatient and outpatient care.

Posttraumatic stress, anxiety, or depression frequently manifest after severe burns. Whereas involvement of burns that involve the hands or face can be anticipated to induce these symptoms, they cannot be otherwise predicted based on burn size or location. Preinjury psychiatric conditions, family dysfunction, or substance abuse further complicate psychosocial recovery. The major impact that psychological recovery has on the burn patient's ability to recover functionally underscores the need for coordinated participation of burn psychologists and social workers in the multidisciplinary care of burn patients. These staff typically interact with the patient, family, and local outpatient support services throughout hospitalization and assist with coordinating discharge plans.

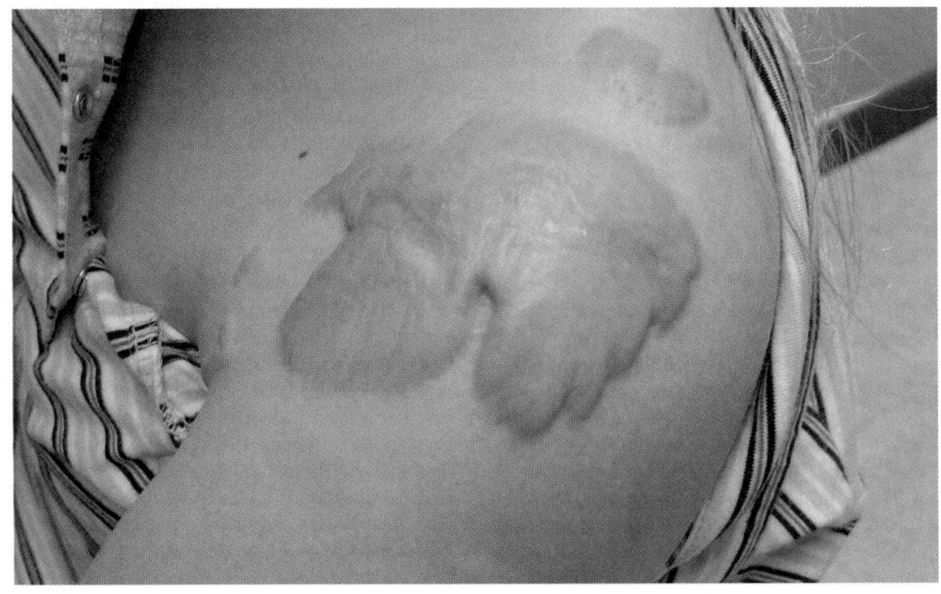

FIGURE 11.16 Hypertrophic scars in healed deep partial-thickness burns cause considerable patient discomfort and misery due to the itching, warmth, raised appearance, and often functional limitations.

KEY POINTS

- **A well-coordinated burn center team, including surgeons, nurses, physical/occupational therapists, social workers, psychologists, and pain specialists, is required to both optimize survival and minimize dysfunction in the burn patient.**
- **Skin is a complex organ of specialized cells that, in addition to loss of barrier function, causes a systemic immunoinflammatory response with risk of MOF following thermal damage.**
- **Increased prevention (smoke alarms, lower temperature hot water heaters, etc.) and advances in care, including early excision, grafting, and use of new artificial skin substitutes have greatly increased survival and functional recovery following thermal injury.**
- **Airway injury from inhalation of steam or toxic burn products greatly increases morbidity and mortality from any associated injury or comorbidity.**
- **Fluid resuscitation must be appropriate to maintain perfusion (e.g., urine output) and prevent progression of burn-induced tissue loss but not excessive, causing tissue swelling, abdominal and extremity compartment syndrome, or ARDS.**
- **Enteral nutritional support should begin within 12 hours of injury to meet the extreme metabolic needs of the burn patient (i.e., two times basal metabolic needs for >40% TBSA burns).**

References

1. **Gibran NS, Klein MB, Engrav LH, Heimbach DM. UW Burn Center A model for regional delivery of burn care. *Burns* 2005;31[Suppl 1]:S36.**
2. Baux S, Mimoun M, Saade H, et al. Burns in the elderly. *Burns* 1989;15:239.
3. **Ryan CM, Schoenfeld DA, Thorpe WP, et al. Objective estimates of the probability of death from burn injuries. *N Engl J Med.* 1998;338:362.**
4. Erdmann TC, Feldman KW, Rivara FP, et al. Tap water burn prevention: the effect of legislation. *Pediatrics* 1991;88:572.
5. Bennett B, Gamelli R. Profile of an abused burned child. *J Burn Care Rehab.* 1998;19(1 Pt 1):88; discussion 87.
6. Barillo DJ, Brigham PA, Kayden DA, et al. The fire-safe cigarette: a burn prevention tool. *J Burn Care Rehab.* 2000;21:162.
7. Jackson D. The diagnosis of the depth of burning. *J Br Surg.* 1953;40:588.
8. Isik S, Sahin U, Ilgan S, et al. Saving the zone of stasis in burns with recombinant tissue-type plasminogen activator (r-tPA): an experimental study in rats. *Burns* 1998;24:217.
9. Payan D, Levine J, Goetzl E. Modulation of immunity and hypersensitivity by sensory neuropeptides. *J Immunol.* 1984;132:1601.
10. Ansel JC, Kaynard AH, Armstrong CA, et al. Skin-nervous system interactions. *J Invest Dermatol.* 1996;106:198–.
11. Arturson G. Pathophysiology of the burn wound. *Ann Chir Gynaecol.* 1980;69:178.
12. Streilein J, Tigelaar R. SALT: skin-associated lymphoid tissue. In: Daynes R, Spikes J, eds. *Experimental and clinical photoimmunology.* Boca Raton, FL: CRC Press; 1983:151.
13. Kupper TS, Deitch EA, Baker CC, Wong WC. The human burn wound as a primary source of interleukin-1 activity. *Surgery* 1986;100:409.
14. Nijsten MW, Hack CE, Helle M, et al. Interleukin-6 and its relation to the humoral immune response and clinical parameters in burned patients. *Surgery* 1991;109:761.
15. Rennekampff HO, Hansbrough JF, Kiessig V, et al. Bioactive interleukin-8 is expressed in wounds and enhances wound healing. *J Surg Res.* 2000;93:41.
16. Sehgal PB. Interleukin-6: molecular pathophysiology. *J Invest Dermatol.* 1990;94[6 Suppl]:2S.
17. Nickoloff BJ, Karabin GD, Barker JN, et al. Cellular localization of interleukin-8 and its inducer, tumor necrosis factor-alpha in psoriasis. *Am J Pathol.* 1991;138:129.
18. Gibran NS, Ferguson M, Heimbach DM, Isik FF. Monocyte chemoattractant protein-1 mRNA expression in the human burn wound. *J Surg Res.* 1997;70:1.
19. Kock A, Schwarz T, Kirnbauer R, et al. Human keratinocytes are a source for tumor necrosis factor alpha: evidence for synthesis and release upon stimulation with endotoxin or ultraviolet light. *J Exp Med.* 1990;172:1609.
20. Rodriguez JL, Miller CG, Garner WL, et al. Correlation of the local and systemic cytokine response with clinical outcome following thermal injury. *J Trauma* 1993;34:684.
21. Bucky LP, Vedder NB, Hong HZ, et al. Reduction of burn injury by inhibiting CD18-mediated leukocyte adherence in rabbits. *Plast Reconstr Surg.* 1994;93:1473.
22. Jang YC, Arumugam S, Gibran NS, Isik FF. Role of alpha(v) integrins and angiogenesis during wound repair. *Wound Repair Regen.* 1999;7:375.
23. Bloch W, Huggel K, Sasaki T, et al. The angiogenesis inhibitor endostatin impairs blood vessel maturation during wound healing. *Faseb J.* 2000;14:2373.
24. Kischer CW, Pindur J, Krasovitch P, Kischer E. Characteristics of granulation tissue which promote hypertrophic scarring. *Scanning Microsc.* 1990;4:877.
25. Gabbiani G. The cellular derivation and the life span of the myofibroblast. *Pathol Res Pract.* 1996;192:708.
26. Wu L, Pierce GF, Galiano RD, Mustoe TA. Keratinocyte growth factor induces granulation tissue in ischemic dermal wounds: importance of epithelial-mesenchymal cell interactions. *Arch Surg.* 1996;131:660.
27. Kaplan ED, Holbrook KA. Dynamic expression patterns of tenascin, proteoglycans, and cell adhesion molecules during human hair follicle morphogenesis. *Dev Dyn.* 1994;199:141.
28. Bohnert A, Hornung J, Mackenzie IC, Fusenig NE. Epithelial-mesenchymal interactions control basement membrane production and differentiation in cultured and transplanted mouse keratinocytes. *Cell Tissue Res.* 1986;244:413.
29. **Garner WL. Epidermal regulation of dermal fibroblast activity. *Plast Reconstr Surg.* 1998;102:135.**
30. Kirsner RS, Falanga V, Eaglstein WH. The biology of skin grafts. Skin grafts as pharmacologic agents. *Arch Dermatol.* 1993;129:481.
31. Ashcroft GS, Horan MA, Herrick SE, et al. Age-related differences in the temporal and spatial regulation of matrix metalloproteinases (MMPs) in normal skin and acute cutaneous wounds of healthy humans. *Cell Tissue Res.* 1997;290:581.
32. Raza SL, Cornelius LA. Matrix metalloproteinases: pro- and anti-angiogenic activities. *J Investig Dermatol Symp Proc.* 2000;5:47.
33. Stricklin GP, Li L, Jancic V, et al. Localization of mRNAs representing collagenase and TIMP in sections of healing human burn wounds. *Am J Pathol.* 1993;143:1657.
34. Hembry RM, Ehrlich HP. Immunolocalization of collagenase and tissue inhibitor of metalloproteinases (TIMP) in hypertrophic scar tissue. *Br J Dermatol.* 1986;115:409.
35. Dasu MR, Hawkins HK, Barrow RE, et al. Gene expression profiles from hypertrophic scar fibroblasts before and after IL-6 stimulation. *J Pathol.* 2004;202:476.
36. Crowe R, Parkhouse N, McGrouther D, Burnstock G. Neuropeptide-containing nerves in painful hypertrophic human scar tissue. *Br J Dermatol.* 1994;130:444.
37. Liang Z, Engrav LH, Muangman P, et al. Nerve quantification in female red Duroc pig (FRDP) scar compared to human hypertrophic scar. *Burns* 2004;30:57.
38. Afromowitz MA, Callis JB, Heimbach DM, et al. Multispectral imaging of burn wounds: a new clinical instrument for evaluating burn depth. *IEEE Trans Biomed Eng.* 1988;35:842.
39. **Heimbach D, Engrav L, Grube B, Marvin J. Burn depth: a review. *World J Surg.* 1992;16:10.**
40. Atiles L, Mileski W, Purdue G, et al. Laser Doppler flowmetry in burn wounds. *J Burn Care Rehab.* 1995;16:388.
41. Rue LW III, Cioffi WG, Mason AD, et al. Improved survival of burned patients with inhalation injury. *Arch Surg.* 1993;128:772; discussion 8.
42. Stassen NA, Lukan JK, Mizuguchi NN, et al. Thermal injury in the elderly: when is comfort care the right choice? *Am Surg.* 2001;67:704.
43. Muller MJ, Pegg SP, Rule MR. Determinants of death following burn injury. *Br J Surg.* 2001;88:583.
44. Jurkovich GJ, Moylan JA. Inhalation injury—a major burn complication. *Physician Assist.* 1983;7:59-62, 5-8.
45. **Heimbach DM, Waeckerle JF. Inhalation injuries. *Ann Emerg Med.* 1988;17:1316.**
46. Hantson P, Butera R, Clemessy JL, et al. Early complications and value of initial clinical and paraclinical observations in victims of smoke inhalation without burns. *Chest* 1997;111:671.
47. Hampson NB, Zmaeff JL. Outcome of patients experiencing cardiac arrest with carbon monoxide poisoning treated with hyperbaric oxygen. *Ann Emerg Med.* 2001;38:36.
48. Hampson NB, Mathieu D, Piantadosi CA, et al. Carbon monoxide poisoning: interpretation of randomized clinical trials and unresolved treatment issues. *Undersea Hyperb Med.* 2001;28:157.
49. Juurlink DN, Stanbrook MB, McGuigan MA. Hyperbaric oxygen for carbon monoxide poisoning. *Cochrane Database Syst Rev.* 2000: CD002041.
50. Grube BJ, Marvin JA, Heimbach DM. Therapeutic hyperbaric oxygen: help or hindrance in burn patients with carbon monoxide poisoning? *J Burn Care Rehab.* 1988;9:249.
51. Hampson NB, Zmaeff JL. Outcome of patients experiencing cardiac arrest with carbon monoxide poisoning treated with hyperbaric oxygen. *Ann Emerg Med.* 2001;38:36.

52. Barillo DJ, Goode R, Esch V. Cyanide poisoning in victims of fire: analysis of 364 cases and review of the literature. *J Burn Care Rehab.* 1994;15:46.
53. Schall GL, McDonald HD, Carr LB, Capozzi A. Xenon ventilation-perfusion lung scans. The early diagnosis of inhalation injury. *JAMA* 1978;240:2441.
54. Bingham HG, Gallagher TJ, Powell MD. Early bronchoscopy as a predictor of ventilatory support for burned patients. *J Trauma* 1987;27:1286.
55. Darling GE, Keresteci MA, Ibanez D, et al. Pulmonary complications in inhalation injuries with associated cutaneous burn. *J Trauma* 1996;40:83.
56. Bulger EM, Jurkovich GJ, Gentilello LM, Maier RV. Current clinical options for the treatment and management of acute respiratory distress syndrome. *J Trauma* 2000;48:562.
57. Ashbaugh DG, Bigelow DB, Petty TL, Levine BE. Acute respiratory distress in adults. *Lancet* 1967;2:319.
58. Hollingsed TC, Saffle JR, Barton RG, et al. Etiology and consequences of respiratory failure in thermally injured patients. *Am J Surg.* 1993;166:592; discussion 6–7.
59. Dancey DR, Hayes J, Gomez M, et al. ARDS in patients with thermal injury. *Intensive Care Med.* 1999;25:1231.
60. Tasaki O, Goodwin CW, Saitoh D, et al. Effects of burns on inhalation injury. *J Trauma* 1997;43:603.
61. Sharar SR, Heimbach DM, Green M, et al. Effects of body surface thermal injury on apparent renal and cutaneous blood flow in goats. *J Burn Care Rehab.* 1988;9:26.
62. Graves TA, Cioffi WG, McManus WF, et al. Fluid resuscitation of infants and children with massive thermal injury. *J Trauma* 1988;28:1656.
63. Greenhalgh DG, Warden GD. The importance of intra-abdominal pressure measurements in burned children. *J Trauma* 1994;36:685.
64. Hobson KG, Young KM, Ciraulo A, et al. Release of abdominal compartment syndrome improves survival in patients with burn injury. *J Trauma* 2002;53:1129; discussion 33.
65. Durtschi MB, Orgain C, Counts GW, Heimbach DM. A prospective study of prophylactic penicillin in acutely burned hospitalized patients. *J Trauma* 1982;22:11.
66. Engrav LH, Richey KJ, Walkinshaw MD, Gottlieb JR. Chondritis of the burned ear: a preventable complication if. *Ann Plast Surg.* 1989;23:1.
67. Chou TD, Gibran NS, Urdahl K, et al. Methemoglobinemia secondary to topical silver nitrate therapy—a case report. *Burns* 1999;25:549.
68. Jackson D, Stone P. Tangential excision and grafting of burns: the method and a report of 50 consecutive cases. *Br J Plastic Surg.* 1972;25:416.
69. Burke JF, Quinby WC, Bondoc CC. Early excision and prompt wound closure supplemented with immunosuppression. *Surg Clin North Am.* 1978;58:1141.
70. Gray DT, Pine RW, Harnar TJ, et al. Early surgical excision versus conventional therapy in patients with 20 to 40 percent burns. A comparative study. *Am J Surg.* 1982;144:76.
71. **Janzekovic Z. A new concept in the early excision and immediate grafting of burns. *J Trauma* 1970;10:1103.**
72. Herndon DN, Barrow RE, Rutan RL, et al. A comparison of conservative versus early excision. Therapies in severely burned patients. *Ann Surg.* 1989;209:547; discussion 52.
73. Merrell SW, Saffle JR, Sullivan JJ, et al. Increased survival after major thermal injury. A nine year review. *Am J Surg.* 1987;154:623.
74. Engrav L, Heimbach D, Reus J, et al. Early excision and grafting vs. nonoperative treatment of burns of indeterminant depth: a randomized prospective study. *J Trauma* 1983;23:1001.
75. Monafo W, Aulenbacher C, Pappalardo C. Early tangential excision of the eschars of major burns. *Arch Surg.* 1972;104:503.
76. Alexander J, MacMillan B, Law E, Kittu RD. Treatment of severe burns with widely meshed skin autograft and meshed skin allograft overlay. *J Trauma* 1981;21:433.
77. Compton CC, Gill JM, Bradford DA, et al. Skin regenerated from cultured epithelial autografts on full-thickness burn wounds from 6 days to 5 years after grafting. A light, electron microscopic and immunohistochemical study. *Lab Invest.* 1989;60:600.
78. Boyce ST, Kagan RJ, Yakuboff KP, et al. Cultured skin substitutes reduce donor skin harvesting for closure of excised, full-thickness burns. *Ann Surg.* 2002;235:269.
79. Boyce ST, Warden GD. Principles and practices for treatment of cutaneous wounds with cultured skin substitutes. *Am J Surg.* 2002;183:445.
80. **Heimbach D, Luterman A, Burke J, et al. Artificial dermis for major burns. A multi-center randomized clinical trial. *Ann Surg.* 1988;208:313.**
81. Heimbach DM, Warden GD, Luterman A, et al. Multicenter postapproval clinical trial of Integra dermal regeneration template for burn treatment. *J Burn Care Rehab.* 2003;24:42.
82. Fang P, Engrav LH, Gibran NS, et al. Dermatome setting for autografts to cover INTEGRA(R). *J Burn Care Rehab.* 2002;23:327.
83. Yannas IV, Burke JF, Orgill DP, Skrabut EM. Wound tissue can utilize a polymeric template to synthesize a functional extension of skin. *Science* 1982;215:174.
84. Burke JF, Yannas IV, Quinby WC Jr, et al. Successful use of a physiologically acceptable artificial skin in the treatment of extensive burn injury. *Ann Surg.* 1981;194:413.
85. Holmes J, Honari S, Gibran N. Excision and grafting of the large burn wound. In: Saffle J, ed. *Problems in general surgery.* Philadelphia: Lippincott Williams & Wilkins; 2003.
86. Sheridan R, Choucair R, Donelan M, et al. Acellular allodermis in burns surgery: 1-year results of a pilot trial. *J Burn Care Rehab.* 1998;19:528.
87. Curreri PW, Luterman A. Nutritional support of the burned patient. *Surg Clin North Am.* 1978;58:1151.
88. Waxman K, Rebello T, Pinderski L, et al. Protein loss across burn wounds. *J Trauma* 1987;27:136.
89. Demling RH, Orgill DP. The anticatabolic and wound healing effects of the testosterone analog oxandrolone after severe burn injury. *J Crit Care* 2000;15:12.
90. **Hart DW, Wolf SE, Mlcak R, et al. Persistence of muscle catabolism after severe burn. *Surgery* 2000;128:312.**
91. Curreri PW, Richmond D, Marvin J, Baxter CR. Dietary requirements of patients with major burns. *J Am Diet Assoc.* 1974;65:415.
92. Schane J, Goede M, Silverstein P. Comparison of energy expenditure measurement techniques in severely burned patients. *J Burn Care Rehab.* 1987;8:366.
93. Gore DC, Rutan RL, Hildreth M, et al. Comparison of resting energy expenditures and caloric intake in children with severe burns. *J Burn Care Rehab.* 1990;11:400.
94. Khorram-Sefat R, Behrendt W, Heiden A, Hettich R. Long-term measurements of energy expenditure in severe burn injury. *World J Surg.* 1999;23:115.
95. Sheridan RL, Prelack K, Cunningham JJ. Physiologic hypoalbuminemia is well tolerated by severely burned children. *J Trauma* 1997;43:448.
96. Rettmer RL, Williamson JC, Labbé RF, Heimbach DM. Laboratory monitoring of nutritional status in burn patients. *Clin Chem.* 1992;38:334.
97. Manelli JC, Badetti C, Botti G, et al. A reference standard for plasma proteins is required for nutritional assessment of adult burn patients. *Burns* 1998;24:337.
98. Saffle JR, Larson CM, Sullivan J. A randomized trial of indirect calorimetry-based feedings in thermal injury. *J Trauma* 1990;30:776; discussion 82.
99. Raff T, Hartmann B, Germann G. Early intragastric feeding of seriously burned and long-term ventilated patients: a review of 55 patients. *Burns* 1997;23:19.
100. Esparza J, Boivin MA, Hartshorne MF, Levy H. Equal aspiration rates in gastrically and transpylorically fed critically ill patients. *Intensive Care Med.* 2001;27:660.
101. Jenkins ME, Gottschlich MM, Warden GD. Enteral feeding during operative procedures in thermal injuries. *J Burn Care Rehab.* 1994;15:199.
102. Mayes T, Gottschlich MM, Warden GD. Nutrition intervention in pediatric patients with thermal injuries who require laparotomy. *J Burn Care Rehab.* 2000;21:451.
103. Van Den Berghe G, Wouters PJ, Bouillon R, et al. Outcome benefit of intensive insulin therapy in the critically ill: Insulin dose versus glycemic control. *Crit Care Med.* 2003;31:359.
104. Gore DC, Chinkes D, Heggers J, et al. Association of hyperglycemia with increased mortality after severe burn injury. *J Trauma* 2001;51:540.
105. van den Berghe G, Wouters P, Weekers F, et al. Intensive insulin therapy in the critically ill patients. *N Engl J Med.* 2001;345:1359.
106. Greenhalgh DG, Housinger TA, Kagan RJ, et al. Maintenance of serum albumin levels in pediatric burn patients: a prospective, randomized trial. *J Trauma* 1995;39:67.
107. Saffle J, Wiebke G, Jennings K, et al. Randomized trial of immune-enhancing enteral nutrition in burn patients. *J Trauma* 1997;42:793.
108. Garrel D, Patenaude J, Nedelec B, et al. Decreased mortality and infectious morbidity in adult burn patients given enteral glutamine supplements: a prospective, controlled, randomized clinical trial. *Crit Care Med.* 2003;31:2444.
109. **Herndon DN. Nutritional and pharmacological support of the metabolic response to injury. *Minerva Anestesiol.* 2003;69:264.**
110. Demling RH, DeSanti L. Oxandrolone induced lean mass gain during recovery from severe burns is maintained after discontinuation of the anabolic steroid. *Burns* 2003;29:793.
111. Nathens AB, Neff MJ, Jurkovich GJ, et al. Randomized, prospective trial of antioxidant supplementation in critically ill surgical patients. *Ann Surg.* 2002;236:814.
112. Karyoute SM, Badran IZ. Tetanus following a burn injury. *Burns Incl Therm Inj.* 1988;14:241.
113. Wahl WL, Brandt MM, Ahrns KS, et al. Venous thrombosis incidence in burn patients: preliminary results of a prospective study. *J Burn Care Rehab.* 2002;23:97.
114. Rue LW III, Cioffi WG Jr, Rush R, et al. Thromboembolic complications in thermally injured patients. *World J Surg.* 1992;16:1151.
115. Still JM, Jr., Belcher K, Law EJ, et al. A double-blinded prospective evaluation of recombinant human erythropoietin in acutely burned patients. *J Trauma* 1995;38:233.
116. Sharar SR, Carrougher GJ, Selzer K, et al. A comparison of oral transmucosal fentanyl citrate and oral oxycodone for pediatric outpatient wound care. *J Burn Care Rehab.* 2002;23:27.
117. Honari S, Patterson DR, Gibbons J, et al. Comparison of pain control medication in three age groups of elderly patients. *J Burn Care Rehab.* 1997;18:500.
118. **Martin-Herz SP, Patterson DR, Honari S, et al. Pediatric pain control practices of North American burn centers. *J Burn Care Rehab.* 2003;24:26.**

119. Ohrbach R, Patterson DR, Carrougher G, Gibran N. Hypnosis after an adverse response to opioids in an ICU burn patient. *Clin J Pain* 1998;14:167.
120. Groene D, Martus P, Heyer G. Doxepin affects acetylcholine induced cutaneous reactions in atopic eczema. *Exp Dermatol.* 2001;10:110.
121. Klein MB, Moore ML, Costa B, Engrav LH. Primer on the management of face burns at the University of Washington. *J Burn Care Rehab.* 2005;26:2.
122. Cole JK, Engrav LH, Heimbach DM, et al. Early excision and grafting of face and neck burns in patients over 20 years. *Plast Reconstr Surg.* 2002;109:1266.
123. Mills DC 2nd, Roberts LW, Mason AD Jr, et al. Suppurative chondritis: its incidence, prevention, and treatment in burn patients. *Plast Reconstr Surg.* 1988;82:267.
124. Matsumura H, Engrav LH, Nakamura DY, Vedder NB. The use of the Millard "crane" flap for deep hand burns with exposed tendons and joints. *J Burn Care Rehab.* 1999;20:316.
125. Caravati EM. Acute hydrofluoric acid exposure. *Am J Emerg Med.* 1988;6:143.
126. Chick LR, Borah G. Calcium carbonate gel therapy for hydrofluoric acid burns of the hand. *Plast Reconstr Surg.* 1990;86:935.
127. Vance MV, Curry SC, Kunkel DB, et al. Digital hydrofluoric acid burns: treatment with intraarterial calcium infusion. *Ann Emerg Med.* 1986;15:890.
128. Bird PE, Harrington DT, Barillo DJ, et al. Elder abuse: a call to action. *J Burn Care Rehab.* 1998;19:522.
129. Bowden ML, Grant ST, Vogel B, Prasad JK. The elderly, disabled and handicapped adult burned through abuse and neglect. *Burns Incl Therm Inj.* 1988;14:447.
130. Assin WD. Multiple cigarette burn wounds in a chronic paranoid schizophrenic. *S Afr Med J.* 1996;86:1437.
131. Barillo DJ, Hallock GG, Mastropieri CJ, et al. Utilization of the burn unit for nonburn patients: the "wound intensive care unit". *Ann Plast Surg.* 1989;23:426.
132. Barillo DJ, McManus AT, Cancio LC, et al. Burn center management of necrotizing fasciitis. *J Burn Care Rehab.* 2003;24:127.
133. Marvin JA, Heimbach DM, Engrav LH, Harnar TJ. Improved treatment of the Stevens-Johnson syndrome. *Arch Surg.* 1984;119:601.
134. Palmieri TL, Greenhalgh DG, Saffle JR, et al. A multicenter review of toxic epidermal necrolysis treated in U.S. burn centers at the end of the twentieth century. *J Burn Care Rehab.* 2002;23:87.
135. Viard I, Wehrli P, Bullani R, et al. Inhibition of toxic epidermal necrolysis by blockade of CD95 with human intravenous immunoglobulin. *Science* 1998;282:490.
136. Warner PM, Kagan RJ, Yakuboff KP, et al. Current management of purpura fulminans: a multicenter study. *J Burn Care Rehab.* 2003; 24:119.
137. Zhu KQ, Engrav LH, Gibran NS, et al. The female, red Duroc pig as an animal model of hypertrophic scarring and the potential role of the cones of skin. *Burns* 2003;29:649.

CHAPTER 12 ■ ANESTHESIOLOGY AND PAIN MANAGEMENT

TIMOTHY W. RUTTER AND KEVIN K. TREMPER

Anesthesia is a combination of amnesia, analgesia, and muscle relaxation. This state can be achieved by inhaling various vapors that produce each of these conditions in proportion to the concentration achieved in the central nervous system. Anesthesia can also be achieved by using one of three pharmacologic agents that are each targeted to produce a specific effect. These are the amnesics, analgesics, and neuromuscular blocking agents. As the concentration of inhalation anesthetics increases, cardiovascular and respiratory functions are progressively depressed. Because of the surgical procedure's requirements or the patient's preexisting cardiac disease, the concentration of inhalation agent that is required to produce sufficient muscle relaxation may be a relative overdose with respect to its effect on the cardiovascular system. For this reason, modern anesthetics usually require titration of these agents to optimize conditions for the surgery while maintaining cardiovascular stability.

The goals of modern anesthesia are (a) to achieve this state quickly and safely by choosing the appropriate techniques and agents considering the patient's medical condition; (b) to maintain this state throughout the surgical procedure while compensating for the effects of varying degrees of painful stimuli and blood and fluid loss; and (c) to reverse the muscle relaxation and amnesia, bringing the patient back to physiologic control while maintaining sufficient analgesia to minimize postoperative pain. This process is accomplished with a high degree of safety 30 to 40 million times a year in the United States, despite the serious potential complications of technical or judgment errors. The high degree of success of both surgical and anesthetic outcomes is due to the efforts of thousands of surgeons and anesthesiologists who have advanced the art and science of their field.[1] Although modern techniques and analgesics have made it possible to nearly eliminate perioperative pain, judgmental feelings about patients who complain of pain still remain. Pain not only is unpleasant, it also has significant adverse physiologic effects and physicians should encourage patients to alert health-care personnel when pain is felt.

ANESTHETIC AGENTS AND THEIR PHYSIOLOGIC EFFECTS

Inhalation Agents

Anesthetics are generalized depressants of consciousness, pain, cardiopulmonary function, motor function, and recall. The potent inhalation agents (e.g., isoflurane, sevoflurane, desflurane) produce these effects in a dose-dependent fashion with about 1% inhaled concentration. The measurement used to compare the potency of inhalation agents is the percentage minimum alveolar concentration (MAC) (measured in percent) that prevents movement on painful stimulation (incision) in half of the subjects. There is significant patient-to-patient variability even when patients possess a similar degree of health. Compounding this variability are the effects of age, weight, preexisting heart disease, liver disease, and medications other than the anesthetics. Table 12.1 lists the commonly used inhalation agents and their MACs and side effects. In general, all agents depress blood pressure by myocardial depression and vasodilation. There is a generalized depression of cerebral function and cerebral metabolic

TABLE 12.1

COMMON INHALATION AGENTS: MINIMUM ALVEOLAR CONCENTRATIONS AND EFFECTS

Agent	Minimum alveolar concentration (%)	Strengths	Weaknesses
Nitrous oxide	105	Analgesia Rapid uptake and elimination Little cardiac or respiratory depression	Sympathetic stimulation Expansion of closed air spaces Interference with vitamin B_{12} metabolism Limitation of FiO_2
Halothane	0.75	Low cost Effectiveness in low concentrations Little airway irritability Uterine relaxation	Less chemical stability Slow uptake and elimination Biodegradability Hepatic necrosis Cardiac depression and arrhythmias
Enflurane	1.68	Good muscle relaxation Stable cardiac rate and rhythm	Pungent odor Seizure activity on electroencephalography
Isoflurane	1.15	Good muscle relaxation Stable cardiac rate and rhythm Usability in neurosurgery	Pungent odor
Desflurane	6	Rapid induction and emergence	Pungent odor Causes coughing High vapor pressure (Boiling point 23.5°C) Requires special pressurized vaporizer High cost
Sevoflurane	1.71	Rapid induction and emergence Less pungent Good for mask induction	High cost Metabolized in liver produces increased plasma fluoride Canister fires with baralyme

FiO_2, fraction of inspired oxygen.
Adapted from Miller FL, Marshall BE. The inhaled anesthetics. In: Longnecker DE, Murphy FL, eds. *Introduction to anesthesia,* 8th ed. Philadelphia: WB Saunders; 1992:77.

rate of oxygen consumption, although cerebral blood flow may increase because of vascular dilatation and a loss of autoregulation. Renal blood flow and glomerular filtration rate are reduced by 20% to 50%. Blood flow to the skin increases and cutaneous autoregulation is reduced, impairing the body's ability to conserve heat. The combination of these effects, the cold environment of the operating room, and open body cavities make the patient extremely vulnerable to hypothermia.

Muscle Relaxants

To prevent movement and to facilitate the surgical exposure, neuromuscular blocking agents are generally used. These drugs are competitive or noncompetitive inhibitors of the neurotransmitter acetylcholine at the neuromuscular junction. The only noncompetitive inhibitor used clinically is succinylcholine. This drug rapidly binds to the neuromuscular junction and produces depolarization, clinically obvious as fine muscle fasciculations occurring about 60 seconds after injection. Succinylcholine cannot be reversed, but its effects are short acting because it is quickly hydrolyzed in the plasma by cholinesterase. Because of rapid onset, succinylcholine is frequently used to facilitate endotracheal intubation when it must be accomplished quickly.

All other clinically useful muscle relaxants are termed *competitive inhibitors* and do not cause depolarization when they attach at the neuromuscular junction. Because these agents compete with acetylcholine, the block produced is in direct proportion to the concentration of the agent relative to the concentration of acetylcholine. If the concentration ratio is low enough, competitive relaxants can be reversed if the concentration of acetylcholine is artificially elevated. Acetylcholine concentration can be increased by giving a drug that blocks its metabolism, an anticholinesterase (neostigmine). The neuromuscular blocking agent is still present, but motor function returns if the acetylcholine concentration is high enough to outcompete the blocking agent. There is a ceiling to which anticholinesterase drugs can elevate acetylcholine; therefore, high levels of nondepolarizing relaxants cannot be reversed. Reversing neuromuscular relaxants is not analogous to using naloxone to reverse the effects of opioids. The reversal agent neostigmine does not compete or combine with the relaxant.

Unfortunately, there are systemic consequences to increasing the plasma concentration of acetylcholine. Acetylcholine is the predominant neurotransmitter in the preganglionic sympathetic and parasympathetic nervous systems and in the postganglionic parasympathetic nervous system. For this reason, an anticholinergic drug (atropine or glycopyrrolate) must be given with the anticholinesterase to prevent the undesirable effects of a generalized acetylcholine overdose. The common neuromuscular blocking drugs and their doses, durations, and side effects are listed in Table 12.2; common regimens of reversal agents are shown in Table 12.3.

TABLE 12.2

COMMON NEUROMUSCULAR BLOCKING DRUGS AND REVERSAL AGENTS

Muscle relaxant	Intubating dose (mg/kg)	Infusion dose (mg/kg/min)	Strengths	Weaknesses
DEPOLARIZING				
Succinylcholine	1.0	100[a]	Fastest onset (30 to 60 s) Short duration[b] (5 min)	Associated with malignant hyperthermia, dysrhythmias, bradycardia, and hyperkalemia, especially in patients with burns or neurologic injury
NONDEPOLARIZING				
Long acting (>1 h)				
Pancuronium	0.1	0.3	No histamine release	Tachycardia Slow onset Long duration
Pipecuronium	0.08	—	Similar to pancuronium, no cardiovascular effects	—
Doxacurium	0.07	—	Similar to pancuronium, minimal cardiovascular effects	—
Intermediate acting (≈1 h)				
Atracurium	0.5	10	Spontaneous breakdown in plasma	Histamine release
Vecuronium	0.1	1	No cardiovascular effects	
Rocuronium	0.8	10	Fast onset, no cardiovascular effects	
Mivacurium	0.2	10	Fast onset, short duration	Histamine release

[a]This should not be used for longer than 1 hour.
[b]Duration is dramatically increased in patients with abnormal plasma pseudocholinesterase.

TABLE 12.3

DRUGS FOR ANTAGONIZING NONDEPOLARIZING NEUROMUSCULAR BLOCKADE[a]

Dose	Time to peak effect (min)	Dose	Use with	Comments
ANTICHOLINESTERASES				
Edrophonium	1–2	0.5–1.0 mg/kg	—	Very fast onset, not commonly used
Neostigmine	3–5	0.04–0.07 mg/kg	—	Most commonly used
Pyridostigmine	10–12	0.2–0.3 mg/kg	—	Not used clinically for neuromuscular reversal
ANTICHOLINERGICS				
Glycopyrrolate	—	0.008 mg/kg (0.5–0.6 mg/70 kg)	Neostigmine Pyridostigmine	Not commonly used in adults CNS effects because it crosses the blood–brain barrier
Atropine	—	0.007–0.02 mg/kg (0.05–1.5 mg/70 kg)	Edrophonium	

[a]For reliable results in reversing the effects of nondepolarizing muscle relaxants, administration of anticholinesterases is delayed until spontaneous recovery permits three of four responses to a train-of-four stimulus. For patients with more profound blockade, larger amounts of anticholinesterases may be required, but doses of neostigmine higher than 0.14 mg/kg are unlikely to produce additional improvement. CNS, central nervous system.
Adapted from Watling SM, Dasta JF. Prolonged paralysis in intensive care unit patients after the use of neuromuscular blocking agents: a review of the literature. *Crit Care Med.* 1994;22:884.

TABLE 12.4

ANALGESICS

	Potency	Sedation dose	Duration	Infusion dose
OPIOIDS				
Morphine	1	0.02–0.1 mg/kg IV	2–7 h	—
Meperidine	0.1	0.2–1 mg/kg IV	2–4 h	—
Fentanyl	100	0.5–1 mg/kg IV	30–60 min	—
Sufentanil	1,000	Not recommended		
Alfentanil	25	10–20 mg/kg IV	10–15 min	
Remifentanil[b]	—	Not recommended	10 min	0.1–0.2 mg/kg/min
OTHER ANALGESICS AND ANESTHETICS				
Propofol		0.1–0.5 mg/kg IV[ac]		25–50 mg/kg/min
Ketamine		0.1–0.5 mg/kg IV[a]		−80 mg/kg/min
		1.0–2.0 mg/kg IM		

IM, intramuscular; IV, intravenous.
[a]May produce apnea.
[b]Will produce apnea.
[c]Produces pain on injection that can be reduced by treatment with 20 mg of lidocaine IV.

Nondepolarizing relaxants are frequently used in critically ill patients who are difficult to manage otherwise, for example, head-injured patients who require hyperventilation or patients with adult respiratory distress syndrome who require complex modes of ventilation. It is imperative that these drugs be given in conjunction with analgesics and amnesic agents. Neuromuscular blocking agents have no analgesic or amnesic properties and only prevent motion of voluntary muscles. Patients can be totally aware and in pain but unable to communicate. When prolonged muscle relaxation is required, it is best to administer the relaxant by continuous infusion and then monitor the effect with a nerve stimulator. For these settings, relaxants should be administered only to achieve the degree of relaxation necessary and in a dose that allows reversal at any time. Table 12.2 includes the recommended ranges of infusion rates. In recent years, there have been reports of patients who have prolonged residual motor weakness after the muscle relaxant is cleared.[2] These problems have been primarily noted with the drug pancuronium bromide (Pavulon), especially when the patients are also being treated with steroids. It is therefore recommended that pancuronium bromide not be used for longer than 2 days.

All muscles in the body are not equally sensitive to muscle relaxants. The diaphragm is most resistant to neuromuscular blockade, whereas the neck and pharyngeal muscles that support the airway are most sensitive. It is possible for an intubated patient to spontaneously ventilate and even to produce a large negative inspiratory effort and yet develop complete airway obstruction when extubated because of the effects of residual muscle relaxant on the upper airway muscles. The definitive clinical test for complete reversal of neuromuscular blockage is the patient's ability to sustain a head lift from the bed for 5 seconds.

Opioids (Narcotics) and Other Intravenous Analgesics

Narcotics and synthetic analogues belong to the class of drugs called *opioids*. The most commonly used drugs in this family are morphine, meperidine, and codeine. Since the mid-1980s, a series of synthetic opioids have been developed with fentanyl as the prototype. More recently developed synthetics (sufentanil, alfentanil, and remifentanil) are more potent and of shorter duration (Table 12.4). Opioids produce profound analgesia and respiratory depression. They have no amnesic properties, no direct myocardial depressive effects, and no muscle-relaxant properties. Opioids can produce significant hemodynamic effects indirectly by releasing histamine or blunting the patient's sympathetic vascular tone because of analgesic properties. The latter effect depends on the degree of sympathetic tone that is present. Acutely injured patients may be hypovolemic and in pain, with high sympathetic tone and peripheral vascular resistance. Patients in this condition can experience dramatic drops in systemic blood pressure with minimal doses of opioids. For this reason, it is important to titrate narcotics in small incremental doses. Because of the lack of direct myocardial depression and the absence of histamine release with the synthetic opioids, they are frequently used as the primary anesthetic in combination with an amnesic agent and a muscle relaxant in patients with significant myocardial dysfunction.

When opioids are titrated intravenously, patients first become apneic because of the respiratory depressive effect (shifting the CO_2 response curve), but they still breathe on command. As the dose increases, patients become apneic and unresponsive. An unusual side effect of high-dose intravenous (IV) opioids is chest-wall muscle rigidity, which can make it extremely difficult to ventilate a patient without the assistance of a muscle relaxant.

Opioids are primarily analgesic and not amnesic. Patients can be totally aware and have substantial recall of conversations despite appearing completely anesthetized. All opioids can be reversed with naloxone. The duration of action of naloxone can be shorter than that of the opioid, and patients must be observed carefully after they have been treated with naloxone. Naloxone reversal of opioids can be dangerous because the agent acutely reverses not only the analgesic effects of the opioid but also the analgesic effects of native endorphins. Naloxone treatment has been associated with acute pulmonary edema and myocardial ischemia and should not be used electively to reverse the effects of a narcotic. It is appropriately used in an emergency situation when the airway is not controlled and the patient is not ventilating because of an opioid overdose.

Propofol

Propofol is a lipid-soluble substituted isopropyl phenol that produces a rapid induction of anesthesia in 30 seconds followed by awakening in 4 to 8 minutes. IV propofol can effectively produce total anesthesia (for less stimulating procedures), including amnesia, analgesia, and some degree of muscle relaxation. This agent is unique because it is rapidly cleared through hepatic metabolism to inactive metabolites in a way that the patient becomes alert very quickly after cessation of infusion. Propofol causes a lower incidence of nausea and vomiting when compared to opioid or inhalation anesthetics. It has important roles in intensive care units when used as a continuous infusion sedative at dosages of 25 to 50 μg/kg/minute. When the infusion is discontinued, the patient becomes alert within minutes. Propofol can produce significant hypotension when IV induction doses are administered. It also produces significant pain on injection. Pain can be diminished or eliminated by pretreatment with IV lidocaine, 0.5 mg/kg. Propofol is insoluble in aqueous solution and therefore comes dissolved in a lipid emulsion that has the associated risk of bacterial contamination. Once a vial of propofol is opened, it is not recommended that it be used after 6 hours.

Ketamine

Ketamine is a phencyclidine derivative that produces anesthesia characterized by dissociation between the thalamus and limbic systems. Induction of anesthesia is achieved within 60 seconds after IV injection of 1 to 2 mg/kg or within 2 to 4 minutes of intramuscular (IM) injection of 5 to 10 mg/kg. Patients appear to be in a cataleptic state in which their eyes remain open with a slow nystagmic gaze. The drug produces intense amnesia and analgesia but has been associated with unpleasant visual and auditory hallucinations that can progress to delirium. The incidence of these problems can be significantly reduced if benzodiazepines are also administered with the drug. At low doses (0.1 to 0.2 mg/kg IV or 2 mg/kg IM), patients continue to spontaneously ventilate but cannot be expected to protect the airway should vomiting occur. At higher doses, ketamine acts as a respiratory depressant and produces complete apnea. Ketamine also has direct and indirect sympathetic nervous system stimulatory effects, which can be useful in hypovolemic patients. These effects are diminished or absent in patients who are catecholamine depleted. The sympathetic stimulatory effect increases myocardial oxygen consumption and intracranial pressure, and ketamine is relatively contraindicated in patients with ischemic heart disease or space-occupying intracerebral lesions. Ketamine is frequently used as an IV analgesic during débridement procedures, at doses listed in Table 12.4. IM ketamine (1.0 to 2.0 mg/kg) is also very useful for sedating patients who are difficult to manage (e.g., combative adult or mentally retarded patient) so IV access can be obtained.

Amnesics and Anxiolytics

Benzodiazepines are the primary class of agents used as amnesics and anxiolytics. The prototype drug, diazepam, has been more recently replaced by its water-soluble analogue of shorter duration, midazolam. Lorazepam also belongs in this family of agents, but because it has a very long duration of action, it is not routinely used intraoperatively. Lorazepam has intensive care unit applications (Table 12.5). Benzodiazepines produce anxiolysis and some degree of amnesia but have no analgesic properties. Intraoperatively, midazolam is always used in conjunction with an opioid or inhalation agent. Midazolam can be used in combination with the short-acting opioid, fentanyl, to produce conscious sedation for minor procedures. Benzodiazepines can produce apnea and have synergistic effects with narcotics. Very small doses of midazolam and fentanyl can quickly produce an unconscious apneic patient. As with all anesthetics, benzodiazepines used as IV agents for

TABLE 12.5

ANXIOLYTICS AND AMNESICS (BENZODIAZEPINES)

Name	Dose (mg/kg)	Duration (h)	Strengths	Weaknesses
Midazolam (Versed)	0.05 (infusion dose 0.25 mg/kg/min)	0.5	Water soluble Short duration Good for sedation for short procedures	Acute respiratory depression
Diazepam (Valium)	0.1	1	Intermediate duration	Irritation on IV injection Phlebitis Acute respiratory depression after IV overdose
Lorazepam (Ativan)	0.02–0.08	6–8	Long duration	—
BENZODIAZEPINE REVERSAL				
Flumazenil (Romazicon)	4–20 mg/kg (0.2 mg repeated every 2 to 10 min until reversal is achieved) Maximum dose 1 mg	45–90 min	—	May produce seizures, panic, arrhythmias

IV, intravenous.

sedation should be given in small incremental doses to achieve the desired effect. A reversal agent is also available for benzodiazepines (flumazenil). The recommended dosages of these drugs and the reversal agents appear in Table 12.5.

Local Anesthetics

Local anesthetics constitute a class of drugs that temporarily block nerve conduction by binding to neuronal sodium channels. As the concentration of the local anesthetic increases around the nerve, autonomic transmission will be blocked first, followed by sensory transmission, and then motor nerve transmission. These drugs can be injected locally into tissue to produce a field block around peripheral nerves to produce a specific dermatome block, around nerve plexuses to produce a major conductive block, or into the spinal or epidural space to produce extensive neuroaxial blockade. All the methods have been used to assist in the provision of an alternative form of balanced anesthesia by supplementing analgesia and muscle relaxation.

Adverse consequences associated with the use of local anesthetics fall into three categories: acute central nervous system toxicity due to excessive plasma concentration, hemodynamic and respiratory consequences due to excessive conduction block of the sympathetic or motor nerves, and allergic reactions. Whenever a local anesthetic is injected, there can be inadvertent intravascular injection or an overdose of the drug because of rapid uptake from the tissues. All can produce seizures. Complications can be minimized by withdrawing before injection to avoid an intravascular injection and limiting dosages to the safe range (Table 12.6).

When local anesthetics are administered for a spinal or epidural block, they produce a progressive blockade of the sympathetic nervous system, which produces systemic vasodilation. Sympathetic nerves travel along the thoracolumbar region with the first four thoracic branches, including the cardiac sympathetic accelerators. A sympathetic blockade of this entire region produces profound systemic vasodilatation and bradycardia. This condition is referred to as *total sympathectomy,* and the hypotension that ensues is usually below the minimal cerebral perfusion pressure required to maintain consciousness. Affected patients are bradycardic, hypotensive, unconscious, and usually apneic. This disastrous situation is easily remedied if treated quickly with a vasopressor (phenylephrine or ephedrine) and atropine. If not treated promptly, the situation proceeds to cardiac arrest. In this emergency situation, the treatment of high doses of epinephrine are 10 to 40 μ/kg, or 1 to 4 mg for an adult. The doses of epinephrine are higher than a usual cardiac arrest because of the total sympathectomy.[3] Because the level of sympathetic block is two to six dermatomal levels higher than the sensory block, it is often difficult to obtain a high spinal sensory level without approaching a total sympathectomy.

Local anesthetics are chemically divided into two groups, esters and amides. The esters (2-chloroprocaine and tetracaine) produce metabolites that are related to *p*-aminobenzoic acid and have been associated with allergic reactions. Amides (lidocaine and bupivacaine) are rarely associated with allergic reactions. If an allergic reaction does occur, it is most likely due to the preservative (methyl paraben) used in multidose vials of lidocaine.

SEDATION ANALGESIA FOR MINOR SURGICAL PROCEDURES

There are a variety of minor surgical procedures which can be accomplished safely and comfortably with anesthesia provided by infiltration of local anesthetics (most commonly 1% lidocaine) and mild sedation/anxiolysis provided by IV benzodiazepines. All IV benzodiazepines, narcotics, and other IV anesthetics produce apnea if given in a high enough dose. Because there is a substantial patient-to-patient variability in response to a given dose, it is important that IV anxiolytics be given in small incremental doses slowly to achieve a safe sedated state. Another important factor to remember is that the anesthesia is provided by infiltration of the local anesthetic and not by the IV sedative. IV agents including narcotics cannot overcome the pain associated with a surgical incision. If large doses of narcotics are given for this purpose, once the

TABLE 12.6

LOCAL ANESTHETICS

	Maximum single dose (mg)	Duration (h)	Comments
AMIDES			
Lidocaine	500	1[a]	Fast onset
Ropivacaine	200	4–12[a]	Less cardiac toxicity than bupivacaine
Bupivacaine	200	4–12[a]	Exaggerated cardiotoxicity with IV injection Slow onset Long duration
ESTERS[b]			
2-Chloroprocaine	1,000	0.5–1[a]	Fast onset Lowest toxicity
Tetracaine	80	0.5–1	Slow onset

IV, intravenous.
[a]Addition of 100 μg of epinephrine (0.1 mL of 1:1,000) lowers the toxicity and increases the duration of the local anesthetic.
[b]Metabolism to paraaminobenzoic acid may cause allergic reactions.

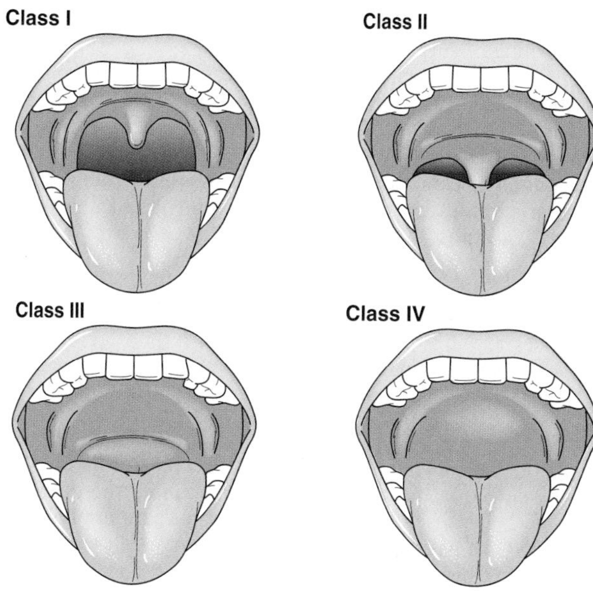

FIGURE 12.1 Classification of the patient's upper airway based on the size of the tongue and the pharyngeal structures visible on mouth opening. Class I, soft palate and anterior/posterior tonsillar pillars, and uvula visible; Class II, tonsillar pillars and part of uvula hidden by base of tongue; Class III, soft and hard palate visible; Class IV, soft palate not visible, only hard palate visibile. (After Stoetling RK, Miller RD. *Basics of anesthesia,* 3rd ed. New York: Churchill Livingston; 1994;146.)

surgical stimulus ends the patient may quickly become apneic. The duration of the respiratory depression for even short-acting narcotics is much longer than the painful stimulus of the incision. Because of the potentially serious consequences of an apneic episode, the Joint Commission for Accreditation of Health Care Organizations (JCAHO) has required that all patients undergoing sedation for minor surgical or medical procedures have the following:[4]

1. A preprocedure evaluation including an airway examination (Fig. 12.1)
2. Appropriate monitoring: pulse oximetry as a minimum
3. Documentation of the patient's vital signs and arterial saturation as well as the dose and timing of sedatives provided during the procedure
4. Documentation of a recovery period and a return to a safe recovered state

The preprocedure evaluation should include current medications, coexisting disease, and a brief physical examination including an evaluation of the airway. It is important to determine how difficult it may be to obtain control of the airway if a patient should become apneic. Although there is no absolute standard to predict a difficult intubation, a simple four-step examination helps to determine the likelihood. First, the patient should have a normal mouth opening, ≥3 cm. Second, the patient should have normal neck flexion and extension. Third, the physician should be able to fit three finger widths under the patient's chin between the thyroid cartilage and the mentum. Finally, when the patient opens the mouth and is asked to stick out the tongue, the airway can be classified depending on whether the uvulae can be completely seen (class 1), only partly seen (class 2), or not seen, with only the hard and soft palate visible (class 3), or only hard palate visible (class 4; see Fig. 12.1). This classification roughly predicts progressive difficulty in intubating due to difficulty in visualizing the larynx.[5]

TABLE 12.7

SEDATION SCALE

Sedation scale	Description
1	Awake and alert
2	Awake and sedated
3	Asleep but arousable to touch or verbal stimuli
4	Asleep but arousable to painful stimulus
5	Asleep and not arousable to painful stimulus

The most common drug used to provide sedation is midazolam. This is a fast onset, relatively short-acting benzodiazepine that can be easily titrated to produce a sedated yet cooperative arousable state. It is usually given to adults in incremental doses of 1 mg (0.01 mg/kg in children). Narcotics such as fentanyl even in small doses act synergistically with benzodiazepines to cause a more sedated state with a much higher incidence of apnea. To assess the effect of the drug, a sedation scale can be of value. The scale used at the University of Michigan is presented in Table 12.7.[6]

RISKS ASSOCIATED WITH ANESTHESIA

Because the anesthetic agents effectively obtund or completely block nearly all physiologic protective mechanisms, there is an associated risk even without a surgical procedure. Fortunately, with the advent of newer agents and monitoring techniques, it is estimated that the mortality rate due to anesthesia alone has decreased from about 1 in 10,000 patients in the 1950s to as low as 1 in 100,000 or less for healthy patients today.[7] Although a 1 in 100,000 risk of death or serious neurologic impairment may appear small, when dire consequences occur in a young patient undergoing a purely elective procedure, the consequences are devastating for everyone involved. When patients are placed in a condition in which they cannot breathe, there is always the possibility of a technical or judgmental error resulting in hypoxia and brain damage or death. It has been estimated that between 50% and 75% of anesthetic-related deaths are due to human error and are preventable. Because the consequences of an anesthetic mishap are usually severe, the emotional and financial costs are high.

The most common problems associated with adverse outcomes are related to the airway and include inadequate ventilation, unrecognized esophageal intubation, unrecognized extubation, and unrecognized disconnection from the ventilator. The incidence of these problems has been significantly reduced by including capnometry and pulse oximetry in addition to other noninvasive monitors, although a cause-and-effect relation has been difficult to prove. Efforts to improve outcome can be approached at three levels: (a) reduction of the incidence of rare but catastrophic anesthetic-related problems, (b) improvement of the care and experience of every patient undergoing anesthesia and surgery, and (c) improvement of the preparation and management of patients with preexisting medical conditions who have higher morbidity and mortality rates. The first goal has been addressed in part with improved monitoring techniques and anesthesia training. Others have been advanced by the addition of comprehensive pain management, as discussed later in this chapter. Issues of preexisting medical disease and how they affect the anesthetic plan are also briefly discussed later in this chapter.

Cardiovascular Diseases

Hypertension

Hypertension is the most common preexisting medical disease in patients presenting for surgery and is a major risk factor for renal, cerebrovascular, peripheral vascular, and coronary artery diseases, as well as congestive heart failure (CHF). It is particularly associated with lipid disorders, diabetes, and obesity. It is these associated comorbidities that are most likely to lead to morbidity and mortality in the perioperative period and therefore the presence of hypertension should prompt the surgeon to review the history and physical examination for them. Hypertensive patients should be treated medically to render them normotensive before elective surgery. Major outcome studies strongly suggest that hypertensive patients with coronary artery disease benefit from the introduction of perioperative selective β-1 blockers, so reducing the incidence of significant myocardial ischemia during the perioperative period.[8] In general, antihypertension medications should be continued throughout the perioperative period. Recently this strategy has been questioned for patients treated with angiotensin II (AIIAs) receptor blockers (e.g., valsartan, candesartan, losartan).[9] Patients treated with these medications have experienced substantial intraoperative hypotension, which is unresponsive to standard vasopressors. This AIIA-associated hypotension has been treated successfully with terlipressin.[10–12] Some now recommend withholding AIIAs the morning of surgery.[9]

The incidence of hypotension and myocardial ischemia intraoperatively is higher in untreated hypertensive patients than in adequately treated hypertensive patients if the preoperative diastolic pressure is 110 mmHg or higher.[13] Inadequately treated hypertensive patients undergoing carotid endarterectomies have an increased incidence of neurologic deficits, and those with a history of prior myocardial infarctions have an increased incidence of reinfarction. Patients commonly have an elevated blood pressure on admission to the hospital. Hypertensive patients can have exaggerated responses to painful stimuli and have a higher incidence of perioperative ischemia.

Coronary Artery Disease

Much of the anesthetic preoperative evaluation is directed toward detecting the presence and determining the degree of ischemic heart disease. Coronary artery disease is present in about 25% of patients who undergo surgery each year.[13] It is the leading cause of death in the United States and continues to be a major cause of postoperative morbidity and mortality. The goal of the preoperative cardiac evaluation is to identify patients who are at increased risk of perioperative cardiac morbidity. Although perioperative cardiac events are the leading cause of death following anesthesia and surgery, it has been difficult to define patient characteristics that accurately predict a high risk of adverse outcome.[14] Preoperative CHF is clearly a significant risk factor, as is recent myocardial infarction or unstable angina (Table 12.8). Diabetes mellitus,

TABLE 12.8

CLINICAL PREDICTORS OF INCREASED PERIOPERATIVE CARDIOVASCULAR RISK (MYOCARDIAL INFARCTION, HEART FAILURE, DEATH)

Major
Unstable coronary syndromes
■ Acute or recent MI[a] with evidence of important ischemic risk by clinical symptoms or noninvasive study
■ Unstable or severe[b] angina (Canadian class III or IV)[c]
Decompensated heart failure
Significant arrhythmias
■ High-grade atrioventricular block
■ Symptomatic ventricular arrhythmias in the presence of underlying heart disease
■ Supraventricular arrhythmias with uncontrolled ventricular rate
Severe valvular disease
Intermediate
Mild angina pectoris (Canadian class I or II)
Previous MI by history or pathologic Q waves
Compensated or prior heart failure
Diabetes mellitus (particularly insulin-dependent)
Renal insufficiency
Minor
Advanced age
Abnormal ECG (left ventricular hypertrophy, left bundle-branch block, ST-T abnormalities)
Rhythm other than sinus (e.g., atrial fibrillation)
Low functional capacity (e.g., inability to climb one flight of stairs with a bag of groceries)
History of stroke
Uncontrolled systemic hypertension

ECG, electrocardiogram; MI, myocardial infarction.
[a]The American College of Cardiology National Database Library defines recent MI as greater than 7 days but less than or equal to 1 month (30 days); acute MI is within 7 days.
[b]May include "stable" angina in patients who are unusually sedentary.
[c]Campeau L. Grading of angina pectoris. *Circulation* 1976;54:522.

TABLE 12.9

CARDIAC RISK[a] STRATIFICATION FOR NONCARDIAC SURGICAL PROCEDURES

High (reported cardiac risk often greater than 5%)
- Emergent major operations, particularly in the elderly
- Aortic and other major vascular surgery
- Peripheral vascular surgery
- Anticipated prolonged surgical procedures associated with large fluid shifts and/or blood loss

Intermediate (reported cardiac risk generally less than 5%)
- Carotid endarterectomy
- Head and neck surgery
- Intraperitoneal and intrathoracic surgery
- Orthopedic surgery
- Prostate surgery

Low[b] (reported cardiac risk generally less than 1%)
- Endoscopic procedures
- Superficial procedures
- Cataract surgery
- Breast surgery

[a]Combined incidence of cardiac death and nonfatal myocardial infarction.
[b]Do not generally require further preoperative cardiac testing.

atherosclerotic vascular disease, and hypertension also appear to confer risk, although less than with CHF or unstable angina. Perioperative risk in patients with valvular heart disease varies with the severity of the disease as represented by CHF, pulmonary hypertension, and dysrhythmias. Dysrhythmias are also a concern in the presence of coronary artery disease. Age and stable angina remain controversial as predictors of perioperative risk, with equal numbers of supporting and refuting studies. Previous coronary artery bypass grafting appears to confer protection against perioperative cardiac events. Because of the incidence of silent ischemia, especially in patients with diabetes melitis, patients in high-risk groups (i.e., men older than age 40, women older than age 50) should be evaluated with preoperative electrocardiography (ECG). In patients without significant pulmonary disease, the ability to climb two flights of stairs without stopping or experiencing symptoms of angina or shortness of breath is considered a good practical test of cardiac reserve. Unfortunately, many patients with ischemic heart disease have concomitant pulmonary disease or other medical problems that limit their activity. The resting 12-lead ECG remains the most cost-effective screening test for ischemic heart disease. ECG may be normal in patients with extensive ischemic heart disease and does not detect the presence of prior subendocardial myocardial infarction. For patients in high-risk groups, further stress evaluations may be required.

A history of myocardial infarction is important information. Large retrospective studies have found that the incidence of reinfarction is related to the time elapsed since the previous myocardial infarction.[15–17] The incidence of reinfarction appears to stabilize at about 6% after 6 months. The highest rate of reinfarction occurs in the 0- to 3-month period. Mortality from reinfarction, for patients undergoing noncardiac surgery (Table 12.9), has been reported to be between 20% and 50% and usually occurs within the first 48 hours after surgery. Invasive hemodynamic monitoring with a pulmonary artery catheter and aggressive pharmacologic intervention has been shown to reduce reinfarction rates (Table 12.10). The incidence of reinfarction is also increased in patients undergoing intrathoracic or intraabdominal procedures lasting longer than 3 hours.[14] The site of surgery and anesthetic technique have not been shown to change the incidence of reinfarction if the procedure is shorter than 3 hours.[13] Patients with known three-vessel or left main coronary artery disease

TABLE 12.10

RISK OF MYOCARDIAL REINFARCTION AFTER SURGERY WITH AGGRESSIVE HEMODYNAMIC MONITORING AND INTERVENTIONS AND POSTOPERATIVE ICU ADMISSION

Age of previous infarction (mo)	Reinfarction rate (%)
7–12	1.0
3–6	2.3
0–3	5.8

ICU, intensive care unit.
From Rao TKL, Jacobs KH, El Etr AA. Reinfarction following anesthesia in patients with myocardial infarction. *Anesthesiology* 1983;59:499, with permission.

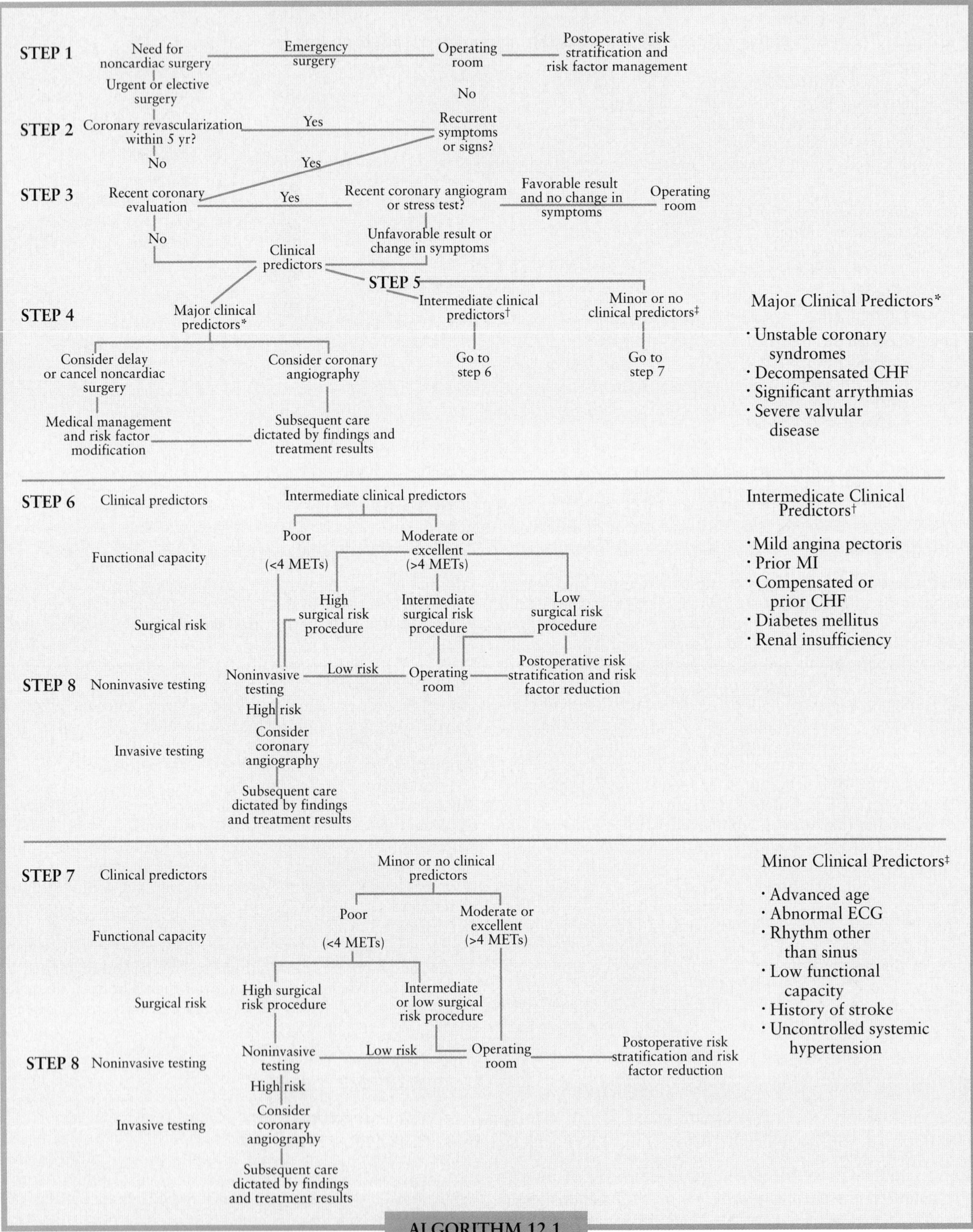

ALGORITHM 12.1 Decision aid for assessing coronary risk for noncardiac surgery. This decision tree for preoperative evaluation takes into account not only the patient's physical status but also the severity of the surgical procedure.

are at increased risk, whereas those who have undergone prior coronary artery bypass grafting are at a substantially decreased risk of reinfarction. Although prophylactic therapy with β blockers, calcium-channel agents, and nitrates have not been proved beneficial, withdrawal of these agents has been associated with perioperative ischemia, myocardial infarction, and death.[14]

All patients in high-risk groups or with a history of ischemic heart disease must be evaluated and properly treated before elective surgery. All elective surgery should be delayed for 6 months after myocardial infarction. If this is not feasible, invasive monitoring should be considered in the perioperative period and intensive postoperative observation should continue for at least 48 hours.

The intrusiveness of the surgical procedure also plays a part in the overall risk and need for preoperative workup of heart disease.[5] The American Heart Association has produced an algorithm for the recommended preoperative workup[18] (Algorithm 12.1).

Congestive Heart Failure

CHF has been described as the single most important factor predicting postoperative cardiac morbidity[19] (Table 12.11). All elective surgical procedures should be deferred until congestive failure is treated. If surgery cannot be deferred, aggressive perioperative management is warranted with a goal of optimizing cardiac output. In contrast to isolated ischemic heart disease, CHF is more easily diagnosed by history, physical examination, and basic preoperative laboratory workup, including ECG and chest radiography. Because patients with left, right, or both left and right ventricular dysfunction are less tolerant of the fluid shifts associated with surgery and the myocardial depression associated with the anesthetic, they constitute the highest-risk group for postoperative cardiac complications.

Pulmonary Disease

Pulmonary disease is divided into acute and chronic restrictive and obstructive disease. Restrictive disease is defined by processes that reduce lung volumes, and obstructive disease is characterized by reduced flow rates on pulmonary function tests. Restrictive diseases are further subdivided into intrinsic and extrinsic forms. Intrinsic disease includes adult respiratory distress syndrome, and extrinsic disease is usually due to external restriction of lung volume by chest wall deformities or the patient's excessive weight. Although restrictive diseases can produce significant pulmonary dysfunction, less anesthetic preparation is necessary for these patients. A more sophisticated ventilator may be needed in the perioperative period.

Obstructive diseases are present in patients with forced expiratory volume in 1 second (FEV_1)/forced vital capacity (FVC) ratios of less than 50%. Obstructive pulmonary disease can be either chronic or acute (asthma). In either case, the reversible component of obstruction should be reversed before elective surgery. Patients are maintained on bronchodilator medications, and those with chronic secretions are appropriately hydrated and receive therapy to mobilize secretions. In patients with reactive airway disease, the endotracheal tube can induce severe bronchospasm. Even in patients who are well-treated preoperatively, reactive bronchospasm can complicate anesthetic induction and the emergence from anesthesia. The principal method used to prevent or diminish this "foreign body" induced bronchospasm is intubation of the patient at a deep level of anesthesia when reflexes are blunted. The classic way to manage a patient with severe asthma is to induce with an agent that produces bronchodilation and to ventilate the patient with an inhalation agent until the patient is deeply anesthetized before performing laryngoscopy and intubation. The patient should be extubated while spontaneously ventilating but with the inhalation agent still in effect.

TABLE 12.11

CLINICAL FACTORS INDEPENDENTLY RELATED TO PERIOPERATIVE CARDIAC COMPLICATIONS

Criteria	Points
S_3 gallop or jugular venous distention on preoperative physical examination	11
Transmural or subendocardial myocardial infarction in the previous 6 mo	10
Premature ventricular beats, more than 5 beats/min documented at any time	7
Rhythm other than sinus or presence of premature atrial contractions on last preoperative ECG	5
Age over 70 y	4
Emergency operations	3
Intrathoracic, intraperitoneal, or aortic site of surgery	3
Evidence for important valvular aortic stenosis	3
Poor general medical condition[a]	3

Total points	Risks of cardiac complication (%)	Risk of death (%)
0–5	0.7	0.2
6–12	5	2
13–25	11	2
≥26	22	5

ECG, electrocardiogram.
[a]As evidenced by electrolyte abnormalities, renal insufficiency, abnormal blood gases, abnormal liver status, or any condition that has caused the patient to become chronically bedridden.
From Goldman L, Caldera DC, Nussbaum SR, et al. Multifactoral index of cardiac risk in noncardiac surgical procedures. *N Engl J Med.* 1977;297:845, with permission.

The patient is brought back to consciousness while ventilating by mask. Unfortunately, this technique may not be feasible in patients who have a full stomach because of the risk of aspiration or who are difficult to intubate or ventilate.

For elective surgery, patients should not be wheezing, and patients with chronic pulmonary disease should have no signs of bacterial infection, such as purulent sputum. Chest physiotherapy combined with hydration helps to remove secretions from the airways. The preoperative use of intermittent positive pressure breathing has not been shown to decrease the incidence of postoperative pulmonary complications.

Regional anesthetics can be useful in these patients for peripheral surgery or for procedures that require an anesthetic sensory level below T6. As the sensory and motor levels rise to T6 and above, patients lose significant accessory motor function that can decrease expiratory reserve volume and the ability to cough and clear secretions. Because of tenuous pulmonary status and the high incidence of postoperative pulmonary complications, pulmonary patients should be extubated with caution only when they meet adequate extubation criteria relative to preoperative test data. Changes in pulmonary mechanics and frequency of postoperative pulmonary complications are greatest after upper abdominal surgery. Both vital capacity and functional residual capacity are reduced, reaching lowest levels in the first 24 hours postoperatively. In the high-risk groups, therapy should be directed toward restoring functional residual capacity to preoperative levels. Such therapy improves compliance and gas exchange. Because of the potential adverse effects of systemic narcotics on respiratory drive, the use of epidural narcotics and local anesthetics for postoperative pain control is very popular. These techniques allow the patients to be extubated earlier and, in patients with intrathoracic and upper abdominal surgery, help restore pulmonary function toward preoperative values.[20]

Obesity

Obesity causes a host of problems on both sides of the surgical drapes. Obesity is defined as being 20% over ideal body weight. Ideal body weight can be easily estimated as height (cm) − 100 = ideal body weight (kg). The pathophysiologic changes associated with morbid obesity (twice the ideal body weight) affect the respiratory, cardiovascular, and gastrointestinal systems. Patients have an external restrictive disease that reduces functional residual capacity and worsens with the supine position. Breathing effort increases and ventilation becomes diaphragmatic and position dependent. Obese patients frequently desaturate at night and have a high incidence of sleep apnea. Because of increased blood volume and frequent desaturations, obese patients can develop pulmonary hypertension and right-sided heart failure. Obese individuals have a high incidence of coronary artery disease. Because of size alone, they have increased cardiovascular demands with limited cardiac reserve and exercise tolerance. Obese patients have a high incidence of hiatal hernia and gastroesophageal reflux, increasing the risk for aspiration on induction and emergence from anesthesia. Because of fatty liver infiltration and fat deposits elsewhere, these patients may experience prolonged effects of anesthetics and other analgesics. Issues as mundane as venous access can cause significant problems in this patient group.

The primary concern of the anesthesiologist is gaining adequate control of the airway. The combined problems of aspiration risk, rapid desaturation caused by reduced functional residual capacity and increased oxygen demand, as well as technical difficulties associated with intubation due to anatomic fat deposits, make intubation a high-risk procedure. If problems occur, there can be significant technical difficulties in obtaining a rapid cricothyrotomy. For these reasons, a nasal or oral awake intubation can be useful. All patients should receive prophylactic administration of H_2-receptor antagonists and metachlopromide to decrease the volume of gastric contents. If intubations are to be done after induction of anesthesia, they should be performed in a rapid sequence using cycroid pressure. To prevent aspiration on emergence, obese patients should be extubated when fully awake, preferably in the sitting position. Regional anesthetics can be very useful when peripheral procedures are planned. Unfortunately, morbidly obese patients can develop pulmonary failure just by lying flat, making it difficult to use epidural or spinal anesthetics for abdominal procedures. Epidural analgesics for postoperative pain management allow earlier extubation and ambulation of these patients.[20]

Overall, hospital mortality rate increases when several chronic diseases are present. Investigators have found that renal failure and CHF are associated with the highest increases in hospital mortality rates, especially in the elderly undergoing emergency procedures[21] (Table 12.12).

TABLE 12.12 RESULTS

HOSPITAL MORTALITY RATES IN RELATION TO AGE, PREOPERATIVE DISEASE, AND SURGERY

	Age (y)		
Preoperative disease and surgery	<50[a]	50–69[a]	>70[a]
Chronic heart failure	0.1%/0.5%	0.4%/2%	0.8%/4%
Renal failure	0.2%/1%	0.9%/2%	2%/9%
Abdominal surgery	0.3%/2%	1%/6%	3%/12%
Chronic heart failure and renal failure	0.7%/3%	3%/13%	6%/24%
Chronic heart failure and abdominal surgery	0.9%/4%	4%/17%	7%/30%
Renal failure and abdominal surgery	2%/8%	2%/32%	16%/50%
Chronic heart failure, renal failure, and abdominal surgery	6%/26%	22%/60%	37%/76%

[a]Figures are for elective surgery (first number) and emergency surgery (second number).
From Pedersen T, Eliasen K, Henriksen E. A prospective study of mortality associated with anesthesia and surgery: risk indicators of mortality in hospitals. *Acta Anaesthesiol Scand.* 1990;34:176, with permission.

Diabetes Mellitus

The incidence of diabetes mellitus (DM) is rising, particularly type 2 DM in the elderly. This is a systemic disorder that has particular relevance for the anesthesiologist because of its effect on the vascular, renal, and nervous systems. Patients with DM should be investigated for the presence of coronary artery disease, peripheral vascular occlusive disease, renal failure, and autonomic and peripheral neuropathy. Problems with cardiovascular instability, fluid balance, and aspiration due to gastroparesis should be expected. In addition, these patients are more prone to infection and have problems with temperature control. The management of the diabetic state in these patients is important and complicated. Hypoglycemia during the anesthetic state is a feared complication. Long-acting antidiabetic agents (e.g., chlorpropamide) should be stopped several days prior to surgery and substituted with shorter-acting agents. Newer oral antidiabetics, such as troglitazone, do not have the same propensity to cause hypoglycemia in the fasting patient. Brittle diabetics, those prone to ketoacidosis or hypoglycemia, should probably be admitted the night before surgery or at least scheduled as the first case of the day. Insulin-dependent diabetics for same day admission or outpatient surgery should take one half of their usual morning dose of long-acting insulin. After the establishment of an IV line, laboratory blood samples are drawn and infusion of dextrose is started. Additional insulin is then given according to the results of the blood sugar monitoring. Alternatively, simultaneous IV infusion of glucose and insulin may be used to keep the blood sugar in the range of 120 to 180 mg/dL. Again, these patients, whenever possible, should be done as the first case of the day to interfere as little as possible with the diabetic regimen.

RISKS ASSOCIATED WITH REGIONAL TECHNIQUES IN PATIENTS BEING TREATED WITH LOW-MOLECULAR-WEIGHT HEPARIN

Low-molecular-weight heparin (LMWH) has become a routine method of prophylactically treating patients who are at risk for deep venous thrombosis (Chapter 5). It has several advantages over traditional heparin and has therefore been adopted in Europe and the United States over the past few years. Unfortunately, there has been an increased number of reported cases of epidural hematoma formation when regional anesthetics are provided in patients who are being treated with LMWH.[22] For that reason, the Society of Regional Anesthesia has published the following guidelines for central conduction block (spinal and epidural anesthesia) to try to minimize the incidence of this devastating complication:

1. The presence of blood during needle and catheter placement will require a delay of 24 hours, postoperatively, before initiation of LMWH therapy.
2. For patients on LMWH (once a day dosing) needle placement should occur at least 12 hours after last LMWH dose. For patients receiving higher dosing (e.g., enoxaparin 1 mg/kg twice a day) placement should occur at least 24 hours after last LMWH dose.
3. It is recommended that patients who have an indwelling epidural catheter will receive LMWH only when there is an extreme risk of deep vein thrombosis (DVT), there is frequent monitoring of the patient's neurologic status (every hour), and the catheter should not be removed within 12 hours of last dose.
4. Following removal of an epidural catheter, LMWH dosing should not occur for at least 2 hours.[22]

PREOPERATIVE EVALUATION

The three goals of the preoperative evaluation are (a) to develop an anesthetic plan that considers the patient's medical condition, the requirements of the surgical procedure, and the patient's preferences; (b) to ensure that the patient's chronic disease is under appropriate medical therapy before an elective procedure; and (c) to gain rapport with and the confidence of the patient, answer any questions, and allay fears.

Optimally, to complete this task, an anesthesiologist would meet every patient before the planned surgical procedure to review the medical history, complete a physical examination, discuss the options and associated anesthetic risks, and develop an anesthetic plan. The anesthesiologist prefers to have a comprehensive evaluation of the medical status by the patient's family practitioner or internist, including the results of pertinent laboratory studies. In the past, this was accomplished when the anesthesiologist visited the patient in the hospital the night before surgery. Currently, it is rare to have patients admitted the night before surgery even before the most comprehensive and complex surgical procedures. The evaluation must still be accomplished, but it must be done on an ambulatory basis, which creates associated logistical problems.

A patient's medical condition should be optimized before an elective surgical procedure. This optimization is best performed by the primary care physician, with medical specialty consultation if necessary. If the procedure is deemed a surgical emergency, the anesthesiologist is responsible for assessing the patient quickly, developing the appropriate anesthetic plan, and proceeding to the operating room as soon as possible. In an emergency situation, the anesthesiologist is not obligated to seek medical consultation to evaluate chronic medical problems because time is essential. The following questions must be answered when evaluating a patient undergoing an elective surgical procedure. What must be included in the preoperative evaluation? Second, who is involved in this process? When and where are all the steps in this process to be conducted? How should all the information be coordinated so that it is available to the appropriate personnel at the appropriate time?

The following steps must be completed before moving the patient into the operating room:

1. A history and physical examination
2. Appropriate laboratory studies and medical consultations
3. An anesthesiologist preoperative evaluation with assignment of an American Society of Anesthesiologists (ASA) physical status
4. Discussion with the patient of the options and risks
5. Development of an anesthetic plan

The history and physical examination have repeatedly been shown to be the most valuable parts of the preoperative assessment. It is primarily the surgeon's responsibility to obtain a history that includes current medical conditions, current medication, and previous surgical and anesthetic history. Questions that are of unique interest to the anesthesiologist are those that involve previous anesthetic problems experienced by the patient or blood relatives and the patient's exercise tolerance. This evaluation not only determines the laboratory tests that may be required but also allows for the assignment of ASA physical status (Table 12.13). The classification serves as a general measure of the patient's state of well being, taking into account all problems the patient brings to the operating room, including systemic disturbances caused by

TABLE 12.13 CLASSIFICATION

PHYSICAL STATUS CLASSIFICATION OF THE AMERICAN SOCIETY OF ANESTHESIOLOGISTS

Physical status classification	Description
PS-1	A normal, healthy patient
PS-2	A patient with mild systemic disease that results in no functional limitation *Examples:* Hypertension, diabetes mellitus, chronic bronchitis, morbid obesity, extremes of age
PS-3	A patient with severe systemic disease that results in functional limitation *Examples:* Poorly controlled hypertension, diabetes mellitus with vascular complications, angina pectoris, prior myocardial infarction, pulmonary disease that limits activity
PS-4	A patient with severe systemic disease that is a constant threat to life *Examples:* Congestive heart failure, unstable angina pectoris, advanced pulmonary, renal, or hepatic dysfunction
PS-5	A moribund patient who is not expected to survive without the operation *Examples:* Ruptured abdominal aneurysm, pulmonary embolus, head injury with increased intracranial pressure
PS-6	A declared brain-dead patient whose organs are being removed for donor purposes
Emergency operation (E)	Any patient in whom an emergency operation is required *Example:* An otherwise healthy 30-year-old woman who requires dilation and curettage for moderate but persistent vaginal bleeding (PS-1E)

the surgical illness. Although studies of anesthetic mortality show a correlation with the physical status classification, this categorization does not describe the risk directly. The risk of any operation is determined not only by patient-related factors but also by procedure-specific ones. For patients with complex medical problems, it is frequently helpful to supplement the surgical history and physical examination with a recent assessment by the patient's primary physician.

The value of preoperative laboratory studies has undergone substantial reevaluation since the mid-1980s. In the past, a surgical procedure was an opportunity to obtain a battery of baseline laboratory tests, even for ASA PS-I patients. The current thinking is that a laboratory test should not be ordered unless a change in the surgical or anesthetic plan is anticipated. The only preoperative screening test required at the University of Michigan, for instance, is an ECG within a year of the planned surgical procedure for men older than 40 and women older than 50 years of age. Pregnancy tests should be obtained only for women who state that they could be pregnant. For procedures with significant anticipated blood loss, a type and cross match is ordered, and a preoperative hematocrit (Hct) is also required. All other tests should have an indication based on history and physical examination. A current strategy for selecting tests indicated by patient history is presented in Table 12.14. Electronic patient questionnaires have also been developed, allowing the appropriate laboratories to be selected based on the patient's response to questions.[23]

TABLE 12.14

SIMPLIFIED STRATEGY FOR PREOPERATIVE TESTING

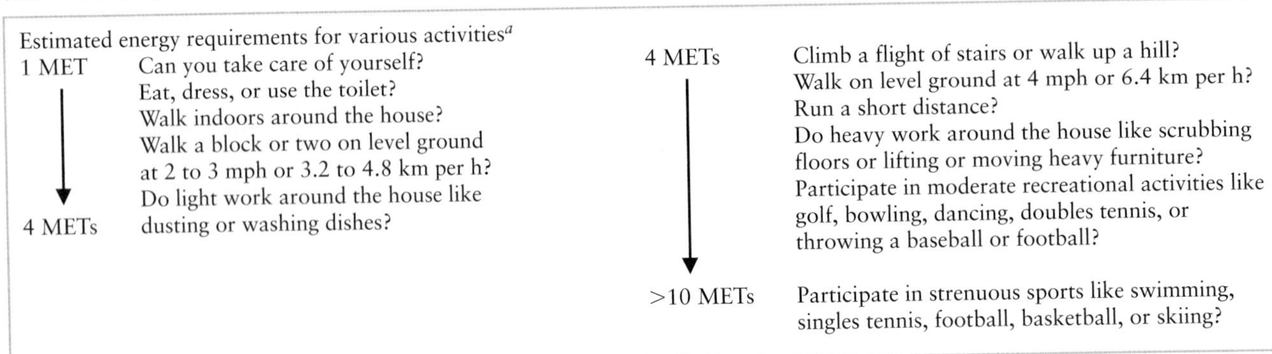

Estimated energy requirements for various activities[a]

1 MET	Can you take care of yourself? Eat, dress, or use the toilet? Walk indoors around the house? Walk a block or two on level ground at 2 to 3 mph or 3.2 to 4.8 km per h? Do light work around the house like dusting or washing dishes?
↓ 4 METs	
4 METs	Climb a flight of stairs or walk up a hill? Walk on level ground at 4 mph or 6.4 km per h? Run a short distance? Do heavy work around the house like scrubbing floors or lifting or moving heavy furniture? Participate in moderate recreational activities like golf, bowling, dancing, doubles tennis, or throwing a baseball or football?
↓ >10 METs	Participate in strenuous sports like swimming, singles tennis, football, basketball, or skiing?

MET, metabolic equivalent.
[a]Adapted from the Duke Activity Status Index[7] and AHA Exercise Standards[27].

There has been significant controversy regarding the minimum level for potassium for elective surgical procedures. In the mid-1980s, several studies noted that patients undergoing procedures with lower than normal potassium levels did not show an increased incidence of rhythm disturbances.[24,25] Although these studies were relatively small, 150 patients and 447 patients, respectively, they did conclude that potassium levels of less than 3.5 mmol/L did not appear to increase the intraoperative risk of arrhythmias. Recently a large study of 2,402 patients undergoing elective coronary artery bypass surgery noted significantly different results.[26] Wahr et al.[26] found that perioperative arrhythmia and the need for cardiopulmonary resuscitation (CPR) increased as preoperative serum potassium level decreased below 3.5 mmol/L. It is known that the ischemic myocardium is more prone to dysrhythmias, but this is the first time that increased morbidity has clearly been demonstrated.[26] It is not known if these results should be extrapolated to patients without ischemic heart disease but it does raise the question of the advisability of proceeding with elective surgery with a potassium level below 3.5 mmol/L.

Discussions of the options of anesthetic techniques and anesthetic risks are best performed by the anesthesiologist who will provide the anesthetic. If the surgeon prefers a specific anesthetic technique, this is best communicated directly to the anesthesiologist rather than recommended to the patient. The development of the anesthetic plan must be determined by the anesthesiologist.

The history, physical examination, and laboratory studies should be performed by the surgeon as soon as the surgical procedure is scheduled. The results of the laboratory studies must be evaluated well in advance of the day of surgery so that positive findings can be attended to in a timely manner. For healthy patients (ASA PS-I and PS-II), the preoperative anesthetic assessment can be conducted by the anesthesiologist on the day of the procedure. If the patients have complex medical problems (ASA PS-III or greater) or have significant concerns they want to discuss with an anesthesiologist, they should be evaluated before the day of surgery. Because of the logistical problems of scheduling, most institutions have developed preoperative anesthesia clinics where this process can take place. When specialty medical consultation is considered, the following questions should be answered. Does this patient have ischemic heart disease that requires further medical management or workup? What is the degree of functional improvement of the organ system in question? Is medical treatment of these problems optimized? If not, what needs to be done and how long will it take?

An obvious problem that concerns anesthesiologists is the potential of a difficult intubation. This can be quickly assessed as discussed earlier (see Fig. 12.1). Even if a patient has no medical problem, the possibility of a difficult airway warrants that the patient be seen preoperatively and evaluated. These patients can always be approached by an awake fiberoptic technique, but this takes planning and can cause a significant delay if there is no prior warning.

MONITORING THE SURGICAL PATIENT

One of the more obvious changes in anesthesia care has been the routine use of an array of electronic monitoring devices to provide continuous surveillance of physiologic status. Because the art and science of anesthesiology involves titrating pharmacologic agents to produce desired physiologic effects, there must be a measured parameter to which drug dosages are titrated. Depending on the severity of preexisting disease and the extent and duration of the surgical procedure, invasive techniques can be used to provide comprehensive continuous data to guide the titration of fluid therapy and cardiovascular agents.

Monitors of Oxygenation

Pulse oximetry has been called the most significant advance in patient monitoring to date. This device continuously, noninvasively, and inexpensively provides arterial hemoglobin saturation (SaO_2) and peripheral pulse by measuring light absorption in a manner similar to that of a laboratory cooximeter. A cooximeter shines light through a cuvette filled with a blood sample. Each hemoglobin species absorbs light in direct proportion to its concentration (Beer-Lambert law). A cooximeter requires one wavelength of light for each hemoglobin species to be measured, that is one wavelength for oxyhemoglobin and one for reduced hemoglobin. To measure other hemoglobins, such as carboxyhemoglobin or methemoglobin, the device requires four wavelengths of light.

The pulse oximeter uses two wavelengths of light, one red and one infrared, that shine through a tissue bed, usually a finger. Opposite the light sources is a photodiode that measures the transmitted light intensity. A large proportion of the light absorbed as it passes through the tissues is not associated with arterial blood but with other components of the tissue, such as skin, muscle, bone, and venous blood. Therefore, the device analyzes only the pulsatile component of absorption and assumes that anything that pulses within the tissue bed is arterial blood, hence the name *pulse oximeter.* Actually, the pulse oximeter measures the ratio of the pulsatile component of red light absorbed to the pulsatile component of the infrared light absorbed. This ratio changes with SaO_2. The exact relation between this ratio and SaO_2 has been empirically determined from volunteer studies and is programmed into the electronics of the oximeter. If any artifacts occur in a pulsatile nature, they may be erroneously integrated into the equation, causing erroneous SaO_2 estimates.

Several things should be remembered when using the pulse oximeter. First, the device measures SaO_2 and not arterial oxygen tension (PaO_2). The PaO_2 must drop below 80 mm Hg before any significant change in SaO_2 occurs. As the PaO_2 drops below 60 mm Hg, the SaO_2 rapidly falls as the inflection point of the sigmoidal oxyhemoglobin dissociation curve is approached. As a rough rule of thumb, as SaO_2 drops below 90%, the PaO_2 can be estimated by subtracting 30 points from the SaO_2. For example, a SaO_2 of 85% corresponds to a PaO_2 of 55 mm Hg. Second, the pulse oximeter measures saturation (milliliters of oxygen per deciliters of blood) and not arterial content or CaO_2. Although the dissolved oxygen is ignored because of its small contribution, the oxygen content is directly proportional to the SaO_2 and the hemoglobin concentration. Because the hemoglobin concentration is about one third of the Hct, the following equation can be used to estimate CaO_2:

$$CaO_2 = 0.45 \text{ Hct} \times SaO_2$$

or, if SaO_2 is 100%:

$$CaO_2 \cdot \tfrac{1}{2} \text{ Hct}$$

The oxygen-carrying capacity of blood can be quickly assessed by spinning a Hct and measuring the arterial saturation with a pulse oximeter.

Because the pulse oximeter uses only two wavelengths of light, it cannot detect the presence of carboxyhemoglobin (carbon monoxide poisoning) or methemoglobin. Because the absorption characteristics of carboxyhemoglobin are similar to those of oxyhemoglobin, the pulse oximeter will register approximately the sum of both these gases. A pulse-oximeter reading of 100% saturation for a patient with smoke inhalation injury may actually indicate severe carbon monoxide poisoning. The only method of determining carbon monoxide poisoning is to send an arterial blood sample for laboratory cooximeter measurement of carboxyhemoglobin. The only clinically accepted device for invasive monitoring of oxygen saturation is the pulmonary arterial oximeter catheter (Chapter 10).

Despite the potential drawbacks, the pulse oximeter has been shown to be impressively accurate in a wide variety of patients with a tremendous variation in pulse amplitude.[27]

Ventilation Monitors

By definition, a patient is appropriately ventilated when arterial carbon dioxide tension ($PaCO_2$) is 40 mm Hg. Measuring the respiratory rate can document only the presence of ventilations not its adequacy. Capnography, or end-tidal CO_2 monitoring, is the visual display of the CO_2 concentration at the airway. To understand the utility of capnography, one must understand dead-space components and how they affect CO_2 removal from the body.[28] Dead space (DS) is defined as the portion of the tidal volume (VT) that does not participate in gas exchange.

$$VT = DS + VA$$

The alveolar volume (VA) is the volume of the inspired gas that reaches well-perfused alveoli. The remainder of the VT, which equals the DS, can be divided into three subcomponents: apparatus dead space (DS_{ap}), anatomic dead space (DS_{an}), and alveolar dead space (DS_{al}).

$$DS = DS_{ap} + DS_{an} + Ds_{al}$$

At the end of inspiration, the respiratory apparatus (e.g., endotracheal tube) is filled with inspired gas that should not contain CO_2. Similarly, all the anatomic airways (trachea, bronchi, and all conducting airways down to the alveoli) should be filled with inspired gas and should therefore contain no CO_2. In this model, there are two types of alveoli: those that are well-perfused alveolar gas and those that are not perfused DS_{al} gas. At the end of inspiration, the DS_{al} gas, because it is not perfused, does not pick up CO_2 and again contains inspired gas and no CO_2. The alveolar gas should completely equilibrate with the arterial blood and contain CO_2 at the same tension as the arterial blood; ideally $PaCO_2$ should equal 40 mm Hg. As the patient expires, the CO_2 detected at the patient's mouth first reflects the DS_{ap} gas having no CO_2, followed by the DS_{an} gas, again with no CO_2, and finally the alveolar gases, containing both dead space and well-perfused alveolar gas. When mixed alveolar gas reaches the airway, it produces a rapid rise in the CO_2 concentration to a level somewhere between the concentration in the alveolar gas (40 mm Hg) and the DS_{al} (0 mm Hg), depending on each component's proportion of volume. For example, if half of the alveoli are DS_{al} and $PaCO_2$ equals 40 mm Hg, then the plateau value of the capnogram should be 20 mm Hg, implying that half of the alveoli are not being perfused. With inspiration, the CO_2 value again drops to 0 until another expiration, and a square wave appears again as the alveolar gas is detected at the mouth. With each breath, there should be a square wave, whose height approaches the $PaCO_2$ value as the amount of the DS_{al} gas approaches 0.

In a healthy young adult, there is no significant DS_{al} gas, and the end-tidal CO_2 value equals the $PaCO_2$. Therefore, the difference between these values indicates the proportion of DS_{al} in the patient. The presence of a capnogram itself implies there is metabolism (the production of CO_2), circulation (blood flow to the lungs), and ventilation (respiratory rate and an intact ventilator circuit).

Providing this information on a breath-to-breath basis, the continuous capnogram is extremely useful in many critical situations. It can be used as a surveillance monitor of both the respiratory circuit and the cardiovascular system. Any acute decrease in cardiac output will decrease blood flow to the lungs and increase the DS_{al}, causing an acute drop in end-tidal CO_2. For this reason, the device was originally used during neurosurgical procedures in the sitting position to detect the presence of air emboli. This principle also allows the detection of pulmonary emboli or any acute drop in cardiac output. In fact, the only acute catastrophic cardiopulmonary problem that will not be detected by the capnometer is arterial desaturation. Therefore, the combination of the capnometer and the pulse oximeter creates a dynamic duo for beat-to-beat and breath-to-breath surveillance of metabolism, circulation, ventilation, and oxygenation.

Circulation Monitors

Hemodynamic stability can be monitored by a variety of methods, the most basic of which is systemic arterial blood pressure. Intermittent, noninvasive measurement of systemic blood pressure with an oscillometric blood pressure cuff is the standard in the operating room, and its accuracy equals that of clinical measurements by auscultation. Circulation monitors can be cycled as quickly as once per minute, but when used for an extended duration, they should be cycled no more than once every 3 to 5 minutes. When tighter control is required in patients with significant hypertension or serious heart disease or in those who may suffer acute blood loss, invasive arterial monitoring is used. Although pressure measurements provided by invasive techniques are different from those of noninvasive techniques, they usually coincide closely. A continuous invasive arterial tracing can also be used to assess the adequacy of fluid resuscitation by following the systolic pressure variation (SPV) with positive-pressure ventilation. The normal range of SPV is 5 to 10 mm Hg. A systolic pressure decrease of greater than 10 mm Hg during positive pressure inspiration implies inadequate preload and the need for more aggressive fluid resuscitation.[29] In patients without left ventricular dysfunction, who are undergoing extended surgical procedures with significant fluid shifts and potential blood loss, central venous pressure monitoring is frequently used, with pulmonary arterial catheter monitoring reserved for more critically ill patients and those with significant left ventricular dysfunction. The adequacy of circulation can be objectively documented by thermodilution cardiac output measurements and mixed venous oxygen saturation monitoring. Transesophageal echocardiography is now commonly used to assess cardiac function. This technique is easily used in the anesthetized, intubated patient and can quickly assess systolic and diastolic function as well as valvular dysfunction.

COMMON PROBLEMS IN THE POSTOPERATIVE PERIOD

Postanesthesia care units are required in any setting where surgical procedures are conducted. The increased scope of surgery and the invasive technology used to monitor sicker patients has increased the service at and training required to operate these facilities. In 1994, the ASA revised the 1988 Standards for Postanesthesia Care (Table 12.15).

TABLE 12.15

STANDARDS FOR POSTANESTHESIA CARE

Standards		Criteria to be fulfilled
Standard I[a]	All patients who have received general, regional, or monitored anesthesia care shall receive appropriate postanesthesia management.	1. A PACU or an area that provides equivalent postanesth care shall be available to receive patients after anesthesia care. All patients who receive anesthesia care shall be admitted to the PACU or its equivalent *except* by specific order of the anesthesiologist responsible for the patient's care. 2. The medical aspects of care in the PACU shall be governed by policies and procedures that have been reviewed and approved by the department of anesthesiology. 3. The design, equipment, and staffing of the PACU shall meet requirements of the facility's accrediting and licensing bodies.
Standard II	A patient transported to the PACU shall be accompanied by a member of the anesthesia care team who is knowledgeable about the patient's condition. The patient shall be continually evaluated and treated during transport with monitoring and support appropriate to the patient's condition.	
Standard III	On arrival in the PACU, the patient shall be reevaluated and a verbal report provided to the responsible PACU nurse by the member of the anesthesia care team who accompanies the patient.	1. The patient's status on arrival in the PACU shall be documented. 2. Information concerning the preoperative condition and the surgical/anesthetic course shall be transmitted to the PACU nurse. 3. The member of the anesthesia care team shall remain in the PACU until the PACU nurse accepts responsibility for the nursing care of the patient.
Standard IV	The patient's condition shall be evaluated continually in the PACU.	1. The patient shall be observed and monitored by the methods appropriate to the patient's medical condition. Particular attention shall be given to monitoring oxygenation, ventilation, circulation, and temperature. During recovery from all anesthetics, a quantitative method of assessing oxygenation such as pulse oximetry shall be employed in the initial phase of recovery. This is not intended for application during the recovery of the obstetric patient in whom regional anesthesia was used for labor and vaginal delivery. 2. An accurate written report of the PACU period shall be maintained. Use of an appropriate PACU scoring system is encouraged for each patient on admission, at appropriate intervals prior to discharge, and at the time of discharge. 3. General medical supervision and coordination of patient care in the PACU should be the responsibility of an anesthesiologist. 4. There shall be a policy to ensure the availability in the facility of a physician capable of managing complications and providing cardiopulmonary resuscitation for patients in the PACU.
Standard V	A physician is responsible for discharging the patient from the PACU.	1. When discharge criteria are used, they must be approved by the department of anesthesiology and the medical staff. They may vary depending on whether the patient is discharged to a hospital room, to the ICU, to a short stay unit, or home. 2. In the absence of the physician responsible for the discharge, the PACU nurse shall determine that the patient meets the discharge criteria. The name of the physician accepting responsibility for discharge shall be noted on the record.

ICU, intensive care unit; PACU, postanesthesia care unit.
Based on ASA's Standards for Postanesthesia Care. A copy of the full text can be obtained from ASA, 520 N. Northwest Highway, Park Ridge, IL 60068-2573.
[a]For nursing care issues, refer to Standards of Postanesthesia Nursing Practice, published by the American Society of Postanesthesia Nurses.

TABLE 12.16

POSTANESTHESIA RECOVERY SCORE[a]

Parameter	Score
ACTIVITY	
Voluntary movement of all limbs to command	2
Voluntary movement of 2 extremities to command	1
Unable to move	0
RESPIRATION	
Breathes deeply and coughs	2
Dyspnea, hypoventilation	1
Apneic	0
CIRCULATION	
Blood pressure equals 80% of preanesthetic level	2
Blood pressure equals 50%–80% of preanesthetic level	1
Blood pressure equals <50% of preanesthetic level	0
CONSCIOUSNESS	
Fully awake	2
Arousable	1
Unresponsive	0
COLOR	
Pink	2
Pale, blotchy	1
Cyanotic	0

[a]Patients should score at least 7 before discharge from the postanesthesia care unit.

The scoring systems used to assess the postoperative patient direct attention to the primary areas of concern. The postanesthesia recovery score is an attempt to evaluate postanesthesia patient status[30] (Table 12.16). This basic information should be incorporated in a record that provides clear documentation of postoperative events. Documentation should also include details of postoperative outpatient care, with a note indicating postoperative telephone contact made to elucidate problems. Problems should receive appropriate follow-up, and written postoperative discharge instructions should be provided for the patient.

Investigators have reported that 24% of patients experience a postanesthesia care unit complication. Nausea, vomiting, and the need for airway support constitute 70% of these complications[31] (Fig. 12.2). The need to maintain airway support was by far the most common respiratory complication. The duration of the procedure as well as ASA classification and type of procedure had a significant bearing on the incidence of complications in this study. Hypothermia was also a common problem that prolonged postoperative postanesthesia care unit stay (Fig. 12.3). Hypothermia has the deleterious effects of altering drug metabolism and delaying recovery. Furthermore, it causes shivering, which increases the metabolic demand for oxygen.

Among cardiovascular complications in the postoperative period, none is more important or more difficult to diagnose than myocardial ischemia. The association of perioperative myocardial ischemia with cardiac morbidity has been clearly documented.[15] In a series of high-risk patients undergoing noncardiac surgery, researchers noted that "early postoperative myocardial ischemia is an important correlate of adverse cardiac outcomes."[15] Diagnosis is complicated by the fact that only 10% to 30% of patients suffering documented myocardial infarction have pain and that postoperative ECG T-wave changes are often nonspecific.[32] Instead, one must seek secondary indications of ongoing ischemia or "angina equivalents," such as hypotension, arrhythmias, elevated filling pressures, or postoperative oliguria. Arrhythmias are common and are significant primarily because of the association with myocardial ischemia or hypoxemia.

Nausea and vomiting are rarely unifactorial and cause considerable discomfort to patients. Opioids are responsible for stimulating the emesis center in a significant cohort of patients. These patients may provide a clear history of opioid sensitivity and anesthetic and analgesic regimens may be tailored to limit the exposure of these patients to these drugs. In general, however, there is little evidence to favor one anesthetic or anesthetic technique over another, although propofol appears to have an antiemetic effect. Nitrous oxide, often considered causative, does not appear to increase the incidence of nausea according to well-documented studies. It is not unusual for an antiemetic agent to be included preoperatively or as part of the anesthetic technique, especially in patients with a positive history or those deemed to be at risk, such as menstruating young women undergoing laparoscopy. Standard usage includes phenothiazines, butyrophenones, metoclopramide, and scopolamine. Recently, the Food and Drug Administration approved the use of the selective $5HT_3$ antagonist (e.g., ondansetron), which was shown in several studies to be superior to other agents.[33] An algorithm for the treatment of postoperative nausea and vomiting is illustrated in Algorithm 12.2.

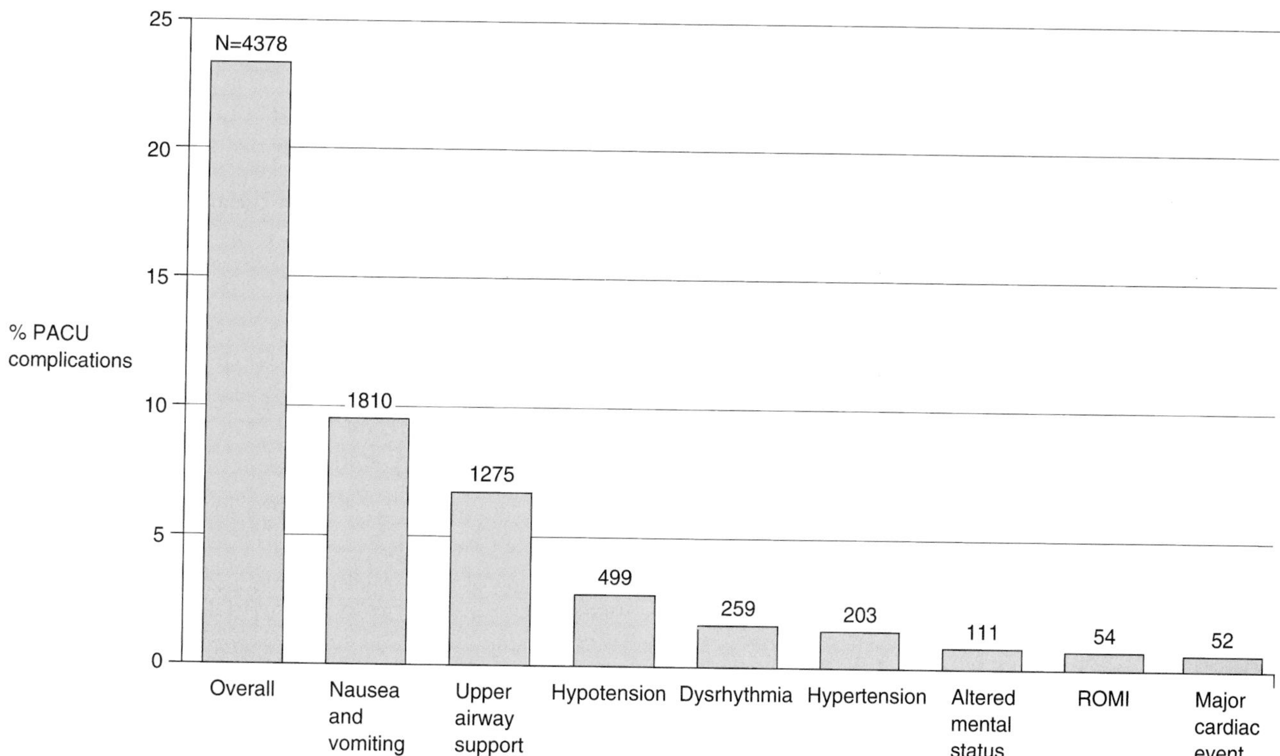

FIGURE 12.2 Major postanesthesia care unit complications by percentage of occurrence and number of patients experiencing each complication. Nausea and vomiting were the most frequently observed complications. ROMI, rule out myocardial infarction. (After Hines R, Barash PG, Watrous G, et al. Complications occurring in the postanesthesia care unit: a survey. *Anesth Analg.* 1992;74:505.)

The most common cause of delayed emergence is the residual effects of anesthesia. The differential diagnosis of delayed emergence is best approached by ruling out physiologic, pharmacologic, and neurologic cases in this order (Table 12.17). There should be little confusion about the implication of muscle relaxants because physical indications of ventilatory distress, combined with the readings of the blockade monitor, should clearly indicate the role of these drugs. Where appropriate, opioids can be reversed using titrated doses of naloxone. Flumazenil can be used for reversal of benzodiazepines.

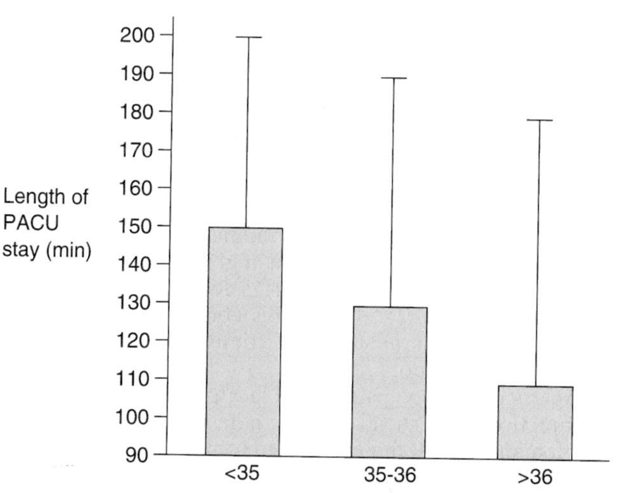

FIGURE 12.3 Patient body temperature at admission also affects the development of postanesthesia care unit (PACU) complications. The duration of PACU stay as a function of temperature at admission is shown. Stay was significantly reduced in patients whose temperature at admission was 36EC or higher (P <.01). (After Hines R, Barash PG, Watrous G, et al. Complications occurring in the postanesthesia care unit: a survey. *Anesth Analg.* 1992;74:506.)

TABLE 12.17

DIFFERENTIAL DIAGNOSIS OF DELAYED EMERGENCE

DIFFERENTIAL DIAGNOSIS OF DELAYED EMERGENCE
METABOLIC ABNORMALITIES
Hypoxia
Hypercarbia
Hypoglycemia
Hypotension
Hypothermia
Hyponatremia
DRUG EFFECTS
Muscle relaxants
Opioids
Barbiturates
Benzodiazepines
Ketamine
Anticholinergics
Inhalational anesthetics
NEUROLOGIC INJURY
Ischemia
Mass lesions
Seizure disorders

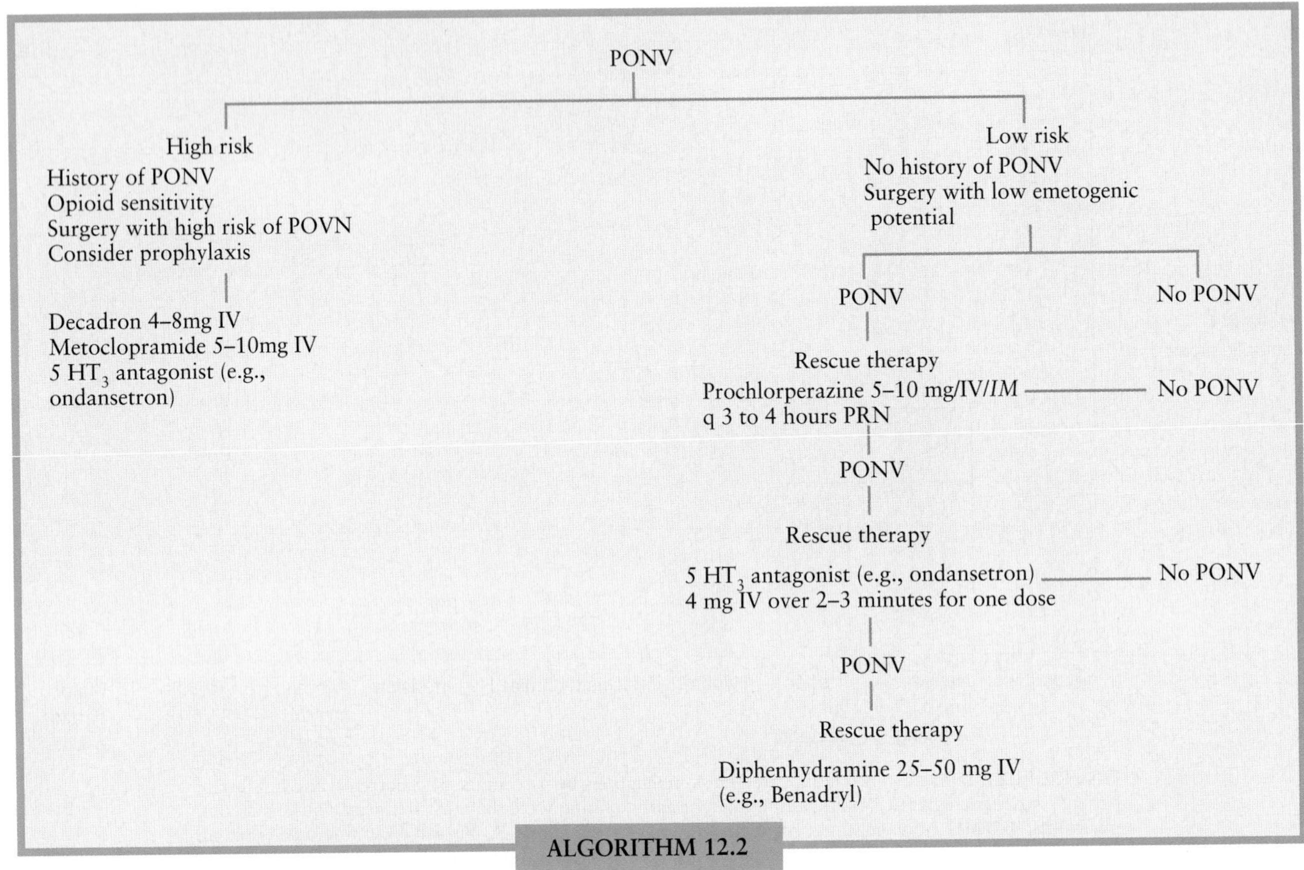

ALGORITHM 12.2 Algorithm for preventing and treating postoperative nausea and vomiting (PONV) in adults.

POSTOPERATIVE ACUTE PAIN MANAGEMENT

Postoperative pain is an inevitable consequence of surgery. Its severity is site dependent (Table 12.18), but the magnitude of the pain experienced by individual patients after similar surgical procedures is influenced by a multitude of factors. Variation in patient experience has been clearly demonstrated by several authors and is reflected in deficiencies in postoperative pain control.[34] The recognition of this clinical problem has prompted interest in underlying pain mechanisms and in innovative ways to alleviate postoperative suffering.

TABLE 12.18

PERCENTAGE OF PATIENTS WHO REQUIRE ANALGESIC INJECTIONS

Operation	No analgesic needed (%)	Three or more analgesic injections (%)
Minor chest wall	82	0
Inguinal hernia	52	0
Appendectomy	25	10
Lower abdominal surgery	18	40
Upper abdominal surgery	10	45–65

In 1965, the crucial role of nociceptive C fiber feedback behavior and its modulation by cells in the substantia gelatinosa of the dorsal horn was recognized.[35] Repetitive stimulation of these fibers by cellular mediators, such as kinins and catecholamines, promotes neural excitation, prolongs repetitive firing, and lowers the threshold to further excitation. As a result, C fibers do not show fatigue, and the stage is set for continuous pain. Counterirritation of large afferent activity has been shown empirically to have beneficial effects. The gate-control theory provides an explanation for the inhibition of C fiber-mediated pain. Serotonergic and enkephalinergic descending inhibitory pathways modulate activity in the dorsal horn before information is relayed to the somatosensory cortex through the spinothalamic tract. The common observation that pain is worse at night, when less sensory information is processed, and that it decreases with daytime activity is an example of how this complex neural system functions. Transcutaneous nerve stimulation is a technical attempt to use this principle.

Superficial somatic pain is well localized and has a protective function. Superficial somatic pain is readily treated by common analgesic techniques. Deep somatic pain may not be well localized; may have some protective function, as in joint immobilization; and is fairly responsive to a variety of analgesics. Visceral pain, served almost entirely by C fiber activity, is poorly localized, often referred, and difficult to treat. In major operations, all modes can be activated, compounding the clinical challenge of providing adequate pain management. These clinical observations direct the focus of postoperative pain management to the treatment of somatic pain by

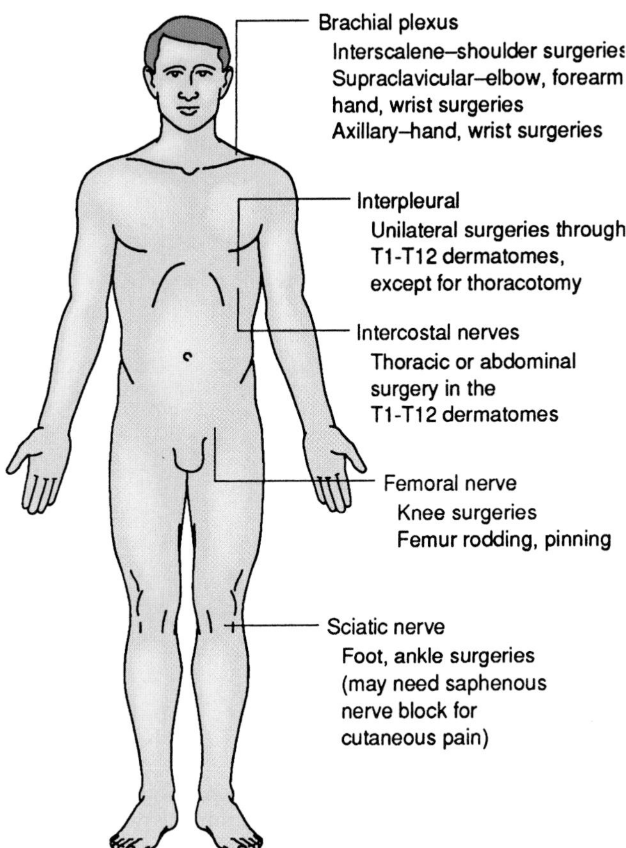

FIGURE 12.4 Surgical procedures in which peripheral nerve blockade can provide postoperative pain relief.

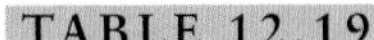

TABLE 12.19

PROBLEMS THAT CAN OCCUR DURING PATIENT-CONTROLLED ANALGESIA (PCA) THERAPY

OPERATOR ERRORS
Misprogramming PCA device
Failure to clamp or unclamp tubing
Improperly loading syringe or cartridge
Inability to respond to safety alarms
Misplacing PCA pump key
PATIENT ERRORS
Failure to understand PCA therapy
Misunderstanding PCA pump device
Intentional analgesic abuse
MECHANICAL ERRORS
Failure to deliver on demand
Defective one-way valve at Y-connector
Faulty alarm system
Device malfunctions

attacking the nociceptor and the subsequent transmission of the painful impulse by the nerve fiber. The use of nonsteroidal antiinflammatory drugs with or without the injection of local anesthetics into the wound is very effective. If done preemptively at the time of surgery, this approach can significantly benefit the patient's postoperative experience.[36] Examples of nerve blocks for various procedures are shown in Figure 12.4.

Including potent opioids in the treatment of deep pain, both somatic and visceral, has been routine. However, the responses to standard regimens have been notoriously unreliable, from inadequate pain relief to narcosis, with complications at both ends of the scale. It was not until the 1980s that variations in response were linked to variable serum concentrations of analgesic drugs. Interpatient variation in serum levels to any standard dose can be fivefold, and interpatient therapeutic concentrations can vary on a similar scale. When factored together, there is the potential for a 25-fold variation in patient response to a standard drug prescription. Each patient has an individual therapeutic window (Fig. 12.5). The clinical implications are enormous.

In 1968, investigators demonstrated the virtue of small IV doses given on demand.[36] As a result, the patient experienced greater pain relief, yet used the same or less total narcotic. Although there was significant patient variation, the demand from any individual patient, though cyclic, was constant. Patient-controlled analgesia (PCA) and the technologic and administrative systems to provide it have developed to a point of some sophistication, requiring servicing and a support structure with its own set of problems (Table 12.19). PCA administration requires a receptive environment, education of all personnel, and adequate patient instruction. PCA has received widespread acceptance by patients, nursing staff, and physicians because it provides more prompt and painless analgesia that more closely matches the patient's need over time.

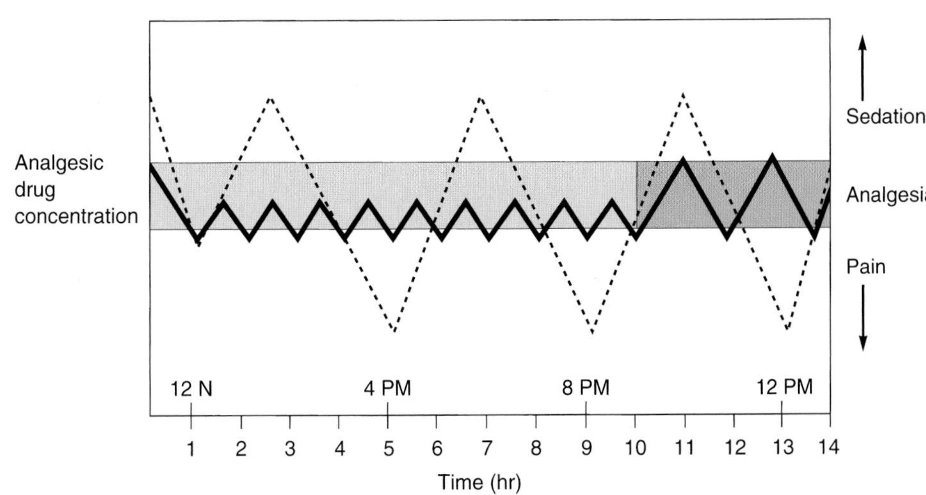

FIGURE 12.5 Theoretical relation among dosing interval, analgesic drug concentration, and clinical effects when comparing a patient-controlled analgesia system (*solid line*) to conventional intramuscular therapy (*dashed line*). (After White PF. Patient-controlled analgesia: a new approach to the management of postoperative pain. *Semin Anesth.* 1985;4:261.)

TABLE 12.20

EXAMPLE OF ORDERS FOR PATIENT-CONTROLLED ANALGESIA (PCA)

1. Patient is to be initiated on PCA with standard monitoring protocol.		
2. Drug selection	Morphine 1 mg/mL	Hydromorphone 0.2 mg/mL
3. Loading II Initial dose (start PRN for pain)	2–4 mg	0.2–0.4 mg
Incremental dose, q 5–10 min PRN	1–2 mg	0.1–0.2 mg
Maximum total loading dose	10 mg	1 mg
Other	____ mg	____ mg
4. Pump setting II PCA dose	____ mg	____ mg
Lockout interval	____ min	____ mg
4-Hour limit	____ mg	____ mg

University of Michigan Hospitals form RP-2044330/982, Rev. 7/93, Acute Pain Service, Patient Controlled Analgesia Standard Orders.

PCA is as safe as conventional IM medication. Morphine and meperidine are commonly used drugs, and an example of orders is shown in Table 12.20.

Transdermal narcotic delivery is receiving attention and may become available for postoperative pain. The method is both practical and inexpensive and aims to maintain continuous delivery and constant blood levels. Fentanyl has been the drug of choice and has been well received by patients. The method appears to be safe, but there is a significant lag time between application and the attainment of therapeutic blood levels.

The discovery of endorphins in the 1970s and recognition of their importance in modulating pain at spinal sites lead to the supposition that it would be possible to selectively apply opioids directly to receptors. This led to the development of epidural opiate analgesia, in which opioids are applied directly to the receptors at spinal sites. The goal of epidural opiate analgesia is to obtain maximal analgesia while minimizing systemic side effects. For severe acute postoperative pain caused by major surgery, epidural opiate analgesia has proved to be a superior modality for pain control. In high-risk cases, there is evidence that it has an overall beneficial effect on morbidity.[20]

The effective use of this sophisticated modality requires education and the establishment of protocols with rigorous attention to detail. The potential for respiratory depression demands adherence to monitoring standards. Morphine and fentanyl, often in combination with a dilute local anesthetic solution, are most often prescribed. A typical order form with monitored parameters is shown in Table 12.21.

A comprehensive postoperative pain management service demands resources and must use the physical and pharmacologic modalities available, while recognizing the significant subjective component of any individual's pain problem. The ability to recognize the impact of acute pain or an underlying chronic pain disorder requires that experience be brought to bear on difficult problems. The active involvement of nursing staff and surgeons is essential for the patient to achieve maximal benefit. It is incumbent on the pain-management service to render efficient, continuous, and cost-effective care.

TABLE 12.21

OPIOID PROTOCOLS IN EPIDURAL OPIATE ANALGESIA

	Morphine[a]	Fentanyl[b]
Length of onset	Longer (30–60 min)	Shorter (15–30 min)
Duration	Longer (6–24 h for single bolus)	Shorter (1–2 h for single bolus)
Cephalad spread and side effects	More prone	Less prone
Indication	Favored for lumbar administration after abdominal surgery	Favored for thoracic administration after chest surgery
Dose	Typically 3–5 mg, q 6–8 h	Typically 50–75 mg/h (± dilute bupivacaine)

[a]Hydrophilic: slow in, slow out.
[b]Lipophilic: fast in, fast out.

One of the most difficult problems in postoperative pain is the care for patients with a preoperative history of chronic pain treated with opioids. These patients require very large doses of IV analgesics and need to be maintained orally. The best way to evaluate an appropriate starting dose is to convert the preoperative opioid regimen to an IV morphine equivalent then add what would be required to treat the acute surgical pain (see Table 12.4).

KEY POINTS

- **Anesthetics are generalized depressants of consciousness, pain, cardiopulmonary function, motor function, and recall.**
- **To prevent movement and to facilitate the surgical exposure, neuromuscular blocking agents are generally used. These drugs are competitive or noncompetitive inhibitors of the neurotransmitter acetylcholine at the neuromuscular junction.**
- **Hypertension is the most common preexisting medical disease in patients presenting for surgery and is a major risk factor for renal, cerebrovascular, peripheral vascular, and coronary artery diseases as well as for congestive heart failure.**
- **The three goals of the preoperative evaluation are (a) to develop an anesthetic plan that considers the patient's medical condition, the requirements of the surgical procedure, and the patient's preferences; (b) to ensure that the patient's chronic disease is under appropriate medical therapy before an elective procedure; and (c) to gain rapport with and the confidence of the patient, answer any questions, and allay fears.**
- **Postanesthesia care units are required in any setting where surgical procedures are conducted.**

References

1. Calverly R. Anesthesia as a specialty: past, present, and future. In: Barash P, Cullen BF, Stoelting RK, eds. *Clinical anesthesia.* Philadelphia: JB Lippincott; 1992.
2. Watling SM, Dasta JF. Prolonged paralysis in intensive care unit patients after the use of neuromuscular blocking agents: a review of the literature. *Crit Care Med.* 1994;22:884.
3. Rosenberg JM, et al. Coronary perfusion pressure during cardiopulmonary resuscitation after spinal anesthesia in dogs. *Anesth Analg.* 1996;82:84.
4. JCAHO. *Comprehensive accreditation manual for hospitals: the official handbook: Conscious sedations.* Oakbrook Terrace, IL: JCAHO; 1999:73–77.
5. Mallampati SR, et al. A clinical sign to predict difficult tracheal intubation: a prospective study. *Can Anaesth Soc J.* 1985;32:429.
6. **Naughton NN, et al. Sedation analgesia for diagnostic and therapeutic procedures. In: Naughton NN, Tremper KK, eds. *Contemporary Clinical Neuroscience Series.* 2003, New Jersey: Human Press; 2003:xx.**
7. Miller R. *Anesthesia,* 3rd ed. New York: Churchill Livingstone; 1990.
8. Mangano DT, et al. Effect of atenolol on mortality and cardiovascular morbidity after noncardiac surgery. Multicenter Study of Perioperative Ischemia Research Group. *N Engl J Med.* 1996;335:1713.
9. Bertrand M, et al. Should the angiotensin II antagonists be discontinued before surgery. *Anesth Analg.* 2001;92:26.
10. Boccara G. et al. Terlipressin versus norepinephrine to correct refractory arterial hypotension after general anesthesia in patients chronically treated with renin-angiotensin system inhibitors. *Anesthesiology* 2003;98:1338.
11. Meersschaert K, et al. Terlipressin-ephedrine versus ephedrine to treat hypotension at the induction of anesthesia in patients chronically treated with angiotensin converting-enzyme inhibitors: a prospective, randomized, double-blinded, crossover study. *Anesth Analg.* 2002;94:835.
12. Colson P, Ryckwaert F, Coriat P. Renin angiotensin system antagonists and anesthesia. *Anesth Analg.* 1999;89:1143.
13. Stoelting RK, DS. *Anesthesia and co-existing disease,* 3rd ed. New York: Churchill Livingstone; 1993.
14. Mangano DT. Perioperative cardiac morbidity. *Anesthesiology* 1990;72:153.
15. **Mangano DT, et al. Association of perioperative myocardial ischemia with cardiac morbidity and mortality in men undergoing noncardiac surgery. The Study of Perioperative Ischemia Research Group. *N Engl J Med.* 1990;323:1781.**
16. Rao TL, Jacobs KH, El-Etr AA. Reinfarction following anesthesia in patients with myocardial infarction. *Anesthesiology* 1983;59:499.
17. Tarhan S, et al. Myocardial infarction after general anesthesia. *JAMA* 1972;220:1451.
18. **Eagle KA, et al. ACC/AHA guideline update for perioperative cardiovascular evaluation for noncardiac surgery—executive summary: a report of the American College of Cardiology/American Heart Association Task Force on Practice Guidelines (Committee to Update the 1996 Guidelines on Perioperative Cardiovascular Evaluation for Noncardiac Surgery). *J Am Coll Cardiol.* 2002;39:542.**
19. Goldman L, et al. Multifactorial index of cardiac risk in noncardiac surgical procedures. *N Engl J Med* 1977;297:845.
20. Yeager MP, et al. Epidural anesthesia and analgesia in high-risk surgical patients. *Anesthesiology* 1987;66:729.
21. **Pedersen T, Eliasen K, Henriksen E. A prospective study of mortality associated with anaesthesia and surgery: risk indicators of mortality in hospital. *Acta Anaesthesiol Scand.* 1990;34:176.**
22. Horlocker TT, Wedel DJ. Neuraxial block and low-molecular-weight heparin: balancing perioperative analgesia and thromboprophylaxis. *Reg Anesth Pain Med.* 1998;23[6 Suppl 2]:164.
23. WWW.HEALTHQUIZ.COM.
24. Hirsch IA, et al. The overstated risk of preoperative hypokalemia. *Anesth Analg.* 1988;67:131.
25. Vitez TS, et al. Chronic hypokalemia and intraoperative dysrhythmias. *Anesthesiology* 1985;63:130.
26. Wahr JA, et al. Preoperative serum potassium levels and perioperative outcomes in cardiac surgery patients. Multicenter Study of Perioperative Ischemia Research Group. *JAMA* 1999;281:2203.
27. Wahr J, Parks R, Boisvert D. Pulse oximetry. In: Blitt HRCD, ed. *Monitoring in anesthesia and critical care medicine,* 3rd ed. New York: Churchill Livingstone; 1994:385.
28. Nunn J. Respiratory dead space and distribution of inspired gases. In: *Applied respiratory physiology,* 2nd ed. London: Butterworths; 1977:213.
29. Coriat P, et al. A comparison of systolic blood pressure variations and echocardiographic estimates of end-diastolic left ventricular size in patients after aortic surgery. *Anesth Analg.* 1994;78:46.
30. Bonner S. *Admission and discharge criteria. Post anesthesia care.* Connecticut: Prentice Hall International; 1990.
31. Hines R, et al. Complications occurring in the postanesthesia care unit: a survey. *Anesth Analg.* 1992;74:503.
32. Breslow MJ, et al. Changes in T-wave morphology following anesthesia and surgery: a common recovery-room phenomenon. *Anesthesiology* 1986;64:398.
33. Alon E, Himmelseher S. Ondansetron in the treatment of postoperative vomiting: a randomized, double-blind comparison with droperidol and metoclopramide. *Anesth Analg.* 1992;75:561.
34. Marks RM, Sachar EJ. Undertreatment of medical inpatients with narcotic analgesics. *Ann Intern Med.* 1973;78:173.
35. Melzack R, Wall PD. Pain mechanisms: a new theory. *Science* 1965;150:971.
36. Tverskoy M, et al. Postoperative pain after inguinal herniorrhaphy with different types of anesthesia. *Anesth Analg.* 1990;70:29.

CHAPTER 13 ■ CANCER

STEVEN K. LIBUTTI

Few medical diagnoses carry with them the fear and dread that a diagnosis of cancer brings to the patient. Historically, Hippocrates is credited with first distinguishing between benign and malignant tumors. Hippocrates described invasive carcinoma using the Greek term for crab, *karkinos,* based on the similarities between the invasive tongue of solid tumors and the claws of the crab. *Karkinos* forms the root for the term *carcinoma*. The word *cancer* is derived from the Latin, *cancrum,* for crab.

The term has come to represent a constellation of malignant processes involving a host of tissue types, each with differing potentials for invasion and metastases. Each pathologic type of cancer has different approaches for its diagnosis and management. However, there are certain basic characteristics that define the transition from normal cell division and proliferation into abnormal, unregulated growth and invasion, which is the hallmark of cancer. The breadth and depth of information regarding the processes involved in the development, diagnosis, and treatment of cancer are complex; this chapter gives an overview to provide a basis for further investigation and discovery.

EPIDEMIOLOGY

The earliest recorded writings related to cancer were made in the Edwin Smith Papyrus in Egypt around 1600 BC. Since that time and throughout recorded history, references are made to various malignancies of the bone and soft tissue that were attributed to sources as varied as vital humors and parasites. Cancer affects approximately 9.6 million Americans, and a total of 1.4 million new cancer diagnoses and 570,000 cancer-related deaths are expected in the United States in the year 2005. For persons younger than the age of 85, cancer is the leading cause of death in the United States and has been since 1999. Although overall mortality rates from cancer have declined in both men and women, the rate of decline in deaths due to heart disease has been much more rapid (Fig. 13.1).

Between 1995 and 2001 the cancer incidence rates in men stabilized, whereas incidence rates in women continued to increase by 0.3% per year from 1987 through 2001. Cancers differ in men and women by both type and incidence.

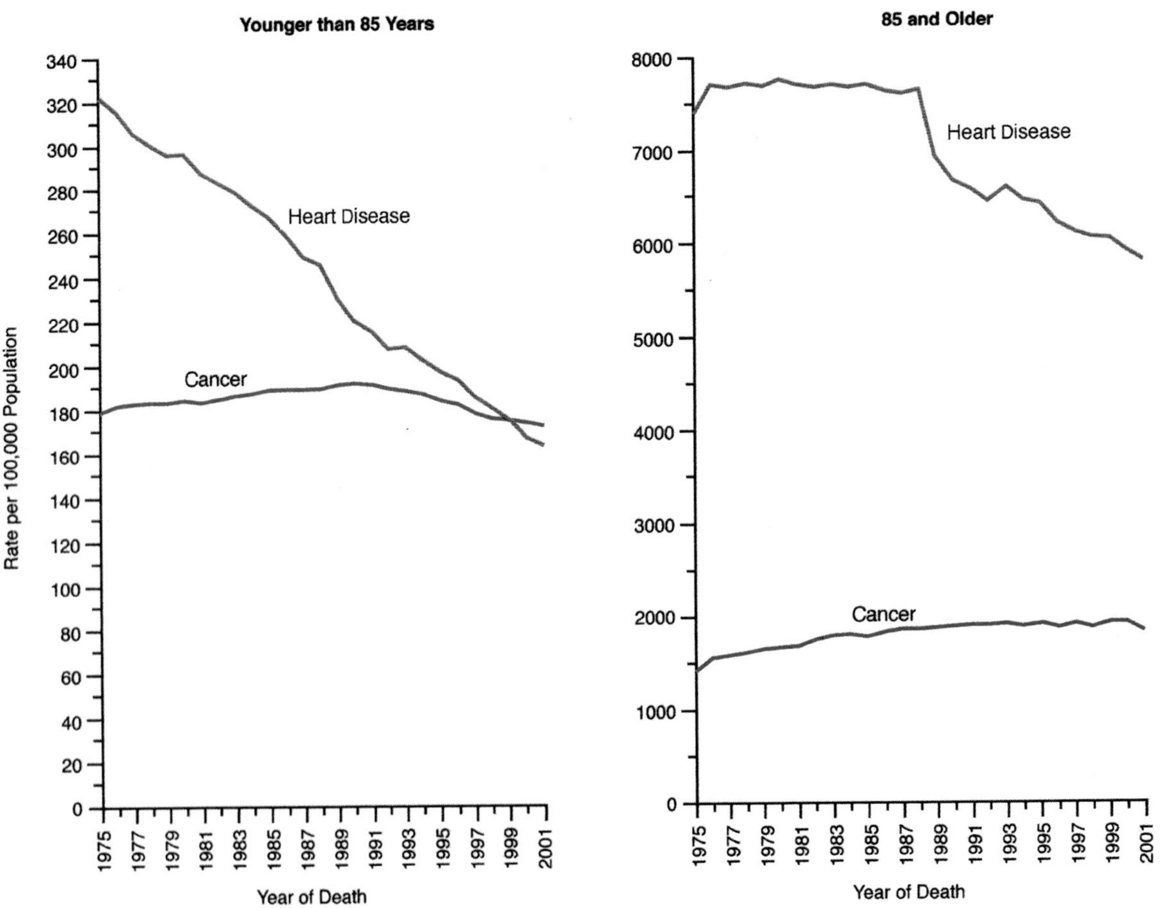

FIGURE 13.1 Age-adjusted death rates from cancer and heart disease. (Jemal A, Murray T, Ward E, et al. Cancer Statistics, 2005. *CA Cancer J Clin.* 2005;55;10.)

The most common cancers in men by incidence are prostate (33%), lung and bronchus (13%), and colon and rectum (10%). In women, the most common cancers by incidence are breast (32%), lung and bronchus (12%), and colon and rectum (11%). In both men and women, lung and bronchial cancers continue to account for the largest number of cancer-related deaths (31% men; 27% women). This is followed by prostate cancer in men (10%) and breast cancer in women (15%) accounting for the second most common histologies resulting in death. Colon and rectal cancer remains the third most common cause of cancer-related deaths in both men (10%) and women (10%) (Table 13.1). Although the overall incidence of cancer, as well as mortality due to cancer, decreased over the decade between 1994 and 2004, for several tumor types there has been either an increase in incidence or relatively little change over that time. For example, melanoma of the skin increased in incidence among men from 3% to 5% and among women from 3% to 4% between 1994 and 2004. The incidence of thyroid cancer doubled from 1% to 2% between 1994 and 2004. For women, in whom thyroid cancer occurs more frequently than in men (3:1), the incidence increased from 1.7% to 2.9% during the decade. Despite the decline in incidence and associated death among the top three cancer types in both men and women, cancer continues to pose a significant cost to the United States in both human and financial terms.

In 2003, cancer cost the United States an estimated $189.5 billion. Roughly one third of these costs were due to direct medical costs, and more than two thirds were related to nonmedical costs, including lost productivity and lost workdays. The Centers for Disease Control and Prevention (CDC) has estimated that cancer screening and early detection could reduce colorectal cancer deaths by 30%, breast cancer deaths by 16%, and cervical cancer deaths by 60%. Further, it is estimated that in the year 2003 more than 180,000 cancer deaths were due to the consequences of tobacco use. Although the connection between cigarette smoking and lung cancer is an obvious and well-established one, smoking plays a role in approximately 30% of all other cancer deaths (e.g., kidney, oral, bladder).

Major efforts are under way in cancer prevention. Some causative agents, such as tobacco, are obvious. Other factors that influence the development of cancer include genetic predisposition, diet and exercise, and environmental factors. For several cancer types, environmental influences have a complex interaction with other known and unknown factors leading to the development of the disease. For example, chronic hepatitis (both hepatitis B and hepatitis C) increases the incidence of hepatocellular carcinoma, but not all patients with hepatocellular carcinoma have chronic hepatitis, and not all patients with chronic hepatitis develop hepatocellular carcinoma. The relationship of cervical cancer to human papillomavirus (HPV) infection is well established. Estimates for the impact of screening demonstrate that reducing the transmission of HPV could have a significant impact on reducing the incidence of cervical cancer. Sun exposure [or artificial ultraviolet (UV) light exposure] influences the incidence of melanoma skin cancer; however, melanoma can develop in patients without a significant history of sun or UV exposure. Although some genetic factors, such as mutations in the *BRCA1* or *BRCA2* genes, significantly increase the risk of developing breast cancer, the

TABLE 13.1

THE TEN LEADING CANCER TYPES FOR THE ESTIMATED NEW CANCER CASES AND DEATHS, BY GENDER, FOR THE UNITED STATES IN 2005

Males		Females	
Cancer	Incidence	Cancer	Incidence
ESTIMATED NEW CASES*			
Prostate	232,090 (33%)	Breast	211,240 (32%)
Lung and bronchus	93,010 (13%)	Lung and bronchus	79,560 (12%)
Colon and rectum	71,820 (10%)	Colon and rectum	73,470 (11%)
Urinary bladder	47,010 (7%)	Uterine corpus	40,880 (6%)
Melanoma of the skin	33,580 (5%)	Non-Hodgkin lymphoma	27,320 (4%)
Non-Hodgkin lymphoma	29,070 (4%)	Melanoma of the skin	26,000 (4%)
Kidney and renal pelvis	22,490 (3%)	Ovary	22,220 (3%)
Leukemia	19,640 (3%)	Thyroid	19,190 (3%)
Oral cavity and pharynx	19,100 (3%)	Urinary bladder	16,200 (2%)
Pancreas	16,100 (2%)	Pancreas	16,080 (2%)
All sites	**710,040 100%**	**All sites**	**662,870 100%**
ESTIMATED DEATHS			
Lung and bronchus	90,490 (31%)	Lung and bronchus	73,020 (27%)
Prostate	30,350 (10%)	Breast	40,410 (15%)
Colon and rectum	28,540 (10%)	Colon and rectum	25,750 (10%)
Pancreas	15,820 (5%)	Ovary	16,210 (6%)
Leukemia	12,540 (4%)	Pancreas	15,980 (6%)
Esophagus	10,530 (4%)	Leukemia	10,030 (4%)
Liver and intrahepatic bile duct	10,330 (3%)	Non-Hodgkin lymphoma	9,050 (3%)
Non-Hodgkin lymphoma	10,150 (3%)	Uterine corpus	7,310 (3%)
Urinary bladder	8,970 (3%)	Multiple myeloma	5,640 (2%)
Kidney and renal pelvis	8,020 (3%)	Brain and other nervous system	5,480 (2%)
All sites	**295,280 100%**	**All sites**	**275,000 100%**

*Excludes basal and squamous cell skin cancers and in situ carcinoma except urinary bladder. Estimates are rounded to nearest 10.
(Adapted from Jemal A, Murray T, Ward E, et al. Cancer statistics, 2005. *CA Cancer J Clin* 2005;55:1.)

majority of patients with breast cancer have no such germline mutations. More work is needed to understand the complex interactions of genetics and environment on the cell to better identify avoidable risk factors. This may help to prevent the development of cancer.

ETIOLOGY

At its most basic, cancer can be defined as abnormal cell growth. Often described as a foreign invader in the body, it is more accurate to think of cancer as the body's own cellular growth machinery gone wrong. Throughout history, a variety of theories emerged in an attempt to explain the findings of abnormal tissue growth and invasion. Hippocrates ascribed the formation of cancer to an excess of black bile (one of the four humors or body fluids) collecting in various body sites. This theory was unchallenged through the Middle Ages. In the 18th century, John Hunter was a proponent of the concept that cancer derived from the lymph system. The notion was that tumors arose from lymph, which is constantly expressed by the blood.

In the 19th century, Yohans Mueller dispelled the lymph theory by demonstrating that cancer was made up of cells. However, Mueller did not believe that cancer arose from normal cells but rather from "budding elements" (blastema) that arose between normal tissues. This theory was later rejected by Mueller's student Rudolph Virchow, who demonstrated that all cells, including cancer cells, had their origin from other cells. Virchow proposed that chronic irritation led to the formation of cancer and that cancers could spread through tissues like a fluid. The idea that cancer resulted from irritation and trauma persisted into the 20th century.

Modern thinking recognizes a series of important events that are required for a cell to become cancerous and to grow, invade, and metastasize. Hanahan and Weinberg described six important capabilities that a cell or a group of cells must acquire to be capable of growing, invading, and metastasizing and thus becoming a cancer. These six properties are as follows (Fig. 13.2):

1. Self-sufficiency in growth signals
2. Insensitivity to antigrowth signals
3. Evading apoptosis
4. Limitless replicative potential
5. Sustained angiogenesis
6. Tissue invasion and metastases

Each of these capabilities is placed in the perspective of current research efforts in the sections that follow.

CANCER BIOLOGY

The basic unit of tissues and organs is the cell. The control of cell growth and differentiation is the focal point in understanding the processes involved in malignant transformation. Cells normally grow, divide, perform necessary functions to maintain homeostasis, and die in a programmed fashion throughout most tissues and organs. A cancer cell is one that has alterations in this carefully controlled program that lead to the phenotype of cancer. Hanahan and Weinberg's model describes four of the six functional capabilities, which directly relate to changes within the cell itself. These are the acquired ability for self-sufficient growth, insensitivity to antigrowth signals, ability to evade apoptosis, and limitless replicative potential. The other two functional capabilities—sustained angiogenesis and tissue invasion and metastases—involve not only changes within the individual cancer cell but also in the interaction and relationship with other host elements.

Oncogenes and Tumor Suppressor Genes

The ability of a cell to become self-sufficient in its growth and no longer rely on the normal temporal sequences of programmed cell growth is often the result of mutations in the genes involved in growth regulation and control. Activating mutations of protooncogenes create oncogenes. For example, a point mutation of a single nucleotide in the *ras* gene can result in cell-transforming activity. Approximately one half of human colon cancers have a mutation in the *ras* oncogene.

The three Ras proteins (h-, k-, and n-ras) are members of a large superfamily of Ras-related proteins that share significant structural homology as well as GTPase activity. All known *ras* genes include an identical nine amino acid domain in the N-terminal half of the protein. This undergoes a conformational shift when Ras binds to GTP. These Ras-related proteins function as molecular switches, involved in the control of a variety of cellular functions including growth, organization, and transport. The biologic activity of

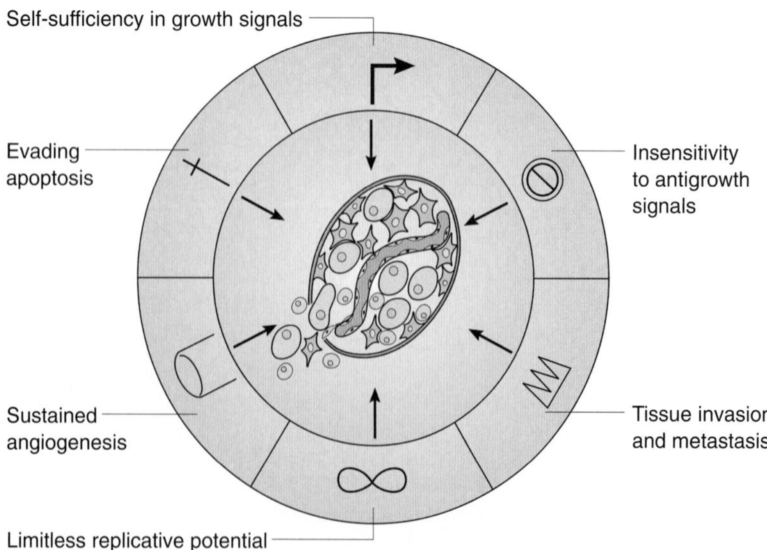

FIGURE 13.2 Acquired capabilities of cancer. (After Hanahan D, Weinberg R. The hallmarks of cancer. *Cell* 2000;100:57.)

Ras is controlled by a number of factors known as guanine nucleotide exchange factors that promote the formation of the active GTP-bound state (e.g., SOS), and the GTPase-activating proteins (e.g., NF1-GAP) that promote formation of the inactive GDP-bound state. Structural mutations involving codons 12, 13, and 61 result in mutant ras proteins that lack this GTPase activity. These oncogenic ras proteins are locked in the active GTP-bound conformation, leading to constitutive activation of downstream targets. This can be thought of as an "on-off" switch for cell growth that is locked in the "on" position due to the mutation in the *ras* oncogene. In addition to stimulating growth signals, mutant Ras proteins can also facilitate survival signals within the cell allowing the cell to evade programmed cell death.

Oncogenes can also be activated through chromosomal rearrangements known as translocations that involve the transfer of one segment of a chromosome to another. The resulting shift in position of genes can change the way in which those genes are regulated. An example of this is the Philadelphia chromosome that appears in chronic myelogenous leukemia (CML). This chromosomal rearrangement results when the small c-*abl* proto-oncogene is translocated from chromosome 9 to the small *bcr* locus on chromosome 22. The result of this creates the small *bcr/abl* oncogene. This oncogene leads to an increase in tyrosine-kinase activity and therefore downstream signaling in the cell leading to uncontrolled cell growth.

Oncogenes also affect the development of familial endocrine tumors. An activating mutation of the RET proto-oncogene on chromosome 10 causes the development of medullary thyroid cancer in patients suffering from multiple endocrine neoplasia (MEN) 2a and MEN 2b. Patients with MEN 2 uniformly develop medullary thyroid cancer, and many also develop other tumors (such as adrenal pheochromocytomas) due to the constitutive activation of this gene.

Another class of genetic change that predisposes to cancer, both sporadically and within inherited cancer syndrome families, is inactivating mutations of tumor suppressor genes. Tumor suppressor genes typically code for proteins that play an important role in cellular growth control. When these genes are mutated growth dysregulation can occur. In the familial setting, these mutations inactivate one allele of a growth control gene in the germline. An inactivating mutation of the second allele of the gene in a susceptible cell causes loss of the growth control function in that cell, contributing to the development of the characteristic tumor. Tumors that develop sporadically due to mutations of tumor suppressor genes require accumulation of inactivating changes in both copies of the gene within a single cell. This explanation of tumor suppressor genes is known as the Knudsen hypothesis. Examples of this include mutations of the *BRCA1* or *BRCA2* genes, which together account for 75% of familial breast cancer cases. *BRCA1* acts as a tumor suppressor gene in that mutation of one copy followed by inactivation of the second copy of the gene in a cell results in malignant transformation. Another examples of tumor suppressor genes are the *MEN1* gene that is inactivated in MEN type 1, the *vHL* gene inactivated in von Hippel-Lindau syndrome, and the adenomatous polyposis coli (*APC*) gene locus that can lead to the development of colorectal cancers when mutated.

Myc Regulation of Cellular Differentiation

In human neoplasia, many components of the dedifferentiated phenotype appear to involve regulation by helix-loop-helix motif (HLH) proteins. At least three major pathways have been identified that impact on HLH-regulated cellular differentiation. These include amplification/overexpression of the c-*myc* protooncogene, overexpression of Id transcriptional repressors, and activation of Notch signaling. With respect to Myc, the c-*myc* protooncogene is amplified in many human tumors, including lung cancer, breast cancer, cervical cancer, and ovarian cancer. In addition, increased expression of c-*myc* is noted in up to one third of breast and colon carcinomas. c-*myc* appears to represent a central switch through which a number of oncogenic pathways including BCR-ABL, b-catenin, and c-*src* converge to stimulate neoplasia (Fig. 13.3). c-*myc* impacts many cellular events relevant to neoplasia including proliferation, apoptosis, adhesion, immortalization, and differentiation. These effects appear to be mediated primarily through formation of heterodimers with the class IV HLH factor Max, leading to activation of Myc target genes (Fig. 13.4). Both during normal development as well as during neoplastic transformation, Myc/Max heterodimers appear to inhibit expression of differentiation-related genes.

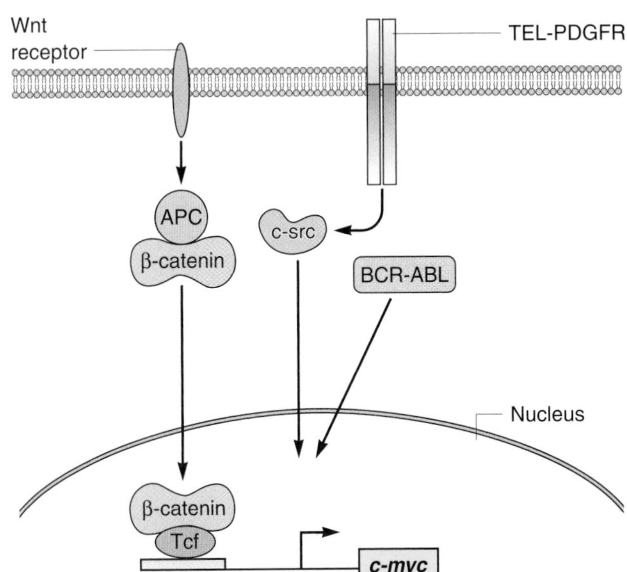

FIGURE 13.3 The *c-myc* gene is a central oncogenic switch for oncogenes and the tumor suppressor adenomatous polyposis coli (APC). The APC tumor suppressor protein mediates the degradation of β-catenin. The Wnt oncoprotein is shown activating its receptor, which results in the stabilization of free β-catenin, which sustains activating mutations in human cancers; β-catenin is a cofactor for the transcription factor Tcf. Tcf activates *c-myc* expression through specific DNA binding sites. The oncogenic fusion protein TEL-PDGFR hypothetically activates *c-src*, as does native PDGFR, resulting in the activation of *c-myc*. The BRC-ABL oncoprotein likewise requires *c-myc* for its activity. (After Dang CV. *c-Myc* target genes involved in cell growth, apoptosis, and metabolism. *Mol Cell Biol.* 1999;19:1.)

Inhibition of Differentiation by Notch Signaling

Another major pathway influencing HLH-regulated cellular differentiation involves the Notch signaling pathway. Notch signaling appears to play a critical role in regulating cellular differentiation during both normal development and during malignant transformation. The pathway is highly conserved, with homologous components in *Caenorhabditis elegans*, *Drosophila*, zebrafish, mice, and humans (Table 13.2).

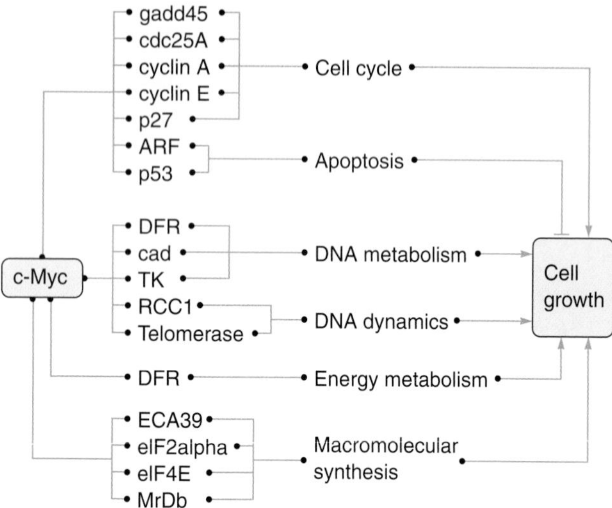

FIGURE 13.4 Links between c-Myc, selected putative target genes, cellular functions, and cell growth. The diagram illustrates the complexity of the connections between c-Myc and its putative target genes, which are shown clustered according to their functions. The various cellular functions cooperate to promote cell growth. It should be noted that this diagram does not reflect the controversies over the authentication of the various target genes. (After Dang CV. c-Myc target genes involved in cell growth, apoptosis, and metabolism. *Mol Cell Biol.* 1999;19:1.)

Four human Notch family members have been identified. Notch proteins are transmembrane receptors containing extracellular tandem epidermal growth factor (EGF)-like repeats as well as three Lin/Notch repeats that function in ligand binding and Notch activation. As transmembrane receptors, Notch proteins are unique in apparently lacking any enzymatic activity. Instead, Notch proteins undergo proteolytic cleavage on activation by binding to DSL ligands (e.g., Delta, Serrate, Lag-2). Recent data suggest that proteolytic cleavage of Notch may be accomplished by g-secretase, an enzyme also responsible for proteolytic production of b-amyloid from amyloid precursor protein. Following proteolytic cleavage, the Notch intracellular domain (Notch-IC) is released to interact with a number of cytoplasmic and nuclear proteins, including CSL proteins such as *Drosophila Suppressor of Hairless* and mammalian CBF-1. Interactions between Notch-IC and CSL proteins results in transcriptional activation of Hairy/Enhancer of Split (HES) class VI HLH protein. Once bound to DNA, HES proteins recruit a corepressor known as Groucho, thereby preventing expression of a number of cell lineage–specific class II bHLH proteins, including MyoD, neurogenin 3, and achaete-scute homologues (Fig. 13.5).

Notch signaling therefore represents a mechanism to prevent lineage-specific cellular differentiation. During development, this function plays a critical role in lateral inhibition as well as in boundary formation. Notch signaling is also implicated in various forms of neoplasia. Notch-IC is capable of transforming rat kidney cells in cooperation with adenoviral E1A and substitutes for activated ras in this assay. Notch receptors and ligands are up-regulated in human cervical cancer, and activating translocations involving Notch family members have been identified in acute T-cell leukemia. Notch also appears to be required for immortalization of B lymphocytes by Epstein-Barr virus and represents a site for activating integration by the mouse mammary tumor virus. Additional studies have identified an important role of the Notch target gene HES-1 in regulating differentiation status in non–small cell lung cancer.

Telomerase and Cell Immortalization/Senescence

Senescence is the process during which a normal cell ages and dies. This process is controlled, in part, by specialized heterochromatic structures at the ends of eukaryotic chromosomes called telomeres that function to stabilize and protect the chromosome. During normal somatic cell replication, telomeres become progressively shorter with each cell division, resulting in chromosome instability. It has been postulated that the shortening of telomeres represents a checkpoint

TABLE 13.2

CONSERVED COMPONENTS OF THE NOTCH SIGNALING PATHWAY

	Caenorhabditis elegans	Drosophila	Mammals
Notch receptors	Lin-12 Glp-1	Notch	Notch1 Notch3 Notch2 Notch4
Extracellular ligands (DSL proteins)	Lag-2 Apx-1	Delta	Delta-1 Delta-1 Delta-like 1 (Dll-1) Delta-like 3 (Dll-3)
		Serrate	Jagged1 (Serrate1) Jagged2 (Serrate2)
Intracellular effectors	Lag-1	Suppressor of hairless [Su(H)] Deltex	CBF-1/RBP-J_K Deltex NF_KB
Target genes		Enhancer of split [E(spl)] bHLH Groucho	HES (Hairy/enhancer of split) bHLH TLE
Processing molecules	SUP-17	Kuzbanian	Kuzbanian
Modifiers		Fringe	Lunatic fringe Manic fringe Radical fringe
		Numb	Numb Numb like
		Disheveled	Disheveled 1,2,3

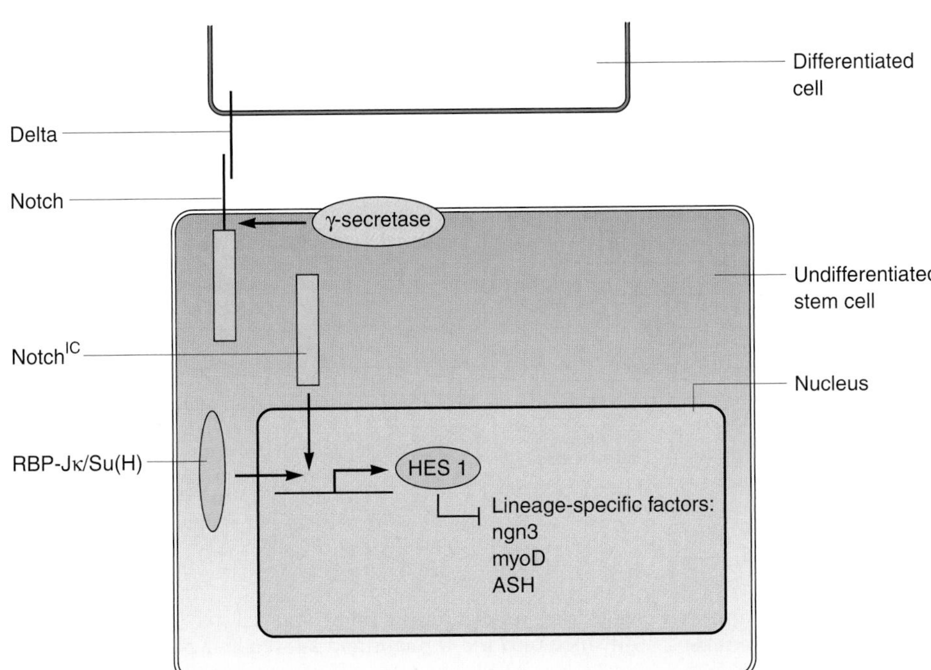

FIGURE 13.5 Notch signaling inhibits lineage-specific cellular differentiation. Ligands presented by adjacent differentiated cells lead to Notch receptor activation. Following intramembrane cleavage of Notch by g-secretase, the intracellular domain of Notch (Notch-IC) translocates to nucleus and cooperates with RBP-Jk (mammalian homologue of *Drosophila Suppressor of Hairless*) to induce HES1. HES1 represses transcription of lineage-specific transcription factors, including neurogenin3, myoD, and the achaete-scute homologue (ASH). Activation of Notch signaling thereby maintains cells in an undifferentiated, stem cell–like state.

mechanism by which cellular senescence is signaled in normal replicating cell populations.

Telomerase is an RNA-dependent DNA polymerase that stabilizes telomeres by synthesizing the six oligonucleotide repeat TTAGGG. This stabilization can allow indefinite replication and thus "cell immortalization." Although inactive in most somatic cells, telomerase remains activated in germ cells and lymphocytes. A unique characteristic of the cancer cell is immortality with the ability to divide repeatedly without undergoing normal cellular senescence. A correlation between telomerase and cancer has recently been documented by the detection of telomerase activity in a high percentage of primary human malignancies including cancer of the lung, colon, breast, and prostate. By remaining in the activated state, telomerase may contribute to the uncontrolled replicative capacity of the cancer cell. This finding has stimulated much discussion of the potential diagnostic, prognostic, and therapeutic implications of telomerase in the management of cancer.

Cell Survival/Programmed Cell Death

Virtually all cell populations are controlled through a balance of cell survival and cell death. Under certain conditions, such as terminal differentiation, growth factor deprivation, or DNA damage, survival signals to the cell are overtaken by death signals. Cell death can occur in a variety of forms, but the most common forms of cell death are necrosis and apoptosis. Necrotic cell death takes place primarily from noxious stimuli to the cell due to chemical or heat exposure, ischemia, or other insults. In contrast, apoptosis, or programmed cell death, occurs via a complex, genetically determined process. Apoptosis is a continual process in many normal as well as altered cell populations. For instance, during embryogenesis, organ formation occurs through a series of remolding events that include apoptosis. Apoptosis is also an active process in many disease states. Following myocardial infarction, induction of apoptosis can occur in the damaged cardiac muscle cells.

The process of apoptosis is described as a cascade of events, each mediated by intracellular proteins, ultimately leading to apoptotic cell death. After receiving a cell death stimulus, induction of genes that promote apoptosis occurs, thereby shifting the intercellular balance toward proteins with proapoptotic activity. Two of the best studied apoptotic genes are *Bcl-2* and *Bax*. Normally, the levels of antiapoptotic *Bcl-2* allow for continued cell survival. During the apoptotic state, *Bcl-2* levels are down-regulated shifting the balance toward proapoptotic proteins such as *Bax*. Downstream regulators of the apoptotic cascade are recruited including endonucleases, which cleave chromatin, resulting in nuclear fragmentation. This results in the formation of apoptotic bodies and other morphologic characteristics of apoptosis such as cell shrinkage and loss of contact with adjacent cells. In contrast, necrotic cell death is characterized by cellular swelling and ultimate rupture of the cell membrane. Just as apoptosis is active in embryogenesis and the molding of organ structure and function, it is also important in disease states such as cancer. In general, cancer cells that are resistant to cell death have altered their balance of apoptotic regulators. For instance, cancer cells that are resistant to conventional therapies such as radiation and chemotherapy often have increased levels of antiapoptotic proteins such as Bcl-2. To change the balance toward apoptotic cell death, some newer therapies attempt to upregulate pro-apoptotic proteins such as Bax or conversely down-regulate antiapoptotic proteins such as Bcl-2.

In addition to the induction of apoptosis by these proteins, programmed cell death can also occur via recognition events of the immune system. Specifically, the Fas antigen (CD-95, APO-1) is a cell surface protein of the tumor necrosis factor (TNF) family. When stimulated by its ligand (FasL) under certain conditions, Fas-bearing cells can undergo apoptotic cell death. This is a possible mechanism of cytotoxic T-cell–and natural killer cell–mediated death as well as other autoimmune responses.

Abnormal Growth Regulation in Cancer

Transformation from the normal phenotype to invasive malignancy appears to involve a loss of normal tumor suppressive and growth inhibitory responses as well as the acquisition of

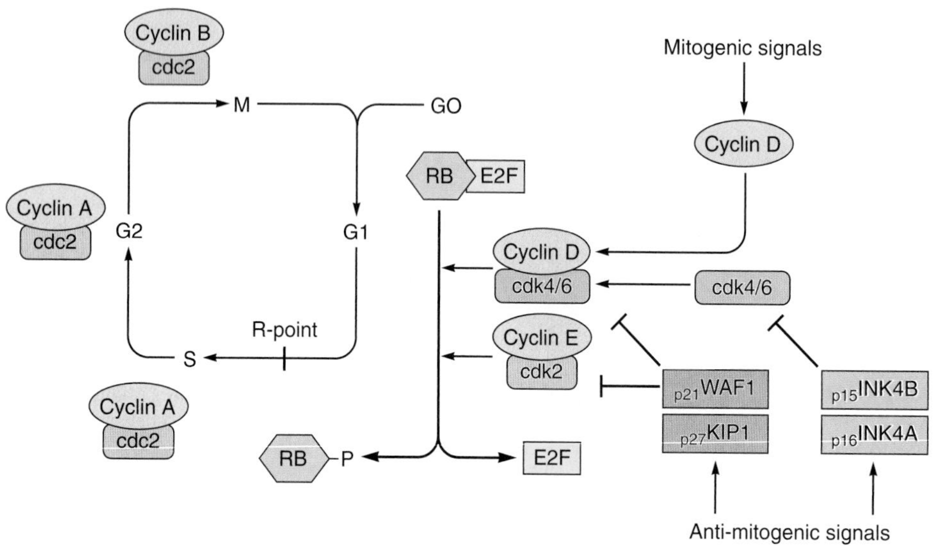

FIGURE 13.6 The cell cycle clock machinery. G0, M, G1, S, and G2 refer to the quiescence, mitosis, first gap, DNA synthesis, and second gap phases of the cell cycle, respectively. The restriction point (R-point) is shown preceding S phase entry. RB and RB-p represent unphosphorylated and hyperphosphorylated forms of the retinoblastoma protein. (After Lundberg AS, Weinberg RA. Control of the cell cycle and apoptosis. *Eur J Cancer* 1999;35:531.)

inappropriate proliferative signals. The presence of inappropriate proliferative signals has been well-documented in most malignancies and includes overexpression of peptide growth factors [transforming growth factor β (TGF-β), amphiregulin, heparin-binding EGF] and of growth factor receptors (e.g., HER2/neu). Alternatively, there may be mutational activation of the signal transduction pathways for the growth factors (e.g., *ras* and *src* oncogenes), activation of oncogenes that are directly involved in stimulating progression of the cell cycle regulation (*myc, cyclin D1,* etc.), or inactivation of genes that provide checkpoint control on cell cycle progression (e.g., the retinoblastoma gene *p53*).

Cell Cycle Regulation in Cancer

The cell cycle involves cellular events controlling replication of chromosomal DNA during the S phase and the separation of replicated chromosomes during cell division (mitosis or meiosis, M phase). The cell cycle is an indispensable process for survival of an organism and is highly conserved throughout evolution. The S phase and M phase are separated by gap periods, or G phases. The G1 phase precedes the S phase and the G2 phase precedes the M phase (Fig. 13.6). G0 describes cells that are in a nonreplicating, quiescent state. G0 cells are often differentiated cells that may be metabolically active, but are not involved in the process of cellular replication. The cell has mechanisms for responding to extracellular signals to recruit G0 cells into the cell cycle.

The process of cell cycle progression is tightly regulated. The factors responsible for advancing cell cycle progression were initially described in yeast and in amphibian eggs. Cyclins were discovered as proteins that oscillated during specific periods of the cell cycle. Subsequent work led to the identification of the catalytic partners of the cyclins, called cyclin-dependent kinases (CDKs). Specific sets of cyclins with their partner CDKs drive progression through specific periods of the cell cycle (Fig. 13.7). Mistakes in DNA replication or in chromosomal segregation are detected and prevented from propagation. This function, termed cell cycle checkpoint control, involves regulation of the levels and activities of the cyclins and CDKs and also involves the regulation of programmed cell death (apoptosis).

Quiescent cells may be recruited to the cell cycle by mitogenic stimulation (e.g., growth factor exposure). Normal cells depend on exogenous mitogenic stimulation only during the first two thirds of the G1 phase. At this two-thirds point, also called the restriction (R) point, the cell may commit itself to advance into the S phase and subsequent phases of the cell cycle (Fig. 13.8). The retinoblastoma protein (pRB) is the molecular switch that controls passage through the R point. Unphosphorylated or hypophosphorylated pRB blocks R point transition, whereas phosphorylation of pRB prevents it from blocking cell cycle progression.

Expression of a specific subset of the cyclins called D-type cyclins (D1, D2, and D3) is increased in early to mid-G1 in response to mitogenic signals. The D-type cyclins assemble with their catalytic partners, CDK4 and CDK6, and the cyclin D/CDK complex enters the cell nucleus where it becomes phosphorylated by a CDK-activating kinase (CAK). A critical function of the cyclin D–dependent kinases is the phosphorylation of the Rb protein. Growth factor activation of Ras signaling and the MAPK cascade induces transcription of the cyclin D1 gene, decreases the turnover of the cyclin D1 protein, and regulates cyclin D-CDK assembly. Expression of the D-type cyclins is dependent on continuous mitogenic stimulation. Progression through the mid to late G1 phase of the mammalian cell cycle is dependent on the cyclin D–dependent protein kinases.

Cyclin D–dependent kinases initiate the phosphorylation of Rb in mid-G1, then subsequent activation of the cyclin E/CDK2 complex leads to further phosphorylation of Rb on additional sites. Cyclin A–dependent CDK (CDK2) becomes

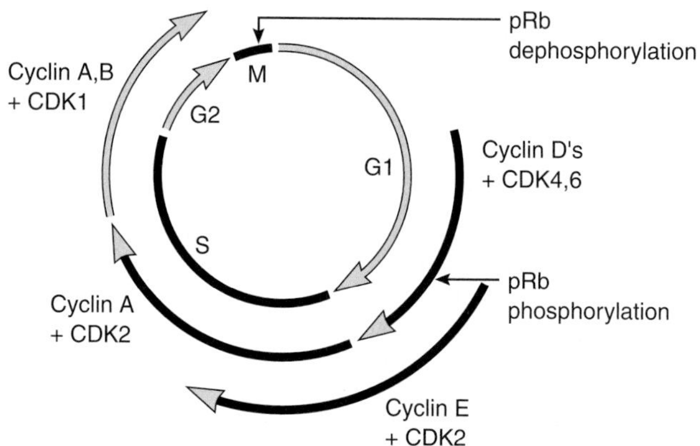

FIGURE 13.7 The cell cycle clock. This version of the cell cycle shows where the RB (pRB) protein is either phosphorylated or dephosphorylated to regulate cell cycle transit.

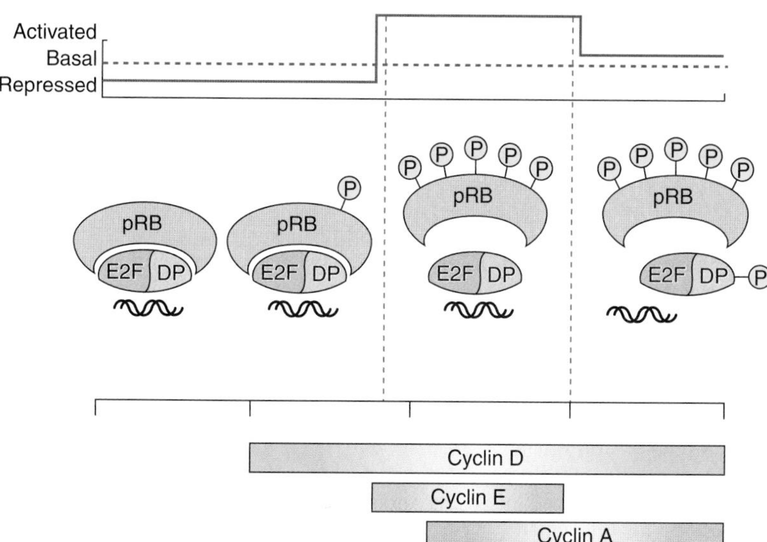

FIGURE 13.8 Interactions of the retinoblastoma protein (pRB). The interaction of pRB and E2F is regulated by cell cycle–dependent phosphorylation by specific cyclins acting with their partner cyclin-dependent kinases (CDKs). Underphosphorylated pRB forms stable complexes with E2F/DP heterodimers and this complex actively represses transcription. pRB becomes hyperphosphorylated in late G1, thereby releasing E2F/DP, which is transcriptionally active when unbound from pRB. Late in S-phase, DP becomes phosphorylated, thereby neutralizing the DNA-binding capability of the E2F/DP heterodimer. (After Kaelin WG Jr. Functions of the retinoblastoma protein. *Bioessays* 1999;21:950.)

activated during the S phase and cyclin B–dependent CDK (CDC2) becomes activated during G2 and M. These cyclin-dependent kinases help to maintain Rb in a hyperphosphorylated state until mitosis has been completed and Rb is returned to its hypophosphorylated state at the beginning of G1. Hypophosphorylated Rb inhibits the transcriptional activity of E2F protein family members. Hyperphosphorylation of Rb in late G1 phase disrupts its association with E2F family members, thereby enabling them to express their activity as transcription factors. The activation of the E2F transcription factor complex is required for the expression of a set of genes whose activities are required for S phase progression. These include gene products that regulate nucleotide metabolism and DNA synthesis, as well as cyclins E and A.

The activities of CDKs are governed by other proteins called CDK inhibitors (CKIs). There are two families of CKIs based on structure and their CDK targets. One class includes the INK4 proteins (inhibitors of CDK4), which specifically bind and inhibit the activities of CDK4 and CDK6. This family is composed of four such proteins ($p16^{INK4a}$, $p15^{INK4b}$, $p18^{INK4c}$, and $p19^{INK4d}$). The Cip/Kip family comprises the other family of CKIs. This family includes the proteins $p21^{Cip1}$, $p27^{Kip1}$, and $p57^{Kip2}$. The CKIs of the Cip/Kip family were originally thought to interfere with the activities of cyclin D–, cyclin E–, and cyclin A–dependent kinases. This view has now evolved with further data confirming that the Cip/Kip proteins are potent inhibitors of cyclin E– and cyclin A–dependent CDK2 activity; however, this family of CKIs appears to act as positive regulators of cyclin D–dependent kinases. Increased levels of cyclin D-CDK4 during the G1 phase results in sequestration of the Cip/Kip CKIs, thereby preventing them from associating with and inhibiting cyclin E– and cyclin A–dependent CDK2. Activated CDK2 catalyzes hyperphosphorylation of Rb and also triggers the proteolytic destruction of $p27^{Kip1}$.

In addition to transcriptional activation and induction of cyclin gene expression, proteolysis is a critical function in the regulation of the cell cycle. As mentioned previously, proteolytic destruction of $p27^{Kip1}$ is triggered during the S phase. Once the S phase has been initiated, the cell is no longer reliant on mitogenic signals or the D-dependent cyclins for progression through the remainder of the cell cycle. Cyclin E is degraded as cells progress through the S phase, cyclin A is degraded during G2, and cyclin B is degraded by the completion of the M phase to reset the system and thereby reestablish a period of mitogen dependence in the next G1 phase (Fig. 13.9).

Disruption of the growth suppressive function of Rb is a common event in cancer. This may occur as the result of mutational inactivation of Rb itself or because of the disruption of p16 function. Increased expression and activation of cyclin D and CDK4 (via amplification or transcriptional activation) are also common events in human cancer and result in the same type of inactivation of growth inhibitory function of Rb. Interestingly, complete loss of Cip/Kip function has not been observed in cancer nor have cyclin E gene amplification or mutations resulted in increased cyclin E–dependent CDK activity.

The CKIs appear to function as checkpoint controls to ensure that cell cycle progression occurs under the proper environmental conditions and that the proper intracellular

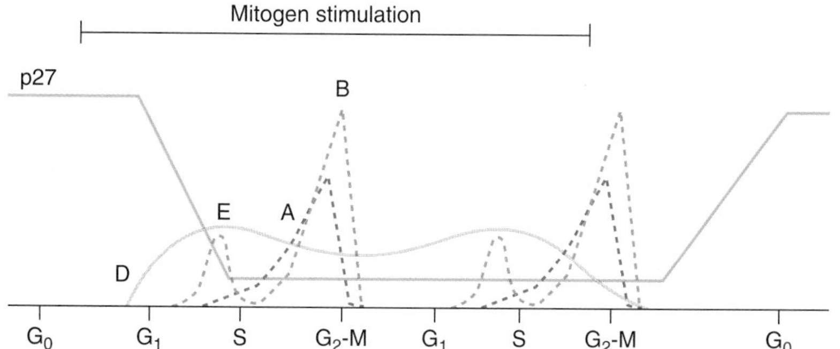

FIGURE 13.9 Fluctuations of cyclins and cyclin kinase inhibitors during the cell cycle. Cyclins E, A, and B undergo periodic oscillation during each cell cycle. In contrast, the D-type cyclins tend to remain elevated in cycling cells under the influence of growth stimuli. Levels of the inhibitor $p27^{Kip1}$ tend to remain high in quiescent cells but are decreased in proliferating cells. (After Sherr CJ. Cancer cell cycles. *Science* 1996; 274:1672.)

signaling has been completed prior to the initiation of DNA synthesis. Further checkpoints are the DNA damage and replication controls that block mitosis when DNA is damaged or DNA replication is incomplete. These checkpoint controls are essential for maintaining genomic stability, the failure of which allows cells to divide when DNA is damaged or DNA synthesis is incomplete or in the presence of faulty chromosomal segregation.

All cancer cells have abnormalities in one or more of the components of cell cycle control involved in G1 to S phase transition. In some cases, loss of Rb function itself is the event that releases the cells from extracellular signaling constraints. Mutational loss of Rb function occurs in the vast majority of retinoblastomas and less frequently in other tumor types such as lung cancers and soft tissue sarcomas. In the absence of functional Rb protein, E2F is active and there is no requirement for activation of cyclin D/Cdk4 to initiate DNA synthesis. Amplification of the cyclin D1 gene is common in several types of human tumors such as breast, head and neck, esophageal, and hepatic malignancies. Increased expression of cyclin D1 without gene amplification is common in colorectal cancer. Deletion of the $p16^{INK4a}$ gene is also common in human cancers, particularly in melanomas and in a subset of pancreatic cancers. Hereditary loss of $p16^{INK4a}$ function is associated with increased risk for melanoma and pancreatic cancer. All of the previous defects in cell cycle regulators result in loss of the same G1/S checkpoint control. It is rare for more than one of the previously mentioned defects to be identified in the same tumor.

Genomic Instability in Cancer

Genomic instability, with a high frequency of chromosomal loss and gain, genome doubling, and subtler genetic mutations, is a common characteristic of cancer cells. Genomic instability increases the chance of specific gene mutations that are ultimately responsible for the various phenotypes of cancer cells. Cancer cells acquire defects in the checkpoints that control normal mitosis, with its equal distribution of chromosomes into daughter cells and cytokinesis. Failure of this checkpoint may result in unequal distribution of chromosomes or failure to undergo cytokinesis, and either polyploidy (4N, 8N, etc.) or aneuploidy.

The tumor suppressor protein p53 plays a critical role in maintaining genomic stability. p53 function is required to initiate checkpoint-activated cell cycle arrest and programmed cell death in response to DNA damage. This function of p53 is necessary to ensure the integrity of the cellular genome by protecting it from the adverse effects of DNA damage. The p53 protein functions as an important transcription factor mediating expression of a variety of genes whose products may directly regulate growth arrest or apoptosis. Growth arrest induced by p53 may enable a cell to repair DNA that has been damaged. Alternatively, p53 also functions to induce apoptosis to prevent propagation of a cell lineage containing mutated DNA sequences.

Expression of p53 may be induced by either DNA damage or by inappropriate mitogenic signaling. An example of an important p53-responsive gene product involved in cell cycle arrest is the cyclin kinase inhibitor protein $p21^{Cip1}$. Several p53-responsive gene products appear to be involved in the apoptotic response. These include Bax, Fas/Apo, Killer/Dr5, and the redox regulator gene products known as PIGs (p53-induced genes). The expression of Mdm2 is also induced on activation of the p53 gene. Mdm2 is a negative feedback regulator of p53 whose function is to target p53 for rapid degradation. Interestingly, one of the two products of the *INK4a/ARF* locus, $p14^{ARF}$ inhibits the function of Mdm2, thereby stabilizing and activating p53 and promoting cell cycle arrest and apoptosis in response to inappropriate mitogenic signals. The other product of the *INK4a/ARF* locus is $p16^{Ink4a}$, the important inhibitor of CDKs 4 and 6, and a mediator of G1 cell cycle.

The protein product of the *Myc* proto-oncogene also regulates both cell proliferation and apoptosis in cell culture systems. *Myc* expression is capable of preventing cells from exiting the cell cycle and of promoting continuous cell cycle progression. Expression of *Myc* also inhibits differentiation in certain cell types. Similar to the situation in which inappropriately increased E2F triggers apoptosis, inappropriate *Myc* expression can also trigger apoptosis. Both increased E2F and *Myc* increase the expression of the ARF protein (p14 and p19), and as described previously, increased expression of ARF stabilizes p53, leading to both growth arrest and apoptosis.

There is a growing list of additional proteins that are involved in sensing and repairing DNA damage, or in ensuring correct chromosomal segregation during mitosis. Loss of function of these important genomic "caretaker" systems appears to be common in cancer cells, and this loss facilitates genomic instability with the accumulation of additional genetic lesions. The cumulative genetic mutations lead to tumor cells with selective advantages for aggressive biologic behavior including invasiveness and metastatic capacity, resistance to immunosurveillance, resistance to apoptosis, and the ability to resist cancer therapeutic interventions.

Loss of Growth Inhibitory Effects of TGF-β in Cancer

TGF-β regulation of epithelial cell proliferation is altered by transformation. Loss of responsiveness to the growth-inhibitory effects of TGF-β occurs in many cancer cell types, including pancreatic, breast, and colorectal carcinoma cells. Thus, loss of growth-inhibitory responses to TGF-β appears to be a common and important event that attends malignant transformation of epithelial cells (Fig. 13.10).

TGF-β Signaling Abnormalities in Cancer

The association of colorectal cancers, pancreatic carcinomas, and breast cancers with genetic lesions in the TGF-β signal transduction pathway underscores the importance of TGF-β in maintaining homeostasis in the digestive tract and in the breast. One of the mechanisms by which tumor cells become resistant to the growth inhibitory actions of TGF-β is through down-regulation or mutation of TGF-β type II receptor (TβRII). Loss of TGF-β receptor function causes cellular loss of negative growth regulation by TGF-β. Several studies have suggested that a decrease in expression or inactivation of TβRII is a key step for the neoplastic transformation of epithelial cells in both the breast and the colon. Activation of Ras protein, which occurs frequently in colorectal cancer, results in a decreased expression of the TβRII.

TβRII inactivation has been detected in a subgroup of colorectal carcinomas associated with the microsatellite instability or RER (replication error) phenotype identified in approximately 13% of all colorectal cancers. Recent studies have also confirmed the presence of TβRII mutations in an additional 15% of microsatellite stable (MSS) colon cancers and TGF-β signaling abnormalities distal to TβRII in an additional 55% of these MSS colon cancers. It is of interest and seemingly paradoxical that the subset of colorectal cancers that exhibit microsatellite instability (and TβRII mutations) tend to be

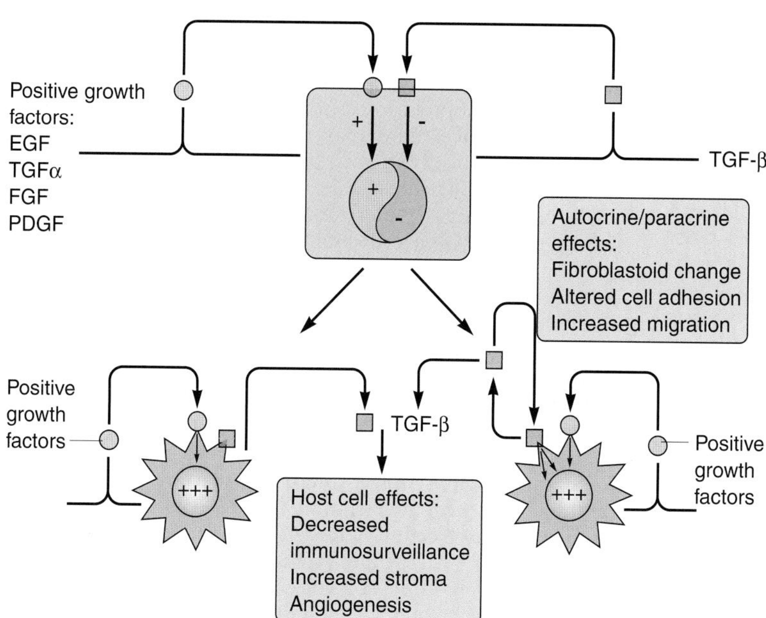

FIGURE 13.10 The effect of the transforming growth factor *β* TGF-*β* signaling pathway on cells is context-dependent. Normal cells respond to TGF-*β* with growth inhibition and TGF-*β* appears to function as a tumor suppressor under normal conditions. Although complete loss of the TGF-*β* receptors is expected to eliminate all autocrine (but not paracrine) effects of tumor-derived TGF-*β*, postreceptor mutations should not. Tumor cells often lose the ability to undergo growth arrest in response to TGF-*β*. Despite this loss of growth inhibitory effect, TGF-*β* autocrine effects on cell morphologic change and cell adhesion and cell migration (all likely to be advantageous for tumor cells) appear to be retained along with the paracrine effects.

proximal colon cancers and have a better prognosis (stage for stage) than the majority of sporadic colorectal cancers that do not share these genetic defects.

Mutational loss of function of TGF-*β* signal transduction proteins has been identified in human colorectal cancer. Madr2 (Smad2) mutation was observed in 4%, and DPC4 (Smad4) mutation has been reported in up to 30% of human colorectal cancers. Also, loss of heterozygosity (LOH) of Smad3 has been detected in two (one sporadic and one HNPCC) of 17 cancers examined. These types of mutations may have a significantly different phenotypic outcome as compared with that resulting from loss of the T*β*RII. Smad4 mutation has also been identified in familial juvenile polyposis, a syndrome characterized by a predisposition to hamartomatous polyps and gastrointestinal cancer. These studies suggest that disruption of Smad signaling may be involved in either the initiation or progression of certain cancers.

TGF-*β* as a Tumor Promoting Factor

There are several lines of evidence that TGF-*β* may actually promote malignant transformation and tumor progression for several different cell types and under selected circumstances. TGF-*β* expression tends to be increased in a wide variety of cancers (including colon cancer) relative to adjacent normal tissues. Transformation of cells with dominant oncogenes (e.g., Ha-*ras* or v-*src*) activates transcription of the TGF-*β*1 gene. Studies of human colorectal cancers have demonstrated that high-level expression of TGF-*β* in the primary tumor is associated with advanced stages and is an independent predictor of risk for recurrence and decreased survival.

There are several potential mechanisms for this tumor-promoting effect. For example, TGF-*β* may suppress tumor immunosurveillance. TGF-*β* exhibits growth-inhibitory effects on moderate to well-differentiated primary colon carcinomas but stimulates the proliferation and invasion of poorly differentiated and metastatic colonic carcinomas. Treatment with TGF-*β* can induce estrogen-independent tumorigenicity of human breast cancer cells. TGF-*β* treatment can also substitute for wounding as a promoter of fibrosarcomas in chickens infected with the Rous sarcoma virus.

Transformation of preinvasive epithelial neoplasm to the invasive phenotype with metastatic potential is characterized by several profound changes in gene expression and in cellular and tissue morphology. The changes in cellular morphology and tissue architecture can be observed histologically and are accompanied by dramatic changes in the behavior of the transformed cells. The metastatic phenotype is associated with the acquisition of fibroblastoid features and the ability of the cells to invade stroma and blood vessels. There is mounting evidence that autocrine TGF-*β* expression by tumor cells can play a major role in the epithelial-to-fibroblastoid conversion that accompanies malignant transformation in mammary cells and in keratinocytes. TGF-*β*1 overexpression enhanced progression of carcinogen-induced skin cancers toward the malignant spindle-cell phenotype in transgenic mice expressing high levels of TGF-*β* in the skin. The TGF-*β*–induced epithelial to mesenchymal transition in Ha-*ras* transformed mammary epithelial cells involves disrupted cell-cell adhesion and the loss of epithelial cell polarity in addition to causing the cells to become more spindle-shaped and invasive. The loss of cell polarity in response to TGF-*β* appears to be the result of a disruption of ZO-1 and F-actin proteins comprising the tight junctions in mammary epithelial cells.

There also is an important regulatory interaction between the TGF-*β* and cyclooxygenase-2 (COX-2) pathways. Forced overexpression of COX-2 in the nontransformed RIE-1 cells results in down-regulation of the T*β*RII, and forced overexpression of COX-2 in a human colon cancer cell line results in increased secretion of TGF-*β*1 from those cells. TGF-*β* synergistically enhances the expression of COX-2 in conditionally Ha-*ras* transformed RIE-1 cells, and the increase in COX-2 expression by TGF-*β* in the context of *ras* transformation occurs primarily through a marked increase in the stability of the COX-2 mRNA.

The predominant effect of TGF-*β* appears to be dependent on the context of the responding cell. Thus, the divergent effects of TGF-*β* in carcinogenesis may depend on the proliferative capacity and state of differentiation of the epithelial cell, both of which may be altered during the process of neoplastic transformation. Clearly, TGF-*β* signaling has an important tumor suppressive role; however, after transformation has occurred, TGF-*β* effects may be detrimental and may actually promote tumor cell survival, invasion, and metastasis. Recent work suggests that these effects may involve TGF-*β* regulation of COX-2 and other pathways that may contribute to tumor cell aggressiveness.

TUMOR HOST INTERACTIONS

There are many complex pathways within the tumor cell that allow it to express a phenotype different from that of normal replicating cells. There are important interactions between the tumor cell and surrounding normal cells that enhance the attributes normally ascribed to cancer. In the Hanahan and Weinberg six capability model, the two capabilities most involved in these tumor interactions are sustained angiogenesis and tissue invasion and metastasis. Both of these processes involve a carefully coordinated interplay between a variety of cell types, each influencing the others' growth and development.

Tumor Angiogenesis

The observation that tumors require the establishment of a vasculature to grow larger than several millimeters is one that was clearly elucidated by Judah Folkman in 1971. Since that time there has been a growing realization that tumors must develop a network of vessels to grow, invade, and metastasize. A variety of signals allow tumor cells to stimulate vessel ingrowth. One of the more commonly studied cytokines is vascular endothelial growth factor (VEGF). Many studies have linked the ability of a tumor to produce VEGF with its malignant potential. This has been shown in breast cancer, colon cancer, kidney cancer, as well as others. VEGF is actually a family of cytokines, which act on the endothelial cell through a variety of surface receptors. The most common VEGF isotypes (A, B, and C) act on predominantly three endothelial cell receptors (VEGF-R 1, 2, and 3). VEGF receptors 1 and 2 bind VEGF and act predominantly to modulate endothelial cell proliferation and maturation in blood vessels. VEGF-C, working through VEGF receptor 3, exerts its effects predominantly on the endothelial cells of the lymphoid system.

Several lines of evidence have demonstrated the importance of VEGF as a tumor derived factor for stimulating and recruiting a blood supply. Models have been developed that demonstrate the importance of VEGF in tumorigenesis. Using a transgenic mouse model of pancreatic islet carcinoma (RIP1-Tag2), Hanahan and colleagues demonstrated that five VEGF lineage genes are expressed in normal islets and throughout islet tumorigenesis. When this group produced an islet beta cell-specific knockout of VEGF-A, the resulting islets in these animals had reduced vascularity but retained their normal physiology. In RIP1-Tag2 mice in which most of the oncogene expressing cells had deleted the VEGF-A gene, both angiogenic switching and tumor growth were disrupted, as was the degree of neovessel formation. This elegant work demonstrates the crucial role of VEGF in angiogenesis. Although such experimental work is compelling, clinical data support this notion further.

A humanized mouse monoclonal antibody against VEGF (Bevacizumab, Avastin, Genentec, Inc.) has recently completed phase III clinical trails and has received Food and Drug Administration (FDA) approval based on its activity in patients with colon cancer. In a prospective randomized phase III trial in renal cancer, James Yang and his colleagues demonstrated that systemic administration of anti-VEGF antibody to patients with metastatic renal cell carcinoma resulted in a significant prolongation in the time to disease progression when compared with patients receiving a placebo. Herb Hurwitz and his colleagues combined anti-VEGF antibody with a three-drug chemotherapy regimen consisting of 5-fluorouracil (5FU), leucovorin and irinotecan for patients with metastatic colorectal carcinoma and compared this combination with the three-drug chemotherapy regimen alone. The addition of the anti-VEGF antibody to the standard chemotherapy regimen resulted in an improved response rate and an improved disease-free and overall survival. This clear relationship between blockade of factors known to induce tumor vasculature leading to antitumor effects seen clinically in patients underscores the importance of the angiogenic process in human tumors.

To gain a better understanding of the complex relationships between tumor cells and the surrounding stromal cells, including the endothelium, a basic understanding of the molecular processes involved in endothelial cell growth and differentiation is important. Indeed, regulation of vessel growth and proliferation is an important component of normal homeostatic mechanisms. Following embryogenesis and tissue formation, the growth of new blood vessels in normal tissues is carefully controlled and regulated. In addition to VEGF there are a number of other regulatory cytokines both initiators of vessel formation as well as inhibitors that are regulated in a careful balance. An understanding of this balance may allow a more informed selection of targets for future cancer therapies. In addition to VEGF, other stimulatory cytokines have been shown to play an important role in a tumor's ability to recruit a vasculature. Among these, acidic fibroblast growth factor (aFGF) and basic fibroblast growth factor (bFGF) as well as placental derived growth factors play important roles.

In addition to a careful balance of cytokines, integrin signaling also plays an important role in regulating angiogenesis. When quiescent blood vessels are compared to activated or actively proliferating blood vessels, the panel of expressed integrins differs. Integrins such as alphav $\beta3$, which plays an important role in endothelial cell adhesion to vitronectin (a component of the extra cellular matrix), is differentially expressed in the vasculature of certain tumors when compared to other histologies and to normal tissues. Endothelial cells differ in their expression of various surface proteins depending on the tissue in which they reside. Work by investigators such as Pasqualini and Arap has demonstrated the diversity of endothelial cells and underscores the important observation that not all endothelial cells are the same.

In landmark studies using phage display techniques, Pasqualini and Arap have demonstrated that endothelial cells have unique surface markers that define their differences based on their tissue of origin. These so-called endothelial cell zip codes may provide a unique target for delivering endothelial cell directed therapies. This diversity may also explain, in part, the differences in response rates of various tumors to different angiogenesis inhibitors.

A series of elegant experiments performed by Kalluri and his colleagues focused on the relationship of endothelial cell surface integrin expression to the response of those endothelial cells to the effects of various angiogenesis inhibitors. Kalluri showed that endothelial cells expressing alphav$\beta3$ responded to the collagen IV derivative tumstatin and not to endostatin. Conversely, endothelial cells expressing the integrin alpha5$\beta1$ responded to endostatin rather than tumstatin. This was confirmed in animals bearing tumors. This specificity for certain integrin profiles is a critical observation in choosing the appropriate angiogenesis inhibitor and may explain, in part, the early clinical results with this class of agents.

A host of counter-regulatory angiogenesis inhibitors have also been elucidated. These include thrombospondin 1, angiostatin, endostatin, and a series of collagen IV derivatives known as canstatin, arresten, and tumstatin. Table 13.3 lists some of these angiogenesis inhibitors; however, the field is rapidly growing and evolving and therefore any list must be considered representative rather than all-inclusive. The balance between proangiogenic factors and angiogenesis inhibitors was termed the "angiogenic switch" by Hanahan and Folkman. Tumors can activate this switch by changing the

TABLE 13.3

ENDOGENOUS NATURALLY OCCURRING ANGIOGENESIS INHIBITORS

Angiostatin/other plasminogen kringles	IP-10
Antithrombin (cleaved)	METH-1 and -2
Endostatin	MIG
Fibronectin fragments	p16
PEX	P53
16-kDa Prolactin	Canstatin
Prothrombin kringle-2	PEDF
Maspin	Platelet factor-4
Restin	Proliferin-related protein
Vasostatin	PSA
IL-1, -4, -10, -12, -18	Protamine
Arresten	Retinoic acid
IFNs	Soluble FGF receptor
TIMPs	TGF-β1
1,25-$(OH)_2$-vitamin D	TNF-α
2-Methoxyestradiol	Troponin I
Angiopoietin-2	TSP-1 and -2
EMAP-II	
gro-β	

EMAP, endothelial monocyte octivating polypeptide; FGF, fibroblast growth factor; IFNs, interferons; IL, interleukin; MIG, ; PSA, prostate-specific antigen; TGF, transforming growth factor; TIMPs, tissue inhibitor of metalloproteinases; TNF, tumor necrosis factor; TSP, thrombospondin.

relative balance between inducers and inhibitors. How this balance is altered is the subject of ongoing study.

An intriguing possibility is that naturally occurring angiogenesis inhibitors play a gatekeeper function by inhibiting the progression of premalignant lesions by preventing their ability to recruit a blood supply. Thrombospondin 1 (TSP-1) has been implicated as a putative regulator of such a process. Preclinical mouse models as well as studies of clinical samples have shown an inverse relationship between the level of TSP-1 expressed and the invasive potential of the tumor. This relationship has also been identified in cervical cancer specimens.

Both endostatin and tumstatin have also been implicated in such a gatekeeping role. A curious clinical observation is that patients suffering from Down syndrome have a distinctly lower incidence of the common solid tumors than the general population. As Down syndrome patients have lived longer, they have a much lower rate of lung, breast, and colon cancers. Down syndrome is caused by trisomy of chromosome 21, which is the location of the gene coding for collagen XVIII, the precursor of endostatin. Down syndrome patients have higher circulating levels of endostatin than the normal population, perhaps due to the extra copy of the collagen XVIII gene on the additional chromosome 21. Kalluri has postulated that these elevated levels of circulating endogenous angiogenesis inhibitors may function as endothelium-specific tumor suppressors. An attractive future strategy for tumor prevention might involve exogenous administration of these inhibitors or alternatively, administration of small molecules that raise the circulating levels of endogenous inhibitors thus decreasing the ability of noninvasive lesions from developing an invasive phenotype.

Tissue Invasion and Metastasis

Although the primary tumor can cause significant morbidity and even death, by far the majority of deaths due to cancer result from metastatic disease. Metastatic disease remains the most difficult component of cancer to treat and therefore a thorough understanding of the processes that lead to the ability of cancer cells to spread to and grow in distant sites is critical. In the past, much work focused on the complex process of metastasis was observational; however, new tools now make it possible to study the pathways involved at a molecular level.

For tumor cells to invade into surrounding tissue and gain access to the lymphatics and blood vessels, a number of changes must take place. The normal cell surface proteins, which mediate contact inhibition and allow for normal anchoring to the extracellular matrix (ECM), must be perturbed. Two classes of such proteins are the cell-cell adhesion molecules (CAMs) and the integrins.

One example of an important CAM is E-cadherin, a member of the calcium-dependent cadherin family. E-cadherin is expressed on epithelial cells and helps to mediate antigrowth signals between cells. E-cadherin forms bridges between cells and transmits antigrowth signals via contact with β-catenin in the cytoplasm and downstream signaling via Lef/Tcf transcription factor. Mutations in E-cadherin or β-catenin can result in the loss of antigrowth signals and contact inhibition leading to epithelial carcinomas.

A member of the immunoglobulin super family, N-CAM, is another example of a CAM that plays a pivotal role in preventing invasion and metastasis. Mutations in N-CAM can result in a change in isoform from an adhesive to a poorly adhesive phenotype. These mutations have been identified in small cell lung cancer and Wilms' tumor.

Integrins play a critical role in anchoring cells to the ECM. Different cell types rely on different integrins to perform this function. Successful interaction between an integrin and the ECM can suppress growth signals. Integrins are often made up of an α and β subunit. The switching between these subunits can result in differing phenotypes with respect to cell growth and invasion.

Beyond contact inhibition and anchorage dependence, cells must also shift in their ability to produce enzymes, which allow for the degradation of the basement membrane and ECM to allow invasion and migration. Differential expression of proteases can allow for tissue invasion and access to lymphatics and vessels, which can provide a conduit to distant organ sites.

Once a tumor cell loses contact inhibition and expresses proteases, there is no guarantee that it will be able to grow in a distant organ such as the lung or liver. In addition to surviving the trip to the distant site, it must be able to take up residence in the organ and grow. Not every tumor cell that successfully reaches a distant site will be able to multiply and grow successfully. Some organs do not readily allow for the growth of cells of certain histologies (e.g., colon cancer does not commonly metastasize to the kidney). In some very elegant experiments, Fidler has studied this "seed and soil" phenomenon.

Fidler and his group looked at the ability of orthotopically placed colon cancer cells implanted in the cecum of mice to effectively metastasize to other organs. When these cells were implanted in the cecum and normal mesenteric vascular anatomy drained the site through the mesenteric vein to the portal vein and into the liver, liver metastases were seen to develop in these animals. However, when Fidler rerouted the venous drainage from the colon by reimplanting the mesenteric vein into the renal vein, metastases did not develop in the kidney. Clearly, some growth factors were present in the target organ or cell surface interactions between the tumor cell and the cells of the target organ that allowed colon cancer to grow in the liver but not in the kidney. Such organ predilection for tumor metastases has also been observed clinically.

Ocular melanoma, melanoma that develops from the pigmented cells within the eye, can metastasize systemically. The most common site of metastases for ocular melanoma is the liver. In fact, the majority of patients with metastatic ocular melanoma present initially with isolated liver metastasis. There is no clear-cut anatomic drainage pattern from the eye to the liver. In fact, when liver metastases are successfully treated, ocular melanoma can grow in other sites, such as the lungs and subcutaneous tissues. However, the liver as a first site for the spread of ocular melanoma clearly indicates some "seed and soil" relationship that promotes the ability of these cells to grow in a specific site.

Other examples of specific sites for metastatic disease are more easily understood based on venous drainage. Colon cancers arising above the peritoneal reflection often metastasize to the liver consistent with the mesenteric venous drainage via the portal system. Rectal cancers below the peritoneal reflection, which are drained by the pudendal veins into the caval system, often metastasize first to the lungs.

Although much of the focus of understanding tumor invasion and metastasis has focused on the tumor cells themselves, there is increasing evidence that the host may play a facilitative role in the ability of cells to invade and metastasize. Kent Hunter and his group at the National Cancer Institute (NCI) have investigated the role of host genetics and tumor metastasis. Hunter's group observed that, although a typical tumor can shed millions of cells into the bloodstream daily, very few clinically relevant metastases are ultimately formed. Using transgenic mouse models, Hunter has demonstrated that tumor cells carrying mutations in key metastasis-associated genes may demonstrate the ability to metastasize in certain strains of mice while they are unable to metastasize in other strains despite their ability to form tumor nodules. Expression of genes that are important for the ability of tumor cells to metastasize has also been shown to be altered in the host tissues themselves. The hypothesis that particular genetic mutations or polymorphisms in the host may make one patient more prone to metastatic disease than another is an intriguing one that warrants further investigation. If such markers could be identified, then patients at higher risk for metastases could be treated with more aggressive adjuvant therapies following surgical resection. By contrast those patients without such a predisposition may do well with surgical resection of the primary lesion alone.

THE FUTURE OF CANCER THERAPY

Throughout the 20th century, the standard approaches for the treatment of cancer included surgical resection, radiation therapy, and chemotherapy. Although advances in specific technical applications and in combinations of therapies were made, these three broad modalities remained the foundation of therapeutic approaches. This section focuses on novel strategies for treating cancer that may serve to complement and in some cases replace the traditional paradigm of surgery, radiation, and chemotherapy.

Targeted Molecular Therapies

The explosion in information and the increase in our understanding of the basic pathways involved in the transformation of normal cells into invasive cancers have ushered in a new field of oncologic research. The concept behind molecular therapeutics is that a more thorough understanding of the alterations in specific pathways that result in the cancer phenotype may allow for the development of agents that either block a precancer phenotype or replace factors that inhibit the transformation to cancer. It could be argued that many standard chemotherapies work in this manner. Alkylating agents as well as antimetabolites indeed target specific structures such as DNA, which are critical for tumor cells to divide and proliferate. However, these agents for the most part do not distinguish between normal cells and tumor cells. The promise of molecular therapy is the ability to make such a distinction. The importance of this is obvious. By distinguishing normal cells from neoplastic cells, toxicity may be reduced and efficacy increased.

One example of this strategy is the development, application, and subsequent FDA approval of the agent imatinib (Gleevec). Imatinib is an inhibitor of the Bcr-Abl kinase and was initially developed as a treatment for Bcr-Abl-positive leukemias. Imatinib was also found to inhibit other receptors, which signaled through kinases such as PDGF-receptor as well as c-Kit. This observation lead to the application of imatinib to tumors beyond leukemias such as gastrointestinal stromal tumors (GISTs). The understanding of the importance of receptor signaling in the transformation of neoplastic cells allowed for the development of an agent that targeted these receptor kinases thus blocking their activity.

Additional receptor kinase inhibitors have been developed against other receptors that have been shown to play an important role in cancer invasion and metastasis. EGF-R has been shown to play an important role in head and neck cancers, non–small cell lung cancers, and pancreatic cancers. Several agents have been developed which block the activity of this receptor. The small molecule tyrosine kinase inhibitor gefitinib (Iressa) has received FDA approval for the treatment of non–small cell lung carcinoma. Cetuximab (Erbitux) has been used for head and neck cancers as well as colon cancer. Table 13.4 gives a representative list of a number of targets and the agents that have been developed to inhibit them. The VEGF receptors also signal through kinases and can be blocked

TABLE 13.4

MOLECULAR TARGETS AND THE AGENTS DEVELOPED TO MODULATE THEM

Target	Agent	Manufacturer
Bcr-abl	Gleevec	Novartis
Her-2 (neu)	Herceptin	Genentech
Ras	R11577	Johnson & Johnson
VEGF	Avastin	Genentech
VEGF	VEGF Trap	Regeneron
EGFR	Iressa	AstraZeneca
EGF	ABX-EGF	Abgenix
Cyclin-dependent kinase	Flavopiridol	Aventis
Protein Kinase C	Affinitak	Isis Pharmaceuticals

EGF, endothelial growth factor; EGFR, epidermal growth factor receptor; VEGF, vascular endothelial growth factor.
Adapted from Becker J. Signal transduction inhibitors: a work in progress. *Nature Biotechnol.* 2004;22:15.

by a variety of agents still in clinical trials. These agents have been utilized alone and in combination with more conventional cytotoxic chemotherapies.

The expression of HER-2 (neu) in breast cancer has been shown to influence the aggressiveness of these tumors. For those patients with breast cancer that expresses HER-2, the agent transtuzumab (Herceptin), a humanized monoclonal antibody, has been used with success to block HER-2 signaling. Herceptin in combination with chemotherapy for patients with tumors expressing HER-2 has been shown to be superior to chemotherapy alone.

These targeted agents represent an important new strategy, and the number of new agents in the study is likely to increase as new targets are identified. In many cases, the evaluation of these agents will require the development of novel monitoring techniques that can reveal if the targeted pathway is being effectively modulated. One example of this is the use of fluorodeoxyglucose (FDG) positron emission tomography (PET) scans and imatinib in the monitoring and treatment of patients with GISTs.

Another area of active investigation is the development of agents that modulate the methylation status of DNA. DNA methylation is an epigenetic event, which commonly occurs in the cell and allows for the control of gene expression. Methyl groups added to specific sequences (known as CpG islands) generally in the region of promoters results in the silencing of gene expression.

Hypermethylation often occurs in cancer. Most often, the genes that are susceptible in to hypermethylation are those involved in cell cycle regulation, DNA repair, apoptosis, drug resistance, differentiation, angiogenesis, and metastasis. Hypermethylation can result in the inactivation of normally reactive tumor suppressors, which would otherwise prevent malignant transformation. Agents that result in DNA demethylation are undergoing active study as anticancer therapies. Agents such as decitabine reverse methylation in a number of tumor lines and have been shown to act on solid tumors as well in clinical trials. Other strategies involve targeting histone-deacetylase (HDAC). HDAC is an important enzyme that is activated by DNA methylation to repress gene expression. HDAC inhibitors have been shown to increase gene expression from methylated genes.

Although the majority of cancers demonstrate hypermethylation, there are some that have evidence of hypomethylation, such as breast, cervical, and brain tumors. Hypomethylation is thought to activate tumorigenesis by turning on oncogenes such as cMYC and H-RAS. Clearly, agents that result in demethylation will not be universally applicable to all cancers, and site-specific methylating agents may also be needed.

Another exciting field of investigation is in the ability to silence specific gene transcripts. If a tumor is known to overexpress K-RAS, having the ability to turn off this expression would be advantageous. Small interfering RNA (siRNA) is a type of RNA designed to bind to messenger RNA, resulting in the degradation and removal of the message. RNA interference can be incorporated into a strategy to decrease the available message for subsequent translation. These siRNA can be generated as short oligonucleotide DNA fragments or delivered in a plasmid form for expression within a cell. *In vitro* and *in vivo* experiments have demonstrated the efficiency of this strategy of gene silencing and efforts are under way to develop methods for delivering siRNA in a clinical setting.

Gene Therapy

Despite the controversy surrounding human clinical trials using gene therapy, this strategy remains a promising approach for the treatment of patients with cancer. Gene therapy involves the delivery of a cDNA coding sequence for a particular gene of interest via a vector to a host organism with subsequent expression of that gene and production of the gene product. The gene product can provide a missing protein whose function in the case of cancer results in the suppression of the neoplastic phenotype or the protein can result in the lysis or destruction of the tumor or the tumors associated vasculature. Many genes have been considered as likely candidates for gene delivery strategies to treat tumors. There are also several different vector systems, which can be utilized to deliver these genes.

Vectors

The choice of a vector, which is a term used to describe the carrier for the gene sequence that is being delivered, depends to a certain degree on the route of administration, the target tissue, the amount of gene product one hopes to produce, and finally the duration of expression of the gene that is necessary to effect a response. Vectors tend to be categorized in two major classes. Nonviral vectors including plasmid DNA, liposomes, nanoparticles, and other synthetic carriers are attractive in that there is generally little to no immune response from the host and no endogenous viral proteins produced. In addition, these vector systems tend to be transient in their expression and, unless otherwise engineered, do not integrate into the host genome. The downside of nonviral vectors is that both the level of gene product expression and the duration of expression tend to be less than with viral vector systems. Viral vectors have the advantage of efficient transfection or transduction of host cells and sustained elevated levels of gene expression. The disadvantage is their potential immunogenicity, which may render multiple administrations less successful as well as increase the potential for host tissue toxicity.

Both nonviral and viral vector systems can be engineered to target specific tissue beds or tissue types and be delivered in a nontargeted way to host organs such as the liver. The choice between a targeted or nontargeted vector generally depends on the particular gene to be expressed and the ultimate goals of the therapy. This strategy has been illustrated by the application of antiangiogenic gene therapy to the treatment of cancer.

The goal of antiangiogenic gene therapy is to deliver an angiogenesis inhibitor in such a way that the body produces the protein of interest thus eliminating the difficulties in recombinant production and the need for repeat administration of these proteins. Two strategies have been employed to deliver antiangiogenic agents via gene therapy (Fig. 13.11). The first is to engineer the vector system to target the gene of interest to the tumor cell or the tumor-associated vasculature. The advantage here is that relative tissue levels of the agent of interest can be significantly higher than those that are achieved through systemic production. In addition, genes that produce a product with direct cytotoxicity to the cancer cell or the tumors associated vasculature can be administered in a targeted way so as to reduce potential toxicity to normal tissues.

An alternative strategy is to deliver a vector to an organ such as the liver resulting in efficient transfection of hepatocytes with the gene for the angiogenesis inhibitor. The goal in this strategy is to harness the liver as a "factory" to produce circulating levels of the angiogenesis inhibitor to prevent the further growth and spread of micrometastatic disease throughout the body. Viral vectors such as adenovirus or adeno-associated virus with their native predilection for liver infection owing to CAR receptor uptake have been the vectors of choice for this approach. However, nonviral vectors such as liposomes tend to be taken up by the reticular endothelial system in the liver as well, and they also result in sustained gene

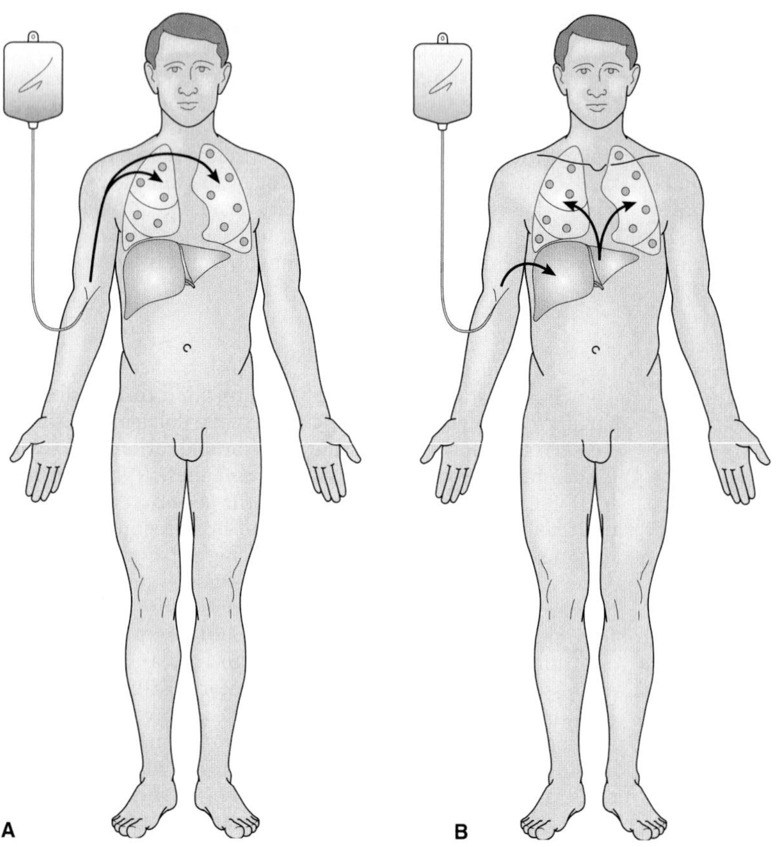

FIGURE 13.11 Strategies for antiangiogenic gene therapy. (*A*) Tumor-directed antiangiogenic gene therapy facilitates paracrine activity and avoids systemic toxicity. (*B*) Systemic antiangiogenic gene therapy utilizes normal host tissue such as the liver as a "factory" to elevate systemic levels of the gene product. (Adapted from Feldman AL, Libutti SK. Progress in antiangiogenic gene therapy of cancer. *Cancer* 2000; 89;1181.)

expression and circulating levels of the protein. Table 13.5 lists various genes coding for angiogenesis inhibitors as well as the vectors used for their delivery that have been studied.

In addition to gene therapy strategies that employ the replacement of a gene such as p53 or the delivery of a cytotoxic gene such as thymidine kinase and ganciclovir therapy, the use of cytotoxic vectors alone has shown some promise. Vaccinia virus is a cytoplasmic virus that is related to the virus causing smallpox. Vaccinia virus delivery results in the infection and subsequent lysis of the cells infected. Studies utilizing vaccinia targeted to tumors have demonstrated the potential for this strategy in inhibiting the growth and spread of tumors.

Several clinical trials have been conducted utilizing gene therapy for cancer. Adenovirus carrying p53 has been studied in both direct arterial infusion into the liver as well as the treatment of glioma, lung cancer, ovarian cancer, and breast cancer. Recurrent head and neck cancer has also been studied. So-called suicide gene therapy utilizing the herpes simplex virus thymidine kinase gene and the prodrug ganciclovir has been studied in the clinic. Patients with mesothelioma have been studied in a phase I trial using this strategy, as have patients with prostate adenocarcinoma using direct injection of an adenovirus expressing hsv-tk followed by ganciclovir exposure. These studies have demonstrated the safety of this strategy, although studies to evaluate efficacy are still under way.

The future of gene therapy for cancer is dependent on several important lines of investigation. Improved vectors are needed that minimize toxicity, allow for specific targeting, decrease the host's immune response or prevent a host immune response, and can be produced efficiently for clinical use. The judicious selection of the appropriate genes to deliver in such a strategy is dependent on further investigation into the molecular pathways that are important to the malignant phenotype.

Immunotherapy

Harnessing the body's immune system to attack cancer is an attractive strategy and area of investigation. Tumors express antigens that are often different from the antigens expressed by the normal cells. There are two main approaches for the use of immunotherapy to treat patients with cancer. The first involves the use of vaccine therapy to stimulate the body's native immune system, mainly antigen presenting cells and lymphocytes, to react specifically against the tumor antigens resulting in tumor regression. The second is the transfer of lymphocytes isolated from the patient's tumor tissue [tumor infiltrating lymphocytes (TIL)] that have been selected for their immunoreactivity against the patient's tumor.

Vaccine therapy may utilize peptides derived from the protein sequence of the cancer antigen, gene therapy with vectors carrying a coding sequence for the peptide or antigen, or alternatively the delivery of whole tumor lysate providing a variety of antigenic stimuli. Once vaccinated, the protein or peptide is processed by antigen-presenting cells in the context of the patient's class I major histocompatibility complex (MHC) molecule, thus stimulating a lymphocyte response to the tumor.

Cancer vaccines have been utilized in clinical trials studying a variety of human tumors. Patients with melanoma, breast cancer, colon cancer, head and neck cancer, and renal cancers have been studied. Although several studies have demonstrated successful immunization of patients to tumor antigens, to date there have been no successful trials demonstrating significant cancer regression to vaccine therapy alone.

Cell transfer therapy has demonstrated antitumor activity in patients. To date, the most effective immunotherapy that has been utilized for patients with melanoma and renal cell cancer has been the infusion of interleukin-2 (IL-2). IL-2 is a

TABLE 13.5

ANTIANGIOGENIC GENE THERAPY: GENES AND VECTORS

Gene	Delivery vector	Findings
Angiostatin	Adeno-associated virus	Supernatant fluid from transduced tumor cells inhibited endothelial cell proliferation *in vitro*
	Cationic liposome: DNA complex	Supernatant fluid from transfected tumor cells inhibited angiogenesis in the *in vivo* Matrigel model
	In vitro transfection	Transfection of murine fibrosarcoma cells inhibited their growth as primary or metastatic tumors in mice
	In vitro transfection Retrovirus	Transfection of murine B16F10 melanoma cells inhibited their growth as primary or metastatic tumors in mice. *In vitro* transduction of glioma cells inhibited their growth in mice
	Adenovirus	Stereotactic injection into intracerebral gliomas inhibited tumor growth in mice
	Adenovirus	Pretreatment with intravenous adenovirus inhibited establishment and growth of C6 rat gliomas in mice
	Cationic liposome: DNA complex	Intravenous injection of liposome:DNA complexes reduced B16F10 murine melanoma metastasis
Endostatin	Adeno-associated virus	Supernatant fluid from transduced tumor cells inhibited endothelial cell proliferation *in vitro*
	In vitro transfection	Stable transfection of mouse and human tumor cell lines inhibited formation of lung and liver metastases in mice
	Polymerized plasmid DNA	Intramuscular injection of endostatin plasmid inhibited syngeneic tumor growth and tumor metastases in mice
	Cationic liposome: DNA complex	Intravenous injection of liposome:DNA complexes inhibited growth of human breast carcinoma in nude mice
	Adenovirus	Intravenous injection of recombinant adenovirus inhibited growth of subcutaneous tumors in nude mice
	Adenovirus	Intravenous injection of recombinant adenovirus inhibited subcutaneous tumor growth and prevented lung metastases in nude mice
IL-4	Retroviral packaging cells	Stereotactic injection inhibited angiogenesis and growth of intracerebral rat gliomas and was immunostimulatory
IL-10	*In vitro* transfection	Transfection of human melanoma cells inhibited angiogenesis, tumor growth, and establishment of metastases
	In vitro transfection	Transfection of human prostate cancer cells inhibited their growth in nude mice
IL-12	Semliki Forest virus	Intratumoral injection inhibited B16 melanoma angiogenesis and growth in mice independent of immune response
IFN-a TIMP-1	*In vitro* retroviral transduction Adenovirus	Transduction of human prostate carcinoma cells inhibited their ability to form tumors and lymph node metastases in nude mice. Adenoviral infection of endothelial cells inhibited their migration *in vitro*
TIMP-2	*In vitro* transfection	Transfection of B16F10 murine melanoma cells inhibited angiogenesis, tumor growth, and metastases in mice
TSP-1	Liposome:DNA complex	Intravenous injection of DNA complexes encoding a TSP-1 fragment inhibited human breast carcinoma growth in mice
p16	Adenovirus	Pretreatment with virus inhibited the ability of glioma cells to induce angiogenesis in a dorsal air sac model in nude mice
p53	Liposome:DNA complex	Intravenous injection inhibited human breast carcinoma growth associated with decreased blood vessel density in nude mice
	Liposome:DNA complex	Intravenous injection reduced angiogenesis and inhibited establishment of B16F10 lung metastases in C57BL/6 mice
PF-4	Adenovirus	Coinjection of adenovirus with glioma cells under renal capsule of nude mice inhibited tumor growth and vascularity
EMAP-II	Vaccinia	Intravenous injection of vaccinia enhanced tumor sensitivity to TNF associated with endothelial cell TNF receptor up-regulation

From Feldman AL, Libutti SK. Progress in antiangiogenic gene therapy of cancer. *Cancer* 2000;89:1181, with permission.

lymphocyte-stimulating cytokine that has a variety of effects on T cells. Response rates to the systemic administration of IL-2 for patients with both melanoma and kidney cancer are 15% to 20% with complete responses being approximately 9%. Complete responses are often durable with a majority of patients enjoying a long-term disease-free survival beyond 10 years. Therefore, any new immunotherapy strategy must improve on these IL-2 results.

TIL can be grown successfully from melanoma. These lymphocytes can then be tested for their reactivity against the melanoma using cell lysis assays. The advantage of cell transfer approaches is the ability to administer extremely large numbers of highly selective cells that have demonstrated avidity for the tumor antigens as well as the ability to affect tumor cell lyses. In studies at the NCI, Rosenberg and his colleagues have demonstrated the ability to effect regression of metastatic melanoma refractory to standard treatment in patients receiving a nonmyeloablative preparative chemotherapy regimen followed by the administration of selected TIL and IL-2. Response rates of 40% have been achieved with such an approach.

Clearly, there is a role for immunotherapy in the treatment of cancer. The future involves a better understanding of the complex interactions that lead to the immune response so as to better harness this knowledge for the development for more effective therapies. Such an understanding of the molecules that suppress or activate the immune response has led to the identification of lymphocyte surface molecules such as CTLA-4. CTLA-4 is an important regulator of T-lymphocyte proliferation and function. When active, CTLA-4 suppresses lymphocyte activation. Antibodies against CTLA-4 have been utilized in clinical trials demonstrating that inhibition of this suppression can result in an immune response against tumors.

ROLE OF THE SURGEON IN CANCER TREATMENT

Modern cancer therapy involves a multidisciplinary approach consisting of a variety of specialists with diverse talents. These individuals can be physicians, nurses, physical therapists, pain and palliative care specialists, dietitians, and clergy. The cancer patient often presents with a complex series of medical and nonmedical issues that require a coordinated approach for the optimal delivery of care. The surgeon's role in this coordinated effort is critical. For many patients, their first experience with the health-care team is with a surgeon for the management of their primary tumor. This requires that the surgeon have a good understanding of the roles of the other members of the team and an ability to coordinate their interactions to provide the patient with the best possible outcome.

Typically, surgeons are associated with the management of early stage disease and are usually called on only to manage the complications of stage IV disease, such as bowel obstruction or bleeding. This paradigm is changing as it has become increasingly evident that aggressive surgical approaches may be of benefit to patients with advanced stage tumors. Throughout this text are descriptions of the role of surgeons for the management of early stage disease. Therefore, this section focuses on surgeons impact in the management and care of cancer patients with metastatic tumors.

Surgical resection of metastatic disease has been practiced for decades. For certain tumor types, most notably, colorectal cancer and sarcoma, surgical resection of metastases in the lung or liver has been associated with improved survival. This approach relies on the fact that metastatic disease is well localized to one or two organs and that resection of those sites can be done safely and completely.

In 2005, it is estimated that there will be approximately 150,000 new cases of colorectal cancer. Of these patients, 20% to 40% will develop liver metastases as the sole or dominant site of their disease progression. Approximately 10% to 20% of patients with liver metastases will have disease that can be resected and patients may potentially benefit from the intervention. For patients with metastatic colorectal cancer confined to the liver, the options for therapy include resection for those with resectable disease with or without the addition of the adjuvant therapy and systemic therapies for those with unresectable disease relying on combinations of irinotecan, 5FU, leucovorin, oxaliplatin, and now most recently bevacizumab (Avastin). Bevacizumab is an antiangiogenic agent that blocks VEGF. It was recently approved by the FDA for the treatment of advanced colon cancer. Regional therapies involving hepatic artery infusion or isolated hepatic perfusion are also options for patients with unresectable disease as are radiofrequency ablation and cryotherapy.

For patients with resectable metastatic colon cancer involving the liver (similar results exist for isolated disease involving the lung), resection of disease is followed by 5-year survival in a significant fraction. A variety of studies evaluating the outcome and operative mortality for patients undergoing complete resection of isolated colorectal cancer metastasis to the liver demonstrate 5-year survival ranging from 26% to 40%. There is at present no systemic chemotherapy regimen that significantly improves on the 10% 5-year survival observed in the earliest 5FU and leucovorin studies. Therefore, it is important to identify those patients with metastatic colorectal cancer isolated to the liver who would be candidates for surgical resection and therefore potentially a cure.

It is important to properly stratify patients to determine which ones will likely derive the greatest benefit from resection. In a 1999 study, Fong and colleagues at Memorial Sloan-Kettering Cancer Center reported on the results of an analysis of more than 1,000 patients treated by surgical resection for stage IV colon cancer isolated to the liver. They analyzed prognostic factors using univariate and multivariate statistics and determined the factors that predicted a positive outcome for their patients. Among the influential factors were disease-free interval between resection of the primary tumor and first sign of liver metastasis, number of tumors in the liver, carcinoembryonic antigen (CEA) value, size of the largest liver lesion, and the nodal status of the primary tumor. Depending on the number of these factors, a prediction of the 5-year survival and median overall survival in months could be determined (Table 13.6).

This type of information is critical in deciding which patients would most likely benefit from an aggressive surgical resection for their liver lesions. These outcomes are improved by the ability to accurately stage patients preoperatively with modalities such as high-resolution computed tomography (CT), magnetic resonance imaging (MRI), and PET using FDG. Intraoperative ultrasound is also critical to the careful intraoperative staging of these patients not only for the detection of additional liver lesions but also for the accurate determination of anatomic relationships to choose the appropriate resection to perform. Improved operative techniques such as segmental resections, use of stapling devices and coagulation devices, minimization of blood loss by extrahepatic ligation of the hepatic vein prior to dissection, and intermittent inflow occlusion of the portahepatis have led to a significant reduction in morbidity and mortality. However, despite these advances, many patients are not candidates for surgical resection. The surgeon can still play a role in the aggressive management of these patients.

Regional therapies for cancer have been the subject of study for more than 50 years. A variety of regional therapies are presently available to treat isolated hepatic metastases that might not otherwise be amenable to surgical resection due to

TABLE 13.6

PREDICTORS OF MORTALITY AND SURVIVAL FOLLOWING RESECTION OF HEPATIC COLORECTAL METASTASES

Prognostic factor	P value	RR death
Disease-free interval <12 mo	0.002	1.56
Tumor number >3	0.01	1.56
CEA >200 μg/L	0.05	1.45
Size >5 cm	0.01	1.46
Node positive primary	0.05	1.34
SURVIVAL BASED ON NUMBER OF FACTORS		
Number of factors	**5-yr survival (%)**	**Median OS**
0	57	74
1	57	73
2	47	50
3	16	30
4	8	15

CEA, carcinoembryonic antigen; OS, overall survival; RR, relative risk.
Adapted from Fong Y, Fortner J, Sun RL, et al. Clinical score for predicting recurrence after hepatic resection for metastatic colorectal cancer: analysis of 1001 consecutive cases. *Ann Surg*. 1999;230:309.

the number of lesions, underlying liver disease, or other comorbid medical conditions. These techniques include cryoablation, radiofrequency ablation, intraarterial hepatic infusion chemotherapy, chemoembolization of tumors, intralesional injection of chemotherapy or alcohol, and regional perfusion through operative or percutaneous techniques. Isolated operative hepatic perfusion and percutaneous hepatic perfusion are two promising strategies for the treatment of patients with isolated hepatic colorectal cancer metastasis.

Isolated hepatic perfusion (IHP) is a complex surgical procedure that was first reported in the early 1960s. It involves the complete isolation of the vascular inflow and outflow of the liver to deliver, via the hepatic arterial circulation, high doses of chemotherapy or cytokines to treat lesions within the liver but to spare the rest of the body from potential toxicity. The liver is ideally suited to such an approach because the majority of liver tumors (approaching 100%) derive their blood supply from the hepatic arterial vessels, whereas the normal liver receives 75% of its blood flow from the portal system. This allows the differential delivery of chemotherapy to the liver tumor by infusing the agent directly into the hepatic arterial circulation. The venous effluent from the hepatic veins is collected in an isolated segment of retrohepatic vena cava and this blood is recirculated back through a perfusion circuit that maintains a constant perfusion of oxygenated blood carrying chemotherapy and cytokines to the liver.

Extrahepatic circulation is maintained by shunting the infrahepatic caval blood as well as the portal circulation through a pump to the axillary vein to maintain systemic blood pressure (Fig. 13.12). Careful dissection of the liver with special attention to the retrohepatic vena cava is required to divide collaterals and prevent systemic exposure to the perfusion agent (Fig. 13.13). The portal structures must also be completely dissected to isolate the portal vein and hepatic vessels for cannulation (Fig. 13.14). The advantages of such an approach are the complete separation of the regional and systemic circulation eliminating or significantly reducing systemic toxicity. Dose escalation of the chemotherapeutic agents is now limited only by the liver's tolerance to these agents as opposed to bone marrow or other systemic sites. The liver generally has a much greater reserve and ability to recover than the bone marrow. This technique also allows the utilization of hyperthermia via this closed circulatory system that can be heated and oxygenated by an extracorporeal heart lung machine.

A number of centers both in the United States and in Europe have explored this technique; the largest experience has been in the Surgery Branch of the NCI. Alexander and coworkers have reported results for 51 patients with unresectable colorectal cancer metastases treated with an IHP using the chemotherapy melphalan (with or without TNF) with or without follow-up hepatic arterial infusion (HAI) with FUDR/LV. Results included a response rate of approximately 75% with a median survival of 16 months for those patients not receiving follow-up HAI therapy and 27 months for those receiving HAI therapy following their IHP. These results demonstrate that significant responses and an acceptable duration of response can be achieved for an aggressive surgical approach for patients with significant liver disease (Fig. 13.15).

The application of IHP to unresectable liver metastases demonstrates the potential role for the surgeon in the management of patients with metastatic cancer. Clearly, however, such an intervention requires significant resources and skill, which may not be available at every major medical center. Therefore, a need to adapt this strategy to a therapy that can be more safely and easily administered and that allows repeated administrations (IHP can only be performed once) would be desirable. Investigators are therefore evaluating whether or not a percutaneous approach to hepatic isolation can be utilized.

This technique relies on the use of balloons placed via a catheter percutaneously introduced into the vena cava through the femoral vein. The balloons can occlude above the hepatic veins and above the renal veins to isolate a segment of the vena cava. The catheter isolates hepatic venous effluent to allow for extra corporeal filtration of chemotherapy delivered

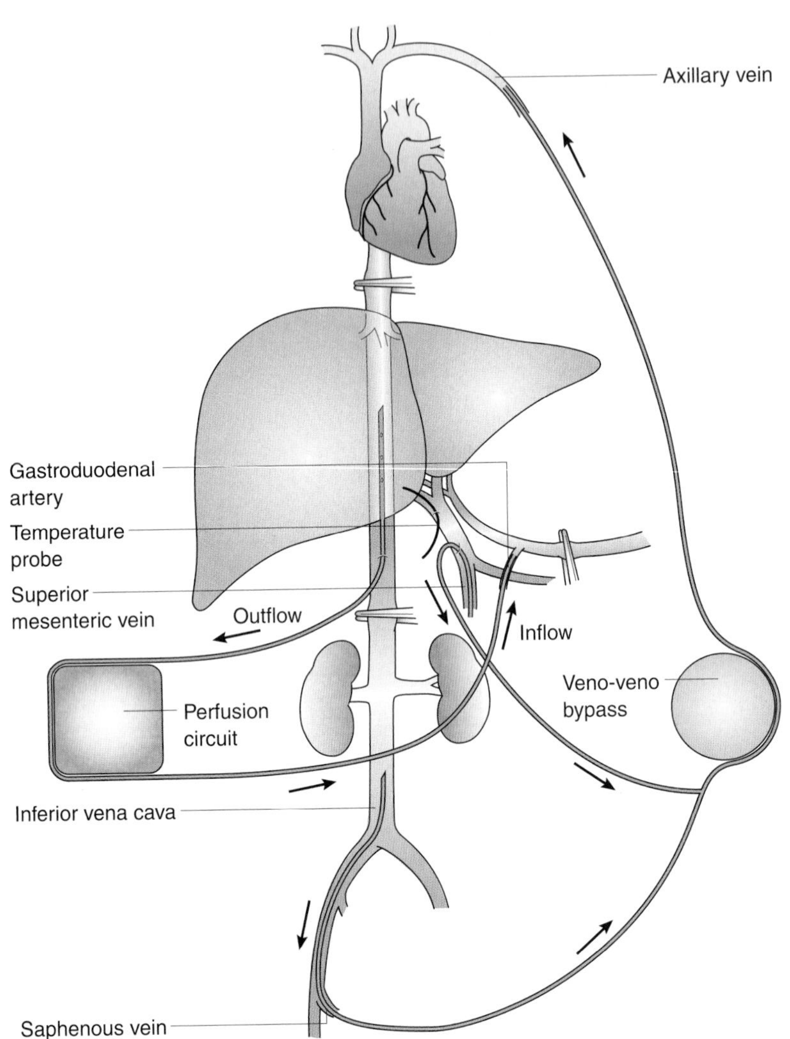

FIGURE 13.12 Schematic diagram of the perfusion and veno-veno bypass circuits used during an isolated hepatic perfusion (IHP). For the perfusion circuit, blood is collected from the hepatic veins via an isolated segment of retrohepatic vena cava that has been carefully prepared by ligating dividing venous tributaries and the adrenal vein. This blood is returned to a heat-oxygenator and is perfused back into the liver via the common hepatic artery (through a catheter in the GDA). The perfusate consists of PRBCs and chemotherapy in a crystalloid solution. Infrahepatic blood and portal blood is shunted via an extracorporeal bypass circuit to the axillary vein to maintain venous return to the heart.

to the liver through a separate catheter introduced into the hepatic artery (Fig. 13.16). The filtered blood is then returned via the internal jugular vein to maintain venous return. A phase I trial was recently completed at the NCI demonstrating a safe dose of melphalan that can be delivered in this fashion. Phase II studies are now under way to evaluate the utility of this approach.

Regional therapy can be applied to other locations in the body such as the limb (isolated limb perfusion for melanoma or sarcoma) and the peritoneal cavity. Peritoneal carcinomatosis secondary to a number of histologies including colorectal cancer, gastric cancer, pancreatic cancer, and malignant mesothelioma can be addressed. Traditionally, surgeons have played a role in managing the complications of this entity such as ascites and obstruction. However, techniques such as surgical debulking and intraperitoneal chemotherapy are gaining prominence as a viable management strategy for treating patients with peritoneal carcinomatosis. Surgeons have a unique role to play and can make a significant impact in treating this condition.

Malignant peritoneal mesothelioma can result in significant abdominal pain and distention accompanied by anorexia and weight loss, ascites, and bowel obstruction. These complications can lead to death and there are no effective systemic treatment options. Although agents such as cisplatin and carboplatin as well as paclitaxel (Taxol) and doxorubicin (Adriamycin) have been used to treat this condition, response rates are low (less than 20%) and survival is poor. The technique of continuous hyperthermic peritoneal perfusion (CHPP) involves an exploratory laparotomy with lysis of adhesions, tumor resection, omentectomy, and peritonectomy of involved peritoneal surfaces (Fig. 13.17). Organs such as the spleen, if significantly involved with tumor, are also resected. At the completion of resection, the abdomen is closed after the insertion of inflow and outflow catheters and temperature probes. Carcinomatosis can involve the surfaces of the mesentery, which can be very difficult to resect (Fig. 13.18). Best efforts are made to strip the peritoneal surface over the mesentery and to fulgurate small lesions with ball electrocautery.

These catheters are connected to a perfusion circuit with a roller pump and heat exchange coil to circulate hyperthermic intraperitoneal chemotherapy agents. At the completion of the perfusion the abdomen is irrigated, and a peritoneal dialysis catheter can be inserted for postoperative dwell therapy with additional regional chemotherapy.

In a study of CHPP for intraperitoneal mesothelioma, Park and coworkers summarized the results of 18 patients with peritoneal mesothelioma treated with CHPP from 1993 through 1998. Of these 18 patients, 13 had clinically significant ascites. Patients were treated with operative debulking and CHPP with cisplatin. After a median follow-up of 19 months, there were no operative or treatment-related mortalities, and the overall operative morbidity was 24%. Morbidity included wound infection, atrial fibrillation, pancreatitis, ileus, and line sepsis.

Nine of 13 patients with ascites had complete resolution of their ascites following a single procedure. Three other patients had resolution of their ascites after a second CHPP.

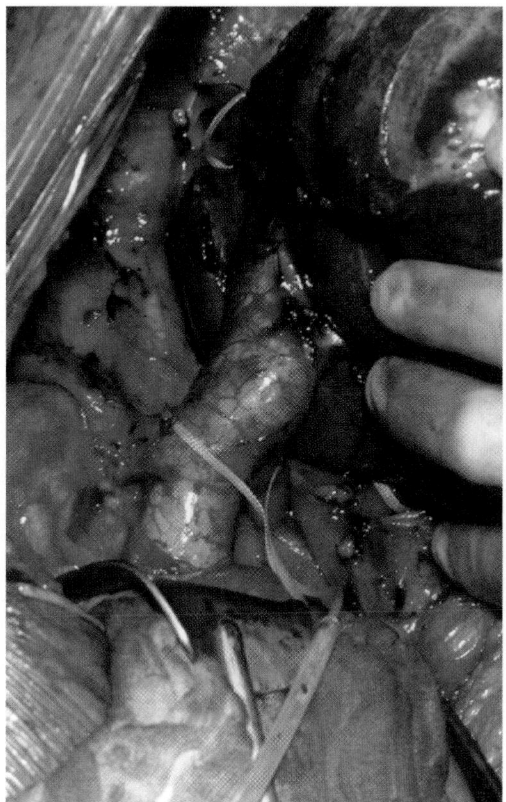

FIGURE 13.13 A view of the retrohepatic vena cava following dissection for an isolated hepatic perfusion (IHP).

The median progression-free survival was 26 months, and the overall 2-year survival was 80%. Although this study did not prospectively compare CHPP to systemic cisplatin, trials of intravenous cisplatin report survival data that is similar to untreated patients. The results of CHPP can be dramatic for patients suffering with the very morbid condition of abdominal ascites (Fig. 13.19).

Thus, the surgeon can play an important role not only in the management of patients with primary tumors but also in the management of patients with stage IV disease. Surgeons must familiarize themselves with the other available nonoperative options for their patients with cancer so the correct therapy can be selected for the appropriate patient. Further study is needed to identify therapies that will benefit patients with advanced disease.

CANCER DETECTION AND BIOMARKERS

Methods to enable more accurate early detection of cancer are an active area of investigation. Some of these methods are amenable to cancer screening, allowing assessment of large populations of at-risk patients to detect disease at its earliest possible time. Other methods are best applied to patients who have already been treated for their cancer and are being followed for signs of recurrence. This section highlights three areas that illustrate the possibilities for early cancer detection.

Imaging

Standard imaging techniques such as CT, MRI, and ultrasound have been applied to patients as a means of both screening and follow-up. Standard plain x-rays have also been used in this setting. As CT scans and MRIs have become more advanced with higher resolution and shorter scanning times, the sensitivity for lesion detection has been dramatically improved. One example has been the development of both CT and magnetic resonance (MR) colonography.

Colonography has been proposed as a means to screen patients for colon polyps and tumors in an effort to avoid the need for an optical endoscopic colonoscopy. Virtual colonoscopy using CT scanning was evaluated as a screening procedure for colorectal neoplasia in asymptomatic adults at the National Naval Medical Center in Bethesda Maryland. A total of 1,233 asymptomatic adults (mean age 58 years) underwent a same-day CT colonography as well as an optical colonoscopy. The radiologist used a three-dimensional endoluminal display for the detection of polyps on the virtual colonoscopy. The physicians performing the optical colonoscopy did not know the results of the virtual colonoscopy for the initial examination. The sensitivity and specificity of virtual colonoscopy compared to optical colonoscopy were then compared to the findings of a final unblinded optical colonoscopy, which was used as the reference standard.

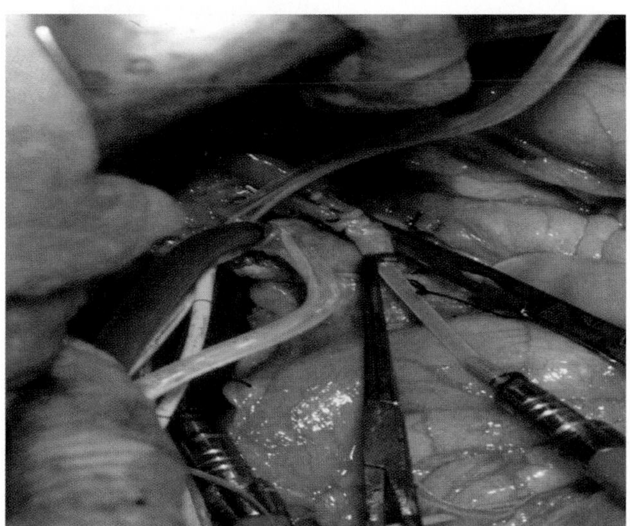

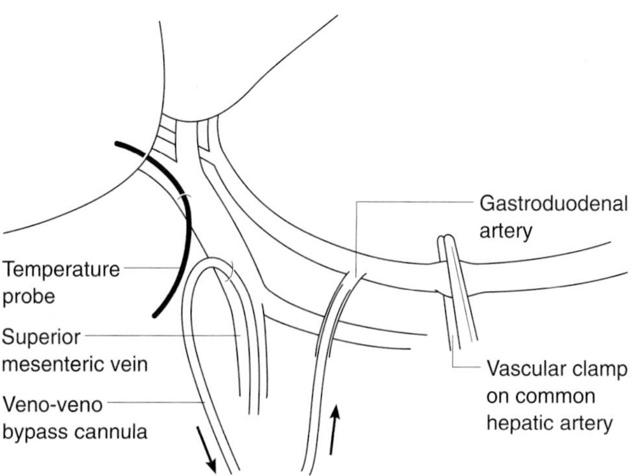

FIGURE 13.14 Complete portal dissection for isolated hepatic perfusion (IHP).

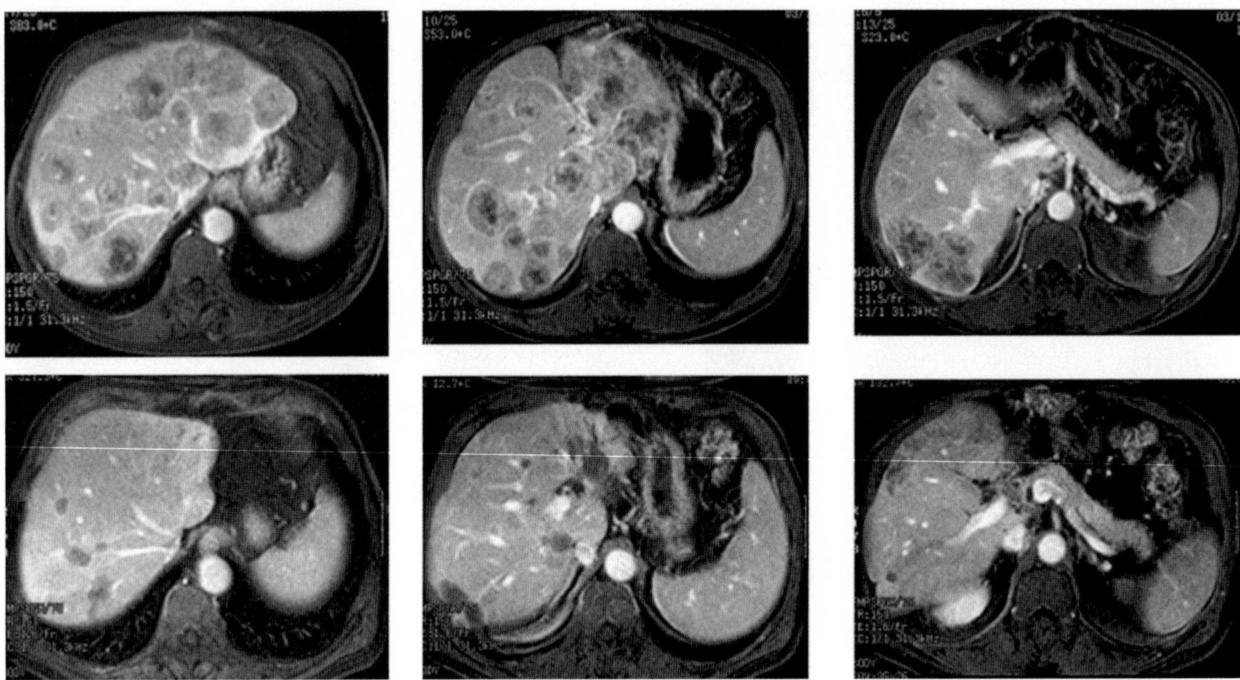

FIGURE 13.15 A magnetic resonance imaging (MRI) of the liver for a patient with colorectal cancer metastatic to the liver before (top) and after (bottom) an isolated hepatic perfusion (IHP).

Sensitivity of the virtual colonoscopy for adenomatous polyps was 94% for polyps greater than 8 mm in diameter and 89% for polyps that measured at least 6 mm in diameter. The sensitivity of optical colonoscopy for adenomatous polyps was 88% to 92% for polyps greater than 8 mm in diameter and 92% for polyps measuring at least 6 mm in diameter. Of the patients screened, two polyps were found to be malignant and both of them were detected by virtual colonoscopy. With sensitivities and specificities that are approaching or better than those of optical colonoscopy, virtual colonoscopy using CT may become a screening procedure of choice. When lesions are detected, a follow-up optical colonoscopy can be performed to biopsy the lesion.

Noninvasive imaging can also be utilized in patients following the treatment of a cancer to detect early recurrence. In a study at the NCI, standard imaging techniques such as CT, MRI, and ultrasound were compared to PET using FDG, anti-CEA antibody immunoscintigraphy, and a blind second-look laparotomy for patients with a rising serum CEA following definitive management of colorectal cancer. In this

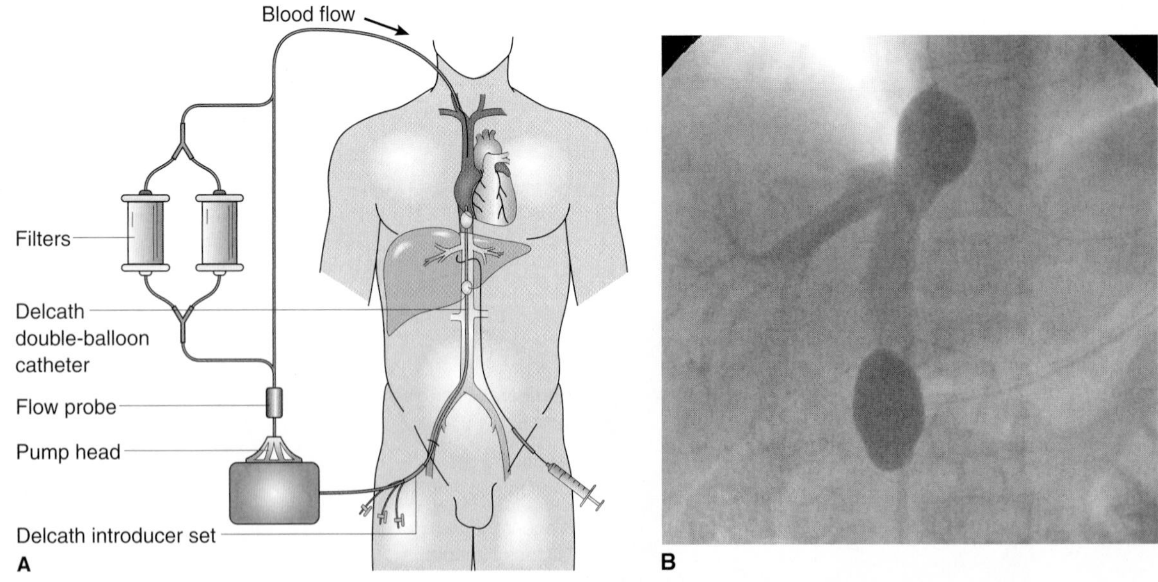

FIGURE 13.16 Schematic diagram (*A*) and fluoroscopic image (*B*) depicting the technique of percutaneous hepatic perfusion (PHP).

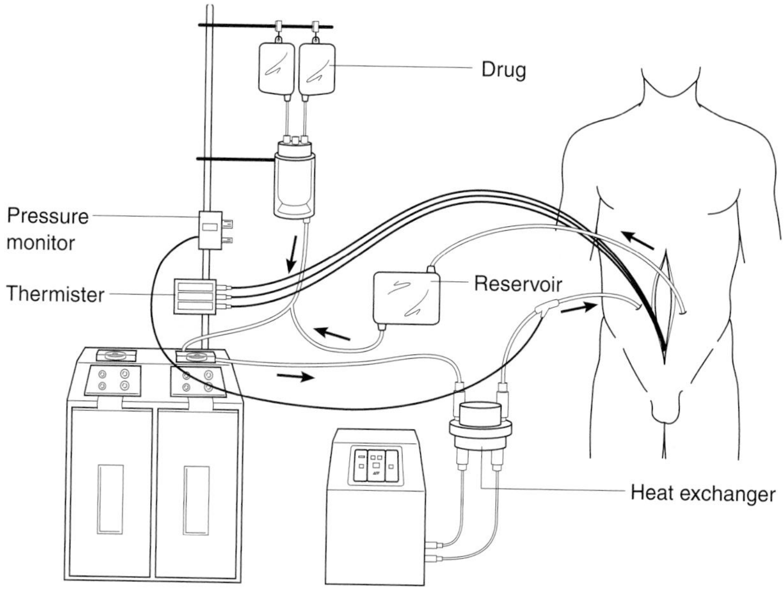

FIGURE 13.17 Diagram of the setup for continuous hyperthermic peritoneal perfusion (CHPP).

study FDG-PET and blind second-look laparotomy were found to be the most sensitive methods for detection of recurrent disease. As a noninvasive screening method, FDG-PET was both sensitive and specific for the detection of recurrent disease in patients with a rising serum CEA and therefore is now recommended as an appropriate screening modality prior to any planned surgical management (Fig. 13.20). FDG-PET is also useful in the metastatic workup of patients with malignant melanoma, primary lung carcinoma, and esophageal cancers.

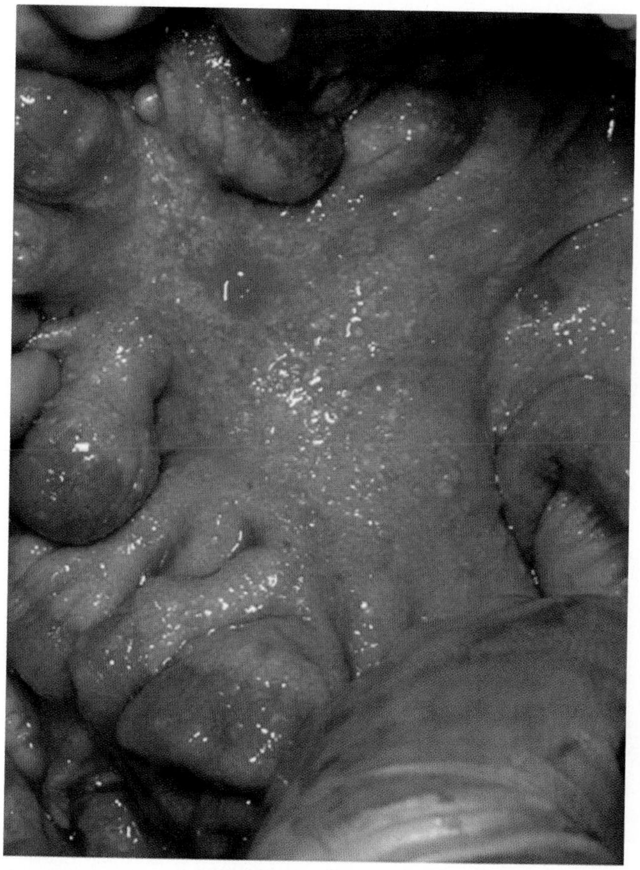

FIGURE 13.18 Intraoperative photo demonstrating significant carcinomatosis involving the mesentery of the small bowel.

Dynamic enhanced MRI (DEMRI) has become a useful noninvasive imaging modality for the evaluation of the functional status of a tumor. Tumor blood flow and blood volume can be calculated from DEMRI images and thus this noninvasive imaging method can be used to follow the response of a tumor to a variety of therapies. DEMRI has been successfully utilized for imaging primary breast cancers as well as for imaging metastatic sites from a variety of histologies. Images obtained from DEMRI can be utilized to determine residual areas of tumor activity following therapies to more accurately guide biopsies and further regional treatment.

The new frontier for cancer imaging is so-called molecular imaging. Although this term can encompass a variety of imaging approaches and methods, it is most commonly used to categorize techniques that rely on imaging a tissue based on specific expression of receptors or pathways. In combination with molecular therapies such imaging methods may allow for noninvasive monitoring of the activity of targeted agents.

A number of preclinical models have been developed to test molecular imaging strategies. Weissleder and his group have designed a number of noninvasive methods for imaging the activity of enzymes and pathways to predict the efficacy of molecular agents. One example is their use of iron oxide nanoparticles cross-linked to Cy-3 and Cy-5 fluorescent dyes. Using cathepsin-B cleavable linking peptides, activity can be measured via cleavage and determination of the ratio of the various fluorophores. By using fluorophores as well as iron particles, both fluorescent imaging and MR imaging of the tissue in question can be performed.

Specific tissue receptors can also be imaged noninvasively. Tumor vasculature is known to have an increased expression of integrins such as alphavbeta 3. Using RGD cyclic pentapeptides labeled with PET positron emitters, tissues with enhanced alphavbeta 3 expression can be imaged. Such techniques can be used to locate areas of increased tumor neovascular density and can also be utilized to follow the targeting or activity of alphavbeta3 specific agents.

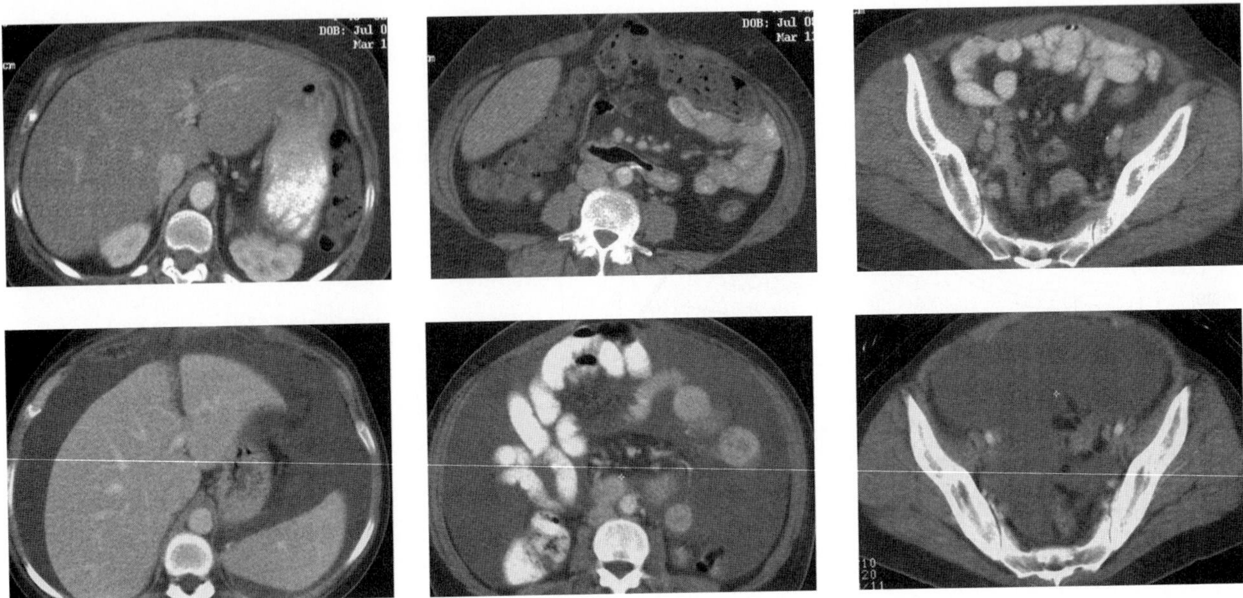

FIGURE 13.19 Computed tomography (CT) scan of a patient with ascites from peritoneal mesothelioma before (*top*) and after (*bottom*) a tumor debulking and continuous hyperthermic peritoneal perfusion (CHPP).

Gene Expression Profiling

With the completion of the sequencing of the human genome, a wealth of information is now available regarding the roughly 30,000 genes that code for various proteins involved in normal cellular homeostasis. The dysregulation of these genes that occurs in neoplastic tissue can now be studied using microarray-based technologies.

Microarrays for the study of gene expression can utilize a variety of platforms, the most common of which are cDNA and oligonucleotide sequences. Nucleic acid sequences can be spotted on glass slides or on proprietary chips, allowing 20,000 or more coding sequences to be placed on a single slide (chip). These techniques allow high throughput screening of these genes from a variety of sources capable of yielding substrate RNA. Using linear RNA amplification techniques, even the smallest samples of RNA from fine needle aspirates (FNAs) or microdissected tissues can be utilized for profiling. Gene expression profiling can be used to answer a variety of questions including the differences in gene expression pathways between malignant and normal tissues. Expression profiles can also be determined in tissues prior to and following therapies to better understand mechanism of action of a treatment.

Complex bioinformatics software programs have been developed to allow a more thorough analysis of the data sets obtained through these studies. The National Institutes of

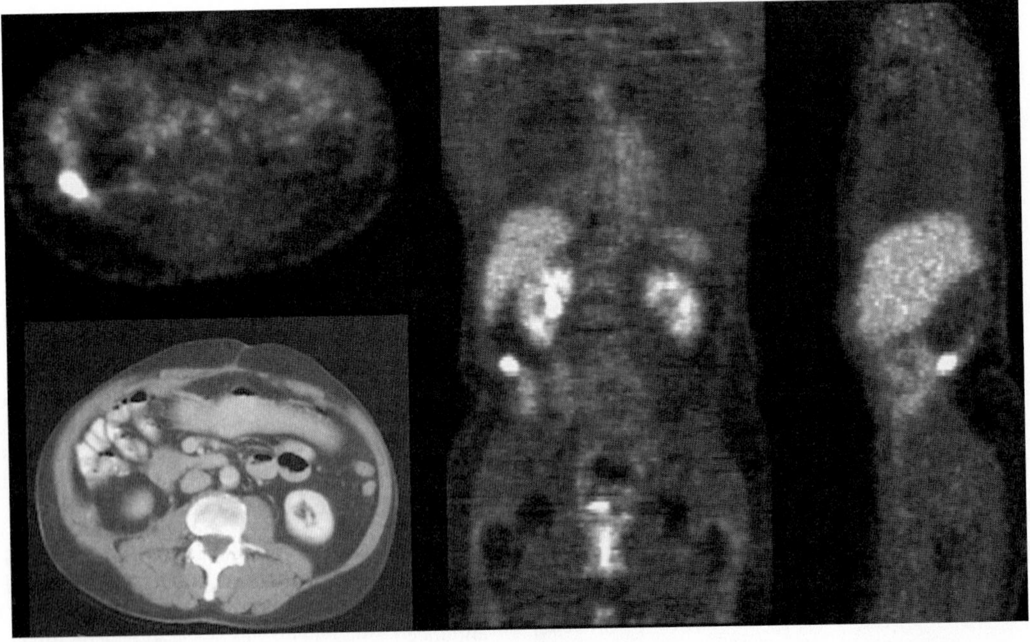

FIGURE 13.20 Fluorodeoxyglucose positron emission tomography (FDG-PET) scan demonstrates a recurrent colon cancer in the bed of a previous right hemicolectomy that was not detected on computed tomography (CT) scan in a patient with a rising serum carcinoembryonic antigen (CEA).

Health (NIH) Center for Information Technology and the NCI have posted a series of bioinformatics tools to allow investigators to better study and understand the results of their microarray experiments. This Web site can be found at http://nciarray.nci.nih.gov/.

One example of the utility of microarray approaches for the diagnosis of cancer is the differentiation of benign versus malignant thyroid lesions. Approximately 10 million new thyroid lesions are diagnosed each year in the United States. Only 5% of these lesions are malignant. Although fine needle aspiration has been utilized in an attempt to identify those patients with a thyroid cancer who require further management, straightforward cytologic examination of FNA samples often leads to indeterminate or nondiagnostic studies. A molecular method for distinguishing benign from malignant thyroid lesions would be helpful in identifying those patients who would most benefit from a surgical intervention.

Utilizing cDNA microarray, our group compared expression profiles of thyroid cancers (papillary thyroid cancers and follicular variant papillary thyroid cancers) to benign thyroid lesions. Cluster analysis developed a model to predict the malignant potential of the tissue. Using this strategy, we identified 10 genes capable of differentiating a benign lesion from a malignant lesion. By using this technique, the diagnosis of thyroid cancer from FNA may be improved.

Microarray approaches have also been used to grade lymphoma as well as predict potential response to therapies. Childhood sarcomas have also been subclassified using a similar molecular approach. As these technologies improve, more widespread use of these molecular-based diagnostics will be feasible.

Proteomics

Genes mainly code for proteins that perform the various structural and functional roles in the cell. Proteins undergo a series of modifications to perform these jobs, most importantly glycosylation and phosphorylation. Although cDNA and oligonucleotide microarrays can determine levels of gene expression, they cannot elucidate the modifications that take place at the protein level.

Proteomics, or the direct study of proteins, allows for not only a quantification of the levels of proteins present in tissues but also for a determination of the phosphorylation status of these proteins. Serum proteomics is an exciting new technology, which holds promise for the diagnosis of cancer from a sample of blood. Such an approach is now being applied to clinical samples.

Based on the assumption that patients harboring a malignancy have circulating proteins in their serum that are not present in unaffected patients, serum proteomics endeavors to distinguish a "biosignature" profile of human cancer. By taking samples from a population of patients with cancer and comparing the proteomic profile of their serum to that of a population of people without cancer, a pattern can be elucidated that identifies the at-risk population. The novelty of this approach is that, unlike investigating single specific biomarkers such as CEA for colon cancer or CA 19-9 for pancreas cancer, a serum proteomic approach requires no hypotheses about which proteins will be important to identify. In fact, thousands of proteins can be queried and utilized to form the biosignature. The most informative of these can be determined using various bioinformatics strategies to reduce the number to a manageable assay.

Applying this approach to patients with ovarian cancer, high-resolution spectral data have been obtained that demonstrated a specific pattern capable of distinguishing patients with stage 1 ovarian cancer from patients with more advanced ovarian cancer, as well as from normal healthy controls. As these techniques improve, they will no doubt be applied to other tumor histologies and will add to the armamentarium of diagnostic tests available to the clinician.

CLINICAL TRIALS

As knowledge increases regarding the pathways involved in tumorigenesis, novel agents will be identified that show promise in treating cancer. Although much can be learned about these agents in preclinical models, the ultimate evaluation of a new cancer therapeutic requires carefully conducted clinical trials.

Clinical trials involve the participation of patient volunteers. These volunteers agree to participate in studies that pose specific scientific questions to find improved strategies to prevent, diagnose, screen for, or treat a particular disease process. There are a number of types of clinical trials.

Prevention trials are designed to evaluate strategies or therapies aimed at preventing the development of cancer. These studies are most often conducted with healthy patient volunteers who have not yet developed cancer but may or may not have a predisposition to develop cancer. Screening trials are aimed at finding improved ways to determine which patients or populations of patients are most at risk for developing cancer and therefore detect cancers in these patients at the earliest time point to be more effective in treating their disease.

Diagnostic trials are geared toward the study of procedures or tests that can identify cancer at its earliest possible stage. The testing of new diagnostics is often performed on patients who are already known to have cancer based on standard diagnostic tests. Supportive care (quality of life) trials are designed to investigate ways to improve the quality of life of patients in whom further therapies may not be available. These trials are of critical importance as they can often determine where new therapies may have a dramatic improvement in the symptoms of cancer and therefore decrease the suffering due to cancer in those patients.

Genetic studies can be stand-alone trials or a part of another trial. These studies may rely on the analyses of germline mutations in patients (e.g., studies of patients with familial cancer syndromes) or may rely on studies of somatic mutations in the tumor tissues themselves to understand pathways involved in tumor growth invasion and metastasis. Special considerations must be made when performing genetic studies that involve germline analysis as the findings of such studies may have far-reaching implications for the patient. Appropriate genetic counseling must be a part of the informed consent process for these studies.

The most common and familiar types of clinical trial are treatment trials, which are designed to evaluate new cancer therapies. Treatment trials are divided into different phases of evaluation for new anticancer agents. Phase I trials are performed to evaluate the safety and toxicity profile of a compound and are generally conducted in a dose escalation format. Patients receive progressively higher doses of the agent to determine the maximum tolerated dose and any dose-related toxicities. This allows for determination of the safe dose for evaluation in the next phase. Pharmacokinetics and pharmacodynamics can also be studied. These studies generally enroll 20 to 30 patients in cohorts of three patients per study dose level.

Phase II trials are focused on determining the efficacy of a given agent at its maximum tolerated dose (MTD). These trials generally focus on a given histology (or small number of histologies) to define the response rate and duration of response for the test compound. Responses are generally scored by measuring changes in the size of measurable lesions, typically using imaging studies or physical measurements of accessible

TABLE 13.7

BEST OVERALL RESPONSE CALCULATIONS BASED ON RECIST CRITERIA

Target lesions	Nontarget lesions	New lesions	Overall response
CR	CR	No	CR
CR	Incomplete response/SD	No	PR
PR	Non-PD	No	PR
SD	Non-PD	No	SD
PD	Any	Yes or no	PD
Any	PD	Yes or no	PD
Any	Any	Yes	PD

CR, complete response; PD, progressive disease; PR, partial response; RECIST, response evaluation criteria in solid tumors; SD, stable disease.

tumors. Responses can also utilize changes in circulating biomarkers or other functional measures of tumor activity.

Most current treatment trials rely on the response evaluation criteria in solid tumors (RECIST) criteria for determining the activity of the test agent. When objective tumor response is the primary endpoint of the trial, only patients with measurable disease at baseline are generally included. Measurable disease is defined as the presence of at least one measurable lesion. Measurable lesions must allow for the accurate measurement in at least one dimension with the longest diameter greater than 20 mm using conventional techniques or 10 mm or larger utilizing spiral-CT scan.

Nonmeasurable lesions are defined as all other lesions including smaller lesions, bone lesions, leptomeningeal disease, ascites, effusions, and so forth. Lesions can be measured utilizing best available methods such CT and MRI or in the case of accessible lesions such as cutaneous lesions by direct caliper measurements. The RECIST criteria does not allow for the measurement of tumor markers alone to assess response.

The RECIST criteria call for the documentation of both target and nontarget lesions. The target lesions are defined as all measurable lesions up to a maximum of five lesions per organ and ten organs in total that are representative of all involved organs. These should be measured at baseline. The criteria define, for the purpose of measurements, the total size of target lesions. This is defined as a sum of the longest diameter (LD) for all target lesions, which is calculated and reported as the baseline sum LD. This baseline sum LD is what is used as the point of reference to characterize all subsequent measurements and therefore objective responses. All other lesions that are not designated target lesions are defined as nontarget lesions and are scored only based on presence or absence rather than directed measurements.

Based on changes from the sum LD, the following response criteria are defined. For the evaluation of target lesions a complete response (CR) is defined as the disappearance of all target lesions. A partial response (PR) is defined as at least a 30% decrease in the sum of the LD of target lesions when compared to the reference baseline sum LD. Progressive disease (PD) is defined as at least a 20% increase in the sum of the LD of target lesions or the appearance of one or more new lesions. Stable disease (SD) is defined as neither a sufficient shrinkage to qualify for PR nor a sufficient increase to qualify for PD.

With respect to the evaluation of nontarget lesions, a CR is defined as the disappearance of all target lesions and normalization of a tumor marker if measured. An incomplete response or stable disease is defined as persistence of one or more nontarget lesions and or maintenance of tumor marker levels above the normal limits. Progressive disease is defined as one or more new lesions or the unequivocal progression of existing nontarget lesions.

The evaluation of response is generally recorded as the best overall response. Table 13.7 defines how best overall response is calculated based on both target and nontarget lesions. Once an overall response is calculated, the duration of this response is measured from the time that measurement criteria are met for CR or PR until the first date that recurrence or PD is objectively documented.

Strict approaches to the definition of response are critically important in evaluating the efficacy of agents in phase II trials. Notions such as "marginal response," although potentially descriptive, are not rigorously supported and therefore not interpretable with respect to the activity of an agent. Adherence to the strict definitions allows for a more critical evaluation and therefore more useful decision making with respect to the development of a new cancer therapy. Once a response rate and duration of response are determined for an agent, a decision is made on whether or not to take that agent to further clinical evaluations.

Phase III clinical trials are conducted once the maximum tolerated dose of an agent has been tested in the phase II trial in a variety of histologies and has demonstrated reasonable response and duration of response data. Although phase I and phase II trials can often be conducted with fewer than 30 patients, phase III trials generally require hundreds or thousands of patients to have the appropriate statistical power and a sufficient variety of patient types to demonstrate definitive activity.

Phase III trials are typically designed to compare the test agent to standard therapy. The strongest design is a prospective randomized trial, in some cases blinding of the investigators and/or the patient to the receipt of the experimental therapy. Although phase III trials are the definitive studies to demonstrate the superiority of a new therapy over the previous standard, the majority of new cancer agents approved by the FDA are approved after successful phase II studies.

In addition to understanding the basic mechanics and nomenclature for clinical trials, research with human subjects must be conducted according to strict scientific and ethical principals. All federally supported clinical trials and trials evaluating new drugs or devices that are subject to FDA regulation are required to be reviewed and approved by an Institutional Review Board (IRB). Most institutions require that all clinical trials and all human subjects research, regardless of funding, be reviewed and approved by their IRB.

The IRB is typically made up of physicians, nonphysician health professionals, laypersons, and statisticians who have the capacity to critically evaluate research studies or protocols to determine relative risk benefit for the patient volunteers. The IRB has the power to stop or hold clinical trials secondary to questions regarding patient safety. It is important that the IRB consider, in its evaluation of the risks and benefits of a particular protocol, the scientific design and questions being asked to determine if they are likely to be answered with the patient population under study. It is also important for the IRB to determine whether any conflicts of interest may exist with regard to the investigator conducting the trial and the agents being tested. If such conflicts exist, they should be clearly delineated in the protocol and consent document so that potential patient volunteers are given a complete disclosure of any potential conflicting motivations for the investigators conducting the study.

As newer agents are identified and new classes of agents defined (biologic agents, molecularly targeted agents, antiangiogenic agents, etc.), modifications and adaptations of the traditional clinical trial phases may be implemented. As agents are identified that impact on a particular pathway, methods for measuring the activity of that pathway may need to be incorporated into the response criteria. Classic stopping rules for traditional chemotherapeutic agents, such as evidence of progressive disease, may need to be adjusted for agents that have a slow onset of activity and require prolonged administration to have an antitumor effect. Issues such as these are under constant evaluation by the FDA and the NIH, and updated information is constantly evaluated. For up-to-date changes in clinical trial strategies as well as access to searches for available clinical trials the URL http://www.cancer.gov is a useful on-line reference.

KEY POINTS

- **There are six important capabilities that a cell or a group of cells must acquire to be capable of growing, invading, and metastasizing and thus becoming a cancer: (1) self-sufficiency in growth signals, (2) insensitivity to antigrowth signals, (3) evading apoptosis, (4) limitless replicative potential, (5) sustained angiogenesis, and (6) tissue invasion and metastases.**
- **Transformation from the normal phenotype to invasive malignancy appears to involve a loss of normal tumor suppressive and growth inhibitory responses as well as the acquisition of inappropriate proliferative signals.**
- **The ability of a cell to become self-sufficient in its growth and no longer rely on the normal temporal sequences of programmed cell growth is often the result of mutations in the genes involved in growth regulation and control.**
- **Angiogenesis is necessary for tumor growth and progression and is a potential site for targeted molecular therapy.**
- **Gene therapy and immunotherapy for cancer are areas of active investigation that have not yet reached standard practice.**
- **Operative resection or regional therapy of metastatic disease can be helpful for patients.**

Bibliography

Anisimov VN. The relationship between aging and carcinogenesis: a critical appraisal. *Crit Rev Oncol Hematol.* 2003;45:277.

Anisimov VN. Aging and cancer in transgenic and mutant mice. *Front Biosci.* 2003;8:s883.

Artavanis-Tsakonas S, Rand MD, Lake RJ. Notch signaling: cell fate control and signal integration in development. *Science* 1999;284:770.

Bartlett DL, Libutti SK, Figg WD, et al. Isolated hepatic perfusion for unresectable hepatic metastases from colorectal cancer. *Surgery* 2001;129:176.

Blagosklonny MV. How cancer could be cured by 2015. *Cell Cycle* 2005;4.

Boguski MS, McCormick F. Proteins regulating Ras and its relatives. *Nature* 1993;366:643.

Costouros NG, Diehn FE, Libutti SK. Molecular imaging of tumor angiogenesis. *J Cell Biochem Suppl.* 2002;39:72.

Dang CV. c-Myc target genes involved in cell growth, apoptosis, and metabolism. *Mol Cell Biol.* 1999;19:1.

Diamandopoulos GT. Cancer: an historical perspective. *Anticancer Res.* 1996;16:1595.

Feldman AL, Libutti SK. Progress in antiangiogenic gene therapy of cancer. *Cancer* 2000;89:1181.

Fidler IJ. The pathogenesis of cancer metastasis: the 'seed and soil' hypothesis revisited. *Nat Rev Cancer* 2003;3:453.

Finkelstein SE, Heimann DM, Klebanoff CA, et al. Bedside to bench and back again: how animal models are guiding the development of new immunotherapies for cancer. *J Leukoc Biol.* 2004;76:333.

Folkman J, Kalluri R. Cancer without disease. *Nature* 2004;427:787.

Fong Y, Fortner J, Sun RL, et al. Clinical score for predicting recurrence after hepatic resection for metastatic colorectal cancer: analysis of 1001 consecutive cases. *Ann Surg.* 1999;230:309; discussion 318.

Forman MR, Hursting SD, Umar A, Barrett JC. Nutrition and cancer prevention: a multidisciplinary perspective on human trials. *Annu Rev Nutr.* 2004;24:223.

Frijhoff AF, Conti CJ, Senderowicz AM. Advances in molecular carcinogenesis: current and future use of mouse models to screen and validate molecularly targeted anticancer drugs. *Mol Carcinog.* 2004;39:183.

Hackel PO, Zwick E, Prenzel N, Ullrich A. Epidermal growth factor receptors: critical mediators of multiple receptor pathways. *Curr Opin Cell Biol.* 1999;11:184.

Hanahan D, Weinberg RA. The hallmarks of cancer. *Cell* 2000;100:57.

Hunter KW. Host genetics and tumour metastasis. *Br J Cancer* 2004;90:752.

Jemal A, Murray T, Ward E, et al. Cancer statistics, 2005. *CA Cancer J Clin.* 2005;55:10.

Kurdziel KA, Figg WD, Carrasquillo JA, et al. Using positron emission tomography 2-deoxy-2-[18F]fluoro-D-glucose, 11CO, and 15O-water for monitoring androgen independent prostate cancer. *Mol Imaging Biol.* 2003;5:86.

Libutti SK, Alexander HR Jr, Choyke P, et al. A prospective study of 2-[18F] fluoro-2-deoxy-D-glucose/positron emission tomography scan, 99mTc-labeled arcitumomab (CEA-scan), and blind second-look laparotomy for detecting colon cancer recurrence in patients with increasing carcinoembryonic antigen levels. *Ann Surg Oncol.* 2001;8:779.

Libutti SK, Barlett DL, Fraker DL, Alexander HR. Technique and results of hyperthermic isolated hepatic perfusion with tumor necrosis factor and melphalan for the treatment of unresectable hepatic malignancies. *J Am Coll Surg.* 2000;191:519.

Libutti SK, Choyke P, Carrasquillo JA, et al. Monitoring responses to antiangiogenic agents using noninvasive imaging tests. *Cancer J Sci Am.* 1999;5:252.

Mazzanti C, Zeiger MA, Costouros NG, et al. Using gene expression profiling to differentiate benign versus malignant thyroid tumors. *Cancer Res.* 2004;64:2898.

Park BJ, Alexander HR, Libutti SK, et al. Treatment of primary peritoneal mesothelioma by continuous hyperthermic peritoneal perfusion (CHPP). *Ann Surg Oncol.* 1999;6:582.

Park JW, Kerbel RS, Kelloff GJ, et al. Rationale for biomarkers and surrogate end points in mechanism-driven oncology drug development. *Clin Cancer Res.* 2004;10:3885.

Petricoin E, Wulfkuhle J, Espina V, Liotta LA. Clinical proteomics: revolutionizing disease detection and patient tailoring therapy. *J Proteome Res.* 2004;3:209.

Preston RJ. Quantitation of molecular endpoints for the dose-response component of cancer risk assessment. *Toxicol Pathol.* 2002;30:112.

Rosenberg SA. Shedding light on immunotherapy for cancer. *N Engl J Med.* 2004;350:1461.

Rosenberg SA, Yang JC, Restifo NP. Cancer immunotherapy: moving beyond current vaccines. *Nat Med.* 2004;10:909.

Rosenblatt KP, Bryant-Greenwood P, Killian JK, et al. Serum proteomics in cancer diagnosis and management. *Annu Rev Med.* 2004;55:97.

Rye PD, Stigbrand T. Interfering with cancer: a brief outline of advances in RNA interference in oncology. *Tumour Biol.* 2004;25:329.

Sekiguchi M, Sakumi K. Roles of DNA repair methyltransferase in mutagenesis and carcinogenesis. *Jpn J Hum Genet.* 1997;42:389.

Selkirk SM. Gene therapy in clinical medicine. *Postgrad Med J.* 2004; 80:560.

Sudhakar A, Sugimoto H, Yang C, et al. Human tumstatin and human endostatin exhibit distinct antiangiogenic activities mediated by alpha v beta 3 and alpha 5 beta 1 integrins. *Proc Natl Acad Sci USA.* 2003; 100:4766.

Sund M, Hamano Y, Sugimoto H, et al. Function of endogenous inhibitors of angiogenesis as endothelium-specific tumor suppressors. *Proc Natl Acad Sci USA.* 2005.

Tandle A, Blazer DG 3rd, Libutti SK. Antiangiogenic gene therapy of cancer: recent developments. *J Transl Med.* 2004;2:22.

Thomas DM, Fleming NI, Holloway AJ, Bowtell DD. Molecular medicine: a clinician's primer on microarrays. *Intern Med J.* 2004;34:565.

Widschwendter M, Jones PA. DNA methylation and breast carcinogenesis. *Oncogene* 2002;21:5462.

Zurita AJ, Arap W, Pasqualini R. Mapping tumor vascular diversity by screening phage display libraries. *J Control Release* 2003;91:183.

Zwick E, Hackel PO, Prenzel N, Ullrich A. The EGF receptor as central transducer of heterologous signalling systems. *Trends Pharmacol Sci.* 1999; 20:408.

CHAPTER 14 ■ EVIDENCE-BASED SURGERY

TOBY A. GORDON

With the national focus on patient safety, the importance of understanding the principles of evidence-based surgical practice and outcomes research has never been greater. The surgery literature manifests the continuous striving of the surgical profession to improve the delivery of healthcare and develop and incorporate new technologies into practice. Advances such as imaging and minimally invasive interventions have blurred boundaries among some specialties. Patient safety has become an area of national focus and priority. These trends, coupled with the rising demand for surgical services, the close scrutiny of health-care costs by government and managed care, consumers' increasing independence in selecting their own care, and, especially of late, the malpractice crisis in the United States, require all surgeons to understand the development and application of evidence-based surgery and surgical outcomes research.

Evidence-based surgery draws from the fields of medicine and public health and centers on the acquisition, evaluation, and application of evidence for the care of the individual patient. More broadly defined beyond the care of the single patient, evidence-based surgery also encompasses population-based outcomes research focused on clinical, economic, and patient-reported data. This chapter was written to assist surgeons in producing and interpreting "evidence" related to surgical practice, for use in educational and patient care forums alike.

SURGICAL EVIDENCE: A HISTORICAL PERSPECTIVE

Throughout the history of surgery, surgical evidence has progressed from anecdotes and observations, case studies and reports of patient series, to sophisticated laboratory, clinical, and epidemiologic research. The modern surgical era began in the mid-19th century, when major obstacles to the progress of surgery—pain, infection, and hemorrhage—were eliminated.

The proceedings of the American Surgical Association (ASA), founded in 1880, serve as a record of the development of surgery in America and allow a historical perspective on the types of surgical "evidence" in use. Major advances in surgery reported from 1880 to 1930 reflect the shifting focus of the surgical research. Technologic developments such as radiation, direct examination of the urinary tract by cystoscopy, blood transfusion, and electric cautery and improvements in operations such as thyroidectomy, gastric resection, and craniotomy resulted in decreased mortality.[1] Early research reports were descriptive and anecdotal but reflected interest in outcomes of surgical treatment. From 1880 to 1942, new operative approaches often were developed on the basis of intuition and insight and evaluated primarily on the basis of trial and error.

The turning point in the evolution of evidence-based surgery can be attributed to Ernest Amory Codman who, in 1910, began efforts to reform clinical medicine and surgery. With his surgical mentor, F. B. Harrington, Codman created a case monitoring system in 1900 to record outcomes. Codman's "end-results" system proposed individual patient cards for data collection, on which a determination regarding outcome would be recorded. Cases in which "perfection" was not obtained would be classified according to his "nosology of errors." By using his system of comparison, Codman reasoned, surgeons could specialize in operations they did best. His approach exemplified the application of scientific management principles of industrial efficiency to the practice of medicine.[2]

Major influences on evidence-based surgery since World War I include the public health movement and the evolution of public policy related to health-care delivery, military medicine's contributions from World War II, and clinical and health services research in practice variation. The introduction of employer- and government-sponsored health insurance had an important impact on evidence-based medicine. Following World War II, the government freeze on wages brought about the provision of health insurance as a form of additional compensation. By 1966, much of the nonworking population had been given the basic right to health benefits under the federally sponsored Medicare coverage for the elderly and the joint federal and state Medicaid program for the poor. The Medicare program brought about peer review, which gave way to performance improvement activities under the mandate of the Joint Commission on Accreditation of Healthcare Organizations, further stimulating interest in outcomes research. The Medicare prospective payment system, implemented in 1983, led to the widespread use of diagnosis-related groups; the creation of comprehensive claims databases now used for economic and clinical outcomes research; and the institution of "centers of excellence," designated cost-effective providers for coronary artery bypass surgery and organ transplantation, based on clinical and outcomes measures. In the 1980s, the Centers for Medicare and Medicaid Services (then the Health Care Financing Administration) publicly disseminated mortality data developed from Medicare claims files, a practice ultimately discontinued following debate over risk adjustment of data.

In the 1920s and 1930s, tonsillectomies came under scrutiny, due to the widespread use of this procedure and the anesthesia-related mortality risks. The next notable study of variation in practice was Wennberg's 1973 research comparing surgical procedure rates in 13 hospital service areas in Vermont. He found that physicians' preferences were the greatest influence on rates of tonsillectomies, appendectomies, hysterectomies, mastectomies, hemorrhoidectomies, and surgeries for other common conditions, with considerable variation in rates of surgery across service areas.[3]

Since the 1960s, increased federal and private-sector funding has supported further clinical research. Surgical outcomes research in the 1980s and 1990s tested the efficacy and effectiveness of new surgical procedures; examined clinical outcomes and cost-effectiveness of new procedures versus existing ones; compared surgical treatment with medical treatment; analyzed the relationship between volume and outcome; and, increasingly, focused on quality-of-life considerations. Refinements in clinical and quality-of-life outcomes measurements have contributed to these areas of study. Other burgeoning areas of research include the use and evaluation of critical pathways and practice guidelines. The managed care movement provided a powerful stimulus for quality and outcomes measurement.

The most significant recent influence on evidence-based surgery comes from the Institute of Medicine's (IOM's) 1996 health-care quality initiative and its 1998 report documenting "the serious and pervasive nature of the nation's overall quality problem."[4] The IOM has identified the overuse, misuse, and underuse of health-care services and laid out a vision for the transformation of the health-care system and health policy to achieve quality care.

Evidence-based surgery in its current form manifests the influences of historic public health concerns, the IOM quality initiative, ever more sophisticated medical treatments and interventions, the increasing application of information technologies in medical care, the economic and political forces that shape health insurance, managed care and health-care reform, and the growing interest of consumers in self-directing their personal care. Ultimately, evidence-based surgical research should enable stakeholders in the health-care delivery process—patients, physicians, payers, and policymakers—to provide the highest quality, most appropriate, and most cost-effective care possible.

FRAMEWORK FOR EVIDENCE-BASED SURGERY

Quality Defined

The IOM defines quality as the degree to which health services for individuals and populations increase the likelihood of desired health outcomes and are consistent with current professional knowledge.[5] Surgical outcomes research studies the quality of surgical care, from the selected treatment approaches and clinical interventions to systems of care delivery, with results of interest to physicians, patients, and policymakers alike.

Measures of the Performance of Health-Care Delivery

Traditional measures of the performance of health-care delivery systems focus on access to care, quality, and cost. Donabedian, the foremost researcher in medical quality assessment, defined a conceptual model in which the outcomes of healthcare are measured by examining the structures and processes of care as well as patient factors and risks.[6] Structural features comprise patient, provider, and payer characteristics; process-of-care measures describe what was done to and for the patient; and outcomes are classified as clinical and physiologic, patient-reported, and economic.[6] Key considerations in evidence-based surgery include the measurement and interpretation of outcomes and the design of studies to obtain them.

Outcomes Measurement

Guice[7] described successful outcomes measurement as documenting changes in clinical condition as a result of medical intervention; collecting data in a common format; maintaining data collected from multiple clinical sites in a single site to facilitate comparison of outcomes; incorporating standardized and validated methods of accounting for a health-care organization's effect on health and quality; enabling physicians to assess and select medical treatments and accurately predict the resources needed for care on the basis of the actual results and cost of a treatment; providing data to establish standards or guidelines for treatment; and providing patients with specific facts to help them make medical decisions, including facts concerning treatments and their cost, efficacy, and impact on quality of life.

Comprehensive measurement of outcomes includes clinical, economic, and patient-reported data.

CLINICAL OUTCOMES MEASUREMENT

Much of the evidence-based surgery literature assesses clinical and physiologic measures, which may include symptoms, anatomic descriptors and physical signs, physiologic or functional data as measured or observed by clinicians at a specific point in time or within a specified time period, and the end results of clinical care as measured by morbidity and mortality. Outcomes measures can be taken at the patient, study group, or population level. The most commonly used clinical measures of the consequences of surgical therapy are rates of mortality and morbidity, gains in life expectancy, relative risk, relative and absolute risk reduction, and potential impact in absolute numbers.

Mortality

Mortality is the most reliably measured clinical outcome. It is most meaningfully expressed as the proportion of deaths from a particular cause over a defined time interval and most reliably measured from death certificates. *Postoperative mortality* generally refers to death within 30 days after a procedure. However, because patients today commonly have hospital stays that are far shorter than a month, care must be taken to differentiate between *in-hospital* and *postoperative* mortality. In *mortality rates,* the denominator represents the entire population at risk of dying from the disease, that is, those with a disease or condition or at risk for the condition. *Case fatality rate* includes only those with the disease in the denominator. *Gain in life expectancy* is generally discerned from life-table analysis, but its interpretation can be problematic without carefully designed clinical trials that control for competing explanations for the gains.

The *relative risk* is the ratio of probabilities of adverse outcomes in two treatments being compared. We interpret relative risk and the odds ratio the same way, and under certain conditions the two rates approximate each other. Alternatively, retrospective study designs commonly measure odds ratios rather than relative risk. *Relative risk reduction* is a treatment's reduction of adverse clinical outcomes due to the progression of disease. It is expressed in the difference in event rates between the control and treatment groups, divided by the event rate in the control group. Relative risk reduction does not reflect the magnitude of the risk without therapy, and thus it will overestimate or underestimate the effect of therapy when adverse events in untreated patients are very rare or very common, respectively. The *absolute risk reduction* (also known as the attributable risk reduction) is the difference in event rates between the control and treatment groups. As an expression of the consequences of giving no treatment, it provides an additional measure of clinical effect. Last, the *number needed to treat* is the number of patients who must be treated to prevent one adverse event. The shortcomings of the foregoing measures of clinical benefit result from the properties of the measures themselves, as well as from the data used. Any measure of the benefit of treatment may vary considerably in different trials of the same or similar therapy because of different patient populations, study design, or chance; thus, the applicability of results of a study must be evaluated carefully. Because trials are of finite duration, the effects of continuing therapy beyond the period of the trial are not known. Some treatments may not be effective until long after they have been started, and there needs to be an adequate duration of follow-up.[8]

Morbidity

Mortality has less meaning in the study of surgical procedures in which death is an extremely rare event; therefore, it is more meaningful to report morbidity, often referred to in the surgical literature as complications. *Morbidity* measures the presence of illness and the degree of dysfunction, which can be assessed as days of work missed or bed-disability days. Because surgical *complications* can range in severity from simple wound infections to life-threatening conditions, they should be reported separately, considering the underlying procedure or treatment of study. Generic surgical complications—such as wound infection, pneumonia, urinary tract infection, and bleeding requiring blood transfusion—should be examined in addition to disease- or procedure-specific complications. Complications are coded according to the International Classification of Diseases (ICD), now in its tenth revision. Because coding categories and regulations change from one revision to another, any study of time trends in morbidity that spans more than one revision must examine the possibility that observed changes could be due entirely or in part to changes in the ICD. Changes in disease definition can also have a significant effect on the number of cases of the disease that are reported or that are reported and subsequently classified as meeting the diagnostic criteria for the disease.

Clinical signs and symptoms are important but subjective measures of morbidity. Care must be taken to standardize definitions. When reporting a test value as a clinical outcome, it is essential to define the normal range for the test, because definitions might vary among laboratories or institutions. In addition, it is important to define clearly the clinical context in which the test was ordered, so that interpretation of the result is appropriate. *Trends* in test results are as important as their absolute values, because changes over time may represent return of disease and poor clinical outcome.

ECONOMIC OUTCOMES MEASUREMENT

Concerns about the costs of healthcare have dramatically increased the demand for economic outcome measures, which quantify the costs and/or benefits of medical and surgical care. In the evidence-based surgery literature, clinical measures of outcome such as mortality or treatment complications are reported much more frequently than are economic measures, either alone or in combination with clinical measures. This scarcity of information may be attributed not only to the interests of investigators but also the difficulties in measuring economic outcomes.

Key parameters for economic analysis include the time period for analysis, the breadth of services provided, and the perspective from which costs are defined, that is, the patient's, the provider's, or the payer's. Ideally, an economic analysis would include long-term comparisons of the costs of all services from the perspectives of all stakeholders (patient, provider, payer, and society). In actuality, the scope of analysis is much narrower; for example, an examination of the perioperative mortality for high-risk surgical procedures may limit the cost analysis to inpatient length of stay, as a proxy for cost.[9] Because the benefits and ultimate costs of a surgical intervention may not be realized until years later, studies taking only hospitalization into account do not reflect all societal costs. Thus, a longer time frame of analysis is desirable, such as an episode of illness, or 1-year or longer periods. The ideal economic measure of costs from the societal perspective is the social opportunity cost of the inputs to the health-care process, that is, the highest value the inputs could earn if used for other purposes.[10] Analyses that compare the utility of additional spending for health-care services with the utility of other societal needs are infrequently reported. Such economic research is generally performed for purposes of making policy. An example is the effort of the Oregon Medicaid program in 1994 to rationalize service delivery by prioritizing all services provided to beneficiaries, based on cost and utility analysis.[11]

Accounting for the costs of health-care services is a complex process. Reimbursement methodologies provide incentives to classify and allocate costs differently than would be desirable for outcomes research. Additionally, the data reflect what providers are paid for services rather than the true economic costs of services. Economic measures for clinical outcomes studies may be developed in several ways. Cost analysis can be completed prospectively as part of a clinical trial. Retrospective cost data can be analyzed typically based on secondary or administrative databases. In other instances, standardized or estimated costs may be applied to models of clinical outcomes. Typically reported costs include hospital and physician charges, obtained from billing data. Administrative databases are also used for standard cost data from Medicare claims and cost reports.

PATIENT-REPORTED OUTCOMES MEASUREMENTS

Surgical procedures aim at improving the quality of life as well as prolonging life, and surgical studies have increasingly examined patient-reported outcome measures such as patient-reported health status or health-related quality of life, including functioning and well-being, and patient satisfaction with healthcare. These data are usually collected using standardized questionnaires or surveys. Most surgical studies before 5 years ago neglected to collect standardized data about patient-reported health status and quality of life.

Health status, functional status, quality of life, and health-related quality of life are terms used almost interchangeably to refer to the concept of patient reports of their own health. In 1948, the World Health Organization defined *health* as "a state of complete physical, mental, and social well-being, and not merely the absence of disease and infirmity."[12] This definition reflects the multidimensional nature of health, and that it has both positive and negative aspects. Bergner identified five dimensions of *health status* (Table 14.1).[13]

TABLE 14.1

BERGNER'S FIVE DIMENSIONS OF HEALTH STATUS

Genetic and inherited characteristics
Biochemical, physiologic, and anatomic condition, including impairment of these systems, disease, signs, and symptoms
Functional status, including performance of the usual activities of daily living, such as self-care, physical activities, cognition, and work
Mental condition, which includes positive and negative emotions
Health potential, including prognosis for longevity and future functioning

Adapted from Bergner M. Measurement of health status. *Med Care.* 1985;23:696.

Quality of life is a broad concept that encompasses a person's experience and assessment of aspects of life. *Health-related quality of life* encompasses several dimensions of health status that are directly experienced by the person, including physical functioning, psychological well-being, cognitive functioning, social and role functioning, and general health perceptions. The patient's symptoms are often also included under this definition.

There are two basic approaches to quality-of-life assessment: generic and disease-specific.[14] *Generic* instruments are designed for use across different diseases, treatments, settings, and patient groups. The major advantage is that they can be used in any population and allow comparisons of the relative impact of various health interventions. However, they may be unresponsive to changes in specific conditions and may be too general to guide clinical decision making. *Disease-specific* measures focus on dimensions of health related to a particular disease, population, symptom, or problem and may be more responsive to a change in the patient's condition than a generic instrument.

Health profiles attempt to measure multiple important dimensions of health-related quality of life. For example, the *Sickness Impact Profile*[15] assesses a physical dimension (including ambulation, mobility, body care, and movement); a psychosocial dimension (including social interaction, alertness behavior, communication, and emotional behavior); and domains such as eating, work, home management, sleep and rest, and recreation and pastimes. The *SF-36 Health Survey* (Ware, 1992) is a brief (36-item), widely used questionnaire that assesses general health perceptions, physical functioning, role limitations due to physical health, role limitations due to mental health, social functioning, pain, mental health, and energy.[16] The *Quality of Well-being Scale*[17] is a widely used instrument that combines questions about various dimensions of functional status to generate a score. The Duke Health Profile is an abbreviated version of the 63-item Duke-UNC Health Profile, developed in 1990, which generically measures patient health status in primary care settings.[18] Intended for use in evaluative studies and policy research, the European Quality of Life (EuroQol) measure, developed in 1990 and revised in 1993, shows health status as a single index score.[18] The European Organization for Research and Treatment of Cancer (EORTC) Quality of Life Questionnaire (QLQ) of 1993 is a standardized system for evaluating the quality of life of cancer patients as research subjects in international clinical trials.[18]

Descriptive or *psychometric measures* are based on the patient's report or rating of their health state on a continuum. *Utility measures,* derived from economic and decision theory,[19] refers to the value placed by the individual on a particular health state. Utility is summarized as a score ranging from 0.0, representing death, to 1.0, representing perfect health. In economic analyses, utilities are used to justify devoting resources to a treatment. Because they weight the duration of life according to its quality, they can be used to generate quality-adjusted life-years. However, because they are expressed as a single score, they do not provide detail about how specific aspects of patients' lives are affected.[12]

Patient satisfaction refers to patients' subjective evaluations of their healthcare.[20] Patient ratings of care reflect what they think is important about the quality of care, including the doctor-patient relationship and their perception of the adequacy of diagnosis and therapy. They predict patients' subsequent behavior, including how well they comply with medications prescribed, whether they return or go elsewhere, and whether they recommend a physician to others.[21] The Patient Satisfaction Questionnaire (PSQ)[22] and the Medical Outcomes Study Nine-Item Visit Rating Form[23] are examples of instruments that assess general medical care and specific physician visits. The Consumer Assessment of Health Plans (CAHPS) surveys are intended to assess health plans and services and help consumers select among them.[24] A new federal initiative, the Hospital CAHPS, or HCAHPS, aims to assess patient satisfaction with inpatient care.[25] The methodology and results of the 25-item survey instrument, developed by the Centers for Medicare and Medicaid Services in partnership with the Agency for Healthcare Research and Quality, will be made available to the public. Although there are no surgery-specific questions, pain control is an area of focus. There are few, if any, established measures of patient satisfaction with surgical care.

Quality-of-life assessments can have relevance to surgical research and practice for defining the indication for surgery, for monitoring the patient, and for evaluating the impact of treatment.[26] Surgical quality-of-life assessments should be made when different treatment alternatives might affect the patient's quality of life differently, when new interventions are implemented, when there is scarcity of resources, when the timing of an operative intervention must be determined, and when improving quality of life is the goal of intervention. When surgery is clearly life-saving or is the only treatment alternative, quality-of-life assessment may be less important. Because early clinical trials that examined the impact of surgical treatment on quality of life, studies have helped to identify treatments that are preferable based on both decreased morbidity and cost-effectiveness. At the present time, quality-of-life assessment has evolved into a crucial component of clinical trials of new and existing treatments, as well as of cohort studies. Selecting an appropriate quality-of-life measure for a specific surgical problem requires a clear formulation of the question to be answered, consideration of the factors that must be assessed, review of available instruments, review of the evidence for usefulness of instruments in a comparable population, and examination of practical considerations.

STUDY DESIGN

The quality of the evidence and the strength of the study design are critical factors in conducting and evaluating outcomes research. Determining causal links between two variables (to establish which procedures are most effective) requires randomized clinical trials or matched-pair experimental studies with blinding. The number of participants needed in a randomized controlled trial is often greater than can be recruited at any one center. The multicenter randomized clinical trial was developed as the means to deal with such circumstances. [27] In this study design, the same randomized clinical trial is conducted simultaneously at several different clinical centers. The clinical centers recruit the participants, collect the data, and administer the treatments, but the randomization of assignment and the data analysis from the trial are performed by a coordinating center. Randomization takes place within each clinical center, and the treatments are distributed at each clinical center.

Randomized clinical trials are generally accepted as the definitive approach for assessing the efficacy of a new treatment. The process of randomization, when properly implemented, provides the means by which the myriad factors that may influence the results of a trial are equally distributed between the experimental treatment group and the control, or "usual care," group. The design may provide information on the natural history of a disease during both usual care and the experimental treatment. It also addresses several weaknesses in the randomized clinical trial. The costs of such studies are generally considerable. It is impossible to subject all new therapies to a randomized clinical trial evaluation, in part because of those costs. Such studies also require considerable time, both for recruitment and, frequently, to obtain the outcomes of interest. There are also instances in which undertaking a randomized trial is simply not ethical—for example, withholding appendectomy after a ruptured appendix to determine whether antibiotic treatment alone was efficacious. Also, randomized clinical trials are not based on random samples of the population of patients. The investigators in a given trial may seek to exclude all but a very specific subset of patients with a particular disease. It is therefore often difficult to generalize the results of a randomized clinical trial to the population of patients with that particular disease. These weaknesses must be carefully weighed against the considerable strengths of this type of study.

With respect to surgery, experimental studies may be impractical because the pace of the introduction of a new surgical technology or technique outstrips the ability of surgical investigators to conduct a randomized controlled trial to evaluate its effectiveness. Experimental study designs may be limited in other ways as well: patients recruited for a clinical study may be dissimilar to the population to which investigators wish to generalize results, and participating centers may have profound differences from nonparticipating centers—for example, centers studying the efficacy of a new surgical procedure may have surgeons more skilled in that procedure.

When clinical trials are impractical or unavailable, quasi-experimental or observational studies can be valuable but must be interpreted with greater caution. Even if recruited randomly, patients may fail to enroll or respond due to factors that may be related to outcomes, such as the effect of illness on compliance with the study protocol.

Observational studies differ from randomized clinical trials in that the investigator merely observes the result of the exposure to the factor of interest, as the investigator does not assign the exposure. There are two varieties of observational studies, cohort studies and case-control studies. In cohort studies, cohorts of individuals exposed to the factor of interest and those not so exposed are recruited and followed by the investigator for a period of time to see whether the outcomes of interest occur. In a case-control study, persons with the outcomes of interest (the "cases") are recruited, as are persons who do not have that outcome (the "controls"). Both groups are queried with regard to their past exposure to the factor(s) of interest. The investigator then determines if an association exists between the exposure and subsequent outcome. The findings may reveal a relationship between exposure and outcome, but a causal link is difficult to determine in this study design, due to compounding variables the study design cannot account for. Cohort studies have been part of the evaluation of surgical procedures for much of the past century.

In the case report, or case series, a major component of clinical research in surgery, the clinician examines the response of a well-characterized disease to a new treatment. Other clinicians can then consider these data in formulating treatment plans for their own patients. Case reports present a variety of advantages, including the speed and ease with which the data may be compiled, the facility with which most clinicians can relate to the information in a given report, and the ability of all clinicians to contribute to the corpus of medical therapeutics without intensive research training. Disadvantages of case reports include the lack of a comparison group, the small sample size, and the lack of risk adjustment for comparisons to other studies and populations.

Levels of Evidence

Regardless of the study design employed, certain fundamentals apply to the analysis of all data. These are best considered within the context of the new evidence-based surgery movement, which has been described as "the conscientious, explicit, and judicious use of the current best evidence in making decisions about the care of individual patients; the integration of individual clinical expertise with the best available external clinical evidence from systematic research."[28] Such "clinical evidence" from systematic research can be of variable quality. One of the most widely used and respected classifications of levels of evidence is that of the United States Preventive Services Task Force (Table 14.2).[29] Much of the clinical decision making performed by the average practicing surgeon falls outside the realm of evidence-based medicine. Thus, the practice of surgery represents the use of extensive clinical experience and contemporaneous research findings to determine the most appropriate treatment for an individual patient.

TABLE 14.2

UNITED STATES PREVENTIVE SERVICES TASK FORCE CLASSIFICATION OF LEVELS OF EVIDENCE

Level	Quality of evidence
I	Evidence obtained from at least one properly conducted, randomized, controlled trial (RCT)
II-1	Evidence obtained from well-designed controlled trials without randomization
II-2	Evidence from well-designed cohort or case control analytic studies, preferably from more than one center or research group
II-3	Evidence obtained from several time series with or without intervention, or dramatic result in uncontrolled experiments
III	Opinions of respected authorities based on clinical experiences, descriptive studies and case reports, or reports of expert committees

As a primer on the critical assessment of outcomes studies, the *Journal of the American Medical Association*'s comprehensive series of articles on evidence design and analysis consideration constitutes an excellent resource.[30–58] Briefly, the recommended framework for critical appraisal of the quality and of a research paper and its applicability to the care of an individual patient is based on the questions in Table 14.3.

Meta-Analysis

In contrast to the study designs discussed previously, in which investigators collect data to answer questions regarding the outcomes of specific surgical procedures or related aspects of those procedures (such as prophylaxis), meta-analysis assembles existing research findings to provide an aggregate view.[59,60] In a meta-analysis, the investigator reviews the literature for all relevant

TABLE 14.3

FRAMEWORK FOR CRITICAL APPRAISAL OF RESEARCH'S APPLICABILITY TO PATIENT CARE

1. Was the assignment of patients to treatment really randomized?
2. Were all clinically relevant outcomes reported?
3. Were the study patients recognizably similar to your own?
4. Were both clinical and statistical significance considered?
5. Is this therapeutic maneuver feasible in your own practice?
6. Were all patients who entered the study accounted for at its conclusion?

studies regarding a given surgical procedure and a specific outcome.[61] The number of subjects and the strength of the association between the procedure and the outcome are recorded for each study. Then, an aggregate strength of the association is calculated using one of the statistical techniques that have been developed for this purpose. Conceptually, the estimates are weighted by the number of subjects in each study; the larger the study, the more weight that is given to that estimate in the calculation.

Meta-analysis is based on the assumptions that the quality of the individual studies are the same, that the factors examined in the studies are the same, that the data missing from any one study will not be prejudicial for the outcomes of interest, that the populations from which the study subjects were drawn are similar, and that the definitions used among the studies are the same.[60–62] There is also the assumption that all studies involving the factor and the outcome are known to the investigators.[60] Frequently, this requirement means that the investigator must know about all studies conducted regarding a factor and an outcome.[63] Because studies that do not attain statistical significance are not published as frequently as those that do reach it, some bias ("publication bias") may attend the results of the meta-analysis. Even when the investigator is aware of such studies and is able to include them in the meta-analysis, it is generally difficult to be certain that all such studies have been included.[64] Because all of these assumptions may not be satisfied, when interpreting the results of any meta-analysis one must consider the degree to which they were violated.

MEASUREMENT

Reliability and Validity

The quality of evidence is determined by the reliability and validity of the outcomes measurement.

Reliability refers to a measure's consistency or repeatability, that is, whether it gives the same result repeatedly when the same thing is measured. For clinical research and quality assessment, reliability is often measured by the criteria in Table 14.4.

TABLE 14.4

CRITERIA FOR MEASURING RELIABILITY

Criterion	Description
Test-retest reliability	Repeated use of the same measure on the same subject, yielding the same value results, when the property measured is something that should be stable over the time between the two measurements
Inter-rater reliability	Consistent results when several observers or judges obtain the information or make judgments
Measurement bias	Prejudicial influences such as investigator hypotheses and beliefs, rater tendencies, recall bias, and others[65]
Random measurement error	

Validity refers to whether or not a measure reflects what it is intended to measure. Validity is a function of reliability, inasmuch as unreliable measures cannot be valid, yet reliable measures may lack validity due to built-in sources of bias. For example, a scale may reliably or repeatedly yield the same weight but be inaccurate, thus invalid. Tests of the validity of measures used to collect evidence about the effectiveness or quality of surgical care are outlined in Table 14.5.

Before acting on evidence, surgical providers should be convinced that it is valid, or accurate. Several aspects of study methods can help determine whether a study is likely to be valid, including the study design, the sampling, the completeness of the conceptual model, the measurement and reporting of confounding variables, and measurement reliability and validity.

TABLE 14.5

TESTS OF THE VALIDITY MEASURES USED TO COLLECT EVIDENCE ABOUT THE EFFECTIVENESS OR QUALITY OF SURGICAL CARE

Criterion	Description
Face validity	Stakeholder perception that the measurement is likely to obtain accurate results
Content validity	Whether all the important content that is part of measuring an outcome is included in the measurements
Predictive validity	Whether the measurement has been demonstrated to predict future events or outcomes
Criterion validity	Similar to predictive validity, but relates subsequent outcomes to a gold standard finding already proven or known
Convergent-discriminant validity	When there is no gold standard or future event for validation, investigators determine whether the measures agree with (or are "convergent with") other similar measures, and disagree with (or can be "discriminated from") measures of states that theoretically should not be related to them

Statistical Analysis and Risk Adjustment

Techniques of statistical analysis are beyond the scope of this chapter, but the univariate versus multivariate distinction merits mention here. Studies using only univariate analyses such as chi-square are limited in strength, whereas multivariate regression, necessary for risk adjustment, is more the gold standard. The risk adjustment process occurs as part of the main statistical analysis, generally multivariate regression analysis. In this method, multivariate regression accounts for the effects of risk variables of interest (the independent variables) on the outcome of interest (the dependent variable). There are many techniques of multivariate regression, a far superior method to another observed analytic approach, that is, multiple chi-square or analysis of variance (ANOVA) analyses, which are fraught with the potential to lead investigators to erroneous conclusions, primarily because with these approaches the variables are studied in isolation and not simultaneously. Simultaneous adjustment of potential confounding variables is critical for "apples to apples" comparisons. Risk adjustment is critical but not the sole component in enhancing a study's validity. Other important study design considerations include sample size and statistical power; the distribution of data, normal or otherwise; and the effect of outliers, to name a few. Adjustment for risk is essential in comparing patient outcomes, because patient-specific risk factors can mask or confound the relationship between interventions or treatments and outcomes.[66] Patient-specific characteristics and many aspects of patient health status, especially disease comorbidities, are causally related to the outcomes of care, as is well documented in the research literature.[67–72] Therefore, risk adjustment—specifically, adjustment for disease comorbidity and severity of illness—is a way to remove the effects of confounding factors before making inferences about the outcomes of care. These adjustments are particularly relevant to surgical studies in which the effectiveness of different procedures or approaches to care is evaluated to guide evidence-based practice.

Risk defines the likelihood of a poor outcome, and the dimensions of risk are manifold. A broad set of patient risk factors can include age; sex; race and ethnicity; clinical stability; principal diagnosis; severity of principal diagnosis; extent and severity of comorbidities; physical functional status; psychological, cognitive, and psychosocial functioning; cultural and socioeconomic attributes and behaviors; health status and quality of life; and patient attitudes and preferences for outcomes.[72]

Comorbidities, or coexisting diagnoses, are usually coded in medical records as the secondary diagnoses, diseases unrelated in etiology to the principal diagnosis. Often comorbidities are chronic conditions, such as diabetes mellitus, chronic obstructive pulmonary disease, or chronic ischemic heart disease. Patients with comorbidities often differ significantly from those without these conditions. In addition to having a higher risk of death and complications, they are less able to tolerate treatment and slower to respond to therapy. In the case of surgery, operative risks often increase due to the presence of comorbidities.[72,73]

Adjustment for severity of illness differs from that for comorbidities. The definition of severity of illness is related to disease prognosis: expectations about patients' clinical outcomes are evaluated according to the extent and nature of diseases. For many diagnoses in which death is not an immediate event, defining severity will involve a subjective standard. Similarly, comparing severity among different diseases or conditions is more of a challenge. However, differentiating by severity among patients within a single diagnostic category is important for describing the illness burden in general, and distinguishing patients by the severity of their principal diagnoses is a necessary first step. Important considerations beyond severity of the primary diagnosis include the number and severity of comorbid diagnoses, acute physiologic stability, functional status, and resource needs[70] secondary to the illness.

Relating severity and comorbidities involves translating different stages of clinical conditions into an overall risk score, which requires sophisticated analysis of very large databases to obtain empirical evidence, as well as clinical judgment and an understanding of the limits of empirical analyses.[74] To begin applying adjustments to surgical outcomes, one must first determine which risk factors need to be accounted for in the study. These could be patient-specific characteristics such as age, sex, race, and medical conditions. In addition, when examining the relationship between interventions and outcomes of care, it is important to adjust for risk factors relating to the patient's condition, such as comorbidities, severity, or other disease-specific conditions, or to the procedure. These factors are generally determined by review of the literature and data analysis examining the correlation between the outcome of interest and each risk factor.

Data Sources

Data sources vary widely depending on the study design, from original primary data collection to extraction of data from clinical databases set up to study the condition of interest or from administrative databases such as Medicare claims files. Types of data generally included for analysis range from clinical signs and symptoms to laboratory results to measures of morbidity and mortality to economic and patient-reported measures as previously described.

Mortality, morbidity, and utilization are the most commonly used clinical measures because they are the most accessible from medical records, health departments, and hospital charts. Detailed clinical information can be collected unobtrusively by retrospective review of medical records. To maximize reliability, trained reviewers with a clinical background must perform abstraction. Patient confidentiality must be assured, and institutional review board (IRB) approval must be secured prior to embarking on such a review.

Morbidity surveys on population samples, such as the National Health Survey and National Cancer Surveys, are helpful because they provide population-based descriptions of frequency of death and complications and can be used to monitor trends over time. Statistical power is obtained with relative ease, and data assembly and analysis are relatively inexpensive. Disease reporting—for communicable diseases and cancer registries—is helpful for the same reasons.

Claims data analysis uses data files, such as those maintained by the Medicare program or accumulated as a byproduct of insurance and prepaid medical care plans, to explore patterns of clinical outcomes at the population level. Several problems limit the value of claims data for assessing medical effectiveness or evaluating the quality of care, however. Because they are intended primarily for financial analysis, claims data may not contain enough detail about clinical features thought to affect prognosis, such as the stage of a disease's progress at the time of diagnosis. Chart audits should be performed to confirm the accuracy of coded information. The description of diagnoses and complications is often constrained by the ICD coding system, and clinical events out of hospital, in the ambulatory setting and at freestanding surgical centers, are frequently excluded from analysis.[75] For confidentiality reasons, patient records tend not to be linked over time or across different settings. As a result, these are often cross-sectional, rather than longitudinal, analyses. Overall, it can be difficult, using claims data, to identify clinically relevant patient groups and to control for clinical factors likely to affect outcomes.

There are three major database sources for most medical and surgical effectiveness research: administrative databases, medical records, and patient-based surveys. Administrative databases, large claims files collected for billing purposes, are very useful for outcomes study of a descriptive nature, such as exploring variations in treatment patterns.

Medical records offer a rich source of information about patients and their care. Generally, medical charts document patients' histories, chief complaints, present symptoms, physical examination results, clinical assessments and diagnoses, diagnostic laboratory results, procedures, medications, in-hospital responses to therapy, clinical courses, and discharge plans. For studies relying on medical records, investigators need to have explicit review criteria; otherwise, interobserver variation and subjectivity could bias the results. Risk adjustment methods that rely on clinical measures obtained from medical records such as vital signs or laboratory findings are able to measure risks not measurable using administrative data systems. However, the costs of primary data collection from medical records may be prohibitive.

Patient surveys can obtain information unavailable in either administrative files or medical records. Survey instruments can be designed to capture subjective information such as the perception of quality, satisfaction, personal preferences, and utility. Currently, there are many survey scales available to measure health behavior and psychosocial characteristics. However, surveying patients for outcomes studies may be expensive. It requires much effort to develop an appropriate instrument and to validate it. In addition to the cost of conducting a survey, there are potential biases and numerous logistical concerns relating to the process of collecting data from patients. Survey-based information should be tested for its reliability and validity.

The practice of evidence-based surgery requires the ability to critically assess and interpret the surgical literature to plan the optimal care of each patient, such as the selection of surgical versus medical treatment, the most appropriate procedure, for example, palliative versus curative, or open versus minimally invasive approaches. Beyond the care of the individual patient, evidence can influence the design of systems of care by identifying structure and process attributes of ideal systems. For example, system design includes minimum procedure volume requirements for facilities and providers, the necessity of dedicated resources such as monitoring capabilities or specialty trained surgeons and staff, or availability of critical pathways and care management protocols. Surgical evidence can greatly contribute to efforts to improve quality and patient safety. In studying outcomes of care, the structural and process attributes of surgeons and facilities can be analyzed to determine those factors that influence outcome to support quality improvement efforts, for example, specialty training, board certification, level of experience, the physical environment, teamwork, and communications. Last, knowledge of the significance of these factors may influence health policy, such as provider and facility licensure requirements, reimbursement for care based on efficacy, effectiveness and quality of care, and planning for manpower and technology requirements.

The most important changes likely to come about in evidence-based surgery include the proliferation of evidence in the literature and the availability of patient data in regional medical record databases. The proliferation of evidence will stem in large part from the efforts of the National Institutes of Health (NIH) to foster more clinical research and quickly promulgate the results and the growing interest and specialty training in surgical outcomes research. If properly designed with sufficient patient and procedural details, regional medical records databases will enable numerous studies of relevance to surgical outcomes research. Knowledge and understanding of the methods and techniques of outcomes research will be increasingly important to all surgeons.

KEY POINTS

- **The most commonly used clinical measures of the consequences of surgical therapy are rates of mortality and morbidity, gains in life expectancy, relative risk, relative and absolute risk reduction, and the potential impact in absolute numbers.**
- **Key parameters for economic analysis include the time period for analysis, the breadth of services provided, and the perspective from which costs are defined, i.e., the patient's, the provider's or the payer's.**
- **Quality-of-life assessment can have relevance to surgical research and practice for defining the indications for surgery, for monitoring the patient, and for evaluating the impact of treatment.**
- **There are two basic approaches to quality-of-life assessment: generic and disease specific.**
- **Randomized clinical trails are generally accepted as the definitive approach for assessing of a new treatment and represent level I evidence.**
- **Observational studies differ from randomized clinical trials in that the investigator merely observes the result of the exposure to the factor of interest, as the investigator does not assign the exposure.**
- **A meta-analysis requires a review of the literature for the outcomes from all relevant studies regarding a given surgical procedure and a specific outcome.**
- **Reliability refers to a measure's consistency or repeatability, that is, whether it gives the same result repeatedly when the same thing is measured.**
- **Validity refers to whether or not a measure reflects what it is intended to measure.**
- **Multivariate regression accounts for the effects of risk variables of interest (independent variables) on the outcome of interest (dependent variable) and is the "gold standard" of statistical analysis for risk adjustment.**

References

1. Ravitch MM. *A century of surgery: the history of the American Surgical Association.* Philadelphia and Toronto: JB Lippincott; 1981.
2. Reverby S. Stealing the golden eggs: Ernest Amory Codman and the science management of medicine. *Bull Hist Med.* 1981;55:156.
3. Wennberg J, Gittelsohn A. Variations in medical care among small areas. *Sci Am.* 1981;245:120.
4. Institute of Medicine. *Crossing the quality chasm: a new health system for the 21st century.* Oregon: National Academies Press; 2001.
5. Lohr KN, ed. *Medicare: a strategy of quality assurance,* Vol. 1. Washington, DC: National Academy Press; 1990. (Institute of Medicine Report available on the Internet at http://www.nap.edu/catalog/1574.html)
6. Donabedian A. *The definition of quality and approaches to its assessment,* Vol. I. Ann Arbor, MI: Health Administration Press; 1980.
7. Guice KS, Lipscomb J. Principles of outcomes analysis. In: Stringer MD, Oldham KT, Mouriquand PDE, Howard ER, eds. *Pediatric surgery and urology: long term outcomes.* Philadelphia: WB Saunders Company; 1998:23–38.
8. Lilienfeld DE. Tools and techniques: study design. In: Gordon TA, Cameron JL, eds. *Evidence-based surgery.* BC Decker; 2000.
9. Gordon TA, Burleyson GP, Shahrokh S, et al. Cost and outcome for complex high-risk gastrointestinal surgical procedures. *Surg Forum* 1996;47:618.
10. Davidoff AJ, Powe NR, The role of perspective in defining economic measures for the evaluation of medical technology. *Int J Technol Assess Health Care* 1996;12(1):9–21.
11. HCFA. Oregon Statewide Health Reform Demonstration Fact Sheet. Available at http://www.hcfa.gov/medicaid/orfact.html, 1999.
12. Wu AW. Patient-reported outcomes measures. In: Gordon TA, Cameron JL, eds. *Evidence-based surgery.* BC Decker; 2000.
13. Bergner M. Measurement of health status. *Med Care* 1985;23:696.
14. Patrick DL, Deyo RA. Generic and disease-specific measures in assessing health status and quality of life. *Med Care* 1989;27:S217.
15. Bergner M, Bobbitt RA, Carter WB, Gilson BS. The sickness impact profile: development and final revision of a health status measure. *Med Care* 1981;19:787.
16. Ware JE, Snow KK, Kosinski M, et al. *SF-36 health survey: manual and interpretation guide.* Boston: The Health Institute; 1993.

17. Kaplan RM, Anderson JP. The quality of well-being scale: rationale for a single quality of life index. In: Walker CS, ed. *Quality of life: assessment and application*. London: MTP Press; 1988:51–77.
18. McDowell I, Newell C. General health status and quality of life. In *Measuring health: a guide to rating scales and questionnaires*. New York: Oxford University Press; 1996:421.
19. Torrance GW, Feeny D. Utilities and quality adjusted life years. *Int J Technol Assess Health Care* 1989;5:559.
20. Ware JE, Snyder MK, Wright WR, Davies AR. Defining and measuring patient satisfaction with medical care. *Evaluation Program Plann*. 1983;6:247.
21. Rubin HR, Wu AW. Patient satisfaction: its importance and how to measure it. In: Gitnick G, ed. *The business of medicine: a physician's guide*. New York: Elsevier Science; 1991:397–409.
22. Ware JE, Hays RD. Methods for measuring patient satisfaction with specific medical encounters. *Med Care* 1998;26:393.
23. Rubin HR, Gandek B, Rogers WH, et al. Patients' ratings of outpatient visits in different practice settings. *JAMA* 1993;270:835.
24. Consumer Assessment of Health Plans (CAHPS). Available at http://www.ahcpr.gov/qual/cahps.
25. Centers for Medicare and Medicaid Services. *Hospital CAHPS fact sheet*, November 5, 2004.
26. Neugebauer E, Troidl H., Wood-Dauphinee S, et al. Quality-of-life assessment in surgery: results of the Meran Consensus Development Conference. *J Theor Surg*. 1991;6:123.
27. Meinert CL. 1986 *clinical trials: design, conduct and analysis*. New York: Oxford University Press.
28. Sackett DL, Rosenberg WMC, Gray JAM, et al. Evidence based medicine: what it is and what it isn't. *BMJ* 1996;312:71.
29. Montz, FJ, Zacur HA, Fox HE, Elkins T. Gynecologic surgery. In: Gordon TA, Cameron JL, eds. *Evidence-based surgery*. BC Decker; 2000.
30. Oxman AD, Sackett DL, Guyatt GH. Users' guides to the medical literature. I. How to get started. *JAMA* 1993;270:2093.
31. Guyatt GH, Sackett DL, Cook DJ. Users' guides to the medical literature. II. How to use an article about therapy or prevention. A. Are the results of the study valid? *JAMA* 1993;270:2598.
32. Guyatt GH, Sackett DL, Cook DJ. Users' guides to the medical literature. II. How to use an article about therapy or prevention. B. What were the results and will they help me in caring for my patients? *JAMA* 1994;271:59.
33. Jaeschke R, Guyatt G, Sackett DL. Users' guides to the medical literature. III. How to use an article about a diagnostic test. A. Are the results of the study valid? *JAMA* 1994;271:389.
34. Jaeschke R, Guyatt GH, Sackett DL. Users' guides to the medical literature. III. How to use an article about a diagnostic test. B. What are the results and will they help me in caring for my patients? *JAMA* 1994;271:703.
35. Levine M, Walter S, Lee H, et al. Users' guides to the medical literature. IV. How to use an article about harm. *JAMA* 1994;271:1615.
36. Laupacis A, Wells G, Richardson WS, Tugwell P. Users' guides to the medical literature. V. How to use an article about prognosis. *JAMA* 1994;272:234.
37. Oxman Ad, Cook DJ, Guyatt GH. Users' guides to the medical literature. VI. How to use an overview. *JAMA* 1994;272:1367.
38. Richardson WS, Detsky AS. Users' guides to the medical literature. VII. How to use a clinical decision analysis. A. Are the results of the study valid? *JAMA* 1995;273:1292.
39. Richardson WS, Detsky AS. Users' guides to the medical literature. VII. How to use a clinical decision analysis. B. What are the results and will they help me in caring for my patients? *JAMA* 1995;273:1610.
40. Hayward R, Wilson M, Tunis S, et al. Users' guides to the medical literature: VIII. How to use clinical practice guidelines. A. Are the recommendations valid? *JAMA* 1995;274:570.
41. Hayward R, Wilson M, Tunis S, et al. Users' guides to the medical literature: VIII. How to use clinical practice guidelines. B. What are the recommendations, and will they help you in caring for your patients? *JAMA* 1995;274:1630.
42. Guyatt GH, Sackett DL, Sinclair JC, et al. Users' guides to the medical literature. IX. A method for grading health care recommendations. *JAMA* 1995;274:1800.
43. Naylor CD, Guyatt GH; for the Evidence-Based Medicine Working Group. Users' guides to the medical literature. X. How to use an article reporting variations in the outcomes of health services. *JAMA* 1996;275:554.
44. Naylor CD, Guyatt GH; for the Evidence-Based Medicine Working Group. Users' guides to the medical literature. XI. How to use an article about a clinical utilization review. *JAMA* 1996;275:1435.
45. Drummond MF, Richardson WS, O'Brien BJ, et al. Users' guides to the medical literature. XIII. How to use an article on economic analysis of clinical practice. A. Are the results of the study valid? *JAMA* 1997; 277:1552.
46. O'Brien BJ, Heyland D, Richardson WS, et al. Users' guides to the medical literature. XIII. How to use an article on economic analysis of clinical practice. B. What are the results and will they help me in caring for my patients? *JAMA* 1997;277:1802.
47. Dans AL, Dans LF, Guyatt GH, Richardson S. Users' guides to the medical literature. XIV. How to decide on the applicability of clinical trial results to your patients. *JAMA* 1998;279:545.
48. Richardson WS, Wilson MC, Guyatt GH, et al. Users' guides to the medical literature. XV. How to use an article about disease probability for differential diagnosis. *JAMA* 1999;281:1214.
49. Guyatt GH, Sinclair J, Cook DJ, Glasziou P. Users' guides to the medical literature. XVI. How to use a treatment recommendation. *JAMA* 1999;281:1836.
50. Barratt A, Irwig L, Glasziou P, et al. XVII. How to use guidelines and recommendations about screening. *JAMA* 1999;281:21.
51. Randolph AG, Haynes RB, Wyatt JC, et al. Users' guides to the medical literature. XVIII. How to use an article evaluating the clinical impact of a computer-based clinical decision support system. *JAMA* 1999;282:1.
52. Bucher HC, Guyatt GH, Cook DJ, et al. Users' guides to the medical literature. XIX. Applying clinical trial results. A. How to use an article measuring the effect of an intervention on surrogate end points. *JAMA* 1999;282:771.
53. McAlister FA, Laupacis A, Wells GA, Sackett DL. Users' guides to the medical literature. XIX. Applying clinical trial results. B. Guidelines for determining whether a drug is exerting (more than) a class effect. *JAMA* 1999;282:4.
54. McAlister FA, Straus SE, Guyatt GH, Haynes RB. Users' guides to the medical literature. XX. Integrating research evidence with the care of the individual patient. *JAMA* 1999;283:21.
55. Hunt DL, Jaeschke R, McKibbon KA. Users' guides to the medical literature. XXI. Using electronic health information resources in evidence-based practice. *JAMA* 2000;283:1875.
56. McGinn TG, Guyatt GH, Wyer PC, et al. Users' guides to the medical literature. XXII: How to use articles about clinical decision rules. *JAMA* 2000;284:1.
57. Giacomini MK, Cook DJ. Users' guides to the medical literature. XXIII. Qualitative research in health care. A. Are the results of the study valid? *JAMA* 2000;284:357.
58. Giacomini MK, Cook DJ. Users' guides to the medical literature. XXIII. Qualitative research in health care. B. What are the results and how do they help me care for my patients? *JAMA* 2000;284:478.
59. Lilienfeld DE, Vlahov D, Tenney JH, McLaughlin JS. On antibiotic prophylaxis in cardiac surgery: a risk factor for wound infection. *Ann Thorac Surg* 1986;42:670.
60. Sacks HS, Berrier J, Reitman D, et al. Meta-analysis of randomized controlled trials. *New Engl J Med*. 1987;316:450.
61. Spector TD, Thompson SG. The potential and limitations of meta-analysis. *J Epidemiol Community Health* 1991;45:89.
62. Meinert CL. Meta-analysis: science or religion? *Controlled Clin Trials* 1989;10:257S.
63. Dickersin K, Berlin JA. Meta-analysis: state-of-the-science. *Epidemiol Rev*. 1992;14:154.
64. Simes RJ. Publication bias: the case for an international registry of clinical trials. *J Clin Oncol*. 1986;4:1529–41.
65. Feinstein AR. *Clinimetircs*. New Haven, CT: Yale University Press; 1987.
66. Iezzoni LI. Risk and outcomes. In: Iezzoni LI, ed. *Risk adjustment for measuring healthcare outcomes*. Chicago: Health Administration Press; 1997:2–3.
67. Blumberg, MS. Risk adjusting health care outcomes: a methodologic review. *Med Care Rev*. 1986;43:351.
68. D'Hoore W, Sicotte C, Tilquin C. Risk adjustment in outcome assessment: the Charlson comorbidity index. *Methods Inf Med*. 1993;32:382.
69. Charlson M. A new method of classifying prognostic comorbidity in longitudinal studies: development and validation. *J Chron Dis*. 1987;40:373.
70. Romano PG. Adapting a clinical comorbidity index for use with ICD-9-CM administrative databases. *J Clin Epidemiol*. 1992;46:613.
71. Deyo R, Cherkin DC, Ciol M. Adapting a clinical comorbidity index for use with ICD-9-CM administrative databases. *J Clin Epidemol*. 1992;46:613.
72. Iezzoni LI. Dimension of risk. In: Iezzoni LI, ed. *Risk adjustment for measuring healthcare outcomes*. Chicago: Health Administration Press; 1997.
73. Deyo R, Cherkin DC, Ciol M. Adapting a clinical comorbidity index for use with ICD-9-CM administrative databases. *J Clin Epidemiol*. 1992;46:613.
74. Schwartz, M, Ash A. Evaluating the performance of risk-adjustment methods: continuous outcomes. In: Iezzoni LI, ed. *Risk adjustment for measuring healthcare outcomes*. Chicago: Health Administration Press; 1997.
75. *International classification of diseases—clinical modification*, 9th rev. Salt Lake City: Med-Index Publications, 1993.

CHAPTER 15 ■ QUALITY ASSESSMENT IN SURGERY

JOHN D. BIRKMEYER AND DARRELL A. CAMPBELL, JR.

From a public health perspective, surgery is associated with considerable morbidity and mortality. Extrapolating from studies on the national Medicare population, more than 25,000 U.S. patients die each year undergoing elective surgery alone.[1] Evidence that mortality rates vary widely across both hospitals and surgeons suggests that many surgical deaths could be avoided. For example, according to recent data from the New York Cardiac Surgery Reporting System, risk-adjusted mortality rates vary widely across both individual hospitals (0% to 4.0%) and individual surgeons (0% to 11%), differences not readily explained by either chance or case mix differences.[2]

In this context, demand for good measures of surgical quality is increasing steadily. Patients and their families are looking to make informed decisions about where to have surgery and turning to Internet-based "scorecards" from proprietary firms (e.g., Healthgrades.com), nonprofit advocacy groups, and departments of health from a growing number of states. Employers and payers are looking for good measures on which to center their value-based purchasing initiatives.[3] Finally, clinical leaders are looking for measures that reliably identify hospitals or surgeons with superior performance, a prerequisite for identifying "best practices" and quality improvement. To meet this demand, a variety of federal agencies, accrediting bodies, and nonprofit trade groups have redoubled efforts to develop suitable quality indicators for surgery (Table 15.1).

As reflected by the heterogeneity of these measures, however, there remains no consensus about which measures should be used to reflect surgical quality. Structural measures—a very broad group of variables that reflect the setting in which care is delivered—have received considerable attention lately. For example, the Leapfrog Group, a large coalition of health-care purchasers, is encouraging patients to seek care at hospitals with high procedure volumes for several operations.[4] Process measures, which reflect the particulars of care that patients actually receive, have long served as quality indicators in primary care and other specialties (e.g., use of beta-blockers after myocardial infarction). The Joint Commission on Accreditation of Healthcare Organizations (JCAHO) has focused its quality assessment efforts in surgery on one process of care measure—appropriate use of perioperative antibiotics.[5] Finally, and most obviously, the quality of surgical care can be assessed by direct outcome measurement. Along these lines, the American College of Surgeons is promoting broad adoption of risk-adjusted morbidity and mortality measures developed by the National Surgical Quality Improvement Program (NSQIP).

Although each has unique strengths, structural, process, and outcome measures of surgical quality have specific limitations[6] (Table 15.2). These include both practical issues (e.g., availability and cost of the necessary data) and conceptual considerations (e.g., how well measures reflect "true" perform-

TABLE 15.1

SAMPLE OF SURGICAL QUALITY INDICATORS ENDORSED BY DIFFERENT GROUPS

Operations	JCAHO/CMS	National Quality Forum	AHRQ	Leapfrog Group
Surgery—general	Appropriate antibiotic prophylaxis	Appropriate antibiotic prophylaxis		Intensivist-managed ICUs
Abdominal aneurysm repair			Volume, mortality	Volume
Carotid endarterectomy			Volume	
Coronary artery bypass grafting		Volume, mortality, IMA use	Volume, mortality	Volume, mortality, IMA use
Esophagectomy			Volume, mortality	Volume
Pancreatic resection			Volume, mortality	Volume
Pediatric heart surgery			Volume, mortality	
Hip replacement			Mortality	
Craniotomy			Mortality	
Cholecystectomy			Use of laparoscopy	
Appendectomy			Avoidance of incidental appendectomy	

JCAHO, Joint Commission on Accreditation of Healthcare Organizations; CMS, Center for Medicare and Medicaid Services; AHRQ, Agency for Healthcare Research and Quality; ICUs, intensive care units.

TABLE 15.2

TRADEOFFS OF USING STRUCTURE, PROCESS, OR OUTCOME MEASURES AS QUALITY INDICATORS

	Structure	Process	Outcomes
Examples	Procedure volume Fellowship-trained surgeons Intensivist-staffed ICUs	Perioperative beta-blockers in high-risk surgical patients Perioperative antibiotics as wound infection prophylaxis	Morbidity and mortality rates Functional health status Patient satisfaction
Primary advantage(s)	Expedient, inexpensive proxies of surgical outcomes Some measures (i.e., volume) resonate with patients	Reflect care that patients actually receive—may seem "fairer" to providers Actionable from provider perspective, clear link to quality improvement activities	Buy in from surgeons—the "bottom line" of what they do Outcomes measurement alone may improve quality
Disadvantages	Most not actionable from provider perspective Limited value for lower risk, more common surgical procedures	Often relate to secondary outcomes (e.g., antibiotics and wound infection) Little information about technical processes related to procedure-specific complications	Limited risk adjustment of outcome measures from administrative data Inadequate caseloads at most hospitals for measuring procedure-specific outcomes with adequate precision

ICUs, intensive care units.

ance). In laying out the tradeoffs associated with the three measures, we make the case that the optimal measure depends on both the clinical and policy context. We close with recommendations for moving forward the field of surgical quality assessment.

STRUCTURAL MEASURES OF SURGICAL QUALITY

Structural measures include a broad list of variables reflecting the setting or system in which care is delivered. Many of these variables are best considered at the hospital level, reflecting, directly or indirectly, its physical plant and resources or staff coordination and organization. Other structural variables describe attributes associated with the relative expertise of individual physicians.

Evidence Linking Structural Measures to Surgical Outcomes

Volume

Procedure volume—the frequency by which a given procedure is performed by the surgeon or hospital—is by far the most recognizable structural variable. Over the past 20 years, hundreds of articles have examined the relative importance of hospital volume with different procedures. Recently, two structured literature reviews have synthesized this large body of work,[7,8] each supporting the premise that high-volume hospitals have lower mortality rates with many surgical procedures. Dudley et al.[8] performed a systematic literature search to identify all studies published between 1988 and 1998 examining correlations between hospital volume and mortality for numerous surgical and medical conditions. After applying several additional methodologic criteria, 72 articles addressing 40 different procedures and diagnoses were identified. Because some articles examined more than one procedure/diagnosis, a total of 127 unique volume-outcome analyses were represented in these studies. The large majority of studies suggested better outcomes at high-volume hospitals. Of the 127 analyses, 123 (96%) noted lower mortality at high-volume hospitals, 80% of which were statistically significant. Only 4 (3%) found higher mortality rates at high-volume hospitals, but none of these findings were statistically significant.

For each procedure/diagnosis, Dudley et al. identified the single highest quality study based on explicit criteria. Factors considered included quality of case mix adjustment, sample size and number of hospitals included, data currency, and other variables. Based on findings from the single best studies, mortality was found to be significantly lower at high-volume hospitals for elective abdominal aortic aneurysm repair, lower extremity bypass, coronary artery bypass graft (CABG), coronary angioplasty, heart transplantation, pediatric cardiac surgery, pancreatic cancer surgery, esophageal cancer surgery, and cerebral aneurysm surgery.

A second structured literature review was performed by Halm et al.[7] in a report commissioned by the Institute of Medicine. The authors identified all volume-outcome studies for six procedure groups: CABG, pediatric cardiac surgery, carotid endarterectomy, abdominal aortic aneurysm repair, and cancer surgery. Of the 88 studies identified, 77% found statistically significant associations between higher volume and better outcomes. The remaining 23% did not, but no study demonstrated statistically significant associations in the opposite direction. The authors described wide variation in the methodologic quality of volume-outcome studies and noted the predominance of studies based on administrative data (with attendant concerns about the adequacy of risk adjustment). However, the 16 studies with the highest quality scores in the Halm review—each using clinical data for risk adjustment—all demonstrated statistically significant lower mortality rates at high-volume hospitals.

Although the conclusions of these two reviews are consistent and compelling, many of the volume-outcome studies on which they are based are outdated or restricted to specific states or regions that may not be broadly representative. To provide a national view of the relative importance of hospital volume with different procedures, Birkmeyer et al.[9] examined operative mortality in 2.5 million Medicare patients undergoing one of 14 different cancer or cardiovascular procedures between 1994 and 1999. Hospital volume was related to both observed and adjusted operative mortality rates for all 14 procedures ($p < 0.001$). The importance of hospital volume varied markedly by procedure (Fig. 15.1). For example, with pancreatic resection, adjusted mortality rates at very low volume hospitals were 12.5% higher (in absolute terms) than at very high volume hospitals (16.3% vs. 3.8%, respectively). Relatively large risk differences were also observed for esophagectomy (11.9%) and pneumonectomy (5.4%). Absolute differences in adjusted mortality rates between very low and very high volume hospitals were between 2% and 5% for gastrectomy, cystectomy, (nonruptured) abdominal aneurysm repair, and aortic and mitral valve replacement and less than 2% for CABG, lower extremity bypass, colectomy, lobectomy, nephrectomy, and carotid endarterectomy.

Although most volume-outcome studies have focused primarily on operative mortality, volume has also been linked to other outcomes, including risks of nonfatal complications. For example, studies have reported that higher volume hospitals (or surgeons) have lower rates of late urinary stricture after radical prostatectomy, nonfatal complications after total hip replacement, and stroke after carotid endarterectomy.[10–12] Hospital volume also seems to be related to improved long-term survival after cancer surgery. Recent studies, most relying on the Medicare-SEER linked databases, have demonstrated that patients receiving care at high-volume hospitals have better late survival after cancer surgery than patients at lower volume centers.[13–18]

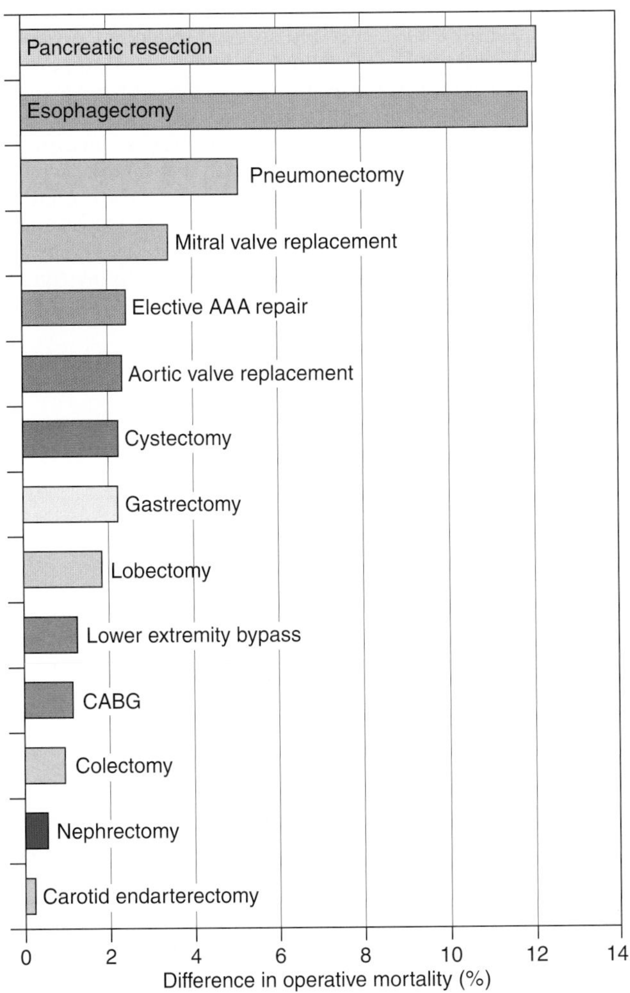

FIGURE 15.1 Absolute differences in adjusted operative mortality rates between very low and very high volume hospitals. Based on U.S. Medicare population, 1994–1999. (From Birkmeyer JD. Assessing surgical quality with structure and process of care measures. In: Mulholland MW, ed. *Complications of surgery,* 2nd ed. Philadelphia: Lippincott Williams & Wilkins; 2005.)

Surgeon Volume. Although most research has focused on hospital volume, a large number of studies have explored associations between surgeon volume and mortality with various procedures. Most have documented significant (inverse) relationships between the two.[10,19–22] For example, in New York state, patients undergoing carotid endarterectomy by low-volume surgeons were twice as likely to die perioperatively (2.0%) than patients treated by high-volume surgeons (0.9%).[22]

In the largest study to date, Birkmeyer et al.[23] used national Medicare data to examine the relationship between surgeon volume and operative mortality with eight different cardiovascular procedures and cancer resections in the national Medicare population. Surgeon volume was inversely related to operative mortality with all eight procedures ($p = 0.003$ for lung resection, $p < 0.001$ for all other procedures). As with hospital volume, the magnitude of surgeon volume-outcome relationships varied markedly by procedure in terms of both absolute mortality rates and adjusted odds ratios of mortality. Comparing low- to high-volume surgeons, adjusted odds ratios of mortality ranged from only 1.24 (lung resection) to 3.61 (pancreatic resection).

This study also suggested that apparent hospital volume effects are often mediated largely by surgeon volume. Without accounting for surgeon volume, hospital volume was inversely related to operative mortality with seven of the eight procedures ($p = 0.20$ for carotid endarterectomy, $p < 0.001$ for others). After adjusting for surgeon volume, however, higher hospital volume remained a significant predictor of decreased mortality for only four procedures. For many procedures, surgeon volume accounted for a large proportion of apparent differences in operative mortality between high- and low-volume hospitals. With elective abdominal aortic aneurysm repair, for example, adjusted odds ratios of mortality by hospital volume fell from 1.40 to 1.17 after adjusting for surgeon volume. Thus, surgeon volume accounted for 57% of the apparent difference in mortality between low- and high-volume hospitals. The proportion of the apparent hospital volume effect attributable to surgeon volume varied by procedure, from 100% with carotid endarterectomy and aortic valve replacement, to only 24% with lung resection.

Subspecialty Training

There is also a growing body of research examining the importance of surgeon training, particularly subspecialty fellowship training and/or board certification.[24,25] For example, patients with rectal cancer managed by board-certified colorectal surgeons had lower recurrence rates and improved long-term survival relative to patients managed by other general surgeons.[24] Many studies in this area have failed to account adequately for potentially confounding variables. Fellowship-trained subspecialists are more likely to have more specialized practices and thus higher volume with specific procedures. They are also more likely to practice in higher volume tertiary care centers, which may also have better patients outcomes.

However, several studies suggest that subspecialty training may be an independent predictor of favorable outcomes. For example, Goodney et al.[25] studied operative mortality in U.S. Medicare patients undergoing resection for lung cancer. Board-certified cardiothoracic surgeons had lower overall mortality rates (5.9%) than general surgeons (7.6%). These specialty-related differences were partly attenuated by surgeon volume, hospital volume, and other characteristics but did not disappear after controlling for these other variables. In another study of carotid endarterectomy in New York state, vascular surgeons had lower rates of 30-day stroke or death than did neurosurgeons or general surgeons, differences that persisted after controlling for their higher procedure volumes.[26]

Intensive Care Unit Staffing

A large proportion of surgical patients, particularly those experiencing serious complications, receive care in the intensive care unit (ICU). Because these patients have high mortality rates, it should not be surprising that structural variables reflecting the quality of ICU care may affect surgical outcomes. The most prevalent studies in this area have focused on ICU staffing and, in particular, the importance of board-certified intensivists. In one systematic review of the literature, Pronovost et al.[27] assessed mortality at hospitals with so-called low-intensity ICU physician staffing (no intensivist or elective intensivist consultation only) and those with high-intensity staffing (mandatory intensivist consultation or "closed" ICU with all care directed by intensivist). High-intensity staffing was associated with lower hospital mortality in 16 of 17 studies (94%) (Fig. 15.2). Studies included in this review were very heterogeneous and all observational in nature. Many were based on comparisons of mortality rates before and after establishment of staffing changes at individual hospitals; other relied on "cross sectional" designs, comparing mortality rates at hospitals with different staffing patterns during a single period of time. Despite their heterogeneity, these studies are remarkable in the consistency of their findings.

Nurse Staffing

Evidence is growing that high nurse staffing levels are associated with better surgical outcomes.[28–30] Aiken et al.[31] studied relationships between nurse staffing and operative mortality in a broad population of more than 230,000 general, vascular, and orthopedic surgery patients. After controlling for both patient and other hospital characteristics, patients treated in hospitals with eight patients or more per nurse were 31% more likely to die perioperatively in relative terms (0.5% higher in absolute terms) than patients in hospitals with four patients per nurse. Nurse staffing levels were more strongly related to mortality among patients experiencing complications. In a follow-up study by the same authors, hospitals in which a high proportion of nurses held a bachelor's degree or higher also had lower operative mortality rates.[32]

Structural Measures as Surgical Quality Indicators: Strengths and Weaknesses

Structural measures have several attractive features as surgical quality indicators. Procedure volume, in particular, has strong face validity for patients, essential for measures used in public reporting efforts. Thus, patients rarely ask their surgeons about their morbidity and mortality rates but frequently ask, "Do you do this procedure often?" The most important strength of structural measures, however, is expediency. Unlike process and outcome measures, many structural variables can be assessed easily and inexpensively with administrative data.

Among the downsides, the literature assessing relationships between structural measures and surgical outcomes is based entirely on observational studies. In some cases, apparent associations between structural measures and outcomes may be attributable to unmeasured differences in patient case mix across providers. Second, in contrast to process measures, many structural measures are not readily actionable, which limits their ultimate effectiveness as a means toward quality improvement. For example, a small hospital can increase the number of its surgical patients receiving perioperative antibiotics, but it cannot readily make itself a high-volume center for a given procedure or, unless it has sufficient staff, convert

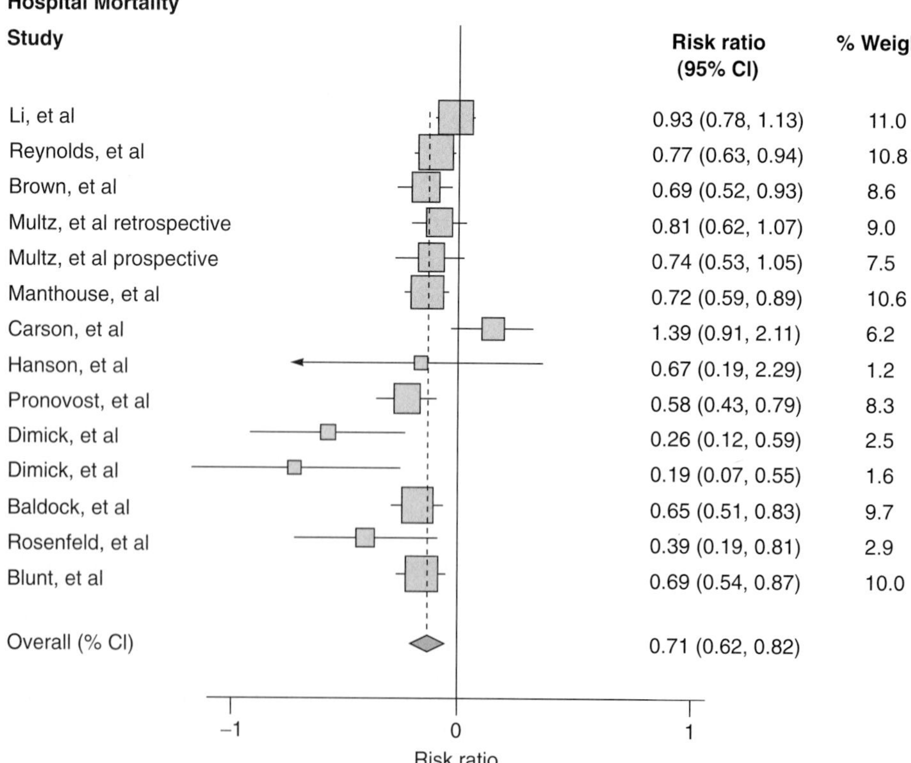

FIGURE 15.2 In-hospital mortality associated with high-intensity versus low-intensity intensive care unit (ICU) physician staffing. (From Birkmeyer JD. Assessing surgical quality with structure and process of care measures. In: Mulholland MW, ed. *Complications of surgery,* 2nd ed. Philadelphia: Lippincott Williams & Wilkins; 2005.)

to a closed-model ICU. Finally, and most importantly, structural variables like procedure volume are strong predictors of surgical performance for a small number of high-risk procedures, like esophagectomy and pancreatic resection. Thus, structural measures have limited value for lower risk (and much more common) surgical procedures.

PROCESS OF CARE MEASURES

Process of care variables reflect different components of the care that patients actually receive before, during, or after a surgical intervention. A full accounting of processes of care related to surgical outcomes is beyond the scope of this chapter. Many procedure-specific processes are considered elsewhere in this text. Among processes that cut across procedures, many have high levels of evidence supporting their effectiveness.

Evidence Linking Processes of Care to Surgical Outcomes

The Agency for Healthcare Research and Quality (AHRQ) recently commissioned a critical review of hospital-based practices related to patient safety.[33] Many practices identified by this review pertain to perioperative care, which are summarized in Table 15.3 according to strength of evidence supporting their effectiveness and the magnitude of their potential benefits. These include the use of sterile barriers and ultrasound guidance in preventing complications with central venous lines; early enteral nutrition and gut decontamination in critically ill patients; stress ulcer prophylaxis; and practices aimed at reducing wrong-site procedures.

A few specific processes of care warrant additional comment because of their wide applicability and/or their high potential to reduce rates of serious complications. Not surprisingly, some of these processes are also used widely as quality indicators in both public reporting and quality improvement initiatives.

Venous Thromboembolism Prophylaxis

The risks of postoperative deep venous thromboembolism (DVT) and pulmonary embolism (PE) vary widely according to both procedure and patient risk factors. In high-risk general surgery patients, however, rates of proximal DVT and PE may exceed 20% and 10%, respectively.[34] Numerous studies show that both low-dose unfractionated heparin (LDUH) and low-molecular-weight heparin (LMWH) reduce the risk of clinically important venous thromboembolism.[35] Pooled results from 46 randomized trials show that prophylaxis of general surgical patients with LDUH compared with placebo reduced the risk of DVT (as determined by imaging) by 68%, from 25% to 8%.[34] LMWH had comparable efficacy to LDUH overall but was possibly more effective for preventing proximal DVT and PE. In the same meta-analysis, both intermittent pneumatic compression and elastic stockings significantly reduced the overall incidence of DVT, but not proximal DVT or PE, in general surgical patients.

Prophylactic Antibiotics

A large body of Level 1A evidence supports the premise that surgical site infections can be prevented through administration of appropriate prophylactic antibiotics. As summarized in the AHRQ report on patient safety,[36] seven meta-analyses and two structured literature reviews have synthesized over 100 randomized controlled clinical trials assessing the effectiveness of prophylactic antibiotics. Although these studies focused on different antibiotic regimens and surgical populations, all concluded that perioperative antibiotics prevent surgical site infection. When compared with single-dose prophylaxis, multiple-dose prophylaxis generally did not result in significant additional benefit. Two national organizations, the Centers for Disease Control and Prevention and the American Society for Health System Pharmacists, have compiled detailed guidelines regarding the administration of prophylactic antibiotics across a broad range of procedures.[37,38]

Prophylactic Beta-Blockers

Cardiac events, including myocardial infarction, are among the most common causes of mortality in patients undergoing major surgery, particularly peripheral vascular surgery. As summarized in one recent review,[39] five randomized clinical trials have assessed the effectiveness of perioperative beta-blockers, generally consisting of therapeutic dosing prior to induction of anesthesia and continuation of targeted, postoperative therapy (generally to heart rates less than 70 per minute). Although the trials varied markedly in terms of study populations and intervention protocols, four of the five showed substantial reductions in rates of perioperative cardiac ischemia. Two of the three focusing on mortality as a primary endpoint also found substantial risk reductions. For example, in one study of male veterans undergoing major noncardiac surgery, patients receiving perioperative beta-blockers had a nearly 55% relative reduction in all-cause mortality at 2 years.[40] The sole trial not to report significant benefits with perioperative beta-blockers was relatively small and enrolled lower risk patients than the other trials.[41]

Intensive Insulin Therapy for Critically Ill Patients

Postoperative hyperglycemia is common in surgical patients, particularly those who are critically ill. However, the clinical importance of hyperglycemia had not been well established until a recent randomized controlled trial of intensive insulin therapy in critically ill patients. In that study, 1,548 patients in the ICU were randomized to traditional therapy (subcutaneous insulin dosed on a "sliding scale") or intensive insulin therapy (continuous, intravenous insulin dosed to maintain blood glucose between 80 and 110 mg/dL).[42] Intensive insulin therapy reduced mortality almost 50%, from 8.0% with conventional treatment to 4.6%. Benefits of a similar magnitude have been reported in a nonrandomized study of cardiac surgery patients.[43] Although randomized clinical trials focusing on other patient groups are clearly needed, the potential benefit of tight perioperative glucose control could be substantial.

Process of Care Measures as Surgical Quality Indicators: Strengths and Weaknesses

As potential quality indicators, process of care measures have several attractive features. First, process variables reflect the care that patients actually receive and thus tend to be perceived by providers as "fairer" measures of quality than structural measures. Second, and more importantly, process of care measures are directly actionable and link directly to quality improvement activities. For example, investigators and clinicians at six hospitals in northern New England have maintained a prospective clinical registry for CABG and other cardiac procedures since 1987. They identified numerous process of care measures linked to lower operative mortality, including use of an internal mammary graft, continuing aspirin through surgery, and maintaining a hematocrit of

24% or higher while "on pump."[44] As a result of systematic efforts to increase the use of these practices and timely feedback of performance data to clinicians, operative mortality rates across the region fell by almost half during the 1990s, a decline significantly greater than observed in regions of the United States without similar quality improvement initiatives in place.[45]

Among their disadvantages, process measures imply the need to accurately identify eligible patient populations, that is, the right denominator. Many processes known to be effective in general may not be appropriate for all patients undergoing a given procedure. For example, beta-blockers may be effective for most high-risk patients undergoing noncardiac surgery, but they are contraindicated in patients with bradyarrhythmias or severe left ventricular dysfunction. Thus, process measures often involve relatively expensive data from medical records.

Second, high-leverage process of care measures are in short supply for most procedures. High-level evidence about specific processes of care is limited primarily to the medical management of surgical patients (see Table 15.3), many of which relate to secondary outcomes. For example, wound infection is clearly associated with patient morbidity and cost, but it is clearly not as important as patient death. A large proportion of serious adverse events occurring after surgery are nonmedical in nature, arising from technical problems associated with the procedure itself—anastomotic leaks, bleeding, stroke, graft thrombosis, and so forth. Although high-leverage technical processes have been elucidated for some procedures (notably CABG and carotid endarterectomy), few procedures have been as carefully studied and thus major knowledge gaps remain.

DIRECT OUTCOME MEASURES

Since surgeon Ernest A. Codman began tracking the "end results" of surgical procedures in the early 20th century,[46] direct outcome measures have long been a staple in surgical quality assessment. Although operative mortality is most commonly used, other outcome measures that could be considered quality indicators include complication rates, length of stay, readmission rates, patient satisfaction, functional health status, and other measures of health-related quality of life. Ongoing efforts in this area vary widely in their scope (regional vs. national), clinical focus (one procedure vs. many), data source (administrative vs. clinical), and primary purpose (public reporting vs. quality improvement).

Among many examples, the Texas Health Care Information Council reports risk-adjusted mortality rates for several surgical procedures based on its hospital discharge abstract database.[47] More broadly, Healthgrades, a for-profit health reporting company, uses Medicare claims data to determine and report risk-adjusted mortality rates for a wide range of procedures and conditions.[48] There are also several ongoing large-scale initiatives aimed specifically at measuring (and improving) surgical outcomes using clinical data. Clinical outcomes registries in cardiac surgery, including those launched in New York, Pennsylvania, and northern New England in the 1980s, were among the earliest.[44,49] Several additional states

TABLE 15.3

EXAMPLES OF PROCESS MEASURES ASSOCIATED WITH SURGICAL OUTCOMES, ACCORDING TO STRENGTH OF SCIENTIFIC EVIDENCE SUPPORTING THEM AND THE COST AND COMPLEXITY OF IMPLEMENTING THEM

Implementation cost/complexity	Strength of the evidence/magnitude of potential benefit				
	Greatest	High	Medium	Lower	Lowest
Low	Appropriate venous thromboembolism prophylaxis Use of perioperative beta-blockers in patients at risk for cardiac events Appropriate use of antibiotic wound prophylaxis Antibiotic-impregnated central venous catheters	Use of supplemental perioperative oxygen Selective decontamination of digestive tract Use of silver alloy-coated urinary catheters	H_2 antagonists for stress ulcer prophylaxis Protocols/nomograms for intravenous heparin titration Maintenance of perioperative normothermia	Early analgesics in patients with acute abdomen (without compromising diagnostic accuracy) Intraoperative monitoring of vital signs/oxygenation	Use of preanesthesia check lists Counting sharps, instruments, and sponges Sucralfate for stress ulcer prophylaxis
Medium or high	Early nutritional support in critically ill patients Use of real-time ultrasound guidance during central line insertion		Barrier precautions (via gowns and gloves; dedicated equipment; dedicated personnel) Perioperative glucose control	Tunneling short-term central venous catheters	"Sign your site" protocols Catheter changes as prophylaxis against central line infections

Adapted from Making health care safer: a critical analysis of patient safety practices, from the Agency for Healthcare Quality and Research. Reprinted from Birkmeyer JD. Assessing surgical quality with structure and process of care measures. In: Mulholland MW, ed. *Complications of surgery*, 2nd ed. Philadelphia: Lippincott Williams & Wilkins; 2005.

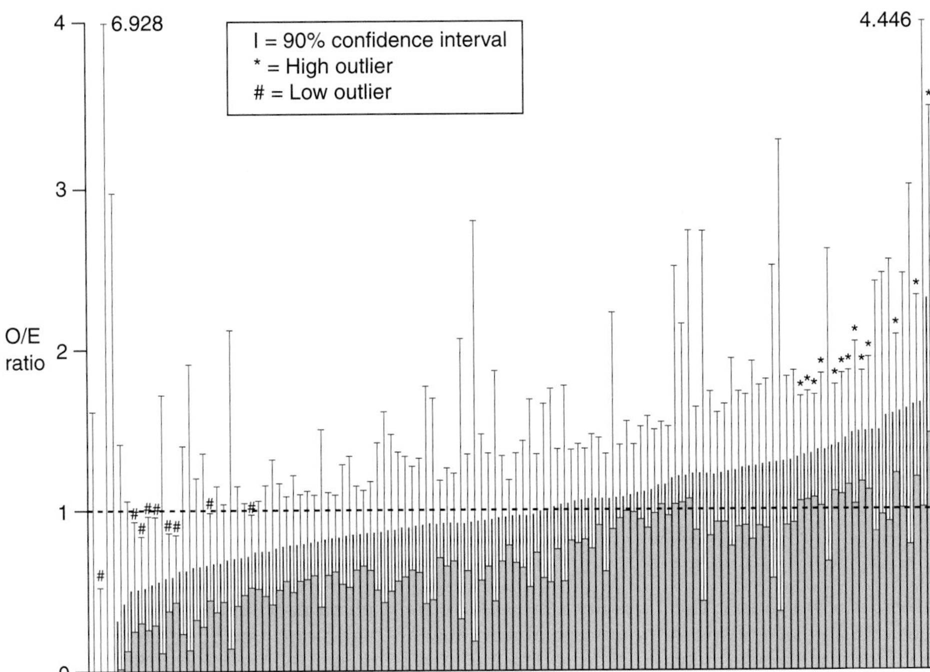

FIGURE 15.3 Observed-expected (O/E) mortality ratios for hospitals of the Department of Veterans Affairs. Each hospital is represented individually on the horizontal axis. The ratio of each hospital's observed and expected mortality rates, with accompanying 95% confidence intervals, is indicated on the vertical axis. (From Campbell DA Jr. Assessing surgical quality with clinical outcomes measures. In: Mulholland MW, ed. *Complications of surgery*, 2nd ed. Philadelphia: Lippincott Williams & Wilkins; 2005.)

and one national organization (the Society for Thoracic Surgeons) have since implemented similar data collection systems. Although these registries vary in many respects, all provide hospitals and cardiac surgeons with feedback on their risk-adjusted mortality rates.

Outside cardiac surgery, the most visible effort aimed at measuring surgical outcomes systematically has been the NSQIP.[50] Originally implemented in 132 Department of Veterans Affairs (VA) hospitals in 1991, NSQIP gathers prospective, clinically detailed data on predetermined samples of patients undergoing cardiac, general, vascular, orthopedic, and urologic procedures. It then provides individual hospitals with regular reports on their risk-adjusted morbidity and mortality rates (expressed in terms of observed/expected ratios), relative to other hospitals in the VA system (Fig. 15.3). Morbidity and mortality are assessed at the hospital level, not for individual surgeons. In addition, morbidity and mortality rates are not procedure-specific and instead reflect hospital performance across all surgical procedures. In 1999, NSQIP methodology was first adopted in the private sector by three major academic centers.[51] The program was later expanded to include 11 additional academic centers and 3 community hospitals. With the American College of Surgeons as champion, efforts are under way to expand the NSQIP into many more hospitals in the private sector.

Direct Outcome Measures as Surgical Quality Indicators: Strengths and Weaknesses

Direct outcome measures have at least two major advantages. First, because most surgeons consider patient outcomes the "bottom line" of surgical quality, efforts focused on direct outcome measures have obvious face validity and are likely to get the greatest buy-in from surgeons. Second, measurement alone may improve outcomes—the so-called Hawthorne effect. Surgical morbidity and mortality rates in VA hospitals have fallen dramatically since implementation of NSQIP in 1991.[52] No doubt many surgical leaders at individual hospitals made specific organizational or process improvements after they began receiving feedback on their hospitals' performance. However, it is very unlikely that even a full inventory of these specific changes would explain such broad-based and substantial improvements in morbidity and mortality rates.

Problems Specific to Administrative Data

Administrative data have obvious limitations with respect to risk adjustment. Claims and other administrative datasets are generally quite accurate in identifying patients undergoing a specific procedure and determining their vital status after surgery. However, these datasets provide relatively limited information with which to estimate patients' baseline operative risks. Comorbidities (e.g., diabetes, congestive heart failure) tend to be systematically underreported. Other variables are absent altogether, including physiologic data (e.g., preoperative hemodynamics, serum albumin) and acuity of the procedure (i.e., elective, urgent, or emergent).

Whether these limitations invalidate the use of administrative data for assessing procedure-specific mortality rates is a matter of debate. Simply put, risk adjustment only matters if, among patients undergoing the same procedure, some hospitals systematically treated "healthier" (or sicker) patients than other hospitals. Studies in this area are inconclusive. For example, NSQIP researchers compared surgical mortality rankings for 44 VA hospitals based on both unadjusted and adjusted mortality rates. The apparent rankings of several hospitals changed dramatically as a result of risk adjustment (Fig. 15.4). However, the marked differences between unadjusted and adjusted mortality rates in this study may have been less attributable to patient factors than to heterogeneity in the types of procedures performed by VA hospitals. Studies focusing on a single procedure are less compelling. In CABG surgery, for example, state- and regional-level studies based on prospective, clinical data suggest relatively close agreement between unadjusted and adjusted hospital mortality rates.[49,53] At least one study, also focusing on CABG, has compared risk-adjusted hospital mortality rates based on clinical data and

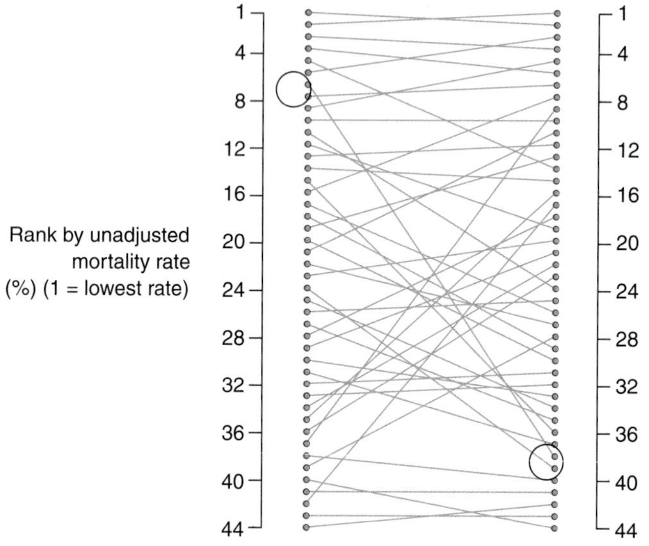

FIGURE 15.4 Hospital rankings based on unadjusted (left axis) and adjusted (right axis) mortality rates for 44 Department of Veterans Affairs hospitals. (From Campbell DA Jr. Assessing surgical quality with clinical outcomes measures. In: Mulholland MW, ed. *Complications of surgery,* 2nd ed. Philadelphia: Lippincott Williams & Wilkins; 2005.)

administrative (hospital discharge abstract) data during the same time period. Correlations between risk-adjusted hospital mortality rates from the two data sources were moderately high (0.75 to 80).[54]

Controversies in risk adjustment aside, administrative data are clearly limited in their usefulness for assessing morbidity rates. They often fail to distinguish between preexisting conditions and postoperative complications (e.g., congestive heart failure). Less ambiguous complications also seem to be consistently undercoded.[55]

Problems with Any Data Source

The most important limitation of direct outcomes measurement relates to sample size. For the large majority of surgical procedures, very few hospitals (or surgeons) have sufficient adverse events (numerators) and cases (denominators) for meaningful, procedure-specific measures of morbidity or mortality. Consider a hypothetical hospital with an observed mortality rate of 10% for a given procedure, twice the national average of 5%. That hospital's rate would need to be based on at least 185 cases to be reasonably confident (95%) that its performance was significantly worse than the national average and not simply random variation. Most common operations tend to be associated with low baseline risk, which substantially compounds problems with statistical power in measuring outcomes at the provider level.

Recent work by Dimick et al.[56] illustrates still further the problems of small sample sizes in interpreting hospital mortality rates. They used data from the Nationwide Inpatient Sample to study seven procedures for which mortality rates have been advocated as quality indicators by the Agency for Healthcare Quality and Research. For only one procedure (CABG) did a majority of U.S. hospitals have adequate caseloads to rule out a mortality rate twice the national average (Fig. 15.5). With the other six procedures, very few hospitals had sufficient caseloads to distinguish between quality problems and simple bad luck.

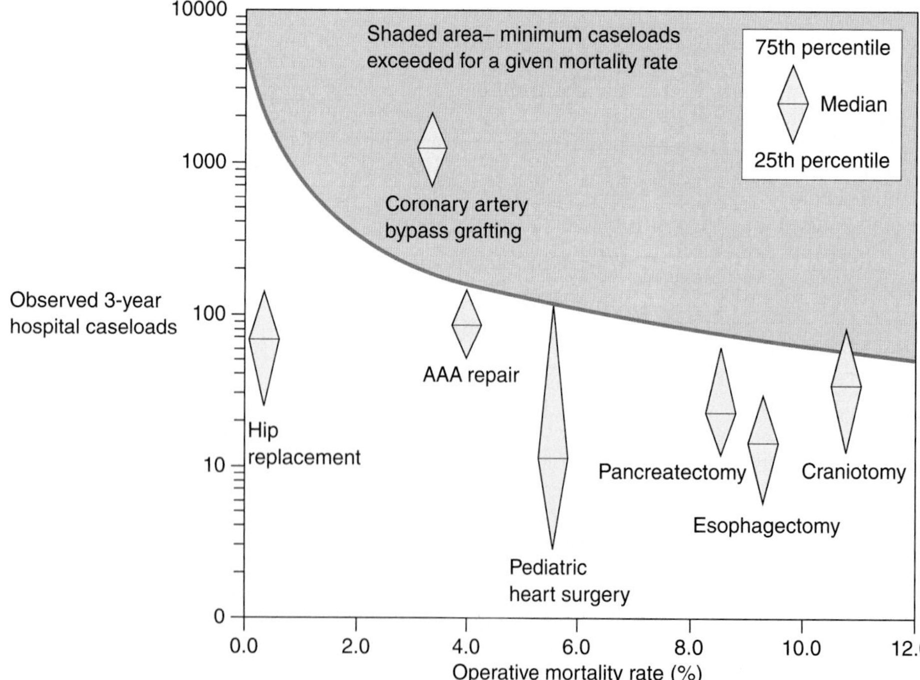

FIGURE 15.5 Distribution of actual hospital caseloads and the minimum caseload needed to detect a doubling of the mortality rate for various operations. Based on data from the 2000 Nationwide Inpatient Sample. (After Dimick JB, Welch HG, Birkmeyer JD. Surgical mortality as an indicator of hospital quality. The problem with small sample size. *JAMA* 2004;292:847. Copyright © 2004, American Medical Association. All rights reserved.)

Sample size problems can be minimized by aggregating a wide range of procedures across different surgical specialties (i.e., the NSQIP approach). However, understanding and improving processes related to a given procedure may require measures specific to that operation. Thus, aggregated measures are less satisfying from a quality improvement perspective. Moreover, aggregated measures of surgical morbidity and mortality may be suboptimal for patients (and payers) interested in identifying excellence with individual operations. Outcome measures weighted toward more common, low-risk operations (e.g., hernia repairs, cholecystectomies) may not be very informative for patients deciding where to undergo a Whipple operation.

RECOMMENDATIONS

Selecting the Right Measure

As this chapter suggests, no single measure of surgical quality is optimal for every situation. The value of structure, process, and outcome measures depends on the policy context, that is, whether the primary goal is redirecting patients to the best hospitals (evidence-based referral) or improving care everywhere (quality improvement). Structural measures, like procedure volume, may be appropriate for the former, but only process and outcome measures will be useful for the latter.

It is also important to consider the attributes of the surgical procedure being assessed. Two factors are particularly important: (a) the baseline risks of the procedure and (b) how commonly it is performed at individual hospitals (Fig. 15.6). Measuring quality for procedures that are both low risk and uncommonly performed (Quadrant III) should receive low priority. Many high-risk procedures, such as esophagectomy and pancreatic resection (Quadrant IV), are performed too infrequently at the vast majority of hospitals to support direct outcomes assessment. Thus, procedure volume, a structural measure highly correlated with mortality for many of these procedures, is likely the only practical quality indicator. Quality for procedures that are both common and relatively high risk (e.g., CABG, Quadrant II) is best assessed directly using risk-adjusted measures of morbidity and mortality. Quality improvement consortiums designed to accomplish this task are also ideal platforms for measuring process variables and linking them to outcomes. Measuring quality is perhaps most problematic for common but relatively low-risk procedures (e.g., laparoscopic cholecystectomy, Quadrant I). For these procedures, volume and other structural measures are not known to be major determinants of outcomes. Low baseline rates of mortality or other serious complications preclude measuring outcomes with sufficient precision. Thus, quality for these procedures is best judged by process measures, where available, or by patient-centered outcome measures (e.g., functional health status).

Improving the Quality of Quality Assessment

Moving the field of surgical quality assessment forward will require progress in several areas. As described earlier, high-leverage, procedure-specific processes of care must be identified. As described earlier, most high-level evidence linking process to surgical outcomes pertains to the medical aspects of perioperative care and, frequently, secondary outcomes. Less is known about the technical aspects of specific procedures that underlie wide variation in mortality rates across both hospitals and surgeons. A better understanding of such processes is essential if successes achieved with CABG are to be replicated in other areas.

Progress in outcomes measurement will simply require better data. One way to achieve this goal would be to improve the accuracy and detail of administrative data, which are relatively standardized, inexpensive, and already collected at every hospital for billing purposes. To improve their usefulness for risk adjustment, hospital discharge abstracts could be modified to include a small number of "clinical" variables most related to surgical risks with specific procedures. For example, with CABG, Hannan et al.[54] noted that risk adjustment models derived from administrative data would

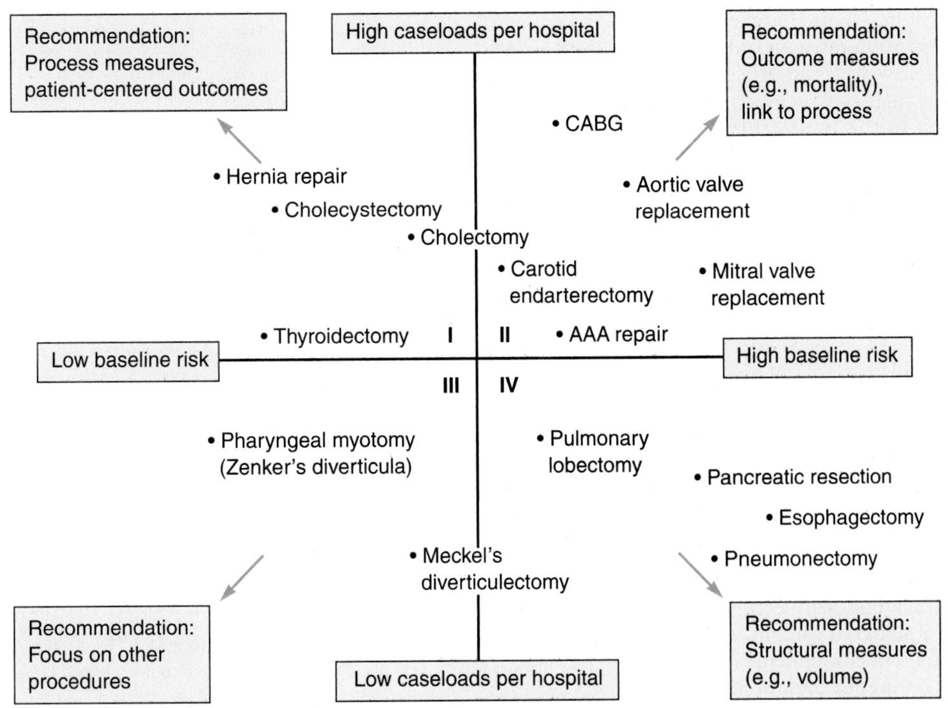

FIGURE 15.6 Recommendations for when to focus on structure, process, or outcomes. (After Birkmeyer JD, Birkmeyer NJ, Dimick JB. Measuring the quality of surgical care: structure, process, or outcomes? *J Am Coll Surg.* 2004;198:626.)

approach the reliability of those from clinical data with the addition of only three variables: ejection fraction, reoperation, and greater than 90% stenosis of the left main coronary artery. Such variables could be defined unambiguously and routinely audited to ensure accuracy. Before this approach could be recommended, however, more research would be needed to clarify the "flat of the curve" for risk adjustment models with different procedures.

A second approach to getting better outcomes data would be to disseminate NSQIP or similar clinical measurement programs across the United States. Unfortunately, gathering prospective, detailed clinical information is expensive. For example, NSQIP participation by private sector hospitals costs over $100,000 annually, which may discourage many centers from participating. Costs associated with outcomes registries may decline over time as more clinical data are collected electronically or as more participating hospitals share in the fixed infrastructure costs. Costs could be further reduced by limiting data collection to only those elements necessary for adequate risk adjustment with specific procedures. Ultimately, however, payers will need to get involved if NSQIP or similar efforts are to be employed widely. Payers can not only leverage participation by providers, they can also help foot the bill. Given the high cost of surgical complications, the business case for surgical outcomes registries and quality improvement may ultimately be very persuasive to payers and purchasers.

Whether ultimately based on clinical or administrative data, efforts to improve the reliability of surgical quality assessment will need to go beyond individual measures. After all, any individual measure of structure, process, or prior outcomes is simply a proxy for "true" hospital performance and the outcomes patients can expect in the future. "Integrative" measures that simultaneously account for multiple quality indicators may be more robust and better at predicting future performance. Such measures would incorporate information on both structural variables and processes of care shown to be related to better surgical outcomes. They would capture hospital mortality rates with the procedure of interest, as well as mortality with other, related procedures. Finally, they would incorporate information on nonfatal outcomes.

Last, we must be careful to ensure that surgical quality is not considered too narrowly. Quality in healthcare can be described as "doing the right things right." This chapter (and debates about surgical quality in general) focuses on only the latter component of this aphorism—how well the procedure was performed (i.e., doing things right). However, as suggested by wide geographic variation in the use of different procedures in the United States,[57] the quality of the decision to operate in the first place (i.e., doing the right thing) may be an equally important issue in surgical care. Thus, a full accounting of surgical quality will require measures of appropriateness and how well patient preferences are incorporated in clinical decisions, not just how well they do after surgery.

KEY POINTS

- **Structural measures include a broad list of variables reflecting the setting or system in which care is delivered.**
- **The large majority of studies suggested better outcomes for surgical procedures at high-volume hospitals.**
- **Although most volume-outcome studies have focused primarily on operative mortality, volume has also been linked to other outcomes, including risks of nonfatal complications.**
- **Process of care variables reflect different components of the care that patients actually receive before, during, or after a surgical intervention. Among processes that cut across procedures, many have high levels of evidence supporting their effectiveness.**
- **The most visible effort aimed at measuring surgical outcomes systematically has been the NSQIP, originally implemented in 132 VA hospitals in 1991. The NSQIP gathers prospective, clinically detailed data on predetermined samples of patients undergoing cardiac, general, vascular, orthopedic, and urologic procedures.**

References

1. Finlayson EVA, Birkmeyer JD. Operative mortality with elective surgery in older adults. *Effective Clin Pract.* 2001;4(4):172.
2. http://www.health.state.ny.us/nysdoh/heart/heart_disease.htm. Last accessed August 31, 2004.
3. Galvin R, Milstein A. Large employers' new strategies in health care. *N Engl J Med.* 2002;347:939.
4. **Birkmeyer JD, Dimick JB. Potential benefits of the new Leapfrog standards: effects of process and outcome measures. *Surgery* 2004;135:569.**
5. www.qualitymeasures.ahrq.gov/summary/. Last accessed August 31, 2004.
6. **Birkmeyer JD, Birkmeyer NJ, Dimick JB. Measuring the quality of surgical care: structure, process, or outcomes? *J Am Coll Surg.* 2004;198:626.**
7. Halm EA, Lee C, Chassin MR. Is volume related to outcome in health care? A systematic review and methodologic critique of the literature. *Ann Intern Med.* 2002;137:511.
8. Dudley RA, Johansen KL, Brand R, et al. Selective referral to high volume hospitals: estimating potentially avoidable deaths. *JAMA* 2000;283:1159.
9. **Birkmeyer JD, Siewers AE, Finlayson EVA, et al. Hospital volume and surgical mortality in the United States. *N Engl J Med.* 2002;346:1128.**
10. Begg CB, Reidel ER, Bach PB, et al. Variations in morbidity after radical prostatectomy. *N Engl J Med.* 2002;346:1138.
11. Cebul RD, Snow RJ, Pine R, et al. Indications, outcomes, and provider volumes for carotid endarterectomy. *JAMA* 1998;279:1282.
12. Katz JN, Losina E, Barrett J. Association between hospital and surgeon procedure volume and outcomes of total hip replacement in the United States Medicare population. *J Bone Joint Surg.* 2001;83:1622.
13. Bach PB, Cramer LD, Schrag D, et al. The influence of hospital volume on survival after resection for lung cancer. *N Engl J Med.* 2001;345:181.
14. Birkmeyer JD, Warshaw AL, Finlayson SR, et al. Relationship between hospital volume and late survival after pancreaticoduodenectomy. *Surgery* 1999;126:178.
15. Gillis CR, Hole DJ. Survival outcome of care by specialist surgeons in breast cancer: a study of 3786 patients in the west of Scotland. *BMJ* 1996;312:145.
16. Hodgson DC, Fuchs CS, Ayanian JZ. Impact of patient and provider characteristics on the treatment and outcomes of colorectal cancer. *J Natl Cancer Inst.* 2001;93:501.
17. Sainsbury R, Haward B, Rider L, et al. Influence of clinician workload and patterns of treatment on survival from breast cancer. *Lancet* 1995;345:1265.
18. Schrag D, Cramer LD, Bach PB, et al. Influence of hospital procedure volume on outcomes following surgery for colon cancer. *JAMA* 2000;284: 3028.
19. Schrag D, Panageas KS, Riedel E, et al. Hospital and surgeon procedure volume as predictors of outcome following rectal cancer resection. *Ann Surg.* 2002;236:583-92.
20. Harmon JW, Tang DG, Gordon TA, et al. Hospital volume can serve as a surrogate for surgeon volume for achieving excellent outcomes in colorectal resection. *Ann Surg.* 1999;230:404; discussion 411.
21. **Hannan EL, Siu AL, Kumar D, et al. The decline in coronary artery bypass graft surgery mortality in New York State: the role of surgeon volume. *JAMA* 1995;273:209.**
22. Hannan EL, Popp AJ, Tranmer B, et al. Relationship between provider volume and mortality for carotid endarterectomies in New York state. *Stroke* 1998;29:2292.
23. **Birkmeyer J, Stukel T, Siewers A, et al. Surgeon volume and operative mortality in the United States. *N Engl J Med.* 2003;349:2117.**
24. Porter GA SC, Yakimets WW, Newman SC. Surgeon-related factors and outcome in rectal cancer. *Ann Surg.* 1998;227:157.
25. Goodney P, Lucas FL, Stukel T, Birkmeyer JD. Surgeon specialty and operative mortality with lung resection. *Ann Thorac Surg.* 2004 (in press).
26. Hannan EL, Popp AJ, Feustel P, et al. Association of surgical specialty and processes of care with patient outcomes for carotid endarterectomy. *Stroke* 2001;32:2890.
27. Pronovost PJ, Angus DC, Dorman T, et al. Physician staffing patterns and clinical outcomes in critically ill patients: a systematic review. *JAMA* 2002;288:2151.
28. Dang D, Johantgen ME, Pronovost PJ, et al. Postoperative complications: does intensive care unit staff nursing make a difference? *Heart Lung* 2002;31:219.

29. Dimick JB, Swoboda SM, Pronovost PJ, Lipsett PA. Effect of nurse-to-patient ratio in the intensive care unit on pulmonary complications and resource use after hepatectomy. *Am J Crit Care* 2001;10:376.
30. Pronovost PJ, Dang D, Dorman T, et al. Intensive care unit nurse staffing and the risk for complications after abdominal aortic surgery.[comment]. *Effective Clin Pract.* 2001;4(5):199.
31. Aiken LH, Clarke SP, Sloane DM, et al. Hospital nurse staffing and patient mortality, nurse burnout, and job dissatisfaction.[comment]. *JAMA* 2002;288:1987.
32. Aiken LH, Clarke SP, Cheung RB, et al. Educational levels of hospital nurses and surgical patient mortality. *JAMA* 2003;290:1617.
33. *Making health care safer: a critical analysis of patient safety practices.* Rockville, MD: Agency for Healthcare Research and Quality; 2001.
34. Geerts WH, Heit JA, Clagett GP, et al. Prevention of venous thromboembolism. *Chest* 2001;119:132S.
35. Kleinbart J, Williams MV, Rask K. Prevention of venous thromboembolism. *Making health care safer: a critical analysis of patient safety practices.* Rockville, MD: Agency for Healthcare Research and Quality; 2001:333–348.
36. Auerbach AD. Prevention of surgical site infections. *Making health care safer: a critical analysis of patient safety practices.* Rockville, MD: Agency for Healthcare Research and Quality; 2001:231–243.
37. ASHP therapeutic guidelines on antimicrobial prophylaxis in surgery. American Society of Health-System Pharmacists. *Am J Health Syst Pharm.* 1999;56:1839.
38. Mangram AJ, Horan TC, Pearson ML, et al. Guideline for prevention of surgical site infection, 1999. Centers for Disease Control and Prevention (CDC) Hospital Infection Control Practices Advisory Committee. *Am J Infect Control* 1999;27:97.
39. Auerbach AD, Goldman L. beta-Blockers and reduction of cardiac events in noncardiac surgery: scientific review.[comment]. *JAMA* 2002;287:1435.
40. Mangano DT, Layug EL, Wallace A, Tateo I. Effect of atenolol on mortality and cardiovascular morbidity after noncardiac surgery. Multicenter Study of Perioperative Ischemia Research Group.[comment] [erratum appears in N Engl J Med 1997;336:1039]. *N Engl J Med.* 1996;335:1713.
41. Urban MK, Markowitz SM, Gordon MA, et al. Postoperative prophylactic administration of beta-adrenergic blockers in patients at risk for myocardial ischemia. *Anesth Analg.* 2000;90:1257.
42. **van den Berghe G, Wouters P, Weekers F, et al. Intensive insulin therapy in the critically ill patients.[comment].** ***N Engl J Med.*** **2001;345:1359.**
43. Furnary AP, Zerr KJ, Grunkemeier GL, Starr A. Continuous intravenous insulin infusion reduces the incidence of deep sternal wound infection in diabetic patients after cardiac surgical procedures. *Ann Thorac Surg.* 1999;67:352.
44. O'Connor GT, Plume SK, Morton JR, et al. Results of a regional prospective study to improve the in-hospital mortality associated with coronary artery bypass grafting. *JAMA* 1996;275:841.
45. Peterson ED, DeLong ER, Jollis JG, et al. The effects of New York's bypass surgery provider profiling on access to care and patient outcomes in the elderly. [comment]. *J Am Coll Cardiol.* 1998;32:993.
46. Neuhauser D. Ernest Amory Codman MD. *Quality Health Care* 2002;11(1):104.
47. http://www.thcic.state.tx.us/. Last accessed August 31. 2004.
48. www.healthgrades.com. Last accessed August 31, 2004.
49. Hannan EL, Kilburn H Jr, O'Donnell JF, et al. Adult open heart surgery in New York State. An analysis of risk factors and hospital mortality rates. *JAMA* 1990;264:2768.
50. **Khuri SF, Daley J, Henderson W. The Department of Veterans Affairs' NSQIP: the first national, validated, outcome-based, risk-adjusted, and peer-controlled program for the measurement and enhancement of the quality of surgical care. National VA Surgical Quality Improvement Program.** ***Ann Surg.*** **1998;228:491.**
51. Fink AS, Campbell DA Jr, Mentzer RM Jr, et al. The National Surgical Quality Improvement Program in non-veterans administration hospitals: initial demonstration of feasibility. *Ann Surg.* 2002;236:344; discussion 353.
52. Khuri SF, Daley J, Henderson WG. The comparative assessment and improvement of quality of surgical care in the Department of Veterans Affairs. *Arch Surg.* 2002;137:20.
53. O'Connor GT, Plume SK, Olmstead EM, et al. A regional prospective study of in-hospital mortality associated with coronary artery bypass grafting. *JAMA* 1991;266:803.
54. Hannan EL, Kilburn H Jr, Lindsey ML, Lewis R. Clinical versus administrative data bases for CABG surgery. Does it matter? *Medical Care* 1992;30:892.
55. Romano PS, Chan BK, Schembri ME, Rainwater JA. Can administrative data be used to compare postoperative complication rates across hospitals?[see comment]. *Medical Care* 2002;40:856.
56. Dimick JB, Welch HG, Birkmeyer JD. Surgical mortality as an indicator of hospital quality. The problem with small sample size. *JAMA* 2004; 292:847.
57. **Wennberg JE.** ***Dartmouth atlas of health care.*** **Chicago: American Hospital Publishing, Inc; 1996.**
58. Birkmeyer JD. Assessing surgical quality with structure and process of care measures. In: Mulholland MW DG, ed. *Complications of surgery.* Philadelphia: Lippincott Williams & Wilkins; 2004.
59. Campbell DA Jr. Assessing surgical quality with clinical outcomes measures. In: Mulholland MW, ed. *Complications of surgery,* 2nd ed. Philadelphia: Lippincott Williams & Wilkins, 2005.

PART TWO

SURGICAL PRACTICE

SECTION A
TRAUMA Background to Trauma Care

CHAPTER 16 ■ TRAUMA: INTRODUCTION

GREGORY J. JURKOVICH AND RONALD V. MAIER

Injury has been a frequent cause of death in the United States since accurate statistics were first collected in the middle of the nineteenth century. With decreases in infectious diseases and the industrialization of society, injury became a leading public health concern, which shows little sign of abating. Perhaps the single most responsible factor for the increase in the incidence of trauma has been the motor vehicle. Deaths from motor vehicle crashes (MVCs) skyrocketed during the 1910s through 1920s, rising from an infrequent occurrence to a peak of 30 deaths per 100,000 per year during the 1930s and 1940s. During this time, trauma achieved its current status as the leading cause of death and disability among young Americans. Trauma (intentional and unintentional injury) is currently the leading cause of death up to the age of 44 years and the fourth leading cause of death overall (after heart disease, cancer, and stroke). As a result of its effect on younger age groups, injury is the leading contributor to years of potential life lost (YPLL) before age 65 in the United States.[1]

According to the most recent Centers for Disease Control National Center for Injury Prevention and Control (CDC-NCIPC) statistics, 157,070 deaths resulted from injury in the United States in 2001 and approximately 29 million nonfatal injuries occurred (Fig. 16.1).[2] Unintentional injuries account for about two thirds of these deaths (101,537 in 2001) and nearly one half of these were caused by MVCs, including occupant, pedestrian, and motorcyclist. Falls, occurring primarily among the elderly, are the second major cause of death from unintentional injuries. In 2002, there were 3,482 unintentional drownings and 14,050 burn injuries, with 2,670 deaths. Intentional injuries are responsible for just over 50,000 deaths per year, of which 60% are suicides and 40% homicides. Firearms account for 60% of all suicides and 72% of all homicides.[3] Injury causes not only mortality but also significant morbidity. Each year, 37 million people are treated in emergency departments for injury, and approximately 10% will require hospitalization.[2] It is estimated that the direct costs associated with fatal and nonfatal injuries total over $60 billion per year.[3] Of the 16 million people living with impairments in the United States, 44% cite injury as the cause of their disability.[4] More than one half of all hospitalized trauma patients have fractures, dislocations, or ligamentous injuries. Orthopedic injuries are particularly problematic for the elderly.

Although its position as the leading killer of young people has not changed, the overall trauma mortality rate has gradually decreased during the past two decades. Prevention efforts have been especially notable in the field of transportation safety. Motor vehicle-related injuries have declined to 20/100,000/year, their lowest level since the 1920s. Moreover, deaths per mile traveled have declined to the lowest levels ever measured. Improved safety standards for vehicles, better roads, and a moderate decrease in alcohol-related crashes are the dominant contributing factors to this decline. Some of the success in combating motor vehicle-related trauma has been offset by increases in death from intentional injury, principally that related to firearms. Deaths from firearms now outnumber those from traffic injuries in several states.

Spurred by two sentinel publications by the National Academy of Sciences and the National Research Council (NAS-NRC), injury became recognized as a public health problem that had a greater impact than cancer or cardiovascular disease. In 1966, the NAS-NRC published a "white paper" entitled, "Accidental Death and Disability: The Neglected Disease of Modern Society."[5] Many have identified this publication as the inaugural event of what has become a sustained effort sponsored by the U.S. government at control of accidental injury. A 20-year follow-up study, entitled, "Injury in America: A Continuing Public Health Problem," appeared in 1985, outlining further efforts that would be needed to address the persistent problem of injury.[6] Over the past four decades and especially since the development of the National Center for Injury Prevention and Control (NCIPC) at the Centers for Disease Control and Prevention, the healthcare community has assumed a larger role in injury control. Medical and surgical specialists, epidemiologists, statisticians, biomechanical engineers, public health practitioners, and economists have all collaborated to develop a sophisticated interdisciplinary science of injury control.

Few areas exist in which public health interests so closely overlap those of direct delivery of care. Trauma care providers

Rank	<1	1-4	5-9	10-14	15-24	25-34	35-44	45-54	55-64	65+	All Ages
1	Congenital Anomalies 5,513	Unintentional Injury 1,714	Unintentional Injury 1,283	Unintentional Injury 1,553	Unintentional Injury 14,411	Unintentional Injury 11,839	Malignant Neoplasms 16,569	Malignant Neoplasms 49,562	Malignant Neoplasms 90,223	Heart Disease 582,730	Heart Disease 700,142
2	Short Gestation 4,410	Congenital Anomalies 567	Malignant Neoplasms 493	Malignant Neoplasms 515	Homicide 5,297	Homicide 5,204	Unintentional Injury 15,945	Heart Disease 36,399	Heart Disease 62,486	Malignant Neoplasms 390,214	Malignant Neoplasms 553,768
3	SIDS 2,234	Malignant Neoplasms 420	Congenital Anomalies 182	Suicide 272	Suicide 3,971	Suicide 5,070	Heart Disease 13,326	Unintentional Injury 13,344	Chronic Low. Respiratory Disease 11,166	Cerebro-vascular 144,486	Cerebro-vascular 163,538
4	Maternal Pregnancy Comp. 1,499	Homicide 415	Homicide 137	Congenital Anomalies 194	Malignant Neoplasms 1,704	Malignant Neoplasms 3,994	Suicide 6,635	Liver Disease 7,259	Cerebro-vascular 9,608	Chronic Low. Respiratory Disease 106,904	Chronic Low. Respiratory Disease 123,013
5	Placenta Cord Membranes 1,018	Heart Disease 225	Heart Disease 98	Homicide 189	Heart Disease 999	Heart Disease 3,160	HIV 5,867	Suicide 5,942	Diabetes Mellitus 9,570	Influenza & Pneumonia 55,518	Unintentional Injury 101,537
6	Respiratory Distress 1,011	Influenza & Pneumonia 112	Benign Neoplasms 52	Heart Disease 174	Congenital Anomalies 505	HIV 2,101	Homicide 4,268	Cerebro-vascular 5,910	Unintentional Injury 7,658	Diabetes Mellitus 53,707	Diabetes Mellitus 71,372
7	Unintentional Injury 976	Septicemia 108	Influenza & Pneumonia 46	Chronic Low. Respiratory Disease 62	HIV 225	Cerebro-vascular 601	Liver Disease 3,336	Diabetes Mellitus 5,343	Liver Disease 5,750	Alzheimer's Disease 53,245	Influenza & Pneumonia 62,034
8	Bacterial Sepsis 696	Perinatal Period 72	Chronic Low. Respiratory Disease 42	Benign Neoplasms 53	Cerebro-vascular 196	Diabetes Melllilus 595	Cerebro-vascular 2,491	HIV 4,120	Suicide 3,317	Nephritis 33,121	Alzheimer's Disease 53,852
9	Circulatory System Disease 622	Benign Neoplasms 58	Cerebro-vascular 38	Influenza & Pneumonia 46	Influenza & Pneumonia 181	Congenital Anomalies 458	Diabetes Mellitus 1,958	Chronic Low. Respiratory Disease 3,324	Nephritis 3,284	Unintentional Injury 32,694	Nephritis 39,480
10	Intrauterine Hypoxia 534	Cerebre-vascular 54	Septicemia 29	Cerebro-vascular 42	Chronic Low. Respiratory Disease 171	Liver Disease 387	Influenza & Pneumonia 983	Homicide 2,467	Septicemia 3,111	Septicemia 25,418	Septicemia 32,238

FIGURE 16.1 Top ten leading causes of death by age group, United States, 2001. Produced by the Office of Statistics and Programming, National Center for Injury Prevention and Control, CDC. Data from the National Center for Health Statistics Vital Statistics System.

have an important role in combating the injury epidemic in the United States. The most significant advances in the care of the injured patient that have occurred in the past 50 years are in surgery, anesthesia, imaging technology, and a better understanding of the basic cellular and genomic responses to shock and inflammation. But unique to trauma care has been the coordinated societal effort at developing a trauma *system* of care, one that spans the continuum from injury occurrence, notification, transportation, emergency and critical care, rehabilitation, and eventual community reincorporation. These advances are highlighted both in the treatment of individual patients and in the establishment of effective systems of prehospital, hospital, and rehabilitative care. Trauma systems have been called a paradigm for healthcare of the 21st century.[7]

These trauma systems have become more inclusive, including all appropriate institutions, at all levels of resources, to optimize access to care for all injured patients. The ideal system, however, is selective to avoid expensive duplication resulting from excessive designation of institutions that exceed the needs of society and the injured patient population. This approach produces both efficient utilization of expensive resources and optimization of volume and experience, leading to improved patient outcome while responding to the needs of each injured member of the society. Each system has a lead authority, usually in the department of health of the state, which is able to designate institutions that meet the various levels of standards and hold those institutions to those standards. A triage plan is in place that optimizes delivery of the right patient to the right institution, in the right time, as dictated by the patient's injuries. The ongoing quality assurance (QA) in the system to assess what is perceived to be the correct approach is truly the best approach in providing an increase in survival and decrease in morbidity and long-term disability. The system should be universal and this has been the greatest challenge, particularly in the great rural areas of America, but one that can be met and overcome with persistence and ongoing societal support. The development of this paradigm has been politically charged with perceived loss of patients and revenue and a mystique based on triage and bypass to optimize patient care. Both this resistance and inherent inertia have led to significant delays in the full deployment of the system. The quality of care, improvement in outcome, and recognized decrease in morbidity and disability continue to support and move system development forward as more and more states and regions become fully accessible to the injured patient.

HISTORICAL DEVELOPMENT OF TRAUMA CARE

Our approach to modern trauma has grown out of the care of wounds and casualty management resulting from war. Advances in rapid transport, volume resuscitation, wound management (both debridement and infection control), blood banking, enteric injury management, vascular surgery, and surgical critical care and the need for early nutritional management have all grown out of military experience. Salient historical events are shown in Table 16.1. Although by no means complete, this table provides

TABLE 16.1

SIGNIFICANT HISTORICAL DEVELOPMENTS RELATES TO TRAUMA CARE

Period or person	Contribution
Greek medicine	Wound care and fracture management
Roman Empire	Realization that laudable pus was undesirable Healing by second intention
16th-century, Paré	Use of dressing and ligature in wound management
French and Indian War, John Hunter	Differentiation between primary and secondary wound healing
Early 1800s, Dominique Jean Larrey	Developed the principle of the ambulance and the concept of triage
Crimean War, 1853–1856	Demonstrated value of nursing care (Florence Nightingale)
Samuel Gross, 1862	Described shock as the root unhinging of the machinery of life
Civil War	Rediscovery of importance of field ambulance, nonsuppurative wound care Initial use of antiseptics Further development of nursing care by Clara Barton, American Red Cross founder
World War I	Principle of débridement and delayed closure for wounds more than 8 hours old Established primary closure for wounds less than 8 hours old only Field ambulance mechanized with automobile availability Recognition that shock was due to blood or fluid loss and use of seawater to replace blood volume Introduction of Dakin solution
World War II	Débridement and delayed closure practiced Diverting colostomies standard care Blood transfusion, rapid evacuation, specialized surgical units close to the front
Korean War	Development of Mobile Army Surgical Headquarters (MASH) units, use of helicopters, development of vascular surgery, field research leading to better understanding of posttraumatic renal failure
Vietnam War	Development of an airbase regional emergency medical system with transport from injury to intervention in 1 hour Better fluid resuscitation Understanding of adult respiratory distress syndrome

examples of the many and significant contributions derived from extensive military experiences with multiple injuries.

Civilian progress, in general, has followed the evolution of military systems with regard to trauma care. In 1922, the importance of orthopedic trauma was first recognized in the United States with the establishment of the Committee on the Treatment of Fractures. This evolved into the Committee on Trauma of the American College of Surgeons in 1949. Increased awareness of traffic injuries and fatalities during the 1950s and 1960s began to raise surgical awareness and public concern. A dedicated trauma unit was opened in 1961 at the University of Maryland and the concept of the "golden hour" was established. In 1966, the National Academy of Sciences and the National Research Council's important white paper entitled, "Accidental Death and Disability: The Neglected Disease of Modern Society," increased public awareness and led to a federal agenda for the general improvement in trauma care.[5] Coupled with leadership from key academic centers and often by surgeons with recent military experience, the spread of advanced trauma systems began. The Maryland Institute of Emergency Medicine became the fist organized, statewide, regionalized system in 1973. Prehospital provider programs were formalized, emergency medical technicians (EMT) and other paramedical personnel were identified, and training programs were established. In 1973, the Emergency Medical Service Act became law, providing specific endorsement and financial assistance for the development of comprehensive prehospital emergency medical service systems. In addition to federal efforts, state and local legislatures began to organize strategies to care for injured patients by using prehospital care systems to stabilize and deliver patients to major hospitals where appropriate care could be given.

Two other factors influenced the rapid development of regionalized systems of trauma care in the late 1970s. First, major teaching hospitals in large cities had become regional trauma centers by default because of their experience and involvement in the trauma care of indigent patients. With strong academic leadership, these centers were able to develop regionalization of systems of trauma care by setting examples.

Of at least equal importance, the American College of Surgeons Committee on Trauma developed a task force to publish "Optimal Hospital Resources for the Care of the Seriously Injured" in 1976, thus establishing a standard for evaluation of care. The current version was published in 1999 and is the most comprehensive of these reports.[8] It establishes criteria for prehospital and trauma care personnel and emphasizes the importance of ongoing quality assessment. In addition, the American College of Surgeons Committee on Trauma developed the Advanced Trauma Life Support course in 1980, which has contributed to uniformity of initial care and the development of a common language for all care providers.[9]

In summary, the current awareness of trauma is the result of many historical factors, both military and civilian in origin. The prevalence and economic impact of trauma and the commitment required to provide optimal care make it a significant, ongoing challenge.

MORTALITY PEAKS AFTER TRAUMA INJURY

Trauma deaths occur at three traditionally recognized times after injury (Fig. 16.2). Approximately half of all trauma-related deaths occur within seconds or minutes of injury and are related to lacerations of the aorta, heart, brainstem, brain, and spinal cord. Few of these patients are saved by health-care systems, regardless of efficacy. In general, these injuries are best addressed using prevention strategies, either devices that prevent injury or laws that limit certain behavior patterns.[10]

The second mortality peak occurs within hours of injury and accounts for approximately 30% of deaths, half of which result from hemorrhage and half from central nervous system (CNS) injuries. Important reductions in mortality rates during this period have resulted from the development of trauma and rapid transport systems. Overall, trauma mortality rates have been reduced from approximately 25% to 30% to 2% to 5% where well-organized trauma care systems exist.[11,12] Only approximately 25% of the United States, however, is served by such systems. Further development of trauma systems, organized care protocols, and expansion of these systems to rural areas will undoubtedly result in further reductions in mortality rates during this early postinjury period.

The third mortality peak includes deaths that occur from day 1 to 2 after trauma to weeks later. This late mortality usually is attributed to infection and multiple organ failure.[13] Of trauma deaths, 10% to 20% occur during this period. The development of efficient trauma systems, however, has changed the epidemiology of these deaths. During the first week after trauma, refractory intracranial hypertension after severe head injury now accounts for a significant number of these deaths. The incidence of sepsis and multiple organ failure has diminished as a result of aggressive and better early

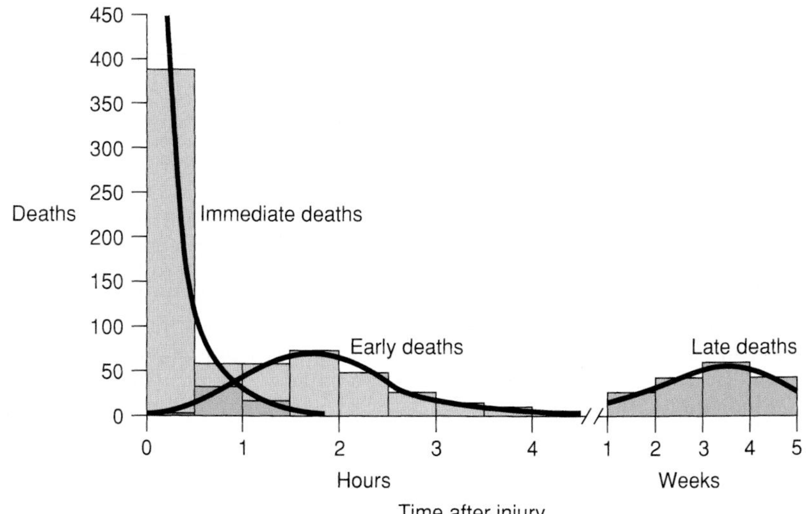

FIGURE 16.2 Three periods of peak mortality after injury.

resuscitation and care. Sepsis and multiple organ failure now account for approximately 5% of overall mortality and only 30% of later mortality where organized trauma systems exist. Finally, fatal pulmonary embolism accounts for a significant number of these late deaths.[14]

Efforts to reduce the morbidity and mortality of trauma must include specific programs for each of the three different mortality peaks. Early deaths can best be reduced with injury prevention programs or legislated protective devices. Focus on the regional planning of trauma system development will affect the number of avoidable deaths during the second mortality peak. Finally, late deaths will be diminished as research generates better understanding of the processes related to inflammation, sepsis, coagulopathy, multiple organ failure, and CNS injury.[6,7]

KEY POINTS

- **Trauma is the leading cause of death to age 45 years, the fourth leading cause overall, and leading contributor to YPLL before age 65.**
- **The interdisciplinary science of injury control requires a team approach that involves medical and surgical specialists, epidemiologists, statisticians, biomechanical engineers, public health practitioners, and economists.**
- **Modern trauma care is derived from care of wounds and casualty management during major wars.**
- **Trauma deaths occur at three time periods following injury, each having a unique pattern and etiology: 50% at the scene, 30% within the "golden hour" or acute resuscitation phase, and 20% delayed from several days to several weeks after injury.**

References

1. Baker S, O'Neill B, Ginsburg M. *The Injury Fact Book*, 2nd ed. New York: Oxford University Press, 1992.
2. **Vital Statistics: Mortality Data; 2001. National Center for Health Statistics, Center for Disease Control. http://www.cdc.gov/ncipc/osp/data.htm.**
3. Injury Fact Sheets; 1999. National Center for Injury Prevention and Control, Center for Disease Control. http://www.cdc.gov/ncipc/cmprfact.htm.
4. LaPlante M, Carlson D. *Disability in the United States: Prevalence and Causes, 1992*. San Francisco: Disability Statistics Center, University of California, 1996.
5. *Accidental Death and Disability: The Neglected Disease of Modern Society*; 1966. Washington, DC: National Research Council (US), Committee on Trauma; National Research Council (US), Committee on Shock. National Academy of Sciences, National Research Council.
6. *Injury in America: A Continuing Public Health Problem*; 1985. Washington, DC: Committee on Trauma Research (US), National Academy Press.
7. **Maier RV. Trauma: the paradigm for medical care in the 21st century. *J Trauma* 2003;54(5):803–813.**
8. ***Resources for Optimal Care of the Injured Patient: 1999*. Chicago: American College of Surgeons Committee on Trauma, 1999.**
9. *Advanced Trauma Life Support Course: Instructor Manual*. Chicago: American College of Surgeons Committee on Trauma, 2004.
10. Kraus JF, Peek C, McArthur DL, et al. The effect of the 1992 California motorcycle helmet use law on motorcycle crash fatalities and injuries. *JAMA* 1994;272(19):1506–1151.
11. Lowe DK, Gately HL, Goss JR, et al. Patterns of death, complication, and error in the management of motor vehicle accident victims: implications for a regional system of trauma care. *J Trauma* 1983;23(6):503–509.
12. **Shackford SR, Hollingworth-Fridlund P, Cooper GF, et al. The effect of regionalization upon the quality of trauma care as assessed by concurrent audit before and after institution of a trauma system: a preliminary report. *J Trauma* 1986;26(9):812–820.**
13. **Baker CC, Oppenheimer L, Stephens B, et al. Epidemiology of trauma deaths. *Am J Surg* 1980;140(1):144–150.**
14. Shackford SR, Mackersie RC, Holbrook TL, et al. The epidemiology of traumatic death. A population-based analysis. *Arch Surg* 1993;128(5):571–575.

CHAPTER 17 ■ GENERAL CONSIDERATIONS IN TRAUMA

DAVID B. HOYT AND RAUL COIMBRA

EPIDEMIOLOGY

In the United States, more than 3 million people are hospitalized annually as a result of unintentional injury, and approximately 35 to 40 million Emergency Department visits occur for the evaluation and treatment of injuries.[1] Of these patients, more than 40% are between the ages of 25 and 44 years, and 20% are between 15 and 24 years. People under the age of 45 sustain almost 80% of all injuries and account for 75% of the total lifetime medical costs. Young males are the highest risk group, not because of physiologic distinctions but because of the propensity to engage in high-risk activities. According to data provided by the National Center for Injury and Prevention Control, reported in 2001, considering all injury-related deaths (total of 157,070), 56.6% occurred in the age group of 15 to 49 years, predominantly in the male population. Overall, the risk of dying following injury for the male population is seven times higher than that for the female population.[2]

Although morbidity and mortality figures are important, another important variable related to injury costs for society is measured in years of potential life lost (YPLL) before age 65, which reflects the potential productivity that is lost as a result of premature death. Traumatic deaths result in a higher number of YPLL when compared with deaths associated with either cancer or cardiovascular diseases. This is because injuries are more prevalent in the younger population. In 1996, the age-adjusted YPLL before age 65 (per 100,000 population) was 1,919, 1,554, and 1,223 for injury, cancer, and heart diseases, respectively.[1] On average, for each traumatic deaths, there are 36 YPLL, compared with 16 for cancer and 12 for cardiovascular diseases.[3]

The leading causes of injury in decreasing rank include motor vehicle crashes, firearms, falls, those related to cutting or piercing instruments, and burns. Fatalities after injury are mainly caused by motor vehicle crashes (MVCs) (32%), gunshot wounds (22%), and falls (9%).[4]

Several important differences are found among the various ethnic groups in the United States in terms of the epidemiology of injury. The three leading causes of traumatic death for persons younger than 35 years are the same for all groups: MVCs, homicide, and suicide. However, in the African American population, the leading cause of death in this age group is homicide. The mortality rate from MVCs is about 42 of 100,000 among Native Americans, 20 per 100,000 among the white population, and 11 per 100,000 in the Asian population.[3] Similarly, suicide rates are higher for American Indians than for any other group.[1]

The impact of injury in children younger than 15 is also significant. The leading causes of injury in this group are MVCs, burns, drowning, falls, and poisoning. Injury in this age group leads to a significant number of deaths, disabilities, days of missed school, medical costs, and missed workdays for parents.

Adolescents are also at increased risk for injury. In fact, more adolescents die from injuries than from all other diseases combined.[5] Of all deaths in this age group, 40% are caused by intentional injuries, such as homicide and suicide.[6] Considering only adolescents 15 to19 years of age, one fourth of the deaths are caused by firearms.[7]

Alcohol ingestion is a major cause of fatal vehicular crashes. Although significant progress has been made in the prevention of drinking and driving, 39% of all traffic fatalities in 1997 were alcohol related (National Highway Traffic Safety Administration [NHTSA]).[8] More importantly, 60% of the time that a child passenger dies in a car crash, the driver was intoxicated.[9] In addition, other commonly abused drugs, such as marijuana and cocaine, have been implicated in 18% of MVC-related fatalities.[10]

Those who participate in injury research and prevention must take into account both the unique characteristics of the specific target population and other important epidemiologic factors such as alcohol and drug use.

BIOMECHANICS OF INJURY

All traumatic injury occurs as a result of deformation of tissues beyond a threshold that results in structural damage. In general, injury is categorized as either penetrating or nonpenetrating (blunt) trauma and thermal injury. Blunt trauma injury is produced as the tissues are either compressed or as deceleration occurs. In penetrating trauma, the injury is produced by crushing and separation of tissues along the path of the penetrating object.

Energy Transfer

The severity of any injury is directly proportional to the amount of kinetic energy transferred to the tissues, whether by a projectile or by blunt impact. Kinetic energy (KE) is a function of the mass (M) of an object and its velocity (V):

$$KE = M \times V^2/2$$

Changes in velocity alter the kinetic energy transfer more significantly than changes in mass. This fact becomes critical when assessing the extent of damage from high-velocity and low-velocity gunshot wounds. Likewise, a small child and a large adult, though significantly different in size and weight, are subjected to similar levels of energy transfer in a high-speed vehicular collision, the primary determinant being velocity rather than mass.

Cavitation

Cavitation occurs as tissue impacted by a moving body recoils from the point of impact, away from the object. The resulting transient tissue cavity can be caused by rapid acceleration or deceleration. Extreme strain occurs at points of anatomic fixation during the formation of these temporary cavities. Forces can be produced both along the longitudinal axis (tensile or compression strain) and across the transverse axis (shear strain). These types of forces cause deformity, tearing, and soft tissue failure or fracture. With penetrating trauma, transfer of kinetic energy from the projectile causes transient cavitation. A permanent cavity is produced by tissue displacement and destruction.

Biomechanics of Blunt Trauma

Blunt trauma results in two types of forces during impact. First, changes in speed (acceleration or deceleration) create shear strain, and second, deformity changes (stretch or compression) create tensile strain. For example, shear stress to the head secondary to deceleration leads to brainstem stretching, and injury to the spinal cord occurs from shear stress at points of attachment. Contrecoup brain injuries include stretch forces placed on bridging veins, which may lead to hemorrhage and a subdural hematoma.

Differential acceleration in the thorax makes the aorta the most common site of life-threatening shear injuries, the most frequent point of injury being the ligamentum arteriosum. Here, the descending aorta is tightly fixed to the thoracic spine, whereas more proximally it is relatively mobile. Shear stress in this area allows the proximal aorta to move forward in relation to the fixed distal aorta and, therefore, to tear. Abdominal injuries can result as a consequence of acceleration of the viscera at a rate out of proportion to movement of the points of attachment. The kidneys, small intestine, large intestine, and spleen are all vulnerable to this type of shear injury. Similarly, with deceleration, the liver may continue to travel relative to the ligamentum teres, generating shear forces that transect or lacerate the hepatic parenchyma. An inappropriately applied, high-riding lap seatbelt, particularly in a small child, can also produce a shear plane, causing severe intestinal injury during crash-induced deceleration. Rapid deceleration can also place sudden flexion and extension forces on the cervical spine and, with a seatbelt on the lower thoracic and upper lumbar spines, cause fractures, subluxation, or ligamentous injury.

Tensile strain creates injury by directly compressing or stretching the tissue. For the head, tensile strain results in fractures of the skull, which in turn may cause intracranial bleeding or contusions of the underlying brain parenchyma. In the thorax, external chest compression can lead to cardiac contusion, pulmonary contusion, pneumothorax, and fractured ribs or a flail chest. In the abdomen, the pancreas, liver, spleen, and occasionally the kidneys are subject to tensile strain injuries, particularly following a frontal (or, for the kidney, flank) impact. In addition, direct compression of the abdomen may increase intraabdominal pressure, rupturing the diaphragm.

Similarly, external compression of the pelvis is associated with bladder rupture and other pelvic injuries.

MOTOR VEHICLE COLLISIONS

Specific patterns of injury are recognized for various types of motor vehicle collisions. These include: (a) head-on or frontal impact, (b) rear impact, (c) lateral or side impact, (d) rotational impact, and (e) rollover. Some estimate of injury pattern is possible by analysis of damage to the vehicle, but the presumption is usually that any or all of these forces may have been involved. In general, a vehicle's occupant receives a kinetic energy transfer similar to that of the vehicle itself. As an automobile collides with an object, passengers collide with the interior of the automobile, and the internal organs collide with the body wall or are sheared from anatomic attachments.

It has been shown that better automotive design has greatly improved the outcome for occupants when the safety features of the vehicle are in use at the time of the crash. Active safety restraint systems include shoulder and lap seatbelts, air bags (frontal and lateral), and door locks; passive restraint systems include front and rear energy-absorbing collapsible chassis, lateral bars, and improved lateral wall design.

Frontal and Rear Impact

With a frontal impact, the vehicle stops abruptly, and unrestrained front-seat occupants move in one of two predictable pathways: down and under the dashboard or up and over the steering wheel (Fig. 17.1). With the former movement, the knees strike the dashboard and the upper legs absorb the primary energy transfer. Dislocated knees, fractured femurs, and posterior fracture dislocations of the hips are expected. With an "up and over" impact, the upper body flexes forward, moving up and over the steering wheel. The chest or abdomen impacts the steering wheel and the head impacts the windshield. The head stops the forward momentum of the torso and the cervical spine absorbs the kinetic energy.

Predictable injury patterns resulting from the up-and-over component of a frontal impact are given in Table 17.1. Rear impact collisions occur when stationary objects or slow-moving vehicles are struck from behind. The amount of kinetic energy generated depends on the difference between the

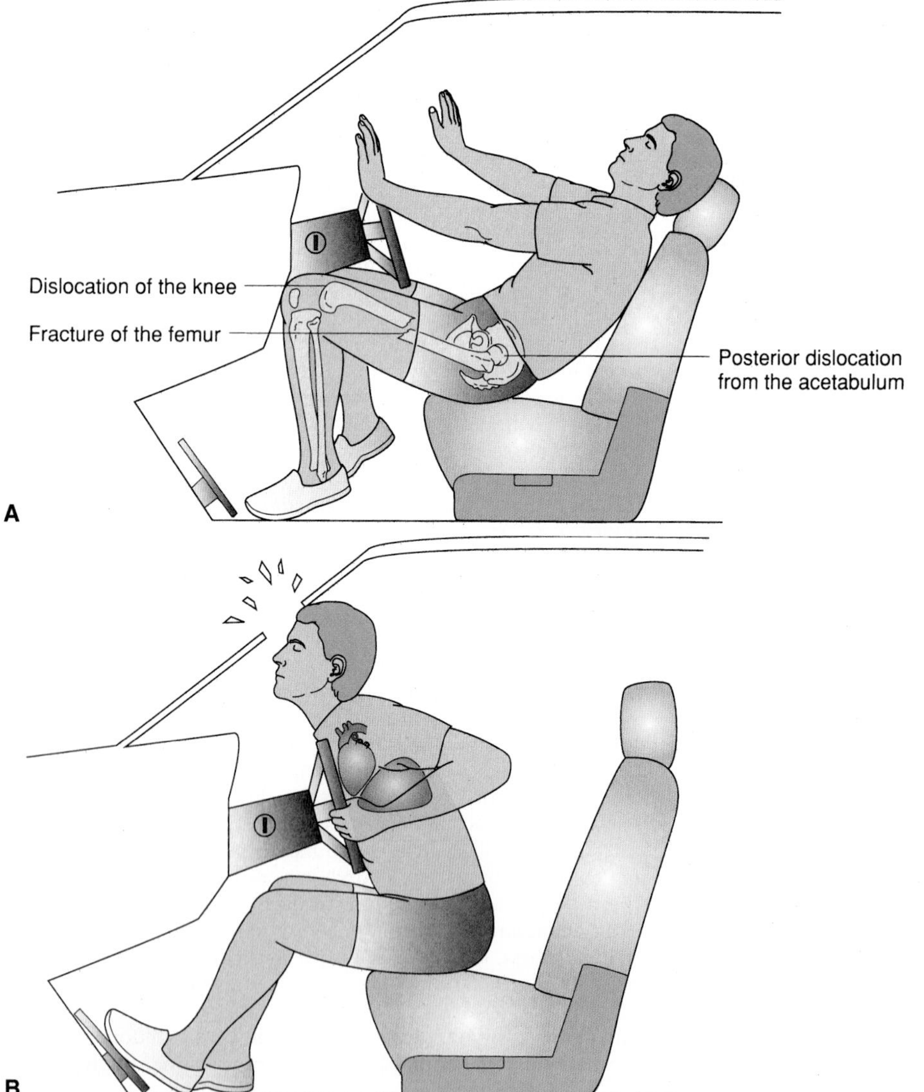

FIGURE 17.1 Down-and-under (*A*) and up-and-over (*B*) mechanisms of injury after frontal deceleration impact.

TABLE 17.1 DIAGNOSIS

PREDICTABLE INJURY PATTERNS RESULTING FROM THE UP-AND-OVER COMPONENT OF FRONTAL IMPACT

- Rib fractures, pulmonary contusion, flail chest, and myocardial contusion from anterior chest wall compression against the steering wheel
- Hollow abdominal viscera and solid organs compression, resulting in intestinal perforation and lacerations of the mesentery and solid organs, with accompanying hemorrhage
- After the anterior chest stops, intrathoracic organs continue to move, resulting in shear injuries such as lacerations of the aorta or liver
- Shear injuries to the kidneys and other solid viscera
- Injury to the brain from direct compression with scalp lacerations, skull fractures, and cerebral contusions, or from deceleration and shear stress, which cause diffuse axonal injury and cerebral contusion or subdural hematoma
- Acute neck flexion, hyperextension, or both, causing a cervical spine injury

velocities of the two vehicles, rather than the sum, as with forward collisions. After a rear impact, the vehicle and its occupants accelerate forward, during which time cervical spine hyperextension with injury may occur. If the vehicle slows to a stop spontaneously, often the occupants are not severely injured. If the car strikes another object, the occupants are thrown forward, with injury potential similar to that seen with a frontal impact. Thus, rear impact collision can potentially cause two types of injury: those from the primary rear impact and those resulting from the secondary frontal impact.

Lateral and Rotational Impact and Rollover

Two patterns of injury result from lateral impact, depending on whether energy is transferred to the vehicle directly or imparts motion to the vehicle. If the target vehicle remains in place or there is significant passenger compartment intrusion, typical injuries include lateral crushing compression injuries to the torso, pelvis, and spine. Energy delivered to the chest with lateral compression can cause a flail chest, pulmonary contusion, and ruptured liver or spleen. Depending on the location of the occupant's arm, humeral and clavicular fractures may occur. The pelvis and femur are often impacted by the door, forcing the femoral head medially, and causing an acetabular impaction fracture. Head injuries range from simple lacerations to cerebral contusions with intracranial hemorrhage.

When the vehicle does not move away from the point of lateral impact, an occupant who is restrained remains fixed in place and is more vulnerable to the intruding vehicle. More commonly, the force of the impact moves the vehicle, and passenger restraints markedly reduce injury. In this case, the occupant begins lateral motion with the car and is pulled away from the impact point by the restraint. As the torso is pushed laterally, the head stays in its original position, producing lateral flexion and rotation to the cervical spine, which leads to fractures and ligamentous injury. Passengers sustaining lateral impact also should be considered for injuries resulting from secondary collisions with other passengers and objects within the vehicle.

Rotational impact injuries occur when the car strikes a moving vehicle laterally. The moving vehicle rotates around the point of impact, resulting in combinations of the injuries seen in head-on and lateral impacts.

During rollover crashes, the automobile may impact many times from many different angles, and as a result, the occupant may have virtually any type of injury. All potential injury mechanisms should be considered. Rollover crashes with passenger ejection are associated with a profound increase in fatality rates, in part because the second impact can cause injuries that compound or exceed those resulting from the initial impact. Rollover crashes with passenger ejection are considered to have the greatest injury potential.

Restraint Device Injury

Theoretically, three-point passenger restraints, when used properly, allow the kinetic energy transferred by the impact to be absorbed by the bony pelvis and chest. If improperly positioned, however, lap belts may rise above the pelvis, delivering the compression force to the soft tissues of the abdominal cavity or retroperitoneum. The number of injuries related to restraint devices is increasing, probably reflecting the broader general use of these systems. Although there is no question of the overall efficacy of these devices, the clinician must recognize specific related injuries.

Common injuries when lap belts are incorrectly strapped above the anterior iliac crest include compression injuries of the intraabdominal organs (liver, pancreas, spleen, small bowel, large bowel), increased intraabdominal pressure and diaphragmatic rupture, and anterior compression of the lumbar spine. Diagonal shoulder straps should be worn in combination with lap belts to prevent forward motion of the trunk. Diagonal shoulder straps should not be worn alone because this can be associated with chest and neck injuries if the pelvis is not secured by the lap belt. Injuries associated with shoulder straps include carotid artery contusion, with or without thrombosis and disruption, and clavicle and rib fractures.

Air bags have enormous potential for injury prevention because they prevent the initial collision of passenger and automobile interior that occurs with frontal impacts. To be effective, air bags must be used in combination with seatbelts because they deflate immediately and therefore do not prevent secondary collisions. Lateral air bags have been recently incorporated in some, but not all vehicles. Injuries such as lateral collisions of the head with the middle column and lateral compression of the chest wall may be, at least in part, prevented by these new devices. Airbags are not effective in rear impact collisions. Given the predominance of frontal impact accidents, however, public health considerations in favor of air bags should be strongly emphasized.

MOTORCYCLES

Motorcycle injuries involve four types of impacts: frontal, angular, ejection, and rear end collision. In a frontal impact, the center of gravity is above and behind the front axle as the motorcycle tips forward and the rider travels over the handlebars. Injuries to the head, chest, or abdomen can occur, depending on which part of the anatomy strikes the handlebars. If the rider's feet are placed on the pegs, the upper leg strikes the handlebars in forward motion, causing bilateral midshaft femur fractures. Angular or lateral impact generally results in crush injuries of the lower extremities. With ejection, the rider is thrown into the air until the head, chest, or extremities strike another object. Injury occurs at the point of impact, and, just as with the occupant ejected from an automobile, the potential for severe injury is high. This mechanism of injury is frequent and contributes importantly to the extraordinary injury potential for motorcycle passengers.

In rear end collisions, the motorcycle is usually at a stop when it is hit by a second vehicle from behind. The injury pattern is that of rapid acceleration with hyperextension and subsequent crush.

PEDESTRIANS

Two general patterns are seen in motor vehicle pedestrian accidents, depending on whether the patient is an adult or a child. In adults, the initial impact is often by the car bumper, producing fractures to the tibia and fibula. As the victim falls over the moving vehicle, the pelvis and upper femur are struck by the front of the vehicle's hood, and the abdomen and thorax continue onto the top of the hood. The secondary strike can result in fractures of the femur or pelvis and produce serious intraabdominal or intrathoracic injury. Injury to the head depends on whether the patient's head strikes the car hood or is protected with the arms. A third impact occurs as the victim falls away, striking the ground. This impact commonly leads to head injury as well.

In children, the initial impact is predictably higher and may produce injury to the pelvis or upper femur. The second impact occurs when the front of the hood strikes the thorax. The final impact may not occur on top of the hood but rather as the child is dragged underneath the vehicle. As the child falls backward, multiple impacts with the ground, underside of the vehicle, and wheels are possible, so virtually any type of injury may occur. Because of the potential for forceful impact and the direct blow to the middle torso, any child struck by a vehicle must be considered to have potentially severe injuries.

FALLS

Falls result in multiple impacts. Energy transfer is a result of the velocity that develops during the fall, so the height of the fall usually determines the magnitude of injury. Falls from more than three times the height of the victim, or from more than 20 feet, are considered severe. The surface on which the victim lands and its degree of compressibility (e.g., water versus concrete) also have an effect on the energy transfer and the types of shear and tensile strain that occur. A typical injury pattern after falls in which the victim lands on the feet is transaxial and includes bilateral calcaneal fractures and multiple compression fractures of the thoracic and lumbar spine (Fig. 17.2).

If the victim falls forward with the arms extended, frequent associated fractures include bilateral Colles' wrist fractures. Hip dislocation and pelvic fractures are common if these structures are impacted, and significant head and torso injuries are always possible, depending on the orientation of the victim at the time of impact.

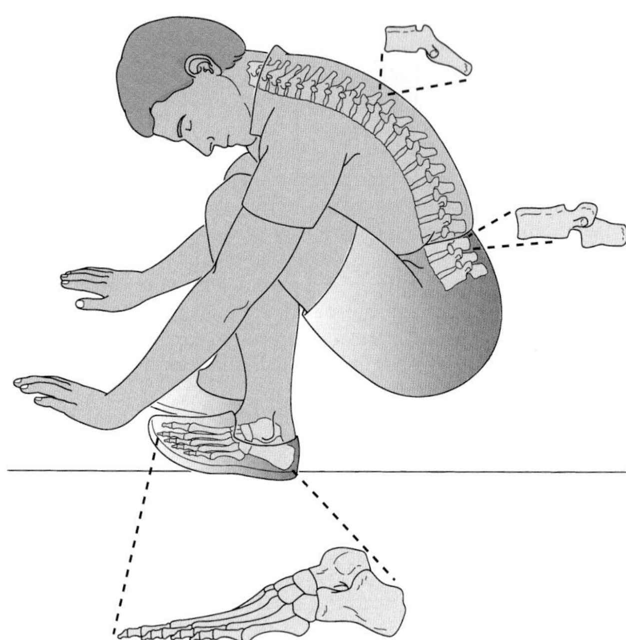

FIGURE 17.2 Hyperflexion and axial loading injury after a fall.

GENERAL ANATOMIC CONSIDERATIONS IN BLUNT INJURY

The first and second ribs, sternum, scapula, and femur are considered to be some of the strongest and least vulnerable bones in the body. Therefore, fractures of these bones are indicators of severe trauma. Clear association exists between first and second rib fractures and injuries to the head, chest, and abdomen. Similarly, fractures to the sternum, though unusual, have a relatively high frequency of associated myocardial contusion. Fractures to the scapula indicate significant thoracic trauma. A femur fracture in a frontal impact injury should raise the concern of acetabular fractures or dislocation of the knee. An inventory of specific orthopedic injuries and their common associated findings is provided in Table 17.2. These associations should be routinely considered during initial evaluation following major blunt trauma.

The anatomic orientation of certain structures also leads to predictable injury patterns. For example, the right ventricle is the most anterior portion of the heart and therefore is the most commonly contused area. The association of splenic injury with rib fractures on the lower left side and liver injuries with rib fractures on the lower right side is also frequently seen after blunt trauma.

TABLE 17.2 DIAGNOSIS

PATTERNS OF INJURY TO THE HEAD, NECK, TRUNK, AND EXTREMITIES ASSOCIATED WITH ORTHOPEDIC INJURIES

Diagnosed injury	Associated injury
Fracture—temporal, parietal bone	Epidural hematoma
Maxillofacial fracture	Cervical spine fracture
Sternal fracture	Cardiac contusion
First and second rib fracture	Descending thoracic aorta, intraabdominal bleeding
Fractured scapula	Pulmonary contusion
Fractured ribs 8–12, right	Lacerated liver
Fractured ribs 8–12, left	Lacerated spleen
Fractured pelvis	Ruptured bladder, urethral transection
Fractured humerus	Radial nerve injury
Supracondylar humerus fracture	Brachial artery injury
Distal radius fracture	Median nerve compression
Supracondylar femur fracture	Popliteal artery thrombosis
Anterior dislocation shoulder	Axillary nerve injury
Posterior dislocation of hip	Sciatic nerve injury
Posterior dislocation of knee	Popliteal artery thrombosis

BIOMECHANICS OF PENETRATING INJURIES

Penetrating trauma involves the transfer of energy to a relatively small tissue area. The velocity of a gunshot wound is exceedingly high compared with any type of blunt trauma. The kinetic energy of a bullet disrupts and fragments cells and tissues, moving them away from the path of the bullet. The actual size of the frontal area of impact is determined by three factors: profile, tumble (spin and yaw), and fragmentation.

The profile, or frontal area, of a knife, screwdriver, or smooth bullet is that of a pointed missile. If the missile is crushed or deformed as a result of impact, the frontal area changes shape and disperses the impact over a wider tissue area, producing greater energy exchange and therefore greater injury. A knife or jacketed bullet does not deform significantly during impact, whereas a hollow-point bullet flattens, spreads, and fragments on impact, enlarging the area of injury.

Tumble results when the center of gravity of a bullet is eccentric, usually because it is located near the base rather than the apex of the bullet. Spin and axial movement (yaw) are bullet movements that occur after a gun is fired (Fig. 17.3). At impact, spin and yaw continue to carry the base of the bullet forward, resulting in end-over-end motion or tumble. This increases the area of energy exchange and results in greater tissue damage. Gunshot wounds are an example of the effect of fragmentation injury. The frontal impact damage can be

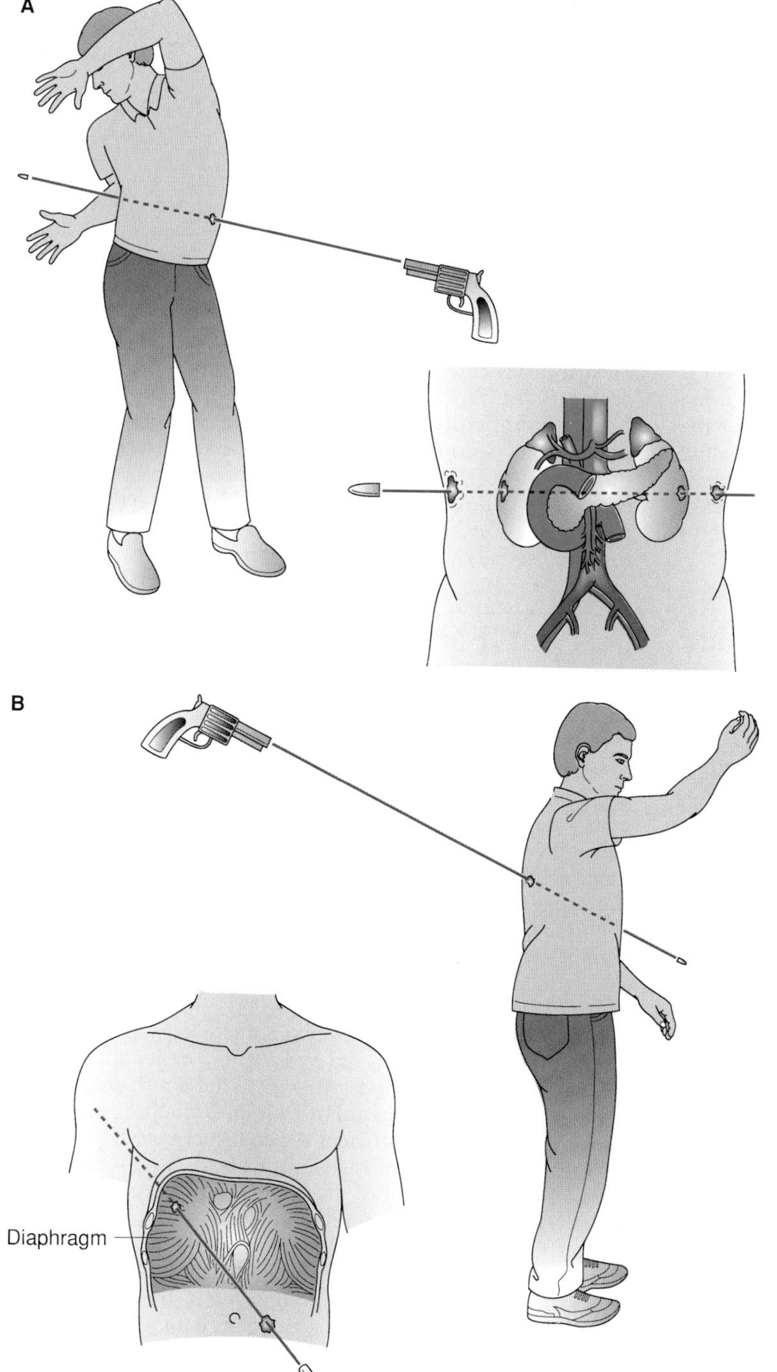

FIGURE 17.3 Axial traverse (*A*) and transdiaphragmatic (*B*) wounding mechanisms with associated injury potential for combined thoracic and abdominal injuries.

TRAUMA

TABLE 17.3

MUZZLE VELOCITY, KINETIC WEIGHT OF PROJECTILE, AND APPROXIMATE MAXIMUM KINETIC ENERGY OF FREQUENTLY USED FIREARMS

Description (caliber)	Projectile weight (g)	Muzzle velocity (ft/s)	Kinetic energy (ft/lb)
Pistols			
.22 Short	29	1,000	72
.38 Special	158	870	263
9-mm Luger	125	1,150	440
.45	250	860	410
.357 Magnum	158	1,430	695
.44 Magnum	240	1,470	1,150
Rifles			
.22 Long	40	1,150	150
.56-mm M-16	55	3,200	1,248
.30-30 Winchester	170	2,200	1,830

estimated by classifying penetrating injuries into low-, medium-, and high-energy capacities.

Low-Energy Stab Wounds

Low-energy missiles include knives and other objects that produce damage only by their sharp cutting edges. Cavitation is minimal and injury can be predicted simply by tracing the pathway of the weapon within the body. Knowledge of the type of weapon is sometimes helpful. The attacker may stab and move the knife or weapon inside the body, which can lead to more injury than that perceived from the cutaneous wound. Judgment of the potential scope of injury by examination of the entrance wound is not reliable.

Low- and Medium-Energy Gunshot Wounds

Low-energy gunshot wounds are defined as those with an initial muzzle velocity of less than 1,200 ft/s. Medium-velocity projectiles have muzzle velocities between 1,200 and 2,000 ft/s. Most handguns and some rifles are low- or medium-energy weapons. Table 17.3 provides a comparison of bullets and initial muzzle velocity for firearms frequently associated with penetrating civilian trauma. The primary point of classification is that these weapons both damage the tissue directly in the path of the missile and produce cavitation injury to tissues in close proximity to the impact. The size of the cavitation injury is directly proportional to the velocity of the bullet. The amount of tumble, fragmentation, and profile change also influence the extent of injury.

High-Energy Weapons

The essential difference between high-energy weapons and the typical civilian gunshot wound is that their projectiles produce a much larger cavity or pressure cone than low- and medium-velocity missiles. The temporary cavity extends well beyond the actual bullet tract, producing a wider injury. The vacuum created by the cavitation pulls clothing, bacteria, and other debris from the surrounding areas into the wound, creating the additional risk of contamination. The proliferation of semiautomatic weapons also has resulted in an increased number of wounds a victim may experience. Instead of a single gunshot wound, the surgeon may be faced with multiple wounds in multiple body locations.

Blast Injuries

Blast injuries caused by close-range shotgun fire constitute devastating injuries comprising extensive tissue destruction. Besides specific organ injury, blast injuries have the highest potential for secondary infection. These injuries, in general, should be surgically explored, devitalized tissue should be extensively debrided, and the wounds should be left open and packed with sterile dressing that should be changed and reviewed serially in the operating room.[11]

GENERAL ANATOMIC CONSIDERATIONS OF PENETRATING INJURIES

Evaluation of entrance and exit wounds is essential to assess the number of projectiles, their courses, and which organs are at risk of injury. Entrance wounds for bullets typically cause tattooing, burning, and abrasion as a result of the spin. Depending on the range, there may be direct burning of skin. Tattooing occurs if the muzzle is within 12 inches of the skin at the time of firing. The range from which a gun is fired is also significant in that the air resistance that slows bullet velocity and reduces kinetic energy is directly proportional to the distance traveled.

Once a missile penetrates tissue, the energy is distributed predictably within a closed space and, depending on the organs impacted and the types of tissue traversed, certain injuries can be anticipated. For example, a bullet penetrating the skull may have insufficient residual energy to traverse and exit the opposite side of the skull. Instead, it may follow the curvature of the interior of the skull, generating a more severe brain injury than would result from a simple linear passage.

In the thorax, lung parenchyma has low mass and, therefore, sustains less damage from penetrating injury than any other thoracic tissue. Similarly, blood vessels that are not fixed may be pushed aside without significant damage. Large fixed vessels, however, such as the aorta and vena cava, are particularly susceptible to fatal injury. If bones are penetrated,

TABLE 17.4 DIAGNOSIS

INJURIES ASSOCIATED WITH SPECIFIC VASCULAR TRAUMA

- Superior mesenteric artery or superior mesenteric vein injury with pancreas and liver
- Renal artery injury with liver, kidney, and colon
- Inferior vena cava injury with liver, small bowel, colon, pancreas, and duodenum
- Portal vein injury with inferior vena cava, liver, pancreas, and duodenum
- Axillary artery injury with brachial plexus trauma

fragments may become secondary missiles and can lacerate the surrounding tissues, including vascular structures. Muscles may expand out of the path of a missile, but this can result in stretching and hemorrhage. Injury to adjacent blood vessels can result in intimal damage with subsequent thrombosis even if the vessel as a whole remains intact. Low-velocity bullets may not follow a straight path but rather ricochet through the body cavity, injuring other organs.

Penetrating injuries also should be evaluated with regard to topography. For example, penetrating wounds of the neck are commonly associated with injury to the jugular veins, trachea, and carotid artery. Injuries to the trachea are commonly associated with injuries to the esophagus, and injuries to the carotid artery are commonly associated with the internal jugular vein. In penetrating wounds to the thorax, consider the possibilities of injury to the heart, lung, and diaphragm. The anterior location of the right ventricle makes it particularly vulnerable to penetrating trauma. All penetrating wounds below the nipple line or inframammary groove must be considered for potential intraabdominal injury (Fig. 17.3B). Similarly, wounds that cross the midline, so-called axial traverse wounds, are important to recognize. In the thorax, this indicates that every mediastinal structure is at risk, and in the abdomen, consider the possibility of major vascular injury, particularly to the aorta and vena cava. Associated abdominal injuries often include hepatic and splenic injuries, as well as diaphragmatic, pulmonary, and gastric injuries. Duodenal and pancreatic injuries are commonly seen with injuries to the liver, inferior vena cava, stomach, and colon. Examples of injuries associated with specific vascular trauma are listed in Table 17.4.

SCORING SYSTEMS AND INJURY ASSESSMENT

Many systems have been developed in an effort to allow comparison of injuries and trauma patients within and among institutions. Although all provide considerable help, none is perfect. The impetus for injury severity scoring systems is provided by the need to identify and classify severely injured patients in the prehospital phase, predict mortality, assess results, and improve communication. These systems also permit tracking of patient outcomes within an institution over time.

One simple way to classify trauma patients is to place them into three groups according to severity of injury: (a) those patients with injuries that are rapidly fatal, (b) those with injuries that are potentially fatal, and (c) those with injuries that are not fatal. The first group includes patients who have exsanguinating injuries, massive head injuries, high cervical spinal cord transection, or major airway disruption producing death in less than 10 minutes. Of traumatic injuries, 5% and half of all injury-related deaths fall within this category. The third group, which accounts for 80% of trauma patients, includes patients with injuries that are minor or confined to soft tissue and isolated extremity fractures. Significant risk to life is seldom seen in this group and urgent treatment is not essential. These patients survive without significant disability even if prolonged delays occur before definitive therapy. The real impact of improved prehospital care and organized trauma systems is on the second category of patients (about 15% to 20% of the total), those who can be saved if effective medical care is provided quickly. It is for this group that scoring systems have been developed.

Revised Trauma Score and Triage

The trauma score developed by Champion and Sacco[12] in 1981 is the most widely applied and the most useful scoring system for the initial evaluation of trauma victims. It mathematically combines the physiologic parameters of blood pressure, respiratory rate, and Glasgow Coma Score to assess injury severity and predict which patients need the most timely and sophisticated medical care. Table 17.5 shows the components of the Revised Trauma Score (RTS).

In addition to physiologic scores, specific anatomic aspects of injury are correlated with high injury potential. Penetrating injuries to the head, neck, torso, and proximal extremities; multiple broken ribs and flail chest; two or more proximal long-bone fractures; pelvic fractures; limb paralysis; and amputation proximal to the wrist have been identified as anatomic indicators of severe injury. Finally, the mechanism of injury is used to identify patients who are at high risk for significant injuries and are best evaluated at a trauma center. These data have been integrated with factors of age and comorbid disease into a triage decision scheme that is recommended by the American College of Surgeons (Algorithm 17.1).

The major criticism of this triage scheme is that it leads to the frequent triage of patients to trauma centers that may not be necessary (i.e., overtriage). On the other hand, it diminishes the number of patients with severe injury who are overlooked and potentially undertreated. Overtriage is the inherent cost of a sufficiently sensitive scoring system.

TABLE 17.5

REVISED TRAUMA SCORE COMPONENTS

Glasgow coma scale	Systolic blood pressure (mm Hg)	Respiratory rate (breaths/min)	Coded value
13–15	>89	10–29	4
9–12	76–89	>29	3
6–8	50–75	6–9	2
4–5	1–49	1–5	1
3	0	0	0

TRAUMA

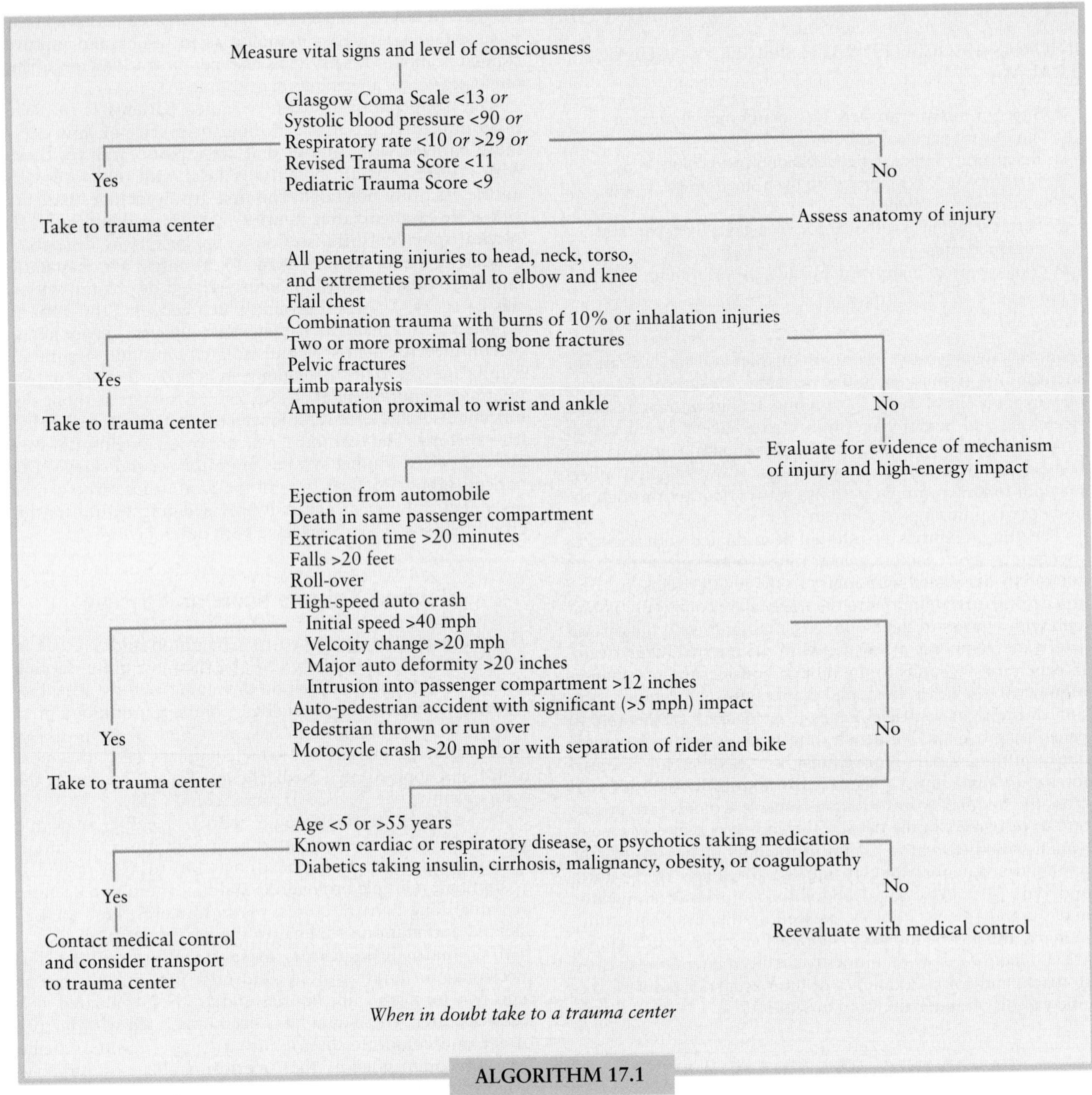

ALGORITHM 17.1 Field triage decision scheme as recommended by the American College of Surgeons.

Outcome Assessment

Also important is the need to accurately compare patients with specific injuries, which requires a scale for rating severity of tissue damage. Outcome analyses based on these parameters is a major objective of these types of scoring systems.[13]

Abbreviated Injury Scale

The Abbreviated Injury Scale (AIS)[14] was developed in 1971 for use in blunt trauma and has subsequently been updated on a periodic basis. The 1990 revision of the AIS includes descriptors for penetrating trauma. Injury severity is determined in six different body areas on a scale of 0 to 6, where 0 indicates no injury, 5 indicates critical injury, and 6 indicates a nonsurvivable injury. The AIS evaluates individual injuries but does not account for multiple injuries. Thus, it is a specific anatomic index.[15] Table 17.6 shows an example of the AIS for abdominal injuries. The shortcoming of the AIS is that it evaluates each injury independently and only the most severe injury in each body area. Thus, AIS scores fail to account for multiple serious injuries within the same body compartment, thereby underscoring the true severity of the injury.

TABLE 17.6

ABBREVIATED INJURY SCALE SCORING SYSTEM FOR ABDOMINAL INJURIES

Score	Injury examples
1	Abdominal wall abrasion
2	Liver, stomach, colon, mesentery contusion
3	Minor liver or spleen laceration Bowel laceration without perforation
4	Major liver or spleen laceration Bowel laceration with perforation
5	Major liver or spleen laceration with tissue loss Bowel laceration with tissue loss

Injury Severity Score

In 1974, Baker[15] developed the Injury Severity Score (ISS), which is calculated by assigning AIS values to the most severe injury in each of six body areas: head and neck (score =1), face (=2), chest (=3), abdomen and pelvic contents (=4), extremities and pelvis (=5), and general and cutaneous (=6). To derive the ISS, the scores for the three most severely injured areas are squared and added. ISS values vary from 0 to 75. If the value of the AIS is 6 (i.e., nonsurvivable injury) in any body area, the ISS is automatically 75.

The result is that substantial quadratic correlation between injury severity based on ISS and death can be developed. The ISS is extremely helpful and has been widely used. However, it does not adjust for patient age or patient-related comorbid risk factors, such as chronic disease. Further, the severity of a head injury is disproportionately underscored in that combinations of injuries in other areas can result in a higher ISS score than a fatal head injury. Despite this drawback, the ISS is an excellent tool for the study of groups of patients with multiple injuries from blunt trauma and allows comparison of outcomes and quality assurance. To address the concern of ignoring the impact of multiple injuries in one body region, a modified new ISS, or NISS, has been developed that includes the three most severe injuries, regardless of body region. Intuitively, this approach has advantages in patients with penetrating trauma where injuries are often concentrated in a single body region. In either blunt or penetrating trauma, this modification improves predictability and appears to better reflect and weight all injuries than the ISS alone.[17]

Trauma and Injury Severity Score

The Trauma and Injury Severity Score (TRISS) methodology[16] is of importance because it attempts to combine the trauma score, or physiologic component, and the ISS, or anatomic component of injury. It also incorporates the patient's age.

The TRISS method yields a specific probability of survival. Adjustments are made for age and mechanism of injury sustained (blunt or penetrating). The methodology allows patient groups to be compared. Individuals with an unexpected outcome, either survival or death, can be specifically identified and investigated. TRISS can be used for quality assurance evaluations both within and between institutions. Typically, a cutoff point (e.g., predictability of survival, Ps = 50%) is chosen, and records of the deaths of patients with a probability of survival greater than the cutoff value are submitted for peer review. TRISS also can be used to examine cases in which the survivors exceeded the cutoff value to help, in part, identify system components that improve outcome. In addition, TRISS has been used to compare trauma outcomes between different institutions.

SUMMARY

Trauma is a major national health-care problem that affects one of four U.S. citizens annually. The cost of trauma injury and treatment to the U.S. society is greater than $200 billion dollars per year when loss of future productivity is considered. The causes of traumatic death vary considerably depending on demographics. Urban and politically unstable areas typically have a higher incidence of penetrating trauma, whereas rural and stable communities have a predominance of blunt injuries, usually vehicular crashes. Nonetheless, causes of death after injury are remarkably similar. Central nervous system (CNS) injury accounts for about half of all fatalities, hemorrhage for 35%, and sepsis, multiple organ failure, and pulmonary embolism for about 15%. With the introduction of trauma systems during the last three decades, the incidence of preventable death has dropped from about 25% to 30% to less than 5%. This is the result of improvements in care both for acute head injuries and for control of hemorrhage. In addition, the incidence of late death attributable to sepsis and multiple organ failure has diminished, in part, as a result of better and early resuscitation. The responsibility of the surgeon for trauma encompasses the early recognition of injury, the resuscitation, and then the definitive care of the patient. As we improve the operative and intensive care rendered to trauma patients, we are beginning to reach the flat portion of the outcome curve.[18,19] The area of injury prevention, however, is still open to substantial improvement. To reduce the morbidity and mortality from trauma, surgeons must take a more active role in the prevention of trauma at the community level.

KEY POINTS

- **Injury is an epidemic in America, killing 150,000 and hospitalizing 3.0+ million while costing more than $250 billion per year.**
- **Injury is the leading cause of death in people under age 45 years and responsible for loss of more years of productive life than any other cause.**
- **The major causes of injury-related death, in decreasing order, are motor vehicle crashes, penetrating trauma, falls, and burns.**
- **Traumatic injury results in deformation and structural damage of tissue dependent on the kinetic energy transferred to the host, which, in turn, is dependent on the mass and, to a much greater extent, the velocity of the injuring force.**
- **Varying mechanisms of injury produce predictable patterns of damage.**
- **Scoring systems allow objective quantification of the injury to assess impact on outcome and to track differences in outcome, both serially within an institution and between institutions.**

References

1. Bonnie RJ, Fulco CE, Liverman CT. Magnitude and costs. In: Bonnie RJ, Fulco CE, Liverman CT, eds. *Reducing the burden of injury, advancing prevention, and treatment.* Washington, DC: National Academy Press, 1999;41–59.
2. National Center for Injury and Prevention Control. Overall injury and adverse-event-related deaths and rate per 100,000. E800-E999.

TRAUMA

www.cdc.gov/ncipc. National Center for Injury and Prevention Control, Centers for Disease Control and Prevention, 2001.
3. Baker S. *The injury fact book.* New York: Oxford University Press, 1992.
4. Rice DP, MacKenzie EJ, and associates, eds. *Cost of Injury in the United States: A Report to Congress.* San Francisco: Institute for Health & Aging, University of California and Injury Prevention Center, Johns Hopkins University, 1989.
5. Centers for Disease Control and Prevention. *Injury mortality: national summary of injury mortality data 1984–1990.* Atlanta: Centers for Disease Control and Prevention, 1993.
6. Runyan CW, Gerken EA. Epidemiology and prevention of adolescent injury: a review and research agenda. *JAMA* 1989;262:2273–2278.
7. Fingerhut LA. *Firearm mortality among children, youth, and young adults 1–34 years of age, trends and current status: U.S., 1985–1990.* Advance data No. 231. Hyattsville, MD: National Center for Health Statistics, Centers for Disease Control and Prevention, 1993.
8. National Highway Traffic Safety Administration (NHTSA). *Traffic safety facts 1997: Alcohol.* Washington, DC: NHTSA, 1998.
9. Centers for Disease Control and Prevention. Alcohol-related traffic fatalities involving children–United States 1985–1996. *MMWR Morb Mortal Wkly Rep* 1997; 46:1130–1133.
10. National Highway Traffic Safety Administration (NHTSA). *The Incidence and Role of Drugs in Fatally Injured Drivers.* Traffic Tech. Washington, DC: NHTSA, 1993.
11. Hoekstra SM, Bender JS, Levison MA. The management of large soft-tissue defects following close-range shotgun injury. *J Trauma* 1990;30: 1489–1493.
12. Champion HR, Fallen WF, Golocovsk M. The trauma score. *Crit Care Med* 1981;9:672.
13. Champion HR, Gainer PS, Yackee E. A progress report on the trauma score in predicting a fatal outcome. *J Trauma* 1986; 26:927.
14. American Association for Automotive Medicine. *The abbreviated injury scale* (AIS), rev. ed. Des Plaines, IL: American Association for Automotive Medicine, 1990.
15. Baker SP, O'Neill B, Haddon W Jr, et al. The Injury Severity Score: a method for describing patients with multiple injuries and evaluating emergency care. *J Trauma* 1974;14:187–196.
16. Boyd CR, Tolson MA, Copes WS. Evaluating trauma care: the TRISS method. *J Trauma* 1987;27:370.
17. Osler T, Baker SP, Long W: A modification of the injury severity score that both improves accuracy and simplifies scoring. *J Trauma* 1997;43(6): 922–925; discussion 925–926.
18. Hoyt DB, Hollingsworth-Fridlund P, Winchell RJ, et al. An analysis of recurrent process errors leading to provider related complications on an organized trauma service: directions for care improvement. *J Trauma* 1994;36:377.
19. U.S. Department of Health and Human Services (DHHS). *Model trauma care system plan.* Washington, DC: U.S. DHHS, September 30, 1992.

CHAPTER 18 ■ TRAUMA SYSTEMS

AVERY B. NATHENS

Care of the trauma patient poses several challenges not encountered in other aspects of surgical care. First, injury might occur at a site remote from medical care. This problem, coupled with the importance of time to definitive care as a critical parameter influencing patient survival, emphasizes the importance of developing means for identifying and transporting critically injured patients quickly. Additionally, the polytrauma patient often requires complex surgical care that crosses specialty lines, requiring that an interdisciplinary team be available with little advanced planning or notification. The primacy of time renders an *ad hoc* approach to the delivery of trauma care unacceptable and is the principal impetus for the development of organized systems of trauma care.

EVOLUTION OF ORGANIZED SYSTEMS OF TRAUMA CARE

It was the American experience in the Korean War that laid the earliest foundation for the current system of trauma care in the United States. The terrain made it difficult to evacuate the wounded along the traditional chain from the front lines to definitive care, as occurred during WWI and WWII.[1] Simultaneously, helicopters had evolved and were used to rapidly move the wounded from combat zones to Mobile Army Surgical Hospitals. Additional experience with rapid evacuation to definitive surgical care was obtained during the Vietnam War, such that mean transport times dropped from 4 hours to 1.25 hours to 27 minutes in World War II, the Korean War, and the Vietnam War, respectively. Over these three conflicts, there was a concomitant reduction in mortality rates from 4.5% in WWII to 1.9% in the Vietnam War. It is likely that several factors contributed to the reduction in mortality over this time interval; first among them is the rapidity with which the injured soldier reached definitive medical care.[1]

In Vietnam, the importance of rapid transport and a prepared receiving facility was well recognized. The distribution of trained personnel, equipment, and medical care was designed such that no soldier in Vietnam was more than 35 minutes away from a medical facility capable of giving definitive, resuscitative lifesaving treatment.[1] This model of prehospital care became the framework for prehospital civilian care in the United States over the next several decades.

In 1966, the National Academy of Science/National Research Council released a report on trauma in which it was explicitly stated that the quality of civilian trauma care in the United States was below the standard achieved in Vietnam, such that "Expert consultants returning from both Korea and Vietnam have publicly asserted that if seriously wounded, the chances of survival would be better in the zone of combat than on the average city street."[2] In response to this report and in an attempt to improve trauma care delivery, the American College of Surgeons and its Committee on Trauma developed criteria for the designation of trauma centers and the establishment of regional trauma systems in 1976.[3]

TRAUMA CENTERS

Trauma centers are the core of an organized system of trauma care. As originally conceived, the trauma center was an institution with all the resources necessary for immediate and definitive care of the critically injured patient. These centers, with their interested and committed staff, also

TABLE 18.1

TRAUMA CENTER DESIGNATION LEVELS IN THE UNITED STATES

Trauma center level	Description	Estimated number
1	Typically located in large urban environments, major cities. Provides full spectrum of trauma care 24 h/d with 24-hour availability of in-house surgeon. Acts as a community leader in trauma research, education, and prevention. Expected to admit >1,200 trauma, >20% of whom are severely injured	190
2	In population-dense areas, supplements the resources of the level 1 center, whereas in more rural environments, may play a lead role in the community. Provides full spectrum of trauma care, 24 h/d. Surgeons must be rapidly available on short notice. Should coordinate outreach programs to incorporate smaller centers within the region.	263
3	Must have the capability to manage the initial care of most injured patients. General surgeon must be promptly available for major resuscitation. Will have transfer agreements in place to rapidly transfer patients to higher levels of care. Will have educational programs for physicians, nurses, and allied health-care workers.	251
4/5	Provide initial evaluation and assessment of injured patients in rural environments. Requires 24-h coverage by a physician (level 4 only). No specific requirement for surgeon or availability of specialists. Most patients will require transfer to larger facilities. Will have transfer agreements in place to rapidly transfer patients to higher levels of care.	450

(Data from reference 4. Table from Nathens AB, Brunet FP, Maier RV. Development of trauma systems and effect on outcomes after injury. *Lancet* 2004;363:1794–1801, with permission from Elsevier.)

TRAUMA

served as the primary teaching sites for those interested in furthering their education in the care of the injured. This description is most consistent with a level 1 trauma center an institution that takes a lead role for the provision of trauma care within a region. With an increasing understanding that it is neither desirable nor efficient that every injured patient must be transported to a center with all necessary resources available, the classification scheme for the designation of centers has evolved to allow a broader range of institutions to participate, while still ensuring standards are met to provide the appropriate level of care for the severity of injury (Table 18.1). This approach improves the efficiency of trauma care by allowing higher resource level centers to focus on the more severely injured patient and reduces the likelihood that patients with minor injuries will be transported outside their community when they might best be cared for closer to home. Currently, more than 1,000 designated trauma centers exist in the United States, with just under half designated as level 1 or 2.[4] The process of trauma center designation begins with on-site verification of resources and commitment by either state health authorities or surveyors from the American College of Surgeons Committee on Trauma (ACSCOT) Verification Review Committee. Hospitals undergo verification at fixed intervals, consistent with either ACSCOT or regional requirements.

TRAUMA SYSTEM COMPONENTS

The trauma center represents the core of the trauma system; however, the system is much broader in scope. Specifically, mechanisms must be in place to ensure that severely injured patients are triaged and ultimately transported to a center where they can receive definitive care. If a patient is injured at a site remote from a level 1 center, agreements must be in place to facilitate interfacility transfer from outlying centers. A quality assurance (QA) program, both at the hospital level and the system level, is critical to ensure optimal patient outcomes. Within a center, these QA programs allow for the evolution of care protocols, whereas at the system level, they ensure adequate triage and the integrity of the triage and interfacility transfer process. These and other critical trauma system components were identified by West and co-workers[5] and then expanded by Bazzoli et al.[6] (Table 18.2)[6] Recently, many have advocated that both injury prevention and postacute hospital care (e.g., rehabilitation) be included under the conceptual umbrella of the trauma system to better reflect the entire continuum of trauma care.[7]

A lead agency with the legal authority to designate trauma centers is critical to the development of an organized system of trauma care. In many regions, the state or regional department of health holds this authority. This authority usually extends beyond the designation of trauma centers to encompass the development of criteria for the triage of

TABLE 18.2

ESSENTIAL TRAUMA SYSTEM COMPONENTS

- Presence of a lead agency with legal authority to designate trauma centers
- Use of a formal process for trauma center designation
- Use of American College of Surgeons (or similar) standards for trauma center verification
- Use of an out-of-area survey team for trauma center designation
- A mechanism to limit the number of designated trauma centers in a community based on community need
- Written triage criteria that form the basis for bypassing nondesignated centers
- Presence of ongoing monitoring systems for quality assurance (e.g., trauma registry)
- Statewide availability of trauma centers

(From Nathens AB, Brunet FP, Maier RV. Development of trauma systems and effect on outcomes after injury. *Lancet* 2004;363:1794–1801, with permission from Elsevier.)

patients. Further, with the instatement of triage criteria potentially nearer, nondesignated centers are bypassed by emergency medical services (EMS) personnel in deference to a regional trauma center. In addition, the number, location, and level of centers should be based on population demographics and geography, rather than mere interest, to meet the needs of the patients and prevent unnecessary duplication of expensive resources. This process is apt to bring with it challenges of monopolistic business practices from the nondesignated centers. The identification of trauma centers in a region results in a loss of market competition among the hospitals within that region, which might result in the loss of income for the nondesignated centers. Ensuring the system is backed by legislation helps to mitigate, but does not eliminate, these issues.

TRAUMA SYSTEM IMPLEMENTATION AND EFFECTIVENESS IN THE UNITED STATES

Progress in the implementation of organized systems of care in the United States has been limited, in part, by the funding required to support the design, implementation, and maintenance of a well-integrated, coordinated regional system of trauma care. Despite this relatively limited funding, considerable progress has been made; now, 38 states have implemented, or are in the process of implementing, organized systems of trauma care (Fig. 18.1).[8]

Several lines of evidence suggest that an organized system of trauma care reduces mortality from injury. West and Trunkey[9] evaluated the preventable death rate caused by trauma in San Francisco County, California, where a single institution was responsible for all trauma care, with the death rate in Orange County, California, where more than 40 centers managed trauma patients. In San Francisco County, only 1% of deaths were considered preventable, whereas almost three quarters of all deaths in Orange County were potentially salvageable. Subsequently, Orange County implemented a trauma system and demonstrated an eightfold reduction in the rate of preventable death as patients were triaged and cared for at designated trauma centers.[10] Population-based studies have also been used to evaluate the benefits of regional trauma centers. For example, Rutledge and coworkers[11] demonstrated that counties with designated trauma centers in North Carolina had a 20% reduction in per capita trauma deaths compared with counties without trauma centers, whereas Nathens et al.[12] demonstrated that states with an organized system of trauma care reduce motor-vehicle crash–related mortality by 10%. These benefits are not instantaneous, taking as long as a decade to manifest.[13,14] It is likely that after formal system implementation a gradual process of quality improvement leads to better outcomes. Presumably, prehospital protocols improve such that the appropriate patients are triaged to centers with adequate resources, whereas the trauma centers themselves evolve as they begin to commit a greater proportion of their resources to trauma and become more experienced and capable of providing optimal care.[15,16]

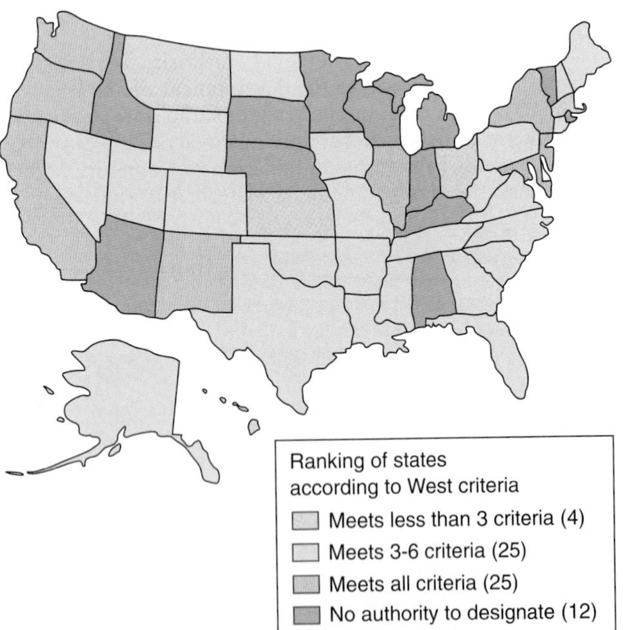

FIGURE 18.1 Regional trauma system in the United States as of 2002. States are ranked by the number of trauma system components implemented in their region. (From U.S. Department of Health and Human Services. A 2002 National Assessment of State Trauma System Development, Emergency Medical Services Resources, and Disaster Readiness for Mass Casualty Events. 2003. ftp://ftp.hrsa.gov/hrsa/trauma/nationalassessment.pdf. Accessed November 2004.)

RURAL TRAUMA SYSTEMS

Rural trauma care has been considered one of the great challenges in trauma system development.[17] Approximately one third of the U.S. population resides in rural areas, yet over half of all deaths caused by motor vehicle crashes (MVCs) occur in this environment. To put this in greater perspective, the rate of death from MVCs is 600 times greater in rural Texas than in New York City.[18] Several factors play into this excess mortality. With a lower population density, discovery times, of necessity, are longer. Further, both EMS response times and transport times are longer; together, these factors increase the risk of prehospital death by as much as sevenfold.[19] In addition, prehospital personnel in rural environments are often volunteers with limited training. For example, in the rural state of Vermont, only 2% of all EMS providers are trained as paramedics capable of providing advanced life support (ALS).[17] Many EMS providers in rural areas attend to fewer than 10 severely injured patients annually, making it virtually impossible for providers to maintain an adequate level of experience despite adequate training. Similarly, physicians working in rural environments have limited exposure to the major trauma patient. Together, these data support the premise that enhanced training (with maintenance of skills), combined with minimal time in the field, provide the best opportunity for optimal outcomes.

Given these impediments to providing adequate and timely trauma care, some rural states have implemented *inclusive* trauma systems such that virtually all hospitals participate as designated trauma centers to the extent that their resources allow.[20] This approach is in contrast to *exclusive* systems, where most severely injured patients are transported to relatively few centers. At a minimum, the structure of an inclusive system ensures that the initial receiving hospital will have a plan as well as appropriate human and material resources in place to provide initial, emergent management of the severely injured patient. Once patients are assessed by the receiving center, they are transferred as indicated to higher-level trauma centers for definitive care.

To facilitate this process, many hospitals (often designated as level 3, 4, or 5 trauma centers) have interfacility transfer protocols and agreements with level 1 or level 2 centers to expedite the transfer process. In the rural settings, these lower level trauma centers play a critical role in initial stabilization and triage.[21] Although conceptually sound, the efficacy of this approach is unproved. For example, when rural centers were designated in Oregon, clear evidence showed that the distribution of trauma patients within the system changed; however, no significant measurable improvements in overall outcome were evident in this limited population of severely injured patients.[22,23]

SUMMARY

There is clear evidence that trauma system implementation reduces injury-related mortality. Despite increasing trauma system implementation across the United States, over one third of major trauma victims are not cared for at regional trauma centers.[24] The reasons for this are multifactorial; however, it is likely that access is not uniformly consistent across states and within regions. For example, the availability of trauma centers varies greatly across states, ranging from 0.9 to 6.6 centers per million population.[4,24] Many of the states have not fulfilled one of the key components of trauma system design-ensuring that populations within more sparsely populated regions have access to high level trauma care. This remains the next challenge in trauma system design.

KEY POINTS

- **Trauma systems in America are based on military experiences of improved survival in injured personnel produced by rapid transport to definitive care.**
- **Regional level 1 trauma centers meet the highest standards for multispecialty manpower readiness, resources, education, and outreach and have triage acceptance agreements with lower level trauma centers.**
- **Trauma systems require a lead agency with designating authority and a formal process utilizing ACS or similar standards. A mechanism should be in place to limit the number of centers based on patient needs and triage criteria, including nontrauma hospital bypass and monitoring for ongoing QA. Statewide availability of trauma centers is necessary.**
- **Trauma systems do work by reducing unnecessary deaths but are politically charged and require years to reach full effectiveness.**
- **The impediments of distance, discovery, training, and maintenance of expertise make rural trauma care a remaining major challenge.**

References

1. Neel S. Army aeromedical evacuation procedures in Vietnam: implications for rural America. *JAMA* 1968;204:99–103.
2. National Committee of Trauma and Committee on Shock. *Accidental Death and Disability: The Neglected Disease of Modern Society.* Washington, DC: National Academy of Sciences/National Research Council, 1966.
3. American College of Surgeons. Optimal hospital resources for care of the seriously injured patient. *Bull Am Coll Surg.* 1976;61:15–22.
4. **MacKenzie EJ, Hoyt DB, et al. National inventory of hospital trauma centers. *JAMA* 2003;289:1515–1522.**
5. **West JG, Williams MJ, Trunkey DD, et al. Trauma systems: current status—future challenges. *JAMA* 1988;259:3597–600.**
6. Bazzoli GJ, Madura KJ, Cooper GF, et al. Progress in the development of trauma systems in the United States: results of a national survey. *JAMA* 1995;273:395–401.
7. American Trauma Society. *Trauma Systems: Agenda for the Future.* United States Department of Transportation, National Highway Traffic Safety Administration, 2002. http://www.nhtsa.dot.gov/people/injury/ems/TRAUMA_SYSTEM/. Accessed November 2004.
8. **U.S. Department of Health and Human Services. *A 2002 National Assessment of State Trauma System Development, Emergency Medical Services Resources, and Disaster Readiness for Mass Casualty Events, 2003.* http://www.hrsa.gov/trauma/survey/default.htm. Accessed November 2004.**
9. **West JG, Trunkey DD, Lim RC. Systems of trauma care: a study of two counties. *Arch Surg.* 1979;114:455–460.**
10. West JG, Cales RH, Gazzaniga AB. Impact of regionalization: the Orange County experience. *Arch Surg.* 1983;118:740–744.
11. Rutledge R, Fakhry SM, Meyer A, et al. An analysis of the association of trauma centers with per capita hospitalizations and death rates from injury. *Ann Surg.* 1993;218:512–524.
12. **Nathens AB, Jurkovich GJ, Rivara FP, et al. Effectiveness of state trauma systems in reducing injury-related mortality: a national evaluation. *J Trauma* 2000;48:25–30.**
13. Mullins RJ, Mann NC, Hedes JR, et al. Preferential benefit of implementation of a statewide trauma system in one of two adjacent states. *J Trauma* 1998;44:609–617.
14. Nathens AB, Jurkovich GJ, Cummings P, et al. The effect of organized systems of trauma care on motor vehicle crash mortality. *JAMA* 2000;283:1990–1994.
15. O'Keefe GE, Jurkovich GJ, Copass MK, et al. Ten-year trend in survival and resource utilization at a Level I trauma center. *Ann Surg.* 1999;229:409–415.
16. Peitzman AB, Courcoulas AP, Stinson C, et al. Trauma center maturation: quantification of process and outcome. *Ann Surg.* 1999;230:87–94.
17. Rogers FB, Shackford SR, Osler TM, et al. Rural trauma: the challenge for the next decade. *J Trauma* 1999;47:802–821.
18. Baker SPH, Whitfield RA, O'Neill B. Geographic variations in mortality from motor vehicle crashes. *N Engl J Med.* 1987;316:1384–1387.
19. Grossman DC, Allegra K, Macdonald SC, et al. Urban-rural differences in prehospital care of major trauma. *J Trauma* 1997;42:723–729.
20. Narad RA, Becker JL, Frecceri C. A decentralized trauma system design for a rural area. *Prehospital Disaster Medicine* 1996;11:134–139.
21. Grossman DC, Hart G, Rivara FP, et al. From roadside to bedside: the regionalization of trauma care in a remote rural county. *J Trauma* 1995;38:14–21.
22. Mann NC, Hedges JR, Mullins RJ, et al. Rural hospital transfer patterns before and after implementation of a statewide trauma system. OHSU Rural Trauma Research Group. *Acad Emerg Med.* 1997;4:764–771.
23. Clay MN, Mullins RJ, Hedges JR, et al. Mortality among seriously injured patients treated in remote rural trauma centers before and after implementation of a statewide trauma system. *Med Care* 2001;39:643–653.
24. **Nathens AB, Jurkovich GJ, MacKenzie EJ, et al. A resource-based assessment of trauma care in the United States. *J Trauma* 2004;56:173–178.**

Initial Care Phase

CHAPTER 19 ■ PREHOSPITAL AND RESUSCITATION CARE

EILEEN M. BULGER

Care of the injured patient begins in the prehospital setting with a tightly integrated multidisciplinary emergency medical service (EMS) system. The goal of the EMS system is to provide immediate access to lifesaving medical care. This care usually entails the use of a first-response team, such as the fire department or other public safety personnel with the capability of providing basic life support (BLS) within minutes of an injury. When available, a rapid transport team capable of providing advanced life support (ALS) moves the injured patient to a trauma center where a multidisciplinary team meets the patient to continue resuscitation, identify injuries, and provide expeditious therapy with the aim of completing all of these processes within 1 hour (called the *golden hour*). The goal of the EMS system is to assess for life-threatening injuries, initiate emergency care, and transport the injured patient as expeditiously and safely as possible to the nearest appropriate trauma center.

PREHOSPITAL CARE

Personnel

The initial goal of any EMS system is to provide a rapid response by personnel trained in BLS skills to the scene of the injured patient. In most cases, this function is performed by an Emergency Medical Technician-Basic (EMT-B). The EMT-B's responsibility is to assess rapidly the patient's airway, breathing, and circulation and look for evidence of obvious external hemorrhage. The EMT-B's skills include extrication, spinal protection, immobilization, splinting, and control of external hemorrhage. In most EMS systems, BLS is followed by ALS. ALS personnel are usually Emergency Medical Technician-Paramedic (EMT-P) or specially trained nurses or physicians and may have air or ground transportation capabilities. ALS personnel are trained in a variety of advanced skills including endotracheal intubation, IV access and drug administration, needle and/or surgical cricothyrotomy, and needle thoracentesis. However, significant variability exists among different ALS systems regarding the procedures permitted and medications allowed for use by an EMT-P.[1,2]

An area of frequent controversy in the literature involves the philosophy of rapid transport ("scoop and run") versus field stabilization ("stay and play") for the injured patient.[3] The choice of approach for the individual patient often requires complex judgments. Decisions made by experienced on-scene EMTs, communicating online with trauma center control that will receive the patient, provide the best patient outcome.[4,5] The procedures performed and the time invested depend on factors such as the patient's hemodynamic stability, level of consciousness, complexity of extrication, distance from the receiving trauma center, and experience of the prehospital personnel. Injured patients who are at risk for progressive deterioration from continued hemorrhage are better served with stabilization procedures done en route rather than at the scene.[4]

Nationally standardized training programs for EMTs, both BLS and ALS, have become popular. These programs, Basic Trauma Life Support (BTLS) and Prehospital Trauma Life Support (PHTLS) provide EMS personnel a curriculum to assist in making these complex decisions.

Assessment and Management Priorities

Airway Assessment

Because the most immediately life-threatening problem to the injured patient is loss of airway patency, this is the first priority of the first-response team on arrival at the injury site. Patients who are awake, alert, and talking obviously have a patent airway, but those who are unconscious or have evidence of respiratory insufficiency require immediate attention. Typical BTLS skills, such as suctioning, chin lift or jaw thrust, the placement of oropharyngeal airways, and the use of bag mask devices, are usually sufficient, at least temporarily, to restore oxygenation. On arrival of ALS personnel, a more definitive airway can be secured by endotracheal intubation. Endotracheal intubation is the best procedure for airway control for patients who are in shock, have abnormal breathing patterns, or are unable to protect the airway because they are unconscious. Endotracheal intubation is a skill that requires proper training and regular use of the technique. In addition, ongoing quality assurance and continuing education are needed to maintain skills over time.

Training of paramedical personnel almost always includes endotracheal intubation, but the indications for intubation vary. The indications for intubation are often dependent on whether ALS providers are allowed to use neuromuscular blocking agents (NMBAs), such as succinylcholine, to facilitate intubation. In systems that do not have clearance to use NMBA, intubation is limited to severely injured patients without airway reflexes. The use of NMBA has been associated with increased success at achieving prehospital intubation with minimal complication rates.[6–12] However, the absolute benefit of prehospital intubation for patients with traumatic brain injury remains controversial. Concerns have been raised that transient hypoxia associated with intubation or inadvertent hyperventilation after intubation could worsen outcome for these patients.[13,14] In contrast, early intubation reduces the risk of gastric aspiration, which can be exacerbated by positive-pressure ventilatory assistance by bag valve mask and cause gastric distention.

Common indications for endotracheal intubation in the field include respiratory distress, unconsciousness, hypovolemic shock, significant head injury, severe chest injury, and facial burns. More liberal indications for endotracheal intubation include all patients with significant mechanism of injury and unstable vital signs or altered mental status. Intubation in an uncontrolled environment such as the prehospital setting can be difficult. Patients with head injuries are at high risk for cervical spine injuries, so in-line mobilization techniques are necessary. In patients in whom intubation is not successful, the use of a pharyngeal lumen airway or *Combitube* may be an option.[15] Nasotracheal intubation is an effective technique if practiced frequently, but requires patient-initiated airflow to open the glottis; most paramedical personnel lack training in this technique, and patients with potential basilar skull fracture are not candidates for this approach. In some cases, needle or surgical cricothyroidotomy in the field may be the only way to establish an airway. Reasonable results have been obtained in the prehospital setting using cricothyroidotomy, but as with endotracheal intubation, mastering this skill requires ongoing training.[16,17]

Breathing

After establishment of a patent and controlled airway, the next priority is to ensure that air exchange is taking place. Immediately life-threatening injuries that preclude air exchange include tension pneumothorax, massive open chest wounds, sucking chest wounds, and tracheal disruption. There are no maneuvers likely to correct tracheal disruption in the field. Both open chest wounds and sucking chest wounds respond to endotracheal intubation and positive-pressure ventilation. Tension pneumothorax occasionally requires field decompression. Field techniques to deal with tension pneumothorax include needle thoracostomy and chest tube thoracostomy in the midclavicular line of the second intercostal space. Some trauma systems allow paramedical personnel to place chest tubes in the field or en route under medical control.[18] Chest tube placement probably is not necessary in urban trauma systems with short response times but may be of value in rural areas.

Circulation

The most common cause of death during the first hour after injury is hemorrhage. Therefore, after establishment of a patent airway and adequate air exchange, the next priority is support of the circulation. Direct pressure controls obvious external hemorrhage. The placement of one or two large-bore intravenous (IV) lines in the upper extremities en route to the trauma center facilitates resuscitation. However, placement of lines must not delay transport unless the patient is undergoing a complex extrication or is more than 30 minutes from a trauma center.[19] The standard of care in the prehospital setting for hypotensive patients is volume replacement and rapid transport to a trauma center. Historically, the pneumatic antishock garment was also used in this setting but has been largely abandoned based on data demonstrating increased mortality particularly in patients with thoracic trauma.[20] The pneumatic antishock garment is still occasionally used as a splint for combined pelvic and lower extremity injuries.

The appropriate volume and type of fluid used for initial resuscitation of the hypotensive trauma patient remains controversial. Recent experimental and clinical evidence raises the possibility that internal hemorrhage from major vascular injuries should not be treated with IV fluid infusion until the bleeding can be controlled in the operating room.[21] In the hypotensive state, major vascular injuries have a chance to clot and temporarily stop hemorrhaging; however, if IV volume restores normal blood pressure, the clot can dislodge and the rate of bleeding can increase significantly. However, the clinical data supporting this approach are based on a single trial that focused on patients with penetrating torso trauma and with a short transport time to the trauma center.[21] The role of limited volume resuscitation in blunt trauma is unknown and could be harmful to patients with traumatic brain injury. Currently the standard resuscitation fluid for trauma patients is a crystalloid solution of either lactated Ringer's solution or normal saline. Several recent studies have suggested that hypertonic saline solutions may be more beneficial as the initial resuscitation fluid for hypotensive trauma patients; clinical trials are ongoing.[22–24]

The controversy between the scoop-and-run philosophy and the field-resuscitation philosophy in seriously injured patients is best resolved by common sense. Patients who are a short distance from a trauma center should be expeditiously transported to the trauma center with attempts made during transport to obtain IV access. This strategy facilitates initiation of resuscitation on arrival at the trauma center. Alternatively, patients who are a long distance from a trauma center or who require long extrication times most likely benefit from the administration of IV fluids. Current standardized training programs (BTLS, PHTLS) for EMS personnel suggest that, at minimum, a trauma patient who does not require extrication should be assessed, treated, and packaged for transportation in less than 8 to 10 minutes.

RESUSCITATION PHASE

Development of trauma centers and trauma systems has produced documented improvement in survival of multiply injured patients in numerous reports. Trauma centers are hospitals committed to the total care of the trauma patient, 24 hours a day. Multidisciplinary trauma teams consist of emergency physicians, general and orthopedic surgeons and neurosurgeons, critical care nurses, and diagnostic technicians. After notification of a major injury from the scene, the trauma team assembles in a specially equipped resuscitation room and waits for the patient to arrive. On arrival, care is immediately transferred to the trauma team, and the resuscitation phase is initiated without a delay. If feasible, seriously injured patients should bypass hospitals without these resources and be taken to the nearest trauma center.

Many patients have relatively minor injuries that do not require mobilization of this expensive team and resources. Therefore, an important function of a trauma system is to allow communication between prehospital personnel and the trauma center to identify those patients who will benefit from trauma center care. A written prehospital report describing the mechanism and extent of injury, vital signs, Glasgow Coma Scale (GCS) score, and treatment started by the prehospital personnel should also be provided. These details alert the trauma center team to look for specific injury patterns based on mechanism of injury and guide further workup. Assessment and treatment then follow a logical sequence based on nationally standardized protocols using the advanced trauma life support (ATLS) format.[25]

Trauma Team Composition

The trauma team consists of members from different disciplines, each of whom sees the patient from a particular point of view. Of necessity, the team must have a single "captain of the ship" whose responsibility it is to organize and prioritize treatment efforts. In a well-orchestrated team, the team leader integrates and coordinates several tasks simultaneously. In most level 1 and 2 trauma centers, the team captain is a general surgeon trained in trauma care. In the ideal situation, the trauma surgeon should be present when the patient arrives. In many rural and nonacademic level 3 trauma centers, the initial team captain is an emergency physician, with a general surgeon assuming the role on arrival. Academic institutions with both emergency medicine and surgical residency programs have the obligation of training both specialties to assume the role of trauma team leadership.

Although responsibilities vary between institutions, anyone involved in the resuscitation of trauma patients must master several procedures: all types of airway management, including cricothyroidotomy; establishment of vascular access through both percutaneous and open approaches; decompression of the pleural space using needle or tube thoracostomy; and decompression of the pericardial space by pericardiocentesis, subxiphoid window, or emergency thoracotomy.

Primary Survey: Initial Assessment

The first priority of the trauma team is to repeat the assessment of the airway, breathing, circulation, and level of consciousness of the patient. This assessment is referred to as the *primary survey*. Although in reality the primary survey is performed in a simultaneous fashion, it is described here into its individual components and their appropriate priorities.

The first priority is reassessment of the airway. Airway obstruction often responds to simple maneuvers such as suctioning, chin lift, jaw thrust, or placement of an oropharyngeal airway. Protection of the cervical spine with in-line immobilization is imperative during these maneuvers. Persistence of respiratory insufficiency requires endotracheal intubation. Unsuccessful intubation necessitates cricothyroidotomy. Occasionally, the anatomy does not allow cricothyroidotomy, as can occur with laryngeal fracture. In these cases, a formal tracheotomy must be performed. After an airway is established, a physician auscultates the chest to confirm air exchange, confirms return of carbon dioxide via the endotracheal tube and obtains a chest radiograph to ensure proper tube position with the tip proximal to the carina. Appropriate placement of endotracheal tubes inserted in the prehospital setting should also be confirmed at this time.

The next priority is to ensure adequate ventilatory exchange by rapid auscultation of both lung fields and assessment for mechanical factors that may interfere with breathing. These factors include compression of the lung from hemothorax, pneumothorax, or visceral herniation; loss of chest wall stability from flail chest; lung damage from pulmonary contusion; and airway obstruction from aspiration. A dramatic presentation with cyanosis, intense respiratory effort without air movement, distended neck veins, and lack of breath sounds on chest auscultation indicates that a tension pneumothorax is present. Clinical diagnosis of tension pneumothorax requires immediate needle thoracostomy followed by chest tube thoracostomy. Sucking chest wounds should be sealed with an occlusive dressing secured on three sides to function as a flap valve. Most other problems become evident on the initial chest radiograph and are relieved by chest tube insertion, suctioning, or repositioning of the endotracheal tube. The optimal position for chest tube insertion is the midaxillary line at the fifth or sixth interspace, avoiding the axilla, the large muscles of the back and chest, and the breast. Insertion of a finger into the chest before chest tube placement ensures entry into the pleural space and provides the opportunity to search digitally for defects in the diaphragm.

After establishment of an airway, ventilation, and appropriate pleural drainage, the next priority is assessment of the patient's circulatory status. Blood pressure, pulse, skin perfusion, temperature, capillary refill, mental status, presence of breath sounds, and neck vein distention are all useful clinical indicators of hemodynamic status. The first issue is to establish whether the patient is in hypovolemic shock and, if so, to determine the source of hemorrhage. Circulatory collapse in the injured patient is almost always caused by hypovolemia secondary to hemorrhage. Occasionally, concurrent heart disease, spinal cord injury, or cardiac tamponade may contribute. The mainstay of treatment for hypotension in the injured patient, regardless of cause, is volume resuscitation with crystalloid solution and, if hypotension is persistent, packed red blood cells (RBCs). A lack of response to IV infusion of 2 L of lactated Ringer's solution indicates significant, ongoing hemorrhage and necessitates immediate blood transfusion.

Effective resuscitation from hemorrhagic shock requires both restoration of intravascular volume and control of hemorrhage. Most hypotensive patients are already compensating maximally on arrival in the emergency department (ED) and many have ongoing hemorrhage. The less responsive a patient is to initial volume resuscitation, the more urgent is the need for hemorrhage control. One need not wait for a response to resuscitation before taking the patient to the operating room. Another situation that requires vigilance is the cool, pale patient with relatively normal vital signs. These patients are compensating maximally and have a normal blood pressure because of intensive peripheral vasoconstriction. However, this compensatory mechanism is of only limited duration, and such patients require immediate rapid volume transfusion, blood transfusion, and operative control of bleeding. A similar trap exists for patients with the mangled extremity syndrome or multiple open fractures. Patients may have lost significant blood volume at the injury scene. Before resuscitation, there may be relatively little hemorrhage from the open wounds; however, initiation of IV fluids may increase blood pressure and cause vasodilation, resulting in increased hemorrhage. These patients require immediate volume resuscitation and operative control of their wounds.

The final priority in the primary survey is a brief neurologic evaluation to assess the components of the GCS (Table 19.1). The GCS is scored by assessing eye opening, verbal responses, and motor responses with a maximal (normal) score of 15. In addition, pupillary size and reactivity and the presence of other lateralizing signs are assessed. Mental status may improve in response to volume resuscitation; however, a patient with a GCS score of 8 or less is assumed to have a significant brain injury. In this case, aggressive resuscitation, including appropriate adequate ventilation, restoration of

TABLE 19.1 DIAGNOSTIC

GLASGOW COMA SCALE (GCS)

EYE OPENING	
Spontaneous	4
To voice	3
To pain	2
None	1
VERBAL RESPONSE	
Oriented	5
Confused	4
Inappropriate words	3
Incomprehensible sounds	2
None	1
MOTOR RESPONSE	
Obeys commands	6
Purposeful movement (pain)	5
Withdraw (pain)	4
Flexion (pain)	3
Extension (pain)	2
None	1
GCS SUBTOTAL	3–15

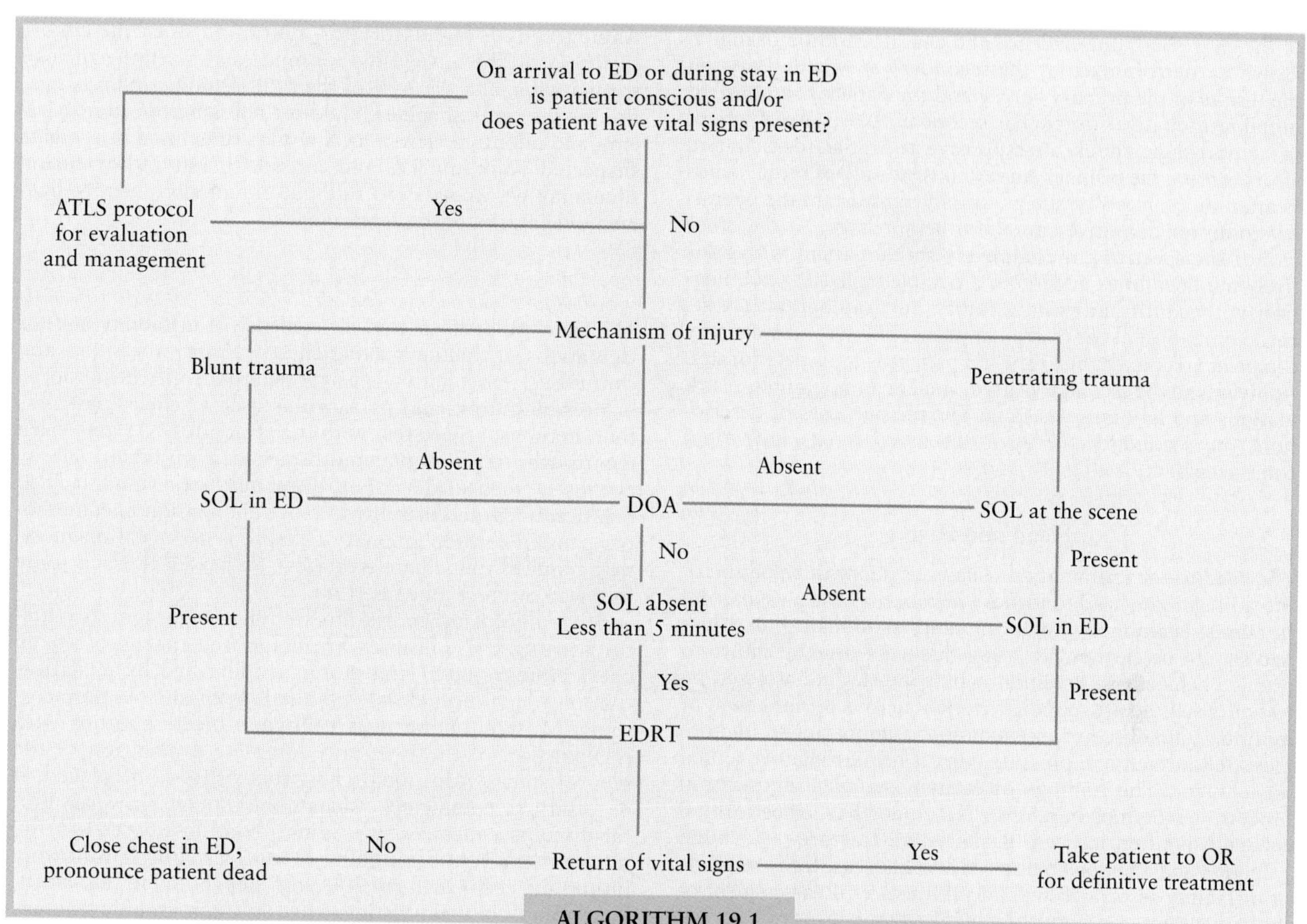

ALGORITHM 19.1 Emergency thoracotomy for penetrating trauma. ED, emergency department; ATLS, advanced trauma life support; SOL, signs of life; DOA, dead on arrival; EDRT, emergency department resuscitative thoracotomy; OR, operating room. (Adapted from Boyd M, Vanek VW, Bourguet CC. "Emergency room resuscitative thoracotomy: when is it indicated?" *J Trauma*. 1992;33:714–721, with permission.)

circulating volume, and the provision of adequate oxygenation, are important considerations.

ED resuscitative thoracotomy is an aggressive, desperate attempt to save a dying patient. The dramatic return to full consciousness of a clinically dead patient after release of a pericardial tamponade from a stab wound to the heart provides complete justification for ED thoracotomy to those who have witnessed it. However, the widespread use of the technique in all patients arriving without vital signs has resulted in an extremely low survival rate at a very high cost. At first glance, the cost of an unsuccessful ED thoracotomy would seem to be nothing more than that of sterilizing the instruments and the physician's time. Many times, however, vital signs are temporarily restored, and the patient dies in the operating room or in the intensive care unit after massive blood transfusion and the use of considerable resources. Even worse is the rare patient who survives in a permanent vegetative state. The cost of the care for these patients must be included in any cost-benefit analysis.

Boyd et al.[26] performed a meta-analysis of 24 reports concerning the outcome of ED thoracotomy. They found that the overall survival rate after ED thoracotomy was 11% (264 of 2,294 patients). There were no survivors among patients with no signs of life at the trauma scene. Signs of life were defined as supraventricular electrical activity, pupillary reaction, and agonal respirations. In addition, there were no neurologically intact survivors among blunt trauma patients who were without signs of life on arrival in the ED. Considering these findings, the researchers proposed an algorithm that would indicate ED thoracotomy for penetrating trauma only if the patient had signs of life at the scene and had lost signs of life less than 5 minutes before arrival in the ED. Blunt trauma patients would be allowed ED thoracotomy only if the patient had signs of life on arrival in the ED. For patients who meet these criteria and lose cardiac function, airway placement and fluid resuscitation are initiated simultaneously with, or are immediately followed by, left anterior thoracotomy, pericardiotomy, and internal cardiac massage (Algorithm 19.1).

Secondary Survey

The secondary survey is directed at specific identification of suspected and unsuspected injuries. It consists of a thorough physical examination that includes observation and palpation of the entire body for evidence and characterization of injury. However, performance of the secondary survey depends on the results of the primary survey and the patient's response to initial resuscitative efforts. The secondary survey for a patient in hemorrhagic shock unresponsive to initial resuscitative efforts during the primary survey consists only of rapid identification of the bleeding site and rapid transport to the operating room for definitive control of hemorrhage. At the other end of the spectrum, a completely stable patient with relatively minor injuries undergoes a complete physical examination with confirmatory laboratory and radiographic tests before initiation of the treatment phase. The secondary survey can be interrupted at any time if a patient's status deteriorates. Adjuvants to the secondary survey include radiographic examinations and laboratory testing. For the purposes of description, the secondary survey is discussed by its individual components.

Head and Face

The head-to-toe examination usually begins with palpation of the skull and the head to identify hematomas, lacerations, and fractures. Scalp lacerations can cause significant blood loss and should be closed with a full-thickness running suture to provide hemostasis. Potential ocular injuries are assessed by testing visual acuity, pupillary function, and ocular range of motion. A funduscopic examination is important to identify increased intracranial pressure, vitreal hemorrhage, or retinal detachment. The findings of ecchymosis over the mastoid process, hemotympanum, otorrhea, rhinorrhea, or periorbital ecchymosis often indicate basilar skull fracture. Thorough palpation and attempts to displace facial bones identify step-offs or instability associated with facial fractures. Reassessment of the airway and a careful bimanual examination of the oral cavity identify loose teeth as well as mandibular and maxillary fractures. Bleeding from nasal fractures may require posterior and anterior packing for hemostasis; transnasal posteriorly placed Foley catheter balloons often work well to stanch bleeding.

Neck

Examination of the cervical region is conducted while axial immobilization of the cervical spine is maintained. The cervical collar is removed and the neck is examined for tracheal deviation, subcutaneous emphysema, hematomas, lacerations, or distended jugular veins. The posterior cervical spine is palpated to elicit tenderness or other signs of obvious fracture. Evidence of laryngeal fracture includes subcutaneous emphysema, tenderness, "step-off" (distortion of the thyroid and cricoid cartilage), and voice change. The presence of a fractured larynx is a relative contraindication to endotracheal intubation because of the possibility of extending the injury or creating a false passage leading to loss of the airway. Patients with suspected laryngeal fractures should be taken to the operating room immediately for formal tracheotomy. Carotid pulses are assessed, and bruits or expanding hematomas that may be suggestive of carotid artery injury are identified.

Penetrating injuries should not be probed, cannulated, or explored past the platysma because uncontrollable hemorrhage may ensue if a clot is dislodged from a major vascular injury. Wounds that have penetrated the platysma are evaluated either by formal operative exploration of the neck or by some combination of angiography, triple endoscopy (pharyngoscopy, laryngoscopy, and esophagoscopy), radiographic contrast study, computed tomography (CT) scan, and observation.[27] Injuries encompassing the area from the cricoid cartilage to the angle of the mandible are usually explored. Angiography is mandatory for injuries between the cricoid cartilage and the clavicle and for injuries between the angle of the mandible and the base of the skull. Radiographic evaluation of the cervical spine should include anteroposterior, lateral, and odontoid views. A CT scan is often used to evaluate suspected bony injuries, and careful flexion and extension films may be necessary to rule out potentially unstable ligamentous injuries of the cervical spine.

Chest

The chest wall is inspected for evidence of instability and for lacerations, including sucking chest wounds, abrasions, and contusions. Auscultation is performed to identify hemothorax or pneumothorax, and palpation is used to elicit tenderness that may be associated with rib fractures. As has been mentioned, tension pneumothorax can be identified by cyanosis, tracheal deviation, distended neck veins, lack of breath sounds, and inability to move air. Tension pneumothorax causing cardiopulmonary collapse is a clinical diagnosis that requires immediate treatment by needle thoracostomy followed by chest tube insertion.

Virtually all other life-threatening and potentially life-threatening chest injuries are diagnosed or suspected on chest radiography. Hemothorax is identified by opacification of a hemithorax and is treated by chest tube thoracostomy. Most pulmonary parenchymal bleeding stops with reexpansion of the lung and complete evacuation of the pleural space. Additional chest tubes should be placed, if necessary, to completely evacuate the thorax. However, thoracotomy is indicated if the initial blood loss exceeds 1,500 mL or if the rate of ongoing blood loss shortly following injury exceeds 200 to 300 mL per hour in an adult. Pulmonary contusion is identified by radiographic findings of an irregular interstitial pattern or frank consolidation in the lung parenchyma. The clinical manifestations of pulmonary contusion vary from mild dyspnea to overt pulmonary failure with development of acute respiratory distress syndrome. The magnitude of the injury is rarely appreciated during the initial evaluation, and it is important to follow up with serial blood gas determinations and a repeat chest radiograph at 6 hours.

All patients with chest trauma should have an electrocardiographic (ECG) evaluation and continuous monitoring during the first hour in the ED. If the ECG is normal, the patient may be discharged, if otherwise appropriate. Patients with ECG changes during the initial hour may have a blunt cardiac injury and should be monitored for at least 24 hours. If there is any sign of myocardial failure, the patient should undergo echocardiography. Most blunt cardiac injuries are self-limited and require only monitoring and treatment of significant dysrhythmias during the first 24 to 48 hours. Rarely, patients have manifestations of overt myocardial failure and require full support, including an intra-aortic balloon pump.

Patients with rapid deceleration blunt injuries to the chest may sustain a transection of the thoracic aorta. The chest radiograph should be evaluated for widening of the mediastinum (more than 8 cm on a 40-inch anteroposterior chest radiograph), apical capping of the lung with blood, tracheal displacement, depression of the left main-stem bronchus, loss of the aortic window, deviation of the nasogastric tube, and loss of the parispinous stripe. Each of these findings suggests the presence of a mediastinal hematoma, which is often associated with a transection of the aorta. Patients with a significant mechanism of injury and suspicion of mediastinal hematoma on chest radiography should undergo diagnostic evaluation with either CT angiography or arch aortography to rule out transection of the aorta. In some centers, transesophageal echocardiography has also been reported to identify these injuries.

Evidence of a ruptured diaphragm on chest radiograph includes the presence of the nasogastric tube or bowel above the normal plane of the diaphragm. If the patient has a diagnosis of ruptured diaphragm and respiratory distress, consideration should be given to careful placement of a chest tube. Placement of the chest tube to water seal instead of suction minimizes the negative intrathoracic pressure and prevents further herniation. These patients should undergo expeditious exploratory laparotomy to repair the defect and address the commonly associated intraabdominal injuries.

Management of penetrating injuries to the chest depends on the trajectory of the missile. Wounds confined to one lung or pleural cavity are usually treated by chest tube placement alone, with reexpansion of the lung. If the missile may have traversed the mediastinum, further evaluation is necessary, potentially including bronchoscopy, esophagoscopy, and aortography. Echocardiography is used to rule out pericardial blood and heart injury. False-negative studies have occurred when blood in the pericardium decompresses into the pleural space. However, echocardiography may be a sufficient screening tool if there are no clinical signs or symptoms and no hemothorax. Gunshot wounds below the nipple line place the abdominal cavity at risk and thus require abdominal exploration as well.

Abdomen

The abdominal examination should attempt to determine whether there is a significant injury requiring surgical intervention. Although physical examination is often accurate and reliable, it can be misleading in 20% to 30% of patients.[28] This inaccuracy is particularly true in patients who are obtunded from head injury, alcohol, drug use, or shock. If patients are hemodynamically unstable, it is important to determine rapidly whether free intraperitoneal hemorrhage is responsible for the hypotension. Diagnostic peritoneal lavage (DPL) or the focused abdominal sonogram for trauma (FAST) accomplish this goal rapidly and safely. Both are reported to be extremely reliable in the hemodynamically unstable patient.[29,30] Both studies are operator dependent, however, and the choice of the best approach may depend on local hospital resources. DPL has the advantage of also being very sensitive for hollow viscous injury and thus is often preferred in the setting of a seatbelt sign with increased concern for bowel perforation.

DPL is considered grossly positive if more than 10 mL of blood is freely aspirated after catheter insertion. If less than 10 mL of blood or no blood is aspirated, 1 L of warmed crystalloid solution is infused into the peritoneum and then drained. A sample of the drained fluid is sent to the laboratory for RBC and leukocyte count (), amylase and bilirubin level, and gram stain for the presence of bacteria. DPL is considered microscopically positive if the RBC count is higher than 100,000/mL. If the goal is to find the source of hemorrhage in a hypotensive patient, then a grossly positive DPL pinpoints the abdomen as at least one source, and the patient should undergo immediate laparotomy. In contrast, a microscopically positive DPL indicates intraabdominal injury that may eventually require laparotomy, but the major source of hemorrhage causing the hypotension is likely elsewhere (chest or pelvis).[31]

In the hemodynamically stable patient, the lack of specificity of the DPL and FAST could lead to nontherapeutic and therefore unnecessary laparotomies. For this reason, CT has become routine for the evaluation of the abdomen in hemodynamically stable patients. Injuries that often have subtle findings during the first several hours after injury but may be found on a delayed CT scan include duodenal rupture, pancreatic transection, and blunt rupture of the intestine. Laboratory evaluations that may be helpful include liver enzyme levels and serial serum amylase levels.

The work-up for patients with penetrating abdominal injuries depends on the missile. Gunshot wounds to the abdomen are an indication for exploratory laparotomy because 90% to 95% of these patients have intraabdominal injuries. The occasional patient with a tangential subcutaneous wound can be evaluated by laparoscopy or even CT to determine whether peritoneal penetration injury has occurred.[32] Stab wounds to the abdomen are often evaluated initially by local exploration of the wound. If the wound traverses the anterior fascia, then the patient can be evaluated by DPL or laparoscopy and should undergo exploratory laparotomy if the results are positive. A lower threshold for a positive RBC count is often set for stab wound injuries because the DPL is designed simply to confirm peritoneal penetration and not significant bleeding. Stab wounds to the flank and back are best evaluated by a triple contrast CT scan and serial observation.[33] CT scan findings that mandate exploratory laparotomy include significant retroperitoneal hematoma, free air, extravasation of contrast material, and free intraperitoneal fluid.

Pelvis

After evaluation of the abdomen, the pelvis is assessed by physical examination. The bones of the pelvis are palpated gently to elicit tenderness that could indicate fracture. Evidence of instability of the pelvic ring warrants placement of a sheet around the pelvis to reduce the pelvic volume and minimize venous bleeding in the retroperitoneum. This procedure can be performed in the field or on arrival in the ED. In some systems the pneumatic antishock garment is used for this purpose, but better reduction can often be achieved with a simple bed sheet tied around the iliac crests. The genitalia should be inspected for scrotal hematoma or blood at the urethral meatus, which indicates probable urethral transection. A bimanual pelvic examination in women identifies evidence of vaginal laceration, indicating an open pelvic fracture. A rectal examination is performed to identify blood indicative of bowel injury and, occasionally, a mobile, "floating" prostate, which indicates urethral transection. Evidence of a free-floating prostate, blood at the urethra, or scrotal hematoma should prompt a retrograde urethrogram before placement of a bladder catheter is attempted. All patients sustaining significant blunt torso trauma should undergo plain radiography of the pelvis to diagnose potential pelvic fracture.

If the patient is hemodynamically unstable, the pelvic fracture must be considered a potential source of hemorrhage. This consideration is important because pelvic fracture bleeding is retroperitoneal and rarely controllable at exploratory laparotomy. Venous bleeding is treated by reducing the volume of the pelvis, and arterial bleeding should be evaluated and treated by early angiography and embolization. If the patient is hemodynamically stable, the pelvic fracture should be evaluated further with additional plain radiographs and CT scans (Algorithm 19.2).

Extremities

Finally, the extremities are evaluated for open wounds with potential sources of hemorrhage or occult open fractures. Evaluation of pulses may indicate vascular injury. Palpation and passive range of motion tests diagnose potential long-bone fractures, dislocations, and ligamentous injuries. Dislocations require prompt reduction, especially if there is any evidence of neurovascular compromise. Penetrating wounds to the extremities necessitate evaluation for potential

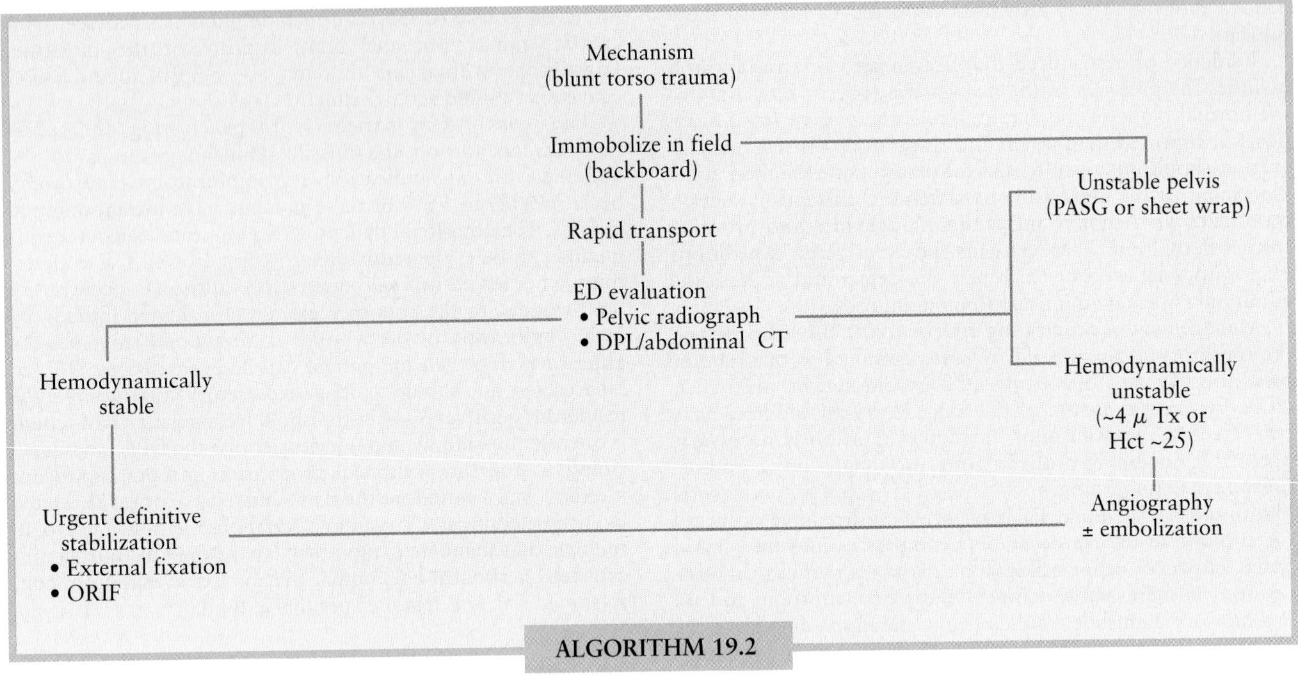

ALGORITHM 19.2 Emergency management of pelvic fractures. PASG, pneumatic antishock garment; ED, emergency department; DPL, diagnostic peritoneal lavage; CT, computed tomography; Tx, Hct, hematocrit; ORIF, open reduction internal fixation.

vascular injury by palpation of pulses, auscultation for bruits, and recognition of expanding hematomas. Proximity wounds can be evaluated by duplex ultrasound scan or arteriography.

SUMMARY

The ideal trauma system consists of a prehospital care team that quickly and safely transports an injured patient to a trauma center where a multidisciplinary trauma team immediately begins resuscitation of the patient. Treatment of immediately life-threatening injuries begins during transport and continues after arrival at the trauma center. Rapid initial evaluation, followed by a more detailed secondary survey, allows identification of injuries while therapy is simultaneously begun. The primary survey focuses on identification and simultaneous treatment of life-threatening injuries, including airway obstruction, mechanical factors in the chest that impair ventilation, and control of hemorrhage. The next priority is assessment and intervention for neurologic injuries including traumatic brain injury and spinal cord injury. Once these issues have been addressed, the secondary survey is performed to identify all other injuries. The secondary survey is interrupted as necessary to treat life-threatening and limb-threatening injuries as they are identified according to this priority list. If interruption occurs, the secondary survey is completed at a later time.

KEY POINTS

- **Emergency medical service systems provide a rapid, tiered response to the injured, beginning with an emergency medical technician-basic (first responder) and followed by an emergency medical technician-paramedic, as needed.**
- **Airway control is paramount and, if required, should be achieved using an orotracheal approach with neck immobilization and neuromuscular blockade, if needed.**
- **Duration at the scene should be individualized to the patient's injuries and physiologic status. "Scoop and run" versus "stay and play" approaches cannot be generalized.**
- **A multidisciplinary team of specialists, led by the "captain of the ship," usually a trauma surgeon, is available in level 1 and 2 trauma centers to provide coordinated optimal care for any and all injuries.**
- **Trauma assessment and care are provided in a logical, consistent manner. The primary survey identifies and simultaneously treats life-threatening injuries, including airway loss, inadequate ventilation, ongoing hemorrhage, and central nervous system damage. The secondary survey identifies all other injuries, including those with potential long-term disability.**

References

1. Lavery RF, Dora J, Tortella BJ, Cody RP. A survey of advanced life support practices in the United States. *Prehospital Disaster Med.* 1992;7:144–150.
2. McDonald CC, Bailey B. Out-of-hospital use of neuromuscular-blocking agents in the United States. *Prehosp Emerg Care* 1998;2:29–32.
3. **Liberman M, Mulder D, Sampalis J. Advanced or basic life support for trauma: meta-analysis and critical review of the literature. *J Trauma* 2000;49:584–599.**
4. Pepe PE, Maio RF. Evolving challenges in prehospital trauma services. Current issues and suggested evaluation tools. *Prehospital Disaster Med.* 1993;8(suppl):25–34.
5. Sampalis JS, Lavoie A, Williams JI, et al. Impact of on-site care, prehospital time, and level of in-hospital care on survival in severely injured patients. *J Trauma* 1993;34:252–261.

6. **Bulger EM, Copass MK, Maier RV, et al. An analysis of advanced prehospital airway management. *J Emerg Med.* 2002;23:183–189.**
7. Hedges JR, Dronen SC, Feero S, et al. Succinylcholine-assisted intubations in prehospital care. *Ann Emerg Med.* 1988;17:469–472.
8. Wayne MA, Friedland E. Prehospital use of succinylcholine: a 20-year review. *Prehosp Emerg Care* 1999;3:107–109.
9. Ochs M, Davis D, Hoyt D, et al. Paramedic-performed rapid sequence intubation of patients with severe head injuries. *Ann Emerg Med.* 2002;40:159–167.
10. Sloane C, Vilke GM, Chan TC, et al. Rapid sequence intubation in the field versus hospital in trauma patients. *J Emerg Med.* 2000;19:259–264.
11. Davis DP, Ochs M, Hoyt DB, et al. Paramedic-administered neuromuscular blockade improves prehospital intubation success in severely head-injured patients. *J Trauma* 2003;55:713–719.
12. Ma OJ, Atchley RB, Hatley T, et al. Intubation success rates improve for an air medical program after implementing the use of neuromuscular blocking agents. *Am J Emerg Med.* 1998;16:125–127.
13. Davis DP, Hoyt DB, Ochs M, et al. The effect of paramedic rapid sequence intubation on outcome in patients with severe traumatic brain injury. *J Trauma* 2003;54:444–453.
14. **Davis DP, Dunford JV, Poste JC, et al. The impact of hypoxia and hyperventilation on outcome after paramedic rapid sequence intubation of severely head-injured patients. *J Trauma* 2004; 57:1–10.**
15. Davis DP, Valentine C, Ochs M, et al. The Combitube as a salvage airway device for paramedic rapid sequence intubation. *Ann Emerg Med.* 2003;42:697–704.
16. Salvino CK, Dries D, Gamelli R, et al. Emergency cricothyroidotomy in trauma victims. *J Trauma* 1993;34:503–505.
17. Boyle MF, Hatton D, Sheets C. Surgical cricothyrotomy performed by air ambulance flight nurses: a 5-year experience. *J Emerg Med.* 1993;11: 41–45.
18. York D, Dudek L, Larson R, et al. A comparison study of chest tube thoracostomy: air medical crew and in-hospital trauma service. *Air Med J.* 1993;12:227–229.
19. Cayten CG, Murphy JG, Stahl WM. Basic life support versus advanced life support for injured patients with an injury severity score of 10 or more. *J Trauma* 1993; 35:460–467.
20. Mattox KL, Bickell W, Pepe PE, et al. Prospective MAST study in 911 patients. *J Trauma* 1989; 29:1104–1112.
21. Bickell WH, Wall MJ, Jr., Pepe PE, et al. Immediate versus delayed fluid resuscitation for hypotensive patients with penetrating torso injuries. *N Engl J Med.* 1994; 331:1105–1109.
22. Wade C, Grady J, Kramer G. Efficacy of hypertonic saline dextran (HSD) in patients with traumatic hypotension: meta-analysis of individual patient data. *Acta Anaesthesiol Scand Suppl.* 1997;110:77–79.
23. Wade CE, Grady JJ, Kramer GC. Efficacy of hypertonic saline dextran fluid resuscitation for patients with hypotension from penetrating trauma. *J Trauma* 2003; 54(5 suppl):S144–S148.
24. **Wade CE, Grady JJ, Kramer GC, et al. Individual patient cohort analysis of the efficacy of hypertonic saline/dextran in patients with traumatic brain injury and hypotension. *J Trauma* 1997;42(5 suppl):S61–S65.**
25. ***Advanced Trauma Life Support Course: Instructor Manual.* Chicago: American College of Surgeons Committee on Trauma; 2004.**
26. Boyd M, Vanek VW, Bourguet CC. Emergency room resuscitative thoracotomy: when is it indicated? *J Trauma* 1992;33:714–721.
27. Jurkovich GJ, Zingarelli W, Wallace J, et al. Penetrating neck trauma: diagnostic studies in the asymptomatic patient. *J Trauma* 1985;25: 819–822.
28. Miller FB, Cryer HM, Chilikuri S, et al. Negative findings on laparotomy for trauma. *South Med J.* 1989;82:1231–1234.
29. Nagy KK, Roberts RR, Joseph KT, et al. Experience with over 2500 diagnostic peritoneal lavages. *Injury* 2000;31:479–482.
30. **Rozycki GS, Ballard RB, Feliciano DV, et al. Surgeon-performed ultrasound for the assessment of truncal injuries: lessons learned from 1540 patients. *Ann Surg.* 1998;228:557–567.**
31. Evers BM, Cryer HM, Miller FB. Pelvic fracture hemorrhage. Priorities in management. *Arch Surg.* 1989;124:422–424.
32. Fabian TC, Croce MA, Stewart RM, et al. A prospective analysis of diagnostic laparoscopy in trauma. *Ann Surg.* 1993; 217:557–564.
33. Boyle EM, Jr., Maier RV, Salazar JD, et al. Diagnosis of injuries after stab wounds to the back and flank. *J Trauma* 1997;42:260–265.

CHAPTER 20 ■ SHOCK

JOSEPH CUSCHIERI

Shock, a condition first described by Walter B. Cannon, is caused by inadequate blood flow that results in cellular hypoxia. Persistence of cellular hypoxia results in cellular and organ dysfunction. This state can result from a variety of insults and was first classified by Blalock as hematogenic, neurogenic, cardiogenic, and vasogenic. Although each is important, hematogenic or hypovolemic shock is the most common type of shock in patients with polytrauma. Successful resuscitation of traumatic shock is most often achieved by obtaining adequate hemostasis.

PATHOPHYSIOLOGY

Due to a decrease in circulating intravascular volume, hemorrhage initiates both a rapid and a sustained compensatory response. Within minutes, a rapid compensatory response occurs, primarily because of adrenergic output. Sustained responses, in contrast, occur more slowly and result in intravascular fluid resorption and renal conservation of water and electrolytes (Algorithm 20.1).

Rapid Response

Hemorrhage results in secretion of epinephrine and norepinephrine from the adrenal gland as a result of decreased afferent impulses from arterial baroreceptors. Catecholamine release is limited to the first 24 hours following injury. Adrenergic-induced vasoconstriction of the systemic capacitance small veins and venules shifts blood back to the central venous circulation, thus increasing right-sided cardiac filling pressures. Concomitantly, selective vasoconstriction occurs in the skin, kidneys, and viscera, effectively shunting blood flow to the heart and brain. In addition to vasoconstriction and increased cardiac filling, adrenergic stimulation causes increased contractility and reflex tachycardia, all of which combine to increase stroke volume and cardiac output.

Adrenergic-mediated vasoconstriction affects arterioles, precapillary and postcapillary sphincters, and small veins and venules. Because of this specific pattern of vasoconstriction, there is a decrease in hydrostatic pressure distal to the precapillary sphincter that leads to resorption of interstitial fluid [water, Na^+, and Cl^-] into the vascular space. This resorption

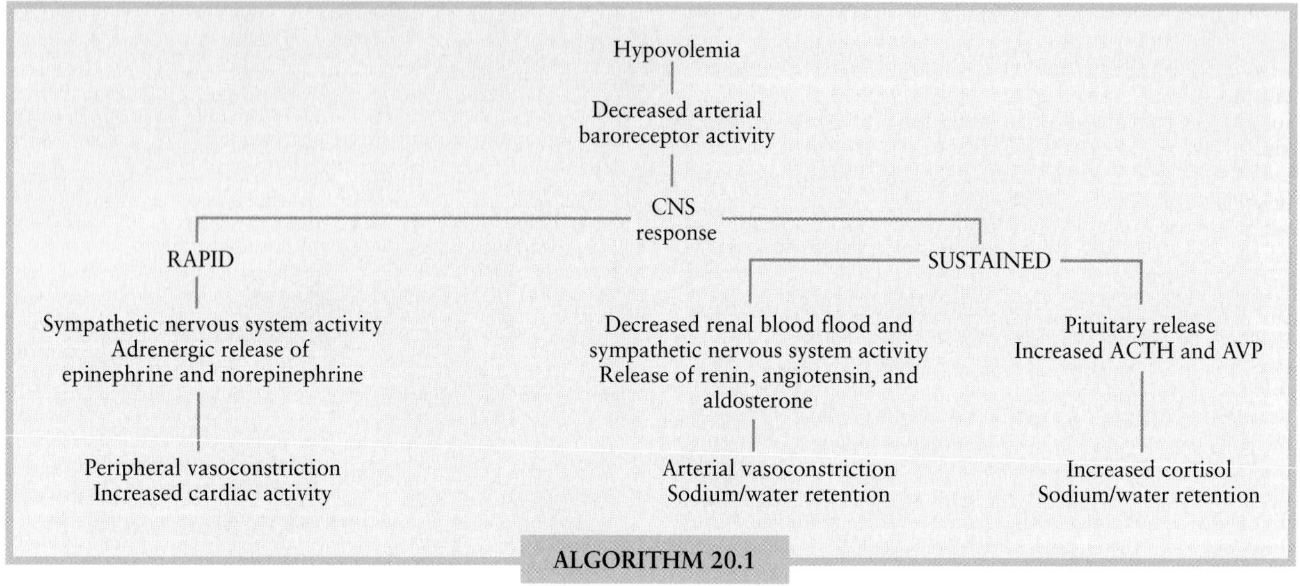

ALGORITHM 20.1 Neurohormonal response to hemorrhage. CNS, central nervous system; ACTH, adrenocorticotropic hormone; AVP, arginine vasopressin.

functions to restore circulating blood volume and is known as *transcapillary refill.*[1]

Sustained Response

Sustained compensatory responses include the release of vasoactive hormones and fluid shifts from the interstitium and the intracellular space to the intravascular compartment. Decreased renal blood flow, increased adrenergic activity and compositional changes in tubular fluid lead to the secretion of renin from the juxtaglomerular complex. Renin results in increased formation of angiotensin I. Circulating angiotensin I is rapidly converted to angiotensin II by the lungs and is the most potent known arterial and arteriolar vasoconstrictor. Angiotensin II also stimulates the release of pituitary adrenocorticotropic hormone (ACTH). Increased circulating levels of both angiotensin II and ACTH result in increased secretion of aldosterone. As a result, resorption of Na^+ in the distal renal tubules in exchange for potassium and hydrogen ions occurs.

Additionally, due to hypovolemia and increased serum osmolarity, reduced stimulation of arterial baroreceptors occurs, leading to the release of arginine vasopressin (AVP), also known as *antidiuretic hormone* (ADH). This hormone not only functions as a potent vasoconstrictor but also causes increased resorption of water by increasing water permeability and passive Na^+ transport in the distal renal tubule. The overall net effect of aldosterone and AVP is to decrease glomerular filtration and increase tubular reabsorption of salt and water in an effort to replace circulating intravascular volume deficits.

Finally, injury stimulates the release of the stress hormones (epinephrine, ACTH, cortisol, and glucagons), which leads to glycogenolysis, lypolysis, and protein catabolism causing a negative nitrogen balance and a high extracellular concentration of glucose due to both decreased insulin release and peripheral insulin resistance. This effect leads to increased glucose utilization by insulin-independent tissues such as the brain and heart. In addition, the hyperglycemia plus products of anaerobic metabolism from hypoperfused cells accumulate in the extracellular compartment, inducing hyperosmolarity. This extracellular hyperosmolarity draws water from the intracellular space, which in turn drives water, Na^+, and Cl^- across the capillary endothelium into the vascular space.

Loss of Compensation

If shock is prolonged, the arteriolar and precapillary sphincters become refractory and relax while the postcapillary sphincter remains in spasm. Therefore, the capillary hydrostatic pressure increases, and Na^+, Cl^-, and water move into the interstitium, leading to depletion of intravascular volume.

Cellular membrane function is also impaired in hemorrhagic shock. The normal, negative membrane potential approaches neutrality, leading to increased permeability and interstitial concentration of K^+. This is caused in part by a decrease in function of the adenosine triphosphate-dependent Na^+-K^+ membrane pump that is induced by cellular hypoxia. This loss of membrane potential leads to Na^+ influx and cellular swelling due to increased intracellular fluid.

In addition to these cellular effects, severe and prolonged hemorrhagic shock results in the development of multiple organ injury, including acute respiratory failure in the postinjury period. Direct injury to the alveolar-capillary interface occurs that results in leakage of proteinaceous fluid from the intravascular space into the interstitium and subsequently into alveolar spaces. This pulmonary injury is clinically referred to as acute respiratory distress syndrome (ARDS).[2,3]

EVALUATION OF SHOCK

Even the most inexperienced caregiver easily recognizes shock after the compensatory mechanisms are overcome. It is more difficult to recognize the patient in compensated shock, who presents with vital signs that are almost normal.

However, it is critical to the patient's ultimate outcome that recognition and treatment of shock occur before decompensation. The clinical assessment must be guided by the knowledge that the severity of the symptoms and signs of shock varies, both between patients and by the volume of blood lost. The patient is evaluated based on clinical appearance, hemodynamic measurements, and biochemical analysis.

The initial vasoconstriction causes the skin to be cool with poor capillary refill. Patients in shock hyperventilate to compensate for metabolic acidosis. As shock progresses, mental status changes occur; decreased cerebral blood flow and increased catecholamine stimulation of the reticular activating formation may lead to anxiety and restlessness. With increasing blood loss, lethargy may result. True coma, however, seldom results from blood loss alone and is most often a sign of concomitant direct brain injury or is coincident with terminal cardiovascular collapse.[4]

The hemodynamic assessment should include evaluation of the rate and character of the pulse, the blood pressure, and, in some cases, the central venous pressure (CVP) and pulmonary artery pressure. Tachycardia is a normal response to volume loss but also to pain, anxiety, and fear, all of which are commonly present. Assessment of the pulse (full and strong or weak and thready) may be helpful in determining the proper diagnosis. Because of the body's ability to compensate for hypovolemia, changes in blood pressure do not occur reliably until 20% to 30% of blood volume has been lost. The pulse pressure usually narrows in compensated shock because of the effects of vasoconstriction on the diastolic blood pressure. In patients with multisystem injuries or significant premorbid medical conditions, more invasive cardiovascular monitoring may be necessary. The CVP reflects the adequacy of the blood volume and the state of the venous tone. Changes in CVP in response to treatment or from continuing hemorrhage are more revealing than a solitary measurement.

An indirect but extremely valuable measure of perfusion and volume status is urine output. A urinary catheter should be inserted in every trauma patient evaluated for shock. Hourly urine output should be 0.5 to 1 mL/kg for adult patients, at least 1 mL/kg for most pediatric patients, and 1 to 2 mL/kg for patients younger than 2 years.

Biochemical analysis of shock is based on the shift from aerobic to anaerobic metabolism in underperfused tissues. Increased lactate production is associated with tissue hypoperfusion.[5] In addition lactate appears to be prognostic: lactate levels are higher in nonsurvivors compared with survivors, and the median lethal level for lactate in hemorrhagic shock is 7.3 mEq/L.[6,7] Resuscitation of hypovolemia results in a decrease in serum lactate levels, and the time required to normalize serum lactate levels appears to be an additional important prognostic factor for survival.[8,9]

Another biochemical marker of shock and resuscitation is the base deficit. This is defined as the amount of a fixed base (or acid) that must be added to an aliquot of blood to restore the pH to 7.40. Base deficit values have been categorized as normal (2 to −2), mild (−3 to −5), moderate (−6 to −9), and severe (<− 10).[10] Changes in the base deficit with volume infusion can be used to judge the efficacy of resuscitation.[11] Further, base deficit has been shown to be superior to pH values in assessing the normalization of acidosis after shock resuscitation, and the time required for normalization of base deficit has perhaps even greater prognostic significance than that for lactate.[12]

These biochemical changes associated with the hypoperfusion of shock occur even with compensation. Because of the potential difficulties in diagnosing compensated shock, an arterial blood gas analysis including base deficit should be obtained for every major trauma patient, and any patient with a base deficit of 6 mEq/L or more should be considered to be in shock until proved otherwise.

Although each of these factors can be used to characterize shock, no single measurement has been determined to be optimal for resuscitation guidance. Currently other measurements that demonstrate promise consist of central and mixed venous oxygen saturations and specific noninvasive end-organ oxygen saturation levels.[13,14] Each of these has demonstrated promise in other shock states and is currently being specifically studied during hemorrhagic shock.

CLASSIFICATION OF HEMORRHAGE

The signs and symptoms of shock vary with both the severity and duration of blood loss. The Advanced Trauma Life Support classification system of the American College of Surgeons is useful to comprehend the manifestations and physiologic changes associated with hemorrhagic shock in adults.[15] Blood volume is estimated at 7% of ideal body weight, or approximately 4,900 mL in a 70-kg patient. (Table 20.1)

TABLE 20.1 CLASSIFICATION

CLASSIFICATION OF SHOCK

	Class I	Class II	Class III	Class IV
Blood loss (mL)	Up to 750	750–1,500	1,500–2,000	>2,000
Blood loss (%)	Up to 15	15–30	30–40	40
Heart rate (bpm)	<100	>100	>120	>140
Blood pressure	Normal	Normal	Decreased	Decreased
Pulse pressure	Normal	Decreased	Decreased	Decreased
Respiratory rate (breath/min)	14–20	20–30	30–40	>35
Urine output (mL/hr)	>30	20–30	5–15	Minimal
Mental status	Normal	Mildly anxious	Anxious and confused	Confused and lethargic
Fluid replacement	Crystalloid	Crystalloid	Crystalloid and blood	Crystalloid and blood

TREATMENT OF HEMORRHAGIC SHOCK

Therapy of hemorrhagic shock requires control and arrest of hemorrhage as well as restitution of the circulating blood volume. Although the causes of traumatic shock may be multifactorial, hemorrhage remains the leading cause. Thus, a diligent search for the source of hemorrhage should occur simultaneously with the institution of volume infusion. Once a source is identified, rapid control should be obtained. Identification and pressure applied to external sources of hemorrhage, such as the scalp or extremity may hasten resuscitative efforts.

A minimum of two large-bore (14- to 16-gauge) intravenous (IV) catheters should be established in adults. Isotonic fluid is then infused at the same time as blood is obtained for arterial blood gas analysis, typing, and screening. Fluid can be infused up to 200 mL/min through a 14-gauge catheter and up to 220 mL/min through a 7-Fr catheter. A fluid challenge of 1 to 2 L is administered to the hypotensive patient and the response is assessed. This therapeutic challenge is an effective trial in determining the amount of preexisting or continuing blood loss. If the blood pressure returns to normal and is stabilized, the blood loss was relatively small, and the only treatment required may be the infusion of isotonic fluid.

If the increase in blood pressure is transient after fluid bolus, the hemorrhage was severe or ongoing. Additional crystalloid is administered, and the need for blood transfusion is assessed. Patients who continue to require large amounts of fluid and blood to support perfusion usually have ongoing hemorrhage and require invasive intervention. No response or a minimal response to apparently adequate infusions of crystalloid solution and blood indicates exsanguinating hemorrhage and the frequent need for urgent surgery.

Although controversy has developed over how much resuscitation should be attempted before definitive control of hemorrhage, animal studies have demonstrated increased blood loss and increased mortality rates after infusion of isotonic and hypertonic solutions in models of uncontrolled hemorrhage.[16] In a similar study, improved survival rates and decreased hemorrhage were achieved by infusion of only enough fluid to maintain a mean arterial pressure of 40 mm Hg (instead of 80 mm Hg).[17] It seems logical that restoration of normal blood volume would lead to increased hemorrhage if the sites of bleeding were not controlled. However, this approach to resuscitation in patients at high risk for ongoing hemorrhage, such as those with penetrating truncal trauma, remains controversial.[18]

The same clinical indicators used to evaluate shock are used to evaluate the patient's response to resuscitative efforts. The commonly considered end points of resuscitation include blood pressure, heart rate, urine output, and CVP. The same compensatory mechanisms that can allow shock to go unrecognized, however, also can lead to underresuscitation. Therefore, none of these end points alone can serve to guide resuscitation, whereas the combination of these parameters is more useful. In addition, metabolic parameters should be used to assess resuscitation. With adequate restoration of volume, metabolic acidosis should resolve and the base deficit and serum lactate level should normalize. Persistent acidosis despite an apparently adequate volume of resuscitation necessitates a diligent search for ongoing hemorrhage or other evidence of inadequate resuscitation.[11]

Monitoring technology for cellular perfusion is currently under development. Because blood flow is not uniformly distributed to all tissue beds, assessment of regional blood flow may indicate tissue beds with hypoperfusion even when the more global indices (base deficit, lactate) are normalizing. Measurement of tissue oxygen tension has significant appeal as an end point of resuscitation. The measurement of tissue oxygen tension during inspired oxygen challenges is both sensitive and specific in determining flow-dependent oxygen consumption.[19] Although this technology has significant potential, the confounding variables of vasoconstriction from hypothermia and catecholamine release have not been resolved. Another approach to assessment of regional perfusion is the measurement of mitochondrial cytochrome a,a_3 redox shifts using near-infrared spectroscopy. Early investigational efforts suggest that this technique may be useful in identifying regional hypoperfusion.[20] However, the use of this technology as an end point for early resuscitation requires further investigation.

Because the splanchnic circulation is one of the first to be compromised and one of the last to be restored, assessing gut perfusion, and specifically gastric mucosal perfusion, has been suggested as an appropriate and accessible regional circulatory bed to be monitored. Low gastric mucosal pH (pH <7.32) has been associated with increased organ failure and a higher mortality rate.[21] Unfortunately, this technology has not proved to be reliable in the acute resuscitation of the injured patient.

RESUSCITATIVE FLUIDS

Crystalloids

Balanced salt solutions are the most commonly used resuscitative fluids, and their use to restore extracellular volume significantly decreases the transfusion requirement after hemorrhagic shock. Lactated Ringer's solution is isotonic, readily available, and inexpensive. It also rapidly replaces the depleted interstitial fluid compartment and does not aggravate any preexisting electrolyte abnormalities. Administration of lactated Ringer's solution does not lead to aggravation of the lactic acidosis that is present in shock.[8] In fact, animal models have demonstrated that the use of blood plus lactated Ringer's solution results in a more rapid return to normal lactate and pH than does shed blood alone. As volume and perfusion are restored, lactate is metabolized to bicarbonate in the liver. Mild metabolic alkalosis may even occur 1 or 2 days after large-volume resuscitations with lactated Ringer's. Normal saline solution is also effective for resuscitation of hypovolemic patients. However, concerns exist about inducing hypernatremic, hyperchloremic metabolic acidosis with massive resuscitation volumes.

Recently several investigations have raised concerns about the proinflammatory effects of resuscitation with lactated Ringer's solution. Some commercially available lactated Ringer's solution contains racemic lactate that is made of equal concentrations of D(−)- and L(+)-isomers of lactate. The D(−)-isomer has been demonstrated *in vitro* to result in enhanced production of reactive oxygen species by neutrophils and inflammatory gene expression by leukocytes.[22,23] In addition, increased apoptosis in both the small intestine and the liver was seen after resuscitation from hemorrhage with lactated Ringer's solution, but not with hypertonic solutions or blood resuscitation.[24] These findings, however, are not consistent and do not appear dissimilar from those for saline resuscitation in other animal models.[25] Thus, further investigations are required to determine the overall inflammatory effect of crystalloid resuscitation.

Colloids

Colloids have the theoretic advantages of increasing the intravascular colloid oncotic pressure and requiring smaller volumes for resuscitation than crystalloids.[26] Colloids commonly used for volume expansion in hypovolemia include albumin, dextran 70, dextran 40, and hydroxyethyl starch. Although each has unique individual characteristics, currently there is little justification for the routine addition of colloids to balanced salt solutions for volume replacement during hemorrhagic shock.

Albumin solutions have been used during resuscitation to increase colloid oncotic pressure and, hypothetically, to protect the lung from interstitial edema; however, there is a relatively rapid flux of albumin across the pulmonary capillary membranes and relatively rapid clearance through the pulmonary lymphatic system. In fact, colloid albumin infusion has been demonstrated to prolong the resuscitation phase and delay postresuscitation diuresis. Additionally, albumin may serve to depress circulating immunoglobulin level, and suppress albumin synthesis.

Dextran 40 and dextran 70 are polysaccharides with molecular weights of 40 and 70 kD, respectively. Dextran 40 (10%) is hyperoncotic and initially exerts a volume-expanding effect. However, because of its lower molecular weight, it is more rapidly excreted. Thus, dextran 40 is most commonly used in cases of peripheral vascular disease and hyperviscosity syndromes. Dextran 70, conversely, is provided as a 6% solution and does not exert a hyperoncotic effect. The volume expansion is somewhat greater than the amount infused, and because of its large molecular size the effect is maintained for up to 48 hours. The dextran preparations, however, cause decreased platelet adhesiveness and decreased factor VIII activity. They also carry an incidence of allergic reaction of up to 5% and anaphylaxis of 0.6%.[26]

Hydroxyethyl starch is an amylopectin with volume-expanding effects for approximately 36 hours. It has side effects similar to those of dextran, but with less frequency. The incidence of anaphylaxis is 0.006%. A new hydroxyethyl starch, pentastarch, has a lower molecular weight and fewer hydroxyethyl groups than hydroxyethyl starch. Pentastarch has a shorter duration of action (2.5 hours) and has been reported to have even fewer side effects.[27, 28]

The controversy regarding use of crystalloids versus colloids in resuscitation has not been resolved. Both types of solutions can restore circulating volume. The effects of the solutions on pulmonary function are a primary issue and are summarized as follows: (a) the use of crystalloid solutions decreases plasma oncotic pressure, thereby leading to lung edema at lower microvascular pressures; and (b) colloids given in the face of pulmonary injury can extravasate, promoting edema because of the reduced plasma interstitial oncotic gradient. In fact, a previous meta-analysis of colloid versus crystalloid resuscitation after hemorrhagic shock demonstrated a higher mortality rate among the colloid-resuscitated patients, partly because of pulmonary complications.[29] Therefore, because colloid infusion has not demonstrated a significant benefit over crystalloid resuscitation alone, it is not currently recommended in the management of hypovolemic shock.

Blood

Most patients with class I or II hemorrhage can be resuscitated with balanced salt solutions alone. Patients who lose more than 25% to 30% of their total blood volume need blood for resuscitation. The decision about the extent of blood cross-matching prior to transfusion is determined in part by the urgency of the situation. Blood that has been fully typed and cross-matched carries the least risk of transfusion reactions, but it also takes the most time to obtain. Other transfusion options include the use of type O or type-specific blood. (Table 20.2)

Type O Blood

Type O (universal donor) blood is immediately available without a cross-match. Because type O blood contains no AB cellular antigens, administration of packed red blood cells (RBCs) is relatively safe for patients of any blood type. Males should be transfused type O Rh-positive blood, while prepubescent females and females of childbearing age should be given type O Rh-negative blood to avoid sensitization that would complicate future pregnancies. The administration of more than four units of type O blood to a non–O blood type patient, however, theoretically can result in an admixture of blood type. A pretransfusion blood specimen should be sent to the blood bank when the patient is admitted, and type-specific blood should be transfused as soon as it is available.

Type-Specific Blood

Type-specific blood is available from most blood banks within 5 to 10 minutes of receipt of the blood specimen, while the patient is being resuscitated with balanced salt solutions. Although not fully cross-matched, this blood can be administered relatively safely, as demonstrated in both military and civilian experiences.[30]

Autotransfusion

Autotransfusion involves collection of the shed blood and its reinfusion through a filter back into the patient. Autotransfusion can be as simple as aspiration of the blood into a citrate-containing collection chamber, followed by reinfusion through a 40-mm filter. A more elaborate system, the Haemonetics autotransfuser (Haemonetics Corp., Braintree, MA) centrifuges the collected blood and delivers washed, packed RBCs for reinfusion. The advantages of

TABLE 20.2

COMPARISON OF BLOOD AVAILABILITY

Blood	Typing	Antibody Screen	Cross-match	Time
Type O	No	No	No	Immediate
Type specific	Yes	No	No	<10 min
Type and screen	Yes	Yes	Yes	20–30 min
Type and cross-match	Yes	Yes	Yes	45–60 min

TRAUMA

autotransfusion include transfusion with warm, compatible blood without delays and with no risk of transmission of hepatitis, human immunodeficiency virus, or other blood-borne pathogens.

Autotransfused blood can produce disseminated intravascular coagulation and activation of fibrinolysis. In addition, collection of blood from the peritoneal cavity after hollow viscus injury, even with cell washing, can lead to bacterial contamination of the autotransfused blood.[31] Successful autotransfusion of contaminated blood has been demonstrated, but blood obtained from enteric-contaminated cavities probably should not be used, except perhaps in extreme circumstances.[32] Despite the potential benefits, investigators have found that the autotransfuser was used in only 26% of the trauma patients for whom it was prepared.[33] Although autotransfusion is cost saving, currently no evidence exists to show that it improves outcome compared to exclusive homologous blood transfusions in trauma patients.

SPECIAL SITUATIONS

Pregnancy

Several hemodynamic changes are associated with pregnancy, which include increased blood volume, decreased hematocrit, increased cardiac output, increased heart rate, and decreased peripheral vascular resistance. Because of these changes, especially the increase in blood volume, pregnant patients may lose a significant amount of blood before signs of hypovolemia and shock develop. However, because placental blood flow is shunted early during shock, the fetus may be in shock while the mother maintains adequate perfusion. Because of these changes and concerns, early aggressive fluid resuscitation is indicated in pregnant patients. Additionally, the pregnant patient should be maintained on her left side to relive pressure of the uterus on the inferior vena cava, thus minimizing compromise of venous return to the heart. Most important, restoration of adequate blood volume to the mother will result in restoration of adequate placental blood flow to the fetus.

Geriatric Patients

The number of geriatric patients suffering severe trauma is increasing.[34] Although the fundamentals of resuscitation are similar between the elderly and young, significant comorbid conditions may be present in elderly patients, and several prescription and over-the counter medications, such as beta-blockers, may be used, making theassessment and monitoring of the elderly more challenging. Early use of invasive monitoring, such as a CVP or pulmonary artery catheter, may be a useful adjunct to gauge fluid resuscitation.

Spinal Cord Injuries

Although spinal cord injury may be associated with neurogenic shock, hemorrhage remains the most common cause of shock. Thus, the search for associated injuries must be performed. Once hemorrhage has been controlled or ruled out, continued hemodynamic instability may then be attributed to neurogenic shock.

Head Injuries

Head injuries remain the leading cause of death and disability in the injured patient. Morbidity and mortality are worsened as a result of secondary brain injury. Secondary brain injury occurs as a result of episodes of hypotension and hypoxemia. Thus, the primary goal of resuscitation is to minimize secondary brain injury secondary to hypotension by using aggressive fluid resuscitation and pharmacologic support directed at maintaining adequate cerebral blood flow. Restoration of cerebral blood flow should be obtained without the use of hypotonic or glucose-containing solutions to minimize the risk of progressive brain edema.[35–37]

EXPERIMENTAL RESUSCITATION FLUIDS

Hypertonic Saline

Hypertonic saline solutions have been used in resuscitation of patients after burn shock, elective vascular surgery, and trauma. Hypertonic fluid resuscitation expands intravascular volume both from the fluid infused and from an osmotically induced shift of intracellular fluid into the intravascular compartment. In addition to expanding volume, hypertonic saline solutions have been shown to increase left ventricular performance, decrease peripheral resistance from arteriolar dilatation, and redistribute cardiac output to the kidneys and viscera.[38–40]

The optimal osmolarity of hypertonic saline solutions for resuscitation from hypovolemia has not been determined. Investigations with 2,400-mOsm saline solutions administered in boluses of 4 mL/kg have shown that this concentration rapidly restores blood pressure to baseline levels after hemorrhagic loss of 40% to 50% of blood volume.[41] However, the response to bolus administration was not sustained. The addition of colloid to the hypertonic saline solution led to sustained increases in arterial pressure, cardiac output, and measured plasma volumes, with the colloid acting to hold the water drawn into the intravascular space by the hypertonic saline. Other reports have described more effective volume replacement with smaller-volume infusions of 500-mOsm solutions than with lactated Ringer's solution, and suggest a mortality advantage in head-injured patients.[42–44] In contrast, studies of hypertonic saline resuscitation in models of uncontrolled hemorrhage have demonstrated increased hemorrhage and increased mortality rates after administration of hypertonic saline solutions compared with resuscitation with normal saline solution.[45] The increased hemorrhage is thought to be caused in part by the peripheral vasodilatation produced by administration of hypertonic saline solutions.

Hypertonic solutions have also been demonstrated to modulate innate immune responses. Among hypertonic saline immunomodulatory effects is a decrease in leukocyte adherence and neutrophil and macrophage activation.[25,46] Although these effects may not be important during immediate resuscitation, they may serve to limit the amount of subsequent organ dysfunction post injury, in particular the development of ARDS. Further studies are required to determine the optimal use of hypertonic solutions for the treatment of hemorrhagic shock.

Blood Substitutes

Readily available oxygen-carrying solutions have tremendous potential for trauma patient resuscitation. The "ideal blood substitute" would be nonantigenic and free of transmissible disease and would have normal or near-normal oxygen-carrying capacity. Efforts to produce this ideal solution have included perfluorocarbon preparations and stroma-free hemoglobins from human, bovine, and recombinant sources.

Perfluorocarbons

Perfluorocarbon preparations were stabilized with emulsifiers and added to solutions of hetastarch and balanced salt solutions as one of the first clinically used blood substitutes. These compounds did improve oxygen delivery and restore volume but had significant side effects, including depression of platelet counts, fibrinogen levels, and the immune system.[47-49] These compounds have been withdrawn from clinical use.

Stroma-Free Hemoglobin

After removal from an erythrocyte, hemoglobin retains its oxygen-carrying capacity. Hemoglobin solutions prepared from lysis of RBCs have been shown to be effective oxygen-carrying resuscitative fluids in animal models.[50] The side effects from the use of hemolyzed blood (e.g., renal dysfunction, coagulopathy) are caused by stromal elements of the erythrocyte. Removal of these stromal elements by lysis decreases the incidence of such problems. However, isolated preparations of stroma-free hemoglobin as a blood substitute have a short half-life and a marked affinity for the oxygen molecule, becoming half-saturated at a PO_2 of 14 mm Hg instead of the normal 27 mm Hg.[30]

Efforts to produce clinically useful stroma-free hemoglobin have included diaspirin cross-linking of the hemoglobin tetramer, glutaraldehyde or pyridoxylated polymerization of human and bovine hemoglobins, and recombinantly cross-linked hemoglobin. Unfortunately, diaspirin cross-linked hemoglobin results in excessive increases in blood pressure, pulmonary hypertension, and increased mortality.[51–53]

Polymerized, pyridoxylated, stroma-free hemoglobin (PolyHeme; Northfield, Evanston, IL) is a different formulation. This substance has been shown to have essentially the same oxygen-carrying capacity and P_{50} as whole blood.[54,55] Clinical phase I and II studies with this substance have demonstrated safety and efficacy in restoration of blood volume and oxygen-carrying capacity in severely injured hypovolemic patients. There have been no adverse consequences from this blood substitute with infusion of volumes up to the equivalent of 10 units of blood.[51,56]

COMPLICATIONS OF SHOCK

Hemorrhagic shock can lead to a cascade of related complications, each requiring its own intervention if the clinician is to achieve the goal of resuscitating the patient from the shock state. The most commonly encountered of these complications are metabolic acidosis, hypothermia, and coagulopathy. Other complications of shock and resuscitation include ischemia—reperfusion, multiorgan system dysfunction or failure, ARDS, and intraabdominal hypertension.

Metabolic Acidosis

The acidosis of hemorrhagic shock results from tissue hypoperfusion, anaerobic metabolism, and lactate accumulation. The treatment for acidosis from shock is restoration of adequate tissue perfusion. Acidosis can lead to cardiac compromise and some therapeutic drugs (e.g., lidocaine) are inactive if pH is less than 7.2. Although severe acidosis can be treated with judicious administration of bicarbonate with frequent monitoring of the pH, extreme caution must be exercised not to overadminister bicarbonate. Overadministration of bicarbonate leads to shifts to the left in the oxyhemoglobin dissociation curve, resulting in greater oxygen affinity for the hemoglobin molecule and less oxygen release into the tissues. Therefore, the best means to treat metabolic acidosis is through restoration of circulating blood volume.

Hypothermia

Hypothermia (core temperature <35°C) is common after severe injury. Heat loss is increased in the trauma patient because of immobilization and both prehospital and postadmission exposure, leading to conductive, convective, and evaporative heat loss, which should all be minimized. In addition, the administration of room-temperature IV fluids and of cold stored blood also contributes to hypothermia.[57] Hypothermia increases fluid requirements and independently increases acute mortality rates after major trauma.[58]

As the core temperature decreases, the rate of oxygen consumption also decreases, to approximately 50% of normal at 28°C. The decrease in oxygen consumption is accompanied by increased production of acid metabolites. A leftward shift in the oxyhemoglobin dissociation curve also occurs with hypothermia but is partially compensated by the acidosis. Central nervous system effects progress from confusion and loss of manual dexterity to obtundation and frank coma as the core temperature decreases from 35° to 26.5°C. The heart rate decreases to approximately half of baseline at 28°C, with a concomitant decrease in cardiac output. All cardiac electrical conduction intervals are prolonged, consistent with the changes in heart rate, and both atrioventricular dissociation and refractory ventricular fibrillation can occur below 28°C. Other physiologic effects include ileus and pancreatitis (from cold enzyme activation) at temperatures lower than 35°C.

Compensatory responses to hypothermia include increased excretion of catecholamines, resulting in doubling of the basal metabolic rate, and increased production of thyroid hormones, further increasing the basal metabolic rate to five times baseline. Shivering can increase heat production as well, but it represents significant energy expenditure and has been shown to be inhibited during episodes of hypotension or hypoxemia.[59] Compensatory responses to hypothermia are lost at temperatures below 30° or 31°C, and a state of complete poikilothermy is reached.

The treatment for hypothermia is rewarming. The core temperature should be obtained on admission of the trauma patient. Patients whose core temperatures are 33° to 35°C can be treated with passive external rewarming, warm blankets, and hot packs. Patients with core temperatures lower than 33°C require active rewarming. If the patient is unconscious, airway control should first be obtained. Because severe hypothermia causes vasoconstriction, noninvasive blood pressure measurements may not be feasible or accurate, and an arterial line should be placed for monitoring and blood gas sampling. The inspired gas through the ventilator should be heated to 41°C and fully saturated with water vapor to increase heat conductance in the lung. All IV fluids should be warmed. Commercially available rapid infusion systems with heating elements should be used. For extreme hypothermia, either continuous mechanical cardiac bypass or cardiac-driven arteriovenous countercurrent rewarming can be used for rewarming and, if necessary, circulatory support. Finally, other warming methods include lavage of heated saline through nasogastric and thoracostomy tubes as well as peritoneal lavage, but they are not as effective.

Coagulopathy

Coagulopathy is a frequent problem in the trauma patient who has received large volumes of crystalloid solution and blood for resuscitation. Although this problem is incompletely understood, it is clear that posttraumatic coagulation defects are multifactorial. The presence of shock, the fluid volume required for resuscitation, massive injury-induced consumption of coagulation components, the presence of hypothermia, and preexisting diseases (e.g., cirrhosis) all influence the likelihood and severity of coagulopathy.[60]

The major factor in coagulopathy has been postulated to be the dilutional thrombocytopenia that occurs after massive volume resuscitation. Although bleeding times can be prolonged with platelet counts of less than 100,000 cells/mL, platelet counts of 50,000 cells/mL or greater are usually adequate for surgical hemostasis. Dilutional thrombocytopenia becomes more likely with infusions of more than one blood volume. Each unit of platelets administered increases the platelet count by 10,000 to 15,000 cells/mL. Control of surgically remediable hemorrhage is preferable, if possible, before platelet transfusion to prevent the loss of the transfused platelets.

Dilution of other coagulation factors also plays a role in development of coagulopathy. Factors V and VIII are the most labile in banked blood, but levels of less than 10% of normal also occur for factors VII, X, XI, XII and XIII and are associated with abnormalities in hemostasis, as demonstrated by prolonged partial thromboplastin time and prothrombin time. Fresh frozen plasma can be administered as a source of all the soluble coagulation factors. The administration of cryoprecipitate may be necessary as a concentrated source of factor VIII and fibrinogen, particularly if adequate hemostasis is not obtained with the use of fresh frozen plasma. In addition, recent support has emerged for the use of recombinant activated factor VIIa. Although developed initially for the use in hemophiliac patients who developed inhibitors to factor VIII, anecdotal evidence has suggested that rFVIIa may serve to quickly reverse hemorrhage-induced coagulopathy if other coagulation components are replaced first and hypothermia or acidosis is not severe.[61] However, no definitive data currently exist on which patients may benefit, and, therefore, further studies are required before its routine use can be advocated.

KEY POINTS

- **Shock describes a clinical syndrome of inadequate tissue perfusion and cellular oxygenation that leads to cellular and organ dysfunction and, ultimately, failure.**
- **Hemorrhagic shock (hypovolemia) produces both acute (adrenergic) and sustained hormonal (renin/angiotensin, aldosterone, antidiuretic hormone, cortisol and glucagon) responses to compensate and restore intravascular volume.**
- **Each level of shock produces a characteristic pattern of physiologic responses, and recognition of early shock, prior to decompensation, is critical to prevent morbidity and improve survival.**
- **Resuscitation requires, at a minimum, crystalloid (preferable) or colloid infusion and, with greater degrees of blood loss, blood transfusion. The extent of blood cross-matching prior to transfusion is dictated by the severity of the shock.**
- **Small-volume hypertonic saline and cross-linked stroma-free hemoglobin may improve resuscitation and outcomes following shock.**
- **The "bloody triad" induced by massive blood loss and transfusion is acidosis, hypothermia, and coagulopathy. Each must be aggressively treated and, preferably, prevented.**

References

1. Gann DS, Carlson DE, Byrnes GJ, et al. Impaired restitution of blood volume after large hemorrhage. *J Trauma* 1981;21(8):598–603.
2. Sladen A. Shock lung syndrome. *Compr Ther.* 1981;7(9):14–24.
3. Rodman GH, Jr., Kirby RR. Post-traumatic respiratory failure: role of fluid therapy. *Contemp Anesth Pract.* 1983;6:119–135.
4. Whittington LK, Roscelli JD, Parry WH. Hemorrhagic shock and encephalopathy: further description of a new syndrome. *J Pediatr.* 1985;106(4):599–602.
5. Huckabee WE. Relationships of pyruvate and lactate during anaerobic metabolism. III. Effect of breathing low-oxygen gases. *J Clin Invest.* 1958;37(2):264–271.
6. Broder G, Weil MH. Excess Lactate: An index of reversibility of shock in human patients. *Science* 1964;143:1457–1459.
7. Vitek V, Cowley RA. Blood lactate in the prognosis of various forms of shock. *Ann Surg.* 1971;173(2):308–313.
8. Canizaro PC, Prager MD, Shires GT. The infusion of Ringer's lactate solution during shock. Changes in lactate, excess lactate, and pH. *Am J Surg.* 1971;122(4):494–501.
9. Abramson D, Scalea TM, Hitchcock R, et al. Lactate clearance and survival following injury. *J Trauma.* 1993;35(4):584–589.
10. Davis JW, Parks SN, Kaups KL, et al. Admission base deficit predicts transfusion requirements and risk of complications. *J Trauma* 1996;41(5):769–774.
11. Davis JW, Shackford SR, Mackersie RC, et al. Base deficit as a guide to volume resuscitation. *J Trauma* 1988;28(10):1464–1467.
12. **Davis JW, Kaups KL, Parks SN. Base deficit is superior to pH in evaluating clearance of acidosis after traumatic shock. *J Trauma* 1998;44(1):114–118.**
13. Rivers E, Nguyen B, Havstad S, et al. Early goal-directed therapy in the treatment of severe sepsis and septic shock. *N Engl J Med.* 2001;345(19):1368–1377.
14. Crookes BA, Cohn SM, Burton EA, et al. Noninvasive muscle oxygenation to guide fluid resuscitation after traumatic shock. *Surgery* 2004;135(6):662–670.
15. American College of Surgeons Committee on Trauma. Advanced trauma life support for doctors. *Shock* 2004;69–85.
16. Krausz MM, Bar-Ziv M, Rabinovici R, et al. "Scoop and run" or stabilize hemorrhagic shock with normal saline or small-volume hypertonic saline? *J Trauma* 1992;33(1):6–10.
17. Kowalenko T, Stern S, Dronen S, et al. Improved outcome with hypotensive resuscitation of uncontrolled hemorrhagic shock in a swine model. *J Trauma* 1992;33(3):349–353,361–362.
18. Bickell WH, Wall MJ, Jr., Pepe PE, et al. Immediate versus delayed fluid resuscitation for hypotensive patients with penetrating torso injuries. *N Engl J Med.* 1994;331(17):1105–1109.
19. Waxman K, Annas C, Daughters K, et al. A method to determine the adequacy of resuscitation using tissue oxygen monitoring. *J Trauma* 1994;36(6):852–858.
20. Rhee P, Langdale L, Mock C, et al. Near-infrared spectroscopy: continuous measurement of cytochrome oxidation during hemorrhagic shock. *Crit Care Med.* 1997;25(1):166–170.
21. Chang MC, Cheatham ML, Nelson LD, et al. Gastric tonometry supplements information provided by systemic indicators of oxygen transport. *J Trauma* 1994;37(3):488–494.
22. **Alam HB, Stanton K, Koustova E, et al. Effect of different resuscitation strategies on neutrophil activation in a swine model of hemorrhagic shock. *Resuscitation* 2004;60(1):91–99.**
23. Koustova E, Stanton K, Gushchin V, et al. Effects of lactated Ringer's solutions on human leukocytes. *J Trauma.* 2002;52(5):872–878.
24. Deb S, Martin B, Sun L, et al. Resuscitation with lactated Ringer's solution in rats with hemorrhagic shock induces immediate apoptosis. *J Trauma* 1999;46(4):582–589.
25. Corso CO, Okamoto S, Ruttinger D, et al. Hypertonic saline dextran attenuates leukocyte accumulation in the liver after hemorrhagic shock and resuscitation. *J Trauma* 1999;46(3):417–423.
26. Ross AD, Angaran DM. Colloids vs. crystalloids—a continuing controversy. *Drug Intell Clin Pharm.* 1984;18(3):202–212.
27. Waxman K, Holness R, Tominaga G, et al. Hemodynamic and oxygen transport effects of pentastarch in burn resuscitation. Ann Surg. 1989;209(3):341–345.
28. London MJ, Ho JS, Triedman JK, et al. A randomized clinical trial of 10% pentastarch (low molecular weight hydroxyethyl starch) versus 5% albumin for plasma volume expansion after cardiac operations. *J Thorac Cardiovasc Surg.* 1989;97(5):785–797.
29. **Velanovich V. Crystalloid versus colloid fluid resuscitation: a meta-analysis of mortality. *Surgery* 1989;105(1):65–71.**

30. Gervin AS, Fischer RP. Resuscitation of trauma patients with type-specific uncrossmatched blood. *J Trauma* 1984;24(4):327–331.
31. Boudreaux JP, Bornside GH, Cohn I Jr. Emergency autotransfusion: partial cleansing of bacteria-laden blood by cell washing. *J Trauma* 1983;23(1): 31–35.
32. Glover JL, Smith R, Yaw PB, et al. Autotransfusion of blood contaminated by intestinal contents. *JACEP*. 1978;7(4):142–144.
33. Jurkovich GJ, Moore EE, Medina G. Autotransfusion in trauma. A pragmatic analysis. *Am J Surg*. 1984;148(6):782–785.
34. Medical expenditures attributable to injuries—United States, 2000. *MMWR Morb Mortal Wkly Rep*. 2004;53(1):1–4.
35. Gurevich B, Talmor D, Artru AA, et al. Brain edema, hemorrhagic necrosis volume, and neurological status with rapid infusion of 0.45% saline or 5% dextrose in 0.9% saline after closed head trauma in rats. *Anesth Analg*. 1997;84(3):554–559.
36. Hovda DA, Becker DP, Katayama Y. Secondary injury and acidosis. *J Neurotrauma*. 1992;9 suppl 1:S47–S60.
37. Trost HA, Gaab MR. Plasma osmolality, osmoregulation and prognosis after head injury. *Acta Neurochir (Wien)*. 1992;116(1):33–37.
38. Wildenthal K, Mierzwiak DS, Mitchell JH. Acute effects of increased serum osmolality on left ventricular performance. *Am J Physiol*. 1969;216(4): 898–904.
39. de Barros LF, Baena RC, Velasco IT, et al. Early hemodynamic effects of the rapid infusion of sodium chloride Dextran-70 hypertonic solution as treatment for hemorrhagic shock in dogs [in Portuguese]. *Arq Bras Cardiol*. 1993;61(4):217–220.
40. Rocha-e-Silva M, Negraes GA, Soares AM, et al. Hypertonic resuscitation from severe hemorrhagic shock: patterns of regional circulation. *Circ Shock* 1986;19(2):165–175.
41. Smith GJ, Kramer GC, Perron P, et al. A comparison of several hypertonic solutions for resuscitation of bled sheep. *J Surg Res*. 1985;39(6):517–528.
42. Shackford SR, Fortlage DA, Peters RM, et al. Serum osmolar and electrolyte changes associated with large infusions of hypertonic sodium lactate for intravascular volume expansion of patients undergoing aortic reconstruction. *Surg Gynecol Obstet*. 1987;164(2):127–136.
43. Vassar MJ, Perry CA, Gannaway WL, et al. 7.5% sodium chloride/dextran for resuscitation of trauma patients undergoing helicopter transport. *Arch Surg*. 1991;126(9):1065–1072.
44. **Vassar MJ, Fischer RP, O'Brien PE, et al. A multicenter trial for resuscitation of injured patients with 7.5% sodium chloride. The effect of added dextran 70. The Multicenter Group for the Study of Hypertonic Saline in Trauma Patients. *Arch Surg*. 1993;128(9):1003–1011.**
45. Gross D, Landau EH, Klin B, et al. Quantitative measurement of bleeding following hypertonic saline therapy in 'uncontrolled' hemorrhagic shock. *J Trauma* 1989;29(1):79–83.
46. Cuschieri J, Gourlay D, Garcia I, et al. Hypertonic preconditioning inhibits macrophage responsiveness to endotoxin. *J Immunol*. 2002;168(3): 1389–1396.
47. Tremper KK, Friedman AE, Levine EM, et al. The preoperative treatment of severely anemic patients with a perfluorochemical oxygen-transport fluid, Fluosol-DA. *N Engl J Med*. 1982; 307:277–283.
48. Elliott LA, Ledgerwood AM, Lucas CE, et al. Role of Fluosol-DA 20% in prehospital resuscitation. *Crit Care Med*. 1989;17:166–172.
49. McCoy LE, Elliott LA, Lucas CE, et al. Regenerative responses to exchange perfusion. *Biomater Artif Cells Artif Organs* 1988;16(1–3): 575–583.
50. Greenburg AG, Hayashi R, Siefert I, et al. Intravascular persistence and oxygen delivery of pyridoxalated, stroma-free hemoglobin during gradations of hypotension. *Surgery*. 1979;86(1):13–16.
51. Cohn SM. Is blood obsolete? *J Trauma* 1997;42(4):730–732.
52. Cohn SM. Alternatives to blood in the 21st century. *Crit Care* 2004; 8 suppl 2:S15–S17.
53. Cohn SM. Oxygen therapeutics in trauma and surgery. *J Trauma* 2003; 54 (suppl):S193–S198.
54. Gould SA, Moss GS. Clinical development of human polymerized hemoglobin as a blood substitute. *World J Surg*. 1996; 20(9):1200–1207.
55. **Gould SA, Moore EE, Hoyt DB, et al. The first randomized trial of human polymerized hemoglobin as a blood substitute in acute trauma and emergent surgery. *J Am Coll Surg*. 1998; 187:113–122.**
56. Johnson JL, Moore EE, Offner PJ, et al. Resuscitation of the injured patient with polymerized stroma-free hemoglobin does not produce systemic or pulmonary hypertension. *Am J Surg*. 1998;176(6):612–617.
57. **Gentilello LM. Advances in the management of hypothermia. *Surg Clin North Am*. 1995;75(2):243–256.**
58. Gentilello LM, Jurkovich GJ, Stark MS, et al. Is hypothermia in the victim of major trauma protective or harmful? A randomized, prospective study. *Ann Surg*. 1997;226(4):439–449.
59. Stoner HB. Studies on the mechanism of shock. The impairment of thermoregulation by trauma. *Br J Exp Pathol*. 1969;50(2):125–138.
60. **Gubler KD, Gentilello LM, Hassantash SA, et al. The impact of hypothermia on dilutional coagulopathy. *J Trauma* 1994;36(6):847–851.**
61. Dutton RP, McCunn M, Hyder M, et al. Factor VIIa for Correction of Traumatic Coagulopathy. *J Trauma* 2004;57(4):709–719.

Definitive Care Phase

CHAPTER 21 ■ HEAD TRAUMA

RANDALL M. CHESNUT

EPIDEMIOLOGY

In trauma, other than gunshot wounds, brain injury is the most common cause of death, accounting for about half of deaths at the injury site. The injuries are generally blunt, occurring most frequently in motor vehicle crashes (MVCs). Of particular significance are motorcycle crashes involving unhelmeted passengers, which produce severe injuries.

As many as two thirds of all MVC victims sustain some head injury. Complications from closed head injuries are the single largest cause of morbidity and mortality in patients who reach the hospital alive. Of patients who require long-term rehabilitation, head trauma is usually the primary injury.

These data are generally applicable to children as well. Although the mechanisms vary, head injuries are the major cause of morbidity and mortality in childhood trauma victims, accounting for an annual mortality rate of 1 per 1,000 in this age group.

In the mid-1990s, gunshot wounds surpassed other mechanisms as the most common cause of brain injuries.[1] Because of a case mortality ratio of approximately 94%, however, they continue to represent only a fraction of the brain injuries that come to definitive hospital care. In addition, because civilian gunshot wounds to the head are frequently isolated injuries, their spectrum of care varies more toward individual neurosurgical management.

PATHOPHYSIOLOGY

Traumatic injury to the brain involves a primary brain injury that occurs at impact and leads to disruption of brain substance and blood vessels. In addition, secondary brain injury may result from hypoxia, hypotension, pyrexia, the effects of increased intracranial pressure (ICP), and altered cellular biochemical processes that are often ongoing long after the primary insult.

Primary Injury

Energy transfer to the head causes direct disruption of neurons, glial cells, and microvasculature localized at the area of impact. As the brain decelerates within the skull, it is also vulnerable to impact with the opposite inner table. Therefore, countercoup injury to the contralateral brain is relatively common, in some cases being the more severe site of damage.

Diffuse injury from brain distortion, particularly when the mechanism includes rotational forces, can lead to damage to deep brain structures, which can then lead to widespread disruption of white matter axons throughout the brain, producing the situation termed "diffuse axonal injury." Such injuries often produce some degree of damage to a large number of neurologic systems. When such injuries involve ascending pathways in both hemispheres, the result is depressed level of consciousness.

The brain is also subject to torsion injury resulting from rotation around the fixed brainstem. This type of injury can damage the reticular activating system, which is the other mechanism of unconsciousness. Intracranial hemorrhage can take many forms. Direct laceration of epidural arteries from impact fractures or bleeding from fracture lines produces epidural hematomas, which damage the brain by compression. Disruption of bridging subdural veins and bleeding from cortical tissue damage produces a subdural hematoma, which is generally associated with disruption of underlying brain tissue. Intracerebral contusions, lacerations, and hematomas are caused by direct tissue disruption with associated vascular injury, producing neuronal damage and intraparenchymal bleeding.

Penetrating injury damages the brain through tissue injury caused directly by the projectile as well as disruption of neural tissue at a greater distance from the track via cavitation injury. In survivors, the extent and degree of the cavitation injury (related linearly to the mass and in a cubed fashion to the velocity of the projectile) is often the primary determinant of outcome. Another source of morbidity is vascular injury, producing aneurysms, pseudoaneurysms, and other vascular anomalies that may present immediately or be delayed.

Whether a projectile or direct impact causes contusion, subdural hematoma, epidural hematoma, or diffuse axonal injury, little can be done therapeutically to change the magnitude or location of the primary injury once it has occurred. As such, most of our present care focus is on secondary injuries.

Secondary Injury

Secondary brain injuries result from events occurring after the primary insult, either from the direct consequences of process initiated by the primary injury or from deleterious outside influences. The occurrence and magnitude of secondary insults is often the determining factor in outcome from brain injury. In contrast to primary injuries, secondary insults are amenable to medical management; they are the focus toward which the medical treatment of brain injury is directed.

Primary tissue injury initiates a variety of biochemical processes, including free-radical mediated lipid peroxidation, excitotoxic "super-activation" of glutamate-aspartate neurotransmitter systems, and alterations in membrane receptor and ionic channel characteristics, among others. A variety of genetic processes are also activated, including apoptosis, which is a focus of much current research. These processes can proceed for significant periods of time following primary injury and often are self-sustaining. The goal of the numerous clinical trials involving treatment of patients with brain trauma with various pharmacologic agents is to determine means by which these processes may be attenuated or reversed.

The primary external secondary injury processes occurring following brain injury are hypotension and hypoxia. Hypotension is the number one treatable determinant of severe head injury. A single episode of systolic blood pressure <90 mm Hg occurring during the period from injury through resuscitation doubles the mortality and significantly increases the morbidity of any given brain injury.[2] Furthermore, an early hypotensive episode strongly increases the probability of later intracranial hypertension. For these reasons, rapid and complete restoration of blood pressure is the most important goal in the resuscitation of the brain-injured patient. Also for this reason, the somewhat unconventional suggestion of using pressors as temporizing agents during volume resuscitation has been incorporated into brain injury care.[2]

Hypoxia (apnea or cyanosis in the field or a Pao_2 <60 mm Hg) is also an independent predictor of poor outcome.[2,3] The frequency and magnitude of hypoxia have been notably decreased by modern airway management techniques, particularly early endotracheal intubation and assisted ventilation, in addition to ensuring adequate oxygen carrying capacity through the avoidance of anemia.

Another important source of secondary injury is pyrexia. Fever is correlated with poorer outcome both by degree and duration.[3] Although the precise mechanism of this effect remains unclear, increased metabolism and the resultant metabolic recruitment of additional blood flow (and blood volume) is presumed to play a role.

Intracranial Pressure

Intracranial pressure results from the aggregate volumes of brain, cerebrospinal fluid (CSF), and blood within the fixed intracranial compartment. Mild or slow expansion of one or two of these compartments can be buffered by compensatory decreases in either the CSF or blood compartments (into the spinal subarachnoid space or the venous sinuses, respectively). When this buffering capacity is exceeded, the compliance of the brain is compromised and small additional increases in intracranial volume will produce marked elevations in ICP.

Intracranial hypertension is considered deleterious via two somewhat separable mechanisms: herniation and ischemia. Herniation occurs when a pressure gradient exists across an incomplete barrier, such as the tentorium, falx cerebri, or foramen magnum. It is deleterious because of the tissue damage when herniation occurs. Transtentorial herniation, the most noted form, is manifest by anisocoria, motor posturing, autonomic disturbances, and death. The specter of herniation is the major determinant of the absolute threshold of ICP management, which is generally accepted as 20 to 25 mm Hg, although this range has not been well determined empirically. A major unanswered question is how ICP should be managed when separated from perfusion, both in terms of measuring the probability of herniation and in determining whether there are detrimental effects of elevated pressure *per se*. It is hoped that ongoing research in the area of cerebral compliance will produce clinically useful information regarding these issues.

The second deleterious aspect of intracranial hypertension is elevated resistance to cerebral blood flow (CBF), resulting in or exacerbating ischemia. This resistance can be roughly approximated by cerebral perfusion pressure (CPP), which is defined as the difference between mean arterial blood pressure and ICP:

$$\text{CPP} = \text{mean arterial pressure} - \text{ICP}$$

Under normal circumstances, cerebral pressure autoregulation maintains CBF stable over a wide range of CPP (approximately 50 to 150 mm Hg) (Fig. 21.1). Following injury to the brain, this autoregulation is generally disrupted. This disruption can be complete, resulting in a pressure-passive system.[4]

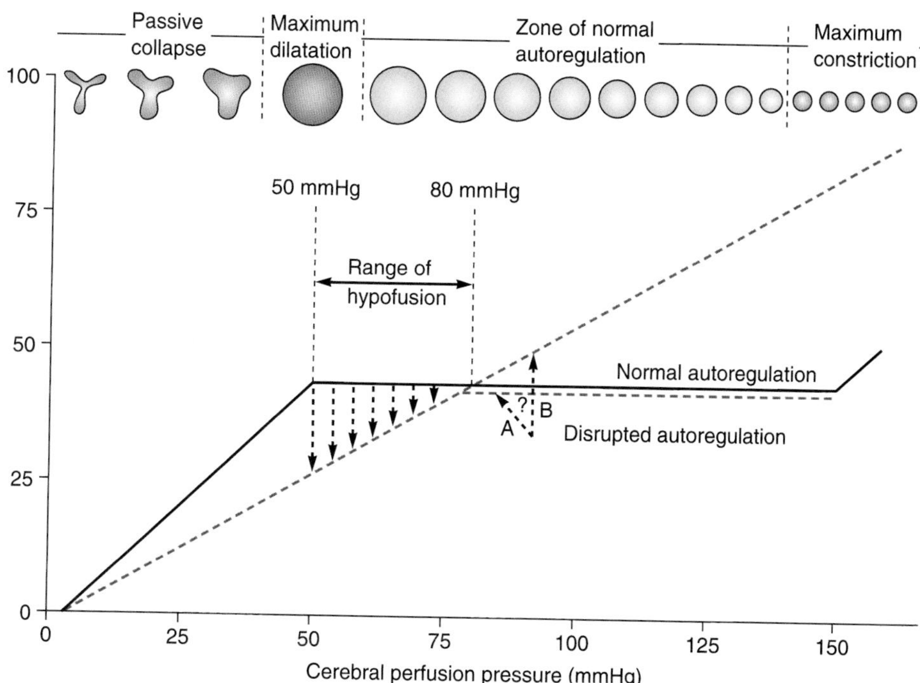

FIGURE 21.1 Cerebral pressure autoregulation. The normal relationship is indicated by the *solid line* with autoregulatory breakpoints at 50 and 150 mm Hg. Two disrupted states are also diagrammed. Complete loss of autoregulation (*straight dashed line B*) results in a pressure-passive system wherein cerebral blood flow (CBF) (and cerebral blood volume [CBV]) increases linearly with cerebral profusion pressure (CPP). The more common form of disruption is indicated by the sigmoid (*dashed line A*) where the major alteration is a right shift in the lower breakpoint. The *circles* at the top of the figure represent the diameters of the resistance vessels in the normal situation. The area of the circles represents CBV. Shifting this relationship to the right by 30 mm Hg would represent the partially disrupted state. (© R.M. Chesnut, M.D., FCCM, reproduced with permission.)

More frequently, the disruption is incomplete, characterized by a normal sigmoid shape but with abnormal elevation of the lower breakpoint above the normal value of 50 mm Hg (sigmoid dashed line). A possible consequence of this disruption is that a CPP that is satisfactory for uninjured patients may be associated with a lower CBF following head trauma (range of hypoperfusion).

In a pressure-passive system, cerebral blood volume (CBV) will increase in proportion to CPP. In such an instance, the goal is to keep the CPP just above the level of cerebral ischemia, thereby minimizing iatrogenic intracranial hypertension driven by increased CBV. In the situation of incomplete disruption, the goal is to keep CPP within the range of autoregulation, because this not only avoids ischemia but also may decrease ICP if autoregulatory vasoconstriction in response to increased CPP serves to decrease CBV.

Confounding this situation is the recent information that CBF may be significantly depressed during the early postinjury period. It is particularly critical, therefore, that CPP be supported assiduously from the first point of patient contact. Because hyperventilation causes vasoconstriction, thereby decreasing CBF, the use of hyperventilation during this early period is somewhat more hazardous than after the first 24 to 48 hours.

The preceding physiologic reasoning gave rise to cerebral perfusion pressure therapy, wherein CPP is elevated to 70 mm Hg or higher throughout the course of intracranial hypertension. The efficacy of CPP therapy has been suggested by studies without internal controls reporting decreased morbidity and mortality associated with CPP therapy compared with historical controls that practiced more conventional ICP-based therapy. The result of such reports has been that CPP-based therapy has become widely accepted as standard practice. Recent reports, however, suggest that such acceptance may have been premature. Potential errors in selecting the historical control groups against which CPP-based therapy results have been compared have prevented differentiating the effects of artificially increasing CPP from those of simply avoiding in-hospital hypotensive episodes. When control groups are selected to address this deficiency, it becomes apparent that CPP-based therapy may simply be a proxy for avoidance of transient ischemia.[5] Such a possibility is further supported by preliminary analysis of data from the National Institutes of Health (NIH)—funded North American Brain Injury Study on Hypothermia, which suggests that dips of CPP below 60 mm Hg are much more highly correlated with outcome than the efficacy of maintaining CPP above 70 mm Hg.[6]

In addition, it appears that elevating CPP may increase the duration of intracranial hypertension.[7,8] This might be caused by the elevation of hydrostatic forces favoring the formation of vasogenic edema, thereby iatrogenically prolonging brain swelling and ICP elevation. Finally, the results of a prospective, randomized investigation of CPP-based versus ICP-based management suggest that there is no overall difference in outcome between the two strategies, with the major effect of CPP-based therapy being the alteration in the mode of exitus from early, ICP-related deaths to delayed mortality from systemic complications (especially acute respiratory distress syndrome [ARDS]).[9] Such considerations imply that, although attention to CPP (and, thus, cerebral perfusion) is important, the proper method of managing CPP remains to be determined. It is clear, however, that routinely elevating CPP to values above 60 mm Hg is not associated with improved outcome.[10]

Ultimately, the goal of managing blood pressure and CBF is to maintain a level of perfusion that meets the metabolic demands of the cell. The major problem with managing traumatic brain injury (TBI) based on pressure measurements is that alterations in cerebral metabolism will be missed. This may be of significant importance because the usual course of cerebral metabolism is to decrease drastically following injury, slowly returning toward normal in patients who improve. One implication of such a metabolic course is that CBF values that would be dangerous under normal metabolic conditions might be satisfactory when cerebral metabolism is depressed. Indeed, because metabolic flow autoregulation is generally preserved following TBI, low values of CBF might often reflect flow:metabolism matching. One result of such a course of metabolic change might be that CPP elevation is reasonable during the early (i.e., first 12 to 24 hours) posttraumatic period when metabolism is near normal and ischemia is both probable and extremely devastating. Subsequently, when metabolism falls, CPP elevation may not be necessary and, indeed, be counterproductive.

Absolute metabolic information is not readily available in the clinical situation. The relative balance between metabolic needs and substrate delivery, however, can often be usefully estimated by monitoring the oxygen saturation in the internal jugular vein ($JVSo_2$) or the tissue oxygen tension in the brain ($Ptio_2$). Although limited by problems of averaging, incomplete sampling of the total cerebral tissue volume, and technical issues of accuracy, the monitoring of $JVSo_2$ is a clinically useful method of detecting some otherwise occult episodes of ischemia as well as tailoring therapy to individual patient needs as they evolve.[11] By adding measurement of the arteriojugular lactate difference (AVDL), occult areas of ischemia or anaerobic metabolism can also be detected that would not be apparent if only $JVSo_2$ were measured.

More recently, it has become possible to measure brain tissue oxygen tension ($Ptio_2$) using implantable Clark electrodes. This makes it possible to follow the balance between oxygen consumption and delivery, thereby providing the potential of detecting actual ischemia. These electrodes are easily implanted, either in a tunneled fashion or through a threaded bolt. Although absolute thresholds have not been rigorously determined, values above 15 to 20 mm Hg are generally considered adequate and values below 5 mm Hg are associated with increasingly poor outcome in a duration-dependent fashion.[12,13] The major limitation of this system is the extremely focal nature of this monitoring. Although there is theoretical attractiveness to monitoring at the border of focal injuries (the "penumbra"), most monitoring is performed within normal brain.

We have found that combining the monitoring of ICP, CPP, $JVSo_2$, AVDL, $Ptio_2$, and quantitative regional CBF (with cold xenon computed tomography [CT] or CT perfusion CBF studies) have allowed us to safely tailor management to cerebral needs, thereby avoiding overtreatment and undertreatment, minimizing the likelihood of iatrogenic systemic toxicity, and shortening intensive care unit (ICU) stay. Most "straightforward" cases of brain injury where ICP control is not difficult and systemic determinants of perfusion are stable and adequate do not require invasive multimodality monitoring. In the approximately 10% of cases where these parameters are problematic, however, expanded monitoring is strongly suggested.

Treatment of hypertension is rarely indicated in the patient with head injury. There is no evidence that hypertension promotes continued intracranial hemorrhage and hypertension related to brain injury generally resolves when the intracranial hypertension is controlled. When profound hypertension requires treatment, short-acting, selective ß-blockers or intravenous (IV) titration of calcium channel blockers should be used. Vasodilators (e.g., sodium nitroprusside) should be avoided because they increase CBV, which can exacerbate ICP.

As noted, metabolic autoregulation is the other and somewhat more fundamental type of intrinsic CBF control. Vasoconstriction is nonlinearly proportional to pH and, therefore, subject to manipulation of $PaCo_2$. As a result, hyperventilation-induced alkalosis produces vasoconstriction, resulting in a decrease of both CBF and CBV. Although the latter is beneficial in controlling ICP, the former is potentially deleterious and mandates caution when using hyperventilation. For reasons outlined above, hyperventilation is best avoided whenever possible during the early postinjury course when the risk of ischemia is extremely high. As well, because of rapid compensatory buffering of iatrogenic hypocapnic alkalosis, the beneficial effects of hyperventilation tend to be relatively short-lived.

Cerebral Edema and Osmolar Therapy (Mannitol)

Cerebral edema during the early postinjury period is generally cytotoxic (intracellular). Later, vasogenic (extracellular) edema may play a role in brain swelling. Although resulting from different mechanisms (cellular membrane dysfunction and blood–brain barrier breakdown), present treatment for cerebral edema is limited to the administration of osmotic agents, most commonly mannitol. Mannitol increases the osmotic gradient, drawing fluid from the interstitial compartment into plasma, thereby reducing brain volume. In regions where the blood–brain barrier has been disrupted, however, mannitol is minimally effective and can actually leak into tissues.[14] The area of blood–brain barrier breakdown is generally much smaller than the area of edema that it creates and mannitol is generally effective in lowering ICP.

Mannitol also has other mechanisms of action. It creates an acute increase in intravascular volume, which may transiently improve cardiac output and CBF. It also appears to cause acute and transient vasoconstriction as a result of its ability to decrease blood viscosity and improve flow. Both of these effects are of more immediate onset than the osmotic effects of mannitol. They may be responsible for its early effects on ICP and may also explain why mannitol is more effective in lowering ICP when administered as a bolus rather than a slow infusion.

Mannitol, however, can produce significant diuresis. The resulting hypovolemia can result in hypotension, not only producing secondary insult to the brain but also causing intracranial hypertension from autoregulatory vasodilatation. Recent evidence suggests that the apparent relationship between early mannitol use and hypotension may be associated with hypotensive episodes that are correlated with increased morbidity and mortality.[15] Therefore, mannitol should be used only for proved or strongly suspected intracranial hypertension; it should be avoided under conditions of hypovolemia, and fluid losses should be diligently replaced. Because smaller doses of mannitol (0.25 g/kg) are equally as efficacious as larger doses (1 g/kg) in lowering ICP, the smaller doses should be used.

More recently, the use of hypertonic saline to elevate serum osmolarity has become increasingly incorporated into TBI management. This approach has been studied best in the pediatric population where it has been demonstrated to be beneficial in controlling intracranial hypertension (although not yet rigorously shown to improve clinical outcome). Three percent sodium chloride (3%) solution is generally used, infused at 0.5 to 1.0 mL/kg per hour.

CLINICAL ASSESSMENT

The objectives during early clinical assessment of the patient with head injury are multiple and must be accomplished simultaneously. These include establishing adequate oxygenation, ventilation, and circulatory stability and evaluating the extent of brain injury while treating ICP elevations. Although some evidence indicates that systemic hypotension may infrequently be the result of a head injury, always initially presume that hypotension in a trauma patient is the result of hypovolemia. It is a significant error to withhold volume resuscitation in a misdirected effort to control cerebral edema.

During initial assessment, mental status changes cannot be presumed to be the result of drugs or alcohol, although routine toxicology screening is appropriate. It should be presumed that any change in mental status or the neurologic examination in general or any evidence of herniation (e.g., anisocoria) suggests an expanding intracranial mass lesion.

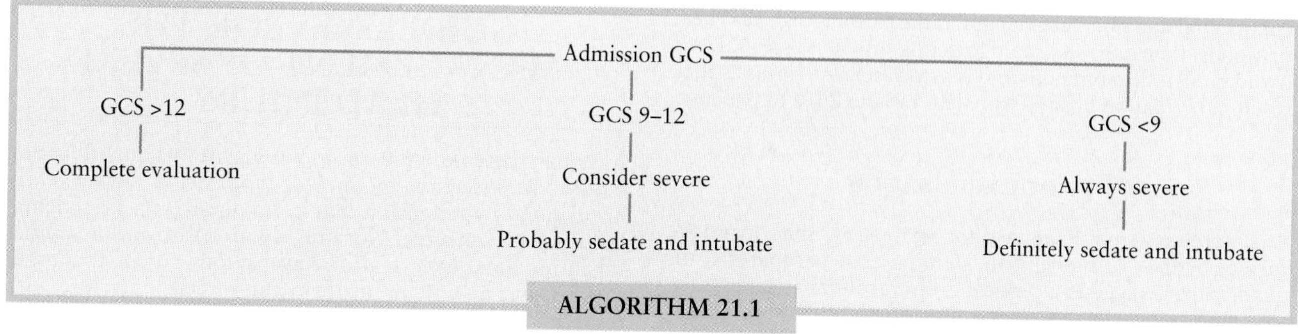

ALGORITHM 21.1 Glasgow Coma Scale (GCS) triage guide for initial evaluation of head injury. For the motor scale, the best response for any limb is recorded.

Under such circumstances, therapeutic ICP reduction becomes the first priority and emergency imaging or surgical decompression must be accomplished emergently.

Do not assume that apparent neurologic unresponsiveness represents a lack of sensitivity to pain. Noxious stimuli, such as placement of urinary drainage catheters, nasogastric tubes, or IV catheters, can precipitate ICP peaks during resuscitation. These procedures should be done quickly and efficiently, optimally after sedation. Endotracheal intubation is particularly susceptible to inducing herniation in borderline cases. Whenever practical, consider premedication with analgesics, sedatives, or IV or endotracheal lidocaine before airway instrumentation.

With regard to the brain injury, several critical assessments are necessary and should be precisely recorded because trends are at least as important as any single observation. The three key parameters are level of consciousness, pupillary reflexes and size, and the motor examination.

Glasgow Coma Scale

The single most important assessment for a patient with head injury is to evaluate the level of consciousness. In this regard, the Glasgow Coma Scale (GCS) has become an international standard that is easily, rapidly, and reliably obtained (Algorithm 21.1). It is not, and was never intended to be, a neurologic examination and should not be substituted for such information.

It has been suggested that early estimations of GCS, done in the field by emergency personnel, are often inaccurate.[16] In some areas, alternate, simpler systems (e.g., the AVPU scale) are accepted for this reason. In the recent *Guidelines for the Prehospital Care of Severe Brain Injury*, however, the continued use of the GCS was supported for all prehospital care providers.[17] Special training has been developed by the Brain Trauma Foundation to optimize its accuracy (http://www.braintrauma.org/).

Components of the GCS include assessment of eye opening, verbal response, and motor response. The routine use of GCS provides a useful measure of initial injury severity and allows stratification for initial therapy as well as for outcome analysis.

Patients can be stratified for triage purposes into those with severe injuries (GCS, <8), moderate injuries (GCS, 8 to 12), or mild injuries (GCS, >12; see Algorithm 21.1). Patients with severe head injuries require immediate endotracheal intubation, mechanical ventilation, and complete resuscitation; any clinical evidence of intracranial hypertension (e.g., signs of herniation) mandates maximal therapy to decrease ICP.

Many significant injuries occur in patients with GCS scores between 8 and 12. Although this is defined as the moderate injury group, all these patients require maximal brain resuscitation until a definitive diagnosis can be made. A patient with a GCS of 12 or more tends to be confused but responsive to verbal stimulation. These patients need serial neurologic evaluations because they are in the group that can "talk and die" because of missed or delayed intracranial pathology. In general, however, and whenever expedient, attention to other major injuries can take priority over cerebral imaging or management.

Pupils

Pupillary asymmetry, dilation, or loss of light reflex in an unconscious patient usually reflects herniation because of the mass effect from intracranial hemorrhage ipsilateral to the dilated pupil. The probability of an intracranial mass lesion can be roughly approximated given the degree of anisocoria (≥1 mm or ≥3 mm), the mechanism of injury (± motor vehicle crash), and age (Fig. 21.2).[18] Occasionally, pupillary signs may indicate direct second or third nerve injury or trauma to the globe, but this must always be a diagnosis of exclusion.

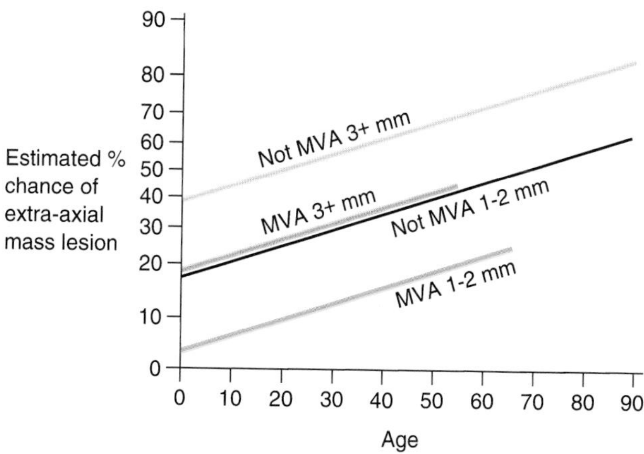

FIGURE 21.2 Estimated percentage chance of an extraaxial intracranial mass lesion greater than 25 mL as a function of degree of anisocoria, age, and mechanism of injury. Mechanism of injury was defined as motor vehicle accident (MVA) or other mechanism (not MVA). (Reproduced from Chesnut RM, Gautille T, Blunt BA, et al. The localizing value of asymmetry in pupillary size in severe head injury: relation to lesion type and location. *Neurosurgery* 1994;34:840–845, with permission.)

An unequal and nonreactive pupil is the cardinal sign that herniation is occurring, and rapid lowering of ICP is essential. An ovoid pupil is also ominous and is associated with injuries that result in herniation in approximately 15% to 20% of patients.

Motor Examination

The motor system is examined for asymmetry, abnormal posturing, or lack of movement. Hemiparesis, paraparesis, or quadriparesis suggests a cervical or thoracolumbar spine fracture with spinal cord injury. Hemiparesis secondary to brainstem herniation from the mass effect may be either ipsilateral or contralateral to the side of the dilated pupil. Hemiparesis may also result from significant brain contusion. In the unconscious patient, a painful stimulus should be used to evaluate motor function. All four extremities should be examined and the results noted, because only the response of the best limb will be reflected in the GCS score.

INITIAL TREATMENT

Evidence-based Medicine and the Management of Traumatic Brain Injury

The publication of *Guidelines for the Management of Severe Brain Injury* represented a significant step in standardizing the management of TBI based on published, peer-reviewed literature.[19] This document represents the application of a strict evidence-based process to 14 topics relevant to TBI care. Following an exhaustive, explicitly defined literature search covering each topic, the recovered literature was carefully classified along a three-point continuum of scientific rigor. As such, each article was ranked as class I, class II, or class III and the analysis of the scientific basis of each topic was predicated on the most scientifically rigorous (highest literature class) reports available. This process produced a set of standards, guidelines, and options for treatment where **standards** (based on class I evidence) represent principles with a high degree of clinical certainty, **guidelines** (based on class II evidence) reflect principles with a moderate degree of clinical certainty, and **options** (based on class III evidence) reflect principles for which unclear clinical certainty exists. By specifically defining the scientific foundation of 14 TBI management issues, *Guidelines for the Management of Severe Brain Injury* provide an unbiased reference focused on facilitating scientific management of TBI.

Since the initial publication of *Guidelines for the Management of Severe Brain Injury*, it has undergone updating and revision[10] and the same evidence-based process has been applied in the generation of other sets of brain injury guidelines. *Guidelines for the Prehospital Management of Traumatic Brain Injury* were published in 2002,[17] spawning the previously noted training efforts. In 2001, *Guidelines for the Management of Penetrating Brain Injury* was published.[20] *Guidelines for the Management of Pediatric Brain Injury* was published in 2003.[21] Finally, *Guidelines for the Surgical Management of Traumatic Brain Injury* has been finished and is in the process of publication. In light of the sensitivity of all evidence-reports to the publication of new literature, the Brain Trauma Foundation has ensured that all of these reports are regularly updated and expanded through the Neurosurgical Evidence-based Medicine Center at the University of Washington.

Wherever applicable, the findings contained in these guidelines have been incorporated into this text. For details, the reader is referred to the source documents.

GUIDELINES FOR THE MANAGEMENT OF SEVERE HEAD INJURY

Although there is no present technology for its quantification before the insertion of an ICP monitoring device, early intracranial hypertension may certainly exert a detrimental influence on outcome. Not only do all treatment modalities for intracranial hypertension have serious potential complications, but also many of them can directly interfere with resuscitation procedures (e.g., use of diuretics). The efficacy of successful systemic resuscitation in improving the likelihood of survival from trauma in general is well accepted. In addition, the acknowledged negative influence of secondary insults (e.g., hypotension and hypoxia) on outcome from severe head injury render systemic resuscitation a *conditio sine qua non*, which provides a vital infrastructure on which treatment of intracranial hypertension must be based. Therefore, all treatment must be consistent with optimal systemic resuscitation. When definite signs of transtentorial herniation occur, they should be interpreted as definitive evidence of intracranial hypertension and prompt, rapid, and definitive treatment specifically focused toward lowering ICP should be implemented consistent with continued physiologic resuscitation.

The composition and volume of the IV fluids used to resuscitate patients with head injuries should be selected with the purpose of restoring intravascular blood volume. Although the widely disseminated but scientifically unsupported adage of "keeping TBI patients dry" has now been discarded, the concept of restricting free water remains desirable. As such, isotonic crystalloid solution in the form of 0.9% NS is preferable to lactated Ringer's solution as a resuscitation fluid for TBI. Furthermore, a growing body of scientific support exists for initiating the use of 250 mL of 7.5% NS as the first resuscitation fluid in TBI victims,[22–24] although a recent randomized controlled trial from Australia suggests that this may not be of benefit under optimal resuscitation conditions.[25]

The end points of resuscitation do not change depending on the presence or absence of a head injury. Blood volume should be normal, with an appropriate blood pressure and continuous venous pressure (CVP), adequate urine output and peripheral perfusion, and progressive improvement of any base deficit. The systolic blood pressure should never be allowed to drop below 90 mm Hg. Some evidence indicates an advantage to targeting a mean arterial pressure of 80 to 90 mm Hg during resuscitation until ICP monitoring can be initiated. Once ICP is available, a minimal CPP of 60 mm Hg should initially be the goal.

Resuscitation in the Absence of Clinical Signs of Herniation

Algorithm 21.2 is based on *Guidelines for the Management of Severe Brain Injury*[10] and *Guidelines for the Prehospital Management of Severe Brain Injury*[17] for use by prehospital and initial at-hospital care providers and emergency physicians to guide decision making in resuscitating TBI victims and determining the necessity of ICP-lowering therapy. "Signs of increased ICP" implies pupillary abnormalities, motor posturing, or neurologic deterioration not related to medications. When these signs are not present, mannitol is not given and the goal of ventilation is eucapnia. When such signs are present, the patient is hyperventilated to a $PaCo_2$ of 30 to 35 mm Hg and mannitol may be given if the patient's volume status is normal.

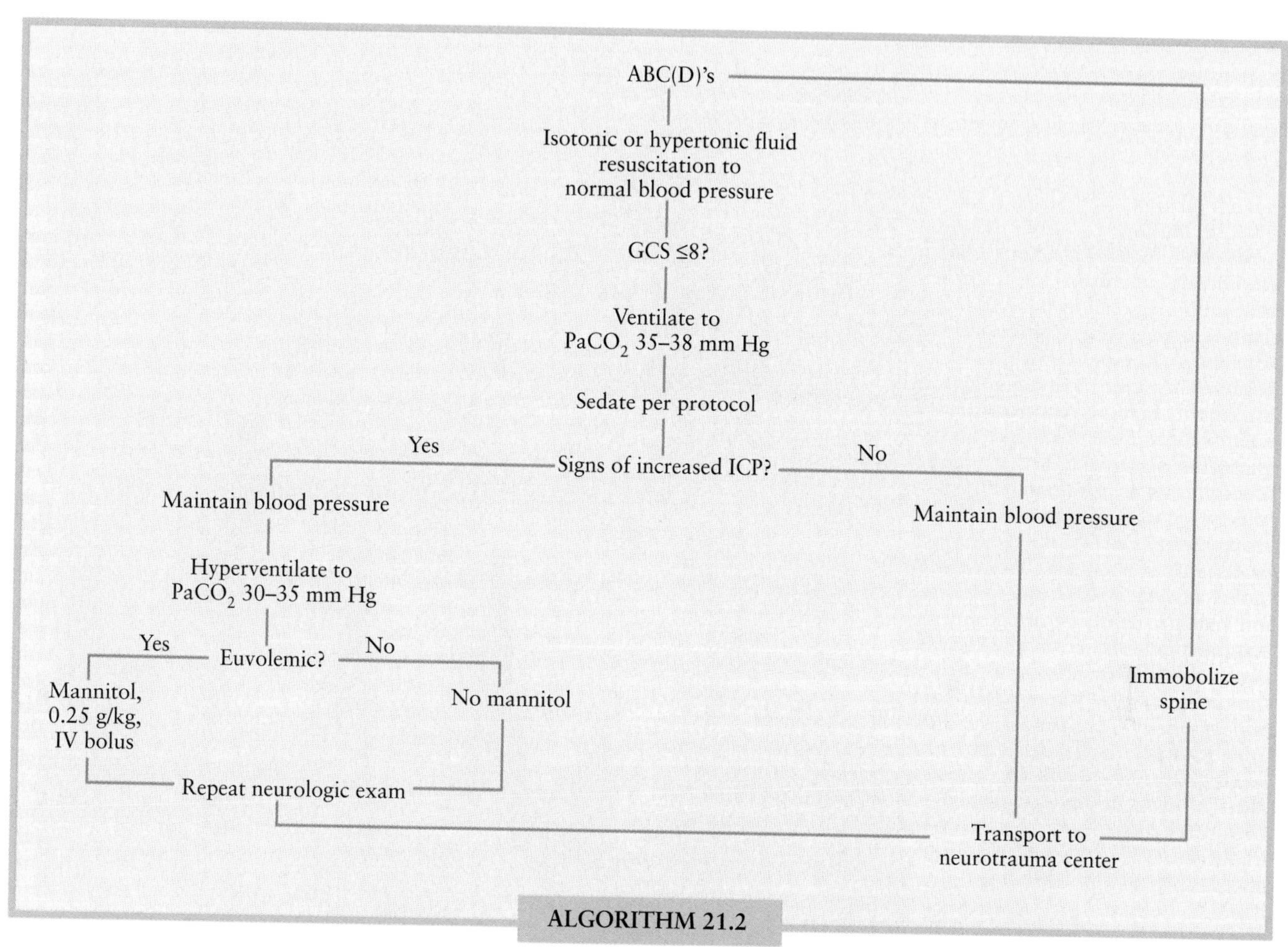

ALGORITHM 21.2 Prehospital evaluation and treatment of a patient with severe traumatic brain injury. "Signs of increased ICP" is the decision point for determining the necessity of ICP-lowering therapy. These signs include pupillary abnormalities, motor posturing, or neurologic deterioration not related to medications. The order of steps is determined by the risk:benefit ratio for individual treatment maneuvers. This algorithm should be viewed as "expert opinion" and used as a framework, which may be useful in guiding an approach to field management of such patients. (© R.M. Chesnut, M.D., FCCM, reproduced with permission.)

Algorithm 21.3 is based on *Guidelines for the Management of Severe Brain Injury*[10] for evaluation and treatment of the severe TBI patient from arrival at the trauma center up to placement of an ICP monitor. As with any trauma patient, the first step is Advanced Trauma Life Support (ATLS) resuscitation. When appropriate, brain-specific therapies are incorporated into the treatment course. Brain-friendly initial ICU management should lead directly to monitoring of ICP.

Elevating the head of the bed (reverse Trendelenburg position in the absence of clearance of the axial skeleton) has been shown to generally lower the CPP in the absence of adequate volume resuscitation.[26] Because this may elevate the ICP *per se*, it is not advised until complete resuscitation has been accomplished.

The confusion and agitation often attendant to head injury often renders sedation desirable and can drive intracranial hypertension. Therefore, patients with suspected head injury should generally receive sedatives and analgesics whenever possible. Short-acting agents are preferable in the interest of following the neurologic examination.

In addition to eliminating any possibility of spontaneous ventilation and mandating complete ventilatory control, pharmacologic relaxation has the undesirable effect of limiting the neurologic examination to the pupils and the CT scan. Its use in the absence of evidence of herniation, therefore, should be limited to situations where sedation alone is not sufficient to optimize safe and efficient patient transport and resuscitation. When sedation is used, short-acting agents are strongly preferred.

The "prophylactic" administration of mannitol is not suggested because of its volume-depleting diuretic effect. In addition, although it is desirable to approximate the lower end of the normal range of $Paco_2$ during transport of a patient suspected of having brain injury, the risk of exacerbating early ischemia by vigorous hyperventilation outweighs the questionable benefit in the patient without evidence of herniation. Therefore, ventilatory parameters consistent with optimal oxygenation and "normal" ventilation are recommended. The minute ventilation should be targeted at 100 mL/kg/min unless quantitative measurement of $Etco_2$ or $Paco_2$ is available. *Guidelines for the Prehospital Management of Severe Brain Injury* suggest the use of $Etco_2$ monitoring during prehospital resuscitation and transport whenever possible. In the absence of signs of intracranial hypertension, ventilation should be adjusted to accomplish a $Paco_2$ of 35 mm Hg when arterial gas values become available.

TRAUMA

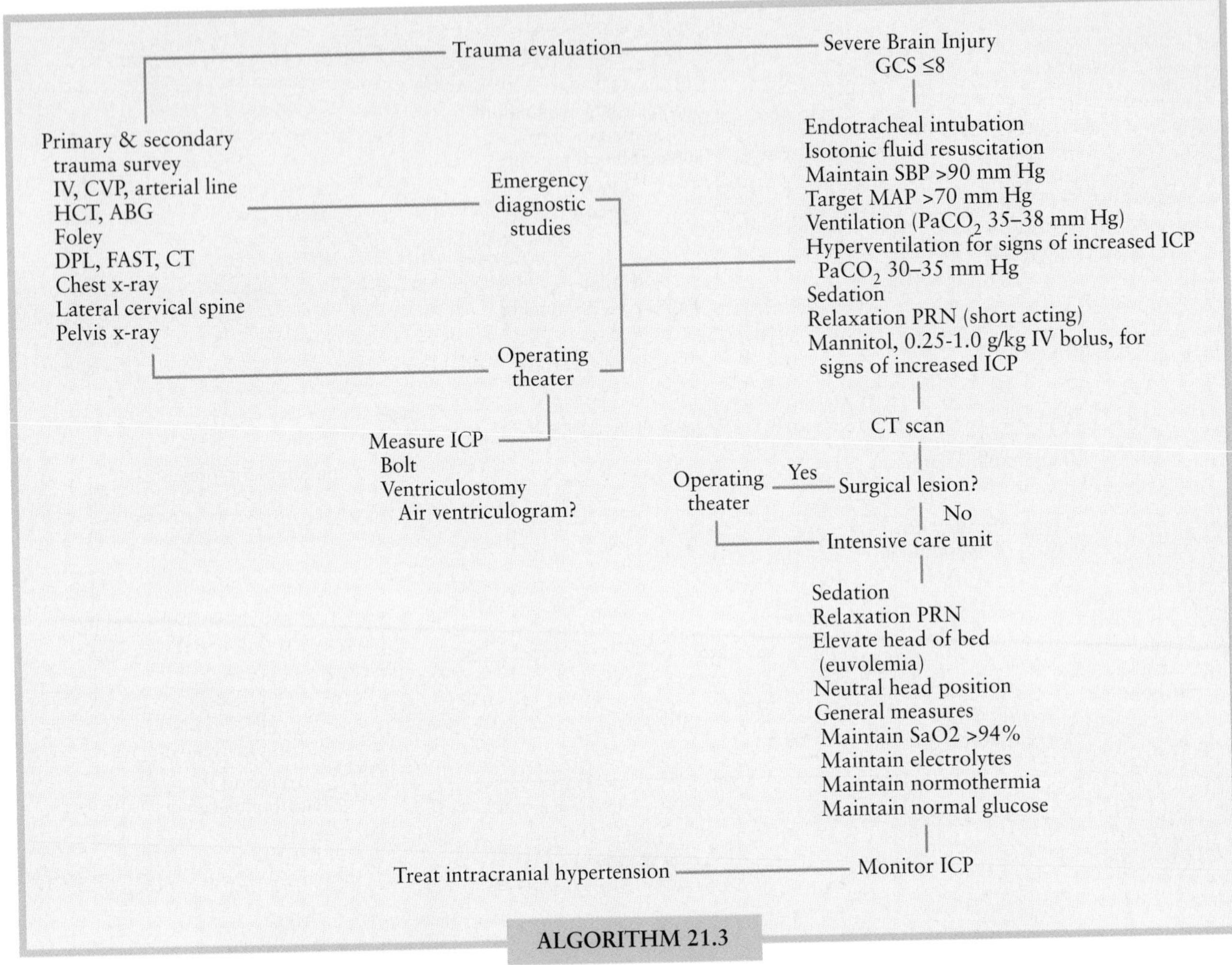

ALGORITHM 21.3 Evaluation and treatment of the patient with severe traumatic brain injury on arrival at the trauma center. The order of steps is determined by the risk:benefit ratio for individual treatment maneuvers. This algorithm should be viewed as "expert opinion" and used as a framework, which may be useful in guiding an approach to initial hospital management of such patients prior to the initiation of ICP monitoring. (© R.M. Chesnut, M.D., FCCM, reproduced with permission.)

Resuscitation in the Presence of Clinical Signs of Herniation

Signs of intracranial hypertension consist of evidence of transtentorial herniation (pupillary dilation or loss of reactivity or motor posturing or flaccidity) or progressive neurologic deterioration not attributable to other causes (e.g., sedation). When such signs occur, aggressive treatment of suspected intracranial hypertension is indicated. Hyperventilation to a $PaCO_2$ target of approximately 30 mm Hg should be accomplished by increasing the minute ventilation to approximately 120 to 140 mL/kg/min or as directed by quantitative CO_2 monitoring. Because hypotension can produce both neurologic deterioration and intracranial hypertension, the use of mannitol is less desirable unless adequate volume resuscitation has been accomplished. If such is the case, however, mannitol should be administered by bolus infusion. Under such circumstances, it is critical that the diagnosis and treatment of the neurologic injury be accomplished with utmost haste. These patients must be transported to a trauma center with neurosurgical coverage.

Radiographic Priorities

Neurosurgical evaluation and assessment is initiated as soon as the potential for significant head injury is realized. Prompt radiographic evaluation is essential and CT scanning is the imaging modality of choice for virtually all acute neurological conditions. Patients with mild head injuries can usually be observed with sequential examinations and radiographic evaluation may be unnecessary unless the results determine whether the patient can be discharged from the hospital. In contrast, however, a cogent argument can be made for the liberal application of CT scanning to even patients with minimal evidence of TBI as a method of making safe, efficient, and economic triage decisions.[27] In any instance, evidence of neurologic deterioration or the occurrence of a situation wherein the neurologic examination cannot be followed (e.g., the need for general anesthesia) mandates CT scanning, intraoperative ICP monitoring, or both. General indications for neurologic imaging (generally, CT scanning) are listed in Table 21.1.

TABLE 21.1 DIAGNOSIS

INDICATIONS FOR NEUROLOGIC IMAGING

Suspected skull penetration by a foreign body
- Discharge of cerebrospinal fluid (CSF), blood, or both from the nose
- Hemotympanum or discharge of blood or CSF from the ear
- Protracted unconsciousness
- Altered state of consciousness at the time of examination
- Focal neurologic signs or symptoms
- Any situation precluding proper surveillance
- Head injury plus additional trauma
- Possible head injury in the presence of additional pathologic findings, such as stroke
- Head injury with alcohol or drug intoxication

Patients with moderate or severe injuries require prompt neurosurgic consultation and rapid radiographic evaluation using the CT scan. Hemodynamically stable patients with significant neurologic deterioration should go to the CT scanner immediately following ATLS resuscitation. In hemodynamically unstable patients who require immediate surgical intervention to sustain intravascular volume, exploratory thoracotomy or laparotomy must take precedence. In such cases, it is a mistake to delay further investigation of the intracranial compartment pending the end of the case and transport to the CT scanner. A number of methods can be employed to evaluate the intracranial compartment during such lifesaving, extracranial surgery, including insertion of an ICP monitor or ventriculostomy (with air ventriculography, if deemed necessary), transcranial Doppler evaluation, or even placement of exploratory burr holes in the instance of herniation. For this reason, neurosurgical consultation should be initiated on arrival in the theatre rather than at the finish of the case.

The spine should be cleared radiographically or immobilized and protected in every patient with a severe head injury. Although only 13% of patients with severe head injuries have spinal cord injuries, the potentially devastating consequences of an overlooked spine injury require constant vigilance.

Plain Skull Radiographs

With the routine availability of CT scanning, plain skull radiography has been criticized. Several authors have concluded that the presence of a fracture on a skull radiograph rarely influences treatment, does not reflect the severity of injury or predict outcome, and has seldom been a legal concern. On the other hand, the likelihood of a surgical intracranial hematoma is strongly correlated with the presence or absence of a skull fracture and the normalcy of the neurologic examination.[28] The utility of skull films in head injury therefore remains controversial.

In general, any patient meeting one of the aforementioned criteria should have CT imaging. Skull radiographs should be reserved for the patient with a mild head injury who has a normal neurologic examination and where the results of the skull radiographic study will alter the care plan (i.e., allow discharge from the hospital without a CT scan or determine the necessity for a CT scan). As noted, a growing body of evidence supports the more liberal use of CT imaging, which will obviate the use of plain skull radiographs except under circumstances where CT scanning is unobtainable.

If a CT scan is unavailable, a lateral displacement of the calcified pineal gland of greater than 2 mm on a skull radiograph suggests mass effect. When intracranial pathology is suggested, more definitive diagnostic maneuvers are indicated.

Linear skull fractures appear as two radiolucent lines with sharp, well-demarcated edges typically coursing from the point of impact on the calvarium toward the base of the skull. Depressed skull fractures are easily seen on plain frontal and lateral skull films. The mechanism of injury is usually a direct blow to the skull by a blunt object. Closed depressed skull fractures that are comminuted and those with a fragmented outer margin displaced beneath the inner table have generally been treated surgically, although growing evidence indicates that many may be treated nonoperatively if there is no neurological dysfunction or CT evidence of underlying tissue injury. Open fractures are also generally treated surgically, although, again, growing evidence indicates that fresh, noncomminuted fractures without neurologic deficit, CSF or brain extrusion, gross contamination, or underlying tissue injury can be closed and treated with prophylactic antibiotics.

Basilar skull fractures are usually diagnosed with CT imaging or on clinical evidence, because they are poorly visualized on plain films. Only about 20% of patients with clinical evidence of basilar skull fractures have discernible injury on plain skull radiographs. These clinical signs include otorrhea or rhinorrhea, subcutaneous ecchymoses overlying the mastoid region (Battle sign), bilateral periorbital ecchymoses (raccoon eyes), or hemotympanum. A basilar skull fracture may involve the paranasal sinuses, piriform sinus, petrous bone, sphenoid sinus, or sella turcica. Injury to adjacent structures, such as the seventh or eighth cranial nerves, brainstem and carotid or basilar artery, are not uncommon. These fractures are generally visualized with CT scanning, although special protocols may be required. In the acute situation, no specific therapy is indicated. The leak should not be tamponaded unless bleeding is brisk and antibiotics should not be administered solely for prophylaxis of meningitis. Most CSF leaks stop spontaneously with minimal treatment (e.g., elevating the head of the bed). Leaks that continue more than 72 hours generally require CSF diversion (e.g., via lumbar drainage or ventriculostomy). CSF drainage that does not respond to diversion will require surgery. Because most instances of rhinorrhea cease without surgery, the most common operation is exploration of the floor of the frontal fossa.

Computed Tomography

The CT finding that correlates most highly with intracranial hypertension is compression or obliteration of the basilar cisterns (Fig. 21.3). Not only does this finding portend a stormy ICP course, but also the primary predictor of outcome in patients with this CT picture is the peak level of intracranial hypertension occurring during the first 72 hours.[29,30] When cisternal compression is paired with a midline shift of more than5 mm, the prognosis is even more ominous. ICP monitoring should be immediately initiated in any patient with cisternal compression, and intracranial hypertension should be vigorously treated. Such patients, particularly those with minimal evidence of contusions, die primarily from secondary insults, which implies that they are potentially salvageable.

Acute epidural hematomas correlate well with skull fractures. The most common association is a linear, nondisplaced fracture in the temporoparietal region, crossing the middle meningeal artery. The classic clinical course involves a lucid interval following a brief loss of consciousness with subsequent neurologic deterioration. However, such a course occurs in less than 50% of epidural hematoma cases, so clinical suspicious must remain high. The typical CT appearance is a high- or mixed-density concave extra-axial hematoma with smooth borders (Fig. 21.4).

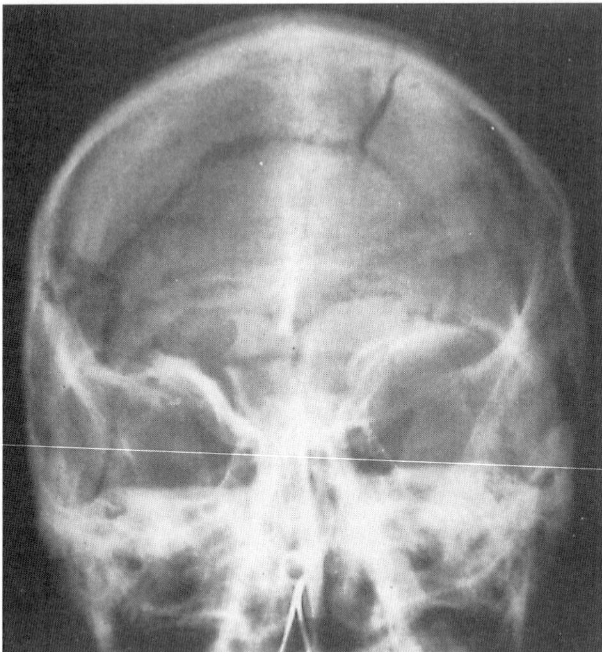

FIGURE 21.3 A computed tomography scan that is highly predictive of intracranial hypertension. The basilar cisterns are obliterated and the sulci are flattened.

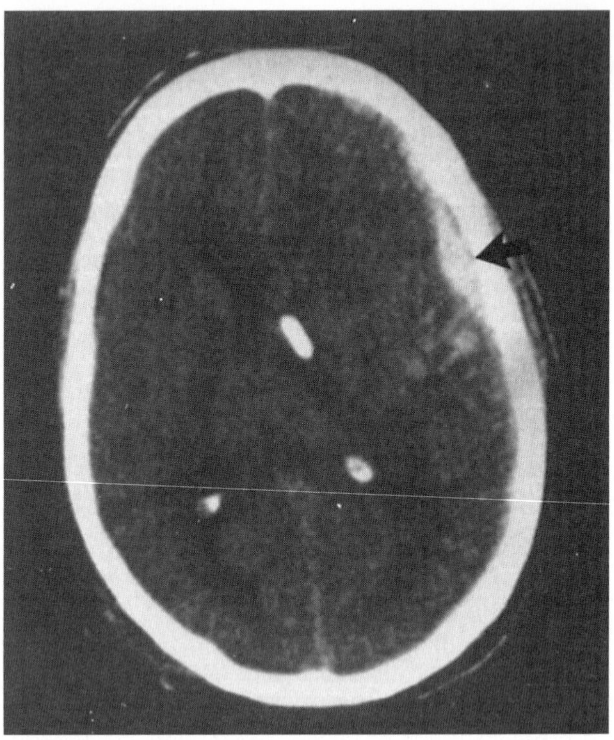

FIGURE 21.5 Usual computed tomography scan appearance of a crescent-shaped, high-density blood collection conforming to the contour of the cerebral hemisphere in a subdural hematoma.

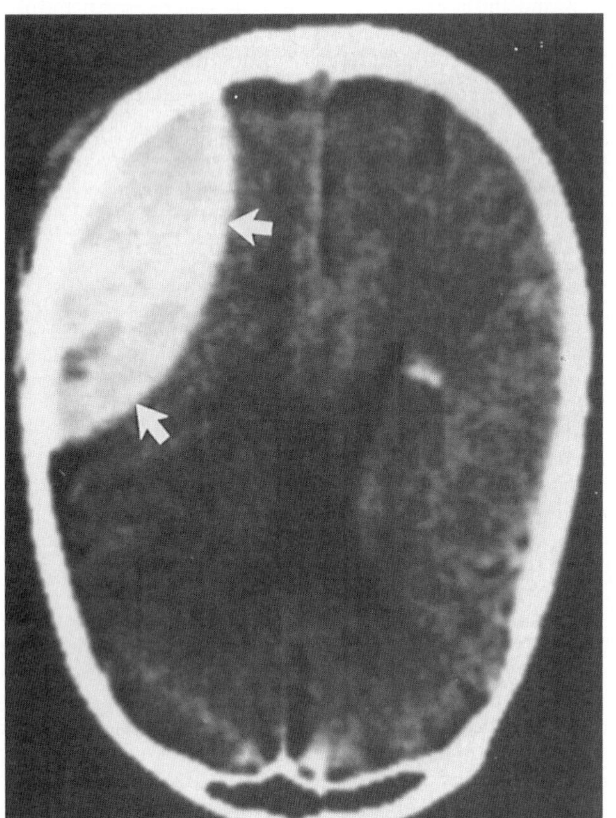

FIGURE 21.4 Typical computed tomography scan appearance of mixed-density, lens-shaped, acute epidural hematoma with mass effect.

Acute subdural hematomas occur over the convexity of the brain. The hematoma may evolve from rupture of bridging cortical veins or bleeding from the underlying parenchymal injury, which is common. It is this subjacent tissue damage that generally determines the neurologic outcome of patients not succumbing to intracranial hypertension. On CT scan, a subdural hematoma appears as an extraaxial high- or mixed-density crescentic mass that spreads out over the hemisphere, following the cortical irregularities (Fig. 21.5). The midline shift may be out of proportion to the size of the hematoma because of the contributing mass effect from an underlying brain contusion or hemispheric swelling.

Intracerebral hemorrhage and cerebral contusion are common after trauma and are readily visualized with CT scanning. Brain contusion appears as a focal, heterogeneous density with hemorrhage interspersed with injured tissue (Fig. 21.6). Intracerebral hematomas are generally more homogenous in their high-density appearance. Both of these lesions tend to "blossom" over time because of some continued hemorrhage and the development of edema. It is important, therefore, to closely observe and monitor the ICP of such patients because significant and hazardous mass effect may evolve, requiring surgical extirpation.

With temporal or deep frontal contusions, late deterioration may occur, generally because of progressive edema development. The peak of such deterioration appears to be around 1 week, although cases have occurred as late as 10 to 14 days. Most of these patients will complain of severe or increasing headache or their CT images will show progressive edema formation. As such, a high index of suspicion must be accompanied by liberal use of follow-up CT imaging and, in particular, not dropping the level of surveillance until both the clinical situation and the CT appearance are stable.

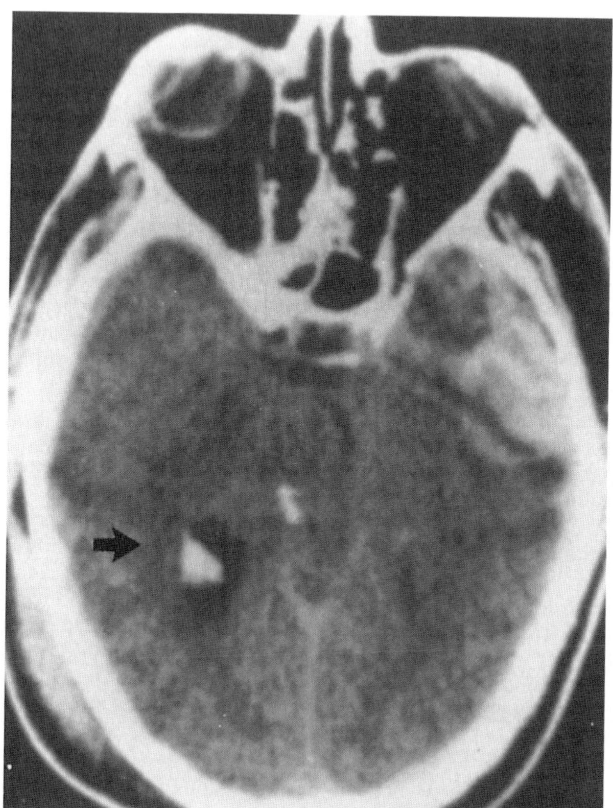

FIGURE 21.6 Contusion and associated intracerebral hematoma in the frontotemporal area.

The typical CT appearance of subarachnoid hemorrhage is a layer of blood over the cerebral cortex, layering over the tentorium and commonly filling the basal cisterns. Cerebral edema appears as areas of decreased density, which may be either focal or diffuse. Posttraumatic edema formation generally takes hours to days to develop unless compounded by hypoxia or hypotension. The "swollen brain" commonly seen in the setting of trauma may be caused by edema or increased CBV (unclotted, intravascular blood is low density). Diffuse axonal injury, typical of acute acceleration-deceleration injury, appears on CT scan as small areas of focal hemorrhage in the brainstem, thalamus or deep nuclear region, corpus callosum, and hemispheric white matter and cerebral swelling. Finally, gunshot wounds or other penetrating injuries can be evaluated with CT scanning to allow accurate preoperative assessment of the anatomic injury for prognostic and therapeutic planning purposes.

One significant issue of recent origin is the "blossoming" or appearance of new lesions subsequent to CT images obtained at very short intervals following injury. Reports as recent as 5 to 10 years ago often presented initial CT data from studies done hours following trauma. With improved prehospital transport and the ready availability of CT imaging, many initial studies are now performed 15 to 30 minutes after injury. As a result of such ultra-early CT scanning, there is now a risk of missing significant intracranial lesions by imaging before their appearance or during an early phase of their evolution. For this reason, in any patient with intracranial pathology or intracranial hypertension, we routinely obtain an early follow-up CT image at 4 to 6 hours after admission. At that time, CT imaging of the cervical spine can also be done in an effort to facilitate its clearance.

Ancillary Imaging

As noted above, there is a significant association between TBI and injury to the axial skeleton, particularly to the cervical spine. In addition, particularly when associated with basilar skull fractures or facial fractures, TBIs suggest the possibility of damage to the major arteries of the neck. As such, particular attention should be given to careful radiographic clearance of the spine and consideration to studies such as CT angiography of great vessels rostral to the aortic arch.

DEFINITIVE MANAGEMENT

Surgical Decompression and Outcome

Mass Lesions

The possibility of a mass lesion must be entertained in any patient who develops evidence of herniation (see Fig. 21.2). Under optimal circumstances, this herniation can be reversed medically (with hyperventilation and mannitol), allowing an emergent CT scan, which will demonstrate the location and size of any intracranial mass lesions and any herniation caused by nonsurgical processes.

When CT scanning is not immediately available or herniation is refractory to medical management, emergency trephination is a useful and lifesaving option. The first burr hole is placed in the ipsilateral temporal region and the dura is opened if an epidural hematoma is not in evidence (Fig. 21.7). If this exploration is negative, a second hole is placed in the opposite temporal region. If this is unrewarding, serial trephines are performed in the region of the parietal boss and the frontal convexity, first on the ipsilateral side, then contralaterally. A burr hole exploration is not negative until six holes have been drilled. A positive trephine is turned into a craniotomy, and the hematoma is thoroughly evacuated.

The upcoming *Guidelines for the Surgical Management of Traumatic Brain Injury* (in press) represents an evidence-based analysis of the present body of literature with respect to surgical indications in the management of TBI. Because this information has not been published yet, it is not presented in detail here. Nevertheless, because of the extreme relevance that the

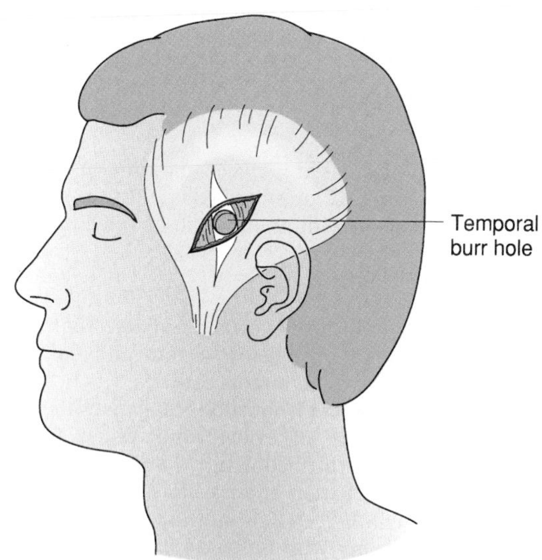

FIGURE 21.7 Location for placement of initial exploratory burr hole in the temporal region for emergency diagnosis and decompression.

indications for neurosurgical operative management have for trauma care, a synopsis follows.

Epidural Hematomas

Epidural hematomas are frequently of arterial origin and have a tendency to expand. Prognosis varies directly with level of consciousness at time of surgery, ranging from 0% mortality for patients conscious throughout, to 27% with the classic lucid interval, to over 50% if the patient never regains consciousness. Aggressive surgical management has resulted in an overall mortality of about 9%.[30]

An epidural hematoma larger than 30 mL, clot thickness greater than 15 mm, or midline shift over 5 mm should be surgically evacuated regardless of the patient's GCS score. In patients with a GCS score of 8 or less, evacuation should be emergent. If the GCS is highter than 8, evacuation should be done as soon as possible but may not interfere with other resuscitative efforts unless there is evidence of progressive deterioration. It is strongly recommended that patients with any acute epidural hematoma with anisocoria undergo surgical evacuation as soon as possible. Epidural hematomas of less than 30 mL, clot thickness below 15 mm, and midline shift less than5 mm should be considered for evacuation because the risk of evacuation appears less than the dangers of enlargement and neurologic injury. Epidural hematomas of this size in patients with GCS scores above 8 may be considered for nonoperative management, including frequent neurologic monitoring in an ICU setting and serial CT imaging. Although the mean time for enlargement of such lesions is approximately 8 hours after trauma, they may occur at intervals up to 36 hours.

Subdural Hematomas

Subdural hematomas are more common, particularly in non–motor-vehicle trauma. For subdural hematomas, the prognosis is less optimistic, with mortality rates of approximately 50%. To a great extent, this is related to the often-significant injury to the underlying brain.

An acute subdural hematoma with a thickness greater than 10 mm or midline shift above 5 mm on CT should be surgically evacuated, regardless of the patient's GCS score. Evacuation should be on an emergency basis if the initial GCS is less than 8. In patients with higher GCS scores, evacuation should be as soon as reasonably possible. A comatose patient (GCS score ≤8) with a subdural hematoma with less than 10 mm thickness and midline shift below 5 mm should undergo surgical evacuation of the lesion if any of the following apply:

- The GCS score decreased between the time of injury and hospital admission by 2 or more GCS points
- The patient presents with asymmetric or fixed and dilated pupil(s)
- The ICP exceeds 20 mm Hg

Patients with subdural hematomas of less than 10 mm thickness and midline shift below 5 mm and GCS scores greater than 8 can be treated nonoperatively.

It appears that outcome from subdural hematomas is proportional to the timing of evacuation. When surgery is planned, it should be performed within 4 hours whenever possible.[31] If surgical evacuation of an acute subdural hematoma in a comatose patient (GCS ≤8) is indicated, it should be done using a full craniotomy with or without bone flap removal and duraplasty.

All patients with acute subdural hematoma in coma (GCS score <9) should undergo ICP monitoring, including in the initial stages following evacuation.

Parenchymal Lesions

Surgery for intraparenchymal mass lesions remains controversial. Arguments against surgery include the risks of the operation itself as well as damage to tissue that may otherwise go on to recover. Arguments for surgery focus on preventing the hazards of intracranial hypertension caused by the lesion itself or progressive edema formation. Much of the difficulty in determining the applicability of surgery in individual situations arises from our inability to consistently predict which patients will rapidly deteriorate (e.g., proceed on to herniation) or fail nonoperative therapy by developing intracranial hypertension refractory to medical therapy. Unfortunately, this controversy has not been adequately addressed by well-done clinical investigations, so recommendations remain based on class III evidence. One thing that does appear consistent is that lesions of the anterior temporal lobe or the deep basilar frontal lobe are particularly dangerous because of the risk of precipitous herniation without impressive ICP elevation.

In general, patients with any lesion greater than 50 mL in volume should be treated operatively. Additionally, patients who have parenchymal mass lesions and signs of progressive neurologic deterioration referable to the lesion, medically refractory intracranial hypertension, or signs of mass effect on CT scan should be considered for surgery.

Patients with GCS scores of 6 to 8 should be treated operatively if they have frontal or temporal contusions greater than 20 mL in volume with either midline shift over 5 mm or cisternal compression on CT scan.

Patients with parenchymal mass lesions may be managed nonoperatively if they do not show evidence for neurologic compromise, have controlled ICP, and have no significant signs of mass effect on CT scan. Such patients should be managed with intensive monitoring and serial imaging. Surgery should be readdressed if difficulties with control of intracranial hypertension lead to consideration of "second tier" therapies (e.g., hypothermia or barbiturate coma) so as to avoid the secondary complications of such therapy. In all nonoperatively treated patients with parenchymal mass lesions, surgery should be considered before reaching the medical "point of failure."

Surgical management may involve decompression to "make room" for the lesion-induced swelling, evacuation or débridement of the offending lesions, or a combination of the two. Because evacuation of such lesions does not always eliminate the development of intracranial hypertension, extensive craniotomy with expansile duraplasty and without replacing the bone flap should be considered at the time of operation.

Diffuse Injury

The mortality rate of diffuse brain injury is directly related to the significance of the associated intracranial hypertension. As such, the mortality rate of diffuse injury with open basilar cisterns is approximately 13%, whereas compression or absence of cisterns has an associated mortality rate of about 38%. Diffuse injuries are not amenable to surgical therapy unless decompressive craniectomy is indicated for control of intractable intracranial hypertension.

Diffuse axonal injury is a reasonably distinct subset of diffuse brain injury. It is characterized on CT scan as small areas of focal hemorrhage in the brainstem, thalamus or deep nuclear region, corpus callosum, and hemispheric white matter which may be associated cerebral swelling. Intracranial hypertension is an inconsistent part of this syndrome. When ICP is elevated, however, successful management improves outcome. These patients tend to recover to varying extents; many of them will significantly improve in their level of consciousness but will generally be left with diffuse neurologic deficits (e.g., spasticity, cognitive impairments). Although a favorable prognosis seems to be correlated with fewer lesions on imaging studies and early improvement in level of consciousness, prognostication is difficult in individual cases of diffuse axonal injury.

Posterior Fossa Lesions

Posterior fossa lesions are particularly protean because the progression from a benign lesion to a critical lesion is so precipitous and deadly. Patients may rapidly deteriorate from awake and alert to comatose, with signs of herniation ("upward" [caused by uncompensated swelling in the posterior fossa] or "downward" [from hydrocephalus]). Because of difficulties with the technology and uncertainly as to what pressures might be critical, monitoring of posterior fossa intracranial pressure is rarely performed. Vigilant clinical observation, tempered with a high degree of preemptive concern, therefore, represents the only form of monitoring currently applicable.

In light of the available published evidence, rapid suboccipital craniectomy for evacuation of acute traumatic posterior fossa mass lesions is recommended in patients with neurologic dysfunction or deterioration referable to the lesion or mass effect on CT scan. Mass effect on CT scan appears as distortion, dislocation, or obliteration of the fourth ventricle, compression or loss of visualization of the basal cisterns, or presence of obstructive hydrocephalus. In general, surgery is recommended for any clot larger than 3 cm in diameter, whereas conservative management may be considered with clots smaller than 3 cm when not associated with acute subdural or epidural hematomas. Because of the potential for rapid, unheralded deterioration, evacuation should be performed as soon as possible in patients with indications for surgical intervention.

Depressed Skull Fractures

Skull fractures are a common result of head trauma and, when closed and not displaced, rarely require treatment *per se*. When displaced (generally defined as beyond the inner table of the skull), surgical intervention should be considered for the management of underlying intracranial pathology or cosmesis. The best available evidence does not support elevation for the prevention or treatment of epilepsy. As such, nonoperative management of closed (simple) depressed skull fractures is a routine treatment option.

Treatment of open, depressed fractures is focused primarily on avoidance of infection Cosmesis is a secondary consideration. In general, patients with open (compound) skull fractures depressed greater than the thickness of the skull should undergo operative intervention to prevent infection. Indications for nonoperative management are given in Table 21.2.

When surgery is indicated, early operation is recommended to reduce the incidence of infection. Elevation and débridement is recommended as the surgical method of choice. Primary bone fragment replacement is a surgical option in the absence of wound infection at the time of surgery.

All management strategies for open (compound), depressed fractures should include antibiotics regardless of whether surgery is undertaken. The exact nature of the antibiotics used and the duration of treatment remain inadequately delineated in the existing literature. The general tendency is the use of broad-spectrum antibiotics (versus gram-positive and gram-negative aerobic and anaerobic bacteria) for 1 to 2 weeks.

Penetrating Injuries

Penetrating injuries to the brain present several unique management problems, including the prophylaxis and treatment of intracranial infection, the possibility of epilepsy, and the risk of occult vascular injuries.

Although plain radiographs may be useful in determining intracranial trajectory, CT scanning of the head is the modality of choice in penetrating brain injury (PBI). In addition to the standard axial views with bone and soft tissue windows, coronal sections may be helpful in patients with skull base or high convexity involvement.

Angiography or CT angiography should be considered in patients with PBI. It is strongly recommended in cases in which the wound's trajectory passes through or near the Sylvian fissure, supraclinoid carotid, cavernous sinus, or a major venous sinus because of the increased risk of traumatic aneurysm or arteriovenous malformation. Sentinel signs of vascular abnormalities are large initial hematomas or the delayed development of substantial and otherwise unexplained subarachnoid hemorrhage or hematoma. When discovered, such vascular lesions should be definitively managed.

A major complication of penetrating injury is infection, both meningitis and abscess. Most infections occur within 3 weeks (55%) to 6 weeks (90%). The major risk factors appear to be CSF leaks, air sinus wounds, or wound dehiscence. The incidence of infection with the use of broad-spectrum antibiotic treatment ranges from 1% to 11%. Although the main causative agent appears to be *Staphylococcus*, gram-negative bacteria are also frequent and *Clostridium* or other anaerobic organisms may be found with appropriate culture techniques. As such, antibiotic prophylaxis is indicated in all penetrating injuries. The choice of antibiotics and the proper duration for their administration have not been formally investigated. Broad-spectrum regimens, including anaerobic coverage, lasting for 7 to 14 days appears to be a reasonable approach.

Seizures are much more frequent following PBI than nonpenetrating injury in general. Between 30% and 50% of patients with PBI develop seizures; 4% to 10% of those have their first seizure within the first week after injury and 80% during the first 2 years. About 18% may not have their first seizure until 5 or more years after injury. The risk decreases markedly with time. When followed for 15 years after a PBI, nearly 50% of patients with epilepsy eventually stop having

TABLE 21.2 INDICATIONS/CONTRAINDICATIONS

INDICATIONS FOR NONOPERATIVE MANAGEMENT OF COMPOUND DEPRESSED SKULL FRACTURES

No clinical or radiographic evidence of:

- Gross wound contamination
- Significant intracranial hematoma
- Gross cosmetic deformity
- Frontal sinus involvement
- Dural penetration
- Depression >1 cm
- Wound infection
- Pneumocephalus

TRAUMA

seizures. Of patients with PBI, 95% remain seizure-free if they have no seizures during the first 3 years after injury.

Although there is a distinct lack of rigorous study, the increased incidence of early seizures has led to the recommendation that antiseizure medications (e.g., phenytoin, carbamazepine, valproate, phenobarbital) should be used during the first week after PBI. Prophylactic treatment with anticonvulsants beyond the first week after PBI has not been shown to prevent the development of new seizures and is not recommended.

The surgical management of penetrating wounds to the brain has undergone significant evolution over the past two decades. In the more distant past (and until recently, in terms of U.S. military policy), it was routine to fully explore penetrating injury tracts to completely remove all foreign substances. Reoperation was common for this purpose. Based on class III evidence from military actions of other countries (most from the Middle East), however, it is now recognized that outcomes are not measurably worse in patients who do not undergo aggressive débridement. At present, surgical débridement of the missile tract in the brain is not recommended in the absence of significant mass effect. As well, routine surgical removal of fragments lodged distant from the entry site or reoperation solely to remove retained bone or missile fragments is not recommended.

Treatment of small bullet entrance wounds to the head in patients whose scalp is not devitalized and have no significant intracranial pathology should consist of local wound care and closure. In more extensive wounds with nonviable scalp, bone, or dura, surgical management with more extensive débridement followed by primary closure or grafting to secure a watertight wound is recommended. Closure of the dura and prevention of CSF leakage are extremely important goals in managing penetrating wounds. In patients with significant fragmentation of the skull, débridement of the cranial wound with either craniectomy or craniotomy is recommended.

Mass lesions should be surgically managed to prevent intracranial hypertension. As such, débridement of necrotic brain tissue and safely accessible bone fragments is recommended when they produce significant mass effect. As well, evacuation of intracranial hematomas is recommended if they produce significant mass effect as defined by the production of midline shift of over 5 mm or intracranial hypertension. This is one of the reasons that monitoring of ICP in penetrating injuries is an important adjunct to surgical decision making.

Repair of an open-air sinus injury with watertight closure of the dura is recommended.

Decompressive Craniectomy for Control of Intracranial Hypertension

Craniectomies done in conjunction with hematoma evacuation (usually on admission) must be separated from craniectomies done only for brain edema treatment (ICP/CPP management). The former consist of "leaving the bone out" and not closing the dura after surgery, which is done to evacuate extraaxial or (more rarely) intracranial mass lesions. The surgery, per se, is not done simply to increase the size and compliance of the cranial compartment to allow for brain swelling.

Craniectomies done to treat brain swelling involve intentionally removing very large bone flaps, leaving them out, and performing duraplasties to prevent the dura from constraining the bulging brain. The most common scenario is that of diffuse swelling wherein bilateral frontotemporoparietal flaps are removed. When edema is localized primary to one hemisphere (producing intracranial hypertension with midline shift), unilateral craniectomy is usually performed. In both cases, the bone flaps are as large as possible and particular attention is paid to removing the temporal squame forming the lateral wall of the middle cranial fossa.

Other surgical approaches to managing the swollen brain include subtemporal decompression and temporal lobectomy. In subtemporal decompression, the procedure is focused entirely on removing the lateral wall of the middle cranial fossa to decompress the temporal lobe. Temporal lobectomy involves removing a portion of the temporal lobe to "make room." The right temporal lobe is generally chosen because of its less elegant nature. By definition, the operation involves removing undamaged or only partially damaged brain, which certainly decreases its attractiveness when alternatives exist. In addition, it is generally realized that the amount of room made by such operation is rapidly filled by swollen brain such that intracranial hypertension often soon returns. In the author's practice, this operation has been completely replaced by decompressive craniectomy.

The goal of decompressive craniectomy is to completely obviate further ICP treatment. To this end, extensive bone removal and duraplasty are recommended.

Although it has not been rigorously studied in well-controlled, prospective fashion, the present evidence base definitely supports decompressive craniotomy within 48 hours of injury as a treatment option for patients with diffuse, medically refractory posttraumatic cerebral edema and resultant intracranial hypertension. One of the difficulties in determining the proper timing for such a procedure is the issue of when intracranial hypertension becomes medically refractory. The point of failure of second tier treatments is a clear but unacceptably late threshold. In general, decompressive craniectomy should be considered as an option to instituting such second tier treatment. In the interest of performing decompression before damage occurs from ICP elevation, many support its use prophylactically as soon as a high degree of suspicion arises that medical management will fail before ICP control is attained. Examples of such decision points are patients with diffuse parenchymal injury with clinical and radiographic evidence for impending transtentorial herniation (e.g., obscuration of the basal cisterns or midline shift >5 mm) where the initial ICP is very high or where early management requires rapid escalation in the intensity of treatment.

Intracranial Pressure Monitoring

All patients with severe brain injuries and a significant percentage of those with moderate injuries require continuous ICP monitoring. *Guidelines for the Management of Severe Brain Injury* indicates that class II evidence supports monitoring of all patients with a postresuscitation GCS score equal to or less than 8 who either have any CT evidence of intracranial pathology or have a normal CT scan but two or three of the following: (a) age greater than 40 years; (b) any history of hypotension; or (c) abnormal motor posturing. ICP monitoring in other patients is left to the discretion of the physician. ICP monitoring should be considered in any patient with a GCS of 12 or less who cannot be closely monitored clinically or whose CT scan demonstrates evidence of intracranial hypertension (i.e., mass lesion, obscured or absent basal cisterns, or midline shift).

Although many techniques are available, the most common involve small fiberoptic or strain gauge catheter tip pressure sensors placed several millimeters into the brain or fluid-coupled catheters placed into the lateral ventricles. The minimally invasive catheters are reliable and have a very low complication rate, making them an ideal choice in instances where a minimum-risk ICP monitoring technique is desired (e.g., in a moderate head injury that needs general anesthetic). They are also useful when the ventricles are too small to cannulate or there is an uncorrected coagulopathy. Ventriculostomy catheters have the added capability of allowing CSF drainage for ICP control. They are technically more difficult to place, however, and the complication rate is somewhat higher. In any case, a monitoring technology is available for any instance in which ICP monitoring is desired.

Monitoring ICP not only provides early warning of herniation but also, by allowing calculation of CPP, opens up the possibility of more precisely optimizing CBF and preventing ischemic secondary brain injury. Because all methods of lowering ICP have potentially harmful side effects, using such agents to treat suspected intracranial hypertension without monitoring ICP is not recommended.

MEDICAL MANAGEMENT

General Measures

Aggressive restoration of intravascular volume, maintenance of adequate cerebral perfusion pressure, and avoidance of hypoxia are the *conditio sine qua non* of medical treatment for intracranial hypertension. Volume resuscitation should be vigorous and thorough, with a target of euvolemia. The poorly founded, dangerous, and outmoded practice of restricting fluid volume should be abandoned. Restrict free water by using isotonic fluids, which makes normal saline preferable to lactated Ringer's solution. Optimally, continuous monitoring of central venous and arterial pressures should be instituted early.

Control of pain and the response to noxious stimuli is necessary to avoid iatrogenic elevation of ICP. It should not be assumed that the comatose patient has a blunted pain response. Analgesia should be combined with sedation, using short-acting agents whenever possible to facilitate repeated neurologic examination. It is preferable to use sedatives that concomitantly decrease cerebral metabolism to increase the margin for hypoperfusion tolerance. Propofol is a good choice for this reason, albeit its use is proscribed in children.

Neuromuscular blockade may be added to sedation and analgesia if further ICP control is desired. It does not always work so a trial is often considered. Blockade to the level of one to two twitches out of a train-of-four is a reasonable target in this population.

Guidelines for the Management of Severe Brain Injury does not support the early administration of antiepileptic medication for the prophylaxis of late seizures.[10] With respect to the prevention of early seizures (e.g., occurring within 10 to 14 days), prophylaxis does decrease their frequency but without proved benefit in outcome. As such, administration of antiepileptic agents for the first 2 weeks is at the discretion of the physician. One reasonable approach is to treat only in cases where seizures could compromise tenuous ICP control or when seizures are likely not to be detected (e.g., during neuromuscular blockade).

Fever will elevate ICP, generally through increasing CBV. Local measures (e.g., cooling blankets, fans) should be used in conjunction with acetaminophen to keep temperatures below 37.5°C to 38°C when ICP requires treatment. Scheduled indomethacin may prove effective in cases where acetaminophen is not.

Venous drainage of the brain should be facilitated by avoiding constriction of the jugular system in the neck and elevating the head of the bed in euvolemic patients. In addition, attention should be paid to intrathoracic pressures, particularly when considering the use of positive end-expiratory pressure (PEEP) or continuous positive airway pressure (CPAP). Finally, meticulous general critical care is important, because the protracted ICU stay and the necessity for intubation, mechanical ventilation, and other artificial support systems significantly increase the risk of nosocomial and iatrogenic complications.

Recent investigations in the trauma population in general have demonstrated an increased risk of complications, such as the acute respiratory distress syndrome and the systemic inflammatory response syndrome in patients who undergo transfusion. This has led to a reticence to transfuse and a strong tendency toward accepting hematocrit levels in the low 20s. On the other hand, evidence indicates that the injured brain is exquisitely sensitive to secondary insults such as ischemia. Unfortunately, there is little evidence that the damage caused by such events can be treated or reversed. As such, the general neurosurgical recommendation is to maintain an oxygen-carrying capacity that is higher than that afforded by such low hemoglobin levels, more commonly striving to values of approximately 30. In the absence of definitive studies, the choice of threshold for transfusion remains nebulous.

Control of Established Intracranial Hypertension

Cerebrospinal fluid drainage, hyperventilation, mannitol, barbiturates, and so on are the mainstays of therapy to control documented intracranial hypertension. Each, however, has significant potential complications, which can obviate their beneficial effects. Therefore, they should not be employed unless intracranial hypertension is established by monitoring and caution and vigilance must attend their usage. Although the treatment of intracranial hypertension is not the primary focus of this chapter, some brief comments will be useful.

As noted, the treatment of intracranial hypertension should be initiated on a base of adequate sedation and analgesia, control of fever, and optimization of systemic physiologic conditions that might exacerbate ICP elevation (e.g., intrathoracic pressure). Treatment for intracranial hypertension from *Guidelines for the Management of Severe Brain Injury* is outlined in Algorithm 21.4. When consulting this algorithm, remember that it represents a consensus opinion (class III evidence). When it was developed, the role of hypertonic saline was not addressed. This algorithm is in the process of revision.

When available via ventriculostomy, CSF drainage should be the first method of managing intracranial hypertension. There is no consensus on what pattern of drainage is most efficacious. It must be noted that ICP measurement cannot be performed when the ventricular catheter is open to drain. For this reason, we generally drain against approximately 10 cm H_2O for 2-minute intervals, then reclamp the catheter and measure the ICP.

As discussed, mannitol is useful for treating intracranial hypertension. There are no specific physiologic indications for the use of mannitol over other agents. Mannitol should be avoided under conditions of hypovolemia or increased serum osmolarity (i.e., >320 mOsm/L). When administered, mannitol should be given as a bolus. It appears that lower doses (e.g., 0.25 g/kg) are equally as effective in lowering ICP as larger doses (e.g., 1 g/kg).[19] No adequate evidence exists to guide the choice between mannitol and hypertonic saline when osmolar treatment is being considered.

Hypertonic saline is becoming an increasingly common tool in the management of traumatic brain injury. Its efficacy in reversing intracranial hypertension has been best demonstrated in children, where administration of 3% NaCl to osmolarity thresholds of up to 360 mOsm/L and serum sodium levels of up to 160 mEq/L are tolerated. Because of a lack of outcome-based studies, however, the independent ability of such treatment to improve outcome remains unclear.

There has been a strong tendency to extrapolate such use of hypertonic saline to the treatment of intracranial hypertension in adults where it has been less well studied. Doses are generally in the 0.5 to 1.0 mEq/kg/hour range. The tolerable limits for serum osmolarity and sodium levels have not been well defined in adults, but the levels used in children appear to be reasonably tolerated. A risk of rebound cerebral edema appears to exist when levels are allowed to drop too quickly after the administration of 3% saline is stopped. Our present practice is to not consider the patient "out of the

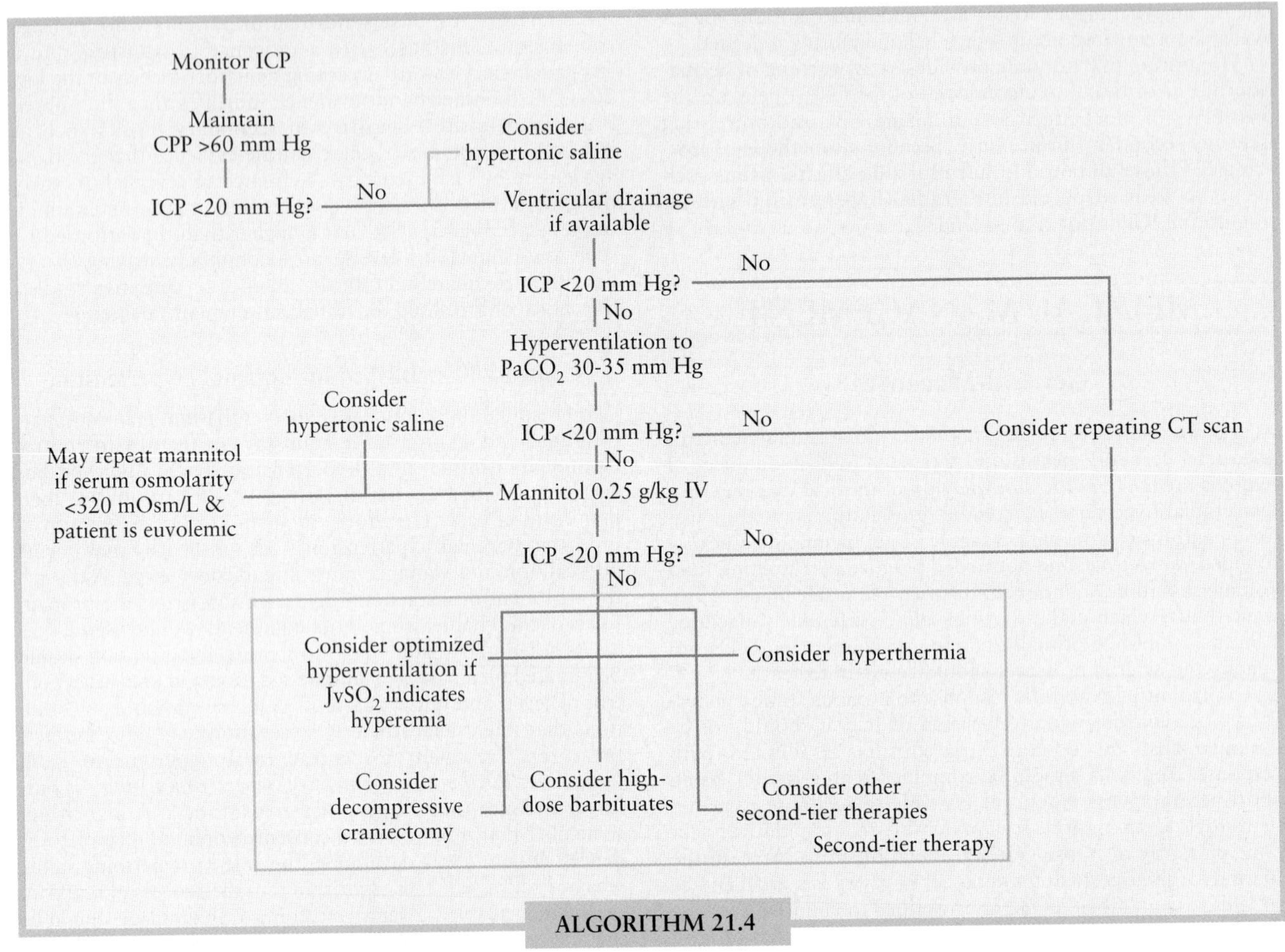

ALGORITHM 21.4 Approach to the early care of the patient with severe traumatic brain injury from the revised *Guidelines for the Management of Severe Brain Injury*. The necessity of the ABCs is stressed, accenting the establishment of a satisfactory cerebral perfusion pressure. The decision tree for employing hyperventilation and administering mannitol is also illustrated. The importance of safely and quickly obtaining a computed tomography scan of the brain in directing the choice between surgery or intracranial pressure monitoring should be noted. (After Bullock R, Chesnut R, Clifton G, et al. The Brain Trauma Foundation. The American Association of Neurological Surgeons. The Joint Section on Neurotrauma and Critical Care. Guidelines for the Management of Severe Head Injury—Revision. *J Neurotrauma* 2000;17:457–627, with permission.)

woods" for such rebound until the serum sodium has returned to within normal limits. As such, we generally leave the ICP monitor in and caution against major, nonemergent surgical cases.

Hyperventilation is generally effective in lowering ICP. As noted, however, it works by vasoconstriction-induced decreases in CBV, which allows the possibility of inducing ischemia by embarrassing CBF. At present, no clinically applicable method exists for measuring CBV, and it is unclear how often elevated CBV *per se* is a primary physiologic abnormality in intracranial hypertension. Therefore, lowering CBV to treat intracranial hypertension includes risks that need be minimized.

In keeping with *Guidelines for the Management of Severe Brain Injury*, hyperventilation ($Pa{CO_2}$ <35 mm Hg) should be avoided during the first 24 hours following TBI.[19] Thereafter, if intracranial hypertension maintains, hyperventilation to $Pa{CO_2}$ values between 30 and 35 mm Hg may be considered. Whenever hyperventilation is used, and certainly when $Pa{CO_2}$ values of less than 30 mm Hg are targeted, methods of monitoring the effects on CBF or flow-perfusion matching should be considered, such as quantitative CBF measurement, jugular venous saturation monitoring, or following cerebral tissue oxygen saturation.

When ICP control does not respond to these management steps, second tier therapies should be considered. These include barbiturate therapy, hypothermia, decompressive craniectomy, and optimized hyperventilation (among other approaches). The details of the choice between second tier agents are beyond the scope of this chapter. In general, the choice should be based on and directed using as much multimodality monitoring as is available, because the risk:benefit ratio of most of these treatments is very narrow.

KEY POINTS

- **Traumatic brain injury (TBI) results from both primary (impact disruption of brain and vascular tissue) and secondary (hypoxia, hypotension, pyrexia, effects of elevated ICP and biochemical processes) insults.**

- Secondary insults are often the determining factor in outcome and, unlike primary injury, are amenable to medical intervention and, thus, the focus of care.
- Increases in ICP are deleterious because of herniation or ischemia (due to decreased cerebral blood flow), and ischemia is primarily prevented by maintaining the cerebral perfusion pressure at greater than 60 mm Hg.
- Initial increases in ICP are treated by removal of mass lesions (blood collections or edematous injured brain) or with osmolar therapy using mannitol or hypertonic saline to decrease edema.
- Persistent ICP elevation may be treated with CSF drainage, hyperventilation, and barbiturates or hypothermia. Hyperventilation should be avoided early ($PaCO_2$ 35 to 38 mm Hg) and used cautiously ($PaCO_2$ 30 to 35 mm Hg) later to treat unresponsive elevated ICP.
- Assessment of the head-injured patient requires evaluation of (a) level of consciousness (using GCS); (b) pupil asymmetry, dilation or loss of light reflex; and (c) best motor response to painful stimulus.
- Computed tomography is the diagnostic test of preference and should be used serially in settings of increased risk of progression of TBI.

References

1. Center for Disease Control. Surveillance data on traumatic brain injury. *MMWR* 1997;46:8–11.
2. **Chesnut RM, Marshall LF, Klauber MR, et al. The role of secondary brain injury in determining outcome from severe head injury. *J Trauma* 1993;34:216–222.**
3. Jones PA, Andrews PJ, Midgley S, et al. Measuring the burden of secondary insults in head-injured patients during intensive care. *J Neurosurg Anesthesiol.* 1994;6:4–14.
4. Lang EW, Chesnut RM. A bedside method for investigating the integrity and critical thresholds of cerebral pressure autoregulation in severe traumatic brain injury patients. *Br J Neurosurg.* 2000;14:117–126.
5. Chesnut RM. Avoidance of hypotension: condition *sine qua non* of successful severe head-injury management. *J Trauma* 1997;42(suppl):S4–S9.
6. **Clifton GL, Miller ER, Choi SC, et al. Fluid thresholds and outcome from severe brain injury. *Crit Care Med.* 2002;30:739–745.**
7. Chesnut RM. Hyperventilation versus cerebral perfusion pressure management: time to change the question. *Crit Care Med.* 1998;26:210–212.
8. Cruz J. The first decade of continuous monitoring of jugular bulb oxyhemoglobin saturation: management strategies and clinical outcome. *Crit Care Med.* 1998;26:344–451.
9. Robertson CS, Valadka AB, Hannay HJ, et al. Prevention of secondary ischemic insults after severe head injury. *Crit Care Med.* 1999;27:2086–2095.
10. **Bullock R, Chesnut RM, Clifton G, et al. The Brain Trauma Foundation. The American Association of Neurological Surgeons. The Joint Section** on Neurotrauma and Critical Care. Guidelines for the Management of Severe Head Injury—Revision. *Journal of Neurotrauma* 2000;17:457–627.
11. Robertson CS, Cormio M. Cerebral metabolic management. *New Horizons* 1995;3(3):410–422.
12. van Santbrink H, Maas AI, Avezaat CJ. Continuous monitoring of partial pressure of brain tissue oxygen in patients with severe head injury. *Neurosurgery* 1996;38:21–31.
13. **Kiening K, Unterberg A, Bardt T, et al. Monitoring of cerebral oxygenation in patients with severe head injuries: brain tissue PO_2 versus jugular vein oxygen saturation. *J Neurosurg.* 1996;85:751–757.**
14. Kaufmann AM, Cardoso ER. Aggravation of vasogenic cerebral edema by multiple-dose mannitol. *J Neurosurg.* 1992;77:584–589.
15. Chesnut RM, Gautille T, Blunt BA, et al. Neurogenic hypotension in patients with severe head injuries. *J Trauma* 1998;44:958–963.
16. Marion DW, Carlier PM. Problems with initial Glasgow Coma Scale assessment caused by prehospital treatment of patients with head injuries: results of a national survey. *J Trauma* 1994;36:89–95.
17. **Gabriel EJ, Ghajar J, Jagoda A, et al. Guidelines for prehospital management of traumatic brain injury. *J Neurotrauma* 2002;19:111–174.**
18. Chesnut RM, Gautille T, Blunt BA, et al. The localizing value of asymmetry in pupillary size in severe head injury: relation to lesion type and location. *Neurosurgery* 1994;34:840–855.
19. **Bullock R, Chesnut R, Clifton G, et al. Guidelines for the Management of Severe Head Injury. *Journal of Neurotrauma* 1996;13:639–734.**
20. **Aarabi B, Alden TD, Chesnut RMD JH, et al. Guidelines for the management of penetrating brain injury. *J Trauma* 2001;51(suppl):S1–S86.**
21. **Adelson PD, Bratton SL, Carney NA, et al. Guidelines for the acute medical management of severe traumatic brain injury in infants, children, and adolescents. *Pediatr Crit Care Med.* 2003;4(suppl):S1–S71.**
22. Vassar MJ, Perry CA, Gannaway WL, et al. 7.5% sodium chloride/dextran for resuscitation of trauma patients undergoing helicopter transport. *Arch Surg.* 1991;126:1065–1072.
23. Vassar MJ, Fischer RP, O'Brien PE, et al. A multicenter trial for resuscitation of injured patients with 7.5% sodium chloride. The effect of added dextran 70. The Multicenter Group for the Study of Hypertonic Saline in Trauma Patients. *Arch Surg.* 1993;128:1003–1011; discussion 11–13.
24. Vassar MJ, Perry CA, Holcroft JW. Prehospital resuscitation of hypotensive trauma patients with 7.5% NaCl versus 7.5% NaCl with added dextran: a controlled trial. *J Trauma* 1993;34(5):622–632; discussion 32–33.
25. Cooper DJ, Myles PS, McDermott FT, et al. Prehospital hypertonic saline resuscitation of patients with hypotension and severe traumatic brain injury: a randomized controlled trial. *JAMA* 2004;291:1350–1357.
26. Rosner MJ, Coley IB. Cerebral perfusion pressure, intracranial pressure, and head elevation. *J Neurosurg.* 1986;65:636–641.
27. **Stein SC, Ross SE. Mild head injury: a plea for routine early CT scanning. *J Trauma* 1992;33:11–13.**
28. Mendelow AD, Teasdale G, Jennett B, et al. Risks of intracranial haematoma in head injured adults. *Br Med J Clin Res Ed.* 1983;287:1173–1176.
29. Marmarou A, Anderson RL, Ward JD, et al. Impact of ICP instability and hypotension on outcome in patients with severe head trauma. *J Neurosurg.* 1991;75(suppl):S159–S166.
30. Marshall LF, Gautille T, Klauber MR, et al. The outcome of severe head injury. *J Neurosurg.* 1991;75(Suppl):S28–S36.
31. Seelig JM, Becker DP, Miller JD, et al. Traumatic acute subdural hematoma: major mortality reduction in comatose patients treated within four hours. *N Engl J Med.* 1981;304:1511–1518.

CHAPTER 22 ■ MAXILLOFACIAL TRAUMA

RICHARD A. HOPPER AND JOSEPH S. GRUSS

Facial trauma often accompanies life-threatening injuries and is a warning of concomitant airway, central nervous system, visceral, and orthopedic injuries.[1] Although the associated life-threatening injuries demand immediate attention, it is the severity of facial trauma that has a direct correlation with the ability of patients to return to preinjury work.[2] Because of the significant role that facial appearance serves in our ability to function daily, and the density of functional units within the craniofacial skeleton, injuries in this region can cause life-long debility that precludes functioning in society.

Current management of complex facial trauma aims to restore and maintain the normal anatomy of the craniofacial skeleton. Comprehensive clinical examination and computerized tomography are used to establish the severity and extent of facial fractures and to identify injuries that require urgent treatment. Definitive operative treatment is performed as soon as the patient is stable to minimize the secondary problems of massive edema, bony collapse, and soft tissue shrinkage. Craniofacial surgical techniques are used to expose the facial skeleton through limited incisions, to achieve anatomic reduction of the fractures, to restore occlusion and orbital volume, and then to use rigid internal fixation to stabilize the reconstructed skeletal framework for uncomplicated fracture healing. Because the long-term results of timely treatment far exceed those of delayed treatment, it is essential that the definitive care phase of a trauma victim include the early detection, evaluation, acute management, and appropriate referral of maxillofacial injuries.

EPIDEMIOLOGY

Maxillofacial trauma includes soft tissue injuries, dentoalveolar damage, facial bone fractures, and combinations of these. The epidemiology of these injuries is directly related to social structure, geography, and economics, all of which influence the activities of a population. Consequently, significant regional and national variability is seen in the etiology and incidence of maxillofacial trauma patterns.[1–3] Despite this epidemiologic variation, maxillofacial injuries are relatively common in all societies and are present in up to one third of seriously injured patients with multisystem trauma.[4]

The incidence of facial trauma as a whole peaks in the first decade of life and slowly degrades over the remaining decades of life.[1–3,5] The incidence of facial bone fractures, in contrast, peaks in the third decade of life. Counter to the trend of increasing incidence of facial bone fractures in the first three decades of life, the actual relative risk per accident of facial bone fractures increases with increasing age (4.4%/year of life) because of the associated decrease in bone density.[1] Most injuries in the first decade of life are isolated soft tissue lacerations or dentoalveolar trauma (tooth impaction, alveolar process fractures, crown fractures, and so on) as opposed to the facial bone fractures seen in the adult population.

The causes of facial trauma include motor vehicle crashes (automobile, motorcycle, bicycle, and pedestrian), interpersonal violence, falls, industrial injuries, sports-related trauma, and ballistic injuries. In the United States and Japan, motor vehicle crashes and interpersonal violence continue to be the major causes of facial bone fractures,[2,5] whereas in European studies, sports and activities of daily life are predominant.[1] A relationship exists between mechanism of injury and age. Falls predominate as a mechanism of injury in the first decade of life and then again after the fifth decade of life. Sports-related injuries and motorcycle crashes occur more often within the second decade of life. Motor vehicle crashes and interpersonal violence predominate in the third and fourth decades of life.

Approximately 20% of all patients with facial soft tissue, dentoalveolar, or facial fracture trauma have associated injury to additional organ systems.[1] Motor vehicle crash victims with facial injuries have a relatively high associated rate of neurologic (32%), orthopedic (31%), visceral (24%), and ophthalmologic (14%) injuries. Personal assault has a lower association with neurologic (11%) and ophthalmologic (4%) injuries.[3] When facial fractures are present in patients suffering an occupational injury, an average of four associated injuries are seen for every facial fracture present and 2.4 associated injuries for every facial fracture present in a victim of a motorcycle crash.

INITIAL EVALUATION

Although maxillofacial injuries can be visually distracting to the trauma team members, they must not cause deviation from the established Advanced Trauma Life Support (ATLS) protocols. Rarely is facial trauma itself directly life threatening; however, it should be viewed as a strong indicator of a significant mechanism of injury with associated injuries. Within the ATLS algorithms, there are considerations specific to maxillofacial injuries.

Airway Management

Airway compromise in maxillofacial injuries can result from direct laryngeal injury, foreign bodies (including aspirated teeth and bone fragments), or active bleeding from an upper airway source. Treatment of the compromised airway is complicated by the likelihood that 10% of patients with facial trauma have a cervical spine injury.[6] As initial treatment, any blood clots should be suctioned from the oropharynx, and a finger sweep is used to remove foreign material from the oral airway. Comminuted fractures of the mandible can lead to loss of support of the hyomandibular complex, and consequent ptosis and retroposition of the tongue. Manual anterior traction on the mandible symphysis often temporarily resolves this obstruction until definitive control of the airway can be achieved.

For definitive control of the airway, an artificial oral or nasal airway is often possible, but blind nasal intubation should be carried out with caution. Nasal intubations can exacerbate bleeding from the nasal and nasopharyngeal regions, and the tube may be inadvertently placed into the cranial fossa in the obtunded patient with a comminuted skull base fracture. In the case of severe maxillofacial injuries (e.g., a gunshot wound to the face), intubation is often easier than expected, because the missing or pathologically mobile jaws allow an unprecedented view of the glottis. As with all patients with facial trauma, those with significant maxillofacial injury should have a secured airway early in the trauma assessment. The secondary swelling that occurs over the first few hours following the trauma can impede, or in some cases prevent, oral intubation.

Emergent tracheotomy is rarely indicated except in the unusual circumstance of laryngeal fracture or the inability to intubate orally because of massive bleeding or swelling. Semielective tracheostomy in the operating room is reserved for those patients requiring prolonged intubation because of massive soft tissue and bony injuries or impaired consciousness.

Massive Hemorrhage

The elaborate vascularity of the head and neck can result in rapid, significant blood loss. The location of the injuries, however, allows sufficient access for direct pressure to control the hemorrhage. When possible, try to expose and visualize the source of bleeding before suture ligature or cautery to avoid collateral damage to adjacent structures.

Nasopharyngeal bleeding is common with maxillofacial injuries. The blood supply to the nose arises from both the internal and external carotid systems. The external carotid artery supplies the internal maxillary artery, whose sphenopalatine branch supplies the posterior nasal septum and lateral nasal walls, and the facial artery, whose superior labial branch supplies the anterior inferior nasal cavity. The internal carotid artery gives off the ophthalmic artery which in turn supplies the anterior and posterior ethmoidal arteries that perfuse the superior and anterior nasal septum. The most common site of epistaxis is at Kiesselbach plexus at the confluence of the anterior ethmoidal and superior labial arteries. Anterior bleeding is best controlled by formal anterior nasal packing of half-inch gauze coated with antibiotic ointment. The tail of the gauze is left exposed, and with the aid of a nasal speculum, good lighting, and bayonet forceps, the gauze is carefully layered and packed back and forth along the nasal floor until the roof is reached. The direction of packing is directly posterior, then inferior. Prefabricated nasal packing is also available.

Posterior nasal bleeding (e.g., from the sphenopalatine artery) requires posterior packing. A 16 or 18 Foley catheter is inserted into the nasopharynx through the nostril. The balloon is then inflated and pulled anteriorly against the vomer and posterior soft palate. The catheter is secured in this position with a clamp at the nostril. A rolled gauze is used to protect the columella from pressure necrosis. Posterior packing will stop the posterior bleeding from draining into the airway but will divert the flow of blood anteriorly out the nose. The posterior packing must therefore be augmented with anterior packing.

Surgical ligation of the external carotid artery will not control bleeding from its injured branches because of the robust collateralization present. Selective ligation, such as of the ethmoidal vessels through a radix incision or of the internal maxillary artery through a Caldwell–Luc incision, is possible but rarely feasible in the emergency department. If the patient is stable enough to undergo general anesthesia, the most effective way to address bleeding that is not controlled by packing is through reduction and rigid fixation of the fractures.

Recalcitrant bleeding is treated by angiographic embolization. The source vessels are identified angiographically and then occluded with embolization material (e.g., Gelfoam). At Harborview Regional Medical Center in Seattle, from 1985 to 2000, of the 62,366 trauma cases, 7,147 had craniofacial trauma. During this same period, of the 3,529 cases of radiographic embolization, only four were performed on patients with craniofacial trauma. This emphasizes that although radiographic embolization is a component of the treatment algorithm of maxillofacial bleeding, the vast majority of cases can be treated with other means.

Ocular Injury

Direct injury to the eyeball should be suspected in all patients with orbital fractures or lacerations to the periorbital region. One prospective study reported a 29% incidence of ocular injury in 49 patients with orbital fractures.[7] Pain, decreased vision, and the appearance of spots before the eyes are all highly suggestive of globe damage. During the neurologic phase of trauma assessment, a brief clinical ophthalmologic examination should be performed, including visual acuity, pupillary response to light and accommodation, extraocular range of motion, globe position, and turgor. If there are any abnormal findings on the examination, an immediate ophthalmologic consult should be obtained for examination of the retina and ocular pressures. Injuries that may require immediate ophthalmologic treatment or result in permanent sequelae include corneoscleral lacerations, lens dislocation, major hyphema, acute glaucoma, and retinal detachment.

Blindness at the time of presentation is rare but is an extremely poor prognostic factor for future sight. Patients who have light perception at the time of presentation but who then demonstrate progressive loss of vision during the trauma assessment must be treated aggressively. The most common cause of this presentation is traumatic optic neuropathy secondary to optic nerve compression from a retrobulbar hematoma, a bone fragment, or edema. The management of progressive vision loss remains controversial, for it is unclear which patients benefit from emergent optic nerve decompression. If the eyeball is tense, then immediate lateral canthotomy is indicated to release the confining force of the lids. If a clear source of compression is visualized on computed tomography (CT) scan, immediate operative decompression is indicated.[8] All other patients are treated with high-dose steroids.[9]

Cerebrospinal Fluid Rhinorrhea

Actively search for cerebrospinal fluid (CSF) leaks in patients with craniofacial or high maxillary fractures. Clear or serosanguineous nasal discharge, anosmia, or a salty taste in the mouth are highly suggestive. A CSF leak into the nasal cavity implies a defect in the pia-arachnoid and an abnormal communication between the subarachnoid space and the external environment. The thin bone in the anterior skull base and the close adherence of the dura to the anterior fossa and cribriform plate predisposes to penetration of fracture fragments into the subarachnoid space. Common associated fracture patterns that are detailed later in the chapter include Le Fort II and III midface fractures, naso-orbital ethmoid (NOE) patterns, orbital roof fractures, and displaced fractures of the posterior table of the frontal sinus. CSF is differentiated from serum on laboratory examination by its low protein concentration and from normal nasal secretions by the presence of glucose but no mucin.

Most CSF fistulas close spontaneously. Morgan et al. reported a 35% incidence of CSF rhinorrhea in 300 patients with severe facial fractures, of which 66% resolved spontaneously by the fifth postinjury day and 87% by the tenth day.[10] Fistulas that do not close spontaneously can be visualized on a metrizamide contrast CT scan, followed by surgical exploration and obliteration of the fistula using a dural patch.

Occlusion

Occlusion is the contact of the posterior masticating (chewing) and anterior incising (cutting) surfaces of the maxillary and mandibular teeth. Malocclusion is an indicator of orthognathic fracture or dental injury. The maxillary teeth should overlap the mandibular teeth in normal occlusion in three ways: (a) overjet describes the horizontal projection of the upper front teeth in front of the lower teeth; (b) overbite describes the vertical overlap of the upper front teeth over the lower teeth; and (c) the posterior maxillary arch should be wider than the mandible arch on both sides by the space of one cusp. Typical malocclusion patterns seen following fractures include an anterior open bite (gap between the upper and lower front teeth) that indicates the fractured maxilla is impacted upward, or that both condyles of the mandible have collapsed; a posterior open bite (gap between the upper and lower back teeth), often associated with a unilateral condylar fracture; or a posterior crossbite (back teeth lateral or medial to the normal arch form) that indicates either a mandible fracture or a comminuted fracture of the maxilla and palate. These malocclusive patterns indicate that surgical intervention is indicated.

Missing or fractured teeth should be documented. If a tooth is missing, the oral cavity and airway should be carefully checked for the foreign body. Securing the tooth to an adjacent one with a wire can often salvage a loose or dislocated tooth. If a tooth is fractured with unstable fragments, the fragments should be removed to prevent entrance into the airway.

Neurologic Injury

Injury to the muscles of facial expression or the seventh cranial nerve can be particularly debilitating because of their importance in interpersonal interactions. The most common cause of facial nerve injury is fracture of the temporal bone in the intraosseous canal.[11] Penetrating injury to the facial branches of the seventh nerve require exploration and repair, whereas nonpenetrating injury is observed for recovery over a period of 3 to 6 months. Injury to the middle branches of the nerve distal to the parotid (zygomatic and buccal) can be masked by cross-innervation with other branches. The marginal mandibular (lower lip depressors) and temporal (brow elevation) branches have the least degree of cross-innervation and, therefore, more commonly result in functional problems.

COMPUTED TOMOGRAPHY DIAGNOSIS OF MAXILLOFACIAL FRACTURES: THE FACIAL BUTTRESSES

The functional units of the face are held together and stabilized by several vertical and horizontal skeletal buttresses (Fig. 22.1). These buttresses represent regions of relatively dense bone that serve to support the functional units of the face in an optimal relation and define the form of the face by projecting the overlying soft tissue envelope.[12] Additionally, the facial buttresses stabilize the face to the cranial base and determine the proper relationship between these two important structural units. Conceptualizing and describing maxillofacial fractures according to the involved buttresses is useful because it is directly related to the definitive surgical treatment. Each buttress can be visualized on the craniofacial CT scan.

There are four transverse and four paired vertical buttresses. Because of the reliance of facial form and function on these buttresses, as well as the mechanical force exerted on them, the craniofacial trauma surgeon typically treats any significant buttress displacement using anatomic reduction and rigid internal fixation.

As structural units that support the face, the buttresses must either directly or indirectly interface with the skull base or cranium as a stable reference. From superior to inferior, the transverse facial buttresses are as follows:

1. **Upper transverse maxillary buttress** runs from the temporal bone across the zygomatic arch and inferior orbital rim, superiorly to the frontal bone via the frontal process of the maxilla and then across to the contralateral temporal bone via a similar path. This buttress crosses the zygomaticotemporal, the zygomaticomaxillary, and the nasofrontal sutures, which are commonly involved in fracture patterns. The sagittal extension of this buttress lies in the orbital floors.
2. **Lower transverse maxillary buttress.** From the pterygoid projection of the skull base, it extends along the bone of the maxillary alveolar arch to the contralateral pterygoids. The sagittal extension of this buttress is the hard palate.
3. **Upper transverse mandibular buttress** is at the level of the mandible's alveolar arch.
4. **Lower transverse mandibular buttress** is at the inferior border of the mandible.

The paired vertical buttresses from lateral to medial are as follows:

1. **Posterior vertical mandibular buttress** is composed of the ascending ramus and condyle of the mandible; this buttress links the transverse mandibular buttresses with the skull base.
2. **Lateral maxillary buttress** is composed of the column of bone from the alveolar bone of the posterior maxillary molars across the zygomaticomaxillary suture and body of the zygoma, extending superiorly to the lateral orbital rim and across the zygomaticofrontal suture. The sagittal projection of this buttress includes the lateral orbital wall as it joins the sphenoid bone of the skull base.
3. **Medial maxillary buttress** comprises the column of bone from the alveolar bone of the anterior maxillary dentition, extending superiorly along the rim of the piriform aperture and frontal process of the maxilla, then across the nasofrontal junction to frontal bone. The sagittal projection of this buttress includes the medial orbital wall.
4. **Posterior maxillary buttress** comprises the column of bone at the pterygomaxillary junction where the pterygoid plates of the sphenoid join the posterior maxilla. These last three vertical buttresses support the transverse buttress of the maxillary occlusion.

Although other anatomic buttresses of the face can be conceptualized, the ones listed here meet the following critical criteria: (a) they are all linked either directly or through another buttress to the cranium or cranial base as a stable reference point; (b) they have sufficient bone thickness to accommodate metal screw fixation; and (c) with the exception of the posterior maxillary buttress, they are surgically accessible through standard limited surgical incisions. Accurate reduction and fixation of these facial buttresses restores projection, width, and height of the facial skeleton relative to the cranial base and, more importantly, establishes a functional support for the teeth and globes.

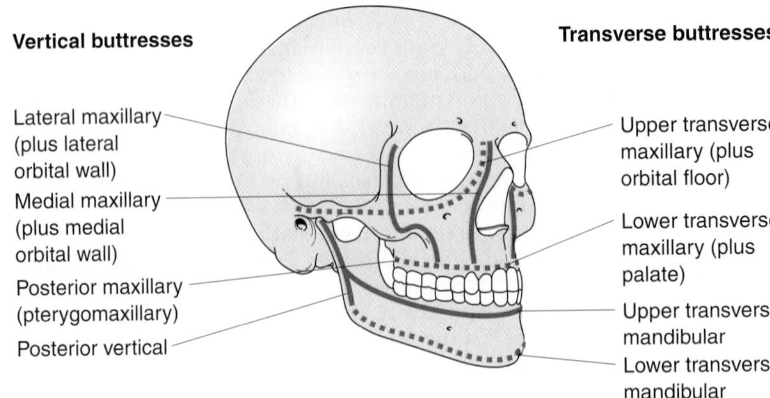

FIGURE 22.1 Illustration of adult skull demonstrating the four paired vertical and four transverse buttresses, all existing in areas of relative increased bone thickness.

PATTERNS OF INJURY

Naso-orbito-ethmoid Fractures

NOE fractures involve the central upper midface between the eyes, disrupting the confluence of the medial maxillary buttress with the upper transverse maxillary buttress. A fracture of the NOE complex can be one of the most difficult fracture patterns to accurately repair. Failure to restore the sagittal projection of this region and correct the rotation of the frontal process of the maxilla (superior portion of the medial maxillary buttress) results in a lack of upper nasal projection and telecanthus (increased distance between the inner corner of the eyes), both of which are difficult to correct as a secondary operation. The eyelids insert around the lacrimal fossa through the medial canthal tendon. If the tendon insertion is not returned to its correct position, the patient loses the normal shadow definition on either side of the nose, the medial corner of the palpebral fissure drifts laterally, and the eyes appear too far apart. If the distance between the medial canthi is greater than 30 mm, a NOE pattern should be suspected.

By definition, NOE fractures include damage to the ethmoid sinus and walls. If there is bilateral comminution and displacement in this region, the nasofrontal ducts that drain the frontal sinus are also likely disrupted. In this situation, the surgeon obliterates the frontal sinus by removing all of the sinus mucosa and filling the sinus with bone, fat, or some other tissue. Failure to diagnose disruption of the nasofrontal ducts and obliterate the sinus increases the risk of the patient developing a frontal sinus mucocele postoperatively.

Zygoma and Orbital Fractures

After nasal fractures, zygomatic fractures are the most common injury resulting from blunt trauma. The zygoma has two attachments to the cranium and two to the maxilla and forms a large portion of the orbital floor and lateral wall. These paired "cornerstone" bones are, therefore, surgically important in establishing orbital volume and in serving as a reference for maxilla reduction in Le Fort type maxillary fractures. The two major buttresses of the zygoma are the upper transverse maxillary (across the zygomaticotemporal and zygomaticomaxillary sutures) and the lateral vertical maxillary (across the zygomaticomaxillary and the frontozygomatic sutures). Fractures typically occur across these three buttress-related sutures, leading to the term "tripod fracture." This term fails to recognize the posterior relationship of the zygoma with the sphenoid bone of the skull base. A displaced orbitozygomatic fracture is really a quadripod fracture. If the two buttresses of the zygoma are reduced and fixated, it is still possible to have a rotational deformity of the zygoma about the zygomaticosphenoid suture. The surgeon pays particular attention to the alignment of the zygoma and sphenoid at the lateral orbital wall because angulation here, after fixation of the remaining buttresses, reflects a residual rotational deformity and an associated increased orbital volume.

If the zygomatic arch component of the transverse buttress is comminuted and is needed as a reference to establish facial projection following a panfacial injury, the only way to access this region is via the coronal scalp degloving approach. This procedure carries with it an associated increased blood loss, increased operating time, and risk of potential complications.

Orbital floor fractures can occur in isolation but are also commonly associated with zygoma fractures through posterior propagation of the fracture from the upper transverse maxillary buttress at the inferior orbital rim. The size and displacement of the orbital floor fragment must be known

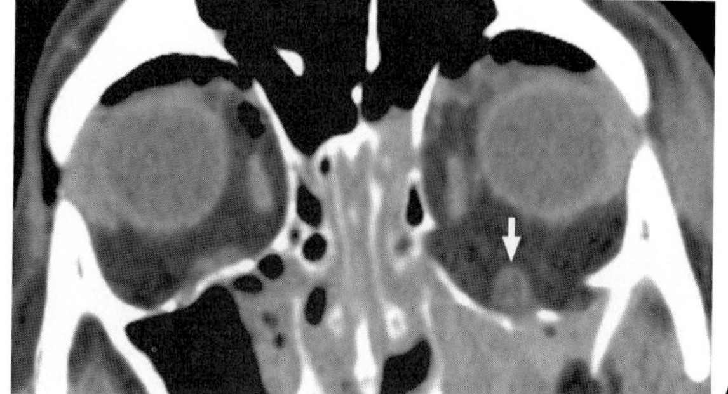

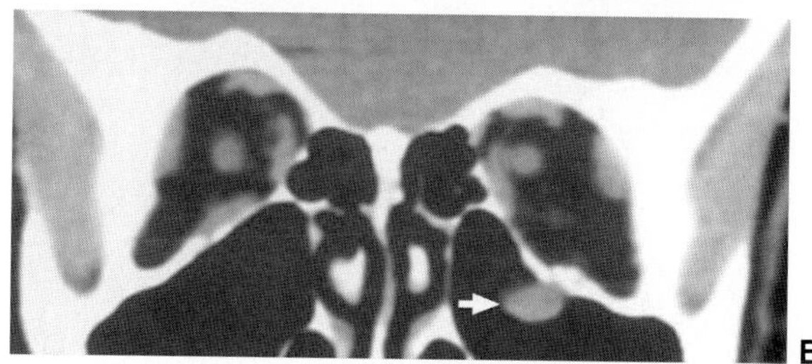

FIGURE 22.2 Computed tomography coronal plane, noncontrast images demonstrating two patterns of orbital floor blowout fractures. *Left:* A left orbital floor fracture with evidence of entrapment of the inferior rectus muscsle. The inferior rectus (*arrow*) is displaced inferiorly into the maxillary sinus. Note how the muscle cross-section has changed from ovoid to circular. The fascial support has been disrupted and the muscle is entrapped. *Right:* A pediatric trapdoor left orbital floor blowout fracture. The orbital floor was disrupted by the impact but then sprung back in place, trapping the inferior rectus muscle (*arrow*) within the maxillary sinus. Because the bone has returned to its anatomic location, this diagnosis can easily be missed unless attention is paid to the location of the extraocular muscles. Trapdoor fractures require emergent treatment to optimize the chance of recovery.

preoperatively to decide what treatment, if any, is required. The width of the defect of the floor can be estimated from the coronal reformat images, and the depth by counting the number of coronal cuts containing the fracture. Multiplying these two numbers gives an estimate of the area of the defect. Attention to the shape and position of the inferior rectus muscle on the coronal CT scan can provide information regarding damage to the fascial sling of the globe. If the rectus remains flattened on cross-section and in the correct position, the surgeon will likely encounter minimal entrapped periorbital tissue. If, however, the inferior rectus is round and inferiorly displaced, the fascial sling is disrupted and the periorbita and muscle have prolapsed into the orbital floor defect (Fig. 22.2A). Entrapment of the inferior rectus in children can be easily missed, because the flexible bone can spring back into place like a trapdoor and look normal on CT scan except for the entrapped muscle beneath it (Fig. 22.2B). This trapdoor fracture requires urgent treatment within 24 to 72 hours to minimize the chance of motility problems.[13]

Maxillary Fractures

With the exception of alveolar and palate fractures, maxillary fractures are commonly described according to the classification described by Rene Le Fort in 1901[14] (Fig. 22.3). Le Fort fractures involve a separation of all or a portion of the maxilla from the skull base. For this to occur, the posterior vertical maxillary buttress at the junction of the posterior maxillary sinus with the pterygoid plates of the sphenoid must be

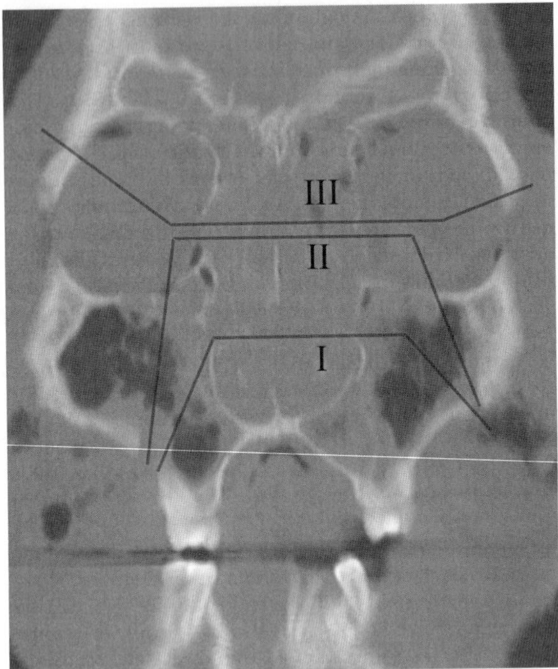

FIGURE 22.3 Computed tomography coronal plane, noncontrast image demonstrating bilateral Le Fort I, II, and III fractures in the same patient. The Le Fort I pattern has fractures through the inferior portions of the medial and lateral maxillary buttresses; the Le Fort II pattern is through the zygomaticomaxillary and frontomaxillary sutures; and the Le Fort III pattern is complete craniofacial dissociation. To confirm the diagnosis, pterygomaxillary disjunction and fractures of the zygomatic arches would need to be observed on axial plane images.

disrupted. This can be either through the posterior walls of the sinus or through the plates themselves as seen on axial CT images. Once a pterygomaxillary disjunction has been diagnosed, the remaining facial buttresses are inspected to determine the class of Le Fort fracture. If the inferior portions of both the lateral and medial maxillary buttresses are fractured, a Le Fort I fracture has occurred, and the maxillary arch (lower transverse maxillary buttress) will move in relation to the rest of the face and skull. If the inferior lateral maxillary buttress (zygomaticomaxillary suture) and the superior medial maxillary buttresses (frontomaxillary sutures) are fractured, then the entire maxilla will move in relation to the skull base as a Le Fort II fragment. If the upper transverse maxillary buttress (zygomatic arch), superior lateral (frontozygomatic), and superior medial (maxillofrontal) maxillary buttresses are fractured, then craniofacial separation has occurred as a Le Fort III pattern, with the entire face moving in relation to the skull base.

For all Le Fort fractures, the maxillary dental arch is mobile; therefore, the patient must be placed in maxillomandibular fixation before plating of the fractures. All buttresses can be plated with the exception of the buttress common to all Le Fort patterns—the pterygomaxillary posterior vertical buttress. Similar to zygomatic fractures, if there is severe comminution of a buttress, bone grafting may be required.

Mandible Fractures

Unlike the rest of the facial buttresses, isolated mandible fractures are typically diagnosed with plain radiograph series. In a trauma patient with multiple injuries, however, the diagnosis is often made on CT scan imaging as a disruption of the mandible arch. Fractures can occur at any point on the mandible, including, in decreasing order of frequency, the body, angle, condylar neck, symphysis and parasymphysis, ramus, and alveolar ridge. The condyles are best visualized on coronal images. Many condylar fractures are not directly fixated because of the difficulty in accessing this region surgically as a result of the proximity of the facial nerve, as well as the risk of iatrogenic temporomandibular joint (TMJ) dysfunction. In cases of bilateral condylar neck fractures associated with a severely comminuted Le Fort fracture, one condyle is typically exposed, reduced, and plated to reestablish a stable vertical buttress for reestablishing facial height. Intracapsular condylar injuries have a high risk of ankylosis and are treated conservatively with early range of motion if occlusion can be established.

TIMING OF DEFINITIVE REPAIR

There are two windows for optimum treatment of maxillofacial injuries. The first is in the first 6 to 12 hours following injury, before the onset of edema. With the exception of emergencies (e.g., optic nerve compression, uncontrollable facial bleeding, pediatric trapdoor orbital fractures), this phase is not feasible in a multisystem trauma victim because of the priority of other injuries. The most common timing for treatment of maxillofacial injuries is after the initial postinjury edema has subsided and the patient is cleared for the operating room. This is typically 3 to 7 days postinjury. Although facial fractures can be reduced up to 3 weeks postinjury, the soft tissue fibrosis and the early fracture callus make the procedure progressively more difficult starting 10 days after the injury. Mandibular fractures have been traditionally treated as open fractures, with definitive treatment within 24 hours.

SUMMARY

Maxillofacial injuries in a trauma victim should be considered an indicator of associated severe injuries. The initial evaluation within the ATLS protocol includes special considerations of airway management, ocular assessment, control of bleeding, identification of CSF leaks, and neurologic injury. The definitive treatment of maxillofacial injuries, following a structured history and physical examination, includes identification of damage to the facial buttresses on CT imaging. Displaced buttress fractures require open reduction and internal fixation in a timely fashion to minimize secondary soft tissue contracture and optimize the final functional and esthetic outcome.

KEY POINTS

- **Facial trauma is common (11% of all trauma patients), is frequently associated with life-threatening injuries, and should provide a warning of potential concomitant airway, central nervous system, and orthopedic injuries.**
- **Maxillofacial trauma is directly related to social structure, geography, and economics. Facial injury patterns vary according to age, risk-taking, and daily activities.**
- **Initial management of maxillofacial trauma follows ATLS principles and involves airway management, control of hemorrhage, and rapid identification of injuries with significant morbidity, ocular injury, CSF leakage, neurologic damage, and malocclusion.**
- **Structured history and physical examination and CT scan–guided diagnosis with reconstruction of major facial buttress damage using open reduction and internal fixation**

in a timely fashion is critical to optimize final functional and esthetic outcome.

Acknowledgment

We would like to acknowledge Dr. Patrick Kelley, our craniofacial fellow, for his contribution to the literature review of this chapter.

References

1. **Gassner R, Tuli T, Hachl O, et al. Cranio-maxillofacial trauma: a 10-year review of 9,543 cases with 21,067 injuries. *J Craniomaxillofac Surg.* 2003;31:51–61.**
2. Girotto JA, MacKenzie E, Fowler C, et al. Long-term physical impairment and functional outcomes after complex facial fractures. *Plast Reconstr Surg.* 2001;108:312–327.
3. **Haug RH, Prather J, Indresano AT. An epidemiologic survey of facial fractures and concomitant injuries. *J Oral Maxillofac Surg.* 1990;48:926–932.**
4. Sastry SM, Sastry CM, Paul BK, et al. Leading causes of facial trauma in the major trauma outcome study. *Plast Reconstr Surg.* 1995;95:196–197.
5. Iida S, Kogo M, Sugiura T, et al. Retrospective analysis of 1502 patients with facial fractures. *Int J Oral Maxillofac Surg.* 2001;30:286–290.
6. Sinclair D, Schwartz M, Gruss J, et al. A retrospective review of the relationship between facial fractures, head injuries, and cervical spine injuries. *J Emerg Med.* 1988;6:109–112.
7. **Jabaley ME, Lerman M, Sanders HJ. Ocular injuries in orbital fractures. A review of 119 cases. *Plast Reconstr Surg.* 1975;56:410–418.**
8. Stanley RB, Jr., Sires BS, Funk GF, et al. Management of displaced lateral orbital wall fractures associated with visual and ocular motility disturbances. *Plast Reconstr Surg.* 1998;102:972–979.
9. **Li KK, Teknos TN, Lai A, et al. Traumatic optic neuropathy: result in 45 consecutive surgically treated patients. *Otolaryngol Head Neck Surg.* 1999;120:5–11.**
10. Morgan BD, Madan DK, Bergerot JP. Fractures of the middle third of the face—a review of 300 cases. *Br J Plast Surg.* 1972;25:147–151.
11. Coker NJ. Management of traumatic injuries to the facial nerve. *Otolaryngol Clin North Am.* 1991;24:215–227.
12. **Gruss JS, Mackinnon SE. Complex maxillary fractures: role of buttress reconstruction and immediate bone grafts. *Plast Reconstr Surg.* 1986;78: 9–22.**
13. Grant JH, 3rd, Patrinely JR, Weiss AH, et al. Trapdoor fracture of the orbit in a pediatric population. *Plast Reconstr Surg.* 2002;109:482–489; discussion 490–495.
14. Le Fort R. Etude experimentale sur les fractures do la machoire siperieuve. *Riv Chir de Paris* 1901;23:208.

CHAPTER 23 ■ NECK TRAUMA

SAMAN ARBABI AND GREGORY J. JURKOVICH

The numerous vital structures of the neck are concentrated in a small anatomic area, generally unprotected by bone or dense muscular covering. Yet, because of its relatively small size, only 5% to 10% of traumatic injuries involve the neck. Although neck injuries occur infrequently, they often require prompt surgical management. Disruption of the airway or carotid circulation is an immediate, life-threatening problem, and esophageal or peripheral nerve injury can cause chronic morbidity. Penetrating injuries are most common and most severe, with fatality rates ranging from 1% to 2% for stab wounds, from 5% to 12% for gunshot wounds, and up to 50% for rifle or shotgun blasts.[1–3] Up to 50% of these deaths are preventable with appropriate early care. Significant blunt neck trauma is less common but can be particularly difficult to manage because it often involves the airway. Carotid or vertebral artery injury can also occur as a consequence of acute cervical spine hyperextension, even in the absence of bony injury. The initial diagnosis of these injuries can be difficult, but the consequences of missing an injury are severe.

As a general guideline, all patients with penetrating neck wounds that traverse the platysma muscle should be admitted to the hospital for evaluation, observation, and treatment. Likewise, all patients with blunt traumatic injuries of the neck should be admitted. This section focuses on the preferred and available diagnostic and treatment options for patients with blunt or penetrating neck trauma.

ANATOMY

The neck is classically divided into a number of anatomic triangles (Fig. 23.1). The two large anterior and posterior triangles are particularly important in neck trauma. Wounds to the posterior triangle rarely involve the esophagus, airway, or major vascular structures, although if the blow is directed inferiorly, intrathoracic injury can occur. In contrast, penetrating wounds that enter through either the sternocleidomastoid muscle or the anterior triangle carry a high likelihood of vascular, airway, or esophageal injury (Fig. 23.2).

The anterior neck is further divided into three zones defined by horizontal planes. Zone I represents the base of the neck and is variably defined. In Roon and Christensen classification,[4] zone I is defined as extending from the sternal notch to the lower border of the cricoid cartilage (Fig. 23.3). Injuries here carry the highest mortality rate because of the risk of major vascular and intrathoracic injury. Zone II is the central and largest portion of the neck. It extends from the top of zone I to the angle of the mandible. Zone II injuries are most common but carry a lower mortality rate than either zone I or III injuries, because injury is usually apparent and exposure of vital structures is readily accomplished. Zone III is that part of the neck above the angle of mandible. The risk of injury to the distal carotid artery, salivary glands, and pharynx is greatest in this zone. Exposure in this region can be particularly difficult.

The other major anatomic landmark in the neck is the platysma muscle. This thin, broad muscle lies just beneath the skin and covers the entire anterior triangle and the anteroinferior aspect of the posterior triangle. Wounds that fail to penetrate the platysma are considered superficial and do not warrant extensive evaluation. Wounds that penetrate the platysma must be considered a serious surgical problem that mandates hospital admission and further evaluation.

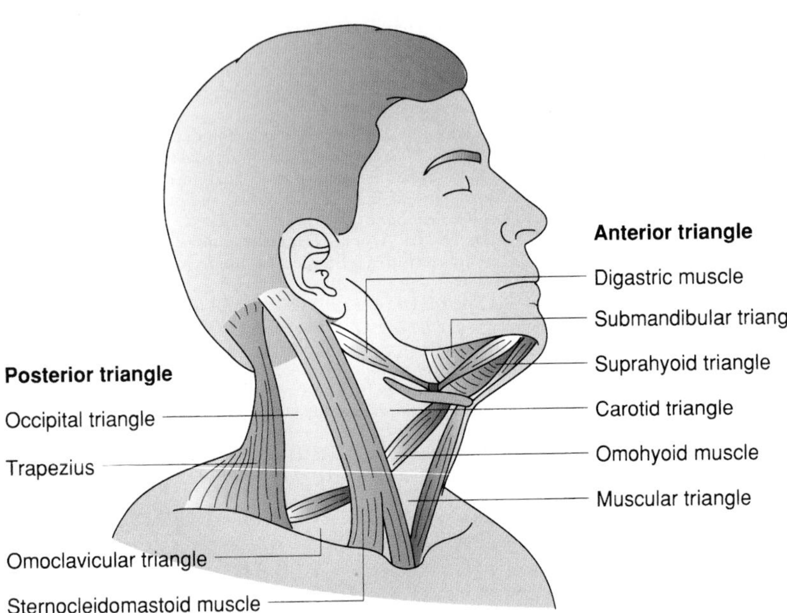

FIGURE 23.1 Anatomic triangles of the neck. The posterior triangle is composed of the smaller occipital and omoclavicular triangles. The anterior triangle has as smaller divisions the carotid, muscular, submandibular, and suprahyoid triangles.

INITIAL MANAGEMENT

The same priorities for initial care of the multiply injured patient apply to the management of isolated neck trauma. Airway control remains the primary tenet of initial trauma care, and it takes precedence over all other aspects of the evaluation and resuscitation. If injury involves the airway itself or surrounding structures, this management task takes on special significance. Rapid inspection for air movement, crepitus, hoarseness, and subcutaneous emphysema is the first step. Supplemental oxygen should always be administered, and adequate lighting and suction are essential. If spontaneous ventilation appears adequate, close observation and pulse oximetry monitoring are suggested, because acute decompensation can occur with little warning. If spontaneous respirations

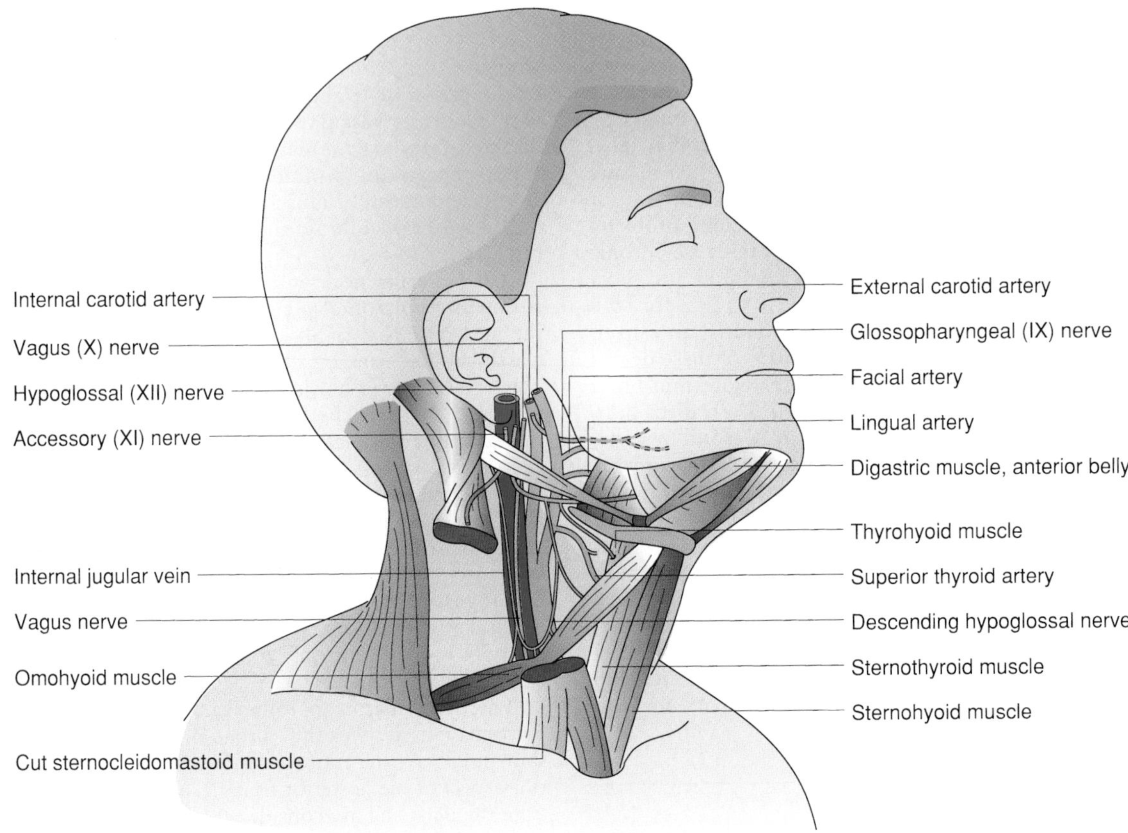

FIGURE 23.2 Proximity of cranial nerves to the carotid arteries of the neck. Trauma resulting in cranial nerve deficits in this region is often associated with vascular injury.

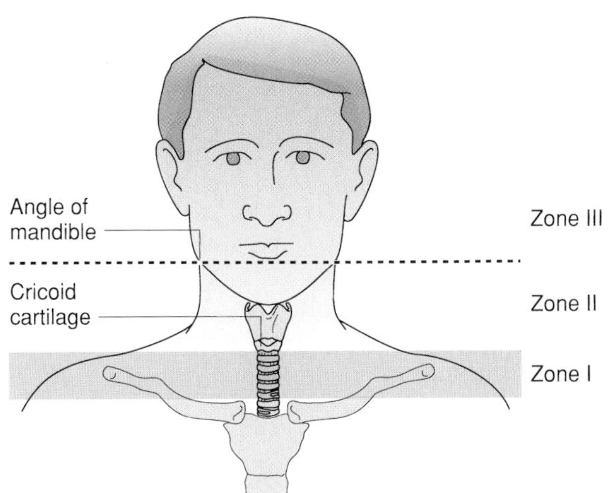

FIGURE 23.3 Zones of the neck. The junction of zones I and II is variously described as being at the cricoid cartilage or at the top of the clavicles. The important implication of a zone I injury is the greater potential for intrathoracic great vessel injury.

are inadequate, if blood or other material obstructs the airway, or if progressive cervical swelling from hemorrhage threatens to occlude the airway, emergency intubation is necessary. Procrastination converts a simple intubation into a potentially difficult and bloody emergency cricothyroidotomy. Direct visualization of the vocal cords and oral endotracheal intubation are usually preferred. If cervical spine injury has not been excluded, hyperextension of the neck must be avoided. Two-man intubation with in-line cervical traction is the preferred alternative to nasotracheal intubation.

A massive pharyngeal or neck hematoma can totally occlude the airway, making direct intubation impossible. Attempts at blind nasotracheal intubation cause further mucosal or laryngeal injury, and an emergency surgical airway (cricothyroidotomy or tracheostomy) is required. Occasionally, blunt laryngeal trauma is so severe as to disrupt and occlude the airway. The preferred method of controlling the airway in this setting is controversial, but provisions for a surgical airway must be at hand. Options include primary tracheostomy or a single attempt at endoscopically assisted endotracheal intubation. Temporization with transtracheal needle-jet insufflation can be a valuable adjunct in these settings.

Concurrent with airway control is awareness of potential cervical spine injury, particularly in unconscious patients who have sustained blunt head and neck trauma. The head and neck should be supported in the neutral position until this possibility is excluded radiographically and by physical examination. In the emergency room, support of the head and neck during manipulation or procedures is best accomplished by a strong, steady assistant rather than by collars, sandbags, or tape. The lateral cervical spine film is an essential component of the initial evaluation of patients with either blunt or penetrating neck trauma, both to assess the bony cervical spine and to evaluate soft tissues for edema or misplaced air.

The initial management subsequent to control of the airway follows the ABC guidelines of trauma care advocated by the Advanced Trauma Life Support course of the American College of Surgeons, with particular attention directed at adequacy of ventilation, treatment of shock, and baseline neurologic examination. Patients with blunt neck trauma often have concomitant thoracic injuries, and penetrating neck wounds may follow a caudal trajectory, injuring lung or intrathoracic great vessels, particularly if the entrance is in zone I.[5] Rapid physical examination of the thorax is, therefore, part of the initial evaluation of patients with neck trauma and should include inspection, palpation, and auscultation. Pneumothorax must be treated rapidly by needle decompression, tube thoracostomy, or both, and treatment should not necessarily be delayed for radiographic confirmation, particularly in the unstable patient. Major neck hemorrhage is treated with direct pressure. Blind clamping of vessels is discouraged to avoid inadvertent injury to adjacent nerve or esophagus. Adequate peripheral intravenous access is required in all patients with neck trauma and usually requires at least two peripheral intravenous catheters lines of 16 gauge or larger. Blood is drawn for typing and crossmatching and routine laboratory evaluations, and fluid resuscitation is initiated based on the degree of shock and anticipated potential ongoing hemorrhage. A rapid yet thorough neurologic examination is also part of the initial management, with particular attention to the patient's level of consciousness and the status of cranial and brachial plexus nerves. Changes in the results of serial neurologic examinations are key indicators of ongoing injury.

After the initial resuscitation, a complete physical examination is performed to detect associated injuries and to better define the extent of neck trauma. Close visual inspection of the neck alerts the physician to the possibility of underlying injuries and the mechanism of injury. For example, an oblique 4- to 6-cm bruise on the neck of a restrained passenger in a motor vehicle accident should alert the physician to the possibility of blunt cervical vascular trauma from a seatbelt injury. Neck wounds should not be probed for fear of dislodging a clot and reinstituting hemorrhage. The neck should be palpated with attention to normal anatomic landmarks and areas of tenderness. Crepitus or subcutaneous emphysema indicates injury to the trachea, esophagus, or lung until proved otherwise. Never assume that a penetrating skin wound itself is responsible for subcutaneous air. If the patient is able to talk, determine the presence of hoarseness, dysphagia, or dysphonia. Hemoptysis and hematemesis are also signs of tracheal or esophageal injury. Table 23.1 lists the clinical signs of significant injury that usually mandate neck exploration to exclude or treat vascular, airway, esophageal, or nerve injuries.

All patients with blunt or penetrating neck trauma should have a chest radiograph to help rule out thoracic trauma. Stable patients should have soft tissue neck films to look for retropharyngeal hematoma, tracheal narrowing or deviation, retained missile fragments and pathways, and subcutaneous or retropharyngeal air. Computed tomography (CT) of the neck is particularly helpful in blunt trauma to evaluate laryngeal structures to look for laryngeal fractures. Patients with blunt neck trauma whose neurologic examination is inconsistent with findings on head CT should undergo studies to evaluate for cervical vascular injury.

TRAUMA

TABLE 23.1 DIAGNOSIS

CLINICAL SIGNS OF SIGNIFICANT INJURY IN PENETRATING NECK TRAUMA

VASCULAR	DIGESTIVE TRACT
Shock	Hemoptysis
Active bleeding	Dysphagia or odynophagia
Large or expanding hematoma	Hematemesis
Pulse deficit	Subcutaneous emphysema
AIRWAY	**NEUROLOGIC**
Dyspnea	Focal or lateralized neurologic deficit
Stridor	
Hoarseness	
Dysphonia or voice change	
Subcutaneous emphysema	

TABLE 23.2

MANDATORY OPERATION COMPARED WITH SELECTIVE MANAGEMENT OF PENETRATING NECK TRAUMA

	Mandatory	Selective
Patients		
Number of series	11	24
Number of patients	1,653	2,540
Outcome		
Mortality rate (range)	5.85% (0.3%–11.0%)	3.75% (0%–9.8%)
Cases explored	1,492 (90.2%)	1,596 (62.8%)
Positive explorations	803 (53.8%)	1,117 (70.0%)
Cases observed	161 (9.8%)	944 (37.2%)
Delayed exploration	3 (1.9%)	20 (2.1%)
System injured		
Arterial injuries	213 (12.9%)	303 (11.9%)
Venous injuries	310 (18.8%)	459 (18.0%)
Esophagus or pharinx	163 (9.9%)	191 (7.5%)
Larynx or trachea	150 (9.1%)	181 (7.1%)

Modified from Asensio J, Valenziano C, Falcone R, et al. Management of penetrating neck injuries: the controversy surrounding zone III injuries. *Surg Clin North Am* 1991;71:267.

SELECTIVE VERSUS MANDATORY EXPLORATION

There is uniform agreement that all unstable patients and all patients with clinical signs of significant neck injury require prompt exploration. All other patients with wounds that penetrate the platysma should at least be admitted to the hospital and observed. Controversy exists, however, in the management of asymptomatic, stable patient with penetrating neck injury. Two distinct schools of thought exist, one advocating mandatory surgical exploration of all wounds that penetrate the platysma[2,6,7] and the other favoring a more selective approach.[8–12] A comprehensive review of selective versus mandatory operative management published in 1991 documents similar rates for injury incidence, overall mortality, and delayed complications, as well as similar hospital costs, but with a significant reduction of negative neck explorations in the selective management group[13] (Table 23.2). Most recent studies have advocated some type of selective management in a clinical setting, with explicit guidelines and involvement of expertise in the appropriate use of various diagnostic modalities.[14–17]

Advocates of a mandatory exploration policy cite the low morbidity and negligible mortality rate after negative neck exploration as justification for the high rate of negative findings (40% to 60%). The disastrous complications of missed injuries further support this stance. A 67% mortality rate is reported after delayed operations for neck vascular injuries, and a 44% mortality rate for delayed operations for esophageal injuries.[3] A 1986 literature review reported an overall mortality rate of 16.7% for patients initially observed after penetrating neck trauma who subsequently required surgical exploration.[18] In addition, a few reports have documented major structural injury in a small percentage of patients who undergo exploratory surgery despite a clinically silent physical examination; in one report, 5.5% of patients with wounds that appeared innocuous but were nevertheless explored had significant injuries.[7] Transcervical gunshot injuries represent a special category of neck wounds, with one report documenting the high likelihood of injuries to cervical structures (83%) and supporting aggressive surgical exploration in all cases.[19]

Supporters of a more selective approach berate the high incidence of negative explorations, the cost of a surgical exploration, and the fact that some injuries are missed despite surgical exploration. They also argue that the original data supporting mandatory neck exploration are based on World War II and Vietnam War experience with large-caliber, high-velocity projectiles, unlike the typical knife or handgun injury observed in civilian trauma. The wide availability and diagnostic accuracy of angiography, endoscopy, and esophagography further support a selective management plan. Merion and colleagues,[12] as part of a review of the cost of managing penetrating neck trauma, analyzed 27 reported series in which the clinical courses of more than 4,000 patients with penetrating neck trauma were documented. Of patients treated by surgeons advocating selective exploration, 52% underwent immediate operation, compared with almost 90% of patients treated by those advocating mandatory exploration. Reexamination of these series revealed that mortality rate was no different in the two groups, and only 2.4% of initially observed patients required subsequent operation.[18]

No uniform policy has been accepted for selective management of patients with penetrating neck injury in the absence of positive clinical findings. There is a general agreement that zone I and III injuries require diagnostic studies such as helical CT angiography, angiography, endoscopy, and esophageal contrast studies.[20] The management of zone II injury, however, is variable and subject to the experience and preference of individual surgeons and trauma centers.[14–17] The disagreement concerns whether patients should routinely undergo surgical neck exploration, undergo extensive diagnostic evaluation similar to zone I and III injuries, or simply be observed. Because a number of clinical reviews demonstrate similar patient outcomes, each institution or surgeon should adopt a management plan most consistent with local resources and experience.

At Harborview Medical Center in Seattle, all patients with neck wounds who are in hypovolemic shock or who have evolving stroke are immediately explored for vascular control. Most of those with neck wounds that penetrate the platysma in zone II undergo exploratory surgery, as do all patients with clinical signs of tracheal, esophageal, or major vascular injury. Preoperative angiography is usually not required for zone II injuries because of the relative ease of exposure and control of critical vascular structures. The track of the offending agent is followed throughout its course to exclude any possible vascular, tracheal, esophageal, or neurologic injury. Endoscopy is usually performed intraoperatively if pharyngeal, esophageal, or tracheal injury is suspected but cannot readily be identified.

Zone I and III penetrating injuries are selectively managed, based on clinical presentation and the results of diagnostic studies. Hemodynamically unstable patients undergo immediate exploratory surgery, with operative incision based on the most likely source of vascular injury. Zone I injuries are managed similar to mediastinal traversing wounds.[19,21] Angiography is performed in hemodynamically stable patients with penetrating wounds to zone I to identify potential injuries to the thoracic outlet vessels or to better plan the operative approach. Cinefluoroesophagography, first with water-soluble contrast material and then with thin barium, is performed after angiography for zone I injuries. Endoscopy is considered a complementary procedure to the esophagography, and should follow if any question of an abnormality exists.[22] Angiography is also performed for zone III injuries, because of the possible inaccessibility of internal carotid artery lesions or to demonstrate a need for systemic anticoagulation. In addition, most of the vascular lesions identified at the base of the skull are best managed by interventional angiography techniques. Esophageal studies are not done for zone III injuries.

EVOLUTION IN DIAGNOSTIC MODALITIES

Hemodynamically stable patients who sustain trauma with potential injury to the neck may be candidates for nonoperative management. Most of these patients lack the "hard" signs of injury such as expanding hematoma, active bleeding, significant air leak, or airway compromise.[23] These patients may be observed with assistance of diagnostic modalities when indicated. Traditionally, the most common studies are radiographic survey of the cervical spine, four-vessel angiography; esophagoscopy and/or esophagography; and bronchoscopy. Performing these studies, however, can be expensive and time-consuming. In addition, four-vessel angiography is an invasive test with potential for complications. A more selective approach to screen for cerebrovascular injuries is, therefore, warranted and has been practiced.[24] Recently with improvement of less invasive diagnostic methods such as helical CT angiography (CTA) or magnetic resonance angiography (MRA), there has been an effort to substitute such modalities for routine angiography.[25,26] A preliminary study demonstrated that helical CT scan may be an excellent early diagnostic tool in penetrating trauma.[23] In fact, high-resolution CTA has replaced angiography in evaluation of selected patients with potential for cerebrovascular injuries in some centers. The allure for helical CT is that it is a relatively fast, noninvasive test that can evaluate cervical spine, trachea, soft tissue, and vascular structures at the same time. Earlier data demonstrated CTA to be inadequate for screening of patients with blunt neck injury. In one of the largest series comparing CTA with traditional angiography in selected patients, the sensitivity and specificity of CTA was 47% and 53%, respectively.[27] The diagnostic accuracy of high-resolution helical CTA, however, has improved with advances in image technology, as well as increasing experience and expertise in evaluating these studies in trauma patients. Helical CT technology is rapidly changing, and the single-detector row is being replaced with a multidetector row configuration, generating 1-mm thick sections that are reconstructed at 0.5-mm intervals.[28] Recent data from the radiology literature are favorable with Munera et al. reporting a sensitivity and specificity of 90% and 100% in the diagnosis of carotid and vertebral artery injuries in selected patients with penetrating neck injury.[28–30]

The accuracy of helical CT scan in detecting esophageal injury has not been studied extensively. In one study, two (50%) of four esophageal injuries in patients with penetrating traumawere missed by CT. It is important to note that esophagography missed the same two esophageal injuries, as well.[31] The conclusion appears to be that CT scan is no better or worse than esophagography in screening for esophageal injury. Additional support for use of helical CT in penetrating trauma is the identification of the trajectory tract. Such findings may increase suspicion of injury to the aerodigestive tract, thus delineating the need for observation, esophagoscopy, or operative exploration.

Evaluation of the cervical spine to identify fractures following blunt trauma has been evolving from the traditional three-view plain film to helical CT scan with sagittal reconstruction. This is especially true in patients who require CT scan of the head. In the past CT was frequently used only to evaluate the cervical spine after incomplete or inadequate plain films. Patients required multiple trips to the radiology suite, increasing the cost, risk of complications, and the time to cervical spine clearance. Obtaining a helical CT scan of the cervical spine as the initial study has expedited time to spine clearance,[32] increased sensitivity,[33] and decreased costs.[34]

The combination of the above findings makes helical CT scan an ideal screening tool for neck injuries. One advantage of helical CTA is that it can be incorporated in the workup of a patient with blunt trauma who is having a head CT to evaluate intracranial structures because of concomitant head injury. Ideally, the cervical spine, soft tissue, and vascular structures are evaluated, without extra trips to plain radiology or the angiography suite. Other modalities (e.g., MRA) do not have the versatility of the helical CT scan and may not be appropriate for trauma patients. However, there remains a lack of data regarding the accuracy of helical CT. In fact, the largest study in the surgical literature raises doubt regarding the sensitivity and specificity of CTA in detecting vascular injury.[27] In addition, although CTA is less invasive than traditional angiography, the volume of contrast material used for helical CTA may be higher.[30] This is especially true when a focused study of the unilateral carotid or vertebral artery is desired rather than the four-vessel angiography. Therefore, a digital subtraction angiography may be preferred in patients with high risk for contrast-induced nephrotoxicity.[30] Further studies of helical CTA in evaluation of trauma patients is warranted before uniform acceptance of this diagnostic modality.

OPERATIVE EXPLORATION

Of patients with penetrating neck trauma (depending on mechanism), 25% to 50% present with obvious signs of injury requiring prompt operation. An additional 10% to 20% of patients without clinical signs of injury are discovered to have significant vascular, esophageal, or airway injury on further diagnostic testing. A physician treating patients with neck trauma must be capable of performing a complete neck exploration and repair of vascular and aerodigestive injuries. Neck exploration should be performed in the operating room under general endotracheal anesthesia. In the hemodynamically stable patient with a patent airway, intubation can be deferred until laryngoscopy and bronchoscopy have been performed in the operating room. A nasogastric tube is usually passed to ensure an empty stomach. Preparation and draping of the patient before induction of anesthesia allows control of hemorrhage if the patient starts to gag at the time of placement of the endotracheal tube. The chest is also auscultated before surgery, and a chest radiograph is routinely performed,

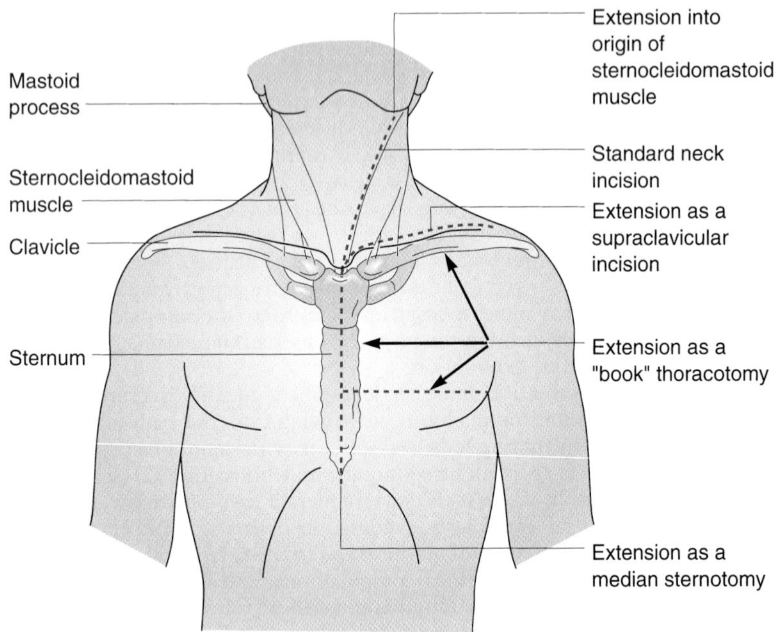

FIGURE 23.4 Neck exploration incisions. Extension of oblique or collar incision into a median sternotomy affords excellent exposure of the great vessels.

because penetrating injuries may follow a downward path with pleural penetration. A pneumothorax may not develop until positive-pressure ventilation is applied, and it may initially present as unexplained hypotension during anesthesia.

The incision is planned to allow full exposure of the tract of the injury (Fig. 23.4). The oblique incision along the anterior border of the sternocleidomastoid muscle is preferred for unilateral and high (zone III) injuries, whereas the transverse collar incision is preferable for bilateral or neck-traversing wounds. Extension of either neck incision into a median sternotomy affords excellent exposure of the thoracic great vessels. Proximal and distal control of the major vessels must also be considered in the length and position of the incision, and the patient is always surgically prepared for a possible median sternotomy. The tract of the injury is followed to its depth, systematically examining each structure in or near the tract.

MANAGEMENT OF SPECIFIC INJURIES

Blood Vessels

Blood vessels are the most commonly injured structures in the neck. Major arterial and venous injuries occur in 18% and 26% of penetrating neck wounds, respectively.[35] Blunt vascular injury accounts for perhaps only 3% of all carotid injuries.[36] An increase in blunt carotid injuries has been reported, perhaps because of better recognition.[37,38] The initial diagnosis, however, remains a difficult one and must always be suspected with appropriate mechanisms of injury.

Carotid Artery

In the largest series reported in English literature, 85 blunt carotid injuries were recognized in 67 patients over 11 years in a level I trauma center.[38] Motor vehicle crashes were the most common injury mechanism (82%), followed by motorcycle crashes (7%), and assaults (6%). All but two of the patients had associated injuries, and combinations of blunt carotid injury with closed head and cervical spine injuries occurred in 48% and 6% of patients, respectively. The initial physical examination demonstrated neurologic findings that were not compatible with brain CT findings in 34% and soft tissue injury in the anterior neck in 14% of the patients. A neurologic deficit developed subsequent to hospital admission in 43% of the patients. The average interval from injury to definitive diagnosis was 53 hours, highlighting the point that, although its recognition is often delayed, blunt carotid trauma must be suspected in patients who develop focal neurologic signs or symptoms after a latent interval. In a multicenter review, 29% of patients developed significant neurologic deficits >12 hours or more after admission.[39] Other physical findings—expanding hematoma, audible bruit, pulsatile neck mass, palpable thrill, Horner's syndrome, or any neurologic symptom not explained by other injuries—may be absent at the initial examination. Because some evidence suggests improved outcome with early diagnosis,[37–39] a high index of suspicion must exist if the mechanism of injury involves a direct blow to or compression of the neck, basilar skull fracture, cervical hyperextension and rotation, or blunt bilateral perioral fractures.[36] Table 23.3 lists screening criteria for blunt cerebrovascular injury in asymptomatic trauma patients.[24,27]

TABLE 23.3 DIAGNOSIS

SCREENING CRITERIA FOR SUSPECTED BLUNT CEREBROVASCULAR INJURY IN ASYMPTOMATIC PATIENTS

Cervical spine fracture in proximity to internal carotid or vertebral artery

- Skull base fracture extending into the carotid canal
- Le Fort II or III facial fracture
- Extensive soft tissue neck injury such as seat belt injury or hanging
- Diffuse axonal injury
- Mechanism associated with severe cervical hyperextension or hyperflexion

Currently, cerebral angiography remains the gold standard for diagnosis. Angiography is invasive, not risk-free, and time-consuming, however, and therefore not a suitable screening test. Helical CTA may soon replace traditional angiography in screening for blunt cervical vascular injury. Also, there is encouraging evidence regarding the use of duplex ultrasound and MRA as additional screening diagnostic tools.[40,41] These modalities, however, still lack sufficient evidence to demonstrate their accuracy and require the presence of around-the-clock expertise. Because of high costs, they may remain impractical to use as mass screening tools for patients with blunt trauma.[27] In a multicenter study, duplex ultrasound demonstrated 86% (12 of 14) of the arterial injuries, but was unable to discern dissection of the internal carotid artery at the base of the skull in two patients; proximal flow characteristics were also normal in both of these patients.[39,40] Use of MRA in screening of trauma patients has been limited because of practical problems such as monitoring in the MRI suite and lack of around-the-clock access. Most data regarding evaluation of cerebrovascular structures by MRA are in non-trauma patients.[42–44] In these studies MRA demonstrated a high accuracy in detecting vascular disease but remained less reliable than the gold standard digital subtraction angiography. The sensitivity of MRA in detecting cerebrovascular injuries in 143 patients with blunt trauma was only 50%.[27] This study, however, utilized a 0.2 Tesla open magnet, and current studies utilize 1.5 Tesla magnets with significantly better image quality. Improving image quality and increasing experience interpreting the findings will improve the accuracy of MRA in detecting cerebrovascular injury.

The mortality rate remains high with blunt carotid injury, ranging from 20% to 40%, with permanent neurologic impairment in 25% to 80% of survivors.[37–39,45] There is a reasonably good neurological outcome, better than 55%, for an uncomplicated arterial dissection and uniformly poor outcome, with close to 100% mortality, for complete arterial disruption or bilateral arterial occlusion.[37–39] Treatment is highly variable and the efficacy has not been proved in a prospective study.[37,38,46] Therapy depends on the type and location of the vascular lesion, concomitant injuries, availability of interventional techniques, and preference of the treating surgeon. Arterial dissections appear best managed by systemic anticoagulation.[38] For patients with contraindication to full anticoagulation, aspirin and antiplatelet therapy have been suggested.[37] The anticoagulation is to prevent thrombosis propagation or embolization. Stenting or primary surgical repair, in anatomically favorable locations, has also been used in the management of arterial dissection in small studies.[37–39,47] If it is anatomically feasible, pseudoaneurysms are resected. Larger inaccessible pseudoaneurysms are a difficult management challenge; the treatment includes anticoagulation, balloon occlusion, stenting, ligation, or extracranial-intracranial bypass.[46,48,49] Patients with carotid-cavernous fistulas have been treated with balloon occlusion with variable results.[38,39] The outcome of an arterial injury with complete vascular thrombosis depends more on the neurologic status than on any treatment regimen. Nonsurgical management seems appropriate for most of these patients.[45] The rare and fortunate patient with complete carotid thrombosis without neurologic deficits can best be treated with anticoagulation to prevent further or contralateral damage.

Patients with penetrating carotid artery injury most commonly present with exsanguinating hemorrhage. The principles of operative repair of vascular structures in the neck are the same as those for other major vessels. What makes neck vascular trauma unique is the intolerance of the perfused end-organ (brain) to even short periods of ischemia. The indication for repair versus ligation of a carotid injury in part depends on the neurologic presentation. Patients without a neurologic deficit should have restoration of vascular continuity, with a good neurologic outcome anticipated. Also, patients with all grades of neurologic deficits short of coma should also have primary vascular repair.[50] Although the experience with revascularization of patients suffering acute stroke from arteriosclerotic occlusive disease suggests that hemorrhagic infarction and death can result from revascularization, several reviews of acute revascularization in the trauma patient note that the combined morbidity and mortality rate is significantly lower in patients undergoing primary repair (15%) compared with those treated with arterial ligation (50%).[51–53] In comatose patients, neither repair nor ligation appears to influence what is a uniformly poor prognosis. Ligation of the carotid artery is indicated in the comatose patient with no prograde flow, in the presence of uncontrollable hemorrhage, or if technical reasons prohibit repair. There currently is little experience or evidence to favor extracranial–intracranial bypass in the patient requiring carotid artery ligation for trauma, although it has been used selectively in patients requiring selective carotid occlusion.[54,55]

Vertebral Artery

Traumatic injury to the vertebral artery, once only rarely diagnosed, is now more commonly identified, certainly because of the liberal application of neck angiography after both penetrating and blunt neck injuries. Blunt vertebral artery injuries occur more commonly than blunt carotid injuries, probably because of the narrow canal and close association of bony and ligamentous structures. Mechanisms reported to cause vertebral artery injury are remarkably diverse, including hyperextension and rotation, direct blows, chiropractic manipulation, yoga exercises, volleyball, and even "head banging"' to heavy metal rock music.[56,57] Unilateral vertebral artery occlusion seldom results in a neurologic deficit, despite a 15% incidence of underlying congenital unilateral hypoplastic vertebral arteries.[58] Treatment of blunt vertebral artery injury with thrombosis usually is nonoperative; systemic anticoagulation (if possible) is recommended to avoid further propagation of existing thrombus. More often with penetrating wounds, acute hemorrhage, pseudoaneurysm, or formation of an arteriovenous fistula are reasons for surgically addressing a known vertebral artery injury. Operative exposure and exploration can be difficult. The extraosseous first portion of the vertebral artery can be exposed by a supraclavicular incision with transection of the sternal head of the sternocleidomastoid muscle (Fig. 23.5). More distal exposure (second or third portion) is best obtained by an anterior approach.[59,60] An incision is made along the anterior border of the sternocleidomastoid muscle, and the carotid sheath is identified and retracted, either anterosuperiorly or posteroinferiorly, to expose the prevertebral space (Fig. 23.6). Hemoclips are blindly applied where the vertebral artery is free of the osseous vertebral canal between the transverse processes, behind the longus cervicis (colli) muscle. High ligation of the vertebral artery at the C1-2 level (fourth portion) is a satisfactory method of obtaining distal control without unroofing the bony canal of the vertebral artery.[1, 58] Percutaneous embolization, both distal and proximal to the site of arterial injury, simplifies the management, but it requires a skilled and experienced interventional angiographer to cross the site of injury without causing further, uncorrectable damage. Contralateral vertebral angiography is recommended to both accurately determine the extent of injury or the adequacy of embolization therapy.

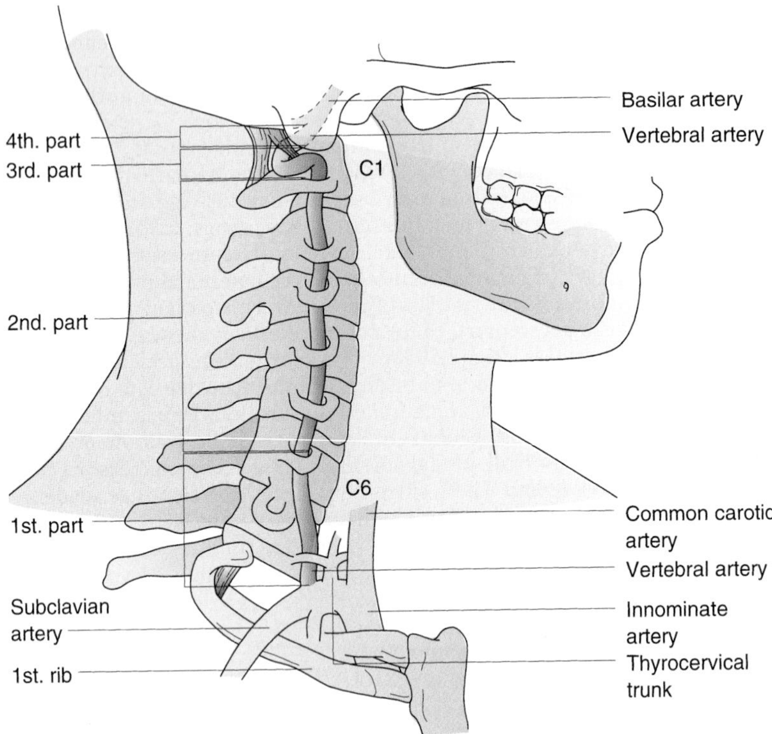

FIGURE 23.5 Normal anatomy of the vertebral artery, showing its division into four parts.

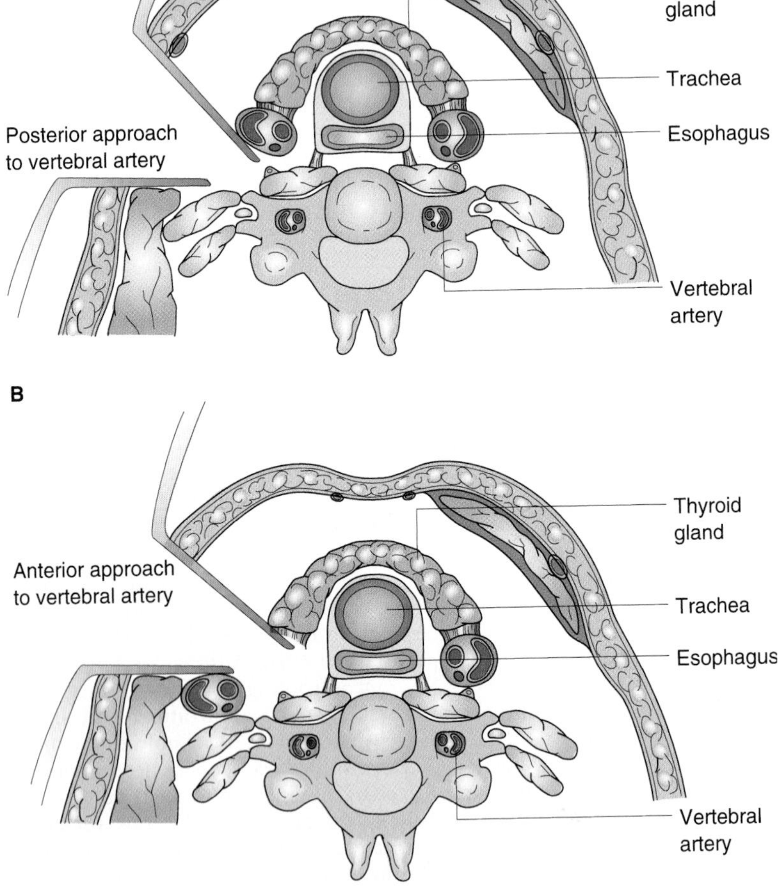

FIGURE 23.6 Operative approach to the vertebral artery. (*A*) Carotid artery and sheath retracted anteriorly. (*B*) Carotid artery and sheath retracted posteriorly.

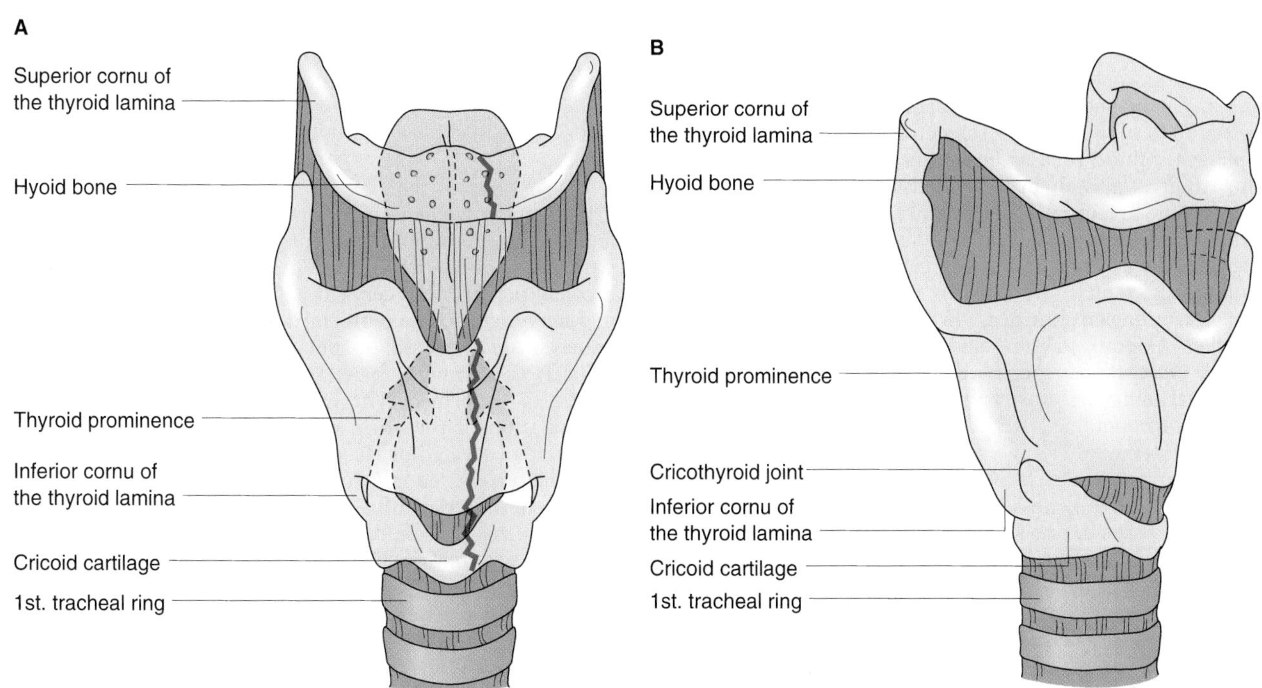

FIGURE 23.7 Frontal view (*A*) and three-quarters view (*B*) of larynx.

Trachea and Larynx

Blunt laryngeal trauma typically results from an anterior impact force (e.g., dashboard, steering wheel) that drives the larynx posteriorly against the rigid cervical spine. The impact can produce a simple or comminuted fracture of laryngeal cartilage, disruption of the mucosa of the endolarynx, or perforation and tears of the hypopharynx. Figure 23.7 depicts the critical laryngeal anatomy and the most common blunt injury pattern. These injuries are frequently occult and are often initially overlooked as attention is directed to injuries of the head, face, and thorax. Delayed recognition of blunt laryngeal trauma is the single greatest contributor to mortality, followed by aspiration of blood, missed esophageal injury, and overlooked concomitant intraabdominal injury. Subtle clinical signs and symptoms of laryngeal injury cannot be ignored. One report identifies hoarseness as the most common symptom, followed by shortness of breath, inability to tolerate the supine position, pain, dysphagia, and aphonia. Tenderness was identified as the most common clinical sign, followed by subcutaneous emphysema, neck contusion, tracheal deviation, and hemoptysis.[61] Liberal use of fiberoptic endoscopy and neck CT aids greatly in the diagnosis.[62]

Unlike blunt laryngeal trauma, penetrating injuries to the trachea and larynx are usually readily apparent and dramatic in their clinical presentation. Subcutaneous emphysema (occasionally massive), pain, hoarseness, and respiratory distress are hallmarks of tracheal injury. Rapid endotracheal intubation by field paramedics, however, can mask a high tracheal injury. Concomitant esophageal, vascular, and thoracic injuries are frequent. A 20-year review of 106 tracheobronchial injuries documented a 22% incidence of concomitant esophageal injuries, a 16% incidence of major vessel injury, and a 40% incidence of hemopneumothorax.[63]

As with any trauma victim, the first treatment priority for those with laryngotracheal injuries is to secure an adequate airway. With a laryngeal injury, this usually straightforward task can be extremely challenging. If an emergency airway is required, direct endotracheal intubation can be attempted initially if the laryngeal structures are well visualized and the endotracheal tube is passed over a flexible endoscope. However, this risks further damage to the trachea even in the most experienced hands. Equipment and preparation for emergency tracheostomy should always be at hand, and tracheostomy is usually recommended if an emergency airway is required, even though it also carries some risk of further injury.[64] Pulse oximetry monitoring is essential, and care must be taken to prevent episodes of hypoxia while alternative airway access techniques are attempted. Transtracheal needle-jet insufflation can temporize a critical situation and allow a more controlled tracheostomy.

Operative repair is usually not required for patients with simple laryngeal edema, hematomas without mucosal disruption, small lacerations of the endolarynx not involving the anterior commissure or the free margin of the vocal fold, and small lacerations of the supraglottic larynx that do not disrupt the integrity of this site.[64] Indications for primary open repair of the larynx include virtually all penetrating tracheal or laryngeal wounds, vocal cord disruption, mucosal tears with exposed cartilage, thyrohyoid separation, thyroid or cricoid cartilage fractures, and hypopharyngeal perforations. The basic tenets of operative care are débridement of devitalized cartilage, reduction of cartilaginous fractures, mucosal coverage of exposed cartilage, and closure of tracheal defects. Tracheostomy is not always required, but it is useful if extensive edema or prolonged airway compression is anticipated. Controversial areas in the surgical care of patients with laryngotracheal trauma include the timing of operation, the role of laryngeal stints, the use of steroids, indications for skin grafting, and the techniques of operative exposure of the larynx.[65]

Pharynx and Esophagus

Esophageal injuries occur in only 5% of patients with penetrating neck wounds. Esophageal perforation from external blunt trauma is rare and accounts for <10% of all esophageal perforations.[66,67] Most blunt injuries are caused by a direct blow to the neck with a hard object, such as steering wheel in high-speed motor vehicle crashes, but it can occur from minor trauma. The diagnosis of an esophageal injury can be difficult and requires high index of suspicion. The clinical signs of esophageal injury, such as hematemesis, odynophagia, neck pain, crepitus, and air in the soft tissues on chest and neck radiographs, are often absent or obscured by concomitant laryngotracheal injury.[68] In one study, the blunt cervicothoracic esophageal injury had a 56% incidence of associated tracheolaryngeal injury.[67] In a review of 77 patients with penetrating esophageal injuries, 45 had cervical esophageal wounds.[69] Overall, physical findings were diagnostic in only 26% of patients. Furthermore, the morbidity of a missed esophageal injury is catastrophic. One review of penetrating neck wounds contained 109 cases of esophageal injuries; the mortality rate was 2% if operation was immediately performed but increased to 44% if operation was delayed because of an initially missed injury and to 100% if no operation was performed.[3] This information is widely used as support for a mandatory neck exploration policy. Other authors, however, have documented a small but significant incidence of missed esophageal injury even after neck exploration. In one report, cervical esophageal injury was initially missed at neck exploration in three patients, and all three died.[69] As a result, an aggressive effort at excluding esophageal injury is warranted, and some authors recommend routine esophagography or esophagoscopy, or both, to aid in the diagnosis of isolated esophageal injuries. The sensitivity of esophagography in detecting esophageal injury varies from approximately 50% to 90%, and the sensitivity of endoscopy varies from 29% to 100%.[18] These modalities should be considered complementary; when combined, they have an accuracy of almost 100%.[22] The choice of rigid or flexible esophagoscopy is controversial and probably reflects individual preferences.

Careful evaluation of the entire tract of the offending penetrating agent or region of blunt hematoma is required to document esophageal integrity. This can be technically challenging and time consuming, but it is a crucial component of the neck exploration. Concomitant intraoperative endoscopy, esophageal air insufflation, or even vital dye instillation can be helpful in excluding injury. Because almost all reported deaths from cervical esophageal injuries are the result of a delayed or missed diagnosis, a particularly high level of suspicion is warranted. The key to successful management of cervical esophageal and pharyngeal injury is early adequate drainage.[70] All such wounds should be drained to avoid deep neck infection or development of a salivary fistula, which occurs in 9% to 18% of these patients.[68,71] Esophagography before drain removal is also recommended, because about half of postrepair fistulas are initially clinically silent. The injured esophagus should be meticulously débrided and repaired primarily, in two layers, with absorbable and nonabsorbable suture. Single-layer closure may be adequate.[68,71] A sternocleidomastoid or strap muscle should always be placed between the trachea and esophagus in a combined repair. If primary closure is not realistic or safe, because of an extensive loss of tissue, as with shotgun blast, it may be necessary to perform a cutaneous esophagostomy for feeding purposes and a cutaneous pharyngostomy for salivary drainage. A secondary reconstructive procedure is then required after the initial healing is complete. Recently, there have been reports of non-operative management of small injuries confined to the upper hypopharynx, above the arytenoid cartilage, if there are no other associated injuries.[70] The treatment includes close observation, intravenous antibiotics, and restricted oral intake. Most surgeons advocate primary repair of all esophageal injuries, if it can be accomplished early. Delays >12 hours significantly increase the risk of repair dehiscence, wound abscess, and death. Neck esophageal injuries diagnosed more than 24 to 48 hours after injury are best managed initially by diversion and drainage.

Nerves

The preoperative determination of level of consciousness and lateralizing gross motor or sensory deficits is required in all patients; a more detailed neurologic examination of the brachial plexus, deep cervical plexus, phrenic nerve, and cranial nerves should be performed in all but the most unstable patients. A hypoglossal or spinal accessory nerve injury is particularly easy to miss unless a preoperative neurologic examination is performed. The vagus nerve can be evaluated by examination of the vocal cords. Primary débridement and repair of all severed or lacerated "named" nerves is preferred, with the use of fine interrupted nonabsorbable suture on the perineurium. Repair of a *single* recurrent nerve injury is controversial. An avulsed recurrent laryngeal nerve (blunt laryngotracheal disruption) should be implanted into the posterior cricoarytenoid muscle.[72] If a motor nerve deficit is apparent, an expendable sensory nerve such as the great auricular can be interposed as a nerve graft to allow anastomosis without tension. If the patient's condition precludes primary repair, the nerve ends should be marked with silver clips or nonabsorbable colored suture. Secondary repair 3 weeks after injury is advised.

KEY POINTS

- **The numerous vital structures in the neck are concentrated in a small anatomic area at risk of injury, unprotected by bone or dense muscular covering.**
- **Anatomically, in addition to large bilateral anterior and posterior triangles, the anterior neck is divided into three zones: (I) extending from sternal notch to cricoid cartilage; (II) from cricoid cartilage to angle of the mandible; and (III) from angle of mandible to base of skull.**
- **Mechanism and anatomic location of trauma are frequently predictive of pattern and number of vital structures injured.**
- **Mandatory versus selective exploration of a penetrating neck injury is determined by anatomic and physical findings in addition to local resources and physician capabilities.**
- **Patterns of fractures of the face, skull, and neck, along with significant soft tissue trauma and subcutaneous emphysema, predict the likelihood of airway or vascular injury, with CT angiography being the most definitive diagnostic test.**
- **Blunt vascular trauma is predominantly treated nonoperatively, whereas any significant injury or disruption of the upper airway or esophagus requires operative repair and drainage.**

References

1. Ordog GJ. Penetrating neck trauma. *J Trauma* 1987;27:543–554.
2. Saletta JD, Lowe RJ, Lim LT, et al. Penetrating trauma of the neck. *J Trauma* 1976;16:579–587.
3. Sankaran S, Walt AJ. Penetrating wounds of the neck: principles and some controversies. *Surg Clin North Am.* 1977;57:139–150.
4. Roon AJ, Christensen N. Evaluation and treatment of penetrating cervical injuries. *J Trauma* 1979;19:391–397.
5. Flint LM, Snyder WH, Perry MO, et al. Management of major vascular injuries in the base of the neck. An 11-year experience with 146 cases. *Arch Surg.* 1973;106:407–413.
6. Bishara RA, Pasch AR, Douglas DD, et al. The necessity of mandatory exploration of penetrating zone II neck injuries. *Surgery* 1986;100:655–660.

7. Jones RF, Terrell JC, Salyer KE. Penetrating wounds of the neck: an analysis of 274 cases. *J Trauma* 1967;7:228–237.
8. Ayuyao AM, Kaledzi YL, Parsa MH, et al. Penetrating neck wounds. Mandatory versus selective exploration. *Ann Surg.* 1985;202:563–567.
9. Demetriades D, Charalambides D, Lakhoo M. Physical examination and selective conservative management in patients with penetrating injuries of the neck. *Br J Surg.* 1993;80:1534–1536.
10. Jurkovich GJ, Zingarelli W, Wallace J, et al. Penetrating neck trauma: diagnostic studies in the asymptomatic patient. *J Trauma* 1985;25:819–822.
11. Mansour MA, Moore EE, Moore FA, et al. Validating the selective management of penetrating neck wounds. *Am J Surg.* 1991;162:517–520; discussion 520–521.
12. Merion RM, Harness JK, Ramsburgh SR, et al. Selective management of penetrating neck trauma. Cost implications. *Arch Surg* 1981;116:691–696.
13. Asensio JA, Valenziano CP, Falcone RE, et al. Management of penetrating neck injuries. The controversy surrounding zone II injuries. *Surg Clin North Am.* 1991;71:267–296.
14. Biffl WL, Moore EE, Rehse DH, et al. Selective management of penetrating neck trauma based on cervical level of injury. *Am J Surg.* 1997;174: 678–682.
15. Irish JC, Hekkenberg R, Gullane PJ, et al. Penetrating and blunt neck trauma: 10-year review of a Canadian experience. *Can J Surg.* 1997;40: 33–38.
16. Klyachkin ML, Rohmiller M, Charash WE, et al. Penetrating injuries of the neck: selective management evolving. *Am Surg.* 1997;63:189–194.
17. Sofianos C, Degiannis E, Van den Aardweg MS, et al. Selective surgical management of zone II gunshot injuries of the neck: a prospective study. *Surgery* 1996;120:785–788.
18. Carducci B, Lowe RA, Dalsey W. Penetrating neck trauma: consensus and controversies. *Ann Emerg Med.* 1986;15:208–215.
19. Hirshberg A, Wall MJ, Johnston RH, Jr., et al. Transcervical gunshot injuries. *Am J Surg.* 1994;167:309–312.
20. Sclafani SJ, Cavaliere G, Atweh N, et al. The role of angiography in penetrating neck trauma. *J Trauma* 1991;31:557–562; discussion 562–563.
21. Richardson JD, Flint LM, Snow NJ, et al. Management of transmediastinal gunshot wounds. *Surgery* 1981;90:671–676.
22. Weigelt JA, Thal ER, Snyder WH, 3rd, et al. Diagnosis of penetrating cervical esophageal injuries. *Am J Surg.* 1987;154:619–622.
23. Gracias VH, Reilly PM, Philpott J, et al. Computed tomography in the evaluation of penetrating neck trauma: a preliminary study. *Arch Surg.* 2001;136:1231–1235.
24. **Biffl WL, Moore EE, Offner PJ, et al. Optimizing screening for blunt cerebrovascular injuries. *Am J Surg.* 1999;178:517–522.**
25. **Rogers FB, Baker EF, Osler TM, et al. Computed tomographic angiography as a screening modality for blunt cervical arterial injuries: preliminary results. *J Trauma* 1999;46:380–385.**
26. LeBlang SD, Nunez DB, Jr. Helical CT of cervical spine and soft tissue injuries of the neck. *Radiol Clin North Am.* 1999;37:515–532, v–vi.
27. Miller PR, Fabian TC, Croce MA, et al. Prospective screening for blunt cerebrovascular injuries: analysis of diagnostic modalities and outcomes. *Ann Surg.* 2002;236:386–393; discussion 393–395.
28. Nunez DB, Jr., Torres-Leon M, Munera F. Vascular injuries of the neck and thoracic inlet: helical CT-angiographic correlation. *Radiographics* 2004;24: 1087–1098; discussion 1099–1100.
29. Munera F, Soto JA, Nunez D. Penetrating injuries of the neck and the increasing role of CTA. *Emergency Radiology* 2004;10:303–309.
30. Munera F, Soto JA, Palacio DM, et al. Penetrating neck injuries: helical CT angiography for initial evaluation. *Radiology* 2002;224:366–372.
31. Gonzalez RP, Falimirski M, Holevar MR, et al. Penetrating zone II neck injury: does dynamic computed tomographic scan contribute to the diagnostic sensitivity of physical examination for surgically significant injury? A prospective blinded study. *J Trauma* 2003;54:61–64; discussion 64–65.
32. Daffner RH. Cervical radiography for trauma patients: a time-effective technique? *AJR Am J Roentgenol.* 2000;175:1309–1311.
33. **Hanson JA, Blackmore CC, Mann FA, et al. Cervical spine injury: a clinical decision rule to identify high-risk patients for helical CT screening. *AJR Am J Roentgenol.* 2000;174:713–717.**
34. Grogan EL, Morris JA, Jr., Dittus RS, et al. Cervical spine evaluation in urban trauma centers: lowering institutional costs and complications through helical CT scan. *J Am Coll Surg.* 2005;200:160–165.
35. Beitsch P, Weigelt JA, Flynn E, et al. Physical examination and arteriography in patients with penetrating zone II neck wounds. *Arch Surg.* 1994;129:577–581.
36. Welling RE, Saul TG, Tew JM, Jr., et al. Management of blunt injury to the internal carotid artery. *J Trauma* 1987;27:1221–1226.
37. Eachempati SR, Vaslef SN, Sebastian MW, et al. Blunt vascular injuries of the head and neck: is heparinization necessary? *J Trauma* 1998;45: 997–1004.
38. **Fabian TC, Patton JH Jr, Croce MA, et al. Blunt carotid injury. Importance of early diagnosis and anticoagulant therapy. *Ann Surg.* 1996;223:513–522; discussion 522–525.**
39. Cogbill TH, Moore EE, Meissner M, et al. The spectrum of blunt injury to the carotid artery: a multicenter perspective. *J Trauma* 1994;37:473–479.
40. Davis JW, Holbrook TL, Hoyt DB, et al. Blunt carotid artery dissection: incidence, associated injuries, screening, and treatment. *J Trauma* 1990;30:1514–1517.
41. Mascalchi M, Bianchi MC, Mangiafico S, et al. MRI and MR angiography of vertebral artery dissection. *Neuroradiology* 1997;39:329–340.
42. JM UK-I, Trivedi RA, Graves MJ, et al. Contrast-enhanced MR angiography for carotid disease: diagnostic and potential clinical impact. *Neurology* 2004;62:1282–1290.
43. Ho KY. MR angiography of carotid arteries. *Jbr-Btr* 2004;87:29–32.
44. Hathout GM, Duh MJ, El-Saden SM. Accuracy of contrast-enhanced MR angiography in predicting angiographic stenosis of the internal carotid artery: linear regression analysis. *AJNR Am J Neuroradiol.* 2003;24: 1747–1756.
45. Fakhry SM, Jaques PF, Proctor HJ. Cervical vessel injury after blunt trauma. *J Vasc Surg.* 1988;8:501–508.
46. Pretre R, Reverdin A, Kalonji T, et al. Blunt carotid artery injury: difficult therapeutic approaches for an underrecognized entity. *Surgery* 1994;115: 375–381.
47. Okada Y, Shima T, Nishida M, et al. Traumatic dissection of the common carotid artery after blunt injury to the neck. *Surg Neurol.* 1999;51: 513–519; discussion 519–520.
48. Gewertz BL, Samson DS, Ditmore QM, et al. Management of penetrating injuries of the internal carotid artery at the base of the skull utilizing extracranial-intracranial bypass. *J Trauma* 1980;20:365–369.
49. Sundt TM, Jr., Pearson BW, Piepgras DG, et al. Surgical management of aneurysms of the distal extracranial internal carotid artery. *J Neurosurg* 1986;64:169–182.
50. Brown MF, Graham JM, Feliciano DV, et al. Carotid artery injuries. *Am J Surg.* 1982;144:748–753.
51. Liekweg WG, Jr., Greenfield LJ. Management of penetrating carotid arterial injury. *Ann Surg.* 1978;188:587–592.
52. Unger SW, Tucker WS J, Mrdeza MA, et al. Carotid arterial trauma. *Surgery* 1980;87:477–487.
53. Weaver FA, Yellin AE, Wagner WH, et al. The role of arterial reconstruction in penetrating carotid injuries. *Arch Surg.* 1988;123:1106–1111.
54. Martin WS, Gussack GS. Pediatric penetrating head and neck trauma. *Laryngoscope* 1990;100:1288–1291.
55. Vazquez Anon V, Aymard A, Gobin YP, et al. Balloon occlusion of the internal carotid artery in 40 cases of giant intracavernous aneurysm: technical aspects, cerebral monitoring, and results. *Neuroradiology* 1992;34: 245–251.
56. DeBehnke DJ, Brady W. Vertebral artery dissection due to minor neck trauma. *J Emerg Med.* 1994;12:27–31.
57. Egnor MR, Page LK, David C. Vertebral artery aneurysm—a unique hazard of head banging by heavy metal rockers. Case report. *Pediatr Neurosurg.* 1991;17:135–138.
58. Golueke P, Sclafani S, Phillips T, et al. Vertebral artery injury—diagnosis and management. *J Trauma* 1987;27:856–865.
59. Hatzitheofilou C, Strahlendorf C, Kakoyiannis S, et al. Penetrating external injuries of the oesophagus and pharynx. *Br J Surg.* 1993;80:1147–1149.
60. Meier DE, Brink BE, Fry WJ. Vertebral artery trauma: acute recognition and treatment. *Arch Surg.* 1981;116:236–239.
61. Myers EM, Iko BO. The management of acute laryngeal trauma. *J Trauma* 1987;27:448–452.
62. Fuhrman GM, Stieg FH III, Buerk CA. Blunt laryngeal trauma: classification and management protocol. *J Trauma* 1990;30:87–92.
63. Kelly JP, Webb WR, Moulder PV, et al. Management of airway trauma. I: Tracheobronchial injuries. *Ann Thorac Surg.* 1985;40:551–555.
64. **Schaefer SD. The acute management of external laryngeal trauma. A 27-year experience. *Arch Otolaryngol Head Neck Surg.* 1992;118:598–604.**
65. Gussack GS, Jurkovich GJ. Treatment dilemmas in laryngotracheal trauma. *J Trauma* 1988;28:1439–1444.
66. Beal SL, Pottmeyer EW, Spisso JM. Esophageal perforation following external blunt trauma. *J Trauma* 1988;28:1425–1432.
67. Jacobs I, Niknejad G, Kelly K, et al. Hypopharyngeal perforation after blunt neck trauma: case report and review of the literature. *J Trauma* 1999;46:957–958.
68. Glatterer MS, Jr., Toon RS, Ellestad C, et al. Management of blunt and penetrating external esophageal trauma. *J Trauma* 1985;25:784–792.
69. Defore WW Jr, Mattox KL, Hansen HA, et al. Surgical management of penetrating injuries of the esophagus. *Am J Surg.* 1977;134:734–738.
70. **Stanley RB Jr, Armstrong WB, Fetterman BL, et al. Management of external penetrating injuries into the hypopharyngeal-cervical esophageal funnel. *J Trauma* 1997;42:675–679.**
71. Winter RP, Weigelt JA. Cervical esophageal trauma. Incidence and cause of esophageal fistulas. *Arch Surg.* 1990;125:849–851; discussion 851–852.
72. Snow JB, Jr. Diagnosis and therapy for acute laryngeal and tracheal trauma. *Otolaryngol Clin North Am.* 1984;17:101–106.

CHAPTER 24 ■ CHEST TRAUMA

RIYAD KARMY-JONES AND GREGORY JURKOVICH

Chest injuries are primarily responsible for at least 25% of fatalities following injury and play a major contributing factor in as many as a further 50% of fatal cases.[1] Although in most cases the major technical procedure is tube thoracostomy, attention to detail is critical because there are often delayed complications and interventions are often both hazardous and immediate.

PROCEDURES

Tube Thoracostomy

Tube thoracostomy is the primary invasive treatment for managing chest injury. In patients at risk of developing tension pneumothorax (e.g., during air transport with chest injuries or those who are requiring significant ventilator support), prophylactic tubes are also indicated. It is critical to recognize that in 20% of cases the physical examination is misleading.[2] Unstable patients with chest injuries or those with decreased breath sounds and increased tympany should have tubes placed without delay. Stable patients without distress should be allowed the benefit of a chest radiograph, if available, before tube placement.

In stable patients, attention to anesthesia (including local and, if appropriate, conscious sedation) and sterile technique is important. The usual landmark is the anterior to midaxillary line at or above the inframammary crease. If there is a thoracotomy scar, the tube should be placed superior to it because the diaphragm usually is scarred to the level of the previous incision. Two basic methods are used, the "Kelly clamp" and the "sharp" approach. Using scissors or a scalpel to incise down to the intercostal muscles, rather than blunt dissection, may be quicker and less painful. Tunneling should not be done more than one to two ribs higher than the skin incision.[2]

Pain is the most common complication and can lead to splinting, atelectasis, and pneumonia. Laceration of underlying structures can occur because of high airway pressure or prior adhesions (present in 15% to 20% of patients de novo). Careful determination of intrapleural placement can avoid this problem, as can controlling the dissection device carefully. Tubes can become displaced (1.7% to 5.2% incidence), usually because they are not pushed in far enough, and when such patients sit up or lower their arm, tubes are pulled out 1 to 3 cm on average.[3] Misplacement at the time of insertion into the extrathoracic space can occur in patients with larger body habitus, thick parietal pleura (e.g., empyema), and if significant soft tissue edema is present. Chest radiography may not be clear but persistent pneumothorax with lack of respiratory variation suggests the diagnosis. The tube should be removed and a new one placed through a new incision. Empyema occurs in 2% to 10% of patients who undergo emergency room tube thoracostomy. Risk factors include retained hemothorax, poor sterile technique, shock, extrathoracic infectious sites, pain, and pneumonia.[4] In the trauma setting, gram-positive organisms are particularly prevalent and prophylactic antibiotics for 24 hours or less compared with no antibiotics appears to reduce empyema.[5]

Thoracoscopy

Rigid thoracoscopy advantages are that lung isolation is not required, blood and other debris can be evacuated through the larger port, pleural exploration is possible, and in many cases a single port can complete the procedure.[6] Video-thoracoscopy (VATS) usually requires that the lung on the operative side be collapsed, but offers a more panoramic view and allows advanced procedures, such as repairing the diaphragm or resecting injured lung parenchyma.[7] Resolution of persistent airleak (>3 days) does appear to be shorter with VATS resection compared with placing additional chest tubes.[8] Thoracoscopy has also been used successfully to diagnose cardiac and diaphragmatic injuries and, in some instances, repair the latter.

When entering the chest, it is important to avoid parenchymal injury by bluntly pushing through the intercostal space. Placing the ports as anteriorly as possible (where the rib spaces are wider) and minimizing the use of ports (which increase nerve trauma) can reduce the incidence of postoperative persistent pain, which occurs in up to 7% of patients.

Thoracotomy

The choice of operative approach is influenced by injury pattern, patient stability, available equipment, and experience of the surgeon. The initial exposure may prove to be inadequate, and recognizing this and making modifications or closing and repositioning is far better than continuing to struggle.

The most common "urgent" incision is the anterolateral thoracotomy. This incision should be made in the inframammary crease (not nipple line), with the incision turning superiorly in the medial aspect after crossing over the midclavicular line for possible extension across the sternum. The ribs and costal cartilages change course dramatically at this point also, acutely rising superior-medially. If, on entering the chest, high apical bleeding consistent with great vessel injury is encountered, packing the apex and holding pressure while performing an appropriate counterincision can be lifesaving.

The heart, pulmonary hilum, and ascending aorta are all easily accessible with a median sternotomy. Sternotomy is most likely to provide adequate exposure for penetrating injuries between the nipple lines compared with other approaches.[9] The midline is indicated by a line between the suprasternal notch and the root of the xiphoid. Crossing veins at the suprasternal notch and just superior to the sternal-xiphoid junction often need to be ligated. The origin of the great vessels can be controlled through this approach, and dissection should start within the pericardium particularly if there is extensive superior mediastinal hematoma.[10] The innominate vein can be divided or mobilized to expose the innominate artery as it passes beneath it. Sternotomy in conjunction with supraclavicular

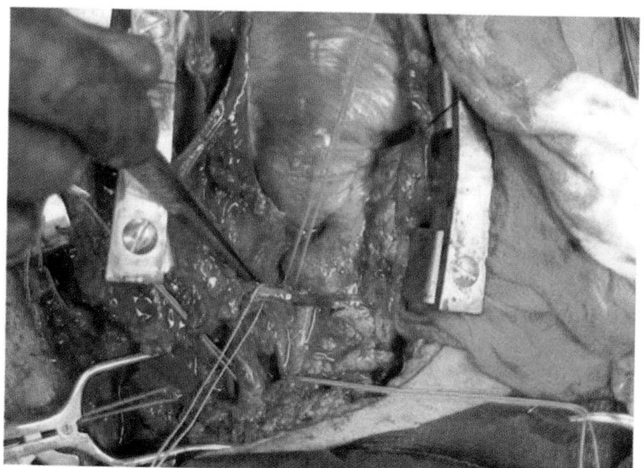

FIGURE 24.1 View from the head. Patient had suffered an impalement injury through the left clavicle, rupturing the intrathoracic left subclavian artery. Through a sternotomy, with left supraclavicular extension, the origin of the great vessels has been controlled and the axillary artery controlled.

extension offers equal exposure to the left subclavian artery as does the "trap-door" approach with less morbidity. On either side, the midportion of the subclavian vessels is best accessed through a supraclavicular incision (Fig. 24.1).[11] This incision can be further extended across the mid aspect of the clavicle, curving down toward the deltopectoral groove for access to the distal subclavian and axillary artery junction. Sufficient exposure usually requires division of the sternocleidomastoid muscle attachments to the clavicle, as well as the attachments of the anterior scalenus muscle onto the first rib. In addition, the attachments of the pectoralis major muscle laterally may need to be divided. Great care must be exercised to avoid injury to the phrenic nerve, vagus nerve, and cords of the brachial plexus with this approach. Resection of the medial portion of the clavicle can potentially increase exposure of the subclavian artery. Performing a subperiosteal resection with repair of the periosteum at the conclusion of the case provides adequate cosmetic and functional results without the risks of malunion and persistent pain. Alternatively, if exposure of the midsubclavian vessels is all that is required, a supraclavicular approach, splitting the clavicle in the middle, is often adequate. Plating the clavicle at the end preserves shoulder girdle stability.

A clamshell incision has many of the advantages of sternotomy, with the additional benefit of providing better posterolateral exposure. A rolled towel is placed longitudinally in the midline with the arms raised above the head to allow the incision to be made across the sternum at the fourth intercostal space (as opposed to the usual "extension of anterolateral thoracotomy," which is usually at the fifth space). Having divided the internal mammary arteries, the sternum is split and the intercostal spaces opened laterally. Placing bilateral rib spreaders, which are sutured in place, and dividing the retrosternal areolar tissue provides access to all central structures. The carina and right main pulmonary artery can be reached between the ascending aorta and superior vena cava by incising the posterior pericardium.

Posterolateral thoracotomy can be performed using a variety of muscle-sparing techniques. The latissimus can be mobilized, but often simply preserving the serratus anterior by mobilizing it anteriorly will provide adequate support to shoulder function postoperatively. In most cases, a fifth intercostal incision is the best, entering the chest at the level of the major fissure. The rib spaces can be counted, with the second rib most often palpated and recognized by the insertions of the strap muscles posteriorly near the spinous ligament. Resecting the rib is helpful if extensive pleural inflammation is present. This method may be associated with reduced postoperative pain, because the pleural edges can be sutured without pericostal sutures, which can entrap nerve bundles of the ribs above and below the incision. The fourth intercostal approach is used for descending aortic injuries (left) or tracheal injuries (right), and seventh or eighth left intercostal approaches for lower esophageal injuries. Posterolateral thoracotomy provides dramatically better exposure than anterolateral approaches do but obviously prevents exploration across the midline and, except for splenectomy from the left, prevents management of intraabdominal injuries.

CHEST WALL TRAUMA

Rib Fractures and Flail Chest

Chest wall trauma is a marker of significant injury and is associated with increased need for laparotomy, thoracotomy, or both.[12] Apart from associated injuries, rib fractures (with or without flail segments) are associated with significant morbidity owing to pain and subsequent atelectasis as well as underlying pulmonary contusion.

The primary therapy for rib injuries is pain control in conjunction with aggressive pulmonary toilet.[13] A variety of techniques are available, ranging from rib blocks to epidural catheters; the latter are associated with improvement in functional volumes and reduction in respiratory failure.[12] Epidural approaches appear to more reliably improve respiratory function compared with intravenous pain medicine, but the latter is clearly appropriate if other approaches are not possible.[14,15]

Stabilization of flail segments has been studied extensively. Internal stabilization using positive pressure ventilation has been superseded by pain management because routine intubation increases risk of pneumonia.[13,16] Most patients will demonstrate some fibrosis and stabilization of the flail segment within 3 weeks, and the presence of a flail segment is not an indication, in and of itself, to continue mechanical ventilation. Occasionally, however, the chest wall instability is so great or there are other indications for operation, that fixation may be indicated (Fig. 24.2). The question of early rib fixation leading to improved outcomes has been studied only in small series. A major problem is the lack of consistently reliable tools for fixation.[12] In addition, during fixation, intercostal nerves can be trapped, thus increasing the pain. Frequently, the bone is too thin to hold hardware and the normal rib movement is not only up and down but also outward with respiratory effort, placing tension on any repair. Flail chest, however, is associated with significant late morbidity in terms of chronic pain and sensation of decreased ventilator capacity. Early fixation may reduce this late debility and deserves study.[17]

Sternal Fractures

Because of the force required, sternal fractures have been associated with an increased incidence of both cardiac and great vessel injury. However, there is debate about how prevalent these injuries are. One study found an incidence of cardiac injury in 18%, another found 62%.[18,19] As with rib fractures, management is primarily supportive. Most fractures are transverse, involve the sternal manubrial junction or upper one third of the sternum, and stabilize with pain control. Unstable fractures, fractures associated with chronic pain, or those associated with infection (indicated by new sternal click in the setting of fever or erythema) require operative intervention. Options include wires in figure-of-eight fashion, plates, or both. Longitudinal fractures may require closure similar to

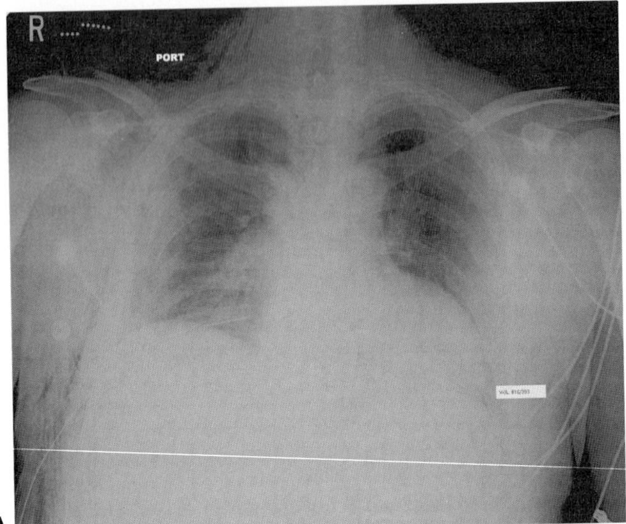

A

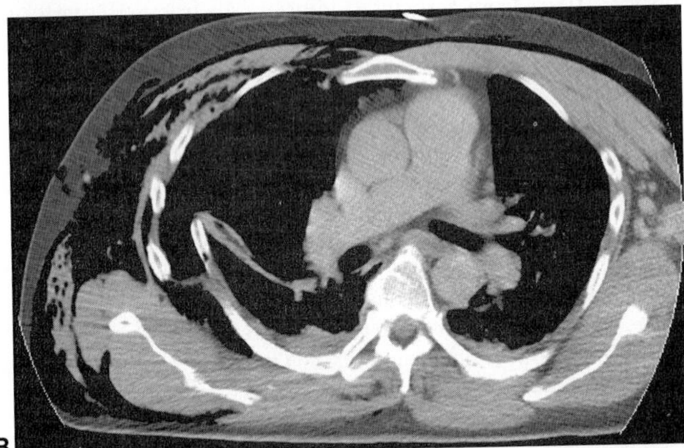

B

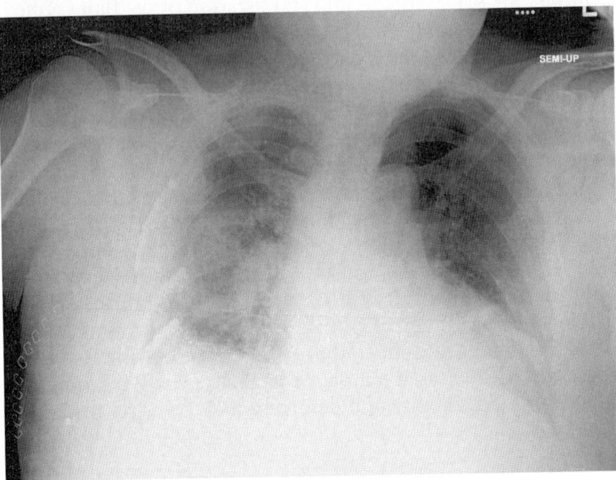

C

FIGURE 24.2 (*A*) Chest radiographic study (CXR) after blunt trauma. Multiple posterior fractured ribs. Patient had severe pain and increasing atelectasis despite epidural catheter and persistent effusion and air leak. (*B*) Computed tomography scan demonstrating intrusion of ribs and potential parenchymal injury. (C) Postoperative CXR. Patient was rapidly weaned from pain medication and had marked respiratory improvement.

that for closing a sternotomy incision. Sternal fractures complicated by mediastinal abscess require débridement. Simple approaches include placement of an irrigation system, but recalcitrant or widespread infection requires closure with muscle or omental flaps after widespread débridement.[20]

Chest Wall Defects

Large, complex open wounds require a multidisciplinary approach. Initially, aggressive wound débridement, drainage of hemothorax, and simple packing are appropriate.[4] Subsequent management depends on which levels are involved, as well as on location (ribs, muscle, intrathoracic, skin, and so on).[21] A dreaded complication of chest wounds is necrotizing infection, characterized by rapidly progressive sepsis with local erythema and, at times, minimal superficial evidence of infection.[22] These infectious complications require wide débridement and reconstruction. If sepsis is not a concern, stability can be achieved, depending on the size of the defect, with a variety of meshes or methylmethacrylate "sandwiches." Probably the most important factor is the use of vascularized tissue flaps.

Traumatic lung hernia, characterized by protrusion of lung parenchyma outside the ribs, is uncommon but has been described as a complication of chest tubes, thoracotomy, or traumatic defects.[23] As long as no evidence of incarceration or infarction is seen, immediate repair is not needed. With evidence of lung necrosis, early repair (using mesh or other techniques) accompanied by resection of the involved lung will be required.[23]

PLEURAL SPACE

Urgent Thoracotomy for Ongoing Hemorrhage

In 1970, McNamara and associates described a reduction in mortality when thoracotomy was performed early following penetrating trauma.[24] The current Advanced Trauma Life Support (ATLS) guidelines list "initial chest tube output exceeding 1,500 milliliters or a continued hourly output of more than 250 milliliters for three consecutive hours" as criteria for surgical exploration following chest trauma, regardless of hemodynamic stability. Evacuating the hemithorax completely and enabling visceral-parietal pleural apposition provides an opportunity for the lung to "tamponade" bleeding. Prolonging the interval before this is achieved can result in an insidious cycle of further blood loss, increasing coagulopathy, and metabolic derangement. There tends to be a low threshold for operation following penetrating injury, but following blunt trauma significant delays can occur. The reasons include distraction by multiple associated injuries, need for complex radiologic tests, and dissatisfaction with operating for multiple chest wall bleeders. This has led to a tendency to watch hourly outputs or attempt interventional approaches. The risk with monitoring chest tube output is that the tubes can be plugged or not properly monitored or transient decreases in output can lead to critical delays. A retrospective multicenter study of patients who underwent thoracotomy within 48 hours of injury because of ongoing bleeding noted that, independent of mechanism, each 500 mL of tube output was associated with a 60% increase in mortality.[25] Planning operation whenever the *total* output exceeds 1,500 mL over a 24-hour period is appropriate. If patients are stable and not coagulopathic, "mini" thoracotomy or thoracoscopic approaches may be feasible.

Retained Hemothorax

Tube thoracostomy fails to completely evacuate hemothorax in approximately 5% of cases.[26] Complications that may arise include empyema and fibrothorax. Conditions that predispose patients to both include prolonged ventilation, development of pneumonia, break in the pleura (as is the case following tube thoracostomy), and other sites of infection.[27] On the other hand, stable, nonventilated patients with small effusions (<one fourth hemothorax) following blunt trauma with no obvious pleural disruption usually will resolve without sequelae and should be observed.

Early evacuation of hemothorax has been shown to reduce the incidence of complications, preferably within 7 days, before loculations begin to complicate pleural débridement.[28] Recognizing the extent of hemothorax, however, can be difficult. Although chest radiography can underestimate it, chest computed tomography (CT) is much more accurate.[29] Moderate effusions in ventilated patients or those with other risk factors should be aggressively drained.[27,30] When recognized acutely following injury, the most expeditious treatment is to place a second chest tube. When recognized after 1 to 2 days, this may not be helpful in that it may simply increase pain, splinting, and the risk of pneumonia. Intrapleural streptokinase (250,000 U) or urokinase (40,000 U) has efficacy of 65% to 90%.[31] Complications include fever and pain, but the risk of rebleeding is negligible. However, it takes several days longer than direct operative drainage and will not break down loculations.

Thoracoscopy offers the advantage of complete removal of all clot without the excess morbidity of a formal thoracotomy. Patients undergoing thoracoscopy had a shortened length of time requiring chest tube drainage, a shortened hospital stay (2.7 days less), and a decreased total hospital cost ($6,000 less) compared with patients treated with a second chest tube.[32] There were no failures or complications, and no patients required conversion to a formal thoracotomy with early thoracoscopy. In contrast, a second chest tube failed to completely evacuate the retained hemothorax, requiring operative treatment in over 40% of the patients. Thoracotomies through mini approaches are often sufficient to allow removal of soft, gelatinous visceral and pleural rind, permitting full lung expansion. The denser the adhesions, the greater the exposure must be, and if a formal decortication of a formed visceral peel is anticipated, a standard approach is required. Patients who present late (usually >3 months following injury) with an element of fibrothorax (but with no infection) should be managed nonoperatively, because at 6 to 9 months in most cases there is remodeling and adaptation and, if surgery is required, there is no increased difficulty if it is undertaken at a later date.

Empyema

Posttraumatic empyema is likely to require surgical intervention because the blood and inflammation create a vigorous inflammatory reaction and aggressive management of retained or contaminated hemothorax may reduce morbidity.[4,33,34] Patients with hemothoraces after chest tube placement with opacification of more than one third hemithorax on chest radiographic study (CXR) should be considered for drainage. Other risk factors include ventilation, splinting secondary to pain, hollow viscus injury, and chest tube placed in the emergency room. The primary reason that simple drainage or thoracoscopic approaches may fail in treating empyema in the trauma population is the presence of a dense visceral peel preventing parenchymal reexpansion. Early and aggressive approaches are thus warranted in the trauma population.

PARENCHYMAL INJURIES

Pulmonary Contusion

Pulmonary contusion is the most common potentially life-threatening chest injury. Transmission of kinetic energy (with or without overlying rib fractures and subsequent laceration) results in bruising of the lung characterized by interstitial and alveolar edema, hemorrhage, and subsequent alveolar collapse.[35] Contrecoup injuries can occur, and the extent of bony injuries depends on the compliance of the chest wall. Clinically, hypoxia and ventilatory embarrassment develop within 24 to 48 hours, although changes can occur in a much shorter time, depending on the extent of injury and the need for volume replacement, which aggravates the process.[36] Initial chest films may be normal or, at most, patchy, but as resuscitation continues a "blossoming" is noted with opacification and air bronchograms. If significant changes are noted on an initial radiograph taken shortly after injury, in general the course will be severe. Chest CT can grade the degree of injury more accurately but does not lead to significant improvement in outcome.[37]

The treatment is generally supportive.[35] Oxygen (including continuous positive airway pressure [CPAP] mask, if needed) should be applied early. If intravenous volume can be restricted (i.e., in a stable patient), it should, because the associated capillary leak leads to worsening pulmonary edema. Diuresis may help, particularly with evidence of volume overload (pulmonary occlusion pressure >18 mm Hg or end-diastolic volume index >135 mL/m^2). Colloid solutions appear to aggravate pulmonary dysfunction because the obligatory leak results in the colloidal agents themselves leaking into the interstitial and alveolar spaces, further promoting edema.

Intubation should be performed for the usual indications. Flail chest is not, of itself, an indication for mechanical ventilation.[16] Aggressive pain control should be attempted first. A significant early complication linked to the need for intubation and mechanical ventilation is pneumonia, increasing from as low as 6% in nonintubated patients to 44% in those requiring ventilation.[38] No role is seen for prophylactic antibiotics. Of all patients admitted with a diagnosis of contusion, nearly 50% develop pneumonia, barotrauma, or major atelectasis and 25% develop acute respiratory distress syndrome (ARDS). Long-term disability occurs with focal fibrosis.[39,40] Mortality is primarily dictated by associated injuries, in particular closed head injury.[41] However, there is some correlation with extent of contusion, as defined by chest CT.[42] Most reviews report a mortality of 5% to 30%, and contusion is the direct cause of death in 25% to 50% of fatalities.

Parenchymal Injury

It has been estimated that 20% to 30% of patients who undergo thoracotomy following trauma will require some form of lung resection.[43,44] Considering all patients with chest trauma, however, as few as 2% of all blunt and 6% of penetrating injuries will require resection. Most patients who present with penetrating injuries have peripheral injuries that are simple to manage, whereas extensive blast or blunt trauma often results in combinations of diffuse contusion and lung maceration that is extremely difficult to salvage.[51] The most common procedures required are simple suture repair or wedge resection. Tractotomy is used to either define deep injuries or to manage peripheral injuries that pass through the parenchyma. Mortality rates as high as 3% to 50% following lobectomy and 70% to 100% following pneumonectomy reflect the severity of lung and overall injury in patients requiring extensive resection.[43,45,46] The use of nonanatomic and stapling techniques has been advocated as a method of both damage control and rapid definitive resection with reduced operative time and blood loss and increased parenchymal salvage.[44,47–50]

Minimal peripheral injuries are often encountered when operating for associated injuries.[51,52] Typically, the patient is taken to surgery for ongoing hemorrhage secondary to intercostal vessel damage. The intercostal arteries are perfused at systemic pressures and as a result can bleed profusely. Peripheral bullet tracts may spontaneously stop bleeding because of the relatively low pressure in the pulmonary circuit. To eliminate potential bleeding or air leaks, however, a wedge resection is performed. Standard stapling devices may be safely used without pledgets or oversewing of the edges.[50] The entire bullet tract must be contained within the excised specimen.

The management of deep lobar injuries is controversial. Simple oversewing of the entry and exit sites is insufficient, because of invariably continued deep parenchymal hemorrhage that results in aspiration, pneumonia, and unremitting ARDS. In general, tractotomy should be performed with either stapler or between clamps. This will expose deep bleeding vessels and allow definitive control.[44,48,50] It is not uncommon after tractotomy for diffuse bleeding to require placing large pledgeted mattress sutures, similar to liver stitches, from the depth of the wound to the edge to provide control. A minority of patients will have significant air leaks or long tracts of devitalized tissue. If these patients are stable, they should be considered for resection up to and including lobectomy.

Patients with perihilar injuries or extensive lung maceration generally present with severe shock, and survival correlates with the rapidity of control.[51] Thus, on entering the chest, if large central bleeding is encountered, the pulmonary ligament is taken down to the level of the inferior pulmonary vein, which allows torsion of the entire lung as a temporizing method. Rarely, very proximal injuries may require intrapericardial control of the pulmonary artery. When both artery and vein are injured or a significant length of vessel is damaged, a linear stapler is fired across the hilum and a simultaneous stapled pneumonectomy (SSP) performed.[53] Trauma pneumonectomy is generally associated with 50% to 100% mortality and, although it should not be delayed, should not be performed without assessing lesser options. A common cause for acute mortality is sudden right ventricular failure. Supportive efforts using diuretics, vasodilators, and occasionally extracorporeal membrane oxygenation (ECMO), in addition to stopping fluid boluses when the hilum is controlled, avoid aggravating the right heart strain. A second pitfall is the potential for increased bronchial stump leak and empyema.[53] Elective reexploration, washout, and stump reinforcement with viable tissue should be performed as soon as the patient is stable. Rarely, elective resection may be required. Lobectomy may be needed for persistent hemoptysis or progressive respiratory failure following high-velocity gunshot wounds or other focal devastating but relatively isolated injuries.[54]

Hematoma, Pneumatocele, and Persistent Air Leak

Hematoma and pneumatoceles represent small parenchymal lacerations that are usually clinically insignificant. Hematomas tend to be discrete and usually resolve, although in some instances they may remain and be mistaken for coin lesions. Pneumatoceles also have discrete margins, can be associated with air–fluid levels, and rarely require intervention. They do not require prophylactic antibiotics, but in the rare circumstances when they become infected, standard treatment as for lung abscess, including antibiotics, postural drainage, or percutaneous drainage, is usually sufficient. Even more rarely, the pneumatocele can be the source of persistent air leak requiring resection. Any persistent air leak requires a workup for airway injury, but in most cases represents a small parenchymal laceration that may be exacerbated by high airway pressures, incomplete drainage of pneumothorax, or parenchymal consolidation. In most cases, adjusting or adding chest drains, weaning from the ventilator, or reducing peak airway pressure, and, most often, the passage of time, will allow healing. Thoracoscopy can allow quicker resolution if imaging identifies a discrete lesion. Patients with underlying lung disease, particularly emphysema, present additional difficulties. Resection, similar to lung volume reduction surgery with adjunctive use of peristrips, may be required but should be used as a last resort, because these patients often have underlying pneumonia and staple lines often fail, resulting in even worse leaks.

MEDIASTINAL INJURIES

Transmediastinal Gunshot Wounds

Transmediastinal gunshot wounds can cause numerous potentially immediately life-threatening injuries. The key to managing these injuries is to determine the tract of the missile and whether the victim is stable or unstable. The former seems self-evident, but in numerous cases the missile is not truly transmediastinal, defined as crossing from one hemithorax through the visceral mediastinum, which contains heart, airway, esophagus, and aorta. It is not uncommon for missiles to tract posteriorly, hit the posterior elements of the spine, and end up in the extrathoracic soft tissue of the opposite hemithorax.

Approximately one third of patients are unstable, requiring immediate thoracotomy or sternotomy, and have an acute mortality of 35% owing to cardiovascular injuries.[55] Patients not in frank arrest should have bilateral chest tubes placed, and the side with the most blood should be opened first. The workup of stable patients remains controversial. Richardson noted that 62% of these patients had life-threatening injuries, including cardiac (14%), aorta or great vessel (26%), esophagus (21%), or tracheobronchial (14%).[55] Nagy also noted that stability did not preclude significant injury, although only 16% had injuries requiring urgent operation.[56] Significantly, no differences in vital signs, hemothorax, or arterial blood gas analysis were noted between those with or without injuries. This has prompted a classic workup, including aortography, esophagoscopy, esophagogram, and bronchoscopy.[57,58] Other methods to evaluate the mediastinum include transthoracic or transesophageal ultrasound, and CT angiography appears to be the most definitive test to document the tract of the missile, identify injuries, and prompt a directed evaluation.[59,60]

Tracheobronchial Injury

Blunt tracheobronchial disruption occurs in only 1% to 3% of motor vehicle crashes, and more than 80% of victims die before reaching the hospital.[61,62] The injury is within 2 cm of the carina in 76% of cases, within 1 cm in 58%, and specifically in the right main stem within 2 cm of the carina in 43%.[62,64] Approximately 50% of injuries are circumferential.[63] Penetrating injuries involve the cervical trachea in more than 80% of cases.

Clinical evidence suggestive of tracheobronchial disruption includes subcutaneous emphysema, persistent air leak, and hemoptysis.[65] Chest radiography can demonstrate pneumothorax (60%), cervical emphysema or pneumomediastinum (70%), or occasionally the "fallen lung sign," in which the lung is seen to drop away from the hilum.[66] CT can also demonstrate avulsion of the airway (Fig. 24.3).[67] Diagnosis can be difficult, however, because many patients have underlying lung injury that could lead to air leak. In addition, mediastinal tissue, blood clot, or airway enfolding results in partial or complete occlusion preventing significant air leak. This may result in radiographic appearance of a persistent pneumothorax despite a well-placed chest tube.[66] CT bronchography

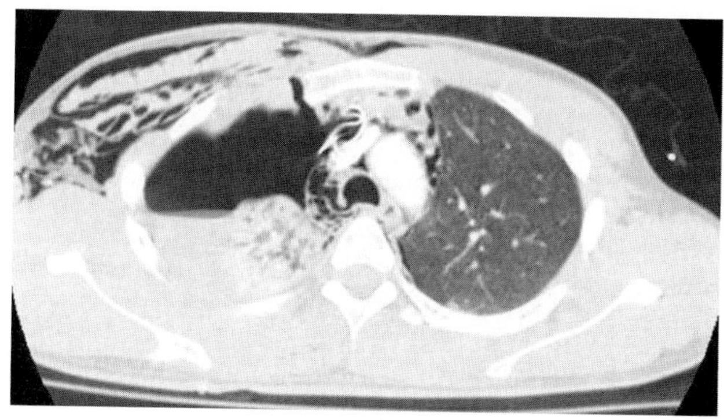

FIGURE 24.3 Computed tomography scan in patient following blunt trauma demonstrating distal tracheal laceration.

may be more sensitive for evaluating airway anatomy and has been used both for diagnostic purposes and for planning and may be helpful in selected cases.[68,69] Penetrating cervical perforation may present with a "bubbling" neck wound that stops after intubation. This is virtually diagnostic because it implies that the endotracheal tube has been passed distal to the injury site.

In the acute setting the initial priority is airway control. Flexible bronchoscopy can provide diagnosis, be performed in a stable sedated patient or in a patient whose neck cannot be cleared, and act as an obturator to pass an endotracheal tube and assess vocal cord function. The rigid bronchoscope can maintain an airway and has a larger lumen to allow suctioning of blood or other debris.[70] If acute surgical airway is needed and a question of blunt laryngeal fracture exists, tracheostomy, as opposed to cricothyroidotomy, is favored because the latter can lead to complete upper airway separation. Incases of a large slash wound in the neck, the distal trachea often retracts into the chest. It can be grabbed with clamps and elevated and the airway intubated directly.

Bronchial injuries are frequently diagnosed late (>24 hours) and manifest as obstructive pneumonitis with hemoptysis and signs of pulmonary sepsis. At least 20% of patients with such injuries will present with late stricture formation and symptoms varying from asthma to dyspnea to recurrent pneumonia.[66] If parenchymal destruction has not occurred, airway reconstruction should be attempted, although stents may be possible as a temporizing or even definitive approach in some settings where the airway distal to the injury can be clearly seen at bronchoscopy.[63]

Intraoperative airway management depends on the acuity of the injury as well as its location. In elective situations, a double-lumen tube may be appropriate. In acute settings, especially if the diagnosis is not certain, an "uncut" endotracheal tube, preferably at least 8.0 French should be used. This allows bronchoscopy and adequate suctioning, reduces the risk of aggravating the airway tear, is easier to place, can be passed across the injury site, and can be manipulated during surgery. On occasion, the distal airway must be intubated through the operative field to allow adequate exposure. Jet ventilation, with tubes passed through the injury into one or both mainstem bronchi, is also useful at times.

Operative exposure depends on site of injury and associated injuries. The proximal two thirds of the trachea is best approached via a low-lying collar incision.[70] This also allows access to associated esophageal or vascular injuries in the neck. Extending this into a "T" into the manubrium will increase exposure of the middle one third of the trachea and allow proximal control of the innominate artery and vein. If there is a question of major great vessel, ascending aortic, or cardiac injury, sternotomy should be employed.[62] The distal one third of the trachea, carina, and right mainstem bronchus are most easily approached through a right fourth intercostal space posterolateral thoracotomy. The left mainstem bronchus can be approached through a left fourth or fifth intercostal incision, which also exposes the proximal left subclavian artery, the descending thoracic aorta, and the lower esophagus. The very proximal left mainstem is difficult to expose and requires mobilization of the arch by dividing the ligamentum arteriosum.[70] Finally, a clamshell approach can provide exposure of the distal trachea and carina.

Operative repair varies depending on timing of surgery and extent of injury. Distal airway injuries associated with lobar destruction (either acutely from trauma or chronically from infection) can be managed by simple lobectomy.[71] Small injuries, usually ones in which the membrane has torn away from the cartilage, can be primarily repaired. Simple lacerations can be closed with interrupted absorbable sutures of either monofilament or braided varieties. Dissection should be limited to the region to be resected to preserve blood supply. Muscle flaps can be used as an adjunct.[72] In cases where there has been complete disruption or significant airway injury, resection and end-to-end anastomosis are required. Cervical resections should be buttressed with sternocleidomastoid in cases of associated carotid or esophageal injury. End-to-end reconstructions in the chest should be buttressed with viable tissue, such as pericostal flap, thymic pedicle flap, or omentum.[66] Stricture and dehiscence occur in 3% of patients following tracheobronchial reconstruction, the former presenting in many instances as new onset wheezing.[66] If the stricture is limited, dilation and temporary stenting to allow remodeling can provide a permanently patent and functioning airway. In selected cases, endobronchial techniques or resuspension of the injured bronchus may be feasible.[73,74]

CARDIAC INJURY

The significance of cardiac injury varies widely depending on the mechanism. Blunt cardiac injury usually is considered "silent" or fatal. Penetrating injury can, even under primitive conditions, be salvageable by relatively simple techniques.[75]

Contusion

Myocardial contusion represents a wide spectrum of conditions, and the incidence following blunt chest trauma has been estimated to be 10% to 20%.[76–79] The significance of making the diagnosis in asymptomatic patients is not clear, nor is the best method. As few as 1% to 20% of patients develop complications that require treatment (life-threatening arrhythmias or pump failure) and these are usually self-evident.[79–81] Symptoms, however, are often masked by associated injuries.

A simple screen in asymptomatic patients is a routine electrocardiogram (ECG). If it is normal at admission and 4 hours later, the risk of developing life-threatening arrhythmia is essentially nil. Nonspecific changes, however, may require monitoring for a 24-hour period.[81] This latter recommendation is vague and treating physicians need to determine whether sinus tachycardia, for example, represents such a rhythm. Cardiac enzymes have been used to define the presence or absence of contusion. Creatinine phosphokinase myocardial bands (CPK-MB) have proved to be "irrelevant" as they do not predict the risk of complications.[81] Both cardiac-specific troponin I and T have been studied and it appears that cTNI may be more specific than cTnT, although with both there is little independent correlation with clinically relevant risk for developing complications, or at least complications that are not self-evident.[82–86]

Nevertheless, elevation of cTnI or T probably warrants 24-hour monitoring and consideration for early transthoracic echocardiography.

The management of arrhythmias follows standard algorithms. No evidence supports prophylaxis and benign rhythm disturbances [e.g., occasional unifocal premature ventricular contractions (PVC)] do not need to be treated.[80] Low cardiac output, caused by left ventricular failure, may require support with an intraaortic balloon pump, especially in patients requiring major orthopedic or general surgery procedures.[87] Transthoracic or transesophageal echocardiography can be critical in determining the best therapy and its impact. Right ventricular dysfunction can be assisted by both increasing preload and reducing pulmonary afterload.[80] Echocardiography can help determine the impact of ventilatory changes on cardiac function in those with coexisting acute lung injury or ARDS.

Blunt Cardiac Rupture

Blunt cardiac rupture is acutely fatal in more than 90% of victims.[88] The mechanisms are varied and include laceration from bony fractures, acute right atrial distension secondary to compression of the abdomen, deceleration resulting in motion and tension at the caval atrial junctions, and direct compression or delayed necrosis as a complication of contusion or coronary artery injury.[76,78,88,89] The right side is most commonly affected (right atrium 33% to 41%; right ventricle 30% to 39%) and is associated with the greatest chance of survival as compared with left-sided ruptures (left atrium 17% to 25%; left ventricle 6% to 13%).[88] Survival is reduced in the setting of multichamber rupture. Of patients with blunt rupture who survive to reach a trauma center with some vital signs, survival rates of 20% to 50% have been recorded.[88,90] The diagnosis is usually made by emergency thoracotomy in patients who arrive in extremis but can be made because of persistent hypotension by pericardial window or ultrasound.[78] Rarely, a CT performed to evaluate a widened mediastinum will reveal a "floating heart" suggestive of a small laceration.[91]

Management requires immediate exploration. Sternotomy offers the best overall exposure, followed by right anterolateral thoracotomy, because *two thirds or more* of injuries are right sided. Simple atrial ruptures or superior vena caval–atrial junction tears can be managed by clamping and suturing. Complex tears involving the inferior vena caval junction with the right atrium often require circulatory arrest or at least cardiopulmonary bypass. Digital control and rapid suture closure are the best method for ventricular lacerations.[10]

Complex Blunt Cardiac Injuries

The most common form of complex injury is valve rupture, noted in 5% of autopsies. The mitral valve is the most common valvar injury noted in autopsy series, whereas the aortic valve is the most commonly described valve injured in clinical series.[76] The left-sided valves are presumably at greater risk than those on the right side because of higher pressures. Mitral, tricuspid, and the rare pulmonary dehiscence can be diagnosed by echocardiography, and often patients have multiple injuries, including acute lung injury, that preclude immediate repair. Temporization with medical management is often possible.[92,93] Aortic injury usually results in significant insufficiency, which precludes intraaortic counterpulsation, and urgent repair is often required.[94,95] Rarely, tricuspid insufficiency can be complicated by shunting through a patent foramen ovale leading to recalcitrant right-to-left shunt. This can require earlier repair and closure of the foramen ovale.[76] Repair usually implies valve replacement, but, at times, particularly after papillary rupture, various repair techniques can be used.[96] Coronary occlusion, dissection, and aneurysm have all been described after blunt trauma with late ventricular aneurysm, septal defect, and myocardial infarction.[97-99] Coronary lesions can be treated by formal bypass or, depending on anatomy, coronary stents.

Penetrating Cardiovascular Injury

The incidence of penetrating cardiac injuries varies between centers and overall affects, ranging from 0.5% to 6% of patients admitted after penetrating injury.[100,101] Survival is linked to rapidity of prehospital transport, recognition of the injury, and operative intervention.[100,102,103]

Signs of cardiac tamponade remain elusive. Beck's triad of muffled heart sounds, jugular venous distention, and pulsus paradoxus is present in only 15% of patients who are later judged to have tamponade.[104] One reason is that hypovolemic patients do not require much compression to be functionally compromised. Pulsus paradoxus can be difficult to detect in a noisy emergency room with a tachypneic patient. One method of detecting pulsus paradoxus is to allow the blood pressure cuff to deflate slowly. The difference in pressure between the points when the systolic "pings" are heard intermittently (i.e., during expiration only) and more consistently (i.e., during all phases of respiration) represents the gradient. Differences greater than 10 mm Hg suggest accentuation of the physiologic drop in pressure associated with inspiration. CXR can occasionally demonstrate a widened cardiac shadow. Central venous pressure (CVP) reflecting elevated pressures can lead to the diagnosis. The focused abdominal ultrasound for trauma (FAST) or transthoracic echocardiogram has been advocated as a rapid and accurate method of evaluation.[105] Whereas evidence of obvious effusion is diagnostic, a normal findings will not absolutely rule out injury.[106] In particular, echo cannot reliably exclude cardiac injury in the setting of left-sided effusion. This is because the effusion can obscure the pericardium or may represent blood that has escaped through a rent, thus resulting in an empty pericardial sac (Fig. 24.4).

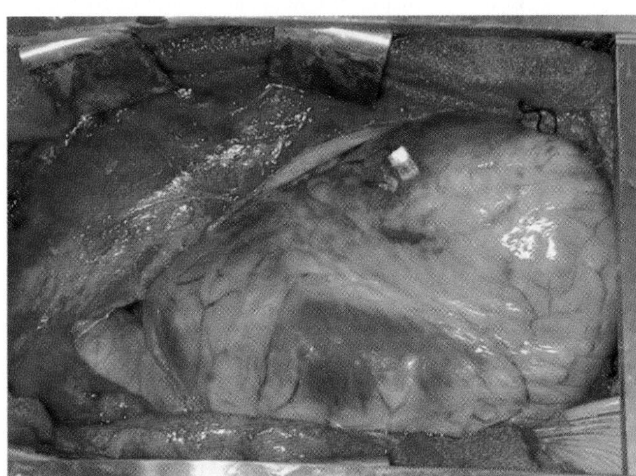

FIGURE 24.4 Thoracic surgery was consulted 24 hours after admission for self-inflicted stab wounds. The patient had a negative focused abdominal ultrasound for trauma study and transthoracic echocardiogram (TTE) but had a left hemothorax. The patient developed low-grade fevers and elevated erythrocyte sedimentation rate and electrocardiogram, suggesting pericarditis. Rigid thoracoscopy identified two lacerations in the pericardium with myocardium protruding. The anterior injury was easily repaired. A posterior injury was repaired using adenosine to reduce tension on the left atrial-ventricular junction during rotation to expose the injury.

Pericardiocentesis should not be used as a diagnostic tool, but in patients who do have findings suggesting tamponade, pericardiocentesis before induction does appear to reduce the risk of cardiac arrest at the time of intubation.[107] A low threshold for performing a pericardial window has been advocated by multiple centers. Thoracoscopy can be an option in stable patients in the setting of hemothorax or if there is abdominal contamination that raises the concern of possibly seeding the pericardium if a window is performed.[108]

The basic operative approaches include left anterolateral thoracotomy or sternotomy. The latter is more versatile for penetrating injuries between the anterior axillary lines. It provides exposure to the great vessels, aorta, and entire surface of the heart. In the rare instance that cardiopulmonary bypass is required, it can be established rapidly. The proximal portions of the great vessels can be controlled by advancing along the ascending aorta from within the pericardium.[10] Posterior cardiac injuries can be exposed by placing surgical pads to elevate the apex of the heart or by elevating the pericardium using stay sutures. Occasionally, patients will present with right-sided stab wounds, in extremis, and in these cases it is reasonable to perform a right anterolateral thoracotomy. Temporary cardiac arrest can be achieved using adenosine, starting at 6-mg doses and increasing until a transient arrest of 10 to 15 seconds is achieved.

Initial control includes using digital pressure and a stapler or by carefully placing a Foley catheter into the wound.[109,110] Fortunately, the majority of penetrating injuries are anatomically simple to correct (Figs. 24.4 and 24.5). Care must be given when manipulating the thin-walled right ventricle. Side biting vascular clamps can be applied to the atrial appendages or portions of the superior vena cava. Horizontal mattress sutures are the preferred technique of repair. Pledgets can be made from pericardium. With this technique, it is important to place the sutures through the pericardium, the wound, and then the opposite pericardium before cutting the pericardium, so as to avoid having to deal with floppy tissue that is easily tangled. Injuries that are close to coronary arteries should be managed by placing the sutures deep to the artery. It is important to remember that the proximal right coronary artery lies in the groove between the right atrial appendage and the right ventricle, and it is at risk of injury in this location. Injuries that are massively bleeding, whether from heart or proximal aorta, may require caval occlusion to allow exposure. By allowing the heart to "beat empty," a number of advantages are derived: a drop in blood loss; the ability to place initial sutures; and decreased pulmonary congestion with reduced lung injury.

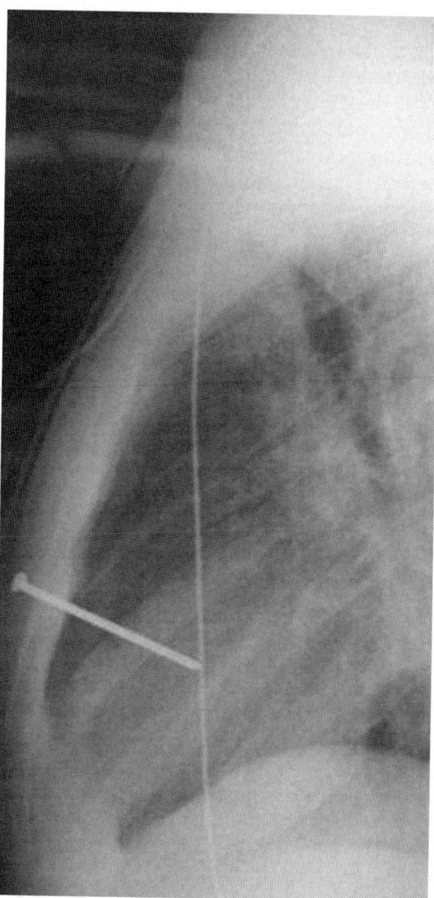

FIGURE 24.5 Nail gun injury to the heart. Although such injuries can be associated with significant periinjury contusion, they usually require simple pledgeted sutures.

Complex Penetrating Cardiac Injuries

Between 10% and 20% of survivors of penetrating cardiac injury sustain injuries that may require more than simple suture control.[111] These include coronary artery injuries, septal defects, and rare valvular injuries. In general, patients with these injuries are best managed by temporizing, because most are coagulopathic and hypothermic, and the best hope of survival is to end the operation as quickly as possible. The primary indication for immediate repair is inability to sustain cardiac output despite use of the intraaortic balloon pump. Overall, cardiopulmonary bypass is needed in 2% of patients with penetrating cardiac injuries and in as few as 10% of complex injuries acutely.[49,112] Rarely, bypass may be used as an adjunct to resuscitation.[113]

The most common coronary artery injured is the left anterior descending (LAD). Distal LAD and most other coronary lacerations can be managed by simple ligation.[49] There is an advantage to repairing selected coronary artery lacerations, because the postoperative morbidity of a myocardial infarction, particularly with proximal LAD injuries, can be significant. It may be immediately obvious in the operating room that there is significant myocardial ischemia developing. Small injuries may be primarily repaired. More complex injuries in stable patients who are not coagulopathic can be managed by bypass grafting, either on or off cardiopulmonary bypass.[114] Recent techniques in nonpump coronary surgery have facilitated this approach with the development of stabilization devices.[115,116]

A rare complication is coronary artery fistula, usually to the right ventricle, which can be associated with ischemia, low cardiac output, cardiac failure, or subacute bacterial endocarditis. They can be managed by stenting or operative repair depending on location and severity. Valve defects are uncommon. Aortic valve injuries resulting in severe insufficiency are noted by a wide pulse pressure, dilated left ventricle, and a palpable thrill at the aortic root. Intraaortic balloon pump is contraindicated in this situation. Most injuries in survivors are small, and the valve may be primarily repaired.

Ventricular septal defects (VSDs) should be suspected in any injury that involves both right and left ventricles as well as any injury close to the LAD, which marks the anterior septum.[49] Diagnosis can be suggested by a thrill and right ventricular dilation. Evidence of an oxygen step-up or echo will confirm the diagnosis. Most VSDs are small and many will close spontaneously. VSDs associated with a large shunt or those causing prolapse of the noncoronary cusp of the aortic valve require repair. The optimal approach is through the site of injury.

GREAT VESSEL INJURY

The great vessels and their major branches traverse the superior mediastinum, thoracic outlet, and the neck. Vascular injuries in this area constitute approximately 12% of all vascular trauma. Adjacent vital structures are often injured, accounting not only for the high mortality at the scene or in transit but also for severe hypotension of patients on arrival.[11,117] Blunt trauma is less common but can be particularly difficult to manage when it involves the airway. The sudden deceleration forces involved in vehicular crashes result in hyperextension injuries of the carotid and vertebral arteries, which may occur in the absence of bony injury. Diagnosis of these injuries can be difficult, because initially they are often unaccompanied by neurologic deficits and the consequences of missing such injuries can be devastating. Neurologic deficits, when present, may include cranial nerve palsies and Horner's syndrome in addition to hemispheric ischemia.[11]

In cases of blunt trauma, chest films may reveal classic widened mediastinum, occasionally associated with fractures of the clavicle and first and second ribs. In penetrating injury, mediastinal emphysema and hemopneumothorax may be noted.[117] In a stable patient, progression to angiography will accurately define arterial injury and assist the surgeon in planning for operative control and repair. When time permits, angiography is desirable in the assessment of zone 1 and zone 3 injuries. Duplex scanning may provide rapid, noninvasive assessment of a wide variety of carotid and vertebral injuries.[118] Transcranial Doppler monitoring can provide evidence of hypoperfusion and thromboembolism in intracranial vessels, indicating injury in major vessels more proximally.

Certain injuries require immediate operative exploration. These include injuries associated with active hemorrhage and hemodynamic instability. Large or expanding hematoma at the base of the neck, weak or nonpalpable pulses in the neck or upper limbs, and presence of a thrill or bruit also necessitate early surgical management. Most patients do not require cardiopulmonary bypass. If, when performing sternotomy for penetrating injury, a rapidly expanding hematoma is found, exploration initially should be performed within the pericardium.[10] Careful exposure allows the origins of the great vessels to be controlled before entering the hematoma. If there is active bleeding from arch or ascending aorta, performing bicaval occlusion allows the heart to "beat empty," reduces blood loss, allows exposure of the bleeding site, and may reduce the incidence of fatal postoperative respiratory failure.[10]

Median sternotomy provides the best approach to the innominate artery and the origins of the right common carotid and right subclavian arteries, as well as the left common carotid artery (see Fig. 24.1).[10] There is also good access to the superior vena cava, innominate veins, pulmonary artery, and heart, enabling expeditious control of a difficult situation.[118] Exposure of the left subclavian artery is best established through a left anterior thoracotomy, usually through the third intercostal space. Addition of a left supraclavicular incision and detachment of the insertions of the sternocleidomastoid and strap muscles creates a trapdoor for approach to the subclavian artery.[10] Further access to vessels in the neck can be established by extending the upper end of the median sternotomy into standard oblique incisions along the sternocleidomastoid. Mobilization of the clavicle or subperiosteal-resection may be necessary to access some subclavian injuries. When the clavicle is divided, subperiosteal resection should be performed and careful repair with orthopedic fixation, if necessary, performed attentively. Median sternotomy with supraclavicular extension is an alternative to the trap door approach and appears to offer as effective exposure with less morbidity.

Innominate artery injuries comprised 0.7% of 5,760 cardiovascular injuries in 4,459 patients in the extensive Baylor University experience.[119] Nonoperative management can be performed in patients with small intimal defects and no contraindications to anticoagulation,without surrounding hematoma.[120] In some settings, stent grafts may be applicable.[121] In all other settings, surgical intervention is warranted. In blunt trauma to the innominate artery, the most common site of injury is its origin.[117,122] Associated aortic injury is common. Inability to secure swift control is the most common cause of intraoperative mortality. When the patient has a hematoma, firm digital compression may be required while adequate exposure is being secured. The innominate vein may be clamped and divided with impunity to gain access to life-threatening arterial bleeding beneath. Avulsions and tears at the origin of the great vessels can be controlled by partially occluding C-clamps. Anomalous anatomy should always be kept in mind. Common origin of the innominate and left common carotid arteries (bovine arch) occurs in 5% of individuals. Lacerations within the innominate and left common carotid arteries may be controlled by simple distal and proximal clamping. Use of indwelling shunts to maintain cerebral blood flow remains variable. Occasionally, they are mandatory for cerebral perfusion, particularly in hypotensive patients and in cases of simultaneous innominate and left common carotid artery injury. Ligation of both the innominate and left common carotid arteries is generally fatal. In general, if the artery can be clamped proximal to its bifurcation, there is usually enough back perfusion via vertebral and portions of the circle of Willis to maintain cerebral perfusion. If concerned, stump pressures can be easily measured. Placement of a temporary prosthetic shunt from the ascending aorta to more distal potions of these vessels is facilitated by extending the sternotomy along the sternocleidomastoid on either side. Care must be taken to avoid injury to the recurrent laryngeal nerve. In cases of laceration, lateral suture may be effective, but if a defect persists, patch angioplasty is preferable. Occasionally, simple transection and end-to-end anastomosis is possible, but commonly vessel retraction and anastomotic tension results and prosthetic graft interposition is preferable.[117] Injury at the origin of the innominate artery necessitates aortoinnominate bypass. A contained hematoma at the arch is best left undisturbed while the bypass is performed. Bifurcated grafts may restore flow to both the innominate and left common carotid arteries, or the limbs can be extended to both subclavians.

The subclavian artery is relatively protected by the sternum and clavicles. In cases of penetrating injury to the subclavian, external bleeding at the root of the neck or into the pleural cavity may cause shock that fails to respond to blood transfusion. A cold, pulseless hand associated with neurologic deficits, supraclavicular bruits, or expanding pulsatile hematoma may be a feature of blunt trauma to the subclavian artery; however, presence of distal pulses does not rule out significant proximal injury. Traumatic occlusion of the first portion of the subclavian artery proximal to the vertebral takeoff may give rise to subclavian steal. Dyspnea may be an indication of an expanding hematoma at the base of the neck, a large hemothorax, or a hemopneumothorax. Occlusive thrombosis may be complicated by distal embolization, requiring thromboembolectomy. Associated brachial plexus injury is common and may result in a chronic, painful extremity; however, early amputation is not advised unless the nerve roots are completely avulsed.[117] In extremities, the artery may be ligated because there is good collateral supply around the shoulder.

The underlying consideration in management of carotid artery injuries is cerebral protection. Whereas many patients with penetrating carotid artery injury present with exsanguinating hemorrhage, ligation should, if possible, be reserved for patients with established neurologic deficits in the presence of complete occlusion of the entire carotid. Although the view was once held that ligation is preferable to repair in all patients with neurologic deficits so as to avoid mortality, the consensus is now firmly in favor of carotid reconstruction in cases of both blunt and penetrating injuries, as long as antegrade flow is present. Combined morbidity and mortality is significantly lower in patients undergoing primary repair compared with ligation (15% vs. 50%).[118] The role of anticoagulation in these situations remains variable. Cerebral CT with contrast or diffusion magnetic resonance imaging (MRI) is helpful in assessing the potential risk for hemorrhagic conversion of an infarct. Remove established thrombus by balloon catheter before repair or insertion of a shunt.

Blunt Rupture of the Thoracic Aorta

The primary mechanism of injury is acute deceleration with a variety of forces applied to the descending thoracic aorta near the ligamentum arteriosum. Traumatic rupture had been considered an absolute surgical emergency with immediate repair being the standard of care. This philosophy arose from Parmley's 1958 study documenting a death rate at the scene of up to 85% and a subsequent mortality rate in nonoperated survivors of 1% per hour for the first 48 hours.[123] Currently, although the scene mortality remains similar, it appears that of patients who survive to be admitted, one third (roughly 5% of the whole) present unstable or become acutely unstable within a short period. The mortality in this group approaches 100%. The remaining two thirds (10% of the whole) remain stable, and if treated appropriately, the mortality is approximately 25%, the primary cause of death being associated injuries.[124] The mortality of patients who present with a systolic blood pressure of less than 90 mm Hg or whose pressure drops to below this level within 1 hour of admission is approximately 70% to 98%, whereas for those who remain stable, the mortality is approximately 20%.[125]

In most cases, the diagnosis is suggested by plain chest radiographic evidence of mediastinal blood (Fig. 24.6).

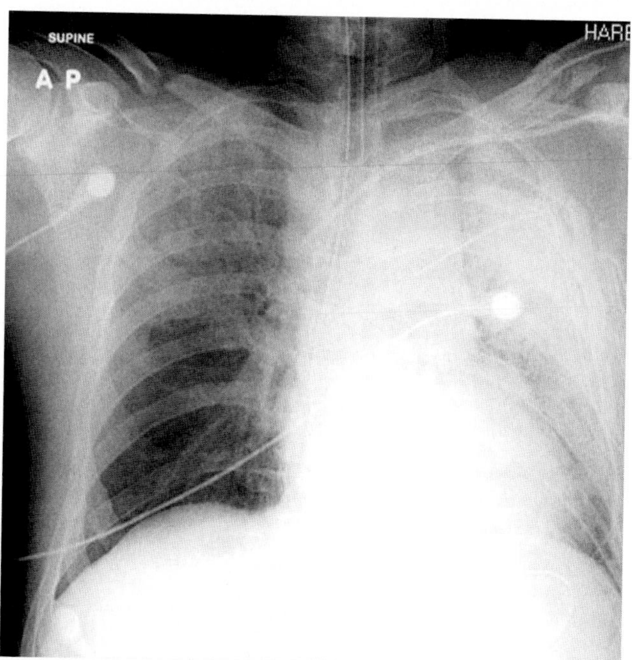

FIGURE 24.6 Plain chest radiographic study of patient with traumatic aortic rupture. Noted are widening of the superior mediastinum, loss of anteroposterior window, and blurring of the aortic knob.

Although sternal and first-rib fractures have been used as criteria for angiography, they have very low association with thoracic aortic rupture and, in isolation, do not warrant routine angiography.[126] When combined with a high degree of clinical suspicion based on mechanism, plain CXR has a 98% or greater sensitivity, although specificity can be as low as 10% to 45%.[127] Up to 7% of patients with aortic rupture have normal CXR findings initially.[128] Thoracic aortography has a sensitivity of nearly 100% and specificity of 98%.[129] False-negative findings have been attributed to small intimal lesions and false-positive findings to atheromatous plaques or anatomic variants. CT scanning has been advocated as a screening tool but has recently been superseded by CTA (angiography). This should be considered a combination of angiography and helical scanning and has a sensitivity and specificity approaching that of angiography.[130,131] In addition, three-dimensional reconstructions give valuable data on which to plan operative or endovascular approaches. If both modalities are available, angiography is ideally utilized when it is required for another reason (e.g., pelvic embolization, concern for cerebrovascular injury), whereas CTA can be used if there is indication for CT scan (to assess the abdomen for example) or as the primary workup after CXR. Transesophageal echocardiography (TEE) has sensitivity and specificity of 57% to 63% and 84% to 91%, respectively.[132] The arch extending to an area between the left common carotid and left subclavian arteries is often obscured by the trachea. Advantages of TEE include its abilities to be performed during laparotomy, obviating the need for further workup, and to discriminate between ulcerated plaques and true injuries the ability to perform, and the ability to perform concomitant assessment of cardiac function. Intravascular ultrasound (IVUS) has been used in a similar fashion. Both modalities appear to have their greatest utility in assessing equivocal findings on CTA or angiography, for following lesions that are not deemed immediately operable, and, in the case of IVUS, assisting in placing stent grafts.

When the diagnosis is suspected on the basis of CXR, immediate control of blood pressure is critical.[131] The target pressure has been described as "less than 120 mm Hg," but more recently it has been argued that a pressure "lower than admission" is sufficient to significantly reduce the risk of rupture during workup.[124] Short-acting ß-blockers, such as Esmolol, or combination agents, such as Labetolol, are excellent. Pure vasodilating agents (Nipride principally) are not favored because the reflex increased heart rate increases $\Delta P/\Delta T$ and may aggravate spinal ischemia by causing shunting of blood away from the cord. Pain control is often all that is required.

Nearly 75% of patients have associated injuries. The triage of associated injuries can be difficult, but, in general, hypotensive patients are much more likely to become unstable because of associated injuries (principally pelvic and intraabdominal hemorrhage).[125,133] Patients who have grossly positive diagnostic peritoneal lavage (DPL) or negative FAST should undergo laparotomy first, whereas stable patients with only count-positive DPL or negative FAST should have their aortic injury addressed first.[134] Although the vast majority of patients who present with stable blood pressure and are immediately started on ß-blockade remain stable, patients with hemothorax greater than 500 mL without pneumothorax, supraclavicular hematoma, or "psuedocoarcation" are at high risk of early free rupture and should be operated on immediately unless there are significant contraindications.[135] Of patients, 20% to 50% may not be candidates for immediate operative repair because of associated injuries.[125,136] The primary contraindications are pulmonary injury preventing single-lung ventilation, deep lung lacerations, cardiac ischemia, and cardiac "contusion" requiring inotropic support.

The risk of rupture when ß-blockade is possible appears to be less than 5%, but it can occur even with minimal injury.[124,131,136,137] One review noted that the risk of expansion or rupture was greatest in the first 5 to 7 days, following which the natural history of aortic rupture was similar to that of nontraumatic aneurysmal disease, presumably resulting from the secondary fibrotic reaction.[137] Serial studies (e.g., helical CTA) every 48 to 72 hours for the first 7 days can be used to follow the lesion and ensure stability. Evidence of growth would prompt earlier intervention, even if the risk were greater. Hypotensive therapy can itself be associated with complications. Patients with closed head injury and elevated intracranial pressure may have pressure-affected cerebral perfusion, leading to secondary brain injury. Prolonged lower pressure may also result in end-organ dysfunction. Thus, urgent repair should still be considered the standard of care, unless there are specific indications to delay surgery.

Endovascular Approaches

Endovascular stent grafting has become an attractive alternative to open repair or nonoperative management. Most patients with traumatic aortic lesions have small-diameter (20 mm or less) aortas, and thus commercially available cuff extenders designed for infrarenal aortic disease may be appropriate.[138] A number of anatomic considerations, however, make it difficult to apply the experience gained from infrarenal aortic disease to the thoracic aorta.[139] Most aortic injuries are close to the origin of the left subclavian artery, and, to gain appropriate landing zones, often the stents must be placed into the arch across the origin of the artery.[140] This does not pose a risk of limb loss, but rather the risk of endoleak from retrograde flow. In addition, placing the stent into the curvature can affect the ability of the tension to be placed uniformly against the aortic wall, resulting in increased risk for telescoping and late migration. Another source of telescoping is short landing zones. If the tear is large, lateral expansion of the stent graft can result in shortening, in turn leading to the risk of endoleak and migration.[141]

Operative Management

In contrast to autopsy studies, less than 1% of injuries in clinical series involve the ascending aorta or arch.[142] These lesions require an approach via sternotomy utilizing hypothermic circulatory arrest. Associated vascular or multiple injury sites are present in approximately 10% of cases. In up to 20% of cases, anatomic anomalies are present, including bovine arch and aberrant origin of the vertebral artery.[140] Injuries in the descending thoracic aorta, within 1 cm of the origin of the subclavian artery, present subtle but at times critical differences compared with those more distal.[143] The more proximal injuries require control proximal to the left subclavian artery, an important source of collateral blood supply to the spinal cord. Finally, there is increased risk of rupture during proximal dissection. In stable patients, therefore, it is often advisable to institute left heart bypass before proximal exposure. Usually grafts are required, but in up to 20% of cases primary anastomosis can be used (with shorter cross clamp times).[144] Primary repair of small lesions has been reported.

Paralysis is the dreaded complication of aortic reconstruction. Factors that appear to be related and not in isolation include preoperative hypotension, cross clamp time (>30 minutes), and not using mechanical circulatory support.[125,145,146] In addition to reducing the risk of paralysis, however, left heart bypass appears to reduce stress on the heart and maintain splanchnic perfusion.[147] Using the superior or inferior pulmonary veins for pump inflow reduces the risk of left atrial rupture and postoperative cardiac complications.[145,148] Heparin-bonded circuits allow minimal use of heparin and can reduce bleeding risk.

DIAPHRAGMATIC INJURIES

Injuries to the diaphragm make up only 3% of the total number of injuries sustained from trauma. Blunt injuries usually occur secondary to high-speed motor vehicle crashes.[149] Penetrating injuries, such as gunshot wounds and stab wounds, probably occur more frequently but have been cited less often in the literature. Overall, the associated injury rate has been reported to be as high as 80% to 100%, particularly after blunt trauma.[150]

The anatomic location appears to be more often left sided than right sided for two reasons. Most assailants are right-handed and, therefore, are more likely to injure their victims on the left side. In blunt injury, the liver probably affords some degree of protection to lacerations of the diaphragm. The radiographic signs of a left-sided injury are much easier to see and more likely to be detected.[149] Bilateral injuries to the diaphragm occur in only 2% of all patients sustaining diaphragmatic trauma. Tears of the central tendon of the diaphragm with herniation of abdominal contents into the pericardium are extremely rare but have been reported.[149]

Patients may present with symptoms that are abdominal or thoracic in nature, or both. They may present with marked hemodynamic instability and require an emergency laparotomy. Chest or abdominal pain, dyspnea, and orthopnea are frequent complaints. Initial CXR findings are usually normal in 50% of patients and show a pneumothorax or hemothorax in most of the remaining 50% of patients with diaphragmatic injury. Abnormalities that can be detected that suggest diaphragmatic tears include elevation or obscuration of the diaphragm and visceral herniation. The finding of the nasogastric tube coiling in the left hemithorax is rarely seen but is pathognomic for diaphragmatic injury.[150–152] One scenario in which plain CXR can overlook a diaphragmatic injury, even a large left-sided one, is when a patient arrives intubated or is intubated shortly thereafter and requires more than 5 cm H_2O of positive end-expiratory pressure (PEEP). As a patient is weaned from ventilator support, progressive herniation of abdominal contents occurs.[153] This underlines the importance of serial chest films. CT has become the primary diagnostic modality (Fig. 24.7).

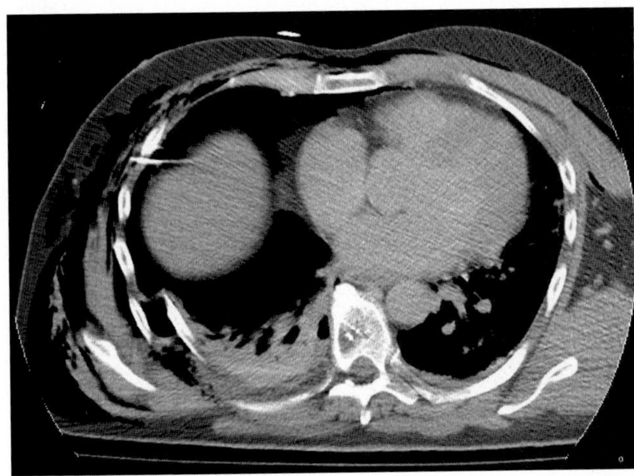

FIGURE 24.7 Same patient as in Figure 24.2. The lowermost displaced ribs are close to the diaphragm–pleural interface, and there is a suggestion of pleural elevation. At surgery, a 2-cm diameter defect was found.

It is very accurate in detecting intraabdominal fluid, solid organ injury, fractures, intraperitoneal air, pneumothorax, and retroperitoneal injury. Unfortunately, according to a number of reports in the literature, it has not been able to consistently demonstrate diaphragmatic lacerations.[150]

Failure to diagnose diaphragmatic injury by radiographic means has led some surgeons to utilize newer surgical techniques to improve accuracy. Reports of the use of both diagnostic laparoscopy and videothoracoscopy have documented high rates of injury identification.[6,108,154] An occasional patient's small, accessible defect has been successfully repaired by these methods as well.

Most acute diaphragmatic injuries are best approached by a laparotomy. A chest tube is often required before operation in those patients with either hemothorax or pneumothorax. It should be inserted carefully in patients with suspected diaphragmatic injury to avoid inadvertent injury to any potentially herniated abdominal viscera. Injuries without tissue loss (class I to III) are best repaired with a continuous monofilament suture of 1-0 or larger.[149] The edges of the diaphragm need to be grasped and elevated by long Allis clamps before suturing. This helps prevent inadvertent suturing of the underlying lung and facilitates identification of the full extent of the injury. Class IV injury repairs may be made easier by placing interrupted sutures first to realign the edges before repair with a continuous suture. On occasion, the defect along the lateral chest wall can be extensive or there may be combined loss of chest wall integrity. In this setting, resuspending the diaphragm from the ribs at a higher level can allow closure.[149]

TRAUMATIC ESOPHAGEAL PERFORATION

Diagnosis, management, and outcome for traumatic esophageal perforation are critically affected by etiology, location, and duration between event and intervention. In trauma, there is a tendency for the diagnosis to be delayed.[155] There has been a trend away from "time-based" therapy, with injuries diagnosed more than 24 hours after injury being managed by exclusion-diversion to therapy based on the clinical stability of the patient, underlying esophageal pathology, and quality of the mediastinal tissues, with an emphasis on primary repair, usually with some form of tissue buttressing.

Traumatic injuries, because they tend to involve the cervical esophagus in younger patients, have a mortality rate ranging from 9% to 19%.[155] The most common traumatic injury occurs following penetrating neck injury, accounting for more than 80% of all traumatic perforations.[155] Only 0.5% to 5% of penetrating neck injuries, however, are associated with esophageal involvement. Blunt trauma leads to esophageal perforation in less than 0.1% of cases; most in the cervical area are caused by a sudden blow to the anterior hyperextended neck.[156] Virtually all thoracic traumatic perforations are a consequence of penetrating trauma. Other causes described include blast injury (particularly compressed air) and acute gastric compression resulting in complex lower third intrathoracic esophageal tears. Transmediastinal gunshot wounds involving "low-velocity" missiles that course close to the spine can result in through-and-through injuries (Fig. 24.8). Stab wounds to the abdomen, particularly through the back, are rarely associated with intraabdominal esophageal perforation.

Most traumatic esophageal injuries are discovered because the mechanism of injury suggests the possibility, but they may present in a more occult fashion.[155] Initial symptoms

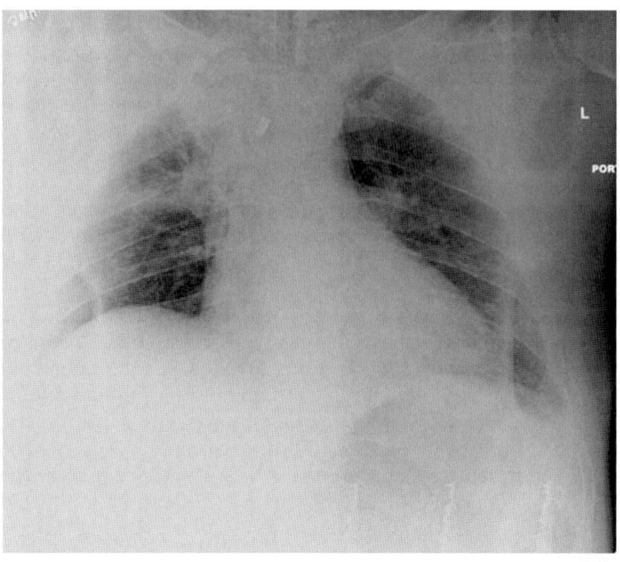

FIGURE 24.8 Gunshot wound to the base of the left neck. The bullet is lying just to the right of the midline structures. Computed tomography scan suggested the possibility of esophageal injury because of proximity and ruled out vascular injury. Esophagoscopy confirmed the injury.

of cervical perforations may be simply hoarseness, spitting up blood, subcutaneous air, or anterior tracheal deviation. Untreated, fever, erythema, swelling, increasing crepitus, airway distress, and, finally, frank abscess formation occur. Infection often spreads along the precervical plane to involve upper mediastinal structures, leading to signs and symptoms of mediastinitis. Patients who present with zone II injuries that are associated with penetration of the platys should be considered at risk for esophageal injury. Thoracic perforations usually are initially silent. Patients may complain of ill-defined substernal pain after iatrogenic perforation. Many patients with spontaneous perforation have acute tearing pain unless they are severely intoxicated, in which case they present in a delayed fashion. Usually, within 24 hours, mediastinitis and empyema result in unrelenting septic shock. Pleural fluid that is foul-smelling, associated with pH below 6.0 or with elevated amylase, should raise the possibility.[157] Subdiaphragmatic injuries present with abdominal tenderness, referred shoulder tip pain, and, ultimately, in over 50% of cases, peritonitis and sepsis.[156]

Conventional radiographs may demonstrate subcutaneous emphysema, hydropneumothorax, hydro-pneumomediastinum, or free abdominal air, depending on location of perforation and duration of injury. Occasionally, a nasogastric tube is noted to be lying extraesophageal. Radiologists, who fear barium contamination, favor Gastrograffin swallows. Gastrograffin, however, can miss up to 15% of perforations and, therefore, if negative should be followed by barium. We prefer to use "thin" barium as the initial study. The advantage of a contrast study is that it confirms location of leak, to which side of the esophagus the leak predominantly tends, and determines if significant stricture or other pathology needs to be addressed. Overall, the false-negative rate using combined gastrograffin-tin barium is as high as 10%.[156] CT scan, which may demonstrate contrast or air in the surrounding mediastinum and reveal pleural effusions, can be used to follow up. Sensitivity rates of 90% have been reported.

Esophagoscopy and contrast studies are complementary in the trauma setting.[155] Esophagoscopy can miss 15% to 40% of traumatic injuries, but when combined with contrast studies the sensitivity approaches 100%. Flexible and rigid esophagoscopy are both acceptable in the trauma setting. Flexible endoscopy tends to be less sensitive for detecting injuries in the most proximal cervical esophagus, because blind passage of the scope through the cricopharyngeus tends to miss the most proximal 2 to 4 cm. Rigid esophagoscopy is limited by the need for anesthesia and the requirement that the patient's neck be cleared for flexion.

Basic principles include control of leak, débridement and drainage of all areas of suppuration, nutritional support (with emphasis on gastric or jejunostomy tubes, or both) and early use of broad-spectrum antibiotics. Most traumatic perforations require operative therapy, and most cases should be approached with the intention of performing primary repair.[157] However, the presence of significant underlying esophageal pathology, extreme inflammation of tissues and/or degree of shock may mandate other approaches. Most injuries can be repaired primarily. Additional protection can be achieved by buttressing the repair.[158] In the cervical area, the sternocleidomastoid or other strap muscles can be mobilized as an onlay patch. In the chest, intercostal muscle flap can be laid onto the repair. It may not be advisable to circumferentially wrap the esophagus because late calcification can result in an unyielding extrinsic stricture. Other options include diaphragm, pericardium, or pericardial fat pad flaps. In the abdomen, omentum, fundoplication, or Thal (gastric tube) patches are options.

Primary repair should still be considered, even in the setting where diagnosis has been delayed for more than 24 hours.[157,158] The limiting factors in these circumstances are tissue quality and patient stability. In fact, in a field of moderate inflammation, repair with tissue flaps (either as primary method or to reinforce primary repair) may be even more effective. The "Grillo" pleural flap appears to be particularly effective when pleural inflammation is present.[157,158] It is critical, however one attempts to deal with the delayed perforation, that a thorough decortication is performed to allow full lung expansion. Some authors feel that if the tissue is tenuous, primary repair can still be performed if either a diversion (cervical fistula or drainage with T-tube) or exclusion (absorbable suture or staples at E-G junction) is performed to "protect" the repair.[156]

Occasionally, in the cervical or thoracic esophagus, through-and-through wounds are significant enough that primary repair would lead to critical narrowing. Short (1- to 2-cm) circumferential resection and end-to-end anastomosis can be performed for penetrating traumatic injuries in the neck or chest. When the tear or perforation is very large, resection can be performed expeditiously. A long cervical esophagostomy can be brought out onto the anterior chest wall below the clavicle.[156] This procedure has the advantages of being more comfortable for the patient and maximizing the length of residual esophagus for later reconstruction.

Drainage is best suited for the management of late-diagnosed cervical perforations.[155,156] Drainage of complex thoracic aortic perforation that, because of size of injury, inadequate tissue, or patient instability, is not a candidate for primary repair or resection is best achieved with a tracheal T-tube into which a 28 French chest tube can be intussuscepted. At least two other chest tubes should be placed nearby. This creates a controlled fistula that, once the patient recovers, can be downsized by removing the T-tube via esophagoscopy and then slowly changing the chest tube to smaller and smaller caliber tubes. Simple drainage with a chest tube is associated with nearly 70% mortality. On the other hand, in hemodynamically unstable patients with other injuries, simple drainage with or without stapling or ligating the esophagus above and below the injury may be needed simply to "get the patient off the table."[155,156]

KEY POINTS

- **Chest injuries are primarily responsible for 25% of fatalities and contribute to a further 50% of fatalities following trauma.**
- **Most chest injuries do not require thoracotomy and, in 85% of cases, are resolved with chest tube thoracostomy.**
- **Unrecognized hemothorax and delayed recognition of retained hemothorax leading to infection and lung volume loss are persistent complications of thoracic injury.**
- **Large or persistent air leaks require bronchoscopy and frequently either thorascopic or open repair, tractotomy, or resection.**
- **Blunt cardiac injury is usually "silent" and requires supportive care only.**
- **The great vessels of the upper mediastinum are best repaired by primary stent or interposition graft approached through a median sternotomy with initial proximal control.**
- **Rupture of the thoracic aorta usually results from deceleration and shear at the fixation point of the ligamentum arteriosum, may or may not require immediate repair, and can frequently be maintained with "hypotensive therapy" and repaired with stent placement rather than formal open repair.**
- **Diaphragmatic and esophageal injuries are often diagnosed late, should be evaluated aggressively based on risk, and require repair or operative drainage to prevent significant morbidity and mortality.**

References

1. **Calhoon JH, Trinkle JK. Pathophysiology of chest trauma. *Chest Surg Clin N Am.* 1997;7:199–211.**
2. Cuschieri J. Tube thoracostomy. In: Karmy-Jones R, Nathens A, Stern E, eds. *Thoracic Trauma and Critical Care.* Boston: Kluwer Academic Publishers, 2002;45–47.
3. Bailey RC. Complications of tube thoracostomy in trauma. *Journal of Accident Emergency Medicine* 2000;17:111–114.
4. Romanoff H. Prevention of infection in war chest injuries. *Ann Surg.* 1975;182:144–149.
5. Luchette FA, Barrie PS, Oswanski MF, et al. Practice Management Guidelines for Prophylactic Antibiotic Use in Tube Thoracostomy for Traumatic Hemopneumothorax: the EAST Practice Management Guidelines Work Group. Eastern Association for Trauma. *J Trauma* 2000;48:753–757.
6. **Karmy-Jones R, Vallieres E, Kralovich K, et al. A comparison of rigid –v– video thoracoscopy in the management of chest trauma. *Injury* 1998;29:655–659.**
7. Brusov PG, Kuritsyn AN, Urazovsky NY, et al. Operative videothoracoscopy in the surgical treatment of penetrating firearms wounds of the chest. *Mil Med.* 1998;163:603–607.
8. Schermer CR, Matteson BD, Demarest GB III, et al. A prospective evaluation of video-assisted thoracic surgery for persistent air leak due to trauma. *Am J Surg.* 1999;177:480–484.
9. Mitchell ME, Muakkassa FF, Poole GV, et al. Surgical approach of choice for penetrating cardiac wounds. *J Trauma* 1993;34:17–20.
10. **Pate JW, Cole FH, Walker WA, et al. Penetrating injuries of the aortic arch and its branches. *Ann Thorac Surg.* 1993;55:586–592.**
11. Abouljoud MS, Obeid FN, Horst HM, et al. Arterial injuries of the thoracic outlet: a ten-year experience. *Am Surg.* 1993;59:590–595.
12. Mayberry JC, Trunkey DD. The fractured rib in chest wall trauma. *Chest Surg Clin N Am.* 1997;7:239–261.
13. Easter A. Management of patients with multiple rib fractures. *Am J Crit Care* 2001;10:320–327; quiz 328–329.
14. Mackersie RC, Shackford SR, Hoyt DB, et al. Continuous epidural fentanyl analgesia: ventilatory function improvement with routine use in treatment of blunt chest injury. *J Trauma* 1987;27:1207–1212.
15. Mackersie RC, Karagianes TG, Hoyt DB, et al. Prospective evaluation of epidural and intravenous administration of fentanyl for pain control and restoration of ventilatory function following multiple rib fractures. *J Trauma* 1991;31:443–449; discussion 449–451.
16. Shackford SR, Smith DE, Zarins CK, et al. The management of flail chest. A comparison of ventilatory and nonventilatory treatment. *Am J Surg.* 1976;132:759–762.
17. Tanaka H, Yukioka T, Yamaguti Y, et al. Surgical stabilization of internal pneumatic stabilization? A prospective randomized study of management of severe flail chest patients. *J Trauma* 2002;52:727–732; discussion 732.

18. Buckman R, Trooskin SZ, Flancbaum L, et al. The significance of stable patients with sternal fractures. *Surg Gynecol Obstet.* 1987;164:261–265.
19. Wojcik JB, Morgan AS. Sternal fractures—the natural history. *Ann Emerg Med.* 1988;17:912–914.
20. Cuschieri J, Kralovich KA, Patton JH, et al. Anterior mediastinal abscess after closed sternal fracture. *J Trauma* 1999;47:551–554.
21. White C, Isik F. Reconstruction of complex chest wall defects. In: Karmy-Jones R, Nathens A, Stern E, eds. *Thoracic Trauma and Critical Care.* Boston: Kluwer Academic Publishers, 2002;247–251.
22. Losanoff JE, Metzler MH, Richman BW, et al. Necrotizing chest wall infection after blunt trauma: case report and review of the literature. *J Trauma* 2002;53:787–789.
23. Kao L. Traumatic lung hernia. In: Karmy-Jones R, Nathens A, Stern E, eds. *Thoracic Trauma and Critical Care.* Boston: Kluwer Academic Publishers, 2002;257–259.
24. **McNamara JJ, Messersmith JK, Dunn RA, et al. Thoracic injuries in combat casualties in Vietnam. *Ann Thorac Surg.* 1970;10:389–401.**
25. **Karmy-Jones R, Jurkovich GJ, Nathens AB, et al. Timing of urgent thoracotomy for hemorrhage after trauma: a multicenter study. *Arch Surg.* 2001;136:513–518.**
26. Eddy AC, Luna GK, Copass M. Empyema thoracis in patients undergoing emergent closed tube thoracostomy for thoracic trauma. *Am J Surg.* 1989;157:494–497.
27. Coselli JS, Mattox KL, Beall AC, Jr. Reevaluation of early evacuation of clotted hemothorax. *Am J Surg.* 1984;148:786–790.
28. Rosenblatt M, Lemer J, Best LA, et al. Thoracic wounds in Israeli battle casualties during the 1982 evacuation of wounded from Lebanon. *J Trauma* 1985;25:350–354.
29. Velmahos GC, Demetriades D, Chan L, et al. Predicting the need for thoracoscopic evacuation of residual traumatic hemothorax: chest radiograph is insufficient. *J Trauma* 1999;46:65–70.
30. Karmy-Jones R, Sorenson V, Horst HM, et al. Rigid thorascopic debridement and continuous pleural irrigation in the management of empyema. *Chest* 1997;111:272–274.
31. Inci I, Ozcelik C, Ulku R, et al. Intrapleural fibrinolytic treatment of traumatic clotted hemothorax. *Chest* 1998;114:160–165.
32. Meyer DM, Jessen ME, Wait MA, et al. Early evacuation of traumatic retained hemothoraces using thoracoscopy: a prospective, randomized trial. *Ann Thorac Surg.* 1997;64:1396–1400;discussion 1400–1391.
33. **Richardson JD, Carrillo E. Thoracic infection after trauma. *Chest Surg Clin N Am.* 1997;7:401–427.**
34. Weissberg D, Refaely Y. Pleural empyema: 24-year experience. *Ann Thorac Surg.* 1996;62:1026–1029.
35. Cohn SM. Pulmonary contusion: review of the clinical entity. *J Trauma* 1997;42:973–979.
36. Tranbaugh RF, Elings VB, Christensen J, et al. Determinants of pulmonary interstitial fluid accumulation after trauma. *J Trauma* 1982;22: 820–826.
37. Guerrero-Lopez F, Vazquez-Mata G, Alcazar-Romero PP, et al. Evaluation of the utility of computed tomography in the initial assessment of the critical care patient with chest trauma. *Crit Care Med.* 2000;28: 1370–1375.
38. Richardson JD, Adams L, Flint LM. Selective management of flail chest and pulmonary contusion. *Ann Surg.* 1982;196:481–487.
39. Kishikawa M, Yoshioka T, Shimazu T, et al. Pulmonary contusion causes long-term respiratory dysfunction with decreased functional residual capacity. *J Trauma* 1991;31:1203–1208;discussion 1208–1210.
40. Hanning CD, Ledingham E, Ledingham IM. Late respiratory sequelae of blunt chest injury: a preliminary report. *Thorax* 1981;36:204–207.
41. Johnson JA, Cogbill TH, Winga ER. Determinants of outcome after pulmonary contusion. *J Trauma* 1986;26:695–697.
42. Tyburski JG, Collinge JD, Wilson RF, et al. Pulmonary contusions: quantifying the lesions on chest X-ray films and the factors affecting prognosis. *J Trauma* 1999;46:833–838.
43. Carrillo EH, Block EF, Zeppa R, et al. Urgent lobectomy and pneumonectomy. *Eur J Emerg Med.* 1994;1:126–130.
44. Asensio JA, Demetriades D, Berne JD, et al. Stapled pulmonary tractotomy: a rapid way to control hemorrhage in penetrating pulmonary injuries. *J Am Coll Surg.* 1997;185:486–487.
45. Robison PD, Harman PK, Trinkle JK, et al. Management of penetrating lung injuries in civilian practice. *J Thorac Cardiovasc Surg.* 1988;95: 184–190.
46. Stewart KC, Urschel JD, Nakai SS, et al. Pulmonary resection for lung trauma. *Ann Thorac Surg.* 1997;63:1587–1588.
47. Stanic V. The advantages of limited resection vs. suture in the primary management of penetrating lung war wounds. *Vojnosanit Pregl.* 1998;55: 583–590.
48. **Cothren C, Moore EE, Biffl WL, et al. Lung-sparing techniques are associated with improved outcome compared with anatomic resection for severe lung injuries. *J Trauma* 2002;53:483–487.**
49. Wall MJ, Jr., Soltero E. Damage control for thoracic injuries. *Surg Clin North Am.* 1997;77:863–878.
50. Wall MJ, Jr., Villavicencio RT, Miller CC, 3rd, et al. Pulmonary tractotomy as an abbreviated thoracotomy technique. *J Trauma* 1998;45: 1015–1023.
51. **Karmy-Jones R, Jurkovich GJ, Shatz DV, et al. Management of traumatic lung injury: a Western Trauma Association Multicenter review. *J Trauma* 2001;51:1049–1053.**
52. Gasparri M, Karmy-Jones R, Kralovich KA, et al. Pulmonary tractotomy versus lung resection: viable options in penetrating lung injury. *J Trauma* 2001;51:1092–1095;discussion 1096–1097.
53. Wagner JW, Obeid FN, Karmy-Jones RC, et al. Trauma pneumonectomy revisited: the role of simultaneously stapled pneumonectomy. *J Trauma* 1996;40:590–594.
54. Geiger JP, Fischer RP, Guernsey JM, et al. Pulmonary resection: the treatment of choice for pulmonary contusion due to high velocity thoracic wounds. *US Army Vietnam Medical Bulletin* 1971.
55. Richardson JD, Flint LM, Snow NJ, et al. Management of transmediastinal gunshot wounds. *Surgery* 1981;90:671–676.
56. Nagy KK, Roberts RR, Smith RF, et al. Trans-mediastinal gunshot wounds: are "stable" patients really stable? *World J Surg.* 2002;26: 1247–1250.
57. Cornwell EE, 3rd, Kennedy F, Ayad IA, et al. Transmediastinal gunshot wounds. A reconsideration of the role of aortography. *Arch Surg.* 1996;131:949–952;discussion 952–943.
58. **Degiannis E, Benn CA, Leandros E, et al. Transmediastinal gunshot injuries. *Surgery* 2000;128:54–58.**
59. McIntyre RC, Jr., Moore EE, Read RR, et al. Transesophageal echocardiography in the evaluation of a transmediastinal gunshot wound: case report. *J Trauma* 1994;36:125–127.
60. Stassen NA, Lukan JK, Spain DA, et al. Reevaluation of diagnostic procedures for transmediastinal gunshot wounds. *J Trauma* 2002;53:635–638.
61. Kirsh MM, Orringer MB, Behrendt DM, et al. Management of tracheobronchial disruption secondary to nonpenetrating trauma. *Ann Thorac Surg.* 1976;22:93–101.
62. **Kiser AC, O'Brien SM, Detterbeck FC. Blunt tracheobronchial injuries: treatment and outcomes. *Ann Thorac Surg.* 2001;71:2059–2065.**
63. Velly JF, Martigne C, Moreau JM, et al. Post traumatic tracheobronchial lesions. A follow-up study of 47 cases. *Eur J Cardiothorac Surg.* 1991;5: 352–355.
64. Taskinen SO, Salo JA, Halttunen PE, et al. Tracheobronchial rupture due to blunt chest trauma: a follow-up study. *Ann Thorac Surg.* 1989;48: 846–849.
65. Jones WS, Mavroudis C, Richardson JD, et al. Management of tracheobronchial disruption resulting from blunt trauma. *Surgery* 1984;95:319–323.
66. Sattler S, Canty TG, Jr., Mulligan MS, et al. Chronic traumatic and congenital diaphragmatic hernias: presentation and surgical management. *Can Respir J.* 2002;9:135–139.
67. Wintermark M, Schnyder P, Wicky S. Blunt traumatic rupture of a mainstem bronchus: spiral CT demonstration of the "fallen lung" sign. *Eur Radiol.* 2001;11:409–411.
68. Ferretti GR, Thony F, Bosson JL, et al. Benign abnormalities and carcinoid tumors of the central airways: diagnostic impact of CT bronchography. *AJR Am J Roentgenol.* 2000;174:1307–1313.
69. Kawamoto S, Yuasa M, Tsukuda S, et al. Bronchial atresia: three-dimensional CT bronchography using volume rendering technique. *Radiat Med.* 2001;19:107–110.
70. Wood D. Tracheobronchial trauma. In: Karmy-Jones R, Nathens A, Stern E, eds. *Thoracic Trauma and Critical Care.* Boston: Kluwer Academic Publishers, 2002;109–122.
71. **Rossbach MM, Johnson SB, Gomez MA, et al. Management of major tracheobronchial injuries: a 28-year experience. *Ann Thorac Surg.* 1998;65: 182–186.**
72. Crouch RD, Nelson LE, Hawley PC, et al. Onlay patch repair of tracheobronchial rupture. *Ann Thorac Surg.* 1997;64:1158–1160.
73. Hira HS, Kumar D, Sondhi V, et al. Bronchial stenosis after blunt chest trauma. *J Assoc Physicians India* 2002;50:1189–1191.
74. Pilcher JA, Jr., Ishitani MB, Rodgers BM. Left upper lobe bronchus reimplantation for nonpenetrating thoracic trauma. *Ann Thorac Surg.* 2000;69:273–275.
75. Zakharia AT. Cardiovascular and thoracic battle injuries in the Lebanon War. Analysis of 3,000 personal cases. *J Thorac Cardiovasc Surg.* 1985;89:723–733.
76. Pretre R, Bednarkiewicz M, Faidutti B. Blunt cardiac injury: in achieving a practical diagnostic classification. *J Trauma* 1994;36:462–463.
77. Mattox KL, Flint LM, Carrico CJ, et al. Blunt cardiac injury. *J Trauma* 1992;33:649–650.
78. **Brown J, Grover FL. Trauma to the heart. *Chest Surg Clin N Am.* 1997;7:325–341.**
79. Lindstaedt M, Germing A, Lawo T, et al. Acute and long-term clinical significance of myocardial contusion following blunt thoracic trauma: results of a prospective study. *J Trauma* 2002;52:479–485.
80. van Wijngaarden MH, Karmy-Jones R, Talwar MK, et al. Blunt cardiac injury: a 10 year institutional review. *Injury* 1997;28:51–55.
81. Biffl WL, Moore FA, Moore EE, et al. Cardiac enzymes are irrelevant in the patient with suspected myocardial contusion. *Am J Surg.* 1994;168: 523–527;discussion 527–528.
82. Robert E, de La Coussaye JE, Aya AG, et al. Mechanisms of ventricular arrhythmias induced by myocardial contusion: a high-resolution

mapping study in left ventricular rabbit heart. *Anesthesiology* 2000;92:1132–1143.
83. Bertinchant JP, Robert E, Polge A, et al. Comparison of the diagnostic value of cardiac troponin I and T determinations for detecting early myocardial damage and the relationship with histological findings after isoprenaline-induced cardiac injury in rats. *Clin Chim Acta* 2000; 298:13–28.
84. Bertinchant JP, Polge A, Mohty D, et al. Evaluation of incidence, clinical significance, and prognostic value of circulating cardiac troponin I and T elevation in hemodynamically stable patients with suspected myocardial contusion after blunt chest trauma. *J Trauma* 2000;48:924–931.
85. Ferjani M, Droc G, Dreux S, et al. Circulating cardiac troponin T in myocardial contusion. *Chest* 1997;111:427–433.
86. Helm M, Hauke J, Weiss A, et al. [Cardiac troponin T as a biochemical marker of myocardial injury early after trauma. Diagnostic value of a qualitative bedside test]. *Chirurg* 1999;70:1347–1352.
87. Flancbaum L, Wright J, Siegel JH. Emergency surgery in patients with post–traumatic myocardial contusion. *J Trauma* 1986;26:795–803.
88. Biffle WL, Moore EE. Blunt cardiac injury. In: Karmy-Jones R, Nathens A, Stern E, eds. *Thoracic Trauma and Critical Care*. Boston: Kluwer Academic Publishers, 2002;281–288.
89. Pretre R, Chilcott M. Blunt trauma to the heart and great vessels. *N Engl J Med*. 1997;336:626–632.
90. Fulda G, Brathwaite CE, Rodriguez A, et al. Blunt traumatic rupture of the heart and pericardium: a ten-year experience (1979–1989). *J Trauma* 1991;31:167–172;discussion 172–163.
91. Krejci CS, Blackmore CC, Nathens A. Hemopericardium: an emergent finding in a case of blunt cardiac injury. *AJR Am J Roentgenol*. 2000;175: 250.
92. Cuadros CL, Hutchinson JE, Mogtader AH. Laceration of a mitral papillary muscle and the aortic root as a result of blunt trauma to the chest. Case report and review of the literature. *J Thorac Cardiovasc Surg*. 1984;88:134–140.
93. End A, Rodler S, Oturanlar D, et al. Surgery of blunt heart trauma. *Chirurg* 1992;63:641–646.
94. Hanna KM, Weiman DS, Pate JW, et al. Aortic valve injury secondary to blunt trauma from an air bag. *Tenn Med*. 1997;90:195–196.
95. Pretre R, Faidutti B. Aortic valve rupture in closed trauma: the extent of the damage. *J Thorac Cardiovasc Surg*. 1993;106:371–373.
96. End A, Rodler S, Oturanlar D, et al. Elective surgery for blunt cardiac trauma. *J Trauma* 1994;37:798–802.
97. Pretre R, Kursteiner K, Khatchatourian G, et al. Traumatic occlusion of the left anterior descending artery and rupture of the aortic isthmus. *J Trauma* 1995;39:388–390.
98. Gillebert T, van de Werf F, Piessens J, et al. Post-traumatic infarction due to blunt chest trauma. Report of two cases. *Acta Cardiol*. 1980;35: 445–453.
99. Gaspard P, Clermont A, Villard J, et al. Non-iatrogenic trauma of the coronary arteries and myocardium: contribution of angiography—report of six cases and literature review. *Cardiovasc Intervent Radiol*. 1983;6: 20–29.
100. Rhee PM, Foy H, Kaufmann C, et al. Penetrating cardiac injuries: a population-based study. *J Trauma* 1998;45:366–370.
101. Campbell NC, Thomson SR, Muckart DJ, et al. Review of 1198 cases of penetrating cardiac trauma. *Br J Surg*. 1997;84:1737–1740.
102. Asensio JA, Murray J, Demetriades D, et al. Penetrating cardiac injuries: a prospective study of variables predicting outcomes. *J Am Coll Surg*. 1998;186:24–34.
103. Tyburski JG, Astra L, Wilson RF, et al. Factors affecting prognosis with penetrating wounds of the heart. *J Trauma* 2000;48:587–590; discussion 590–581.
104. Knott-Craig CJ, Dalton RP, Rossouw GJ, et al. Penetrating cardiac trauma: management strategy based on 129 surgical emergencies over 2 years. *Ann Thorac Surg*. 1992;53:1006–1009.
105. Kirkpatrick AW, Brown DR, Crickmer S, et al. Hand-held portable sonography for the on-mountain exclusion of a pneumothorax. *Wilderness Environ Med*. 2001;12:270–272.
106. Aaland MO, Bryan FC, 3rd, Sherman R. Two-dimensional echocardiogram in hemodynamically stable victims of penetrating precordial trauma. *Am Surg*. 1994;60:412–415.
107. Callaham M. Pericardiocentesis in traumatic and nontraumatic cardiac tamponade. *Ann Emerg Med*. 1984;13:924–945.
108. Villavicencio RT, Aucar JA, Wall MJ, Jr. Analysis of thoracoscopy in trauma. *Surg Endosc*. 1999;13:3–9.
109. Macho JR, Markison RE, Schecter WP. Cardiac stapling in the management of penetrating injuries of the heart: rapid control of hemorrhage and decreased risk of personal contamination. *J Trauma* 1993;34:711–715; discussion 715–716.
110. Bowman MR, King RM. Comparison of staples and sutures for cardiorrhaphy in traumatic puncture wounds of the heart. *J Emerg Med*. 1996;14:615–618.
111. Wall MJ, Mattox KL, Chen CD, et al. Acute management of complex cardiac injuries. *J Trauma* 1997;42:905–912.
112. Reissman P, Rivkind A, Jurim O, et al. Case report: the management of penetrating cardiac trauma with major coronary artery injury—is cardiopulmonary bypass essential? *J Trauma* 1992;33:773–775.
113. Karmy-Jones R, van Wijngaarden MH, Talwar MK, et al. Cardiopulmonary bypass for resuscitation after penetrating cardiac trauma. *Ann Thorac Surg*. 1996;61:1244–1245.
114. Karmy-Jones R, van Wijngaarden MH, Talwar MK, et al. Penetrating cardiac injuries. *Injury* 1997;28:57–61.
115. Narayan P, Caputo M, Roidl M, et al. The use of off pump surgery for management of penetrating coronary artery injury. *Eur J Cardiothorac Surg*. 2002;21:361–362.
116. Bowley DMG, Saeed M, Somwe D, et al. Off-pump cardiac revascularization after a complex stab wound. *Ann Thorac Surg*. 2002;74: 2192–2193.
117. Rosenberg JM, Bredenberg CE, Marvasti MA, et al. Blunt injuries to the aortic arch vessels. *Ann Thorac Surg*. 1989;48:508–513.
118. Nicholls SC. Management of great vessel injury. In: Karmy-Jones R, Nathens A, Stern E, eds. *Thoracic Trauma and Critical Care*. Boston: Kluwer Academic Publishers, 2002;303–313.
119. Mattox KL, Feliciano DV, Burch J, et al. Five thousand seven hundred sixty cardiovascular injuries in 4459 patients. Epidemiologic evolution 1958 to 1987. *Ann Surg*. 1989;209:698–705;discussion 706–697.
120. Rhee RY, Gloviczki P, Cherry KJ, Jr. Management of injuries to branches of the aortic arch. *Semin Vasc Surg*. 1996;9:147–155.
121. Patel AV, Marin ML, Veith FJ, et al. Endovascular graft repair of penetrating subclavian artery injuries. *J Endovasc Surg*. 1996;3:382–388.
122. Turney SZ. Blunt trauma of the thoracic aorta and its branches. *Semin Thorac Cardiovasc Surg*. 1992;4:209–216.
123. Parmley L, Mattingly T, Manion W, et al. Nonpenetrating traumatic injury of the aorta. *Circulation* 1959;17:1086–1101.
124. Mattox KL, Wall MJ, Jr. Historical review of blunt injury to the thoracic aorta. *Chest Surg Clin N Am*. 2000;10:167–182.
125. Karmy-Jones R, Carter YM, Nathens A, et al. Impact of presenting physiology and associated injuries on outcome following traumatic rupture of the thoracic aorta. *Am Surg*. 2001;67:61–66.
126. Sturm JT, Luxenberg MG, Moudry BM, et al. Does sternal fracture increase the risk for aortic rupture? *Ann Thorac Surg*. 1989;48:697–698.
127. Mirvis SE, Bidwell JK, Buddemeyer EU, et al. Value of chest radiography in excluding traumatic aortic rupture. *Radiology* 1987;163: 487–493.
128. Mattox KL. Red River anthology. *J Trauma* 1997;42:353–368.
129. Sturm JT, Hankins DG, Young G. Thoracic aortography following blunt chest trauma. *Am J Emerg Med*. 1990;8:92–96.
130. Downing SW, Sperling JS, Mirvis SE, et al. Experience with spiral computed tomography as the sole diagnostic method for traumatic aortic rupture. *Ann Thorac Surg*. 2001;72:495–501; discussion 501–492.
131. Fabian TC, Davis KA, Gavant ML, et al. Prospective study of blunt aortic injury: helical CT is diagnostic and antihypertensive therapy reduces rupture. *Ann Surg*. 1998;227:666–676; discussion 676–667.
132. Smith MD, Cassidy JM, Souther S, et al. Transesophageal echocardiography in the diagnosis of traumatic rupture of the aorta. *N Engl J Med*. 1995;332:356–362.
133. Borman KR, Aurbakken CM, Weigelt JA. Treatment priorities in combined blunt abdominal and aortic trauma. *Am J Surg*. 1982;144:728–732.
134. Hudson HM, 2nd, Woodson J, Hirsch E. The management of traumatic aortic tear in the multiply-injured patient. *Ann Vasc Surg*. 1991;5:445–448.
135. Clark DE, Zeiger MA, Wallace KL, et al. Blunt aortic trauma: signs of high risk. *J Trauma* 1990;30:701–705.
136. Maggisano R, Nathens A, Alexandrova NA, et al. Traumatic rupture of the thoracic aorta: should one always operate immediately? *Ann Vasc Surg*. 1995;9:44–52.
137. Holmes JHT, Bloch RD, Hall RA, et al. Natural history of traumatic rupture of the thoracic aorta managed nonoperatively: a longitudinal analysis. *Ann Thorac Surg*. 2002;73:1149–1154.
138. Hoffer EK, Karmy-Jones R, Bloch RD, et al. Treatment of acute thoracic aortic injury with commercially available abdominal aortic stent-grafts. *Journal of Vascular Interventional Radiology* 2002;13:1037–1041.
139. Karmy-Jones R., Hoffer EK, Meissner M, et al. Endovascular stent grafts and aortic rupture: a case series. *J Trauma* 2003;55:805–810.
140. Borsa JJ, Hoffer EK, Karmy-Jones R, et al. Angiographic description of blunt traumatic injuries to the thoracic aorta with specific relevance to endograft repair. *J Endovasc Ther*. 2002;9(suppl. 2):II84–II91.
141. Orford VP, Atkinson NR, Thompson K, et al. Blunt traumatic aortic transection: The endovascular experience. *Ann Thorac Surg*. 2003;75: 106–112.
142. Feczko JD, Lynch L, Pless JE, et al. An autopsy case review of 142 nonpenetrating (blunt) injuries of the aorta. *J Trauma* 1992;33:846–849.
143. Carter Y, Meissner M, Bulger E, et al. Anatomical considerations in the surgical management of blunt thoracic aortic injury. *J Vasc Surg*. 2001;34:628–633.
144. McBride LR, Tidik S, Stothert JC, et al. Primary repair of traumatic aortic disruption. *Ann Thorac Surg*. 1987;43:65–67.
145. Karmy-Jones R, Carter Y, Meissner M, et al. Choice of venous cannulation for bypass during repair of traumatic rupture of the aorta. *Ann Thorac Surg*. 2001;71:39–41; discussion 41–32.
146. Fabian TC, Richardson JD, Croce MA, et al. Prospective study of blunt aortic injury: Multicenter Trial of the American Association for the Surgery of Trauma. *J Trauma* 1997;42:374–380; discussion 380–373.

147. Forbes AD, Ashbaugh DG. Mechanical circulatory support during repair of thoracic aortic injuries improves morbidity and prevents spinal cord injury. *Arch Surg*. 1994;129:494–497; discussion 497–498.
148. Fullerton DA. Simplified technique for left heart bypass to repair aortic transection. *Ann Thorac Surg*. 1993;56:579–580.
149. Sorensen VJ. Diaphragmatic Injuries. In: Karmy-Jones R, Nathens A, Stern E, eds. *Thoracic Trauma and Critical Care*. Boston: Kluwer Academic Publishers, 2002;261–266.
150. Mansour KA. Trauma to the diaphragm. *Chest Surg Clin N Am*. 1997;7:373–383.
151. Sharma OP. Traumatic diaphragmatic rupture: not an uncommon entity—personal experience with collective review of the 1980's. *J Trauma* 1989;29:678–682.
152. Shah R, Sabanathan S, Mearns AJ, et al. Traumatic rupture of diaphragm. *Ann Thorac Surg*. 1995;60:1444–1449.
153. Karmy-Jones R, Carter Y, Stern E. The impact of positive pressure ventilation on the diagnosis of traumatic diaphragmatic injury. *Am Surg*. 2002;68:167–172.
154. Lindsey I, Woods SD, Nottle PD. Laparoscopic management of blunt diaphragmatic injury. *Aust N Z J Surg*. 1997;67:619–621.
155. Asensio JA, Chahwan S, Forno W, et al. Penetrating esophageal injuries: multicenter study of the American Association for the Surgery of Trauma. *J Trauma* 2001;50:289–296.
156. Kao L, Karmy-Jones R. Esophageal injury and perforation. In: Karmy-Jones R, Nathens A, Stern E, eds. *Thoracic Trauma and Critical Care*. Boston: Kluwer Medical Publishers, 2002;271–280.
157. Whyte RI, Iannettoni MD, Orringer MB. Intrathoracic esophageal perforation. The merit of primary repair. *J Thorac Cardiovasc Surg*. 1995;109:140–144.
158. Gouge TH, Depan HJ, Spencer FC. Experience with the Grillo pleural wrap procedure in 18 patients with perforation of the thoracic esophagus. *Ann Surg*. 1989;209:612–617.

CHAPTER 25 ■ ABDOMINAL TRAUMA

DAVID H. WISNER AND DAVID B. HOYT

Most civilian abdominal injuries are caused by blunt trauma secondary to high-speed automobile crashes, although penetrating injuries are common in urban environments. The failure to successfully manage abdominal injuries accounts for most of the preventable deaths that follow multiple trauma. Failure to recognize occult abdominal hemorrhage and to control bleeding from intraabdominal organs leads to significant morbidity, and such injuries account for approximately 10% of the traumatic deaths that occur annually in the United States.

ANATOMIC CONSIDERATIONS

The abdomen is defined by the diaphragm at its superior aspect and by the infragluteal fold at its caudal aspect; it includes the entire circumference of the torso. Abdominal injury is often accompanied by trauma to other sites, such as the central nervous system, the chest, and the musculoskeletal system. To simplify the initial trauma evaluation, the abdomen can be divided into four areas: intrathoracic abdomen, true abdomen, elvic abdomen, and retroperitoneal abdomen (Fig. 25.1). With the exception of the true abdomen, all of these areas are difficult to assess by physical examination alone.

The intrathoracic abdomen is the portion of the upper abdomen that lies beneath the rib cage (Fig. 25.1A). Bony and cartilaginous structures make this area essentially inaccessible to palpation. Its contents include the diaphragm, liver, spleen, and stomach. Each of these organs can be injured when blunt or penetrating impact is delivered to the rib cage.

The pelvic abdomen is defined by the bony pelvis (Fig. 25.1B). Its contents include the rectum, bladder, urethra, small intestine, and, in female patients, the uterus, fallopian tubes, and ovaries. Trauma to the pelvis, particularly pelvic fractures, can damage the organs within, and penetrating injuries of the buttocks can injure any or all of the pelvic organs. Injury to these structures may be extraperitoneal and, therefore, difficult to diagnose. For this reason, suspected injuries may require adjunctive procedures such as bladder catheterization, urethrocystography, and sigmoidoscopy for diagnosis.

The retroperitoneal abdomen contains the kidneys, ureters, pancreas, second and third portions of the duodenum, great vessels, aorta, and vena cava (Fig. 25.1C). Injury to these structures can also occur secondary to penetrating or blunt trauma. The kidneys can be damaged by injury to the lower ribs posteriorly, and any of these structures can be damaged by crushing injuries to the front or side of the torso. Again, injury to these structures may result in few physical findings, and physical examination and diagnostic peritoneal lavage (DPL) are of little use.[1] Evaluation of the retroperitoneal abdomen requires use of radiographic imaging procedures, including computed tomography (CT), angiography, ultrasound, and intravenous pyelography.

The true abdomen contains the small and large intestines, the bladder when distended, and the uterus when gravid. Perforation of these organs is usually manifested by pain from peritonitis and is associated with significant abdominal physical findings. DPL is a useful adjunct if injury is suspected, and a plain abdominal film can be helpful if free air is present.

PENETRATING INJURY

Handguns are the most common cause of serious penetrating injury to the abdomen. Significant intraabdominal injury occurs in approximately 80% of patients who sustain abdominal gunshot wounds but in only 20% to 30% of patients with stab wounds. The frequency of organ injury after penetrating abdominal trauma is shown in Table 25.1.

Injuries to both thoracic and abdominal cavities occur in 25% of patients with penetrating wounds of the abdomen. Patients with penetrating wounds of the thorax also may have significant intraabdominal injury because a bullet can readily traverse the diaphragm. Patients with gunshot wounds to the abdomen and lower chest should routinely undergo laparotomy

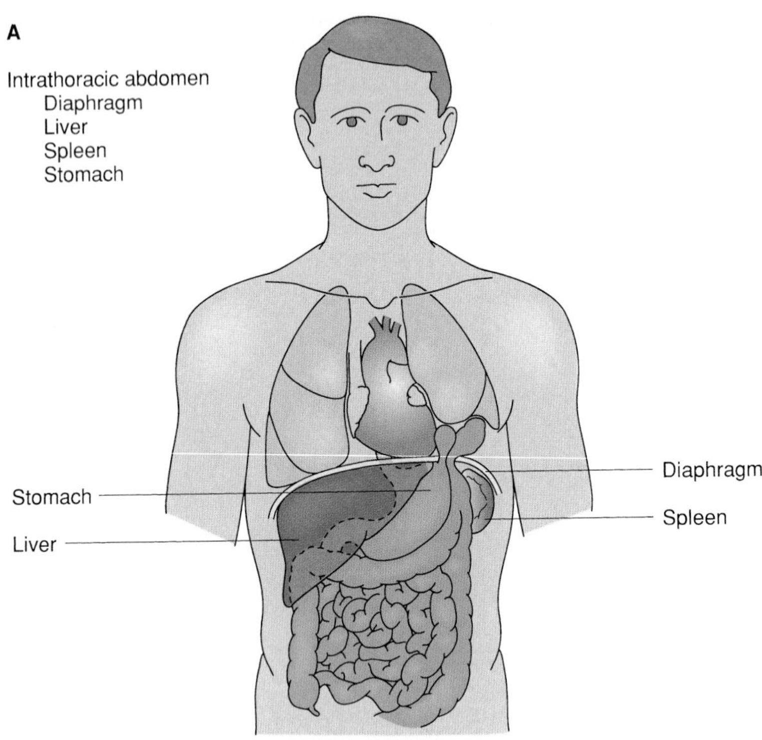

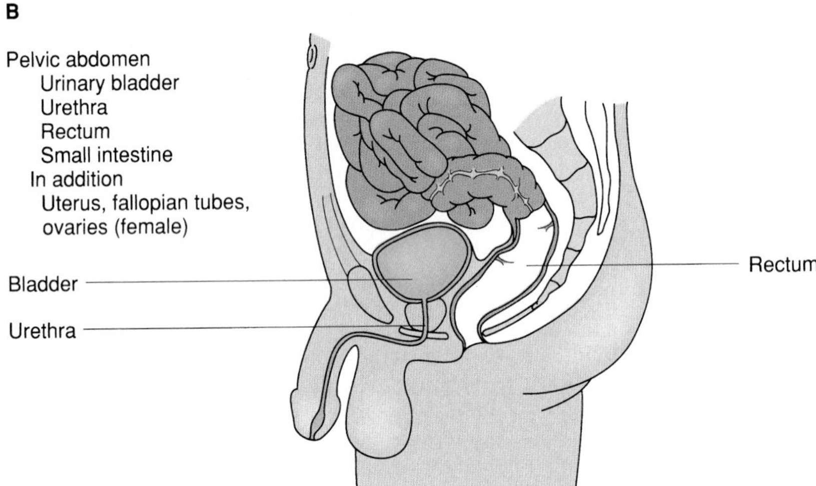

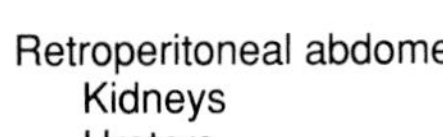

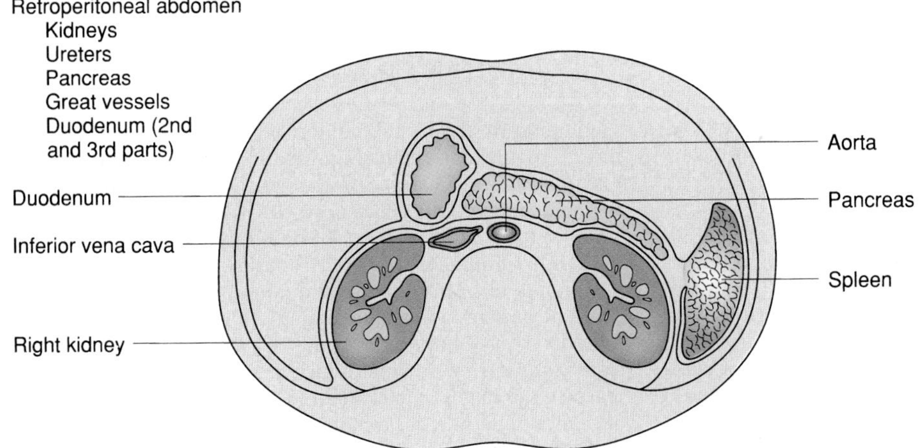

FIGURE 25.1 Four traditional anatomic divisions of the abdomen. (*A*) Intrathoracic abdomen. Contents of this area are subdiaphragmatic but cephalad to the costal margin. With respiration, the diaphragm is presumed to ascend to the level of the nipples (fourth intercostal space anteriorly). A ruptured left hemidiaphragm is illustrated with herniation of the stomach and distal transverse colon into the left hemithorax. (*B*) Similarly, the contents of the pelvic abdomen are within the bony pelvis. (*C*) The structures in the retroperitoneal abdomen. The true (intraperitoneal) abdomen contains the remainder of the viscera, and the inventory of its contents is dynamic, depending on body position and respiration (not shown).

TABLE 25.1

FREQUENCY OF ORGAN INJURY IN PENETRATING ABDOMINAL TRAUMA

Organ	Occurrence (%)
Liver	37
Small bowel	26
Stomach	19
Colon	17
Major vascular	13
Retroperitoneal	10
Mesentery and omentum	10
Spleen	7
Diaphragm	5
Kidney	4
Pancreas	4
Duodenum	2
Biliary system	1
Other	1

because the probability of intraabdominal injury is high. The difference in injury potential between gunshot wounds and stab wounds is a function of the higher kinetic energy associated with gunshot wounds, and selective management may be the best method for treating stab wounds.

BLUNT TRAUMA

Automobile crashes are the cause of at least 60% of all traumatic injuries. Table 25.2 shows the frequency with which specific organs are injured by blunt abdominal trauma. Some series list the liver rather than the spleen as the most commonly injured intraabdominal organ; this difference probably reflects the means of diagnosis. Small liver injuries are often detected in patients who undergo CT scan of the abdomen, whereas splenic injuries in adults are more likely to be clinically significant and to require surgical intervention.

Solid organs are most frequently injured from blunt trauma. The sudden application of pressure to the abdomen is more likely to rupture a solid organ than a hollow viscus. The more elastic tissues of young people tolerate trauma better than those of older people, and this accounts in part for the differences in incidence and pattern of injuries between children and adults with blunt abdominal trauma.

TABLE 25.2

FREQUENCY OF ORGAN INJURY IN BLUNT ABDOMINAL TRAUMA IN ADULTS

Organ	Occurrence (%)
Liver	30
Spleen	25
Retroperitoneal hematoma	13
Kidney	7
Urinary bladder	6
Intestine	5
Mesentery	5
Pancreas	3
Diaphragm	2
Urethra	2
Vascular	2

PREHOSPITAL CARE

Little can be done outside a hospital for patients with abdominal injuries. For penetrating wounds, sterile dressings should be applied and the patient should be carefully monitored. Foreign bodies embedded in the trunk should not be removed because major bleeding can follow. Evisceration is best left undisturbed except for application of a moist sterile dressing and protection of the patient from further injury. General principles of stabilization and evaluation should be followed, including ensuring an adequately functioning airway, inserting intravenous lines (preferably in the upper extremity), beginning fluid resuscitation, and providing rapid transport to a trauma facility. Recent controversy surrounding the issue of the value of fluid resuscitation in the early posttraumatic period has arisen. Although fluid resuscitation in the prehospital phase of care is still indicated, preoccupation with fluid resuscitation should not delay rapid transport to a trauma center. The prehospital application of the pneumatic antishock garment is usually not indicated for severe abdominal hemorrhage but may play a role in the temporary stabilization of severe pelvic fractures, particularly if prolonged transport times are anticipated.

HOSPITAL RESUSCITATION AND DIAGNOSIS

Diagnosis and treatment should proceed concurrently according to established protocols. A functioning airway must be established, particularly in the comatose patient, before evaluation of the abdomen occurs. If necessary, an endotracheal tube is placed and assisted ventilation is begun. Upper extremity, large-bore intravenous catheters are initiated, and resuscitation is begun with a balanced salt solution (e.g., lactated Ringer's or normal saline). Early crystalloid resuscitation is indicated, especially in the presence of a head injury, despite theoretic considerations that instillation of intravenous fluids increases bleeding and causes a dilutional coagulopathy.[1] When operative intervention is necessary, however, it should not be delayed by overzealous and prolonged attempts at fluid resuscitation.

HISTORY AND PATTERN OF INJURY

Penetrating injuries present little diagnostic challenge other than the question of whether to explore the abdomen operatively. An attempt should be made to establish details of the trauma event and the weapon used. The blunt trauma assessment can be aided considerably by an accurate history. If the patient was involved in an automobile crash in which he or she struck the steering wheel or if no seatbelt was used, specific thoracic and epigastric abdominal trauma should be suspected. If the patient was restrained, it can be helpful to determine whether the restraint was a two-point lap belt or a three-point shoulder belt. The patient who sustains rib fractures involving the lower left chest has a 15% chance of associated splenic injury; the patient with rib fractures on the right has a 10% chance of liver injury. A compression fracture of the lumbosacral region carries a 20% risk of significant renal parenchymal injury.

PHYSICAL EXAMINATION

The objective of the physical examination in abdominal trauma is to rapidly identify the patient who needs laparotomy. Precise definition of specific organ injury is unnecessary.

The specificity and sensitivity of physical examination alone, however, are not adequate to make these determinations. Associated injuries often cause tenderness and spasm in the abdominal wall and make diagnosis difficult. Lower rib fractures, pelvic fractures, or abdominal wall contusions can mimic the signs of peritonitis.

In patients with gunshot wounds, no presumptions should be made about entrance and exit wounds. Unfounded presumptions can lead to inaccurate estimations about the number of times a patient was shot and the course of the bullets. If time permits, radiographs should be obtained to determine the location of any bullets or bullet fragments that remain in the patient.

Because the primary manifestation of blunt solid organ injury is hemorrhage, the patient should be monitored closely during the initial assessment, and continuing or refractory shock is presumed to result from continuing or massive hemorrhage. The patient should be examined from head to toe for signs of blunt trauma and for penetrating wounds. Small abrasions or areas of ecchymosis suggest significant local intraabdominal injury. Penetrating wounds should be marked with radiopaque clips to allow radiographic delineation of the injury tract. The abdominal wall and back should be carefully inspected, and posterior ecchymosis should raise the possibility of retroperitoneal injury. The absence of bowel sounds is consistent with an ileus, but it is a nonspecific finding and, in the context of a busy emergency department, it is insensitive for discriminating between patients who do and do not need laparotomy.

Palpation can reveal localized tenderness, spasm, or rigidity of the abdominal wall. These findings and the finding of rebound tenderness are consistent with peritonitis and perforation of hollow viscera. Exploratory laparotomy is required for this presumed diagnosis. Suprapubic tenderness and pelvic lateral wall tenderness, which can indicate a pelvic fracture, are assessed in the conscious patient. Inspection of the perineum and urethral meatus for blood is routine to look for signs of pelvic fracture and possible urethral injury.

As assessment continues, rectal examination is performed and sphincter tone is evaluated. The integrity of the rectal wall and the position and mobility of the prostate associated with urethral injury are evaluated. The stool should be tested for the presence of gross or occult blood. A urinary catheter is placed, and a urine sample is sent for analysis for microscopic hematuria. If injury to the urethra is suspected, retrograde urethrography (RUG) should be performed before catheterization and a suprapubic catheter placed if necessary.

The physical findings for injuries to these different structures are sometimes a function of the time between injury and examination. Hollow viscus perforations may require several hours before peritonitis becomes apparent. Colonic or gastric perforations produce peritonitis more rapidly, small bowel perforations less so. Hematomas and bruising from retroperitoneal or pelvic fracture bleeding may not be apparent initially. Frequent reevaluation is an essential strategy in the treatment of patients with blunt abdominal trauma.

LABORATORY STUDIES

The hematocrit is the primary blood study of value in the initial evaluation of a patient with abdominal trauma. Leukocyte counts, serum creatinine, glucose, serum amylase/lipase, and serum electrolyte determinations are often obtained for reference but usually have little value in the immediate management period.

The diagnosis of massive hemorrhage is usually obvious from hemodynamic parameters, and the hematocrit merely confirms the diagnosis. Iatrogenic dilutional anemia is common and, in the presence of hemodynamic stability, is well tolerated. Urinalysis confirms the presence of microscopic hematuria. For blunt trauma, radiographic evaluation of the kidneys and bladder should be initiated if the patient has gross hematuria or microscopic hematuria and shock (systolic blood pressure <90 mm Hg in an adult) at any point during the prehospital or emergency department course.

The serum amylase is insensitive and nonspecific as a marker for major pancreatic or enteric injury. Injuries to the head and face commonly cause increased plasma amylase concentrations. Serum lipase levels are not elevated by facial trauma and are possibly more specific than amylase levels. Sensitivity and specificity of lipase levels, however, especially in the early postinjury period, are still relatively low. Sensitivity and specifity of both the amylase and lipase improve with time. Persistent or increasing elevations of the amylase or lipase should, therefore, raise concern of significant intraabdominal injury and are an indication for aggressive radiographic or surgical investigation.

RADIOGRAPHIC EVALUATION

Radiologic studies of potential value in the evaluation of abdominal trauma include a chest radiograph, retrograde urethrography and cystography, CT scans, ultrasound, and angiography. In addition, all injuries from penetrating trauma should be evaluated with a plain radiograph with the use of radiodense markers on the wound sites to allow evaluation of the missile trajectory. With blunt trauma, an anteroposterior film of the pelvis can delineate pelvic fractures not detectable on physical examination. The initial pelvic film or chest radiograph can also demonstrate fractures of the thoracic or lumbar spine. A transverse fracture of the vertebral bodies, or Chance fracture, should increase the search for serious blunt intestinal injury. The value of plain abdominal films after blunt trauma is extremely limited and they should not be routinely obtained.

Of greater value are CT scans, ultrasound, and angiography. CT has real value in the accurate assessment of solid organ injuries, particularly of the liver, kidney, and spleen; contrast-enhanced CT has great accuracy in the delineation of intraabdominal bleeding. The accuracy of CT scan in evaluation of hollow viscus injury is somewhat more limited, but improvements in CT technology have led to increasing sensitivity of CT in the detection of the more subtle signs of injury to the intestine.[2,3] CT is also highly specific in the evaluation of retroperitoneal injuries and is the single most useful and informative diagnostic study for patients with abdominal trauma.

CT scanning can also be used on occasion for penetrating injuries when it is uncertain whether the track of the knife or bullet violated the retroperitoneum or the peritoneal cavity. Such an approach is most useful in patients with back and flank wounds but is also occasionally helpful in patients with anterior wounds if it is likely that the knife did not reach the peritoneal cavity or the bullet traversed a tangential path. Patients with any signs of peritonitis or hemodynamic instability after penetrating trauma are obviously not candidates for diagnostic CT scanning.

Angiography is reserved for specific situations, such as suspected aortic or renal arterial injuries, or ongoing hemorrhage from hepatic or splenic injuries. It is not considered an initial screening investigation.

Laparoscopy has been used for both diagnosis and treatment of trauma patients.[4] Although limited to evaluation of the diaphragm in blunt trauma, after penetrating trauma laparoscopy is helpful when it is unclear whether the peritoneum has been penetrated. In patients in whom peritoneal penetration is seen, the use of laparoscopy to further explore the peritoneal cavity and repair injuries is more controversial. The adequacy of abdominal exploration, particularly examination of the bowel and retroperitoneum, has been questioned, and repair of large injuries through the laparoscope can be tedious. In patients with a lower chest wound, however, laparoscopy can identify both peritoneal penetration and diaphragmatic injury. An isolated diaphragmatic injury or associated nonbleeding liver laceration is one area in which repair of the diaphragm through the laparoscope has proved feasible. When laparoscopy is used in patients with potential diaphragmatic injury, positive pressure in the peritoneal cavity can lead to tension pneumothorax if the chest is not adequately vented.

DIAGNOSTIC PERITONEAL LAVAGE AND ABDOMINAL ULTRASOUND

Diagnostic peritoneal lavage and focused abdominal sonography for trauma (FAST) are standard techniques to detect significant intraabdominal hemorrhage after blunt trauma. FAST is less useful after penetrating trauma for potential intestinal injury.

The specific indications for DPL or FAST in blunt trauma include the following:

- Unconscious patient with question of potential abdominal injury
- Patient with a high-energy injury, suspected intraabdominal injury, and equivocal physical findings
- Patient with multiple injuries and unexplained shock
- Patient with major noncontiguous or thoracoabdominal injuries
- Patient with spinal cord injury
- Intoxicated patient in whom abdominal injury is suspected
- Patient who has a suspected intraabdominal injury with equivocal diagnostic findings and who will be undergoing prolonged general anesthesia for another injury, making continued reevaluation impossible

Relative contraindications to DPL but not to FAST are previous abdominal operations, pregnancy, and morbid obesity. Obvious peritonitis is a contraindication to either study. If the patient is hemodynamically stable, CT scan is prudent, and if the patient is unstable immediate exploratory laparotomy, rapid abdominal tap, or FAST to confirm gross hemoperitoneum is indicated.

Diagnostic peritoneal lavage is not generally useful for patients with abdominal gunshot wounds, most of whom require laparotomy.[5] If local exploration of a stab wound suggests penetration of the fascia or peritoneum, DPL can help distinguish significant and insignificant injuries. It is most sensitive in the diagnosis of hemoperitoneum, but significant hemoperitoneum does not necessarily accompany hollow viscus lacerations. In blunt trauma, DPL is considered positive if 10 mL of grossly bloody aspirate is obtained before instillation of lavage fluid or if the siphoned lavage fluid has more than 100,000 red blood cells (RBCs) per milliliter. Evaluation of lavage fluid in stab wounds should be based on a more sensitive protocol. In general, more than 1,000 RBCs/mL is considered a positive DPL, and laparotomy should follow. In both cases, presence of bile, amylase, bacteria, or particulate matter should indicate visceral injury and need for laparotomy.

Diagnostic peritoneal lavage and CT scan are both satisfactory tests for the diagnosis of visceral injury after blunt abdominal trauma. DPL has some advantages, including rapidity, higher sensitivity, lower cost, and immediate interpretation (Table 25.3). The major disadvantages are a 1% to 3% risk of iatrogenic intraperitoneal injury and the high sensitivity of the test. The high sensitivity can lead to nontherapeutic laparotomies (i.e., when there are no injuries requiring repair). False-positive DPL findings may result from traversing a pelvic hematoma that has dissected into the anterior infraumbilical abdominal wall if an infraumbilical approach is used in a patient with a pelvic fracture. A pelvic radiograph should be obtained before DPL, and if a pelvic fracture is present, the incision is placed cephalad to the umbilicus.

TABLE 25.3 DIAGNOSIS

COMPARISON OF DIAGNOSTIC PERITONEAL LAVAGE AND COMPUTED TOMOGRAPHY IN THE DIAGNOSIS OF VISCERAL INJURY AFTER BLUNT ABDOMINAL TRAUMA

	Diagnostic peritoneal lavage	Computed tomography
False-negative result	<1%	5%–20%
False-positive result	5%–12%	5%
Time to complete	5 min	55 min
Cost	$125	$900

Before DPL, the bladder should be emptied with a Foley catheter. The abdomen is prepared with povidone–iodine solution and draped with sterile towels. The infraumbilical midline is infiltrated using lidocaine with epinephrine, and a 3-cm incision is carried down to the linea alba. This is opened, and a peritoneal dialysis catheter is placed through the peritoneum under direct vision. After peritoneal entry, the catheter is directed at a 45-degree angle into the pelvis and aspirated. If the aspirate returns 10 mL of bloody fluid, the study is considered positive and is terminated. If little or no blood is aspirated, 1,000 mL of warm normal saline (or 10 mL/kg in a child) is rapidly infused into the peritoneal cavity. After the infusion is complete, the empty intravenous bottle is placed on the floor, allowing the intraperitoneal fluid to be siphoned into the bottle for analysis.

Ultrasound (FAST) has become increasingly popular in the initial diagnostic management of abdominal trauma and, when available, can be used in the circumstances outlined earlier for DPL.[6] FAST has been used as a screening modality for all patients with blunt trauma to determine which stable patients should undergo further diagnostic imaging with CT scanning.[7–9] It has also been used in hemodynamically unstable patients to rapidly determine presence of intraperitoneal fluid and the need for immediate surgery analogous to the use of gross blood on DPL.[10]

In FAST, the ultrasound probe is used to interrogate serially the subhepatic space, the pericolic gutters, the left upper quadrant, the pericystic area in the pelvis, and the pericardial space. A small amount of physiologic fluid is occasionally seen in the pelvis, but anything more should be considered abnormal and should prompt either operative exploration or further investigation.

There is a steep learning curve for the use of FAST in the emergency department, but in the hands of experienced personnel it is effective in determining the presence or absence of intraperitoneal blood. Emergency department ultrasound is not very sensitive for the identification of specific organ injuries and is relatively insensitive for the diagnosis of bowel injuries. It has proved much better for the evaluation of blunt trauma than for penetrating trauma, although interrogation of

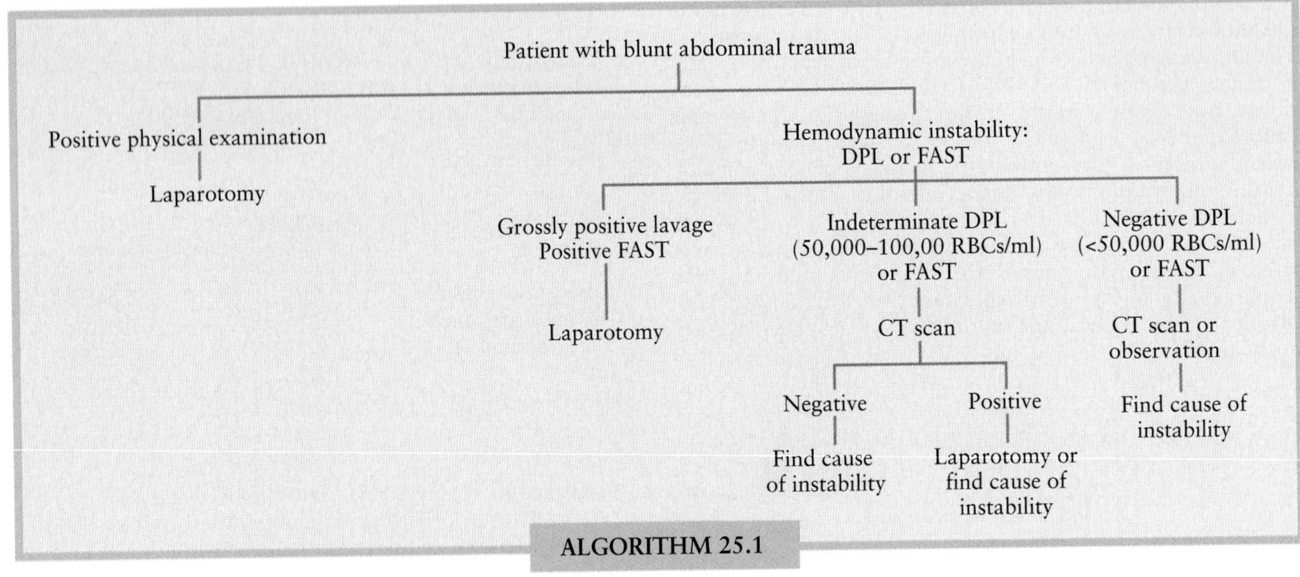

ALGORITHM 25.1 Diagnosis of blunt abdominal trauma.

the pericardial space with an ultrasound probe placed in the subxiphoid position is sensitive for the presence of pericardial blood in patients with potential penetrating cardiac injuries.

The general approaches to the diagnosis of blunt and penetrating trauma are outlined in Algorithms 25.1 and 25.2.

INDICATIONS FOR SURGERY

It is the job of the general surgeon directing a trauma team to integrate the various specialties involved in the care of the multiply injured patient. Judgments about specialized procedures for problems that are not life threatening need to be made with an overall view of the patient's physiologic status. Indications for laparotomy include signs of peritonitis, evisceration, clinical deterioration during observation, and, in the presence of hemodynamically instability, a DPL or FAST examination consistent with hemoperitoneum.

Broad-spectrum antibiotics are given as soon as the decision to perform a laparotomy is made. The spectrum of coverage should include anaerobic, in addition to aerobic, organisms. Good evidence suggests that antibiotics do not need to be

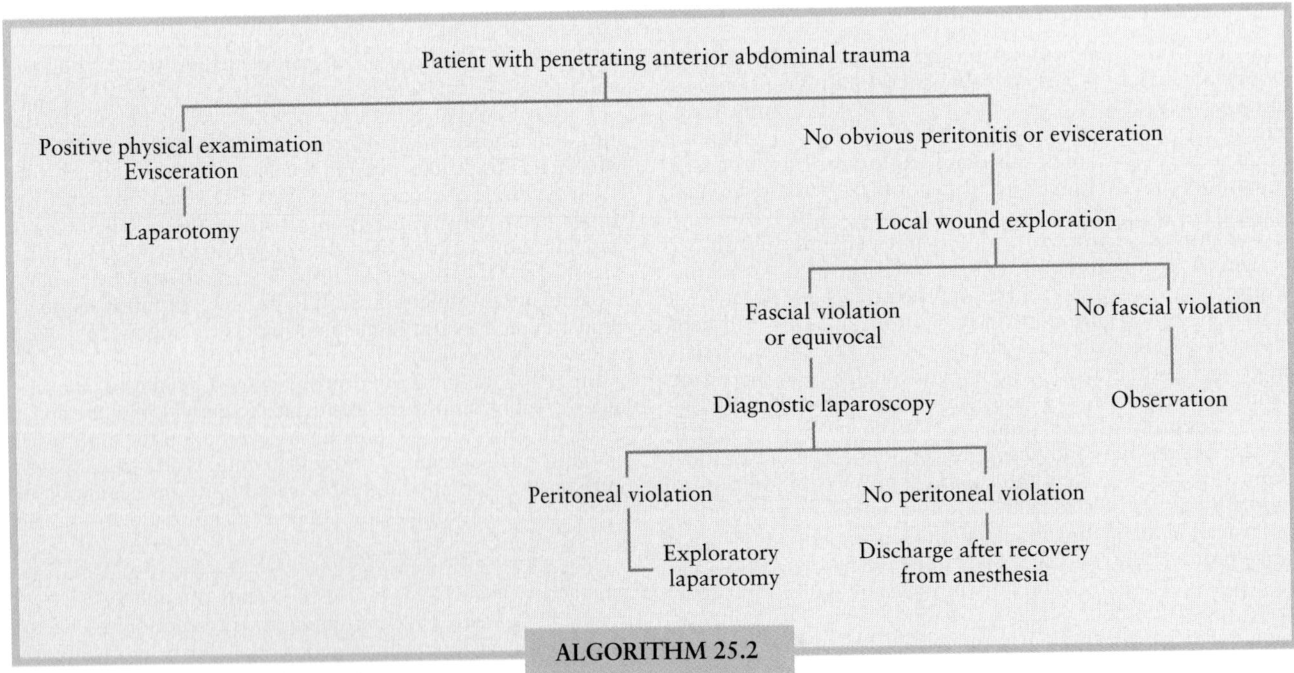

ALGORITHM 25.2 Diagnosis of low-velocity penetrating abdominal trauma.

continued for longer than 24 hours postoperatively, even if contamination from an injured hollow viscus has occurred.[11,12] Tetanus prophylaxis should be administered. If fully immunized as a child, a patient is adequately treated with a booster immunization. If adequate childhood immunization is absent, unlikely, or unknown, then passive immunization should be provided with hyperimmune globulin.

OPERATIVE APPROACH

The patient should be placed supine on the operating room table and the entire anterior torso from the sternal notch to the middle thighs should be prepared and draped to allow for maximum exposure and harvesting of the saphenous vein, if necessary for vascular repair. A midline incision is preferred and there are few reasons to deviate from this choice. This incision also allows extension into a median sternotomy in the event that more proximal control of the vena cava is needed or if the patient is found to have a cardiac injury.

After the abdomen is opened, obvious blood and clot are removed, and packing of the four quadrants is accomplished as indicated by ongoing bleeding. If the peritoneal cavity is full of blood, the location of clot is often a clue to the site of bleeding. Inflow occlusion can be accomplished, if needed, by clamping the aorta at the diaphragmatic hiatus adjacent to the esophagus. Obvious hollow viscus wounds should be rapidly controlled by sutures, clamps, or staples. This initial closure does not need to be definitive and is done primarily to minimize contamination during the course of the operation. Retroperitoneal bleeding may be the source of exsanguinating hemorrhage if rupture into the free peritoneal cavity has occurred. If not, these hematomas can be left for investigation at a later time, depending on their location. Hematomas of the pelvis that are associated with pelvic fractures should not be disturbed. Stable hematomas in the perinephric space lateral to the midline are also best left undisturbed. Central hematomas that can involve injury to the major vascular structures, pancreas, or duodenum are noted and explored after control of injuries within the peritoneal cavity.

After packing has controlled hemorrhage and ongoing contamination has been stopped, time is taken to allow resuscitation of the patient's circulating blood volume. Warming is necessary if massive blood loss has occurred and all fluids must be infused through warming devices, such as the level I. Sustained periods of hypotension should be avoided at all costs, which usually can be accomplished with packing. A complete and thorough exploratory laparotomy is performed methodically to investigate the entire contents of the abdomen for occult injuries.

In some patients, a temporizing approach to intraabdominal injuries, or "damage control," is appropriate.[13] Minimizing operative time is emphasized and the definitive management of all injuries is not necessary. Appropriate candidates for damage control laparotomy are patients with profound coagulopathy, severe acidosis, hypothermia, massive intraabdominal injuries, or severe associated nonabdominal injuries. Hollow viscus injuries should be temporarily controlled to prevent ongoing contamination, but restoration of gastrointestinal continuity is not performed. The abdominal wall is either left open because of excessive tension or closed temporarily, and resuscitative efforts are continued with particular emphasis on correcting coagulopathy, acidosis, and hypothermia. A variety of techniques are available to temporarily avoid abdominal wall closure and still adequately cover the abdominal viscera. Temporary vacuum dressing of the abdominal wall with plastic sheets, dressings, suction drarins, and iobane drapes or commercial devices has shown promise as a means of protecting the viscera and while maintaining the pliability of the abdominal wall to allow for later fascial closure.[14] A planned reoperation is then undertaken when the patient's condition permits and definitive injury repair is undertaken at that time.

SPECIFIC INJURIES

Diaphragm

Injuries to the diaphragm after blunt trauma involve predominantly the left hemidiaphragm. All diaphragmatic injuries must be repaired to avoid the long-term potential for herniation, incarceration, and strangulation of abdominal viscera. Strangulation can occur months or even years after the injury if the hole in the diaphragm is not diagnosed and treated. The diagnosis of diaphragm injury should be suspected if respiratory distress and radiologic evidence of pleural effusion are not relieved by tube thoracostomy or if an upright radiograph demonstrates obvious visceral herniation into the thorax (Fig. 25.2). Chest radiograph (CXR) findings in patients with blunt diaphragmatic rupture are sometimes subtle, particularly in the face of positive pressure ventilation, and may appear only as a blurring of the costophrenic angle or the line of the hemidiaphragm. Serial CXRs may demonstrate evidence of delayed herniation. Low-thoracic (below the level of the nipples) penetrating injuries should be presumed to have traversed the diaphragm. During exploratory laparotomy, the entire diaphragmatic surface should be exposed and directly visualized. Linear lacerations can be repaired with a simple running suture or interrupted horizontal mattress sutures, whereas larger lacerations and tissue deficits occasionally

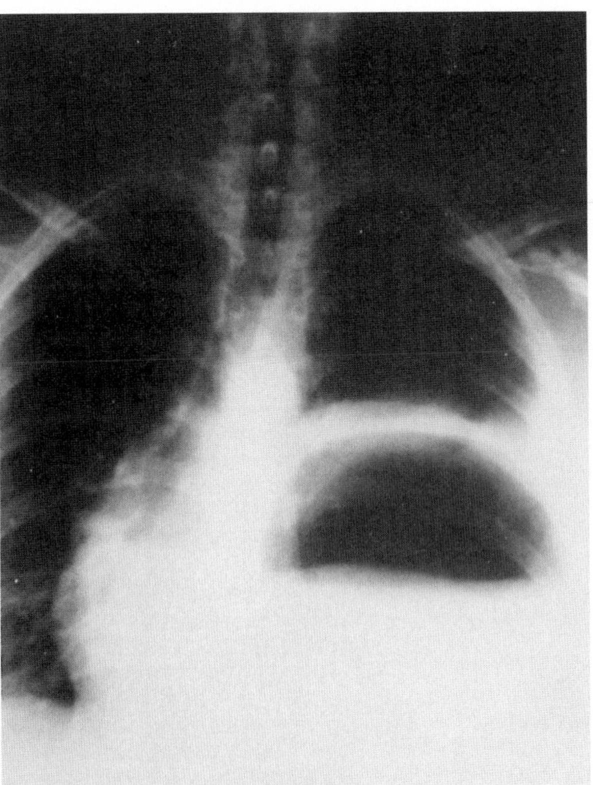

FIGURE 25.2 Chest radiograph showing gastric bubble in the left chest consistent with a rupture of the left hemidiaphragm.

require repair with prosthetic material or resuspension of the diaphragm to higher ribs. Exploration of acute traumatic diaphragmatic rupture is usually accomplished through the abdomen because of the high potential for associated intraperitoneal injury and because the lack of adhesions makes reduction of the abdominal viscera back into the peritoneal cavity relatively easy. Defects discovered at a later date can be addressed satisfactorily by a transthoracic approach, which facilitates lysis of adhesions.

Spleen

Splenic injury is often heralded by lower rib fractures on the left because the spleen lies in the left upper quadrant just to the left and slightly posterior to the stomach. The history is helpful if the patient describes a direct blow to the left chest, flank, or abdomen. For penetrating trauma, a wound entry or exit in this area should raise the suspicion of splenic injury. The clinical signs may be few and subtle; a high level of suspicion must be maintained simply on the basis of mechanism of injury. Clinical evidence of splenic injury includes signs of blood loss, left upper quadrant abdominal pain or tenderness, and pain referred to the left shoulder (Kehr's sign).

In general, laboratory studies are of limited help. CT scan is useful in hemodynamically stable patients for demonstrating splenic injury. Ultrasound can confirm hemoperitoneum, if present, with splenic injury.

Historically, splenic injury was routinely treated with splenectomy. During the last few decades, several factors have contributed to a change in this management strategy. Postsplenectomy sepsis, with its high attendant mortality rate, has been characterized, particularly in the treatment of children. In addition, the relative success rates for splenic salvage techniques and nonoperative management are well established. Nonoperative approaches focus on the clinical presentation of the patient rather than the CT scan appearance, although the presence of a "blush" on the CT scan is indicative of potential ongoing bleeding and an increased likelihood of need for operative intervention[15] (Fig. 25.3). The presence of a "blush" has also been used as a trigger for angiographic embolization in hemodynamically stable patients to prevent ongoing or recurrent bleeding. Although increasingly practiced, nonoperative management is not without dangers and limitations. Potential disadvantages include a more prolonged hospitalization and possibly more exposure to transfused blood, but the principal risks are ongoing hemorrhage and missed associated intraabdominal injuries, particularly to the pancreas or bowel.

The spleen is evaluated for hemorrhage during the course of laparotomy. If hemorrhage is noted, a decision must be made regarding splenic salvage. This assessment requires complete mobilization of the spleen from its lateral and posterior attachments, and care must be taken to prevent further injury. The spleen and tail of the pancreas must be mobilized together to evaluate adequately the extent of splenic injury. Ongoing bleeding is controlled during mobilization by manual compression. Topical hemostatic agents usually control capsular tears of the spleen. Lacerations of the splenic substance can be controlled with interlocking absorbable sutures. Major lacerations of the splenic substance can be treated with segmental splenic resection or wrapped in absorbable mesh. Splenic salvage should not be attempted if the patient has protracted hypotension or other severe injuries or if undue delays are encountered in the attempt to repair the spleen. With penetrating injury, damage to adjacent structures, such as the stomach, pancreas, colon, and diaphragm, must be anticipated and investigated.

The nonoperative management of splenic trauma is most attractive if the diagnosis has been made with an abdominal CT scan, the patient is hemodynamically stable, and no other signs of abdominal injury are present. Nonoperative management is successful in such circumstances approximately 90% of the time in adults, and even more often in children. Followup CT scans are routinely obtained by some surgeons, but they are probably not necessary if the patient is doing well clinically.[16] In general, nonoperative management should be carried out for the initial 24 to 48 hours in an intensive care unit, and patients should remain hospitalized until the hematocrit remains stable postmobilization. The maximum risk of continued or recurrent bleeding is within the first 48 hours after injury, but there is a decreasing risk of delayed bleeding within the first week postinjury and cases of delayed bleeding even months after injury have been reported.[17]

Complications after splenectomy include early transient thrombocytosis, which usually resolves spontaneously within 2 or 3 months. Anticoagulation is neither necessary nor helpful. Delayed hemorrhage, pancreatitis, pancreatic leak, and subphrenic abscess also may occur. Subphrenic abscess is primarily related to associated hollow viscus injuries and is uncommon. Routine "prophylactic" drainage of the subphrenic space should not be done; it is associated with an increased incidence of abscess.

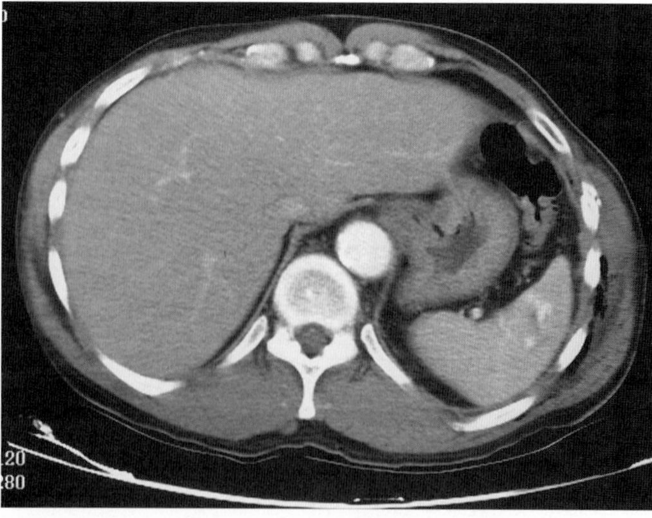

FIGURE 25.3 A cut from a computed tomography scan through the upper abdomen of a patient with a splenic injury. The spleen has evidence of several areas of contrast "blush."

Postsplenectomy Sepsis

Fatal pneumococcal septicemia after splenectomy was first noted in the mid 1950s in children. Postsplenectomy sepsis syndrome is caused by failure to clear one of several encapsulated bacteria in the absence of the spleen. The incidence is inversely related to age and is higher with underlying hematologic disorders such as lymphoma or thalassemia. The incidence of life-threatening sepsis in adult trauma patients is low and the overall clinical significance is not easily defined. Concern about the possibility of postsplenectomy sepsis should not obscure the fact that the initial priority is to arrest hemorrhage and deal with the patient's immediate life-threatening injuries.

If splenectomy is performed, postoperative followup is important.[18] Immunization with the polyvalent pneumococcal vaccine has become the standard of care, and booster immunization is recommended every 3 years. Immunization for *Hemophilus influenzae*, meningococcus, and annually for influenza virus is also recommended. In addition, prophylactic antibiotics, usually oral penicillin, should be given any time the patient is to undergo instrumentation, such as during dental repair or surgery. Postsplenectomy patients should be advised of their increased potential for postsplenectomy sepsis and should carry an identification card to alert healthcare workers of this possibility if they develop an infection. Also recommended is that they should be given a several-day supply or prescription of oral antibiotics to be taken at the first sign of infection. All infections should be considered emergencies and treated aggressively with intravenous antibiotics in the hospital.

Liver

The liver, the largest organ in the abdominal cavity, is commonly damaged in blunt and penetrating abdominal trauma as well as in thoracoabdominal injuries. Some series have found that the incidence of liver injuries exceeds that of injuries to the spleen. In any case, the two together account for approximately 75% of all blunt intraabdominal injuries. Trauma sufficient to lacerate the liver is often associated with injuries to other organs. Spontaneous hemostatic mechanisms are sufficiently effective that approximately 85% of patients with liver injuries are not actively bleeding at the time of laparotomy, and these injuries are predictably well tolerated. At laparotomy, most liver injuries require no specific therapy, and drainage is usually unnecessary. Injuries that do require definitive surgical care present a complex and life-threatening series of problems.

Patients with significant liver injuries usually have a history of major blunt energy transfer to the right thorax or upper abdomen. Physical findings may be minimal because early bleeding may not cause peritoneal irritation or abdominal distention. Any patient with unexplained hypotension or a history of shock at the scene after blunt abdominal trauma must be considered at risk for a severe liver injury. DPL or FAST is most helpful in establishing the diagnosis of hemoperitoneum, and if the results are positive, laparotomy is appropriate. In hemodynamically stable patients, a CT scan is precise in evaluating subcapsular hematomas, lacerations, and other hepatic parenchymal injuries. The use of nonoperative management has increased significantly over the last 10 years. Liver injuries seen on CT scan in hemodynamically stable patients can be treated nonoperatively as long as the patient is followed closely and the possibility of associated hollow viscus or pancreatic injury is borne in mind.[19] A CT scan with contrast medium enhancement should be obtained, and if extravasation is demonstrated, then attempting angiographic embolization should be considered along with the need for operative intervention. The absence of contrast agent extravasation during the arterial phase of the CT indicates a liver injury, which generally can be treated nonoperatively. Overall reported success of nonoperative management is greater than 90% in most series. When broken down by grade of injury, the success rate of nonoperative management for injuries grades I through III approaches 95%. In stable patients with ongoing bleeding, angiographic embolization as an adjuvant to a protocol of nonoperative management is successful in lowering the number of blood transfusions and the number of operations.

Patients are generally admitted to the ICU for monitoring of vital signs and serial hematocrit determinations. When no evidence of further bleeding is seen, patients can be mobilized and started on a diet. A repeat CT scan before discharge is not imperative and normal physical activity can be resumed 3 months postinjury.

Operative Management

Injuries vary from simple capsular tears and nonbleeding lacerations, to complex fractures with lobar destruction and extensive parenchymal disruption, to bile duct disruption, to hepatic artery and central venous injuries. The principles of liver injury management are the same regardless of the severity of injury. They involve control of bleeding, removal of devitalized tissue, and establishment of adequate drainage.

Simple lacerations that have stopped bleeding at the time of surgery do not require drainage unless they are deep into the parenchyma, in which case they have an increased probability of postoperative biliary leakage. Subcapsular hematomas can be simply evacuated or, preferably, left intact if there is no associated parenchymal injury. Lacerations that continue to bleed despite attempts at local control, including packing, require exploration of the liver wound, and specific vessels and biliary radicals are individually ligated. In the event that bleeding continues, the structures of the porta hepatis should be compressed as a diagnostic maneuver (Pringle maneuver; Fig. 25.4). If the bleeding stops, it is presumed to originate from the portal veins or the hepatic artery. If the bleeding continues, it is presumed to arise principally from the main hepatic veins or inferior vena cava, although this distinction is seldom clear-cut in the operating room. The portal triad can be intermittently occluded to allow improved visualization during placement of sutures as parenchymal vessels are ligated. When selective parenchymal ligation fails, ligation of the hepatic artery is an alternative if the trial Pringle occlusion has had a salutary effect. This is rarely necessary but can occasionally produce dramatic hemostasis. The vessel is occluded as close to the liver injury as possible and after initial efforts at hemostasis have failed.

An alternative for deep lacerations with persistent bleeding is resectional débridement of the involved segment of the liver. This is accomplished by the finger fracture technique, removing devitalized liver or the appropriate portion of the liver. This is required in approximately 5% to 8% of all patients with liver injuries. Subsegmental resection is usually adequate; if segmentectomy or lobectomy is required, a knowledge of the anatomy is imperative so as not to compromise inflow or outflow of the remaining segments. This decision should be made early in the exploration, the blood bank notified, adequate help procured, and exposure obtained. Exposure is best accomplished by complete division of the capsular attachments of the liver. This alternative is associated with operative mortality rates as high as 30% and as such should be avoided unless absolutely necessary.

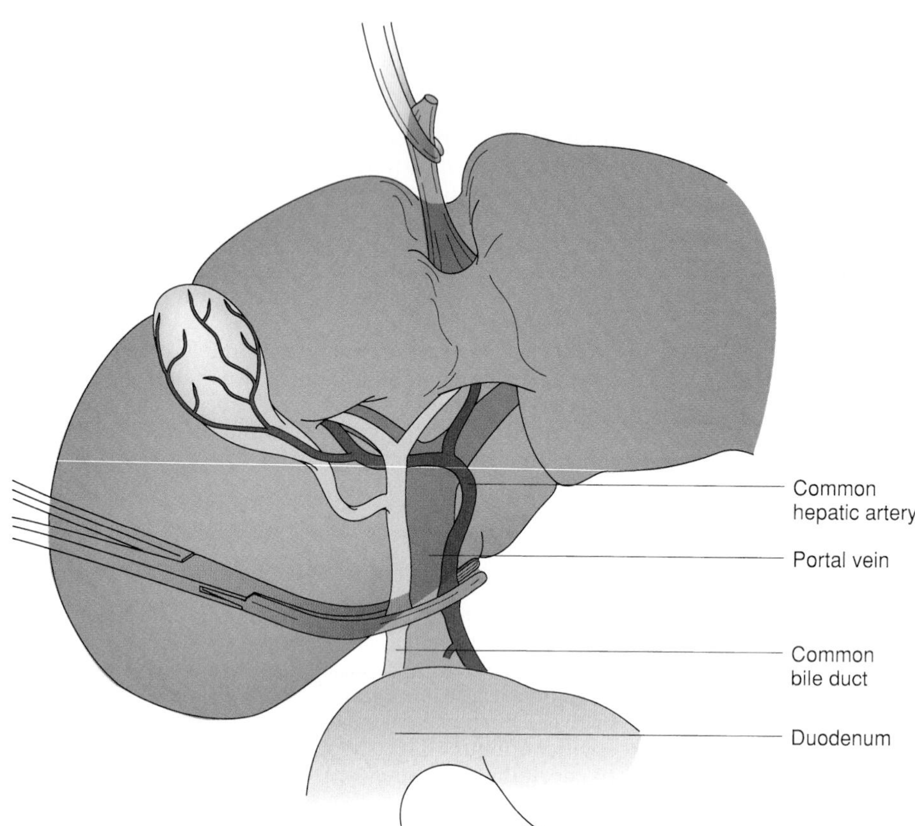

FIGURE 25.4 Pringle maneuver compression of the portal triad structures with a noncrushing vascular clamp for hepatic inflow control. If possible, clamp times should be limited to 15- to 20-minute intervals.

An additional technique uses an absorbable mesh individually wrapping each lobe of the liver and attaching the mesh to the falciform ligament. This technique is useful, with or without packing, when there are multiple superficial lacerations of the liver with active bleeding and can be used as an alternative to parenchymal debridement. If blood loss is significant and the patient remains difficult to resuscitate, is hypothermic or acidotic, and has a coagulopathy from massive transfusion, however, an early decision to pack the injury and perform further resuscitation after the abdomen is closed is most appropriate. Packing is done to significantly compress the injured liver with laparotomy pads placed above and below the liver. An absorbable mesh can be placed over the raw surface and left in place to preserve hemostasis when the packs are removed. For packing to be successful, it should be used early, before coagulopathy has become too severe. Subsequent operative removal of the packs 24 to 72 hours later can be accompanied occasionally by resection and suture ligation as needed. After hemostasis has been achieved, the area should be drained, preferably with sump drainage.

Inability to control bleeding by any of the previously described techniques suggests significant retrohepatic vena caval bleeding or adjacent hepatic veins. Early consideration should be given to complete vascular isolation or the placement of an intracaval shunt. This approach is rarely necessary and should be undertaken only if packing has not controlled hemorrhage from the liver and appropriate expertise is available (Fig. 25.5). To accomplish this, the midline laparotomy incision is extended into the chest, either by a right anterior thoracotomy or, preferably, by a median sternotomy. Infrahepatic (cephalad to the renal veins) and suprahepatic (usually intrapericardial) control of the vena cava is obtained. A shunt or other large conduit is then inserted through a right atrial purse-string suture into the vena cava, and vascular occlusion around the conduit at these sites is obtained. The resultant vascular isolation is always imperfect but may allow better visualization of hepatic vein and vena cava lacerations for direct suture ligation or repair. Total venous occlusion may be equally effective and serves the same general purpose. The risk of hypotension is significant with either approach, in the former because of significant blood loss during atrial cannulation, and with the latter owing to diminished venous return to the right atrium. Last, in select institutions the availability of venous bypass may be an alternative.

The major complications after liver injury include hemorrhage, respiratory insufficiency, coagulopathy, hypoglycemia, biliary fistula or other bile duct injury, hemobilia, and subdiaphragmatic or intraparenchymal abscess formation. The coagulopathy after liver resection is usually the result of hypothermia and inadequate replacement of blood components. In addition to aggressive component replacement, addition of activated factor VII (FVIIa) has anecdotally been lifesaving. Patients undergoing major hepatic resection or liver destruction need continuous glucose infusion, often 10% dextrose, during the early postoperative period. Hypoalbuminemia is common but does not usually require albumin administration and should be treated simply with aggressive nutritional support. Hyperbilirubinemia is transient and usually peaks in 2 to 3 weeks after major resection. Intrahepatic and subphrenic abscesses can develop, particularly if significant débridement has been necessary. They are diagnosed by clinical evidence of sepsis combined with ultrasound or CT scan and often can be treated with percutaneous drainage. When percutaneous drainage is unsuccessful, drainage can be effected surgically either transperitoneally or posteriorly through the bed of the

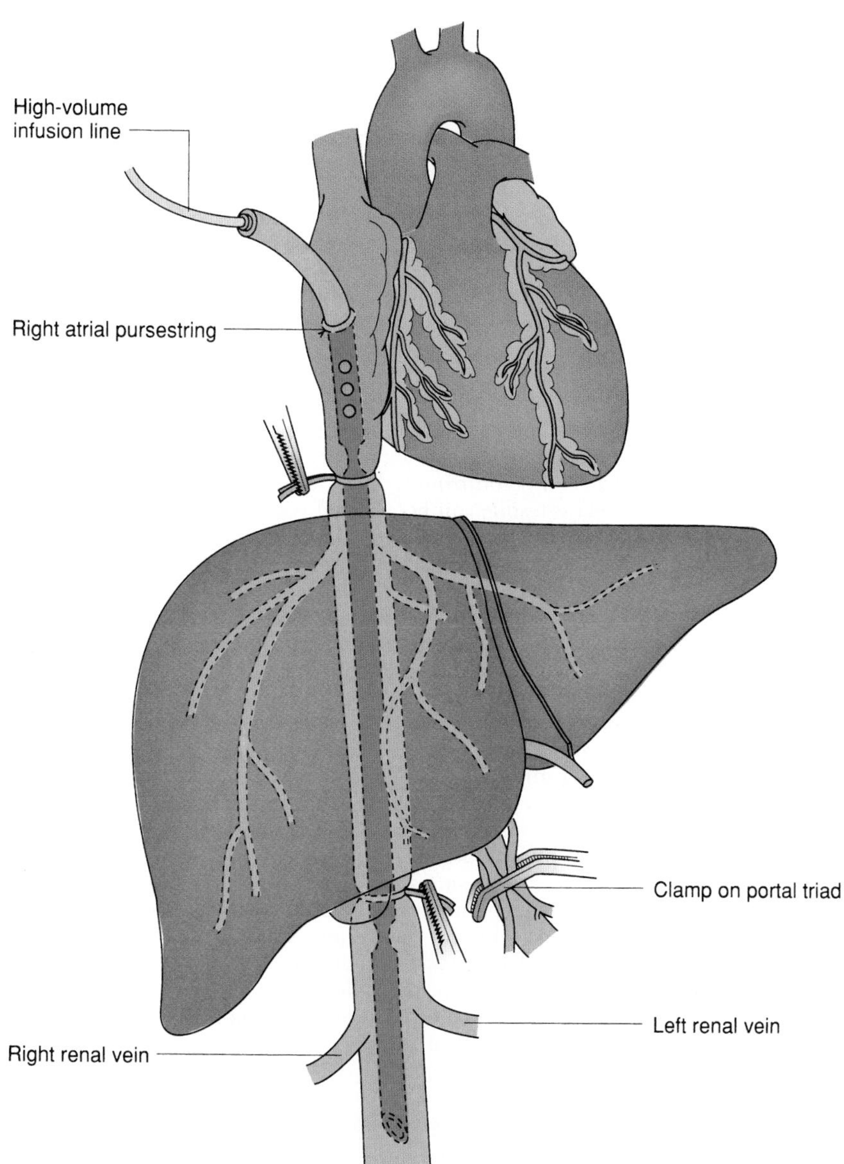

FIGURE 25.5 Intracaval shunt used for retrohepatic venous injuries, combined with a Pringle maneuver for isolation of the retrohepatic vena cava for operative repair.

TRAUMA

12th rib. Biliary fistulas or bilomas usually resolve spontaneously, and major extrahepatic ductal injuries are rare. For the rare biliary leak or fistula that does not close spontaneously, placement of a temporary intrabiliary stent either at the site of injury or, preferably, via the sphincter of Oddi (to decrease intrabiliary pressure) is recommended. A T-tube placed in an otherwise normal common bile duct is inappropriate unless the extrahepatic biliary tree is injured. Hemobilia is a rare complication, occurring with intrahepatic bleeding into the bile ducts, and is best diagnosed with angiography or endoscopy. Angiographic embolization is the treatment of choice.

Stomach

The stomach is vulnerable to penetrating injuries of the upper abdomen and lower chest. The upper abdominal viscera underlie the lower ribs to a level as high as the fourth intercostal space. The stomach is injured in 5% to 10% of patients with penetrating abdominal trauma. Hematemesis or blood found on aspiration of the stomach with a nasogastric tube is a finding suggestive of gastric injury. Although many patients with blood in the stomach after penetrating abdominal trauma have a gastric injury, the absence of blood in the gastric aspirate does not rule out such an injury.

At laparotomy, adequate exposure requires mobilization and visualization of the entire stomach. Most of the anterior surface of the stomach can be adequately visualized without extensive mobilization by grasping the edge of the greater curve of the stomach with fingers or Babcock clamps, and the stomach is pulled down and spread. Exposure of the gastroesophageal junction can be difficult if the flare of the costal margin is narrow or if the left lobe of the liver is in the way. Improved exposure is accomplished with extension of the midline incision as high as possible by creating a paraxiphoid extension. The left hepatic lobe is retracted to the right after division of the left triangular ligament. Mobilization of the gastroesophageal junction, encirclement with a tape or drain, and caudal traction into the operative field improves visualization and the performance of any necessary repairs. The posterior wall of the stomach should also be examined for the presence of injuries, particularly if there is an injury on the anterior surface. The posterior stomach is exposed by opening the gastrocolic ligament bluntly to the left of the midline approximately halfway between the stomach and the transverse colon in a relatively avascular area. The lesser sac is entered and the posterior wall of the stomach examined.

Injuries to the stomach are usually easy to repair, primarily in two layers, with an inner layer of 3-0 or 4-0 absorbable sutures followed by an outer layer of 3-0 or 4-0 permanent Lembert sutures. Because of the ample blood supply and large lumen of the stomach in all areas except the gastroesophageal junction and pylorus, there is minimal concern for excessive inversion and luminal compromise. On rare occasions, especially after shotgun wounds, large injuries of the stomach may require resection. Injuries to the pylorus are rare. If viable tissue is present, it should be closed with a Heineke-Mikulicz pyloroplasty; a concomitant vagotomy is not necessary.

Because of the stomach's position high in the abdomen, penetrating injuries to the stomach are frequently associated with lacerations of the diaphragm. During spontaneous ventilation, there is negative pressure in the pleural cavity and positive pressure in the abdomen, and the resultant pressure gradient causes movement of gastric fluid and particulate matter from the abdomen into the chest. The degree of contamination can be deceptive in the operating room because most occurs before the institution of positive-pressure ventilation and laparotomy. Because even small amounts of contamination can result in an empyema, combined injuries to the stomach and diaphragm require the pleural cavity to be lavaged before closure of the diaphragm. The diaphragmatic laceration should be enlarged enough to allow lavage from the abdomen. The course of the phrenic nerve in the diaphragm should be borne in mind, and enlargement of the diaphragmatic laceration should be done either radially or as peripherally as possible. Occasionally, adequate lavage is difficult because of the amount of pleural contamination or if enlargement of the diaphragmatic laceration cannot be done without risk of denervation. In such instances, the patient should be closely followed postoperatively for evidence of the development of an empyema or undergo "prophylactic" video-assisted thoracic surgery (VATS) to lavage the chest. If empyema develops, it can usually be managed with a VATS approach.[20]

Blunt injuries to the stomach are rarer than penetrating injuries. The stomach is large, distensible, and mobile. A great deal of force is necessary to cause a blowout of the gastric wall. As a consequence, the mortality rate from associated injuries is high in patients with blunt stomach injuries. Blowout injuries of the stomach also tend to be large and the stomach is more likely to be full at the time of the injury. Thus, blunt trauma injuries are often associated with significant intraperitoneal contamination. Principles of operative exposure and repair are the same as for penetrating injuries.

Duodenum

Penetrating Injuries

Because of the retroperitoneal location of the duodenum close to a number of other viscera and major vascular structures, isolated penetrating injuries to the duodenum are rare. The need for abdominal exploration is usually dictated by associated injuries, and the diagnosis of duodenal injury is usually made in the operating room.[21] With blunt trauma, gastrointestingal (GI) contrast CT scans are frequently diagnostic

Diagnosis and treatment of duodenal injuries in the operating room depend on adequate exposure. Exposure is obtained by incising the lateral peritoneal reflection of the duodenum and mobilizing the duodenum from right to left with a combination of blunt and cautery dissection. This technique is known as the Kocher maneuver, and it can be carried well across the midline to the level of the abdominal aorta, providing exposure of the underlying vena cava and aorta. Entry into the lesser sac by way of the gastrocolic ligament provides exposure of the caudal aspect of the first portion of the duodenum and the medial aspect of the second portion. Exposure of the third and fourth portions of the duodenum, if necessary, is carried out by incising the ligament of Treitz and mobilizing the right colon from right to left so that the right colon and small intestine can be elevated (Cattell maneuver). With this combination of maneuvers, the entire duodenum can be mobilized and exposed for evaluation of any injury. It is critical to identify all injuries at the time of the initial exploration, because overlooked injuries are associated with a significant increase in subsequent morbidity.

Grading systems have been devised to characterize duodenal injuries. Although useful for research purposes, the specifics of the grading systems are less important than several simple aspects of the duodenal injury (Table 25.4). Most penetrating injuries to the duodenum are simple lacerations that can be repaired primarily. Such repairs should be done in two layers, with an inner absorbable layer of 3-0 or 4-0 sutures followed by an outer layer of 3-0 or 4-0 permanent Lembert sutures. The closure should be oriented transversely, if possible, to avoid luminal compromise, but transverse orientation is not as critical in the duodenum as it is in the rest of the small intestine. The biliary tract does not require drainage in such cases unless an associated biliary tract injury is present, and the duodenum does not require tube decompression, although both of these maneuvers have been advocated in the past. The periduodenal area should be drained with closed suction drainage.

Injuries that encompass as much as 40% or 50% of the duodenal wall can be successfully closed primarily. Primary repair of injuries larger than this, however, can lead to luminal compromise. If the duodenum has been transected or almost transected, the edges should be débrided and a two-layer primary anastomosis done without tension after mobilization of the duodenum, provided that the transection is not close to the ampulla of Vater. Large injuries of the duodenum can be repaired with a jejunal patch by bringing up a loop of jejunum and laying it onto the area of injury so that

TABLE 25.4 DIAGNOSIS

IMPORTANT ASPECTS TO NOTE FOR DUODENAL INJURIES

- Anatomic relation to the ampulla of Vater
- Character of the injury (e.g., a simple laceration versus destruction of the duodenal wall)
- Involved circumference of the duodenum
- Associated injuries to the biliary tract, pancreas, or major vascular structures

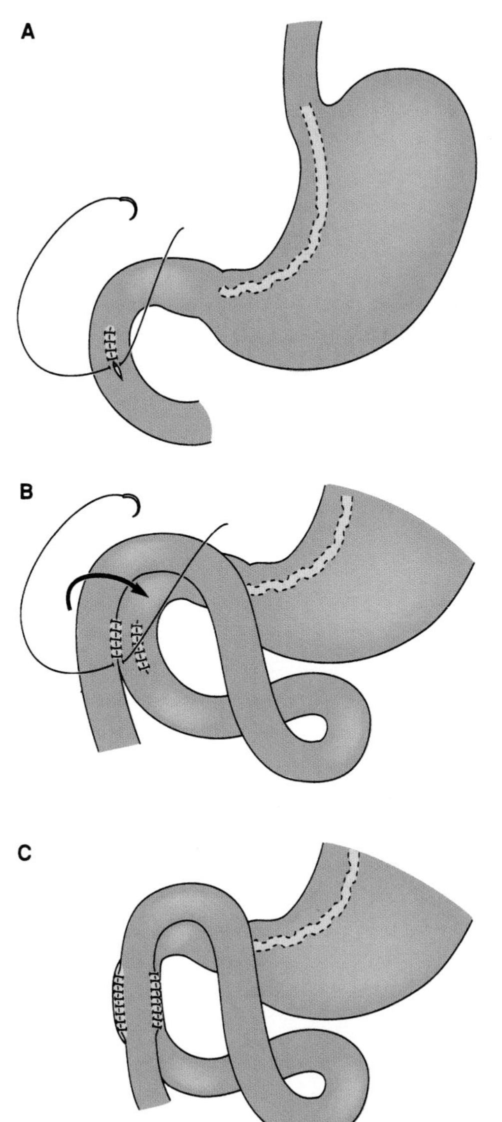

FIGURE 25.6 A jejunoileal patch can be used to reinforce repairs of the duodenum. (*A*) The duodenum is first repaired. (*B*) The retrocolic loop of jejunum is brought up to the area of repair. (*C*) The serosa is sewn over the repair.

the serosa of the jejunum buttresses the duodenal repair (Fig. 25.6). Alternatively, a Roux-en-Y duodenojejunostomy can drain a large defect internally. If there are severe associated injuries to the pancreas or biliary tract, pancreaticoduodenectomy may be necessary. The morbidity associated with pancreaticoduodenectomy is substantial, and this operation is indicated only if the extent of injury is so great that the necessary resection has, in essence, been done by the injury.

Some duodenal repairs are tenuous. This is a particular problem if there is associated pancreatic injury, raising concern about the digestive action of activated pancreatic enzymes on the repair. Pyloric exclusion defunctionalizes the duodenum and protects the repair from activated pancreatic enzymes until it has had time to heal. A gastrotomy along the greater curvature of the stomach provides access to the pylorus, which is closed with a large running suture or, alternatively, the pylorus is stapled shut. GI continuity is restored by a gastrojejunostomy (Fig. 25.7). Tube decompression of the duodenum should be performed in severe duodenal injuries, but the biliary tract does not require decompression except in cases of an associated biliary tract injury. As with all duodenal injuries, the periduodenal area should be externally drained to control postoperative leak as a controlled fistula. With creation of a gastrojejunal anastomosis and no concomitant procedure to decrease gastric acid production, H_2 blockers or proton pump inhibitors should be given in the postoperative period to prevent marginal ulceration. After a number of weeks, most patients have reconstituted normal GI continuity. The closure of the pylorus breaks down, regardless of whether the pylorus was closed with absorbable or nonabsorbable suture. As the pylorus reopens, the inherently ulcerogenic gastrojejunostomy gradually closes of its own accord and, thus, does not require a concomitant vagotomy.

Blunt Injuries

Blunt injuries to the duodenum are less common and more difficult to diagnose than penetrating injuries. They can occur in isolation or with pancreatic injury. The need for immediate abdominal exploration is frequently not obvious. Because the duodenum is located in the retroperitoneum, findings on physical examination of the abdomen may be subtle except in cases of associated intraabdominal injuries. Nonetheless, the physical examination is still one of the best methods for determining the presence of a duodenal injury. This is particularly true if the admission examination is indeterminate, emphasizing the need for serial abdominal examinations.

The serum amylase concentration is helpful in the diagnosis of blunt duodenal injuries; however, the test lacks sensitivity. The duodenum is retroperitoneal, the concentration of amylase in the fluid that leaks is variable, and amylase concentrations often take hours, even days, to increase after injury. Although serial determinations of serum amylase are better than a single, isolated determination on admission, sensitivity is still poor and delays are inherent in serial determinations.

Upper GI series and CT scans with GI contrast are reasonably sensitive for the presence of duodenal injury after blunt trauma. Performance of these tests requires a stable patient without any other obvious indications for abdominal exploration. An advantage of CT over upper GI series is that the rest of the retroperitoneum and peritoneal viscera are also visualized. With either study, extravasation of contrast material from the duodenum constitutes an absolute indication for surgical intervention and repair.

Operative exposure and repair of the duodenum after blunt trauma are the same as for penetrating injuries. Crush injuries are more common after blunt trauma and occasionally require extensive resection, but the injuries can be treated frequently by simple techniques of repair if they are diagnosed in a timely fashion.

Intramural hematoma of the duodenum is a rare injury specific to patients with blunt trauma. It is most common in children after isolated localized force to the upper abdomen (e.g., bicycle handlebars). Intramural hematomas occur when the duodenum is crushed and bleeding occurs in the submucosal or subserosal layers of the duodenum. The duodenum is not perforated. Such hematomas can lead to obstruction of the lumen. If the diagnosis is not made at the time of the initial injury, the obstruction usually takes several days to develop, presumably because of increased accumulation of intramural water as the hemoglobin in the

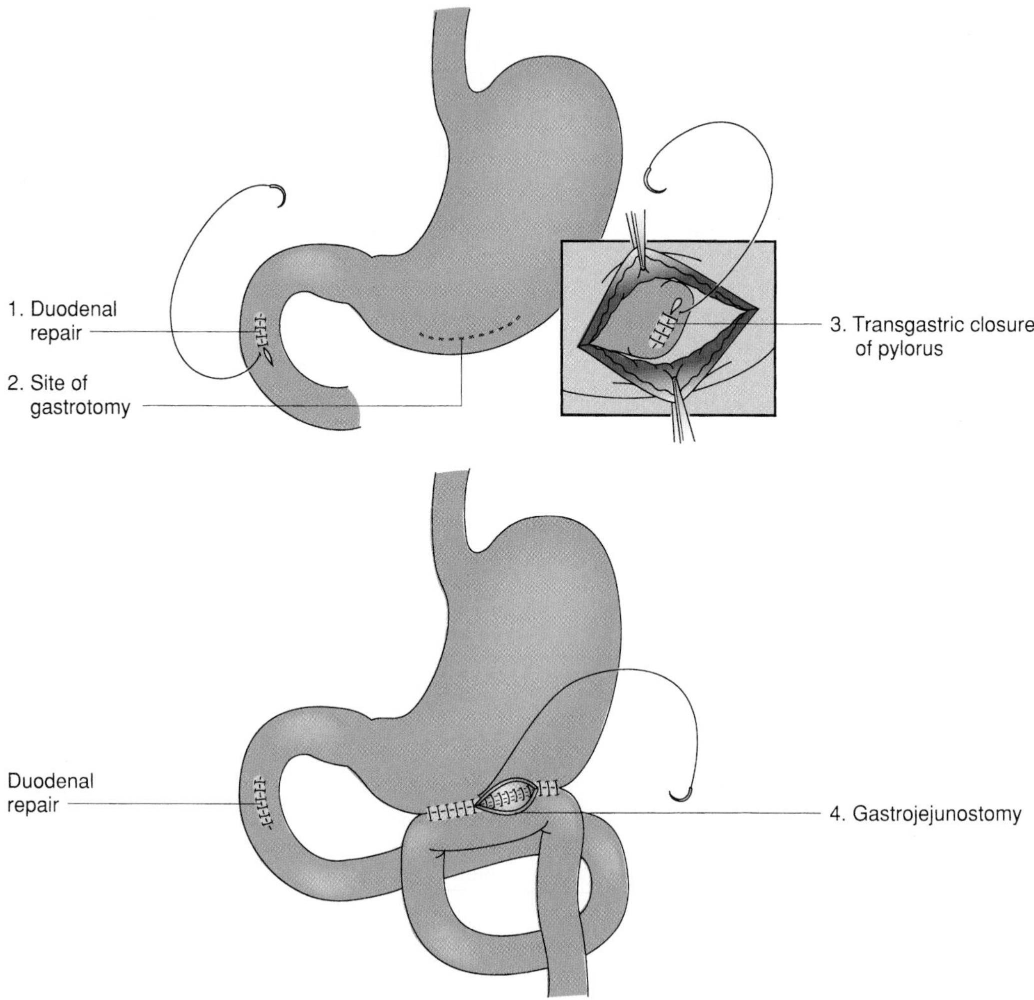

FIGURE 25.7 Technique of pyloric exclusion for complex duodenal injury.

hematoma begins to break down and osmotic forces increase absorption of water. If exploration takes place shortly after injury, intramural hematomas of the duodenum are seen as periduodenal hematomas. All hematomas in the area of the duodenum should be explored to rule out the possibility of perforation. Such exploration includes a Kocher maneuver and mobilization of the duodenum, which in most instances successfully drains subserosal hematomas. Submucosal hematomas may require drainage with a deeper, separate myotomy-type incision. If surgery does not occur shortly after injury, obstructive symptoms become manifest after a number of days. An upper GI series or CT scan should be performed to demonstrate obstruction. The obstruction is usually in the second portion of the duodenum and, in the classic picture, demonstrates a coiled-spring appearance. Debate surrounds the treatment of intramural hematomas of the duodenum if the diagnosis is delayed, but the weight of opinion argues for initial nonoperative treatment. This strategy is usually successful because the hematoma gradually resolves and the obstructive symptoms subside without long-term residual sequelae. If obstructive symptoms persist beyond 10 to 14 days from the time of diagnosis, abdominal exploration should be undertaken to drain the hematoma, relieve the obstruction, and rule out a missed injury.

Complications

The duodenum is particularly susceptible to leak of repairs because of the presence of intraluminal digestive enzymes. Adequate drainage of the periduodenal area helps to ensure that such leaks are controlled and do not result in an intraabdominal abscess. Placement of a decompressive duodenal tube to protect duodenal repairs is not necessary. If a duodenal repair breaks down and the duodenum is adequately drained, a duodenal fistula results. In the absence of distal obstruction, foreign body, or persistent infection (the chances of which are minimized by adequate drainage), most of these controlled fistulas ultimately close. They may be slow to resolve, and a wait of several months is advised to allow them to resolve spontaneously. Support with total parenteral nutrition increases the rate of spontaneous closure. If a fistula fails to close after an appropriate waiting period, further surgical intervention is warranted. It consists of reexploration of the abdomen and construction of a defunctionalized Roux-en-Y duodenojejunostomy as a form of internal drainage.

Pancreas

Penetrating Injuries

Penetrating injuries to the pancreas are usually diagnosed in the operating room.[22] The pancreas is located in the retroperitoneum, surrounded by a number of other viscera and major vascular structures. As a result, an isolated injury to the pancreas is unusual, and patients with penetrating pancreatic trauma usually have obvious indications for abdominal exploration. Preoperative serum amylase and lipase concentrations are not helpful; they are elevated only in a few patients with penetrating pancreatic injuries.

On abdominal exploration, signs of pancreatic injury include a projectile path that passes near the pancreas, a central hematoma in the upper abdomen, and injuries to the duodenum, vena cava, suprarenal aorta, or mesenteric vessels. In all these instances, the pancreas should be thoroughly explored.

The anterior surface of the pancreas is visualized by entry into the lesser sac of the peritoneal cavity. This is done in the same fashion as outlined previously for exposure of the posterior aspect of the stomach, with division of the gastrocolic ligament in a relatively avascular area to the left of the midline. A thin layer of peritoneum overlies the anterior surface of the pancreas at this point, and complete visualization of the surface sometimes requires incision of this layer.

The tail of the pancreas can be more fully visualized, especially in its posterior aspect, by mobilization of the spleen and the tail of the pancreas as a unit. This is accomplished by incision of any lateral attachments of the spleen to the abdominal wall and mobilization of the spleen with blunt dissection laterally to medially by development of the plane between the anterior surface of the left kidney and the posterior aspect of the spleen. This brings the spleen into the abdominal wound and elevates the posterior aspect of the pancreatic tail for inspection. The posterior aspect of the body of the pancreas is visualized by opening the avascular area at the inferior margin of the body and tail of the pancreas with a combination of sharp and blunt dissection. The pancreas can then be mobilized inferiorly to superiorly. This maneuver is also important to mobilize the pancreas in preparation for distal pancreatic resection.

The posterior aspect of the head of the pancreas can be exposed by an extensive Kocher maneuver. In combination with entry into the lesser sac, this also allows for bimanual palpation of the pancreatic head, with one hand placed on the anterior surface of the pancreas through the hole in the lesser sac and the other hand placed behind the pancreas in the plane developed by the Kocher maneuver.

In the evaluation of penetrating pancreatic injuries, an important key to operative management is whether a ductal injury is present. Transduodenal intraoperative pancreatography has been recommended. The advantage of this maneuver is that it allows for more definitive determination of the type of operative intervention that should be undertaken. The major disadvantage is that it necessitates entry into the duodenum when there is no associated duodenal injury, which turns simple pancreatic injuries into combined pancreaticoduodenal injuries, with an attendant increase in potential postoperative morbidity. A further argument against intraoperative pancreatography is that most injuries to the pancreas can be adequately evaluated and decisions made about appropriate operative treatment without radiographic examination of ductal anatomy. In rare circumstances in which the patient's condition permits and the necessary equipment and expertise are available, the use of intraoperative endoscopic retrograde cholangiopancreatography (ERCP) provides an excellent option.

The operative management of penetrating pancreatic injuries depends on both the location and severity of the injury.[23] With respect to location, injuries can be subdivided into those of the head, body, and tail of the pancreas. With respect to severity, injuries can be classified by the degree of parenchymal disruption and the presence or absence of ductal injury.

Contusions of the pancreas, regardless of location, should be either simply observed or drained. The optimal type of drainage is a matter of some debate, and a variety of different drainage methods have been espoused. The type of drain used after pancreatic injury is probably not as important as ensuring that adequate drainage has been effected. If drains are used, they should be left in place for at least 5 to 7 days to ensure that a drain tract develops. Pancreatic fistulas can develop on a delayed basis 3 to 7 days after injury, and if the drains are removed before that time, drainage may be inadequate. The morbidity rate for patients with undrained pancreatic secretions is much greater than for those with drained pancreatic secretions.

The timing of drain removal should be based on both the amount and character of the pancreatic drainage. Drain outputs in excess of 150 to 200 mL/day are suggestive of pancreatic fistulas. Determinations of drain amylase concentration are helpful, but amylase concentrations within a few days of injury, even if very high levels (>50,000 IU/L), do not correlate with the development of a pancreatic fistula or other complications. Determinations at 7 days after injury correlate with the persistence of a pancreatic fistula or other pancreatic complication only if the level is higher than 100,000 IU/L, whereas the negative predictive value of a concentration below 100,000 IU/L is poor and does not rule out the presence or subsequent development of a pancreatic complication.

Treatment of major parenchymal disruptions depends on location and the presence of ductal injury. Injuries to the body or tail of the pancreas should be evaluated for possible ductal disruption. It can be difficult to determine definitively whether an injury has occurred to the duct by inspection of the parenchymal injury. If a ductal injury is obvious or likely, the distal pancreas should be resected and the proximal pancreas and pancreatic duct oversewn. Distal resection can include up to 80% of the gland, if necessary. Subsequent endocrine or exocrine insufficiency is rare if the pancreas is normal. If a ductal injury is not present or is unlikely, the pancreas should be drained. Major parenchymal disruptions of the head of the pancreas should be drained, regardless of the presence of ductal disruption, because the morbidity of pancreaticoduodenectomy or attempts at internal drainage is greater than the morbidity of simply draining the area of injury. If a pancreatic fistula develops, drains can control it. If the fistula does not resolve with time, the pancreas can be drained internally or resected at a later date.

For massive injuries to the duodenum and head of the pancreas, pancreaticoduodenectomy with reconstruction should be reserved for cases in which débridement of devitalized tissue results in a *de facto* removal of the duodenum and head of the pancreas. Penetrating injuries to the ampulla of Vater also may require formal pancreaticoduodenectomy.

Internal drainage of the pancreas has been suggested as a means of treating ductal injuries without the need for resection of viable and functional pancreatic tissue. Although in theory this approach preserves pancreatic function and minimizes the risk of postoperative pancreatic insufficiency, it has major risks. The pancreaticojejunal anastomosis is susceptible to break down and leak, especially if suboptimal conditions of associated injury and hemodynamic instability exist. The construction of a Roux-en-Y jejunal limb requires the opening of the intestine and the creation of a small bowel anastomosis. If the intestine has not been injured, this procedure increases the amount of contamination associated with the injury as well as the likelihood of postoperative morbidity. For these reasons, most major trauma centers rarely carry out internal drainage procedures in the early postinjury period, relying instead on either resection or drainage. Internal drainage is usually reserved for cases in which persistent pancreatic fistulas or pseudocysts develop late[24] and is done on a delayed basis.

Distal pancreatectomy for traumatic injuries should be performed only after the pancreas has been thoroughly mobilized and exposed. In some cases, the pancreas has already been transected, and the site of resection has therefore already been determined for the surgeon. If this is not the case, the pancreas should be transected just proximal to the site of known or presumed ductal injury. If associated splenectomy is planned, elaborate dissection is unnecessary. The splenic artery can be identified near the superior margin of the pancreas and ligated. The splenic vein also can be individually ligated at this point. Commonly, the splenic vein lies behind the body and tail of the pancreas, and its isolation requires more dissection. As an alternative to extensive dissection to isolate the splenic vein behind the pancreas, the vein can be transected along with the pancreatic parenchyma. Individual ligation of the splenic vein stump can be done after the distal pancreas and spleen have been removed. It is helpful first to mobilize the spleen and tail of the pancreas.

The pancreas should be mobilized at the site of transection and can be encircled with a rubber drain. Mobilization and encirclement are best done by an approach to the pancreas along its inferior margin and mobilization inferiorly to superiorly. The pancreas can be divided either distal to a bowel clamp or with a stapler. There are some indications that a sutured closure is less likely to break down and lead to fistula formation than a stapled closure. If a bowel clamp is used, the pancreatic stump should be oversewn with a nonabsorbable running suture. It is recommended that an individual figure-of-eight suture be placed in the cut end of the pancreatic duct. This proves exceedingly difficult in patients with normal pancreatic ductal systems because the duct is small and not easily identified in the cut edge of the pancreatic stump. A pancreatic duct that can be seen easily may indicate preexisting proximal ductal obstruction. In this case, the duct should be individually ligated. If the cut end of the duct is not immediately apparent, time and effort should not be taken to locate and individually ligate it.

It is possible to perform a distal pancreatectomy without a concomitant splenectomy. Splenic salvage involves individual ligation and division of the branches of the splenic artery and vein that supply the body and tail of the pancreas. This adds to operative time and can increase the risk of bleeding, particularly if there is an associated injury to the spleen treated with splenorrhaphy. Splenic salvage should be attempted, therefore, only in hemodynamically stable patients with minimal or no associated intraabdominal or extraabdominal injuries.

Pancreatic injuries can lead to a number of complications, including pancreatic fistulas, pseudocysts, bleeding in the area of the pancreatic bed, and pancreatitis. Pancreatic fistulas after trauma are characterized by persistent drainage of pancreatic enzymes and secretions from the pancreatic injury for a number of weeks after injury. Most of these fistulas close spontaneously, especially if there is no proximal obstruction of the pancreatic ductal system. A trial of total parenteral nutrition may improve the rate and incidence of spontaneous closure. Experience with the use of somatostatin in patients with posttraumatic pancreatic fistulas is limited. Somatostatin given to patients with pancreatic fistulas after elective pancreatic resections seems to decrease the amount of fistula drainage but has not consistently decreased the time to fistula closure.

Pseudocysts that develop after pancreatic trauma often resolve on their own or with percutaneous aspiration or drainage. If, after 4 to 6 weeks of observation with serial ultrasound or CT scans, the pseudocyst does not show signs of resolution, it should be drained internally, into either the stomach or a defunctionalized limb of jejunum, depending on its location.

Bleeding in the area of the pancreatic bed is usually an early complication caused by inadequate drainage with resultant autodigestion of the pancreas and surrounding tissue. Bleeding can be avoided by identifying all injuries at the time of exploration and ensuring adequate drainage. If massive bleeding does occur, it should be dealt with through angiographic or operative intervention.

Pancreatitis is another complication of pancreatic injury and is worsened by inadequate drainage of pancreatic secretions. Treatment consists of provision of adequate drainage and supportive care. If the pancreatitis is localized to the distal pancreas and a trial of conservative management fails, distal pancreatectomy should be considered.

Blunt Injuries

The major difference between penetrating and blunt injuries of the pancreas concerns diagnosis. Penetrating injuries are usually discovered on abdominal exploration for associated injuries, but blunt injuries can occur in isolation and the preoperative diagnosis can be difficult. Blunt pancreatic injuries are relatively rare, which increases the difficulty of diagnosis. In one series of pancreatic injuries, delays in diagnosis of blunt injuries ranged up to several days. Making the diagnosis as quickly as possible is important because delays in diagnosis are associated with significantly increased morbidity and mortality.

The body of the pancreas lies directly anterior to the vertebral column and is vulnerable to crush injuries when the anterior abdominal wall is forcibly compressed, as can occur from a seatbelt, steering wheel, or sharp blow to the epigastrium. In such instances, the pancreas may be the only intraabdominal organ injured.

Physical examination of the abdomen is useful, but because of the retroperitoneal location of the pancreas the results can be misleadingly benign until a number of hours to days after injury. This emphasizes the importance of serial examinations. In most cases, the abdomen becomes progressively more tender to palpation during the first 24 to 48 hours after injury and the need for abdominal exploration becomes more obvious. The physical examination of the abdomen is much less reliable in young children and in patients with head injuries.

Serum amylase and lipase concentrations drawn on admission have low positive and negative predictive values but are helpful in providing an initial value of these enzymes for comparison with subsequent serial determinations. Serial amylase and lipase concentrations are occasionally helpful in monitoring the courses of patients with normal or only mildly elevated admission values, but overreliance on these methods can result in dangerous delays in diagnosis.

Computed tomography scan of the abdomen allows for visualization of the retroperitoneum, including the pancreas. In the case of isolated injury to the pancreas, the sensitivity of the CT scan is at its lowest shortly after injury. Although CT diagnosis of pancreatic injury improves greatly after a number of hours have passed, immediate CT scan of the abdomen sometimes misses pancreatic injuries, particularly if expert interpretation is not available. Serial CT scans, with GI contrast to evaluate the duodenum, should be performed if pancreatic injury is of concern.

Endoscopic retrograde cholangiopancreatography is an attractive diagnostic method for pancreatic injury because it is less invasive than abdominal exploration and also provides information about the status of the ductal system, but there are several practical disadvantages to the technique. Most successful studies using ERCP have involved stable patients studied hours to days after injury at a referral center specifically because of suspicion of a pancreatic injury. These patients are a select group, different from patients who are recently injured. In addition, ERCP is not universally available and, even in large centers, is often unavailable at the odd hours necessary for early diagnosis in acutely injured patients. Many endoscopists are also fearful of inducing an exacerbation of pancreatitis in patients with mild pancreatic injuries lacking ductal involvement. Magnetic resonance cholangiopancreatography (MRCP) is a newer possibility for diagnosis of pancreatic ductal injury in patients with blunt trauma and has also been used as an alternative to ERCP for the investigation of possible postinjury or postoperative complications.[25] Experience to date with MRCP is limited, but it has the advantage of being noninvasive and does not cause pancreatitis. Further experience will be necessary to determine whether the false-negative and false-positive rates of MRCP are acceptable in the diagnosis of pancreatic injury.

Basic principles of exposure and operative management of blunt injuries of the pancreas are the same as for penetrating injuries. In many instances of severe injury, the pancreas already has been transected by the trauma, making the pancreatic resection somewhat simpler to carry out. Isolated injuries of the pancreas from blunt trauma also lend themselves to distal pancreatectomy with splenic preservation. As in penetrating injury, splenic salvage should be attempted only in stable patients without associated splenic rupture or severe associated intraabdominal or extraabdominal injuries. Complications of blunt pancreatic injury are similar to those outlined for penetrating injuries.

Small Intestine

Because the small intestine occupies more volume in the peritoneal cavity than any other organ, it is the intraabdominal viscus most frequently injured by penetrating abdominal trauma. The severity of injury ranges from trivial rents in the bowel serosa or mesentery to massive perforation or devascularization injuries requiring extensive resection.

Diagnosis of small bowel injury can be made by a number of methods. Physical examination of the abdomen reveals peritoneal signs in many patients with penetrating small bowel injuries. Patients with gunshot wounds should routinely undergo laparotomy. In stable patients, exploration for other penetrating anterior abdominal injuries that violate the abdominal wall fascia is more selective. One alternative is to use serial abdominal examinations, hematocrits, and leukocyte counts. If the patient shows increasing signs of intraperitoneal injury, abdominal exploration is performed. Another approach is DPL, with a variety of criteria for positivity in patients with anterior abdominal wounds, ranging from 1,000 RBCs/mL of lavage fluid up to the conventional 100,000 RBCs/mL used in patients with blunt trauma. Recently, CT has been used to determine the track of the wound and potential peritoneal penetration with or without evidence of intestinal or other visceral injury.

Regardless of the approach taken for the preoperative diagnosis of penetrating injuries of the small intestine, the operative approach is the same. The abdomen should be explored through a standard midline incision, and initial attention should be directed toward bleeding from associated injuries or from the small bowel mesentery. Bleeding from the mesentery usually can be controlled with suture ligation or with a rapid running closure of the mesenteric rent. This closure does not need to constitute definitive repair, but it temporarily controls bleeding until definitive treatment is delineated.

After bleeding has been controlled, steps to prevent ongoing leakage of intestinal contents from the injured small bowel should be taken. This is done by rapid examination of the small intestine and by application of Babcock or Allis clamps, a temporizing running single-layer closure, or stapled control of the injured areas. Definitive repair or resection should not be done until the entire length of the intestine has been carefully examined because knowledge of the extent of injury is necessary for a logical and rational approach to operative management. It makes no sense, for example, to repair a segment of small intestine, only to determine after further exploration that injuries to adjacent segments of the bowel dictate resection of an entire larger segment.

The entire length of the small intestine should be carefully examined, starting at the ligament of Treitz and moving sequentially, proximally to distally, to each successive loop. This should be done in a systematic manner and should include inspection of the small bowel mesentery by fanning out the mesentery and examining each new loop. When a suspect area is seen along the mesenteric border of the intestine, the mesentery should be cleared away to allow adequate visualization. The small intestine has a good blood supply and easily tolerates this maneuver. Any blood or other debris found on the serosa of the bowel should be wiped away. Sometimes, such debris overlies an otherwise unsuspected area of injury. Compression of the intestine in areas of suspected injury may also demonstrate a leak that would otherwise be missed.

In theory, the number of holes found in the small intestine should add up to an even number because the number of entrance and exit wounds should be identical. This rule is sometimes violated in practice, however, because the intestine is extensively coiled in the peritoneal cavity and tangential wounds of the bowel are common. Rather than focusing on the number of holes in the bowel, attention should be directed to a close inspection of the entire length of the intestine. After all areas of injury have been identified, a decision about repair or resection is made. Areas of massive destruction of the bowel or the mesentery, with associated ischemia, should be treated with resection. If after débridement more than 40% to 50% of the circumference of the wall of the small intestine is missing, that segment also should be resected. Stapled anastomoses in trauma patients should not be performed if extensive bowel wall edema, significant ischemia, or hypoperfusion has occurred. With normal intestinal wall thickness, however, stapled anastomoses are particularly useful when time is of the essence and should be constructed in a side-to-side, functional end-to-end fashion.

Knife wounds to the small intestine are usually easy to manage and rarely require extensive débridement or resection. On rare occasions, a large rent in the small bowel mesentery results in enough devascularization to require resection of a segment of intestine.

Minor mesenteric lacerations should be treated with suture ligation of bleeding points and closure of the rent. Major lacerations with devascularization should be treated with resection and primary anastomosis. Small bowel anastomoses, when properly done and after adequate débridement of devitalized tissue, have an excellent rate of healing even with severe associated injuries, shock, and peritonitis.

Shotgun wounds to the abdomen from close range are often associated with massive tissue destruction, which should be débrided and anastomosis completed as appropriate. Medium- or longer-range shotgun wounds sometimes result in a diffuse pattern of shot injury, creating multiple small perforations of the small intestine. In such instances, the general principles outlined should be followed and obvious areas of injury repaired. It is sometimes impossible to ensure closure of all the numerous areas of perforation, and planned repeat laparotomy may be required to rule out occult injuries.

On rare occasions, injuries to the small intestine occur in patients who are hemodynamically unstable as a result of associated injuries. In such instances, the small intestine can be treated most expeditiously by application of the gastrointestinal anastomosis stapler as necessary to remove the injured areas of bowel as a "damage control" technique. A second operation is planned and definitive anastomosis is deferred with the stapled ends of the intestine returned to the abdomen until the second procedure is performed.

Blunt injuries to the small intestine are much less common than penetrating injuries. As with other blunt intraabdominal injuries, they are more difficult to diagnose because the need for urgent intraabdominal intervention is not always obvious. Blunt perforations and devascularizations of the small intestine often occur in isolation, either as the only injury or as the only intraabdominal injury present. This makes early diagnosis even more difficult.[26]

Seatbelts, in particular high-riding lap belts, have been implicated in the pathogenesis of blunt injuries of the small intestine. The intestine or mesentery is sheared across the seatbelt to the point of rupture or disruption of its mesentery, resulting in either perforation or devascularization. Because of the severe degree of force necessary to produce a blunt intestinal injury, there is a frequent association with transverse fractures of a lumbar vertebral body (Chance fracture), caused by flexion or distraction over the seatbelt.

Abdominal examination is usually positive shortly after injury, but initial findings in some cases can be subtle, resulting in delays in diagnosis. Presence of a Chance fracture and lower abdominal "lap belt" transverse contusion should warrant laparotomy. If head injury or intoxication makes physical examination of the abdomen unreliable, DPL should be performed. The false-negative rate of DPL for this injury is less than 5%. CT and ultrasound, particularly if done early after injury, are not reliable in ruling out blunt intestinal injury. The injury itself may not be obvious, and small amounts of intraperitoneal fluid from the injury may not be detectable. If either is used instead of DPL, then it should be repeated at regular intervals to look for changes indicative of a perforation.

Blunt injuries to the small intestine are most common in either the proximal jejunum or the distal ileum, probably because the intestine is fixed at these two points and more vulnerable to shear and stretch injuries. Multiple injuries to the small intestine from blunt trauma occur in approximately 25% of cases. Second or even third areas of injury should be carefully sought if a blunt intestinal injury is discovered on abdominal exploration.

After the suspicion of blunt intestinal or other intraabdominal injury has been raised and the decision to explore the abdomen has been made, the basic principles of abdominal exploration and operative management of blunt small bowel injuries are the same as for penetrating injuries. Because of the nature of the mechanism of injury, the perforations are usually amenable to primary repair. Mesenteric rents that cause devascularization and require resection are relatively more common after blunt injury than after penetrating injury.

Colon and Rectum

Most injuries to the colon and rectum are the result of penetrating or perforating trauma. Blunt trauma accounts for only approximately 5% of colonic injuries. Rectal injuries can occur in association with pelvic fractures and the possibility of rectal injury must be considered in any patient with a significant pelvic fracture, in addition to evaluation of other pelvic viscera such as the bladder, distal ureters, uterus, and vagina.

Signs and symptoms of peritonitis result from injury to the colon and rectum but are not specific. Injury to the extraperitoneal rectum is particularly difficult to recognize because peritonitis does not result. Conventional laboratory studies usually are not helpful. Plain radiographs may show free air in the peritoneal cavity, but this finding is relatively uncommon; when it is not present, the patient cannot be assumed to be free of bowel perforation. DPL may be of value if intraperitoneal colonic injury is present, yielding lavage fluid with blood, bacteria, or fecal material. If the injury is confined to the extraperitoneal colon and rectum, however, DPL is of no value. Extraperitoneal colonic or rectal injury is extremely difficult to diagnose. The possibility of rectal injury must be considered in any patient with penetrating trauma to the lower abdomen or buttocks. Digital examination is essential. The presence of blood on examination is strong evidence for colon or rectal injury, and proctoscopic and sigmoidoscopic examinations should be performed. Water-soluble contrast studies also may be useful, but direct bowel examination usually is preferable. Approximately 95% of colon injuries are caused by gunshot, shotgun, or stab wounds, and, whenever the possibility of colonic injury is entertained, broad-spectrum intravenous prophylactic antibiotics should be started immediately and continued postoperatively using a standard protocol limiting their use to no more than 2 to 3 days.

The longstanding controversy between primary repair of low-risk colonic injuries and repair or resection with exteriorization has been largely resolved.[27] Primary repair is preferred after additional risk factors that increase the incidence of complications have been excluded, such as preoperative hypotension, intraperitoneal hemorrhage exceeding 1 L, more than two additional injured organs (hepatic, pancreatic, and splenic injuries have the highest morbidity rates), gross fecal spillage, or an elapsed time since injury of more than 6 hours. Many patients with penetrating colon injuries, however, can be treated with primary closure even in the presence of these risk factors. Resection and colostomy are an overly conservative approach, and recent series indicate that primary repair may be safe even in the presence of some risk factors. Exteriorization of the repaired segment has also been advocated, but the success of this technique is low and has little benefit over diverting colostomy alone. Overall primary repair is indicated for most colon wounds, but each surgeon must decide in the context of the individual patient's risks. Postoperative complications include abscess formation, anastomotic leak, peristomal hernia, and the morbidity and mortality associated with colostomy closure.

The morbidity and mortality from rectal injuries is primarily a result of inadequate initial therapy and the complications associated with delayed sepsis. Rectal injury must be suspected in any penetrating injury that enters the buttocks or tracks into the true pelvis, or if a pelvic fracture produces a ring disruption or large displaced bone fragments. Sigmoidoscopic examination is essential. The principles of operative

TABLE 25.5 MANAGEMENT

PRINCIPLES OF OPERATIVE MANAGEMENT OF COLON AND RECTAL INJURIES

- Placement of the patient in the lithotomy position to provide simultaneous exposure of both the perineum and abdomen
- Wide débridement of all dead and devitalized tissue
- A totally defunctioning colostomy (simple loop colostomy may be inadequate)
- Rectal wall closure, if the injury is easily accessible
- Retrorectal drainage, primarily in severe injuries
- Distal rectal stump washout if feasible
- Broad-spectrum intravenous antibiotics, nutritional support, and serial débridement

management of colon and rectal injuries are outlined in Table 25.5.

Complete rectal destruction is a rare injury for which primary abdominoperineal resection with packing may be necessary. If done, the packing should be removed operatively in approximately 48 hours. Complications of rectal injuries include pelvic abscesses, urinary or rectal fistulas, rectal incontinence and stricture, urinary incontinence, and loss of sexual function.

Retroperitoneal Hematoma

The optimal management of retroperitoneal hematoma depends on a number of factors, including its cause, its location, and the presence of associated injuries. The retroperitoneum can be divided into anatomic zones for purposes of decision making (Fig. 25.8 and Table 25.6). Retroperitoneal hematomas in zone 1, regardless of cause or size, are formally explored with inspection of each of the relevant structures. This is required because of the high incidence of associated major vascular, pancreatic, or duodenal injuries and the high morbidity and mortality rates if these are overlooked.

Zone 2 hematomas caused by penetrating injuries are routinely explored if encountered in the operating room. Whether proximal control of the renal pedicle should be obtained before exploration of a perinephric hematoma is controversial. In cases of severe ongoing hemorrhage, time should not be taken to obtain proximal control, and the kidney should be mobilized directly. If time and the degree of hemorrhage permit, however, it is acceptable to obtain vascular control before mobilization of the kidney. Zone 2 hematomas caused by blunt trauma can be left alone if they are not expanding.

Zone 3 retroperitoneal hematomas in patients with penetrating injuries should be explored to exclude major vascular

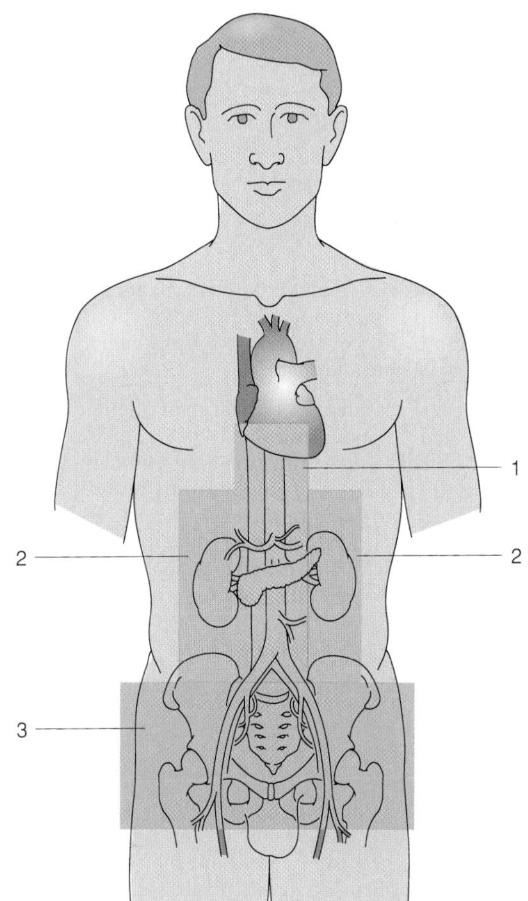

FIGURE 25.8 Zones of the retroperitoneum.

injuries. Bleeding from iliac vessels can be challenging and have a significant mortality. Venous control with direct pressure and dissection allows exposure for diagnosis, ligation, or repair. Arterial injuries are controlled proximally and occasionally require distal control below the inguinal ligament. Patients with zone 3 hematomas secondary to blunt trauma usually have associated pelvic fractures. Exploration of the hematoma can be hazardous and difficult to control and is usually avoided. There is often extensive injury to the rich presacral venous and arterial circulation. Incision of the peritoneum releases the tamponade, and dissection within the hematoma can produce catastrophic bleeding. Discrete bleeding points rarely can be identified. Exploration of these hematomas is associated with an increased requirement for transfusion and a higher mortality rate.

TABLE 25.6

ZONES OF THE PERITONEUM

Zone	Location	Associated injuries
1	Central retroperitoneum	Pancreaticoduodenal injuries or major abdominal vascular injury
2	Flank or perinephric area	Injuries to the genitourinary tract or to the colon (i.e., with penetrating trauma)
3	Pelvis	Pelvic fractures

KEY POINTS

- To aid in the evaluation for injury, the abdomen can be divided into four areas:
  1. Intrathoracic (diaphragm, liver, spleen, stomach),
  2. True (small and large intestines, distended bladder, gravid uterus),
  3. Pelvic (rectum, bladder, urethra, small intestine, female reproductive organs), and
  4. Retroperitoneal (kidneys, ureters, pancreas, second and third duodenum, aorta, vena cava) abdomen, all of which are difficult to assess by physical examination, except the true abdomen.
- Adjunctive assessment is critical using hematocrit, white blood cell count, biochemical markers (amylase, lipase, creatinine, bilirubin, liver function tests), imaging, including ultrasound (FAST), CT, angiography, and DPL, as indicated by mechanism, pattern, and risk.
- The top three patterns of injury are liver, intestines and spleen caused by blunt (usually vehicular crashes, vehicle versus pedestrian, and falls), and penetrating (gunshot and shotgun) trauma.
- The objective is to determine who needs an operation—not what organ is injured. The primary effect of solid organ injury is bleeding (monitored by hematocrit and FAST, DPL, or CT) and visceral injury, peritonitis (diagnosed by physical examination, laboratory, or DPL and, increasingly, CT).
- Specific pattern of injury (e.g., lower abdominal lap belt bruising along with lumbar spine fracture) indicates need for operative intervention for intestinal injury and should be recognized early to minimize morbidity.
- Operative treatment of specific injuries is dictated by pattern, extent, and overall stability of patient and associated injuries. Blunt and penetrating injuries are, in large part, treated by similar principles. Grossly unstable patients require a "damage control" approach and return on a later day, when stable.
- Approach to retroperitoneal hematoma depends on cause, location, and other injuries. The retroperitoneum is divided into zones to aid decision making: central (zone 1) is associated with pancreaticoduodenal injuries or major vascular injury and must be explored; flank (zone 2) is associated with perinephric bleeding and injuries are explored if enlarging, pulsatile, or caused by penetrating trauma; and pelvic (zone 3) is associated with pelvic fractures, entered at great risk, and best left alone.

References

1. Bickell WH, Wall MJ Jr, Pepe PE, et al. Immediate versus delayed fluid resuscitation for hypotensive patients with penetrating torso injuries. *N Engl J Med.* 1994;331:1105–1109.
2. **Malhotra AK, Fabian TC, Katsis SB, et al. Blunt bowel and mesenteric injuries: the role of screening computer tomography. *J Trauma* 2000;48: 991–1000.**
3. Killeen KL, Shanmuganathan K, Poletti PA, et al. Helical computed tomography of bowel and mesenteric injuries. *J Trauma* 2001;51:26–36.
4. Villavicencio RT, Aucar JA. Analysis of laparoscopy in trauma. *J Am Coll Surg.* 1999;189:11–20.
5. Moore E, Moore J, Van Duzer-Moore S, et al. Mandatory laparotomy for gunshot wounds penetrating the abdomen. *Am J Surg.* 1980;140:847–851.
6. **Rozycki GS, Ballard RB, Feliciano DV, et al. Surgeon-performed ultrasound for the assessment of truncal injuries: lessons learned from 1,540 patients. *Ann Surg.* 1998;228:557–567.**
7. McKenny MG, Martin L, Lentz K, et al. 1,000 Consecutive ultrasounds for blunt abdominal trauma. *J Trauma* 1996;40:607–612.
8. Branney SW, Moore EE, Cantrill SV, et al. Ultrasound based key clinical pathway reduces the use of hospital resources for the evaluation of blunt abdominal trauma. *J Trauma* 1997;42:1086–1090.
9. Shackford SR, Rogers FB, Osler TM, et al. Focused abdominal sonogram for trauma: the learning curve of nonradiologist clinicians in detecting hemoperitoneum. *J Trauma* 1999;46:553–564.
10. Wherrett LJ, Boulanger BR, McLellan BA, et al. Hypotension after blunt abdominal trauma: the Role of emergent abdominal sonography in surgical triage. *J Trauma* 1996;41:815–820.
11. **Luchette FA, Borzotta AP, Croce MA, et al. Practice management guidelines for prophylactic antibiotic use in penetrating abdominal trauma: The EAST Practice Management Guidelines Work Group. *J Trauma* 2000;48: 508–518.**
12. Kirton OC, O'Neill PA, Kestner M, et al. Perioperative antibiotic use in high-risk penetrating hollow viscus injury: a prospective randomized, double-blind, placebo-control trial of 24 hours versus 5 days. *J Trauma* 2000; 49:822–832.
13. **Rotondo MF, Schwab CW, McGonigal MD, et al. "Damage control": an approach for improved survival in exsanguinating penetrating abdominal injury. *J Trauma* 1993;35:375–382.**
14. **Suliburk JW, Ware DN, Balogh Z, et al. Vacuum-assisted wound closure achieves early fascial closure of open abdomens after severe trauma. *J Trauma* 2003;55:1155–1160.**
15. Schurr MJ, Fabian TC, Gavant M, et al. Management of blunt splenic trauma: computed tomographic contrast blush predicts failure of nonoperative management. *J Trauma* 1995;39:507–512.
16. Thaemert BC, Cogbill TH, Lambert PJ. Nonoperative management of splenic injury: are follow-up computed tomographic scans of any value? *J Trauma* 1997;43:748–751.
17. **Peitzman AB, Heil B, Rivera L, et al. Blunt splenic injury in adults: multi-institutional study of the eastern association for the surgery of trauma. *J Trauma* 2000;49:177–189.**
18. Davidson RN, Wall RA. Prevention and management of infections in patients without a spleen. *Clin Microbiol Infect.* 2001;7:657–660.
19. **Croce MA, Fabian TC, Menke PG, et al. Nonoperative management of blunt hepatic trauma is the treatment of choice for hemodynamically stable patients: results of a prospective trial. *Ann Surg.* 1995;221:744–753.**
20. Scherer LA, Battistella FD, Owings JT, et al. Video-assisted thoracic surgery in the treatment of posttraumatic empyema. *Arch Surg.* 1998;133: 637–642.
21. Levison MA, Peterson SR, Sheldon GF, et al. Duodenal trauma: experience of a trauma center. *J Trauma* 1984;24:475–480.
22. Wisner DH, Wold RL, Frey CF. Diagnosis and treatment of pancreatic injuries: an analysis of management principles. *Arch Surg.* 1990;125: 1109–1113.
23. **Patton JH, Lyden SP, Croce MA, et al. Pancreatic trauma: a simplified management guideline. *J Trauma* 1997;43:234–240.**
24. Lucas CE. Diagnosis and treatment of pancreatic and duodenal injury. *Surg Clin North Am.* 1977;57:49–65.
25. Fulcher AS, Turner, MA, Yelon JA, et al. Magnetic resonance cholangiopancreatography (MRCP) in the assessment of pancreatic duct trauma and its sequelae: preliminary findings. *J Trauma* 2000;48:1001–1007.
26. Wisner DH, Chun Y, Blaisdell FW. Blunt intestinal injury: keys to diagnosis and management. *Arch Surg.* 1990;125:1319–1322.
27. **Stone HH, Fabian TC. Management of perforating colon trauma: randomization between primary closure and exteriorization. *Ann Surg.* 1979; 190:430–436.**

CHAPTER 26 ■ GENITOURINARY AND PELVIC TRAUMA

JAMES K. KUAN, MILTON L. ROUTT, JR., AND HUNTER WESSELLS

Genitourinary and pelvic injuries rarely occur in isolation and thus afford an opportunity for multidisciplinary collaboration to provide lifesaving, as well as definitive, reconstruction for these complex injuries. Reliable, recognizable clinical presentations and improved diagnostic ability have improved the care of these traumatized individuals. Much of what we know, however, comes from retrospective or case control series, because few prospective, randomized studies examining genitourinary (GU) or pelvic trauma management exist. Fundamental principles now exist for the management of each GU and pelvic trauma. These treatments are reviewed and the American Association for the Surgery of Trauma (AAST) Organ Injury Scale is outlined (Table 26.1).

UPPER URINARY TRACT INJURY

Injury to the upper urinary tract (kidney, ureter) is rare following trauma. The widespread use of contrast-enhanced computed tomography (CT) provides accurate staging of upper urinary tract injuries.[1] Unfortunately, ureteric injuries, though rare (1%), frequently are missed at the initial assessment and delayed diagnosis is common.[2] Recognizing the factors that predispose to upper urinary tract injury facilitates early diagnosis and management, which is associated with improved outcomes.

TABLE 26.1 CLASSIFICATION

AMERICAN ASSOCIATION FOR THE SURGERY OF TRAUMA (AAST) ORGAN INJURY SCALES FOR URINARY TRACT

Injured structure	AAST grade	Characteristics of injury
Kidney[a]	I	Contusion with microscopic or gross hematuria, urologic studies normal; nonexpanding subcapsular hematoma without parenchymal laceration
	II	Nonexpanding perirenal hematoma confined to renal retroperitoneum; laceration <1.0 cm parenchymal depth of renal cortex without urinary extravasation
	III	Laceration >1.0 cm parenchymal depth of renal cortex without collecting system rupture or urinary extravasation
	IV	Parenchymal laceration extending through renal cortex, medulla, and collecting system with urinary extravasation; injury to main renal artery or vein with contained hemorrhage
	V	Completely shattered kidney; avulsion of renal hilum that devascularizes kidney
Ureter[a]	I	Contusion or hematoma without devascularization
	II	<50% transection
	III	= 50% transection
	IV	Complete transection with <2 cm devascularization
	V	Avulsion with >2 cm devascularization
Bladder[b]	I	Contusion, intramural hematoma; partial-thickness laceration
	II	Extraperitoneal bladder wall laceration <2 cm
	III	Extraperitoneal bladder wall laceration >2 cm or intraperitoneal bladder wall laceration <2 cm
	IV	Intraperitoneal bladder wall laceration >2 cm
	V	Intraperitoneal or extraperitoneal bladder wall laceration extending into bladder neck or ureteral orifice (trigone)
Urethra	I	Contusion with blood at urethral meatus and normal urethrography
	II	Stretch injury with elongation of urethra, but without extravasation of urethrography contrast material
	III	Partial disruption with extravasation of urethrography contrast material at injury site with visualization in the bladder
	IV	Complete disruption with <2 cm urethral separation and extravasation of urethrography contrast material at injury site, without visualization in the bladder
	V	Complete transection with = 2 cm urethral separation or extension into the prostate or vagina

[a]Advance one grade for bilateral injuries, up to grade III.
[b]Advance one grade for multiple injuries, up to grade III.
(Adapted from *ACS Surgery: Principles and Practice: Injuries to the Urogenital Tract* 2002;10:3; copyright 2002 WebMD.)

The kidneys lie in the retroperitoneum, protected by the ribcage, retroperitoneal fat, perirenal fat within Gerota's capsule, and overlying viscera (right; liver, colon, duodenum, adrenal; left: spleen, colon, adrenal, pancreas). Currently, a rate of renal injury of 4.89 per 100,000 persons is reported and occurs in 1.2% to 3.25% of trauma patients.[3–6] These injuries occur predominantly in males aged 20 to 30 years, following blunt (71%) or penetrating (16%) trauma. Motor vehicle collision was the primary mechanism in 47.8% of injuries in a large population-based study.[7] Geographically these proportions vary, and in areas where war is a factor penetrating injuries may prevail.

Anatomically, the ureter extends from the renal pelvis (ureteropelvic junction [UPJ]) and traverses the retroperitoneum protected by retroperitoneal fat and psoas muscle. It crosses over the common iliac vessels to enter the pelvis, coursing caudad to the base of the bladder, entering the trigone obliquely (ureterovesical junction [UVJ]). The most common injury to the ureter is iatrogenic during hysterectomy and usually occurs at the level of infundibulopelvic ligament ligation. UPJ avulsion injury, though rare, is more common in children, who are susceptible because of increased hyperextensibility of the spine. In general, ureteric injury following external trauma is usually from gunshot wounds and should be suspected when organs anatomically related to the ureter sustain injury: iliac vessels, bladder, sigmoid colon, and lumbar spine transverse processes. The blood supply is segmental, arising laterally (upper), medially (mid to true pelvis), and posterolaterally (lower).

Hematuria is the most sensitive clinical sign of renal injury, yet the degree does not predict injury severity. Thus, its presence should prompt radiographic investigation for renal injury in selected patients.[8] There are, however, no unique physical signs of ureteric trauma and hematuria is unreliable. All pediatric-aged patients with hematuria should undergo imaging and in adults the guidelines in Table 26.2 are suggested[9]: Contrast-enhanced CT is the preferred imaging modality in stable patients, and injuries can be accurately staged using the AAST scale (Fig 26.1). The scan consists of scout and contrast-enhanced images, detecting arterial blush, parenchymal integrity, retroperitoneal fluid collections, and renal perfusion. Delayed (10 minutes) imaging is essential for detecting collecting system injury (extravasation, hydronephrosis) and ureteral continuity to the bladder. Conventional intravenous urography (IVU) with tomography, though inferior to CT, can be used for staging when CT is not available.[10] The ability of a single-shot urography to stage injuries is limited and should not be used for this purpose. Focused abdominal ultrasound for trauma (FAST) remains inferior to CT scanning and thus remains investigational.[11] Renal arterial angiography is rarely used diagnostically but therapeutically is indicated to treat isolated, symptomatic early or late renal bleeding, arteriovenous fistula, or pseudoaneurysm using embolization.

If renal exploration is contemplated or necessary (gunshot wound, hypotension from renal bleeding, expanding hematoma in blunt trauma),[12] demonstration of contralateral renal function is important, in the event ipsilateral nephrectomy is performed. If immediate laparotomy is performed without preoperative imaging, an intraoperative single-shot IVU (KUB at 10 minutes following intravenous injection of 2 mL/kg contrast) can provide this information.[13] Failure to demonstrate contrast excretion from the contralateral kidney may indicate a solitary kidney, hilar injury, hypoperfusion, or global renal insufficiency secondary to chronic renal disease. Exploration of a solitary kidney should be performed only when absolute indications exist, to avoid rendering the patient anephric, requiring hemodialysis or tedious autotransplantation.

Most injuries are managed nonoperatively.[7] Grade I and II injuries, as well as grade III and nonvascular grade IV injuries, can be managed expectantly. Exploration should be undertaken, however, for grade III and IV injuries in patients undergoing laparotomy for other indications, reducing the potential for complications.[15] The absolute indications for renal exploration include symptomatic renal hemorrhage, penetrating injury, expanding or pulsatile retroperitoneal hematoma at laparotomy, and grade V injury (Fig 26.2). Invariably, patients with ureteric injuries undergo surgical exploration for associated injuries, allowing the ureter to be inspected directly. The upper urinary tract is accessed through a midline abdominal incision. Using the inferior mesenteric vein (IMV) as a landmark, a posterior peritoneal window is created medial to the IMV overlying the aorta, which allows access, dissection, and control of the proximal renal vasculature. If urgency does not permit time for dissection to obtain proximal control, direct rapid mobilization of the kidney permits vascular control at the hilum. The retroperitoneum is entered by mobilizing the colon, which exposes Gerota's fascia, which is then opened, allowing one to strip away the perinephric fat. Manual compression followed by vascular clamping may be required. Cooling is not routinely employed, thus allowing 30 to 45 minutes of tolerated warm ischemia time. For ureteric injuries occurring in the mid to distal ureter without associated renal injury, simple mobilization of the colon without hilar control can be used to gain access to the ureters.

During renal exploration, débridement, hemostasis, collecting system repair, and pledgeted, bolstered closure using renal capsule are performed using absorbable suture, unless nephrectomy is required (grade V, progressive hemodynamic instability). A perinephric suction drain is placed away from the repair in the retroperitoneum.[16] In the case of renal artery thrombosis, surgical revascularization is rarely helpful because of the time delay from injury to exploration. Isolated left renal vein injuries can be managed by controlling and oversewing the caval stump. Adequate left renal vein collateral drainage is present via the gonadal, adrenal, and lumbar veins. Postoperatively, drains remain *in situ* until acceptable drainage, usually less than 50 mL/day, is observed. Frequent monitoring for ongoing bleeding is essential. Postoperative complications of ileus, urinoma, atelectasis, and infection can occur. Secondary bleeding of nonoperatively managed and explored kidneys should be managed angiographically, because nephrectomy is likely with exploration. Renin-mediated hypertension from chronic renal ischemia is rare, as are arteriovenous malformations, pseudoaneurysm, and renal calculus formation.

For ureteric injuries, definitive reconstruction should be performed only if the patient is stable. If not, damage control involves débridement, ligation, bladder and retroperitoneal

TABLE 26.2 DIAGNOSIS

GUIDELINES FOR IMAGING TO DETERMINE RENAL INJURY IN ADULTS WITH HEMATURIA

Radiographic investigation required

- Gross hematuria
- Microscopic hematuria and episode of systolic BP <90 mm Hg
- Microscopic hematuria with systolic BP >90 mm Hg and index of suspicion based on physical exam (rib fracture, flank ecchymosis) or mechanism of injury (flank impact, deceleration injury, penetrating injury)

Radiographic investigation not required

- Microscopic hematuria, systolic BP >90 mm Hg and absence of other indications

BP, blood pressure.

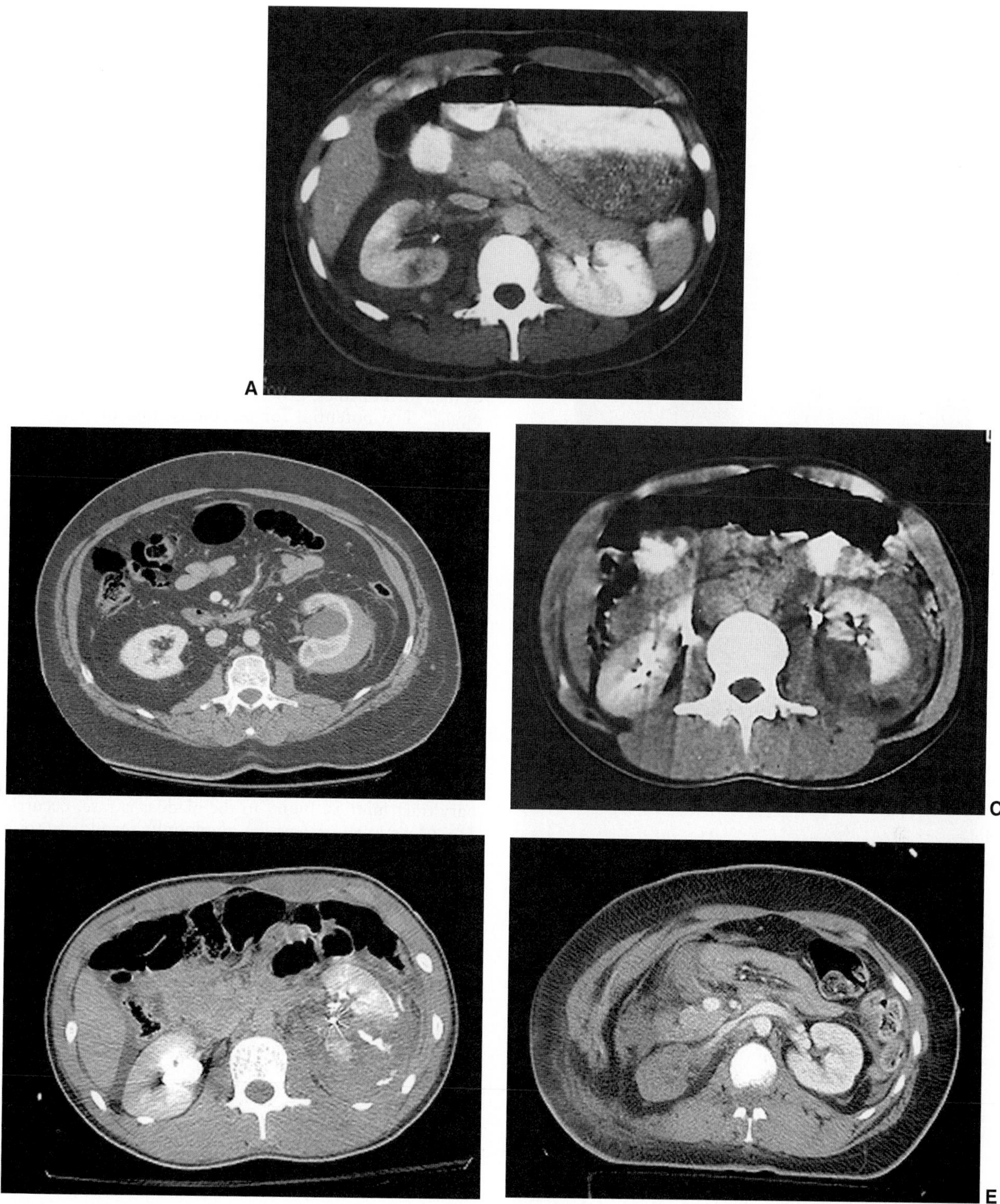

FIGURE 26.1 AAST grading of renal injury by computed tomography. (*A*) Grade I: contusion. (*B*) Grade II. (*C*) Grade III. (*D*) Grade IV: contrast extravasation. (*E*) Grade V: devascularized.

drainage, and percutaneous placement of a nephrostomy tube. Complete débridement precedes ureter reconstruction, and the level and length of ureter dictates the type of repair (Figs. 26.3 and 26.4). Low pelvic ureteric injuries are best repaired by nonrefluxing ureterocystostomy in children; however, refluxing implant is acceptable in adults. When the defect is too long for primary repair, a vesicopsoas-hitch reconstruction or Boari flap is performed. Short midureteric injuries are repaired by spatulated end-to-end anastomosis or end-to-side transureteroureterostomy. Ureteropelvic junction (UPJ) disruptions demand formal reconstruction by reanastomosis or ureteropyelostomy. Ileal interposition and autotransplantation have little role in the acute trauma setting, because they are long procedures, which is prohibitive. Patients presenting with ureteric injury in a delayed fashion may show evidence of fever, flank pain, fullness, tenderness, atelectasis, or oliguria.[17] Immediate operative intervention at the time of delayed diagnosis frequently results in nephrectomy and, thus, is avoided. A "less is

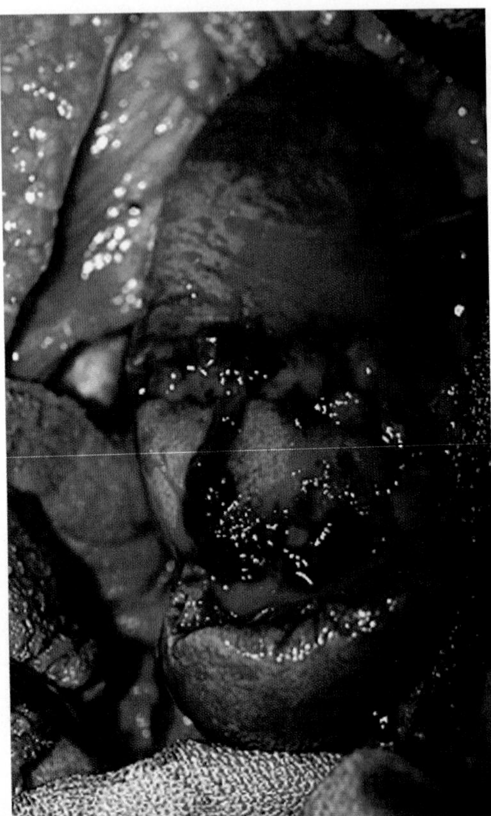

FIGURE 26.2 Grade V renal injury at exploration.

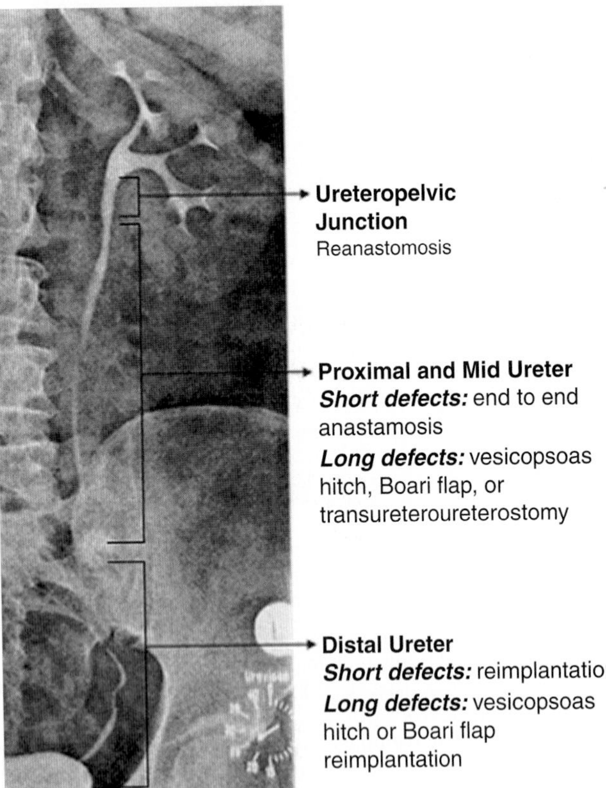

FIGURE 26.3 Ureteral reconstruction by location of injury.

more" approach is adopted, securing a nephrostomy tube fluoroscopically, and bladder and fluid collection drainage. Stenting across an injury in this setting should be delayed for 1 to 2 weeks. Delayed reconstruction is planned beyond 3 months. Complications of ureteric injury include fistula, fluid collections, ureteral stricture, and obstructive uropathy.

All individuals who have sustained injury to the upper urinary tract require follow-up, performing imaging in the form of radionuclide scanning or IVU at 3 and 12 months to evaluate for hydronephrosis and potential functional loss.[18]

PELVIC AND LOWER URINARY TRACT INJURY

Blunt trauma causing disruption of the pelvic ring is a challenging clinical problem, requiring the expertise of many specialties (orthopedics, general surgery, neurosurgery, and urology).[19] The potential for morbidity, loss of function, and death (approximately 50%) is significant.[20] Particular attention is paid to thorough evaluation of the lower urinary tract for concurrent injury, because of the frequency of these injuries with pelvic fracture. Penetrating and iatrogenic trauma to the pelvis or perineum is less common and generally results in visceral (bladder, bowel), urethral, or genital injuries, but without the morbidity of pelvic disruption.

High-energy pelvic trauma, secondary to rapid deceleration during motor vehicle collision, pedestrian–vehicle impact, or falls, places the bony pelvis, comprising two innominate bones and the sacrococcygeal unit, at risk for an array of injuries, including pubic symphysis diastasis, displaced pubic rami fractures, fractures of the iliac wings, sacroiliac disruption, and displaced sacral fractures. The vector of impact determines the injury type and the subsequent risk of visceral injury (Table 26.3).[21,22]

Pelvic fractures are frequently associated with lower urinary tract injuries. Injury to the bladder is rare, occurring in 1% of trauma patients,[23] commonly secondary to blunt trauma. An associated pelvic fracture is present in nearly 90% of cases, though only 9% of pelvic fractures result in bladder injury. Following rapid deceleration intravesical pressures rise significantly, causing a "burst" type injury with extravasation of urine intraperitoneally (30%), extraperitoneally (60%), or both (10%).[24] Additionally, shearing forces at deceleration may cause injury at the fixed sites of pelvic fascial attachment. Direct injury from pelvic bone fragments may also cause laceration of the bladder. A larger proportion of pediatric injuries are intraperitoneal because of the relative intraabdominal location of their bladders. Concomitant urethra injury is encountered in 10% to 29%.[25] Blunt trauma is the most common mechanism of injury, consisting of straddle injuries to the anterior urethra (bulbous, pendulous) and prostatomembranous disruption occurring in the posterior urethra (membranous, prostatic) after pelvic fracture. Failure to recognize these

TABLE 26.3 ETIOLOGY

INJURIES FROM HIGH-ENERGY PELVIC TRAUMA

Injury type	Area of impact
Anteroposterior compression	Spleen, liver, bowel, pelvic vascular injury, retroperitoneal hematoma
Lateral compression	Brain, lung, or upper abdominal viscera
Vertical shear	Most unstable

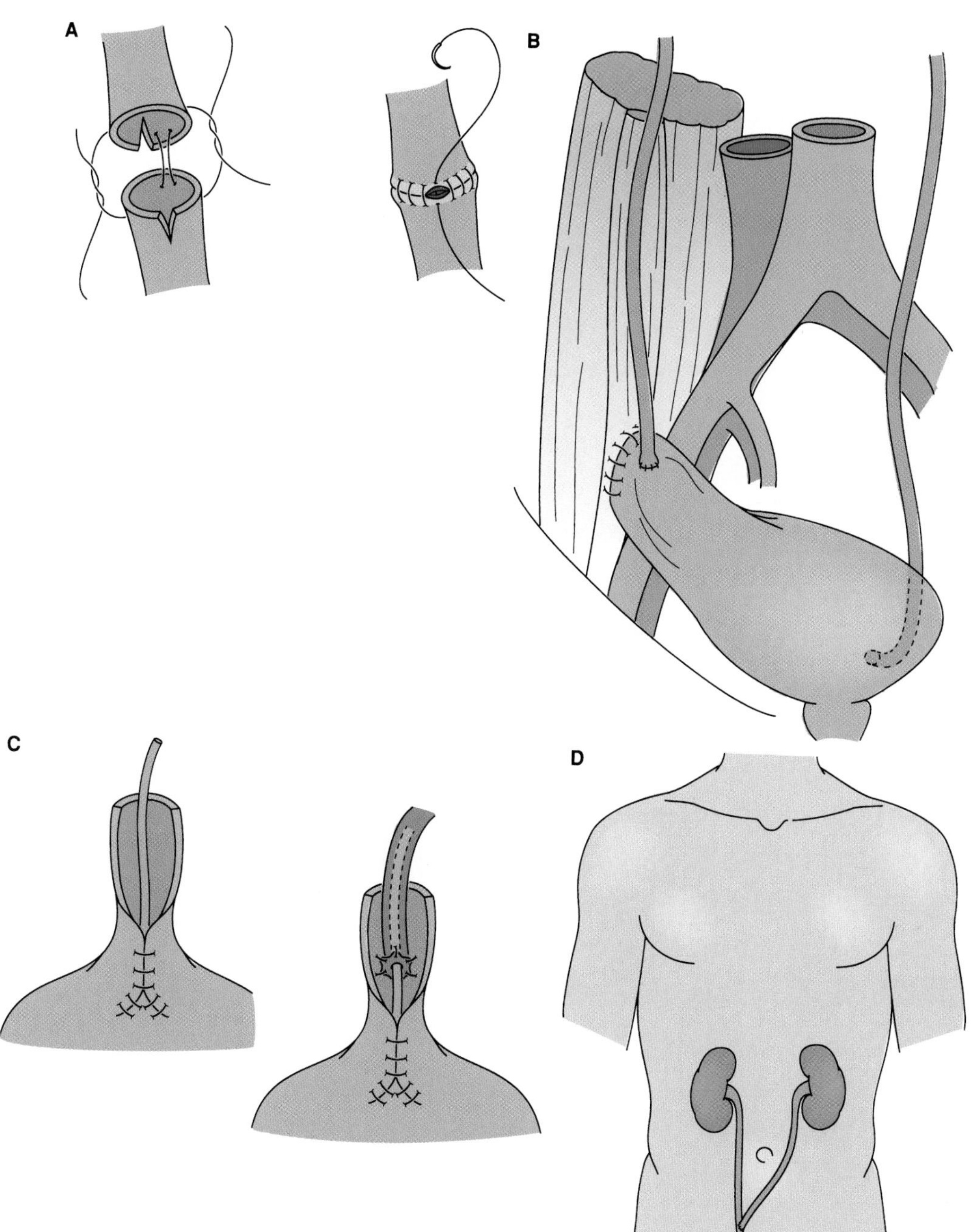

FIGURE 26.4 Techniques of ureteral repair. (*A*) End-to-end ureteroureterostomy. (*B*) Vesicopsoas hitch reconstruction with reimplantation performed by suturing of the bladder to psoas tendon after mobilization of both obliterated umbilical, plus or minus contralateral superior vesical pedicles, avoiding the genitofemoral nerve. (*C*) Boari flap performed using an anterior tubularized bladder flap based on the ipsilateral superior vesical artery. (*D*) Transureteroureterostomy (TUU). For all repairs the principles include tension free, watertight, stented, spatulated, mucosa-to-mucosa anastomosis using absorbable suture with drain placement.

types of injuries can result in conversion of a partial injury to a complete injury if blind catheter placement is performed.[26]

Numerous management algorithms exist for pelvic fractures, but these vary among institutions. The central principle is early pelvic stabilization and aggressive hemodynamic support. Initially, Advanced Trauma Life Support (ATLS) protocols are followed. Signs of pelvic fracture (lacerations of the perineum, rectum, buttocks, iliac wings, and external genitalia; leg length discrepancies, gross rotational deformities of the legs, and hip asymmetry)[27] and associated injuries are sought on physical examination. Acutely, patients presenting with bladder injury may complain of inability to void or suprapubic pain, though these symptoms may be masked by pain from more significant injuries.[28] Gross hematuria is a reliable sign of bladder injury, occurring in 95% of patients[25] and in the setting of blunt or penetrating trauma should prompt evaluation using cystography, urethrography, or both. At delayed presentation, abdominal distension, ileus, fever, or urinary ascites may be present. Biochemically acidosis, hyperkalemia, hyperchloremia, hypernatremia, and uremia may be present with intraperitoneal bladder injuries. Neurologic screening and a digital rectal examination (DRE) for hematoma, bony

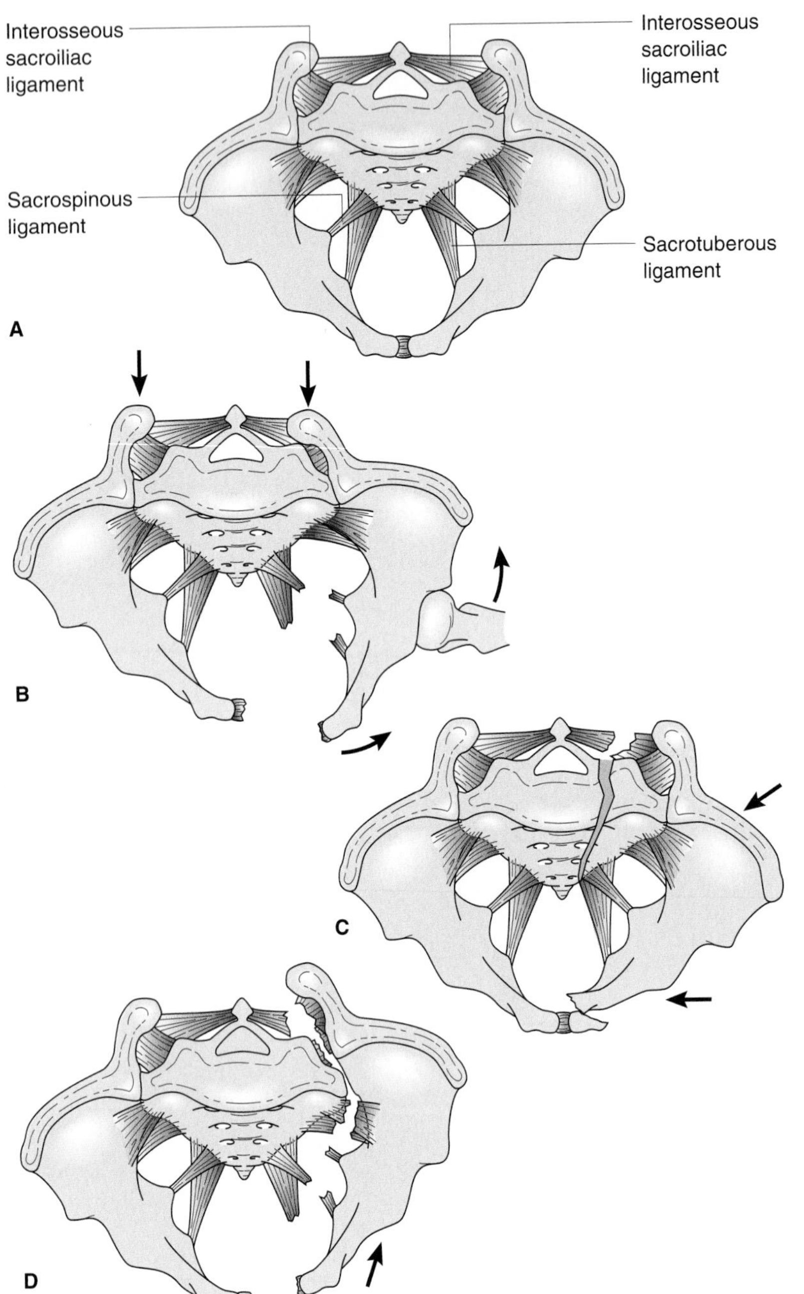

FIGURE 26.5 Pennal and Tile classification for pelvic ring injuries. (*A*) Normal pelvis. (*B*) Anteroposterior compression injury. (*C*) Lateral compression injury. (*D*) Vertical shear injury. (From Tile M. Acute pelvic fractures: I. Causation and classification. *J Am Acad Orthop Surg*. 1996;4:143–151.)

spicules, hemoccult blood, or a high-riding prostate is performed. These findings on DRE and the presence of perineal ecchymosis or scrotal hematoma suggest anterior pelvic disruption and urethral injury. Gross blood at the external urethral meatus is the most reliable sign and warrants evaluation for injury. Females with vaginal bleeding are evaluated for gynecologic as well as urethral injuries (found in 6%).[29] Applying gentle lateral pressure to the iliac wings may reveal anteroposterior (AP) rotational instability. Aggressive palpation may only worsen instability, aggravating pelvic bleeding. Early pelvic stabilization using a vacuum bean bag, large circumferential sheet, or military antishock trousers (MAST) is recommended as a temporary measure to minimize hemorrhage and has been shown to improve survival following pelvic injury.[19] These maneuvers reduce the pelvic volume, and by reapproximating displaced bone fragments, the exposed bleeding surface is minimized, achieving a tamponade effect until definitive fixation is performed.

Anteroposterior, inlet, outlet, and lateral sacral radiographic imaging is obtained acutely. Multiple classification schemes for pelvic fractures have been based on these studies (Fig. 26.5). The most commonly used is the Tile and Pennal scheme, which classifies pelvic injuries based on the vector of force.[30] Contrast-enhanced abdominopelvic CT scanning is also obtained, screening for arterial bleeding (contrast blush), concurrent intraabdominal or retroperitoneal injuries, and size and location of the pelvic hematoma.

Definitive imaging of the urethra and bladder, if indicated, is usually withheld until the patient is stable. When gross blood is present at the urethral meatus, retrograde urethrography (RUG) is indicated before catheterization.[26] RUG is easily performed using portable fluoroscopy. The fossa navicularis is occluded with the partially filled (2- to 3-mL) balloon tip of the catheter, the penis is stretched, and contrast is gently injected opacifying the urethra. Oblique images are taken to establish the absence of or the presence and location of

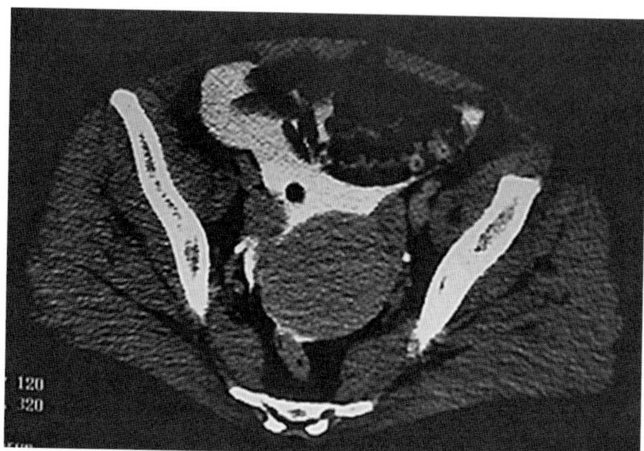

FIGURE 26.6 Computed tomography cystography for intraperitoneal bladder injury.

extravasation, which is indicative of injury. If no extravasation is present, the catheter is advanced into the bladder and cystography is performed. Static cystography traditionally has been performed and remains an acceptable means of assessing for bladder rupture. However, CT cystography is used more liberally because of the central role of CT scanning in trauma assessment. For CT cystography, retrograde filling of the bladder with contrast is begun. Scanning is performed at 300 to 400 mL of contrast. A scout image and imaging at 300 to 400 mL of retrograde filling with contrast constitutes static cystography.[31] Postdrainage films are essential for and static cystography, and oblique images may identify posterior defects. Characteristic patterns of extravasation on CT (pooling in cul-de-sac, paracolic gutter, or retrohepatic space) and on static cystography (outlining of bowel loops) will be diagnostic of intraperitoneal rupture (Fig 26.6). Extraperitoneal extravasation is confined to the pelvis on CT and appears "flame-shaped" on cystography (Fig 26.7).

In unstable patients, prioritization of pelvic versus intraabdominal hemorrhage remains a challenge (Algorithm 26.1). In the setting of pelvic trauma, the indications for laparotomy remain unchanged in the unstable patient and adjunctive studies (e.g., supraumbilical diagnostic peritoneal lavage [DPL] or FAST ultrasound) are helpful in differentiating among abdominal, pelvic, and retroperitoneal hemorrhage. In the stable patient requiring laparotomy, some centers recommend external fixation before laparotomy to avoid release of the pelvic tamponade following incision.[32] Others advocate immediate

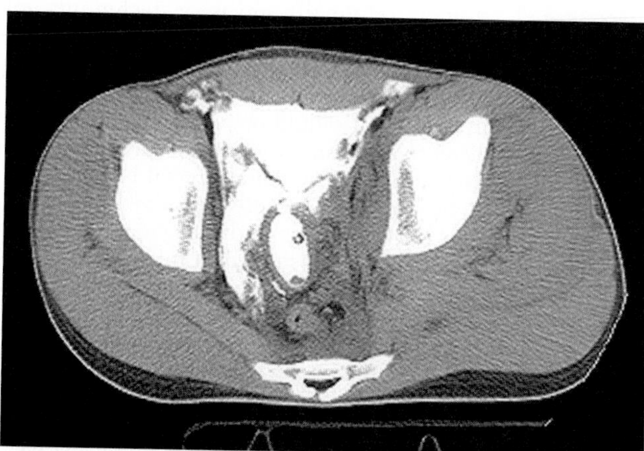

FIGURE 26.7 Computed tomography cystography for extraperitoneal bladder injury.

laparotomy followed by external fixation for individuals with indications for laparotomy at initial evaluation. In this instance, the pelvis may be packed in an effort to minimize hemorrhage. All intraperitoneal, penetrating, and selected extraperitoneal bladder injuries (e.g., concomitant vaginal or rectal injury, bladder neck injury or avulsion, foreign body, or bony spicule at site of injury, to avoid secondary contamination with internal fixation of orthopedic hardware, and stable patients undergoing laparotomy for other indications) are repaired and a suprapubic (SP) catheter is placed, if indicated (significant hematuria warranting irrigation or urethral injury). The pelvis can be primarily managed by applying an external fixating device (e.g., a C-clamp).[33] Increasingly, however, the initial approach to ongoing bleeding associated with pelvic fracture or disruption is selective angioembolization. Also, because of frequent failure of C-clamps resulting from complex combined anterior and posterior pelvic instability, definitive stabilization is preferred. Attempts at open hypogastric ligation are generally futile, and bleeding persists through rich collaterals and venous plexi. The most common source of pelvic arterial bleeding is the internal pudendal, superior gluteal, obturator, and lateral sacral arteries, which can be selectively targeted radiographically. This can also be helpful when isolated pelvic trauma with ongoing bleeding is experienced after pelvic fixation.

Definitive management of unstable pelvic fractures in stable patients can be performed urgently, but generally it is delayed until adequate resuscitation and hemostasis has occurred (usually 2 to 10 days).[34] A delay often provides an opportunity for other operative procedures to be performed (e.g., urethral realignment). Open reduction with internal fixation (ORIF), using plates and screws, is standard for anterior pelvic fractures. ORIF alone is also used for posterior sacroiliac fractures, in combination, or preferably with percutaneous sacroiliac screws alone. Use of percutaneous sacroiliac screws has greatly reduced the impact and morbidity associated with traditional ORIF approaches to posterior pelvic fractures. These decisions are based on factors such as patient age, body habitus, bone quality, injury pattern, and other clinical factors.[19] Postoperatively, patients generally receive non–weight-bearing rehabilitation initially and then full weight-bearing by 3 months. Mortality from pelvic fractures is high (secondary to associated injuries, including those of the central nervous system, and subsequent development of multiple organ failure syndrome), and long-term morbidity from permanent nerve injury, gait abnormalities, chronic pain, and associated injuries is common.[19]

Repair of bladder injury, as indicated previously and in cases of penetrating injury, is generally performed at the time of exploratory laparotomy for concomitant injuries, penetrating bladder trauma, or ORIF for pelvic fractures. Care is taken to avoid disruption of a pelvic hematoma, which may cause significant hemorrhage, although adequate reduction of concomitant pelvic injury is the most important measure to control bleeding. The ureteral orifices and bladder wall are inspected through an anterior cystotomy or the laceration itself. Sites of injury within the bladder are repaired with interrupted full-thickness absorbable sutures (e.g., 3-0 Vicryl), and a two-layer running 3-0 or 2-0 Vicryl is used to close the cystotomy and anterior lacerations. SP catheter diversion using a Malecot catheter (22 to 24 Fr) is used when irrigation for heavy bleeding is required.[35] Closed suction drains are placed away from the sites of repair and can be removed in 48 hours or when drainage is minimal. Bladder drainage is continued for 10 to 14 days, and the catheter is removed only after no leak is observed on cystography (Fig. 26.8). Complications following bladder injury are rare but include persistent leakage, pelvic urinoma or abscess formation, and voiding dysfunction in the case of bladder neck injury. Delayed exploration, repair, recon-

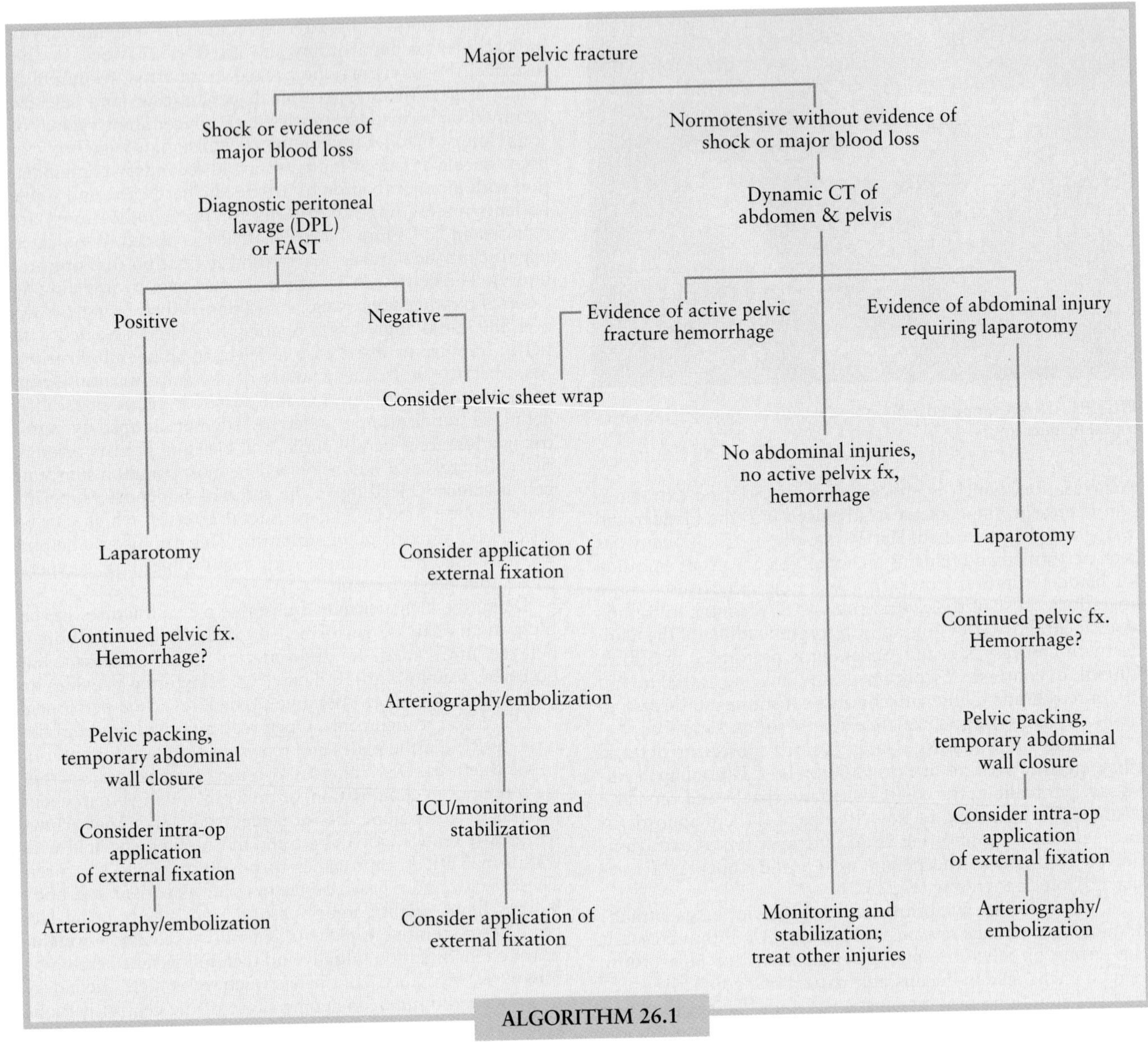

ALGORITHM 26.1

struction, or drainage may be required to remedy problems that fail to resolve with conservative measures.

Early management of most urethral injuries involves urinary diversion with an SP diverting catheter, and the decision to primarily realign or defer reconstruction is based on the type and location of the injury. Grades I and II urethral injuries are managed without a catheter, provided the patient can void. Partial anterior injuries are managed with a urethral catheter alone, and a pericatheter urethrogram is done at 7 to 10 days to confirm healing before its removal. Whereas primary débridement and closure with diversion are advocated for anterior stab wounds or low-velocity gunshot wounds (Fig 26.8), high-velocity injuries should be managed with an SP catheter and delayed reconstruction. Most posterior injuries can be managed with urinary diversion and delayed (3 to 6 months) reconstruction following resorption of the pelvic hematoma. At this time antegrade voiding cystography and RUG is performed, and definitive reconstruction is planned. Aggressive early operative reconstruction is discouraged, though minimally invasive techniques of realignment may obviate the need for future urethroplasty (53% vs. 97%).[36] Early realignment is achieved using a Seldinger technique or magnetic sounds[37] employing endoscopes and fluoroscopy and should be performed only by an experienced surgeon to avoid inadvertent infection or disruption of a pelvic hematoma. Concomitant rectal injury, placement of orthopedic hardware, severe vascular injury, and bladder neck injury are exceptions to this approach, and primary realignment should be considered to minimize complications of fistula, infection, hemorrhage, or incontinence, respectively.[38] Urethral catheters remain in place until healing is confirmed radiographically at 3 to 6 weeks, depending on the degree of injury or repair performed, and suprapubic catheters remain in place until satisfactory voiding without urethral catheter or reconstruction is achieved. Failure to execute an appropriate plan of followup for tube changes, removals, and definitive reconstructive efforts is regrettable, because significant morbidity (infection, encrustation,

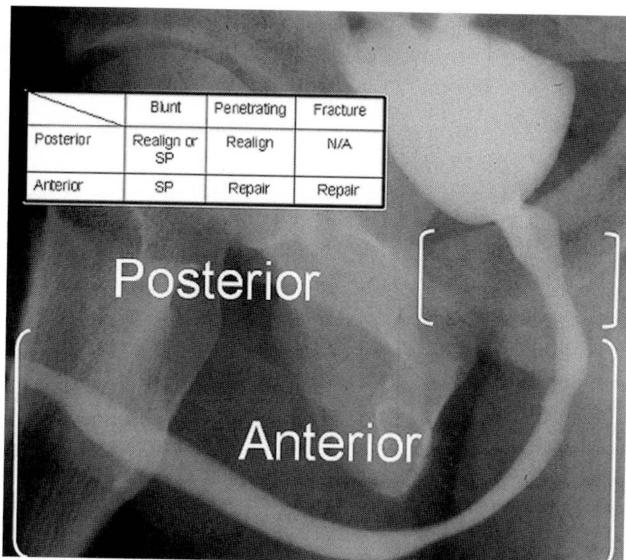

FIGURE 26.8 Normal retrograde urethrogram and management by segment and mechanism of injury.

hematuria, obstructive uropathy) can ensue. Overall, erectile dysfunction occurs in 30% to 50%; neurogenic erectile dysfunction in 20%, whereas vasculogenic impotence predominates in 80%.[39]

KEY POINTS

- **Upper urinary tract injury is rare and nearly one half of such injuries are caused by vehicular collisions.**
- **Risk of renal injury requiring further evaluation is indicated by (a) gross hematuria; (b) microscopic hematuria with an episode of systolic blood pressure less than 90 mm Hg; or (c) microscopic hematuria and physical findings or mechanism of trauma to the flank.**
- **Most renal injuries are managed nonoperatively, with indications for exploration being symptomatic renal hemorrhage, penetrating injury, expanding or pulsatile retroperitoneal hematoma at laparotomy, and grade V injury.**
- **Definitive management of unstable pelvic injuries can be done urgently but should be delayed until adequate resuscitation and hemostasis are achieved.**
- **For pelvic injuries, the vector of the impact determines the injury type and the subsequent risk of visceral injury.**
- **Pelvic fractures should undergo definitive early stabilization using ORIF plates and screws anteriorly and ORIF, preferably with percutaneous sacroiliac screws, posteriorly.**
- **In the unstable patient, DPL or FAST should be used to assess potential intraabdominal blood loss to plan timing of angiographic evaluation and embolization of associated pelvic fracture bleeding.**
- **Injuries to the bladder and urethra require prompt diagnosis, and early management of urethral injuries involves urinary diversion with an SP tube. Primary reconstruction of posterior urethral injuries secondary to pelvic fracture is discouraged, and primary realignment should be undertaken only by a surgeon experienced with this technique.**

References

1. **Bretan PN, McAninch JW, Federle MP, et al. Computerized tomographic staging of renal trauma: 85 consecutive cases. *J Urol.* 1986;136:561.**
2. Boone TB, Gilling PJ, Jusmann DA. Ureteropelvic junction disruption following blunt abdominal trauma. *J Urol.* 1993;150:33.
3. Krieger JN, Algood CB, Mason JT. Urologic trauma in the Pacific Northwest: etiology, distribution, management, and outcome. *J Urol.* 1984;132:70-73.
4. Herschorn S, Radomski SB, Shoskes DA, et al. Evaluation and treatment of blunt renal trauma. *J Urol.* 1991;146:274–277.
5. Miller KS, McAninch JW. Radiographic assessment of renal trauma: our 15-year experience. *J Urol.* 1995;154:352–355.
6. Baverstock R, Simons R, McLoughlin M. Severe blunt renal trauma: a 7-year retrospective review from a provincial trauma center. *Can J Urol.* 2001;8:1372–1376.
7. **Wessells H, Suh D, Porter JR, et al. Renal injury and operative management in the United States: results of a population-based study. *J Trauma* 2003;54:423–430.**
8. Bright TC, White K, Peters PC. Significance of hematuria after trauma. *J Urol.* 1978;120:145.
9. **Miller KS, McAninch JW. Radiographic assessment of renal trauma: our 15 year experience. *J Urol.* 1995;154:352.**
10. Pollack HM. Renal trauma: imaging and intervention. *Problems in Urology* 1994;8:199.
11. McAninch JW, Carroll PR, Klosterman PW, et al. Renal reconstruction after injury. *J Urol.* 1991;145:932.
12. Morey AF, McAninch JW, Tiller BK, et al. Single shot intraoperative excretory urography for the immediate evaluation of renal trauma. *J Urol.* 1999;161:1088–1092.
13. McGahan JP, Richards JR, Jones CD, et al. Use of ultrasonography in the patient with acute renal trauma. *J Ultrasound Med.* 1999;18:207–216.
14. **Husmann DA, Gilling PJ, Perry MO, et al. Major renal lacerations with a devitalized fragment following blunt abdominal trauma: comparison between nonoperative (expectant) versus surgical management. *J Urol.* 1993;150:1774.**
15. Corriere JN Jr, McAndrew JD, Benson GS. Intraoperative decision-making in renal trauma. *J Trauma* 1991;31:1390.
16. Elliott SP, McAninch JW. Ureteral injuries from external violence: the 25-year experience at San Francisco General Hospital. *J Urol.* 2003;170(4 Pt 1): 1213–1216.
17. Blankenship JC, Gavant ML, Cox CE, et al. Importance of delayed imaging for blunt renal trauma. *World J Surg.* 2001;25:1561–1564.
18. **Kregor PJ, Routt MLC Jr. Unstable pelvic ring disruptions in unstable patients. *Injury* 1999;30(suppl 2):B19–28.**
19. Tile M. Classification. In: Tile M, ed. *Fractures of the Pelvis and Acetabulum.* Baltimore: Williams & Williams, 1984:66–101.
20. Tile M. Pelvic ring fractures: should they be fixed? *J Bone Joint Surg Br.* 1988;70:1.
21. **Dalal SA, Burgess AR, Siegel JH, et al. Pelvic fracture in multiple trauma: classification by mechanism is key to pattern of organ injury, resuscitative requirements, and outcome. *J Trauma* 1989;16:283.**
22. Freid FA, Rutledge R. A statewide population-based analysis of the frequency and outcome of genitourinary injury in a series of 215,220 trauma patients. *J Urol.* 1995;153:314A.
23. Corriere JN Jr, Sandler CM. Management of the ruptured bladder: seven years of experience with 111 cases. *J Trauma* 1986;26:830.
24. Cass AS, Gleich P, Smith C. Simultaneous bladder and prostatomembranous urethral rupture from external trauma. *J Urol.* 1984;132:907–908.
25. **Sandler CM, Corriere JN Jr. Urethrography in the diagnosis of acute urethral injuries. *Urol Clin North Am.* 1989;16:283.**
26. Brandes S, Borrelli J. Pelvic fracture and associated urologic injuries. *World J Surg.* 2001;25:1578–1587.
27. Peters PC. Intraperitoneal rupture of the bladder. *Urol Clin North Am.* 1989;16:279.
28. Perry MO, Husmann DA. Urethral injuries in female subjects following pelvic fractures. *J Urol.* 1992;147:139.
29. **Tile M. Pennal GF. Pelvic disruption: principles of management. *Clin Orthop.* 1980;51:56.**
30. Deck AJ, Shaves S, Talner L, et al. Computerized tomography cystography for the diagnosis of traumatic bladder rupture. *J Urol.* 2000;164:43.
31. Taffet R. Management of pelvic fractures with concomitant urologic injuries. *Orthop Clin North Am.* 1997;28:389.
32. Riemer BL, Butterfield SL, Diamond DL, et al. Acute mortality associated with injuries to the pelvic ring: the role of early patient mobilization and external fixation. *J Trauma* 1993;35:671.
33. Browner BD,, Cole JD, Graham JM, et al. Delayed posterior internal fixation of unstable pelvic fractures. *J Trauma* 1987;27:998.
34. Parry NG, Rozycki GS, Feliciano, et al. Traumatic rupture of the urinary bladder: is the suprapubic tube necessary? *J Trauma* 2003;54(3): 431–436.
35. Patterson BM. Pelvic ring injury and associated urologic trauma: an orthopedic perspective. *Semin Urol.* 1995;13:25.
36. **Porter JR, Takayama TK, Defalco AJ. Traumatic posterior urethral injury and early realignment using magnetic urethral catheters. *J Urol.* 1997;158:425.**
37. Webster GD. Perineal repair of membranous urethral stricture. *Urol Clin North Am.* 1989;16:303.
38. Armenakas NA, McAninch JW, Lue TF, et al. Posttraumatic impotence: magnetic resonance imaging and duplex ultrasound in diagnosis and management. *J Urol.* 1993;149:1272.

CHAPTER 27 ■ VASCULAR TRAUMA

MICHAEL J. SISE AND STEVEN R. SHACKFORD

Vascular injuries have become increasingly common because of the epidemic of urban violence and the increasingly common use of endoluminal vascular procedures for diagnosis and therapy. Improved prehospital care and rapid transport have also contributed to the increased prevalence of vascular injuries by delivering patients with previously fatal injuries to the hospital in a timely fashion. Early diagnosis and successful management require a thorough examination with a focus on both the mechanism and location of injury, an efficient use of diagnostic modalities, and a timely application of an evidence-based approach to management.

EPIDEMIOLOGY

In urban environments, vascular trauma is usually penetrating, mostly caused by gunshot wounds, and typically affects men between the ages of 20 and 40.[1] In rural environments, vascular injury is usually blunt, caused by motor vehicle crash, and white males predominate. However, a higher proportion of females in rural areas receive such injuries than in urban centers.[2]

Endovascular therapies have increased the number of iatrogenic injuries, which now account for about one third of the vascular trauma seen in many centers. Iatrogenic vascular injury is usually the result of catheter-site occlusive complications in the femoral, axillary, and brachial arteries. Less common, but more morbid, are perforations of more proximal vessels that occur during the passage of large endovascular device delivery catheters.[3] This population is usually in the seventh, eighth, and ninth decades of life and has significant multiple comorbidities.

PATHOPHYSIOLOGY

The principal physiologic consequences of vascular injury result from either hemorrhage or inadequate perfusion distal to an arterial injury. Great vessel injury in the chest or abdomen is more likely to result in the former, whereas arterial injury of the limb is usually associated with the latter. Extremity trauma, however, can produce life-threatening hypovolemia when it is not tamponaded or controlled or when it is combined with other injuries.

Local consequences of vascular injuries are usually related to acute arterial occlusion from thrombosis after injury. This results in ischemia distal to the injury site and can lead to limb or organ loss. The degree of tissue loss is related to the adequacy of collateral flow, the sensitivity of the distal tissue to ischemia, and the delay involved in repairing the injury and restoring blood flow. The variability in these factors is great. The brain is most sensitive to ischemia because of high basal energy requirements and the absence of glycogen stores. Brain ischemia lasting longer than 4 minutes results in irreversible injury. Peripheral nerves and muscles can tolerate ischemia for up to 4 hours without permanent damage. An important principle of vascular repairs, however, is that outcome is time-dependent, necessitating a sense of urgency in management.

Protracted arterial ischemia produces anoxic cell death. The restoration of arterial flow after complete ischemia often results in a reperfusion injury that is mediated by oxygen-free radicals.[4] The free radicals initiate lipid peroxidation, which injures the microvascular endothelium, resulting in interstitial edema formation and increased interstitial fluid pressure. The increased interstitial pressure compresses capillaries and venules, ultimately leading to vascular stasis and a "no reflow" phenomenon. The increased interstitial pressure, venous congestion, and lack of capillary flow leads to ischemia of nerves, initially, and muscle, subsequently, resulting in a compartment syndrome. If untreated, compartment syndrome will lead to rhabdomyolysis and the release of potassium and myoglobin into the systemic circulation. Acidosis, hyperkalemia, and myoglobin-induced renal failure can occur as a result. Beyond the immediate threat of limb loss, the systemic effects of muscle necrosis can ultimately prove fatal.

Simple lacerations are the most common penetrating injuries to both arteries and veins. Incomplete lacerations often cause more hemorrhage than complete transections because partially transected vessels cannot retract and vasoconstrict as they would if completely transected. Blunt trauma can produce complete or partial disruption of the vessel wall. As the arterial wall is deformed, the elastic adventitia and muscular layers remain intact, whereas the intima fractures. Blood dissects beneath the fractured intima, which prolapses into the lumen and obstructs the artery, leading to thrombosis. Partial disruption of the vascular wall that leaves the adventitia intact will result in an acute pseudoaneurysm, which has the potential to rupture during the acute phase of care.

The increasing incidence of high-velocity wounds in the setting of urban violence has led to the appearance of "shock-wave" vessel injuries. The high-velocity projectile produces a shock wave that displaces tissues in a 90-degree direction away from the path of the bullet. A temporary cavity is created that significantly distorts adjacent tissue several centimeters away from the bullet tract. The shock wave can stretch and disrupt blood vessels and create intimal tears with localized dissection, thrombosis, or embolization. Although these injuries are usually immediately apparent, partial intimal disruption can lead to delayed thrombosis or embolization.

DIAGNOSIS

Vascular trauma may be immediately apparent on initial presentation or remain occult. The timely diagnosis of vascular injury requires a high index of suspicion, a rapid and thorough history and physical examination supplemented by Doppler pressure measurements when indicated, and the thoughtful and selective application of radiographic imaging. Although the assessment of blood loss during the prehospital phase of care is frequently unreliable, a history of pulsatile arterial bleeding or a large amount of hemorrhage surrounding the site of penetrating injury strongly suggests vascular injury. High-velocity crash victims and those who fall from

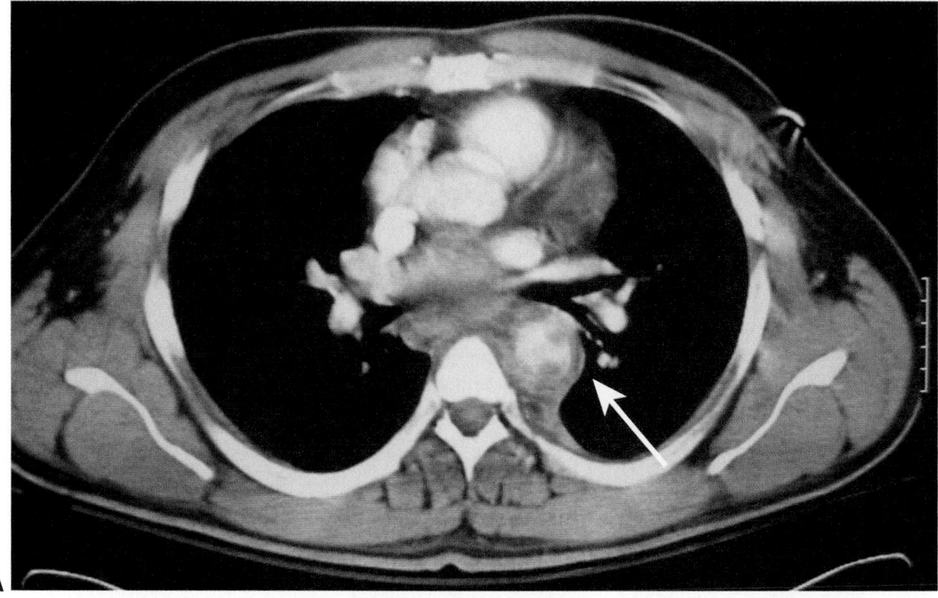

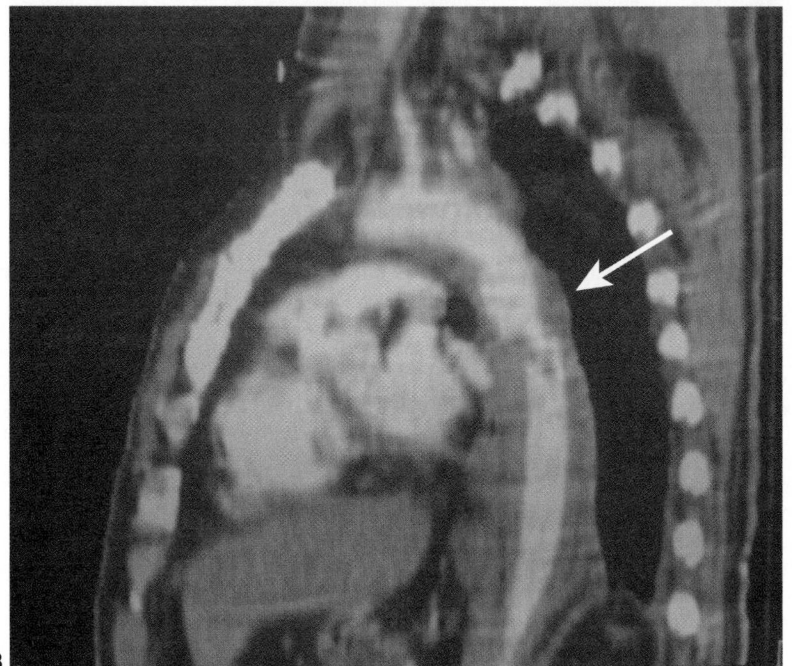

FIGURE 27.1 (*A*) Spiral computed tomography cross-sectional image of traumatic aortic aneurysm (*arrow*). (*B*) Aortic injury in left anterior-oblique view (*arrow*).

significant heights must be assumed to be at risk for vascular injury until proved otherwise.

Intraabdominal or intrathoracic vascular injuries should be suspected in hypotensive victims of penetrating injuries of the torso. Blunt aortic and great vessel injury in the chest should be considered whenever there is external evidence of major thoracic trauma or a history of rapid deceleration. The injuries that should raise the index of suspicion of associated aortic injury include sternal fracture, flail chest, thoracic spine fracture, and first-rib fracture. Physical findings associated with intrathoracic vascular trauma include differential arm blood pressures or differential arm-to-lower-extremity blood pressures. Chest radiographic study, although not definitive, may be used as a screening tool. A widened mediastinum (more than 8 cm on an anterior-posterior exposure), loss of normal aortic contour, and thoracic outlet hematoma suggest aortic injury.[5] Spiral computed tomographic (CT) angiography of the chest is also effective in the diagnosis of aortic injury and has results similar to catheter angiography with high rates of accuracy[6] (Fig. 27.1).

Limb ischemia produces the classic physical findings ("hard signs") of pain, pallor, pulse deficit, paresthesia, and diminished perfusion. Partial occlusions produce lesser signs and symptoms and are, therefore, more likely to be missed. The course of a penetrating injury should be estimated, both visually and radiographically, using plain films with radiopaque markers for entrance and exit wounds. Segmental arterial pressure determination using a continuous wave Doppler device is a valuable adjunct in the detection of arterial injury of an extremity. This is accomplished by placing the probe over the selected artery in the foot or at the wrist

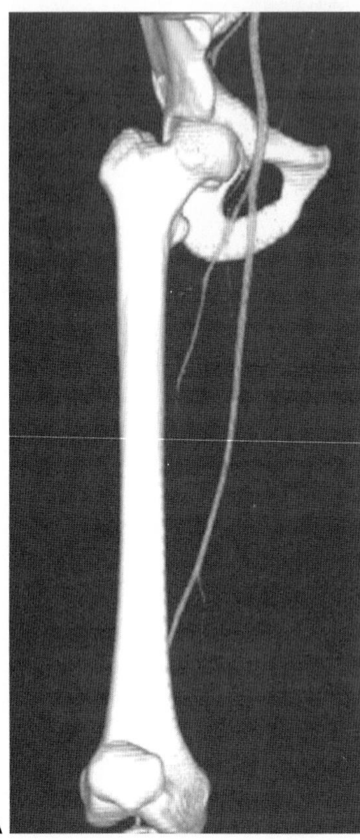

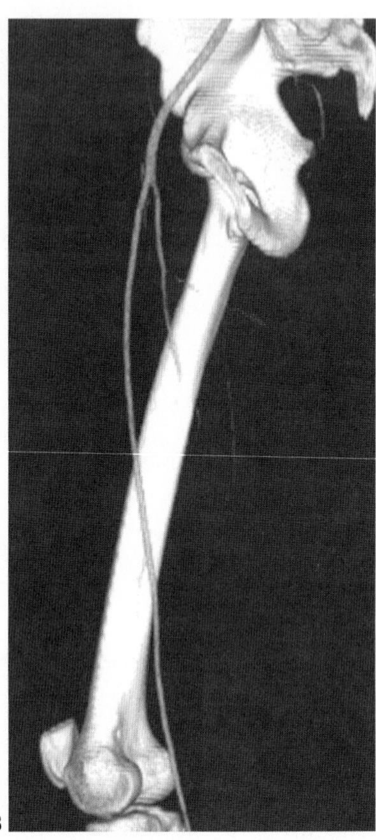

FIGURE 27.2 Three-dimensional spiral computed tomography reconstruction anteroposterior (*A*) and medial (*B*) views of the femoral artery in a patient with penetrating thigh injury.

and slowly inflating the blood pressure cuff at the ankle or the forearm. The pressure at which Doppler signals cease indicates the perfusion pressure at the level of the blood pressure cuff. This pressure should be compared with the other extremity in upper extremity evaluation or with the highest upper extremity pressure in lower extremity evaluation. In a healthy person, the ankle/brachial index is 1.1. A ratio of less than 0.9 or a 20-mm difference between extremities should arouse suspicion of significant arterial trauma. In hypovolemic patients, both lower extremity ankle/brachial indices may be diminished to as low as 0.75. Reevaluation after resuscitation is essential if both lower extremity indices are similarly diminished. It is important to note that the presence of audible Doppler signals over an artery in the extremity does not rule out an arterial injury or indicate adequate perfusion.

Some patients need operative intervention simultaneously with diagnosis. These patients are identified early in the acute phase of care by being hemodynamically unstable from cavitary or extremity hemorrhage or by having an advanced ischemia of an extremity (i.e., they manifest the "hard signs"). Many preventable deaths following vascular trauma result from inappropriate delays to obtain diagnostic studies.

High-speed, multidetector spiral CT scanning is useful in the timely diagnosis of vascular trauma caused by blunt force injury. Although catheter-based contrast arteriography is currently the gold standard for vascular imaging, spiral CT is less invasive and faster and has fewer complications. Three-dimensional reconstructions rapidly provide a high degree of anatomic definition (Fig. 27.2).

Multiarray spiral CT angiography is extremely effective in screening victims of deceleration injury for major vessel injury in the chest and abdomen. Four- and sixteen-array scanners provide equally accurate results compared with traditional catheter angiography in the diagnosis of thoracic aortic injury. Its effectiveness in the diagnosis of arch vessel and abdominal great vessel injury, however, has yet to be proved. Sixteen-array and the soon to be available 64-array CT scanners provide two- and three-dimensional anatomic reconstruction views that are exceptionally clear in their detail and provide rapid, accurate visualization of torso and extremity vessels.

Arteriography is not indicated for patients with hard signs but should be considered for patients suspected by history and physical examination of being at high risk for vascular trauma. Ample evidence shows that physical examination and the ankle/brachial or wrist/brachial index are reliable indicators of the need for angiography in patients with penetrating extremity trauma and has suggested limiting its use to only those patients without hard signs and a pulse deficit or an index of less than 1.0.[7,8] Formal arteriography, using the Seldinger technique or high-definition spiral CT angiography, is preferred in stable patients. In unstable patients with other major injuries and suspected occult extremity arterial trauma, arteriography can be performed in the emergency department or on the operating table. In these cases, a rapid bolus injection of sufficient contrast material without inflow occlusion is sufficient to produce adequate visualization of extremity vessels.

The appropriate use of arteriography can significantly reduce the rate of negative exploration for suspected vascular trauma. Arteriography has a sensitivity and specificity of 97% to 100% and an overall accuracy of 92% to 98% in vascular trauma. It has a minor complication rate of 2% to 4% (i.e., hematoma at the access site) and a major complication rate of 0.6% (i.e., embolus, arterial injury, or frank thrombosis).

NONOPERATIVE MANAGEMENT

The aggressive application of arteriography for suspected occult vascular trauma results in the detection of clinically insignificant lesions that can be treated nonoperatively. These include intimal irregularity, focal spasm with minimal narrowing, and small pseudoaneurysms. Ongoing surveillance for subsequent occlusion or hemorrhage is mandatory. Operative therapy is indicated for thrombosis, for chronic symptoms of occlusive disease, and for failure of small pseudoaneurysms to undergo thrombosis. Nonoperative therapy may also be indicated for clinically insignificant lesions in patients with multiple injuries for whom vascular repair would present a prohibitive risk. Dennis et al. have demonstrated that nonoperative therapy with appropriate follow-up is highly successful in patients with penetrating injuries of the extremity.[7]

ENDOVASCULAR MANAGEMENT

Effective endovascular treatment of vascular injuries requires special training and expertise by either interventional radiologists or vascular surgeons. Collaboration between these specialties and the trauma surgeon is necessary to optimize patient selection and management. Planning for endovascular treatment should include the option to perform a more traditional open operative approach as soon as possible, should the endovascular attempt fail. Many centers have operating rooms equipped to function as interventional radiology suites to deal efficiently with this occurrence.

The indications for endovascular treatment include the following: (a) branch vessel hemorrhage, which may be occluded without producing significant ischemia; (b) acute pseudoaneurysm without active hemorrhage; (c) intimal flap without significant underlying thrombosis, and (d) acute arteriovenous fistula. Complete arterial disruption or thrombosis, particularly in the presence of multiple other injuries, is not appropriate for endovascular management. Endovascular placement of stent grafts for vascular trauma in certain settings can be both safe and effective.[9,10,16,17] Increasing numbers of centers are using these stent grafts in both blunt and penetrating vascular injures, but the accumulated experience and the long-term follow-up of treated patients remains small (Fig. 27.3).

Endovascular embolization is particularly effective in branch vessel hemorrhage. A pelvic fracture with hemorrhage from the hypogastric artery responds well to this technique. Extremity trauma with significant hemorrhage from branch vessels can also be successfully managed by embolization. Coils may be placed with thrombotic protein foam material. Biologic glues have also been used effectively. Balloon catheter occlusion of the underlying artery distal to branch vessels is an important adjunct and is frequently effective in preventing distal embolization.

ULTRASOUND-GUIDED THERAPY

Pseudoaneurysms of the extremity arteries, particularly those that are iatrogenic, can be successfully treated with ultrasound-directed thrombin injection (0.5 to 1.0 mL containing 1,000 (μ/mL). Color flow imaging is necessary to differentiate

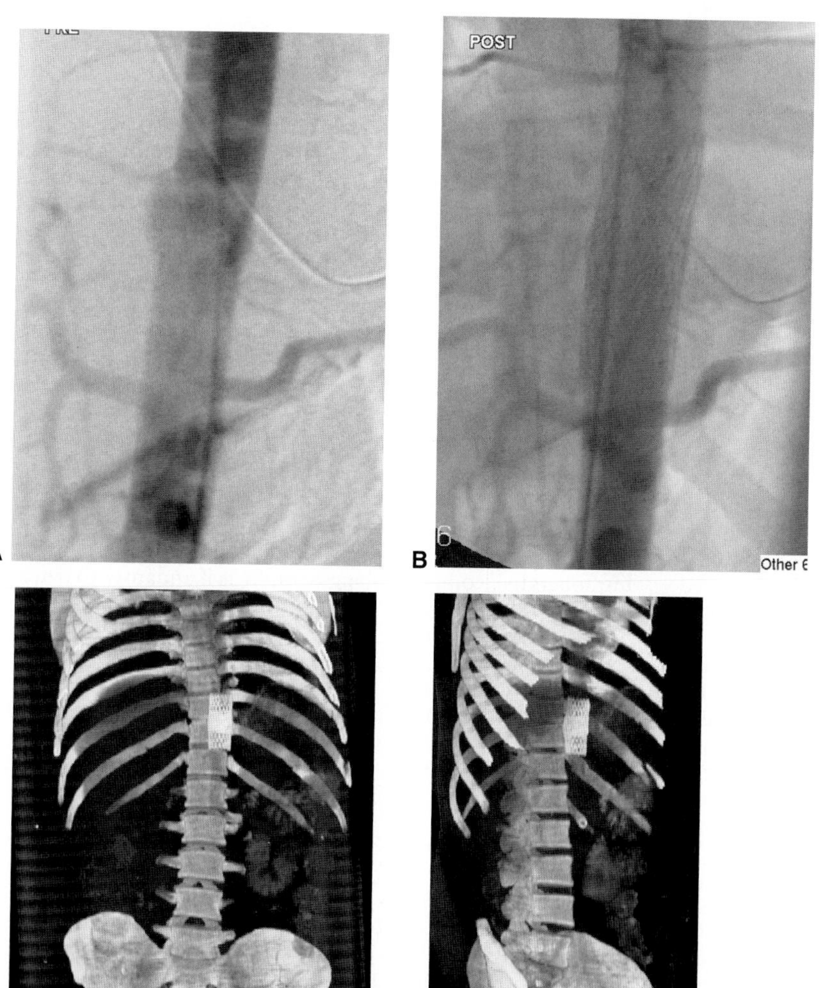

FIGURE 27.3 Distal thoracic aortic pseudoaneurysm (*A*) managed with two overlapping aortic stents (*B*). (*C* and *D*) Three-dimensional spiral computed tomography scans demonstrate stent placement.

a hematoma from a pseudoaneurysm, to assist in guiding the injection needle into the pseudoaneurysm and to ensure that thrombosis of the pseudoaneurysm has occurred. The procedure requires little time and is superior to ultrasound-guided compression. Thrombin injection has a success rate of 97% and a complication rate of less than 1% and is durable on long-term follow-up.[11,12]

OPERATIVE MANAGEMENT

Preoperative Care

The guiding principle in the management of vascular trauma is "life over limb." As such, initial attention should be directed to restoring and maintaining blood volume. External bleeding should be controlled by direct pressure. Blind clamp placement into hemorrhaging wounds is unsafe because visualization is always poor and clamping may cause injury to adjacent structures. Tourniquets may be necessary to control hemorrhage if the injury is extensive. Remember that tourniquets occlude collateral vessels, making distal ischemia worse. Improperly applied tourniquets allow arterial inflow, occlude venous outflow, and increase bleeding.

In the setting of multiple injuries, the management of vascular injuries must be orchestrated with the overall care of the patient's other injuries. Although life-threatening cranial, abdominal, or thoracic injuries take priority over limb-threatening arterial injuries, preoperative planning should allow for simultaneous vascular repairs using a second operating team. Preoperative consultations with orthopedists and plastic surgeons should be sought for complex injuries involving bone and soft tissue.

Prophylactic intravenous antibiotics should be administered as preparations for surgery are being made and tetanus prophylaxis added if there is a penetrating wound. In a patient with an isolated extremity vascular injury with arterial occlusion, intravenous heparin should be administered to avoid propagation of thrombus in the injured vessel. Heparin has been shown to limit ischemia-reperfusion injury and to reduce the volume of myonecrosis in an experimental model of extremity ischemia.[12,13] However, heparin is inappropriate in multiply injured patients, especially those with central nervous system trauma.

Intraoperative Care

A wide sterile field should be prepared to allow for adequate exposure. An uninjured leg should be prepared as a potential site for saphenous vein harvest. For patients with suspected major vessel injury of the neck or abdomen, the chest should be prepared to allow access to the aorta and its branches.

For combined skeletal and vascular trauma of the extremity, reperfusion of the ischemic limb is the first priority. This can be done by performing a formal vascular repair or inserting a temporary intraluminal shunt (see later) and then allowing the orthopedic surgeon to proceed with stabilization.[14] During the orthopedic procedure the vascular surgeon should remain in attendance to ensure that skeletal fixators do not obstruct the arterial repair or dislodge the temporary shunt. A few patients will present with a mangled extremity in which there is vascular injury associated with extensive soft tissue trauma, neurologic deficit, and complex fractures. Usually, there is little hope for functional recovery, and careful consideration should be given to primary amputation. An objective scoring system has been developed to aid decision making when the surgeon is presented with this difficult problem.[15] However, any system should be used only as a general guide, and ultimately the decision to primarily amputate or reconstruct must be made in consultation with orthopedic and reconstructive surgical colleagues and should consider the patient's overall status. Complex reconstruction to save a limb should not be undertaken in patients whose lives are threatened by other injuries that make them physiologically and metabolically unstable. Further, patients with lower extremities at high risk for amputation who undergo reconstruction have similar functional outcomes at 2 years to those who undergo amputation.[16]

Vascular reconstruction for trauma should be performed with sedulous attention to proper technique. The use of fine monofilament sutures on the appropriately sized needles, vascular instruments, coaxial lighting, and loupe magnification are all appropriate. For the best outcome, surgeons unfamiliar with techniques of vascular reconstruction should obtain assistance from experienced colleagues.

The initial technical step is to obtain proximal and distal control of the injured vessel. This is most easily accomplished through uninjured areas adjacent to the injury, using incisions normally used for elective exposure of these vessels. Direct approach through the site of injury is fraught with the hazards of severe hemorrhage and iatrogenic trauma to the vessel itself or to adjacent nerves. Balloon-tipped catheters can be valuable in obtaining proximal and distal control when they are inserted carefully through the site of injury and inflated. Subsequent dissection then establishes proximal and distal control.

After control has been established, gentle catheter thrombectomy of the proximal and distal arteries is repeated until no evidence of thrombus remains. Heparinized saline (10 IU/mL) is then flushed proximally and distally into the lumen of the artery.

The technique for arterial repair should not be selected until the entire extent of the injury is known and the injured vessel has been débrided. The extent of arterial injury is inevitably greater than appreciated at first inspection. After adequate débridement of the injured vessel, end-to-end anastomosis without tension may not be possible and interposition grafting is often required. Reversed saphenous vein from an uninjured lower extremity is the first choice for conduit. Polytetrafluoroethylene (PTFE) grafts are occasionally indicated in large vessel injuries because a vein is either unavailable or of inadequate size. Although PTFE grafts have been used with success in the iliac and common femoral arteries at many centers,[17] saphenous vein remains the primary choice for interposition grafting, particularly for vessels below the axilla and groin crease. Anastomoses should be spatulated to avoid stenosis, and care must be taken to avoid either kinking from a redundant graft or stretching from undue tension. Intraoperative completion angiography is mandatory to determine the adequacy of repair, confirm patency, and visualize the distal arterial runoff.

The repair of concomitant venous injuries is controversial. Repair is recommended in the stable patient. Techniques of repair vary from simple suture closure to saphenous vein patch or graft interposition. Although most complex repairs will undergo thrombosis within several days, many recanalize. In the unstable patient, ligation should be performed to expedite the operation.

The use of intraluminal shunts provides a valuable adjunct for patients in need of complex arterial reconstructive procedures.[17] Standard shunts used in elective carotid operation or intravenous tubing cut to fit the defect function well in the early restoration of both arterial and venous flow if extensive grafting or limb reimplantation is required. Limb ischemia time is significantly reduced when shunts are used properly. Interposition grafting can be performed by placing the interposition graft over the shunt. Shunts effectively restore flow to injured extremities in patients who are too unstable initially to undergo completion of peripheral arterial repair. Shunts have been left in place for extended periods with ultimate salvage of the extremity.[17]

Extraanatomic bypass plays a limited but important role in arterial trauma. Penetrating abdominal trauma with aortic or iliac artery disruption associated with extensive bowel injury and contamination by enteric contents can make *in situ* arterial repair highly susceptible to infection and disruption. In this situation, arterial ligation and extraanatomic bypass through the axillofemoral or femorofemoral route may be the only acceptable means to restore distal perfusion. The long-term patency rate of such grafts may be inferior to *in situ* reconstruction, but they do provide a means to maintain perfusion and avoid life-threatening complications.

The development of an extremity compartment syndrome following reperfusion is a devastating complication after arterial trauma. The syndrome is uncommon in the thigh and forearm and is most often seen in the calf. Because of the grave consequences of compartment syndrome, many trauma surgeons perform four-compartment fasciotomy whenever there is extensive soft tissue injury or skeletal trauma in the lower leg combined with vascular trauma or the history of prolonged ischemia (Fig. 27.4). In any patient with lower extremity trauma who exhibits signs of pain or distal ischemia, the compartment pressure should be measured and fasciotomy performed as needed. Controversy exists regarding the degree of compartment pressure elevation that should necessitate fasciotomy; a pressure greater than 30 mm Hg is abnormal and requires repetitive measurement or fasciotomy, whereas a pressure greater than 45 mm Hg, or a gradient of less than 30 mm Hg between the compartment pressure and the diastolic blood pressure, mandates fasciotomy. In general, factors suggesting the need for fasciotomy are prolonged ischemia (>6 hours), associated crush injury, preoperative swelling, combined arterial and venous injuries, major venous ligation, loss of sensation or motor function, severe pain on active or passive motion, and elevated compartment pressure.

Proper management of contamination is essential to successful limb salvage after vascular trauma. Aggressive wound débridement and pulse irrigation with copious antibiotic solution should be performed routinely. Coverage of the vascular repair with viable muscle or fascia and subcutaneous tissue is necessary to prevent desiccation and infection. Such coverage may require the use of rotation flaps or free tissue transfer; if so, the assistance of a plastic and reconstructive surgeon is essential.

Postoperative Care

The use of low-molecular-weight dextran can prevent early thrombosis and improve microvascular circulation in patients with prolonged ischemia. Dextran 40 at 40 to

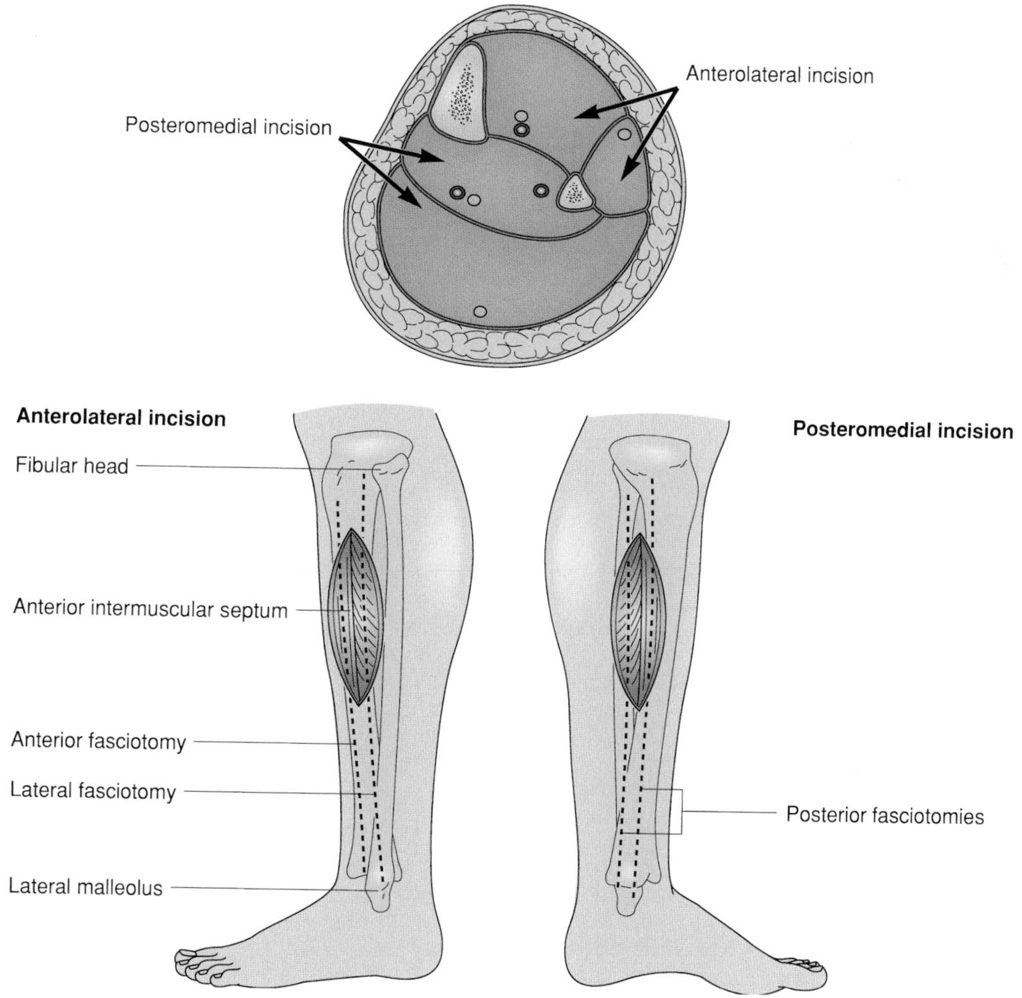

FIGURE 27.4 Surgical approach for four compartment fasciotomies through incisions on the medial and lateral aspects of the calf.

TABLE 27.1

COMPARISON OF VASCULAR INJURIES FROM THE VIETNAM EXPERIENCE WITH TWO MODERN URBAN EXPERIENCES

Site	Vietnam	Houston	San Diego	Total
Neck	50 (5%)	17 (8%)	53 (8%)	120 (6%)
Chest	11 (1%)	40 (18%)	194 (29%)	245 (13%)
Abdomen	29 (3%)	41 (18%)	154 (23%)	197 (11%)
Upper extremity	342 (34%)	64 (29%)	102 (16%)	508 (28%)
Lower extremity	568 (57%)	59 (27%)	161 (24%)	788 (42%)
Total	1,000	221	664	1,858

50 mL/hour for 24 hours does not cause significant bleeding complications and may maintain the patency of arterial reconstructions, especially in small arteries. The routine use of a postoperative heparin infusion, however, significantly increases the incidence of wound hematoma. Heparin should be reserved for patients with documented thrombotic complications or hypercoagulable states. Vasodilators are of limited value in the perioperative management of vascular injuries.

The immediate challenges after operation are restoration of adequate intravascular volume and rewarming of the patient. Evaluation of distal circulation is difficult until the patient is normovolemic and normothermic. In the early postoperative period, palpable pulses are frequently absent and pressure indices or ratios are decreased, despite a patent repair; however, audible Doppler signals should be present over the distal arteries. Normal pulses may not return for several hours after reconstruction. Early reoperation should be performed if Doppler signals become inaudible or if initially palpable pulses become nonpalpable. The salvage rate for reoperation after initially successful reconstruction is more than 90% if performed in a timely fashion. Delay in reoperation dooms the reconstruction to almost certain failure.

COMPLICATIONS

Early thrombosis of the vascular reconstruction is the most immediate potential postoperative complication. Careful surveillance, as outlined previously, allows for prompt recognition and reoperation. Significant swelling in the early postoperative period suggests venous thrombosis. A duplex scan should be obtained to confirm the presence of venous thrombus. If the popliteal or more proximal veins are involved, heparin should be started and continued until the patient has been therapeutically anticoagulated with warfarin.

Infection of a vascular reconstruction is a devastating complication. Disruption of the suture line and hemorrhage frequently follow. Suture repair of the disrupted anastomosis is doomed to failure. The safest course is ligation of the artery in an area free of infection, combined with extraanatomic bypass in uninvolved tissue to restore the distal perfusion. If possible, the bypass should be performed first to avoid any protracted ischemia.

Late complications include stenosis or occlusion of the arterial repair, aneurysmal changes in vein grafts, and postthrombotic syndrome after venous thrombosis or ligation. Arteriovenous fistulas may manifest many years after vascular trauma as pain, leg swelling caused by venous insufficiency, or arterial insufficiency. These usually are caused by missed injuries. All patients who require surgical treatment of vascular trauma should be monitored regularly on a long-term basis because of the potential for late complications.

MANAGEMENT OF SPECIFIC VASCULAR INJURIES

Most patients presenting to trauma centers with penetrating vascular trauma have injuries of the extremities. Penetrating injuries of the head, neck, chest, and abdomen are often immediately fatal. In contrast to the military experience, in which many of the wounds are from high-velocity missiles, civilians' penetrating injuries tend to result from low-velocity weapons. As a result, more patients with torso, head, and neck injuries survive to reach the hospital. Table 27.1 compares the civilian experience with the military experience with regard to the distribution of vascular injuries. The increased use of body armor by the military has led to significantly fewer deaths from torso wounds. Most military vascular injuries occur in the lower extremity and are inflicted by antipersonnel weapons. In contrast, civilian trauma more frequently involves the upper extremity.

Injury to the Thoracic Great Vessels

Both penetrating and blunt injuries of the great vessels in the chest are predictably life threatening because of the associated hemorrhage and the high frequency of concomitant injury to major adjacent structures.[17] Because these injuries are discussed in the broader context elsewhere, focus here is on the management of injuries to the aorta and its main branches.

Penetrating injuries of the great vessels usually are associated with hemothorax and evidence of hypovolemia. Tube thoracostomy reveals severe ongoing hemorrhage and requires either emergency department thoracotomy or an urgent transfer to the operating room. In patients with penetrating trauma who remain stable and who do not have significant ongoing hemorrhage after tube thoracostomy, a number of signs suggest the need for spiral CT or arteriography to rule out great vessel injury. These include missile emboli to peripheral vessels, the presence of missiles or missile trajectories in proximity to great vessels, and a mediastinal hematoma on chest radiograph. Significant active hemorrhage may well preclude any maneuver other than immediate thoracotomy.

Penetrating wounds to the ascending aorta, innominate artery, and right subclavian artery are best approached by a median sternotomy. Extrathoracic extensions may be necessary to obtain proximal and distal vascular control. The approach to a penetrating wound of the innominate vein and left common carotid artery is shown in Figures 27.5 and 27.6. In general,

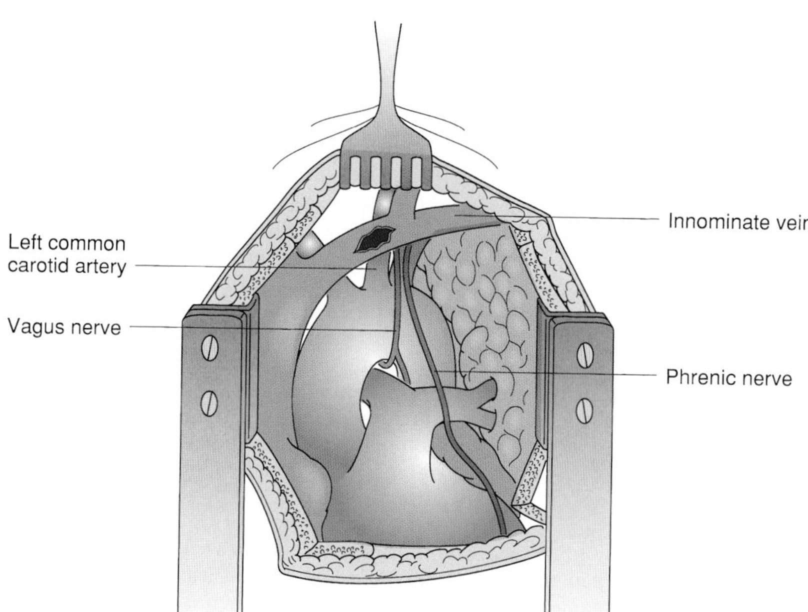

FIGURE 27.5 Proximal and distal control of both venous and arterial injuries must be obtained without injury to the adjacent structures (e.g., the phrenic, vagus, or recurrent laryngeal nerves).

venous ligation is well tolerated and arterial repair is performed. Proximal left subclavian and descending thoracic aortic injuries require a left thoracotomy for exposure. Distal subclavian injuries can be approached by removal of the clavicle or with a supraclavicular approach. If an emergency department thoracotomy is required, exposure of all but the apex of the mediastinum can be obtained by carrying the incision across the sternum into the right chest.

Almost all survivable blunt great vessel injuries result in acute pseudoaneurysms of the aortic isthmus or the proximal arch vessels. The aortic isthmus (the area of the descending aorta between the ligamentum arteriosum and the origin of the left subclavian artery) is susceptible to shear injury in deceleration trauma. Such injuries typically involve transection of the intima and media, with containment of hemorrhage by the adventitia. The mortality rate from delayed rupture of this lesion approaches 50% in the first 24 hours if left untreated.

Stent graft repair of traumatic aortic pseudoaneurysms has been successful in a number of centers that are staffed by personnel with special training and expertise who use well-developed preexisting protocols and that have an active stent graft program for elective infrarenal aortic aneurysm repair.[10]

Conventional surgical management of aortic injuries consists of direct suture repair or synthetic graft interposition. If possible, cardiopulmonary bypass capability, preferably from pulmonary vein to femoral artery, should be available in the event that aortic clamping is necessary for repair. Paraplegia, caused by cord ischemia during repair, occurs in approximately

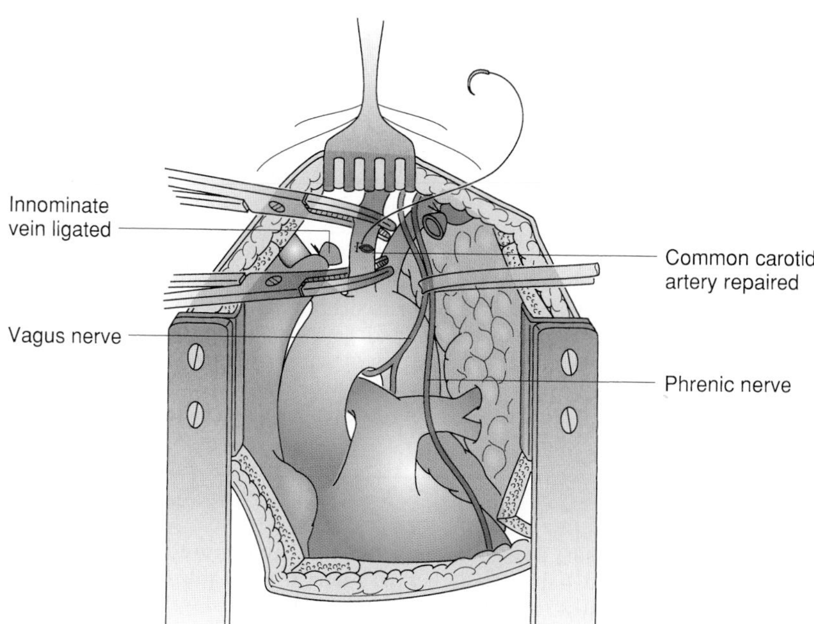

FIGURE 27.6 Combined arterial and venous injuries often are best treated with ligation of the vein, whereas isolated venous injuries may be safely repaired. Common carotid arterial repair is shown.

8% of patients and is more common in the presence of preoperative hypotension and extensive aortic injury.[18]

Abdominal Vascular Injury

The diagnosis of major intraabdominal vascular injury is most often made at celiotomy. Blunt renal artery injury, however, is most frequently diagnosed at the time of spiral CT scanning of the abdomen. The priorities in the management of abdominal vascular trauma are similar to those employed in other areas. If active bleeding is encountered at celiotomy, it is controlled by direct pressure. If contained retroperitoneal hemorrhage is encountered, proximal and distal vascular control is obtained before the hematoma is opened. Associated bowel injury should be closed expeditiously to avoid ongoing contamination from enteric contents. The most common finding at celiotomy in patients with blunt abdominal trauma is either retroperitoneal or intramesenteric hematoma. Less commonly, intestinal ischemia may be present as a result of thrombosis or avulsion of mesenteric vessels.

Exposure of the great vessels of the posterior abdomen is essential in the management of significant abdominal vascular trauma. If active hemorrhage is encountered, precise identification of the source of bleeding can be difficult. If it is necessary, exposure of the aorta at the diaphragmatic hiatus for clamp placement is best performed by entering the lesser sac and longitudinally splitting the crural fibers.

The infrarenal aorta and its bifurcation are best approached by mobilization of the small intestine to the right upper quadrant and opening the retroperitoneum in the midline, medial to the inferior mesenteric vein or lateral to either the ascending or the descending colon. The superior and inferior mesenteric arteries, the left renal hilum, and the left iliac artery can be exposed by reflection of the spleen and entire left colon for entry into the retroperitoneum. Similarly, the vena cava, right renal hilum, and right iliac artery can be exposed by a Kocher maneuver combined with mobilization of the right colon. The portal area is best exposed by the combination of a Kocher maneuver and mobilization of the hepatic flexure of the colon from the underlying duodenum and head of the pancreas.

Arterial and venous repair in the abdomen employ the same general principles of vascular technique used elsewhere. Primary suture repair, patch angioplasty, and saphenous vein interposition are used selectively to restore adequate flow. The use of synthetic graft material should be avoided if there is associated bowel or pancreatic injury. All mesenteric arterial repairs should include a careful inspection of the intestine for evidence of ischemia. Completion of angiography after abdominal vascular repair is difficult and suboptimal. Therefore, documentation of patency of the repair is best achieved using Doppler ultrasound or, possibly, intraoperative duplex scanning. If there is any doubt about the viability of the intestine, a second-look operation should be scheduled within the next 24 hours.

Injuries to the vena cava or the portal vein present significant management challenges because of the insidious nature of ongoing blood loss, the difficulty of obtaining proximal and distal control, and the high risk of subsequent thrombosis. These vessels should be ligated only as a desperate measure in unstable patients. Massive lower-extremity edema accompanies ligation of the infrarenal vena cava, and ligation above the renal veins is uniformly fatal. Portal venous ligation should be avoided if at all possible because the portal vein provides 80% of the oxygen and nutrient blood flow to the liver.[14] Direct suture and patch angioplasty are the most effective means to repair injuries of the great veins. Mesenteric venous injury can be managed by ligation without significant complications in most patients.

Extremity Vascular Trauma

The most common sites of extremity arterial trauma are the brachial and the superficial femoral arteries. Penetrating injuries are more common than blunt injuries. If they do occur, blunt injuries are usually associated with major fractures or dislocations. Supracondylar humeral fractures and posterior dislocations of the knee are associated with significant risks of brachial and popliteal artery injury, respectively. Concomitant peripheral nerve injuries occur in 60% of patients with vascular injuries in the extremities.

The extensive collateral circulation and the smaller muscle mass in the arm make acute arterial occlusion in the arm less likely to cause limb-threatening ischemia than when it occurs in the leg. The priorities of prompt diagnosis and timely restoration of perfusion, however, remain applicable to upper-extremity arterial trauma. A potentially limb-threatening situation is caused by injury to the brachial artery proximal to the origin of the profunda brachii artery or by occlusion of both the ulnar and radial arteries in the forearm; prompt arterial repair should be undertaken. In contrast, if isolated radial or ulnar artery occlusion occurs, reconstruction is not required as long as adequate flow into the hand through the remaining vessel can be documented. Fasciotomy in the forearm is rarely required and is necessary only after prolonged delays in restoration of flow or if there is extensive soft tissue injury.

In the lower extremity, vascular trauma is a significant management challenge. The large muscle mass of the leg and the lack of significant arterial collaterals increase the risk of limb loss whenever arterial occlusion occurs. Early diagnosis, timely operation, and proper vascular technique are therefore essential. Injuries to the femoral arteries, whether blunt or penetrating, often can be successfully managed by direct repair. Popliteal artery injuries usually require interposition grafting.[17] Isolated tibial vessel injury does not require treatment if one of the other leg arteries is patent. The liberal use of fasciotomy in the lower leg is necessary to avoid compartment syndrome.

OUTCOME

The results of properly diagnosed and expeditiously treated vascular trauma are encouraging. The mortality rate after isolated peripheral vascular trauma is low, with no mortalities reported in many series. The mortality rate for suprarenal aortic injuries remains at approximately 50% to 70%. Infrarenal aortic injuries have mortality rates of 20% to 40%.

The amputation rate after peripheral vascular trauma continues to decrease, with several series reporting amputation rates of less than 2%. The recent improvement in limb salvage is a result of a combination of factors, most of which decrease the warm ischemia time, such as rapid transport, immediate operation, placement of intraluminal shunts, and so forth. Early amputation is more frequent following blunt trauma and when delays occur in diagnosis or treatment. Late amputation is done primarily for severe pain, disability, or infection. Long-term functional outcome of extremity vascular trauma is not dependent on patency of the vascular graft, but rather on the integrity of the neuromuscular and skeletal elements.[16]

KEY POINTS

- **The consequences of vascular injury are hemorrhage and distal tissue ischemia; many preventable deaths and limb loss occur because of inappropriate delays in diagnosis.**
- **Vascular injury requires a high index of suspicion and thorough primary and secondary physical examination**

supplemented with Doppler pressure measurements and selective radiographic imaging. Angiography is the gold standard, whereas CT angiography is less invasive and more rapid and has fewer complications.

- Endovascular therapy is indicated for branch vessel hemorrhage, which can be occluded without significant ischemia, acute pseudoaneurysm, intimal flap without significant thrombosis, and acute arteriovenous fistula.
- Extremity vascular trauma management requires "life over limb," with the basic approach of local pressure, as required, followed by proximal and distal control. Thrombectomy is followed by repair, patch, or graft (preferably autologous), without tension or redundancy. Temporary shunting permits safe orthopedic fixation before definitive repair.
- The ascending aorta, innominate and right subclavian arteries are approached by median sternotomy. Proximal left subclavian artery and descending aorta are accessed via a left thoracotomy. Contained injuries can be treated by endovascular stent grafting.
- In the abdomen, retroperitoneal control is achieved by left colon mobilization for the infrarenal aorta and left iliac artery, along with spleen and pancreas for superior and inferior mesenteric and left renal arteries. Similarly, the vena cava, right renal hilum, and right iliac artery are approached by Kocher maneuver and mobilization of right colon, as is the portal area by lifting the hepatic flexure off the duodenum.

References

1. Mattox KL, Feliciano DV, Burch J, et al. 5,760 cardiovascular injuries in 4,459 patients: epidemiologic evolution 1958–1987. *Ann Surg.* 1989;209:698–705.
2. Oller DW, Rutledge R, Clancy T, et al. Vascular injuries in a rural state: a review of 978 patients from a state trauma registry. *J Trauma* 1992;32:740–745.
3. Ricci MA, Trevisani GT, Pilcher DB. Vascular complications of cardiac catheterization. *Am J Surg.* 1994;167:375–378.
4. Odeh M. The role of reperfusion-induced injury in the pathogenesis of the crush syndrome. *N Engl J Med.* 1991;324:1417–1422.
5. Cook AD, Klein JS, Rogers FB, et al. Chest radiographs of limited utility in the diagnosis of blunt aortic traumatic laceration. *J Trauma* 2001;50:843.
6. Downing SW, Sperling JS, Mirvisw SE, et al. Experience with spiral computed tomography as the sole diagnostic method for traumatic aortic rupture. *Ann Thorac Surg.* 2001;72:495–502.
7. Dennis JW, Frykberg ER, Veldenz HC, et al. Validation of nonoperative management of occult vascular injuries and accuracy of physical examination alone in penetrating extremity trauma: 5- to 10-year follow up. *J Trauma* 1998;44:243–252.
8. Schwartz MR, Waever FA, Bauer M, et al. Refining the indications for arteriography in penetrating extremity trauma: a prospective analysis. *J Vasc Surg.* 1993;17:116–124.
9. Weiss VJ, Chaikof EL. Endovascular treatment of vascular injuries. *Surg Clin North Am.* 1999;79:653–655.
10. Karmy-Jones R, Hoffer E, Meissner MH, et al. Endovascular stent grafts and aortic rupture: a case series. *J Trauma* 2003;55:805–810.
11. Khoury M, Rebecca A, Greene K, et al. Duplex scanning-guided thrombin injection for the treatment of iatrogenic pseudoaneurysms. *J Vasc Surg.* 2002;35:517–521.
12. Powell A, Benenati JF, Becker GJ, et al. Percutaneous ultrasound-guided thrombin injection for the treatment of pseudoaneurysms. *J Am Coll Surg.* 2002;194:s53–s57.
13. Wright JG, Kerry JC, Hobson RW. Heparin decreases ischemia-reperfusion injury in isolated canine gracilis muscle. *Arch Surg.* 1988;123:470–472.
14. Hossny A. Blunt popliteal artery injury with complete lower limb ischemia: is routine use of temporary intraluminal shunt justified? *J Vasc Surg.* 2004;40:61–66.
15. Johansen K, Daines M, Howie T, et al. Objective criteria accurately predicting amputation following lower extremity trauma. *J Trauma* 1990;30:568–572.
16. Bosse MJ, MacKenzie EJ, Kellam JF, et al. An analysis of outcomes of reconstruction or amputation of leg threatening injuries. *N Engl J Med.* 2002;347:1924–1931.
17. Rozycki GS, Tremblay LN, Feliciano DV, et al. Blunt vascular trauma in the extremity: diagnosis, management, and outcome. *J Trauma* 2003;55:814–824.
18. Mattox KL, Wall MJ. Injury to the thoracic great vessels. In: Feliciano DV, Moore EE, Mattox KL, eds. *Trauma*, 3rd ed. Norwalk, CT: Appleton & Lange, 1996.

CHAPTER 28 ■ ORTHOPAEDIC TRAUMA

JASON THOMPSON AND JENS R. CHAPMAN

The initial resuscitation of the trauma patient is directed at identifying and treating the immediately life-threatening conditions that affect the airway, breathing, and circulation. Commonly, injuries to the head, chest, and abdomen take precedence when constructing a treatment plan. However, orthopaedic injuries may occur in over 70% of multiply injured trauma patients and may greatly impact the initial and subsequent management of this patient population.[1] Accurately diagnosing and expeditiously treating these orthopaedic injuries may lead to diminished morbidity and mortality. On a conceptual basis, orthopaedic injuries can be differentiated into the three general impact categories: (a) life-threatening injuries; (b) limb-threatening injuries; and (c) injuries with adverse long-term functional implications.

To minimize the effects of musculoskeletal injuries on the care of trauma patients, implementation of a formal approach is helpful. Because approximately 75% of missed injuries are orthopaedic in nature, a systematic musculoskeletal systems evaluation is recommended.[2–6] The most common cause of missed injury seems to be failure to adequately visualize the region of injury or failure to perform a secondary or tertiary survey.

Initial orthopaedic assessment of an acutely injured patient is performed concurrently with general trauma patient evaluation, which should include vital signs monitoring, determination of mental status, and radiographic evaluation with anteroposterior radiograph of the pelvis, lateral radiograph of the cervical spine, and an anteroposterior roentgenogram of the chest. Additional orthopaedic workup continues with exposure of the patient, palpation of the trunk and extremities, manual realignment of misaligned extremities, palpation of pulses, and detailed neurologic examination. Open injuries and penetrating wounds are evaluated for their impact on the patient's vital function and limb survival and then are dressed sterile until definitive care is rendered. Appropriate antibiotic management and Tetanus immunization should be administered in the emergency setting. The neurologic examination is performed in accordance with the American Spinal Cord Injury Association and recorded accordingly and should include perianal and rectal examination for presence of blood, voluntary contraction, sensation, and reflexes. For all trauma patients a protocol for secondary and tertiary evaluation should be in place to minimize the impact of delayed injuries. This is particularly important for patients with cognitive impairment and patients who have been taken out of the normal care trauma evaluation algorithm because of their emergent care needs.

LIFE-THREATENING INJURIES

Musculoskeletal trauma may lead to patient demise on an acute, subacute, or delayed basis. Acutely life-threatening conditions may arise from large-scale blood loss such as that encountered with major arterial injuries in conjunction with long bone fractures, pelvic ring disruption, or spine fracture dislocations. Subacute life-threatening circumstances may result from occult blood loss with delayed recognition and response. Postprimary or delayed patient loss of life may occur as an indirect result of injuries and subsequent resuscitation circumstances encountered. Secondary pulmonary deterioration and sepsis after multiple fractures are leading causes of such postprimary patient loss of life. Although the exact cause of posttraumatic sepsis and pulmonary deterioration remains incompletely understood and is likely multifactorial, the timing and technique of resuscitation and musculoskeletal injury treatment, including factors such as duration of recumbence, undoubtedly play a considerable role in onset as well as prevention of these serious events.

Injuries to the musculoskeletal system may be of sufficient severity to cause acutely life-threatening hemodynamic instability because of hypovolemia or neurologic alterations. Injuries with disruption of vascular structures leading to acute or subacute hypovolemia include pelvic ring disruptions, multiple long bone fractures, traumatic forequarter or hindquarter amputations, scapulothoracic dissociations, and upper- to mid-thoracic level fracture dislocations as well as any form of distractive spinal column injury.[7–16] The blood loss in each of these injuries may be occult if the injury is closed. The source of bleeding may be of arterial, venous, or combined origin with relatively large volumes entering soft tissue planes such as the retroperitoneal pelvis, thigh, chest, or subcutaneous tissues at relatively low pressures. Suspicion of hypovolemia must remain high, therefore, as musculoskeletal injuries as listed are encountered, and aggressive countermeasures should be taken. Simple bedside measures such as pressure dressings, pelvic sheet application, and limb realignment may be all that is required to assist the trauma team in regaining hemodynamic stability.

If preliminary physical or radiographic examination reveals musculoskeletal injuries as listed, further investigation may be indicated during the initial evaluation phase. During subsequent imaging evaluation, such as with magnetic resonance imaging (MRI) and computed tomography (CT) scans, adequate monitoring for hemodynamic instability and hypoxia should be provided.

Pelvic Ring Disruption

Open book pelvic injuries, which characteristically have a distractive disruption of the anterior pelvic ring and external rotation of the pelvic wings, can be associated with diffuse venous plexus bleeding into the traumatically expanded lower abdominal cavity. Because of the typically venous nature of the associated substantial volume loss, attempts at stopping the hemorrhage with interventional angiographic embolization may be futile. Emergent reduction and compression of this traumatically expanded space may, however, be an effective emergent management strategy. This procedure can be achieved with a number of percutaneous surgical intervention measures, such as external fixation or a pelvic clamp, which can be placed in an emergency room setting. More recently, application of a "pelvic sheet" has been introduced as a similarly effective means to achieve lower abdominal and pelvic volume reduction. Although we describe a number of techniques, in principle a simple folded linen sheet is wrapped around the affected patient's pelvic ring from posterior to anterior and then clamped tightly in front (Fig. 28.1).[2] The realignment of the injured pelvis can be assessed with an anteroposterior radiograph. Definitive surgical stabilization can be deferred to a later time; a variety of definitive management options, ranging from minimally invasive to open instrumentation techniques, are available.

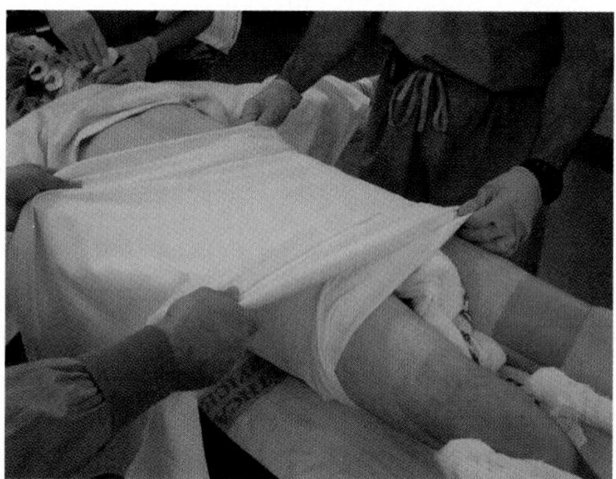
A

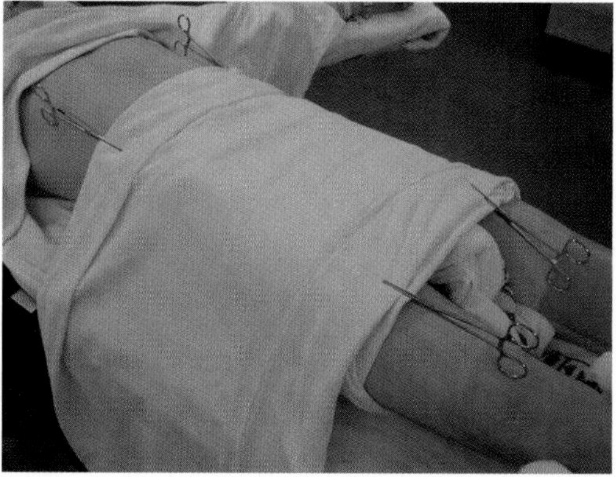
B

FIGURE 28.1 (*A*) Application of pelvic sheet to provide external stability and reduce pelvic volume. (*B*) Pelvic sheet in place swaddling patient's pelvis with application of pressure over both iliac wings and trochanteric area. The clamps are applied as cephalad and caudal and lateral as possible to prevent obfuscation of subsequent imaging. Should groin access be necessary, the sheet may be fenestrated without significant compromise of the pelvic binding ability.

Major Limb Injuries

Major sources of blood loss may stem from proximal limb trauma, such as open fractures; traumatic amputations, such as forequarter amputations; and closed disruptive injuries, such as scapulothoracic dissociation. Because bleeding may come from arterial sources, emergent embolization following attempts at closed injury reduction and application of nonconstrictive compression dressing may reduce further volume loss. Emergent operative intervention to control bleeding may have to be considered, especially in the presence of patients with proximal limb or forequarter amputations. Scapulothoracic dissociation injuries can be commonly identified on chest radiographs but can elude casual observation. A combination of arterial injuries with venous bleeding, in addition to brachial plexus disruption, may pose a significant source of hemorrhage. If possible, application of a chest–arm compressive spica dressing may limit fluid extravasation into the soft tissue planes of the torso. Should these measures prove unsuccessful, interventional angiography should be considered. Surgical exploration of the injured shoulder girdle in a patient with known scapulothoracic dissociation is prone to significant hemorrhage in the acute setting and should be weighed carefully.

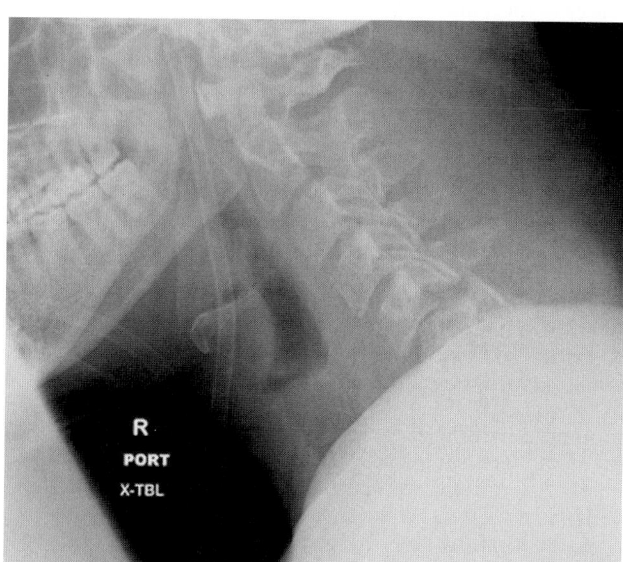

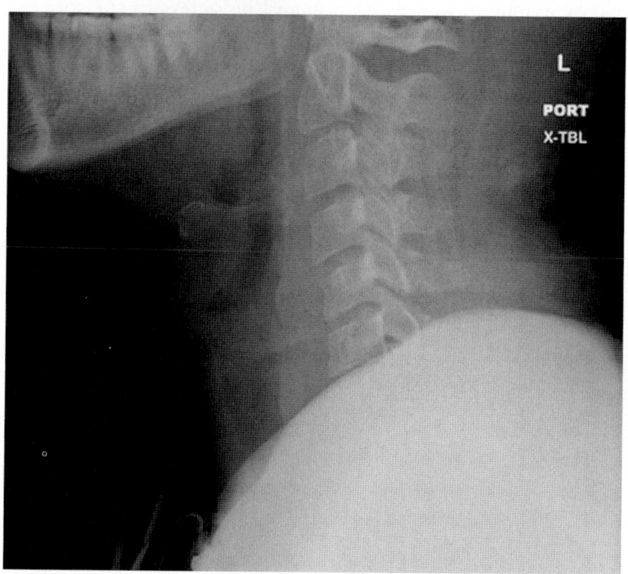

FIGURE 28.2 (*A*) Initial lateral cervical radiograph of a young man after a motorcycle crash. He presented with paraplegia and neurogenic shock. Once the shock was under control, the next phase in care was rapid closed reduction of the cervical spine. (*B*) Postreduction radiograph. This patient went on to have definitive surgical stabilization in 2 days once he was fully stabilized medically.

Spine Injuries

Life-threatening circumstances may follow spinal column injury with neurologic injury as well. Injuries to the upper cervical spinal cord or brainstem may be caused by traumatic bony or ligamentous disruption from the craniocervical junction through the C4 level. Patients with craniocervical injuries in particular are at risk for anoxia because of primary lack of breathing impulse secondary to lack of neural input. As in any musculoskeletal injury, the potential exists for an unstable ligamentous disruption to go unrecognized on initial imaging tests because of a partial "rebounding mechanism" leading to an apparent, yet unstable skeletal reduction. Patients have sustained catastrophic secondary deterioration after surviving the initial assessment phase due to such occult distractive-type injuries or high cervical spinal cord injuries. Should a distractive-type cervical spine injury be considered or identified, immediate efforts should be undertaken to protect the spinal cord and column. Such temporizing measures can include placement of sandbags around the head and immobilizing the head with tape or application of a halo ring and vest, unless contraindicated.

Severe hypotension may also result from neurogenic shock. This condition can result from fracture dislocations of the subaxial cervical spine or the upper thoracic spine with spinal cord injury and direct disruption of sympathetic input (Fig. 28.2). Neurogenic shock is typically manifested by systemic hypotension with low peripheral vascular resistance, normal to high urine output, and relative bradycardia with warm and flush extremities (Table 28.1). Protracted efforts at treating this condition with intravascular fluid administration are usually unsuccessful and may lead to fluid overload and cardiopulmonary deterioration. Neurogenic hypotension or shock is best counteracted with intravenous pressors in addition to judicious fluid resuscitation to fill dilated capacitance vessels. By correcting neurogenic hypotension, the remainder of the workup may be completed safely, and blood circulation and oxygenation of a distressed or damaged spinal cord is enhanced, thereby reducing the potential for permanent spinal cord injury.[18] Should the initial lateral cervical radiograph demonstrate cervical fracture dislocation,

TABLE 28.1

COMPARISON OF NEUROGENIC AND HEMORRHAGIC SHOCK

Parameter	Hemorrhagic shock	Neurogenic shock
Blood pressure	⇓	⇓
Heart rate	⇑	⇓
Urine output	⇓	⇔
Skin	Pale, clammy	Warm, pink
Mental status	Anxious	Normal
Central venous pressure	⇓	⇓

strong consideration should be given to urgent closed skeletal reduction under controlled circumstances.[17]

In case of cervical fracture dislocations, acute reduction in an emergency room setting has been shown to be an effective and safe intervention with improved neurologic outcome in the presence of spinal cord injury and may decrease the incidence and severity of pulmonary insufficiency. Respiratory failure as a result of prolonged recumbence in cervical traction and misguided mobilization efforts may occur as late as 7 to 10 days following spinal cord injury.[19] Cervical traction to accomplish reduction of cervical fractures is most commonly performed by application of Gardner-Wells head tongs using a controlled setup, including fluoroscopy, automated vital sign monitoring, and with sequential increase of weights and intermittent neurologic evaluations. Contraindications to application of Gardner-Wells tongs include the presence of a skull fracture in the area of intended pin application or the presence of distractive-type neck injuries. Timing of surgical intervention to definitively stabilize the orthopaedic injury is often a matter of judgment, but in general surgery is preferred in the early postinjury phase, provided the patient's resuscitation status allows it. This should be determined by all services involved in the care of the multiply injured patient.

Timing of Surgical Intervention

There remains a lack of consensus as to the ideal timing of fracture stabilization in the multiply injured patient. There is little doubt that early definitive skeletal stabilization can reduce secondary "fracture disease," such as pulmonary decompensation, decubitus ulcers, and soft tissue compromise in the injured limb. However, untimely and prolonged early surgical procedures may aggravate lung trauma. Perioperative secondary hypotension may aggravate central nervous system and spinal cord injury. In general, every attempt should be made to provide surgical débridement to high-grade open or open long bone and joint injuries. Temporary stabilization of the pelvic ring—as outlined above—can be a major resuscitation aid in an "open book type" pelvic ring injury.[2] Stabilization of femoral shaft fractures within 24 hours specifically has been shown to reduce the rate of adult respiratory distress syndrome (ARDS).[37]

The success of treatment of open fractures is strongly related to the severity of soft tissue injury and the amount of primary bone loss. Timing to surgical débridement within 8 hours is another important variable in reducing the rate of osteomyelitis and delayed fracture union in the tibia.[38] Timing of stabilization of thoracolumbar surgery for acute fractures with or without spinal cord injury has been the subject of many divergent opinions in the past. Aside from the prospect of optimizing chances for spinal cord recovery, the chance to mobilize a patient rapidly into an upright position has been shown to be safe, to reduce the risk of pulmonary decompensation, and to provide improved neurologic outcomes.[39] Early surgical intervention for musculoskeletal trauma should follow the principle of being expedient and effective in stabilization while minimizing exposure and dissection-related blood loss.

LIMB-THREATENING INJURIES

Although the majority of orthopaedic injuries in major trauma patients are not life threatening, they may be a significant source of morbidity.[20] This is particularly true when the injury may directly lead to loss of limb or, if unrecognized, lead to severe morbidity in which limb salvage is no longer a viable alternative or will leave the affected patient with an essentially nonfunctional limb. Injuries in which the limb is immediately threatened include any injury with major arterial supply disruption, such as is seen in open or closed long bone fractures secondary to high-energy or penetrating trauma (Figs. 28.3 and 28.4). Furthermore, any crushing or mangling-type limb injury may result in loss of blood supply on a delayed basis even in the absence of an actual arterial separation by diffuse intimal damage or through development of a compartment syndrome.

Efforts to identify limb-threatening conditions early and initiate appropriate treatment include focused evaluation of the limbs both clinically and radiographically. Distraction prompted by other injuries or impaired cognitive function should not prevent a systematic evaluation of the torso and all limbs. Any trauma evaluation should include a formal secondary survey.

Aside from the physical examination standards of inspection for lacerations, bruising, and skin discoloration, for instance, palpation for crepitus and tenseness of the soft tissue envelope should be accompanied by functional testing of joints and their respective stability. Clinical vascular testing of perfusion of a traumatized limb ranges from simple palpation of pulses, assessing skin color, temperature, capillary refill and blanching to determining ankle-brachial indices (ABI), and ultrasound probing of blood flow to angiography techniques.

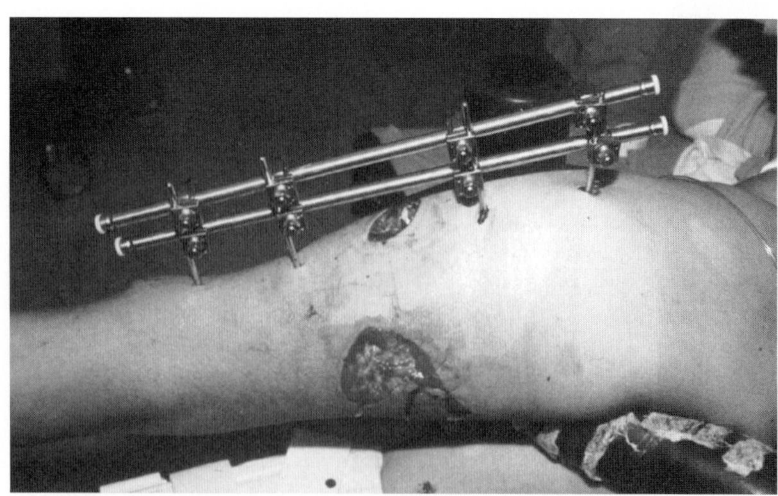

FIGURE 28.3 External fixation may be thought of as portable traction. This method can rapidly stabilize any extremity and allow for patient mobilization while awaiting definitive internal or external stabilization.

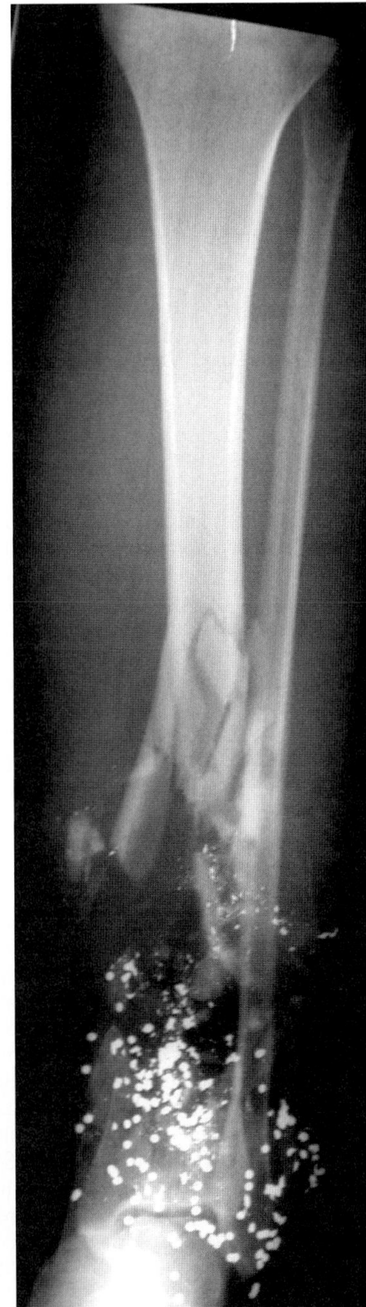

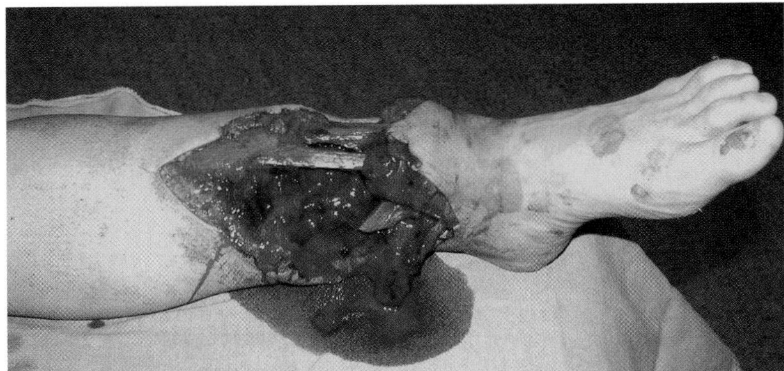

FIGURE 28.4 (*A*) Clinical photo of a mangled lower extremity. This young woman sustained a high-velocity gunshot wound to her tibia. MESS equaled 8. (*B*) Injury radiograph. Note soft tissue defects and extensive bone loss with comminution. She went on to definitive below-knee amputation and good functional results.

Although the general goal of treatment is directed at limb preservation, a timely and well-performed amputation may be in a patient's best interest. With medical advances, scenarios where limb salvage is a distinct technical feasibility have become more commonplace, leaving the patient, however, with multiple surgeries over a protracted period of time and, in the end, with a painful extremity of little functional use. In contrast, excellent functional results can be obtained, especially in lower extremity amputations, with state-of-the-art amputee care. Therefore, amputation may not constitute a treatment failure but rather a prudent treatment choice. This stands in contrast to loss of limb resulting from an avoidable delay of diagnosis of a limb-threatening condition or failure to institute timely treatment.[30]

Vascular Injuries

After realignment of misaligned limbs in a trauma patient, any potentially injured limb should have its vascular and neurologic status evaluated. Diagnosis of clinically significant vascular injury may be made by using the ABI and confirming by angiography. An ABI of greater than 0.9 is considered low risk for arterial injury, and immediate arteriography is not

TABLE 28.2

RISK OF VASCULAR INJURY

Location and type of injury	Risk of vascular injury
Proximal humerus fracture (open or closed, high energy)	<1%
Femur shaft fracture (closed)	<1%
Femur shaft fracture (open)	1.9%
Tibia/fibula fracture (closed)	1%
Tibia/fibula fracture (open)	10%
Supracondylar femur fracture	1%–2%
Knee dislocation	16%–40%
Floating knee (ipsilateral femur and tibia fractures)	29%

indicated.[21,22] Delay in diagnosis of vascular injury in limb trauma with a warm ischemia time of 6 hours or more leads to an increased rate of amputation.[23] Typical extremity trauma associated with an increased risk of vascular injury includes any penetrating injury or open fracture, any high-energy long bone fracture as evidenced by history or fracture pattern seen on radiographs, knee dislocations, supracondylar femur fractures, and displaced proximal humerus fractures in metabolically healthy patients.

In certain locations, such as the supracondylar femur, the major arterial vessel lies in direct contact with bone and is tethered by fascia and soft tissue structures. This constellation increases the vascular injury risk by fracture laceration of the vessel or through distractive intimal damage (Table 28.2).

TABLE 28.3

MANGLED EXTREMITY SEVERITY SCORE (MESS)

Parameter	Points[a,b]
Skeletal/soft tissue injury	
Low energy (stab, simple fracture, civilian GSW)	1
Medium energy (open/multiple fractures, dislocations)	2
High energy (crush injury, military GSW)	3
Very high energy (above + gross contamination, avulsion)	4
Limb ischemia	
Pulse reduced or absent, perfusion normal	1*
Pulseless, paresthesias, reduced cap refill	2*
Cool, paralyzed, insensate, numb	3*
Shock	
Systolic BP always >90 mm Hg	0
Hypotensive transiently	1
Persistent hypotension	2
Age (yr)	
30	0
30–50	1
>50	2

[a]MESS greater ≥7 predictive of amputation.
[b]Score doubled for ischemia >6 hr.
GSW, gunshot wound; BP, blood pressure.

Mangled Extremity

The descriptive term "mangled extremity" is commonly attached to a limb that has sustained a combination of significant soft tissue and osseous damage with or without vascular injury of such magnitude that limb survival is questionable even under the best of circumstances. The diagnosis of a mangled extremity is usually readily made because of the dramatic nature of its clinical presentation. Feasibility of limb salvage, however, is far more difficult to ascertain. Several scoring systems have been proposed to help the clinician determine whether or not the limb is amenable for reconstruction at a reasonable risk to the patient. The most widely used of these is the Mangled Extremity Severity Score (MESS; Tables 28.3 and 28.4).[24]

When the MESS is calculated to be greater than 7, consideration of primary amputation has been recommended. Attempts to salvage limbs with prolonged warm ischemia time, massive soft tissue contamination, neurologic injury, and skeletal instability may lead to increased morbidity and even to overwhelming sepsis and death.[25] Even if limb salvage has been successfully accomplished, long-term quality of life and functional outcomes scores have called into question the reconstruction of highly traumatized limbs.[30]

Factors to consider before embarking on the reconstruction of a severely injured lower extremity are age and injury load of the patient, presence of comorbidities, severity of soft tissue injury and type of contamination, time to débridement, warm ischemia time, and integrity of neurologic function. In the lower extremity, the presence of severe ipsilateral foot trauma has been associated with poor outcome and thus may sway a treating surgeon toward primary amputation.[40] Similarly, disruption of lower extremity nerves below the knee level with loss of protective sensation usually indicates a poor outlook for most afflicted patients, regardless of reconstruction method.

Diagnosis of neurologic injury in the extremity is often difficult in a multiply injured patient, and it may elude even the most thorough physical examination if the patient has an impaired cognitive status. Unfortunately, even advanced imaging studies such as MRI or electrophysiologic studies rarely provide diagnostic data in acute trauma. Specifically electromyography is not expected to show signs of neurologic injury until 3 weeks after injury.[41] Therefore, clinical evaluation and direct surgical exploration of neural elements in case of surgical exposure of an affected nerve can be all the decision-making help that a treating physician may have to rely on. In contrast to the upper extremity repair of transected or avulsed neural elements, in the lower extremity this has been

TABLE 28.4

MANGLED EXTREMITY SCORING SYSTEMS

Author, year	Scoring system
Johansen et al., 1990	Mangled extremity severity score (MESS)
Howe et al., 1987	Predictive salvage index (PSI)
Russell et al., 1991	Limb salvage index (LSI)
McNamara et al., 1994	Nerve injury, ischemia, soft tissue injury, skeletal injury, shock, and age score (NISSA)
Tscherne et al., 1982	Hannover fracture scale-97 (HFS-97)

associated with poor rates of neurologic outcomes. Therefore, in general, the boundaries of replantation or limb salvage attempts can be pushed further in upper extremity trauma compared to in the lower extremities with relatively greater chances at functional recovery.

Compartment Syndrome

Compartment syndromes are defined as a mismatch of tissue perfusion to tissue oxygen requirements secondary to elevation of tissue perfusion pressure in an anatomically confined space. The most common site for compartmental syndromes is the lower leg with the superficial and anterior compartments being most affected. Other locations include the thigh, foot, and forearm. On occasion it can also be seen in the gluteal and psoas compartments. Pain medication, multiple injuries, altered mental status, and bulky splints may hinder accurate physical examination and thus prevent or delay detection of this condition. The earliest and most relevant warning sign of an evolving compartmental syndrome is severe pain out of proportion to that which is expected with passive stretch maneuvers of the muscles of the fascial compartment. Other signs, such as tenseness and local tenderness of the fascial compartment are variable and clinically not apparent in the thigh and gluteal region. Pallor, pulselessness, or neurologic signs such as paresthesia or weakness are ominous late signs of compartmental syndrome and indicate prolonged ischemia in most circumstances. In patients for whom compliance with physical examination is diminished, a high degree of suspicion and vigilant monitoring is required. Invasive monitoring of intracompartmental pressures may provide information critical to surgical decision making if clinical examination is unobtainable, unreliable, or equivocal. The perfusion gradient (diastolic blood pressure minus compartmental pressure) in the monitored compartment should be greater than 30 mmHg. If the perfusion gradient falls below 30 mmHg, then the compartment is at a considerably elevated risk for ischemia and fasciotomy should be considered. The definitive treatment of pathologically elevated compartment pressure consists of a decompressive fasciotomy performed in a timely fashion. Presently, there are no fixed time guidelines regarding decompression of an evolving compartment syndrome. Depending on the affected anatomic region and a number of other variables, decompression within 6 hours from time of insult is necessary for preservation of tissue. Routine fasciotomies should also be considered after revascularization of an extremity or under other reperfusion conditions.[26–29]

Infection

There are multiple causes for posttraumatic infection. Aside from primary inoculation at the site of injury, the most common cause of infection in a trauma situation is presence of devitalized tissue. Adequate resuscitation efforts with maintenance of oxygenation and tissue perfusion pressures and judicious surgical débridement are important first steps in preventing musculoskeletal infection. Aside from host factors, effective early skeletal stabilization in combination with meaningful surgical débridement and supplemental antibiotic prophylaxis can decrease the likelihood of musculoskeletal infection. From an orthopaedic perspective, expedient initial skeletal stabilization in an acutely injured patient may be an important adjuvant to decreasing the injury burden of a multiply injured patient. Specifically the advent of intramedullary nails and joint-crossing external fixation techniques can expedite care of patients with long bone trauma.

INJURIES ASSOCIATED WITH LONG-TERM MORBIDITY

Certain injuries of the musculoskeletal system have strong associations with increased long-term morbidity if they are not treated as urgently as possible. Though not life threatening or limb threatening, these injuries may represent a considerable source of disability for the traumatized patient after many of the injuries to the major organ systems have healed. Major joint dislocations such as of the hip, femoral neck fractures, open fractures with contamination, talar neck fractures with displacement or dislocation, and thoracic fracture dislocations are examples of injuries with potential significant long-term illness impact.

Hip dislocations can be identified on the advanced trauma life support (ATLS) recommended initial anteroposterior pelvic trauma screening radiograph. For dislocations of the hip or fractures surrounding the femoral head and neck, early reduction and stabilization are desirable. Hip dislocations specifically should be viewed with urgency. Earliest possible closed reduction followed by CT scan is the standard of care. Vascular supply to the femoral head is tenuous and is derived largely from the vessels that reach the head after branching from the medial femoral circumflex artery. These vessels then travel through the posterior lateral aspect of the hip joint capsule as the posterior superior retinacular arteries. Prolonged dislocation of the femoral head leads to disruption of these retinacular arteries and gives rise to avascular necrosis (AVN) of the femoral head.[42] Delay of reduction of this major joint dislocation also makes reduction progressively harder because of muscular contractions. CT of the pelvis following closed reduction of the hip is required to assess for articular debris. Presence of debris within the weight-bearing portion of the hip may lead to accelerated cartilage wear and arthrosis and should prompt consideration for early joint débridement through a suitable arthrotomy. Larger acetabular fragments may require stabilization through internal fixation to ensure congruent joint alignment.

Femoral neck fractures may also compromise perfusion of the femoral head by virtue of traumatic disruption of vascular supply and outflow.[43] Early stable internal fixation with anatomic reduction and release of an intracapsular hematoma is associated with decreased incidence of AVN or nonunion of femoral neck fractures. In younger patients, few satisfactory reconstructive surgery options exist for either scenario. For elderly patients, eventual hip arthroplasty may be a viable alternative when AVN leads to joint destruction; however, posttraumatic hip arthroplasty in younger patients rarely provides a lasting treatment option.

In general, any open fracture, regardless of contamination, requires some type of formal débridement and irrigation. Removal of all foreign material and devitalized tissue at the earliest possible time has been shown to decrease the overall infection rate, both for acute wound infection and chronic osteomyelitis.[44–46] If the patient is too ill to have adequate débridement in an operating room environment, it should be done as thoroughly as possible in the resuscitation or intensive care area. Internal fixation of fractures can be safely performed after appropriate soft tissue management and can aid soft tissue healing.[31–33]

Displaced fractures of the talar neck with or without dislocation of the talar body are associated with a poor prognosis. Urgent reduction of the fracture or dislocation should be undertaken as soon as the diagnosis is made. Operative débridement of open wounds and internal fixation of these injuries should also be performed at the earliest reasonable time.[34–36] Delay of reduction of peritalar fractures or dislocations can be expected to lead to soft tissue breakdown of the very vulnerable lower half of the extremity, leading to subsequent reconstruction challenges. Neglect of these fractures has also been consistently associated with a higher incidence of AVN of the talus, subsequent severe hindfoot arthrosis, and disability.

Neurologic Injury

Presence of a neurologic deficit can be a major source of poor outcomes. Annually there are approximately 11,000 new spinal cord injuries in the United States. Considerable long-term morbidity can arise from neurologic injury following trauma. On the whole no other condition affects patient outcome as adversely as spinal cord injury. Thus, it seems reasonable to aggressively diagnose and treat spinal cord injuries according the following philosophies: minimize the occurrence of preventable spinal cord injuries through education of the population at large and target groups, specifically

- avoid secondary spinal cord injuries through minimizing the occurrence of missed spinal column injuries;
- optimize chances for spinal cord recovery through a number of measures including adequate resuscitation, timely decompression and stabilization of the spine, and pharmacologic measures;
- implement a formal spinal cord rehabilitation program at the earliest possible time.

Recovery from spinal cord injury is a highly variable and somewhat unpredictable occurrence. Injury mechanism, age, and health of patient are factors influencing the outcomes of spinal cord injury. To date there are no reproducible methods to achieve spinal cord regeneration. Pharmacologic treatment with methylprednisolone has been a widely followed practice in North America after several prominent studies.[51] The recommended dose of 30 mg/kg methylprednisolone bolus given over 1 hour followed by a drip of 5.4 mg/kg/hour over 23 hours has remained a widely used regimen despite numerous criticisms about the scientific merits of this treatment regimen.[47–50]

SUMMARY

The diagnosis and management of orthopaedic injuries in the multiply injured patient population are often complex. Early recognition of certain injuries may lead to diminished morbidity (both early and late), earlier stability of patient hemodynamics, decreased length of stay in intensive care settings, decreased rates of transfusion, more rapid institution of appropriate treatment, earlier patient mobilization, and decreased mortality. Improved understanding of how each component of multisystem trauma impacts overall patient well-being can improve patient outcomes through collaborative care by many specialists. While orthopaedic consultation may be readily available at major level 1 trauma centers, this may not be true in the greater community. It behooves the orthopaedist to understand the basics of general surgery; the converse is certainly true, so that initial appropriate management takes place.

KEY POINTS

- **Orthopaedic injuries occur in 70% of multiply injured patients and, of missed injuries, 75% are orthopaedic, which mandates systematic, thorough secondary and tertiary surveys. Delayed recognition leads to potential ongoing blood loss and secondary insult, such as pulmonary failure.**
- **Life-threatening blood loss can occur secondary to long bone fractures, which are treated by realignment, splinting, and compression wrapping; pelvic ring disruption, treated by sheet wrapping to decrease pelvic volume and stabilize fractures; and spine fracture dislocations, treated with immobilization, realignment, and airway and vascular support. Open, bleeding wounds require direct intervention, including potential amputation or complete amputation.**
- **Making the decision to amputate is difficult but preferable to saving a disabling, nonfunctional, or painful extremity. Loss of significant tissue, prolonged ischemia, and disruption of nerves plus scores, such as the MESS, aid in this decision.**
- **Compartment syndromes are inadequate tissue perfusion to meet oxygen requirements resulting from increased pressure in a confined anatomical space. The earliest reliable sign is excessive pain to passive or active movement of muscles in the compartment. Pressure monitoring with pressure differences between the compartment and diastolic pressure of less than 30 mmHg require decompression.**
- **Major joint dislocations such as of the hip, femoral neck fracture, open fractures with contamination, talar neck fracture with dislocation, and thoracic fracture dislocations are examples of injuries with potential long-term disability that require aggressive early intervention.**
- **Spinal cord injuries create long-term morbidity and mortality. Aggressive prevention programs, adequate recognition and resuscitation to optimize perfusion, timely decompression, and treatment acutely with steroids are required to optimize recovery.**

References

1. Court-Brown CM. Care of accident victims. *Br Med J.* 1989;298:115.
2. Davis JW, et al. The etiology of missed cervical spine injuries. *J Trauma* 1993;34:342.
3. Hanson DA, et al. *Am J Roentgenol.* 2000;174:713.
4. Soundappand SV, et al. Role of an extended tertiary survey in detecting missed injuries in children. *J Trauma* 2004;57:114.
5. **Brooks A, et al. Missed injury in major trauma patients. *Injury* 2004;35:407.**
6. Stephen DJG, et al. Early detection of arterial bleeding in acute pelvic trauma. *J Trauma* 1999;47:638.
7. Evers BM, et al. Pelvic fracture hemorrhage: priorities in management. *Arch Surg.* 1989;124:422.
8. **Pape HC, et al. The timing of fracture treatment in polytrauma patients: relevance of damage control orthopedic surgery. *Am J Surg.* 2002; 183:622.**
9. Hildebrand F, et al. Damage control: extremities. *Injury* 2004;35:678.
10. Olson SA. Pulmonary aspects of treatment of long bone fractures in the polytrauma patient. *Clin Orthop.* 2004;422:66.
11. Johansen K, et al. Traumatic scapulothoracic dissociation: a case report. *J Trauma* 1991;31:147.
12. Ebraheim NA, et al. Scapulothoracic dissociation (closed avulsion of the scapula, subclavian artery, and brachial plexus): a newly recognized variant, a new classification, and a review of the literature and treatment options. *J Orthop Trauma* 1987;1:18.
13. Hovius SE, et al. Acute management of traumatic forequarter amputations: case reports. *J Trauma* 1991; 31:1415.
14. Dendrinos G, et al. Traumatic hemipelvectomy: a case report and comments on associated injuries. *Acta Orthop Trauma Surg.* 1992;111:293
15. **Rout ML, et al. Circumferential pelvic anti-shock sheeting: A temporary resuscitation aid. *J Orthop Trauma* 2002;16:45.**
16. Krengel WF, et al. Early stabilization and decompression for incomplete paraplegia due to thoracic-level spinal cord injury. *Spine* 1993;18:2080.
17. Grant GA, et al. Risk of early closed reduction in cervical spine subluxation injuries. *J Neurosurg.* 1999;90(suppl 1):13.
18. **Vale FL, et al. Combined medical and surgical treatment after acute spinal cord injury: Results of a prospective pilot study to assess the merits of aggressive medical resuscitation and blood pressure management. *J Neurosurg.* 1997;87:239.**
19. Tator CH, et al. Management of acute spinal cord injuries. *Can J Surg.* 1984;27:289.
20. Myerson MS, et al. Morbidity after crush injuries to the foot. *J Orthop Trauma* 1994;8:343.

21. Mills WJ, et al. The value of the ankle-brachial index for diagnosing arterial injury after knee dislocation: a prospective study. *J Trauma* 2004;56:1261.
22. Klineberg EO, et al. The role of arteriography in assessing popliteal artery injury in knee dislocations. *J Trauma* 2004;56:786.
23. Subasi M, et al. Popliteal artery injuries associated with fractures and dislocations about the knee. *Acta Orthop Belg.* 2001;67:259.
24. **Johansen K, et al. Objective criteria accurately predict amputation following lower extremity trauma. *J Trauma* 1990;30:568.**
25. Bondurant FJ, et al. The medical and economic impact of severely injured lower extremities. *J Trauma* 1988;28:1270.
26. McQueen M. Acute compartment syndrome. *Acta Chir Belg.* 1998;98:166.
27. McQueen M, et al. Compartment monitoring in tibial fractures. The pressure threshold for decompression. *J Bone Joint Surg Br.* 1996;78:99.
28. Heckman MM, et al. Compartment pressure in association with closed tibial fractures. The relationship between tissue pressure, compartment, and the distance from the site of the fracture. *J Bone Joint Surg Am.* 1994;76:1285.
29. Brostrom LA, et al. Acute compartment syndrome in forearm fractures. *Acta Orthop Scand.* 1990;61:50.
30. **MacKenzie EJ, et al. Functional outcomes following trauma-related lower-extremity amputation. *J Bone Joint Surg Am.* 2004(Aug);86-A(8):1636-45. Erratum in: *J Bone Joint Surg Am.* 2004(Nov);86-A(11):2503.**
31. Gustilo RB, et al. The management of open fractures. *J Bone Joint Surg Am* 1990;72:299.
32. Gustilo RB. Use of antimicrobials in the management of open fractures. *Arch Surg.* 1979;114:805.
33. Gustilo RB, et al. Problems in the management of type III (severe) open fractures: a new classification of type III open fractures. *J Trauma* 1984;24:742.
34. Vallier HA, et al. Talar neck fractures: results and outcomes. *J Bone Joint Surg Am.* 2004;86:1616.
35. Canale ST, et al. Fractures of the neck of the talus. Long-term evaluation of seventy-one cases. *J Bone Joint Surg Am.* 1978;60:143.
36. Hawkins LG. Fractures of the neck of the talus. *J Bone Joint Surg Am.* 1970;52:991.
37. **Bone LB, et al. Early versus delayed stabilization of femoral fractures: a prospective randomized study.1989 *Clin Orthop.* 2004;422:11–16.**
38. **Harvery, EG, et al. Deleterious effect of smoking on healing of open tibia-shaft fractures. *Am J Orthop.* 2002;31:518.**
39. **McLain RF. Functional outcomes after surgery for spinal fractures: return to work and activity. *Spine* 2004(Feb 15);29(4):470-477; discussion Z6.**
40. Hansen, ST Jr. Salvage or amputation after complex foot and ankle trauma. *Orthop Clin North Am.* 2001(Jan);32(1):181–186.
41. Grant GA, et al. Evaluation and surgical management of peripheral nerve problems. *Neurosurgery* 1999(Apr);44:825–839; discussion 839–840. Review.
42. Tornetta P 3rd. Hip dislocation: current treatment regimens. *J Am Acad Orthop Surg.* 1997;5(1):27–36.
43. Kregor PJ. The effect of femoral neck fractures on femoral head blood flow. Orthopedics 1996(Dec);19:1031–1036.
44. Henley MB, et al. Treatment of type II, IIIA, and IIIB open fractures of the tibial shaft: a prospective comparison of unreamed interlocking intramedullary nails and half-pin external fixators. *J Orthop Trauma* 1998(Jan);12:1–7.
45. Gosselin RA, et al. Antibiotics for preventing infection in open limb fractures. *Cochrane Database Syst Rev.* 2004;(1):CD003764.
46. Verhelle N, et al. How to deal with bone exposure and osteomyelitis: an overview. *Acta Orthop Belg.* 2003(Dec);69:481–494.
47. Bracken MB, et al. Clinical measurement, statistical analysis, and risk-benefit: controversies from trials of spinal injury. *J Trauma* 2000(Mar); 48:558–561.
48. Bracken MB. Methylprednisolone and acute spinal cord injury: an update of the randomized evidence. *Spine* 2001(Dec 15);26(24 Suppl):S47–S54.
49. Bracken MB, et al. Neurological and functional status 1 year after acute spinal cord injury: estimates of functional recovery in National Acute Spinal Cord Injury Study II from results modeled in National Acute Spinal Cord Injury Study III. J *Neurosurg Spine* 2002;96(3):259–266.
50. Coleman WP, et al. A critical appraisal of the reporting of the National Acute Spinal Cord Injury Studies (II and III) of methylprednisolone in acute spinal cord injury. *J Spinal Disord.* 2000;13(3):185–199.
51. **Bracken MB, et al. Administration of methylprednisolone for 24 or 48 hours or tirilazad mesylate for 48 hours in the treatment of acute spinal cord injury. Results of the Third National Acute Spinal Cord Injury Randomized Controlled Trial. National Acute Spinal Cord Injury Study. *JAMA.* 1997(May 28);277:1597–1604.**

CHAPTER 29 ■ PEDIATRIC TRAUMA

MARY E. FALLAT

EPIDEMIOLOGY

Unintentional injury is the leading cause of death among children ages 14 years and under in the United States and remains the greatest public health problem affecting these young people.[1] The cost of injury in America is estimated at 12% of the total health care cost.[2] Despite the fact that death and disability resulting from trauma surpass all major diseases in young Americans, far more federal funding is spent each year to reduce the incidence of cancer, stroke, heart disease, and AIDS than for injury prevention.

Injury prevention is the most effective method of reducing deaths in children and adolescents. The science of injury prevention is complex and involves societal decisions that trade safety for other benefits. For example, individual states have chosen both to raise the speed limit past 55 miles per hour to reduce travel time and to rescind motorcycle helmet laws to preserve individual freedom, rather than to protect the populace from increased death and disability due to vehicular crashes.[2] Healthcare workers can ultimately play a pivotal role in injury prevention by carefully documenting and collecting data regarding how injuries occur, which will serve the dual roles of identifying populations at risk and providing compelling evidence to lawmakers in support of effective injury prevention legislation.

Trauma registries are one way to show trends or patterns of specific injuries and to use cumulative data to build a case for legislation. The National Pediatric Trauma Registry (NTPR) and the National Trauma Registry of the American College of Surgeons (NTRACS) are examples of national registries that have identified and can elucidate areas to target for prevention initiatives. The predominant mechanism of injury varies by age, with falls more common in young children, pedestrian injuries most common in toddlers and elementary school age children, and motor vehicle trauma most common in adolescents.

Mortality rates for all types of trauma are greater in rural parts of the country than in cities and suburbs. The reasons for this are protean and include longer times from injury to definitive care,[3] in-hospital delays to definitive treatment,[4] less time for injury prevention education in schools and primary care offices, and socioeconomic and ethnic factors. Other associations have been identified that increase susceptibility to trauma. For example, children with behavioral disorders such as attention–deficit hyperactivity disorder (ADHD) have one and one half times the odds of sustaining a variety of injuries from multiple causes than those without behavioral disorders, even after controlling for known demographic correlates.[5]

The "trimodal" mortality curve described in adults is not seen in children. Children who die from injury do so either at the scene or within a few hours of hospital admission. Late deaths due to sepsis or organ failure are rare.[6] After injury control, prompt recognition and emergent treatment of all life-threatening injuries are the most important way to decrease death and disability after pediatric trauma.

PREHOSPITAL CARE

Pediatric runs represent approximately 10% of all prehospital emergency calls in the United States. Although educational courses such as Pediatric Education for the Prehospital Professional (PEPP)[7] and Pediatric Advanced Life Support (PALS)[8] have augmented the knowledge base of some prehospital providers, the recommended amount of pediatric training included in the Department of Transportation's national standard curriculum for emergency medical technicians and paramedics is temporally limited and basic. The adequacy of prehospital airway management and the ability to obtain venous access in children are associated with proper training, experience, skill maintainance, and medical oversight for individual prehospital care providers.[9,10]

All ambulances must be equipped with pediatric equipment in various sizes, including blood pressure cuffs, masks, endotracheal tubes, and intravenous (IV) access devices. Prehospital care of injured pediatric patients may be limited to maintaining spinal precautions, assurance of an adequate airway, administration of oxygen, and rapid transport to definitive care for short transports. Establishment of IV or intraosseous access (IO) is recommended for longer transport times. The goal is to prevent secondary brain injury associated with hypoxia or hypotension by controlling the airway and striving for normotension with appropriate fluid resuscitation.

An inclusive trauma system must provide for the needs of injured children as well as adults, with triage by the prehospital provider to the closest appropriate facility with the capabilities of caring for major trauma. This may be a pediatric trauma center or a regional trauma center with pediatric commitment.[11] The receiving center must have the necessary personnel and equipment to care for the injured child, as outlined in *Resources for Optimal Care of the Injured Patient: 1999* by the Committee on Trauma, American College of Surgeons.[12]

INITIAL RESUSCITATION AND EVALUATION

Preparation is the key to a successful pediatric trauma resuscitation. In institutions using a team approach, interventions may be done simultaneously (i.e., for airway and circulation).

The best protection for the airway in the child who is breathing spontaneously is maintainance of a superior and anterior position of the middle face (sniffing position), while keeping the cervical spine immobilized. If the airway is inadequate, it can be opened with a gentle jaw thrust. The mouth is cleared of blood and foreign material and supplemental oxygen used. In a young child, respiratory compromise can result from gastric dilatation or from compression of the diaphragm by intraabdominal blood or air, necessitating the use of a gastric tube. The tube should be inserted orally if there is concern for a basilar skull or midface fracture.

Children with obvious respiratory distress, a Glasgow Coma Scale (GCS) score of 8 or lower, or those who arrive in shock must have immediate tracheal intubation. The proper-sized endotracheal tube can be estimated by choosing one that corresponds to the diameter of the child's small finger or the nares or using an appropriate reference as a guide. An excellent approach is the use of color-coded drawers containing all of the equipment necessary for a certain size child and using a length-based pediatric resuscitation tape to estimate the child's weight.[13] In children younger than 8 years, nasotracheal intubation is avoided because of the more anterior and cephalad positioned airway, relatively large adenoids and tonsils, a soft short trachea, and the potentially serious complications associated with blind nasal passage. After preoxygenation, a drug-assisted intubation using a neuromuscular blocker and a sedative is performed, unless the child has a GCS of 3 or has arrested. A chest radiograph should be obtained to confirm proper position of the endotracheal tube. If the airway cannot be secured by the most senior person in the resuscitation room, a temporizing needle cricothyrotomy is placed and jet insufflation initiated until an airway can be established in the operating room. Tracheostomy in young children is reserved for experienced surgeons under operating room conditions only.

Because of small blood volumes in children, shock can occur rapidly from blood loss from external wounds (Fig. 29.1). Bleeding should be controlled with pressure bandages. Preferred sites for percutaneous IV access in the child are the back of the hand, the antecubital fossa, and the saphenous vein at the ankle. If a child is in shock, and no IV line can be established after two attempts, an IO needle is placed in an uninjured proximal tibia. Alternatively, a percutaneous femoral venous line can be placed by an experienced physician. It is important to follow a protocol so that time is not wasted with too many attempts at percutaneous IV access before resuscitation can begin. Baseline laboratory work can be drawn concurrent with establishing IV access, including at least a complete blood count (CBC), serum aspartate aminotransferase or alanine aminotransferase, amylase, and urine dip for blood. A urinalysis is done if there is occult blood in the urine specimen. A clot to hold or type and cross-match is sent to the blood bank as indicated by the physiologic status of the child. An arterial blood gas is sent if the child required tracheal intubation. A prothrombin time (PT) and partial thromboplastin time (PTT) are indicated for a GCS below 13, low systolic blood pressure, open/multiple bony fractures, and major soft tissue wounds.[14]

A child's systolic blood pressure should be at least 70 mm Hg plus twice his or her age in years.[8] In general, a blood pressure of less than 70 mm Hg systolic is considered shock in a child, with the exception of small infants. Hypotension is a late sign of shock because of the increased physiologic reserve in children compared with adults. The initial signs of shock can be subtle in a child and manifested only by tachycardia or lethargy. Once hypotension has developed, a child has already lost approximately 40% of the circulating blood volume and traumatic arrest is imminent if treatment is delayed.

Fluid resuscitation begins with 20 mL/kg of warmed lactated Ringer's solution given by rapid IV/IO push. This is approximately one fourth of the blood volume of a child. This fluid bolus can be repeated twice, but if the child remains in shock, the source of bleeding should be quickly identified and addressed. Transfusion of O negative packed red blood cells may be needed at an initial volume of 10 mL/kg. A Foley catheter should be inserted, assuming no blood at the urethral meatus or an unstable pelvic fracture. In addition to reestablishing normotension, a proper response to resuscitation includes slowing of the heart rate, return of extremity skin color and warmth, clearing of the sensorium, and a sustained urine output of 1 to 2 mL/kg/hour.

Small children are especially prone to hypothermia, which may render the child unresponsive to resuscitation efforts. Use

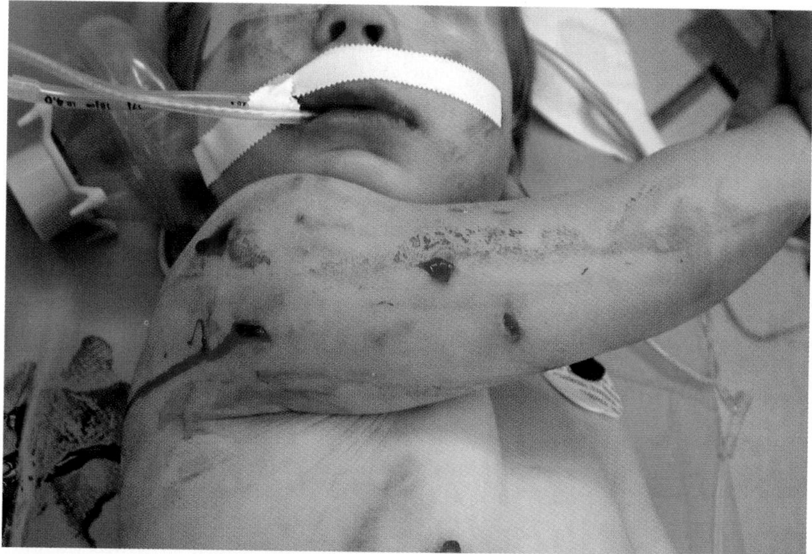

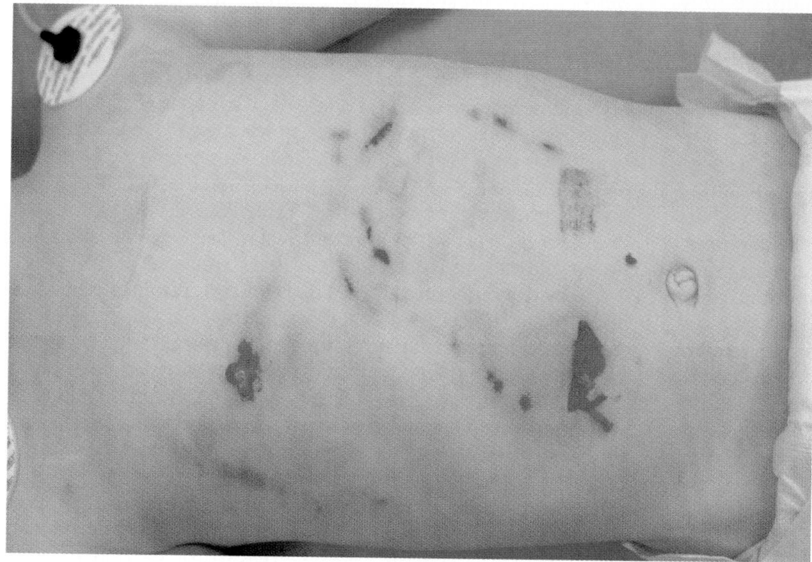

FIGURE 29.1 Child with multiple dog bites on face, extremities, and torso.

of convective air blankets, warm IV fluids, and warm blankets is indicated as soon as feasible.

During the resuscitation, radiographic studies of the chest and pelvis are performed and cervical spine protection is maintained until at least three views can be obtained (anteroposterior, lateral, and odontoid). Clearing of the cervical spine is relatively elective; time should not be wasted on these films if other injuries take priority. In the unstable child, a quick sonographic evaluation of the pericardium and the peritoneum [the focused sonographic assessment for trauma (FAST) examination] for blood can be helpful in establishing the priorities of treatment. Blood in the pericardial or peritoneal cavity in the persistently unstable child demands surgical intervention. In the stable child, a computed tomography (CT) scan of the abdomen and pelvis with IV contrast is indicated in certain situations (Table 29.1).

Although ultrasound is reasonably sensitive in detecting the presence of fluid in the abdomen, its accuracy is highly dependent

TABLE 29.1 ■ INDICATIONS/CONTRAINDICATIONS

INDICATIONS FOR COMPUTED TOMOGRAPHY OF THE ABDOMEN AND PELVIS

- History of shock but now stable
- Unexplained drop in hematocrit
- Positive FAST examination
- Presence of hematuria
- Presence of lower rib or pelvic fractures
- Unreliable abdominal examination because of head injury
- Presence of abdominal pain/ecchymosis
- Uncorrected base deficit

FAST, focused sonographic assessment for trauma.

on the operator. Some data suggest that hospital resources are conserved when the FAST examination is incorporated into the algorithm in the evaluation of the pediatric abdomen after blunt trauma.[15] Ultrasound, however, may not detect the presence of intraparenchymal solid organ injuries without free blood, may miss small amounts of blood early in the resuscitation, cannot be used to grade the degree of injury to a solid organ, and cannot exclude pancreatic injury. In addition, the finding of blood in the peritoneum in a stable child does not dictate laparotomy. For all these reasons, the role of FAST in pediatric trauma patients remains controversial. Neither ultrasound nor CT reliably detects the presence of a bowel injury. Serial abdominal examinations and, potentially, DPL are indicated.

Throughout this critical period of resuscitation and evaluation, the emotional needs of the child must be kept constantly in mind. A frightened child is emotionally labile and may regress to infantile behavior. A calm and reassuring approach with attempted explanation of procedures gains the most cooperation. There is evidence that the psychological effects surrounding a traumatic event are long lasting, even if the trauma is relatively minor. The needs of the "injured" family must be met by providing a continual flow of information to the distressed parents or guardian during the resuscitation. A chaplain or member of the family support services staff can admirably serve this vital role on a pediatric trauma team.

With the shift in medical training from disease-centered to patient-centered and family-centered care, there has also been increasing interest in and tolerance of family presence during invasive procedures and cardiopulmonary resuscitation[16,17] Although this concept has had limited exposure in the emergency pediatric trauma setting, family members often desire to be present and are more accepting of death and more satisfied with the level of care that their loved one received if they witness the events of the resuscitation.[18] Pediatric healthcare workers who have more frequent contact with seriously ill children are more likely to accept parental presence.[17]

MANAGEMENT OF SPECIFIC INJURIES

Neurologic and Extracranial Head Trauma

Traumatic brain injury (TBI) is the leading cause of traumatic death and disability in children. Unique to infants is the large number of traumatic brain injuries resulting from child maltreatment. The aim of neurosurgical care is to minimize secondary brain damage that may occur after a severe TBI.

TABLE 29.2

PEDIATRIC VERBAL SCORE

Verbal response	Verbal score
Appropriate words or social smile, fixes and follows	5
Cries but consolable	4
Persistently irritable	3
Restless, agitated	2
None	1

Adapted from American College of Surgeons Committee on Trauma. Advanced trauma life support course for doctors: student course manual, 7th ed), Chapter 10.A, p. 257. Chicago: American College of Surgeons, 2004.

Primary treatment of a child with a TBI begins with correction of hypoxemia and shock by restoring oxygenation, ventilation, and perfusion. A thorough neurologic examination is performed and documented, including the GCS score. The verbal portion of the score has been adapted for application in infants and toddlers, but it is the motor score that correlates best with outcome (Table 29.2). Except for the most minor cases, a head CT scan is performed in all children with evidence of neurologic injury (Fig. 29.2).

Guidelines for the acute medical management of severe traumatic brain injury in infants, children, and adolescents were published in 2003. The goal of the document was to assimilate the data that exists and present it within an evidence-based framework to provide treatment guidelines.[19] The guidelines address key issues relating to the management of severe TBI in pediatric patients with a GCS score of 3 to 8. *Pediatric* is defined as less than 18 years of age, and *TBI* is defined as primary or secondary injury to the brain resulting from a traumatic cause (includes abusive head injury). For purposes of defining the guidelines, class I evidence included only randomized controlled trials, class II evidence was clinical studies in which the data were collected prospectively and retrospective analyses that were based on clearly reliable data, and class III evidence was most studies based on retrospectively collected data. The guidelines were proposed as standards, or accepted principles of patient management that reflect a high degree of clinical certainty; guidelines, or a particular strategy or range of management strategies that reflect a moderate clinical certainty; and options, or the remaining strategies for patient management for which there is unclear clinical certainty. Table 29.3 lists recommendations based on topics. If no pediatric data were given, extrapolation of indications from adult guidelines are listed.

Secondary measures to treat TBI in children include evacuation of an intracranial space occupying hematoma, normalization of intracranial pressure and maintainance of tissue oxygen, external ventricular drainage, and decompressive craniectomy in rare cases of conservative treatment failure.[20] Although mass lesions from hemorrhage requiring surgical intervention are relatively uncommon in children, cerebral edema is common. Children with a GCS score of 8 or less and those with evidence of cerebral edema on CT scan require sedation, paralysis, endotracheal intubation, and mechanical ventilation to keep the partial pressure of carbon dioxide ($Paco_2$) at approximately 35 mm Hg. An intracranial pressure monitor (or ventriculostomy catheter) is placed, with the exception of infants with open cranial sutures, so that a cerebral perfusion pressure of at least 50 to 70 mm Hg can be maintained. Brain metabolism is minimized by treating fever and avoiding seizures. Despite aggressive treatment, the overall mortality rate from severe head injury in pediatric patients is approximately 8%, and the coexistence of extracranial injury significantly reduces recovery potential.[21] There is significant reported variation in the use of paralytic agents, seizure medications, induced hypothermia, and intracranial pressure monitoring across pediatric critical care units.[22] Interestingly, the use of anticonvulsants may be associated with reduced mortality.[22] A study in patients with severe head injuries found that survival was associated with a maximum systolic blood pressure greater than or equal to 135 mm Hg.[23]

There is an exponential rise in the incidence of facial fractures associated with skull fractures between infancy and adolescence.[24] The GCS of children with combined facial and skull fractures is lower than in those with skull fractures only, suggesting that a higher energy injury may be required for combined skull and facial fractures in the pediatric population.

Although children in general have a higher survival rate after head injury, they may be more vulnerable to long-term disability than adults. For the child with long-term disabilities resulting from traumatic brain injury, there is a major

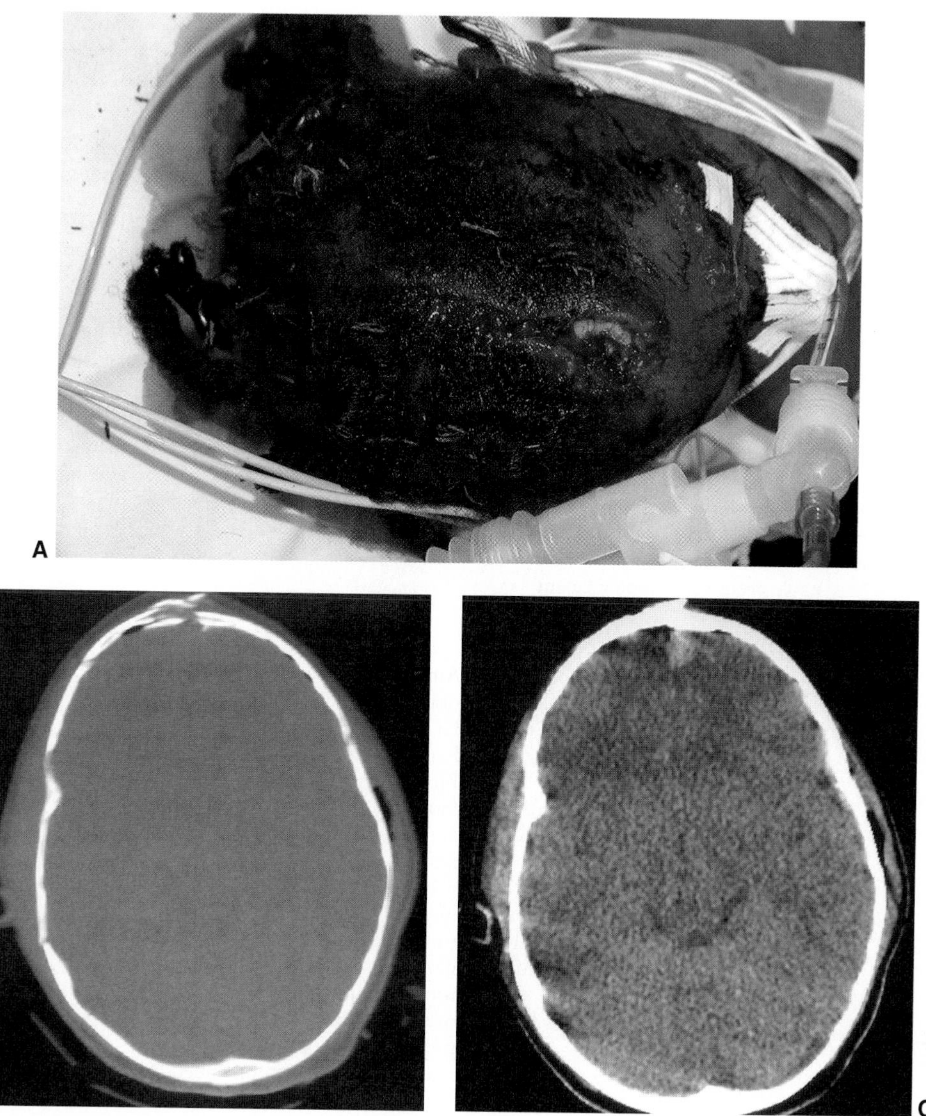

FIGURE 29.2 (*A*) Scalp wound with underlying open frontal skull fracture. (*B*) Bone window CT image showing comminuted frontal skull fracture, pneumocephaly and multiple additional skull fractures. (C) A small frontal contusion is seen beneath the skull fracture.

impact on both their personal quality of life and that of their family.[25]

Spinal Trauma

The incidence of pediatric spine injuries has been reported as 2% to 5% of all spine injuries.[26] Spine injuries in children are less common than in adults because of the greater mobility and elasticity of the pediatric spine and the smaller mass of the child's body.

Certain anatomic features predispose younger children (age less than 8 years) to injury of the upper cervical spine, from the occiput to the base of C-2.[26,27] These include a proportionately heavier head and weak ligaments that permit greater mobility of C-1 on C-2 compared with the lower spine; horizontally inclined articulating facets and immature vertebral joints that facilitate sliding; growth centers that are susceptible to shear forces during rapid deceleration or hyperflexion–extension; and a higher fulcrum of flexion.[27] In children less than 8 years old, cervical spine fractures are seen primarily at C-5 to C-6, resulting from motor vehicle trauma or diving mishaps.

Some normal anatomic variables make interpretation of cervical spine films in children challenging.[27,28] Pseudo-subluxation occurs normally in approximately 40% of children and is most commonly seen as anterior displacement of C-2 on C-3. An increased distance between the dens and the anterior arch of C-1 may also occur without any pathologic consequences. Skeletal growth centers may resemble fractures, especially involving the odontoid and the spinous processes. If there is doubt over whether an abnormality exists, it is wise to protect the spine until expert consultation can be arranged.

An abnormality seen more commonly in children is spinal cord injury without radiographic abnormality (SCIWORA).[29] This phenomenon is attributed to the elastic nature of the child's spine and may result from longitudinal distraction, hyperflexion, hyperextension, or spinal cord ischemia. The diagnosis is established by magnetic resonance imaging.

High-dose steroid therapy should be initiated immediately if spinal cord injury is suspected.[30,31] Long-term results of management of spinal injuries in children confirm the validity of conservative treatment for stable fractures and the need for early surgical treatment for unstable fractures and fractures with associated spinal cord injury.[26]

TABLE 29.3

GUIDELINES FOR PREHOSPITAL MANAGEMENT OF PEDIATRIC TRAUMATIC BRAIN INJURY

TOPICS	RECOMMENDATIONS Standards	Guidelines	Options	Indications from adult guidelines
Trauma systems, pediatric trauma centers, and the neurosurgeon	None	In a metropolitan area, pediatric patients with severe TBI should be transported directly to a PTC if available	Pediatric patients with severe TBI should be treated in a PTC or in an ATC with added qualifications for pediatrics in preference to a level I or II ATC	There is an overall reduction in mortality rate for individuals with severe TBI after implementation of an organized trauma system
Prehospital airway management	None	Hypoxia must be avoided if possible and attempts made to correct it immediately. Supplemental oxygen should be administered. There is no evidence to support an advantage of ETI over BVM ventilation for the prehospital management of the airway in children with TBI	If prehospital ETI is instituted for pediatric TBI patients, specialized training and use of end-tidal CO_2 detectors is necessary	The airway should be secured in patients who have severe head injury (GCS <9), the inability to maintain an adequate airway, or hypoxemia not corrected by supplemental oxygen
Resuscitation of blood pressure and oxygenation and prehospital brain-specific therapies for the severe pediatric traumatic brain injury patient	None	Hypotension should be identified and corrected as rapidly as possible with fluid resuscitation. Hypotension is defined as systolic blood pressure below the 5th percentile for age or by clinical signs of shock. The lower limit of systolic blood pressure (5th percentile) for age may be estimated by the formula: 70 mm of mercury + (2 × age in years)[a]	Airway control should be obtained in children with a GCS ≤ 8 to avoid hypoxemia, hypercarbia and aspiration. Blood pressure should be monitored frequently and accurately. Timely fluid administration should be provided to maintain systolic blood pressure in the normal range. Sedation, analgesia, and neuromuscular blockade can be useful to optimize transport of the patient with TBI. The prophylactic administration of mannitol is not recommended.[b] Mild prophylactic hyperventilation is not recommended.[c]	

[a]American Heart Association: Pediatric Advanced Life Support. American Heart Association, 2000.
[b]Mannitol may be considered for use in euvolemic patients who show signs of cerebral herniation or acute neurologic deterioration.
[c]Hyperventilation may be considered in patients who show signs of cerebral herniation or acute neurologic deterioration, after correcting hypotension or hypoxemia.
TBI, traumatic brain injury; PTC, pediatric trauma center; ATC, adult trauma center; BVM, bag-valve-mask; ETI, endotracheal intubation; GSC, Glasgow Coma Score
Adapted from Adelson PD, Bratton SL, Carney NA, et al. Guidelines for the acute medical management of severe traumatic brain injury in infants, children and adolescents. *Pediatr Crit Care Med.* 2003;4(suppl):S1–S18.

Thoracic Trauma

There are important anatomic and physiologic differences between children and adults who present with thoracic injury. Rib fractures are uncommon in children because both bone and cartilage in the chest wall are more pliable. Multiple fractures are associated with increased morbidity and mortality, and displaced rib fractures can occasionally cause thoracic or abdominal injury. Posterior rib fractures in infants have a high association with child maltreatment. Aortic and great vessel injury are uncommon because of greater vessel elasticity and mobility of mediastinal structures. Enhanced pulmonary vasoconstriction results in less bleeding.

The most common injuries in children are pulmonary contusion, hemothorax, and pneumothorax because of the increased pliability of the chest wall. Pulmonary parenchymal injury following blunt trauma may result from direct compression, shearing forces, contrecoup compression, or laceration from fractured ribs. Chest radiography is the primary screening modality for thoracic injury. It is used to identify life-threatening injuries and to locate tubes and catheters (Fig. 29.3). Pulmonary contusion is characterized by areas of alveolar and interstitial hemorrhage and edema that appear as ill-defined opacities that do not follow anatomic boundaries.[32] Secondary edema from disruption of the alveolar-capillary interface peaks at 24 to 36 hours following injury, and the radiographic appearance of the lungs

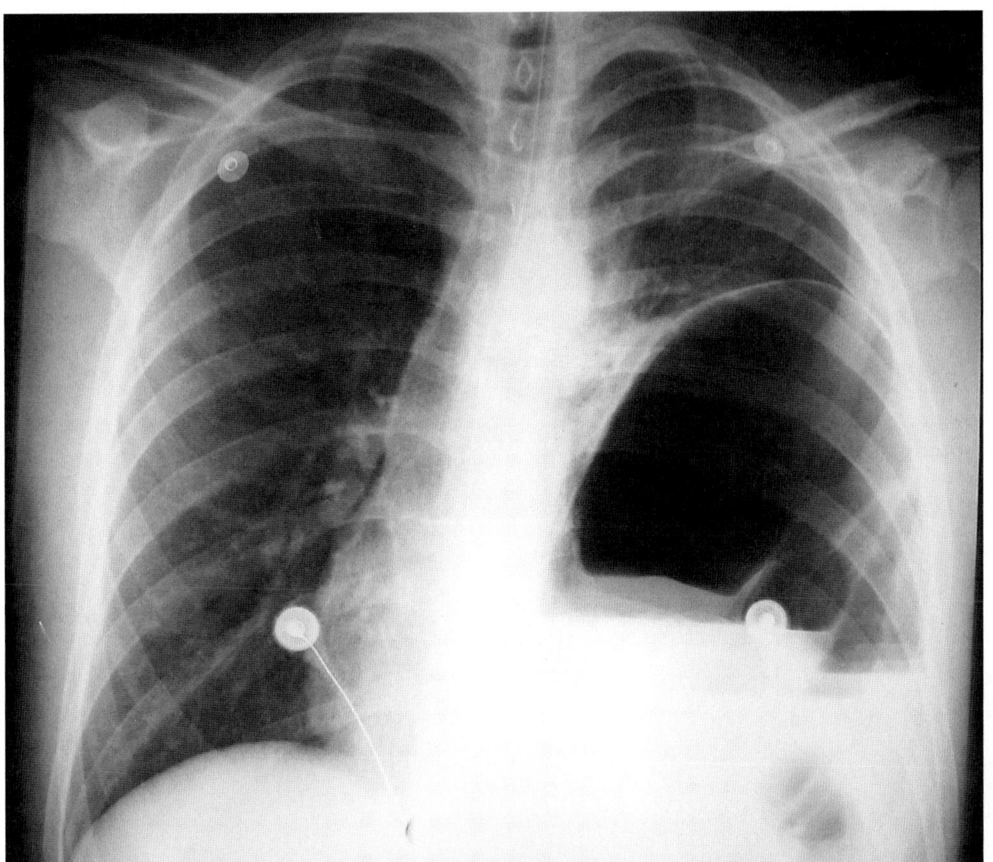

FIGURE 29.3 Anteroposterior chest x-ray showing an air-fluid level in the left chest and diaphragm elevation indicative of a traumatic diaphragmatic hernia. The cardiac silhouette is deviated into the right chest.

may worsen over the first several days. Pneumothorax and pneumomediastinum most commonly occur following alveolar or small airway rupture. Air dissects medially along peribronchial tissues toward the mediastinum or pleural space. If the air dissection is extensive, increased air pressure shifts the flexible mediastinum, compressing the contralateral lung and twisting the great vessels (tension pneumothorax).[32] If this condition is not emergently corrected, venous return to the heart is decreased and shock may ensue.

Pulmonary contusion may not be obvious on the initial chest radiograph but may be seen on CT scan. Hemothoraces and pneumothoraces are managed as in adults. Tracheobronchial disruption should be suspected in a child with a tension pneumothorax, massive subcutaneous emphysema, and a continuing air leak or persistent collapse of the lung despite a functioning chest tube. The diagnosis is confirmed by bronchoscopy. Dynamic chest CT provides improved detection and detail of pleural, parenchymal, mediastinal, and chest wall injury. It lacks specificity for esophageal, tracheal, and main stem bronchial disruption or for cardiac injury.

Blunt cardiac injuries can occur in children and range from mild to lethal.[33] The primary mechanisms of injury associated with this diagnosis are motor vehicle and pedestrian-related trauma. It is extremely rare for a hemodynamically stable patient with a normal sinus rhythm to develop a subsequent cardiac dysrhythmia or cardiac failure.[33] Significant cardiac injuries rarely occur in isolation, and most of these children die at the scene.[34] A few survive and are transported to trauma centers. Use of the FAST examination of the pericardium can readily identify these children and allow for prompt treatment.

Thoracic aortic rupture is a rare injury in children but is highly lethal if undiagnosed. A report from the National Pediatric Trauma Registry described 28 patients (from a total of 25,301) with traumatic aortic disruptions and a mortality rate of 57%.[35] Multisystem trauma from motor vehicle crashes or pedestrian collisions are the most common mechanisms. An appropriate mechanism of injury in conjunction with a chest radiograph demonstrating a wide mediastinum should raise suspicion and prompt investigation. Dynamic spiral CT scan of the chest may be used as a screening test, but arch angiography remains the most definitive method of diagnosis. Good outcomes can be expected from early diagnosis, antihypertensive therapy, and definitive operative management.

Abdominal Trauma

Twenty-five percent of children who sustain trauma have abdominal injuries. Unstable patients should undergo a FAST examination in the trauma room, and those with positive findings in the setting of continued hemodynamic abnormality despite fluid resuscitation should be taken straight to the operating room. The FAST examination will miss solid organ intraparenchymal injuries without free fluid, and stable pediatric trauma patients with major injury mechanisms or abdominal tenderness are evaluated with an abdominal and pelvic CT scan using IV contrast and then serial physical examinations during inpatient observation.[36–38] Six findings have been independently associated with intraabdominal injury, including systolic blood pressure below normal for age, abdominal tenderness, associated femur fracture, serum

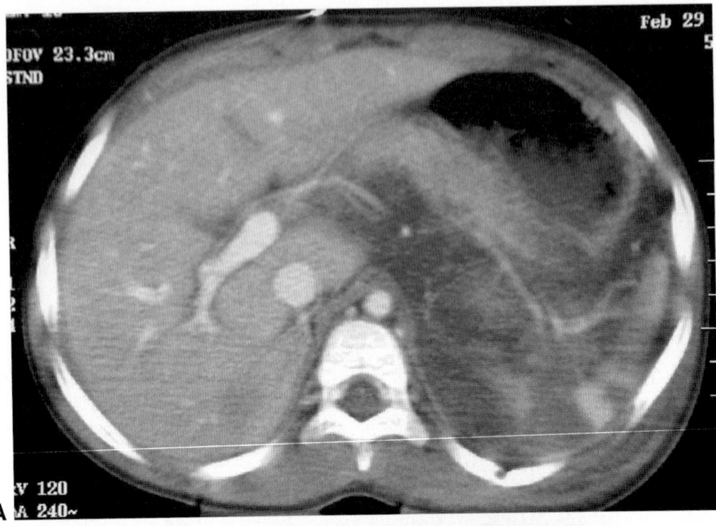

A

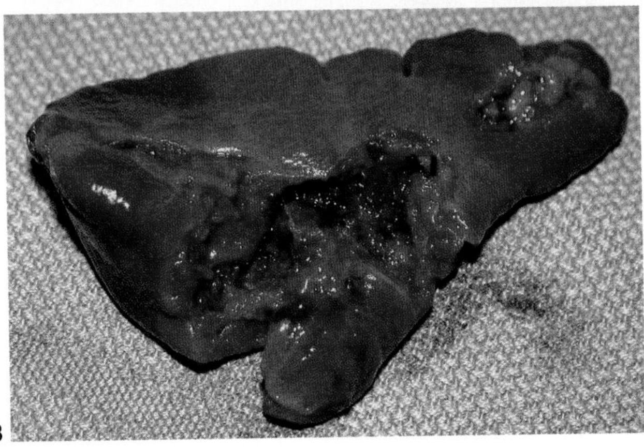

B

FIGURE 29.4 (*A*) Abdominal computed tomography image showing grade V splenic rupture with extravasation of contrast. (*B*) Ruptured spleen.

aspartate aminotransferase concentration greater than 200 IU/L or serum alanine aminotrasferase concentration above 125 IU/L, urinalysis showing more than 5 RBCs per high power field, and an initial hematocrit of less than 30%.[39]

The approach to solid organ injuries (liver, spleen, kidney) discovered on CT scan is primarily observational. Most (more than 90%) of these injuries heal without operation. The kidney is relatively large and anterior, and a significant abdominal blow often manifests with hematuria. However, hematuria is more often associated with a liver or spleen injury than with a significant renal injury. The indications for operation in children with solid organ injury include evidence of ongoing bleeding, uncorrected base deficit, persistent hemodynamic abnormality, the development of peritoneal signs or other signs and symptoms of an associated gastrointestinal (GI) injury, or major urinary extravasation with a renal injury. Although most pediatric patients with blunt abdominal trauma do not require operation, the need for surgical judgment in determining which children fail nonoperative therapy is critical (Fig. 29.4).

Until recently, there has been little consensus on the need for intensive care, the amount of transfusion considered acceptable, the need for and timing of follow-up imaging procedures, and the activities allowed after discharge of a child with a liver or spleen injury.[40,41] A prospective study by the American Pediatric Surgical Association of stable patients with traumatic liver and spleen injuries revealed a very low incidence of nonoperative failures (zero in some centers), a general agreement that transfusions were not required unless the hemoglobin fell to 7 to 8 g/dL, and that only children with grade IV injuries needed observation in an intensive care unit (ICU) setting for 24 to 48 hours.[42] Children may be allowed out of bed when the hematocrit stabilizes, abdominal pain resolves, and hematuria is no longer present (renal injuries). Routine follow-up imaging is unnecessary in the absence of recurrent signs or symptoms of an abdominal complication. Recommendations on activity level after discharge have been tested prospectively with a very low failure rate (Table 29.4). A reasonable approach to the stable child with a solid organ injury is outlined in Table 29.5.

Pancreatic injuries occur in less than 1% of pediatric trauma patients but carry a high morbidity and mortality risk if

TABLE 29.4

EVIDENCE-BASED STANDARDS FOR RESOURCE UTILIZATION IN CHILDREN WITH ISOLATED BLUNT SPLEEN AND LIVER INJURIES

	CT Grade			
	I	II	III	IV
ICU stay	None	None	None	1 day
Hospital stay	2 days	3 days	4 days	5 days
Predischarge imaging	None	None	None	None
Postdischarge imaging	None	None	None	None
Activity restriction	3 wk	4 wk	5 wk	6 wk

Reprinted with permission from Stylianos S. Evidence-based guidelines for resource utilization in children with isolated spleen or liver injury. APSA Trauma Committee. *J Pediatr Surg* 2000;35:164–169.

TABLE 29.5 TREATMENT

APPROACH TO THE STABLE CHILD WITH A SOLID ORGAN INJURY

- Documentation of the degree of injury by computed tomography scan
- A brief hospital stay based on physiologic status
- Allow ambulation when pain and tenderness resolve
- Allow oral intake when pain and tenderness resolve
- Discharge when eating, ambulating without pain, and stable hematocrit
- Selectively repeat computed tomography scan for those with recurrent signs or symptoms following initial resolution
- Office follow-up before release to return to contact sports and physical education at school

overlooked. The mechanism of injury is usually a blow to the epigastrium, such as with the handlebars of a bicycle. Pancreatic injuries also may be the result of child maltreatment. Abdominal tenderness frequently is absent initially. The most sensitive diagnostic study is an abdominal CT scan with oral and IV contrast, but this injury can be missed on the initial scan. The approach to a blunt pancreatic injury is conservative unless major ductal disruption is present.[43] Postinjury complications include pancreatic fistula or pseudocyst. Both may resolve with drainage alone.

With abdominal and pelvic CT scan as the cornerstone of diagnosis after blunt abdominal trauma in children, and a general nonoperative approach to solid organ injuries, much attention has been directed toward the diagnosis of small intestinal injuries in these patients.[44–46] Blunt intestinal injuries occur in 1% to 5% of pediatric patients with abdominal trauma. Mechanisms of injury involve intrusion type blows and can include restrained or unrestrained motor vehicle passengers involved in crashes, pedestrians struck by motor vehicles, child maltreatment, bike handlebar injuries, and direct blows to the abdomen or back (Fig. 29.5). The initial findings on physical examination may be subtle.

A

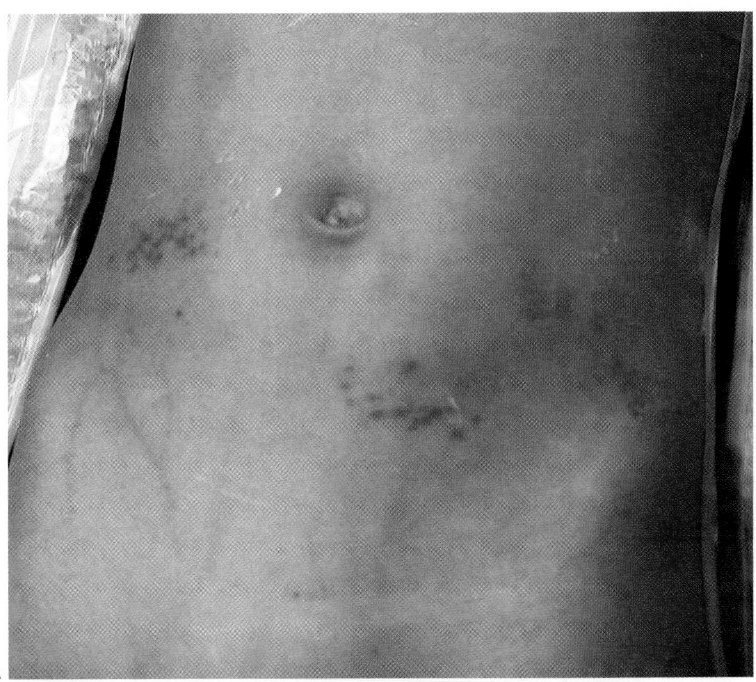

B

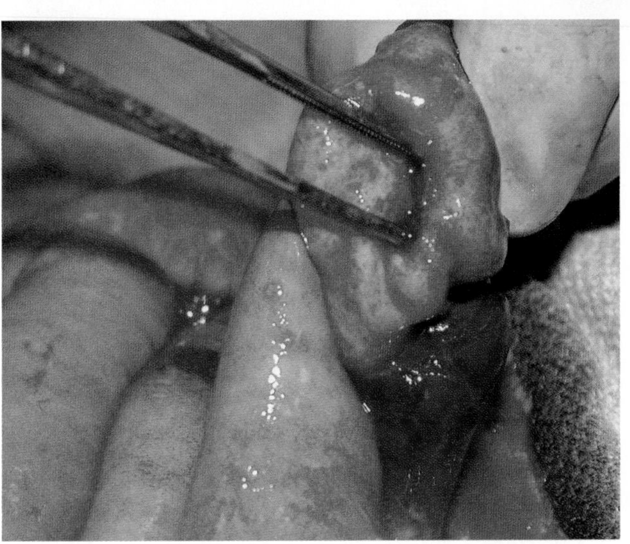

FIGURE 29.5 (*A*) Ecchymosis of the abdominal wall resulting from improperly positioned seatbelt on the torso of a small child. (*B*) Deserosalized segment of jejunum containing enterotomy.

Findings on CT scan may be equally subtle and include extravasation of *per os* (PO) contrast material, free intraabdominal air, localized bowel wall thickening or dilatation or signs of a mesenteric hematoma.[45] The presence of free pelvic fluid that is not associated with a solid organ injury is especially concerning for an intestinal injury. The presence of a small intestinal injury also should be suspected when there are associated spinal fractures caused by the use of a lap belt (lap belt complex, or Chance fractures) without a shoulder harness.[47] Occasionally, a blunt injury to the abdomen results in a hematoma that causes obstruction but not a full-thickness injury. This is most common in the duodenum and usually resolves with conservative treatment.[44] At least one study in children with a missed or delayed diagnosis of GI tract injury showed no significant differences in ICU stay, total length of stay, associated injuries, and mortality compared with children who had a timely diagnosis. However, there was a significant increase in complications including abscess, fistula, wound infection, and delayed intestinal obstruction. Signs and symptoms in children whose injuries are initially missed exhibit evolving signs of peritonitis including fever, increasing abdominal pain, leukocytosis, and tachycardia (Fig. 29.6).[46]

Pelvic Fractures and Extremity Trauma

Fractures are the second most common injury occurring in pediatric trauma patients. Blood loss associated with bony injuries, especially in the pelvis, is proportionately greater in the child than in the adult, and this fact must be considered during volume resuscitation. Depending on age, location, and type of fracture, options for stabilization and alignment include casting, traction followed by casting, various methods of internal fixation including flexible rods and plates, and external fixation.[48] External fixation is particularly well suited for open complex fractures, fractures complicated by extensive soft tissue injury, open fractures complicated by a vascular injury, or fractures in multiple trauma victims who will require prolonged rehabilitation.

Trauma to the growing extremity of a child can cause a bend without complete fracture of the bone (greenstick fracture). If the epiphysis of a long bone is involved, there may be long-term consequences in bone growth and development. Supracondylar fractures at the elbow are relatively common in children and may be associated with vascular injury. All injured extremities must be monitored carefully with frequent

A

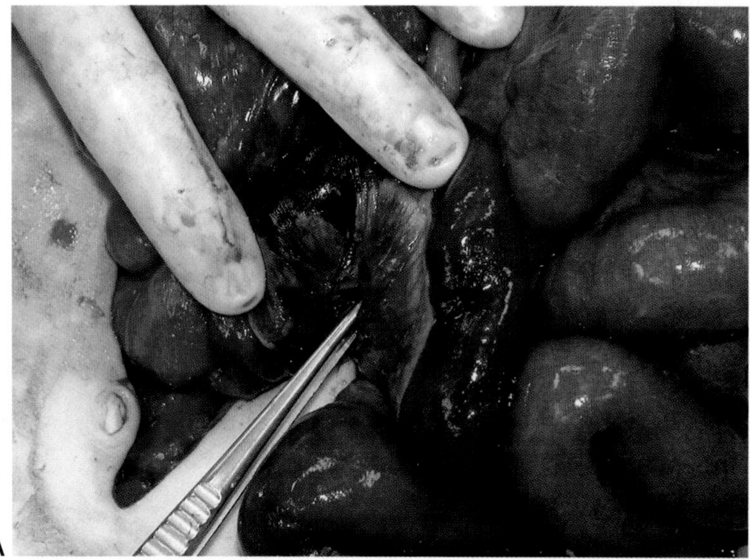

B

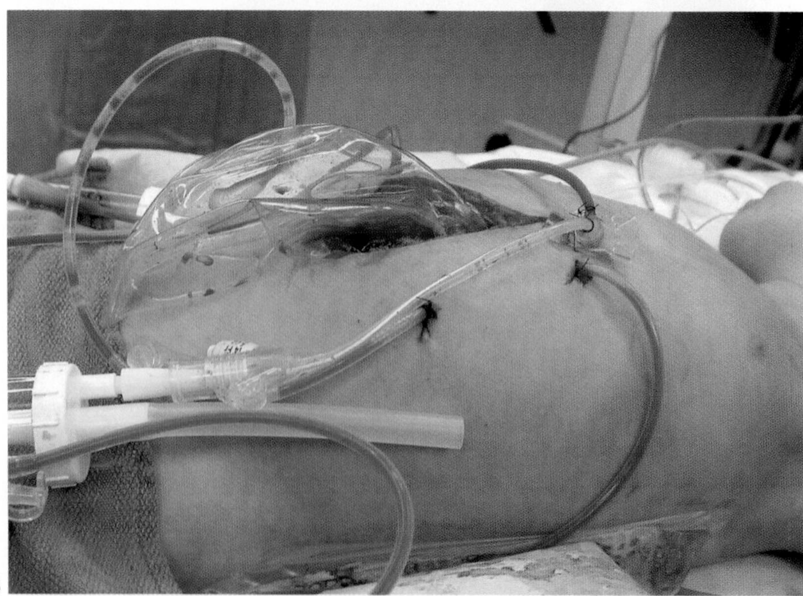

FIGURE 29.6 (*A*) Jejunal hematoma and perforation at the ligament of Treitz resulting from child maltreatment. This child presented in hypovolemic shock. (*B*) The abdomen was treated open for several days using a conventional, commercially available pediatric silo.

neurovascular examinations for possible development of a compartment syndrome.

Children with pelvic fractures are at risk for life-threatening hemorrhage and associated abdominal injuries.[49] At significant risk for hemorrhage are patients with bilateral anterior and posterior fractures.[50] The presence of multiple pelvic fractures also predicts the presence of associated genitourinary and abdominal injuries.

Delay in diagnosis of fractures is common in both the minimally and the multiply injured child.[51] A representative study of 149 multiply injured Canadian children with 494 total injuries reported a 6% incidence of delayed fracture diagnosis (46% of the 13 missed injuries).[52] Children who are evaluated in emergency departments after trauma and subsequently discharged home should be asked to ambulate first, to avoid missing an occult fracture.

CHILD MALTREATMENT

All physicians caring for injured children have an ethical and legal responsibility to recognize and report the possibility of child maltreatment. The Centers for Disease Control and Prevention estimates that abuse and neglect is responsible for 4.5 of every 10,000 deaths in children 4 years of age and younger. Sadly, most children who die or sustain serious injury from child maltreatment have a history of previous injury. Deaths or additional injuries are potentially preventable if the abusive behavior is recognized and remediated or the child is removed to foster care. Inconsistency between the history and the anatomic injury or discrepancies in injury mechanism reported by involved adults should alert the medical provider to suspect maltreatment. Frequently, the child has been taken to several different emergency departments to avoid raising suspicion. Physical signs of child abuse include laceration or tear of the upper frenulum, retinal hemorrhages, multiple subdural hematomas without an acute skull fracture, genital or perianal injuries, burns in unusual areas (including burns caused by cigarettes), multiple torso bruises, and radiographic evidence of multiple old or healed fractures. If maltreatment is suspected, hospital admission is mandatory and a formal report is required by law in most states.

PERFORMANCE INDICATORS

The pediatric trauma system requires constant reevaluation. Because death after trauma is relatively less common in children who are brought to the hospital alive (compared with adults), pediatric performance filters are aimed at reducing morbidity after injury. Participation in systemwide reviews and a commitment to correction of identified problems is required of all professionals caring for injured children to ensure the best possible outcomes.

FUNCTIONAL RECOVERY

Children who survive trauma may experience long-term problems related to both physical and psychological impairment. A subset of children with mild traumatic brain injury display increased hyperactivity or inattention and conduct disorders, particularly if injured before the age of 5 years.[53] Cognitive or behavioral changes may be evident as well as problems with school performance or sleep disorders. Many children with persistent disability noted at the time of hospital discharge do not receive appropriate rehabilitation services (physical therapy, occupational therapy, and speech services) because of lack of availability, insurance coverage, or parental perception of need.[54] When availability of rehabilitative resources for injured children are lacking, full recovery from injury is limited.[55]

Within the first month after a traumatic event, individuals may display reexperiencing, avoidance, hyperarousal symptoms, and dissociation (feelings of unreality or emotional numbing).[56] Brief education is appropriate to explain that these symptoms are normal reactions that are likely to resolve. Symptoms that persist for more than a month or are particularly distressing in their intensity may be indicative of post-traumatic stress disorder (PTSD). Symptoms of this disorder in young children include sleep disturbances and nightmares, separation anxiety, difficulties in concentration, intrusive thoughts, difficulties in talking with parents and friends, mood disturbance, deterioration in academic performance, specific fears, and accident-related play. PTSD was reported in 35% of children involved in motor vehicle crashes compared with only 3% of children injured while playing sports.[57] Interventional programs that are aimed at both recognition and treatment of PTSD symptoms have the potenial to improve functional recovery after injury in children.

INJURY PREVENTION

Public health experts recommend that injury prevention efforts focus on injuries that are common, severe, and readily preventable. Examples include mechanisms likely to result in head or spinal cord injuries, where there is a high mortality or hospitalization rate and a long-term disability rate and effective countermeasures exist. The national Emergency Medical Services for Children (EMSC) program emphasizes a step-by-step approach to injury prevention by establishing goals and objectives with measurable outcomes[58] (Table 29.6).

TABLE 29.6

NATIONAL EMSC PROGRAM APPROACH TO INJURY PREVENTION

1. **Conduct a community assessment.** Bring individuals and groups who represent the community at large together to assess regional accomplishments and determine available resources.
2. **Define the injury problem.** Based on the community assessment and any available data, define a problem in specific, quantifiable terms.
3. **Set goals and objectives.** Make your goal a broad, general statement about the long-term changes the prevention initiatives are designed to make and the objective(s) specific, time-limited, and quantifiable, in terms of either a *process* or an *outcome*.
4. **Plan and test interventions.** Interventions are the actions that you take to accomplish your goals and objectives. Use the E's of prevention to design options:
   - *Engineering* of products and environments
   - *Enactment* of legislation to promote safety
   - *Education* of children, caregivers, health care professionals, legislators
   - *Evaluation* of the efficacy of specific interventions
5. **Implement and evaluate interventions.** Quantitate your results to determine whether your goals and objectives have been met.

After EMS for Children. Preventing childhood emergencies: A guide to developing effective injury prevention initiatives. www.ems-c.org.

TRAUMA

Physicians have been cited as the parent's first choice for information on injury control and child safety, but most physicians know little about injury prevention.[59] Major educational programs must be aimed at all caregivers to have a significant impact on pediatric trauma mortality rates.

Methods aimed at reducing childhood injury can be described as active or passive. The most successful prevention strategies are those that work automatically (i.e., are passive). Making roadways and vehicles safer has done more to decrease injuries from motor vehicle crashes than asking drivers to adhere to the speed limit or refrain from drinking alcohol before driving. Active intervention requires a behavioral change to be effective, such as securing a child in a safety seat.

Successful injury prevention programs have resulted in a significant reduction in the number of burn injuries in children, specifically with the development of fire-retardant sleepwear and working smoke detectors. There has been less success in reducing injuries to pediatric pedestrians: risk factors for pedestrian injuries in children include an age of 5 to 9 years, male sex, poverty, household crowding, inadequate parental supervision, family stress, and minority race or ethnic group.[1] Environmental contributions include living on streets with high traffic, lack of pedestrian-control devices, absence of alternatives to the street for play, and a high density of curbside parking. Successful environmental modifications, termed *traffic calming,* have been pioneered in Europe and include diversion of high-speed traffic away from the core of the city and residential areas and decreasing the speed limit to 10 to 20 mph. These changes reduce the risk of injury for all pedestrians, but especially for children. Bicycle helmets are effective in reducing the risk of head injuries by 85% and the risk of brain injuries by 88%. There is evidence that educating pediatricians improves the use of car seats for children. Although the rate of use of car seats for newborns and infants is approximately 75%, their use in toddlers is estimated at only 29%, and more than half of car seats for children are not used correctly.

In the child over 4 years or 40 pounds, there is ample evidence that booster seats should be used rather than adult type restraints. Few states have legislation aimed at this high-risk population.

A substantial proportion of motor vehicle crashes are alcohol related, and alcohol-related crashes are a serious problem even for the youngest drivers. Drivers aged under 21 years are more likely than older drivers to be involved in fatal crashes, and their added risk for fatal crash involvement increases more sharply at all levels of alcohol use.[60] This group has been the target of several interventions to reduce alcohol-impaired driving. These interventions include "zero-tolerance" blood alcohol concentration (BAC) standards for drivers under the legal drinking age; graduated driver licensing programs that require new drivers to progress through stages and allow them increased driving privileges as they gain experience; and the 1984 Uniform Drinking Age Act, which required states to adopt a minimum legal drinking age of 21 years. Collectively, these and other targeted interventions have contributed to a decrease in alcohol-related fatal crashes across all age groups during 1982 to 2001, with the largest decrease among drivers aged under 21 years.[60,61]

Preventing penetrating trauma is more complicated but still can be done effectively. Laws that make gun owners responsible for storing firearms in a manner that makes them inaccessible to children have resulted in a 23% reduction in unintentional shooting deaths among children where they are in effect.[62] An injury prevention program in Harlem that included improving environmental safety, supporting community development, providing safe and supervised activities for children and adolescents, and providing effective health education resulted in a 50% reduction in assault and gun injuries in the intervention community, compared with inceased injuries in a neighboring community.[63] Thus, there is hope for curbing the epidemic of pediatric injuries, but it will require a combination of legislative efforts, education of all child care providers, enforcement of existing safety laws, and use of widespread, community-based prevention programs using methods that have proved effective. Comprehensive injury data will allow us to direct our efforts into programs that target serious, common injuries with practical interventions.

KEY POINTS

- **Injury is the leading cause of death in children under 14 years and prevention, utilizing a public health model, is the most effective method to reduce deaths in children.**
- **Injuries and host response to injury in children is similar to that in adults. However, there are critical select patterns and physiologic responses unique to the child that must be recognized and understood, including: the upper airway is anterior and susceptible to iatrogenic injury; the blood volume is small and easily depleted by external bleeding, long bone and soft tissue injury, and due to occult processes; and the child is able to compensate more effectively than an adult, but when the ability to compensate is exceeded recovery is usually unsuccessful.**
- **The approach to TBI is similar to that for adults and although the child may have a higher survival rate, the long-term negative impact of a minor TBI on learning and personal quality of life is much greater. The upper cervical spine is at more risk of injury in the child because of increased relative head mass and underdeveloped ligaments, and diagnosis is more challenging due to normal anatomic variants.**
- **Pulmonary contusion is more likely the result of plasticity of the thorax, transmitting kinetic energy to the lung. Abdominal solid organ injury is unlikely to require surgery, but hollow viscus injury is difficult to diagnose and requires a high index of suspicion, serial abdominal examinations, and select diagnostic studies, particularly with patterns of injury such as a "lap belt" sign.**
- **Children with unusual patterns of injury, such as retinal hemorrhages, multiple subdural hematomas without skull fracture, genital or perianal injury, burns in unusual places (including cigarette pattern), and multiple new and old fractures, mandate follow-up for child maltreatment.**
- **The injured child, even more than an adult, requires a patient- and family-centered approach to care. Increasingly, family members should be permitted during all phases of resuscitation and care. In addition, children are emotionally vulnerable and every effort should be made to protect them; follow-ups should provide support to recognize and care for PTSD in this population.**

References

1. Rivara FP, Grossman DC, Cummings P. Injury prevention. *N Engl J Med.* 1997;337:543–548, 613–618.
2. Griffiths K. Best practices in injury prevention —national award highlights programs across the nation. *JEMS Online* 2002;27:1–22.
3. Svenson JE, Spurlock C, Nypaver M. Factors associated with the higher traumatic death rate among rural children. *Ann Emerg Med.* 1996;27:625–632.
4. Esposito TJ, Sanddal ND, Dean JM, et al. Analysis of preventable pediatric trauma deaths and inappropriate trauma care in Montana. *J Trauma* 1999;47:243–253.
5. Brehaut JC, Miller A, Raina P, et al. Childhood behavior disorders and injuries among children and youth: a population based study. *Pediatrics* 2003;111(2):262–269.
6. Calkins C, Bensard DD, Moore EE, et al. The injured child is resistant to multiple organ failure: a different inflammatory response? *J Trauma* 2002;53(6):1058–1063.

7. Pediatric Education for the Prehospital Professional, American Academy of Pediatrics, 2001.
8. Pediatric Advanced Life Support, American Heart Association 2002.
9. Nakayama DK, Gardner MJ, Rowe MI. Emergency endotracheal intubation in pediatric trauma. *Ann Surg.* 1990;211:218–223.
10. Paul TR, Marias M, Pons PT, et al. Adult versus pediatric prehospital trauma care: is there a difference? *J Trauma* 1999;47:455–459.
11. Potoka DA, Schall LC, Gardner MJ, et al. Impact of pediatric trauma centers on mortality in a statewide system. *J Trauma* 2000;49:237–245.
12. Resources for Optimal Care of the Injured Patient. American College of Surgeons (eds). Chicago, American College of Surgeons, 1999.
13. **Luten R, Wears RL, Broselow J, et al. Managing the unique size-related issues of pediatric resuscitation: reducing cognitive load with resuscitation aids. *Acad Emerg Med.* 2002;9(8):840–847.**
14. Holmes JF, Goodwin HC, Land C, et al. Coagulation testing in pediatric blunt trauma patients. *Ped Emerg Care* 2001;17(5):324–328.
15. Partrick DA, Bensard DD, Moore EE, et al. Ultrasound in an effective triage tool to evaluate blunt abdominal trauma in the pediatric population. *J Trauma* 1998;45:57–63.
16. Meyers TA, Eichhorn DJ, Guzzetta C, et al. Family presence during invasive procedures and resuscitation. *Am J Nurs.* 2000;100:32–41.
17. O'Brien MM, Creamer KM, Hill EE, et al. Tolerance of family presence during pediatric cardiopulmonary resuscitation: a snapshot of military and civilian pediatricians, nurses, and residents. *Ped Emerg Care* 2002;18(6):409–413.
18. **Hanson C, Strawser D. Family presence during cardiopulmonary resuscitation: Foote Hospital emergency department's nine-year perspective. *J Emerg Nurs.* 2002;18:104–106.**
19. **Adelson PD, Bratton SL, Carney NA, et al. Guidelines for the acute medical management of severe traumatic brain injury in infants, children and adolescents. *Pediatr Crit Care Med.* 2003;4(3) (Suppl):S1–S18.**
20. Meier U, Zeilinger FS, Henzka O. The use of decompressive craniectomy for the management of severe head injuries. *Acta Neurochir.* 2000;76: 475–478.
21. Tepas JJ III, DiScala C, Ramenofsky MLO, et al. Mortality and head injury: the pediatric perspective. *J Pediatr Surg.* 1990;25:92–96.
22. Tilford JM, Simpson PM, Yeh TS, et al. Variation in therapy and outcome for pediatric head trauma patients. *Crit Care Med.* 2001;29(5):1056–1061.
23. White JRM, Farukhi Z, Bull C, et al. Predictors of outcome in severely head-injured children. *Crit Care Med.* 2001;29(3):534–540.
24. Chan J, Putnam MA, Feustel PJ, et al. The age dependent relationship between facial fractures and skull fractures. *Intl J Pediatr Otorhinolaryngology* 2004;68:877–881.
25. Montgomery V, Oliver R, Reisner A, et al. The effect of severe traumatic brain injury on the family. *J Trauma* 2002;52(6):1121–1124.
26. Parisini P, DiSilvestre M, Greggi T. Treatment of spinal fractures in children and adolescents: long-term results in 44 patients. *Spine* 2002;27(18):1989–1994.
27. Orenstein JB, Klein BL, Gotschall CS, et al. Age and outcome in pediatric cervical spine injury: 11-year experience. *Pediatr Emerg Care* 1994;10:132–137.
28. Givens TG, Polley KA, Smieth GR, et al. Pediatric cervical spine injury: a three-year experience. *J Trauma* 1996;41:310–314.
29. Kriss VM, Kriss TC. SCIWORA (spinal cord injury without radiographic abnormality) in infants and children. *Clin Pediatr* 1996;35:119–124.
30. Bracken MB, Collins WF, Freeman DF, et al. Efficacy of methylprednisolone in acute spinal cord injury. *JAMA* 1984;251:45–52.
31. Bracken MB, Shephard MJ, Collins WF, et al. A randomized, controlled trial of methylprednisolone or naloxone in the treatment of acute spinal-cord injury: results of the Second National Acute Spinal Cord Injury Study. *N Engl J Med* 1990;322:1405–1411.
32. Sivit C. Pediatric thoracic trauma: imaging considerations. *Emerg Radiol.* 2002;9:21–25.
33. Dowd MD, Krug S. Pediatric blunt cardiac injury: epidemiology, clinical features, and diagnosis. *J Trauma* 1996;40:61–67.
34. Scorpio RJ, Wesson DE, Smith CR, et al. Blunt cardiac injuries in children: a postmortem study. *J Trauma* 1996;41:306–309.
35. Cooper A, Barlow B, DiScala C, et al. Mortality and truncal injury: the pediatric perspective. *J Pediatr Surg.* 1994;29:33–38.
36. Murphy R, Ghosh A, Mackway-Jones K. Ultrasound or computed tomography in paediatric blunt abdominal trauma. *Emerg Med J.* 2002;19: 554–556.
37. Baka AG, Delgado CA, Simon HK. Current use and perceived utility of ultrasound for evaluation of pediatric compared with adult trauma patients. *Ped Emerg Care* 2002;18(3):163–167.
38. Taylor GA, Fallat ME, Potter BA, et al. The role of computed tomography in blunt abdominal trauma in children. *J Trauma* 1988;28:1660–1664.
39. Holmes JF, Sokolove PE, Brant WE, et al. Identification of children with intra-abdominal injuries after blunt trauma. *Ann Emerg Med.* 2002;39(5); 500–509.
40. Fallat ME, Casale AJ. Practice patterns of pediatric surgeons caring for stable patients with traumatic solid organ injury. *J Trauma* 1997;43:820–824.
41. Stylianos S, APSA Trauma Committee: Evidence-based guidelines for resource utilization in children with isolated spleen or liver injury. *J Pediatr Surg.* 2000;35:164-169.
42. **Stylianos S, APSA Liver/Spleen Trauma Study Group: Compliance with evidence-based guidelines in children with isolated spleen or liver injury. *J Pediatr Surg.* 2002; 37:453–456.**
43. Keller MS, Stafford PW, Vane DW. Conservative management of pancreatic trauma in children. *J Trauma* 1997;42:1097–1100.
44. Grosfeld JL, Rescorla FJ, West KW, et al. Gastrointestinal injuries in childhood: analysis of 53 patients. *J Pediatr Surg.* 1989; 24(6):580–583.
45. **Jamieson DH, Babyn PS, Pearl R. Imaging gastrointestinal perforation in pediatric blunt trauma. *Pediatr Radiol* 1996; 26:188–194.**
46. Canty TG, Canty TC Jr, Brown C. Injuries of the gastrointestinal tract from blunt trauma in children: a 12-year experience at a designated pediatric trauma center. *J Trauma* 1999;46:234–240.
47. Newman KD, Bowman LM, Eichelberger MR, et al. The lap belt complex: intestinal and lumbar spine injury in children. *J Trauma* 1990;30: 1133–1140.
48. Norman D, Peskin B, Ehrenraich A, et al. The use of external fixators in the immobilization of pediatric fractures. *Arch Orthop Trauma Surg.* 2002; 122:379–382.
49. Bond SJ, Gotshall CS, Eichelberger MR. Predictors of abdominal injury in children with pelvic fracture. *J Trauma* 1991;31:1169–1173.
50. McIntyre RC, Bensard DD, Moore EE, et al. Pelvic fracture geometry predicts risk of life-threatening hemorrhage in children. *J Trauma* 1993;35:423–429.
51. Connors JM, Ruddy RM, McCall J, et al. Delayed diagnosis in pediatric blunt trauma. *Ped Emerg Care* 2001;17(1):1–4.
52. Letts M, Davidson D, Lapner P. Multiple trauma in children: predicting outcome and long- term results. *Can J Surg.* 2002; 45(2):126–131.
53. **McKinlay A, Dalrymple-Alford JC, Horwood LJ, et al. Long term psychosocial outcomes after mild head injury in early childhood. *JNNP* 2002; 73(3):281–288.**
54. Nakayama DK, Gardner MJ, Rogers KD. Disability from bicycle-related injuries in children. *J Trauma* 1990;30:1390–1394.
55. Wesson DE, Scorpio RJ, Spence LJ, et al. The physical, psychological, and socioeconomic costs of pediatric trauma. *J Trauma* 1992;33:252–257.
56. Winston FK, Kassam-Adams N, Vivarelli-O'Neill C, et al. Acute stress disorder symptoms in children and their parents after pediatric traffic injury. *Pediatrics* 2002;109(6):e90.
57. **Stallard P, Velleman R, Baldwin S. Prospective study of post-traumatic stress disorder in children involved in road traffic accidents. *BMJ* 1998;317:1619–1623.**
58. **EMS for Children. Preventing childhood emergencies: a guide to developing effective injury prevention initiatives. www.ems-c.org.**
59. Eichelberger MR, Gotschall CS, Feely HB, et al. Parental attitudes and knowledge of child safety: a national survey. *Am J Dis Child* 1990;144:714–720.
60. Elder RW, Shults RA. Involvement by young drivers in fatal alcohol-related motor-vehicle crashes—United States, 1982–2001. *MMWR* 2002;519480: 1089–1091.
61. Hedlund JH, Ulmer RG, Preusser DF. Determine why there are fewer young alcohol- impaired drivers. Washington, DC: National Highway Traffic Safety Administration, 2001 (publication no. DOT-HS-809-348).
62. Cummings P, Grossman DC, Rivara FP, et al. State gun safe storage laws and child mortality due to firearms. *JAMA* 1997;278:1084–1086.
63. Durkin MS, Kuhn L, Davidson LL, et al. Epidemiology and prevention of severe assault and gun injuries to children in an urban community. *J Trauma* 1996;41:667–673.

CHAPTER 30 ■ GERIATRIC TRAUMA

DAVID W. SCAFF, DONALD R. KAUDER, AND C. WILLIAM SCHWAB

DEMOGRAPHICS

Although traditionally viewed as an affliction of youth, injury in older individuals is common and will grow as a healthcare issue as this segment of our population increases. In 2002, unintentional injury was the fifth leading cause of death in the United States. For the portion of the population aged 65 and older, unintentional injuries were the ninth leading cause of death, accounting for more than 33,000 victims.[1] The expected growth of our elder population poses a major challenge for healthcare professionals. With improved health care, the U.S. life expectancy has increased from 69.7 years in 1960 to 76.9 years in 2000. Those who live to 65 years can be expected to survive until the age of 85.[1] According to the 2000 census, 35 million (12.4%) Americans were over 65; this figure is projected to reach 86 million (20.7%) by 2050. By far the fastest growing subset is the over 85 group, expected to quintuple from 4 million to 20 million by 2050.[2] Paralleling this rapid population growth, hospitals are treating increased numbers of geriatric trauma patients. In 2001, more than 3.2 million elderly patients who sustained unintentional injuries were evaluated in U.S. emergency departments, and 2.2 million (68.7%) of them were admitted.[3] The average cost of hospitalization for such a patient was $15,700 in 1989;[4] the impact in terms of current healthcare dollars is staggering. The 2001 National Hospital Discharge Survey estimates that elderly injured patients accrued over 8.5 million hospital days nationwide.[3] In a setting of continued reductions in reimbursement, a contributing factor to rising healthcare costs is an ever increasing length of stay because of the difficulty in placing patients in nursing facilities or rehabilitation centers.[5] It is thus easy to understand why geriatric trauma patients account for almost one third of all trauma-related expenses.[4,6,7] Faced with this reality, trauma centers and healthcare providers must become more cognizant of the nuances involved in the care of our injured elders so that efficient, compassionate healthcare can be provided.

PHYSIOLOGY

Normal physiologic changes of the elderly, coupled with preexisting comorbidities create a unique challenge in caring for older trauma patients. Healthcare providers must be aware of older patients' decreased physiologic reserve and inability to mount a normal physiologic response to the stress of injury. With advancing age, there is a progressive loss of functional reserve in each organ system. The degree of loss varies among organs and individuals.

Diminution in renal function can be subtle but significant. Renal glomeruli are progressively lost, resulting in decreased renal mass and glomerular filtration rate. Renal blood flow may decrease because of atherosclerotic changes. These changes lead to an impaired ability to concentrate urine and conserve water and solute. Accompanying fluid and electrolyte changes coupled with a decreased thirst response predispose patients to hypovolemia.[8] Reduction in muscle mass may result in a normal serum creatinine despite a reduced creatinine clearance. Age-adjusted formulas for creatinine clearance provide better estimates of renal function than serum creatinine in the elderly population.

With the loss of lean tissue mass, thermoregulation is disrupted due to less efficient mechanisms of heat conservation and production, predisposing the elderly patient to hypothermia. Shivering results in increased oxygen consumption and cardiopulmonary demands. Fever may be absent despite serious infection because of altered thermoregulation. The loss of muscle mass has negative effects on other organs systems as well.

The respiratory muscles lose strength and endurance. Combined with decreased compliance of the chest wall and loss of normal lung parenchyma, hypoxemia and respiratory failure may develop with even minimal chest wall injury. Another common reduction in pulmonary function involves alterations in the ability to clear secretions and mucus, contributing to an increased risk of aspiration and development of pneumonia.

Significant age-related changes also occur in the central nervous system (CNS). With advancing cerebral atrophy, there is an increase in the size and volume of the subdural space. Thus, older patients who sustain a closed head injury may take more time than younger individuals to develop neurologic signs of brain injury, intracranial bleeding, or intracranial hypertension. Preexisting conditions such as stroke or dementia may further confound the clinical picture.

Alterations in the cardiovascular system are frequent as well. The myocardium has a blunted inotropic and chronotropic response to endogenous catecholamines, leading to a decrease in maximal heart rate, cardiac output, and ejection fraction. To overcome this, there is an increased reliance on end-diastolic volume to increase cardiac output in times of stress. Coronary vasculature relies on diastolic filling time and pressures for myocardial perfusion. In the setting of coronary atherosclerosis, relatively mild or brief periods of hypotension or tachycardia may result in myocardial ischemia or infarction. Prescription of beta-blockers is very common and may mask the normal physiologic response to stress or hypovolemia.

MECHANISM OF INJURY

Today's elderly population enjoys a degree of freedom and activity unmatched by prior generations. Improved access to healthcare and injury prevention programs, as well as access to assisted living communities allows many older Americans to function relatively independently well into their ninth decade. Traumatic injuries often impact this autonomy, creating dependence on relatives or caregivers.

Blunt trauma accounts for the vast majority of geriatric injuries. Falls are the most common mechanism of injury. It is estimated that 28% to 45% of the elderly in the community and 45% to 61% of nursing home patients will fall each year.[9,10]

In 2003, the Centers for Disease Control reported more than 3.6 million fall-related injuries among the elderly. Falls are the leading cause of injury-related death in those over 75 years of age and are second only to motor vehicle crashes in those aged 65 to 74 years.[11] Elderly fall victims sustain more severe injuries over multiple body regions when compared to their younger counterparts given the same mechanism of injury. The morbidity of even minor falls is significant. In the older population, ground-level falls appear to have the same injury severity as falls from a height.[12] A gender difference is also seen, and females are injured by falling more frequently than men (69.6% vs. 30.4%).[13] Common risk factors for falls include inappropriate use of assist devices, changes in gait, peripheral neuropathies, alterations in balance, and overall deconditioning and loss of strength.

Although falls take a terrible toll on this population, injuries sustained in motor vehicle crashes are also very common. In 2001, there were 19 million older licensed drivers in the United States, a 32% increase since 1991.[14] Motor vehicle crashes are the second most common mechanism of injury leading to death in elder trauma, resulting in over 7,200 deaths in 2001.[11] Crash data from the National Highway Traffic Safety Administration shows that drivers aged 65 to 74 years old have very high rates of crash fatalities, second only to drivers aged 16 to 20. Drivers older than 75 years have the highest incidence of traffic fatalities per mile driven.[14] Most traffic fatalities involving older drivers occur during the daytime (81%), on weekdays (72%), and involve another vehicle (75%).[15] Changes in visual acuity, delayed reaction times, and impaired judgment may all contribute to this increased rate of motor vehicle crashes.

The older person struck by a motor vehicle represents only 10% of auto versus pedestrian accidents. Although the younger population is more likely to be struck, older victims sustain higher rates of moderate and severe injuries. Closed head injuries predominate; however, injuries to the chest and abdomen are also frequent, as are extremity fractures. Mortality approaches 25% for those over age 65.[16] Hearing impairments, neurological disorders, altered visual acuity, gait disturbances, diminished strength and balance, and impairments in judgment may all be contributing factors leading to this mechanism of injury.

Injury related to assault is more common in younger individuals, but the elderly also fall victim to this mechanism of injury. In fact, the elderly account for 5.7% of all persons injured in this manner. Although this is a relatively small number of victims, elderly patients who are assaulted are five times as likely to die as their younger counterparts. Over 50% of assault-related fatal injuries result from firearms, whereas 80% of nonfatal injuries result from blunt assault.[17] Lack of mobility, overall physical decline, and a solitary lifestyle all contribute to the elderly being easy targets for assailants. Depression, physical illness, death of a loved one, and uncontrolled pain are common causes of self-inflicted injury in the elderly. Of the more than 11,000 self-inflicted geriatric injuries seen in 2001, 48% resulted in a mortality and more than 50% resulted from firearms.[17]

PREVENTION

The random nature of unintentional injuries is a fact of life. Unintentional injury, however, may be preventable, and in many cases, this can be accomplished with relatively simple and inexpensive interventions.

The National Committee for the Prevention of Elder Abuse defines elder abuse as: neglect, domestic violence, and physical, psychological, financial, or sexual abuse of elderly persons. Elder abuse affects 4% to 6% of the geriatric population. It is estimated that 450,000 incidents of elder abuse occurred in 1996, with only 20 percent incidents reported.[18] Females are more often at risk for abuse than males, and persons older than 80 are abused two to three times more often than those aged 65 to 80. A critical step in preventing elder abuse is education of primary healthcare providers and the public about this growing problem. Assessment tools such as the KAMA (knowledge and management of abuse) instrument have been developed to identify education and management strategies for the prevention of elder abuse. The KAMA instrument utilizes a series of vignettes to assess a caregiver's knowledge and thought process of the identification, treatment, and prevention of elder abuse.[19]

The prevention of falls has the potential to reap the greatest benefits for our elderly population. Implementation of fall-intervention programs, modification of environmental hazards (removal of loose carpets, improved lighting, provision of grip bars), use of mobility aids (walkers, appropriate footwear, wheelchairs), and improved physical strength reduce fall incidence rates from 2.9 to 1.7 per person-year for active seniors.[20] Using alternative medications rather than benzodiazepines, antidepressants, and neuroleptics may improve cognition, balance, and stamina.

As experienced drivers grow older, changes in their vision, attention, and physical abilities may cause them to drive less safely than when they were younger. Sometimes these changes happen so gradually that the drivers are unaware that their ability to drive safely has become impaired. Geriatric drivers involved in a motor vehicle crash should be evaluated as to their physical and cognitive abilities and counseled on driving restrictions and the need for ongoing assessment. Driving rehabilitation programs are available to assess driving skills and provide rehabilitation to enable the elderly to resume or continue driving safely. Senior transit shuttles, public transportation, and volunteer driver programs are alternative forms of transportation available to maintain a person's relative independence and reduce their risk of further motor vehicle–related injury.

OUTCOMES

Despite improved technology and access to trauma centers, when compared with their younger counterparts, geriatric trauma patients have an overall increased mortality, even for less severe injuries.[21,22] Age, independent of other variables, contributes a 5% increase in mortality for each additional year beyond 65.[23] The elevated mortality rate is also in part the result of the effects of comorbidities and preexisting conditions. These conditions may reflect a patient's "physiologic" rather than chronologic age. Considering that up to 33% of patients over 65 have at least one chronic medical condition, it is logical to assume some effect.[24] When comparing patients with preexisting conditions to patients without, comorbities increased the risk of mortality during the 5 years following an injury between 2.0 and 8.4 times.[25] Grossman et al. found hepatic disease, renal disease, malignancy, and congestive heart failure to be independent predictors of mortality. Hepatic, renal, and heart disease along with a prior spinal injury have the greatest negative impact, increasing the risk of death in all forms of geriatric trauma.[13,24] These comorbidities appear to have the greatest consequence in patients with less severe injuries. As a patient's injury severity score (ISS) rises above 15, chronic medical conditions have a lesser effect on outcomes and, above 25, survival becomes a function of the severity of the injury.[24]

Geriatric trauma patients have increased rates of cardiac, infectious, respiratory, and renal complications during hospitalization.[26,27] Complications occur more often in the most severely injured patients and patients with preexisting conditions.[23] As one might imagine, the development of complications negatively impacts survival. Smith et al. showed that mortality increased from 5.6% in patients without complications to 8.6% for one complication and 30% for two or more.[28]

The high mortality rate in geriatric trauma warrants an aggressive diagnostic and therapeutic approach. Patients who have sustained hypotension, have multiple comorbidities or an ISS above 9 may benefit from admission to the intensive care unit and invasive hemodynamic monitoring. Work by Scalea et al. has shown that geriatric patients who appear clinically stable after initial evaluation benefited from early invasive monitoring and goal-directed resuscitation. Forty-three percent of patients were found to be in cardiogenic shock with an associated low flow state despite "normal" vital signs. With early intervention, mortality was reduced from 93% to 47%.[29] This benefit has also been shown in less severely injured patients. In a study by Schultz et al., mortality in geriatric patients undergoing open reduction and internal fixation of the hip was reduced from 29% to 2.9% with the use of invasive monitoring.[30]

For the elderly, the adverse effects of trauma often persist far beyond hospital discharge. Discharge disposition is spread evenly among home, short-term rehabilitation, and skilled nursing facilities (SNF). There is a predisposition for patients older than 80 to require SNFs (37%), while patients aged 65 to 79 more frequently return home (53%).[31] Over time, 50% of patients discharged to an SNF return home and 50% of patients discharged home with assistance will become independent.[32] Health surveys show that although up to 63% of patients ultimately return to independent living, there is a transient decline in psychological well-being that improves over the ensuing year.[22,33]

SPECIAL CONSIDERATIONS

Although even minor injury may have a significantly negative impact on the elder patient, several specific injuries or disease states bear special comment. They are addressed next.

Blunt Splenic Injury

Management of splenic injuries has evolved over the last 20 years. It is now well accepted that pediatric patients have a 70% to 80% splenic salvage rate using nonoperative management. This approach has been extrapolated to the adult population with variable success. Early reports by Smith and Godley reviewing nonoperative management in the elderly have demonstrated poor results.[34,35] More recently, several groups studying the injured elderly have reported results comparable to those in the pediatric population.[36–38] Although nonoperative management of blunt splenic injury may be successful in up to 80% of geriatric trauma patients, older patients fail this approach more often than their younger counterparts, and those who do so suffer increased mortality and morbidity.[39] Factors that increase the odds of a splenectomy include a higher grade of splenic injury, contrast extravasation or pseudoaneurysm seen on CT scan, combined hepatic and splenic injuries, and the need for multiple blood transfusions.[38,40] Although the optimal management of geriatric blunt splenic injuries is still a matter of some debate, surgeons caring for this population would be wise to remember that these patients have little physiologic reserve and that the most "conservative" approach may actually be surgical.

Central Cord Syndrome

Spinal cord injury is devastating, regardless of the age of the patient. However, the patient's age can have a significant bearing not only on the outcome but also on the injury pattern itself. Age-related cervical spinal stenosis and increased osteophyte formation puts older patients at especially high risk of central cord syndrome. The etiology is often associated with a forward fall with striking of the chin, resulting in cervical hyperextension. This results in bleeding in the more central regions of the spinal cord, leading to preferential neurologic deficits in the upper extremities. The diagnosis can be missed unless meticulous attention is paid to the neurologic examination. The findings can be subtle and varied, at times appearing only as mild weakness of the distal arms or hands, with sparing of the lower extremities.[41] Because this injury complex frequently occurs in the absence of bony injury, magnetic resonance imaging is extremely helpful in elucidating the hemorrhagic necrosis and compression of the spinal cord that can be missed with computed tomography (CT) scanning. Initiating therapy with methylprednisolone should proceed in standard fashion, as with younger individuals, and in accordance with the Third National Acute Spinal Cord Injury Study (NASCIS III).[42] Prognosis for complete recovery following central cord syndrome is poor for older patients. In patients over 70 years, bladder control and ambulatory function are restored only 20% and 40% of the time, respectively.[43] Mortality rates in excess of 50% are common.[44]

Rib Fractures

Rib fractures are commonly seen in blunt injury to the torso and can occur in isolation or in association with more severe chest or abdominal injuries. Aside from the serious sequelae of hemothorax and pneumothorax, managing the chest wall pain associated with rib fractures or chest wall contusions in the older individual presents unique challenges. Inadequate pain control in the setting of decreased pulmonary reserve or underlying intrinsic lung disease, such as chronic obstructive pulmonary disease, can have devastating consequences. Elderly patients with isolated thoracic trauma have increased rates of adult respiratory distress syndrome and pleural effusions and three times the risk of contracting pneumonia when compared with younger patients.[45,46] Mortality increases in a linear fashion with the number of rib fractures. An elderly patient's mortality with one to two fractures is 12.3%, whereas the chance of death with more than six fractures approaches 40%.[47] Adequate analgesia is the mainstay of care, but the use of intravenous or oral narcotics, although effective, can be dangerous if not closely monitored. Oversedation can result in hypoventilation, with resultant hypercarbia and hypoxia. In a population with a predisposition to coronary ischemia, this can be lethal. It can also promote loss of airway protection and lead to aspiration. Ileus is also commonly seen. The use of epidural analgesia for geriatric thoracic trauma has been a great advance and has been shown to decrease mortality from 16% to 10%.[46] However, even this therapy occurs at the expense of increased complication rates. Common complications include excessive sedation, hypotension, catheter migration, and insertion site soft tissue infections. An awareness of the serious nature of "just a rib fracture" and attention paid to aggressive pulmonary toilet, supplemental oxygen, and adequate pain control, frequently in the ICU setting, will maximize the elder trauma patient's chance of survival.

Anticoagulation

Anticoagulant medications and antiplatelet agents are commonly prescribed for a variety of prophylactic and therapeutic indications, including treatment of deep venous thrombosis, chronic atrial fibrillation, mechanical cardiac valves, and atherosclerotic coronary vascular disease. Use of anticoagulation agents has been found to be especially effective in reducing the risk of stroke.[48] Patients with an elevated international normalized ratio (INR) who present to the hospital following injury pose a unique and complex problem for the surgeon. Common sense would dictate that such patients would suffer more severe bleeding and worse outcomes than patients with a normal coagulation profile, but such a general statement cannot yet be supported in the literature.[49,50] However, the subset of anticoagulated older patients who have sustained traumatic intracranial bleeding clearly fare worse. When other confounding variables are excluded, studies by Lavoie and Mina both showed statistically significant increases in mortality rate compared with similarly injured patients with normal coagulation states.[51,52] Anticoagulated patients presenting with suspected closed head injury should undergo expedient head CT scan and receive fresh frozen plasma if pathology is identified. Although no current data recommend the empiric use of plasma to treat the elevations in INR in this group, it is a therapy that should receive serious consideration by the clinician.

Injury in our elders is an issue with which our healthcare system must come to grips. It is a huge problem now and will only grow in volume, scope, and complexity as the aging population burgeons. A working knowledge of the common mechanisms of injury, physiologic changes of aging, and the complexities of providing care for this vibrant, yet fragile population will serve the clinician well.

KEY POINTS

- **The growth of the elder population poses a major challenge. In 2001, 2.2 million injured elderly were admitted for care and account for one third of all trauma-related expenses.**
- **With age comes a progressive loss in functional reserve in every organ system, with impaired ability to concentrate urine and conserve water and solute; thermoregulation is poor because of decreased heat conservation and heat generation predisposing to hypothermia; respiratory muscles lose strength and endurance coupled with decreased chest wall compliance and loss of functional parenchyma; the myocardium is blunted to inotropic and chronotropic stimuli with decreased maximal heart rate, output, and ejection fraction; and the CNS atrophies with an increased subdural space and an increased risk of bleeding due to tethering of bulging vessels, able to hold an increased volume of blood.**
- **The most common cause of injury is falls resulting from instability, with significant morbidity to even ground-level falls; next are vehicular crashes due to a highly mobile population with decreasing sight, reflexes, and judgment; and also intentional trauma, including a significant incidence of elder abuse and suicide.**
- **Prevention is critical; modifying the environment to prevent falls and retraining to improve driving skills, along with reduction in unnecessary mind-altering prescription medications, are important.**
- **Mortality is higher for any given severity of injury, with comorbidities having most impact in less severe trauma, and requires aggressive intervention for monitoring, including PAC lines, resuscitation to adequate elevated preloads, balanced treatment of pain to avoid sedation and attendant risks, and careful timing of invasive procedures, such as orthopedic open reduction internal fixation.**

References

1. Available at: http://www.cdc.gov/nchs/data/hus/hus04.pdf. Centers for Disease Control, National Center for Injury Prevention and Control. Health, United States, 2004. Accessed February 1, 2005.
2. Available at: http://www.aoa.gov/prof/Statistics/online_stat_data/AgePop2050.asp Administration on Aging. Dept. of Health and Human Services. Accessed February 1, 2005.
3. National Hospital Discharge Survey: 2001 Annual summary with detailed diagnosis and procedure data. National Center for Health Statistics. Series 13, No. 156.
4. Ross N, Timberlake GA, Rubino LJ, et al. High costs of trauma care in the elderly. *South Med J*. 1989;82:857–859.
5. Fath JJ, Ammonn AA, Cohen MM. Urban trauma care is threatened by inadequate reimbursement. *Am J Surg*. 1999;177:371–374.
6. **MacKenzie EJ, Morris JA, Smith GS, et al. Acute hospital costs of trauma in the United States: Implications for regionalized systems of care. *J Trauma* 1990;30:1096–1103.**
7. Covington DL, Maxwell J, Clancey TV. Hospital resources used to treat the injured elderly at North Carolina trauma centers. *J Am Geriatr Soc*. 1993;41:847–852.
8. Watters JM, McClaran JC. The elderly surgical patient. In Wilmore DW, Cheung LY, Harken AH, eds. et al. *ACS surgery: principles and practice 2003*. New York: WebMD Professional Publishing; 2003.
9. Tinetti ME, Speechley M, Gineter SF. Risk factors for falls among elderly persons living in the community. *N Engl J Med*. 1988;319:1701–1707.
10. Rubenstein LZ, Josephson KR, Robbins AS. Falls in the nursing home. *Ann Intern Med*. 1994;121:442–451.
11. Web-based Injury Statistics Query and Reporting System. National Center for Injury Prevention and Control. CDC. Accessed February 1, 2005
12. Sterling DA, O'Connor JA, Bonadies J. Geriatric Falls: Injury severity is high and disproportionate to mechanism. *J Trauma*. 2001;50:116–119.
13. Grossman MD, Miller D, Scaff DW, et al. When is an elder old? Effect of preexisting conditions on mortality in geriatric trauma. *J Trauma*. 2002;52:242–246.
14. **Zwerling C, Peek-Asa C, Whitten PS, et al. Fatal motor vehicle crashes in rural and urban areas: decomposing rates into contributing factors. *Injury Prevention* 2005;11:24–28.**
15. National Highway Traffic Safety Administration. Traffic safety facts 2002. U.S. Department of Transportation.
16. Demetriades D, Murray J, Martin M, et al. Pedestrians injured by automobiles: Relationship of age to injury type and severity. *J Am Coll Surg*. 2004;199:382–387.
17. **Vyrostek SB, Annest JL, Ryan GW. Surveillance for fatal and nonfatal injuries—United States, 2001. *MMWR Surveill Summ*. 2004;53:1–57.**
18. Tatara T, Kuzmeskus LB, Duckhorn E, et al. The national elder abuse incidence study—1998. National Center on Elder Abuse. The American Public Human Services Association.
19. **Richardson B, Kitchen G, Livingston G. Developing the KAMA instrument. *Age and Ageing* 2003;32:286–291.**
20. **Jensen J, Nyberg L, Gustafson Y, et al. Fall and injury prevention in residential care— Effects in residents with higher and lower levels of cognition. *J Am Geriatr Soc*. 2003;51:627–635.**
21. Hannan EL, Waller CH, Farrell LS, et al. Elderly trauma inpatients in New York state: 1994–1998. *J Trauma* 2004;56:1297–1304.
22. Inaba K, Goecke M, Sharkey P, et al. Long-term outcomes after injury in the elderly. *J Trauma*. 2003;54:486–491.
23. Richmond TS, Kauder D, Strumpf N, et al. Characteristics and outcomes of serious traumatic injury in older adults. *J Am Geriatr Soc*. 2002;50: 215–222.
24. McGwin G, MacLennan PA, Fife JB, et al. Preexisting conditions and mortality in older trauma patients. *J Trauma*. 2004;56:1291–1296.
25. Gubler KD, Davis R, Koepsell T, et al. Long-term survival of elderly trauma patients. *Arch Surg*. 1997;132:1010–1014.
26. Perdue PW, Watts DD, Kaufmann CR, et al. Differences in mortality between elderly and younger adult trauma patients: Geriatric status increases risk of delayed death. *J Trauma* 1998;45:805–810.
27. Tornetta P, Mostafavi H, Riina J, et al. Morbidity and mortality in elderly trauma patients. *J Trauma* 1999;46:702–706.
28. Smith DP, Enderson BL, Maull KI. Trauma in the elderly: determinants of outcome. *South Med J*. 1990;83:171–177.
29. **Scalea TM, Simon HM, Duncan AO, et al. Geriatric blunt multiple trauma: Improved survival with invasive monitoring. *J Trauma* 1990;30:129–136.**
30. Schultz RJ, Whitfield GF, LaMura JJ, et al. The role of physiologic monitoring in patients with fractures of the hip. *J Trauma* 1985;25:309–316.
31. Grossman MD, Scaff DW, Miller D, et al. Functional outcomes in octogenarian trauma. *J Trauma* 2003;55:26–32
32. DeMaria EJ, Kenney PR, Merriam MA, et al. Aggressive trauma care benefits the elderly. *J Trauma* 1987;27:1200–1206.

33. Scaf-Klomp W, Sanderman R, Ormel J, et al. Depression in older people after fall-related injuries: a prospective study. *Age and Ageing* 2003;32:88–94.
34. Smith JS Jr, Wengrovitz MA, Delong BS. Prospective validation of the ruptured spleen. *J Trauma* 1992;33:363–369.
35. Godley CD, Warren RL, Sheridan RL, et al. Nonoperative management of blunt splenic injuries in adults: age over 55 years as a powerful indicator for failure. *J Am Coll Surg*. 1996;183:133–139.
36. Barone JE, Burns G, Svehlak SA, et al. Management of blunt splenic trauma in patients older than 55 years. *J Trauma* 1999;46:87–90.
37. Cocanour CS, Moore FA, Ware DN, et al. Age should not be a consideration for nonoperative management of blunt splenic injury. *J Trauma* 2000;48:606–610.
38. Nix JA, Costanza M, Daley BJ, et al. Outcome of the current management of splenic injuries. *J Trauma* 2001;50:835–842.
39. Harbrecht BG, Peitzman AB, Rivera L, et al. Contribution of age and gender to outcome of blunt splenic injury in adults: Multicenter study of the Eastern Association for the Surgery of Trauma. *J Trauma* 2001;51:887–895.
40. Malhotra AK, Latifi R, Fabian TC, et al. Multiplicity of solid organ injury: Influence on management and outcomes after blunt abdominal trauma. *J Trauma* 2003;54:925–929.
41. Marion DW. Injuries of the spinal cord and spinal column. In: Peitzman AB, Rhodes M, Schwab CW, et al., eds. *The Trauma Manual*. Philadelphia: Lippincott-Raven; 1998.
42. Bracken MB, Shepard MJ, Holford TR, et al. Administration of methylprednisolone for 24 or 48 hours or tirilazad mesylate for 48 hours in the treatment of acute spinal cord injury: Results of the Third National Acute Spinal Cord Injury Randomized Controlled Trial: National Acute Spinal Cord Injury Study. *JAMA*. 1997;277:1597–1604.
43. **Newey ML, Sen PK, Fraser RD. The long-term outcome after central cord syndrome: a study of the natural history. *J Bone Joint Surg Br.* 2000;82:851–855.**
44. Alander DH, Parker J, Stauffer ESF. Intermediate-term outcome of cervical cord-injured patients older than 50 years of age. *Spine* 1997;22(11): 1189–1192.
45. Bergeron E, Lavoie A, Clas D, et al. Elderly trauma patients with rib fractures are at greater risk of death and pneumonia. *J Trauma* 2003;54:478–485.
46. **Bulger EM, Arneson MA, Mock CN, et al. Rib fractures in the elderly. *J Trauma* 2000;48:1040–1046.**
47. Stawicki SP, Grossman MD, Hoey BA, et al. Rib fractures in the elderly: a marker of injury severity. *J Am Geriatr Soc*. 2004;52:805–808.
48. Man-Son-Hing M, Laupacis A. Anticoaulant-related bleeding in older persons with atrial fibrillation. *Arch Internal Med*. 2003;163:1580–1586.
49. Kennedy DM, Cipolle MD, Pasquale MD, et al. Impact of preinjury warfarin use in elderly trauma patients. *J Trauma* 2000;48:451–453.
50. Mina AA, Bair HA, Howells GA, et al. Complications of preinjury warfarin use in the trauma patient. *J Trauma* 2003;54:842–847.
51. **Lavoie A, Ratte S, Clas D, et al. Preinjury warfarin use among elderly patients with closed head injuries in a trauma center. *J Trauma* 2004;56: 802–807.**
52. Mina AA, Knipfer JF, Park DY, et al. Intracranial complications of preinjury anticoagulation in trauma patients with head injury. *J Trauma* 2002;53:668–672.

CHAPTER 31 ■ TRAUMA IN PREGNANCY

GRACE S. ROZYCKI

Although injured pregnant patients make up only approximately 1% of all trauma admissions,[1–6] the magnitude of the problem is much greater because two patients are being cared for simultaneously. The overall maternal mortality rate continues to decline in the United States, but trauma accounts for a significant number of deaths in pregnant women.[2,7] In fact, this problem may be underestimated because the gravid status may not be routinely recorded on death certificates.[8]

In several series,[3,9,10] the rate of fetal death parallels the extent of maternal injury, yet it also has been reported to be three to four times greater than the maternal death rate, implying that the survival of the mother is not always sufficient to ensure fetal well-being.[1,2,5,11] Although most trauma involving pregnant patients occurs during the second or third trimester,[1,9,11–13] some reports of domestic abuse show this occurs frequently before 18 weeks' gestation and then diminishes between 20 and 30 weeks' gestation. Motor vehicle crashes occur with equal frequency throughout the gestational period.[13–15] Fetal demise is directly related to birth weight and gestational age. Fifty percent of fetuses die after serious maternal trauma if they are no older than 26 weeks' gestational age. Ninety percent of fetuses die after significant maternal trauma if their weight is less than 750 g, compared with a 40% mortality rate when the weight is greater than 750 g.[16,17]

An understanding of the anatomic and physiologic changes unique to pregnancy as well as of the principles of resuscitation and treatment after trauma is important to provide the best care for both the injured mother and her unborn child.

ANATOMY AND PHYSIOLOGY UNIQUE TO THE GRAVID PATIENT

Anatomic and physiologic changes of pregnancy can alter the injury response, necessitating a modified approach to resuscitation and therapy (Table 31.1). Knowledge of these changes should be kept in mind as the evaluation and resuscitation of the pregnant trauma patient proceeds.

Anatomic Changes

By the twelfth week of gestation, the gravid uterus is considered an intraabdominal organ. With the ascent of the enlarged uterus out of the pelvis, it undergoes dextrorotation because of the presence of the rectosigmoid colon.[18] Important marks for estimating gestational age include the umbilicus (20 weeks' gestation) and the costal margins (34 to 36 weeks' gestation). During the final 2 weeks of normal gestation, the fetal head descends into the pelvis, accounting for the fetal skull fractures or traumatic brain injuries that are often associated with maternal pelvic fractures. With increasing gestational age, the uterus also becomes relatively thin (1.5 cm at term) and the amount of amniotic fluid decreases.[18] As a result, the fetus is more vulnerable to injury, especially when the mother receives a direct blow to the abdomen. Although the myometrium is relatively elastic, the placenta is not, predisposing it to shear

TABLE 31.1

PHYSIOLOGIC ALTERATIONS IN PREGNANCY

System	Change	Implication
Neurologic	Eclampsia may mimic traumatic brain injury (headache, seizures, hypertension)	Exclude traumatic brain injury (head computed tomography scan) May mask shock
Cardiovascular	Cardiac output increased by 1.0 to 1.5 L/min Heart rate ↑ 10–15 bpm Blood pressure ↓ 5–15 mm Hg in second trimester but returns to normal in third trimester Plasma volume increase by 50% Vena caval compression	Delayed signs of shock Supine hypotension syndrome
Respiratory	Residual lung volume decreased Decreased Po_2 Chronic respiratory alkalosis	Decreased buffering capacity
Gastrointestinal	Decreased gastrointestinal motility	Increased propensity toward aspiration and vomiting Urinary stasis
Genitourinary	Dilatation of renal system	Physiologic hydronephrosis and urinary stasis
Laboratory values	Increased white blood cell count Decreased hematocrit Increased fibrinogen and factors VII, VIII, X, XII	Difficulty interpreting clinical picture regarding hemorrhage Hypercoagulable stage

forces at the uteroplacental interface, which may lead to *abruptio placentae*.

Placental perfusion depends on the blood flow through the uterus and ovarian arteries. It is estimated to be approximately 500 mL/min[19] but varies with position and hormonal changes.[20] In early pregnancy, there is a softening and cyanosis of the cervix with an eversion of the proliferating columnar endocervical glands.[18] These changes make the cervix friable and prone to bleed even with minor trauma. There is also enlargement of ovarian veins and increased vascularity of the maternal vagina with advancing gestational age.

Cardiovascular

Maternal blood volume (plasma and erythrocytes) begins to increase during the first trimester but expands most rapidly during the second trimester, reaching approximately 45% above nonpregnant levels.[21–23] The increase in plasma volume is proportionally greater than the enlarged erythrocyte volume and results in the anemia of pregnancy. Near term, the plasma volume continues to expand, but the red cell mass begins to increase, resulting in a near-normal hematocrit. Pregnancy-induced hypervolemia supplies the extraordinary demands of the enlarged uterus, allows for fewer red blood cells to be lost during parturition, minimizes the loss of oxygen-carrying capacity associated with hemoglobin, and protects the mother from the hypotensive effects of impaired venous return.[24] This physiologic hypervolemia masks volume loss after trauma and may give the clinician an unfounded sense of security about the patient's hemodynamic stability. Almost 35% of the mother's blood volume may be lost before clinical signs of shock are noted.[25]

As pregnancy progresses, cardiac output increases up to 50% above normal until the 24th week of gestation, after which it plateaus (Table 31.2). This increase in cardiac output is a result of a modest rise in heart rate and stroke volume that relates to the expanded blood volume and the direct inotropic effect of estrogen.[26]

If the pregnant patient is in the supine position, the inferior vena cava is partially obstructed by the gravid uterus, which decreases venous blood return to the heart, lowers cardiac output, and causes supine hypotension. The enlarged uterus also compresses the abdominal aorta, reducing blood flow to the fetus through diminished uterine arterial flow. Turning the pregnant patient onto her left side improves venous return and increases cardiac output by approximately 30%.[27]

Overall, cardiac work is increased with pregnancy because of the volume load and estrogen effect, despite a decrease in systemic vascular resistance mediated by prostaglandin, progestin, intracellular calcium flux, and endothelial-derived factors.[28] Early in pregnancy, the blood pressure, especially the diastolic level, decreases but then slowly returns to normal by term. Mean normal values for the first trimester are 105 mm Hg systolic and 60 mm Hg diastolic; for the second trimester, 102 and 55 mm Hg; and for the third trimester, 108 and 67 mm Hg. Significant elevation above these levels may indicate pregnancy-induced hypertension.[29]

Finally, the enlarged uterus causes the heart to be displaced upward and to the left. This change, along with the common development of a serous pericardial effusion,[30] results in an enlarged cardiac silhouette and increased pulmonary vascular markings on the chest radiograph.[31]

Pulmonary Changes

As the uterus enlarges during pregnancy, the diaphragm rises approximately 4 cm, which results in a lower residual lung volume, diminished ventilatory reserve, and decreased resting arterial oxygen tension. Both diaphragmatic excursion and thoracic circumference increase, resulting in larger tidal volumes (Table 31.3). A chronic respiratory alkalosis shifts the oxyhemoglobin dissociation curve to the left, thereby increasing the affinity of maternal hemoglobin for oxygen. Simultaneously, however, this slight increase in pH stimulates an increase in 2,3-diphosphoglycerate, which shifts the curve to the right, facilitating oxygen release to the fetus.[18,32]

TABLE 31.2

CENTRAL HEMODYNAMIC CHANGES IN 10 NORMAL NULLIPARIOUS WOMEN BETWEEN 35 WEEKS' GESTATION AND AGAIN WHEN 11 TO 13 WEEKS' POSTPARTUM

	Pregnant[a]	Postpartum	Change
Mean arterial pressure (mm Hg)	90 ± 6	86 ± 8	No change
Pulmonary capillary wedge pressure (mm Hg)	8 ± 2	6 ± 2	No change
Central venous pressure	4 ± 3	4 ± 3	No change
Heart rate (beats/min)	83 ± 10	71 ± 10	+17%
Cardiac output (L/min)	6.2 ± 1.0	4.3 ± 0.9	+43%
Systemic vascular resistance (dyne/s/cm^{-5})	1,210 ± 266	1,530 ± 520	−21%
Pulmonary vascular resistance (dyne/s/cm^{-5})	78 ± 22	119 ± 47	−34%
Serum colloid osmotic pressure (mm Hg)	18.0 ± 1.5	20.8 ± 1.0	−14%
COP–PCWP gradient (mm Hg)	10.5 ± 2.7	14.5 ± 2.5	−28%
Left ventricular stroke work index (g/m/m^2)	48 ± 6	41 ± 8	No change

[a]Made in lateral recumbent position.
COP, colloid osmotic pressure; PCWP, pulmonary capillary wedge pressure.
Adapted from Maternal adaptions to pregnancy. In: Cunningham FG, MacDonald PC, Gant NF, et al., eds. *Williams obstetrics,* 20th ed. Norwalk, CT: Appleton & Lange, 1997:191–225, with permission.
Adapted from Jurkovich GJ. Hypothermia in the trauma patient. *Adv Trauma* 1989;4:111.

Pulmonary artery pressures remain normal, but pulmonary vascular resistance decreases to accommodate the incremental change in blood volume and cardiac output[26,33]

Gastrointestinal

As pregnancy progresses, the enlarged uterus stretches the abdominal wall and compresses the viscera. This results in a diminished response to peritoneal irritation and altered or referred pain perception, making the clinical examination unreliable. An increased propensity toward aspiration occurs because of compression of the intraabdominal organs, which decreases gastrointestinal motility. Also, the relaxant effect of progesterone and estrogen on smooth muscle diminishes lower esophageal sphincter competency. Alkaline phosphatase levels are almost doubled, most likely from placental alkaline phosphatase enzymes. Progesterone inhibits gallbladder contractility by inhibition of cholecystokinin, leading to bile stasis and a propensity for the development of gallstones.[34] Finally, gastrin is produced by the placenta, which lowers gastric pH during pregnancy.

Nutrient changes during pregnancy include decreased nitrogen use (demanding more protein intake) and a diabetogenic state characterized by a mild fasting hyperglycemia, postprandial hyperglycemia, and hyperinsulinemia.[22] Progesterone and estrogen may contribute to a peripheral resistance to insulin.[22] Also noted are increased plasma lipid levels that may correlate with estradiol, progesterone, and human placental lactogen levels.

Renal

Throughout pregnancy, the renal collection system enlarges to meet the demands of the increased blood volume and urine formation. The renal pelvis and ureter dilate early in the first trimester, resulting in a mild hydronephrosis (1.5 cm longer) and hydroureter.[35] Urinary stasis in the collecting system predisposes the pregnant woman to pyelonephritis. In the first trimester, the renal blood flow and the glomerular filtration rate increase by up to 50%; consequently, the levels of creatinine and blood urea nitrogen (BUN) decrease.[36] This event precedes significant increases in cardiac output or blood volume. The clinical significance is that normal or slightly elevated levels of creatinine or BUN may signify renal dysfunction. Davison and Hytten noted the presence of glucosuria in the gravid patient as a result of the increase in glomerular filtration rate and the decrease in reabsorptive capacity for filtered glucose.[37] Because of hormonal and osmoreceptor alterations, the normal serum sodium concentration for a pregnant woman is approximately 132 mEq/L. Increased clearance of

TABLE 31.3

VENTILATORY FUNCTION IN PREGNANT WOMEN COMPARED WITH NONPREGNANT WOMEN

Function	Nonpregnant	Pregnant	Change (%)
Respiratory rate	15	16	
Tidal volume (mL)	485	680	+39[a]
Minute ventilation (mL)	7,270	10,340	+42[a]
Vital capacity (mL)	3,260	3,310	+1
Residual volume (mL)	965	770	20[a]

[a]Significant differences.
Adapted from Maternal adaptions to pregnancy. In: Cunningham FG, MacDonald PC, Gant NF, et al., eds. *Williams obstetrics,* 20th ed. Norwalk, CT: Appleton & Lange, 1997.

TABLE 31.4

RENAL CHANGES IN NORMAL PREGNANCY

Alteration	Manifestation	Clinical relevance
Increased renal size	Approximately 1 cm greater on radiographs	Postpartum decreases in size should not be mistaken for parenchymal loss
Dilation of pelvis, calyces, and ureters	Resembles hydronephrosis on ultrasound or intravenous pyelography (more marked on right)	
Increased renal hemodynamics	Glomerular filtration rate and renal plasma flow increase ~50%	Serum creatinine and urea nitrogen values decrease during normal gestation; an increase >0.8 mg/dL creatinine may be sign of renal insufficiency; protein, amino acid, and glucose excretion all increase
Changes in acid–base metabolism	Renal bicarbonate threshold decreases; progesterone stimulates respiratory center	Serum bicarbonate is 4 to 5 mEq/L lower P_{CO_2} is 10 mm hg lower, (a P_{CO_2} of 40 mm Hg already represents CO_2 retention)
Renal	Osmoregulation altered: osmotic thresholds for vasopressin release and thirst decrease	Serum osmolarity decreases ~10 mOsm/L (serum Na ~5 mEq/L) during normal gestations

Adapted from Maternal adaptations to pregnancy. In: Cunningham FG, MacDonald PC, Gant NF, et al., eds. *Williams obstetrics*, 20th ed. Norwalk, CT: Appleton & Lange, 1997.

uric acid occurs in the first and second trimesters, but reabsorption becomes normal later. An elevated serum uric acid level in the first or second trimester may portend toxemia even in the normotensive gravida[38] (Table 31.4).

Musculoskeletal

The relaxation of the interosseous ligaments during pregnancy causes increased mobility of the sacroiliac and sacrococcygeal joints and widening of the symphysis pubis. These changes, coupled with an enlarged uterus, result in lordosis, disrupt the maternal center of gravity, and increase the risk for falls.

Laboratory Values

The peripheral blood leukocyte count increases to approximately 12,000 cells/mL during gestation and may be as high as 25,000 cells/mL during labor.[39] The platelet count may appear falsely low because of dilution from increases in plasma volume. Fibrinogen (factor I) and factors VII, VIII, IX, and X are increased considerably during pregnancy, but prothrombin (factor II) is increased only slightly. Although there is a slight decrease in the protein S level and its activity,[40] levels of antithrombin III and protein C show no significant change during the pregnancy. The level of plasminogen (profibrinolysin) in plasma increases significantly, most likely induced by estrogen.

INITIAL ASSESSMENT AND MANAGEMENT

Priorities for the resuscitation of the injured pregnant patient are the same as for any other trauma patient. Patient care, however, is altered to accommodate the unique anatomic and physiologic characteristics of the gravid woman.[41]

The best therapy for the unborn child is expedient maternal resuscitation. An adequate airway with supplemental oxygenation is essential to prevent fetal hypoxemia. The release of maternal catecholamines causes uteroplacental vasoconstriction, compromising fetal circulation.[42,43] Because fetal blood functions on a different oxyhemoglobin dissociation curve, small positive increments in oxygen concentration improve oxygen content and physiologic reserve for the fetus, even if maternal arterial oxygen content does not change appreciably. Maternal hemorrhagic shock, with its resultant release of catecholamines, causes uterine artery vasoconstriction, reducing uterine perfusion and compromising fetal viability. Hence, vigorous crystalloid resuscitation is encouraged, even for patients who appear normotensive. In late pregnancy, compromised cardiac output and blood pressure secondary to vena cava compression can be relieved by placing the patient in the left lateral decubitus or right hip-flexed position. A nasogastric tube should be inserted because of the pregnant patient's increased propensity toward vomiting and aspiration. Urinary volume per hour should be monitored to provide some indication of perfusion status.

History and Physical Examination

The secondary survey consists of a thorough history (including obstetric history), physical examination, and fetal monitoring.[44] Maternal prenatal history is crucial and may alter management decisions if medical problems such as preeclampsia, diabetes, essential hypertension, or congenital heart disease are present. Obstetric history includes the date of the last menstrual period, the expected date of confinement, the perception of fetal movement, and the status of the current and previous pregnancies. Gestational age (fetal maturity) can be estimated from the fundal height, as measured by palpation. (Fundal height at the umbilicus represents approximately 20 weeks' gestation.) These factors help in the decision matrix if emergent delivery is necessary. For example, a 26-week-old fetus is considered viable and has a good chance of survival if given neonatal intensive care support. Pelvic and rectal examinations are performed with special attention to vaginal discharge (amniotic fluid or blood), effacement, dilation, and fetal station.[45]

Fetomaternal hemorrhage occurs in 6% of all pregnancies but in 20% of injured pregnant patients. Although 0.01 mL of fetal blood (1 to 3 fetal cells per 500,000 maternal red blood cells) sensitizes 70% of Rh-negative patients, the remainder require up to 40 mL, or one third of fetal blood volume. The Kleihauer-Betke (KB) test detects fetal cells in the maternal circulation, indicating fetomaternal hemorrhage, although recently it has been shown to be less reliable because a positive

KB test alone does not necessarily indicate fetal-maternal hemorrhage in these patients.[46–48] Because this test can determine the risk of isosensitization in Rh-negative gravid women, it is recommended for injured Rh-negative pregnant patients in the second or third trimester to detect impending fetal exsanguination. If positive, the Kleihauer-Betke test should be repeated 24 hours later to identify ongoing fetomaternal hemorrhage. Treatment consists of an initial dose of Rh immune globulin with an additional dose administered for every 30 mL of fetomaternal transfusion estimated by this test.

Fetal Assessment and Monitoring

Fetal evaluation consists of uterine assessment, fundal height measurement, and recording of heart tones, heart rate, and movement. A heart rate of 100 beats/min or less is considered bradycardia. Uterine tenderness and contraction may be related to *abruptio placentae,* which can occur in the absence of vaginal bleeding. Auscultation for a complete minute determines regularity (acceleration and deceleration) of the fetal heartbeat. However, continuous fetal monitoring is the best predictor of a healthy or distressed fetus.[16] There is still no consensus on the indications for fetal monitoring in trauma patients. A guideline for patients with major injuries, including shock, is to provide continuous fetal monitoring for at least 24 hours.

Fetal heart rate and uterine activity can be monitored by either external (indirect) or internal (direct) methods. The external method is noninvasive and has wider clinical application. Internal monitoring requires insertion of an intrauterine catheter and application of a fetal scalp electrode. The normal fetal heart rate ranges between 120 and 160 beats/min. Abnormalities in variability may signal hypoxia or dysrhythmia in the fetus. Early decelerations of fetal heart rate, which conform closely to uterine contractions, are vagal nerve–mediated and not of significance. Similarly, variable decelerations secondary to transient umbilical cord compression are not of great concern. The presence of late deceleration of fetal heart rate after uterine contractions is thought to be related to uteroplacental insufficiency and may warrant routine monitoring after injury.[16]

Ultrasonography is not only a valuable adjunct in determining fetal viability, it also has been shown to detect the fetus in a very focused examination.[49] Ultrasound detects the changes of pregnancy 3 to 4 weeks after ovulation and is therefore useful in the gestational period, especially because it involves no radiation exposure. During the first trimester, an endovaginal ultrasound probe provides close approximation of the transducer to the uterus through cervical tissue. This method does not require bladder catheterization or filling and thus allows for a rapid examination.[50–52] Real-time B-mode ultrasound demonstrates fetal cardiac movement and determines fetal size and placental location. *Abruptio placentae* may be identified as a retroplacental lucency (blood clot) or an echogenic structure in the amniotic fluid.

DIAGNOSTIC MODALITIES

After patient stabilization, several diagnostic modalities are used to define the extent and type of injury for the mother and her unborn child. Initially, laboratory studies are obtained. If blood is urgently needed, type O, Rh-negative blood is chosen. Evaluation of the abdomen may be performed by diagnostic peritoneal lavage, computed tomography (CT) scan, or ultrasound.[53] There is an increasing role for ultrasound in the diagnosis of hemoperitoneum secondary to blunt abdominal trauma. Diagnostic peritoneal lavage may be performed in the pregnant patient, but the open, supraumbilical technique is recommended. Reliance on ultrasound to evaluate both the mother and the fetus obviates the need to perform a CT scan or diagnostic peritoneal lavage and can provide valuable information on fetal motion, heart tones, location, and placement.

Liberal but judicious use of radiographic studies is advised for the evaluation of the pregnant trauma patient. A diagnostic modality deemed necessary should not be withheld for fear of potential hazard to the fetus. Factors contributing to the sequelae of prenatal exposure to ionizing radiation are the stage of development, the exposure time, the dose delivered, and the dose absorbed. The absorbed radiation dose varies according to many factors, including instrument model, desired image quality, and distance from the radioactive source. The developmental stages are the preimplantation phase (0 to 8 days after conception), major organogenesis (9 to 60 days), and the fetal period (61 to 270 days). The roentgen (R) is the unit of exposure, and the centigray (cGy) or rad is the unit of absorbed dose. Approximate absorbed fetal doses for radiographic tests are presented in Table 31.5. No estimates have been made of radiation risk during the first few days of human development. Because the natural prevalence of congenital anomalies is approximately 6%, any effects of such tests are undetectable at low radiologic doses. There is no medical justification for terminating pregnancy in women exposed to 5 cGy or less.[54] A 0.1% increase in the rate of spontaneous abortion during the first 2 weeks of development follows a dose of 10 cGy, and there is a 1% increase in congenital abnormalities at the same dose.[55] Another concern is the potential for late neoplasia development. The risks for radiation-induced cancer after *in utero* exposure (during the second and third trimesters) are estimated to be 1 in 15,000 children if exposed to 1 mGy x-radiation.[56] If the fetus receives 50 mGy, the risk is increased to 1 in approximately 300 children. Combined studies, such as CT scan of the abdomen with oral and intravenous contrast, obviate the need for multiple studies such as an intravenous

TABLE 31.5

APPROXIMATE FETAL DOSES FROM COMMON DIAGNOSTIC PROCEDURES

Examination	Mean exposure (mGy)	Maximum dose (mGy)
CONVENTIONAL X-RAY EXAMINATIONS		
Abdomen	1.4	4.2
Chest	<0.01	<0.01
Intravenous pyelogram	1.7	10
Lumbar spine	1.7	10
Pelvis	1.1	4
Skull	<0.01	<0.01
Thoracic spine	<0.01	<0.01
FLUOROSCOPIC EXAMINATIONS		
Upper GI	1.1	5.8
Barium enema	6.8	24
COMPUTED TOMOGRAPHY		
Abdomen	8.0	49
Chest	0.06	0.96
Head	<0.005	<0.005
Lumbar spine	2.4	8.6
Pelvis	25	79

Adapted from Sharp C, Shrimpton JA, Bury RF. *Diagnostic Medical Exposures,* 1998.

pyelography. Prudent judgment and foresight by the physician should ensure that specific radiographic studies are ordered and accurately performed to avoid repetition.

BLUNT TRAUMA

Motor vehicle crashes remain the chief cause of blunt trauma in the pregnant patient. As pregnancy progresses, the uterus becomes more vulnerable, rising out of the protective bony pelvis, and it absorbs most of the impact of blunt abdominal trauma. These factors often result in direct fetal injury, usually skull fracture or intracerebral hemorrhage. Pelvic fractures in the gravid patient may cause extensive maternal retroperitoneal hemorrhage as a result of engorged pelvic veins.

Uterine rupture from blunt trauma occurs most often at the site of prior cesarean section or at the posterior fundus. It can present with massive hemorrhage or more insidiously with minimal vaginal bleeding if rupture occurs at the fundus, far from the uterine vessels. Repair can be either primary in two layers or with a polytetrafluoroethylene patch.[57] Avulsion of the uterus has been reported, with bladder rupture being an associated finding.

Abruptio placentae is the most common cause of fetal death after maternal injury. This carries a 30% to 70% rate of fetal death and a 1% maternal mortality rate. Over 50% placental separation invariably results in fetal demise[58] *Abruptio placentae* can occur in the absence of obvious abdominal injury, because maternal shock is a far greater stimulus for abruption than are the mechanical forces of trauma disrupting the placenta.[45] Abruptio placentae is more common in the presence of hypertension, diabetes mellitus, advanced age, multiparity, and maternal use of tobacco or cocaine. *Abruptio placentae* presents with vaginal bleeding (in 80% of cases), abdominal pain, disseminated intravascular coagulation due to thromboplastin release, and inexplicable maternal hypovolemia. It invariably occurs within 48 hours after trauma, and pregnant patients who are at risk should be monitored accordingly.

The pregnant patient with minor injury should be observed for several hours. Most patients with insignificant trauma do not require admission unless specific signs and symptoms, such as vaginal bleeding, abdominal cramps, or leakage of amniotic fluid, are present. In one series,[6] only 1 of 11 patients had symptoms after minor trauma, and pregnancy outcome was successful. Occult *abruptio placentae* has been reported after motor vehicle accidents in which the patient displayed only subtle clinical signs and symptoms. Because placental separation can occur with rapid deceleration injuries, a three-point restraint system appropriately applied is recommended for pregnant automobile passengers.[59–61] The mechanism of injury may provide invaluable information regarding potential injuries in even a healthy-appearing patient. At a minimum, a prompt and thorough maternal assessment, fetal assessment, and comprehensive search for injuries are necessary for evaluating the pregnant patient with minor trauma.

PENETRATING TRAUMA

The perinatal mortality rate from penetrating injury to the mother has been reported to range from 47% to 71%.[62] In general, pregnant women with gunshot wounds to the abdomen should undergo celiotomy. For those who sustain stab wounds to the abdomen, management is based on the likelihood of intraabdominal injury. The abdominal examination may be unreliable because of a diminished response to peritoneal irritation and altered or referred pain perception. If the clinical presentation is unclear (e.g., absence of peritonitis or evisceration), then a diagnostic peritoneal lavage performed with the open technique in the supraumbilical area may be diagnostic.

OPERATIVE MANAGEMENT

General anesthesia is preferred for the gravid patient with multisystem injury. The risks of anesthesia are related to the physiologic changes that accompany pregnancy. For example, because aspiration is more likely, rapid-sequence induction is preferred. The effects of anesthetics are related to the stage of fetal development and the dose of the agent administered. Because premature labor has been shown to be associated with surgery and with various anesthetic regimens, intraoperative fetal monitoring is recommended. One study reported an increase in fetal demise after celiotomy, especially if the operation was performed in the first trimester or in the presence of peritonitis.[63] In a multicenter study, fetal death occurred in 35% of cases in which the pregnant women underwent general anesthesia and surgery, compared with 11% of cases in which general anesthesia was not used. However, the mean Injury Severity Score in the surgery group was 18.0, compared with 5.5 in the nonsurgery group.

The standard vertical midline incision is used for maternal celiotomy. Adequate visualization of viscera is mandatory, and the pregnant uterus should not interfere with abdominal exploration or repair of an injury. If labor ensues, vaginal delivery is almost always encouraged. Even early in the postoperative period, vaginal delivery is still preferred and does not appear harmful to the mother or the neonate. Cesarean section prolongs the operative time and increases blood loss, generally by approximately 1 L. Algorithm 31.1 provides a suggested plan for the management of the uterus during a

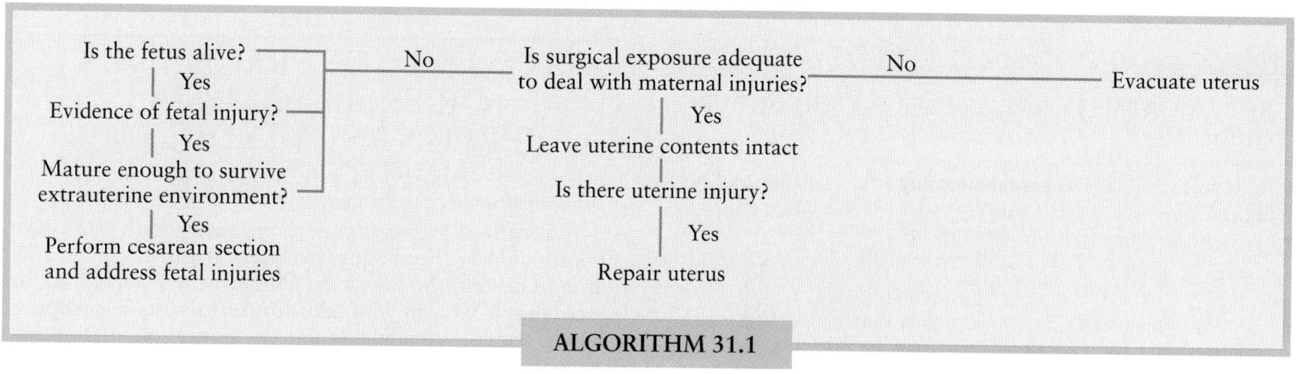

ALGORITHM 31.1 Assessment of the pregnant uterus during celiostomy.

TRAUMA

TABLE 31.6 INDICATIONS/CONTRAINDICATIONS

INDICATIONS FOR CESAREAN SECTION DURING CELIOTOMY FOR TRAUMA

- Maternal shock, pregnancy near term
- Threat to life from exsanguination (injury or disseminated intravascular coagulation)
- Mechanical limitation of maternal treatment
- Risk of fetal distress exceeding risk of prematurity
- Unstable thoracolumbar spinal injury

celiotomy.[64] Indications for cesarean section during celiotomy for trauma are listed in Table 31.6.

If fetal delivery is cesarean, the uterus is incised longitudinally. After the amniotic membranes are ruptured, the fetus is delivered, and the placenta is removed. The uterus is closed in a running-locking fashion using large, absorbable suture. Once the uterus is evacuated, postpartum hemostasis begins. In cases of uterine atony, bimanual compression of the uterus and the intravenous administration of oxytocin are begun. In addition, the surgeon should examine the uterus and cervix for any lacerations and ensure that the uterus is thoroughly evacuated. Other measures to control severe hemorrhage include intravenous methyl ergonovine, or intramyometrial injection of 15-methyl prostaglandin F_{2a}. For the most part, massive hemorrhage associated with emergent cesarean section in the injured women is associated with a pelvic fracture. Packing of the pelvis or embolization of the internal iliac arteries may be needed as well.

Successful outcome of a postmortem cesarean section depends on the duration of the gestation and the time interval between maternal death and delivery. Under optimal conditions, at 26 to 28 weeks' gestation, the estimated fetal survival rate is approximately 50%. Therefore, postmortem cesarean section is justified if the estimated gestational age is at least approximately 26 to 28 weeks. If the time between maternal death and delivery is less than 5 minutes, the fetal prognosis is considered excellent. If the time since maternal death is prolonged to approximately 20 minutes, fetal prognosis is poor. Uncertainty about maternal death time is not a contraindication for this procedure.[65]

BURNS

Fewer than 0.1% of pregnant patients sustain severe burns. The successful approach to the management of the burn victim relies on maintaining a normal intravascular volume and avoiding hypoxia. In these patients, inadequate initial resuscitation is often responsible for the loss of the pregnancy. In a review of 15 pregnant victims of electric shock, 4 fetuses were viable and only 1 was normal.[66] Because the fetus is much less resistant to electrical shock, fetal monitoring is strongly recommended after this type of injury. Table 31.7 delineates the estimates of body surface area burned and associated mortality rates in pregnant patients.

TABLE 31.7

CRUDE MORTALITY RATES AFTER MATERNAL BURN INJURIES

Body surface injured (%)	Maternal mortality rate (%)	Fetal mortality rate (%)
<40	3	22
50	25	53
>80	100	100

From Taylor JW, Plunkett GD, McManus WF, et al. Thermal injury during pregnancy. *Obstet Gynecol.* 1976;47:434–438.

CRITICAL CARE MANAGEMENT

Critical care management of the traumatized pregnant patient covers a wide range of topics. The basic principles of hemodynamic monitoring, adequate ventilatory support, nutrition, and careful assessment of volume status apply to the injured pregnant patient and are covered in more detail in other chapters. Knowledge of the disease processes that can arise in the pregnant patient within the first 24 hours after injury allows the physician to render high-quality critical care to the traumatized patient and her unborn child.[67]

When administrating medication to the gravid patient, potential risk versus therapeutic benefit must be considered especially carefully. Prophylactic tetanus immunization should be given appropriately, with anti-D globulin for patients who are Rh negative and at risk for isoimmunization. Prophylactic antibiotics are administered if needed, but tetracycline and most sulfa drugs should be avoided.

CARDIOPULMONARY RESUSCITATION

The enlarged uterus compresses the vena cava, resulting in a 25% decrease in cardiac output as a result of decreased venous return. To improve the effects of cardiopulmonary resuscitation (CPR), patients before 24 weeks' gestation can be maintained in the supine position but with manual displacement of the uterus laterally. After 24 weeks' gestation, a procedure table with a 30-degree left lateral tilt is helpful, although CPR is only 80% effective when performed with the patient in this position. Emergent cesarean section may be needed if the patient does not respond to CPR within approximately 5 minutes.[68,69] Morris et al. found that if the fetus is viable (presence of fetal heart tones) and is at least 26 weeks' gestation, emergent cesarean section is justified;[70] they found that infants who met these criteria had a survival rate of 75%.

TOXEMIA OF PREGNANCY OR PREECLAMPSIA (PREGNANCY-INDUCED HYPERTENSION)

Any traumatized pregnant patient presenting with seizures or coma should have head injury excluded. If antiseizure medication is indicated, the following should be considered before prescribing it. Women who take anticonvulsants during pregnancy have approximately double the general population risk of malformations (i.e., about a 5% increase).[71] Phenytoin (Dilantin) decreases folate absorption, which has been implicated in birth defects.[72] Therefore, it is recommended that supplemental folic acid be given to these patients.[73] In general, the blood levels of the drugs should be monitored carefully, and the neonatologist should be notified when a patient is taking anticonvulsants because most affect the vitamin K–dependent clotting factors in the newborn. In the severe state, eclampsia is manifested by hypertension, pulmonary edema, elevated liver function enzymes, proteinuria (i.e., HELLP syndrome), and seizure activity. The pathophysiologic cause is vasospasm, which affects hepatic, renal, cerebral, and placental blood flow. Despite the presence of pulmonary edema, intravascular volume depletion is often present, and a fluid challenge may be appropriate. Rapid control of the hypertension is achieved with hydralazine.[74] However, elevated maternal oxygen consumption disrupts uterine vascular oxygen supply and maternal equilibrium, resulting in fetal distress. Smoother control of reduction in blood pressure and myocardial oxygen consumption is accomplished by achieving volume expansion before vasodilation. Inotropic support, in combination with vasodilator treatment, maximizes oxygen delivery and affects afterload reduction. Magnesium sulfate has a slight hypotensive effect but does not decrease systemic vascular resistance. The hemodynamic parameters illustrated in Table 31.2 are guidelines for optimizing maternal hemodynamics, uteroplacental perfusion, and, ultimately, fetal well-being.

THROMBOEMBOLISM

Pregnant patients are at increased risk of thromboembolism from all three components of Virchow's triad: stasis, intimal damage, and hypercoagulability. Increased venous capacitance, vena cava compression, and weight gain promote venous stasis. Labor and trauma cause intimal damage, and hypercoagulability results from elevated levels of fibrinogen and intrinsic coagulation factors with the gravid state. Advanced age and multiparity further increase these risks. No method of prophylaxis has been demonstrated to be both safe and universally effective in preventing thromboembolism, either in the patient with multiple injuries or in the pregnant patient. In general, warfarin is avoided because it is associated with congenital anomalies if given to the mother in the first trimester and has been shown to cause serious fetal bleeding when administered during the second and third trimesters.[75,76] The American College of Cardiology/American Heart Association guidelines recommend subcutaneous heparin if prophylaxis is indicated until after delivery.[77]

AMNIOTIC FLUID EMBOLISM

Amniotic fluid embolism after trauma in pregnancy or parturition is characterized by hypotension, hypoxemia, and coagulopathy. The diagnosis is often difficult, and an 80% mortality rate has been reported. Amniotic fluid debris enters the maternal venous circulation, causing sudden dyspnea and hypotension. A mixed metabolic acidosis and respiratory alkalosis ensue. The chest radiograph shows characteristic pulmonary edema or an acute respiratory distress syndrome (ARDS) pattern. Hemodynamically, the patient has an elevated pulmonary capillary wedge pressure and a low systemic vascular resistance. Disseminated intravascular coagulation develops in approximately 30% of these patients. Although most cases of amniotic fluid embolism occur during labor, it has been reported to occur after abdominal trauma[78] and *abruptio placentae*. This diagnosis is established on clinical findings, and the treatment consists of supportive care (i.e., oxygenation, maximization of hemodynamic parameters, and correction of coagulopathy).

INTERPERSONAL VIOLENCE

Although motor vehicle crashes and falls are the most common causes of trauma during pregnancy, reports indicate that 4% to 17% of pregnant women are victims of interpersonal violence.[2–4] In fact, this number may be underestimated because population-based prevalence estimates are often unavailable, pregnancy is not consistently recorded on death certificates,[8] and, as with many abuse crimes, it is not always reported.

Poole et al. reported that 64 (31.5%) of 203 injured pregnant patients experienced interpersonal violence.[11] Of the eight fetal deaths in this series, three occurred 7 days after injury and five occurred in women with an Injury Severity Score of zero. These findings indicate that severe trauma to the fetus may occur without obvious injury to the mother, emphasizing the need for the physician to question the patient directly about abuse. Furthermore, physicians should be encouraged to take measures for early intervention, such as establishing a link with agencies that deal with battered women, so that physical protection, emotional support, and information about legal rights are readily available.

SUMMARY

The pregnant trauma victim presents a unique challenge to the resuscitating physician. Two patients are being treated, and a high degree of expertise is needed to treat both. Initially, evaluation should involve the cooperative efforts of the emergency physician, trauma surgeon, obstetrician, and obstetric nurse. If the pregnancy is near term or delivery is anticipated, a pediatrician and pediatric surgeon should be consulted. The pregnancy should not distract the surgeon from initiating basic resuscitation. Equally important, the injury should not confound the obstetrician. The expertise of the obstetric nurse is useful in coordinating the overall care plan for the mother and her unborn child. Expedient, accurate resuscitation of the mother takes priority because the best chance for fetal survival is maternal survival.

KEY POINTS

- **Care of the injured pregnant patient brings the challenge of treating two patients, both with unique physiologic responses to the trauma. The mortality risk to the fetus is three to four times greater than that of the mother.**
- **By the twelfth week of gestation, the gravid uterus is intraabdominal and it reaches the umbilicus by the twentieth week. The uterus thins but remains elastic, whereas the placenta does not, leading to risk of *abruptio placentae* following injury, which is the most common cause of fetal demise and may present as an occult process.**
- **Multiple physiologic changes occur during pregnancy with increased uterine/pelvic blood flow, increased blood volume with a relative anemia, increased cardiac output, decreased venous return when supine (because of uterine compression of the vena cava), mild hypotension, increased tidal volume and respiratory alkalosis with increased 2,3-DPG, increased risk of aspiration and gallstones, mild hydronephrosis with increased glomerular filtration and decreased creatinine, a diabetogenic state, and an enhanced coagulant risk with increased fibrinogen and factors VII, VIII, IX, and X levels.**
- **Following injury, the fetus is highly susceptible to hypoxia and decreased perfusion, particularly in response to catecholamines released in response to hypovolemia. Fetal**

evaluation includes fundal height measurement and recording heart tones, heart rate and movement. Focused abdominal sonogram for trauma (FAST) is an excellent noninvasive, radiation-free method of evaluating the mother, uterus, and fetus.

- **Trauma can lead to urgent transfusion, which should be of Type O, Rh negative; fetomaternal hemorrhage (as confirmed by Kleihauer-Betke test), which causes isosensitization in Rh-negative women and requires Rh immune globulin; toxemia of pregnancy, which requires volume resuscitation and smooth control of hypertension; an increased risk of venous thromboembolism, which should be treated with heparin, avoiding Coumadin because of teratogenicity; and amniotic fluid embolism with acute hypoxia, hypotension, and coagulopathy.**

References

1. Rogers FB, Rozycki GS, Osler TM, et al. A multi-institutional study of factors associated with fetal death in injured pregnant patients. *Arch Surg.* 1999;134:1274–1277.
2. Kissinger DP, Rozycki GS, Morris JA, et al. Trauma in pregnancy: predicting pregnancy outcome. *Arch Surg.* 1991;126:1079–1086.
3. Drost TF, Rosemurgy AS, Sherman HF, et al. Major trauma in pregnant women: maternal/fetal outcome. *J Trauma* 1990;30:574–578.
4. Hoff WS, D'Amelio LF, Tinkoff GH, et al. Maternal predictors of fetal demise in trauma during pregnancy. *Surg Gynecol Obstet.* 1991;172: 175–180.
5. Esposito TJ, Gens DR, Smith LG, et al. Trauma during pregnancy: a review of 79 cases. *Arch Surg.* 1991;126:1073–1078.
6. Pearlman MD, Tintinalli JE, Lorenz RP. A prospective controlled study of outcome after trauma during pregnancy. *Am J Obstet Gynecol.* 1990;162: 1502–1510.
7. Fildes J, Reed L, Jones N, et al. Trauma: the leading cause of maternal death. *J Trauma* 1992;32:643–645.
8. Dietz P, Rochat R, Goldner T, et al. Osewe PL, ed. Pregnancy status poorly reported on death certificates. In: *Georgia epidemiology report.* Atlanta: Department of Human Resources, 1995:Report #11-6, pp. 1–4.
9. Shah KH, Simons RK, Holbrook T, et al. Trauma in pregnancy: maternal and fetal outcomes. *J Trauma* 1998;45:83–86.
10. Scorpio RJ, Esposito TJ, Smith LG, et al. Blunt trauma during pregnancy: factors affecting fetal outcome. *J Trauma* 1992;32:213–216.
11. **Poole GV, Martin JN Jr, Perry KG Jr, et al. Trauma in pregnancy: the role of interpersonal violence. *Am J Obstet Gynecol.* 1996;174:1873–1878.**
12. Biester EM, Tomich PG, Esposito TJ, et al. Trauma in pregnancy: normal revised trauma score in relation to other markers of maternofetal status—a preliminary study. *Am J Obstet Gynecol.* 1997;176:1206–1212.
13. Connolly A, Katz VL, Bash KL, et al. Trauma and pregnancy. *Am J Perinatol.* 1997;14:331–336.
14. Weiss HB, Songer TJ, Fabio A. Fetal deaths related to maternal injury. *JAMA.* 2001;286:1863–1868.
15. Weiss HB, Lawrence B, Miller T. Prevalence and risk of hospitalized pregnant occupants in car crashes. In: *Annual Proceedings/Association for the Advancement of Automotive Medicine* 2002;46:355–366.
16. Depp R. Clinical evaluation of fetal status. In: Scott JR, DiSaia PJ, Hammond CB, et al., eds. *Danforth's obstetrics and gynecology*, 6th ed. Philadelphia: JB Lippincott, 1990:315–334.
17. Thedorou DA, Velmahos GC, Chan LS, Vassiliu P, et al. Fetal death after trauma in pregnancy. Am Surg. 2000;66:809–812.
18. Cunningham FG, MacDonald PC. Maternal adaptations to pregnancy. In: Gant NF, et al., eds. *Williams obstetrics*, 20th ed. Norwalk, CT: Appleton & Lange, 1997;191–225.
19. Edman CD, Toofanian A, MacDonald PC, et al. Placental clearance rate of maternal plasma androstenedione through placental estradiol formation: an indirect method of assessing uteroplacental blood flow. *Am J Obstet Gynecol.* 1981;69:851.
20. Kauppila A, Koskinen M, Puolakka J, et al. Decreased intervillous and unchanged myometrial blood flow in supine recumbency. *Obstet Gynecol.* 1980;55:203.
21. Pritchard JA. Changes in blood during pregnancy and delivery. *Anesthesiology* 1965;26:393.
22. Whittaker PG, MacPhail S, Lind T. Serial hematologic changes and pregnancy outcome. *Obstet Gynecol* 1996;88:33.
23. Scott DE. Anemia during pregnancy. *Obstet Gynecol Ann.* 1972;48:638.
24. Smith CV, Phelan JP. Trauma in pregnancy. In: Clark SL, Cotton DB, Hankins GDV, et al., eds. *Critical care obstetrics,* 2nd ed. Boston: Blackwell, 1991:498.
25. Brinkman CRI, Mofid M, Assali NS. Circulatory shock in pregnant sheep: effects of hemorrhage on uteroplacental and fetal circulation and oxygenation. *Am J Obstet Gynecol.* 1974;118:77–90.
26. Gonick B. Intensive care monitoring of the critically ill pregnant patient. In: Creasy RK, Resnick R, eds. *Maternal-fetal medicine: principles and practice,* 2nd ed. Philadelphia: WB Saunders, 1989:845.
27. Bieniarz J, Branda LA, Maqueda E. Aortocaval compression by the uterus in late pregnancy: III. Unreliability of the sphygmomanometric method in estimating uterine artery pressure. *Am J Obstet Gynecol.* 1968;102:1106.
28. Greiss FC, Anderson SG. Effect of ovarian hormones on the uterine vascular bed. *Am J Obstet Gynecol.* 1970;107:829.
29. Clark SL, Cotton DB, Lee W. Central hemodynamic assessment of normal term pregnancy. *Am J Obstet Gynecol.* 1989;161:1439.
30. Enein M, Zina AAA, Kassem M, et al. Echocardiography of the pericardium in pregnancy. *Obstet Gynecol.* 1987;69:851.
31. Lee W, Cotton DB. Cardiorespiratory changes during pregnancy. In: Clark SL, Cotton DB, Hankins GDV, et al., eds. *Critical care obstetrics,* 2nd ed. Boston: Blackwell, 1991:2.
32. Tsia CH, deLeeuw NKM. Changes in 2,3-diphosphoglycerate during pregnancy and puerperium in normal women and in B-thalassemia heterozygous women. *Am J Obstet Gynecol.* 1982;142:520.
33. Hume RF, Killam AP. Maternal physiology. In: Scott JR, DiSaia J, Hammon DB, et al., eds. *Obstetrics and gynecology.* Philadelphia: JB Lippincott, 1990:93.
34. Braverman DZ, Johnson ML, Kern F Jr. Effects of pregnancy and contraceptive steroids on gallbladder function. *N Engl J Med.* 1980;302:362.
35. Bailey RR, Rollerston GL. Kidney length and ureteric dilatation in the puerperium. *Br J Obstet Gynaecol.* 1971;78:55.
36. Chesley LC. Renal function during pregnancy. In: Carey HM, ed. *Modern trends in human reproductive physiology* 1963;1:205–214.
37. Davison JM, Hytten FF. The effects of pregnancy on the renal handling of glucose. *Br J Obstet Gynaecol.* 1975;82:374.
38. Lindheimer MD, Grunfeld JP, Davison JM. Renal disorders. In: Barron WM, Lindheimer MD, ed. *Medical disorders during pregnancy,* 2nd ed. St. Louis: Mosby, 1995:37.
39. Taylor DJ, Phillips P, Lind T. Puerperal hematological indices. *Br J Obstet Gynaecol.* 1981;88:601.
40. Bremme K, Ostlund E, Almqvist I, et al. Enhanced thrombin generation and fibrinolytic activity in normal pregnancy and the puerperium. *Obstet Gynecol.* 1992;80:132.
41. Advanced Trauma Life Support. American College of Surgeons Committee on Trauma. *Trauma in women,* 6th ed. Chicago: American College of Surgeons, 1997:313–324.
42. Rosenfeld CR, Barton MD, Meschia G. Effects of epinephrine on distribution of blood flow in the pregnant ewe. *Am J Obstet Gynecol.* 1976;124:156.
43. Rosenfeld CR, West J. Circulatory response to systemic infusion of norepinephrine in the pregnant ewe. *Am J Obstet Gynecol.* 1977;127:376.
44. Higgins SD. Perinatal protocol: trauma in pregnancy. *J Perinatol.* 1988;8: 288–292.
45. **Neufeld JDG, Moore EE, Marx JA, et al. Trauma in pregnancy. *Emerg Med Clin North Am.* 1987;5:623–640.**
46. Kleihauer E, Braun H, Betke K. Demonstration von fetalem hamoglobin in den erythrocyten eines blutausstrichs. *Klin Wochenschr.* 1957;35:637.
47. Scott JR, Beer AE, Guy LR. Pathogenesis of Rh immunization in primigravidas: fetomaternal versus maternal-fetal bleeding. *Obstet Gynecol.* 1977;49:9.
48. **Dhanraj D, Lambers D. The incidences of positive Kleihaour-Betke test in low-risk pregnancies and maternal trauma patients. *Am J Obstet Gynecol.* 2004; 190:1461–1463.**
49. Bochicchio GV, Haan J, Scalea T. Surgeon-Performed Focus Assessment with Sonography for Trauma as an Early Screening Tool for Pregnancy after Trauma. *J Trauma* 2002;52:1125–1128.
50. Thorsen MK, Lawson TL, Aiman EJ, et al. Diagnosis of ectopic pregnancy: endovaginal vs. transabdominal sonography. *AJR Am J Roentgenol.* 1990;155:307–310.
51. Timor-Tritsch I, Greenidge S, Admon D, et al. Emergency room use of transvaginal ultrasonography by obstetrics and gynecology residents. *Am J Obstet Gynecol.* 1992;166:866–872.
52. Mateer JR, Valley VT, Aiman EJ, et al. Outcome analysis of a protocol including bedside endovaginal sonography inpatients at risk of ectopic pregnancy. *Ann Emerg Med.* 1996;27:283–289.
53. Reed KL. Ultrasound in obstetrics. In: Scott JR, DiSaia PJ, Hammond CB, et al., eds. *Danforth's obstetrics and gynecology,* 6th ed. Philadelphia: JB Lippincott, 1990:297–314.
54. Brent RL. The effect of embryonic and fetal exposure to x-ray, microwaves, and ultrasound: counseling the pregnant and nonpregnant patient about these risks. *Semin Oncol.* 1989;16:347–368.
55. Bushong SC. *Radiologic science for technologists.* Washington, DC: Mosby, 1983:550.
56. Stovall M, Blackwell CR, Novada DH, et al. Fetal dose from radiotherapy with photon beams: report of AAPM Radiation Therapy Committee Task Group No. 36. *Med Phys.* 1995;22:63–82.
57. Martin JN, Brewer DW. Successful pregnancy outcome following mid-gestational uterine rupture and repair using Gore-Tex soft tissue patch. Obstet Gynecol. 1990;75:518.
58. Higgins SD, Garite TJ. Late abruptio placentae in trauma patients: implications for monitoring. *Obstet Gynecol.* 1984; 63(3)[Suppl]:10S–12S.
59. Crosby WM. Automobile trauma in pregnancy: prevention and treatment. *Prim Care Update Ob/Gyn.* 1996;3:6.

60. Crosby WM, Costiloe J. Safety of lap-belt restraint for pregnant victims of automobile collisions. *N Engl J Med.* 1971;284:632.
61. Pearlman MD, Viano D. Automobile crash simulation with the first pregnant crash test dummy. *Am J Obstet Gynecol.* 1996;175:977–981.
62. Franger AL, Buchsbaum HJ, Peaceman AM. Abdominal gunshot wounds in pregnancy. *Am J Obstet Gynecol.* 1989;160:1124–1128.
63. Saunders P, Milton PJ. Laparotomy during pregnancy: an assessment of diagnostic accuracy and fetal wastage. *BMJ* 1973;3:165–167.
64. Eddy VA, Morris JA Jr, Rozycki GS. Trauma and pregnancy. In: Ivatury RR, Cayten CG, eds. *Penetrating trauma.* Baltimore: Williams & Wilkins, 1996:695–701.
65. Rothenberger D, Quattlebaum FW, Perry JF. Blunt maternal trauma: a review of 103 cases. *J Trauma* 1978;18:173.
66. Fatovich DM. Electric shock in pregnancy. *J Emerg Med.* 1993;11:175.
67. **Naylor DF Jr., Olson MM. Critical care obstetrics and gynecology. *Critical Care Clinics* 2003;19:127–149.**
68. Marx GF. Cardiopulmonary resuscitation of late-pregnant women. *Anesthesiology* 1982;56:156.
69. Oates S, Williams GL, Rees GA. Cardiopulmonary resuscitation in late pregnancy. *BMJ* 1988;297:40.
70. **Morris JA, Rosenbower TJ, Jurkovich GJ, et al. Infant survival after cesarean section for trauma. *Ann Surg.* 1996;223:481–449.**
71. **Niebyl J. Drugs in pregnancy and lactation. In: Gabbe SG, Niebyl JR, Simpson, JL eds. *Obstetrics normal and problem pregnancies.* Philadelphia: Churchill Livingstone, 2002; 9,224.**
72. Dansky LV, Rosenblatt DS, Andermann E: Mechanisms of teratogenesis: folic acid and antiepileptic therapy. *Neurology* 1992;42:32.
73. Biale Y, Lewenthal H. Effect of folic acid supplementation on congenital malformations due to anticonvulsive drugs. *Eur J Obstet Gynecol Reprod Biol.* 1984;18:211.
74. Common complications of pregnancy: hypertensive disorders in pregnancy. In: Cunningham FG, MacDonald PC, Gant NF, et al., eds. *Williams obstetrics,* 20th ed. Norwalk, CT: Appleton & Lange, 1997:693–744.
75. **Ginsberg JS, Hirsch J. Use of antithrombotic agents during pregnancy. *Chest* 1998;114:524S–530S.**
76. Easterling TR, Otto C. Heart Disease. In: Gabbe SG, Niebyl JR, Simpson, JL, eds. *Obstetrics normal and problem pregnancies.* Philadelphia: Churchill Livingstone, 2002:29,1016.
77. Bonow R, Carabello B, de Leon A, et al. ACC/AGA guidelines for the management of patients with valvular heart disease. Executive summary: A report of the American College of Cardiology/American Heart Association Task Force on practice guidelines (committee on management of patients with valvular heart disease). *J Heart Valve Dis.* 1998;7:672.
78. **Judich A, Kuriansky J, Engelberg I, et al. Amniotic fluid embolism following blunt abdominal trauma in pregnancy. *Injury* 1998;29:475–477.**

CHAPTER 32 ■ CRITICAL CARE AND POSTINJURY MANAGEMENT

GRANT E. O'KEEFE

The majority of deaths occurring in trauma patients who survive to reach a trauma center occur in the intensive care unit (ICU); furthermore, the most costly complications occur in and require treatment in the ICU.[1,2] Many of these deaths and complications are related to injury-induced alterations in inflammatory and innate immune responses. Understanding their biology, epidemiology, and clinical features helps to focus our resuscitative and definitive care efforts in these patients.[3,4] Although these patients experience many changes and complications common to other, noninjured critically ill patients, this chapter focuses on those that are of particular importance to trauma victims.

The topics in this chapter are addressed according to the temporal order in which they are generally encountered. Overlap occurs and these time periods should not be considered exclusive. However, they provide an important framework within which to think about the challenges these patients present as they arrive in the ICU from the operating room, emergency department, and elsewhere.

STABILIZATION AND SECONDARY SURVEY (INITIAL 24 HOURS POSTINJURY)

This phase is often a continuation of emergency department or operating room stabilization of vital functions and the ongoing diagnosis and management of life-threatening injuries. In other circumstances, resuscitation is complete, but secondary or "tertiary" surveys to search for occult injuries are undertaken, support of vital organ function is continued, and careful monitoring for deterioration is required.

Hemodynamic Resuscitation: Monitoring and Targets

Tissue injury, local and global ischemia, and hypoxia are well-known contributors to subsequent organ dysfunction, nosocomial infection, and other complications after severe injury.[5,6] The duration and degree of shock both increase the risk for subsequent organ dysfunction and severe nosocomial infection after various types of trauma (blunt, penetrating, and burn injury).[6,7] Therefore, rapid and adequate hemodynamic resuscitation is a critical component of the initial ICU care of trauma patients. Unfortunately, there are no definitive markers of adequate resuscitation. Arterial blood base deficit and lactate concentration are good indicators of the degree of injury, but they correlate poorly with other measures of inadequate tissue perfusion and do not function well as tools to monitor the progress of resuscitation. These markers may remain elevated after perfusion is appropriately restored, in part because they reflect adrenergic stimulation of Na^+-K^+ ATPase, which increases lactate production unrelated to tissue hypoxia.[8,9] Other biochemical or physiological markers may be obtained only by invasive means, which may not be warranted in all cases. Therefore, this early phase of resuscitation should initally be guided by the objectives of normalizing heart rate and blood pressure, achieving adequate urine output (0.5 mL/kg per hour in adults and 1.0 mL/kg per hour in

TABLE 32.1

HEMODYNAMIC RESUSCITATION PARAMETERS DURING INITIAL 24 HOURS AFTER INJURY

Parameter	Goal
Urine output	30 mL/kg/hr
Hemoglobin	12–15 g/dL
Heart rate	100/min
Arterial blood pressure	≥120 mHg
Central venous pressure	12–15 mHg
Cardiac index	4.0 L/min/m^2
Oxygen delivery	500–550 mL O_2/min/m^2
Mixed venous oxyhemoglobin saturation	≥65%
Central venous oxyhemoglobin saturation	≥70%

children) while approximating normal central venous pressure (8 to 12 mm Hg), measurements that can be obtained simply from an indwelling bladder catheter, an arterial line, and central venous line. Overall, more invasive hemodynamic monitoring, such as with a pulmonary artery catheter (PAC), and aggressive resuscitation to end points based on this monitoring does not improve survival consistently or reduce complications in critically ill patients.[10,11] Although less information is available regarding the role of the PAC in trauma patients, attempting to achieve relatively high cardiac index (equal to or greater than 4.5 L/min/m^2) and oxygen delivery index (equal to or greater than 600 mL/min/m^2) is of no benefit over resuscitation to more modest goals.[12,13] Nevertheless, there may be certain circumstances where additional information is needed to guide appropriate resuscitation, such as shock accompanied by hypoxemia or oliguria, and the appropriate use of either continued volume resuscitation or vasoactive drug support must be balanced. Therefore, in patients who arrive in the ICU after receiving large-volume resuscitation in the operating room or emergency department, invasive monitoring may be helpful in avoiding subsequent overresuscitation by targeting more modest end points (cardiac index ~3.5 to 4.0 L/min/m^2 and oxygen delivery index ~500 mL/min/m^2). In addition, there are a number of potential alternatives to invasive monitoring with a PAC. These include continuous measurement of central venous oxyhemoglobin saturation ($ScvO_2$) (rather than mixed venous oxyhemoglobin saturation [$SmvO_2$] with a PAC), which has been shown to improve survival when used early in the management of patients with sepsis.[14] Less invasive estimates of cardiac output, based on thoracic bioimpedance, have been combined with blood pressure, arterial oxygen saturation (SaO_2), and transcutaneous measures of tissue oxygenation to identify trauma patients likely to survive or to die.[15] These less-invasive options are especially attractive outside of the ICU setting (e.g., emergency department), but they may also be applicable in the ICU. Incorporating these newer methods into more aggressive monitoring and resuscitation protocols has not been shown to improve survival but may reduce organ failure in critically ill trauma patients.[16] A summary of resuscitation targets is included in Table 32.1.

Hypothermia

Thermoregulation may be compromised in severely injured patients by shock and failure of cellular metabolism. Resulting hypothermia is often exacerbated by ongoing heat loss through the four general mechanisms of energy transfer: radiation, convection, evaporation, and conduction.[17] Minimizing additional heat loss through careful attention to the patient's environment is central to preventing hypothermia and its consequences. An example of the energy required to restore normothermia is illustrated in Table 32.2.[17,18] In contrast to treating established hypothermia, prevention simply requires the elimination or minimization of heat loss, which is a comparatively easier task. Although warm air contains little heat (specific heat = 0.25 kcal/kg/°C) and is therefore of little help in actively warming a patient, a warm air environment or air-circulating blanket can prevent hypothermia by avoiding heat transfer (loss) from the patient. Therefore, it is critical to minimize exposure of the patient to a cool environment.

To warm a hypothermic patient requires the addition of energy, which, when hypothermia is marked, must be done actively, rather than relying on metabolism by the patient (termed *passive warming*). A number of techniques are used for actively rewarming patients. These include overhead radiant heat warmers, whose effectiveness requires that they be placed relatively close to the patient (within 70 cm) and that the patient be fully exposed to the radiant heat. Body cavity lavage (pleural or peritoneal) can transfer large amounts of energy but may not be practical in the multiply-injured patient. Airway warming with heated, humidified oxygen

TABLE 32.2

MATHEMATICAL ILLUSTRATION OF ENERGY REQUIRED TO WARM A HYPOTHERMIC 70-KG TRAUMA VICTIM

Heat (energy) loss must be replaced to restore normothermia (defined here as 37°C). The body's only intrinsic mechanism for generating heat is through metabolism and oxygen consumption. The following example illustrates the amount of heat that must be generated to restore a trauma patient at 34°C to 37°C.

The specific heat (c) is defined as the amount of energy (measured in kilocalories) required to raise the temperature of 1 kg of a substance by 1°C. The specific heat of the human body is 0.83 kcal/kg/°C (that of water is 1 kcal/kg/°C). The following equation defines the amount of heat lost by the hypothermic patient:

$$Q\text{ (heat)} = m\text{ (in kg)} \times 0.83\text{ kcal/kg/°C} \times [\text{Temp}_1 - \text{Temp}_2\ (\Delta\text{Temp})]$$

$$Q\text{ (heat)} = 70\text{ kg} \times 0.83\text{ kcal/kg/°C} \times [37°C - 34°C] = \mathbf{181\ kcal}$$

This heat must be generated by consuming oxygen, and approximately 1 kcal is generated by the consumption of approximately 200 mL of oxygen. Therefore, this degree of hypothermia requires the consumption of 36,000 mL of oxygen. Assuming a resting oxygen consumption of approximately 200 mL/min, this patient would have to double oxygen delivery for 3 hours (or increase by 50% for 6 hours) to return to normothermia. Clearly in a patient in shock or recovering from shock, such demands are impossible to meet and the patient will remain hypothermic.

Adapted from the work of Gentilello.[17,18]

transfers relatively little energy and should not be relied on for treatment of hypothermia. The most effective method for rewarming is full cardiopulmonary bypass, which has been used successfully in hypothermic trauma victims. Although a heparin-bonded system avoids the need for systemic anticoagulation, limited availability hampers its usefulness.[19,20] A more useful form of extracorporeal rewarming is continuous arteriovenous rewarming, in which blood is circulated through a countercurrent exchange warmer using commercially available blood and intravenous fluid warmers, relying on the patient's blood pressure to drive the system, and has been demonstrated to reduce blood and intravenous fluid requirements, and prolong survival after trauma-associated hypothermia.[21] Venovenous bypass systems, which rely on an extracorporeal pump, not the patient's own blood pressure, can also be used to treat hypothermia associated with trauma.[22] Given the consequences of moderate to severe hypothermia, active rewarming should be used in any patient with a temperature of 34.5°C or below. Extracorporeal rewarming is the most effective option, and radiant heat warmers are a reasonable alternative. Recently, induced hypothermia has been advocated to increase survival after out-of-hospital cardiac arrest.[23] However, these findings should not be generalized to the critically ill trauma patient, in whom hypothermia is, on balance, harmful.

Hemostatic Abnormalities

Hemostatic complications are common in critically injured trauma patients and are the result of many processes (Table 32.3). Treatment does not require, and in the event of coagulopathic bleeding must not wait for, precise laboratory characterization of the defect(s). Clinical evidence of coagulopathic bleeding, such as the development of diffuse hemorrhage intraoperatively, abnormal bleeding from intravenous sites, and marked bloody drain (e.g., thoracostomy, other surgically placed drains) output, suggest hemostatic defects and mandate empiric treatment. Review of the likely contributing factors will help direct appropriate blood component therapy while waiting for definitive laboratory diagnosis of the specific abnormalities. Laboratory characterization and treatment can be based on four tests: platelet count, prothrombin time (PT), activated partial thromboplastin time (aPTT), and fibrinogen levels. It is evident that hemorrhage accompanied by crystalloid and red blood cell transfusion results in dilution of coagulation factors, yet the implications of this dilution are not clear. Correlation between the amount of blood transfused and specific factor levels, or the global measures of coagulation (aPTT, PT), are relatively low; however, coagulopathy seems to generally occur after rather large transfusions (10 to 12 units of packed red blood cells).[24,25] The effect on platelet counts produces wide variations in the incidence of thrombocytopenia.[26]

Factors other than dilution contribute to hemostatic abnormalities. Tissue trauma leads to platelet aggregation and activation of coagulation. Variable induction of these processes, depending on the nature and severity of the trauma, likely explains the lack of correlation of measured hemostatic deficits with blood loss, resuscitation, and blood transfusion volumes. For example, traumatic brain injury can result in coagulopathy that is independent of blood loss and transfusion volumes.[27] This coagulopathy is likely due to the exposure of circulating platelets and capillary endothelial cells to brain tissue thromboplastin and is often reflected by marked reductions in circulating fibrinogen concentrations (less than 50 mg/dL). The effect of hypothermia on hemostasis is multifactorial but for the most part demands achieving near normothermia in addition to treatment with required blood components.

In the severely injured, a combination of platelet, plasma, and cryoprecipitate transfusions are usually required. However, there are no definitive platelet count, aPTT, or PT thresholds that require treatment. Isolated, minor abnormalities in the PT (equal to or less than 1.8 times control) do not warrant treatment. Similarly, isolated increases in the aPTT (with a normal PT) should not be treated with blood products because they are not due to deficiencies in the common pathway factors (X, V, II, and I). The results may be spurious (blood drawn through heparinized tubing) or due to a lupus anticoagulant or hemophilia. In the initial postinjury period, platelet counts should be maintained above 50,000/µL, and above 100,000/µL in the presence of an injury with major hemorrhage (e.g., severe liver injury requiring packing, pelvis fracture with large hematoma) or when the consequence of ongoing bleeding is devastating, such as in the case of an intracranial hemorrhage or contusion. Combined moderate abnormalities in the aPTT and PT (1.5 to 3.0 times the upper limit of normal) should be treated with 2 to 4 units of plasma. Marked elevations in PT and aPTT may also reflect very low fibrinogen levels. In this case or when measured fibrinogen is 100 mg/dL or lower, cryoprecipitate should also be given. A normal aPTT should be the target. In the presence of a traumatic intracranial bleed (epidural, subdural, or intracerebral hematoma), the risk for hemorrhage progression has been associated with the aPTT, but because there is no particular threshold where bleeding clearly increases, the treatment goal should be to maintain the aPTT within the normal range.[28]

Recombinant factor VIIa has been used in severely coagulopathic trauma patients, although this use is not approved by the FDA. Factor VIIa binds to tissue factor exposed at the site of injury and rapidly stimulates coagulation. Small studies have reported its usefulness in coagulopathic trauma patients who continue to bleed despite treatment with platelets, plasma, and cryoprecipitate.[29–31] Factor VIIa may also be indicated in bleeding trauma patients who have been receiving warfarin and for the rare trauma patient with hemophilia A who also has factor VIII inhibitors.

TABLE 32.3 ETIOLOGY

ETIOLOGY OF HEMOSTASIS DEFECTS IN TRAUMA

Dilution of coagulation factors
Hypothermia (impaired enzyme activity, platelet dysfunction, enhanced fibrinolysis)
Traumatic brain injury (exposure of blood to brain tissue thromboplastin)
Preexisting hemostatic defects (von Willebrand disease, hemophilia, chronic liver disease)
Medications (Warfarin, antiplatelet agents)

Management of Traumatic Brain Injury and Intracranial Hypertension

Severely injured patients, particularly those who have sustained their injuries by a blunt mechanism, often have a traumatic brain injury (TBI) in additon to torso and extremity injuries. The three principal challenges in the management of TBI are: (a) avoiding secondary brain injury, (b) control of elevated intracranial pressure (ICP), and (c) early identification of any progression of mass lesions that would require surgical decompression. Management of severely head-injured patients requires the use of various monitoring and therapeutic strategies based on clinical course, computed tomography (CT) scan findings, and response to treatment. Significant deterioration in clinical course or ICP should be considered an absolute indication for repeat CT scan. This is the only practical method for the prompt identification of patients in whom surgically correctable mass lesions develop during the initial phase of care.

Important additional and avoidable causes of secondary brain injury include hypotension, hyperthermia, seizure activity, hyperglycemia, and hypoxemia. Taken together, these contribute to deterioration in brain function and are often preventable. Hypotension at any point (even for brief periods) approximately doubles the likelihood of death from a given brain injury and must be avoided.[32,33] Posttraumatic seizures increase cerebral metabolic rate, may increase ICP, and may cause important secondary brain injury. Prevention with intravenous phenytoin for the first 7 days after injury is indicated and effective.[34] Normocapnea ($PaCO_2$ 35 to 40 mm Hg) should be maintained to avoid cerebral vasoconstriction. However, brief but not excessive hyperventilation (keep $PaCO_2$ higher than 25 mm Hg) as a temporizing measure to treat sudden increases in ICP or herniation may be necessary while preparing for definitive treatment (e.g., craniotomy, ventriculostomy for CSF drainage).

Mechanical Ventilation

There are a number of important considerations in the delivery of mechanical ventilation during the ongoing resuscitative and diagnostic phase. First, abnormal gas exchange, leading to hypoxemia, commonly exists in patients who are being resuscitated from hemorrhagic shock. Pulmonary edema may arise more as a consequence of aggressive crystalloid resuscitation and transiently increased endothelial permeability consequent to shock. The transient hypoxemic respiratory failure observed in trauma patients may reflect a somewhat different pathophysiological process than that which exists in the more prolonged hypoxemic respiratory failure seen with the acute respiratory distress syndrome (ARDS).[35] Furthermore, the goals of support at this point are primarily to assist in resuscitation from shock by supporting oxygen delivery and restoring normal metabolism. Therefore, it is important to distinguish the approach to mechanical ventilation (including potential use of high peak and plateau pressures, as required) in these first hours from the approach used once the patient has been successfully resuscitated and may have developed moderate to severe acute lung injury (ALI).

Abdominal Compartment Syndrome

Elevated intraabdominal pressure (intraabdominal hypertension) leading to critical pulmonary, renal, or cardiac dysfunction is termed *abdominal compartment syndrome* (ACS). Death is frequently associated with significantly increased pressure.[36] Intraabdominal hypertension has been variably defined as intraabdominal pressures of 20 cm H_2O or greater.[37] Experimental data indicates that hepatic arterial, portal venous, and hepatic microcirculatory blood flows are markedly reduced when intraabdominal pressure is increased to 20 cm H_2O or greater.[38] Typically, it is observed after severe abdominal trauma that requires celiotomy and control of intraabdominal hemorrhage.[39,40] It has also been described in the setting of intraabdominal injuries that were initially managed nonoperatively (e.g., severe liver or kidney injuries).[41] Injury victims without intraabdominal injuries, such as with severe burns, who receive large-volume resuscitations are also at risk for ACS.[42–44]

The diagnosis often begins with a triad of clinical findings: (a) tense, distended abdomen; (b) increased end-inspiration airway pressures; and (c) oliguria despite appropriate volume resuscitation. Additional clinical measurements, particularly those that reflect poor cardiac performance, may be helpful in making the diagnosis. Signs consistent with ACS are reduced cardiac output, elevated systemic vascular resistance, and elevated pulmonary capillary wedge pressure with simultaneous low or normal calculated estimates of end-diastolic volume. The addition of corroborative findings from invasive hemodynamic monitoring may help clarify the diagnosis and direct the appropriate treatment.

Bladder pressure is the most widely used surrogate for intraabdominal pressure. It is measured with the patient supine by distending the bladder with 100 mL of sterile saline. The tubing is then occluded and connected to the pressure transducer through the aspiration port on the catheter tubing. An adequate pressure "tracing" is indicated by visible respiratory variation, which is usually less than 5 to 10 mm Hg.[45] The mean pressure should be used as an estimate of the intraabdominal pressure, although this aspect of the procedure is not well characterized. A simpler method (although not validated) involves filling the bladder with 100 mL of sterile saline and elevating the clear tubing vertically above the pubic symphysis. The height of the fluid column is measured and converted to mm Hg (1.3 cm H_2O = 1 mm Hg).

Established ACS is treated with surgical decompression of the abdomen.[37] Elevated intraabdominal pressures, regardless of the actual measured value, in the absence of physiologic derangement is not an indication for decompressive celiotomy. Similarly, high intrathoracic pressures, marked FiO_2 and PEEP requirements are not sufficient to warrant decompression. Progressive renal dysfunction (oliguria, rising creatinine) despite adequate preload and ongoing resuscitation should warrant abdominal decompression. Persistent shock, particularly when vasopressor agents are required to supplement fluid resuscitation, also warrants decompressive celiotomy. There are no airway pressure, urine output, or arterial blood lactate concentration thresholds that indicate or contraindicate decompressive celiotomy. ACS can also occur in patients whose fascia has been "left open." One factor that seems common to all cases of ACS is the use of aggressive crystalloid resuscitation. Therefore, attempts to achieve "supranormal" end points (cardiac index of 4 L/min/m^2 or greater or oxygen delivery index of 600 mL/min/m^2 or greater), which often requires large resuscitation volumes, may contribute to ACS and should be avoided.[46]

ORGAN SYSTEM SUPPORT AND DEFINITIVE CARE (1 TO 7 DAYS POSTINJURY)

Mechanical Ventilation and Acute Respiratory Failure

Within 24 to 48 hours, many severely injured patients can be rapidly liberated from mechanical ventilation, are able to adequately protect their airway, and can be extubated. Prompt recognition of when the patient is ready to be liberated from mechanical ventilation can be best accomplished by performing a trial of spontaneous breathing, rather than relying on any single measure (or even a combination of measures) of respiratory muscle strength or endurance.[47,48] Many patients require more prolonged mechanical ventilation, either for respiratory failure or often because they are unable to protect their airway, particularly in cases of TBI. In some cases, mechanical ventilation is supportive, gas exchange is not particularly impaired, and the lung fields on chest radiography are relatively normal. In these circumstances, mandatory volume-controlled (also termed *assist-controlled*) ventilation aimed at maintaining the PaO_2 at 80 to 100 mm Hg and the $PaCO_2$ at 35 to 45 mm Hg is appropriate. This can be accomplished using tidal volumes of 8 to 10 mL/kg of predicted body weight, positive end-expiratory pressure of 5 to 10 cm H_2O, an FiO_2 of 40 to 60 mm Hg and a respiratory rate of 12 to 24 breaths per minute. Slight adjustments above or below any of these thresholds are acceptable to achieve these targets. There is no proved advantage to using any other mode or technique of delivering positive pressure ventilation.

Severe acute lung injury (ALI) and ARDS develop in a substantial fraction of critically ill trauma patients and contribute to prolonged and costly ICU care.[4,49] ALI and ARDS are defined by the following set of clinical criteria: (a) diffuse, bilateral patchy pulmonary infiltrates on chest radiograph; (b) PaO_2/FiO_2 equal to or less than 300 (ARDS equal to or less than 200); and (c) cardiac failure excluded as a cause for pulmonary edema. Although the pathophysiology is not entirely clear, an intense underlying alveolar inflammatory response exists in these patients that may be aggravated by positive pressure ventilation.[50–52] Combining high end-inspiratory and low end-expiratory pressures increases interstitial and alveolar edema that can be reduced by preventing end-expiratory collapse with sufficient PEEP.[53] In addition, a marked inflammatory response can be induced in otherwise normal lungs in experimental animals exposed to positive pressure ventilation, particularly when alveoli are allowed to repeatedly collapse (0 cm H_2O PEEP) and repeatedly overexpand.[54] A similar inflammatory response is seen in patients with ARDS, and this inflammatory response can be reduced by a strategy that prevents end-expiratory collapse (PEEP) and end-inspiratory distention (low tidal volumes).[52] In randomized controlled trials, mortality was reduced when patients were treated with protocols designed to limit alveolar stretch using tidal volumes of 6 mL/kg compared with subjects ventilated with higher tidal volumes (~12 mL/kg).[55,56] These trials included patients with ALI and ARDS due to many different risk factors, including trauma and massive transfusion. This approach is applicable to trauma patients with ALI and ARDS. Judicious use of PEEP and moderate FiO_2 levels should typically be employed. An acceptable approach is based on PEEP and FiO_2 combinations used by the ARDS Network.[55] There is no proved benefit to using relatively higher or lower levels of PEEP or FiO_2 in these patients.[57]

Nutritional and Metabolic Support

Nutritional and metabolic support is an important but often neglected component of caring for critically injured patients. Once resuscitation from shock is complete, a hypermetabolic and hyperdynamic cardiovascular response ensues, which has features characteristic of the more general acute phase response. Important changes include increased energy expenditure and protein breakdown, with a shift in metabolic priorities to favor the production of proteins characterized as acute phase reactants and produced primarily by the liver.[58] Although the initial injury and subsequent complications are the prime drivers, the type and timing of nutritional and metabolic support are important modifiers of this response and can help reduce the loss of nitrogen derived from structural protein catabolism.

The route of administration, timing, amount, and nutrient composition of nutritional support are of particular relevance to critically injured patients. When compared to parenteral nutrition (TPN), enteral nutrition (EN) is associated with greater constitutive protein concentrations (prealbumin and albumin) and lower acute phase reactant proteins (such as C-reactive protein) in the initial days after trauma. These effects may be due to a direct effect of the route of nutrient delivery or to an associated reduction in infectious complications seen with EN.[59] Small randomized clinical trials and subsequent meta-analyses have shown that enteral nutrition results in fewer nosocomial infections than does parenteral nutrition. Therefore, nutritional support should be delivered enterally when possible. The evidence is more complete in patients with severe torso trauma but can be generalized to those with severe extremity injuries.[60,61]

The optimal time to institute EN is not definitively known. However, it is important to ensure that the patient has been fully resuscitated because intestinal ischemia and infarction may be the consequence of feeding in the case of shock-induced splanchnic hypoperfusion. Beginning EN feeding once shock has resolved is safe, but there is no proved definitive advantage of a very aggressive approach to feeding (6 to 12 hours after injury) when compared to EN delayed until 48 to 72 hours after injury. Nevertheless, it has been demonstrated that starting EN within 12 hours of being resuscitated from shock is safe and tolerated by approximately 80% of patients when a defined protocol for EN was used.[62]

The amount and composition of nutritional support, whether delivered enterally or parenterally, can be estimated or directly measured, and the metabolic response to this support should be monitored. Caloric requirement estimates are derived from the Harris-Benedict equation (HBE) in which basal energy expenditure (BEE) and, thus, caloric needs are calculated from an equation based on the patient's age, height, weight, and gender. The equations are as follow:

$$\text{Females: BEE} = 655 + 9.7\,(\text{wt in kg}) + 1.8\,(\text{ht in cm}) - 4.7\,(\text{age})$$

$$\text{Males: BEE} = 66 + 13.75\,(\text{wt in kg}) + 5\,(\text{ht in cm}) - 6.8\,(\text{age})$$

Depending on the severity of injury, the BEE expenditure is multiplied by a "stress" factor that estimates the energy expenditure above basal requirements. On average, this factor is approximately 1.3 to 1.4. Caloric needs according to this formula are approximately 25 to 30 kcal/kg per day. Head-injured patients typically have higher energy expenditures than other trauma patients (140% BEE), whereas spinal cord–injured patients often have lower metabolic demands (94% BEE). It is reasonable to estimate the initial caloric requirements using the HBE, but when critical illness is prolonged beyond 5 to 7 days direct measurements should be used to determine energy expenditure and refine nutritional support. Metabolism consumes oxygen and produces carbon dioxide. Therefore, oxygen consumption (VO_2) and carbon dioxide production (VCO_2) can be used to calculate caloric needs using the abbreviated de Weir equation: $EE = 1.44 \times [(3.9 \times VO_2) + (1.1 \times VCO_2)]$. Measuring VCO_2 requires a metabolic cart and is often inaccurate when FiO_2 requirements are high. It is possible to estimate energy expenditure from the VO_2 alone. Assuming a mixed-fuel energy source, the respiratory quotient ($RQ = 0.85 = VCO_2/VO_2$) can be used to replace the VCO_2 in the Weir equation as follows: $EE = 6.9 \times VO_2$. Thus, energy expenditure and caloric needs can be estimated using a pulmonary artery catheter (PAC).[63] Protein calories are excluded from these calculations because it is hoped that delivered protein is not broken down as an energy source but, rather, used as a source of amino acids. Protein or nitrogen requirements are generally determined relative to caloric goals. A kilocalorie/nitrogen (mg) ratio of 100:1 is considered appropriate for critically injured, catabolic patients. Elemental formulas may be better tolerated in patients who have been without EN for more than a few days, although there is no definitive advantage over nonelemental ones. The use of "immune-enhancing" formulas, in which additional amino acids such as arginine, omega-3 fatty acids, and various antioxidants are added, are not clearly better than standard nonelemental EN. However, the addition of antioxidants, delivered enterally and intravenously, commenced early in the postinjury phase, may reduce postinjury organ failure.[64]

Prevention of Gastric Stress Ulcer Hemorrhage

The incidence of clinically relevant stress ulceration or gastritis appears to be much lower now than before the 1990s. Whether this is a function of overall better general supportive care or due to specific preventive measures is uncertain. Nevertheless, trauma patients in the ICU receiving mechanical ventilation for over 48 to 72 hours constitute a high-risk group in whom the risk for upper gastrointestinal hemorrhage is reported to be from 4% to 12%.[65,66] Histamine-2 receptor antagonists may be the most effective agent for preventing upper gastrointestinal hemorrhage in the ICU, and many practitioners choose them for prophylaxis.[67,68] Nevertheless, consequences of gastric acid neutralization and possibly also of unintended alterations in inflammatory responses by systemically delivered histamine-2 antagonists, must be considered given the relative rarity of stress ulcer hemorrhage. Nosocomial pneumonia and, in trauma patients, other nosocomial infections as well are increased in patients receiving histamine-2 antagonists when compared to those given sucralfate.[69,70] The use of sucralfate avoids gastric acid neutralization and the potential systemic effects of histamine-2 receptor antagonists. Although gastric acid secretion can be markedly reduced by proton pump inhibitors, there is no evidence supporting their use as prophylactic agents.

Pain Relief

Approaches to pain relief and sedation assume great importance in the care of the critically ill trauma patient. In particular, adequate pharmacologic relief of thoracic pain resulting from multiple rib fractures may be critical to avoiding intubation or to hastening liberation and extubation. It appears that, when possible, thoracic epidural analgesia results in fewer cases of nosocomial pneumonia and fewer days of mechanical ventilation than systemically administered opioid analgesia.[71] Given the multiple painful stimuli experienced by trauma patients in the ICU (e.g., fractures, surgical incisions, lacerations), it is reasonable to consider regional analgesia. However, contraindications to the use of epidural analgesia are commonly encounterd and include severe traumatic brain injury, spinal fracture, coagulopathy, or any injury that precludes appropriate positioning for accessing the epidural space.

Venous Thromboembolic Disease

Deep venous thrombosis (DVT) and its lethal counterpart, pulmonary embolism (PE), are frequent complications after severe injury. PE remains an important cause of delayed posttraumatic death. DVT and PE can occur at any time after injury and a minority occur in the initial 48 hours.[72] Spinal cord injuries and lower extremity fractures are strong risk factors for DVT and PE.[73] Other important risk factors include increasing age, pelvis fracture, and the need for blood transfusions.[73,74]

Low-molecular-weight heparin appears to be more effective than unfractionated heparin for prophylaxis. One large randomized trial demonstrated that DVT and, more importantly, proximal DVT risk was approximately 30% lower in patients receiving low-molecular-weight heparin (30 mg twice daily) than in those receiving unfractionated heparin (5,000 IU twice daily). Furthermore, the results of that study suggested that unfractionated heparin is not better than no prophylaxis in preventing DVT.[73,75] Nevertheless, others have demonstrated that both unfractionated and low-molecular-weight heparins are effective in preventing DVTs in critically ill (not necessarily injured) patients.[76] The risk of bleeding may be higher when patients are given low-molecular-weight heparin, and it is not recommended for use in those with intracranial hemorrhage or ongoing extracranial bleeding. Alternative prophylactic methods exist to address the risk of DVT in patients who cannot receive prophylactic or therapeutic heparin. Intermittent pneumatic compression devices can be used in patients with contraindications to heparin prophylaxis. Although it was once thought that these devices increased local and regional fibrinolysis by increasing tissue factor pathway inhibitor and decreasing plasminogen activator inhibitor activities, recent evidence suggests that this is not the case. Any benefit from pneumatic compression is likely due to improved venous blood flow.[77,78] Prophylactic placement of inferior vena cava (IVC) filters has been recommended for patients at high risk for PE who cannot receive prophylactic anticoagulation.[79] This practice, however, is not widely used. Alternatively, routine sonographic screening followed by IVC filter placement in those with documented DVT can be used in patients with a contraindication to prophylactic and therapeutic anticoagulation.[80] These approaches will likely evolve with the use of retrievable filters and with increased experience in bedside placement.[81]

MANAGEMENT OF INFECTIOUS COMPLICATIONS (8 DAYS AND BEYOND)

Infectious complications can occur earlier in the postinjury period, but they assume heightened importance as patients remain in the ICU beyond the first week. At this point, prevention, surveillance, rapid diagnosis, and effective treatment become an important focus of the critical care team.

Nosocomial Pneumonia

Pneumonia is the most common pulmonary complication and the most common infection in trauma victims. It most often occurs in association with tracheal intubation and, when associated with mechanical ventilation, is referred to as ventilator-associated pneumonia (VAP). Posttraumatic VAP occurs due to a combination of factors, including alterations in host-defense mechanisms and concomitant colonization with pathogenic bacteria. Taken together with supine, recumbent positioning translaryngeal intubation bypasses glottic defense mechanisms and facilitates microaspiration of secretions that have pooled in the hypopharynx. Although gastric bacterial colonization, often associated with treatment-induced increases in gastric pH, may lead to oropharyngeal and tracheal colonization, oropharyngeal colonization frequently precedes both gastric and tracheal colonization.[66] Alterations in host innate immune mechanisms likely contribute to the risk for pneumonia by impairing cellular immune responses to aspirated bacteria. A number of lines of evidence suggest alterations in host innate immunity exist in critically ill patients. Examples include reductions in immune cell expression of bacterial antigen receptors (Toll-like receptors 2 and 4) and alterations in intracellular signaling (decreased nuclear factor (B heterodimer formation) leading to reduced cytokine responses.[82,83]

Posttraumatic nosocomial pneumonia is caused by a range of gram-negative and gram-positive organisms. *Pseudomonas* species and *Staphylococcus aureus* are the two most common pathogens and together are responsible for up to 40% of cases.[84,85] Multidrug-resistant bacteria have become a great challenge. Both gram-negative organisms, such as *Acinetobacter* species and gram-positive organisms, such as methicillin- and vancomycin-resistant staphylococci and enterococci have emerged as important pathogens.

Potential preventive strategies include selective digestive decontamination, continuous aspiration of subglottic secretions, and semirecumbent positioning to minimize aspiration events.[86] Elevating the head of the bed to 45 degrees has been shown to reduce the incidence of nosocomial pneumonia in mixed cohorts of critically ill patients, including trauma patients, presumably by minimizing gastroesophageal reflux.[87] While generally safe and inexpensive, head elevation may be contraindicated in certain patients with vertebral or spinal cord injuries. Selective digestive decontamination has been studied in a number of clinical trials and sytematic reviews, and has been variably shown to reduce nosocomial pneumonia but to affect mortality only in certain subgroups of patients.[88] It is generally not recommended, because it is resource intensive and may contribute to the selection of antibiotic-resistant bacteria. Finally, specialized endotracheal tubes have been designed with a small aspiration port located just above the cuff. These tubes have been compared to standard endotracheal tubes for their effect on reducing the incidence of microaspiration and, thus, nosocomial pneumonia. Data are not conclusive and the increased cost of these tubes is currently not justified until more definitive evidence is available.[86]

The diagnosis and treatment of VAP is ideally based on direct sampling and quantitative cultures of distal pulmonary secretions, typically with bronchoscopic guidance, when the clinical suspicion of pneumonia is raised. Clinical factors indicating possible pneumonia are leukocytosis, fever, purulent tracheal secretions, and persistent or progressive pulmonary infiltrates on chest radiography. Although not sufficient to diagnose VAP, these criteria should prompt bronchoscopic sampling for quantitative cultures that can be obtained from bronchoalveolar lavage (BAL) or with a protected specimen brush (PSB). The threshold for diagnosis of pneumonia based on BAL is equal to or greater than 10^4 colony-forming units/mL and equal to or greater than d10^3 colony-forming units/mL based on PSB samples. An approach using bronchoscopically obtained specimens leads to more appropriate antibiotic use, shorter ICU stays, and lower mortality in patients with pneumonia, including trauma patients.[89]

Treatment is initially empiric and choice of antibiotic depends on initial Gram's stain identification of predominant organisms and the knowledge of prevailing antibiotic sensitivities and organisms specific to the unit or hospital. This principle is critical because inadequate initial antibiotic coverage has been shown to be associated with higher mortality in patients with VAP.[90] Once the organism and specific antibiotic sensitivities are identified, treatment should be modified accordingly, using the most appropriate antibiotic or combination for the specific organism. The duration of antibiotic therapy is controversial. An inadequate duration of treatment may increase the risk for recurrent VAP with resistant organisms, whereas excessive treatment is costly, may result in the selection of other resistant organisms, and does not seem to improve outcome. Generally, antibiotic treatment for 8 days, assuming adequate initial treatment, is as effective as a 15-day course of treatment. However, for VAP caused by nonlactose fermenting gram-negative rods (e.g., *Acinetobacter* and *Pseudomonas*) a 15-day course results in lower recurrence.[85]

Vascular Catheter-related Infections

Intravascular catheters are an important source of nosocomial infections. These infections can be classified as primary bloodstream infections, catheter-related bloodstream infections (in which cultures of the blood and of the catheter reveal the same pathogen), and exit site infection, in which there is local evidence of infection but without positive blood or catheter cultures.[91] Approximately 10% of critically ill patients develop a vascular catheter-related infection during their ICU stay, and this translates into approximately nine infections per 1,000 patient-days.[91] In the absence of infection at the site of insertion, the diagnosis of catheter-related infection is difficult. A number of options exist and include culture of a catheter segment or of blood drawn through the catheter, alone or simultaneously with blood drawn from a peripheral vein. These specimens can be quantitatively, semiquantitatively, or qualitatively cultured. In general, quantitative catheter segment cultures are the most accurate (highest combined sensitivity and specificity) for the diagnosis of infection. Unpaired quantitative culture of blood (drawn via the vascular catheter alone, without paired peripheral samples) is slightly less accurate.[92] Therefore, when infection is suspected but the insertion site is not inflamed and is without purulent drainage, the catheter should be removed for segmental culture or blood should be drawn from the catheter for quantitative culture.[92]

Preventive strategies can lower the incidence of catheter-related infections in the ICU. Full sterile barriers are appropriate for insertion of central venous catheters and reduce infection rates, but they may not be required for the insertion of peripheral arterial catheters.[93,94] Chlorhexidine gluconate results in fewer bloodstream infections in comparison to povidone-iodine when used for insertion site disinfection.[95] Impregnated catheters with antimicrobials (rifampin-minocyclin) may reduce the risk of catheter-related infections but raise the spectre of antibiotic resistance. A better alternative is a silver-impregnated antimicrobial subcutaneous cuff attached to a central venous catheter to decrease the incidence of associated line infections.

Other Infections

Other infections are less common but are still of considerable importance and reflect the spectrum of infections seen in other cohorts of critically ill patients. Wound and urinary tract infections, intraabdominal abscesses, and less commonly considered complications such as *Clostridium difficile* colitis and acalculous cholecystitis must be considered in the days to weeks after injury.

Fungal infection is an uncommon but serious complication in critically ill trauma victims. It typically develops after a prolonged ICU course in patients who have received multiple antibiotics for nosocomial bacterial infections. Fungal infections are responsible for approximately 5% to 17% of bloodstream infections in critically ill patients and various *Candida* spp. are responsible for the majority of these infections.[96,97] Candidemia is to the growth of *Candida* from blood cultures, and systemic candidiasis is the situation in which microabscesses are present in multiple organs and tissues and are extremely difficult to eradicate.

The single most relevant risk factor for the development of candidemia in nonneutropenic trauma patients is the use of broad-spectrum antibiotics. Colonization with *Candida* organisms is another important risk factor that can be useful in identifying the highest risk patients.[97,98] Fungal infections acquired in the ICU are an important risk factor for death in critically ill patients in general, as well as in trauma patients.[96] Although antifungal prophylaxis with fluconazole seems safe and may reduce the incidence of invasive fungal infections in high-risk surgical patients, its use is not widespread, particularly in trauma patients, who do not seem to be at as high a risk as neutropenic patients or transplant recipients.[98] The diagnosis of candidemia is challenging and the clinical presentation is neither sensitive nor specific for fungal infection. Candidemia is an indication for antifungal therapy; however, systemic disease may exist despite negative blood cultures. Therefore, treatment may need to be empiric, based on a high clinical suspicion, typically in a patient colonized by *Candida* who has signs of sepsis that are not responding to antibiotic therapy. Treatment is generally with fluconazole unless hospital resistance patterns indicate a high likelihood of resistance. In such circumstances, Amphoteracin is the appropriate agent.

KEY POINTS

- **The majority of deaths, complications, and costs following admission for injury occur in the ICU.**
- **The goal of resuscitation is to restore perfusion and organ function and should not be driven by arbitrary or isolated individual parameters, such as supranormal oxygen delivery.**
- **Hypothermia and coagulopathy are major complications of severe injury that must be monitored closely and, when indicated, aggressively treated by active extracorporeal blood warming and multiple-component treatment of specific coagulation defects, including activated factor VII in extreme situations.**
- **Abdominal compartment syndrome (ACS) occurs from elevated intraabdominal pressure causing critical pulmonary, renal, and cardiac dysfunction following severe injury and requires large-volume resuscitation. There are no absolute criteria to open the abdomen, and surgery should be considered based on impact on organ dysfunction.**
- **Ventilatory support is frequently required by severely injured patients. Optimal support for acute lung injury requires low tidal volume and adequate PEEP to decrease FiO_2 requirements. Daily testing by spontaneous breathing trial should be used to expedite extubation.**
- **Nutrition in the critically ill is essential. The enteral route is preferred and shown to decrease complications. Support should be based on estimated needs, monitored and modified to support caloric needs and replace protein catabolism.**
- **Infectious complications are major sources of morbidity and resource consumption. Ventilator-associated pneumonia (VAP) is the most common infectious complication in the critically injured. Therapy is begun empirically, following direct sampling via bronchoscopy, based on institutional predominant organisms and sensitivities, and modified to the narrowest appropriate treatment following identification and sensitivities. Duration of therapy should fit physiologic responses, not arbitrary time intervals.**

References

1. Sauaia A, Moore FA, Moore EE, et al. Epidemiology of trauma deaths: a reassessment. *J Trauma* 1995;38:185–193.
2. O'Keefe GE, Jurkovich GJ, Copass M, et al. Ten-year trend in survival and resource utilization at a level I trauma center. *Ann Surg.* 1999;229: 409–415.
3. Acosta JA, Yang JC, Winchell RJ, et al. Lethal injuries and time to death in a level I trauma center. *J Am Coll Surg.* 1998;186:528–533.
4. O'Keefe GE, Maier RV, Diehr P, et al. The complications of trauma and their associated costs in a level I trauma center. *Arch Surg.* 1997;132:920–924.
5. **Sauaia A, Moore FA, Moore EE, et al. Early predictors of postinjury multiple organ failure. *Arch Surg.* 1994;129:39–45.**
6. Fitzwater J, Purdue GF, Hunt JL, et al. The risk factors and time course of sepsis and organ dysfunction after burn trauma. *J Trauma* 2003;54:959–966.
7. Moore FA, Moore EE, Sauaia A. Blood transfusion. An independent risk factor for postinjury multiple organ failure. *Arch Surg.* 1997;132:620–624.
8. Luchette FA, Jenkins WA, Friend LA, et al. Hypoxia is not the sole cause of lactate production during shock. *J Trauma* 2002;52:415–419.
9. James JH, Luchette FA, McCarter FD, et al. Lactate is an unreliable indicator of tissue hypoxia in injury or sepsis. *Lancet* 1999;354:505–508.
10. Gattinoni L, Brazzi L, Pelosi P, et al. A trial of goal-oriented hemodynamic therapy in critically ill patients. SvO2 Collaborative Group. *N Engl J Med.* 1995;333:1025–1032.
11. Sandham JD, Hull RD, Brant RF, et al. A randomized, controlled trial of the use of pulmonary-artery catheters in high-risk surgical patients. *N Engl J Med.* 2003;348:5–14.
12. McKinley BA, Kozar RA, Cocanour CS, et al. Normal versus supranormal oxygen delivery goals in shock resuscitation: the response is the same. *J Trauma* 2002;53:825–832.
13. Balogh Z, McKinley BA, Cocanour CS, et al. Secondary abdominal compartment syndrome is an elusive early complication of traumatic shock resuscitation. *Am J Surg.* 2002;184:538–543.
14. **Rivers E, Nguyen B, Havstad S, et al. Early goal-directed therapy in the treatment of severe sepsis and septic shock. *N Engl J Med.* 2001;345: 1368–1377.**
15. Shoemaker WC, Wo CC, Chan L, et al. Outcome prediction of emergency patients by noninvasive hemodynamic monitoring. *Chest* 2001;120:528–537.
16. Velmahos GC, Demetriades D, Shoemaker WC, et al. Endpoints of resuscitation of critically injured patients: normal or supranormal? A prospective randomized trial. *Ann Surg.* 2000;232:409–418.
17. Gentilello LM. Advances in the management of hypothermia. *Surg Clin North Am.* 1995;75:243–256.
18. Gentilello LM, Moujaes S. Treatment of hypothermia in trauma victims: thermodynamic considerations. *J Intensive Care Med.* 1995;10:5–14.
19. Chughtai TS, Gilardino MS, Fleiszer DM, et al. An expanding role for cardiopulmonary bypass in trauma. *Can J Surg.* 2002;45:95–103.
20. Perchinsky MJ, Long WB, Hill JG, et al. Extracorporeal cardiopulmonary life support with heparin-bonded circuitry in the resuscitation of massively injured trauma patients. *Am J Surg.* 1995;169:488–491.
21. **Gentilello LM, Jurkovich GJ, Stark MS, et al. Is hypothermia in the victim of major trauma protective or harmful? A randomized, prospective study. *Ann Surg.* 1997;226:439–447.**
22. Knight DA, Manifold CA, Blue J, King JA. A randomized, controlled trial comparing arteriovenous to venovenous rewarming of severe hypothermia in a porcine model. *J Trauma* 2003;55:741–746.
23. Mild therapeutic hypothermia to improve the neurologic outcome after cardiac arrest. *N Engl J Med.* 2002;346:549–556.
24. Harvey MP, Greenfield TP, Sugrue ME, et al. Massive blood transfusion in a tertiary referral hospital. Clinical outcomes and haemostatic complications. *Med J Aust.* 1995;163:356–359.
25. Counts RB, Haisch C, Simon TL, et al. Hemostasis in massively transfused trauma patients. *Ann Surg.* 1979;190:91–99.
26. Ciavarella D, Reed RL, Counts RB, et al. Clotting factor levels and the risk of diffuse microvascular bleeding in the massively transfused patient. *Br J Haematol.* 1987;67:365–368.
27. Hulka F, Mullins RJ, Frank EH. Blunt brain injury activates the coagulation process. *Arch Surg.* 1996;131:923–927.
28. Oertel M, Kelly DF, McArthur D, et al. Progressive hemorrhage after head trauma: predictors and consequences of the evolving injury. *J Neurosurg.* 2002;96:109–116.
29. Dutton RP, McCunn M, Hyder M, et al. Factor VIIa for Correction of Traumatic Coagulopathy. *J Trauma* 2004;57:709–719.
30. Grounds M. Recombinant factor VIIa (rFVIIa) and its use in severe bleeding in surgery and trauma: a review. *Blood Rev.* 2003;17(suppl 1):S11–S21.
31. Hedner U, Erhardtsen E. Potential role for rFVIIa in transfusion medicine. *Transfusion* 2002;42:114–124.
32. Winchell RJ, Simons RK, Hoyt DB. Transient systolic hypotension. A serious problem in the management of head injury. *Arch Surg.* 1996;131:533–539.
33. **Manley G, Knudson MM, Morabito D, et al. Hypotension, hypoxia, and head injury: frequency, duration, and consequences. *Arch Surg.* 2001;136: 1118–1123.**
34. Temkin NR, Dikmen SS, Wilensky AJ, et al. A randomized, double-blind study of phenytoin for the prevention of post-traumatic seizures. *N Engl J Med.* 1990;323:497–502.
35. Dicker RA, Morabito DJ, Pittet JF, et al. Acute respiratory distress syndrome criteria in trauma patients: why the definitions do not work. *J Trauma* 2004;57:522–526.
36. Ivatury RR, Porter JM, Simon RJ, et al. Intra-abdominal hypertension after life-threatening penetrating abdominal trauma: prophylaxis, incidence, and clinical relevance to gastric mucosal pH and abdominal compartment syndrome. *J Trauma* 1998;44:1016–1021.
37. Hong JJ, Cohn SM, Perez JM, et al. Prospective study of the incidence and outcome of intra-abdominal hypertension and the abdominal compartment syndrome. *Br J Surg.* 2002;89:591–596.
38. Diebel LN, Wilson RF, Dulchavsky SA, Saxe J. Effect of increased intra-abdominal pressure on hepatic arterial, portal venous, and hepatic microcirculatory blood flow. *J Trauma* 1992;33:279–282.
39. Morris JA, Jr., Eddy VA, Blinman TA, et al. The staged celiotomy for trauma. Issues in unpacking and reconstruction. *Ann Surg.* 1993;217:576–584.
40. Chen RJ, Fang JF, Chen MF. Intra-abdominal pressure monitoring as a guideline in the nonoperative management of blunt hepatic trauma. *J Trauma* 2001;51:44–50.

41. Yang EY, Marder SR, Hastings G, et al. The abdominal compartment syndrome complicating nonoperative management of major blunt liver injuries: recognition and treatment using multimodality therapy. *J Trauma* 2002;52:982–986.
42. Balogh Z, McKinley BA, Cocanour CS, et al. Secondary abdominal compartment syndrome is an elusive early complication of traumatic shock resuscitation. *Am J Surg.* 2002;184:538–543.
43. Hobson KG, Young KM, Ciraulo A, et al. Release of abdominal compartment syndrome improves survival in patients with burn injury. *J Trauma* 2002;53:1129–1133.
44. **Biffl WL, Moore EE, Burch JM, et al. Secondary abdominal compartment syndrome is a highly lethal event. *Am J Surg.* 2001;182:645–648.**
45. Kron IL, Harman PK, Nolan SP. The measurement of intra-abdominal pressure as a criterion for abdominal re-exploration. *Ann Surg.* 1984;199:28–30.
46. McKinley BA, Kozar RA, Cocanour CS, et al. Normal versus supranormal oxygen delivery goals in shock resuscitation: the response is the same. *J Trauma* 2002;53:825–832.
47. Ely EW, Baker AM, Dunagan DP, et al. Effect on the duration of mechanical ventilation of identifying patients capable of breathing spontaneously. *N Engl J Med.* 1996;335:1864–1869.
48. O'Keefe GE, Hawkins K, Boynton J, et al. Indicators of fatigue and of prolonged weaning from mechanical ventilation in surgical patients. *World J Surg.* 2001;25:98–103.
49. Treggiari MM, Hudson LD, Martin DP, et al. Effect of acute lung injury and acute respiratory distress syndrome on outcome in critically ill trauma patients. *Crit Care Med.* 2004;32:327–331.
50. Pugin J, Ricou B, Steinberg KP, et al. Proinflammatory activity in bronchoalveolar lavage fluids from patients with ARDS, a prominent role for interleukin-1. *Am J Respir Crit Care Med.* 1996;153(6 Pt 1):1850–1856.
51. Pugin J, Verghese G, Widmer MC, et al. The alveolar space is the site of intense inflammatory and profibrotic reactions in the early phase of acute respiratory distress syndrome. *Crit Care Med.* 1999;27:304–312.
52. Ranieri VM, Suter PM, Tortorella C, et al. Effect of mechanical ventilation on inflammatory mediators in patients with acute respiratory distress syndrome: a randomized controlled trial. *JAMA* 1999;282:54–61.
53. Dreyfuss D, Soler P, Basset G, et al. High inflation pressure pulmonary edema. Respective effects of high airway pressure, high tidal volume, and positive end-expiratory pressure. *Am Rev Respir Dis.* 1988;137: 1159–1164.
54. Chu EK, Whitehead T, Slutsky AS. Effects of cyclic opening and closing at low- and high-volume ventilation on bronchoalveolar lavage cytokines. *Crit Care Med.* 2004;32:168–174.
55. **ARDS Network. Ventilation with lower tidal volumes as compared with traditional tidal volumes for acute lung injury and the acute respiratory distress syndrome. *N Engl J Med.* 2000;342:1301–1308.**
56. Amato MB, Barbas CS, Medeiros DM, et al. Effect of a protective-ventilation strategy on mortality in the acute respiratory distress syndrome. *N Engl J Med.* 1998;338:347–354.
57. Brower RG, Lanken PN, MacIntyre N, et al. Higher versus lower positive end-expiratory pressures in patients with the acute respiratory distress syndrome. *N Engl J Med.* 2004;351:327–336.
58. Gabay C, Kushner I. Acute-phase proteins and other systemic responses to inflammation. *N Engl J Med.* 1999;340:448–454.
59. Kudsk KA, Minard G, Wojtysiak SL, et al. Visceral protein response to enteral versus parenteral nutrition and sepsis in patients with trauma. *Surgery* 1994;116:516–523.
60. **Moore FA, Feliciano DV, Andrassy RJ, et al. Early enteral feeding, compared with parenteral, reduces postoperative septic complications. The results of a meta-analysis. *Ann Surg.* 1992;216:172–183.**
61. Kudsk KA, Croce MA, Fabian TC, et al. Enteral versus parenteral feeding. Effects on septic morbidity after blunt and penetrating abdominal trauma. *Ann Surg.* 1992;215:503–511.
62. Kozar RA, McQuiggan MM, Moore EE, et al. Postinjury enteral tolerance is reliably achieved by a standardized protocol. *J Surg Res.* 2002;104:70–75.
63. Cobean RA, Gentilello LM, Parker A, et al. Nutritional assessment using a pulmonary artery catheter. *J Trauma* 1992;33:452–456.
64. Nathens AB, Neff MJ, Jurkovich GJ, et al. Randomized, prospective trial of antioxidant supplementation in critically ill surgical patients. *Ann Surg.* 2002;236:814–822.
65. Cook DJ, Fuller HD, Guyatt GH, et al. Risk factors for gastrointestinal bleeding in critically ill patients. Canadian Critical Care Trials Group. *N Engl J Med.* 1994;330:377–381.
66. Maier RV, Mitchell D, Gentilello L. Optimal therapy for stress gastritis. *Ann Surg.* 1994;220:353–360.
67. Cook D, Guyatt G, Marshall J, et al. A comparison of sucralfate and ranitidine for the prevention of upper gastrointestinal bleeding in patients requiring mechanical ventilation. Canadian Critical Care Trials Group. *N Engl J Med.* 1998;338:791–797.
68. Daley RJ, Rebuck JA, Welage LS, et al. Prevention of stress ulceration: Current trends in critical care. *Crit Care Med.* 2004;32:2008–2013.
69. Cook DJ, Reeve BK, Guyatt GH, et al. Stress ulcer prophylaxis in critically ill patients. Resolving discordant meta-analyses. *JAMA* 1996;275:308–314.
70. O'Keefe GE, Gentilello LM, Maier RV. Incidence of infectious complications associated with the use of histamine2-receptor antagonists in critically ill trauma patients. *Ann Surg.* 1998;227:120–125.
71. **Bulger EM, Edwards T, Klotz P, et al. Epidural analgesia improves outcome after multiple rib fractures. *Surgery* 2004;136:426–430.**
72. Owings JT, Kraut E, Battistella F, et al. Timing of the occurrence of pulmonary embolism in trauma patients. *Arch Surg.* 1997;132:862–866.
73. Geerts WH, Code KI, Jay RM, et al. A prospective study of venous thromboembolism after major trauma. *N Engl J Med.* 1994;331:1601–1606.
74. Montgomery KD, Geerts WH, Potter HG, et al. Practical management of venous thromboembolism following pelvic fractures. *Orthop Clin North Am.* 1997;28:397–404.
75. **Geerts WH, Jay RM, Code KI, et al. A comparison of low-dose heparin with low-molecular-weight heparin as prophylaxis against venous thromboembolism after major trauma. *N Engl J Med.* 1996;335:701–707.**
76. Geerts W, Selby R. Prevention of venous thromboembolism in the ICU. *Chest* 2003;124(6 suppl):357S–363S.
77. Macaulay W, Westrich G, Sharrock N, et al. Effect of pneumatic compression on fibrinolysis after total hip arthroplasty. *Clin Orthop,* 2002;399: 168–176.
78. Killewich LA, Cahan MA, Hanna DJ, et al. The effect of external pneumatic compression on regional fibrinolysis in a prospective randomized trial. *J Vasc Surg.* 2002;36:953–958.
79. Rogers FB, Shackford SR, Ricci MA, et al. Routine prophylactic vena cava filter insertion in severely injured trauma patients decreases the incidence of pulmonary embolism. *J Am Coll Surg.* 1995;180:641–647.
80. Knudson MM, Ikossi DG. Venous thromboembolism after trauma. *Curr Opin Crit Care* 2004;10:539–548.
81. Ashley DW, Gamblin TC, McCampbell BL, et al. Bedside insertion of vena cava filters in the intensive care unit using intravascular ultrasound to locate renal veins. *J Trauma* 2004;57:26–31.
82. Ikushima H, Nishida T, Takeda K, et al. Expression of Toll-like receptors 2 and 4 is downregulated after operation. *Surgery* 2004;135:376–385.
83. Adib-Conquy M, Adrie C, Moine P, et al. NF-kappaB expression in mononuclear cells of patients with sepsis resembles that observed in lipopolysaccharide tolerance. *Am J Respir Crit Care Med.* 2000;162: 1877–1883.
84. Singh N, Rogers P, Atwood CW, et al. Short-course empiric antibiotic therapy for patients with pulmonary infiltrates in the intensive care unit. A proposed solution for indiscriminate antibiotic prescription. *Am J Respir Crit Care Med.* 2000;162(2 pt 1):505–511.
85. Chastre J, Wolff M, Fagon JY, et al. Comparison of 8 vs 15 days of antibiotic therapy for ventilator-associated pneumonia in adults: a randomized trial. *JAMA* 2003;290:2588–2598.
86. **Collard HR, Saint S, Matthay MA. Prevention of ventilator-associated pneumonia: an evidence-based systematic review. *Ann Intern Med.* 2003; 138:494–501.**
87. Drakulovic MB, Torres A, Bauer TT, et al. Supine body position as a risk factor for nosocomial pneumonia in mechanically ventilated patients: a randomised trial. *Lancet* 1999;354:1851–1858.
88. Nathens AB, Marshall JC. Selective decontamination of the digestive tract in surgical patients: a systematic review of the evidence. *Arch Surg.* 1999;134:170–176.
89. Fagon JY, Chastre J. Diagnosis and treatment of nosocomial pneumonia in ALI/ARDS patients. *Eur Respir J Suppl.* 2003;42:77s–83s.
90. Clec'h C, Timsit JF, De Lassence A, et al. Efficacy of adequate early antibiotic therapy in ventilator-associated pneumonia: influence of disease severity. *Intensive Care Med.*2004;30:1327–1333.
91. Eggimann P, Harbarth S, Constantin MN, et al. Impact of a prevention strategy targeted at vascular-access care on incidence of infections acquired in intensive care. *Lancet* 2000;355:1864–1868.
92. Siegman-Igra Y, Anglim AM, Shapiro DE, et al. Diagnosis of vascular catheter-related bloodstream infection: a meta-analysis. *J Clin Microbiol.* 1997;35:928–936.
93. Rijnders BJ, Van Wijngaerden E, Wilmer A, et al. Use of full sterile barrier precautions during insertion of arterial catheters: a randomized trial. *Clin Infect Dis.* 2003;36:743–748.
94. Raad II, Hohn DC, Gilbreath BJ, et al. Prevention of central venous catheter-related infections by using maximal sterile barrier precautions during insertion. *Infect Control Hosp Epidemiol.* 1994;15(4 pt 1):231–238.
95. Chaiyakunapruk N, Veenstra DL, Lipsky BA, et al. Chlorhexidine compared with povidone-iodine solution for vascular catheter-site care: a meta-analysis. *Ann Intern Med.* 2002;136:792–801.
96. Laupland KB, Kirkpatrick AW, Church DL, et al. Intensive-care-unit-acquired bloodstream infections in a regional critically ill population. *J Hosp Infect.* 2004;58:137–145.
97. Vincent JL, Anaissie E, Bruining H, et al. Epidemiology, diagnosis and treatment of systemic Candida infection in surgical patients under intensive care. *Intensive Care Med,* 1998;24:206–216.
98. Pelz RK, Hendrix CW, Swoboda SM, et al. Double-blind placebo-controlled trial of fluconazole to prevent candidal infections in critically ill surgical patients. *Ann Surg.* 2001;233:542–548.

CHAPTER 33 ■ ENVENOMATION AND ENVIRONMENTAL INJURIES

GREGORY J. JURKOVICH

ENVENOMATION

Snakes and Snakebites

There are more than 3,000 species of snakes worldwide, of which approximately 375 are venomous. Although estimates vary greatly, possibly 300,000 venomous bites each year are responsible for 30,000 deaths annually worldwide. In the United States, an estimated 45,000 snakebites occur annually, of which 7,000 are from venomous snakes, resulting in 14 to 20 deaths each year.[1–4] The American Association of Poison Control Centers provides an annual report of documented snakebites in the United States that can be accessed at the Web site http://www.aapcc.org/; however, many snakebites are likely unreported because some victims do not seek treatment, reporting is not mandatory, and physicians do not always contact a poison center.

The five main families of poisonous snakes found worldwide are the Colubridae, Elapidae, Hydrophidae, Viperidae, and Crotalidae. The Colubridae family consists primarily of the boomslang and the bird snake, which are mainly found in Africa. The Elapidae family includes the cobras, the coral snakes, and the adders, which are found throughout Asia, Africa, the Americas, and Australia. The Hydrophidae family consists of the sea snakes, which are found throughout the Pacific and along the west coast of South America. The Viperidae family consists of Old World vipers, which are found throughout Africa, Europe, and the Middle East, and are noted by their lack of a heat-sensing pit. The Crotalidae are the true pit vipers and are found worldwide. Some classification systems note the pit vipers as a subfamily of the Viperidae.[5]

The native venomous snakes of North America are members of the phylum Chordata, class Reptilia, order Squamata, suborder Serpentes, and of the two families Crotalidae and Elapidae (Table 33.1).

Rattlesnakes are members of the family Crotalidae and the genus *Crotalus* or *Sistrurus*. Water moccasins (or cottonmouths) and copperheads are also members of the Crotalidae family, but of the genus *Agkistrodon*. The coral snake is the major representative of the Elapidae family and of the genus *Micrurus* or *Micruroides*. Other well-known members of the Elapidae family that are not indigenous to North America are the cobras and mambas. The distribution of venomous snakes in the United States is extensive, with at least one native species found in every state except Maine, Alaska, and Hawaii. Rattlesnakes are particularly widely distributed, whereas the water moccasin is found in the southeastern United States, Mississippi Valley, Illinois, and Indiana. The copperhead's range is primarily from central Massachusetts to northern Florida and west to Illinois and Texas.

The Crotalidae, or pit vipers, have a number of characteristics that help distinguish them from benign snakes (Fig. 33.1). Their unique and characteristic thermoreceptor "pit" is an infrared sensor located between the nostril and the eye that helps the snake localize its prey. Pit vipers also have a vertical elliptical pupil, a triangular head, and retractable fangs. Venomous snakes have a single row of plates distal to the anal plate on their ventral surface, whereas harmless snakes have a double row of caudal plates.

Coloration is so variable that it is nearly useless as a distinguishing characteristic. An exception is the coloration of the Elapidae coral snake, which can be identified by the simple rhyme, "Red on yellow kill a fellow; red on black venom lack." Coral snakes have circular bands of colors with red adjacent to yellow, whereas the nonvenomous but similar-looking king snake has red on black bands that do not completely encircle it. The eastern coral snake has a completely black nose, whereas the king snake usually does not.

Most snakebites in the United States occur in the Sunbelt region between April and October, with the peak incidence occurring in the summer months of July and August. Prehibernation and posthibernation snakes appear to be more

TABLE 33.1

SNAKES OF THE FAMILY CROTALIDAE

Genus	Common name	Characteristics	Range
Agkistrodon	Water moccasin and copperhead	No rattles; large plates on crown	North America, southeastern Europe, Asia
Bothrops	New World pit vipers	No rattles; small scales on crown; large scales on ventral tail	Mexico to South America
Crotalus	Rattlesnakes	Rattles; small scales on crown	North, Central, and South America
Lachesis	Bushmaster	No rattles; small scales on crown; small scales on ventral tail	Central and South America
Sistrurus	Massasaugas and pygmy rattlesnakes	Rattles; large plates on crown	North America
Trimeresurus		No rattles; small scales on crown	Asia

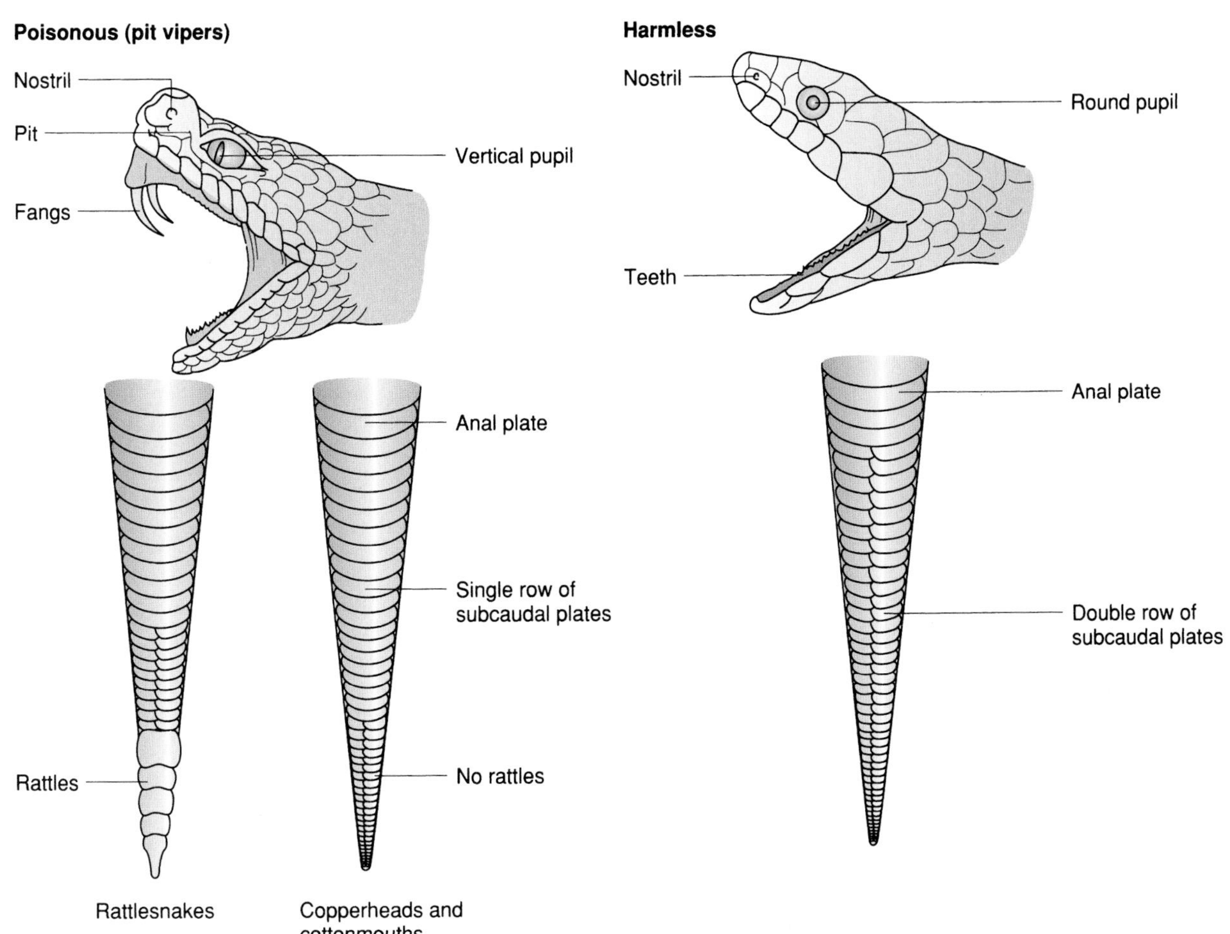

FIGURE 33.1 Characteristics of snakes that differentiate poisonous pit vipers from harmless snakes.

aggressive. The victims of snakebites are typically men between 18 and 50 years of age. Up to 60% of snakebite victims are deliberately handling snakes,[6] and alcohol consumption in snakebite victims is common.[7]

Not every poisonous snakebite results in envenomation, and even the presence of fang marks does not necessarily correlate with envenomation. Venom is produced in Duvernoy's glands, which are located on the dorsal sides of the head and correspond to the parotid glands. The location of this large gland gives the head its characteristic triangular shape. During the bite, the venom is forced through the hollow fangs by the palatine muscles and extruded out the orifices, which are located just proximal to the tip. Therefore, clothing, gloves, and shoes may significantly diminish the depth of penetration and limit the amount of envenomation.

The severity of envenomation is related to the amount of venom injected, the concentration of the venom, and the size of the snake. Direct intravenous envenomation is unusual but particularly severe.[8] Snakebites with a distance between the fangs of more than 15 mm are representative of a large snake and therefore suggest a potentially more significant envenomation. Hibernation also seems to play a role in severity. After hibernation, snakes are relatively dehydrated because they have been in a prolonged fasting state, and therefore they produce a more potent, concentrated venom. The degree of envenomation also varies because 10% to 25% of bites have no significant envenomation, even when fang marks are noted on the victim. With each strike, the snake may discharge between 25% and 75% of its venom, so that successive or repetitive strikes tend to diminish the amount of venom available. Snakes that are angered or fearful may discharge greater amounts of venom. Table 33.2 lists the grading scale for pit viper bites.[24–28]

TABLE 33.2 CLASSIFICATION

GRADING OF PIT VIPER BITES

Grade	Description of bite
0	Visible bite but no envenomation; swelling/erythema around the fang mark <2.5 cm; minimal pain and tenderness; no systemic symptoms
I	History of immediate pain with bite; swelling and erythema 5 to 15 cm from fang marks; no systemic signs or symptoms
II	Moderate pain; erythema and edema of 15 to 40 cm; mild systemic signs such as weakness and emesis; may have abnormal laboratory findings
III	Severe pain; erythema and edema >40 cm, with petechiae and bullae; systemic signs and symptoms such as vertigo, DIC, or coagulopathy; abnormal laboratory values
IV	Lethal envenomation with widespread edema, shock, seizures, coma, renal failure, bleeding, DIC, paralysis

DIC, disseminated intravascular coagulation.

TABLE 33.3

ENZYMES OF SNAKE VENOMS

Proteolytic enzymes
Arginine ester hydrolase
Thrombin-like enzyme
Collagenase
Hyaluronidase
Phospholipase A_2 (A)
Phospholipase C
Lactate dehydrogenase
Phosphomonoesterase
Phosphodiesterase
Acetylcholinesterase
RNase
DNase
5′-Nucleotidase
L-Amino acid oxidase

Snake Venom

The function of venom is to kill or immobilize prey and to aid in digestion. Venom consists of a complex array of proteins and enzymes that have historically been characterized as neurotoxins, hemotoxins, and cardiotoxins.[9] The components of pit viper venom, however, affect almost every organ system, thus labeling snake venom as a specific organ toxin is probably inaccurate.[5] More than 26 different proteins and nonenzymatic peptides have been isolated from various venoms.[2,5] The Crotalidae venom consists of approximately 90% water, five to 15 enzymes, three to 12 nonenzymatic proteins and peptides, and more than six other unidentified substances. A partial list of these enzymes is shown in Table 33.3 and includes several proteolytic enzymes, phospholipase, nucleotidase, acetylcholinesterase, and amino acid oxidase.

These low-molecular-weight peptides and polypeptides (6 to 100 kD) appear to act by damaging vascular endothelial cells. Electron microscopic analysis of tissue from human snakebite victims has demonstrated disruption of the vascular endothelium and other plasma membranes. Microangiopathic vascular injury leads to increased permeability, peripheral edema, pulmonary edema and hemorrhage, significant interstitial fluid sequestration, and hypotension. Other venom proteins appear to induce a neuromuscular blockade or coagulopathy. Procoagulant venom factors seem to dominate, primarily exerting their effect late in the clotting cascade by activating factor X or prothrombin or by directly converting fibrinogen to fibrin.[10] Tissue destruction is aided by several different proteins. L-Amino acid oxidase causes extensive tissue destruction and splits fibrinogen, leading to platelet trapping and unstable clot formation, thus contributing to the genesis of disseminated intravascular coagulation (DIC). Phospholipase A2 causes hydrolysis of lecithin at the C-2 position, resulting in the formation of lysolecithin. This event alters the permeability of erythrocyte membranes and muscle cell plasma membranes, leading to hemolysis and tissue edema. Hyaluronidase induces the lysis of ground substance and thereby aids in the distribution of the venom throughout body tissues.

The Elapidae snake venom also contains specific and unique neurotoxins and cardiotoxins, which have a more direct effect on the neuroactivity of the prey. Coral snake venom directly blocks action of acetylcholine receptor sites that do not appear to be responsive to neostigmine. This blockade results in ptosis, dysphagia, and slurred speech and can lead to seizures, coma, and death within 8 to 72 hours.

Signs and Symptoms of Envenomation by Snakebite

The important signs and symptoms of snakebites include both local and systemic effects. Immediate pain and progressive edema and erythema at the site of the bite are the norm. Local signs and symptoms progressing at a rate of greater than 30 cm/hour, in addition to microscopic hematuria and bleeding from the puncture sites, indicate significant envenomation.[11] Delayed toxicity has been observed on occasion, and rarely severe toxicity has followed resolution of initial local symptoms.[12] Occasionally a bite by a nonpoisonous garter snake (*Thamnophis* species) can be confused at an early stage with the bite of a poisonous snake of the Crotalidae family. Edema and erythema can be produced by toxic salivary secretions of a parotidlike gland (Duvernoy's glands) if the skin has been broken.[13] Systemic signs fail to develop, however, and the local signs resolve spontaneously within a few days.

Myonecrosis at or near the bite site is affected by both the direct toxic effects of the venom and the added ischemia of edema and increased compartment pressures. The development of a frank compartment syndrome after a snakebite of the extremity can occur but is unusual, occurring in only one of 272 Eastern diamondback and water moccasin bites in one report.[14] Studies using purified venom injected into the anterolateral leg compartment of mongrel dogs determined that only intramuscular injection leads to an increase in compartmental pressure.[15] Compartment syndromes are unusual because most snakebites do not penetrate through the superficial fascia; the principal cause of myonecrosis is probably direct toxicity of the venom rather than ischemia from elevated compartment pressure. Nonetheless, in one report of 36 rattlesnake bites, three definitive diagnoses of compartment syndrome were made on the basis of elevated compartment pressures.[16] The indication for fasciotomy remains controversial, with some authors recommending fasciotomy in nearly all cases,[17] but others believing that aggressive use of antivenin precludes the need for fasciotomy in most instances.

Shock is a common finding with significant systemic envenomation, resulting from increased microvascular permeability and the loss of plasma volume. Bradycardia and arrhythmia result from the cardiotoxins. Renal failure may occur from hypoperfusion and shock, DIC with renal tubular necrosis, or as a direct toxic effect of the venom. Sheehan syndrome of pituitary necrosis has been reported after a Russell viper bite, likely a result of the procoagulant activity of the viper's venom.[18]

The hematologic effects of venom cause both local and systemic problems. Venom appears to activate factor X as well as factors V and IX or directly converts fibrinogen to fibrin, leading to activation of the coagulation cascade and a consumptive coagulopathy.[18] The prothrombin time (PT) and partial thromboplastin time (PTT) are commonly increased, which may result in persistent bleeding, ecchymosis, or petechiae at the puncture site or affected extremity. Microscopic hematuria and bleeding from any preexisting condition, such as peptic ulcer or menstrual bleeding, may aggravate the situation. Venom also causes a mild defibrinogenation state, with unstable clot formation using fibrinogen but sparing platelets. This state may contribute to DIC.

Venom also appears to cause myriad neurologic effects, especially the venom from the Elapidae family. The venom of coral snakes, cobras, and sea snakes contains an acetylcholinesterase receptor antagonist that causes ptosis, slurred speech, and impaired swallowing leading to hypersalivation. This venom also has central nervous system activity that results in progressive weakness, paresthesia, and eventually respiratory muscle failure and respiratory arrest. Seizures and psychotic behavior may develop that can lead to coma or death in 8 to 72 hours. The toxins responsible include neurotoxin A, which appears to act on the central nervous system, and neurotoxin B, which acts at the myoneural junction.

Clinical Evaluation of Snakebites

Victims of snakebites require the same aggressive supportive and resuscitative care as any trauma patient. Attention to airway and breathing are the first priority, followed by cardiovascular assessment and resuscitation. A detailed history is often helpful in determining the type and size of snake, the circumstances of the bite, and timing. Key points should include snake description, first-aid measures applied, known allergies and comorbidities, and history of snakebites or use of antivenin. A complete and detailed physical examination should specifically look for fang marks (usually a single pair, rarely more than one strike), distance between fang marks (indicates size of the snake), and measurement of the zone of erythema and edema initially surrounding the fang marks and subsequently over time. Signs of systemic toxicity to be searched for include petechiae, bruises, bullae, or blisters. Measurements at the same site should be repeated every 15 minutes until edema and erythema progression has ceased. Frequent clinical examinations should focus on neurologic, hematologic, and hemodynamic profiles.

Initial laboratory testing should include electrolytes, complete blood count with platelet count, PT, PTT, fibrinogen level, blood urea nitrogen, and serum creatine plus urinalysis. Depending on the patient's age and comorbidities, an electrocardiogram and chest radiograph should be included. Type and cross-matching for blood is advised, particularly if the patient presents with a more severe grade of injury. Tetanus immunization status should be queried and brought up to date if needed. Enzyme-linked immunosorbent assays (ELISAs) have been developed to directly measure serum venom antigens in patients and to help identify the species of snake.[18] ELISA is sensitive to 5 mg/L of venom and can assess serum, urine, blister fluid, or aspiration fluid. This test is helpful when attempting to determine the specific snake to direct monovalent antivenin therapy. Radioimmunoassay is extremely sensitive, with some venoms being detected to levels of 0.4 mg/L. The applicability of this assay is limited because of its expense and the fact that it may take 24 hours to produce a definitive result.[19] In the United States, however, there is only one Crotalidae antivenin and only one coral snake antivenin; therefore, this more detailed identification is usually unnecessary.

Treatment of Snakebite Envenomation

First aid begins with immobilization and splinting of the infected part at the level of the heart or at a slightly dependent position, much as a fracture of the extremity would be treated. The utility of incision and suction at the puncture site has been debated for years. In dogs, up to half of the venom can be removed if incision and suction are begun within 3 minutes of the bite,[19] and in rabbits, a suction device (the Sawyer extractor pump) has been shown to remove up to 37% of radiolabeled venom in rabbits when applied 3 minutes after envenomation;[34] however, these results have not been verified in humans. Russell[2] has indicated that if immediate incision and suction is started and continued for 1 hour, at best 11% of the venom may be removed.[20] Most authorities do not recommend incision and suction therapy.[1,20,21]

The use of a proximal tourniquet should also be discouraged because it may lead to venous congestion and increased ischemia without demonstrated benefit. Cryotherapy (ice pack) is discouraged universally because it increases tissue ischemia. The effects of cryotherapy and steroids were studied in envenomated mongrel dogs, and it was found that no added benefit could be demonstrated by using corticosteroids or cryotherapy as adjuvants to antivenin alone.[22]

Tetanus prophylaxis and the prevention of secondary infections are important objectives of snakebite treatment. Species of the gram-negative bacteria *Aerobacter, Proteus,* and *Pseudomonas* are particularly common causes of bacterial infection, and appropriate systemic antibiotics are given routinely. Cholinergic agonists may be of benefit after an Elapidae bite because this venom has a significant effect on acetylcholine receptors. Calcium gluconate may also be of benefit after an Elapidae bite to control the onset of seizures. Some snake venoms have been shown to contain metallopeptides, and for this reason, ethylenediaminetetra-acetic acid has been tried experimentally in animals as a chelator to inactivate these proteins. The use of this agent is to be discouraged, however, because it appears to hasten death in laboratory animals for unknown reasons.[16] Systemic steroids have no effect in the initial treatment of snakebites, but they play a significant role in treatment of serum sickness that often follows antivenin therapy.[23]

Antivenin is the mainstay of treatment of significant envenomation throughout the world.[1] More than 100 antivenin* products are available worldwide. Most recent attention has focused on the sheep (ovine)-produced antivenin, which contains only the venom-binding portion of immunoglobulin G. One product, CroFab (Crotalidae Polyvalent Immune Fab–Ovine Fougera, Melville, NY) is a sterile, nonpyrogenic, purified, lyophilized preparation of ovine Fab (monovalent) immunoglobulin fragments obtained from the blood of healthy sheep immunized with one of the following North American snake venoms: *Crotalus atrox* (western diamondback rattlesnake), *Crotalus adamanteus* (eastern diamondback rattlesnake), *Crotalus scutulatus* (Mojave rattlesnake), and *Agkistrodon piscivorus* (cottonmouth or water moccasin). To obtain the final antivenin product, the four different monospecific antivenins are mixed. Each monospecific antivenin is prepared by fractionating the immunoglobulin from the ovine serum, digesting it with papain, and isolating the venom-specific Fab fragments on ion exchange and affinity chromatography columns.[33]

CroFab is standardized by its ability to neutralize the lethal action of each of the four venom immunogens following intravenous injection in mice. The potency of the product varies with each batch; however, a minimum number of mouse LD50 neutralizing units against each of the four venoms is included in every vial of final product. A schema for using CroFab to treat snakebites is given in Algorithm 33.1. This product is roughly five times more potent than the older equine Crotalidae polyvalent antivenin; it has rapidly replaced the equine antivenin once widely used against all North American crotalids, primarily because of fewer allergic reactions.[5,29,30] Recurrence of the effects of venom after an initial response to antivenin has been well recognized, hence the subsequent smaller doses 6, 12, and 18 hours following an effective initial response. As the algorithm illustrates, however, the equine antivenin may still have a role in the patient who is a nonresponder to CroFab, and an equine antivenin remains the most effective antivenin for coral snake bites.

The Crotalidae equine antivenin by Wyeth-Ayerst (St. David's, PA) is a polyvalent, hyperimmune equine serum produced by horse envenomation with the eastern diamondback, western diamondback, tropical rattlesnake, and fer-de-lance. The horse serum, before being administered to humans, is partially purified using ammonium sulfate

*Regarding the terminology for envenomation, the term *venom* describes the poisonous fluid produced by snakes, spiders, scorpions, etc.; the term *venin* describes any poisonous substance found in venom; antivenin is the term used by both *Stedman's Medical Dictionary* and *Webster's English Dictionary* to describe an antitoxin or antiserum against an animal or insect venom.

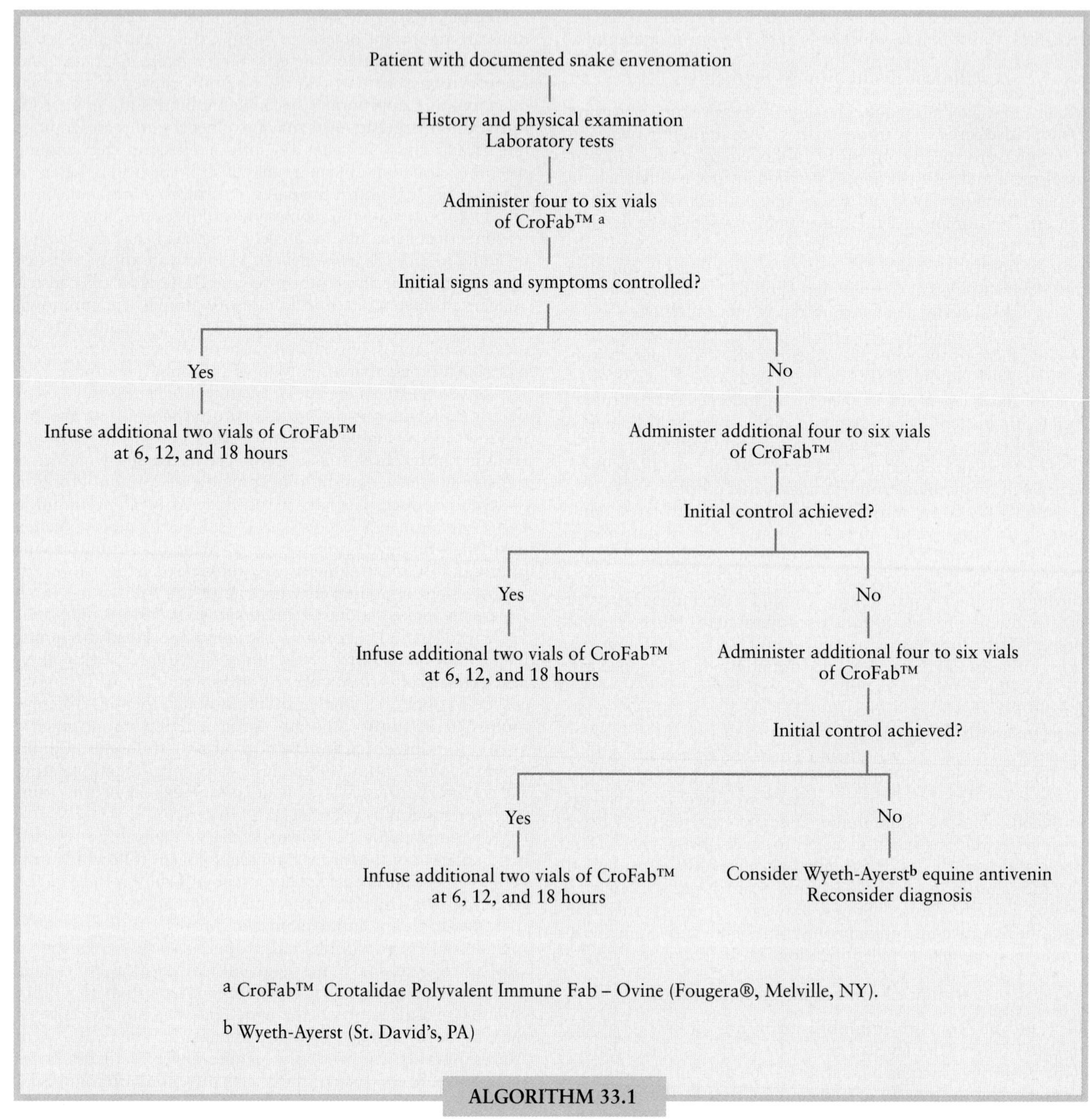

ALGORITHM 33.1 Treatment of snakebite envenomation with antivenin. (Adapted from Gold BS, Dart RC, Barish RA: Bites of venomous snakes. *N Engl J Med.* 2002;347:347–356; and Cribari, C: Management of poisonous snakebites. American College of Surgeons Committee on Trauma Poster, Chicago, Ill., 2004.)

precipitation followed by freeze-drying. The other available antivenin is the eastern coral snake antivenin, also manufactured by Wyeth-Ayerst.

Before administration of equine antivenin, the patient must be tested for sensitivity. Intradermal testing with 0.2 mL of a 1:10 or 1:100 serum dilution should be performed in all patients, with a positive test consisting of a wheal or erythema within the first 15 to 30 minutes. Similarly, two drops in the conjunctiva with a 1:1,000 dilution serum give a positive result with the production of itching and erythema in the conjunctiva. These sensitivity tests have a false-positive rate of approximately 50% and a false-negative rate of 8% to 10%. Anaphylaxis is reported in 3% to 54% of patients treated with equine antivenin, but only 14% of those treated with ovine CroFab[5,25] The anaphylaxis is a type I immunoglobulin E–mediated reaction to the horse serum, which results in mast cell degranulation.

The occurrence of anaphylaxis during or after administration of antivenin mandates immediate cessation of therapy and countermeasures, including antihistamines (oral diphenhydramine), epinephrine infusion, or corticosteroids. The adequacy of the airway and volume status must be ensured. The risk of continuing antivenin must be weighed against the potentially fatal consequences of severe envenomation.

The Wyeth-Ayerst antivenin product brochure describes a lengthy desensitization schedule. Concomitant administration of intravenous antihistamine and epinephrine in small, titrated microdrip doses to prevent the most severe manifestations of systemic anaphylaxis has been described in an allergic patient in whom antivenin therapy was deemed essential. This technique requires close physician observation because there are risks from both anaphylaxis and the treatment itself.

The other major complication of any antivenin therapy is serum sickness. Serum sickness occurs in approximately 50% to 75% of all patients treated with an equine-based antivenin but only 16% with the ovine source antivenin.[5,24] Serum sickness is a type III hypersensitivity reaction in which soluble antigen–antibody complexes are deposited diffusely in the presence of antigen access. In 26 patients who were treated with a total of 507 vials of Crotalidae antivenin, there was a 23% incidence of immediate hypersensitivity reaction and a 50% incidence of serum sickness.[24] Of patients who received more than eight vials of antivenin, 83% experienced serum sickness compared with 38% of patients who received fewer than eight vials. Serum sickness symptoms of urticaria, itching, nephritis, and arthralgia can occur at any time up to 3 weeks after antivenin therapy. The exact number of vials of antivenin required to induce serum sickness is unknown, but it appears that increasing amounts of antivenin lead to a higher incidence of serum sickness, with almost universal occurrence after the administration of seven to 10 vials of antivenin. The treatment for serum sickness is systemic corticosteroids in decreasing doses over a 7- to 14-day period.

Treatment of snakebites with antivenin has changed with the more widespread use of the ovine polyvalent CroFab. As illustrated in Algorithm 33.1, patients with a suspected or confirmed envenomation are recommended to receive an initial four to six vials of CroFab. If signs and symptoms of envenomation are controlled, additional vials are administered in a delayed fashion to prevent recurrence of symptoms. However, if the initial treatment fails to control envenomation, an additional four to six vials of CroFab are repeated twice, and then consideration should be given to using the "older" Wyeth-Ayerst polyvalent equine antivenin. The estimated initial amount of Crotalidae antivenin needed should correlate with the presenting clinical grade of envenomation. The package insert for Wyeth-Ayerst Crotalidae Antivenin Polyvalent provides detailed instructions for preparing, administering, and dosing this agent.

Although early surgical excision of the bite wound has been advocated by some, most authorities regard antivenin as the primary therapy and reserve surgery for the occasional compartment syndrome or débridement of necrotic tissue at the site of the bite several days after envenomation. Unless deep intramuscular envenomation has occurred and antivenin therapy has been delayed, fasciotomy is rarely required. Because the musculature and deep compartments of the hand are relatively superficial, however, intramuscular penetration may occur at these sites. Myonecrosis and interstitial edema may cause enough compartmental hypertension in these sites that linear finger fasciotomy and digital release are helpful. Fasciotomy may help reduce the ischemic tissue damage caused by increased pressure but does not alleviate the myonecrosis caused by the direct toxic effect of the venom.[31,32] Noninvasive arterial studies may help select patients who require special surgical intervention for ischemia.[33]

Venomous Lizards and Lizard Bites

Two species of venomous lizards exist, *Heloderma suspectum* and *Heloderma horridum*. *H. suspectum*, or the Gila monster, is found in the southwestern United States, and *H. horridum*, or the Mexican beaded lizard, is found in central and southern Mexico.[35] Physicians may, however, encounter a bite victim anywhere in the world because these colorful animals are common in zoos and often are kept illegally as pets. Nonetheless, human envenomation is very unusual, with only a few case reports of Gila monster or Mexican beaded lizard envenomation, and occurs most often from captive animals.[35,36]

Gila monsters grow up to 55 cm in length. They characteristically have slow, lingering movements, but they also have surprisingly quick reflexes and incredibly powerful jaws. Although usually docile, the medical literature reports suggest they can strike without warning or provocation. The mechanism of envenomation is fairly inefficient. The lizard has eight pairs of inferior labial glands located on either side of the lower jaw that secrete venom into the floor of the mouth. By capillary action alone, the venom travels out of the glands and into grooves of the posteriorly curved lower canines (teeth 4 through 7, counting from the central incisor). Only approximately 60% of bites have significant envenomation because prolonged chewing is required to disperse the venom adequately into the prey. Dislodging the animal from its prey, however, may be difficult because of its extremely powerful jaws. It may be necessary to cut the powerful masseter muscles to pry open the lizard's mouth. More ill-advised techniques of grabbing the tail or igniting the lizard (flame under the lower jaw) have also been attempted. The teeth of the Gila monster are poorly anchored, and periodically shed. Wounds must be thoroughly explored for the teeth because soft-tissue radiographs often fail to demonstrate these foreign bodies.[35]

In general, Gila monster bites have local effects, with direct tissue destruction and capillary membrane injury by serotonin, amine oxidases, phospholipase A, hyaluronidase, and a variety of proteases. The exact composition of Gila monster venom has not been elucidated, although the U.S. Food and Drug administration in April 2005 approved the use of a new injectable drug for the treatment of type II diabetes derived from Gila monster venom. Amylin Pharmaceuticals, Inc. (San Diego, CA) and Eli Lilly and Company (Indianapolis, IN) codeveloped Byetta, a 39-amino acid, glucagonlike peptide-1 agonist derived from the venom of *H. suspectum* and the first approved drug of a class called *incretin mimetics*, hormones secreted by the gut that help spur insulin production. The peptide appears to spur insulin production only when blood glucose levels are high, decreasing the risk of hypoglycemia. Clinical trials have been initiated comparing this drug alone and in combination with metformin and sulfonylureas.[37]

The most common clinical symptom of a Gila monster bite is pain, usually subsiding in 8 to 10 hours, although it may persist for several days. Generalized weakness, dizziness, perspiration, and anxiety are other common symptoms. Hypotension is a common clinical finding with envenomation, usually responding to fluid resuscitation alone. There has been one reported case of significant systemic hypotension and myocardial infarction in a 23-year-old man after a Gila monster bite.[38] Other common signs include erythema, edema, and even lymphangitis, probably from pathogens injected at the time of the bite because injection of sterile venom produces none of these clinical signs. Rather severe nausea and vomiting can also be seen. Laboratory abnormalities are rare. The treatment of Gila monster bites is largely local wound care and systemic support of the patient (fluids, pain relief, antibiotics, antiemetics). No antivenin is available. Tetanus immunization should be current. A period of observation after the bite to assess the potential for systemic toxicity is warranted.

Venomous Spiders and Spider Bites

More than six genera of spiders in the United States can inflict painful bites and necrotic ulceration, but most widely known

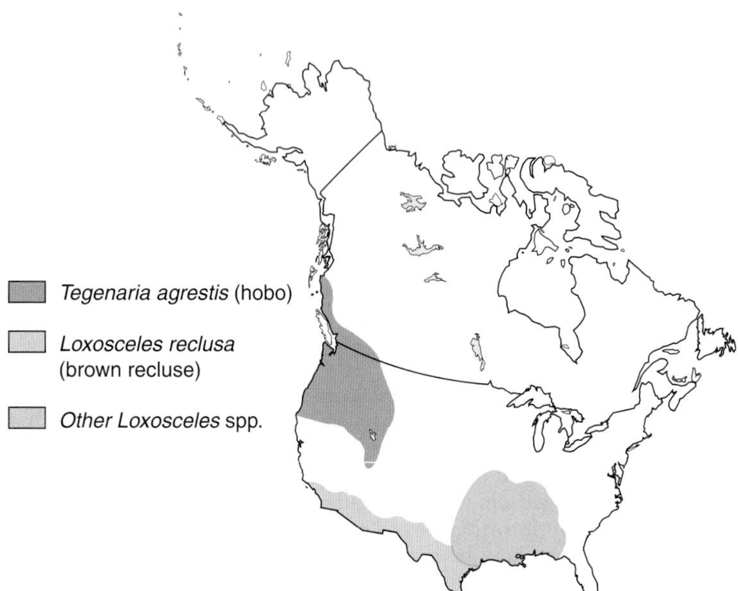

FIGURE 33.2 The geographic distribution of medically relevant spiders in North America.

and ones of medical significance are *Loxosceles reclusa* (brown recluse spider), *Tegenaria agrestis* (hobo spider), and *Latrodectus mactans* (black widow spider).[60] In the United States, the brown recluse spider is native to the central South, whereas other *Loxosceles* species exist in the southwestern border state regions.[39] (Fig. 33.2). Sighting of the brown recluse outside its native region is rare, is usually attributed to shipping of the spider in boxes of possessions or commerce, and is a single specimen only, not the typical large populations of spiders that exist when the habitat is conducive to their survival. The hobo spider is indigenous to the Northwest, whereas the black widow spider resides throughout the United States, except for Alaska.[40]

All three of these spiders can cause a painful, slow-healing, necrotic ulceration, but not all painful ulcerations should be attributed to spider bites. When a spider has not been positively identified as the offending agent, consideration should be given to other possible causes of necrotic ulceration.[39,41–42] Lyme disease *(Borrelia burgdorferi)* in particular can present with the classic "bull's-eye" patterning characteristic of the brown recluse bite.[43] Lyme disease is caused by an *Ixodes* tick-borne spirochete and is most common in the Northeast, Middle Atlantic area and the upper Midwest. Lyme disease is important to distinguish because early treatment with antibiotics (doxycycline) is usually curative, whereas unrecognized infections can cause late arthritic and neurologic symptoms that may not respond to antibiotics.

T. agrestis was introduced to the Pacific Northwest in the early 1900s from Europe. It was first reported from Seattle in the 1930s and had become common by the 1960s. *T. agrestis* is long-legged (40 mm resting length), hairy, and ranges in color from light tan to dark brown. The cephalothorax (10 to 12 mm) is distinguished by two stripes and "butterfly" markings on the dorsal surface and two stripes marking the ventral surface. *T. agrestis* is a poor climber and hence is usually found in low places. Sometimes referred to as an "aggressive house spider," the hobo builds a funnel-shaped web that can be found in woodpiles, crawl spaces, barns, haystacks, and objects that have not been moved in a long time. The hobo spiders are active from spring through fall, and although not overtly aggressive, the most dangerous time to encounter the hobo spider is during the fall mating season; the nests should be avoided and not probed with a finger. A bite of the hobo spider causes a necrotic wound similar to that of the brown recluse spider, along with a characteristic persistent headache.[39] The ulcer is slow to heal, often leaving a central crater.

The brown recluse spider is so named because it lives in dark, dry places, emerging only at night. This spider does not spin a web but catches prey by pursuit. It is small (body, 0.5 to 1 cm wide; leg span, 3 to 4 cm) and recognizable by the characteristic violin-shaped mark on the cephalothorax. When viewed under a microscope, it has three pairs of eyes rather than the two pairs most spiders have. Like most biting spiders, the brown recluse spider bites humans only when trapped or crushed against the skin. Brown recluse spider bites cause a complex and chronic soft tissue ulcer. Clinical signs begin first with an erythematous papule (2 to 8 hours), followed by white vasoconstriction (8 to 72 hours), ecchymosis (24 to 72 hours), and a hemorrhagic vesicle (48 to 96 hours).[39,41] Two to 7 days after the bite, an eschar develops over a characteristic crateriform ulcer, with surrounding soft tissue induration.[44] The eschar may conceal a progressive undermining necrosis that can persist for months. These wounds are most severe in the fatty parts of the body, such as the thighs and buttocks, perhaps because of the relatively poor blood supply to these tissues. There may also be a particular dermonecrotic factor in brown recluse venom. Sphingomyelinase D is present in the venom and appears to interact with the sphingomyelin of the red blood cell membrane and perhaps capillary endothelial cell membranes, causing cell destruction[45] Histologically, the site of the bite is said to resemble a cutaneous Arthus reaction, with the mechanism involving interactions between complement neutrophils and the clotting system.[46] Investigations suggest the necrosis is completely dependent on the victim's neutrophils, yet these neutrophils are not activated by the venom. *Loxosceles* venom appears to be a novel yet potent endothelial cell agonist, stimulating the release of interleukin-8 and granulocyte–macrophage colony-stimulating factor and E-selectin expression.[47]

Significant systemic symptoms after a brown recluse bite occur infrequently, in less than 10% of cutaneous manifestations. The clinical spectrum includes fever, chills, malaise, arthralgia, nausea and vomiting, and a scarlatiniform rash but can progress to hemolytic anemia, renal failure, and DIC in rare cases, perhaps more commonly in children than adults.[48]

Treatment of brown recluse spider bites includes analgesics, wound care, antitetanus therapy, avoidance of early surgical débridement, and perhaps oral dapsone. Antibiotics are reserved for true associated cellulitis. Dapsone is thought to work as an inhibitor of polymorphonuclear leukocyte chemotaxis, but it can cause hemolysis in glucose-6-phosphate dehydrogenase-deficient patients and can produce methemoglobinemia. Some studies show dapsone effective in reducing the size of the skin lesion and limiting the need for surgical débridement,[49,50] whereas other studies demonstrate no benefit in animal models,[51] and no prospective study in humans supports its use.[52] The most common dose is 50 to 100 mg (0.7 mg/kg) twice daily for 3 days to 2 weeks, although it is not approved for this use by the U.S. Food and Drug Administration. One controlled trial of dapsone, electric shock therapy, or no therapy in guinea pigs injected with 30 mg of spider venom demonstrated efficacy of dapsone in reducing lesion induration and necrosis area 72 hours after envenomation.[53] Electric shock therapy had no benefit. Hyperbaric oxygen treatment of model envenomation in rabbits and pigs also failed to demonstrate any effect on lesion healing time or superficial appearance, although hyperbaric treatments seemed to have decreased the amount of undermining necrosis visualized histologically on day 24 after envenomation.[54,55] A trial of hyperbaric oxygen, dapsone, and cyproheptadine in rabbits also failed to demonstrate any significant difference in lesion size, ulcer size, or histopathologic ranking up to 10 days after injection of toxin.[55] Local injections of lidocaine, phentolamine, and systemic steroids and antihistamines have been widely used in the past but have no demonstrable benefit. Systemic corticosteroids probably have a role only in the rare case of systemic loxoscelism, which has minimal skin changes but produces massive hemolysis.[44] Surgical excision of the lesion itself has no clear benefit.[56]

Commercial antivenin for the brown recluse spider is not available in the United States, although a rabbit antivenin for *L. laeta* is available in South America.[39] Equine-derived antivenin has been shown effective in mice and rabbits, and pepsin treatment to isolate the $F(ab')_2$ monoclonal fragment has been attempted. However, studies to date fail to demonstrate any advantage to antivenin, with or without dapsone, particularly if there is a few hour delay in administering the antivenin. In areas where loxosceles spiders are endemic, vaccination might hold promise.[60]

Few living creatures invite such poetic fascination and fear as the black widow spider. Its name, coloring, carnivore diet, and the disconcerting habit of the female eating her sexual partner invite such fascination. And although both the male and female spider possess potent venom, only the female is dangerous to humans because the male is smaller and thus its bite cannot penetrate human skin. The mature female has a black body, approximately 6 mm in diameter, with a characteristic red hourglass mark on the ventral aspect of the thorax. This mark is not always present and may consist only of two red dots. The black widow prefers a dry, protected, dimly lit area with access to flies and other insects, such as an outdoor privy. During the period in which the female *L. mactans* is guarding an egg sac, she is particularly aggressive and will attack the male if he disturbs the web, hence earning the particularly dark and descriptive common name *black widow*.[49] The diet most commonly consists of insects of any size, but reportedly includes mice, toads, and tarantulas that wander into the dense web and succumb to the poisonous bite and organ liquefication.

Black widow venom has a systemic neurotoxin, the primary effect of which is chest pain and abdominal pain. The abdominal pain may mimic an abdominal crisis, with marked cramping and a rigid abdomen. The neurologic signs of hyperreflexia, paresthesia, and cutaneous hyperesthesia help distinguish this from a true intraabdominal catastrophe. Profuse sweating, hypertension, and tachycardia are also common.[57] The primary treatment is supportive care and narcotics and muscle relaxants (methocarbamol or benzodiazepam) for pain control, although antivenin therapy also provides effective pain relief in patients with severe envenomations.[58] Antivenin is a horse serum–derived immunoglobulin therapy, usually suggested for use in young patients (<6 years of age), very infirm patients, and patients with a severe reaction. The usual dose is 1 ampule in 50 mL of normal saline. Calcium gluconate, 10 mL of a 10% solution given intravenously over 15 to 20 minutes, has usually been considered the first-line treatment of severe envenomations, although one report disputes its efficacy at pain relief.[58] Most black widow spider bite symptoms resolve within 1 day, but recurrent symptoms may persist for 2 to 3 days. Antivenin has been reported to be effective up to 30 hours after a bite.[59] The reported mortality rate is 2% to 6%, usually as a result of severe acute or delayed hypersensitivity reactions with paralysis, hemolysis, renal failure, and coma.

Venomous *Hymenoptera* Species and Bites

The more than 100,000 species of Hymenoptera consist of the well-known families of bees, wasps, and hornets but also include the fire ants, a nonwinged Hymenoptera present in the southeastern United States.[61] More envenomations and deaths (approximately 40 annually) in the United States are caused by Hymenoptera stings than by snakebites, emphasizing the fact that the venom of most Hymenoptera is as toxic as the rattlesnake's venom, the difference being the volume administered. The venom is primarily a hemolysin and neurotoxin, known for triggering anaphylactic reactions. Bee venom also contains melittin, phospholipase A_2, and hyaluronidase, which when given in adequate volume can cause endothelial disruption, cell breakdown, and tissue necrosis. It is estimated that approximately 0.4% of the human population is at risk for anaphylaxis from Hymenoptera stings.[62] Fortunately, most sting reactions are mild, involving dermal manifestations (e.g., hives, edema) only. The clinical effects are related both to the local toxic effects and the anaphylactic systemic effects. The local toxic effects include significant pain, swelling, and pruritus. If a significant amount of toxin is injected, the patient may experience nausea, emesis, and muscle spasms.

Most deaths from Hymenoptera stings are a result of severe anaphylactic reaction, which can occur at any age, but is relatively more common in adults. In this reaction, a preformed immunoglobulin E antibody activates mast cells, leading to degranulation with massive histamine release and prompting laryngeal and pulmonary edema, vasodilation, and vascular collapse. The treatment for Hymenoptera bites and stings is to remove the stinger, treat the local wound with ice and possibly an enzymatic meat tenderizer, and treat the anaphylactic reactions aggressively with antihistamines (diphenylhydramine, 50 to 100 mg intramuscularly or intravenously) or epinephrine (1:1,000 dilution, 0.3 to 0.5 mL intramuscularly or subcutaneously). Patients also require supplemental oxygen and intravenous fluids.

After sting anaphylaxis, approximately 50% of patients remain allergic to subsequent stings, in part determined by the severity of the initial anaphylactic symptoms. Children with benign dermal reactions only are unlikely to have recurrent reactions. Patients with more severe reactions are at risk for repeat anaphylaxis. Patients with a history of insect sting anaphylaxis and positive venom skin tests should have epinephrine available and are candidates for subsequent venom immunotherapy, which provides almost 100% protection against subsequent sting reactions. Such desensitization can take more than 3 years.[62]

Africanized bees *(Apis mellifera scutellata)* are a more aggressive subspecies than the native European bees of North and South America. Initially imported from Africa to Brazil in 1956 in the hope that they would hybridize with the better honey-producing European bee, some escaped and began interbreeding with domestic bees, proliferated, and migrated through Central America and the Yucatan peninsula of Mexico, first detected near Hidalgo, Texas, in 1993 and reportedly advancing at a rate of 100 miles per year.[63,64] Currently located primarily in the arid southwestern United States, these bees now pose a significant threat because massive envenomations (more than 50 bites) have occurred, resulting in nausea, vomiting, shock, hemolysis, rhabdomyolysis, and DIC; coma and renal failure can follow. Rarely, in patients initially complaining only of pain after multiple bee stings, a delayed (6 to 48 hours) toxic reaction has been reported, and some poison centers now recommend a 24-hour hospitalization for pediatric patients, older patients, and patients with underlying medical problems after an envenomation of 50 or more stings because such patients have an increased risk of delayed severe systemic reaction.[65] Laboratory studies on patients sustaining massive envenomations should be performed on presentation and 6 hours later to rule out hemolysis, thrombocytopenia, liver function abnormalities, and rhabdomyolysis.

Two species of imported fire ants now infest large areas of the Gulf Coast states.[66] The most aggressive species, *Solenopsis invicta,* has adapted well to environmental conditions in the southern United States, where it has become a considerable agricultural pest and a significant public health problem. Sting reactions typically include a dermal wheal-and-flare reaction followed by sterile pustules at sting sites. Occasionally, large local dermal reactions and pyoderma, or even life-threatening anaphylaxis, can occur. Caplan et al.[67] have shown that residents of Augusta, Georgia, an endemic area, had a 17% incidence of fire ant–specific immunoglobulin E compared with a 7.5% incidence of peanut-specific immunoglobulin E, posing a significant risk of potential fatal anaphylaxis.[67] Four venom allergens have been isolated and characterized. Clinical studies under way are designed to compare the safety and efficacy of fire ant venom with whole-body extract for diagnosis and treatment of fire ant allergy.[66] Additionally, biologic control of fire ants by the release of multiple species of decapitating flies has shown promise of keeping the fire ant population under control.[68]

Scorpions and Scorpion Stings

More than 650 types of scorpions can be found worldwide. In the United States, most scorpion stings are not lethal and the sting results primarily in local effects. In parts of Brazil, Mexico, North Africa, India, and Israel, however, the scorpion sting may be lethal. The venom toxicity depends greatly on species, season, and the age of the scorpion. In a fatal response, the venom induces a sympathetic storm, resulting in hypertension, tachycardia, and high-output cardiac failure.[69] Serum biochemistry reveals increased potassium and glucose, decreased sodium, and markedly elevated catecholamine levels. The treatment is specific antivenin therapy and systemic support directed at controlling hypertension and acute pulmonary edema. The outcome in the United States is usually excellent, with complete resolution of local effects; however, in some parts of Brazil, the mortality rates for a scorpion sting have been reported to be as high as 12% in adults and 60% in children.[70] In India, of 34 children admitted to a hospital after scorpion sting, 14 had hypertension, nine had acute pulmonary edema, five had myocardial failure, and four died.[69] In one report from Israel, respiratory distress was the main feature in 17 of 54 children with scorpion stings, but only three required mechanical ventilation; two patients died, but both failed to receive antivenin.[71] However, another report from Israel evaluated the treatment of 104 children with scorpion envenomation, noting that since 1989 they had discontinued using antivenin, with similar, if not better results in the no-antivenin group.[72] The antivenin in this report, however, is prepared from donkeys treated with the venom of the yellow scorpion *(Leiurus quinquestriatus),* which is not the same as that of the North American bark scorpion *(Centuroides exilicauda)* antivenin.

ENVIRONMENTAL INJURIES

Hypothermia

Because humans are homeotherms, we attempt to maintain a constant body temperature despite changes in environmental temperature. Normal body temperature depends on the site of measurement and is 37°C sublingually, 38°C in the rectum, 32°C at the skin, and 38.5°C deep in the liver. Even minor deviation from normal leads to important symptoms and disability.[73] Humans have a remarkable capacity to dissipate heat by evaporating body water; however, our tropical evolutionary heritage has provided us with far less ability to cope with cold conditions. As a result, hypothermia can occur in a variety of clinical settings and from a number of causes (Table 33.4).

To allow for the normal circadian temperature variation of 0.5° to 1°C, hypothermia is considered to be present in humans if the core temperature drops below 35°C (95°F). Hypothermia is usually classified by temperature zones as mild (32° to 35°C), moderate (28° to 32°C), or severe (<28°C).[73] Primary accidental hypothermia is defined as a decrease in core temperature that occurs as a result of overwhelming environmental cold stress. It most often occurs as a result of recreational misadventures that lead to cold-water

TABLE 33.4

CLINICAL DEFINITIONS OF HYPOTHERMIA AND EXAMPLES OF SETTINGS IN WHICH THEY OCCUR

Type	Settings
Accidental	Recreational environmental exposure, cold water immersion
Therapeutic	Treatment of Reye's syndrome, cardiopulmonary bypass, organ preservation
Drug induced	Alcohol, anesthetics, barbiturates, phenothiazines, morphine, other drugs
Central nervous system dysfunction	Transection of spinal cord, hypopituitarism, cerebrovascular accidents
Hypothalamic dysfunction	Wernicke's encephalopathy, anorexia nervosa, head trauma, pinealoma, other tumors
Metabolic	Hypoglycemia, hypothyroidism, hypoadrenalism, malnutrition
Dermal dysfunction	Burns, erythrodermas
Traumatic	Occurs after any major injury

Adapted with permission from Jurkovich GJ. Hypothermia in the trauma patient. *Adv Trauma* 1989;4:111–140.

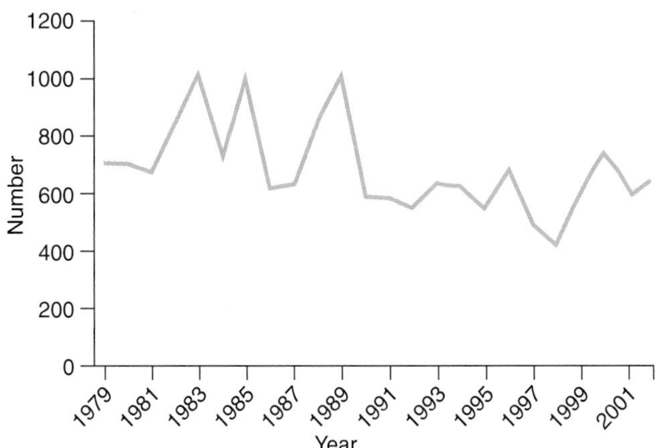

FIGURE 33.3 Number of hypothermia-related deaths by year in the United States, 1979–2002. (After Hypothermia-related deaths—United States, 2003–2004. *MMWR Morb Mortal Wkly Rep*. 2005; 54:173–175.)

immersion or prolonged environmental exposure. Secondary accidental hypothermia occurs in patients with abnormal heat production or thermoregulation, who become cold despite only mild cold stress. The most significant risk factors are advanced age, mental impairment, and substance abuse, in particular, of alcohol, although hypothyroidism, hypoadrenalism, trauma, and hypoglycemia are other risk factors.[74,75] Chronic hypothermia develops in patients with impaired heat generation (i.e., the elderly and infirm) who live in unheated apartments, are under continual cold stress, and after a time are found always to have a low temperature as if they have autoregulated to a new set temperature. A multicenter review of 428 cases of accidental hypothermia reported an overall mortality rate of 17%,[76] although other reports document mortality rates as high as 80%, primarily a result of infection and underlying illness.

From 1979 to 2002, a total of 16,555 deaths in the United States, an average of 689 per year (range 417 to 1,021), were attributed to exposure to excessive natural cold (Fig. 33.3).[75] In 2002, a total of 646 hypothermia-related deaths were reported, with an annual death rate of 0.2 per 100,000 population. Most reported hypothermia-related deaths (66%) occurred in males (Fig. 33.4), but the overall death rate (0.5 per 100,000 population) was the same for both males and females. Hypothermia-related deaths were reported by states with characteristically milder climates that experience rapid

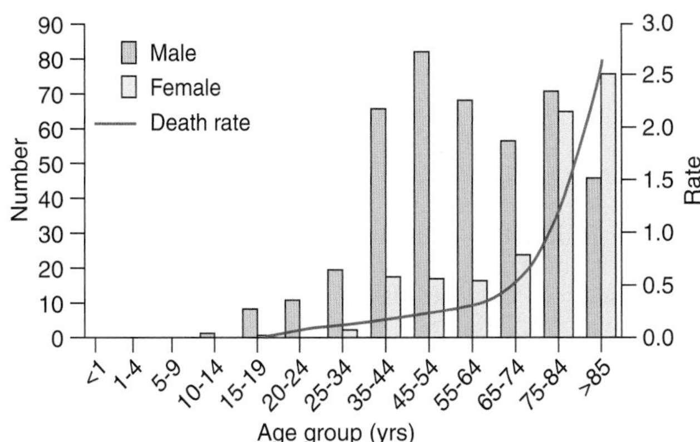

FIGURE 33.4 Number and rate (per 100,000 population) of hypothermia-related deaths, by age group and gender, in the United States. 1979–2002. (After Hypothermia-related deaths United States, 2003–2004. *MMWR Morb Mortal Wkly Rep*. 2005;54:173–175.)

temperature changes [e.g., North Carolina (0.4) and South Carolina (0.4)] and by western states that have high elevations and experience considerable changes from daytime to nighttime temperatures [e.g., Arizona (0.3)]. States with the greatest overall death rates caused by hypothermia are Alaska, New Mexico, North Dakota, and Montana.

The physiologic response to hypothermia is one of transitional changes, with few exact temperature-dependent responses (Fig. 33.5). Broadly speaking, the transition from a "safe zone" of hypothermia (in which physiologic adaptations to heat loss are working) to a "danger zone" of hypothermia (in which shivering is abolished, metabolism decreases, and heat loss is passively accepted) occurs between 33° and 30°C. The initial effects of hypothermia mimic intense sympathetic stimulation, with tremulousness, profound vasoconstriction, tremendous increases in oxygen consumption, and acceleration of heart rate and minute ventilation.[77]

The cardiovascular response includes tachycardia, followed by progressive bradycardia, which starts at approximately 34°C and results in a 50% heart rate decrease at 28°C. Cardiac output initially increases with the tachycardia, then progressively decreases, with a concomitant fall in blood pressure. The conduction system is particularly sensitive to hypothermia: the PR interval, then the QRS complex, and finally the QT interval become progressively prolonged.[78] As temperature falls below 30°C, atrial fibrillation, bradycardia, and ventricular dysrhythmia become common, with asystole occurring at temperatures below 25°C.[79] Because palpating pulses or measuring blood pressure in cold, stiff, hypothermic patients is difficult, the presence of an organized cardiac electrical rhythm should be taken as a sign of life that contraindicates cardiopulmonary resuscitation chest compressions, despite the absence of a palpable pulse. Such a rhythm may provide diminished but sufficient circulation in patients with severely reduced metabolism, and it is likely that vigorous chest compressions will convert this perfusing rhythm to fibrillation. Rewarming with close monitoring of rhythm, pulse, and blood pressure is indicated. If cardiac arrest occurs, extracorporeal cardiopulmonary bypass for perfusion and rewarming is indicated.[80–82] One report noted excellent long-term functional outcomes in 15 of 32 young patients successfully rewarmed in this manner.[81] All patients were intubated and ventilated and had received ongoing cardiac massage during transportation, and all 15 survivors had documented circulatory arrest (ventricular fibrillation or asystole) and fixed, dilated pupils. The mean interval from discovery of the patient to rewarming with cardiopulmonary bypass was 141 ± 50 minutes; the mean temperature was 21.8° ± 2.5°C. A recent report from Finland documents a 61% (14 of 23) survival to hospital discharge for adults undergoing cardiopulmonary bypass after a mean of 70 minutes of cardiopulmonary resuscitation following hypothermic arrest primarily from cold water immersion or exposure.[82]

Respiratory drive is increased during the early stages of hypothermia, but below 33°C progressive respiratory depression occurs, resulting in a decrease in minute ventilation. This decrease is not usually a significant problem until temperatures below 29°C are reached. Occasionally, hypothermia results in the production of a large amount of mucus (cold bronchorrhea).[83] This development predisposes to atelectasis and aspiration because ciliary action and the cough reflex are also depressed. Noncardiogenic pulmonary edema is also occasionally reported, especially in elderly patients and especially after prolonged periods of hypothermia.[84]

The effect of core hypothermia on arterial blood gas interpretation warrants a comment. Arterial blood gas samples are typically warmed to 37°C before measurement. A nomogram of Severinghaus mathematical corrections is then used to estimate the blood gas values at the patient's actual body

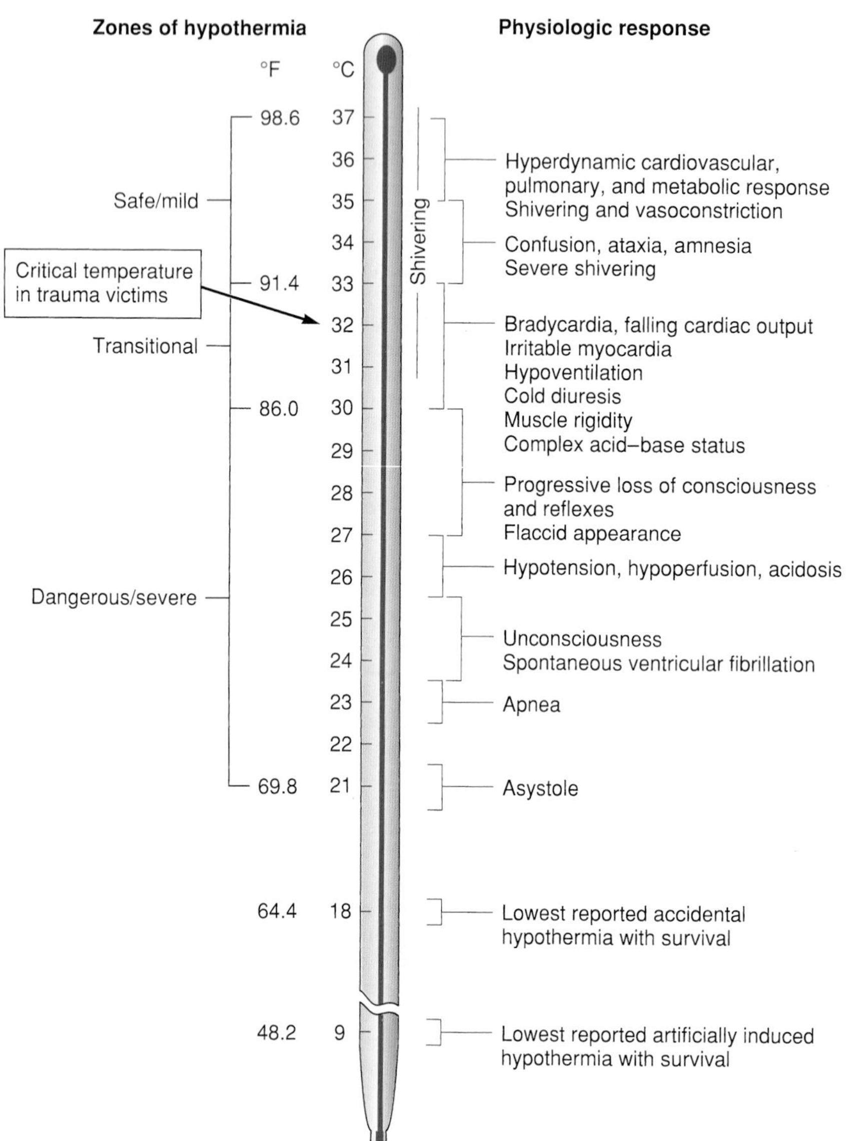

FIGURE 33.5 Zones of hypothermia and corresponding physiologic responses. Wide biologic variability accounts for physiologic changes rarely occurring at the exact temperatures noted. (After Jurkovich GJ. Hypothermia in the trauma patient. *Adv Trauma* 1989;4:111–140.)

temperature. With each 1°C temperature reduction, the PCO_2 decreases by 4.4% and the PO_2 decreases by 7.2%. Thus, a blood gas measured at 37°C with a PCO_2 of 40 mm Hg and a PO_2 of 70 mm Hg in a 32°C patient is reported as having a PCO_2 of 32 mm Hg and a PO_2 of 48 mm Hg after temperature correction.

The decrease in partial pressure is related to the increased solubility of gases in cold fluids and is not a result of a change in carbon dioxide content, oxygen content, or serum bicarbonate level. Clinicians often assume that the normal PCO_2 and PO_2 at 37°C are the values that should be attained at all temperatures. However, if normothermic end points for PCO_2 are attained in a hypothermic patient, they would have increased total body CO_2 stores, which would manifest by a rising PCO_2 and a falling pH during rewarming. Likewise, attempts at increasing a PO_2 that reflects normal oxygen content at a lower temperature are also inappropriate. A far simpler strategy is to assess the blood gases at 37°C without temperature correction. Values that are normal and acceptable when reported at 37°C correspond to normal values and contents when "corrected" for hypothermic temperatures.

Temperature correction of blood gases for pH management is also unnecessary. A pH of 7.40 at 37°C would be temperature corrected to 7.47 in a 32°C patient. At 37°C, the acid–base balance of water is neutral (pH is equal to pOH) when the pH is 6.8, and the body functions optimally when its pH is offset 0.6 pH units above the neutral point of water and has a relatively alkaline pH of 7.40. The pH of water rises with cooling, causing the pH of blood to rise by 0.015 pH units/°C, without a change in bicarbonate content.[86,87] Treating a patient with a temperature of 30°C with a pH of 7.40 instead of 7.47 fails to maintain the normal pH offset above the neutral point of water (relative alkalinity) and results in an acidotic cellular and chemical environment that has a multiplicity of effects on enzyme systems. Because blood with a pH of 7.40 assessed at 37°C is reported as having a pH of 7.47 when temperature corrected to 32°C, the simplest strategy when confronted with a patient with a temperature of 32°C is to assess the blood gas at 37°C only and to use the 37°C uncorrected pH value for management.[87,88]

The neurologic response to hypothermia is heralded by progressive loss of lucidity and deep tendon reflexes and, eventually, by flaccid muscular tone. Patients are often amnestic below 32°C, and between 31° and 27°C they usually lose consciousness. Pupillary dilatation and loss of cerebral autoregulation occur at temperatures below 26°C, and electroencephalography becomes silent at 19° to 20°C.[89] These findings, combined with an unobtainable pulse and apparent rigor mortis, may cause the patient to appear dead. It is important to remember that patients have been revived from core temperatures as low as 14°C,[90] and hence the saying "No one is dead until warm and dead." An exception to this admonition probably includes the patient who has sustained an anoxic event while still normothermic and has a serum potassium level greater than 10 mmol/L.[82,91] Reduction in blood pressure and cardiac output decreases glomerular filtration rate, but urinary output is maintained because of an impairment in renal tubular Na^+ reabsorption (cold diuresis).[92,93] Vasoconstriction also results in an initial increase in central blood volume that prompts a diuresis. Ileus, bowel wall edema, depressed hepatic drug detoxification, punctate gastric erosions (Wischnevsky ulcers), hyperamylasemia, and, rarely, hemorrhagic pancreatitis are hallmarks of the intestinal response to hypothermia. Hypothermia inhibits insulin release and insulin uptake at receptor sites, making hyperglycemia a relatively common finding, especially at temperatures below 30°C.[94] Exogenous insulin administration is unwarranted because it may result in rebound hypoglycemia during rewarming. Serum electrolyte changes are unpredictable, but serum potassium is often slightly increased in hypothermic patients because of renal tubular dysfunction, acidosis, and the breakdown of liver glycogen.[95] Hypothermia also appears to affect endothelial cell adhesion molecule function, which may partially explain increased infectious complications in hypothermic patients.[96] Only 1.9° C core hypothermia triples the incidence of surgical wound infection following colon resection and increases the duration of hospitalization by 20%.[97]

Body temperature has a significant effect on oxygen uptake. Oxygen consumption (VO_2) increases dramatically with any fall in body temperature. When involuntary muscle contractions in the form of shivering occur, oxygen consumption increases by as much as threefold to fivefold.[98,99] This process is inefficient because shivering produces heat near the surface of the body, causing most of the heat to be lost to the environment, with less than 45% being retained by the patient.

The thermoregulatory drive is such a powerful one that it takes precedence over many other homeostatic functions. The resultant increase in oxygen utilization may result in anaerobic metabolism, acidosis, and significant cardiopulmonary stress. One study noted a 35% increase in oxygen consumption and a 65% increase in CO_2 production in postoperative patients after resolution of anesthesia, when the thermostatic drive reappeared.[100] In another study, a core temperature decrease of as little as 0.3°C in postoperative patients was associated with a 7% increase in VO_2, and temperature reductions between 0.3° and 1.2°C were associated with a 92% increase in VO_2, with proportional increases in minute ventilation.[101] Further details of the specific organ system responses to hypothermia are beyond the scope of this chapter, but the interested reader is referred to several excellent in-depth monographs.[73,101–103]

Hypothermia in Trauma Patients

Mild hypothermia is very common after traumatic injury. When ambient temperature falls below the thermoneutral temperature (i.e., the temperature at which no thermogenesis or heat dissipation is necessary), which is 28°C (82.5°F) for humans, an increase in heat production is required to maintain a normal body temperature. Combustion is the only source of endogenous heat production, and this process requires an increase in oxygen utilization. After shock or injury, however, oxygen supplies are often limited and further heat loss occurs owing to cold emergency department and operating room environments, cold fluid resuscitation, and open thoracic and abdominal cavities. This is further aggravated by anesthetic and neuromuscular blocking agents that prevent the heat-producing shivering response. Thus, the occurrence of hypothermia in surgical or critically injured patients is most often a form of secondary accidental hypothermia.

One study found that 57% of trauma patients admitted to a level 1 trauma center were hypothermic at some time and that temperature loss was most significant in the emergency department[104] Another study reported that the average initial temperature for 94 intubated major trauma victims was 35°C, with no seasonal variation.[105] Of patients in this study, 66% were hypothermic on admission: 43% were mildly hypothermic (34° to 36°C) and 23% had temperatures below 34°C. Likewise, Jurkovich et al.[106] reported that 42% of 71 adult trauma victims with an Injury Severity Score (ISS) of 25 or higher had core temperatures below 34°C and in 13% the core temperature fell below 32°C. Importantly, there were no survivors when core body temperature was below 32°C. Both mortality rate and the incidence of hypothermia increase with higher ISS, massive fluid resuscitation, and the presence of shock, but controlling for these variables still demonstrates that the mortality rate of the hypothermic trauma patient is greater than that of the warm trauma patient.[106,107] Although the mortality rate for moderate (28° to 32°C) degrees of primary accidental hypothermia is approximately 20%,[76] moderate levels of hypothermia in trauma and critically ill patients are associated with a much higher mortality rate. Rutherford et al.[108] reported that 9.4% of surgical intensive care unit patients had a core body temperature less than 35°C; the mortality rate of the hypothermic trauma patients was 53%. In fact, compared with other patient populations, the mortality rate associated with hypothermia in the trauma victim is so high that the definition of mild, moderate, and severe hypothermia in the trauma patient warrants special classification (Table 33.5).[73]

Hypothermia appears to occur primarily in victims of relatively severe trauma. Little and Stoner,[109] reporting on a heterogeneous group of 82 trauma patients, observed that hypothermia occurred only in those patients with an ISS greater than 12. Skin temperature fell from 32.0°C to 31.7°C, whereas core temperature fell from 37.3°C to 36.5°C. Hypothermia did not occur in less severely injured patients, and shivering, which should be expected, was noted in only one of the hypothermic patients. Mild degrees of injury have, in fact, been associated with small elevations in core body temperature, particularly when the shivering response mechanism has not been abated.[73,110]

The detrimental effect of hypothermia in the human trauma victim is contrasted by a large body of experimental evidence in animals suggesting that hypothermia has a protective role in shock. This extensive body of literature is reviewed

TABLE 33.5 CLASSIFICATION

ZONES OF SEVERITY FOR HYPOTHERMIA

Zone	Temperature
Mild hypothermia	36° to 34°C (<96.8° to 93.2°F)
Moderate hypothermia	34° to 32°C (<93.2° to 89.6°F)
Severe hypothermia	<32°C (<89.6°F)

elsewhere,[73] but in general, animals subjected to combined hypothermia and shock (hemorrhage, burn, blunt trauma) usually survive longer than similarly injured but actively warmed animals. Blalock and Mason[111] (1941) were among the first in modern times to recognize the ability of hypothermia to prolong survival times after shock, but they emphasized that the overall survival rate was unchanged, an observation reaffirmed in 2003.[112] However, increases in both survival times and survival rates have been shown in a number of animal models of induced hypothermia after hemorrhagic shock.[113,114] The protective effects of hypothermia in preventing ischemia–reperfusion injury have been described in a number of models, including muscle, intestine, and rabbit ear.[115–118]

Hypothermia has also been suggested to protect the traumatically injured brain. The use of therapeutic hypothermia in a patient with traumatic brain injury was first reported in 1943[119] and sporadically over the ensuing two decades[120] More recently, a randomized, multicenter, controlled trial of core body hypothermia in trauma patients with severe closed head injury (Glasgow Coma Scale scores of 3 to 7) was conducted.[121] Select trauma patients with severe head injury were intentionally cooled within 6 hours of injury to 32° to 33°C for 48 hours after injury and then rewarmed. The outcome was poor (defined as severe disability, a vegetative state, or death) in 57% of the patients in both groups. Mortality was 28% in the hypothermia group and 27% in the normothermia group ($P = 0.79$). The patients in the hypothermia group had more hospital days with complications than the patients in the normothermia group. The authors concluded that treatment with hypothermia is not effective in improving outcomes in patients with severe brain injury. Other authors have also reported higher rates of pneumonia and diabetes insipidus in a small study of induced hypothermia in severely head-injured patients (Glasgow Coma Scale scores of 3 to 7) was conducted.[121] Select trauma patients with severe head injury were intentionally cooled within 6 hours of injury to 32° to 33°C for 48 hours after injury and then rewarmed. The outcome was poor (defined as severe disability, a vegetative state, or death) in 57% of the patients in both groups. Mortality was 28% in the hypothermia group and 27% in the normothermia group ($P = 0.79$). The patients in the hypothermia group had more hospital days with complications than the patients in the normothermia group. The authors concluded that treatment with hypothermia is not effective in improving outcomes in patients with severe brain injury. Other authors have also reported higher rates of pneumonia and diabetes insipidus in a small study of induced hypothermia in severely head-injured patients (Glasgow Coma Scale score <8), with no effect on neurologic outcome.[122] Evidence further supporting the harmful effect of hypothermia in the trauma patient is provided by a prospective, randomized trial of rapid rewarming versus conventional rewarming of 57 multiple-trauma patients.[123] In this study, trauma patients who were rapidly rewarmed with continuous arteriovenous rewarming from less than 34.5°C to greater than 36°C required less resuscitation fluid volume and had a lower early mortality rate than those rewarmed more slowly. Failure to rewarm in either group was uniformly fatal. The survival rate at 3 days after injury was 82% in the rapid rewarm group versus 62% in conventionally managed patients. Approximately 50% of the patients in both groups had a severe head injury, defined as a head Abbreviated Injury Severity score of 3 or greater. In this well-controlled study, maintenance of hypothermia not only failed to confer an advantage but also was detrimental to early survival.

The role of hypothermia in the injured patient remains unresolved. It is apparent that the physiologic consequence of severe trauma is a drop in core body temperature. It remains unclear, however, whether this response is a protective response to shock or the result of diminished heat production caused by failing metabolism. The frequent presence of lactic acid accumulation in cold, seriously injured patients supports the latter hypothesis. Clinical studies indicate that even mild hypothermia in the trauma patient is predictive of a poor outcome. Hypothermia does diminish metabolic demands and oxygen consumption in anesthetized patients, but the price appears to be malfunction of enzymes and physiologic systems necessary to recover from injury.

The systems most affected by hypothermia in victims of injury are those involved in clotting. Reports of coagulation abnormalities in patients with apparently normal clotting factor levels surfaced shortly after the introduction of hypothermic cardioplegia for cardiac surgery.[124,125] Although hemodilution with volume expanders deficient in clotting factors and platelets is the usual cause of nonsurgical bleeding, cold platelets are known to undergo morphologic changes that affect adherence, including loss of shape, cytoplasmic swelling, and dissolution of cytoplasmic microtubules necessary for normal motility.[126] Platelet activation is also associated with activation of cell membrane phospholipases that hydrolyze phospholipids to arachidonic acid, a precursor to prostaglandin endoperoxides and thromboxane A_2, a potent vasoconstrictor necessary for normal platelet aggregation[127] Valeri et al.[128] induced systemic hypothermia to 32°C in baboons, but kept one forearm warm using heating lamps and a warming blanket. Simultaneous bleeding time measurements in the warm and cold arm were 2.4 and 5.8 minutes, respectively. This effect, which was reversible with rewarming, appeared to be mediated by cold-induced slowing of the enzymatic reaction rate of thromboxane synthetase, which resulted in decreased production of thromboxane A_2. A recent report suggests that bleeding observed at mildly reduced temperatures (33° to 37°C) results primarily from a platelet adhesion defect and not reduced enzyme activity or platelet activation; however, at temperatures below 33°C, both reduced platelet function and enzyme activity likely contribute to the coagulopathy,[129] perhaps helping to explain why 32°C is such a critical temperature in the coagulopathic injured patient.

As with blood gases, clinical tests of coagulation are temperature standardized to 37°C. Fibrometers contain a thermal block that heats the plasma and reagents to 37°C before initiating the assay. Thus, tests of coagulation reflect clotting factor deficiencies but are corrected for any potential effect of hypothermia on clotting factor function. A detailed study of the kinetic effects of hypothermia on clotting factor function has been undertaken by Reed et al.,[130] who performed clotting tests (PT, PTT, and thrombin time) on reference human plasma-containing normal clotting factor levels at temperatures ranging from 25° to 37°C. The results showed a significant slowing of all coagulation tests at temperatures below 35°C that was proportional to the degree of hypothermia. The prolongation of clot formation occurred at clinically relevant levels of hypothermia and was equivalent to that seen in normothermic patients with significant clotting factor depletion. For example, assays conducted at 35°C, 33°C, and 31°C prolonged the PTT to the same extent as would occur in a euthermic patient with reductions in factor IX levels to 66%, 32%, and 7% of normal, respectively.

Clotting factor supplementation is not the answer to a hypothermia-induced coagulopathy; rewarming is. However, in many seriously injured patients, clotting factor depletion exists in conjunction with hypothermia. A potentiating effect of hypothermia on coagulation dysfunction occurs in plasma of patients with deficient clotting factor levels, although there does not appear to be synergy between the two conditions.[131] Hypothermic, coagulopathic trauma patients still benefit from coagulation profile testing. If prolongation of PT and PTT is evident in plasma warmed to 37°C, clotting factor replacement is indicated. If PT and PTT are near normal, rewarming alone reverses the clinically apparent coagulopathy.

Treatment

Rewarming techniques are usually classified as passive external rewarming, active external rewarming, or active core rewarming.[132] Passive external rewarming simply implies allowing spontaneous rewarming to occur with the patient removed from a hypothermic environment and is usually used only for the mildly hypothermic patient. Active external rewarming techniques include surrounding the patient with warm blankets or heating pads, infrared heating lights, and immersion in warm water. Active core rewarming includes heated intravenous fluids, as well as heated peritoneal or thoracic lavage; heated gastric, bladder, or colonic lavage; heated and water-saturated inhaled air; and extracorporeal circulatory rewarming. Blood rewarming is currently limited to a maximum temperature of 42°C by the American Association of Blood Banks, but rewarming to 49°C with inline microwave blood rewarmers has been reported as safe, as has intravenous fluid rewarming to 65°C.[133,134]

The advantages and disadvantages of each technique are regularly debated, particularly regarding the role of external versus core rewarming. It is clear, however, that the rate of heat transfer to the hypothermic patient is greatest using active core rewarming, particularly extracorporeal circulation rewarming. This may be a critical factor in surgical patients for whom rapid restoration of clotting and cardiac function is necessary.

The technique of rewarming the hypothermic victim by extracorporeal circulation has been described by numerous authors, based primarily on small personal experiences.[81,82] This technique has appeal in cases of primary accidental hypothermia, in which maintenance of circulation, correction of hypoxia, and replenishment of intravascular volume may play a role as large as correcting the temperature change itself. The need for systemic anticoagulation has, however, generally limited the usefulness of full cardiopulmonary bypass rewarming in the trauma patient.

A simplified technique of extracorporeal active core rewarming is continuous arteriovenous rewarming.[135] This technique makes use of the patient's own blood pressure to drive an extracorporeal circuit through an efficient, but small countercurrent heat-exchange device. Systemic anticoagulation is not necessary because the tubing is heparin bonded and trauma patients are relatively anticoagulated. The relative ease of use makes this device widely applicable in rewarming severely hypothermic patients with an intact circulation and, in a prospective, randomized trial of rewarming trauma patients, demonstrated its efficacy.[123]

The use of body cavity lavage with warm solutions is a simple, less invasive method of accomplishing active core rewarming; however, rewarming rates with body cavity lavage vary greatly based on initial core temperature, dialysate temperature, infusion rate, and dwell time. Several studies support the notion that active core rewarming by peritoneal lavage is preferable to active external rewarming.[136] Moss[74] examined three techniques of rewarming hypothermic and cardiac-arrested dogs, concluding that both peritoneal lavage (55°C dialysate) and partial extracorporeal circulation were faster than active external rewarming with a heating blanket.[74] A frequently stated disadvantage of external rewarming is that the peripheral tissues are rewarmed in advance of the still cool "core," resulting in peripheral vasodilation. In the presence of inadequate volume resuscitation, this rewarming method may result in vascular collapse ("rewarming shock") and a subsequent fall in central temperature ("afterdrop") as the cold peripheral blood returns to the core. Whether this process is the mechanism of the core afterdrop is debatable because a core afterdrop has been noted to occur in animal models even during complete circulatory arrest. Volume contraction caused by vasoconstriction, cold diuresis, and cellular swelling coupled with inadequate fluid resuscitation may be a more appropriate explanation for circulatory collapse during rewarming.

The thermodynamic principles of heat transfer to the hypothermic patient are reviewed in greater detail elsewhere, but a sense of rewarming rates and quantity of heat transferred by various techniques is instructional.[132,137] Ventilating a patient with a core temperature of 32°C with water-saturated air at 41°C results in a maximum heat transfer rate of 9 kcal/hour. For comparison, basal metabolic heat generation produces approximately 70 kcal/hour, and shivering produces up to 250 kcal/hour. Given the specific heat of the body (0.083 kcal/kg/°C), 58 kcal is required to raise the temperature of a 70-kg patient by 1°C. Thus, more than 6 hours would be required to warm a 32°C patient using 41°C humidified inspired air.

Heat transfer rates using body cavity lavage can be similarly calculated based on the specific heat of water (1 kcal/kg/°C). If 1 L of 44°C water infused into a body cavity dwells long enough to exit at 40°C, 4 kcal of heat will have been transferred to the patient. Thus, over 14 L of fluid is needed to increase core temperature by 1°C. However, warming becomes less efficient as the patient rewarms because a longer dwell time is required to reduce the temperature of the infusate to 40°C.

Warming by cardiopulmonary bypass or continuous arteriovenous rewarming is the most efficient method of core heating. With flow rates of 15 to 30 L/hour, it is possible to deliver 120 to 240 kcal/hour if the reinfused blood is heated to 40°C, a rate of heat transfer over 10 times that of the other methods. In any case, the urgency with which rewarming must be accomplished depends on how adversely the hypothermia is affecting the patient. With the exception of extracorporeal circulatory methods, most rewarming techniques serve primarily to prevent loss of endogenously generated heat and are ineffective in circumstances during which rapid rewarming is indicated. Early and direct attention to the mechanisms of heat loss is necessary to prevent the metabolic and hemorrhagic complications associated with hypothermia in surgical patients.

Cold Injury and Frostbite

Cold injuries limited to digits, extremities, or exposed surfaces are the result of either direct tissue freezing (frostbite) or more chronic exposure to an environment just above freezing (chilblain [pernio], trench foot). Cold injury has been a major cause of morbidity during war experiences. It resulted in more than 7 million lost soldier fighting days by Allied forces in World War II and was reportedly the most common major injury sustained by British soldiers in the Falklands expedition.[138]

The terms *chilblain* and *pernio* describe a form of local cold injury characterized by pruritic, red-purple papules, macules, plaques, or nodules on the skin. The lesions are often associated with edema or blistering and are caused by a chronic vasculitis of the dermis;[139] this entity does not appear to be related to hereditary protein C or S deficiency.[140] This pathologic process is provoked by repeated exposure to cold, but not freezing, temperatures. This injury typically occurs on the face, the anterior surface of the tibia, or the dorsum of the hands and feet, areas poorly protected or chronically exposed to the environment. With continued exposure, ulcerative or

TABLE 33.6 CLASSIFICATION

CLASSIFICATION OF FROSTBITE

Degree	Description of Frostbite
First	Tissue freezing with hyperemia and edema but without blistering
Second	Tissue freezing with hyperemia, edema, and characteristic large, clear blisters
Third	Tissue freezing with death of subcutaneous tissues and skin, resulting in hemorrhagic vesicles that are in general smaller than second-degree blisters
Fourth	Tissue necrosis, gangrene, and eventual full-thickness tissue loss

hemorrhagic lesions may appear and progress to scarring, fibrosis, and atrophy. Treatment consists of sheltering the patient, elevating the affected part on sheepskin, and allowing gradual rewarming at room temperature. Rubbing and massage are contraindicated because they can cause further damage and secondary infection.

Trench foot or cold immersion foot (or hand) describes a nonfreezing injury of the hands or feet, typically in sailors, fishermen, or soldiers, that is caused by chronic exposure to wet conditions and temperatures just above freezing.[141] It appears to involve an alternating arterial vasospasm and vasodilatation, with the affected tissue first cold and anesthetic and then hyperemic after 24 to 48 hours of exposure. With the hyperemia comes an intense, painful burning and dysesthesia, and tissue damage is characterized by edema, blistering, redness, ecchymosis, and ulceration. Complications of local infection or cellulitis, lymphangitis, and gangrene may occur. A posthyperemic phase occurs 2 to 6 weeks later and is characterized by tissue cyanosis with increased sensitivity to cold. Treatment is best started during or before the reactive hyperemia state and consists of immediate removal of the extremity from the cold, wet environment with exposure of the feet (or hands) to warm, dry air. Elevation to minimize edema, protection of pressure spots, and local and systemic measures to combat infection are indicated. Massage, soaking of the feet, or rapid rewarming is not indicated. Demyelination of nerves, muscle atrophy, fallen arches, and osteoporosis may all present long-term complications, and a tendency toward marked vasospasm during subsequent exposure to cold develops in some patients.[142]

Frostnip is the mildest form of cold injury. It is characterized by initial pain and pallor, with subsequent numbness of the affected body part. Skiers and other winter outdoor enthusiasts are most likely to experience this cold injury to the nose, ears, or tips of digits. The injury is reversible and warming of the cold tissue results in return of sensation and function with no tissue loss.

Frostbite is a more severe and common form of cold injury. Frostbite damage is caused by direct ice crystal formation at the cellular level with cellular dehydration and microvascular occlusion. Frostbite is traditionally classified into four grades of injury severity (Table 33.6).

The affected body part nearly always initially appears hard, cold, white, and anesthetic, regardless of the depth of injury. Because the appearance of the lesion changes frequently during the course of treatment and because the initial treatment regimen is applicable for all degrees of insult,[143] some authorities suggest discarding this classification as a prognostic impossibility and simply classifying frostbite as either superficial or deep.[144]

Weather conditions, altitude, degree of protective clothing, duration of exposure, and degree of tissue wetness are all contributing external factors to the development of frostbite injury. Because sensory nerve activity is abolished at 7° to 9°C, the disappearance of pain is an early warning sign of cold injury. Acclimation to cold may be protective, whereas a previous history of frostbite probably predisposes to another cold tissue injury. Smoking and a history of arterial disease also are contributing factors. In urban environments, more than 50% of frostbite injuries are alcohol related and a significant portion of these patients (16%) have an underlying psychiatric illness.[145]

Evidence suggests that frostbite injury has two components—the initial freeze injury and a reperfusion injury that occurs during rewarming. The initial response to tissue cooling is vasoconstriction and arteriovenous shunting, intermittently relieved (every 5 to 7 minutes) by vasodilation, the so-called hunting response.[146] With prolonged exposure, this response fails, and the temperature of the freezing tissue approximates ambient temperature until −2°C. At this point, extracellular ice crystals form, and as these crystals enlarge the osmotic pressure of the interstitium increases, resulting in movement of intracellular water into the interstitium. Cells begin to shrink and become hyperosmolar, disrupting cellular enzyme function. If freezing is rapid (>10°C/min), intracellular ice crystal formation occurs, resulting in immediate cell death.[138] Intravascularly, endothelial cell disruption and red cell sludging result in cessation of circulation.

During rewarming, red cell, platelet, and leukocyte aggregation is known to occur and results in patchy thrombosis of the microcirculation. These accumulated blood elements are thought to release, among other products, the toxic oxygen free radicals and the arachidonic acid metabolites PGF_{2a} and thromboxane A_2, which further aggravate vasoconstriction and platelet and leukocyte aggregation.[147,148] However, the exact mechanism of tissue destruction and death after freeze injury remains poorly defined. Animal studies suggest that vascular injury in the form of endothelial cell damage and subsequent interstitial edema, but not vessel thrombosis, predominate as initial events in rewarming injury.[149,150] A substantial component of severe cold injury may be neutrophil mediated, as suggested by the observation that a monoclonal antibody to neutrophil–endothelial and neutrophil–neutrophil adherence can markedly ameliorate the pathologic process of a severe cold injury.[151] In this rabbit model, animals treated with anti-CD11/CD18 adhesion molecule after cold injury (30 minutes at −15°C) but before rewarming (39°C water bath) had significantly less tissue loss and edema. The implication of these observations is that much of the injury of severe frostbite occurs during rewarming or reperfusion. Clinical application of these experimental observations remains untested.

Treatment

Prehospital or field care of the victim of cold injury should focus on removing the patient from the hostile environment and protecting the injured body part from further damage. Rubbing or exercising the affected tissue does not augment blood flow and risks further cold injury or mechanical trauma. Because repeated bouts of freezing and thawing worsen the injury, it is preferable for the patient with frostbite of the hands or feet immediately to seek definitive shelter and care rather than rewarm the tissue in the field and risk refreezing. Although the initial symptoms may be mild and overlooked by the patient, severe pain, burning, edema, and even necrosis and gangrene may appear with rewarming. With severe injury the range of motion progressively decreases and edema becomes prominent. The injury may progress to numbness and, eventually, to loss of all sensation in the affected tissue.

The emergency room treatment of a frostbite victim should first focus on the basic ABCs (airway, breathing, and circulation) of trauma resuscitation and then systemic hypothermia should be identified and corrected. Most patients are dehydrated, and resuscitation with warm fluids is an important part of early management. Fractures are often accompanied by frostbite in mountaineers, and although manipulation may be required to treat vascular compromise, open reduction is hazardous, and application of traction should be delayed until after postthawing edema has been assessed.

Rapid rewarming is the goal. Gradual, spontaneous rewarming is inadequate, particularly for deeper injuries, and rubbing the injured part in ice or snow often delays warming and results in marked tissue loss.[152] Rapid rewarming should be achieved by immersing the tissue in a large water bath of 40° to 42°C (104° to 108°F). The water should feel warm, but not hot, to the normal hand. The bath should be large enough to prevent rapid loss of heat, and the water temperature should be maintained. Dry heat is not advocated because it is difficult to regulate, and the result of using excessive heat is often disastrous. The rewarming process should take approximately 30 to 45 minutes for digits, with the affected area appearing flushed when rewarming is complete and good circulation has been reestablished. Narcotics are required because the rewarming process can be quite painful.

The skin should be gently but meticulously cleansed and air dried and the affected area elevated to minimize edema. A tetanus toxoid booster should be administered as indicated by immunization history. Sterile cotton is placed between toes or fingers to prevent skin maceration and extreme care taken to prevent infection and avoid even the slightest abrasion. The affected tissue should be protected by a tent or cradle, and pressure spots must be prevented. In one review, infection developed in 13% of urban frostbite victims, but one half of these infections were present at time of admission.[145] Most clinicians reserve antibiotics for identified infections.[153]

After rewarming, the treatment goals are to prevent further injury while awaiting the demarcation of irreversible tissue destruction. All patients should be hospitalized and affected tissue gently cleansed once or twice a day in warm (38°C) whirlpool baths, with some clinicians adding an antiseptic such as chlorhexidine or an iodophor to the bath. Based on the findings of arachidonic acid metabolites in the blisters of frostbite victims, some authors advocate the use of topical aloe vera (thromboxane inhibitor) and systemic ibuprofen or aspirin. Heggers et al.[154] report on a nonrandomized trial in which 56 patients treated with these agents, plus prophylactic penicillin, had less tissue loss, a lower amputation rate, and a shorter hospital stay than 98 patients treated with warm saline, silver sulfadiazine, or Sulfamylon dressings (Bertek Pharmaceuticals, Research Triangle Park, N.C.).[154] Another report on frostbite treatment in rabbits demonstrated improved tissue viability when systemic pentoxifylline and topical aloe vera cream were used.[155] Uninfected blebs should be left intact because they provide a sterile biologic dressing for 7 to 10 days and protect underlying epithelialization. After resolution of edema, digits should be exercised during the whirlpool bath and physical therapy begun. Tobacco, nicotine, and other vasoconstrictive agents must be withheld. Weight bearing is prohibited until complete resolution of edema.

Numerous adjuvants have been suggested and tried in an effort to restore blood supply to frostbitten areas. The intense vasoconstrictive effect of cold injury has focused attention on increased sympathetic tone. Sympathetic blockade and even surgical sympathectomy continues to be advocated by some authors based on the theory that it releases the vasospasm that precipitates thrombosis in the affected tissue.[156,157] This method of treatment has produced inconsistent results and is difficult to evaluate clinically, with no prospective, randomized trials available. Although sympathectomy appears to mollify the pain, hyperhidrosis, and vasospasm of cold injuries, it may increase vascular shunting and adversely affect healing. In one series, a more proximal demarcation of injury in sympathectomized limbs was noted than in nonsympathectomized ones, despite apparently equal bilateral injury.[152]

Experience with intraarterial vasodilating drugs such as reserpine and tolazoline has also been unrewarding. Bouwman et al.[157] demonstrated in a controlled clinical study that immediate (mean 3 hours) ipsilateral intraarterial reserpine infusion coupled with early (mean 3 days) ipsilateral operative sympathectomy failed to alter the natural history of acute frostbite injury compared with the contralateral limb. Heparin, thrombolytic agents, and hyperbaric oxygen have also failed to demonstrate any substantial treatment benefit, whereas low-molecular-weight dextran alleviated postthawing circulatory obstruction as late as 2 hours after thawing and markedly reduced tissue loss in rabbit feet.[158]

The difficulty in determining the depth of tissue destruction in cold injury has led to a conservative approach to the care of frostbite injuries.[153,159,160] As a general rule, amputation and surgical débridement are delayed for 2 to 3 months unless infection with sepsis intervenes. The natural history of a full-thickness frostbite injury is the gradual demarcation of the injured area with dry gangrene or mummification clearly delineating nonviable tissue. Often the permanent tissue loss is much less than originally suspected. In an Alaskan series, only 10.5% of patients required amputation, usually involving only phalanges or portions of phalanges.[141] The need for emergency surgery is unusual, but vigilance should be maintained during the rewarming phase for the development of a compartment syndrome requiring fasciotomy. Open amputations are indicated in patients with persistent infection and sepsis that is refractory to débridement and antibiotics. Mills[161] convincingly demonstrated that of all the factors in the treatment of frostbite that may influence outcome, premature surgical intervention by any means, in any amount, was by far the greatest contributor to poor results.

The use of technetium 99 m methylene diphosphonate bone scanning has shown some promise in the early detection of eventual bone and soft tissue viability,[162] as has the use of magnetic resonance imaging.[163] Technetium 99m "triple-phase" scanning (at 1 minute, 2 hours, and 7 hours) performed beginning 48 hours after admission has been used to assess early tissue perfusion and viability, in an attempt to define the extent of fatally damaged tissues and to allow for early débridement and wound closure.[164,165] The utility of this diagnostic modality continues to evolve, however, with one recent study suggesting that the moderate to severe frostbite lesion identified by technetium 99 m scans can be "hibernating" (viable) tissue, which can show improvement up to 6 months following injury.[153,166]

Frostbitten tissues seldom recover completely. Some degree of cold insensitivity invariably remains. Hyperhidrosis (in up to 72% of patients), neuropathy, decreased nail and hair growth, and a persistent Raynaud's phenomenon in the affected part are frequent sequelae to cold injury.[167] The affected tissue remains at risk for reinjury and should be carefully protected during any cold exposure. As mentioned previously, chilblain (or chronic pernio) is a specific form of a dermopathy secondary to cold-induced skin vasculitis. Treatment with antiadrenergic agents (prazosin hydrochloride, 1 to 2 mg/day) or calcium channel blockers (nifedipine, 30 to 60 mg/day) and careful protection from further exposure is often helpful.[139,167] However, few therapies afford significant relief to the chronic symptoms after tissue freeze injury, although β- and α-adrenergic blocking agents, calcium channel blockers, topical and systemic steroids, and a host of home remedies have been tried with occasional individual success.

KEY POINTS

- **Of 3,000 species of snakes worldwide, only 375 are venomous, with approximately 20 deaths per year in the United States caused by snakebites compared with 100,000 species of Hymenoptera that cause approximately 40 deaths per year, mostly as a result of severe anaphylactic reactions.**
- **Snakebite morbidity is a result of venom composition, time of year, size of snake, and depth and amount of envenomation. Venoms consist of numerous (up to 30 or more) proteins that disrupt endothelial cells and blood flow, produce neuromuscular blockade, or generate a coagulopathy via procoagulants. Coral snake venom also has direct neurotoxins and cardiotoxins.**
- **Snakebite induces immediate pain, edema, and erythema at the site, and spread at greater than 30 cm/hour indicates severe envenomation. Initial incision and suction provides little benefit, as does a proximal tourniquet, which may cause harm. Use of purified ovine antivenin is effective and has replaced equine antivenin with its associated risk of serum sickness.**
- **Most spider bite toxicity is local tissue necrosis caused by brown recluse, hobo, and black widow spiders in the United States. Deaths may be caused by stinging Hymenoptera, including bees (particularly aggressive Africanized bees), fire ants, and scorpions.**
- **Hypothermia risk is high in the severely injured patient as a result of exposure, loss of normal protective metabolism (i.e., shivering), rapid massive infusion of cold fluids/blood, and open thoracic and abdominal cavities.**
- **Loss of protective responses to hypothermia occurs between 33° and 30°C with an initial intensive sympathetic type reaction with tremulousness, profound vasoconstriction, tremendous increases in oxygen consumption and accelerated heart rate and minute ventilation.**
- **Hypothermia affects both blood gases and coagulation parameters with increased pAO_2 and decreased PCO_2, whereas coagulopathy is aggravated as a result of platelet dysfunction and impaired enzyme activity. However, both blood gases and coagulation parameters should be assessed at 37°C because if the arterial blood gas value is normal at 37°C, it will be acceptable at lower temperatures, whereas coagulopathy at 37°C requires blood component therapy separate from warming to correct the cold-induced coagulopathy.**
- **Hypothermia increases risk of mortality at every level of injury. And, although hypothermia delays mortality in experimental shock models, there is no improvement in outcome when applied to the severe TBI, and patients rapidly rewarmed require less resuscitation volume and have improved survival.**
- **Hypothermia is treated either passively by preventing further losses and allowing endogenous rewarming, or actively either externally by use of warm blankets, heating pads, or lights and immersion in warm water or internally by core rewarming, which includes heated intravenous fluids; heated peritoneal, thoracic, gastric, bladder, or colonic lavage; heated moist inhaled air; and extracorporeal circulatory rewarming, preferably using the patient's own circulation (continuous arteriovenous rewarming).**
- **Frostbite involves ice crystal formation and unpredictable loss of tissue. Early definitive rewarming (avoiding refreezing) by submersion in 40° to 42°C water is preferable with subsequent meticulous care, awaiting demarcation and avoidance of early débridement to optimize outcomes and tissue salvage.**

References

1. **Gold BS, Barish RA, Dart RC. North American snake envenomation: diagnosis, treatment, and management. *Emerg Med Clin North Am.* 2004;22(2):423–443.**
2. Russell FE. Medical problems of snakebite: epidemiology. In: Russell FE, ed. *Snake venom poisoning.* Great Neck, NY: Scholium International, 1983:250–258.
3. Litovitz TL, Klein-Schwartz W, White S, et al. Annual report of the American Association of Poison Control Centers Toxic Exposure Surveillance System. *Am J Emerg Med.* 2001;19:337–395.
4. Centers for Disease Control, http://www.cdc.gov. Accessed May 28, 2005.
5. **Gold BS, Dart RC, Barish RA: Bites of venomous snakes. *N Engl J Med.* 2002;347(5):347–356.**
6. Curry SC, Horning D, Brady P, et al. The legitimacy of rattlesnake bites in central Arizona. *Ann Emerg Med.* 1989;18:658–663.
7. Wingert WA, Chan L. Rattlesnake bites in southern California and rationale for recommended treatment. *West J Med.* 1988;148:37–44.
8. Davidson TM. Intravenous rattlesnake envenomation. *West J Med.* 1988;148:37–44.
9. Russell FE. Snake venom poisoning in the United States. *Annu Rev Med.* 1980;31:247–259.
10. Hutton RA, Warrell DA. Action of snake venom components on the haemostatic system. *Blood Rev.* 1993;7:176–189.
11. Arnold R. Treatment of venomous snakebites in the Western Hemisphere. *Mil Med.* 1984;149:361–365.
12. Guisto JA. Severe toxicity from crotalid envenomation after early resolution of symptoms. *Ann Emerg Med.* 1995;26:387–388.
13. Gomez HF, Davis M, Phillips S, et al. Human envenomation from a wandering garter snake. *Ann Emerg Med.* 1994;23:1119–1122.
14. White RR, Weber RA. Discussion of poisonous snakebite in central Texas: possible indicators for antivenin treatment. *Ann Surg.* 1991;213:466–472.
15. Garfin SR, Castilonia RR, Mubarak SJ, et al. Rattlesnake bites and surgical decompression: results using a laboratory model. *Toxicon* 1984; 22:177–184.
16. Downey DJ, Omer GE, Moneim MS. New Mexico rattlesnake bites: demographic review and guidelines for treatment. *J Trauma.* 1991;31: 1380–1386.
17. Glass TJ Jr. Early débridement in pit viper bites. *JAMA* 1976;235: 2513–2516.
18. Nelson BK. Snake envenomation: incidence, clinical presentation, and management. *Med Toxicol.* 1989;4:17–431.
19. Bucher B, Canonge D, Thomas L, et al: Clinical indicators of envenoming and serum levels of venom antigens in patients bitten by Bothrops lanceolatus in Martinique. *Trans R Soc Trop Med Hyg.* 1997;91:186–190.
20. Minton SA. Present tests for detection of snake venom: clinical applications. *Ann Emerg Med.* 1987;16:932–937.
20. McCullough N, Gennaro J. Evaluation of venomous snake bite in southern United States. *J Fla Med Assoc.* 1963;40:959–967.
21. Kunkel DB. Bites of venomous reptiles. *Emerg Med Clin North Am.* 1984;2:563–577.
22. Treatment of snakebite in the United States. *Med Lett.* 1982:87–90.
23. Clark RW. Cryotherapy and corticosteroids in the treatment of rattlesnake bite. *Mil Med.* 1971;136:42–44.
24. Jurkovich GJ, Luterman A, McCullar K, et al. Complications of Crotalidae antivenin therapy. *J Trauma* 1988;28:1032–1037.
25. Cribari C: Management of poisonous snakebites. American College of Surgeons Committee on Trauma Poster, Chicago, Ill., 2004.
26. McCullough N, Gennaro J Jr. Treatment of venomous snake bites in the United States. *Clin Toxicol.* 1970;3:483–500.
27. Wood JT, Hoback WW, Green TW. Treatment of snake venom poisoning with ACTH and cortisone. *Va Med Monthly* 1955; 82:130–135.
28. Dart RC, Hurlbut KM, Garcia RA, Boren JL. Validation of a severity score for the assessment of crotalid snakebite. *Ann Emerg Med.* 1996; 27:321–326.
29. Dart RC, Seifert SA, Boyer LV, et al. A randomized multicenter trial of crotalinae polyvalent immune Fab (ovine) antivenom for the treatment of crotaline snakebite in the United States. *Arch Intern Med.* 2001; 161:2030–2036.
30. Consroe P, Egen NB, Russell FE, et al. Comparison of a new ovine antigen binding fragment (Fab) antivenin for United States Crotalidae with the

commercial antivenin for protection against venom-induced lethality in mice. *Am J Trop Med Hyg.* 1995;53:507–510.
31. Garfin SR, Castilonia RR, Mubarak SJ, et al. The effect of antivenin on intramuscular pressure elevations induced by rattlesnake venom. *Toxicon.* 1985;23:677–680.
33. Garfin SR, Castilonia RR, Mubarak SJ, et al. Rattlesnake bites and surgical decompression: results using a laboratory model. Toxicon 1984; 22:177–182.
32. Curry SC, Kraner JC, Kunkel DB, et al. Noninvasive vascular studies in management of rattlesnake envenomations to extremities. *Ann Emerg Med.* 1985;14:1081–1084.
33. **Chippaux JP, Goyffon M. Venoms, antivenoms, and immunotherapy. *Toxicon.* 1998;36:823–846.**
34. Bornstein AC, Russell, Sullivan JB. Negative pressure suction in field treatment of rattlesnake bite. *Vet Hum Toxicol.* 1985; 25:297–299.
35. Hooker KR, Caravati EM, Hartsell SC. Gila monster envenomation. *Ann Emerg Med.* 1994;24:731–735.
36. Cantrell FL. Envenomation by the Mexican beaded lizard: a case report. *J Toxicol Clin Toxicol.* 2003;41:241–244.
36a. *Wall Street Journal*, April 30, 2005, page B3
37. Giannoukakis N. Exenatide. Amylin/Eli Lilly. *Curr Opin Investig Drugs.* 2003;4:459–465.
38. Preston CA. Hypotension, myocardial infarction, and coagulopathy following Gila monster bite. *J Emerg Med.* 1989;7:37–40.
39. Swanson DL, Vetter RS: Bites of brown recluse spiders and suspected necrotic arachnidism. *N Eng J Med.* 2005;352:700–707.
40. Necrotic arachnidism—Pacific Northwest, 1988–1996. *MMWR Morb Mortal Wkly Rep* 1996;45:433–436.
41. Walker JS, Hogan DE. Bite to the left leg: clinical pearls. *Acad Emerg Med.* 1995;2:223–237.
42. Russell F. A confusion of spiders. *Emerg Med.* 1986;18:8–13.
43. Edlow JA. Lyme disease and related tick-borne illnesses. *Ann Emerg Med.* 1999;33:680–693.
44. Wilson DC, King LE Jr. Spiders and spider bites. *Dermatol Clin.* 1990;8:277–286.
45. Wasserman G. Wound care of spider and snake envenomations. *Ann Emerg Med.* 1988;17:1331–1335.
46. Futrell JM. Loxoscelism. *Am J Med Sci.* 1992;304:261–267.
47. Patel KD, Modur V, Zimmerman GA, et al. The necrotic venom of the brown recluse spider induces dysregulated endothelial cell-dependent neutrophil activation: differential induction of GM-CSF, IL-8, and E-selectin expression. *J Clin Invest* 1994;94:631–642.
48. Ginsberg C, Weinberg A. Hemolytic anemia and mulitorgan failure associated with localized cutaneous lesion. *J Pediatr* 1988;112:496–499.
49. Pennell TC, Babu SS, Meredith JW. The management of snake and spider bites in the southeastern United States. *Am Surg.* 1987;53:198–204.
50. DeLozier JB, Reaves L, King LE, et al. Brown recluse spider bites of the upper extremity. *South Med J.* 1988;81:181–184.
51. Hobbs GD, Anderson AR, Greene TJ, et al. Comparison of hyperbaric oxygen and dapsone therapy for *Loxosceles* envenomation. *Acad Emerg Med.* 1996;3:758–761.
52. Bryant SM, Pittman LM. Dapsone use in *Loxosceles reclusa* envenomations: is there an indication? *Am J Emerg Med.* 2003;21:89–90.
53. Barrett SM, Romine-Jenkins M, Fisher DE. Dapsone or electric shock therapy of brown recluse spider envenomation? *Ann Emerg Med.* 1994;24:21–25.
54. Strain GM, Snider TG, Tedford BL, et al. Hyperbaric oxygen effects on brown recluse spider *(Loxosceles reclusa)* envenomation in rabbits. *Toxicol.* 1991;29:989–996.
55. Phillips S, Kohn M, Baker D, et al. Therapy of brown spider envenomation: a controlled trial of hyperbaric oxygen, dapsone, and cyproheptadine. *Ann Emerg Med.* 1995;25:363–368.
56. Rees R, Altenbern D, Lynch J, et al. Brown recluse spider bites: a comparison of early surgical excision versus dapsone and delayed surgical excision. *Ann Surg.* 1985;202:659–663.
57. Muller GJ. Black and brown widow spider bites in South Africa: a series of 45 cases. *S Afr Med J.* 1993;83:399–405.
58. **Clark RF, Wethern-Kestner S, Vance MV, et al. Clinical presentation and treatment of black widow spider envenomation: a review of 163 cases. *Ann Emerg Med.* 1992;21:782–787.**
59. Suntorntham S, Roberts J, Nilsen G. Dramatic clinical response to the delayed administration of black widow spider antivenin [Letter]. *Ann Emerg Med.* 1994;24:1198–1199.
60. Saucier JR: Arachnid envenomation. *Emerg Med Clin North Am.* 2004; 22:405–422.
61. Freeman TM. Imported fire ants: the ants from hell! *Allergy Proc.* 1994;15:11–15.
62. **Reisman RE. Stinging insect allergy. *Med Clin North Am.* 1992;76: 883–894.**
63. Schumacher M. Significance of Africanized bees for public health: a review. *Arch Intern Med.* 1995;155:2038–2043.
64. Kim KT, Oguro J. Update on the status of Africanized honey bees in the western states., *West J Med.* 1999;170:220–222.
65. Kolecki P. Delayed toxic reaction following massive bee envenomation. *Ann Emerg Med.* 1999;33:114–116.
66. Stafford CT. Fire ant allergy. *Allergy Proc* 1992;13:11–16.
67. Caplan EL, Ford JL, Young PF, Ownby DR: Fire ants represent an important risk for anaphylaxis among residents of an endemic region. *J Allergy Clin Immunol.* 2003;111:1274–1277.
68. Williams DF, deShazo RD. Biological control of fire ants: an update on new techniques. Ann Allergy *Asthma Immunol.* 2004;93:15–22.
69. Bawaskar HS, Bawaskar PH. Cardiovascular manifestations of severe scorpion sting in India (review of 34 children). *Ann Trop Paediatr.* 1991;11:381–387.
70. Yarom R. Scorpion venom: a tutorial review of its effects in man and experimental animals. *Clin Toxicol* 1970;3:561–569.
71. Dudin AA, Rambaud-Cousson A, Thalji A, et al. Scorpion sting in children in the Jerusalem area: a review of 54 cases. *Ann Trop Paediatr.* 1991;11:217–223.
72. Sofer S, Shahak E, Gueron M. Scorpion envenomation and antivenom therapy. *J Pediatr.* 1994;124:973–978.
73. **Jurkovich GJ. Hypothermia in the trauma patient. *Adv Trauma.* 1989;4: 111–140.**
74. Moss J. Accidental severe hypothermia. *Surg Gynecol Obstet.* 1986;162:501–513.
75. Hypothermia-related deaths—United States, 2003–2004. *MMWR Morb Mortal Wkly Rep.* 2005;54(7):173–175.
76. Danzl D, Pozos R, Auerbach P, et al. Multicenter hypothermia survey. *Ann Emerg Med.* 1987;16:1042–1055.
77. Brantigan C, Patton B. Clinical hypothermia, accidental hypothermia, and frostbite. In: Goldsmith H, ed. *Lewis' practice of surgery.* New York: Harper & Row, 1978.
78. Trevino A, Razi B, Beller BM. The characteristic electrocardiogram of accidental hypothermia. *Arch Intern Med.* 1971;127:470–473.
79. Ferguson N. Urban hypothermia. *Anaesthesia* 1985;40:651–654.
80. Hauty MG, Esrig BC, Hill JG, et al. Prognostic factors in severe accidental hypothermia: experience from the Mt. Hood tragedy. *J Trauma* 1987;27:1107–1112.
81. Walpoth BH, Walpoth-Aslan BN, Mattle HP, et al. Outcome of survivors of accidental deep hypothermia and circulatory arrest treated with extracorporeal blood warming. *N Engl J Med.* 1997;337:1500–1505.
82. Silfvast T, Pettila V. Outcome from severe accidental hypothermia in Southern Finland—a 10-year review. *Resuscitation* 2003;59(3):285–290.
83. Cohen DJ, Cline JR, Lepinski SM, et al. Resuscitation of the hypothermic patient. *Am J Emerg Med.* 1988;6:475–478.
84. Ledingham IM, Mone JG. Treatment of accidental hypothermia: a prospective clinical study. *BMJ.* 1980;1:1102–1105.
85. Rahn H, Reeves RB, Howell BJ. Hydrogen ion regulation, temperature, and evolution. *Am Rev Respir Dis.* 1975;112:165–172.
86. Ream AK, Reitz BA, Silverberg G. Temperature correction of $PaCO_2$ and pH in estimating acid-base status: an example of emperor's new clothes? *Anesthesiology* 1982;56:41–44.
87. White FN. A comparative physiologic approach to hypothermia. *J Thorac Cardiovasc Surg,* 1982;82:821–831.
88. Hansen JE, Sue DY. Should blood gas measurements be corrected for the patient's temperature? [Letter]. *N Engl J Med* 1980;303:341.
89. Orlowski JP, Erenberg G, Lüders H, et al. Hypothermia and barbiturate coma for refractory status epilepticus. *Crit Care Med.* 1984;12:367–372.
90. Dobson JA, Burgess JJ. Resuscitation of severe hypothermia by extracorporeal rewarming in a child. *J Trauma.* 1996;40:483–485.
91. Schaller MD, Fischer AP, Perret CH. Hyperkalemia: a prognostic factor during acute severe hypothermia. *JAMA.* 1990;264:1842–1845.
92. Moyer J, Morris GJ, DeBakey M. Effect on renal hemodynamics and excretion of water and electrolytes in dog and man. *Ann Surg.* 1957;145:26.
93. Anderson M, Nielsen K. Renal function under experimental hypothermia in rabbits. *Acta Med Scand.* 1955;151:191.
94. Curry DL, Curry KP. Hypothermia and insulin secretion. *Endocrinology* 1970;87:750–755.
95. Axelrod DR, Bass DE. Electrolytes and acid base balance in hypothermia. *Am J Physiol.* 1956;186:31–34.
96. Haddix TL, Pohlman TH, Noel RF, et al. Hypothermia inhibits human E-selectin transcription. *J Surg Res.* 1996;64:176–182.
97. Kurz A, Sessler DI, Lenhardt R, et al. Perioperative normothermia to reduce the incidence of surgical-wound infection and shorten hospitalization. *N Eng J Med.* 1996;334:1209–1215.
98. Iampietro PF, Vaughan JA, Goldman RF, et al. Heat production from shivering. *J Appl Physiol.* 1960;15:632–634.
99. Pozos R, Wittmers L. *The nature and treatment of hypothermia.* Minneapolis: University of Minnesota Press, 1983.
100. Zwischenberger JB, Kirsh MM, Dechert RE, et al. Suppression of shivering decreases oxygen consumption and improves hemodynamic stability during postoperative rewarming. *Ann Thorac Surg.* 1987;43:428–431.
101. Roe C, Goldberg M, Blair C, et al. The influence of body temperature on early postoperative oxygen consumption. *Surgery* 1966;60:85–92.
102. **Gentilello L. Practical approaches to hypothermia. *Adv Trauma Crit Care.* 1994:39–79.**
103. Paton B. Accidental hypothermia. *Pharmacol Ther.* 1983;22:331–337.
103. Reuler J. Hypothermia: pathophysiology, clinical settings, and management. *Ann Intern Med.* 1978;89:519–527.
104. Gregory J, Townsend M, Cloutier C, et al. Timing and incidence of hypothermia (T < 36°C) in operated trauma patients. Paper presented at

the American Association for the Surgery of Trauma 50th Annual Meeting; 1990; Tucson, AZ.
105. Luna GK, Maier RV, Pavlin EG, et al. Incidence and effect of hypothermia in seriously injured patients. *J Trauma.* 1987;27:1014–1018.
106. Jurkovich GJ, Greiser WB, Luterman A, et al. Hypothermia in trauma victims: an ominous predictor of survival. *J Trauma.* 1987;27:1019–1024.
107. Psarras P, Ivatury R, Rohman M, et al. Hypothermia in trauma: incidence and prognostic significance. Paper presented at the meeting of the Eastern Association for the Surgery of Trauma; 1988; Longboat Key, FL.
108. Rutherford EJ, Fusco MA, Nunn CR, et al. Hypothermia in critically ill trauma patients. *Injury* 1998;29:605–608.
109. Little RA, Stoner HB. Body temperature after accidental injury. *Br J Surg.* 1981;68:221–224.
110. Hardy J, Randini I. Some physiologic aspects of surgical trauma. *Am Surg.* 1952;136:345.
111. Blalock A, Mason M. A comparison of the effects of heat and those of cold in the prevention and treatment of shock. *Arch Surg.* 1945;42:1054–1059.
112. Wu X, Stezoski J, Safar P, et al. After spontaneous hypothermia during hemorrhagic shock, continuing mild hypothermia (34 degrees C) improves early but not late survival in rats. *J Trauma.* 2003; 55(2):308–316.
113. Sori AJ, El-Assuooty A, Rush BF, et al. The effect of temperature on survival in hemorrhagic shock. *Am Surg.* 1987;53:706–710.
114. Alam HB, Bowyer MW, Koustova E, et al. Learning and memory is preserved after induced asanguineous hyperkalemic hypothermic arrest in a swine model of traumatic exsanguination. *Surgery* 2002;132(2): 278–288.
115. Cornejo CJ, Kierney PC, Vedder NB, et al. Mild hypothermia during reperfusion reduces injury following ischemia of the rabbit ear. *Shock* 1998;9:116–120.
116. Jurkovich GL, Pitt RM, Curreri PW, et al. Hypothermia prevents increased capillary permeability following ischemia-reperfusion injury. *J Surg Res.* 1988;44:514–521.
117. Wright J, Kerr J, Valeri C, et al. Regional hypothermia protects against ischemia-reperfusion injury in isolated canine gracilis muscle. *J Trauma.* 1988;28:1027–1031.
118. Childs EW, Udobi KF, Hunter FA. Hypothermia reduces microvascular permeability and reactive oxygen species expression after hemorrhagic shock. *J Trauma.* 2005;58:271–277.
119. Fay T. Observations on generalized refrigeration in cases of severe cerebral trauma. *Assoc Res Nerv Ment Dis Proc.* 1943;24:611–619.
120. Milde LN. Clinical use of mild hypothermia for brain protection: a dream revisited. *J Neurosurg Anesthesiol.* 1992;4:211–215.
121. Clifton GL, Miller ER, Choi SC, et al. Lack of effect of induction of hypothermia after acute brain injury *N Engl J Med.* 2001; 344:556–563.
122. Shiozaki T, Kato A, Taneda M, et al. Little benefit from mild hypothermia therapy for severely head injured patients with low intracranial pressure. *J Neurosurg.* 1999;91:185–191.
123. Gentilello LM, Jurkovich GJ, Stark MS, et al. Is hypothermia in the victim of major trauma protective or harmful? A randomized, prospective study. *Ann Surg.* 1997;226:439–449.
124. Bachmann F, McKenna, Cole ER, et al. The hemostatic mechanism after open heart surgery: I. studies on plasma coagulation factors and fibrinolysis in 512 patients after extracorporeal circulation. *J Thorac Cardiovasc Surg.* 1975;79:76–85.
125. Harker LA, Malpass TW, Branson HE, et al. Mechanism of abnormal bleeding in patients undergoing cardiopulmonary bypass: acquired transient platelet dysfunction associated with selective alpha-granule release. *Blood* 1980;56:824–834.
126. Kattlove HE, Alexander B. The effect of cold on platelets: 1. cold-induced platelet aggregation. *Blood* 1971;38:39–48.
127. Patt A, McCroskey BL, Moore EE. Hypothermia-induced coagulopathies in trauma. *Surg Clin North Am.* 1988;68:775–785.
128. Valeri CR, Feingold H, Cassidy G, et al. Hypothermia induced reversible platelet dysfunction. *Ann Surg.* 1987;205:175–181.
129. Wolberg AS, Meng ZH, Monroe DH III, et al. A systematic evaluation of the effect of temperature on coagulation enzyme activity and platelet function. *J Trauma.* 2004;56:1221–1228.
130. Reed RL II, Bracey AW Jr, Hudson JD, et al. Hypothermia and blood coagulation: dissociation between enzyme activity and clotting factor levels. *Circ Shock.* 1990;32:141–152.
131. Gubler KD, Gentilello LM, Hassantash SE, et al. The impact of hypothermia on dilutional coagulopathy. *J Trauma.* 1994;36:847–851.
132. Gentilello L, Jurkovich G, Moujaes S. Hypothermia and injury: thermodynamic principles of prevention and treatment. In: Levine B, ed. *Perspectives in surgery.* St. Louis: Quality Medical, 1991.
133. Sheaff CM, Fildes JJ, Keogh P, et al. Safety of 65°C intravenous fluid for the treatment of hypothermia. *Am J Surg.* 1996;172:52–55.
134. Herron DM, Grabowy R, Connolly R, et al. The limits of bloodwarming: maximally heating blood with an inline microwave bloodwarmer. *J Trauma.* 1997;43:219–228.
135. Gentilello LM, Cortes V, Moujaes S, et al. Continuous arteriovenous rewarming: experimental results and thermodynamic model simulation of treatment for hypothermia. *J Trauma.* 1990;30:1436–1449.
136. Patton JF, Doolittle WH. Core rewarming by peritoneal dialysis following induced hypothermia in the dog. *J Appl Physiol.* 1972;33:800–804.
137. Gentilello LM, Moujaes S. Treatment of hypothermia in trauma victims: thermodynamic considerations. *J Intensive Care Med.* 1995;10:5–14.
138. Britt LD, Dascombe WH, Rodriguez A. New horizons in management of hypothermia and frostbite injury. *Surg Clin North Am.* 1991;71:345–370.
139. Jacob JR, Weisman MH, Rosenblatt SI, et al. Chronic pernio: a historical perspective of cold-induced vascular disease. *Arch Intern Med.* 1986;146:1589–1592.
140. Benchikhi H, Roujeau JC, Levent M, et al. Chilblains and Raynaud phenomenon are usually not a sign of hereditary protein C and S deficiencies. *Acta Derm Venereol.* 1998;78:351–352.
141. Auerbach P. Disorders due to physical and environmental agents. In: Mills J, et al., eds. *Current Emergency Diagnosis and Treatment.* Los Altos, CA: Lange Medical, 1985.
142. Francis T, Golden FSC. Non-freezing cold injury: the pathogenesis. *J R Nav Med Serv.* 1985;71:3–8.
143. Lloyd E. *Hypothermia and Cold Stress.* Rockville, MD: Aspen Publications, 1986:84–85.
144. Mills WJ Jr. Frostbite: a discussion of the problem and a review of the Alaskan experience. [1973 classical article.] *Alaska Med.* 1993;35:28–49.
145. Urschel JD. Frostbite: predisposing factors and predictors of poor outcome. *J Trauma.* 1990;30:340–342.
146. Dana H, Rex I, Samitz M. The hunting reaction. *Arch Dermatol.* 1969;99:441.
147. Mjurphy JV, Banwell PE, Roberts AH, et al. Frostbite: pathogenesis and treatment. *J Trauma.* 2000; 48:171–178.
148. Ozyazgan I, Tercan M, Melli M, et al. Eicosanoids and inflammatory cells in frostbitten tissue: prostacyclin, thromboxane, polymorphonuclear leukocytes, and mast cells. *Plast Reconstr Surg.* 1998;101:1881–1886.
149. Bourne M, Piepkorn M, Clayton F, et al. Analysis of microvascular changes in frostbite injury. *J Surg Res.* 1986;40:26–35.
150. Zook H, Hussmann J, Brown R, et al. Microcirculatory studies of frostbite injury. *Ann Plast Surg.* 1998;40:246–253.
151. Mileski WJ, Raymond JF, Winn RK, et al. Inhibition of leukocyte adherence and aggregation for treatment of severe cold injury in rabbits. *J Appl Physiol.* 1993;74:1432–1436.
152. Mills WJ Jr, Whaley R. Frostbite: experience with rapid rewarming and ultrasonic therapy: part I and II. [1960 classical article.] *Alaska Med.* 1993;35:6–18.
153. Petrone P, Kuncir EJ, Asensio JA: Surgical management and strategies in the treatment of hypothermia and cold injury. *Emerg Med Clin North Am.* 2003; 21:1165–1178.
154. Heggers J, Robson M, Weingarten M, et al. Experimental and clinical observations on frostbite. *Ann Emerg Med.* 1987;16:1056–1062.
155. Miller MB, Koltai PJ. Treatment of experimental frostbite with pentoxifylline and aloe vera cream. *Arch Otolaryngol Head Neck Surg.* 1995;121:678–680.
156. Rakower S, Shahgoli S, Wong SL. Doppler ultrasound and digital plethysmography to determine the need for sympathetic blockade after frostbite. *J Trauma.* 1978;18:713–718.
157. Bouwman DL, Morrison S, Lucas CE, et al. Early sympathetic blockade for frostbite—is it of value? *J Trauma.* 1980;20:744–749.
158. Purdue G, Hunt J. Cold injury: a collective review. *J Burn Care Rehabil.* 1986;7:331–342.
159. Edlich R, Chang D, Birk K, et al. Cold injuries: comprehensive therapy. *Compr Ther.* 1989;15:13–21.
160. Mills W Jr. Comment and recapitulation. *Alaska Med.* 1993;35:69–87.
161. Mills W Jr. Summary of treatment of the cold injured patient: hypothermia. [1980 classical article.] *Alaska Med.* 1993;35:50–53.
162. Mehta RC, Wilson MA. Frostbite injury: prediction of tissue viability with triple-phase bone scanning. *Radiology* 1989;170:511–514.
163. Barker JR, Haws MJ, Brown RE, et al. Magnetic resonance imaging of severe frostbite injuries. *Ann Plast Surg.* 1997;38:275–279.
164. Greenwald D, Cooper B, Gottlieb L. An algorithm for early aggressive treatment of frostbite with limb salvage directed by triple-phase scanning. *Plast Reconstr Surg.* 1998;102:1069–1074.
165. Cauchy E, Marsigny B, Allamel G, et al. The value of technetium 99 scintigraphy in the prognosis of amputation in severe frostbite injuries of the extremities: A retrospective study of 92 severe frostbite injuries. *J Hand Surg.* 2000;25:969–978.
166. Bhatnagar A, Sarker BB, Sawroop K, et al. Diagnosis, characterisation and evaluation of treatment response of frostbite using pertechnetate scintigraphy: a prospective study. *Eur J Nucl Med Mol Imaging.* 2002; 29:170–175.
167. Rustin M, Newton J, Smith N, et al. The treatment of chilblains with nifedipine: the results of a pilot study, a double-blind placebo-controlled randomized study and a long-term open trial. *Br J Dermatol.* 1989;120:267–275.

CHAPTER 34 ■ TERRORISM

ERIC R. FRYKBERG

THE CHALLENGE

Terrorism is defined as the unlawful exercise of random and ruthless violence against people, usually innocent civilians including women and children, and property to intimidate governments or societies for political or ideological purposes[1] Over the past few decades, terrorist attacks on civilian populations worldwide rank among the most common and most prominent causes of mass casualty disasters. These attacks have increasingly confronted health-care providers with the unique demands of mass casualty management and have demonstrated the importance of developing a basic knowledge and skill set for disaster planning and management within the medical community.

Among the greatest impediments to a successful response to terrorist-related disasters are the complacency and apathy that pervade the mindset of most health-care providers in the United States because of the low probability of these events and the belief that this country is well protected from such attacks. Disaster and mass casualty management has never been included in medical school or residency training. Even though most terrorist attacks involve bodily injury, surgeons in particular have largely abrogated their natural leadership role in disaster planning and management to other nonsurgical specialists and even to nonmedical organizations, agencies, and personnel.[2] The inaccuracy of these perceptions has been repeatedly demonstrated by the suboptimal medical response to such prominent disasters as the 1993 World Trade Center bombing in New York City, the 1995 bombing of the Alfred P. Murrah Federal Building in Oklahoma City, the Centennial Olympics bombing in Atlanta, Georgia, in 1996, and the jetliner attacks on and collapse of the World Trade Center twin towers on September 11, 2001, among many others.[3–6]

The two major goals of most terrorist attacks are maximal casualty generation and maximal lethality.[7] These goals are best achieved by the "weapons of mass destruction" of biological, nuclear or radiologic, incendiary, chemical, and explosive (BNICE) agents. Even the mere threat of these weapons is sufficient in many settings to achieve the public chaos and societal disruption that terrorists seek. It is essential that surgeons be fully prepared to meet these threats by learning the associated history, epidemiology, pathophysiology, and injury patterns, so as to allow appropriate preparation and practice for their medical management.

BIOLOGICAL WEAPONS

The term *biological weapons* as agents of terrorism refers to the deliberate use of microorganisms, or toxins derived from them, to intentionally inflict disease and death on large populations.[8] Biological agents have a number of features that theoretically make them useful weapons. The most prominent such feature is that they can easily be deployed silently and anonymously over wide areas. Their incubation period results in a delayed time interval after initial exposure before the effects, and any suspicion of a terrorist attack, become manifest. A large number of casualties may occur before the medical community is able to initiate containment measures. Also, most biological pathogens are widely available, readily disseminated over large geographic areas, and have a historically proved capability to cause widespread disease and death (i.e., bubonic plague and influenza epidemics). In contrast, only a relatively few pathogens are believed to be suitable for potential use in terrorist attacks, and their development into effective weapons is quite expensive and difficult, which is confirmed by the extreme rarity of their use for this purpose.[9]

There is a long history of the use of biological pathogens as weapons of war and terrorism. The contamination of drinking water with animal carcasses or human feces dates back at least as far as the Roman Empire. In 1346, the corpses of victims of an outbreak of bubonic plague among Tartar invaders of the port city of Caffa (now Feodosiya, Ukraine) on the Black Sea were catapulted into the city, which spread the disease among the Genoese defenders. It is believed that these Genoese carried this disease back to Europe to begin the Black Death epidemic that killed one third of Europe's population. During the French and Indian War in North America, the British caused an outbreak of smallpox among Native Americans by giving them gifts of disease-ridden blankets. In recent decades, countries such as Japan, Iraq, the United States, and the Soviet Union developed large-scale weaponization of anthrax, smallpox, and botulinum toxin.[9–14]

The level of threat of any biological agent for use as a bioterrorist weapon is dependent on four factors: (a) the public health impact, in terms of its virulence, communicability, and susceptibility in exposed populations and its lethality; (b) the ease of production, delivery, and dissemination to large populations; (c) the requirements for surveillance, diagnosis, and stockpiling of treatments and antidotes; (d) the potential for fear, panic, and societal disruption based on public perceptions. The U.S. Centers for Disease Control and Prevention (CDC) have developed three categories of threat of bioterrorist agents (A, B, and C), with the six pathogens in category A posing the greatest risks.[15] Frontline medical providers must be aware of the clinical manifestations and treatment of these six organisms and should have a high index of suspicion for their deliberate use to contain an attack as early as possible.

High-risk Biological Agents

Anthrax is carried by the gram-positive rod *Bacillus anthracis* and is considered the most likely agent to be used in a bioterrorist attack. Its spores can be produced easily in large quantities with little training, they can be stored for many years without loss of potency, they are undetectable by human senses, and they are easily spread in air by such delivery mechanisms as sprayers, bombs, and missiles. Conversely, a relatively high dose of 10,000 to 50,000 spores is necessary to cause infection, and the infection cannot be transmitted from person to person.[16,17] An accidental release of anthrax spores from a Soviet military facility in 1979 led to 66 human deaths within a 4-km radius.[18] One report estimates that an aerosolized release of 100 kg of anthrax spores could result in 130,000 to 3 million deaths in the Washington, D.C. area.[17] Reports conflict as to how easily or cheaply weapons-grade anthrax can be produced, because the most virulent form requires that the anthrax particles be less than 5 microns in size with minimal clumping, which is difficult and expensive to achieve.

The incubation period of anthrax is between 2 and 6 days and manifests in three clinical forms: cutaneous, gastrointestinal, and pulmonary. The cutaneous form is the most common, representing 95% of all reported cases. It occurs naturally, from exposure to infected animals, and has a 20% case fatality rate. The gastrointestinal form results from ingestion of contaminated meat and has a higher mortality rate due to its delayed recognition. It manifests nonspecific symptoms of abdominal pain, fever, nausea, vomiting, and gastrointestinal bleeding and peritonitis. The pulmonary form is the most lethal and is believed to be the most likely form to be used in a terrorist attack from an aerosolized spread. This form is 100% fatal if untreated and 80% fatal if treated after the onset of symptoms. The antibiotics ciprofloxacin and doxycycline are the treatments of choice for both active infection and prophylaxis. Vaccination is considered to be 92% effective when given after exposure.[17]

Botulinum toxin is a highly lethal neurotoxin produced by the organism *Clostridium botulinum*, causing a neuromuscular blockade that leads to respiratory failure. Although most commonly contracted from ingestion of contaminated food, aerosolized forms have been developed that could be especially effective as lethal weapons through inhalation. Standard gas masks provide protection from this agent, and treatment involves supportive care with mechanical ventilation until the effects subside. Antitoxins may shorten the duration of clinical effects, and vaccines are available for high-risk individuals in research and the military.[18]

Bubonic plague and tularemia are bacterial diseases, and smallpox is a virulent viral pathogen; all have a high case fatality rate and an established history of causing millions of deaths. Although bubonic plague and tularemia are usually spread through the bite of infected organisms (i.e., mosquitoes, fleas) and smallpox is spread by contact with infected body fluids, all can be effectively transmitted by aerosolized airborne dissemination. Bubonic plague and tularemia are treated with streptomycin as the antibiotic of choice. Vaccination is the only effective measure against smallpox and must be administered as soon as possible after exposure to prevent or minimize its consequences.[17,19–21]

Viral hemorrhagic fever is a clinical syndrome that manifests symptoms of fever, myalgias, headaches, and malaise in association with evidence of neurovascular collapse (shock, mucus membrane hemorrhages). Viral hemorrhagic fever is caused by the four major viral groups of filoviruses (Ebola and Marburg), arenaviruses (Lassa fever), bunyaviruses (Rift Valley fever), and flaviviruses (yellow fever and dengue). Filoviruses are considered bioterrorist threats because of their ability to infect via aerosolized dissemination, their ease of replication in culture for large-scale production, and their virulence, with mortality rates ranging up to 90%. Treatment is supportive, and contact and droplet precautions are generally adequate for infection control. Antiviral drugs have shown some promise, and a vaccine is available only for yellow fever.[22]

CHEMICAL WEAPONS

Toxic chemicals have a proven capability to cause widespread morbidity, mortality, and societal disruption among large populations and thus pose a major threat as terrorist weapons. Their deadly effects could be imparted through inhalation of aerosolized and gaseous agents, ingestion of contaminated foods, and direct contact with the skin, mucus membranes, and eyes (Table 34.1).

Poison gases have been used extensively in warfare, especially in the 20th century. In World War I, about 4% of all casualties (about one million people) were caused by these agents, which included 26% of all American casualties.[23] The worst chemical disaster in history involved the accidental release of 40 tons of methyl isocyanate gas in Bhopal, India in 1984, resulting in 2,500 deaths and an additional 200,000 casualties.[24] These devastating results demonstrate how effective these agents could be in the hands of terrorists. The bomb that exploded in the World Trade Center in New York City in 1993 contained enough cyanide to contaminate the entire building, but it was destroyed by the blast.[25] In 1995, the gaseous release of the nerve agent sarin in the Tokyo subway system caused 12 deaths and 5,000 injuries, representing the first terrorist use of this agent on a civilian population.[26]

The initial phase of response to intentional chemical attacks such as biological and radiologic attacks, is known as *consequence detection*. Early detection is essential if casualties and death are to be minimized and can occur from either the discovery of the source of environmental release or exposure or the diagnosis of the afflicted casualties. Patterns of large numbers of patients with similar symptom clusters must be recognized, which requires a knowledge of the classic symptoms of chemical poisoning, including coughing and choking, dry mouth and mucus membranes, seizures, eye irritation, and the cholinergic symptoms described by the mnemonic DUMBBELS (diarrhea, urination, miosis, bronchospasm, bronchorrhea, emesis, lacrimation, and salivation).

TABLE 34.1

CHEMICAL AGENTS THAT POSE A THREAT AS TERRORIST WEAPONS

Category	Agents	Treatment/antidote
Pulmonary irritants	Phosgene, chlorine, ammonia, mace	Decontamination, water cleansing, bronchodilators, mechanical ventilation
Incapacitating agents (anticholinergics)	Benzene	Intravenous hydration, physostigmine
Vesicants (blistering agents)	Mustard, lewisite, phosgene oxime	Decontamination, hypochlorite, dimercaprol
Nerve agents	Tabun, sarin, soman, *VX*	Atropine, 2-Pam, diazepam, airway control, decontamination
Blood agents	Cyanide	Decontamination, hyperbaric oxygen, amyl nitrite

The response phase that involves organization and cleanup of the disaster scene and medical and psychological treatment of the casualties is termed *consequence management.* The identified source of contamination and exposure must be neutralized to prevent further damage. Health-care workers must wear personal protective equipment to prevent their exposure to hazardous materials (HAZMAT), including the prevention of inhalation of toxic fumes from offgassing that may emanate from the tissues of afflicted victims. Triage and decontamination of casualties must be established outside the hospital, and away from the disaster scene, to prevent health-care providers and hospital facilities from being contaminated and rendered useless for further treatment of casualties. All casualties must undergo decontamination as early as possible to minimize adverse effects. Simply removing their clothing and showering with soap and water removes more than 90% of all contaminating agents, a process known as *gross decontamination.* The more intensive *technical decontamination* then follows for specific forms of exposure, such as hypochlorite solutions for mustard agents, and copious eye irrigation with saline solution. Poison control centers, public health officials, pharmacologists, and toxicologists are important resources and personnel who should be involved in the planning and management of chemical terrorist disasters.

NUCLEAR/RADIOLOGIC WEAPONS

Dispersal of radioactive substances poses a significant potential for a terrorist attack because of the theoretical damage that could be inflicted on large populations, although such a deliberate attack on civilian populations has never occurred outside of war. These agents also carry the potential of widespread psychosocial effects and panic caused by the mystique that is associated with radiation among the general population. The dangers of these agents are largely overestimated, however, and result from poor understanding of radiation biology. These misperceptions are as common among health-care providers as among the lay public and represent a major barrier to effective management. In fact, major radiation exposure from a terrorist attack should be easier to manage than biological or chemical events because of easy detection methods with Geiger counters and dose-rate meters; the large number of hospital, industrial, and government personnel who regularly deal with radiation; and the well-known clinical effects that can be monitored with simple laboratory tests.[27,28]

Ionizing radiation causes damage to living cells and tissues from its direct energy as well as from the indirect effects of the unstable and toxic hyperoxide molecules it creates. Gamma rays and X-rays (called *wave radiation*) in addition to neutron particles have high tissue penetrance and cause the greatest tissue damage, especially to rapidly dividing cells (gastrointestinal tract and bone marrow). Alpha (helium nuclei) and beta (electrons) particle radiation have low tissue penetrance and damage potential, are easily shielded, and cause damage only if ingested or if they gain access through open wounds. The major factors that determine the severity of radiation exposure are time, distance, and shielding. The absorbed radiation dose rapidly decreases with shortened duration of exposure and with the square of the distance from the source, so that quadrupling the distance reduces the dose-rate to one-sixteenth of the original exposure.[29]

In doses of less than 1 Gy (1 Gy = 100 rads) the effects are not clinically significant, although long-term malignant transformation is always possible. The handling of highly radioactive sources or fallout of radioactive dust from alpha or beta particles results in local skin exposure with thermal burns that are characterized by erythema, desquamation, and blistering. Treatment of these low levels of exposure includes prophylactic antibiotics and standard burn wound care. The effects of whole-body exposure from highly penetrating wave and particle sources (gamma rays, X-rays, and neutrons) are dose and duration dependent. Nausea, vomiting, diarrhea, and blood cell count depression (termed *acute radiation syndrome*) begin at doses greater than 1.0 Gy. A dose of 10 Gy is considered to be the highest survivable dose if maximal medical therapy is provided. Symptoms develop in less than 5 minutes following doses greater than 10 Gy, and doses greater than 30 Gy inevitably lead to death from cardiovascular and nervous system collapse in 24 to 72 hours.[30]

The two major forms that a nuclear or radiologic terrorist attack could take are the dispersal of radioactive materials that are commonly used in industry and medicine (i.e., cobalt-60, cesium-137, iridium-192, iodine-131), most likely using conventional explosives (*dirty bombs*), and the atmospheric release of large amounts of intense ionizing radiation through the sabotage of nuclear power plants or the detonation of nuclear bombs. Dirty bombs are easy to construct with little training. They could spread contamination over a few city blocks at most and cause bodily injuries from the blast as well as fear and panic in the population. Property damage and radiation exposure are unlikely to be extensive, and the relatively small area of contamination should be easily monitored and contained for long-term cleanup. In contrast, nuclear sabotage and explosions require significant technical expertise and money to develop and execute and are therefore considered relatively unlikely to be used by terrorists. However, they threaten substantial property destruction as well as injury and death to people over a range of hundreds of miles because of the physical effects of the blast, the thermal and blinding effects of the ensuing fireball, and the high levels of ionizing radiation thrown into the atmosphere.[29]

The appropriate medical care of casualties from a radiologic incident first requires an understanding of the distinction between radiation *exposure* and radiologic *contamination.* Exposure to ionizing radiation results in damage to body tissues, and the clinical manifestations of the victim and their timing provides a reliable guide to their absorbed dose. Exposure alone does not make a casualty "radioactive," does not require decontamination, and offers no danger whatever to medical providers. *Contamination* refers to radioactive material that is found on the clothing or body of a victim, which can be spread to medical providers and the environment and requires decontamination to reduce such spread. Treatment of these casualties is largely supportive, involving the management of the skin, gastrointestinal, and hematopoietic signs and symptoms, after removing them from the source. Internal contamination through inhalation, ingestion, or skin or open wound absorption is treated by minimizing absorption and through the use of dilution, blockage, displacement, stimulation of renal and gastrointestinal elimination, and chelation methods. Most of these approaches are largely unproved and ineffective, including bone marrow transplantation or stem cell augmentation, or they have some beneficial effect only against specific radioisotopes. There is no "antiradiation" drug or agent. Potassium iodide does effectively block thyroid uptake of radioactive iodine, but this isotope is found only after nuclear explosions or nuclear plant leaks. Also, potassium iodide is effective only if given within 4 hours of exposure and is of benefit only in children.[28,31]

External contamination of clothing and exposed skin is easily managed by simply removing clothing and showering with water and detergent, which should remove more than 90% of the contamination. Technical decontamination can then follow with removal or intensive cleansing of all hair and through scrubbing of the body, guided by the use of radiation dose meters to detect residual radiation. All clothing and fluid runoff is bagged and carefully disposed of to control the spread of radioactive materials. Open contaminated wounds must be washed and débrided according to standard aseptic principles, and wound excision should be considered for contamination with long-lived radionuclides (e.g., alpha-emitters). After whole-body exposure of greater than 1.0 Gy, open wounds should be closed as soon as possible to prevent them from becoming portals of entry for lethal internal contamination. External radiologic contamination does not constitute a medical emergency for either victims or medical providers. It is best to consider radioactive contamination as nothing more than dirt, something that is preferably cleaned off before treatment or hospitalization but that should *not* cause any delay in treatment of life-threatening injuries or the withholding of appropriate medical care for fear of exposure. Life-threatening injuries that require urgent medical management should not await extensive decontamination, although removal of clothing and a quick shower can usually be accommodated. Medical personnel and hospital facilities will not be overexposed even with the highest levels of exposure and contamination of casualties and personnel should simply wear protective clothing and gloves in accordance with standard universal precautions.[27–30,32]

The overall response to a radiologic or nuclear disaster should include proper planning and preparation, training of personnel, and on-scene triage and evacuation of casualties on the assumption of hazardous internal exposure. Triage officers must be familiar with the clinical effects and treatment of radiation injury.[33] National government resources should be contacted for guidance on the recognition and management of radiation exposure.[28] Severely injured casualties with radiation exposure should be triaged for definitive care to different facilities from those who are not seriously injured, and all possible measures to contain further contamination should be undertaken. Medical personnel should wear standard protective gear and treat all emergent medical and surgical problems without consideration of the radioactive contamination and exposure. Resources and procedures for dealing with the stress and psychosocial effects that are inevitably associated with radiologic incidents, in both casualties and medical providers, should be in place.

EXPLOSIVE WEAPONS

Explosive attacks by terrorists have typically been characterized among conventional weapons, but the magnitude of energy that terrorist bombings have achieved over the past three decades and the thousands of resulting casualties make it clear that these agents belong as much in the category of unconventional weapons of mass destruction as those discussed previously. Furthermore, explosive devices have historically been and currently are the most common weapons of terrorism by far and therefore remain overwhelmingly the most prominent and most likely threat for which civilian populations must be prepared in the future. This has important implications for the role of surgeons in disaster planning and management because the casualties of explosive disasters will be afflicted predominantly with traumatic injuries for which surgical expertise and support are necessary. The technology required for large-scale casualty generation and lethality with this mechanism is easily learned, and its cost effectiveness is unsurpassed by any other method.[34,35] These factors have resulted in a dramatic worldwide increase in frequency of these incidents with each passing year (Table 34.2).[7]

Historical Perspective

An analysis of two major accidental explosions of the 20th century serves to demonstrate the devastation of civilian populations that can result from large-magnitude explosive agents and provides important lessons in the planning for and prevention of their disastrous consequences. On December 6, 1917, in Halifax harbor, Nova Scotia, the Belgian ship *Imo* collided with the French munitions ship *Mont Blanc*, causing a fire on the top deck of *Mont Blanc* from the ignition of 35 tons of benzene. Hundreds of first-responder city firefighters and civilian onlookers then flocked to the scene. After 15 minutes, the fire ignited a cargo below decks consisting of 2,300 tons of picric acid, 10 tons of gun cotton, 300 rounds of ammunition, and 200 tons of trinitrotoluene (TNT). The ensuing explosion, the largest non-nuclear manmade explosion ever to occur, was followed by a 150-foot tidal wave,

TABLE 34.2

PROMINENT TERRORIST BOMBINGS WORLDWIDE

Event	Year(s)	Explosive agent (*building collapse)
Irish Republican Army bombings, U.K.	1970s	TNT, dynamite
Bologna train terminal	1980	TNT
Beirut Airport	1983	Ammonium nitrate(*)
Paris bombings	1986	TNT
World Trade Center, NY	1993	Ammonium nitrate
AMIA building, Buenos Aires	1994	Ammonium nitrate(*)
Oklahoma City	1995	Ammonium nitrate(*)
Atlanta Olympics	1996	TNT
U.S. Embassies, Africa	1998	TNT(*)
USS Cole, Yemen	2000	TNT
World Trade Center, NY; Pentagon, VA	2001	Jet air liner crashes (*)
Israel suicide bombings	2001–Present	TNT, C-4
U.N. Baghdad headquarters	2003	Ammonium nitrate(*)
Madrid train terminals, Spain	2004	TNT

which leveled more than 2.5 square km of the city, blew the ship 1 mile high and vaporized it, threw its 1,100 pound anchor 2 miles away and a cannon 3.5 miles away, shattered windows 100 km away, and wiped out the hundreds of initially responding citizens and firefighters. There were 2,000 deaths, 9,000 injured, and more than 20,000 left homeless in a city of only 50,000 population.[36]

In the port of Texas City, TX, on April 16, 1947, the freighter *Grand Camp* caught fire, again attracting the entire city's firefighters and hundreds of onlookers. Its cargo of several tons of ammonium nitrate fertilizer was ignited 20 minutes later, creating an explosion with a 2,000-foot high smoke plume and hurling the ship's anchor 2 miles away. A second more powerful blast occurred a short time later, causing widespread fires and a 150-foot tidal wave. This disaster resulted in 600 deaths in a city of only 16,000 population, including, again, the city's entire fire department and dozens of citizens initially attracted to the fire.[37]

These disasters demonstrate how devastating explosions can be and how effectively they can achieve the terrorist aims of casualty generation and lethality with relatively little cost or training. In Texas City, simple ammonium nitrate fertilizer caused one of the largest manmade explosions ever. It is quite likely that terrorists have studied these and similar events. With the ever-increasing use of bombings as instruments of terror in subsequent years, it is clear that lessons learned from these accidental disasters have been used. Ammonium nitrate–based fuel-air explosives have been used in several major terrorist attacks to generate explosions of great magnitude (see Table 34.2). Another effective and commonly used technique in terrorist bombings has been the "second hit," so well demonstrated in both Halifax and Texas City, in which an initial event draws in onlookers and first responders, who are then wiped out by a second deliberate event—another explosion, sniper fire, or a building collapse.[6,35,38 39] In this way, to further expand injury, death, and panic among their target population, terrorists exploit the natural and predictable urge of people to help others. This second hit phenomenon is best combated by restricting access to any disaster scene, especially to medical personnel who have no training to manage that scene, whose help and skills are best used in the protected and resource-rich environment of hospitals, and whose deaths will further and needlessly magnify the risk to surviving casualties. The noble but emotional, ego-driven, and misguided urge to run to a scene to "help" must be restrained by a disciplined and rational analysis of how help can best be delivered.

Terrorist bombings increased dramatically in the 20th century, with 5,075 such events documented worldwide between 1973 and 1983, causing 3,689 deaths and 7,991 injuries. There was a tenfold increase in these incidents between 1968 and 1980 as their success became evident.[40] In the United States alone, 12,216 terrorist bombings occurred between 1980 and 1990, with 1,582 bombings causing 222 injuries and 27 deaths occurring in 1990 alone.[41] From 1988 to 1997, the number of actual and attempted terrorist bombings increased by 127% within the United States, with 17,579 incidents causing 4,063 injuries and 427 deaths.[42] Since then, major bombings of U.S. embassies in Tanzania and Kenya in 1998, the USS *Cole* in Yemen in 2000, the jet airliner crashes into the World Trade Center and Pentagon in 2001, and the Madrid train terminal bombings in 2004, as well as the ongoing suicide bombings in Israel and Iraq have shown that explosive weapons remain the most likely threat that must be confronted by surgeons in coming years. Analysis of these many events, and an understanding of the pathophysiology of blast, provide a valuable insight into the patterns of injury around which planning and management can be formulated.

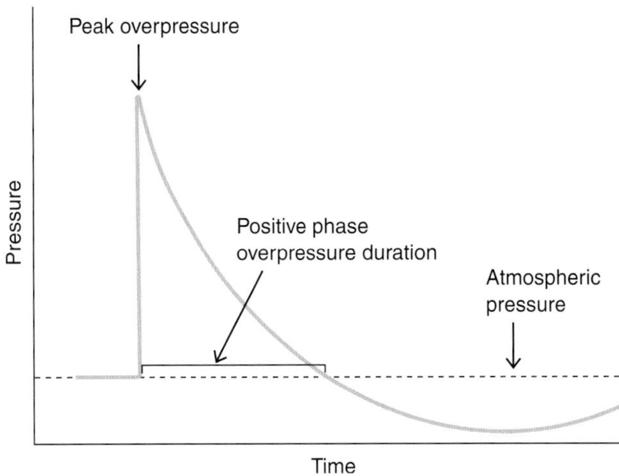

FIGURE 34.1 Graph of the pressure characteristics of a blast wave over time.

Biodynamics of Blast

Terrorist bombings typically employ high-energy detonations that generate a pressure pulse wave, called a *blast wave*, which travels through air at supersonic speeds. The edge of this radially propagating wave is known as the *blast front*. Immediately following detonation, a *peak overpressure* phase, lasting only a fraction of a second, involves the sudden rise of air pressure far above ambient levels. This instantaneous rise in pressure imparts to the blast wave the characteristic of *brisance*, or shattering ability. The peak overpressure is followed by a more gradual ebbing of pressure lasting up to ten times longer, which ends in a negative pressure phase into which air and debris can be sucked (Fig. 34.1). This negative pressure phase accounts for the implosion of some surrounding structures, as well as the creation of tidal waves in coastal areas, as happened after both the Halifax and Texas City explosions. The term *blast wind* refers to these rapid back-and-forth movements of air. Underwater blasts are generally three times more powerful in blast wave propagation than those in air because of the greater density of water.[43–45]

The four factors that determine the force of a blast and the severity of injuries it causes are the size of the explosive charge, the distance from the blast, indoor or outdoor location, and the surrounding medium of air or water. The magnitude of an air blast tends to dissipate rapidly according to the cube of the distance from the blast, so that moving three times the distance away reduces the energy by 27-fold. Indoor detonations cause the blast energy to be magnified rather than dissipated as the blast wave is reflected off walls, floors, and ceilings, causing greater damage than open air blasts. This magnification explains why terrorists seek to detonate bombs in confined spaces, such as in buses in Israel, rather than open air.[46,47]

The medical management of casualties of terrorist bombings requires an understanding of the three categories of injury that result from explosions. Primary blast injury is caused by the passage of the blast wave through the body, which causes a disruptive turbulence, called *spalling*, in the tissues of organs with air-to-liquid interfaces, such as the lung, bowels, eyes, and ears. For this reason, tympanic membrane rupture is quite common among casualties of explosive events and should be viewed as a sensitive marker for more severe internal effects of primary blast injury.[48] The lung is the most common visceral organ damaged in air blasts, whereas bowel disruption is found primarily in underwater blasts. Most victims of primary

TABLE 34.3

IMPACT OF BUILDING COLLAPSE ON THE OUTCOME OF THE 1995 TERRORIST BOMBING IN OKLAHOMA CITY, OK[a]

Casualty location	No. casualties	No. dead	No. survivors	No. survivors hospitalized
Collapsed	175	153 (87%)	22	18 (82%)
Uncollapsed	186	10 (5%)	176	32 (18%)
Total	361	163 (45%)	168	50 (25%)

[a]Includes only 361 casualties inside the Alfred P. Murrah Federal Building stratified by portion of building in which they were located.
Adapted with permission from Mallonee S, Shariat S, Stennies G, et al. Physical injuries and fatalities resulting from the Oklahoma City bombing, *JAMA* 1996;276:382–387.

blast lung injury die immediately because such injuries require that they be so close to the blast that they suffer lethal bodily harm. Only 0.6% of survivors of major terrorist bombings have been found to have blast lung injury, but more than 10% of these victims ultimately die, indicating that this injury should also be considered a marker of severity that requires urgent treatment.[34] Blast lung is characterized by progressive pulmonary insufficiency, with radiologic and pathologic findings typical of blunt pulmonary contusion. Death is caused by cerebral and coronary air embolism.[43,49] A higher incidence of blast lung injury is found among survivors of urban bombings as compared with bombings in rural and isolated locales as a result of the rapid triage and transport of victims and abundant medical resources available in larger cities.[50]

Secondary blast injury is caused by the impact on the body of flying objects and debris set in motion by the blast. Tertiary blast injury involves the displacement of the victim's body to impact other objects. Both of these forms of blast injury cause the standard forms of blunt trauma that predominate among survivors of terrorist bombings and that surgeons typically manage in routine practice.[45,46,49,51] Secondary blast injury has also increasingly included penetrating trauma from destructive shrapnel placed in the bombs, as well as from body parts of suicide bombers that become embedded in the victim.[5,52,53] An especially bizarre implication of these latter injuries to both casualties and medical care providers is that the embedded terrorist body parts have been shown to carry chronic diseases, such as hepatitis and AIDS, that are transmitted to surviving casualties and serve to further magnify the level of injury and terror.[54]

Quaternary, or miscellaneous, blast injuries are indirect consequences of explosive events, including burns, crush injuries from falling debris or structural collapse, inhalational injuries from dust and toxic chemicals, penetrating wounds from shrapnel placed in the bomb, and ocular injuries. The dissemination of biological, chemical, and radiologic agents in dirty bombs falls into this category and is also called *combined blast injury*.[2]

Patterns of Injury, Severity, and Mortality

Terrorist bombings result in consistent and predictable patterns of injury and mortality in all published reports.[3,34,35,51,55] The incidence of immediate deaths and critical injuries among survivors is related to the magnitude of the explosion, whether it occurs indoors or outdoors or in urban or isolated locales, and the association with building collapse. By exploding a bomb within a large building, the probability of complete structural collapse is increased, which greatly magnifies the casualty generation and lethality beyond the blast itself. This magnification is another reason why terrorists seek to place explosives in buildings. In the suicide bombing of the U.S. Marine barracks in Beirut, Lebanon, in 1983, with an ammonium nitrate fuel-air explosive imparting an estimated explosive force of 6 tons of TNT, the complete collapse of the four-story building resulted in the immediate death of 68% of all 346 casualties.[56] A terrorist bombing in Buenos Aires, Argentina, in 1994, caused the complete collapse of a seven-story building, resulting in the immediate death of 29% of all casualties but of 94% of casualties within the building.[55] In the 1995 bombing in Oklahoma City, the partial collapse of the nine-story Alfred P. Murrah Federal Building, also caused by an ammonium nitrate bomb constructed as a fuel-air explosive imparting a 2-ton TNT equivalent blast force,[3] resulted in significantly greater injury and death among victims in the collapsed portion of the building (Table 34.3). This is remarkably different from the 3.3% immediate death rate among the 574 casualties of the Khobar Towers bombing in Saudi Arabia in 1996, in which there was no building collapse.[57] These observations emphasize the preventive value of both barricading major buildings to prevent vehicular access and improving structural design of buildings to withstand major blasts without collapsing.

Most survivors of terrorist bombings are not critically injured. Generally only 10% to 20% of survivors require urgent treatment for severe injuries, a pattern that is typical of most mass casualty disasters from any mechanism. The most common injuries found in immediate fatalities involve the head, chest, abdomen, blast lung, and traumatic amputation. These same severe injuries are found in only a small minority of survivors (0.5% to 2%) but contribute to a disproportionately high mortality among those survivors (10% to 50%) and therefore must be considered important markers of severity that require urgent attention. The great majority of survivors have noncritical soft tissue and skeletal injuries, for which care may be delayed for hours or days if necessary to maximize casualty flow and the immediate care of critical injuries.[3,5,6,34,35,57,58]

TRIAGE

The prioritizing of patients according to injury severity, their need for immediate care, and available resources is called *triage*. In societies and geographic areas with an abundance of medical resources, such as the United States, triage is seldom necessary or practical because all injured individuals are brought to hospitals and provided with maximal care. In true mass-casualty disasters, however, such as those resulting from terrorism, triage must assume major importance on the part of medical providers because of the limited resources available to the large casualty numbers. The difficulty of triage in this setting lies in the need to rapidly identify that small minority of critically injured casualties who require immediate care among the large majority of casualties who have noncritical injuries, but who tend to rapidly inundate medical facilities. Although this rationing of care, and the possibility of denying care to some victims because of limited resources, is antithetical to current medical training and moral values, it may nonetheless be essential to maximize casualty survival. Disaster triage thus requires a paradigm change in mindset and approach to medical care, which in turn mandates that medical providers be educated in these principles that are so different from the routine approach to medical care.[35] The goal of management must shift from the greatest good for each individual to the greatest good for the greatest number, with the population taking priority over the individual. Triage officers not only must be experienced in the care of those injuries expected in any form of disaster (i.e., trauma in explosive events), but also must understand how to assess and treat these injuries within the unique context of mass casualties.

The five categories of triage that are generally accepted are immediate, delayed, minimal or walking wounded, expectant, and dead. In the first triage performed at a disaster scene, the only decision made is that of who needs immediate care and hospital transport and who does not.[39] As secondary and tertiary triage is performed later, more discrimination can be applied. The expectant category includes those casualties with such severe and extensive injuries that more time and resources would be required than is justified by the limited resources, which can better be applied to more salvageable victims. This category best illustrates the change in mindset required in mass casualty management and why special training and experience are needed to serve in the role of triage officer. A physician may be appropriate for this role, but any healthcare provider could fulfill this role with the proper training. In fact, physicians may be too scarce and valuable a resource to spare for this duty.[59] Exactly what constitutes an expectant casualty must be decided early in each disaster and cannot be predicted because the definition depends on the specific types of injuries, casualty numbers, and what resources are available.

The accuracy of triage could certainly affect the ultimate outcome of surviving casualties. Improper assignment to a delayed category of critically ill or injured casualties who require urgent care, termed *undertriage,* is the most important to avoid and imparts an obvious potential for preventable death in all settings. The term *overtriage* describes the assignment of noncritical casualties to immediate care. In the routine management of trauma patients, with small numbers arriving at any given time, overtriage is an economic, logistical, and administrative burden that does not affect casualty outcome and is considered necessary to minimize undertriage.[60] However, the published results of 10 major mass casualty disasters from terrorist bombings that relate the overtriage rate to the mortality among critically injured survivors (Table 34.4) confirms a direct impact of overtriage on the *critical mortality rate* in this setting (Fig. 34.2).[3,45,51,55,56,61–65] This impact occurs because the inundation of a hospital with large numbers of casualties all at once, most of whom are not critically injured, impedes the ability of medical personnel to rapidly detect that small minority who require immediate care, thus increasing the risk of preventable deaths.[35] It is reasonable to postulate that this principle probably applies to all mass casualty events of any mechanism and emphasizes the importance of accurate triage discrimination in these events to minimize both overtriage and undertriage.

TRAUMA

TABLE 34.4

RELATION OF OVERTRIAGE TO CRITICAL MORTALITY IN TERRORIST BOMBING SURVIVORS

Event	Year	No. survivors	No. critically injured (%)[a]	No. overtriage (%)[b]	No. critical mortality (%)[c]
Cu Chi, Vietnam [65]	1969	34	3 (9)	9 (75)	1 (33)
Craigavon, Northern Ireland[64]	1970's	339	113 (33)	29 (20)	5 (4)
Old Bailey, London, U.K.[61]	1973	160	4 (2.5)	15 (79)	1 (25)
Guildford pubs, U.K.[45]	1974	64	22 (34)	2 (8.3)	0
Birmingham, U.K.[63]	1974	119	9 (8)	12 (57)	2 (22)
Tower of London, U.K.[62]	1974	37	10 (27)	9 (47)	1 (10)
Bologna train station, Italy[51]	1980	218	48 (22)	133 (73.5)	11 (23)
Beirut, Lebanon[56]	1983	112	19 (17)	77 (80)	7 (37)
AMIA building, Buenos Aires, Argentina[55]	1994	200	14 (7)	47 (56)	4 (29)
Oklahoma City, OK[3]	1995	597	52 (9)	31 (37)	5 (10)
Total		**1880**	**294 (16)**	**364 (53)**	**37 (12.6)**

[a]Percentage of total survivors.
[b]Number of noncritical survivors triaged to immediate care as a percentage of all casualties triaged to immediate care.
[c]Number and percentage of all critically injured survivors who died.
Adapted with permission from Frykberg, ER. Medical management of disasters and mass casualties from terrorist bombings: How can we cope? *J Trauma* 2002;53:201–212.

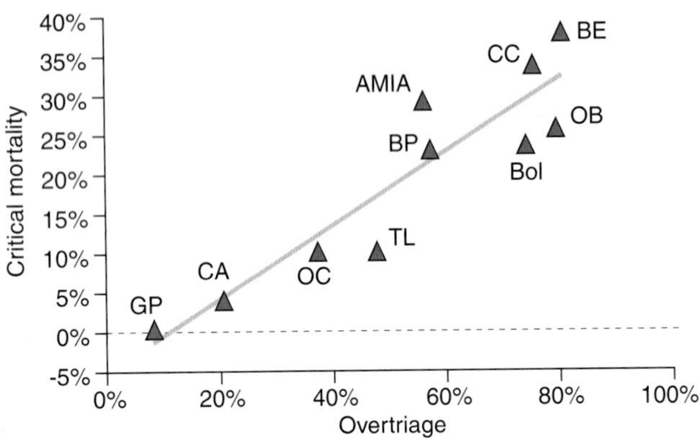

FIGURE 34.2 Relationship of overtriage to critical mortality rate in survivors of major terrorist bombings, from data in Table 34.4 (r = 0.92). GP, Guildford pubs U.K.; CA, Craigavon, Northern Ireland; OC, Alfred P. Murrah Federal Building, Oklahoma City, OK, U.S.; TL, Tower of London, U.K.; BP, Birmingham pubs, U.K.; AMIA building, Buenos Aires, Argentina; Bol, Bologna train terminal, Italy; OB, Old Bailey, London, U.K.; CC, Cu Chi, Vietnam; BE, Beirut airport, Lebanon. (After Frykberg, ER. Medical management of disasters and mass casualties from terrorist bombings: How can we cope? *J Trauma* 2002;53:201–12.)

PLANNING AND REPORTING

Advance preparations are immensely important for the success of any disaster response because disasters are completely random, unexpected, and unpredictable. However, their magnitude requires a rapid, organized, and comprehensive response involving a number of disparate elements that do not usually work together and a medical approach that is quite different from routine patient care. Such a response cannot occur without plans in place that have been extensively rehearsed.

Disasters are rare events, requiring that planning be based on the abundant literature that documents experience from past disasters. Although every disaster is different in several specific factors, consistent patterns have clearly been established that are common to most disasters, allowing for realistic planning. Every plan must also have a built-in flexibility to allow adaptation to unique contingencies of a specific event. Terrorist bombings, in view of their frequency, should be considered as the universal model for disaster management, and planning can be based on the well-established patterns of injury and mortality previously described. It is possible to anticipate resource needs and distribution from knowledge of the prognostic factors of these events that can be gleaned from the literature (Table 34.5).[35]

TABLE 34.5

PROGNOSTIC FACTORS THAT AFFECT THE CASUALTY OUTCOME FOR TERRORIST BOMBINGS

Magnitude of explosion
Triage accuracy
Time interval to treatment
Anatomic injuries
Location
Confined space vs. open air
Rural vs urban
Building collapse
Immediate presence of surgical capability

The Incident Command System has been widely adopted as the best organizational and functional scheme for a comprehensive and successful disaster response. The five major components of this system are command, planning, logistics, operations, and finance/administration (Fig. 34.3). This integration of resources into a unified command has been shown to avoid the major barriers and to promote the most effective interaction of the several components of a disaster response.[66,67]

It is essential that surgeons be integrally involved in disaster planning and management by participating in their local hospital disaster committee, their hospital disaster drills, and community disaster exercises. The care of trauma patients and rapid decision making for large numbers of patients are what surgeons are trained to do and what they regularly practice. In fact, U.S. trauma centers and the nationwide trauma systems should logically serve as the template for a national disaster response system in view of their extensive resources, collective expertise, and already established liaisons with most of the elements necessary in a disaster response (i.e., prehospital assets, search and rescue, air medical transport, law enforcement, fire services, public health, media, local and state government health services).[68–70] It is also important that the results of a disaster be analyzed and reported in the surgical literature as the only means by which healthcare providers can be educated. This analysis also allows a postevent debriefing on the part of those involved in a disaster, which should result in a revision of the disaster plan to correct any deficiencies identified. These goals all require that an effective method of record keeping be in place to allow patient tracking and data accumulation during the disaster, from which a comprehensive analysis of results can be derived. A successful disaster response can be achieved only through intensive education, research, self-analysis, reassessment, and practice.

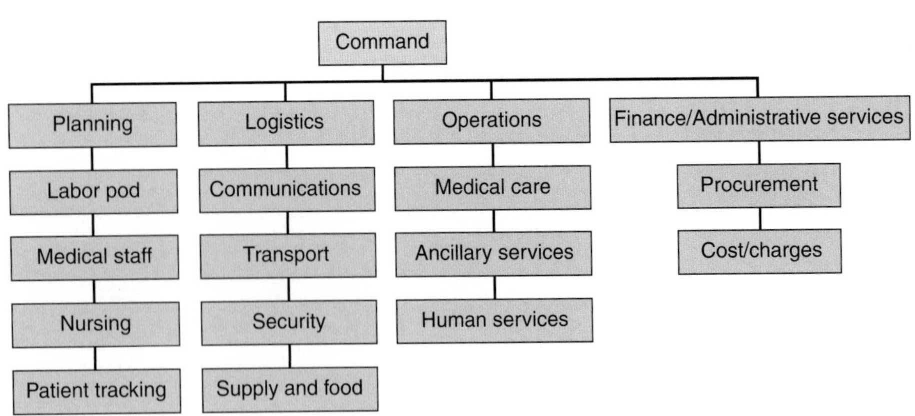

FIGURE 34.3 Structure of the Incident Command System.

KEY POINTS

- Terrorism is random and ruthless violence against people—usually innocent civilians—and property, to intimidate societies and governments for political or ideological purposes. Terrorism has increased greatly and is the most common cause of mass casualties today. In the United States, complacency and apathy of healthcare providers is the greatest impediment to effective response to terrorism.
- The major goals of terrorism are maximal casualties and lethality using, most frequently, "weapons of mass destruction" of biological, nuclear or radiological, incendiary, chemical, and explosive (BNICE) agents.
- Biological weapons use microorganisms or their toxins to inflict disease. Useful because of easy deployment over wide areas, delay in onset, variability in recognition for containment, and proven effectiveness in nature (e.g., influenza epidemics), biological weapons have been used in war since at least the Roman Empire.
- Major biological agents include anthrax (*Bacillus anthracis*), botulinum toxin (*Clostridium botulinum*), bubonic plague, tularemia, small pox, and viral hemorrhagic fever, caused by four viral groups. However, their development is dangerous, expensive, and difficult, explaining their rare use.
- Chemical agents are aerosolized or gaseous, ingested as contaminated food, or absorbed by direct contact and have been used frequently during wars in the 20th century. Response requires recognition, treatment (including decontamination and protection of caregivers), and specific antidotes.
- Dispersal of radioactive agents has severe theoretical risk but is primarily a psychological and panic effect. Penetration by ionizing radiation causes severe damage but is limited in range, (square of the distance) and containment is relatively easy and nontransmittable. Care is supportive, treating dermal burns and gastrointestinal and hematopoietic damage.
- Terrorist attacks are, by far, implemented most commonly using conventional weapons and confirm the need of a system to treat the casualties of bombings. The magnitude of energy achieved, the ease of technology required, and cost effectiveness support an ongoing increase in risk of mass casualties.
- Explosion injuries are caused by the primary blast wave–induced disruption of organs with air-liquid interfaces (lung, bowels, eyes, and ears); secondary blast injury from flying objects, particularly shrapnel placed in bombs and suicide bomber body parts; tertiary blast injury from displacement of the victim's body; and quaternary blast injury from indirect causes such as building collapse.
- Response to mass casualty events requires triage of victims to effectively utilize resources, including the paradigm shift from greatest good for the individual to greatest good for the greatest number, with need for preemptive planning, coordination, and practice of an Incident Command System to respond optimally.

References

1. US Department of State. *International Terrorism. Selected Documents, No. 24.* Washington: US Government Printing Office; 1986.
2. **Ciraulo DL, Frykberg ER, Feliciano DV, et al. A survey assessment of the level of preparedness for domestic terrorism and mass casualty incidents among Eastern Association for the Surgery of Trauma members. *J Trauma* 2004;56:1033–1041.**
3. Mallonee S, Shariat S, Stennies G, et al. Physical injuries and fatalities resulting from the Oklahoma City bombing. *JAMA* 1996;276:382–387.
4. Quenemoen LE, Davis YM, Malilay J, et al. The World Trade Center bombing : injury prevention strategies for high-rise building fires. *Disasters* 1996;20:125–132.
5. Feliciano DV, Anderson GV, Rozycki GS, et al. Management of casualties from the bombing at the Centennial Olympics. *Am J Surg.* 1998;176:538–543.
6. Cushman JG, Pachter HL, Beaton HL. Two New York City hospitals' surgical response to the September 11, 2001 terrorist attack in New York City. *J Trauma* 2003;54:147–155.
7. Slater MS, Trunkey DD. Terrorism in America: an evolving threat. *Arch Surg.* 1997;132:1059–1066.
8. Mobley JA. Biological warfare in the twentieth century: Lessons from the past, challenges for the future. *Mil Med.* 1995;160:547–553.
9. **Kortepeter MG, Parker GW. Potential biological weapons threats. *Emerging Inf Dis.* 1999;5:523–527.**
10. Derbes VJ. DeMussis and the Great Plague of 1348, a forgotten episode of bacteriological warfare. *JAMA.* 1966;196:179–182.
11. Christopher GW, Cieslak TJ, Pavlin JJ, et al. Biological warfare, a historical perspective. *JAMA.* 1997;278:412–417.
12. Zilinskas RA. Iraq's biological weapons, the past as future? *JAMA* 1997;278: 418–424.
13. Alibek K, Handelman S. *Biohazard.* New York, Random House, 1999.
14. Green MS, Kaufman Z. Syndromic surveillance for early detection and monitoring of infectious disease outbreaks associated with bioterrorism. In: Shemer J, Shoenfeld J eds. *Terror and medicine: medical aspects of biological, chemical and radiological terrorism.* Lengerich, Germany: Pabst Science Publishers; 2003:81–95.
15. **Khan AS, Ashford DA, Craven RB, et al. Biological and chemical terrorism: Strategic plan for preparedness and response. Recommendations of the CDC strategic planning workgroup. *MMWR Morb Mortal Wkly Rep.* 2000;49:1–14.**
16. **Inglesby TV, Henderson DA, Bartlett JG, et al. Anthrax as a biological weapon: medical and public health management. *JAMA* 1999;281: 1735–1745**
17. Eachempati SR, Flomenbaum N, Barie PS. Biological warfare : current concerns for the health care provider. *J Trauma.* 2002;52:179–186.
18. Meselson M, Gillemin J, Hugh-Jones M, et al. The Sverdlovsk anthrax outbreak of 1979. *Science* 1994;209:1202–1208
19. Henderson DA, Inglesby TV, Bartlett JG, et al. Smallpox as a biological weapon: medical and public health management. *JAMA* 1999;281: 2127–2137.
20. Inglesby TV, Dennis DT, Henderson DA, et al. Plague as a biological weapon: medical and public health management. *JAMA* 2000;283:2281–2290.
21. Dennis DT, Inglesby TV, Henderson DA, et al. Tularemia as a biological weapon. *JAMA* 2001;285:2763–2773.
22. Centers for Disease Control and Prevention. Management of patients with suspected viral hemorrhagic fever. MMWR *Morb Mortal Wkly Rep.* 1988;37:1–16.
23. Smart JK. History of chemical and biological warfare: an American perspective. In: *Medical Aspects of Chemical and Biological Warfare.* Bethesda, MD: Office of the Surgeon General, 1997:11–42.
24. Anderson N. Disaster epidemiology: lessons from Bhopal. In: Murray V, ed. *Major Chemical Disasters—Medical aspects of Management.* London: Royal Society of Medicine Services, Limited; 1990:183–195.
25. Jenkins BM. Understanding the link between motives and methods. In: Roberts B, ed. *Terrorism with chemical and biological weapons: calibrating risks and responses.* Alexandria, VA: Chemical and Biological Arms Control Institute; 1997:43–52.
26. Lillibridge SR, Sidell FR. A report on the casualties from the Tokyo subway incident by the U.S. medical team. Atlanta: Centers for Disease Control and Prevention; 1995.
27. Management of terrorist events involving radioactive material. NCRP report no. 138. Bethesda, MD: National Council on Radiation Protection and Measurement, 2001.
28. **Mettler FA, Voelz GL. Major radiation exposure—what to expect and how to respond. *N Engl J Med.* 2002;346:1554–1560.**
29. Yehezkelli Y, Lehavi O, Dushnitsky T, et al. Radiation terrorism—the medical challenge. In: Shemer J, Shoenfeld Y, ed. *Terror and medicine, medical aspects of biological, chemical and radiological terrorism.* Lengerich, Germany: Pabst Science Publishers; 2003:335–46.
30. Brill AB, ed. *Low dose radiation effects: a fact book.* New York: Society of Nuclear Medicine; 1982.
31. Reeves GI. Radiation injuries. *Crit Care Clin North Am.* 1999;2:457–472.
32. Fong F, Schrader DC. Radiation disasters and emergency department preparedness. *Emerg Med Clin North Am.* 1996;14:349–369.
33. Reeves GI, Jarrett DG, Seed TM, et al, eds. *Triage of irradiated personnel.* Bethesda: Armed Forces Radiology Research Institute; 1998.
34. Frykberg ER, Tepas JJ. Terrorist bombings: lessons learned from Belfast to Beirut. *Ann Surg.* 1988;208:569–576.
35. **Frykberg, ER. Medical management of disasters and mass casualties from terrorist bombings: how can we cope? *J Trauma* 2002;53:201–212.**
36. Bird M. *The Town That Died: The True Story of the Greatest Man-Made Explosion Before Hiroshima.* Halifax, NS; Nimbus Publishing, 1995.
37. Stephens HW. *Texas city disaster, 1947.* Austin: University of Texas Press; 1996.

38. Jacobs LM, Ramp JM, Breay JM. An emergency medical system approach to disaster planning. *J Trauma* 1979;19:157–162.
39. **Stein M, Hirshberg A. Medical consequences of terrorism: the conventional weapon threat. *Surg Clin North Am.* 1999;79:1537–1552.**
40. Rignault DP, Deligny MC. The 1986 terrorist bombing experience in Paris. *Ann Surg.* 1989;209:368–373.
41. Karmy-Jones R, Kissinger D, Golocovsky M, et al. Bomb-related injuries. *Mil Med.* 1994;159:536–539.
42. Federal Bureau of Investigation. *1997 Bomb summary.* Washington, D.C.: U.S. Department of Justice; 1997.
43. Clemedsson CJ. Blast injury. *Physiol Rev.* 1956;36:336–54.
44. Hill JF. Blast injury with particular reference to recent terrorist bombing incidents. *Ann R Coll Surg Engl.* 1979;61:4–11.
45. Cooper GJ, Maynard RL, Cross NL et al. Casualties from terrorist bombings. *J Trauma* 1983;23:955–967.
46. Candole CA. Blast injury. *Can Med Assoc J.* 1967;96:207–214.
47. Lebovici D, Gofrit ON, Stein M, et al. Blast injuries: bus versus open-air-bombings—a comparative study of injuries in survivors of open-air versus confined-space explosions. *J Trauma* 1996;41:1030–1035.
48. **Phillips YY. Primary blast injuries. *Ann Emerg Med.* 1986;15:1446–1450.**
49. Rawlins JSP. Physical and pathophysiological effects of blast. *Injury* 1977;9:313–320.
50. Gutierrez de Caballos JP, Turegano-Ruentes F, Perez-Diaz D, et al. Casualties treated at the closest hospital in the Madrid, March 11, terrorist bombings. *Crit Care.* 2004;9:104–111.
51. Brismar B, Bergenwald L. The terrorist bomb explosion in Bologna, Italy, 1980: an analysis of the effects and injuries sustained. *J Trauma* 1982;22:216–220.
52. Boffard KD, MacFarlane C. Urban bomb blast injuries: patterns of injury and treatment. *Surg Ann.* 1993;25:29–47.
53. Almogy G, Belzberg H, Mintz Y, et al. Suicide bombing attacks: update and modifications to the protocol. *Ann Surg.* 2004;239:295–303.
54. Stein M, Hirshberg A. Limited mass casualties due to conventional weapons—the daily reality of a level 1 trauma center. In: Shemer Y, Shoenfield Y, eds. *Terror and medicine, medical aspects of biological, chemical and radiological terrorism.* Lengerich, Germany: Pabst Science Publishers 2003:378–393.
55. Biancolini, CA, Del Bosco CG, Jorge MA. Argentine Jewish Community Institution bomb explosion. *J Trauma* 1999;47:728–732.
56. Frykberg ER, Tepas JJ, Alexander RH. The 1983 Beirut airport terrorist bombing: injury patterns and implications for disaster management. *Am Surg.* 1989;55:134–141.
57. Thompson D, Brown S, Mallonee S, et al. Fatal and non-fatal injuries among U.S. Air Force personnel resulting from the terrorist bombing of the Khobar Towers. *J Trauma* 2004;57:208–215.
58. Davis TP, Alexander BA, Lambert EW, et al. Distribution and care of shipboard blast injuries (USS Cole DDG-67). *J Trauma* 2003;55:1022–1028.
59. Hirshberg A, Stein M, Walden R. Surgical resource utilization in urban terrorist bombing: a computer simulation. *J Trauma* 1999;47:545–550.
60. American College of Surgeons Committee on Trauma. Field categorization of trauma patients (field triage). *Bull Am Coll Surg.* 1986;71:17–21.
61. Caro D, Irving M. The Old Bailey bomb explosion. *Lancet* 1973;1:1433–1435.
62. Tucker K, Lettin A. The Tower of London bomb explosion. *Brit Med J.* 1975;3:287–290.
63. Waterworth TA, Carr MJT. Report on injuries sustained by patients treated at the Birmingham General Hospital following the recent bomb explosions. *Brit Med J.* 1975;2:25–27.
64. Pyper PC, Graham WJH. Analysis of terrorist injuries treated at Craigavon Area Hospital, Northern Ireland, 1972–1980. *Injury* 1982;14:332–338.
65. Henderson JV. Anatomy of a terrorist attack: the Cu Chi mess hall incident. *J World Assoc Emerg Dis Med.* 1986;2:69–73.
66. Klein JS, Weigelt JA. Disaster management: lessons learned. *Surg Clin North Am.* 1991;71:257–266.
67. Irwin RL. The Incident Command System (ICS). In: Auf der Heide E, ed. *Disaster response: principles of preparation and coordination.* St. Louis: Mosby;1989:133–163.
68. Jacobs LM, Goody M, Sinclair A. The role of a trauma center in disaster management. *J Trauma* 1983;23:697–701.
69. Ammons MA, Moore EE, Pons PT, et al. The role of a regional trauma system in the management of a mass disaster: an analysis of the Keystone Colorado chairlift accident. *J Trauma* 1988;28:1468–1471.
70. **Jacobs LM, Burns KJ, Gross RI. Terrorism: a public health threat with a trauma system response. *J Trauma* 2003;55:1014–1021.**

SECTION B
TRANSPLANTATION

CHAPTER 35 ■ TRANSPLANT IMMUNOLOGY

JONATHAN S. BROMBERG AND JOHN C. MAGEE

The major impediment to universal, long-term allograft function in transplant recipients is the host immune response. Various manifestations of host antidonor immune reactivity result in allograft dysfunction and loss. To prevent these adverse outcomes, systemic immunosuppression is required. Current immunosuppression, however, is not completely reliable in preventing or reversing rejection, and immunosuppression itself results in several undesirable complications. To control the events that occur during clinical organ allografting, it is important to understand the processes of antigen recognition, the effector mechanisms of immune reactivity, and the cellular and molecular interactions that control and regulate the fate of antigen.

INITIATION OF THE IMMUNE RESPONSE

Recognition of Antigen

For allografts to be recognized as foreign and subsequently rejected, or as self and therefore accepted, the potential antigenic determinants of the graft must come into contact with a variety of specific receptors of the immune system. Antigen–receptor interactions are the first steps in a series that ultimately determines the fate of an antigen or an organ. The molecular and cellular participants in these processes are the immunoglobulin receptors of B cells, the antigen or T-cell receptors (TCRs) of T cells, and major histocompatibility complex (MHC) antigens of antigen-presenting cells (APCs).

Direct Recognition of Antigen by Immunoglobulin

Conceptually, the easiest interaction to understand is the direct binding of antigen to immunoglobulin. In this case, antigen can be any cellular constituent (e.g., protein, carbohydrate, lipid, nucleic acid) that is bound by high affinity to a specific immunoglobulin, or antibody. Antibody molecules usually comprise two heavy (H) chains and two light (L) chains. Each chain has an amino-terminal variable (V) region domain, which differs from antibody to antibody. Each chain also has a few to several carboxy-terminal constant (C) region domains, which different antibody molecules may share. There are several different classes of immunoglobulins. The typical IgG dimer, comprising two L chains and two H chains, is shown in Fig. 35.1. Other classes of antibodies differ from IgG in their polymeric structure, number of H-chain constant region domains, and soluble or cell membrane location of the molecules. These features are listed in Table 35.1. Membrane-bound immunoglobulin usually serves as an antigen-specific receptor for stimulating naive or memory B cells, whereas soluble antibodies

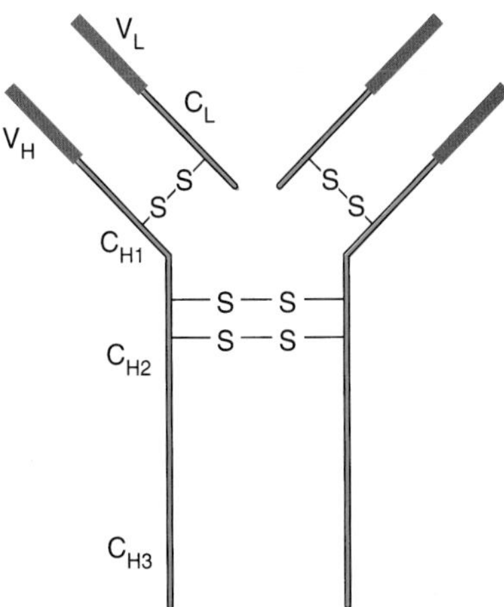

FIGURE 35.1 Structure of immunoglobulin (IgG). Variable (*V*) and constant (*C*) regions of heavy (*H*) and light (*L*) chains are joined by disulfide bonds.

TABLE 35.1

STRUCTURAL PROPERTIES OF IMMUNOGLOBULIN CLASSES AND SUBCLASSES

Immunoglobulin	IgD	IgM	IgG	IgA	IgE
Subclasses	—	—	G1, G2, G3, G4	A1, A2	—
Molecular weight (kd)	184	970	146–170	160	188
Polymeric Structure	Dimer	Pentamer	Dimer	Monomer, dimer or trimer	Dimer
Additional Chains	—	J chain	—	J chain	—
Functional Associations	Membrane-bound receptor	Primary antibody, membrane receptor	Secondary antibody	Mucosal antibody	Immediate hypersensitivity

usually perform effector functions of antigen recognition, opsonization, complement-mediated lysis, or activation of effector cells through Fc receptor interactions. The generation of membrane versus soluble forms of immunoglobulin is usually the result of alternative splicing of messenger (mRNA).

Genetic analysis of immunoglobulin gene structure reveals several features that demonstrate how antibody diversity is generated and maintained. The H-chain gene complex is encoded on chromosome 14 in humans; k L chains are encoded by chromosome 2 and l L chains by chromosome 22. A single B cell can produce only a single type of L chain from only one of its chromosomes, a process termed *allelic exclusion.* The molecular determinants of allelic exclusion are just beginning to be elucidated. There appears to be a complex interaction between positive and negative regulatory transcription factors at the level of chromatin structure, and these factors are in turn regulated by membrane-initiated signaling events in response to specific antigens.[1]

Heavy- and light-chain loci have a common structural motif of the V regions located upstream, or 5′, of the C region. Furthermore, there are many V regions. These have been sequenced and further subdivided into unique or related classes and subclasses. Presumably, these multiple V region families arose by an evolutionary process of gene duplication followed by mutation of individual family members. Further analysis has shown that between the V and C regions are multiple additional genetic elements that provide further structural variation. These elements are termed *joining* (J) and *diversity* (D) regions. J regions are present in both H- and L-chain genes, whereas D regions are present only in H-chain genes. During the process of B-cell maturation, these separate regions are physically brought together in a stochastic process that excises the intervening DNA sequences, including other V, D, and J genes (Fig. 35.2). Because there are many different V-, D-, and J-region genes for each H- and L-chain locus, which all may independently associate, the combinatorial possibilities are extremely large, showing why the immune system is able to generate antibodies for virtually all known antigenic determinants. The general process of gene rearrangement in B cells involves the complex interaction of membrane-initiated differentiating signals, cytoplasmic transcriptional factors, and nucleic acid excisional machinery at the level of chromatin structure.[1–5]

Further diversity is also generated by the nucleic acid template-independent addition of nucleotides (N regions) at the V-D, V-J, and D-J junctions. N regions increase the diversity of

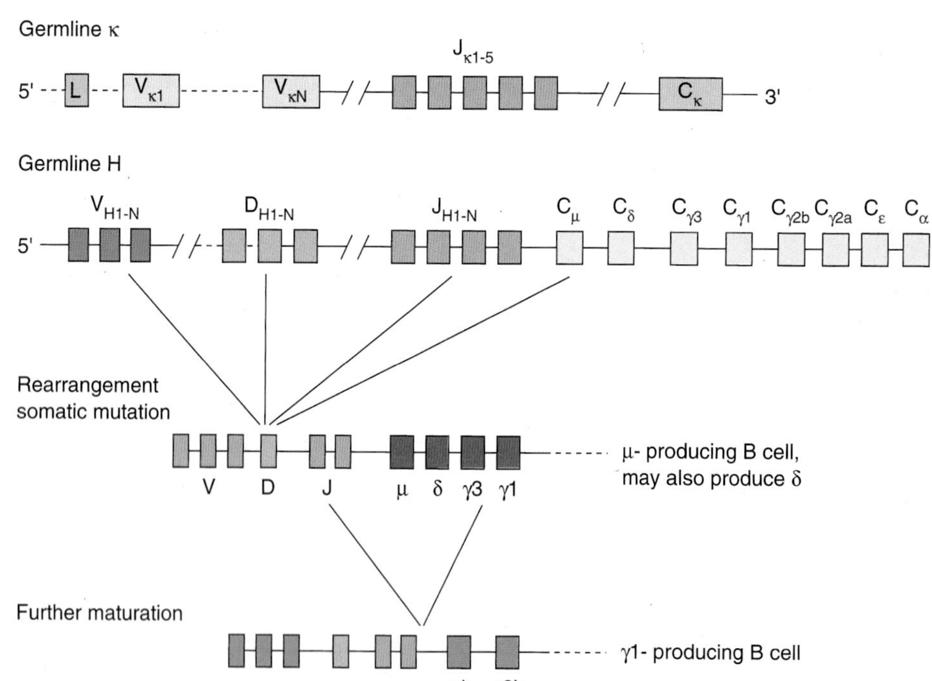

FIGURE 35.2 Structure of germline immunoglobulin heavy- and light-chain loci showing V, D, J, and C region genes. Maturation results in approximation of specific genes.

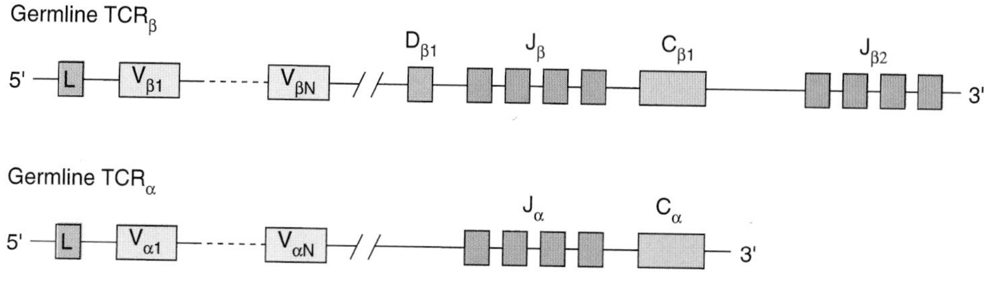

FIGURE 35.3 Structure of T-cell receptor (TCR) β- and α-chain loci.

immunoglobulin sequences and antibody specificity by another few orders of magnitude. Thus, what is known about the immunoglobulin gene structure explains the presence of diversity at the protein level. Importantly, the regions of greatest nucleotide diversity correspond to the three hypervariable regions of the antibody molecule, which are the amino acid contact residues responsible for direct antigen–antibody or receptor–ligand interactions.

It was previously concluded that a single B cell expresses only a single isotype, or H chain. However, molecular analysis shows that alternative mRNA splicing may allow a single B cell to express different H chains. It was also previously considered that membrane-bound forms of immunoglobulin functioned independently as antigen receptors. However, biochemical analysis demonstrates that at least three invariant chains, Ig-α, Ig-β, and Ig-γ, must associate with surface immunoglobulin for efficient expression and signal transduction.[6,7]

Recognition of Antigen by the T-Cell Receptor in the Context of the Major Histocompatibility Complex

T cells do not bind and recognize antigen directly. T cells recognize a complex composed of a peptide fragment of antigen bound to an MHC molecule. In other words, T cells recognize antigen in the context of MHC, a process termed *MHC restriction*. Structural and genetic analysis of the TCR reveals that it shares many principles with B-cell immunoglobulin receptors. The TCR is composed of separate α and β chains encoded by loci on chromosomes 14 and 7, respectively. Each locus comprises a series of V, D, J, and C segments (Fig. 35.3). The α-chain locus has only V and J genes, whereas the β locus has D regions. These loci undergo rearrangements during T-cell development, maturation, and differentiation, following the principles of gene rearrangement and allelic exclusion. This results in the generation of enormous receptor diversity and the potential to recognize the entire universe of antigens. Diversity is further increased by the insertion of N regions at V-D-J junctions.

T cells may also express alternative TCR γ and δ chains encoded on chromosomes 7 and 14, respectively. These chains are similar to α and β but show somewhat less diversity and are structurally more similar to immunoglobulins than ab TCRs. Further, $\gamma\delta$ T cells recognize not only peptide but also nonpeptide antigens,[8] and they may play unique roles in recognizing certain intracellular pathogens (e.g., *Mycobacteria, Listeria*).[9,10] $\gamma\delta$ TCR T cells are particularly concentrated among intraepithelial lymphocytes of the gastrointestinal tract, further reinforcing the notion that gd T cells perform functions related to surveillance of certain pathogens. Soluble forms of the TCR exist, resulting from alternative mRNA splicing or from proteolytic cleavage of surface receptors. The function of soluble TCR is not understood; studies show these molecules behave as suppressor factors or proinflammatory mediators.

Similar to surface immunoglobulin, the TCR is not expressed alone in the membrane. The TCR requires the coexpression of a complex of invariant chains termed *cluster determinant 3* (CD3). CD3 is a complex of five transmembrane proteins (γ, δ, ε, ζ, η), as shown in Fig. 35.4, which are important for the assembly of the TCR and its transport and insertion into the cell membrane. The CD3 complex plays an essential role in signal transduction by the TCR, particularly the cytoplasmic domains of the ζ and η chains.[11] Additional molecules also function in tandem with the ab TCR. In particular, the CD4 and CD8 molecules, transmembrane proteins that are likewise members of the immunoglobulin gene superfamily, physically associate with the $\alpha\beta$ TCR and bind to the same MHC molecules as the TCR. This association increases the affinity and avidity of TCR and T cells for antigen. CD4 binds to class II MHC [i.e., human leukocyte antigen (HLA)-DR, DP, and DQ] and is generally considered a cell surface marker for helper T cells (T_H). This explains why T_H are MHC class II restricted. CD8 binds to class I MHC (i.e., HLA-A, B, and C) and is generally considered a cell surface marker for cytotoxic (T_C) or suppressor (T_S) T cells. This explains why T_C are generally MHC class I restricted.

There are two major classes of MHC molecules encoded by linked loci on chromosome 6 and defined by structural and functional associations (Table 35.2). Class I MHC molecules result from the noncovalent association between a polymorphic, transmembrane α chain and a nonpolymorphic soluble β chain, termed *β_2-microglobulin*. Thus, α chains encoded by diverse HLA-A, B, or C alleles each associate with β_2-microglobulin on the cell surface (Fig. 35.5). Class II molecules result from the noncovalent association of polymorphic transmembrane α and β chains encoded by HLA-DP, DQ, or

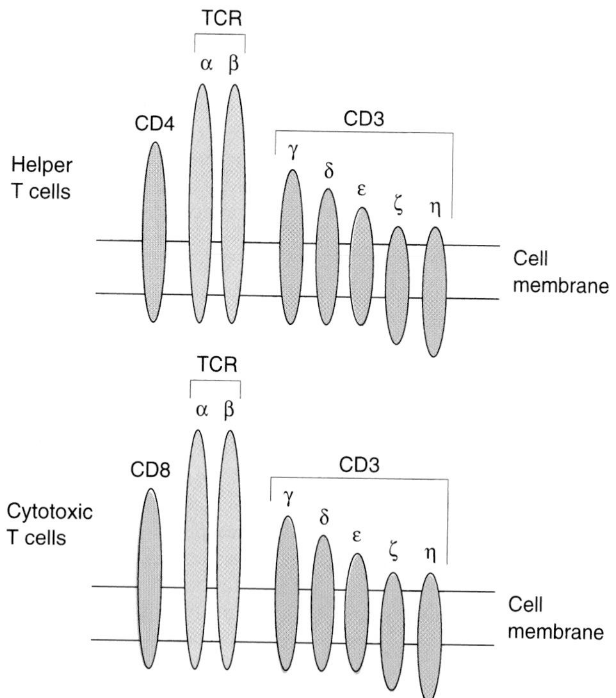

FIGURE 35.4 T-cell receptor (TCR) complex in the cell membrane composed of TCR $\alpha\beta$, CD3, CD4, and CD8 chains.

DR (Fig. 35.6). There are separate α and β chains encoded within each separate class II subregion. Despite some structural differences, these class I and II dimers all have four major extracellular domains, with two of the domains contributing the major amino acid side chains to the walls of the peptide binding groove.

The TCR binds to a complex of MHC plus antigen. X-ray crystallography has determined the three-dimensional structure of these complexes and provided a firm structural and biochemical basis for understanding the cellular process of MHC restriction.[12,13] Figure 35.7 shows that the α_1 and β_2 domains of an MHC class I molecule form a groove on the surface of the MHC molecule. Peptide antigens are loaded into this groove when the functions of antigen processing and presentation are performed. The α_1 and β_1 domains of class II MHC perform a similar function. The TCR residues come in contact with residues of both antigen and MHC. Therefore, polymorphisms of the TCR generated by gene arrangement, and polymorphisms of MHC resulting from allelic variation within the population and the expression of several different class I or II molecules, provide the structural variation required to accommodate the potential universe of antigenic determinants. Some of the most important recent advances in immunology have been the determination of the three-dimensional structure of the MHC, peptide binding groove, and TCR and the unequivocal demonstration of the loading of peptide antigen into the MHC molecules. Precise, structurally based approaches to altering the T cell's initial recognition of antigen are now possible and are being investigated experimentally to determine their application to clinical transplantation.

TABLE 35.2

CLASS I AND CLASS II ANTIGENS: STRUCTURE AND FUNCTION

Class I antigens	Class II antigens
STRUCTURE	
Encoded by HLA-A, -B, -C loci in humans	Encoded by HLA-D locus (DR, DP, DO)
Single polymorphic heavy chain (45 kd)	Two chains α (29 kd) β (34 kd)
Associated with β_2-microglobulin (12 kd)	—
Five domains α_1, α_2, α_3 extracellular Transmembrane Cystoplasmic	Four domains α_1, α_2 or β_1, β_2 extracellular Transmembrane Cytoplasmic
Expressed on all nucleated cells	Expressed on B cells, antigen-presenting cells, and vascular endothelium
MAJOR FUNCTIONS	
Activator and target for cytotoxic T (CD8+) lymphocytes	Activator of helper T cells (CD4+) and stimulator in mixed lymphocyte reaction
Target for antibody-mediated rejection	Possible target for antibody-mediated
Stimulate antibody response	Stimulator of antibody response (unknown significance)

HLA, human leukocyte antigen

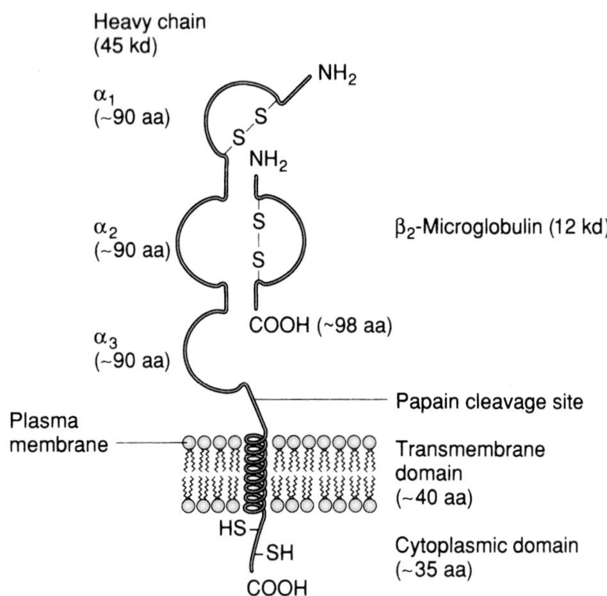

FIGURE 35.5 Human leukocyte antigen (HLA) class I molecule. The polymorphic heavy chain (45 kd) of the class I polypeptide is noncovalently bound to the invariant light chain, b_2-microglobulin (12 kd). The heavy chain consists of five domains—three extracellular domains (α_1, α_2, and α_3), a transmembrane domain, and a cytoplasmic domain. The α_1 and α_2 domains contain the most polymorphic residues responsible for antigen binding and form the side walls of the peptide binding groove; the transmembrane portion anchors the molecule to the plasma membrane; and the β_2-microglobulin stabilizes the conformation of the extracellular domains.

Antigen Processing

Identifying the MHC–antigen complex structure has also initiated much recent study toward defining the pathways by which antigen is loaded onto MHC molecules. The pathways of antigen processing encompass a wide variety of cellular functions, including the receptor-mediated endocytosis of

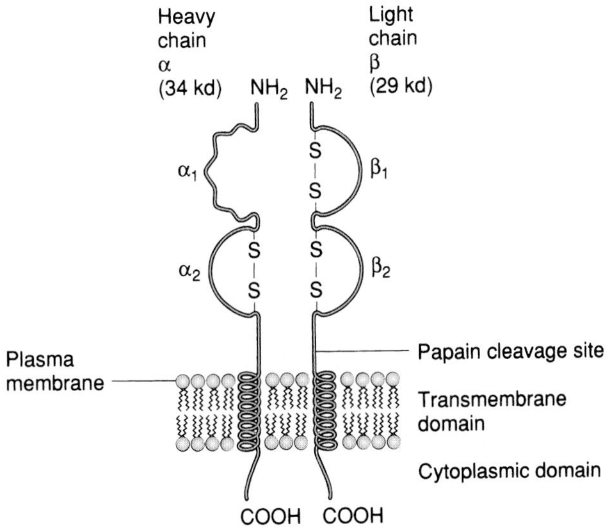

FIGURE 35.6 Human leukocyte antigen (HLA) class II molecule. The two chains, α (29 kd) and β (34 kd), are noncovalently associated and are made up of four domains—two extracellular domains, a transmembrane domain, and a cytoplasmic domain. Most of the allelic variance is contained in the β chain. The peptide binding site is believed to be in the groove between the α_1 and β_1 domains.

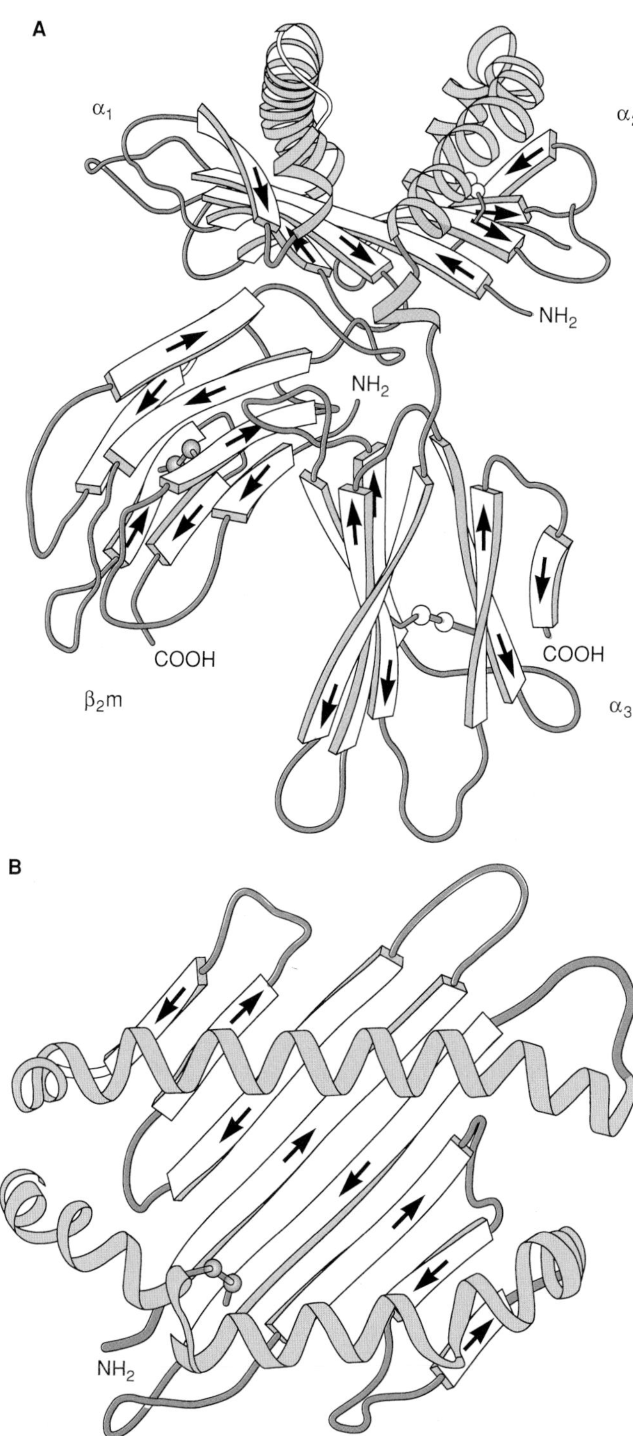

FIGURE 35.7 Human leukocyte antigen (HLA)-A2 class I molecule. (*A*) There are four domains with the polymorphic α_1 and α_2 on top presenting themselves to the T-cell receptor and α_3 and β_2 below close to the cell membrane. (*B*) Looking at the top of the molecule, the peptide binding groove is shown as made up of the α_1 and α_2 domains forming the side walls and the β pleated sheet forming the floor.

antigen, transfer of cytoplasmic or endosomal antigen to proteolytic organelles, translocation of proteolyzed peptide into the endoplastic reticulum to nascent "naked" MHC molecules, correct folding of new MHC molecules around antigen, transport of antigen–MHC by the *cis*- and *trans*-Golgi apparatus to the cell surface, and recycling of cell surface MHC molecules to endosomal and Golgi compartments to exchange one antigenic peptide for another (Fig. 35.8). This brief list of some of the defined steps of antigen processing and presentation reveals that many of the normal cellular housekeeping processes are coopted during the handling of antigen. These processes include vesicle transport and fusion, microtubule and microfilament function, correct folding and localization of nascent polypeptides coming off the ribosome by chaperonins, and control of intracellular proteolysis. Therefore, the study and eventual understanding of antigen processing and presentation requires knowledge of most normal cellular functions. Immunosuppression may eventually be directed not at T cells or B cells, as is currently the case, but may alter the functions of chaperones, Golgi apparatus, or proteolytic controls.

Figure 35.8 provides a general picture of the major processes, which include antigen uptake, proteolysis, translocation to the endoplasmic reticulum or Golgi, and presentation on the cell surface.[14–37] A number of important features should be mentioned. The source of antigen determines how and where it comes into contact with the processing machinery and onto which MHC molecules it is loaded. Thus, endogenously synthesized proteins, such as self-proteins or viral antigens in the cytoplasm, are degraded in the cytoplasm, transported to the endoplasmic reticulum, and loaded onto nascent class I MHC.[38] Conversely, exogenously synthesized antigens are taken up in endosomes through receptor-mediated processes, degraded in an endosomal compartment (e.g., lysosome, Golgi apparatus, or a unique structure), transported to the Golgi, and loaded onto nascent class II MHC.[39] Although this general scheme for the processing and presentation of endogenous versus exogenous antigens will likely remain intact, there are numerous exceptions where endogenous antigens may be presented by class II MHC or exogenous antigens presented by class I MHC. This undoubtedly reflects the incomplete understanding of vesicle transport, proteolytic control, partitioning of molecules to various endosomal compartments, and the molecular control of MHC folding and peptide loading.

Proteolytic degradation of antigens may be accomplished either in endosomal compartments, probably through fusion with lysosomes, or in the cytoplasm. The latter process seems to be accomplished by a large multiprotein complex called the *proteasome*.[40,41] In addition, some of the proteasome subunits are encoded in the MHC region. Thus, the MHC provides the information to degrade antigen and to determine the carrier onto which antigenic peptides are loaded. The control of proteolysis is poorly understood; it is not clear if all cellular constituents have equal access to proteolytic components or if antigens are somehow preferentially shunted into the system. Proteolytic enzymes have specificity for particular peptide bonds; therefore, not all proteins should be equally susceptible to the processing apparatus and some should make "better" antigens than others. This has been confirmed experimentally using amino acid–substituted antigens. In addition, there is allelic variation among the MHC-encoded proteasome subunits so that antigen is processed into different peptides by different alleles. Allelic variation in MHC class I and II peptide binding grooves also determines what set of peptides can be bound by MHC molecules. Thus, heterogeneity of antigens, proteolytic enzymes, and MHC molecules all determine the nature of the peptide ultimately presented to the TCR.

Further molecular analysis demonstrates that the MHC class I peptide binding groove is a fairly closed structure and can accommodate peptides of a relatively restricted size, ranging from 8 to 10 amino acids in length. Conversely, the class II groove is larger and more open ended. It can tolerate more length heterogeneity in the peptide that it binds so that a modal distribution of 12 to 24 amino acids is found loaded onto these molecules. These structural constraints suggest that certain types of antigens may be presented only by certain MHC molecules. Indeed, there is evidence that certain microbial antigens are

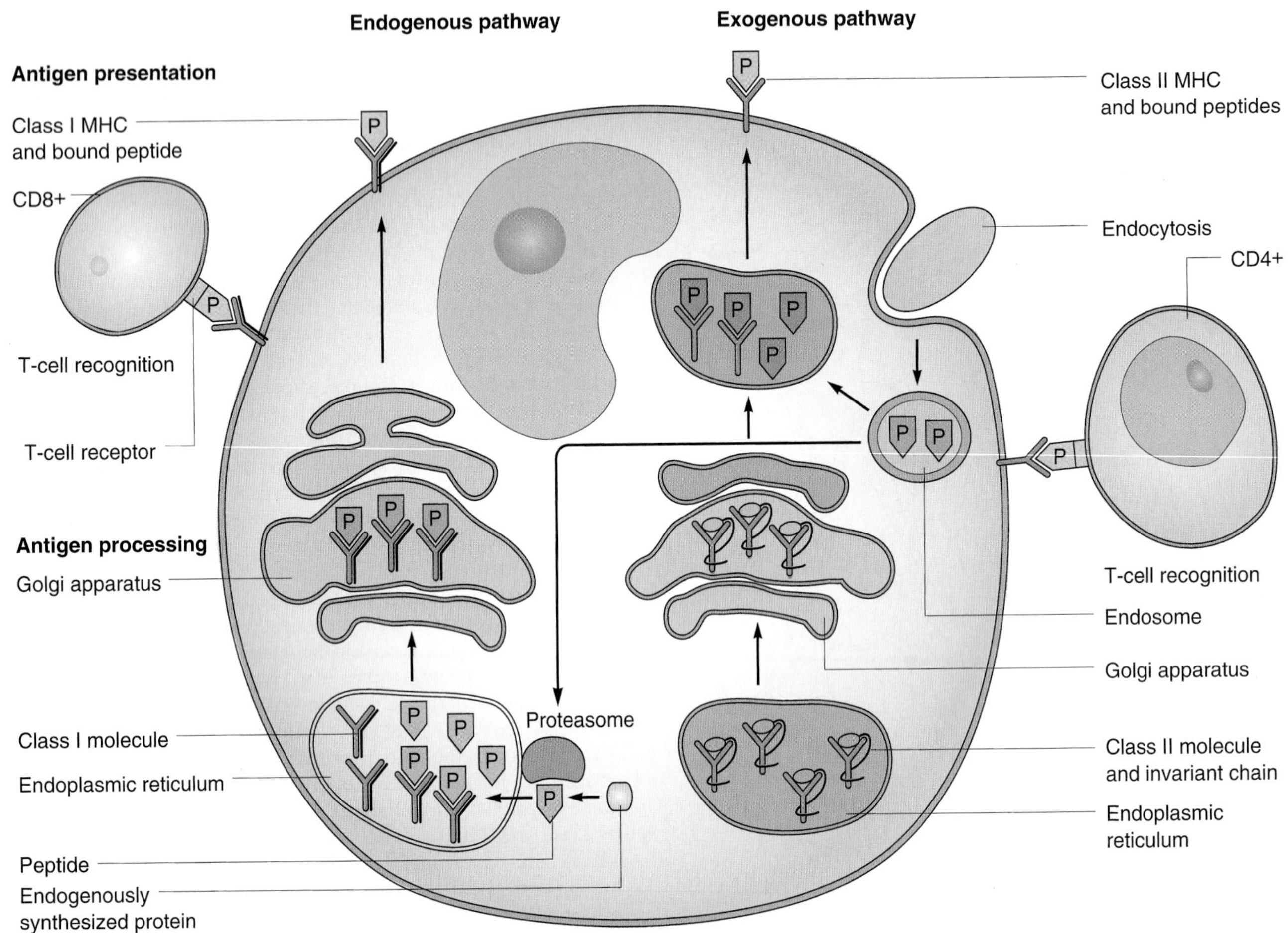

FIGURE 35.8 Antigen processing and presentation. Endogenously synthesized or intracellular proteins (e.g., viral gene products) are degraded into peptides that are transported to the endoplasmic reticulum. These peptides bind to class I major histocompatibility complex (MHC) molecules and are transported to the surface of the antigen-presenting cell. CD8+ T cells recognize the foreign peptide bound to class I MHC by way of the T-cell receptor complex. Exogenous antigen (e.g., bacterial) is endocytosed and broken down into peptide fragments in endosomes. Class II molecules are transported to the endosome in association with the invariant chain, bound to the peptide, and delivered to the surface of the antigen-presenting cell, where they are recognized by CD4+ cells.

preferentially presented by class I MHC.[42,43] This example also represents one exception where exogenously synthesized antigens are presented by class I. Although the discussion to this point has focused on protein antigens, it is not known whether or how nonprotein antigens are loaded into the antigen-binding groove of MHC molecules.

Another important issue is how antigen is transported into the endoplasmic reticulum or Golgi apparatus. The determinants of endosomal transport and its specificity are not defined. The determinants of cytoplasmic transport seem dependent on a transporter complex that physically links the proteasome to the endoplasmic reticulum. Furthermore, this transporter complex is at least partly MHC encoded. Current models suggest that as a peptide antigen is degraded, it is immediately transported from the proteasome to the lumen of the endoplasmic reticulum, where it is loaded onto class I MHC. The fact that the MHC encodes the transporter and that allelic variation is also present in these molecules provides another level of variation in the ability ultimately to recognize any antigen.

Another noteworthy issue is how peptide is loaded into the binding groove of MHC molecules. Experimental evidence suggests that class I and II dimers are incompletely assembled in the endoplasmic reticulum and are also bound by chaperone proteins. In the case of class II MHC, this chaperone is called the *invariant chain.* Failure to load peptide results in retention of MHC molecules within the endoplasmic reticulum and markedly decreases cell surface MHC expression. Loading of peptide causes the release of MHC by chaperones, completion of folding and assembly, and transport to the cell surface. A related issue is the fate and recycling of cell surface antigen–MHC complexes. There is evidence of endocytosis and reloading of both class I and II molecules with new peptide antigens. The molecular determinants of these processes are still poorly defined.

Antigen Presentation and Antigen-presenting Cells

Based on the previous discussion, it is apparent that antigen processing and presentation depend on a large number of coordinated intracellular events. Many of these events, however, seem to depend on normal cellular processes of transport, proteolysis, and posttranslational modification of proteins. Antigen presentation also depends on the expression of MHC-encoded class I, class II, proteasome, and transporter molecules. All nucleated cells express MHC class I, and many cell types can also express the other loci. This suggests that many different cell types are capable of presenting antigens. In fact, this has been proved in a number of experimental and clinical analyses. Nonetheless, certain cell types are more efficient at processing and presenting antigen and are localized to certain tissues or organs that increase the likelihood that they will participate in antigen presentation. These so-called *professional APCs* are generally considered to be monocytes and macrophages. In addition, closely related interstitial dendritic cells and Langerhans cells of the dermis are extremely efficient APCs. These cells constitutively express class I and II MHC and the other MHC-encoded components. All these products can be up-regulated in response to proinflammatory cytokines, such as interferon-γ (IFN-γ). These cells are also localized to regions such as the lymph nodes, spleen, and skin where they are most likely to encounter antigen. Other cell types, such as vascular endothelium, organ parenchymal cells, and tumor cells, can act as APCs under many conditions. The nature of the responding T cell, the cytokine milieu, and the expression of other cell surface adhesion receptors determine APC function.

Alloreactivity

The discussion to this point has centered on general considerations of antigenic recognition. In transplantation, the response to alloantigens is most germane. The immune response to alloantigens is extraordinarily strong, and the immune system seems obsessed by allelic variations in MHC antigens. Thus, in a culture of human T lymphocytes stimulated with a purified protein antigen (e.g., murine cytochrome C), far less than 1% of the T cells respond to the antigen. Conversely, if the same culture is stimulated with human allogenic cells expressing different MHC alleles, up to 10% of the T cells respond to the antigenic stimulation. In terms of clinical transplantation, this suggests that the immune system is specifically directed against foreign MHC and that any attempts to improve immunosuppression, prevent rejection, and prolong allograft survival depend on a detailed understanding of alloreactivity.

Current cellular and molecular models of alloreactivity rely on the understanding of TCR and MHC structural interactions. The TCR does not recognize MHC alone but as a complex of antigen plus MHC. During T-cell maturation, autoreactive T cells are eliminated or tolerized (see Development of Lymphocytes). Thus, T cells that recognize self-peptides loaded into self-MHC are no longer present or able to respond to antigen. The remaining T cells have TCR specificities that enable them to recognize foreign peptides loaded onto self-MHC molecules, a concept termed *recognition of altered self.* These same T cells may also fortuitously recognize foreign peptides loaded onto allo-MHC or even self-peptides loaded onto allo-MHC. The reason for these other types of recognition is that TCR–antigen–MHC interactions ultimately rely on the three-dimensional interaction of amino acid side chains of the molecules.

Figure 35.9 shows these potential TCR–MHC interactions, including recognition of self-peptides on self-MHC, or an autoimmune response, and various types of alloantigenic responses. The recognition of foreign or self-peptides loaded onto allo-MHC is termed *direct recognition* because intact allo-MHC is being recognized. The response to foreign MHC peptides loaded onto self-MHC is termed *indirect recognition* because

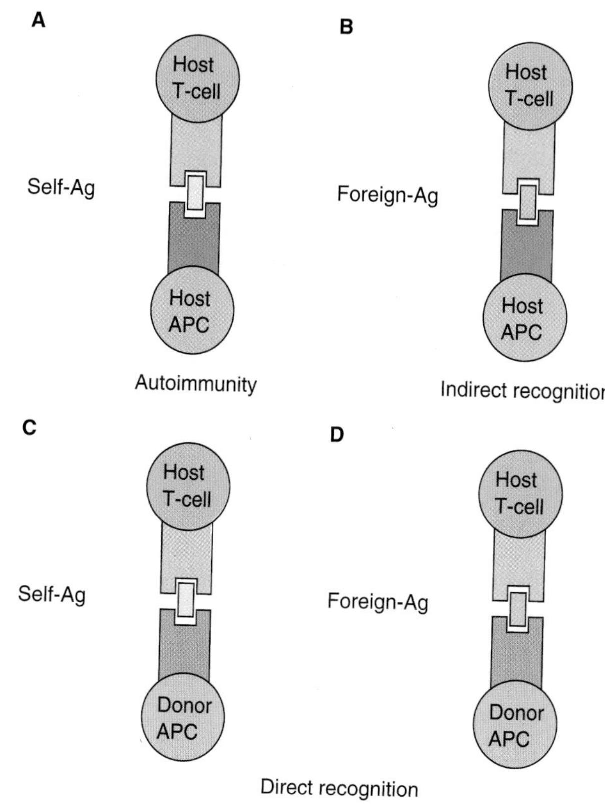

FIGURE 35.9 T-cell receptor recognition of self- and foreign peptide antigen (Ag) in the context of self- or foreign major histocompatibility complex molecules. (*A*) represents autoimmunity; (*B*), (*C*), and (*D*) are aspects of alloimmunity. APC, antigen-presenting cell.

intact allo-MHC is not being recognized. These terms and concepts apply to both class I and class II MHC as well as CD4+ and CD8+ T cells. Most alloreactivity is due to allogenic cells of the donor organ acting as APCs and presenting endogenous peptides in the context of allogenic class I MHC to host CD8+ T cells. However, all permutations of self- and foreign peptides and MHC, and class I and II MHC, have been demonstrated to occur experimentally or clinically. A single T cell may be capable of recognizing one peptide in the context of self-MHC and another peptide in the context of allo-MHC.

Antigenicity

The structural and cellular information in the previous section provides a foundation for considering what determines whether a molecule is perceived as an antigen and how strong an immune response it elicits. In the case of a protein antigen, it must be correctly transported, proteolyzed, loaded onto MHC molecules, and interact with the TCR. Failure to achieve any one of these steps may prevent an appropriate immune response. Immunosuppressive strategies based on this new information are being experimentally evaluated and are discussed later in this chapter. There are many other determinants of antigenicity, such as antigen quaternary structure,[44] location of cell types involved in presenting antigen,[45] the types of T cells present, and the types of cytokines present during the response. These issues are also discussed later in this chapter. The molecular pathways for antigen processing and presentation are defined for *peptide* antigens. Pathways for carbohydrates, lipids, nucleic acids, or derivatives of these are undefined and may have novel interactions with APC pathways or be incapable of eliciting T-cell immunity. The complexity of the response to antigen demonstrates that many potential loci for immunosuppression exist and that to achieve timely, effective immunosuppression, many of these loci may have to be simultaneously disrupted.

Sites of Antigen Recognition

Anatomic Organization of the Immune Response

In vitro experimental studies of immune function often juxtapose stimulator and responder cells in an environment where all possible cellular interactions may take place more or less equally. *In vivo*, the situation is quite different because cells and antigen are sequestered or compartmentalized. Thus, interactions among cells are more restricted, resulting in a channeling of immune responses in certain directions. There are several intersecting levels of anatomic organization of the immune system. First, immature T cells, B cells, and APCs arise centrally in the bone marrow. The initial interaction of T and B cells with the bone marrow microenvironment may determine whether these cells are tolerized to self-antigens expressed in the bone marrow. T cells undergo further maturation and selection in the thymus (see Development of Lymphocytes). Interactions with thymic medullary and cortical tissues determine that self-reactive cells are tolerized, whereas altered-self-reactive cells remain fully functional.

Second, mature cells circulate in the periphery through the lymphatic and vascular systems, passing through lymph nodes. Lymph nodes are highly organized juxtapositions of T cells, B cells, and APCs, which concentrate antigen in the vicinity of responding lymphocytes. For example, a wound infection or a skin graft introduces bacterial antigens or alloantigens, respectively, into the dermis. Antigen is taken up by APCs and transported to regional lymph nodes by lymphatic channels. APCs present antigen to T and B cells, which either reside in the node or recirculate through it. This highly organized and stereotyped sequence of events results in antibody production by B cells and priming of T cells to antigen.

Third, regional collections of lymphoid tissue serve specialized functions. The gut-associated lymphoid tissue (GALT) and bronchial-associated lymphoid tissue (BALT) are collections of lymph nodes (e.g., Peyer's patches) and specialized T and B cells, localized to the gut lumen and tracheobronchial tree, areas expected to have a very high burden of antigen and microbial contamination. Most B cells can secrete IgA in these tissues. IgA, or secretory immunoglobulin, is structurally capable of retaining its functions of opsonization and antimicrobial activity within gut and bronchial secretions. There are also intraepithelial gd TCR T cells of the gut. As mentioned earlier, these cells may have specialized roles in responding to certain microorganisms by virtue of TCR specificity for evolutionarily conserved microbial antigens. The signals that localize IgA+ B cells or $\gamma\delta$+ T cells or that induce cells already present in these regions to express the relevant receptors are not understood.

Fourth, there is a division between the function of central and peripheral lymphoid tissue. Antigen presented peripherally (i.e., subcutaneously or intradermally) localizes to regional lymph nodes and induces long-lived T- and B-cell immunity. Antigen presented centrally (i.e., orally, intrabronchially, or intravenously) may induce transient or local immunity (e.g., intestinal IgA secretion) but also tends to induce systemic unresponsiveness or tolerance to the antigen. This may be an adaptive response to prevent severe, debilitating inflammatory responses to what we ingest or breathe. From the standpoint of transplantation, it may be possible to take advantage of this central versus peripheral difference in antigen presentation to help induce tolerance. What determines this difference is unknown. The possibility that the nature of the APCs in central compartments (e.g., liver, spleen, BALT, GALT) is different from that in the peripheral lymph node has been considered. No such differences, however, have been unequivocally demonstrated. More recent inquiries suggest that the microenvironments (e.g., cytokine levels) differ between central and peripheral compartments and that these differences interact with APCs to channel immune responses in various directions.

Homing and Trafficking

It has long been known that lymphocytes traffic between the vascular and lymphatic compartments and localize to sites of inflammation and that specialized subsets can home to specific anatomic sites (e.g., IgA+ B cells to the gut). Many of the determinants of lymphocyte homing and trafficking have been defined by molecular and cellular techniques, and determining the physiologic roles of these components is now a much more tractable problem. The major issue to understand in homing and trafficking is leukocyte–vascular endothelial cell interactions. This is the initial interaction required in any immune or inflammatory response. It is not possible for a lymphocyte to home, localize, or circulate without first passing through the vascular endothelial layer. Studies using videomicroscopy and blocking specific molecules with antibodies or genetic techniques have shown that this initial interaction can be divided into several steps.[46] Many of these studies have examined neutrophils and monocytes in addition to lymphocytes. In the first step, leukocytes come in contact with the vascular endothelium and adhere to the surface. The cell attaches to and then rolls over the endothelial surface as a result of hemodynamic shear forces. In the second step, the leukocyte is activated to express other receptors and secretes cytokines. The endothelial cell may also become activated and alter receptor expression and cytokine production. In the third step, the leukocyte stops on the endothelial surface, and the adhesive interaction between the cells increases. The final step is transendothelial cell migration.

Each step is associated with several specific interactions between receptors on the leukocyte cell surface and ligands on the endothelial surface or soluble cytokine ligands. Because so many cytokines and surface receptors or ligands have been identified, with many more reported regularly in the literature, the current challenge is to understand how all these signals are integrated in a coherent and specific fashion. Modeling suggests that specific classes of molecules are associated with each of the first three steps of the trafficking process and that these molecules are restricted by cell type.[46] The result is a three-digit "zip code," which may specifically direct neutrophils, monocytes, or lymphocytes to the correct anatomic location. This model is illustrated in Figure 35.10. Different subsets of lymphocytes or other leukocytes can express different receptor and cytokine arrays. Likewise, different subsets of endothelial cells also express different molecular arrays. These differences could account for fine tuning and further specificity of the system.

Cells and Molecules that Participate in Antigen Recognition

T Cells

The central paradigm for the initiation of an immune response is that antigen is taken up by an APC, processed, and then presented to a T cell (Fig. 35.11). The T cell is activated in

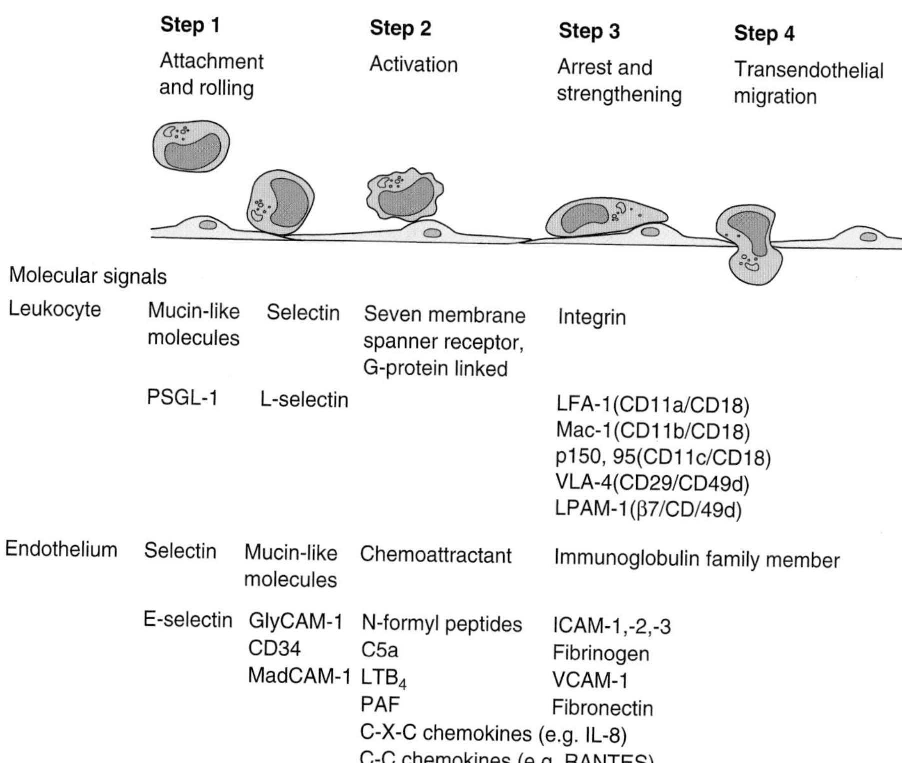

FIGURE 35.10 Model of leukocyte–vascular endothelial cell interactions important for specific trafficking and homing. The three major classes of cellular adhesion receptors—selectins, integrins, immunoglobulin gene superfamily members—play distinct temporal and functional roles. See Table 35.4 for abbreviations.

response to appropriately processed and presented antigen. The activated T cell may become an effector T cell and may also provide help to B cells, other T cells, or even macrophages, which then proceed to act as immune effectors. In this paradigm, the T cell plays a central and indispensable role. For this reason, much of transplantation immunology is directed toward understanding and manipulating T-cell responses.

T cells are divided into two main subclasses: CD4+ and CD8+. CD4+8+ double-positive cells are usually immature T cells or thymocytes, whereas the fully differentiated T cell is usually single positive. Because of the molecular interactions

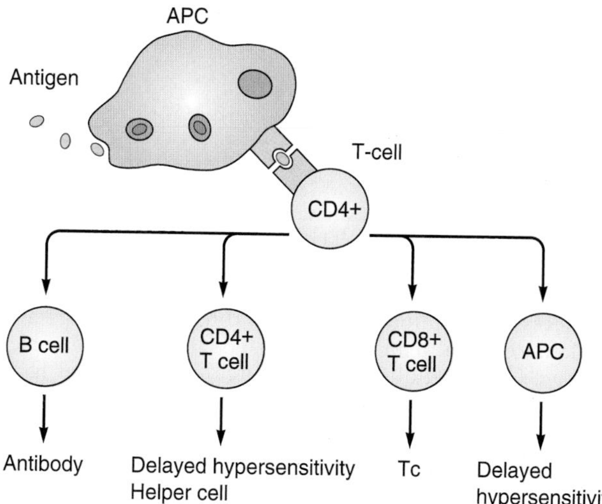

FIGURE 35.11 Central paradigm for cellular initiation of an immune response. CD4+ T cells respond to appropriately presented antigen on antigen-presenting cells (APCs) and in turn help other T cells, B cells, and APCs.

described earlier,[47,48] CD4+ T cells are restricted to recognizing antigen in the context of class II MHC and usually perform roles related to B-cell help, T-cell help, and inflammatory responses, such as delayed and contact hypersensitivity. CD8+ T cells are restricted to class I MHC and often perform cytotoxic functions. Under certain circumstances, particularly experimental conditions with transgenic or knockout-derived cells, CD4+ cells can be class I restricted or perform cytotoxic functions. Conversely, CD8+ cells can be class II restricted or perform helper or inflammatory functions. These findings suggest there is sufficient plasticity in TCR structure and cellular programming that a single T-cell subset can perform the functions of other subsets. This may also imply that blocking or ablating the function of a single T-cell subset may not provide reliable immunosuppression from the standpoint of clinical transplantation. However, the complexity of immunoregulatory systems might permit the manipulation of a single T-cell subset to determine the responses of other T-cell subsets.

The CD4+ T cells fall into one of two major subsets, termed *T helper type 1* (T_H1) and *type 2* (T_H2) (Table 35.3). T_H1 cells are characterized by proinflammatory, delayed-type hypersensitivity effector functions and the release of IFN-g. T_H2 cells are characterized by providing B-cell help, suppressing T-cell responses, and releasing interleukin (IL)-4, IL-5, and IL-10. IL-4 and IL-5 promote B-cell differentiation, maturation, and immunoglobulin production, and IL-4 may act as a feedback cytokine to promote further T_H2 proliferation and inhibit T_H1 and IFN-γ. IL-10 may also inhibit IFN-γ production. Conversely, IFN-γ may promote T_H1 and inhibit T_H2 production. Furthermore, the potent macrophage-derived T-cell-stimulatory cytokine, IL-12, also promotes T_H1 production. Current models suggest that T_H1 and T_H2 form a regulatory circuit in which one subset inhibits the activity of the other (Fig. 35.12). These models imply that the channeling of an immune response occurs early and is determined by the relative balance of T_H subsets and their cytokines.

TABLE 35.3

T_H1 AND T_H2 SUBCLASSES

Subclass	Function	Cytokines produced
T_H1	Effect delayed-type hypersensitivity	IL-2
	Effect contact sensitivity	IFN-τ
	Provide T_c help	(Respond to IL-12)
T_H2	Provide B-cell help	IL-2
	Suppress T-cell responses	IL-4
		IL-5
		IL-10

IFN, interferon; IL, interleukin.

Several uncertainties about the T_H1/T_H2 model remain.[49,50] Although these subsets have been repeatedly demonstrated in murine experimental systems, it is not clear whether the human subsets are so well defined and compartmentalized. There may be more overlap in humans. Second, it is not clear if T_H1 and T_H2 interconvert or if their phenotype represents terminal differentiation. A related issue is whether T_H1 and T_H2 are derived from a common T_H0 precursor or if they represent more distant and distinct lineages. Third, the amount and ratio of IL-12, IL-4, IL-2, and IFN-γ at the initiation of an immune response determine whether T_H1 or T_H2 predominate, yet the initial determinants of these cytokine levels are not well known. Nonetheless, the recognition that distinct cytokines can channel immunity has led to much current experimental and clinical work in which these cytokines are used to drive responses. IL-12 is being considered as a way to boost tumor immunity, and IL-10 is being used to suppress allograft responses.

In many texts, CD8+ T cells are also said to perform suppressor functions. The situation is more complicated than this. Experimental results demonstrate that both CD4+ and CD8+ T cells can act as T_S.[51–55] In addition, non-T cells may also act as suppressor cells in some circumstances.[56] The major problem with most descriptions of suppressor cells is that a phenotypically well-defined population has not been isolated. Thus, only vague descriptions of suppressor cells and their phenotypes have been available. The notion of T_H1 and T_H2 subsets has provided a new context in which to view T_S. Instead of supposing that T_S down-regulate all responses, it is now considered more likely that T_S channel immunity in one direction or another. Thus, T_H2 cells suppress T_H1 and T_C function while supporting B-cell responses.

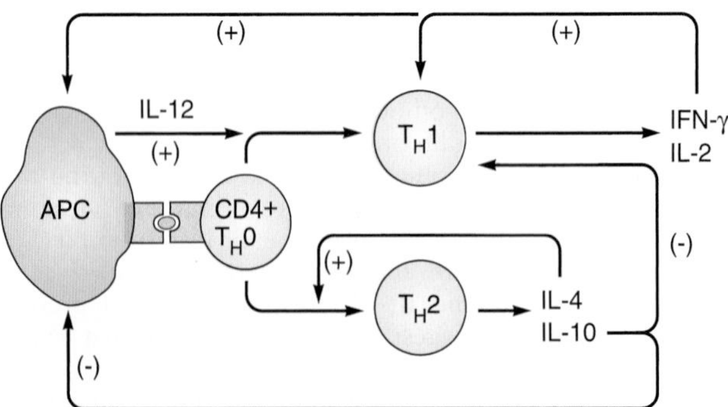

FIGURE 35.12 T helper type 1 (T_H1)/T_H2 paradigm of CD4+ T-cell subsets. APC, antigen-presenting cell; IFN-γ, interferon-γ; IL, interleukin.

Current models suggest that T_H2 cells are the relevant T_S of cell-mediated immunity, and attempts to boost T_H2 responses during organ allografting are seen as a way to promote graft survival.[52]

B Cells

B cells develop initially in the bone marrow, recirculate throughout the vascular and lymphatic systems, and initiate primary and secondary antibody responses, particularly in the germinal centers of lymph nodes. B cells, T cells, and APC-type dendritic cells are brought into close juxtaposition in germinal centers, concentrating antigen to the relevant cells and receptors of the immune system. B cells primarily produce IgM antibody for primary responses and other isotypes for secondary responses. Antibody then performs effector functions of complement fixation, opsonization, clearance, or feedback immune regulation through idiotype–antiidiotype interactions. B-cell responses may be *T independent,* in which B cells respond to antigen in the absence of T_H. These are usually, but not exclusively, IgM responses to polymeric antigens bearing multiple identical epitopes, such as bacterial cell wall polysaccharides. T-independent responses may occur after transplantation and result in graft damage or loss. T-independent responses are also responsible for much of the natural antibody found in graft recipients. Natural antibody is preformed immunoglobulin directed toward alloantigens, despite no previous exposure of the individual to the alloantigen. The antibody putatively arises from exposure to cross-reactive environmental antigens.

T-dependent responses require the T-cell–APC–B-cell interaction. This interaction requires coordinated signaling among these cells of numerous cell surface and soluble ligands. The specificity of the interaction is ensured by the specificity of the T- and B-cell receptors for antigen. Thereafter, a series of nonclonally distributed receptors and ligands interact to amplify and modulate these signals. Figure 35.13 shows some of the important cell surface receptor interactions that take place during T-cell stimulation of B cells. Because so many potential interactions may occur, it is unclear which signals are absolutely required or how any one receptor or group of receptors may alter the function of other receptors. Nonetheless, current models[57–61] suggest that the interactions of primary importance are as follows:

- TCR–antigen–class II MHC–CD4
- Antigen–sIgM (B-cell antigen receptor)
- CD28–CD80 (B7-1)/CD86 (B7-2)
- CD40–CD40L

Failure to engage these receptors severely or completely inhibits appropriate responses. Secondary receptor–ligand interactions of importance include CD11a/18 [leukocyte functional antigen-1 (LFA-1)]–CD54 [intercellular adhesion molecule-1 (ICAM-1)], CD2–CD58 (LFA-3), and CD19–(unknown ligand). Failure to achieve these interactions, however, does not necessarily inhibit the B-cell response. Cytokines also required for T and B interactions include IL-4 and IL-5, which promote immunoglobulin class switching to IgE and IgG4 production, and IL-10 and IL-12, which promote switching to IgG1, IgG2, IgG3, and IgA.

The molecular signaling between T and B cells demonstrates that the B cell is not a passive member of the pair that merely receives T-cell–derived signals and then secretes immunoglobulin. As T cells become activated, they express CD40 ligand (CD40L), which binds to CD40 on B cells and activates B cells. B cells in turn then express more CD80 (B7/BB1), which binds to the T cell CD28 receptor. CD28

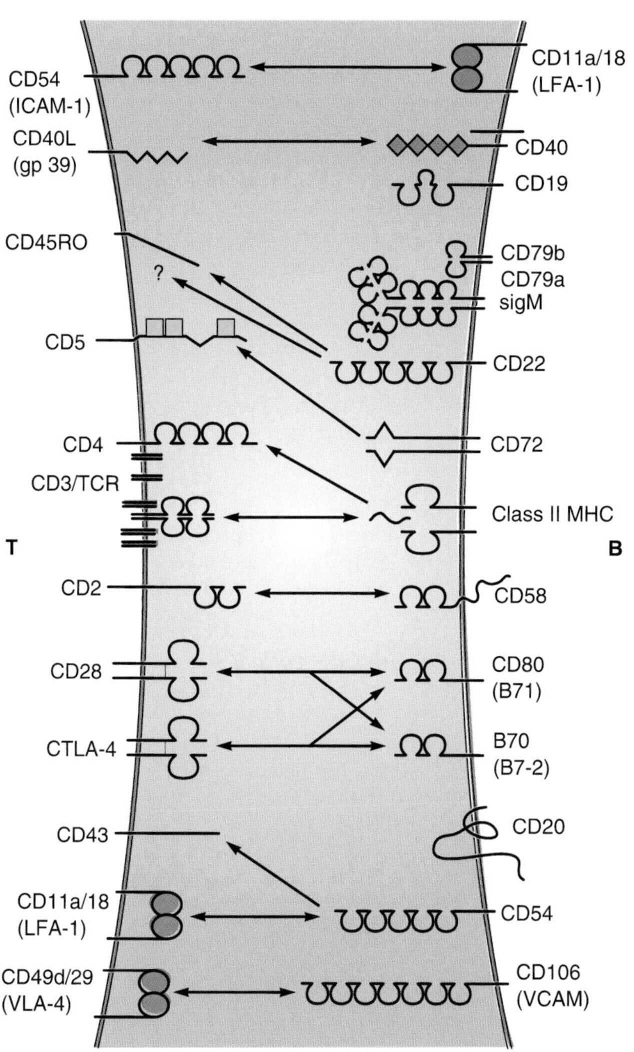

FIGURE 35.13 Adhesion receptors that may mediate interactions between CD4+ T cells and B cells. ICAM-1, intercellular adhesion molecule-1; LFA-1, leukocyte functional antigen-1; MHC, major histocompatibility complex; TCR, T-cell receptor; VCAM, vascular cell adhesion molecule; VLA-4, very late antigen-4.

ligation provides a potent costimulatory signal to T cells, which synergizes with TCR/CD3-derived activational signals. Therefore, there is important bidirectional T and B communication. B-cell–derived immunoglobulins may also regulate T and B immunity through idiotype–antiidiotype interactions. In this case, an antibody recognizes and binds to the polymorphic antigen-binding region of B- or T-cell antigen receptors. The interaction can positively or negatively regulate immunity. Last, the B cell itself may act as an APC. The ability of surface immunoglobulin to bind low concentrations of antigen with high affinity makes B cells particularly efficient APCs. As Fig. 35.13 shows, B cells express the relevant ligands and receptors for direct T-cell interactions. Thus, the T–APC–B ternary complex may really be a T–B binary complex. This is probably the major interaction during secondary responses, when T and B cells are already partially activated and express many of the relevant receptors. For primary responses, CD40L, CD80, CD86, and other receptors are not yet upregulated, and direct T–B interactions are less efficient. In this case, professional APCs are likely required to initiate appropriate immunity.

Antigen-presenting Cells

It has already been mentioned that virtually any cell type may perform the functions of an APC because many of the steps of processing and presentation take advantage of ubiquitous, constitutive cellular pathways. Most frequently, the term *antigen-presenting cell* is applied to monocyte/macrophage or dendritic cells because both express class I and class II MHC, the cells are specialized to take up extracellular components and catabolize them, and these cells are histologically and anatomically located at sites most relevant for antigen entry and recognition. Based on these criteria, B cells are also efficient APCs and are usually most relevant for secondary responses when T cells are already primed or partially activated.

Another cell type of major importance for APC function, particularly in organ allografting, is the vascular endothelial cell.[62–71] As discussed earlier, this is the cell with which the immune system first comes in contact and that directs the homing, trafficking, and egress of lymphocytes into regions of inflammation. Vascular endothelial cells are dynamic in their ability to process and present antigen and direct lymphocyte function. Quiescent endothelial cells are far less efficient and active with these processes than activated cells are. Activation usually occurs as a result of antigen nonspecific signals during inflammation. Trauma, burns, ischemia, infection, allografting, or any other proinflammatory condition can activate endothelial cells. The signals most relevant for endothelial activation are the cytokines IL-1 and IL-4, tumor necrosis factor (TNF), and bacterial lipopolysaccharide. In turn, activated endothelial cells produce cytokines [IL-1, IL-6, IL-8, IFN-γ, and transforming growth factor (TGF-β)] and display cell surface receptors important for presentation or trafficking [class II MHC, increased class I MHC, vascular cell adhesion molecule-1 (VCAM-1), ELAM-1, and P-selectin]. From the standpoint of transplantation, nonimmunologic events, such as prolonged cold ischemic time or the type of preservation solution, can profoundly affect endothelial cell function and integrity and subsequent lymphocyte–endothelial cell interactions. Despite close tissue matching and good immunosuppression, these nonimmunologic events can activate endothelium, which in turn activates lymphocytes and other leukocytes and facilitates the development of antigen-dependent, immunologic organ rejection.

Adhesion Receptors

An essential feature of lymphocyte communication is the interaction of cell surface receptors with specific ligands.[72–78] As shown in Figures 35.10 and 35.13, a large number of potential interactions among T cells, B cells, APCs, and vascular endothelial cells can occur. Several features are important. First, although these molecules have often been called *adhesion molecules,* most are transmembrane proteins linked to cytoplasmic second messengers. Therefore, receptor engagement is likely to lead to a series of second signals that may alter the transcriptional activation of a wide array of genes and subsequently cellular function. Adhesion is only one function of these molecules.

Although it is possible to describe in detail the individual function of any single receptor–ligand pair, the issue of understanding the integration of many different signals has been a less tractable problem. Figure 35.10 shows current models that assign these receptors to a few related molecular groups and to a few functionally separate steps. Clearly, the immune system has an extraordinary amount of redundancy, so that if a single pathway or receptor–ligand pair is compromised, it is likely that other processes circumvent the block.

Adhesion receptors are classified into three major groups based on structural similarities. The *selectins* are transmembrane glycoproteins. The amino-terminal domain is lectinlike in structure. Lectins are molecules that bind carbohydrates. The amino-terminal domain is followed by a domain with homology to epidermal growth factor. This domain is followed by two to nine repeated domains with homology to complement-binding proteins. The ligands for selectins are mucin-like molecules containing large amounts of carbohydrate presumably bound by the lectin domain. Distinct selectins are recognized on leukocytes, platelets, and endothelial cells and termed L-selectins, P-selectins, and E-selectins (Table 35.4). *Integrins* are heterodimeric transmembrane proteins. There are at least eight known integrin β chains that can associate with a wide variety of α chains, generating a large number of possible combinations. The ligands for integrins include many basement membrane components and immunoglobulin gene superfamily members. *Immunoglobulin gene superfamily*

TABLE 35.4

ADHESION RECEPTORS

Molecule	Primary expression	Ligand
SELECTINS		
L-selectin (CD62L)	PMN, lymphocytes	CD34, GlyCAM-1, MAdCAM-1
P-selectin (CD62P)	EC, platelets	P-selectin glycoprotein ligand (PSGL-1) Sialyl Lewis* and others
E-selectin (CD62E)	EC	Sialyl Lewis* and others
INTEGRINS		
LFA-1 (CD11a/CD18) (β_2, αL)	PMN, lymphocytes	ICAM-1, ICAM-2
Mac-1 (CD11b/CD18) (β_2/αM)	PMN	ICAM-1, IC3b, Fibrinogen, LPS
VLA-4 ($\alpha_4\beta_1$ integrin)	Eosinophils, lymphocytes	VCAM-1, FN
Integrin subunits	**Ligands and counterreceptors**	**Integrin name**
β_1 α_1	Collagens, laminin	VLA-1
α_2	Collagens, laminin	VLA-2
α_3	Fibronectin, laminin, collagens	VLA-3
α_4	Fibronectin, VCAM-1	VLA-4
α_5	Fibronectin	VLA-5
α_6	Laminin	VLA-6
α_7	Laminin	VLA-7
α_8	7	
α_V	Vitronectin, fibronectin	
β_2 α_L	ICAM-1, ICAM-2, ICAM-3	LFA-1
α_M	IC3b, fibrinogen, factor X, ICAM-1	Mac-1
α_X	Fibrinogen	p150, 95
β_3 α_{IIb}	Fibrinogen, fibronectin, von Willebrand factor, vitronectin, thrombospondin	
α_V	Vitronectin, fibrinogen, von Willebrand factor, thrombospondin, fibronectin, osteopontin, collagen	
β_4 α_4	?	
β_5 α_V	Vitronectin	
β_6 α_V	Fibronectin	
β_7 (=β_p?) α_4	Fibronectin, VCAM-1, MAdCAM-1	LPAM-1
α_{IEL}	?	
β_8 α_V	?	
IMMUNOGLOBULIN SUPERFAMILY		
ICAM-1 (CD54)	Lymphocytes, EC	LFA-1, Mac-1
ICAM-2 (CD102)	Lymphocytes, EC	LFA-1
VCAM-1 (CD106)	EC	VLA-4
PECAM-1	EC, PMN, lymphocytes, platelets	?
MAdCAM-1	EC	LPAM-1
CD28	T	CD80 (B7/BB1)
CTLA4	T	CD80, B70/B7-2, B7-3
CD2	T, NK, some B	CD58 (LFA-3), possibly CD59

PMN, polymorphonuclear cell; EC, endothelial cells; T, T cells; NK, natural killer cells; B, B cells; ICAM, intercellular adhesion molecule; PECAM, platelet–endothelial cell adhesion molecule; VCAM, vascular cell adhesion molecule.

members share structural similarities to antibody, particularly tandem extracellular domains each containing a disulfide bond. The ligands for these molecules are often integrin family members. Many cells express both members of the receptor and ligand pair simultaneously. For example, both T and B cells express the selectin LFA-1 (CD11a/CD18) and the immunoglobulin family member ICAM-1 (CD54). How receptor function is regulated such that a cell does not bind to its own surface is not known. Adhesion receptors do not play passive adhesive roles, merely binding ligands that are presented to them. They are involved in more active regulatory processes.

Cytokines and Cytokine Receptors

Immune cells communicate not only by direct cell–cell contact but also by soluble factors called *cytokines*. The problem with understanding cytokine action is similar to the problem of defining receptor function. There are so many known cytokines (Table 35.5) that although individual detailed actions are defined, many of these actions overlap and it is not yet possible to integrate these signals into a unified model.[79–102] Furthermore, many different cell types are capable of expressing each cytokine or cytokine receptor. This makes it difficult to define any specificity of cytokine function. Nonetheless, several generalizations have practical implications.

First, the chemoattractant cytokines are important for leukocyte homing and trafficking (see Fig. 35.10). Table 35.5 shows that these molecules are categorized according to structural criteria.

Second, the central paradigm of T-cell–APC–B-cell interaction (Fig. 35.11) relies on the production of a few cytokines (Fig. 35.14). The initial CD4+ T-cell–APC interaction results in IL-1 production by APCs, which stimulates CD4+ T cells. These cells then produce IL-2, IL-4, and IL-5. IL-2 and IL-4 help stimulate CD8+ T cells and B cells or even self-stimulate CD4+ T cells by a mechanism termed *autocrine stimulation*. IL-5 primarily helps B cells. Many other cytokines, however, are involved even in this central paradigm (Fig. 35.12). Blockade of any single cytokine rarely impairs the stimulatory process because other cytokines tend to be redundant.

Third, the distinction between receptors and cytokines is often blurred. Alternative mRNA splicing, posttranslational modifications, or cell surface endopeptidases can convert cell

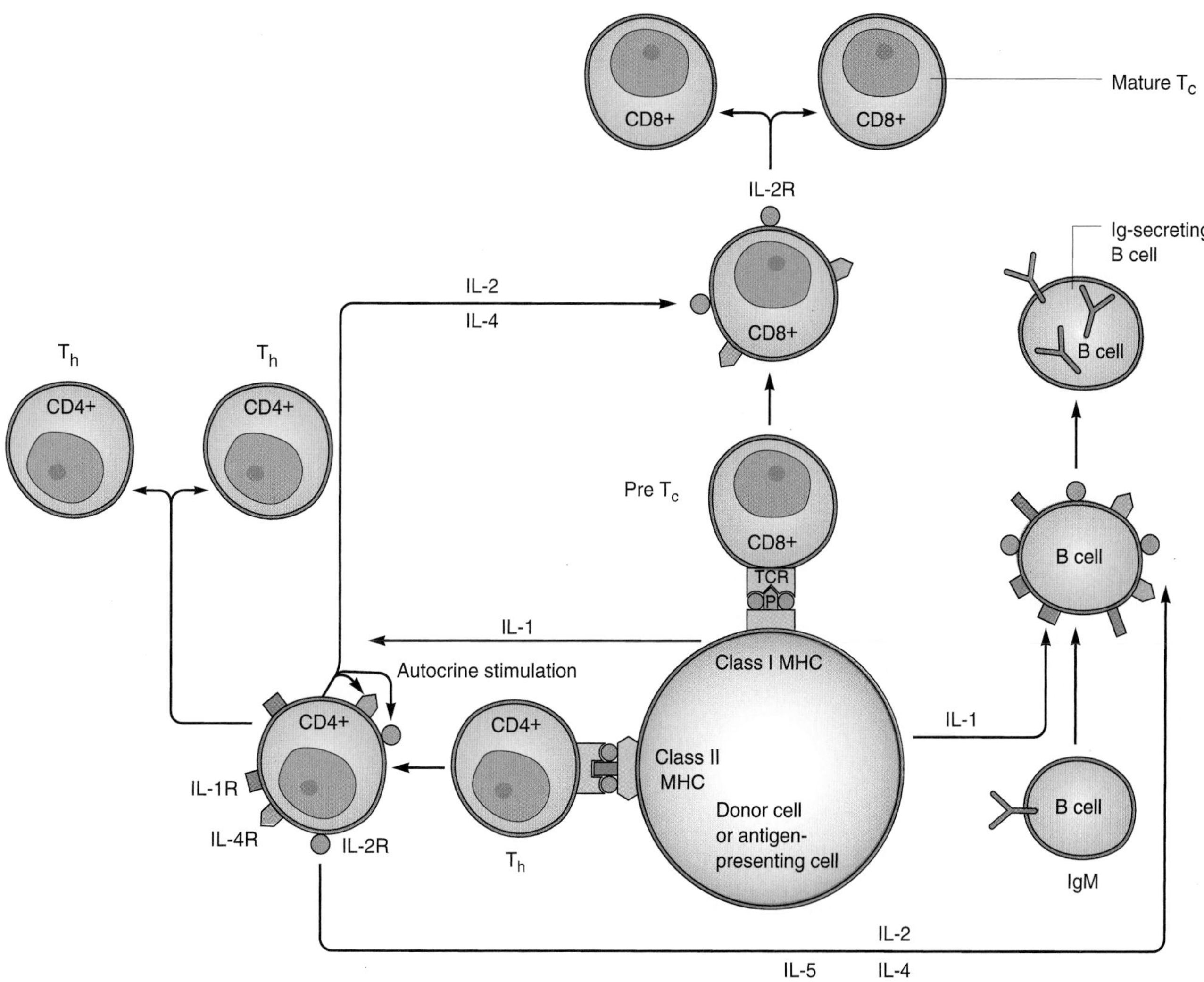

FIGURE 35.14 T- and B-cell activation. Two signals are required. First, alloantigen binds to antigen-specific receptors–the T-cell receptor (TCR; T cells) or surface immunoglobulin M (IgM; B cells). The second, or costimulatory, signal is provided by interleukin (IL)-1 released by the antigen-presenting cell. CD4+ helper T cells (T_H) release IL-2, IL-4, and IL-5, which provide help for CD8+ cytotoxic T cells (T_C) and for B-cell activation. MHC, major histocompatibility complex.

TABLE 35.5

CYTOKINE AND CYTOKINE RECEPTORS

	Origin	Responding cells
CYTOKINE		
IL-1α or -β	Monocytes, EC	T, B, EC
IL-2	T, B	T, B, monocytes, EC
IL-3	T	T
IL-4	T	T, B, monocytes, mast cells, EC, eosinophils
IL-5	T	T, B, eosinophils
IL-6	T, B, monocytes, EC	T, B, EC
IL-7	T	T, B, monocytes
IL-8	T, EC, monocytes	T, EC, neutrophils
IL-9	T	T, mast cells
IL-10	T	T, B, monocytes
IL-11	Fibroblasts	B, megakaryocytes
IL-12	Monocytes	T, B, NK
IL-13	?	B, monocytes
IL-14	?	B
IFN-α or -β	EC	T, B, EC
IFN-t	T, B	T, B, EC
TNF-α	T, B, EC	T, B, EC
TNF-β	T	T, B, EC
G-CSF	Fibroblasts, osteoblasts	Granulocytes
GM-CSF	T	Granulocytes, monocytes
M-CSF	Fibroblasts, monocytes	Monocytes
Classic Chemoattractants		
N-formyl peptide	Bacterial	Monocytes, granulocytes
C5a	Complement activation	Monocytes, granulocytes
LTB4	Arachidonate metabolism	Monocytes, neutrophils
PAF	Phosphotidylcholine metabolism	Monocytes, granulocytes
C-X-C Chemokines		
IL-B	T, EC, monocytes	T, EC, neutrophils
β-Thromboglobulin	Platelets	T, granulocytes
C-C Chemokines		
MCP-1	T, EC, monocytes	Monocytes
MIP-1α, β	T, monocytes	T, monocytes, granulocytes
RANTES	T, platelets	Monocytes
CYTOKINE RECEPTORS		
Type 1 Cytokine Receptors (Hematopoietin Receptors)		
IL-2, -4, -7, -9, -13, -15 receptors (share γ-chain)		
IL-3, -5, GM-CSF receptors (share KH97 subunit)		
LIF, OSM, CNTF, IL-6, IL-1 1 receptors (share gp130 subunit)		
GH, PRL		
EPO, G-CSF		
Type II Cytokine Receptors		
IFN-α, -β, -γ		
TNF-Like Receptors		
TNF-α, TNF-β receptors		
gp39 (CD30-L)		
CD27-L, CD30-L		
NGF, 4-1 BB		
Fas		
TGF-β Receptor Family		
TGF-β1, TGF-βII receptors (share common ISR-1 subunit)		
Activin receptor-II, -IIβ		
IL-8 Receptor Family (Seven-Membrane Spanner, G-Linked Proteins)		
IL-8R		
C5α-R		
PAF-R		
fMLP-R		

EC, endothelial cells; T, T cells; B, B cells; (G, GM, M)-CSF, (granulocyte, granulocyte–monocyte, macrophage) colony-stimulating factor; IL, interleukin; IFN, interferon; TNF, tumor necrosis factor; NGF, nerve growth factor; PAF, plateplet activating factor; GH, growth hormone; PRL, prolactin; EPO, erythropoletin; LIF, leukocyte inhibitory factors; OSM, oncostatin M; CNTF, ciliary neutrophic factor.

bond receptors into soluble mediators or vice versa. For example, TNF-α can be found as a soluble or cell surface molecule. Cytokine receptors can be processed into soluble fragments that still bind the relevant cytokine. In this case, the soluble receptor may act as an inhibitor of cytokine function because it prevents the interaction of the cytokine with its specific cell surface receptor. Alternatively, these same soluble receptors may prolong the serum half-life of cytokines by preventing proteolytic degradation and may transport the active cytokine to regions of inflammation or antigen presentation. In this case, the soluble receptor potentiates rather than inhibits cytokine function. This situation occurs with a soluble TNF receptor. Soluble forms of the TCR and class I MHC molecules have also been described. Although their physiologic roles are uncertain, both suppressor and activator functions have been ascribed to these molecules. Likewise, B-cell immunoglobulin may be cell bound and act as the B-cell antigen-specific receptor or circulate freely as soluble antibody performing a variety of immune regulatory or effector functions.

Fourth, cytokine receptors are often heteromeric complexes sharing common subunits with other cytokine receptors and possessing unique but related subunits that confer specificity for an individual cytokine. Genetic or pharmacologic interference with receptor function may therefore impair the effects of only one or of several cytokines. For example, the IL-2, IL-4, IL-7, IL-9, IL-13, and IL-15 receptors all have related cytokine-specific subunits and share a common g subunit. The same is true for the IL-6, IL-11, leukemia inhibitory factor (LIF), oncostatin M (OSM), and ciliary neurotrophic factor (CNTF) receptors, and the IL-3, IL-5, and granulocyte–monocyte colony-stimulating factor (GM-CSF) receptors.

EFFECTOR MECHANISMS OF THE IMMUNE RESPONSE

Cellular Effectors

Once primed and activated, T cells, B cells, and APCs perform the effector functions of graft rejection.[103–110] B cells secrete specific antibody that binds to the allograft cell surface and can kill cells by complement-mediated lysis. Antibody may also alter graft cell function by binding to and cross-linking important cell surface receptors, causing receptor blockade, receptor activation, or inappropriate cellular responses. Antibody may also direct other cells, which possess receptors for the constant region of the immunoglobulin molecule, termed *Fc receptors* (FcRs), to the allogenic cells. Many cell types express FcRs, including T cells, APCs, natural killer (NK) cells, and granulocytes. These FcR+ cells may damage or kill cells with antibody bound to the cell surface by a process called *antibody-dependent cellular cytotoxicity.*

Monocytes and macrophages, the prototypical APCs, become activated by CD4+ T cells during the initial encounter with antigen (Fig. 35.11). These activated APCs can then cause local tissue destruction through direct cell lysis and phagocytosis or indirectly through release of cytotoxic cytokines (e.g., TNF and lymphotoxin). CD4+ T cells can also generate local tissue destruction through inflammatory processes similar to delayed-type hypersensitivity. Cytotoxic lymphokines are released and other inflammatory cells, such as APCs, are recruited to the local environment.

Cytotoxic CD8+ T lymphocytes kill target cells through direct cell contact. Killer T cells have cytoplasmic granules containing a series of cytotoxic proteins. Contact with a target cell causes the release of these granules onto or into the target. Granule contents include perforins, which assemble to form pores in the target cell membrane, making the cells leaky and susceptible to osmotic death. Granzymes are a series of serine proteases that can disrupt normal intracellular proteins. Cytotoxic T cells also kill cells by engaging a target cell surface receptor called *Fas*, a member of the TNF receptor family (see Table 35.5). The interaction of the Fas ligand on the T-cell surface with Fas on the target cell surface leads to apoptotic target cell death. Fas and Fas ligand are distributed not only throughout the immune system but also on many other cell types. Fas is probably a general mechanism for determining cellular responses to development, immune activation, and oncogenesis. The regulation and control of the cellular response to engagement of Fas by its ligand involves a poorly understood series of cytoplasmic events comprising second messenger pathways and transcriptional regulators. Delineation of these events will probably lead to important methods for controlling cytotoxic responses.

In addition to the aforementioned cells, a number of other cell types probably also participate in the process of graft destruction and rejection, although their precise roles are not well understood. NK cells are large granular lymphocytes lacking immunoglobulin and most T-cell surface markers.[111,112] They do, however, express CD2 (characteristic of T cells) and a subclass of FcR known as CD16, which is characteristic of some B cells. NK cells also express the IL-2 receptor, secrete numerous cytokines (IL-1, IL-2, IL-3, IL-4, IL-6, GM-CSF, TNF, IFN-α, IFN-γ), and produce cytotoxic granzymes and phospholipases. NK cells function by lysing target cells that lack MHC class I. The mechanism by which NK cells recognize targets is through a series of nonclonally distributed receptors that inhibit NK cells if MHC class I is bound, while permitting NK mediated lysis if the receptor is unoccupied. The precise role of NK cells in allograft rejection is not understood, but these cells may be found infiltrating rejecting grafts, and it is presumed they are recruited to the inflammatory site.

Eosinophils are classically found throughout acutely rejecting allografts. Their role and function in graft rejection is also not understood, but they do perform potent cytotoxic effector functions. IL-5, which is secreted by CD4+ T_H2 cells, is a potent trophic cytokine for eosinophils. The process of T-cell activation may therefore recruit eosinophils to rejecting grafts.[113]

Other cell types, including neutrophils, basophils, and mast cells, can also be found in rejecting grafts or other inflammatory processes.[114,115] These cells are presumably recruited to regions of inflammation by cytokines and changes in vascular endothelium. These cells have direct cytotoxic effects, produce cytotoxic cytokines, and recruit additional cells to their locality.

Soluble Effectors

The soluble cytokines have been discussed thus far in terms of promoting homing and trafficking, inducing antigen-specific immunity, and amplifying immune responses. Cytokines also participate directly in the process of inflammation or graft destruction.[116–124] TNF-α and TNF-β have direct cytotoxic effects on parenchymal cells and may help mediate the final effector pathway. Many other cytokines (e.g., IL-2, IL-4, IL-5, IL-6, IL-10, and IFN-γ) can be found in rejecting allografts. These cytokines are probably not directly cytotoxic, but recruit additional cells and amplify those already present.

Many other soluble mediators are probably also involved in allograft destruction. Antibody-directed, complement-mediated lysis is an important mechanism in hyperacute and some forms of acute rejection.[125] Clotting factors are activated when vascular endothelium is compromised by antibody, cytokines, or cell-mediated injury. Obviously, vascular thrombosis is lethal to vascularized organ allografts. Injured vessels may also release the potent vasoconstricting peptide endothelin, further decreasing blood flow to injured grafts.[126] Kinins, prostaglandins, and prostacyclins may all participate in the effector stage of the inflammatory response, serving to potentiate cellular injury or recruit more proinflammatory cells.[127] Oxygen intermediates, such as nitric oxide and oxygen free radicals, are also likely important mediators of tissue destruction in transplantation.[128–131] So many potential mediators of cellular death make it difficult to control the process at the effector stage. Strategies that interfere with only a single cytotoxic pathway are unlikely to have major therapeutic effects. It will be necessary to subvert many effector pathways or to block initiation processes further upstream of effector mechanisms.

Clinical Syndromes

The wide variety of immune effector mechanisms results in a limited number of defined presentations in clinical transplantation (Figs. 35.15 to 35.18). The pathologic definition of these presentations is defined by the Banff classification system. *Hyperacute rejection* is the result of preformed antibody binding to the allograft at the time of revascularization in the operating room. Complement is activated, resulting in endothelial cell activation, vascular leak, recruitment of platelets and neutrophils, thrombosis of vessels, and destruction of the graft within minutes to hours. Hyperacute rejection can occur if transplantations are performed across an ABO incompatibility or if the recipient possesses high-titer anti-donor class I HLA antibodies.[132] Because current clinical protocols test for the presence of such incompatibilities or antibodies (see Important Aspects of Antigenicity and Immunity for Clinical Transplantation), hyperacute rejection should not occur. Kidney, heart, pancreas, and lung allografts are all susceptible to hyperacute rejection; however, liver grafts are relatively resistant to this process and are often transplanted across antibody differences (termed a *positive crossmatch*) and even across an ABO difference. The reason for this resistance is not understood but may relate to the large mass of hepatic parenchyma and its ability to absorb antibody and complement or to the way antibody and complement interact with hepatic endothelium and its dual blood supply. In addition, hyperacute rejection is responsible for the major barrier to xenotransplantation (across-species barrier).[133] Most mammals

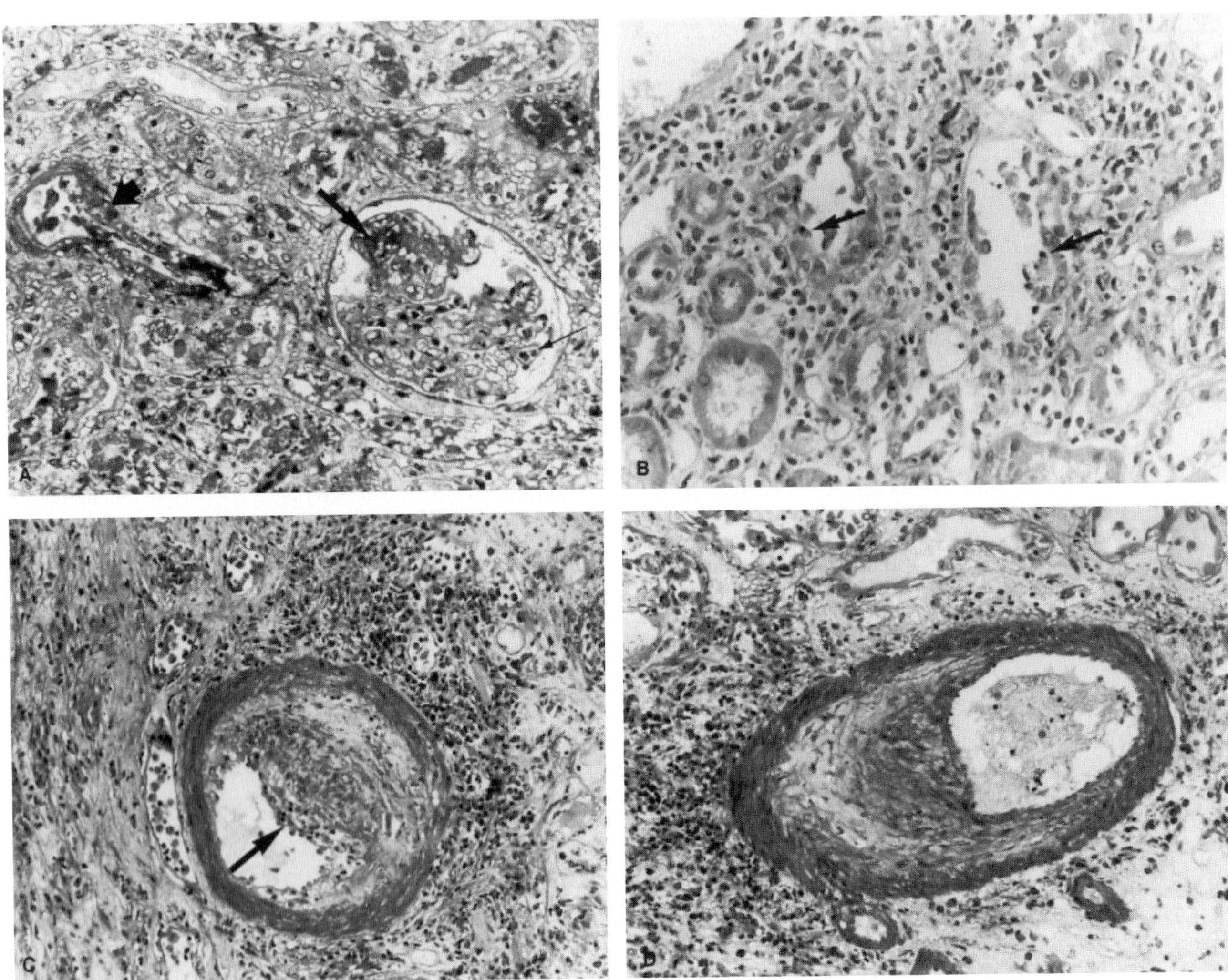

FIGURE 35.15 Kidney rejection. (*A*) Hyperacute rejection characterized by microthrombi in the glomerular capillaries (*large arrow*), infiltration with neutrophils (*small thin arrow*), and endothelial destruction (*thick arrow*). (*B*) Acute tubulointerstitial rejection showing an interstitial lymphocytic infiltrate, interstitial edema, and infiltration of lymphocytes into the epithelium of the tubules (tubulitis; *arrows*). (*C*) Acute vascular rejection with a subendothelial lymphocytic infiltrate (*arrow*), along with some evidence of chronic vascular rejection. (*D*) Chronic rejection with severe proliferative endarteritis. (Courtesy of Roger D. Smith, M.D.).

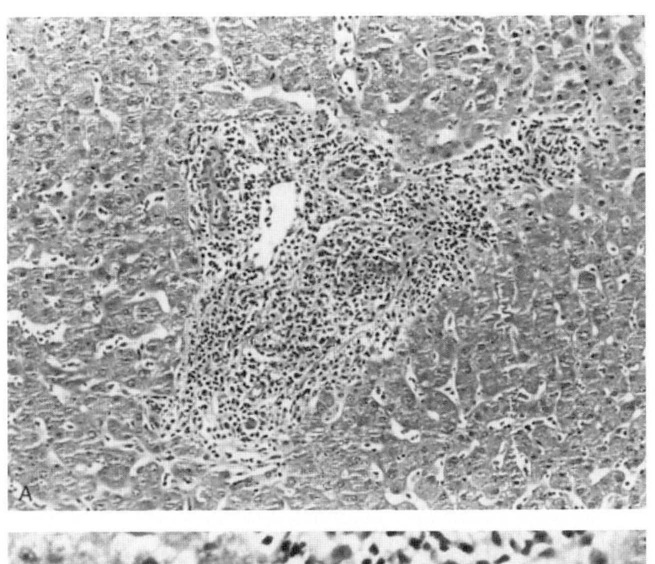

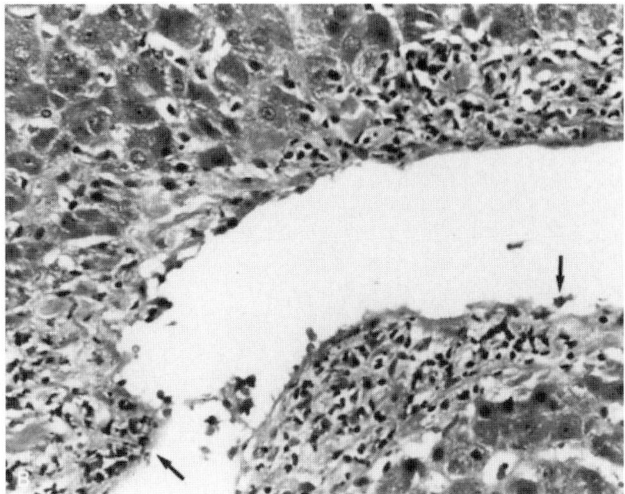

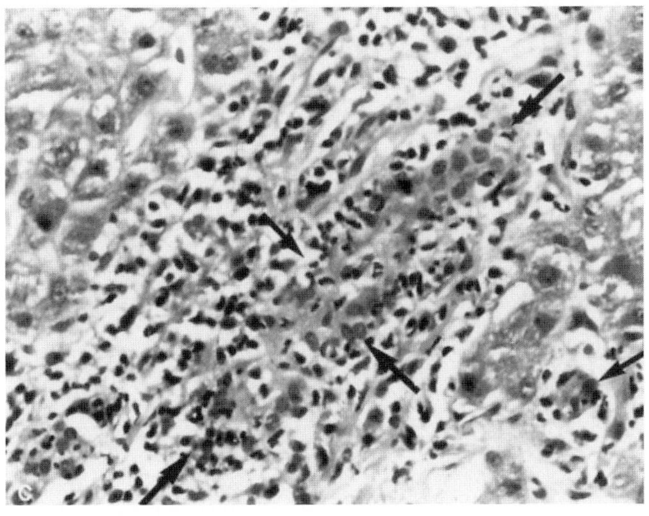

FIGURE 35.16 Liver rejection. (*A*) Acute rejection is characterized by a mixed portal inflammatory infiltrate of lymphocytes, plasma cells, eosinophils, and neutrophils. (*B*) The portal vein shows subendothelial inflammation and endothelialitis (*arrows*). (*C*) Bile duct destruction has occurred as a result of infiltrating mononuclear cells. (Courtesy of Makunda Ray, M.D.)

have high-titer, preformed antibodies directed against cell surface antigens of other species. The current challenge in experimental xenotransplantation is to control antibody and complement function and prevent hyperacute rejection.

Acute rejection usually occurs days to weeks after transplantation; it rarely occurs months or years later. Acute rejection is initiated by T-cell–dependent immunity and is characterized microscopically by a lymphocytic infiltrate accompanied by plasma cells, eosinophils, and a few mast cells or neutrophils. In the kidney, the infiltrate is in the tubular interstitium, causing a tubulitis. Particularly severe forms also cause a vasculitis or vascular rejection. Hepatic acute cellular rejection is typically a mixed cellular infiltrate in the portal triad with eosinophils, disruption of biliary endothelium, and portal venous endothelialitis. The heart demonstrates an interstitial lymphocytic myositis, whereas the lung shows varying degrees

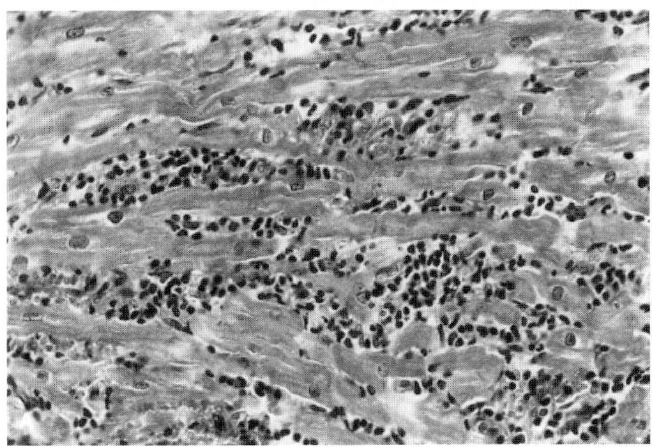

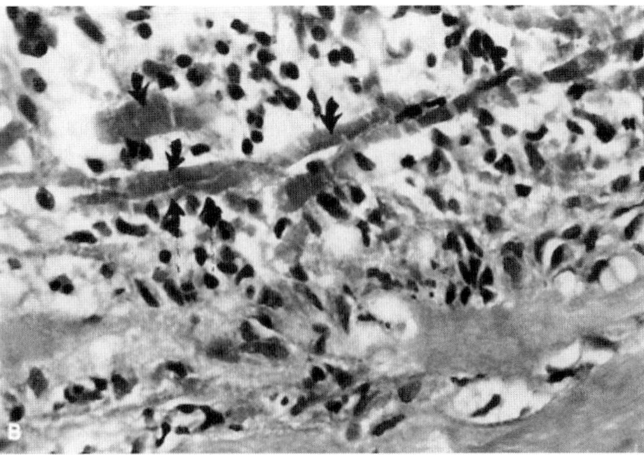

FIGURE 35.17 Heart rejection. Severe rejection manifests as a diffuse lymphocytic infiltrate with neutrophils and hemorrhage in the interstitium and myocyte necrosis (*arrows*). (Courtesy of Jeff Safitz, M.D.)

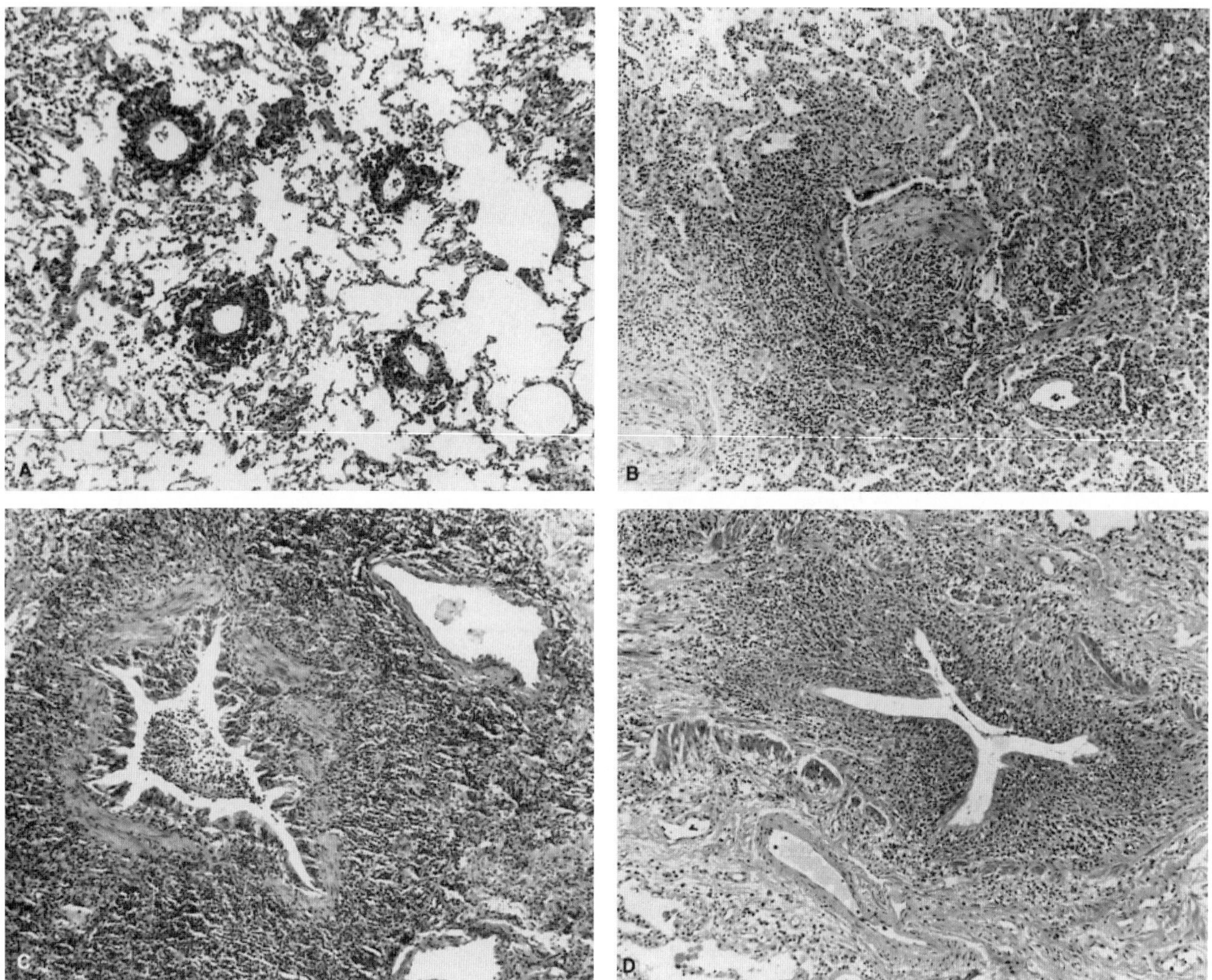

FIGURE 35.18 Lung rejection. (*A*) Mild acute rejection with a perivascular mononuclear infiltrate around small venules and arterioles. (*B*) With progression to moderate rejection, extension of the infiltrate into the alveolar septa occurs. (*C*) In severe rejection, there is a diffuse perivascular, interstitial, and peribronchiolar infiltrate with abundant fibrin, red blood cells, and neutrophils in the air spaces. (*D*) Bronchiolitis obliterans is the result of chronic rejection and is characterized by narrowing of the bronchioles from scarring. A mild mononuclear infiltrate is still present. (Courtesy of Samuel A. Yousem, M.D., University of Pittsburgh, Pittsburgh, PA.)

of peribronchiolar and perivascular lymphocytic infiltration. Most clinical immunosuppressive agents are directed toward T cells and preventing or treating acute rejections.

Chronic rejection usually occurs months to years after transplantation. It is characterized by loss of normal histologic structure, fibrosis, and atherosclerosis. Renal chronic rejection demonstrates interstitial fibrosis, tubular and glomerular loss, and vascular obliteration. Hepatic chronic rejection is characterized by portal fibrosis and the disappearance of bile ducts (ductopenia or vanishing bile duct syndrome). Accelerated graft atherosclerosis is the cardinal manifestation with hearts, and bronchiolitis obliterans indicates chronic pulmonary rejection. Chronic rejection is a major cause of graft failure and patient loss with all organs.[134] The problem with understanding and eventually treating and preventing chronic rejection is that it undoubtedly represents the final common pathologic pathway of a variety of insults. Thus, repeated bouts of rejection, drug toxicity, recurrent infections (e.g., pneumonias in lung transplants or cholangitis in liver transplants), chronic obstruction (ureter, bile ducts, pancreatic duct), severe ischemic damage to donor organs at the time of transplantation, use of older or suboptimal organ donors, or patient noncompliance with the immunosuppressive regimen can all contribute to a pathologic diagnosis of chronic rejection. Preventing chronic rejection requires attention to each of these problems. Nonetheless, a feature common to all types of chronic rejection is vascular atherosclerosis and obliteration with intragraft expression of certain cytokines and adhesion molecules, such as IL-1, IL-6, TNF-α, and ICAM-1.[135] Methods to prevent chronic rejection may come from a better understanding of vascular biology and how cytokines affect the process of atherosclerosis.[136]

REGULATION OF THE IMMUNE RESPONSE

Development of Lymphocytes

The preceding sections have outlined the major molecular and cellular interactions that occur on primary antigenic stimulation and show that different responses, cell types, and molecular entities may be involved. Superimposed on these pathways, however, are several layers of complex immune regulation that result from a variety of cellular interactions. It is important not only that the immune system respond to antigen but that the response is of the appropriate magnitude, type, and duration and that responses to self (i.e., autoimmunity) are avoided.[137] The regulatory processes that control these parameters have important implications for transplantation tolerance and immunosuppression.

The primary determinants of T- and B-cell receptor specificity occur during early lymphocyte development in the bone marrow and thymus.[138–144] When developing, immature T or B cells come in contact with self-antigen in these compartments, antigen binds to those cells that possess receptors for self, and the cells are tolerized. The next problem to consider is what happens to cells that are not exposed to self-antigens in these central lymphoid compartments because the antigen is expressed only in the periphery. When lymphocytes mature, migrate to the periphery, and come in contact with these antigens, what prevents subsequent autoimmune responses? There are several levels of control of this process. First, newly emerging lymphocytes are susceptible to tolerizing signals in the periphery, so contact with self-antigen shortly after egress from the bone marrow or thymus can also lead to appropriate nonresponsiveness. Second, because B-cell responses are T-cell dependent, if the T cell is tolerant, the B cell does not respond to the autoantigen. Third, many autoantigens are not expressed on, and therefore not presented by, professional APCs. This results in a failure of appropriate presentation so that T cells cannot "see" the antigen; TCRs may be engaged but tolerance, instead of immunity, ensues.

The problem of T-cell maturation is actually more complex than what was discussed earlier in this chapter. As noted, the TCR is selected to recognize altered self or a foreign peptide loaded into the antigen-binding groove of class I or II self-MHC. The cellular and molecular processes by which this occurs are the subject of intense current investigations and represent one of the major intellectual challenges in immunology. As T cells mature in the thymus, they sequentially acquire β TCR, α TCR, and CD4 and CD8 cell surface receptors. This is accompanied by migration from medullary to cortical regions of the thymus and by extensive proliferation and *loss* of most thymocytes. Numerous experimental studies have revealed that the maturing T cell expresses TCRs of multitudinous specificities and that these cells interact with class I and II molecules on the thymic epithelium. A very strong interaction between a developing T cell and the thymic epithelium indicates autoimmunity and leads to negative selection of those T cells by a process called *programmed cell death,* or *apoptosis.* This is probably responsible for the massive thymocyte loss seen in the normal thymus. Alternatively, complete failure of the T cell to interact with the thymic epithelium probably also results in negative selection by failure to stimulate these developing T cells.

However, a low-affinity interaction between the T cell and the thymic epithelium results in T-cell stimulation, positive selection, and proliferative expansion of those T cells. Thus, these regulatory processes select T cells that have a low affinity for self-peptides and self-MHC (Fig. 35.19). Presumably then, these cells have a higher affinity for allogenic peptides and self-MHC and are able to respond appropriately to antigen. These same cells are also able fortuitously to recognize self-peptides in the context of allo-MHC and allogenic peptides in the context of allo-MHC. This focuses attention again on the fact that T cells are obsessed with the MHC and on why such a high percentage of T cells in an unselected population responds to a single allogenic MHC.

A major unresolved issue in thymic selection of T cells is TCR expression. The process of assortment and rearrangement of α and β V-D-J regions, accompanied by the addition of N regions, must interact with the maturation, proliferation,

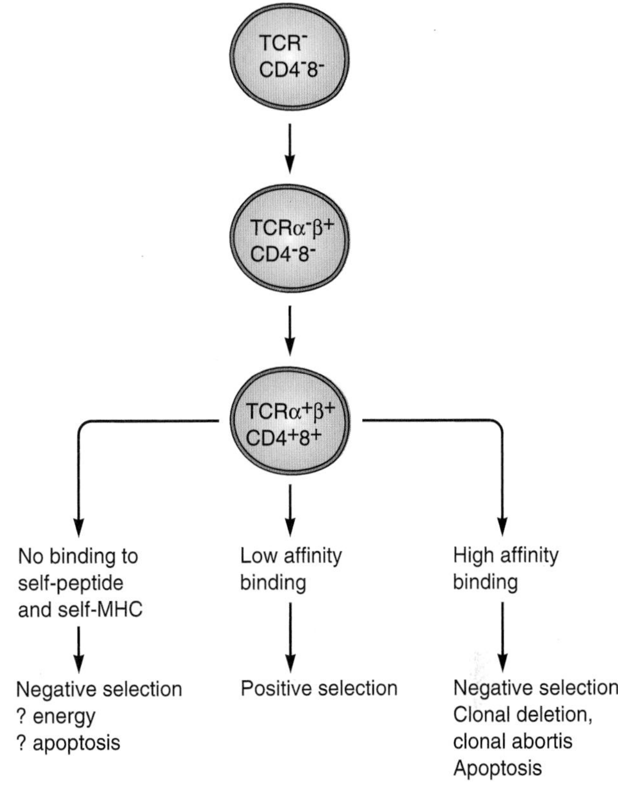

FIGURE 35.19 Thymic selection of developing T cells. MHC, major histocompatibility complex; TCR, T-cell receptor.

and selection processes at the level of the thymic epithelium. It is unclear whether TCR expression is an entirely random, stochastic process with subsequent positive or negative selection of T cells or whether there may be an instructional component such that as TCR β and α chains are expressed, they interact with epithelial ligands and direct further assortment and rearrangement of receptor genes. There is evidence for both of these mechanisms; however, a definitive answer requires a more detailed understanding of the precise regulatory and transcriptional mechanisms that connect cell surface TCR receptors to TCR gene rearrangements and expression in the nucleus.

Receptor-driven Stimulation of T and B Responses

The ultimate control of all antigen- and developmentally driven responses depends on a series of receptor–ligand interactions at the cell surface. For B cells, this comprises antigen and cell surface immunoglobulin. For T cells, this includes antigen, TCR, MHC, CD4, and CD8 interactions. However, these signals usually are not enough to completely stimulate T- and B-cell proliferation, maturation, and effector function. B cells require additional ligands, such as the soluble cytokines IL-2, IL-4, and IL-5. Likewise, T cells also require cytokines, such as IL-1, IL-2, IL-4, IFN-γ, IL-10, and IL-12 (Figs. 35.12 and 35.14). T cells also require the simultaneous or sequential engagement of multiple coreceptors (Fig. 35.13) to become fully activated. CD4 and CD8 are the primary coreceptors, and their engagement is usually absolutely required for T-cell responses. Another major coreceptor is CD28 and the closely related receptor CTLA4.[145,146] The ligands for these receptors are CD80 (B7-1) and CD86 (B7-2). Both receptors can bind both ligands. Blockade of these particular receptor–ligand interactions can prevent T-cell stimulation and cause tolerance to antigen. These pathways are being investigated as a way to

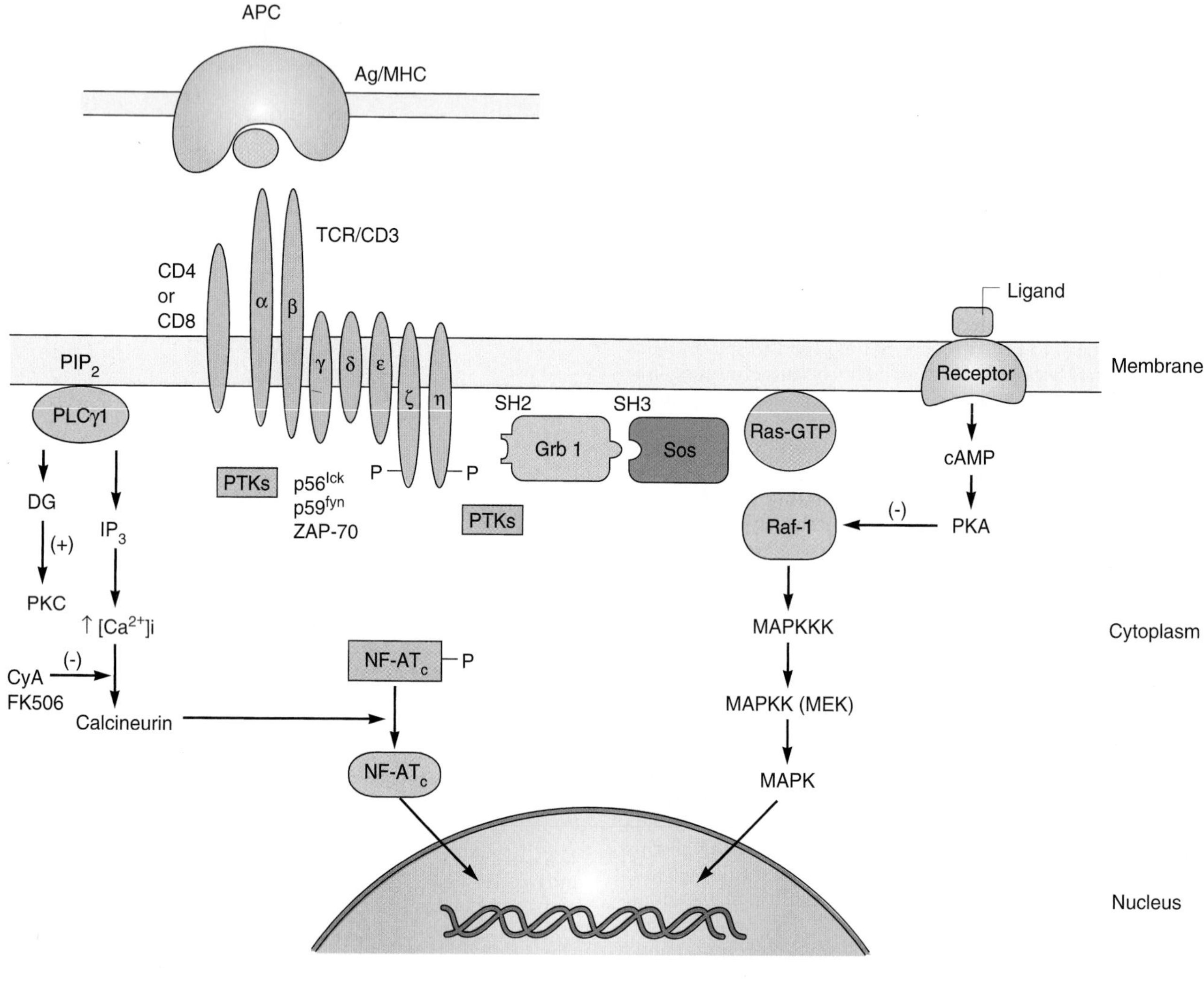

FIGURE 35.20 Signaling pathways of activated T cells. Ag, antigen; APC, antigen-presenting cell; cAMP, cyclic adenosine monophosphate; CyA, cyclosporine; DG, diacylglycerol; FK506, tacrolimus; IP_3, inositol triphosphate; MAPK, microtubule-associated protein kinase; MHC, major histocompatibility complex; $NF\text{-}AT_c$, inactive cytoplasmic nuclear factor of activated T cells; PIP_2, phosphatidylinositol biphosphate; PKA, protein kinase A; PKC, protein kinase C; PLCγ1, phospholipase Cγ1; PTK, protein tyrosine kinase; SH, Src-homology domain; TCR, T-cell receptor.

produce clinical transplantation tolerance. Additional coreceptors that are important for activation include CD2, CD29/CD49d [very late antigen-4 (VLA-4)], and CD11a/CD18 (LFA-1). Their ligands are CD58 (LFA-3), VCAM-1, and CD54 (ICAM-1), respectively. Despite the description of a large number of important receptor–ligand interactions, there is no unified view of hierarchy among the receptors or of combinations of stimulated receptors that may eventuate a given type of response.

Understanding receptor-driven stimulation and engagement of multiple coreceptors is ultimately the biochemical problem of elucidating the cytoplasmic second messenger pathways and transcriptional transactivators and repressors activated by each receptor or receptor combination. Numerous second messenger pathways, including G proteins, phospholipid and inositol phosphate metabolism, calcium currents, protein phosphorylation, and cyclic adenosine monophosphate (cAMP) metabolism have been described, and many of these are addressed in other chapters in this text.

For T cells, recent investigations have outlined major signaling pathways important for cellular activation[147–150] (Fig. 35.20). Engagement of TCR/CD3–CD4/8 by antigen–MHC results in the activation and phosphorylation of TCR/CD3 by associated protein tyrosine kinases (PTKs) called $p56^{lck}$, $p59^{fyn}$, and ZAP-70. ZAP-70 is a member of the Syk family of PTKs, whereas $p56^{lck}$ and $p59^{fyn}$ are members of the Src family. Phosphorylation of specific cytoplasmic tyrosines of the TCR/CD3 complex enables the receptor to bind an adapter protein, Grb2. Grb2 binds specific phosphorylated tyrosine residues by its Src-homology two (SH2) domain. Grb2 then binds to another protein, Sos, by its SH3 domain. The Grb2 SH3 domain recognizes a proline-rich region on Sos. This complex in turn activates the Ras–guanosine diphosphate complex, causing nucleotide exchange to the activated Ras–guanosine triphosphate (GTP) form. Ras–GTP then activates the Raf-1 serine-threonine kinase. Raf-1 then activates a series of downstream serine-threonine kinases termed MAPKKK, MAPKK (or MEK), and MAPK (for microtubule-associated protein kinase). These downstream kinases serve effector functions by modifying cytoplasmic structural or enzymatic proteins or modifying cytoplasmic transcriptional factors that subsequently translocate to the nucleus. Several levels of control of this cascade are beginning to be elucidated; in particular, cAMP negatively regulates Raf-1 kinase. Thus, two major signaling systems are linked by this recently described interaction. Once an understanding is achieved about what signaling pathways are activated by each T-cell coreceptor, a hierarchy or classification scheme may be possible in which blockade or activation of particular receptors or combinations of receptors will reliably produce specific gene activation or inactivation and tolerance.

The PTKs activate phospholipase Cg1 (PLC-g1), which catalyzes the hydrolysis of phosphatidylinositol biphosphate (PIP_2) to inositol triphosphate (IP_3) and diacylglycerol (DG). IP_3 increases intracellular calcium and activates the cytoplasmic protein tyrosine phosphatase, calcineurin. Calcineurin dephosphorylates tyrosines on the inactive cytoplasmic nuclear factor of activated T cells ($NF\text{-}AT_c$). The now activated, dephosphorylated $NF\text{-}AT_c$ is translocated to the nucleus, where it complexes with nuclear subunits ($NF\text{-}AT_n$) and acts as a transcriptional regulator. This pathway not only is linked to the other important pathways but also is blocked by the immunosuppressive agents cyclosporine and tacrolimus.

Tolerance

The term *tolerance* is applied to a variety of different circumstances and therefore presents a semantic problem depending on context. Tolerance usually refers to whole-animal or -organism responses observed experimentally or clinically. It is a functional and not a mechanistic observation. The usual criteria for tolerance include long-term graft acceptance without the need for chronic immunosuppression. In addition, a second donor-specific allograft (i.e., of the same MHC type as the original donor) should also be accepted without the need for additional immunosuppression. The most desirable end point from a clinical view would be true tolerance; however, this is virtually never achieved clinically and achieved only with difficulty experimentally. From a practical standpoint, long-term graft acceptance with minimal chronic immunosuppression, regardless of responses to subsequent second grafts, is highly desirable and would be of enormous clinical benefit.

When the term *tolerance* is applied to cellular analyses of lymphocytes, it is again a functional and not a mechanistic description. T and B lymphocytes can be tolerant or nonresponsive to antigen in a variety of specific ways.[150–157] *Clonal abortion* refers to the developmental process whereby nascent T- and B-cell clones that recognize autoantigen with high affinity are eliminated. Evidence suggests that at this developmental stage, high-affinity engagement of the antigen-specific receptor and coreceptors leads to second messenger events resulting in apoptosis. In the case of T cells, the complete failure to engage the TCR/CD3 complex may likewise lead to apoptotic clonal elimination.

Clonal deletion can encompass the process of clonal abortion, but it also refers to the elimination of mature T and B cell clones. Probably several specific cellular and molecular mechanisms are responsible for this process. Prolonged or excessive stimulation of the antigen receptor can eventually cause lymphocyte death. Antiidiotype antibodies can eliminate idiotype-positive clones. Suppressor cells may kill or deliver cytotoxic signals to certain antigen-reactive clones. Costimulatory blockade may also result in clonal deletion.

Clonal anergy is a state in which potentially reactive clones and their receptors are physically present but fail to respond to antigen. Anergy may also be the result of several distinct mechanisms, including prolonged receptor stimulation, receptor down-modulation, idiotype–antiidiotype interactions, suppressor cells, and inappropriate APC function in which coreceptor or cytokine function is blocked.

Suppression usually refers to an active process in which a leukocyte or its soluble products inhibit the development or effector function of immune lymphocytes. CD8+ and CD4+ T cells, B cells, macrophages, NK cells, and other cell types have all been shown to act as suppressor cells in certain experimental systems. Given the cellular interactions that can take place during lymphocyte recruitment (Figs. 35.11 and 35.14), it could be anticipated that each interactive site could be a locus for suppression. Given the number of mechanistic possibilities for clonal deletion and clonal anergy, it is also likely that numerous cells could be involved in suppression. Current models of immune regulation suggest that the T_H1/T_H2 dichotomy (Fig. 35.12) may explain much of suppression and be used in practical clinical settings. Thus, IL-10 can be used to suppress allograft responses, and IL-12 can be used to boost anticancer responses.

The term *split tolerance* is used to describe a state in which some responses to alloantigen are suppressed or deleted while other responses remain intact. This is likely a reflection of more detailed cellular analyses of tolerant states where anergy or suppression are dominant mechanisms. Likewise, T cells may proliferate or produce some cytokines, such as IL-2, in response to specific alloantigen but may be unable to generate cytotoxic effector cells because of anergy.

The major problem in clinical transplantation is that despite the detailed description of a large number of potential molecular and cellular mechanisms for inducing and maintaining tolerance, or some type of relative nonresponsiveness, it is not yet possible reliably and reproducibly to control any of these mechanisms in clinical settings. Our ability to induce tolerance will likely rely on a complete understanding of intracellular activational pathways (Fig. 35.20).

Potential Loci for Inducing Nonresponsiveness

The molecular, cellular, and tissue-specific organization of immune development and responses suggests there are a number of discrete steps suitable for interventions designed to promote tolerance or immunosuppression. The thymus is the primary site for T-cell development and for positive and negative selection of specific T-cell clones, depending on the clonotypic expression of the TCR. If specific alloantigen could be placed in the thymus, this could redirect TCR selection and produce tolerance. This has been achieved in experimental models by injecting the recipient thymus with donor-derived cells.[158–160] The problem with applying this to humans is the relatively involuted characteristic of the adult thymus. This may be approachable with thymotropic hormones. Nonetheless, the principle remains that thymic presentation of alloantigen "teaches" developing T cells to recognize that alloantigen as self.

The bone marrow is the primary site for B-cell development, and there is some evidence that precursor T cells can be tolerized to some antigens at this stage. In addition, bone marrow precursors populate the thymus. Protocols that attempt to replace part or all of the bone marrow stem cell and precursor population with donor-derived cells should induce tolerance to donor alloantigen.[161] In addition, partial replacement of the stem cell compartment results in chimerism, or a state in which both donor- and recipient-derived cells coexist in lymphoid organs. There is much interest in protocols that combine parenchymal organ grafting with bone marrow or stem cell transplantation.[162–164] Although these approaches are still experimental, there is evidence that some patients with very long-surviving allografts, who receive minimal or no immunosuppression, have stable low-level chimerism of lymphoid cells.[165]

The APC is an absolute requirement for proper T-cell activation. Techniques that alter APC function may induce T_H2 suppressor cells, anergy, or tolerance rather than T_H1 helper cells, CD8+ cytotoxic T cells, or graft rejection. One approach to this is the isolation of specialized APC subpopulations that channel T-cell responses in one direction or another.[166] Another approach is the use of ultraviolet B irradiation, which can disrupt APC function and produce suppression or anergy. The problem with both of these methods is that it is not possible to replace, or expose to physical agents, all the APCs in an individual. A more rational approach will be the use of APC receptor-ligand–disrupting agents.

The major intellectual and scientific directions in immunology have been the understanding of the molecular events of receptor–ligand interactions, second messenger pathways, and transcriptional regulation. New immunosuppressive drugs will likely be designed to interact with these pathways. For example, it is now known that cyclosporine and tacrolimus act primarily by inhibiting the NF-AT transcriptional activator. Other potentially promising agents under development are molecules that block the major CD28/CTLA4–CD80/CD86 and CD40–CD40L costimulatory pathways of T cells.[167–171] Approaches to support the preferential production of the T_H2 immunosuppressive cytokine IL-10 or disrupt the TCR–antigen–MHC interaction are also under investigation.

Clinical Immunosuppression

Despite the tremendous knowledge of immune regulation, current immunosuppressive regimens used for clinical transplantation are based on empirically derived protocols, using agents such as azathioprine and corticosteroids developed in the 1960s, cyclosporine A developed in the 1970s, and mycophenolate and tacrolimus developed in the 1980s and 1990s (Table 35.6). Newer, more rationally designed drugs are being subjected to clinical trials, and several may soon receive approval. Protocols for immunosuppression vary widely from one transplantation center to another and even within a center from one organ to another. The major principle of immunosuppression is to *induce* the patient with high doses of drugs at the time of allografting to prevent rejection. The drugs are then reduced rapidly, within days to weeks, to less toxic *maintenance* levels. Patients are examined frequently, and multiple laboratory tests are obtained to detect rejection or organ dysfunction early for effective treatment. Induction regimens rely on three or four drugs (mycophenolate, corticosteroids, cyclosporine or tacrolimus, antibodies), whereas maintenance regimens rely on two or three of these drugs. Treatment of first or mild rejections is usually accomplished with high-dose "pulse" steroids, whereas steroid-unresponsive, very severe, or secondary rejections are often treated with antibodies, especially OKT3.

The antimetabolites include azathioprine, cyclophosphamide (Cytoxan), and mycophenolate. By interfering with nucleic acid metabolism, these agents inhibit proliferation and clonal expansion of activated lymphocytes, limiting alloantigen-specific immune responses. Many immunosuppressive regimens use these drugs during induction immunosuppression at the time of allografting or for maintenance immunosuppression. They are most useful for preventing rejection but have little role for treating an acute, ongoing rejection. A more recent pharmaceutical, the morpholinoethyl ester of mycophenolic acid, also called CellCept (Roche Laboratories, Nutley, N.J.), inhibits *de novo* purine synthesis. It is more lymphocyte selective than azathioprine. Current data suggest it has important roles in inducing and maintaining immunosuppression and treating ongoing, particularly resistant rejections.[172,173]

Glucocorticoids are mainstays of virtually all immunosuppressive regimens and are used for induction and maintenance and for treating rejections. Glucocorticoids are primarily transcriptional regulators, binding to cytoplasmic steroid receptors, which are then translocated to the nucleus, where the complex binds specific gene promoters and other regulatory regions. The glucocorticoids all have similar immunosuppressive actions, and none is more effective than any other at equipotent doses. The relative potency on a milligram basis for the most commonly used drugs are hydrocortisone and cortisol, 1 mg; prednisone, 4 mg; and prednisolone and methylprednisolone, 5 mg. Steroid use is associated with several significant complications and side effects (see Table 35.6), and at equipotent doses all have equivalent toxicities. Although the use of multiple-drug regimens has decreased the overall dosing of glucocorticoids, the goal of steroid-free regimens for inducing and maintaining immunosuppression and for treating rejection in all patients has not been achieved.

Cyclosporine is a hydrophobic, cyclic undecapeptide that binds to a cytoplasmic protein, cyclophilin. The major immunosuppressive activity of cyclosporine appears to be related to the ability of the cyclosporine–cyclophilin complex to bind and inhibit the cytoplasmic protein tyrosine phosphatase calcineurin (Fig. 35.20). This in turn inhibits activation of the NF-AT_c transcriptional factor. In essence, cyclosporine is a transcriptional regulator. Cyclosporine is an integral part of all immunosuppressive regimens for induction and maintenance therapy but seems to have little role in reversing an ongoing acute rejection. The addition of cyclosporine to routine immunosuppressive regimens in 1983 allowed for the exponential growth of transplantation over the following decade. The 1-year graft and patient survival rates for the various organs increased from the 30% to 60% range to the 70% to 90% range. Cyclosporine has several significant toxicities (see Table 35.6), but attempts to design congeners with less toxicity but equal immunosuppression have not been successful.

The search for additional immunosuppressive agents led to the discovery of tacrolimus, or FK 506, approved by the U.S. Food and Drug Administration (FDA) in 1994. This macrolide antibiotic binds to a series of related cytoplasmic receptors termed *FK-binding protein* (FKBP). The tacrolimus–FKBP complex inhibits calcineurin. Thus, cyclosporine and tacrolimus have similar mechanisms of action. Tacrolimus is 10 to 100 times more potent than cyclosporine on a molar basis, but it too is associated with a number of significant and similar toxicities (see Table 35.6). Tacrolimus has roles in inducing and maintaining immunosuppression and may also be particularly useful for treating resistant rejections. A structurally similar compound, called rapamycin or sirolimus, has recently completed clinical trials and is currently approved.[174,175] This macrolide binds to and inhibits FKBP; however, it does not complex to calcineurin. Its molecular mechanism is under investigation. The existence of compounds such as cyclosporine, tacrolimus, and sirolimus suggests that there must be normal cellular constituents that regulate calcineurin function. These regulatory factors are unknown; their purification and isolation will presumably lead to more rational drug design for immunosuppression.

Antimetabolites, glucocorticoids, and calcineurin inhibitors are universally applied both to induction and to maintenance immunosuppression, and any of these agents may be administered chronically to patients. The fourth major group of reagents is antibodies. These may be given for only short periods because of their extreme potency and because of host anti-immunoglobulin responses that limit their efficacy. Antibodies are used for induction to prevent rejection and for treatment

TABLE 35.6

CURRENTLY APPROVED IMMUNOSUPPRESSIVE AGENTS

Agent (Brand name)	Mechanism of action	Dosage	Monitoring	Clinical uses	Adverse effects
Azathioprine (Imuran)	Inhibits purine synthesis by active metabolites 6-thioinocinic acid (by conversion to 6-mercaptopurine) and 6-thioguanine nucleotides; inhibits DNA and RNA synthesis; has greater effect on T cells than B cells	1–3 mg/kg/d IV or PO	Maintain WBCs >3,000/μl	Part of regimens to lower doses of cyclosporine or prednisone	Myelosuppression (leukopenia, occasionally thrombocytopenia and megaloblastic anemia), hepatitis, cholestatis, hepatic vein thrombosis, pancreatitis dermatitis, alopecia, increased susceptibility to infection
Cytoxan	Alkylates DNA	0.5–1.5 mg/kg/d	Maintain WBCs >3,000/μL	Substitution for azathioprine if adverse effects occur	Leukopenia, thrombocytopenia, hemorrhagic cystitis, nausea, vomiting, increased susceptibility to infections
Glucocorticoids	Complex; affects T cells and macrophages; has little effect on antibody production by B cells. Steroid–receptor complex binds to DNA; alters transcription of genes responsible for cytokine synthesis; blocks MLR and development of CTL; inhibits IL-1 and IL-6 synthesis	Prednisolone, 1–2 mg/kg/d induction; 0.1–0.2 mg/kg/d maintenance bid, qd, or qod dosing Prednisolone, 2 mg/kg/d for rejection; tapering schedule Solu-Medrol 5–15 mg/kg/d IV for rejection	No objective means to monitor; adjustment done by protocol; adverse effects	Foundation of most multidrug protocols; treatment of rejection	Cushingoid features (moon facies, acne, centripetal obesity, striae), hypertension, weight gain, (increased appetite), hyperglycemia, osteoporosis, type II diabetes, poor wound healing, pancreatitis, peptic ulcer, colonic perforation, psychosis, increased susceptibility to infection
Cyclosporine (Sandimmune)	Binds to cyclophilin; blocks transcription of several early T-cell activation genes, including IL-2, II-3, IL-4, and interferon-γ; inhibits IL-1 production by macrophages	8–10 mg/kg/d PO qd, bid, or tid or 2.5–3 mg/kg/d IV	Trough levels (usually 12 h); serum creatinine; mg/kg dose (protocol); biopsy (histologic evidence of cyclosporine toxicity)	Induction therapy with prednisolone or azathioprine in most multidrug regimens	Nephrotoxicity, hypertension, hyperkalemia, hyperuricemia and gout, gingival hypertrophy, hepatotoxicity, hirsutism, tremors, seizures, hyperglycemia; hemolytic uremic syndrome increased susceptibility to infection
FK 506, Tacrolimus (Prograf)	Similar to cyclosporine (10–100 times more potent); binds to FK-binding protein; blocks expression of IL-2 receptors on allostimulated T cells	0.15 mg/kg/d PO qd or bid or 0.075 mg/kg IV q 12 h	Trough levels; serum creatinine; dose mg/kg dose (protocol); adverse effects (neurologic)	Induction therapy with prednisone; treatment of rejection; maintenance without prednisolone	Nephrotoxicity, headache, weight loss, tremors, paresthesia, increased sensitivity to light, insomnia and mood changes, increased susceptibility to infections

MLR, mixed lymphocyte response; CTL, cytotoxic T lymphocytes; IL, interleukin; WBCs, white blood cells.

TABLE 35.7

POLYCLONAL AND MONOCLONAL ANTIBODIES

Antibody	Source	Mechanism of action	Dosage	Monitoring	Clinical uses	Adverse effects
ALG or ATG	Horse, goat, rabbit	Depletes T cells more than B cells as a result of complement-dependent lysis and opsonization	10–30 mg/kg/d IV qd over 6 h; must be given in central line	Peripheral T-cell levels; monitor for antihorse or antigoat antibody development; platelets; white blood cell count	Induction with azathioprine or prednisone as part of triple or quadruple therapy protocols; treatment of rejection with or without steroids	Fever, chills, leukopenia, thrombocytopenia, nausea, vomiting, diarrhea, arthralgia, headache, myalgia, rash, pruritus, urticaria, chest pain, phlebitis, rarely anaphylaxis or serum sickness
OKT3	Mouse	Reacts with CD3 recognition complex on T cells; blocks recognition of class I or II antigens; inhibits generation and function of effector T cells; opsonizes CD3+ cells; modulates CD3 antigen-recognition complex; renders T cells anergetic or kills them by apoptosis	2.5–10 mg/d IV over 30 min; can be given in peripheral vein	Peripheral CD3 levels; monitor for antimouse antibody development	Same as ALG, ATG	Usually with first dose: fever, chills, diarrhea, headache, nausea, vomiting, dyspnea, wheezing, pulmonary edema, tachycardia, hypotension, aseptic meningitis, seizures, coma; markedly reduced with pretreatment with steroids, acetaminophen, indomethacin, and diphenhydramine hydrochloride

ALG, antilymphocyte globulin; ALT, antithymocyte globulin.

of acute, ongoing rejections. There are two major types of antibody preparations (Table 35.7). Polyclonal antibodies, such as antilymphocyte globulin, thymoglobulin, and antithymoctye globulin, are prepared by immunizing animals with human lymphocytes or lymphoid lines, bleeding the animals to obtain serum, and purifying whole immunoglobulin from serum. These preparations are directed against many different antigens present on T cells (e.g., CD2, CD3, CD4, CD8) but also recognize B-cell, monocyte, platelet, and granulocyte antigens. Polyclonal antibodies are very useful for induction[176] but tend to be less effective for treatment of acute rejection. They are associated with a number of side effects related either to their depleting effect on cell populations (leukopenia, thrombocytopenia) or to allergic reactions related to host antiimmunoglobulin responses (urticaria, rash, pruritus).

The second type of antibody preparation is monoclonal antibody, derived from cloned hybridoma cells of a single specificity. OKT3, approved by the FDA in 1985, is a mouse monoclonal directed against the nonpolymorphic ε chain of the CD3 complex of the TCR. OKT3 therefore recognizes all T cells (both $\alpha\beta$ TCR and $\gamma\delta$ TCR) and interferes with their antigen recognition functions in the context of either class I or II MHC. OKT3 is used for both induction and the treatment of rejection. The antibody is used either as first-line treatment for rejection or as treatment for rejections unresponsive to high-dose steroids or polyclonal antibodies. Anti-IL-2 receptor (IL-2R) monoclonal antibodies, basiliximab (Simulect; Novartis, East Hanover, N.J.)[177] and daclizumab (Zenapax; Roche Laboratories),[178] were FDA approved in 1998 and are used for induction immunosuppression.

It has previously been considered that polyclonal or monoclonal antibodies function by inhibiting T-cell function through opsonization, complement-mediated lysis, or steric hindrance of the TCR. Although these mechanisms certainly do occur, it is now clear that other effects may be even more important for immunosuppression. When OKT3 is first administered to a patient, a significant clinical response often occurs within 30 minutes to 4 hours, consisting of fevers, chills, rigors, myalgias, arthralgias, and vascular leak. This has been called the *cytokine syndrome* and is due to OKT3 binding to and cross-linking T-cell CD3, which activates all T cells, thereby causing massive release of IL-2. The IL-2 in turn causes other cells to release IL-1, IL-6, IFN-γ, and TNF-α. These cytokines can be found at very high concentrations throughout the serum, and blocking cytokine production or action can ameliorate the cytokine syndrome. When T cells are stimulated, they lose cell surface CD3, CD4, and CD8 as a result of the antibody. This process is termed *antigenic modulation* and results in naked T cells that are refractory to antigenic stimulation because they lack receptors. Because OKT3 binds CD3 in the absence of other T-cell costimulatory signals (e.g., CD28, CD2, CD29/49d, CD11a/18), this is the equivalent of inappropriate antigen presentation, which experimentally can result in anergy or apoptosis. There is now evidence that because of OKT3, these T cells may also be rendered anergic or even killed by apoptotic mechanisms. The effects of cytokine stimulation, antigenic modulation, anergy, and apoptosis may be separable, and experimental work to produce a form of OKT3 that lacks the clinically deleterious cytokine-inducing properties while preserving the other immunosuppressive characteristics is of significant interest. Polyclonal antibodies also have anti-CD3 specificities and may therefore have a similar mechanism of action. In addition, because polyclonals have many other antireceptor specificities, they may produce a variety of other effects related to receptor cross-linking, antigenic modulation, anergy, and apoptosis.

Other monoclonal antibodies are undergoing clinical evaluation, including anti-CD4, anti-CD8, and anti-CD3. All seem to have some efficacy, but none has yet proved superior to OKT3. Consideration has also been given to toxin-conjugated monoclonal antibodies, but none has reached phase II or III clinical transplantation trials.

Several dozen other compounds of diverse structure and mechanistic activity have been or are being evaluated in experimental and clinical allografting protocols. Several, discussed here briefly, may find a role in clinical transplantation during the next decade. The bacterial product 15-deoxyspergualin is a potent immunosuppressive with mild side effects, including neurotoxicity, anorexia, and bone marrow depression.[179] Its mechanism may be related to binding to cytoplasmic members of the heat-shock protein 70 (Hsp 70) family[180] Hsp members are often involved as chaperones in protein folding and transport; therefore, 15-deoxyspergualin may interfere with antigen presentation or the translocation of transcription factors into the nucleus.[181] Leflunomide, an isoxazol derivative, has potent immunosuppressive activities and synergizes with cyclosporine.[182,183] Its mechanism may be related to inhibiting intracellular messengers and second signals generated by IL-2 and costimulatory receptors such as CD28. Studies suggests that leflunomide may inhibit protein kinases and *de novo* pyrimidine biosynthesis.[184] Molecules aimed at effector mechanisms of cellular destruction have also had some activity in experimental analyses. Thus, inhibitors of complement, platelet-activating factor, nitric oxide synthesis, superoxide synthesis, granzymes, perforins, and interleukins can all prolong graft survival. These latter agents will probably have only adjunctive roles because the most important processes to regulate are probably the initiation of immune responses, immunologic priming, and immunologic memory.

Recent investigations have focused on the design of soluble molecules that mimic various parts of the TCR–antigen–MHC–CD4/CD8 complex. A molecule with high enough affinity for the recognition complex could inhibit T-cell activation and immunity. Analogues of CD4 can perform such a function.[185] Likewise, analogues of peptide antigen seem to complete with antigen at the level of binding to the peptide groove of MHC. Furthermore, antigen analogues may induce a negative regulatory signal in T cells and actually anergize T cells as a result of altered receptor affinities and kinetics.[186–188] This form of immunosuppression also has the advantage of being strictly antigen specific. One envisions transplanting a patient and then injecting the patient with mimics of the immunodominant peptides corresponding to the mismatched MHC molecules of donor origin to promote selective anergy.

A variety of physical methods have been considered for immunosuppression. Total lymphoid irradiation is successful in experimental transplantation.[189] Total lymphoid irradiation ablates much of the immune system and also seems to generate suppressor cells. There is concern that total lymphoid irradiation markedly increases the risk of systemic infection and lymphoid malignancies. It has been known since the early 1970s that prior blood transfusions are associated with a decreased risk of renal allograft rejection and increased graft survival.[190] Furthermore, donor-specific transfusions have an antigen-specific protective effect. The cellular and molecular consequences of transfusion or donor-specific transfusion are not certain; however, the presentation of antigen to central lymphoid compartments (e.g., intravenous injection of cells) can generate suppression, anergy, and tolerance (see Sites of Antigen Recognition). Problems with transfusion include the fact that high-titer anti-HLA antibodies develop in 10% to 30% of transfused recipients. These highly sensitized recipients cannot be transplanted. In this respect, transfusions may merely be "selecting" potential high- versus low-reacting recipients. Transfusions and donor-specific transfusions were widely used until the 1980s. The advent of cyclosporine

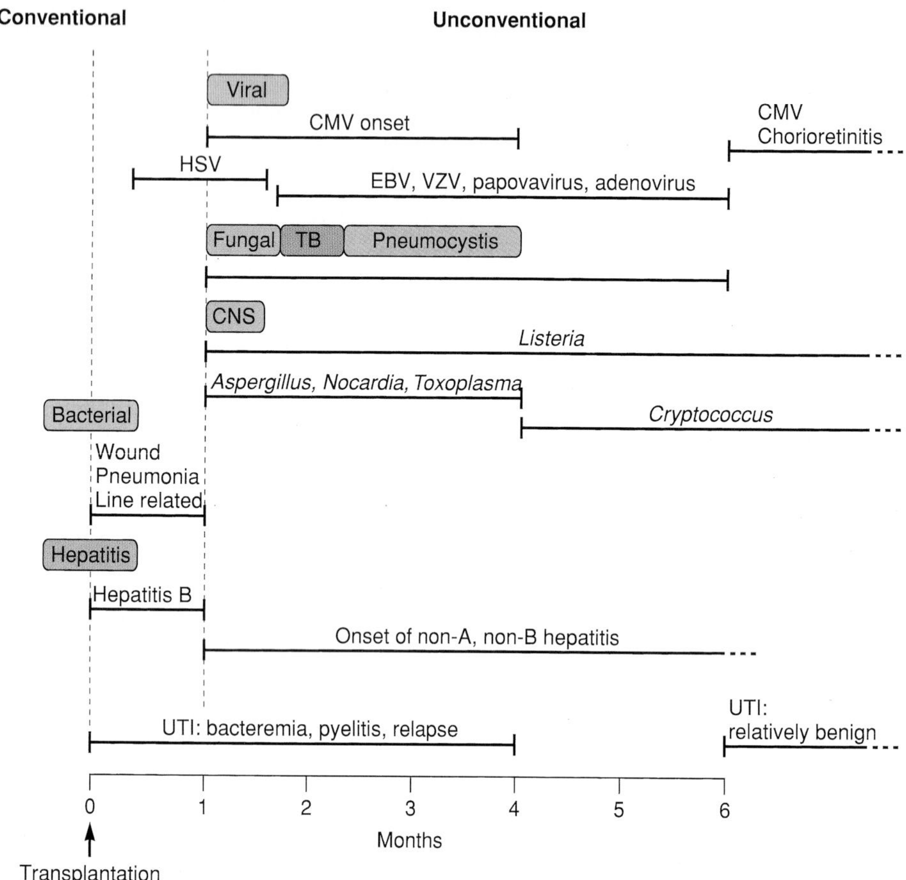

FIGURE 35.21 Timing of posttransplantation infections. CMV, cytomegalovirus; EBV, Epstein-Barr virus; CNS, central nervous system; HSV, herpes simplex virus; UTI, urinary tract infection; VZV, varicella-zoster virus. (After Rubin RH, Wolfson JS, Cosimi AB, et al. Infection in the renal transplant patient. *Am J Med.* 1981;70:405.)

erased much of the benefit that transfusions conferred; they are now only rarely used. Oral feeding of antigen or peptide can also produce suppression, anergy, and tolerance.[191,192] A trial of oral peptides in patients with multiple sclerosis suggested they conferred some clinically beneficial immunosuppressive effect.[191] It remains to be seen if the same can be accomplished with clinical allografting.

Complications of Immunosuppression

The therapeutic index for immunosuppressives is very low. As a result, numerous toxicities and adverse effects occur, and they are an integral part of treating transplant recipients (see Tables 35.6 and 35.7). The most obvious complication is infection. As immunosuppression becomes stronger and more effective, the recipient's ability to resist infection diminishes. Allograft recipients are susceptible both to typical bacterial infections (e.g., urinary tract infection, pneumonia, wound infections) and to infections with unusual organisms (e.g., fungus, virus, atypical bacteria). Immunosuppressives also blunt the inflammatory response to infection so that patients present with very subtle signs and symptoms or very late in the infectious process. The tenets of patient care are the judicious management of immunosuppression to prevent infectious complications, the use of prophylactic antibiotics (i.e., acyclovir or ganciclovir for herpesviruses; sulfamethoxazole for *Pneumocystis;* and nystatin, clotrimazole, or fluconazole for candidiasis), and a low threshold of suspicion for examining, culturing, and treating patients with suspected infections.

Figure 35.21 diagrams the typical transplant-related infections and when they occur. Of particular concern is cytomegalovirus (CMV). CMV, a member of the herpes family, which can infect any cell in the body and produce cytopathic effects. CMV infection in immunocompetent people is often clinically inapparent and results in the viral genome persisting in the patient's lymphocytes for life. As a result, organ transplantation almost invariably results in the transfer of viral genomes to the recipient. Evidence of past infection is indicated by elevated serum IgG anti-CMV titers; approximately 70% of the population is CMV seropositive. When seropositive (i.e., previously infected) patients are transplanted and immunosuppressed, CMV virus from their own lymphocytes may be reexpressed and reactivate disease. Reactivation disease is usually mild and self-limited and presents approximately 6 weeks after transplantation as fevers, myalgias, arthralgias, leukopenia, mild elevation of liver enzymes, and mild, nonspecific abdominal complaints. A more serious situation occurs when a previously uninfected, CMV-seronegative patient receives an organ from a CMV-seropositive donor. This situation occurs in 10% to 30% of transplant recipients. The recipient has almost a 100% chance of contracting CMV infection and greater than a 70% chance of having clinically significant or even life-threatening disease, including CMV encephalitis, pneumonitis, hepatitis, and necrotizing gastroenteropathy with perforation and bleeding. Effective prophylactic regimens now include the following: acyclovir, 800 mg four times a day orally for 3 months; ganciclovir, 2.5 mg/kg twice a day intravenously for 2 weeks; and CMV hyperimmune globulin, 150 mg/kg for five doses over

6 to 8 weeks. Therapeutic regimens for established disease include ganciclovir and CMV IgG.

Another complication in allograft recipients is malignancy. There is an increased incidence for only a few histologic types of tumors. The immunosuppressive drugs do not appear to be directly mitogenic or transforming, but rather suppress immune mechanisms that keep transformed cells in check. Squamous cell carcinomas of the exposed areas of the skin are by far the most common. These usually are not aggressive or invasive tumors and can be cured with simple local excision. Avoiding ultraviolet exposure from the sun is the best preventive measure.

Lymphomas are the next most common tumor and are 10 to 100 times more common in transplant recipients than in the general population. These are usually non-Hodgkin's B-cell lymphomas and are often related to malignant transformation by Epstein-Barr virus (EBV).[193] In immunocompetent people, EBV normally infects B cells and causes polyclonal proliferation of infected cells. The infection is eventually controlled by cytotoxic CD8+ T cells, which recognize and kill viral antigens on the surface of infected B cells. In immunosuppressed patients, T-cell–mediated immunity is impaired, allowing EBV-directed polyclonal B-cell proliferation to continue. Some of the B-cell clones eventually acquire additional mutations, and a benign polyclonal expansion of B cells becomes a more aggressive oligoclonal proliferation. One of these clones can accumulate even more mutations and become an autonomous, monoclonal lymphoma. At this stage, the lymphoma may even lose viral antigens and become insusceptible to immune control. The incidence of lymphoma is directly related to the amount of immunosuppression received over time. Thus, avoiding overimmunosuppression prevents this malignancy. Management of established disease consists primarily of reducing or withdrawing immunosuppression, even to the point of allograft rejection and loss. Although the latter maneuver is possible with renal and pancreatic transplants, where the patient may return to dialysis or insulin, it is not possible with hepatic or cardiac grafts. High-dose intravenous ganciclovir is sometimes effective for treatment and may have a role in prophylaxis. Conventional chemotherapy for lymphoma usually is ineffective for these tumors.

Other tumors with a higher incidence in transplant recipients include Kaposi's sarcoma and a slight increase in cervical carcinoma. The causative agent of Kaposi's sarcoma is human herpesvirus 8, also now called Kaposi's sarcoma herpesvirus. Cervical carcinomas are related to papilloma viruses. This association suggests that immunosuppression primarily interferes with normal antiviral responses in the case of some tumors. Common neoplasms, such as breast, lung, and colon cancer, are *not* more common in transplant recipients than in the general population, suggesting that immune mechanisms are generally irrelevant for these tumors. The effect of immunosuppression on the recurrence of a preexisting or a previously treated cancer is controversial. Data suggest that immunosuppression either has no effect or may slightly increase the incidence of recurrent carcinoma. Current clinical recommendations suggest that after a curative resection, patients should wait at least 2 years before undergoing transplantation.[194] It is also possible to transplant a tumor to a recipient from a donor with metastatic disease. Therefore, a history of malignancy excludes potential organ donors. The one exception to this rule is malignant central nervous system tumors that usually do not metastasize. Unfortunately, even these tumors have been transferred by organ transplantation despite no clinical evidence of metastatic disease.[195]

Tables 35.6 and 35.7 also show a large number of drug-specific toxicities, many of which are clinically common. This again stresses the point that the therapeutic index for immunosuppression is very narrow and that frequent monitoring of laboratory tests is required for patients receiving these agents. Of particular concern is atherosclerotic vascular disease. Since the late 1970s, organ failure and infection have become less significant causes of morbidity and mortality, whereas various manifestations of vascular disease have become more important. In fact, coronary artery disease is the primary cause of mortality in the renal transplant population. Many factors related to immunosuppression contribute to vascular disease. Glucocorticoids alter serum lipid components and ratios to unfavorable varieties. They also promote glucose intolerance and insulin resistance. Cyclosporine unfavorably alters serum lipids and contributes to insulin resistance. Cyclosporine also causes hypertension by mechanisms related to vascular endothelial cell–induced release of endothelin and interferes with renal function by altering glomerular hemodynamics and renal prostaglandin production. Prolonged cyclosporine administration may lead to permanent renal damage and eventually the need for dialysis. Sirolimus and tacrolimus share the same toxicities as cyclosporine, causing hypercholesterolemia, insulin resistance, hypertension, and renal insufficiency. Renal insufficiency itself further contributes to hypertension and dyslipidemia. All these variables contribute to atherosclerosis of cerebral, coronary, renal, and peripheral vascular beds. The care of transplant recipients now requires careful monitoring of individual drug doses and levels to reduce their toxicities. Close attention to serum lipid profiles, hypertension, weight, diet, and exercise are also major factors in the long-term treatment of these patients.

Another complication of organ allografting is graft-versus-host disease (GVHD). All vascularized allografts contain lymph nodes and mature lymphocytes. These donor-derived T and B cells can be stimulated by host alloantigen and transiently repopulate the host. The antihost reactive cells can cause T-cell–mediated lesions, such as hepatitis, dermatitis, or gastrointestinal mucosal lesions, as seen in bone marrow transplant recipients with GVHD. The B cells can produce antihost antibodies; an ABO incompatibility can even result in a hemolytic anemia. GVHD is usually self-limited as the donor cells are eliminated either by immunosuppression or by host antidonor responses.

Important Aspects of Antigenicity and Immunity for Clinical Transplantation

Current clinical protocols determine a limited number of variables and parameters for matching and allocating donor organs to potential recipients. ABO compatibility is obviously required for successful transplantation. Placing an A donor organ in an O recipient results in hyperacute rejection because of the presence of preformed anti-A antibodies. It is possible to transplant A2 donor organs into O recipients because most anti-A antibodies do not bind to the A2 ligand. It is also possible to place O organs into A or B recipients; however, because of the severe organ shortage and long waiting lists, this is not usually performed.

The central position of MHC in immune regulation suggests that HLA matching is very important for allografting. Significant data prove that HLA matching is important for kidney and pancreas transplantation. A well-matched organ has up to a 10% long-term survival advantage over a poorly matched graft. However, as the overall success rate for renal allografting approaches 90%, there is debate over the magnitude of this advantage and what defines poor versus good matching. Good data show that HLA matching is *not* important for liver transplantation and does not affect graft survival. The immunologic reasons for this are not known. The data for cardiac grafting are more controversial; there is probably a small advantage for HLA matching with this organ.

Most laboratories use serologic-based, or antibody-based, techniques to type potential donors and recipients for HLA. The main loci typed are HLA-A, HLA-B, and HLA-DR. For a normal, completely heterozygous person, this results in six antigens typed, and a complete donor–recipient match is referred to as a *six-antigen match* or a *zero-antigen mismatch*. Newer nucleic acid- and polymerase chain reaction–based techniques are being used by an increasing number of HLA laboratories. This technology is more accurate than serology-based techniques and types for additional loci, including HLA-DP and HLA-DQ and separate α and β chains. Typing for more loci may allow for better matching. However, because HLA heterogeneity is so enormous and because there is such a severe shortage of donor organs, technical advances in typing may confer no benefit on clinical results.

An important test for graft compatibility is the cross-match. This assay determines whether there are preformed antibodies in the potential recipient's serum that react with antigens on the cell surface of the potential donor's lymphocytes (Fig. 35.22). A positive cross-match means that such antibodies are present and that hyperacute rejection will ensue if the transplantation is performed. Appropriate controls are always performed to exclude autoantibodies. Cross-matching is important for kidney, pancreas, lung, and heart allografting, whereas hepatic allografts resist hyperacute rejection. The reasons for this resistance are not known but may relate to the large mass of hepatic tissue that can absorb antibody and complement and still preserve sufficient functioning cellular mass.

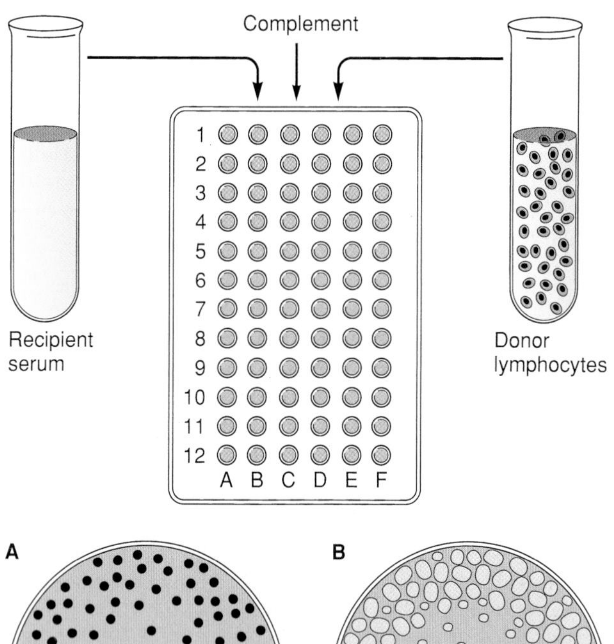

FIGURE 35.22 Lymphocytotoxicity cross-match. Recipient serum is incubated with donor lymphocytes and complement in microtiter plates. If donor-specific lymphocytotoxic antibodies are present in the recipient serum, antibody binding results in complement fixation and lysis of the donor lymphocytes. This is detected by the addition of a dye that is taken up through the damaged cell membrane, and a positive cross-match is noted (*A*). If no antibodies are present, cells remain viable and do not take up the dye (*B*). This is a negative cross-match.

Figure 35.22 shows that the standard cross-match detects high-titer complement-fixing antibodies. If the recipient has antidonor antibodies that inefficiently fix complement, a positive cross-match could be missed. Some laboratories use enhancing techniques, such as secondary antibodies or fluorescent flow cytometry, to increase the sensitivity of the cross-match. The problem with these modifications is that increased sensitivity is accompanied by decreased specificity; therefore, some positive cross-matches could be clinically acceptable. Clinical experience has shown that positive cross-matches from IgG antibodies are the most significant, whereas positive testing from IgM antibodies is not clinically relevant. IgM antibodies can be eliminated from serum specimens by adding a reducing agent such as dithiothreitol.

Figure 35.22 also shows that the standard cross-match tests donor-derived lymphocytes for the presence of antigen. Because the most relevant antibodies are anti-HLA and because HLA is expressed by essentially all cell types, the experimental design is appropriate. However, if the recipient has antibodies that are cell or organ specific, these antibodies may be missed by the standard cross-match. Some recipients do occasionally possess cell- or organ-specific antibodies, and hyperacute or severe accelerated acute rejection can ensue in these situations. Experimental studies have also demonstrated a distinct vascular endothelial cell-specific antigen system, which can be a target for hyperacute rejection. This endothelial cell system is, however, still poorly defined and reagents are not available for widespread clinical use. The practical consequence of all these limitations is that hyperacute rejections rarely occur because of noncomplement fixation or antibodies with unusual specificities. Conversely, some positive cross-matches that have precluded a transplantation may have been determined by too sensitive a technique.

Another important test that also reflects the presence of host antidonor antibodies is the panel-reactive antibody (PRA). Most recipients on transplant waiting lists send serum samples to the transplantation center on a regular basis. These sera are then periodically tested against a panel of typing cells of known HLA specificities using techniques identical to those for the cross-match (see Fig. 35.22). The percentage of cells with which recipient serum reacts is determined, and this number is the PRA. Most normal people have no anti-HLA antibodies and a low PRA (0% to 5%). Patients who have been transfused, pregnant or previously transplanted or who have an autoimmune disorder that induces a lot of antibodies may have a high PRA (50% to 99%). The presence of a very high PRA suggests a patient is likely to have a positive cross-match. This information is useful for determining the logistics of organ allocation when cadaveric donor organs become available and have to be transplanted within a short time frame.

A matching technique used in living-related transplantation is the mixed lymphocyte culture or mixed lymphocyte reaction. Lymphocytes are isolated from peripheral blood specimens from both donor and recipient. The donor cells are gamma-irradiated to prevent mitosis, and the two cell populations are placed in culture together. Recipient cells recognize donor antigen in culture, are activated, and proliferate rapidly. After a few days of culture, the amount of proliferation is measured by incorporating radiolabeled nucleic acids into the cells. The amount or degree of proliferation compared with appropriate positive and negative controls is assumed to represent the potential for a host antidonor response and the chance of allograft rejection. Unfortunately, the correlation between the mixed lymphocyte reaction and clinical outcome is poor and most centers no longer use this test. Further, because this assay requires several days to complete, it is not useful for cadaveric grafting.

FUTURE DIRECTIONS

Xenotransplantation

One of the most critical problems in clinical transplantation is a shortage of donor organs. There has been continued liberalization of criteria for acceptable cadaveric donors and improvements in operative techniques and preservation solutions. Despite this, only 20% to 30% of potentially suitable donors are ever used. In addition, societal enforcement of mandatory seat belt and helmet laws as well as reduced tolerance for drunk driving have substantially reduced the number of donors available from trauma. At the same time, the increasing success of organ transplantation has increased the indications for transplantation and subsequently the demands for organs. As a result, the number of people waiting for organs in the United States alone is currently more than 70,000 and growing by approximately 10% to 15% each year. One approach to this shortage of organs is xenotransplantation, or the use of organs from different species.[196] The successful application of this modality could potentially provide an unlimited supply of organs and make all transplantation operations elective procedures. Unfortunately, a number of significant issues impede the clinical application of xenotransplantation.

The choice of donor species is limited. Primate donors, although phylogenetically similar to humans, are difficult to breed in captivity, and many species are even endangered. In addition, there are significant ethical ramifications of using such closely related species. Furthermore, the transmission of viruses from primates, such as simian retroviruses, could be potentially life threatening. Because of these concerns, attention has been focused on the pig as a suitable donor. The pig is viewed as a good donor because of its size, physiology, acceptance by the public, an extensive knowledge of porcine genetics, and the ability to make inbred and transgenic swine.

The first major hurdle to xenotransplantation between such widely disparate species such as human and pig is hyperacute rejection.[197] Humans and many primates have high-titer natural antibodies directed against cell surface determinants present on other species. In the case of pig-to-human xenotransplantation, these antibodies appear to be primarily IgM and are directed against galactose α1-3 galactose present on the porcine cells.[198] These natural antibodies are present because humans do not have the enzyme a-galactosyl transferase and do not put these terminal sugar residues on their cell surface. Because of these natural antibodies, pig-to-human transplantation results in hyperacute rejection after these antibodies bind to the endothelium of the porcine organ and activate complement. Several approaches to solving this problem have proved successful in the laboratory. One approach is to deplete serum antibody levels by either plasmapheresis or immunoabsorption while concurrently suppressing B-cell function. Another approach is to eliminate the primary antigenic determinant on the porcine cells by either creating pigs "knocked out" for α-galactosyl transferase or enzymatically removing the sugar moieties from the graft before transplantation. An alternative tactic is to regulate complement activation,[199] which also prevents hyperacute rejection. One such approach is the use of soluble inhibitors of complement activation, such as soluble complement receptor-1. Other approaches have focused on the construction of transgenic pigs that express human complement regulatory proteins on the cell surface.[200]

Although the hyperacute rejection barrier to discordant xenotransplantation is relatively severe, it can be overcome.[201] Unfortunately, none of these current approaches produces long-term graft survival. This most likely reflects return of humoral immunity and complement function to the recipient as well as generation of a specific cellular immune responses. The relative importance of these processes, and strategies to avert them, is the subject of ongoing investigation.

Another problem with xenotransplantation is the physiologic incompatibility between proteins synthesized by the graft and the recipient. For example, the inability of inhibitors of thrombosis to function adequately on the endothelium surface may predispose a xenograft to thrombosis in the absence of any immune response. In addition, organs such as the liver secrete many serum proteins that might be unable to function in their new host environment. For other organs, such as the heart, this might be less of a barrier.

The final and perhaps most daunting hurdle in xenotransplantation is the transmission of unusual pathogenic organisms to humans, or zoonoses.[202] Recent concern has focused on the transmission of porcine retroviruses.[203] The subject of zoonoses and xenotransplantation is still in its infancy and appropriate studies must be performed to devise the appropriate clinical protocols for preventing the introduction of any such pathogens into the human population.

Gene Therapy

Technical advances in the delivery and expression of exogenous genetic elements have made gene transfer and gene therapy practical approaches to managing many diseases. In transplantation, gene therapy has at least two potential roles. First, liver transplantation is performed for a number of inborn errors of metabolism (e.g., Wilson's disease). If these diseases are diagnosed before irreversible liver damage, the missing enzyme could be transfected into the patient's own liver and the disease cured without the need for transplantation. The newly introduced gene may be immunogenic and represent an autoantigen or alloantigen. In that case, the patient would still require immunosuppression, but probably not of the magnitude normally administered to organ recipients. A variation in this approach is to remove tissue from the patient, grow single-cell suspensions in culture, stably transfect the cells in culture, and return the cells to the patient. Fibroblasts, vascular endothelial cells, lymphocytes, and hepatocytes are all good candidates for this technique and have proved successful in experimental protocols. The second role for gene therapy is in the actual delivery of immunosuppression. Cytokines, receptors, antisense RNA, or transcriptional regulators could all be engineered into appropriate delivery vectors and introduced directly into the graft. Experimental protocols have successfully demonstrated the utility of these approaches in animals.[204–206]

Gene transfer and gene therapy are such new modalities that it is not yet clear how they will eventually be used. A number of difficult technical problems remain to be solved.[207] Current transfer vectors result in only transient, low-level expression of the transferred gene within a few cells in the target organ. Sustained, high-level gene expression throughout the graft has not yet been reliably achieved in any system. The transfer vectors and the transferred gene may be highly immunogenic. Additional immunosuppressive strategies are therefore required to circumvent those responses that would limit gene transfer efficacy. The transfer vectors also have potential pathogenic effects that may limit their utility. For example, adenoviral vectors can induce direct cytopathic effects by disrupting lysosomal membranes. Retroviral vectors can incorporate into genomic DNA and therefore have the potential for malignant transformation. Candidate genes for gene therapy have been evaluated in experimental systems, but it is not certain which will be most useful. For example, transforming growth factor-β is a soluble immunosuppressive cytokine; however, it can also induce exuberant fibrosis of the vasculature. IL-10, another immunosuppressive cytokine, can also activate T and B cells in some circumstances. Cytoplasmic or membrane-bound gene transfer products may be better candidates, but unless they can be expressed uniformly throughout the graft, their utility is doubtful. Some of the problems with gene transfer may make it particularly suited to transplantation. The transient expression of an immunosuppressive molecule in a graft at the time of transplantation may be the immunoregulatory signal that would permit the induction of tolerance without the need for long-term, systemic administration of conventional immunosuppression. Low-level expression of gene transfer products may also limit the immunosuppressive effect solely to the target organ, preventing systemic immunosuppression and its deleterious side effects.

Cellular Transplants

There are several situations in which cellular transplantation would better serve the potential recipient than whole-organ transplantation. As mentioned earlier, liver transplantation for certain inborn errors of metabolism could be supplanted by providing a specific gene product. This could be accomplished by infusing liver cells from a normal donor into the portal vein of the recipient and allowing them to populate the recipient liver. Such protocols have been successful clinically but require conventional immunosuppression.[208] In addition, the ability to detect rejection would be difficult by either biochemical or histologic means. An alternative is to obtain recipient hepatocytes by partial liver resection, grow them in culture, stably transfect them with the appropriate gene or genes, and reinfuse them into the recipient's portal circulation. Immunosuppression may be required because the new gene product would be recognized as foreign. Similar approaches with fibroblasts, smooth muscle, skeletal muscle, lymphocytes, and vascular endothelial cells have been demonstrated in experimental models.

Pancreas transplantation is performed for type 1 diabetes mellitus, so only the endocrine tissue is required by the recipient. The exocrine tissue in conventional whole-organ pancreas transplantation is often the source of a variety of complications related to the exocrine secretions. Therefore, pancreatic islet transplantation would be preferable. Some islet transplantations have been performed in humans, and the overall success rate for this highly experimental process is still poor, although there are a few notable exceptions. There are two major barriers to islet cell transplantation. First, the physical and mechanical means to separate islets from the whole organ are expensive and inefficient. With current technology, it may be necessary to use several donors for each recipient. With the current donor shortage, this is not a long-term solution to the problem. Xenotransplantation, with the use of porcine islets, may circumvent this problem but introduces the immunologic difficulties of xenoantigens. The second major barrier is immunosuppression and rejection. The success of any organ or cell transplant relies on the ability to detect rejections at an early stage with a simple biochemical or histologic test. None is known for islet transplants, and this is hampering current attempts to provide appropriate immunosuppression for these patients. These issues will likely yield to further experimental endeavors, and islet transplantation will likely supplant whole-organ pancreas transplantation.

KEY POINTS

- **The molecular and cellular participants in these processes are the immunoglobulin receptors of B cells, the antigen or T-cell receptors (TCRs) of T cells, and major histocompatibility complex (MHC) antigens of antigen-presenting cells (APCs).**
- **T cells do not bind and recognize antigen directly. T cells recognize a complex composed of a peptide fragment of antigen bound to an MHC molecule.**
- **Antigen is taken up by an APC, processed, and then presented to a T cell. The T cell is activated in response to appropriately processed and presented antigen.**
- **B cells primarily produce IgM antibody for primary responses and other isotypes for secondary responses.**
- **Immune cells communicate not only by direct cell–cell contact but by soluble factors called cytokines.**
- **Hyperacute rejection is the result of preformed antibody binding to the allograft at the time of revascularization in the operating room.**
- **Acute rejection usually occurs days to weeks after transplantation; it rarely occurs months or years later. Acute rejection is initiated by T-cell-dependent immunity and is characterized microscopically by a lymphocytic infiltrate accompanied by plasma cells, eosinophils, and a few mast cells or neutrophils.**
- **Chronic rejection usually occurs months to years after transplantation. It is characterized by loss of normal histologic structure, fibrosis, and atherosclerosis**

References

1. Eckhardt LA. Immunoglobulin gene expression only in the right cells at the right time. *FASEB J.* 1992;6:2553.
2. Komori T, Okada A, Stewart V, et al. Lack of N regions in antigen receptor variable region genes of TdT-deficient lymphocytes. *Science* 1993;261:1171.
3. Gilfillan S, Dierich A, Lemeur M, et al. Mice lacking TdT: mature animals with an immature lymphocyte repertoire. *Science* 1993;261:1175.
4. Aldhouse P. Transgenic mice display a class (switching) act. *Science* 1993;262:1212.
5. Papavasiliou F, Jankovic M, Gong S, et al. Control of immunoglobulin gene rearrangements in developing B cells. *Curr Opin Immunol.* 1997;9:233.
6. Cambier JC, Campbell KS. Membrane immunoglobulin and its accomplices: new lessons from an old receptor. *FASEB J.* 1992;6:3207.
7. Clark MR, Campbell KS, Kazalauskas A, et al. The B cell antigen receptor complex: association of Ig-α and Ig-β with distinct cytoplasmic effectors. *Science* 1992;258:123.
8. Constant P, Davodeau F, Peyrat M, et al. Stimulation of human gdT cells by nonpeptidic mycobacterial ligands. *Science* 1994;264:267.
9. Momvaerts P, Arnoldi J, Russ, F, et al. Different roles of and T cells in immunity against an intracellular bacterial pathogen. *Nature* 1993;365:53.
10. Schild H, Mavaddat N, Litzenberger C, et al. The nature of major histocompatibility complex recognition by gd T cells. *Cell* 1994;76:29–37.
11. Weiss A. T cell antigen receptor signal transduction: a tale of tails and cytoplasmic protein-tyrosine kinases. *Cell* 1993;73:209.
12. Williams AF, Beyers AD. At grips with interactions. *Nature* 1992;356:746.
13. Barinage M. Getting some "backbone": how MHC binds peptides. *Science* 1992;257:880.
14. **Germain RN. MHC-dependent antigen processing and peptide presentation: providing ligands for T lymphocyte activation. *Cell* 1994;76:287.**
15. Townsend A. A new presentation pathway? *Nature* 1992;356:386.
16. Schmid SL, Jackson MR. Making class II presentable. *Nature* 1994;368:103.
17. Howard JC, Seelig A. Peptides and the proteasome. *Nature* 1993;365:211.
18. Powis SJ, Deverson EV, Coadwell WJ, et al. Effect of polymorphism of an MHC-linked transporter on the peptides assembled in a class I molecule. *Nature* 1992;357:211.
19. Lanzavecchia A, Reid PA, Watts C. Irreversible association of peptides with class II MHC molecules in living cells. *Nature* 1992;357:249.
20. Peterson M, Miller J. Antigen presentation enhanced by the alternatively spliced invariant chain gene product p41. *Nature* 1992;357:596.
21. Malnati MS, Marti M, LaVaute T, et al. Processing pathways for presentation of cytosolic antigen to MHC class II-restricted T cells. *Nature* 1992;357:702.
22. Riberdy JM, Newcomb JR, Surman MJ, et al. HLA-DR molecules from an antigen-processing mutant cell line are associated with invariant chain peptides. *Nature* 1992;360:474.
23. Eisenlohr LC, Bacik I, Bennink JR, et al. Expression of a membrane protease enhances presentation of endogenous antigens to MHC class IB restricted T lymphocytes. *Cell* 1992;71:963.
24. Kaer LV, Ashton-Rickardt PG, Ploegh HL, et al. TAP-1 mutant mice are deficient in antigen presentation, surface class I molecules, and $CD4^{-}8^{+}$ T cells. *Cell* 1992;71:1205.
25. Pfeifer JD, Wick MJ, Roberts RL, et al. Phagocytic processing of bacterial antigens for class I MHC presentation to T cells. *Nature* 1993; 361:359.
26. Michalek MT, Grant EP, Gramm C, et al. A role for the ubiquitin-dependent proteolytic pathway in MHC class I-restricted antigen presentation. *Nature* 1993;363:552.

27. Germain RN, Rinker AG. Peptide binding inhibits protein aggregation of invariant-chain free class II dimers and promotes surface expression of occupied molecules. *Nature* 1993;373:725.
28. Driscoll J, Brown MG, Finley D. MHC-linked LMP gene products specifically alter peptidase activities of the proteasome. *Nature* 1993;365:262.
29. Gaczynska M, Rock KL, Goldberg AL. γ-Interferon and expression of MHC genes regulate peptide hydrolysis by proteasomes. *Nature* 1993;365:264.
30. Heemels MT, Schumacher TN, Wonigeit K, et al. Peptide translocation by variants of the transporter associated with antigen processing. *Science* 1993;262:2059.
31. Jackson MR, Cohen-Doyle MF, Peterson PA, et al. Regulation of MHC class I transport by the molecular chaperone, calnexin (p88, IP90). *Science* 1994;263:384.
32. Chicz RM, Urban RG, Lane WS, et al. Predominant naturally processed peptides bound to HLA-DR1 are derived from MHC-related molecules and are heterogeneous in size. *Nature* 1992;358:764.
33. Momburg F, Roelse J, Howard JC, et al. Selectivity of MHC-encoded peptide transporters from human, mouse and rat. *Nature* 1994;367:648.
34. Bodmer H, Viville S, Benoist C, et al. Diversity of endogenous epitopes bound to MHC class II molecules limited by invariant chain. *Science* 1994;263:1284.
35. Ortmann B, Androlewicz MJ, Cresswell P. MHC class I/β_2-microglobulin complexes associate with TAP transporters before peptide binding. *Nature* 1994;368:864.
36. Suh WK, Cohen-Doyle MF, Fruh K, et al. Interaction of MHC class I molecules with the transporter associated with antigen processing. *Science* 1994;264:1322.
37. Hunt DF, Michel H, Dickinson TA. Peptides presented to the immune system by the murine class II major histocompatibility complex molecule I-A^d. *Science* 1992;256:1817.
38. **Pamer E, Cresswell P. Mechanisms of MHC class I-restricted antigen processing. *Annu Rev Immunol.* 1998;16:323.**
39. Wolf PR, Ploegh HL. How MHC class II molecules acquire peptide cargo: biosynthesis and trafficking through the endocytic pathway. *Annu Rev Cell Dev Biol.* 1995;11:267.
40. Groettrup M, Soza A, Kuckelkorn U, et al. Peptide antigen production by the proteasome: complexity provides efficiency. *Immunol Today* 1996;17:429.
41. Rock KL, Goldberg AL. Degradation of cell proteins and the generation of MHC class I–presented peptides. *Annu Rev Immunol.* 1999;17:739.
42. Kurlander RJ, Shawar SM, Brown ML, et al. Specialized role for a murine class I-b MHC molecule in prokaryotic host defenses. *Science* 1992;257:678.
43. Rotzschke O, Falk K, Stevanovic S, et al. Qa-2 molecules are peptide receptors of higher stringency than ordinary class I molecules. *Nature* 1993;361:642.
44. Bachmann MF, Rohrer UH, Kundig TM, et al. The influence of antigen organization on B cell responsiveness. *Science* 1993;262:1448.
45. Guymer RH, Mandel TE. A comparison of corneal, pancreas, and skin grafts in mice. *Transplantation* 1994;57:1251.
46. Springer TA. Traffic signals for lymphocyte recirculation and leukocyte emigration: the multistep paradigm. *Cell* 1994;76:301.
47. Parham P. The box and the rod. *Nature* 1992;357:538.
48. Konig R, Huang L, Germain RN. MHC class II interaction with CD4 mediated by a region analogous to the MHC class I binding site for CD8. *Nature* 1992;356:796.
49. Kelso A. Th1 and Th2 subsets: paradigms lost? *Immunol Today* 1995;16:374.
50. Piccotti JR, Chan SY, VanBuskirk AM, et al. Are Th2 helper T lymphocytes beneficial, deleterious, or irrelevant in promoting allograft survival? *Transplantation* 1997;63:619.
51. Reiner SL, Wang Z, Hatam F, et al. T_H1 and T_H2 cell antigen receptors in experimental leishmaniasis. *Science* 1993;259:1457.
52. Takeuchi T, Lowry RP, Konieczny B. Heart allografts in murine systems. *Transplantation* 1992;53:1281.
53. Gaur A, Haspel R, Mayer J, et al. Requirement for CD8+ cells in T cell receptor peptide-induced clonal unresponsiveness. *Science* 1993;259:91.
54. LaRosa FG, Smilek D, Talmage DW, et al. Evidence that tolerance to cultured thyroid allografts is an active immunological process. *Transplantation* 1992;53:903.
55. Qin S, Cobbold SP, Pope H, et al. "Infectious" transplantation tolerance. *Science* 1993;259:974.
56. Halwani F, Guttmann RD, Ste. Croix H, et al. Identification of natural suppressor cells in long-term renal allograft recipients. *Transplantation* 1992;54:973.
57. **Clark EA, Ledbetter JA. How B and T cells talk to each other. *Nature* 1994;367:425.**
58. Marx J. Cell communication failure leads to immune disorder. *Science* 1993;259:896.
59. Hill A, Chapel H. The fruits of cooperation. *Nature* 1993;361:494.
60. Tsubata T, Wu J, Honjo T. B-cell apoptosis induced by antigen receptor crosslinking is blocked by a T-cell signal through CD40. *Nature* 1993;364:645.
61. Carter RH, Fearon DT. CD19: lowering the threshold for antigen receptor simulation of B lymphocytes. *Science* 1992;256:105.
62. Mantovani A, Bussolino F, Dejana E. Cytokine regulation of endothelial cell function. *FASEB J* 1992;6:2591.
63. Gerritsen ME, Bloor CM. Endothelial cell gene expression in response to injury. *FASEB J.* 1993;7:523.
64. Willebrand E, Salmela K, Isoniemi H, et al. Induction of HLA class II antigen and interleukin-2 receptor expression in acute vascular rejection of human kidney allografts. *Transplantation* 1992;53:1077.
65. Fuggle SV, Sanderson JB, Gray DW, et al. Variation in expression of endothelial adhesion molecules in pretransplant and transplanted kidneys: correlation with intragraft events. *Transplantation* 1993;55:1170.
66. Wuthrich RP, Jenkins TA, Snyder TL. Regulation of cytokine-stimulated vascular cell adhesion molecule-1 expression in renal tubular epithelial cells. *Transplantation* 1993;55:172.
67. Pelletier RP, Morgan CJ, Sedmak DD, et al. Analysis of inflammatory endothelial changes, including VCAM-1 expression, in murine cardiac grafts. *Transplantation* 1993;55:315.
68. Hoffmann MW, Wonigeit K, Steinhoff G, et al. Production of cytokines (TNFα, IL-1β) and endothelial cell activation in human liver allograft rejection. *Transplantation* 1993;55:329.
69. Morgan CJ, Pelletier RP, Hernandez CJ, et al. Alloantigen-dependent endothelial phenotype and lymphokine mRNA expression in rejecting murine cardiac allografts. *Transplantation* 1993;55:919.
70. Pober JS, Orosz CG, Rose ML, et al. Can graft endothelial cells initiate a host anti-graft immune response? *Transplantation* 1996;61:343.
71. Briscoe DM, Alexander SI, Lichtman AH. Interactions between T lymphocytes and endothelial cells in allograft rejection. *Curr Opin Immunol.* 1998;10:525.
72. Albelda SM, Smith CM, Ward PA. Adhesion molecules and inflammatory injury. *FASEB J.* 1994;8:504.
73. Hynes RO. Integrins: versatility, modulation, and signaling in cell adhesion. *Cell* 1992;69:11.
74. Lasky LA. Selectins: interpreters of cell-specific carbohydrate information during inflammation. *Science* 1992;258:964.
75. Shimizu Y, Shaw S. Mucins in the mainstream. *Nature* 1993;366:630.
76. Baumhueter S, Singer MS, Henzel W, et al. Binding of L-selectin to the vascular sialomucin CD34. *Science* 1993;262:436.
77. Berg EL, McEvoy LM, Berlin C, et al. L-selectin–mediated lymphocyte rolling on MAdCAM-1. *Nature* 1993;366:695.
78. Taylor PM, Rose ML, Yacoub MH, et al. Induction of vascular adhesion molecules during rejection of human cardiac allografts. *Transplantation* 1992; 54:451.
79. **Paul WE, Seder RA. Lymphocyte responses and cytokines. *Cell* 1994;76:241.**
80. Nowak R. Bubble boy paradox resolved. *Science* 1993;262:1818.
81. Kondo M, Takeshita T, Higuchi M, et al. Functional participation of the IL-2 receptor γ chain in IL-7 receptor complexes. *Science* 1994;263:1453.
82. Kishimoto T, Akira S, Taga T. Interleukin-6 and its receptor: a paradigm for cytokines. *Science* 1992;258:593.
83. Kishimoto T, Taga T, Akira S. Cytokine signal transduction. *Cell* 1994;76:253.
84. Taga T, Kishimoto T. Cytokine receptors and signal transduction. *FASEB J* 1993;7:3387.
85. Stahl N, Yancopoulos GD. The alphas, betas, and kinases of cytokine receptor complexes. *Cell* 1993;74:587.
86. Hunter T. Cytokine connections. *Nature* 1993;366:114.
87. Stahl N, Boulton TG, Farruggella T, et al. Association and activation of Jak-Tyk kinases by CNTF-LIF-OSM-IL-6 β receptor components. *Science* 1994; 263:92.
88. Ramsay AJ, Husband AJ, Ramshaw IA, et al. The role of interleukin-6 in mucosal IgA antibody responses in vivo. *Science* 1994;264:561.
89. Scott, P. IL-12: initiation cytokine for cell-mediated immunity. *Science* 1993;260:496.
90. Afonso LC, Scharton TM, Vieira LQ, et al. The adjuvant effect of interleukin-12 in a vaccine against leishmania major. *Science* 1994;263:235.
91. Massague J. Receptors for the TGFβ family. *Cell* 1992;69:1067.
92. Wrana JL, Attisano L, Carcamo J, et al. TGFβ signals through a heteromeric protein kinase receptor complex. *Cell* 1992;71:1003.
93. Barral-Netto M, Barral A, Brownell CE, et al. Transforming growth factor-β in leishmanial infection: a parasite escape mechanism. *Science* 1992; 257:545.
94. Attisano L, Carcamo J, Ventura F, et al. Identification of human activin and TGFβ type I receptors that form heteromeric kinase complexes with type II receptors. *Cell* 1993;75:671.
95. Smith CA, Farrah T, Goodwin RG. The TNF receptor superfamily of cellular and viral proteins: activation, constimulation, and death. *Cell* 1994;76:959.
96. Cohen J. New protein steals the show as "costimulator" of T cells. *Science* 1993;262:844.
97. Beutler B, van Huffel C. Unraveling function in the TNF ligand and receptor families. *Science* 1994;264:667.
98. Suda T, Takahashi T, Golstein P, et al. Molecular cloning and expression of the Fas ligand, a novel member of the tumor necrosis factor family. *Cell* 1993;75:1169.
99. Barinaga M. Interfering with interferon. *Science* 1993;259:1693.
100. Huang S, Hendriks W, Althage A, et al. Immune response in mice that lack the interferon-g receptor. *Science* 1993;259:1742.

101. Darnell JE, Kerr IM, Stark GR. Jak-STAT pathways and transcriptional activation in response to IFNs and other extracellular signaling proteins. *Science* 1994;264:1415.
102. Wu CJ, Lovett M, Wong-Lee J, et al. Cytokine gene expression in rejecting cardiac allografts. *Transplantation* 1992;54:326.
103. Halloran PF, Broski AP, Batiuk TD, et al. The molecular immunology of acute rejection: an overview. *Transplant Immunol.* 1993;1:3.
104. Bishop DK, Shelby J, Eichwald E. Mobilization of T lymphocytes following cardiac transplantation. *Transplantation* 1992;53:849.
105. Doherty PC. Cell-mediated cytotoxicity. *Cell* 1993;75:607.
106. Kagi D, Vignaux F, Ledermann B, et al. Fas and perforin pathways as major mechanisms of T cell–mediated cytotoxicity. *Science* 1994; 265:528.
107. Mueller C, Shao Y, Altermatt HJ, et al. The effect of cyclosporine treatment on the expression of genes encoding granzyme A and perforin in the infiltrate of mouse heart transplants. *Transplantation* 1993;55:139.
108. Clement MV, Legros-Maida S, Isreal-Bib D, et al. Perforin and granzyme B expression is associated with severe acute rejection. *Transplantation* 1994;57:322.
109. Clark WR. The hole truth about perforin. *Nature* 1994;369:16–17.
110. Kagi D, Ledermann B, Burki K, et al. Cytotoxicity mediated by T cells and natural killer cells is greatly impaired in perforin-deficient mice. *Nature* 1994;369:31.
111. Whiteside TL, Herberman RB. Role of human natural killer cells in health and disease. *Clin Diagn Lab Immunol.* 1994;1:125.
112. Raulet DH. A sense of something missing. *Nature* 1992;358:21.
113. Martinez OM, Ascher NL, Ferrell L, et al. Evidence for a nonclassical pathway of graft rejection involving interleukin 5 and eosinophils. *Transplantation* 1993;55:909.
114. Zhang Y, Ramos BF, Jakschik BA. Neutrophil recruitment by tumor necrosis factor from mast cells in immune complex peritonitis. *Science* 1992;258:1957.
115. Baggiolini M, Boulay F, Badwey JA, et al. Activation of neutrophil leukocytes: chemoattractant receptors and respiratory burst. *FASEB J.* 1993;7:1004.
116. Morel D, Norman E, Lemoine C, et al. Tumor necrosis factor alpha in human kidney transplant rejection: analysis by in situ hybridization. *Transplantation* 1993;55:773.
117. Pizarro TT, Malinowska K, Kovacs E, et al. Induction of TNFα and TNFβ gene expression in rat cardiac transplants during allograft rejection. *Transplantation* 1993;56:399.
118. Saito R, Prehn J, Zuo X, et al. The participation of tumor necrosis factor in the pathogenesis of lung allograft rejection in the rat. *Transplantation* 1993;55:967.
119. Martinez OM, Villanueva JC, Lake J, et al. IL-2 and IL-5 gene expression in response to alloantigen in liver allograft recipients and in vitro. *Transplantation* 1993;55:1159.
120. Merville P, Pouteil-Noble C, Wijdenes J, et al. Detection of single cells secreting IFN-gamma, IL-6, and IL-10 in irreversibly rejected human kidney allografts, and their modulation by IL-2 and IL-4. *Transplantation* 1993; 55:639.
121. Kopf M, Baumann H, Freer G, et al. Impaired immune and acute-phase responses in interleukin-6–deficient mice. *Nature* 1994;368:339.
122. Blancho G, Moreau JF, Chabannes D, et al. HILDA/LIF, G-CSF, IL-1β, and TNFα production during acute rejection of human kidney allografts. *Transplantation* 1993;56:597.
123. Bentouimou N, Moreau JF, Peyrat MA, et al. The effects of cyclosporine on HILDA/LIF gene expression in human T cells. *Transplantation* 1993;55:163.
124. Blotnick S, Peoples GE, Freeman MR, et al. T lymphocytes synthesize and export heparin-binding epidermal growth factor-like growth factor and basic fibroblast growth factor, mitogens for vascular cells and fibroblasts: differential production and release by CD4$^+$ and CD8$^+$ T cells. *Proc Natl Acad Sci USA* 1994;91:2890.
125. Johnston PS, Wang MW, Lim SM, et al. Discordant xenograft rejection in an antibody-free model. *Transplantation* 1992;54:573.
126. Stansby G, Fuller B, Jeremy J, et al. Endothelin release: a facet of reperfusion injury in clinical liver transplantation? *Transplantation* 1993;56:239.
127. Spurney RF, Ibrahim S, Butterly D, et al. Leukotrienes in renal transplant rejection in rats. *J Immunol.* 1994;152:867.
128. Langreher JM, Hoffman RA, Lancaster JR, et al. Nitric oxide: a new endogenous immunomodulator. *Transplantation* 1993;55:1205.
129. Xenos ES, Stevens RB, Sutherland DE, et al. The role of nitric oxide in IL-1β–mediated dysfunction of rodent islets of Langerhans. *Transplantation* 1994;57:1208.
130. Connor HD, Gao W, Nukina S, et al. Evidence that free radicals are involved in graft failure following orthotopic liver transplantation in the rat: an electron paramagnetic resonance spin trapping study. *Transplantation* 1992;54:199.
131. Land W, Schneeberg H, Schleibner S, et al. The beneficial effect of human recombinant superoxide dismutase on acute and chronic rejection events in recipients of cadaveric renal transplants. *Transplantation* 1994;57:211.
132. Alexandre GP, Latinne D, Gianello P, et al. Preformed cytotoxic antibodies and ABO-incompatible grafts. *Clin Transpl.* 1991;5:583.
133. Bach FH. Xenotransplantation: problems for consideration. *Clin Transpl.* 1991;5:595.
134. Paul LC, Fellstrom B. Chronic vascular rejection of the heart and the kidney: have rational treatment options emerged? *Transplantation* 1992;53:1169.
135. Hancock WH, Whitely WD, Tullius SG, et al. Cytokines, adhesion molecules, and the pathogenesis of chronic rejection of rat renal allografts. *Transplantation* 1993;56:643.
136. Hajar DP, Pomerantz KB. Signal transduction in atherosclerosis: integration of cytokines and the eicosanoid network. *FASEB J.* 1992;6:2933.
137. Van Parijs L, Abbas AK. Homeostasis and self-tolerance in the immune system: turning lymphocytes off. *Science* 1998;280:243.
138. Weissman IL. Developmental switches in the immune system. *Cell* 1994;76:207.
139. vonBoehmer H. Positive selection of lymphocytes. *Cell* 1994;76:219.
140. Nossal GJ. Negative selection of lymphocytes. *Cell* 1994;76:229.
141. Allen PM. Peptides in positive and negative selection: a delicate balance. *Cell* 1994;76:593.
142. Marrack P, Parker DC. A little of what you fancy. *Nature* 1994;368:397.
143. Janeway CA. Thymic selection: two pathways to life and two to death. *Immunity* 1994;1:3.
144. vonBoehmer H, Kisielow P. Lymphocyte lineage commitment: instruction versus selection. *Cell* 1993;73:207.
145. Schwartz RH. Costimulation of T lymphocytes: the role of CD28, CTLA-4, and B7/BB1 in interleukin-2 production and immunotherapy. *Cell* 1992;71:1065.
146. Harding FA, McArthur JG, Gross JA, et al. CD28-mediated signaling co-stimulates murine T cells and prevents induction of anergy in T-cell clones. *Nature* 1992;356:607.
147. McCormick F. How receptors turn Ras on. *Nature* 1993;363:15.
148. Marx J. Two major signal pathways linked. *Science* 1993;262:988.
149. Clements JL, Koretzky GA. Recent developments in lymphocyte activation: linking kinases to downstream signaling events. *J Clin Invest.* 1999;103:925.
150. Schillance RV, Scott JD. Organization of kinases, phosphatases and receptor signaling complexes. *J Clin Invest.* 1999;106:761.
151. Jenkins MK, Miller RA. Memory and anergy: challenges to traditional models of T lymphocyte differentiation. *FASEB J.* 1992;6:2428.
152. Sprent J. T and B memory cells. *Cell* 1994;76:315.
153. vonBoehmer H. Tolerance by exhaustion. *Nature* 1993;362:696.
154. Ferber I, Schonrich G, Schenkel J, et al. Levels of peripheral T cell tolerance by different doses of tolerogen. *Science* 1994;263:674.
155. Critchfield JM, Racke MK, Zuniga-Pflucker J, et al. T cell deletion in high antigen dose therapy of autoimmune encephalomyelitis. *Science* 1994;263:1139.
156. Ramsdell F, Fowlkes BJ. Maintenance of in vivo tolerance by persistence of antigen. *Science* 1992;257:1130.
157. Lombardi G, Sidhu S, Batchelor R, et al. Anergic T cells as suppressor cells in vitro. *Science* 1994;264:1587.
158. Araten DJ, Lawton T, Ferrara J, et al. In vitro alloreactivity against host antigens in an adult HLA-mismatched bone marrow transplant recipient despite in vivo host tolerance. *Transplantation* 1993;55:76.
159. Posselt AM, Barker CF, Friedman AL, et al. Prevention of autoimmune diabetes in the BB rat by intrathymic islet transplantation at birth. *Science* 1992;256:1321.
160. Campos L, Alfrey EJ, Posselt AM, et al. Prolonged survival of rat orthotopic liver allografts after intrathymic inoculation of donor-strain cells. *Transplantation* 1993;55:866.
161. Markmann JF, Odorico JS, Bassiri H, et al. Deletion of donor-reactive T lymphocytes in adult mice after intrathymic inoculation with lymphoid cells. *Transplantation* 1993;55:871.
162. Spitzer TR, Delmonico F, Tolkoff-Rubin N, et al. Combined histocompatibility leukocyte antigen matched donor bone marrow and renal transplantation for multiple myeloma with end stage renal disease: the induction of allograft tolerance through mixed lymphohematopoietic chimerism. *Transplantation* 1999;68:480.
163. Wekerle T, Sykes M. Mixed chimerism as an approach for the induction of transplantation tolerance. *Transplantation* 1999;68:459.
164. Miller J, Mathew J, Garcia-Morales R, et al. The human bone marrow as an immunoregulatory organ. *Transplantation* 1999;68:1079.
165. Starzl TE, Demetris AJ, Trucco M, et al. Chimerism and donor-specific nonreactivity 27 to 2 years after kidney allotransplantation. *Transplantation* 1993;55:1272.
166. Fuchs EJ, Matzingert P. B cells turn off virgin but not memory T cells. *Science* 1992;258:1156.
167. Larsen CP, Elwood ET, Alexander DZ, et al. Long-term acceptance of skin and cardiac allografts after blocking CD40 and CD28 pathways. *Nature* 1996;381:434.
168. Kirk AD, Harlan DM, et al. CTLA4-Ig and anti-CD40 ligand prevent renal allograft rejection in primates. *Proc Natl Acad Sci USA* 1997;94:8789.
169. Sayegh MH, Turka LA. The role of T-cell costimulatory activation pathways in transplant rejection. *N Engl J Med.* 1998;338:1813.
170. Kirk AD, Burkly LC, Batty DS, et al. Treatment with humanized monoclonal antibody against CD154 prevents acute renal allograft rejection in nonhuman primates. *Nat Med.* 1999;5:686.
171. Harlan DM, Kirk AD. The future of organ and tissue transplantation: can T-cell costimulatory pathway modifiers revolutionize the prevention of graft rejection? *JAMA* 1999;282:1076.
172. Halloran P, Mathew T, Tomlanovich S, et al. Mycophenolate mofetil in renal allograft recipients. *Transplantation* 1997;63:39.
173. The Mycophenolate mofetil acute renal rejection study group. Mycophenolate mofetil for the treatment of a first acute renal allograft rejection. *Transplantation* 1998;65:235.

174. Groth CG, Backman L, Morales JM, et al. Sirolimus (Rapamycin)-based therapy in human renal transplantation. *Transplantation* 1999;67:1036.
175. Kahan BD, Julian BA, Pescovitz MD, et al. Sirolimus reduces the incidence of acute rejection episodes despite lower cyclosporin doses in Caucasian recipients of mismatched primary renal allografts: a phase II trial. *Transplantation* 1999;68:1526.
176. Brennan DC, Flavin K, Lowell JA, et al. A randomized, double-blinded comparison of Thymoglobulin versus Atgam for induction immunosuppressive therapy in adult renal transplant recipients [published erratum appears in *Transplantation* 1999;67:1386] *Transplantation* 1999;67: 1011.
177. Kahan BD, Rajagopalan PR, Hall M, et al. Reduction of the occurrence of acute cellular rejection among renal allograft recipients treated with basiliximab, a chimeric anti-interleukin-2 receptor monoclonal antibody. *Transplantation* 1999;67:276.
178. Vincenti F, Kirkman R, Light S, et al. Interleukin-2-receptor blockade with daclizumab to prevent acute rejection in renal transplantation. *N Engl J Med.* 1998;338:161.
179. Morris RE. ±15-Deoxyspergualin: a mystery wrapped within an enigma. *Clin Transpl.* 1991; 5:530.
180. Nadler SG, Tepper MA, Schacter B, et al. Interaction of the immunosuppressant deoxyspergualin with a member of the Hsp70 family of heat shock proteins. *Science* 1992;258:484.
181. Ramos EL, Nadler SG, Grasela DM, et al. Deoxyspergualin: mechanism of action and pharmacokinetics. *Transplant Proc.* 1996;28:873.
182. Chong AS, Finnegan A, Jiang X, et al. Leflunomide, a novel immunosuppressive agent. *Transplantation* 1993;55:1361.
183. Williams JW, Xiao F, Foster P, et al. Leflunomide in experimental transplantation. *Transplantation* 1994;57:1223.
184. Chong AS, Huang W, Liu W, et al. In vivo activity of leflunomide: pharmacokinetic analyses and mechanism of immunosuppression. *Transplantation* 1999;68:100.
185. Jameson BA, McDonnell JM, Marini JC, et al. A rationally designed CD4 analogue inhibits experimental allergic encephalomyelitis. *Nature* 1994;368:744.
186. Travers P. Immunological agnosia. *Nature* 1993;363:117.
187. Weber S, Traunecker A, Oliveri F, et al. Specific low-affinity recognition of major histocompatibility complex plus peptide by soluble T-cell receptor. *Nature* 1992;356:793.
188. Sloan-Lancaster J, Evavold BD, Allen PM. Induction of T-cell anergy by altered T cell-receptor ligand on live antigen-presenting cells. *Nature* 1993;363:156.
189. Roslin MS, Tranbaugh RE, Panza A, et al. One-year monkey heart xenograft survival in cyclosporine-treated baboons. *Transplantation* 1992;54:949.
190. Hardy MA, Reed E, Suciu-Foca N. Antiidiotypic antibodies and pretreatment with blood transfusions in organ transplantation. *Clin Transpl.* 1991;5:501.
191. Weiner HL, Mackin GA, Matsui M, et al. Double-blind pilot trial of oral tolerization with myelin antigens in multiple sclerosis. *Science* 1993;259:1321.
192. Hancock WW, Sayegh MH, Kwok CA, et al. Oral, but not intravenous, alloantigen prevents accelerated allograft rejection by selective intragraft T_H2 cell activation. *Transplantation* 1993;55:1112.
193. Paya CV, Fung JJ, Nalesnik MA, et al. Epstein-Barr virus-induced post-transplant lymphoproliferative disorders. ASTS/ASTP EBV-PTLD Task Force and The Mayo Clinic Organized International Consensus Development Meeting. *Transplantation* 1999;68:1517.
194. Penn I. The effect of immunosuppression on pre-existing cancers. *Transplantation* 1993;55:742.
195. Colquhoun SD, Robert ME, Shaked A, et al. Transmission of CNS malignancy by organ transplantation. *Transplantation* 1994;57:970.
196. **Auchincloss H, Sachs DH. Xenogeneic transplantation. *Annu Rev Immunol.* 1998;16:433.**
197. Leventhal JR, Matas AJ. Xenotransplantation in rodents: a review and reclassification. *Transplant Rev.* 1994;8:80.
198. Gorski A, Grieb P, Makula J, et al. Human xenoreactive natural antibodies: avidity and targets on porcine endothelial cells. *Transplantation* 1993;56:1251.
199. Dalmasso AP, Platt JL. Prevention of complement-mediated activation of xenogeneic endothelial cells in an in vitro model of xenograft hyperacute rejection by C1 inhibitor. *Transplantation* 1993;56:1171.
200. McCurry KR, Kooyman DL, Alvarado CG, et al. Human complement regulatory proteins protect swine-to-primate cardiac xenografts from humoral injury. *Nat Med.* 1995;1:423.
201. Lambrigts D, Sachs DH, Cooper DK. Discordant organ xenotransplantation in primates: world experience and current status. *Transplantation* 1998;66:547.
202. Michaels MG, Simmons RL. Xenotransplant-associated zoonoses. *Transplantation* 1994;57:1.
203. Patience C, Takeuchi Y, Weiss RA. Infection of human cells by an endogenous retrovirus of pigs. *Nat Med.* 1997;3:282.
204. Shaked A, Csete ME, Shiraishi M, et al. Retroviral-mediated gene transfer into rat experimental liver transplant. *Transplantation* 1994;57:32.
205. Fedoseyeva EV, Li Y, Huey B, et al. Inhibition of interferon-γ-mediated immune functions by oligonucleotides. *Transplantation* 1994;57:606.
206. Ramanathan M, Lantz M, MacGregor RD, et al. Inhibition of interferon-γ-induced major histocompatibility complex class I expression by certain oligodeoxynucleotides. *Transplantation* 1994;57:612.
207. Magee JC, Sung RS, Bromberg JS. Gene therapy in organ transplantation: applicabilities and shortcomings. In: Sayegh MH, Remuzzi G, eds. *Current and future immunosuppression therapies following transplantation.* Dordrecht, The Netherlands: Kluwer Academic (in press).
208. Fox JJ, Chowdhury JR, Kaufmann SS, et al. Treatment of the Crigler-Najjar syndrome type I with hepatocyte transplantation. *N Engl J Med.* 1998;338:1422.

CHAPTER 36 ■ ORGAN PRESERVATION

ROBERT M. MERION

PATHOPHYSIOLOGY OF ORGAN PRESERVATION INJURY

The removal, storage, and transplantation of a solid organ from a donor results in profound alterations in homeostatic control of the *milieu interieur* of that organ. These effects manifest themselves in the degree to which the return of normal organ function is delayed or prevented once the recipient transplantation procedure is completed. The injury sustained by an organ during the processes of procurement, preservation, and transplantation occurs primarily as a result of ischemia and hypothermia, the former being customarily classified as warm or cold ischemia. Warm ischemia and its consequences are associated with normothermic events that occur before removal of the organ from the body. Cold ischemia refers to events occurring during the interval between initial organ cooling and revascularization in the recipient.

The principles of modern organ preservation are to provide for hypothermia, prevention of cellular swelling, and avoidance of biochemical injury.[1,2] These principles are intended to interfere with the loss of cellular integrity, changes in ionic composition, and disruption of cellular energy systems that occur during organ storage. The following discussion describes these phenomena. Finally, the effects of oxygen-derived free radicals, cytokines, and nitric oxide at the time of reperfusion are discussed.

Structural Integrity

The cell membrane plays a crucial physical protective role and provides an active interface with the extracellular environment. Receptors, ion regulation, and enzyme systems linked to the cell membrane complex contain extracellular, transmembrane, and intracellular components essential to their function. The interrelation of such systems with the membrane itself is highly dependent on a stable configuration of the lipid bilayer and on tight control of temperature, pH, and osmolarity. Organ ischemia and preservation disrupt all these relations. Lowering the temperature through the phase transition of lipids results in profound changes in conformation and stability of the membrane in addition to drastically altering the function of membrane-bound enzymes. Physicochemical membrane changes induced by hypothermia result in increased permeability, which in turn adds to the burden of maintaining a stable intracellular environment and contributes to cell swelling. Organ preservation solutions have historically therefore been hypertonic to minimize these alterations.

Ionic Composition

The foregoing membrane changes are compounded by crippling of the Na^+-K^+-adenosine triphosphatase (ATPase) pump caused by the lack of ATP production and by generation of excess hydrogen ion resulting from anaerobic metabolism during ischemia. When the Na^+-K^+-ATPase pump is paralyzed, potassium diffuses down its concentration gradient to the extracellular environment while sodium, normally present at a low concentration in the cell, pours in. Modern preservation solutions have typically had electrolyte compositions similar to that inside the cell with high potassium and low sodium concentrations. Osmotic gradients are, therefore, minimized, and the cellular ionic charge remains relatively constant.

Hydrogen ion production continues in ischemic organs and may result in cellular damage. Intracellular pH gradually falls without replenishment of buffering capabilities, and under conditions requiring a switch from aerobic to anaerobic glycolysis, the production of lactic acid also increases. The liver appears to be especially susceptible to this type of injury. A plausible mechanism has been described whereby glucokinase in the liver phosphorylates glucose (endogenous or provided in preservation solution) to glucose-6-phosphate.[3] The normal metabolic pathway for glucose-6-phosphate results in production of pyruvate and ultimately lactate by lactic dehydrogenase (Fig. 36.1). Unlike the kidney, the hepatic isozyme of lactic dehydrogenase, M4, functions particularly well under acidotic conditions in the presence of high concentrations of lactic acid. These biochemical differences underlie the range of acceptable cold ischemia time for various organs.

Calcium ion permeability is increased with ischemia, and a rapid influx of calcium may overwhelm mitochondrial buffering capacity. There is increased activity of calmodulin, a cytoplasmic calcium-binding protein, and a cascade of enzyme

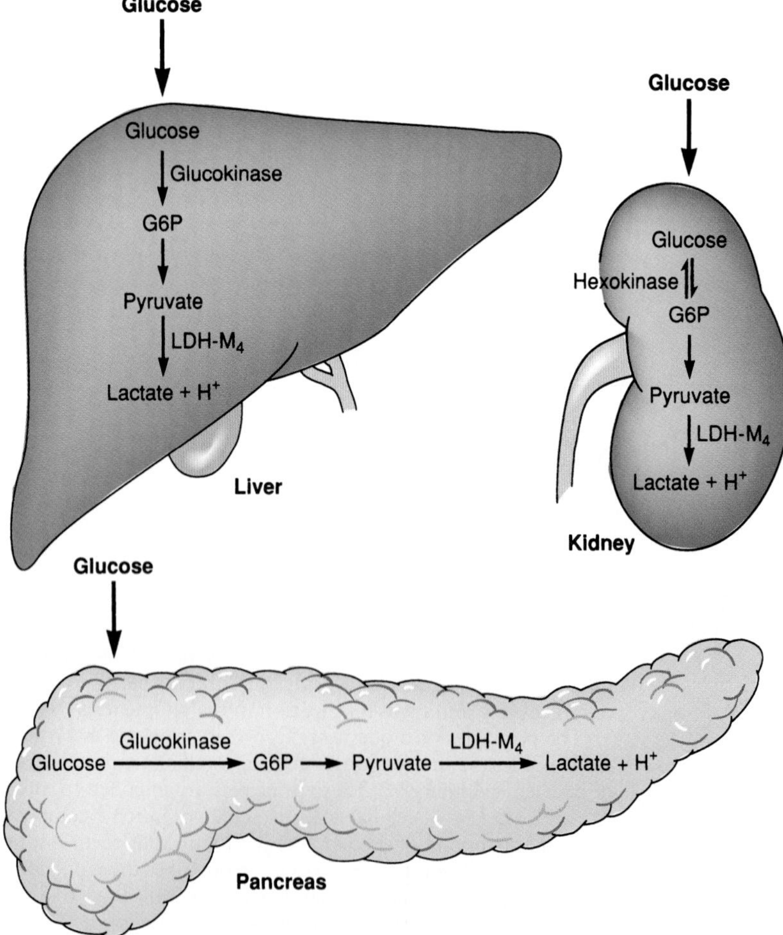

FIGURE 36.1 The effects of acidosis on glucose metabolism are organ specific. For example, the M4 isozyme of lactate dehydrogenase (LDH) functions well in an acidotic environment in the presence of high concentrations of lactic acid. G6P, glucose-6-phosphate. (Adapted with permission from Belzer FO, Southard JH. Principles of solid-organ preservation by cold storage. *Transplantation* 1988;45:673–676.)

activation events, including the upregulation of phospholipases and subsequent production of prostaglandin derivatives, results in mitochondrial and cell membrane injury. Vascular smooth muscle myofibrillar contraction may be initiated by increased cellular calcium concentrations, with the resulting vasospasm contributing to ischemic damage. Endothelin, a 21 amino-acid peptide with potent vasoconstrictor properties has been recognized as another factor that plays a role in preservation injury by inducing vasospasm after revascularization.[4,5]

Cellular Energy

The energy requirements of aerobic cells are provided by a combination of the enzymatic breakdown of glucose (glycolysis) and by the process of cellular respiration, encompassing the transfer of electrons from organic molecules to molecular oxygen (electron transport and oxidative phosphorylation) (Fig. 36.2). Hypothermia results in decreased metabolic rate and slows the rate at which enzymes degrade cellular components but metabolism is not completely suppressed. It has been calculated that cooling from 37°C to 0°C results in a 12-fold reduction of cellular metabolism.[1] Although metabolism is slowed and utilization of cellular energy stores is slowed, ATP and adenosine diphosphate (ADP), the major sources of cellular metabolic energy, are gradually depleted during hypothermia. This depletion is presumably a result of residual energy requirements that exceed the capacity of the cell to produce ATP.

During ischemia and organ preservation, the glycolytic pathway is sidetracked to lactate production as the Krebs tricarboxylic acid cycle and mitochondrial respiration are impaired. Although some of the enzymes of the Krebs cycle may be found in the extramitochondrial cytoplasm, the inner compartment of the mitochondrion is where the enzymatic reactions of the cycle occur. Mitochondrial dysfunction, therefore, is responsible for most of the changes in cellular energy associated with ischemia and organ preservation.

Hypothermic preservation results in reduced activity of mitochondrial enzymes. Cellular respiration, which requires adenine nucleotide substrates, is reduced. For ADP to be transported into the mitochondrion as a substrate for conversion to high-energy ATP, a membrane adenine nucleotide translocase is required. Hypothermia unfavorably alters the relation between the enzyme and the inner mitochondrial membrane within which it resides, reducing substrate delivery.[6] Phospholipid hydrolysis by phospholipases increases levels of free fatty acids, acyl derivatives of which may also affect membrane structure and the function of the translocase. Cannibalization of ADP sequestered in the extramitochondrial cytoplasm by adenylate kinase for conversion to ATP results in accumulation of adenosine monophosphate as a byproduct, which reduces purine synthesis and results in the loss of ATP precursors from the cell.

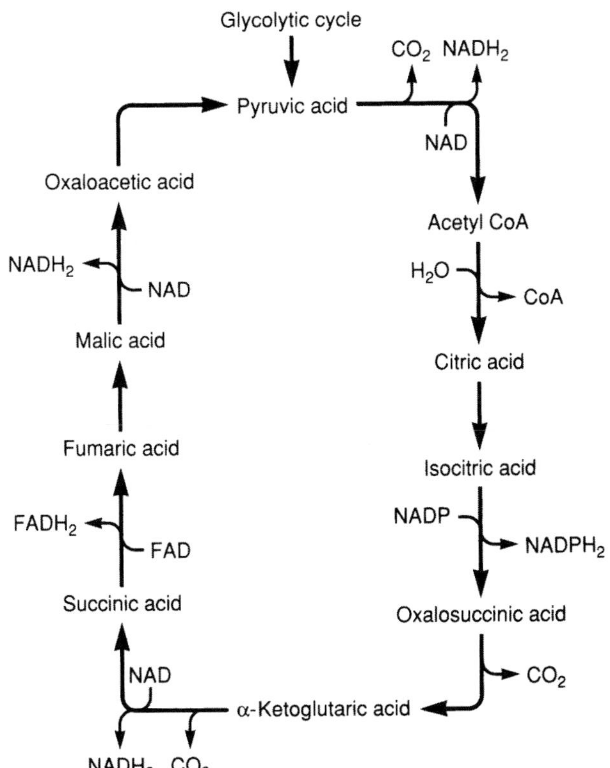

FIGURE 36.2 Cellular energy requirements are met largely through the processes of glycolysis, the Krebs tricarboxylic acid cycle, and oxidative phosphorylation. CoA, coenzyme A; $NADH_2$, reduced form of nicotinamide adenine dinucleotide; NAD, nicotinamide adenine dinucleotide; NADP, nicotinamide-adenine dinucleotide phosphate ; $NADPH_2$; FAD, flavin adenine dinucleotide; $FADH_2$, reduced form of FAD.

Reperfusion Injury

It is apparent that much of the injury to transplanted organs occurs not during the period of ischemia per se but on organ reperfusion. This realization has led to many advances in organ preservation. Furthermore, some of the events that occur during reperfusion may result in enhanced immunogenicity of the graft. A better understanding of these events will hopefully lead to the development of preservation methods that decrease the propensity for allograft rejection at a later date.

Oxygen Free Radical–Mediated Effects

The mechanisms by which reactive species of oxygen are produced in biologic systems and the effects of these molecules on various cells and tissues were elucidated in the 1970s and 1980s.[7] The best studied model involves the production of superoxide anion (O_2^-) as a by-product of the enzymatic catabolism of the purine metabolites hypoxanthine and xanthine to uric acid by xanthine oxidase (Fig. 36.3). During ischemic states a cytosolic enzyme is activated by increased

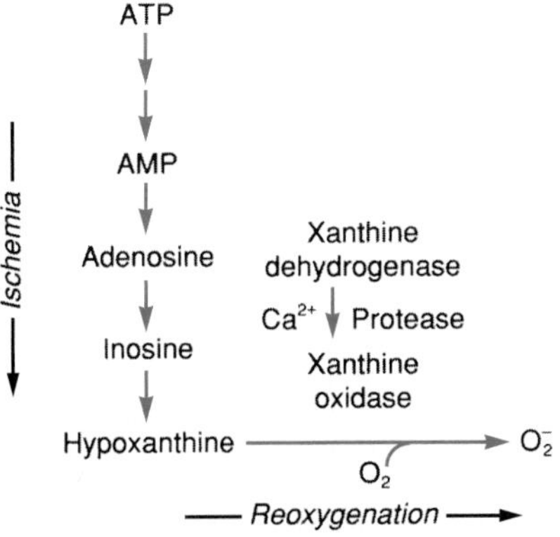

FIGURE 36.3 The classic pathway of superoxide anion generation by the metabolism of purines by xanthine oxidase. ATP, adenosine triphosphate; AMP, adenosine monophosphate; Ca_2, O_2, oxygen.

intracellular calcium resulting in the conversion of xanthine dehydrogenase to xanthine oxidase. Both xanthine dehydrogenase and xanthine oxidase catabolize hypoxanthine and xanthine to uric acid. Xanthine oxidase utilizes molecular oxygen as an electron acceptor and forms O_2^- as a result. Superoxide anion rapidly reacts with itself to form hydrogen peroxide, a potent oxidant capable of injuring the cell by oxidizing lipid membranes and cellular proteins. Hydrogen peroxide then produces a cascade of oxygen free radicals, including hydroxyl radical (OH•) and singlet oxygen, that are even more potent oxidants. The damaging effects of oxygen free radicals begin upon reperfusion of the organ. During ischemic conditions, tissue oxygen levels fall below the threshold needed to allow xanthine oxidase to metabolize xanthine and hypoxanthine. This allows the intracellular concentration of these metabolites to rise. Upon reperfusion, oxygen is suddenly available and metabolism proceeds rapidly, resulting in a dramatic and sudden production of reactive oxygen intermediates. The cellular defenses against peroxidation are overwhelmed and injury occurs.[8]

Agents that reduce oxygen free radical generation, or scavenge them once they are formed, have been used to determine the contribution of these molecular species to preservation-related reperfusion injury and have the ability to decrease peroxidation due to oxygen free radicals during reperfusion. Allopurinol, an inhibitor of xanthine oxidase, has been shown to have protective effects when used before the ischemic insult in a variety of experimental systems. Unfortunately, allopurinol has other effects, such as vasodilatation and preservation of the purine nucleotide pool, making it a less-than-ideal agent for defining oxygen free radical effects. Other studies using superoxide dismutase have clearly demonstrated a role for oxygen radicals in reperfusion injury in transplantation.[9] Similarly, desferroxamine, an iron chelator, removes an essential metal cofactor for the generation of the extremely reactive hydroxyl radical resulting in decreased oxidative injury.

Indirect evidence of oxygen free radical effects rests on the documentation of lipid peroxidation. In this process, interaction of highly reactive oxygen species with polyunsaturated fatty acids in the cell membrane starts a chain reaction that may ultimately destroy cellular integrity and result in cell death. The products of this reaction can be measured by several different assays. The magnitude of lipid peroxidation appears to be inversely related to levels of glutathione, which functions as an endogenous free radical scavenger. Glutathione and other agents that protect against peroxidation are, therefore, useful in organ preservation solutions to attenuate reperfusion injury.

Production of oxygen free radicals also initiates production of prostaglandins including leukotriene B_4 by direct activation of phospholipase A_2. This chemoattractant causes leukocyte adherence to vascular endothelium. These neutrophils may contribute to local injury by plugging the microcirculation and by degranulation resulting in proteolytic damage to the organ.

Cytokine-Mediated Effects

Cytokines are a recently described group of intercellular messenger molecules that may be produced in a variety of normal and pathophysiologic states. Ischemia and reperfusion are known to be associated with marked release of tumor necrosis factor-α, a cytokine with profound systemic effects.[10] Other cytokines, including interferon-γ, interleukin-1 and interleukin-8 (neutrophil chemotactic factor) may also be released during organ reperfusion and cause upregulation of adhesion molecule expression on vascular endothelium. These changes as well as adhesion molecule upregulation may lead to leukocyte adherence and platelet plugging following revascularization resulting in graft failure and an increased risk of later rejection.

Nitric Oxide–Mediated Effects

Nitric oxide (NO) is an extremely labile autocoid generated by nitric oxide synthase from L-arginine. It has potent vasodilatory effects on microvasculature and is responsible for a wide variety of physiologic effects. Evidence suggests that NO production is induced by inflammatory cytokines including tumor necrosis factor-α, interferon-γ, and interleukin-1. In the setting of ischemia-reperfusion, NO may, therefore, mediate injury to organs directly as a result of cytokine release. Inhaled nitric oxide has been demonstrated to attenuate reperfusion injury in transplanted lungs.[11] Increased NO synthesis also correlates with acute rejection.[12]

CONTEMPORARY CLINICAL PRACTICE

The science of transplantation has developed rapidly during the past 40 years. Improved understanding of the immune response to allografts and better appreciation of the complexity of organ ischemia and preservation related injury have contributed to greatly improved graft and patient survival results. Most solid organ transplants are now performed as the therapeutic option of choice, and in many cases transplantation offers the only definitive treatment for a given disease entity. As a result, an ever-widening list of indications for solid organ transplantation has emerged, placing increasing pressure on an already limited supply of donor organs. As of December 2003, there were 86,355 patients awaiting deceased donor organ transplantation in the United States, almost double the number listed in 1996.[13] Each year, more patients are placed on the waiting lists than are transplanted, resulting in thousands of waiting list deaths and increasing waiting time.

Determination of Suitability for Deceased Donor Organ Donation

General Considerations

The characteristics of a suitable deceased donor organ donor can be divided into those that are general in nature and those that are organ specific. Broadly stated, the general attributes of an acceptable organ donor include pronouncement of donor death, previously good general health, and relative hemodynamic stability from the time of the precipitating event leading to death until organ procurement is complete. Informed consent from the donor's next of kin is required before organ procurement. The concepts of brain death and the renewed practice of donation after cardiac death (DCD) are discussed in detail later. A detailed understanding of these conditions and their associated pathophysiology is essential for the successful procurement and subsequent transplantation of solid organs from deceased donors. A detailed medical history should be sought by contacting family members or friends of the potential donor.

Age

As experience has been gained with donors considered less than ideal, it has become apparent that arbitrarily defined chronologic age limits for organ donors are unnecessary.

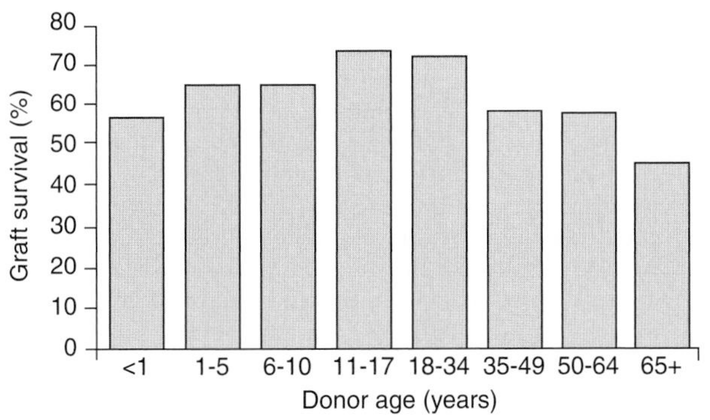

FIGURE 36.4 Kidneys transplanted from deceased pediatric donors age 5 years and younger have lower graft survival rates than those from older pediatric and young adult donors. At the older extreme of age, graft survival rates are also lower. (Adapted with permission from 2003 U.S. Organ Procurement and Transplantation Network and the Scientific Registry for Transplant Recipients Annual Report: Transplant Data 1993–2002: Department of Health and Human Services, Health Resources and Services Administration, Office of Special Programs, Division of Transplantation, Rockville, MD; United Network for Organ Sharing, Richmond, VA; University Renal Research and Education Association. Ann Arbor, MI; 2003: Table 5.9a. The cohort is transplants performed during 1996–1997.)

Ample evidence supports the relaxation of upper age limits for most abdominal organs. For example, kidney procurement from deceased donors older than age 65 years is routinely considered, and successful renal transplantation has been reported from a deceased donor of 84 years.[14] Donor age has been similarly deemphasized in liver transplantation, where almost one-third of deceased donors are older than 50. The acceptable upper donor age limit for cardiac transplantation has been cautiously but steadily increased, and approximately 10% of heart donors are older than 50.

Transplantation of organs from donors at the younger extreme of life is similarly successful. Some controversy exists with regard to the advisability of transplanting kidneys from infants and children younger than 5 years (Figs. 36.4 and 36.5).[13,15] Lower graft survival rates have been reported when kidneys from very young donors have been transplanted.[13] However, some centers report extremely good short-term results using en-bloc transplantation of both kidneys from pediatric donors to adults.[16,17]

Overall Premorbid Health

Because most deceased organ donors have acute cerebral trauma or intracerebral catastrophe as the cause of death, serious associated systemic diseases are relatively uncommon in this population. As the donor population ages, however, the effects of hypertension, atherosclerosis, and other diseases associated with advancing age are more common. Thus, careful screening to ascertain that the donor was previously in good health is mandatory. Common disorders, such as hypertension and diabetes mellitus, do not automatically disqualify a person from organ donation, but the duration, severity, and treatment of such conditions should be evaluated for their potential effects on individual organs.

Hemodynamic Stability

Cardiovascular instability and eventual cardiopulmonary collapse eventually occur in all brain dead patients. Thus, hemodynamic management is one of the most important aspects of donor management once brain death has been established and consent for organ donation has been obtained. Many potential organ donors sustain significant hypotension or even cardiac arrest during the initial stages of their illness or as the presenting signs of intracerebral catastrophe. Knowledge of the course and management of these episodes is helpful in predicting damage to the various organs and in guiding the work-up of the donor for suitability of the organs for transplantation. In terms of specific organs, the kidneys appear to tolerate transient hypotension best, whereas the liver and pancreas may be more severely damaged by such episodes. The cardiac response to hypotension or actual cardiac arrest depends on the cause of the hemodynamic instability and the magnitude of direct cardiac injury sustained as a result of cardiac compressions during cardiopulmonary resuscitation.

Contraindications

Sepsis. Active systemic infection has traditionally been an absolute contraindication to organ donation. However, these tenets are being reexamined because of the current organ shortage. A history of diseases such as tuberculosis or HIV infection clearly renders a person unsuitable for donation. Pneumonia (except for lung donors) and urinary tract infection are no longer considered to be problematic in the absence of systemic sepsis. Even in the presence of bacteremia, the risk of transmission of infectious agents by organ transplantation

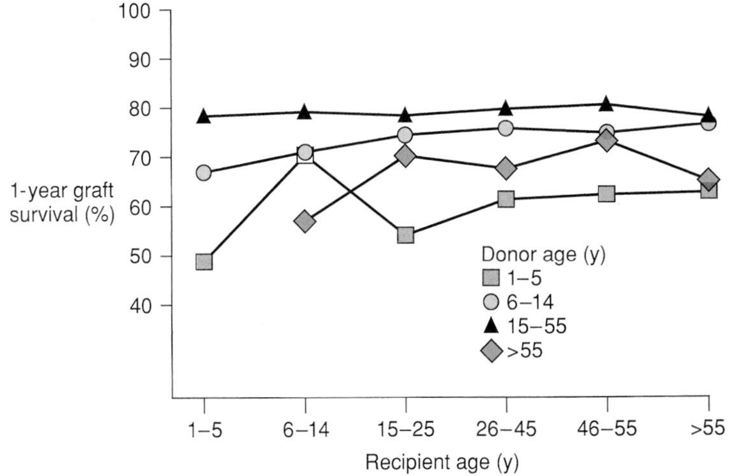

FIGURE 36.5 Relation between donor and recipient age and 1-year kidney graft survival. (Adapted with permission from Zhou YC, Cecka JM. Effect of age on kidney transplants. In: Terasaki PI, ed. *Clinical transplantation 1989*. Los Angeles: UCLA Tissue Typing Laboratory, 1989:369–378.)

appears to be small.[18] In all cases, appropriate antibiotic therapy should be initiated before the procurement procedure.

Viral Infection. All potential organ donors, regardless of whether they are considered high-risk, are tested for evidence of infection with HIV. Under most circumstances, this test is carried out using an enzyme-linked immunosorbent assay. Although the incidence of false-positive results may be a problem, the high sensitivity of the test ensures that the potential for transmission of this virus is minimized. Testing is also routinely performed for evidence of hepatitis B and C. History of viral hepatitis or serologic evidence of past infection has previously been considered an absolute contraindication to organ donation. Many centers are now reconsidering this issue, however, in selected situations. Some organs from donors who have evidence of past infection with the hepatitis B virus are able to transmit the virus. However, these organs may be considered for recipients that have long-standing infection with this virus or have received the recombinant hepatitis B vaccine and have serologic immunity. Similarly, organs from donors with evidence of past infection with the hepatitis C virus are possible sources of infectious virus. The risk of infection is small, however, and these organs are now being considered for patients with known preexisting exposure to the hepatitis C virus.[19] Other viral titers that are frequently determined during workup of a donor include members of the herpesvirus family, such as cytomegalovirus (CMV), Epstein-Barr virus, and herpes simplex virus. Evidence of previous infection with these viruses does not preclude organ donation but may require additional therapy in the recipient, such as valganciclovir prophylaxis or hyperimmune globulin administration in the case of CMV.

Cancer. Cancer, whether treated or not, has long been considered to contravene organ donation based on the knowledge that tumor cells may circulate widely even in patients with malignant lesions thought to be localized. The transplantation of even a small number of malignant cells into a recipient who is heavily immunosuppressed carries the threat of dissemination and a disastrous outcome. The only exception to this rule has been the donor with a primary malignancy of the central nervous system. It has long been thought that as long as the blood–brain barrier is intact, these tumors are rarely capable of systemic spread. Although transmission of a central nervous system tumor of donor origin to a liver transplant recipient has been reported, the rate of transmission is dependent on the organ transplanted and the type of malignancy involved.[20] These cases must be considered on an individual basis.

Specific Organ Dysfunction

The condition of particular organs of interest in great measure dictates their individual suitability for transplantation. With appropriate emphasis on the overall maintenance of donor homeostasis, most if not all transplantable organs should be procured from most donors. A history of longstanding hypertension may result in fixed damage to the kidneys as a result of hypertensive scarring and secondary to the effects of aortic and renal atherosclerosis. Similarly, insulin-dependent diabetes mellitus produces a well-known renal lesion. These changes may be reversible, however, after transplantation into a nondiabetic recipient.[21] The kidneys are relatively resilient organs, and simple measures usually suffice to identify serious renal dysfunction. Measurements of hourly urinary output, coupled with determinations of the central venous pressure, are useful monitors of the adequacy of volume repletion in potential donors. Significant volume depletion is the combined result of intentional volume contraction to treat cerebral edema and the effects of diabetes insipidus accompanying lethal brain injury. Serum creatinine is measured as a global, if imperfect, indicator of renal function. Significant elevation of the serum creatinine level during the course of the donor hospitalization may be a sign of renal injury, predisposing to delayed graft function after transplantation.[22]

Preexisting liver disease usually can be identified before organ procurement. A history of cirrhosis precludes donation. Prior cholecystectomy for uncomplicated cholelithiasis is not a contraindication to liver donation. Standard liver function tests, such as serum alanine aminotransferase, aspartate aminotransferase, alkaline phosphatase, and bilirubin may be helpful in identifying gross injury to the donor liver resulting from traumatic, metabolic, or hemodynamic causes, but the absolute levels of these tests are poor indicators of the likelihood of immediate, life-sustaining graft function in the recipient. Hepatic synthetic function as assessed by prothrombin time may also be deceiving because of the effects of severe brain injury on the coagulation cascade.[23]

The pancreas may be difficult to assess until the time of organ procurement. Hyperglycemia and hyperamylasemia are common in patients who sustain brain death, particularly if the cause is traumatic. A careful history establishing the absence of preexisting diabetes mellitus and pancreatitis provides the most useful information. A history of alcohol abuse alone does not correlate well with the finding of chronic pancreatitis pathology at laparotomy. Computed tomographic examination of the abdomen may be indicated if the donor sustained any abdominal injury. It is more appropriate to examine the organ at the time of multiple organ procurement to determine if it is suitable for transplantation rather than making a decision on the basis of historical or laboratory information alone.

Cardiac dysfunction resulting in arrhythmia or the need for high dose inotropic support suggests that the heart may be unsuitable for transplantation. Transient supraventricular tachycardias, ventricular arrhythmia associated with severe hemodynamic instability or cardiac arrest require investigation before acceptance as a cardiac donor. Significant valvular disease and wall motion abnormalities can be readily identified by bedside echocardiographic examination, a study that is routinely obtained by many transplant centers. In many cases the fluid management of the donor radically affects the apparent cardiac function since over or under hydration will markedly reduce effective cardiac output. Urine output can be extremely misleading due to the loss of antidiuretic hormone secretion from the hypothalamus. Measurements of central venous pressure or pulmonary artery wedge pressure may allow for more accurate management of fluid replacement. Determination of cardiac output using a flow-directed balloon-tipped pulmonary artery catheter is also helpful and complements echocardiographic findings. In questionable cases, cardiac catheterization may be required to exclude significant coronary artery disease.

Brain Death

Definition

The concept of brain death was crystallized in the 1968 Report of the Ad Hoc Committee of Harvard Medical School developed to examine the definition of brain death.[24] This document established the following clearly defined criteria that were reliably predictive of irreversibility: (a) unreceptivity and unresponsivity, (b) absence of spontaneous muscular movement, (c) absence of reflexes, and (d) silent electroencephalogram. Since the publication of the so-called Harvard

Criteria, the prerequisites for the diagnosis of brain death have been refined. Most hospitals have constituted a Brain Death Committee that is responsible for making uniform determinations of brain death according to locally established specific criteria, while conforming generally to the Harvard Criteria. The following requirements must be met to make a firm diagnosis of brain death: (a) the presence of reversible causes of coma should be excluded; (b) clinical criteria establishing the loss of all functions of the entire brain must be met (deep coma, absence of brain-stem function, absence of spontaneous respiration); (c) a confirmatory diagnostic test must be carried out (electroencephalogram, nuclear brain blood flow study, four-vessel cerebral arteriography).

Reversible causes of coma include sedation, hypothermia below 32.2°C, neuromuscular blockade, and shock. Coma should be deep and fixed, without perception or response to external stimuli, including deep pain. Decerebrate and decorticate responses should not be present. Occasionally, spinal reflexes may be present. Absence of brain-stem function can be documented by confirming the absence of pupillary light response, corneal reflex, oculocephalic reflex, oculovestibular reflex, and spontaneous respiration.

An apnea test should be performed to assess spontaneous respiration. Ventilation of the patient with 100% oxygen for 10 minutes before the test reduces the risk of hypoxemia and subsequent cardiovascular collapse. After the period of preoxygenation, passive flow of oxygen into the endotracheal tube is continued, and the patient is monitored for evidence of respiratory effort. During this interval, hypercarbia with a $PaCO_2$ greater than 60 mm Hg should be documented by arterial blood gas testing.

The confirmatory test of choice is an electroencephalogram documenting electrocerebral silence or absence of brain blood flow by nuclear scintigraphy. The electroencephalogram may be done 6 hours after the initial clinical determination of brain death and, when accompanied by a second clinical determination, is diagnostic of brain death. Nuclear scintigraphic determination of brain blood flow is a satisfactory method to provide definitive confirmation of brain death. This test has the advantage that it can be done as a portable examination at the patient's bedside in the intensive care unit (ICU) or emergency department, avoiding the risk of unnecessarily transporting a potentially unstable patient. Alternatively, four-vessel cerebral arteriography demonstrating cessation of blood flow to the brain may be used within an hour of the clinical brain death declaration.

Etiology

Any condition that results in an overwhelming cerebral insult may be sufficient to cause brain death. In general, these conditions fall into the broad categories of subarachnoid or intracerebral hemorrhage, direct cerebral trauma, primary malignancy of the central nervous system, and other rare and miscellaneous entities. Subarachnoid hemorrhage may result from rupture of an intracranial aneurysm. Other cerebrovascular accidents including hypertensive hemorrhagic stroke be lethal. These entities are responsible for most cases of brain death that lead to organ donation. Brain injury after trauma, either vehicular or related to firearms, is also common.

Pathophysiology

Cardiovascular Instability. During the events that lead to brain death, there is usually progressive intracranial hypertension. Important pathophysiologic responses are evident before the actual occurrence of brain death, including the development of marked systemic hypertension associated with vastly increased sympathetic activity and the massive release of catecholamines. Arrhythmia may become manifest at any time during the process of tentorial herniation. Bradyarrhythmia may be associated with the systemic hypertensive response to intracranial hypertension (Cushing reflex), but ventricular and supraventricular tachyarrhythmia may also be seen in the presence of high levels of catecholamines.

Once herniation is complete and brain death has occurred, a high proportion of donors manifest a hypotensive response related to the loss of sympathetic tone and the failure to maintain circulating catecholamine levels. It has been reported that 62% of brain-dead patients sustain cardiac arrest within 24 hours and 87% by 72 hours in the absence of specific donor maintenance measures.[25] Even with aggressive donor support, about 10% of donors manifest cardiopulmonary arrest during the interval between the determination of brain death and the procurement of organs.[26]

Central Hormonal Failure. As the brain and brain stem cease to function, failure of the central hormonal axis occurs. Pituitary hormones cease to be produced, and diabetes insipidus ensues. Without antidiuretic hormone, urinary output may increase to astonishing rates, sometimes well in excess of 1 L/h. The urine becomes extremely dilute, resulting in increasing serum osmolarity and hypernatremia. The resultant hypovolemia may contribute to cardiovascular collapse if untreated.

The influence of other aspects of central hormonal function is less well understood. There is experimental evidence of reduced circulating levels of triiodothyronine, cortisol, and insulin after brain death in pigs and baboons.[27,28] These factors may contribute to the hemodynamic instability, cardiovascular collapse, and hyperglycemia so often seen in association with brain death and have led some to advocate using combinations of these compounds before organ procurement. Confirmatory studies in humans have not shown these hormonal systems to play major roles in the pathophysiology of the hypotensive state following brain death, although use of these agents is still common in clinical practice.

Request for Permission From Next of Kin

All states and the federal government have passed legislation requiring that relatives of deceased patients be asked whether they are willing to permit organ or tissue donation. Unfortunately, the contribution of such laws to an increase in the actual supply of donor organs is less than clear. What is far more important than required request is the careful training, uniform deployment, and empathetic demeanor of the individuals who actually approach the family. In many hospitals, trained donor coordinators are on call to discuss the option of organ donation with bereaved families. Such people may come from a variety of fields, including medicine, nursing, social work, or pastoral care. Refusal of consent by the family is one of the biggest stumbling blocks to increasing the supply of organs actually donated. It has also been suggested that the discussion of possible organ donation should occur at a time subsequent to and separate from informing the family of the patient's death.

The use of the term *brain death* may be confusing to lay people and professionals alike; it implies that brain death is different from other kinds of death. Obviously, the distinction is intended to differentiate this modality of dying from cardiac death but not to indicate that the person is any less dead. Phrases such as "keeping the organs alive so they can be transplanted" are as misleading and confusing as they are incorrect.

According to the Uniform Anatomical Gift Act, a signed and witnessed organ donor card is a legally binding indication of the decedent's wishes, but throughout North America and most European countries, the family's consent is routinely obtained before organ procurement. Although it is desirable

TABLE 36.1

HIERARCHY FOR PERMISSION FOR ORGAN DONATION FROM NEXT OF KIN

1. Spouse
2. Adult son or daughter
3. Either parent
4. Adult brother or sister
5. Guardian
6. Any other person authorized to dispose of the body

that the entire family be in agreement about donating, the legal next of kin is required to agree to the donation and grant signed permission (Table 36.1).

Donor Maintenance

Tissue Perfusion

Most donors are maintained with a minimum of fluids to prevent increased cerebral edema, and, therefore, one of the first priorities in donor maintenance should be the prompt restoration of intravascular volume. Depending on the duration of the donor's underlying illness, this process may require from 3 to 10 L of volume resuscitation. In general, the dosage of pressor agents required to support blood pressure can be progressively decreased as the central venous pressure is raised to 10 to 12 cm H_2O. Crystalloid may be used, and lactated Ringer solution is often given because its slightly lower sodium concentration counteracts the concentrating effects of diabetes insipidus. If the latter condition has resulted in severe hypernatremia, the addition of free water may be necessary. Colloid and blood should be used to restore and maintain osmotic pressure and normovolemia. The hematocrit should be kept around 35 volume percent to replace traumatic losses and to maintain oxygen-carrying capacity. Enough volume should be administered to achieve a urine output of at least 100 ml/h and a systolic arterial pressure of 90 to 120 mmHg. Higher levels of arterial blood pressure are usually unnecessary because the loss of sympathetic tone accompanying brain death facilitates tissue perfusion at lower pressure.

If diabetes insipidus is severe, exogenous vasopressin must be given. Available in a variety of forms, desmopressin acetate, a synthetic analog of 8-arginine vasopressin, appears to have the least splanchnic vasoconstrictive effect compared with its antidiuretic action. This agent can be given by a variety of routes, including intranasally, subcutaneously, or intravenously. The usual dosage is 20 μg intranasally or 2 to 4 μg intravenously or subcutaneously.

Oxygenation and Ventilation

Arterial blood gases should be checked regularly and appropriate adjustments of the ventilator made to optimize gas exchange and acid-base balance. Oxygen supply should be adequate to maintain an arterial oxygen saturation of greater than 95% and mixed venous oxygen saturation above 70%. Low levels of positive end-expiratory pressure may facilitate achieving a balanced oxygen supply and demand.

Inotropic Support

Most donors are hypovolemic at the time of brain death and are receiving inotropic support in lieu of volume to support their blood pressure. Dopamine hydrochloride is the most commonly used agent. The need for dosages of this drug in excess of 10 μg/kg/min usually indicates persistent hypovolemia, and the restoration of normovolemia is almost always accompanied by a reduction in dopamine requirements. High doses of dopamine maintained for long periods before organ procurement may be associated with increased rates of acute tubular necrosis and hepatic allograft failure. Cardiac procurement is often abandoned if high doses of inotropic support are required despite adequate volume status.

Other inotropic agents, such as isoproterenol, epinephrine, norepinephrine, and phenylephrine, are occasionally used, but the use of these agents should be discouraged because of their peripheral vasoconstrictive effects. Dobutamine is sometimes used in conjunction with low doses of dopamine.

Prevention of Hypothermia

Thermoregulatory homeostatic mechanisms are destroyed with the occurrence of brain death, and the development of severe hypothermia may lead to ventricular arrhythmia and cardiac arrest. Warming blankets should be used above and below the donor to keep body temperature above 35°C, and exposure for the purposes of examination or intervention should be kept to a minimum. If maintenance of normal body temperature is problematic, intravenous fluids may be prewarmed before administration, and a heated humidifier circuit can be added to the ventilator.

Multiple-Organ Procurement

The Organ Procurement and Transplantation Network and the Coordination of Surgical Teams

When brain death has been declared, the person has been identified as a suitable organ donor, and permission has been given by the next of kin, the logistics of organ procurement must be arranged. Since passage of the National Organ Transplantation Act, a national Organ Procurement and Transplantation Network has been organized. The federal contract for this important function is held by the United Network for Organ Sharing (UNOS). UNOS is responsible for the fair and equitable distribution of deceased donor organs throughout the United States. The 50 states are divided into 11 regions (Fig. 36.6). Within each region, federally certified local organ procurement organizations (OPOs) are responsible for maintaining the list of potential recipients for their catchment area. All transplant candidates within the United States are entered into a computer system, and an allocation system is used to determine the appropriate potential recipient for a given donor organ. In general, offers are made first to candidates listed with transplant centers in the local OPO service area, then to suitable candidates in the region, and finally to any candidate in the nation. In each case, priority is ordered by the existing allocation system designed for that organ.[29] An important exception to these general rules relates to renal transplant recipients who share six antigens with the donor. These kidneys are automatically shared nationwide even if suitable local recipients are available.

Recipients of the various organs may reside in geographically distant locations. Because the recipient transplantation teams must be given considerable detailed information about the donor to decide whether to use a particular organ for a particular recipient, a finite period of time is required to assemble the necessary donor retrieval teams. When all teams are on site at the donor hospital, the donor is transferred to the operating room for the actual procurement procedure.

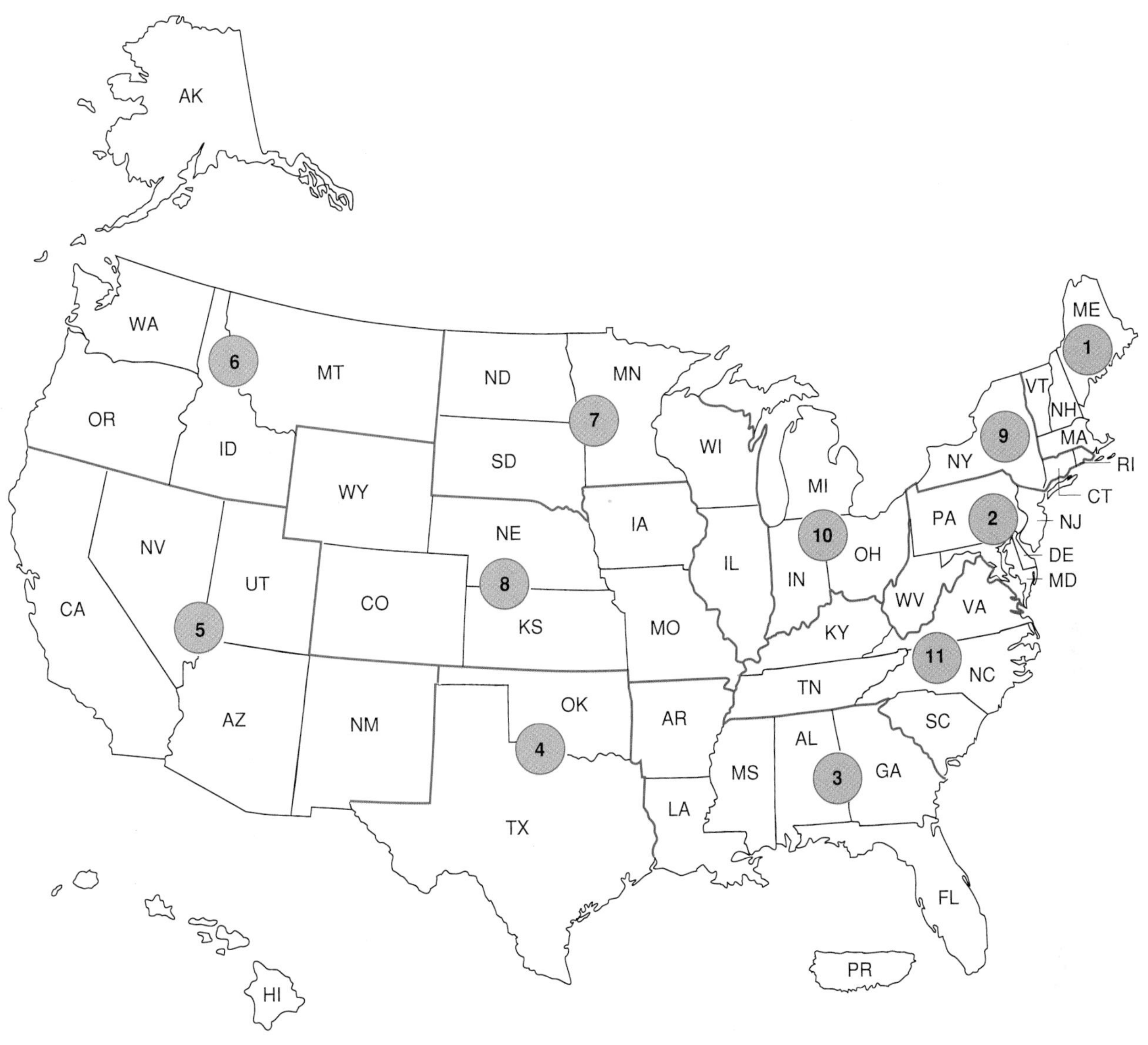

FIGURE 36.6 The United Network for Organ Sharing has divided the 50 United States into 11 regions of approximately equal populations for purposes of administration of organ procurement, distribution, and educational objectives.

Surgical Technique for Multiple Organ Procurement

Techniques of multiple organ procurement allow for the removal of the heart, lungs, kidneys, liver, intestine, and pancreas from a single donor for transplantation into multiple recipients. The following discussion details the methods used to remove all these organs from a donor.

The heart-beating donor is brought to the operating room from the ICU or emergency department with appropriate hemodynamic and electrocardiographic monitoring. Oxygen is delivered by hand bagging at 100% inspired concentration. Inotropic drug infusions are continued during transport and procurement. The anesthesiologist should maintain close communication with the procurement teams to avoid the development of cardiac arrhythmia, hypotension, and hypoxemia.

The steps in the procedure can be categorized as follows: (i) incision, (ii) exploration and inspection, (iii) individual organ mobilization, (iv) *in situ* perfusion, (v) removal of organs, and (vi) closure of the incision. Postprocurement processing, packaging, and transport to the recipient centers are the final steps.

The entire torso is prepared with an iodine-containing solution, and a field is draped from the neck to the pubis. A long, midline incision is made from the suprasternal notch to the pubis. The sternum is split with an electrical or air-powered saw if available, although manual methods using a Lebsche knife or Gigli saw work perfectly well. Exposure of the abdominal organs may be facilitated by the addition of cruciate incisions (Fig. 36.7). A general exploration is carried out to ascertain that no unexpected conditions are present that would preclude donation, such as tumor, infection, or specific organ damage. In general, a "no-touch" technique is used to minimize trauma to the organs during the procurement procedure.

For the so-called rapid technique of organ procurement, relatively little in the way of mobilization of individual organs is necessary. Preparation for *in situ* perfusion consists of a complete Kocher maneuver, with mobilization of the right colon, duodenum, and small bowel in a cephalad direction to the patient's left (Fig. 36.8). The aorta is exposed from the bifurcation distally to the level of the left renal vein proximally. The inferior mesenteric artery may be divided. Lumbar branches may be ligated and divided at this point. The inferior vena cava is similarly exposed. Next, the left triangular ligament of the liver is taken down, exposing the crural fibers at

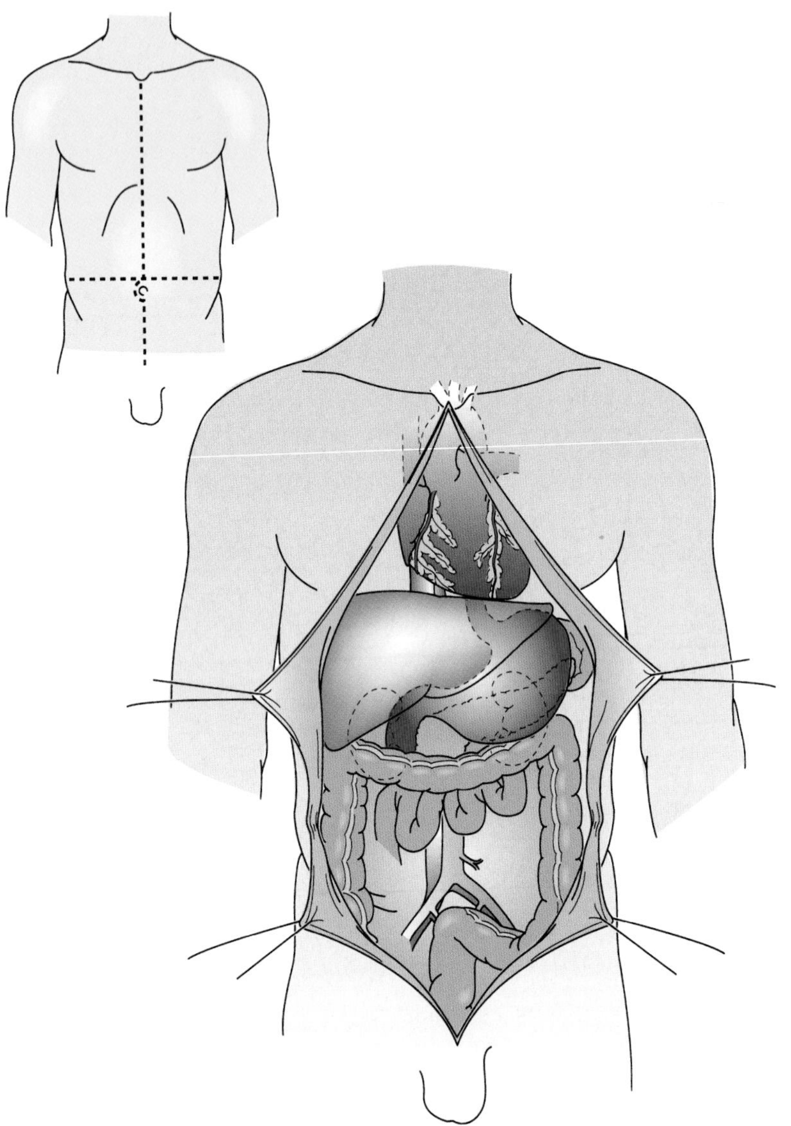

FIGURE 36.7 A complete midline incision from suprasternal notch to pubis is made for multiple organ procurement. The sternum is split. If necessary, cruciate abdominal incisions are added to facilitate exposure of the intraabdominal organs.

the aortic hiatus. The aorta is encircled with a tape at the diaphragm (Fig. 36.9A). These maneuvers can be accomplished in 10 to 15 minutes and allow *in situ* perfusion through the distal aorta and cross clamping of the proximal aorta to begin immediately in the event that the donor becomes hemodynamically unstable or sustains cardiac arrest. Warm ischemia is completely prevented by *in situ* perfusion.

Stable donors afford the luxury of further preparation before *in situ* flushing. The inferior mesenteric vein is isolated as it enters the retroperitoneum behind the pancreas. This vein provides convenient access for *in situ* portal flushing by means of a small catheter. If pancreas and/or intestinal procurement is also planned, the portal flush can be done after removal. The pars flaccida of the lesser omentum should be inspected for evidence of a replaced left hepatic artery arising from the left gastric artery, and minimal dissection of the hepatic artery is necessary (Fig. 36.9B). The portal triad should be palpated carefully for evidence of a replaced right hepatic artery arising from the superior mesenteric artery. This vessel, when present, can be palpated as it courses toward the liver posterior to the common bile duct and along the right side of the portal vein as it emerges from its origin off the superior mesenteric artery posterior to the pancreas (Fig. 36.10).

If the pancreas is to be procured, 250 mL of an iodine-containing solution, followed by a similar volume of amphotericin B solution (50 mg/L) is administered via the nasogastric tube into the duodenum. After the gastrocolic omentum is divided, the short gastric vessels are carefully divided between ligatures or hemostatic clips. The left and right gastric branches to the stomach are then divided. After the nasogastric tube is withdrawn from the duodenum, a stapling device is applied just beyond the pylorus (Fig. 36.11). The spleen is delivered anteriorly, dividing its attachments to the body wall and diaphragm. Using the spleen as a handle, the retroperitoneal attachments of the pancreas are divided from lateral to medial, until the superior mesenteric vessels are reached (Fig. 36.12). The distal duodenum is divided with a stapler near the Treitz ligament just before or after aortic cross clamping.

If the intestine is to be procured for an isolated small bowel transplant, the only additional dissection required is to separate the distal ileum near the ileocecal valve from the colon. The small bowel is transected here using a stapling device.[30]

The course of the ureters should be identified. The Gerota fascia is widely incised to allow topical cooling with iced slush solution to supplement the *in situ* perfusion. Complete mobilization of the kidneys before *in situ* flushing is unnecessary

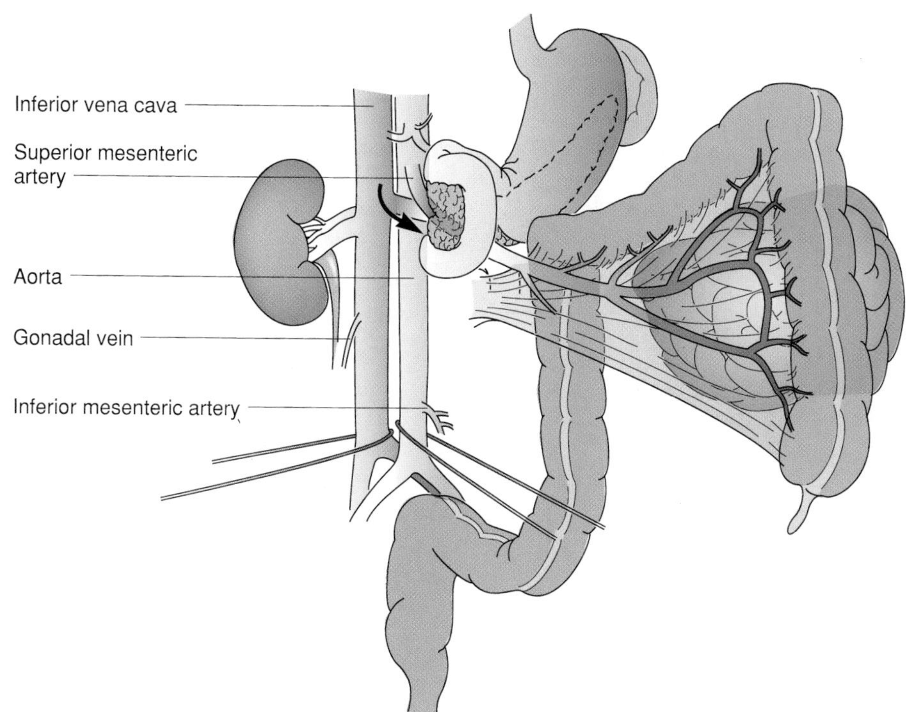

FIGURE 36.8 The Kocher maneuver is used to mobilize completely the right colon and duodenum, exposing the retroperitoneum, including the aorta, from the level of the superior mesenteric artery to the bifurcation and the inferior vena cava from the iliac veins to the edge of the liver.

and risks damage to the renal vessels or inadvertent division of accessory renal arteries.

The heart and lungs can be readied for removal by a team working simultaneously with the abdominal retrieval team. The superior and inferior vena cavae are mobilized, and the aortic arch is dissected sufficiently for the placement of a crossclamp at the time of infusion of aortic root cardioplegia (Fig. 36.13). Preliminary mobilization of the lungs is usually performed, and access to the pulmonary artery is necessary for pulmonary preservation.

When all teams are ready, a coordinated sequence of events ensures that all organs are simultaneously cooled and protected. The donor is systemically heparinized. At this point, if *in situ* portal flushing is desired, a catheter is advanced through the inferior mesenteric vein near the pancreas into the portal vein (Fig. 36.14A). A cardioplegia needle is positioned in the aortic arch (Fig. 36-14B). The distal abdominal aorta is cannulated for retrograde *in situ* perfusion of the kidneys, liver, pancreas, and intestine, and an exsanguination cannula is placed in the distal inferior vena cava (Fig. 36-14C). Alternatively, the inferior vena caval-right atrial junction may be divided in the chest with suction catheters placed in the caval lumen and right thoracic cavity to decompress the venous circulation at the moment of aortic cross clamping.

The aortic arch and the abdominal aorta at the diaphragm are simultaneously cross clamped. Cardioplegia solution is infused under pressure into the aortic root, perfusing the coronary arteries and arresting the heart. Ventilation is ceased. Portal and distal aortic perfusion are initiated with ice cold preservation solution. Topical iced slush is placed in the abdomen and chest to assist the cooling process. The heart and lungs are then removed. The clamp is removed from the distal vena caval cannula for exsanguination and to preclude venous congestion. The liver and pancreas are removed en bloc. The diaphragm surrounding the suprahepatic inferior vena cava and adjacent to the bare area of the liver is divided. The infrahepatic inferior vena cava is divided just cephalad to the left renal vein. The liver and pancreas unit is now attached only by the distal superior mesenteric vessels coursing to the small bowel and by the aortic origins of the superior mesenteric artery and celiac axis. The superior mesenteric artery and vein emerging from the uncinate process are ligated and divided, and a cylinder of aorta is removed encompassing the superior mesenteric artery and celiac axis. The distal superior mesenteric artery and vein provide blood supply to the small intestinal graft, which is removed next. The liver and pancreas are separated as a bench procedure, retaining the celiac axis with the liver (Fig. 36.15). The splenic artery is divided at its origin. This vessel and the superior mesenteric artery are reconstructed with a bifurcated donor iliac artery graft. The portal vein is divided about 1 cm from the pancreas. The common bile duct is divided at the superior edge of the pancreas.

The kidneys are also removed en bloc. The ureters are given wide berth to avoid devascularization and are divided near their entrance into the bladder. Dissection is carried out posterior to the aorta and vena cava in the plane of the prevertebral fascia. Once removed, the left renal vein is divided flush with the vena cava (Fig. 36.16). The aorta is opened in the midline to identify the orifices of the renal arteries from within the lumen. In this way, multiple renal arteries can be readily identified and kept on a single aortic Carrel patch. Once the abdominal and thoracic organs have been removed, a sampling of lymph nodes and spleen are taken for tissue typing and crossmatch testing. The chest and abdomen are closed, and standard postmortem care is given.

Donation after Cardiac Death

The profound shortage of organs has led to efforts aimed at utilizing organs from patients who die as a result of cardiac standstill rather than brain death. This process is referred to as *donation after cardiac death* (DCD). Individuals who are declared dead in the emergency department without cardiac function are not generally used as donors because the hemodynamic situation

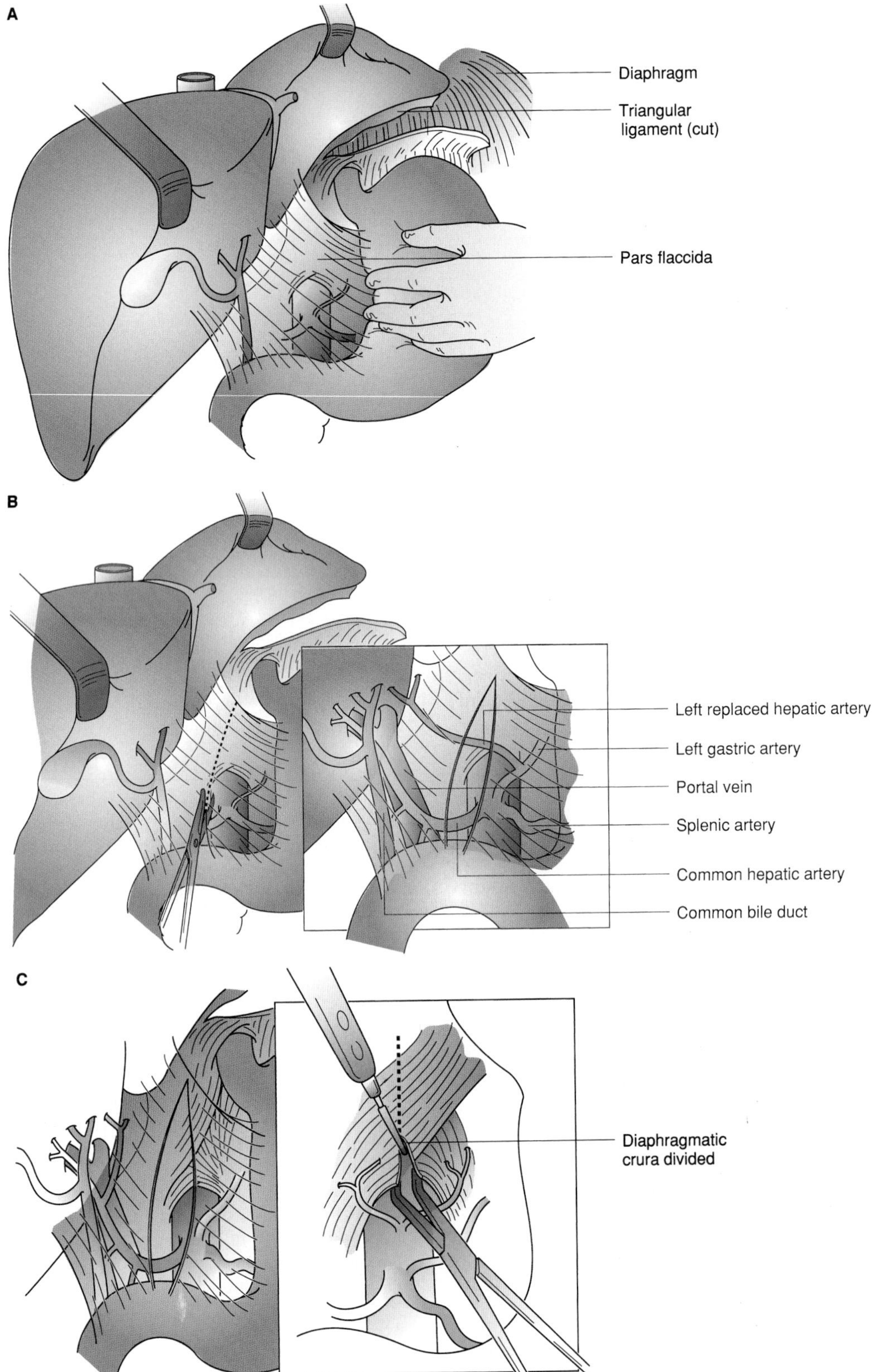

FIGURE 36.9 (*A*) The left triangular ligament is divided and the left lateral segment of the liver is retracted to expose the esophagus and aortic hiatus. (*B*) The pars flaccida of the lesser omentum is widely opened after checking for the presence of a replaced left hepatic artery arising from the left gastric artery. (*C*) After division of the diaphragmatic crura, the supraceliac aorta is encircled at the level of the diaphragm.

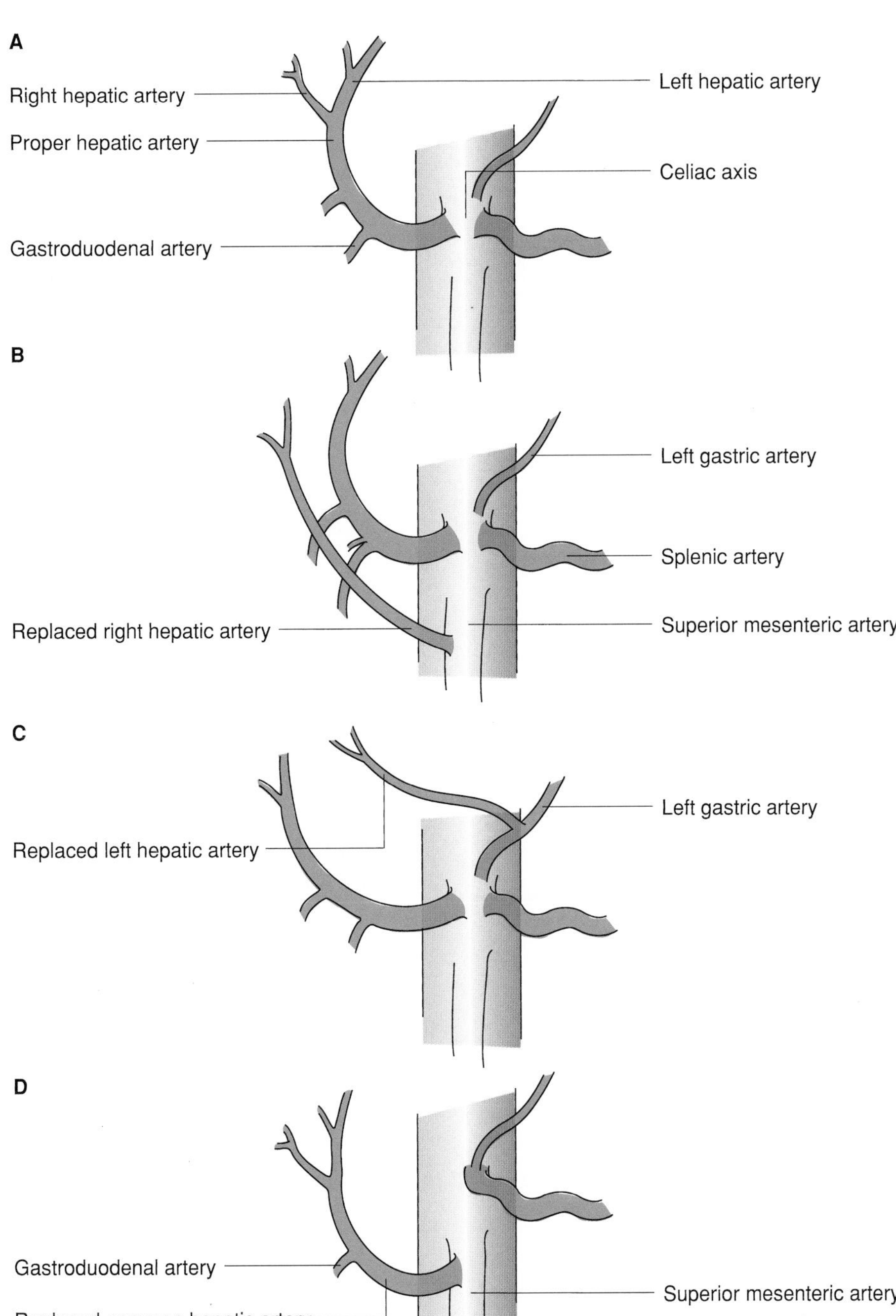

FIGURE 36.10 (*A*) Standard hepatic arterial anatomy, with the artery arising as a single vessel as a branch of the celiac axis. (*B*) Aberrant hepatic arterial anatomy, with a replaced right hepatic artery arising from the superior mesenteric artery and ascending posterior to the common bile duct and anterolateral to the portal vein. (*C*) A replaced left hepatic artery arising from the left gastric artery is usually visible and palpable crossing the pars flaccida of the lesser omentum from the lesser curvature of the stomach. (*D*) A completely replaced common hepatic artery arising from the superior mesenteric artery.

is uncontrolled. In contrast, patients who have severe brain injury but who do not meet brain death criteria can be considered as controlled DCD donors. In this setting, a decision to withdraw further life support measures has already been made by the family and the treating team of physicians. DCD, especially of kidneys and increasingly of livers, has become one of the fastest growing sources of donor organs.[31] Once the decision to withdraw support has been made, organ donation can be considered. The Institute of Medicine has studied the issues surrounding the utilization of DCD donors and recommends that: "the recovery of organs from non-heartbeating donors is an important medically effective and ethically acceptable approach to reducing the gap that exists now and will continue to exist in the future between the demand for and available supply of for transplantation."[32]

Following informed consent, perfusion and exsanguination cannulae are placed in the femoral artery and vein, respectively. The patient is then extubated and must expire within 60 minutes in order for the donation to proceed. The Institute of Medicine recommends waiting an additional 5 minutes after cessation of effective cardiac function and pronouncement of death before proceeding with organ procurement.

At this point, the organs are rapidly cooled by infusing cold preservation fluid via the previously placed cannula. Simultaneously, the abdomen and chest are opened and a standard organ procurement procedure is carried out. Growing experience demonstrates that outcomes of kidneys transplanted from DCD donors are comparable with those from brain-dead donors, with the exception of a higher incidence of delayed graft function.[33]

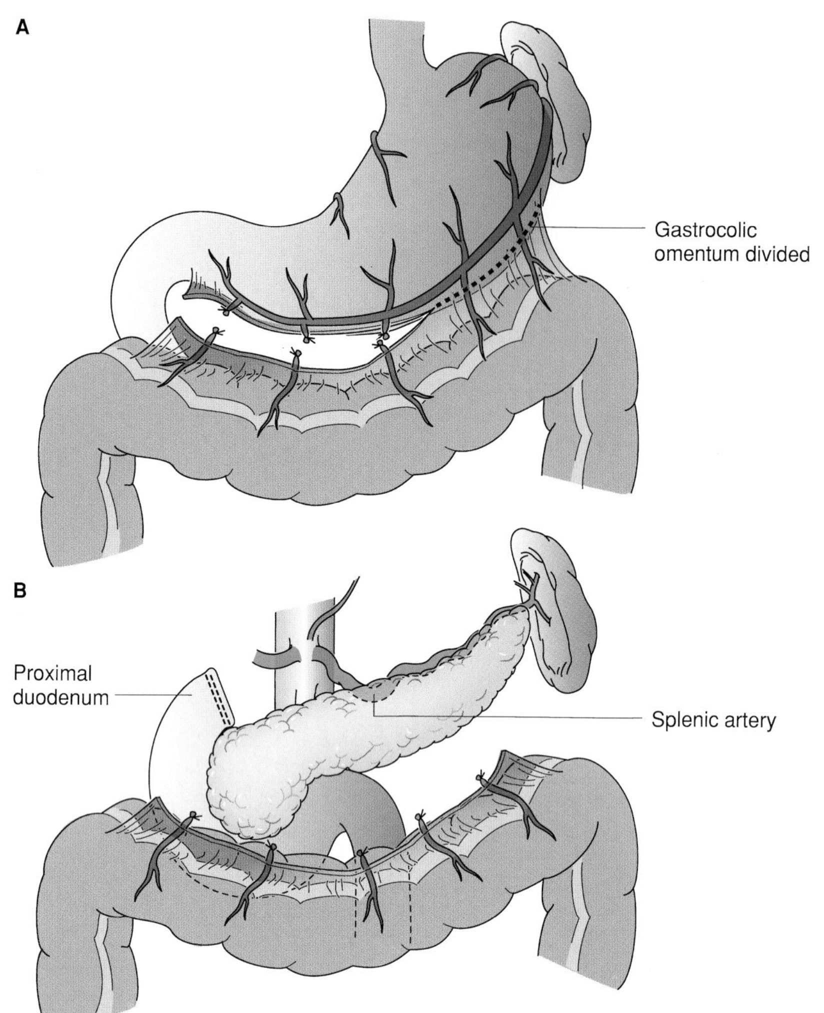

FIGURE 36.11 (*A*) Division of the gastrocolic omentum exposes the pancreas. The short gastric vessels are ligated and divided, separating the spleen from the stomach. (*B*) After completion of gastric devascularization, the duodenum is stapled just beyond the pylorus and the stomach is retracted superolaterally to facilitate exposure and mobilization of the pancreas.

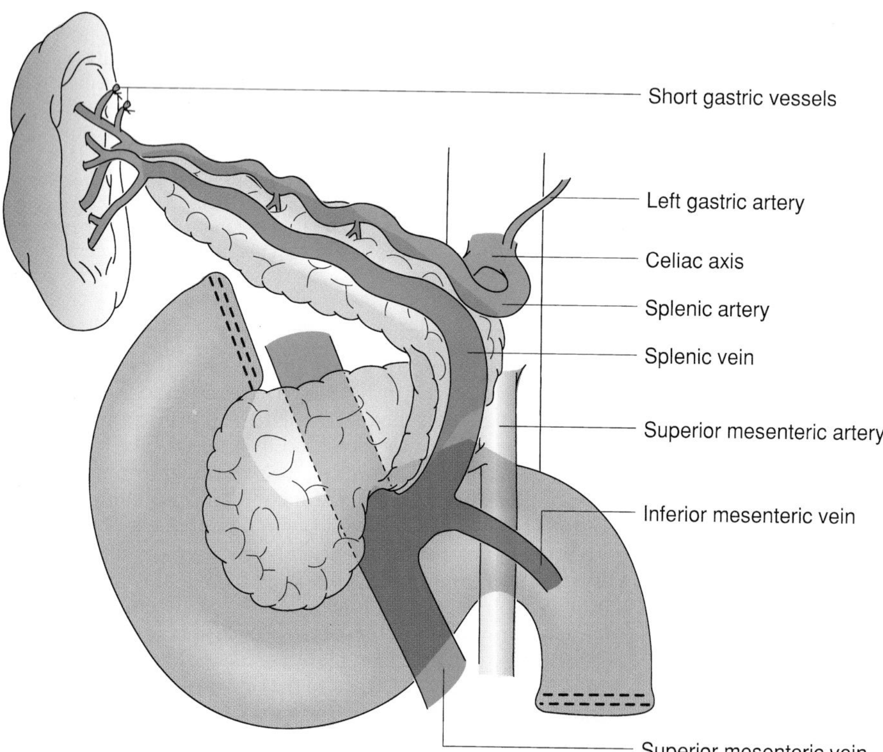

FIGURE 36.12 The pancreas is reflected anteriorly and to the right to the level of the superior mesenteric vein near the confluence with the splenic vein. The aortic origins of the celiac axis and superior mesenteric arteries are identified.

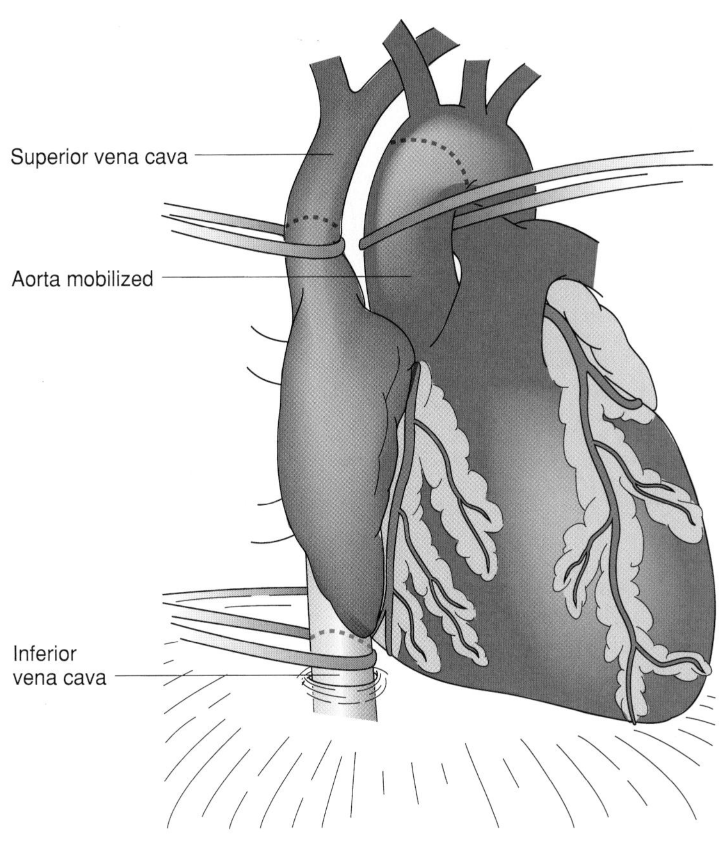

FIGURE 36.13 Preparation of the heart for cardioplegia. Minimal dissection is necessary. The venae cavae are encircled, and the aorta is separated from the pulmonary artery.

Current Preservation Techniques and Results

Kidneys, Liver, and Pancreas

For many years, the primary solution used for cold storage preservation of the kidneys was Euro-Collins solution (Table 36.2). This formulation provides a hyperosmolar environment with intracellular electrolyte composition that is intended to reduce cellular swelling. In combination with hypothermia, kidneys can be safely stored in this solution for 36 to 48 hours before transplantation.

In the 1980s, the advent of new immunosuppressive agents, such as cyclosporine, meant that for the first time extrarenal organs could be transplanted with good success rates, and the need for more effective preservation became apparent. Cold ischemia limitations of about 8 hours for the liver and pancreas meant that donor and recipient teams had to be exquisitely coordinated; complex recipient operations requiring a multitude of ancillary support services had to be organized in the middle of the night; and all personnel involved in the procedure, including the surgeons, were starting the operation in a fatigued condition.

At the University of Wisconsin (UW), a solution was developed that transformed the practice of hepatic and pancreatic transplantation. This solution includes lactobionate, raffinose, hydroxyethyl starch, and a host of other ingredients designed to provide high-energy phosphate precursors, hydrogen ion buffering capacity, and antioxidant properties. It is unclear how many of these components are truly necessary. Lactobionate, an impermeant anion to prevent cellular swelling, is used in place of the glucose that is contained in Euro-Collins solution; raffinose, a naturally occurring trisaccharide of fructose, glucose, and galactose, which is found in abundance in sugar beets, provides additional osmotic activity; and hydroxyethyl starch is a colloid

TABLE 36.2

COMPOSITION OF HYPOTHERMIC ORGAN PRESERVATION SOLUTIONS

Component	Amount per liter
Euro-Collins Solution	
KH_2PO_4	2.05 g
K_2HPO_4	7.4 g
KCl	1.12 g
$NaHCO_3$	0.84 g
Glucose	35 g
University of Wisconsin Solution	
K^+-lactobionate	100 mmol
KH_2PO_4	25 mmol
$MgSO_4$	5 mmol
Raffinose	30 mmol
Adenosine	5 mmol
Glutathione	3 mmol
Insulin	100 IU
Penicillin	40 IU
Dexamethasone	8 mg
Allopurinol	1 mmol
HTK Solution	
NaCl	15 mmol
KCl	9 mmol
KH-2-ketoglutarate	1 mmol
$MgCl_2$	4 mmol
Histidine hydrochloride	18 mmol
Histidine	180 mmol
Tryptophan	2 mmol
Mannitol	30 mmol
$CaCl_2$	0.015 mmol

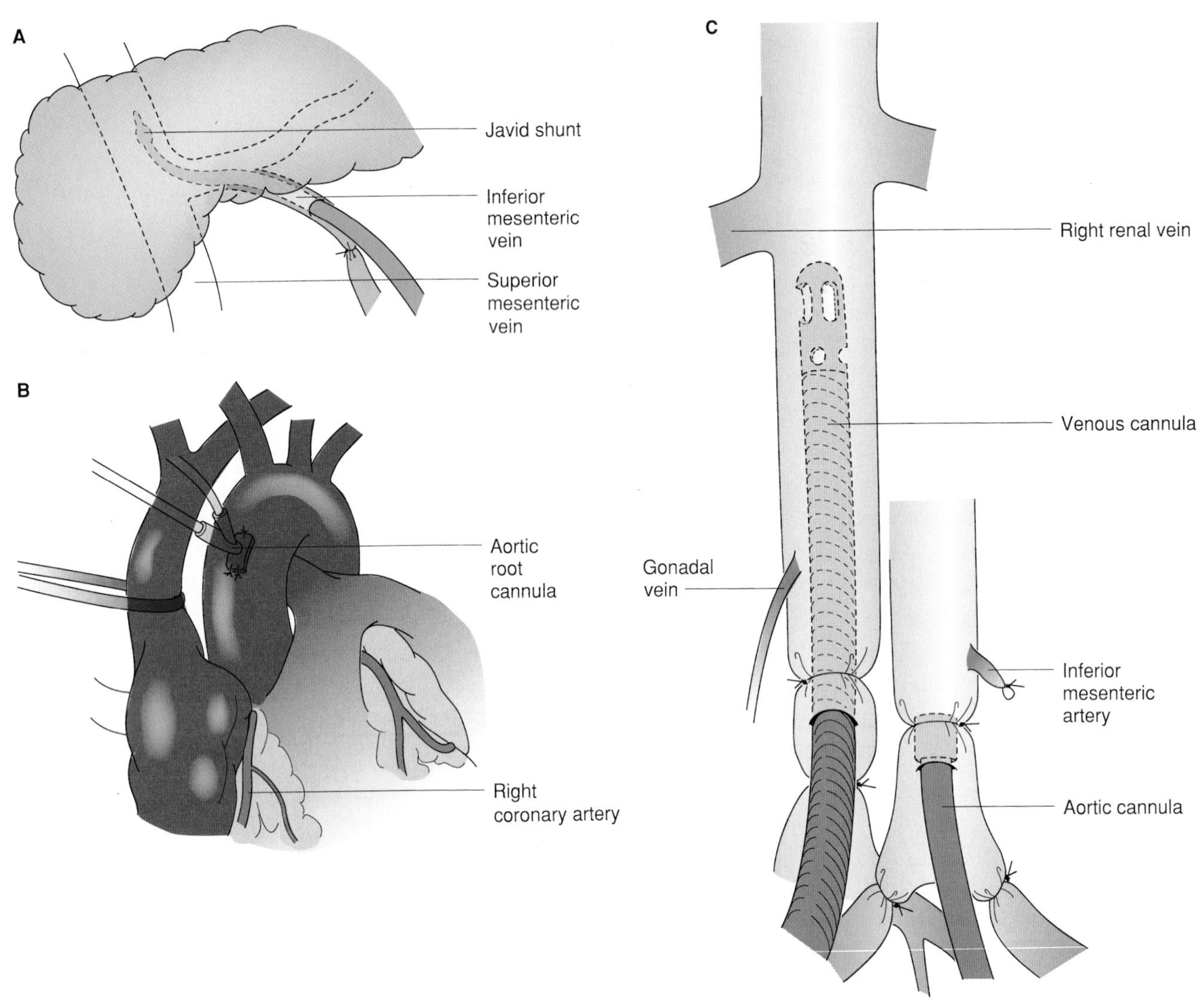

FIGURE 36.14 *In situ* perfusion set-up. (*A*) A cannula is placed into the portal vein through the inferior mesenteric vein for portal venous perfusion. (*B*) A needle is placed in the aortic root for perfusion of the coronary arteries with cardioplegia solution. (*C*) A cannula is placed in the distal aorta for retrograde perfusion with cold preservation solution. Another cannula is placed in the distal vena cava for venous decompression and exsanguination.

intended to prevent an increase in the extracellular space. UW solution is used to preserve most organs in the United States. Livers and pancreata can be stored for up to 24 hours, and isolated clinical cases with total cold ischemia times in excess of 30 hours have been reported.[34,35] However, although livers will function in terms of hepatocellular metabolism, evidence is accumulating that cold ischemia times of greater than 12 hours may be associated with a higher incidence of biliary strictures.

It is not clear whether UW cold storage solution has any significant advantages over Euro-Collins solution for the preservation of kidneys. In a large, randomized, multicenter European trial, patient and graft survival rates were similar among recipients of the two solutions, but the incidence of delayed graft function requiring dialysis was reduced by about one third in the UW group. The results of other ongoing trials are needed before a definitive statement can be made about the relative merits of the two solutions in renal preservation. This point may be moot, however, because the majority of deceased donors are used for the procurement of extrarenal organs as well as kidneys, so UW solution is generally used for all of the abdominal organs. Newer preservatives, including histidine-triptophane-ketoglutarate (HTK) solution, are appearing and may have advantages over UW solution in terms of reduced viscosity.[36]

Heart and Lungs

Cardiac preservation has changed relatively little in recent years. Hyperkalemic, crystalloid cardioplegia solution is used at 4°C, and 4 hours is the generally accepted limit of cold ischemia. For this reason, donor and recipient operations must be finely coordinated.

A comprehensive review of pulmonary preservation has recently been published.[37] Hypothermia is used along with intracellular-type solutions such as Euro-Collins. Pulmonary inflation also appears to be important. The optimal vascular perfusate for the lungs remains unknown, however, and results with pulmonary transplantation are still limited by

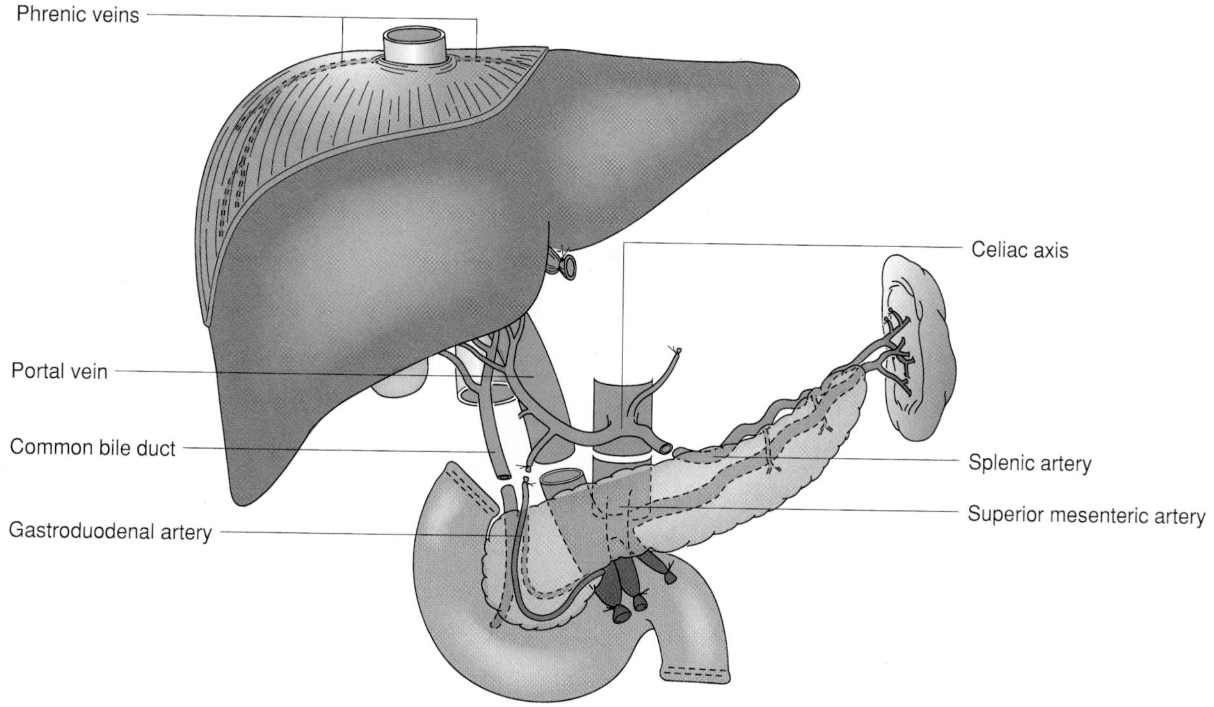

FIGURE 36.15 The liver and pancreas are removed *en bloc*. Separation of the two organs is accomplished as a bench procedure. The celiac axis is retained with the liver, dividing the splenic artery just beyond its origin. The gastroduodenal artery is ligated and divided. The portal vein is divided approximately 1 cm from the superior edge of the pancreas, and the common bile duct is divided just superior to its entrance into the pancreas.

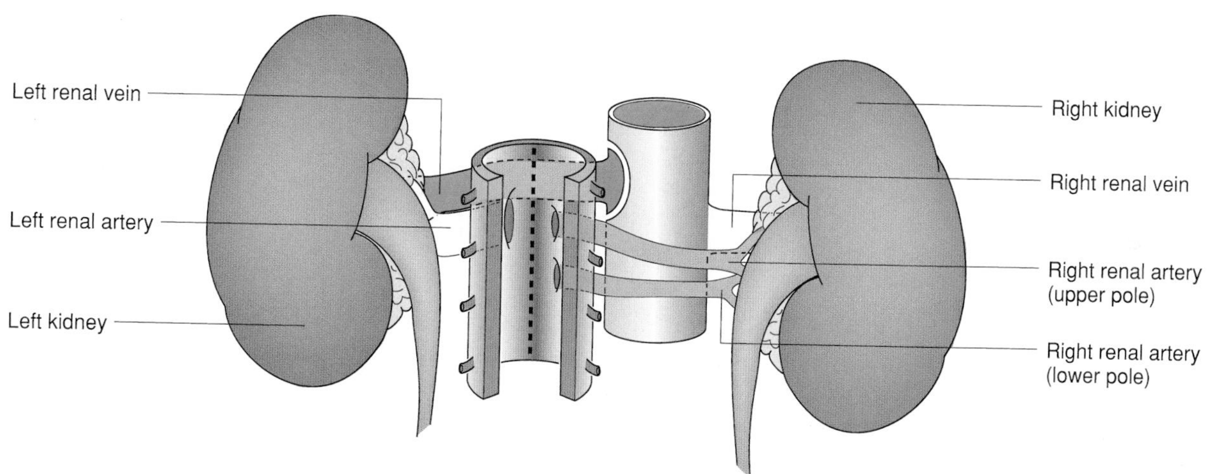

FIGURE 36.16 The kidneys are removed *en bloc* and separated on the back bench. Safe division is ensured by viewing the kidneys posteriorly. The aorta is divided between the paired lumbar arteries, and renal arterial orifices can be viewed directly from within the aortic lumen. This avoids any hilar dissection with the accompanying risk of injury to renal arteries. The left renal vein is divided at its entrance to the inferior vena cava, leaving the entire vena cava with the shorter right renal vein.

deficiencies in the quality and duration of preservation. UW solution has been used recently.

Small Bowel

The transplantation of small bowel segments with or without concomitant liver transplant is being performed with more and more regularity as the treatment of choice for short-gut syndrome. Preservation of the bowel is generally performed with UW solution or HTK solution, although experimental evidence does not indicate that these offer any advantage over simple hypothermia.[38] Most small bowel procurements, however, are from donors that have multiple useful organs, hence the use of standard intra-aortic preservation techniques. The current limit of cold ischemia time for small bowel is approximately 12 hours.[39]

KEY POINTS

- **Much of the injury to transplanted organs occurs not during the period of ischemia but during organ reperfusion.**
- **The general attributes of an acceptable organ donor include pronouncement of donor death, previously good general health, and relative hemodynamic stability from the time of the precipitating event leading to death until organ procurement is complete.**
- **The following requirements must be met to make a firm diagnosis of brain death: the presence of reversible causes of coma should be excluded; clinical criteria establishing the loss of all functions of the entire brain must be met (deep coma, absence of brainstem function, absence of spontaneous respiration); and a confirmatory diagnostic test must be carried out (electroencephalogram, nuclear brain blood flow study, four-vessel cerebral arteriography).**
- **All transplant candidates within the United States are entered into a computer system, and an allocation system is used to determine the appropriate potential recipient for a given donor organ.**

References

1. Belzer FO. Evaluation of preservation of the intra-abdominal organs. *Transplant Proc.* 1993;25:2527–2531.
2. McLaren AJ, Friend PJ. Trends in organ preservation. *Transpl Int.* 2003;16:701–708.
3. Belzer FO, Southard JH. Principles of solid-organ preservation by cold storage. *Transplantation* 1988;45:673–676.
4. Simonson MS, Dunn MJ. Endothelins: A family of regulator peptides. State-of-the-art lecture. *Hypertension* 1991;17:856–863.
5. Wilhelm SM, Simonson MS, Robinson AV, et al. Cold ischemia induces endothelin gene upregulation in the preserved kidney. *J Surg Res* 1999; 85:101–108.
6. Southard JH, Senzig KA, Belzer FO. Effects of hypothermia on canine kidney mitochondria. *Cryobiology* 1980;17:148–153.
7. McCord JM. Oxygen-derived free radicals in postischemic tissue injury. *N Engl J Med.* 1985;312:159–163.
8. Clavien PA, Harvey RP, Strasberg SM. Preservation and reperfusion injuries in liver allografts. *Transplantation* 1992;53 :957–978.
9. Koyama I, Bulkley GB, Williams GM, et al. The role of oxygen free radicals in mediating the reperfusion injury of cold preserved ischemic kidneys. *Transplantation* 1985;40:590–595.
10. Colletti LM, Burtch GD, Remick DG, et al. The production of tumor necrosis factor alpha and the development of a pulmonary capillary injury following hepatic ischemia/reperfusion. *Transplantation* 1990;49:268–272.
11. Sturber M, Harringer W, Ernst M, et al. Inhaled nitric oxide as a prophylactic treatment against reperfusion injury. *Thorac Cardiovasc Surg.* 1999;47:179–182.
12. Devlin J, Palmer RMJ, Gonde CE, et al. Nitric oxide generation. *Transplantation* 1994: 58:592–595
13. **2003 U.S. Organ Procurement and Transplantation Network and the Scientific Registry for Transplant Recipients Annual Report: Transplant Data 1993–2002: Department of Health and Human Services, Health Resources and Services Administration, Office of Special Programs, Division of Transplantation, Rockville, MD; United Network for Organ Sharing, Richmond, VA; University Renal Research and Education Association. Ann Arbor, MI; 2003.**
14. The 11th report of the human renal transplant registry. *JAMA* 1973;226:1197–1204.
15. Zhou YC, Cecka JM. Effect of age on kidney transplants. In: Terasaki PI, ed. *Clinical transplants* 1989. Los Angeles: UCLA Tissue Typing Laboratory; 1989:369–378.
16. Bergmeijer JH, Cransberg K, Nijman JM, et al. Functional adaptation of en-bloc-transplanted pediatric kidneys into pediatric recipients. *Transplantation* 1994;58:623–624.
17. Sanchez-Fructuoso AI, Prats D, Perez-Contin MJ, et al. Increasing the donor pool using en bloc pediatric kidneys for transplant. *Transplantation* 2003;76:1180–1184.
18. Freeman RB, Giatras I, Falagas ME, et al. Outcome of transplantation of organs procured from bacteremic donors. *Transplantation* 1999;68:1107–1111.
19. Roth D, Fernandez JA, Babischkin S, et al. Detection of hepatitis C virus among cadaver organ donors: evidence for low transmission of disease. *Ann Intern Med.* 1992;117:470–475.
20. Morse JH, Turcotte JG, Merion RM, et al. Development of a malignant tumor in a liver transplant graft procured from a donor with a cerebral neoplasm. *Transplantation* 1990;50:875–877.
21. Abouna GM, Al-Adnani MS, Kremer GD. Reversal of diabetic nephropathy in human cadaveric kidneys after transplantation into non-diabetic recipients. *Lancet* 1983;2:1274–1276.
22. **Port FK, Bragg-Gresham JL, Metzger RA, et al. Donor characteristics associated with reduced graft survival: an approach to expanding the pool of kidney donors. *Transplantation* 2002;74:1281–1286.**
23. Kaufman HH, Hui KS, Mattson JC, et al. Clinicopathologic correlations of disseminated intravascular coagulation in patients with head injury. *Neurosurgery* 1984;15:34–42.
24. **A definition of irreversible coma: report of the Ad Hoc Committee of Harvard Medical School to examine the definition of brain death. *JAMA.* 1968;205:337–340.**
25. Jorgensen EO. Spinal man after brain death. *Acta Neurochir (Wien).* 1973;28:259–273.
26. Emery RW, Cork RC, Levinson MM, et al. The cardiac donor: a six-year experience. *Ann Thorac Surg.* 1986;41:356–362.
27. Novitzky D, Wicomb WN, Cooper DKC, et al. Electrocardiographic, hemodynamic and endocrine changes occurring during experimental brain death in the Chacma baboon. *Heart Transplant.* 1984;4:63–69.
28. Novitzky D, Wicomb WN, Cooper DKC, et al. Improved cardiac function following hormonal therapy in brain dead pigs: relevance to organ donation. *Cryobiology* 1987;24:1–10.
29. The Organ Procurement and Transplantation Network. Policies. Available at: http://www.optn.org/policiesAndBylaws/.
30. Yersiz H, Renz JF, Hisatake GM, et al. Multivisceral and isolated intestinal procurement techniques. *Liver Transpl.* 2003;9:881–886.
31. Cooper JT, Chin LT, Krieger NR, et al. Donation after cardiac death: the University of Wisconsin experience with renal transplantation. *Am J Transplant.* 2004;4:1490–1494.
32. The Institute of Medicine. *Non-heartbeating Organ Transplantation: Medical and Ethical Issues in Procurement.* Washington: National Academy Press; 1997:1.
33. **Cho YW, Terasaki PI, Cecka JM, et al. Transplantation of kidneys from donors whose hearts have stopped beating. *N Engl J Med.* 1999;338:221–225.**
34. Todo S, Nery J, Yanaga K, et al. Extended preservation of human liver grafts with UW solution. *JAMA.* 1989;261:711–714.
35. D'Alessandro AM, Sollinger HW, Hoffmann RM, et al. Experience with Belzer UW cold storage solution in simultaneous pancreas-kidney transplantation. *Transplant Proc.* 1990;22:532–534.
36. Pokorny H, Rasoul-Rockenschaub S, Langer F, et al. Histidine-tryptophan-ketoglutarate solution for organ preservation in human liver transplantation-a prospective multi-centre observation study. *Transpl Int.* 2004;17:256–260.
37. Conte JV, Baumgartner WA. Overview and future practice patterns in cardiac and pulmonary preservation. *J Card Surg.* 2000;15:91–107.
38. Kokudo Y, Furuya T, Takeyochi I, et al. Comparison of University of Wisconsin, Euro-Collins, and lactated Ringer's solutions in rat small bowel preservation for orthotopic small bowel transplantation. *Transplant Proc.* 1994;26:1492–1493
39. Furukawa H, Casavilla A, Abu-Elmagd K, et al. Basic considerations for the procurement of intestinal grafts. *Transplant Proc.* 1994;26:1470.

CHAPTER 37 ■ RENAL TRANSPLANTATION

CHRIS FREISE AND PETER STOCK

Renal transplantation has evolved to become the preferred therapeutic modality for patients with end-stage renal failure. Improved patient survival and quality of life as compared with dialysis has been established, with cost effectiveness achieved after a minimum of 18 months of allograft function. The importance of minimizing time on dialysis, compounded by the exponential growth of patients on the waiting list has led to several strategies to increase the number of deceased and living donor organs. These new strategies have been the focus of clinical research in kidney transplantation, and will be discussed in this chapter. Other important topics that will be reviewed include immunologic considerations specific to kidney transplantation; preoperative assessment of kidney allograft recipients; the standard surgical approach in kidney transplantation and advances in laparoscopic technology for the donor; current strategies in immunosuppression; management of the technical and immunosuppressive complications; and future trends.

IMMUNOLOGY OF RENAL TRANSPLANTATION

The immunologic response to allografted tissue is well defined and under the influence of both T-cell and B-cell derived reactions. The cells and cytokines responsible for rejection vary with time post-transplant (hyperacute, acute, and chronic rejection) and have a differential response to currently available immunosuppressive agents.

The major barriers to successful renal transplantation include ABO compatibility and the human leukocyte antigen (HLA) system. In general, renal transplantation is done between ABO compatible donor and recipients using the same guidelines as for blood transfusion. However, because of the shortage of donors, cadaver kidneys are nearly always used in recipients of identical blood type. Recently, ABO incompatible living-donor transplants have been performed on an experimental basis secondary to excessive wait times for ABO-compatible deceased-donor transplants.[1,2]

The HLA system is made up of well-defined antigens present on most cell types that are genetically determined for each patient and are termed the *major histocompatibility complex*. These genes reside on chromosome 6 and are distributed in a Mendelian fashion to offspring. The HLA system includes several loci, but the most commonly characterized are the HLA-A, HLA-B, and HLA-D regions. Given that each human has two alleles for each locus, there are six potential HLA antigens of clinical significance. These are characterized using tissue typing techniques and can be used to determine the degree of matching between a donor and potential recipient, i.e., one-antigen match to six-antigen match. Improved results of graft survival are seen when the degree of matching reaches the six-antigen level, and long-term results may be better with matching to a lesser degree.

Class I antigens include the HLA antigens A, B, and C whereas Class II antigens include the D and DR loci. Class I antigens act as targets for cytotoxic T lymphocytes, and Class II antigens are important for antigen presentation. Class II antigens are also responsible for triggering lymphocyte proliferation in the mixed lymphocyte culture system.

Before a renal transplant is undertaken, histocompatibility of the donor and recipient are determined. Standard testing consists of two procedures. Donors and recipients first undergo tissue typing which involves characterization of their respective HLA type. Recipient serum is tested against a panel of antigens that contain the known HLA types, to identify anti-HLA antibodies. The amount of reactivity of a potential recipient to this panel of antigens is indicative of the degree of sensitization. Sensitization occurs as a result of previous exposure to foreign HLA antigen either from pregnancy, previous blood transfusion, or a previous organ transplant. A patient who is highly sensitized is more difficult to transplant because of the greater likelihood of having antibodies to a potential donor.

The second test performed prior to transplantation is commonly known as the *final cross-match*. Several recipient serum samples collected at different times are mixed with donor lymphocytes in a culture system. This assay will detect preformed cytotoxic antibodies that would result in a hyperacute rejection if the transplantation were performed (see Rejection, later). A more sensitive method of detecting these antibodies utilizes a fluorescent activated cell scanner and is commonly used when evaluating potential recipients who are highly sensitized or receiving second transplants.

THE DONOR POOL: LIVING DONORS, DECEASED DONORS, NON–HEART BEATING DONORS

There is marked improvement in graft survival for both living-related and deceased donors when a transplant can be completed before the initiation of dialysis.[3] The significantly better outcomes achieved with preemptive transplantation and minimization of dialysis times have given rise to several strategies to increase the number of available kidneys.

Living Donors

The first long-term success in renal transplantation nearly 50 years ago involved a live donor transplant between twin brothers. The number of living donors has increased significantly in the last few years, in part as a result of the increased use of the laparoscopic technique for donor nephrectomies. For the first time in 2001, the number of living donors exceeded the number of deceased donors, although deceased donor transplants still represent the majority of kidney transplants done today.[4] This trend toward increased live donation may also be the result of the excessive waiting times for deceased donor transplants, now more than 5 years for blood type O and B recipients in many parts of the United States.

Despite initial concerns about the safety and efficacy of the laparoscopic technique for the donor procedure, morbidity and mortality rates (0.03%) remain low and comparable with those of the open technique.[5,6]

The evaluation of a potential living kidney donor begins with a brief overall assessment of physical condition because potential donors must be in good health with normal kidney function. Diabetes, hypertension, and cardiovascular disease generally rule out a potential donor. ABO is also determined before further workup, because ABO incompatibility has been a relative contraindication to donation. A cross-match test is usually performed at this time to ensure donor and recipient immunologic compatibility. After this initial screen, a careful medical and psychosocial screen takes place to confirm donor suitability. Following a normal physical examination, further studies should include: chest radiography, electrocardiogram, urinalysis, and blood work. During this phase, any conditions that could predispose to later renal insufficiency need to be ruled out. For example, donors from families with a history of type II diabetes are at a significant risk for the development of diabetes, and glucose tolerance testing is justified as part of the screening process. A history of renal stones warrants stone analysis to assess likelihood for recurrent stones. Any inherited disorders of kidney disease must also be ruled out, particularly in potential living-related donors when the recipient has polycystic kidney disease.

The psychosocial history is directed at ensuring a genuine emotional bond between the donor and the recipient. The establishment of a true relationship can be challenging but is particularly important in this era of increased donation from unrelated donors and the occasional donor found over the Internet. The motivation for donation should be clear and not be connected in any way to financial gain. It is also the duty of the physician evaluating the potential donor to review the current statistics on morbidity and mortality, and the potential donor should be provided with the opportunity to speak to the transplantation team privately to address issues of reluctance or coercion.

The final testing of a potential donor involves anatomic definition of the two kidneys and is typically done with either an intravenous pyelogram in combination with a renal arteriogram, or more recently a computed tomography angiogram alone, which avoids the needle stick and catheters associated with a conventional angiogram. The results of these studies are used to detect any anatomic abnormalities that would exclude a donor and to decide which kidney will be removed. In general, the left kidney is favored for transplant because it has a longer renal vein.

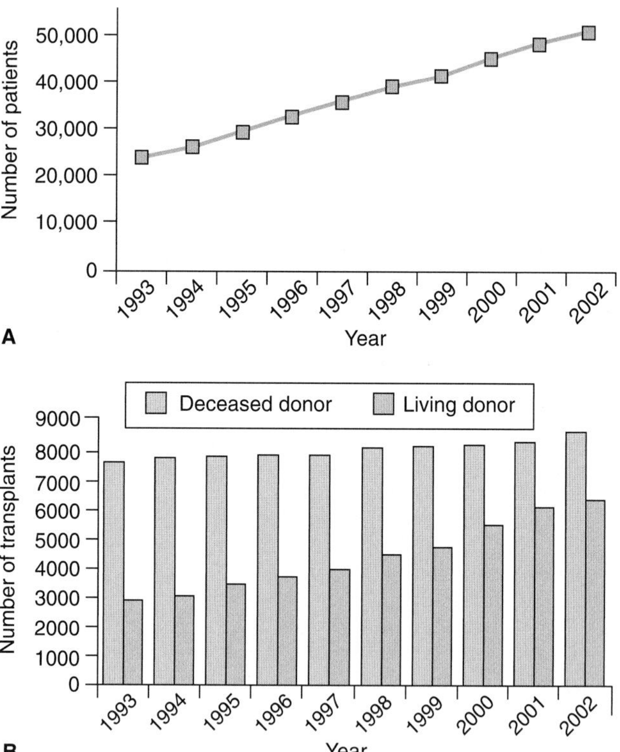

FIGURE 37.1 The growth in the number of patients awaiting transplant (*A*) has exceeded the relatively stagnant rate of deceased donation (*B*), leading to increased waiting times for deceased donor kidneys. Living donors have had a slight increase, which may be in part due to the introduction of the laparoscopic donation procedure. (Adapted with permission from Wynn JJ, Distant DA, Pirsch JD, et al. Kidney and pancreas transplantation. *Am J Transplant.* 2004;4 (suppl 9):72–80.)

Deceased Donors

Procurement of kidneys from brain-dead deceased donors has not increased at the same pace as the rapid growth of the national wait list (Fig. 37.1). Although most deceased donors are brain dead, there has been an increased utilization of kidneys from donors who do not meet the strict definitions of brain death but have cardiopulmonary support withdrawn because of a severe brain injury or high spinal cord injury, with little hope of living without the use of ongoing mechanical ventilation and/or the possibility of existing in a persistent vegetative state. Organs are recovered after withdrawal of support, once the heart stops beating, hence the terminology of *donors by cardiac death* or *DCD donors*. Usually support is withdrawn in a controlled setting so that the time of warm ischemia and poor organ perfusion can be minimized. The time from cessation of the heart to perfusion of organs with preservation fluid requires an experienced procurement team, and the successful use of these organs is dependent on rapid procurement. Several studies from the United States and Japan have demonstrated comparable graft success between kidneys procured from DCD donors and brain-dead donors. Although the use of livers from DCD donors appears to be associated with a higher incidence of biliary tract complications following transplantation, kidneys procured from DCD donors are proving to be an important source of donor kidneys.[7]

Placement of deceased-donor kidneys is guided by a series of allocation rules established by the United Network for Organ Sharing (UNOS). When a suitable deceased-donor kidney becomes available, it is first offered nationally to any potential recipient who shares the same antigens as the donor. This zero-mismatch kidney is then shipped to the center where the matched recipient is listed. This initial allocation is done because of the superior short- and long-term results of zero-mismatched kidneys. Allocation then follows a complex set of rules but is basically first offered to a patient who is listed at a center in the same geographic region as the donor, based on the best degree of HLA matching. If no suitable recipient is found, the kidney can then be offered outside the local region and eventually at the national level to an interested center. Several situations can raise a patient's priority on the list, including pediatric status, need for emergency kidney transplant because of failing dialysis access, or desire of a donor family to direct the kidney to a specific recipient. In addition, some regions apply for a variance to the usual allocation scheme and may use strict waiting time as the sole determinant of which patient receives the next available kidney. The use of HLA matching versus waiting time as a determinant for kidney allocation continues to be a hot topic of debate at UNOS.[8]

Further Strategies for Increasing the Number of Donor Kidneys

Many of the unique approaches for increasing the number of potential donors have come from Japan, where cultural beliefs have limited the number of available deceased donor transplants. Several groups have reported successful kidney transplantation across ABO blood group barriers, utilizing aggressive pretransplant immunosuppression, plasmapheresis to decrease anti-ABO titers, and in some cases splenectomy.[1,2] This strategy has been implemented with increasing frequency in the United States as a result of the marked increases in the waiting times for blood group O and B recipients.[9]

An important strategy currently being implemented in the United States as well as internationally involves the use of intravenous gammaglobulin to facilitate transplantation across a known positive anti-HLA cross-match. This protocol could potentially impact the increasing number of sensitized patients on waiting lists with little hope of finding a compatible donor.[10]

Further strategies have recently been implemented to expand the availability of kidneys procured from deceased donors. In addition to the use of kidneys from DCD donors described earlier, another strategy recently implemented by UNOS involves expedited placement of kidneys at risk for delayed graft function. These kidneys are designated as *extended-criteria donors* and are expected to have decreased longevity compared with kidneys procured from the standard pool of deceased donor kidneys designated as *standard criteria donors*. The classification as an extended criteria donors kidney is based on the relative risk of delayed graft function; the risk is increased by the presence of older donor age, higher donor creatinine at the time of organ procurement, cerebrovascular accident as the cause of brain death, and a history of hypertension in the donor. The kidneys that fall into the category of extended criteria donors kidneys are generally allocated to older recipients to decrease time on waiting lists that are now exceeding 5 to 6 years. Expedited placement and transplantation of older recipients minimizes the potential for delayed graft function and increases use of organs that otherwise would be discarded.[11,12]

TABLE 37.1 ETIOLOGY

ETIOLOGY OF RENAL DISEASE AS INDICATIONS FOR RENAL TRANSPLANTATION, RANKED IN ORDER OF PREVALENCE

Diabetes mellitus (type I and II)
Hypertension
Polycystic kidney disease
IgA nephropathy
Chronic glomerulonephritis
Focal sclerosis
Systemic lupus
Membranous glomerulonephritis
Pyelonephritis
Focal segmental glomerulosclerosis
Congenital obstructive uropathy
Nephritis
Alport syndrome
Hypoplasia, dysplasia
Wegener granulomatosis
Postinfectious glomerulonephritis
Obstructive uropathy
Hemolytic uremia
Membranoproliferative glomerulonephritis
Goodpasture syndrome
Membranous nephropathy
Analgesic nephropathy
Prune belly syndrome
Medullary cystic disease
Henoch-Schönlein purpura
Nephronophthisis
Scleroderma
Sickle cell anemia
Amyloidosis
Oxalosis

Adapted with permission from Cecka JM. The OPTN/UNOS Renal Transplant Registry. In Cecka JM, Terasaki PI, eds. *Clinical Transplants 2003*. Los Angeles: UCLA Immunogenetics Center; 2004:1–12.

THE TRANSPLANT PROCEDURE

Preoperative Assessment

The etiology of kidney disease resulting in end-stage failure and the necessity for transplantation are led by glomerulonephritis, diabetes, and hypertension (Table 37.1).[13] Because of the high incidence of cardiovascular disease associated with many of these diseases, most notably diabetes, a careful assessment of the cardiovascular status of the potential recipient is critical. For patients at risk, this assessment should minimally include an echocardiogram and an exercise or pharmacologic stress test as a screen for reversible ischemia requiring cardiac catheterization. Controversy remains with regard to the accuracy of noninvasive studies in terms of identifying significant occlusion of the coronary arteries, particularly in diabetic patients. Nonetheless, for most centers this remains the standard screen, and updated studies should be obtained within 1 year of the transplant procedure. If either coronary artery bypass or stenting has taken place in preparation for renal transplantation, follow-up angiograms and/or stress tests should be repeated within 1 year of the actual transplant.

Although the evaluation of potential recipients is focused on the assessment of cardiovascular status, further studies must exclude malignancies and infections that would contraindicate transplantation and immunosuppression. Potential kidney recipients who are infected with hepatitis C should be evaluated by a hepatologist to determine the risks of immunosuppression causing progression to end-stage liver disease. Potential kidney recipients with evidence of advanced liver disease should be evaluated for a combined liver and kidney transplant. For patients with less advanced liver disease, consideration should be given to interferon therapy before proceeding with kidney transplantation to provide the opportunity for viral clearance. Kidney transplantation was previously contraindicated in people with HIV infection secondary to concerns of exacerbating an already immunologically compromised state. Recent advances in antiretroviral therapy and the ability to provide effective prophylaxis against opportunistic infections has prompted several centers to perform transplantation in people with end-stage renal disease and HIV infection. Early results suggest that progression of HIV to AIDS has not been seen following transplantation and immunosuppression, with early allograft success rates comparable to those in non–HIV-positive recipients.[14] Potential patients with a previous history of tuberculosis or conversion to purified protein derivative positivity should be evaluated for active disease.

Colonoscopy, mammography, and Pap smear should be performed as dictated by age-specific standard guidelines.

For most malignancies, with the exception of nonmelanoma skin cancers, a disease-free interval of 5 years is recommended before kidney transplantation.

For patients with congenital abnormalities as the cause of renal failure, a complete workup of the genitourinary systems is necessary, including urodynamics and voiding cystourethrograms. These studies are particularly important in children with end-stage disease resulting from posterior urethral valves, to ensure that the bladder will serve as an adequate conduit for the kidney transplant. For patients with severe reflux disease and chronic pyelonephritis, native ureteronephrectomy may be required to prevent posttransplant infection secondary to chronic reflux into the native ureters. For patients with inadequate bladder capacity and function, pretransplant reconstructive procedures such as ileal augmentation or ileal conduits may be required.

For patients with suspected clotting disorders based on a previous history of thromboembolic events (frequently clotting problems with dialysis access) or diseases associated with an increased frequency of clotting disorders (i.e., lupus), a hematologic workup is necessary to determine the necessity for anticoagulation at the time of the transplant. This workup should include a determination of serum levels of protein C, protein S, anticardiolipin antibody, factor V Leiden, antithrombin III levels, and the G20210A prothrombin gene mutation.

Donor Nephrectomy: Open and Laparoscopic

A living kidney donor operation is a unique surgical procedure for two reasons. First, the donor has no medical reason to be in the operating room, and the process is driven only by his or her willingness to help another person with their gift of donation. Second, the removed tissue must be in perfect condition because it will be reimplanted into the recipient. These two features, therefore, necessitate that the donor operation is done safely and done well. The original donor operation was done through a generous flank incision, allowing for good exposure and careful dissection of the renal vessels. Unfortunately, this flank approach generally left a large incision, with its accompanying morbidity, pain, and sometimes adverse cosmetic result. The development of the laparoscopic procedure to remove kidneys has revolutionized the field, although its initial introduction was met with trepidation because of concerns over donor safety. With the explosive growth and dissemination of this procedure, it has now become the standard for donor nephrectomy.

The procedure is most commonly done through a transperitoneal approach, although some surgeons prefer to remain retroperitoneal. Once the operative space is expanded with carbon dioxide gas and the scope is inserted , two to three additional ports are placed to allow for the passage of instruments to dissect the kidney (Fig. 37.2). Some centers also favor the use of a gastight "hand-port," which allows placement of the surgeon's hand in the operative space to assist in exposure and to have available if sudden bleeding is encountered. Once the kidney vessels are transected and the vessels stumps are controlled by clips or laparoscopic staples, the kidney can be removed through a 2- to 3-inch incision, which can be placed in a position that leaves minimal scarring and avoids cutting muscle tissue. Donors who undergo the laparoscopic procedure typically have reduced pain medicine requirements, have a slightly shorter hospital stay, and are able to return to their usual activities sooner.[5,6]

12 mm port for stapler
Extraction incision
11 mm ports
Camera port
A

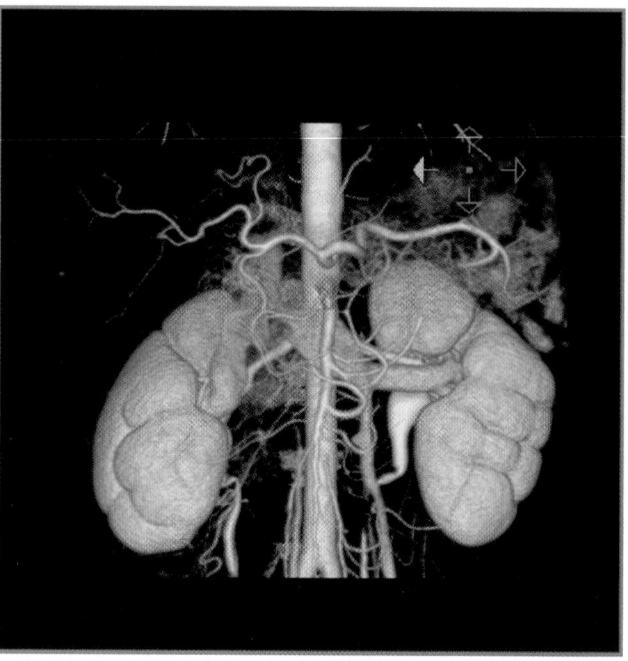
B

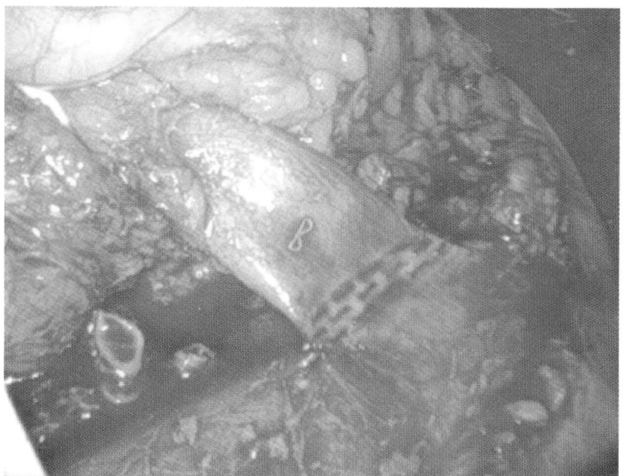
C

FIGURE 37.2 (*A*) The laparoscopic donor procedure is performed with the donor in a lateral position, typically using three to four ports, with extraction of the kidney through a 6- to 8-cm incision. (*B*) Preoperative computed tomography angiogram revealing the arterial and venous anatomy. (*C*) Intraoperative photograph of laparoscopic view of right kidney just prior to transection of the renal vein. The artery has already been divided.

The safety of this relatively new procedure has been established, in addition to the demonstration that the function of kidneys recovered through a laparoscopic approach function as well as kidneys removed in an open operation. Importantly, there seems to have been an increased interest in live donation, coincident with the introduction of the laparoscopic procedure, suggesting that this procedure has removed some of the disincentives of the donation process.

Recipient Operative Procedure

The kidney transplant is heterotopically placed in the extraperitoneal iliac fossa. Although this is a less technically demanding procedure than either liver or pancreas transplants, attention to detail is imperative to optimize immediate graft function and avoid technical complications resulting in loss of the kidney transplant.

The operation is initiated by exposure of the iliac fossa through a curvilinear incision and can be done on either the right or left side. The incision extends from 1 cm above the symphysis pubis to approximately 2 cm lateral to the anterior iliac spine (Fig. 37.3). The fascia is divided along the lateral border of the rectus sheath, and the contents of the peritoneal cavity are reflected cephalad and medially, exposing the iliac vessels in the retroperitoneum. Lymphatics overlying the iliac vessels are suture ligated and divided to prevent the development of lymphoceles. In males, the spermatic cord is secured with a vessel loop and can be retracted away from the operative field. In females, the round ligament is suture ligated and divided. The inferior epigastric artery and vein are divided to prevent potential compression of the transplanted ureter. Placement of a mechanical retractor should avoid compression of iliac artery and vein as well as the femoral nerve to prevent neuropraxias.

The living or deceased donor kidney is inspected for the presence of multiple vessels, duplication of the urinary collecting system, and parenchymal abnormalities. The artery and vein are dissected from surrounding structures to provide the necessary length for transplantation. In the case of multiple arteries, a decision must be made as to whether to perform *ex vivo* reconstruction to achieve a single implantable conduit versus implanting the vessels separately. This decision is in part dependent on the quality of the recipient vessels and an assessment as to whether the anastomosis of multiple vessels directly into the recipient would require an unacceptable period of warm ischemia to the kidney. In general, in an adult the anastomosis of the renal artery and vein are performed in an end-to-side fashion to the external iliac vessels, although occasionally the presence of atherosclerotic disease requires transplantation to the common iliac vessels. In children who weigh less than 20 kg, or for third transplants in adults, an intraperitoneal approach is used and the vascular anastomoses are frequently performed to the aorta and inferior vena cava. For kidneys from deceased donors, a Carrel patch of aorta is used to prevent stenosis and to provide a common patch for multiple arteries. Warm ischemia time should be minimized to prevent delayed graft function. Ensuring adequate intravascular volume and stable hemodynamics at the time of reperfusion is extremely important to achieve optimal function of the transplant.

The reimplantation of the ureter is most frequently performed through an extravesicular technique. Following positioning of the revascularized kidney in the iliac fossa and assurance of hemostasis, the ureter is shortened to permit a tension-free anastomosis with adequate blood supply to the distal ureter. In men, the ureter is placed under the spermatic cord to prevent ureteral obstruction. The bladder is distended with an antibiotic solution to identify a suitable area for ureteral implantation on the dome of the bladder, and a cystotomy is made at this site. An anastomosis between the mucosa of the bladder and transplanted ureter is constructed using an absorbable suture to prevent stone formation. A second layer of the bladder musculature is closed over distal portion of the ureter to prevent reflux during micturation.

There are alternative techniques to reimplant the ureter, including the Politano-Leadbetter transvesical ureteroneocystostomy. This technique involves tunneling the ureter through the bladder wall from the inside of the bladder. This technique is still preferred by some surgeons who believe the long-term prevention of reflux is superior with the transvesicular approach. However, this technique requires a second cystotomy, and posttransplant hematuria is more common than with the extravesicular technique. A third technique for ureteral implantation in recipients with normal native ureters is ureteroureterostomy over a double-J stent. In general, this technique is reserved for reimplantation of transplanted ureters with distal strictures secondary to ischemia. It can also be used as a primary technique if there are questions regarding

TRANSPLANTATION

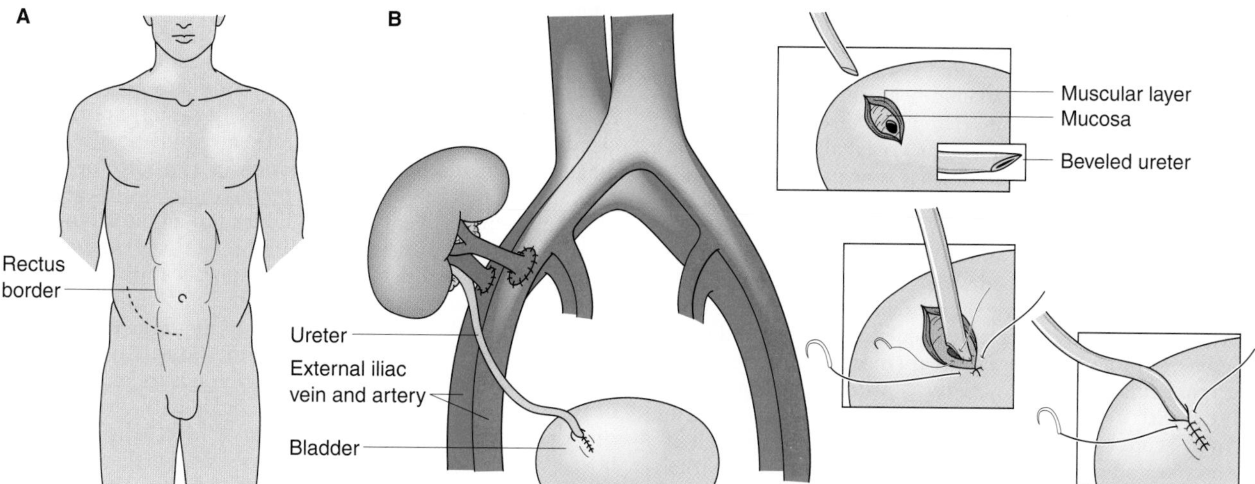

Figure 37.3 (*A*) Curvilinear iliac fossa incision used for the kidney transplant recipient procedure. (*B*) Vascular anastomoses completed between the recipient external iliac artery and vein and donor renal artery and vein. *Insets:* ureteral anastomosis performed using the external ureteroneocystostomy technique.

the blood supply to the distal ureter at the time of transplant. This technique is preferred if the donor ureter was damaged or inadvertently stripped of its blood supply at the time of procurement but is dependent on the availability of normal native ureters to serve as an adequate conduit.

COMPLICATIONS

Early Graft Dysfunction

The majority of kidneys begin to function right after implantation, especially in the case of a living donor. When the initial function results in only a slow drop in serum creatinine, the diagnosis of slow graft function is made. When dialysis is needed in the first week because of poor function, the diagnosis of delayed graft function is made. Delayed graft function typically occurs in 15% to 30% of deceased donor transplants. The diagnosis of slow graft function or delayed graft function is important to establish because other problems, such as rejection, vascular occlusion, or ureteral obstruction, can also result in low urine output and need for dialysis. These other causes must be eliminated before the diagnosis of slow graft function or delayed graft function can be made.

In the immediate postoperative period, careful attention to fluid status is critical. In cases of immediate graft function, fluid orders should include replacement for urine output as well as a maintenance fluid rate. This policy ensures that the patient does not become volume depleted and compromise perfusion to the new kidney. In cases of delayed graft function, fluid should be restricted and dialysis instituted when electrolyte imbalance or fluid overload are evident.

A decrease in urine output in the early postoperative period requires immediate diagnostic and therapeutic intervention. Once mechanical obstruction of the indwelling Foley catheter has been excluded by irrigation, the volume status of the patient should be assessed, preferably with a central venous pressure line or pulmonary artery catheter. Fluid replacement to restore intravascular volume should be initiated in the volume-depleted patient.

Radiologic evaluation using various imaging techniques is required if urine output remains low in the face of adequate volume status. Ultrasonography is most helpful to diagnose ureteral obstruction caused by technical complications at the anastomosis or fluid collections that may be obstructing the ureter by extrinsic compression. With the addition of duplex and color Doppler imaging, blood flow to the kidney can be evaluated, and technical problems with the vessels can be assessed. Nuclear medicine techniques are also valuable for assessing renal function. Technetium 99m diethylenetriamine pentaacetic acid (DTPA) and iodine-131 iodohippurate (Hippuran) are the two major radionuclides used in the evaluation of renal allograft function. DTPA renal scans evaluate the vascular flow pattern of the kidney as well as the gross anatomy of the ureter and bladder. Scans are performed over 30 minutes, with uptake of contrast within 6 seconds indicating adequate flow to the graft. Peak activity in the parenchyma should be reached within 2 minutes, followed by a gradual decline in radioactivity in the renal parenchyma and an increase in radioactivity in the urinary collecting system and bladder. Iodine-131 iodohippurate scans are more sensitive in evaluating renal function. Peak activity is also reached in 2 to 4 minutes, with gradual decline over the next 30 minutes. In rejection, acute tubular necrosis and drug toxicity as well as poor uptake and poor excretion are the typical findings with a nuclear medicine scan.

If these imaging techniques do not indicate an explanation for the poor urine output, the diagnosis of delayed graft function is made. Immunosuppression can then be adjusted to minimize or avoid the calcineurin inhibitors, which can prolong the recovery from delayed graft function and also to initiate antibody therapy to protect the kidney from rejection. The combination of delayed graft function and early rejection is clearly associated with worse outcome in the long term, and an early biopsy of the kidney that is functioning poorly is helpful to diagnose rejection and guide therapy.

Technical Complications

The majority of surgical complications are experienced in the immediate postoperative period. The two main types of complications can be classified as vascular and urologic.

Renal artery thrombosis is a rare complication occurring in about 1% of transplants. The risk of this complication is higher with size mismatch of donor renal artery and recipient internal iliac artery when an end-to-end anastomosis is performed, in kidneys with multiple renal arteries, in kidneys traumatized because of rough handling, and in the presence of an unidentified renal artery intimal flap. Sudden loss of urinary output, not the result of an obstructed Foley catheter or inadequate vascular volume, should necessitate a workup with duplex Doppler ultrasound. Loss of signal is indicative of no flow to the kidney. Alternatively, a nuclear medicine renal scan is informative, with lack of isotope uptake by the kidney indicating no blood flow. Prompt return to the operating room for correction of a technical problem is imperative, but often the diagnosis is not made quickly enough to salvage the kidney.

Renal artery stenosis occurs in up to 15% of transplanted kidneys. Difficult-to-control hypertension should suggest the possibility of stenosis. Diagnosis with renal Duplex ultrasound followed by arteriography to better define the anatomy and degree of stenosis should be done before operative repair or angioplasty. Initial success rates for both methods are similar (75% to 80%), but the restenosis rate following angioplasty is not well defined. Anastomotic strictures respond less well to angioplasty and probably should be repaired by operative intervention.

Aneurysms that occur in the renal artery are either pseudoaneurysms at the anastomotic site or mycotic aneurysms secondary to bacterial or fungal infection. A rapidly expanding, tender pulsatile mass in the region of the kidney suggests a mycotic aneurysm. Arteriography is confirmatory for diagnosis. Treatment consists of appropriate antibiotics and removal of the transplanted kidney.

Venous complications are less frequent, with thrombosis occurring in 1% to 4% of transplants. Causative factors include intimal damage during retrieval, kinking at the iliac vein anastomosis, or pressure secondary to a lymphocele, urinoma, or hematoma. Occasionally, severe rejection can result in venous occlusion. Heparin infusion for incomplete occlusion and transplant nephrectomy for complete occlusion are the indicated therapies. Occasionally, graft salvage is possible if the diagnosis is made before progression of clot into the kidney itself. The classic sign of new hematuria may be an early hint of a renal vein problem and should lead to an ultrasound.

Urologic complications include ureteral obstruction, urinary fistula, or bladder leak. These complications all present with decreased urine output and a rise in serum creatinine. With a urine leak, pain in the region of the transplant may be severe. Mechanical obstruction of the Foley catheter must first be eliminated. Ureteral obstruction occurs in 1% to 9% of transplants, and diagnosis can be made with ultrasonography demonstrating hydronephrosis. A leak is usually diagnosed with a nuclear medicine renal scan. Further definition of a leak or stricture can be obtained via an antegrade pyelogram (Fig. 37.4). Early obstruction of the transplant ureter at the site of the bladder anastomosis may respond to internal stenting. Late strictures usually require reoperation, and urine and blood polymerase chain reaction for the polyoma

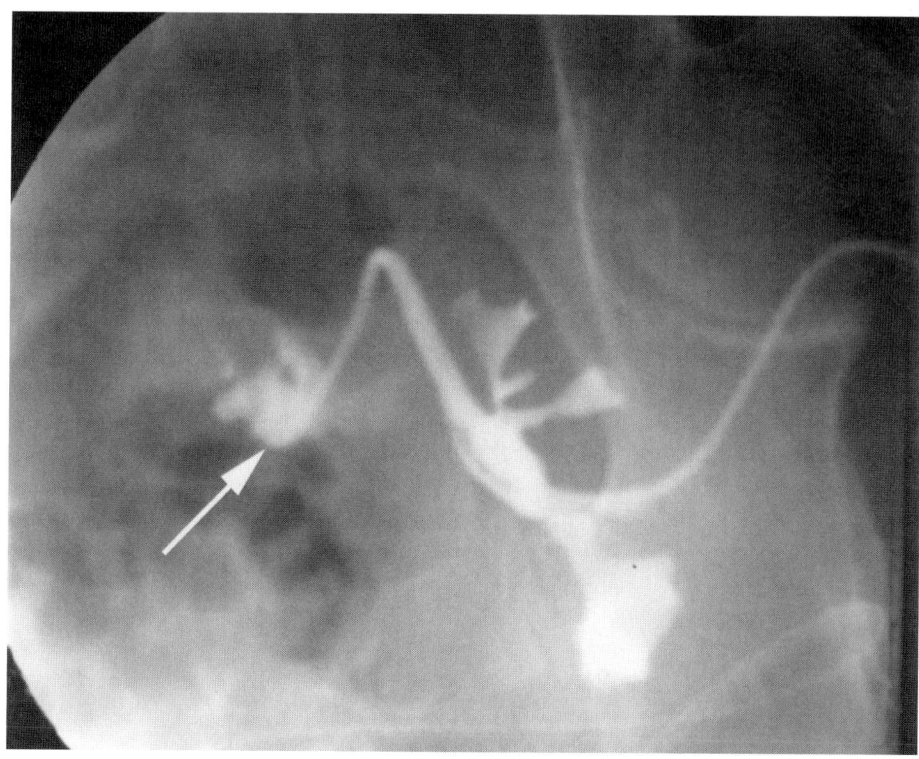

FIGURE 37.4 Percutaneous nephrostogram revealing a urine leak from the ureterovesical anastomosis.

virus should be done in that circumstance, because polyoma viral infection can lead to ureteral stricture. The surgical correction of a ureteral stricture may require reimplantation of the ureter into the bladder, the creation of a Boari flap, or the use of the recipient's native ureter for a ureteroureterostomy. (Fig. 37.5)

IMMUNOSUPPRESSION, REJECTION, AND IMMUNOSUPPRESSIVE COMPLICATIONS

Immunosuppression

Major advances in the ability to block immune-mediated destruction of the kidney have taken place in the past few years, resulting in a significant decrease in the incidence of acute rejection and improvement in long-term allograft survival rates.[13] This advance is the result of numerous agents that have been added during the past decade to the immunosuppressive armamentarium of prednisone, azathioprine, and cyclosporine A. These agents include tacrolimus, mycophenolate mofetil, sirolimus, anti-interleukin-2 receptor blockers, antithymocyte globulin (a polyclonal anti-T-cell agent), rituximab (an anti-CD20 monoclonal agent), and most recently costimulatory blockade with CTLA4-Ig. The addition of a variety of newer drugs targeting different pathways in the alloimmune cascade has permitted the development of regimens that are less dependent on the calcineurin inhibitors cyclosporine A and tacrolimus or on prednisone. Minimization of calcineurin inhibitors is an important aspect of many of the newer regimens, because long-term nephrotoxicity from calcineurin inhibitors is in part responsible for the chronic damage leading to poor long-term function.[15] In addition, both calcineurin inhibitors and prednisone are associated with the development of posttransplant diabetes mellitus, which in turn is associated with greater risks of graft failure and mortality.[16] New strategies using mycophenolate mofetil, sirolimus, and induction therapy with either interluekin-2 receptor inhibitors or antithymocyte globulin have permitted reduction in the levels of calcineurin inhibitors required to protect the allograft from rejection. Similarly, the addition of these agents has permitted the early withdrawal of prednisone, another diabetogenic agent that also results in long-term musculoskeletal problems. A further long-term concern associated with both calcineurin inhibitors and prednisone is their association with atherogenesis, adversely effecting long-term graft and patient survival.

Rejection

Hyperacute rejection is extremely rare and is humorally mediated by preformed anti-HLA antibodies. Hyperacute rejection occurs within minutes to hours following reperfusion of the kidney, whereas classic cell-mediated rejection typically does not occur until 1 to 2 weeks after the transplant. In hyperacute rejection, the anti-HLA antigens bind to the vascular endothelium of the kidney transplant, resulting in activation of the complement cascade and rapid graft thrombosis. The kidney appears blue-black with poor tissue turgor despite adequate blood flow. The characteristic histologic appearance includes the triad of polymorphonuclear leukocytes in the glomerular capillary loops, fibrin deposition, and platelet thrombi. The kidney cannot be salvaged, and a transplant nephrectomy is necessary. The presence of anti-HLA antibodies should be detected in the pretransplant cross-match and with the sensitivity of current immunologic assays, hyperacute rejection is usually a result of technical or clerical errors in the cross-match procedure. A more common and less intense form of humoral rejection occurring within a few days of transplantation is a result of reactivation of memory B-cells following reexposure to alloantigen. The histologic findings are defined by positive C4d staining on vascular endothelium, although lymphocytic infiltrates consistent with classic cell-mediated rejection can be present. Treatment of this aggressive rejection can include plasmapheresis, the anti B-cell agent rituximab

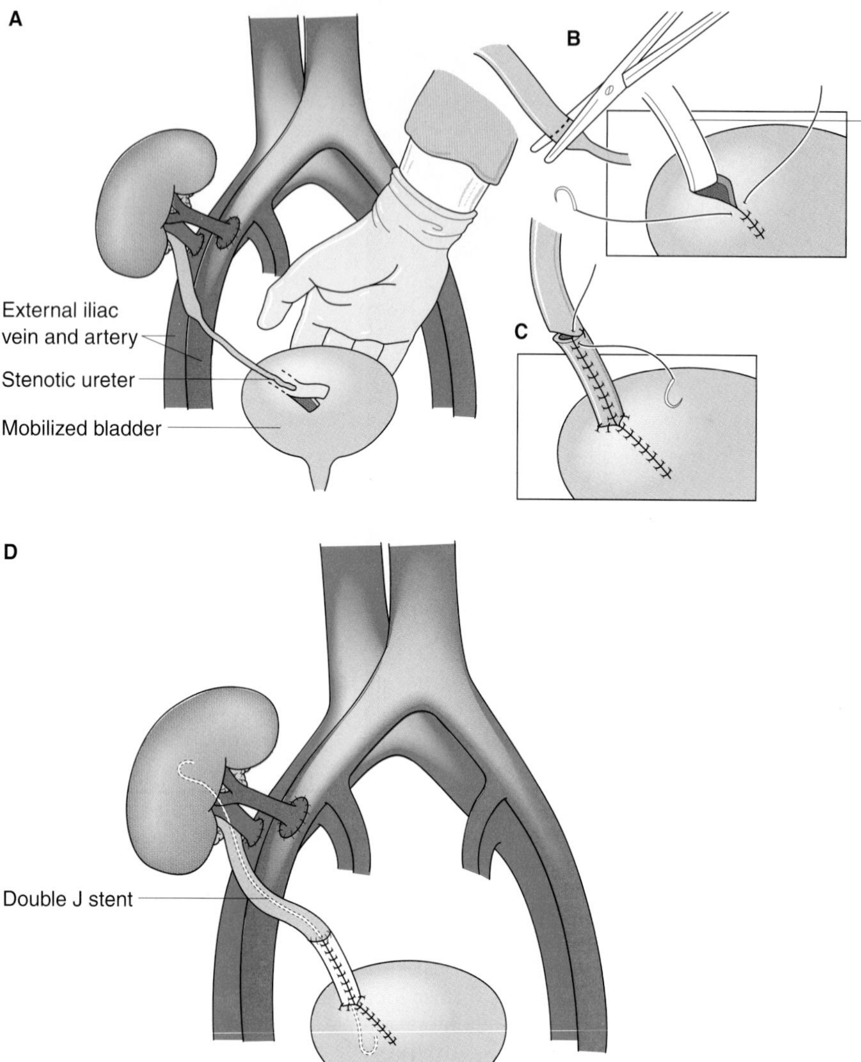

FIGURE 37.5 (*A*) Reconstruction of a stenotic donor ureter, showing resection of the stenotic segment and mobilization of the bladder. (*B*) to (*D*) A Boari flap is constructed from a tabularized segment of bladder wall and anastomosed end-to-end to the proximal donor ureter.

(anti-CD20 monoclonal antibody), and polyclonal antilymphocyte preparations (antithymocyte globulin).

Classic acute cell-mediated rejection typically occurs between 1 week and 3 months following transplantation. Most patients with rejection episodes present with decreasing urine volumes and increases in serum creatinine values. Low-grade fever and allograft tenderness may be present, but significant physical symptoms frequently are absent. Immediate workup of increasing serum creatinine should be initiated, beginning with an ultrasound to rule out ureteral obstruction or technical vascular complications as the cause of the deteriorating function. Similarly, toxicity from calcineurin inhibitors needs to be determined by checking drug levels. A percutaneous kidney biopsy is performed to confirm rejection. The severity of the rejection episode is based on the presence of lymphocytes in renal tubules (tubulitis) and vascular endothelium (vasculitis). Mild rejection is generally treated with pulse corticosteroids and maximizing the maintenance immunosuppression to ensure therapeutic levels of calcineurin inhibitors. More severe rejection with both tubulitis and vasculitis, as well as steroid-resistant rejection, is treated with antilymphocyte antibody preparations, most frequently muromonab-CD3 (a monoclonal agent directed against the CD3 receptor) or rabbit polyclonal antilymphocyte preparations. If the rejection episode occurred while the patients had therapeutic drug levels, maintenance therapy is frequently altered following the antibody therapy. For example, if maintenance therapy consisted of cyclosporine A, the calcineurin inhibitor could be switched to tacrolimus. Other potential strategies include the addition of sirolimus to the immunosuppressive regimen, particularly for cases where there is evidence of calcineurin inhibitor toxicity on biopsy.

Each rejection episode takes a toll on long-term function of the kidney transplant. Even well-controlled acute rejection episodes initiate a cascade of events leading to interstitial fibrosis and proliferative changes affecting the vascular endothelium. These histologic and progressive degenerative changes are classified as chronic rejection or chronic allograft nephropathy. These changes lead to loss of graft function over the course of months to several years. Current strategies minimizing calcineurin inhibitor nephrotoxicity are being used to prolong function in kidneys with these chronic changes and involve the addition of sirolimus to replace the calcineurin inhibitors. It remains unclear whether the marked decrease in acute rejection episodes, from greater than 50% to less than 20% observed in the past 5 years, will translate to better long-term function of transplants. Nonetheless, it is evident that immunosuppression strategies minimizing prednisone and calcineurin inhibitors are providing safer and more effective immunosuppression for kidney transplant recipients while decreasing long-term toxicities associated with immunosuppression.

Immunosuppressive Complications

It would be naïve to assume that the intensification of immunosuppressive regimens resulting in decreased acute and chronic rejection rates can be accomplished without sequelae. Infections and malignancy remain significant complications associated with long-term immunosuppression and are the driving force for drug-minimization strategies. Early infections during the perioperative period are commonly iatrogenic and involve bladder infections or intravenous catheter use. Higher doses of immunosuppressive drugs used in the early postoperative period predispose patients to these infections and emphasize the importance of maintaining sterility during Foley catheter placement and insertion of intravenous catheters. Pneumonia related to mechanical ventilation and poor postoperative inspiratory effort can occur in the early postoperative period, and early incentive spirometry should be encouraged to decrease the potential for this infection. Wound infections are relatively uncommon, although diabetes and obesity are both associated with a much higher incidence of wound complications. Weight reduction to achieve a body mass index of less than 35 is strongly recommended to facilitate the operative procedure and minimize the risks of wound complications, particularly in the recipient with diabetes mellitus.

Cytomegalovirus (CMV), a herpesvirus, remains a problematic infection in the immunosuppressed patient and can become symptomatic 1 to 2 months following the transplant. CMV seronegative patients who receive a kidney from a CMV seropositive donor are at the highest risk for infection, although prophylaxis with acyclovir or ganciclovir is generally provided for all recipients for a period of 3 to 6 months following the transplant. Despite prophylaxis, activation of CMV can occur, accompanied by fever, malaise, pneumonia, gastrointestinal distress, or dysfunction of the kidney transplant. The effective treatment of blood or tissue invasive CMV has been one of the major advances in the management of kidney transplant patients within the past decade. What was a life-threatening disease in the early era of solid organ transplantation can today be effectively managed with oral antibiotics.

Prophylaxis against *Candida albicans* with fluconazole and *Pneumocystis carinii* with trimethoprim-sulfamethoxazole is also part of most management strategies posttransplant. Other potentially life threatening opportunistic organisms that can affect the chronically immunosuppressed transplant recipient include *Aspergillus, Cryptococcus, Listeria, Nocardia,* and *Mycobacterium.*

More potent immunosuppression regimens used in the current era have been associated with the emergence of BK virus, a previously rare infection that may cause graft loss in up to 5% of infected patients. Reduction in immunosuppression is necessary to prevent progression of viral tubulitis. Unfortunately, the use of cidofovir, a nucleotide analogue that inhibits viral DNA polymerase, is also nephrotoxic and its *in vivo* efficacy has not been proved. Patients with a previous history of active tuberculosis or conversion to purified protein derivative positivity should receive appropriate prophylaxis for 6 months to 1 year following the transplant procedure.

More potent immunosuppression regimens will also have an impact on the development of neoplasms following transplantation.[17] Skin cancers are the most common malignancy following transplantation, with more than 90% being squamous or basal cell cancers. The incidence of skin cancers is staggering, with 50% or more of white recipients ultimately developing lesions. The immunosuppressed patient also has a higher incidence of nodal spread, and educating the patient about the importance of avoiding direct sun exposure is essential. Other malignancies that have a particularly high incidence in transplant recipients include non-Hodgkin lymphomas and carcinomas of the anogenital areas. The etiology of anogenital carcinoma is related to the presence of human papilloma virus.

Posttransplant lymphoproliferative disease is the second most common form of malignancy in transplant recipients and is associated with Epstein-Barr virus. These lymphoproliferative syndromes present as a spectrum of pathology, extending from polyclonal lymphoproliferation to monoclonal B-cell lymphomas. Polyclonal disease has been managed by decreasing or withdrawing immunosuppression, whereas progression to monoclonal lymphomas has required chemotherapy. CD20-positive lymphomas have been successfully managed with rituximab, an anti-CD20 antibody, with no significant side effects.

CURRENT RESULT AND FUTURE TRENDS

Over the past three decades, progressive improvement has been made in patient and graft survival, independent of donor source. This progression is best shown in Figure 37.6 for the period of time spanning 1992 to 2002. Overall graft survival, as well as the half-life of the graft, improved incrementally for live donor transplants, standard deceased donor transplants, and even deceased donor transplants utilizing suboptimal or extended criteria donors.[13] This change is related to improved organ preservation, perfected operative technique, and most importantly, improved immunosuppressive agents. Current 1-year actuarial graft survival for living and deceased donor transplants is 94.8% and 88.9%, respectively.[18] These remarkable 1-year results continue to be overshadowed by the specter of late graft loss due to chronic rejection. This problem remains unsolved in renal transplantation, and future improvement in long-term survival will be achieved only when the mechanisms of this process are understood.

The exponential growth in waiting lists compounded by the ongoing critical shortage of organs will continue to stimulate creative means of increasing both the living and deceased donor pools. Expansion in the number and types of immunosuppressive agents has resulted in marked decreases in the incidence of acute rejection, which it is hoped will translate to prolongation in the long-term function of kidney transplants. Newer strategies in immunosuppressive regimens that minimize nephrotoxic cyclosporine and tacrolimus by adding nonnephrotoxic agents will also benefit the long-term function of transplanted kidneys.

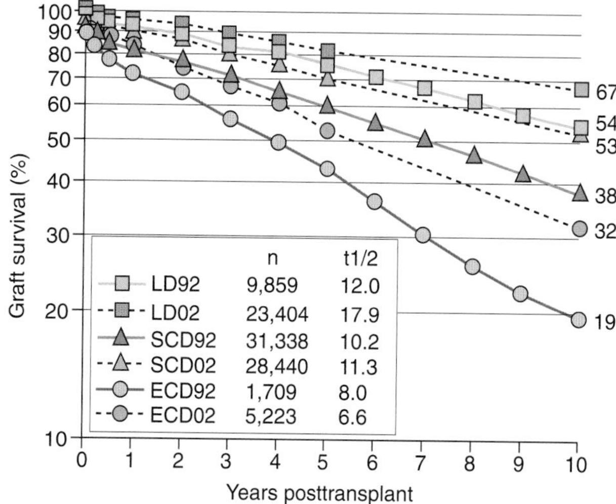

FIGURE 37.6 Comparison of graft survival and graft half-life ($t_{1/2}$) in 1992 and 2002 for different donor types (age >60 years in 1992 group, age >50 years with hypertension, elevated creatinine, or donor death from cerebrovascular accident in 2002 group). There has been an improvement in survival for all donor types, with the best long-term results with living donor kidneys. LD, living donor; SCD, standard deceased donor; ECD, extended criteria donor.

TRANSPLANTATION

The effect of ischemia-reperfusion injury on both early and late graft function, as well as its impact on the development of chronic rejection and transplant glomerulopathy, is an area of active research, and potential therapeutic interventions to minimize this injury are being evaluated. The induction of tolerance to foreign antigen remains the "Holy Grail" of transplantation. A paucity of tolerizing regimens have been applied clinically, although the use of donor bone marrow or stem cells will likely have a future role in achieving the elusive goal of transplantation tolerance.

KEY POINTS

- **The major barriers to successful renal transplantation include ABO compatibility and the HLA system.**
- **Before a renal transplant is undertaken, histocompatibility of the donor and recipient are determined.**
- **The etiology of kidney disease resulting in end-stage failure and the necessity for transplantation are led by glomerulonephritis, diabetes, and hypertension.**
- **The kidney transplant is heterotopically placed in the extraperitoneal iliac fossa.**
- **Hyperacute rejection is humorally mediated by preformed anti-HLA antibodies. Hyperacute rejection occurs within minutes to hours following reperfusion of the kidney.**
- **Acute cell-mediated rejection most typically occurs between 1 week and 3 months following transplantation.**
- **Chronic rejection leads to loss of graft function over the course of months to several years.**

References

1. Tanabe K, Tokumoto T, Ishida H, et al. Excellent outcome of ABO-incompatible living kidney transplantation under pretransplantation immunosuppression with tacrolimus, mycophenolate mofetil, and steroid. *Transplant Proc.* 2004;36:2175–2177.
2. Takahashi K, Saito K, Takahara S, et al. Excellent long-term outcome of ABO-incompatible living donor kidney transplantation in Japan. *Am J Transplant.* 2004;4:1089–1096.
3. Meier-Kriesche HU, Kaplan B. Waiting time on dialysis as the strongest modifiable risk factor for renal transplant outcomes: a paired donor kidney analysis. *Transplantation* 2002;74:1377–1381.
4. **Rosendale JD. Organ Donation in the United States: 1998–2002. In Cecka JM, Terasaki PI, eds. *Clinical Transplants 2003.* Los Angeles: UCLA Immunogenetics Center; 2004:65–76.**
5. Leventhal JR, Kocak B, Salvalaggio PR, et al. Laparoscopic donor nephrectomy 1997 to 2003: lessons learned with 500 cases at a single institution. *Surgery.*2004;136:881–890.
6. Jacobs SC, Cho E, Foster C, et al. Laparoscopic donor nephrectomy: the University of Maryland 6-year experience. *J Urol.* 2004;171:47–51.
7. Cooper JT, Chin LT, Krieger NR, et al. Donation after cardiac death: the University of Wisconsin experience with renal transplantation. *Am J Transplant.* 2004;4:1490–494.
8. Roberts JP, Wolfe RA, Bragg-Gresham JL, et al. Effect of changing the priority for HLA matching on the rates and outcomes of kidney transplantation in minority groups. *N Engl J Med.* 2004;350:545–551.
9. Warren DS, Zachary AA, Sonnenday CJ, et al. Successful renal transplantation across simultaneous ABO incompatible and positive crossmatch barriers. *Am J Transplant.* 2004;4:561–568.
10. Jordan SC, Tyan D, Stablein D, et al. Evaluation of intravenous immunoglobulin as an agent to lower allosensitization and improve transplantation in highly sensitized adult patients with end-stage renal disease: report of the NIH IG02 trial. *J Am Soc Nephrol.* 2004;15:3256–3262.
11. Metzger RA, Delmonico FL, Feng S, et al. Expanded criteria donors for kidney transplantation. *Am J Transplant.* 2003;3 (suppl 4):114–125.
12. Port FK, Bragg-Gresham JL, Metzger RA, et al. Donor characteristics associated with reduced graft survival: an approach to expanding the pool of kidney donors. *Transplantation* 2002;74:1281–1286.
13. **Cecka JM. The OPTN/UNOS Renal Transplant Registry. In Cecka JM, Terasaki PI, eds. *Clinical Transplants 2003.* Los Angeles: UCLA Immunogenetics Center; 2004:1–12.14.**
14. Stock PG, Roland ME, Carlson L, et al. Kidney and liver transplantation in human immunodeficiency virus-infected patients: a pilot safety and efficacy study. *Transplantation* 2003;76:370–375.
15. Vincenti F. Immunosuppression minimization: current and future trends in transplant immunosuppression. *J Am Soc Nephrol.* 2003;14:1940–1948.
16. Kasiske BL, Snyder JJ, Gilbertson D, Matas AJ. Diabetes mellitus after kidney transplantation in the United States. *Am J Transplant.* 2003;3:178–185.
17. **Morath C, Mueller M, Goldschmidt H, et al. Malignancy in renal transplantation. *J Am Soc Nephrol.* 2004;15:1582–1588.**
18. Wynn JJ, Distant DA, Pirsch JD, et al. Kidney and pancreas transplantation. *Am J Transplant.* 2004;4 (suppl 9):72–80.

CHAPTER 38 ■ HEPATIC TRANSPLANTATION

JEFFREY D. PUNCH

Liver transplantation has evolved over the past four decades to be the standard treatment for patients with a variety of acute and chronic liver diseases. The first successful liver transplant was performed on a moribund child with a hepatoma by Thomas Starzl when he was at the University of Colorado in 1967.[1] This child lived more than a year before succumbing to recurrent tumor. Over the next 12 years, liver transplants continued to be performed at a modest rate. Despite 1-year survival rates of less than 50%, it was clear that some patients benefited from the procedure.

In 1979 cyclosporine was introduced into clinical organ transplantation by Sir Roy Calne.[2] Almost immediately 1-year patient survival rates jumped to over 70%. As a result, liver transplantation programs began to appear worldwide. Today more than 6,000 liver transplants are performed annually in the United States, and survival rates exceed 85%.

The clinical success of liver transplantation is now primarily limited by the availability of suitable donor organs. Every year more patients are listed for liver transplantation than receive transplants. In the future it is likely that this problem will worsen because of the large number of individuals with chronic hepatitis C infection, a significant portion of whom will eventually develop cirrhosis and either hepatoma or liver failure. Attention continues to be focused on methods to increase the available supply of livers for transplantation. Notable efforts to improve the supply of available organs include the work by the

Department of Health and Human Services, which recently took up the cause of organ donation vigorously. This effort, termed the Organ Donation Breakthrough Collaborative, focused on improving the success rate of organ donation efforts at the hospitals that have most potential organ donors nationwide. The Center for Medicare and Medicaid Services also joined the effort by declaring specific Conditions of Participation for all hospitals that treat Medicare patients in the United States. This effort focused on encouraging methods of approaching donor families that have been shown to be optimally effective.

Many other methods to increase the organ supply are currently being practiced. These methods include the utilization of organs from older donors and donors with fatty livers that were once routinely discarded, the development of techniques to allow a single liver graft to be split into two grafts, and the utilization of liver grafts from donors that die of cardiac death. Recently, areas of the world where the shortage of transplantable liver is most acute have seen the development of safe surgical techniques that allow healthy, living volunteers to donate a segment of their liver to a recipient in need of a liver transplant.[3]

INDICATIONS FOR HEPATIC TRANSPLANTATION

General Considerations

The most common indication for liver transplantation is end-stage liver disease. The term *end-stage* refers to the clinical scenario in which a pathological process or multiple processes have resulted in a damaged liver that has minimal function and no potential for recovery. The diagnosis of end-stage liver disease is made primarily on the basis of clinical findings. Additional information about the etiology of the liver disease and thus its natural history can often be obtained by supplementary investigations including serologic studies and histologic examination of a liver biopsy specimen. It is important that potential liver transplant recipients are evaluated by a specialist with expertise in end-stage liver disease, because many other diseases may present similar clinical pictures.

The severity of liver disease in an individual is highly variable, from mild cirrhosis resulting in minor symptoms to severe decompensation resulting in deterioration of mental status and frank renal failure. The rate of progression of liver disease from a functional state to invalidism to death is variable and may be rapid or may last several years. The challenge facing transplant professionals is to identify patients who will benefit from transplantation. Hepatic transplantation may result in wonderful and dramatic results, but at the same time it is always a highly risky procedure. In situations in which patients are fully functional, or only minimally symptomatic, transplantation is an inappropriate therapeutic measure. A liver transplant is a major surgical procedure on a profoundly ill individual with unavoidable risk. It cannot be reversed. Even when patients survive the procedure and recover from the effects of chronic liver disease, a necessary component of organ donation is chronic, lifelong immunosuppression. Despite advances in immunosuppressive technology developed over the past four decades, immunosuppression remains a treatment that induces a state of vulnerability in the recipient by virtue of the fact that the recipient's natural resistance to infection is compromised. It is thus critical that patients be selected who will benefit from the procedure.

How is it possible to properly select patients and properly time transplantation so that the benefit of transplantation is assured? In 2002, the Organ Procurement and Transplantation Network began using the Model of End-stage Liver Disease (MELD) score as a method of prioritizing liver transplant recipients. The MELD score is an integer value based on three objective laboratory studies: creatinine, bilirubin, and the international normalized ratio (INR).[4] Work done by the Scientific Registry of Transplant Recipients has shown that patients with MELD scores of less than 17 have a mortality rate on the waiting list that is less than the mortality of the transplant procedure in the same population.[5] This suggests that patients with a MELD score of less than 17 do not receive an absolute survival benefit from transplantation. Patients who have higher MELD scores clearly do receive a definite survival benefit, and there appears to be no upper limit of MELD that is associated with benefit. In other words, there is no evidence that patients who are too sick to benefit from liver transplantation are being transplanted, but patients who have stable, mild liver disease should not receive a transplant until their disease has progressed to a more severe state.

Surprisingly, MELD more accurately predicts mortality than clinical factors that were previously thought to be ominous signs of reduced (6 months or less) survival. Such factors, including the presence of ascites or hepatic encephalopathy, the development of spontaneous bacterial peritonitis, or recurrent variceal hemorrhage, do not add to the predictive value of MELD. This finding may be related to the difficult nature of accurately quantifying clinical variables in registry databases or to the fact that MELD is such an accurate way of measuring functional hepatic capacity that no additional clinical variables are relevant.

The improved ability to predict mortality for patients with liver failure allowed the development of new national allocation policies that direct organs to those patients that will benefit. Importantly, the implementation of the MELD system of allocation for livers from deceased donors has been associated with a decrease in the death rate on the waiting list. Further refinements of our understanding will undoubtedly occur as improved long-term follow-up data on waiting list mortality become available and as quality of life considerations are added to the analysis.

These considerations apply to the chronic forms of liver failure, but not to the important emergency decisions about transplantation that must be made when a patient presents with fulminant hepatic failure, which is defined as the progression from good health to liver failure with hepatic encephalopathy within 8 weeks. Without transplantation, the mortality rate for fulminant hepatic failure is approximately 75%. Death frequently occurs rapidly once patients progress to stage II (confusion), stage III, (stuporous), or stage IV (unresponsive) hepatic encephalopathy. In these cases, the decision to perform transplantation is based on clinical grounds. Current liver transplant allocation policy allows for the rapid transplantation of patients with fulminant hepatic failure. These patients can be listed as "status 1," which gives them higher priority for available livers than patients with chronic liver disease who are prioritized based on MELD score.

Contraindications to Liver Transplantation

The number of absolute contraindications to hepatic transplantation has steadily decreased during the past several years as experience with the procedure has increased. Many clinical situations once considered to be absolute contraindications for transplantation are now either no longer considered to be contraindications or to be only relative contraindications. A thrombosed portal vein is no longer a contraindication to transplantation because techniques have been devised to effectively deal with this condition (see later). The associated comorbidity of juvenile-onset diabetes mellitus formerly precluded transplantation. In current practice, this is not necessarily the case, depending on the patient's physiologic status at the time of evaluation. Similarly, advanced age causes concern, but in most centers the physiologic state of the patient is a more important consideration than the chronologic age.

The inability to withstand the operative procedure, usually for cardiovascular or pulmonary reasons, is still generally considered to be a contraindication to liver transplantation. Cardiac disease that is not amenable to percutaneous therapy poses a particular problem because these patients are frequently unable to withstand a corrective cardiac procedure because of their severe liver disease. Today these problems can sometimes be treated by performing the corrective cardiac procedure immediately preceding the liver transplant, once a donor organ has been identified. In highly select patients it may also be possible to perform combined heart and liver transplantation or combined lung and liver transplantation.

Recent intracranial hemorrhage is almost always a contraindication because during the liver transplant procedure, coagulopathy is invariable due to the anhepatic phase following hepatectomy. The risk of a catastrophic exacerbation of intracranial bleeding during a transplant is therefore high in this setting. However, the meaning of "recent" is not defined in either the transplant or the neurosurgical literature. Profound, irreversible neurologic impairment is also considered to be a contraindication, but mild mental retardation is not necessarily problematic as long as a loving support network exists to ensure compliance with posttransplant regimens. Active substance abuse remains a contraindication, as is the lack of the necessary social support network.

Evidence of infection with HIV, long considered a contraindication, is no longer an absolute exclusion because of the development of highly effective antiretroviral therapies. Active sepsis and active extrahepatic malignancy continue to be contraindications.

Although renal insufficiency increases the risk of liver transplantation, it is not a contraindication. Patients who have hepatorenal syndrome frequently experience recovery of renal function following liver transplantation. Patients who have long-standing hepatorenal failure and patients with known renal parenchymal disease can be treated by combined liver/kidney transplantation.

SPECIFIC DISEASES FOR WHICH TRANSPLANTATION IS APPROPRIATE

Alcoholic Liver Disease

Excessive alcohol consumption can lead to several abnormalities in the liver, ranging from alcoholic hepatitis to steatosis, hepatic fibrosis, and cirrhosis. Alcoholic liver disease was once thought to occur only in individuals who consumed large quantities of alcohol over long periods of time. It has recently become recognized that even moderate amounts of alcohol consumption can induce liver injury, suggesting that hereditary and or environmental factors are probably important. Hepatitis C viral infection, found in 15% to 25% of patients with alcoholic liver disease, appears to exacerbate alcohol-induced liver injury and vice versa.

When liver transplantation emerged as a standard therapy for end-stage liver disease in the 1980s, intense debates occurred surrounding the issue of offering liver transplantation. There were two broad areas of concern. First, many were skeptical that patients with a history of long-standing alcoholism would be able to successfully comply with the rigorous long-term medical treatment required of patients who receive lifelong immunosuppression. On a broader level, concern was expressed that scarce societal resources should not be used to treat patients with "self-induced" diseases. With more experience in this area, it has been recognized that the incidence of recidivism after transplantation is low, and both short- and long-term results in this category are as good as for non-alcohol-related categories. It has also become understood that determining worthiness for receiving a lifesaving organ by making a judgment about past behavior is neither ethical nor possible.

Today, the same methods of determining suitability for transplantation are used for patients with alcoholic liver disease as with other diagnoses with one proviso. Unlike other disorders that tend to be universally progressive, alcohol-induced liver injury frequently regresses following cessation of alcohol consumption as long as cirrhosis is not yet present. Patients with a history of recent alcohol abuse should therefore be observed for a minimum of 6 months to ensure that their hepatic dysfunction is not reversible. In addition, all patients with a history of substance abuse must be evaluated by individuals with expertise in addiction and found to have good insight into their past self-destructive behavior and a stable support network for the posttransplant phase.

Hepatitis B

Most patients who become infected with hepatitis B develop an immunologic response to the virus that results in complete viral clearance. Patients who do not clear the hepatitis viral antigen may persist as carriers or may develop chronic hepatitis, which progresses to fibrosis and cirrhosis. In the 1980s, transplantation for hepatitis B was associated with universal recurrence of viral infection posttransplant and survival rates were poor. Fortunately, transplantation for this indication was revolutionized by the development of effective posttransplant prophylaxis using long-term, high-dose, hepatitis B immune globulin or the nucleoside inhibitor lamivudine, or both. Today, outcomes for transplantation for hepatitis B–induced liver failure are equivalent to or better than those for other conditions.

Hepatitis C

Hepatitis C has become the most common etiology among patients receiving liver transplants. Effective antiviral therapy is now available for early hepatitis C infection, with clinically important responses seen in nearly half of patients treated. However, complete clearance of hepatitis C from serum can only be achieved in a minority of patients and significant toxicity often limits therapy. Once cirrhosis develops, the progression to end-stage liver failure appears to be relentless. Recurrence of viral hepatitis in the transplanted liver occurs universally. Although most patients experience an indolent course, some develop early and severe recurrence. These patients can progress to end-stage liver failure within 6 months posttransplant. Short-term results of transplantation for this disease are comparable to those for the other noninfectious conditions. However, approximately 25% of patients develop recurrent cirrhosis within 5 years posttransplant, and long-term survival is less likely compared with patients who do not have hepatitis C infection. Despite recurrence, transplantation appears to provide a substantial and worthwhile survival benefit to patients with hepatitis C.

Primary Biliary Cirrhosis

Primary biliary cirrhosis, thought to be autoimmune in nature, has a relatively predictable clinical course that is characterized by gradually increasing serum bilirubin levels and progressive fatigue. Early stages of the disease are usually asymptomatic, and disease progression may evolve over 20 years. Treatment with ursodeoxycholic acid appears to slow the progression of the disease, but immunosuppression does not. It was once thought that primary biliary cirrhosis does not recur. Careful histologic analysis has shown that the incidence of recurrence is approximately 15% within 5 years of transplantation.[6] Eventual progression to graft failure requiring retransplantation is possible.

Primary Sclerosing Cholangitis

Primary sclerosing cholangitis is an autoimmune disease that is characterized by gradually progressive inflammation of the biliary tree, eventually resulting in cirrhosis. It is associated with ulcerative colitis, but removal of the colon does not affect progression of the disease. In most cases, colectomy for associated inflammatory bowel disease is done after successful transplantation because the failing liver makes the patient a poor candidate for a large abdominal procedure. Sclerosing cholangitis is also associated with the development of cholangiocarcinoma. Patients who experience a course that suddenly becomes rapidly progressive should be examined by endoscopic retrograde cholangiopancreatography (ERCP) with brushings to exclude cholangiocarcinoma. In addition to the usual considerations about the timing of transplantation, it is important to note that these patients are susceptible to bacterial cholangitis, which can cause systemic sepsis and rapid decompensation of hepatic dysfunction. Bouts of cholangitis that do not respond to suppressive antibiotic therapy should prompt early consideration for transplantation

Biliary Atresia

Biliary atresia is a disorder of infants that is characterized by biliary obstruction resulting from obliteration or discontinuity of the extrahepatic biliary system. Obstruction of bile flow, if untreated, results in cholestasis followed by progressive hyperbilirubinemia, cirrhosis, and hepatic failure. The etiology of biliary atresia is unknown. It is the most common indication for hepatic transplantation in pediatric patients. Standard treatment includes creation of a portoenterostomy (Kasai procedure), if this can be done before 3 months of age. After this point, success rates diminish markedly. Response to the portoenterostomy procedure is highly variable. Patients may develop cirrhosis within the first 6 months of life or live into their twenties before developing synthetic dysfunction and portal hypertension. Approximately 75% of children will require transplantation by 6 years of age.

It is critical that these patients are managed by an experienced pediatric gastroenterologist so that the correct window for effective transplantation can be identified and so they receive appropriate attention to their specialized nutritional needs. Specifically, deficiencies of fat-soluble vitamins that depend on bile for absorption are common and treatable. Transplantation is appropriate when children manifest growth and nutritional failure, when ascites develops, and when portal hypertension progresses to the point of variceal hemorrhage. Recurrent cholangitis is also thought to be an indication for hepatic transplantation.

Inherited Metabolic Disorders

Numerous inherited metabolic disorders are treatable by liver transplantation. Some enzymatic deficiencies in this group result in destruction of the liver, so transplantation may resolve the liver failure as well as supply the missing enzyme. Disorders in this category include Wilson disease, α_1-antitrypsin deficiency, tyrosinemia, and type I glycogen storage disease. In other cases, the liver is not affected by the disease, either structurally or functionally. In these circumstances transplantation is undertaken solely as enzyme replacement therapy. Diseases that have been cured by hepatic transplantation in this category include hemophilia A or B, homozygous familial hypercholesterolemia, Niemann-Pick disease, oxalosis, familial amyloid polyneuropathy, and numerous enzymatic deficiencies of urea cycle metabolism.[7] Determination of eligibility for transplantation depends on determining that transplantation will cure the disease, or at least halt its progression, and that the consequences of the disease without transplantation are devastating, and therefore a risky procedure with uncertain long-term prognosis is appropriate.

Fulminant Hepatic Failure

Acute hepatic failure, defined as the development of altered mental status, coagulopathy and hepatic dysfunction within 8 weeks of the onset of an acute hepatic disease, is a rare, but lethal disease.[8] There are approximately 2,000 cases of acute hepatic failure per year in the United States. The mortality rate approaches 80% in patients who do not receive liver transplants. The causes of acute hepatic failure include viral hepatitis, toxins such as aflatoxins from the poisonous mushroom family *Amanita phalloides*, acute fatty liver of pregnancy, acute Budd-Chiari syndrome, and drug toxicities. Drug toxicities include both idiosyncratic reactions and drugs with predictable toxicity when taken in excess. Drugs that have been reported to induce idiosyncratic liver failure include isoniazid, halothane, valproate, disulfram and phenytoin, among many others. The over-the-counter analgesic acetaminophen causes dose-dependent hepatic failure and is now the single most common cause of acute hepatic failure in the United States.

Acute hepatic failure causes death by producing cerebral edema, which leads to uncal herniation and brain death. The most generally accepted criteria for transplantation of patients with fulminant hepatic failure were described by the group at the King's College hospital in London, England.[9]

Budd-Chiari Syndrome

Budd-Chiari syndrome is characterized by obliteration of the hepatic veins. It may be to the result of congenital webs of the hepatic veins or suprahepatic cava or may be caused by spontaneous thrombosis of the hepatic veins. The latter condition is associated with polycythemia vera and other hypercoagulable states. Diagnosis is made by inferior vena cavagram or magnetic resonance venography. The classic presentation is a triad of right upper quadrant pain, hepatomegaly, and ascites. Patients may present with acute liver failure and have symptoms of encephalopathy and coagulopathy, or they may present in a more indolent fashion with ascites as the predominant feature. The natural history of the indolent form of Budd-Chiari syndrome is the eventual development of cirrhosis.

Patient who present with evidence of severe, acute hepatic dysfunction require urgent transplantation and should be treated the same as other patients with fulminant liver failure.

Patients who present with intact hepatic dysfunction should undergo an assessment to determine whether the liver has been irreversibly injured by the development of cirrhosis. A side-to-side portocaval shunt, in which the portal vein serves as an outflow tract for the congested liver, is the preferred therapy for patients who do not have evidence of synthetic failure and have not yet developed cirrhosis. Transcutaneous portal cava shunt (TIPS) may also be an option if an experienced interventional radiologist is available. In patients with the indolent presentation, transplantation is reserved for cases where portal decompressive shunting is not possible or for patients who have already developed cirrhosis by the time they present. Long-term anticoagulation to prevent recurrent hepatic vein thrombosis in the liver graft is routinely recommended.

Transplantation for Hepatocellular Carcinoma

Cirrhosis is a major risk factor for the development of hepatocellular carcinoma, and the majority of hepatocellular carcinomas develop in patients who have cirrhosis. At one time, transplantation was considered an appropriate therapy for any patient with hepatocellular carcinoma in the setting of cirrhosis. Curative resection is unsafe in the setting of cirrhosis, and it does not eliminate the high likelihood of recurrent malignancy. Because most patients with hepatocellular carcinoma die of liver failure, rather than metastatic disease, it was reasoned that transplantation would be potentially curative. This approach yielded poor survival rates, and during the early 1990s primary hepatic malignancy was considered a contraindication to liver transplantation by many centers. This circumstance changed when Matazafarro reported excellent survival rates for patients who had cirrhosis and either stage I or stage II hepatoma (Table 38.1). Transplantation is now considered standard therapy for hepatocellular carcinoma associated with cirrhosis of the liver if there is no evidence of extrahepatic malignant spread and if tumor burden does not exceed stage II disease (a single tumor more than 5 cm in diameter, or multiple tumors with one tumor larger than 3 cm in diameter). Transplantation of patients with larger tumors is more controversial due to the markedly lower rate of disease-free survival. Transplantation is clearly not beneficial in the presence of known positive nodal or distant metastases (stage IV disease).

Transplantation for Other Hepatic Malignancy

Other primary tumors of the liver include hepatoblastoma, cholangiocarcinoma, and primary sarcoma. Hepatoblastoma occurs primarily in children. Resection is curative, so transplantation is reserved for patients who are unresectable because of bilobar disease. The tumor often responds partially to chemotherapy, but complete and sustained tumor regression is uncommon. Patients are often treated with chemotherapy until the time of transplantation to prevent extrahepatic growth prior to the definitive treatment. Hepatoma is relatively unique among liver tumors in that long-term survival has been reported even in children who have had distant metastatic spread. Evidence of pulmonary or other resectable metastases, therefore, is not necessarily a contraindication to transplantation for this disease.

Cholangiocarcinoma has historically been considered a contraindication to transplantation because 5-year survival rates have been reported at less than 20%. Recently, success has been reported for patients who have limited disease and receive both preoperative and postoperative adjuvant therapies. Transplantation in this setting is still considered experimental. Although there are anecdotal reports of long-term survival following transplantation for primary sarcoma of the liver, the majority of the experiences indicate that transplantation is not a curative therapy for this condition. Liver transplantation is generally not appropriate for patients who have secondary (metastatic) malignancy of the liver, because long-term survival rates are very poor due in part to the observation that immunosuppression promotes tumor growth. The possible exception to this rule is patients who have metastatic carcinoid that is limited the liver. This tumor grows very slowly and local cure of the primary tumor is frequently possible. A subset of patients who have a period of years without evidence of tumor growth anywhere else but in the liver will have long-term disease-free survival following liver transplantation.

TABLE 38.1 CLASSIFICATION AND STAGING

TNM CLASSIFICATION AND STAGING OF HEPATOCELLULAR CARCINOMA

CLASSIFICATION	
T1	1 nodule †1.9 cm
T2	1 nodule 2.0–5.0 cm; 2 or 3 nodules, all <3.0 cm
T3	One nodule >5.0 cm; 2 or 3 nodules, at least one >3.0 cm
T4a	4 or more nodules, any size
T4b	T2,T3, or T4a plus gross intrahepatic portal or hepatic vein involvement on imaging
N0	No evidence of regional nodal involvement
N1	Regional (porta hepatitis) nodal involvement
M0	No evidence of metastatic disease
M1	Evidence of metastatic disease
STAGE GROUPING	
Stage I	T1
Stage II	T2
Stage III	T3
Stage IV A1	T4a
Stage IV A2	T4b
Stage IV B	Any N1, any M1

Nonalcoholic Fatty Liver Disease

Nonalcoholic fatty liver disease may be the most common disease in the United States. It has a high incidence in obese patients and those with adult-onset diabetes mellitus. The disease resembles alcoholic liver disease, but the patients do not report a significant history of alcohol use. The degree of hepatic injury varies from benign elevations of hepatic transaminase serum levels in association with hepatic statotsis to fibrosis and cirrhosis. A majority of patients previously classified as having cryptogenic cirrhosis probably have long-standing steatohepatitis. It is estimated that at least two thirds of the obese population in the United States has hepatic steatosis and close to one fifth have steatohepatitis.[11] Currently we lack a good understanding of the natural history of the benign forms of the disease. The mainstay of treatment is weight reduction through diet and exercise. An effective medical therapy has been elusive.[12] Patients who develop cirrhosis and progress to end-stage liver disease are appropriate candidates for liver transplantation. Recurrence of steatohepatitis leading to graft failure is possible.

TRANSPLANTATION PROCEDURE

Anesthetic Management

Many patients report for liver transplantation procedures without an opportunity for extensive preoperative preparation; therefore, induction of anesthesia is generally conducted with rapid sequence technique, assuming that the patient has a full stomach. After intubation, anesthesia is maintained with a combination of inhalation agent and intravenous infusions of paralytic and analgesic drugs. Multiple vascular access lines are placed for monitoring and administration of blood and blood products. A balloon-tipped flow-directed pulmonary artery catheter is inserted in adult patients, and arterial catheters for pressure monitoring are placed. Although modern liver transplantation entails much less use of blood products compared to in the past, it is advisable that some method of rapidly infusing warmed blood and plasma is available.

Intraoperative Management of Coagulopathy

The liver transplant procedure involves a severe physiologic stress on the patient. The intraoperative management of anesthetics as well as blood and coagulation factor replacement has truly become a specialty. An anesthesiologist with experience in liver transplantation is invaluable to the transplant team.

Patients undergoing liver transplantation have multiple reasons to experience large amounts of blood loss. They frequently have severe portal hypertension, as well as synthetic deficiencies in circulating coagulation factors. Portal hypertension invariably causes splenomegaly and splenic sequestration of platelets, leading to thrombocytopenia. Even the occasional patient who lacks hepatocellular liver failure and portal hypertension undergoes an anhepatic phase between the time when the liver has been devascularized and/or resected and the time that the donor liver has begun to function. Despite the fact that liver transplant procedures today tend to involve considerably less blood loss compared to those in the early years of liver transplantation, it is still possible for bleeding during a liver transplant to be torrential. Blood loss is more likely to be substantial if the patient has had prior upper abdominal procedures, and especially if the patient has previously undergone liver transplantation.

Evaluating the patient's coagulation status during the transplant procedure often requires frequent determinations of standard parameters, including prothrombin time (PT), partial thromboplastin time (PTT), and platelet count. Measurements of individual factor levels are no longer used routinely, but are occasionally helpful. Intraoperative thromboelastography facilitates decision making by rapidly identifying which components of the coagulation cascade are deficient and by easily identifying the presence of a fibrinolytic state. The major problem associated with thromboelastography is that the instrument is fragile and results are not accurate if it is jostled or if its base is not perfectly level and stable. The decreased overall need for coagulation factor replacement has therefore led many programs to abandon the routine use of thromboelastography.

A relatively unique circumstance occurs in the latter phases of liver transplant procedures due to the failure of production of fibrinolysis inhibitors during the anhepatic phase and to the inability of the liver to metabolize profibrinolytic compounds. Coagulopathy that develops following revascularization of the donor liver may be due to primary fibrinolysis. When fibrinolysis is unusually severe or persistent, anti-fibrinolytic therapy with ε-aminocaproic acid is helpful. A loading dose of 5 g is given intravenously, and further doses of 1 g per hour may be given if necessary until the period of fibrinolysis has passed. Therapy with ε-aminocaproic acid has been associated with intravascular thrombus formation therefore it should be used with caution and discontinued when no longer needed.

Surgical Technique

Transplantation of the liver is among the most technically demanding surgical procedures. Conceptually, hepatic transplantation may be thought of as comprising three distinct sequential phases. The first phase involves the preliminary dissection and skeletonization of the recipient's diseased liver. The second phase, known as the anhepatic phase, refers to the period starting with devascularization of the recipient's liver and ending with revascularization of the newly implanted organ. The third phase is the period after revascularization that includes biliary reconstruction and abdominal closure. The following sections describe the surgical technique of hepatic transplantation, emphasizing the potential pitfalls and detailing various strategies for circumventing the many technical challenges that may confront the transplantation surgeon during this formidable procedure.

Dissection of Recipient Liver

After the anesthetic preparation, the patient's chest, abdomen, and left groin are prepared with an anesthetic solution and draped as a single large surgical field. The most commonly used incision is a bilateral subcostal incision with an upper midline extension to the xiphoid process (Fig. 38.1). The incision is carried into the peritoneal cavity and is held open with a mechanical retractor, providing excellent exposure of the entire upper abdomen. Accumulated ascitic fluid is aspirated. If possible without extensive dissection of adhesions from prior abdominal procedures, the abdomen is then explored to rule out evidence of unsuspected intraabdominal malignancy or any other process that would preclude safe liver transplantation. The *ligamentum teres hepatis* is carefully divided between clamps and tied, because a large recanalized umbilical vein is often present in patients with severe portal hypertension.

After inspection of the liver for unforeseen abnormalities, such as an unsuspected hepatoma in a cirrhotic liver, or evidence of extrahepatic spread of a known malignancy, attention is directed to dissecting and skeletonizing the structures of the portal triad. This is accomplished primarily using electrocautery dissection to minimize bleeding. Large collateral veins may need to be ligated with sutures. Periodically the argon beam coagulator is used to restore hemostasis. The hepatic artery can usually be palpated in the anteromedial aspect of the portal triad. Palpation posterior to the common bile duct and lateral to the portal vein reveals the presence of a replaced right hepatic artery, the most common variation from "standard anatomy." Inspection of the *pars flaccida* of the lesser omentum along the lesser curvature of the stomach will demonstrate a replaced left hepatic artery arising from the left gastric artery if it is present (Fig. 38.2). The proper hepatic artery is freed from the gastroduodenal artery to its bifurcation into the left and right hepatic arterial branches. At this point each branch may be ligated and divided. Once the hepatic artery is divided, the patient is effectively anhepatic in most cases because portal flow to the liver tends to be hepatofugal (away from the liver) in the presence of cirrhosis and end-stage liver disease. Division of the hepatic artery may also be deferred until a later stage to allow whatever synthetic capacity the liver has to continue.

The common bile duct is dissected from below the level of the cystic duct entrance to the bifurcation of the common hepatic duct in the hilum of the liver. The cystic duct and proximal common hepatic duct are divided. Collateral venous channels frequently are present running along the course of the bile duct. Care must be exercised during dissection in this area, or significant hemorrhage may occur. In addition, the major blood supply to the distal recipient common bile duct comes from branches of the hepatic artery, so extensive skeletonization of the distal duct should be avoided.

Once the bile duct and the hepatic artery are freed from surrounding tissues, the portal vein can be easily approached from its anterior, medial, and lateral aspects. Again, dissection is performed primarily using electrocautery. Anterior branches are rarely found in the portal vein, even in the presence of

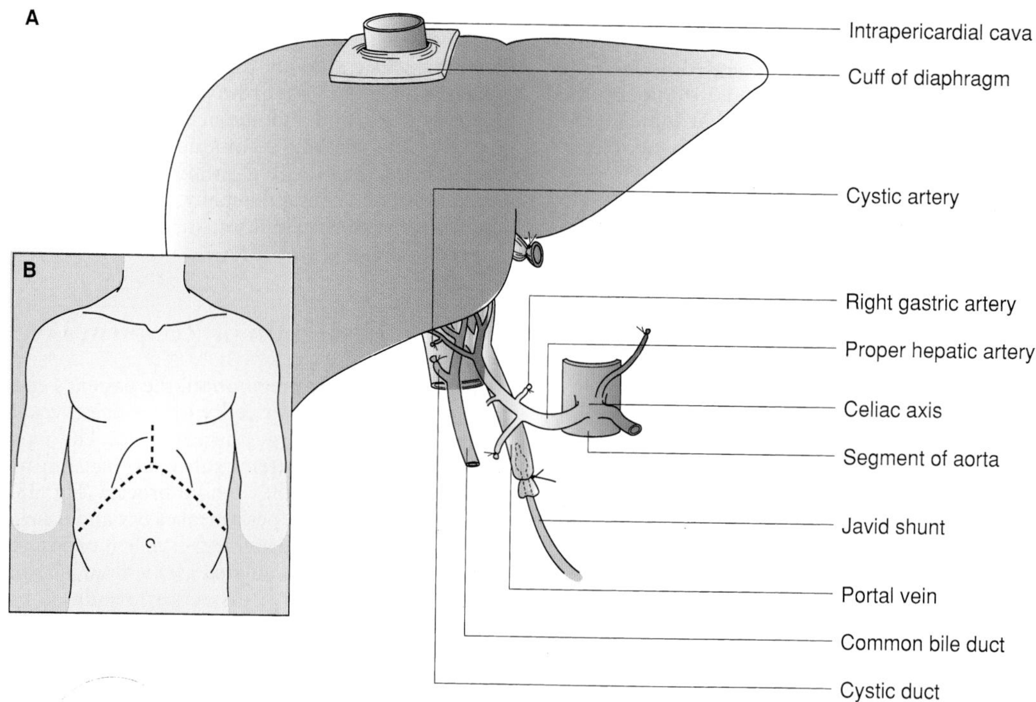

FIGURE 38.1 (*A*) The donor liver after excision and before transplantation. (*B*) Bilateral subcostal incision with a subxiphoid extension.

severe portal hypertension. Thus, dissection is commenced anteriorly between the bile duct and the hepatic artery. The portal vein should be freed over most of its length from the pancreas to the bifurcation in the hepatic hilum. Dissection to the confluence of the superior mesenteric and splenic veins may be necessary if the main portal vein is thrombosed and cannot be disobliterated. This step is frequently necessary in children because the caliber of the portal vein in the porta hepatus may be very small. The portal vein may or may not be divided at this point. Patients with severe, long-standing portal hypertension generally tolerate having their portal vein divided without developing hypotension due to engorgement of the portal circulation with blood. It is wise to wait until the last possible moment before dividing the portal vein if the patient has minimal or no portal hypertension.

The ligamentous attachments of the liver including the falciform, and the left and right triangular ligaments are then divided using electrocautery. The bare area of the liver is dissected along a plane just superficial to the capsule of the liver. Care must be taken to avoid injury to the phrenic or hepatic veins when freeing the suprahepatic inferior vena cava where it traverses the diaphragm. During mobilization of the bare area, the right lobe of the liver is displaced medially to expose, ligate, and divide the right adrenal vein as it enters the retrohepatic vena cava.

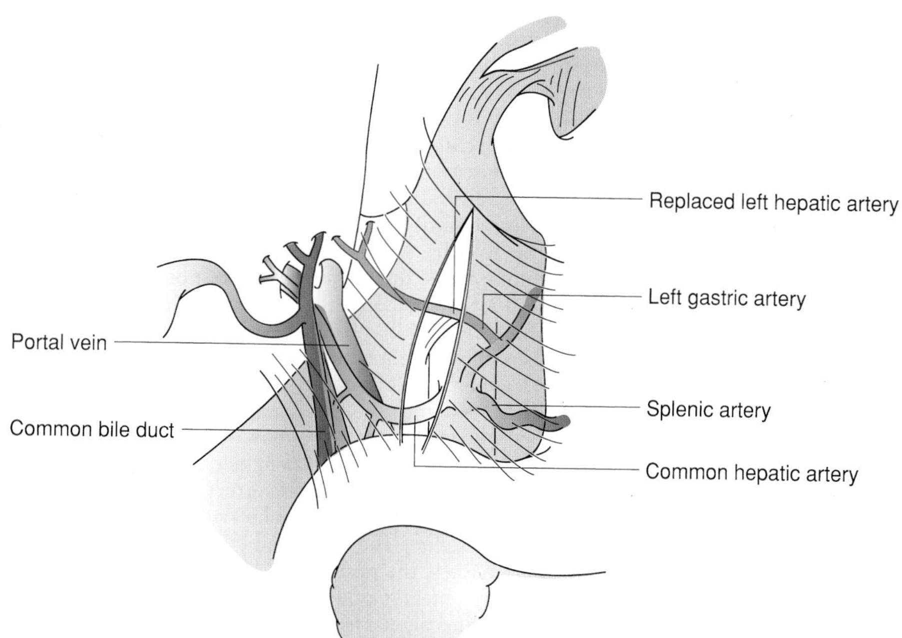

FIGURE 38.2 A replaced left hepatic artery usually arises as a branch of the left gastric artery, traversing the pars flaccida of the lesser omentum from left to right toward the left lobe of the liver.

Next, the infrahepatic inferior vena cava is exposed anteriorly. The liver is then retracted superiorly, laterally, and medially to allow individual hepatic veins draining the caudate lobe to be divided and ligated. In this way, the liver may be gradually retracted superiorly until the right, middle, and left hepatic veins are reached. Division of the portal vein facilitates this dissection but is not required.

Anhepatic Phase and Implantation of the Donor Liver

At this stage, the liver has been skeletonized sufficiently to permit its rapid removal. The decision should now be made whether to use venovenous bypass. If the dissection has gone smoothly to this point, most patients will tolerate clamping of both the portal vein and the inferior vena cava without a problem.[13] It is necessary to work closely with the anesthesiologist at this point, and the cava should be test clamped to make sure that adequate cardiac filling will still be available. If the patient becomes hypotensive during test clamping of the cava, the clamp can be removed and additional intravenous fluids administered. Occasional patients will require venovenous bypass, but its use is no longer routine at most centers.

If necessary, venovenous bypass can be accomplished from both the portal vein and inferior vena cava simultaneously, or a single cannula in either the portal vein or the inferior vena cava may be used (Fig. 38.3). There are several accepted methods of placing cannulas for venovenous bypass. Cannulas may be placed percutaneously in the internal jugular vein and femoral vein prior to beginning the procedure. These cannulas are advanced into the superior and inferior vena cava, respectively. Alternatively, one or both of the bypass cannulas may also be placed by cutdown on the axillary and/or the saphenous vein. Inferior vena caval and mesenteric blood is delivered to the superior vena cava by a centrifugal pump. The cannulas, tubing, and centrifugal pump head are heparin-bonded to reduce the chances of thrombus formation and subsequent embolism without the use of anticoagulation. Flow rates of 1 to 2 L per minute are usual.

Once venovenous bypass has been established or the decision has been made to forgo bypass, the recipient hepatectomy is completed. The portal vein is now divided as high in the hilum as possible, if this has not already been done, and a decision is made regarding the method of liver replacement. Three methods are commonly used for orthotopic liver transplantation: the bicaval technique, the piggyback technique, and the side-to-side caval technique. The bicaval technique involves excision of the recipient liver *en bloc* with the recipient cava. This requires clamping the cava above and below the liver. The hepatic veins are divided within the substance of the liver to allow the creation of a large suprahepatic cuff comprising the left, middle, and right hepatic veins (Fig. 38.4). The piggyback and the side-to-side caval techniques are accomplished by clamping of the hepatic veins and excision of the recipient liver, leaving the recipient cava *in situ*. This can sometimes be accomplished without occluding the vena cava completely, allowing blood from the lower body to return to the heart unimpeded. Each method—bi-caval, piggyback, and side-to-side caval anastamosis—has advantages and disadvantages. The piggyback and side-to-side techniques can often be accomplished without occlusion of caval flow, thus making venovenous bypass unnecessary. Because only one caval anastamosis is required, these techniques may be quicker than the bicaval technique, thus minimizing warm ischemia time. However, in some patients the necessary dissection to allow leaving the cava *in situ* may be so difficult and time-consuming that the bicaval technique is the best option.

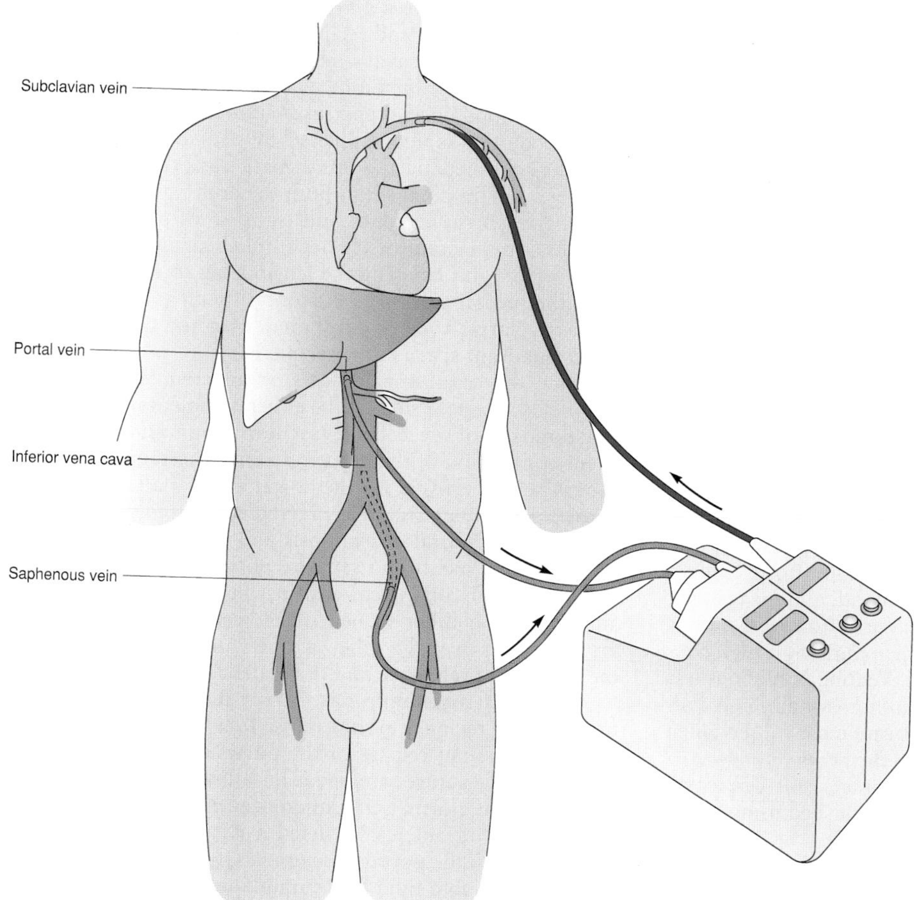

FIGURE 38.3 Setup for venovenous bypass during hepatic transplantation. Cannulas are placed into the portal vein to decompress the splanchnic bed and inferior vena cava (through the greater saphenous vein) to decompress the lower extremities and kidneys during the anhepatic phase of the transplantation. A centrifugal pump is used to deliver bypassed blood to the central circulation by means of a cannula passed into the axillary vein.

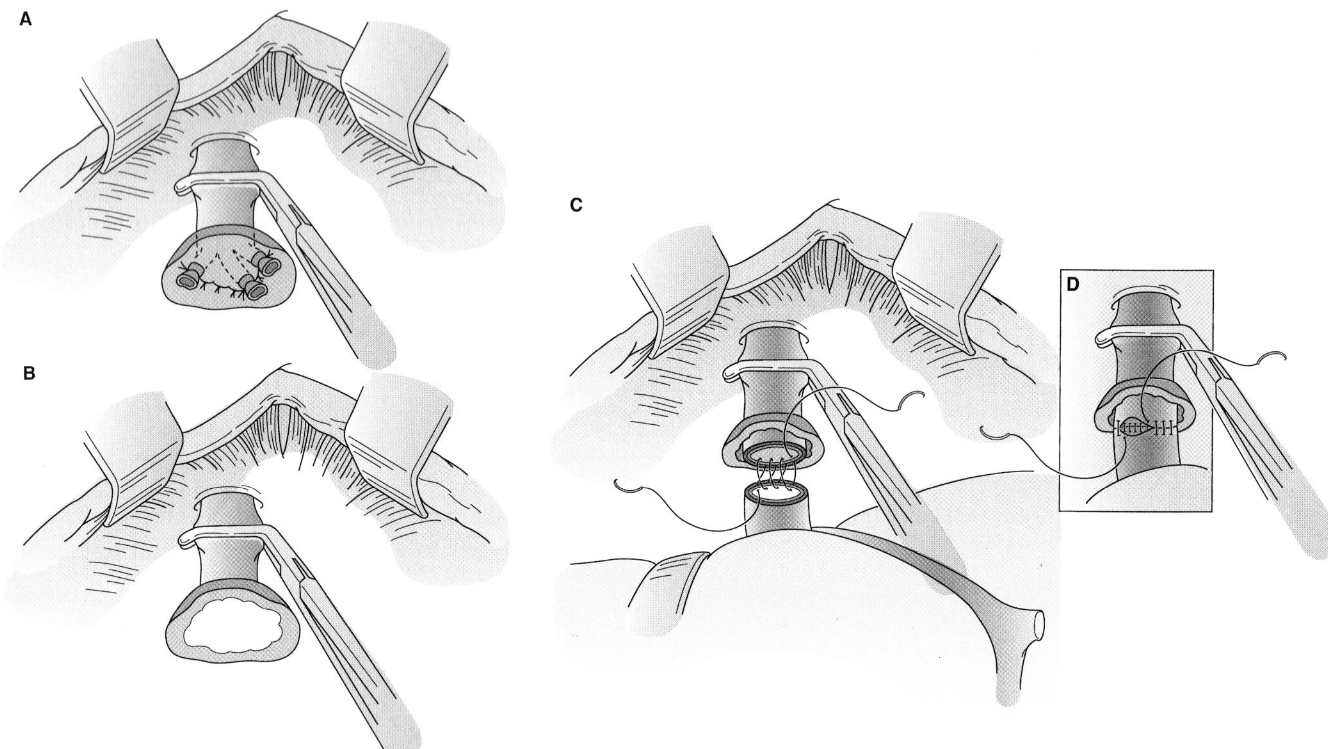

FIGURE 38.4 (*A*) The diseased recipient liver is removed by incising the liver below the level of the hepatic veins. (*B*) The hepatic veins are then opened to form a large suprahepatic cuff for anastomosis. The suprahepatic vena caval anastomosis: (*C*) posterior suture line; (*D*) anterior suture line.

After removal of the recipient liver, the right upper quadrant is carefully inspected, and hemostasis is obtained. Complete hemostasis in the bare area is essential because this region may be relatively inaccessible once the donor liver is implanted, especially if the donor liver is large. Reperitonealization of the bare area can be accomplished if there is significant bleeding from this area using the posterior peritoneum, and it tamponades venous oozing that may occur after transplantation.

The donor liver is brought to the operative field. Bench preparation performed previously includes meticulous ligation of tributaries of the vena cava (right adrenal and phrenic veins), portal vein, and hepatic artery. A Carrel patch of donor aorta is prepared for the arterial anastomotic site if the aorta is not diseased (Fig. 38.5). The gallbladder may be removed at this stage or following reperfusion. The vascular anastomoses are carried out using monofilament polypropylene suture. If the recipient cava has been removed, and bicaval technique is planned, two caval anastomoses will be required. The suprahepatic vena caval anastomosis is performed first by suturing the posterior wall from within the lumen using an imbricating technique (see Fig. 38.4). The anterior aspect of the anastomosis is then completed. The infrahepatic vena caval anastomosis is performed next. The completion of the anastomosis may be left until the time of hepatic revascularization to provide a vent for air, for acidotic, hyperkalemic blood, and for residual preservation solution. Venting of blood prior to reperfusion is most important if preservative solution containing a high concentration of potassium has been used. Venting of blood is less critical if preservative solutions that do not contain high concentrations of potassium are used, but care must still be taken to avoid a rapid bolus of cold blood to the heart.

If the recipient cava has been left intact, only one caval anastamosis is needed. This can be accomplished using either the piggyback or side-to-side caval technique. The piggyback reconstruction is accomplished by suturing the donor suprahepatic cava to the orifice created by combining the three main hepatic veins into a single patch (Fig. 38.6). As above, an imbricating suture technique is often helpful, both to prevent gaps in the anastamosis and to compensate for inequality in the size of the donor and recipient segments of the anastamosis. The infrahepatic cava is then either stapled or oversewn. A segment of the infrahepatic cava may be left open to allow venting of blood during reperfusion if desired. The side-to-side caval technique is accomplished by oversewing or stapling both the suprahepatic and infrahepatic cava on the donor and making a longitudinal slit in both the donor and the recipient cava between the caudate and right lobes posteriorly. The side-to-side anastamosis is accomplished by retracting the liver to the right, bringing the left lobe up to expose the cava from the medial side. This is more difficult to do if the liver graft is relatively large compared with the available right upper quadrant space in the recipient.

Once the caval anastamosis or anastamoses have been completed, the next step can be either completion of the portal anastamosis followed by revascularization and then subsequent completion of the hepatic arterial anastamosis once the liver is being perfused via the portal vein, or alternatively the hepatic arterial anastamosis may be completed prior to completion of the portal anastamosis and prior to reperfusion. If portal bypass has been used, the portal limb of the venovenous bypass circuit is removed just before the portal venous anastamosis. Neither sequence has been clearly shown to be an advantage over the other, so the choice is made based on the surgeon's preference and the patient's anatomy.

The portal anastamosis is usually made end to end from the donor to recipient portal veins. To avoid anastamotic narrowing following release of the portal clamp, air knots are used when the sutures are tied. This allows the anastamosis to expand to the normal circumference of the portal vein. The arterial anastomosis is completed using a branch-patch technique. Prior to the portal anastamosis, the donor liver may be perfused with cold fluid by a cannula in the donor portal vein

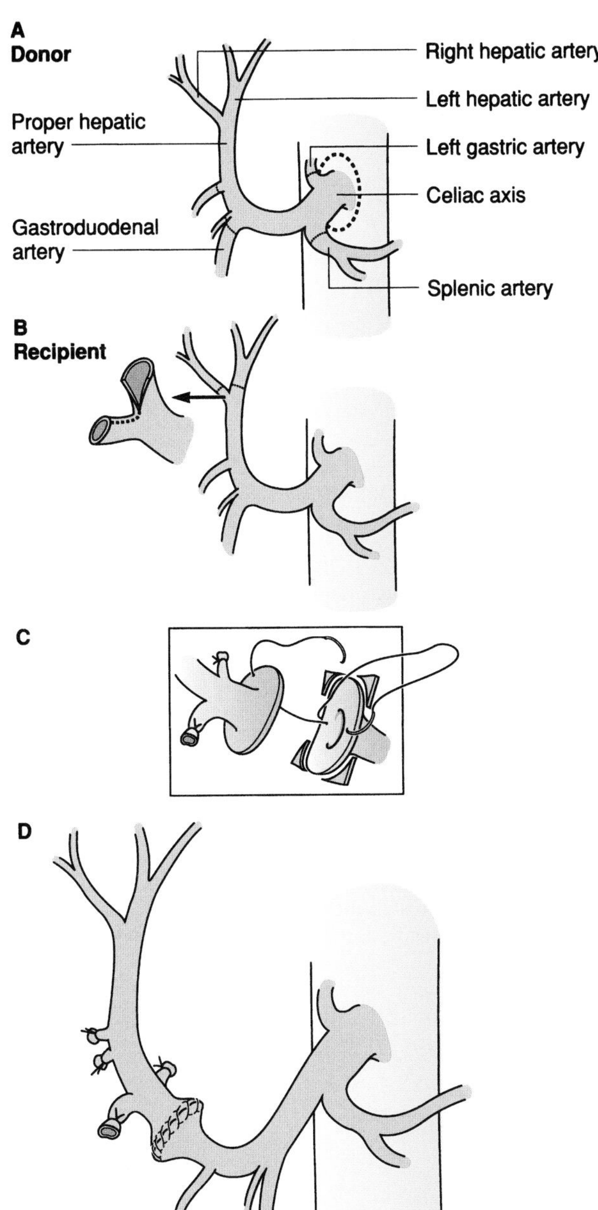

FIGURE 38.5 (*A*) The donor hepatic artery is procured with a Carrel patch of aorta. (*B*) The recipient hepatic artery bifurcation is used to fashion a branch patch for a larger anastomosis. (*C*) The anastomosis is carried out using continuous monofilament suture material. (*D*) The completed anastomosis.

to wash out the preservation solution and to keep the organ at a cryoprotective temperature. This step is not absolutely required but may be advisable if the liver contains preservative solution containing high concentrations of potassium or if a long warm ischemic time is anticipated.

At the time of revascularization, inflow is restored to the liver through the portal vein and/or the hepatic artery. The first 200 to 300 mL of blood may be vented through the infrahepatic vena cava. The final suture is then tied, and the suprahepatic caval clamp is removed. Alternatively, in the case of the piggyback or side-to-side technique, the caval clamp can be removed first and any anastamotic bleeding sutured before restoring portal flow to the liver. If blood is not vented through the infrahepatic cava, portal flow should be restored gradually to avoid cardiac irritability, bradycardia, or hypotension as the result of a sudden bolus of cold blood from the donor liver directly into the right atrium. Close coordination between the surgeon and the anesthesiologist is important during the reperfusion phase.

Postrevascularization Phase

After revascularization, the donor liver usually assumes a normal color and consistency within 10 to 15 minutes. Identifying and controlling surgical bleeding entails a meticulous examination of each of the vascular anastomoses as well as a search for branches of the major vessels that have not been ligated. If venovenous bypass has been used during the anhepatic phase, it is now discontinued. If the arterial reconstruction has not yet been performed, it is now completed as described above. If the gallbladder has not been removed it is removed at this point.

There are several options for biliary reconstruction. In the past, the donor gallbladder was sometimes retained with the graft and used as a conduit. This technique has been abandoned due to the high rate of biliary complications associated with it. The most common technique is currently an end-to-end choledochocholedochostomy from the donor to the recipient duct. If one or both of the ducts are small, spatulation may be used to ensure that the anastamosis is not narrowed by the sutures. Running or interrupted sutures may be used. Absorbable monofilament suture is preferred to avoid a nidus for future stone formation within the bile duct. The anastamosis may be stented with a T tube that exits through the recipient common bile duct or with a smaller straight tube introduced through the donor cystic duct and advanced across the anastamosis, but a stent is not required (Fig 38.7). Patients with a diseased biliary tract, such as those with primary sclerosing cholangitis or those who have a recipient duct of inadequate size or quality, require reconstruction with a choledochoenteric anastamosis. Most commonly, a standard Roux-en-Y choledochojejeunostomy is carried out. No attempt is made to stent this anastomosis (Fig. 38.8). If the patient has biliary atresia and has previously undergone the Kasai procedure, the limb of small bowel used for the portoeneterostomy may often be salvaged and used for biliary drainage of the new liver. Under ordinary circumstances, bile is produced immediately. Placement of a drain is optional because there is no hard data that it alters either the rate of biliary leakage or the morbidity of leaks that occur.

Abdominal closure may be accomplished with either nonabsorbable or absorbable polydioxanone fascial suture. In children who receive large grafts relative to their ideal liver volume, it is sometimes necessary to use a prosthetic material to facilitate closure. This works well, and, as tissue edema resolves and the abdominal wall gradually stretches, the prosthetic patch can usually be removed and the incision closed completely within 7 days of the transplant.[14]

Technique for Reduced-size and Split Hepatic Transplantation

The numbers of available suitably sized donors for pediatric hepatic transplantation are inadequate to meet the needs of children awaiting organs. As a result, techniques for reducing the size of an adult liver were developed in the 1980s whereby a single lobe or segment of an adult liver from a deceased donor could be used for a recipient more than 10 times smaller by weight than the donor.[15,16] Initially the entire liver was removed from the donor, transported to the recipient hospital, and with the liver resting in ice cold slush, the whole liver was reduced to a right lobe, a left lobe, or a left lateral segment graft by resecting the remaining liver (Fig. 38.9). All of the vessels were typically left attached to

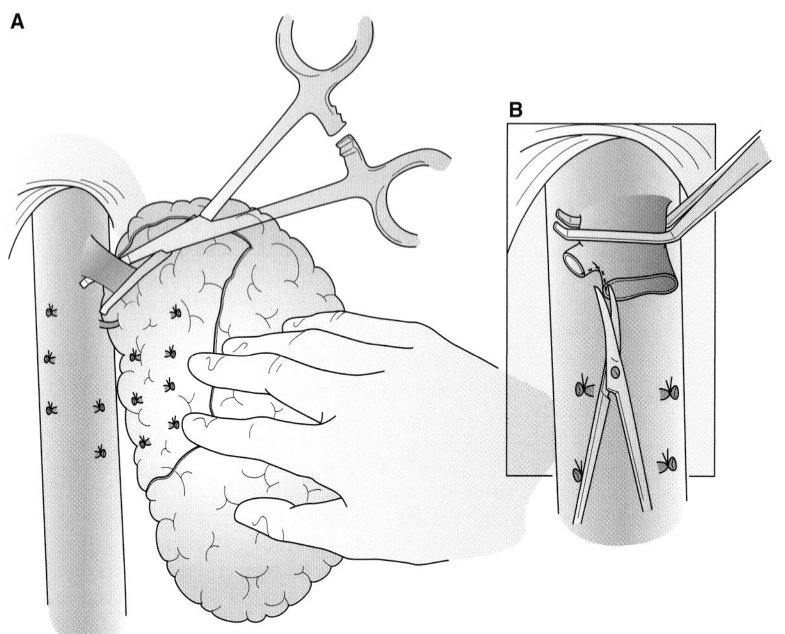

FIGURE 38.6 (*A*) Recipient liver is dissected off native inferior vena cava by dividing veins draining directly into the inferior vena cava up to the level of the hepatic veins. (*B*) Clamp placed on recipient hepatic veins in preparation of excision of the recipient's native liver.

the donor graft, and the remaining liver was discarded. This technique was quite successful and led to the development of techniques that allow two portions of a single liver to be used to transplant two recipients. Initial success was primarily reported using the left lateral segment for a pediatric recipient and the right trisegment graft for an adult (Fig. 38.10A).[17] More recently, success has been reported using the right lobe and the left lobe to transplant two adults.[18] A reason for the recent success reported with split liver transplantation has been the recognition that only livers from "ideal donors" are suitable for this form of transplantation. Livers are generally considered suitable for splitting if the following criteria are met: donor age is between 14 and 50; the donor has been in the intensive care unit for no more than 3 days; body weight is greater than 45 kg and body mass index is less than 27 kg/m^2; mean arterial pressure is at least 60 mm Hg; serum sodium is no higher than 160 mEq/L; SGPT is no higher than 60 IU/L; GGTP is less than 50 IU/L; and no significant steatosis is present.[19]

It has been proposed that widespread adoption of allocation policies that encourage a greater utilization of adult livers as split grafts would result in a net benefit to the population of all patients on the liver transplant waiting list.[20] However, this technique is still in evolution and several technical and practical issues remain unresolved, including whether the splitting procedure should occur while the liver is still *in situ* in the deceased donor or following cold perfusion. In addition, the survival rate for adult recipients of split liver grafts is

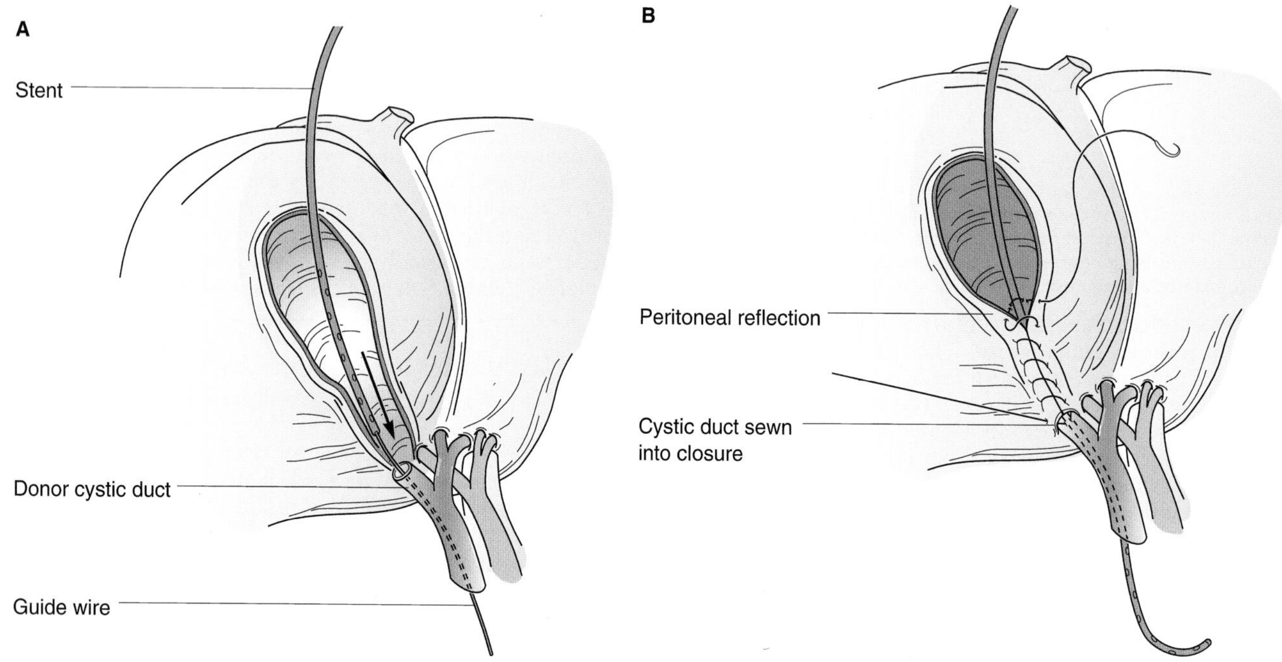

FIGURE 38.7 Catheter in biliary tree of liver transplant. (*A*) The catheter is passed through the donor cystic duct into the common bile duct. (*B*) The peritoneal reflection is closed over the catheter. The catheter is brought out through the anterior abdominal wall and fixed to the skin.

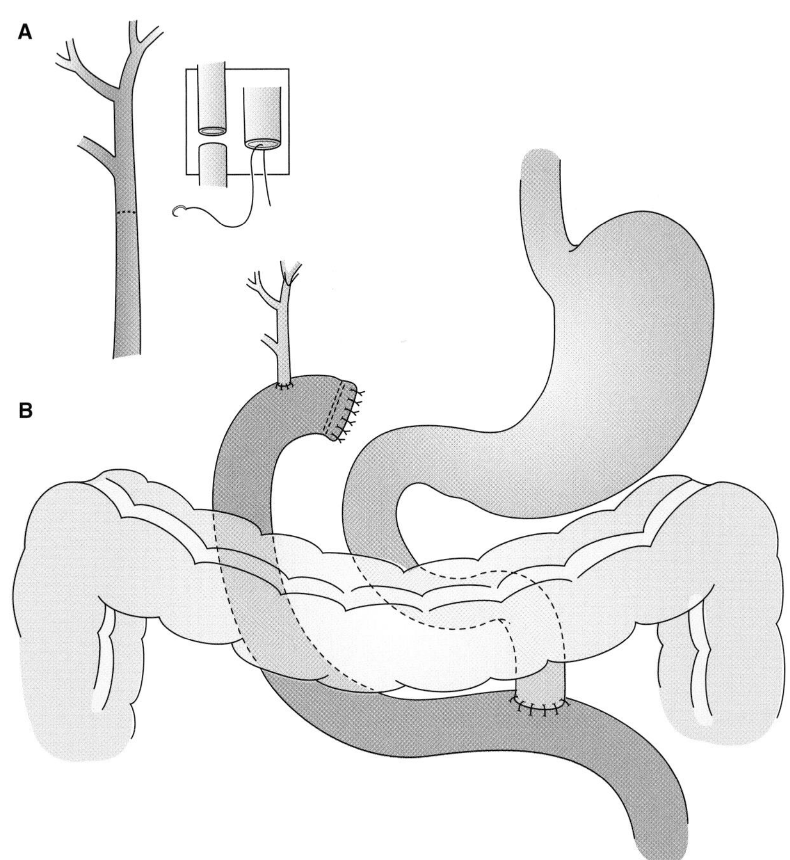

FIGURE 38.8 (*A*) In most cases, a choledocho-choledochostomy is performed over a small drainage tube introduced through the donor cystic duct. (*B*) Patients with a diseased or unsuitable common bile duct require biliary reconstruction with a Roux-en-Y choledochoenterostomy.

still inferior to that obtained with whole-organ transplants, thus discouraging widespread adoption of the technique.

Living Donor Liver Transplantation

The development of techniques to transplant segments of adult livers into children led naturally to the application of this technique to living donors. This technique was first used to allow an adult volunteer to donate the left lateral segment of the liver to a child. The success of these procedures in children, together with the growing waiting list mortality rate, fueled the application of the living donor technique to adult recipients using the right lobe of an adult volunteer.[21] This procedure now accounts for approximately 5% of liver transplants in the United States. In Japan and the Far East, where deceased donor transplantation has not developed because of cultural difficulties with the concept of brain death, living donor transplants are the rule, rather than the exception.

The recipient operation for living donor procedures is identical to that of the deceased donor procedure, except that the recipient cava must be left *in situ* and a direct hepatic vein to vena caval anastamosis is used (Figs. 38.10B and 38.11). Care must be taken to ensure that adequate recipient portal vein and hepatic artery are preserved. The biliary reconstruction can be either duct to duct or using a choledochojejeunostomy.

The development of this technique has been hindered by two factors. First is the concern over donor safety. Even in

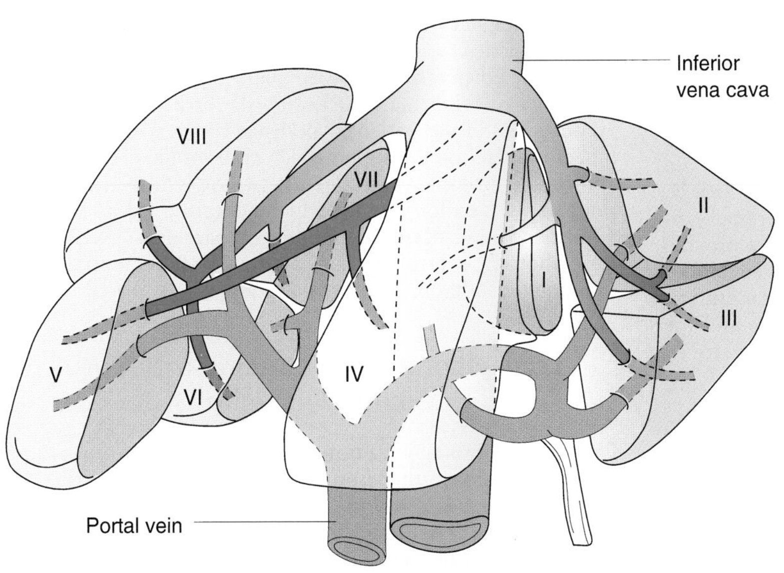

FIGURE 38.9 Segmental anatomy of the liver as based on Couinaud's nomenclature.

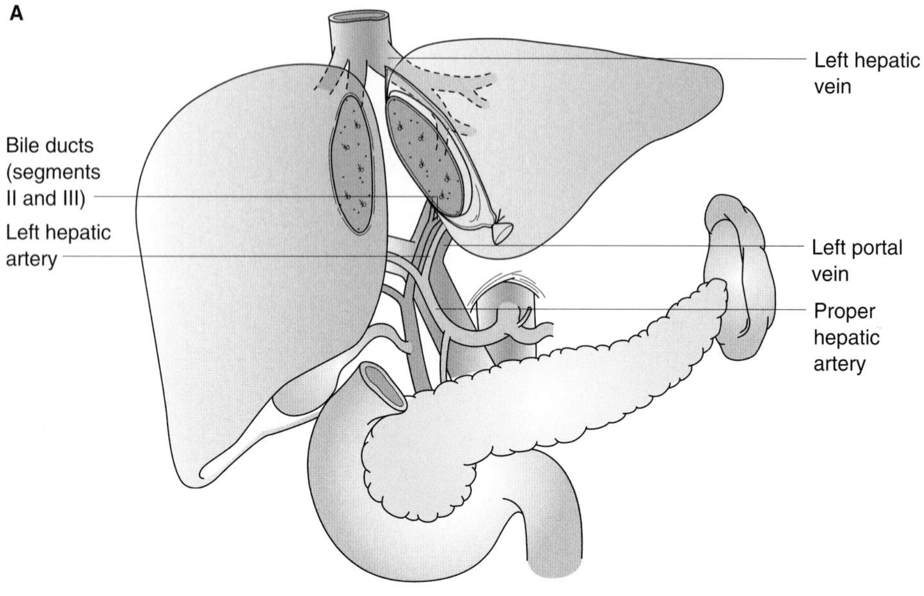

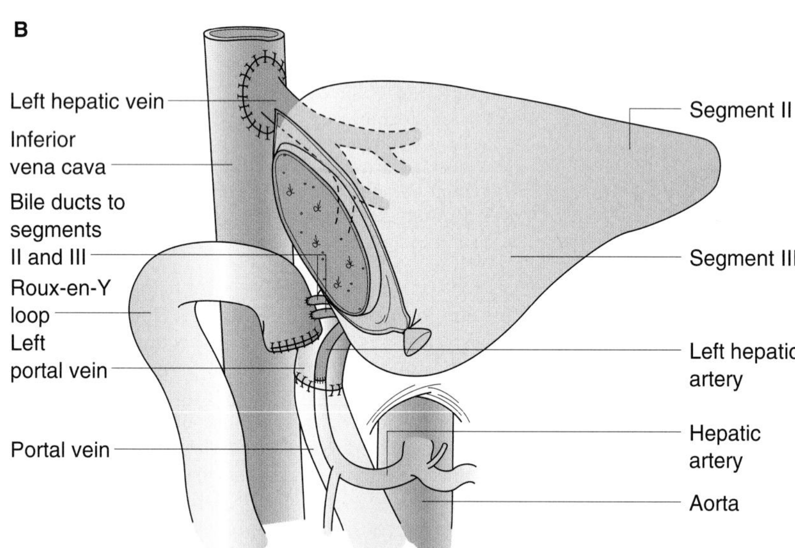

FIGURE 38.10 Left lateral segment (segments II and III) living donor transplantation. (*A*) Donor operation. (*B*) Recipient operation completed.

experienced hands, a major hepatic resection entails significant risks. Mortality is estimated at between 0.1% and 1%. In addition, complications are common, particularly bile leaks from the bile duct stump or the cut edge of the liver. This morbidity may alter long-term quality of life in donors. The current paucity of long-term data on the effects of having donated a portion of one's liver has led to the initiation of several long-term studies that will help define more precisely the nature of the risks. The second factor hindering the development of this procedure is that it does not appear appropriate for patients who are profoundly ill. Patients with advanced end-organ dysfunction, such as those with hepatorenal syndrome, appear to benefit from having an entire liver to provide for an optimal chance of recovery from chronic liver failure. Despite these limitations, living donor liver transplantation has become a standard option for pediatric patients and for adult patients in areas where deceased donor livers are in short supply.

Auxiliary Liver Transplantation

Under some circumstances, there is a good rationale for placing the donor allograft in a heterotopic rather than orthotopic position, leaving the diseased liver in place. This procedure is referred to as an *auxiliary liver transplant.* It is used occasionally for cases in which transplantation is indicated for enzymatic deficiency but the native liver functions well in all other respects. It is also used in cases of fulminant hepatic failure in which there is a reasonable chance for recovery of the native liver. There are two major advantages of the auxiliary procedure. First, it is a procedure of lesser magnitude than the orthotopic procedure. Second, should the patient experience recovery of native liver function, then immunosuppression can be gradually withdrawn and the heterotopic graft allowed to slowly involute. Success rates of the auxiliary transplant have improved as technical refinements have occurred and are comparable to success rates for orthotopic transplantation. Figure 38.12 demonstrates the technique used in one institution.

Transplantation in Patients with Portal Venous Thrombosis

Patients undergoing liver transplantation are sometimes found to have portal vein thrombosis intraoperatively, or this condition may have been identified preoperatively. Historically, this situation was considered to be a contraindication to liver transplantation because portal flow is necessary for allograft

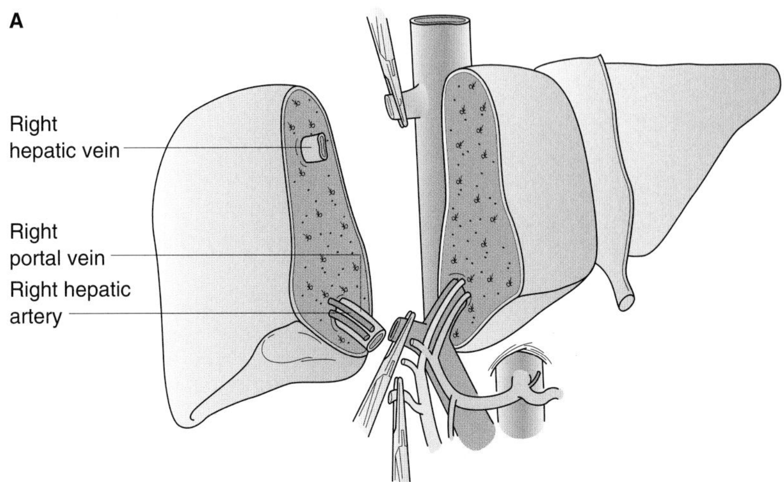

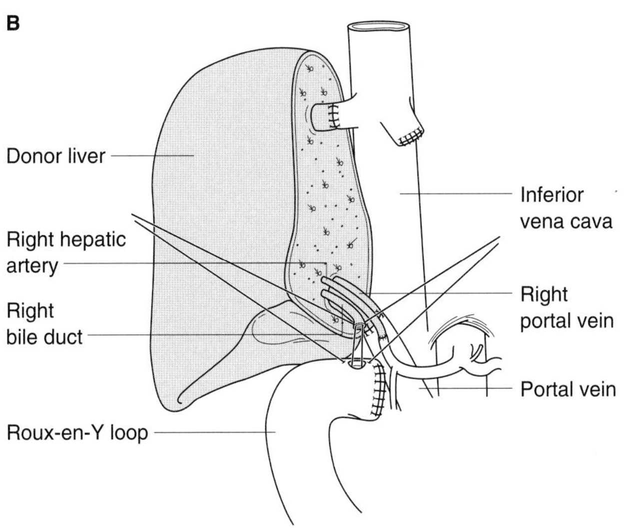

FIGURE 38.11 Right lobe (segments V to VIII) living donor transplantation. (*A*) Donor operation. (*B*) Recipient operation completed.

survival. Recently many methods of dealing with this fairly common clinical circumstance have been devised. The preferred method of dealing with portal vein thrombosis is thrombectomy. If the portal vein has not undergone cavernous transformation, the thrombus in the portal vein can usually be removed by eversion endarterectomy.[22] If endarterectomy is not possible, another option is to use donor iliac vein as a conduit to the recipient superior mesenteric vein. If the superior mesenteric vein is also occluded, the inferior vena cava can be used for portal inflow, a procedure termed *cavoportal hemitransposition*.[23] This procedure is associated with acceptable outcome despite the fact that some degree of portal hypertension remains in the recipient. A fourth option is arterialization of the portal vein, using a conduit created by anastomosing donor iliac vessels to the recipient aorta and connecting this to the donor portal vein.[24]

POSTOPERATIVE COMPLICATIONS

The degree of preoperative debilitation and the complexity of the operative procedure make complications following hepatic transplantation very common. As always, prompt recognition and treatment are essential. In transplantation, however, the additional burden of immunosuppression predisposes to problems not usually encountered in other areas of surgery. Complications associated with immunosuppression, which are predominantly infectious, are detailed in another chapter. In the following sections, some of the major surgical complications that occur after hepatic transplantation are described.

Primary Nonfunction

For reasons that are not completely understood, about 5% to 10% of transplanted livers function so poorly in the immediate postoperative period that death is likely in the absence of retransplantation. This is referred to as primary nonfunction of the allograft. It is thought that most cases of nonfunction are related to ischemic injury during cold preservation. Recipient factors as well as donor factors are important.[25] Donor factors known to predispose to primary nonfunction include steatosis of the liver graft and donor age, as well as prolonged cold ischemia.

Patients with primary nonfunction rapidly become exceedingly ill, developing profound coagulopathy and hepatic encephalopathy, followed swiftly by progressive renal failure and eventually cardiopulmonary collapse. Patients in the United States with primary nonfunction are currently eligible to be listed as UNOS status 1. This emergency transplant status is reserved for patients who are judged to have fewer than 7 days to live without a transplant. Status 1 patients receive

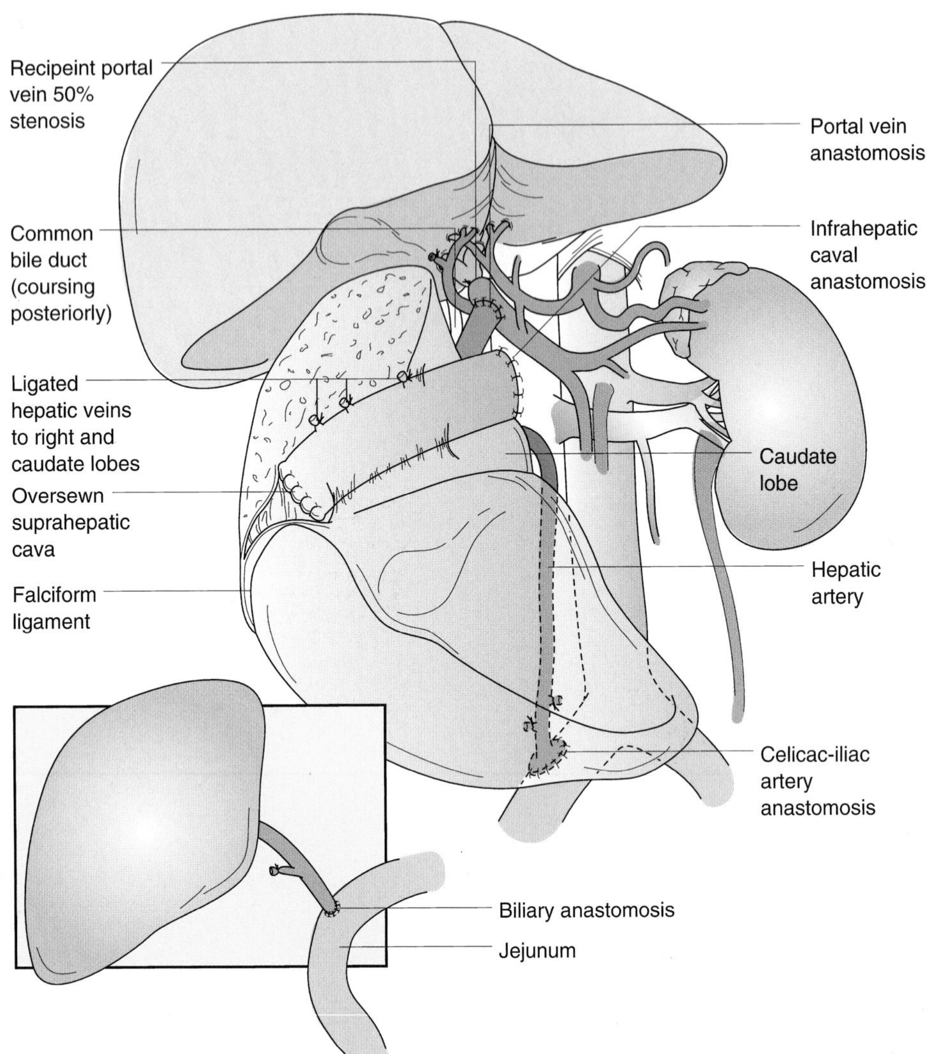

FIGURE 38.12 Heterotopic auxiliary liver transplantation using a reduced-size allograft.

regional priority over less ill patients and frequently wait only a day or two for a liver graft.

The diagnosis of primary nonfunction should be suspected whenever the patient does not regain consciousness following liver transplantation or when a period of lucidity is followed by the rapid development of encephalopathy and coma. Almost all patients with this condition will have AST and ALT values greater than 5,000 and INR values greater than 2.5. Factor V level is occasionally helpful in determining how well the liver is functioning when the patient has been given a large volume of fresh frozen plasma. In this setting the INR may reflect transfused coagulation factors rather than factors synthesized by the liver graft. Fresh frozen plasma contains relatively little factor V because the factor is relatively unstable in cold storage. Therefore, factor V levels can be followed serially as a measure of hepatic synthetic function that is relatively insensitive to the effects of exogenous administration of coagulation factors.

Biliary Leak or Obstruction

Biliary leak or obstruction is a common surgical complication encountered after hepatic transplantation with an incidence of approximately 10% to 30%.[26] Most biliary complications probably relate to ischemia of the donor biliary tree (Fig. 38.13). The transected donor bile duct is totally dependent on arterial flow from the liver graft. Therefore, when a biliary leak is identified, it is appropriate to interrogate the hepatic vasculature to rule out the presence of hepatic artery stenosis or thrombosis.

Although biliary complications can result in mortality from sepsis, most commonly they are merely an expensive annoyance. The initial management of biliary complications can generally be nonoperative. In most cases, the problem can be both diagnosed and treated by endoscopic retrograde cholangiopancreatography (ERCP). If the biliary reconstruction was made using a Roux-en-Y hepaticojejeunostomy, of if ERCP is unsuccessful, biliary leaks must be diagnosed and treated by interventional radiology using percutaneous transhepatic cholangiography and percutaneous placement of a biliary stent. In addition to stenting the anastamosis, it may be necessary to place a percutaneous drain if there is a significant extrahepatic collection of bile. In cases where initial studies show a large defect and in cases where the leak is not controlled through percutaneous measures, operative repair using a Roux-en-Y hepaticojejunostomy may be indicated.

Biliary obstruction resulting from anastamotic strictures can also generally be managed nonoperatively by using percutaneous cholangioplasty or ERCP. When anastomotic strictures persist beyond two attempts at balloon dilatation and stent replacement, operative repair may be an option as long as the entire biliary stricture is extrahepatic and there are no intrahepatic strictures.

Hemorrhage

Laparotomy to control postoperative bleeding is required after 5% to 15% of liver transplants. The most sensitive indication of bleeding is lack of urine output. Any patient who develops oliguria in the first 24 hours postoperatively should be suspected of having bleeding. A dependence on diuretics is not a physiologic explanation for diminished urine output, but hypovolemia is!

In many patients a specific bleeding point cannot be identified at reoperation, suggesting that bleeding is often related more to coagulopathy than to failure of surgical hemostasis. It is thus wise to wait until the coagulopathy has been corrected before reoperating. In many cases where the patient needs some postprocedure transfusions, the bleeding will cease spontaneously due to intraabdominal pressure and to the restoration of normal synthetic function by the new liver.

Hepatic Artery Thrombosis

Hepatic artery thrombosis occurs in approximately 5% to 10% of liver transplants and is more common in children.[27] It is usually suspected clinically based on abnormally elevated transaminases or evidence of biliary problems. The diagnosis is made using Doppler ultrasonography, magnetic resonance imaging, or standard arteriography. When hepatic artery thrombosis occurs in the first week after a liver transplant, the patient invariably develops complete biliary necrosis and graft failure. On identification of acute hepatic artery thrombosis, thrombectomy should be attempted. In this setting thrombectomy is successful in approximately half of cases.[28]

Hepatic artery thrombosis that occurs months to years following liver transplantation does not always lead to graft failure. Although some patients develop biliary strictures and/or hepatic abscesses, approximately a third of patients do well without intervention.[29]

Risk factors for hepatic artery thrombosis include a donor who is significantly smaller than the recipient, as well as the need for reconstructive arterioplasty in the presence of nonstandard donor anatomy, present in a significant percentage of donor livers. Other associated factors include acute rejection within the first week posttransplant, placement of CMV-positive organs into CMV-negative recipients, and a history of smoking.[30] The association between rejection and hepatic artery thrombosis may be to the result of a decrease in hepatic arterial flow that occurs when the liver is swollen and edematous or to release of procoagulations into the microcirculation in association with the inflammatory injury of graft rejection.

The rate of arterial blood flow in the reconstructed hepatic artery is an important determinant of long-term patency with reduced flow. It is believed that children are predisposed to hepatic artery thrombosis because they have smaller vessels and lower mean arterial blood pressure than adults. Pediatric patients with an arterial diameter of less than 3 mm have the highest incidence of hepatic artery thrombosis. However, the experience with pediatric living donor transplantation, where very small arteries are routinely encountered, has indicated that with microsurgical technique it is possible to achieve a low hepatic artery thrombosis rate.[31]

A postoperative hypercoagulable state associated with hepatic transplantation may predispose to hepatic artery thrombosis. Relatively poor hepatic production of natural regulatory anticoagulants, such as proteins C and S and antithrombin III, immediately after transplantation promotes coagulation because production of procoagulant factors, such as factor V and VII, occurs more rapidly after revascularization.[32] This observation has prompted some centers to administer fresh frozen plasma as a source of antithrombin III and proteins C and S in the postoperative period. Most centers recommend prophylactic aspirin to prevent hepatic artery thrombosis in children, although no objective data demonstrate the value of this practice.

Portal Vein Thrombosis

Postoperative portal vein thrombosis is much less common than hepatic artery thrombosis, occurring in 1% to 3% of cases. A higher incidence of portal vein problems is seen in patients that have had previous portal vein operations or prior thrombosis of the portal system. Factors that decrease antegrade portal flow also predispose to portal vein thrombosis. Patients with chronic portal hypertension often spontaneously develop large retroperitoneal collaterals from the portal venous system to the renal vein and inferior vena cava. A previous surgically created splenorenal shunt should be disconnected at the time of transplantation because it usually is associated with reduced flow through the portal vein. This can be accomplished easily during a liver transplant by dissecting down the vena cava and ligating the left renal vein at its origin. This maneuver does not compromise the function of the left kidney. This maneuver can also be useful to improve portal flow if preoperative imaging discloses large spontaneous portal-systemic shunts to the left renal vein.

Portal vein thrombosis should be suspected when the recipient develops symptoms of portal hypertension or ascites that is unusually difficult to control. Doppler ultrasound examination is usually the first diagnostic tool, but magnetic resonance imaging is also an option, as are standard mesenteric arteriography with portal phase views and direct percutaneous transhepatic portography. Transhepatic portography is particularly useful if a stenosis, rather than thrombosis, is identified because it is possible to both measure the pressure gradient across a stenotic area and treat a stenotic area with angioplasty and/or stent placement.

When portal vein thrombosis is identified in the immediate postoperative period, reexploration and attempted thrombectomy are usually indicated. Thrombectomy is more likely to be successful if a technical flaw in the anastamosis is present and can be corrected. When performing thrombectomy, it is advisable to avoid using balloon embolectomy catheters to remove clot from the mesenteric venous system, because these veins are very fragile and rupture of mesenteric veins deep in the mesentery can be catastrophic.

Complications of the Inferior Vena Cava Anastamosis

Thrombosis of the inferior vena cava is a rare complication after liver transplantation, but hepatic vein outflow obstruction occurs in 2% to 4% of patients. Restrictions of hepatic blood flow may result from kinking of the suprahepatic cava. This is particularly problematic when the donor is small relative to the recipient and when the suprahepatic anastamosis is left long. Hepatic outflow problems can present with ascites and renal dysfunction. Presentation may be early in the first week after transplantation or months later. The diagnosis may be suspected on the basis of Doppler ultrasonography, but definitive diagnosis usually requires inferior cavography with measurement of pressure gradients. The incidence of caval complications utilizing the piggyback technique appears to be higher than the incidence with the bicaval technique, at approximately 4%.[33] Outflow stenosis appears to be more common if the combined orifice of two, rather than three, hepatic veins is used for the anastamotic site on the recipient when the piggyback technique is used. In many cases, hepatic vein or suprahepatic caval stenosis can be successfully treated noninvasively with the use of balloon angioplasty and stenting.[34,35]

Intraabdominal Sepsis

Intraabdominal sepsis presents as diffuse peritonitis or localized abscess and occurs in about 5% of patients who undergo liver transplantation. The most common cause of peritonitis is leakage of the biliary anastamosis. Abscesses may also develop spontaneously in the right upper quadrant or elsewhere in the abdomen. Most isolated infected fluid collections can be managed by percutaneous placement of drains guided by ultrasound or CT scanning, along with broad-spectrum intravenous antibiotics. Generalized infected ascitic fluid is managed with peritoneocentesis and antibiotics. Surgical drainage may be necessary if leakage of enteric contents is suspected based on the finding of extravasated oral contrast in the peritoneal cavity on CT scan, or if the patient does not respond to percutaneous drainage.

Neurologic Complications

A number of preoperative and postoperative factors predispose to impaired consciousness and seizure activity after transplantation. Patients who have significant preoperative encephalopathy are more likely to suffer from postoperative neurologic symptoms. In the extreme, patients who are in hepatic coma from fulminant liver failure can sometimes take weeks to regain complete consciousness. Patients undergoing liver transplants are also at risk for watershed infarcts if significant intraoperative hypotension occurs. The effects of transient cerebral ischemia are worsened by the large amount of intravenous fluids that are often necessary during and after transplantation, which can exacerbate cerebral edema. Air embolism is also a risk if venous bleeding occurs from the cava or hepatic veins at a time when the patient is relatively hypovolemic. If the patient has a patent foramen ovale, air embolism can result in cerebral ischemia if large bubbles lodge in the cerebral circulation. If the patient fails to awaken promptly after transplantation, and particularly if the transplant is functioning well, an urgent CT scan of the head should be obtained to rule out intracranial hemorrhage and to assess the degree of cerebral edema.

Seizures are reasonably common after transplantation. The calcineurin inhibitors cyclosporine and tacrolimus both lower seizure threshold and are associated with seizures following liver transplantation. Patients with a history of seizures are particularly predisposed to postoperative seizure activity. Seizures are treated with benzodiazepines acutely followed by intravenous phenytoin. To prevent recurrence of seizure activity it is usually necessary to decrease the dosage of calcineurin inhibitor to a lower target blood level. Frequently it is also necessary to change to a different calcineurin inhibitor altogether, or even to change the patient's maintenance immunosuppression to a regimen that does not include a calcineurin inhibitor.

REJECTION AND IMMUNOSUPPRESSION

For reasons that are not understood, liver transplant recipients require less immune suppression than patients with other types of allografts, such as heart, lung, and kidney recipients. This is somewhat surprising given that the mass of the liver is so great compared with the mass of the other organs. With current immunosuppressive therapy, graft loss from rejection is rare.

Antibody-mediated Rejection

The liver is relatively resistant to injury from recipient antibodies, regardless of whether they are present at the time of transplant or develop later. This is very different compared with renal and cardiac recipients who experience rapid graft destruction, termed *hyperacute rejection*, if performed in a patient who has complement fixing antibodies directed against the donor organ in significant concentrations at the time of transplantation. Hepatic graft injury from preexisting directed at donor ABO determinants does occur, but in a much less pronounced fashion than in the context of renal transplantation. The overall results of ABO-incompatible liver transplants are somewhat inferior to those of ABO-compatible transplantations, but only by about a 10% to 20% decrease in 1-year graft survival rates compared to ABO-compatible grafts. Some of this decrease in graft survival rate may be due to the fact that ABO-incompatible transplants are usually performed only in dire circumstances where the patient is so ill that he or she may not survive the wait for a compatible organ. Because preformed antibodies do not seem to be clinically important, most transplantation programs do not perform prospective crossmatches between recipient serum and donor cells before transplantation, and determination of recipient and donor HLA type is no longer considered mandatory.

Why the liver is less susceptible to antibody-mediated destruction than the kidney is not clearly understood. One factor may be the vastly different microcirculation that the liver has compared with the kidney, with a preponderance of sinusoidal channels and a smaller capillary network. It is probable that antibody-mediated injury affects blood flow through the delicate capillary network of the kidney more than it does liver sinusoids. In addition, each hepatocyte is exposed to two sinusoidal channels, presumably permitting survival if only one sinusoid is occluded. Finally, differences in HLA antigen expression are known to exist in the two organs, with the kidney the more antigenic of the two.

Cell-mediated Rejection

Typical acute rejection in liver transplant recipients is usually cell mediated and occurs frequently but is effectively blunted by antirejection therapy. Acute rejection occurs most commonly in the first 2 postoperative months. In modern practice, cell-mediated rejection is a less common cause of graft loss than are primary nonfunction or hepatic artery thrombosis. Still, the effectiveness of antirejection treatment assumes a relatively early diagnosis and treatment of acute rejection, which is in turn the result of careful monitoring by the transplantation physician and compliance by the patient with frequent laboratory testing. Treatment of acute rejection with enhanced immunosuppressive therapy is highly effective, and an episode of rejection does not affect long-term graft survival. This is very different from renal transplantation, where an episode of rejection decreases long-term graft survival markedly.

The diagnosis of cell-mediated rejection is made primarily on histologic grounds. Clinical features can include low-grade fever and malaise, but frequently the patient is completely asymptomatic. Laboratory evaluation of peripheral blood may demonstrate leukocytosis and occasionally eosinophilia. Biochemical changes associated with rejection include elevated and rising levels of serum transaminases and alkaline phosphatase. A prolonged serum prothrombin time and an

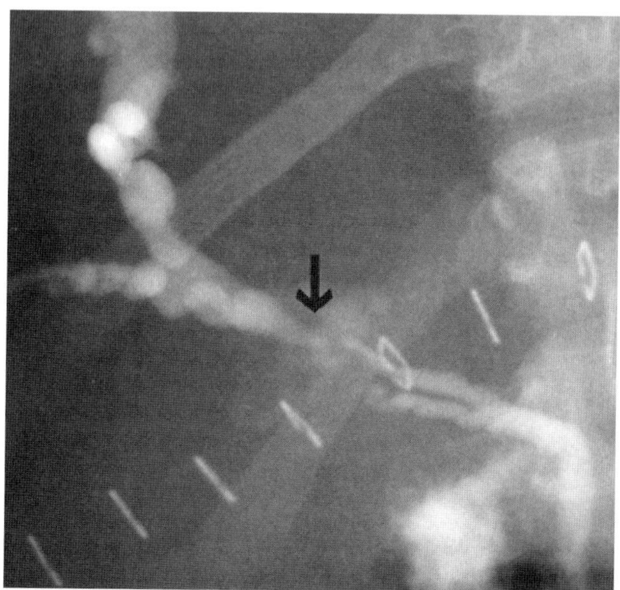

FIGURE 38.13 Bile leak (*arrow*) from the choledochocholedochostomy after hepatic transplantation.

abnormal serum bilirubin also suggest the possibility of rejection, but frequently these parameters are normal if rejection is detected early. Any of these findings should prompt a biopsy.

The diagnosis of cell-mediated rejection rests on the finding of a triad of portal lymphocytosis, endotheliitis (subendothelial deposits of mononuclear cells), and bile duct infiltration and damage (Figs. 38.14 and 38.15). Various classification schemes have been devised to grade the severity of the rejection process based on the degree of cellular involvement or injury in these areas. Cell characterization studies have documented that the cells in the portal triads are primarily T cells, with fewer macrophages and neutrophils. Bile duct epithelial cells appear to be a prime target of immune attack, and they are known to express large amounts of class II HLA antigen.

If the recipient has hepatitis C, it is critical that recurrent hepatitis C is differentiated from acute rejection. At times the difference can be subtle, and a pathologist with experience in the interpretation of allograft biopsies is extremely valuable. Enhanced immunosuppression is associated with accelerated rates of hepatitis C viral replication; it is, therefore, important that immunosuppression is kept to a minimum for these patients.

Chronic Rejection

Chronic rejection is characterized by relentless immune attack on small bile ducts. Clinically, the pattern is one of gradual elevation of alkaline phosphatase and bilirubin, in the absence of obstruction of the large bile ducts. Histologically, small bile ducts are obliterated or completely absent, with a less pronounced cellular infiltrate than is seen with acute rejection. This finding has been termed *vanishing bile duct syndrome* when bile ducts are absent in 15 of 20 portal triads examined.[36] The loss of small bile ducts is partly the result of lymphocyte-directed attack on biliary epithelium. Relative to other cells in the liver, biliary epithelium tends to express more class I antigen. Thus, biliary epithelial cells are vulnerable targets for host attack because of their antigenicity. Loss of bile ducts may also occur indirectly as the result of ischemia secondary to immune-mediated obliteration of small to medium arteries. As in the case of renal transplantations, there is no effective treatment for chronic rejection except retransplantation.

Immunosuppression Induction and Maintenance

Multiple immunosuppressive protocols achieve acceptable suppression of allograft rejection for liver transplant recipients. Induction with antithymocyte globulin is no longer considered to be mandatory but is used at some centers. Similarly prednisone therapy, once considered a mainstay of a successful immunosuppressive protocol, is no longer considered absolutely necessary and when used is often tapered off rapidly. Treatment with a calcineurin inhibitor, either cyclosporine or tacrolimus is still considered to be imperative for most liver transplant recipients. These agents are associated with significant long-term morbidity, particularly the development of chronic renal failure. Dosages of these agents have gradually been reduced both to prevent renal insufficiency and to avoid the rapid and aggressive recurrence of hepatitis C infection. Induction antibody therapy with either polyclonal antilymphocyte preparations or with inhibitors of the receptor for IL-2 are still used commonly in the perioperative setting to avoid the nephrotoxicity associated with the immediate use of calcineurin inhibitors.

Because immunosuppression predisposes to infection, prophylactic antiinfective drugs are usually administered. Trimethoprim-sulfamethoxazole, dapsone, or pentamidine is recommended to prevent *Pneumocystis carinii* infection. Oral Mycostatin or fluconazole therapy is used to prevent fungal infections, particularly esophageal *Candida albicans*. Either ganciclovir or valganciclovir is prescribed for patients who are at risk for cytomegalovirus (CMV) infection, which includes any patient exposed to CMV in the past and any patient transplanted with organs from a donor who has been exposed to CMV. Patients who are CMV negative who receive CMV-negative organs are not at risk for CMV infection but should still receive prophylaxis against disseminated herpes simplex infections with acyclovir therapy. The duration of prophylactic antiinfective therapy has not been rigorously defined by evidenced-based trials and is therefore dependent on each center's experience with the prevalence of these infections in its patient population.

Treatment of Acute Rejection

Despite the overall effectiveness of the regimen described, acute rejection does occur and must be treated promptly. Several options are available for treatment of acute rejection, depending on the clinical circumstances. Traditionally, high doses of methylprednisolone are administered (usually 500 mg to 1 g) intravenously on a daily basis for 3 days. This treatment is effective in reversing most acute rejection episodes. Alternatively, increased doses of a calcineurin inhibitor or the addition of an antimetabolite drug, such as mycophenolate mofetil, will also reverse most episodes of rejection, particularly if the rejection is mild. Rejection that is resistant to these maneuvers is treated with antilymphocyte therapy, either a monoclonal antibody directed at the T3 determinant common to all mature T cells (Orthoclone, OKT3) or polyclonal antilymphocyte treatments such as Atgam or Thymoglobulin. These treatments are typically administered daily for 5 to 10 days. These agents are highly effective, and it is unusual to lose an allograft secondary to acute rejection. However, these treatments are associated with profound and long-lasting Immunosuppression, and it is usually advisable to restart prophylactic antiinfective therapies when they are initiated.

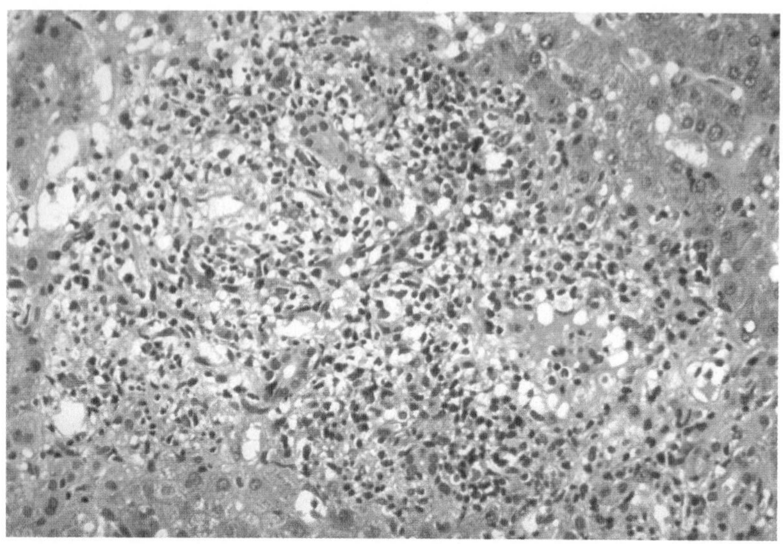

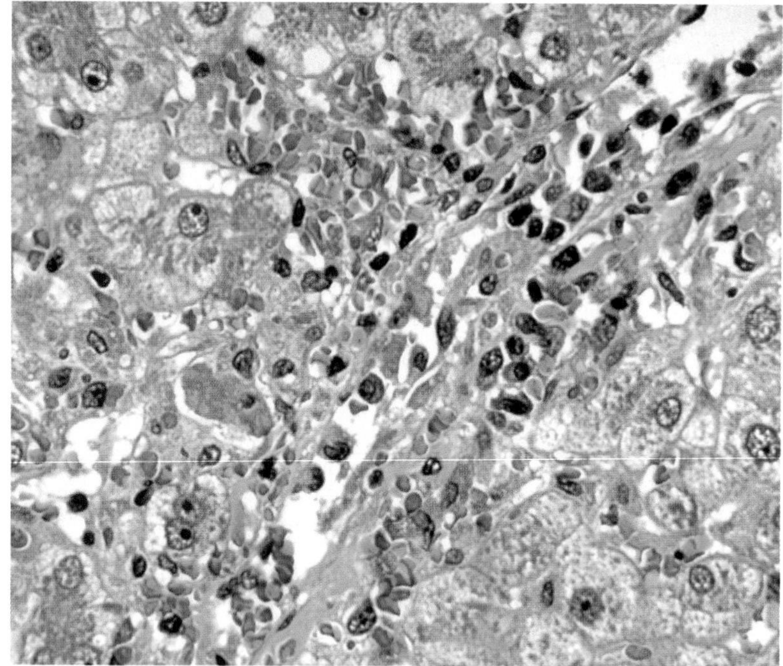

FIGURE 38.14 Acute rejection of a liver transplant. (*A*) A portal tract is expanded by a polymorphous inflammatory infiltrate consisting of large and small lymphocytes, plasma cells, macrophages, and neutrophils. The bile ducts (*arrows*) are damaged and inflamed. (*B*) A central vein from the same biopsy exhibits endothelialitis, characterized by swollen endothelial cells and infiltrating lymphocytes. (From Thung SN, Gerber MA. Histopathology of liver transplantation. In Fabry TL, Klion FM [eds]: *Guide to liver transplantation.* New York: Igaku-Shoin Medical Publishers, 1988.)

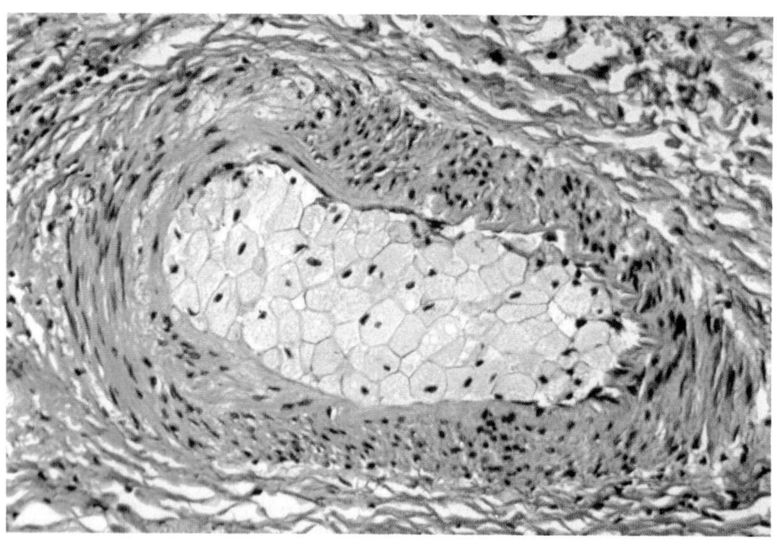

FIGURE 38.15 Arterial lesion of chronic hepatic rejection. Subintimal foam cells, intimal sclerosis, and myointimal hyperplasia obliterate the arterial lumen. (From Rubin E, Farber JL. *Pathology*, 3rd edition. Philadelphia: Lippincott Williams & Wilkins, 1999.)

RESULTS

The patient survival rate following liver transplantation in the United States at 1 year is more than 85% for adults and nearly 90% for children. Patients who survive the first year following a liver transplantation experience approximately a 3% annual mortality rate thereafter, so 3-year survival rates for adults and children are currently 78% and 83%, respectively.

The most important predictors of survival following liver transplantation are whether the patient has previously undergone transplantation and whether the patient was in the intensive care unit at the time of transplantation. Although not as important as the condition of the patient at transplantation, the cause of liver failure is also an important determinant of success. Five-year survival varies from approximately 60% for patients transplanted for malignancy to 70% for patients transplanted for viral and alcoholic cirrhosis. The best 5-year survival rates of around 80% are seen with patients transplanted for metabolic liver disease, biliary atresia, and cholestatic liver diseases (primary biliary cirrhosis and primary sclerosing cholangitis).[37] The volume of liver transplants performed at a given transplant center is also associated with patient survival, with higher-volume programs exhibiting higher adjusted overall patients survival rates.[38]

KEY POINTS

- **The main indication for liver transplantation is end-stage liver disease, defined as the clinical scenario in which a pathological process or multiple processes have resulted in a damaged liver that has minimal function and no potential for recovery.**
- **The Organ Procurement and Transplantation Network uses the Model of End-stage Liver Disease score as a method of prioritizing liver transplant recipients. The MELD score is an integer value based on three objective laboratory studies: creatinine, bilirubin, and the INR.**
- **The degree of preoperative debilitation and the complexity of the operative procedure make complications following hepatic transplantation very common.**
- **Approximately 5% to 10% of transplanted livers function so poorly in the immediate postoperative period that death is likely in the absence of retransplantation, a condition referred to as primary nonfunction of the allograft.**
- **For reasons that are not understood, liver transplant recipients require less immune suppression than patients with other types of allografts, such as heart, lung, and kidney recipients.**
- **Typical acute rejection in liver transplant recipients is usually cell mediated.**
- **Chronic rejection is characterized by relentless immune attack on small bile ducts. Histologically, small bile ducts are obliterated or completely absent, termed *vanishing bile duct syndrome.***
- **The patient survival rate following liver transplantation in the United States at 1 year is more than 85% for adults and nearly 90% for children.**

References

1. **Starzl TE, Groth CG, Brettschneider L, et al. Orthotopic homotransplantations of the human liver. *Ann Surg.* 1968;168:392–415.**
2. **Calne RY, Rolles K, White DJGG, et al. Cyclosporine A initially as the only immunosuppressant in 34 recipients of cadaveric organs: 32 kidneys, 2 pancreases, and 2 livers. *Lancet* 1979;2:1033–1036.**
3. Trotter JF, Wachs M, Everson GT, et al. Adult-to-adult transplantation of the right hepatic lobe from a living donor. *N Engl J Med.* 2002; 346: 1074–1082.
4. **Kamath PS, Wiesner RH, Malinchoc M, et al. A model to predict survival in patients with end-stage liver disease. *Hepatology* 2001;33:464–470.**
5. Freeman RB Jr, Wiesner RH, Roberts JP, et al. Improving liver allocation: MELD and PELD. *Am J Transplant.* 2004;4 (suppl 9):114–131.
6. Sylvestre PB, Batts KP, Burgart LJ, et al. Recurrence of primary biliary cirrhosis after liver transplantation: Histologic estimate of incidence and natural history. *Liver Transpl.* 2003;9:1086–1093.
7. Kayler LK, Rasmussen CS, Dykstra DM, et al. Liver transplantation in children with metabolic disorders in the United States. *Am J Transplant.* 2003;3(3):334–339.
8. Lee WM. Acute liver failure. *N Engl J Med.* 1993;329(25):1862–1872.
9. Shakil AO, Kramer D, Mazariegos GV, et al. Acute liver failure: clinical features, outcome analysis, and applicability of prognostic criteria. *Liver Transpl.* 2000;6(2):163–169.
10. Mazzaferro V, Regalia E, Doci R, et al. Liver transplantation for the treatment of small hepatocellular carcinomas in patients with cirrhosis. *N Engl J Med.* 1996;334:693–700.
11. Wanless IR, Lentz JS. Fatty liver hepatitis (steatohepatitis) and obesity: an autopsy study with analysis of risk factors. *Hepatology* 1990;12(5);1106–1110.
12. Sass DA, Chang P, Chopra KB. Nonalcoholic fatty liver disease: a clinical review. *Dig Dis Sci.* 2005;50(1):171–180.
13. Lerut J, Ciccarelli O, Roggen F, et al. Cavocaval adult liver transplantation and retransplantation without venovenous bypass and without portocaval shunting: a prospective feasibility study in adult liver transplantation. *Transplantation* 2003;75(10):1740–4175.
14. Ong TH, Strong R, Zahari Z, et al. The management of difficult abdominal closure after pediatric liver transplantation. *J Pediatr Surg.* 1996; 31(2):295–296.
15. Otte JB, de Ville de Goyet J, et al. The concept and technique of the split liver in clinical transplantation. *Surgery* 1990;107(6):605–612.
16. **Broelsch CE, Stevens LH, Whitington PF. The use of reduced-size liver transplants in children, including spit livers and living related liver transplants. *Eur J Pediatri Surg.* 1991;1(3):166–171.**
17. Goss JA, Yersiz H, Shackleton CR, et al. In situ splitting of the cadaveric liver for transplantation. *Transplantation* 1997;64(6):871–877.
18. Humar A, Khwaja K, Sielaff TD, et al. Technique of split-liver transplant for two adult recipients. *Liver Transpl.* 2002;8(8):725–729.
19. Toso C, Ris F, Mentha G, et al. Potential impact of in situ liver splitting on the number of available grafts. *Transplantation* 2002;74(2):222–226.
20. **Merion RM, Rush SH, Dykstra DM, et al. Predicted lifetimes for adult and pediatric split liver versus adult whole liver transplant recipients. *Am J Transplant.* 2004;4(11):1792–1797.**
21 Marcos A, Fisher RA, Ham JM, et al. Right lobe living donor liver transplantation. *Transplantation* 1999;68(6):798–803.
22. Dumortier J, Czyglik O, Poncet G, et al. Eversion thrombectomy for portal vein thrombosis during liver transplantation. *Am J Transplant.* 2002;2(10):934–938.
23. Tzakis AG, Kirkegaard P, Pinna AD, et al. Liver transplantation with cavoportal hemitransposition in the presence of diffuse portal vein thrombosis. *Transplantation* 1998;65(5):619–624.
24. Charco R, Margarit C, Lopez-Talavera JC, et al. Outcome and hepatic hemodynamics in liver transplant patients with portal vein arterialization. *Am J Transplant.* 2001;1(2):146–151.
25. Strasberg SM, Howard TK, Molmenti EP, et al. Selecting the donor liver: risk factors for poor function after orthotopic liver transplantation. *Hepatology* 1994;20(4 Pt 1):829–838.
26. Feller RB, Waugh RC, Selby WS, et al. Biliary strictures after liver transplantation: clinical picture, correlates and outcomes. *J Gastroenterol Hepatol.* 1996;11(1):21–25.
27. Oh CK, Pelletier SJ, Sawyer RG, et al. Uni- and multi-variate analysis of risk factors for early and late hepatic artery thrombosis after liver transplantation. *Transplantation* 2001;71(6):767–772.
28. Abbasoglu O, Levy MF, Vodapally MS, et al. Hepatic artery stenosis after liver transplantation—incidence, presentation, treatment, and long term outcome. *Transplantation* 1997;63(2):250–255.
29. Bhattacharjya S, Gunson BK, Mirza DF, et al. Delayed hepatic artery thrombosis in adult orthotopic liver transplantation—a 12-year experience. *Transplantation* 2001;71(11):1592–1596.
30. Pungpapong S, Manzarbeitia C, Ortiz J, et al. Cigarette smoking is associated with an increased incidence of vascular complications after liver transplantation. *Liver Transpl.* 2002;8(7):582–57l.
31. Furuta S, Ikegami T, Nakazawa Y, et al. Hepatic artery reconstruction in living donor liver transplantation from the microsurgeon's point of view. *Liver Transpl.* 1997;3(4):388–393.
32. Stahl RL, Duncan A, Hooks MA, et al. A hypercoagulable state follows orthotopic liver transplantation. *Hepatology* 1990;12(3 Pt 1):553–558.
33. Parrilla P, Sanchez-Bueno F, Figueras J, et al. Analysis of the complications of the piggy-back technique in 1,112 liver transplants. *Transplantation* 1999;67(9):1214–1217.
34. Borsa JJ, Daly CP, Fontaine AB, et al. Treatment of inferior vena cava anastomotic stenoses with the Wallstent endoprosthesis after orthotopic liver transplantation. *Journal of Vascular and Interventional Radiology* 1999;10(1):17–22.
35. Frazer CK, Gupta A. Stenosis of the hepatic vein anastomosis after liver transplantation: treatment with a heparin-coated metal stent. *Australas Radiol.* 2002;46(4):422–425.
36. Wiesner RH, Batts KP, Krom RA. Evolving concepts in the diagnosis, pathogenesis, and treatment of chronic hepatic allograft rejection. *Liver Transpl Surg.* 1999;5:388.
37. Brown RS, Rush SH, Rosen HR, et al. Liver and intestine transplantation. *Am J Transplant.* 2004;4 (suppl 9):81–92.
38. Axelrod DA, Guidinger MK, McCullough KP, et al. Association of center volume with outcome after liver and kidney transplantation. *Am J Transplant.* 2004;4(6):920–927.

CHAPTER 39 ■ CARDIAC TRANSPLANTATION

RICHARD N. PIERSON III

Since 1964, cardiac transplantation has evolved from a sensational, perilous experiment to become conventional therapy for end-stage heart disease, the paradigm of successful but expensive high-tech medicine. This remarkable transformation stemmed from fundamental surgical innovations supported by incremental improvements in the diagnosis and management of common problems. Current challenges revolve around donor supply and allocation, improving longterm outcomes, developing alternative therapies, and related ethical issues.

HISTORICAL PERSPECTIVE

Based on significant contributions by many surgical pioneers,[1–8] the first clinical heart transplant was performed in 1964 by Hardy et al.,[9] who attempted to salvage a man dying from cardiogenic shock by replacing his heart with the heart of a chimpanzee. Then, before the concept of brain death achieved wide social or legal acceptance, in 1967 Barnard et al. captured the imagination of the world with the first operative survival, using the heart of a resuscitated cadaveric donor.[10] This case, and many others that were performed shortly thereafter, demonstrated not only the physiologic capacity of the transplanted human heart allograft to support the recipient's circulation but also the difficulty of managing subsequent immunologic and infectious complications. After a worldwide flurry of activity, generally dismal outcomes at many prominent cardiac surgery centers made clear the need for more thoughtful approaches to what was clearly a difficult constellation of problems beyond effective circulatory support.

A few pioneering programs persisted in cautious clinical application supported by parallel laboratory investigation. Recognizing the need for a more sensitive and specific diagnostic technique to diagnose rejection, Caves et al.[11] developed the technique of transvenous endomyocardial biopsy. Frequent, representative surveillance sampling of the graft allowed early detection of pathogenic host immune responses. Perivascular lymphocytic infiltrates were found to accurately diagnose acute cellular rejection in its presymptomatic phase; when detected early, rejection usually responded to enhanced immunosuppression. Equally important, when rejection was not seen, immunosuppression could be tapered to minimize drug toxicities and reduce the incidence of opportunistic infection. Coupled with important advances in the diagnosis, prevention, and treatment of infectious pathogens in immunosuppressed patients and in selection and management of patients with end-stage heart failure, patient survival at 1 year improved gradually, from about 20% in the 1960s to approximately 70% by 1980.[12]

Even as recently as the early 1980s, however, when rejection persisted or recurred despite high-dose steroids, alternative treatments (total lymphoid irradiation, intramuscular antilymphocyte preparations, thoracic duct ligation, splenectomy) were often toxic or invasive and accompanied by a high incidence of major short- and long-term complications. In this context the discovery and clinical development of cyclosporin A catalyzed the next major improvement in outcomes.[13,14] Because its primary mechanism of action (inhibition of calcineurin-dependent cellular activation events) and toxicity profile were fundamentally different from those of azathioprine, an antimitotic agent, or antiinflammatory steroids, combination "triple" therapy allowed each agent to be used more safely. Meanwhile antithymocyte and antilymphocyte preparations were adapted for safe intravenous use, either as prophylactic induction therapy ("quadruple therapy") or as treatment for steroid-resistant rejection. Based primarily on these pharmacologic innovations in the regulation of the immune response, expected 1-year survival following heart transplant gradually rose from about 70% to almost 90% between 1980 and 2000[15] in older and sicker recipients.[16,17]

CANDIDATE EVALUATION

End-stage heart failure is the primary indication for heart transplantation in adults, with coronary artery occlusive disease and myopathy of various etiologies each accounting for about 45% of cases. Congenital heart disease is the primary indication for infants, whereas myopathy predominates in older children.

The heart transplant evaluation process seeks to identify patients for whom no other reasonable treatment options exist and who are at higher risk of death without transplant than with it, while excluding patients whose comorbid conditions are likely to significantly limit length or quality of life. In 1993, a National Institutes of Health consensus conference developed recipient selection guidelines for cardiac transplantation, based on objective criteria known to predict poor outcome without transplantation;[18] these guidelines (Tables 39.1 to 39.3) continue to evolve in the context of improving heart failure therapy.[19,20] Among patients with heart failure symptoms, maximal oxygen consumption is more sensitive and specific than ejection fraction in gauging prognosis, and blunted cardiac output response to exercise may further stratify patients into high- and low-risk groups.[19]

When no alternative management strategy is available and no clear survival advantage is apparent for transplantation, quality of life and other subjective factors are weighed. Contemporary studies defining relative risks, along with basic considerations in the medical management of end-stage heart failure, are well summarized in recent reviews.[21–23]

DONOR SELECTION AND MANAGEMENT

The ideal donor is a young, previously healthy individual without cardiac disease or hypertension, who is well matched in size to the intended recipient and whose hemodynamics

TABLE 39.1 INDICATIONS/CONTRAINDICATIONS

INDICATIONS FOR HEART TRANSPLANT

General Indications

End-stage heart disease without lower-risk alternative

Absence of any noncardiac condition likely to:

- Limit survival independent of cardiac function
- Preclude safe administration of adequate immunosuppression
- Predispose to life-threatening infection with immunosuppression

Specific Indications

Heart failure of various etiologies

- Myopathy: ischemic, idiopathic, viral, familial, restrictive
- Valvular
- Congenital
- Failed transplant
  - Early: primary nonfunction, acute rejection
  - Late: cardiac allograft vasculopathy

Other Indications

- Angina not amenable to revascularization
- Arrhythmia, failed conventional therapy
- Hypertrophic cardiomyopathy
- Restrictive cardiomyopathy
- Primary cardiac tumor (completely resectable)

TABLE 39.2

SELECTION CRITERIA FOR STRATIFYING RISK AND SURVIVAL

Survival Benefit Established

- Maximal oxygen consumption <10 mL/kg/min
- Class IV chronic heart failure symptoms despite maximal medical therapy
- Mechanical circulatory support required
- Refractory angina without therapeutic alternative
- Refractory ventricular arrhythmia without alternative

Survival Benefit Likely

- Maximal oxygen consumption 10–14 mL/kg/min with blunted cardiac output response to exercise
- Instability of fluid balance or renal function despite documented compliance
- Ejection fraction <20% with class III heart failure symptoms on maximal medical therapy

Survival Benefit Not Established

- Maximal oxygen consumption 10–14 mL/kg/min with preserved cardiac output response to exercise
- Maximal oxygen consumption >14 mL/kg/min, ejection fraction <20% without other indication
- History of chronic heart failure or arrhythmia controlled with medical therapy
- Quality-of-life considerations may influence selection of recipients for whom survival benefit is not established.

TABLE 39.3 INDICATIONS/CONTRAINDICATIONS

CONTRAINDICATIONS TO CARDIAC TRANSPLANTATION

Absolute Contraindications

- High pulmonary vascular resistance*
  - Transpulmonary gradient >15, fixed
  - Pulmonary vascular resistance index >5–6 Woods units
- Irreversible renal insufficiency (CrCl <40)*
- Active infection (viral or bacterial)
- Active peptic ulcer disease
- Diabetes with end-organ damage
  - Renal insufficiency, neuropathy, retinopathy
- Symptomatic extracardiac vascular disease
  - Cerebrovascular obstructive disease with recent transient ischemic attack, cardiovascular accident
  - Pulmonary veno-occlusive disease with claudication, rest pain, or tissue loss
- Current malignancy, or recent treatment (<2 years) for life-threatening malignancy
- Disease of another organ system that would probably limit survival
  - Established cirrhosis, cardiac or other etiology
- Symptomatic chronic obstructive pulmonary disease; chronic bronchitis
- High risk for inability to comply with complex medical regimen
  - Not firmly committed to transplantation
  - Inadequate cognitive capacity to comply with postoperative regimen, coupled with inadequate compensatory social support
  - Documented psychiatric instability
  - Recurrent drug or alcohol abuse
  - Demonstrated noncompliance with therapeutic recommendations

Relative Contraindications

- Age older than 65 years
- Established renal failure
- Diabetes without end-organ disease
- Asymptomatic or previously treated extracardiac vascular disease
- Chronic obstructive pulmonary disease with forced expiratory volume in 1 second or carbon monoxide diffusion in the lung <60% predicted without referable symptoms
- Remote malignancy, in remission (>4 years with no evidence of disease)
- High pulmonary vascular resistance, reversible
- Disease of another organ system that would limit quality of life
- Difficulty complying with complex medical regimen

*On optimal medical therapy.

have been carefully managed during the evolution of their lethal central nervous system injury. Some programs have advocated use of older donors, donors who may transmit infection or malignancy to the recipient, and grafts with hypertensive myocardial hypertrophy for particular recipients.[24] Some aggressive programs have even proposed that hemodynamically significant coronary stenoses can be bypassed at the time of transplant.[25] These approaches to donor selection are associated with less favorable short- and long-term outcomes,[15,26,27] but the increased risk may be considered acceptable for patients for whom the short-term prognosis is poor without transplant.

Donor management requires skill and experience to successfully address the complex physiologic perturbations associated with brain death. Reflex hypertensive and hypotensive responses to intracranial pressure changes, fluid and electrolyte imbalances consequent to the diabetes insipidus from pituitary death, and additional stresses related to hemorrhage, trauma, and surgery often cause hemodynamic and metabolic instability, which may injure a previously healthy heart. The neurohumoral *milieu* of central nervous system catastrophe may also adversely affect other fundamental cell regulatory functions, such as those dependent on thyroid hormone. Despite controversy regarding the mechanisms involved, thyroid hormone is often administered to the donor as a continuous infusion, hoping to correct a "sick euthyroid" syndrome and optimize cardiac metabolism prior to explant. Although evidence to date is largely anecdotal, inotrope requirements can often be reduced after thyroid infusion is begun, and donor hemodynamic lability is less common, suggesting improved cardiac and vasoregulatory function.[28,29]

Cardiac echocardiography has become a standard component of donor assessment, to measure ejection fraction and to exclude structural abnormalities or hypertrophy suggestive of hypertensive myopathy. Cardiac catheterization may be requested for donors older than 45 years, and especially for donors with a strong family history of coronary artery disease, for donors who smoke, or when regional wall motion abnormalities are appreciated on echocardiography.

MATCHING DONOR TO RECIPIENT

Once a potential donor is identified, priority among blood-type-compatible recipients is determined first by relative severity of illness ("status") and then by length of time on the waiting list among recipients at each status in the donor's geographic area. This information is currently tracked and collated by a central, national registry operated by the United Network for Organ Sharing. The heart is first offered to the program whose candidate has seniority on the list and whose registered height and weight range include the potential donor. Donor inotrope requirements and functional assessment, recipient pulmonary vascular resistance, possible infection transmission risks (known hepatitis or potential HIV exposure in the donor), and other logistical considerations (expected graft ischemic time) influence the recipient team's decision regarding acceptance of an organ for an individual patient. If the first program declines the offer for the first patient, the process is repeated for the patient next on the list until the heart is accepted.

Tissue typing, the time-consuming process by which donor and recipient are matched for shared transplant antigens, is not currently used for hearts. The probability is low of identifying a "close" match among the relatively small number of blood-type-compatible potential recipients within the geographic radius (usually less than 1,500 miles) defined by a 4-hour projected ischemic time. In addition, the demonstrated benefit of partial human leukocyte antigen matching is small relative to the added risk of prolonged graft ischemia, a risk augmented by increasing donor age.[30]

RECIPIENT MANAGEMENT BEFORE TRANSPLANT

The medical therapy of patients awaiting transplantation has improved significantly over the past decade, centered around aggressive afterload reduction and diuresis, anticoagulation, and beta blockade.[18–20] This trend, coupled with improved mechanical support, has reduced the mortality rate for patients awaiting transplant. As waiting lists have grown faster than the donor pool, the average time waiting has similarly escalated and cardiac decompensation among patients on the waiting list is frequent. In most areas of the country, the majority of hearts go to patients who are sick enough to require hospitalization for intensive diuresis and intravenous inotrope administration.[27]

When inotropic therapy proves inadequate, as gauged by progressive deterioration in renal and other end-organ function, temporary intraaortic balloon pump counterpulsation and mechanical ventilation can stabilize some patients. These interventions are associated with important risks; the relative risk of death is increased threefold in patients who are ventilator dependent at the time of transplant.[15]

In contrast, mechanical circulatory support using ventricular assist devices has emerged as an effective bridging strategy. Although some bridged patients incur serious complications (stroke, renal or hepatic failure, systemic infection) that preclude transplantation, about two thirds are successfully transplanted, with excellent outcomes relative to patients not requiring this intervention. Patients with biventricular failure can be supported with either implanted or paracorporeal pulsatile left ventricular support, with or without the addition of temporary right heart support.[31] Various total artificial heart devices can be implanted in place of the native heart and have been applied successfully in small numbers.[31] This approach is most likely to find a niche as an alternative to heart transplantation in patients who cannot be supported with a left ventricular assist device, such as those with fixed pulmonary hypertension. Intravascular axial flow devices and other nonpulsatile assist systems have shown promise in clinical trials.[32,33]

HEART PROCUREMENT

Cardiac allograft protection depends primarily on hypothermia, which reduces myocardial energy requirements while the heart graft has no nutritive coronary blood flow. Other important principles include avoidance of distention and warm ischemia in both the donor and the recipient and induction of diastolic (flaccid) cardiac arrest. These goals are accomplished by interrupting systemic venous return for decompression, placing a clamp across the distal ascending aorta, and infusing a hyperkalemic preservation solution proximal to the clamp and thus selectively into the coronary arteries. Both the inferior vena cava and left atrium are incised ("vented") to prevent distention of either ventricle. Some preservation solutions incorporating free radical scavenging molecules or other cytoprotective agents are associated with improved early graft function.[34,35]

Every effort is made to limit the ischemic interval, the time between initial interruption of coronary flow by aortic cross-clamping in the donor and removal of the cross-clamp in the recipient, to less than 4 hours. Although laboratory studies and isolated clinical reports suggest that good results may be expected with storage times of 8 hours or more using various preservation solutions, increased ischemic time remains a strong and important independent risk factor for poor recipient outcome.[15]

OPERATIVE RECIPIENT MANAGEMENT

Timing of the recipient operation requires careful coordination with the procurement team. Anesthesia is induced after the donor heart is visually inspected and found suitable. Venous access is obtained, which will permit rapid volume

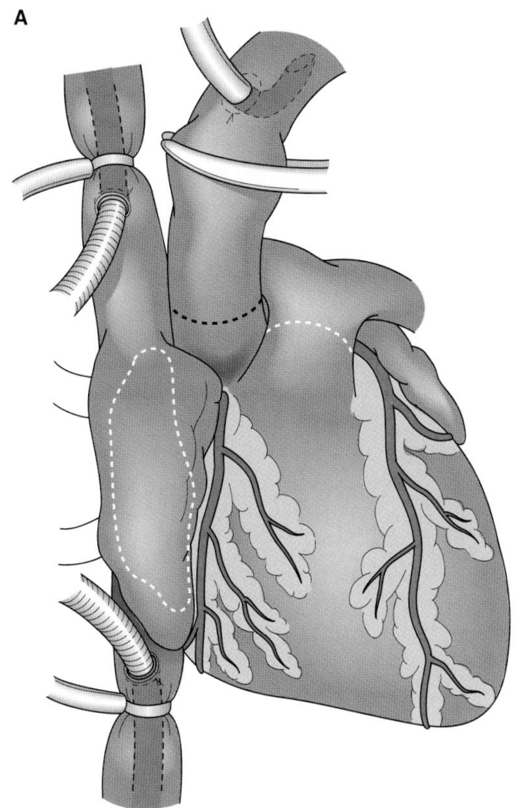

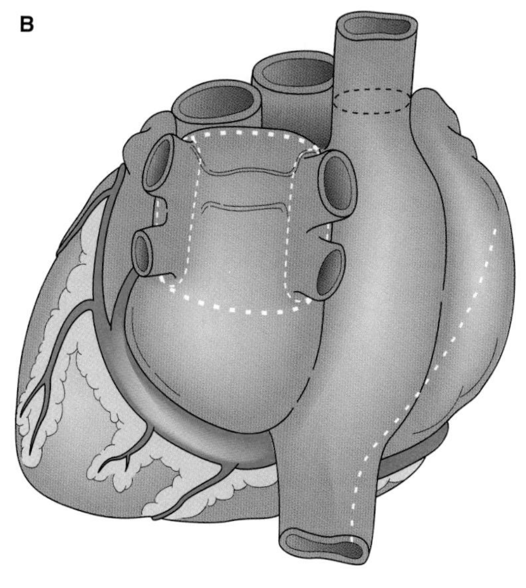

FIGURE 39.1 Native cardiectomy and donor graft preparation. (*A*) Recipient pericardium after institution of cardiopulmonary bypass and ascending aortic occlusion, with caval snares secured. The diseased native heart can then be safely excised by transecting the recipient aorta and pulmonary artery, and the atria divided as appropriate for the intended implant technique. Shown is the right atrial incision for the traditional Lower/Shumway right atrial cuff. (*B*) Posterior view of the explanted donor heart, indicating various incisions used for atrial cuff preparation. Donor atrial cuff incisions made in preparation for traditional Lower/Shumway biatrial implant are indicated by the heavy gray dashed line. The superior vena cava (SVC) is ligated or oversewn. Right and left pulmonary vein (light gray dashed line) and superior vena cava (black dashed line) incisions are indicated for the total atrioventricular implant technique. For the bicaval technique, the donor SVC and inferior vena cava (IVC) are retained as for the total atrioventricular technique (black dashed line), and the donor left atrial cuff trimmed as for the traditional biatrial approach (heavy gray dashed line).

resuscitation and invasive cardiac monitoring after the new heart is implanted. Prior cardiac surgery may complicate coordination of operative timing and is associated with increased risk of bleeding.

If appropriate, coumadin effect is reversed with fresh frozen plasma and vitamin K. Aprotinin or epsilon aminocaproic acid is often used to inhibit fibrinolysis and prevent coagulopathic bleeding after prior cardiac surgery or associated with hepatic congestion. Increased inotropic infusion, antiarrhythmic agents, or mechanical circulatory support may be required to maintain adequate systemic perfusion prior to institution of cardiopulmonary bypass.

Vascular access for bypass is accomplished by cannulation of the superior and inferior vena cavae so as to completely divert systemic venous blood to the cardiopulmonary bypass circuit. The ascending aorta or common femoral artery is used for arterial return from the circuit to the patient. Technical misadventures, such as entry into the heart or great vessels before bypass is established or induction of ventricular arrhythmias, are more common with reoperative procedures and can greatly complicate the intraoperative course and postoperative management.

Once the proximate arrival of the donor heart is ensured, the recipient is placed on bypass and cooled. Snares are secured around the caval cannulae, the ascending aorta is clamped, and the native heart is excised (Fig. 39.1A). Vascular cuffs, which are appropriate for implantation of the donor heart, are preserved (Figs. 39.2A, 39.3A, 39.4A). The donor heart is then prepared according to the implant technique to be used (Fig. 39.1B).

Implant techniques and the sequence of vascular anastomosis vary widely between surgeons, as do strategies used to protect the ischemic organ during implantation. The biatrial orthotopic heart transplant technique is simple, easy to teach, and still used by many surgeons (Fig. 39.2).[8] The donor atria are spatulated open, trimmed if necessary, and laid over the recipient's atrial remnants. The left atrial suture line is everted to achieve endothelial apposition and to avoid leaving epicardial fat or muscle exposed in the lumen as a potential nidus for thromboemboli. Sinoatrial node dysfunction can usually be prevented by keeping the donor right atriotomy anterior to the sinoatrial node and its blood supply (Fig. 39.2B) and by optimizing graft preservation.[35] Even if most of the dilated native atrium is excised, atrioventricular valve annular geometry may be distorted, causing regurgitation, or the area around the sinus node may be placed under tension, leading to atrial arrhythmias or sinus node dysfunction.

During the 1990s, these considerations led to evaluation of alternate atrial anastomotic techniques, including bicaval right atrial connections (Fig. 39.3) and total atrioventricular

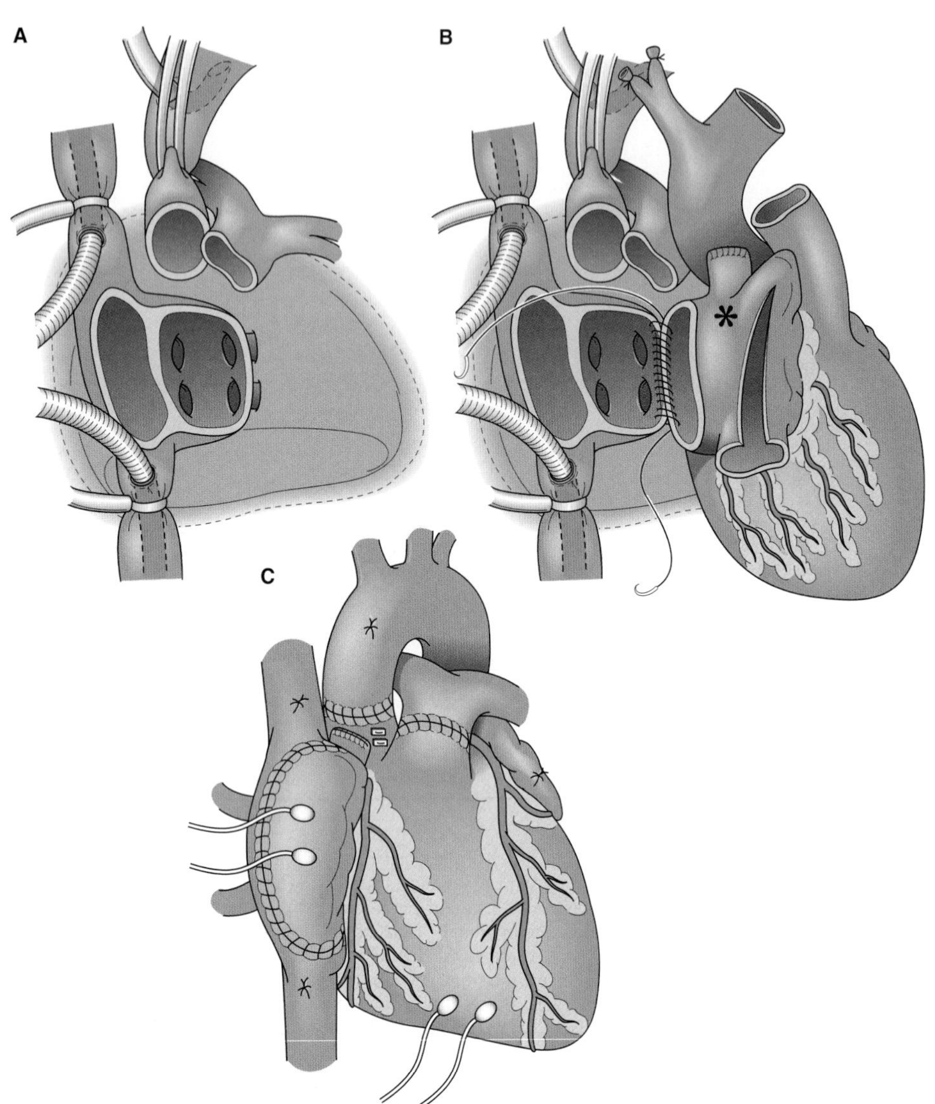

FIGURE 39.2 Traditional Lower/Shumway biatrial technique. (*A*) Recipient cuffs, prepared for bicaval atrial implant technique. After completion of the left atrial anastomosis (*B*), the right atrial (RA) cuffs are joined. Care is taken to avoid carrying the right atrial incision or suture line close to the donor sinoatrial node, at the SVC/RA junction (asterisk). (C) Appearance of the operative field after completion of great vessel anastomoses, weaning from cardiopulmonary bypass, and decannulation.

replacement (two caval and two pulmonary vein anastomoses) (Fig. 39.4). In a prospective, randomized trial (bicaval)[36] and several retrospective analyses,[37,38] the incidence of atrial arrhythmias and atrioventricular valve regurgitation were reduced and hemodynamic results and survival were improved with either the bicaval or total atrioventricular technique.

Independent of whether the aorta or pulmonary artery connection is performed first, the anterior aspect of the pulmonary artery anastomosis is usually left open or vented, to allow decompression of the right heart after reperfusion (Fig. 39.3C). The size mismatch between donor and recipient aortas is often dramatic but can usually be accommodated by beveling the smaller vessel (usually the more pliable donor) to increase its effective circumference and by distributing the discrepancy evenly over the length of each anastomosis. Occasionally it is necessary to tailor down the larger vessel or to replace an aneurysmal ascending aorta with donor tissue or a prosthetic graft. Functional pulmonary stenosis is avoided by trimming back both donor and recipient sufficiently to prevent redundancy.

An alternative "heterotopic" implantation technique places a second heart in the circulation, in parallel with the retained native heart.[39] In principle, leaving the native heart affords protection in the event that the graft fails. The operation is technically demanding, usually produces compressive atelectasis in the right lung, and is associated with a high risk of stroke, perhaps because of stasis of blood in the native heart.[40] Notwithstanding these problems, this surgical approach may be considered for patients with high pulmonary vascular resistance unresponsive to vasodilators and may in the future also find a role in the initial application of cardiac xenografts.

After completion of the anastomoses, the heart is reperfused and allowed to resume contracting without being required to function as a pump ("rested") as the recipient is rewarmed. Atrial and ventricular pacing wires are placed. Cardiac output of the denervated transplant is highly dependent on rate. In addition, the shorter cardiac filling time associated with higher heart rate prevents graft distention. Isoproterenol is initiated prior to weaning from bypass at a dose of 0.005 to 0.02 mg/kg/min and titrated to achieve a heart rate of about 110 beats per minute.

Patients with high preoperative pulmonary vascular resistance may be particularly difficult to wean from cardiopulmonary bypass, even with excellent function of the donor heart, because the "normal" donor right ventricle may acutely dilate and fail when confronted by a high-resistance pulmonary vascular bed. Resting the recently ischemic heart on cardiopulmonary bypass, establishing a stable sinus or atrioventricular sequentially paced rhythm, instituting inotropic support, and intraaortic balloon counterpulsation

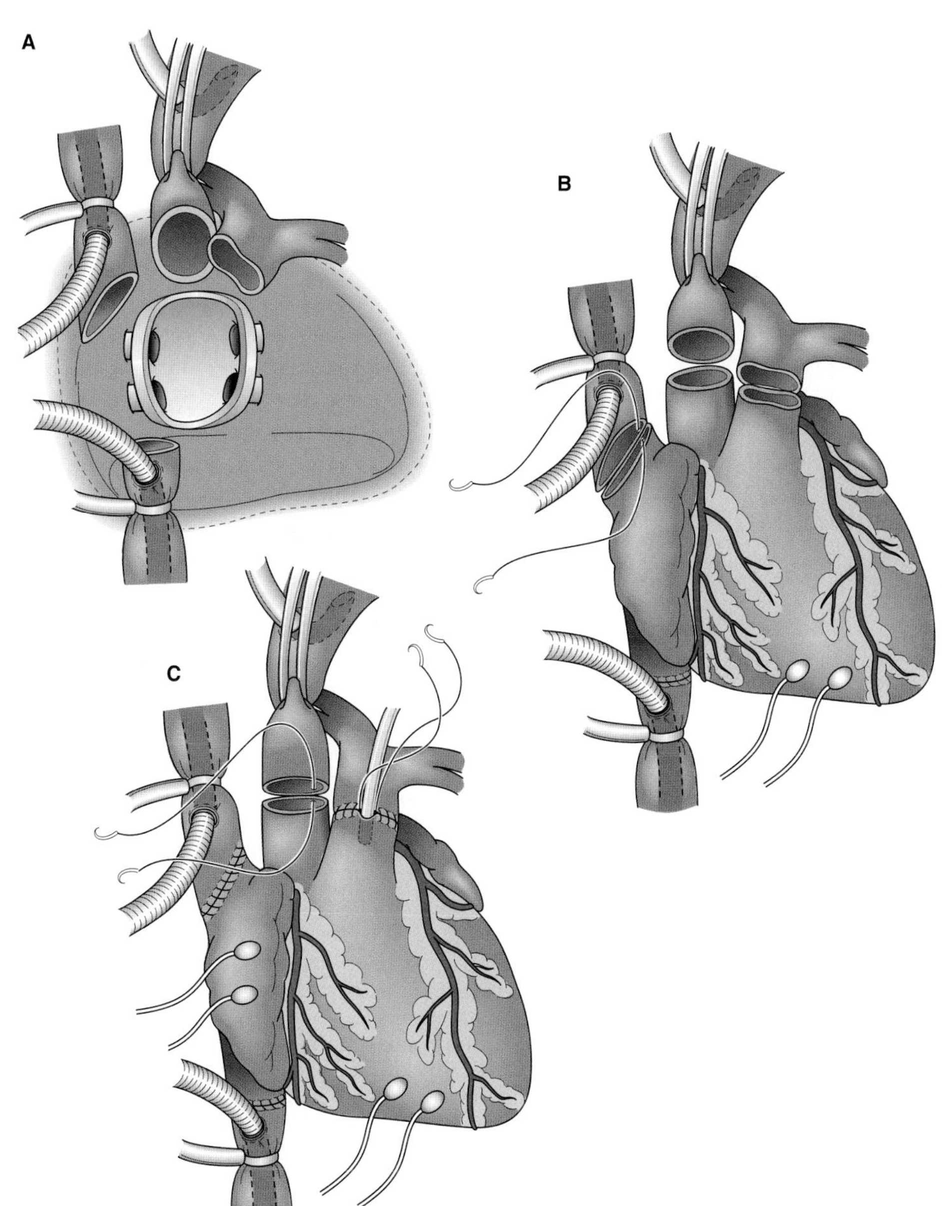

FIGURE 39.3 Bicaval right atrial implant technique. (*A*) During explantation of the native heart, the interatrial septum may be excised, for end-to-end anastomosis of the cavae (*B*), or left in place, allowing the back walls of the donor cavae to be laid into those of the recipient. (*C*) Technique for pulmonary artery venting through an opening in the anterior aspect of this anastomosis, which is useful for deairing and decompressing the right heart. Alternatively, the aorta may be anastomosed earlier in the operation, to minimized graft ischemic time.

are useful in managing this problem. Traditional pharmacologic approaches to reducing pulmonary vascular resistance, such as prostaglandins E_1 or I_2 and sodium nitroprusside, may cause transpulmonary shunting of deoxygenated blood; these agents also reduce systemic vascular resistance and thus coronary perfusion pressure. Inhaled nitric oxide selectively dilates the pulmonary vascular bed before being rapidly inactivated by hemoglobin in the blood. Many surgeons have found this technique very helpful to selectively reduce pulmonary vascular resistance without adverse effects on oxygenation or heart function, and this drug has recently been approved by the U.S. Food and Drug Administration for clinical use.[41] Poor function of either or both ventricles may necessitate institution of mechanical support as a bridge to graft recovery or to retransplantation.

Postoperatively, ventilator and inotropic support is weaned, immunosuppression is instituted, and diuretic and antihypertensive agents are initiated as necessary. Isoproterenol is continued for about 5 days and replaced with theophylline if needed to sustain a resting heart rate over 70 beats per minute. The first surveillance endomyocardial biopsy is performed 7 to 10 days after surgery and biopsy is repeated as an outpatient procedure about every 2 weeks for the first 3 months. Patient and caregiver education with regard to medication schedules and physiologic monitoring facilitate early discharge for patients without complications. Biologic monitoring of peripheral blood gene or protein expression and electrical approaches to monitor the immune response to the graft have shown promise to supplant routine invasive monitoring.[42,43]

IMMUNOSUPPRESSION

The goal of immunosuppressive therapy is to prevent immune-mediated injury to the graft while minimizing associated complications, including opportunistic infection. Most programs employ a "triple-drug" regimen, including a calcineurin inhibitor, an antimitotic agent, and steroids. This approach allows each individual drug to be used within its therapeutic window (Table 39.4). Some centers add antibody "induction" with anti-CD3, polyclonal antilymphocyte serum,

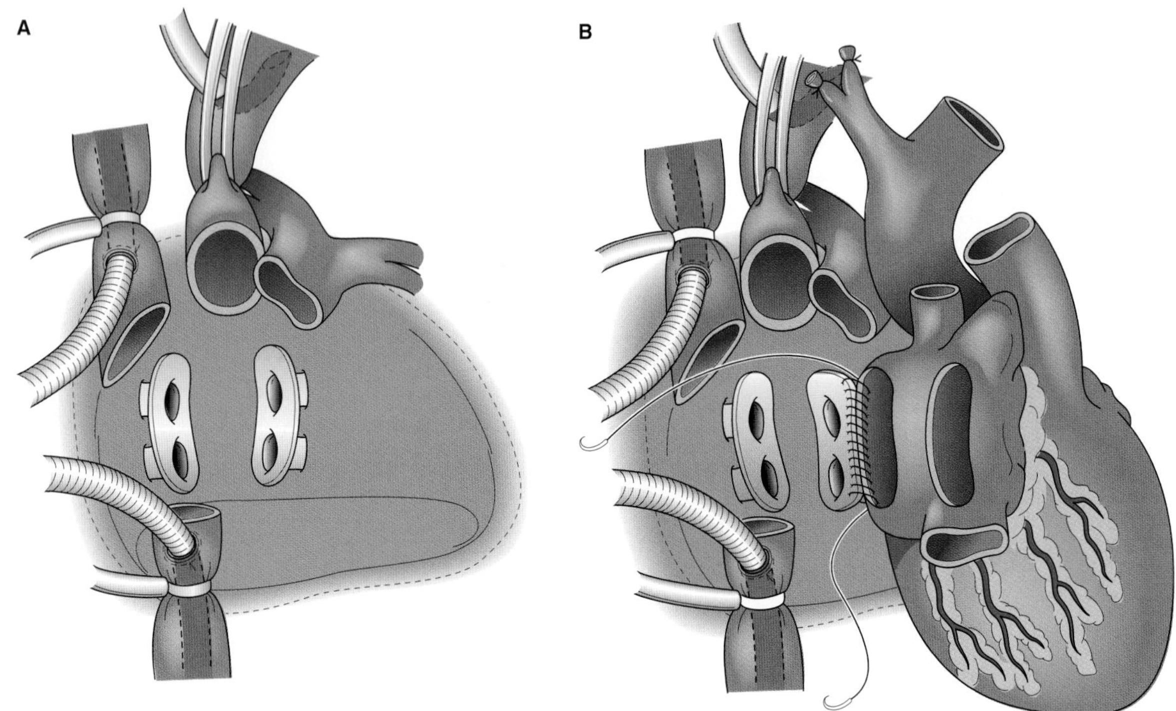

FIGURE 39.4 Total atrioventricular transplant technique. (*A*) Recipient pericardial well after preparation of bilateral pulmonary vein pedicles and caval cuffs, for total atrioventricular heart transplant. (*B*) Construction of left pulmonary vein anastomosis. As with other left atrial anastomotic approaches, atrial walls or vein cuffs are everted to minimize exposure of thrombogenic fat or muscle to the blood.

or anti-interleukin-2-receptor antibodies.[44–49] The mechanisms of action and side effect profiles of these agents are well described in an earlier section of this chapter.

Medical management after heart transplantation is focused on anticipation and prevention of common complications. Hypertension and hyperlipidemia are prevalent because of predisposition in the recipient patient population and as side effects of various immunosuppressive agents. Prophylaxis against opportunistic infections includes agents targeted at common protozoal and viral pathogens (Table 39.4). Surveillance biopsies are performed according to a scheduled routine, and additional biopsies are performed to exclude rejection in the event of hemodynamic instability or unexplained fever. Typically, patients are able to leave the hospital within 10 days of uncomplicated operation, to be followed regularly in outpatient clinic. Monitored physical rehabilitation facilitates optimal cardiovascular and musculoskeletal recuperation,[50] and occupational rehabilitation may offer important psychological and social benefits.

COMPLICATIONS

Complications of antirejection therapy relate primarily to the side effects of the specific immunosuppressive agents currently used. Infections tend to occur in patients with the greatest degree of preoperative debility and malnutrition or in conjunction with additional stressors such as perioperative bleeding or hepatorenal dysfunction. Bacterial pathogens are common in the first several weeks, particularly in the lung and related to surgical or vascular access sites. Opportunistic viral and fungal infections usually predominate later. Increasingly effective prophylaxis for cytomegalovirus and herpes infections have markedly reduced the morbidity associated with these common pathogens. When infection occurs, immunosuppression is tapered as aggressively as possible based on myocardial biopsy results.

Acute rejection occurs in the majority of patients and is graded histologically according to standardized criteria developed by the International Society for Heart and Lung Transplantation. When detected at an early histologic stage (grade 1) (Fig. 39.5) in an asymptomatic patient on surveillance biopsy, rejection often responds to augmented oral steroids or an increased dose of calcineurin inhibitor. When a higher grade of rejection is found (Fig. 39.6), when the infiltrate fails to resolve in response to initial interventions, or in the setting of depressed cardiac function or shock, high-dose intravenous steroids are administered and antilymphocyte therapy is often added. Inotropic or mechanical support is instituted as needed in hope of rescuing graft and patient. Antibody-mediated "vascular" rejection is a controversial entity that, when documented by immunohistochemical techniques, may warrant introduction of cyclophosphamide or other agents with increased activity against B-cells.

Bradycardia is prevalent in the denervated heart for the first weeks after transplant, but a resting heart rate over 70 can usually be achieved by initiating a beta agonist such as theophylline. Persistent bradycardia may be caused by ischemic, surgical, or immunologic injury to the sinus or atrioventricular nodes, or by amiodarone leaching from stores accumulated preoperatively in body fat; pacemaker implantation may be necessary. Atrial flutter or fibrillation may occur spontaneously or herald acute rejection. This dysrhythmia can be difficult to manage because vagal denervation attenuates digoxin's modulation of the typical rapid ventricular response. Most other agents traditionally used to treat atrial arrhythmias depress atrioventricular node conduction or myocardial contractility, particularly undesirable side effects in a recent

TABLE 39.4 MANAGEMENT

TYPICAL IMMUNOSUPPRESSIVE PROTOCOL AND ASSOCIATED MEDICAL THERAPY FOLLOWING HEART TRANSPLANTATION

Calcineurin Inhibitors
Cyclosporine, 2–4 mg/kg po bid or 1–4 mg per hour IV
Tacrolimus, 0.025–0.15 mg/kg po bid
Side effects: Hypertension, renal insufficiency, tremor, hirsutism (cyclosporine A only), gingival hyperplasia, diabetes (tacrolimus only)

Antimitotic Agents
Azathioprine, 1–2 mg/kg/day qd
Mycophenolate mofetil, 500–1,500 mg/day bid
Side effects: Bone marrow suppression, nausea, abdominal cramps, diarrhea

Glucocorticoids
Methylprednisolone IV, *then*
Prednisone PO
Side effects: Hypertension, insulin resistance, osteoporosis, mood swings, central obesity, cushingoid habitus

Antiprotozoal
Trimethoprim-sulfamethoxazole (pneumocystis, toxoplasmosis)

Antiviral
Acyclovir (herpes)
Ganciclovir (cytomegalovirus)

Antihypertensives
Angiotensin-converting enzyme inhibitor or angiotensin-converting enzyme-receptor blocker
Diltiazem (retards cyclosporine A metabolism, reducing drug requirement)
Alpha-receptor blockers

Antilipid Agents
Statin class agent

heart recipient. Amiodarone is generally better tolerated, controls heart rate, promotes conversion to sinus rhythm, and has been used widely in this circumstance.

Among patients who survive beyond the first year, the primary limits to longterm survival are cardiac allograft vasculopathy and malignancy (Fig. 39.7).[27] Current understanding of the pathogenesis of cardiac allograft vasculopathy is incomplete.[51] Widely presumed to be a consequence of "chronic rejection," this process has an incidence of approximately 5% per year. Cardiac allograft vasculopathy may cause progressive insufficiency of coronary flow, myocardial infarction, and ultimately death. Recent research has drawn attention to the importance of donor stress associated with brain death and ischemia/reperfusion injury in the incidence and severity of cardiac allograft vasculopathy in animal models.[52] In contrast to the usual pattern of focal proximal lesions in conventional atherosclerosis, coronary arteries are diffusely involved and conventional revascularization techniques are not generally feasible. In the future, new immunosuppressive or antiproliferative agents may prevent this process or delay its progression.[53] Both cardiac allograft vasculopathy and increased risk of malignancy would likely be prevented if efforts to accomplish durable tolerance are successful, but this obstacle is proving stubborn.[54]

RESULTS

The number of heart transplants performed worldwide has declined from a peak of approximately 4,070 in 1995 to fewer than 3,200 reported in each year since 2000, a 20% decrease. Although some decrease in reporting from European centers may have contributed because of the absence of an incentive to contribute to international registries, reported U.S. activity—which is federally mandated by organ allocation regulations—has decreased by about 10% despite a steady increase in average donor age.[15,27]

Operative survival in adults is over 90%, and both patient and graft 1-year survival rates exceed 80% (Fig. 39.8).[15] The most important risk factors for death within the first year include previous transplant, increased donor age (with age 60 years or more conferring greater risk than age 45 years to 60 years), need for ventilator or left ventricular assist device support before transplant, and recipient age older than 60 years. Rejection and infection together account for most of the mortality during the first year and contribute approximately equally. Beyond the first year, malignancy, including posttransplant lymphoproliferative disease, and chronic rejection emerge as prominent additional factors limiting long-term survival. Extrapolating from current early results, more than 50% of recent recipients can expect to be alive 10 years after transplant, with actuarial graft half-life of 12.3 years.[27,30]

Repeat heart transplantation accounts for less than 2% of all heart transplants done. When performed within the first 6 months, typically for early failure of the first graft, 1-year survival is less than 40%. When performed later, usually for cardiac allograft vasculopathy, 1-year survival is approximately 60%.

Adolescent pediatric heart transplantation recipients (ages 11 to 17 years) fare better (greater than 80% 1-year survival) than do younger children (ages 1 to10 years: approximately 77%) or infants (younger than age 1 year: approximately 68%). Less favorable short-term outcomes may be ascribed to pulmonary hypertension and anatomic challenges posed by congenital heart disease and to monitoring and compliance challenges characteristic of these age groups. Nonetheless, the graft half-life for pediatric patients (11.4 to 13 years) is similar to that for adults.[15,27,30]

ETHICS

Ethical considerations are important in every aspect of heart transplantation. The donor pool is limited and appears to be shrinking despite extended donor acceptance criteria, restricting the number of patients who can undergo transplantation. This shortage forces consideration of ways to limit recipient candidacy (age limits), to increase the donor pool (presumed consent, advertising initiatives, community outreach), and to develop alternatives (mechanical devices; xenografts).[55–57]

The heart transplant community has taken the lead in standardizing patient selection and management guidelines and has established policies for equitable organ allocation. Those given an opportunity to receive the "gift of life" are chosen from a much larger population who might benefit. Recipient candidacy decisions are made by a multidisciplinary group based on objective and subjective input from many individuals who come to know the patient and family in depth. Some recipient selection criteria are fundamentally arbitrary: age is retained as a criterion because of the limited supply of donor organs and based on the consensus view that younger patients deserve preferred access. Recipient selection criteria become

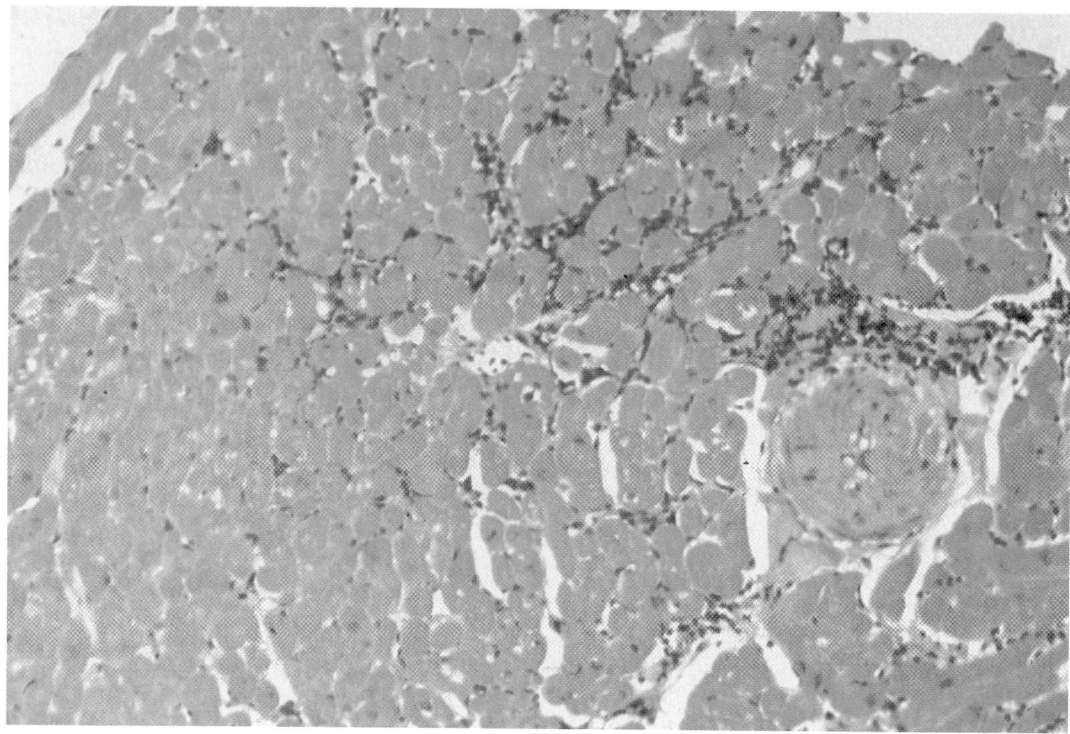

FIGURE 39.5 International Society for Heart and Lung Transplantation grade 1B—diffuse mild acute cellular rejection. (Courtesy of Dr. James Atkinson, Vanderbilt University School of Medicine, Nashville, TN.)

unfair only if they are applied unequally or inconsistently within different programs or among various regions of the country.

Some of the most difficult decisions made by the heart transplant team involve medically marginal candidates with outstanding and effective social support or medically suitable candidates with marginal social support. Although the majority of such patients will do well, outcomes in either case can, on average, be expected to fall below outcome benchmarks. For every marginal patient transplanted, a candidate who meets all the criteria may die. Thus the "right" decision for an individual patient is difficult or impossible to know in advance and may conflict with the best interests of the population of potential recipients.

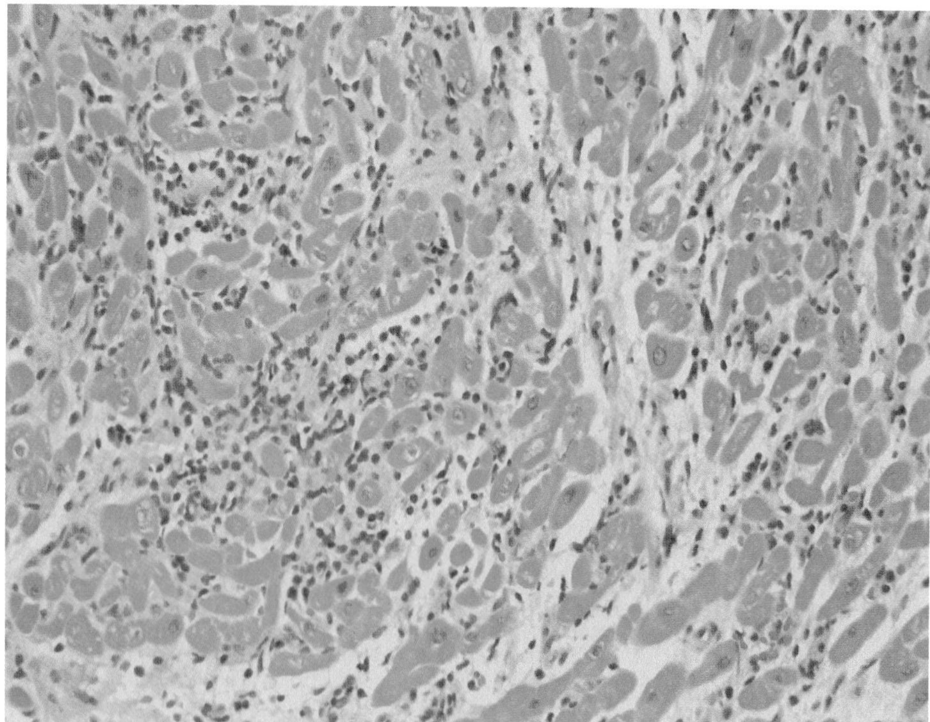

FIGURE 39.6 International Society for Heart and Lung Transplantation grade 3A—multifocal cellular infiltrate with focal myocyte necrosis, typical of moderate to severe acute cellular rejection. (Courtesy of Dr. James Atkinson, Vanderbilt University School of Medicine, Nashville, TN.)

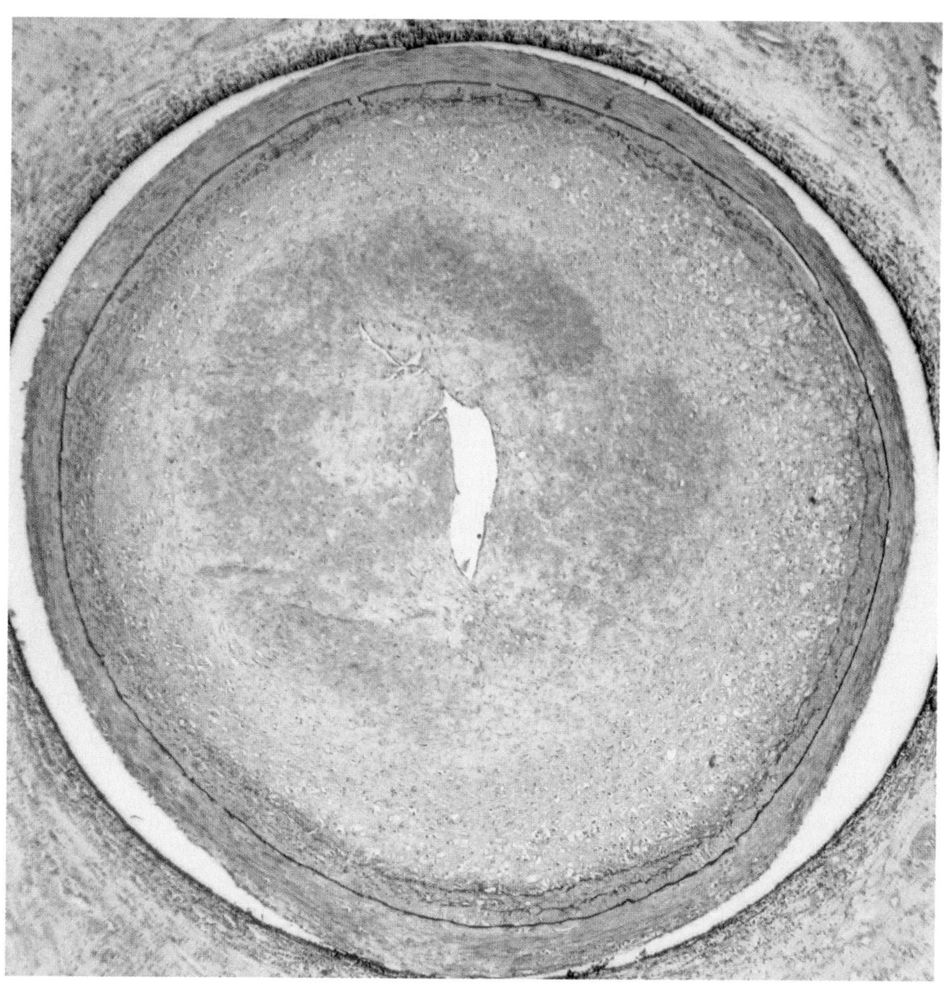

FIGURE 39.7 Autopsy specimen of an epicardial coronary artery demonstrating a moderately severe concentric fibroproliferative intimal lesion characteristic of cardiac allograft vasculopathy. (Courtesy of Dr. James Atkinson, Vanderbilt University School of Medicine, Nashville, TN.)

CURRENT ISSUES

Quantifiable, objective measures of efficacy beyond survival, such as improvement in exercise capacity, freedom from complications, and reduced costs, are becoming the standards by which individual heart transplantation programs are judged. Most important to the patient are subjective factors such as quality of life and productivity, for which standardized measurement tools are being developed. Meanwhile, the efficacy of any proposed alternative to transplantation must be measured against survival, cost, and quality-of-life benchmarks established by this once-experimental procedure.[58]

The most important factor currently restricting the application of heart transplantation is the limited supply of donor organs. Consent is obtained from the donor's legal representatives in only about 25% to 50% of cases in which hearts are appropriate based on acceptable physiologic parameters. Various proactive approaches, such as institution of presumed consent, have been associated with high per-capita donation rates in some countries. However, presumed consent is ethically dubious and may violate basic cultural or religious precepts of individuals or ethnic groups. An adverse societal response to imposition of this unpopular approach as national policy might paradoxically cripple efforts to maintain organ donation even at current levels. Well-conceived efforts to increase the rate of consent by passing laws requiring hospitals to facilitate and document the request, by allowing trained individuals to manage the request process, and by educating the public about "the gift of life," have boosted per-capita donation in several U.S. organ procurement regions.

Efforts to develop improved immunosuppressive drugs are important and are likely to yield incremental near-term improvements in the incidence of chronic rejection. Ideally one could induce tolerance–permanent graft acceptance without requirement for indefinite immunosuppressive therapy. Modulation, rather than suppression, of host responses to donor antigens may allow achievement of this goal.[59,60]

Even if every physiologically suitable donor heart were available, only a minority of patients for whom transplantation would offer a survival advantage could be cared for using this modality. As technical issues related to transcutaneous power delivery, thromboembolism, infection risk, and reliability are addressed, mechanical assist devices are likely to emerge as definitive therapy for some patients.[55] Progress has also been made toward use of porcine "xenografts" in man, and the initial immunologic barrier, hyperacute rejection, appears surmountable using organs from pigs that are genetically modified to express human complement regulatory proteins or "knocked out" for the gene encoding Gal1, 3aGal, the main carbohydrate target recognized by human anti-pig antibodies.[61–63] Control of subsequent cellular and antibody responses has proved difficult in animals models, but life-supporting function of renal xenografts for 3 months and heart xenografts for 1 month have been demonstrated in primates using an intensive regimen of "conventional" immunosuppressive agents.[64,65]

Heart transplantation is one of the most resource-intensive modalities in modern medicine when assessed as cost per year of life saved. The procedure itself, the in-hospital care before transplantation, and maintenance of program infrastructure

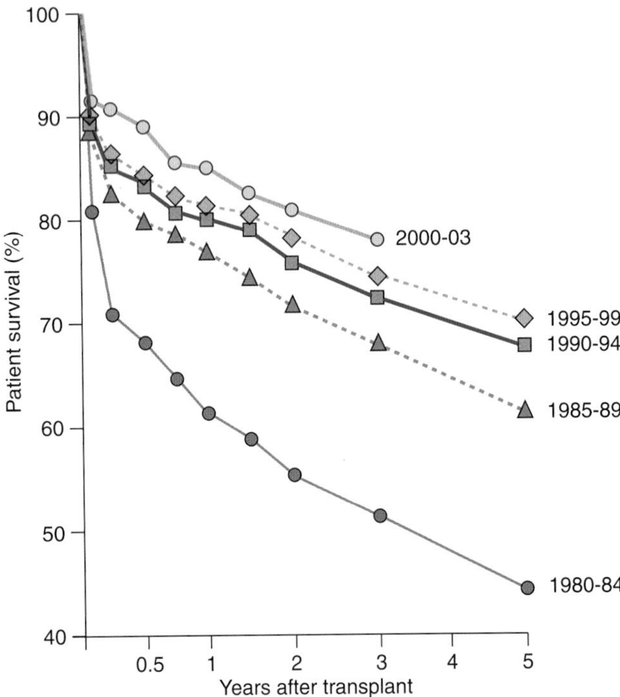

FIGURE 39.8 Heart Transplant Survival, 1980–2003. Survival following heart transplantation in recipients, grouped by era of operation, analyzed by Kaplan-Meier method. Operative survival accounts for much of the steady improvement in outcomes over the past two decades. The subsequent rate of attrition appears to have changed little over the past 20 years, likely reflecting the effect of competing influences such as an older recipient population and improving patient management strategies. (Data from United Network for Organ Sharing, updated 12/10/04.)

are very expensive. Ongoing pharmacy charges and surveillance procedure costs are also substantial. Paradoxically, patients who are physically able to return to work often cannot do so because they rely on medical disability benefits to pay for medications and follow-up care. Whether heart transplantation will continue to receive wide support is a function of societal acceptance of these costs, as currently reflected by coverage policies established by public and private health care insurers.[47] In the future the application of heart transplantation and related technologies may be limited more by what society chooses to afford, rather than what is medically possible.

KEY POINTS

- **End-stage heart failure is the primary indication for heart transplantation in adults, with coronary artery occlusive disease and myopathy of various etiologies each accounting for about 45% of cases.**
- **The ideal donor is a young, previously healthy individual without cardiac disease or hypertension, who is well matched in size to the intended recipient and whose hemodynamics have been carefully managed during the evolution of his or her lethal central nervous system injury.**
- **Cardiac allograft protection depends primarily on hypothermia, which reduces myocardial energy requirements while the heart graft has no nutritive coronary blood flow.**
- **Operative survival in adults is more than 90%, and both patient and graft 1-year survival rates exceed 80%.**

References

1. Carrel A, Guthrie CC. The transplantation of veins and organs. *Am Med (Philadelphia)*. 1905;10:1101.
2. Carrel A. The surgery of blood vessels. *Bull Johns Hopkins Hosp.* 1907;18:18.
3. Neptune WB, Cookson BA, Bailey CP, et al. Complete homologous heart transplantation. *Arch Surg.* 1953;66:174–178.
4. Webb WR, Howard HS, Neely WA. Practical methods of homologous cardiac transplantation. *J Thorac Surg.* 1959;37:361–366.
5. Goldberg M, Berman EF, Akman LC. Homologous transplantation of the canine heart. *J Int Coll Surg.* 1958;30:575.
6. Cass MH, Brock R. Heart excision and replacement. *Guy's Hosp Rep.* 1959;108:285–290.
7. Demikhov VP. Experimental transplantation of vital organs: Authorized translation from the Russian by Haigh B. New York Consultant's Bureau: 1962.
8. Lower RR, Stofer RC, Shumway NE. Homovital transplantation of the heart. *J Thorac Cardiovasc Surg.* 1961;41:196–204.
9. Hardy JD, Chavez CM, Kurrus FE, et al. Heart transplantation in man: developmental studies and report of a case. *JAMA.* 1964;188:1132–1140.
10. **Barnard CN. The operation. A human cardiac transplant: in interim report of a successful operation preformed at Groote Schuur Hospital, Cape Town. *S Afr Med J.* 1967;41:1271.**
11. Caves PK, Stinson EB, Graham AF, et al. Percutaneous transvenous endomyocardial biopsy. *JAMA.* 1973;225:288–291.
12. Kaye MP, Elcombe SA, O'Fallon WM. The International Heart Transplantation Registry. The 1984 report. *J Heart Transplant.* 1985;4:290–292.
13. Calne RY, White DJ, Rolles K, et al. Prolonged survival of pig orthotopic heart grafts treated with cyclosporin A. *Lancet* 1978;1:1183–1185.
14. Reitz BA, Bieber CP, Raney AA, et al. Orthotopic heart and combined heart and lung transplantation with cyclosporin-A immune suppression. *Transplant Proc.* 1981;13:393–396.
15. **Hosenpud JD, Bennet LE, Keck BM, et al. The Registry of the International Society for Heart and Lung Transplantation: Sixteenth official report. *J Heart Lung Transplant.* 1999;18:611–626.**
16. Everett JE, Djalilian AR, Kubo SH, Ket al. Heart transplantation for patients over age 60. *Clin Transplant.* 1996;10:478–481.
17. Blanche C, Takkenberg JJ, Nessim S, et al. Heart transplantation in patients 65 years of age and older: a comparative analysis of 40 patients. *Ann Thorac Surg.* 1996;62:1442–1446.
18. O'Connell JB, Gunnar RM, Evans RW, et al. Task force 1: organization of heart transplantaion in the US. *J Am Coll Cardiol.* 1993;22:8–14.
19. Chomsky DB, Lang CC, Rayos GH, et al. Hemodynamic exercise testing. A valuable tool in the selection of cardiac transplantation candidates. *Circulation* 1996;94:3176–3183.
20. Butler J, Khadim G, Paul KM, et al. Selection criteria for cardiac transplantation in the current era of heart failure therapy. *J Am Coll Cardiol.* 2004;43:787–793.
21. Stevenson LW. Selection and management of the potential candidate for cardiac transplantation. In: *Transplantation and replacement of thoracic organs*, Cooper DKC, Miller LW, Patterson GA, eds, 2nd ed. Kluwer Academic Press,1996:161–176.
22. Massie BM. 15 years of heart-failure trials: what have we learned? *Lancet* 1998; 352 (suppl 1): SI29–133.
23. Sackner-Bernstein JD. Use of carvedilol in chronic heart failure: challenges in therapeutic management. *Prog Cardiovasc Dis.* 1998;41(suppl 1):53–58.
24. Jeevanandam V, Furukawa S, Prendergast TW, et al. Standard criteria for an acceptable donor heart are restricting heart transplantation. *Ann Thorac Surg.* 1996;62:1268–1275.
25. Drinkwater DC, Laks H, Blitz A, et al. Outcomes of patients undergoing transplantation with older donor hearts. *J Heart Lung Transplant.* 1996;15:684–691.
26. Tenderich G, Koerner MM, Stuettgen B, et al. Extended donor criteria: hemodynamic follow-up of heart transplant recipients receiving a cardiac allograft from donors > or = 60 years of age. *Transplantation* 1998; 66:1109–1113.
27. **Pierson RN III, Barr ML, McCullough KP, et al. SRTR Report on the State of Transplantation: Thoracic Organ Transplantation. *Am J Transplant.* 2004;4(suppl 9):93–105.**
28. Novitsky D, Cooper DKC, Reichart B. Hemodynamic and metabolic responses to hormonal therapy in brain-dead potential organ donors. *Transplantation* 1987;43:852–854.
29. Rosengard BR. Donor Management Initiative. *The Chimera* 1999;10:12–13.
30. Opelz G. Results of cardiac transplantation and factors influencing survival based on the collaborative heart transplant study. In: *Transplantation and replacement of thoracic organs.* Cooper DKC, Miller LW, Patterson GA, eds., 2nd ed. Kluwer Academic Press, 1996: 417–427.
31. Sapirstein JS, Pae WE Jr. Mechanical circulatory support before heart transplantation. In: *Transplantation and replacement of thoracic organs.* Cooper DKC, Miller LW, Patterson GA, eds., 2nd ed. Kluwer Academic Press, 1996;185–94.
32. Salzberg S, Lachat M, Zund G, et al. Left ventricular assist device as bridge to heart transplantation—lessons learned with the MicroMed DeBakey axial blood flow pump. *Eur J Cardiothorac Surg.* 2003; 24: 113–118.

33. Letsou GV, Myers TJ, Gregoric ID, et al. Continuous axial-flow left ventricular assist device (Jarvik 2000) maintains kidney and liver perfusion for up to 6 months. *Ann Thorac Surg*. 2003;76:1167–1170.
34. Wieselthaler GM, Chevtchik O, Konetschny R, et al. Improved graft function using a new myocardial preservation solution: Celsior. Preliminary data from a randomized prospective study. *Transplant Proc*. 1999;31:2067–2068.
35. Jeevanandam V, Barr ML, Auteri JS, et al. University of Wisconsin solution versus crystalloid cardioplegia for human donor heart preservation. A randomized blinded prospective clinical trial. *J Thorac Cardiovasc Surg*. 1992;103:194–198.
36. el Gamel A, Yonan NA, Grant S, et al. Orthotopic cardiac transplantation: a comparison of standard and bicaval Wythenshawe techniques. *J Thorac Cardiovasc Surg*. 1995;109:721–729.
37. Aziz T, Burgess M, Khafagy R, et al. Bicaval and standard techniques in orthotopic heart transplantation: medium-term experience in cardiac performance and survival. *J Thorac Cardiovasc Surg*. 1999;118:115–122.
38. Trento A, Takkenberg JM, Czer LS, et al. Clinical experience with one hundred consecutive patients undergoing orthotopic heart transplantation with bicaval and pulmonary venous anastomoses. *J Thorac Cardiovasc Surg*. 1996;112:1496–1450.
39. Cooper DKC, Taniguchi S. Heterotopic heart transplantation – indications, surgical techniques and special considerations. In: *Transplantation and replacement of thoracic organs*. Cooper DKC, Miller LW, Patterson GA, eds, 2nd ed. Kluwer Academic Press, 1996, 353–365.
40. Tagusari O, Kormos RL, Kawai A, et al. Native heart complications after heterotopic heart transplantation: insight into the potential risk of left ventricular assist device. *J Heart Lung Transplant*. 1999;18:1111–1119.
41. Maxey TS, Smith CD, Kern JA, et al. Beneficial effects of inhaled nitric oxide in adult cardiac surgical patients. *Ann Thorac Surg*. 2002;73:529–532.
42. Marboe CC, Billingham M, Eisen HJ, et al. Reigning pathological classification of acute rejection in cardiac allograft recipients: A multicenter study using peripheral blood gene expression profiling. *J Heart Lung Transplant*. 2004;23(suppl):S42.
43. Knosalla C, Grauhan O, Muller J, et al. Intramyocardial electrogram recordings (IMEG) for diagnosis of cellular and humoral mediated cardiac allograft rejection. *Ann Thorac Cardiovasc Surg*. 2000;6:89–94.
44. Starnes VA, Oyer PE, Stinson EB, et al. Prophylactic OKT3 used as induction therapy for heart transplantation. *Circulation* 1989;80: III 79–83.
45. van Gelder T, Baan CC, Balk AH, et al. Blockade of the interleukin (IL)-2/IL-2 receptor pathway with a monoclonal anti-IL-2 receptor antibody (BT563) does not prevent the development of acute heart allograft rejection in humans. *Transplantation* 1998;65:405–410.
46. Carey JA, Frist WH. Use of polyclonal antilymphocytic preparations for prophylaxis in heart transplantation. *J Heart Transplant*. 1990;9:297–300.
47. Miller LW, Naftel DC, Bourge RC, et al. Infection after heart transplantation: a multiinstitutional study. Cardiac Transplant Research Database Group. *J Heart Lung Transplant*. 1994;13:381–392.
48. Swinnen LJ, Costanzo-Nordin MR, Fisher SG, et al. Increased incidence of lymphoproliferative disorder after immunosuppression with the monoclonal antibody OKT3 in cardiac-transplant recipients. *N Engl J Med*. 1990;323:1723–1728.
49. Hammond EH, Wittwer CT, Greenwood J, et al. Relationship of OKT3 sensitization and vascular rejection in cardiac transplant patients receiving OKT3 rejection prophylaxis. *Transplantation* 1990;50:776–782.
50. Kobashigawa JA, Leaf DA, Lee N, et al. A controlled trial of exercise rehabilitation after heart transplantation. *N Engl J Med*. 1999;340:272–277.
51. Pierson RN III, Miller GM. Late graft failure: lessons from clinical and experimental thoracic organ transplantation. *Graft* 3:88–93.
52. Schmid C, Heemann U, Tilney NL. Factors contributing to the development of chronic rejection in heterotopic rat heart transplantation. *Transplantation* 1997;64:222–228.
53. Kaufman DB, Shapiro R, Lucey MR, et al. Immunosuppression: practice and trends. *Am J Transplant*. 2004;4(suppl 9):38–53.
54. Madsen JC. Are the Gods of Tolerance Angry? American Society of Transplantation March/April Newsletter 2004;10:6–13.
55. **Rose EA, Gelijns AC, Moskowitz AJ, et al. Randomized Evaluation of Mechanical Assistance for the Treatment of Congestive Heart Failure (REMATCH) Study Group. Long-term mechanical left ventricular assistance for end-stage heart failure. *N Engl J Med*. 2001; 345: 1435–1443.**
56. Cooper DKC, Keogh AM, Brink J, et al. Report of the Xenotransplantation Advisory Committee of the International Society for Heart and Lung Transplantation: The present status of xenotransplantation and its potential role in the treatment of end-stage cardiac and pulmonary diseases. *J Heart Lung Transplant*. 2000;19:1125–1165.
57. Pierson RN III. Xenotransplantation at the crossroads. *Xenotransplantation* 2004;12:391–393.
58. Evans RW. Socioeconomic aspects of heart transplantation. *Curr Opin Cardiol*. 1995;10:169–179.
59. Harlan DM, Kirk AD. The future of organ and tissue transplantation: can T-cell costimulatory pathway modifiers revolutionize the prevention of graft rejection? *JAMA* 1999;282:1076–1082.
60. Matthews JB, Ramos E, Bluestone JA. Clinical trials of transplant tolerance: slow but steady progress. *Am J Transplant*. 2003;3:794–803.
61. Cozzi E, White DJ. The generation of transgenic pigs as potential organ donors for humans. *Nat Med*. 1995;1:964–966.
62. McGregor CGA, Teotia SS, Byrne GW, et al. Cardiac xenotransplantation: Progress towards the clinic. *Transplantation* 2005. In press.
63. Kuwaki K, Tseng YL, Dor FJMF, et al. Transplantation of hearts from α1,3-galactosyl-transferase gene-knockout (GalT-KO) pigs into baboons. *Nature Medicine* 2005. In press.
64. Zaidi A, Schmoeckel M, Bhatti F, et al. Life-supporting pig-to-primate renal xenotransplantation using genetically modified donors. *Transplantation* 1998;65:1584–1590.
65. Schmoeckel M, Bhatti FN, Zaidi A, et al. Orthotopic heart transplantation in a transgenic pig-to-primate model. *Transplantation* 1998;65:1570–1577; Schmoeckel M, Bhatti FN, Zaidi A, et al. Orthotopic heart transplantation in a transgenic pig-to-primate model [abstract]. 5th International Congress of the International Xenotransplantation Association, Nagoya, Japan, October 25, 1999.

CHAPTER 40 ■ PULMONARY TRANSPLANTATION

LARRY R. KAISER AND THOMAS G. GLEASON

Transplantation of the lung represents one of the last horizons in solid organ transplantation. After an initial effort at human pulmonary transplant in 1963, there was considerable excitement but little activity in this area until 1967, when a flurry of pulmonary transplantations followed the first successful human cardiac transplantation. The longest lung transplant survivor during this early period lived 10 months, most of that time spent in the hospital. The major problems preventing successful pulmonary transplantation have been infection, rejection, and the failure of the bronchial anastomosis to heal.[1]

Unlike other solid organs, the lung has no major systemic arterial blood supply except the small bronchial arteries. Bronchial artery anatomy varies greatly, and the size of bronchial arteries, even when they can be identified, generally precludes direct anastomosis. Therefore, the bronchial anastomosis is immediately ischemic after transplantation, and airway dehiscence may occur, typically 3 weeks after transplantation. The combination of anastomotic ischemia and other factors, including the susceptibility of the lung to infection because of its direct contact with the outside environment, prevented successful transplantation despite the efforts of many investigators.[2]

The first combined heart and lung transplantation was performed successfully in 1981, but the procedure sometimes required removal of an otherwise normal heart from the recipient. Combined cardiac and pulmonary transplantation introduced a series of new problems related to transplanting two organs, including those associated with heart transplantation and, especially, accelerated coronary artery atherosclerosis. With combined cardiac and pulmonary transplantation, tracheal anastomotic healing presents less of a problem, probably because the bronchial artery collaterals in the subcarinal space are preserved.

Recognizing the potential advantage of single-lung transplantation, investigators experimentally defined the factors contributing to failure in pulmonary transplantation.[3] They demonstrated the significant detrimental effect that corticosteroids exert on airway healing and showed that cyclosporine did not have this adverse effect. Delaying the administration of maintenance corticosteroids proved advantageous. It was later suggested that wrapping the bronchial anastomosis with a pedicle of gastrocolic omentum resulted in early capillary ingrowth and revascularization of the airway promoting healing, although this practice has not correlated with a reduction in anastomotic dehiscence.[4]

Another significant factor contributing to the improved success of single-lung transplantation was the recognition of the importance of careful recipient selection. Most early attempts at pulmonary transplantation involved desperately ill, ventilator-dependent patients. It then became apparent that a more suitable candidate for single-lung transplantation was an individual with end-stage restrictive disease (pulmonary fibrosis), a situation that would lead to preferential ventilation and perfusion of the graft because of the increased compliance and relatively decreased pulmonary vascular resistance of the transplanted lung. However, lung replacement in a moribund patient who has already suffered significant nutritional depletion and muscle wasting was doomed to fail, and did fail. Ultimately, the importance of selecting individuals who are ambulatory and undergoing an intense pretransplantation pulmonary rehabilitation program was recognized. Improvement in patient selection may indeed be the single most important factor responsible for the eventual success of pulmonary transplantation. Advances in our understanding of the technical aspects, better patient selection, and better immunosuppression regimens, have considerably broadened the indications for pulmonary transplantation.

INDICATIONS

A patient should be referred for transplantation at a point in the course of the disease at which death is considered likely within several years, so that transplantation would be expected to confer a survival advantage. The patient's perception of an unacceptably poor quality of life is an important additional consideration, but the prognosis must be the overriding impetus for referral. Integrated into the decision must be an anticipated waiting time of up to 2 years, during which the candidate's condition must remain functionally suitable for transplantation.[5] Patients usually have either predominantly obstructive or restrictive disease, although occasionally they may have a mixed defect. Patients with end-stage obstructive physiology may demonstrate changes of emphysema, either nonbullous or bullous, or changes secondary to chronic infection (bronchitic). Patients with cystic fibrosis fall into the latter category, their lung disease resulting from the ravages of chronic, persistent infection (bronchiectasis). Patients with cystic fibrosis may also present with a mixed obstructive/restrictive pattern

TABLE 40.1 INDICATIONS/CONTRAINDICATIONS

GENERAL INDICATIONS FOR PULMONARY TRANSPLANTATION

Advanced obstructive, fibrotic, or pulmonary vascular disease with a high risk of death within 2 to 3 years
Lack of success or availability of alternative therapies
Severe functional limitation, but preserved ability to walk
Less than 60 years for bilateral lung transplantation
Less than 65 years for single-lung transplantation

on pulmonary function testing. Patients with idiopathic pulmonary fibrosis have restrictive physiology. Patients with a congenital deficiency of the α_1-antitrypsin protease commonly present with bullous emphysema, most noticeable at the lung bases. A number of patients also have radiographic and physiologic changes that are similar to those seen in α_1-antitrypsin deficiency, but their levels of α_1-antitrypsin are normal, suggesting the absence of other, as yet undescribed, proteases.

Patients with pulmonary vascular disease are a separate and distinct group. Patients with end-stage disease have either primary pulmonary hypertension, a disease of unknown cause, or secondary pulmonary hypertension, resulting from increased pulmonary perfusion caused by a shunt at the cardiac or supracardiac level. When pulmonary vascular resistance increases sufficiently, the resultant increase in pulmonary artery pressure reverses shunt flow from right to left; this is known as the *Eisenmenger syndrome*. When shunt reversal occurs, patients are typically considered inoperable because, at this point, the mortality associated with primary cardiac operations is prohibitive. Theoretically, it is feasible to close the cardiac shunt if one inserts a new lung or lungs, thus unloading the right ventricle with the subsequent decrease in pulmonary vascular resistance to normal levels yielding an improvement of right ventricular function. Otherwise, *en bloc* heart-lung transplantation is required.

Because of problems with donor availability, lung transplantation is limited to patients 60 to 65 years or younger who have no other systemic disease and who have no significant coronary artery disease. The criteria used in selecting pulmonary transplant recipients are outlined in Table 40.1.

Candidates for pulmonary transplantation ordinarily have significant functional impairment that interferes with activities of daily living. In patients with restrictive or obstructive disease, abnormal gas exchange is the major problem, and essentially they all require supplemental oxygen 24 hours a day. In patients with pulmonary vascular disease, the manifestations of right ventricular failure predominate, and these patients may or may not require oxygen.

Disease-specific guidelines for timely referral, which are based on available prognostic indices, have been published (Table 40.2).[5] Of all patients referred for transplant consideration, about 30% are ultimately accepted.

Potential candidates must be extremely well motivated to cope with the stresses associated with both the pretransplantation and posttransplantation periods and with the lifelong care they require after transplantation. Transplantation trades one chronic disease for another—the posttransplantation state. Patients require daily medication to maintain their transplanted organ and are constantly at risk for infection.

CONTRAINDICATIONS

Absolute and relative contraindications to lung transplantation are listed in Table 40.3.[6] The latter category, consisting of characteristics requiring individualized consideration, merits

TABLE 40.2 INDICATIONS/CONTRAINDICATIONS

DISEASE-SPECIFIC INDICATIONS FOR PULMONARY TRANSPLANTATION

Chronic Obstructive Pulmonary Disease
FEV_1<25% of predicted value after bronchodilator therapy
Clinically significant hypoxemia, hypercapnia, or pulmonary hypertension; rapid decline in lung function; or frequent severe exacerbations

Idiopathic Pulmonary Fibrosis
Symptomatic disease unresponsive to medical therapy
Vital capacity <60% to 70% of predicted value
Evidence of resting or exercise-induced hypoxemia

Cystic Fibrosis
FEV_1 ≤30% of predicted value
FEV_1 >30% with rapidly declining lung function, frequent severe exacerbations, or progressive weight loss
- Female sex and age of less than 18 years with FEV_1 >30%*

Primary Pulmonary Hypertension
- NYHA functional class III or IV
- Mean pulmonary-artery pressure >55 mm Hg
- Mean right atrial pressure >15 mm Hg
- Cardiac index <2 liters/min/m^2
- Failure of medical therapy, especially intravenous epoprostenol, to improve NYHA functional class or hemodynamic indices.

Eisenmenger Syndrome
- NYHA functional class III or IV despite optimal medical management

FEV_1 = forced expiratory volume in 1 second; NYHA = New York Heart Association.
*These factors are associated with a poorer prognosis; therefore, early referral may be indicated.
Adapted with permission from Arcasoy SM, Kotloff RM. Lung transplantation. *N Engl J Med.* 1999;340:1081–1091.

TABLE 40.3 INDICATIONS/CONTRAINDICATIONS

CONTRAINDICATIONS TO PULMONARY TRANSPLANTATIONS

Absolute Contraindications
Severe extrapulmonary organ dysfunction, including renal insufficiency with a creatinine clearance below 50 mL/min, hepatic dysfunction with coagulopathy or portal hypertension, and left ventricular dysfunction or severe coronary artery disease (consider heart-lung transplantation)
Acute, critical illness
Active cancer or recent history of cancer with substantial likelihood of recurrence (except for basal cell and squamous cell carcinoma of the skin)
Active extrapulmonary infection (including infection with human immunodeficiency virus; hepatitis B, indicated by the presence of hepatitis B surface antigen; and hepatitis C with evidence of liver disease on biopsy)
Severe psychiatric illness, noncompliance with therapy, and drug or alcohol dependence
Active or recent (preceding 3 to 6 months) cigarette smoking
Severe malnutrition (<70% of ideal body weight) or marked obesity (>130% of ideal body weight)
Inability of walk, with poor rehabilitation potential

Relative Contraindications
Chronic medical conditions that are poorly controlled or associated with target organ damage
Daily requirement for more than 20 mg of prednisone (or equivalent)
Mechanical ventilation (excluding noninvasive ventilation)
Extensive pleural thickening from prior thoracic surgery or infection

Adapted with permission from Khaghani A, Tadjkarimi S, al-Kattan K, et al. Wrapping the anastomosis with omentum or an internal mammary artery pedicle does not improve bronchial healing after single lung transplantation: results of a randomized clinical trial. *J Heart Lung Transplant.* 1994;13:767–773.

further elaboration. Included in this category are chronic medical conditions such as osteoporosis, hypertension, diabetes mellitus, and coronary artery disease that may worsen after transplantation and are acceptable in a candidate only if they have not resulted in end-organ damage and are well controlled with standard therapy. Preoperative corticosteroid therapy was once considered an absolute contraindication because it was thought to be associated with impaired bronchial anastomotic healing.[7] Because of improved surgical techniques, transplantation can now be performed safely in patients who take moderate doses of corticosteroids.[8] Although patients requiring mechanical ventilation have undergone successful transplantation, as a group they have a significantly higher mortality rate.[5,9]

DONOR CONSIDERATIONS

Unlike other solid organs for transplantation, potential donor lungs can be assessed with plain chest radiographs. Bronchoscopy allows for direct examination of the bronchial tree and for microbiologic examination of bronchial secretions, the results of which may influence later treatment of the recipient. Unlike other solid organ transplants, lungs are unique in carrying a relatively high risk of intrinsic infection (i.e., pneumonia) following transplant. Infiltrates typically preclude donor candidacy. A small infiltrate in one lung without evidence of purulent secretions may still allow this lung to be used in conjunction with a contralateral normal lung in a bilateral lung transplant. Moreover, a pulmonary infiltrate does not necessarily preclude use of the contralateral lung for single-lung transplant.[10] Not infrequently, the lungs of a particular donor may not be suitable because of infiltrates when all other organs are acceptable. Because all brain-dead patients have endotracheal tubes and are on mechanical ventilation, there is a high likelihood that the airway is either colonized with bacteria or that there is ongoing invasive pulmonary infection. With pulmonary infection, an infiltrate often is present on the screening chest radiograph. However, despite a clear chest radiograph, the presence of purulent secretions contraindicates use of the donor lungs for transplantation.

Aspiration at the time of the insult that resulted in brain death is a common cause of pulmonary infiltrates in potential donors. Signs of aspiration may not be evident on a chest radiograph for 24 to 48 hours, underscoring the importance of the bronchoscopic examination when evaluating donor candidacy. Characteristic early bronchoscopic evidence of aspiration includes erythematous tracheobronchial mucosa, purulent secretions, and occasionally the presence of food particles.

Major pulmonary contusion resulting from blunt chest trauma also may eliminate lungs from donor consideration, but minor to moderate contusions unilaterally are often acceptable. Evaluating the full extent of contusion at the time

TABLE 40.4

DONOR MANAGEMENT PROTOCOLS THAT CAN COMPLICATE PULMONARY EDEMA

Maintenance of mean arterial blood pressure above 70 mm Hg
Preference of inotropic support over massive volumes of crystalloid solution to maintain blood pressure (dopamine, 2.5 to 10 μg/kg/min)
Replacement of fluid at the rate of the previous hour's urine output plus insensible losses
Maintenance of normothermia
Maintenance of positive end-expiratory pressure at 5 cm
Frequent endotracheal suctioning
Gram staining of sputum
Monitoring of arterial blood gases every 2 hours

of donor retrieval can be difficult because the interval from injury to determination of brain death and donation may be short. Although the detrimental effect on gas exchange caused by a pulmonary contusion is usually transient, further bleeding into the lung parenchyma could occur if cardiopulmonary bypass is required to perform the transplantation. Pulmonary edema may occur as a result of massive head injury and may be further complicated by certain donor management protocols (Table 40.4).

Traditionally, renal transplantation teams have tried to ensure that adequate urine output is preserved; therefore, they preferentially infuse large volumes of crystalloid solutions. Cardiac transplantation teams prefer to avoid using high doses of inotropic agents to maintain blood pressure and also tend to administer large amounts of crystalloid solutions (Fig. 40.1). The importance of coordinating donor management to prevent pulmonary edema, especially in patients with significant intracranial pathology that predisposes patients to pulmonary edema, cannot be overstated. It can be difficult eliminating pulmonary edema in freshly transplanted lungs that have had their lymphatic vessels divided at the hilar level. The contribution of pulmonary lymphatics (severed during the donor retrieval) to the clearing of edema in the pulmonary parenchyma is not well delineated.

A review of experience with lung donors shows that in 1 year, 174 potential donors were identified, and of these, 128 were rejected outright. After the retrieval team reached the donor hospital, 14 more were refused for a variety of reasons. Most commonly, the lungs were refused after an initial acceptance because bronchoscopy revealed purulent secretions or because arterial blood gases significantly deteriorated between the time of acceptance and the time the retrieval team reached the donor hospital. Size of the donor lungs is less important when the recipient suffers from emphysema, in which each hemithorax is very large, compared with pulmonary fibrosis, in which the hemithorax is contracted. The most important size consideration is a reasonable match between donor and recipient height.

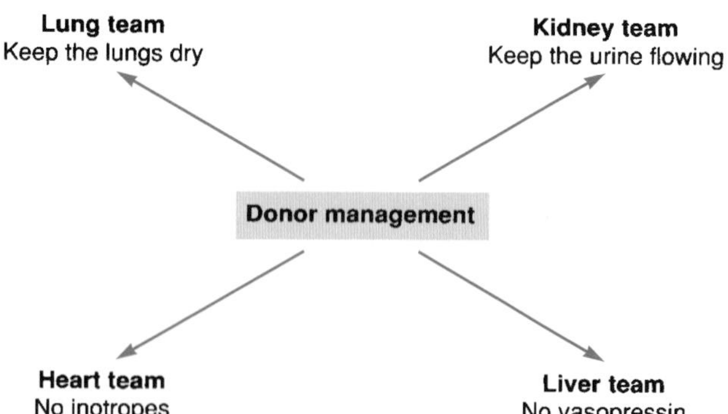

FIGURE 40.1 Each organ retrieval team has its own set of donor management protocols that often conflict.

LUNG PRESERVATION

An important area of investigation involves the optimal preservation technique for the ischemic lung. The donor lung must not only remain viable, it must also participate actively in gas exchange immediately after implantation. A protocol is employed that uses both a flush technique with cold crystalloid solution and topical cooling to 4°C by immersion. At the time of donor lung retrieval, just before cross clamping of the aorta, prostaglandin E_1 is injected directly into the right atrium or pulmonary artery to vasodilate the pulmonary vascular bed. Vasodilatation allows for more uniform distribution of the flush solution and for more uniform and rapid cooling. Prostaglandin E_1 may also serve a cytoprotective role by a mechanism yet to be determined. Crystalloid solution (Euro-Collins) at 4°C is rapidly flushed into the pulmonary artery. After removal of the donor heart, leaving a cuff of left atrium around the pulmonary veins; the lungs are removed by dividing the trachea above the carina and the pulmonary artery just proximal to the bifurcation.

The maximal safe interval for the lung to remain ischemic even when cooled has not been defined. Based on empiric observation, 6 hours has been selected as the limit. This time constraint places limits on the distance that one may travel to procure lungs. The limits of donor lung ischemia have been expanded because of efforts to develop bilateral, sequential lung replacement. The second lung to be implanted perforce is ischemic for a longer time because the lungs are not implanted simultaneously. The longest cold ischemic time has been in the range of 9 to 10 hours, and the lung functioned well within 24 hours after implantation. Although donor lung dysfunction occasionally occurs (5% to 10% incidence), it is usually reversible. Also, the development of this problem has not correlated with prolonged donor lung ischemic time.

Whether one type of preservation solution is superior remains to be determined. A low potassium dextran solution may be better for early lung function than the standard Euro-Collins solution. A recent clinical study demonstrated less reperfusion injury, better immediate and intermediate function, and better early and longterm survival for donor lungs preserved with low potassium dextran solution compared with Euro-Collins.[11] Other methods of preservation have also been used experimentally. Core cooling of the donor with an extracorporeal circuit has been used extensively in Great Britain for cardiopulmonary transplantation. Others have used an immersion technique without flushing the pulmonary artery.

It is believed that lung injury results not only from the ischemic insult but also from reperfusion of the ischemic organ. Several experimental models of acute lung injury implicate oxygen free radicals as a factor in the genesis of reperfusion injury. A significant early increase in lung permeability is seen after an ischemic period followed by reperfusion, which improves within several hours. Changes in the contralateral, nonischemic lung are presumably to the result of substances released during reperfusion of the ischemic lung. Efforts are directed at identifying techniques to attenuate the reperfusion injury.

Most experimental studies in lung preservation to date have been largely empiric, evaluating the effects of various techniques on subsequent lung function. Further progress requires a more detailed understanding of events at the cellular level during ischemia and reperfusion so that a rational approach to reduce or eliminate these changes may evolve. Satisfactory preservation techniques must protect not only cell structure and metabolism but also functional integrity of the lung as a whole to maintain normal gas exchange. In addition, methods of preservation that allow for a prolonged ischemic time must also preserve the viability and microcirculation of the airway to prevent subsequent complications of airway healing. It would serve no useful purpose to extend the ischemic time only to have the airway fail to heal because of thrombosis in small vessels. Given the ability to safely preserve livers and kidneys for 24 hours or longer, it seems likely that donor lung preservation times will be extended in the near future.

TRANSPLANTATION OPERATION

Whether one lung or both lungs are replaced depends on recipient factors, including the cause of the end-stage pulmonary disease as well as donor lung availability. It is clear that patients with chronic infection, such as cystic fibrosis, require replacement of both lungs. Patients with restrictive physiology (pulmonary fibrosis) do well with single-lung replacement. The situation in patients with end-stage obstructive disease, specifically emphysema, offers considerably more variability. Early in the pulmonary transplantation experience, it became evident that problems resulted from leaving the native emphysematous lung in situ. Specifically, air trapping in the remaining native lung, with resultant mediastinal shift, significantly crowded the transplanted lung, resulting in poor expansion and minimal function. Ventilation (V) preferentially went to the overly compliant native lung, while most of the perfusion (Q) went to the newly transplanted lung, creating a significant V/Q mismatch that further worsened an already precarious situation. Despite these concerns, it has been conclusively demonstrated over the past few years that single-lung transplantation not only is an acceptable operation for patients with emphysema but also may be the operation of choice for patients older than 50 years.[12] Recent data from our institution demonstrates improved forced expiratory volume in 1 second (FEV_1) and 6-minute walk results in emphysema patients undergoing double- versus single-lung transplantation at 1 year. Whether this data translates into improved longterm survival or functional level remains to be seen. From a donor standpoint, single-lung transplantation, when acceptable, is a more efficient use of donor organs. The decision to use single-lung transplantation for emphysema evolved mainly from experience with the original *en bloc* double-lung operation, which involved a tracheal anastomosis and routine cardiopulmonary bypass and resulted in significant perioperative cardiac morbidity and mortality. Some emphysema patients may be able to delay or even avoid lung transplantation if they are candidates for lung volume reduction surgery.

Replacement of both lungs, when indicated, was greatly simplified by the development and refinement of the bilateral, sequential lung transplant procedure. Bilateral sequential lung transplant can be approached either by median sternotomy or bilateral thoracotomies and with or without cardiopulmonary bypass depending on the indication for transplantation. A bilateral thoracosternotomy incision ("clamshell") permits easier completion of the recipient pneumonectomies than median sternotomy, but the clamshell incision tends to be more painful. Even previous chest operations are not contraindications for this procedure. This operation has replaced the original *en bloc* double-lung procedure and the heart–lung transplantation as the operation of choice for patients with end-stage pulmonary disease who need both lungs and for those with pulmonary vascular disease.

In patients with pulmonary hypertension, it is questionable whether to replace one or both lungs. Originally single-lung transplantation was chosen because replacing one lung allowed adequate unloading of the right ventricle with immediate improvement in right ventricular function and normalization of pulmonary artery pressures (Table 40.5). It soon became apparent, however, that replacing both lungs in this patient population offers a better margin of safety in the perioperative period and probably results in better hemodynamics in the long term. Whether replacement of both lungs is absolutely required remains to be determined but currently is preferred in most transplant centers for patients with pulmonary hypertension, despite the donor limitations.

TABLE 40.5

TYPICAL HEMODYNAMICS DATA FOR SINGLE LUNG TRANSPLANTATION IN PATIENTS WITH PULMONARY HYPERTENSION

Measurement	Pretransplant	Posttransplant
Pulmonary artery pressure		
Mean	58 mm Hg	16 mm Hg
Systolic	94 mm Hg	28 mm Hg
Right ventricular ejection fraction	25%	52%
Cardiac output	4 L/min	7 L/min
Pulmonary vascular resistance	1302 dyne/cm^5/s	161 dyne/cm^5/s

OPERATIVE TECHNIQUE

Single-Lung Transplantation

The performance of the donor operation does not vary because one always attempts to use both lungs, either for single-lung replacement on two recipients or for distribution to another transplant medical center. This practice provides the most efficient use of limited donor organs. In the recipient operation, a standard posterolateral or muscle-sparing axillary thoracotomy is performed, with dissection of the hilar structures as usual for a pneumonectomy (Fig. 40.2). The dissection mobilizes the main pulmonary artery, both superior and inferior pulmonary veins, and the mainstem bronchus. When the donor lung arrives in the operating room, the recipient pneumonectomy is performed by dividing the hilar vessels as far *distally* as possible and the bronchus at the level of the upper lobe take-off.

The implantation operation begins with construction of an anastomosis between the donor and recipient bronchus. This anastomosis has typically been done in a telescoping fashion with one end brought up inside the other by placing horizontal mattress sutures using nonabsorbable material, More recently, however, standard end-to-end anastomoses with figure-of-eight sutures is gaining popularity because it may reduce bronchial anastomotic complications.[13,14] The bronchial anastomosis, formerly wrapped with a pedicle of gastrocolic omentum, now is typically left unwrapped because bronchial anastomotic wrapping has not been shown to decrease anastomotic leak rate. Bronchial arterial bypass with a native internal mammary artery has been championed by a few groups and shown to decrease bronchial anastomotic complications by these groups, but this technique has not received widespread acceptance or popularity.[15–17] The bronchial anastomosis is followed by a left atrial cuff anastomosis. The pulmonary artery anastomosis is then performed last. Once the vascular anastomoses are constructed, clamps are removed and blood flow is reestablished as the lung is inflated. The chest is closed in standard fashion. Either the

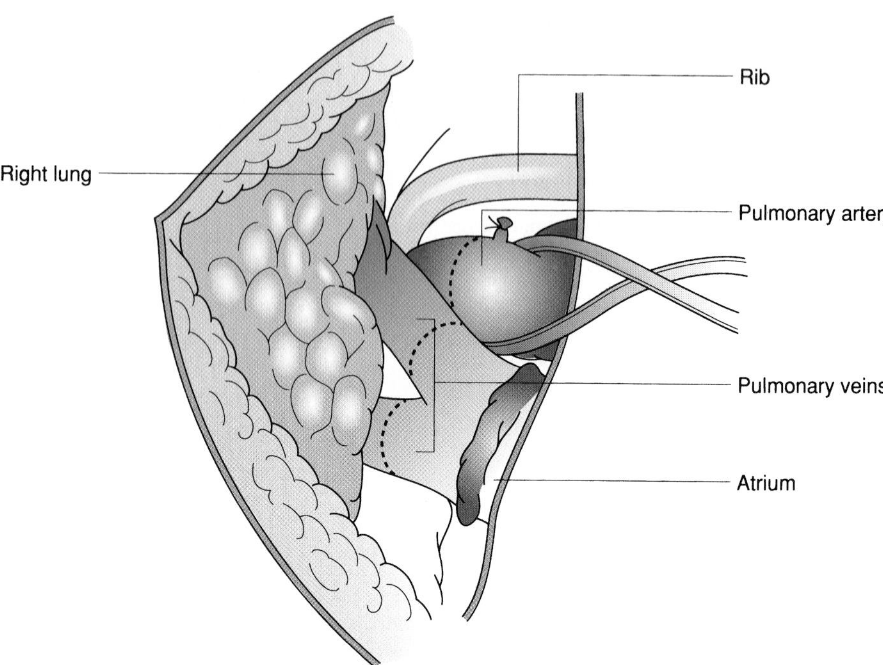

FIGURE 40.2 Mobilization of the hilum of the right lung demonstrating the encircled pulmonary artery with the first branch ligated and divided. The superior and inferior pulmonary veins have been exposed. Both the artery and veins are taken as close to the lung as possible. The bronchus is divided at the level of the take-off of the upper lobe.

right or left lung can be transplanted, and the decision of which side to transplant is based on both donor lung availability and recipient perfusion lung scan data. If one lung receives most of the perfusion, the opposite lung is transplanted.

Double-Lung Transplantation

The technique of double-lung transplantation has evolved considerably since the late 1980s. The favored approach is bilateral, sequential lung replacement.[18] With the patient in the supine position; this operation is performed through sternotomy, bilateral thoracosternotomy (clamshell) incision (Fig. 40.3), bilateral anterior thoracotomies without sternal division or bilateral muscle-sparing, axillary thoracotomies. The bilateral thoracosternotomy incision provides the most exposure to both hemithoraces, facilitating dissection and mobilization of hilar structures. This exposure is particularly important in recipients with diffuse dense adhesions between the visceral and parietal pleural surfaces, as is often seen in patients with chronic infection and bronchiectasis, such as cystic fibrosis.

Although both lungs are replaced, the operation can usually be performed without cardiopulmonary bypass. By first replacing the lung with the least function, the oxygenation and ventilation are maintained by the lung that receives the major fraction of perfusion. If the patient is unable to tolerate single-lung ventilation because of inadequate gas exchange or because of rising pulmonary artery pressures with right ventricular dysfunction, then cardiopulmonary bypass is instituted. The donor lungs are separated as for single-lung transplantation, leaving a cuff of left atrium around the pulmonary veins on each side. The recipient pneumonectomy is carried out with the patient maintained on one-lung ventilation. Each donor lung is implanted using essentially the same technique as described for single-lung transplantation. The bronchial anastomosis is completed first, followed by the left atrial and then the pulmonary arterial anastomoses. Flow and ventilation are restored to the newly implanted lung, and this lung then supports the patient while the opposite lung is removed and the second lung is implanted. Although all cardiac output is going through the newly implanted lung once the opposite

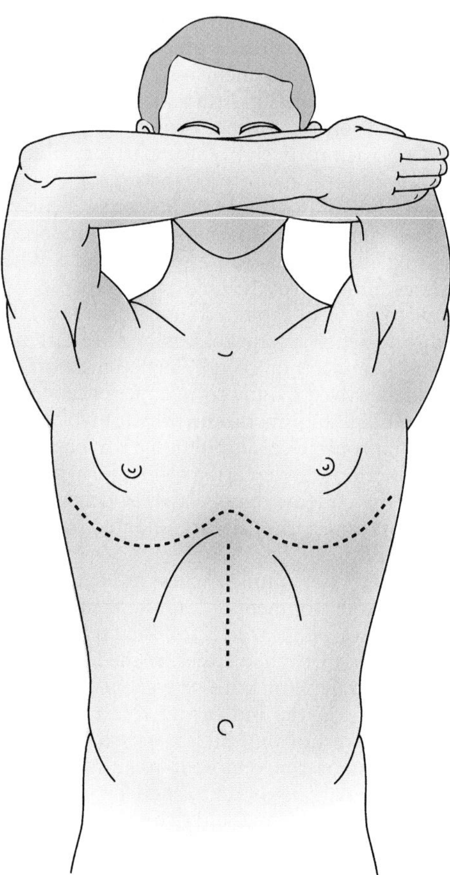

FIGURE 40.3 The position of the patient on the operating table before the start of the bilateral, sequential pulmonary transplantation operation. The chest incision, a bilateral thoracosternotomy, is seen, as is the separate midline incision used to expose the omentum. The sternum is divided transversely, and the fifth intercostal space on each side is entered.

pulmonary artery is ligated, clinically significant pulmonary edema has not been a problem.

Other than procedures performed in patients with pulmonary hypertension or those with bilateral septic pulmonary disease (e.g., cystic fibrosis), essentially all these procedures can be done without the need for cardiopulmonary bypass. The operation has afforded the opportunity to compare function between lungs with different ischemic times. Lungs may remain ischemic from 7 to 9 hours and still actively participate in gas exchange. Immediate postoperative perfusion scans usually show that the lung with the longer ischemic time receives less of the perfusion initially, although perfusion normalizes between the two lungs by 24 to 48 hours.

RESULTS

The Registry of the International Society of Heart and Lung Transplantation has recorded 17,039 lung transplants between January 1985 and June 2003.[19] Currently 142 centers actively perform lung transplants, but only 13 centers perform more than 30 per year. Today roughly 50% of patients transplanted receive bilateral-lung transplants, and the other 50% receive single-lung transplant. The single most common indication for transplant was emphysema either as a result of α_1-antitrypsin deficiency (9% of cases) or idiopathy (39% of cases). Most of the so-called idiopathic cases of emphysema are related to cigarette smoking. Pulmonary fibrosis, the indication first treated successfully by lung transplantation accounted for 17%.[19] Other indications are summarized in Table 40.6.

The overall 1-year survival rate following lung transplant is 75%. The 5-year survival is 45% to 50%. Survival curves for single- and double-lung transplants diverge after 3 years. Patients with emphysema have the best survival rate, whereas those with pulmonary hypertension have the worst (odds ratio 2.24). Patients with cystic fibrosis do almost as well as patients with emphysema. In a given single institution, survival data may be somewhat better than that observed in the Registry Data. Only a small number of lung transplant patients have survived as long as 7 years, but it was only in 1988 that significant numbers of transplants began to be performed. Improved results occurred through 1992 but have plateaued since that time. The longterm outlook for patients undergoing lung transplantation remains unknown, but some insight can be gained by examining the factors responsible for longterm morbidity and mortality in this patient population.

TABLE 40.6 INDICATIONS/CONTRAINDICATIONS

INDICATIONS FOR PULMONARY TRANSPLANTATION

	Single lung (%)	Double lung (%)
Emphysema	53	23
α-1 antitrypsin	8.5	9.5
Cystic fibrosis	2.3	31
Idiopathic pulmonary fibrosis	24	9.7
Primary pulmonary hypertension	1.1	7.6
Retransplant	2.0	1.7

Adapted with permission from Trulock EP, Edwards LB, Taylor DO, et al. The Registry of the International Society for Heart and Lung Transplantation: twenty-first official adult heart transplant report—2004. *J Heart Lung Transplant.* 2004;23:804–815.

IMMUNOSUPPRESSION

Immunosuppression is initiated in the immediate perioperative period and continued for the rest of the recipient's life. Standard regimens consist of cyclosporine or tacrolimus, azathioprine or mycophenolate mofetil, and prednisone. Some centers also use antilymphocyte-antibody preparations or anti-interleukin-2 receptor (CD25) antibodies during the induction phase, but there is not sufficient evidence in humans that this approach diminishes the incidence of acute or chronic rejection. Two important issues regarding standard immunosuppressive therapy are the myriad side effects associated with these agents and their numerous interactions with other commonly prescribed medications.[5]

COMPLICATIONS

Complications resulting from pulmonary transplantation occur frequently, may be severe, and occasionally result in death. Intraoperative complications include technical problems with the vascular or bronchial anastomoses, injury to the phrenic or recurrent laryngeal nerves, and myocardial infarction. Postoperative complications include primary graft dysfunction, infection, and problems with airway healing, acute rejection, and bronchiolitis obliterans (chronic rejection). Intraabdominal complications are not uncommon. Wound infection is noted rarely.

Causes of recipient death can be categorized according to the time frame in which they occur. Early deaths (sooner than 90 days following transplant) most commonly result from primary graft failure (31%).[19] Infection is the second most common cause of early death (24%), followed by heart failure (12%). Rejection accounts for 5% of deaths in the early posttransplantation period. Hemorrhage and airway dehiscence each are responsible for 8% of early postoperative deaths. Infection accounts for about 40% of late deaths (after 90 days). About one third of deaths result from manifestations of chronic rejection and obliterative bronchiolitis, the single biggest impediment to longterm survival following lung transplantation. Respiratory failure and malignancy are the next most common causes of late mortality. Despite the major strides made in the operation itself and early postoperative care, the complications resulting from chronic immunosuppression continue to plague transplant patients.

PRIMARY GRAFT DYSFUNCTION

Mild, transient pulmonary edema is a common feature of the freshly transplanted allograft. In approximately 15% of cases, the injury is sufficiently severe to cause a form of acute respiratory distress syndrome termed *primary graft failure*. Primary graft failure is presumed to reflect ischemia-reperfusion injury, but surgical trauma and lymphatic disruption may be contributing factors. The diagnosis rests on the presence of widespread infiltrates on chest radiographs and severe hypoxemia within 72 hours after transplantation and the exclusion of other causes of graft dysfunction, such as volume overload, pneumonia, rejection, occlusion of the venous anastomosis, and aspiration. Treatment is supportive, relying principally on conventional mechanical ventilation. Independent lung ventilation, inhaled nitric oxide, and extracorporeal membrane oxygenation have been used as adjunctive measures. Mortality rates of up to 60% have been reported, and among those who survive, the recovery period is often protracted, but achievement of normal allograft function is possible. The results of emergency retransplantation in such cases have been poor.[5,20,21]

REJECTION

With few exceptions, acute rejection episodes occur soon after transplantation, usually between posttransplantation days five and seven. Often, two or three rejection episodes occur within the first month. Mild temperature elevation, perihilar fluffy infiltrates, or a minimal decrease in blood oxygenation as measured by arterial oxygen tension may herald rejection. Because rejection occurs so frequently during this period, the distinction between infection and rejection may be difficult. Often, the distinguishing factor between these two entities is that rejection noticeably responds positively to the administration of corticosteroids. Treatment of early rejection episodes involves the use of bolus corticosteroid administration given on 3 consecutive days. Within 12 to 18 hours after the first corticosteroid dose, symptoms relating to rejection usually resolve, including clearing of infiltrates on chest radiograph.

The diagnostic experience using transbronchial biopsy to diagnose and monitor rejection at some centers after cardiopulmonary transplantation is impressive, but the number of biopsies required to maximize specificity is large. One group recommends obtaining 18 separate transbronchial biopsy specimens to achieve 95% specificity. The risks and potential complications of transbronchial lung biopsy do not justify their routine performance because suspected rejection episodes respond so well to corticosteroids. Transbronchial lung biopsy can be used when the issue of rejection versus infection is not resolved after steroid administration. Flexible bronchoscopy can be performed at the bedside, and 6 to 10 separate biopsies can be obtained under fluoroscopic guidance. When symptoms or signs of rejection persist despite adequate treatment, open lung biopsy may be considered.

INFECTION

Infection in the posttransplantation period continues to be a significant cause of morbidity and mortality. Bacterial pneumonia usually responds to appropriate antibiotic therapy, and patients are maintained on specific antibiotics as dictated by sputum culture and results of bronchial washings obtained at bronchoscopy. Antibiotic administration is particularly important if one predominant organism is grown from the donor lung cultures obtained at organ harvest. If a specific organism is grown from donor bronchial washings, the recipient is maintained on an appropriate antibiotic or combination of antibiotics for at least 1 week. The most common organism recovered from donor bronchial washings is *Staphylococcus aureus*. In a series of 32 transplants, this organism was recovered from donors 11 times and subsequently from 4 transplant recipients.[22] Other commonly recovered pathogens include *Enterobacter* species and *Candida albicans*. The presence of organisms cultured from donor bronchial washings, however, does not absolutely predict the development of invasive infection in recipients. Less than half of recipients from whom organisms were recovered went on to develop invasive infection.

The second most significant pathogen is cytomegalovirus (CMV). The diagnosis of CMV is usually made from culture of bronchoalveolar lavage fluid or tissue obtained from transbronchial lung biopsy. In the pulmonary transplantation population, CMV pneumonitis is the predominant form of CMV infection, although CMV enteritis and retinitis also occur. This experience corresponds to that seen in cardiac and cardiopulmonary transplant recipients. About half of lung recipients develop documented CMV infection. Ganciclovir has proved particularly effective and is the drug of choice for CMV infection in this circumstance. The drug is well tolerated in most patients, with neutropenia accounting for most of the toxicity. The mortality rate from life-threatening CMV infections treated with ganciclovir has been reported at 10%, far better than the 40% or greater mortality reported before this agent was available.[23] Major difficulties with life-threatening CMV infection have occurred in CMV-negative recipients who receive a lung from a CMV-positive donor (primary infection) or in recipients who are already CMV positive (secondary infection). Current practice is to attempt to place only a CMV-negative donor lung in a CMV-negative recipient, but this often proves to be unrealistic given the shortage of donor organs. Despite initial thoughts to the contrary, data from the St. Louis International Lung Transplant Registry fails to demonstrate any survival advantage at 1 or 2 years posttransplantation by avoiding donor–recipient CMV mismatching. Cytolytic therapy especially with muromonab-CD3 is associated with an increased risk and severity of CMV infection. CMV prophylaxis with ganciclovir is used in some centers for CMV-positive recipients or in those recipients who receive a lung from a CMV-positive donor.

AIRWAY COMPLICATIONS

Other than infection, a major concern after pulmonary transplantation is airway anastomotic healing. During the early pulmonary transplantation experience, problems with airway healing resulted in a significant percentage of deaths. Patients often did well for the first 3 weeks after transplantation, and then the bronchial anastomosis split, often with erosion into the pulmonary artery. Bronchial anastomotic healing initially was facilitated by withholding maintenance corticosteroids until after the first posttransplantation week and using an omental pedicle wrapped around the anastomosis. Historically, most problems with airway healing occurred after the *en bloc* double-lung operation, which involves a tracheal anastomosis. Double-lung transplantation required extensive dissection in the subcarinal space, resulting in the disruption of a number of bronchial collateral vessels. Since this operation was modified to one involving bilateral, sequential lung replacement using two bronchial anastomoses, airway problems are infrequent and now are rarely if ever implicated in recipient deaths. Partial bronchial dehiscences often heal without sequelae. The use of a telescoping bronchial anastomosis, in which the donor bronchus is intussuscepted into the recipient bronchus or vice versa, obviated the need for the omental pedicle wrap, allowed for immediate use of corticosteroids, and reduced anastomotic dehiscence rates. However, the telescoping anastomosis may actually increase the rate of anastomotic stenosis. Therefore, more recently there has been a trend toward the use of primary end-to-end anastomosis using figure-of-eight sutures, and initial results demonstrate a lower incidence of stenosis with an equivalent rate of dehiscence (about 2%).[13,14]

BRONCHIOLITIS OBLITERANS

About 20% of pulmonary transplant recipients develop progressive deterioration in pulmonary function because of obliterative bronchiolitis. The incidence of this complication reportedly approaches 50% after heart–lung transplantation. This complication is seen with approximately the same incidence following pulmonary transplantation as well. The lesion is characterized histologically by progressive small airway destruction, filling of these small airways with an inflammatory exudate and finally fibrosis. It is first manifested clinically by a subtle decrease in pulmonary function reflected in a decreased FEV_1. This complication is likely a form of chronic rejection although its exact etiology remains unknown. A good animal model of obliterative bronchiolitis does not exist, making study of this entity difficult. If diagnosed early, enhancing immunosuppression may either halt the process or slow the progression. It has been hypothesized that the development of obliterative bronchiolitis in cardiopulmonary transplantation patients is related to a human major histocompatibility complex (human leukocyte antigen)–A2 antigen mismatch. Others postulate that CMV infection may be implicated. Once diagnosed, it is imperative to increase immunosuppression to prevent what is usually an insidiously progressive disorder. Unfortunately, in patients who have developed obliterative bronchiolitis and then undergo retransplantation, the pathology recurs in the newly transplanted lungs. Obliterative bronchiolitis remains the major problem in patients surviving for greater than 2 years following transplantation. Overall, longterm survival for lung transplantation is not likely to change until this problem is solved.

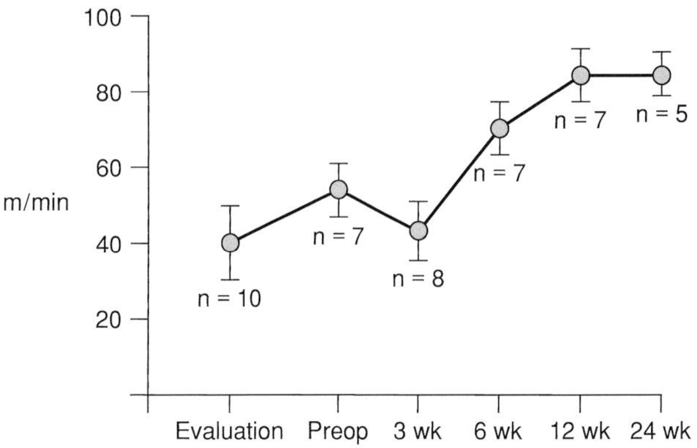

FIGURE 40.4 Mean 6-minute walk data for a group of patients undergoing single-lung transplantations for emphysema. Marked improvement is seen at the 6-week level, with continued improvement at 12 weeks.

POSTTRANSPLANTATION PHYSIOLOGY

Pulmonary transplantation has afforded an opportunity to observe changes in pulmonary physiology that are not seen under ordinary circumstances. It is important to examine these changes relative to the type of transplantation operation.

The development of bilateral, sequential lung replacement provides the opportunity to indirectly assess lung function by perfusion lung scan. Because the newly implanted lungs have different ischemic times, the immediate posttransplantation perfusion scan would be expected to demonstrate less perfusion to the side with the longer ischemic time. Indeed, this situation does occur, especially when ischemic times exceed 6 hours; however, the relative perfusion to each side usually equalizes within 24 to 48 hours.

Performing single-lung transplants in patients with pulmonary hypertension has been particularly illustrative in demonstrating the potential for reversing right ventricular dysfunction. As soon as the lung is implanted, the morphology of the right ventricle changes significantly, as assessed by transesophageal echocardiography. The interventricular septum, previously bulging into the left ventricle, immediately assumes a normal position. An increase in contractility of the right ventricle occurs with significant decrease in dilatation. The pulmonary artery pressure immediately decreases and is essentially normal by the time the patient leaves the operating room (Table 40.5). Late catheterization studies (2 years posttransplantation) in patients undergoing this operation show continued normal hemodynamics.

The situation after single-lung transplantation in patients with emphysema is also illustrative. One would expect a significant V/Q mismatch to occur, with ventilation to the native lung occurring preferentially because the native lung is significantly more compliant. Conversely, perfusion should preferentially go to the newly transplanted lung because of lower pulmonary vascular resistance. Despite this occurrence, patients undergoing this operation do well from a functional standpoint (Fig. 40.4). Early data show that physiologic dead space (V_D/V_T) decreases with work, with a shift in ventilation toward the transplanted side. By 3 months after transplantation, the ventilation/perfusion mismatch narrows (Fig. 40.5). Despite the mismatch, patients generally do not have persistent carbon dioxide retention after transplantation.

From a clinical standpoint, improvement in pulmonary function is seen almost immediately after transplantation. The measurement most often used is FEV_1, and marked improvement is seen within 2 weeks. The FEV_1 essentially triples and then remains fairly stable (Fig. 40.6). This observation holds true for both single- and double-lung replacement in patients with obstructive disease. Improvement after bilateral lung replacement is slightly better.

Likewise, exercise studies show significant improvement after lung transplantation. Though patients who receive two lungs may do better on pulmonary function studies, this benefit is not translated into significantly better exercise capacity. Maximum oxygen consumption, maximum work, peak ventilation, and anaerobic threshold are increased after lung transplantation but remain well below normal values. This may be due in large part to an accompanying abnormal cardiovascular response to exercise.

When exercise testing is performed, no difference is noted between emphysema patients who receive one lung compared with patients who receive two. This finding may be because emphysema sufferers receiving a single lung do better than we would predict because of the effect of the transplant operation on the remaining native lung. Specifically, the shift in the mediastinum toward the transplanted side results in a relative "volume reduction" on the contralateral side with repositioning of the contralateral hemidiaphragm to a more normal location and to a normal concave configuration. This reconfiguration of the hemidiaphragm allows for significantly better diaphragm excursion and improved lung mechanics and gas exchange. Exercise capacity improves sufficiently to allow the majority of transplant recipients to resume an active and unencumbered lifestyle. By the end of the first year after transplantation,

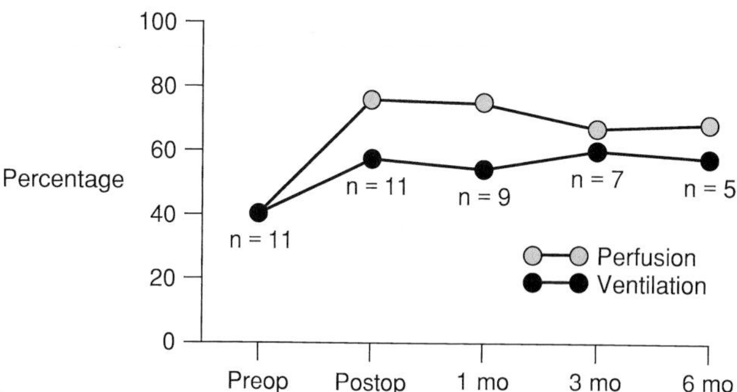

FIGURE 40.5 Mean values for ventilation and perfusion for patients undergoing single-lung transplantation for emphysema. Note the ventilation-perfusion mismatch that occurs, as expected, after transplantation.

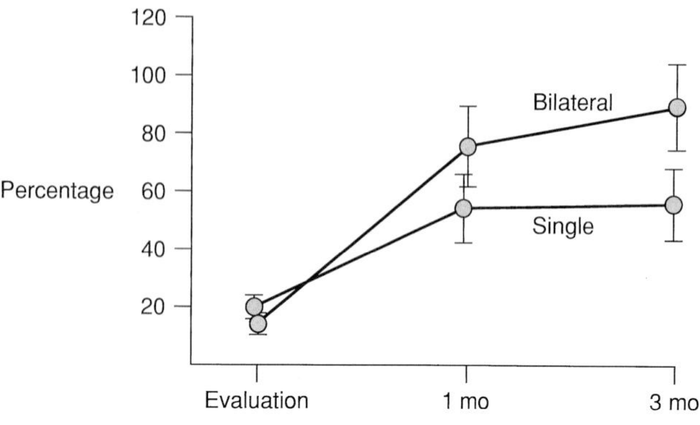

FIGURE 40.6 Comparison of percentage of predicted forced expiratory volume in 1 second in 14 patients undergoing single and 10 patients undergoing bilateral sequential pulmonary transplantation for chronic obstructive pulmonary disease.

approximately 80% of recipients report no limitations in activity.[5] At the other extreme, only 4% require total assistance. On average, after transplantation the distance a patient can cover during a standard 6-minute walk test is double that achieved preoperatively. Recipients of bilateral lung transplants can walk farther in 6 minutes than recipients of single-lung transplants, but this difference may reflect the younger age of the bilateral-transplant recipients.[5,24]

FUTURE CONSIDERATIONS

Pulmonary transplantation has slowly evolved from an experimental therapy. The number of these operations performed is still small compared with other solid organ replacements. Donor availability is still a major issue and will likely continue to be an obstacle. Lung volume reduction surgery has demonstrated some benefit in a select group of chronic obstructive pulmonary disease patients but has not had as significant an impact on quality of life as lung transplant has for patients with emphysema. Questions about longterm impact and preservation of lung function remain to be answered. Pulmonary transplantation has joined other solid organ transplants as a viable alternative in patients with end-stage disease. Cost considerations and managed care will likely continue to impact the number of lung transplants performed despite the accomplishments of the past 30 years.

KEY POINTS

- **Candidates for pulmonary transplantation have significant functional impairment that interferes with activities of daily living. In patients with restrictive or obstructive disease, abnormal gas exchange is the major problem and essentially all require supplemental oxygen. In patients with pulmonary vascular disease, the manifestations of right ventricular failure predominate.**
- **It is believed that lung injury results not only from the ischemic insult but also from reperfusion of the ischemic organ.**
- **Other than infection, the major concern after pulmonary transplantation is airway anastomotic healing.**
- **By the end of the first year after transplantation, approximately 80% of recipients report no limitations in activity.**

References

1. Egan TM, Cooper JD. Lung transplantation. *Ann Thorac Surg.* 1989;48:741–742.
2. Wildevuur CR, Benfield JR. A review of 23 human lung transplantations by 20 surgeons. *Ann Thorac Surg.* 1970;9:489–515.
3. Lima O, Cooper JD, Peters WJ, et al. Effects of *methylprednisolone and azathioprine on bronchial healing following lung autotransplantation. J Thorac Cardiovasc Surg.* 1981;82:211–215.
4. Khaghani A, Tadjkarimi S, al-Kattan K, et al. Wrapping the anastomosis with omentum or an internal mammary artery pedicle does not improve bronchial healing after single lung transplantation: results of a randomized clinical trial. *J Heart Lung Transplant.* 1994;13:767–773.
5. **Arcasoy SM, Kotloff RM. Lung transplantation. *N Engl J Med.* 1999; 340:1081–1091.**
6. **Maurer JR, Frost AE, Estenne M, et al. International guidelines for the selection of lung transplant candidates. The International Society for Heart and Lung Transplantation, the American Thoracic Society, the American Society of Transplant Physicians, the European Respiratory Society. *Transplantation* 1998;66:951–956.**
7. Goldberg M, Lima O, Morgan E, et al. A comparison between cyclosporin A and methylprednisolone plus azathioprine on bronchial healing following canine lung autotransplantation. *J Thorac Cardiovasc Surg.* 1983; 85:821–826.
8. Schafers HJ, Wagner TO, Demertzis S, et al. Preoperative corticosteroids. A contraindication to lung transplantation? *Chest* 1992;102:1522–1525.
9. Low DE, Trulock EP, Kaiser LR, et al. Lung transplantation of ventilator-dependent patients. The Washington University Lung Transplantation Group. *Chest* 1992;101:8–11.
10. Puskas JD, Winton TL, Miller JD, et al. Unilateral donor lung dysfunction does not preclude successful contralateral single lung transplantation. *J Thorac Cardiovasc Surg.* 1992;103:1015–1017; discussion, 1017–1018.
11. Muller C, Furst H, Reichenspurner H, et al. Lung procurement by low-potassium dextran and the effect on preservation injury. Munich Lung Transplant Group. *Transplantation* 1999;68:1139–1143.
12. Kaiser LR, Cooper JD, Trulock EP, et al. The evolution of single lung transplantation for emphysema. The Washington University Lung Transplant Group. *J Thorac Cardiovasc Surg.* 1991;102:333–339; discussion 339–341.
13. Garfein ES, Ginsberg ME, Gorenstein L, et al. Superiority of end-to-end versus telescoped bronchial anastomosis in single lung transplantation for pulmonary emphysema. *J Thorac Cardiovasc Surg.* 2001;121:149–154.
14. Schroder C, Scholl F, Daon E, et al. A modified bronchial anastomosis technique for lung transplantation. *Ann Thorac Surg.* 2003; 75:1697–1704.
15. Baudet EM, Dromer C, Dubrez J, et al. Intermediate-term results after en bloc double-lung transplantation with bronchial arterial revascularization. Bordeaux Lung and Heart-Lung Transplant Group. *J Thorac Cardiovasc Surg.* 1996;112:1292–1299; discussion 1299–1300.
16. Sundset A, Tadjkarimi S, Khaghani A, et al. Human en bloc double-lung transplantation: bronchial artery revascularization improves airway perfusion. *Ann Thorac Surg.* 1997;63:790–795.
17. Pettersson G, Norgaard MA, Arendrup H, et al. Direct bronchial artery revascularization and en bloc double lung transplantation—surgical techniques and early outcome. *J Heart Lung Transplant.* 1997; 16:320–333.
18. Pasque MK, Cooper JD, Kaiser LR, et al. Improved technique for bilateral lung transplantation: rationale and initial clinical experience. *Ann Thorac Surg.* 1990;49:785 –791.
19. **Trulock EP, Edwards LB, Taylor DO, et al. The Registry of the International Society for Heart and Lung Transplantation: twenty-first official adult heart transplant report—2004. *J Heart Lung Transplant.* 2004;23:804 –815.**
20. Novick RJ, Kaye MP, Patterson GA, et al. Redo lung transplantation: a North American-European experience. *J Heart Lung Transplant.* 1993;12:515; discussion 15–16.
21. Christie JD, Bavaria JE, Palevsky HI, et al. Primary graft failure following lung transplantation. *Chest* 1998;114:51–60.
22. Low DE, Kaiser LR, Haydock DA, et al. The donor lung: infectious and pathologic factors affecting outcome in lung transplantation. *J Thorac Cardiovasc Surg.* 1993;106:614–621.
23. Keay S, Petersen E, Icenogle T, et al. Ganciclovir treatment of serious cytomegalovirus infection in heart and heart-lung transplant recipients. *Rev Infect Dis.* 1988;10 (suppl 3):S563–572.
24. Bavaria JE, Kotloff R, Palevsky H, et al. Bilateral versus single lung transplantation for chronic obstructive pulmonary disease. *J Thorac Cardiovasc Surg.* 1997;113:520–527.

CHAPTER 41 ■ PANCREAS AND ISLET TRANSPLANTATION

RANDALL S. SUNG

Diabetes mellitus is a disease that represents a spectrum of impaired glucose tolerance, ranging from gestational glucose intolerance to severe hyperglycemia and ketoacidosis. Diabetes can be divided into two major classifications. Type 1, or insulin-dependent diabetes, is an autoimmune disease characterized by the eventual loss of all pancreatic β-cell function. Although the mean age of onset is in the early teenage years, the disease may present as early as the first year of life. Type 1 diabetes afflicts approximately one in every 400 to 500 children and adolescents.[1] Patients may present as late as the fourth decade of life, and these patients may be misclassified as having type 2 diabetes, despite clearly possessing the physiology of type 1 diabetes. The disease typically occurs in a lean patient with the symptoms of polyuria, polydipsia, and polyphagia. The disease may present at the time of a concurrent illness. Although there is a brief "honeymoon" period in which insulin is not required, eventually exogenous insulin is always needed to replace that lost by the complete destruction of β-cell mass. Type 2 diabetes, previously referred to as non-insulin–dependent diabetes or adult-onset diabetes, affects approximately 6% of the U.S. population, and characteristically presents in obese patients over age 40.[2] The incidence of type 2 diabetes is increasing as the prevalence of obesity increases, especially in younger age groups. There is a prominent genetic component.

PATHOPHYSIOLOGY

The pathophysiology of type 2 diabetes is characterized by peripheral insulin resistance. Patients with type 2 diabetes display hypersecretion of insulin by β-cells. Whereas insulin resistance is thought to be the primary defect, whether insulin resistance leads to β-cell hypersecretion or vice versa is unproved. Although most type 2 diabetic patients may be treated initially with agents that enhance the sensitivity of insulin receptors and augment the action of insulin on target cells, in many patients the ability of the β-cells to secrete insulin is exhausted and exogenous insulin is required. Because of peripheral insulin resistance, many patients require insulin in amounts that exceed 1 unit/kg, far greater than typically required by Type 1 diabetic patients.

Type 1 diabetes has a known autoimmune etiology. Genetic susceptibility to type 1 diabetes is related to human leukocyte antigen (HLA) class II genotype; 90% of people with type 1 diabetes have DR3, DQ2 or DR4, DQ8 haplotypes.[3] DR3 or DR4 heterozygosity is highest in children who develop diabetes before age 5 years and lowest in adults who develop type 1 diabetes.[4] Of identical twins, 50% are concordant for type 1 diabetes, and the risk for a first-degree relative is 5%.[5] It is believed that an environmental event is necessary to trigger the autoimmune destruction of β-cells in genetically susceptible individuals. The environmental influence, possibly viral infection of the β-cell, provokes an autoimmune response, presumably initiated by a foreign antigen that mimics β chain sequences. The inflammatory response in type 1 diabetes is characterized by infiltration of islets by activated T lymphocytes (insulitis), an increase in the helper to suppressor T-cell ratio, and the expression of class II human leukocyte antigen molecules on the surface of β-cells. β-cell destruction involves both humoral and cell-mediated mechanisms. Patients with type 1 diabetes have antibodies to glutamic acid decarboxylase, carboxypeptidase A, ganglioside antigens, and islet cell antigens. These antibodies have the ability to fix complement and lyse β-cells, and can cause β-cell dysfunction prior to cell death. This observation suggests that these antibodies have a primary etiologic role, rather than developing as a consequence of autoimmune islet destruction.

SECONDARY COMPLICATIONS OF DIABETES

Diabetes mellitus is responsible for tens of thousands of deaths each year in the United States. The high incidence of cardiovascular complications in diabetic patients is primarily responsible for the twofold increase in the risk of death in diabetic patients compared with patients without diabetes.[2] Complications of diabetes include end-stage renal disease, retinopathy, peripheral vascular disease, coronary artery disease, and neuropathy. Diabetic nephropathy is responsible for nearly half of all cases of end-stage renal disease; diabetes is also the leading cause of blindness and amputation in the United States.[6] The estimated cost of providing care for patients with diabetes and its complications is over $100 billion per year.[7]

Although diabetic complications have a multifactorial etiology, they are ultimately secondary to structural alterations in nerves, blood vessels, and connective tissue. Excess glucose is converted to sorbitol by aldose reductase, leading to the reduction of cellular content of myoinositol, abnormal phosphoinositide metabolism, and reduction in Na^+-K^+-adenosine triphosphatas (ATPase) activity. In experimental animals, aldose reductase inhibitors prevent diabetic neuropathy, cataracts, and retinopathy.[8] The accumulation of advanced glycosylation end products, resulting from abnormal nonenzymatic glycosylation of proteins, and extensive cross linking of these proteins is likely to be pathogenic.[9] Ligation of endothelial cell receptors by advanced glycosylation end products results in the release of proinflammatory cytokines and activation of the coagulation cascade. Microangiopathy is characterized by thickening of capillary basement membranes, which increases with the duration of disease, and altered capillary permeability.

The Diabetes Control and Complications Trial clearly demonstrated that tight control of blood glucose and minimization of hemoglobin A1c prevents and delays the progression of secondary complications of diabetes.[10] This study, in which patients with type 1 diabetes were randomized to conventional treatment with one or two doses of daily insulin versus intensive treatment with three or more injections per day or continuous delivery with an insulin pump, demonstrated a dramatic reduction in the risk of progression of retinopathy, microalbuminuria, albuminuria, and peripheral neuropathy in the subjects randomized to intensive treatment. The major side effect of intensive treatment was a threefold increase in the risk of severe hypoglycemic episodes; approximately 10% of patients in the intensive insulin therapy cohort experienced five or more episodes of seizure or coma during the study period. Even in the absence of overt brain injury, multiple episodes of severe hypoglycemia have been associated with cerebral perfusion abnormalities and poor neuropsychiatric performance. In addition, there is a significant risk of accident during hypoglycemic episodes. Frequently, especially as hypoglycemia becomes more frequent, a syndrome of hypoglycemic unawareness results in which the typical symptoms of tremor and anxiety do not occur. Patients with hypoglycemia unawareness may develop profound hypoglycemia, and risk severe neurologic injury.

Although the overall management of diabetes is focused on maintaining blood glucose as close to normal range as possible while attempting to minimize significant hypoglycemic episodes, in practice it is a rare diabetic patient who can maintain tight glucose control without significant hypoglycemic complications. Even type 1 diabetic patients on the most intensive insulin therapy are rarely able to maintain hemoglobin A1c levels in the normal range, and most patients will ultimately develop progressive diabetic complications.

PANCREAS TRANSPLANTATION

Pancreas transplantation for many years represented the only cure for type 1 diabetes. Recipients with functioning pancreas transplants have normal glycemic control without the need for exogenous insulin. Initial experience with pancreas transplantation was marked by low success rates and high mortality.[11] In 1980, the 1-year graft survival rate for pancreas transplantation was only 21%. Consequently, there was skepticism about the utility of the procedure prior to the advent of cyclosporine. Significant advances in technique and in immunosuppression have dramatically improved graft survival rates to greater than 85% at 1 year. In addition to the development of cyclosporine, the advent of bladder drainage of the donor pancreas improved the results of pancreas transplantation (Fig. 41.1).[12,13] Graft survival has continued to improve throughout the past two decades, especially for isolated pancreas transplantation [pancreas transplant alone (PTA) or pancreas after kidney transplantation (PAK)], the results of which have been historically inferior to simultaneous kidney–pancreas transplants (SPK).

Because of the morbidity associated with bladder drainage, in recent years there has been a shift toward enteric drainage. The current trend is to perform pancreas transplantation with enteric exocrine drainage and systemic venous drainage. However, an increasing number of groups now perform pancreas transplantation by draining venous blood into the recipient portal circulation, usually via the superior mesenteric vein (Fig. 41.2). This technique avoids systemic hyperinsulinemia following systemically drained pancreas transplantation. Hyperinsulinemia has been associated with dyslipidemia and accelerated atherosclerosis, and portal venous drainage theoretically should decrease cardiovascular risk compared with systemic drainage.[14] However, despite a nearly 10-year experience with the procedure, no effect on cardiac morbidity or mortality has yet been shown, although equivalent graft and patient survival have been demonstrated.[15]

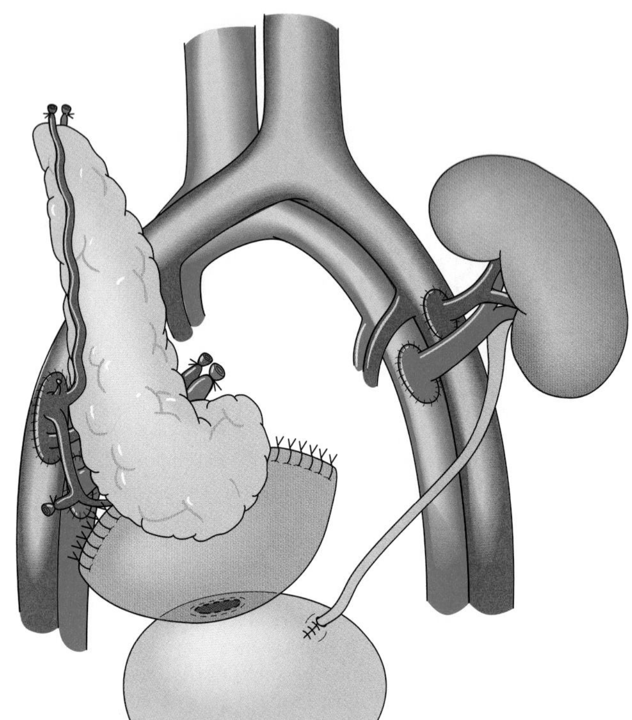

FIGURE 41.1 Simultaneous pancreas kidney transplantation performed with drainage of the pancreatic exocrine secretions into the ruinary bladder (bladder drainage). This technique has been predominant until recently. Note that a segment of the second portion of the duodenum is left attached to the pancreas. Despite its heterotopic isolation, the transplanted pancreas responds to gastrointestinal hormones with a marked increase in secretion of pancreatic juice that has a very high bicarbonate content. With bladder drainage, recipients must consume as many as 40 tablets of sodium bicarbonate daily. Also note that the portal vein drains into the iliac vein (i.e., systemic venous drainage). In healthy individuals 50% of the secreted insulin is extracted from the circulation in the first pass through the liver. Transplant recipients with systemic venous drainage have peripheral insulin levels two to two and one half times higher than normal.

Patient Selection

Pancreas transplantation is generally reserved for patients with type 1 diabetes. The diagnosis of type 1 diabetes is relatively straightforward for most individuals. A history of juvenile onset, diabetic ketoacidosis, a lean body habitus, and a low insulin requirement (less than 0.7 units/kg) all support the diagnosis of type 1 diabetes. In contrast, adult age of onset, obesity, an interval of treatment with diet or oral agents, or high insulin requirements are all suggestive of type 2 diabetes. A subset of adult-onset diabetic patients display characteristics otherwise associated with type 1 diabetes, including absence of insulin production. Whether these individuals are properly classified as type 1 or type 2 diabetic patients is uncertain, but these individuals may benefit from pancreas transplantation. Similarly, there are individuals with type 1 physiology but adult age of onset and low but detectable C-peptide secretion who may be considered for pancreas transplantation. Approximately 5% of pancreas transplant recipients are reported to have type 2 diabetes, and outcomes are similar to those for patients with type 1 diabetes. Most type 2 diabetic patients are not candidates for pancreatic transplantations.

Most individuals evaluated for pancreas transplantation have end-stage renal disease. These patients may present prior to onset of dialysis, while currently receiving dialysis, or following kidney transplantation. For individuals without a

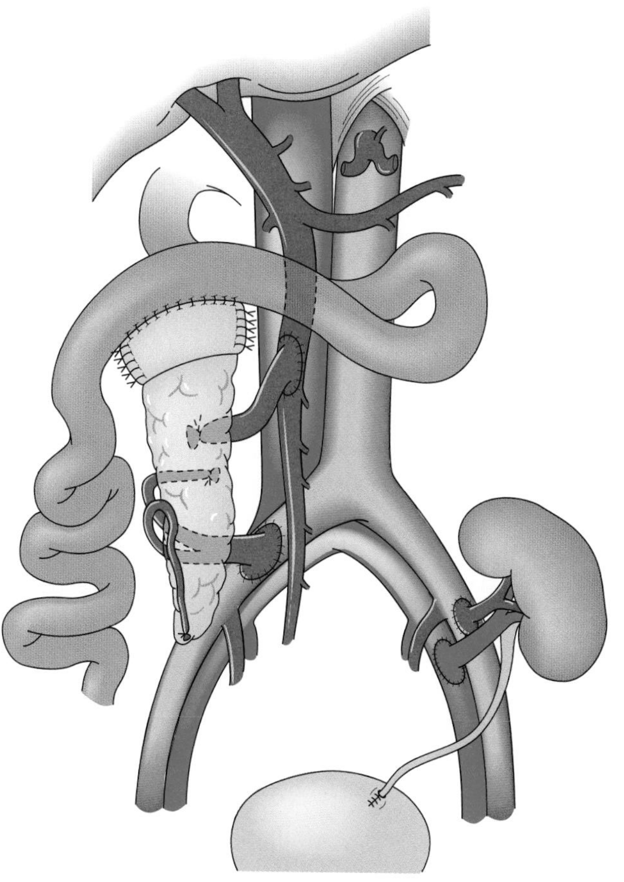

FIGURE 41.2 Simultaneous pancreas kidney transplantation performed with drainage of the pancreatic exocrine secretions into the proximal jejunum (enteric drainage). This technique has been adopted by most transplant centers in the United States for simultaneous pancreas kidney transplant cases. For solitary pancreas transplantation, some centers still utilize bladder drainage to allow monitoring of the urinary amylase. Note that the donor portal vein drains into the recipient superior mesenteric vein (portal venous drainage), preventing peripheral hyperinsulinemia. This technique appears to be associated with a lower incidence of rejection. Many centers continue to place the pancreas in the pelvis, combining enteric drainage and systemic venous drainage. This placement requires enteric anastomosis to a more distal segment of jejunum or ileum.

functioning kidney transplant, potential options include simultaneous cadaveric kidney–pancreas transplantation (SPK), living donor kidney transplantation followed by cadaveric pancreas transplantation (PAK), simultaneous living donor kidney–cadaver pancreas transplantation (SPLK), or simultaneous living donor kidney/pancreas transplantation. Of these options, the first two are by far the most common.

Simultaneous Kidney–Pancreas Transplantation

SPK is the most commonly performed pancreas transplant option, with the number exceeding all other types combined. SPK transplantation has the advantage of requiring only one operation for both transplants. Because alloreactivity against the transplanted pancreas tends to be concordant with activity against the kidney, pancreas rejection may be heralded by signs of kidney rejection, which are more sensitive and present earlier. Consequently, SPK pancreas outcomes have been historically superior to those of solitary pancreas transplants.

Pancreas after Kidney Transplantation

If a living kidney donor is available, candidates have the option of receiving a living donor renal transplant, followed by a deceased donor pancreas transplant. This approach has the disadvantage of requiring two separate operations, but the recipient enjoys the benefit of a living donor kidney transplant that may occur sooner than would an SPK. Because the primary benefit of kidney–pancreas transplant comes from the restoration of renal function, this is a significant advantage. Because a PAK is essentially a solitary pancreas transplant, however, pancreas outcomes are worse than for SPK.

Simultaneous Living Donor Kidney–Deceased Donor Pancreas Transplantation

Simultaneous living donor kidney/deceased donor pancreas transplantation (SPLK) is another option performed at a few centers.[16] Candidates with identified living donors are listed for deceased donor pancreas transplantation. When a deceased donor pancreas becomes available, the living kidney donor transplant is performed at the same time as the pancreas transplant. This approach has the advantages of PAK transplants but requires only one operation. This option does require that the potential living donor be available around the clock, a requirement that excludes some donors from this approach.

Living Donor Kidney–Pancreas Transplantation

A few centers perform living donor kidney–pancreas transplantation, with a single living donor donating the tail of the pancreas as well as the kidney (Fig. 41.3). This approach has the advantages of a single operation, a single donor, and no waiting time. Results have been comparable to SPK transplants.[17,18] Widespread adoption of this approach has been limited by concerns about donor morbidity from the pancreatectomy. Serious complications such as pancreatitis, fistula, abscess or pseudocyst occur in nearly 10% of pancreas donors. Glucose intolerance and frank diabetes have occurred, although this problem has largely abated with more stringent donor selection criteria.[18]

Patients may be counseled in a variety of ways depending on the availability of a living donor. How individuals are counseled depends on factors particular to the potential living donor and recipient and also on the expected waiting time for SPK and PAK transplantation, which vary greatly by geographic region. Because the mortality benefit of a kidney–pancreas transplant derives primarily from the kidney transplant, priority is generally given to achieving kidney transplantation expeditiously. In regions where the waiting time for SPK is long (5 years is not unusual), living donor kidney transplantation is advised. Recipients of living donor kidney transplant can then be listed for PAK which can be performed following recovery from the living donor kidney transplant. Individuals without living donors or those with borderline living donors in areas with short waiting times can be listed for SPK.

Pancreas Transplantation Alone

A small number of type 1 diabetic patients are evaluated for pancreas transplantation alone. These individuals are generally extremely labile diabetic patients who have progressive complications, excluding nephropathy. In these individuals the risk-benefit equation is quite different than for uremic diabetic patients.

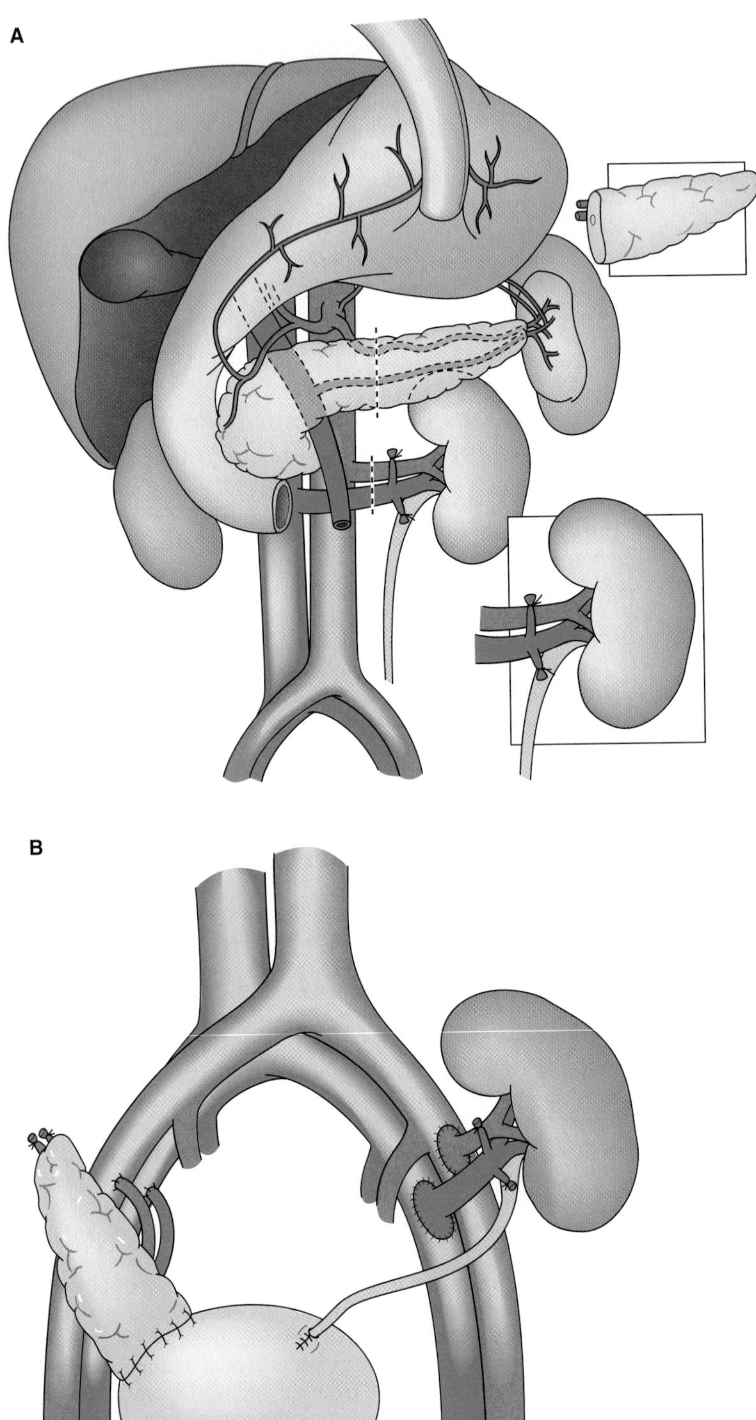

FIGURE 41.3 Live donor pancreas and kidney transplantation. (*A*) Provided that the donor has a normal or supranormal glucose tolerance test, a living donor may donate the segment of the pancreas that is to the left of the superior mesenteric vessels. (*B*) Transplantation of tail of the pancreas is based on the splenic artery and vein.

For nonuremic diabetic patients the risk of immunosuppression in addition to the surgical procedure must be weighed against the potential benefits from transplantation. In contrast, for uremic diabetic patients, the risk of immunosuppression is already assumed by virtue of the need for a kidney transplant. Whether PTA for type 1 diabetes results in a significant mortality benefit is controversial. For this reason, PTA in most centers is offered only in the most exceptional cases, usually for frequent life-threatening hypoglycemic events. Most PTA organs are from deceased donors, with a small number of centers offering living-donor PTA.

Evaluation and Screening

In general, eligibility criteria for pancreas transplantation are more stringent than for kidney transplantation alone because the operation and potential complications are more stressful and the benefits less pronounced. All candidates should have noninvasive cardiac stress testing such as dobutamine stress echocardiography or adenosine thallium stress scintigraphy. Potential candidates with reversible myocardial defects should undergo coronary angiography. The decision to perform pretransplantation coronary revascularization with angioplasty, stenting, or bypass must be made with consideration of both peritransplant mortality and long-term survival. Individuals with extensive myocardium at risk and without revascularization options are frequently excluded from consideration for pancreas transplantation.

Screening for peripheral vascular occlusive disease should be performed. Although distal peripheral vascular occlusive disease is characteristic of longstanding diabetes, aortoiliac disease and femoral popliteal vascular disease may also be present. Mild femoral popliteal disease is not a contraindication to transplantation, unless there are clinical signs of arterial insufficiency such as severe claudication or nonhealing ulcers. The presence of iliac disease is more problematic, because disease in this location can compromise inflow to the transplanted organs. Diabetic patients may have significant vascular calcification, which could preclude transplantation even in the absence of flow abnormalities. Screening for peripheral vascular occlusive disease, in addition to a thorough physical examination, may include noninvasive flow studies, magnetic resonance angiography, conventional angiography, and pelvic radiographs or computed tomography (CT) scanning to detect vascular calcification. Candidates with a history suggestive of cerebrovascular disease should be screened for hemodynamically significant carotid occlusive lesions.

Other evaluations are tailored to the individual medical history and differ among centers. Screening for malignancy commonly includes mammography and Pap smears for women, prostate-specific antigen levels in men, and colonoscopy. Individuals with a history of treated cancer are usually candidates following an appropriate disease-free interval. This interval is decreasing as greater experience with transplantation in individuals with a history of cancer has accumulated and can be as little as 2 years for many solid epithelial tumors to none for carcinoma *in situ*.[19] Screening for chronic viral infections such as hepatitis B, hepatitis C, and HIV is commonly performed. Although these infections were previously considered contraindications to pancreas transplantation, transplants in selected individuals with chronic hepatitis are being performed with increasing frequency.[20,21] Early experience with liver and kidney transplantation in carefully selected individuals with HIV infection has been encouraging.[22] Whether this practice eventually extends to pancreas transplantation is undetermined. Social and psychiatric evaluations are performed to exclude psychiatric disease, inadequate social environments, and other issues that may impair cooperation with posttransplantation management.

The Kidney–Pancreas Waiting List and Recipients

The number of patients on the waiting list for an SPK increased from 989 in 1994 to 2,366 in 2000.[23] The majority of patients are white (79%), though the percentages of African American (19%) and Hispanic-Latino patients (9%) continue to increase. The number of patients on the waiting list has increased over the past decade for all adult age groups, though the age distribution has shifted upward. Although the majority of patients are ages 35 to 49 years (60% in 2003), the percentage of patients who are ages 50 to 64 years is increasing and the percentage of patients who are ages 18 to 34 years is decreasing. The annual death rate on the SPK waiting list was 88 per 1,000 patient-years in 2003.

There has been a steady decrease in the number of SPK transplants performed, from a peak of 970 in 1998 to 867 in 2003 (Fig. 41.4). Since 1998, the decline in the number of SPK transplants has been accompanied by an increase in PAK transplants. Median times to SPK have decreased from a peak of 543 days for registrants listed in 2000 to 472 days for registrants listed in 2002. Time to transplant is longer for African American and Hispanic-Latino recipients. The majority of SPK recipients are white and male. The percentage of SPK recipients who are African Americans increased from 9% in 2000 to 16% in 2003; SPK recipients who are Hispanic increased from 5% to 9% over the same period. The age distribution of recipients parallels that of the waiting list.

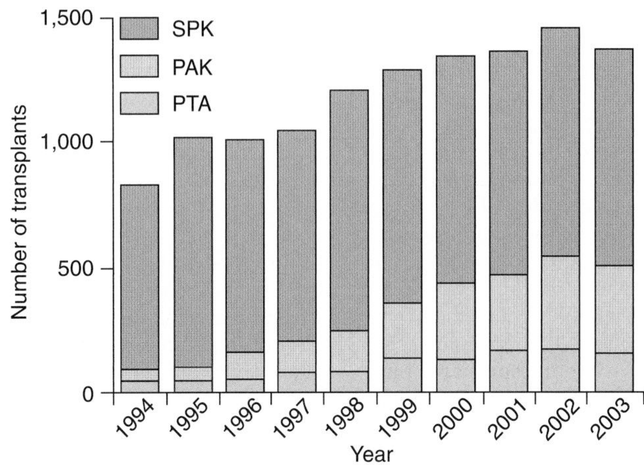

FIGURE 41.4 Number of U.S. simultaneous pancreas–kidney (SPK), pancreas after kidney transplantation (PAK), and pancreas transplantation alone (PTA) pancreas transplants performed by year. Data from Scientific Registry of Transplant Recipients. 2004 Annual Report. Rockville, MD: Health Resources and Services Administration, Department of Health and Human Services; 2004.

The Pancreas Transplant Waiting List and Recipients

The number of patients awaiting isolated pancreas transplants in 2003 continues to increase and was 784 in 2002.[23] The increase in the number of patients listed for isolated pancreas transplant in the last 5 years is largely responsible for the increase in the number of pancreas transplants being performed nationally. This may reflect improved results in isolated pancreas transplants, increase in the number of people receiving living donor kidneys, and Medicare coverage for PAK since 1999. The majority of patients awaiting isolated pancreas transplants are white (94% for PTA, 90% for PAK); unlike with SPK, there have not been significant changes in the racial distribution over the last several years. The majority of patients awaiting both PTA and PAK are between 35 and 49 years old. The number of older patients listed for PAK has increased somewhat, with 20% of the waiting list in 2003 being between the ages of 50 and 64 years.

The median time to transplant for PAK has gradually increased over the last 5 years, with the mean waiting time for 2002 being 651 days. PAK and PTA patients with blood groups type O and B have historically had longer waiting times than those with type A and AB, a pattern observed in both kidney and SPK recipients. The ages and races of recipients of solitary pancreas transplants reflect the waiting list.

Donor Evaluation

The selection of appropriate pancreas donors is a crucial determinant of successful pancreas transplantation. Many of the early complications of pancreas transplantation are secondary to processes related to organ quality and preservation, rather than to the technical conduct of the recipient operation. Whereas the ideal donor is young, nonalcoholic, and nonobese, too few donors meet this description, and the surgeon frequently needs to consider pancreata from imperfect donors. As with other organs, there are rarely absolute contraindications, and the decision to transplant a pancreas is made after consideration of a large number of donor and recipient factors.

Increased donor age increases the risk for graft failure, and the maximum age threshold is significantly lower than for liver and kidney transplantation.[24] Because of higher risk of thrombotic complications in pancreas transplantation compared to other organs, the presence of hypotension or the use of vasopressors is of more concern with the pancreas than with other organs. A history of ethanol abuse can lead to fatty changes or fibrosis within the pancreas. Risk factors for atherosclerosis such as hyperlipidemia, hypertension, and cigarette smoking may affect the pancreas transplant by causing atherosclerosis in the arteries supplying the pancreas and in the donor iliac artery, which is required for vascular reconstruction of the pancreas. A cerebrovascular cause of death (versus trauma) and elevated body mass index (BMI) greater than 30 have also been associated with adverse outcome. Although the presence of donor hyperglycemia may raise concerns about latent diabetes, in most donors this reflects the rapid administration of dextrose-containing solutions, corticosteroids for cerebral edema, and high-dose catecholamines for blood pressure support, rather than pancreatic endocrine insufficiency. Similarly, although elevations of the pancreatic enzymes, such as amylase and lipase, may suggest pancreatic injury or inflammation, these markers are nonspecific and of no consequence if the pancreas is normal on inspection.

The most important component of the donor pancreas evaluation is visual and tactile inspection by an experienced pancreas transplant surgeon. The pancreas should be soft and free of fibrosis, which is an indicator of previous pancreatitis. The gland should be salmon pink in appearance and have no fat within the interlobular septa. Peripancreatic fat is acceptable. Traumatic injury to the pancreas or hematoma within the substance of the pancreas precludes transplantation. Prior splenectomy is not a contraindication, provided that the tail can be dissected atraumatically.

Procurement Technique

The importance of pancreatic procurement cannot be overstated. Procurement is thought by many pancreas transplant surgeons to be more critical to the success of the transplant than the recipient procedure. Because the pancreas is susceptible to traumatic injury, it must be carefully dissected and manipulated to avoid injury to the pancreatic parenchyma. Typically the pancreas is procured along with the liver and kidneys through a midline incision that extends from the sternal notch to the pubic symphysis. After a Kocher maneuver, mobilization of the right colon, and isolation of the distal and supraceliac aorta, the pancreas is mobilized. Pancreatic mobilization is achieved by entering the lesser sac, dividing the gastrocolic omentum. Dissection continues with division of the short gastric vessels and the avascular gastrosplenic ligament. The pancreas is dissected from the pancreatic bed using the spleen as a handle. The tail is lifted from the pancreatic bed using blunt dissection and occasional electrocautery. The proximal jejunum is dissected at the ligament of Treitz. An antibiotic- or betadine-containing solution is frequently instilled into the duodenum through a nasogastric tube for decontamination. The duodenum is divided at the ligament of Treitz and at the pylorus using a stapler. Division of the middle colic vessels permits exposure of the proximal small bowel mesentery, which is divided distal to the pancreas with a vascular stapler.

Perfusion of the pancreas is achieved through an intraarterial cannula placed in the distal aorta following clamping of the supraceliac aorta and the aortic bifurcation. Pancreatic perfusion is typically performed with approximately 3 L of University of Wisconsin solution, while the entire abdominal organs are packed in saline slush. Recent experience with histidine-tryptophan-ketoglutarate in pancreas transplantation suggests that use of this preservation solution is safe, with no increase in risk of adverse outcomes.[25] Some centers also perfuse the abdominal viscera with a portal perfusion cannula, typically through the inferior mesenteric vein. The pancreas can be removed either *en bloc* with the liver and kidneys, *en bloc* with the liver, or separately, following removal of the liver. Whatever the technique, the portal triad is dissected out in cooperation with the liver procurement team. Typically the portal vein is shared by dividing it at the level of the coronary vein. In the presence of a replaced right hepatic artery, the superior mesenteric artery can be divided just distal to the replaced right hepatic artery, leaving a very short cuff of superior mesenteric artery on the pancreas with which to place a Y-graft of donor iliac artery. Alternatively, the replaced right hepatic artery, if large enough to be safely reconstructed by the liver transplant team without a cuff of superior mesenteric artery, can be transected as it exists superiorly from behind the head of the pancreas. The bile duct is ligated on the pancreas side and divided on the liver side, as is the gastroduodenal artery. The splenic artery, which constitutes the other arterial blood supply to the pancreas, is divided a few millimeters from its origin. Once the pancreas is removed or split from the liver, the gland is packed in preservation solution and the entire common iliac artery and its two main branches, the internal and external iliac arteries, are packaged along with the pancreas for back table reconstruction. A graft of donor iliac vein is also included in case the portal vein needs to be extended. Although most centers transplant the pancreas as soon as possible, up to 24 hours of cold ischemia time (time between perfusate infusion and organ reperfusion) has not been associated with reduced graft survival.[26]

Back Table Preparation of the Pancreas

The pancreas is placed on ice and remains cold at all times. The spleen is removed by dividing all vessels in continuity near the spleen, taking care to avoid injury to the tail of the pancreas. Significant peripancreatic fat should be trimmed. Both ends of the distal duodenum are shortened to a point immediately adjacent to the head of the pancreas. The iliac artery Y-graft is typically attached by anastomosis of the internal iliac artery to the splenic artery stump and anastomosis of the external iliac artery to the superior mesenteric artery (Fig. 41.5). In the absence of a Y-graft, the splenic artery may be implanted in end-to-side fashion to the superior mesenteric artery. The portal vein is mobilized to the confluence of the splenic and superior mesenteric veins. This maneuver allows adequate length of portal vein for anastomosis.

Recipient Operation

The pancreas transplant is typically performed through a midline incision, although a lower quadrant incision similar to that used for a kidney transplant incision may be used. The recipient should receive broad-spectrum antibiotics preoperatively. The pancreas transplant, for systemic venous drainage, is placed in the iliac fossa, preferably on the right side. After dissection of the iliac artery and vein, the portal vein is anastomosed in end-to-side

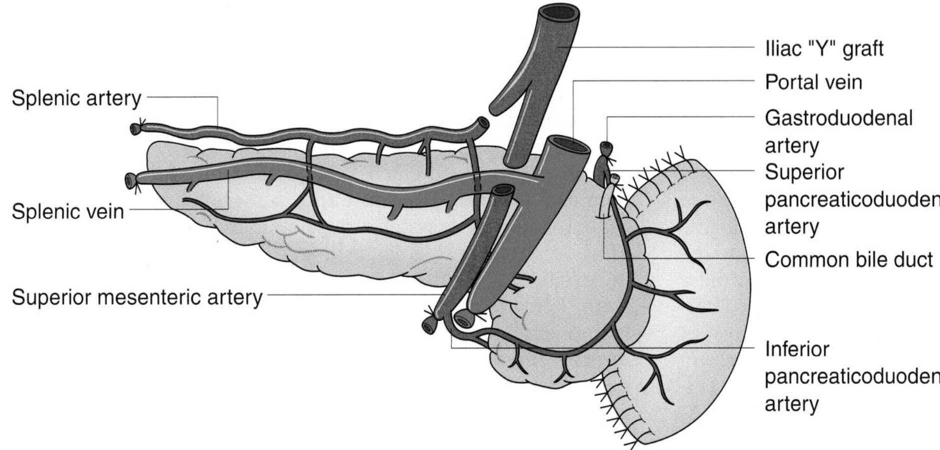

FIGURE 41.5 Back table preparation of the pancreas. Before transplantation, the pancreas must be prepared in a slush-filled basin to maintain cryopreservation. Preparation includes unifying the arterial blood supply of the pancreas by anastomosis of the donor external iliac artery to the superior mesenteric artery and the donor internal iliac artery to the splenic artery. The donor common iliac artery is used for anastomosis to the recipient iliac artery. During back table preparation, donor splenectomy is performed and both ends of the duodenum are inverted.

fashion to the external iliac vein. The common iliac vein or distal inferior vena cava can also be used; the recipient vein segment should be mobile enough for the portal vein to reach without tension. The common iliac artery component of the donor Y-graft is then anastomosed in end-to-side fashion to either the recipient external iliac artery or common iliac artery; the distal aorta can also serve as the site of anastomosis. A left-sided pancreas may be placed either medial or lateral to the sigmoid colon. Multiple variations have been described.

Because of concerns about systemic hyperinsulinemia that develops with systemically drained pancreas transplants, portal venous drainage is increasing in popularity. As 50% of insulin is removed with the first pass through the liver, systemic drainage leads to elevated peripheral insulin levels, which are not observed following portal venous drainage. The decision to perform portal or systemic drainage may depend on the anatomy of an individual patient. Patients with previous abdominal operations or those with thickened mesentery may be better suited for systemic venous drainage. Alternatively, patients who have had multiple transplants or other operations on the iliac vessels may be candidates for portal venous drainage.

For portal venous drainage, the superior mesenteric vein is dissected just below the transverse mesocolon.[27] The right common iliac artery is dissected. An end-to-side anastomosis of the donor portal vein to the recipient superior mesenteric vein is performed with the duodenum oriented superiorly and the tail pointed inferiorly. The iliac artery graft of the donor is then passed through a hole created in the small bowel mesentery and anastomosed to the recipient common iliac artery.

Most centers currently use enteric exocrine drainage for pancreas transplantation. This shift to enteric drainage has occurred as a reaction to the significant complications associated with bladder drainage. These problems include recurrent urinary tract infection, hematuria, chemical urethritis, severe bicarbonate wasting, and dehydration. Approximately 25% of individuals who receive a bladder-drained pancreas transplant require enteric conversion because of persistent complications.[28] The major advantage of bladder drainage is the ability to monitor urinary amylase, a decrease in which can be associated with rejection. This sign can be helpful in solitary pancreas transplants but is not as important for simultaneous pancreas–kidney transplants where pancreatic graft function may be monitored by serum creatinine determination. Improved immunosuppression and an increased utilization of biopsy to diagnose rejection have led to a decreased reliance on urinary amylase.[29]

Enteric drainage is achieved by creating a side-to-side or end-to-side anastomosis of donor duodenum to recipient jejunum. This may be a loop of jejunum, or a Roux-en-Y configuration may be created. For bladder drainage, a side-to-side anastomosis between the donor duodenum and the bladder is performed. Enteric drainage is always used for pancreas transplants with portal venous drainage, because the orientation of the pancreas precludes anastomosis of the duodenum to the bladder.

If an SPK is performed, the kidney transplant is usually placed in the left iliac fossa. The anastomoses, as with a kidney transplant via a retroperitoneal incision, are typically to the external iliac artery and external iliac vein. One consideration in placing a kidney in an intraperitoneal location is the potential for torsion of the kidney on its vascular pedicle. Some surgeons prefer to raise a retroperitoneal flap to place the kidney retroperitoneally after implantation. The retroperitoneal location improves percutaneous access, should biopsy be required, and decreases the risk of postbiopsy hemorrhage.

Following revascularization of the pancreas, attention is paid to bleeding from the pancreas. Anticoagulation in the perioperative period to prevent thrombosis is frequently employed, particularly for solitary pancreas transplantation. Thrombosis is less of a concern in simultaneous pancreas–kidney transplantation, where uremic platelet dysfunction is protective. The extent of anticoagulation may range from the intraoperative administration of heparin followed by low-dose heparin infusion and warfarin anticoagulation, to low-dose heparin for a limited interval postoperatively, to aspirin or other antiplatelet agents. Whatever the approach, patients should be monitored for bleeding; 5% of patients experience postoperative hemorrhage requiring reoperation.[30]

Dextrose-containing fluids are not given before revascularization of the pancreas. Following revascularization, serum glucose levels are obtained hourly. It is common for the blood glucose to decline significantly following revascularization and not uncommon for serum glucose to fall to normal levels soon after the patient's arrival in the recovery room. At some point, intravenous fluids should be converted to dextrose-containing solution to prevent hypoglycemia. Pancreas transplant recipients with enteric drainage require only maintenance fluid with consideration of third space losses. SPK recipients require fluid replacement that would be administered following kidney transplantation alone. Individuals who receive bladder-drained pancreas transplants require replacement of pancreatic exocrine losses, which can be quite profound in the early postoperative period.

Immunosuppression

The immunogenicity of a pancreas transplant is considered to be greater than the majority of solid organ transplants because of the extensive lymphoid component of the gland. In addition, the difficulty in diagnosing rejection compared to that of other solid organ transplants makes the choice of immunosuppression especially significant. Most centers use some form of triple-drug maintenance therapy, including a calcineurin inhibitor, an antiproliferative agent, and steroids, although steroid-free regimens are becoming more common. Early concerns about the diabetogenicity of tacrolimus have dissipated with greater experience, and the use of tacrolimus in pancreas transplantation has increased dramatically. According to data from the Scientific Registry of Transplant Recipients, 84% of kidney–pancreas recipients received tacrolimus as maintenance therapy, compared with only 9% who received cyclosporine.[23] Mycophenolate mofetil has largely supplanted azathioprine as the antiproliferative agent of choice in pancreas transplantation. The use of sirolimus has increased from virtually nil in 1999 to nearly 20% in 2003. The use of steroids for combined kidney transplantation is decreasing; whereas in 1999, 97% of kidney–pancreas recipients received steroids as part of initial maintenance immunosuppression, this rate has decreased to 84% in 2003. This pattern of usage is similar to that employed for solitary pancreas transplantation, either PTA or PAK.

The use of induction therapy to inhibit lymphocyte function is controversial. Two large randomized multicenter trials utilizing diverse agents such as T-cell depleting antibody induction (muromonab-CD3 and antithymocyte globulin) and interleukin-2 receptor antibody inhibition (daclizumab and basiliximab) have failed to demonstrate a significant effect on patient or graft survival.[31,32] However, in both studies a beneficial impact on the incidence of acute rejection was demonstrated. Despite the modest impact on overall graft outcome, most centers use induction therapy as part of standard immunosuppression for pancreas transplantation.[23] In 2003, 72% of kidney–pancreas transplant recipients received induction therapy. Of these, approximately two thirds received antithymocyte globulin, the remaining one third received anti- interleukin-2 receptor induction therapy. For pancreas after kidney transplants, fewer recipients received induction (64%), with a greater proportion receiving antithymocyte globulin than anti-interleukin-2 receptor agents. Multivariate analysis from the International Pancreas Transplant Registry has demonstrated a lower risk of pancreas graft loss in all categories of pancreas transplantation with the use of tacrolimus and also demonstrated similar associations with the use of mycophenolate mofetil.[26] Consistent with the multicenter trials, these analyses failed to demonstrate a beneficial effect of induction therapy on patient and graft survival.

Several recent reports have documented excellent patient and graft outcomes utilizing steroid minimization protocols.[33,34] These protocols generally employ an induction agent, usually a depleting T-cell antibody, tacrolimus and either mycophenolate mofetil or sirolimus. Steroids are given for a maximum of 3 days. These steroid minimization protocols aim to avoid the significant short- and long-term side effects associated with corticosteroids.

Complications

Thrombosis of the pancreas transplant is the most common cause of graft loss in the early postoperative period. The factors that make pancreas transplants more prone to thrombosis than other solid organ transplants are uncertain. The most likely mechanism is that ischemia reperfusion injury in the pancreas, characterized by the release of cytokines and activation of pancreatic enzymes, leads to accelerated injury and a procoagulant state. Diabetic patients have impaired fibrinolysis and are therefore relatively hypercoagulable. The relatively low venous flow through the portal vein, which leads to diminished flow velocity, may be contributory. Thrombosis is more common in solitary pancreas transplantation than in SPK, probably because of the absence of uremic platelet dysfunction. The risk of thrombosis has been associated with donor factors such as older patient age, BMI, and cerebrovascular cause of death.[35,37]

Pancreas transplant thrombosis is usually heralded by a sudden rise in blood glucose. Confirmation of the diagnosis is obtained with duplex ultrasound. Although anecdotal reports have described successful surgical and angiographic thrombectomy or thrombolysis in restoring flow to the pancreas,[36,38] the usual treatment is immediate removal of the infarcted pancreas. Because of the high risk of thrombosis, anticoagulation is frequently employed. Because of these efforts and improvements in immunosuppression, the thrombosis rate has decreased to less than 5% for simultaneous pancreas–kidney transplants and to less than 10% for isolated pancreas transplants.

Bleeding is a frequent cause for reoperation in the early postoperative period. Because of the large number of vessels that enter and exit the pancreas, bleeding following reperfusion is not unusual. Hemorrhage can be minimized by meticulous ligation of vascular structures during pancreas procurement. The use of anticoagulation in the perioperative period adds to bleeding risk. Pancreas transplant recipients are monitored carefully in the early postoperative period for signs and symptoms of intraabdominal hemorrhage.

The other major early complication is leak from the donor duodenum. Duodenal leaks occur in approximately 10% of cases, usually 1 to 2 weeks after the transplant.[39] A leak may present as fever, abdominal pain, leucocytosis, lower abdominal tenderness, and persistent ileus. The diagnosis is supported by the finding of a focal fluid collection near the head of the pancreas on CT scanning or ultrasonography. Diffuse peritonitis may reflect disseminated contamination. For bladder-drained pancreas transplants, the diagnosis may be made by cystography. Occasionally peripancreatic sepsis can occur in the absence of a duodenal leak, caused by the growth of organisms transmitted to the peritoneal cavity during performance of the duodenal-enteric or duodenal-bladder anastomosis.

The management of duodenal leak is operative. The peritoneum should be lavaged and all necrotic debris removed. If a leak is present it is usually at the stapled end of the duodenum rather than at the anastomosis. Successful repair depends on viability of the duodenum at the point of leak, hemodynamic stability, and the degree of surrounding inflammation. Usually one attempt at repair is made, but failure may necessitate removal of the pancreas. Some surgeons have adopted a practice of managing leaks from duodenal enteric anastomosis by conversion to bladder drainage. This minimizes the risk of recurrent contamination of the peritoneal cavity with enteric contents and allows for Foley catheter decompression of the duodenum but has the morbidity associated with bladder drainage. Occasionally a fluid collection that presents late can be treated with percutaneous CT-guided drainage. In addition, drainage of infection without primary repair of the duodenal leak has been successfully employed in situations where inflammation is so profound that the leak could not be primarily repaired.

Diagnosis and Treatment of Rejection

The timely and accurate diagnosis of pancreas transplant rejection is one of the most important and challenging aspects of posttransplant management. Because noninvasive means of diagnosing rejection are neither sensitive nor specific, the diagnosis of rejection is best made by histologic examination of a pancreatic biopsy specimen.[40] Although the pancreas graft in SPK transplants can be monitored by following the serum creatinine, the concordance rate for rejection between kidney and pancreas grafts is only about two thirds.[41] Improvements in the outcome of solitary pancreas transplants are attributable not only to improvements in the overall quality of immunosuppression but also in the ability to more accurately treat pancreas rejection.

The technique of pancreas transplant biopsy has evolved over the years. In the era of bladder-drained pancreas transplants, cystoscopic biopsy of both the pancreas and transplant duodenum was common.[42] As more enteric-drained pancreas transplants have been performed, a greater reliance on percutaneous biopsy has developed, using either ultrasound or CT-guided techniques.[43] Laparoscopic-assisted pancreas biopsy has proved successful for patients whose pancreas transplant may not be accessible to percutaneous approaches.[44] The indications for pancreatic biopsy include hyperamylasemia, hyperlipasemia, hyperglycemia, or unexplained pain in the vicinity of the pancreas transplant. The differential diagnosis includes toxicity from calcineurin inhibitors, pancreatitis, cytomegalovirus infection, and, in the early postoperative period, peripancreatic infection. A major advance in the success of solitary pancreas transplantation is the development of a histologic grading system for pancreas biopsies.[45] Mild rejection grades (2 and 3) are usually treated with pulse corticosteroids, whereas moderate and severe rejection may be treated with either muromonab-CD3 or antithymocyte globulin.

As long-term survival of pancreas transplants becomes more commonplace, chronic rejection is emerging as an important problem.[46] Chronic rejection is histologically characterized as expansion of fibrous septa within the pancreatic parenchyma, progressing to lobular atrophy or loss of both acini and β-cells. Although there are parallels to chronic allograft nephropathy, whether chronic calcineurin inhibitor toxicity contributes to chronic pancreas rejection is unknown (Table 41.1).

Recurrent Autoimmunity

Selective β-cell destruction in pancreas transplants may occur in a pattern similar to the insulitis seen in type 1 diabetes. This pattern is histologically distinct from cellular rejection. Although recurrent autoimmunity has been documented in both immunosuppressed pancreas transplant recipients and nonimmunosuppressed living donor recipients from identical twin siblings, well-documented case series have been infrequent. A variety of

TABLE 41.1

ANTIREJECTION METHODS IN THE ABSENCE OF CONTINUOUS IMMUNOSUPPRESSION IN RODENTS THAT LEAD TO INDEFINITE SURVIVAL

Method	Species	Reference
24°C culture pretreatment of donor islets combined with single injection of antilymphocyte serum	Rat	Lacy PE, et al. Science 1979;204:312–313.
95% O_2 pretreatment of donor islets	Mouse	Bowen KM, et al. Aust J Exp Biol Med Sci 1980;58:441–447.
Microencapsulation of islets	Rat	Lim F, Sun AM. Science 1980;210:908–910.
Donor-specific blood transfusions treated with ultraviolet irradiation	Rat	Lau H, et al. Science 1984;221:754–756.
Ultraviolet irradiation of donor islets combined with a 3-day course of cyclosporine	Rat	Lau H, et al. Science 1984;223:607–609.
Transplantation of islets into the intraabdominally placed testis	Rat	Selawry HJ, Whittington K. Diabetes 1984;33:405–406.
Gamma irradiation pretreatment of donor islets combined with a 3-day course of cyclosporine	Rat	James R, et al. Transplantation 1989;47:929–933.
Intrathymic islet transplantation combined with a single injection of antilymphocyte serum	Rat	Posselt A, et al. Science 1990;249:1293–1295.
Selective costimulatory blockade by anti-CD154 treatment combined with pretransplantation infusion of donor lymphocytes	Mouse	Parker, et al. Proc Nat Acad Sci USA 1995;96:9560–9564.
Cotransplantation of syngeneic myoblasts engineered to express the Fas liquid	Mouse	Lau H, et al. Science 1996;273:109–112.
Contranspiantation of allogeneic testicular cell aggregates	Rat	Korbutt GS, et al. Diabetes 1997;46:317–322.
Antibody-mediated targeting of CD45 isoforms	Mouse	Basadonna GP, et al. Proc Natl Acad Sci USA 1998;95:3821–3826.

Adapted with permission from Hering BJ, Ricordi C. Islet transplantation for patients with type 1 diabetes. *Graft* 1999;2:23.

associations have been suggested with autoantibodies to glutamic acid decarboxylase (GAD-65) and islet cells (IA-2), but patterns of autoantibody expression have not established etiologic relevance or prognostic value.

Results of Kidney–Pancreas Transplantation

There were 6,861 recipients of SPK transplants alive with functioning grafts at the end of 2003.[23] Current kidney graft survival at 1 and 5 years following SPK transplantation is 91% and 77%, respectively. African Americans have somewhat poorer 5-year graft survival (72%) than whites (77%). Kidneys from older donors have the poorest graft survival; 5-year graft survival from donors older than 50 is 68% compared with approximately 79% from donors age 11 to 34 years. Recipients with a previous kidney transplant have graft survival that is worse than for those without. Five-year kidney graft survival tends to decrease with increasing levels of HLA mismatch.

Pancreas graft survival at 1 and 5 years following SPK transplantation is 86% and 70%, respectively (Fig. 41.6). Worse 5-year graft survival is seen in African American and Asian recipients compared with white recipients. Five-year graft survival from donors over age 50 years is significantly lower than that from donors less than 35 years, including those younger than age 10 years. Recipients with a previous transplant (kidney, pancreas, or both) have worse pancreas graft survival. There is a trend toward decreased 5-year pancreas graft survival with increasing levels of HLA mismatch.

Registry analyses demonstrate a mortality benefit of SPK transplantation compared with dialysis[47] or kidney transplantation alone.[48] Patient survival at 1 year and 5 years following SPK transplantation is 95% and 85%, respectively (Fig. 41.7). Race, ethnicity, sex, and transplant center volume are not associated with decreased patient survival at 5 years, and patient survival has not changed significantly since 1995. Death rates for recipients in the first year following transplant have steadily decreased, from 93 per 1,000 patient-years at risk in 1994 to 52 per thousand patient-years at risk in 2002. These rates continue to be lower than the corresponding death rates for candidates on the SPK waiting list. Older (ages 50 to 64 years) and African-American recipients tend to have higher death rates in the first year following transplantation.

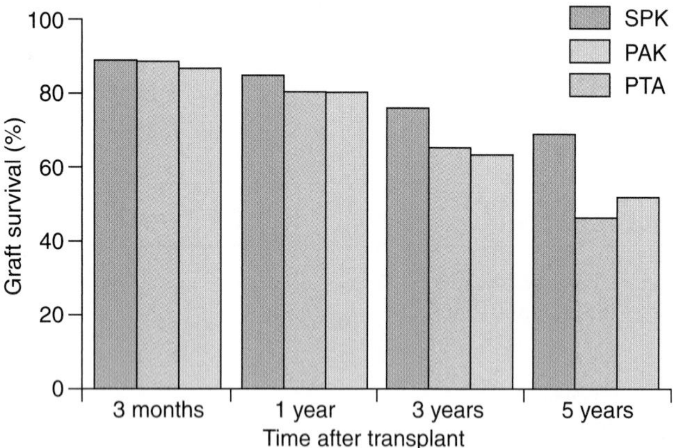

FIGURE 41.6 Pancreas graft survival for U.S. transplants. Cohorts are transplants performed during 2001 to 2002 for 3-month and 1-year survival; 1999 to 2000 for 3-year survival; and 1997 to 1998 for 5-year survival. (Data from Scientific Registry of Transplant Recipients. 2004 Annual Report. Rockville, MD: Health Resources and Services Administration, Department of Health and Human Services; 2004. From Danovitch GM, Cohen DJ, Weir MR, et al. Current status of kidney and pancreas transplantation in the United States, 1994–2003. *Am J Transplant.* 2005;5:904–915.)

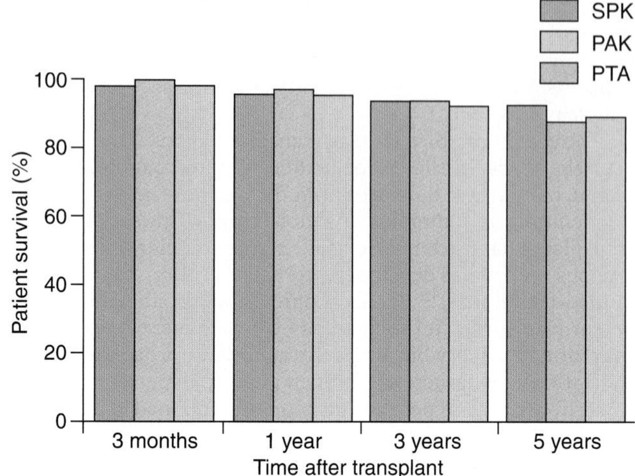

FIGURE 41.7 Patient survival for U.S. pancreas transplant recipients. Cohorts are transplants performed during 2001 to 2002 for 3-month and 1-year survival; 1999 to 2000 for 3-year survival; and 1997 to 1998 for 5-year survival. (Data from Scientific Registry of Transplant Recipients. 2004 Annual Report. Rockville, MD: Health Resources and Services Administration, Department of Health and Human Services; 2004. From Danovitch GM, Cohen DJ, Weir MR, et al. Current status of kidney and pancreas transplantation in the United States, 1994–2003. *Am J Transplant.* 2005;5:904–915.)

Results of Solitary Pancreas Transplantation

The 1-year pancreas graft survival for recipients of a PAK transplant has improved in the last 5 years, although the 1-year unadjusted graft survival decreased from 84% for PAK transplants performed in 2001 to 78% for PAK transplants performed in 2002.[32] The 1-year graft survival for PAK has ranged between 72% and 84% since 1998, and this success may have prompted the overall increase in the number of PAK transplants being performed nationally. The graft survival for PAK at 3 years and 5 years is currently 65%, and 53%, respectively. Patient survival for PAK recipients is excellent, 96% and 82% at 1 year and 5 years, respectively.

One-year pancreas graft survival for PTA has improved in the last 5 years to 83% for transplants performed in 2002. The unadjusted graft survival for PTA at 3 and 5 years is 66% and 47%, respectively. Overall the results of PTA now approximate those observed for PAK. Patient survival rates for PTA recipients are 98% at 1 year and 80% at 5 years, respectively.

Whether pancreas transplantation positively impacts patient mortality is controversial. Recently, investigators reported that registrants on the waiting lists for PAK and PTA had better survival rates than recipients who underwent these procedures.[47] These findings have been challenged by others[49] who reported better survival rates for recipients of solitary pancreas transplantation than registrants on the waiting list. These discrepancies are in part related to variability in the year-to-year death rates on the waiting list and may reflect the inherent difficulties in using data obtained from large registries.

Effect of Pancreas Transplantation on Secondary Complications of Diabetes Mellitus

Pancreas transplantation has an impact on diabetic complications. Whereas type 1 diabetic recipients of kidney transplants alone show typical findings of diabetic nephropathy following transplantation, SPK transplantation prevents the development of recurrent diabetic nephropathy.[50] In addition, native diabetic nephropathy has been demonstrated to reverse 10 years following successful isolated pancreas transplantation.[51] These reports demonstrate convincingly that pancreas transplantation has a significant impact on diabetic nephropathy.

Effects on diabetic neuropathy have also been documented using nerve conduction studies, which are significantly improved following pancreas transplantation.[52] Progression of diabetic neuropathy is significantly diminished compared with non-transplanted controls. However, no study has been able to demonstrate clinical improvement in existing diabetic neuropathy following transplantation. There is also an impact on autonomic neuropathy, with clinical improvement in epinephrine responses to hypoglycemia.[53] The effect of pancreas transplantation on retinopathy is only modest. Stabilization of moderate retinopathy has been demonstrated, although long-term graft function (greater than 3 years) is required.[54] Many pancreas transplant candidates have advanced retinopathy, and an effect has not been demonstrated in these individuals. Early acceleration of retinopathy, a phenomenon that has been noted with other methods of improving glycemic control, can occur in the first 6 to 12 months following transplant. An assessment of the impact of pancreas transplantation on the progression of atherosclerosis is lacking a definitive large-scale study. Smaller single-center studies are mixed, with some centers demonstrating a positive impact on peripheral vascular occlusive disease, and others demonstrating a worsening of disease.[55,56]

Irrespective of the magnitude of objectively demonstrable benefits of pancreas transplantation, most recipients enjoy a dramatic improvement in quality of life.[57,58] Although many diabetic patients adapt quite well to the dramatic glucose fluctuations and the associated morbidity of diabetes, the freedom from insulin and the avoidance of hyperglycemia and hypoglycemia offered by a functioning pancreas transplant is a primary motivator for many recipients. The fervor with which many candidates pursue pancreas transplantation, especially retransplantation, is an indication of the enormous benefit on quality of life.

ISLET TRANSPLANTATION

The notion that insulin-producing β-cells could be physically separated from the pancreas and transplanted for the treatment of diabetes has long been recognized. Islet transplantation, as a cellular transplant, has significant potential advantages over whole-organ pancreas transplantation. Islet transplantation does not require an operative procedure.[59] The potential to preserve islets without impairment of graft function, through culture or cryopreservation, opens new possibilities with regard to distribution, allocation, transportation, and preparation of the islet recipient. Pretreatment of the graft to reduce immunogenicity or enhance survival and function is also possible.[60] Recipients of successful islet transplants have glucose metabolism and insulin secretion profiles that are close to normal and maintain long-term metabolic control in a manner equivalent to whole-pancreas transplantation.[61] Although effects on mortality and progression of diabetic complications are unproved, these benefits are also anticipated. From a long-range perspective, the development of islet transplantation sets some of the procedural, technical, and regulatory groundwork for the eventual establishment of stem-cell derived β-cell transplantation.

HISTORY

The development of islet transplantation was historically limited by poor graft survival. The first human islet allograft in a type 1 diabetic patient was performed in 1974.[62] The first islet autograft for the treatment of chronic pancreatitis was performed in 1977. Despite intense research over three decades, until 2000, clinical islet transplantation met with minimal success.[63] While the transplanted islets were capable of physiologic function, as evidenced by the 66% rate of insulin independence at 1 year in the 163 recipients of islet autografts from 1974 to 1995, even these recipients had significantly reduced functional β-secretory reserve.[64] Alloimmunity to the islets presented an even greater hurdle; in the 96 islet allograft recipients with type 1 diabetes from 1990 to 1994, C-peptide production and insulin independence at 1 year were 25% and 7%, respectively.[63] Of the 270 recipients until 1999, only 6 had achieved insulin independence for greater than 2 years.

The dramatic improvement in islet transplant outcome reported in 2000 sparked a resurgence of interest in islet transplantation and islet transplant activity.[65] Important refinements in islet isolation and immunosuppression, collectively referred to as the *Edmonton Protocol*, have largely been adopted by all islet programs. Important features include careful attention to pancreas procurement, minimization of cold ischemia time of the pancreas prior to isolation, avoidance of xenoproteins in the islet isolation process, and avoidance of steroids in the immunosuppressive regimen. More than 15 centers are actively performing islet transplantation in North America, and at least that many aspire to develop islet transplant programs. Consequently, the significant recent increase in the number of islet transplants is expected to continue.

Islet Isolation

The precise separation of the islets from the other tissues of the pancreas (exocrine cells, lymphatics, vascular structures), is perhaps the most important determinant of successful islet transplantation (Fig. 41.8). One of the limitations of islet isolation is the difficulty in obtaining a large number of high-quality islets, and consistent success in islet isolation is a combination of science, art, and experience. Although a variety of methods have been used, most currently employ combined mechanical distension with enzymatic digestion of the pancreas.[66] After cleaning the pancreas of surrounding fat, the pancreatic duct is cannulated and the pancreas is distended with warm collagenase solution, which digests the pancreas.[67] The pancreas is then placed into a sterile stainless steel chamber, which also contains a number of stainless steel or glass spheres. Additional collagenase solution is added, and the chamber is attached to a shaking apparatus. Agitation of the chamber allows the spheres to disrupt the structural integrity of the pancreas as it digests. Following digestion, separation of islets from non-islet tissue is performed through density gradient centrifugation. After suspension in culture media, islets are counted and assessed for sterility, purity, viability, and functional capacity. The percentage of islet isolations that result in a transplantable preparation varies widely among centers, between 25% and 70%, and depends both on donor selection practices and the experience and expertise of the particular center.

Patient Selection

Candidates for islet transplantation are selected in a similar manner as for whole-organ pancreas transplantation. Islet transplantation is currently limited to adult type 1 diabetic patients with progressive diabetic complications who have failed intensive insulin therapy. Because islet transplantation remains experimental therapy with limited availability, and because of widespread patient interest in the procedure, the

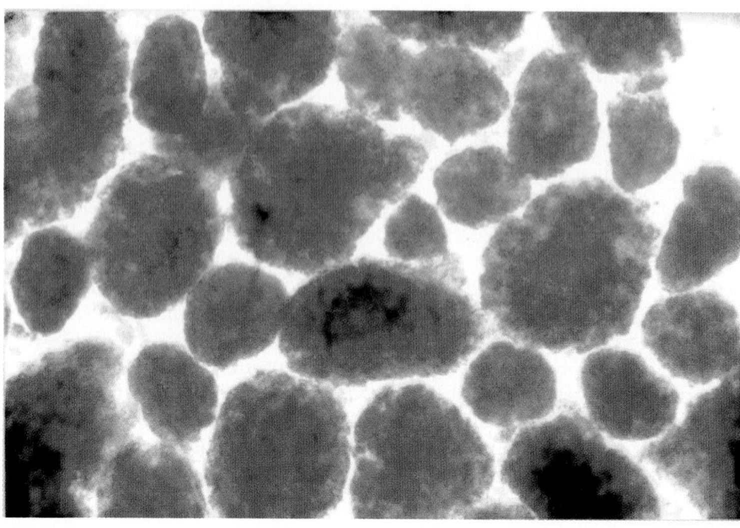

FIGURE 41.8 Isolated, purified human islets. Islets are stained red with diphenylthiocarbazone. (Adapted with permission from Robertson PR. Islet transplantation as a treatment for diabetes: A work in progress. *N Engl J Med.* 2004;350:694–705.)

therapy is offered only to ideal candidates with minimal medical conditions other than diabetes. Most centers require evaluation and a period of treatment by an experienced endocrinologist specializing in diabetes. Candidates with coronary artery disease; chronic infections, including hepatitis B and C; or prior solid organ transplant are excluded. Nonuremic candidates must be free of renal insufficiency because of concerns about aggravation of nephropathy by calcineurin inhibitors. Because efficacy of the islet transplant appears to be related to the number of islets transplanted per kilogram of recipient body weight, only lean recipients (less than 70 kg or BMI below 28) are selected. Although most islet transplants are currently performed in nonuremic diabetic patients, islet transplantation either concurrent with or following kidney transplantation is being performed more frequently than in the past.

Donor Selection, Procurement, and Preservation

Donor selection for islet isolation differs from that for whole-pancreas transplantation in several respects. Whereas the ideal donor for islet isolation is still young and healthy, the age and weight criteria are far less stringent than for whole-pancreas transplantation. Donors older than age 50, those on vasopressors, and obese donors are all suitable for islet isolation. Because the ideal pancreas is easily distensible and digestible, fatty pancreata are thought to be suitable, whereas fibrotic pancreata are not suitable. A recent U.S. Organ Procurement and Transplantation Network policy preferentially allocates pancreata from older and obese donors (which are infrequently used for whole pancreas) for islet transplantation rather than for regional and national sharing for whole-pancreas transplantation.[68] This policy change should lead to more expeditious placement of suitable pancreata for islet transplantation without adversely affecting the overall volume of whole-pancreas transplants.

The pancreas is procured in a manner similar to whole-pancreas transplantation. Less attention to preservation of vascular structures is required. Attention is paid to surface cooling following flushing of preservation solution and to avoidance of pancreatic injury. A number of reports have highlighted the importance of a dedicated team trained in pancreas procurement in the success of islet isolation.[69,70] Expanded use of the two-layer technique of pancreas preservation, using both standard preservation solution (University of Wisconsin solution or histidine-tryptophan-ketoglutarate) and oxygenated perfluorocarbon solution, has resulted in increased islet yields.[71–73] The two-layer technique also permits the successful use for islet transplantation of pancreata subjected to cold ischemia prolonged for as long as 18 hours. Success with pancreata from donors after cardiac death has been reported.[74] As overall utilization of organs from donors after cardiac death increases, more pancreata suitable for islet isolation can be expected.

Transplant Techniques

The portal circulation of the liver is currently the preferred site for islet transplantation (Fig. 41.9).[75] The portal system can be accessed by a minilaparotomy, with infusion of the islets into a peripheral mesenteric vein. Most centers use interventional radiology techniques, avoiding both a surgical incision and general anaesthesia. Percutaneous transhepatic portal vein catheterization is done under ultrasound and fluoroscopic guidance, usually with a small-gauge (4-Fr) catheter. The islets are infused into the portal vein through the catheter by either gravity from an infusion bag or by hand injection, and the islets lodge in the hepatic parenchyma. Portal vein pressure is monitored intermittently throughout the procedure. Following infusion of islets, hemostasis is achieved using a combination of coils and gelfoam. Recipients receive heparin in the islet preparation, systemically during the procedure, and in the perioperative period as prophylaxis against portal vein thrombosis.

Because of concerns about the short- and long-term complications of portal vein islet transplantation, alternative techniques have been explored. Sites underneath the kidney capsule, within an omental pouch, and in subcutaneous and intramuscular locations have been employed experimentally.[76–78] Technologies that encapsulate islets with synthetic polymers designed to allow diffusion of small molecules but provide immunoprotection and bioartificial pancreas, which function similarly but contain a large number of islets in a single device, are under development.[79,80]

Perioperative Care

It is common for recipients to receive a few days of inpatient care for monitoring purposes. Immediately following the islet transplant, patients are maintained on bed rest for a short

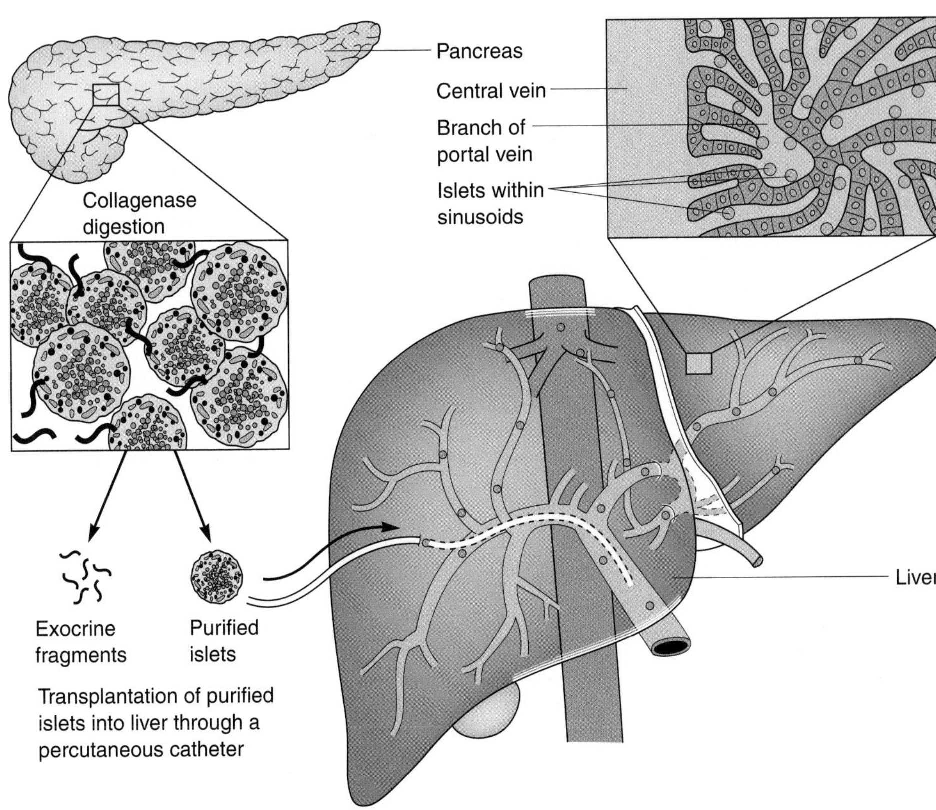

FIGURE 41.9 Islet transplantation. The pancreas is procured as a whole organ from the donor. The islets are isolated from the pancreas and are purified and infused into a cannula placed in a branch of the recipient's portal vein.

interval and monitored for bleeding. Liver function tests are monitored, and a liver ultrasound is frequently performed to assess portal venous flow and to check for hematoma. Intensive glycemic control with insulin in the immediate post-transplant period is beneficial for islet function.[81] Hence, many centers administer insulin postoperatively to keep the serum glucose tightly controlled, to "rest" the islets. Additional adjuncts to prevent nonspecific inflammation include antioxidants such as vitamin E, antibodies against tumor necrosis factor-α, pentoxifylline, and others.

Immunosuppression

The defining feature of the Edmonton Protocol was the elimination of steroids from the immunosuppressive regimen, which also included basiliximab induction, and maintenance therapy with low-dose tacrolimus and sirolimus. Although most immunosuppressive regimens are still based on these agents, those employing mycophenolate mofetil and cyclosporine are becoming more common. Induction agents range from polyclonal or monoclonal antibodies directed against lymphocytes to the immunotoxin alemtuzumab. Islet transplantation is being employed with increasing success in uremic diabetic patients, either in combination with (simultaneous islet–kidney) or following a kidney transplant (islet after kidney).[82,83] In general, the best results for islet–kidney transplantation continue to be cases in which steroids are avoided or eliminated at the time of islet transplantation. Long-term effects of either the islet transplant or steroid elimination on kidney function are not known, although short-term outcomes of steroid avoidance in kidney transplant recipients are promising.[84]

Metabolic Control

All centers report significant improvement in metabolic function and glycemic reserve. Although hormonal counterregulation to hypoglycemia is diminished, actual hypoglycemic events are rare.[85] Analyses of the impact on diabetic complications and mortality await further experience. Preliminary data demonstrate potentially beneficial effects on endothelial function and markers of coagulation,[86] which could positively affect microvascular complications.

Complications

Morbidity from islet transplantation is substantial but less frequent than had been once feared and much less than that for whole-pancreas transplantation. The most common serious complication remains bleeding (1% to 5%), as the importance of anticoagulation to prevent portal vein thrombosis has become recognized. Most cases of bleeding can be managed nonoperatively with adjustments in anticoagulation, though occasionally laparotomy is required. Branch or main portal vein thrombosis was encountered more commonly in the past (approximately 1%), with significant morbidity. The side effects of immunosuppression, such as hyperlipidemia and mouth ulcers in sirolimus-containing regimens, are much more common and can significantly affect quality of life.[87] Renal insufficiency occasionally has been encountered. Transient elevations of portal venous pressure during islet infusion and elevations of liver function tests following infusion are common and usually well tolerated.[88,89] Recently, the demonstration of late steatosis has raised concerns about chronic liver disease; to date this has not occurred.[90] Other common adverse consequences in whole-organ transplantation, such as cytomegalovirus infection and sensitization to alloantigen, have not materialized. Mortality is virtually nil.

Results

The results of islet transplantation at high-volume centers are approaching that of whole-pancreas transplantation.

The University of Alberta has reported insulin independence rates of 80% at 1 year.[91] Both the University of Miami and the University of Minnesota recently have reported insulin independence rates of greater than 90%, with sustained insulin independence of greater than 80% at 1 year.[92,93] Unfortunately, the successes of the largest islet centers have been replicated inconsistently elsewhere. The Immune Tolerance Network multicenter trial of the Edmonton Protocol, which features steroid avoidance and uses of fresh islets and avoidance of xenoproteins, has completed enrollment.[94] Interim analyses demonstrated success rates at three of the centers (Edmonton, Minnesota, Miami) that were significantly higher than at the other centers.[95] Nevertheless, some other groups have demonstrated success equivalent to that of the larger centers,[87,96] and it is anticipated that outcomes will continue to improve with experience.

One of the ongoing shortcomings of islet transplantation compared with whole-pancreas transplantation is the inability to reverse diabetes with the islets from one pancreas. Most of the recipients in the modern era have required two or more islet infusions to achieve insulin independence. Because only 50% to 70% of all islet isolations lead to a transplantable islet preparation, as many as four pancreata may be necessary to reverse diabetes in one recipient. Clearly, the total number of islets transplanted is an important determinant of the success of transplantation. Some centers have successfully employed single-donor islet transplantation by using careful donor and recipient selection, usually by transplanting islets from pancreata of large donors into small recipients.[92,96] The ability to maximize the use of islets and minimize islet requirements for an individual recipient is critical if islet transplantation is to compare favorably with whole-pancreas transplantation from an organ utilization perspective.

As more centers report successful experience with cultured islets, a shift has taken place toward less rapid transplantation following islet isolation.[91–93] This trend has significant implications for many aspects of transplantation. The ability of islets to be sustained in culture for several days permits an adequate period of pretransplant immunosuppression. It also may encourage the further development of islet networks, where islets are shipped from the isolation center to a different transplant center. Existing collaborations of this sort have been highly successful.[97,98]

Graft Failure

Graft failure appears to occur earlier in islet transplantation than in whole-pancreas transplants. Approximately 20% to 30% of recent recipients return to insulin within 2 years. Failure may be related to the inability to histologically diagnose and treat islet rejection because the islets are scattered about the liver parenchyma. Attempts to identify immunologic markers of rejection or recurrent autoimmunity, or metabolic indicators of impending graft failure are not sufficiently predictive for clinical application.[99,100] Recipients with prior graft function who have returned to insulin are candidates for retransplantation. In fact, some centers have used islets from isolations in which the yields are insufficient for a primary transplant as retransplants because the islet requirement may be less.

The Future of Pancreas and Islet Transplantation

Many challenges remain in determining the ideal insulin replacement therapy for type 1 diabetic patients. Although the current allocation system designed to maximize whole-pancreas transplantation ensures the most efficient use of donor pancreata, improvements in the efficiency of islet isolation may require that further refinements be made to allocation policy. Current candidate selection criteria are more liberal for whole-pancreas transplantation than for islet transplantation, but as islet transplantation moves further into the mainstream, the reduced morbidity of islet transplantation may mean that a large number of candidates who are not surgical candidates for pancreas transplantation may be islet candidates in the future. Many centers have taken the philosophical step to offer islet transplantation primarily to diabetic patients who would not otherwise receive immunosuppression, for example, nonuremic diabetic patients. Taken further, islet transplantation could theoretically be open to a large number of type 1 diabetic patients who would surely exhaust the limited supply of donor pancreata. Experience gained by the development of islet transplantation would surely apply to technologies not affected by donor supply, such as islet xenografts or engineered β-cells, which could theoretically have a profound impact on the devastating effects of diabetes on the public health worldwide.

KEY POINTS

- **The Diabetes Control and Complications Trial demonstrated that tight control of blood glucose and minimization of hemoglobin A1C delays the progression of secondary complications of diabetes.**
- **Recipients with functioning pancreas transplants have normal glycemic control without the need for exogenous insulin, and pancreas transplantation has a beneficial impact on a number of diabetic complications.**
- **Most pancreas transplants are performed in patients with end-stage renal disease, either concomitant with or following a kidney transplant.**
- **Pancreas graft survival rates are greater than 80% at 1 year.**
- **Pancreas transplant outcome is dependent on the careful selection of donors and on meticulous pancreas procurement technique.**
- **Islet transplantation does not require an operative procedure.**

References

1. American Diabetes Association. National Diabetes Fact Sheet 2002. Available at http://www.diabetes.org/diabetes-statistics/national-diabetes-fact-sheet.jsp.
2. Engelgau MM, Geiss LS, Saaddine JB, et al. The evolving diabetes burden in the United States. *Ann Intern Med.* 2004;140:945–950.
3. Atkinson MA, Eisenbarth GS. Type 1A diabetes: new perspectives on disease pathogenesis and treatment. *Lancet* 2001;358:221–229.
4. Bennett ST, Todd JA. Human type 1A diabetes and the insulin gene: principles of mapping polygenes. *Annu Rev Genet.* 1996;30:343–370.
5. Redondo MJ, Rewers M, Yu L, et al. Genetic determination of islet cell autoimmunity in monozygotic twin, dizygotic twin, and non-twin siblings of patients with type 1A diabetes: prospective twin study. *BMJ* 1999;318:698–702.
6. Nathan DM. Clinical practice Initial management of glycemia in type 2 diabetes mellitus. *N Engl J Med.* 2002;347:1342–1349.
7. Rubin RJ, Altman WM, Mendelson DN. Health care expenditures for people with diabetes mellitus, 1992. *J Clin Endocrinol Metab.* 1994;78:809A–809F.
8. Greene DA, Lattimer S, Ulbrecht J, et al. Glucose-induced alterations in nerve metabolism: current perspective on the pathogenesis of diabetic neuropathy and future directions for research and therapy. *Diabetes Care* 1985;8:290–299.
9. Sheetz MJ, King GL. Molecular understanding of hyperglycemia's adverse effects for diabetic complications. *JAMA.* 2002;288:2579–2588.
10. **DCCT Research Group. The effect of intensive treatment of diabetes on the development and progression of long-term complications in insulin-dependent diabetes mellitus. *N Engl J Med.* 1993; 329:977–986.**
11. Kelly WD, Lillehei R, Merkel F, et al. Allotransplantation of the pancreas and duodenum along with the kidney in diabetic nephropathy. *Surgery* 1967;61:827–837.
12. Sollinger HW, Cook K, Kamps D, et al. Clinical and experimental experience with pancreaticocystostomy for exocrine pancreatic drainage in pancreas transplantation. *Transplant Proc.* 1984;16:749–751.

13. Nghiem DD, Corry RJ. Technique of simultaneous renal pancreatoduodenal transplantation with urinary drainage of pancreatic secretion. *Am J Surg*. 1987;153:405–406.
14. Rosenlof LK, Earnhardt RC, Pruett TL, et al. Pancreas transplantation. An initial experience with systemic and portal drainage of pancreatic allografts. *Ann Surg*. 1992;215:586–597.
15. Stratta RJ, Shokouh-Amiri MH, Egidi MF, et al. A prospective comparison of simultaneous kidney-pancreas transplantation with systemic-enteric versus portal-enteric drainage. *Ann Surg*. 2001; 233:740–751.
16. Farney AC, Cho E, Schweitzer EJ, et al. Simultaneous cadaver pancreas living-donor kidney transplantation: a new approach for the type 1 diabetic uremic patient. *Ann Surg*. 2000;232:696–703.
17. Gruessner RW. Kendall DM, Drangstveit MB, et al. Simultaneous pancreas-kidney transplantation from live donors. *Ann Surg*. 1997;226:471–482.
18. Gruessner RWG. Living donor pancreas transplantation. In: *Transplantation of the pancreas*. Gruessner RWG, Sutherland DER, eds. New York: Springer, 2004, p. 429.
19. Morath C, Mueller M, Goldschmidt H, et al. Malignancy in renal transplantation. *J Am Soc Nephrol*. 2004;15:1582–1588.
20. Stehman-Breen CO, Psaty BM, Emerson S, et al. Association of hepatitis C virus infection with mortality and graft survival in kidney-pancreas transplant recipients. *Transplantation* 1997;64:281–286.
21. Honaker MR, Stratta RJ, Lo A, et al. Impact of hepatitis C virus status in pancreas transplantation: a case controlled study. *Clin Transplant*. 2002;16:243–251.
22. Stock P, Roland M, Carlson L, et al. Solid organ transplantation in HIV-positive patients. *Transplant Proc*. 2001;33:3646–3648.
23. Scientific Registry of Transplant Recipients. *2004 Annual Report*. Rockville, MD: Health Resources and Services Administration, Department of Health and Human Services; 2004.
24. Douzdjian V, Gugliuzza KG, Fish JC. Multivariate analysis of donor risk factors for pancreas allograft failure after simultaneous pancreas-kidney transplantation. *Surgery* 1995;118:73–81.
25. Fridell JA, Agarwal A, Milgrom ML, et al. Comparison of histidine-tryptophan-ketoglutarate solution and University of Wisconsin solution for organ preservation in clinical pancreas transplantation. *Transplantation* 2004;77:1304–1306.
26. **Gruessner AC, Sutherland DE. Analysis of United States (US) and non-US pancreas transplants reported to the United Network for Organ Sharing (UNOS) and the international pancreas transplant registry (IPTR) as of October 2001. *Clin Transplant*. 2001;5:41–72.**
27. Gaber AO, Shokouh-Amiri H, Grewal HP, et al. A technique for portal pancreatic transplantation with enteric drainage. *Surg Gynecol Obstet*. 1993;177:417–419.
28. Sollinger HW, Sasaki TM, D'Alessandro AM, et al. Indications for enteric conversion after pancreas transplantation with bladder drainage. *Surgery* 1992;112:842–846.
29. Benedetti E, Najarian JS, Gruessner AC, et al. Correlation between cystoscopic biopsy results and hypoamylasuria in bladder-drained pancreas transplants. *Surgery* 1995;118:864–872.
30. Troppmann C, Gruessner AC, Dunn DL, et al. Surgical complications requiring early relaparotomy after pancreas transplantation: a multivariate risk factor and economic impact analysis of the cyclosporine era. *Ann Surg*. 1998;227:255–268.
31. Stratta RJ, Alloway RR, Lo A, et al. Two-dose daclizumab regimen in simultaneous kidney-pancreas transplant recipients: primary endpoint analysis of a multicenter, randomized study. *Transplantation* 2003;75:1260–1266.
32. **Kaufman DB, Iii GW, Bruce DS, et al. Prospective, randomized, multi-center trial of antibody induction therapy in simultaneous pancreas-kidney transplantation. *Am J Transplant*. 2003;3:855–864.**
33. Freise CE, Kang SM, Feng S, et al. Excellent short-term results with steroid-free maintenance immunosuppression in low-risk simultaneous pancreas-kidney transplantation. *Arch Surg*. 2003;138:1121–1126.
34. Kaufman DB, Leventhal JR, Koffron AJ, et al. A prospective study of rapid corticosteroid elimination in simultaneous pancreas-kidney transplantation: comparison of two maintenance immunosuppression protocols: tacrolimus/mycophenolate mofetil versus tacrolimus/sirolimus. *Transplantation* 2002;73:169–177.
35. Troppmann C, Gruessner AC, Benedetti E, et al. Vascular graft thrombosis after pancreatic transplantation: univariate and multivariate operative and nonoperative risk factor analysis. *J Am Coll Surg*. 1996;182:285–316.
36. Humar A, Ramcharan T, Kandaswamy R, et al. The impact of donor obesity on outcomes after cadaver pancreas transplants. *Am J Transplant*. 2004;4:605–610.
37. Gilabert R, Fernandez-Cruz L, Real MI, et al. Treatment and outcome of pancreatic venous graft thrombosis after kidney-pancreas transplantation. *Br J Surg*. 2002;89:355–360.
38. Ciancio G, Julian JF, Fernandez L, et al. Successful surgical salvage of pancreas allografts after complete venous thrombosis. *Transplantation* 2000; 70:126–131.
39. **Sollinger HW, Odorico JS, Knechtle SJ, et al. Experience with 500 simultaneous pancreas-kidney transplants. *Ann Surg*. 1998;228:284–296.**
40. Kuo PC, Johnson LB, Schweitzer EJ, et al. Solitary pancreas allografts. The role of percutaneous biopsy and standardized histologic grading of rejection. *Arch Surg*. 1997;132:52–57.
41. Bartlett ST, Schweitzer EJ, Johnson LB, et al. Equivalent success of simultaneous pancreas kidney and solitary pancreas transplantation. A prospective trial of tacrolimus immunosuppression with percutaneous biopsy. *Ann Surg*. 1996;224:440–452.
42. Carpenter HA, Engen DE, Munn SR, et al. Histologic diagnosis of rejection by using cystoscopically directed needle biopsy specimens from dysfunctional pancreatoduodenal allografts with exocrine drainage into the bladder. *Am J Surg Pathol*. 1990;14:837–846.
43. Atwell TD, Gorman B, Larson TS, et al. Pancreas transplants: experience with 232 percutaneous US-guided biopsy procedures in 88 patients. *Radiology* 2004;231:845–849.
44. Kayler LK, Merion RM, Rudich SM, et al. Evaluation of pancreatic allograft dysfunction by laparoscopic biopsy. *Transplantation* 2002;74:1287–1289.
45. Drachenberg CB, Papadimitriou JC, Klassen DK, et al. Evaluation of pancreas transplant needle biopsy: reproducibility and revision of histologic grading system. *Transplantation* 1997;63:1579–1586.
46. Humar A, Khwaja K, Ramcharan T, et al. Chronic rejection: the next major challenge for pancreas transplant recipients. *Transplantation* 2003;76:918–923.
47. Venstrom JM, McBride MA, Rother KI, et al. Survival after pancreas transplantation in patients with diabetes and preserved kidney function. *JAMA*. 2003;290:2817–2823.
48. Reddy KS, Stablein D, Taranto S, et al. Long-term survival following simultaneous kidney-pancreas transplantation versus kidney transplantation alone in patients with type 1 diabetes mellitus and renal failure. *Am J Kidney Dis*. 2003;41:464–470.
49. Gruessner RW, Sutherland DE, Gruessner AC. Increased survival after solitary pancreas transplants. *Am J Transplant*. 2004;4(suppl 8):582 [abstract].
50. Bilous RW, Mauer SM, Sutherland DE, et al. The effects of pancreas transplantation on the glomerular structure of renal allografts in patients with insulin-dependent diabetes. *N Engl J Med*. 1989;321:80–85.
51. Fioretto P, Steffes MW, Sutherland DE, et al. Reversal of lesions of diabetic nephropathy after pancreas transplantation. *N Engl J Med*. 1998;339: 69–75.
52. Kennedy WR, Navarro X, Goetz FC, et al. Effects of pancreatic transplantation on diabetic neuropathy. *N Engl J Med*. 1990;322:1031–1037.
53. Kendall DM, Rooney DP, Smets YF, et al. Pancreas transplantation restores epinephrine response and symptom recognition during hypoglycemia in patients with long-standing type I diabetes and autonomic neuropathy. *Diabetes* 1997;46:249–257.
54. Walsh AW. Effects of pancreas transplantation on secondary complications of diabetes: retinopathy. In: *Transplantation of the pancreas*, Gruessner RWG, Sutherland DER, eds. New York:Springer, 2004, pp. 462–470.
55. Morrissey PE, Shaffer D, Monaco AP, et al. Peripheral vascular disease after kidney-pancreas transplantation in diabetic patients with end-stage renal disease. *Arch Surg*. 1997;132:358–362.
56. Knight RJ, Schanzer H, Guy S, et al. Impact of kidney-pancreas transplantation on the progression of peripheral vascular disease in diabetic patients with end-stage renal disease. *Transplant Proc*. 1998;30:1947–1949.
57. Nakache R, Tyden G, Groth CG. Quality of life in diabetic patients after combined pancreas-kidney or kidney transplantation. *Diabetes* 1989; 38(suppl 1):40–42.
58. Gross CR, Limwattananon C, Matthees BJ. Quality of life after pancreas transplantation: a review. *Clin Transplant*. 1998;12:351–361.
59. Owen RJ, Ryan EA, O'Kelly K, et al. Percutaneous transhepatic pancreatic islet cell transplantation in type 1 diabetes mellitus: radiologic aspects. *Radiology* 2003;229:165–170.
60. Lau H, Reemtsma K, Hardy MA. Prolongation of rat islet allograft survival by direct ultraviolet irradiation of the graft. *Science* 1984;223:607–609.
61. Ryan EA, Lakey JR, Paty BW, et al. Successful islet transplantation: continued insulin reserve provides long-term glycemic control. *Diabetes* 2002;51:2148–2157.
62. Sutherland DE, Matas AJ, Goetz FC, et al. Transplantation of dispersed pancreatic islet tissue in humans: autografts and allografts. *Diabetes* 1980;29(suppl 1):31–44.
63. Brendel MD, Hering BJ, Schultz AO, et al, eds. *International Islet Transplant Registry 2001*. 2001;8:1.
64. Teuscher AU, Kendall DM, Smets YF, et al. Successful islet autotransplantation in humans: functional insulin secretory reserve as an estimate of surviving islet cell mass. *Diabetes* 1998;47:324–340.
65. **Shapiro AM, Lakey JR, Ryan EA, et al. Islet transplantation in seven patients with type 1 diabetes mellitus using a glucocorticoid-free immunosuppressive regimen. *N Engl J Med*. 2000;343:230–238.**
66. **Ricordi C, Lacy PE, Firike EH, et al. Automated method for isolation of human pancreatic islets. *Diabetes* 1988;37:413–420.**
67. Linetsky E, Bottino R, Lehmann R, et al. Improved human islet isolation using a new enzyme blend, Liberase^{TM}. *Diabetes* 1997;46:1120–1123.
68. Organ Procurement and Transplantation Network. Organ Distribution: Pancreas Allocation. Policy 3.8.1.4, November 19, 2004.
69. Lakey JR, Warnock GL, Rajotte RV, et al. Variables in organ donors that affect the recovery of human islets of Langerhans. *Transplantation* 1996; 61:1047–1053.
70. Kneteman NM, Lakey JR, Kizilisik TA, et al. Cadaver pancreas recovery technique. Impact on islet recovery and in vitro function. *Transplantation* 1994;58:1114–119.
71. Lakey JR, Tsujimura T, Shapiro AM, Kuroda Y. Preservation of the human pancreas before islet isolation using a two-layer (UW solution-perfluorochemical) cold storage method. *Transplantation* 2002;74: 1809–1811.

72. Ricordi C, Fraker C, Szust J, et al. Improved human islet isolation outcome from marginal donors following addition of oxygenated perfluorocarbon to the cold-storage solution. *Transplantation* 2003;75:1524–1527.
73. Hering BJ, Matsumoto I, Sawada T, et al. Impact of two-layer pancreas preservation on islet isolation and transplantation. *Transplantation* 2002;74:1813–1816.
74. Markmann JF, Deng S, Desai NM, et al. The use of non-heart-beating donors for isolated pancreatic islet transplantation. *Transplantation* 2003; 75:1423–1429.
75. Weimar B, Rauber K, Brendel MD, et al. Percutaneous transhepatic catheterization of the portal vein: A combined CT- and fluoroscopy-guided technique. *Cardiovasc Intervent Radiol.* 1999;22:342–344.
76. Simeonovic CJ, Dhall DP, Wilson JD, et al. A comparative study of transplant sites for endocrine tissue transplantation in the pig. *Aust J Exp Biol Med Sci.* 1986;64:37–41.
77. Kramp RC, Cuche R, Renold AE. Subcutaneous, isogeneic transplantation of either duct-ligated pancreas or isolated islets in streptozotocin diabetic mice. *Endocrinology* 1976;99:1161–1167.
78. Weber CJ, Hardy MA, Pi-Sunyer F, et al. Tissue culture preservation and intramuscular transplantation of pancreatic islets. *Surgery* 1978;84: 166–174.
79. Scharp DW, Swanson CJ, Olack BJ, et al. Protection of encapsulated human islets implanted without immunosuppression in patients with type I or type II diabetes and in nondiabetic control subjects. *Diabetes* 1994; 43:1167–1170.
80. Maki T, Otsu I, O'Neil JJ, et al. Treatment of diabetes by xenogeneic islets without immunosuppression. Use of a vascularized bioartificial pancreas. *Diabetes* 1996;45:342–347.
81. Bretzel RG, Brandhorst D, Brandhorst H, et al. Improved survival of intraportal pancreatic islet cell allografts in patients with type-1 diabetes mellitus by refined peritransplant management. *J Mol Med.* 1999; 77:140–143.
82. Lehmann R, Weber M, Zullig R, et al. Simultaneous islet-kidney transplantation under glucocorticoid-free immunosuppression (Edmonton Protocol): Single center experience [abstract]. Dublin, Ireland: 9th Congress of the International Pancreas and Islet Association: July 8–11, 2003.
83. Kaufman DB, Baker MS, Chen X, et al. Sequential kidney/islet transplantation using prednisone-free immunosuppression. *Am J Transplant.* 2002;2:674–677.
84. Matas AJ, Ramcharan T, Paraskevas S, et al. Rapid discontinuation of steroids in living donor kidney transplantation: A pilot study. *Am J Transplant.* 2001;1:278–283.
85. Paty BW, Ryan EA, Shapiro AM, et al. Intrahepatic islet transplantation in type 1 diabetic patients does not restore hypoglycemic hormonal counterregulation or symptom recognition after insulin independence. *Diabetes* 2002;51:3428–3434.
86. Fiorina P, Folli F, Maffi P, et al. Islet transplantation improves vascular diabetic complications in patients with diabetes who underwent kidney transplantation: a comparison between kidney-pancreas and kidney-alone transplantation. *Transplantation* 2003;75:1296–1301.
87. Hirshberg B, Rother KI, Digon BJ III, et al. Benefits and risks of solitary islet transplantation for type 1 diabetes using steroid-sparing immunosuppression: The National Institutes of Health experience. *Diabetes Care* 2003;26:3288–3295.
88. Casey JJ, Lakey JR, Ryan EA, et al. Portal venous pressure changes after sequential clinical islet transplantation. *Transplantation* 2002;74: 913–915.
89. Rafael E, Ryan EA, Paty BW, et al. Changes in liver enzymes after clinical islet transplantation. *Transplantation* 2003;76:1280–1284.
90. Markmann JF, Rosen M, Siegelman ES, et al. Magnetic resonance-defined periportal steatosis following intraportal islet transplantation: A functional footprint of islet graft survival? *Diabetes* 2003;52:1591–1594.
91. Shapiro J, Ryan E, McGhee-Wilson D, et al. Prospective comparison of clinical outcomes with fresh vs cultured islets at a single institution. *Am J Transplant.* 2004;4(suppl 8):553 [abstract].
92. Hering BJ, Kandaswamy R, Harmon JV, et al. Transplantation of cultured islets from two-layer preserved pancreases in type 1 diabetes with anti-CD3 antibody. *Am J Transplant.* 2004;4:390–401.
93. Alejandro R, Ferreira JV, Froud T, et al. Insulin independence following transplantation of cultured human islets in patients with type 1 diabetes: The Miami experience. *Am J Transplant.* 2004;4:553 [abstract].
94. Shapiro J, Ricordi C, Hering B, et al. International multicenter trial of islet transplantation using the Edmonton protocol in patients with type 1 diabetes. *Am J Transplant.* 2004; 4(suppl 8):552 [abstract]).
95. Ault A. Edmonton's islet success tough to duplicate elsewhere. *Lancet* 2003;361:2054.
96. Markmann JF, Deng S, Huang X, et al. Insulin independence following isolated islet transplantation and single islet infusions. *Ann Surg.* 2003;237:741–750.
97. Kessler L, Bucher P, Milliat-Guittard L, et al. Influence of islet transportation on pancreatic islet allotransplantation in type 1 diabetic patients within the Swiss-French GRAGIL network. *Transplantation* 2004;77: 1301–1304.
98. Goss JA, Schock AP, Brunicardi FC, et al. Achievement of insulin independence in three consecutive type-1 diabetic patients via pancreatic islet transplantation using islets isolated at a remote islet isolation center. *Transplantation* 2002;74:1761–1766.
99. Han D, Xu X, Pastori RL, et al. Elevation of cytotoxic lymphocyte gene expression is predictive of islet allograft rejection in nonhuman primates. *Diabetes* 2002;51:562–566.
100. Shapiro AM, Hao EG, Lakey JR, et al. Novel approaches toward early diagnosis of islet allograft rejection. *Transplantation* 2001;71:1709–1718.

SECTION C
HEAD AND NECK

CHAPTER 42 ■ HEAD AND NECK

JEFFREY S. MOYER AND THEODOROS N. TEKNOS

The head and neck are a beautifully complex region of the human body, with an equally complex range of disease processes affecting it. To adequately cover the entire subject matter in a brief chapter is impossible; therefore, highlights of the most common disease states are outlined. Specifically, discussions in this chapter center around the evaluation of patients presenting with head and neck complaints, clinically relevant head and neck anatomy, common infectious processes, and benign and malignant tumors as well as treatment approaches.

DIAGNOSTIC EVALUATION

Every patient with a complaint referable to the head and neck must have a complete history and physical examination to better characterize the presenting complaint and aid in making the proper diagnosis. History-taking when dealing with a head and neck patient is similar to history-taking when dealing with any other patient in general medicine; more mistakes are made because of errors of omission than errors of commission.[1,2] Therefore, a thorough history with direct questioning regarding the symptoms outlined in Table 42.1 is critical. In any smoker aged 35 or older, the presence of any signs and symptoms outlined in this table is considered indicative of head and neck cancer until proved otherwise.

After the presenting symptoms have been fully characterized, the patient must be questioned regarding potential risk factors for head and neck cancer. The best recognized carcinogens are tobacco use and alcohol consumption. These behaviors account for approximately 80% of all cancers in the upper aerodigestive tract, and users of these drugs present a 15-fold greater increase of developing squamous cell carcinoma than nonsmokers and nondrinkers.[1,3] In addition to smoking and drinking, other, less recognized risk factors for malignancy of the head and neck exist, and these should be included in the complete history[1,4] (Table 42.2). Once all the pertinent history of the present illness has been obtained, the remaining aspects of the history, as well as the review of systems, should be elicited. A host-performance scale must also be assessed for each patient by inquiring about daily activities and current levels of impairment.[5,6] Although time-consuming to obtain, this information is critical in assessing the patient's perioperative risk status and identifying any medical illnesses that would require treatment prior to initiating any therapeutic intervention.

Physical Examination

After completing a detailed history, the next step in appropriate management of a patient with a head and neck complaint is a complete physical examination. Adequate examination of the head and neck can often be difficult to perform. It requires a certain amount of skill and mastery of specialized

TABLE 42.1 ■ DIAGNOSIS

PROGRESSIVE SIGNS AND SYMPTOMS INDICATING HEAD AND NECK CANCER

Odynophagia
Dysphagia
Weight loss
Loose dentition
Oral fetor
Trismus
Otalgia
Neck mass
Serous otitis media
Nasal obstruction
Epistaxis
Facial pain
Cranial neuropathies
Secondary infections
Aspiration
Fistulization
Hemorrhage
Airway obstruction

TABLE 42.2 ETIOLOGY

RISK FACTORS FOR MALIGNANCY OF THE HEAD AND NECK

SKIN CANCERS
Ultraviolet and ionizing radiation
Neoprene inorganic arsenics
Burns
Riboflavin deficiencies

NOSE AND PARANASAL SINUS CANCER
Wood dust
Leather manufacturing
Nickel refining
Radium dial painting
Thorotrast and mustard gas

NASOPHARYNGEAL CARCINOMA
Nitrosamine
Salted fish
Epstein-Barr virus types II and III
Vitamin deficiency

ORAL CARCINOMA
Betel nut chewing
Snuff
Tobacco chewing
Reverse smoking
Syphilis
Vitamin B and riboflavin deficiencies
Chronic irritation

LARYNGEAL AND HYPOPHARYNGEAL CARCINOMA
Asbestos
Coke oven exposure
Wood dust
Riboflavin deficiency

THYROID CANCER
Radiation exposure
Iodine deficiency
Genetic inheritance

SALIVARY GLAND NEOPLASMS
Radiation exposure
Eskimo heritage

instrumentation, inasmuch as the upper aerodigestive tract is not accessible to direct visualization.[1,7] An important tenet, however, is that no head and neck examination should be considered complete until all mucosal surfaces of the nasal cavity, nasopharynx, oropharynx, oral cavity, hypopharynx, and larynx have been clearly visualized. In addition to inspection of the skin and scalp, pneumatic otoscopy and a complete cranial nerve examination must clearly be documented as well. Finally, inspection, palpation, and auscultation of the neck as well as bimanual palpation of the oral cavity and oropharynx must be accomplished in each case. Performing all these steps in a routine, systematic manner will provide the surgeon with the maximum amount of information and limit any errors of omission. Furthermore, any complete physical examination should be able to characterize the primary tumor if there is one, define and characterize any neck disease, rule out any synchronous tumors or other disease processes, and rule out the presence of a neoplastic process and lead the surgeon toward a diagnosis that would most likely be infectious in etiology. If there is a primary malignancy, it is characterized with regard to its size and extent, as manifested by bony involvement, soft tissue extension, and cranial neuropathies. Neck disease, on the other hand, is described by nodal size, number of nodes, level of

TABLE 42.3 CLASSIFICATION

REGIONAL LYMPH NODE (N) STAGING FOR HEAD AND NECK CANCER

Stage	Description
NX	Regional lymph nodes cannot be assessed
N0	No regional lymph node metastasis
N1	Metastasis in a single ipsilateral lymph node ≤3 cm
N2a	Metastasis in a single ipsilateral lymph node >3 cm but ≤6 cm
N2b	Metastasis in multiple ipsilateral lymph nodes, none >6 cm
N2c	Metastasis in bilateral or contralateral lymph nodes, none >6 cm
N3	Metastasis in a lymph node >6 cm

Data from American Joint Committee on Cancer. *Cancer staging manual*, 6th ed. New York: Springer-Verlag; 2002, with permission.

nodes in the neck (Table 42.3), and fixation to skin or vascular structures. The astute examiner has a thorough understanding of the anatomy of each nodal group and the patterns of spread for a particular primary site. This knowledge is critical for identifying an unknown primary tumor in a patient with known neck disease. Conversely, finding an unusual drainage pattern for a known primary tumor can alert the examiner to the presence of a second primary lesion[8,9] (Table 42.4). Clearly, a well-performed and thorough examination can provide the physician with a tremendous amount of information with far-reaching therapeutic implications (Table 42.5).

A synthesis of the information obtained from the history and physical examination will then allow the head and neck surgeon, in a vast majority of cases, to make the appropriate diagnosis. The most common diagnoses that will be encountered by the surgeon in the head and neck are listed in the following sections.

INFECTIOUS PROCESSES

Infectious processes of the head and neck are among the most common complaints seen by the medical practitioner. In a vast majority of cases, the diagnosis and treatment of these conditions are fairly straightforward. However, these seemingly innocuous infections, if left undetected or untreated, can lead to profound complications including blindness, airway obstruction, and death.

TABLE 42.4

MOST COMMON PRIMARY SITES IN PATIENTS PRESENTING WITH NECK MASSES

Nodal level	Primary site
I	Oral cavity
II	Oropharynx
	Nasopharynx
	Supraglottic larynx
III	Hypopharynx
	Larynx
IV	Thyroid
	Hypopharynx
	Larynx
	Subclavicular sites
V	Scalp
	Nasopharynx

TABLE 42.5

CORRELATION OF PRIMARY SITE AND STAGE OF HEAD AND NECK CANCER WITH SURVIVAL RATES

	Survival rate (%)[a]			
Primary site	Stage I	Stage II	Stage III	Stage IV
ORAL CAVITY				
Tongue	70	50	40	20
Floor of mouth	70	50	25	10
Buccal mucosa	75	65	30	20
Alveolar ridge	80	65	35	15
PHARYNX				
Nasopharynx	80	60	40	20
Oropharynx	80	60	30	20
Hypopharynx	60	50	30	10
LARYNX				
Supraglottic	75	60	50	25
Glottic	95	80	50	30
Subglottic[b]				

[a]These numbers represent approximate averages; wide ranges have been reported for all sites and stages.
[b]Too rare for meaningful survival data.

Sinusitis

Sinusitis is a common complaint that is usually self-limited, with infrequent complications. Typically, patients complain of vague discomfort in the infected cheek/upper molar region (maxillary sinusitis), forehead (frontal sinusitis), medial canthal region (ethmoid sinusitis), or retro-orbital/vertex regions (sphenoid sinusitis). Often there is a purulent nasal discharge, nasal obstruction, a positional character to the discomfort, and accompanying aural complaints. Diagnosis of this condition is made by history and nasal endoscopy, with visualization of purulent material at the sinus ostia. In adult patients, fever does not accompany sinusitis, and when temperature elevation is noted, a complication of sinusitis must be suspected. Other warning signs of impending orbital and intracranial complications include severe headache, facial swelling, proptosis, or visual changes (Fig. 42.1). If any of these take place, the patient must be immediately evaluated by nasal endoscopy and high-resolution computed tomography (CT) scanning of the brain and sinuses in both the axial and coronal planes. The potential complications and emergencies related to sinusitis are listed in Table 42.6. These complications require immediate surgical intervention for abscess drainage.

A specific subgroup of patients that must always be evaluated extensively with sinusitis are those who are immunodeficient, who have insulin-dependent diabetes, or who are transplant recipients and severely neutropenic individuals on chemotherapy. These patients are at risk for invasive fungal sinusitis secondary to Zygomycetes (*Mucor, Rhizopus,* and *Absidia* species) or *Aspergillus* species. These are fulminant, rapidly fatal diseases that must be promptly diagnosed and treated with radical surgical débridement and postoperative antifungal therapy. The classic finding in these patients on endoscopy is a necrotic, blackened mucosal lining along the lateral nasal wall. The survival rate for these infections varies from 30% to 80%, with patients with granulocytopenia faring worse than those with insulin-dependent diabetes.

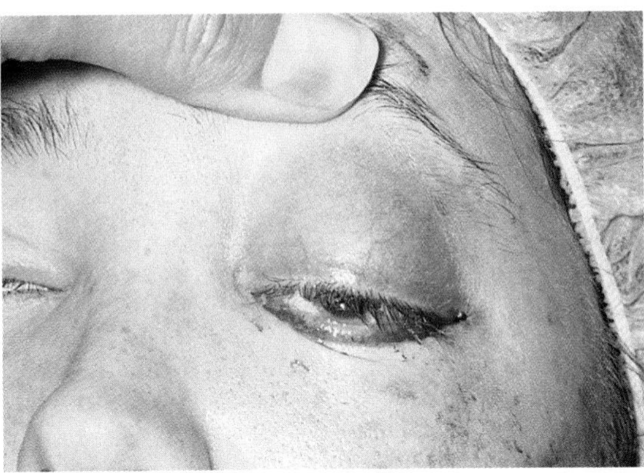

FIGURE 42.1 This 19-year-old woman suddenly developed proptosis and no light perception in her left eye after 2 weeks of preseptal cellulitis and ethmoid sinusitis. (From Tasman W, Jaeger E. *The Wills Eye Hospital atlas of clinical ophthalmology,* 2nd edition. Philadelphia: Lippincott Williams & Wilkins; 2001, with permission.)

Pharyngitis

Pharyngitis is the most common complaint that a general practitioner will encounter in his or her practice. It is an inflammatory disease of the mucosal and submucosal structures of the throat. Infected tissues include the tonsils, adenoids, oropharynx, and hypopharynx. Most pharyngitides are diagnosed by history and physical examination and can be secondary to bacterial, viral, or fungal causes. Bacterial pharyngitis is typically secondary to gram-positive alpha and gamma hemolytic streptococci and several anaerobic organisms. Symptoms include sore throat, fever, and odynophagia. On physical examination, there is typically intense erythema of the tonsils, with purulent exudate, symmetric tonsillar enlargement, and tender, palpable lymphadenopathy bilaterally. Effective treatment includes oral penicillin or clindamycin therapy. A dangerous and common complication of tonsillitis is the peritonsillar abscess. Specifically, a peritonsillar abscess is a collection of pus between the capsule of the tonsil and the muscle of the lateral pharyngeal wall (Fig. 42.2). Warning signs that one may be dealing with a peritonsillar abscess include unilateral throat discomfort with severe odynophagia, hyponasal voice (hot potato voice), and trismus. Physical examination findings include a medialization of the affected tonsil, unilateral palatal swelling, and trismus. The diagnosis is confirmed by aspirating pus from the abscess pocket. Once the pocket has been localized, a formal incision and drainage must be performed as appropriate treatment. The mucosal surface overlying the abscess is incised with a guarded no. 11 blade, and the abscess pocket is bluntly dissected and marsupialized with a tonsil clamp. Cultures are obtained from the purulence expressed, and the patient is begun on clindamycin or augmented penicillin therapy.

TABLE 42.6

COMPLICATIONS OF ACUTE SUPPURATIVE SINUSITIS

OPHTHALMOLOGIC
Orbital cellulitis
Subperiosteal abscess
Orbital abscess
Ophthalmoplegia, blindness

NEUROLOGIC
Subdural, epidural abscess
Meningitis
Brain abscess
Cavernous sinus thrombosis

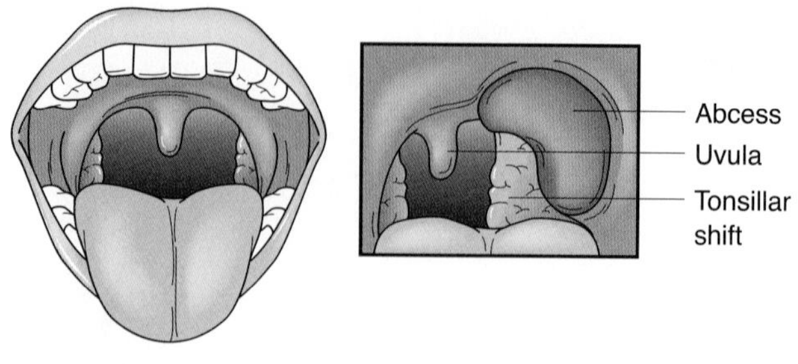

Abcess
Uvula
Tonsillar shift

FIGURE 42.2 Schematic representation of peritonsillar abscess. Purulence develops between the tonsillar capsule and the superior pharyngeal constriction. As a result, the tonsil is medialized, there is a bulge in the palate, and trismus develops.

Another important consideration in evaluating a patient with complaints of a sore throat is not to miss an occult supraglottitis (epiglottitis being its more limited form). Adults with this condition are often misdiagnosed with pharyngitis; however, suspicion should be heightened when the patient states that the sore throat is lower than usual or when the patient has impressive odynophagia and hoarseness, which rarely accompany uncomplicated pharyngitis. Since the universal institution of *Haemophilus influenzae* B vaccine, the epidemiology of epiglottitis and supraglottitis has changed. Currently, more cases are diagnosed in adults than in children, and the dominant organism has shifted from *Haemophilus* to *Staphylococcus aureus* and *Streptococcus pyogenes*. The disease is usually more indolent in adults. If, however, there is a rapid onset of symptoms (less than 4 hours) accompanied with a high fever (greater than 102.5°F) and a white blood cell count greater than 20,000 cells/dL, these patients should have their airway secured immediately, because they are most likely to develop rapid airway compromise.[10] If these criteria are not met, adults can typically be treated with intravenous augmented penicillin therapy, humidification, and steroid therapy in an intensive care unit setting. The acute phase of inflammation responds to therapy within 48 to 72 hours.

Deep Neck Infections

The advent of antibiotics has significantly decreased the incidence and mortality of deep neck infections. Despite this progress, deep neck infections remain life-threatening conditions and demand prompt diagnosis and treatment. In the years before antibiotics, 70% of deep neck infections resulted from direct spread of localized abscesses from the pharyngeal-tonsillar areas. Consequently, the parapharyngeal space was the most frequently involved space in deep neck infections. An increasing percentage of currently treated infections, however, are secondary to dental and salivary gland origin, which results in submaxillary space abscesses. The various deep neck spaces are listed in Table 42.7. Any patient with a recent history of tonsillitis, pharyngitis, an odontogenic infection, or recent dental work with onset of neck swelling and pain must be assumed to have a deep neck infection until proved otherwise. Other common findings include odynophagia, trismus, and respiratory compromise. If the diagnosis is suspected, a high-resolution CT scan must be obtained to confirm the diagnosis.

The first step in caring for these patients is securing and maintaining an adequate airway. If intubation is not possible due to airway edema or trismus, a tracheotomy under local anesthesia must be performed, remembering that the trachea may be deviated due to the inflammation (Fig. 42.3). Wide surgical drainage of the entire involved space is the required treatment for the abscess itself. Postoperatively, the patient is treated with intravenous ampicillin/sulbactam therapy or clindamycin with a third-generation cephalosporin.

TABLE 42.7 CLASSIFICATION

DEEP NECK SPACES

SPACES INVOLVING ENTIRE LENGTH OF NECK
Danger space (prevertebral space)
Retropharyngeal space
Visceral vascular space
SPACES LIMITED TO ABOVE THE HYOID BONE
Pharyngomaxillary space
Submandibular space
Parotid space
Masticator space
Peritonsillar space
Temporal space
SPACES BELOW HYOID BONE
Anterior visceral space

Adapted from Teknos TN, Coniglio JU, Netterville JL. Guidelines for patient management. In: Bailey BJ, ed. *Head and neck surgery—otolaryngology.* Philadelphia: JB Lippincott; 1993:80.

If a salivary gland is believed to be the source of the abscess, patients are treated empirically with antistaphylococcal penicillins until culture results return.

NEOPLASMS OF THE HEAD AND NECK

Despite increasing public awareness concerning the detrimental effects of tobacco and alcohol abuse, head and neck cancer remains a major contributor to the annual incidence of cancer in the United States. Each year, 78,000 people will be diagnosed with a head and neck malignancy; 17,500 will succumb to this disease.[1,11] This constitutes 7% of all cancers diagnosed and 4% of all cancer deaths annually.[11] Recent advances in tumor recognition, diagnosis, and treatment have offered hope for increased survival and functional outcomes in these patients. In truth, however, survivorship has not improved over the last 30 years, and 33% of all patients with head and neck malignancies eventually die of their disease.[12] Much of this can be attributed to delays in diagnosis and inadequate initial treatment; therefore, it is imperative for the head and neck surgeon to recognize this disease process early and have a well-organized plan of care. The most common neoplasms and treatment approaches for each region of the head and neck are outlined in the following sections.

Nose and Paranasal Sinuses

The neoplasms found in this region of the head and neck are among the most diverse in terms of histologic tissue of origin. They include both epithelial and nonepithelial tumors, with the former accounting for approximately 80% of all lesions. The most common symptoms associated with nasal and paranasal sinus tumors are unilateral nasal obstruction and epistaxis. The most common benign lesion is the inverting papilloma or Schneiderian papilloma. These lesions arise from the lateral nasal wall and have a propensity for local recurrence. Approximately 5% to 15% of inverting papillomas contain a component of squamous cell carcinoma. For these reasons, the treatment for inverting papilloma is *en bloc* surgical resection via medial maxillectomy. More conservative resections have been attempted, but, the recurrence rates have been high compared with the medial maxillectomy approach—60% and 16%, respectively.[13]

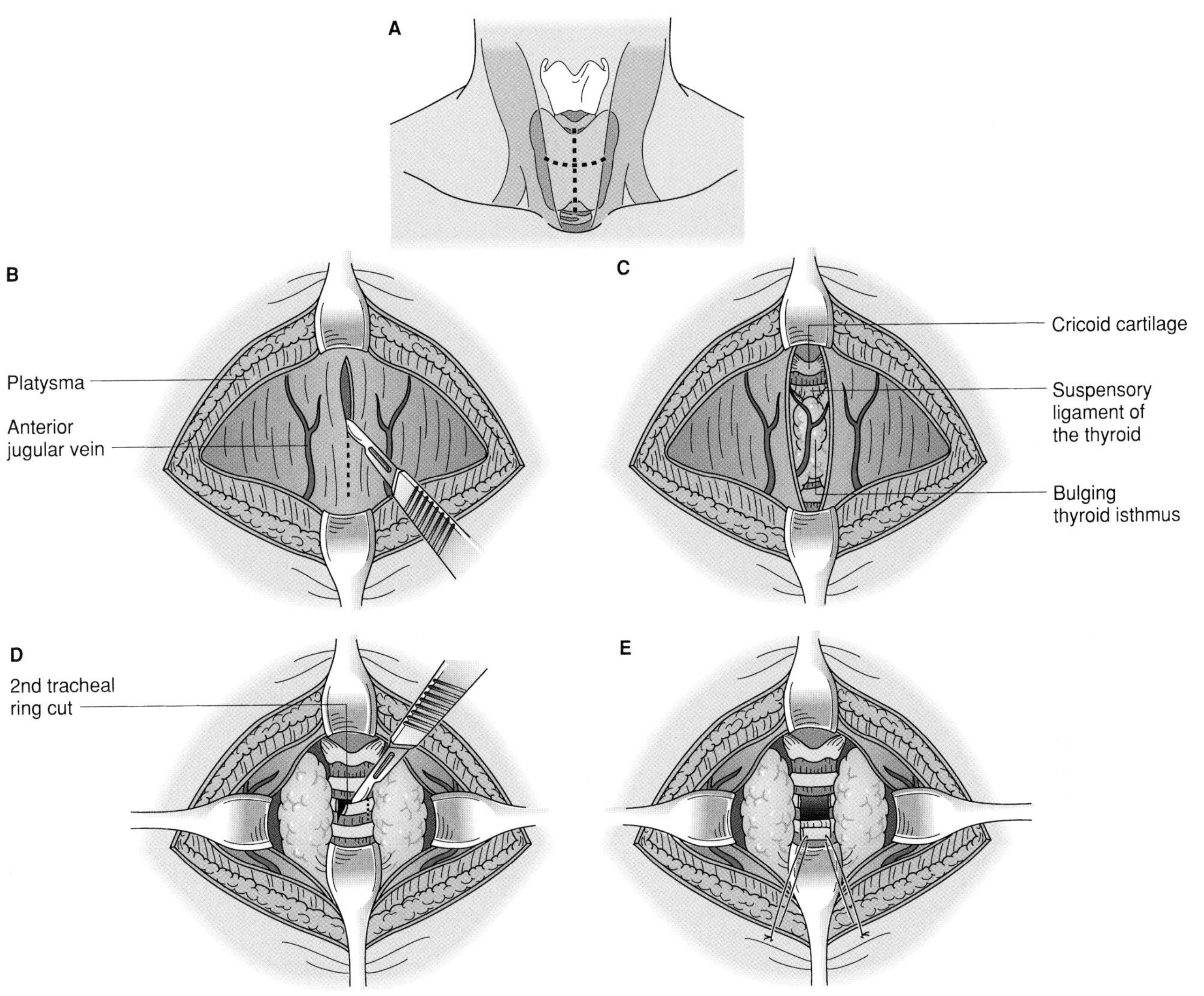

FIGURE 42.3 Tracheostomy. (*A*) Incision is usually made transversely for elective tracheostomy, but a vertical incision allows for less bleeding when the procedure must be performed emergently. (*B*) The strap muscles are separated in the midline. The thyroid isthmus may bulge into the wound (*C*), necessitating inferior retraction (*D*). (*E*) After the second tracheal ring is cleaned off, an inferiorly based flap is developed in the tracheal wall and sutured to the skin to allow easy access to the trachea while the tract is maturing.

Squamous cell carcinoma is the most prevalent malignant tumor of the nose and paranasal sinuses. Approximately two thirds of these tumors arise in the maxillary sinus and one third in the ethmoid sinuses. Malignant tumors arising in the frontal or sphenoid sinuses are exceedingly rare. Cross-sectional imaging with high-resolution CT scanning or magnetic resonance imaging (MRI) is mandatory for accurate staging in these lesions as well as for planning the surgical approach. Primary tumor staging in the maxillary and ethmoid sinuses is shown in Table 42.8. Curative treatment for paranasal sinus squamous cell carcinoma is primarily surgical. Maxillary sinus cancers, depending on their stage, are treated by medial maxillectomy, preserving the hard palate; subtotal maxillectomy; or total maxillectomy with or without orbital exenteration. Orbital exenteration is indicated for tumors that invade the periorbita, orbital fat, or orbital apex. Ethmoid sinus tumors, on the other hand, often involve the anterior skull base and require (upstairs-downstairs) resection via frontal craniotomy and lateral rhinotomy. Subcranial/midface degloving approaches can also be used effectively in such cases. The intracranial and intranasal spaces are separated by reconstructing the anterior skull base with pericranial flaps and/or microvascular free flaps. Postoperative radiotherapy is given in advanced lesions, with improved long-term survival. Overall survival in paranasal sinus carcinoma is approximately 45%. A particularly poor prognostic sign is neck metastasis, which decreases 5-year survival to 10%.[14]

Salivary Gland Neoplasms

The salivary glands are divided into the major salivary glands (which include the parotid, submandibular, and sublingual glands) and the minor salivary glands (which include several thousand glands distributed through the upper aerodigestive tract). Approximately 80% of salivary gland neoplasms originate in the parotid gland, 10% to 15% in the submandibular gland, and the remaining in the sublingual and minor salivary glands.[15] Additionally, approximately 80% of parotid neoplasms are benign, and approximately 50% of submandibular neoplasms are benign. In contrast, less than 40% of sublingual and minor salivary lesions are benign.[15] Malignancies are often asymptomatic, but signs and symptoms indicative of a malignancy include rapid tumor enlargement, pain, trismus, and facial or other cranial nerve paralyses. A key diagnostic test, which has 95% sensitivity in salivary gland neoplasms, is fine needle aspiration.[15,16] As a result, any patient with a mass in the salivary glands should undergo fine needle aspiration for histologic diagnosis and surgical planning. A CT or MRI

TABLE 42.8 CLASSIFICATION

PRIMARY TUMOR STAGING OF MAXILLARY SINUS, NASAL CAVITY, AND ETHMOID SINUS CANCERS

Stage	Description
MAXILLARY SINUS	
T1	Tumor limited to maxillary sinus mucosa with no erosion or destruction of bone
T2	Tumor causing bone erosion or destruction including extension into the hard palate and/or middle nasal meatus, except extension to posterior wall of maxillary sinus and pterygoid plates
T3	Tumor invades any of the following: bone of the posterior wall of maxillary sinus, subcutaneous tissues, floor or medial wall of orbit, pterygoid fossa, ethmoid sinuses
T4a	Tumor invades anterior orbital contents, skin of cheek, pterygoid plates, infratemporal fossa, cribriform plate, sphenoid or frontal sinuses
T4b	Tumor invades any of the following: orbital apex, dura, brain, middle cranial fossa, cranial nerves other than maxillary division of trigeminal nerve (V_2), nasopharynx, or clivus
NASAL CAVITY AND ETHMOID SINUS	
T1	Tumor restricted to any one subsite, with or without bony invasion
T2	Tumor invading two subsites in a single region or extending to involve an adjacent region within the nasoethmoidal complex, with or without bony invasion
T3	Tumor extends to invade the medial wall or floor of the orbit, maxillary sinus, palate, or cribriform plate
T4a	Tumor invades any of the following: anterior orbital contents, skin of nose or cheek, minimal extension to the anterior cranial fossa, pterygoid plates, sphenoid or frontal sinuses
T4b	Tumor invades any of the following: orbital apex, dura, brain, middle cranial fossa, cranial nerves other than maxillary division of trigeminal nerve (V_2), nasopharynx, or clivus

Data from American Joint Committee on Cancer. *Cancer staging manual*, 6th ed. New York: Springer-Verlag; 2002, with permission.

TABLE 42.9 CLASSIFICATION

PRIMARY TUMOR STAGING FOR SALIVARY GLAND CANCER

Stage	Description
T1	Tumor ≤2 cm in greatest dimension without extraparenchymal extension
T2	Tumor more than 2 cm but ≤4 cm in greatest dimension without extraparenchymal extension
T3	Tumor >4 cm and/or having extraparenchymal extension
T4a	Tumor invades skin, mandible, ear canal, and/or facial nerve
T4b	Tumor invades skull base and/or pterygoid plates and/or encases carotid artery

Malignant tumors account for 20% of tumors arising in the parotid gland, 50% of tumors arising in the submandibular gland, and 75% of tumors arising in minor salivary glands.
Data from American Joint Committee on Cancer. *Cancer staging manual*, 6th ed. New York: Springer-Verlag; 2002, with permission.

scan can also be useful in determining whether a tumor is in the superficial or deep lobe of the parotid gland and can frequently suggest whether a lesion is locally aggressive. This is often helpful in preoperative planning as well as in preparing the patient for possible surgical outcomes.

The most common benign lesion of the major salivary glands is pleomorphic adenoma or benign mixed tumor. Grossly, these lesions appear smooth and lobular, with a well-defined capsule. Histologically, however, they have epithelial and mesenchymal components but incomplete encapsulation with pseudopod extension beyond the apparent borders of the mass. These features account for the high recurrence rate when tumors are removed by enucleation alone. Appropriate surgical therapy involves resection of the tumor with a margin of normal gland surrounding it. The intimate relationship between the parotid gland and the facial nerve necessitates facial nerve identification and dissection to ensure its preservation and complete tumor extirpation (Fig. 42.4). A second benign lesion that deserves mention is Warthin's tumor (papillary cystadenoma lymphomatosum). Warthin's tumors are typically cystic lesions in the tail of the parotid gland, occurring primarily in men between their fourth and seventh decades of life. They are often multicentric, and approximately 10% are bilateral. Treatment includes superficial parotidectomy, similar to pleomorphic adenoma.

Malignant lesions of the salivary glands are staged according to size and extent of local tissue invasion (Table 42.9). The most common malignant tumor of the parotid gland is mucoepidermoid carcinoma, which histologically consists of epidermoid and mucous cells. These tumors are characterized as low-, intermediate-, or high-grade, directly related to the proportion of epidermoid to mucoid cells found on histologic examination. High-grade mucoepidermoid carcinomas are highly aggressive, with a local recurrence rate of 60%, regional metastatic rate of 50%, and distant metastatic rate of 30%. These tumors are treated with total parotidectomy, neck dissection, and postoperative radiotherapy, with a 5-year survival of 50%. The most common malignancy of the submandibular gland (Fig. 42.5), and the second most common of the parotid gland is adenoid cystic carcinoma. Adenoid cystic carcinomas account for 58% of malignant submandibular and minor salivary gland tumors and 12% of malignant parotid tumors. This tumor has a propensity for perineural invasion and spread, as well as distant metastases. Surgical management of these tumors includes radical resection, sacrificing nerves only for direct tumor extension and postoperative radiation therapy. Despite this aggressive therapy, these tumors, which follow an indolent course, develop regional and distant metastases 40% of the time over a 10- to 20-year course.

General principles for surgical treatment of salivary gland malignancies are given in Table 42.10. Much has been written recently considering fast neutron radiation beam therapy in inoperable salivary gland tumors or in adenoid cystic carcinomas of the skull base and paranasal sinuses. There are no effective chemotherapeutic regimens for parotid neoplasms.

Squamous Cell Carcinomas of the Head and Neck

The neoplasm most commonly affecting the remaining regions of the head and neck is squamous cell carcinoma. Greater than 90% of head and neck cancers are of this histologic type.

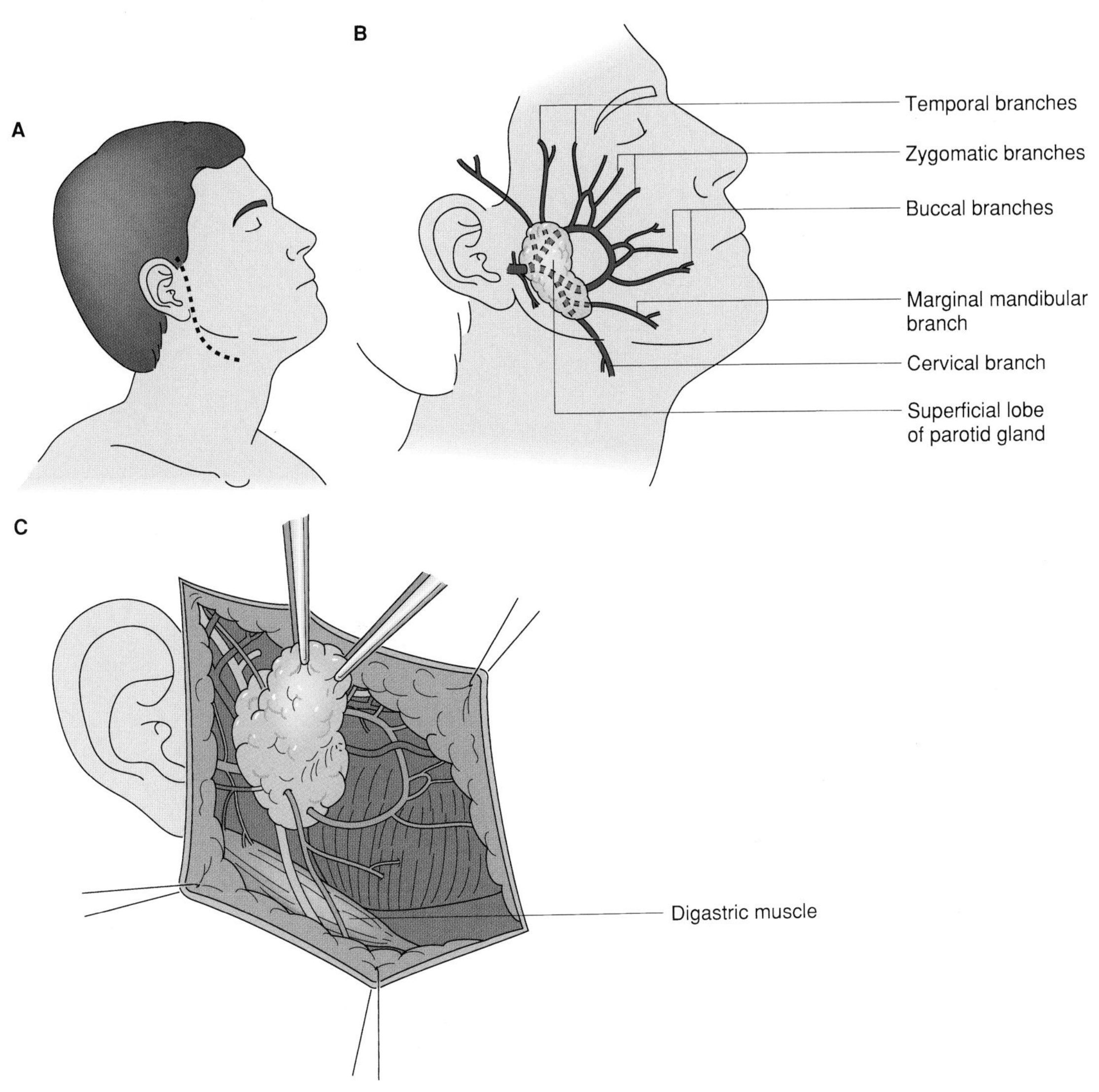

FIGURE 42.4 Superficial parotidectomy. (*A*) The standard Blair incision or the cosmetically superior face lift incision can be used. (*B*) Branches of the facial nerve course between the superficial and deep lobes of the parotid (*C*). The main trunk of the facial nerve is identified 8 mm deep to the tympanomastoid suture line and at the same level as the digastric muscle. (*D*) The nerve is then dissected anteriorly, separating it from the substance of the parotid. (*E*) Schematic representation of the relationship between the parotid and surrounding structures.

Early identification and treatment of squamous cell carcinoma of the upper aerodigestive tract is the most important component in reducing mortality from this devastating disease. The first step in successful treatment of these tumors is tissue confirmation of malignancy. Frequently this can be obtained by direct biopsy of the primary lesion in the office when the tumor is in the oral cavity or oropharynx. Alternatively, fine needle aspiration of an enlarged lymph node can also confirm squamous cell carcinoma of the head and neck if the primary lesion is inaccessible. Once the diagnosis has been confirmed, the patient must then be adequately staged. Although the use of flexible video-laryngoscopy and thorough office examination often provides an accurate staging of the tumor, there is no substitute for a thorough examination and biopsy under general anesthesia. This operative endoscopy, called panendoscopy, should include direct laryngoscopy (with or without microscopic assistance), esophagoscopy, and tracheobronchoscopy. The operative examination under anesthesia should include a thorough inspection of all mucous membranes of the aerodigestive tract. This is a critical part of the evaluation and is imperative because of the fairly high incidence of simultaneous primary lesions. The incidence of synchronous primary tumors varies from 2.5% to as high as 25% in the literature.[17] The general consensus among otolaryngologists, however, is a synchronous tumor rate of 5% to 15%, which is highest in patients with tumors of the hypopharynx.[17] Because these tumors are

TABLE 42.10 MANAGEMENT

GENERAL PRINCIPLES FOR SURGICAL TREATMENT OF SALIVARY GLAND MALIGNANCIES

- Malignant tumors of the parotid gland warrant total parotidectomy.
- The facial nerve should be sacrificed only for direct tumor invasion or for preexisting facial paralyses.
- Patients with high-grade tumors should undergo elective neck dissection if there is no clinical neck disease or a modified neck dissection for palpable adenopathy.
- Postoperative radiotherapy is indicated for all high-grade tumors; close margins; recurrent disease; skin, bone, nerve, or extraparotid involvement; positive nodes; or unresectable disease.

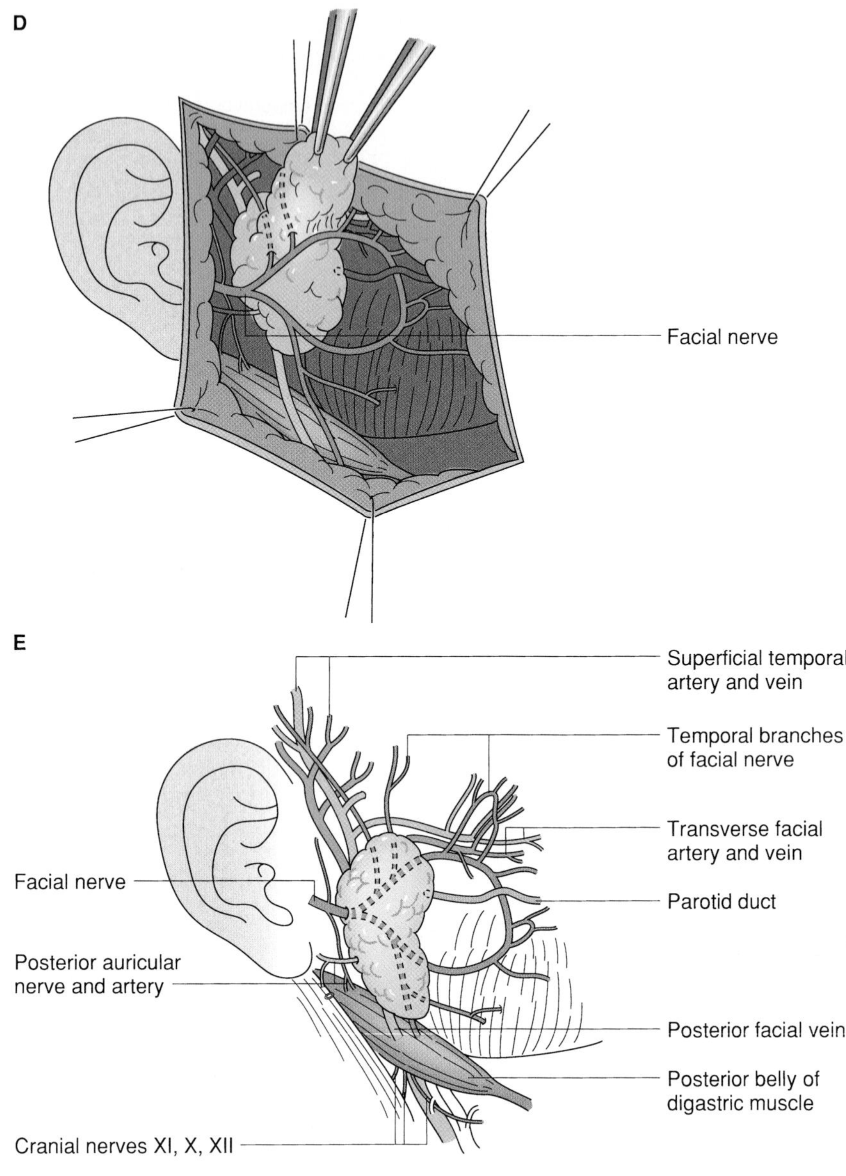

FIGURE 42.4 *(Continued)*

TABLE 42.11 CLASSIFICATION

STAGING OF HEAD AND NECK CANCER

Stage	Stage grouping
0	Tis, N0, M0
I	T1, N0, M0
II	T2, N0, M0
III	T3, N0, M0
	T1–T3, N1, M0
IVA	T4a, N0–1, M0
	T1–T4a, N2, M0
IVB	T4b, Any N, M0
	Any T, N3, M0
IVC	Any T, Any N, M1

Data from American Joint Committee on Cancer. *Cancer staging manual*, 6th ed. New York: Springer-Verlag; 2002, with permission.

frequently asymptomatic, panendoscopy is the only way to detect these tumors in roughly half of the cases. Retrospective studies in the head and neck literature reveal that tumors in the digestive tract, that is, oral cavity, oropharynx, or hypopharynx, tend to have second primary lesions in other regions of the digestive tract. Conversely, laryngeal lesions tend to have second primary tumors in other portions of the respiratory tract, predominantly the lungs and mainstem bronchi.[18] Based on these data, some argue that esophagoscopy is not necessary in laryngeal carcinomas, and instead a barium swallow should be used as a screening tool, with much less morbidity and equal yield.

Regardless of the endoscopic method utilized, adequate biopsies of the tumor must be taken to ensure accurate histologic diagnosis. In addition, based on the panendoscopy, an accurate and detailed tumor diagram must be created and entered in the patient's permanent record. With the information gleaned from the office examination and panendoscopy, the patient's tumor is staged according to the TNM classification and staging system of the American Joint Committee for Cancer[19] (Table 42.11).

TREATMENT GUIDELINES

Patients with head and neck cancer present a challenge to everyone involved in their clinical care. With all the complexities of modern-day head and neck cancer treatment, including multiple treatment modalities available, patients are best served by presenting each individual case at a multidisciplinary tumor board. After considering the tumor stage, prognostic variables,

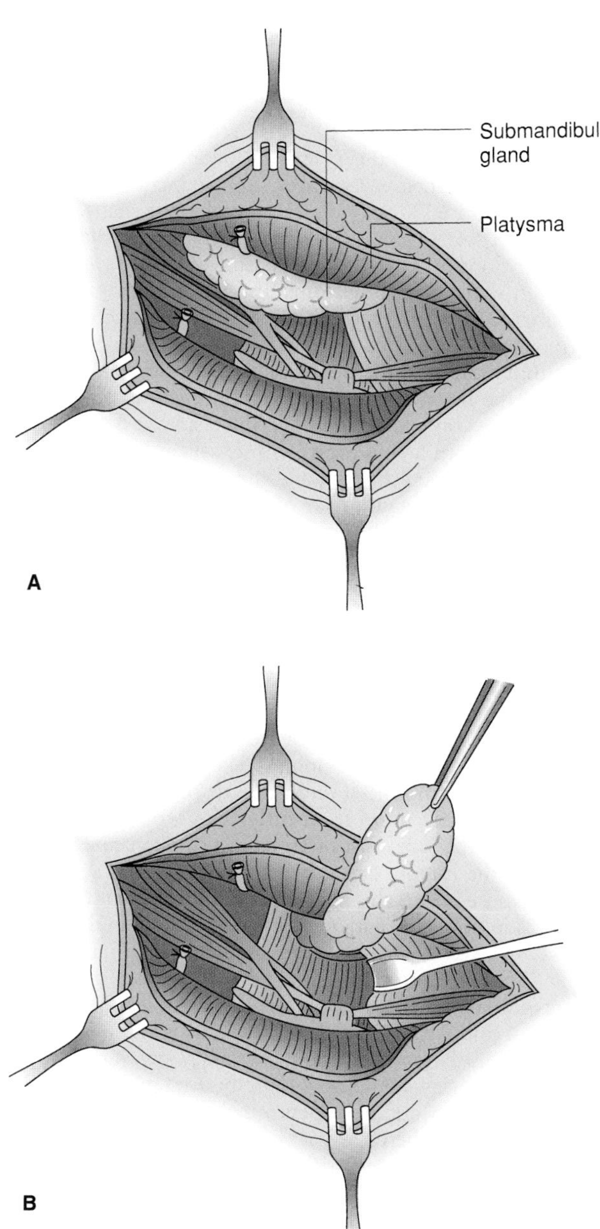

FIGURE 42.5 Resection of submandibular gland. The skin incision usually is placed in a skin crease. (*A*) After division of platysma, the ramus mandibularis is identified and retracted superiorly. (*B*) Elevation of the gland allows identification of the lingual nerve. After removal of the gland, the lingual nerve is in the base of the wound.

performance status of the patient, and medical and psychosocial issues, a treatment plan is formulated that is agreeable to all caregivers. The objective of any treatment is to cure the patient while maintaining optimal form and function. The specific treatments for different regions of the head and neck are discussed in the sections that follow, but overall treatment guidelines are essentially the same in most regions and are discussed here. The first goal of any successful treatment for head and neck cancer is to curtail alcohol and tobacco use. No therapy for the head and neck cancer can be expected to have long-term success unless this goal is accomplished. If the patient continues to abuse tobacco and alcohol, there is an approximately 40% risk of local regional recurrence and a 10% to 40% risk of developing a second primary tumor[4]. In addition, before initiating any therapy, the patient's medical, nutritional, and psychosocial status should be optimized. These steps will maximize treatment benefit and limit the number of complications.

In general, stage 1 and 2 lesions can be managed equally successfully by either primary surgery or radiation therapy. For these early lesions, there is an 80% to 100% cure rate with minimal morbidity.[1] The treatment modality of choice depends on tumor location and the surgeon's experience as well as on the patient's preference. The advantages of a surgical approach to stage 1 and 2 tumors include the ability to fully resect the tumor while eradicating occult or palpable nodal disease in a relatively short period of time. In addition, successful primary surgery reserves radiation therapy for any recurrences or second primary tumors that may develop over the patient's lifetime. On the other hand, radiation therapy has the advantage of resulting in minimal functional disturbance with a comparable rate of control. For these reasons, it is ideally suited for tumors that would result in significant functional disturbance, such as those of the larynx or hypopharynx.

In contrast, stage 3 and 4 lesions typically require multimodality therapy. Initial treatment is usually surgical; however, tumors in these categories typically have more aggressive biologic behavior and can be multicentric. As a result, large areas of the upper aerodigestive tract need to be resected to completely clear the tumor. Despite the surgeon's best efforts and often massive resection, these advanced lesions tend to have close margins and frequent regional metastases with extracapsular and nodal spread. Based on these factors, postoperative radiation therapy with or without adjunctive chemotherapy has been the approach employed for these high-risk patients. Importantly, two recent studies have demonstrated that postoperative chemotherapy and radiation in high-risk patients (histologic evidence of invasion of two or more regional lymph nodes, extracapsular extension of nodal disease, or microscopically positive margins) improves locoregional control and probably improves overall survival.[20,21]

There are relatively few absolute contraindications to surgery for advanced lesions of the head and neck. Some of these contraindications include randomly scattered dermal metastases that cannot be completely encompassed by a full-thickness resection, solid fixation to the skull base with intracranial extension, and fixation to the cervical spine. Relative contraindications include fixation to the common or internal carotid artery, periosteal invasion of the skull base, or a clinically positive node in the root of the neck.[8]

Despite our best efforts to diagnose these tumors early, patients will often present with or develop distant metastases from head and neck cancer. The mainstay of therapy in these cases is palliative chemotherapy such as cis-platinum and 5-fluorouracil. A more easily tolerated regimen is of methotrexate, which can be taken with minimal side effects but equally minimal effects on tumor regression. In most cases, a low-dose minimally toxic chemotherapeutic agent combined with analgesics is the best form of palliative care. There have been valiant attempts at surgical resection of isolated lung metastases, with essentially unchanged long-term survival.[22] As a result, this is not recommended therapy unless the thoracic surgeon believes this represents a second primary rather than a true metastasis.

TREATMENT BY SITE

Oral Cavity

Malignant tumors of the oral cavity can be devastating with regard to speech and swallowing impairment following successful treatment. Principles of treatment vary according to stage. The current primary tumor staging is shown in Table 42.12.

Lip

Squamous cell carcinoma is the most common lip cancer. It arises secondary to smoking and alcohol as well as to extensive

TABLE 42.12 CLASSIFICATION

PRIMARY TUMOR STAGING OF LIP AND ORAL CAVITY CANCER

Stage	Description
TX	Primary tumor cannot be assessed
T0	No evidence of primary tumor
Tis	Carcinoma *in situ*
T1	Tumor 2 cm or less in greatest dimension
T2	Tumor >2 cm but not more than 4 cm in greatest dimension
T3	Tumor >4 cm in greatest dimension
T4	(Lip) Tumor invades through cortical bone, inferior alveolar nerve, floor of mouth, or skin of face (i.e., chin or nose)
T4a	(Oral cavity) Tumor invades adjacent structures [e.g., through cortical bone, into deep (extrinsic) muscle of tongue (genioglossus, hyoglossus, palatoglossus, styloglossus), maxillary sinus, skin of face]
T4b	(Oral cavity) Tumor invades masticator space, pterygoid plates, or skull base and/or encases internal carotid artery

Data from American Joint Committee on Cancer. *Cancer staging manual*, 6th ed. New York: Springer-Verlag; 2002, with permission.

sun exposure. Approximately 90% of these lesions occur on the lower lip between the midline and lateral commissure. Stage 1 and 2 lesions of the lip can be treated with wide local excision and closure. Up to one half of the lip can be resected and closed primarily with minimal cosmetic defect. Neck dissection should be performed for known nodal disease or tumors that are stage T3 or greater. Only 10% of lip cancers develop neck metastases, and this frequently portends a very poor prognosis. Overall, lip malignancies are among the most readily cured head and neck tumors, with a 5-year survival of 89%.[23] This survival rate, however, drops to 25% to 50% when neck metastases are present. Aside from surgical treatment, postoperative radiation therapy should be given to patients with stage 3 and 4 disease or perineural or perivascular spread as well as in recurrent tumors.

Tongue

Due to its rich vascularity, lesions of the oral tongue tend to grow rapidly and develop early occult nodal metastases. Approximately 30% to 40% of early T1 and T2 oral tongue lesions have occult nodal metastases at the time of presentation.[24] For this reason, treatment of tongue tumors involves not only wide local excision with 2-cm margins but the appropriate neck dissection as well. Tumors that are minimally invasive (2 mm or less) probably do not require neck dissection because of the low risk of regional metastasis.[25] Locally advanced oral tongue lesions may involve the mandible, and a composite resection with mandibulectomy may be required for adequate resection. In such instances, microvascular free tissue transfer is necessary for optimal functional outcome. In general, lateral lesions of the tongue that do not involve resection of the floor of mouth can be reconstructed with split-thickness skin grafting. If, however, the floor of the mouth, the entire hemi-tongue, or the mandible is involved in the resection, optimal reconstruction is obtained with microvascular free–tissue transfer. Five-year survival for oral tongue carcinomas is approximately 75% for stage 1 and stage 2 tumors and less than 40% for stage 3 and stage 4 tumors.[26]

Floor of Mouth

Surgery is the treatment of choice for patients with cancer of the floor of mouth. Similar to tongue cancer, there is a nodal, occult metastatic rate approaching 40% in T2 tumors and 70% in T3 lesions.[27] In addition, floor of mouth lesions often involve the mandible even in their early stages. Approximately 7% of T1, 55% of T2, and 63% of T3 lesions involve the mandible and require some sort of mandibulectomy.[28] Based on these facts, surgery for floor of mouth carcinomas involves wide local excision, often with mandibulectomy and bilateral primary neck dissections. The reason for the bilateral neck dissections is an approximately 50% occult metastatic rate to lymph nodes in both submandibular regions. Following resection of these tumors, if the floor of mouth musculature is intact and separated from the contents of the neck, the resultant defect can be reconstructed with a skin graft, with excellent functional outcome. When there are through-and-through defects of the floor of mouth, or when mandibular defects are accompanying the floor of mouth defect, a composite microvascular flap is the most reliable and successful reconstruction in restoring form and function. Five-year survival rates for floor of mouth squamous cell carcinomas, stages 1, 2, 3, and 4, are approximately 90%, 80%, 65%, and 30%, respectively.[29]

Buccal Mucosa

Carcinomas of the buccal mucosa are uncommon and make up only 5% of oral cavity carcinomas. The mean age for buccal carcinomas is during the seventh decade of life, and men are affected four times more frequently than women. Although buccal carcinomas are most often seen in smokers and chewers of tobacco, the use of betel nut and a history of lichen planus also predispose one to this aggressive tumor. Due to the lack of symptoms in this area, patients often present late in the disease process with trismus, involvement of the bony mandible or maxilla, and neck metastases. Cervical metastases are present in approximately 50% of cases. Recent studies have shown that stage 1 and 2 tumors of the buccal mucosa are best treated with radiation therapy to both the primary site and the neck. Advanced lesions, stages 3 and 4, are best treated with a combination of surgery and postoperative radiation therapy.[30] Due to the thinness of the cheek, it is often necessary to perform through-and-through resections of the cheek, and these are best reconstructed with microvascular free-tissue transfer. Approximate 5-year survival rates for stages 1, 2, 3, and 4 are 75%, 65%, 30%, and 20%, respectively.[31]

Oropharynx

The confines of the oropharynx extend from the soft palate to the level of the hyoid bone and include the soft palate, tonsils, lateral and posterior pharyngeal walls, and the base of tongue. The current primary tumor staging is shown in Table 42.13. Squamous cell carcinoma of the oropharynx most commonly occurs in the fourth and fifth decades of life, with a male-to-female ratio of approximately 4:1. Traditionally, the cure rates for oropharyngeal carcinoma have been poor because most of these lesions are diagnosed at an advanced stage and they tend to metastasize early. Further clinical features of oropharyngeal carcinomas are that they spread submucosally, with early spread to the regional lymphatics. The rate of regional metastases varies from 40% for the soft palate to as high as 70% for the base of tongue. In addition, due to the rich vascularity of this region as well as the bilaterality of this vascularity, it is not unusual for patients to have bilateral cervical metastases. The tonsil and tonsillar fossa are the most common site for primary tumors of the oropharynx. These are also the easiest tumors to

TABLE 42.13 CLASSIFICATION

PRIMARY TUMOR STAGING OF OROPHARYNX CANCER

Stage	Description
T1	Tumor 2 cm or less in greatest dimension
T2	Tumor >2 cm but not more than 4 cm in greatest dimension
T3	Tumor >4 cm in greatest dimension
T4a	Tumor invades the larynx, deep/extrinsic muscle of tongue, medial pterygoid, hard palate, or mandible
T4b	Tumor invades the lateral pterygoid muscle, pterygoid plates, lateral nasopharynx, or skull bases or encases carotid artery

Data from American Joint Committee on Cancer. *Cancer staging manual*, 6th ed. New York: Springer-Verlag; 2002, with permission.

diagnose due to their easy visualization. On the other hand, patients with a tongue-base tumor typically present with a neck mass, and the primary is identified on careful examination and palpation of the tongue base. Early lesions of the oropharynx (stages 1 and 2) are best treated with radiation therapy. This form of treatment results in less functional disturbance and an equivalent cure rate. Advanced tumors are treated with multimodality therapy including surgery and radiotherapy. Survival rates for oropharyngeal tumors vary from site to site, with the best long-term prognosis seen in tonsillar cancers. The 5-year survival rate for stages 1 and 2 tonsillar carcinoma approaches 80%, whereas it decreases to 50% in stage 3 tumors. The prognosis for tongue-base tumors is somewhat worse, with 70% survival in stages 1 and 2 tumors, decreasing to approximately 40% in stage 3 and 30% in stage 4.[32]

Surgical resections of the oropharynx are the most likely of any region of the head and neck to leave the patient with impaired ability to swallow and protect their airway from secretions. Primary closure is rarely achievable, and a major advance in reconstructing these defects occurred with the use of pedicled myocutaneous flaps. The pectoralis myocutaneous flap was the workhorse of head and neck reconstruction for the oropharynx in the 1970s and 1980s. However, due to pedicle retraction, unpredictability of residual bulk, and the insensate nature of these flaps, they yielded in the mid to late 1980s and the 1990s to microvascularfree tissue reconstruction. Currently, microvascular free flaps, predominantly the radial forearm free flap, are used to reconstruct complex defects in the oropharynx. These flaps have the ability to reliably provide bulk, contour, and sensate capabilities to improve overall swallowing. Microvascular free flaps have resulted in approximately 80% to 90% of patients returning to a normal diet, whereas this figure is approximately 40% to 50% in myocutaneous free flaps.

Alternatively, combined chemotherapy and radiation strategies are being increasingly utilized to improve functional outcomes and improve survival in patients with advanced oropharyngeal cancer. Calais et al.[33] reported on a randomized trial of 222 patients with advanced resectable oropharyngeal cancer treated with either radiation or concurrent chemoradiation. With median follow-up of 35 months, overall survival and disease-free survival were statistically greater in the chemoradiation arm (51% and 42%) compared with the radiation-alone arm (31% and 20%). These numbers compare quite favorably to the historical controls of surgery with radiation.

Nasopharynx

The anatomic confines of the nasopharynx extend from the skull base superiorly to the level of the hard palate inferiorly. Carcinoma of the nasopharynx occurs infrequently in the United States; however, it is quite common in China and Hong Kong. A number of etiologic factors have been identified in this increased incidence, and they include nitrosamines from the ingestion of salted fish, chronic sinusitis, nickel exposure, and polycyclic hydrocarbons. Furthermore, carcinoma of the nasopharynx is closely associated with Epstein-Barr virus infections. High levels of the antibodies to this virus can be identified in approximately 70% of patients with this disease.[34,35] The peak incidence of nasopharynx carcinoma is bimodal, either in the teens or between the ages of 45 and 55. Undifferentiated carcinomas tend to occur in a younger age group, whereas the well-differentiated squamous cell carcinomas are more common in the more elderly group. The World Health Organization has defined three histologic classes of nasopharyngeal carcinoma, denoted WHO types 1, 2, and 3. WHO type 1 tumors most closely resemble squamous cell carcinoma in the other regions of the head and neck, and they represent 25% of all nasopharyngeal carcinomas and are the most common histologic type found in the United States. WHO type 2 tumors are known as transitional cell carcinomas, which include both lymphoepithelial elements and squamous elements. There is no keratinization in these tumors, and this allows for their identification. These tumors account for approximately 12% of all nasopharyngeal carcinomas. Finally, the most common type of nasopharyngeal carcinoma is the WHO type 3, which is endemic in southeast Asia. This is also known as undifferentiated carcinoma or lymphoepithelioma. These tumors are the most radiosensitive and represent 63% of nasopharyngeal carcinomas. Due to their location, the first sign that a patient may have a nasopharyngeal carcinoma is a neck mass, and this is the presenting symptom in approximately 65% of patients.[36] The next most common symptoms are ear fullness, a hearing loss, and epistaxis. Furthermore, approximately one fifth of patients have bilateral neck nodes at the time of presentation, but only 3% have distant metastases.[35] For all forms of nasopharyngeal carcinoma, the initial treatment is radiation therapy. These tumors are unusually radiosensitive and, even with neck metastases, the treatment should involve radiotherapy. More recently, improved long-term survival has been found with patients receiving combined chemotherapy and radiation therapy for advanced nasopharyngeal carcinoma.[37] Five-year survival for patients with nasopharyngeal carcinoma is directly related to the type of nasopharyngeal carcinoma they possess. WHO type 1 tumors have an approximately 20% survival, whereas WHO type 3 have a better prognosis, with approximately 60% 5-year survival.[35]

Hypopharynx

The hypopharynx is the anatomic region defined as the mucosal area lateral to the larynx inferior to the hyoid bone down to the level of the cricopharyngeus muscle. Squamous cell carcinoma of this region is an extremely aggressive disease with a poor prognosis, irrespective of the therapeutic regimen instituted. Aside from smoking and drinking, etiologic factors for squamous cell carcinomas in this area include Plummer-Vinson syndrome and gastroesophageal reflux disease. This tumor most commonly occurs in men between the ages of 60 and 80, and the pyriform fossa is the most frequently involved site. Interestingly, symptoms are not present until very late in the course of this disease. Symptoms include odynophagia, referred otalgia, dysphagia, and a neck mass. Occult cervical metastasis is very common and occurs in approximately 75% of these lesions at the time of presentation. Most lesions are diagnosed at stages 3 and 4 because they are often very difficult to visualize in the office.

TABLE 42.14 CLASSIFICATION

PRIMARY TUMOR STAGING OF HYPOPHARYNX CANCER

Stage	Description
T1	Tumor limited to one subsite of hypopharynx and 2 cm or less in greatest dimension
T2	Tumor involves more than one subsite of hypopharynx or adjacent site or measures >2 cm but not more than 4 cm in greatest diameter without fixation of hemilarynx
T3	Tumor measures >4 cm in greatest dimension or with fixation of hemilarynx
T4	Tumor invades thyroid/cricoid cartilage, hyoid bone, thyroid gland, esophagus, or central compartment soft tissue

Data from American Joint Committee on Cancer. *Cancer staging manual*, 6th ed. New York: Springer-Verlag; 2002, with permission.

The staging of a hypopharyngeal cancer is based primarily on the subsite of the pharynx that is involved, the presence of vocal cord fixation, and the extent of lymph node metastases (Table 42.14). Surgical treatment of any hypopharyngeal lesion involves laryngectomy; therefore, early lesions, stages 1 and 2, are typically treated by primary radiotherapy. Advanced lesions are standardly treated with surgery and postoperative radiation therapy. The surgical procedure typically involves a total laryngopharyngectomy with microvascular free tissue reconstruction of the neopharynx. Because of the morbidity of this procedure, many alternative approaches for treatment have been investigated. Lefebre et al.[38] in France have published the results of a European cooperative study using induction chemotherapy followed by radiation therapy for advanced hypopharyngeal tumors. They have found comparable survival rates between the organ preservation arm and the surgery arm. This allows patients to preserve their larynx without a decrease in survival. Regardless of the treatment type, however, 5-year survival rates for hypopharyngeal cancer remain dismal. The overall 5-year survival rates in stages 1, 2, 3, and 4 are 50%, 40%, 25%, and 5%, respectively.[39]

Larynx

The site of the head and neck that has received the greatest attention with regard to cancer therapy is the larynx. The larynx is divided into three portions, including the supraglottic, glottic, and subglottic regions. The supraglottic larynx extends from the vallecula to the laryngeal ventricles. The glottis includes the true vocal cords as well as the inferior portion of the ventricles and approximately 1 cm below the true vocal cords in the superior subglottis. The subglottic larynx includes the region from 1 cm below the level of the glottis to the first tracheal ring. The hallmark symptom of laryngeal cancer is persistent hoarseness. Due to the early onset of this symptom, many laryngeal cancers are diagnosed early in their disease course, particularly at the glottic level. Other symptoms associated with laryngeal cancers include referred otalgia, dysphagia, a neck mass, weight loss, airway obstruction, hemoptysis, and odynophagia. Because of the significant role that the larynx plays in speech, swallowing, and airway, treatment decisions about cancer of the larynx involve significant quality of life issues. For this reason, every attempt is made to spare the patient's larynx, while providing adequate cure.

As a general rule, stages 1 and 2 disease in any region of the larynx can be managed with radiotherapy or surgery, with equal cure rates. Due to the improved functional outcome of patients following radiotherapy, this is typically the primary treatment option. Furthermore, in stages 3 and 4 disease, surgical treatment frequently requires total laryngectomy with bilateral neck dissections and postoperative radiation therapy. Due to the significant emotional and functional deficits that a total laryngectomy can cause the patient, other forms of treatment have been investigated and proved successful in stages 3 and 4 tumors.

The landmark study that was conducted at the Department of Veterans Affairs in advanced laryngeal cancer has changed the treatment of advanced laryngeal tumors significantly. This seminal study utilized induction chemotherapy (cis-platinum and 5-FU) combined with radiation therapy as an alternative to traditional laryngectomy plus radiation therapy for patients with advanced laryngeal squamous carcinoma. Analysis of the 332 patients with 5 years of median follow-up revealed that the larynx was preserved in 66% of surviving patients, without a decrease in survival rate. The estimated survival in both groups was similar at 42% and 46%, respectively.[40] At 12 years of follow-up, 61% of survivors treated with chemoradiation had laryngeal preservation, with survival rates similar to the surgical arm.[41] An alternative approach is the use of concurrent chemoradiation for the primary treatment of advanced laryngeal carcinoma. Forastiere et al.,[42] reporting for the National Cancer Institute Cooperative Trials Head and Neck Intergroup (R91-11), demonstrated that concurrent chemoradiation had greater laryngeal preservation rates than the Veterans Affairs protocol of induction chemotherapy followed by radiation.

Supraglottic Carcinoma

Primary supraglottic tumors account for 25% to 50% of all laryngeal cancers. The staging of these tumors is outlined in Table 42.15 and is based on the number of subsites involved, vocal cord fixation, and tumor invasion of laryngeal cartilage and structures outside the larynx. Not uncommonly, supraglottic tumors invade the preepiglottic space, which sits just inferior to the hyoepiglottic ligament. The rich vascularity of the supraglottis, as we have seen in other areas, predisposes this region to a high rate of occult nodal metastases. Approximately 50% to 55% of supraglottic tumors have occult nodal metastases that are bilateral.

Stages 1 and 2 lesions of the supraglottic larynx can be treated with primary radiotherapy, with response rates ranging from 85% to 70%, respectively. Alternatively, these early tumors may be treated with endoscopic laser resection of the supraglottic larynx as well as open supraglottic laryngectomy with neck dissections. In patients who have undergone surgical excision and have no evidence of nodal metastases, postoperative radiation therapy is not necessary and significantly decreases patient morbidity. Stages 3 and 4 tumors may be treated with equal cure rates in one of two ways. Surgical resection requires, in most instances, total laryngectomy with bilateral neck dissections. Induction chemotherapy followed by radiation or concurrent chemoradiation also offers equal survival, rates with laryngeal preservation in more than 50% of patients. Radiation therapy alone can be used in these advanced lesions; however, there is a recurrence rate of 50% to 60% with this unimodality therapy. A fourth alternative for treatment of advanced lesions is the newly described supracricoid laryngectomy for selected T1 to T3 supraglottic and transglottic cancers. These oncologically sound partial laryngeal surgeries involve removing the entire thyroid cartilage, the true vocal cords, and the entire supraglottic larynx, down to the level of the cricoid cartilage. The arytenoid cartilages and the cricoid are then suspended to the base of the tongue to allow for airway protection and phonation. Contraindications to this procedure include tumor extension inferior to the cricoid cartilage, arytenoid fixation, and extralaryngeal spread of tumor. Stages 1 and 2 supraglottic lesions are associated with excellent cure rates approaching 75% using either surgery or radiation alone. Survival, however, decreases

TABLE 42.15 CLASSIFICATION

PRIMARY TUMOR STAGING OF LARYNX CANCER

Stage	Description
SUPRAGLOTTIS	
T1	Tumor limited to one subsite of supraglottis with normal vocal cord mobility
T2	Tumor invades mucosa of more than one adjacent subsite of supraglottis or glottis or region outside supraglottis (e.g., mucosa of base of tongue, vallecula, medial wall of pyriform sinus) without fixation of the larynx
T3	Tumor limited to larynx with vocal cord fixation and/or invades any of the following: postcricoid area, preepiglottic tissues, paraglottic space, and/or minor thyroid cartilage erosion (e.g., inner cortex)
T4a	Tumor invades through the thyroid cartilage and/or invades tissues beyond the larynx (e.g., trachea, soft tissues of neck including deep extrinsic muscle of tongue, strap muscles, thyroid, or esophagus)
T4b	Tumor invades prevertebral space, encases carotid artery, or invades mediastinal structures
GLOTTIS	
T1	Tumor limited to the vocal cord(s) (may involve anterior or posterior commissure) with normal mobility
T1a	Tumor limited to one vocal cord
T1b	Tumor involves both vocal cords
T2	Tumor extends to supraglottis and/or subglottis and/or with impaired vocal cord mobility
T3	Tumor limited to the larynx with vocal cord fixation and/or invades paraglottic space, and/or minor thyroid cartilage erosion (e.g., inner cortex)
T4a	Tumor invades through the thyroid cartilage and/or invades tissues beyond the larynx (e.g., trachea, soft tissues of neck including deep extrinsic muscle of tongue, strap muscles, thyroid, or esophagus)
T4b	Tumor invades prevertebral space, encases carotid artery, or invades mediastinal structures
SUBGLOTTIS	
T1	Tumor limited to subglottis
T2	Tumor extends to vocal cord(s) with normal or impaired mobility
T3	Tumor limited to larynx with vocal cord fixation
T4a	Tumor invades through the thyroid cartilage and/or invades tissues beyond the larynx (e.g., trachea, soft tissues of neck including deep extrinsic muscle of tongue, strap muscles, thyroid, or esophagus)
T4b	Tumor invades prevertebral space, encases carotid artery, or invades mediastinal structures

From American Joint Committee on Cancer. *Cancer staging manual*, 6th ed. New York: Springer-Verlag; 2002, with permission.

dramatically when lymph node metastasis is present. Stage 3 supraglottic tumors have a 5-year survival of approximately 60%, and survival with stage 4 lesions decreases to 40%.[43]

Glottis

Fortunately, due to the early detection afforded by persistent hoarseness, glottic tumors are frequently discovered in their early stages and have among the best cure rates of tumors of the head and neck. Early glottic cancers are amenable to treatment with radiation therapy or microsurgical resection. Vocal results tend to be slightly better with radiation therapy; however, new techniques of microflap dissection of early glottic tumors may provide equal or superior results on prospective analysis. T1 and T2 glottic cancers are also amenable to more traditional open hemilaryngectomy approaches. These cause a significant disruption in normal phonation and are rarely performed for primary lesions. Contraindications to hemilaryngectomy include posterior commissure involvement, transglottic tumor spread, and cricoarytenoid joint involvement as well as subglottic extension. Stage 1 and stage 2 glottic carcinomas are nearly universally treated with radiotherapy, with excellent 5-year survival data. However, some surgeons advocate laser resection with radiation held in reserve for persistent or recurrent disease. Five-year survival in stage 1 lesions is 95%, and in stage 2 lesions it is 87%. Stages 3 and 4 lesions, similarly to the supraglottic larynx, are treated either with total laryngectomy, bilateral neck dissections, and concurrent chemoradiation or with induction chemotherapy with radiotherapy. Survival rates in stages 3 and 4 are 66% and 50%, respectively.[44]

Subglottis

Primary subglottic carcinomas account for less than 5% of all laryngeal cancers. Limited data support the role of radiation therapy in stages 1 and 2 disease treatment. More advanced tumors require total laryngectomy, partial tracheal resection, bilateral neck dissections, paratracheal neck dissections, and superior mediastinal dissection. Subglottic tumors have occult metastases in approximately 65% of cases; therefore, the assessment of nodes is critical in appropriate treatment. Overall survival in stages 1 and 2 is 70%, but in more advanced tumors survival is dismal.[45]

Unknown Primary Tumors

Occasionally a patient will present to the surgeon with a neck mass in which a primary lesion cannot be identified. The regions most likely to present in this manner include the nasopharynx, tonsillar fossa, base of tongue, and hypopharynx. In evaluating these patients, special attention must be paid to these areas to identify an occult primary lesion. Of the lesions that present in this manner, approximately 80% will have a primary tumor identified during some point in the treatment process.

Treatment of the neck for both known and unknown primary tumors is a point of significant controversy in head and neck surgery. In a known primary with a high rate of occult metastases but no clinical evidence of metastases (N0 neck), the neck is addressed during surgical therapy via a selective neck dissection (Table 42.16). This includes a resection of only the lymph node–bearing tissues in the regions to be staged, preserving all other structures.

In the case of known nodal metastases (N-positive neck), selective neck dissections can be used as oncologic procedures if the node is small (less than 3 cm) and not infiltrative of any nonvital structures (sternocleidomastoid, internal jugular vein, or spinal accessory nerve). However, this is a controversial principle, and many head and neck surgeons advocate a modified radical neck dissection for anyone with known neck disease. The modified radical neck dissection is the most commonly performed for known neck disease and includes resection of the sternocleidomastoid

TABLE 42.16 MANAGEMENT

TYPES OF SELECTIVE NECK DISSECTION

Type	Levels	Commonly used for
Supraomohyoid neck dissection	1–3	Oral cavity primary tumors
Anterolateral neck dissection	1–4	Oropharyngeal primary tumors
Lateral neck dissection	2–4	N0 disease of the larynx
Functional or Bocca neck dissection	1–5	Melanoma and primary thyroid malignancies with known metastases

muscle and internal jugular in addition to levels 1 to 5 of lymph nodes. The difference between a modified radical neck dissection and a radical neck dissection is that the radical neck dissection includes removal of the spinal accessory nerve, which is spared in other forms of neck dissections. Any patient with a node larger than 3 cm, multiple lymph nodes, or a node with extracapsular spread must be treated with postoperative radiation therapy. In the case of an unknown primary, the areas of greatest risk, namely, the nasopharynx, tonsillar fossa, base of tongue, and hypopharynx (Waldeyer's ring), are included in the radiation field. Overall survival in patients with an unknown primary is approximately 50%.

KEY POINTS

- **In any smoker aged 35 or older, the presence of any signs, neck mass, or airway compromise is considered indicative of head and neck cancer until proved otherwise.**
- **The best recognized carcinogens are tobacco use and alcohol consumption.**
- **After completing a detailed history, the next step in management of a patient with a head and neck complaint is a complete physical examination. No head and neck examination should be considered complete until all mucosal surfaces of the nasal cavity, nasopharynx, oropharynx, oral cavity, hypopharynx, and larynx have been clearly visualized.**
- **The neoplasm most commonly affecting the head and neck is squamous cell carcinoma.**

References

1. Teknos TN, Coniglio JU, Netterville JL. Guidelines for patient management. In: Bailey BJ, ed. *Head and neck surgery—otolaryngology.* Philadelphia: JB Lippincott; 1993:80.
2. **Gluckman JL, Waner M. Physical examination of the head and neck. In: Caparella MM, Schumrick DA, Gluckman JL, et al., eds. *Otolaryngology*, vol. 3. Philadelphia: WB Saunders; 1991:1.**
3. Rice DH, Spiro RH. General management guidelines. In: *Current concepts in head and neck cancer.* New York: The American Cancer Society; 1989:1.
4. Jessie RH. General considerations. In: Suen JY, Myers EN, eds. *Cancer of the head and neck.* London: Churchill Livingston; 1981:1.
5. Goldman L, Hashimoto B, Cook EF, et al. Comparative reproducibility and validity of systems for assessing cardiovascular functional class: advantages of a new specific activity scale. *Circulation* 1981;64:1227.
6. Snow GB. Evaluation and staging. In: Snow GB, Clark JR, eds. *Multimodality therapy for head and neck cancer.* New York: Thieme Medical; 1992:1.
7. McQuarry DG, Adams GL, Shons AR, et al. Objectives of care in head and neck malignancy. In: McQuarry DG, ed. *Head and neck: clinical decisions and management principles.* Chicago: Year Book Medical; 1986:1.
8. Million RR, Cassissi NJ. General principles for treatment of cancer in the head and neck. In: Million RR, Cassissi NJ, eds. *Management of head and neck cancer.* Philadelphia: JB Lippincott; 1984:64.
9. **Shaw JP. Patterns of cervical lymph node metastasis from squamous carcinomas of the upper aerodigestive tract. *Am J Surg.* 1990;160:405.**
10. Senior DA, Redkowski D, McArthur D, et al. Changing patterns in pediatric supraglottitis: a multi-institutional review, 1980–1992. *Laryngoscope* 1994;104:1314.
11. Goine CC, Squires TS, Tawn T. Cancer statistics, 1991. *CA Cancer J Clin.* 1991;41:19.
12. McQuarry DG, Adams GL, Shons AR, et al. Objectives of care in head and neck malignancy. In: McQuarry DG, ed. *Head and neck: clinical decisions and management principles.* Chicago: Year Book Medical; 1986:1.
13. Vrabec DP. The inverted schneiderian papilloma. *Laryngoscope* 1994;104: 582.
14. Myers EN, Fernau JL, Johnson JT, et al. Management of inverted papilloma. *Laryngoscope* 1990;100:481.
15. Eilele DW, Johns ME. Salivary gland neoplasms. In: Bailey BJ, ed. *Head and neck surgery—otolaryngology.* Philadelphia: JB Lippincott; 1993: 1485.
16. Frable MAS, Frable WJ. Fine needle aspiration biopsy of salivary gland. *Laryngoscope* 1991;101:245.
17. Savary M, Passche R, Monner P. Endoscopic screening for multiple squamous cell carcinomas of the upper digestive and respiratory tracts. In: Wygand ME, Steiner W, Stell PM, eds. *Functional partial laryngectomy: conservation surgery for carcinoma of the larynx.* Berlin: Springer-Verlag; 1984:51.
18. **Sturgis EM, Miller RH. Second primary malignancies in the head and neck cancer patient. *Ann Otol Rhinol Laryngol.* 1995;104:946.**
19. American Joint Committee on Cancer (AJCC). *Cancer staging manual*, 6th ed. New York: Springer-Verlag; 2002.
20. Bernier J, Domenge C, Ozsahin M, et al. Postoperative irradiation with or without concomitant chemotherapy for locally advanced head and neck cancer. *N Engl J Med.* 2004;350:1945.
21. Cooper JS, Pajak TF, Forastiere AA, et al. Postoperative concurrent radiotherapy and chemotherapy in high-risk squamous-cell carcinoma of the head and neck. *N Engl J Med.* 2004;350:1937.
22. Masard G, Roeslin N, Jung GM, et al. Bronchiogenic cancer associated with head and neck tumors. *J Thorac Cardiovasc Surg.* 1993;103:218.
23. Jesse RH. Cancer of the oral cavity: is elective neck dissection beneficial? *Am J Surg.* 1970;120:505.
24. Spiro RH, Alfonso AE, Farr HW, et al. Cervical node metastases from epidermoid carcinoma of the oral cavity and oral pharynx: a critical assessment of current staging. *Am J Surg.* 1974;128:562.
25. Spiro RH, Huvos AG, Wong GY, et al. Predictive value of tumor thickness in squamous carcinoma confined to the tongue and floor of the mouth. *Am J Surg.* 1986;152:345.
26. Faranceschi D. Improved survival in the treatment of squamous cell carcinoma of the oral tongue. *Am J Surg.* 1993;166:360.
27. Ditroia JF. Nodal metastasis and prognosis in carcinoma of the oral cavity. *Otolaryngol Clin North Am.* 1972;5:333.
28. Bradford CR, Krause CJ. Floor mouth cancer. In: Gates G, ed. *Current therapy of head and neck cancer,* 5th ed. St. Louis: Mosby; 1994:266.
29. Shaha AR, et al. Squamous carcinoma of the floor of the mouth. *Am J Surg.* 1984;184:455.
30. Strome SE, Towaiyat, Strauderman M, et al. Squamous cell carcinoma of the buccal mucosa: the role of parotidectomy. *Otolaryngol Head Neck Surg.* 1999;120:375.
31. Bloom ND, Spiro RH. Carcinoma of the cheek mucosa: a retrospective analysis. *Am J Surg.* 1980;140:556.
32. Perez CA, Carmichael T, Devineni VR, et al. Carcinoma of the tonsillar fossa: a non-randomized comparison of irradiation alone or combined with surgery—long-term results. *Head Neck Surg.* 1991;13:282.
33. **Calais G, Alfonsi M, Bardet E, et al. Randomized trial of radiation therapy versus concomitant chemotherapy and radiation therapy for advanced-staged oropharynx carcinoma. *J Natl Cancer Inst.* 1999;91:2081.**
34. Dickson RI. Nasopharyngeal carcinoma: an evaluation of 209 patients. *Laryngoscope* 1981;91:333.
35. Neal HB, et al. Antibodies to Epstein-Barr virus in patients with nasopharyngeal carcinoma in comparison groups. *Ann Otol Rhinol Laryngol.* 1984;93:477.
36. Neal HB. Nasopharyngeal carcinoma: clinical presentation, diagnosis, treatment, and prognosis. *Otolaryngol Clin North Am.* 1985;18:479.
37. **Al-Sarraf M, LeBlan M, Giri PGS, et al. Chemoradiotherapy versus radiotherapy in patients with advanced nasopharyngeal cancer: phase III randomized intergroup study 0099. *J Clin Oncol.* 1998;16:1310.**
38. Lefebre JL, Chevalier D, Luboinski B, et al. Larynx preservation in pyriform sinus cancer: preliminary results of the European Organization for Research and Treatment of Cancer Phase III Trial. *J Natl Cancer Inst.* 1996;88:890.
39. Elbadawi SA, et al. Squamous carcinoma of the pyriform sinus. *Laryngoscope* 1982;92:357.
40. Wolf GT, Hawn WK, Fisher SG, et al. Induction chemotherapy plus radiation compared with surgery plus radiation in patients with advanced laryngeal cancer. *N Engl J Med.* 1991;324:1685.
41. Wolf GT. Chemotherapy for laryngeal cancer. In: Ferlito A, ed. *Diseases of the larynx.* London: Arnold Publishers; 2000:709.
42. **Forastiere AA, Goepfert H, Maor M, et al. Concurrent chemotherapy and radiotherapy for organ preservation in advanced laryngeal cancer. *N Engl J Med.* 2003;349:2091.**
43. Hoekstra CJ, Lovendag PC, VanPolten WL. Squamous cell carcinoma of the supraglottic larynx without clinically detectable lymph node metastasis: problem of local relapse and influence of overall treatment time. *Int J Radiat Oncol Biol Phys.* 1990;18:13.
44. Wang CC, Schulz MD, Miller D. Combined radiation therapy and surgery for carcinoma of the supraglottis and pyriform sinus. *Am J Surg.* 1972;124:551.
45. Ward P, Harwood A. Carcinoma of the subglottis. *Arch Otolaryngol.* 1987;113:1.

SECTION D
ESOPHAGUS

CHAPTER 43 ■ ESOPHAGEAL ANATOMY AND PHYSIOLOGY AND GASTROESOPHAGEAL REFLUX DISEASE

JEFFREY H. PETERS, THOMAS J. WATSON, AND THOMAS R. DEMEESTER

ANATOMY

A detailed knowledge of the anatomic relationships of the esophagus is essential for the surgeon to plan and perform safe surgery, as well as to understand the significance of abnormalities detected on studies such as upper endoscopy, barium roentgenography, or computed tomography.[1] In this section, the embryology of the esophagus is first described, then the topographic relations of the esophagus are covered, and finally the conduct of investigations that yield anatomic information are addressed.

The embryology of the esophagus is important in understanding the pathogenesis of congenital malformations of the esophagus and trachea. The embryonic esophagus forms when paired longitudinal grooves appear on each side of the laryngotracheal diverticulum. These grooves subsequently grow medially and fuse to form the tracheoesophageal septum. This septum divides the foregut into the ventral laryngotracheal tube and the dorsal esophagus. Incomplete fusion of the two lateral grooves was thought to be the major factor in the pathogenesis of congenital tracheoesophageal fistula, but the anomaly is now attributed to abnormal growth and differentiation of the lung buds. Initially the esophagus is short, but elongation occurs rapidly, and the final relative length is attained by the seventh gestational week. This is followed by endodermal proliferation, resulting in near obliteration of the esophageal lumen and subsequent recanalization by the development of large vacuoles that coalesce. The striated muscle of the upper esophagus is derived from the caudal branchial arches and is innervated by the vagus nerve and its recurrent laryngeal branches. The smooth muscle of the lower esophagus arises from splanchnic mesenchyme and is supplied by a visceral nerve plexus derived from neural crest cells. The adult position of the vagus nerves on the esophagus is the result of unequal growth of the greater curve of the stomach relative to the lesser curve, resulting in rotation of the left vagus anteriorly and the right vagus posteriorly.

The *cervical esophagus* begins below the cricopharyngeus muscle, which itself is a continuation of the inferior constrictor of the pharynx. The potential space between these muscles posteriorly is the site where Zenker's diverticulum develops. The cervical esophagus is about 5 cm long. It begins at the level of C6 and extends to the lower border of T1, curving slightly to the left in its descent. Anteriorly, it abuts against the trachea and posterior larynx and can be dissected off both organs if necessary. Posteriorly, the retroesophageal space is continuous with the retropharyngeal space above and the superior mediastinum below. Laterally, the omohyoid muscle crosses it obliquely and is usually divided to gain access to the esophagus. The carotid sheaths lie laterally and the lobes of the thyroid and the strap muscles anteriorly. The recurrent laryngeal nerves lie in the grooves between the esophagus and the trachea. The right recurrent nerve runs a more oblique course and is more prone to anatomic variants. Consequently, although the surgical approach to this portion of the esophagus may be from either side of the neck through an incision along the anterior border of sternocleidomastoid muscle, the left side is chosen if possible.

The *thoracic esophagus* in its upper part is closely related to the posterior wall of the trachea. This close relation is responsible for the early spread of cancer of the upper esophagus into the trachea, and it limits the ability of the surgeon to perform an *en bloc* resection of such a tumor. Above the level of the tracheal bifurcation, the esophagus moves to the right of the descending aorta. It then moves to the left, passes behind the tracheal bifurcation and the left main bronchus, and descends to the diaphragm. In its lower third, the esophagus courses anteriorly and to the left to pass through the diaphragmatic hiatus. The lower esophagus is covered only by flimsy mediastinal pleura on the left, and it is this portion that is most commonly the site of perforation in Boerhaave's syndrome. The azygos vein is closely related to the esophagus as it arches from its paraspinal position over the right main bronchus to enter the superior vena cava. The thoracic duct ascends behind and to the right of the distal esophagus, but at the level of T5 it passes posterior to the aorta and ascends on the left side of the esophagus and posterior to the left subclavian artery.

Throughout its length, the attachments of the esophagus to its adjacent structures other than the posterior trachea are flimsy. This accounts for the ease with which the esophagus may be bluntly mobilized out of the mediastinum during transhiatal esophagectomy. In general, the lower esophagus is most easily approached through the left chest, but access to the supraaortic esophagus is restricted. Thus, a left thoracotomy is most useful for performing Heller's myotomy, transthoracic fundoplication, or resection of an epiphrenic diverticulum. Access to the entire thoracic esophagus can be obtained only from the right chest, but access to the intraabdominal organs is restricted by the liver and normally requires a separate upper abdominal incision.

The abdominal esophagus begins as the esophagus enters the abdomen through the diaphragmatic hiatus (Fig. 43.1). It is surrounded by a fibroelastic membrane, the phrenoesophageal ligament, which arises from the subdiaphragmatic fascia (Fig. 43.2). The lower limit of the phrenoesophageal membrane anteriorly is marked by a prominent fat pad, which corresponds to the gastroesophageal (GE) junction. The lower esophageal sphincter (LES) is a zone of high pressure 3 to 5 cm long at the lower end of the esophagus.[2] Although it does not correspond to any macroscopic anatomic structure, its function appears to be related to the microscopic architecture of the muscle fibers. The esophageal hiatus is formed by the right and left crura, which form a sling of muscular fibers arising by

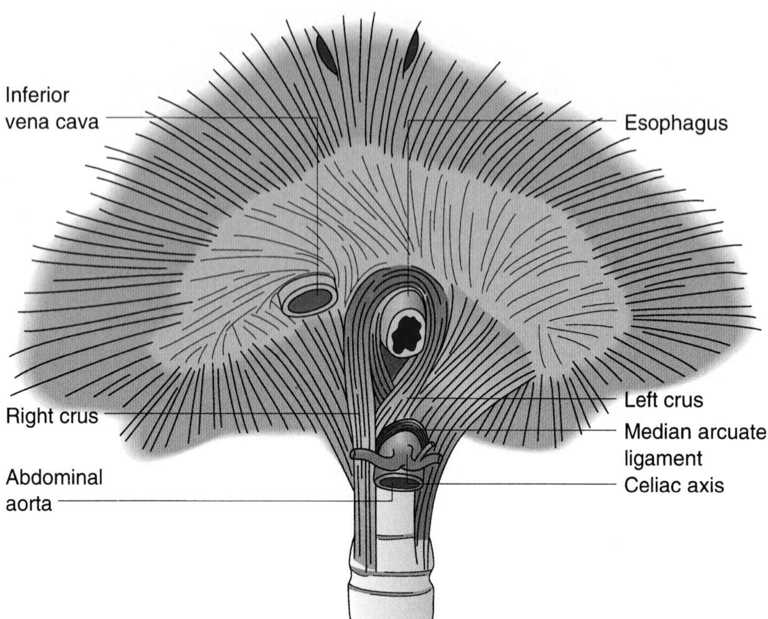

FIGURE 43.1 The diaphragm and esophageal hiatus viewed from below.

tendinous bands from the anterolateral surface of the first four lumbar vertebrae. The relative contributions of the right and left crura to the sling are variable. Surgeons name the crura from their relation to the esophagus, whereas anatomists name them from their relation to the aorta. Thus, both right and left "surgical" crura originate from the right "anatomic" crus. Caudally, the crura are united by a tendinous arch, the median arcuate ligament, just anterior to the aorta at the level of the celiac axis.

The blood supply and venous drainage are largely segmental. The inferior thyroid artery provides the main blood supply to the cervical portion of the esophagus. This becomes important in a patient with a previous thyroidectomy, although ligation is usually performed distal to the esophageal branch. The thoracic portion of the esophagus receives its blood supply from two sources. Usually, branches from two to three bronchial arteries provide the proximal arterial supply, and branches directly from the aorta supply the more distal thoracic esophagus. The upper of these aortic branches arises between the sixth and seventh thoracic vertebrae; the lower one arises between the eighth and ninth thoracic vertebrae. Intrathoracic mobilization of the esophagus during the performance of antireflux procedures often requires ligation of these branches. The abdominal esophagus receives its blood supply from branches of the left gastric artery and inferior phrenic arteries (Fig. 43.3). A particularly constant artery at the base of the left surgical crus connects the inferior phrenic artery to branches of the left gastric artery and is sometimes called Belsey's artery. It is often seen during the crural dissection in performing laparoscopic fundoplication. Once the vessels have entered the muscular wall of the esophagus, branching occurs at right angles to provide a longitudinal vascular plexus. This anatomic arrangement allows for mobilization of the esophagus from the stomach to the aortic arch without ischemic injury.

A venous plexus in the submucosa collects capillary blood and delivers it into a periesophageal venous plexus. From this plexus, esophageal veins arise that empty into the inferior thyroid vein proximally; into the bronchial, azygos, or hemiazygos veins in the thorax; and into the left gastric vein in the abdominal region (Fig. 43.4). The left gastric vein, or coronary vein, provides the principal collateral in portal hypertension when esophageal varices develop. The submucosal veins become much more superficial in the most distal esophagus, 1 to 2 cm above the GE junction and are consequently the most common site of bleeding in portal hypertension. The continuity between the submucosal venous networks of the esophagus and stomach provides an additional collateral pathway for portal blood to enter the superior vena cava through the azygos vein in patients with portal hypertension.

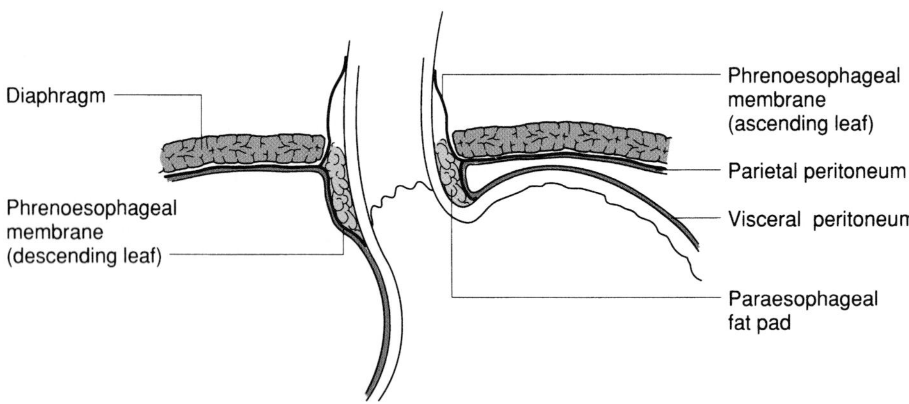

FIGURE 43.2 Attachments of the phrenoesophageal membrane.

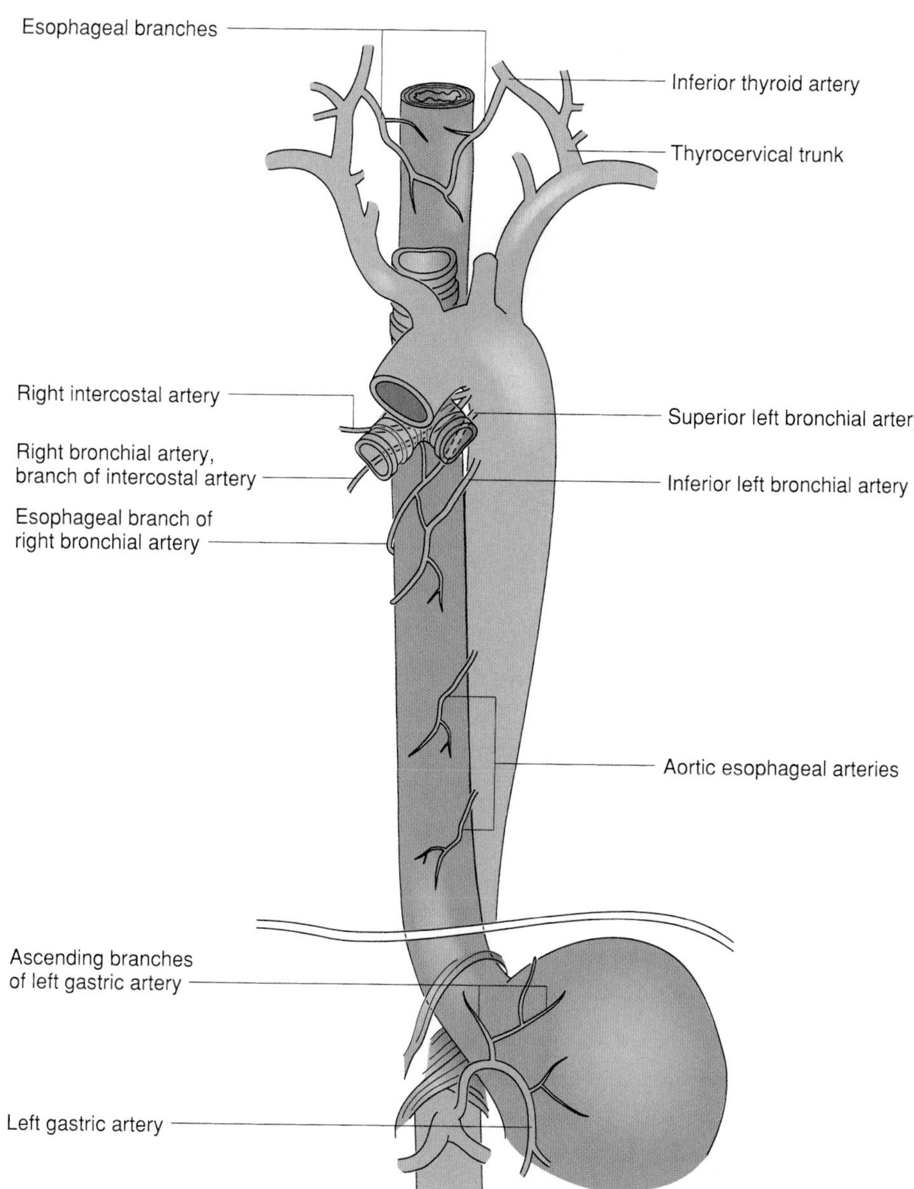

FIGURE 43.3 Arterial blood supply of the esophagus.

The *lymphatics* of the esophagus form a rich submucosal network draining into regional lymph nodes in the periesophageal connective tissue (Fig. 43.5). Thus, little barrier exists to longitudinal spread of cancer in the esophagus; it is estimated that for every 1 cm of axial spread, there are 6 cm of longitudinal spread. Lymphatic drainage from the upper two thirds of the esophagus is usually cephalad, but drainage from the lower one third is in both directions. In the cervical region, esophageal lymphatic drainage is toward the internal jugular and upper tracheal nodes. Posterior mediastinal nodes drain the thoracic portion of the esophagus dorsally. Drainage from the anterior portion of the thoracic esophagus is most often to tracheal nodes superiorly and subcarinal and paraesophageal nodes inferiorly. In the abdomen, the esophageal lymph drains to cardiac and celiac nodes, which may eventually drain into the cisterna chyli or the thoracic duct. Although lymphatic metastases in the esophagus generally involve the regional nodes in proximity, nodal involvement may occur several centimeters away from the primary lesion because of the rich intramural lymphatic anastomotic channels. When a carcinoma is limited to the mucosa (above the muscularis mucosae), the incidence of lymphatic metastases is low, but once it spreads into the submucosa the incidence rises to 50% to 60%. The results of three-field lymph node dissection for esophageal carcinoma have emphasized the widespread lymphatic connections within the esophagus.

The *innervation* of the cricopharyngeal sphincter and cervical portion of the esophagus is from both the right and left recurrent laryngeal nerves.[2] These nerves, arising from the vagus, travel dorsally around the subclavian artery on the right and the arch of the aorta on the left. Branching to both the esophagus and trachea occurs as these nerves ascend in the tracheoesophageal groove. The nerve may be injured during dissection of the upper esophagus in the neck or during the mediastinal dissection in transhiatal esophagectomy. Although much attention is given to the vocal cord dysfunction that accompanies recurrent laryngeal nerve damage, it is also clear that cricopharyngeal sphincter dysfunction and motility problems of the cervical esophagus can occur with injury to these nerves. Serious aspiration following recurrent nerve injury is caused not only by cricopharyngeal dysfunction, but also by the additional morbidity incurred because of inability to close the glottis during swallowing and loss of the protection afforded by effective coughing.

Branches from the left recurrent laryngeal nerve and from both vagus nerves provide innervation of the upper thoracic esophagus.

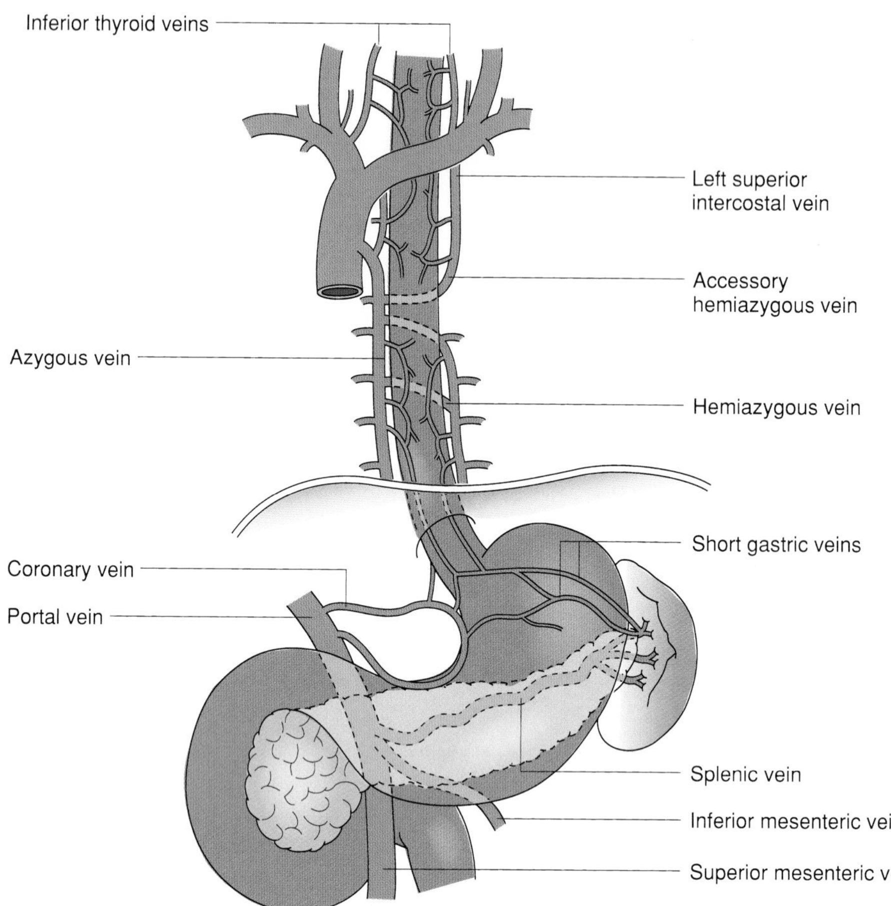

FIGURE 43.4 Venous drainage of the esophagus.

The esophageal plexus on the anterior and posterior wall of the esophagus provides innervation for the lower esophagus. The esophageal plexus also receives fibers from the thoracic sympathetic chain. The single trunks located distally contain fibers from both right and left original vagus nerves.

Efferent preganglionic sympathetic fibers supplying the esophagus arise from the fourth to sixth thoracic spinal cord segments and terminate in the cervical and thoracic sympathetic ganglions. Fibers from the superior cervical ganglion arrive at the pharyngeal plexus by way of vagal nerves. The postganglionic fibers reach the esophagus by branches from the cervical and thoracic sympathetic chain. The distal esophageal segments also receive direct sympathetic fibers from the celiac ganglion.

Afferent visceral sensory pain fibers from the esophagus terminate without synapsing in the first four segments of the thoracic spinal cord, following both sympathetic and vagal pathways. Pain fibers from the heart also travel in this same pathway, which explains the similarity of the symptoms in many esophageal and cardiac diseases.

PHYSIOLOGY

The act of alimentation requires the passage of food and drink from the mouth into the stomach. Food is taken into the mouth in a variety of bite sizes, where it is broken up, mixed with saliva, and lubricated. Swallowing, once initiated, is entirely a reflex. When food is ready for swallowing, the tongue, acting like a piston, moves the bolus into the posterior oropharynx and forces it into the hypopharynx.[3] Concomitantly with the posterior movement of the tongue, the soft palate is elevated, thereby closing the passage between the oropharynx and nasopharynx. This partitioning prevents pressure generated in the oropharynx from being dissipated through the nose. When the soft palate is paralyzed, as following a cerebral vascular accident, food is commonly regurgitated into the nasopharynx. During swallowing, the hyoid bone moves upward and anteriorly, elevating the larynx and opening the retrolaryngeal space, bringing the epiglottis under the tongue. The backward tilt of the epiglottis covers the opening of the larynx to prevent aspiration. The whole pharyngeal part of swallowing occurs within 1.5 seconds.

During swallowing, the pressure in the hypopharynx rises abruptly to at least 60 mm Hg because of the backward movement of the tongue and contraction of the posterior pharyngeal constrictors. A sizable pressure difference develops between the hypopharyngeal pressure and the less-than-atmospheric midesophageal or intrathoracic pressure. This pressure gradient speeds the movement of food from the hypopharynx into the esophagus when the cricopharyngeus or upper esophageal sphincter relaxes. The bolus is both propelled by peristaltic contraction of the posterior pharyngeal constrictors and sucked into the thoracic esophagus. Critical to receiving the bolus is the compliance of the cervical esophagus; when compliance is lost due to muscle pathology, dysphagia can result. The upper esophageal sphincter closes within 0.5 second of the initiation of the swallow, with the immediate closing pressure reaching approximately twice the resting level of 30 mm Hg. The postrelaxation contraction continues down the esophagus as a peristaltic wave (Fig. 43.6). The high closing pressure and the initiation of the peristaltic wave prevents reflux of the bolus from the esophagus back into the pharynx. After the peristaltic wave has passed further down the esophagus, the pressure in the upper esophageal sphincter returns to its resting level.

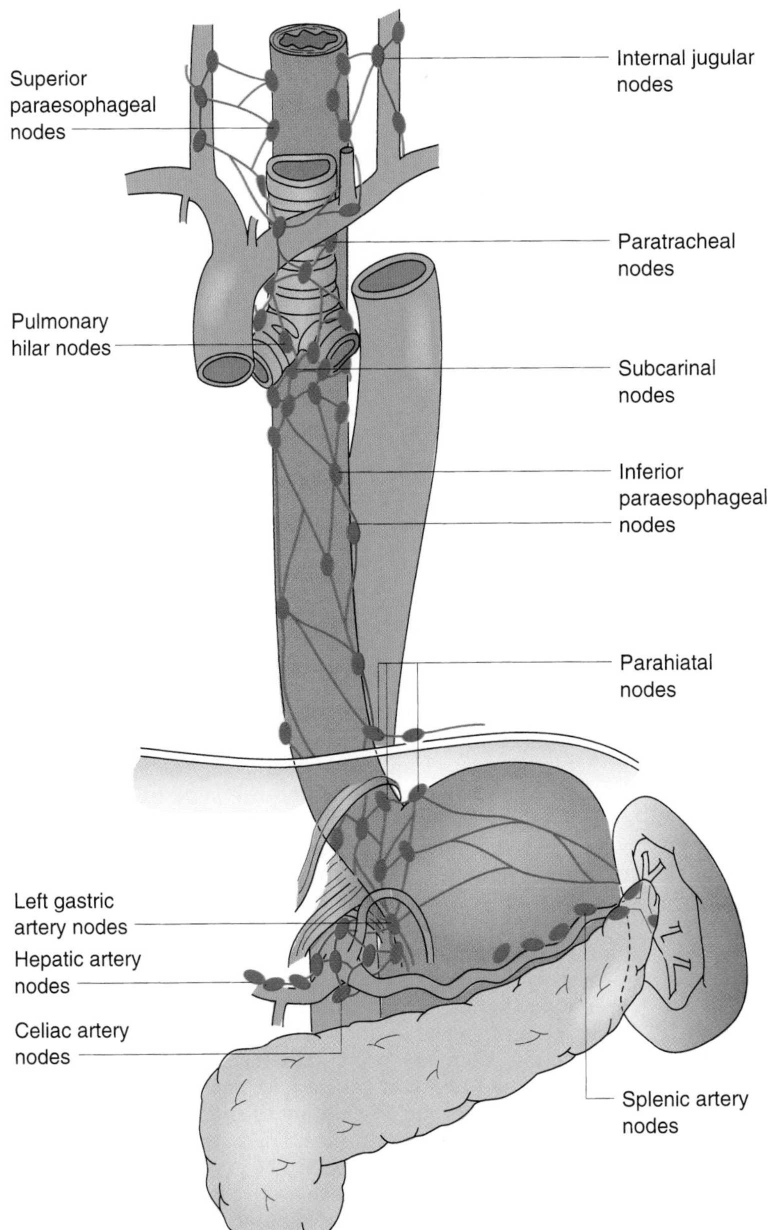

FIGURE 43.5 Lymphatic drainage of the esophagus.

Swallowing can be started at will, or it can be elicited as a reflex by the stimulation of areas in the mouth and pharynx, among them the anterior and posterior tonsillar pillars or the posterior lateral walls of the hypopharynx. The afferent sensory nerves of the pharynx are the glossopharyngeal nerves and the superior laryngeal branches of the vagus nerves. Once aroused by stimuli entering via these nerves, the swallowing center in the medulla coordinates the complete act of swallowing by discharging impulses through the fifth, seventh, tenth, eleventh, and twelfth cranial nerves, as well as the motor neurons of C1 to C3. Discharges through these nerves occur in a rather specific pattern and last for approximately 0.5 second. Little is known about the organization of the swallowing center except that it can trigger swallowing after a variety of different inputs, but the response is always a rigidly ordered pattern of outflow. Following a cerebral vascular accident, this coordinated outflow may be altered, causing mild to severe abnormalities of swallowing. In more severe injury, swallowing can be grossly disrupted, leading to repetitive aspiration.

The striated muscles of the cricopharyngeus and the upper third of the esophagus are activated by efferent motor fibers distributed through the vagus nerve and its recurrent laryngeal branches. The integrity of innervation is required for the cricopharyngeus to relax in coordination with the pharyngeal contraction and resume its resting tone once a bolus has entered the upper esophagus. Operative damage to the innervation can interfere with laryngeal, cricopharyngeal, and upper esophageal function and predispose the patient to aspiration.

Pharyngeal activity in swallowing initiates the esophageal phase. Owing to the helical arrangement of its circular muscles, the body of the esophagus functions as a worm drive propulsive pump and is responsible for transmitting a bolus of food into the stomach. The esophageal phase of swallowing represents esophageal work done during alimentation in that food is moved into the stomach from a negative-pressure environment of −6 mm Hg intrathoracic pressure to a positive-pressure environment of 6 mm Hg intraabdominal pressure or over a gradient of 12 mm Hg. Effective and coordinated smooth

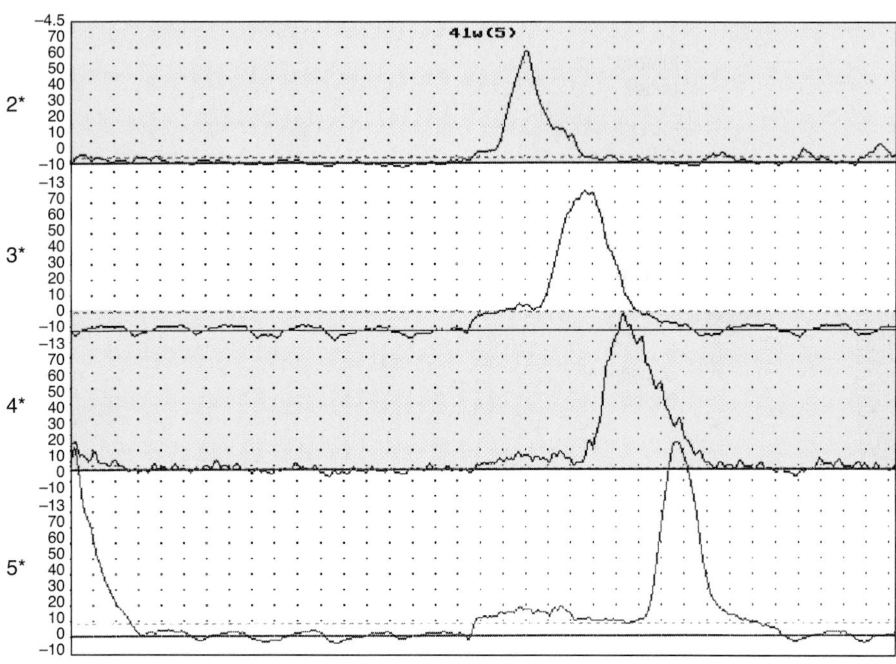

FIGURE 43.6 Representative example of manometric tracing of an esophageal peristaltic wave. Channel 2 is in the proximal esophagus and channel 5 is in the distal esophagus. The channels are 5 cm apart. The wave can be seen to progress in time down the esophagus.

muscle function in the lower third of the esophagus is, therefore, important in pumping the food across this gradient.

The peristaltic wave generates an occlusive pressure varying from 30 to 120 mm Hg. The wave rises to a peak in 1 second, lasts at the peak for about 0.5 second, and then subsides in about 1.5 seconds (Fig. 43.6). The whole course of the rise and fall of occlusive pressure may occupy one point in the esophagus for 3 to 5 seconds.[4,5] The peak of a primary peristaltic contraction initiated by a swallow (primary peristalsis) moves down the esophagus at 2 to 4 cm per second and reaches the distal esophagus about 9 seconds after swallowing starts. Consecutive swallows produce similar primary peristaltic waves, but when the act of swallowing is rapidly repeated, the esophagus remains relaxed and the peristaltic wave occurs only after the last movement of the pharynx. Progress of the wave in the esophagus is caused by sequential activation of its muscles initiated by efferent vagal nerve fibers arising in the swallowing center.

Continuity of the esophageal muscle is not necessary for sequential activation if the nerves are intact. If the muscles, but not the nerves, are cut transversely, the pressure wave begins distally below the cut as it dies out at the proximal end above the cut. For this reason a sleeve resection of the esophagus can be performed without destroying its normal function. Afferent impulses from receptors within the esophageal wall are not essential for progress of the coordinated wave. Afferent nerves, however, do go to the swallowing center from the esophagus, because if the esophagus is distended at any point, a contractual wave begins with a forceful closure of the upper esophageal sphincter and sweeps down the esophagus. This secondary contraction occurs without any movements of the mouth or pharynx. Secondary peristalsis can occur as an independent local reflex to clear the esophagus of ingested material left behind after the passage of the primary wave. Current studies suggest that secondary peristalsis is not as common as once thought.

Despite the rather powerful occlusive pressure, the propulsive force of the esophagus is relatively feeble. If a subject attempts to swallow a bolus attached by a string to a counterweight, the maximum weight that can be overcome is 5 to 10 g. Orderly contractions of the muscular wall and anchoring of the esophagus at its inferior end are necessary for efficient aboral propulsion to occur. Loss of the inferior anchor, as occurs with a large hiatal hernia, can lead to inefficient propulsion.

The LES provides a pressure barrier between the esophagus and stomach. Although an anatomically distinct LES has been difficult to identify, microdissection studies show that, in humans, the sphincterlike function is related to the architecture of the muscle fibers at the junction of the esophageal tube with the gastric pouch. The sphincter actively remains closed to prevent reflux of gastric contents into the esophagus and opens by a relaxation that coincides with a pharyngeal swallow (Fig. 43.7). The LES pressure returns to its resting level after the peristaltic wave has passed through the esophagus. Consequently, reflux of gastric juice that may occur through the open valve during a swallow is cleared back into the stomach.

If the pharyngeal swallow does not initiate a peristaltic contraction, then the coincident relaxation of the LES is unguarded and reflux of gastric juice can occur. This may be an explanation for the observation of spontaneous LES relaxation, thought by some to be a causative factor in gastroesophageal reflux disease (GERD). The power of the esophageal body is insufficient to force open a valve that does not relax. In dogs, a bilateral cervical parasympathetic blockade abolishes the relaxation of the LES that occurs with pharyngeal swallowing or distention of the esophagus. Consequently, vagal function appears to be important in coordinating the relaxation of the LES with esophageal contraction.

The LES has intrinsic myogenic tone, which is modulated by neural and hormonal mechanisms.[6,7] Alpha-adrenergic neurotransmitters or beta-blockers stimulate the LES, and alpha blockers and beta stimulants decrease its pressure. It is not clear to what extent cholinergic nerve activity controls LES pressure. The vagus nerve carries both excitatory and inhibitory fibers to the esophagus and sphincter. The hormones gastrin and motilin have been shown to increase LES pressure; and cholecystokinin, estrogen, glucagon, progesterone, somatostatin, and secretin decrease LES pressure. The peptides bombesin, B-enkephalin, and substance P increase LES pressure; and calcitonin gene-related peptide, gastric inhibitory peptide, neuropeptide Y, and vasoactive intestinal polypeptide decrease LES pressure. Some pharmacologic agents such as antacids, cholinergics, domperidone, metoclopramide, and prostaglandin F_2 are known to increase LES pressure; and anticholinergics, barbiturates, calcium channel blockers, caffeine, diazepam, dopamine, meperidine, prostaglandin E_1 and E_2, and theophylline decrease LES pressure. Peppermint, chocolate,

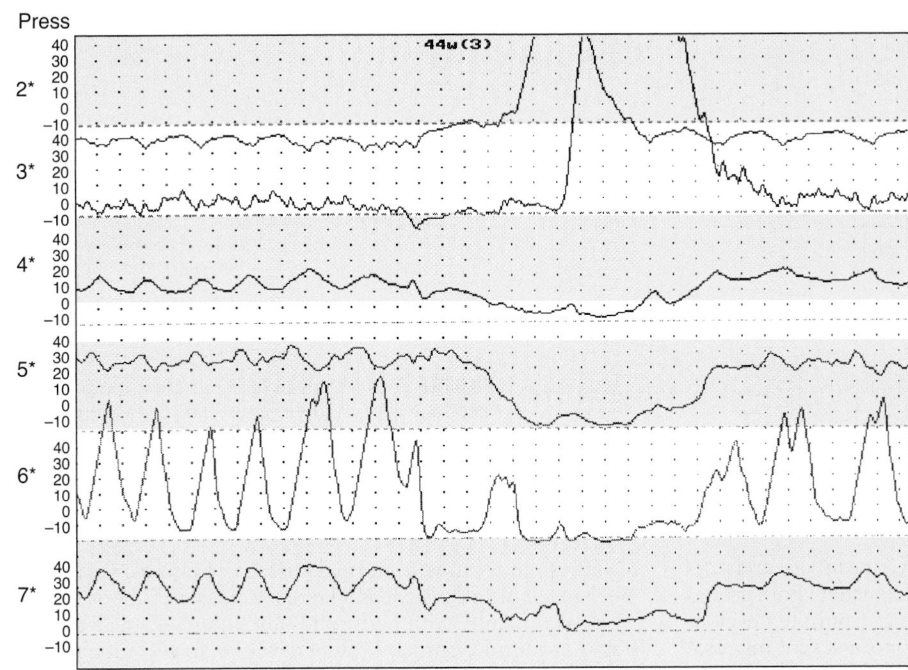

FIGURE 43.7 Representative example of a manometric tracing of lower esophageal sphincter relaxation. Channels 2 and 3 are in the distal esophagus and show a peristaltic wave progressing downward. The lower four channels are all at the same level within the lower esophageal sphincter and oriented radially at 12, 3, 6, and 9 o'clock. The dotted lines below each tracing represent gastric baseline pressures. The lower four tracings each relax to gastric baseline at the initiation of the swallow.

coffee, ethanol, and fat are all associated with decreased LES pressure and may be responsible for esophageal symptoms after a sumptuous meal.

During 24-hour esophageal pH monitoring, healthy individuals have occasional episodes of GE reflux. This physiologic reflux is more common when a person is awake and in the upright position than during sleep in the supine position. When reflux of gastric juice occurs, normal subjects rapidly clear the acid gastric juice from the esophagus regardless of their position.

GASTROESOPHAGEAL REFLUX DISEASE

Epidemiology

Population-based studies have reported that one third of Western populations experience the symptoms of GERD at least once a month, with 4% to 7% of the population experiencing daily symptoms.[8,9] Judging from the high prevalence of heartburn in the general population, GERD is a very common condition. Most patients with mild symptoms carry out self-medication, whereas those with more severe and persistent symptoms seek out medical attention. Further, the prevalence and severity of GERD is likely increasing. This is in contrast to duodenal ulcer disease where the prevalence has markedly decreased (Fig. 43.8).[10] These trends may be in part related to the effects of *Helicobacter pylori* (see later). The diagnosis of a columnar-lined esophagus is also increasing at a rapid rate, and deaths from end-stage benign esophageal disease are on an upward trend.[11] These epidemiologic changes have occurred despite dramatic improvements in the efficacy of treatment options.

Studies on the natural history of GERD are rare.[12,13] The few that do exist usually involve patients who were receiving some form of therapy. One of the most detailed studies on the natural history of the disease comes from Lausanne, Switzerland, where an intensive endoscopic follow-up of a defined population of 959 patients was performed over a 30-year period.[12] The study involved only patients who had endoscopic esophagitis and did not include those who had symptoms without mucosal injury. It showed that in about 45% of patients esophagitis developed as an isolated episode and does not return while on acid suppression therapy. In the remaining patients esophagitis intermittently recurs on acid suppression therapy, and in 42% it progressed on therapy to more severe mucosal injury. This latter group makes up about 23% of the initial population of patients with esophagitis. The study also showed that 18% of the initial population acquired, while on therapy and within as short a period of 6 weeks, a columnar-lined lower esophagus with intestinal metaplasia.

The Role of *H. pylori*

Recent studies suggest that colonization with *H. pylori* may have a protective effect against the development of GE reflux and that the gradual eradication of *H. pylori* from the Western population may be an underlying reason for the increasing prevalence of GERD.[14] Labenz et al.[15] have shown that patients with duodenal ulcer and successful eradication of *H. pylori* developed esophagitis significantly more frequently over the ensuing 3 years than those who remained positive for *H. pylori*. They suggested that the increased frequency of esophagitis may result from increased gastric acid secretion following eradication therapy. Others have suggested, however, that gastric acid secretion may decrease following *H. pylori* eradication and questioned the association between eradication therapy and GERD with and without erosive esophagitis. *H. pylori* is not involved in the pathophysiology of GERD or the development of erosive esophagitis. Studying patients in Los Angeles, Oberg et al.[19] found the prevalence of *H. pylori* to be similar in patients with and without erosive esophagitis. Furthermore, there was no difference in the prevalence of esophagitis in patients with pH-positive reflux disease when grouped according to the presence or absence of *H. pylori* infection.

Investigations focused on the role of subpopulations of *H. pylori* have implicated cagA$^+$ strains as particularly relevant to the development of GE reflux and its complications.[16] Vicari et al.[17] demonstrated that in patients with *H. pylori* infection the prevalence of cagA$^+$ strains progressively decreased with the severity of GERD, including Barrett's esophagus and esophageal adenocarcinoma. Chow et al.[18] confirmed an inverse

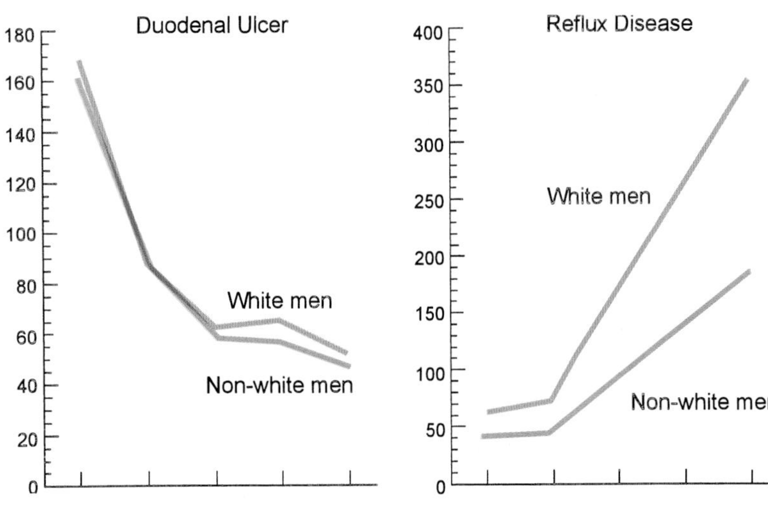

FIGURE 43.8 Trends in hospitalization for duodenal ulcer and gastroesophageal reflux disease from the 1970s to 1990s in U.S. veterans. (From El-Serag HB, Sonnenberg A. Opposing time trends of peptic ulcer and reflux disease. *Gut* 1998;43:327, with permission.)

relationship between the presence of cagA positivity and adenocarcinoma of the esophagus and the GE junction. Both groups postulated that cagA$^+$ strains may protect from the development of adenocarcinoma by inducing more severe mucosal inflammation and atrophic gastritis and thereby decreasing acid reflux. Present data regarding gastric acid secretion are conflicting, however, and further studies are required to test whether this hypothesis is true.

Clinical Presentation

The most common complaints in patients with GERD are heartburn; regurgitation; and, occasionally, dysphagia or difficult swallowing. These represent the so-called typical symptoms of GERD. Although none of these are specific to GERD, the latter is more commonly a sign of serious underlying pathology, including esophageal carcinoma. Dysphagia should always be investigated promptly and thoroughly.

Heartburn is characterized as a substernal "burning" discomfort often radiating from epigastrium to sternal notch. Occasionally patients will refer to it as "chest pain" rather than heartburn, and the two can be difficult to distinguish. Even the location can be variable with patients occasionally experiencing discomfort in the epigastrium, base of the neck, back, or other areas. Heartburn is typically made worse by "spicy" foods such as tomato sauce, citrus juices, chocolate, coffee, and alcohol. It occurs 1 to 2 hours after eating, often at night and is relieved by antacids and antisecretory agents such as the over-the-counter histamine-2 blockers. It is well recognized that the severity of symptoms is not necessarily related to the severity of the underlying disease (Fig. 43.9).

Regurgitation is the spontaneous return of gastric contents proximal to the GE junction. Its spontaneous nature distinguishes it from vomiting. The patient often gets a sensation that fluid or food is returning into the esophagus, even if it does not reach as high as the pharynx or mouth. It is typically worse at night in the recumbent position or when lying down after a meal. Patients commonly compensate by not eating late at night or by sleeping partially upright with several pillows or in a chair. This symptom is often less well relieved with antacids and antisecretory agents, although it may change in character from acid to a more "bland" nature.

Dysphagia is present in up to 40% of patients with GERD. It is generally manifested by a sensation of food hanging up in the lower esophagus (esophageal dysphagia) rather than difficulty transferring the bolus from the mouth to the esophageal inlet (oropharyngeal dysphagia). Classically dysphagia limited to only solid food, with normal passage of liquids, suggests a mechanical disorder such as a large hernia, stricture, or tumor, whereas difficulty with both solids and liquids suggest a functional or motor disorder. It often develops slowly enough that the patient may adjust his or her eating habits and not necessarily notice that it is happening. Thus, a thorough esophageal history includes an assessment of the patient's dietary history. Questions should be asked regarding the consistency of food that is typically eaten; whether the patient requires liquids with the meal; is the last to finish; has interrupted a social meal; chokes or vomits with eating; or whether he or she has been admitted on an emergency basis for food impaction. These assessments, in addition to the ability to maintain nutrition, help to quantify the dysphagia and are important in determining the indications for surgical therapy.

Many patients with GE reflux often manifest "atypical" symptoms, such as cough, asthma, hoarseness, and noncardiac chest pain. Atypical symptoms are the primary complaint in 20% to 25% of patients with GERD and are secondarily present in association with heartburn and regurgitation in many more. It is considerably more difficult to prove a cause-and-effect relationship between atypical symptoms and GE reflux than it is to do so for the typical symptoms. Consequently, the results of surgical therapy have been correspondingly less good. That is not to say that patients with atypical symptoms are not good candidates for antireflux surgery, because many will benefit greatly, but that in these patients it should be applied cautiously. Often a trial of high-dose proton pump inhibitors (PPIs) is helpful. Given atypical symptoms, the outcome of antireflux surgery is optimal in patients with a good response to medical treatment rather than in those who fail to respond.

The diagnosis of GERD based on symptoms alone is correct in only approximately two thirds of patients.[20] This is because these symptoms are not specific for GE reflux and can be caused by other diseases such as achalasia, diffuse spasm, esophageal carcinoma, pyloric stenosis, cholelithiasis, gastritis, gastric or duodenal ulcer, and coronary artery disease. This fact underscores the need for objective diagnosis before the decision is made for surgical treatment.

Physiology of the Antireflux Barrier

In humans, a zone of high pressure can be identified at the junction of the esophagus and stomach. This lower esophageal "sphincter" provides the barrier between the esophagus and stomach that normally prevents gastric contents from entering the esophagus. It has no anatomic landmarks, but its presence

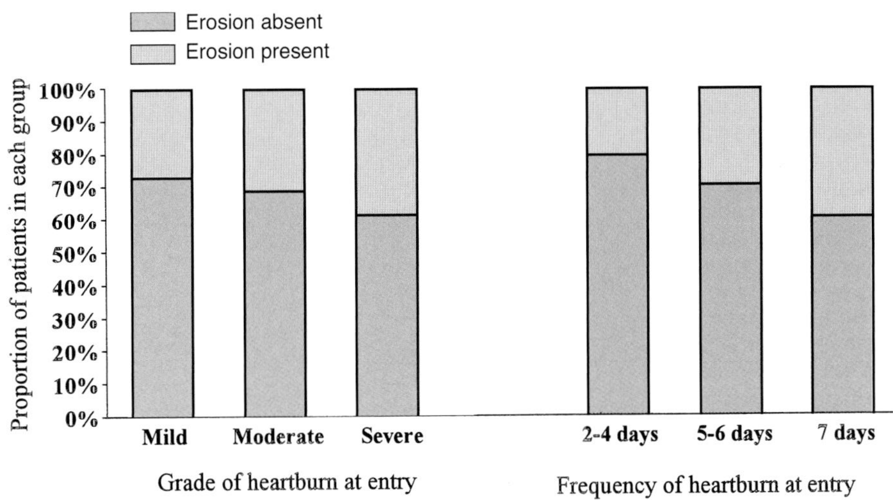

FIGURE 43.9 Prevalence of erosive esophagitis in 994 patients with varying severity and frequency of reflux symptoms. (From Venables TL, Newland RD, Patel AC, et al. Omeprazole 10 milligrams once daily, omeprazole 20 milligrams once daily, or Ranitidine 150 milligrams twice daily, evaluated as initial therapy for the relief of symptoms of gastro-oesophageal reflux disease in general practice. *Scand J Gastroenterol.* 1997;32: 965, with permission.)

can be identified by a rise in pressure over gastric baseline pressure as a pressure transducer is pulled from the stomach into the esophagus. This high-pressure zone is normally present except in two situations: (a) after a swallow, when it momentarily relaxes to allow passage of food into the stomach and (b) when the fundus is distended with gas, it is eliminated to allow venting of the gas (a belch). The common denominator for virtually all episodes of GE reflux, whether physiologic or pathologic, is the loss of the normal high-pressure zone and the resistance it imposes to the flow of gastric juice from an environment of higher pressure, the stomach, to an environment of lower pressure, the esophagus. In severe disease, this is usually due to the permanent nonexistent or a reduced high-pressure zone. In early disease or normal subjects, loss of the high-pressure zone is transient.

Three characteristics of the LES maintain its resistance or "barrier" function to intragastric and intraabdominal pressure challenges. These are its pressure, its overall length, and the length exposed to the positive-pressure environment of the abdomen (Table 43.1). The tonic resistance of the LES is a function of both its pressure and the length over which this pressure is exerted.[21] The shorter the overall length of the high-pressure zone, the higher the pressure must be to maintain sufficient resistance to remain competent (Fig. 43.10). Consequently, a normal sphincter pressure can be nullified by a short overall sphincter length. Further, as the stomach fills, the length of the sphincter decreases, rather like the neck of a balloon shortening as the balloon is inflated. If the overall length of the sphincter is abnormally short when the stomach is empty, then with minimal gastric distention there will be insufficient sphincter length for the existing pressure to maintain sphincter competency, and reflux will occur.

The third characteristic of the LES is its position, in that a portion of the overall length of the high-pressure zone should be exposed to positive intraabdominal pressure. During periods of increased intraabdominal pressure, the resistance of the LES would be overcome if the abdominal pressure were not applied equally to the high-pressure zone and stomach.[22] Think of sucking on a soft soda straw immersed in a bottle of carbonated beverage; the hydrostatic pressure of the fluid and the negative pressure inside the straw due to sucking cause the straw to collapse instead of allowing the liquid to flow up the straw in the direction of the negative pressure. If the abdominal length is inadequate, the sphincter cannot respond to an increase in applied intraabdominal pressure by collapsing and reflux is more likely to result.

If the pressure in the high-pressure zone is abnormally low, the overall length is short, or the zone is minimally exposed to the abdominal pressure environment in the fasting state, then the LES resistance is permanently lost, and the reflux of gastric contents into the esophagus is unhampered throughout the circadian cycle. A *permanently defective sphincter* is thus identified by one or more of the following characteristics: a high-pressure zone with an average pressure of less than 6 mm Hg, an average overall length of 2 cm or less, and an average length exposed to the positive-pressure environment

TABLE 43.1

NORMAL MANOMETRIC VALUES OF THE DISTAL ESOPHAGEAL SPHINCTER IN 50 SUBJECTS

Parameter	Median value	2.5th percentile	97.5th percentile
Pressure (mm Hg)	13	5.8	27.7
Overall length (cm)	3.6	2.1	5.6
Abdominal length (cm)	2	0.9	4.7

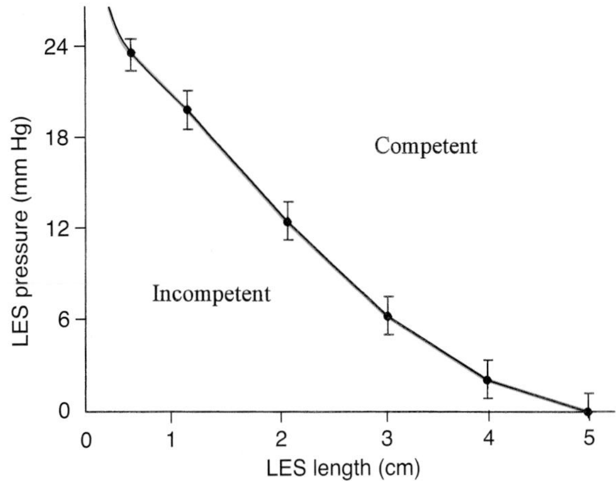

FIGURE 43.10 The relationship between the magnitude of pressure in the high-pressure zone measured at the respiratory inversion point and the overall length of the zone to the resistance to the flow of fluid through the zone. Competent, no flow. Incomplete, flow of varied volumes. Note that the shorter the overall length of the high-pressure zone, the higher the pressures must be to maintain sufficient resistance to remain competent.

of the abdomen of 1 cm or less.[23] In comparison with values in normal subjects, these values are below the 2.5 percentile for each parameter. The most common cause of a permanently defective sphincter is an inadequate abdominal length, likely secondary to the near ubiquitous presence of a hiatal hernia in patients with GERD.

For the clinician, the finding of a permanently defective sphincter has several implications. Foremost, it is almost always associated with esophageal mucosal injury[24] and predicts that the patient symptoms will be difficult to control with medical therapy.[25] It is a signal that surgical therapy is likely to be needed for consistent and long-term control of the patient's symptoms. It is now accepted that when the sphincter is permanently defective, it is irreversible, even when the associated esophagitis is healed. The presence of a permanently defective sphincter is commonly associated with reduced esophageal body function, and if the disease is not brought under control, the progressive loss of effective esophageal clearance can lead to severe mucosal injury, repetitive regurgitation, aspiration, and pulmonary failure.[26,27,32]

A transient loss of the high-pressure zone can also occur and usually results from a functional problem of the gastric reservoir.[28] Excessive air swallowing or food can result in gastric dilatation, and if the active relaxation reflex has been lost, an increased intragastric pressure. When the stomach is distended, the vectors produced by gastric wall tension pull on the GE junction with a force that varies according to the geometry of the cardia; that is, the forces are applied more directly when a hiatal hernia exists than when a proper angle of His is present. The forces pull on the terminal esophagus, causing it to be "taken up" into the stretched fundus and thereby reducing the length of the high-pressure zone or "sphincter." This process continues until a critical length is reached, usually about 1 to 2 cm, when the pressure drops precipitously and reflux occurs. The mechanism by which gastric distention contributes to shortening of the length of the high-pressure zone, so that its pressure drops and reflux occurs, provides a mechanical explanation for "transient relaxations" of the LES without invoking a neuromuscular reflex. Rather than a "spontaneous" muscular relaxation, there is a mechanical shortening of the high-pressure zone, secondary to progressive gastric distention, to the point where it becomes incompetent. These "transient sphincter" shortenings occur in the initial stages of GERD and are the mechanism for the early complaint of excessive postprandial reflux. After gastric venting, the length of the high-pressure zone is restored and competence returns until distention again shortens it and encourages further venting and reflux. This sequence results in the common complaints of repetitive belching and bloating in patients with GERD. The increased swallowing frequency seen in patients with GERD contributes to gastric distention and is due to their repetitive ingestion of saliva in an effort to neutralize the acid refluxed into their esophagus.[29] Thus, GERD may begin in the stomach, secondary to gastric distention resulting from overeating and the increased ingestion of fried foods, which delay gastric emptying. Both characteristics are common in Western society and may explain the high prevalence of the disease in the Western world.

The Importance of a Hiatal Hernia

If mechanical forces set in play by gastric distention are important in pulling on the terminal esophagus and shortening the length of the high-pressure zone or "sphincter," then the geometry of the cardia, that is, the presence of a normal acute angle of His or the abnormal dome architecture of a sliding hiatus hernia, should influence the ease with which the sphincter is pulled open. A close relationship exists between the degree of gastric distention necessary to overcome the high-pressure zone and the morphology of the cardia (Fig. 43.11).[30]

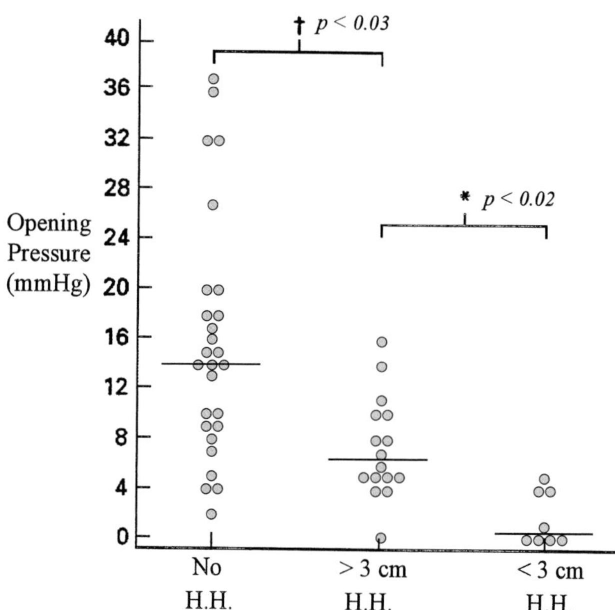

FIGURE 43.11 The intragastric pressure at which the lower esophagus endoscopically opened in response to gastric distention by air during endoscopy. Note that the dome architecture of a hiatus hernia (HH) influenced the ease with which the sphincter can be pulled open by gastric distention. (From Ismail T, Bancewicz J, Barlow J. Yield pressure, anatomy of the cardia and gastro-oesophageal reflux. *Br J Surg.* 1995;82:943, with permission.)

Greater gastric dilatation, as reflected by a higher intragastric pressure, is necessary to "open" the sphincter in patients with an intact angle of His compared to those with a hiatus hernia.[31] This is what would be expected if the high-pressure zone were shortened by mechanical forces and accounts for why a hiatal hernia is often associated with the presence of GERD.

A recent series of studies from Glasgow assesses the nature of the acid environment at the GE junction,[33] including possible inciting factors in the development of cardia and distal esophageal adenocarcinoma. The studies were initiated to investigate a long-recognized observation that esophageal pH monitoring reveals postprandial esophageal acidification at the same time as the gastric contents are alkalinized. This paradox is hard to explain given that reflux of gastric content into the esophagus is the primary mechanism underlying GERD. Hypothesizing that acidic material must be present somewhere in the upper stomach, the investigators studied luminal pH at 1 cm increments across the upper stomach and lower esophagus in healthy volunteers before and after meals. Surprisingly, they identified a "pocket" of acid at the GE junction unaffected by the buffering action of the meal, which extended across the squamocolumnar junction an average of 1.8 cm into the lumen of the esophagus (Fig. 43.12). The authors concluded that this was the source of postprandial esophageal acid exposure. They expanded these initial studies, confirming that the same process occurs in patients with endoscopy-negative dyspepsia and normal conventional esophageal pH monitoring 5 cm above the upper border of the LES.[34] Perhaps more important, they also identified that dietary nitrate consumed in the form of green vegetables results in the generation of concentrations of nitric oxide at the GE junction high enough to be potentially mutagenic (Fig. 43.13).[35] These observations provide the fundamental basis for the observations of inflammation and other alterations in the epithelium long known to occur at the squamocolumnar junction in both overt and unrecognized GERD.

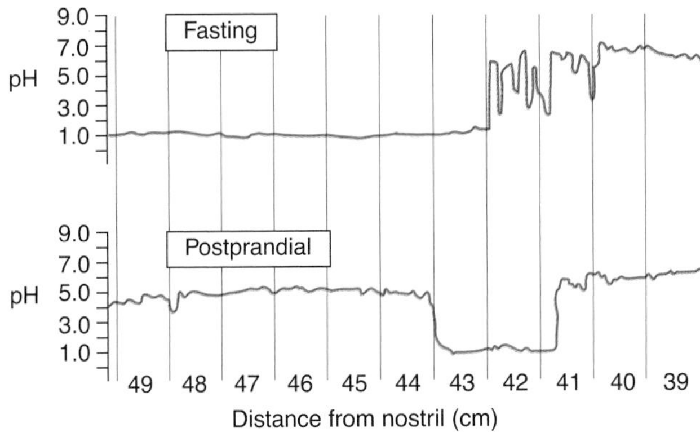

FIGURE 43.12 Fasting and postprandial gastric and esophageal pH measurements in 1-cm increments during a pull through the gastroesophageal junction. The postprandial tracing reveals an "acid pocket" from 44 to 41 cm from the nares. The fasting tracing reveals this to be the same area as the pH "step up" corresponding to the transition from stomach to esophagus. (From Fletcher J, Wirz A, Young J, et al. Unbuffered highly acidic gastric juice exists at the gastroesophageal junction after a meal. *Gastroenterology* 2001;121:775, with permission.)

Integrated Hypothesis of the Pathophysiology of Gastroesophageal Reflux Disease

The data support the likelihood that GERD begins in the stomach. Fundic distention occurs because of overeating and delayed gastric emptying secondary to the high-fat Western diet. The distention causes the sphincter to be "taken up" by the expanding fundus, exposing the squamous epithelium with the high-pressure zone, which is the distal 3 cm of the esophagus, to gastric juice. Repeated exposure causes inflammation of the squamous epithelium, columnarization, and carditis. This is the initial step and explains why in early disease the esophagitis is mild and commonly limited to the very distal esophagus. The patient compensates by increased swallowing, allowing saliva to bathe the injured mucosa and alleviate the discomfort induced by exposure to gastric acid. Increased swallowing results in aerophagia, bloating, and repetitive belching. The distention induced by aerophagia leads to further exposure and repetitive injury to the terminal squamous epithelium and the development of cardiac-type mucosa. This is an inflammatory process, commonly referred to as "carditis" and explains the complaint of epigastric pain so often registered by patients with early disease. The process can lead to a fibrotic mucosal ring at the squamocolumnar junction and explains the origin of a Schatzki ring. Extension of the inflammatory process into the muscularis propria causes a progressive loss in the length and pressure of the distal esophageal high-pressure zone associated with an increased esophageal exposure to gastric juice and the symptoms of heartburn and regurgitation. The loss of the barrier occurs in a distal to proximal direction and eventually results in the permanent loss of LES resistance and the explosion of the disease into the esophagus with all the clinical manifestations of severe esophagitis. This accounts for the observation that severe esophageal mucosal injury is almost always associated with a permanently defective sphincter. At any time during this process and under specific luminal conditions or stimuli, such as exposure time to a specific pH range, intestinalization of the cardiac-type mucosa can occur and set the stage for malignant degeneration.

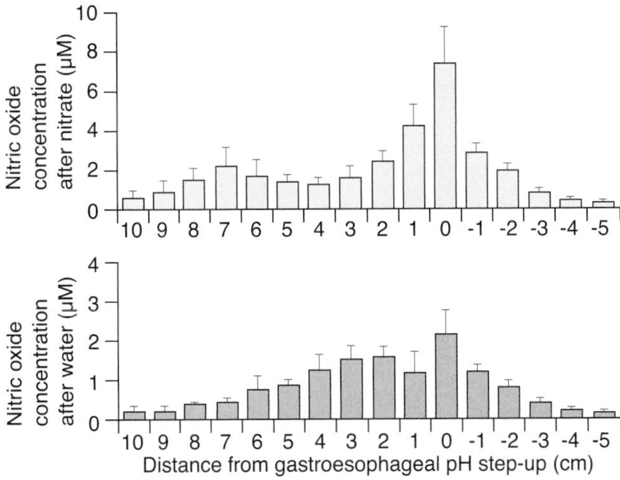

FIGURE 43.13 Mean (±SEM) nitric oxide concentrations in the upper stomach and lower esophagus after administration of water with 2 mmol nitrate (upper tracing) and water alone (lower tracing). (**$p < 0.01$, *$p < 0.05$ compared with value at gastroesophageal junction pH stepup). (From Iljima K, Henry E, Moriya A, et al. Dietary nitrate generates potentially mutagenic concentrations of nitric oxide at the gastroesophageal junction. *Gastroenterology* 2002;122:1248, with permission.)

Complications of Gastroesophageal Reflux Disease

The complications of GE reflux result from the damage inflicted by gastric juice on the esophageal mucosa and laryngeal or respiratory epithelium (Fig. 43.14). These can be conceptually divided into (a) mucosal complications, such as esophagitis and stricture; (b) extraesophageal or respiratory complications, such as laryngitis, recurrent pneumonia, and progressive pulmonary fibrosis; and (c) metaplastic and neoplastic complications, such as Barrett's esophagus and esophageal adenocarcinoma. The prevalence and severity of complications is related to the degree of loss of the GE barrier, defects in esophageal clearance, and the content of refluxed gastric juice (Fig. 43.15).[24]

Mucosal Complications

The potential injurious components that reflux into the esophagus include gastric secretions, such as acid and pepsin, biliary and pancreatic secretions that regurgitate from the duodenum into the stomach, and toxic compounds generated in the mouth, esophagus, and stomach by the action of bacteria on dietary substances.

Our current understanding of the role of the various ingredients of gastric juice in the development of esophagitis is based on classic animal studies performed by Lillemoe, Harmon, and others.[36,37] These studies have shown that acid alone does minimal damage to the esophageal mucosa, but the combination of acid and pepsin is highly deleterious. Hydrogen ion injury to the esophageal squamous mucosa occurs only at a pH below 2. In acid refluxate, the enzyme pepsin appears to be the major injurious agent. Similarly, the reflux of duodenal juice alone does little damage to the mucosa, whereas the combination of duodenal juice and gastric acid is particularly noxious. Reflux of bile and pancreatic enzymes into the stomach can either protect against or augment esophageal mucosal injury. For instance, the reflux of duodenal contents into the stomach may prevent the development of peptic esophagitis in a patient whose gastric acid secretion maintains an acid environment, because the bile salts would attenuate the injurious effect of pepsin and the acid would inactivate the trypsin. Such a patient would have bile-containing acid gastric juice that, when refluxed, would irritate

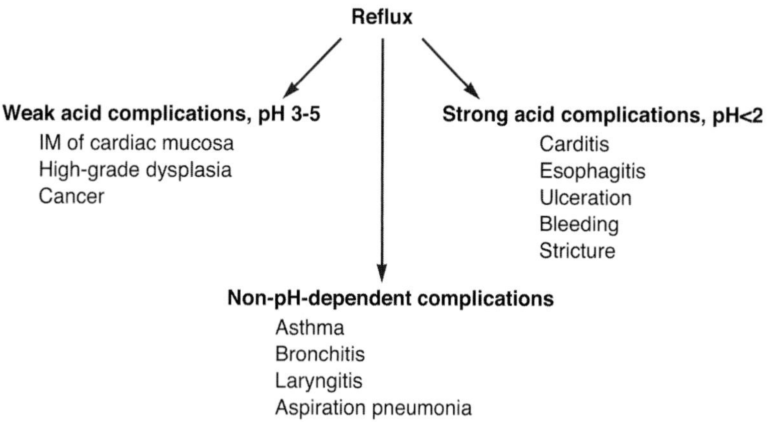

FIGURE 43.14 Schematic representation of the types of complications of gastroesophageal reflux disease.

the esophageal mucosa but cause less esophagitis than if it were acid gastric juice containing pepsin. In contrast, the reflux of duodenal contents into the stomach of a patient with limited gastric acid secretion can result in esophagitis, because the alkaline intragastric environment would support optimal trypsin activity, and the soluble bile salts with a high pK_a would potentiate the enzyme's effect. Hence, duodenal-gastric reflux and the acid secretory capacity of the stomach interrelate by altering the pH and enzymatic activity of the refluxed gastric juice to modulate the injurious effects of enzymes on the esophageal mucosa.

This disparity in injury caused by acid and bile alone, as opposed to the gross esophagitis caused by pepsin and trypsin, provides an explanation for the poor correlation between the symptom of heartburn and endoscopic esophagitis. The reflux of acid gastric juice contaminated with duodenal contents could break the esophageal mucosal barrier, irritate nerve endings in the papillae close to the luminal surface, and cause severe heartburn. Despite the presence of intense heartburn, the bile salts present would inhibit pepsin, the acid pH would inactivate trypsin, and the patient would have little or no gross evidence of esophagitis. In contrast, the patient who refluxed alkaline gastric juice may have minimal heartburn because of the absence of hydrogen ions in the refluxate but have endoscopic esophagitis because of the bile salt potentiation of trypsin activity on the esophageal mucosa. This is supported by recent clinical studies which indicate that the presence of alkaline reflux is associated with the development of mucosal injury.[38]

Although numerous studies have suggested the reflux of duodenal contents into the esophagus in patients with GERD, few have measured this directly. The components of duodenal juice thought to be most damaging are the bile acids and, as such, they have been the most commonly studied. Most studies have implied the presence of bile acids using pH measurements. Studies using either prolonged ambulatory aspiration techniques (Fig. 43.16) or spectrophotometric bilirubin measurement (Fig. 43.17) have shown that, as a group, patients with GERD have greater and more concentrated bile acid exposure to the esophageal mucosa than do normal subjects.[39,40] This increased exposure occurs most commonly during the supine period while asleep and during the upright period following meals. Most studies have identified the glycine conjugates of cholic, deoxycholic, and chenodeoxycholic acids as the predominant bile acids aspirated from the esophagus of patients with GERD, although appreciable amounts of taurine conjugates of these bile acids were also found. Other bile salts were identified but in

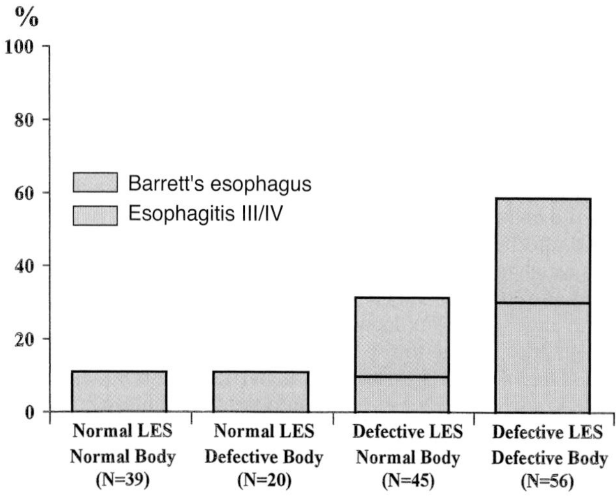

FIGURE 43.15 Prevalence of esophageal mucosal injury related to the presence of a defective lower esophageal sphincter, esophageal body motility, or both.

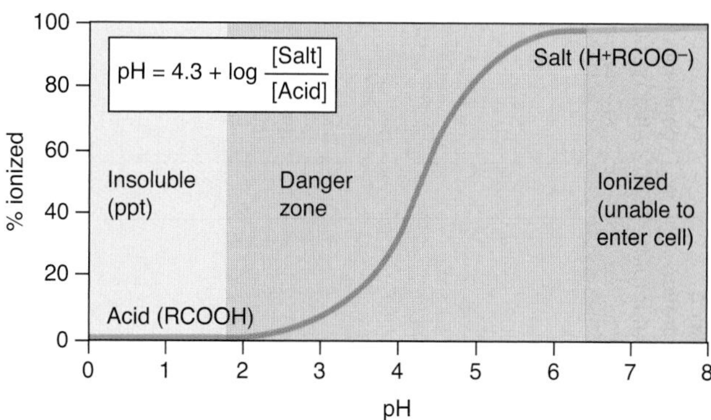

FIGURE 43.16 A representative ionization curve for bile acid. At a pH of 2 or below, bile acids are in their associated form (un-ionized RCOOH), insoluble and precipitate. Once precipitated, they are difficult to redissolve. At a pH of 6.5 or above, bile acids are completely dissociated (ionized H^+ + $RCOO^-$), soluble, and nontoxic to the cells because their polarity prevents them crossing the cell membrane. Between these extremes, bile acids can exist in their associated form and remain soluble. In this form, they can enter the cell with detrimental effects. Hence, the pH range between 2 and 6.5 is called the "danger zone."

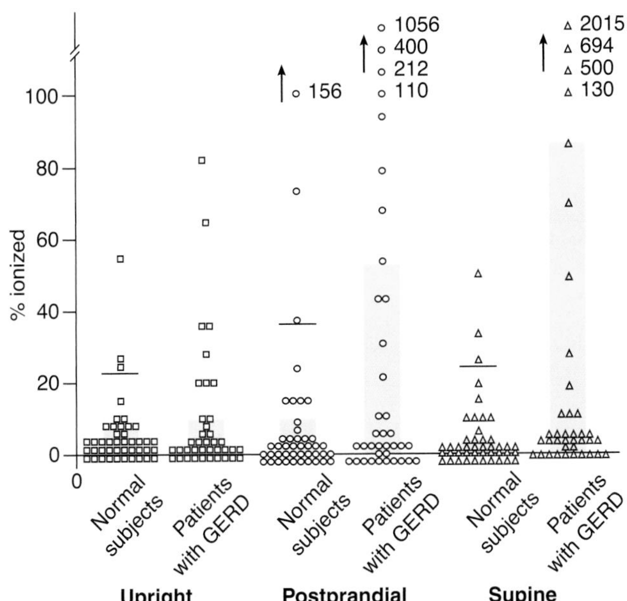

FIGURE 43.17 Peak bile acid concentration (μmol/L) for patients and normal subjects during upright, postprandial, and supine aspiration periods. The shaded area represents the mean and the bar the 95th percentile values.

small concentrations. This is as one would expect because glycine conjugates are three times more prevalent than taurine conjugates in normal human bile.

The potentially injurious action of toxic compounds either ingested or newly formed on the mucosa of the GE junction and distal esophagus has long been postulated. Until recently, however, few studies have substantiated this possibility. Expanding on studies of acid exposure at the GE junction, investigators from Glasgow, Scotland, have recently shown that dietary nitrate consumed in the form of green vegetables and food contaminated by nitrate-containing fertilizers results in the generation of nitric oxide at the GE junction in concentrations high enough to be potentially mutagenic.[35] Previous studies have shown that nitrate ingested in food is reabsorbed in the small bowel with approximately 25% resecreted into the mouth via the salivary glands. Oral bacteria chemically transform the relatively innocuous nitrate to the more toxic nitrite, which is swallowed and subsequently converted to nitric oxide and other toxic nitroso-compounds by acid and ascorbic acid in the stomach. Whether this mechanism in fact contributes to injury and or neoplastic transformation in the upper stomach, GE junction, and distal esophagus is currently unknown.

Respiratory Complications

It is increasingly recognized that a significant proportion of patients with GE reflux will have either primary respiratory symptoms or respiratory symptoms in association with more prominent heartburn and regurgitation.[41] For example, numerous studies have shown that up to 50% of patients with asthma have either endoscopic evidence of esophagitis or increased esophageal acid exposure on 24-hour ambulatory pH monitoring.[42] This suggests that the frequency of dual pathology is higher than would be expected by chance alone.[43]

Pathophysiology of Reflux-Induced Respiratory Symptoms. Two mechanisms have been proposed as the pathogenesis of reflux-induced respiratory symptoms. The first, the so-called reflux theory, maintains that respiratory symptoms are the result of the aspiration of gastric contents. The second or "reflex" theory maintains that vagally mediated bronchoconstriction follows acidification of the lower esophagus. The evidence supporting a reflux mechanism is fivefold. First, clinical studies have documented a strong correlation between idiopathic pulmonary fibrosis and hiatal hernia. The presence of GERD was shown to be highly associated with several pulmonary diseases, including asthma, in a recent Department of Veterans Affairs study.[41] Second, pathologic acid exposure in the proximal esophagus is often identified in patients with respiratory symptoms and reflux disease. Third, scintigraphic studies have shown aspiration of ingested radioisotope in some patients with reflux and respiratory symptoms. Fourth, simultaneous tracheal and esophageal pH monitoring in patients with reflux disease has documented tracheal acidification in concert with esophageal acidification. Finally, animal studies have shown that tracheal instillation of hydrochloric acid profoundly increases airways resistance.[44]

A reflex mechanism is primarily supported by the fact that bronchoconstriction occurs following the infusion of acid into the lower esophagus.[45] This can be explained by the common embryologic origin of the tracheoesophageal tract and its shared vagal innervation. Second, patients with respiratory symptoms and pathologic distal esophageal acid exposure but normal proximal esophageal acid exposure may experience an improvement in their respiratory symptoms after antireflux therapy.

The primary challenge in implementing treatment for reflux-associated respiratory symptoms lies in establishing the diagnosis. In patients with predominantly typical reflux symptoms and secondary respiratory complaints, the diagnosis may be straightforward. However, in a substantial number of patients with reflux-induced respiratory symptoms, the respiratory symptoms dominate the clinical scenario. GE reflux in these patients is often silent and is uncovered only when investigation is initiated. A high index of suspicion is required, notably in patients with poorly controlled asthma despite appropriate bronchodilator therapy. Supportive evidence for the diagnosis can be gleaned from endoscopy and stationary esophageal manometry. Endoscopy may show erosive esophagitis or Barrett's esophagus. Manometry may indicate a hypotensive LES or ineffective body motility, defined by 30% or more contractions in the distal esophagus of less than 30 mm Hg in amplitude.

The gold standard for the diagnosis of reflux-induced respiratory complaints is ambulatory dual-probe pH monitoring. One probe is positioned in the distal esophagus and the other at a more proximal location. Sites for proximal probe placement have included the trachea, pharynx, and proximal esophagus. Most authorities would agree that the proximal esophagus is the preferred site for proximal probe placement. Although ambulatory esophageal pH monitoring allows a direct correlation between esophageal acidification and respiratory symptoms, the chronologic relationship between reflux events and bronchoconstriction is complex.

Treatment. Once GE reflux is suspected or thought to be responsible for respiratory symptoms, treatment may be with either prolonged PPI therapy or antireflux surgery. A 3- to 6-month trial of high-dose PPI therapy [twice a day (b.i.d.) or three times a day (t.i.d.) dosing] may help confirm (by virtue of symptom resolution) that reflux is partly or completely responsible for the respiratory symptoms. The persistence of symptoms despite PPI treatment, however, does not necessarily rule out reflux as a potential contributor. Algorithm 43.1 bases clinical decisions on the results of dual-probe 24-hour pH monitoring and is a useful starting point.

Based on reported observations, relief of respiratory symptoms can be anticipated for 25% to 50% of patients with reflux-induced asthma treated with antisecretory medications.[46–48]

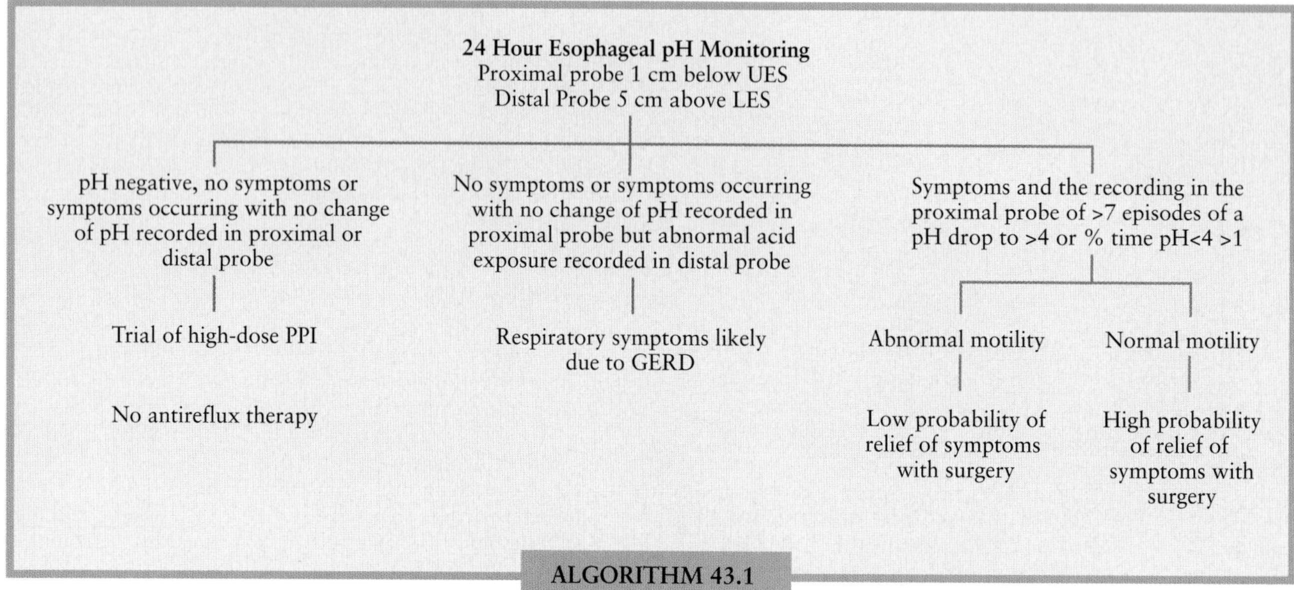

ALGORITHM 43.1 Algorithm of clinical decision making based on outcome of dual-probe 24-hour pH testing and esophageal manometry in patients with respiratory symptoms thought secondary to gastroesophageal reflux disease.

Fewer than 15%, however, can be expected to have objective improvements in their pulmonary function. The reason for this apparent paradox may be that most studies employed relatively short courses of antisecretory therapy (less than 3 months). This time period may have been sufficient for symptomatic improvement but insufficient for recovery of pulmonary function. The chances of success with medical treatment are likely directly related to the extent of reflux elimination. The conflicting findings of reports of antisecretory therapy may well be to the result of inadequate control of GE reflux in some studies. The literature indicates that antireflux surgery improves respiratory symptoms in nearly 90% of children and 70% of adults with asthma and reflux disease.[48–50] Improvements in pulmonary function were demonstrated in around one third of patients. Comparison of the results of uncontrolled studies of each form of therapy and the evidence from the two randomized controlled trials of medical versus surgical therapy indicate that fundoplication is the most effective therapy for reflux-induced asthma.[49] The superiority of the surgical antireflux barrier over medical therapy is probably most noticeable in the supine posture, which corresponds with the period of acid breakthrough with PPI therapy and is the time in the circadian cycle when asthma symptoms and peak expiratory flow rates are at their worst.

It is also important to realize that, in asthmatic patients with a nonreflux—induced motility abnormality of the esophageal body, performing an antireflux operation may not prevent the aspiration of orally regurgitated, swallowed liquid or food. This can result in respiratory symptoms and airway irritation that may elicit an asthmatic reaction. This factor may explain why surgical results appear to be better in children than adults, because disturbance of esophageal body motility is more likely in adult patients.

Metaplastic (Barrett's) and Neoplastic (Adenocarcinoma) Complications

The condition whereby the tubular esophagus is lined with columnar epithelium rather than squamous epithelium was first described by Norman Barrett in 1950 (Fig. 43.18).[51] He incorrectly believed it to be congenital in origin. It is now realized that it is an acquired abnormality, occurring in 7% to 10% of patients with GERD, and represents the end stage of the natural history of this disease.[52] It is also understood to be distinctly different from the congenital condition in which islands of mature gastric columnar epithelium are found in the upper half of the esophagus.

The definition of Barrett's esophagus has evolved considerably over the past decade.[51–53] Traditionally, Barrett's esophagus was identified by the presence of any columnar mucosa extending at least 3 cm into the esophagus. Recent data indicating that specialized intestinal-type epithelium is the only

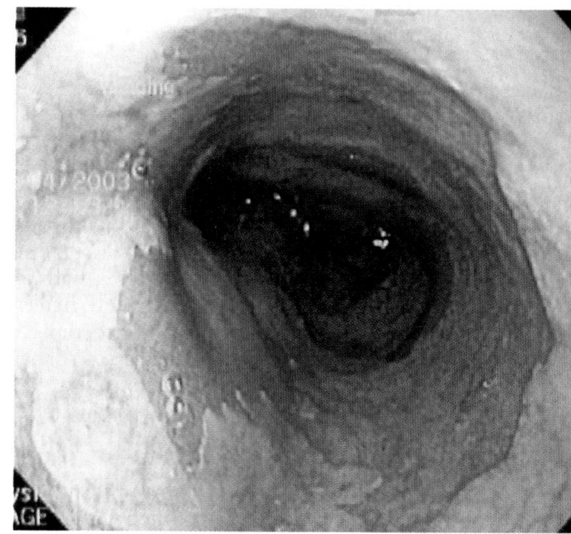

FIGURE 43.18 Endoscopic appearance of Barrett's esophagus. Note the pink metaplastic mucosa as opposed to the normal whitish squamous lining of the esophagus.

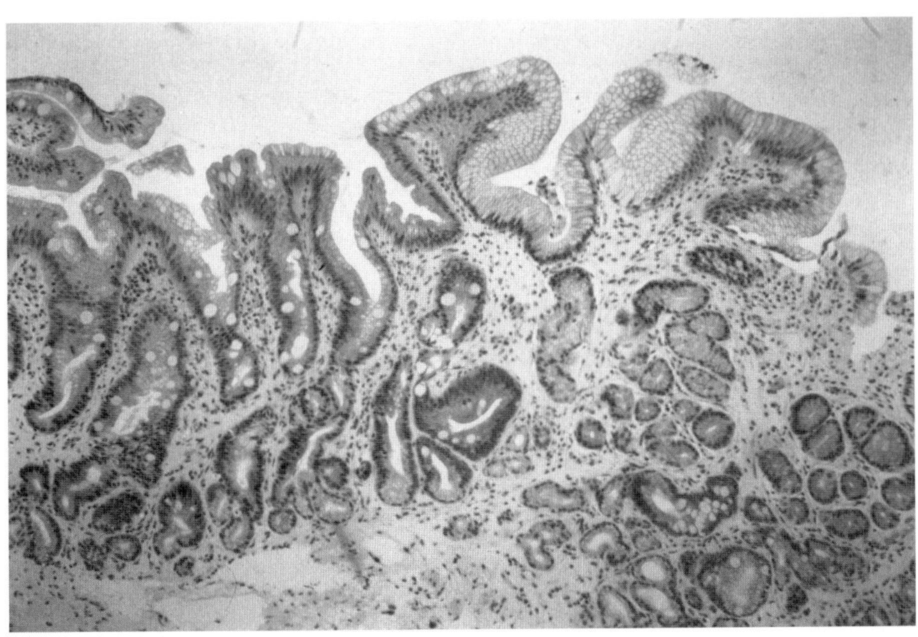

FIGURE 43.19 Histologic appearance of Barrett's esophagus. To the left of the photograph, columnar mucosa with abundant goblet cells is seen. This is intestinal metaplasia, which is the histologic hallmark of Barrett's esophagus. To the right of the photomicrograph, cardiac epithelium is present.

tissue predisposed to malignant degeneration, coupled with the finding of a similar risk of malignancy in segments of intestinal metaplasia less than 3 cm long, have resulted in the diagnosis of Barrett's esophagus, given any length of endoscopically visible tissue that is intestinal metaplasia on histology (Fig. 43.19). Whether to call long segments of columnar mucosa without intestinal metaplasia Barrett's esophagus is unclear. The hallmark of intestinal metaplasia is the presence of goblet cells. Recent studies have identified a high prevalence of biopsy-proved intestinal metaplasia at the cardia, in the absence of endoscopic evidence of a columnar-lined esophagus. The significance and natural history of this finding remains unknown. The term *Barrett's esophagus* should currently be used in the setting of an endoscopically visible segment of intestinal metaplasia of any length or columnar replacement of the esophagus of 3 cm or more.

Factors predisposing to the development of Barrett's esophagus include early-onset GERD, abnormal LES and esophageal body physiology, and mixed reflux of gastric and duodenal contents into the esophagus.[54] Direct measurement of esophageal bilirubin exposure as a marker for duodenal juice has shown that 58% of the patients with GERD have increased esophageal exposure to duodenal juice and that this exposure is most dramatically related to Barrett's esophagus.

Pathophysiology of Barrett's Metaplasia. Recent studies suggest that the metaplastic process at the GE junction may begin by conversion of distal esophageal squamous mucosa to cardiac-type epithelium, heretofore presumed to be a normal finding.[53] This is likely due to exposure of the distal esophagus to excess acid and gastric contents via prolapse of esophageal squamous mucosa into the gastric environment. This results in inflammatory changes at the GE junction or a metaplastic process, both of which may result in the loss of muscle function and a mechanically defective sphincter allowing free reflux with progressively higher degrees of mucosal injury. Intestinal metaplasia within the sphincter may result, as in Barrett's metaplasia of the esophageal body. This mechanism is supported by the finding that as the severity of GERD progresses, the length of columnar lining above the anatomic GE junction is increased.

Treatment. The relief of symptoms remains the primary force driving antireflux surgery in patients with Barrett's esophagus. Healing of esophageal mucosal injury and the prevention of disease progression are important secondary goals. In this regard, patients with Barrett's esophagus are no different than the broader population of patients with GE reflux. Antireflux surgery should be considered when patient factors suggest severe disease or predict the need for long-term medical management, both of which are almost always true in patients with Barrett's esophagus.

PPI therapy, both to relieve symptoms and to control any coexistent esophagitis or stricture, is an acceptable treatment option in patients with Barrett's esophagus. Once initiated, however, most patients with Barrett's will require lifelong treatment. Complete control of reflux with PPI therapy can be difficult, however, as has been highlighted by studies of acid breakthrough while on therapy. Katzka, Castell, Triadafilopoulos, and others have shown that 40% to 80% of patients with Barrett's esophagus continue to experience abnormal esophageal acid exposure despite up to 20 mg twice daily of PPI.[55,56] Ablation trials have shown that mean doses of 56 mg of omeprazole are necessary to normalize 24-hour esophageal pH studies.[57] Antireflux surgery likely results in more reproducible and reliable elimination of reflux of both acid and duodenal content, although long-term outcome studies suggest that as many as 25% of patients postfundoplication have persistent pathologic esophageal acid exposure confirmed by 24-hour pH studies.[58]

An important consideration is that patients with Barrett's esophagus generally have severe GERD, with its attendant sequelae such as large hiatal hernia, stricture, shortened esophagus, and poor motility. These anatomic and physiologic features make successful antireflux surgery a particular challenge in this population. Indeed, recent data suggest that antireflux surgery in patients with Barrett's esophagus may not be as successful in the long term as in those without Barrett's.

Studies focusing on the symptomatic outcome following antireflux surgery in patients with Barrett's esophagus document excellent to good results in 72% to 95% of patients at 5 years following surgery.[58,59] The outcome of laparoscopic Nissen fundoplication in patients with Barrett's esophagus has been assessed at 1 to 3 years after surgery. Hofstetter et al.[58] reported the experience at the University of Southern California in 85 patients with Barrett's esophagus at a median of 5 years after surgery. Fifty-nine had long-segment and 26 short-segment Barrett's and 50 underwent a laparoscopic antireflux

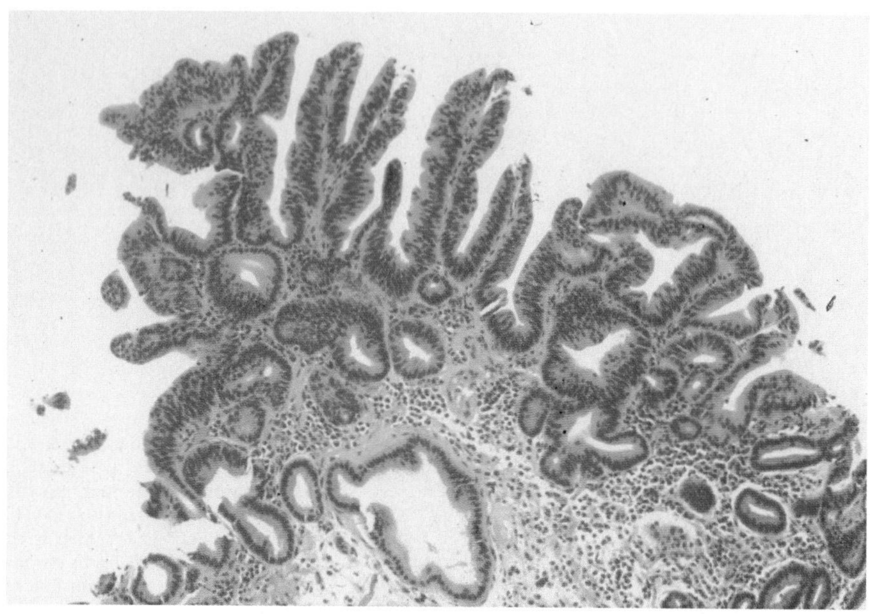

FIGURE 43.20 Histologic appearance of high-grade dysplasia. The cellular architecture and structure of the glands is becoming disorganized.

procedure. Reflux symptoms were absent postoperatively in 79% of the patients. Postoperative 24-hour pH was normal in 17 of 21 (81%) patients. Ninety-nine percent of the patients considered themselves cured or improved, and 97% were satisfied with the surgery. Similar studies have been published from Emory University, University of Washington, and Europe.[59,60]

The Development of Dysplasia in Barrett's Esophagus. The prevalence of dysplasia in patients presenting with Barrett's esophagus ranges from 15% to 25% if low-grade dysplasia is included and 5% to 10% if only high-grade dysplasia is considered. The identification of dysplasia in Barrett's epithelium rests on histologic examination of biopsy specimens. The cytologic and tissue architectural changes are similar to those described in ulcerative colitis (Fig. 43.20). By convention, Barrett's metaplasia is currently classified into four broad categories (Table 43.2).

There are few prospective studies documenting the progression of nondysplastic Barrett's epithelium to low- or high-grade dysplasia. Those that are available suggest that 5% to 10% per year will progress to dysplasia and 0.5% to 1% per year to adenocarcinoma (Table 43.3). Once identified, Barrett's esophagus complicated by dysplasia should undergo aggressive therapy (Table 43.4). Patients whose biopsies are interpreted as indefinite for dysplasia should be treated with a medical regimen consisting of 60 to 80 mg of PPI therapy for 3 months and then rebiopsied. Importantly, esophagitis should be healed before interpretation of the presence or absence of dysplasia. The presence of severe inflammation makes the microscopic interpretation of dysplasia difficult. The purpose of acid suppression therapy is to resolve inflammation that may complicate the interpretation of the biopsy specimen. If the diagnosis

TABLE 43.2 CLASSIFICATION

CLASSIFICATION OF BARRETT'S METAPLASIA

No dysplasia
Indefinite for dysplasia
Low-grade dysplasia
High-grade dysplasia

TABLE 43.3 DIAGNOSIS

DEVELOPMENT OF DYSPLASIA: PROSPECTIVE EVALUATION OF 62 PATIENTS

		Final diagnosis			
Initial diagnosis	No.	Metaplasia	Indeterminate/ LGD	HGD	CA
Metaplasia	39	27	10	1	1
I/LGD	20	4	8	3	2
HGD	3			1	2

I, indeterminate; LGD, low-grade dysplasia; HGD, high-grade dysplasia; CA, carcinoma.
From Reid BJ, Blount PL, Rubin CE, et al. Flow-cytometric and histological progression to malignancy in Barrett's esophagus: prospective endoscopic surveillance of a cohort. *Gastroenterology* 1992;102:1212–1219, with permission.

TABLE 43.4 MANAGEMENT

MANAGEMENT OF BARRETT'S ESOPHAGUS WITH DYSPLASIA

INDEFINITE FOR DYSPLASIA
Aggressive antireflux therapy (60 mg PPI per day)
Repeated biopsy in 3 months

LOW-GRADE DYSPLASIA
Aggressive antireflux therapy
Medical vs. surgical treatment

HIGH-GRADE DYSPLASIA
Confirmation by two experienced pathologists
Esophagectomy (? extent)

PPI, proton pump inhibitor.

remains indefinite, the patient should be treated as if low-grade dysplasia were present with continued medical therapy or antireflux surgery and repeat biopsy every 6 months. Patients with low-grade dysplasia are perhaps the most difficult group. This is because of the potential difficulty in surveillance following antireflux surgery. Biopsies within the fundic wrap may be difficult for the inexperienced endoscopist. Either aggressive medical treatment or, given an experienced endoscopist, antireflux surgery is appropriate.

High-grade dysplasia should be confirmed by two pathologists knowledgeable in gastrointestinal pathology. Corroboration of dysplasia is important prior to consideration of esophagectomy. Most authorities would agree that the current standard of care is to proceed with esophagectomy in patients with high-grade dysplasia who are physiologically fit enough to tolerate a major surgical undertaking. Recent, less invasive options, including photodynamic therapy and endoscopic mucosal resection, have been reported with some success,[61,62] although they remain largely investigational or reserved for high-risk surgical candidates. On average, 45% to 50% of patients with the preoperative diagnosis of Barrett's esophagus with high-grade dysplasia harbor invasive cancer when the specimen is removed and examined in its entirety. Thus, high-grade dysplasia is a marker for the presence of invasive carcinoma in nearly half of patients. This fact has been confirmed in studies from the University of Southern California as well as those from the Mayo Clinic, Johns Hopkins, and many other centers around the world.[63–66] It is not possible with present technology, including endoscopic ultrasound, to differentiate patients who harbor a cancer from those who do not. Furthermore, esophageal adenocarcinoma associated with high-grade dysplasia, identified by surveillance endoscopy, is generally highly curable. We and others have documented 5-year survival rates of 90% in this setting.

Treatment of Gastroesophageal Reflux Disease

Medical Treatment

GERD is such a common condition that most patients with mild symptoms carry out self-medication. Patients when first seen with symptoms of heartburn without obvious complications can reasonably be placed on 8 to 12 weeks of simple antacids before extensive investigations are carried out. In many situations, this successfully aborts the attacks. Patients should be advised to elevate the head of the bed; avoid tight clothing; eat small, frequent meals; avoid eating their nighttime meal shortly before retiring; lose weight; and avoid alcohol, coffee, chocolate, and peppermints, which may aggravate the symptoms.

Alginic acid, used in combination with simple antacids, may augment symptomatic relief by creating a physical barrier to reflux as well as by acid reduction. Alginic acid reacts with sodium bicarbonate in the presence of saliva to form a highly viscous solution that floats like a raft on the surface of the gastric contents. When reflux occurs, this protective layer is refluxed into the esophagus and acts as a protective barrier against the noxious gastric contents. Medications to promote gastric emptying, such as metoclopramide, domperidone, or cisapride, are beneficial in early disease but of little value in more severe disease.

The mainstay of medical therapy is acid suppression. Patients with persistent symptoms should be given hydrogen potassium PPIs, such as omeprazole. In doses as high as 40 mg per day, they can effect an 80% to 90% reduction in gastric acidity. This usually heals mild esophagitis, but healing may occur in only three fourths of patients with severe esophagitis. It is important to realize that in patients who reflux a combination of gastric and duodenal juice, inadequate acid suppression therapy may give symptomatic improvement while still allowing mixed reflux to occur. This can result in an environment that allows persistent mucosal damage in an asymptomatic patient. Unfortunately, within 6 months of discontinuation of any form of medical therapy for GERD, 80% of patients have a recurrence of symptoms.[67]

In patients with reflux disease, esophageal acid exposure is reduced by up to 80% with H_2-receptor antagonists and up to 95% with PPIs. Despite the superiority of the latter class of drug over the former, emerging evidence suggests that periods of acid breakthrough still occur.[68,69] This occurs most commonly at nighttime and is some justification for a split rather than a single dosing regimen. Katzka et al.[68] studied 45 patients with breakthrough reflux symptoms while on omeprazole 20 mg b.i.d. and found that 36 patients were still refluxing, defined by a total distal esophageal acid exposure greater than 1.6%. Peghini et al.[69] employed intragastric pH monitoring in 28 healthy volunteers and 17 patients with reflux disease and found that nocturnal recovery of acid secretion (more than1 hour) occurred in 75% of the individuals. Recovery of acid secretion occurred within 12 hours of the oral evening dose of PPI, the median recovery time being 7.5 hours. This is particularly pertinent because it is during the nighttime and early morning that asthma symptoms are most pronounced and that peak expiratory flow rate is at its lowest. In their latest study, Peghini et al. have shown that ranitidine 300 mg at bedtime is superior to omeprazole 20 mg at bedtime in preventing acid breakthrough. The authors speculated that it was due to the abolition of histamine-mediated acid secretion in the fasting state.

Patients presenting for the first time with symptoms suggestive of GE reflux may be given initial therapy with H_2 blockers. In view of the availability of these as over-the-counter medication, many patients will have already self-medicated their symptoms. Failure of H_2 blockers to control the symptoms or immediate return of symptoms after stopping treatment suggests that either the diagnosis is incorrect or the patient has relatively severe disease. Endoscopic examination at this stage of the patient's evaluation provides the opportunity for assessing the severity of mucosal damage and the presence of Barrett's esophagus. Both of these findings on initial endoscopy predict a high risk for medical failure. A measurement of the degree and pattern of esophageal exposure to gastric and duodenal juice, with 24-hour pH and bilirubin monitoring, should be obtained at this point. The status of the LES and the function of the esophageal body should also be measured. These studies identify features that predict a poor response to medical therapy, frequent relapses, and the development of complications and include supine reflux, poor esophageal contractility, erosive esophagitis or a columnar-lined esophagus at initial presentation, bile in the refluxate, and a structurally defective sphincter. Patients who have these risk factors should be given the option of surgery as a primary therapy with the expectation of long-term control of symptoms and complications.

Antireflux Surgery

Indications. Antireflux surgery is indicated for the treatment of objectively documented, relatively severe GERD. Candidates for surgery include not only patients with erosive esophagitis, stricture, and Barrett's esophagus but also those without severe mucosal injury who are dependent on PPIs for symptom relief. Patients with atypical or respiratory symptoms who have a good response to intensive medical treatment are also candidates. The option of antireflux surgery should be given to all patients who have demonstrated the need for long-term medical therapy, particularly if escalating doses of PPIs are needed to control symptoms. Antireflux surgery may be the preferred

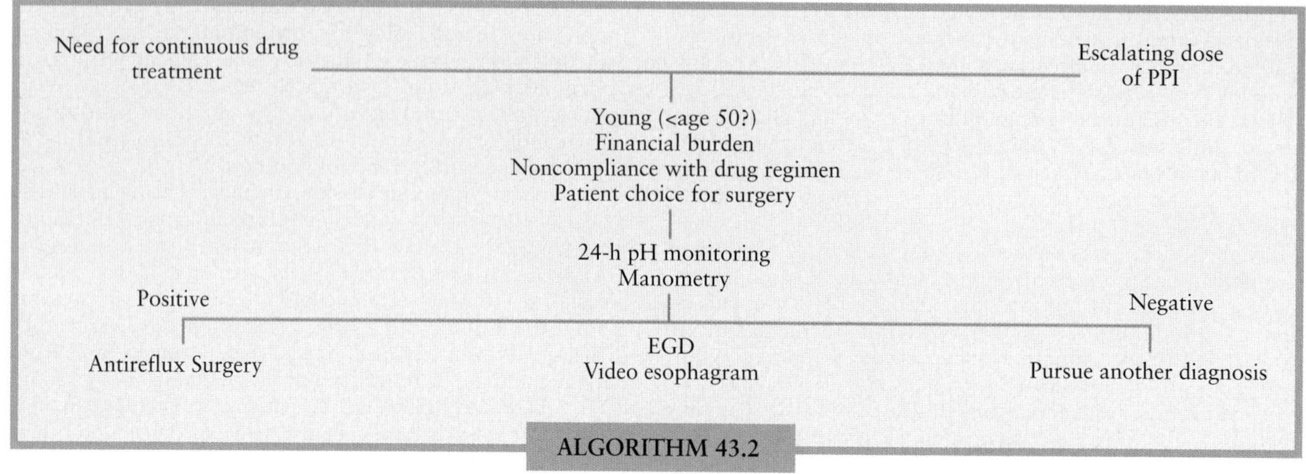

ALGORITHM 43.2 Indications for laparoscopic fundoplication.

option in patients younger than 50 years, those who are noncompliant with their drug regimen, those for whom medications are a financial burden, and those who favor a single intervention over long-term drug treatment (Algorithm 43.2). It may be the treatment of choice in patients who are at high risk of progression despite medical therapy. Although this population is not well defined, risk factors that predict progressive disease and a poor response to medical therapy include (a) nocturnal reflux on 24-hour esophageal pH study, (b) a structurally deficient LES, (c) mixed reflux of gastric and duodenal juice, and (d) mucosal injury at presentation.[70]

Preoperative Evaluation. Successful antireflux surgery is largely defined by two objectives: the achievement of long-term relief of reflux symptoms and the absence of complications or complaints after the operation. In practice, achieving these two deceptively simple goals is difficult. Both are critically dependent on establishing that the symptoms for which the operation is performed are the result of excess esophageal exposure to gastric juice, as well as the proper performance of the appropriate antireflux procedure. Success can be expected in the vast majority of patients if these two criteria are met. The status of the LES is not as important a factor as in the days of open surgery. Patients with normal resting sphincters are often selected for antireflux surgery in the era of laparoscopic fundoplication. The outcome is not dependent on sphincter function.

There are four important goals of the diagnostic approach to patients suspected of having GERD and being considered for antireflux surgery (Table 43.5).

TABLE 43.5 DIAGNOSIS

GOALS OF THE DIAGNOSTIC APPROACH TO PATIENTS SUSPECTED OF HAVING GERD AND BEING CONSIDERED FOR ANTIREFLUX SURGERY

Establish that GERD is the underlying cause of the patient's symptoms.
Estimate the risk of progressive disease.
Determine the presence or absence of esophageal shortening.
Evaluate esophageal body function and, occasionally, gastric emptying function.

GERD, gastroesophageal reflux disease.

Objective Documentation. The introduction of laparoscopic access, coupled with the growing recognition that surgery is a safe and durable treatment for GERD, has dramatically increased the number of patients being referred for laparoscopic fundoplication. The threshold for surgical referral is such that increasing numbers of patients without endoscopic esophagitis or other objective evidence of the presence of reflux are now considered candidates for laparoscopic antireflux surgery. These facts combine to underscore the importance of selecting patients for surgery who are likely to have a successful outcome. Although a Nissen fundoplication will reliably and reproducibly halt the return of gastroduodenal juice into the esophagus, little benefit is likely if the patient's symptoms are not caused by this specific pathophysiologic derangement. Thus, in large part, the anticipated success rate of laparoscopic fundoplication is directly proportional to the degree of certainty that GERD is the underlying cause of the patient's complaints.

Three factors predictive of a successful outcome following antireflux surgery have emerged (Table 43.6).[71] These are (a) an abnormal score on 24-hour esophageal pH monitoring; (b) the presence of typical symptoms of GERD, namely heartburn or regurgitation; and (c) symptomatic improvement in response to acid suppression therapy prior to surgery. It is immediately evident that each of these factors helps to establish that GERD is indeed the cause of the patient's symptoms and that they have little to do with the severity of the disease.

Endoscopic evaluation. Endoscopic visualization of the esophagus equates to the physical examination of the foregut and is a critical part of the preoperative evaluation of patients with GERD. Its main aim is to detect complications of GE reflux, the presence of which may influence therapeutic decisions.

In every patient, the locations of the diaphragmatic crura, the GE junction, and the squamocolumnar junction are determined. These anatomic landmarks are commonly at three different sites in patients with GERD. The crura are usually evident and can be confirmed by having the patient sniff during the examination. The anatomic GE junction is identified as the point where the gastric rugal folds meet the tubular esophagus and is often below the squamocolumnar junction, even in patients without otherwise obvious Barrett's esophagus.

Endoscopic esophagitis is defined by the presence of mucosal erosions (Table 43.7). When present, the grade and length of esophageal mucosal injury are recorded. The presence and

TABLE 43.6

PREDICTORS OF OUTCOME AFTER LAPAROSCOPIC FUNDOPLICATION: STEPWISE LOGISTIC REGRESSION RESULTS OF 199 PATIENTS

Predictor	Status	Adjusted odds ratio (95% confidence intervals)	Wald's p value
Composite acid score	Increased	5.4 (1.9–15.3)	<.001
	Normal	—	—
Symptom	Typical	5.1 (1.9–13.7)	<.001
	Atypical	—	—
Response to medical therapy	Complete/partial	3.3 (1.3–8.7)	.02
	Minor/none	—	—

Odds ratios and corresponding p values are adjusted for age and for all other factors in the model.
From Campos GMR, Peters JH, DeMeester TR, et al. Multivariate analysis of the factors predicting outcome after laparoscopic Nissen fundoplication. *J Gastrointest Surg*. 1999;3:292–300, with permission.

length of columnar epithelium extending above the anatomic GE junction is also noted. It is suspected at endoscopy when there is difficulty in visualizing the squamocolumnar junction at its normal location and by the appearance of a velvety red luxuriant mucosa. The presence of Barrett's esophagus is confirmed by biopsy evidence of specialized intestinal metaplasia and is considered histologic evidence of GERD. Endoscopic visualization of columnar lining without histologic confirmation of specialized intestinal metaplasia is not considered Barrett's esophagus and likely has no premalignant potential. Multiple biopsies should be taken in a cephalad direction to determine the level at which the junction of Barrett's epithelium and normal squamous mucosa occurs. Barrett's esophagus is susceptible to ulceration, bleeding, stricture formation, and malignant degeneration. Dysplasia is the earliest sign of malignant change. Because dysplastic changes typically occur in a random distribution within the distal esophagus, a minimum of four biopsies (each quadrant) every 2 cm should be obtained from the metaplastic epithelium. Particular attention must be paid to the squamocolumnar junction in these patients, where a mass, ulcer, nodularity, or inflammatory tissue is always considered suspicious for malignancy and requires thorough biopsy. The GE junction is defined endoscopically where the tubular esophagus meets gastric rugal folds, and the squamocolumnar junction is where there is an obvious change from the velvety and darker columnar epithelium to the lighter squamous epithelium.

After completion of the esophageal examination, the first and second portions of the duodenum and the stomach are systematically inspected. This is commonly done on withdrawal of the endoscope. When the antrum is visualized, the incisura angularis appears as a constant ridge on the lesser curve. Turning the lens of the scope 180 degrees allows inspection of the fundus and cardia. Attention is paid to the frenulum (angle of His) of the esophagogastric junction and to the closeness with which the cardia grips the scope. Hill et al.[72] have graded the appearance of this valve on a scale from I to IV according to the degree of unfolding or deterioration of the normal valve architecture. This grading system has been correlated with the presence of increased esophageal acid exposure, occurring predominantly in patients with a grade III or IV valve.

A hiatal hernia is endoscopically confirmed by finding a pouch lined with gastric rugal folds lying 2 cm or more above the margins of the diaphragmatic crura. A prominent sliding hernia is frequently associated with increased esophageal exposure to gastric juice. When a paraesophageal hernia exists, particular attention is given to exclude a gastric ulcer or gastritis within the pouch. The intragastric retroflex or "J" maneuver is important in evaluating the full circumference of the mucosal lining of the herniated stomach. As the endoscope is removed, the esophagus is again examined and biopsies taken. The location of the cricopharyngeus is identified and the larynx and vocal cords are visualized. Acid reflux may result in inflammation of the larynx. Vocal cord movement is recorded both as a reference for subsequent surgery and an assessment of the patient's ability to protect the airway.

TABLE 43.7 CLASSIFICATION

MODIFIED LA CLASSIFICATION OF ESOPHAGITIS

Grade	Lesion
A	One (or more) mucosal break of longer than 5 mm that does not extend between the tops of two mucosal folds
B	One (or more) mucosal break more than 5 mm long that does not extend between the tops of two mucosal folds
C	One (or more) mucosal break that is continuous between the tops of two or more mucosal folds but that involves less than 75% of the circumference
D	One (or more) mucosal break that involves at least 75% of the esophageal circumference

Twenty-four hour ambulatory pH monitoring. The most direct method of assessing the relationship between symptoms and GERD is to measure the esophageal exposure to gastric juice with an indwelling pH electrode. Miller[73] first reported prolonged esophageal pH monitoring in 1964, although it was not until 1973 that its clinical applicability and advantages were demonstrated by Johnson and DeMeester.[74] Ambulatory pH testing is considered by many to be the gold standard for the diagnosis of GERD, because it has the highest sensitivity and specificity of all tests currently available. Some experts have suggested that 24-hour pH monitoring be used selectively, limited to patients with atypical symptoms or no endoscopic evidence of GE reflux. Given present-day referral patterns, more than half of the patients referred for antireflux surgery will have no endoscopic evidence of mucosal injury. For these patients, 24-hour pH monitoring provides the only objective measure of the presence of pathologic esophageal acid exposure. Although it is true that most patients with typical symptoms and erosive esophagitis have a positive 24-hour pH result, the study provides other useful information. It quantifies the actual time that the esophageal mucosa is exposed to gastric juice, measures the

TABLE 43.8

NORMAL VALUES FOR ESOPHAGEAL EXPOSURE TO PH <4 IN 50 SUBJECTS

Component	Mean	Standard deviation	95th percentile
Total time pH <4	1.51	1.36	4.45
Upright time pH <4	2.34	2.34	8.42
Supine time pH <4	0.63	1.0	3.45
No. episodes	19.00	12.76	46.9
No. >5 min	0.84	1.18	3.45
Longest episode	6.74	7.85	19.8

From Johnson LF, DeMeester TR. Development of the 24-hour intraesophageal pH monitoring composite scoring system. *J Clin Gastroenterol.* 1986;8[Suppl 1]:52–58. with permission.

ability of the esophagus to clear refluxed acid and correlates esophageal acid exposure with the patient's symptoms. It is the only way to quantitatively express the overall degree and pattern of esophageal acid exposure, both of which may impact the decision toward surgery.[75] Patients with nocturnal or bipositional reflux have a higher prevalence of complications and failure of long-term medical control. For these reasons, we continue to advocate its routine use in clinical practice.

The units used to express esophageal exposure to gastric juice are (a) cumulative time the esophageal pH is below a chosen threshold, expressed as the percent of the total, upright, and supine monitored time; (b) frequency of reflux episodes below a chosen threshold, expressed as number of episodes per 24 hours; and (c) duration of the episodes, expressed as the number of episodes greater than 5 minutes per 24 hours and the time in minutes of the longest episode recorded. Table 43.8 shows the normal values for these components of the 24-hour record at the whole number pH threshold derived from 50 normal, asymptomatic subjects. The upper limits of normal were established at the 95th percentile. Most centers use pH 4 as the threshold. Combining the result of the six components into one expression that reflects the overall esophageal acid exposure below a pH threshold, a pH score was calculated by using the standard deviation of the mean of each of the six components measured.

Assessment of esophageal length. Esophageal shortening is a consequence of scarring and fibrosis associated with repetitive esophageal injury. Anatomic shortening of the esophagus can compromise the ability to perform an adequate tension-free fundoplication and may result in an increased incidence of breakdown or thoracic displacement of the repair. Esophageal length is best assessed preoperatively using video roentgenographic contrast studies and endoscopic findings. Endoscopically, hernia size is measured as the difference between the diaphragmatic crura, identified by having the patient sniff, and the GE junction, identified as the loss of gastric rugal folds. We consider the possibility of a short esophagus in patients with strictures or those with large hiatal hernias (greater than 5 cm), particularly when the latter fail to reduce in the upright position on a video barium esophagram.[76]

The definitive determination of esophageal shortening is made intraoperatively when, after thorough mobilization of the esophagus, the GE junction cannot be reduced below the diaphragmatic hiatus without undue tension on the esophageal body. Surgeons performing fundoplication have reported varying incidences of esophageal shortening, attesting to the judgment inherent in defining and recognizing "undue tension." An advantage of transthoracic fundoplication is the ability to mobilize the esophagus extensively from the diaphragmatic hiatus to the aortic arch. With the GE junction marked with a suture, esophageal shortening is defined by an inability to position the repair beneath the diaphragm without tension. In this situation, a Collis gastroplasty coupled with either a partial or complete fundoplication may be performed.[77]

Potential pitfalls of laparoscopic fundoplication include the elevation of the diaphragm due to pneumoperitoneum, potentially contributing to a false impression that esophageal length is adequate, and the limited ability to mobilize the esophagus relative to the transthoracic approach.[78] In our experience, the failure to appreciate esophageal shortening is a major cause of fundoplication failure and is often the explanation for the "slipped" Nissen fundoplication. In many such instances, the initial repair is incorrectly constructed around the proximal tubularized stomach rather than the terminal esophagus. Surgeons opting to perform fundoplication laparoscopically in the setting of potential esophageal shortening must be vigilant of esophageal tension, technically facile at extensive mediastinal mobilization of the esophagus while preserving vagal integrity, and able to perform a laparoscopic or open transabdominal Collis gastroplasty should esophageal lengthening be necessary.

Radiographic evaluation. Radiographic assessment of the anatomy and function of the esophagus and stomach is one of the most important parts of the preoperative evaluation. Critical issues are assessed, including the presence of esophageal shortening (Fig. 43.21), the size and reducibility of a hiatal hernia, and the propulsive function of the esophagus for both liquids and solids.

The definition of radiographic GE reflux varies depending on whether reflux is spontaneous or induced by various maneuvers. In only about 40% of patients with classic symptoms of GERD is spontaneous reflux observed by the radiologist (i.e., reflux of barium from the stomach into the esophagus with the patient in the upright position). In most patients who show spontaneous reflux on radiography, the diagnosis of increased esophageal acid exposure is confirmed by 24-hour esophageal pH monitoring. Therefore, the radiographic demonstration of spontaneous regurgitation of barium into the esophagus in the upright position is a reliable indicator that reflux is present. Failure to see this does not indicate the absence of disease.

A carefully performed video esophagram can provide an enormous amount of information on the structure and function of the esophagus and stomach. The modern barium swallow emphasizes motion-recording (video), utilizes a tightly controlled examination protocol (Table 43.9), and requires an understanding of esophageal physiology.

Videotaping the study greatly aids the evaluation, providing the surgeon with a real-time assessment of swallowing function, bolus transport, and the size and reducibility of hiatal hernias. Given routine review before antireflux surgery, its value becomes increasingly clear. The study provides structural information including the presence of obstructing lesions and anatomic abnormalities of the foregut. A hiatal hernia is

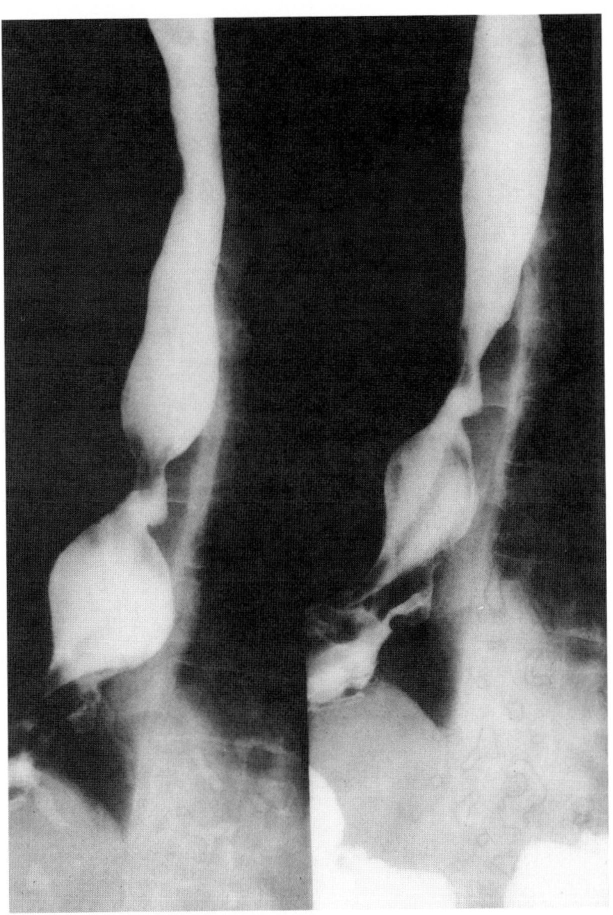

FIGURE 43.21 Barium-filled esophagogastric segment in a patient with a short esophagus. Note that the gastroesophageal junction is well above the hiatus.

present in more than 80% of patients with GE reflux and is best demonstrated with the patient in the prone position, which causes increased abdominal pressure and promotes distention of the hernia above the diaphragm. The presence of a hiatal hernia is an important component of the underlying pathophysiology of GE reflux. Other relevant findings include a large (greater than 5 cm) or irreducible hernia, suggesting the presence of a shortened esophagus; a tight crural "collar" that inhibits barium transit into the stomach, suggesting a possible cause of dysphagia; and the presence of a paraesophageal hernia.

Lower esophageal narrowing resulting from a ring, stricture, or obstructing lesion is optimally viewed with full distention of the esophagogastric region. A full-column technique with distention of the esophageal wall can be used to discern extrinsic compression of the esophagus. Mucosal relief or double-contrast films should be obtained to enhance the detection of small esophageal neoplasms, mild esophagitis, and esophageal varices. The pharynx and upper esophageal sphincter are evaluated in the upright position, and an assessment of the relative timing and coordination of pharyngeal transit is possible.

The assessment of peristalsis on video esophagram often adds to, or complements, the information obtained by esophageal motility studies. This is in part because the video barium study can be done both upright and supine and with liquid and solid bolus material, which is not true of a stationary motility examination. This is particularly true with subtle motility abnormalities. During normal swallowing, a stripping wave (primary peristalsis) is generated that completely clears the bolus. Residual material can stimulate a secondary peristaltic wave, but usually a second pharyngeal swallow is required. Motility disorders with disorganized or simultaneous esophageal contractions have "tertiary waves" and provide a segmented appearance to the barium column, often referred to as beading or corkscrewing. In dysphagic patients, a barium-impregnated marshmallow, bread, or hamburger is a useful adjunct, which can discern a functional esophageal transport disturbance not evident on the liquid barium study. Reflux is not easily seen on video esophagram, and motility disorders that cause retrograde barium transport may be mistaken for reflux.

Assessment of the stomach and duodenum during the barium study is a necessity for proper preoperative evaluation of the patient with GERD. Evidence of gastric or duodenal ulcer, neoplasm, or poor gastroduodenal transit has obvious importance in the proper preoperative evaluation.

Assessment of esophageal body and gastric function. The presence of poor esophageal body function can impact the likelihood

TABLE 43.9 DIAGNOSIS

UNIVERSITY OF SOUTHERN CALIFORNIA PROTOCOL FOR VIDEO ESOPHAGRAM STUDIES

Patient position	Purpose	Technique
Prone RAO	Esophageal body function	Five separate 10-mL swallows, 15 s between each, follow bolus on videotape Video swallow over thoracic inlet and another over distal third of esophagus without panning
	Esophageal diameter	Rapid swallow of several gulps to distend esophagus maximally
	Gastric function	Videorecord activity of stomach and duodenum for 30 s in prone position
Supine	Relationship of GE junction to hiatus	Two or three individual swallows focused on distal esophagus and GE junction
Erect	Cricopharyngeal function	Lateral and anteroposterior views of oropharynx and upper esophagus
	Mucosal injury	Spot of collapsed esophagus for mucosal detail
	Reducibility of hernia	Video images of one or two swallows focused on distal esophagus and GE junction
	Gas distention of distal esophagus	
Erect	Solid bolus transport	Record video images of passage of two contrast-coated hamburger boluses from oropharynx to stomach

GE, gastroesophageal; RAO, right anterior oblique.

HEAD AND NECK

of relief of regurgitation, dysphagia, and respiratory symptoms following surgery and may influence the decision to undertake a partial rather than a complete fundoplication. When peristalsis is absent or severely disordered, many would opt for a partial fundoplication, although recent studies would suggest a complete fundoplication may be appropriate even in this setting. The less favorable response of atypical, compared with typical, reflux symptoms after fundoplication may be related to persistent poor esophageal propulsive function and the continued regurgitation of esophageal contents.[79,80]

The function of the esophageal body is assessed with esophageal manometry. This is performed with five pressure transducers located in the esophagus (Fig. 43.22). To standardize the procedure the most proximal pressure transducer is located 1 cm below the well-defined cricopharyngeal sphincter. With this method a pressure response along the entire esophagus can be obtained during one swallow. The study consists of recording ten standard wet swallows with 5 mL of water. Amplitude, duration, and morphology of contractions following each swallow are all calculated at the five discrete levels within the esophageal body (Fig. 43.23). The delay between onset or peak of esophageal contractions at the various levels of the esophagus is used to calculate the speed of wave propagation and represents the degree of peristaltic activity.

Esophageal disorders are frequently associated with abnormalities of duodenogastric function. Symptoms suggestive of gastroduodenal pathology include nausea, epigastric pain, anorexia, and early satiety. Abnormalities of gastric motility or increased gastric acid secretion can be responsible for increased esophageal exposure to gastric juice. If not identified before surgery, unrecognized gastric motility abnormalities are occasionally "unmasked" by an antireflux procedure, resulting in disabling postoperative symptoms.[81] Considerable experience and judgment are necessary to identify the patient with occult gastroduodenal dysfunction. The surgeon should maintain a keen awareness of this possibility and investigate the stomach given any suggestion of problems. Tests of duodenogastric function that are helpful when investigating the patient with GE reflux include gastric emptying studies, gastric acid analysis, 24-hour gastric pH monitoring, and ambulatory bilirubin monitoring of the esophagus and stomach.

Poor gastric emptying or transit can provide for reflux of gastric contents into the distal esophagus. Standard gastric emptying studies are performed with radionuclide-labeled meals. They are often poorly standardized and difficult to interpret. Emptying of solids and liquids can be assessed simultaneously when both phases are marked with different tracers. After ingestion of a labeled standard meal, gamma camera images of the stomach are obtained at 5- to 15-minute intervals for 1.5 to 2 hours.

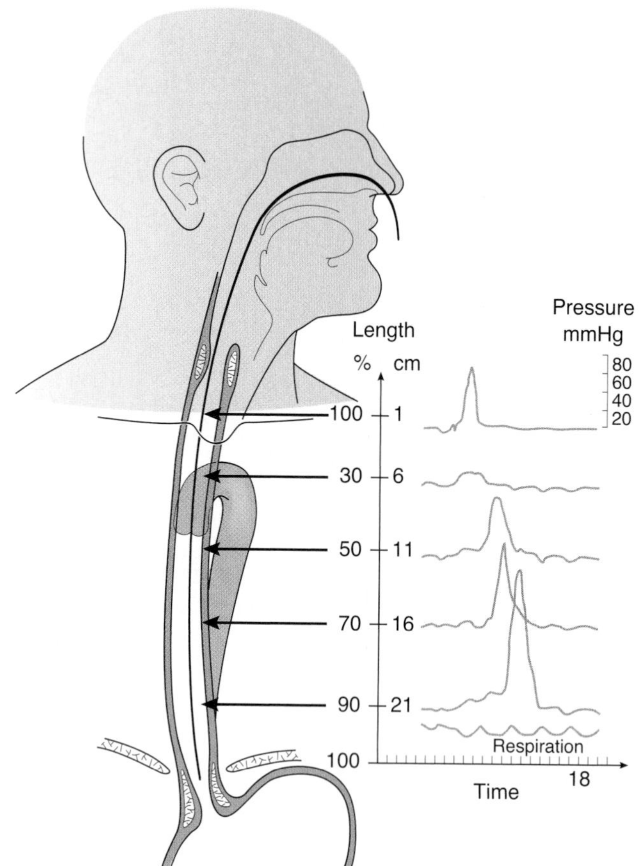

FIGURE 43.22 Illustration of the position of a five-channel esophageal motility catheter during the esophageal body portion of the study.

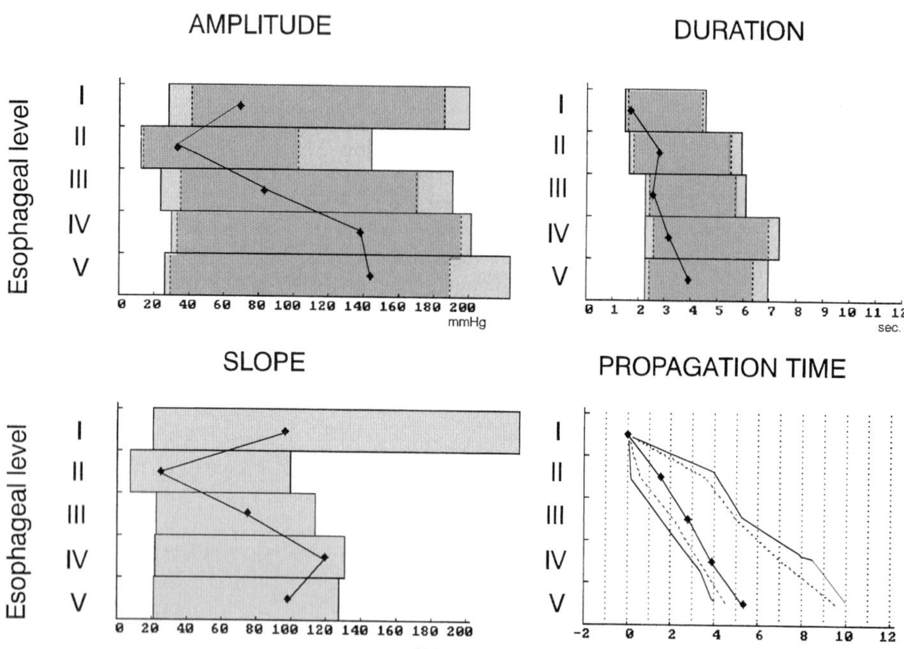

FIGURE 43.23 Computer-generated graphic representation of esophageal body contraction amplitudes, duration of contraction, and wave progression.

After correction for decay, the counts in the gastric area are plotted as percentage of total counts at the start of the imaging. The resulting emptying curve can be compared with data obtained in normal volunteers. In general, normal subjects will empty 59% of a meal within 90 minutes.

Partial Versus Complete Fundoplication. The decision between partial and complete fundoplication and an open or laparoscopic approach requires considerable judgment. Two randomized studies of unselected patients undergoing laparoscopic fundoplication have shown equivalence of complete and partial fundoplications, anterior in one study[82] and posterior in the other,[83] in terms of operative time, perioperative morbidity, and hospital stay. Watson et al.[82] noted that resting and residual LES pressures were greater after complete fundoplication and that esophageal clearance of liquid radioisotope was prolonged in these patients compared with after partial fundoplication. Six months after operation, partial fundoplication was linked to a greater overall level of patient satisfaction manifested by a lower incidence of the symptoms of dysphagia, inability to belch, and excessive flatus. Laws et al.[83] did not identify any difference in symptomatic outcome between patients treated by complete and those treated by posterior partial fundoplication at a mean follow-up time of 27 months.

Hagedorn et al.[84] reported on the results of a randomized, controlled trial comparing total (Nissen–Rosetti) and posterior partial (Toupet) fundoplication in which long-term efficacy was assessed.[84] A total of 110 patients (54 undergoing a total wrap, 56 a partial wrap) completed a median follow-up of 11.5 years. No significant differences were observed between the groups in terms of heartburn, regurgitation, or dysphagia scores. A significant difference, however, was noted in the prevalence of rectal flatus and postprandial fullness, which were reported more often by those having undergone a total fundoplication.

These observations, however, must be tempered by reports questioning the durability of partial fundoplications. Jobe et al.[85] found that 51% of patients studied by 24-hour esophageal pH monitoring after Toupet fundoplication still had pathologic acid exposure. Disturbingly, only 40% of the refluxers were symptomatic. Two studies have identified the presence of a defective LES function, an aperistaltic distal esophagus, and higher grades of esophagitis (Savary-Miller grades 2 to 4) as risk factors for partial fundoplication failure.[84,85] Bell et al.[86] reported recurrent reflux in 14% after Toupet fundoplication. The presence of mild esophagitis and a normal LES were associated with a 3-year success rate of 96%, whereas the presence of complicated esophagitis or a defective LES lowered this value to 50% (Fig. 43.24).

These findings highlight an apparent paradox, in that partial fundoplications afford suboptimal reflux protection in those most at risk from the effects of unabated GERD. The question arises, therefore, whether total fundoplication should be applied more liberally to patients with severe reflux disease and associated esophageal dysmotility. Patti et al.[87] recently reported on 357 patients undergoing antireflux surgery, 235 undergoing a "tailored approach" with either a partial or total fundoplication depending on the results of preoperative manometry, and 122 more recent patients undergoing a total fundoplication regardless of the quality of esophageal peristalsis. In the first group, heartburn from pathologic reflux, confirmed by postoperative ambulatory esophageal pH monitoring, recurred in 19% after partial fundoplication and in 4% after total fundoplication. In the latter group, heartburn recurred in 4% after total fundoplication. Importantly, the incidence of postoperative dysphagia was similar in the two groups. This recent evidence, as well as our own experience, has led us to utilize the complete fundoplication more readily, particularly in patients with Barrett's esophagus. Currently, partial fundoplication is best reserved for patients with severe esophageal

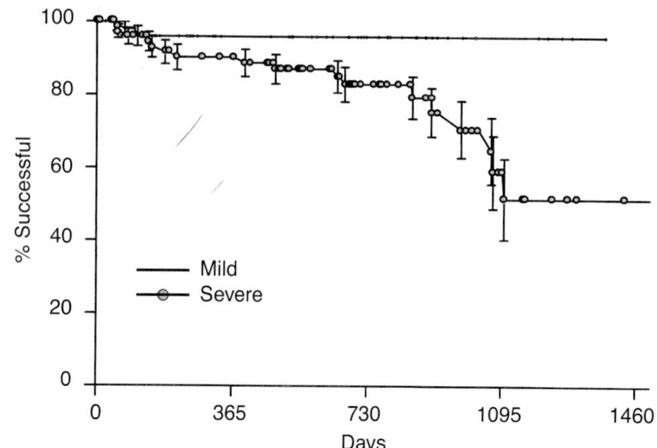

FIGURE 43.24 Kaplan-Meier plot indicating fundoplication success with time. Patients with normal lower esophageal sphincter characteristics and/or mild esophagitis had an actuarial success rate of 96% at 3 years, whereas those with defective lower esophageal sphincter function and/or complicated esophagitis had only a 50% success rate. (From Bell RC, Hanna P. *Surg Endosc.* 1999;13:1189, with permission.)

dysmotility approaching aperistalsis, such as occurs in scleroderma, or in combination with a distal esophageal myotomy for achalasia.[88]

Laparoscopic Nissen Fundoplication. The performance of laparoscopic fundoplication should include the steps identified in Table 43.10.

Port placement. Five ports are used (Fig. 43.25). The camera is placed above and to the left of the umbilicus, roughly one third of the distance to the xiphoid process. In most patients, placement of the camera in the umbilicus is too low to allow adequate visualization of the hiatal strictures once dissected. A transrectus location is preferable to midline to minimize the prevalence of port site hernia formation. Two lateral retracting ports are placed, one for the liver retractor in the right midabdomen (midclavicular line), at or slightly below the camera port. This allows the proper angle toward the left lateral segment of the liver and thus the ability to push the retractor toward the operating table, lifting the liver. A second retraction port is placed slightly above the level of the umbilicus, in the left anterior axillary line. Placement of these ports too far lateral or too low on the abdomen will compromise the excursion of the instruments and thus the ability to retract. The left-sided operating port (surgeon's right hand) is placed 1 to 2 cm below the costal margin approximately at the lateral rectus border. Such placement allows triangulation between the camera and the two instruments and avoids the difficulty associated with the instruments being in direct line with the camera. The right-sided operating port (surgeon's left hand) is placed last, after the left lateral segment of the liver has been retracted.

TABLE 43.10 MANAGEMENT

ELEMENTS OF LAPAROSCOPIC FUNDOPLICATION

1. Crural dissection, identification and preservation of both vagi including the hepatic branch of the anterior vagus
2. Circumferential dissection of the esophagus
3. Crural closure
4. Fundic mobilization by division of short gastric vessels
5. Creation of a short, loose fundoplication by enveloping the anterior and posterior wall of the fundus around the lower esophagus

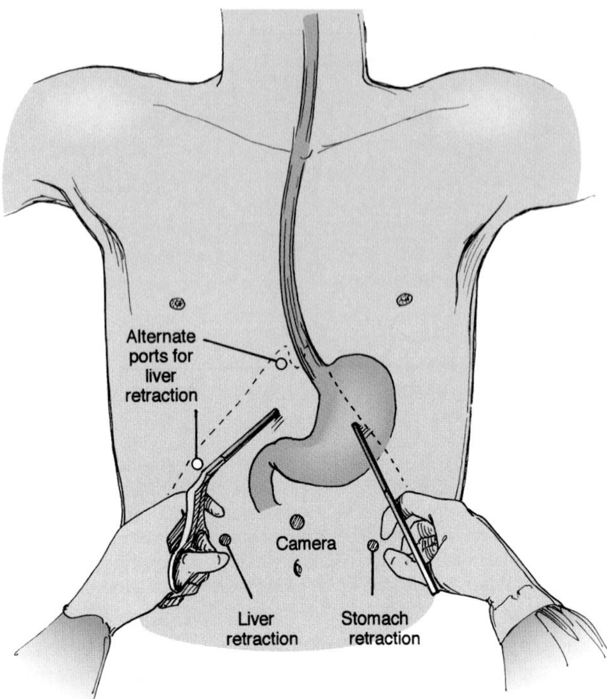

FIGURE 43.25 Trocar placement for laparoscopic antireflux surgery. The patient is placed with the head elevated 45 degrees in the modified lithotomy position. The surgeon stands between the patient's legs and the procedure is completed via five abdominal access ports.

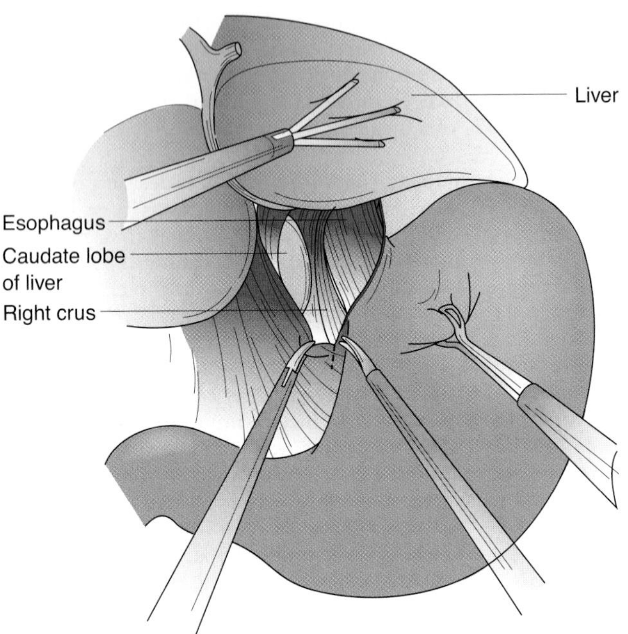

FIGURE 43.26 Illustration of the initial dissection of the esophageal hiatus. The right crus is identified and dissected toward its posterior confluence with the left crus.

This placement prevents "sword fighting" between the liver retractor and the left-handed instrument. The falciform ligament hangs low in many patients and provides a barrier around which the left-handed instrument must be manipulated.

Hiatal dissection. A fan or similar suitable retractor is placed into the right anterior axillary port and positioned to hold the left lateral segment of the liver toward the anterior abdominal wall. We prefer to use a table retractor to hold this instrument once properly positioned. Trauma to the liver should be meticulously avoided, because subsequent bleeding will obscure the field. Mobilization of the left lateral segment by division of the triangular ligament is not necessary. A Babcock or fundus clamp placed through the left anterior axillary port is used to grasp the GE fat pad and retract the stomach toward the patient's left foot. This maneuver exposes the esophageal hiatus. Commonly a hiatal hernia will need to be reduced. Atraumatic clamp should be used and care taken not to grasp the stomach too vigorously, as gastric perforations can occur.

Crural dissection. Crural dissection begins with identification of the right crus. Metzenbaum-type scissors and fine grasping forceps are preferred for dissection. In all except the most obese patients, there is a very thin portion of the gastrohepatic omentum overlying the caudate lobe of the liver. The dissection is begun by incising the portion of the gastrohepatic omentum above and below the hepatic branch of the anterior vagal nerve (which the author routinely spares). A large left hepatic artery arising from the left gastric artery is present in up to 25% of patients (Fig. 43.26); it should be identified and avoided. A right crural branch is occasionally seen, which can be divided. After incising the gastrohepatic omentum, the outside of the right crus will become evident. The peritoneum overlying the anterior aspect of the right crus is incised with scissors and electrocautery, and the right crus dissected from anterior to posterior as far as possible. The medial portion of the right crus leads into the mediastinum and is entered by blunt dissection with both instruments.

At this juncture the esophagus usually becomes evident. The right crus is retracted laterally with the surgeon's left-handed grasper and a modest dissection of the tissues posterior to the esophagus is performed. In most patients it is best not to dissect behind the GE junction at this time. Meticulous hemostasis is critical. Blood and fluid tend to pool in the hiatus and are difficult to remove. Irrigation should be avoided. Modest bleeding can be controlled by placing a 4 × 4 sponge into the abdomen. A large hiatal hernia often makes this portion of the procedure easier because it accentuates the diaphragmatic crura. On the other hand, dissection of a large mediastinal hernia sac can be difficult.

Following dissection of the right crus, attention is turned toward the anterior crural confluence. The tissues anterior to the esophagus are held upward by the left-handed grasper and the esophagus is swept downward and to the right, separating it from the left crus (Fig. 43.27). The anterior crural tissues are then divided and the left crus identified. The anterior vagus nerve often "hugs" the left crus and can be injured in this portion of the dissection if not carefully searched for and protected. The left crus is dissected as completely as possible, including taking down the angle of His and the attachments of the fundus to the left diaphragm (Fig. 43.28). A complete dissection of the lateral and inferior aspect of the left crus and fundus of the stomach is the key maneuver allowing circumferential mobilization of the esophagus. Failure to do so will result in difficulty encircling the esophagus, particularly if approached from the right. Repositioning of the Babcock retractor toward the fundic side of the stomach facilitates retraction for this portion of the procedure. The posterior vagus nerve may be encountered in the low left crural dissection and should be protected.

A window behind the GE junction can generally now be easily created. Attention is returned to the right side of the esophagus where the left-handed instrument is used to retract the esophagus anteriorly. This allows the right hand to perform the dissection behind the esophagus. The posterior vagus nerve should be identified and left on the esophagus. The left crus is identified and the dissection kept caudad to it. There is a tendency to dissect into the mediastinum and left pleura. In the presence of severe esophagitis, transmural inflammation, esophageal shortening, or a large posterior fat pad, this

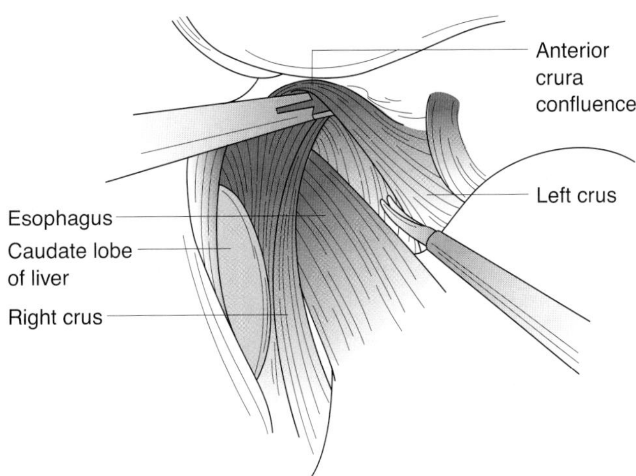

FIGURE 43.27 Artistic depiction of division of the anterior crural fibers and mobilization of the esophagus off the left crus.

dissection may be particularly difficult. If unduly difficult, abandon this route of dissection and approach the hiatus from the left side by dividing the short gastric vessels at this point in the procedure rather than later. After completing the posterior dissection, pass a grasper (through the surgeon's left-handed port) behind the esophagus and over the left crus and pull a Penrose drain around the esophagus to be used as an esophageal retractor for the remainder of the procedure.

Fundic mobilization. Complete fundic mobilization allows construction of a tension-free fundoplication. This is best done by suspending the gastrosplenic omentum anteroposteriorly, in a clothesline fashion via two Babcock forceps, and opening into the lesser sac approximately one third the distance down the greater curvature of the stomach (Fig. 43.29). The short gastric vessels can then be sequentially dissected and divided with the aid of ultrasonic shears (Ethicon Endosurgery, Cincinnati, OH). An anterior-posterior rather than medial to lateral orientation of the vessels is preferred, with the exception of those close to the spleen. The dissection includes pancreaticogastric branches posterior to the upper stomach and continues until the right crus and caudate lobe can be seen

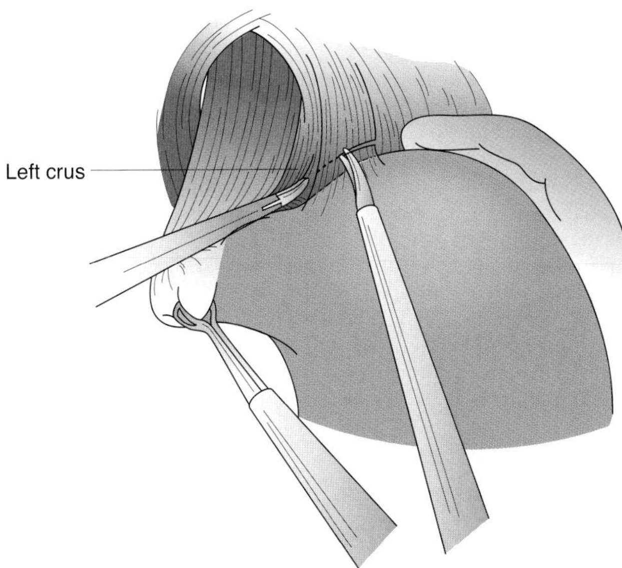

FIGURE 43.28 Left-sided crural dissection. The left crus is dissected as completely as possible and the attachments of the fundus of the stomach to the diaphragm are taken down.

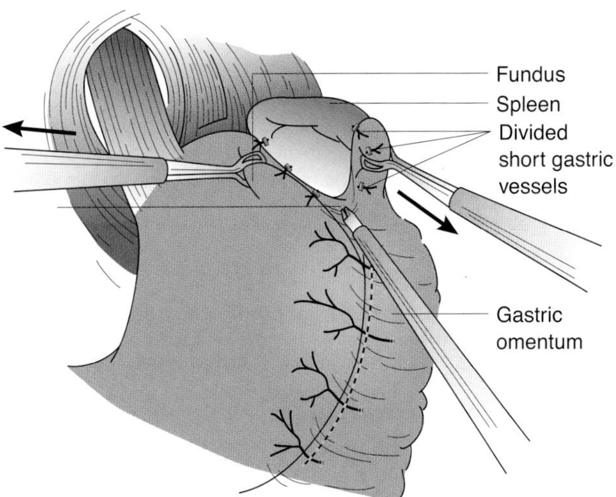

FIGURE 43.29 Illustration of the proper retraction of the gastrosplenic omentum facilitating the initial steps in short gastric division. Complete fundic mobilization is continued by retraction of the stomach rightward and the spleen and omentum left and downward. These maneuvers allow opening of the lesser sac and facilitate division of the high short gastric vessels.

from the left side (Fig. 43.30). With caution and meticulous dissection, the fundus can be completely mobilized in virtually all patients. Although generally possible via the right- and left-handed surgeon's access ports, occasionally this dissection requires removal of the liver retractor and placement of a second Babcock forceps through the right anterior axillary port to facilitate retraction during division of the short gastric vessels.

The relationship between complete fundic mobilization (short gastric vessel division) and postoperative dysphagia is a debate that has continued from the open era, when fundic mobilization was linked to a lower incidence of dysphagia. Two randomized studies have compared fundic mobilization with nonmobilization; one found no difference in outcome[89] and the

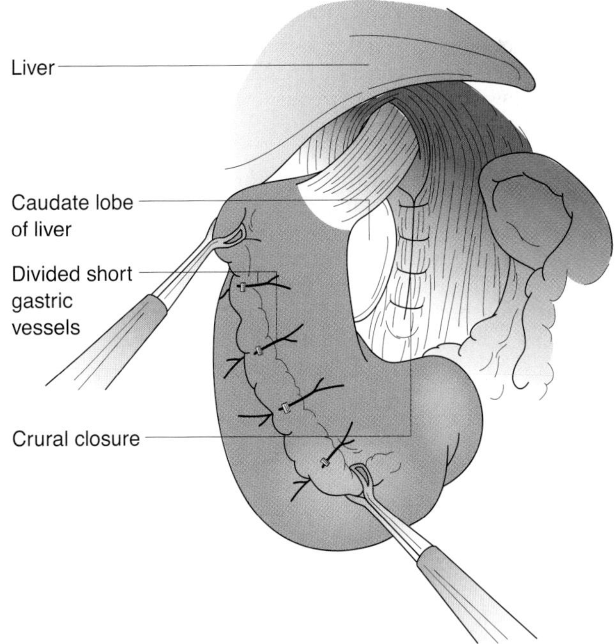

FIGURE 43.30 The fundic mobilization is continued to include pancreaticogastric branches as well as the short gastric branches. Dissection continues until the crura and the caudate lobe can be seen from left posterior.

other showed significant reductions in the incidence of dysphagia, gas bloat, and inability to belch after fundic mobilization.[90] The beneficial effect of fundic mobilization on these parameters has also been noted by other authors.[91] Whether fundic mobilization per se has a direct impact on dysphagia is unclear. It may simply be that mobilization permits better visualization of the procedure, thus ensuring that the repair is constructed with the posterior portion of the fundus.

Esophageal mobilization and crural closure. The esophagus is mobilized into the posterior mediastinum for several centimeters to provide maximal intraabdominal esophageal length. Posterior and right lateral mobilization is readily accomplished. In performing the anterior and left lateral mobilization, the surgeon must take care not to injure the anterior vagus nerve. Gentle traction on the Penrose drain around the GE junction facilitates exposure. The right and left pleural reflection often come into view and should be avoided. Continue the crural dissection to enlarge the space behind the GE junction as much as possible. Following mobilization and an assessment of intraabdominal esophageal length the hiatus is closed in all patients. The esophagus is held anterior and to the left and the crura approximated with two to four interrupted figure-of-eight 0-Ethibond sutures, starting just above the aortic decussation and working anterior. The author prefers a large needle (CT1) passed down the left upper 10-mm port to facilitate a durable crural closure. Because space is limited, it is often necessary to use the surgeon's left-handed (nondominant) instrument as a retractor, facilitating placement of single bites through each crus with the surgeon's right hand. The aorta may be punctured while suturing the left crus. Identification of the anterior aortic surface and retracting the left crus via the left-handed grasper will help avoid inadvertent aortic puncture. The author prefers extracorporeal knot tying using a standard knot pusher or a "tie knot" device (LSI Solutions, Victor, NY), although tying within the abdomen is perfectly appropriate. More recently, we have inspected the crural closure at the completion of the procedure following creation of the fundoplication and removal of the bougie. Doing so will often reveal that the bougie has dilated the hiatal opening such that a final stitch should be placed to further approximate it. Although there have been no randomized studies evaluating the role of routine crural closure, there is compelling evidence to indicate that closure should be standard. Watson et al.[92] identified paraesophageal herniation in 17 of 253 patients (7%), the frequency being 3% in those who had undergone crural repair and 11% in those who had not.

Creation of the fundoplication. A short, loose fundoplication is fashioned with particular attention to the geometry of the wrap (Fig. 43.31). The midposterior fundus is grasped and passed left to right behind the esophagus rather than pulling right to left. This ensures that the posterior fundus is used for the posterior aspect of the fundoplication. This is accomplished by placing a Babcock clamp through the left lower port and grasping the midportion of the posterior fundus (Fig. 43.32). One should gently bring the posterior fundus behind the esophagus to the right side with an upward, rightward, and clockwise twisting motion. This maneuver can be difficult particularly for the novice. If so, placement of a 0-silk suture in the midposterior fundus and grasping it from the right side facilitates bringing the posterior fundus around to create the fundoplication. The anterior wall of the fundus is then folded over the esophagus to meet the posterior at about the 10 to 11 o'clock position above the supporting Penrose drain.

The posterior and anterior fundic lips should be maneuvered (as in a "shoe shine") to allow the fundus to envelope the esophagus without twisting. Laparoscopic visualization has a tendency to exaggerate the size of the posterior opening that has been dissected. Consequently, the space for the passage of the

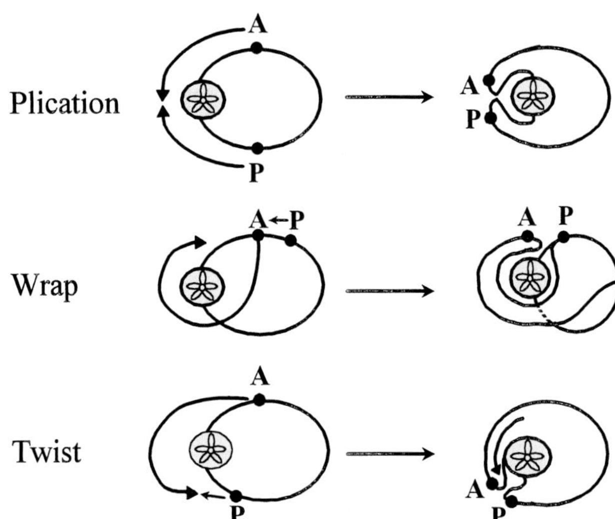

FIGURE 43.31 Schematic representations of the various possibilities of orientation of a Nissen fundoplication. The top set of figures represents the preferred approach, whereas the bottom two sets can be seen to result in twisting of the fundoplication.

fundus behind the esophagus may be tighter than thought and the fundus relatively ischemic when brought around. If the right lip of the fundoplication has a bluish discoloration, the stomach should be returned to its original position and the posterior dissection enlarged. A 60-French bougie is passed to properly size the fundoplication, and the "lips" of the fundoplication sutured utilizing a single U-stitch of 2-0 Prolene buttressed with felt pledgets. The most common error is an attempt to grasp the anterior portion of the stomach to construct the right lip of the fundoplication rather than the posterior fundus. The esophagus should comfortably lie in the untwisted fundus prior to suturing. Finally, two anchoring sutures of 2-0 silk or Ethibond are placed above and below the U-stitch to complete the fundoplication. When finished, the suture line of the fundoplication should be facing in a right anterior direction (Fig. 43.33). The abdomen is then irrigated, hemostasis checked, and the bougie, Penrose drain, and any sponges placed into the abdomen removed.

Transthoracic Nissen Fundoplication. The indications for performing an antireflux procedure by a transthoracic approach are given in Table 43.11.

In the thoracic approach the hiatus is exposed through a left posterior lateral thoracotomy incision in the sixth intercostal space (i.e., over the upper border of the seventh rib). When necessary, the diaphragm is incised circumferentially 2 to 3 cm from the lateral chest wall for a distance of approximately 10 to 15 cm. The esophagus is mobilized from the level of the diaphragm to underneath the aortic arch. Mobilization up to the aortic arch is usually necessary to place the repair in a patient with a shortened esophagus into the abdomen without undue tension. Failure to do this is one of the major causes for subsequent breakdown of a repair and return of symptoms. The cardia is then freed from the diaphragm. When all the attachments between the cardia and diaphragmatic hiatus are divided, the fundus and part of the body of the stomach are drawn up through the hiatus into the chest. The vascular fat pad that lies at the GE junction is excised. Crural sutures are then placed to close the hiatus and the fundoplication constructed by enveloping the fundus around the distal esophagus in a manner similar to that described for the abdominal approach. When complete, the fundoplication is placed into the abdomen by compressing the fundic ball with the hand and manually maneuvering it through the hiatus.

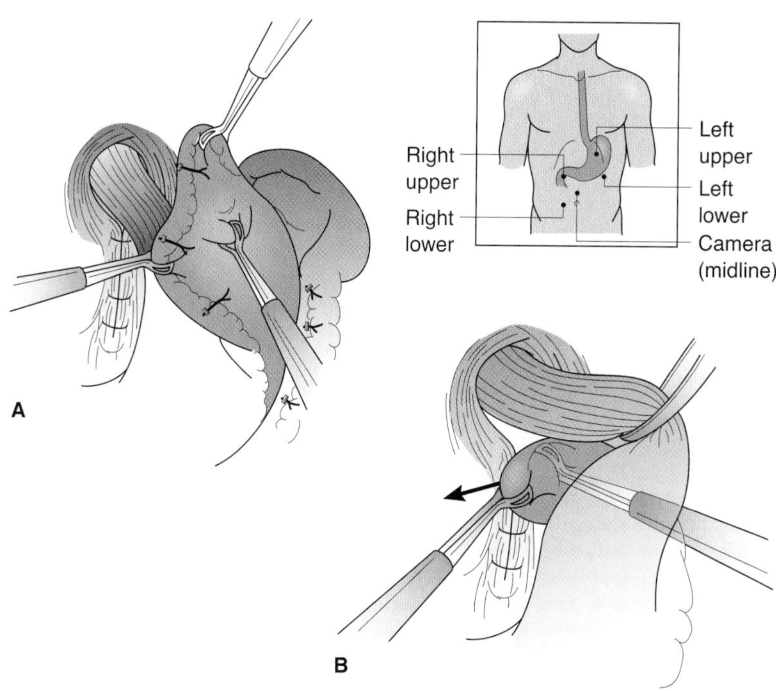

FIGURE 43.32 Placement of Babcock on the posterior fundus in preparation for passing it behind the esophagus to create the posterior or right lip of the fundoplication. (*Inset*) To achieve the proper angle for passage, the Babcock is placed through the left lower trocar. The posterior fundus is passed left to right and grasped from the right via a Babcock through the right upper trocar. (*A*) Location of posterior fundus for passage to the right side. (*B*) The posterior fundus passed underneath the esophagus and grasped on the right.

Collis Gastroplasty. In patients with a short esophagus secondary to a stricture, Barrett's esophagus, or a large hiatal hernia, the esophagus is lengthened with a Collis gastroplasty. The gastroplasty lengthens the esophagus by forming a gastric tube or "neoesophagus" along the lesser curvature. The procedure allows a tension-free construction of a total or partial fundoplication around the newly formed gastric tube, with placement of the repair in the abdomen. A gastroplasty can be readily performed via either an abdominal or thoracic approach. A number of techniques have been reported for the laparoscopic performance of Collis gastroplasty, and the surgeon opting to manage the shortened esophagus laparoscopically must be able to perform such a procedure should the need arise.[93]

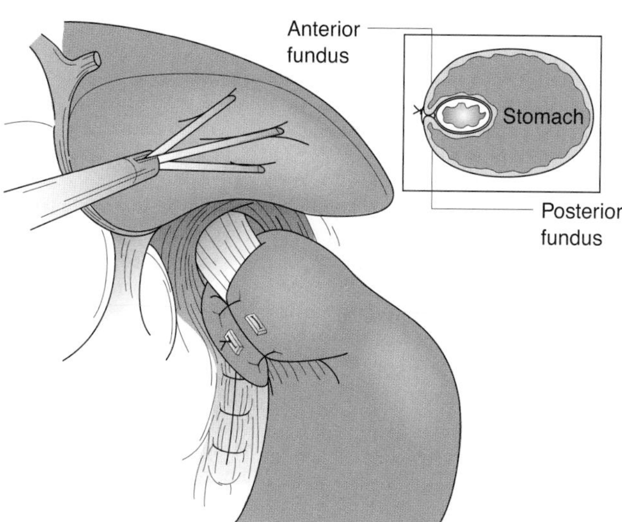

FIGURE 43.33 Fixation of the fundoplication. The fundoplication is sutured in place with a single U-stitch of 2-0 Prolene pledgeted on the outside. A 60-French mercury-weighted bougie is passed through the gastroesophageal junction prior to fixation of the wrap to ensure a floppy fundoplication. Inset illustrates the proper orientation of the fundic wrap.

Complications of Antireflux Surgery. Carlson and Frantzides[94] reported on complications and results of primary minimally invasive antireflux operations based on a literature review. Included in their analysis were 41 papers comprising 10,489 procedures. Postoperative complications were found to occur in approximately 8% of patients, with the rate of conversion to an open procedure of about 4%. The most common perioperative complication was early wrap herniation (1.3%), defined as occurring within 48 hours of surgery. This is one complication that may be more common with the laparoscopic than open approach. The explanation for this is unclear but may be related to the opening of tissue planes by the pneumoperitoneum and the reduced tendency for adhesion formation after laparoscopic compared to open surgery. In an attempt to eliminate this complication, most surgeons routinely perform a crural repair.

Both pneumothorax and pneumomediastinum have been reported. The occurrence of pneumothorax is related to breach of either pleural membrane, usually the left, during the hiatal dissection. Chest drain insertion is usually not required because accumulated carbon dioxide rapidly dissipates following release of pneumoperitoneum by a combination of positive pressure ventilation and absorption.

As with any laparoscopic procedure, instrumental perforation of the hollow viscera may occur. Early esophageal perforation may arise during passage of the bougie, during the retroesophageal dissection, or during suture pull-through. Late esophageal perforation is related to diathermy injury at the time of mobilization. Gastric perforations usually resulted from excessive traction on the fundus for retraction purposes. Recognition of the problem at the time of surgery requires repair, which may be performed either laparoscopically or by an open technique.

Hemorrhage during the course of laparoscopic fundoplication usually arises from the short gastric vessels or spleen. Rarer causes include retractor trauma to the liver, injury to the left inferior phrenic vein, an aberrant left hepatic vein, or the inferior vena cava. Cardiac tamponade as a result of right ventricular trauma has also been reported. Major vascular injury mandates immediate conversion to an open procedure to achieve hemostasis. One complication that has been virtually eliminated since the advent of laparoscopic fundoplication is incidental splenic injury necessitating splenectomy (0.06%), which occurred with

TABLE 43.11 INDICATIONS/CONTRAINDICATIONS

INDICATIONS FOR PERFORMING AN ANTIREFLUX PROCEDURE BY A TRANSTHORACIC APPROACH

Indication	Explanation
Previous hiatal hernia repair	In this situation, a peripheral circumferential incision in the diaphragm is made to provide simultaneous exposure of the upper abdomen. This allows safe dissection of the previous repair from both the abdominal and thoracic sides of the diaphragm.
Concomitant procedure	Concomitant esophageal myotomy for achalasia or diffuse spasm.
Short esophagus	This is usually associated with a stricture or Barrett's esophagus. In this situation, the thoracic approach is preferred to allow maximum mobilization of the esophagus, the performance of a Collis gastroplasty, or, if necessary, to place the repair without tension below the diaphragm.
Sliding hiatal hernia that does not reduce below the diaphragm during a roentgenographic barium study in the upright position	This can indicate esophageal shortening and, again, a thoracic approach is preferred for maximum mobilization of the esophagus and, if necessary, the performance of a Collis gastroplasty.
Associated pulmonary pathology	The nature of the pulmonary pathology can be evaluated and the proper pulmonary surgery, in addition to the antireflux repair, can be performed.
Obesity	The abdominal repair is difficult because of poor exposure, whereas the thoracic approach gives better exposure and allows a more precise repair.

a frequency of around 2% to 5% during the open era. The mortality rate for primary minimally invasive antireflux surgery has fortunately been quite low, reported at 0.08%.

Outcomes Following Antireflux Surgery. Studies of long-term outcome following both open and laparoscopic fundoplication document the ability of laparoscopic fundoplication to relieve typical reflux symptoms (heartburn, regurgitation, and dysphagia) in more than 90% of patients at follow-up intervals averaging 2 to 3 years and 80% to 90% of patients 5 years or more following surgery.[95–100] This includes evidence-based reviews of antireflux surgery,[100] prospective randomized trials comparing antireflux surgery to PPI therapy[101] and open to laparoscopic fundoplication,[102] and analysis of U.S. national trends in utilization and outcomes.[103] Laparoscopic fundoplication results in a significant increase in LES pressure and length, generally restoring these values to normal. Postoperative pH studies indicate that the pH tracings of more than 90% of patients will normalize. The results of laparoscopic fundoplication compare favorably with those of the "modern" era of open fundoplication. They also indicate the less predictable outcome of atypical reflux symptoms (cough, asthma, laryngitis) after surgery being relieved in only two thirds of patients.[104]

Recent reports have called attention to the observation that many patients are prescribed acid-suppression medications after antireflux surgery. Spechler et al. reported on the long-term follow-up of patients with complicated GERD enrolled in the Department of Veterans Affairs randomized trial of medical versus surgical therapies.[105,106] In the first report, almost half (46.9%) of the patients treated by fundoplication had taken acid-suppression medications at some point during the 11- to 13-year follow-up period.[105] In the second report, 62% of the surgically treated patients had used medications.[106]

Lord et al.[107] reported on 86 patients who had symptoms after Nissen fundoplication severe enough to warrant evaluation with 24-hour ambulatory esophageal pH monitoring. Thirty-seven (43%) of these patients were taking acid-suppression medications, and only 9 of them (24%) were found to have abnormal pH scores. Heartburn and regurgitation were the only symptoms that were significantly associated with an abnormal pH study. Multivariable logistic regression analysis showed that patients with a disrupted, abnormally positioned fundoplication had a 52.6 times increased risk of abnormal esophageal acid exposure. Based on these data, most patients using acid-suppression medications after antireflux surgery do not have abnormal esophageal acid exposure. Objective evidence of reflux should be obtained in patients who complain of postoperative symptoms.

The goal of surgical treatment for GERD is to relieve the symptoms of reflux by reestablishing the GE barrier. The challenge is to accomplish this without inducing dysphagia or other untoward side effects. Dysphagia that existed prior to surgery usually improves following laparoscopic fundoplication. Temporary dysphagia is common after surgery and generally resolves within 3 months. Dysphagia persisting beyond 3 months has been reported in up to 10% of patients. In our experience, dysphagia, manifested by occasional difficulty in swallowing solids, was present in 7% of patients at 3 months, 5% at 6 months, 2% at 12 months and in a single patient at 24 months following surgery.[96] Others have observed a similar improvement in postoperative dysphagia with time. Induced dysphagia is usually mild, does not require dilatation, and is temporary. It can be induced by technical misjudgments, but this explanation does not hold in all instances. In experienced hands, its prevalence should be less than 3% at 1 year. Other side effects common to antireflux surgery include the inability to vomit and increased flatulence. Most patients cannot vomit through an intact wrap, though this is rarely clinically relevant. Hyperflatulence is a common and noticeable problem, likely related to increased air swallowing that is present in most patients with reflux disease.

Quality-of-life analyses have become an important part of surgical outcome assessment, with both generic and disease-specific questionnaires in use, in an attempt to quantitate quality of life before and after surgical intervention. In general, these measures relate the effect of disease management to the overall well-being of the patient.[108] Most studies have utilized the Short Form 36 (SF-36) instrument, because it is rapidly administered and well validated. This questionnaire measures 12 different health-related quality-of-life parameters encompassing mental and physical well-being. Data from Los Angeles indicate significant improvements in scores for the area of bodily pain and in a portion of the general health index.[96] Most other measures were improved but failed to achieve statistical significance. Trus et al.[109] have also analyzed SF-36 scores before and after laparoscopic antireflux surgery. In contrast to our data, scores in all fields were significantly better after surgery. In this study, preoperative scores were dramatically lower than were found in our study. Thus, the difference is likely to be secondary to the relatively high scores of our patients prior to surgery (perhaps reflecting good disease control on medical therapy) and to our small sample size.

Other investigators have also reported improvement in quality of life following antireflux surgery. Glise et al.[110] utilized two standardized and validated questionnaires, the Psychological General Well Being Index and the Gastrointestinal Symptom Rating Scale to evaluate quality of life in a cohort of 40 patients following laparoscopic antireflux surgery. Scores with both instruments were improved following antireflux surgery and better than in untreated patients. Of particular note was that scores were as good as or better than those of patients receiving optimal medical therapy. Velonovich et al.,[111] using a 10-item health-related quality-of-life questionnaire specific for GERD, have also shown an improvement in quality of life following antireflux surgery.

Fernando et al.[112] reported on quality of life after antireflux surgery compared with nonoperative management for severe GERD. Follow-up quality of life was measured using the SF-36, and heartburn severity was measured using the Health Related Quality of Life (QOL) scale. Detailed outcomes were available for 101 surgical patients and 37 medical patients. Mean QOL scores were better in the surgical group. More of the medical patients were dissatisfied with therapy. SF-36 scores were better in six of eight domains for surgical patients. These data support the notion that antireflux surgery, performed on properly selected patients, can significantly improve quality of life and may outperform medical therapy in this regard.

KEY POINTS

- **The lymphatics of the esophagus form a rich submucosal network draining into regional lymph nodes in the periesophageal connective tissue; thus, little barrier exists to the longitudinal spread of esophageal cancer.**
- **The diagnosis of GE reflux based on symptoms alone is correct in only approximately two thirds of patients because the symptoms are often nonspecific and can be caused by other conditions.**
- **The three characteristics of the LES that maintains its resistance or "barrier" function to intragastric and intraabdominal pressure challenges are pressure, overall length, and length exposed to the positive pressure environment of the abdomen.**
- **An important complication of GE reflux is the development of reflux-induced respiratory symptoms either with or without heartburn.**
- **Antireflux surgery improves respiratory symptoms in nearly 90% of children and 70% of adults with asthma and reflux disease.**
- **Factors predisposing to the development of Barrett's esophagus include early-onset GERD, abnormal lower esophageal and esophageal body physiology, and mixed reflux of gastric and duodenal contents into the esophagus.**
- **PPI therapy, both to relieve symptoms and to control esophagitis, is an acceptable treatment, although most patients will require life-long treatment.**
- **Progression of nondysplastic Barrett's epithelium occurs with 5% to 10% of patients per year progressing to dysplasia and 0.5% to 1% per year progressing to adenocarcinoma.**
- **The standard of care of the treatment of confirmed Barrett's esophagus with high-grade dysplasia is esophagectomy because approximately 50% will harbor invasive adenocarcinoma.**
- **Three factors predictive of a successful outcome following antireflux surgery are (a) an abnormal score on 24-hour esophageal pH monitoring; (b) the presence of typical symptoms of GERD, namely heartburn or regurgitation; and (c) symptomatic improvement in response to acid-suppression therapy prior to surgery.**

References

1. Patti MG, Gantert W, Way LW. Surgery of the esophagus; anatomy and physiology. *Surg Clin North Am.* 1997;77:959.
2. Gray SW, Rowe JS Jr, Skandalakis JE. Surgical anatomy of the gastroesophageal junction. *Am Surg.* 1979;45:575.
3. Dua KS, Ren J, Bardan E, et al. Coordination of deglutitive glottal function and pharyngeal bolus transport during normal eating. *Gastroenterology* 1997;112:73.
4. Pouderoux P, Shi G, Tatum RP, et al. Esophageal solid bolus transport; studies using concurrent videofluoroscopy and manometry. *Am J Gastroenterol.* 1999;94:1457.
5. Pouderoux P, Lin S, Kahrilis PJ. Timing, propagation, coordination and effect of esophageal shortening during peristalsis. *Gastroenterology* 1997;112:1147.
6. Mittal RK, Balaban DH. The esophagogastric junction. *N Engl J Med.* 1997;336:924.
7. Clave P, Gonzalez A, Moreno A, et al. Endogenous cholecystokinin enhances postprandial gastroesophageal reflux in humans through extrasphincteric receptors. *Gastroenterology* 1998;115:597.
8. Locke GR, Talley NJ, Fett SL, et al. Prevalence and clinical spectrum of gastroesophageal reflux; a population-based study in Olmsted County Minnesota. *Gastroenterology* 1997;112:1448.
9. Isolauri J, Laippala P. Prevalence of symptoms suggestive of gastroesophageal reflux disease in an adult population. *Ann Med.* 1995;27:67.
10. El-Serag HB, Sonnenberg A. Opposing time trends of peptic ulcer and reflux disease. *Gut* 1998;43:327.
11. Panos MZ, Walt RP, Stevenson C, et al. Rising death rate from non-malignant disease of the oesophagus (NMOD) in England and Wales. *Gut* 1995;36:488.
12. Monnier Ph, Ollyo JB, Fontolliet C, et al. Epidemiology and natural history of reflux esophagitis. *Semin Laparosc Surg.* 1995;2:2.
13. Spechler SJ. Epidemiology and natural history of gastro-oesophageal reflux disease. *Digestion* 1992;51:24.
14. Graham DY. The changing epidemiology of GERD: Geography and *Helicobacter pylori. Am J Gastroenterol.* 2003;98:1462.
15. Labenz J, Blum AL, Bayerdorffer E, et al. Curing *Helicobacter pylori* infection in patients with duodenal ulcer may provoke reflux esophagitis. *Gastroenterology* 1997;112:1442.
16. Ackermark P, Kuipers EJ, Woldf C, et al. Colonization with cag-A positive Helicobacter pylori strains in intestinal metaplasia of the esophagus and the esophagogastric junction. *Am J Gastroenterol.* 2003; 98:1719.
17. Vicari JJ, Peek RM, Falk GW, et al. The seroprevalence of cag-A positive Helicobacter pylori strains in the spectrum of gastroesophageal reflux disease. *Gastroenterology* 1998;115:50.
18. Chow WH, Blaser MJ, Blot WJ, et al. An inverse relation between cagA+ strains of *Helicobacter pylori* infection and risk of esophageal and gastric carcinoma. *Cancer Res.* 1998;58:588.
19. Oberg S, Peters JH, DeMeester TR. Helicobacter pylori is not associated with the manifestations of gastroesophageal reflux disease. *Arch Surg.* 1999;134:722.
20. Costantini M, Crookes PF, Bremner RM, et al. The value of physiologic assessment of foregut symptoms in a surgical practice. *Surgery* 1993; 114:780.
21. Bonavina L, Evander A, DeMeester TR, et al. Length of the distal esophageal sphincter and competency of the cardia. *Am J Surg.* 1986; 151:25.
22. O'Sullivan GC, DeMeester TR, Joelsson BE, et al. The interaction of the lower esophageal sphincter pressure and length of sphincter in the abdomen as determinants of gastroesophageal competence. *Am J Surg.* 1982;143:40.
23. Zaninotto G, DeMeester TR, Schwizer W, et al. The lower esophageal sphincter in health and disease. *Am J Surg.* 1988;155:104.
24. Stein HJ, Barlow AP, DeMeester TR, Hinder RA. Complications of gastroesophageal reflux disease: role of the lower esophageal sphincter, esophageal acid and acid/alkaline exposure, and duodenogastric reflux. *Ann Surg.* 1992;216:35.
25. Kuster E, Ros E, Toledo-Pimentel V, et al. Predictive factors of the long term outcome in gastro-oesophageal reflux disease: six year follow up of 107 patients. *Gut* 1994;35:8.
26. Stein HJ, Eypasch EP, DeMeester TR, Smyrk TC. Circadian esophageal motor function in patients with gastroesophageal reflux disease. *Surgery* 1990;108:769.
27. DeMeester TR, Johnson WE. Outcome of respiratory symptoms after surgical treatment of swallowing disorders. *Semin Resp Crit Care Med.* 1995;16:514.
28. DeMeester TR, Ireland AP. Gastric pathology as an initiator and potentiator of gastroesophageal reflux disease. *Dis Esoph.* 1997;10:1.
29. Bremner RM, Hoeft SF, Costantini M, et al. Pharyngeal swallowing: the major factor in clearance of esophageal reflux episodes. *Ann Surg.* 1993;218:364.
30. Ismail T, Bancewicz J, Barlow J. Yield pressure, anatomy of the cardia and gastroesophageal reflux. *Br J Surg.* 1995;82:943.
31. Pandolfino JE, Shi G, Trueworthy B, Kahrilas PJ. Esophagogastric junction opening pressure during relaxation distinguishes nonhernia reflux patients, hernia patients and normal subjects. *Gastroenterology* 2003;125:1018.

32. Rakic S, Stein HJ, DeMeester TR, et al. Role of esophageal body function in gastroesophageal reflux disease: implications for surgical management. *J Am Coll Surg.* 1997;185:380.
33. Fletcher J, Wirz A, Young J, et al. Unbuffered highly acidic gastric juice exists at the gastroesophageal junction after a meal. *Gastroenterology* 2001;121:775.
34. Fletcher J, Wirz A, Henry E, et al. Studies of acid exposure immediately above the gastroesophageal squamocolumnar junction; evidence of short segment reflux. *Gut* 2004;53:168.
35. Iljima K. Henry E, Moriya A, et al. Dietary nitrate generates potentially mutagenic concentrations of nitric oxide at the gastroesophageal junction. *Gastroenterology* 2002;122:1248.
36. Lillemoe KD, Johnson LF, Harmon JW. Role of the components of the gastroduodenal contents in experimental acid esophagitis. *Surgery* 1982;92:276.
37. Lillemoe KD, Johnson LF, Harmon JW. Alkaline esophagitis: a comparison of the ability of components of gastroduodenal contents to injure the rabbit esophagus. *Gastroenterology* 1983;85:621.
38. Kauer WKH, Peters JH, DeMeester TR, et al. Mixed reflux of gastric juice is more harmful to the esophagus than gastric juice alone. The need for surgical therapy reemphasized. *Ann Surg.* 1995;222:525.
39. Stein HJ, Feussner H, Kauer W, et al: Alkaline gastroesophageal reflux: assessment by ambulatory esophageal aspiration and pH monitoring. *Am J Surg.* 1994;167:163.
40. Kauer WKH, Burdiles P, Ireland A, et al. Does duodenal juice reflux into the esophagus in patients with complicated GERD? Evaluation of a fiberoptic sensor for bilirubin. *Am J Surg.* 1995;169:98.
41. El-Serag HB, Sonnenberg A. Comorbid occurrence of laryngeal or pulmonary disease with esophagitis in United States Military Veterans. *Gastroenterology* 1997;113:755.
42. Sontag SJ, O'Connell S, Khandewal S, et al. Most asthmatics have gastroesophageal reflux with or without bronchodilator therapy. *Gastroenterology* 1990;99:613.
43. Gastal OL, Castell JA, Castell DO. Frequency and site of gastroesophageal reflux in patients with chest symptoms. *Chest* 1994;106:1793.
44. Tuchman DN, Boyle JT, Pack AI, et al. Comparison of airway responses following tracheal or esophageal acidification in the cat. *Gastroenterology* 1984;87:872.
45. Mansfield LE, Hameister HH, Spaulding HS, et al. The role of the vagus nerve in airway narrowing caused by intraesophageal hydrochloric acid provocation and esophageal distention. *Ann Allergy* 1981;47:431.
46. Levin TR, Sperling RM, McQuaid KR. Omeprazole improves peak expiratory flow rate and quality of life in asthmatics with gastroesophageal reflux. *Am J Gastroenterol.* 1998;93:1060.
47. Boeree MJ, Peters FTM, Postma DS, et al. No effects of high-dose omeprazole in patients with severe airway hyperresponsiveness and symptomatic gastro-oesophageal reflux. *Eur Respir J.* 1998;11:1070.
48. Harding SM, Richter JE, Guzzo MR, et al. Asthma and gastroesophageal reflux: acid suppressive therapy improves asthma outcome. *Am J Med.* 1996;100:395.
49. Sontag SJ, O'Connell S, Khandelwal S, et al. Asthmatics with gastroesophageal reflux; Long term results of a randomized trial of medical and surgical antireflux therapies. *Am J Gastroenterol.* 2003;98:987.
50. Perrin-Fayolle M, Gormand F, Braillon G, et al. Long-term results of surgical treatment for gastroesophageal reflux in asthmatic patients. *Chest* 1989;96:40.
51. Spechler SJ. The Columnar lined esophagus: history, terminology and clinical issues. *Gastroenterol Clin North Am.* 1997;26:455.
52. Peters JH, Hagen JA, DeMeester SR. Barrett's esophagus. *J Gastrointest Surg.* 2004 ;8:1.
53. Chandrasoma P. Norman Barrett: so close, yet 50 years away from the truth. *J Gastrointest Surg.* 1999;3:7.
54. Campos GMR, DeMeester SR, Peters JH, et al. Predictive factors of Barrett's esophagus; multivariate analyses of 502 patients with GERD. *Arch Surg.* 2001;136:1267.
55. Katzka DA, Castell DO. Successful elimination of reflux symptoms does not insure adequate control of acid reflux in patients with Barrett's esophagus. *Am J Gastroenterol.* 1994;89:989.
56. Ouatu-Lascar R, Triadafilopolous G. Complete elimination of reflux symptoms does not guarantee normalization of intraesophageal acid reflux in patients with Barrett's esophagus. *Am J Gastroenterol.* 1998; 93:711.
57. Sampliner RE, Fennerty B, Garewal HS. Reversal of Barrett's esophagus with acid suppression and multipolar electrocoagulation: preliminary results. *Gastrointest Endosc.* 1996;44:532.
58. Hofstetter WA, Peters JH, DeMeester TR, et al. Long term outcome of antireflux surgery in patients with Barrett's esophagus. *Ann Surg.* 2001;234:532.
59. Farrell TM, Smith CD, Metreveli RE, et al. Fundoplication provides effective and durable symptom relief in patients with Barrett's esophagus. *Am J Surg.* 1999;178:18.
60. Oelschlager BK, Barreca M, Chang L, et al. Clinical and pathologic response of Barrett's esophagus to laparoscopic antireflux surgery. *Ann Surg.* 2003;238:458.
61. Overholt BF, Panjehpour M, Halberg DL. Photodynamic therapy for Barrett's esophagus with dysplasia and/or early stage carcinoma; long term results. *Gastrointest Endosc.* 2003;58:183.
62. Pacifico RJ, Wang KK, Wongkeesong LM, et al. Combined endoscopic mucosal resection and photodynamic therapy versus esophagectomy for management of early adenocarcinoma in Barrett's esophagus. *Clin Gastroenterol Hepatol.* 2003;1:252.
63. Peters JH, Clark GWB, Ireland AP, et al. Outcome of adenocarcinoma arising in Barrett's esophagus in endoscopically surveyed and non-surveyed patients. *J Thorac Cardiovasc Surg.* 1994;108:813.
64. Altorki NK, Sunagawa M, Little AG, Skinner DB. High-grad dysplasia in the columnar-lined esophagus. *Am J Surg.* 1991;161:99.
65. Pera M, Trastek VF, Carpenter HA, et al. Barrett's esophagus with high grade dysplasia; an indication for esophagectomy. *Ann Thorac Surg.* 1992;54:199.
66. Ferguson MK, Naunheim KS. Resection for Barrett's mucosa with high-grade dysplasia: implications for prophylactic photodynamic therapy. *J Thorac Cardiovasc Surg.* 1997;114:824.
67. Sandmark S, Carlsson R, Fausa O, et al. Omeprozole or Ranitidine in the treatment of reflux esophagitis. *Scand J Gastroenterol.* 1988;23:625.
68. Katzka DA, Paoletti V, Leite L, et al. Prolonged ambulatory pH monitoring in patients with persistent gastroesophageal reflux disease symptoms: testing while on therapy identifies the need for more aggressive anti-reflux therapy. *Am J Gastroenterol.* 1996;91:2110.
69. Peghini PL, Katz PO, Bracy NA, et al. Nocturnal recovery of gastric acid secretion with twice-daily dosing of proton pump inhibitors. *Am J Gastroenterol.* 1998;93:763.
70. Campos GM, Peters JH, DeMeester TR, et al. The pattern of esophageal acid exposure in GERD influences the severity of the disease. *Arch Surg.* 1999;134:882.
71. Campos GMR, Peters JH, DeMeester TR, et al. Multivariate analysis of the factors predicting outcome after Laparoscopic Nissen fundoplication. *J Gastrointest Surg.* 1999;3:292.
72. Hill LD, Kozarek RA, Kraemer SJM, et al. The gastroesophageal flap valve. In vitro and in vivo observations. *Gastrointest Endosc.* 1996; 44:541.
73. Miller FA. Utilization of inlying pH-probe for evaluation of acid-peptic diathesis. *Arch Surg.* 1964;89:199.
74. Johnson LF, DeMeester TR. Development of the 24-hour intraesophageal pH monitoring composite scoring system. *J Clin Gastroenterol.* 1986; 8[Suppl 1]:52.
75. Jamieson JR, Stein HJ, DeMeester TR, et al. Ambulatory 24-h esophageal pH monitoring: normal values, optimal thresholds, specificity, sensitivity, and reproducibility. *Am J Gastroenterol.* 1992;87:1102.
76. Gastal OL, Hagen JA, Peters JH, et al. Short esophagus: analysis of predictors and clinical implications. *Arch Surg.* 1999;134:633.
77. Ritter MP, Peters JH, DeMeester TR, et al. Treatment of advanced gastroesophageal reflux disease with Collis gastroplasty and Belsey partial fundoplication. *Arch Surg.* 1998;133:523.
78. DeMeester SR, Sillin LF, Lin HW, et al. Increasing esophageal length: a comparison of laparoscopic versus transthoracic esophageal mobilization with and without vagal trunk division in pigs. *J Am Coll Surg.* 2003; 197:558.
79. Stein HJ, Feussner H, Siewart JR. Failure of antireflux surgery; causes and management. *Am J Surg.* 1996;171:36.
80. Johnson WE, Hagen JA, DeMeester TR, et al. Outcome of respiratory symptoms after antireflux surgery on patients with gastroesophageal reflux disease. *Arch Surg.* 1996;131:489.
81. Schwizer W, Hinder RA, DeMeester TR. Does delayed gastric emptying contribute to gastroesophageal reflux disease? *Am J Surg.* 1989;157:74.
82. Watson DI, Jamieson GG, Pike GK, et al. Prospective randomized double-blind trial between laparoscopic Nissen and anterior partial fundoplication. *Br J Surg.* 1999;86:123.
83. Laws HL, Clements RH, Swillie CM. A randomized, prospective comparison of the Nissen fundoplication versus the Toupet fundoplication for gastroesophageal reflux disease. *Ann Surg.* 1997;225:647.
84. Hagedorn C, Lonroth H, Rydberg L, et al. Long-term efficacy of total (Nissen-Rossetti) and posterior partial (Toupet) fundoplication: results of a randomized clinical trial. *J Gastrointest Surg.* 2002;6:540.
85. Jobe BA, Wallace J, Hansen PD, et al. Evaluation of laparoscopic Toupet fundoplication as a primary repair for all patients with medically resistant gastroesophageal reflux. *Surg Endosc.* 1997; 11:1080.
86. Bell RC, Hanna P, Mills MR, et al. Patterns of success and failure with laparoscopic partial fundoplication. *Surg Endosc.* 1999;13:1189.
87. Patti MG, Robinson T, Galvani C, et al. Total fundoplication is superior to partial fundoplication even when esophageal peristalsis is weak. *J Am Coll Surg.* 2004;198:863.
88. Horvath KD, Jobe BA, Herron DM, et al. Laparoscopic Toupet is an inadequate procedure for patients with severe reflux disease. *J Gastrointest Surg.* 1999;3:583.
89. Watson DI, Pike GK, Baigrie RJ, et al. Prospective double-blind randomized trial of laparoscopic Nissen fundoplication with division and without division of short gastric vessels. *Ann Surg.* 1997;226:642.
90. Dalenbäck J, Lönroth H, Blomqvist A, et al. Improved functional outcome after laparoscopic fundoplication by complete gastric fundus mobilization. *Gastroenterology* 1998;114:A1384.
91. Hunter JG, Swanstrom L, Waring JP. Dysphagia after laparoscopic antireflux surgery. The impact of operative technique. *Ann Surg.* 1996;224:51.

92. Watson DI, Jamieson GG, Devitt PG, et al. Paraoesophageal hiatus hernia: an important complication of laparoscopic Nissen fundoplication. *Br J Surg*. 1995;82:521.
93. Terry ML, Vernon A, Hunter JG. Stapled-wedge Collis gastroplasty for the shortened esophagus. *Am J Surg*. 2004;188:195.
94. Carlson MA, Frantzides CT. Complications and results of primary minimally invasive antireflux procedures: a review of 10,735 reported cases. *J Am Coll Surg*. 2001;193:429.
95. Hinder RA, Filipi CJ, Wetscher G, et al. Laparoscopic Nissen fundoplication is an effective treatment for gastroesophageal reflux disease. *Ann Surg*. 1994;220:472.
96. Peters JH, DeMeester TR, Crookes P, et al. The treatment of gastroesophageal reflux disease with laparoscopic Nissen fundoplication. Prospective evaluation of 100 patients with "typical" symptoms. *Ann Surg*. 1998;228:40.
97. DeMeester TR, Bonavina L, Albertucci M. Nissen fundoplication for gastroesophageal reflux disease—evaluation of primary repair in 100 consecutive patients. *Ann Surg*. 1986;204:9.
98. Bammer T, Hinder RA, Klaus A, et al. Five-to eight year outcome of the first laparoscopic Nissen fundoplications. *J Gastrointest Surg*. 2001;5:42.
99. Granderath FA, Kamolz T, Schweiger UM, et al. Long-term results of laparoscopic antireflux surgery; surgical outcomes and analysis of failure after 500 laparoscopic antireflux procedures. *Surg Endosc*. 2002; 16:753.
100. **Catarci M, Gentileschi P, Papi C, et al. Evidence-based appraisal of antireflux fundopplicaion. *Ann Surg*. 2004;239:325.**
101. Lundell L., Miettinen P, Myrvold HE, et al. Continued (5-year) follow-up of a randomized clinical study comparing antireflux surgery and omeprozole in gastroesophageal reflux diesease. *J Am Coll Surg*. 2001;192:172.
102. Nilsson G, Wenner J, Larsson S, et al. Randomized clinical trial of laparoscopic versus open fundoplication for gastroesophageal reflux. *Br J Surg*. 2004;91:552.
103. Finlayson SRG, Laycock WS, Birkmeyer JD. National trends in utilization and outcomes of antireflux surgery. *Surg Endosc*. 2003;17:864.
104. So JB, Zeitels SM, Rattner DW. Outcomes of atypical symptoms attributed to gastroesophageal reflux treated by laparoscopic fundoplication. *Surgery* 1998;124:28.
105. Spechler SJ. Comparison of medical and surgical therapy for complicated gastroesophageal reflux disease in veterans. The Department of Veterans Affairs Gastroesophageal Reflux Disease Study Group. *N Engl J Med*. 1992;326:786.
106. Spechler SJ, Lee E, Ahnen D, et al. Long-term outcome of medical and surgical therapies for gastroesophageal reflux disease: follow-up of a randomized controlled trial. *JAMA* 2001;285:2331.
107. Lord RVN, Kaminski A, Oberg S, et al. Absence of gastroesophageal reflux disease in a majority of patients taking acid suppression medications after Nissen fundoplication. *J Gastrointest Surg*. 2002;6:3.
108. Testa MA, Simonson DC. Assessment of quality-of-life outcomes. *N Engl J Med*. 1996;334:835.
109. Trus TL, Laycock WS, Waring JP, et al. Improvement in quality of life measures following laparoscopic antireflux surgery. *Ann Surg*. 1999;229:331.
110. Glise H, Hallerbäck B, Johansson B. Quality-of-life assessments in evaluation of laparoscopic Rosetti fundoplication. *Surg Endosc*. 1995;9:183.
111. Velonovich V, Vallance SR, Gusz JR, et al. Quality of life scale for gastroesophageal reflux disease. *J Am Coll Surg*. 1996;183:217.
112. Fernando HC, Schauer PR, Rosenblatt M, et al. Quality of life after antireflux surgery compared with nonoperative management for severe gastroesophageal reflux disease. *J Am Coll Surg*. 2002;194:23.

CHAPTER 44 ■ ESOPHAGEAL INJURY, DIVERTICULA, AND NEOPLASMS

JOHN C. KUCHARCZUK AND LARRY R. KAISER

The role of the esophagus is to propel food and secretions from the pharynx to the stomach. As such, it is primarily an organ of motility with no absorptive capacity. It also provides an important barrier function, isolating the mediastinum from the bacteria present in the mouth and external environment.

The esophageal anatomy is discussed in previous chapters. Nevertheless, several specific anatomic points need to be highlighted when discussing surgery for injuries and tumors or the esophagus. First, indentations made on the esophagus by external mediastinal structures are clinically important. These indentations can readily be seen on esophagram (Fig. 44.1). The cricopharyngeus causes the first constriction of the esophagus and is a common location for iatrogenic perforations caused by instrumentation. The second indentation seen to the left of the esophagus is the aortic arch, which is a common location for food or foreign body impaction. The third indentation is the left mainstem bronchus.

In the adult, esophageal length is variable depending on upper body length. Nevertheless, the overall average length from the upper esophageal sphincter to the lower one approximates 24 cm or 10 inches. Because endoscopy plays an important role in the localization of esophageal injuries and tumors, esophageal locations are usually referenced relative to the distance from the incisors. Thus, on average, the esophagus begins at 16 cm from the incisors and ends at 38 to 40 cm from the incisors.

Externally, the esophagus is composed of an outer layer of longitudinal muscle and an inner layer of circular muscle. There is no serosal layer as ensheaths all other parts of the gastrointestinal tract. Transmural invasion by esophageal carcinoma is common because the tumor is not limited by overlying serosa or pleura. This is in contrast to other gastrointestinal cancers, which usually extend to, but not through, the peritoneum. Another important anatomic feature of the esophagus is the unique submucosal layer. This layer has a high fat content, which accounts for the mobility of the overlying mucosa. Because of this arrangement, care must be taken to ensure that every anastomotic suture transfixes the submucosa; if it does not "an anastomotic leak will occur when the mucosa retracts proximally and an accurate apposition of the mucosa is not achieved."[1]

The esophageal blood supply is segmental. The esophagus is vascularized by numerous arteries coursing through the lateral attachments, and it has an extensive submucosal collateral circulation. The cervical esophagus receives blood from the superior and inferior thyroid arteries. Multiple aortic esophageal arteries supply the intrathoracic esophagus and through collaterals connect with the inferior thyroid, intercostal, bronchial, inferior phrenic, and left gastric arteries. Improper control of these vessels during a transhiatal esophagectomy can result in significant blood loss.

The esophagus is innervated by the autonomic nervous system. The cervical esophagus receives parasympathetic innervation through the recurrent laryngeal branches of the vagus nerve. Thus, injury to the recurrent laryngeal nerve not only produces hoarseness and a poor cough but may also result in upper esophageal sphincter dysfunction predisposing to life-threatening aspiration following esophagectomy.

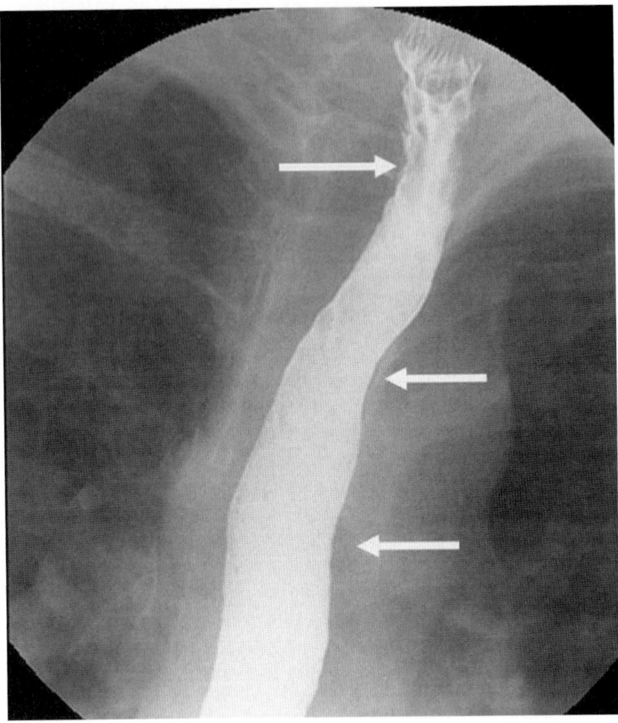

FIGURE 44.1 Barium contrast esophagography showing the constriction caused by the cricopharyngeal muscle, aortic arch, and the left mainstem bronchus. Indentations of the esophagus made by external structures are important anatomic landmarks and are often the sites of perforation due to instrumentation.

SURGICAL APPROACHES TO THE ESOPHAGUS

Multiple factors influence the surgical approach to the esophagus. These include the nature of the injury or neoplasm (benign vs. malignant), the overall health of the patient, and the expertise of the surgeon.

A complete working knowledge of the anatomic relationships between the esophagus and adjacent structures is vital to planning surgical therapy. The upper thoracic esophagus is in contact with the posterior membranous trachea, the left mainstem bronchus, and the aortic arch. Patients with cancers involving the upper thoracic esophagus must undergo preoperative bronchoscopy to rule out invasion of the posterior membranous trachea, because this precludes resection. Although flexible bronchoscopy may demonstrate gross airway invasion, rigid bronchoscopy is much more sensitive in determining adherence to the membranous trachea. Loss of the normal "ripple" effect as the rigid scope slides over the membranous trachea suggests the tumor is fixed to the airway and is not resectable. This is equally important where the esophagus passes under the left mainstem bronchus.

From a surgical perspective, the esophagus is divided into thirds. The upper third can be reached through a cervical incision. The middle third is best approached through the right chest; access to the middle third of the esophagus from the left chest is obscured by the aorta. The distal third of the esophagus is best approached through the left chest. The short segment of intraabdominal esophagus may be approached through the upper abdomen.

When esophagectomy is required, several surgical approaches have been described. These include the transhiatal approach,[2] the transabdominal transthoracic approach (Ivor-Lewis),[3] the "three stage" approach (McKeown),[4] the thoracoabdominal approach, and the "minimally invasive" approach. These approaches are described in detail. Each approach has its own set of risks and benefits as well as outspoken opponents and proponents. Selection of the appropriate approach requires experienced surgical judgment. Despite the rhetoric, several studies have shown equivalent outcomes among the multiple approaches. It appears that the experience of the surgeon[5] and the number of cases performed at a particular institution are the leading factors determining outcome.[6] Clearly, failures in technique that occur during the performance of an esophagectomy are associated with increased length of hospital stay and increased in-hospital mortality and are predictive of a poorer overall long-term survival.[7]

ESOPHAGEAL INJURY

Perforation

Despite decades of clinical experience and surgical innovation, perforation of the esophagus continues to present diagnostic and therapeutic challenges. Accurate diagnosis and early treatment are essential to the successful management of patients with esophageal perforation. Outcome is determined by the cause and location of the injury, the presence of concomitant esophageal disease, and the interval between perforation and initiation of therapy.

The causes of esophageal perforation are listed in Table 44.1. Over the past decade, the incidence of esophageal perforation has increased and the most common etiology has changed from spontaneous and traumatic to iatrogenic. This is due to the increasing use of invasive diagnostic and therapeutic endoscopic procedures. In our review of the literature, we found that iatrogenic injury to the esophagus by instrumentation accounted for 59% of all cases and spontaneous perforations accounted for only 15%.[8]

Other, less common injuries include foreign body ingestion (12%) and trauma (9%). Ingestion of foreign bodies or caustic materials can produce perforation in areas of anatomic narrowing including the cricopharyngeus, the segment where the aortic arch and left mainstem bronchus impinge on the

TABLE 44.1 ETIOLOGY

CAUSES OF ESOPHAGEAL PERFORATION

INSTRUMENTAL
- Endoscopy
- Dilation
- Intubation
- Sclerotherapy
- Laser therapy

NONINSTRUMENTAL
- Barogenic trauma
  - Postemetic (Boerhaave's syndrome)
  - Blunt chest or abdominal trauma
  - Other (e.g., labor, convulsions, defecation)
- Penetrating neck, chest, or abdominal trauma
- Operative trauma
  - Esophageal reconstruction (anastomotic disruption)
  - Vagotomy, pulmonary resection, hiatal hernia repair, esophagomyotomy
- Corrosive injuries (acid or alkali ingestion)
- Erosion by adjacent infection
- Swallowed foreign body

esophagus, and at the distal esophageal sphincter. External penetrating trauma causes perforations mainly in the cervical esophagus, the portion not protected by the thoracic cage. The morbidity and mortality of penetrating esophageal trauma is usually the result of the associated injuries including major vascular and airway injuries.[9] Blunt traumatic perforation is exceedingly rare but may be evident following motor vehicle accident or performance of the Heimlich maneuver.

Spontaneous, or barogenic, esophageal perforation results from a sudden increase in intraesophageal pressure. This has been associated with hyperemesis, childbirth, seizure, prolonged coughing, or weightlifting. Of special historical note are patients with Boerhaave's syndrome. These patients develop spontaneous perforation of the distal esophagus after the excessive ingestion of food and alcohol followed by violent emesis resulting in disruption of the distal esophagus with soilage into the left pleural cavity. This syndrome is named after Herman Boerhaave who, in 1723, provided a detailed account with postmortem correlation of the spontaneous perforation of the esophagus of the High Admiral of the Dutch Navy, Baron Van Wassenaer.[10]

Clinical Features

The presenting clinical features of esophageal perforation depend on the location of the perforation and the time interval between injury and presentation. Patients with cervical perforations generally present with cervical dysphagia, neck pain, dysphonia, and subcutaneous cervical emphysema. This is in distinction to patients with intrathoracic perforations, who often present with signs and symptoms of mediastinitis. These include tachycardia, tachypnea, fever, and leukocytosis. Perforations of the intraabdominal esophagus result in soilage of the peritoneal cavity and present as an acute abdomen. As with thoracic perforations, patients present with tachycardia, tachypnea, fever, and leukocytosis. Systemic sepsis, rapid deterioration, and shock are common.

Diagnosis

The diagnosis of esophageal perforation begins with a high level of suspicion. Esophageal perforation must be ruled out in any patient presenting with cervical, thoracic, or abdominal pain following endoscopy. Contrast esophagography remains the gold standard for diagnosis. Water-soluble contrast (e.g., Gastrografin) is the initial agent used for contrast esophagography. These agents demonstrate extravasation in 50% of cervical perforations and 80% of perforations located within the chest.[11] If no extravasation is seen with Gastrografin, thin barium should be used because it will demonstrate 60% of cervical perforations and 90% of intrathoracic perforations.[12] In patients known to have problems with aspiration or in cases of suspected airway-esophageal fistula, barium contrast should be used alone because the hyperosmolar water-soluble contrast agents may cause rapid pulmonary edema and ventilatory collapse.

Flexible esophagoscopy may be used to directly visualize and localize the area of perforation. It has a sensitivity of 100% and a specificity of 80%.[13] Proponents of flexible esophagoscopy use this technique for confirmation of the injury and in planning the surgical approach. Opponents of this practice argue that air insufflation enlarges the injury and results in further bacterial contamination. One particular case that warrants special discussion is a mucosal or submucosal tear without perforation. Clearly, endoscopy is contraindicated in these patients as air insufflation may convert this to a full-thickness injury, thus converting a problem that could be managed conservatively to one that requires surgical intervention. We routinely perform flexible endoscopy for localization in patients requiring operative management of their perforation. In the small subset of patients who will be treated conservatively, we avoid the practice.

Computed tomography (CT) scan is useful in localizing collections in the pleural space or mediastinum; it is not used to localize the primary site of perforation. We do not generally obtain this study on presentation, although many patients have this study performed prior to surgical consultation. The real value of CT scanning is in the patient who remains septic following drainage and repair. The CT scan may reveal a collection requiring percutaneous or operative drainage.

Management

The treatment of esophageal perforation is dictated by the location of the perforation, the amount of soilage present, the clinical condition of the patient, and the presence of underlying esophageal pathology. The goal of treatment is to stabilize the patient, stop ongoing soilage, control infection, and reestablish esophageal continuity. Our current protocol for management of esophageal perforations is outlined in Algorithm 44.1.

Nonoperative Treatment. In practice, only a very small subset of patients with esophageal perforation are appropriate for nonoperative treatment. The successful use of nonoperative therapy requires careful patient selection, sound surgical judgment, and repeated clinical evaluation. Because the stakes are so high, it must be recognized that operative treatment really is the more "conservative" approach. Selecting the wrong patient or making a poor judgment will lead to local complications, continued sepsis, and a potentially devastating outcome.

The first reported series of the nonoperative treatment of esophageal perforation appeared in 1965 and included 18 patients with instrument perforations of the thoracic esophagus; there was only one death.[14] In 1979, Cameron et al.[15] established a set of criteria to aid in the selection of patients for nonoperative management. Currently, nonoperative management is appropriate for the treatment of all intramural dissections without evidence of frank full-thickness perforation. For transmural perforations, however, the approach can be considered only if (a) the perforation is well contained, (b) there is no associated esophageal malignancy, (c) the perforation is not in the abdominal cavity, (d) there is no simultaneous obstructive esophageal disease, and (e) there are no signs or symptoms of systemic sepsis.[16]

Nonoperative management begins with the administration of broad-spectrum antibiotics, the suspension of oral intake, and the institution of alternative nutrition either parenterally or enteral via a gastric or jejunal feeding tube. Vigilant monitoring for fever, tachycardia, and leukocytosis suggesting impending sepsis is necessary. Any clinical deterioration suggests failure of this approach should prompt expedient operative intervention. From a practical standpoint, it is best to think in terms of operative management whenever esophageal perforation is suspected.

Operative Treatment. The operative management of esophageal perforation is dictated by the location of the perforation, the extent of injury, and the presence or absence of underlying esophageal pathology. Approaches include primary reinforced repair, esophagectomy with immediate reconstruction, and exclusion or resection with diversion.

The typical radiographic studies of a patient with cervical esophageal perforation are shown in Figure 44.2. Perforations of the upper third of the esophagus down to the level of the carina are treated by cervical drainage. This is easily performed through a left neck incision as depicted in Figure 44.3. Usually it is not necessary to find or close the perforation. However, ensuring complete drainage by opening the prevertebral fascia is of paramount importance. If the perforation is easily seen, it can be sutured with minimal difficulty. A small open gastrostomy tube or jejunostomy tube is placed for enteral feeding during the recovery period. Oral intake is prohibited for 1 week, and then the patient is restudied with contrast esophagography. If no extravasation is noted, the diet is advanced, the drain is removed, and the patient is discharged. If a leak persists, oral intake is again prohibited, enteral feeding is continued, and the patient is studied at 1-week intervals until resolution occurs. As long as there is no underlying distal esophageal pathology, essentially all adequately drained esophageal perforations will heal spontaneously.

Perforations of the middle third are best approached through a right fifth intercostal space thoracotomy. We favor a buttressed primary repair whenever possible, even in delayed presentations.[17] Material for buttressing the repair includes flaps of pleura, pericardium, diaphragm, omentum, or muscle. For small- to moderate-size repairs, we prefer an intercostal muscle flap. This is a reliable pedicled muscle flap based on the intercostal vessels. It should be harvested at the start of the procedure prior to the placement of retractors to avoid damage to the vascular pedicle. Once harvested, the chest is opened, all pleural collections are drained, and the perforation is localized. Necrotic tissue around the perforation is débrided. A vertical myotomy is performed to fully expose the rent in the mucosa, which almost always extends beyond the tear in the muscularis. The proximal and distal extent of the mucosal tear must be fully visualized and repaired; failure to do so will result in persistent leakage. We repair the mucosa with interrupted absorbable sutures and then reapproximate the muscular layer with interrupted fine silk suture. The intercostal muscle is then secured as an onlay patch. The steps involved in the operation are depicted in Figure 44.4. Large chest tubes are placed and the patient is recovered. Enteral access either via a gastrostomy tube or jejunostomy tube aides in postoperative nutrition. A contrast swallow is performed on postoperative day 7. If there is no ongoing leakage, an oral diet is restarted

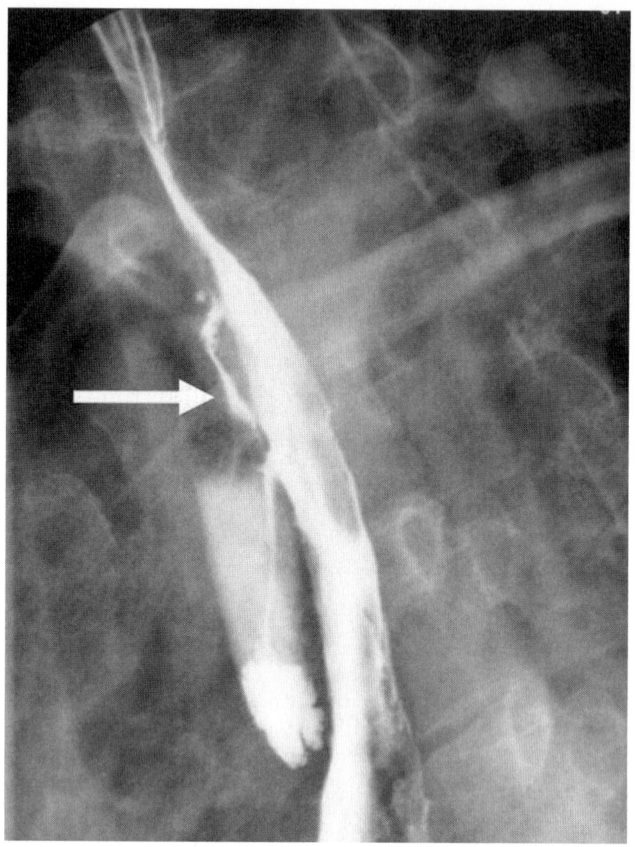

FIGURE 44.2 (*A*) Barium swallow and (*B*) computed tomography scan showing cervical esophageal perforation. The patient was treated with drainage and 1 week of gastrostomy tube feeding. The follow-up swallow at 1 week showed resolution.

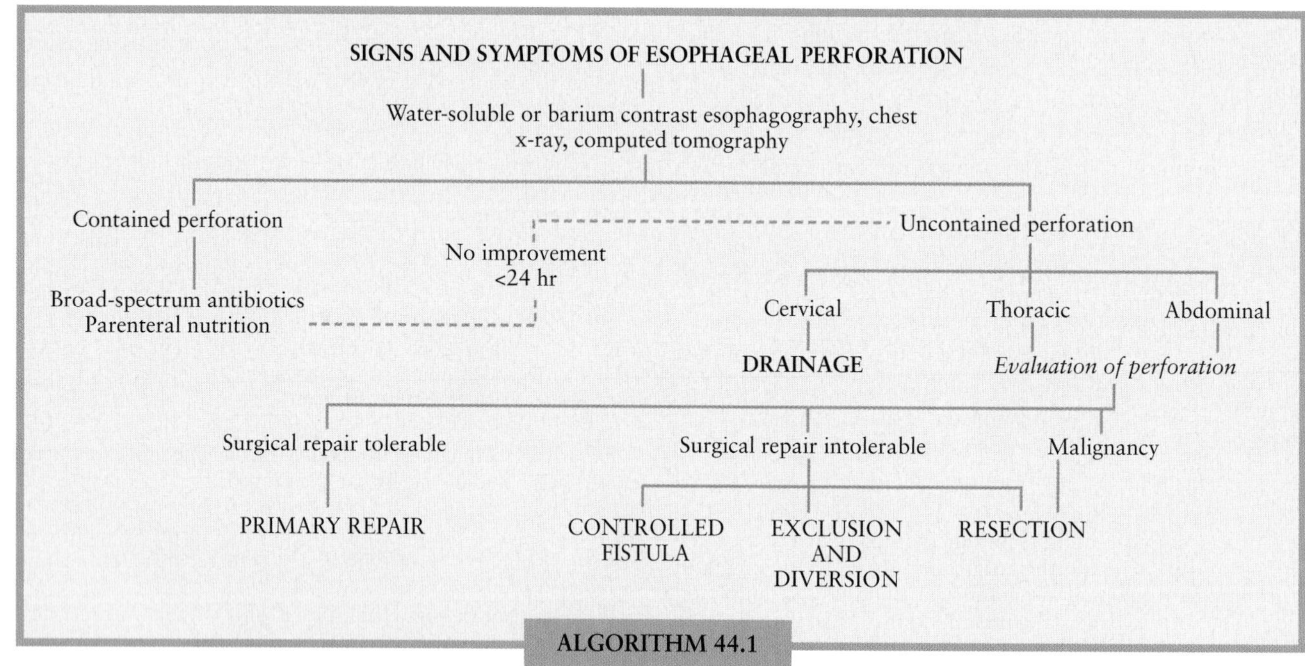

ALGORITHM 44.1 Evaluation and treatment of esophageal perforation. (After Brinster CJ, Singhal S, Lawrence L, et al. Evolving options in the management of esophageal perforation. *Ann Thorac Surg*. 2004;77:1475.)

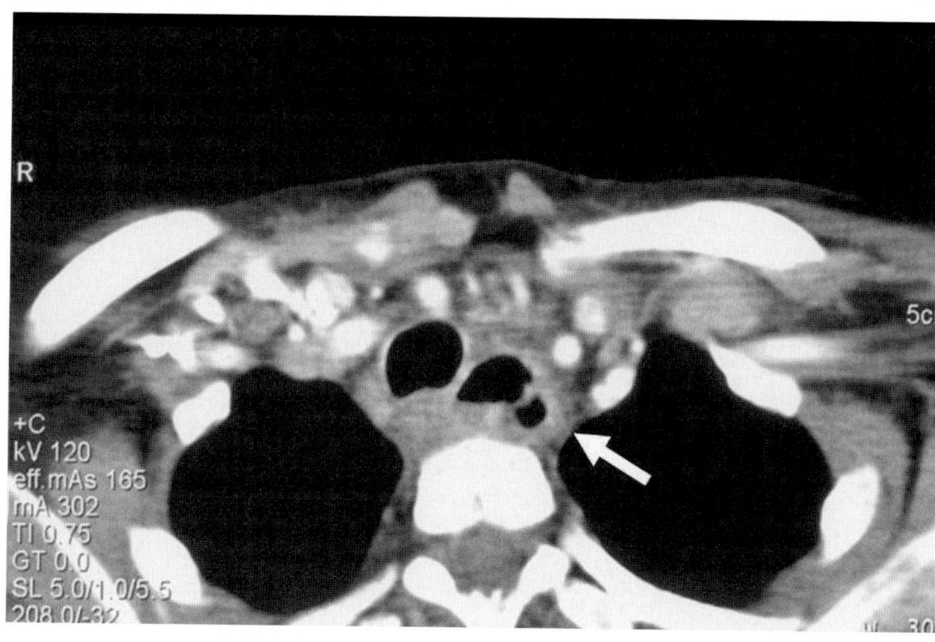

FIGURE 44.2 (*Continued*)

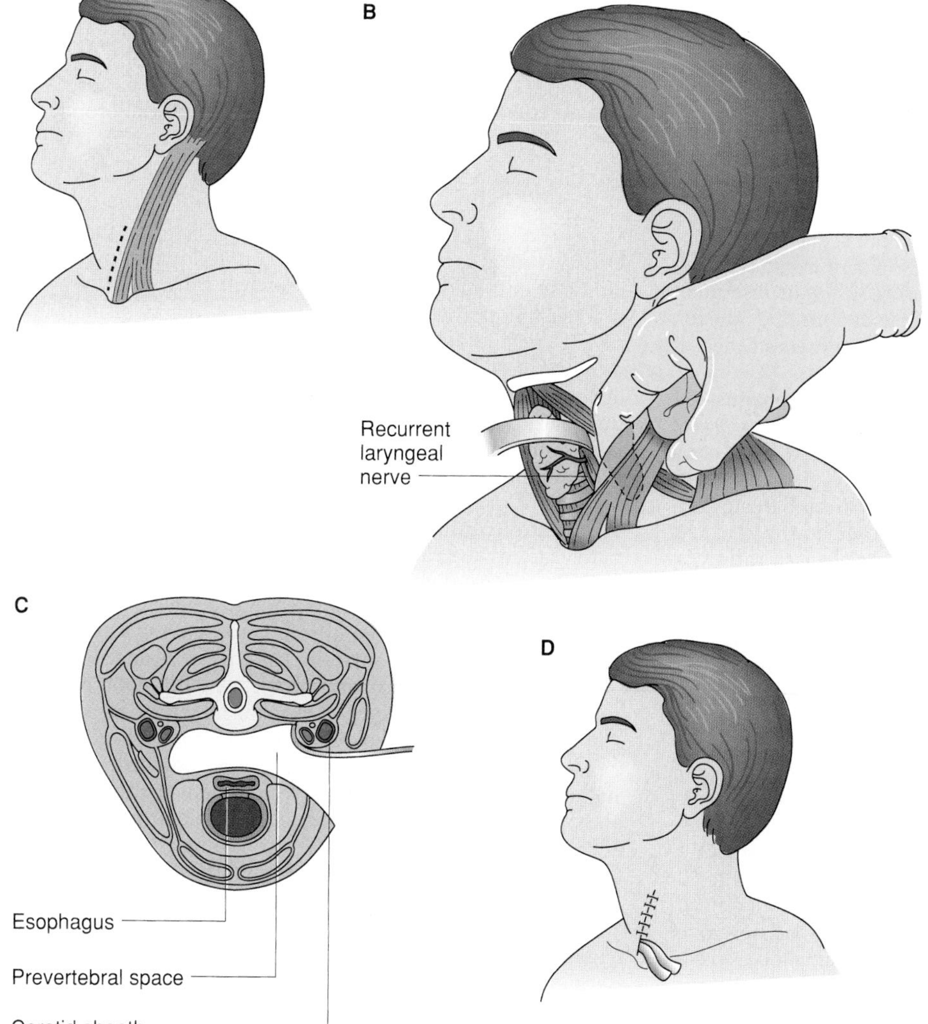

FIGURE 44.3 Approach for drainage of a cervical esophageal perforation. (*A*) Skin incision parallel to the anterior border of the left sternocleidomastoid muscle, extending from the level of the cricoid cartilage to the sternal notch. (*B*) With the sternocleidomastoid muscle and carotid sheath retracted laterally and the trachea and thyroid gland medially, blunt dissection along the prevertebral fascia in the superior mediastinum is carried out. Injury to the recurrent laryngeal nerve in the tracheoesophageal groove must be avoided. (*C*) Schematic drawing of the prevertebral space drained by this cervical approach. (*D*) Two 1-in rubber drains placed into the superior mediastinum are brought out through the neck wound to allow establishment of an esophagocutaneous fistula, which usually heals spontaneously. (After Orringer MB. The mediastinum. In: Nora PH, ed. *Operative surgery,* 3rd ed. Philadelphia: WB Saunders; 1990:370.)

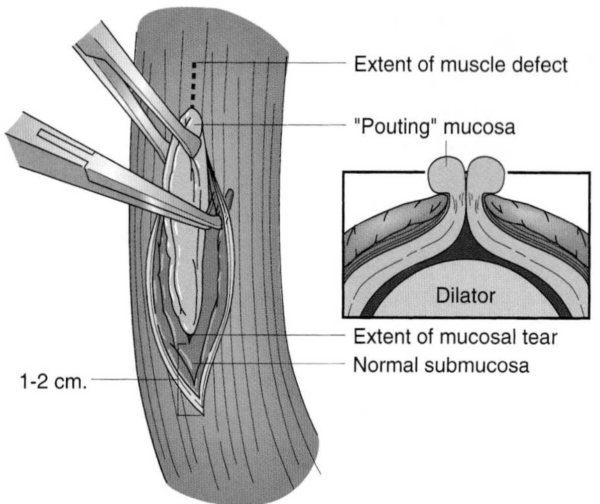

FIGURE 44.4 Primary repair of esophageal perforation. The edematous mucosa pouting through the muscular defect (inset) is grasped with Allis clamps and elevated. A 1-cm vertical esophagomyotomy is made at either end of the muscular defect to expose the entire limits of the tear. This is facilitated by using a right-angle clamp to direct muscularis away from underlying submucosa around the entire circumference of the tear. The result of this mobilization is exposure of a circumferential rim of normal submucosa that can then be closed. (After Whyte RI, Iannettoni MD, Orringer MB. Intrathoracic esophageal perforation: the merit of primary repair. *J Thorac Cardiovasc Surg*. 1995;109:140.)

and the chest tubes are removed. Persistent leaks are treated conservatively with chest tube drainage and alternative nutrition as long as the leak is well drained and there is no sign of clinical instability. If such a patient becomes systemically ill, CT scanning is indicated to identify any undrained collections. Reoperation with the goal of obtaining better and more complete drainage may be required on occasion. Depending on the findings of the CT scan and reexploration, the leaking repair may need to be taken down, and the esophagus excluded with a cervical esophagostomy. If this is required, subsequent reconstruction can be very challenging; therefore, exclusion with diversion is reserved for those patients in whom there is no other viable alternative.

Perforations of the distal third of the esophagus are approached via a left seventh intercostal space thoracotomy. Again a pedicled intercostal muscle flap is harvested, the chest is opened, the mediastinum is drained, and the perforation site is identified. The technique for primary repair and postoperative management is the same as described previously.

The operative treatment of esophageal perforation in patients with underlying esophageal pathology deserves special consideration. Repair of a proximal perforation with distal obstruction will fail, and the obstructing lesion must be addressed at the initial procedure. For distal strictures, simple intraoperative dilation will usually decompress the esophagus to allow healing of a proximal perforation.

Patients with achalasia who are perforated during pneumatic dilation warrant separate discussion. Most have small, asymptomatic mucosal tears or well-contained small perforations and as such are candidates for nonoperative management as long as the dilation has successfully relieved the distal obstruction. For those that fail nonoperative management or do not qualify for it, the decision on how to proceed surgically requires thought and discussion. In patients with achalasia and preserved esophageal motility, the perforation should be repaired primarily, a vertical esophageal myotomy should be performed 180 degrees opposite the injury, and a noncircumferential wrap such as a modified Belsey should be performed. Recently it has been demonstrated that a "floppy" or loose Nissen fundoplication or 360-degree wrap may be just as acceptable and likely to be more familiar to the surgeon who does esophageal surgery only on an occasional basis. For patients with decompensated achalasia, a sigmoid nonfunctional esophagus, and a perforation who are hemodynamically stable, consideration should be given to performance of esophagectomy with immediate restoration of gastrointestinal continuity.

Unstable patients with thoracic esophageal perforation and associated severe underlying esophageal pathology should be treated with exclusion and diversion. This includes a cervical esophagostomy, pleural drainage, stapled division of the gastroesophageal (GE) junction, and placement of gastrostomy and jejunostomy tubes. If the patient survives, he or she can be brought back to the operating room at a later time for restoration of gastrointestinal continuity, usually following 6 to 8 weeks of recovery.

Foreign Body

Foreign body ingestion typically occurs in pediatric, psychiatric, alcoholic, and elderly patients. Most objects remain in the cervical esophagus; blunt objects as well as small sharp objects usually can be removed either by flexible and/or rigid esophagoscopy. Objects such as fish and chicken bones can be "reoriented" with a long grasper and easily brought out through a rigid esophagoscope. Large, rigid foreign bodies with sharp edges embedded in the mucosa and those that exceed the diameter of the rigid endoscope in all orientations pose a particularly difficult problem and may require esophagotomy for removal. Following endoscopic removal of a foreign body, completion esophagoscopy and contrast esophagography should be performed to rule out esophageal perforation. If a perforation is present, the patient is managed according to the esophageal protocol presented in Algorithm 44.1.

Caustic Injury

Caustic injury to the esophagus occurs following ingestion of either strong acids or strong base chemicals, usually household cleaning products. Ingestions in children are usually accidental and the quantities involved small. Ingestions in adults are often associated with a suicide attempt or other psychiatric illness. The quantities swallowed in this group can be quite large and the injury extensive. Fortunately, these types of ingestion injuries are relatively rare today when compared to the number formerly seen.

Management of caustic ingestion injuries requires experienced surgical judgment.[18] The first step in caring for any patient following caustic ingestion is airway protection. Burns to the oropharynx result in ongoing edema and may cause loss of the airway. A tracheostomy should be performed early if this is suspected. The second step is to determine the type of agent, the approximate quantity, and the time since ingestion.

Unfortunately, history and physical examination alone are not predictive of the degree of esophageal injury. Severe injury can occur in the absence of significant oropharyngeal burns; thus, examination of the esophagus is required. When the ingestion is minor or questionable and there are no symptoms, the patient should be observed and flexible upper endoscopy is carried out at 24 to 48 hours. This timing allows for an adequate endoscopic evaluation of the injury, whereas immediate endoscopy may underestimate the extent of esophageal damage. In symptomatic patients or those with suspected large ingestions of strong caustic agents, immediate esophagoscopy should be performed. The esophageal injury is graded endoscopically as shown in Table 44.2. This information is used to determine the appropriate treatment. The acute management is summarized in Algorithm 44.2.

TABLE 44.2 CLASSIFICATION

ENDOSCOPIC GRADING OF ACUTE CAUSTIC INJURY TO THE ESOPHAGUS

Injury grade	Endoscopic appearance	Depth of injury
I	Superficial hyperemia	Mucosal
II A	Sloughing mucosa, superficial ulceration	Patch partial thickness
II B	Deep ulceration	Circumferential
III	Eschar, necrosis	Full thickness

ESOPHAGEAL DIVERTICULA

Esophageal diverticula may arise at any location along the length of the esophagus. True esophageal diverticula contain all layers of the esophageal wall and are unusual. If present, they are caused by traction on the esophageal wall and occur in regions of periesophageal inflammation, typically the midthoracic portion of the esophagus adjacent to the inflamed subcarinal lymph nodes. Pseudo or false diverticula are caused by pulsion. They are a manifestation of underlying motility disorders that include hypertonic esophageal peristalsis, failure of sphincter relaxation, or both. Pseudodiverticula contain only mucosa and submucosal layers of the esophageal wall.

Diverticula of the esophagus are usually discovered and confirmed on esophagram. Those found incidentally in asymptomatic patients do not require surgical intervention. The symptomatic patient may present with dysphagia, regurgitation, choking, weight loss, and recurrent pneumonia. The specific surgical intervention in symptomatic patients depends on the location and associated underlying esophageal abnormalities. From a surgical perspective, esophageal diverticula are best discussed by division into three separate categories based on anatomic location: cervical, midthoracic, and epiphrenic diverticula.

Cervical Pharyngoesophageal Diverticulum

A Zenker's or pharyngoesophageal diverticula are the most common type of the esophagus. They occur at Killian's triangle, which is an anatomic weakness in the posterior pharyngeal constrictor muscle just above the cricopharyngeus muscle. These are pulsion-type pseudodiverticula and result from a combination of the anatomic weakness at Killian's triangle and an underlying motility disorder manifested by incoordinated or incomplete relaxation of the upper esophageal sphincter (cricopharyngeus) during swallowing (Fig. 44.5). Symptoms are an indication for surgical intervention.

Any surgical approach to a Zenker's diverticulum must address the underlying motility disorder to be successful. Diverticulectomy alone has an unacceptably high recurrence rate. A cricopharyngeal myotomy is required to produce a durable result. The traditional surgical approach is via a left cervical incision along the border of the sternocleidomastoid muscle. The omohyoid muscle is divided and dissection is continued down to the prevertebral fascia. The diverticulum is located and carefully dissected from the surrounding tissues down to its base. Small diverticula (less than 2 cm) can be suspended to provide drainage; however, larger diverticula should be excised with

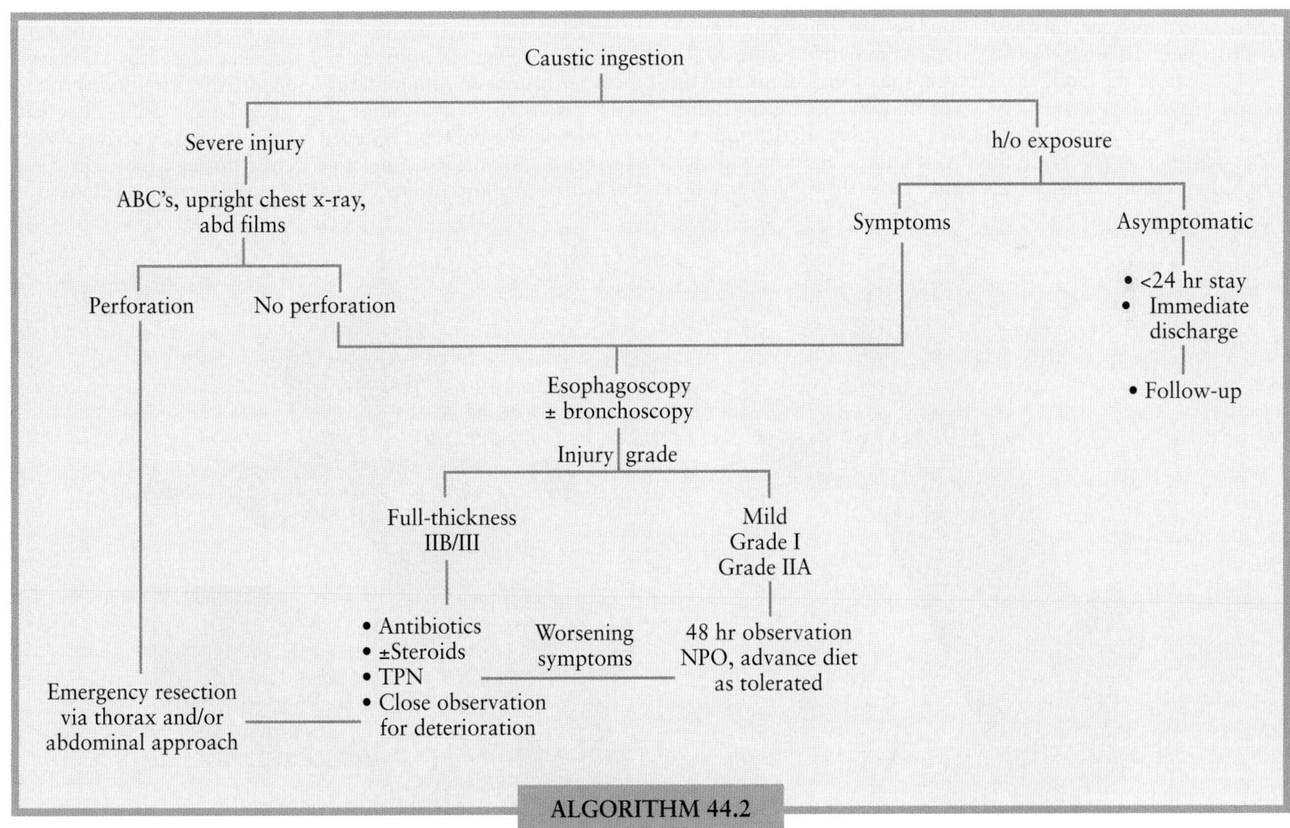

ALGORITHM 44.2 Evaluation and management of acute caustic ingestion. (After Paidas, Charles N. Caustic burns of the esophagus. In: Yang, Cameron, eds. *Current therapy in thoracic and cardiovascular surgery.* Philadelphia: Mosby; 2004:99.)

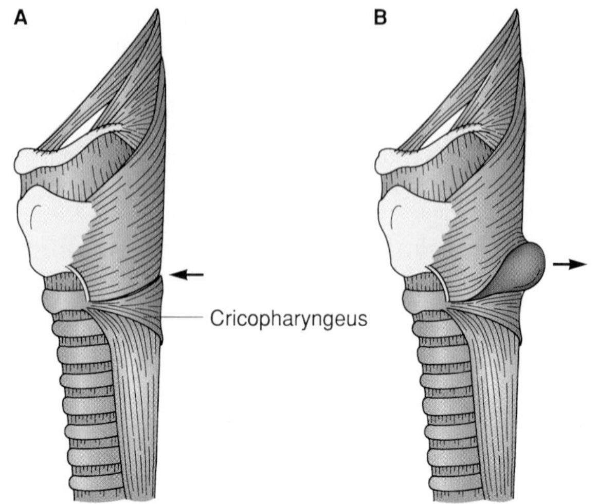

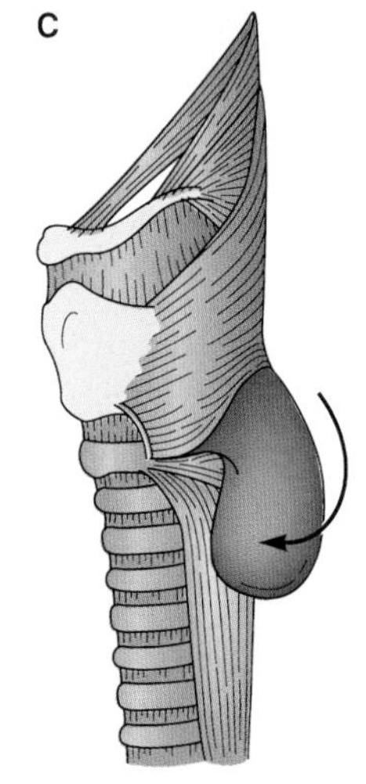

FIGURE 44.5 Formation of pharyngoesophageal (Zenker's) diverticulum. (*A*) Herniation of the pharyngeal mucosa and submucosa occurs at the point of potential weakness (Killian's triangle) (*arrow*) between the oblique fibers of the thyropharyngeus muscle and the more horizontal fibers of the cricopharyngeus muscle. (*B*) and (*C*): As the diverticulum enlarges, it drapes over the cricopharyngeus sphincter and descends into the superior mediastinum in the prevertebral space. (After Orringer MB. Diverticula and miscellaneous conditions of the esophagus. In: Sabiston DC Jr, ed. *Textbook of surgery*, 13th ed. Philadelphia: WB Saunders; 1986:726.)

a gastrointestinal stapler (Fig. 44.6). A 40-Fr bougie is placed prior to staple excision to avoid narrowing the esophagus. A vertical myotomy is performed through the entire length of the cricopharyngeus. A small drain is placed and the neck is closed. The largest surgical series of open transcervical diverticulectomy was reported from the Mayo Clinic.[19] The series included more than 900 patients and reported 93% durable resolution of symptoms with an 8% perioperative complication rate.

An alternative approach is transoral stapling, which creates a common channel between the esophagus and the diverticulum while dividing the cricopharyngeus muscle. This approach was simultaneously reported in 1993 by independent groups in the United Kingdom[20] and Belgium.[21] The transoral procedure is performed under general anesthesia. The Weerda bivalved diverticuloscope (Karl Storz, Culver City, CA) shown in Figure 44.7 is used to expose the esophageal lumen, the diverticulum, and the common wall between the two. An Endo-GIA surgical stapler (U.S. Surgical Corp. Norwalk, CT) is inserted through the diverticuloscope to divide the diverticular common wall and cricopharyngeus muscle. A large U.S. series from Duke University Medical Center reports on 71 patients undergoing transoral stapling with 97% relief of symptoms and a low complication rate.[22] This approach is more widely used in Europe and is the most commonly performed technique employed by U.K. otolaryngologists in the management of these patients.[23]

Midthoracic Diverticulum

Most midthoracic diverticula are asymptomatic and do not require surgical treatment. Barium swallow is the diagnostic study of choice to demonstrate a midthoracic diverticula. These can be true or false diverticula depending on their etiology. Those arising within a few centimeters of the carina are likely to be traction-type true diverticula caused by subcarinal or peribronchial inflammatory adenopathy. Pseudodiverticula can also occur in association with underlying motility disorders. Surgical intervention is reserved for symptomatic patients. When resection is indicated, the approach is through the right chest. The diverticulum is resected with a gastrointestinal stapler over

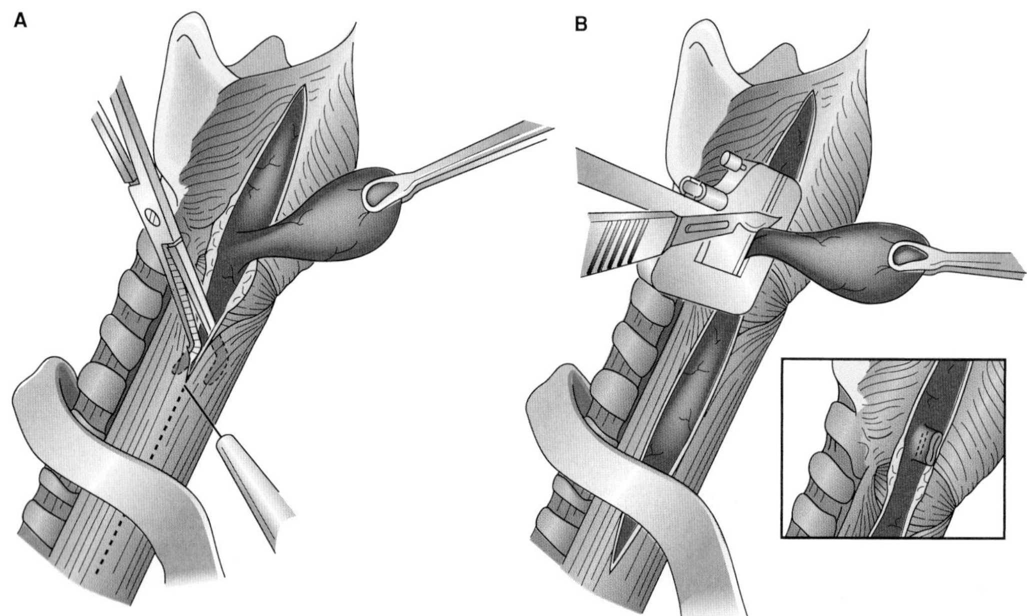

FIGURE 44.6 Cervical esophagomyotomy and concomitant resection of a pharyngoesophageal diverticulum. (*A*) An esophagomyotomy is performed for several centimeters in either vertical direction from the base of the mobilized diverticulum. (*B*) After completion of the esophagomyotomy, the base of the pouch is crossed with a TA-30 stapler and amputated. (After Orringer MB. Extended cervical esophagomyotomy for cricopharyngeal dysfunction. *J Thorac Cardiovasc Surg*. 1980;80:669.)

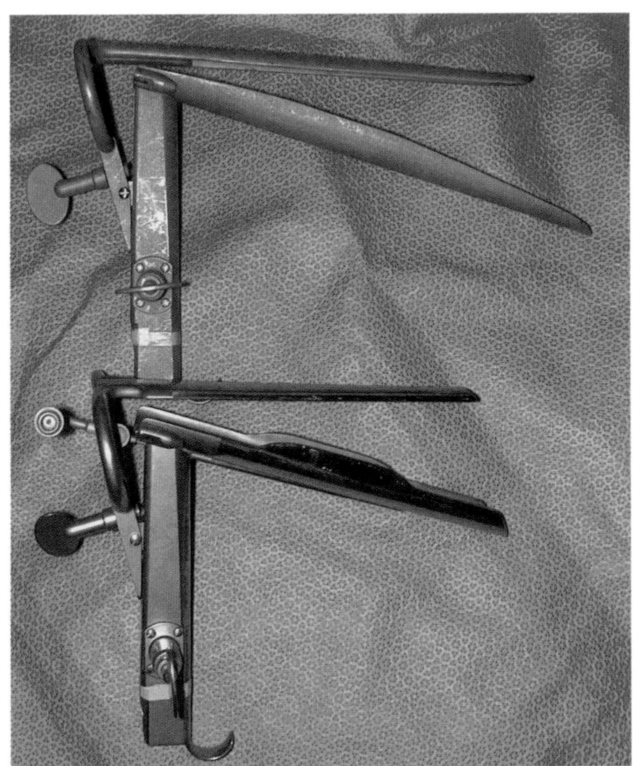

FIGURE 44.7 Weerda diverticuloscopes (Karl Storz, Tuttlingen, Germany) used to expose the common wall between the esophagus and a Zenker's diverticulum for transoral stapling.

a bougie to avoid narrowing of the esophageal lumen. The muscularis is reapproximated over the staple line with interrupted sutures and a myotomy is performed 180 degrees opposite the excision site to protect the staple line from high pressures.

Epiphrenic Diverticulum

Epiphrenic diverticula are pseudodiverticula caused by pulsion. They occur in the distal 10 cm of the esophagus and are associated with an underlying motility disorder. As with other types of esophageal diverticula, surgery is reserved for symptomatic patients.

Barium esophagram is the gold standard radiographic study for diagnosis. Esophageal manometry complements the study by more precisely identifying the underlying motility disorder.

The traditional surgical approach to epiphrenic diverticula is via a seventh interspace left thoracotomy, even if the diverticulum is projecting into the right chest. The inferior pulmonary ligament is incised up to the level of the inferior pulmonary vein, and the lung is retracted in a cephalad position. The pleura overlying the esophagus is incised and the esophagus is circumferentially dissected. A Penrose drain can be placed around the esophagus for retraction. The hiatus is opened and the fat pad at the GE junction is removed. This allows mobilization of the proximal stomach into the chest. The diverticulum is dissected free and excised with a stapler over a bougie to avoid narrowing of the esophagus. The muscularis is reapproximated with interrupted sutures over the staple line. Diverticulectomy alone is associated with a high primary leak and recurrence rate. Therefore, a longitudinal myotomy should be performed 180 degrees opposite the excision site. It is carried down onto the stomach for 1 to 2 cm and includes any manometrically defined abnormal segments.[24] Whether or not to perform an antireflux procedure remains debated. The authors prefer a modified Belsey-type partial wrap to avoid symptomatic postoperative reflux.

Recently, several case series have reported on the safety and efficacy of minimally invasive approaches to epiphrenic diverticula. These have included thoracoscopic[25] and laparoscopic approaches.[26] These reports demonstrate that minimally invasive approaches are feasible; however, whether or not this procedure has a durable result with fewer postoperative complications remains to be seen.

BENIGN NEOPLASMS

Table 44.3 shows a complete listing of the benign neoplasms of the esophagus. All are rare. Leiomyoma is the most common benign esophageal neoplasm and is discussed later. Esophageal polyps are also seen with some frequency at referral centers and deserve mention. The remainder of the benign neoplasms occur so infrequently that they are not individually discussed in this chapter.

Leiomyoma

Leiomyomas account for roughly two thirds of all benign tumors of the esophagus.[27] The incidence of leiomyoma reported in autopsy series ranges from 0.005% to 5.1%.[28] Approximately 80% of leiomyomas are located intramurally and originate in the muscularis propria. They are slow-growing tumors and therefore the size of the lesion may not change for many years. Leiomyomas usually presents as single lesions, although cases of multiple lesions have been reported.[29]

TABLE 44.3 CLASSIFICATION

CLASSIFICATION OF BENIGN ESOPHAGEAL TUMORS

EPITHELIAL TUMORS
Papillomas
Polyps
Adenomas
Cysts
NONEPITHELIAL TUMORS
Myomas
Leiomyomas
Fibromyomas
Lipomyomas
Fibromas
Vascular tumors
Hemangiomas
Lymphangiomas
Mesenchymal and other tumors
Reticuloendothelial tumors
Lipomas
Myxofibromas
Giant cell tumors
Neurofibromas
Osteochondromas
HETEROTOPIC TUMORS
Gastric mucosal tumors
Melanoblastic tumors
Sebaceous gland tumors
Granular cell myoblastomas
Pancreatic gland tumors
Thyroid nodules

From Nemir P Jr, Wallace HW, Fallahnejad M. Diagnosis and surgical management of benign disease of the esophagus. *Curr Probl Surg.* 1976;13:1, with permission.

Figure 44.8 shows the typical esophagogram of a midthoracic esophageal leiomyoma; note the smooth-walled appearance of the lesion, indicating that the mucosa is not involved by this submucosal lesion. Figure 44.9 shows the endoscopic appearance of a distal esophageal leiomyoma.

Evaluation of a patient with a suspected leiomyoma usually includes a barium swallow, endoscopy, endoscopic ultrasound (EUS), and a CT scan of the chest. Indications for resection of an esophageal leiomyoma include symptoms of dysphagia, increase in tumor size, mucosal ulceration, and definitive establishment of a diagnosis ruling out a malignant process such as a leiomyosarcoma. The surgical approach to these lesions depends on the size, location, and character of the leiomyoma. Leiomyomas less than 8 cm without annular characteristics are best treated by surgical extramucosal enucleation. Those greater than 8 cm or annular in character usually require esophageal resection. Treatment of the asymptomatic patient with a small leiomyoma (less than 3 cm) is controversial and can include either nonoperative surveillance or resection.[30] The process we employ for evaluation and treatment of esophageal leiomyomas is shown in Algorithm 44.3.

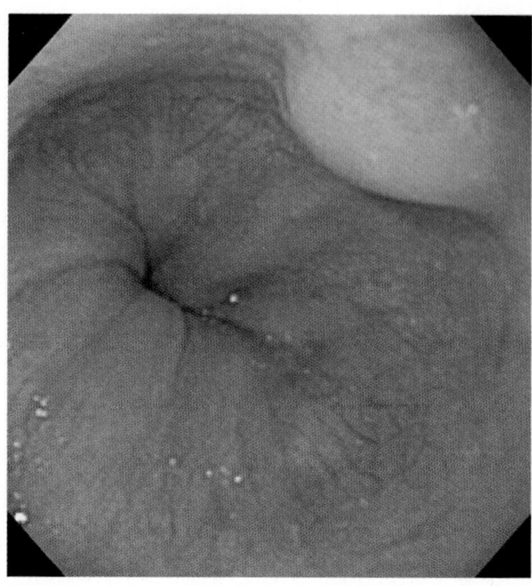

FIGURE 44.9 Endoscopic appearance of an esophageal leiomyoma at the level of the gastroesophageal junction. (Courtesy of Dr. Michael Kochman, Hospital of the University of Pennsylvania, Philadelphia.)

Fibrolipomas and Fibrovascular Polyps

Esophageal fibrolipomas present as intraluminal cervical esophageal polyps. The peristaltic action of the esophagus may cause this lesion to elongate over time and reach extraordinary lengths.[31] Patients present with dysphagia. The lesion almost always originates in the cervical esophagus; it is usually on a stalk and can be removed endoscopically. Very large lesions may require cervical esophagotomy or occasionally right thoracotomy for removal. With large polyps, asphyxiation has been reported when the stalked polyp "flips" into the airway and becomes trapped. They should be excised.

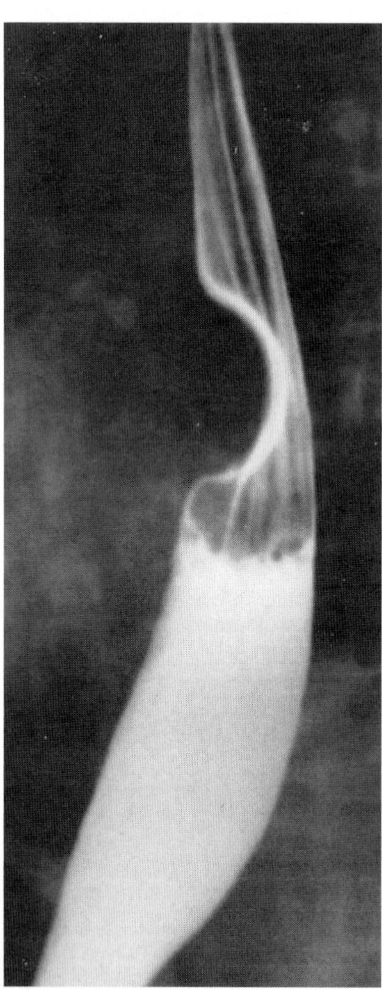

FIGURE 44.8 Esophagogram of a leiomyoma. The acute angle at its junction with the esophageal wall is typical. (From Orringer MB. Tumors of the esophagus. In: Sabiston DC Jr, ed. *Textbook of surgery*, 13th ed. Philadelphia: WB Saunders; 1986:736.)

MALIGNANT NEOPLASMS

Malignant neoplasms of the esophagus include adenocarcinoma, squamous cell carcinoma, small cell carcinoma, leiomyosarcoma, rhabdomyosarcoma, fibrosarcoma, liposarcoma, lymphomas, and metastatic lesions from distant primary sites. Adenocarcinoma and squamous cell carcinoma are the most frequent malignant lesions, and adenocarcinoma has emerged in recent years as the more common lesion. Most thoracic surgeons will complete an entire career without seeing the less common types of esophageal malignancies.

The goal of esophageal resection, whether as primary treatment or as part of a multimodality plan, is cure, though this goal remains elusive. Palliative esophagectomy is associated with mortality rates in excess of 20% and morbidity rates as high as 50% and should be avoided.[32] Very effective palliation can be obtained with chemotherapy, radiation therapy, and endoscopic interventions such as stenting. Unfortunately, there will be more than 14,000 new cases of esophageal cancer and essentially the same number of deaths from this disease this year in the United States.[33] The lifetime risk of developing esophageal cancer is about 0.5%, being slightly higher for men and slightly lower for woman.

Tobacco, alcohol, and obesity are all risk factors associated with the development of esophageal cancer. Table 44.4 shows the additional risk factors associated with esophageal cancer and their contributions to the development of either squamous cell carcinoma or adenocarcinoma.

Although many have postulated a genetic predisposition to esophageal cancer, tylosis is the only recognized familial syndrome that predisposes to the development of esophageal cancer. This is an autosomal dominant disorder, which has been mapped to chromosome 17q25.[34] Patients have hyperkeratosis of the palms of their hands and the soles of their feet.

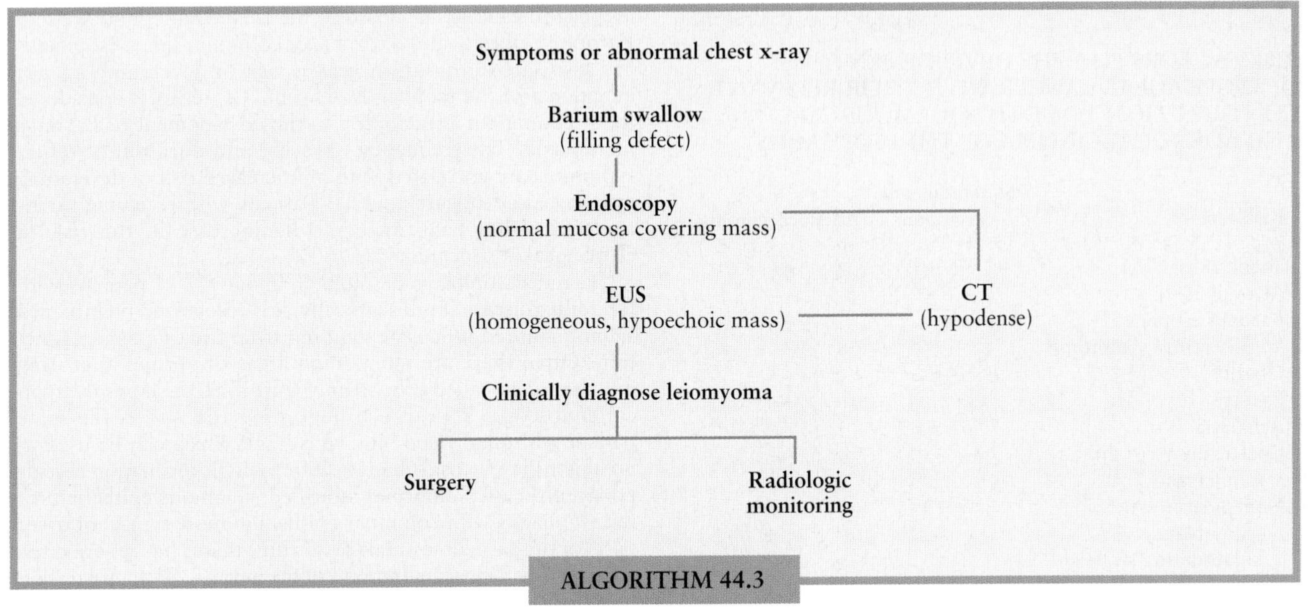

ALGORITHM 44.3 Evaluation and treatment of esophageal leiomyoma. (After Lee LS, Singhal S, Brinster CJ, et al. Current management of esophageal leiomyoma. *J Am Coll Surg.* 2004;198:136.)

The risk of developing squamous cell carcinoma of the esophagus by age 70 is 95% in this cohort of patients.[35]

Diagnosis

Unfortunately, early esophageal carcinomas are largely asymptomatic. As a distensible muscular tube, a significant portion of the esophageal lumen must be obstructed to impede passage of a food bolus and produce symptoms. Dysphasia is the primary manifestation of esophageal cancer in 80% of patients and up to 20% have odynophagia. Vague symptoms of retrosternal discomfort and transient dysphasia are often overlooked by the patient and the physician. On retrospective evaluation, many patients have significantly altered their eating habits by avoiding foods such as meats and breads and at the same time increasing liquid intake. About one half of patients have significant weight loss. Weight loss of more than 10% of body mass is an independent predictor of poor prognosis.[36]

Occasionally, other medical conditions need to be considered in the differential diagnosis of dysphagia. Cardiomegaly, hepatomegaly, and enlarged thoracic aorta have all been reported to cause dysphagia by compression of the esophagus. Large substernal thyroid goiters can produce cervical dysphagia and airway compression. Cervical dysphagia is an indication for thyroidectomy in these patients.

Pulmonary symptoms may be caused by aspiration of regurgitated food or by direct invasion of the airway by esophageal tumor. Direct airway invasion can occur with locally advanced lesions at the location where the left mainstem bronchus passes over the esophagus. New hoarseness due to vocal cord paralysis is indicative of left recurrent nerve involvement and suggests unresectability. Virchow's node, a palpable left supraclavicular lymph node, may be apparent in some patients. Fine-needle aspiration with positive cytology confirms the pathologic involvement of Virchow's node and confirms the diagnosis of distant metastatic disease.

The evaluation of a patient with suspected esophageal cancer centers involves securing the diagnosis, clinically staging the patient, and determining the medical operability in patients with stage-appropriate lesions for resection. Barium swallow and esophagoscopy remain the most important diagnostic tools for assessing the patient with esophageal symptoms. Barium swallow is usually the first study obtained. It provides both anatomic and functional information. Flexible esophagoscopy is used to precisely locate the lesion and provide tissue confirmation of malignancy. In patients considered for surgical resection, EUS is the single most valuable test in determining the tumor size and the depth of penetration (T stage). Regional lymph nodes are also visualized during EUS and can be sampled to determine the cytologic presence or absence of metastatic nodal disease. CT scanning of the chest and abdomen is valuable for assessing lung and liver metastasis; it is not accurate for determining T stage or assessing regional lymph node involvement.

Positron emission tomography (PET) is a physiologic test under investigation in patients with esophageal carcinoma. Preliminary studies suggest that PET can detect otherwise radiographically occult metastatic disease.[37] It has been reported that PET will detect disease in up to 15% of patients who were thought to have only localized disease by conventional studies.[38] At present, these findings await confirmation in larger studies.

The use of combined thoracoscopy and laparoscopy for preoperative staging has been advocated by some centers. Periesophageal mediastinal lymph nodes and celiac lymph nodes can be sampled with a high degree of accuracy using these techniques.[39] Whether or not this will correlate with improved outcomes remains to be seen. We currently do not use these techniques as part of our standard evaluation.

Unfortunately, no serum tumor markers have been consistently found in patients with esophageal cancers. Standard serum cancer markers including CEA, CA 19-9, and CA 125 have no value in the preoperative evaluation of patients with esophageal cancer.

Adenocarcinoma

Adenocarcinoma of the esophagus was once considered rare; however, over the past 30 years, the incidence has risen faster than that of any other cancer in the United States. Adenocarcinoma of the esophagus currently accounts for more than 50% of the

TABLE 44.4 ETIOLOGY

RISK FACTORS FOR THE DEVELOPMENT OF ESOPHAGEAL CANCER WITH THEIR RELEVANT CONTRIBUTION TO BOTH SQUAMOUS CELL AND ADENOCARCINOMA OF THE ESOPHAGUS

Risk factor	Squamous cell carcinoma	Adenocarcinoma
Tobacco use	+++	++
Alcohol use	+++	—
Barrett's esophagus	—	++++
Weekly reflux symptoms	—	+++
Obesity	—	++
Poverty	++	—
Achalasia	+++	—
Caustic injury to the esophagus	++++	—
Nonepidermolytic palmoplantar keratoderma (tylosis)	++++	—
Plummer-Vinson syndrome	++++	—
History of head and neck cancer	++++	—
History of breast cancer treated with radiotherapy	+++	+++
Frequent consumption of extremely hot beverages	+	—
Prior use of beta-blockers, anticholinergic agents, or aminophyllines	—	±

+, Increase in the risk by a factor of less than two; ++, increase by a factor of two to four; +++, increase by a factor of more than four to eight; ++++, increase by a factor of more than eight; ±, conflicting results have been reported; —, no proven risk.

From Enzinger C, Mayer J. Esophageal cancer. *N Engl J Med.* 2003; 349:2241 Copyright © 2003 Massachusetts Medical Society. All rights reserved.

esophageal cancers diagnosed in the United States and Western Europe.[40] Obesity and Barrett's, or columnar-lined, esophagus are associated with an increased risk of developing adenocarcinoma of the esophagus. Chronic GE reflux is considered the predominant contributor to the development of Barrett's metaplasia. The frequency, severity, and duration of reflux symptoms are correlated with an increased risk of developing esophageal adenocarcinoma.[41] Patients with recurring symptoms of reflux have an eightfold increase in the risk of esophageal adenocarcinoma.[42]

Barrett's esophagus develops in about 5% of patients with GE reflux disease. Endoscopically, it is recognized by inflamed salmon-colored mucosa extending from the esophageal junction. Often there are intervening areas of normal appearing mucosa, or so-called skip areas. Figure 44.10A shows the typical endoscopic appearance; Figure 44.10B shows the same patient with methylene blue vital stain, which can be used to highlight the mucosal changes. Microscopic evaluation reveals replacement of the normal stratified squamous epithelium of the esophagus with columnar epithelium more typical of other parts of the gastrointestinal tract. Thus, these changes are often referred to as "intestinalization" of the mucosa. With progression to dysplasia, the nuclei become "crowded" and the normal glandular architecture is lost. Histologically, patients with high-grade dysplasia carry a significant risk for esophageal carcinoma and should be considered candidates for resection. Barrett's esophagus increases the risk of esophageal adenocarcinoma when compared with the general population.[43] The annual rate of neoplastic transformation to adenocarcinoma in patients with Barrett's is 0.5%.[44]

Squamous Cell Carcinoma

The primary risk factor for squamous cell carcinoma of the esophagus is chronic irritation of the esophageal mucosa. Prolonged alcohol consumption, especially in combination with tobacco exposure, appears to be the major contributing factor. Nitrosamines and other nitrosyl compounds found in smoked meats also are important factors in native populations who rely on them for their main source of nutrition. In some Asian countries, there appears to be strong correlation between the development of squamous cell cancer of the esophagus and ingestion of hot beverages. Medical conditions

A

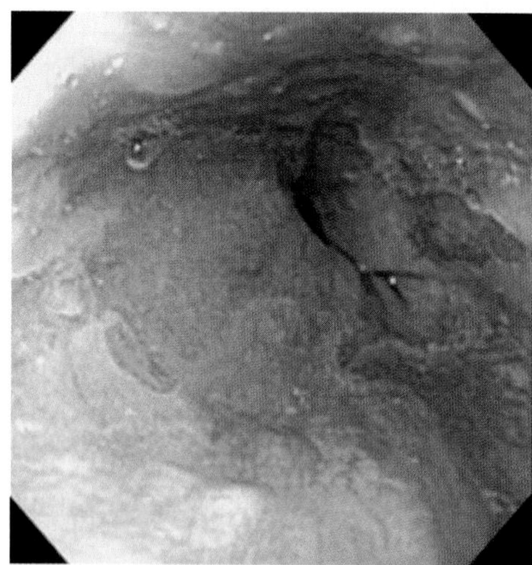

B

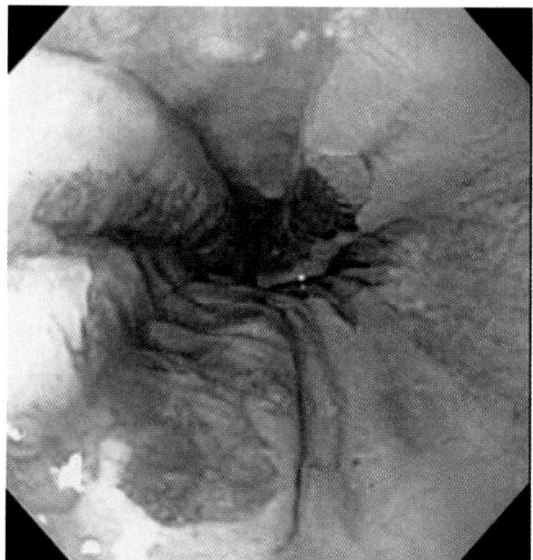

FIGURE 44.10 (*A*) The typical endoscopic appearance of Barrett's changes at the gastroesophageal (GE) junction. Note the salmon-colored areas of erosion extending from the GE junction. Also note the intervening areas of normal appearing mucosa. (*B*) Vital staining with methylene blue. Vital stains are used to highlight the mucosal changes at the time of endoscopy. (Courtesy of Micheal L. Kochman, M.D., University of Pennsylvania, Philadelphia.)

including achalasia, caustic strictures, Plummer-Vinson syndrome, and tylosis also increase the risk of squamous cell carcinoma. Patients with tylosis have a risk as high as 40% of developing a squamous cell carcinoma of the esophagus.[45] The risk with long-standing achalasia approximates 7%.[46]

Staging of Esophageal Cancers

Esophageal cancers are staged according to the American Joint Committee on Cancer (AJCC) TNM staging system.[47] The current AJCC definitions are shown in Table 44.5. The stage groupings and current recommended treatment strategy for each stage are displayed in Table 44.6.

It is clear that the outcome in esophageal cancer is strongly associated with the stage of the disease. Thus, accurate clinical staging is of paramount importance in formulating an appropriate treatment plan and providing the patient with information regarding prognosis. The preoperative evaluation is intended to define the extent of disease and thus the clinical stage. All patients should have a CT scan of the chest and abdomen. In the absence of lung, liver, or other distant metastatic disease, an EUS is performed to define the depth of tumor invasion and assess regional lymph nodes. Recently, we have added PET scanning to the preoperative evaluation because it appears that the PET scan is a complementary modality to the CT scan and in conjunction with CT is very sensitive at detecting distant metastatic disease. In stage-appropriate candidates, plans are made to optimize the patient from a medical standpoint and proceed to resection. The role of preoperative therapy followed by operation remains ill defined and hotly debated.

The current information on neoadjuvant treatment can be divided into studies evaluating preoperative radiation, preoperative chemotherapy, and combined preoperative radiochemotherapy. In operable patients with resectable tumors, the results of any preoperative therapy followed by resection must be compared with the results of primary resection alone. Importantly, this analysis must take into account the toxicities associated with multimodality therapy and the impact on the intended resection and quality of life.

A number of randomized trials have failed to show any benefit from preoperative radiation therapy alone. Proponents of preoperative radiotherapy argue that the trials are too small to demonstrate the advantages of this approach. A meta-analysis of available randomized trials comprising 1,147 patients, however, found no improvement in survival with preoperative radiotherapy alone in patients with resectable esophageal cancer.[48] At this time, there is no indication for preoperative radiation therapy alone followed by resection.

The utility of preoperative chemotherapy alone is much more poorly defined. A large multicenter randomized trial in the United States (Intergroup Trial) of 440 patients failed to show any improvement in survival after three cycles of combined cisplatin and fluorouracil followed by surgery and two postoperative cycles when compared to surgery alone.[49] This is in contrast to a large randomized European study (Medical Research Council), which suggested that neoadjuvant chemotherapy resulted in nearly a 10% improvement in survival at 2 years.[50] Unfortunately, the preoperative staging techniques and duration of treatments were quite different, making the two studies difficult to compare. From an evidence-based perspective, a recent review of 11 randomized controlled trials with 2,051 patients suggested that there was improved survival in patients who underwent preoperative chemotherapy followed by resection; however, it did not reach statistical significance until 5 years and there was increased toxicity and mortality in the chemotherapy group.[51] This issue remains unresolved, and operation remains the standard treatment for esophageal cancer outside of a clinical trial. At this time we consider neoadjuvant chemotherapy to be investigational.

TABLE 44.5 STAGING

AMERICAN JOINT COMMITTEE ON CANCER (AJCC) STAGING OF ESOPHAGEAL CANCER

Stage	Description
PRIMARY TUMOR (T)	
TX	Primary tumor cannot be assessed
T0	No evidence of primary tumor
Tis	Carcinoma in situ
T1	Tumor invades lamina propria or submucosa
T2	Tumor invades muscularis propria
T3	Tumor invades adventitia
T4	Tumor invades adjacent structures
REGIONAL LYMPH NODES (N)	
NX	Regional lymph nodes cannot be assessed
N0	No regional lymph node metastasis
N1	Regional lymph node metastasis
DISTANT METASTASIS (M)	
MX	Distant metastasis cannot be assessed
M0	No distant metastasis
M1	Distant metastasis
TUMORS OF THE LOWER THORACIC ESOPHAGUS	
M1a	Metastasis in celiac lymph nodes
M1b	Other distant metastasis
TUMORS OF THE MIDTHORACIC ESOPHAGUS[a]	
M1a	Not applicable
M1b	Nonregional lymph nodes and/or other distant metastasis
TUMORS OF THE UPPER THORACIC ESOPHAGUS	
M1a	Metastasis in cervical nodes
M1b	Other distant metastasis

[a]For tumors of midthoracic esophagus, use only M1b because these tumors with metastasis in nonregional lymph nodes have an equally poor prognosis as those with metastasis in other distant sites.

From American Joint Committee on Cancer. *AJCC cancer staging manual,* 6th ed. New York: Springer; 2002:91–98.

Several small randomized trials have evaluated combined preoperative chemoradiation followed by surgical resection. The most widely cited trial to justify the use of combined treatment followed by surgery was published by Walsh et al. in 1996.[52] This study projected a 3-year survival of 32% in the neoadjuvant treatment group as compared to 6% in the surgery alone group for patients with adenocarcinoma. Critics were quick to point out the lack of appropriate staging, the poor survival in the surgical group as compared with other surgical series, and the small study size. A more recent study found equivalent median and 3-year survival rate in patients with squamous cell carcinoma of the esophagus randomized to either preoperative chemoradiation followed by surgery or surgery alone.[53] An increased complication rate was noted in the patients undergoing preoperative chemoradiation therapy. Unfortunately, a large intergroup trial designed to answer this question was closed because of poor accrual.

Management

Approaches to Esophagectomy

There are several surgical approaches to esophagectomy. Selecting the appropriate procedure for an individual patient depends on the overall medical condition of the patient, the

TABLE 44.6 STAGING

AMERICAN JOINT COMMITTEE ON CANCER (AJCC) STAGE GROUPING WITH RECOMMENDED TREATMENT STRATEGY AND PREDICTED 5-YEAR SURVIVAL

Stage	TNM designation	Treatment	5-yr survival (%)
0	Tis, N0, M0	Surgery alone	95
I	T1, N0, M0	Surgery alone	75
IIA	T2, N0, M0 T3, N0, M0	Surgery alone	30
IIB	T1, N1, M0 T2, N1, M0	Surgery alone or surgery +/− preop chemo/XRT under investigation	20
III	T3, N1, M0	Surgery for T3 lesions with or without preoperative chemo/XRT under investigation	10–15
	T4, any N, M0	Palliation (chemo, XRT, stenting, or combination)	
IVA	Any T, any N, M1a	Palliation (chemo, XRT, stenting, or combination)	5
IVB	Any T, any N, M1b	Palliation (chemo, XRT, stenting, or combination)	1

chemo, chemotherapy; XRT, radiation therapy.

location of the tumor, and the expertise and experience of the surgeon. Possible approaches include the transhiatal approach, the transabdominal transthoracic approach (Ivor-Lewis), the "three stage" approach (McKeown), the thoracoabdominal approach, and the "minimally invasive" approach. Options for reconstruction include a gastric tube, a colonic interposition, and in selected cases small intestinal free graft. Because of its good blood supply, ease of mobilization, and ability to reach the neck, the gastric tube is the usual conduit of choice for reconstruction. The use of colon is more complex and has an increased morbidity when compared to gastric pullup.[54] We reserve the use of colon or jejunum for patients with an unusable stomach due to previous surgery, tumor extension, or other technical considerations.

The esophageal anastomosis requires meticulous attention. Many esophageal operations are plagued by high anastomotic leak rates and a significant number of postoperative strictures. At present, the modified stapled anastomosis[55] as described by Orringer appears to have the lowest leak rate, about 2% as compared with sutured techniques, which are as high as 15%. The technique is shown in Figure 44.11; many thoracic surgeons have adopted this anastomotic technique.

The Transhiatal Approach. The transhiatal esophagectomy was reintroduced by Orringer and Sloan[56] in 1978 and continues to be refined.[57] The procedure is performed through an upper midline laparotomy and left cervical incision as shown in Figure 44.12. A gastric conduit based on the right gastroepiploic artery is used to establish intestinal continuity. The completed operation is depicted in Figure 44.13. If the stomach is unusable, a colonic interposition can be performed.

Today, the transhiatal esophagectomy is the preferred approach by many surgeons. Nevertheless, debate continues over whether this approach has lower morbidity and mortality than other approaches involving thoracotomy and whether it provides an optimal cancer operation. Proponents argue that this approach results in less surgical trauma by avoiding thoracotomy and thus less postoperative morbidity, especially pulmonary complications. Furthermore, with placement of the anastomosis in the neck, a leak, should it occur, can be treated by simple bedside cervical drainage. In contrast, a leak in the chest is far more likely to result in the severe mediastinitis and more devastating complications.

The Ivor Lewis Approach. The transabdominal, transthoracic approach to esophagectomy as initially described is often referred to as the Ivor Lewis Esophagectomy.[58] This approach includes an upper midline laparotomy for mobilization of the stomach with creation of a gastric tube in the same manner employed for the transhiatal esophagectomy. Once the stomach has been mobilized, the hiatus is opened and the GE junction and distal esophagus are mobilized. At this point the abdomen is closed, the patient is repositioned, and a right fifth intercostal space thoracotomy is performed. The intrathoracic esophagus is mobilized under direct vision up to the level of the azygous vein. The esophagogastric anastomosis is performed at the level of the divided azygous vein. The advantage of this approach is that the intrathoracic esophagus is mobilized directly with full exposure of the mediastinum and surrounding structures. This may be of value in avoiding injury to the airway or other mediastinal structures, especially with bulky tumors in the middle third of the esophagus at the level of the carina. Unfortunately, these patients are subject to increased early postoperative pulmonary complications due to the thoracotomy incision. In addition placing the anastomosis in the chest can lead to life-threatening mediastinitis should an anastomotic leak occur. Additionally, a large amount of thoracic esophagus is retained with this approach and may be at risk of recurrent disease, specifically in the setting of severe Barrett's esophagus.

Three-Field Esophagectomy. This approach is carried out through separate laparotomy, right thoracotomy, and cervical incisions.[59] Proponents of this approach fall into two categories. The first group utilizes this approach to resect large intrathoracic lesions of the midesophagus. Exposure especially at the level of the carina and left mainstem bronchus is superior as compared with the transhiatal approach. Because visualization is improved, the injury rate to nearby structures, especially the airway and azygous vein, is lower. The second group utilizes this approach to perform a complete two- or three-field lymph node dissection, suggesting that this approach provides a more complete resection and thus improves long-term survival. This approach has been shown to have acceptable morbidity and mortality as compared with other approaches; however, the often-cited report was from a single U.S. center.[60] On the other hand, a large randomized Dutch trial comparing transhiatal resection with extended transthoracic resection showed

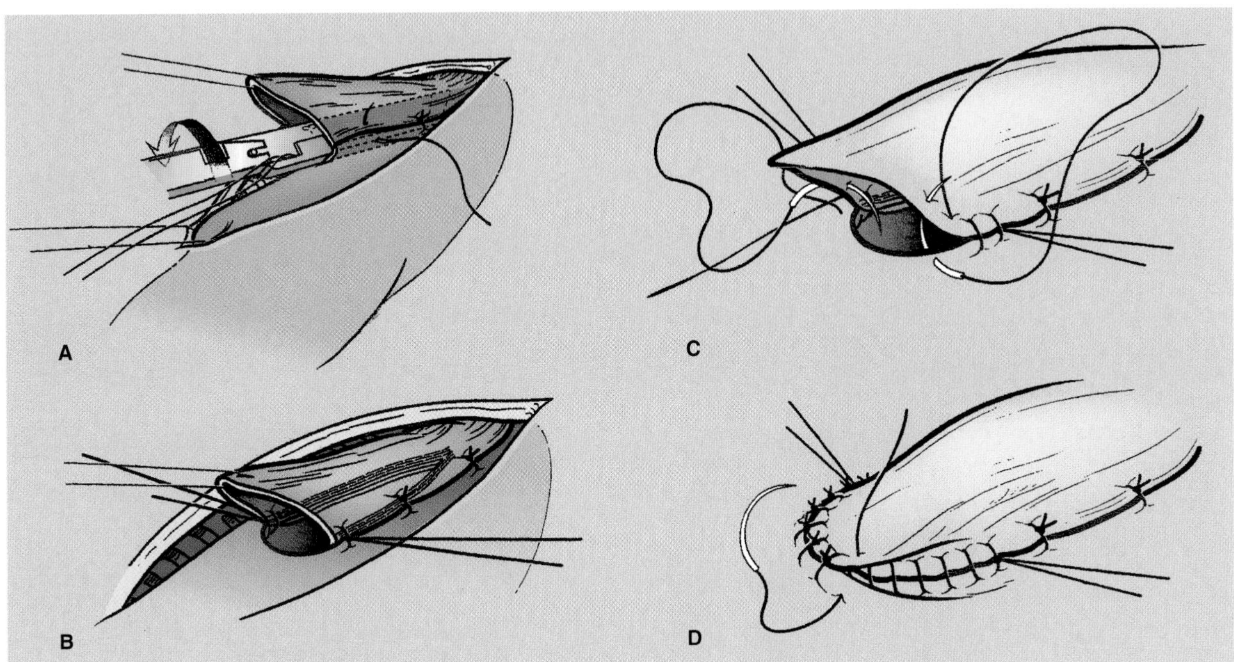

FIGURE 44.11 The stapled technique for cervical esophageal anastomosis. This technique results in lower anastomotic leak rates and less postoperative strictures. (From Orringer MB, Marshall B, Iannettoni MD. Eliminating the cervical esophagogastric anastomotic leak with a side-to-side stapled anastomosis. *J Thorac Cardiovasc Surg*. 2000;119:277.)

that the transhiatal approach was associated with a lower morbidity and no statistically different overall, disease-free, and quality-adjusted survival.[61] The true value of extensive nodal dissection remains undefined.

The Thoracoabdominal Approach. The left thoracoabdominal approach is probably the least utilized of all approaches to the esophagus. It is performed by making an oblique incision from the midpoint between the xiphoid and umbilicus across the costal arch to the tip of the scapula. The abdomen is opened, the costal arch is divided, and the chest is entered through the seventh intercostal space. The diaphragm is opened in a circumferential manner along the chest wall to avoid any damage to the phrenic nerve branches. At least a 2-cm rim of diaphragm is preserved on the chest wall to aid in reconstruction of the diaphragm at the completion of the procedure. This approach offers superior exposure to the left upper quadrant, including the hiatus, and is our approach of choice in patients with previous extensive hiatal or proximal gastric surgery. For patients with distal tumors and inadequate conduit for total esophageal replacement, the anastomosis can be placed in the left chest below the inferior pulmonary vein or up to the level of the aortic arch. For those with adequate conduit, a separate left cervical incision can be made and the cervical esophagastric anastomosis can be placed in the neck. A consecutive case series of 64 thoracoabdominal esophagectomies reported no anastomotic leaks and a 2% mortality rate.[62]

The Minimally Invasive Approach. A number of minimally invasive techniques to esophagectomy have been described. These include laparoscopic, hand-assisted, thoracoscopic, and robotic-assisted esophagectomy. The hope of these procedures is that minimizing the incision size will decrease the morbidity of the operation while at the same time providing adequate resection. The largest study included 217 patients from the University of Pittsburgh who underwent esophagectomy via thoracoscopy, laparoscopy, and a left neck incision.[63] The investigators observed equivalent results as compared to open techniques and suggest development of a multicenter trial to define the role of minimally invasive esophagectomy. At present, the advantage of this approach remains to be determined.

Cervical Esophageal Cancer

Cervical esophageal cancer represents a very small subset of primary esophageal cancers. Direct extension into the cervical esophagus from a primary laryngeal or thyroid malignancy is much more common. Unfortunately, all are difficult to treat. Traditional methods of treatment have relied on radiation therapy. A small subset of patients may be candidates for salvage resection, which usually includes laryngectomy with permanent tracheostomy, esophagectomy, and gastric transposition to reconstitute the gastrointestinal tract.

Palliation

Several palliative therapies are available for patients who have unresectable disease, have metastatic disease, or are medically unfit for surgery. The intent of palliation is to maintain comfort, restore swallowing function if possible, and support nutrition.

Establishment of alternative enteral access is helpful in maintaining nutritional status and hydration. When possible, this is provided by a percutaneous gastrostomy (PEG) tube placed under endoscopic guidance. For patients with bulky obstructing lesions who cannot undergo PEG, an open gastrostomy or jejunostomy tube is required.

Chemotherapy

Esophageal cancers are usually responsive to chemotherapeutic drugs providing some palliation. Agents currently in use include fluorouracil and taxanes either alone or in combination with platin-based agents. Palliative chemotherapy requires time to effectively reduce symptoms of dysphagia and must be balanced with the associated risks of systemic treatment in usually debilitated, malnourished patients.

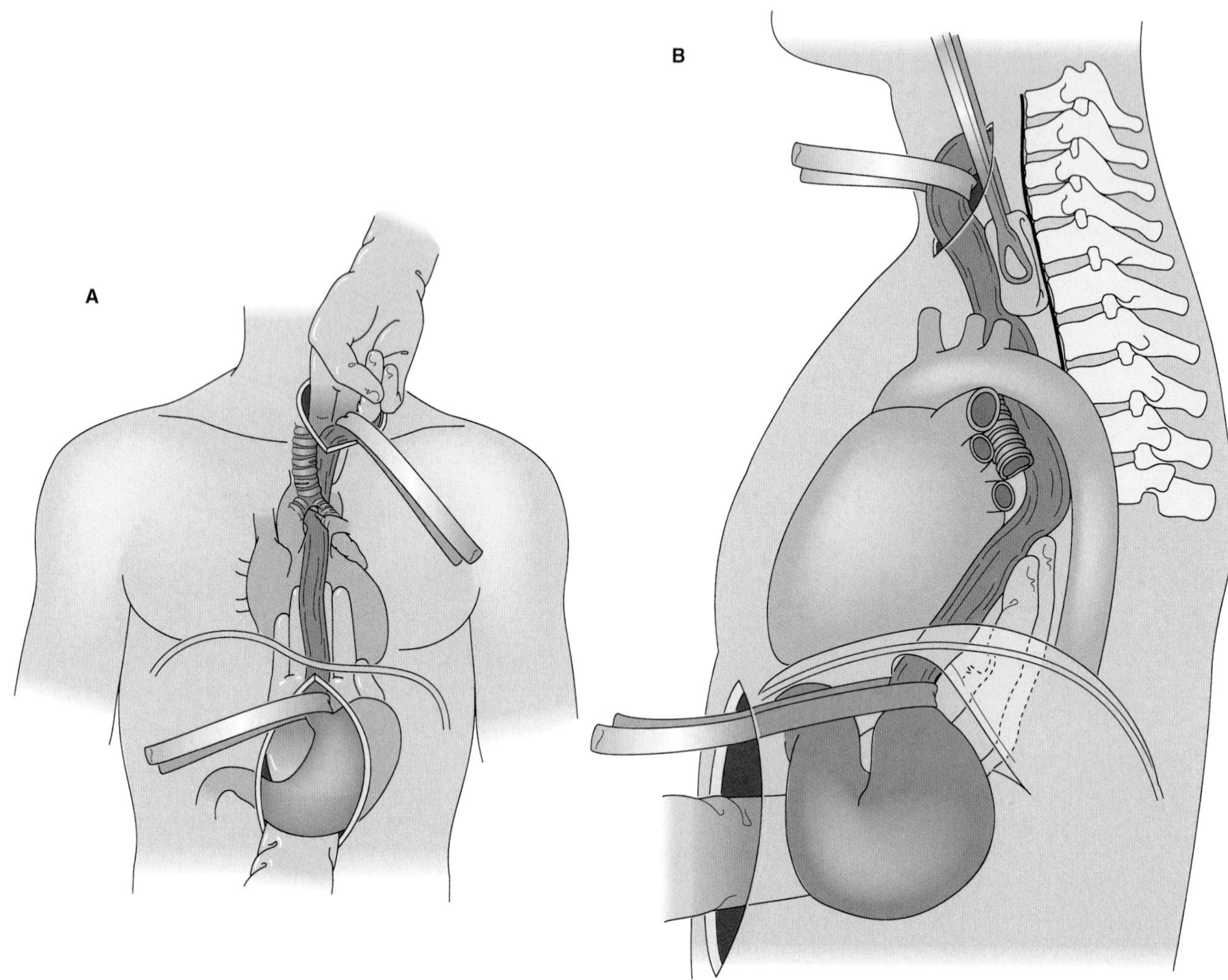

FIGURE 44.12 (*A*) Transhiatal mobilization of the thoracic esophagus from the posterior mediastinum with the use of blunt dissection and traction on rubber drains placed around the esophagogastric junction and cervical esophagus. The volar aspects of the fingers are kept against the esophagus to reduce the risk for injury to adjacent structures. (*B*) Lateral view showing transhiatal mobilization of the esophagus away from the prevertebral fascia. Half of a sponge on a stick is inserted through the cervical incision and advanced until it makes contact with the hand inserted from below through the diaphragmatic hiatus. Arterial pressure is monitored as the heart is displaced forward by the hand in the posterior mediastinum. (After Orringer MB. Surgical options for esophageal resection and reconstruction with stomach. In: Baue AE, Geha AS, Hammond GL, eds. *Glenn's thoracic and cardiovascular surgery*, 5th ed. Norwalk, CT: Appleton & Lange; 1991:799.)

Radiation

Palliative radiotherapy relieves dysphagia in up to 75% of patients. The dose is 4,000 to 5,000 cGy delivered over 4 weeks. This allows patients with advanced disease and severe dysphagia to handle secretions and to swallow liquids as well as dietary supplements. Unfortunately, relief is not immediate and maximal improvement occurs at about 4 weeks following completion of treatment. In patients with a life expectancy greater than 3 months, combined chemotherapy with radiation is utilized. Short-term side effects from radiation therapy include skin irritation and erythema. Esophagitis with painful swallowing also occurs with frequency. Additional complications include stricture formation, radiation pneumonitis, and fistulization to the airway.

Intubation and Stenting

A number of endoesophageal tubes have been used to provide palliation for patients with esophageal carcinoma. The tubes are divided into *pulsion* tubes, which are pushed through the tumor, and *traction* tubes, which are pulled by downward traction from a gastrotomy. Unfortunately, esophageal tubes are plagued with problems including migration, erosion into adjacent structures, obstruction, and pain. The average survival following palliative intubation for esophageal carcinoma is less than 6 months due to progression of disease.

Recently, self-expanding coated and uncoated nitinol stents have been utilized for palliation. These stents can be inserted either radiologically or endoscopically on an outpatient basis. Following insertion, the lumen can be balloon dilated to an acceptable diameter to provide palliation.

Neodymium:Yttrium-Aluminum-Garnet Laser Fulguration

Endoscopic neodymium:yttrium-aluminum-garnet (Nd:YAG) laser fulguration can be used to provide temporary relief of esophageal obstruction in patients with unresectable obstructing tumors. A flexible quartz fiber is passed through the working channel of the esophagoscope to deliver the laser energy at the fiber tip. Multiple sessions are usually required to achieve debulking and functional success. Laser fulguration is often combined with endoluminal stenting and radiation therapy. It

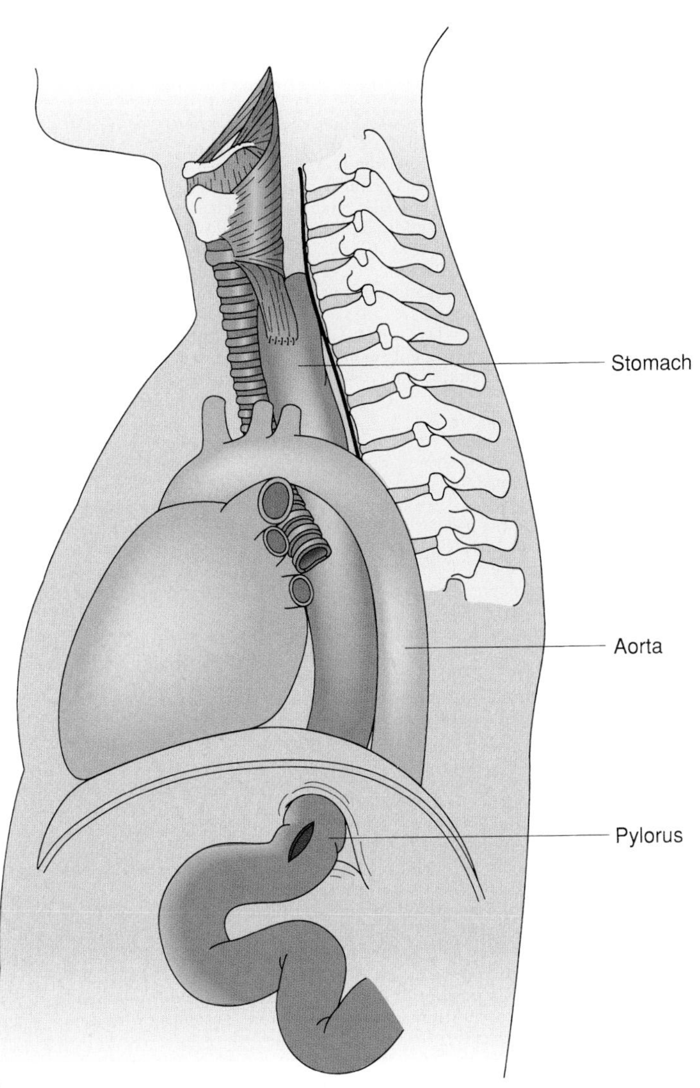

FIGURE 44.13 Final position of the mobilized stomach in the posterior mediastinum after transhiatal esophagectomy and cervical esophagogastric anastomosis. The gastric fundus has been suspended from the cervical prevertebral fascia, and an end-to-side cervical esophagogastrostomy has been performed. The pylorus is now located several centimeters below the level of the diaphragmatic hiatus. (After Orringer MB, Sloan H. Esophagectomy without thoracotomy. *J Thorac Cardiovasc Surg*. 1978;76:643.)

can also be useful in patients who have undergone uncovered stenting procedures with ingrow of tumor through the stent.

Photodynamic Therapy

Intraluminal photodynamic therapy (PDT) is a nonthermal ablative technique that can be used to palliate patients. This technique requires the systemic administration of a hematoporphyrin, which is concentrated within the malignant cells. Approximately 48 hours after administration of the photosensitizer, patients undergo endoscopy and an argon-pump dye-laser is used to deliver endoluminal light at a wavelength of 630 nm. This results in the generation of oxygen radicals, which quickly lead to tumor necrosis. The depth of penetration is relatively limited and this decreases the risk of full-thickness necrosis with perforation. Unfortunately, the photosensitizing agents are retained by the reticuloendothelial system in skin; thus, patients are sensitive to infrared wavelength light, including sunlight, radiant heat, fluorescent light, and strong incandescent light. Depending on the photosensitizing agent used, this sensitivity can persist up to 3 months, a challenging problem in patients with short life expectancies.

A recent series of 215 patients treated with palliative endoluminal PDT revealed a procedure-related mortality rate of 1.8%, effective palliation for patients with obstructing cancers in 85% of the treatment courses, and median survival of 4.8 months.[64] A number of patients in this series also required stenting, suggesting that PDT has a role in multimodality palliation of obstructing esophageal cancers.

KEY POINTS

- **The high fat content of the esophageal submucosa leads to mobility of the overlying mucosa; therefore, care must be taken that every anastomotic suture transfixes the submucosa to prevent anastomotic leak.**
- **The incidence of esophageal perforation has increased over recent decades due to the increasing use of invasive endoscopic procedures, such that iatrogenic injury by instrumentation accounts for more than 50% of all cases.**
- **The operative management of esophageal perforation is dictated by the location of the perforation, the extent of injury, and the presence or absence of underlying esophageal pathology.**
- **The management of an esophageal perforation associated with endoscopic dilatation for achalasia includes primary repair of the injury, a vertical esophageal myotomy performed 180 degrees opposite the injury, and a noncircumferential wrap such as a Belsey procedure.**
- **A Zenker's or pharyngoesophageal diverticulum is a pulsion-type pseudodiverticulum resulting from the anatomic weakness at Killian's triangle and an underlying motility disorder manifested by incoordinated or incomplete relaxation of the upper esophageal sphincter.**
- **The goal of surgical resection for esophageal cancer is cure, as effective palliation can be obtained with chemotherapy, radiation therapy, and endoscopic interventions such as stents.**
- **Over the last 30 years, the incidence of adenocarcinoma of the esophagus has risen faster than that of any other cancer in the United States.**

- **Advantages of the transhiatal esophagectomy are less surgical trauma by avoidance of a thoracotomy and placement of the anastomosis in the neck, which minimize the morbidity of an anastomotic leak.**
- **The data concerning improved survival following neoadjuvant treatment for esophageal cancer are inconclusive and must be considered in light of the associated toxicity of the multimodality therapy.**
- **The intent of palliation of unresectable esophageal cancer is to maintain comfort, restore swallowing function if possible, and support nutrition.**

References

1. Orringer MB. Complications of esophageal surgery and trauma. In: Greenfield LJ, ed. *Complications in surgery and trauma*, 3rd ed. Philadelphia: JB Lippincott; 1990:302.
2. Orringer MB, Sloan H. Esophagectomy without thoracotomy. *J Thorac Cardiovasc Surg*. 1978;76:643.
3. Lewis I. The surgical treatment of carcinoma of the esophagus with special reference to a new operation for growths of the middle third. *Br J Surg*. 1946;34:18.
4. McKeown KC. Total three-stage esophagectomy for cancer of the esophagus. *Br J Surg*. 1976;51:259.
5. Bolten JS. Teng S. Transthoracic or transhiatal esophagectomy for cancer of the esophagus—does it matter. *Surg Oncol Clin North Am*. 2002;11:365.
6. Dimick JB, Pronovost PJ, Cowan JA, et al. Surgical volume and quality of care for esophageal resection: do high-volume hospitals have fewer complications? *Ann Thor Surg*. 2003;75:337.
7. Rizk NP, Bach PB, Schrag D, et al. The impact of complications on outcomes after resection for esophageal and gastroesophageal junction carcinoma. *J Am Coll Surg*. 2004;198:42.
8. Brinster CJ, Singhal S, Lawrence L, et al. Evolving options in the management of esophageal perforation. *Ann Thorac Surg*. 2004;77:1475.
9. Weiman DS, Walker WA, Brosnan KM, et al. Noniatrogenic esophageal trauma. *Ann Thorac Surg*. 1995;59:845; discussion 849.
10. Barrett N. Spontaneous perforation of the esophagus: review of the literature and a report of three new cases. *Thorax* 1946;1:48.
11. Foley MJ, Ghahremani GG, Rogers LF. Reappraisal of contrast media used to detect upper gastrointestinal perforations: comparison of ionic water-soluble media with barium sulfate. *Radiology* 1982;144:231.
12. Gollub MJ, Bains MS. Barium sulfate: a new (old) contrast agent for diagnosis of postoperative esophageal leaks. *Radiology* 1997;202:360.
13. Horwitz B, Krevsky B, Buckman RF Jr, et al. Endoscopic evaluation of penetrating esophageal injuries. *Am J Gastroenterol*. 1993;88:1249.
14. Mengold L, Klassen KP. Conservative management of esophageal perforation. *Arch Surg*. 1965;91:232.
15. Cameron JL, Kieffer RF, Hendrix TR, et al. Selective nonoperative management of contained intrathoracic esophageal disruptions. *Ann Thorac Surg*. 1979;27:404.
16. Altorjay A, Kiss J, Voros A, et al. Nonoperative management of esophageal perforations. Is it justified? *Ann Surg*. 1997;225:415.
17. Port JL, Kent MS, Korst RJ, et al. Thoracic esophageal perforations: a decade of experience. *Ann Thorac Surg*. 2003;75:1071.
18. Hugh TB, Kelly MD. Corrosive ingestion and the surgeon. *J Am Coll Surg*. 1999;189:508.
19. Payne WS. The Treatment of pharyngeoesophgeal diverticulum: the simple and complex. *Hepatogastroenterology* 1994;39:109.
20. Martin-Hirsch DP, Newbegin CJ. Autosuture GIA gun: a new application in the treatment of hypopharyngeal diverticula. *J Laryngol Otol*. 1993;107:723.
21. Collard JM, Otte JB, Kestens PJ. Endoscopic stapling technique of esophagodiverticulostomy for Zenker's diverticulum. *Ann Thorac Surg*. 1993;56:573.
22. Cook RD, Huang PC, Richstmeier WJ, et al. Endoscopic staple-assisted esophagodiverticulostomy: an excellent treatment choice for Zenker diverticulum. *Laryngoscope* 2000;110:2020.
23. Siddiq MA, Sood S. Current management in pharyngeal pouch surgery by UK otorhinolaryngologists. *Ann R Coll Surg Engl*. 2004;86:247.
24. Nehra D, Lord R, DeMeester TR, et al. Physiologic basis for the treatment of epiphrenic diverticulum. *Ann Surg*. 2002;235:346.
25. Van der Peet DL, Klinkenberg-Knol EC, Berends FJ, Cuesta MA. Epiphrenic diverticula: minimal invasive approach and repair in five patients. *Dis Esophagus* 2001;14:60.
26. DelGenio A, Rossetti G, Maffettone V, et al. Laparoscopic approach in the treatment of epiphrenic diverticula: long-term results. *Surg Endosc*. 2004.
27. Seremetis MG, Lyons WS, deGuzman VC, Peabody JW Jr. Leiomyomata of the esophagus. An analysis of 838 cases. *Cancer* 1976;38:2166.
28. Postlethwait RW, Musser AW. Changes in the esophagus in 1,000 autopsy specimens. *J Thorac Cardiovasc Surg*. 1974;68:953.
29. Taylor FH, Christenson W, Zollinger RW 2nd, et al. Multiple leiomyomas of the esophagus. *Ann Thorac Surg*. 1995;60:182.
30. Lee LS, Singhal S, Brinster CJ, et al. Current management of esophageal leiomyoma. *J Am Coll Surg*. 2004;198:136.
31. Schuhmacher C, Becker K, Dittler HJ, et al. Fibrovascular esophageal polyp as a diagnostic challenge. *Dis Esophagus* 2000;13:324.
32. Orringer MB. Substernal gastric bypass of the excluded esophagus-results of an ill-advised operation. *Surgery* 1984;96:467.
33. American Cancer Society. *Cancer facts and figures 2004*. Atlanta, GA: American Cancer Society; 2004.
34. Risk JM, Mills HS, Garde J, et al. The tylosis esophageal cancer (TOC) locus: more than just a familial cancer gene. *Dis Esophagus* 1999;12:173.
35. Ellis A, Field JK, Field EA, et al. Tylosis associated with carcinoma of the oesophagus and oral leukoplakia in a large Liverpool family—a review of six generations. *Eur J Cancer B Oral Oncol*. 1994;30:102.
36. Fein R, Kelsen DP, Geller N, et al. Adenocarcinoma of the esophagus and gastroesophageal junction: prognostic factors and results of therapy. *Cancer* 1985;56:2512.
37. Liberale G, Van Laethem JL, Gay F, et al. The role of PET scan in the preoperative management of oesophageal cancer. *Eur J Surg Oncol*. 2004;30:942.
38. Flamen P, Lerut A, Van Cutsem E, et al. Utility of positron emission tomography for the staging of patients with potentially operable esophageal carcinoma. *J Clin Oncol*. 2000;18:3202.
39. Krasna MJ, Flowers JL, Attar S, et al. Combined thoracoscopic/laparoscopic staging of esophageal cancer. *J Thorac Cardiovasc Surg*. 1996;111:800; discussion 806.
40. Bollschweiler E, Wolfgarten E, Gutschow Ch, et al. Demographic variations in the rising incidence of esophageal adenocarcinoma in white males. *Cancer* 2001;92:549.
41. Lagergren J, Bergström R, Lindgren A, et al. Symptomatic gastroesophageal reflux as a risk factor for esophageal adenocarcinoma. *N Engl J Med*. 1999;340:825.
42. Lagergren J, Bergström R, Lindgren A, et al. Symptomatic gastroesophageal reflux as a risk factor for esophageal adenocarcinoma. *N Engl J Med*. 1999;340:825.
43. Solaymani-Dodaran M, Logan RF, West J, et al. Risk of oesophageal cancer in Barrett's oesophagus and gastro-oesophageal reflux. *Gut* 2004;53:1070.
44. Shaheen N, Ransohoff DF. Gastroesophageal reflux, Barrett esophagus, and esophageal cancer: scientific review. *JAMA* 2002;287:1972.
45. Risk JM, Mills HS, Garde J, et al. The tylosis esophageal cancer (TOC) locus: more than just a familial cancer gene. *Dis Esophagus* 1999;12:173.
46. Aggestrup S, Holm JC, Sørensen HR. Does achalasia predispose to cancer of the esophagus? *Chest* 1992;102:1013.
47. Esophagus. In: American Joint Committee on Cancer. *AJCC cancer staging manual*, 6th ed. New York: Springer; 2002:91–98.
48. Arnott SJ, Duncan W, Gignoux M, et al. (Oeosphageal Cancer Collaborative Group). Preoperative radiotherapy for esophageal carcinoma (Cochrane Review). In: *The Cochrane Library*, Issue 4. Chichester, UK: John Wiley & Sons, Ltd.; 2004.
49. Kelsen DP, Ginsberg R, Pajak TF, et al. Chemotherapy followed by surgery compared with surgery alone for localized esophageal cancer. *N Engl J Med*. 1998;339:1979.
50. Medical Research Council Oesophageal Cancer Working Group. Surgical resection with or without postoperative chemotherapy in oesophageal cancer: a randomised controlled trial. *Lancet* 2002;359:1727.
51. Malthaner R, Fenlon D. Preoperative chemotherapy for resectable thoracic esophageal cancer. *Cochrane Database Syst Rev*. 2003;Issue 4, Art. No. CD001556, DOI 10.1002/14651858.CD001556.
52. Walsh T, Noonan N, Hollywood D, et al. A comparison of multimodal therapy and surgery for esophageal adenocarcinoma. *N Engl J Med*. 1996;335:462.
53. Bosset J-F, Gignoux M, Triboulet J-P, et al. Chemoradiotherapy followed by surgery compared with surgery alone in squamous-cell cancer of the esophagus. *N Engl J Med*. 1997;337:161.
54. Davis PA, Law S, Wong J. Colonic Interposition after esophagectomy for cancer. *Arch Surg*. 2003;138:303.
55. Orringer MB, Marshall B, Iannettoni MD. Eliminating the cervical esophagogastric anastomotic leak with a side-to-side stapled anastomosis. *J Thorac Cardiovasc Surg*. 2000;119:277.
56. Orringer MB, Sloan H. Esophagectomy without thoracotomy. *J Thorac Cardiovasc Surg*. 1978;76:643.
57. Orringer MB. Marshall B. Iannettoni MD. Transhiatal esophagectomy: clinical experience and refinements. *Ann Surg*. 1999;230:392; discussion 400.
58. Lewis I. The surgical treatment of carcinoma of the esophagus with special reference to a new operation for growths of the middle third. *Br J Surg*. 1946;34:18.
59. McKeown KC. Total three-stage oesphagectomy for cancer of the esophagus. *Br J Surg*. 1976;51:259.
60. Altorki N, Kent M, Ferrara C, Port J. Three-field lymph node dissection for squamous cell and adenocarcinoma of the esophagus. *Ann Surg*. 2002;236:177.
61. Hulscher JB, van Sandick JW, de Boer AG, et al. Extended transthoracic resection compared with limited transhiatal resection for adenocarcinoma of the esophagus. *N Engl J Med*. 2002;374:1662.
62. Heitmiller RF. Results of standard left thoracoabdominal esophagogastrectomy. *Semin Thorac Cardiovasc Surg*. 1992;4:314.
63. Luketich JD, Alvelo-Rivera M, Buenaventura PO, et al. Minimally invasive esophagectomy: outcomes in 222 patients. *Ann Surg*. 2003;238:486.
64. Litle VR, Luketich JD, Christie NA, et al. Photodynamic therapy as palliation for esophageal cancer: experience in 215 patients. *Ann Thorac Surg*. 2003;76:1687.

SECTION E

STOMACH AND DUODENUM

CHAPTER 45 ■ GASTRIC ANATOMY AND PHYSIOLOGY

MICHAEL W. MULHOLLAND

GROSS ANATOMY

The stomach and duodenum, along with the esophagus, liver, bile ducts, and pancreas, are derived from the embryonic foregut. During the fifth week of gestation, the future stomach is marked as a dilation in the caudal portion of the foregut. Cranial to this dilation, the trachea forms as a bud from the future esophagus. At this time, the primitive stomach is invested with both ventral and dorsal mesenteries. The embryonic ventral mesentery is represented in postnatal life by the falciform ligament and by the gastrohepatic and hepatoduodenal mesenteries that form the lesser omentum. The celiac artery, the major blood supply to the foregut, passes within the dorsal mesentery. The primitive dorsal mesentery ultimately forms three structures: the gastrocolic ligament, the gastrosplenic ligament, and the gastrophrenic ligament.

During the sixth and seventh weeks of gestation, the typical morphology of the stomach is established. Accelerated growth of the left gastric wall, relative to the right, establishes the greater and lesser curvatures. This unequal growth also rotates the stomach and causes the left vagal nerve trunk to assume its anterior position, whereas the right vagal trunk is located posteriorly. The growth of structures cephalad to the stomach causes the organ to descend. During the sixth week, the primitive stomach lies between the T10 and T12 vertebral segments. By the eighth week, the stomach is located between the T11 and the L4 segments. In adult life, the stomach is most commonly located between the T10 and the L3 vertebral segments.

The stomach can be divided into anatomic regions based on external landmarks (Fig. 45.1). Although this division is commonly referred to in surgical texts and is useful in discussing gastric resective procedures, it does not necessarily reflect the secretory or motor functions of the mucosal and muscular layers of the stomach. The gastric cardia is the region of the stomach just distal to the gastroesophageal junction. The fundus is the portion of the stomach above and to the left of the gastroesophageal junction. The corpus constitutes the region between the fundus and the antrum. The margin between corpus and antrum is not distinct externally but can be defined arbitrarily by a line from the incisura angularis on the lesser curvature to a point one fourth of the distance from the pylorus to the esophagus along the greater curvature. The gastric antrum is bounded distally by the pylorus, which can be appreciated by palpation as a thickened ring of smooth muscle.

The stomach is mobile in most people and is fixed at only two points, proximally by the gastroesophageal junction and distally by the retroperitoneal duodenum. Therefore, the position of the stomach varies and depends on the habitus of the person, the degree of gastric distention, and the position of the other abdominal organs. Anteriorly, the stomach is in contact with the left hemidiaphragm, the left lobe and the anterior segment of the right lobe of the liver, and the anterior parietal surface of the abdominal wall. The posterior surface of the stomach is related to the left diaphragm; the left kidney and left adrenal gland; the neck, tail, and body of the pancreas; the aorta and celiac trunk; and the periaortic nerve plexuses. The greater curvature of the stomach is near the transverse colon and the transverse colonic mesentery. The concavity of the spleen contacts the left lateral portion of the stomach.

The stomach is an extremely well-vascularized organ, supplied by a number of major arteries and protected by a large number of extramural and intramural collaterals. Gastric viability can be preserved after ligation of all but one primary artery, an advantage that can be exploited during gastric reconstructive procedures. Also, the rich network of anastomosing vessels means that gastric hemorrhage cannot be controlled by the extramural ligation of gastric arteries. Most gastric blood flow is ordinarily derived from the celiac trunk (Fig. 45.2). The lesser curvature is supplied by the left gastric artery, which is the first major branch of the celiac trunk, and by the right gastric artery, which is derived from the hepatic artery. Branches of the left gastric artery also supply the lowermost portion of the esophagus. The greater curvature is supplied by the short gastric

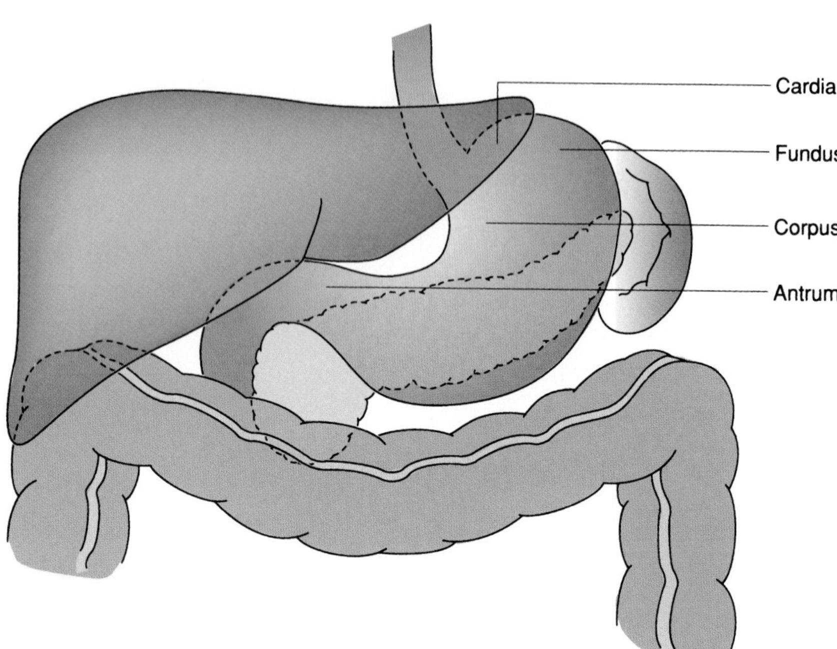

FIGURE 45.1 Topographic relations of the stomach.

and left gastroepiploic arteries, which are branches of the splenic artery, and by the right gastroepiploic artery, a branch of the gastroduodenal artery. In instances of celiac trunk occlusion, gastric blood flow is usually maintained from the superior mesenteric artery collaterally by way of the pancreaticoduodenal arcade. In general, venous effluent from the stomach parallels the arterial supply. The venous equivalent of the left gastric artery is the coronary vein.

As a first approximation, the lymphatic drainage of the stomach parallels gastric venous return (Fig. 45.3). Lymph from the proximal portion of the stomach along the lesser curvature first drains into superior gastric lymph nodes surrounding the left gastric artery. The distal portion of the lesser curvature drains through suprapyloric nodes. The proximal portion of the greater curvature is supplied by lymphatic vessels that traverse pancreaticosplenic nodes, whereas the antral portion of the greater curvature drains into the subpyloric and omental nodal groups. Secondary drainage from each of these systems eventually traverses nodes at the base of the celiac axis. These discrete anatomic groupings are misleading. The lymphatic drainage of the human stomach, like its blood supply, exhibits extensive intramural ramifications and a number of extramural communications. As a consequence, disease processes that involve the gastric lymphatics often spread intramurally beyond the region of origin and to nodal groups at a distance from the primary lymphatic zone.

The left and right vagal nerves descend parallel to the esophagus within the thorax before forming a periesophageal plexus between the tracheal bifurcation and the diaphragm. From this plexus, two vagal trunks coalesce before passing through the esophageal hiatus of the diaphragm (Fig. 45.4). The left vagal trunk is usually closely applied to the anterior

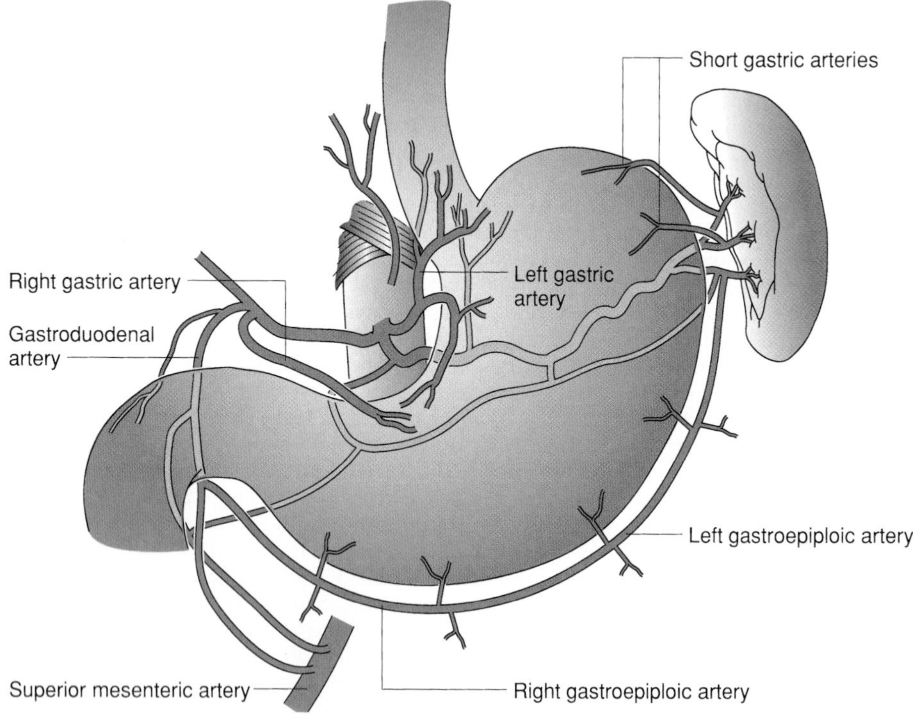

FIGURE 45.2 Arterial blood supply of the stomach.

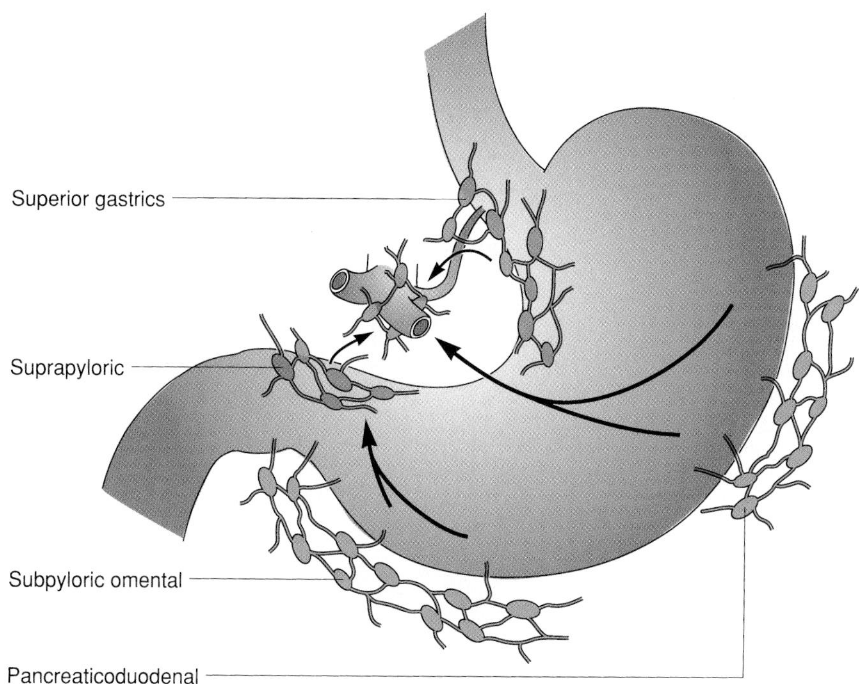

FIGURE 45.3 Lymphatic drainage of the stomach.

surface of the esophagus, whereas the posterior vagal trunk is often midway between the esophagus and the aorta. The anterior vagus supplies a hepatic division, which passes to the right in the lesser omentum before innervating the liver and biliary tract. The remainder of the anterior vagal fibers parallel the lesser curvature of the stomach, branching to the anterior gastric wall. The posterior vagus nerve branches into the celiac division, which passes to the celiac plexus, and a posterior gastric division, which innervates the posterior gastric wall.

Approximately 90% of the fibers in the vagal trunks are afferent, transmitting information from the gastrointestinal tract to the central nervous system (CNS). Parasympathetic afferent fibers are not responsible for the sensation of gastric pain. Only 10% of vagal nerve fibers are motor or secretory efferents. Parasympathetic efferent fibers contained in the vagus originate in the dorsal nucleus of the medulla. Vagal efferent fibers pass without synapse to contact postsynaptic neurons in the gastric wall in the myenteric and submucous plexuses. Secondary neurons directly innervate gastric smooth muscle or epithelial cells. Acetylcholine is the neurotransmitter of primary vagal efferent neurons.

The gastric sympathetic innervation is derived from spinal segments T5 through T10. Sympathetic fibers leave the corresponding spinal nerve roots by way of gray rami communicantes and enter a series of bilateral prevertebral ganglia (Fig. 45.5). From these ganglia, presynaptic fibers pass through the greater splanchnic nerves to the celiac plexus, where they synapse with secondary sympathetic neurons. Postsynaptic sympathetic nerve fibers enter the stomach in association with blood vessels. Afferent sympathetic fibers pass without synapse from the stomach to dorsal spinal roots. Pain of gastroduodenal origin is sensed through afferent fibers of sympathetic origin.

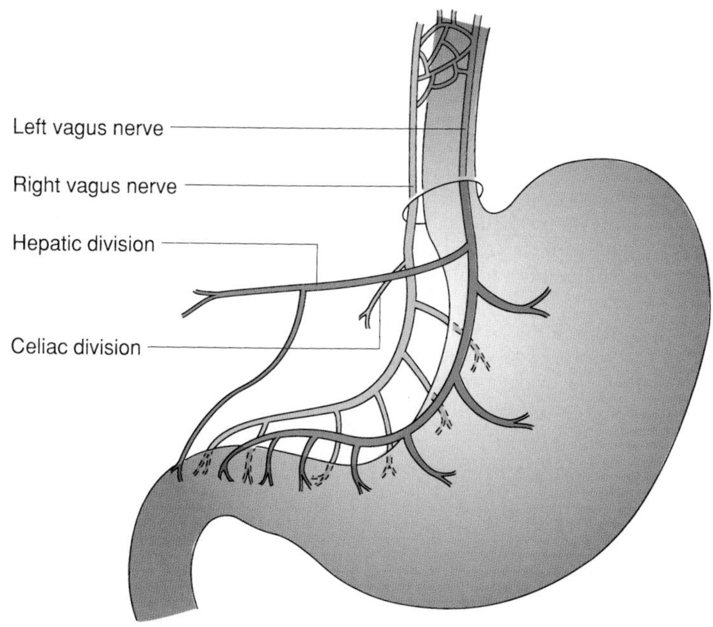

FIGURE 45.4 Vagal innervation of the stomach.

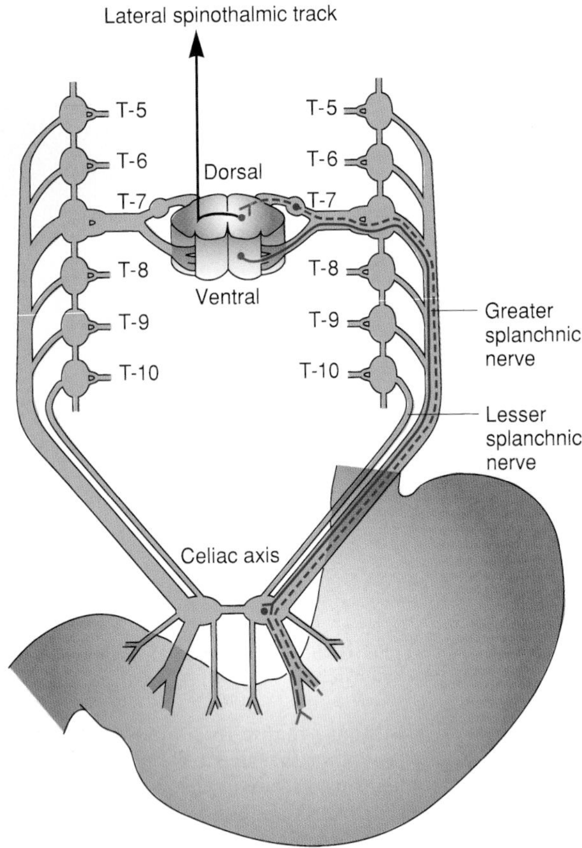

FIGURE 45.5 Derivation of gastric sympathetic innervation.

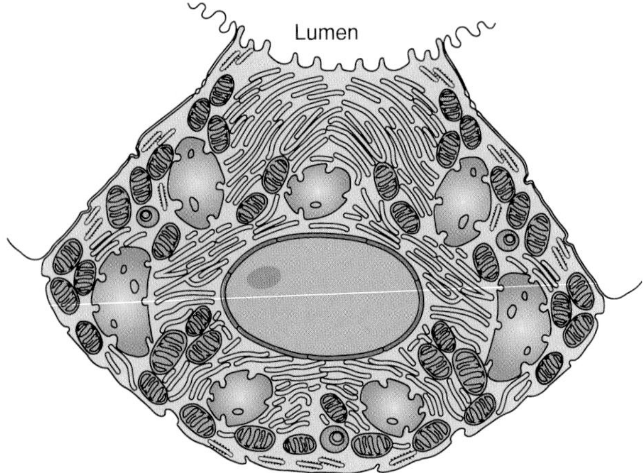

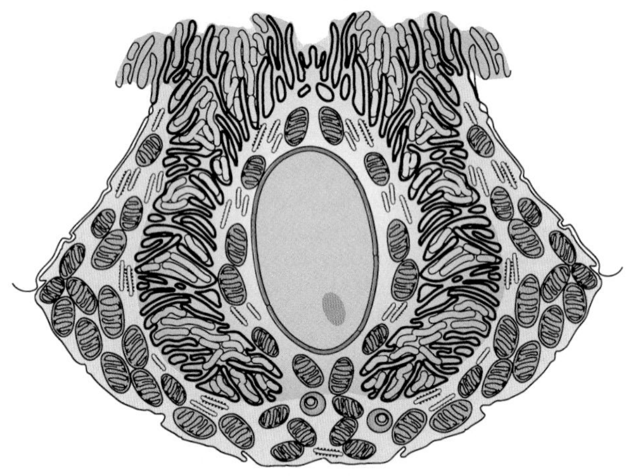

FIGURE 45.6 Resting and stimulated parietal cell, emphasizing morphologic transformation with increase in secretory canalicular membrane surface area that occurs with acid secretion.

MICROSCOPIC ANATOMY

The glandular portions of the stomach are lined by a simple columnar epithelium composed of surface mucous cells. The luminal surface, visualized by scanning electron microscopy, appears cobblestoned, interrupted at intervals by gastric pits. Opening into the gastric pits are one or more gastric glands that impart functional significance to the gastric mucosa. The mucosa of the human stomach is composed of three distinct types of gastric glands—cardiac, oxyntic, and antral.

In humans, cardiac glands occupy a narrow zone adjacent to the esophagus and mark a transition from the stratified squamous epithelium of the esophagus to the simple columnar epithelium of the stomach. The surface and gastric pit mucous cells of the cardia are not distinguishable from those in other areas of the stomach. Cardiac glands contain mucous and undifferentiated and endocrine cells but not the parietal or chief cells that are prominent in the adjacent oxyntic mucosa. Cardiac glands are usually branched and connect with relatively short gastric pits. The functional properties of cardiac glands include the secretion of mucus.

Oxyntic glands are the most distinctive feature of the human stomach. They occupy the fundus and body of the stomach and contain the oxyntic or parietal cells, which are the sites of acid production. Oxyntic glands also contain chief cells, the site of gastric pepsinogen synthesis. The tubular oxyntic glands are usually relatively straight but sometimes branch; several glands may empty into a single gastric pit. The glands are divided into three regions: (a) the isthmus, containing surface mucous cells and a few scattered parietal cells; (b) the neck, with a heavy concentration of parietal cells and a few neck mucous cells; and (c) the base of the gland, containing chief cells, undifferentiated cells, a few parietal cells, and some mucous neck cells. Endocrine cells are scattered throughout all three regions of oxyntic glands.

The most distinctive cell of the gastric mucosa is the acid-secreting parietal cell. Parietal cells have an unusual ultrastructural specialization in the form of intracellular canaliculi, a network of clefts extending to the basal cytoplasm and often encircling the nucleus, which is continuous with the gland lumen (Fig. 45.6). The surface area provided by the intracellular secretory canaliculi is large and is further magnified by microvilli lining the canaliculi. In parietal cells that are not stimulated to secrete acid, the secretory canaliculi are collapsed and inconspicuous. On stimulation, a severalfold increase in canalicular surface area occurs, the intracellular clefts become prominent, and the communication with the luminal surface is readily identified. These changes create an intracellular space in communication with the gastric lumen into which hydrogen ions are secreted at high concentration.

The cytoplasm of the parietal cell also contains an abundance of large mitochondria. Mitochondria are estimated to occupy 30% to 40% of the cytoplasmic volume of unstimulated parietal cells, reflecting the extremely high oxidative activity of these cells. The oxygen consumption rate of isolated parietal cells is approximately five times higher than that of gastric mucous cells. The cytoplasm also contains a limited amount of rough endoplasmic reticulum, presumed to be the production site of intrinsic factor, which is also secreted by parietal cells.

In addition to parietal cells, the oxyntic glands contain the gastric chief cells, which synthesize and secrete pepsinogen.

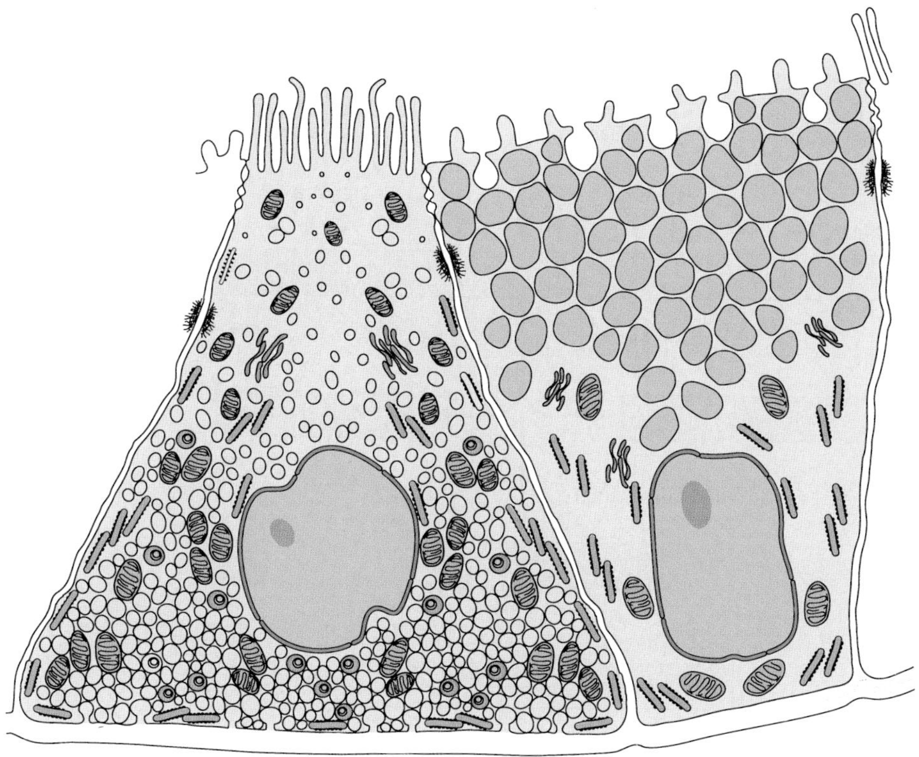

FIGURE 45.7 Contrasting morphology of antral gastrin cell (*left*) with basally oriented secretory granules, and gastric mucous cell (*right*) with apical mucous granules.

Chief cells are most abundant in the basal region of the oxyntic glands. The cells have a morphology typical of protein-secreting exocrine cells and are similar in ultrastructural appearance to pancreatic acinar cells. Rough endoplasmic reticulum is abundant in the cytoplasm and extends between secretory granules. Zymogen granules containing pepsinogen are most concentrated in the apical cytoplasm. Pepsinogen is released by exocytosis from secretory granules at the apical surface of chief cells.

Antral glands occupy the mucosa of the distal stomach and pyloric channel. Antral glands are relatively straight and often empty through deep gastric pits. Although most cells in the antral glands are mucus secreting, gastrin cells are the distinctive feature of this mucosa. Gastrin cells are pyramid shaped, with a narrow area of luminal contact apically and a broad surface overlying the lamina propria basally (Fig. 45.7). Gastrin cells are identified immunocytochemically by the presence of the peptide. Granules ranging from 150 to 400 nm in diameter are the sites of gastrin storage and are most numerous in the basal cytoplasm. Gastrin is released by exocytotic fusion of the secretory granule with the plasma membrane. In contrast to secretion from chief cells, emptying of gastrin-containing granules occurs at the basal membrane rather than at the apical region of the cell. Gastrin thus released diffuses to and enters submucosal capillaries in close apposition to the lamina propria.

GASTRIC PEPTIDES

The stomach contains a number of biologically active peptides in nerves and mucosal endocrine cells, including gastrin, somatostatin, ghrelin, gastrin-releasing peptide, vasoactive intestinal polypeptide (VIP), substance P, glucagon, and calcitonin gene-related peptide. The two peptides with the greatest importance to human disease and clinical surgery are gastrin and somatostatin.

Gastrin

The synthesis, secretion, and action of gastrin have been extensively studied, and many aspects of the biology of gastrin appear to be shared by other gastrointestinal peptide hormones.[1] The gene that encodes for gastrin has been isolated using a human DNA library. The human gastrin gene contains three exons; two exons consist of coding sequences. The major active product is encoded by a single exon. In adults, the gastrin gene is expressed primarily in mucosa cells of the gastric antrum, with lower levels of expression in the duodenum, pituitary, and testis. During embryonic development, the gastrin gene is transiently active in pancreatic islets and colonic mucosa.

The human gene encompasses approximately 4,100 base pairs and directs the synthesis of a peptide of 101 amino acids (Fig. 45.8). The resulting peptide, preprogastrin, contains the sequence of gastrin within its amino acid sequence. Preprogastrin consists of a signal peptide of 21 amino acids, an intervening peptide of 37 amino acids, the 34-residue region of the gastrin molecule, and a carboxyl-terminal extension of nine amino acids. Gastrin is derived from its preprohormone by the sequential enzymatic cleavage of the signal peptide, the intervening peptide, and the carboxyl-terminal extension.

The signal peptide region of preprogastrin consists of a series of hydrophobic amino acids that direct the nascent peptide into the endoplasmic reticulum as it is translated from messenger RNA. After directing the preprogastrin molecule into the rough endoplasmic reticulum, the signal peptide is removed. The remaining peptide is termed *progastrin.* Progastrin is further processed as it traverses the endoplasmic reticulum to mature secretory vesicles. Enzymatic cleavage at a pair of basic amino acid residues proximal to the gastrin 34 (G_{34}) sequence removes the intervening peptide. A similar cleavage removes a six-amino-acid fragment at the carboxyl-terminal end. The peptide that remains has a Gly-Arg-Arg sequence at the carboxyl terminus. Carboxypeptidase cleaves the Arg residues, and the peptide that results is termed *glycine-*

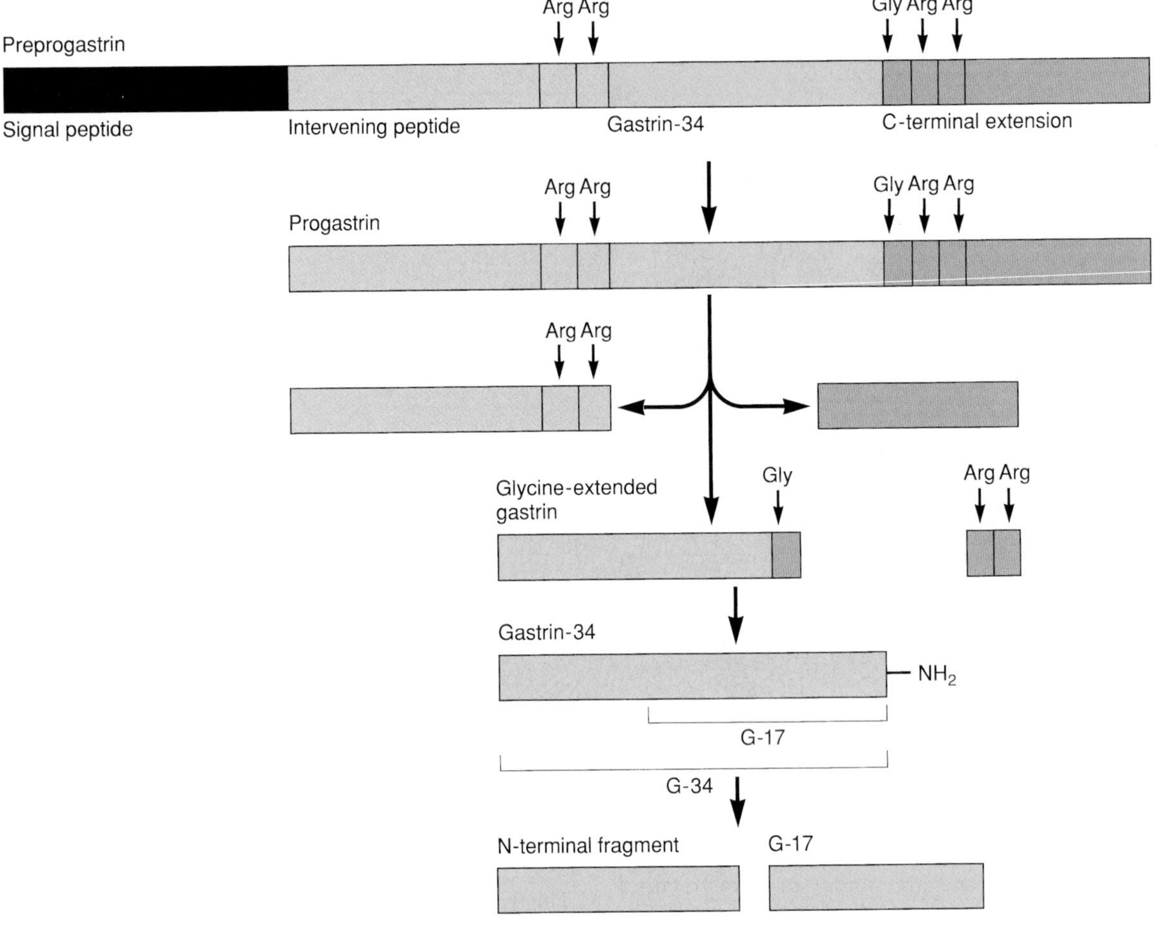

FIGURE 45.8 Sequential processing of preprogastrin molecule.

extended gastrin. G_{34} is formed by cleavage of the Gly-Arg-Arg sequence and amidation of the carboxyl-terminal phenylalanine. Gastrin, like most gastrointestinal peptide hormones, requires terminal amidation for biologic activity. Gastrin 17 (G_{17}), the most abundant form of gastrin in the human antrum, is formed by further processing that removes the first 17 amino acids at the amino terminus of G_{34}. G_{34} is the predominate molecular form of gastrin in the duodenum.

The most important stimulant of gastrin release is a meal. Small peptide fragments and amino acids that result from intragastric proteolysis are the most important food components that stimulate gastrin release. The most potent gastrin-releasing activities are demonstrated by the amino acids tryptophan and phenylalanine. Ingested fat and glucose do not cause gastrin release. Gastric distention by a meal activates cholinergic neurons and stimulates gastrin release. As the meal empties and distention diminishes, VIP-containing neurons are activated, which stimulate somatostatin secretion and thus attenuate gastrin secretion.

Postprandial luminal pH also strongly affects gastrin secretion. Gastrin release is inhibited when acidification of an ingested meal causes the intraluminal pH to fall below 3.0. Conversely, maintaining intragastric pH above 3.0 potentiates gastrin secretion after ingestion of protein or amino acids.[2] Pernicious anemia and atrophic gastritis, which produce chronic achlorhydria, are associated with fasting hypergastrinemia and an exaggerated gastrin meal response. Release of mucosal somatostatin occurs with gastric acidification, and this peptide has been implicated in the inhibited gastrin release that occurs when luminal pH falls.

The vagus nerve appears to both stimulate and inhibit gastrin release.[3] In humans, vagally mediated stimulation of gastrin release can be demonstrated by sham feeding, insulin-induced hypoglycemia, and administration of the vagal stimulant γ-aminobutyric acid. In contrast to these stimulatory vagal effects, hypergastrinemia, observed after vagotomy, suggests that inhibitory vagal effects on gastrin release may also exist. Cholinergic neurons stimulate gastrin secretion directly by actions on gastrin cells. By decreasing somatostatin secretion, cholinergic neurons also indirectly stimulate gastrin release. Evidence suggests that vagal stimulation of gastrin release is mediated by bombesin or its mammalian equivalent, gastrin-releasing peptide, acting as a neurotransmitter in the gastric wall. Adrenergic stimulation has also been noted to increase gastrin release.

Chronic gastric infection with *Helicobacter pylori* causes increased acid secretion by altering gastrin release.[4,5] *H. pylori* has been observed to upregulate proinflammatory cytokines, including interleukin (IL)-6, IL-8, and tumor necrosis factor-α (TNF-α). Several inflammatory mediators have been demonstrated to stimulate gastrin release from isolated gastrin cells. The putative gastrin secretagogues include IL-1, IL-8, TNF-α, interferon-γ, and leukotrienes C4 and D4. The same factors that affect gastrin release also influence gastrin mRNA expression. Food ingestion increases gastrin mRNA abundance, whereas fasting and somatostatin decrease gastrin mRNA production. Chronic achlorhydria, as seen in pernicious anemia, increases gastrin mRNA production.

In addition to stimulating acid secretion from gastric parietal cells (detailed later in this chapter), gastrin has important physiologic actions in the control of gastrointestinal mucosal growth. The acid-secreting oxyntic mucosa is particularly sensitive to the trophic actions of gastrin, but the mucous membranes of the duodenum, colon, and pancreatic parenchyma

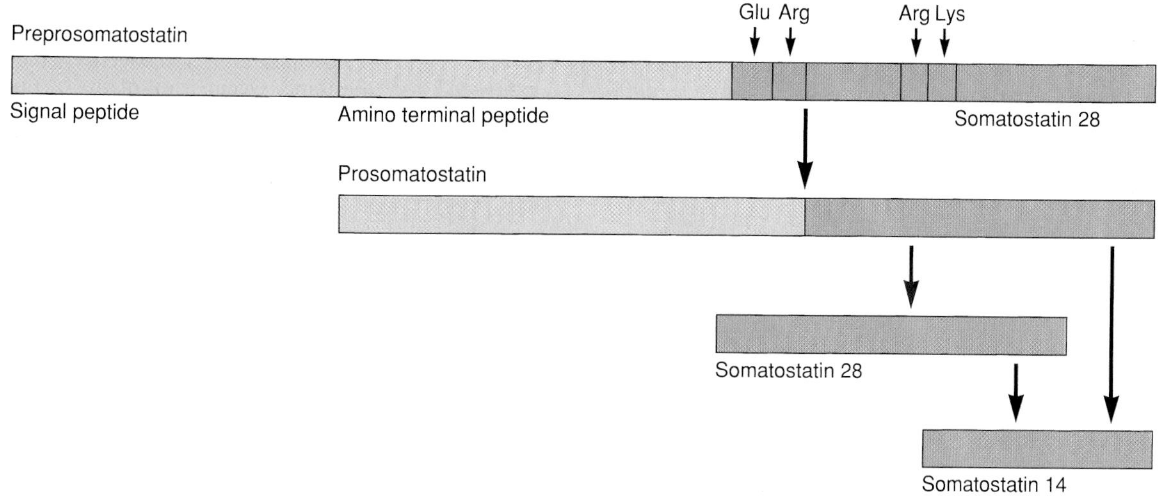

FIGURE 45.9 Derivation of somatostatin 14 from preprosomatostatin precursor.

are also affected. Stimulation of mucosal growth by gastrin is enhanced by the presence of solid food in the diet. The 17- and 34-amino acid forms of gastrin are equipotent in stimulating mucosal growth. In humans, the relative importance of gastrin and other influences, such as the composition and form of the diet and the actions of other trophic hormones, have not been completely established. Prolonged stimulation by high levels of gastrin, as seen in the Zollinger-Ellison syndrome, is associated with hypertrophy of the gastric mucosa. Smaller increases in circulating gastrin, such as those that follow vagotomy, do not cause mucosal hypertrophy.

Somatostatin

Somatostatin, like gastrin, is very significant in gastric physiology. Somatostatin was first isolated from hypothalamic tissues and was named for its ability to inhibit the release of growth hormone. The peptide was subsequently localized in neurons in central and peripheral nervous systems, and in endocrine cells in the pancreas, stomach, and intestine. The wide tissue distribution of somatostatin suggested important regulatory functions, a concept validated by many investigations.

The human somatostatin gene is located on chromosome 3 and encodes for a precursor of 116 amino acids (Fig. 45.9). The somatostatin molecule is contained in the carboxyl-terminal sequence of this preprohormone. The first 24 amino acids of the amino terminus of preprosomatostatin constitute a signal peptide; cleavage of this signal peptide leaves prosomatostatin. Enzymatic cleavage of an additional 64-amino acid segment from prosomatostatin forms somatostatin 28. Further processing of somatostatin 28 to somatostatin 14 is tissue-specifically regulated. In the stomach, most somatostatin exists as the shorter peptide.

Gastric somatostatin release responds to luminal, hormonal, and neural signals. Luminal acidification is associated with increased somatostatin release, whereas somatostatin release decreases when luminal pH is increased. A number of peptides have been demonstrated experimentally to release somatostatin from the stomach, including gastrin, cholecystokinin, and secretin. β-Adrenergic agonists have also been shown to release somatostatin. In contrast, electrical stimulation of vagal nerves inhibits somatostatin release, as does the cholinergic agonist methacholine.

The most important gastric function of somatostatin appears to be regulation of acid secretion and gastrin release. Circulating somatostatin appears to be important in modulating gastric acid secretion; locally released somatostatin functions to regulate gastrin release. In each instance, somatostatin serves an inhibitory function, decreasing acid secretion and diminishing the release of gastrin. In animals, antral or duodenal acidification has been associated with an increase in circulating somatostatin. Increases in circulating somatostatin are followed, in turn, by decreased gastric acid secretion. Infusion of exogenous somatostatin in doses that produce somatostatin levels similar to those observed postprandially has also been shown to inhibit acid secretion. In humans, concentrations of somatostatin capable of inhibiting acid secretion can do so without altering serum gastrin levels, indicating a direct action on the acid-secreting fundic mucosa.

Somatostatin is believed to influence gastrin secretion through a locally active intramucosal mechanism. Local actions of somatostatin are supported by ultrastructural studies of antral somatostatin cells, which demonstrate long cytoplasmic processes that make intimate cell-to-cell contact with antral gastrin cells. The presence of somatostatin at these sites of cellular contact implies that somatostatin cells influence the function of gastrin cells through local release of the peptide. Somatostatin can also reach neighboring gastrin cells through diffusion or local blood flow. A number of experiments have suggested that release of somatostatin and gastrin is functionally, although reciprocally, linked. For example, in anesthetized animals, an increase in gastric pH or ingestion of a meal is associated with increases in gastrin and decreases in somatostatin in antral venous blood. Cholinergic agents stimulate gastrin release while inhibiting somatostatin release. Prostaglandin E_2, in contrast, inhibits gastrin release and stimulates somatostatin secretion. These and similar observations suggest that increases in somatostatin release are often associated with decreased gastrin secretion. A family of five somatostatin receptors has been cloned. Inhibition of gastrin-stimulated gastric acid secretion is mediated by somatostatin receptor subtype 2.

Ghrelin

Ghrelin is a gastric peptide that is localized to oxyntic glands.[8] The hormone is also produced in the hypothalamus. The ghrelin receptor is a member of the family of G-protein-coupled receptors and contains seven transmembrane domains. Ghrelin receptors are widely distributed among both central and peripheral tissues, including pituitary gland, hypothalamus, pancreas, stomach and intestine. Ghrelin causes growth hormone secretion following either peripheral or central administration and release of growth hormone from cultured pituitary cells.

Ghrelin plays an important role in the control of food intake and energy metabolism.[9] Ghrelin secretion is increased by weight loss and by restriction of caloric intake. Ghrelin administration has been found to stimulate food intake, to induce growth of adipose tissues, and to increase body weight. Administration of ghrelin antibody or ghrelin receptor antagonists blunts ghrelin-induced weight gain and positive energy balance.

Ghrelin is a circulationg hormone with CNS effects. Although ghrelin is secreted from the stomach and circulates in the blood, the ability of ghrelin to stimulate appetite, termed the orexigenic effect, is mediated by hypothalamic circuits in the central nervous system. Direct peripheral effects of ghrelin on peripheral tissues that contribute to the regulation of body weight and energy homeostasis may also exist.

GASTRIC ACID SECRETION

Cellular Events

An appreciation of the mechanisms that control the stomach's acid formation is essential to a discussion of gastric disease. An understanding of the cellular basis of acid secretion by the gastric parietal cell also provides a foundation for discussing the pharmacologic treatment of acid–peptic diseases. The basolateral membrane of the parietal cell contains specific receptors for histamine, gastrin, and acetylcholine, the three major stimulants of acid production.[6] Each stimulant reaches the parietal cell by a different route. Histamine is released from mastlike cells within the lamina propria and diffuses to the mucosa, acetylcholine is released close to the parietal cells from cholinergic nerve terminals, and gastrin is delivered by the systemic circulation to the fundic mucosa from its source in the antrum and proximal duodenum (Fig. 45.10).

Histamine receptors in the gastric mucosa are classified pharmacologically as H_2 receptors because they may be stimulated by agonists such as 4-methylhistamine and selectively blocked by agents such as cimetidine. Occupation of the histamine receptor activates a membrane-bound enzyme called *adenylate cyclase* (Fig. 45.11). Activated adenylate cyclase catalyzes the conversion of intracellular adenosine triphosphate (ATP) to cyclic adenosine monophosphate (cAMP), and enhancement of cAMP production by histamine is closely linked to stimulation of parietal cell acid production. cAMP mediates histamine-stimulated acid production by activating protein kinase A, which in turn catalyzes protein phosphorylation. The target protein molecules for this phosphorylation, in turn, stimulate acid production.

Acetylcholine and related cholinergic agonists activate parietal cells after binding to muscarinic receptors. The stimulatory effects of acetylcholine and its congeners can be abolished by atropine. The action of acetylcholine is mediated by muscarinic receptor subtype 3 (M_3). Studies suggest that cholinergic stimulation of parietal cell function is coupled to enhanced mobilization of intracellular calcium. The resultant transient increases in intracellular calcium activate mechanisms that stimulate acid secretion (Fig. 45.11). Evidence also indicates that occupation of acetylcholine receptors increases turnover of specific membrane phospholipids termed *phosphatidylinositides*. Acetylcholine–receptor binding is followed by activation of membrane-associated phospholipase C. Phospholipase C acts on phosphatidylinositol-4,5 bisphosphate (PIP_2) within the plasma membrane to liberate water-soluble inositol triphosphate (IP_3) and diacylglycerol. A major action of IP_3 is to increase intracellular calcium, mainly from intracellular stores in the endoplasmic reticulum. The resulting increased cytosolic calcium interacts with calmodulin or other calcium-binding proteins. Calmodulin kinase type II is involved in parietal cell activation by acetylcholine. Intracellular calcium in this form is postulated to modulate parietal cell function through protein phosphorylation or enzyme activation. Diacylglycerol,

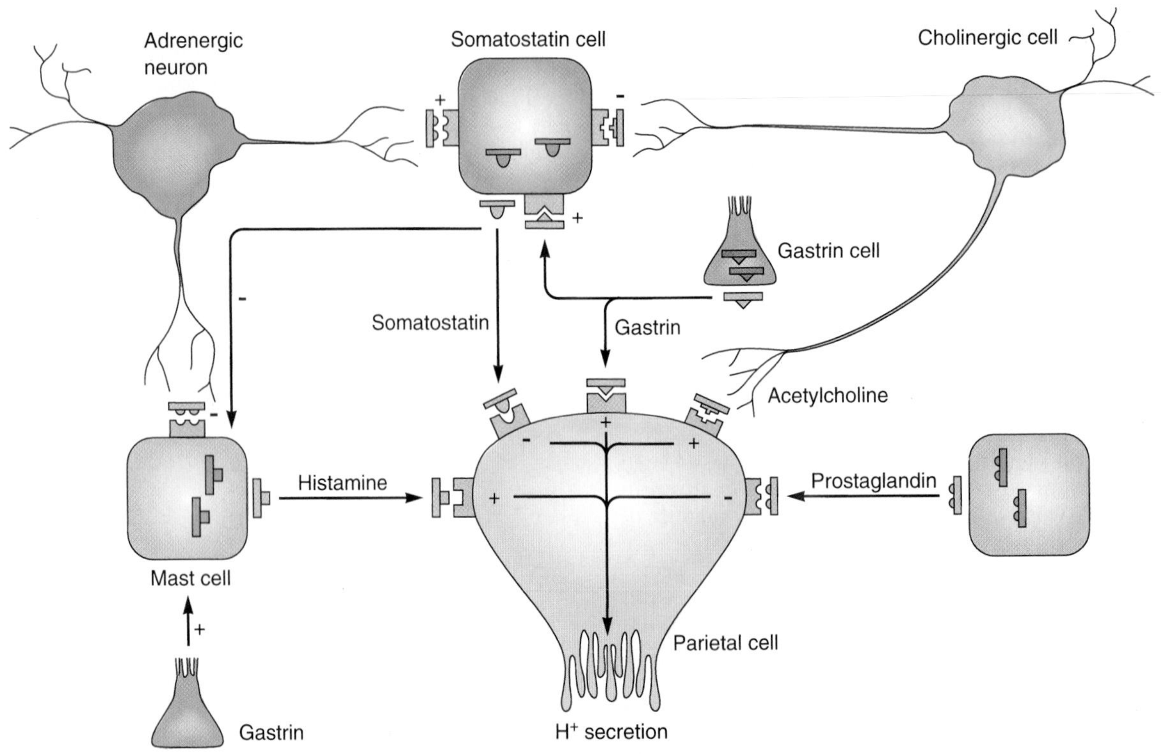

FIGURE 45.10 Interactions of cell types that affect parietal cell acid secretion.

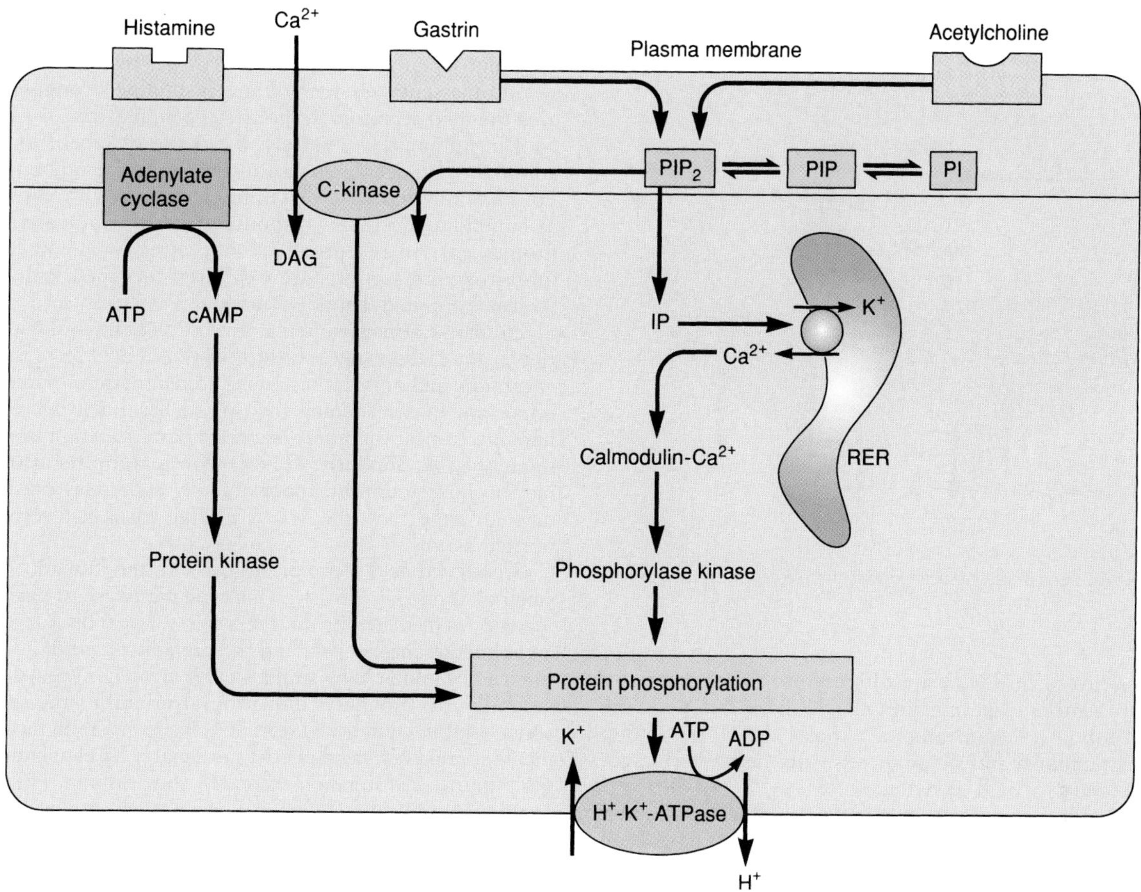

FIGURE 45.11 Cellular mechanisms controlling parietal cell acid secretion.

the second product released by hydrolysis of PIP_2, activates a class of protein kinases that are phospholipid dependent and Ca^{2+} activated, protein kinase C. Protein kinase C in turn acts to phosphorylate a set of proteins that are distinct from those affected by the calmodulin-dependent system. The ultimate result of this protein phosphorylation is parietal cell activation and hydrogen ion secretion.

Parietal cells can also be activated by occupation of specific gastrin receptors. As with cholinergic stimulation, gastrin exposure increases membrane PIP_2 turnover (see Fig. 45.11). Like acetylcholine, the actions of gastrin depend highly on increases in intracellular calcium and activation of protein kinase C.

Although histamine, acetylcholine, and gastrin occupy separate receptors on the parietal cell and activate differing second-messenger systems, each secretagogue ultimately acts by means of a specialized ion transport system called the *parietal cell proton pump*. This membrane-bound protein is located in the secretory canaliculus of the parietal cell; the peptide has not been identified in other gastric cells or in significant amounts in other organs. The proton pump is an H^+-K^+-adenosine triphosphatase (ATPase) that electroneutrally exchanges cytosolic H^+ for luminal K^+. Hydrogen ions are concentrated 2.5-million-fold within the secretory canaliculus, and the hydrolysis of ATP is the energy source for transport against the steep electrochemical gradient generated. For each H^+ ion transported to the luminal surface of the canalicular membrane, one K^+ ion is transported to the cytosolic surface (Fig. 45.12). This cotransport requires that K^+ be continuously supplied to the luminal surface of the secretory membrane. This requirement is satisfied by conductance of K^+ across the canalicular membrane from intracellular stores. Chloride ions also enter the secretory canaliculus by diffusion.

Activation of the H^+-K^+-ATPase significantly increases intracellular OH^- generation, with potential cellular toxicity. Carbonic anhydrase, which is associated with the canalicular membrane, converts OH^- to HCO_3^-. The HCO_3^- produced is disposed of by exchange for Cl^- at the basolateral membrane. Intracellular Cl^- thus acquired supplies the necessary Cl^- on a one-to-one basis for each H^+ secreted. The transcellular exchange of H^+ for HCO_3^- ensures that the voluminous secretion of hydrochloride at the luminal surface of the gastric mucosa is matched by an equivalent delivery of base to submucosal capillaries. Parietal cell ionic transport pathways are shown in Fig. 45.13.

The function of the proton pump is highly regulated. In the unstimulated state, the enzyme is sequestered in cytoplasmic structures termed *tubulovesicles* that are not connected to the gastric lumen. Tubulovesicle membranes in this state have a low permeability to KCl. Stimulation of acid secretion causes

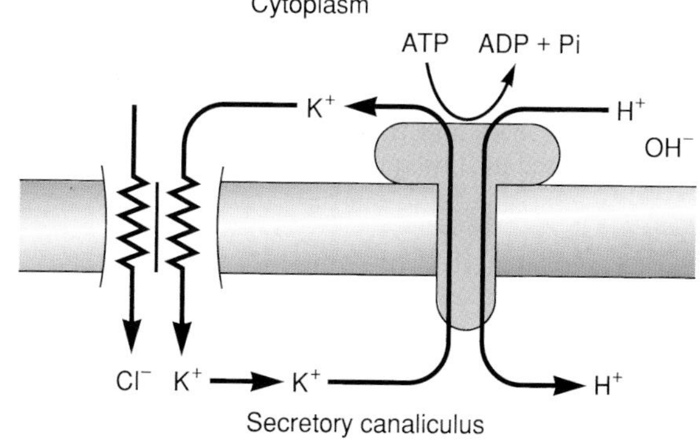

FIGURE 45.12 Gastric H^+-K^+-adenosine triphosphatase (ATPase).

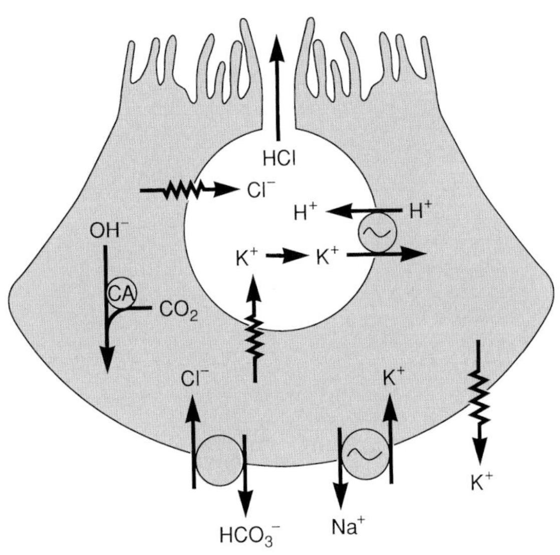

FIGURE 45.13 Ionic fluxes associated with acid secretion by the parietal cell.

tubulovesicles to fuse with apical secretory membranes and increases membrane permeability to KCl. In this way, the fusion of tubulovesicle membrane exposes the H^+-K^+ pump to the gastric lumen and simultaneously provides the K^+ substrate necessary for acid secretion.

Parietal cells also contain membrane receptors that inhibit acid secretion. Specific receptors for somatostatin have been identified using isolated gastric cells. Activation of isolated parietal cells by histamine, pentagastrin, or the cholinergic agonist carbachol can be blocked by somatostatin 28. In the case of histamine activation, the inhibitory effects appear to be mediated by the ability of somatostatin to block the production of cAMP. The mechanisms by which somatostatin interferes with activation by pentagastrin or carbachol are not completely defined. Somatostatin appears to inhibit the actions of these agonists at a point distal to second-messenger generation. Gastric parietal cells also contain receptors for prostaglandins, notably prostaglandin E_2 and its derivatives. Prostaglandin E_2 is a potent inhibitor of histamine-stimulated parietal cell activation, probably by a mechanism that inhibits formation of cAMP. Prostaglandin inhibition is specific for histamine; the actions of gastrin or carbachol are not affected. Epidermal growth factor and transforming growth factor-α also inhibit histamine-stimulated acid secretion through effects on cAMP production.

These considerations of the cellular basis of acid production demonstrate how parietal cell function can be altered pharmacologically. Gastric acid production can be blocked by receptor antagonists for each of the three primary stimulants—gastrin, acetylcholine, and histamine. Direct inhibition of acid production can be effected by derivatives of somatostatin or prostaglandin E_2. All forms of stimulated acid production could be blocked by agents that act as inhibitors of the parietal cell proton pump. Agents that act at each of these points have been developed, and their appropriate clinical applications are discussed in subsequent chapters.

Regulation of Acid Secretion

Given the multiple receptors on parietal cells, it is not surprising that a great deal of secretagogue interdependence, both stimulatory and inhibitory, exists in humans. Parietal cell activation and the resultant acid secretion is greater in response to a combination of agonists than it is in response to the total effect of agents used singly. This increase in responsiveness is defined as *potentiation.* Potentiating interactions are most apparent when agents are used that act by way of different second-messenger systems. Thus, histamine strongly potentiates the acid-secretory response to pentagastrin or to carbachol in humans. Conversely, blockade of receptors to one stimulant also decreases responsiveness to the other agonists. For example, blocking histamine receptors with agents such as cimetidine decreases responsiveness to pentagastrin, even though gastrin receptors are not directly affected. These inhibitory interactions are exploited therapeutically in the treatment of acid–peptic diseases.

Humans normally secrete 2 to 5 mEq per hour of hydrochloride in the fasting state, constituting basal acid secretion. Both vagal tone and ambient histamine secretion are presumed to be important in determining the rate of basal acid secretion. In humans, truncal vagotomy decreases basal secretion by approximately 85%. Similarly, H_2 receptor antagonists also inhibit basal acid secretion by approximately 80%. Gastrin does not have an important role in determining basal acid secretion in normal people.

Stimulated acid secretion begins with the thought, sight, or smell of food (Fig. 45.14). This cephalic phase of gastric acid secretion is mediated by the vagus nerve. Vagal discharge directs a cholinergic mechanism, and the cephalic phase of acid secretion can be inhibited by administering atropine. Vagal discharge secondary to cephalic stimulation also inhibits the release of somatostatin. Diminished secretion of somatostatin further augments stimulatory vagal effects, presumably by eliminating tonic inhibition of acid secretion exerted by somatostatin. The cephalic component of acid secretion can be measured in normal people by sham feeding and is approximately 10 mEq per hour. The cephalic phase approximates 40% of the maximal acid-secretory response to gastrin infusion.

The gastric phase of acid secretion begins when food enters the stomach. The presence of partially hydrolyzed food constituents, gastric distention, and the buffering capacity of food all stimulate acid secretion. Gastrin is the most important mediator of the gastric phase of acid secretion. In normal humans, acid-secretory rates after a mixed meal average 15 to 25 mEq per hour, approximately 75% of the maximal response achieved with infusion of exogenous gastrin or histamine. The meal response is less than the maximal response to exogenous stimulants because food also causes the release of somatostatin and initiates other inhibitory responses. In humans, 90% of meal-stimulated acid secretion is mediated by gastrin release.[7]

The inhibitory regulation of gastric acid secretion is accomplished by CNS, gastric, and intestinal mechanisms. Stimulated acid secretion can be inhibited experimentally by administering various neuropeptides into the lateral cerebral ventricles, including gastrin-releasing peptide (bombesin), corticotropin-releasing factor, and calcitonin gene-related peptide. Although the relevance of these observations to human physiology remains to be determined, it is likely that CNS inhibition of acid secretion exists in humans. In this regard, the vagus nerve has both a stimulatory and an inhibitory role in acid secretion and gastrin release. Vagotomy causes fasting and postprandial hypergastrinemia, indicating that an inhibitory regulation of gastrin release normally exists. Hypergastrinemia is sustained long term after vagotomy by hyperplasia of antral gastrin cells. The vagal fibers to the oxyntic region of the stomach appear to mediate this inhibitory effect.

In humans, the most important and clearly established gastric inhibitory influence is the suppression of gastrin release when the antral mucosa is exposed to acid. When luminal pH falls to 2.0, gastrin release stops. Antral acidification also suppresses the gastrin response to an ingested meal. Somatostatin acting locally in the gastric mucosa as a paracrine agent may mediate this important inhibitory response. Release of gastric somatostatin is reciprocally linked to that of gastrin; acidification of the antrum causes

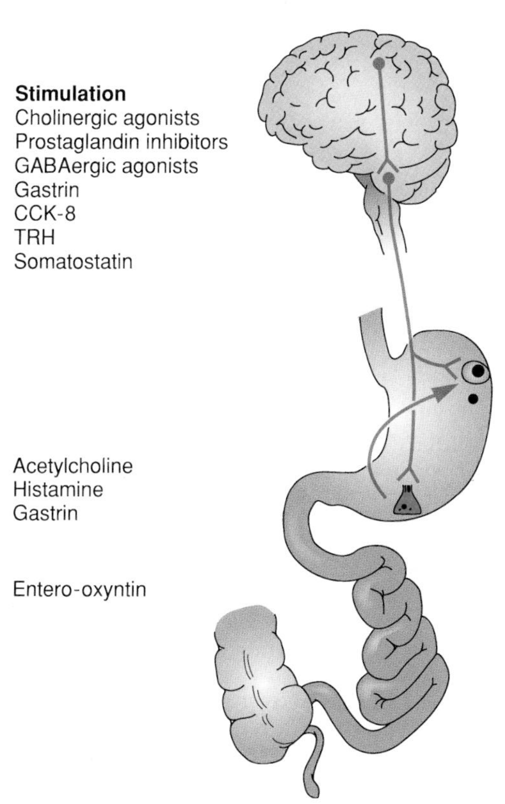

FIGURE 45.14 Regulation of acid secretion *in vivo*.

increases in somatostatin release and decreases in gastrin secretion. Antral distention also inhibits stimulated acid secretion.

The entry of digestive products into the intestine begins intestinal-phase inhibition of gastric acid secretion. Acidification of the duodenal bulb inhibits acid secretion, and although exogenous secretin also can inhibit acid secretion, this effect appears to be independent of the release of secretin from the duodenal mucosa. Hyperosmolar solutions and those containing fat also potently inhibit acid secretion. Several peptides, including secretin, somatostatin, peptide YY, gastric inhibitory peptide, and neurotensin, have been proposed as mediators of the intestinal phase effects.

PEPSIN

Pepsins are a heterogeneous group of proteolytic enzymes that are secreted by the gastric chief cells. Pepsin is derived under acidic conditions from pepsinogen by the autocatalytic loss of a variable amino-terminal sequence of the parent compound. This conversion occurs slowly at pH values of 5.0 to 6.0 and occurs rapidly when luminal pH approximates 2.0. Pepsin catalyzes the hydrolysis of a wide variety of peptide bonds that contain acidic residues, with a pH optimum for hydrolysis between 1.5 and 2.5. Once activated, pepsin is sensitive to ambient pH values; it is irreversibly denatured at pH 7.0 or greater.

The most important stimulus for pepsinogen secretion is cholinergic stimulation. Acetylcholine and its derivatives stimulate pepsinogen secretion by a mechanism that can be antagonized by atropine, indicating a muscarinic receptor. The receptor appears to have a high affinity for the selective muscarinic antagonist pirenzepine and therefore appears to be an M_1 type. Endogenous cholinergic stimulation through the vagal nerve results in the formation of a gastric secretion that is rich in pepsin. Although both exogenous histamine and gastrin can stimulate pepsin secretion, their actions appear to be indirectly due to the concomitant secretion of gastric acid rather than to direct stimulation of chief cells. Chief cells have also been shown to possess cholecystokinin receptors, and cholecystokininlike peptides appear to have a direct stimulatory action on chief cells. The oxyntic mucosa contains somatostatin cells near chief cells. Pepsinogen secretion in response to a variety of stimuli has been demonstrated to be inhibited by somatostatin.

The major physiologic function of pepsin is to initiate protein digestion. Pepsin is highly active against collagen and may be important in the digestion of animal protein. Intragastric protein hydrolysis by pepsin is incomplete, and relatively large peptides enter the intestine, although amino acids and small peptide fragments are released. These products of partial hydrolysis are important signals for gastrin and cholecystokinin release, which in turn regulates digestive processes. In this way, pepsin also contributes to the overall coordination of the digestive process.

INTRINSIC FACTOR

Autoradiographic and immunocytochemical techniques have confirmed the parietal cell as the site of intrinsic factor synthesis and storage in humans. Intrinsic factor secretion, like acid secretion, is stimulated by histamine, acetylcholine, and gastrin. Unlike acid production, intrinsic factor secretion peaks rapidly after stimulation and then returns to baseline. The amount of intrinsic factor secreted usually greatly exceeds the amount needed to bind and absorb available dietary cobalamin.

GASTRIC BICARBONATE PRODUCTION

It is generally agreed that the gastric mucosa secretes HCO_3^- in addition to acid. The cells responsible for HCO_3^- production are presumed to be the surface mucous cells facing the gastric lumen, and HCO_3^- transport has been postulated to protect against damage from luminal acid. In theory, H^+ ions diffusing from luminal bulk fluids toward the gastric mucosa could be

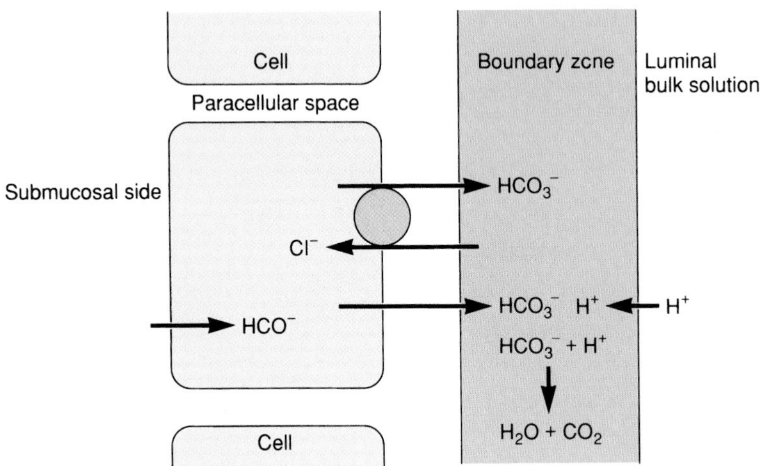

FIGURE 45.15 Schematic representation of mucosal bicarbonate secretion showing neutralization of luminal hydrogen ions immediately above the mucosal surface.

neutralized by secreted HCO_3 near the surface (Fig. 45.15). In this way, nearly neutral pH can be maintained at the mucosal surface, even if the total amount of hydrochloride secreted greatly exceeds gastric HCO_3^- production. The occurrence of pH gradients at the surface of the gastric mucosa have been demonstrated in humans using microelectrodes. Drugs or chemicals that inhibit bicarbonate secretion result in acidification of the mucosal surface.

The degree of luminal acidity, reflected by pH, required to stimulate bicarbonate secretion is greater in the stomach than in the duodenum. Direct exposure of the gastric mucosa to pH levels of 2.0 or more increases bicarbonate secretion. In the duodenum, exposure of the mucosa to pH 5.0 doubles bicarbonate secretion, whereas exposure to pH 2.0 increases alkaline secretion 10-fold.

Cholinergic agonists, vagal nerve stimulation, and sham feeding have all been shown to increase gastric HCO_3^- production. The effects of cholinergic stimulation can be blocked by atropine. In the human stomach, exposure to luminal perfusates at pH 2.0 has been associated with increased release of prostaglandin E_2. Prostaglandin E_2 and its synthetic derivatives are also potent stimulants of gastric bicarbonate secretion. Because mucosal bicarbonate production can be decreased in experimental models by indomethacin, endogenous prostaglandins are thought to be important in the mucosal alkaline response.

GASTRIC BLOOD FLOW

Because the gastric mucosa is metabolically highly active, control of mucosal blood flow is of great physiologic importance. In addition, studies have implicated perfusion abnormalities in the development of mucosal lesions during periods of stress. Mucosal blood flow is regulated by neural, hormonal, and locally active influences.

Postganglionic sympathetic nerve fibers reach the stomach in association with its blood supply and richly innervate small mucosal arteries. Mucosal capillaries do not receive adrenergic innervation. Electrical stimulation of sympathetic nerves supplying the stomach is followed by decreased total gastric blood flow, decreased flow in celiac and gastroepiploic vessels, and diminished blood flow to the mucosa. Studies in animals demonstrate that vasoconstriction of the gastric vascular bed is mediated by α-adrenergic receptors and that vasodilation is mediated by β-adrenergic receptors.

Stimulation of the vagus nerve is followed by a prompt increase in blood flow, suggesting a dilatory effect of parasympathetic nerves. The effects of vagal stimulation on mucosal blood flow are complicated by accompanying increases in acid secretion. Almost all stimuli that increase acid production also increase blood flow secondarily.

A number of gastrointestinal peptide hormones affect gastric blood flow, most because of their ability to increase or decrease acid secretion. Thus, gastrin, because it is a potent stimulant of acid secretion, also increases mucosal blood flow. Cholecystokinin appears to have direct vasodilatory effects on the gastric vasculature. Vasopressin has been well demonstrated to have direct vasoconstrictor activity.

Nitric oxide modulates basal gastric vascular tone and controls gastric vasodilation and hyperemia. Nitric oxide mediates the hyperemic response that accompanies increases in acid secretion, although the molecule has no direct stimulatory role in acid production.

Prostaglandins are important mucosally produced compounds that have clear effects on the gastric vasculature. Prostaglandins of the E class have been shown in animals and humans to increase gastric blood flow at doses that decrease acid secretion. Indomethacin, in doses sufficient to inhibit prostaglandin formation, decreases the diameter of submucosal blood vessels and reduces basal blood flow. Complete inhibition of cyclooxygenase activity causes an approximate 50% reduction in resting blood flow. These studies suggest that endogenous, locally produced prostaglandins are crucial to maintaining basal gastric blood flow in humans and probably act in concert with endogenous nitric oxide.

GASTRIC MOTILITY

Gastric Smooth Muscle

Consideration of gastric motility requires that the stomach be viewed in functional terms as two different regions, the proximal one third and the distal two thirds. These areas are distinct in terms of smooth muscle anatomy, electrical activity, and contractile function. The regions do not correspond to the traditional anatomic divisions of fundus, corpus, and antrum.

In the proximal stomach, three layers of gastric smooth muscle can be distinguished: an outer longitudinal layer, a middle circular layer, and an inner oblique layer. In the distal two thirds of the stomach the longitudinal layer is most clearly defined, and the inner oblique layer is usually not distinct. The gastric smooth muscle ends at the pylorus.

The smooth muscle of the proximal stomach is electrically stable, whereas the smooth muscle of the distal stomach demonstrates spontaneous, repeated electrical discharges. Gastric smooth muscle exhibits myoelectric activity that is based on a highly regular pattern called the *slow wave*.[10] In the stomach, slow waves occur with a frequency of three cycles per minute. Slow waves do not, by themselves, lead to gastric contractions, but they do set the maximum rate of contractions at three per minute. Gastric contractions occur when action potentials are phase locked with the crest of the slow wave.

Extracellular electrical recording from the serosal surface of the stomach also demonstrates the intrinsic electrical activity of the distal stomach in the form of pacesetter potentials. Pacesetter potentials reflect partial depolarization of the gastric smooth muscle cell and are recorded during relatively long periods (2 or 3 seconds). Pacesetters originate along the greater curvature at a point in the proximal third of the stomach. Pacesetter potentials, discharging at a rate of three times per minute in humans, drive cells located distally. Spread of the pacesetter potentials is faster along the greater curvature, so that a ring of electrical activity reaches the pylorus simultaneously along both curvatures. The pacesetter potentials do not result in smooth muscle contraction unless an additional depolarization is superimposed in the form of an action potential. When action potentials occur, a ring of smooth muscle contraction moves peristaltically along the distal stomach toward the pylorus.

Duodenal slow-wave frequency and maximum rate of phasic contractions are higher than those observed in the stomach. The duodenal rate is approximately 12 cycles per minute; the contraction rate declines progressively to nine cycles per minute in the distal ileum.

The smooth muscle activity of the proximal stomach is fundamentally different from that of the distal stomach. There are no pacesetter or action potentials in the proximal stomach. As a result, peristalsis does not occur. Proximal gastric contraction is tonic and prolonged, and increases in luminal pressure are often sustained for several minutes.

Coordination of Contraction

Important vagally mediated reflexes influence intragastric pressure, presumably by affecting contractile activity of smooth muscle in the proximal stomach. The most important reflex is termed *receptive relaxation* and occurs with ingestion of a meal. Increasing gastric volumes are accommodated with little increase in intragastric pressure by relaxation of the proximal stomach. This receptive relaxation allows the proximal stomach to act as a storage site for ingested food in the immediate postprandial period. Afferent impulses, presumed to originate from stretch receptors in the gastric wall, are carried along vagal fibers; efferent vagal discharges are inhibitory. Receptive gastric accommodation is lost after either truncal or proximal gastric vagotomy. After the meal has been ingested, proximal contractile activity increases; alterations in proximal gastric tone cause the compressive movement of gastric content from the fundus to the antrum.

Food that enters the antrum from the proximal stomach is propelled peristaltically toward the pylorus. A number of observations indicate that the pylorus closes 2 or 3 seconds before the arrival of the antral contraction ring. This coordinate closing of the pylorus allows a small bolus of liquid and suspended food particles to pass while retropulsing the main mass of gastric contents back into the proximal antrum. The churning action that results mixes ingested food particles, gastric acid, and pepsin, and contributes to the grinding function of the stomach. Solid food particles do not ordinarily pass the pylorus unless they are no larger than 1 mm.

A consistent finding in humans ingesting a mixed solid–liquid meal is that liquids empty more quickly than solids. Characteristically, solid food empties only after a lag period, whereas liquid emptying begins almost immediately. A traditional interpretation of these human observations has been that the proximal stomach is the dominant force in determining how quickly a liquid meal empties by the gastroduodenal pressure gradient generated by proximal gastric contractions. The actions of the proximal stomach in liquid emptying are also regulated by the sieving actions of the antropyloric segment and are modified by the nutrient composition of the ingested meal. The distal gastric segment has been postulated to control solid emptying through its grinding and peristaltic actions. This traditional concept of the two-component stomach is useful in considering observations in patients who have undergone gastric operative procedures. Patients who have undergone proximal gastric vagotomy exhibit accelerated emptying of liquids but have normal solid emptying. Because of loss of receptive relaxation, the denervation of the proximal stomach is presumed to increase intragastric pressure and accelerate liquid emptying while leaving the distal gastric segment unaffected. Conversely, vagal denervation of the antrum interrupts gastric emptying of solids to a greater degree than liquids. Although this model of gastric emptying oversimplifies the many mechanisms (gastric, pyloric, and intestinal) that work in concert to control gastric emptying, it provides a useful framework for considering the effects of gastric surgical procedures.

KEY POINTS

- **The stomach is an extremely well-vascularized organ, supplied by a number of major arteries and protected by a large number of extramural and intramural collaterals.**
- **Oxyntic glands occupy the fundus and body of the stomach and contain the oxyntic or parietal cells, which are the sites of acid production. Oxyntic glands also contain chief cells, the site of gastric pepsinogen synthesis.**
- **The most important stimulant of gastrin release is a meal. Postprandial luminal pH also strongly affects gastrin secretion.**
- **The basolateral membrane of the parietal cell contains specific receptors for histamine, gastrin, and acetylcholine, the three major stimulants of acid production.**
- **Pepsins are a heterogeneous group of proteolytic enzymes that are secreted by the gastric chief cells.**
- **The gastric mucosa is the site of production of intrinsic factor, which is necessary for the absorption of cobalamin from the ileal mucosa. Total gastrectomy is regularly followed by cobalamin malabsorption, as is resection of the proximal stomach or atrophic gastritis that involves the oxyntic mucosa.**

References

1. Dockray GJ, Varro A, Dimaline R. Gastric endocrine cells: gene expression, processing, and targeting of active products. *Am Phys Soc.* 1996;76:767–798.
2. Magee DF. Pyloric antral inhibition of gastrin release. *J Gastroenterol.* 1996;31:758–763.
3. Debas HT, Carvajal SH. Vagal regulation of acid secretion and gastrin release. *Yale J Biol Med.* 1994;67:145–151.
4. DeValle J. The stomach as an endocrine organ. *Digestion* 1997;58[suppl 1]: 4–7.
5. Sachs G, Meyer-Rosberg K, Scott DR, et al. Acid secretion and Helicobacter pylori. *Digestion* 1997;58[suppl 1]:8–13.
6. Urushidani T, Forte JG. Signal transduction and activation of acid secretion in the parietal cell. *J Membr Biol.* 1997;59:99–111.
7. Waldum HL, Brenna E, Kleveland PM, et al. Gastrin—physiological and pathophysiological role: clinical consequences. *Dig Dis.* 1995;13:25–38.
8. Date, Y, Kojima, M, Hosoda, H, et al. Ghrelin, a novel growth hormone-releasing acylated peptide, is synthesized in a distinct endocrine cell type in the gastrointestinal tracts of rats and humans. *Endocrinology* 2000;141:4255–4261.
9. Tschop, M, Smiley, DL, Heiman, ML Ghrelin induces adiposity in rodents. *Nature* 2000;407:908–913.
10. Quigley EM. Gastric and small intestinal motility in health and disease. *Gastroenterol Clin North Am.* 1996;25:113–145.

CHAPTER 46 ■ GASTRODUODENAL ULCERATION

MICHAEL W. MULHOLLAND

EPIDEMIOLOGY

Peptic ulceration remains a major public health problem worldwide.[1] Some 300,000 new cases of peptic ulcer are diagnosed in the United States each year, and 4 million people receive some form of ulcer treatment. In the United States, ulcer mortality and hospitalization rates have fallen since the early 1980s, but physicians are now treating a cohort of older patients with frequent comorbidity and ulcer disease of greater chronicity. Mortality attributed to peptic ulceration remains substantial; ulcer disease is listed as a contributing cause of death in more than 10,000 cases annually.

The surgical treatment of peptic ulcer has changed fundamentally. New insights into disease pathogenesis, especially the realization that gastric infection has a role in most cases of peptic ulceration, have been especially exciting. Antibiotics have become front-line antiulcer therapy. A number of powerful antisecretory drugs have been introduced into clinical practice. Medical, endoscopic, and surgical therapies are frequently integrated in the care of individual patients.

No clear racial predilection for the development of duodenal ulceration exists, but genetic factors can be important. Hyperpepsinogenemia I, with autosomal dominant inheritance, is common in duodenal ulcer, although the relation of this trait to the development of ulceration remains obscure. A number of rare familial syndromes associated with peptic ulceration have been described.

PATHOPHYSIOLOGY

The pathogenesis of peptic ulceration is complex and multifactorial but increasingly understood. The development of peptic ulceration is often depicted as a balance between acid–peptic secretion and mucosal defense, with the equilibrium shifted toward disease. Although large increases in acid secretion alone can occasionally cause ulceration, and although acid–peptic secretion is crucial in the development of ulcers, usually a defect in mucosal defense also exists to tip the balance away from health. Mucosal infection with *Helicobacter pylori* is the factor that contributes to ulcer pathogenesis in most patients.

Helicobacter pylori

The relation between *H. pylori* infection and ulceration is inferential but overwhelmingly strong; a causal relation between *H. pylori* infection and peptic ulceration has not been tested directly.[2] Because *H. pylori* infection is difficult to eradicate with certainty, and because of the potentially serious consequences of infection, the intentional exposure of humans to the organism to establish such a relation is not justified.

Many lines of circumstantial evidence establish *H. pylori* as a factor in the pathogenesis of duodenal ulceration:[3–6]

1. *H. pylori* is the primary cause of chronic active gastritis, characterized by nonerosive inflammation of the gastric mucosa. Antral gastritis is nearly always present histologically in patients with duodenal ulcer, and *H. pylori* can be isolated from gastric mucosa in almost all cases.
2. Gastric metaplasia is extremely common in duodenal epithelium surrounding areas of ulceration. *H. pylori* binds only to gastric-type epithelium, regardless of location; metaplastic gastric epithelium can become colonized by *H. pylori* from gastric sources. Gastric metaplasia of the duodenal bulb is a nonspecific response to damage and is the means by which antral gastritis with *H. pylori* is converted to active chronic duodenitis.
3. Eradication of *H. pylori* with antimicrobials that have no effect on acid secretion leads to ulcer healing rates equivalent to those seen with histamine type 2 (H_2) receptor antagonists.
4. Therapy with bismuth compounds, which eradicate *H. pylori*, is associated with reduced rates of ulcer relapse relative to conventional therapy.
5. Relapse of duodenal ulcer after antimicrobial therapy is preceded by reinfection of the gastric mucosa by *H. pylori*.

However, half of patients evaluated for dyspepsia, but without ulceration, have histologic evidence of mucosal bacterial infection. Furthermore, 20% of healthy volunteers harbor the bacteria; the incidence of bacterial carriage in the healthy, asymptomatic population increases with age. The occurrence of peptic ulcers in only a small proportion of people who carry the organism suggests that other factors must also act to induce ulceration. The ability of *H. pylori* infection to induce alterations in gastric acid secretion is a prerequisite for ulcer development in most patients.

Acid Secretory Status

The formation of duodenal ulcers depends on gastric secretion of acid and pepsin. The dictum "no acid–no ulcer" properly focuses on the importance of luminal acid in the development of the disease, although a more complete statement might be "no acid and no *H. pylori*–no ulcer." As a group, patients with duodenal ulcers have an increased capacity for gastric acid secretion relative to normal people (Table 46.1). The maximal acid output of normal men is approximately 20 mEq per hour in response to intravenous histamine stimulation, whereas patients with duodenal ulcer secrete an average of approximately 40 mEq per hour. Considerable overlap exists between these two groups, and the values for most people with duodenal ulcer fall within the normal range. The increase in acid secretion in some patients with duodenal ulcer has been postulated to be due to an increase in the mass of parietal cells in the acid-secreting gastric mucosa or to an increased sensitivity to circulating gastrin.

Groups of patients with duodenal ulcer demonstrate a prolonged and larger acid-secretory response to a mixed meal than do groups of normal subjects. As with histamine-stimulated acid output, overlap exists between patients with duodenal ulcer and normal subjects. Disturbances in gastric motility can exacerbate meal-stimulated acid-secretory abnormalities.

TABLE 46.1 ETIOLOGY

PATHOGENESIS OF PEPTIC ULCER

Helicobacter pylori infection
ENDOCRINE CONSEQUENCES ■ Increased basal serum gastrin ■ Increased gastrin response to a meal ■ Increased responsiveness to gastrin-releasing peptide ■ Production of Nα-methylhistamine ■ Decreased density of somatostatin cells ■ Decreased mucosal somatostatin content
GASTRIC ACID SECRETION ■ Increased acid secretory capacity ■ Increased basal secretion ■ Increased pentagastrin-stimulated output ■ Increased meal response ■ Abnormal gastric emptying
MUCOSAL DEFENSE ■ Decreased duodenal bicarbonate production ■ Decreased gastric mucosal prostaglandin production
Environment
Cigarette smoking Nonsteroidal antiinflammatory drugs

Patients with duodenal ulcer have accelerated emptying of gastric contents, particularly liquids, after a meal, and duodenal acidification fails to slow emptying appropriately. In such patients, the duodenal mucosa can be exposed to low pH for prolonged periods relative to normal subjects.

Groups of patients with duodenal ulcer also demonstrate increased basal secretion of acid. Increased basal secretion can be demonstrated by nocturnal collection of gastric secretions. Increased vagal discharge has been postulated as the responsible mechanism. In support of this contention, basal acid secretion in patients with duodenal ulcer correlates with circulating concentrations of vagally released pancreatic polypeptide. In addition, sham feeding, which is vagally mediated, does not increase acid output above basal secretion in these patients.

Studies indicate that most of these secretory abnormalities are a direct consequence of *H. pylori* infection.[7] Ironically, the earliest stages of *H. pylori* infection are accompanied by a marked decrease in gastric acid secretion.[8] Acute antral gastritis is followed by fundal inflammation. Fundal inflammation is associated with mucosal production of a number of cytokines, including interleukin (IL)-1β, IL-6, IL-8, and tumor necrosis factor-α (TNF-α). IL-1β is a potent inhibitor of gastric acid secretion.[9] Investigators have postulated that acute reduction in gastric acid secretion facilitates further gastric colonization with *H. pylori*. Acute hypochlorhydria resolves despite persistence of *H. pylori* and is followed by a state of chronically increased acid secretion.

Basal and peak acid output are increased in patients with duodenal ulcer infected with *H. pylori* relative to uninfected healthy volunteers.[10] With eradication of *H. pylori* infection, basal acid output returns to normal within 4 weeks, and peak acid output declines to the normal range by 6 months. Peak acid output reflects parietal cell mass; the slow return to normal levels suggests that *H. pylori* infection may stimulate increases in the parietal cell mass.

Abnormalities in acid secretion and parietal cell mass appear to be due to *H. pylori*–induced hypergastrinemia. *H. pylori*–infected patients have increased basal serum gastrin levels, increased gastrin responses to meal stimulation, and an augmented gastrin response to intravenous gastrin-releasing peptide. Eradication of *H. pylori* infection causes serum gastrin levels to return to baseline. Gastric mucosal inflammatory cells and epithelial cells are activated by *H. pylori* infection to release cytokines such as IL-8, interferon-γ, and TNF-α. These cytokines are stimulants of gastrin release from cultured canine gastrin cells.

Helicobacter pylori expresses N^{α}-histamine methyltransferase activity. This enzyme produces N^{α}-methylhistamine, an abnormal analogue of histamine that can act as a gastric acid secretory stimulant.[12]

The concentration of somatostatin in the antral mucosa and the number of somatostatin-producing cells in the antrum are diminished in *H. pylori*–infected patients. Treatment of *H. pylori* infection is followed by increases in numbers of somatostatin cells and in mucosal somatostatin messenger RNA levels.[13] These observations suggest that alterations in mucosal somatostatin metabolism may also contribute to the hypergastrinemia seen in *H. pylori*–infected patients by removing the inhibitory effects that somatostatin exerts on gastrin release. Somatostatin release is also suppressed by N^{α}-methylhistamine.

Mucosal Defense against Peptic Injury

Investigative attention has also focused on the ability of the duodenal mucosa to resist the injurious effects of luminal acid and pepsin. Because many patients with duodenal ulcer secrete normal amounts of acid and pepsin, it is attractive to postulate that abnormalities of mucosal defense might result in ulceration. In addition, several agents that are useful in the treatment of peptic ulceration are cytoprotective, which is defined as the ability to protect the mucosa from injury at doses lower than the threshold dose needed to inhibit acid secretion. The ability of cytoprotective agents to heal ulcers has suggested that abnormalities in mucosal defense are responsible for some instances of ulceration. Most investigative efforts have focused on the role of mucosally secreted bicarbonate and on mucosal prostaglandin production.

Gastric surface epithelial cells secrete mucus and bicarbonate, creating a pH gradient within the mucus layer that is nearly neutral at the mucous cell surface, even when the lumen is highly acidic. Failure of normal bicarbonate secretion locally would, in theory, result in exposure of surface epithelial cells to the peptic activity of gastric secretions at low pH. Patients with duodenal ulcers have been demonstrated to have significantly lower basal bicarbonate secretion in the proximal duodenum than normal subjects. In addition, in response to a physiologically relevant amount of hydrochloric acid instilled into the duodenal bulb, stimulated bicarbonate output was approximately 40% of the normal response.[14] Abnormalities in duodenal bicarbonate secretion normalize after elimination of *H. pylori* in infected patients. These results suggest one mechanism by which ulceration could occur, even in patients secreting normal amounts of acid.

Diminished mucosal prostaglandin production has also been proposed to exist in subsets of patients with duodenal ulcer.[15] Prostaglandins and prostaglandin analogues have been shown to exert cytoprotective effects, to accelerate healing of established duodenal ulcers, and to decrease acid secretion. In the duodenum, locally produced prostaglandins stimulate mucosal bicarbonate secretion. In patients with active duodenal ulceration, gastric mucosal production of prostaglandin E_2 and other prostanoids has been shown to be diminished. An increase in prostanoid synthesis within the gastric mucosa characterizes ulcer healing. Duodenal bicarbonate responses to prostaglandin E_2 are impaired in patients with duodenal ulcer.

Environmental Factors

Substantial evidence implicates cigarette smoking as an additive risk factor in the development of duodenal ulcers. Cigarette smoking impairs ulcer healing and increases the recurrence of ulcers. Continued smoking attenuates the effectiveness of active ulcer therapy. Cigarette smoking increases both the probability that surgery will be required and the risks of operative therapy. Cessation of smoking is a key element of antiulcer therapy.

Nonsteroidal antiinflammatory drugs (NSAIDs) have emerged as a significant risk factor for the development of acute ulceration. Although acute mucosal injury caused by NSAIDs is more common in the stomach than in the duodenum, NSAID-induced ulcer complications occur with equal frequency in these two sites. NSAIDs produce a variety of lesions, ranging from hemorrhage, to superficial mucosal erosions, to deeper ulcerations. In the duodenum, it appears likely that invasive NSAID-associated ulcers result from underlying peptic ulcer diathesis compounded by the direct injurious effects of these drugs.

The ulcerogenic actions of NSAIDs have been attributed to their systemic suppression of prostaglandin production. Numerous experimental models have demonstrated the ability of NSAIDs to injure the gastroduodenal mucosa. Ulcers resembling those caused by NSAIDs can be produced experimentally by antibodies to prostaglandins. Conversely, NSAID-associated gastric ulcers can be prevented by the coadministration of prostaglandin analogues. Ulcers associated with NSAIDs usually heal rapidly when the drug is withdrawn, corresponding to the reversal of antiprostaglandin effects. All available NSAIDs appear to pose the hazard of gastroduodenal ulceration. Clinically important ulceration (of both the stomach and duodenum) is estimated by the U.S. Food and Drug Administration to occur at a rate of 2% to 4% per patient-year. The risks inherent with NSAID use appear to be increased by a history of *H. pylori* infection, by cigarette smoking, and by alcohol use. The incidence of NSAID-caused ulcer complications is highest in older patients, as is the attendant mortality rate. Peptic ulcer disease is rare in individuals who are *H. pylori*–negative and who are not receiving NSAID medications.

DIAGNOSIS

The cardinal feature of duodenal ulceration is epigastric pain. The pain is usually confined to the upper abdomen and is described as burning, stabbing, or gnawing. Unless perforation or penetration into the head of the pancreas has occurred, referral of pain is not common. Many patients report pain on arising in the morning. Ingestion of food or antacids usually provides prompt relief. In uncomplicated cases, abnormal physical findings are minimal. The differential diagnosis is broad and includes a variety of diseases originating in the upper gastrointestinal tract. The most common disorders to be distinguished include nonulcerative dyspepsia, gastric neoplasia, cholelithiasis and related diseases of the biliary system, and both inflammatory and neoplastic disorders of the pancreas. In dyspeptic patients, the principal diagnoses that must be differentiated definitively are peptic ulceration and gastric cancer.

The evaluation of patients with suspected peptic ulceration usually involves either barium contrast examination of the stomach and duodenum or endoscopy. In most circumstances, endoscopy is the preferred method and has become the standard against which other diagnostic modalities are measured. Endoscopy is recommended because it eliminates the need for radiation, is safe, is preferred by elderly patients, and permits biopsy of the esophagus, stomach, and duodenum. In a controlled trial comparing endoscopy and barium radiography, endoscopy was both more sensitive (92% vs. 54%) and more specific (100% vs. 91%) than radiographic examination.[18] Endoscopy must be recommended with discretion because of associated morbidity (approximately 1 per 5,000 cases) and higher costs.

Duodenal ulcer is characterized by lesions that are erosive to the bowel wall. When viewed endoscopically, the ulcers have a typical appearance. The edges are usually sharply demarcated and the underlying submucosa is exposed. The ulcer base is often clean and smooth, although acute ulcers and those with recent hemorrhage can demonstrate eschar or adherent exudate. Surrounding mucosal inflammation is common. The most frequent site for peptic ulceration is the first portion of the duodenum, with the second portion less commonly involved. Ulceration of the third or fourth portions of the duodenum is unusual, and its occurrence should arouse suspicion of an underlying gastrinoma. Ulceration in the pyloric channel or the prepyloric area is similar in endoscopic appearance to duodenal ulceration, and ulcers in these areas demonstrate other clinical features similar to duodenal ulcers. Endoscopic demonstration of a duodenal ulcer should prompt mucosal biopsy of the gastric antrum to demonstrate the presence of *H. pylori* and guide subsequent therapy.

Barium meal radiographs demonstrate retention of contrast in the ulcer. When viewed in profile, the ulcer can be seen to project beyond the level of the duodenal mucosa. Distortion of the duodenal bulb by spasm or cicatrization is a secondary sign of current or previous ulceration.

The hallmarks of the histologic appearance of duodenal ulcers are chronicity and invasiveness. Chronic injury is suggested by surrounding fibrosis; collagen is deposited in the submucosa during each round of ulcer relapse and healing. The adjacent mucosa often demonstrates evidence of chronic injury with infiltration of acute and chronic inflammatory cells. Gastric metaplasia, in which the duodenum exhibits histologic features of gastric mucosa, is common in the surrounding nonulcerated mucosa. The ulcer can extend for a variable distance through the wall of the duodenum, including the full thickness of the bowel in cases of perforation.

DRUG TREATMENT OF ULCER DISEASE

In the absence of active treatment, *H. pylori* infection is lifelong. Spontaneous healing of infected mucosa is very rare, occurrng in fewer than 0.5% per patient-year. Current treatment of peptic ulceration involves a combination of an antisecretory drug, usually a proton pump inhibitor, with antibiotics. This therapy is rational for most patients who are *H. pylori* positive and results in a high rate of sustained ulcer healing.

A large number of drug regimens have been described, but the most widely used treatment protocols combine a proton pump inhibitor, usually omeprazole, with two antibiotics, usually clarithromycin and metronidazole or amoxicillin.[19] A combination of antibiotics is more effective than one antibiotic alone in almost all series. This triple therapy is administered for 7 or 14 days. Triple-drug therapy is cost effective and associated with a low rate of side effects, low rates of antibiotic resistance, and acceptable levels of patient compliance. *H. pylori* eradication rates of greater than 90% have been reported.

After elimination of *H. pylori,* ulcer recurrence rates reflect the rate of reinfection. In developed countries, reinfection rates of less than 10% at 5 years have been reported. Eradication of *H. pylori* improves quality of life, as measured by symptoms, drug prescriptions, physician visits, and days of missed employment. To date, antibiotic resistance has been low, approximately 5% worldwide, but it is likely to increase with ongoing use of macrolide antibiotics.[20]

HISTAMINE RECEPTOR ANTAGONISTS

Histamine, released into the interstitial fluid by cells in the fundic mucosa, diffuses to the mucosal parietal cell. Histamine stimulates acid production by occupying a membrane-bound receptor and activating parietal cell adenylate cyclase. Histamine is released in response to a number of physiologic stimuli; blockade of histamine receptors inhibits most forms of stimulated acid secretion in humans. Parietal cell histamine receptors are classified as H_2 receptors because they are activated by agonists such as 4-methylhistamine and are selectively blocked by agents such as cimetidine. Some H_2 receptor antagonists also possess nongastric actions by binding to androgen receptors, by interacting with the hepatic microsomal oxidase system, and by crossing the blood–brain barrier. All clinically useful gastric histamine receptor antagonists are of the H_2 type.

H_2 receptor antagonists bind competitively to parietal cell H_2 receptors to produce a reversible inhibition of acid secretion. An enormous worldwide experience has accumulated with the use of H_2 receptor antagonists. The agents are effective and safe when used in the treatment of peptic ulcer. The various compounds have similar efficacy in terms of ulcer healing when used in doses that produce similar reductions in acid output. When endoscopic criteria are used to determine healing, approximately 70% of patients are ulcer free within 4 weeks of therapy. By 8 weeks, 85% to 90% of patients are pain free and without endoscopic evidence of ulceration. Most studies of maintenance therapy have used single nocturnal doses of cimetidine or ranitidine; ulcer relapse during maintenance therapy occurs in approximately 15% of patients under these circumstances. It is clear that H_2 receptor blockers do not affect the underlying ulcer diathesis; if H_2 receptor antagonists are stopped, recurrent ulceration occurs in more than half of patients within 1 year. The current understanding of the role of *H. pylori* in ulcer pathogenesis has changed the role of H_2 receptor antagonists from primary therapy to that of a substitute for proton pump inhibitors in conjunction with antibiotic treatment.

PROTON PUMP BLOCKERS

Acid secretion by the gastric parietal cells is due to the active transport of hydrogen ions from the parietal cell cytoplasm into the secretory canaliculus in exchange for potassium. Because this so-called *proton pump* is tissue specific, being present only in gastric mucosa, its blockade would be expected to have minimal effects on nongastric functions. Omeprazole is representative of a family of compounds that selectively block the parietal cell proton pump.

Omeprazole is a weak base, with a pKa of approximately 4. The drug is nonionized and lipid soluble at neutral pH, but it becomes ionized and activated at a pH of less than 3. In its activated state, omeprazole binds to the membrane-bound H^+-K^+-adenosine triphosphatase (ATPase) of the parietal cell. Because the compound is a weak base, omeprazole accumulates selectively within the acidic environment of the parietal cell secretory canaliculus; 4 hours after administration, the drug is detectable in appreciable quantities only in the gastric mucosa. If enough drug is administered to occupy all parietal cell binding sites, anacidity can be produced. Omeprazole, in doses from 20 to 30 mg, causes nearly complete inhibition of stimulated gastric acid secretion within 6 hours. At 24 hours after drug administration, 60% to 70% reduction in acid secretion persists.

Repeated daily dosing with omeprazole results in increasing inhibitory action on gastric secretion and thus in decreased intragastric degradation of the drug. Acid suppression stabilizes after approximately 3 days. Because of tissue accumulation, the secretory actions of omeprazole do not correlate with plasma levels. Several studies have demonstrated a significant inhibition of peak acid output, marked relief of epigastric pain, and decreased use of supplemental antacids during omeprazole therapy. Direct comparisons with H_2 receptor antagonists have generally favored omeprazole in terms of pain relief and rate of ulcer healing.

SUCRALFATE

Sucralfate is the aluminum salt of sulfated sucrose. In the acidic environment of the stomach, sucralfate polymerizes, becoming viscous and adhering to the gastroduodenal mucosa. Coating of the ulcer base by the polymer has been claimed to provide a protective barrier, binding bile salts and inhibiting the actions of pepsin. Sucralfate also stimulates the production of mucus. Sucralfate stimulates increased mucosal prostaglandin E_2 production and increases bicarbonate secretion. Sucralfate binds epidermal growth factor and may protect the mitogen from acid degradation. Sucralfate stimulates epithelial proliferation at the ulcer margin. The drug has almost no buffering capacity. Virtually no systemic absorption occurs, and because of this property, sucralfate is the recommended agent for the treatment of peptic ulcer in pregnancy.

ANTACIDS

The availability of compounds that effectively suppress acid production, combined with their greater convenience, has greatly reduced the use of antacids as the primary treatment for acute ulceration. Nonetheless, when properly used, antacids can effectively heal ulcers. Intensive treatment of acute ulcers with antacids (30 mL of liquid antacid taken seven times daily, providing approximately 1,000 mEq of buffering capacity) has been shown to heal ulcers in 78% of patients at 4 weeks.[21] Although this rate compares favorably with the healing rates observed with other forms of therapy, the large and frequent dosages are unacceptable to many patients. In addition, a significant proportion of patients have diarrhea on such a regimen.

BISMUTH COMPOUNDS

Many successful antibiotic regimens are based on a bismuth compound (colloidal bismuth subsalicylate or colloidal bismuth subcitrate) plus metronidazole, alone or in combination with amoxicillin or tetracycline. Bismuth compounds act locally and achieve gastric concentrations above the minimum inhibitory concentration for 90% of *H. pylori* isolates.

OPERATIVE TREATMENT OF ULCER DISEASE

Surgical Goals

Operative intervention is reserved for the treatment of complicated ulcer disease. Three complications are most common and constitute the indications for peptic ulcer surgery—hemorrhage, perforation, and obstruction. The first goal in the surgical treatment of the complications of ulcer disease should be alteration of the ulcer diathesis so that ulcer healing is achieved and recurrence is minimized. The second goal is treatment of coexisting anatomic complications, such as pyloric stenosis or perforation. The third major goal should be patient safety and freedom from undesirable chronic side effects. To achieve these goals, the gastric surgeon can direct therapy through endoscopic, radiologic, or operative means, the appropriate choice depending on the clinical circumstances.

Operative Procedures

A number of operative procedures have been used to treat peptic ulcer, but with decreasing frequency in the past decade. There is currently no indication for surgical treatment of uncomplicated ulcer disease. Operative treatment of gastric outlet obstruction has decreased by approximately 50%. Most surgical patients are now treated emergently for the complications of bleeding or perforation.

Three procedures—truncal vagotomy and drainage, truncal vagotomy and antrectomy, and proximal gastric vagotomy—have been most widely used in the operative treatment of peptic ulcer disease. With increasing frequency, surgical therapy of peptic ulcer is directed exclusively at correction of the immediate problem (e.g., closure of duodenal perforation) without gastric denervation. The underlying ulcer diathesis is then addressed after surgery by antibiotic therapy directed at *H. pylori*. This approach is applicable to most patients with peptic ulcer undergoing emergent operation and predicts a greatly diminished role for vagotomy in the future.

Division of both vagal trunks at the esophageal hiatus—truncal vagotomy—denervates the acid-producing fundic mucosa as well as the remainder of the vagally supplied viscera (Fig. 46.1). Because denervation impedes normal pyloric coordination and can result in impairment of gastric emptying, truncal vagotomy must be combined with a procedure to eliminate pyloric sphincteric function. Usually, gastric drainage is ensured by performance of a pyloroplasty. Several methods of pyloroplasty have been described; often they are referred to eponymously (Fig. 46.2). The Heineke-Mikulicz pyloroplasty is performed by making a longitudinal incision of the pyloric sphincter extending into the antrum and the duodenum for approximately 2 cm on either side. The incision is closed transversely, thereby increasing the lumen of the pyloric channel.

Truncal vagotomy can also be combined with resection of the gastric antrum to effect a further reduction in acid secretion, presumably by removing antral sources of gastrin. The limits of antral resection are usually defined by external landmarks, rather than the histologic transition from fundic to antral mucosae. The stomach is divided proximally along a line from a point above the incisura angularis to a point along the greater curvature midway from the pylorus to the gastroesophageal junction. Restoration of gastrointestinal continuity by a gastroduodenostomy is termed a Billroth I reconstruction. A Billroth II procedure uses a gastrojejunostomy (Fig. 46.3).

Proximal gastric vagotomy differs from truncal vagotomy in that only the nerve fibers to the acid-secreting fundic mucosa are divided (see Fig. 46.1). Vagal nerve fibers to the antrum and pylorus are left intact, and the hepatic and celiac divisions are not transected. The operation has also been called parietal cell vagotomy to emphasize its most important functional consequence.

The role of vagotomy in clinical surgery diminished significantly in the 1990s. In 1998, only 7,000 vagotomies were performed in the United States, of more than 41 million operative procedures.[23]

Physiologic Consequences of Operation

Division of efferent vagal fibers directly affects acid secretion by reducing cholinergic stimulation of parietal cells. In addition, vagotomy also diminishes parietal cell responsiveness to

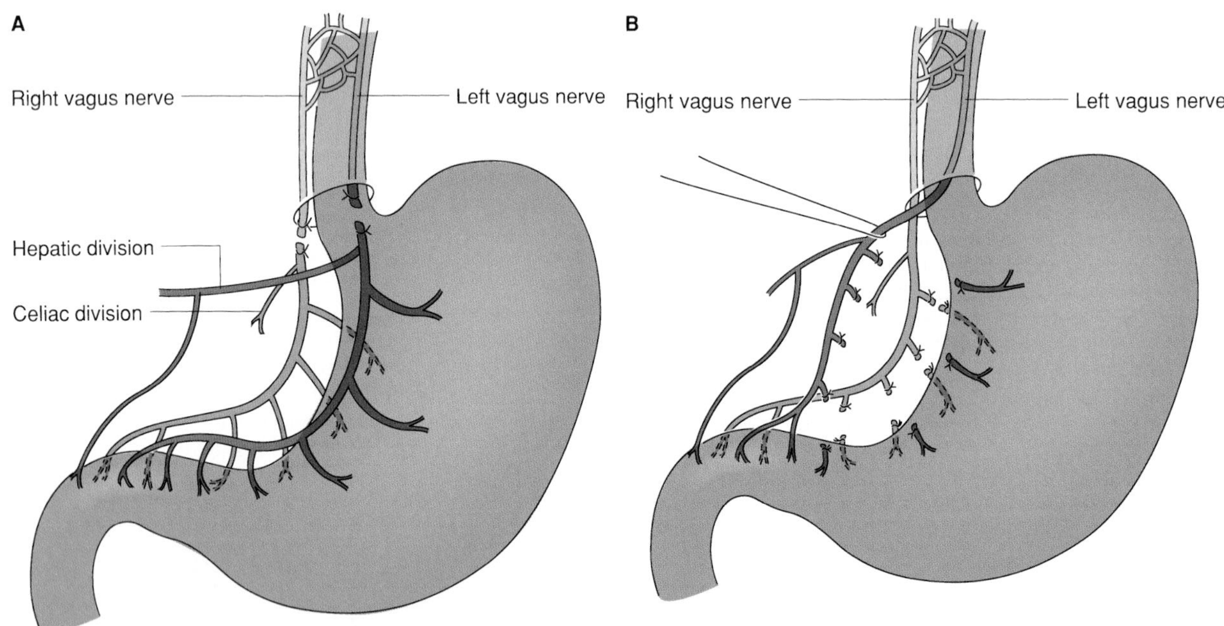

FIGURE 46.1 Truncal vagotomy and proximal gastric vagotomy. (*A*) With truncal vagotomy, both nerve trunks are divided at the level of the diaphragmatic hiatus. (*B*) Proximal gastric vagotomy involves division of the vagal fibers that supply the gastric fundus. Branches to the antropyloric region of the stomach are not transected, and the hepatic and celiac divisions of the vagus nerves remain intact.

gastrin and histamine. Basal acid secretion is reduced by approximately 80% in the immediate postoperative period. It increases slightly within months of surgery but remains unchanged thereafter. The maximal acid output in response to exogenously administered stimulants such as pentagastrin is reduced by approximately 70% in the early period after surgery. After 1 year, pentagastrin-stimulated maximal acid output rebounds to 50% of prevagotomy values but remains at this level on subsequent testing. Acid secretion due to endogenous stimulation by a liquid meal is reduced by 60% to 70% relative to normal subjects.

The inclusion of antrectomy with truncal vagotomy causes further reductions in acid secretion. Pentagastrin-stimulated maximal acid output is reduced by 85% relative to values recorded before surgery. Little rebound in acid secretion occurs with the passage of time.

Truncal vagotomy and proximal gastric vagotomy both cause postoperative hypergastrinemia. Fasting gastrin values are elevated to approximately twice preoperative levels, and the postprandial response is exaggerated. Immediately after vagotomy, hypergastrinemia appears to be due to decreased luminal acid, with loss of feedback inhibition of gastrin release. Loss of vagal inhibitory pathways can also be important. Chronic hypergastrinemia, sustained long term in most cases, is caused by gastrin cell hyperplasia in addition to loss of inhibitory feedback. When antrectomy is added to vagotomy, circulating gastrin levels are decreased. Basal gastrin values are reduced by approximately half and postprandial gastrin levels by two thirds. The major form of circulating hormone after antrectomy is gastrin 34, released from the duodenum.

Operations that involve vagotomy alter gastric emptying. Proximal gastric denervation abolishes vagally mediated receptive relaxation. Thus, for any given volume ingested, the intragastric pressure rise is greater and the gastroduodenal pressure gradient higher than in normal subjects. As a result, emptying of liquids, which depends critically on the gastroduodenal pressure gradient, is accelerated after proximal gastric vagotomy. Because nerve fibers to the antrum and pylorus are preserved, the function of the distal stomach to mix and triturate solid food is preserved, and emptying of solids is nearly normal in patients who have undergone proximal gastric vagotomy. Truncal vagotomy affects the motor activities of both proximal and distal stomach. Solid and liquid emptying rates are usually increased when truncal vagotomy is accompanied by pyloroplasty.

A number of prospective, randomized trials have compared the various surgical options in terms of postoperative symptoms, including dumping, diarrhea, weight loss, and disturbance of lifestyle (Table 46.2). In most comparisons, proximal gastric vagotomy has proved superior to other operations in these measures. Dumping, a postprandial symptom complex of abdominal discomfort, weakness, and vasomotor symptoms of sweating and dizziness, occurs in 10% to 15% of patients with truncal vagotomy and antrectomy in the early postoperative period and is chronically disabling in 1% to 2%. After truncal vagotomy and pyloroplasty, dumping is present initially in 10%, and remains severe in approximately 1%. Permanent symptoms of dumping are rare after proximal gastric vagotomy. The incidence of diarrhea, which is presumably caused by denervation of the pylorus and small bowel and by elimination of pyloric function, parallels the incidence of dumping after truncal vagotomy and antrectomy or pyloroplasty. Persistent or disabling diarrhea is present in less than 1% of patients after proximal gastric vagotomy.

Proximal gastric vagotomy has the lowest operative mortality rate, the lowest incidence of postoperative symptoms, and an acceptable risk of recurrent ulcer. Collected series of proximal gastric vagotomies have reported an operative mortality rate of less than 0.05%, lower than the reported mortality rate for any other gastric procedure for peptic ulcer. Truncal vagotomy and pyloroplasty has a reported mortality rate of 0.5% to 0.8%, whereas the mortality rate after truncal vagotomy and antrectomy approximates 1.5%.

Most prospective surgical series examining ulcer recurrence rates were reported in the era before the pathogenic role of *H. pylori* was appreciated. With appropriate use of postoperative antimicrobials directed against *H. pylori,* these ulcer recurrence rates are currently expected to be much lower. Although recurrence rates (without *H. pylori* treatment) as low as 5% have been reported, a more generally accepted figure is 10%. This rate is similar to that of reinfection with *H. pylori* after its succesful eradication. The reported ulcer recurrence rates after proximal gastric vagotomy can be adversely affected by the inclusion of prepyloric and pyloric channel ulcers. For reasons that are not clear, proximal gastric vagotomy is significantly less effective when used to treat ulcers in this position than when used for duodenal ulceration.

Hemorrhage

Hemorrhage is the leading cause of death associated with peptic ulcer, and the incidence of this complication has not changed since the introduction of H_2 receptor antagonists.[23] The lifetime risk of hemorrhage for patients with duodenal ulcer who have not had surgery and who do not receive continuing maintenance drug therapy approximates 35%. Most hemorrhages

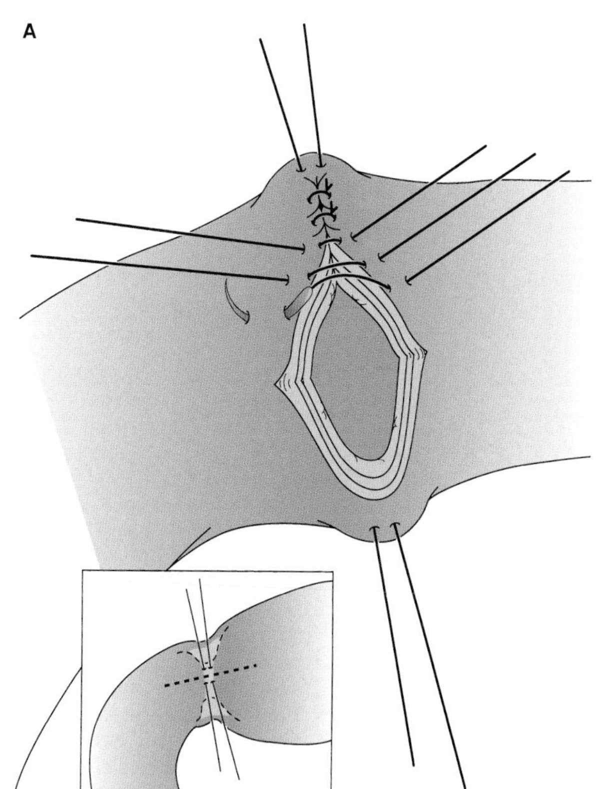

FIGURE 46.2 Pyloroplasty formation. A Heineke-Mikulicz pyloroplasty (*A*) involves a longitudinal incision of the pyloric sphincter followed by a transverse closure. The Finney pyloroplasty (*B*) is performed as a gastroduodenostomy with division of the pylorus. The Jaboulay pyloroplasty (C) differs from the Finney procedure in that the pylorus is not transected.

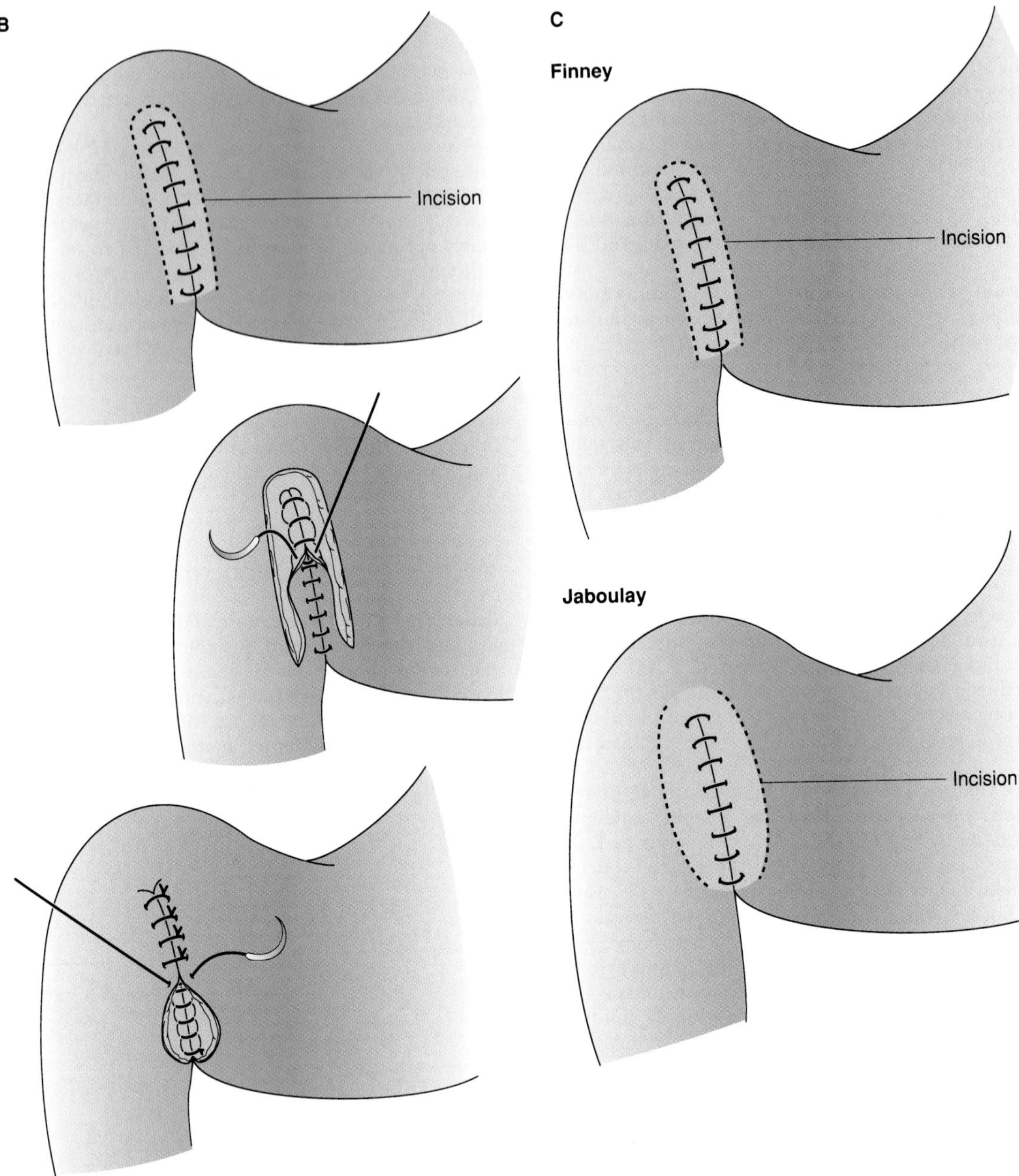

FIGURE 46.2 (*Continued*)

occur during the initial episode of ulceration or during a relapse, and patients who have hemorrhaged previously have a higher risk of bleeding again. Patients with recurrent hemorrhage and elderly patients are at greatest risk of death, and these two groups should be resuscitated vigorously, investigated promptly, and treated aggressively.[24,25]

The contemporary risk of mortality from bleeding ulcer approximates 10% to 20%. Operative risk is increased in patients who have shock at admission, recurrent bleeding, delay in operative intervention, or coexisting medical illnesses. Surgical delay may lead to recurrent hypovolemia and, subsequently, multisystem organ failure.

Upper gastrointestinal endoscopy is the appropriate initial diagnostic test when hemorrhage from duodenal ulceration is suspected. Endoscopy can correctly determine the site and cause of bleeding in more than 90% of patients. An ulcer should be accepted as the bleeding source only if it has one of the stigmata of active or recent hemorrhage. Active hemorrhage is defined by an arterial jet, active oozing, or oozing beneath an adherent clot. The signs of recent hemorrhage include an adherent clot without oozing, an adherent slough in the ulcer base, or a visible vessel in the ulcer. The ability of these endoscopic findings to accurately predict recurrent hemorrhage has been extensively validated. Approximately 30% of patients who have stigmata of recent hemorrhage experience rebleeding, and most of the patients who experience recurrent hemorrhage require emergency treatment. These stigmata are not sufficiently accurate to be used alone as indications for surgery. Rather, they serve as a warning that aggressive therapy is needed and close follow-up mandatory. The occurrence of hypovolemic shock, rebleeding during hospitalization, and a posteroinferior location of the ulcer are additional clinical

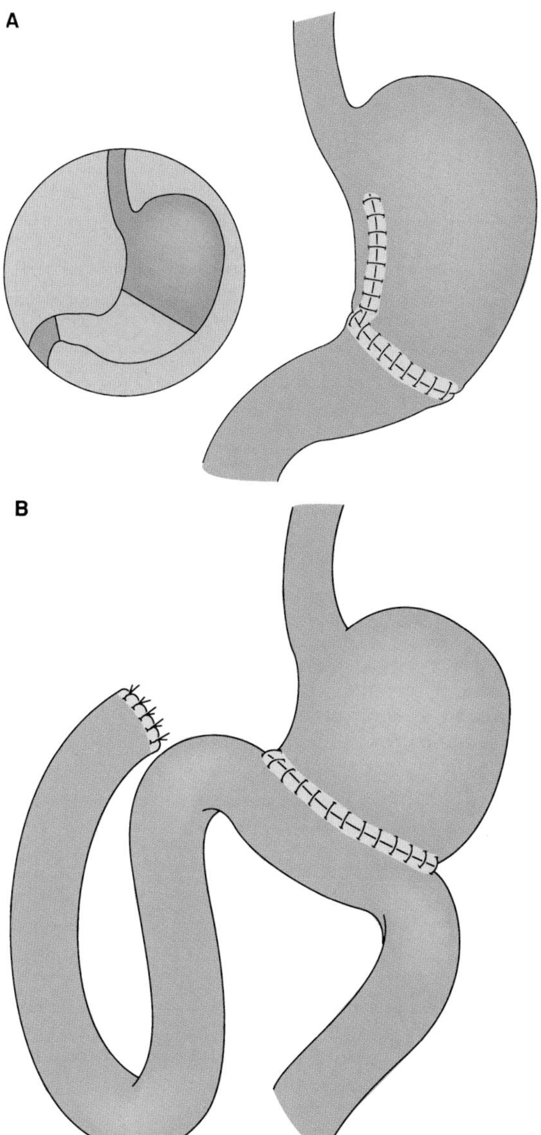

FIGURE 46.3 Antrectomy involves resection of the distal stomach (*pink area in inset*). Restoration of gastrointestinal continuity may be accomplished as a Billroth I gastroduodenostomy (*A*) or Billroth II gastrojejunostomy (*B*) reconstruction.

features that have been associated with increased risks of recurrent bleeding. The role of gastric acidity as a cause for in-hospital rebleeding appears to be inconsequential, and reduction of acid secretion by H_2 receptor antagonists or omeprazole is not sufficient to prevent recurrent hemorrhage.[26]

The ability to visualize bleeding duodenal ulcers endoscopically has led to attempts to treat hemorrhage endoscopically. There are many different methods of endoscopic therapy, but the most established consist of thermal coagulation. Thermal coagulation can be achieved by bipolar electrocoagulation or direct application of heat through a heater probe.[27] Injection of epinephrine into the base of the bleeding ulcer is also effective in control of ulcer hemorrhage.

Proof of efficacy, in the form of lowered rebleeding rates and avoidance of operation, has been convincingly demonstrated for all of these methods of endoscopic hemostasis.[27,28] The analysis of reports of endoscopic treatment of hemorrhage is complicated by the 70% rate of spontaneous, although sometimes temporary, cessation of bleeding without intervention. In addition to endoscopic stigmata, hemodynamic instability, need for continuing transfusion, red stool or hematemesis, age older than 60 years, and serious medical comorbidity are clinical features that mandate endoscopic therapy. Rebleeding during hospitalization and the endoscopic findings of visible vessel, oozing, or bleeding associated with an adherent clot are other indications for endoscopic hemostasis. Ulcers with clean bases require no treatment. Failure of endoscopic hemostasis is usually due to inaccessibility because of scarring, to rapid active bleeding, or to an adherent clot. Patients treated endoscopically should be observed closely for further hemorrhage. Patients who rebleed within 72 hours of initial endoscopic control may be successfully retreated without increasing the risk of mortality.[28]

The efficacy of endoscopy is dependent on timing. Early endoscopy correctly identifies pateints at low risk for recurrent hemorrhage and permits safe avoidance of hospitalization. Early endoscopy also benefits high-risk patients by directing active hemostatic therapy. Patients treated in this way have been demonstrated to have fewer episodes of rebleeding, lower rates of operation, and shorter hospitalizations.[30]

Table 46.3 lists situations in which operative intervention is appropriate. The need for emergency surgery significantly increases surgical risks; mortality rates are increased approximately 10-fold. Operative therapy should consist of duodenotomy with direct ligation of the bleeding vessel in the ulcer base.

TABLE 46.2 RESULTS

CLINICAL RESULTS OF DUODENAL ULCER SURGERY

	PGV (%)	TV + P (%)	TV + A (%)
Mortality rate	0	0.5–1	1–2
Acid reduction			
Basal	80	70	85
Stimulated	50	50	85
Ulcer recurrence	10	12	1–2
Gastric emptying			
Liquids	Accelerated	Accelerated	Accelerated
Solids	No change	Accelerated	Slowed
Dumping			
Mild	<5	10	10–15
Disabling	0	1	1–2
Diarrhea			
Mild	<5	25	20
Disabling	0	2	1–2

PGV, proximal gastric vagotomy; TV + P, truncal vagotomy and pyloroplasty; TV + A, truncal vagotomy and antrectomy.

TABLE 46.3 INDICATIONS/CONTRAINDICATIONS

SITUATIONS IN WHICH OPERATIVE INTERVENTION IS APPROPRIATE

- Massive hemorrhage leading to shock or cardiovascular instability
- Prolonged blood loss requiring continuing transfusion
- Recurrent bleeding during medical therapy or after endoscopic therapy
- Recurrent hemorrhage requiring hospitalization

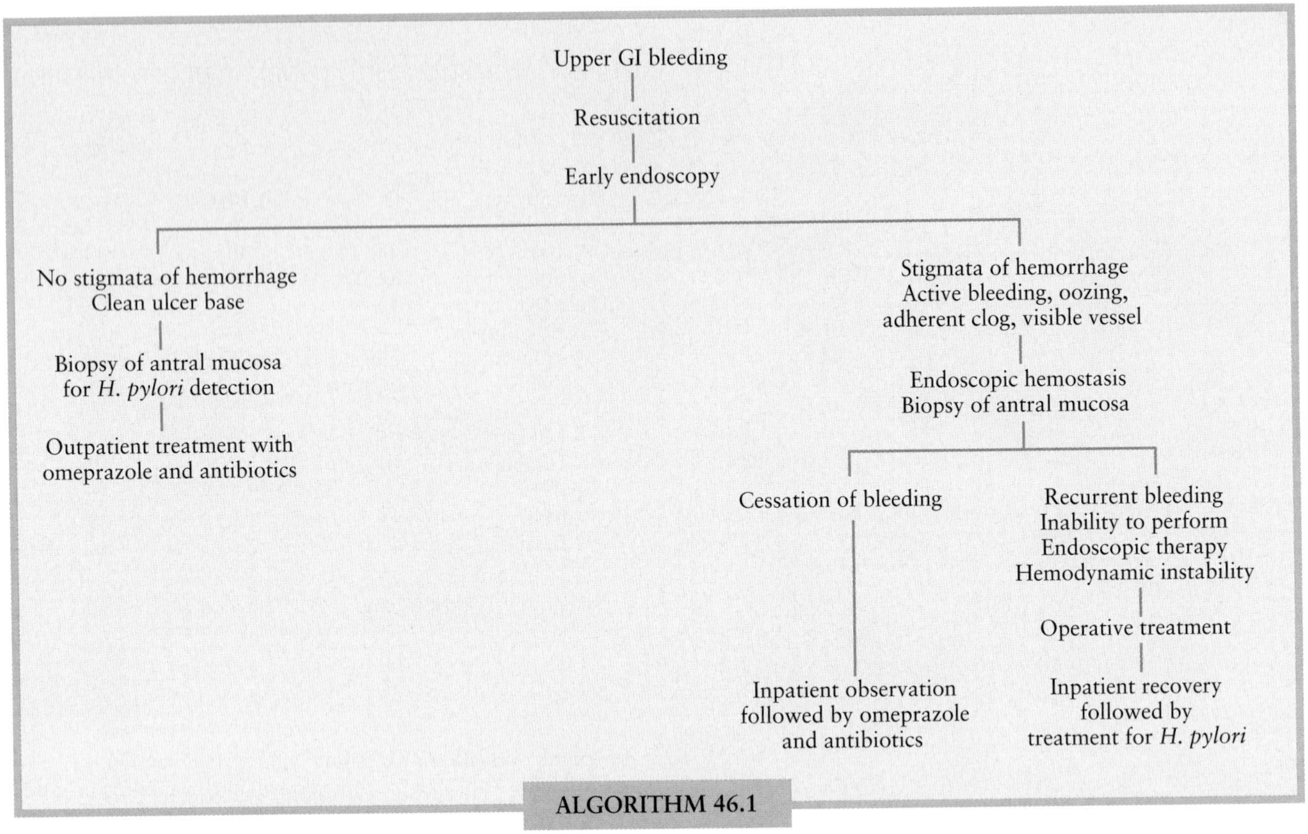

Upper GI bleeding

Resuscitation

Early endoscopy

- No stigmata of hemorrhage
Clean ulcer base
  - Biopsy of antral mucosa for *H. pylori* detection
    - Outpatient treatment with omeprazole and antibiotics
- Stigmata of hemorrhage
Active bleeding, oozing, adherent clog, visible vessel
  - Endoscopic hemostasis
Biopsy of antral mucosa
    - Cessation of bleeding
      - Inpatient observation followed by omeprazole and antibiotics
    - Recurrent bleeding
Inability to perform Endoscopic therapy
Hemodynamic instability
      - Operative treatment
        - Inpatient recovery followed by treatment for *H. pylori*

ALGORITHM 46.1

ALGORITHM 46.1 Treatment of bleeding duodenal ulceration.

Postoperatively, patients should receive antibiotics directed against *H. pylori*. This treatment paradigm is based on the observation that peptic ulcer hemorrhage recurs in 20% of patients in whom *H. pylori* is not eradicated, whereas rebleeding is reduced to 3% in patients who receive *H. pylori* eradication therapy.[31,32] (Algorithm 46.1). The studies that support this practice were not specifically designed to evaluate postoperative hemorrhage, but the results are so definitive that they support this application (Fig. 46.4).

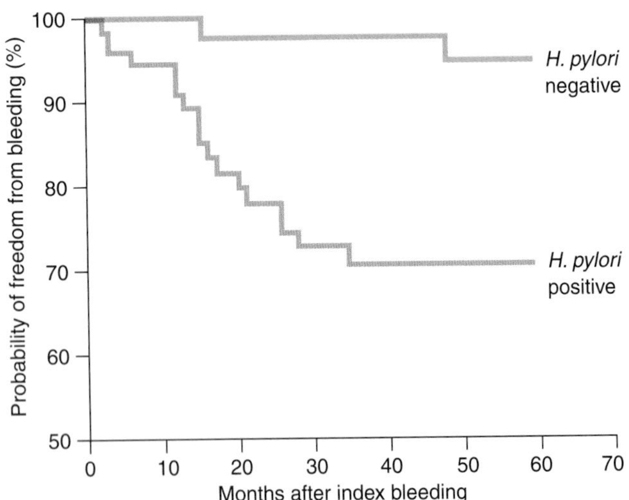

FIGURE 46.4 Probability of freedom from recurrent hemorrhage according to posttreatment *H. pylori* status.

Perforation

The lifetime risk for perforation in patients with duodenal ulceration who do not receive therapy approximates 10%. In contrast, ulcer perforation is unusual if initial ulcer healing has been achieved.

Perforation of a duodenal ulcer is usually accompanied by sudden and severe epigastric pain. The pain, caused by the spillage of highly caustic gastric secretions into the peritoneum, rapidly reaches peak intensity and remains constant. Radiation to the right scapular region is common because of right subphrenic collection of gastric contents. Occasionally, pain is sensed in the lower abdomen if gastric contents travel caudally through the paracolic gutter. Peritoneal irritation is usually intense, and most patients avoid movement to minimize discomfort.

Physical examination reveals low-grade fever, diminished bowel sounds, and rigidity of the abdominal musculature. Usually, upright abdominal radiographs reveal pneumoperitoneum, but up to 20% of perforated ulcers do not show free intraperitoneal air. Computed tomography of the abdomen is very sensitive for demonstrating perforation if pneumoperitoneum is not demonstrated but perforation is still suspected.

Although occasional reports have described the nonoperative treatment of this complication, perforation remains a strong indication for surgery in most circumstances. Laparotomy or laparoscopy affords the opportunity to relieve intraperitoneal contamination and to close the perforation (Fig. 46.5).

Signs of antecedent duodenal ulceration, in terms of history of prior symptoms and anatomic evidence of duodenal scarring, should be sought. A lack of antecedent symptoms is not protective. Reports suggest that patients without antecedent symptoms are also at risk for recurrent ulceration. By 5 to 6 years, symptomatic ulcer recurrence in patients with acute ulcer perforation is similar

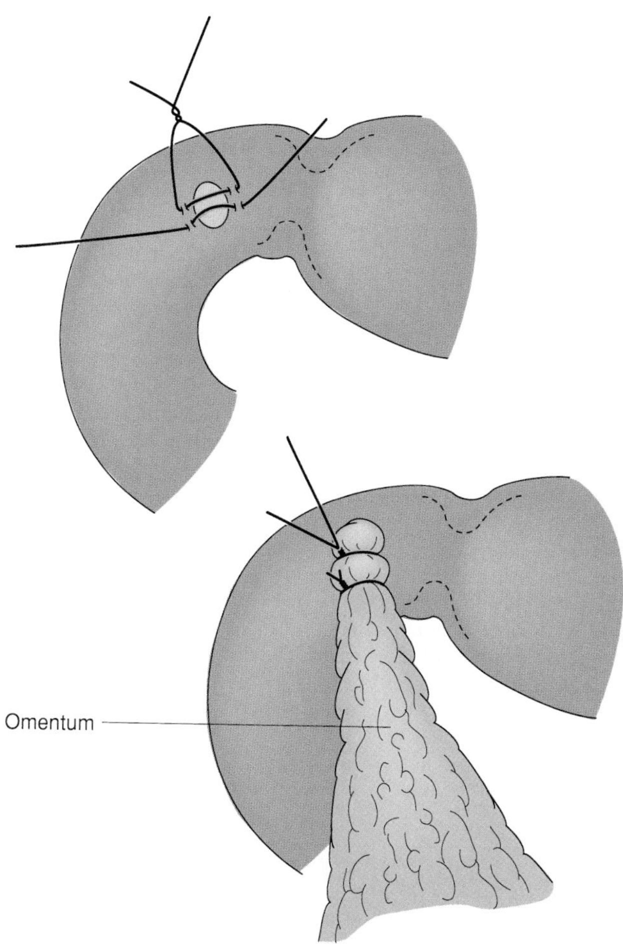

FIGURE 46.5 Omental patching of perforated duodenal ulcer.

to that for patients with chronic disease. Before the role of *H. pylori* was appreciated, simple omental closure of duodenal perforation resulting from chronic ulceration did not provide satisfactory long-term results; up to 80% of patients so treated had recurrent ulceration, and 10% experienced reperforation if untreated. Approximately four fifths of all patients with perforation have *H. pylori* infestation and therefore are at risk of recurrent disease.

The mortality of emergent ulcer operations is most clearly correlated with the following circumstances:[33,34] preoperative shock, coexisting medical illness, and presence of perforation for more than 48 hours.

For most patients receiving prompt surgical attention, antiulcer therapy can be performed with a risk equivalent to that of simple closure. Proximal gastric vagotomy with patch closure of the perforation is an option in this circumstance and has been shown to be both safe and effective in preventing ulcer relapse. Incorporation of the perforation as part of a pyloroplasty or resection of the site of perforation during antrectomy can also be combined with truncal vagotomy with favorable results. The need for these operations has declined significantly with the focus on *H. pylori* as the cause of most ulcer recurrences.

Current reports advocate omental patch closure only, often laparoscopically, with postoperative anti–*H. pylori* therapy.[35–39] This approach presumes that most duodenal ulcers are caused by *H. pylori,* that secure closure of the perforation can be obtained, and that further surgical therapy will be obviated by the effects of medical therapy. Minimally invasive approaches are becoming standard practice.

Obstruction

Gastric outlet obstruction can occur acutely or chronically in patients with duodenal ulcer disease. Acute obstruction is caused by edema and inflammation associated with ulcers in the pyloric channel and the first portion of the duodenum. Pyloric obstruction is suggested by recurrent vomiting, dehydration, and hypochloremic alkalosis due to loss of gastric secretions. Acute gastric outlet obstruction is treated with nasogastric suction, rehydration, and intravenous administration of antisecretory agents. In most instances, acute obstruction resolves with such supportive measures within 72 hours.

Repeated episodes of ulceration and healing can lead to pyloric scarring and a fixed stenosis with chronic gastric outlet obstruction. In cases of untreated duodenal ulceration, the lifetime risk of chronic pyloric stenosis approximates 10%.

Upper endoscopy is indicated to confirm the nature of the obstruction and to exclude neoplasm. Endoscopic hydrostatic balloon dilatation of pyloric stenoses can also be attempted at this time (Fig. 46.6). Approximately 85% of pyloric stenoses are amenable to balloon dilatation.[41] Only 40% of patients

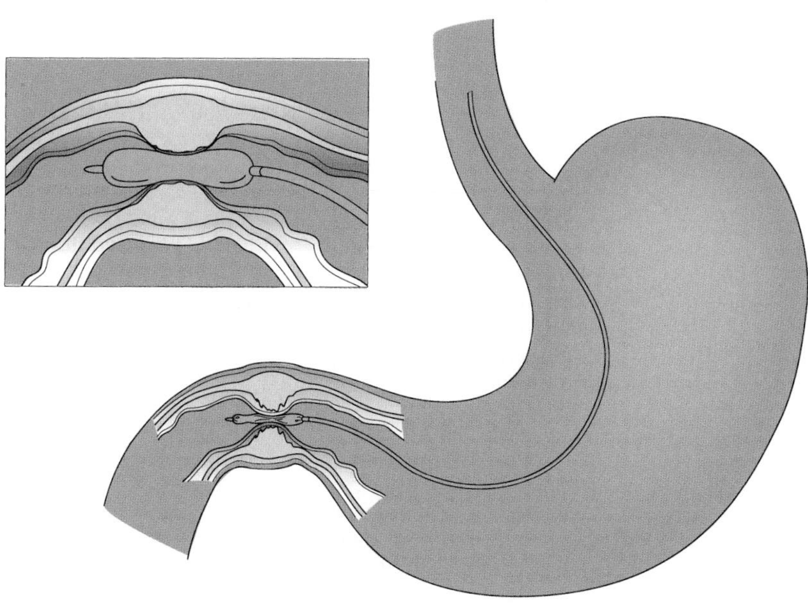

FIGURE 46.6 Schematic representation of balloon dilatation of pyloric stenosis.

with gastric stenoses have sustained improvement by 3 months after balloon dilatation. Recurrent stenoses are presumably due to residual scarring in the pyloric channel. Thus, although pyloric dilatation is occasionally palliative, in most cases operative correction is required.

Operative management of gastric outlet obstruction should include treatment of the underlying ulcer disease and relief of the anatomic abnormality. Truncal vagotomy with antrectomy and truncal vagotomy with drainage have both been used with success in this circumstance, with low ulcer recurrence rates and with satisfactory restoration of gastric emptying.

GASTRIC ULCER

Benign gastric ulcers are a form of peptic ulcer disease, occurring with one third the frequency of benign duodenal ulceration. In the United States, gastric ulcer is somewhat more common in men than in women and occurs in a patient cohort approximately 10 years older than for duodenal ulceration.

Endoscopic Diagnosis

Upper gastrointestinal endoscopy is the preferred method for diagnosing gastric ulceration. The ulcer base in benign disease is commonly smooth and flat and often covered by a gray, fibrous exudate. The margin is usually slightly raised, erythematous, and friable. Differentiation of benign and malignant gastric ulcers is reliably made only by histologic examination. Visual endoscopic differentiation of benign from malignant ulcers is not reliable. All gastric ulcers should have multiple biopsies taken from the perimeter of the lesion. The addition of lesional brushings to biopsy increases diagnostic accuracy to approximately 95%.

Benign gastric ulcers may occur in any location in the stomach, but approximately 60% are located along the lesser curvature proximal to the incisura angularis. Less than 10% of benign gastric ulcers are located on the greater curvature. Virtually all gastric ulcers lie within 2 cm of the histologic transition between fundic and antral mucosa. With increasing age, this mucosal transition zone moves proximally along the lesser curvature. Movement of this transition zone is reflected by the greater prevalence of proximal ulcers in elderly patients.

As with benign duodenal ulceration, *H. pylori* plays a central role in the pathogenesis of benign gastric ulcers. Benign gastric ulcers associated with *H. pylori* respond to antibiotic therapy at a rate equivalent to that of duodenal ulceration. The recurrence rate of ulcerations in these patients after *H. pylori* eradication is equal to the rate of reinfection.

In addition to *H. pylori* infection, alterations in gastric motility have been demonstrated in a small subset of patients with benign ulcers. A variety of defects have been identified, including delayed gastric emptying, incompetent pyloric sphincter function, prolonged high-amplitude gastric contractions, duodenogastric reflux, and alterations in the migrating motor complex. No defect has been demonstrated to be definitely pathogenic. A strong association of benign gastric ulceration with the use of NSAIDs has been recognized. Cigarette smoking is associated with development of gastric ulceration, and continued smoking impedes medical therapy. Gastric and duodenal ulcers have been noted in patients receiving hepatic artery chemotherapy in whom improper placement of the catheter permits perfusion of gastric and duodenal mucosae. A variety of agents, including 5-fluorouracil, cisplatin, doxorubicin, and mitomycin C, have been implicated.

Therapy

The primary therapy for benign gastric ulceration in most patients is antimicrobial treatment of *H. pylori* infection. The treatment protocols are similar to those used for benign duodenal ulceration. For many patients, cessation of NSAID therapy is also required.

Indications for surgical treatment of gastric ulcer include hemorrhage, perforation, failure of a recurrent ulcer to respond to medical therapy, and inability to exclude malignant disease.

For benign gastric ulcers, the elective operation of choice is usually a distal gastrectomy with gastroduodenal (Billroth I) anastomosis. The ulcer should be included in the gastrectomy specimen. With this approach, operative mortality rates of 2% to 3%, with ulcer recurrence rates of less than 5%, have been reported. Because benign gastric ulcers are not associated with gastric acid hypersecretion, inclusion of vagotomy does not improve recurrence rates.

The occurrence of a gastric ulcer near the gastroesophageal junction represents a difficult surgical problem. When possible, the ulcer should be excised. This usually requires a distal gastrectomy with an extension along the lesser curvature near the esophageal wall and reconstruction with gastrojejunostomy.

Emergency operations performed for hemorrhage or perforation require ulcer excision. Distal gastrectomy, performed with gastroduodenal reconstruction, is usually the procedure of choice. Operative mortality rates average 10% to 20% in the presence of hemorrhage or perforation.

POSTGASTRECTOMY SYNDROMES

A number of syndromes have been described that are associated with distressing symptoms after gastric operations performed for peptic ulcer or gastric neoplasm. The occurrence of severe postoperative symptoms is fortunately low, perhaps 1% to 3% of cases, but the disturbances can be disabling. The two most common postgastrectomy syndromes, categorized according to predominant manifestation, are dumping and alkaline reflux gastritis.

Dumping

The term *dumping* denotes a clinical syndrome with both gastrointestinal and vasomotor symptoms. The precise cause of dumping is not known but is believed to relate to the unmetered entry of ingested food into the proximal small bowel after vagotomy and either resection or division of the pyloric sphincter. Early dumping symptoms occur immediately after a meal and include nausea, epigastric discomfort, borborygmi, palpitations, and, in extreme cases, dizziness or syncope. Late dumping symptoms follow a meal by 1 to 3 hours and can include reactive hypoglycemia in addition to the aforementioned symptoms.

Although a relatively large number of patients experience mild dumping symptoms in the early postoperative period, minor dietary alterations and the passage of time bring improvement in all but approximately 1%. The somatostatin analogue octreotide has been reported to improve dumping symptoms when 50 to 100 mg is administered subcutaneously before a meal.[42] The beneficial effects of somatostatin on the vasomotor symptoms of dumping are postulated to be due to pressor effects of the compound on splanchnic vessels. In addition, somatostatin analogues inhibit the release of vasoactive peptides from the gut, decrease peak plasma insulin levels, and slow intestinal transit, all effects that might be expected to ameliorate dumping symptoms. Octreotide administration before meal ingestion has been shown to prevent changes in pulse, systolic blood pressure, and packed red cell volume during early dumping and blood glucose levels during late dumping.

Alkaline Reflux Gastritis

The term *alkaline reflux gastritis* should be reserved for patients who demonstrate the clinical triad of postprandial epigastric pain often associated with nausea and vomiting, evidence of reflux of bile into the stomach, and histologic evidence of gastritis. One or more of these findings occur transiently in 10% to 20% of patients after truncal vagotomy and drainage or resection, but they persist in only 1% to 2%.

The differential diagnosis for a patient with postoperative epigastric pain includes recurrent ulceration, biliary and pancreatic disease, afferent loop obstruction, and esophagitis in addition to alkaline reflux gastritis. Gastric acid analysis shows basal hypochlorhydria with little increase with pentagastrin stimulation. Serum gastrin measurements should be determined to exclude Zollinger-Ellison syndrome and retained gastric antrum. Endoscopic examination is essential to exclude recurrent ulcer.

Endoscopically, the gastric mucosa appears red, friable, and edematous. Gastric inflammation is patchy and nonulcerative. Histologic examination shows mucosal and submucosal edema and infiltration of acute and chronic inflammatory cells into the lamina propria. Glandular atrophy and intestinal metaplasia are frequent accompaniments.

No perfect solution to alkaline reflux gastritis exists. Antacids, H_2 receptor antagonists, bile acid chelators, and dietary manipulations have not been demonstrated definitely to be beneficial. The only proved treatment for alkaline reflux gastritis is operative diversion of intestinal contents from contact with the gastric mucosa. The most common surgical procedure used for this purpose is a Roux-en-Y gastrojejunostomy with an intestinal limb of 50 to 60 cm constructed to prevent reflux of intestinal contents (Fig. 46.7). This procedure is effective in eliminating bilious vomiting (nearly 100%), but recurrent or persistent pain is reported in up to 30% of patients, and up to 20% of patients are troubled with postoperative delayed gastric emptying.

STRESS GASTRITIS

Major trauma accompanied by shock, sepsis, respiratory failure, hemorrhage, or multiorgan injury is often accompanied by acute stress gastritis. Acute stress gastritis is particularly prevalent after thermal injury with greater than 35% total surface area burned. A similar entity is also observed as a result of central nervous system injury or intracranial hypertension. Multiple superficial ulcerations and erosions are noted in the proximal, acid-secreting portion of the stomach, with fewer lesions in the antrum and only rare ulcerations in the duodenum.

The most sensitive diagnostic test for stress ulceration is endoscopic examination. If patients are examined within 12 hours of the onset of injury, acute mucosal ulcerations may be observed that appear as multiple, shallow areas of erythema and friability, often accompanied by focal hemorrhage. The lesions are progressive during the first 72 hours after injury. When lesions are examined histologically, they are seen to consist of coagulation necrosis of the superficial endothelium with infiltration of leukocytes into the lamina propria. Chronic disease, characterized by fibrosis and scarring, is not observed. With resolution of the underlying injury or sepsis, healing is accompanying by mucosal restitution and regeneration.

Clinical observations and a large number of experimental studies suggest that mucosal ischemia is the central event underlying the development of stress gastritis. In clinical practice, most patients who contract stress gastritis do so after an episode of sepsis, hemorrhage, or cardiac dysfunction accompanied by shock. Experimental studies that cause depletion of high-energy phosphate compounds such at ATP predispose to the development of stress gastritis. Luminal gastric acid secretion, although not the sole cause of stress gastritis, appears to be a necessary concomitant process. A number of experimental observations suggest that a critical concentration of luminal acid is required to initiate injury in the setting of mucosal ischemia. The fall in mucosal energy supply permits proton back-diffusion into the mucosa; the resultant decrease in mucosal pH exacerbates ischemic damage.

Clinical risk factors that predict development of stress gastritis include adult respiratory distress syndrome, multiple long-bone fractures, a major burn over 35% of the body surface, transfusion requirement above 6 units, hepatic dysfunction, sepsis, hypotension, and oliguric renal failure. Scoring systems of critical illness, exemplified by the Acute Physiology and Chronic Health Evaluation (APACHE) system, accurately predict risk for acute stress gastritis.

The major complication of stress gastritis is hemorrhage. Admission to an intensive care unit is not an independent risk factor for bleeding. However, the development of respiratory failure or coagulopathy [platelet count less than 50,000/mm^3, international normalized ratio (INR) greater than 1.5, or partial thromboplastin time (PTT) greater than two times normal] imparts the greatest risk for hemorrhage.[43,44]

Diagnosis

Clinical studies that use bloody nasogastric discharge as a sign of stress gastritis probably underestimate its incidence in critically ill patients. Conversely, studies based on endoscopy overestimate the incidence of clinically important stress gastritis. In one endoscopically controlled study, 100% of patients with life-threatening injuries had evidence of gastric erosions by 24 hours. Severely burned patients have endoscopic evidence of gastric erosions in greater than 90% of cases, whereas significant upper gastrointestinal hemorrhage occurs in between 25% to 50% of patients with burn wound infection.

Barium contrast examinations have no role in the diagnosis of stress gastritis and interfere with subsequent endoscopic examination. Analysis of gastric contents for titration of acid production is not informative.

Treatment and Prophylaxis

All critically ill patients are at risk for development of acute stress gastritis. Because hemorrhage associated with stress gastritis significantly increases mortality, all such patients should be treated prophylactically.

Stress gastritis prophylaxis has focused on control of gastric luminal pH. If intragastric pH can be maintained above 3.5, effective prophylaxis can be obtained. In one study of seriously ill patients, antacid prophylaxis decreased bleeding from 25% to 4% of patients.

A number of prospective studies suggest that administration of H_2 antagonists are as effective as antacids for prophylaxis of stress gastritis.[45] Infusion of an H_2 antagonist at a rate that maintains intraluminal gastric pH at greater than 3.5 is equally effective, relative to antacids, in terms of prevention of bleeding. Continuous-infusion H_2 receptor antagonist therapy appears to be equally effective relative to intermittent dosing with H_2 blockers or antacids. Proton pump inhibitors have also been shown to be effective as stress ulcer prophylaxis.[46]

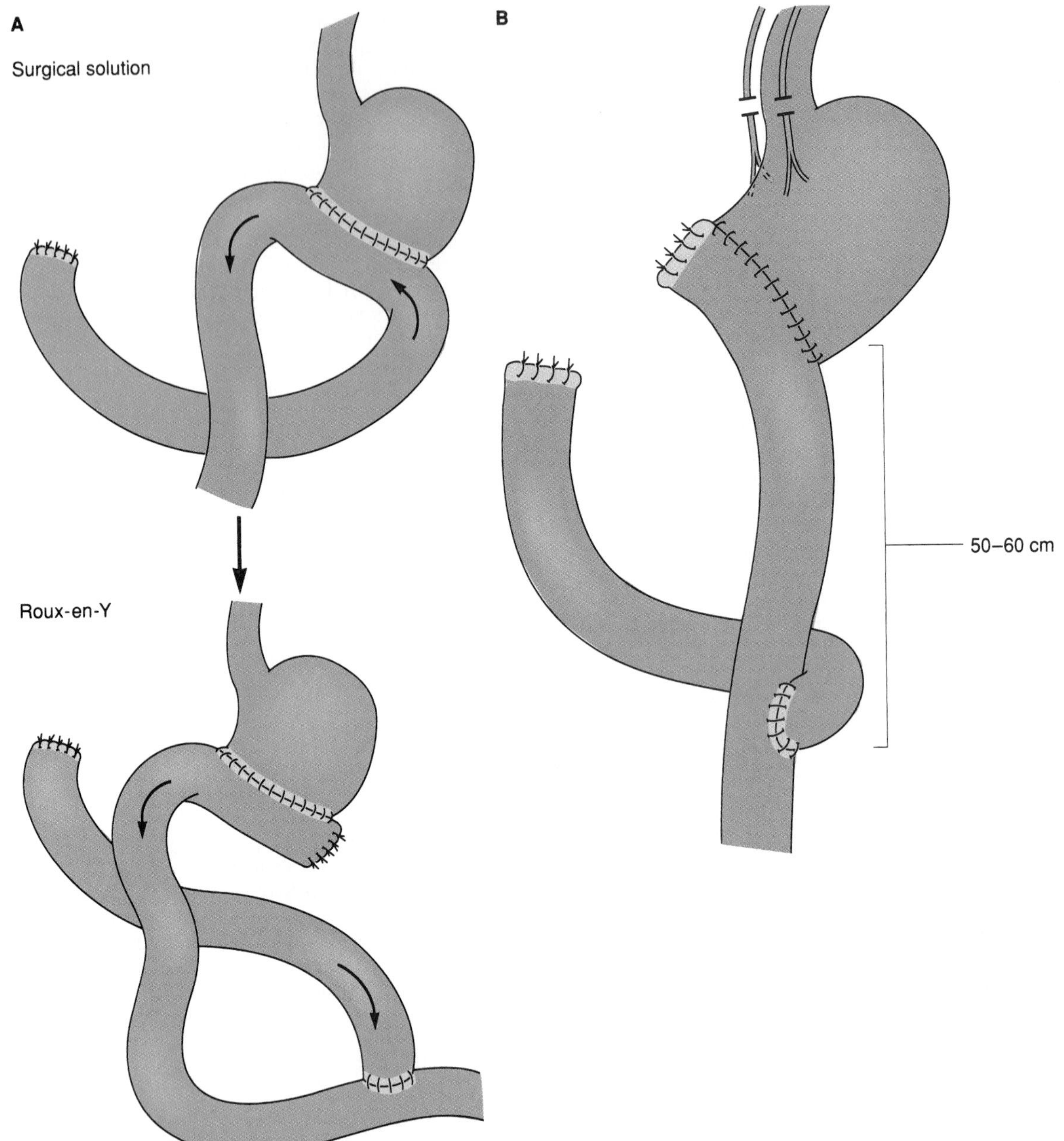

FIGURE 46.7 Conversion of Billroth II gastrojejunostomy to Roux-en-Y gastrojejunostomy. The afferent limb is divided (*A*), and intestinal continuity is reestablished by anastomosis 50 to 60 cm downstream from the original gastrojejunostomy (*B*).

Sucralfate is another antiulcer agent that shows efficacy as prophylactic treatment for stress gastritis. Sucralfate is not absorbed in the gastrointestinal tract and has no antisecretory activity. The agent binds to exposed collagen in areas of epithelial erosions. The mechanism of action of sucralfate is incompletely understood, but the drug prevents bacterial overgrowth by causing intragastric pH to remain low. A lower rate of pneumonia has been observed in patients receiving sucralfate relative to prophylactic H_2 receptor antagonist therapy.

When stress gastritis causes gastrointestinal bleeding, endoscopic therapy is used as first-line treatment. Endoscopic examination is diagnostic and permits application of electrocautery or heater probe hemostasis.

Only a small minority of patients with acute stress gastritis and hemorrhage require operative therapy. The surgical approach should control acute bleeding, have a low risk of recurrent hemorrhage, and be associated with a low operative mortality rate. No procedure meets all of these criteria, and no large clinical experience is available to confirm the superiority of one procedure over another. Total gastrectomy is associated with the lowest risk of recurrent bleeding but has a mortality rate of approximately 20%. Procedures such as vagotomy and pyloroplasty, vagotomy and antrectomy, and vagotomy and subtotal gastrectomy are each associated with high risks of recurrent hemorrhage.

KEY POINTS

- **Mucosal infection with *Helicobacter pylori* is the factor that contributes to ulcer pathogenesis in most patients.**
- **As a group, patients with duodenal ulcers have an increased capacity for gastric acid secretion relative to normal people.**

- **Current treatment of peptic ulceration involves a combination of an antisecretory drug, usually a proton pump inhibitor, with antibiotics.**
- **Hemorrhage is the leading cause of death associated with peptic ulcer.**
- **Major trauma accompanied by shock, sepsis, respiratory failure, hemorrhage, or multiorgan injury is often accompanied by acute stress gastritis.**

References

1. Logan RPH, Hirschl AM. Epidemiology of *Helicobacter pylori* infection. *Curr Opin Gastroenterol.* 1996;12:1–5.
2. ***Helicobacter pylori* in peptic ulcer disease. NIH Consensus Statement 1994;12:1–18.**
3. Suerbaum S, Michetti P: Helicobacter pylori infection. *N Engl J Med.* 347(15):1175-1186, Oct 2002.
4. Kokoska ER, Kauffman, Jr. GL. Helicobacter pylori and the gastroduodenal mucosa. *Surgery* 2001;130:13–16.
5. Blaser MJ. *Helicobacter* are indigenous to the human stomach: duodenal ulceration is due to changes in gastric microecology in the modern era. *Gut* 1998;43:721–727.
6. Atherton JC. The clinical relevance of strain types of *Helicobacter pylori. Gut* 1997;40:701–703.
7. Hatz R, Schildberg FW. Helicobacter pylori infections—are these diseases relevant for surgical treatment? *Arch Surg.* 2003;385:75–83.
8. Morris A, Nicholson G. Ingestion of *Campylobacter pyloridis* causes gastritis and raised fasting gastric pH. *Am J Gastroenterol.* 1987;82:192–199.
9. Crabtree JE, Farmery SM, Lindley IJD, et al. Cag A/cytotoxic strains of *Helicobacter pylori* and interleukin-8 in gastric epithelial cell lines. *J Clin Pathol.* 1994;47:945–950.
10. Peterson WL, Barnett CC, Evans DJ, et al. Acid secretion and serum gastrin in normal subjects and patients with duodenal ulcer: the role of *Helicobacter pylori. Am J Gastroenterol.* 1993;88:2038–2043.
11. Pérez TV, Gisbert JP, García JMP: Geographic differences and the role of cagA gene in gastroduodenal diseases associated with Helicobacter pylori infection. *Rev Esp De Enferm Dig.* 93:476–480, 2001.
12. Parasher G, Eastwood GL: Smoking and peptic ulcer in the Helicobacter pylori era. *Euro J Gastroenterol Hepat.* 2000;12:843–853.
13. Queiroz DM, Mendez EN, Rocha GA, et al. Effect of *Helicobacter pylori* eradication on antral gastrin- and somatostatin-immunoreactive cell density and gastrin and somatostatin concentrations. *Scand J Gastroenterol.* 1993;28:858–864.
14. Isenberg JI, Selling JA, Hogan DL, et al. Impaired proximal duodenal mucosal bicarbonate secretion in patients with duodenal ulcer. *N Engl J Med.* 1987;316:374.
15. Bukhave K, Rask-Madsen J, Hogan DL, et al. Proximal duodenal prostaglandin E_2 release and mucosal bicarbonate secretion are altered in patients with duodenal ulcer. *Gastroenterology* 1990;99:951.
16. Sontag S, Graham DY, Belsito A, et al. Cimetidine, cigarette smoking, and recurrence of duodenal ulcer. *N Engl J Med.* 1984;311:689.
17. Huang JQ, Sridhar S, Hunt RH: Role of *Helicobacter pylori* infection and non-steroidal anti-inflammatory drugs in peptic-ulcer disease: a meta-analysis. *Lancet* 2002;359:14–22.
18. Hopkins RJ, Girardi LS, Turney EA. Relationship between *Helicobacter pylori* eradication and reduced duodenal and gastric ulcer recurrence: a review. *Gastroenterology* 1996;110:1244–1252.
19. **Laheij RJR, Van Rossum LGM, Jansen JBMJ, et al. Evaluation of treatment regimens to cure *Helicobacter pylori* infection—a meta-analysis. *Aliment Pharm Ther.* 1999;13:857–864.**
20. Houben MHMG, Van De Beek D, Hensen EF, et al. A systematic review of *Helicobacter pylori* eradication therapy—the impact of antimicrobial resistance on eradication rates. *Aliment Pharm Ther.* 1999;13:1047—1055.
21. Berstad A, Weberg R. Antacids in the treatment of gastroduodenal ulcer. *Scand J Gastroenterol.* 1986;21:385.
22. Johnson AG: Promimal gastric vagotomy: does it have a place in the future management of peptic ulcer? *World J Surg.* 2000;24:259–-263.
23. Kleeff J, Friess H, Büchler MW: How *Helicobacter pylori* changed the life of surgeons. *Dig Surg.* 2003;20:93–102.
24. Legrand MJ, Jacquet N: Surgical approach in severe bleeding peptic ulcer. *Acta Gastro-Enter Belgica* 1996;59:240–244.
25. Lundell L. Upper gastrointestinal hemorrhage-surgical aspects. *Dig Dis.* 2003;21:16–18.
26. Bustamante M, Stollman N. The efficacy of proton-pump inhibitors in acute ulcer bleeding. A qualitative review. *J Clin Gastroenterol.* 2000;30:7–13.
27. Machicado GA, Jensen DM. Thermal probes alone or with epinephrine for the endoscopic haemostasis of ulcer haemorrhage. *Baillière's Clin Gastroenterol.* 2000;14:443–458.
28. Hepworth CC, Swain CP. Mechanical endoscopic methods of haemostasis for bleeding peptic ulcers: a review. *Baillière's Clin Gastroenterol* 2000;14:467–476.
29. **Boey J, Wong J, Ong GB. A prospective study of operative risk factors in perforated duodenal ulcers. *Ann Surg.* 1982;195:265.**
30. Spiegel BMR, Vakil NB, Ofman JJ. Endoscopy for acute nonvariceal upper gastrointestinal tract hemorrhage: is sooner better? *Arch Intern Med.* 2001;161:1393–1404.
31. Gisbert JP, Khorrami S, Carballo F, et al. *H. pylori* eradication therapy vs. antisecretory non-eradication therapy (with or without long-term maintenance antisecretory therapy) for the prevention of recurrent bleeding from peptic ulcer. The Cochrane Library 2, 2004.
32. Sharma VK, Sahai AV, Corder FA, et al. *Helicobacter pylori* eradication is superior to ulcer healing with or without maintenance therapy to prevent further ulcer haemorrhage. *Ailment Pharmacol Ther.* 2001;15:1939–1947.
33. Matsuda M, Nishiyama M, Hanai T, et al. Laparoscopic omental patch repair for perforated peptic ulcer. *Ann Surg.* 1995;221:236–240.
34. **Lau W-Y, Leung K-L, Kwong K-H, et al. A randomized study comparing laparoscopic versus open repair of perforated peptic ulcer using suture or sutureless technique. *Ann Surg.* 1996;224:131–138.**
35. Dubois F. New surgical strategy for gastroduodenal ulcer: laparoscopic approach. *World J Surg.* 2000;24:270–276.
36. Lagoo S, McMahon RL, Kakihara M, et al. The sixth decision regarding perforated duodenal ulcer. *JSLS* 2002;6:359–368.
37. Donovan AJ, Berne TV, Donovan JA. Perforated duodenal ulcer: an alternative therapeutic plan. *Arch Surg.* 1998;133:1166–1171.
38. Matsuda M, Nishiyama M, Hanai T, et al. Laparoscopic omental patch repair for perforated peptic ulcer. *Ann Surg.* 1995;221:236–240.
39. Lau W-Y, Leung K-L, Kwong K-H, et al. A randomized study comparing laparoscopic versus open repair of perforated peptic ulcer using suture or sutureless technique. *Ann Surg.* 1996;224:131–138.
40. Millat B, Fingerhut A, Borie F. Surgical treatment of complicated duodenal ulcers: controlled trials. *World J Surg.* 2000;24:299–306.
41. Hogan RB, Hamilton JK, Polter DE. Preliminary experience with hydrostatic balloon dilation of gastric outlet obstruction. *Gastointest Endosc.* 1986;32:71.
42. Lamers CBHW, Bijlstra AM, Harris AG. Octreotide, a long-acting somatostatin analog, in the management of postoperative dumping syndrome. *Dig Dis Sci.* 1993;38:359.
43. Hiramoto JS, Terdiman JP, Norton JA. Evidence-based analysis: postoperative gastric bleeding: etiology and prevention. *Surg Oncology* 2003;12:9–19, 2003.
44. Mutlu GM, Mutlu EA, Factor P. GI complications in patients receiving mechanical ventilation. *Chest* 2001;119:1222-1238.
45. Tryba M. Role of acid suppressants in intensive care medicine. *Best Practice Res Clin Gastroenterol.* 2001;15:447–461.
46. Yang Y, Lewis JD. Prevention and treatment of stress ulcers in critically ill patients. *Semin Gastro Dis.* 2003;14:11–19.

CHAPTER 47 ■ MORBID OBESITY

ERIC J. DEMARIA

Obesity and its sequelae have reached epidemic proportions. At least two thirds of the U.S. adult population is considered overweight [body mass index (BMI), calculated as weight in kilograms divided by the square of the height in meters, equal to or greater than 25], and half of those are obese (BMI of 30 or higher).[1] This expansive health issue has now spread beyond the developed world such that the World Health Organization (WHO) estimates that 1.7 billion people worldwide are overweight or obese.[2] Additionally, obesity has become increasingly prevalent in the pediatric population and 30% of U.S. children have a BMI greater than the 85th percentile for their age.[3]

Morbid obesity is defined as a BMI equal to or greater than 40 and is the degree of overweight that is clearly associated with increased morbidity and mortality.[4] The causes of morbid obesity are unknown but likely include genetic factors, abnormalities of neural or humoral transmitters to the hypothalamic hunger or satiety centers, and psychologically induced oral dependency drives. Morbidly obese adults have been found to have a lower basal energy expenditure.[5] A genetic predisposition to obesity has been reported in multiple studies. In adoption studies, the severity of obesity was more concordant with the natural than the adoptive parents.[6,7] Furthermore, monozygotic twins have more similar weights than dizygotic twins, even if they grow up in different environments.[8,9]

Gastrointestinal and neuroendocrine peptides are involved in weight homeostasis. Ghrelin, a potent orexigenic peptide secreted by the stomach, increases in response to fasting and decreases postprandially. Ghrelin levels are decreased in obese individuals.[10] The adipocyte hormone leptin stimulates anorexigenic neuropeptides in the hypothalamus to inhibit food intake; obese individuals often have increased serum levels of leptin and may be resistant to leptin effects on food intake and energy expenditure.[11]

Severe obesity is associated with a large number of problems that give rise to the term *morbid* obesity (Table 47.1). Several of these problems are underlying causes for the earlier mortality associated with obesity; they include coronary artery disease, hypertension, impaired cardiac ventricular function, adult-onset diabetes mellitus, obesity hypoventilation and sleep apnea syndromes, hypercoagulability leading to an increased risk of pulmonary embolism, necrotizing panniculitis, diverticulitis, and necrotizing pancreatitis. Morbidly obese patients can also die as a result of difficulties in recognizing the signs and symptoms of peritonitis. They have an increased risk for development of colon, prostate, breast, and uterine carcinoma. Premature death is much more common: a white male with a BMI of 45 or greater is estimated to have 13 years of life lost due to obesity (a 22% reduction in expected remaining life span).[4]

TABLE 47.1

MORBIDITY OF OBESITY

- Cardiovascular dysfunction
- Hypertension
- Coronary artery disease
- Heart failure
- Type II diabetes mellitus (adult onset or noninsulin dependent)
- Nonalcoholic steatohepatitis
- Respiratory insufficiency of obesity (pickwickian syndrome)
- Obesity hypoventilation syndrome
- Obstructive sleep apnea syndrome
- Increased intraabdominal pressure
- Stress overflow urinary incontinence
  - Gastroesophageal reflux
  - Venous disease
  - Thrombophlebitis
  - Stasis ulcers
  - Pulmonary embolism
  - Nephrotic syndrome
  - Pseudotumor cerebri
- Degenerative osteoarthritis
- Cholelithiasis
- Infectious complications
  - Difficulty recognizing peritonitis
  - Necrotizing subcutaneous infections
  - Wound infections or dehiscence
- Sexual hormone dysfunction
  - Polycystic ovary (Stein-Leventhal) syndrome

CENTRAL VERSUS PERIPHERAL OBESITY

Central obesity (android, or "apple," distribution of fat) is associated with a significantly greater morbidity than peripheral obesity (gynoid, or "pear," distribution of fat). This increased morbidity is secondary to the increased metabolism of visceral fat which leads to increased blood glucose levels, hyperglycemia, increased insulin secretion, insulin resistance, and insulin-induced sodium reabsorption leading to hypertension.

Increased fatty acid and cholesterol turnover with an increased risk of atherosclerosis and gallstones, polycystic ovary (Stein-Leventhal) syndrome, and nonalcoholic steatohepatitis (NASH) also result. This combination of problems is called the metabolic syndrome.[12] Another major complication of central obesity is increased intraabdominal pressure. This condition can lead to venous stasis disease, gastroesophageal reflux, stress or urge urinary incontinence, obesity hypoventilation syndrome, nephrotic syndrome, incisional and inguinal hernia, and elevated pleural pressures that can markedly increase pulmonary artery and pulmonary capillary wedge pressures.[13,14] The latter is probably responsible for pseudotumor cerebri seen in morbid obesity[15,16] and systemic hypertension.

CARDIAC DYSFUNCTION

Morbid obesity is often associated with increased circulating blood volume, left ventricular enlargement and both systolic and diastolic dysfunction, even in patients without overt heart disease.[17] Severe obesity can lead to chronically increased cardiac output, left ventricular dilation, and compensatory eccentric left ventricular hypertrophy. When hypertension accompanies obesity, both eccentric and concentric left ventricular hypertrophy are often present. Obesity cardiomyopathy is the form of congestive heart failure resulting from the compensatory structural cardiac changes associated with morbid obesity (left ventricular dilation, inadequate eccentric left ventricular hypertrophy).[18] Treatment of morbid obesity often improves cardiac function in these patients.[19] These structural cardiac changes also predispose to arrhythmias: obesity is associated with a 50% increase in the risk of developing atrial fibrillation secondary to left atrial enlargement.[20] Morbid obesity is also associated with coronary artery disease, although the exact relationship remains debatable. Although the Honolulu Heart Study revealed an increased risk of coronary atherosclerosis with increasing BMI, only coexistent comorbidities, especially lipid abnormalities, were identified as independent risk factors.[21] Respiratory insufficiency associated with morbid obesity can result in hypoxemic pulmonary artery vasoconstriction, which can lead to right-sided heart failure in severe cases. Correction of respiratory insufficiency after surgically induced weight loss improves pulmonary artery hypertension within 3 months to 1 year.[22] Severe obstructive sleep apnea syndrome can be associated with prolonged sinus arrest, premature ventricular contractions, and sudden death.

PULMONARY DYSFUNCTION

Respiratory insufficiency of obesity is associated with obesity hypoventilation syndrome, obstructive sleep apnea syndrome, or a combination of the two, commonly called the *pickwickian syndrome*. The obesity hypoventilation syndrome arises from the increased weight of the chest wall and increased intraabdominal pressure leading to a high-riding diaphragm. As a result, the lungs are compressed, producing a restrictive pulmonary defect. These patients have a markedly decreased expiratory reserve volume as well as smaller reductions in all other lung volumes. They have hypoxemia and hypercarbia while awake and a blunted ventilatory response to carbon dioxide. Chronic hypoxemia leads to pulmonary artery vasoconstriction and both right and left heart failure, as well as an increased risk of fatal arrhythmias and pulmonary embolism.

The obstructive sleep apnea syndrome is associated with severe obesity. These patients snore very loudly while asleep and have severe daytime somnolence with tendencies to fall asleep while driving or at work. Daytime somnolence is probably secondary to impaired nighttime stage III and IV and rapid-eye-movement stage sleep. The diagnosis of obstructive sleep apnea is suggested by a history of severe daytime somnolence, frequent nocturnal awakening, loud snoring, and morning headaches; it is confirmed with sleep polysomnography. This technique documents cessation of airflow during sleep associated with persistent respiratory efforts. This syndrome can be associated with sudden death and should always be considered in trauma victims who have fallen asleep while driving. The prevalence of obstructive sleep apnea in morbidly obese patients is as high as 71%, but no correlation has been identified between BMI and presence of sleep-related obstructive disorders.[23] Obstructive sleep apnea and obesity hypoventilation syndromes are associated with high mortality and serious morbidity rates; weight reduction corrects both.

DIABETES

Obesity is a frequent etiologic factor in the development of type II (adult-onset, noninsulin-dependent) diabetes mellitus. Morbidly obese patients can be resistant to insulin because of downregulation of insulin receptors. Most of these patients are able to discontinue medications and maintain normal serum glucose levels following surgery-induced weight loss.[24] Malabsorptive procedures appear to be more successful than purely restrictive procedures (gastric banding) in resolution of diabetes; this effect is likely related to alterations in gastrointestinal hormones associated with the former procedure.[25] The tendency toward hyperglycemia and hyperinsulinemia manifested by obese patients is another risk factor for coronary artery disease, as well as for severe, even fatal, soft tissue infections. Insulin resistance is also thought to be responsible for the Stein-Leventhal syndrome and NASH.

VENOUS STASIS DISEASE

Morbidly obese patients have an increased risk for deep venous thrombosis, venous stasis ulcers, and pulmonary embolism secondary to the increased intraabdominal pressure associated with central obesity. Low levels of antithrombin III can increase risk of blood clots. The increased weight in the abdomen raises inferior vena caval pressure and resistance to venous return, increasing the tendency for thrombosis. A similar mechanism may be responsible for the increased risk of pulmonary embolism in patients with right heart failure secondary to hypoxemic pulmonary artery vasoconstriction. Stasis ulcers are common in morbidly obese patients. These can be incapacitating and extremely difficult to treat; weight reduction can be the critical factor for healing because pressure stockings and wound care are often ineffective.[26]

DEGENERATIVE JOINT DISEASE

The increased weight in the morbidly obese leads to early degenerative arthritic changes of the weight-bearing joints, including ankles, knees, hips, and spine. These patients are poor candidates for total joint replacement because of the inability of the artificial joint—bone interface to withstand the abnormal pressures. Many orthopedic surgeons refuse to insert total hip or knee prostheses in patients weighing more than 250 pounds because of an unacceptable incidence of prosthetic loosening. Weight reduction after gastric surgery for obesity can permit subsequent successful joint replacement. In some instances, the decrease in pain after weight loss obviates joint surgery.

OTHER OBESITY-RELATED CONDITIONS

Morbidly obese patients frequently have gastroesophageal reflux. Women often have problems with stress overflow urinary incontinence. Both of these problems are probably related to an increased intraabdominal pressure.[27] Pseudotumor cerebri, also known as idiopathic intracranial hypertension, can be associated with morbid obesity. Weight loss after gastric surgery for obesity is accompanied by a significant reduction in cerebrospinal fluid pressure and associated headaches.[16] Pseudotumor has also been shown to be secondary to increased intraabdominal pressure leading to increased intrathoracic and central venous pressures.[16] Women often have sexual dysfunction as a result of excessive levels of both the virilizing hormone androstenedione and the feminizing hormone estradiol. These abnormalities can produce infertility, hirsutism, ovarian cysts (Stein-Leventhal syndrome), hypermenorrhea, and endometrial carcinoma. These hormonal abnormalities also resolve after weight loss.

MEDICAL MANAGEMENT OF MORBID OBESITY

There are a number of dietary programs for weight reduction, including hospital-supervised programs, psychiatric behavioral modification programs, commercial organizations, commercial diets, protein-sparing fast programs, and medications. Unfortunately, no dietary approach has achieved uniform, long-term success for the morbidly obese. Although many people can lose weight successfully through dietary manipulation, only 5% to 10% of patients with extreme obesity are able to sustain significant weight reduction.[28] A National Institutes of Health (NIH) Technology Assessment Conference in 1992 concluded that dietary management of severe obesity, with or without behavioral modification, failed to provide acceptable evidence of long-term efficacy.[29] Pharmacotherapy includes orlistat, a pancreatic lipase inhibitor that blocks fat absorption, and sibutramine, which works as an appetite suppressant. These agents provide only modest weight loss and are inadequate therapy for the morbidly obese patient.[30]

SURGICAL MANAGEMENT OF MORBID OBESITY

Surgical Eligibility

According to a 1991 NIH Consensus Panel (Table 47.2), patients are considered eligible for surgical management if they have a BMI of 40 or over without comorbidity or a BMI of 35 or over with comorbidity (e.g., diabetes, respiratory insufficiency, pseudotumor cerebri).

Jejunoileal Bypass

The first popular surgical procedure for morbid obesity was the jejunoileal bypass. This operation produced an obligatory malabsorption state through bypass of a major portion of the absorptive surface of the small intestine. The procedure connected a short length of proximal jejunum (8 to 14 inches) to the distal ileum (4 to 12 inches) as an end-to-end or end-to-side anastomosis. The end-to-end procedures, which were associated with a better weight loss, required decompression of the bypassed small intestine into the colon. The jejunoileal bypass was associated with a number of early and late complications. The most serious postoperative complication was cirrhosis due to either protein—calorie malnutrition or absorption of degradation products from bacterial overgrowth in the bypassed intestine. Other complications include cholelithiasis, urolithiasis, metabolic acidosis, chronic diarrhea with electrolye depletion, iron deficiency anemia, and vitamin K deficiency resulting from bacterial overgrowth.[30] Randomized, prospective studies have shown that the gastric bypass operation is associated with a comparable weight loss and a significantly lower complication rate than jejunoileal bypass.[31] Because of the significant complication rate, standard jejunoileal bypass should no longer be performed.

TABLE 47.2 INDICATIONS/CONTRAINDICATIONS

CRITERIA FOR PATIENT SELECTION FOR BARIATRIC SURGERY

- Body mass index >40 kg/m^2
- Body mass index >35 kg/m^2 with coexisting comorbidities
- Failure of nonsurgical methods of weight reduction
- Psychological stability
- Absence of drug and alcohol abuse

Gastric Procedures for Morbid Obesity

In 1969, investigators reported the results of weight loss after division of the stomach into a small upper pouch connected to a loop gastroenterostomy. The concept for this procedure was based on the observation of weight loss that sometimes followed subtotal gastrectomy for duodenal ulcer disease. There was initial concern that peptic ulcers would develop in the bypassed stomach or duodenum, and although these have occurred, the incidence is low. The technique for gastric bypass was simplified with the use of stapling instruments. The concept of gastroplasty was then proposed as a safer, easier method for restricting food intake. In gastroplasty, the stomach is only stapled and not divided, leaving a small opening to permit the normal passage of food into the distal stomach and duodenum. Thus, weight loss can be assisted through pure restrictive gastric procedures (gastroplasty or gastric banding) or a combination of restriction and malabsorption (gastric bypass, biliopancreatic diversion). (See Chapter 85, Mastery of Surgery.)

Gastroplasty

Gastroplasties are purely restrictive procedures which have been performed with either horizontal or vertical placement of the staples. Horizontal gastroplasty usually requires ligation and division of the short gastric vessels between the stomach and spleen, and it carries the risk of devascularization of the gastric pouch or splenic injury. The failure rate (loss of less than 40% of excess weight) of horizontal gastroplasty ranges from 42% to 71%.[32] The vertical banded gastroplasty is a procedure in which a stapled opening is made in the stomach with a circular stapler 5 cm from the cardioesophageal junction. Two applications of a 90-mm stapling device are made between this opening and the angle of His, and a 1.5 × 5-cm strip of polypropylene mesh is wrapped around the stoma on the lesser curvature and sutured to itself but not to the stomach. Erosion of the mesh into the stomach has been an unusual complication of this procedure. Pouch enlargement and stomal dilation are less common with the vertical technique, although staple line disruption occurs in up to 35% of cases. Some surgeons now recommend transecting the stomach to decrease the incidence of this complication (Table 47.3).

Gastric Bypass

Gastric bypass combines restriction and malabsorption to assist weight loss. A small (15- to 30-mL) gastric pouch is created along the lesser curve with staplers, followed by construction of a gastrojejunostomy (most commonly Roux-en-Y configuration) with a 1-cm stoma to drain the pouch. With the Roux technique, a 40- to 50-cm jejunal limb provides moderate malabsorption and limits bile reflux (Fig. 47.1). Significantly improved weight loss has been achieved in the superobese population (BMI equal to or greater than 50 kg/m^2) with a 150-cm Roux limb (long-limb gastric bypass).[33]

Gastroplasty Versus Gastric Bypass

Roux-en-Y gastric bypass provides significantly improved weight loss over vertical banded gastroplasty. Reduction in excess body weight at 2 years ranges from 60% to 70% with gastric bypass compared with 40% to 50% with vertical banded gastroplasty. Gastric bypass carries a higher incidence of stomal ulcer, stomal stenosis, vitamin B_{12} deficiency, and, in menstruating

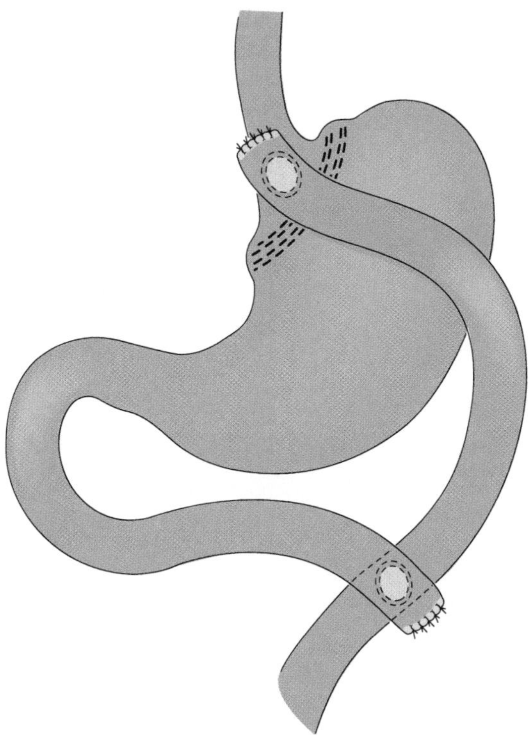

FIGURE 47.1 Open proximal Roux-en-Y gastric bypass.

women, iron-deficiency anemia than does gastroplasty. Gastric bypass is, however, more effective than vertical banded gastroplasty in correcting glucose intolerance in patients without overt type II diabetes mellitus. "Sweet eaters" tend to achieve greater weight reduction with gastric bypass, and this finding likely results from the development of dumping syndrome symptoms.[34]

Weight reduction failures nonethless occur with gastric bypass. Although regained weight could be the result of staple disruption, pouch expansion, or stomal dilation, these findings are not observed in the majority of patients. Approximately 10% to 15% regain lost weight or fail to achieve an acceptable weight loss. The cause for this failure appears to be excessive, constant nibbling on foods with high caloric density.

Partial Biopancreatic Diversion

The partial biliopancreatic diversion was developed as both a gastric restrictive procedure and a malabsorptive procedure that does not have a blind intestinal limb for bacterial overgrowth.[35] In this operation (Fig. 47.2), the quantity of food ingested is partially restricted and then passes down the intestine mostly undigested and unabsorbed until it reaches the bile and pancreatic juices, 0.5 meter from the ileocecal valve, where digestion and absorption take place. Treated patients usually pass four to six stools per day, which are foul smelling and float, reflecting malabsorption of fat. Reduction in excess weight approximates 70% to 80%.

As with the proximal or standard gastric bypass, patients with the biliopancreatic diversion are at risk for iron deficiency anemia and vitamin B_{12} deficiency. In addition, they are at risk for protein deficiency, osteoporosis secondary to calcium and vitamin D malabsorption, night blindness and skin eruptions secondary to vitamin A deficiency, and problems with the other fat-soluble vitamins, E and K.[35] Italian patients—the operation was developed in Italy—appear to have less malabsorption and nutritional deficiencies than U.S. patients, probably because of a much lower fat content in the Italian diet. The duodenal switch operation is a modification of the partial biliopancreatic bypass but still may be associated with malnutrition and fat-soluble vitamin and calcium deficiencies.[37]

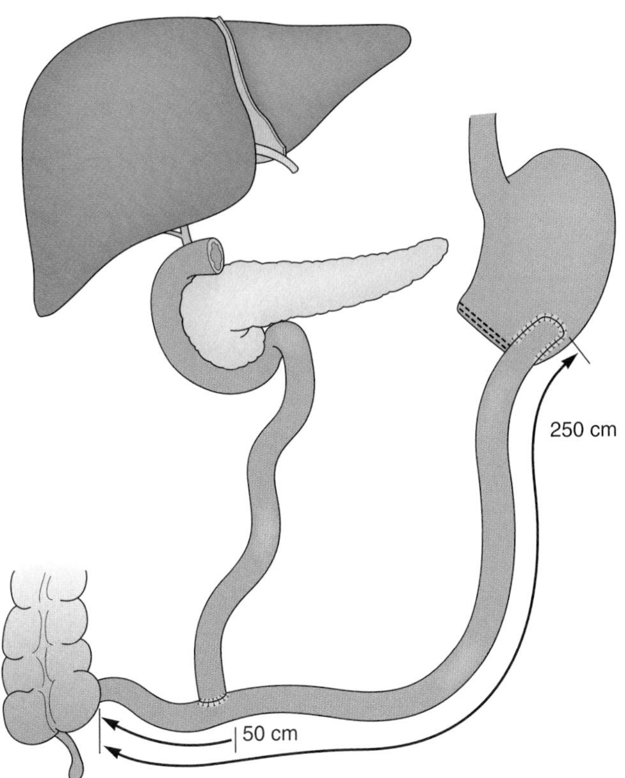

FIGURE 47.2 Biliopancreatic diversion. A distal gastrectomy is performed, followed by division of the distal small bowel 250 cm proximal to the ileocecal valve. The proximal bypassed bowel is anastamosed to the ileum 50 cm from the ileocecal valve.

Laparoscopic Obesity Surgery

The adjustable silicone gastric band has been developed to be placed laparoscopically. The procedure involves placing the band around the proximal stomach to create a 15-mL pouch. The amount of restriction is adjusted by injecting saline into a subcutaneously implanted port (Fig. 47.3). This procedure has

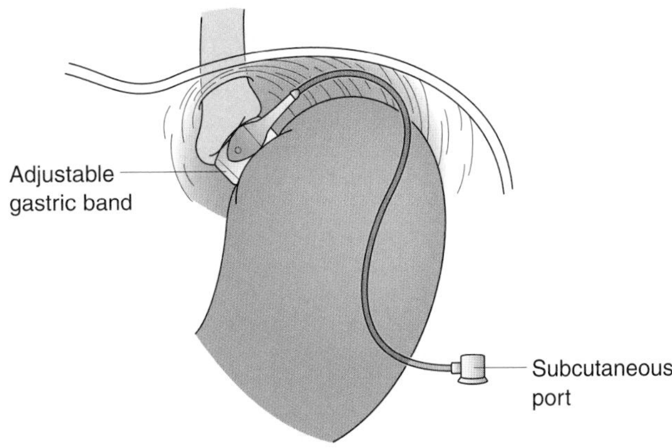

FIGURE 47.3 Schematic representing laparoscopic adjustable gastric banding. The buckle would be oriented medially, and anterior gastrogastric sutures would be placed proximal and distal to the band to prevent gastric herniation.

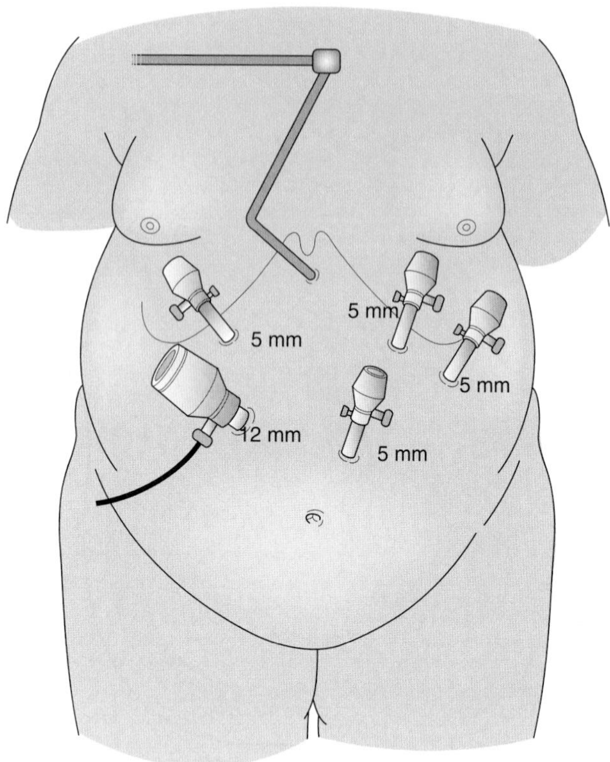

FIGURE 47.4 Trocar placement for laparoscopic Roux-en-Y gastric bypass.

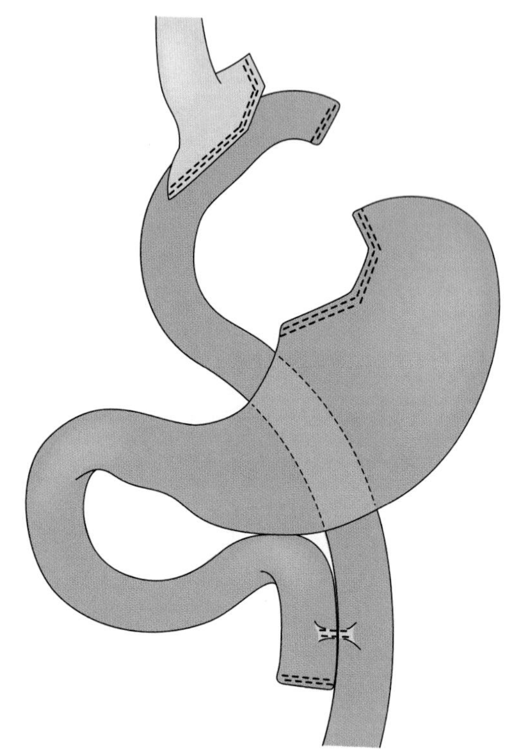

FIGURE 47.5 Laparoscopic proximal Roux-en-Y gastric bypass (retrocolic, retrogastric).

become very popular in Europe, where loss of up to 50% of excess weight at 2 years has been reported. This device was approved by the U.S. Food and Drug Administration approval in 2001, but American trials have yielded varied results.[38,39] Long-term studies validating its safety and efficacy are needed. Complications include band slippage, gastric obstruction, port malfunction or infection, and band erosion.

Laparoscopic Roux-en-Y gastric bypass is being performed with increasing frequency in the United States. This is a technically demanding procedure with a steep learning curve. Five or six ports are utilized (Fig. 47.4). A linear cutting stapler is used to create a stapled side-to-side jejunojejunostomy after measuring a 50-cm Roux limb. This alimentary limb can be tunneled through the mesocolon (retrocolic) or allowed to pass anterior to the colon and stomach (antecolic). The proximal lesser curvature 15- to 20-mL gastric pouch is created with the linear cutting stapler with care to avoid injury to the spleen or esophagus. The gastrojejunostomy is formed with a stapled posterior row and a hand-sewn anterior row (Fig. 47.5). The anastamosis is tested with insufflation via a gastroscope. Drainage and postoperative radiographs to assess for leaks can be performed routinely or selectively according to surgeon preference.

Although the laparoscopic technique is associated with increases in operative time, operative cost, and incidence of gastrojejunal stricture, advantages include decreased hospital length of stay, decreased incidence of wound infection and incisional hernia, and reductions in perioperative blood transfusions. Internal hernias may increase in frequency with the laparoscopic technique as a result of decreased severity of adhesions (Fig. 47.6). In terms of weight loss, laparoscopic gastric bypass offers similar short-term reductions in excess body weight when compared with the open technique in randomized prospective trials;[40] additional trials are needed to validate its long-term efficacy.

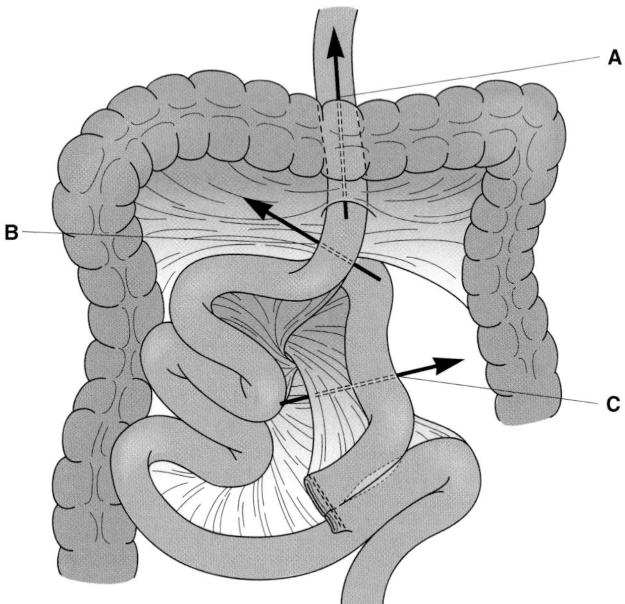

FIGURE 47.6 Potential sites of internal hernia following Roux-en-Y gastric bypass: mesocolic defect (*A*), Petersen's defect (*B*), and jejunojejunal (*C*)

TABLE 47.3 RESULTS

RESOLUTION OF COMORBIDITIES FOLLOWING GASTRIC BYPASS

Comorbidity	Resolution rate (%)
Diabetes	73
Obstructive sleep apnea (mild/moderate)	100
Obstructive sleep apnea (severe)	75
Hypertension (high blood presure)	56
Urinary stress incontinence	91
Gastroesophageal reflux disease	90
Venous stasis ulcers	94
Pseudotumor cerebri	100
Joint pain	71

COMPLICATIONS OF GASTRIC SURGERY FOR MORBID OBESITY

The most feared complication of gastric surgery for morbid obesity is gastrointestinal leak (Algorithm 47.1). This occurs most commonly at the gastrojejunostomy, although other potential sites include the jejunojejunostomy, excluded stomach, and inadvertent enterotomies. Following gastric bypass, the excluded stomach can perforate because of marked dilatation resulting from biliopancreatic limb obstruction. This complication is often heralded by frequent hiccups and can be diagnosed by noting a large gastric bubble on abdominal radiographs. Impending gastric perforation requires urgent percutaneous or operative decompression. In patients undergoing revisional gastric surgery for obesity, a gastrostomy tube should be inserted prophylactically for decompression.

Leaks can be extremely difficult to detect in the morbidly obese patient. If patients complain of increasing pain in the abdomen, back, or shoulder (consistent with irritation of the left hemidiaphragm) or of pelvic pressure or hiccups, the clinician must suspect a leak. Tachycardia, tachypnea, fever, anxiety, and leukocytosis are often present, although it is not uncommon for a leak to manifest as unexplained persistent tachycardia in an asymptomatic patient. This complication can often be confirmed with an emergent upper gastrointestinal series using water-soluble contrast. If the study is negative but suspicion is high, the patient's abdomen should be reexplored urgently. An attempt to repair the leak should be made, and a large sump drain should be placed nearby because the repair frequenty breaks down. This leads to a controlled fistula, which usually heals with total parenteral nutrition or tube feeds via gastrostomy or jejunostomy. Some gastrojejunal leaks can be managed nonperatively in situations where the leak is drained (via a drain placed at time of operation or radiographically guided) or contained; in either circumstance, Algorithm 47.1 is appropriate only in stable patients without signs of systemic toxicity. Factors associated with leak include increasing age, revisional surgery, male gender, and sleep apnea.[41]

Marginal ulcers develop in approximately 10% of patients with gastric bypass even when treated with postoperative acid suppression. This complication usually responds to additional medical therapy with proton pump inhibitors. Stomal stenosis can occur following gastric bypass or vertical banded gastroplasty. Outpatient endoscopic dilatation is usually successful in patients with gastric bypass, although more than one treatment may be necessary.

Rapid weight loss following bariatric surgery is associated with a high incidence (up to 35%) of gallstone formation and need for subsequent cholecystectomy for biliary colic or acute cholecystitis. Some surgeons recommend prophylactic cholecystectomy at the time of bariatric surgery, whereas others perform cholecystectomy only if sonographic evidence of gallstones is identified. Ursodeoxycholic acid (300 mg orally twice daily) administered for 6 months following gastric bypass (the period of rapid weight loss) reduces the risk of gallstone formation to 2%.[42] Compliance with this medication can be difficult secondary to adverse side effects (nausea, diarrhea, and pruritus).

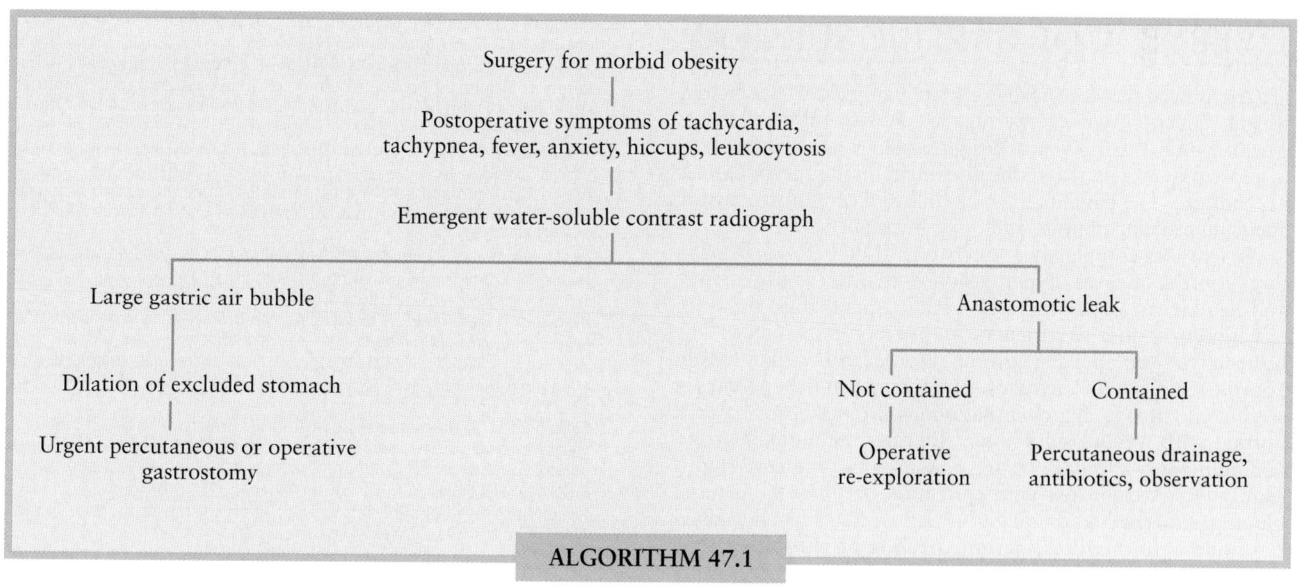

ALGORITHM 47.1 Management of anastomotic leak after gastric surgery for obesity.

Nutritional follow-up is mandatory after gastric bypass because these patients are at risk for deficiency states and their sequelae. Vitamin B_{12}, iron, and calcium supplements are often necessary along with routine administration of multivitamins. A high-protein diet (50 g/day for women and 65 g/day for men) is required to avoid protein malnutrition.

The incidence of perioperative venous thrombosis and pulmonary embolism can be reduced with prophylactic subcutaneous heparin, sequential compression boots, and early ambulation. Pulmonary embolism nonetheless occurs in 0.9% of patients despite these measures; independent risk factors include extreme obesity (BMI of 50 kg/m^2 or greater), obesity hypoventilation syndrome, and venous stasis. It has been receommended that prophylactic vena caval filters be placed in these high-risk patients at the time of obesity surgery.

The operative mortality rate after gastric surgery is now approximately 0.5% in most series. Independent risk factors associated with increased risk of death include gastrointestinal leak, pulmonary embolus, hypertension, and preoperative weight.[43]

FAILED GASTRIC SURGERY FOR OBESITY

Revision of a failed gastroplasty is often unsuccessful because of recurrence of stomal dilation and problems with gastric emptying; conversion to gastric bypass provides better results. Laparoscopic gastric banding with ineffective weight loss can likewise be converted to gastric bypass, but the complication rate with this and any revision is higher than for a primary gastric bypass. Revision of a dilated gastrojejunal stoma has not been effective, but application of an adjustable band to the pouch above the stoma has been suggested as an option for this problem. Most patients who fail a gastric bypass do so as a result of dietary indiscretion. If a patient has significant obesity-related comorbidities that have failed to resolve or have returned with weight gain, conversion to long-limb gastric bypass can be performed. This modification can be associated with steatorrhea, fat-soluble vitamin deficiency, and osteoporosis.

OVERVIEW OF GASTRIC SURGERY

Gastric procedures for morbid obesity can yield a satisfactory weight reduction, with an average loss of two thirds of excess weight within 1 to 1.5 years. Weight becomes stable at this level in most patients as the reduced caloric intake meets caloric expenditure. The patients must be followed carefully to ensure adequate protein, vitamin, and other micronutrient levels.

Weight loss completely corrects type II diabetes mellitus in three fourths of cases, hypertension in two thirds of patients, and headaches associated with cerebrospinal fluid pressure elevation in almost all patients with pseudotumor cerebri. The obstructive sleep apnea syndrome resolves with weight loss in approximately 80% of cases. Hypoxemia and hypercarbia seen in the obesity hypoventilation syndrome return toward normal with weight reduction.[24] Elevated pulmonary artery and pulmonary capillary wedge pressures also improve significantly after weight loss with correction of abnormal arterial blood gases. The loss of weight usually corrects female sexual hormone abnormalities, permits healing of chronic venous stasis ulcers associated with venous insufficiency, prevents reflux esophagitis, relieves stress overflow urinary incontinence, and improves low back pain as well as joint-related pain. Weight loss can permit successful total artificial joint replacement. Patient self-image is often markedly improved after gastric surgery for obesity.

Treatment of morbidly obese patients requires a multidisciplinary approach including psychologists, nutritionists, and experienced physicians and ward personnel. Patients must be willing to make a lifelong commitment to behavioral modification, regular exercise, and long-term medical follow-up.

KEY POINTS

- **At least two thirds of the U.S. adult population is considered overweight [body mass index (BMI), calculated as weight in kilograms divided by the square of the height in meters, equal to or greater than], and half of those are obese (BMI of 30 or higher).**
- **A National Institutes of Health (NIH) Technology Assessment Conference in 1992 concluded that dietary management of severe obesity, with or without behavioral modification, failed to provide acceptable evidence of long-term efficacy.**
- **Patients are considered eligible for surgical treatment of obesity if they have a BMI of 40 or over without comorbidity or a BMI of 35 or over with comorbidity (e.g., diabetes, respiratory insufficiency, pseudotumor cerebri).**
- **Gastroplasties are restrictive procedures that have been performed with either horizontal or vertical placement of the staples.**
- **Gastric bypass combines restriction and malabsorption to assist weight loss.**

References

1. National Center for Health Statistics NHANES IV Report. Available at http://www.cdc.gov/nchs/product/pubs/pubd/hestats/obes/obese99.htm2002. Accessed November 29, 2004.
2. Deitel M. Overweight and obesity worldwide now estimated to involve 1.7 billion people. *Obes Surg.* 2003;13:329–330.
3. **Ogden CL, Flegal KM, Carroll MD, et al. Prevalence and trends in overweight among US children and adolescents, 1999–2000. *JAMA* 2002; 288:1728–1732.**
4. **Fontaine KR, Redden DT, Wang C, et al. Years of life lost due to obesity. *JAMA* 2003;289:187–193.**
5. van Gemert WG, Westerterp KR, van Acker BA, et al. Energy, substrate and protein metabolism in morbid obesity before, during and after massive weight loss. *Int J Obes Relat Metab Disord.* 2000;24:711–718.
6. Stunkard AJ, Sorensen TA, Hanis C, et al. An adoptive study of human obesity. *New Engl J Med.* 1986;314:193–198.
7. Vogler GP, Sorensen TI, Stunkard AJ, et al. Influences of genes and shared family environment on adult body mass index assessed in an adoption study by a comprehensive path model. *Int J Obes Relat Metab Disord.* 1995;19:40–45.
8. Stunkard AJ, Harris JR, Pedersen NL, et al. The body-mass index of twins who have been reared apart. *N Engl J Med.* 1990;322:1483–1487.
9. Austin MA, Friedlander Y, Newman B, et al. Genetic influences on changes in body mass index: a longitudinal analysis of women twins. *Obes Res.* 1997;5:326–331.
10. Neary NM, Small CJ, Bloom SR. Gut and mind. *Gut* 2003;52:918–921.
11. Jequier E. Leptin signaling, adiposity, and energy balance. *Ann N Y Acad Sci.* 2002;967:379–88.
12. Bjorntorp P, Rosmond R. The metabolic syndrome—a neuroendocrine disorder? *Br J Nutr.* 2000;83:S49–57.
13. Sugerman H, Windsor A, Bessos M, et al. Intra-abdominal pressure, sagittal abdominal diameter, and obesity co-morbidity. *J Intern Med.* 1997;241: 71–79.
14. Sugerman H, Windsor A, Bessos M, et al. Effects of surgically induced weight loss on urinary bladder pressure, sagittal abdominal diameter, and obesity co-morbidity. *Int J Obes Relat Metab Disord.* 1998;22:230–235.
15. Sugerman HJ, Felton WL III, Salvant JB, et al. Effects of surgically induced weight loss on idiopathic intracranial hypertension in morbid obesity. *Neurology* 1995;45:1655–1659.
16. Sugerman HJ, DeMaria EJ, Felton WL III, et al. Increased intra-abdominal pressure and cardiac filling pressures in obesity associated pseudotumor cerebri. *Neurology* 1997;49:507–511.
17. Wong CY, O'Moore-Sullivan T, et al. Alterations of left ventricular myocardial characteristics associated with obesity. *Circulation* 2004;110: 3081–3087.
18. Alpert MA. Obesity cardiomyopathy: pathophysiology and evolution of the clinical syndrome. *Am J Med Sci.* 2001;321:225–236.

19. Alpert MA, Terry BE, Mulekar M, et al. Cardiac morphology and left ventricular function in normotensive morbidly obese patients with and without congestive heart failure, and effect of weight loss. *Am J Cardiol.* 1997;80:736–740.
20. Wang TJ, Parise H, Levy D, et al. Obesity and the risk of new-onset atrial fibrillation. *JAMA* 2004;292:2471–2477.
21. Huang B, Rodreiguez BL, Burchfiel CM, et al. Associations of adiposity with prevalent coronary heart disease among elderly men: the Honolulu Heart Program. *Int J Obes Relat Metab Disord.* 1997;21:340–348.
22. Sugerman HJ, Baron PL, Fairman RP, et al. Hemodynamic dysfunction in obesity hypoventilation syndrome and the effects of treatment with surgically induced weight loss. *Ann Surg.* 1988;207:604–613.
23. Frey WC, Pilcher J. Obstructive sleep-related breathing disorders in patients evaluated for bariatric surgery. *Obes Surg.* 2003;13:676–683.
24. **Buchwald H, Avidor Y, Braunwald E, et al. Bariatric surgery: a systematic review and meta-analysis. *JAMA* 2004;292:1724–1737.**
25. **Rubino F, Gagner M, Gentileschi P, et al. The early effect of the Roux-en-Y gastric bypass on hormones involved in body weight regulation and glucose metabolism. *Ann Surg.* 2004;240:236–242.**
26. Sugerman HJ, Sugerman EL, Wolfe L, et al. Risks and benefits of gastric bypass in morbidly obese patients with severe venous stasis disease. *Ann Surg.* 2001;234:41–46.
27. Bump RC, Sugerman HJ, Fantl JA, et al. Obesity and lower urinary tract function in women: effect of surgically induced weight loss. *Am J Obstet Gynecol.* 1992;167:392–397.
28. Fisher BL, Schauer P. Medical and surgical options in the treatment of severe obesity. *Am J Surg.* 2002;184:9S–16S.
29. **NIH Technology Assessment Conference Panel. NIH conference: methods for voluntary weight loss and control. *Ann Intern Med.* 1992;116:942–949.**
30. Hocking MP, Duerson MC, O'Leary JP, et al. Jejunoileal bypass for morbid obesity. Late follow-up in 100 cases. *N Engl J Med.* 1983;308:995–999.
31. Griffen WO Jr, Young VL, Stevenson CC. A prospective comparison of gastric and jejunoileal bypass procedures for morbid obesity. *Ann Surg.* 1977;186:500–509.
32. Sugerman HJ, Wolper JL. Failed gastroplasty for morbid obesity. Revised gastroplasty versus Roux-Y gastric bypass. *Am J Surg.* 1984;148:331–336.
33. Brolin RE, Kenler HA, Gorman JH, et al. Long-limb gastric bypass in the superobese. A prospective randomized study. *Ann Surg.* 1992;215:387–395.
34. Sugerman HJ, Starkey J, Birkenhauer R. A randomized prospective trial of gastric bypass versus vertical banded gastroplasty for morbid obesity and their effects on sweets versus non-sweets eaters. *Ann Surg.* 1987; 205:613–624.
35. Scopinaro N, Gianetta E, Civalleri D, et al. Two years of clinical experience with biliopancreatic bypass for obesity. *Am J Clin Nutr.* 1980;33:506–514.
36. Jones DB, Provost DA, DeMaria EJ, et al. Optimal management of the morbidly obese patient SAGES appropriateness conference statement. *Surg Endosc.* 2004;18:1029–1037.
37. Hess DS, Hess DW. Biliopancreatic diversion with a duodenal switch. *Obes Surg.* 1998;8:267–282.
38. Ren CJ, Weiner M, Allen JW. Favorable early results of gastric banding for morbid obesity: the American experience. *Surg Endosc.* 2004;18:543–546.
39. DeMaria EJ, Sugerman HJ, Meador JG, et al. High failure rate after laparoscopic adjustable silicone gastric banding for treatment of morbid obesity. *Ann Surg.* 2001;233:809–818.
40. Nguyen NT, Goldman C, Rosenquist CJ, et al. Laparoscopic versus open gastric bypass: a randomized study of outcomes, quality of life, and costs. *Ann Surg.* 2001;234:279–289.
41. Fernandez AZ Jr, DeMaria EJ, Tichansky DS, et al. Experience with over 3,000 open and laparoscopic bariatric procedures: multivariate analysis of factors related to leak and resultant mortality. *Surg Endosc.* 2004;18:193–197.
42. Sugerman HJ, Brewer WH, Shiffman ML, et al. A multicenter, placebo-controlled, randomized, double-blind, prospective trial of prophylactic ursodiol for the prevention of gallstone formation following gastric-bypass-induced rapid weight loss. *Am J Surg.* 1995;169:91–96.
43. Fernandez AZ Jr, Demaria EJ, Tichansky DS, et al. Multivariate analysis of risk factors for death following gastric bypass for treatment of morbid obesity. *Ann Surg.* 2004;239:698–702.

CHAPTER 48 ■ GASTRIC NEOPLASMS

MICHAEL W. MULHOLLAND

Gastric cancer is a relatively common, frequently lethal affliction and remains a serious and unsolved problem in general surgery. The disease often is not recognized until it is at an advanced stage. Gastric cancer usually cannot be controlled by surgery alone, and surgical cure rates have remained disappointingly low. Technical innovations and basic scientific investigations continue to be applied to this disease, however, and cautious optimism for the future is appropriate.

ADENOCARCINOMA

Epidemiology

Starting in 1930, the incidence of gastric cancer declined dramatically in the United States (Fig. 48.1). By 1980, the incidence of gastric cancer (10 cases per 100,000 population) was approximately one fourth the incidence recorded in 1930. The incidence of the disease remained relatively constant in the decades from 1980 to 2000.[1] By 1997, reported new cases of gastric cancer had declined to 22,000, a small number relative to the 150,000 estimated deaths from cancer of the lung.[2] Gastric cancer remains among the top 10 causes of cancer-related deaths for both men and women in the United States. The reasons for the early decline in the incidence of gastric cancer are unknown, but the factors contributing to its persistence are now better understood.

The worldwide incidence and death rates for gastric cancer vary markedly. The highest age-adjusted death rate for gastric cancer occurs in Japan, where the disease accounts for approximately 50% of cancer-related deaths in men and 40% of cancer deaths in women. High incidence rates are also reported in Chile, Costa Rica, Hungary, Portugal, Singapore, and Romania, a geographically and ethnically diverse group. It had been widely assumed that exposure to environmental carcinogens, probably in the diet, accounted for the increased disease frequency observed in these populations. This supposition is supported by studies of immigrant populations. Migration from an area at high risk to one at low risk is associated with a decreased probability of development of gastric cancer. However, early infection with the organism *Helicobacter pylori* now appears to be the predominant risk factor which predisposes to subsequent development of gastric carcinoma. In animal models, ingested nitrites and metabolic derivatives such as nitrosamines can promote gastric carcinogenesis. Although nitrites in the diet have been postulated to have a role in gastric carcinogenesis in humans, specific dietary constituents that promote tumor formation in humans have not been identified.

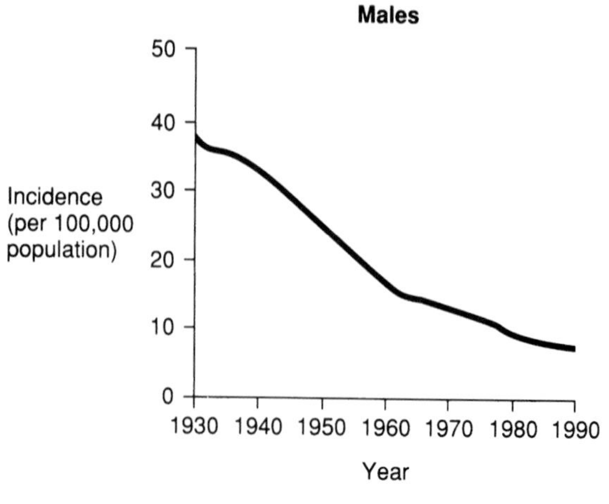

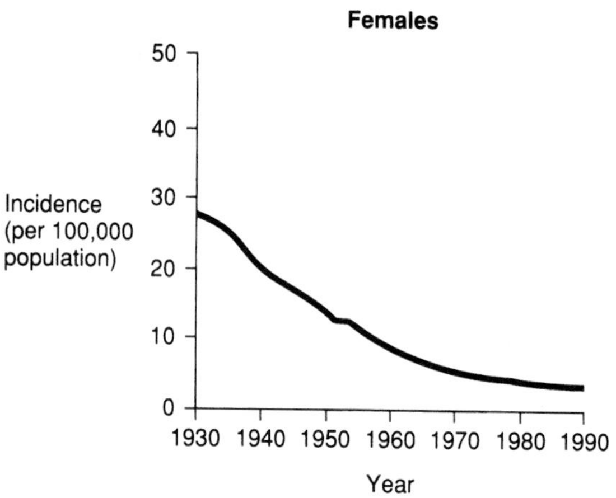

FIGURE 48.1 Incidence of gastric cancer deaths in the United States.

Premalignant Lesions

The risk for development of gastric cancer is greater in stomachs that harbor polyps. This risk is related most closely to polyp histologic type, size, and number. Variations in these three factors account for the wide range in reported risk associated with gastric polyps. In terms of malignant potential, gastric polyps can be divided into two broad categories—hyperplastic polyps and adenomatous polyps.

Hyperplastic polyps are common, occurring in 0.5% to 1% of the general population and accounting for 70% to 80% of all gastric polyps. The hyperplastic polyp contains an overgrowth of histologically normal-appearing gastric epithelium. Atypia is rare. Hyperplastic gastric polyps are considered to have no neoplastic potential.

Most people with hyperplastic polyps are asymptomatic. Dyspepsia and vague epigastric discomfort are the most common complaints, although coexistent gastroduodenal disease is also frequently identified. Complications are unusual, and gastrointestinal hemorrhage occurs in less than 20% of patients. When hyperplastic polyps are discovered, endoscopic removal for histologic examination is indicated and is sufficient treatment.

Adenomatous polyps, in contrast, have a distinct risk for the development of malignancy.[3] Mucosal atypia is frequent, and mitotic figures are more common than in hyperplastic polyps. Dysplasia and carcinoma *in situ* have developed in adenomatous polyps observed over time. The risk for the development of carcinoma has been estimated at 10% to 20% and is greatest for polyps more than 2 cm in diameter. Multiple adenomatous polyps increase the risk of cancer. The presence of an adenomatous polyp is also a marker indicating an increased risk for the development of cancer in the remainder of the gastric mucosa.

Symptoms are similar to those for hyperplastic polyps. Endoscopic removal is indicated for pedunculated lesions and is sufficient if the polyp is completely removed and shows no evidence of invasive cancer on histologic examination. Operative excision is recommended for sessile lesions larger than 2 cm, for polyps with biopsy-proved invasive carcinoma, and for polyps complicated by pain or bleeding. After removal, endoscopic surveillance of the gastric mucosa is indicated.

Gastritis

The incidence of both gastric cancer and atrophic gastritis increases with age. Chronic gastritis is frequently associated with intestinal metaplasia and mucosal dysplasia, and these histologic features are often observed in mucosa adjacent to gastric cancer. Gastritis is frequently progressive and severe in the gastric mucosa of patients with cancer.

Gastric malignancy seems to be increased in patients with chronic gastritis associated with pernicious anemia, although the risk appears to have been overstated in the past. This disease, characterized by fundic mucosal atrophy, loss of parietal and chief cells, hypochlorhydria, and hypergastrinemia, is present in 3% of people older than 60 years. For people in whom pernicious anemia has been active for more than 5 years, the risk of gastric cancer is twice that of age-matched control subjects. Evidence also indicates an increased risk of gastric carcinoid development in patients with pernicious anemia. This increased risk warrants aggressive investigation of new symptoms in patients with long-standing pernicious anemia, but it is not high enough to justify repeated endoscopic surveillance.

Intestinal metaplasia, the presence of intestinal glands within the gastric mucosa, is also commonly associated with both gastritis and gastric cancer. The evolution from metaplasia to dysplasia to carcinoma to invasive cancer has been demonstrated in other organs, but no direct evidence can be provided for this progression in gastric cancer.

Helicobacter Pylori

Helicobacter pylori has been unequivocally associated with chronic inflammatory conditions in the stomach; this association has stimulated interest in the role of chronic infection by this organism in gastric carcinogenesis. Those areas of the world with high rates of gastric adenocarcinoma also have a high prevalence of *H. pylori* infection. Childhood acquisition of *H. pylori* infection is frequent in areas of high gastric cancer incidence, and high rates of infection have been identified in patients with premalignant lesions and invasive cancer.

In the United States, seropositivity for *H. pylori* increases the risk for cancer development approximately threefold.[4] Infection with *H. pylori* is associated with an increased risk of adenocarcinoma of both major histologic types and for tumors arising in the body or antrum of the stomach. In contrast, *H. pylori* infection is not a risk factor for cancers of the gastroesophageal junction, which are frequently associated with mucosal abnormalities of Barrett's esophagus. In a separate study of Japanese-American men in Honolulu, *H. pylori*—positive subjects had an odds ratio of 6 for gastric cancer development.[5]

Infection with *H. pylori* alone cannot explain the development of gastric cancer. In North America, approximately 50% of adults older than 50 years are seropositive for *H. pylori,* yet gastric cancer develops in only a small fraction. In several Asian populations, seropositivity of *H. pylori* approaches 70% to 90%. Several investigators have postulated that long-term gastric inflammation, consequent to childhood acquisition of *H. pylori,* makes the gastric mucosa more susceptible to the effects of environmental carcinogens. Dietary cofactors have been supposed to increase cancer risk, but specific carcinogens have not yet been identified. If *H. pylori* infection predisposes to gastric cancer development, then the widespread practice of treating peptic ulcer disease with antibiotics may eventually reduce cancer incidence further.

Previous Gastric Surgery

A number of uncontrolled reports have suggested that gastric cancer is more likely to develop in people who have undergone previous partial gastrectomy. The so-called *gastric remnant cancer* is a true clinical entity, although the risk for development of this gastric neoplasm appears to have been overestimated. Several large, prospective studies with long-term follow-up indicate that the relative risk is not increased for up to 15 years after gastric resection, likely due to surgical removal of mucosa at risk for development of gastric cancer, followed by modest increases in cancer risk (three times the control value) observed only after 25 years.[6–9]

The cellular mechanisms that contribute to the development of neoplasia in the remnant stomach are unknown. Decreased luminal pH, bacterial overgrowth with increased production of *N*-nitroso carcinogens, and reflux of bile acids into the stomach have been postulated to promote cancer development, but this remain unproved. Vagotomy, often performed in conjunction with gastric surgery for benign disease, does not appear to promote cancer development. A population-based study from Sweden of 7,198 vagotomized patients followed for up to 18 years did not report increased risk.[8] Most gastric remnant cancers are diagnosed at advanced stage, and, consequently, prognosis is poor. Reported 5-year survival ranges from 7% to 33%.

Clinical Features

The symptoms produced by gastric cancer are not specific and unfortunately can closely mimic those associated with a number of nonneoplastic gastroduodenal diseases, especially benign gastric ulcer (Fig. 48.2). In early gastric cancers, epigastric pain is present in over 70% of patients.[10] The pain is often constant, nonradiating, and unrelieved by food ingestion. In a surprising number of patients, pain can be relieved, at least temporarily, by antacids or gastric antisecretory drugs. Anorexia, nausea, and weight loss are present in less than 50% of patients with

TABLE 48.1 DIAGNOSIS

COMMON SYMPTOMS AND PHYSICAL FINDINGS IN GASTRIC CANCER

Symptoms	Physical findings
Weight loss	Guaiac-positive stool
Pain	Cachexia
Nausea and vomiting	Abdominal mass
Anorexia	Abdominal tenderness
Dysphagia	Hepatomegaly
Melena	—

early gastric cancers but become increasingly common with disease progression. Dysphagia is present in 20% of patients with proximal gastric lesions. Overt gastrointestinal hemorrhage is present in only 5%. Perforation is rare (1%).

In most patients with early gastric cancers, physical examination is negative. Stool is guaiac positive in one third. Abnormal physical findings usually reflect advanced disease (Table 48.1). Cachexia, abdominal mass, hepatomegaly, and supraclavicular adenopathy usually indicate metastasis.[11] There are no simple laboratory tests specific for gastric neoplasms.

Diagnosis and Screening

Fiberoptic endoscopy is the most definitive diagnostic method when gastric neoplasm is suspected. In the initial stages, gastric cancers can appear polypoid, as flat, plaquelike lesions, or as shallow ulcers. Advanced lesions are typically ulcerated. The ulcer border can have an irregular, beaded appearance because of infiltrating cancer cells, and the base is frequently necrotic and shaggy. The ulcer can appear to arise from an underlying mass. Although each of these features suggests a malignant ulcer, differentiation of benign from malignant gastric ulcers can be made definitively only with gastric biopsy. Accuracy of diagnosis can exceed 95% if multiple biopsy specimens are obtained. False-negative results occur in approximately 10% of patients, usually as the result of sampling error; false-positive results are rare. Diagnostic accuracy can be further enhanced by the addition of direct brush cytology.

The ability to diagnose gastric adenocarcinoma endoscopically has prompted screening programs for populations at high risk. Mass screening has been performed in Japan since the 1960s with the use of fiberoptic endoscopy. The overall

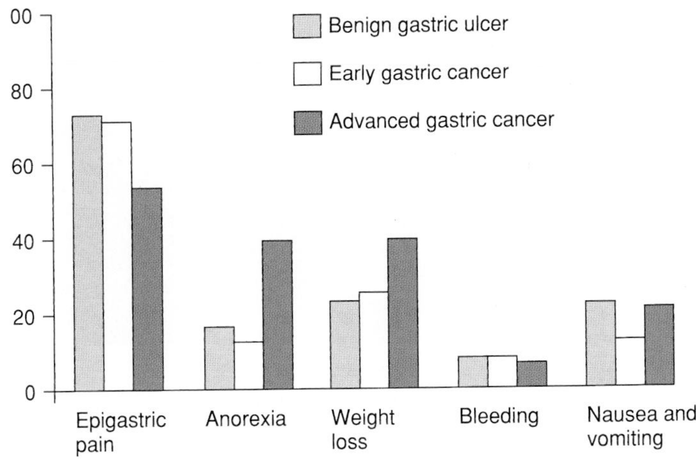

FIGURE 48.2 Clinical symptom frequency in benign gastric ulcer, early gastric cancer, and advanced gastric cancer. (After Meyer WC, Damiano RJ, Postlethwait RW, et al. Adenocarcinoma of the stomach: changing patterns over the past four decades. *Ann Surg* 1987;205:18.)

yield for the Japanese screening program has been 0.12%.[12] The proportion of early cancers, defined as tumors whose growth is confined to the mucosa and submucosa regardless of the presence or absence of metastatic disease in the perigastric lymph nodes, steadily increased during the study period. Currently, greater than 60% of gastric malignancies detected by this program are early cancers. Early detection translates directly into improved survival (Fig. 48.3). The Japanese findings that early detection can improve survival have been confirmed by European investigations, in which patients with early gastric cancers had survival rates equivalent to those of patients with benign gastric ulcer[10] (Fig. 48.4). Mass screening for gastric adenocarcinoma has not been advocated in the United States or Canada. With incidence rates approximately one fifth of those observed in Japan, detection rates are too low to justify such a program economically.

Barium contrast radiographs have, in the past, been the standard method for diagnosing gastric neoplasm. Single-contrast examinations have a diagnostic accuracy of 80%. This diagnostic yield increases to approximately 90% when double-contrast (air and barium) techniques are used. Typical findings include ulceration, the presence of a gastric mass, loss of mucosal detail, and distortion of the gastric silhouette (Fig. 48.5). Contrast radiography has been largely supplanted by endoscopy because of the ability to obtain biopsy material by the latter technique.

Computed tomography (CT) has been used both as a primary diagnostic method and to assess extragastric spread.

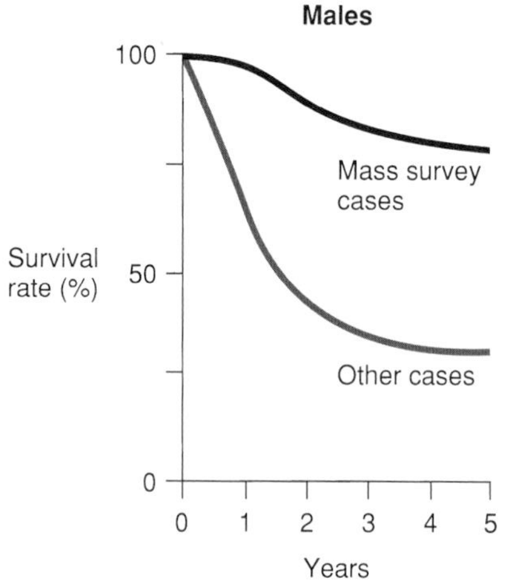

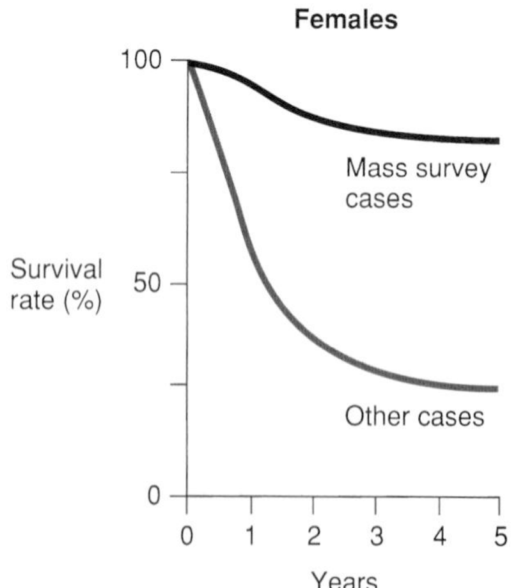

FIGURE 48.3 Early cancer survival rate in Japan.

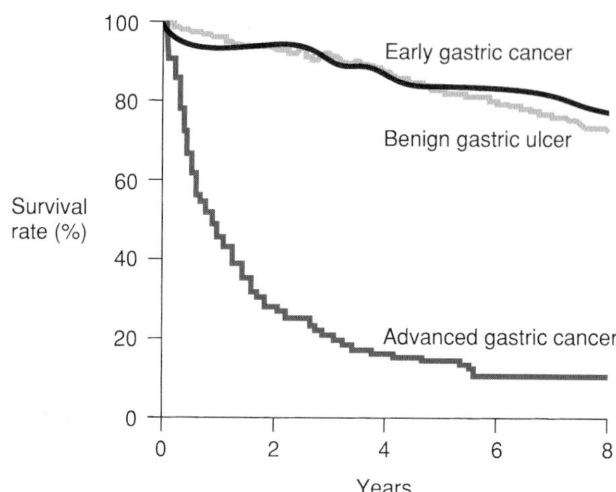

FIGURE 48.4 Early cancer survival rate in Europe.

When performed with intraluminal contrast, CT can reliably demonstrate infiltration of the gastric wall by tumor, gastric ulceration, and hepatic metastasis (Figs. 48.6 and 48.7). The technique is less reliable with regard to invasion of adjacent organs or the presence of lymphatic metastases. In most series, involvement of adjacent organs has been overestimated by CT scanning (false-positive). Conversely, metastases to regional or distant lymph nodes have been underestimated (false-negative). One review estimated a 40% to 50% accuracy rate for CT scanning in preoperative local staging of gastric carcinoma.[13] Because of these limitations, CT does not usually eliminate the necessity for laparoscopy or laparotomy.

Endoscopically directed ultrasound is another method of preoperative evaluation. Endoscopic ultrasound is excellent at

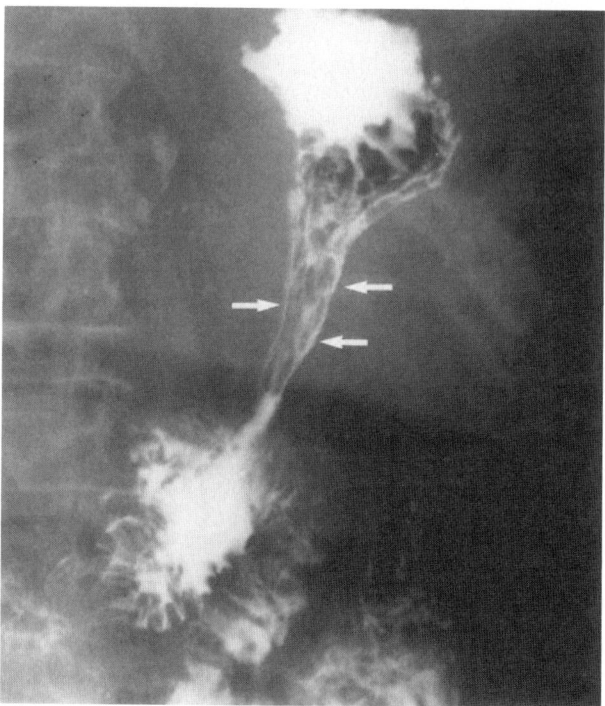

FIGURE 48.5 Barium contrast radiograph demonstrating extensive involvement of the gastric body by infiltrating adenocarcinoma (linitis plastica). The gastric silhouette is narrowed (*arrows*), and the stomach is nondistensible.

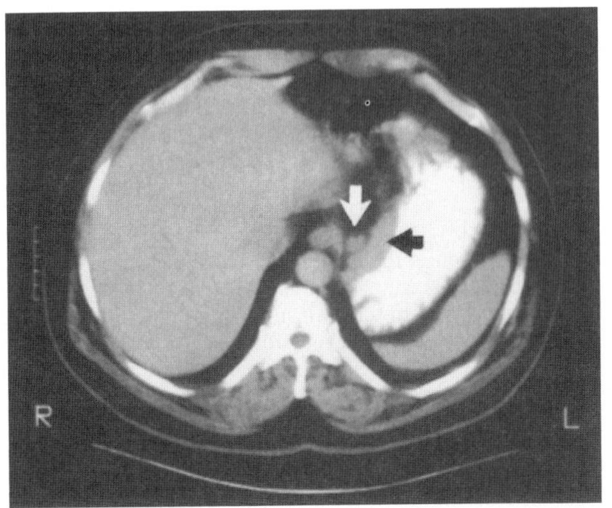

FIGURE 48.6 Computed tomography scan demonstrating mass along lesser curvature of the stomach (*black arrow*) and associated lymph node enlargement (*white arrow*).

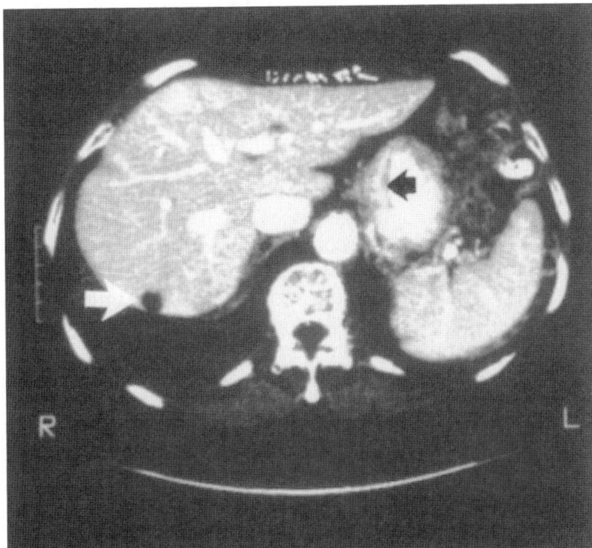

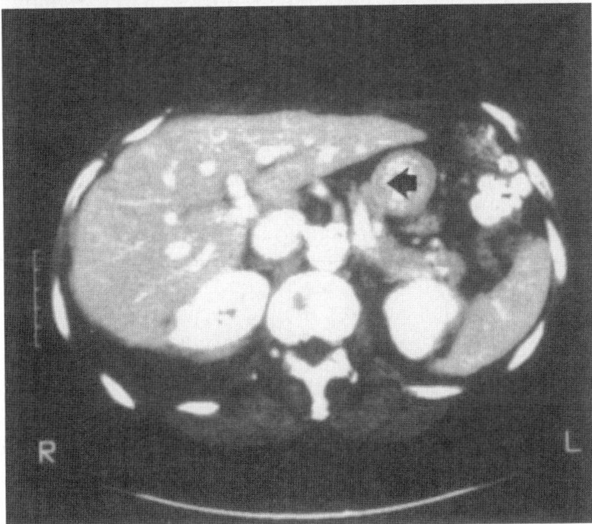

FIGURE 48.7 Computed tomography scans of the upper abdomen showing extensive thickening of the gastric wall (*black arrows*) caused by infiltrating adenocarcinoma and associated hepatic metastasis (*white arrow*).

delineating subepithelial lesions that may be confused with gastric cancer. Ultrasound-guided biopsy of subepithelial tumors is possible. Investigation of infiltrative gastric disorders, enlarged gastric epithelial folds, and differentiation of gastric lymphoma from gastric adenocarcinoma are each aided by endoscopic ultrasound. The technique has the ability to assess the depth and pattern of gastric wall penetration by gastric cancer and has good correlation with intraoperative assessment and histologic findings. Perigastric lymph nodes involved with tumor are reliably identified by endoscopic ultrasound. Because of a limited depth of tissue penetration, however, endoscopic ultrasound is unable to detect hepatic metastases; this inability is a major limitation in preoperative staging of patients with gastric cancer. Because of the inability to detect liver metastases, this method serves as an adjunct to cross-sectional methods of radiologic imaging.

Pathology

Gastric adenocarcinoma occurs in two distinct histologic subtypes—intestinal and diffuse. These subtypes are characterized by differing pathologic and clinical features and by differing patterns of metastatic spread.

In the intestinal form of gastric cancer, the malignant cells tend to form glands. The intestinal form of malignancy is more frequently associated with gastric mucosal atrophy, chronic gastritis, intestinal metaplasia, and dysplasia. Gastric cancer with the intestinal histologic subtype is more common in populations at high risk (e.g., Japan), and it occurs with increased frequency in men and older patients. Clinical studies suggest that this subtype more frequently demonstrates bloodborne metastases.

The diffuse form of gastric adenocarcinoma does not demonstrate gland formation and tends to infiltrate tissues as a sheet of loosely adherent cells. Lymphatic invasion is common. Intraperitoneal metastases are frequent. The diffuse form of gastric adenocarcinoma tends to occur in younger patients, in women, and in populations with a relatively low incidence of gastric cancer (e.g., the United States). The prognosis is less favorable for patients with the diffuse histologic subtype.

Efforts have been made to grade tumors on histologic criteria. Progressively anaplastic carcinomas are assigned higher grades. Not surprisingly, histologic grade correlates closely with 5-year survival; only 11% of grade IV patients survive 5 years, whereas 66% of grade I patients are alive 5 years after operation.

Gastric adenocarcinomas demonstrate a number of chromosomal and genetic abnormalities. Cytometric analysis reveals that gastric tumors with a large fraction of aneuploid cells (with a greater-than-normal amount of nuclear DNA) tend to be more highly infiltrative and have a poorer prognosis. Amplifications of both the HER-2/*neu* and K-*ras* protooncogenes have been consistently detected in gastric adenocarcinomas. The mechanisms by which these genetic abnormalities contribute to gastric oncogenesis remain unclear. A number of growth factors, including epidermal growth factor, platelet-derived growth factor, and transforming growth factor-β, are overexpressed in gastric carcinoma cells.[14]

In the United States, gastric adenocarcinomas occur with equal frequency in the proximal and distal regions of the stomach. In 2000, approximately one third of cases involved the proximal stomach, which is defined as the esophagogastric junction, fundus, or body, and an equal proportion arose in the antrum. In 10% of cases, the stomach is diffusely involved at the time of diagnosis.[11] Proximal involvement is more common in elderly patients. The proportion of tumors involving the proximal stomach has dramatically increased over the past decades; in the 1960s, only 16% involved this region.

TABLE 48.2 CLASSIFICATION AND STAGING

TNM CLASSIFICATION FOR STAGING OF GASTRIC ULCER

TNM definitions	
PRIMARY TUMOR	
T1	Tumor confined to the mucosa
T2	Tumor involves the mucosa and submucosa and extends to but does not penetrate serosa
T3	Tumor penetrates serosa with or without invasion of adjacent structures
T4	Diffuse involvement on gastric wall without obvious boundaries (linitis plastica)
REGIONAL LYMPH NODE INVOLVEMENT	
N0	No nodal metatasis
N1	Metastasis to perigastric lymph nodes in immediate vicinity of tumor
M2	Metastasis to lymph nodes distant from primary tumor or along both curvatures of the stomach
DISTANT METASTASIS	
M0	No distant metastasis
M1	Metastasis beyond regional lymph nodes
Stage grouping	
Stage I	T1, N0, M0
Stage II	T2–3, N0, M0
Stage III	T1–3, N1–3, M0
Stage IV	Tumor unresectable or metastatic

Prognosis is distinctly less favorable for tumors arising from the proximal stomach or for those with diffuse involvement of the organ relative to antral tumors.[15] The need to resect other organs in the upper abdomen, in addition to gastric resection, is also an unfavorable prognostic factor.[16]

The gastric cancer staging format used by the American Joint Committee on Cancer is presented in Table 48.2. The staging system is oriented toward surgical and pathologic examinations but also accurately reflects prognosis (Fig. 48.8).

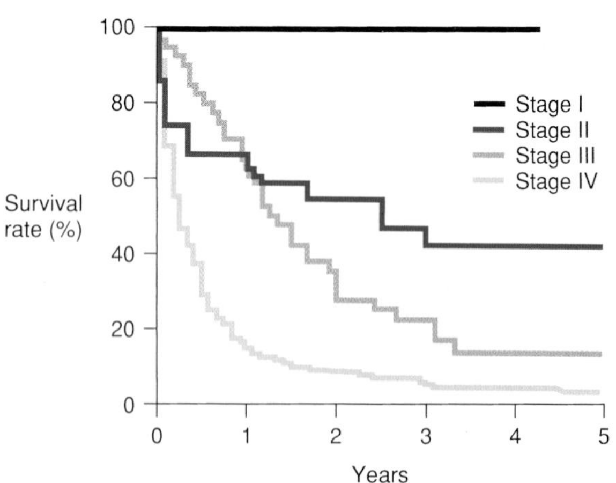

FIGURE 48.8 Survival rates of gastric cancer by stage.

A consideration of staging data illustrates the high frequency with which lymph node metastases are present at the time of diagnosis in the United States and the severe impact lymphatic involvement has on survival. Even early gastric cancers have a 15% prevalence of nodal metastasis.

Curative Treatment

Surgical resection is the only hope for cure in gastric cancer, but an advanced stage of disease at the time of diagnosis precludes curative resection for most patients. The surgical objectives in gastric cancer must, therefore, be two: (a) to maximize chances for cure in patients with localized tumor and (b) to provide effective and safe palliation to patients with advanced malignancy. Evolution of the surgical approach to gastric adenocarcinoma has focused on the following six issues: the ability of preoperative tests to detect metastatic disease, the extent of gastric resection needed for potentially curable lesions, the role of perigastric lymphadenectomy, the adequacy of proximal and distal resection margins, the role of splenectomy, and the implications of involvement of adjacent organs.

Laparoscopy

The ability of CT scanning to detect metastatic disease is limited, especially when tumor deposits are small. The surface of the liver, the omentum, and the peritoneal surfaces are common sites for gastric cancer metastasis that are difficult to evaluate preoperatively by CT scanning. In prospective studies, diagnostic laparoscopy has been superior to preoperative CT or percutaneous ultrasound in detection of peritoneal, hepatic, or lymphatic metastasis. Diagnostic laparoscopy can be combined with laparoscopic ultrasound to further increase diagnostic yield. Preoperative endoscopic ultrasound and operatively performed laparoscopic ultrasound are complementary techniques. When combined, 100% sensitivity in detecting inoperable cancers has been reported.[17]

Accurate staging and detection of incurable lesions is crucial because the mean life expectancy of affected patients is only 3 to 9 months. In 25% to 30% of patients, laparoscopy will detect distant disease that precludes curative resection.[18] Relative to laparotomy, the shorter hospitalization and reduced operative trauma following laparoscopy are obvious benefits to individuals with shortened life expectancy. Most patients with systemic metastasis can be treated without palliative surgical resection. In one study, no patients deemed incurable by laparoscopy required subsequent operation.[19]

Laparotomy

Epidemiological studies demonstrate in the United States that gastric cancer has decreased in incidence over the last two decades. Paralleling this decrease in incidence, the frequency of gastric resection for cancer has also declined.[20] Using nationwide hospital discharge data, the number of patients with a diagnosis of gastric cancer decreased from 25 cases per 100,000 U.S. adults in 1988 to 20 cases per 100,000 in 2000. (Fig. 48.9) The decreased rate of hospitalization reflected decremental rates of gastric resection, with a 29% decrease from 5.6 cases per 100,000 adults in 1988 to 4.0 cases per 100,000 in 2000. (see Fig. 48.9) The overall proportion of hospitalized gastric cancer patients undergoing gastric resection remained constant at 22%.

Gastric resection for cancer has a relatively high rate of postoperative complications and significant operative mortality. From 1988 to 2000, in-hospital mortality did not significantly change, with an overall mortality rate of 7.4% for the nationwide group. Complication rates were not uniform, however, and varied in relation to hospital experience with

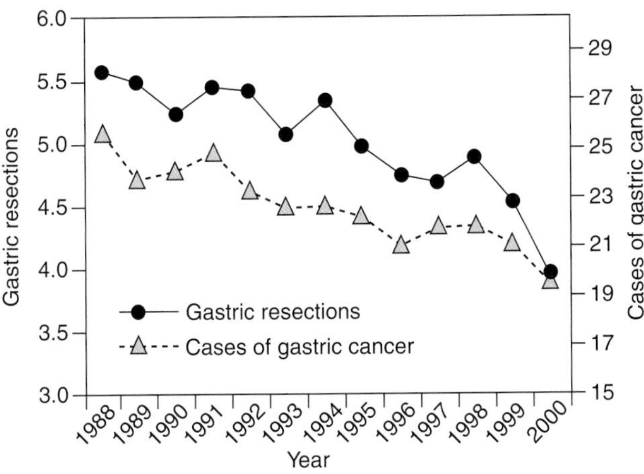

FIGURE 48.9 Incidence of gastric cancer and gastric cancer resection in the United States, per 100,000 adults, over the time period 1988 through 2000.

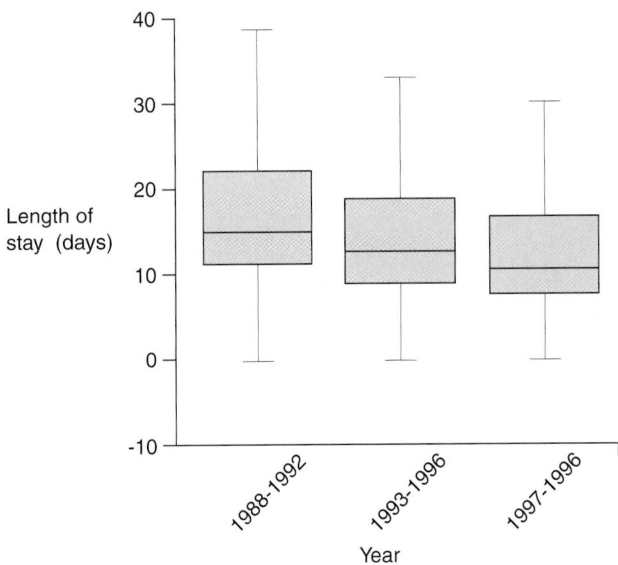

FIGURE 48.11 Length of stay after gastric resection by time period from 1988 through 2000.

gastric surgery. Low-volume centers had an 8.3% mortality rate, medium-volume hospitals had a 7.1% death rate, and high-volume centers had a 6.5% mortality rate (Fig. 48.10). The safety of gastric resection improved progressively from 1988 to 2000 at high-volume medical centers. A decline in mortality was not observed at low- or medium-volume hospitals. Despite significant overall complication rates, patients are spending less time in the hospital after gastric resection (Fig. 48.11). Shorter hospital stays likely reflect improved efficiency with better use of hospital resources but may also derive from societal efforts to curtail health-care costs.

Since the mid-1990s, the surgical treatment of gastric cancer has continued to evolve, with minimally invasive approaches for early cancers and increasingly radical operations for advanced tumors. Japanese surgeons have reported the largest experience with early gastric cancer. The Japanese Gastric Cancer Association defines early gastric cancer as tumor in which invasion is restricted to the mucosa or submucosa.[21] The presence or absence of lymph node metastasis is not considered in this classification. While the presence of lymphatic metastasis cannot be correctly judged by endoscopic findings, it is critically important in prognosis. For tumors confined to the mucosa, lymphatic metastasis is present in 1% to 3% of cases; with submucosal involvement, the rate of nodal positivity increases to 14% to 20%.[22,23]

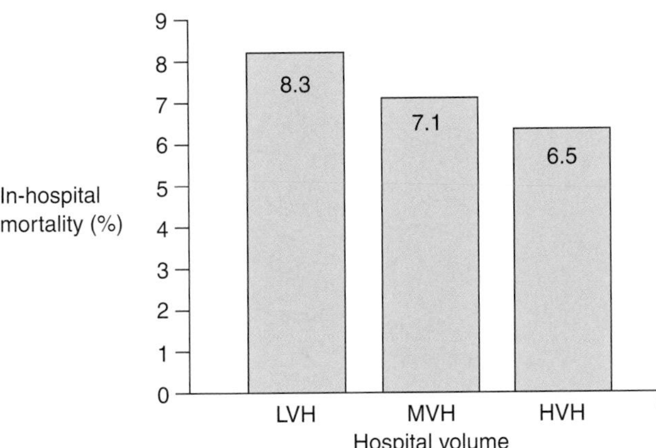

FIGURE 48.10 In-hospital mortality as a function of varying hospital volume. Low-volume hospitals are defined as performing four or fewer resections per year. Medium-volume hospitals are defined as performing five to eight resections per year. High-volume hospitals are defined as performing nine or more resections per year.

For well-differentiated mucosal tumors of less than 3 cm without ulceration, endoscopic mucosal resection has been performed. With this approach, postoperative bleeding or perforation has been reported in 5%, and in 17% histologic examination revealed submucosal invasion that required further operative treatment.[24] Reports that suggest underestimation of tumor invasion in 45% and missed lymphatic metastasis in 9% urge caution before widespread acceptance of this technique.[25]

Laparoscopic gastrectomy has also been reported for treatment of gastric malignancy, with advantages of reduced pain, shorter hospitalization, and improved quality of life.[26] Long-term cancer control rates, the most important criteria, have not yet been reported by controlled clinical trial, however.

Since the early 1980s, radical operations have been performed for the treatment of gastric cancer, including total gastrectomy, extended subtotal gastrectomy with *en bloc* resection of celiac and splenic lymph nodes, splenectomy, and distal pancreatectomy. With time, it has become apparent that radical operations increase operative morbidity but do not improve survival. For early lesions (N0–1, M0) of the antrum or middle stomach, distal subtotal gastrectomy including 80% of the stomach provides satisfactory 5-year survival rates without increasing operative morbidity. Proximal gastric lesions or larger middle stomach lesions may require total gastrectomy or esophagogastrectomy to encompass the tumor (Figs. 48.12 and 48.13). Regardless of the extent of gastric resection, patients with more advanced tumors fare poorly because of the increased likelihood of lymphatic and hematogenous spread (Algorithm 48.1).

The extent of gastric resection is determined, in part, by the need to obtain a resection margin free of microscopic disease. Microscopic involvement of the resection margin by tumor cells is associated with poor prognosis.[11] Patients with positive surgical margins are at high risk for development of recurrent disease, and histologically positive margins are strongly correlated with the development of anastomotic recurrence. In contrast to colon cancer, gastric cancer frequently demonstrates extensive intramural spread. The propensity for intramural

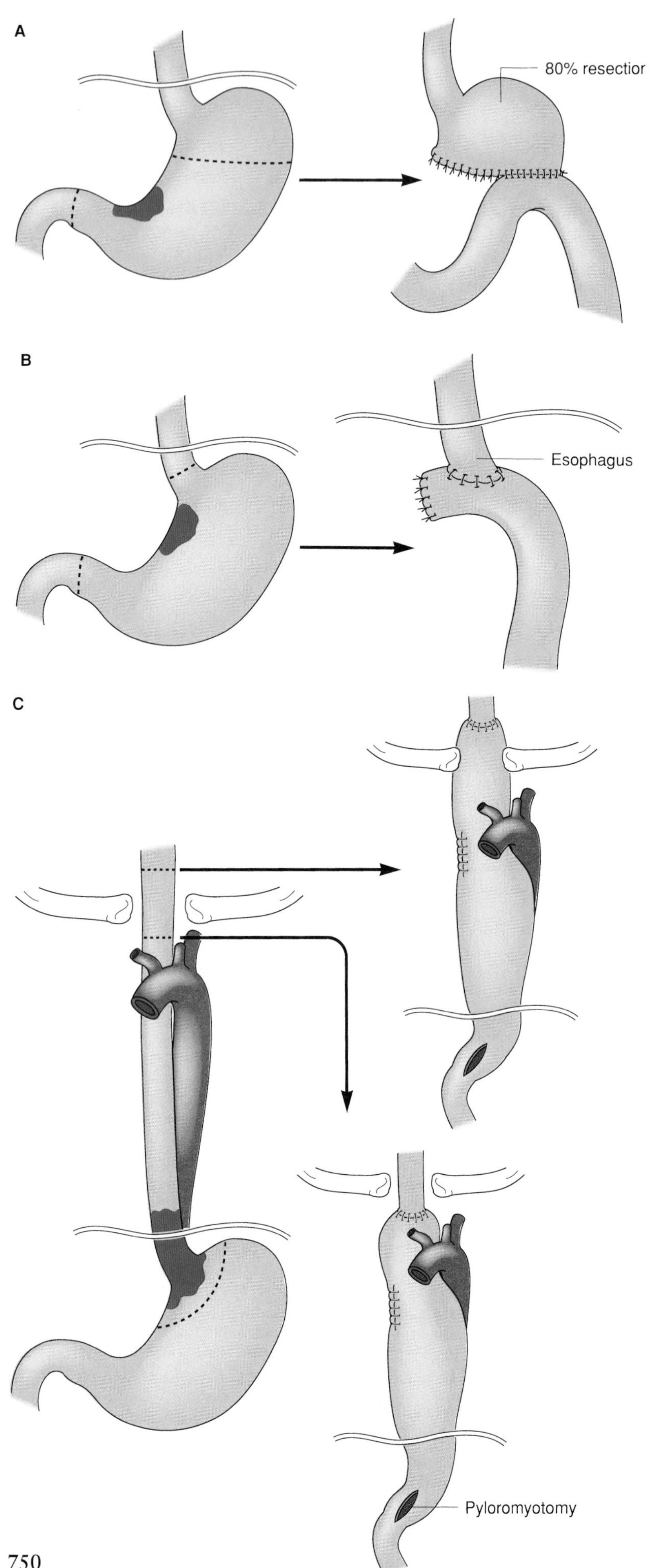

FIGURE 48.12 Surgical options for resection of gastric neoplasms. (*A*) Subtotal gastrectomy with gastrojejunal reconstruction. (*B*) Total gastrectomy with esophagojejunostomy. (*C*) Esophagogastrectomy with anastomosis in cervical or thoracic position.

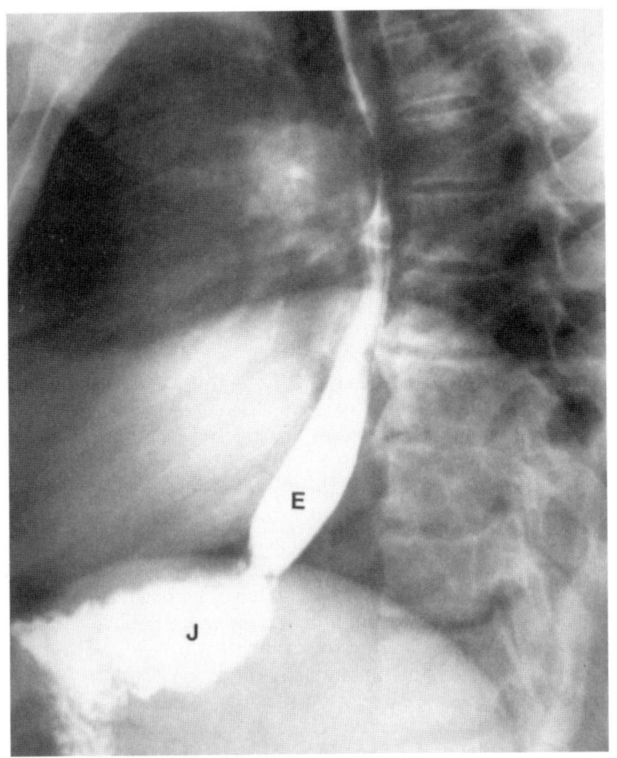

FIGURE 48.13 Postoperative radiograph after total gastrectomy with esophagojejunal anastomosis, showing esophagus (E) and jejunum (J).

metastasis is related, in part, to the extensive anastomosing capillary and lymphatic network in the wall of the stomach. Retrospective studies suggest that a line of resection 6 cm from the tumor mass is necessary to ensure a low rate of anastomotic recurrence. Efforts to achieve even larger margins have not translated into improved survival.

Radical gastric operations can be performed with acceptable morbidity and low mortality rates in the older age groups at greatest risk for gastric cancer. Mortality rates for total gastrectomy range from 3% to 7%.[27] Nutritional support in the immediate postoperative period is an important adjunctive measure as patients resume oral intake.[28] Surgical reconstructions that interpose a small intestinal reservoir between the esophagus and the jejunum have been advocated after total gastrectomy, but provide no clear-cut nutritional benefit.[29–32]

Because gastric cancer metastasizes so frequently to lymph nodes, radical extirpation of draining lymph nodes has been practiced as a therapeutic maneuver.[33] The value of extended lymphadenectomy in the treatment of gastric adenocarcinoma is controversial. The first favorable experience was reported by Japanese surgeons and the Japanese Research Society for Gastric Cancer.[34,35] Resections in the original Japanese system are shown in Table 48.3. Only retrospective studies of extended perigastric lymphadenectomy have been reported from Japan. Initial reports suggested an improvement of approximately 10%, stage for stage, for patients with advanced disease treated with R2 or R3 operations.[34–37] The benefits of extended lymphadenectomy have not been confirmed in non-Japanese centers, and several randomized trials have failed to show a survival benefit for extended lymphadenectomy when the entire patient population was analyzed.[38–42]

The safety of extended lymphadenectomy is disputed. Data from a national Japanese registry indicate a contemporary mortality of less than 1%.[43] Low mortality risks have been reported from multiinstitutional trials conducted in Italy and Germany.[42,44] Investigations from the United States, Britain, and the Netherlands have been less optimistic, indicating increased short-term morbidity and in-hospital mortality.[40,41]

One effect of extended lymphadenectomy appears to be "up-staging" of tumors; as more lymph nodes are removed, additional micrometastatic disease is discovered, and patients

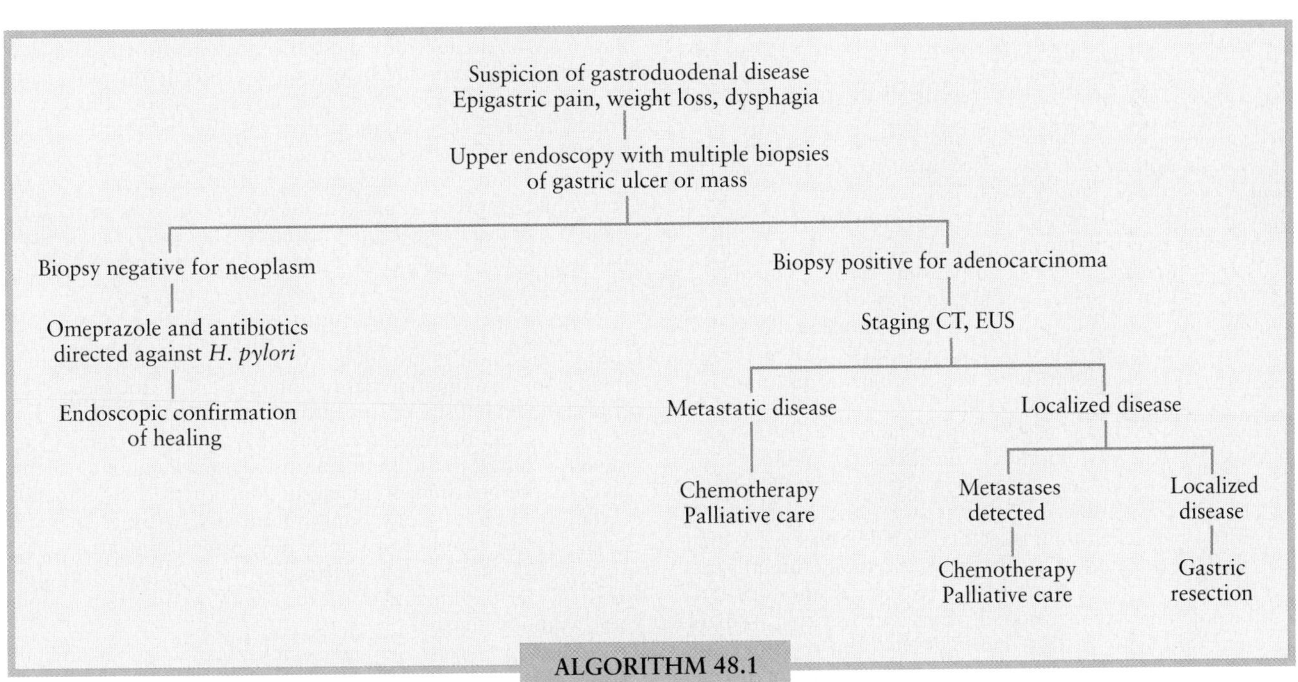

ALGORITHM 48.1 Treatment of gastric adenocarcinoma.

TABLE 48.3 MANAGEMENT

LYMPHADENECTOMY RESECTIONS IN THE ORIGINAL SYSTEM OF THE JAPANESE RESEARCH SOCIETY FOR GASTRIC CANCER

Level	Description
R1	Resection of stomach, omentum, and perigastric lymph nodes
R2	Resection of stomach, omentum, and *en bloc* removal of the superior leaf of the transverse mesocolon, the pancreatic capsule and lymph nodes along the branches of the celiac artery and in the infraduodenal and supraduodenal areas
R3	Resection of the above structures plus lymph nodes along the aorta and esophagus, along with the spleen and the tail of the pancreas, and skeletonization of vessels in the porta hepatis

are correctly placed in higher-stage categories with worse prognoses.[45,46] Reciprocally, some patients who do not undergo extended lymphadenectomy will have undetected micrometastases and, because of progressive disease, will decrease the survivorship of the staging group to which they are assigned.

Histologically positive lymph nodes are frequently present in the splenic hilum and along the splenic artery, and routine splenectomy has been practiced in some centers. Splenectomy has not been demonstrated to improve outcome for similarly staged patients.[47,48] Likewise, resection of the tail or body of the pancreas has not been demonstrated to improve survival. Resection of adjacent organs may be required for local control if direct invasion has occurred. In this circumstance, operative morbidity is increased and the long-term survival rate is approximately 25%.[49]

Palliative Treatment

When preoperative evaluation demonstrates disseminated disease, palliation of symptoms becomes a primary consideration. Palliation does not usually require surgery. Obstruction and bleeding can be managed nonoperatively by the use of endoscopic laser fulguration in selected patients. Dysphagia caused by proximal lesions and bleeding can be controlled in 80% of patients. Successful application of laser treatment requires adequate visualization, and it is hampered by circumferential tumor growth that impedes passage of the endoscope, by sharp angulation of the esophagogastric junction, and by lesions more than 6 cm long.

In the setting of metastatic gastric cancer, palliative resection does not improve survival. Nonetheless, resection appears to provide superior relief of symptoms, particularly dysphagia, compared with surgical bypass. Bypass of obstructing distal gastric cancers without resection provides relief to less than half of patients, and mean survival is less than 6 months. For proximal obstructing lesions, total gastrectomy with Roux-en-Y esophagojejunal reconstruction may be necessary. An operative mortality rate of less than 5% has been reported, and introduction of stapling devices has reduced the rate of anastomotic leaks to less than 5% in several series. Mean survival after palliative gastric resection approximates 9 months. For nonresectable gastric adenocarcinoma, when dysphagia is present, radiation therapy may have a significant palliative role.

Chemotherapy

Chemotherapy has limited efficacy in the treatment of patients with disseminated gastric adenocarcinoma. The drugs most commonly used in single-agent chemotherapy trials have been 5-fluorouracil (5-FU), mitomycin C, and doxorubicin. Few single-agent trials have partial response rates above 25% to 30%, and complete responses have not occurred.[19] Because long-term survival can be expected only in patients who experience complete response, there has been no impact on patient survival from single-drug approaches.

A number of trials have used a combination of 5-FU, doxorubicin, and/or a nitrosourea as adjuvant therapy for the treatment of resected gastric cancer, with an overall partial response rate of approximately 33%, and an absolute reduction in death rate of 4% to 18%. Increases in mean survival have been reported in several prospective trials that utilized multiagent chemotherapy as postoperative adjuvants.

The addition of radiation therapy to chemotherapy has modest benefit. In these circumstances, chemotherapeutic agents may act as radiosensitizers by reducing the threshold for radiation damage, inhibiting DNA repair, or increasing radiation-induced apoptosis. Chemoradiation protocols have demonstrated improvements in local control of tumor in the resectional field. Overall and disease-free survival are improved by 10% to 15% with use of postoperative chemoradiation relative to surgery alone.

GASTRIC LYMPHOMA

Clinical Features

The stomach is the site of more than half of gastrointestinal lymphomas and is the most common organ involved in extranodal lymphomas. Non-Hodgkin's lymphomas account for approximately 5% of malignant gastric tumors; lymphoma represents an increasing proportion of gastric neoplasms diagnosed currently. Patients are considered to have primary gastric lymphoma if initial symptoms are gastric and the stomach is exclusively or predominantly involved with the tumor. Patients who do not fulfill these criteria are considered to have secondary gastric involvement from systemic lymphoma.

Gastric lymphoma is distinctly uncommon in children and young adults. The peak incidence is in the sixth and seventh decades. Symptoms are indistinguishable from those of gastric adenocarcinoma. Epigastric pain, weight loss, anorexia, nausea, and vomiting are common.[50] Although gross bleeding is uncommon, occult hemorrhage and anemia are observed in more than half of patients. Patients rarely have spontaneous perforation.

Diagnosis

Radiologic findings are similar to those for adenocarcinoma. Endoscopic examination has become the diagnostic method of choice. The endoscopic appearance of lesions may be ulcerated, polypoid, or infiltrative. Gastric lymphoma is most commonly localized to the middle or distal stomach and unusually involves the proximal stomach, in contrast to gastric adenocarcinoma. Endoscopic biopsy, combined with endoscopic brush cytology and ultrasonography, provides positive diagnosis in 90% of cases. Submucosal growth without ulceration of the overlying mucosa can occasionally render endoscopic biopsy nondiagnostic.

Endoscopic ultrasound-guided biopsy is useful in this circumstance. When gastric lymphoma is first diagnosed by endoscopic means, evidence of systemic disease should be sought. CT of the chest and abdomen (to detect lymphadenopathy), bone marrow biopsy, and biopsy of enlarged peripheral lymph nodes are all appropriate.

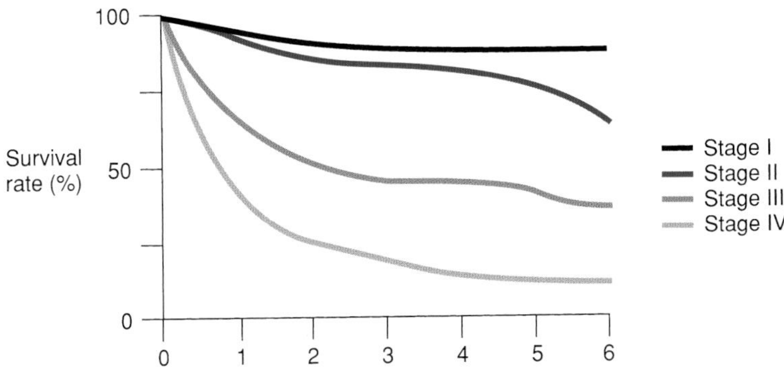

FIGURE 48.14 Survival rates of gastric lymphoma by stage.

Mucosa-associated Lymphoma Tissue

The concept that low-grade gastric lymphomas have features resembling mucosa-associated lymphoid tissue (MALT) is a major advance in the understanding of gastric lymphomas. The gastric submucosa does not ordinarily contain lymphoid tissue, and the development of lymphoid tissue resembling small intestinal Peyer's patches is believed to occur in response to infection with *H. pylori*.[51] A number of observations support a causal relationship between chronic *H. pylori* infection and lymphoma development. *H. pylori* is present in the stomachs of more than half of patients with gastric lymphoma.[52] As with gastric adenocarcinoma, geographic regions with a high prevalence of *H. pylori* also have a high incidence of gastric lymphoma. Infection with *H. pylori* has been noted to precede development of gastric lymphoma.[53]

After development of gastric lymphoid tissue, low-grade lymphoma is postulated to occur as a result of monoclonal B-cell proliferation. Initially, B-cell proliferation depends on interleukin-2 production by antigenically stimulated nonneoplastic T cells. Progressive genetic rearrangements lead to B-cell proliferation that is independent of *H. pylori*—stimulated interleukin-2. With cumulative genetic defects, low-grade MALT lymphoma progresses to high-grade MALT lymphoma.

Low-grade MALT lymphomas resemble Peyer's patches. Lymphoma cells invade between follicles and into gastric epithelium; invasion of gastric glands forms characteristic lymphoepithelial lesions. Low-grade lesions are often multifocal. Low-grade MALT lesions are less likely than high-grade tumors to invade transmurally, involve perigastric lymph nodes, or invade adjacent organs.[53] High-grade MALT lymphomas cannot be distinguished histologically from non-MALT, high-grade B-cell lymphomas.

The concept that low-grade lymphoma depends on continued *H. pylori* antigenic stimulation supports eradication of *H. pylori* with antibiotics as first-line antineoplastic therapy. Complete regression of low-grade MALT lymphomas with antibiotic treatment has been reported in 70% to 100% of cases.[54,55] The median time to complete response averaged 5 months.[56] Most patients with partial responses were subsequently determined also to have foci of high-grade lymphoma. Radiation and chemotherapy have been proposed as salvage for antibiotic treatment failures.

Non-MALT Lymphomas

In the past, a multimodality treatment program was used in most centers for primary gastric lymphomas, with gastrectomy as the first step in the therapeutic strategy.[57] This approach evolved empirically, and prospective data to support it were lacking. Several advantages of this approach had been cited: (a) more accurate histologic evaluation was possible; (b) in cases with localized tumor, the procedure could be curative; and (c) gastrectomy eliminated the risk of life-threatening hemorrhage or perforation, which attended the treatment of tumors involving the full thickness of the gastric wall.[58] The role of resection in the treatment of gastric lymphoma has diminished, with the role of surgery evolving from cure to staging to palliation. Currently, most patients are treated with chemoradiation therapy alone.

The risk of hemorrhage or perforation was frequently alluded to in the past as a motive for operative care, but the risk was overstated. The incidence of perforation in primary gastric lymphomas that are treated with cytolytic agents in unresected patients approximates 5%. The use of endoscopic ultrasonography to detect full-thickness involvement of the gastric wall may be used to identify patients at risk for perforation.

In more than 30% of patients with stage II disease who undergo apparently adequate surgery and radiation therapy, the cancer recurs outside the treatment field. Patients with stage II primary gastric lymphoma should, therefore, be considered to have systemic disease and to require systemic therapy in addition to surgery or radiation therapy. Survival for gastric lymphoma is closely linked to stage at diagnosis (Fig. 48.14). A recent prospective, randomized study has demonstrated that complication-free survival is highest in patients treated with chemotherapy alone consisting of cyclophosphamide, vincristine, doxorubicin and prednisone.[59] (Fig. 48.15).

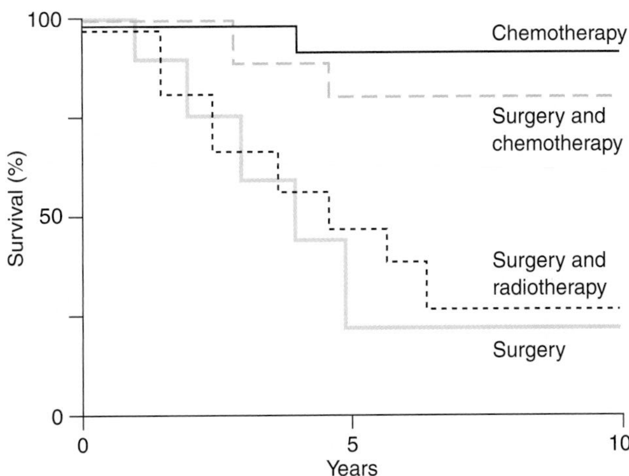

FIGURE 48.15 Actuarial curves of complication-free survival, according to stage.

GASTRIC CARCINOIDS

Gastric carcinoid tumors have been considered to be rare tumors, accounting for 3% to 5% of all gastrointestinal carcinoids and only 0.3% of gastric neoplasms. The number of gastric carcinoids may have been underestimated in the past because of confusion with gastric carcinoma. In addition to an increased risk of adenocarcinoma, patients with pernicious anemia have an increased risk for development of gastric carcinoids. This association has suggested to several investigators that gastric carcinoids can develop as a result of chronic trophic stimulation by hypergastrinemia associated with pernicious anemia.[60] Carcinoid tumors associated with pernicious anemia are localized to the gastric body or fundus. Histologically, the tumors appear as nests of monotonous hyperchromatic cells originating in the submucosa or in the basal area of gastric glands. Invasion, uncommon in small tumors, occurs with increasing frequency in tumors larger than 2 cm.

Most patients with small gastric carcinoids are asymptomatic. When viewed endoscopically at an early stage, carcinoids are reddish-pink to yellow submucosal nodules in the proximal stomach. Tumors are frequently multiple. Larger tumors can cause ulceration of the overlying mucosa; symptoms are similar to those of gastric ulcer or gastric adenocarcinoma. Endoscopic biopsy is usually diagnostic if deep enough to sample submucosal tumor cells. Because of the potential for invasion, attempts at curative resection are indicated in almost all cases.

GASTROINTESTINAL STROMAL TUMORS OF THE STOMACH

Gastrointestinal stromal tumors (GIST) can arise from any of the mesenchymal components of the gastric wall, constituting approximately 3% of gastric malignancies. GIST occur with equal frequency in both sexes in the sixth and seventh decades of life. The tumor frequently has prominent extraluminal growth and attains a large size before causing symptoms (Fig. 48.16). Endoluminal growth or ulceration of the overlying mucosa due to ischemic necrosis can be associated with epigastric pain, weight loss, and gastrointestinal hemorrhage. Clinical symptoms are identical to those produced by adenocarcinoma. With large tumors, an epigastric mass can be detected by physical examination.

Benign smooth muscle tumors are often asymptomatic until they reach a large size. Symptoms related to mass effects with compression of adjacent structures are most frequent. Gastrointestinal hemorrhage can occur as a result of necrosis of overlying gastric mucosa. Endoscopic examination is usually negative if the major component of growth is extraluminal; umbilication of the mucosa can indicate an underlying mass. The presence and nature of symptoms should direct the need for surgical excision.

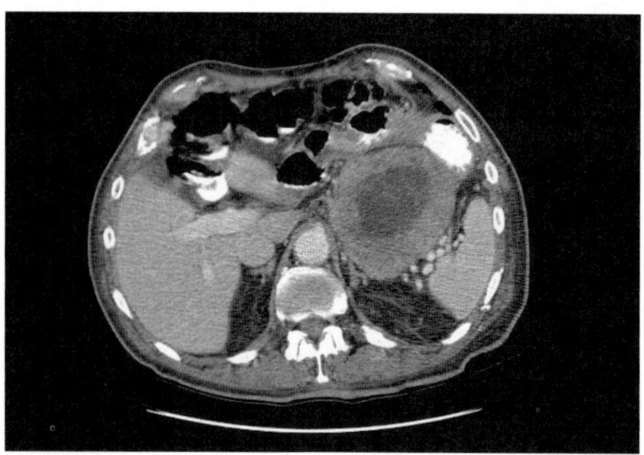

FIGURE 48.16 CT scan of GIST of stomach arising from lesser curvature. The arrow indicates central tumor necrosis. The lesion caused mucosal erosion with gastrointestinal hemorrhage.

Grossly, the tumors are firm, gray-white masses; a pseudocapsule separating tumor from normal smooth muscle can occasionally be present. When the tumors reach a large size, central necrosis is common. GIST are often graded histologically, with the frequency of mitotic figures the prime indicator of aggressive behavior. Lesions with more than 5 to 10 mitoses per 10 high-power fields demonstrate increased metastasis. With benign GIST, mitoses are absent or rare.

Intraperitoneal sarcomatosis is frequent, as is local recurrence after resection. Metastasis occurs by the hematogenous route; thus, hepatic involvement is common. Lymphatic metastasis is observed in less than 10% of patients.

GIST are not radiosensitive, and traditional chemotherapy has not been shown to improve survival. Surgical resection has been the treatment of choice. *En bloc* resection of the tumor and involved structures should be attempted. Negative surgical margins must be ensured histologically, but extensive lymphadenectomy is not indicated because of the low frequency of lymphatic metastasis.

Most gastric stromal tumors express the c-kit receptor. c-kit is the receptor for the kit ligand, also known as cytokine stem cell factor. c-kit is a tyrosine kinase that acts as a growth factor or developmental antigen receptor; occupation of the receptor acts to stimulate cellular proliferation. Imatinib mesylate (Gleevac) is a small molecule inhibitor of the c-kit receptor. The majority of malignant gastric stromal tumors are responsive to imatinib mesylate; the agent holds great promise as the first of a new generation of tumor-specific cytotoxic agents.

KEY POINTS

- **The risk for development of gastric cancer is greater in stomachs that harbor polyps.**
- **Those areas of the world with high rates of gastric adenocarcinoma also have a high prevalence of *H. pylori* infection.**
- **The symptoms produced by gastric cancer are not specific and can mimic those associated with a number of nonneoplastic gastroduodenal diseases, especially benign gastric ulcer.**
- **The extent of gastric resection is determined by the need to obtain a resection margin free of microscopic disease.**
- **The stomach is the site of more than half of gastrointestinal lymphomas and is the most common organ involved in extranodal lymphomas.**
- **Most gastric stromal tumors express the c-kit receptor.**

References

1. Silverberg E, Boring CC, Squires TS. Cancer statistics, 1990. *CA Cancer J Clin.* 1990;40:9–26.
2. Boring CC, Squires TS, Tong T. Cancer statistics, 1993. *CA Cancer J Clin.* 1993;43:19.
3. Harju E. Gastric polyposis and malignancy. *Br J Surg.* 1986;73:532–533.
4. **Parsonnet J, Friedman GD, Vandersteen DP, et al. Helicobacter pylori infection and the risk of gastric carcinoma. *N Engl J Med.* 1991;325:1127–1131.**
5. Nomura A, Stemmermann GN, Chyou P-H, et al. *Helicobacter pylori* infection and gastric carcinoma among Japanese Americans in Hawaii. *N Engl J Med.* 1991;325:1132–1136.
6. Hansson L. Risk of stomach cancer in patients with peptic ulcer disease. *World J Surg.* 2000;24:315–320.
7. Tersmette AC, Giardiello FM, Tytgat GNJ, et al. Carcinogenesis after remote peptic ulcer surgery: the long-term prognosis of partial gastrectomy. *Gastroenterology* 1991;101:148–153.

8. Lundegårdh G, Ekbom A, McLaughlin JK, Nyrén O. Gastric cancer risk after vagotomy. *Gut* 1994;35:946.
9. Holstein C. Long-term prognosis after partial gastrectomy for gastroduodenal ulcer. *World J Surg* 2000;24:307–314.
10. Moreaux J, Bougaran J. Early gastric cancer: a 25-year surgical experience. *Ann Surg* 1993;217:347–355.
11. **Wanebo HJ, Kennedy BJ, Chmiel J, et al. Cancer of the stomach: a patient-care study by the American College of Surgeons. *Ann Surg* 1993;218:583–592.**
12. Endo M, Habu H. Clinical studies of early gastric cancer. *Hepatogastroenterology* 1990;37:408–410.
13. Rosch T, Classen M. Staging gastric cancer: the Munich experience. In: Van Dam J, Sivak MV, eds. *Gastrointestinal endosonography.* New York: WB Saunders, 1999:195–199.
14. Katano M, Nakumura M, Fujimoto K, et al. Prognostic value of platelet-derived growth factor-A (PDGF-A) in gastric carcinoma. *Ann Surg.* 1998;227:365–371.
15. Harrison LE, Karpeh MS, Brennan MF. Proximal gastric cancers resected via a transabdominal-only approach. *Ann Surg.* 1997;225:678–685.
16. Kodama I, Takamiya H, Mizutani K, et al. Gastrectomy with combined resection of other organs for carcinoma of the stomach with invasion to adjacent organs: clinical efficacy in a retrospective study. *J Am Coll Surg.* 1997;184:16–22.
17. Mortensen MB, Scheel-Hincke JD, Madsen MR, et al. Combined endoscopy ultrasonography and laparoscopic ultrasonography in the pretherapeutic assessment of resectability in patients with upper gastrointestinal malignancies. *Scand J Gastroenterol.* 1996;31:1115–1119.
18. **Lowy AM, Mansfield PF, Leach SD, Ajahi J. Laparoscopic staging for gastric cancer. *Surgery* 1996;119:611–614.**
19. Dúgo DM, Coppola R, Persiani R, et al. Immediately preoperative laparoscopic staging for gastric cancer. *Surg Endosc.* 1996;10:996–999.
20. **Wainess RM, Dimick JB, Upchurch GR, et al. Epidemiology of surgically treated gastric cancer in the United States, 1988–2000. *J Gastrointest Surg.* 2003;7:879–883.**
21. Adachi Y, Shiraishi N, Kitano S. Modern treatment of early gastric cancer: Review of the Japanese experience. Dig Surg. 2002;19:333–339.
22. Nakamura K, Morisaki T, Sugitani A, et al. An early gastric carcinoma treatment strategy based on analysis of lymph node metastasis. *Cancer* 1999;85:1500–1505.
23. Kunisaki C, Shimada H, Takahaski M, et al. Prognostic factors in early gastric cancer. *Hepatogastroenterology* 2001;48:294–298.
24. Ono H, Kondo H, Gotoda T, et al. Endoscopic mucosal resection of treatment of early gastric cancer. *Gut* 2001;48:225–229.
25. Korenaga D, Orita H, Mackawa S, et al. Pathological appearance of the stomach after endoscopic mucosal resection for early gastric cancer. *Br J Surg.* 1997;84:1563–1566.
26. Cuschieri A. Laparoscopic gastric resection. *Surg Clin North Am* 2000;80: 1269–1284.
27. Schwarz R, Karpeh MS, Brennan MF. Factors predicting hospitalization after operative treatment for gastric carcinoma in patients older than 70 years. *J Am Coll Surg.* 1997;184:9–15.
28. Daly JM, Weintraub FN, Shou J, et al. Enteral nutrition during multimodality therapy in upper gastrointestinal cancer patients. *Ann Surg.* 1995;221:327–338.
29. de Almeida ACM, dos Santos NM, Aldeia FJ. Long-term clinical and endoscopic assessment after total gastrectomy for cancer. *Surg Endosc.* 1993;7: 518–523.
30. Chareton B, Landen S, Manganus D, et al. Prospective randomized trial comparing Billroth I and Billroth II procedures for carcinoma of the gastric antrum. *J Am Coll Surg.* 1993;183:190–194.
31. Nakane Y, Okumura S, Akehira K, et al. Jejunal pouch reconstruction after total gastrectomy for cancer: a randomized controlled trial. *Ann Surg.* 1995;222:27–35.
32. Bozzetti F, Bonfanti G, Castellani R, et al. Comparing reconstruction with Roux-en-Y to a pouch following total gastrectomy. *J Am Coll Surg.* 1996;183:243–248.
33. Shiu MH, Moore E, Sanders M, et al. Influence of the extent of resection on survival after curative treatment of gastric cancer: a retrospective multivariate analysis. *Arch Surg.* 1987;122:1347–1351.
34. Maruyama K, Okabayashi K, Kinoshita T. Progress in gastric cancer in Japan and its limit of radicality. *World J Surg.* 1987;11:418–425.
35. **Noguchi Y, Imada T, Matsumoto A, et al. Radical surgery for gastric cancer: a review of the Japanese experience. *Cancer* 1989;64:2053–2062.**
36. Adachi Y, Kamakura T, Mori M, et al. Role of lymph node dissection and splenectomy in node-positive gastric carcinoma. *Surgery* 1994;116:837–841.
37. Baba H, Maehara Y, Takeuchi H, et al. Effect of lymph node dissection on the prognosis in patients with node-negative early gastric cancer. *Surgery* 1994;117:165–169.
38. Maeta M, Yamashiro H, Saito S, et al. A prospective plot study of extended (D3) and superextended para-aortic lymphadenectomy (D4) in patients with T3 or T4 gastric cancer managed by total gastrectomy. *Surgery* 1999;125:325–331.
39. Robertson CS, Chung SCS, Woods SDS, et al. A prospective randomized trial comparing R1 subtotal gastrectomy with R3 total gastrectomy for antral cancer. *Ann Surg.* 1994;220;176–182.
40. **Bonekamp JJ, Hermans J, van de Velde CJH. Extended lymph-node dissection for gastric cancer. *N Engl J Med.* 1999;340:908–914.**
41. Cushieri A, Fayers P, Fielding J, et al. Postoperative morbidity and mortality after D1 and D2 resections for gastric cancer. *Lancet* 1996;347:995–999.
42. Siewert JR, Bottcher K, Stein HJ, et al. Relevant prognostic factors in gastric cancer: ten-year results of the German gastric cancer study. *Ann Surg.* 1998;228:449–461.
43. Lee JS, Douglass, HO. D2 dissection for gastric cancer. *Surg Oncol.* 1997;6:215–225.
44. Pacelli F, Doglietto GB, Bellantone R, et al. Extensive versus limited lymph node dissection for gastric cancer: a comparative study of 320 patients. *Br J Surg.* 1993;80:1153–1156.
45. Kodera Y, Yamamura Y, Shimizu Y, et al. The number of metastatic lymph nodes: a promising prognostic determinant for gastric carcinoma in the latest edition of the TNM classification. *J Am Coll Surg.* 1998;187:579–603.
46. Clinical significance of occult micrometastasis in lymph nodes from patients with early gastric cancer who died of recurrence. *Surgery* 1996;119:397–402.
47. Stipa S, DiGiorgio A, Ferri M, et al. Results of curative gastrectomy for carcinoma. *J Am Coll Surg.* 1994;179:567–572.
48. Otsuji E, Yamaguchi T, Sawai K, et al. End results of simultaneous splenectomy in patients undergoing total gastrectomy for gastric cancer. *Surgery* 1996;120:40–44.
49. Shchepotin IB, Chorny VA, Nauta RJ, et al. Extended surgical resection in T4 gastric cancer. *Am J Surg.* 1998;175:123–126.
50. Isaacson PG. Gastrointestinal lymphoma. *Hum Pathol.* 1994;25:1020–1029.
51. **Isaacson PG. Gastric lymphoma and Helicobacter pylori. *N Engl J Med.* 1994;330:1310–1311.**
52. Parsonnet J, Hansen S, Rodriguez L, et al. *Helicobacter pylori* infection and gastric lymphoma. *N Engl J Med.* 1994;330:1267–1271.
53. Montalban C, Castrillo JM, Abriapa V, et al. Gastric B-cell mucosa-associated lymphoid tissue (MALT): clinicopathological study and evaluation of the prognostic factors in patients. *Ann Oncol.* 1995;6:798–799.
54. Bayerdorffer E, Neubauer A, Rudolph B, et al. Regression of primary gastric lymphoma of mucosa-associated lymphoid tissue type after cure of *Helicobacter pylori* infection. *Lancet* 1995;345:1591–1594.
55. Neubauer A, Thiede C, Morgner A, et al. Cure of *Helicobacter pylori* infection and duration of remission of low grade gastric mucosa associated lymphoid tissue lymphoma. *J Natl Cancer Inst.* 1997;89:1350–1355.
56. Pinotti G, Zucca E, Roggero E, et al. Clinical features, treatment and outcome in a series of 93 patients with low grade gastric MALT lymphoma. *Leuk Lymphoma* 1997;26:527–537.
57. Stephens J, Smith J. Treatment of primary gastric lymphoma and gastric mucosa-associated lymphoid tissue lymphoma. *Am Coll Surg.* 1998;178: 312–320.
58. Bartlett DL, Karpeh MS, Filippa DA, et al. Long-term follow-up after curative surgery for early gastric lymphoma. *Ann Surg.* 1996;223:53–62.
59. **Aviles A, Nambo MJ, Neri N, et al. The role of surgery in primary gastric lymphoma: results of a controlled clinical trial. *Ann Surg.* 2004; 240:44–50.**
60. Creutzfeldt W. The achlorhydria—carcinoid sequence: role of gastrin. *Digestion* 1988;39:61–79.

SECTION F

SMALL INTESTINE

CHAPTER 49 ■ ANATOMY AND PHYSIOLOGY OF THE SMALL INTESTINE

DIANE M. SIMEONE

The small intestine is the longest organ of the gastrointestinal tract, extending from the duodenal bulb to the ileocecal valve. The functions of the small intestine are diverse. Two key functions of the small intestine are absorption of nutrients from the intestinal lumen and maintaining a balance between the absorption and secretion of water and electrolytes. By virtue of its vast surface area exposed to the outside environment, the small intestine is an important immunologic defense barrier. In addition, the small intestine serves as the largest and most complex endocrine organ in the body.

GROSS ANATOMY

Duodenum

The duodenum is the first and widest portion of the small intestine, measuring approximately 25 cm from the pylorus to the ligament of Treitz, the site where the jejunum begins. The duodenum is divided into four parts: the bulb, followed by the second (descending), third (transverse), and fourth (ascending) portions. The duodenal bulb, or cap, is invested with mesentery and slopes in a slightly cephalad direction from the pylorus. The mucosal surface of the bulb is smooth. The bulb is 5 cm long and is the site of most duodenal ulcers. Posterior to the bulb are the head of the pancreas, portal vein, common bile duct, and the gastroduodenal artery.

The second (descending) portion of the duodenum courses posteriorly and caudally from the duodenal cap along the right side of the bodies of the L1 and L2 vertebra. The second portion of the duodenum becomes a retroperitoneal structure as it courses posteriorly. The head of the pancreas is in direct contact with the medial portion of the descending duodenum. The descending duodenum directly overlies Gerota's fascia and, more medially, the right renal vein and inferior vena cava. Incision of the peritoneum lateral to the second portion of the duodenum allows elevation of the duodenum and pancreatic head. This mobilization, referred to as the *Kocher maneuver*, allows palpation of the anteroposterior aspect of the head of the pancreas. The descending portion of the duodenum is approximately 10 cm long. The transition from the duodenal bulb to the descending duodenum is marked by the appearance of concentric mucosal folds known as *Kerckring folds* (plicae circulares), which are 1 to 3 mm high and spaced 2 to 4 mm apart with smooth mucosa intervening between the folds. The common bile duct, lying either within the substance of the pancreas or in a retropancreatic position, descends along the posteromedial surface of the duodenum; it is joined by the pancreatic duct before the two traverse the duodenal wall and open into its lumen as the major ampulla of Vater (duct of Wirsung). The ampulla of Vater is typically 7 to 10 cm from the pylorus and appears as a small, nipple-like structure marked by a longitudinal duodenal fold. The minor papilla (duct of Santorini) can be seen endoscopically in approximately half of cases, appearing as a 1- to 3-mm polypoid structure.

The third and fourth portions of the duodenum complete the duodenal sweep. The third part of the duodenum is almost completely retroperitoneal. It is intimately attached to the uncinate process of the pancreas and extends from the second part of the duodenum to the third lumbar vertebra directly over the aorta. The third portion of the duodenum is directly posterior to the hepatic flexure of the colon, and care must be taken to avoid injury to this part of the duodenum during mobilization of the hepatic flexure for colon resection. The third portion of the duodenum passes between the superior mesenteric artery anteriorly and the aorta, which lies posteriorly. This point marks the transition from the third to the fourth part of the duodenum. The fourth portion of the duodenum ascends superiorly and obliquely to the left of the aorta along the lower border of the pancreas, reaching as high as the L2 vertebra. It reaches the ligament of Treitz, which extends downward from the right crus of the diaphragm in front of the aorta and behind the pancreas to attach to the outer wall of

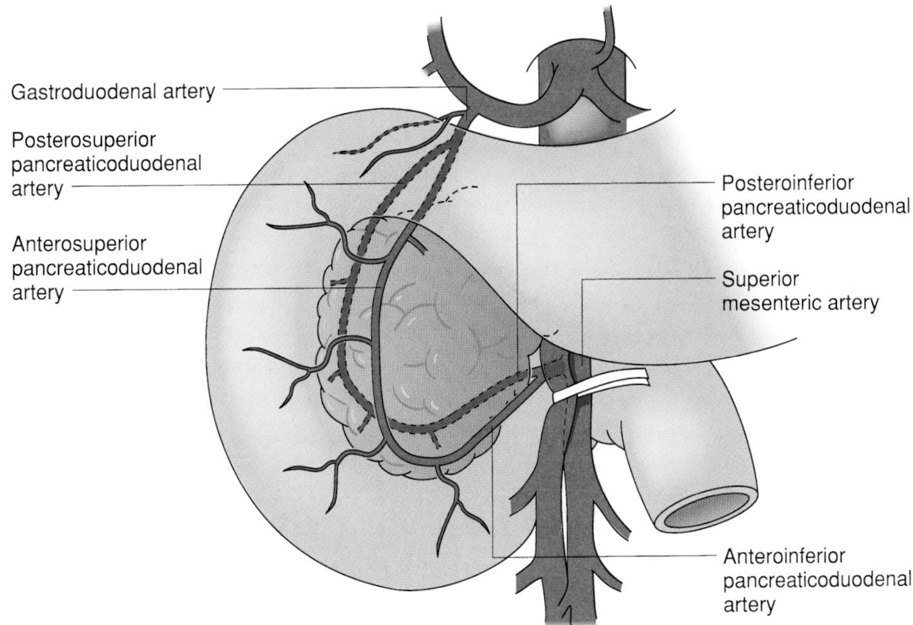

FIGURE 49.1 Arterial supply to the duodenum.

the duodenojejunal flexure. The duodenum is separated from the jejunum by the ligament of Treitz.

Jejunum and Ileum

There is no clear anatomic boundary between the jejunum and ileum, and the proximal two fifths of the small intestine distal to the ligament of Treitz has been arbitrarily defined as *jejunum* and the distal three fifths as *ileum*. Their combined length varies from 5 to 10 meters, with an average length of 7 meters. Both the jejunum and ileum are invested in mesentery. The jejunum is slightly wider than the ileum and has a thicker wall because of its thick mucosal lining. The mucosa of the jejunum is characterized by prominent plicae circulares that become shorter and less frequent in the ileum. The diameter of the ileum progressively decreases as it approaches the ileocecal valve. The ileocecal valve exhibits motor characteristics separate from the terminal ileum and colon, postulated to prevent reflux of fecal material from the colon into the small intestine. The difference in bacterial flora between the terminal ileum and the cecum demonstrates the ability of this region to prevent reflux. In humans, distention of the terminal ileum causes relaxation of the ileocecal valve and distention of the colon causes increased tone, suggesting that the valve may possess sphincteric function.[1]

The mesentery suspends the jejunum and ileum from the posterior abdominal wall. The base, or root, of the mesentery attached to the posterior abdominal wall is approximately 15 cm long and extends from the ligament of Treitz to left of the L2 vertebra down toward the right sacroiliac joint. The broad-based mesentery tethers the small intestine, preventing kinking of its blood supply.

Arterial Blood Supply

The blood supply to the duodenal bulb comes directly from the hepatic artery as well as the gastroduodenal artery as it branches from the hepatic artery. The second and third portions of the duodenum share a common blood supply with the head of the pancreas. The anterosuperior and posterosuperior pancreaticoduodenal arteries arise from the gastroduodenal artery, and the anteroinferior and posteroinferior pancreaticoduodenal arteries branch from the superior mesenteric artery. The first jejunal branch of the superior mesenteric artery supplies the jejunum just beyond the ligament of Treitz and sends small branches back to the fourth portion of the duodenum (Fig. 49.1).

The superior mesenteric artery also supplies the jejunum and ileum through a series of branches that form arcades in the mesentery. The intestinal arteries (vasa recta) arise from the most peripheral arcades and run directly to the intestine without anastomosing. The vasa recta bifurcate as they reach the intestinal wall. The vascular pattern in the mesentery can help distinguish the jejunum from the ileum: in the jejunum, the vasa recta are straight and long, whereas in the ileum, the vasa recta are shorter with greater arborization (Fig. 49.2).

Venous and Lymphatic Drainage

The venous drainage of the duodenum, in general, follows the arterial supply. There are anterior and posterior venous arcades that parallel the arterial arcades. Several small branches that drain the duodenal bulb empty into either the pancreaticoduodenal, right gastroepiploic, or portal vein. One of these venous branches, the prepyloric vein, is a landmark for the pylorus.[2] The general pattern of venous drainage of the jejunum and ileum is the same as the arterial supply. The major venous drainage route is by the superior mesenteric vein, which joins the splenic vein to empty into the portal vein.

The lymphatics of the small intestine follow the blood vessels, and lymph is filtered through several levels of lymph nodes; the first set is located adjacent to the bowel wall, the second set is adjacent to the mesenteric arcades, and the third set lies along the trunk of the superior mesenteric artery. The duodenum may also drain into lymph nodes along the celiac artery. These mesenteric lymph nodes ultimately drain into the cisterna chyli and thoracic duct. Lymphatics of the small intestine are unique because they participate in absorption of fat. Lymphatics in the small intestinal mesentery may appear milky white because of the presence of emulsified fat in the lymph.

Innervation

The small intestine contains a complex, intrinsic nervous system referred to as the *enteric nervous system* (ENS). The ENS

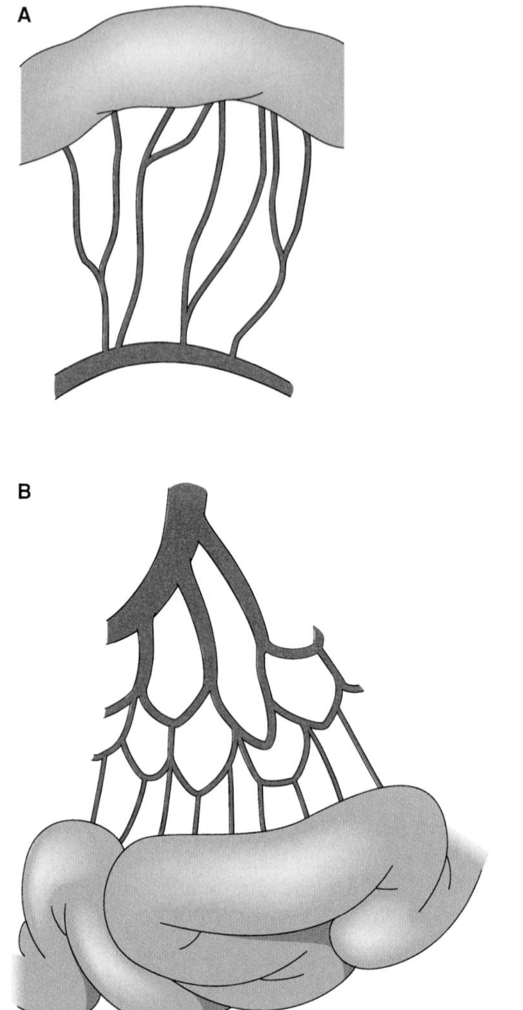

FIGURE 49.2 Contrasting vasa recta of jejunum (*A*) and ileum (*B*).

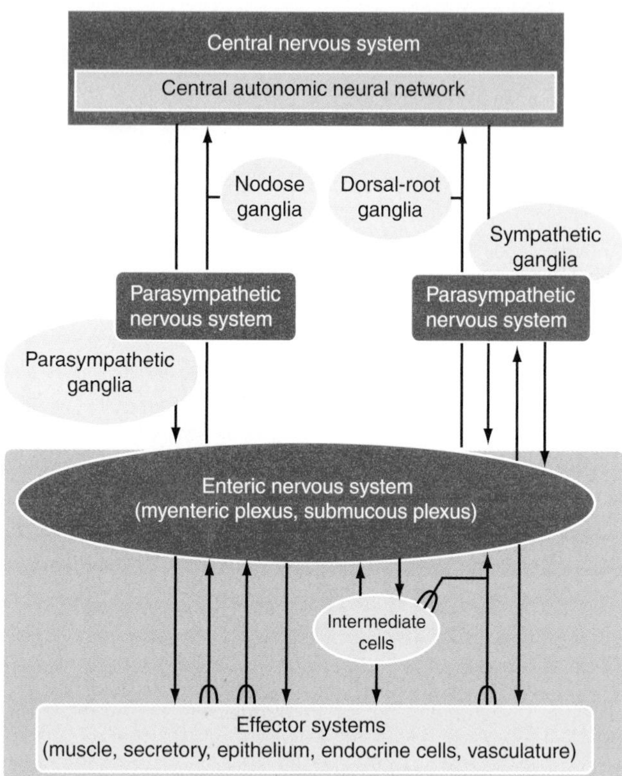

FIGURE 49.3 Innervation of the gastrointestinal tract. The neural plexuses in the gut represent an independently functioning network, the enteric nervous system, which is connected to the central autonomic neural network in the central nervous system by parasympathetic and sympathetic nerves. The enteric nervous system may influence the effector system in the gut directly, or indirectly through its actions on intermediate cells, which include endocrine cells and cells of the immune system. The cell bodies of the primary vagal and primary splanchnic afferent neurons are located in the nodose ganglia and dorsal root ganglia, respectively; each carries distinct information from the gut to the central nervous system. The *pitchfork* symbols represent afferent nerve endings, and the *arrows* show the direction of neural transmission. (Adapted with permission from Goyal RK, Hirano I. Mechanisms of disease: the enteric nervous system. *N Engl J Med.* 1996;334:1106–1115.)

is a network of approximately 10 to 100 million neurons with cell bodies in the bowel wall, containing as many neurons as the spinal cord.[3] The ENS is distinct from the autonomic nervous system and is unique in its ability to mediate reflex activity even when isolated from the central nervous system. The ENS contains two major plexuses, the myenteric (Auerbach's) plexus, located between the longitudinal and circular muscle layers, and the submucous (Meissner's) plexus. Enteric neurons have extensive connections with each other, intestinal smooth muscle cells, epithelial cells, endocrine cells, extrinsic neurons, and the vasculature (Fig. 49.3). Through these connections, the ENS provides neural control of all gastrointestinal functions, including motility, blood flow, secretion, and absorption.[4] The chemical mediators in the ENS were initially thought to be limited to neurotransmitters such as acetylcholine and serotonin; however, subsequent research has added purines to the list, such as adenosine triphosphate (ATP), and peptides, such as vasoactive intestinal peptide, somatostatin, substance P, and neurokinin A. Nitric oxide has also been identified as a neurotransmitter in the ENS. More than 20 candidate neurotransmitters have now been identified in enteric neurons.[5] The extrinsic autonomic innervation of the small intestine consists of components of the parasympathetic and sympathetic systems. Parasympathetic efferent fibers arise from the vagus and pass through the celiac and superior mesenteric ganglia; their postganglionic cell bodies are located in the enteric ganglia. Parasympathetic efferent fibers, in general, increase peristaltic activity and intestinal secretion. The function of the vagal afferent fibers is largely unknown, although they are believed to mediate feelings of nausea and distention and may be involved in visceral reflexes, such as the gastrocecal reflex, which activates discharge of ileal contents into the cecum when food enters the stomach.[2] Sympathetic efferent fibers travel in the splanchnic nerves and synapse in the superior mesenteric ganglia. They function to inhibit motility and secretory activity, although their most marked effect is to cause vasoconstriction. Pain from the intestine is mediated by sympathetic afferent fibers.

MICROSCOPIC ANATOMY

The wall of the small intestine is composed of four concentric layers: the serosa, muscularis, submucosa, and mucosa. The serosa, or outer coat, consists of a thin layer of mesothelial cells overlying loose connective tissue. The serosa covers only the anterior surface of the retroperitoneal segments of small bowel, but it completely covers the portions of small bowel that are invested with mesentery. The muscularis consists of an inner circular and an outer longitudinal muscle layer. Between the muscle layers lies the myenteric (Auerbach's) plexus. The muscular layers are responsible for coordinating peristaltic movements.

The submucosa is a dense connective tissue layer just below the mucosa that has a rich network of blood vessels, nerves, and lymphatics. The submucosa contains Meissner's plexusand is the strongest layer of the intestinal wall. Brunner's glands are found in the submucosa of the duodenum and secrete mucus and bicarbonate into the small bowel lumen. Brunner's glands are thought to be important in neutralizing acid from the stomach. Peyer's patches are localized collections of lymphoid follicles that are most prominent in the submucosa of the ileum. They may be as large as 10 mm in diameter. Peyer's patches are most abundant in early life and gradually disappear with old age.

The innermost layer of the small intestine is the mucosa, which consists of a layer of epithelial cells overlying the connective tissue core or lamina propria and resting on a narrow layer of smooth muscle, the muscularis mucosae. The basic structural unit of the mucosa is the crypt and villus. Villi are fingerlike projections of mucosa 0.5 to 1 mm high extending into the intestinal lumen that have a columnar epithelial surface and a cellular connective tissue core of lamina propria. Each villus contains a central lymphatic (lacteal), a small artery and vein, and a capillary network. Between the villi are the crypts of Lieberkühn.

Anchored stem cells in the crypts of Lieberkühn are the source of the four major types of differentiated cells: the absorptive enterocyte, goblet cells, enteroendocrine cells, and Paneth cells. Absorptive enterocytes differentiate as they migrate from the crypt compartment up toward the tip of the intestinal villus. Cells then undergo programmed apoptotic cell death and are extruded into the intestinal lumen. This process occurs over approximately 4 to 5 days in humans. Thus, most of the epithelial lining of the small intestine is continually renewed at a relatively rapid rate. Despite the rapid rate of cellular turnover, intestinal epithelial cells exhibit complex patterns of gene expression that vary according to their location on the two main spatial axes of the gut, the vertical (crypt-villus) and horizontal (proximal to distal) axes. For example, cells destined to become enterocytes do not begin to express a variety of genes important in digestion and absorption until the cells have migrated out of the crypt and up the villus. In addition, many epithelial cell genes are selectively expressed in the proximal small intestine, whereas other genes are specifically expressed only in the ileum.[6]

Columnar epithelial cells are responsible for absorption and secretion and constitute 90% of the cells on the villus. These cells are 22 to 25 μm high with basally located nuclei. The apices of these cells have microvilli, produced by numerous folds in the apical membrane, that account for the brush border appearance. The surface of the microvilli is covered by a filamental coat called the *glycocalyx*. This coat represents external extensions of proteins and glycoproteins rooted in the cell membrane that are essential for digestion and absorption.[7] The lateral membranes of neighboring enterocytes are connected by tight junctions, an apparent fusion of adjoining plasma membranes just below the level of the brush border. Movement of ions and water can occur by either a transmembrane or a paracellular route through tight junctions, which behave as selective pores.

Mucus-secreting goblet cells are present in both the crypts and villi. They are referred to as *goblet cells* because of their morphologic appearance, with a narrow base and wide apical membrane. Goblet cells have a basal nucleus and a large number of apical granules containing mucin. Mucin secreted by the goblet cell functions as a lubricant and has a cytoprotective function.

Paneth cells are pyramidal cells that reside in the crypt base. They contain large eosinophilic secretory granules located at their apical surface. Their life span is approximately 4 weeks, much longer than the life span of the enterocyte. It has been suggested that Paneth cells play a role in host defense based on their abundant expression of lysozyme and defensins, a family of small peptides that are found in human neutrophils and exhibit microbicidal activity toward many different bacterial organisms *in vitro*. However, examination of the role of Paneth cells in the small intestine by lineage ablation in transgenic mice revealed no alteration in host defense mechanisms, and therefore the exact role of Paneth cells has yet to be determined.[8]

Multiple types of enteroendocrine cells in the mucosa are characterized by their specific hormonal products. Enteroendocrine (also referred to as *amine precursor uptake and decarboxylation*, or *APUD*) cells may reside in the either the crypts or the villi, depending on the particular neuroendocrine substance they produce. Specific areas of the small intestine have higher concentrations of specific neuroendocrine substances than other areas (Fig. 49.4). Unlike exocrine cells, which secrete apically into the lumen, endocrine cells are oriented for secretion toward the basement membrane. Their secretory granules are located below the nucleus near the basement membrane.

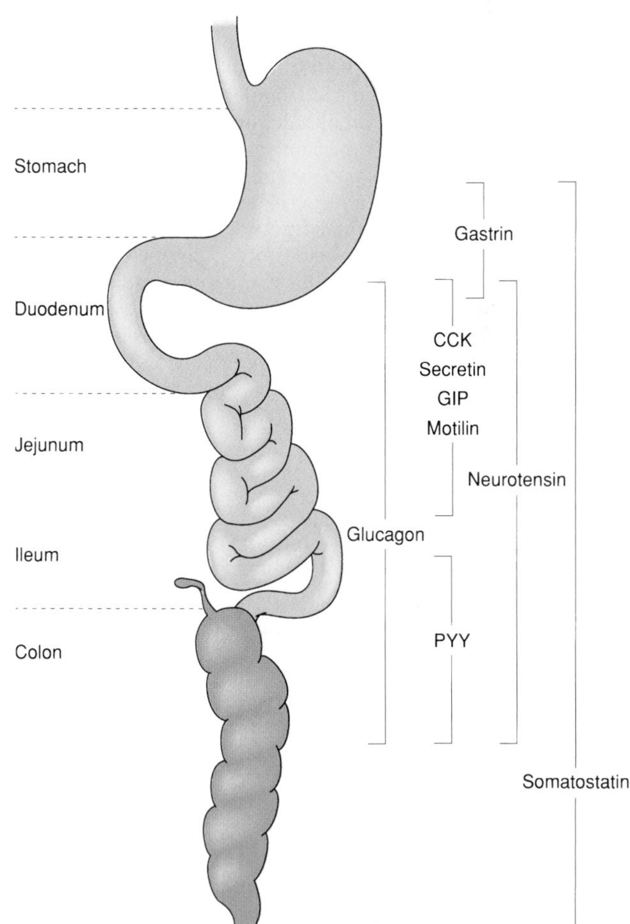

FIGURE 49.4 Distribution of peptide hormones in the gastrointestinal tract.

PHYSIOLOGY

Motility

One of the major functions of the small intestine is to process and absorb nutrients. Although neural and hormonal factors are important in modulating motility, the primary control mechanism is myogenic. The intestinal smooth muscle cell has a normal resting membrane potential of −50 to 70 mV, which is maintained by Na^+-K^+-ATPase activity.[9] In humans, rhythmic fluctuations of the membrane potential of smooth muscle cells occur, resulting in slow-wave activity, also referred to as *basic electrical rhythm* or *pacemaker potential*. The rhythmic depolarizations are thought to be generated by an oscillating electrogenic sodium pump and do not themselves cause muscle contraction. They occur 11 to 13 times per minute in the duodenum and decrease to 8 to 10 times per minute in the ileum. Specialized, low-resistance cell-to-cell connections (gap junctions or nexuses) couple electrical activity between cells, allowing the distal portion of the small intestine to be entrained by the higher frequencies of the proximal small intestine. The regional variation in velocity is advantageous for digestion. In the proximal intestine, nutrients are propelled more rapidly over a large surface area for more rapid absorption and digestion. Propulsion is slower in the ileum to permit absorption of more slowly digested substances, such as bile salts and fats. With neural or chemical stimulation, membrane depolarization exceeds a certain excitation threshold and a contraction results (Fig. 49.5). The electrical correlate of the contraction is called the *spike potential*. Spike potentials occur only during the depolarization phase of the slow-wave activity. Although both the spatial and temporal patterns of contractile activity are under myogenic control, whether a contraction occurs at all depends on local neurochemical stimulation. This relationship allows modulation of the amplitude, duration, frequency, and distance of contractions by mechanisms outside of the gut.

After a meal, two gross patterns of small intestinal contraction result: segmentation and peristalsis. Contraction of the circular muscle divides the small intestine into segments, which allows local churning and circulation of chyme to promote optimal digestion and absorption. Contents of adjacent segments mix, and the process repeats itself. Peristalsis consists of a wavelike propagation of a reflex that consists of contraction proximal and relaxation distal to a bolus of food.[10] Circular muscle also initiates peristalsis, with contractions propelling intestinal contents in an aboral direction. Food empties from the stomach and passes from proximal to distal small intestine.

In healthy humans, the mean transit time in the small intestine documented by scintigraphic studies is 221 ± 49 minutes, with a range of 131 to 322 minutes.[11] The composition of the meal affects the rate of occurrence and propagation of contractions during the postprandial period; frequency of contraction is greatest with meals containing glucose and least after meals high in fat. Therefore, transit is regulated to optimize absorption of nutrients.

During fasting, the bowel undergoes a cyclic pattern of phasic contractions called the *migrating motor complex* (MMC). The MMC originates in either the stomach or proximal small intestine, migrates aborally along the intestine to the distal ileum, and cycles every 90 to 120 minutes. The MMC is referred to as the *intestinal housekeeper*, and the presumed role of the MMC is to propel sloughed enterocytes, undigested food particles, and mucus into the colon.[12,13] The MMC is divided into four distinct phases. Phase I is an interval of contractile quiescence; phase II consists of accelerating, intermittent contractions; phase III consists of a series of high-amplitude contractions that occur at a maximum frequency for 6 to 8 minutes; and phase IV is a short transition of intermittent contractions. The overall control of the MMC seems to reside in periodic activation of the ENS. Simple transection of the small intestine disrupts the normal migration of the MMC along the length of the bowel. The central and autonomic nervous systems only modulate MMC, especially under periods of stress, because MMC cycling is not abolished with vagotomy, interruption of the splanchnic nerves, or even total extrinsic denervation.[14–16]

Available evidence indicates that induction of phase III complexes results from secretion of the peptide motilin by enteroendocrine cells in the duodenum.[17,18] Other peptides that have serum levels that cycle with MMC activity are somatostatin and pancreatic polypeptide; however, it is unclear whether either of these two peptides is a physiologic mediator of the cycle.[19,20] Other substances that may modulate intestinal MMC activity are serotonin, glucagonlike peptide 1, and opioids.

The ENS plays a vital role in the organization of contractile patterns. Most of the neurons controlling contractile activity have their cell bodies in the myenteric plexus. The submucous (Meissner's) plexus also contains ganglia but appears to have a much smaller role in regulating motility, instead playing an important part in secretory control. Several intestinal motility disorders have been attributed to deficient or defective enteric neurons, including chronic intestinal pseudoobstruction and diabetic dysmotility.

Small intestinal motility may be modulated by gastrointestinal hormones, although their exact physiologic role is not well understood. Cholecystokinin (CCK), gastrin, and motilin stimulate intestinal motility. Gut peptides that inhibit intestinal motility include peptide YY (PYY) and enteroglucagon.

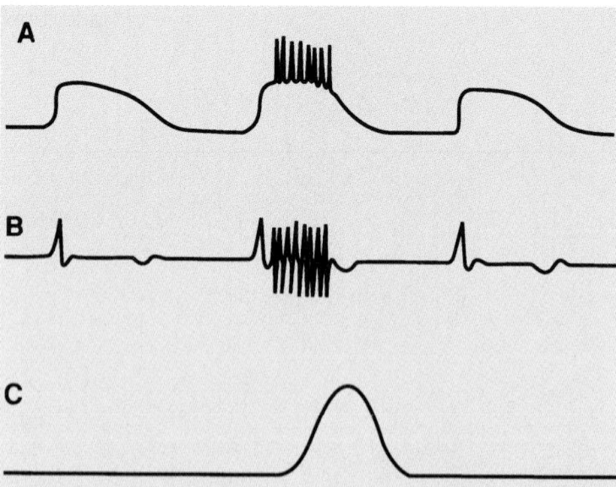

FIGURE 49.5 (*A*) Recording of transmembrane potential showing slow waves and superimposed spike potentials. (*B*) Extracellular recording of electrical activity represented in (*A*). (*C*) Muscular contraction in response to electrical activity in (*A*). (Adapted with permission from Christensen J. The control of gastrointestinal movements: some old and new views. *N Engl J Med* 1971;285:85–98.)

Digestion and Absorption

Absorption of Water and Electrolytes

The intestine has a remarkable ability to absorb and secrete large quantities of fluid. Absorption of water is a net result of fluxes into and out of the intestinal lumen. Approximately 8 to 10 L of fluid is presented to the small intestine each day, of which 1 to 2 L of water is oral intake, with an additional 5 to 10 L in the form of salivary (1 to 2 L), gastric (2 to 3 L), biliary (0.5 L), pancreatic (1 to 2 L), and intestinal secretions (1 L). Eighty percent of this fluid is absorbed in the small intestine, whereas the colon absorbs most of the remaining fluid, with a small amount (0.1 L) excreted in the stool. The balance between intestinal absorption and secretion of water is tightly regulated so that there is normally net absorption of fluid. Alterations in this fine balance, due to either impaired absorption or augmented secretion, can result in overall net secretion of water and diarrhea.

Water absorption is controlled indirectly through regulation of electrolyte transport. Fluid follows the direction of electrolyte movement to maintain isotonicity between the intestinal lumen and the tissue compartments. Water is absorbed passively by either a paracellular route (through tight junctions between enterocytes) or by a transcellular route. Water absorption in the proximal small intestine tends to be by paracellular transit because of higher tight junction permeability. The transcellular route is thought to be more important in the distal small bowel and colon, where tight junction permeability is decreased. Evidence suggests that an important method of transcellular water flux is through direct coupling to active transport of electrolytes and solutes.[21,22]

The three basic mechanisms of sodium absorption are solute-coupled Na^+ absorption, electroneutral NaCl absorption, and electrogenic Na^+ absorption independent of other solutes or ions. Cotransport of Na^+ with organic solutes and electroneutral NaCl absorption account for most or all of Na^+ absorption in the small intestine. Electrogenic Na^+ absorption through Na^+ channels occurs primarily in the colon. In each case, Na^+ absorbed across the apical membrane is extruded across the basolateral membrane by the Na^+-K^+-ATPase pump. In the presence of ATP, the Na^+-K^+-ATPase pump catalyzes the outward movement of three Na^+ ions coupled with the inward movement of two K^+ ions, maintaining a relatively low intracellular Na^+ concentration.

The absorption of many nutrients, including glucose, amino acids, dipeptides and tripeptides, and bile acids is mediated by Na^+ cotransporters in the small intestine (Fig. 49.6A). Luminal Na^+ enters the cell and then exits through the basolateral Na^+-K^+-ATPase. The energy generated by the electrochemical gradient for Na^+ drives intracellular accumulation of the organic solute. Electroneutral NaCl absorption is a process that couples two neutral ion countertransport mechanisms, one that exchanges Na^+ for H^+ and another that exchanges Cl^- for HCO_3^- (Fig. 49.6B). This exchange results in entry of NaCl into the cell in exchange for H^+ and HCO_3^- efflux. This electroneutral exchange reaction is important in intracellular pH regulation as well as Na^+ transport. Less evidence supports direct Na^+/Cl^- cotransport in mammalian small intestinal epithelial cells.[23]

Chloride ion absorption occurs primarily through electroneutral Na^+ absorption. Chloride may also be absorbed through paracellular spaces because the interstitial space is slightly electrically positive compared with the intestinal lumen. Chloride is the principal ion governing secretion. Chloride secretion occurs through apical Cl^- channels and is regulated by the intracellular second messengers cyclic adenosine monophosphate and calcium. Metabolic studies reveal that approximately 85% of ingested K^+ is absorbed in the small intestine, with passive absorption through an H^+-K^+ exchange pathway driven by preexisting electrochemical gradients.[24] The accumulated K^+ may then diffuse across the basolateral membrane by a K^+ channel or K^+ carrier.

Bicarbonate absorption involves formation of carbon dioxide in the intestinal lumen from secreted hydrogen ion and bicarbonate ion. Carbon dioxide levels in the lumen exceed those in the cell, and carbon dioxide diffuses into the cell to reform hydrogen ion and bicarbonate ion through the action of carbonic anhydrase. Bicarbonate ion diffuses into the interstitium and hydrogen ion is resecreted, partly in exchange for sodium. Bicarbonate secretion occurs in the duodenum and ileum by a Cl^--HCO_3^- exchange mechanism. Bicarbonate secretion serves to neutralize gastric acid in the duodenum. The role of HCO_3^- secretion in the distal small intestine is less clear, but it may act to conserve Cl^- at the expense of HCO_3^- secretion, thus playing a role in acid-base homeostasis.

Ion transport by the intestinal epithelium is regulated by a number of different signals, including signals supplied by hormones (both local and distant), the ENS, and the immune system. There is substantial interplay between the mediators produced by the various controlling systems. All regulatory mechanisms ultimately affect ion transport by targeting specific protein components of the transport mechanism and modifying their level of activity, abundance, or localization in the enterocyte.

Carbohydrate Digestion and Absorption

Carbohydrates constitute approximately 50% of the total daily caloric intake in humans. In Western cultures, a typical adult consumes an average of 400 g per day of carbohydrates, which yields approximately 1,600 kcal (4 kcal/g). Three major

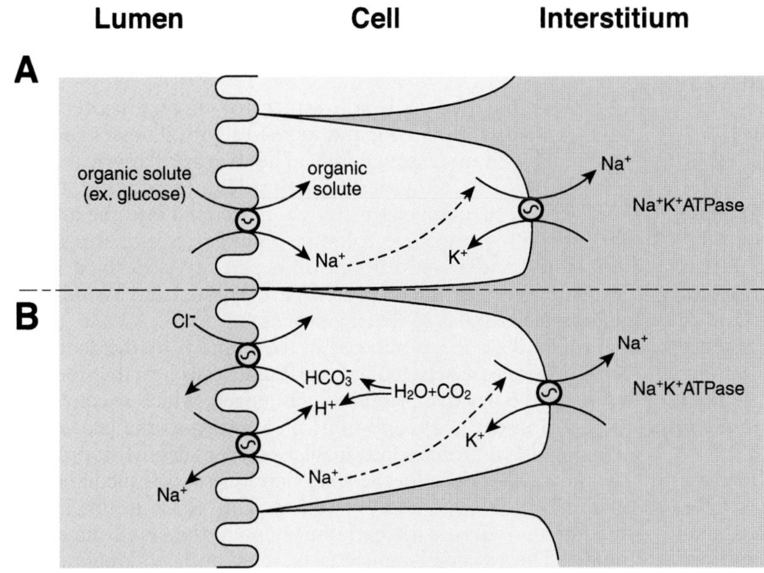

FIGURE 49.6 Mechanisms of sodium absorption in the small intestine: solute-coupled Na^+ absorption (*A*) and electroneutral NaCl absorption (*B*).

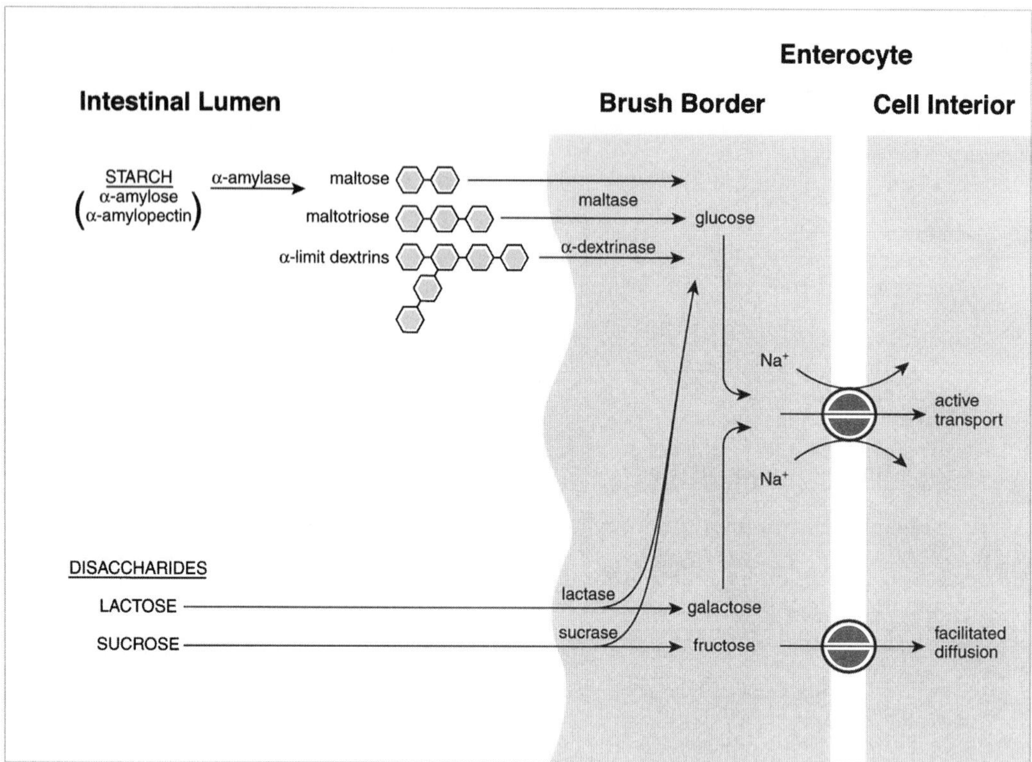

FIGURE 49.7 Digestion and absorption of carbohydrates.

types of digestible carbohydrates are found in our diet: complex starches, the disaccharides sucrose and lactose, and simple sugars, such as glucose, galactose, and fructose. Starch accounts for most of the ingested carbohydrates (approximately 60%) and exists in two basic forms: amylopectin and amylose. Amylose is a linear polymer of glucose joined by α(1,4)-glycosidic bonds. Amylopectin is a branched form of amylose with α(1,6)-glycosidic linkages at branch points, which occur every 20 to 26 molecules. Disaccharides make up approximately one third of dietary carbohydrate. The two principal disaccharides are sucrose (glucose-fructose dimer) and lactose (glucose-galactose dimer). The remainder of dietary carbohydrate consists of undigestible fiber, such as cellulose, hemicellulose, gums, and pectin. Cellulose and hemicellulose are β-linked glucose polymers and are nondigestible because the human gastrointestinal tract does not contain digestive enzymes capable of cleaving β-glucose linkages.

Digestion of starch is initiated by salivary amylase, but this mechanism is of only minor significance because salivary amylase is rapidly inactivated in the acid environment of the stomach. Most intraluminal starch digestion is accomplished by pancreatic amylase, which has a high activity for cleavage of internal $\alpha(1,4)$-glycosidic bonds. Starch digestion by amylase yields maltose (glucose dimer, 1,4 linkage), maltotriose (glucose trimer, 1,4 linkage), and α-limit dextrins, which are a series of four or more glucose molecules containing an $\alpha(1,6)$ linkage. The process of starch hydrolysis is efficient and is usually complete by the time the carbohydrate load reaches the proximal jejunum. These starch hydrolysis products, along with the ingested disaccharides sucrose and lactose, are then presented to brush border saccharidases in the jejunum for further digestion.

Brush border saccharidases are specific enzymes anchored to the apical membrane of enterocytes. They are responsible for the further breakdown of short-chain sugars into the monosaccharides glucose, galactose, and fructose. Only monosaccharides can be transported across the apical membrane of the enterocyte and absorbed into the cell (Fig. 49.7). Transport through the intestinal cell is usually the rate-limiting process for carbohydrate absorption, except for surface hydrolysis of lactose, which occurs more slowly than its transport process. Glucose and galactose compete for the same carrier mechanism and enter the cell by sodium-coupled active transport. Na^+-K^+-ATPase, located on the basolateral membrane, assists in the absorption of monosaccharides by maintaining a low intracellular Na^+ concentration, providing a large gradient for transport from the intestinal lumen into the cell. Fructose is absorbed by carrier-mediated facilitated diffusion. Although the enterocyte may use simple sugars as an energy source, most are transported across the basolateral membrane into the mesenteric venous tributaries of the portal vein.

Protein Digestion and Absorption

The recommended daily allowance for dietary proteins in adult humans is 0.75 g/kg and increases with illnesses such as sepsis, as well as in pregnancy. The average American diet consists of 70 to 100 g per day of protein. In addition, 20 to 30 g per day of endogenous protein is secreted into the intestinal lumen from gastric, biliary, pancreatic, and intestinal secretions, and an additional 30 g per day is derived from desquamated cells. These proteins are digested and assimilated in a manner similar to dietary proteins.

Protein digestion is initiated in the stomach by the action of pepsin, a protease secreted by gastric chief cells into the stomach lumen as the inactive precursor pepsinogen, which is converted to pepsin under acid conditions. Pepsin begins the process of breaking down proteins into smaller polypeptides. Most proteolysis, however, occurs in the small intestine and is mediated by pancreatic proteases and peptidases. This phase begins in the duodenum, where pancreatic juice enters the small intestinal lumen. The exocrine pancreas secretes both endopeptidases (trypsin, chymotrypsin, and elastase), which are capable of cleaving internal peptide bonds, and carboxypeptidases (carboxypeptidase A and B), which hydrolyze the terminal peptide bond on the carboxyl terminus of peptides. Each of these enzymes has distinct substrate specificities. Pancreatic proteases are initially released as inactive precursors, or zymogens. Activation of the inactive zymogens is initiated in the duodenum by enterokinase, a brush border enzyme in the duodenum. Enterokinase cleaves trypsinogen to trypsin. Trypsin is then capable of cleaving additional molecules of trypsinogen as well as the other zymogens to their active forms. The action of these pancreatic enzymes on proteins in the intestinal lumen produces a mixture of short oligopeptides (70%) and free amino acids (30%).

Further hydrolysis of the oligopeptides occurs by a series of peptidases associated with the brush border membrane, resulting in a mixture of free amino acids, dipeptides, and tripeptides before absorption. Enterocytes are capable of absorbing dipeptides and tripeptides as well as free amino acids into the cell. Many amino acids are more efficiently absorbed as constituents of dipeptides or tripeptides rather than as single amino acids. Dipeptides and tripeptides are transported into the cell by a single peptide transport system that uses a transmembrane electrochemical H^+ gradient rather than an Na^+ gradient as the driving force.[25,26] Once inside the cell, the dipeptides and tripeptides are broken down into amino acids by various cytosolic peptidases that differ from those in the brush border. Absorption of free amino acids into the enterocyte is mediated by at least five different transport systems with different substrate sensitivities and is an Na^+-dependent active transport process. Absorbed amino acids can be used by the enterocyte either as an energy source or for protein synthesis, but most are transported across the basolateral membrane by several passive carrier-mediated amino acid transport systems into the portal circulation.

Lipid Digestion and Absorption

The average Western diet consists of 60 to 100 g per day of fat, approximately 40% of the total caloric intake, which is composed primarily of triglycerides (90%), phospholipids, cholesterol, and fat-soluble vitamins. Entry of fat into the small intestine stimulates secretion of CCK from the duodenal mucosa, which is turn promotes release of lipase and its necessary cofactor colipase from the pancreas. Lipase hydrolyzes the first and third positions of triglycerides, yielding two fatty acids and β-monoglyceride (a fatty acid esterified to glycerol). Cholesterol and fat-soluble vitamins are hydrolyzed by pancreatic cholesterol esterase, and phospholipids by phospholipase A_2. The fat hydrolysis products are then solubilized in the aqueous contents of the intestine by aggregating with bile salts to form complexes called *micelles*. The combination of fatty acids, bile salts, and monoglycerides is referred to as *mixed micelles*. Cholesterol, phospholipids, and fat-soluble vitamins can also be solubilized in these micelles. Bile salts possess both hydrophobic and hydrophilic regions and, when placed in an aqueous environment, orient the hydrophilic portions to face outward and the hydrophobic portions of the molecule to face inward. Free fatty acids, β-monoglyceride, as well as cholesterol, phospholipid, and fat-soluble vitamins, reside in the hydrophobic core.

Because micelles are water compatible, they can diffuse through the unstirred water layer next to the brush border membrane and empty their contents, which then traverse the plasma membrane by passive diffusion. The bile salts remain in the intestinal lumen to create new micelles. After cellular uptake, long-chain fatty acids and β-monoglyceride are transported across the cell to the smooth endoplasmic reticulum by cytosolic carrier proteins referred to as *fatty acid-binding proteins*. In the endoplasmic reticulum, resynthesis of triglycerides takes place, and the triglycerides accumulate in the Golgi apparatus. Triglycerides are then packaged into structures called *chylomicrons* before exit from the cell. Chylomicrons are large particles, 80 to 600 nm, that contain a core of hydrophobic lipids, primarily triglycerides, but also cholesterol, phospholipid, and fat-soluble vitamins. The surface is coated with phospholipids and apoproteins, the latter of which are essential for chylomicron formation and transport. Within the Golgi, chylomicrons are packaged into secretory vesicles and exit the cell by exocytosis, where they enter the central lacteal of the villus and the intestinal lymphatic system. Smaller lipoprotein particles, called *very-low-density lipoproteins*, are also produced within enterocytes. They contain a higher cholesterol/triglyceride ratio and are the major route for entry of dietary cholesterol into the lymphatic system. Most dietary fat is absorbed in the duodenum and upper jejunum.

Short-chain fatty acids (less than eight carbon atoms) are water soluble, enter and exit the enterocyte by simple diffusion, and are taken up into the portal circulation without entering lymphatics. Medium-chain triglycerides (6 to 12 carbon atoms) are absorbed into the enterocyte by both simple diffusion and the same absorptive process used by long-chain triglycerides. These fatty acids are not reassembled into complex lipid but rather can enter the portal circulation directly as free fatty acids.

Absorption of Bile Acids

Approximately 95% of bile salts secreted into the intestine are reabsorbed and returned through the portal circulation to the liver. In the liver, bile salts are resecreted and stored in the gallbladder in preparation for release with the next meal. This cycling of bile salts is referred to as the *enterohepatic circulation*. Reabsorption of bile salts occurs by both passive and active mechanisms. A small fraction of the bile acids is absorbed passively along the entire length of the small intestine. Most of the bile salts pass to the terminal ileum, where they are absorbed by an Na^+-dependent active transport mechanism. A small amount of bile salt escapes into the colon and undergoes bacterial modification to increase solubility and promote further passive absorption. High concentrations of bile salts in the colon can promote diarrhea by inhibition of sodium and water absorption. This effect may occur in patients who undergo ileal resection and can be treated with the bile salt-binding resin cholestyramine.

Vitamin Absorption

Fat-soluble vitamins (A, D, E, and K) are solubilized by bile salt micelles and are absorbed into enterocytes along with fats. Fat-soluble vitamins are packaged into chylomicrons and enter the lymph. Water-soluble vitamins are absorbed in the jejunum and ileum by a variety of mechanisms. The absorption of vitamin C (ascorbic acid), biotin, and vitamin B_2 (riboflavin) occurs by separate, Na^+-dependent brush border carriers, whereas thiamine and folate are absorbed by Na^+-independent carrier mechanisms. Niacin and vitamin B_6 (pyridoxine) are absorbed by passive diffusion.

Vitamin B_{12} (cobalamin) absorption requires intrinsic factor, a glycoprotein secreted by gastric parietal cells. In the terminal ileum, free cobalamin forms a complex with intrinsic factor and binds to a highly specific membrane receptor. Once absorbed, free cobalamin is released from the complex and exits from the cell into the portal circulation. Deficiency of cobalamin can lead to megaloblastic anemia. Factors that can inhibit absorption of cobalamin include loss of intrinsic factor, distal ileal resection or disease, and bacterial overgrowth (competition by bacteria for luminal cobalamin).

Mineral Absorption

Approximately 1 g of calcium is ingested each day, mainly in milk and dairy products. The stomach aids in calcium absorption by solubilizing nonionic calcium salts. Ionized calcium is absorbed throughout the small intestine, with greatest absorption in the duodenum. At low levels of calcium intake, calcium absorption is an active three-step process involving transport across the apical membrane by carrier-mediated facilitated diffusion, transport across the cell by calcium-binding proteins, and extrusion of calcium into the interstitium by a Ca^{2+}-ATPase pump. This process is regulated indirectly by parathyroid hormone, which in low-calcium states promotes the conversion of vitamin D to its active form, 1,25 $(OH)_2$ vitamin D. The 1,25 $(OH)_2$ vitamin D acts directly on the intestine to increase Ca^{2+} absorption by increasing expression of both calcium-binding proteins and Ca^{2+}-ATPase.[27,28] At high intraluminal calcium concentrations, the active transport process is saturated and passive Ca^{2+} absorption occurs in the distal small intestine by a paracellular route.

Most dietary iron is complexed (heme) iron that comes from ingested meat as myoglobin or hemoglobin. This form of iron is readily absorbed. Inorganic (nonheme) iron, ingested from vegetables, grains, and fruits, is preferentially absorbed in the ferrous (Fe^{2+}) form. Ascorbic acid promotes iron absorption by reducing the ferric (Fe^{3+}) ion to the more soluble ferrous ion. Absorption of iron across the apical membrane of the enterocyte involves carrier-mediated translocation. Once inside the cell, enzymes release ferrous iron from the heme moiety. Ferrous iron can then be sequestered for intracellular storage by ferritin or transported to plasma by transferrin. Regulation is thought to occur through iron-sensing proteins called *iron-regulatory proteins*.[29] Iron-regulatory peptides promote iron binding to transferrin in low-iron states and binding to ferritin in high-iron states. Iron is absorbed in the duodenum and proximal jejunum.

Immunology

The small intestine represents a vast surface area that must be protected from entry of infectious and toxic materials while allowing the gut to absorb needed nutrients. The small intestine uses immunologic and nonimmunologic mechanisms to achieve this goal. The nonimmunologic defense mechanisms used by the gut to exclude, inactivate, and degrade pathologic substances include (a) gastric acid and enteric proteolytic enzymes; (b) mucin production, which coats and protects epithelial cells as well as inhibits bacterial growth; (c) secretion and peristalsis; (d) competitive inhibition between endogenous and pathologic bacteria; and (e) tight junctions between epithelial cells, which prevent penetration of bacteria.

A major component of intestinal defense against harmful substances involves immunologic mechanisms. In fact, the mucosal immune system of the gastrointestinal tract represents one of the largest immunologic compartments in the body.[30] Gut-associated lymphoid tissue is a major division of the immune system and is organized into aggregated (lymphoid follicles, Peyer's patches) and nonaggregated (luminal, intraepithelial, and lamina propria) cellular components.

Nonaggregated Lymphoid Tissue

The first cells to encounter an antigenic challenge are neutrophils, lymphocytes, and macrophages located in the intestinal lumen. Increased numbers of intraluminal lymphocytes are associated with Peyer's patches during gastrointestinal infections, and there is evidence of trafficking of leukocytes through the mucosa into the lumen in inflammatory states, such as ulcerative colitis.[31] Such luminal cells probably represent an effector mechanism directed toward an antigenic challenge.

The epithelium of the small intestine contains intraepithelial lymphocytes (IELs), which are found between epithelial cells along their basolateral surface. There are an average of 10 to 20 IELs per 100 villus enterocytes in the small bowel in humans.[32] In normal health, their major biologic function is secretion of cytokines that regulate epithelial cell function and responses to luminal antigens.[33] Their high level of CD8 expression suggests that they are T cells that function biologically as cytolytic effectors as a consequence of antigen recognition. In fact, the number of IELs can be increased dramatically in response to bacterial antigens. IELs appear to enter the epithelium from the bloodstream at the crypt, but they do not migrate up the villus with the epithelial cells. It is presumed that they return to the circulation after exposure to luminal antigen.

The lamina propria contains a variety of nonaggregated lymphoid tissue, including B and T cells, macrophages, mast cells, and eosinophils (Fig. 49.8). B cells in the lamina propria are thought to be derived from precursors in Peyer's patches and undergo cytokine-induced differentiation in the lamina propria to become active producers of immunoglobulin A (IgA). In contrast to IELs, most T cells in the lamina propria exert a helper-inducer function for immunoglobulin production rather than a cytolytic function. Mast cells and eosinophils represent less than 1% of the cell population in the lamina propria. Mast cells and eosinophils are activated by a variety of factors, including IgE and IgG immune complexes, and play an important role in allergic and hypersensitivity reactions.

Aggregated Lymphoid Tissue

The aggregated lymphoid tissue in the lamina propria consists of lymphoid follicles and Peyer's patches, which represent large collections of lymphoid follicles found on the antimesenteric border of the ileum. Peyer's patches are critical structures in the recognition and processing of antigen and in the development of mucosal immunity. In Peyer's patches, lymphocytes are compartmentalized with B lymphocytes in the germinal centers and T lymphocytes in the interfollicular area. Follicles have highly specialized epithelium overlying their apical dome area that contains microfold (M) cells (Fig. 49.9). M cells can be differentiated morphologically from absorptive epithelial cells by the presence of fewer, shorter, and wider microvilli. M cells cover lymphoid follicles and provide a site for selective sampling of luminal antigens.[34] M cells are able to transport antigens transcellularly using a endocytotic mechanism into the underlying lymphoid tissues of Peyer's patches. M cells thus facilitate macrophage and dendritic cell processing and antigen presentation to naive lymphocytes in the lymphoid follicle.

Activated lymphocytes from intestinal lymphoid follicles migrate into afferent lymphatics, pass through mesenteric lymph nodes, and enter the circulation through the thoracic duct. During this process, the lymphocytes mature into B and T lymphoblasts with an enriched population of IgA-bearing B cells. The lymphoblasts then home in to the lamina propria of the gastrointestinal mucosa at the site of original antigenic stimulation, where B lymphoblasts mature into IgA-secreting B cells under the control of antigen-stimulated T cells that have completed the same journey. These mature effector cells provide protective immunity in the lamina propria.

In addition to the gastrointestinal mucosa, activated lymphoblasts may also home to the lamina propria of other mucosa-bearing tissues, such as breast, lung, and eye, where antigen-specific antibodies are secreted.[35] For example, IgA-bearing cells preferentially migrate to the mammary gland during lactation. Thus, a breast-feeding mother can passively transfer secretory IgA to her nursing infant. The secretory IgA protects the infant from bacteria and viruses in the mother's gastrointestinal tract.

The ability of activated lymphoblasts to home to specific mucosal sites is regulated by interactions with endothelial cells.

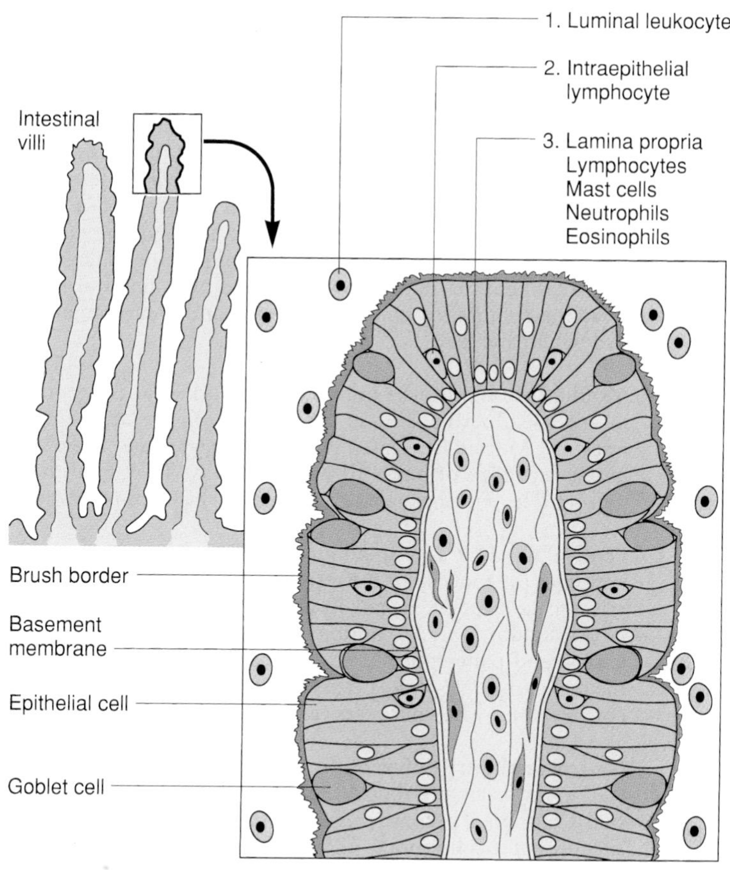

FIGURE 49.8 Small intestinal villus with associated immunologic cells.

Antigenic stimulation and chronic inflammation produce a rapid increase in endothelial venules. Increased expression of adhesion molecules on these endothelial cells is mediated by cytokines and stimulates an influx of antigen-specific, stimulated lymphoblasts to the effector compartment of the nonaggregated lamina propria.

Immunoglobulin Secretion

A major protective mechanism of the intestinal immune system is synthesis and secretion of IgA. Less than 5% of immunoglobulin-producing cells in the gut produce IgG. In serum, IgA exists in monomeric form. In the intestine (and other mucosal surfaces), IgA exists as a dimer that is complexed covalently with two additional molecules-the J chain, which links two IgA molecules, and the polymeric immunoglobulin receptor, which transports the IgA complex across the cell and allows release of the complex, termed *secretory component,* into the intestinal lumen.[36] The J chain is a polypeptide produced in the plasma cell. The polymeric immunoglobulin receptor, a transmembrane glycoprotein, is produced by the intestinal epithelial cell. It is thought that secretory component

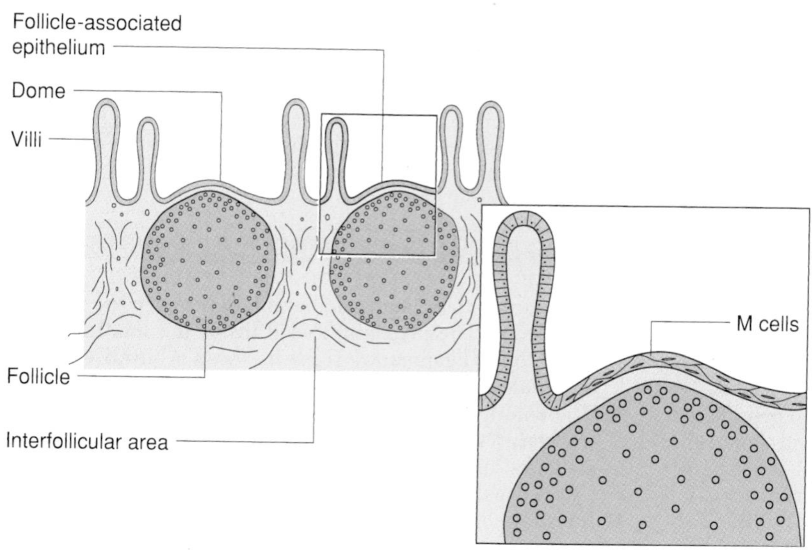

FIGURE 49.9 Epithelial anatomy in the area of Peyer's patches.

may prevent proteolytic degradation of the secretory IgA molecule and may stabilize the structure of the polymeric IgA complex in an environment containing numerous proteolytic enzymes and bacteria that would otherwise rapidly degrade it.[36] IgA possesses functional characteristics that are distinct from other antibodies. Unlike IgG and IgM, IgA does not activate complement and does not promote cell-mediated opsonization. The major function of secretory IgA in host defense is protection against bacteria, viruses, and luminal antigens. The protective effect of secretory IgA results from its ability to effectively bind harmful substances while resisting enzymatic degradation by gut enzymes. Secretory IgA inhibits the adherence of bacteria to epithelial cells, leading to impaired colonization and proliferation. Binding of antigen to secretory IgA stimulates mucus secretion and can prevent uptake of both viruses and bacteria by entrapment in the mucus layer. Secretory IgA also binds to and blocks the absorption of antigens and toxins and may be very important in disease states in which the mucosal barrier is disrupted, such as in inflammatory bowel disease. The ability of IgA to use relatively unobtrusive mechanisms in host defense minimizes the need for an inflammatory response and thus protects the intestinal mucosa against injury.

Endocrine Function

The gastrointestinal tract is the largest endocrine system in the body. Unlike other endocrine organs, which possess a solid mass of hormone-producing cells, the source of gastrointestinal hormones is scattered single cells and enteric neurons along the length of the gastrointestinal tract. These hormones play a key role in all aspects of small bowel function, including motility, secretion and absorption, blood flow, growth, and immunity.

Cholecystokinin. CCK is predominantly produced by endocrine cells in the mucosa of the proximal two thirds of the small intestine. CCK is also present in less abundance in enteric neurons. CCK exists in multiple molecular forms (CCK-8, CCK-33, CCK-39, and CCK-58); however, no differential biologic effects among the different forms have been described. CCK is released from the small bowel mucosa in response to luminal fats and proteins. The major actions of CCK are to stimulate pancreatic acinar cell secretion of zymogens via vagal cholinergic pathways and stimulate gallbladder contractility.[37] The actions of CCK result in delivery of key digestive components into the intestinal lumen. CCK also has trophic effects on small bowel mucosa and pancreas.

Secretin. Secretin is a 27-amino acid peptide synthesized in the endocrine cells (S cells) that are present in the duodenum and jejunum. The main stimulus for secretin release is acid in the duodenum when the luminal pH decreases to 4 or lower. The major effect of secretin is secretion of bicarbonate from pancreatic and biliary ductal epithelium and Brunner's glands. The bicarbonate neutralizes luminal acid and provides a negative feedback loop for release of secretin. The ability of secretin to paradoxically induce gastrin release in patients with gastrinoma while having no effect on gastrin release in normal subjects has made the secretin stimulation test a useful tool in the diagnosis of Zollinger-Ellison syndrome.

Vasoactive intestinal peptide. Vasoactive intestinal peptide is a member of the secretin family of peptides and functions exclusively as a neurotransmitter. It is a potent vasodilator and also functions to stimulate enteric smooth muscle and pancreatic exocrine and intestinal secretion and inhibit gastric acid secretion.

Somatostatin. Somatostatin is synthesized and secreted from both neurons and endocrine cells (D cells) found in small quantities throughout the gut mucosa. Most of the biologic effects of somatostatin are inhibitory. Somatostatin inhibits biliary, gastric, and pancreatic secretion, in addition to inhibiting release of a broad range of gastrointestinal hormones. Somatostatin also inhibits motility, presumably by inhibiting cholinergic neurons. The peptide decreases splanchnic and portal blood flow. A long-acting cyclic analogue of somatostatin, octreotide, is a very useful clinical therapeutic agent in the treatment of patients with gastrointestinal hormone-secreting tumors, carcinoid syndrome, and enterocutaneous and pancreatic fistulas.[38]

Motilin. Motilin is a 22-amino acid peptide that is produced in enteroendocrine cells in the mucosa of the upper small intestine. Motilin is released in the fasting state and is a physiologic regulator of phase III MMC activity. The initiation of motilin release is through a cholinergic-dependent pathway.

Peptide YY. PYY is a 36-amino acid peptide found predominantly in the mucosa of the terminal ileum and colon. PYY is released in response to fats in meals. The actions of PYY are largely inhibitory-PYY inhibits gastrointestinal motility and gastric and pancreatic secretion. The peptide has been given the nickname *ileal brake* because these actions promote longer contact times when nutrients reach the distal small bowel.

Gastric inhibitory polypeptide. Gastric inhibitory polypeptide (GIP) was originally thought to inhibit gastric acid secretion, but it has since become clear that this is not the physiologic function of this hormone. GIP is a 42-amino acid peptide that is found in highest concentration in the mucosa of the duodenum and jejunum. The main physiologic function of GIP is to regulate insulin release in response to a meal (incretion effect). GIP has no effect on insulin release to parenterally administered nutrients.

Neurotensin. Neurotensin, a 13-amino acid peptide, is produced predominantly in the ileal mucosa but is also produced in smaller quantities in the proximal small intestine and colon. It is released by a mixed meal and fats. Neurotensin has been demonstrated to stimulate pancreatic bicarbonate secretion, inhibit gastric secretion, stimulate intestinal motility, and produce trophic effects on the small intestinal mucosa.

Pancreatic glucagon and enteroglucagon. Pancreatic glucagon and enteroglucagon are 29- and 37-amino acid peptides located in the pancreas and small intestine, respectively, and are the products of tissue-specific processing of the propeptide glicentin (69 amino acids). Pancreatic glucagon resides in A cells in the islet and is important in inducing glycogenolysis, lipolysis, gluconeogenesis, and ketogenesis. Enteroglucagon is produced predominantly in the distal small intestine and functions to inhibit small bowel motility.

KEY POINTS

- **There is no clear anatomic boundary between the jejunum and ileum. The proximal two fifths of the small intestine distal to the ligament of Treitz has been arbitrarily defined as *jejunum* and the distal three fifths as *ileum*.**
- **The enteric nervous system contains two major plexuses, the myenteric (Auerbach's) plexus, located between the longitudinal and circular muscle layers, and the submucous (Meissner's) plexus.**
- **Intestinal epithelial cells exhibit complex patterns of gene expression that vary according to their location on the two**

main spatial axes of the gut, the vertical (crypt-villus) and horizontal (proximal to distal) axes.

- Although neural and hormonal factors are important in modulating motility, the primary control mechanism is myogenic.
- Water absorption is controlled indirectly through regulation of electrolyte transport.

References

1. Cohen S, Harris LD, Levitan R. Manometric characteristics of the human ileocecal junction zone. *Gastroenterology* 1968;54:72.
2. Rosse C, Gaddum-Rosse P, eds. *Hollinshead's textbook of anatomy*, 5th ed. Philadelphia: Lippincott-Raven, 1997.
3. Furness JB, Costa M. *The enteric nervous system*. New York: Churchill Livingstone, 1987.
4. Sternini C. Functional organization of the enteric nervous system. *Regul Pept.* 1993;5:25.
5. **Goyal RK, Hirano I. Mechanisms of disease: the enteric nervous system. *N Engl J Med.* 1996;334:1106–1115.**
6. Rubin DC. Spatial analysis of transcriptional activation in fetal rat jejunum and ileal gut epithelium. *Am J Physiol.* 1992;263:G853–863.
7. Holmes R, Lobley RW. Intestinal brush border revisited. *Gut* 1989;30:1667–1668.
8. Garabedian EM, Roberts LJ, Mcnevin MS, et al. Examining the role of Paneth cells in the small intestine by lineage ablation in transgenic mice. *J Biol Chem.* 1997;272:23729–23740.
9. Casteels R. Membrane potential in smooth muscle cells. In: Bulbring E, Brading AF, Jones AF, et al., eds. *Smooth muscle: an assessment of current knowledge*. Austin, TX: University of Texas Press; 1981:105.
10. Furness JB, Bornstein JC, Kunze WA, et al. The enteric nervous system and its extrinsic connections. In: Yamada T, ed. *Textbook of gastroenterology*, 3rd ed., vol 1. Philadelphia: Lippincott-Raven, 1999:11.
11. Argenyi EE, Soffer EE, Madsen MT, et al. Scintigraphic evaluation of small bowel transit in healthy subjects: inter- and intrasubject variability. *Am J Gastroenterol.* 1995;90:938–942.
12. Carlson GM, Bedi BS, Code CF. Mechanism of propagation of intestinal interdigestive myoelectric complex. *Am J Physiol.* 1972;222:1027–1030.
13. Rees WDW, Malagelada JR, Miller LJ, et al. Human interdigestive and postprandial gastrointestinal motor and gastrointestinal hormone patterns. *Dig Dis Sci.* 1982;27:321–329.
14. Weisbrodt NW, Copeland EM, Moore EP, et al. Effect of vagotomy on electrical activity of the small intestine of the dog. *Am J Physiol.* 1975;228:650–654.
15. Marlett JA, Code CF. Effects of celiac and superior mesenteric ganglionectomy on interdigestive myoelectric complex in dogs. *Am J Physiol.* 1979; 237:E432–E433.
16. Sarr MG, Kelly KA. Myoelectric activity of the autotransplanted canine jejunoileum. *Gastroenterology* 1981;81:303–310.
17. Itoh Z. Motilin and clinical application. *Peptides* 1997;18:593–608.
18. Tonini M. Recent advances in the pharmacology of gastrointestinal prokinetics. *Pharmacol Res.* 1996;33:217–226.
19. Von der Ohe M, Layer P, Wollny C, et al. Somatostatin 28 and coupling of human interdigestive intestinal motility and pancreatic secretion. *Gastroenterology* 1992;103:974–981.
20. Owyang C, Achem-Karem SR, Vinik AI. Pancreatic polypeptide and intestinal migrating motor complex in humans. *Gastroenterology* 1983;84:10–17.
21. Loo DD, Zeuthen T, Chandy G, et al. Cotransport of water by the Na^+/glucose cotransporter. *Proc Natl Acad Sci USA.* 1996;93:13367–13370.
22. Wright EM, Loo DD, Turk E, et al. Sodium cotransporters. *Curr Opin Cell Biol.* 1996;8:468–473.
23. Knickerbein R, Aronson PS, Schron CM, et al. Sodium and chloride transport across the rabbit ileal brush border: II. evidence for Cl-HCO_3 exchange and mechanism of coupling. *Am J Physiol.* 1985;249:G236–245.
24. Agarwal R, Afzalpurkar R, Fordtran JS. Pathophysiology of potassium absorption and secretion in the small intestine. *Gastroenterology* 1994;107:548–571.
25. Ganapathy V, Leibach FH. Proton-coupled solute transport in the animal cell plasma membrane. *Curr Opin Cell Biol.* 1991;3:695–701.
26. Leibach FH, Ganapathy V. Peptide transporters in the intestine and the kidney. *Annu Rev Nutr.* 1996;16:99–119.
27. Cai Q, Chandler JS, Wasserman RH, et al. Vitamin D and adaptation to dietary calcium and phosphate deficiencies increase intestinal plasma membrane calcium pump gene expression. *Proc Natl Acad Sci USA* 1993;90:1345–1349.
28. Walters J. Calbindin-D_{9k} stimulates the calcium pump in rat enterocyte basolateral membranes. *Am J Physiol.* 1989;256:G124–G128.
29. Ponka P, Beaumont C, Richardson DR. Function and regulation of transferrin and ferritin. *Semin Hematol.* 1998;35:35–54.
30. Brandtzaeg P, Solli d L, Thrane P, et al. Lymphoepithelial interactions in the mucosal immune system. *Gut* 1988;29:1116–1130.
31. Saverymuttu SH, Camilleri M, Rees H, et al. Indium 111-granulocyte scanning in the assessment of disease extent and disease activity in inflammatory bowel disease: a comparison with colonoscopy, histology, and fecal indium 111-granulocyte excretion. *Gastroenterology* 1986;90;1121–1128.
32. Ferguson A. Intraepithelial lymphocytes of the small intestine. *Gut.* 1977;18:921–937.
33. Boismenu R, Harvan WL. Modulation of epithelial cell growth by intraepithelial T cells. *Science* 1994;266:1253–1255.
34. Neutra M, Frey A, Kraehenbuhl JP. Epithelial M cells: gateways for mucosal infection and immunization. *Cell.* 1996;86:345–348.
35. Blumberg RS. The immune system. In: Yamada T, ed. *Textbook of gastroenterology*, 3rd ed., vol 1. Philadelphia: Lippincott-Raven, 1999:106.
36. McGhee JR, Mestecky J, Dertzbaugh MT, et al. The mucosal immune system: from fundamental concepts to vaccine development. *Vaccine* 1992;10:75–88.
37. **Owyang C, Logsdon CD. New insights into neurohormonal regulation of pancreatic secretion. *Gastroenterology* 2004;127:957–969.**
38. Weckbecker G, Lewis I, Albert R, et al. Opportunities in somatostatin research: biological, chemical and therapeutic aspects. *Nat Rev Drug Discov.* 2003;2:999–1017.

CHAPTER 50 ■ ILEUS AND BOWEL OBSTRUCTION

MANDEEP SAUND AND DAVID I. SOYBEL

INTRODUCTION AND HISTORICAL PERSPECTIVE

The purpose of this chapter is to provide an overview of the pathophysiology, natural history, diagnosis, and management of acute obstruction and ileus of the small and large intestines. The development of the modern approach to intestinal obstruction and ileus paralleled the development of techniques for safe abdominal surgery. Chief among these accomplishments were the discovery of safe general anesthetics, the popularization of aseptic methods in the operating rooms and management of wounds, and the development of techniques for intestinal resection, intestinal anastomosis, and colostomy. The foundations of the recognition and management of intestinal obstruction and ileus are attributed to Frederick Treves.[1–3] In 1884, he published a detailed discussion of the etiologies (including adhesions) and surgical management of mechanical intestinal obstruction.[1] Treves also distinguished mechanical from nonmechanical (i.e., paralytic) causes of intestinal distention, classifying the latter causes under the term *ileus*. From 1880 to 1925, proximal intestinal decompression was recognized to provide relief from the symptoms of

GASTROINTESTINAL

mechanical obstruction or ileus.[3] In 1933, Wangensteen and Paine reported the efficacy of gastrointestinal intubation in relieving symptoms of intestinal distention caused by intestinal obstruction or from the ileus that resulted from laparotomy.[4,5] Subsequently, Wangensteen and Rea provided experimental evidence that the source of gaseous distention in cases of obstruction or ileus was swallowed air.[6] The value of intravenous fluid resuscitation in experimental models of intestinal obstruction was recognized as early as 1912[7] and became a principle of care of the patients with intestinal obstruction in the late 1920s. By 1920, plain abdominal radiographs were used in diagnosis of intestinal obstruction.[3] Thus, the principles of early diagnosis, rapid intravenous fluid resuscitation, gastrointestinal decompression, and early operation to avoid intestinal gangrene and peritonitis, were established well before the advent of antibiotic therapy, invasive hemodynamic monitoring, and parenteral nutrition.[8] These early developments were most important in reducing morbidity and mortality of mechanical intestinal obstruction and ileus.[9]

MECHANICAL OBSTRUCTION OF THE INTESTINES

Terminology and Classification

The term *mechanical obstruction* means that luminal contents cannot pass through the gut tube because the lumen is blocked. This obstruction is in contrast with *neurogenic* or *functional* obstructions in which luminal contents are prevented from passing because of disturbances in gut motility that prevent coordinated peristalsis from one region of the gut to the next. This latter form of obstruction is commonly referred to as *ileus* in the small intestine and *pseudoobstruction* in the large intestine. In *simple* obstruction the intestinal lumen is partially or completely occluded without compromise of intestinal blood flow. Simple obstructions may be *complete*, meaning that the lumen is totally occluded (Fig. 50.1), or *incomplete*, meaning

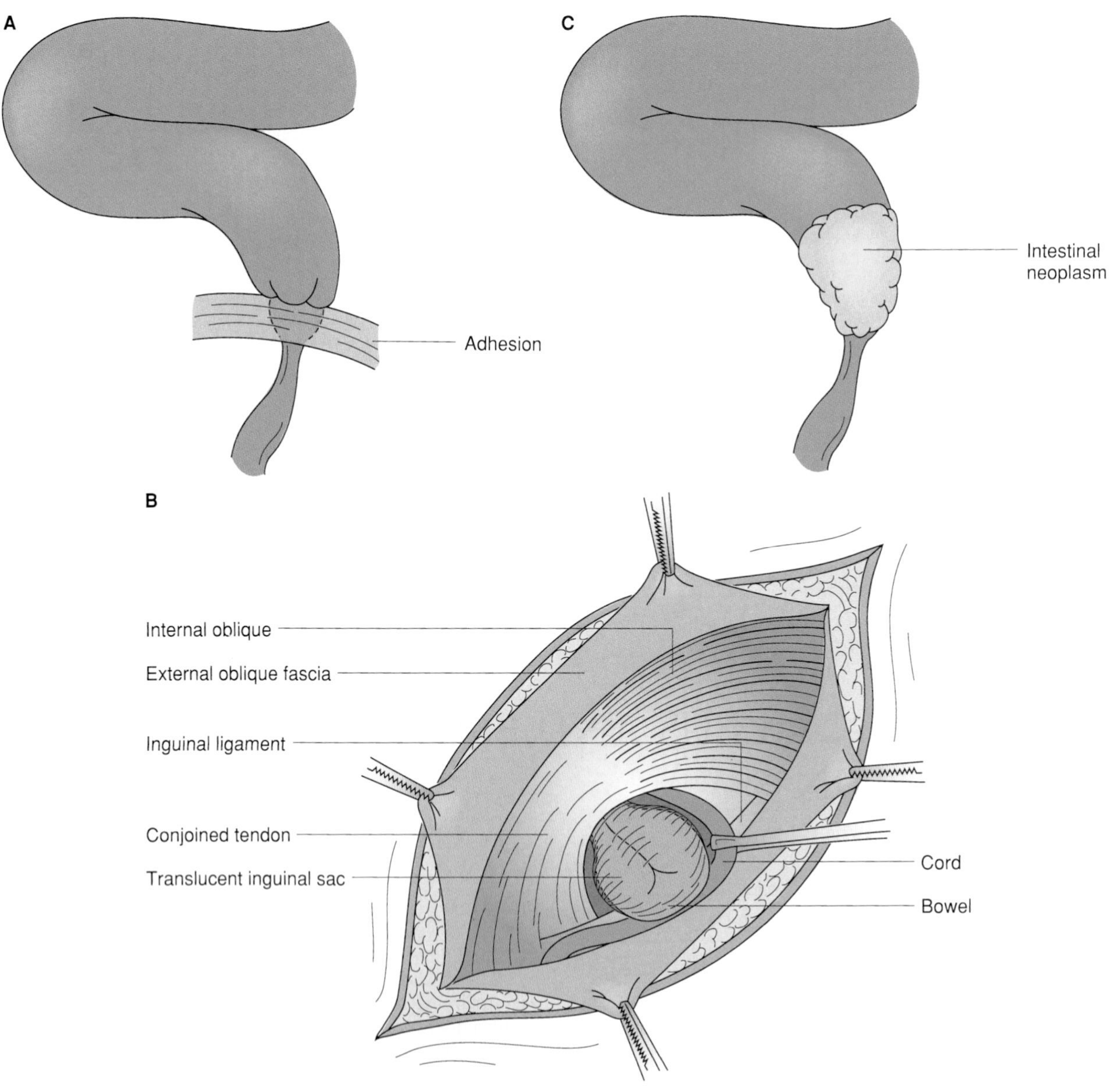

FIGURE 50.1 Schematic illustration of different forms of simple mechanical obstruction. Simple obstruction is most often due to adhesion (*A*), groin hernia (*B*), or neoplasm (C). The hernia can act as a tourniquet, causing a closed-loop obstruction and strangulation.

that the lumen is narrowed but permitting distal passage of some fluid and air. In *strangulation* obstruction, blood flow to the obstructed segment is compromised and tissue necrosis and gangrene are imminent. Strangulation usually implies that the obstruction is complete, but some forms of partial obstruction can also be complicated by strangulation.

The various forms of mechanical intestinal obstruction can be classified according to different but overlapping schemes. Most commonly, obstruction is classified according to etiology. As detailed in Table 50.1, distinctions are drawn between intraluminal obturators such as foreign bodies or gallstones, intramural lesions such as tumors or intussusceptions, and extrinsic or extramural lesions such as adhesions. In order to highlight the pathophysiology, presentation and natural history, however, it is useful to classify obstruction according to the location of the obstructing lesion. Proximal or "high" obstructions involve the pylorus, duodenum and proximal jejunum. Intermediate levels of obstruction involve the intestine from the midjejunum to the midileum. Distal levels of obstruction arise in the distal ileum, ileocecal valve and proximal colon whereas the most distant or "low" obstructions would arise in regions beyond the transverse colon. As shown in Table 50.2, clinical symptoms and signs of obstruction (pain, vomiting, abdominal distention, gas pattern on abdominal radiographs) vary with the level of obstruction.

It is also important to distinguish between *open-loop* and *closed-loop* obstructions. An open-loop obstruction occurs when intestinal flow is blocked but proximal decompression is possible through vomiting. A closed-loop obstruction occurs when inflow to the loop of bowel and outflow from the loop are both blocked. This obstruction permits gas and secretions to accumulate in the loop without a means of decompression, proximally or distally. Examples of closed-loop obstructions are torsion of a loop of small intestine around an adhesive band (Fig. 50.2), incarceration of the bowel in a hernia, volvulus of the cecum or colon, or development of an obstructing carcinoma of the colon with a competent ileocecal valve. The primary symptoms of a closed-loop obstruction of the small intestine are sudden, severe abdominal pain and vomiting whereas symptoms of the large intestine are pain and sudden abdominal distention. This pain often occurs before associated findings of localized abdominal tenderness or involuntary guarding. When physical findings develop, there is a high level of suspicion that the viability of the bowel is compromised. When bowel obstruction is the most likely diagnosis, "abdominal pain out of proportion to physical findings" represents a surgical emergency.

TABLE 50.1 CLASSIFICATION

CLASSIFICATION OF ADULT MECHANICAL INTENSTINAL OBSTRUCTIONS

INTRALUMINAL
Foreign bodies
Barium inspissation (colon)
Bezoar
Inspissated feces
Gallstone
Meconium (cystic fibrosis)
Parasites
Other (e.g., swallowed objects, enteroliths)
Intussusception (usually associated with tumor in adults)
Polypoid, exophytic lesions
INTRAMURAL
Congenital (rare in adults)
Atresia, stricture, or stenosis
Web
Intestinal duplication
Meckel's diverticulum
Inflammatory process
Crohn disease
Diverticulitis
Chronic intestinal ischemia or postischemic stricture
Radiation enteritis
Medication induced (nonsteroidal antiinflammatory drugs, potassium chloride tablets)
Neoplasms
Primary bowel (malignant or benign)
Secondary (metastases, especially melanoma)
Traumatic (e.g., intramural hematoma of duodenum)
EXTRINSIC
Adhesions
Congenital
Ladd or Meckel's bands
Postoperative
Postinflammatory (after PID)
Hernias
External
Internal
Volvulus
External mass effect
Abscess
Annular pancreas
Carcinomatosis
Endometriosis
Pregnancy
Pancreatic pseudocyst

Pathophysiology of Intestinal Obstruction

Local Effects of Bowel Obstruction

When a loop of bowel becomes obstructed, intestinal gas and fluid accumulate. Stasis of luminal content favors bacterial overgrowth, alters intestinal fluid transport properties and motility, and causes variations in intestinal perfusion and lymph flow. Luminal contents and volume, bacterial proliferation, and alterations in motility and perfusion work in concert to determine the rate at which symptoms and complications develop. Each of these factors merits discussion in some detail.

Intestinal gas. Approximately 80% of the gas seen on plain abdominal radiographs is attributable to swallowed air.[6] Approximately 70% of the gas in the obstructed gut is inert nitrogen.[10] Oxygen accounts for 10% to 12%, CO_2 for 6% to 9%, hydrogen 1%, methane 1%, and hydrogen disulfide 1% to 10%. In the setting of acute pain and anxiety, patients with intestinal obstruction may swallow excessive amounts of air. Passage of such swallowed air distally is prevented by nasogastric suction.

Intestinal flora. An important contribution to normal digestive function comes from its bacterial population. In patients with normal gastric acid secretion, the chyme entering the duodenum is sterile. The small numbers of bacteria that are found in stomach and proximal intestine are aerobic, gram-positive species found in the oropharynx. Distally, in the ileum and colon, gram-negative aerobes are present and anaerobic organisms predominate. Total bacterial counts in normal feces reach 10^{11} organisms per gram of fecal matter. Control of the bacterial populations depends on intact motor activity of the intestines and the interactions of all species present. This ecology can be

TABLE 50.2 DIAGNOSIS

SYMPTOMS AND SIGNS OF BOWEL OBSTRUCTION

Symptom or sign	Proximal small bowel (open loop)	Distal small bowel (open loop)	Small bowel (closed loop)	Colon and rectum
Pain	Intermittent, intense, colicky; often relieved by vomiting	Intermittent to constant	Progressive, intermittent to constant; rapidly worsens	Continuous
Vomiting	Large volumes, bilious and frequent	Low volume and frequency; progressively feculent with time	May be prominent (reflex)	Intermittent, not prominent feculent when present
Tenderness	Epigastric or periumbilical; quite mild unless strangulation is present	Diffuse and progressive	Diffuse, progressive	Diffuse
Distention	Absent	Moderate to marked	Often absent	Marked
Obstipation	May not be present	Present	May not be present	Present

Adapted from Schuffler MD, Sinanan MN. Intestinal obstruction and pseudo-obstruction. In: Sleisenger MH, Fordtran JS, eds. *Gastrointestinal disease,* 5th ed. Philadelphia: WB Saunders, 1993:898.

disturbed by antibiotic therapy or by surgical reconstructions that result in stasis within intestinal segments. Intestinal bacteria serve several functions, including metabolism of fecal sterols, releasing the small chain fatty acids that are an important food source for colonocytes; metabolism of fecal bile acids, fat-soluble vitamins (e.g., vitamin K) and vitamin B12; and breakdown of complex carbohydrates and organic matter, leading to formation of CO_2, H_2, and CH_4 gases.[9] Considerable evidence suggests that the normal flora may contribute to baseline levels of intestinal secretion and, perhaps, normal intestinal motility. Under baseline conditions, the small intestines in germfree animals are frequently dilated, fluid filled and without peristalsis.[11,12]

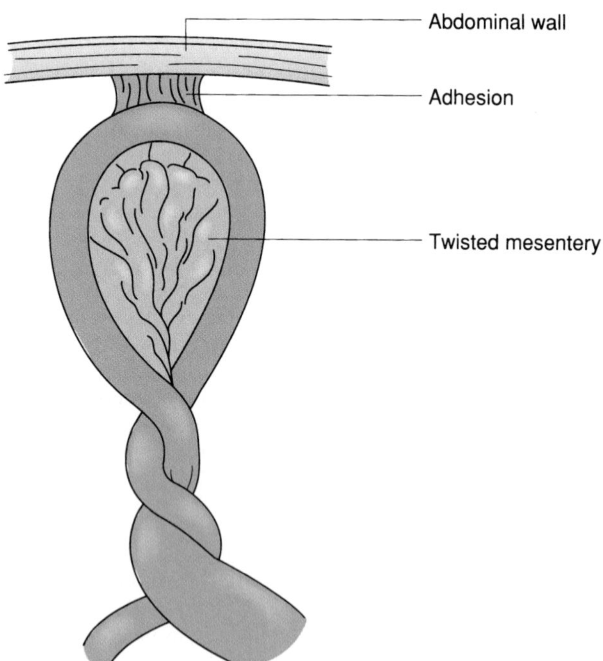

FIGURE 50.2 Schematic illustration of a closed-loop obstruction. The small intestine twists around its mesentery, compromising inflow and outflow of luminal contents from the loop. Also, the vascular supply to the loop may be compromised because of the twisting of the mesentery. The risk of strangulation is high.

In recent years, the role of bacterial toxins in mediating the mucosal response to obstruction has received increasing attention. In germ-free dogs, luminal accumulation of fluid is not observed and absorption continues.[12] In addition, it is well recognized that bacterial endotoxins can stimulate secretion, possibly via release or potentiation of activity of neuroendocrine substances and prostaglandins.[11] Finally, since a substantial part of systemic microvascular and hemodynamic responses to endotoxemia appear to be attributable to heightened synthesis of nitric oxide,[13,14] it seems likely that mucosal response to local inflammation and endotoxin release will also be altered by conditions modifying the synthesis or activity of nitric oxide. The role of nitric oxide in mucosal fluid and electrolyte movements is currently under active investigation.[15,16]

Intestinal fluid. Classical experimental studies established that fluid accumulates intraluminally with open- or closed-loop small intestinal obstruction.[9,17] Factors contributing to the accumulation of fluid include intraluminal distention and pressure, release of prosecretory and antiabsorptive hormones and paracrine substances, changes in mesenteric circulation, and elaboration and luminal release of bacterial toxins. Experimental studies and clinical investigation[18,19] demonstrated that elevation of luminal pressures above 20 cm H_2O inhibits absorption and stimulates secretion of salt and water into the lumen proximal to an obstruction. In closed-loop obstructions, luminal pressures may exceed 50 cm H_2O and may account for a substantial proportion of luminal fluid accumulation.[20] In simple, open-loop obstructions, distention of the lumen by gas rarely leads to luminal pressures higher than 8 to 12 cm H_2O.[21] Thus, in open-loop obstructions, the contributions of high luminal pressures to hypersecretion may not be important.

The release of endocrine/paracrine substances remains relatively uncharacterized in states of mechanical bowel obstruction.[22,23] Suggestions have been made that vasoactive intestinal polypeptide (VIP) may be released from the submucosal and myenteric plexuses within the gut wall, promoting epithelial secretion and inhibiting absorption.[23] Use of prostaglandin synthesis inhibitors has also implicated excess release of prostaglandins.[22] Further work may be expected to focus on the role of luminal factors such as irritative bile acids, proinflammatory agents such as endotoxin and platelet-activating factor, and messengers such as nitric oxide in coordinating responses of mucosal secretory and absorptive functions during intestinal obstruction.

Intestinal blood flow. Microvascular responses to intestinal obstruction may also play an important role in determining the hydrostatic gradients for fluid transfer across the mucosa into the lumen. In response to heightened luminal pressure, total blood flow to the bowel wall may initially increase.[24] The breakdown of epithelial barrier structures and enzymatic breakdown of stagnant intestinal contents leads to increased osmolarity of luminal contents. In addition to secretory stimulation and absorptive inhibition of the mucosa, the simultaneous changes in hydrostatic and osmotic pressures on the blood and lumen sides of the mucosa favor flow of extracellular fluid into the lumen. Perfusion is then compromised as luminal pressures increase, bacteria invade, and inflammation leads to edema within the bowel wall.

Intestinal motility. Obstruction of the intestinal lumen does not simply block distal passage of luminal contents. The accumulation of fluid and gas in the obstructed lumen also elicit changes in myoelectrical function of the gut, proximal and distal to the obstructed segment. In response to this distention, the obstructed segment itself may dilate, a process known as *receptive relaxation*.[25] Such changes ensure that, despite accumulation of air and fluid, intraluminal pressures do not rise easily to the point of compromising blood flow to the intestinal mucosa. At sites proximal and distal to the obstruction, changes in myoelectrical activity are time dependent. Initially, there may be intense periods of activity and peristalsis. Subsequently, myoelectrical activity is diminished and the interdigestive migrating myoelectrical complex pattern, is replaced by ineffectual and seemingly disorganized clusters of contractions.[26–28] Similar alterations have been observed in experimental models of large bowel obstruction. Subsequent patterns of myoelectrical quiescence may correspond to increasing accumulation of fluid and air proximally and the attempt to prevent luminal pressures from rising. It is likely that many factors contribute to the rate at which these changes in myoelectrical activity occur. These factors would include neurohumoral milieu, bacterial products, and luminal constituents.

Complications and Systemic Effects of Bowel Obstruction

Closed-loop obstructions. The complications of closed-loop obstructions evolve rapidly. The reasons for this rapid evolution are best understood by considering the simplest and most common form of closed-loop obstruction, appendicitis. When a fecalith obstructs the blind-ended appendix, secretion of mucus and enhanced peristalsis represent the initial attempt to clear the blockage. Intense crampy abdominal pain focused at the umbilicus results. Nausea and vomiting are not uncommon as a result of luminal obstruction but as a reflexive response to hyperperistalsis and stretching of the mesentery. Over the next 8 to 18 hours, continued secretion of mucus to high intraluminal pressures, stasis, bacterial overgrowth, mucosal disruption, and elevation of luminal pressures convert intermittent cramps to constant and worsening pain. When luminal pressure exceeds mural venous pressure and then capillary perfusion pressures, inflammatory cells are recruited from surrounding peritoneal structures. This sequence of events leads to intense inflammation, release of exudate in the area of the appendix and the first localization of pain from the umbilicus to the area of peritoneum lying nearest the inflamed appendix. Peritoneal findings (localized tenderness, involuntary guarding, rebound or referred tenderness) and fevers appear. Subsequently, 20 to 24 hours into the illness, the blood supply of the appendix is compromised. Gangrene and perforation follow and, if not contained by surrounding structures, free perforation leads to a rigid abdomen. Toxins from necrotic tissue and bacterial overgrowth are released into the systemic circulation and shock ensures. Torsion of a loop of small intestine around an adhesive band or inside a hernia leads to a similar pattern of events. As discussed below, torsions of the large bowel are usually accompanied by massive distention of the loop by air and feces, but the compromise of intestinal wall perfusion and evolution into peritonitis, systemic toxicity, and shock are similar.

Open-loop obstructions. Complications in open-loop obstructions do not necessarily evolve as rapidly as in closed-loop obstructions. Not uncommonly, an open-loop obstruction located in the proximal jejunum can be decompressed by the patient's ability to vomit. Proximal obstruction is characterized by vomiting and loss of gastric, pancreatic, and biliary secretions, with resulting electrolyte disturbances. These disturbances include dehydration, metabolic alkalosis, hypochloremia, hypokalemia, and usually hyponatremia. In contrast, obstructions of the distal ileum may lead only to a slowly progressing distention of the small intestine, with accommodation by intestinal myoelectrical function and minor alterations in fluid and electrolyte balances. Open-loop obstructions located in the midgut are often complicated by events similar to those seen in closed-loop obstructions or combinations of events seen in high and low obstructions (Table 50.2). Patients with distal jejunal obstruction tend to present with a combination of complications resulting from loss of intestinal contents from vomiting, as well as distention and compromise of intestinal wall perfusion.

Clinical Presentation and Differential Diagnosis

The four key symptoms are associated with acute mechanical bowel obstruction include abdominal pain, vomiting, distention, and obstipation. Colon obstruction is usually accompanied by varying levels of pain with massive abdominal distention and obstipation. As noted earlier, the signs and symptoms of acute but simple small intestinal obstructions are related to the level of the obstruction and the closed- or open-loop nature of the obstruction. Other abdominal conditions, such as appendicitis, diverticulitis, perforated peptic ulcer, cholecystitis or choledocholithiasis can usually be distinguished from small bowel obstruction, by clinical examination and basic laboratory data. It should be emphasized that bowel obstruction can complicate any of these abdominal conditions. The presence of another abdominal process does not exclude the complication of small bowel obstruction.

Over the years, numerous attempts have been made to use groupings of clinical criteria to establish the diagnosis of complete and irreversible intestinal obstruction, as distinguished from partial intestinal obstruction that might improve without operative intervention or other abdominal pathology. In recent studies, computer-assisted analysis has been used to identify such criteria.[29]) Key factors in the history and clinical examination include previous abdominal surgery, quality of pain (colic/intermittent versus steady), abdominal distention, and hyperactivity of bowel sounds. Not surprisingly, the use of such computer-assisted algorithms confirms that the most important clues to the diagnosis of simple obstruction of the small intestine are obtained in a complete and careful history and physical examination. As discussed below, the role of plain abdominal radiographs and other imaging studies is to confirm the clinical diagnosis of simple obstruction. It should be emphasized that, in simple obstruction, laboratory studies do not play a direct role in diagnosis, but aid in understanding the extent of complications such as dehydration, strangulation, and sepsis.

Strangulation obstruction is accompanied by symptoms and signs suggesting peritonitis, large fluid shifts, or systemic toxicity. These symptoms and signs include: abdominal tenderness or involuntary guarding localizing to the area of the strangulated loop of bowel, decreasing urine output, fever, and tachycardia. There have been attempts to use common clinical and laboratory test criteria to identify the likelihood that the obstruction is associated with strangulation. Stewardson et al.[30] observed that the risk of strangulation was low in patients with partial (i.e., incomplete) or complete small bowel obstruction if fever, tachycardia, localized abdominal tenderness, or leukocytosis were not present. These authors suggested that, in a setting consistent with bowel obstruction, any one of these four cardinal signs indicated a small risk for strangulation. The presence of any two of these signs increased the risk of strangulation so high as to warrant immediate surgery. These authorities and others have stressed, however, that when complete obstruction is present, no satisfactory criteria are available to reliably exclude the possibility of strangulation.[30–32]

Different laboratory tests have been advocated for early detection of strangulated intestine. Metabolic (i.e., lactic) acidosis and increases in serum amylase, inorganic phosphate, hexosaminidase, intestinal fatty acid binding protein, and serum D-lactate levels have all been associated with intestinal ischemia.[33,34] Such laboratory abnormalities may be helpful in diagnosing established strangulation in a small group of patients where the diagnosis of necrotic bowel is not clear. However, a noninvasive and rapid test has not yet been developed that can provide information to suggest that tissue necrosis is imminent but not yet established.[35]

Radiographs and Imaging

Plain films

The role of plain abdominal radiographs and imaging studies is to confirm the diagnosis of bowel obstruction, locate the site of obstruction, and gain insight into the lesion responsible for the obstruction. On plain radiographs of the abdomen, the key findings of small bowel obstruction reflect the accumulation of air and fluid proximal and clearance of fluid and air distal to the point of obstruction. Dilated loops of small intestine are defined as those greater than 3 cm in diameter. Free air represents perforation of a viscus and mandates immediate operation. Such findings include: dilated loops of small bowel on the flat plate and multiple air-fluid levels located at different levels on the upright film or lateral decubitus film (Fig. 50.3). Based on these criteria plain abdominal radiography is diagnostic in 67% to 80% of patients.[36,37] In complete obstruction of the small intestine, the colon loops do not contain air. If there is air in the colon, the obstruction may be complete, but early, or it may be incomplete.

In the colon, tight closed-loop obstructions (i.e., volvulus of the cecum, transverse colon, or sigmoid colon) are accompanied by distention of the obstructed segment (Fig. 50.4). The proximal colon is considered dilated when it reaches 8 to 10 cm; the sigmoid colon is considered dilated at 4 to 5 cm. In contrast, obstruction by carcinoma or diverticulitis presents with massive distention of the entire colon from the point of obstruction to the ileocecal valve. From this standpoint, any large bowel obstruction may represent a "closed-loop" as long as the ileocecal valve is competent. Although plain film findings

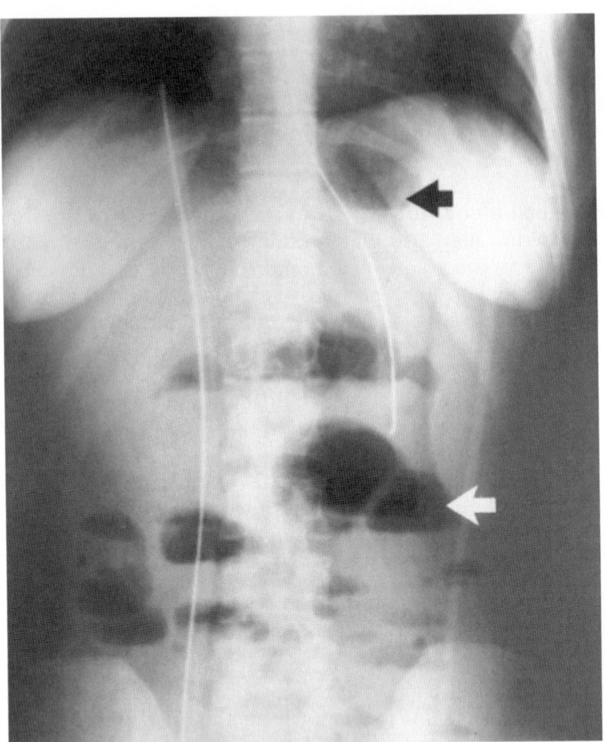

FIGURE 50.3 Plain upright abdominal film of a patient with small intestinal obstruction. Note the air–fluid levels in the stomach (*black arrow*), multiple dilated loops of small intestine (*white arrow*), and absence of air in the colon or rectum.

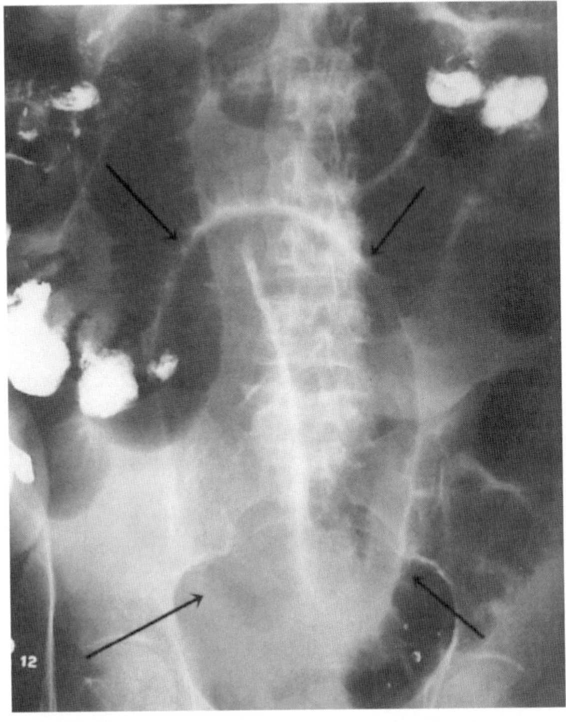

FIGURE 50.4 Plain supine abdominal film of a patient with sigmoid volvulus. The centrally located sigmoid loop is outlined by trapped air. The proximal small intestine is dilated as well, suggesting that the volvulus has been present for sufficient time to cause accumulation of air and fluid proximally. (Courtesy of John Braver, M.D., Department of Radiology, Brigham and Women's Hospital, Harvard Medical School, Boston, MA.)

can be used to differentiate obstruction of the small bowel from that of the large bowel, they are not accurate for localizing the specific site of obstruction.

A number of findings on plain films are highly suggestive of the nature of the offending lesion. These findings will be discussed below in relation to specific causes of intestinal obstruction. One point needs to be stressed, however, and that is the appearance of plain films in the patient with a closed-loop obstruction of the small intestine. Such a loop of bowel may contain fluid and very little gas. Thus, it may not be visible or only barely visible as a minimally dilated "sentinel loop" that remains unchanged in position on films that are performed in different projections. Because such patients generally present early after the onset of symptoms, the loops proximal to the closed-loop will not have had to time to fill with air and the remainder of the abdomen may appear gasless. In the setting of "abdominal pain out of proportion to physical findings," a "normal" plain film does not exclude a closed-loop obstruction.

Contrast studies

The diagnosis of bowel obstruction can generally be made by considering the clinical history, physical examination, laboratory, and plain radiograph findings. Contrast studies (i.e., small bowel follow-through, enteroclysis, contrast enema) may provide specific localization of the point of obstruction and the nature of the underlying lesion. When obstruction of the small intestine is not progressing or resolving, a small bowel follow-through may be performed to confirm the presence and location of the obstruction. Also, even under acute circumstances, diagnosis and management of colonic obstructions are generally enhanced by the use of a contrast enema. Under some circumstances, however, contrast studies are unnecessary and may be contraindicated. For example, in the classic setting of abdominal pain, nausea, vomiting, and a plain film indicating multiple air-fluid levels in the small intestine and colonic collapse, the diagnosis of acute obstruction can be made clinically. Failure to improve in a short period of time will mandate operation and contrast studies are unnecessary. When strangulation or perforations are strongly suspected, contrast studies are contraindicated.

The choice of contrast materials includes water-insoluble suspensions of barium and water-soluble agents such as Gastrografin or Hypaque. Barium studies provide the clearest images, in both small bowel studies where the contrast is given from above and colon/rectum studies in which the contrast is given by enema. If barium leaks into the peritoneum, it elicits intense peritonitis. If there is any possibility of bowel perforation or gangrene, barium should not be used. Water-soluble agents such as sodium amidotrizoate/meglumine amidotrizoate diatrizoate oral solution (Gastrografin) or diatrizoate sodium/diatrizoate meglumine (Hypaque) are hyperosmotic and can elicit fluid translocation into the gut. When the obstruction of the small intestine is incomplete (as discussed later), the use of these agents may facilitate resolution.[38] One small randomized trial, comparing diagnostic and therapeutic use of Gastrografin reduced the need for operation by 74%.[39] Gastrografin is hyperosmolar and causes mobilization of fluid into the bowel lumen and occasionally is therapeutic in cases of incomplete obstruction. In another study, Assalia et al.[38] divided 99 patients including 107 episodes of adhesive partial small bowel obstruction into two groups; conservative management versus administration of 100 mL of Gastrografin via nasogastric tube. The group of patients who received Gastrografin had their first bowel movement, on average, in 6 hours versus 23 hours in the control group. Operative intervention was required in only 10% of the Gastrografin group (six episodes) compared with 21% (10 episodes) in the control group. The mean intervals of hospital stay were 2.2 days and 4.4 days, respectively. The authors suggested that orally administered Gastrografin is safe and therapeutic in adhesive partial small bowel obstruction, though further studies were required to confirm the significance of the reduction in need for an operation.

Computed Tomography and Other Imaging Modalities

The potential benefits of **computed tomography** (CT) scanning in diagnosis of bowel obstruction include the following: [40,41] First, using dilute barium for luminal contrast, the obstructing segment may be localized and characterized as complete or incomplete. Second, the nature of the obstructing lesion, especially if it is malignant, can be established. Third, additional abdominal pathology (e.g., metastases, ascites, parenchymal liver abnormalities) may be identified. There is also evidence that, in special circumstances, CT may improve preoperative detection of strangulation.[42,43]) CT findings indicating the site of obstruction include beaklike narrowing, mesenteric edema, vascular engorgement, moderate to severe intestinal wall thickening (greater than 2 mm). In addition high attenuation of bowel wall on unenhanced CT scans, low or reduced attenuation of bowel wall on intravenous contrast CT scans and presence of intramural air (pneumatosis) or portal venous gas are CT findings suggestive of strangulation. Attenuation reflects increased energy absorption, scattering, beam divergence, and other causes of energy loss. Thus, areas of high attenuation appear darker than areas of low attenuation.

It has also been suggested that real-time abdominal sonography could aid in the diagnosis of strangulation obstruction. Ogata et al.[44] demonstrated that the presence of significant amounts of peritoneal fluid and of an akinetic and dilated loop of bowel were strongly associated with the presence of strangulation. In 15 patients who had strangulation, but were thought to have simple obstruction only, these finding helped to make the preoperative diagnosis of infarction. The role of CT and real-time ultrasound in early detection of strangulation seems promising. Again, it should be emphasized that when the clinical picture suggests strangulation, unnecessary imaging studies should not delay resuscitation or expeditious movement to the operating room. Such studies will not necessarily be helpful when clinical criteria and basic abdominal radiographs have indicated the presence of a simple and complete obstruction. By itself, this diagnosis mandates urgent exploration and the information sought should be weighed against the risk of delay in going to the operating room. In one study, it was suggested that CT improved the diagnosis of strangulation to virtually 100%, compared to about 20% when clinical findings only were utilized.[45] The message of this study was that clinical diagnosis is seldom incorrect—it is highly specific when multiple clinical signs (tenderness, peritoneal signs, leukocytosis, profound dehydration) of strangulation are present. However, such a picture represents advanced disease and use of CT scan may detect strangulation before such signs are manifest. These findings reinforce the dictum that when there are clinical signs of strangulation, surgery should be performed without additional imaging studies. In patients with equivocal findings or uncertain clinical diagnosis, CT can be highly useful in confirming the diagnosis, localizing the site and detecting the cause of intestinal obstruction and strangulation.[46]

General Considerations in Management of the Patient with Bowel Obstruction

Patients with obstruction of the large bowel present with abdominal pain, distention, and obstipation. Vomiting and electrolyte imbalances are sometimes prominent, though usually delayed. Elderly patients, in particular, are prone to dehydration.

TABLE 50.3 DIAGNOSIS

QUESTIONS TO CONSIDER WHEN DIAGNOSING BOWEL OBSTRUCTION

1. Is the pain out of proportion to the physical findings?
2. How rapidly are the symptoms and signs evolving (minutes, hours, or more slowly)?
3. Does the patient suffer from dehydration and serum electrolyte and pH imbalances?
4. Is the obstruction complete or incomplete?
5. Is there a possibility of strangulation?

The presentation of small bowel obstruction depends on level of obstruction, open- or closed-loop nature, and interval since onset of symptoms. Symptoms and signs of pain, vomiting, obstipation, and distention are present in variable degrees. The overall picture, however, is usually one of a patient with abdominal symptoms that are evolving and getting worse. In the settings described previously, the questions in Table 50.3 must be addressed as expeditiously as possible. Clinical data and basic laboratory studies will provide reliable information to answer the first three questions. Answering questions 4 and 5 will often depend on close clinical observation and reexamination in the first hours or days after presentation. Abdominal radiographs and imaging studies are frequently used to provide additional information to help answer these latter questions, as well as providing information to identify the obstructing lesion.

Summarized in Table 50.4 are thumb-nail sketches of different, but typical, kinds of patients presenting with symptoms and signs consistent with bowel obstruction. The principles of diagnosis and management of each of these patients begins with clinical information that indicates the likelihood of a bowel obstruction. Laboratory studies and plain abdominal films are used to confirm the diagnosis of obstruction and determine the extent of physiological impairment. The patient's history and clinical course in the first few hours of observation are used to determine the likelihood of strangulation. Indications for surgery include rapid evolution of symptoms and signs and the diagnosis that the obstruction is complete. Contrast or imaging studies are used only when symptoms are not evolving rapidly and when identification of the underlying lesion might alter the operative strategy (see specific lesions later).

The initial management of all patients with suspected bowel obstruction includes designating the patient "NPO" and starting intravenous fluids comprised of isotonic Ringers or normal saline solutions. Restoration of fluid and electrolyte balance is a priority, often requiring frequent evaluation of serum electrolytes and pH. In rapidly evolving cases or patients with significant dehydration, an indwelling urinary catheter should be placed to monitor urine output. Invasive hemodynamic monitoring (e.g., a Swan-Ganz catheter) may be necessary to monitor the response to fluid resuscitation in patients with underlying cardiac, pulmonary or renal insufficiency. Nasogastric decompression is indicated in most cases. The nasogastric tube, typically a 16- or 18-French sump tube, serves to prevent distal passage of swallowed air and minimizes the discomfort of refluxing intestinal content. The use of longer tubes has been advocated in certain settings, especially for patients with chronic but intermittent

TABLE 50.4 MANAGEMENT

DIAGNOSIS AND MANAGEMENT OF BOWEL OBSTRUCTION IN THREE HYPOTHETICAL PATIENTS

	Patient 1	Patient 2	Patient 3
Clinical	Crampy periumbilical pain worsening over last 12 hours 2 to 3 episodes of emesis. No distension, minimal flatus.	Diffuse, crampy abdominal pain over 2 days with many episodes of vomiting. No bowel movements or flatus. T, 100°F, P, 100, dehydrated. Mild distension; local tenderness lower abdomen.	Progressive abdominal distension over previous 2 weeks. Mild discomfort. No vomiting. Few bowel movements and little flatus. Distension prominent, mild tenderness, no peritoneal findings.
Laboratory	No leukocytosis, no pH or electrolyte disturbances.	WBC 16K, Serum Na^+ Low, K^+ low, Cl^- low, pH alkalotic.	WBC normal, serum electrolytes mildly decreased.
Radiography	Nonspecific gas pattern on plain film.	Multiple dilated loops and air-fluid levels. No gas in colon.	Multiple dilated small bowel loops and air-fluid levels. Some gas and stool in proximal colon.
Differential diagnosis	Broad: includes appendicitis, closed-loop SBO, pancreatitis, nonsurgical conditions.	Narrow: Complete SBO likely, strangulation cannot be excluded.	Narrow: distal small bowel or proximal colon obstruction likely, possibly incomplete.
Initial treatment	Admit with re-evaluation every 3–4 hr by clinical exam, WBC. Repeat films every 8–12 hr. NG tube if vomiting persists. IVFs.	Admit for rapid resuscitation with IVFs, IV antibiotics. Urinary catheter and NG intubation indicated.	Admit for IVFs, NG intubation. Hypaque enema followed by barium to evaluate colon. CT if malignancy suspected.
Indications for surgery	If pain worsens, local tenderness or peritoneal signs evolve, WBC rises, urine output falls.	Already present. Patient should be scheduled and brought to OR after adequate resuscitation (dramatic improvement with resuscitation may permit observation for 4 hr).	Surgery performed when evaluation is complete or if clinical course deteriorates during evaluation.

SBO, small bowel obstruction; WBC, leukocytecount; NG, nasogastric; IVFs, intravenous fluids; T, temperature; P, pulse; IV, intravenous; OR, operating room; CT, computed tomography.

obstruction arising from Crohn disease, peritoneal carcinomatosis, radiation enteritis, or many previous laparotomies for obstruction. The underlying rationale is that advancement of the tip of the long tube to the obstructed loop would permit more effective decompression, perhaps resulting in relaxation of the loop and relief of the obstruction. Although this concept is appealing, no well-designed trials have been performed to support the use of the long tube in such settings.[47]

The use of intravenous antibiotics in the initial management of bowel obstruction should be discussed as well. Clinically, it has been recognized that antibiotics can ameliorate the evolution of symptoms and signs of strangulation in closed-loop obstruction and appendicitis. Studies in humans have demonstrated that, even in simple obstruction, bacteria can translocate across the intestinal mucosa, passing into lymph channels.[48] Further, experimental studies have demonstrated that germ-free animals can survive strangulation obstruction longer than normal animals and that luminal fluid taken from obstructed segments in germ-free animals is much less toxic than fluid taken from normal animals.[49,50] Thus, it is well established that perioperatively administered antibiotics reduce wound infection and abdominal sepsis rates in patients undergoing operation to relieve intestinal obstruction, simple or strangulated. Once the decision has been made to proceed with surgery, broad-spectrum antibiotics, covering gram-negative aerobes and anaerobes should be given. A second-generation cephalosporin or a combination of a first generation cephalosporin and metronidazole is rational practice for perioperative coverage in both simple and strangulation obstruction. Nevertheless, the use of antibiotics in patients who have not yet been committed to operation has not been evaluated systematically. Giving antibiotics to patients who are being observed can obscure the underlying process and, in the end, delay optimal therapy.

The decision to perform abdominal exploration to relieve intestinal obstruction should be made expeditiously, but not in the absence of critical information or before adequate resuscitation. Indications for surgery are given in Table 50.5. It should be emphasized that once a diagnosis of complete obstruction is made, simple or strangulated, the operation should proceed without undue delay. It is reasonable to commit the patient to a period of observation when the diagnosis is uncertain (i.e., there is a possibility of a nonsurgical diagnosis or that the obstruction is not complete). A practical point is that obstruction occurring in a patient without a previous history of laparotomy is not likely to be caused by peritoneal adhesions. This is known as *de novo* obstruction and, whatever the underlying cause, will not usually resolve without operation.

Specific Types of Bowel Obstruction

Chronic Adhesions

Peritoneal adhesions account for more than half of small bowel obstruction cases. Lower abdominal procedures such as appendectomy, hysterectomy, colectomy and abdominoperineal resection are common precursor operations to adhesive obstruction. Adhesions form after any abdominal procedure, however, including cholecystectomy, gastrectomy, and abdominal vascular procedures. In long-term follow-up, about 5% of patients undergoing laparotomy will develop adhesive obstruction; of these, 10% to 30% will suffer from additional episodes.[51] Simple adhesive obstruction is distinguished from most other forms of obstruction by its capacity to resolve without surgical intervention. In recent surveys, up to 80% episodes of small bowel obstruction due to adhesions may resolve nonoperatively.[30,31,38,42,47,52] This observation makes it difficult to distinguish between a complete mechanical obstruction that resolves nonoperatively and a partial obstruction that never was complete. From a practical standpoint, however, the distinction does not matter. The previous history of a laparotomy simply provides a reasonable basis for expectant management of patients in whom it is not yet possible to diagnose a complete obstruction. Ultimately, patients who present with signs and symptoms from bowel obstruction are managed according to the CT findings and clinical course.

The pathobiology of adhesion formation has been the subject of considerable investigation. Histologic examination of chronic adhesions reveals foreign body reaction, usually to talc, starch, lint, intestinal content, or suture. Talc and starch are found less commonly now than previously, because of improvements in techniques of manufacture and sterilization of surgical gloves. Mesothelial cells are the presumed origin of tissue plasminogen activator (TPA). TPA binds fibrin and plasminogen, thereby preventing adhesion formation. Inflammatory cells, including mast cells, appear to be significant in the process that produces adhesions, but the cell biology of their contributions is not yet defined.[53] At present, the most reasonable approach to reducing adhesion formation at the time of the first laparotomy includes meticulous attention to hemostasis, surgical technique, and removal of foreign material from the peritoneal cavity. It is also possible that the use of monofilament sutures for fascial closure and avoidance of closure of the peritoneum as a separate layer may lower the formation of adhesions between viscera and the abdominal wall.[54] Attempts to minimize or prevent adhesion formation have resulted in development of hyaluronic acid–carboxymethylcellulose membrane (Seprafilm, Genzyme, Cambridge, MA). This compound mechanically prevents adhesion formation by physically separating adjoining tissues. It is absorbed by the body in 7 days and thus is present only during the phase of fibrosis, and not as a persistent foreign body. Randomized trials have suggested that this compound prevents, minimizes severity, and decreases density and vascularity of adhesions.[55] Others trials corroborate decreased severity, density, and vascularity of adhesions but not prevention.[56] Seprafilm has been advocated for use in patients in whom a second abdominal procedure is planned or significant adhesions anticipated (e.g., Hartmann's procedure, ileal pouch anal anastomosis with protecting ileostomy, pelvic surgery, gynecologic procedures, and colon surgery) though proposed for all surgeries by the manufacturer.

TABLE 50.5 INDICATIONS/CONTRAINDICATIONS

INDICATIONS FOR SURGERY FOR SUSPECTED BOWEL OBSTRUCTION

- Rapidly progressing abdominal pain or distention, with or without peritoneal findings
- Development of peritoneal findings, fever, diminished urine output, leukocytosis, hyperamylasemia, metabolic acidosis
- Failure of obstructive picture to resolve over 24 to 48 hours, even in the absence of evolving symptoms or peritoneal findings

Early Postoperative Adhesions

Obstruction in the immediate period following abdominal surgery is uncommon but may occur in up to 1% of patients in the 4 weeks following laparotomy. Adhesions are responsible for approximately 90% of such cases and hernias for approximately 7%. Intussusception, abscess, or technical errors may be responsible for the remainder of cases.[57,58] Most cases occur after surgery of the colon, especially abdominoperineal resections, or operations in the lower abdomen. It is rare for upper abdominal surgery to cause such obstructions. A common scenario is that a patient will undergo colectomy uneventfully, pass flatus and have bowel sounds by postoperative day 3. On the fourth

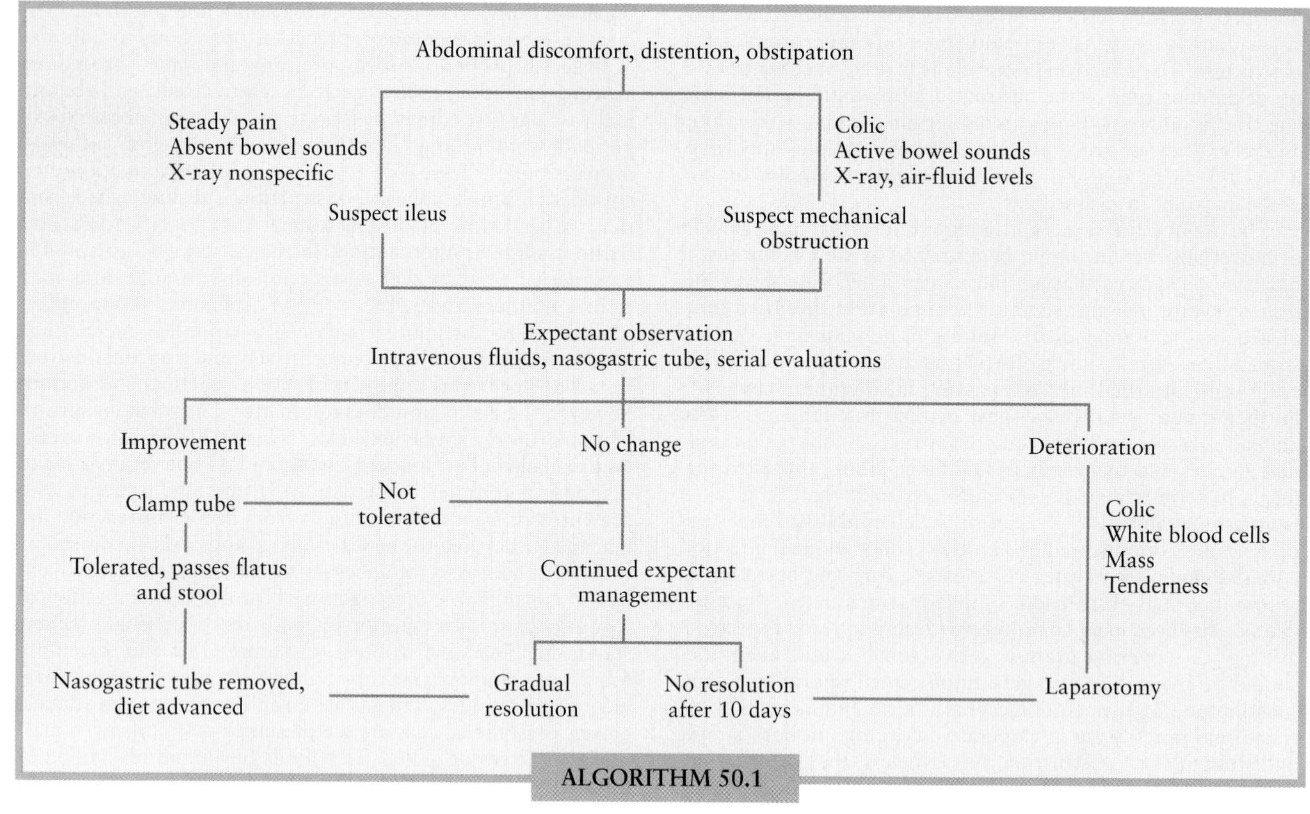

ALGORITHM 50.1 Approach to postoperative intestinal obstruction. (Adapted with permission from Welch JP. *Bowel obstruction: differential diagnosis and clinical management.* Philadelphia: WB Saunders: 1989.)

postoperative day the patient suddenly becomes distended and uncomfortable, and stops passing flatus and stool. Patients with acutely evolving symptoms and signs represent complete obstruction and should be managed as such. In this latter setting, the mortality is may be as high as 15% due to delays in recognition and operative intervention. The loss of bowel sounds after a short period of normal or hyperactive activity is worrisome for ischemia of the obstructed segment. The vast majority of such cases may be treated as partial intestinal obstruction; nasogastric suction and intravenous fluids will help resolve symptoms within a few days (Algorithm 50.1). When the clinical course does not demand earlier intervention, a nonoperative approach may be tried for 10 to 14 days and will resolve the obstruction in over 75% of such cases.[59,60]

Hernia

Hernias of all types are second only to adhesions as the most frequent causes of obstruction in western countries. External hernias such as inguinal or femoral hernias may present with the symptoms of obstruction and will not be diagnosed unless sought. Femoral hernias are particularly prone to incarceration and bowel necrosis due to the small size of the hernia inlet.[56] Other hernias such as umbilical, incisional, paracolostomy, or lumbar hernias are obvious. Still others, such as internal hernias are usually diagnosed at laparotomy for obstruction. These include obturator hernias, paraduodenal hernias (Fig. 50.5), and hernias through the foramen of Winslow or mesenteries. When hernia has been identified as the cause of the obstruction, the patient is quickly resuscitated, given antibiotics, and taken to the operating room. The hernia is then reduced and the viability of the bowel assessed. If viable, the bowel is left alone; if not, it is resected. The hernia defect is then repaired. One important consideration is the Richter's hernia (Fig. 50.6). In this variant, only a portion of the wall of the bowel is incarcerated and thus incarceration and strangulation may not be associated with complete obstruction. These most frequently occur in association with femoral or inguinal hernias. Complete obstruction can occur if more than half of the bowel circumference is incarcerated.

For external hernias, it may be possible to perform *taxis,* that is, the manual reduction of an incarcerated/irreducible hernia. Taxis is usually successful in reduction of an irreducible hernia. Occasionally taxis results in reduction of the contents of the hernia sac *en mass* (still obstructed), reduction of strangulated bowel resulting in generalized peritonitis, or reduction of an obstructed Richter's hernia. This is one reason for using circumspection in relying on taxis as a mode of treatment for incarcerated inguinal, femoral and incisional hernias. In general, taxis should be followed very expeditiously by operative repair.

Gallstone Ileus

As a result of intense inflammation surrounding a gallstone, a fistula may develop between the biliary tree and the small or large intestine. Most fistulae develop between the gallbladder fundus and duodenum. If the stone is greater than 2.5 cm in diameter, it can lodge in the narrowest portion of the terminal ileum, which is just proximal to the ileocecal valve. This complication is rare, accounting for less than 6 in 1000 cases of cholelithiasis and no more than 3% of cases of intestinal obstruction. Typically, the patient is elderly and presents with

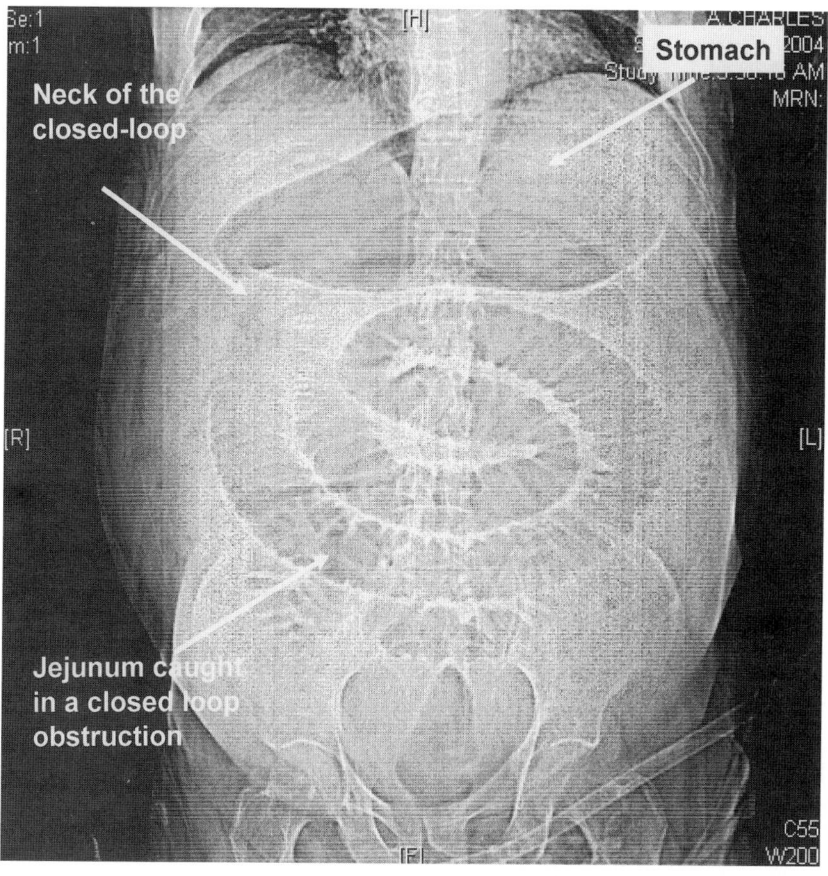

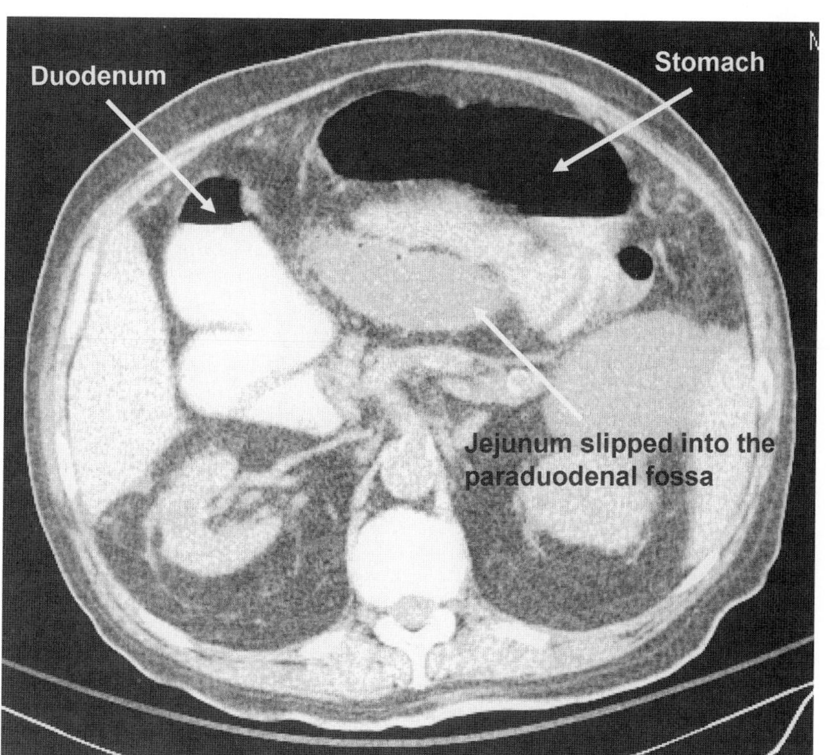

FIGURE 50.5 Paraduodenal hernia. (*A*) Plain film of the closed-loop obstruction with the neck in the right upper abdomen. (*B*) CT scan showing slippage of the jejunum behind the stomach, with dilatation and obstruction of the duodenum as the loop passes behind it. (*C*) Schematic diagram showing relationships of the paraduodenal fossa and transverse mesocolon (Adapted with permission from Skandalakis and Gray. *Embryology for Surgeons,* 2nd edition, Williams and Wilkins, 1994;131–149.)

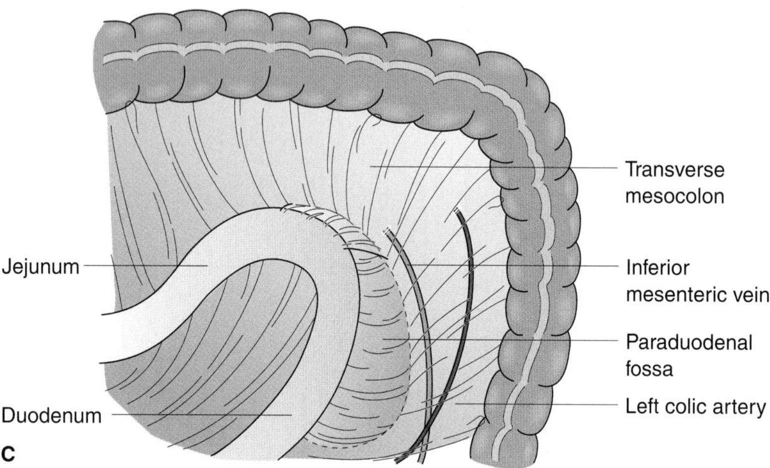

FIGURE 50.5 (*Continued*)

intermittent symptoms over several days, as the stone tumbles distally toward the ileum. The classic findings on plain radiographs include those of intestinal obstruction, a stone lying outside the right upper quadrant, and air in the biliary tree (Fig. 50.7). Treatment includes removal of the stone and resection of the obstructed segment only if there is evidence of tissue necrosis. The risk of a recurrent gallstone ileus is about 5% to 10%.[61] Such recurrences usually occur within 30 days, of the initial episode and are usually due to stones in the small intestine that were missed at the original operation.

The difficult decisions in management of gallstone ileus focus on the fistula. The arguments in favor of disconnecting

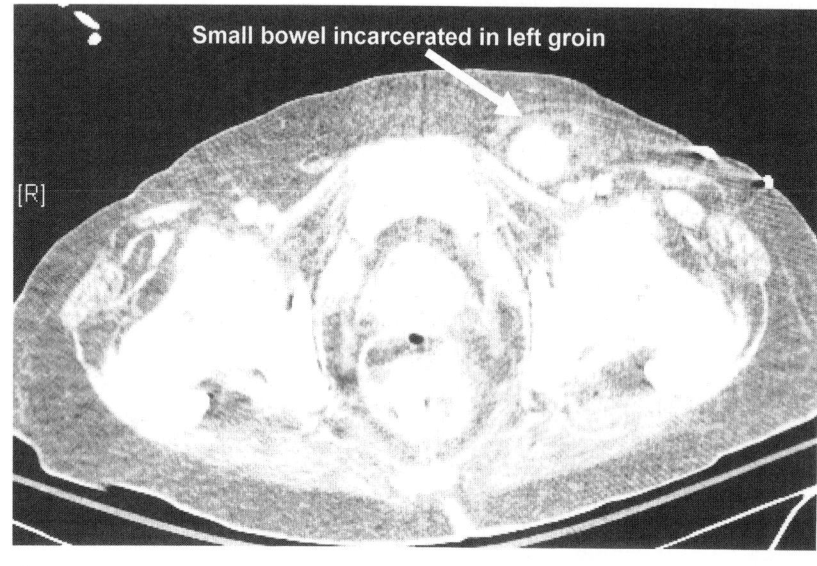

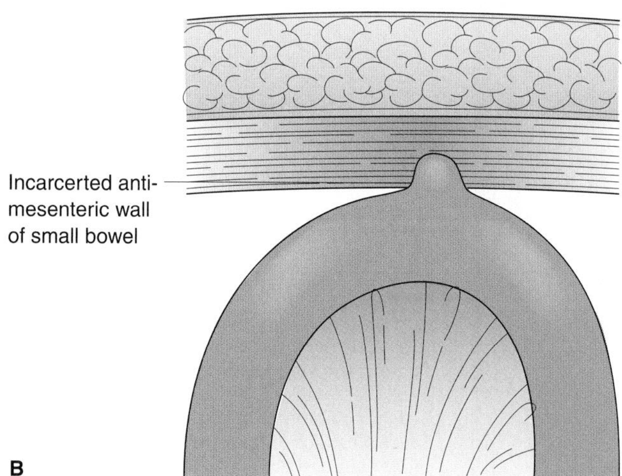

FIGURE 50.6 Richter's hernia. (*A*) CT scan showing contrast and air in the incarcerated segment within the left groin. (*B*) Schematic diagram showing Richter's hernia, in which the antimesenteric border, but not the whole wall, of the bowel is incarcerated.

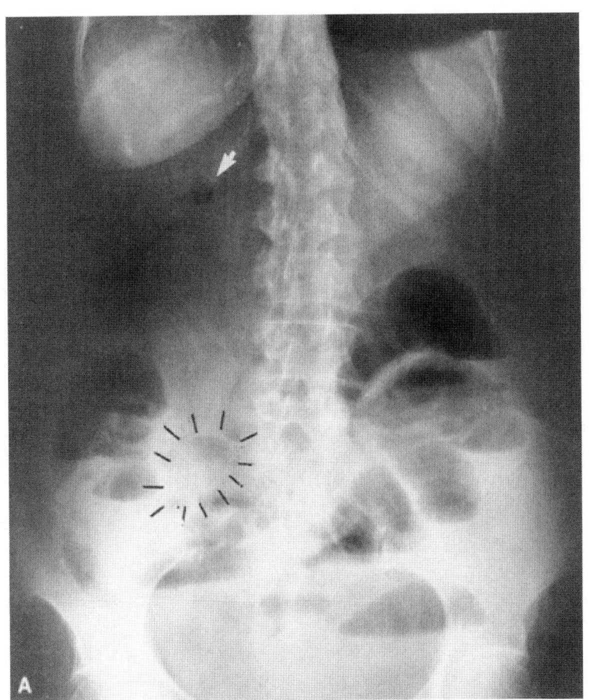

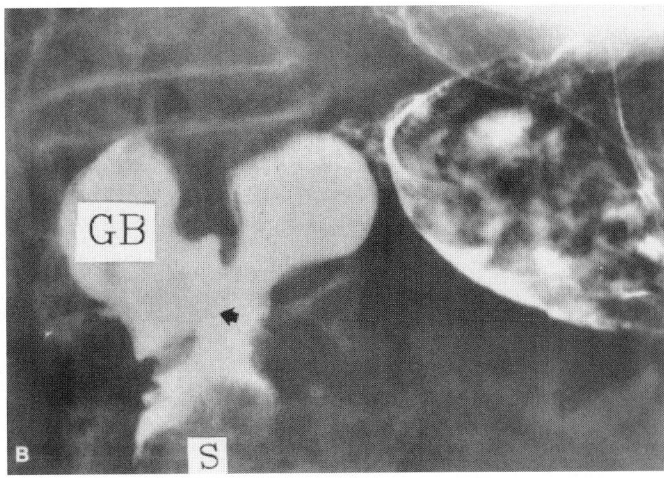

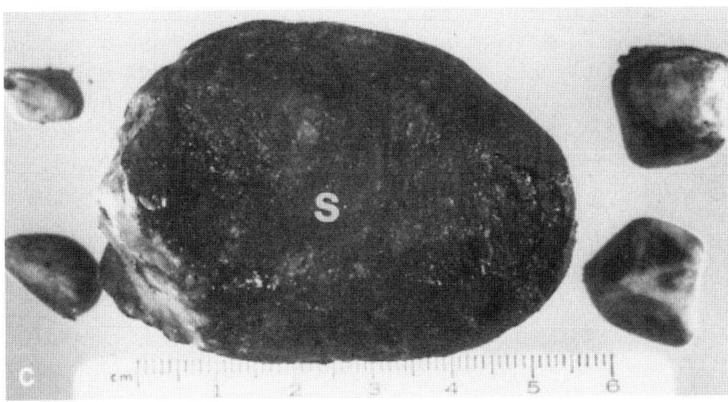

FIGURE 50.7 (*A*) Plain radiograph of a patient with gallstone ileus, showing air in the biliary tree and a gallstone *(highlights)* outside the right upper quadrant. (*B*) Upper gastrointestinal radiograph showing a cholecystoduodenal fistula (*arrow*) with a large stone (S) obstructing the duodenum. (C) Stones recovered from the duodenum and small stones found distally in the small intestine.

the fistula and removing the gallbladder have been the possibility of recurrence of gallstone ileus and the risk of cholangitis due to reflux of intestinal content into the biliary tree. When the latter operation is included, the mortality may be doubled as compared to simple removal of the gallstone. It is used selectively in good-risk patients. The long-term incidence of biliary tract infections has not been common enough to warrant the more aggressive approach at the initial operation. Some authors have advocated cholecystectomy at a second operation, especially if the patient is young and fit. The consensus is that cholecystectomy should not be performed at the initial operation for gallstone ileus, except in highly selected patients. A careful search of the entire intestine should be performed to exclude the possibility of additional large stones.

Intussusception

About 5% of intussusceptions occur in adults. An intussusception occurs when one segment of bowel telescopes into an adjacent segment, resulting in obstruction and ischemic injury to the intussuscepting segment (Fig. 50.8). The obstruction may become complete, particularly if tissue inflammation and necrosis occur. Of adult cases, 90% are associated with pathologic processes. Tumors, benign or malignant, act as the lead point of intussusception in more than 65% of adult cases (Fig. 50.9). A significant proportion of cases have been reported to occur after abdominal surgery for lesions other than neoplasm. In cases not associated with neoplasm, Sarr et al.[62] reported that approximately 20% were related to the suture line, approximately 30% to adhesions, and approximately 60% to intestinal tubes. Intussusception related to long tubes can occur when the tube is withdrawn, but most frequently occurs with the tube in place. Perioperative intussusception frequently subsides without intervention.[62]

Four types of intussusception are recognized: enteric, ileocolic, ileocecal, and colonic. In the ileocolic form, the ileum telescopes into the colon past a fixed ileocecal valve. In the ileocecal form, the valve itself may be the lead point of the intussusception. Radiographic features of intussusception are not specific. Plain films reveal evidence of partial or complete obstruction. Occasionally, a sausage-shaped soft tissue density will be seen, outlined by two strips of air. Recently, in both pediatric and adult cases, it has been suggested that sonography may be useful in diagnosis. Nevertheless, the mainstays of diagnosis are contrast studies or CT scan. Because of the high incidence of tumors, surgery is recommended. Reduction by hydrostatic pressure, which is the standard of care in pediatric cases, is not usually attempted in adults.

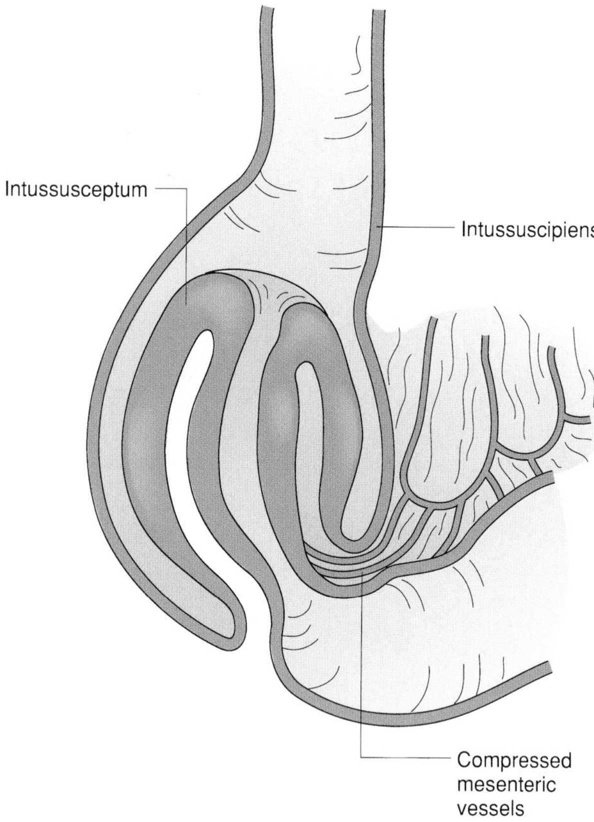

FIGURE 50.8 Anatomy of intussusception. The intussusceptum is the segment of bowel that invaginates into the intussuscipiens.

Crohn Disease

Indications for surgery in Crohn disease are discussed elsewhere in this book. However, it should be noted that intestinal obstruction is the most frequent indication for surgery in patients with Crohn disease.[63,64] In this disease, obstruction occurs under two different sets of circumstances. When the disease has flared acutely, the lumen may be narrowed by a reversible inflammatory process. The result is an open-loop obstruction that may respond, first to intravenous hydration and nasogastric decompression, and ultimately to therapy with corticosteroids or other antiinflammatory regimens. Alternatively, obstruction may occur in the setting of a chronic stricture. Such strictures will not respond to conservative measures and, once diagnosed, operative therapy should not be delayed. One important clinical point is that Crohn-affected bowel may not dilate proximal to the obstruction but can be complicated by a small perforation. Such a microperforation may not be large enough to be associated with free air on plain films. The patient may thus present with significant abdominal pain and tenderness. A CT scan may be most sensitive in providing evidence to differentiate conditions that require immediate surgery (closed-loop obstruction, microperforation) from simple obstruction that would otherwise be observed. In the absence of clinical progression of symptoms and signs, however, extended conservative management is warranted before the patient is committed to surgery.

Malignant Obstruction

Obstruction can complicate malignancies of the small and large bowel in a number of settings. Most commonly, a primary lesion such as an adenocarcinoma or lymphoma will enlarge until the lumen of the intestine is blocked. The lesion then presents with symptoms and signs associated with the level of obstruction and are managed accordingly. A second setting involves a patient who previously has undergone surgery for malignancy and now returns with evidence of bowel obstruction. The likelihood that that the obstruction is due to recurrent disease is based on several factors, including the origin of the primary malignancy and the stage of the primary malignancy and the designation of the original surgery as curative or palliative. Gastric and pancreatic carcinomas often present with or are subsequently complicated by peritoneal carcinomatosis and thus the subsequent obstruction is most likely due to malignancy. With respect to colon and rectal carcinomas, as many as 50% of cases presenting with obstruction after resection of the primary may be due to adhesions and not recurrent malignancy.[65] In addition, even if the obstruction is due to now unresectable disease, significant palliation can be obtained through bypass or enterostomy in up to 75% of patients (Fig. 50.10).

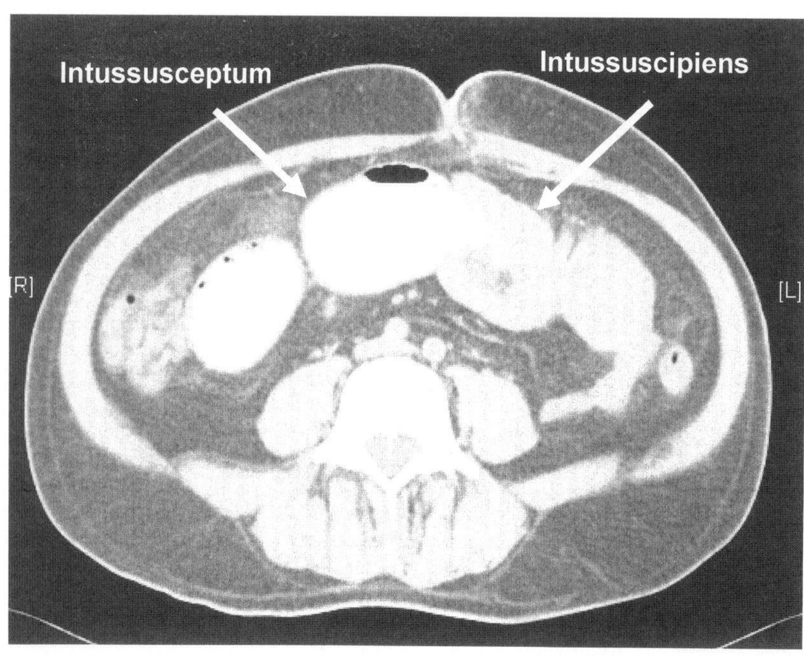

FIGURE 50.9 CT scan showing intussuception of jejunum into jejunum due to metastatic melanoma.

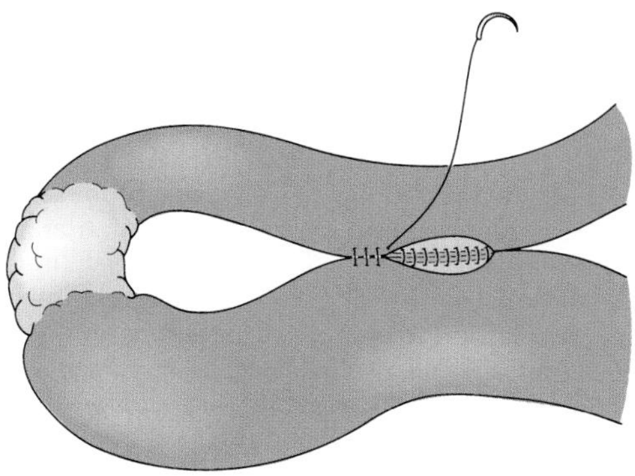

FIGURE 50.10 Significant palliation can be achieved in a patient with obstructing but unresectable malignancy. Enteroenterostomy is performed to bypass the obstructing segment.

Management of incurable malignant obstruction may require an approach that moves away from classical surgical teaching of nil by mouth, nasogastric tube, intravenous fluids, and serial radiographs. Patients with advanced malignant obstruction in the absence of a solitary or correctable obstructing lesion are generally managed without surgery. Patients are managed without a nasogastric tube if possible. They are encouraged to eat as soon as obstructive symptoms resolve using a low-fiber diet. Antiemetics and opioids via continuous subcutaneous infusions are used to manage nausea, vomiting and colic respectively. In addition, octreotide, a somatostatin analogue, is used in palliation of refractory malignant intestinal obstruction by improving intestinal mucosal absorption, improving motility, reducing gastrointestinal hormone levels and intestinal secretions, and having a direct antineoplastic effect on the obstructing tumor.[66,67] This allows true palliative care outside a hospital setting saving patients the pain, discomfort, and complications of hospitalization and unproductive surgery.[68,69]

Volvulus

The term *volvulus* indicates that a loop of bowel is twisted more than 180 degrees about the axis of its mesentery. Volvulus has been reported for the cecum, transverse colon, splenic flexure, and sigmoid colon. A special variant of volvulus, complicating a condition known as *Chiladiti syndrome*, can occur when redundant loops of the transverse colon slip between the liver and diaphragm and then torse.[70] Generally, the condition is asymptomatic, but when associated with volvulus must be relieved surgically. The most common site for volvulus is the sigmoid colon, accounting for 65% of cases.[71] By definition, a volvulus is a form of closed-loop obstruction of the colon. Air is always present in the colon and rectum, and thus volvulus of any segment of the colon is associated with abdominal distention and, usually, severe abdominal pain. As shown in Algorithm 50.1, the most common radiographic features include the "bent inner tube" appearance of the sigmoid, which is located in the upper abdomen. The preferred method of management involves endoscopic decompression. A rigid or flexible proctosigmoidoscope is advanced gently into the rectum until a rush of air and feces indicates that the loop has been untorsed. A rectal tube is then advanced well into the loop as a stent to prevent retorsion. Gangrene of the colon does not usually complicate the picture if the patient is seen and treated promptly. This conservative approach resolves the volvulus in 85% to 90% cases and elective resection or fixation of the redundant segment can then be planned. Following endoscopic decompression, recurrence of the volvulus is higher than 60%.[72] Thus, an operation to remove the sigmoid should be performed if the patient is fit for surgery.[72,73] However, a majority of these patients are elderly and infirm and approximately 15% have a history of psychiatric disorder. As a result, the patient may present with peritoneal findings, sepsis, and shock. In this setting, rapid resuscitation followed by urgent resection and colostomy is warranted. Other forms of volvulus generally cannot be detorsed without operation. Fixation of the torsed segment (e.g., via cecostomy or cecopexy) is generally a less satisfactory solution than resection of the involved segment and is not generally recommended.

Radiation Enteritis

After asymptomatic periods lasting at least 10 years, chronic intestinal obstruction can result. Radiation injury elicits an underlying vasculitis and fibrosis that lead to chronic, recurring low-grade partial obstruction of the small intestine or stricturing and bleeding in the colon and rectum. Operation is indicated for incapacitating symptoms and obstruction not resolved by conservative management. Recurrence of the original tumor as a cause of obstruction should be considered and excluded. However, the diffuse nature of the injury and pathologic responses can lead to massive resections that leave the patient with short-bowel syndrome. Attempts to suture scarred loops can also result in chronic inflammation and formation of interloop abscesses and fistulae. The incidence of suture line leak is high.

Role of Laparoscopy in Management of Small Bowel Obstruction

Since the advent of laparoscopically assisted techniques for general abdominal surgery, a number of investigators have reported the feasibility of laparoscopic approaches to small and large bowel obstruction. Such approaches have been used for lysis of adhesions, enterolithotomy for gallstone ileus, fixation of volvulus segments and so forth. In the initial enthusiasm, laparoscopic approaches to all forms of abdominal surgery has been advocated as a way of reducing formation of adhesions and thus of reducing the long-term risk for adhesive small bowel obstruction. This long-term benefit has not yet been documented.

In anecdotal case reports, bowel obstruction has been observed as a complication of laparoscopic procedures. Specific lesions causing obstruction have included Richter's hernias resulting from entrapment of bowel in trocar entry sites or in unrecognized internal or abdominal wall hernias. The incidence of such complications in large series has not been published but should diminish with improvements in trocar design and operator experience. Obstruction after laparoscopy represents a special circumstance and an exception to the rule that early postoperative obstruction should be managed expectantly. Recent reports confirm that the cause of obstruction is most frequently from incarceration in a port site or internal hernia.[74] This circumstance mandates surgical relief before strangulation occurs.

ILEUS AND PSEUDOOBSTRUCTION

Ileus

Etiologic factors

As noted earlier, ileus reflects underlying alterations in motility of the gastrointestinal tract, leading to functional obstruction. From a practical standpoint, ileus represents the interval between abdominal exploration and return of normal bowel function. Our understanding of the physiology of ileus, however, has been hindered by the insensitivity of techniques for studying gastrointestinal motility and for recognizing the resolution of ileus. Clinically, bowel sounds, passage of flatus, and bowel movements have been used to signal the return of bowel function and coordination of peristalsis. Liquid contrast and radiolabeled marker studies suggest that the effective duration of ileus varies in different regions of the alimentary tract.[75–77] Electromyographic or intraluminal pressure recordings have proved to be reproducible and more objective, but have not necessarily correlated with the ability of the different segments of the bowel to coordinate propulsion of gas and liquid from the stomach to the rectum. When radioactive markers are given orally after laparotomy, it appears that the markers will remain for 12 to 24 hours in the stomach. Although such markers move into the small intestine rapidly and electromyographic activity seem normal by 4 to 6 hours postlaparotomy, the markers may remain in the small intestine for 3 to 5 days before moving to the transverse colon and beyond for defecation.[77] The effective duration of ileus is therefore primarily dependent on the return of colonic motility.

A number of factors have been implicated in development and persistence of ileus (Table 50.6). These factors include sympathetic neuronal hyperactivity and increases in endogenous opioid release and other peptides such calcitonin gene-related peptide, motilin or substance P.[77–80] Peritonitis or spillage of noxious material (acid, bile, stool, blood) is known to delay passage of such markers. Nitric oxide, VIP and substance P have been established as inhibitory neurotransmitters in the intrinsic gut nervous system. Kalff et al.[81]found that nitric oxide synthesis is stimulated in activated macrophages in the muscularis layer of the small intestine following surgical intervention. Activated macrophages were found as early as 3 hours after surgical intervention in muscularis of small bowel studied using immunohistochemistry to identify leukocyte function-associated antigen 1 (LAF-1). LAF-1 mediates cell adhesion and is expressed on activated macrophages that are found in areas of acute and chronic inflammation. Surgical intervention resulted in elevated levels of interleukin-6 (IL-6), cyclooxygenase isoform COX-2, and inducible nitric oxide synthetase (iNOS), all mediators of inflammation. It is likely that such alterations will also be detected in segments of colon. In addition, experimental evidence has demonstrated that antagonists to VIP, substance P and inhibitors of NO synthesis improve postoperative bowel motility.[82,83] Calcitonin gene-related peptide inhibits postoperative gastric emptying and gastrointestinal transit.[78,84] Use of anticholinergic medications and narcotics delays recovery of ileus.[85,86] Opioids are established neurotransmitters in central and peripheral nervous systems, lead to inhibition of gastric emptying and nonpropulsive smooth muscle contraction with an increase in intraluminal pressure throughout the entire gastrointestinal tract.[87,88]

In clinical studies, it appears that the use of intravenously delivered, patient-controlled analgesia, conventional intramuscular administration, and epidural opioid administration may delay recovery of ileus.[87,89] Postoperative epidural analgesia decreases time to recovery from ileus, further improved by providing analgesia without opioids. Also implicated have been solute and electrolyte disturbances such as hypokalemia and hyper or hypocalcemia and magnesemia, uremia, diabetic ketoacidosis, and metabolic conditions such as hypothyroidism. In the current era of laparoscopically assisted general abdominal surgery, it appears that less invasive access and manipulation of the bowel may decrease the interval between operation and the passage of flatus and stool.[90] Laparoscopic surgery reduces the tissue injury and inflammatory response and thus is postulated to reduce duration of postoperative ileus. In colectomy, it has been suggested that laparoscopic approaches are associated with earlier return of gastrointestinal motility, normalization of myoelectric activity and bowel movements in comparison to open colectomy.[91–95] These findings were recently challenged in a study in which open colectomy patients went home after 48 hours with all systems functional.[96] However, there is evidence that the interval to toleration of oral diets may be shorter than previously thought, for patients undergoing laparotomy or laparoscopy,[97] and there may be an inherent bias to feed patients undergoing laparoscopic surgery earlier.[98]

TABLE 50.6 ETIOLOGY

POTENTIAL CONTRIBUTIONS TO PROLONGED ILEUS

NEUROGENIC
Spinal cord lesions or injury
Retroperitoneal process, hematoma, tumor
Ureteral colic

METABOLIC
Hypokalemia
Uremia
Ca^{2+}, Mg^{2+} imbalance
Hypothyroidism
Diabetic coma or ketoacidosis

PHARMACOLOGIC
Anticholinergics
Opiates
Autonomic blockers
Antihistamines
Psychotropics
Phenothiazines
Haloperidol
Tricyclic antidepressants
Clonidine
Vincristine

INFECTIOUS
Systemic sepsis
Pneumonia
Peritonitis
Herpes zoster
Tetanus
Bacterial overgrowth (blind loop)

Diagnosis

Because ileus is a predictable consequence of laparotomy, it is important to distinguish between normal *postoperative ileus* and what some authors have termed *paralytic ileus*. The distinction is predominantly one of time since operation and based on the circumstances. For example, for a patient who has undergone cholecystectomy, the normal period for the ileus should not be more than 48 hours. For the patient who has undergone a low anterior resection of the colon, a period of 3 to 5 days before passage of flatus would not be unexpected. Thus, the absence of bowel sounds, flatus, or bowel movements beyond the expected period indicates delayed resolution.

When the patient's postoperative ileus has extended beyond the expected period, plain films of the abdomen reveals gas in segments of both small and large bowel (Fig. 50.11). At this point, however, the patient may begin to experience some discomfort and distention, as swallowed air fills loops that do not have effective peristalsis. Bowel sounds may be present, if hypoactive. The differential diagnosis now includes the possibility of mechanical obstruction from early postoperative adhesions (see earlier). To differentiate early postoperative

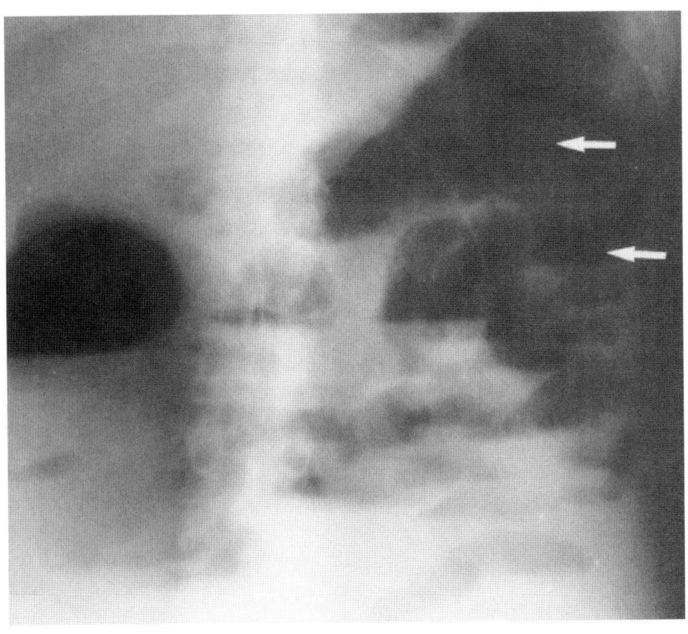

FIGURE 50.11 Plain upright abdominal radiograph of a patient with ileus. Air–fluid levels are present in the stomach and small intestine (*arrows*). Gas is seen in the colon. These findings are characteristic of, but not specific for, ileus.

obstruction from ileus, contrast studies or CT scan are helpful. The latter may be useful if other abdominal pathology such as an abscess could be contributing to the clinical picture. The flow of contrast to the large bowel will exclude the diagnosis of complete small bowel obstruction but does not necessarily exclude a partial obstruction.

Management

The normal postoperative ileus is not necessarily a condition that requires management. Nevertheless, a number of interventions have been advocated for reducing the period of ileus (Table 50.7). Traditionally ileus is managed by not allowing the patient to eat or drink, by maintaining nasogastric suction and supporting hydration with intravenous fluids. In addition correctable conditions such as electrolyte disturbances or uremia are investigated and rectified. Though widely practiced, supportive therapy with nasogastric tube does not reduce time to flatus or time to effective oral intake.[99,100] Randomized trials and meta-analyses have concluded that nasogastric tubes should not be used routinely. Contrary to popular belief, early mobilization and walking does not improve colonic motility or shorten postoperative ileus. Mobilization has other benefits in reducing morbidity.[101,102] Early feeding is thought to stimulate gastrointestinal hormones, secretions and motility, and coordinated propulsive activity. In addition early feeding may improve immune function, reduce infectious and catabolic complications.[103,104] Despite the use of laxatives with prokinetic agents, no controlled trial exists to assess the possible beneficial effects of laxatives on postoperative ileus.[98]

Other treatments such as gum chewing have been tested as simple and inexpensive methods of accelerating return of bowel function. If use of chewing gum is proved to be effective, it may represent forms of sham feeding. Sham feeding stimulating vagal cholinergic pathways that stimulate gastrointestinal hormone secretion like gastrin, pancreatic polypeptide, and neurotensin, all of which effect gastrointestinal motility.[105,106] In one small and underpowered study, gum chewing resulted in earlier passage of flatus and bowel movement in patients undergoing laparoscopic colectomy.[107] This finding will require confirmation but offers the principle that sham feeding and similar strategies may be used to accelerate intestinal recovery.

Salt and water balance in the body also influences bowel motility. In one recent and well-executed study of patients undergoing colectomy, patients receiving a restricted regimen of perioperative fluid resuscitation recovered more quickly than patients who were resuscitated with liberal fluid and salt. The group of patients managed with restricted fluid perioperatively passed flatus and moved their bowels earlier and were discharged earlier from hospital.[108]

Recent experimental studies, have used pharmacologic interventions specifically directed at abnormal release of neurotransmitters or hormones that might prolong ileus. Thus, opioid antagonists, somatostatin analogue, use of sympatholytic methods, injection of local anesthetics into mesenteric nerve roots, or nonsteroidal antiinflammatory agents such as ketorolac appear to promote faster recovery to normal myoelectric activity and intestinal transit times.[78–80,90,109,110] In contrast, nonspecific adrenergic receptor blockers such as propranolol have been found to be ineffective.[111]

Prokinetic agents such as metoclopramide, cisapride (presently not approved by U.S. Food and Drug Administration), and erythromycin have been evaluated for their efficacy in shortening the duration of postoperative ileus. For ileus following upper gastrointestinal procedures (e.g. pancreaticoduodenectomy), such medications may be effective in promoting gastric emptying.[112] For general abdominal procedures involving the small intestine, colon, and retroperitoneal structures such as the aorta, there has been limited success in using such agents to shorten recovery times.[113,114] In multiple controlled studies, metoclopramide did not have significant impact on the duration of ileus.[114,118] In other studies, no benefit was observed when patients were given erythromycin.[113,119] Promising results have been observed with cisapride, which significantly reduced the duration of ileus; results depend on the route of its administration.[120–128] However this medication is no longer approved for use in the United States due to the occurrence of potentially fatal arrhythmias.[129] It is to be hoped that analogous medications can be developed with improved safety profiles.

Perhaps more important than the use of prokinetic agents is the avoidance of agents that hinder motility. Endogenous and exogenous opioids slow gastrointestinal transit through kappa and mu receptors. Their use can be limited perioperatively, using ketorolac as a substitute if it is not contraindicated. Use of nonsteroidal antiinflammatory medications limits use of opioids by 20% to 30%.[130] In addition, in major abdominal surgery, epidural catheters are used for 48 to 72 hours with only

TABLE 50.7 MANAGEMENT

TREATMENT FOR POSTOPERATIVE ILEUS

Treatment	Benefit	Drawback
Nasogastric tube	■ Possible relief of vomiting and bloating	■ Does not shorten duration of ileus ■ May contribute to fever, atelectasis, and aspiration
Early postoperative feeding	■ Stimulates reflex for propulsive bowel motility and enzyme secretion ■ Stimulates immune system ■ Reduces postoperative and posttraumatic infectious complications	■ Data not conclusive ■ Patients may not tolerate feeding
Laparoscopic procedures	■ Earlier return of bowel function and discharge from hospital	■ Not all patients and procedures are amenable to laparoscopic approach
Epidural anesthetics/analgesics	■ Reduced duration of ileus vs. systemic opioid ■ Increases splanchnic blood flow ■ Antiinflammatory	■ Risks associated with epidural catheter placement
Gum chewing	■ May shorten duration of ileus ■ Simple and inexpensive	■ Limited data
Laxatives	■ May shorten duration of ileus ■ Inexpensive	■ Data proving effectiveness lacking
Nonsteroidal anti-inflammatory drugs	■ Decreases opioid needed for pain control ■ May increase motility by acting as an antiinflammatory	■ Possible increased risk of postoperative bleeding ■ Other adverse effects

Adapted from: Table 2 Luckey A, Livingston E, and Tache, Y. Mechanisms and treatment of postoperative ileus. *Arch Surg*, 2003;**138**(2): 206–214.

local anesthetic agents, avoiding opioids. This is beneficial because earlier return of bowel function has been observed in multiple randomized controlled trials.[131–135] Improvement in postoperative ileus may be mediated via blockade of afferent and efferent reflexes, efferent sympathetic blockade with concomitant increase in splanchnic blood flow and antiinflammatory effects mediated via systemic absorption of local anesthetics[134,136–143] Investigational agents, such as kappa receptor agonist (fedotozine) and the mu receptor antagonist (ADL 8-2698), have recently been developed. A randomized trial of ADL 8-2698 was performed in a group of 79 patients undergoing partial colectomy and hysterectomy: use of the drug was associated with improved time to flatus, bowel movement, and shorter hospital stay.[144] In addition, the antagonist methylnaltrexone may reverse the opioid mediated inhibition of gastrointestinal function[145] This agent has not yet been evaluated in the postsurgical setting.

For the present, reasonable measures to prevent prolongation of ileus are given in Table 50.8. Standardization of management within an institution also may play a role, by limiting capricious practice and promoting good communication among health-care providers and discharge coordinators. Clinical pathways evaluating early recovery of bowel function and discharge from hospital in patients undergoing elective colorectal procedures have resulted in satisfactory discharge of patients 48 hours after surgery.[96]

Colonic Pseudoobstruction (Ogilvie Syndrome)

Etiologic Factors

Acute pseudoobstruction of the colon, also known as *Ogilvie syndrome*, is a paralytic ileus of the large bowel, characterized by a rapidly progressive abdominal distention and often without associated pain. Plain radiographs of the abdomen may reveal air in the small bowel and distention of discrete segments of the colon (i.e., cecum or transverse colon) or the entire abdominal colon. Although the distention of the colon is not due to mechanical obstruction, the wall of the bowel, particularly that of the cecum, can become sufficiently distended so that its blood supply is compromised. Gangrene, perforation, peritonitis, and shock can follow. Major risk factors for development of Ogilvie syndrome include severe blunt trauma, orthopedic trauma or procedures, acute cardiac events or coronary bypass surgery, acute neurological events or neurosurgical procedures, and acute metabolic derangements. Only 5% of cases occur in the absence of other conditions. Several lines of evidence suggest that Ogilvie syndrome is related, at least partly, to sympathetic nervous overactivity or interference with sacral parasympathetic efferents. The syndrome usually occurs in hospitalized sick patients over a course of 3 to 7 days, occasionally over 24 to 48 hours, with most patients older than 60 years and 60% male.

TABLE 50.8 MANAGEMENT

MEASURES TO PREVENT PROLONGATION OF ILEUS

- Minimization of trauma to tissues; using proper technique in the operating room
- Minimal use of narcotics for analgesia, for any route of administration (intravenous, intramuscular, epidural)
- Use of nonsteroidal anti-inflammatory agents for analgesia
- Early feeding
- Correction of any electrolyte or metabolic imbalances
- Early recogniton of septic complications (e.g., abdominal abscess, pneumonia, central line sepsis) that may contribute to prolongation beyond the expected period for ileus

Diagnosis

The diagnosis is usually apparent from plain films. In doubtful cases and cases in which bowel necrosis is not a significant worry, a gentle Hypaque contrast enema can establish the nonmechanical nature of the dilatation. Alternatively, colonoscopy can be diagnostic as well as therapeutic. Features suggesting the complication of bowel ischemia include localized tenderness, leukocytosis, metabolic acidosis, evidence of sepsis, or a rapidly deteriorating clinical course.

Management

Initial management includes resuscitation and correction of any underlying metabolic or electrolyte imbalances. A nasogastric tube is helpful if the patient is vomiting and will prevent swallowed air from passing distally. When bowel ischemia is suspected, surgery is indicated. If bowel necrosis is found, the affected segment is resected and an ileostomy or colostomy established. If the bowel is viable, a cecostomy is placed to vent the colon and prevent distention.

If, initially, the distention is painless and the patient shows no signs of toxicity or bowel ischemia, expectant management will be successful in about 50% of cases.[146,147] The risk of spontaneous perforation is approximately 3%, with attendant mortality of 50%.[148] In most patients acute colonic pseudoobstruction will resolve in 3 days.[149] If the distention worsens so that the cecal diameter increases beyond 10 to 12 cm or if it persists for more than 48 hours, intervention is recommended. The duration of distention may be more important than the absolute size of the cecum with respect to spontaneous perforation.[147,150]) Colonoscopy should only be performed by experienced endoscopists. Endoscopic decompression is successful in 60% to 90% of cases,[146,147] but the condition can recur in up to 40%. This rate of recurrence may be decreased by placement of a decompressive tube.[148] Rectal tubes are ineffective as primary modalities in managing distention of the proximal colon. Such tubes may be useful in promoting passage of air and feces after colonoscopy but should not be used as a substitute for colonoscopic decompression.

In anecdotal reports, prokinetic agents such as cisapride and erythromycin have been used to treat Ogilvie syndrome with some success. Also, successful resolution of pseudoobstruction has been reported with sympatholytic agents or spinal sympathetic block. The efficacies of these modalities have not been systematically evaluated. Neostigmine, a parasympathomimmetic, is used in the treatment of acute colonic pseudoobstruction. It acts through nicotinic acetylcholine receptors; has expected cardiovascular side effects such as bradycardia, hypotension, and dizziness; and is excreted via the kidneys. These are a few relative contraindications to its use in treatment of acute colonic pseudoobstruction: a baseline heart rate of less than 60 beats per minute or systolic blood pressure of less than 90 mm Hg; active bronchospasm requiring medication; a history of colon cancer or partial colonic resection; active gastrointestinal bleeding; pregnancy; or a serum creatinine concentration of more than 3 mg/dL (265 μmol/L). Its side effects include increasing airway secretions and bronchospasm, which are reduced by concomitant use of glycopyrrolate without reduction of colonic response.[151] Ponec et al.[152] recommend use of neostigmine prior to colonoscopy, based on its easy administration, lower expense, and superior results in comparison to colonoscopy. Reported rates of response to treatment with neostigmine are 91% (single administration) and 100% (second administration) in a group of 21 randomized patients.[152] Colonoscopy is associated with morbidity of 3% and mortality of 1%.[153] Further study of this combination therapy is warranted. It should be emphasized, however, that patients should undergo immediate exploration if they exhibit signs of clinical deterioration or bowel perforation (peritoneal signs on physical examination or free air on radiographs).

KEY POINTS

- **Peritoneal adhesions account for more than half of small bowel obstruction cases.**
- **The four key symptoms that are associated with acute mechanical bowel obstruction include abdominal pain, vomiting, distention, and obstipation.**
- **In *simple* obstruction the intestinal lumen is partially or completely occluded without compromise of intestinal blood flow. Simple obstructions may be *complete*, meaning that the lumen is totally occluded, or *incomplete*, meaning that the lumen is narrowed but permitting distal passage of some fluid and air. In *strangulation* obstruction, blood flow to the obstructed segment is compromised and tissue necrosis and gangrene are imminent.**
- **Ileus denotes underlying alterations in motility of the gastrointestinal tract, leading to functional obstruction.**

References

1. Treves F. *Intestinal obstruction: its varieties, with their pathology, diagnosis, and treatment.* Philadelphia: H.C. Lea's Son and Co., 1884.
2. Ballantyne GH. The meaning of ileus. Its changing definition over three millennia. *Am J Surg.* 1984;148:252–256.
3. Welch JP. *History.* In: *Bowel obstruction: differential diagnosis and clinical management* Philadelphia: WB Saunders, 1984.
4. Wangensteen OH Paine JR. Treatment of acute intestinal obstruction by suction with a duodenal tube. *JAMA* 1933;101:1532.
5. Paine JR, HA Carlson, OH Wangensteen. Postoperative control of distention, nausea and vomiting; clinical study with reference to employment of narcotics, cathartics, and nasal catheter suction-siphinage. *JAMA* 1933:100.
6. Wangensteen OH, Rea CE. The distention factor in simple intestinal obstruction: an experimental study with exclusion of swallowed air by cervical esophagostomy. *Surgery* 1939;5.
7. Hartwell HJ, Hoguet JP. Experimental intestinal obstruction in dogs with special reference to the cause of death and the treatment by large amounts of normal saline solution. *JAMA* 1912;59.
8. Milamed DR, Hedley-Whyte J. Contributions of the surgical sciences to a reduction of the mortality rate in the United States for the period 1968 to 1988. *Ann Surg.* 1994;219:94–102.
9. Wangensteen OH. *Intestinal obstructions.* Springfield: Charles C Thomas, 1955.
10. Ellis H. *Pathology.* New York: Appleton Crofts, 1982.
11. Roscher R, Oettinger W, Beger HG. Bacterial microflora, endogenous endotoxin, and prostaglandins in small bowel obstruction. *Am J Surg.* 1988;155:348–355.
12. Heneghan JB, Robinson JW, Menge H, et al. Intestinal obstruction in germ-free dogs. *Eur J Clin Invest.*1981;11:285–290.
13. Stark ME, Szurszewski JH. Role of nitric oxide in gastrointestinal and hepatic function and disease. *Gastroenterology.* 1992;103:1928–1949.
14. Caplan MS, Hedlund E, Hill N, et al. The role of endogenous nitric oxide and platelet-activating factor in hypoxia-induced intestinal injury in rats. *Gastroenterology* 1994;106:346–352.
15. Barry MK, Aloisi JD, Pickering SP, et al. Nitric oxide modulates water and electrolyte transport in the ileum. *Ann Surg.* 1994;219:382–388.
16. Kubes P. Nitric oxide modulates epithelial permeability in the feline small intestine. *Am J Physiol.* 1994;262:G1138–1142.
17. Shields R. The absorption and secretion of fluid and electrolytes by the obstructed bowel. *Br J Surg.* 1965;52:774–779.
18. Wright, HK, O'Brien JJ, Tilson MD. Water absorption in experimental closed segment obstruction of the ileum in man. *Am J Surg.* 1971;121:96–99.
19. Sung DT, Williams LF Jr. Intestinal secretion after intravenous fluid infusion in small bowel obstruction. *Am J Surg.* 1971;121:91–95.
20. Ruf W, Suehiro GT, Suehiro A, et al. Intestinal blood flow at various intraluminal pressures in the piglet with closed abdomen. *Ann Surg.* 1980;191:157–163.
21. Ohman U. Studies on small intestinal obstruction. I. Intraluminal pressure in experimental low small bowel obstruction in the cat. *Acta Chir Scand.* 1975;141:413–416.
22. Ohman U. *The effects of luminal distention and obstruction on the intestinal circulation.* New York: Raven Press, 1984.
23. Basson MD, Fielding LP, Bilchik AJ, et al. Does vasoactive intestinal polypeptide mediate the pathophysiology of bowel obstruction? *Am J Surg.* 1989;157:109–115.

24. Enochsson L, Nylander G, Ohman U. Effects of intraluminal pressure on regional blood flow in obstructed and unobstructed small intestines in the rat. *Am J Surg.* 1982;144:558–561.
25. Fondacaro J. *Intestinal blood flow and motility.*, New York: Raven Press, 1984.
26. Frank JW, Sarr MG. Camilleri M. Use of gastroduodenal manometry to differentiate mechanical and functional intestinal obstruction: an analysis of clinical outcome. *Am J Gastroenterol.* 1994;89:339–344.
27. Camilleri M. Jejunal manometry in distal subacute mechanical obstruction: significance of prolonged simultaneous contractions. *Gut* 1989; 30:468–475.
28. Summers RW, Yanda R, Prihoda M, et al. Acute intestinal obstruction: an electromyographic study in dogs. *Gastroenterology.* 1983;85:1301–1306.
29. Eskelinen M, Ikonen J, Lipponen P. Contributions of history-taking, physical examination, and computer assistance to diagnosis of acute small-bowel obstruction. A prospective study of 1333 patients with acute abdominal pain. *Scand J Gastroenterol.* 1994:29;715–721.
30. Stewardson RH, Bombeck CT, Nyhus LM. Critical operative management of small bowel obstruction. *Ann Surg.* 1978;187;189–193.
31. **Sarr MG, Bulkley GB, Zuidema GD. Preoperative recognition of intestinal strangulation obstruction. Prospective evaluation of diagnostic capability. *Am J Surg.* 1983;145:176–182.**
32. Pain JA, Collier DS, Hanka R. Small bowel obstruction: computer-assisted prediction of strangulation at presentation. *Br J Surg.* 1987;74,:981–983.
33. Murray MJ, Barbose JJ, Cobb CF. Serum D(-)-lactate levels as a predictor of acute intestinal ischemia in a rat model. *J Surg Res.* 1993:54;507–509.
34. Gollin G and Marks WH. Early detection of small intestinal ischemia by elevated circulating intestinal fatty acid binding protein (I-FABP). *Surg Forum* 1991:42–44.
35. Kazmierczak SC, Lott JA, Caldwell JH. Acute intestinal infarction or obstruction: search for better laboratory tests in an animal model. *Clin Chem.* 1988:34;281–288.
36. Silen W, Hein MF, Goldman L. Strangulation obstruction of the small intestine. *Arch Surg.* 1962;85:121–129.
37. Maglinte DD, Balthazar EJ, Kelvin FM, et al. The role of radiology in the diagnosis of small-bowel obstruction. *AJR Am J Roentgenol.* 1997; 168:1171–1180.
38. Assalia A, Schein M, Kopelman D, et al. Therapeutic effect of oral Gastrografin in adhesive, partial small-bowel obstruction: a prospective randomized trial. *Surgery* 1994;115:433–437.
39. Choi HK, Chu KW, Law WL. Therapeutic value of Gastrografin in adhesive small bowel obstruction after unsuccessful conservative treatment: a prospective randomized trial. *Ann Surg.* 2002;236:1–6.
40. Balthazar EJ, George W. Holmes Lecture. CT of small bowel obstruction. *AJR Am J Roentgenol* 1994;162:255–261.
41. Frager D, Medwid SW, Baer JW, et al. CT of small-bowel obstruction: value in establishing the diagnosis and determining the degree and cause. *AJR Am J Roentgenol.* 1994;162;37–41.
42. Ha HK, Park CH, Kim SK, et al. CT analysis of intestinal obstruction due to adhesions: early detection of strangulation. *J Comput Assist Tomogr.* 1993;17:386–389.
43. Smerud MJ, Johnson CD, Stephens DH. Diagnosis of bowel infarction: a comparison of plain films and CT scans in 23 cases. *AJR Am J Roentgenol.*1990;154:99–103.
44. Ogata M, Imai S, Hosotani R, et al. Abdominal ultrasonography for the diagnosis of strangulation in small bowel obstruction. *Br J Surg.* 1994;81: 421–424.
45. Donckier V, Closset J, Van Gansbeke D, et al. Contribution of computed tomography to decision making in the management of adhesive small bowel obstruction. *Br J Surg.* 1998;85:1071–1074.
46. **Peck PJ, Milleson T, Phelan J. The role of computed tomography with contrast and small bowel follow-through in management of small bowel obstruction. *Am J Surg.* 1999;177: 375–378.**
47. Brolin RE, Krasna MJ, Mast BA. Use of tubes and radiographs in the management of small bowel obstruction. *Ann Surg.* 1987;206:126–133.
48. Deitch EA. Simple intestinal obstruction causes bacterial translocation in man. *Arch Surg.* 1989;124:699–701.
49. Cohn I Jr, Floyd C E, Dresden C F, et al. Strangulation obstruction in germfree animals. *Ann Surg.* 1962;156:692–702.
50. Amundsen E, Gustafsson BE. Results of experimental intestinal strangulation obstruction in germfree rats. *J Exp Med.* 1963;117:823–832.
51. Landercasper J, Cogbill TH, Merry WH, et al. Long-term outcome after hospitalization for small-bowel obstruction. *Arch Surg.* 1993;128:765–771.
52. Krebs HB, Goplerud DR. Mechanical intestinal obstruction in patients with gynecologic disease: a review of 368 patients. *Am J Obstet Gynecol.* 1987;157:577–583.
53. Liebman SM, Langer JC, Marshall JS, et al. Role of mast cells in peritoneal adhesion formation. *Am J Surg. 1993;*165:127–130.
54. O'Leary DP, Coakley JB. The influence of suturing and sepsis on the development of postoperative peritoneal adhesions. *Ann R Coll Surg Engl.* 1992;74:134–137.
55. Beck DE. The role of Seprafilm bioresorbable membrane in adhesion prevention. *Eur J Surg* 1997(suppl);577:49–55.
56. Vrijland WW, Tseng LN, Eijkman HJ, et al. Fewer intraperitoneal adhesions with use of hyaluronic acid-carboxymethylcellulose membrane: a randomized clinical trial. *Ann Surg.* 2002; 235:193–199.
57. Stewart RM, Page CP, Brender J, et al. The incidence and risk of early postoperative small bowel obstruction. A cohort study. *Am J Surg. 1987;*154: 643–647.
58. Coletti L, Bossart P. Intestinal obstruction during the early postoperative period. *Arch Surg.* 1964; 88:774–778.
59. Pickleman J, Lee RM. The management of patients with suspected early postoperative small bowel obstruction. *Ann Surg.* 1989*;* 210:216–219.
60. Seror D, Feigin E, Szold A, et al. How conservatively can postoperative small bowel obstruction be treated? *Am J Surg.* 1993;165:121–125; discussion 125–126.
61. Reisner RM, Cohen JR. Gallstone ileus: a review of 1001 reported cases. *Am Surg.* 1994; 60:441–446.
62. Sarr MG, Nagorney DM, McIlrath DC. Postoperative intussusception in the adult: a previously unrecognized entity? *Arch Surg.* 1981; 116:144–148.
63. Mekhjian HS, Switz DM, Watts HD, et al. National Cooperative Crohn's Disease Study: factors determining recurrence of Crohn's disease after surgery. *Gastroenterology 1979;*77:907–913.
64. Farmer RG, Whelan G, Fazio VW. Long-term follow-up of patients with Crohn's disease. Relationship between the clinical pattern and prognosis. *Gastroenterology.* 1985;88:1818–1825.
65. Soybel DL Bliss DP Jr, Wells SA Jr. Colon and rectal carcinoma. *Curr Probl Cancer* 1987;11:257–356.
66. Pandha HS, Waxman J. Octreotide in malignant intestinal obstruction. *Anticancer Drugs* 1996;7(suppl 1):5–10.
67. Khoo D. Hall E, Motson R, et al. Palliation of malignant intestinal obstruction using octreotide. *Eur J Cancer* 1994;30A:28–30.
68. Isbister WH, Elder P, Symons L. (1990) Non-operative management of malignant intestinal obstruction. *J R Coll Surg Edin.* 1990;B35;369–372.
69. Hardy JR. Medical management of bowel obstruction. *Br J Surg.* 2000;87:1281–1283.
70. Orangio GR., Fazio VW, Winkelman E, et. al. The Chilaiditi syndrome and associated volvulus of the transverse colon. An indication for surgical therapy. *Dis Colon Rectum* 1986;29:653–656.
71. Gibney EJ. Volvulus of the sigmoid colon. *Surg Gynecol Obstet.* 1991;173:243–255.
72. Wertkin MG, Aufses AH Jr. Management of volvulus of the colon. *Dis Colon Rectum* 1978;21:40–45.
73. Peoples JB, McCafferty JC, Scher KS. Operative therapy for sigmoid volvulus. Identification of risk factors affecting outcome. *Dis Colon Rectum* 1990;33:643–646.
74. **Sajja SB, Schein M. Early postoperative small bowel obstruction. *Br J Surg.* 2004;91:683–691.**
75. Waldhausen JH, Shaffrey ME, Skenderis BS 2nd, et al. Gastrointestinal myoelectric and clinical patterns of recovery after laparotomy. *Ann Surg.* 1990;211:777–784; discussion 785.
76. Condon RE, Cowles VE, Ferraz AA, et al. Human colonic smooth muscle electrical activity during and after recovery from postoperative ileus. *Am J Physiol.* 1995;269:G408–417.
77. Nadrowski L. Paralytic ileus: recent advances in pathophysiology and treatment. *Curr Surg.* 1983;40:260–273.
78. Zittel TT, Reddy SN, Plourde V, et al. Role of spinal afferents and calcitonin gene-related peptide in the postoperative gastric ileus in anesthetized rats. *Ann Surg.* 1994;219:79–87.
79. Riviere PJ, Pascaud X, Chevalier E, et al. Fedotozine reverses ileus induced by surgery or peritonitis: action at peripheral kappa-opioid receptors. *Gastroenterology* 1993;104:724–731.
80. Cullen JJ, Eagon JC, Kelly KA. Gastrointestinal peptide hormones during postoperative ileus. Effect of octreotide. *Dig Dis Sci.* 1994;39:1179–1184.
81. Kalff JC, Turler A, Schwarz NT, et al. Intra-abdominal activation of a local inflammatory response within the human muscularis externa during laparotomy. *Ann Surg.* 2003;237:301–315.
82. Espat NJ, Cheng G, Kelley MC, et al. Vasoactive intestinal peptide and substance P receptor antagonists improve postoperative ileus. *J Surg Res.*1993;58:719–723.
83. De Winter BY, Robberecht P, Boeckxstaens GE, et al. Role of VIP1/PACAP receptors in postoperative ileus in rats. *Br J Pharmacol.* 1998;124:1181–1186.
84. Zittel TT, Lloyd KC, Rothenhofer I, et al. Calcitonin gene-related peptide and spinal afferents partly mediate postoperative colonic ileus in the rat. *Surgery* 1998;123:518–527.
85. Frantzides CT, Cowles V, Salaymeh B, et al. Morphine effects on human colonic myoelectric activity in the postoperative period. *Am J Surg.* 1992;163:144–148; discussion 148–149.
86. Stanley BK, Noble MJ, Gilliland C, et al. Comparison of patient-controlled analgesia versus intramuscular narcotics in resolution of postoperative ileus after radical retropubic prostatectomy. *J Urol.* 1993;150:1434–1436.
87. Thorn SE, Wattwil M, Lindberg G, et al. Systemic and central effects of morphine on gastroduodenal motility. *Acta Anaesthesiol Scand.* 1996;40:177–186.
88. Ferraz AA, Cowles VE, Condon RE, et al. Opioid and nonopioid analgesic drug effects on colon contractions in monkeys. *Dig Dis Sci.* 1995*;*40:1417–1419.
89. Petros JG, Realica R, Ahmad S, et al. Patient-controlled analgesia and prolonged ileus after uncomplicated colectomy. *Am J Surg.* 1995;170:371–374.
90. Garcia-Caballero M, Vara-Thorbeck C. The evolution of postoperative ileus after laparoscopic cholecystectomy. A comparative study with conventional cholecystectomy and sympathetic blockade treatment. *Surg Endosc.* 1993;7:416–419.

91. Bohm B, Milsom JW, Fazio VW. Postoperative intestinal motility following conventional and laparoscopic intestinal surgery. *Arch Surg.* 1995;130:415–419.
92. Davies W, Kollmorgen CF, Tu QM, et al. Laparoscopic colectomy shortens postoperative ileus in a canine model. *Surgery.* 1997;121:550–555.
93. Lacy AM, Garcia-Valdecasas JC, Pique JM, et al. Short-term outcome analysis of a randomized study comparing laparoscopic vs open colectomy for colon cancer. *Surg Endosc.* 1995;9:1101–1105.
94. Schwenk W, Bohm B, Haase O, et al. Laparoscopic versus conventional colorectal resection: a prospective randomised study of postoperative ileus and early postoperative feeding. *Langenbecks Arch Surg.* 1998;383:49–55.
95. Milsom JW, Bohm B, Hammerhofer KA, et al. A prospective, randomized trial comparing laparoscopic versus conventional techniques in colorectal cancer surgery: a preliminary report. *J Am Coll Surg.* 1998;187:46–54; discussion 54–45
96. Basse L, Hjort Jakobsen D, Billesbolle P, et al. A clinical pathway to accelerate recovery after colonic resection. *Ann Surg.* 2000;232:51–57.
97. Binderow SR, Cohen SM, Wexner SD, et al. Must early postoperative oral intake be limited to laparoscopy? *Dis Colon Rectum.* 1994;37:584–589.
98. Holte K, Kehlet H. Postoperative ileus: a preventable event. *Br J Surg.* 2000; 87:1480–1493.
99. Sagar PM, Kruegener G, MacFie J. Nasogastric intubation and elective abdominal surgery. *Br J Surg. 1992;*79:1127–1131.
100. Cheatham ML, Chapman WC, Key SP, et al. A meta-analysis of selective versus routine nasogastric decompression after elective laparotomy. *Ann Surg.* 1995;221:469–476; discussion 476–468.
101. Rao SS, Beaty J, Chamberlain M, et al. Effects of acute graded exercise on human colonic motility. *Am J Physiol.* 1999;276: 1221–1226.
102. Waldhausen JH, Schirmer BD. The effect of ambulation on recovery from postoperative ileus. *Ann Surg.* 1990;212:671–677.
103. Moore FA, Feliciano DV, Andrassy RJ, et al. Early enteral feeding, compared with parenteral, reduces postoperative septic complications. The results of a meta-analysis. *Ann Surg.* 1992;216:172–183.
104. Kehlet H. Multimodal approach to control postoperative pathophysiology and rehabilitation. *Br J Anaesth.* 1997;78:606–617.
105. Soffer EE, Adrian TE. Effect of meal composition and sham feeding on duodenojejunal motility in humans. *Dig Dis Sci.* 1992;37:1009–1014.
106. Katschinski M, Dahmen G, Reinshagen M, et al. Cephalic stimulation of gastrointestinal secretory and motor responses in humans. *Gastroenterology* 1992;103:383–391.
107. Asao T, Kuwano H, Nakamura J, et al. Gum chewing enhances early recovery from postoperative ileus after laparoscopic colectomy. *J Am Coll Surg.* 2002;195:30–32.
108. Lobo DN, Bostock KA, Neal KR, et al. Effect of salt and water balance on recovery of gastrointestinal function after elective colonic resection: a randomised controlled trial. *Lancet* 2002;359:1812–1818.
109. Kelley MC, Hocking MP, Marchand SD, et al. Ketorolac prevents postoperative small intestinal ileus in rats. *Am J Surg.* 1993;165, 107–111; discussion 112.
110. Cullen JJ, Eagon JC, Dozois EJ, et al. Treatment of acute postoperative ileus with octreotide. *Am J Surg.* 1993;165:113–119; discussion 119–120.
111. Ferraz AA, Wanderley GJ, Santos MA, et al. Effects of propranolol on human postoperative ileus. *Dig Surg.* 2001;18:305–310.
112. Yeo CJ, Barry MK, Sauter PK, et al. Erythromycin accelerates gastric emptying after pancreaticoduodenectomy. A prospective, randomized, placebo-controlled trial. *Ann Surg.* 1993; 218:229–237; discussion 237–238.
113. Bonacini M, Quiason S, Reynolds M, et al. Effect of intravenous erythromycin on postoperative ileus. *Am J Gastroenterol.* 1993;88:208–211.
114. Cheape JD, Wexner SD, James K, et al. Does metoclopramide reduce the length of ileus after colorectal surgery? A prospective randomized trial. *Dis Colon Rectum* 1991;34:437–441.
115. Breivik H, Lind B. Anti-emetic and propulsive peristaltic properties of metoclopramide. *Br J Anaesth.* 1971;43:400–403.
116. Jepsen S, Klaerke A, Nielsen PH, et al. Negative effect of Metoclopramide in postoperative adynamic ileus. A prospective, randomized, double blind study. *Br J Surg.* 1986;73:290–291.
117. Davidson ED, Hersh T, Brinner RA, et al. The effects of metoclopramide on postoperative ileus. A randomized double-blind study. *Ann Surg.* 1979;190:27–30.
118. Kivalo I, Miettinen K. The effects of metoclopramide on postoperative nausea and bowel function. *Ann Chir Gynaecol Fenn.* 1970;59:155–158.
119. Smith AJ, Nissan A, Lanouette NM, et al. Prokinetic effect of erythromycin after colorectal surgery: randomized, placebo-controlled, double-blind study. *Dis Colon Rectum.* 2000;43:333–337.
120. Tollesson PO, Cassuto J, Rimback G. Treatment of postoperative paralytic ileus with cisapride. *Scand J Gastroenterol.* 1991;26:477–482.
121. Cheng G, Cassissi C, Drexler PG, et al. Salsalate, morphine, and postoperative ileus. *Am J Surg.* 1996;171:85–88; discussion 88–89.
122. Ferraz AA, Cowles VE, Condon RE, et al. Nonopioid analgesics shorten the duration of postoperative ileus. *Am Surg.* 1995;61:1079–1083.
123. Fanning J, Yu-Brekke S. Prospective trial of aggressive postoperative bowel stimulation following radical hysterectomy. *Gynecol Oncol.* 1999;73:412–414.
124. Ruwart MJ, Klepper MS, Rush BD. Mechanism of stimulation of gastrointestinal propulsion in postoperative ileus rats by 16,16-dimethyl PGE2. *Adv Prostaglandin Thromboxane Res.* 1980;8:1603–1607.
125. Heimbach DM, Crout JR. Treatment of paralytic ileus with adrenergic neuronal blocking drugs. *Surgery* 1971;69:582–587.
126. Furness JB, Costa M. Adynamic ileus, its pathogenesis and treatment. *Med Biol.* 1974;52:82–89.
127. Kleinfeld D. Edrophonium used for vagotonic action. *JAMA.* 1974;223: 922–923.
128. Kreis ME, Kasparek M, Zittel TT, et al. Neostigmine increases postoperative colonic motility in patients undergoing colorectal surgery. *Surgery* 2001;130:449–456.
129. Tonini M, De Ponti F, Di Nucci A. Review article: cardiac adverse effects of gastrointestinal prokinetics. *Aliment Pharmacol Ther.* 1999;13:1585–1591
130. Merry BPW. Perioperative NSAIDs: Towards greater safety. *Pain Reviews.* 1974;2:268–291.
131. Gelman S, Feigenberg Z, Dintzman M. Electroenterography after cholecystectomy. The role of high epidural analgesia. *Arch Surg.* 1977;112: 580–583.
132. Seeling W, Bruckmooser KP, Hufner C, et al. [No reduction in postoperative complications by the use of catheterized epidural analgesia following major abdominal surgery]. *Anaesthesist* 1990;39:33–40.
133. Jayr C, Thomas H, Rey A, et al. Postoperative pulmonary complications. Epidural analgesia using bupivacaine and opioids versus parenteral opioids. *Anesthesiology.* 1993;78:666–676; discussion 622A.
134. Liu SS, Carpenter RL, Mackey DC, et al. Effects of perioperative analgesic technique on rate of recovery after colon surgery. *Anesthesiology* 1995; 83:757–765.
135. de Leon-Casasola OA, Karabella D, Lema MJ. Bowel function recovery after radical hysterectomies: thoracic epidural bupivacaine-morphine versus intravenous patient-controlled analgesia with morphine: a pilot study. *J Clin Anesth. 1996;*8:87–92.
136. Wallin G, Cassuto J, Hogstrom S, et al. Failure of epidural anesthesia to prevent postoperative paralytic ileus. *Anesthesiology* 1986;65:292–297.
137. Scheinin B, Asantila R, Orko R. The effect of bupivacaine and morphine on pain and bowel function after colonic surgery. *Acta Anaesthesiol Scand.* 1987;31:161–164.
138. Ahn H, Bronge A, Johansson K, et al. Effect of continuous postoperative epidural analgesia on intestinal motility. *Br J Surg. 1988;*75:1176–1178.
139. Wattwil M, Thoren T, Hennerdal S, et al. Epidural analgesia with bupivacaine reduces postoperative paralytic ileus after hysterectomy. *Anesth Analg.* 1989;68:353–358.
140. Bredtmann, RD, Herden HN, Teichmann W, et al. Epidural analgesia in colonic surgery: results of a randomized prospective study. *Br J Surg.* 1990;77:638–642.
141. Neudecker J, Schwenk W, Junghans T, et al. Randomized controlled trial to examine the influence of thoracic epidural analgesia on postoperative ileus after laparoscopic sigmoid resection. *Br J Surg.* 1990;86:1292–1295.
142. Thoren T, Sundberg A, Wattwil M, et al. Effects of epidural bupivacaine and epidural morphine on bowel function and pain after hysterectomy. *Acta Anaesthesiol Scand. 1989;*33:181–185.
143. Asantila R, Eklund P, Rosenberg PH. Continuous epidural infusion of bupivacaine and morphine for postoperative analgesia after hysterectomy. *Acta Anaesthesiol Scand.* 1991;35:513–517.
144. Taguchi A, Sharma N, Saleem RM, et al. Selective postoperative inhibition of gastrointestinal opioid receptors. *N Engl J Med.* 2001;345:935–940.
145. Yuan CS, Foss JF, O'Connor M, et al. Methylnaltrexone for reversal of constipation due to chronic methadone use: a randomized controlled trial. *JAMA* 2000;283:367–372.
146. Love R, Starling JR, Sollinger HW, Colonoscopic decompression for acute colonic pseudo-obstruction (Ogilvie's syndrome) in transplant recipients. *Gastrointest Endosc.* 1988;34:426–429.
147. Strodel WE, Nostrant TT, Eckhauser FE, et al. Therapeutic and diagnostic colonoscopy in nonobstructive colonic dilatation. *Ann Surg.* 1983; 197:416–421.
148. Rex DK. Colonoscopy and acute colonic pseudo-obstruction. *Gastrointest Endosc Clin N Am.* 1977;7:499–508.
149. Sloyer AF, Panella VS, Demas BE, et al. Ogilvie's syndrome. Successful management without colonoscopy. *Dig Dis Sci.* 1988;33:1391–1396.
150. Vanek VW, Al-Salti M. Acute pseudo-obstruction of the colon (Ogilvie's syndrome). An analysis of 400 cases. *Dis Colon Rectum* 1986;29:203–210.
151. Child CS. Prevention of neostigmine-induced colonic activity. A comparison of atropine and glycopyrronium. *Anaesthesia* 1984;39;1083–1085.
152. Ponec RJ, Saunders MD, Kimmey MB. Neostigmine for the treatment of acute colonic pseudo-obstruction. *N Engl J Med.* 1999;341:137–141.
153. Vantrappen G. Acute colonic pseudo-obstruction. *Lancet* 1993;341:152–153.

CHAPTER 51 ■ CROHN DISEASE

FABRIZIO MICHELASSI, ROGER D. HURST, AND ALESSANDRO FICHERA

Crohn disease is a chronic intestinal disorder of unknown etiology. Although Crohn disease can present at any age, the peak incidence is in the third decade of life. Originally Crohn disease was described as a chronic granulomatous inflammatory condition limited to the terminal ileum. It later became clear that it can involve any part of the gastrointestinal tract and cause varying symptoms and complications. Medical treatment is administered with the intent of alleviating symptoms and improving the patient's quality of life. Surgical treatment becomes necessary when medical treatment fails or when complications of the underlying disease develop. The surgical options vary according to the location and the extent of the disease and the nature of the complications. The optimal management of Crohn disease requires an understanding of the pathologic characteristics of this entity in addition to the indications for medical and surgical treatment.

EPIDEMIOLOGY

Crohn disease was first identified as a unique clinical entity in 1932.[1] Since the original description, the number of reported cases has increased greatly, and Crohn disease is no longer seen as a rare disorder, although it remains relatively uncommon.[2,3] Precise trends in incidence have been difficult to determine because of limited population-derived epidemiologic data. The first population-based studies were not undertaken until the 1960s. The best available data indicate that within the Western world, the incidence of Crohn disease increased rapidly through the 1980s. More recently, the incidence of Crohn disease appears to have stabilized, with no increase noted during the past 15 years. In the United States, the incidence of Crohn disease currently approximates four new cases per 100,000 population per year. Because Crohn disease is chronic and patients typically live many decades with the disease, the prevalence is much higher than the incidence and is estimated to be between 40 and 160 cases per 100,000 population.[2] It is estimated that approximately 600,000 persons in the United States suffer from Crohn disease.

Crohn disease is most common in North America and Europe. It is seldom seen in Asia, South America, or Japan. Few data are available regarding the incidence of Crohn disease in Africa, but it is also thought to be rare in this part of the world. It has been observed in immigrants from areas with a low incidence of Crohn disease who immigrate to countries where the incidence is higher; their risk for Crohn disease increases to the level of the native population in the new residence. This observation suggests that environmental factors influence the pathogenesis of the disease. Crohn disease appears to be slightly more common in women than in men. The onset occurs most commonly between the ages of 15 and 25 years, with a second, much smaller peak between ages 55 and 65 years of age. Crohn disease is very uncommon in children younger than age 6 years.

Within the United States population the incidence of Crohn disease is highest among whites, lower among blacks, and lowest among Asians. The disease is three to four times more common among ethnic Jews than in non-Jewish whites. This increased risk is greater for Ashkenazi Jews of European descent than for Sephardic Jews of North African or Asian origin. It has been reported that Crohn disease is more common among persons of higher socioeconomic status, although several contradicting epidemiologic studies indicate that there is no predilection of Crohn disease for the affluent or well educated.

Familial clusters of disease have been observed, with a sixfold to 10-fold increase in the risk for Crohn disease in first-order relatives of patients affected by the disorder. Although familial aggregations are common, distributions within families do not indicate a pattern of Mendelian inheritance.

ETIOLOGY AND PATHOGENESIS

The etiology of Crohn disease is not known, and the possible causes for the disease have been the subject of many theories and much speculation.[4] In the past decade, basic scientific research has advanced understanding of the pathophysiology of Crohn disease, but the ultimate cause of this disease remains elusive.[2,5]

An altered immune response contributes to the pathogenesis of Crohn disease. Although no specific primary defect in the systemic or mucosal immune systems has been identified, various immunologic alterations have been described. Lymphocytes within the lamina propria are substantially increased in Crohn disease. This increase in submucosal and mucosal lymphocytes is most pronounced among mast cells producing immunoglobulin G. Proinflammatory cytokines such as interleukin-A and interleukin-6 are also elevated in Crohn disease. The genesis of the immunologic alterations seen in Crohn disease, however, is not known. Specifically, it is unclear whether Crohn disease is a true autoimmune response driven by host antigens or an exaggerated inflammatory response to exogenous antigens or infection.

As suggested by the observed familial aggregations and the variability of risk among differing ethnic and racial groups, a genetic predisposition is likely to play at least a part in the etiology of Crohn disease. The distribution of Crohn disease within families is complex and defies a simple Mendelian transmission of disease, but genome-wide linkage studies have suggested replicated susceptibility regions for Crohn disease on chromosomes 6, 12, and 16.[6] Genome-wide scans have also demonstrated linkage for Crohn disease to several locations with in the human genome. Of particular interest is the pericentromeric region of chromosome 16 known as the *IBD1 locus*. Within this locus polymorphism in the NOD2/CARD15 gene are strongly associated with Crohn disease. The exact function of the NOD2/CARD15 gene is yet to be fully understood, and how alterations in this gene affects the susceptibility to Crohn disease in not known.

Numerous infectious agents have been investigated as potential causes of Crohn disease, with mycobacteria receiving the most attention. Since the original description of Crohn disease, an association with mycobacteria has been postulated. *Mycobacterium paratuberculosis* has been isolated from the resected specimens of some patients with Crohn disease.

Yet, this association has not been a consistent finding, and even sensitive polymerase chain reaction studies have failed to provide definitive evidence of the presence of *M. paratuberculosis*–specific DNA in bowel affected by Crohn disease. Other specific agents that have been extensively studied include measles virus and *Helicobacter pylori*. To date, no single infectious agent has been identified as a cause of Crohn disease[2,8] Environmental factors, including diet and smoking, have also been investigated as potential causes of Crohn disease. Although dietary modification can affect the severity of the symptoms of Crohn disease, no dietary factor has been identified as a cause of the disease. Smokers are at a higher risk for contracting Crohn disease than nonsmokers.[9] Additionally, smoking is known to exacerbate existing disease. The component of cigarette smoke that is responsible for the deleterious affect on the clinical course of Crohn disease is not known, but it seems likely that chemical components of cigarette smoke represent an aggravating factor rather than a causative agent for Crohn disease.

Studies of intestinal transport have demonstrated an increased intestinal permeability in both patients with Crohn disease and their symptom-free first-degree relatives.[10] This finding has led some investigators to speculate that Crohn disease is the result of an altered mucosal barrier function that allows abnormal interactions to take place between the multitude of antigenic substrates normally found in the gut lumen and the immunocompetent tissue of the submucosa.

Epidemiologic data, in addition to clinical observations and the results of basic science investigation, suggest that the pathogenesis of Crohn disease is complex and that no one single genetic abnormality or environmental factor is responsible. Instead, Crohn disease is more likely the result of a combination of multiple predisposing factors and environmental or infectious triggers that set an immunologic derangement into motion.[4]

PATHOLOGY

The gross and microscopic features of Crohn disease can occur in any segment of the gastrointestinal tract. The disease tends to be discontinuous and segmental, affecting isolated segments of the gastrointestinal tract. Disease of the terminal ileum with or without some involvement of the cecum is the most common pattern, representing approximately 60% of cases.[11] Crohn disease is limited to the colon in 15% to 20% of cases. In 10% of cases, the proximal small bowel is involved; in approximately 15% of cases, a pattern of multiple sites of disease is found. Perianal manifestations of Crohn disease, including perianal fistulae, abscesses and stenoses, occur in about one third of Crohn disease patients. In half of these cases, perianal disease occurs simultaneously with active disease elsewhere in the gastrointestinal tract.

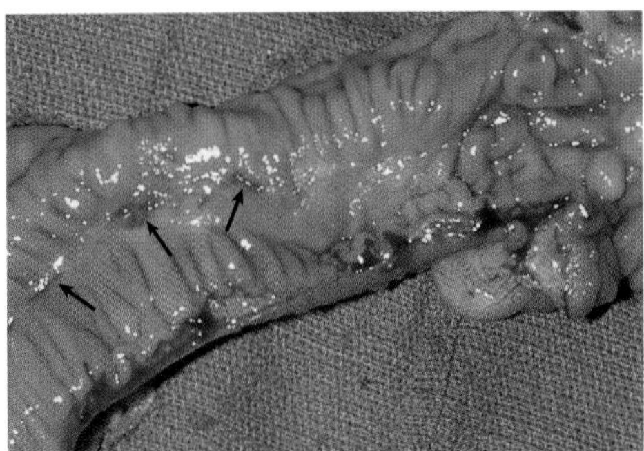

FIGURE 51.1 Mucosal ulcerations (*arrows*) in Crohn disease of the small bowel. (Courtesy of The University of Chicago General Surgery Archives.)

Gross Pathology

The earliest gross manifestation of Crohn disease is the development of small aphthous ulcers.[12] Aphthous ulcers are small areas of mucosal ulceration that generally develop over microscopic lymphoid aggregates. Aphthous ulcers appear as red spots or focal mucosal depressions in the fresh specimen. As the disease progresses, the aphthous ulcers enlarge and become stellate. The ulcerations coalesce to form longitudinal mucosal ulcerations. In Crohn disease of the small bowel, these linear ulcerations almost always occur along the mesenteric aspect of the bowel wall (Fig. 51.1). Further development of disease leads to a serpiginous network of thin, linear ulcerations that surround islands of edematous mucosa; these produce the classic "cobblestone" appearance (Fig. 51.2). Mucosal ulcerations may penetrate through the submucosa and coalesce to form intramural channels that can bore through the bowel wall and produce abscesses, fistulae, or sinuses.

The inflammation of Crohn disease extends through all layers of the bowel wall. The inflammation also involves the mesentery and regional lymph nodes, so that the mesentery can become massively thickened. During early or acute intestinal inflammation, the bowel wall is hyperemic and boggy. As the inflammation progresses, fibrotic scarring develops, and the bowel becomes thickened and leathery (Fig. 51.3). Fatty tissue commonly develops from the mesentery and extends over the serosal surface of the small bowel resulting in a phenomenon known as "fat wrapping" or "creeping fat" (Fig. 51.4).

Microscopic Pathology

Crohn disease results in a transmural inflammation characterized by multiple lymphoid aggregates that thicken and expand the submucosa. In some cases, the lymphoid aggregates are not

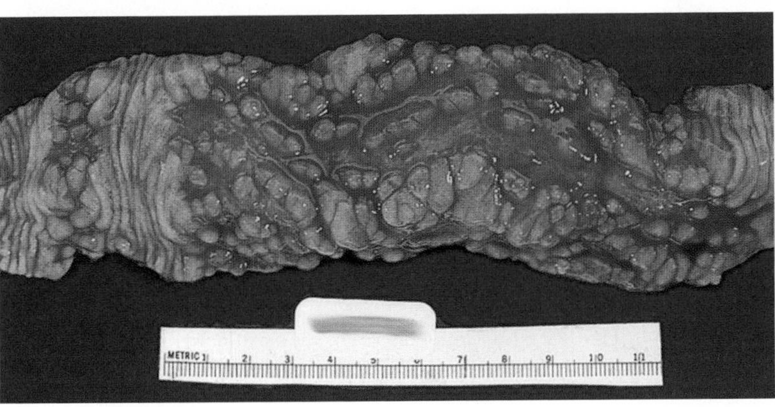

FIGURE 51.2 Islands of edematous mucosa surrounded by linear ulceration showing the classic "cobblestone" appearance of Crohn disease. (Courtesy of The University of Chicago General Surgery Archives.)

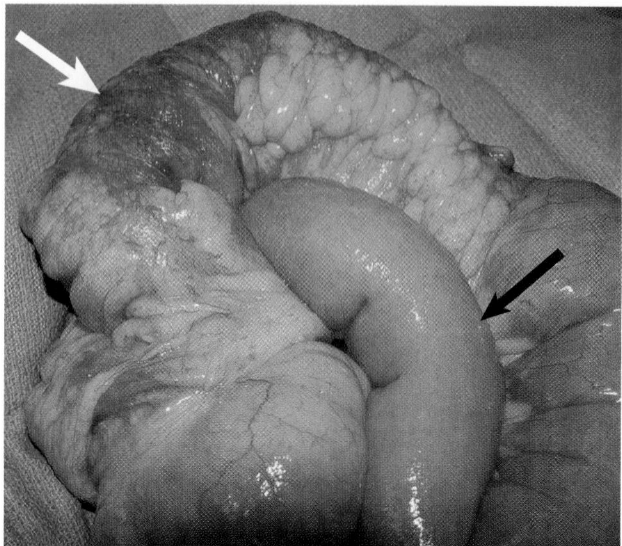

FIGURE 51.3 Severe Crohn disease affecting the terminal ileum (*white arrow*) with normal ileum for comparison (*black arrow*). (Courtesy of The University of Chicago General Surgery Archives.)

limited to the submucosa but extend through the muscularis propria. The presence of well-developed lymphoid aggregates in an edematous or fibrotic submucosa or subserosa is virtually diagnostic of Crohn disease (Fig. 51.5). A sentinel microscopic feature of Crohn disease is the presence of noncaseating granulomas (Fig. 51.6). Granulomas are found in up to 50% of surgically resected specimens but are only rarely seen in specimens obtained endoscopically. Although granulomas are a valuable diagnostic feature of Crohn disease, their presence is not pathognomonic and they do not imply activity.[12]

CLINICAL FEATURES

The clinical features of Crohn disease vary according to the location of the involved intestinal segments and the development of related complications, which include intestinal obstruction, inflammatory mass, fistula, abscess, free perforation, hemorrhage, and cancer.

Patterns of Disease

Crohn disease can be loosely categorized based on the gross pattern of disease that gives rise to the clinical manifestations and associated complications. The three categories of Crohn

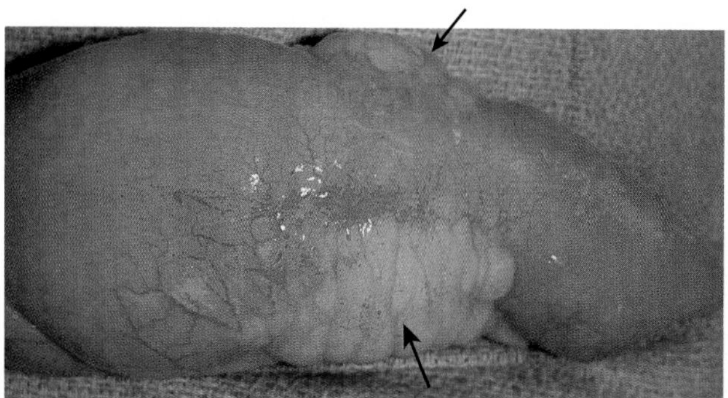

FIGURE 51.4 "Fat wrapping" or "creeping fat" of the terminal ileum (*arrows*). (Courtesy of The University of Chicago General Surgery Archives.)

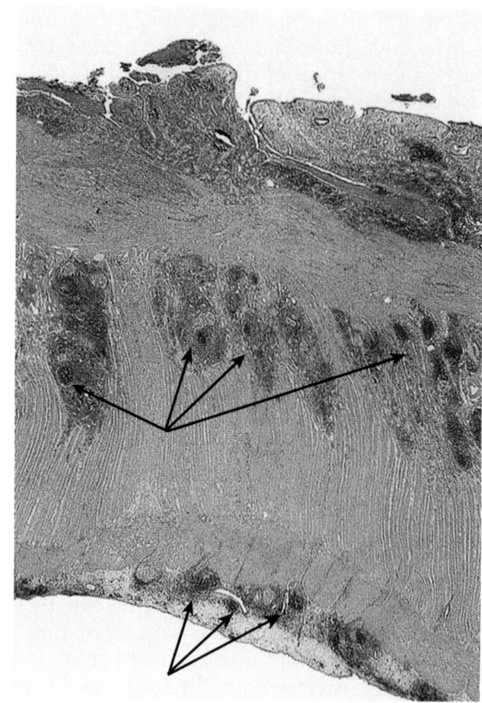

FIGURE 51.5 Classic distribution of lymphoid aggregates in Crohn disease, which are scattered across all layers of the bowel wall (*arrows*). (Courtesy of The University of Chicago General Surgery Archives.)

disease are *stricturing*, *perforating*, and *inflammatory*. These three categories do not represent distinct forms of disease; rather, they provide a means to describe and categorize the predominant gross manifestation of disease.[13] Although features of more than one pattern often occur in the same patient or even in the same segment of intestine, one pattern tends to predominate in most cases. The predominant pattern of disease often determines the clinical presentation and affects management and treatment options.

Inflammatory Pattern

Uncomplicated inflammation is manifested by mucosal ulceration and thickening of the bowel wall caused by inflammatory infiltration and edema. This process can result in narrowing of the intestinal lumen and even partial intestinal obstruction.

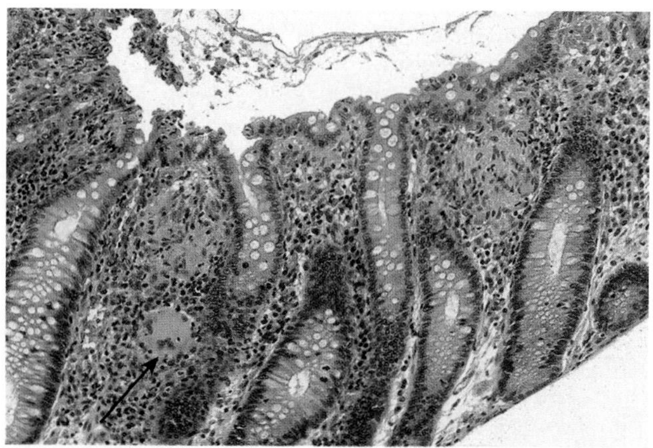

FIGURE 51.6 Crohn disease of the small bowel mucosa showing a noncaseating granuloma (*arrow*). (Courtesy of The University of Chicago General Surgery Archives.)

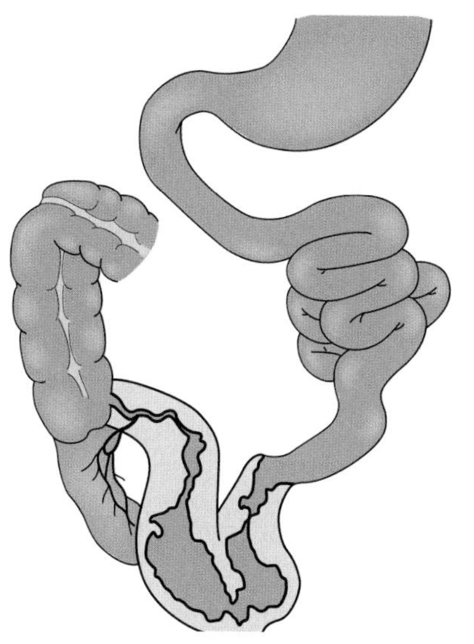

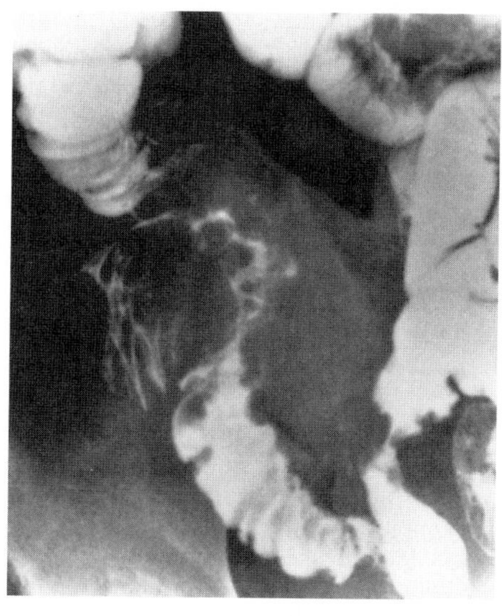

FIGURE 51.7 Small bowel follow-through showing a right psoas abscess originating from a walled-off perforation of the terminal ileum. (From Michelassi F. Crohn's disease. In: Bell RH, Rikkers LF, Mulholland MW, eds. *Digestive tract surgery*. Philadelphia: Lippincott–Raven, 1996, pp. 1201–1227.)

Intestinal luminal narrowing resulting from inflammation and edema can often be relieved with medical treatment.

Stricturing Pattern

In the stricturing pattern of disease, the intestinal lumen is narrowed by fibrotic scar tissue. These cicatricial strictures are referred to as *fibrostenotic lesions*. Patients with a predominantly stricturing pattern of Crohn disease have primarily obstructive symptoms. Fibrotic strictures are not reversible with medical treatment, so symptomatic stricturing disease often requires surgical management.

Perforating Pattern

The perforating pattern of disease is characterized by the development of fistulae and abscesses. Small sinus tracts, which typically originate from the mesenteric portion of the intestinal lumen, bore through the bowel wall. They may simply penetrate for a short distance, in which case they are seen as blind tracts on small bowel radiographs, or they may give rise to abscesses or fistulae (Fig. 51.7). As perforating disease develops, the inflammatory response about the boring sinus typically results in the formation of adhesions, most often to an adjoining segment of intestine, the urinary bladder, or the abdominal wall. The boring sinus then advances through the adhesion and into the adjacent structure, so that a fistula forms. Only rarely does this process result in free perforation with spillage of intestinal contents into the abdominal cavity. Frequently, perforating disease is accompanied by some degree of stricture formation, but the pattern of fistulae and abscesses generally dictates the surgical strategy.

Crohn Disease of the Small Bowel

The symptoms of small bowel Crohn disease include chronic abdominal pain, weight loss, fever, and anorexia.[14] The predominant symptom is pain, which occurs in up to 90% of cases. Abdominal pain related to partial intestinal obstruction is intermittent and cramping and is often brought on by meals. More persistent pain can be the result of acute exacerbations of inflammation or the development of septic complications, such as abscesses. Patients with perforating small bowel disease may have fever or a tender palpable mass associated with abscess or phlegmon. Fistulization to the skin, urinary bladder or vagina may also occur. An enlarged inflammatory mass that adheres to the retroperitoneum can compress the right ureter and cause symptomatic ureteral obstruction and hydronephrosis. Diarrhea, a hallmark of Crohn colitis, is not often a predominant symptom in Crohn disease limited to the small bowel. However, many patients with small bowel Crohn disease report an increased frequency of bowel movements. Many patients with small bowel disease lose weight because of anorexia or avoidance of food for fear of initiating abdominal pain. Malnutrition and weight loss may also result from malabsorption and protein loss in cases of extensive Crohn disease affecting long segments of small bowel.

Crohn Colitis

Patients with Crohn disease of the colon typically have diarrhea in addition to abdominal pain and hematochezia. Crohn colitis can give rise to manifestations of perforating disease, with the formation of abscesses and intestinal fistulae. Stricture can also occur in chronic Crohn colitis and give rise to symptoms of colonic obstruction, including abdominal pain and distention. Toxic megacolon can develop in Crohn colitis, but this potentially life-threatening complication is much less frequent in Crohn colitis than in ulcerative colitis.

Perianal Crohn Disease

Perianal Crohn disease results in the formation of perianal fistulae, abscesses, and strictures that are often associated with hypertrophic perianal skin tags, fissures, and perineal scarring. Perianal manifestations of Crohn disease include acute pain (abscess), purulent drainage and chronic discomfort (fistula), and laborious defecation (anal stenosis).

It is important to distinguish perianal from rectal Crohn disease. In rectal Crohn disease, the rectal mucosa is inflamed and ulcerated, whereas in perianal Crohn disease, inflammation and fistulization develop in the anal crypt glands. This distinction is key in planning therapy for patients with perianal Crohn disease.

Extraintestinal Disease

Crohn disease is associated with a variety of extraintestinal manifestations. They include dermatologic, ocular, hepatobiliary, and joint disorders. Dermatologic disorders in Crohn disease include erythema nodosum and pyoderma gangrenosum. Ocular manifestations include uveitis and episcleritis. Ankylosing spondylitis, sacral ileitis, and a seronegative peripheral polyarthropathy are associated with Crohn disease. Patients with Crohn disease are also at risk for the development of primary sclerosing cholangitis, but this very serious complication is less common in Crohn disease than in ulcerative colitis. The manifestations of peripheral arthritis, uveitis, episcleritis, erythema nodosum, and possibly pyoderma gangrenosum associated with Crohn disease generally parallel the activity of the intestinal disease, and symptoms typically regress with successful medical management or complete surgical resection of the affected segments of bowel. Ankylosing spondylitis and primary sclerosing cholangitis do not correlate with bowel disease activity, and so their clinical course is not attenuated by surgical resection of intestinal Crohn disease.

DIAGNOSIS

Many patients go for months or years after the onset of symptoms before the diagnosis of Crohn disease is made. No specific laboratory test allows the diagnosis of Crohn disease to be made; rather, the diagnosis is most often based on the results of a thorough clinical history, complete physical examination, and small bowel radiography and colonoscopy. Occasionally, tissue obtained during endoscopic biopsy can be diagnostic. Other studies, such as computed tomography (CT), can assist in the detection and diagnosis of the intraabdominal septic complications of Crohn disease.

Radiography of the Small Bowel

Evaluation of the small bowel is best undertaken with contrast radiography, either small bowel follow-through or enteroclysis. The radiographic abnormalities of small bowel Crohn disease are often distinctive.[15] In early disease, mucosal granularity with ulceration and nodularity are typically apparent. Both the mucosal folds and the bowel wall are often thickened. Luminal narrowing, strictures and fissures are radiographically apparent with more severe disease (Fig. 51.8).

Small bowel studies can in many cases demonstrate the complications of Crohn disease, including high-grade strictures and fistulae. It is important to note that many enteric fistulae are not apparent by radiographic contrast studies, and the absence of radiographic evidence of fistulization does not exclude this possibility. Small bowel contrast studies also provide information regarding enlargement of the mesentery by phlegmon and the formation of inflammatory masses or abscesses, demonstrated as a mass effect separating or displacing contrast-filled loops of bowel (Fig. 51.9).

Small bowel radiographs should be studied to determine the location of the disease and to estimate both the length of small intestine affected by the disease process and the length of uninvolved bowel. It is also important to note the pattern of small bowel involvement; small bowel disease may be continuous or it may display a discontinuous pattern in which skip lesions are separated by areas of normal intestine.

Colonoscopy

The colon and rectum are best evaluated with colonoscopy. Colonoscopy allows mucosal disease to be visualized and also provides the opportunity for mucosal biopsy and histologic evaluation. In many cases, the terminal ileum can be entered and evaluated. Characteristic features of Crohn disease seen on colonoscopy include aphthoid ulcers, discrete serpiginous ulcerations that usually track along the long axis of the bowel, diseased mucosa separated by areas of normal mucosa, rectal sparing, and strictures.[16]

Computed Tomography

The most typical CT finding of uncomplicated Crohn disease is thickening of the bowel wall. Bowel wall thickening correlates with disease activity and tends to dissipate with successful medical management.[17] In general, the CT findings of uncomplicated Crohn disease are nonspecific, and routine abdominal CT does not assist in confirming the diagnosis of Crohn disease. CT, however, can be useful in identifying the complications associated with Crohn disease, and when an abscess or inflammatory mass is suspected, CT of the abdomen and pelvis should be performed.[18] Most abscesses related to Crohn disease are readily detectable with CT (Fig. 51.10). Additionally, CT allows for the assessment of possible ureteral obstruction resulting from compression by a retroperitoneal inflammatory mass. Enterovesical fistulae can be detected on CT by the presence of air within the urinary bladder.

DIFFERENTIAL DIAGNOSIS

The differential diagnosis for Crohn disease of the small bowel includes irritable bowel syndrome, acute appendicitis, intestinal ischemia, and gynecologic disorders, such as pelvic

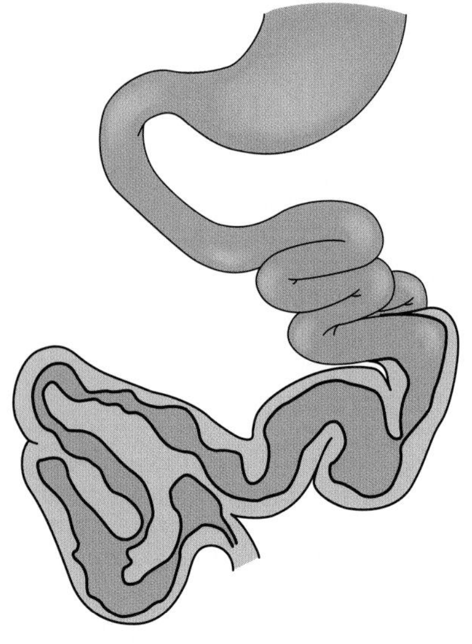

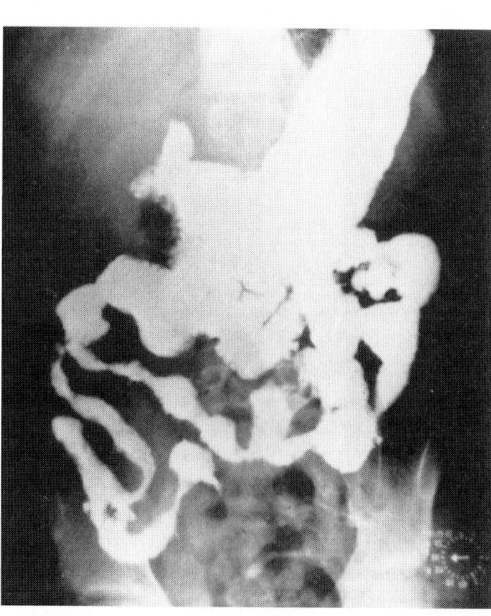

FIGURE 51.8 Typical radiographic appearance of extensive jejunoileal Crohn disease. (Adapted with permission from Block GE, Michelassi F, Tanaka M, et al. Crohn's disease. *Curr Probl Surg.* 1993;30:173–265.)

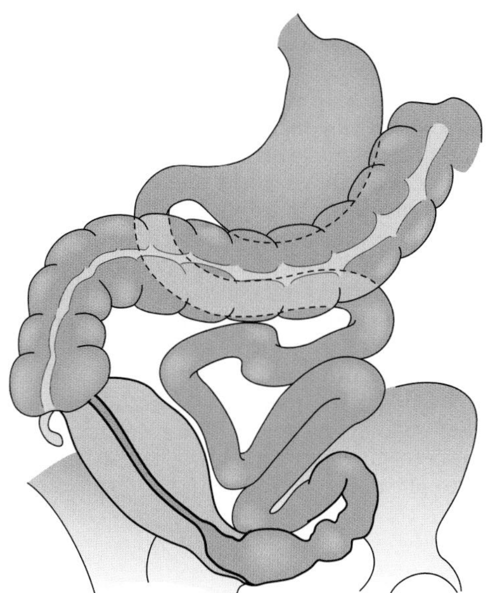

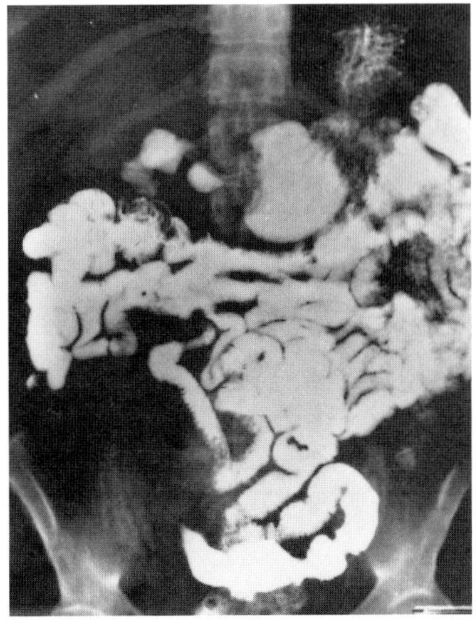

FIGURE 51.9 Crohn disease of the terminal ileum with resultant mass effect resulting in the displacement of several loops of small bowel from the right lower quadrant (Adapted with permission from Michelassi F, Balestracci T, Chappell R, et al. Primary and recurrent Crohn's disease: experience with 1,379 patients. *Ann Surg.* 1991; 214:230–238.)

inflammatory disease, endometriosis, and even gynecologic malignancies. Other entities within the differential diagnosis include radiation enteritis, *Yersinia* infections, intestinal tuberculosis, and small bowel tumors. Occasionally, the distinction between Crohn disease and small bowel malignancies may be difficult to make by small bowel radiograph. When the diagnosis of Crohn disease versus tumors is uncertain, the question should be resolved with surgical resection. Nonsteroidal antiinflammatory drugs (NSAIDs) can cause a focal enteritis with ulceration and stricture formation that can be very difficult to distinguish from Crohn disease.

For Crohn disease limited to the colon, the differential diagnosis includes infectious colitis, microscopic or collagenous colitis, ischemic colitis, diverticular disease, Behçet's disease, colonic neoplasms, solitary rectal ulcer syndrome, and NSAID colopathy. The condition that can be most difficult to distinguish from Crohn colitis is idiopathic ulcerative colitis. In the vast majority of cases of Crohn disease, the unique manifestations of Crohn disease are readily apparent, and the distinction from ulcerative colitis is not difficult. In only a small percentage of patients does Crohn disease present in such a manner that it cannot be distinguished from ulcerative colitis. Evidence to support the diagnosis of Crohn colitis over ulcerative colitis includes small bowel involvement, sparing of the rectal mucosa, cobblestoning of the colonic mucosa, and the presence of skip lesions, perianal abscesses, fistulae or fissures, transmural inflammation, and noncaseating granulomas.

MEDICAL MANAGEMENT

The medical treatment of Crohn disease is often a challenging endeavor. Because the etiology of Crohn disease is unknown, no therapy directed against the primary cause of Crohn disease is available; rather, medical treatment consists of supportive symptomatic care along with a variety of antiinflammatory drugs. Because of the variable course of disease and the differing clinical presentations and associated complications, medical therapy must be individualized to each specific clinical situation.

To assess the relative response to therapy, various systems of scoring clinical disease activity have been utilized to allow some degree of objective assessment of overall disease activity. The most commonly used is the Crohn Disease Activity Index (CDAI).[19,20] Assigned values for the CDAI parameters are weighted by derived regression coefficients (Table 51.1). A CDAI below 150 is indicative of quiescent disease, and a CDAI above 450 signifies severe disease.

Supportive Care

Supportive care includes antidiarrheal agents, antispasmodic agents, and nutritional support. Antidiarrheal agents such as diphenoxylate and loperamide are commonly used. These agents are often effective in relieving diarrhea when the patient has chronic subacute disease or when the diarrhea is related to previous intestinal resection. In the face of a severe acute flare of disease, antidiarrheal agents should be used with caution because they may precipitate intestinal obstruction or even toxic megacolon. Antispasmodic agents lessen cramping abdominal pain by decreasing intestinal hypermotility. In the presence of severe acute colitis, antispasmodic agents should also be avoided because they may precipitate toxic megacolon.

Although no correlation between dietary agents and disease activity has been identified, dietary modification can

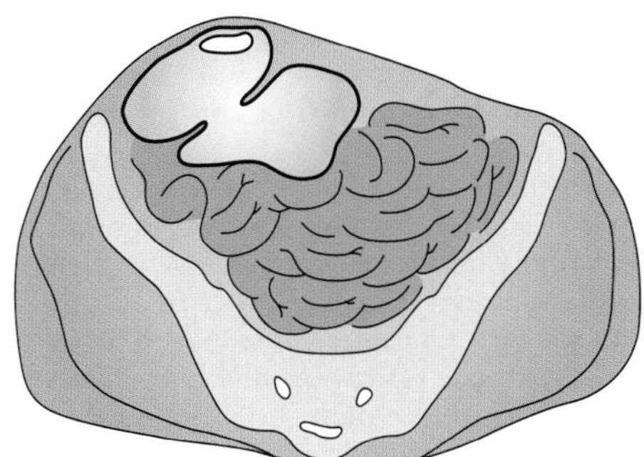

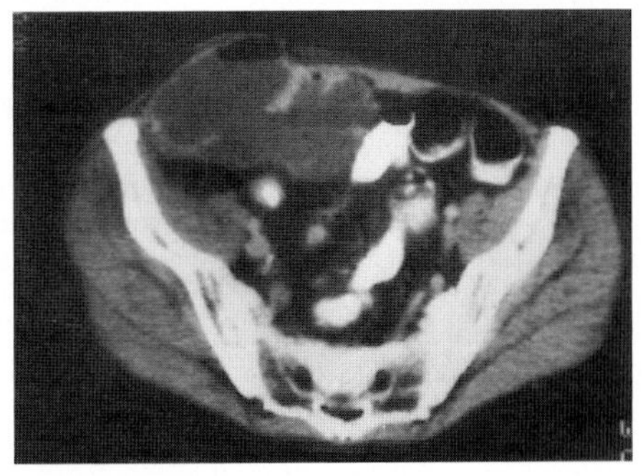

FIGURE 51.10 CT scan showing a right lower quadrant abscess originating from Crohn disease of the terminal ileum (Adapted with permission from Michelassi F, Balestracci T, Chappell R, et al. Primary and recurrent Crohn's disease: experience with 1,379 patients. *Ann Surg.* 1991;214:230–238.)

TABLE 51.1 DIAGNOSIS

CROHN DISEASE ACTIVITY INDEX

Variable	Multiplication factor
Number of liquid or soft stools (each day for 7 days)	2
Sum of 7 daily abdominal pain scores (0, none; 1 or 2, intermediate; 3, severe)	6
Sum of 7 daily general well-being scores (0, good; 1, 2 or 3, intermediate; 4, poor)	6
Number of complications:	30
Arthralgia or arthritis	
Iritis or uveitis	
Erythema nodosum, pyoderma gangrenosum, or aphthous stomatitis	
Anal fissure, fistula, or abscess	
Other fistula	
Fever (>37.8° C) during previous week	
Use of opiates for diarrhea (0, no; 1, yes)	4
Abdominal mass (0, none: 2, questionable; 5, definite	10
47 minus hematocrit (men), 42 minus hematocrit (women)	6
Percentage deviation from standard weight	1
Crohn Disease Activity Index (CDAI)	Sum

lessen the severity of symptoms in some cases. For instance, patients with obstructive symptoms often benefit from a low- or minimal-residue diet as a short-term means of relief. Many patients report fewer symptoms with an exclusionary diet based on personal experience with food.

Nutritional support in the form of total parenteral nutrition (TPN) can be of value in malnourished patients with Crohn disease. TPN has been shown to increase body weight and improve nitrogen balance in patients with severe disease. Prolonged bowel rest combined with TPN can result in a significant reduction in disease activity, and in rare instances, "resting" the gastrointestinal tract with TPN nutritional support is indicated as a means of preparing a malnourished patient for surgery. Although bowel rest may relieve symptomatic Crohn disease, the disease activity frequently recurs when oral intake is resumed.

Corticosteroids

Systemic corticosteroids are the mainstay of treatment in acute exacerbations of Crohn disease. In up to 60% of patients with acutely active small bowel disease, clinical remission can be achieved with a short course of oral prednisone in a dosage of 0.25 to 0.75 mg/kg per day.[21] For adult patients unable to take oral medication, 40 to 60 mg of methylprednisolone can be given as a continuous daily infusion. More than 75% of patients respond within a week to intravenous methylprednisolone.[22]

Long-term systemic corticosteroid therapy is associated with substantial side effects, including osteonecrosis, osteoporosis, cataracts, diabetes, myopathy, systemic infection, and adrenal suppression. Because of the high risk for these serious side effects, systemic steroids should not be given on a long-term basis to treat Crohn disease. Systemic steroids should be utilized to treat acute exacerbations of Crohn disease and then tapered and discontinued within a matter of weeks. If symptoms do not adequately respond to a short course of systemic steroids or if the patient cannot be successfully weaned from steroid therapy during a three to six month period, then alternative treatments or surgery are indicated.

Budesonide, a synthetic glucocorticoid with reduced systemic absorption, has been shown to be effective in moderately acute exacerbations of Crohn disease.[23] Because of its reduced bioavailability, budesonide is less likely to cause the severe side effects observed with systemic corticosteroids. Budesonide can be administered in an oral controlled-release preparation for direct topical application to the ileum and proximal colon. Although the absorption of budesonide is minimal, some systemic absorption through inflamed mucosa does occur, and hypothalamic-pituitary-adrenal suppression may develop. Budesonide is an effective treatment for active disease but has not been shown to have any benefit as a maintenance treatment to prevent recurrent disease.

Aminosalicylates

Aminosalicylates include sulfasalazine and 5-aminosalicylic acid (5-ASA) derivatives (mesalamine). These compounds are commonly used to treat patients with moderately active Crohn disease or quiescent disease. The antiinflammatory mechanisms of the aminosalicylates are not fully understood, but they likely inhibit the cyclooxygenase and lipoxygenase pathways, in addition to thromboxane synthetase and platelet-activating factor synthase. Sulfasalazine at a dosage of 3 to 5 g/d has been shown to be beneficial for mild to moderate ileocolitis or colitis.[21] Sulfasalazine, however, has no beneficial effect when disease is limited to the small bowel.

Mesalamine capsules (encapsulated in ethylcellulose microspheres) provide a continuous release of mesalamine to the small and large intestine and are effective against mild to moderate disease. Continuous-release mesalamine is also effective as maintenance therapy to prevent relapse after medically induced remission or surgical resection.[24]

It is critical to note that the 5-ASA derivatives should not be confused with acetylsalicylic acid (aspirin) or other NSAIDs. Aspirin and other classic NSAIDs have the potential to exacerbate Crohn disease activity and should be avoided in these patients.

Immunomodulators (Azathioprine and 6-Mercaptopurine)

Azathioprine and 6-mercaptopurine (6-MP) are immunosuppressive agents that act by inhibiting DNA synthesis. The result is suppression of cytotoxic T-cell and natural killer cell function. Azathioprine and 6-MP are effective in treating active and quiescent Crohn disease.[25] A 50% to 60% response rate is seen in patients with active Crohn disease when they are given 1.0 to 1.5 mg/kg/day of 6-MP or 2 to 2.5 mg/kg/day of azathioprine.[22,26] Both 6-MP and azathioprine are also effective in maintaining remission and suppressing recurrent disease.

As experience with these agents has increased, concerns over possible long-term side effects have lessened somewhat, and their use is appropriate in selected patients. Nevertheless, many potential and serious side effects can occur, and these agents should be used with caution. Close observation is required. Serious potential side effects include bone marrow suppression, hepatotoxicity, and pancreatitis. Bone marrow suppression with 6-MP and azathioprine is dose related, so that weekly monitoring of blood counts is necessary during initial treatment, and continued monitoring is required every 2 to 3 months during therapy for chronic stable disease. The most concerning toxicity is the potential for iatrogenically induced lymphoma. Accumulating data suggests, however, that the risk for lymphoma in patients with Crohn disease who are taking 6-MP or azathioprine is low.

In addition to the many potential side effects of 6-MP and azathioprine, which limit their use, these agents have a greatly delayed onset of action. Typically, 3 to 6 months of therapy is required before a clinical response occurs, so they are not appropriate to treat acute flares of disease. However, 6-MP and azathioprine are often useful for their steroid-sparing effect, and they can be used to maintain remission as systemic steroid therapy is withdrawn.

Metronidazole

Although no infectious agent has been identified as a cause of Crohn disease, the antibiotic metronidazole is somewhat effective in the treatment of mild to moderately active Crohn disease. The mechanism of action of metronidazole in active Crohn disease is not known. The effects are often marginal, and rarely can active disease be managed with metronidazole alone. The long-term use of metronidazole is associated with many side effects, including peripheral neuropathy, which occurs in up to 50% of patients. In some cases, peripheral neuropathy associated with the long-term use of metronidazole is irreversible. Metronidazole is commonly prescribed as an adjunct in the treatment of Crohn related perianal fistulas.

Tumor Necrosis Factor Antibody

Infliximab, a monoclonal chimeric antitumor necrosis factor antibody, represents a novel approach to the management of Crohn disease. This agent actively blocks tumor necrosis factor (TNF), a proinflammatory cytokine thought to be important in the pathogenesis of Crohn disease. Trials have shown clinical response rates of up to 80% within 1 week of a single infusion of infliximab[27,28] Infliximab is indicated for moderately active Crohn disease that has not adequately responded to more conventional treatment. Infliximab is also effective against persistent perianal fistulae associated with Crohn disease.[29] Initial infusions are typically well tolerated, but a serum sickness–like syndrome can occur after repeated infusions. Additionally, it is thought that infusions of anti-TNF antibody may expose the patient to an increased risk for the development of lymphoma.

Other Medical Therapy

Other medical therapies that have been applied in the treatment of Crohn disease include methotrexate, cyclosporine, ciprofloxacin, omega-3 fatty acids, and thalidomide.

Selecting the optimal medical regimen for each patient requires experience and special expertise. Although most patients respond to initial measures of medical management, ultimately three fourths of patients with Crohn disease require surgery. It is important to emphasize that the goal of medical treatment of Crohn disease is to alleviate symptoms and improve the quality of life and overall health of the patient. This can often be a difficult balance to attain, given the many potential side effects observed with the most commonly utilized therapies. The patient, the gastroenterologist, and the surgeon should not mistakenly assume that avoidance of surgery is a primary goal of medical treatment. Otherwise, the patient may unduly suffer from inadequately controlled Crohn disease, be at risk for side effects and complications related to ineffective medical treatment, and be denied the significant and typically long-term benefits seen in the vast majority of patients who undergo surgical treatment for Crohn disease.

SURGICAL TREATMENT

Crohn disease is a recurring disorder that cannot be cured with surgical resection. As such, surgery is intended to provide palliation. The surgeon must strive to alleviate symptoms as effectively as possible without exposing the patient to excessive morbidity. Nonresectional techniques, such as strictureplasty, may be required to avoid excessive loss of intestine, or it may be necessary to remove only portions of the gastrointestinal tract affected by severe disease while leaving segments with mild, asymptomatic disease intact. To manage Crohn disease optimally, the surgeon must always keep in mind the natural history of the disease, with its high risk for recurrence and the need for repeated surgery.

Indications for Operation

Failure of Medical Management

Failure of medical management to control symptoms and disease activity adequately is the most common indication for surgery.[30] Medical treatment fails when symptoms of an acute flare do not improve or new complications of Crohn disease develop during optimal treatment. Some patients fail medical therapy because significant side effects develop that are related to the medical therapy; in other cases, symptoms may resolve during systemic steroid therapy only to recur with each attempt to withdraw the steroids. Because severe complications are inevitable with prolonged steroid use, surgery is indicated if the patient cannot be weaned from corticosteroids within 3 to 6 months.

Intestinal Obstruction

Partial or complete intestinal obstruction is a common indication for surgery in Crohn disease.[11] Chronic partial obstruction of the small bowel is much more common than acute complete obstruction. Luminal narrowing and partial small bowel obstruction in Crohn disease is the result of acute inflammation and bowel wall thickening or chronic scarring with fixed stricture formation. Partial small bowel obstruction related to acute inflammation and bowel wall edema can often be managed with medical therapy. Failure of medical treatment to relieve obstructive symptoms in these patients obviously indicates a need for surgery. Patients with obstructive symptoms that result from fibrotic, fixed strictures do not benefit from medical therapy and are best treated with surgery.

Enteric Fistulae

Asymptomatic enteroenteric fistulae do not require surgical treatment. However, the presence of asymptomatic fistulae may indicate the presence of severe, complicated disease associated with other indications for surgical treatment. A fistula by itself is can be an indication for surgery if it causes discomfort or embarrasses the patient (e.g., enterocutaneous or enterovaginal fistula) or has the potential to induce significant complications (e.g., enterovesical fistula causing repeated urinary tract infections and deteriorating renal function).[31]

Abscess and Inflammatory Mass

Intraabdominal abscesses and inflammatory masses occur less frequently than fistulae but are more often an indication for surgical therapy. Abscesses do not respond to medical treatment and require drainage. An abscess from Crohn disease that has been drained percutaneously is very likely to recur or result in an enterocutaneous fistula, so that surgical resection is often advised even after successful drainage. Inflammatory masses indicate severe disease and often harbor an unrecognized abscess.[32] Thus, inflammatory masses are considered an indication for surgical treatment.

Hemorrhage

Hemorrhage is an uncommon complication of Crohn disease. Massive gastrointestinal hemorrhage occurs more frequently in Crohn colitis than in small bowel Crohn disease. Hemorrhage in small bowel Crohn disease tends to be more indolent, with episodes of chronic bleeding that require intermittent transfusion.[33]

Perforation

Free perforation with peritonitis is a rare complication of Crohn disease occurring in approximately 1% of patients. Free perforation is a clear indication for urgent operation.

Cancer and Suspected Cancer

Patients with Crohn disease are at increased risk for the development of adenocarcinoma of the colon and small intestine. Current estimates indicate an observed prevalence of 0.3% for small bowel adenocarcinoma and 1.8% for large-intestinal adenocarcinoma.[34,35] The preoperative diagnosis of carcinoma of the small bowel is difficult because the symptoms, physical signs, and radiologic findings of small bowel cancer are similar to those of the underlying Crohn disease. Adenocarcinomas complicating Crohn disease tend to be multifocal (10%) and poorly differentiated. Nonfunctional bowel that has been excluded from the fecal stream seems to be at particular risk for malignancy. Therefore, bypass surgery should not be performed for Crohn disease of the small bowel, and rectal stumps should either be restored to their function or excised.

Small intestinal carcinoma should be suspected in patients with longstanding disease whose symptoms change suddenly, especially after a lengthy quiescent period. Small bowel cancer should also be considered when high-grade obstruction fails to resolve with conservative treatment.

Although surveillance of the large bowel is feasible, it is difficult to distinguish neoplastic from inflammatory stricture and is thus difficult to make an early diagnosis of adenocarcinoma. When adenocarcinoma is suspected or histologically proved, surgical treatment is indicated.

Growth Retardation

Growth is retarded in up to 25% of children affected by Crohn disease.[36] If growth retardation persists despite adequate medical and nutritional therapy, prompt surgical treatment should be carried out before puberty; meaningful growth will not occur after epiphyseal closure.

Preoperative Evaluation and Preparation

A complete preoperative assessment of the gastrointestinal tract should be undertaken before elective surgery for abdominal Crohn disease. The small bowel should be studied with contrast radiography. The colon and rectum are best evaluated with colonoscopy. Patients with suspected abscesses or inflammatory masses should undergo preoperative CT of the abdomen and pelvis to determine the extent of the septic complication, the feasibility of percutaneous drainage, and the relationship of the septic process to retroperitoneal structures. Occasionally, contrast injected into the cutaneous opening of an enterocutaneous fistula can help in determining the extent of disease, the presence of complicating abscess, and the anatomy of diseased segments.

Meticulous mechanical preparation of the colon should be undertaken in all patients before abdominal surgery for Crohn disease. Even in cases thought to be limited to the small bowel, the surgeon must always be prepared to perform surgery on the colon because secondary involvement of the colon by fistulae or an adherent inflammatory mass cannot always be excluded by preoperative studies.

Abdominal Exploration

At initial laparotomy, the contents of the abdomen should be thoroughly examined and the location and extent of disease identified. When exploring the abdomen, the surgeon should closely examine the entire small bowel from the ligament of Treitz to the ileocecal valve, taking note of the precise locations of disease. This practice often requires division of areas of adhesion. The surgeon should make note of areas of possible fistulization. Any inflammatory adhesions should be suspected of harboring a fistulous tract. Although separation of inflammatory adhesions is appropriate, adhesions that may be a result of cancer should be left intact and the affected area resected en bloc.

In most cases, the areas affected by Crohn disease are readily apparent, with the bowel wall thickened and indurated. Serosal hyperemia with a "corkscrew" appearance of the serosal vessels is typical. Also seen in areas of disease is encroachment of the mesentery fat along the serosal surface of the bowel, often referred to as *fat wrapping* or *creeping fat* (see Figs. 51.3 and 51.4). The mesentery of grossly diseased bowel is often massively thickened and stiff. Serosal manifestations of less severe disease are subtler and can be more difficult to identify. In mild Crohn disease, some degree of induration of the mesenteric bowel wall is typically present that can be detected with palpation.

Resection

Small bowel resection is the most common surgical procedure utilized to treat small bowel Crohn disease. For many years, the optimal extent of resection necessary to provide the lowest risk for recurrence has been a subject of controversy. It was once thought that wide resection with generous margins of normal bowel combined with radical mesenteric excision would result in lower recurrence rates. The accumulated clinical data, however, do not support the need for wide or radical resection for Crohn disease. Resection should be wide enough to encompass the limits of gross disease; wider resections offer no benefit in terms of lessening the risk for recurrence, even when the mucosal margins of the resected portion are positive for microscopic features of Crohn disease.[37] The extent of mesenteric resection does not affect the rate of disease recurrence. It is now generally accepted that resection to grossly normal intestinal margins is sufficient and that frozen section to exclude microscopic disease at the resection margins is not warranted because microscopically positive margins do not adversely affect long-term results.

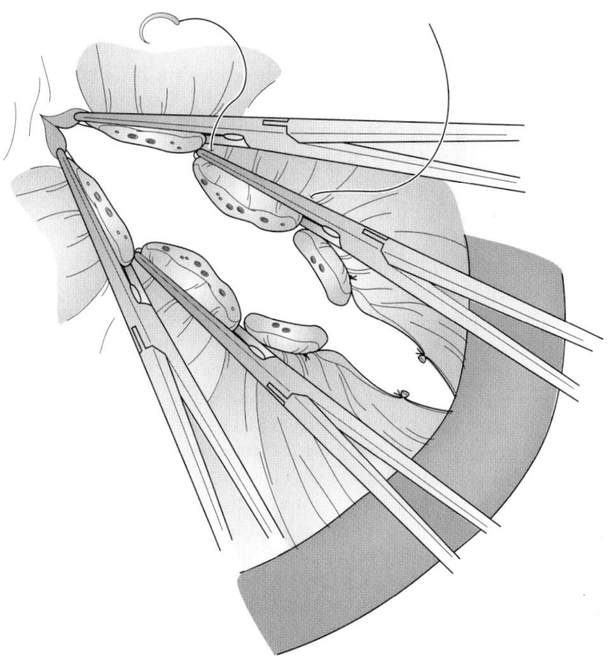

FIGURE 51.11 Technique for suture ligation and division of a thickened and friable Crohn mesentery (After Walsh CJ, Lavery IC. Ileocecectomy. In: Michelassi F, Milsom JW, eds. *Operative strategies in inflammatory bowel disease*. New York: Springer-Verlag, 1999: 294–302.)

Division of the small bowel mesentery that has been affected by Crohn disease is often challenging. The mesentery in Crohn disease is typically massively thickened, with indurated fat, hypertrophied lymphatics, and engorged blood vessels. Standard techniques of simple clamping of mesenteric vessels and ligation are inadequate to handle the thickened mesentery because it is often impossible to fashion vascular pedicles for simple ligation. Inadequate control of mesenteric vessels may result in the development of large mesenteric hematomas, which further complicate the ability to gain vascular control and may even result in a compromise of mesenteric perfusion and resultant bowel ischemia. The preferred technique for dividing the thickened mesentery without losing vascular control is to apply overlapping clamps on either side of the intended line of transection. The mesentery is incised and the tissue within the clamps is suture-ligated (Fig. 51.11). Alternatively the mensenteric vessels can be controlled and mesentery divided with an electrocautery tissue-sealing device. In most cases the use of such device can greatly facilitate the mesenteric dissection. To increase the efficacy and safety of mesenteric control in the case of an extremely thickened mesentery, mattress sutures can be applied through the mesentery on the patient's side of the transection line.

Once the resection is complete, the proximal and distal margins of the resected specimen should be examined to ensure that they are free of gross disease. The entire specimen is closely examined for areas that may be suspected of harboring an occult cancer. Should any areas of the specimen be suspected of harboring an adenocarcinoma, a frozen section should be obtained. If the specimen is found to contain an area of adenocarcinoma, further mesenteric resection may be necessary.

A wide variety of techniques for performing intestinal anastomoses have been applied in the treatment of Crohn disease. These techniques include end-to-end, side-to-end, end-to-side, and side-to-side anastomoses. Standard staple techniques can be utilized on healthy, pliable bowel. Hand sewn techniques provide more versatility for edematous or hypertrophied small intestine. Regardless of the techniques employed, it is important to follow the basic requirements for performing a safe intestinal anastomosis (adequate blood supply, no gross contamination or sepsis, no tension on the anastomosis, no distal obstruction, and adequate bowel cleansing). So long as these basic requirements are met and the patient does not have profound malnutrition, resection and primary anastomosis can be performed in Crohn disease with a high degree of safety.[30]

Minimally Invasive Surgery

Resection of Crohn disease can be performed laparoscopically. To date, the largest experience with laparoscopic resections for Crohn disease have been for ileocecectomy for Crohn disease of the terminal ileum. With a laparoscopic approach the entire small bowel is examined through the laparoscope (Fig. 51.12). To perform the ileocecal resection, the cecum and ascending colon are mobilized laparoscopically. A small incision is made in the abdomen and the mobilized segment of bowel is then delivered through this incision. Vision of the bowel and transection of the mesentery is accomplished extracorporeally and a standard anastomosis performed. The bowel is then returned to the abdominal cavity and the abdominal incision is closed. Multiple nonrandomized studies have reported benefits regarding the length of stay and recovery, smaller wounds and reduced morbidity.[38–44] The demonstrable benefits of this approach, however, have not always been consistently reported.[45] Current available data indicate that laparoscopic ileocecectomy in uncomplicated Crohn disease of the terminal ileum is an acceptable alternative to the standard open surgery and may be superior to standard approaches. The laparoscopic approach is contraindicated in patients who are critically ill and are unable to tolerate a pneumoperitoneum due to hypotension or hypercarbia. Laparoscopic surgery is also to be avoided in patients with dense adhesions, extensive intraabdominal sepsis or complex fistulization.

Strictureplasty

Intestinal strictureplasty is a surgical technique that relieves intestinal obstruction while preserving the length of the small bowel. Although strictureplasty is not appropriate for all surgical cases of Crohn disease, strictureplasty techniques are being utilized with increasing frequency. Strictureplasty is indicated for jejunoileitis with single or multiple fibrotic strictures. Strictureplasty should be considered if the patient has a

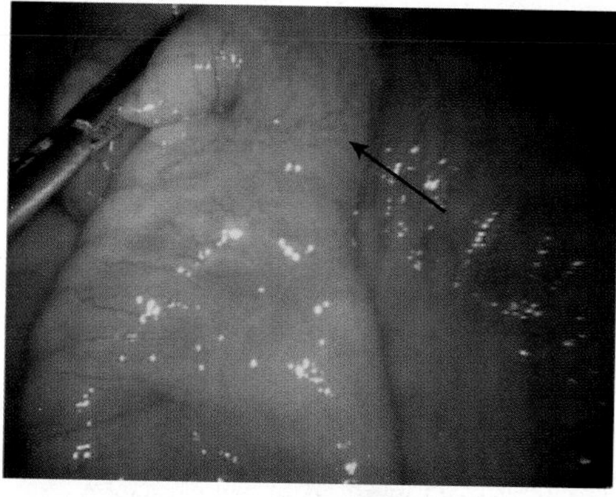

FIGURE 51.12 Crohn disease of the ileum (*arrow*) as seen laparoscopically. (Courtesy of The University of Chicago General Surgery Archives.)

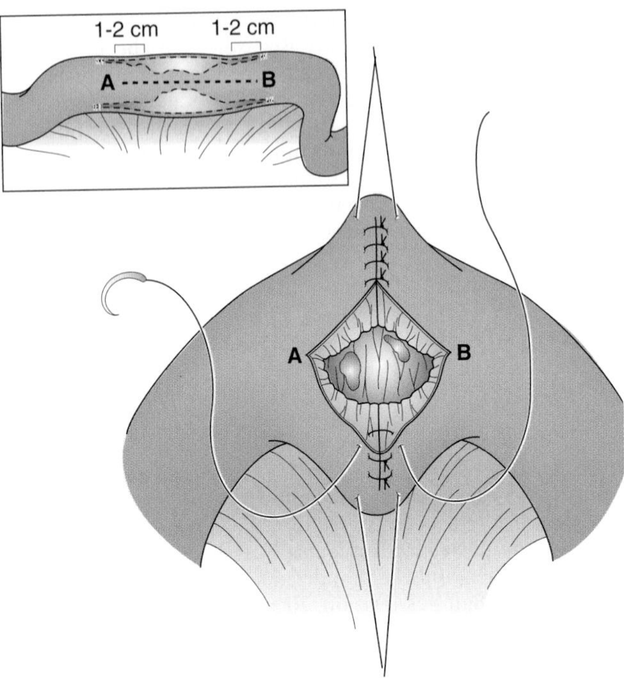

FIGURE 51.13 Heineke-Mikulicz strictureplasty. (After Milsom JW. Strictureplasty and mechanical dilation in strictured Crohn disease. In: Michelassi F, Milsom JW, eds. *Operative strategies in inflammatory bowel disease*. New York: Springer-Verlag, 1999:259–267.)

history of multiple prior resections or rapidly recurring disease. Strictureplasty has also been applied to isolated strictures of the duodenum.

Although strictureplasty is an excellent option in selected cases of small bowel Crohn disease, intestinal resection is required in most cases. Strictureplasty is contraindicated for segments with acute inflammation and phlegmon. It is also contraindicated in patients with generalized peritonitis or profound malnutrition. Additionally, long, high-grade strictures resulting from extremely thickened and rigid intestinal wall are often not amenable to strictureplasty and therefore require resection.

The two most common strictureplasty methods, the *Heineke-Mikulicz* and the *Finney*, are named after the pyloroplasty methods from which they are derived. The Heineke-Mikulicz strictureplasty technique is appropriate for strictures less than 7 cm long.[46] With this technique, a longitudinal incision is made along the antimesenteric border of the stricture. The longitudinal enterotomy is then closed in a transverse fashion to increase the width of the bowel at the point of the stricture (Fig. 51.13). Once the enterotomy is made, the mucosal surface of the stricture is closely examined, and biopsies are taken from areas of the stricture where adenocarcinoma is suspected to rule out the possibility of an occult cancer.

The Finney strictureplasty can be utilized for longer strictures, up to 15 cm in length.[47] With this technique, the affected bowel is folded onto itself in a U-shape and the two limbs are sutured together (Fig. 51.14). A longitudinal enterotomy is then made halfway between the mesenteric and antimesenteric borders, following the course of the U. Again, the mucosal surface is examined and samples are taken as necessary. Sutures are then placed on the posterior wall of the enteroenterostomy, beginning at the apex of the strictureplasty. This suture line is continued anteriorly and is reinforced with an outer layer of interrupted nonabsorbable sutures. For long strictures, the Finney strictureplasty may result in a functional intestinal bypass, with a sizable lateral diverticulum at risk for bacterial overgrowth. For this reason, Finney strictureplasties are utilized far less frequently than Heineke-Mikulicz strictureplasties.

Patients with multiple strictures in close proximity to one another are better treated with a "side-to-side isoperistaltic strictureplasty."[39,48] With this technique, the loop of diseased bowel is divided at its midpoint between bowel clamps, and the mesentery is incised (Fig. 51.15). The proximal intestinal loop is moved over the distal loop in a side-to-side fashion. With the stenotic areas of one loop placed adjacent to dilated areas of the other loop, the two limbs are approximated by a layer of seromuscular interrupted, nonabsorbable sutures. A longitudinal enterostomy is performed on both loops, and the intestinal ends are tapered to avoid blind stumps. Suspected areas of disease are sampled for frozen section to exclude the presence of occult malignancy. The outer suture line is reinforced with an internal row of running, full-thickness absorbable sutures, continued anteriorly. This layer is reinforced by an outer layer of seromuscular interrupted, nonabsorbable sutures (Fig. 51.16). The side-to-side isoperistaltic strictureplasty is a recent advance in the surgical management of difficult cases of extensive Crohn disease, and experience to date with the technique indicates that it is a safe and effective procedure in appropriately selected patients.[49–51]

In resections, diseased tissue is removed and anastomotic sutures are placed in healthy intestine, whereas in strictureplasties, diseased segments are retained and suture lines are placed in diseased tissue. This practice has raised concerns regarding the risk for early postoperative morbidity and recurrent symptomatic disease. The available data indicate that in appropriately selected patients, perioperative morbidity after strictureplasty is similar to that after resection.[50,52–54] The most common postoperative complication directly related to strictureplasty is

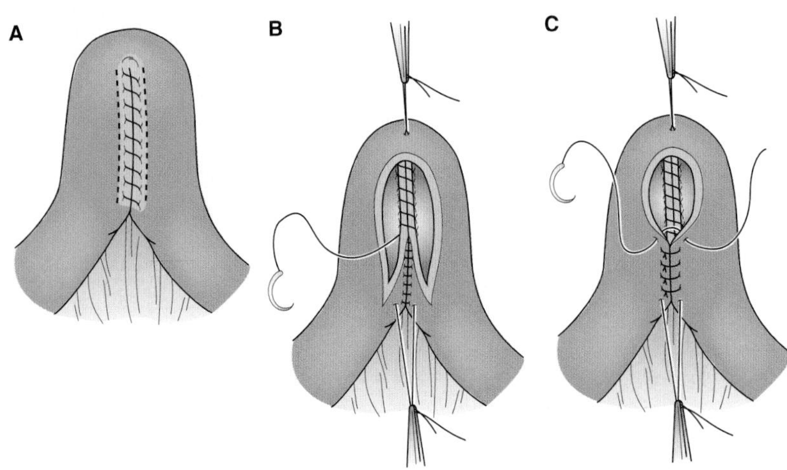

FIGURE 51.14 Finney strictureplasty. (From Hurst RD, Michelassi F. Management of small bowel Crohn's disease. *World J Surg*. 1998;22:359–363.)

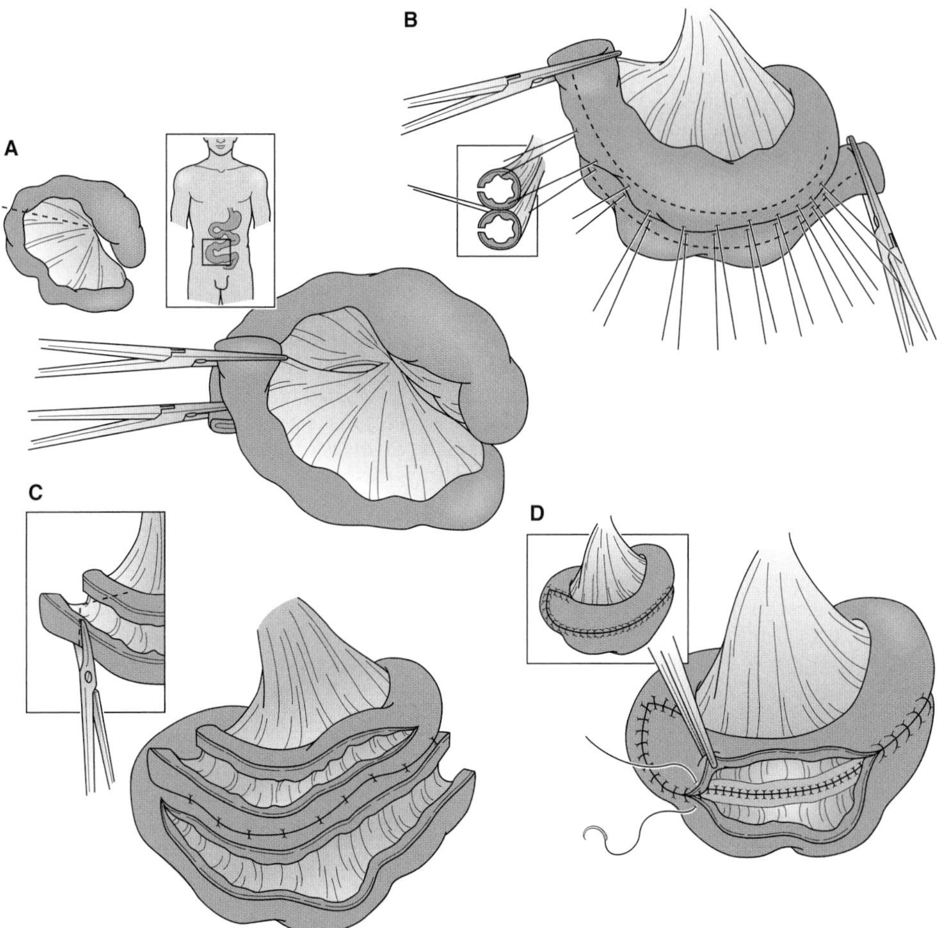

FIGURE 51.15 Side-to-side isoperistaltic strictureplasty. (After Michelassi F. Side-to-side isoperistaltic stricturoplasty for multiple Crohn's strictures. In: *Diseases of the colon and rectum*. Baltimore: Williams & Wilkins, 1996; 39:345–349.)

hemorrhage from the suture line. Hemorrhage occurs in up to 9% of the cases. Fortunately, gastrointestinal hemorrhage following strictureplasty is typically minor and can usually be managed conservatively with blood transfusions alone. Occasionally, arteriography with selected infusion of vasopressin into the branches of the superior mesenteric artery is required to control bleeding. Only in rare instances is reoperation required to control hemorrhage following strictureplasty. Septic complications such as dehiscence, intraabdominal abscess, and fistula formation occur in only 2% to 3% of strictureplasty cases.[52,55] Although no randomized, controlled studies have directly compared recurrence rates after resection versus rates after strictureplasty, the observed recurrence rates after strictureplasty in several reports compare well with published recurrence rates after resection, and rapid recurrence of symptoms following strictureplasty has not proved to be a problem.[50,52,55,56]

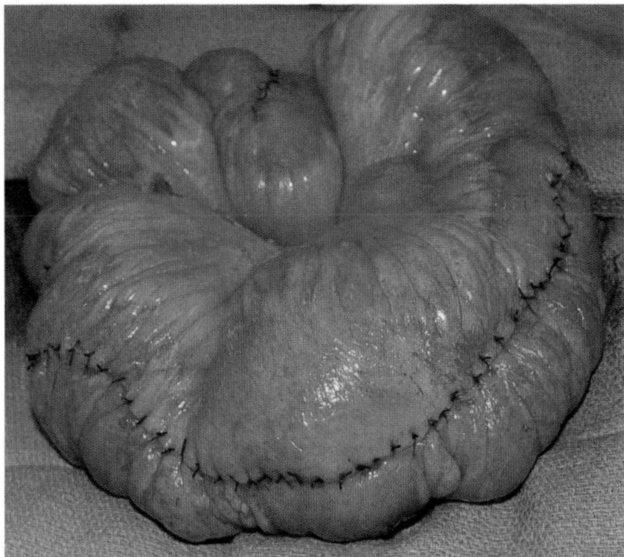

FIGURE 51.16 Appearance of the side-to-side isoperistaltic strictureplasty for management of extensive structuring of the small intestine. (Courtesy of The University of Chicago General Surgery Archives.)

Epidemiologic studies have shown an increased risk for small bowel adenocarcinoma in patients with Crohn disease. Persistently diseased intestine and continued long-term inflammation at the strictureplasty site may increase the risk for adenocarcinoma. Although isolated cases of adenocarcinoma developing close to or at the site of strictureplasty have been reported, the precise risk for neoplastic degeneration is not currently known.

MANAGEMENT OF COMPLICATED CROHN DISEASE

Intestinal Obstruction

Small bowel stricturing disease can range from chronic low-grade obstruction, with symptoms of cramping abdominal pain, bloating, avoidance of food, and weight loss, to high-grade partial or even complete small bowel obstruction.

Intestinal obstruction resulting from Crohn disease does not pose the same degree of surgical urgency as small bowel obstruction caused by adhesions or herniation. Most patients who have high-grade partial or complete small-bowel obstruction associated with Crohn disease can be treated initially with nasogastric decompression, intravenous hydration, and steroid therapy. This regimen, in which acutely distended and edematous bowel is decompressed, in most cases results in resolution of the obstruction, so that appropriate bowel preparation and safer conditions for surgery are possible. When there is concern that the obstruction may not be related to Crohn disease but rather to adhesions or herniation, or if intestinal ischemia or injury is a possibility, then conservative management should be abandoned and the abdomen explored. In addition, if a high-grade or complete bowel obstruction in Crohn disease fails to resolve, one must consider a neoplastic cause.

Patients with complete obstruction who respond well to initial therapy with nasogastric decompression and intravenous steroids remain at high risk for persistent or recurrent symptoms of obstruction and are best managed with surgery once adequate decompression has been achieved.

Stricturing disease of the small intestine can be managed with resection, strictureplasty, or a combination of both techniques.[57] Patients with short-segment stricturing disease are best managed with simple resection and anastomosis because a relatively short resection does not place the patient at risk for the sequelae of short-bowel syndrome. Resection with anastomosis obviates the short-term concern of hemorrhage from the strictureplasty and the long-term concern of cancer risk when diseased tissue is left *in situ*.

Enteric Fistulae

Enteric fistulae in Crohn disease result from full-thickness rupture into an adjacent hollow viscus or through the abdominal wall. Fistulae are present in more than one third of cases of Crohn disease, but only rarely do they represent the primary indication for operative intervention. Most patients with fistulous disease come to surgery with coexisting stricture or abscess. Although fistulae are not often the primary reason for recommending surgery, when they develop in combination with other complications of Crohn disease, they generally pose challenging problems to the surgeon.[58]

Enteroenteric Fistulae

Enteroenteric fistulae are a common manifestation of Crohn disease. They are typically asymptomatic and are often not identified by small bowel radiography. Hence, many are not appreciated before operation and are discovered at the time of abdominal exploration or during inspection of the resected specimen.[59] Many enteroenteric fistulae, especially ileoileal or ileocecal fistulae, are completely contained within the diseased segments of the intestine and can, thus, be managed by simple *en bloc* resection. In cases involving distant fistulization, when *en bloc* resection would require extensive sacrifice of uninvolved intestine, the surgeon should attempt to separate normal loops adherent to the diseased segment and then resect the Crohn-affected segments while retaining normal intestine. The site of distal fistulization can then be managed with either simple closure of the intestinal fistula or by a short segment resection.

Ileosigmoid Fistulae

Because of the proximity of the terminal ileum to the sigmoid colon, ileosigmoid fistulae often develop in Crohn disease of the terminal ileum. Typically, active Crohn disease is limited to the terminal ileum, and the sigmoid colon is only secondarily involved by the ileal inflammatory adhesion and fistulization. Most ileosigmoid fistulae are asymptomatic. However, large-diameter fistulae, particularly those originating proximal to a high-grade stricture, can result in a functional bypass of the colon and cause significant diarrhea.

Two thirds of ileosigmoid fistulae are not recognized before operation.[60] For this reason, the surgeon must always be prepared for the possibility of encountering an ileosigmoid fistula in all cases of small bowel Crohn disease. Most ileosigmoid fistulae can be managed by dividing the fistulous adhesion, resecting the diseased small bowel, and then performing a simple closure of the colonic defect after appropriate débridement of the edges of the colonic fistula opening.[60,61] Sigmoid resection is necessary in the following circumstances: (a) the sigmoid is primarily involved with active Crohn disease, (b) the sigmoid is extensively involved in an inflammatory ileal adhesion and is thus thickened and rigid, (c) débridement of the edges of the fistula results in a large sigmoid defect, and (d) the fistulous opening involves the mesenteric side of the colon and primary closure is difficult.

Ileovesical Fistulae

Ileovesical fistulae are encountered in approximately 5% of patients with Crohn disease.[30] Two thirds of patients with ileovesical fistulae have a history of pneumaturia, fecaluria, or both. Small bowel radiographs and cystograms often do not demonstrate the fistula between the small bowel and the bladder. CT of the pelvis can provide indirect evidence for an enterovesical fistula when air is present within the bladder. Ileosigmoid and ileovesical fistulae often occur together. Up to 60% of patients with an ileovesical fistula also have an ileosigmoid fistula.[61] Thus, the presence of an ileovesical fistula is often an indicator of complex fistulous disease.

The timing of surgery for enterovesical fistulae is controversial. Some physicians consider enteric fistulization to the urinary tract as an absolute indication for surgical treatment, whereas others have argued that patients with enterovesical fistulae can be managed safely with conservative management for extended periods of time.[59] Most surgeons and gastroenterologists agree that the effects of chronic urinary tract infection on renal function, in addition to symptoms of the primary ileal Crohn disease, indicate operation. As with other Crohn fistulae, the surgical treatment is based on resection of the diseased segment of intestine and extirpation of the fistulous tract. With ileovesical fistulae, the connection to the bladder is most commonly located at the dome, and débridement and primary closure can be affected without endangering the trigone.

Enterocutaneous Fistulae

Enterocutaneous fistulae occur in approximately 4% of patients with Crohn disease.[31] Enterocutaneous fistulae result from either direct penetration of a sinus through the abdominal wall or external drainage of an abscess that communicates with the diseased intestinal tract. Common sites of spontaneous drainage of an enterocutaneous fistula in Crohn disease are through a previous abdominal scar or the umbilicus.

The presence of an enterocutaneous fistula does not necessarily dictate the need for surgical intervention. If the patient's underlying disease is under satisfactory control and the output of the enterocutaneous fistula is minimal, then a period of conservative management may be appropriate. The nonoperative management of fistulae related to Crohn disease includes clearance of sepsis, aggressive nutritional support, and appropriate medical therapy. Anti-TNF chimeric monoclonal antibody (infliximab) may be of particular value in this situation.[27,29] Even with aggressive nonoperative management, enterocutaneous fistulae related to Crohn disease are slow to heal, and surgery is often ultimately required. Surgical therapy is based on resection of the diseased intestinal segment, extirpation of the fistula, and débridement of the entire fistulous tract through the abdominal wall.

Enterogenital Fistulae

Enterogenital fistulae, including enterovaginal, enterosalpingeal, and enterouterine fistulae, are very rare complications of Crohn disease. Enterovaginal fistulae most commonly occur in patients who have undergone a previous hysterectomy.[62] Symptoms include a malodorous discharge and the passage of air through the vagina. Surgical treatment involves resection of the diseased intestine and extirpation of the fistulous tract along with drainage of any intervening abscess.

Enterosalpingeal and enterouterine fistulae are extremely rare. They are difficult to identify preoperatively and are most often recognized only at the time of surgical exploration. Enterosalpingeal fistulae should be managed by removal of the affected tube. If the fistula gives rise to a tuboovarian abscess, then resection of both the ovary and the tube is necessary. With enterouterine fistulae, attempts to salvage the uterus may be undertaken should the patient wish to preserve fertility; otherwise, hysterectomy with resection of the affected small bowel is the best surgical option.

Abscesses

Intraabdominal abscesses that form in Crohn disease tend to be chronic, with an indolent clinical course of modest fever, abdominal pain, and leukocytosis. Abscesses related to Crohn disease only rarely present with overwhelming systemic sepsis. A tender palpable abdominal mass is very likely to be an intraabdominal abscess because more than 50% of inflammatory masses harbor an abscess collection. In up to one third of abscesses related to Crohn disease, no preoperative clinical signs of localized infection are present, and the abscesses are discovered only by intraoperative exploration. When an abscess is suspected or a mass palpated, preoperative CT should be performed (see Fig. 51.10). CT provides information regarding the size and location of the abscess, the feasibility of percutaneous drainage, and the relationship of the septic process to retroperitoneal structures, such as the ureters, duodenum, and inferior vena cava.

Many abscesses in Crohn disease are small collections that are nearly completely contained within the area of diseased intestine. This quality is particularly true for intramesenteric and intraloop abscesses (Fig. 51.17). In these cases, resection of the affected segment of intestine extirpates the abscess cavity, so that the placement of drains is not necessary and primary anastomosis can be performed without risk.

Small abscesses can be readily managed at the time of surgical exploration, but larger abscesses are best managed with preoperative CT-guided percutaneous drainage.[63] The preoperative drainage of larger abscesses facilitates subsequent surgical intervention by controlling sepsis that might otherwise result in perioperative hemodynamic instability. Additionally, when a large abscess is adherent to a long segment of normal intestine or to the mesentery of normal intestine, preoperative percutaneous drainage may allow for sufficient healing such that sacrifice of normal intestine can be avoided and a more limited resection accomplished. Percutaneous drainage may also allow for resection and primary anastomosis when the degree of sepsis and inflammation would otherwise dictate the need for a temporary ileostomy.[64]

CROHN DISEASE OF THE DUODENUM

Symptomatic Crohn disease of the duodenum is a rare entity, and the need for surgical intervention is uncommon.[65] When the duodenum is involved with Crohn disease, special surgical strategies must be employed. Unlike jejunal or ileal resections, resection of the duodenum is an extreme undertaking. Fortunately, because of the peculiar manifestations of duodenal Crohn disease, resection of the duodenum is almost never necessary.

The duodenum can be involved either primarily with Crohn disease or secondarily by inflammatory adhesions or fistulae originating from disease elsewhere in the gastrointestinal tract. Primary Crohn disease of the duodenum typically manifests with an inflammatory pattern that results in ulceration and edema. The inflammation may cause strictures to form, but fistulae, sinuses, abscesses, and free perforation almost never develop (Fig. 51.18). Crohn fistulae involving the duodenum are almost always the result of perforating disease originating elsewhere, in the small bowel or colon.[66]

Primary Disease of the Duodenum

Because the predominant complication of duodenal Crohn disease is the formation of strictures rather than fistulae, nonresectional techniques such as strictureplasty and bypass procedures are applicable in most cases. The optimal surgical strategies for

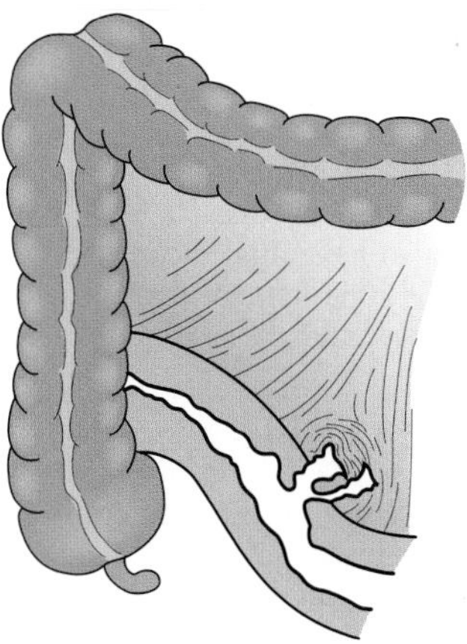

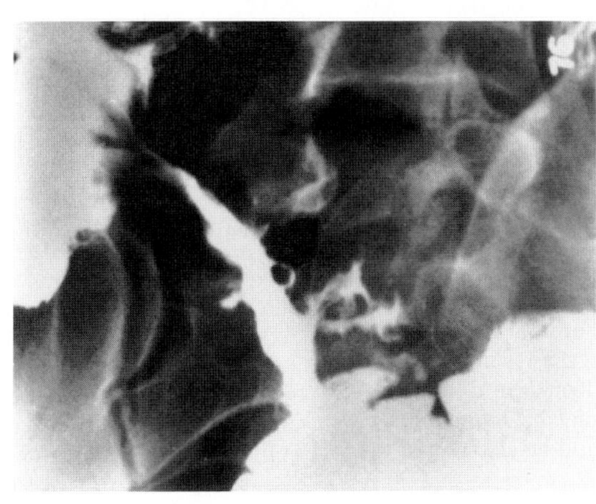

FIGURE 51.17 Small bowel follow-through demonstrating an intra-mesenteric abscess originating from a perforation of the terminal ileum into the mesentery. (From Michelassi F. Crohn's disease. In: Bell RH, Rikkers LF, Mulholland MW, eds. *Digestive tract surgery*. Philadelphia: Lippincott-Raven, 1996:1201–1227.)

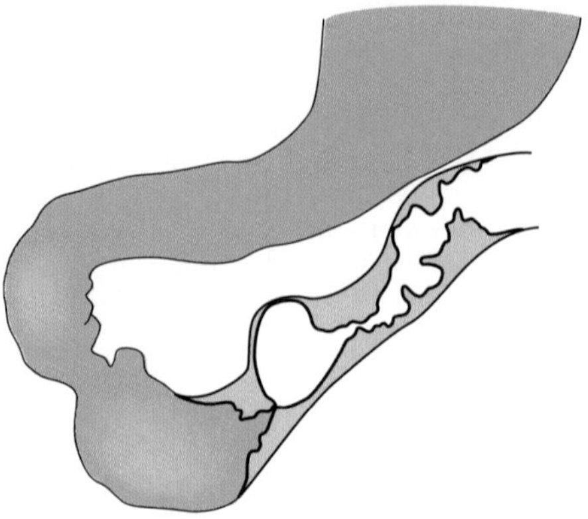

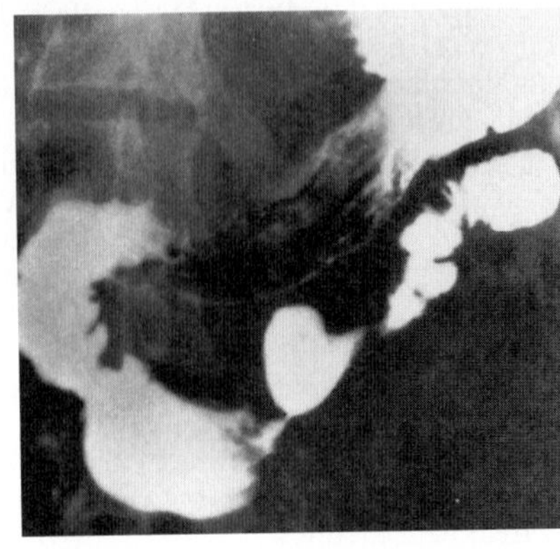

FIGURE 51.18 Crohn disease affecting the third and fourth portions of the duodenum. (From Block GE, Michelassi F, Tanaka M, et. al. Crohn's disease. *Curr Probl Surg.* 1993;30:173–272.)

managing duodenal strictures in Crohn disease depend on the pattern of disease. Most of these strictures are focal and can be managed with a Heineke-Mikulicz strictureplasty.[67]

If the duodenal stricture is lengthy or the tissues are too rigid and unyielding, then strictureplasty is not suitable, and an intestinal bypass procedure should be performed. A simple side-to-side retrocolic gastrojejunostomy can be performed for obstructing disease of the duodenum. This procedure effectively relieves the symptoms of duodenal obstruction but has the drawback of being inherently ulcerogenic. To lessen the likelihood that stomal ulcerations will develop, vagotomy is performed along with the gastrojejunostomy. After truncal vagotomy, the frequency of soft stools is often increased, and in some cases, frank diarrhea develops. This possible side effect is particularly concerning in patients with Crohn disease, who often have an altered baseline bowel function. For this reason, highly selective vagotomy, which is much less likely to cause diarrhea, is preferred over truncal vagotomy.

If the first and second portions of the duodenum are spared from Crohn disease, a Roux-en-Y duodenojejunostomy can be performed to bypass obstructing disease of the more distal duodenum.[68] This procedure allows the strictured duodenum to be bypassed and obviates concerns about acid-induced marginal ulceration and the need for vagotomy.

Secondary Involvement of the Duodenum

Fistulous Crohn disease of the jejunum, ileum, or colon may secondarily involve the duodenum. This involvement is most commonly seen in recurrent Crohn disease at the site of a previous ileocolonic anastomosis that has become adherent to the duodenum (Fig. 51.19). Most duodenal fistulae are asymptomatic; others may shunt duodenal content to the distal small bowel or colon, so that malabsorption and diarrhea result. In a majority of cases, duodenoenteric fistulae are identified with preoperative small bowel radiography, yet many are discovered only at the time of surgery.

The surgical management of duodenal-enteric fistulae entails resection of the primary disease with repair of the duodenal defect. Most duodenal fistulae are located away from the juncture of the duodenal wall with the head of the pancreas, and thus they can be managed by simple débridement and primary closure without difficulty. Larger fistulae or fistulae associated with more significant inflammatory adhesion may require more extensive débridement; the resulting sizable duodenal defects require closure with a Roux-en-Y duodenojejunostomy or with a jejunal serosal patch.[69] Duodenal resections are almost never necessary and should be considered the surgical option of last resort.

CROHN DISEASE OF THE COLON

The surgical management of Crohn disease of the large intestine depends on a variety of factors, including the distribution and pattern of disease, the extent of rectal involvement, and the adequacy of fecal continence. The surgical procedures commonly required include segmental colectomy or ileocolectomy with primary anastomosis, total abdominal colectomy with ileoproctostomy, and total proctocolectomy with permanent end ileostomy. Because of the recurrent nature of Crohn disease, a restorative procedure such as ileal pouch—anal anastomosis or continent ileostomy is often inappropriate for patients with an established diagnosis of Crohn disease.

Ileocolitis

The management of ileocecal or ileocolonic disease is similar to the management of disease limited to the terminal ileum. Resection to grossly normal margins with primary anastomosis is often the beset surgical option. The long-term clinical course of terminal ileal disease with limited involvement of the proximal colon resembles the clinical course of Crohn disease involving only terminal ileum. Disease tends to recur at the anastomosis and preanastomotic ileum. The risk for recurrent disease in the distal colon or rectum is low, so the long-term chance that a permanent stoma will be required is low.

Extensive Crohn Colitis with Rectal Sparing

Crohn disease that predominates in the colon often involves long segments of the colon. Extensive Crohn colitis that does not respond to medical treatment requires total colectomy. Commonly, the rectum is spared, and an ileorectal anastomosis can be performed and a permanent stoma avoided or at least delayed. Unfortunately, recurrence after total abdominal colectomy with ileorectal anastomosis is common, and many of these patients ultimately require proctectomy with permanent ileostomy.[70] Even with a high risk for recurrence, a permanent stoma can be avoided for several years in most patients whose rectum is not affected by disease.[60,71] For patients with Crohn colitis who also have anal incontinence, removal of the colon and rectum with permanent ileostomy is required, even though the rectum itself may be free of disease.

Segmental Crohn Colitis

In segmental Crohn colitis, a short length of diseased colon is surrounded by normal colon both proximally and distally. This is a relatively uncommon pattern. Segmental resection of the diseased portion of the colon with colocolonic anastomosis

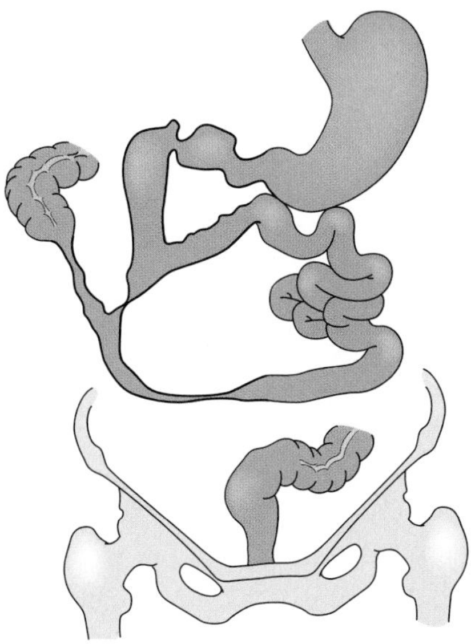

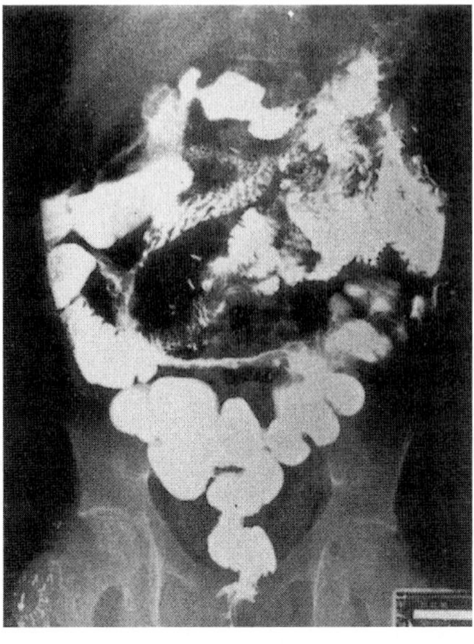

FIGURE 51.19 Upper gastrointestinal series showing an ileoduodenal fistula in patient with recurrent Crohn disease proximal to the ileoascending anastomosis. (From Michelassi F, Balestracci T, Chappell R, et. al. Primary and recurrent Crohn's disease: experience with 1,379 patients. *Ann Surg.* 1991;214:230–238.)

has been advocated, and several reports have demonstrated good long-term results.[71,72] However, segmental colectomy is controversial because of the high risk for recurrence, which at times develops rapidly in the preanastomotic colon. Many believe that the rate of recurrence can be lowered by resecting the entire proximal colon, with subsequent anastomosis of the terminal ileum to the normal colon distal to the area of disease. This approach results in an extensive loss of normal colonic mucosa when disease is limited to the distal left colon or sigmoid, which may result in frequent watery stools or even incontinence. A reasonable approach for the surgical management of segmental Crohn disease of the colon is to perform a segmental resection with colocolonic anastomosis for disease isolated to the distal descending or sigmoid colon and resection to normal ileum with ileocolonic anastomosis for segmental colitis of the more proximal colon. With this approach, the significant absorptive capacity of the proximal colon is not sacrificed in patients with limited left-sided disease, and the risk for rapid recurrence in the proximal colon is avoided in patients with more extensive proximal disease. Regardless of the extent of resection, patients with focal Crohn colitis are at high risk for long-term recurrent Crohn disease of the colon and rectum.

Rectal Crohn Disease

The surgical treatment of Crohn disease of the rectum requires proctectomy with a permanent stoma. Commonly, Crohn proctitis occurs with extensive Crohn colitis, and so a total proctocolectomy is performed. When disease is isolated to the rectum, an abdominoperineal resection with end colostomy will suffice. Unlike removal of the rectum for malignant disease, proctectomy for Crohn disease does not require and should not involve a wide excision of perirectal tissue. To avoid injury to pelvic sympathetic and parasympathetic nerves, the dissection should be undertaken close to the rectal wall.[73] In the absence of significant perianal disease, the perineal dissection is carried out with an intersphincteric dissection between the internal and external anal sphincter muscles. The intersphincteric dissection results in a smaller wound, and healing is faster than after the wide perineal excision required for malignant disease. If significant perianal disease with abscesses, complex fistulae, and dense scarring is present, then a wide perineal excision is required. In more severe cases, the perineal wound may require closure with tissue transfer grafts.

Patients with Crohn disease involving the colon and rectum but without any history of small bowel involvement and without perianal disease can be considered for a restorative proctocolectomy with an ileal pouch—anal anastomosis. This is an unusual pattern of disease, but it has been associated with a relatively low risk for recurrence in the small bowel after proctocolectomy. For this reason, ileoanal anastomosis has been advocated for selected patients with the unusual pattern of Crohn disease strictly limited to colon and rectal involvement.

Perianal Crohn Disease

Perianal manifestations are found in approximately one third of patients with Crohn disease. These manifestations include abscesses, fistulae, fissures, anal stenosis, and hypertrophic skin tags.[74] Except in very rare cases, perianal Crohn disease does not occur in isolation; most patients have some evidence of active or quiescent disease elsewhere in the gastrointestinal tract. Unlike isolated idiopathic perianal abscess or fistula-in-ano, which can occur in patients without Crohn disease, perianal Crohn disease tends to be recurrent, complex, and occasionally progressive (Fig. 51.20). As a general rule, the treatment of perianal Crohn disease should be conservative. Repeated operations with recurring disease can lead to significant injury to the anal sphincters, with a risk for incontinence.

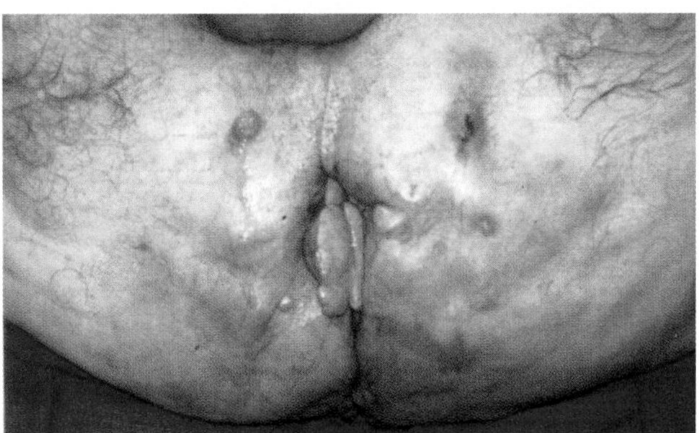

FIGURE 51.20 Severe perianal Crohn disease with multiple draining fistulae-in-ano and enlarged skin tags. (Courtesy of The University of Chicago General Surgery Archives.)

Medical therapies that have been shown to have some effectiveness in the management of perianal Crohn disease include antibiotics, particularly metronidazole and ciprofloxacin; antimetabolites, such as 6-MP and azathioprine; and cyclosporine. Anti-TNF antibody (infliximab) has been shown to be effective in promoting the healing of complex Crohn perianal fistulae, with apparently few side effects.[29] The surgical procedures commonly employed include incision and drainage of abscesses, simple fistulotomy, incision and opening of fistulous tracts, application of "draining" setons or mushroom catheters, and the creation of rectal mucosal advancement flaps.

Surgical incision and drainage are mandated for perianal abscesses. Perianal sepsis requires surgical drainage; attempts at treating purulent collections with medical therapy are invariably unsuccessful. Uncomplicated low-lying fistulae are best treated initially with metronidazole or ciprofloxacin.[75,76] These agents are moderately effective in promoting the healing of fistulae related to Crohn disease and are associated with a very low risk for complications. If the response to antibiotic therapy is inadequate, then simple fistulotomy should be performed for uncomplicated low-lying fistulae. Low-lying Crohn fistulae typically heal well after fistulotomy, and the risk for incontinence is low. More complex perianal fistulae carry a higher risk for postsurgical complications, and so attempts at more aggressive medical treatment with anti-TNF antibody or 6-MP are warranted before surgery is recommended for these more difficult cases.

An option in the treatment of complex perianal fistulae is the cannulation of complex fistulous tracts with setons (Fig. 51.21). In the management of these difficult cases, careful judgment is required, as surgical fistulotomy or the application of cutting setons can result in incontinence with high-lying Crohn fistulae.

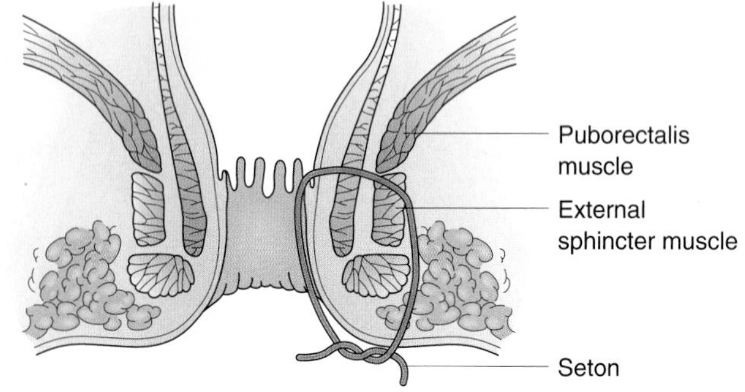

FIGURE 51.21 Placement of a seton suture through a trans-sphincteric fistula-in-ano. (After Gordon PH. Anorectal abscesses and fistula-in-ano. In: Gordon PH, Nivatvongs S, eds. *Principles and practice of surgery for the colon, rectum, and anus*. St. Louis: Quality Medical, 1992:221–265.)

To prevent incontinence in these patients, a rectal mucosal advancement flap procedure is often the best option for high-lying, suprasphincteric, complex fistulae[77] (Fig. 51.22). Rectal advancement flaps are not appropriate when the rectal mucosa itself is affected by active Crohn disease. Patients with active rectal mucosal Crohn disease occurring with complex perianal disease are at high risk for requiring proctectomy with permanent ileostomy.

A temporary stoma to divert the fecal stream is created only in selected cases of complicated perianal disease. Fecal diversion is occasionally appropriate to help in the healing of rectovaginal fistulae. Temporary fecal diversion is sometimes employed in conjunction with rectal advancement flaps to

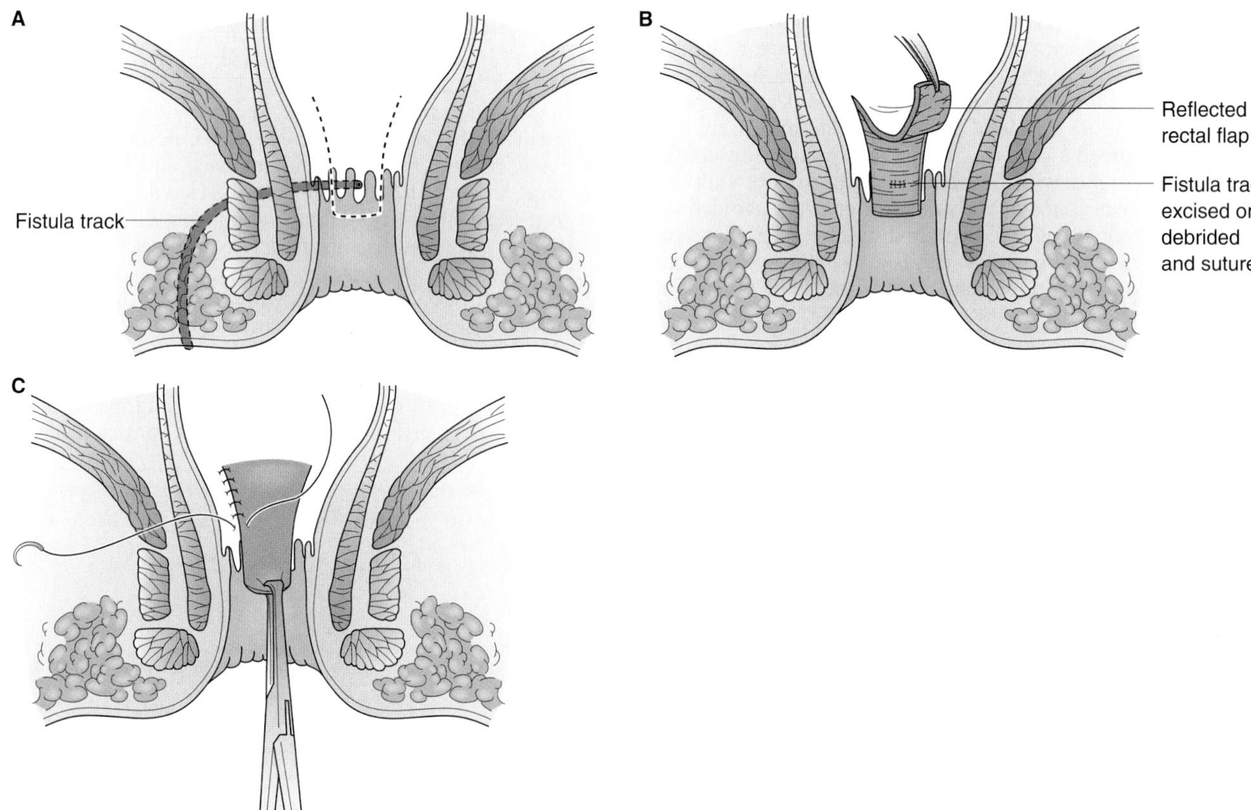

FIGURE 51.22 Rectal advancement flap procedure can be performed for treatment of fistula-in-ano and rectovaginal fistula. (After From Strong S, Fazio VW. The surgical management of Crohn disease. In: Kirsner JB, ed. *Inflammatory bowel disease*, 5th ed. Philadelphia: WB Saunders, 2000, pp. 658–709.)

assist in the healing of particularly difficult cases. In severe cases of perianal disease that do not respond to aggressive medical and surgical treatment, fecal diversion typically results in significant relief of local sepsis and inflammation. Unfortunately, disease activity typically recurs rapidly in these cases after reestablishment of the fecal stream.

LONG-TERM MORBIDITY AND RECURRENCE OF DISEASE

Because of the recurrent nature of Crohn disease, repeated operations are often required. Serial, massive, or injudicious resections of the small bowel in patients with Crohn disease can result in permanent impairment of intestinal absorption. Important factors influencing the absorptive capacity of the bowel include the following:

- Anatomic site of resection
- Length of resection
- Presence of the ileocecal valve
- Condition of the remaining bowel and related digestive organs
- Adaptation of the remaining bowel after resection

Resection of one half to two thirds of the small bowel represents the upper limit of safety. When resections exceed this limit, particularly in the absence of the colon, absorption is markedly altered and poses significant management problems. In addition, loss of the specialized function of the ileum can lead to vexing diarrhea and nutrient-specific malabsorption, even after seemingly "conservative" resections. Fortunately, only in rare instances does a true short-gut syndrome occur. In many such cases, the short-gut syndrome can be managed with dietary manipulations, and less than 1% of patients with Crohn disease become dependent on long-term hyperalimentation.

The loss of ileal function leads directly to malabsorption of bile salts and vitamin B_{12}. After resection of the terminal ileum, particularly if the ileocecal vale is lost, bile salts normally absorbed by the terminal ileum are delivered to the colon. Bile salts interfere with the colonic absorption of fluid and electrolytes. In many patients, this results in an increased frequency of stools, which tend to be soft or pasty. Some patients have frank diarrhea. This so-called bile salt diarrhea may be treated with oral cholestyramine, which binds unabsorbed bile acids so that they do not affect the colon. Significant malabsorption of vitamin B_{12} does not routinely occur in patients who undergo resection of the terminal ileum, but patients who have undergone lengthy or repeated resections of the terminal ileum should be monitored for possible B_{12} deficiency.

The most common long-term complication following surgery for Crohn disease is recurrent disease. Reported crude and cumulative recurrence rates vary greatly. Endoscopic evidence of recurrence has been reported to vary from 28% to 73% at 1 year and from 77% to 85% at 3 years after ileal resection.[78] In most instances, endoscopically detected recurrence is minor and asymptomatic and therefore not of great clinical significance. The recurrence rate of symptomatic Crohn disease is approximately 60% at 5 years, and the recurrence rate increases with time, so that symptomatic recurrence is noted after 20 years in 75% to 95% of cases.[79] Hence, the long-term risk for recurrence of the symptoms of Crohn disease is very high. Reports vary, but the rate of reoperation to treat recurrent disease is approximately 20% at 5 years, 33% at 10 years, and 50% at 20 years.[11,80,81]

Crohn disease is most likely to recur close to the previously resected intestinal segment, typically at the anastomosis and in the preanastomotic bowel. This is particularly true for terminal ileal disease. Additionally, the length of small bowel involved with recurrent disease corresponds to the length of bowel originally resected.[82] Short-segment disease tends to recur within a short segment of the preanastomotic bowel, and lengthy segments of disease typically recur in lengthy segments. Also, with a lesser degree of concordance, stenotic disease tends to recur as stenotic disease and perforating disease tends to recur as perforating disease.

Many putative risk factors for recurrence have been studied. The cumulative literature has validated few of them as true risk factors for postsurgical recurrence of disease. A growing body of evidence indicates that smoking can increase the risk for recurrence. Some evidence indicates that the use of NSAIDs may also promote recurrence of disease. All patients with Crohn disease should be strongly advised to refrain from smoking cigarettes or taking NSAIDs. It does not appear that diet has any influence on the likelihood of recurrence.

The results of recent trials indicate that recurrent disease can be diminished with postoperative maintenance therapy. The most common maintenance therapies recommended are controlled-release 5-ASA (Pentasa) and 6-MP.[24,83,84] Maintenance with 5-ASA is associated with few side effects, but up to 12 pills per day are required, and the drug is expensive. 6-Mercaptopurine is less expensive and is taken on a once-a-day basis, but it is associated with potential bone marrow suppression, so that patients on 6-MP maintenance must be followed with periodic blood cell counts. The degree to which postsurgical maintenance therapy lessens the risk for recurrent disease is in some cases only marginal. The effects on long-term quality of life and the cost-effectiveness of postoperative maintenance therapy have not been fully determined. Thus, the decision to recommend maintenance therapy must be individualized for each patient.

KEY POINTS

- **The etiology of Crohn disease is not known.**
- **The inflammation of Crohn disease extends through all layers of the bowel wall.**
- **The presence of well-developed lymphoid aggregates in an edematous or fibrotic submucosa or subserosa is virtually diagnostic of Crohn disease. Granulomas are a valuable diagnostic feature of Crohn disease, but their presence is not pathognomonic.**
- **Because the etiology of Crohn disease is unknown, no therapy directed against the primary cause of Crohn disease is available; rather, medical treatment consists of supportive symptomatic care along with a variety of antiinflammatory drugs.**
- **Crohn disease is a recurring disorder that cannot be cured with surgical resection. As such, surgery is intended to provide palliation.**
- **Because of the recurrent nature of Crohn disease, repeated operations are often required. Serial resections of the small bowel in patients with Crohn disease can result in permanent impairment of intestinal absorption.**

References

1. Crohn BB, Ginzburg L, Oppenheimer GD. Regional ileitis: a pathological and clinical entity. *JAMA* 1932;99:1323–1329.
2. **Loftus EV, Jr. Clinical epidemiology of inflammatory bowel disease: Incidence, prevalence, and environmental influences. *Gastroenterology* 2004;126:1504–1517.**
3. Sandler RS, Glenn ME. Epidemiology of inflammatory bowel disease. In: Kirsner JB, ed. *Inflammatory bowel disease*, 5th ed. Philadelphia: WB Saunders; 2000:89–112.
4. Kirsner JB. Etiologic concepts of inflammatory bowel disease: past, present, and future. In: Michelassi F, Milsom JW, eds. *Operative strategies in inflammatory bowel disease.* New York: Springer-Verlag, 1999, pp. 3–20.
5. Fiocchi C. Inflammatory bowel disease: etiology and pathogenesis. *Gastroenterology* 1998;115:182–205.

6. Schreiber S, Hampe J. Genomics and inflammatory bowel disease. *Curr Opin Gastroenterol* 2000;16:297–305.
7. Pierik M, Yang H, Barmada MM, et al. The IBD International Genetics Consortium Provides Further Evidence for Linkage to IBD4 and Shows Gene-Environment Interaction. *Inflamm Bowel Dis.* 2005;11:1–7.
8. Mayer L. Current concepts of inflammatory bowel disease etiology and pathogenesis. In: Kirsner JB, ed. *Inflammatory bowel disease*, 5 ed. Philadelphia: WB Saunders., 2000, pp. 280–296.
9. Thomas GA, Rhodes J, Green JT. Inflammatory bowel disease and smoking—a review. *Am J Gastroenterol.* 1998;93:144–149.
10. May GR, Sutherland LR, Meddings JB. Is small intestinal permeability really increased in relatives of patients with Crohn's disease? *Gastroenterology.* 1993;104:1627–1632.
11. Michelassi F, Balestracci T, Chappell R, et al. Primary and recurrent Crohn's disease. Experience with 1379 patients. *Ann Surg.* 1991;214:230–238; discussion 238–240.
12. Block GE, Michelassi F, Tanaka M, et al. Crohn's disease. *Curr Probl Surg.* 1993;30:173–265.
13. Steinhart AH, Girgrah N, McLeod RS. Reliability of a Crohn's disease clinical classification scheme based on disease behavior. *Inflamm Bowel Dis.* 1998;4:228–234.
14. Mekhjian HS, Switz DM, Melnyk CS, et al. Clinical features and natural history of Crohn's disease. *Gastroenterology* 1979;77(4 Pt 2):898–906.
15. Carlson HC. Perspective: the small bowel examination in the diagnosis of Crohn's disease. *AJR Am J Roentgenol.* 1986;147:63–65.
16. Rutgeerts P, Vantrappen G, Geboes K. Endoscopy in inflammatory bowel disease. *Scand J Gastroenterol Suppl.* 1989;170:12–15; discussion 16–19.
17. Gossios KJ, Tsianos EV. Crohn disease: CT findings after treatment. *Abdom Imaging* 1997;22:160–163.
18. Wheeler JG, Slack NF, Duncan A, et al. The diagnosis of intra-abdominal abscesses in patients with severe Crohn's disease. *Q J Med.* 1992;82:159–167.
19. **Best WR, Becktel JM, Singleton JW, et al. Development of a Crohn's disease activity index. National Cooperative Crohn's Disease Study. *Gastroenterology* 1976;70:439–444.**
20. Best WR, Becktel JM, Singleton JW. Rederived values of the eight coefficients of the Crohn's Disease Activity Index (CDAI). Gastroenterology 1979;77(4 Pt 2):843–846.
21. Summers RW, Switz DM, Sessions JT, Jr., et al. National Cooperative Crohn's Disease Study: results of drug treatment. *Gastroenterology.* 1979;77(4 Pt 2): 847–869.
22. Hanauer SB, Stein RB. Medical therapy. In: Michelassi F, Milsom JW, eds. *Operative strategies in inflammatory bowel disease.* New York: Springer-Verlag, 1999, pp. 138–149.
23. Lichtenstein GR, Hanauer SB, Kane SV, et al. Crohn's is not a 6-week disease: lifelong management of mild to moderate Crohn's disease. *Inflamm Bowel Dis.* 2004;10(suppl 2):S2–10.
24. McLeod RS, Wolff BG, Steinhart AH, et al. Prophylactic mesalamine treatment decreases postoperative recurrence of Crohn's disease. *Gastroenterology* 1995;109:404–413.
25. Choi PM, Targan SR. Immunomodulator therapy in inflammatory bowel disease. *Dig Dis Sci.* 1994;39:1885–1892.
26. Pearson DC, May GR, Fick GH, et al. Azathioprine and 6-mercaptopurine in Crohn disease. A meta-analysis. *Ann Intern Med.* 1995;123:132–142.
27. **Targan SR, Hanauer SB, van Deventer SJ, et al. A short-term study of chimeric monoclonal antibody cA2 to tumor necrosis factor alpha for Crohn's disease. Crohn's Disease cA2 Study Group. *N Engl J Med.* 1997;337:1029–1035.**
28. van Dullemen HM, van Deventer SJ, Hommes DW, et al. Treatment of Crohn's disease with anti-tumor necrosis factor chimeric monoclonal antibody (cA2). *Gastroenterology* 1995;109:129–135.
29. Present DH, Rutgeerts P, Targan S, et al. Infliximab for the treatment of fistulas in patients with Crohn's disease. *N Engl J Med.* 1999;340: 1398–1405.
30. Hurst RD, Molinari M, Chung TP, et al. Prospective study of the features, indications, and surgical treatment in 513 consecutive patients affected by Crohn's disease. *Surgery* 1997;122:661–667; discussion 667–668.
31. Michelassi F, Stella M, Balestracci T, et al. Incidence, diagnosis, and treatment of enteric and colorectal fistulae in patients with Crohn's disease. *Ann Surg.* 1993;218:660–666.
32. Michelassi F. Incidence, diagnosis and treatment of abdominal abscesses in Crohn's disease. *Research in Surgery* 1996;8:35–39.
33. Sparberg M, Kirsner JB. Recurrent hemorrhage in regional enteritis. Report of 3 cases. *Am J Dig Dis.* 1966;11:652–657.
34. Ribeiro MB, Greenstein AJ, Sachar DB, et al. Colorectal adenocarcinoma in Crohn's disease. *Ann Surg.* 1996;223:186–193.
35. Darke SG, Parks AG, Grogono JL, et al. Adenocarcinoma and Crohn's disease. A report of 2 cases and analysis of the literature. *Br J Surg.* 1973;60:169–175.
36. Telander RL, Schmeling DJ. Current surgical management of Crohn's disease in childhood. *Semin Pediatr Surg.* 1994;3:19–27.
37. **Fazio VW, Marchetti F, Church M, et al. Effect of resection margins on the recurrence of Crohn's disease in the small bowel. A randomized controlled trial. *Ann Surg.* 1996;224:563–571; discussion 571–573.**
38. Bergamaschi R, Pessaux P, Arnaud JP. Comparison of conventional and laparoscopic ileocolic resection for Crohn's disease. *Dis Colon Rectum* 2003;46:1129–1133.
39. Duepree HJ, Senagore AJ, Delaney CP, et al. Advantages of laparoscopic resection for ileocecal Crohn's disease. *Dis Colon Rectum* 2002;45: 605–610.
40. Tabet J, Hong D, Kim CW, et al. Laparoscopic versus open bowel resection for Crohn's disease. *Can J Gastroenterol.* 2001;15:237–242.
41. Msika S, Iannelli A, Deroide G, et al. Can laparoscopy reduce hospital stay in the treatment of Crohn's disease? *Dis Colon Rectum* 2001;44:1661–1666.
42. Milsom JW, Hammerhofer KA, Bohm B, et al. Prospective, randomized trial comparing laparoscopic vs. conventional surgery for refractory ileocolic Crohn's disease. *Dis Colon Rectum* 2001;44:1–8; discussion 8–9.
43. Bemelman WA, Slors JF, Dunker MS, et al. Laparoscopic-assisted vs. open ileocolic resection for Crohn's disease. A comparative study. *Surg Endosc.* 2000;14:721–725.
44. Alabaz O, Iroatulam AJ, Nessim A, et al. Comparison of laparoscopically assisted and conventional ileocolic resection for Crohn's disease. *Eur J Surg.* 2000;166:213–217.
45. Benoist S, Panis Y, Beaufour A, et al. Laparoscopic ileocecal resection in Crohn's disease: a case-matched comparison with open resection. *Surg Endosc.* 2003;17:814–818.
46. Fazio VW, Galandiuk S, Jagelman DG, et al. Strictureplasty in Crohn's disease. *Ann Surg.* 1989;210:621–625.
47. Sharif H, Alexander-Williams J. The role of strictureplasty in Crohn's disease. *Int Surg.* 1992;77:15–18.
48. Michelassi F. Side-to-side isoperistaltic strictureplasty for multiple Crohn's strictures. *Dis Colon Rectum.* 1996;39:345–349.
49. Tonelli F, Fedi M, Paroli GM, et al. Indications and results of side-to-side isoperistaltic strictureplasty in Crohn's disease. *Dis Colon Rectum* 2004;47:494–501.
50. Roy P, Kumar D. Strictureplasty. *Br J Surg.* 2004;91:1428–1437.
51. Sampietro GM, Cristaldi M, Maconi G, et al. A prospective, longitudinal study of nonconventional strictureplasty in Crohn's disease. *J Am Coll Surg.* 2004;199:8–20; discussion 20–22.
52. Fazio VW, Tjandra JJ, Lavery IC, et al. Long-term follow-up of strictureplasty in Crohn's disease. *Dis Colon Rectum* 1993;36:355–361.
53. Nivatvongs S. Strictureplasty for Crohn's disease of small intestine. Present status in Western countries. *J Gastroenterol.* 1995;30(suppl 8):139–142.
54. Alexander-Williams J, Haynes IG. Conservative operations for Crohn's disease of the small bowel. *World J Surg.* 1985;9:945–951.
55. Hurst RD, Michelassi F. Strictureplasty for Crohn's disease: techniques and long-term results. *World J Surg.* 1998;22:359–363.
56. Spencer MP, Nelson H, Wolff BG, et al. Strictureplasty for obstructive Crohn's disease: the Mayo experience. *Mayo Clin Proc.* 1994;69:33–36.
57. Milsom JW. Strictureplasty and mechanical dilation in strictured Crohn's disease. In: Michelassi F, Milsom JW, eds. *Operative Strategies in Inflammatory Bowel Disease.* New York: Springer-Verlag, 1999, pp. 259– 267.
58. Broe PJ, Bayless TM, Cameron JL. Crohn's disease: are enteroenteral fistulas an indication for surgery? *Surgery* 1982;91:249–253.
59. Glass RE, Ritchie JK, Lennard-Jones JE, et al. Internal fistulas in Crohn's disease. *Dis Colon Rectum* 1985;28:557–561.
60. Block GE, Schraut WH. The operative treatment of Crohn's enteritis complicated by ileosigmoid fistula. *Ann Surg.* 1982;196:356–360.
61. Schraut WH, Chapman C, Abraham VS. Operative treatment of Crohn's ileocolitis complicated by ileosigmoid and ileovesical fistulae. *Ann Surg.* 1988;207:48–51.
62. Heyen F, Winslet MC, Andrews H, et al. Vaginal fistulas in Crohn's disease. *Dis Colon Rectum.* 1989;32:379–383.
63. Doemeny JM, Burke DR, Meranze SG. Percutaneous drainage of abscesses in patients with Crohn's disease. *Gastrointest Radiol.* 1988;13:237–241.
64. Bernini A, Spencer MP, Wong WD, et al. Computed tomography-guided percutaneous abscess drainage in intestinal disease: factors associated with outcome. *Dis Colon Rectum.* 1997;40:1009–1013.
65. Schoetz D. Gastroduodenal Crohn's Disease. In: Michelassi F, JW M, eds. *Operative Strategies in Inflammatory bowel disease.* New York: Springer-Verlag, 1999, pp. 389–393.
66. Harold KL, Kelly KA. Duodenal Crohn Disease. *Problems in general surgery.* 1999;16:50–57.
67. Poggioli G, Stocchi L, Laureti S, et al. Duodenal involvement of Crohn's disease: three different clinicopathologic patterns. *Dis Colon Rectum* 1997;40:179–183.
68. Alexander-Williams J, Haynes IG. Up-to-date management of small-bowel Crohn's disease. *Adv Surg.* 1987;20:245–264.
69. Pichney LS, Fantry GT, Graham SM. Gastrocolic and duodenocolic fistulas in Crohn's disease. *J Clin Gastroenterol.* 1992;15:205–211.
70. Lefton HB, Farmer RG, Fazio V. Ileorectal anastomosis for Crohn's disease of the colon. *Gastroenterology* 1975;69:612–617.
71. Sanfey H, Bayless TM, Cameron JL. Crohn's disease of the colon. Is there a role for limited resection? *Am J Surg.* 1984;147:38–42.
72. Allan A, Andrews H, Hilton CJ, et al. Segmental colonic resection is an appropriate operation for short skip lesions due to Crohn's disease in the colon. *World J Surg.* 1989;13:611–614; discussion 615–616.
73. Berry AR, de Campos R, Lee EC. Perineal and pelvic morbidity following perimuscular excision of the rectum for inflammatory bowel disease. *Br J Surg.* 1986;73:675–677.
74. Homan WP, Tang C, Thorgjarnarson B. Anal lesions complicating Crohn disease. *Arch Surg.* 1976;111:1333–1335.
75. Turunen U, Farkkila M, Seppala K. Long-term treatment of perianal or fistulous Crohn's disease with ciprofloxacin. *Scan J Gastroenterology Suppl.* 1989;24:144.

76. Bernstein LH, Frank MS, Brandt LJ, et al. Healing of perineal Crohn's disease with metronidazole. *Gastroenterology*. 1980;79:599.
77. Kodner IJ, Mazor A, Shemesh EI, et al. Endorectal advancement flap repair of rectovaginal and other complicated anorectal fistulas. *Surgery* 1993; 114:682–990.
78. Rutgeerts P, Geboes K, Vantrappen G, et al. Predictability of the postoperative course of Crohn's disease. *Gastroenterology* 1990;99:956–963.
79. **Mekhjian HS, Switz DM, Watts HD, et al. National Cooperative Crohn's Disease Study: factors determining recurrence of Crohn's disease after surgery. *Gastroenterology* 1979;77(4 Pt 2):907–913.**
80. Post S, Herfarth C, Bohm E, et al. The impact of disease pattern, surgical management, and individual surgeons on the risk for relaparotomy for recurrent Crohn's disease. *Ann Surg*. 1996;223:253–260.
81. Greenstein AJ, Sachar DB, Pasternack BS, et al. Reoperation and recurrence in Crohn's colitis and ileocolitis Crude and cumulative rates. *N Engl J Med*. 1975;293:685–690.
82. D'Haens G, Baert F, Gasparaitis A, et al. Length and type of recurrent ileitis after ileal resection correlate with presurgical features in Crohn's disease. *Inflammatory Bowel Disease* 1997;3:249–253.
83. **Lochs H, Mayer M, Fleig WE, et al. Prophylaxis of postoperative relapse in Crohn's disease with mesalamine: European Cooperative Crohn's Disease Study VI. *Gastroenterology* 2000;118:264–273.**
84. Hanauer SB, Korelitz BI, Rutgeerts P, et al. Postoperative maintenance of Crohn's disease remission with 6-mercaptopurine, mesalamine, or placebo: a 2-year trial. *Gastroenterology* 2004;127:723–729.

CHAPTER 52 ■ SMALL INTESTINAL NEOPLASMS

DOUGLAS J. TURNER AND BARBARA L. BASS

Small bowel tumors, both benign and malignant, are uncommon. Although the small bowel accounts for 75% of the length and 90% of the mucosal surface of the gastrointestinal tract, it is the site of only 1% to 3% of gastrointestinal malignancies. Although they are unusual, autopsy series have demonstrated benign lesions in 0.2% to 0.3% of hospital deaths, a rate 15 times the operative incidence, attesting to the frequently asymptomatic nature of these neoplasms.[1] Table 52.1 shows the wide variety of primary tumors in the small bowel. Small intestinal tumors may originate in cells of the epithelium as adenomas, adenocarcinomas or carcinoids, in the lymphatic tissues as lymphomas or in mesenchymal or neural elements as the gastrointestinal stromal tumors, leiomyomas, lipomas, hemangiomas, neuromas, and a wide variety of sarcomas. The small intestine is also a rare site for metastasis from other primary tumors.

TABLE 52.1 CLASSIFICATION

PRIMARY SMALL BOWEL TUMORS AND REPORTED FREQUENCY RATES

Tumor	Frequency (%)
BENIGN NEOPLASMS	
Leiomyoma	40
Lipoma	13–24
Adenoma	11–18
Lymphangioma	0–12
Fibroma	0–6
Hamartoma	0–6
Hemangioma	0–6
Aberrant pancreas, dermoid cyst, eosinophilic granuloma, angiodysplasias, hyperplastic polyp	Rare
MALIGNANT NEOPLASMS	
Adenocarcinoma	29–50
Carcinoid	10–49
Non-Hodgkin lymphoma	13–42
Gastrointestinal stromal tumors	8–27
Liposarcoma, myxoliposarcoma, lymphangiosarcoma	Rare

EPIDEMIOLOGY

There exists little consensus regarding the relative incidence rates of small bowel tumors in the United States or worldwide. Clearly there are geographic variations around the world. For example, carcinoid tumor is rare to nonexistent in Asian reviews, yet represents 15% to 35% of malignant neoplasms in western series.[2,3] The proportion of small bowel tumors that are benign varies considerably as well, from 14% to 52% in different series, a disparity explained by failure to detect the typically asymptomatic benign lesions. Of malignant tumors, reported rates of non-Hodgkin lymphoma vary from 27% to 72%, a discrepancy due in part to inconsistent categorization of lymphomas as primary or metastatic tumors, but also due partly to true geographic variation. Given the rarity of small bowel tumors and the wide variety of histologies, the actual reported numbers for given histologic types are small even in the largest series, making reliable comparisons difficult and definitive incidence rates impossible to confirm.[4]

Although generalizations regarding these rare tumors can be difficult to formulate, certain patterns can be discerned. Small bowel neoplasms are less common in women than in men. A male preponderance with a 3:2 ratio is reported for both benign and malignant neoplasms. Most patients with small bowel neoplasms present in their sixth to seventh decade of life. Except for adenocarcinoma, which has a predilection for the duodenum, malignant small bowel tumors become more common as one moves more distally in the small bowel. Approximately 20% of tumors arise in the duodenum, 30% in the jejunum, and 50% in the ileum.[5]

PATHOGENESIS

Several hypotheses have been proposed to explain the low incidence of small bowel tumors, particularly those derived from cells of the intestinal epithelium. Although none of these hypotheses have proved true, they provide a plausible explanation relative to the understanding of the pathogenesis of other gastrointestinal tumors. The dilute alkaline liquid contents of the small bowel are potentially less capable of inducing direct mechanical mucosal injury and disruption than the more solid contents of the colon. The luminal content of the healthy small bowel lumen is sterile; bacteria and their potentially toxic metabolites are not present to induce the genetic alterations implicated in colon carcinogenesis. Rapid transit time through the small bowel lumen, normally 30 minutes to 2 hours, may limit mucosal exposure to potential carcinogens whereas the presence of the enzyme benzopyrene hydroxylase in the brush border of the small intestine may provide protection against mucosal damage by detoxifying the carcinogen benzopyrene. The greater concentration and distribution of lymphoid tissue in the intestinal epithelium and submucosa and high levels of luminal immunoglobulin A may provide an immunologic protective mechanism. Some investigators suggest that the high rate of metachronous primary malignancies, observed in up to 20% of patients, and the frequency of multicentric small bowel malignancies support an alteration in host defenses or a breakdown in this immunologic protective mechanism as an important etiologic factor. Unlike the well-defined adenoma-carcinoma genetic sequence described for colorectal malignancy, no consistent pattern of gene mutations or deletions has been identified for small bowel carcinomas.

CONDITIONS ASSOCIATED WITH INCREASED RISK FOR SMALL BOWEL TUMORS

Although the small bowel develops few tumors, risk factors for the development of malignant lesions have been identified. As shown in Table 52.2, several conditions carry an increased risk of neoplasia.

Crohn Disease

Crohn disease is associated with up to an 100-fold increased risk of developing adenocarcinoma, with carcinoma developing in diseased segments of the bowel with preexisting dysplasia.[6]

TABLE 52.2 ETIOLOGY

CONDITIONS ASSOCIATED WITH AN INCREASED RISK OF NEOPLASIA

Preexisting condition	Potential malignancy
Adenomatous polyps	Adenocarcinoma
Familial adenomatous polyposis	Adenocarcinoma
Peutz-Jeghers syndrome/ hamartomatous polyps	Adenocarcinoma
Leiomyomas	Possible leiomyosarcoma
Neurofibromatosis	Leiomyosarcoma, carcinoid, adenocarcinoma
Crohn disease	Adenocarcinoma
Celiac sprue	Lymphoma, adenocarcinoma
Immunosuppression	Lymphoma
HIV infection	Lymphoma, Kaposi sarcoma
Helicobacter pylori infection	Low-grade lymphoma (mucosal-associated lymphoid tissue)
Epstein-Barr virus infection	Lymphoma

Three quarters of these cancers arise in the ileum, the area most commonly involved with Crohn disease, but the segment of small bowel least commonly affected by adenocarcinoma otherwise. The remaining tumors in patients with Crohn disease are found in the duodenum and the jejunum, following the usual distribution of sporadic carcinoma, which tends to develop in the duodenum. Crohn-associated carcinomas carry a particularly poor prognosis because the tumors are frequently diagnosed at an advanced stage, likely because the abdominal symptoms of the tumor are attributed to the underlying inflammatory bowel disease.[7]

Familial Adenomatous Polyposis

Also at risk for the development of adenocarcinoma, primarily of the duodenum, are patients with familial adenomatous polyposis (FAP).[8] Some studies suggest close to 100% of FAP patients will eventually develop adenomatous polyps in the duodenum and that the risk of duodenal carcinoma in these patients has been estimated to be 331-fold over that of the healthy population.[8] Duodenal and periampullary adenocarcinomas are the leading cause of cancer death in patients with FAP previously treated by colectomy. Careful screening with periodic esophagogastroduodenoscopy and prompt local resection of adenomas is of paramount importance in this patient population. Endoscopic polypectomy is appropriate for small or pedunculated lesions, whereas larger villous tumors, particularly in the periampullary region, may require pancreaticoduodenctomy for adequate treatment.

Other Conditions with Increased Risk for Small Bowel Malignancy

Celiac sprue is associated with lymphoma, and to a lesser degree adenocarcinoma, occurring in up to 14% of patients.[9] It remains unclear whether a gluten-free diet decreases this risk, although dietary compliance did not show a decreased risk of malignancy in a recent study.[10] The neurofibromas of von Recklinghausen disease may undergo malignant transformation as may leiomyomas of the small bowel. In Peutz-Jeghers syndrome, hamartomas develop throughout the gastrointestinal tract and may carry a risk of malignant transformation to adenocarcinoma.[11] Whether these malignancies, especially in the duodenum, actually arise from preexisting hamartomas has been poorly documented. Sporadic benign adenomatous polyps are at risk for malignant transformation and should be resected when identified.

Bile acids and their metabolites may have a possible role in the pathogenesis of small bowel adenocarcinoma. In one study of all patients with small intestinal malignancy, 12% had a history of cholecystectomy and of those with duodenal adenocarcinoma, 25% had prior cholecystectomy. A causative relationship between cholecystectomy and small intestinal adenocarcinoma remains unproved, however. Within the duodenum, the periampullary region is the most frequent site of primary carcinoma although a link between this finding and pancreaticobiliary secretions is unexplored.

Immunosuppression, both iatrogenic following organ transplantation or secondary to disease, places a patient at increased risk for small bowel malignancy, primarily lymphoma and sarcoma. After solid organ transplantation, patients maintained on immunosuppressive regimens have an incidence rate 45 to 100 times higher than that of nontransplanted persons for non-Hodgkin's lymphoma (NHL) a condition termed *posttransplant lymphoproliferative disorder* (PTSD).[12] PTSD accounts for 30% of all malignancies in cyclosporine-treated patients but accounts for only 12% of malignancies in patients without cyclosporine in their regimen. PTSD tends to develop rapidly, often within 12 months of transplantation in cyclosporine-treated patients. The level of immunosuppression appears to influence the incidence of PTSD; patients who require high degrees of immunosuppression to sustain their graft, such as those with small bowel, heart, liver, or lung transplants, show rates of lymphoma as high as 30%. In contrast, kidney transplant recipients who generally require less immunosuppression, develop lymphoproliferative tumors in only 5% of cases. Another form of immunosuppression, HIV infection, is also associated with lymphoma. Lymphoma is the second most common malignancy, after Kaposi sarcoma, in these patients. As life expectancy for patients with HIV infection has lengthened with improved antiviral medications, the rates of lymphoma have increased such that the risk at 3 years now approaches 30%. Two thirds of these lymphomas are extranodal and the gastrointestinal tract is involved in 10% to 25% of cases. More than 90% of patients present with stage IV disease and the median survival is only 6 months.

CLINICAL PRESENTATION

There are no pathognomonic signs or symptoms of small bowel tumors. Complaints, if reported at all by the patient, are nonspecific. As shown in Table 52.3, the most common symptoms, abdominal pain, weight loss, anemia, nausea and vomiting, do not suggest specific localization and are usually present in about 45% of patients. These vague complaints have led to diagnostic errors (irritable bowel syndrome or even neurosis) and delay before the correct diagnosis of small bowel neoplasm is established. Location may influence detection, as smaller lesions often present sooner in the ileum as the lumen is narrower and obstruction more likely to develop. As the tumors enlarge, symptoms are more likely to develop. Of all lesions measuring at least 4 cm, 75% will cause symptoms whereas 92% of malignant lesions of that size will be symptomatic. Overall, malignant lesions tend to be more symptomatic than benign lesions, eliciting complaints of abdominal pain and weight loss. In contrast, benign tumors more often present with acute hemorrhage as the primary symptom, or are identified as an incidental finding on a radiologic exam or at laparotomy.

TABLE 52.3 DIAGNOSIS

CLINICAL PRESENTATION OF PRIMARY SMALL BOWEL TUMORS

Signs and symptoms	Frequency (%)
BENIGN NEOPLASMS	
Asymptomatic	47–60
Abdominal pain	24–50
Acute gastrointestinal hemorrhage	29–44
Anemia	28–58
Intermittent obstruction	12–28
MALIGNANT NEOPLASMS	
Asymptomatic	6–12
Abdominal pain	62–83
Weight loss	38–55
Nausea/vomiting	23–64
Acute gastrointestinal hemorrhage	6–31
Anemia	12–38
Abdominal mass	5–32

Because of their ill-defined symptoms, both benign and malignant small bowel tumors frequently present late in their course. Tumors are often diagnosed at the time of emergency surgical exploration for intestinal obstruction, perforation, or massive gastrointestinal hemorrhage. Only in hindsight may a history of abdominal complaints be elicited.

DIAGNOSIS

Many factors contribute to the difficulty in establishing the diagnosis of a small bowel tumor. In most series, the average duration of symptoms prior to diagnosis ranges from weeks to many months. Diagnosis is hindered by the infrequency of these tumors and omission of this diagnosis from the differential diagnosis in patients with nonspecific abdominal complaints. More importantly, diagnosis is delayed because imaging modalities available to study the small bowel are limited. Accurate preoperative diagnosis is rarely established prior to surgery.[13,14]

Plain abdominal radiography is rarely helpful unless the patient presents with obstructive symptoms. For patients being evaluated for gastrointestinal complaints or gastrointestinal bleeding, the diagnosis of possible small bowel tumor is usually considered after unremarkable evaluations of the stomach and colon. For patients presenting with acute of chronic gastrointestinal blood loss, the diagnostic workup should proceed to a computed tomography (CT) scan of the abdomen after negative esophagogastroduodenoscopy and colonoscopy. In addition to readily identifying bulky mass lesions, CT imaging allows detection of subtle findings that are highly suggestive of small bowel tumors. Neoplastic disease must be strongly suspected if the scan shows the small bowel wall to be thicker than 1.5 cm or if there are discrete mesenteric lymph nodes or masses greater than 1.5 cm in diameter. The CT scan may reveal a transition zone, demarcating dilated proximal bowel from decompressed distal bowel. If associated with bowel wall thickening, a tumor is likely, except in patients with clinical presentations more typical of Crohn disease.

Tumors of the distal small bowel may show CT findings of ileocolic or jejunoileal intussusception. This characteristic finding is sufficient to proceed with surgical exploration in adult patients. During intussusception, the small bowel tumor serves as the lead point to pull the small bowel into the distal small bowel or colonic lumen; the mass lesion precludes spontaneous reduction. In adults, radiographic attempts to reduce an intussusception should not be attempted. Rather, prompt surgical exploration and resection of the nonreduced intussuscepted bowel segment with mesenteric resection should be completed.

If abdominal CT imaging fails to reveal evidence of a small bowel tumor, the next diagnostic study should be an upper gastrointestinal contrast series with small bowel follow-through. Barium meals demonstrate a duodenal lesion in 70% to 80% of cases and, when air double-contrast technique is used, the diagnostic rate rises to 85% to 90%, although esophagogastroduodenoscopy has essentially replaced this study for duodenal evaluation. The sensitivity of barium studies declines significantly in the jejunum and ileum. Small bowel follow-through will show an abnormality in 53% to 83% of cases, although direct evidence of a tumor is detected in only 30% to 44%. Given these poor detection rates, some radiologists support enteroclysis as the primary study of choice for imaging the small bowel distal to the ligament of Treitz. Enteroclysis is a dynamic contrast technique that uses a combination of barium and methylcellulose infused into the small bowel via a nasoduodenal tube to uniformly distend the small bowel without abolishing peristalsis. Expertise in this procedure is important for success and may not be available in all radiology departments. Enteroclysis is clearly a superior modality for identification of small luminal tumors. In one series, enteroclysis identified 90% of cases compared to 33% by small bowel follow-through in the same cohort of patients.

Other lesions may mimic small bowel tumors on these imaging studies. An inflammatory reaction secondary to a sealed perforation will thicken the bowel wall and may appear neoplastic. An annular pancreas may appear on an upper gastrointestinal contrast study as an apple-core lesion in the duodenum and be mistaken for a malignancy. Thickening of the bowel wall is common in Crohn disease. The clinical presentation may clarify the diagnosis, although definitive diagnosis may not be confirmed until surgical exploration.

Small Bowel Enteroscopy

Endoscopic modalities are helpful where the expertise is available. "Push" enteroscopy utilizes a pediatric colonoscope for direct examination of the mucosa of the proximal small bowel.[15] Biopsy of identified lesions can be performed with this instrument although the examination is limited to visualization of only the proximal 2 to 3 feet of small bowel. Performed in the endoscopy suite with intravenous sedation, the procedure is not well tolerated by all patients. In contrast, *sonde* (pull) small bowel enteroscopy relies on peristalsis to passively pull a wide-angled lens enteroscope into the distal ileum or colon. Passage requires up to 8 hours after which the enteroscope is slowly withdrawn for visual examination of the tumor. The small diameter of the device precludes a biopsy port for tissue sampling, and the procedure itself is poorly tolerated and has been largely abandoned in the United States.

Intraoperative enteroscopy allows full visualization of the small bowel mucosal surface and the opportunity to surgically treat identified lesions. Rarely, however, is it necessary to resort to this procedure for identification of a tumor. Except in very obese patients, once surgical exploration is initiated, small bowel tumors can usually be readily identified by careful palpation of the bowel.

Video capsule endoscopy (VCE) with a wireless video capsule endoscope is being employed increasingly in the diagnosis of small bowel tumors with otherwise negative diagnostic studies. The device is an ingestible 11 × 26 mm capsule that the patient swallows; it contains a miniature video camera, light source, battery, and transmitter that sends images (up to 50,000 overall) to a recording device worn by the patient.[16] VCE is a good test to identify potential small bowel lesions, however, it does not have the capacity for biopsies nor can precise localizations along the bowel be determined. Relative contraindications to VCE include obstructive symptoms, motility disorders, and pacemakers. The major complication is capsule retention, which can occur at a stricture and has been reported in 5% of cases, although less than 1% of all mandated surgical retrieval.[17]

In addition to these techniques that attempt to visualize intraluminal pathology, other modalities are useful in specific situations. Selective visceral angiography may be helpful in the diagnosis of patients with acute or chronic gastrointestinal hemorrhage. Massive hemorrhage is most common with benign smooth muscle tumors and arteriography may provide both diagnostic and temporizing therapeutic advantages if selective embolization of a bleeding vessel can be achieved. Benign vascular lesions, including hemangioma are more likely to present with occult gastrointestinal blood loss.

Despite these multiple diagnostic modalities, more than half of patients with small bowel neoplasms present with a surgical emergency and more than half of patients with malignant disease have metastatic spread at the time of operation.

BENIGN TUMORS OF THE SMALL INTESTINE

Accounting for 30% to 50% of primary neoplasms of the small bowel, benign tumors are poorly characterized. Half the patients with benign tumors are symptom free, even in retrospect, until the need for emergency surgery. Up to 60% of benign small bowel tumors will be diagnosed at the time of presentation with a surgical emergency including obstruction, massive gastrointestinal hemorrhage or perforation. For patients who do present with symptoms necessitating evaluation, vague abdominal pain and recurrent gastrointestinal bleeding are the most common. In one series,[1] 29% of patients with benign lesions presented with an acute hemorrhage and 40% in another,[5] a feature that may help differentiate benign from malignant lesions, the latter of which bleed less often. Many more lesions are never identified because they elicit no symptoms.

As noted previously, the diagnostic workup is challenging. In patients with symptoms, investigations should proceed as outlined above. The secondary effects of the neoplasms (obstruction, hemorrhage, perforation) will dictate the pathway of evaluation.

Regardless of the location, the treatment of benign small bowel tumors is local excision or limited resection. As gross appearance in the operating room may not definitively establish a small bowel tumor as benign, segmental resection is often the most appropriate surgical approach. Endoscopic resection or submucosal excision via operative enterotomy may be appropriate for small lesions with obvious features of a benign lipoma; however, segmental limited resection is usually the most appropriate intervention. Intraoperative examination of the small bowel with careful palpation, including the possible use of intraoperative enteroscopy for evaluation of suspected abnormalities, is essential to rule out synchronous lesions.

ADENOMAS

Unique to the duodenum, Brunner gland adenomas are rare tumors of the proximal duodenum.[18,19] Brunner glands are normally found in the duodenal submucosa and secrete an alkaline bicarbonate rich fluid and mucus that aids in the neutralization of gastric acid. The pathogenesis of the glandular hyperplasia that is linked to adenoma formation remains unknown. Brunner gland adenomas appear to have minimal if any malignant potential. Once identified, local resection via endoscopic means or duodenotomy with submucosal excision, should be performed to prevent intussusception or biliary obstruction as the adenoma grows.

As in the colon, small bowel adenomas may be histologically classified as tubular, tubulovillous, or villous. Adenomas occur predominantly in the duodenum with the majority found in the periampullary region, but they may also be found in the proximal jejunum. Because roughly 25% of these villous and tubulovillous adenomas harbor malignancy, it is important to identify and resect these tumors when they are identified.[20] All are associated with potential malignant transformation, a risk that likely increases with size, although relative risks of various sized adenomas to undergo this transformation are difficult to determine given the low total number of cases. Adenomas larger than 2 cm should be considered worrisome for malignancy.

Approximately one third of adenomas in the duodenum present with obstructive jaundice or small bowel obstruction, leading to ultrasound and abdominal radiography as the initial diagnostic studies. Without these physical signs to direct the workup, appropriate initial diagnostic studies of the duodenum include double-contrast upper gastrointestinal series or

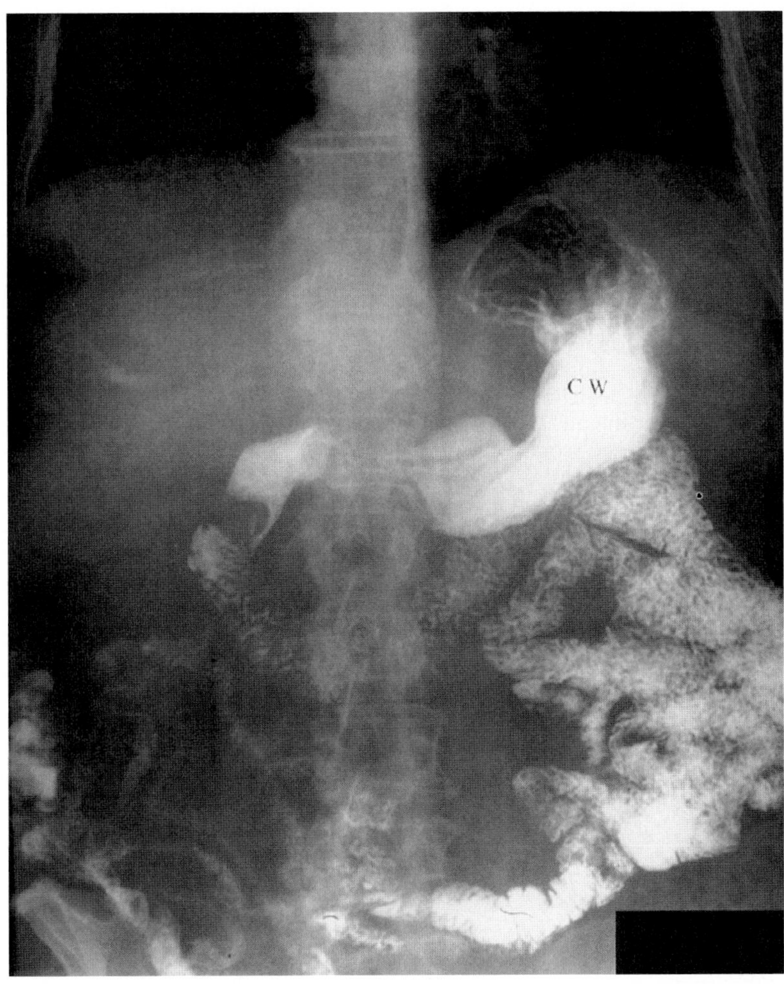

FIGURE 52.1 A 64-year-old woman with a polypoid lesion in the second portion of her duodenum on upper gastrointestinal series, found to be a benign adenoma at operation.

esophagogastroduodenoscopy, both of which are equally sensitive in most series. Adenomas appear usually as small intraluminal filling defects and are frequently pedunculated on a stalk (Fig. 52.1). For those few patients subjected to contrast series prior to esophagogastroduodenoscopy, the pathognomonic finding for villous adenoma is a "soap bubble" or "paint brush" sign, in which rounded radiolucent areas are intermixed with a meshwork of radiopaque material. Esophagogastroduodenoscopy with biopsy is appropriate following a positive upper gastrointestinal study. CT scan may be helpful to differentiate adenoma from carcinoma because the adenoma will not be associated with bowel wall thickening. Similarly, endoscopic ultrasound may detect invasive disease or lymphadenopathy. Treatment requires either endoscopic excision or surgical resection. The surgical choices include transduodenal local excision for small lesions, pancreas sparing duodenectomy, or pylorus preserving pancreaticoduodenectomy for larger lesions or periampullary tumors. A recent review of duodenal villous tumors demonstrated local recurrence rates of 40% at 10 years, 25% of which were malignant. Based on these retrospective data, pancreaticoduodenectomy is recommended as an appropriate surgical option for benign lesions in selected patients. Because of this high risk of local recurrence, those patients in whom local excision is performed require annual surveillance with endoscopy.[21]

LIPOMAS

Fatty tumors that may be found throughout the small bowel; lipomas are typically asymptomatic. Because these tumors are polypoid, compressible intraluminal lesions, they are predisposed to induce intussusception. These tumors are most often found incidentally on abdominal CT scans completed for evaluation of a different clinical condition. Lipomas are identified as well circumscribed lesions of fat density on CT imaging. On barium contrast study they appear as radiolucent lesions. Unless associated with bleeding or obstruction, small tumors under 2 cm can be safely observed, while larger lesions or growing lesions, should be resected to rule out malignant liposarcoma. If surgery is performed either for a complication of the lipoma or for an unrelated condition, local excision is adequate treatment.

HAMARTOMAS

Peutz-Jeghers syndrome is an autosomal dominant condition characterized by multiple gastrointestinal hamartomas and mucocutaneous pigmentation. The polyps arise predominantly in the jejunum and ileum and often present as an intussusception. Although hamartomas rarely if ever undergo malignant transformation, they have been associated with the development of adenocarcinoma.[11] Local resection is indicated for intussusception or bleeding, although the widespread nature of the hamartomas precludes complete extirpation.

HEMANGIOMAS

Hemangiomas are rare lesions of the small bowel, affecting predominantly the jejunum and ileum. They are congenital lesions that grow slowly, typically coming to medical attention in the third decade of life because of acute or chronic blood loss.

Arising from the submucosal vascular plexuses, hemangiomas are classified as capillary, cavernous, or mixed depending on what size vessel primarily is affected. They are usually solitary lesions and malignant degeneration is exceedingly rare. Depending on size, hemangiomas may be locally excised or resected with a limited small bowel resection. Efforts to manage hemangiomas with endoscopic or operative sclerotherapy or coagulation and operative or angiographic interruption of arterial supply have been minimally successful.

MALIGNANT NEOPLASMS

Malignant neoplasms in the small bowel can be either primary or metastatic. Primary malignancies include adenocarcinoma, gastrointestinal stromal tumors (GIST), leiomyosarcoma, NHL, and carcinoid, with rare reports of other lesions including liposarcoma, myxoliposarcoma, and lymphangiosarcoma. Metastatic tumors of the small bowel have been reported from many primary solid tumors, but melanoma and lymphoma are the most common. Compared with benign tumors, malignant lesions are more likely to present with pain, weight loss, and anorexia. Although nonspecific, these findings are more ominous than other symptoms shared with benign tumors, such as nausea and vomiting and acute or chronic blood loss. As a group, patients with malignant small bowel tumors present at advanced stages and have a poor prognosis. High rates of metastatic spread are noted on initial surgical operation.

The diagnosis of small bowel malignancy should prompt a thorough diagnostic evaluation. Second primary malignancies are found in 20% to 30% of patients. This association is especially relevant for carcinoid tumors, where the incidence rate of second primaries is as high as 30% to 50%. The second primary cancer may arise in any organ, but the most frequent second primary sites are the colorectum and breast.[22,23]

ADENOCARCINOMA

Epidemiology

Adenocarcinoma accounts for about 35% of small bowel tumors, making it the most common primary malignancy.[8] Regional prevalence rates correlate with prevalence rates of colon cancer rather than with gastric cancer, a finding that holds true internationally as well. Like adenomas, sporadic adenocarcinomas have a predilection for the duodenum, with a marked decrease in frequency moving axially along the small bowel. Approximately 80% of tumors are located in the duodenum or proximal jejunum. Most studies demonstrate a slight male preference.

There are several risk factors for the development of adenocarcinoma. Malignant transformation of villous and tubulovillous adenomas is likely the most important and occurs predominantly in the periampullary region of the duodenum. Crohn disease increases the risk up to 100-fold and predisposes to cancer in the more distal small bowel in regions of dysplasia.

Clinical Presentation

The presenting symptoms of small bowel adenocarcinoma depend on the location and size of the tumor. Because tumors tend to arise in the proximal small bowel and to encompass the bowel wall, adenocarcinomas cause obstruction with associated anorexia. The majority of tumors cause crampy abdominal pain. Periampullary duodenal adenocarcinomas may cause obstructive jaundice or pancreatitis as they grow. In this case, the physical complaints and findings help guide the direction of the diagnostic evaluation. Often, the only complaint is vague, persistent abdominal pain.

Diagnosis

If obstruction is present, plain abdominal films may reveal gastric distention or near complete proximal small bowel obstruction. More commonly, however, these films are unrevealing. For the jaundiced patient, ultrasound or abdominal CT or magnetic resonance cholangiopancreatography may demonstrate the duodenal mass and site of biliary obstruction. Upper gastrointestinal contrast studies or esophagogastroduodenoscopy demonstrate duodenal adenocarcinomas equally well with diagnostic rates of 85% to 90%. Endoscopy offers the advantage of tissue biopsy. For duodenal lesions, these rates compare favorably to CT scan, which can establish the diagnosis in roughly 50% of cancers.

Of small bowel adenocarcinomas, 70% are polypoid, 20% ulcerated, and 10% infiltrative. Comparable to other segments of the gastrointestinal tract, adenocarcinomas of the jejunum and ileum are usually annular constricting tumors seen as apple core lesions on luminal contrast studies (Fig. 52.2) Such findings may be indistinguishable from metastatic lesions. Compression during fluoroscopic examination shows these tumors are rigid and nondeformable. Long lesions, especially when ulcerated, may be mistaken for lymphomas. On CT scan, adenocarcinomas may attenuate heterogenously and have moderate contrast enhancement. Again, usually only a short segment of small bowel is involved, occasionally associated with an ulcer. Despite the array of diagnostic modalities, preoperative diagnosis remains infrequent, achieved in only 20% to 50% of cancers.

Management

The only potential cure for adenocarcinoma is complete surgical resection. At operation, the resectablility rate for cure is between 50% and 65%. For proximal and midduodenal lesions, pancreaticoduodenectomy is necessary to completely resect the tumor and lymphatic basin. In the third and fourth portions of the duodenum and in the mesenteric small bowel, a segmental resection with lymphadenectomy should be performed to attempt surgical cure. In patients with metastatic or unresectable disease, palliative procedures to relieve obstruction or control hemorrhage should be considered. Segmental resection or intestinal bypass is appropriate pending operative findings. Duodenal obstruction may be palliated with endoscopic placement of expandable stents, although recurrent obstruction and hemorrhage may complicate this procedure. Consideration should be given to placement of gastrojejunal or gastrostomy tubes in patients with carcinomatosis or unresectable disease for long term decompression or nutritional support.

Staging and Prognosis

The American Joint Committee on Cancer (AJCC) staging system for small bowel adenocarcinoma is similar to those for gastric and colon carcinoma.[24] The staging system applies to only to adenocarcinoma of the small bowel and not to other malignant neoplasms of the small intestine. Carcinoma of the ampulla of Vater is also staged separately. As in other gastrointestinal malignancies, the tumor classification (T) describes depth of invasion, with T1 and T2 both contained within the bowel wall and T3 and T4 describe gradations of penetration through the wall. Unlike colon cancer, the node classification (N) in small bowel carcinoma classifies only by presence or absence of lymph node metastases, and not by

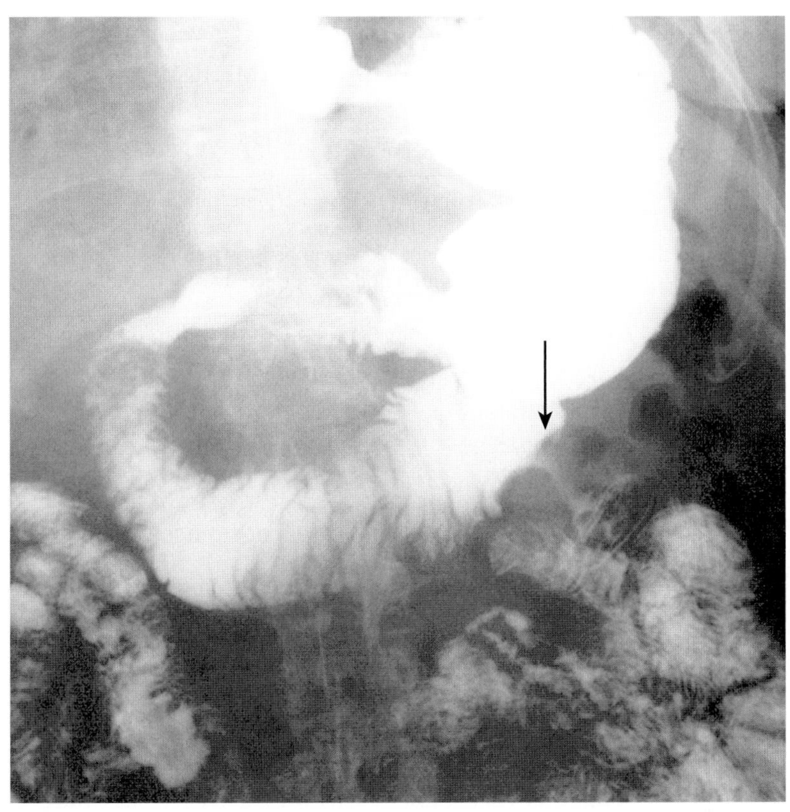

FIGURE 52.2 A 73-year-old woman who presented with gastric outlet obstruction was found on this small bowel follow-through study to have apple core lesion of the proximal jejunum. At exploration, she was found to have jejunal adenocarcinoma.

numbers of positive nodes. Distant metastases are classified (M). Table 52.4 shows the TNM classification and staging system for small bowel adenocarcinoma. As shown, prognosis is grim for patients presenting with stage III or IV disease, the most frequent stages at diagnosis.

Factors that affect long-term survival in small bowel adenocarcinoma vary slightly by study and tumor location. For duodenal tumors, negative resection margins and tumors in the first and second portions seem to favorably affect prognosis, whereas nodal status and size and differentiation of the tumor do not.[25] In contrast, ampullary tumors are associated with better prognosis if lymph nodes are not involved and the tumor does not infiltrate the pancreas.[20] One study evaluating prognostic factors for all small bowel malignancies, exclusive of periampullary lesions, demonstrated poor survival in node positive patients regardless of curative resection. Studies examining cancers of the jejunum and ileum are limited by their small sizes; however, a recent study concluded that among the factors for survival were positive margins, extramural venous spread, positive lymph nodes, and history of Crohn disease.[7]

Chemotherapy and/or radiation therapy has not been shown to confer a survival advantage or prolonged disease

TABLE 52.4 STAGING

TNM CLASSIFICATION AND STAGING OF SMALL BOWEL ADENOCARCINOMA

TNM	Carcinoma penetration	Stage	5-Year survival rate
Tx	Unknown primary		
T0	No evidence of primary		
Tis	Carcinoma-*in-situ*	0	
T1	Tumor invades lamina propria or submucosa	I	70%
T2	Tumor invades muscularis propria		
T3	Tumor extends less than 2 cm into subserosa or into nonperitonealized perimuscular tissue (mesentery in jejunum or ileum, retroperitoneum in duodenum)	II	50%
T4	Tumor penetrates visceral peritoneum or directly invades more than 2 cm into adjacent structures		
Nx	Regional lymph nodes not assessed		
N0	No regional lymph node involvement		
N1	Regional lymph nodes involved		
Mx	Distant metastases not assessed	III	20%
Mo	No distant metastases		
M1	Distant metastases present	IV	10%

free interval.[7] At this time, the role of adjuvant therapies is within clinical trials. Wide surgical resection remains the mainstay of therapy.

NON-HODGKIN LYMPHOMA

NHL of the gastrointestinal tract represents 4% to 20% of all NHL with the gastrointestinal tract being the most common extranodal site. The stomach harbors the most lymphomas, followed by the small bowel and then the colon. Of all gastrointestinal NHL, 25% to 35% of cases occur within the small bowel. The distribution pattern is marked by relative sparing of the duodenum and equal frequency in the jejunum and ileum.

Many retrospective reviews of small bowel malignancy exclude primary NHL from analysis because of the difficulties in differentiating primary from secondary lymphomas in chart review data. Specific criteria must be met to establish the diagnosis of primary gastrointestinal NHL. On physical examination, there may be no superficial adenopathy, and chest radiograph may show no mediastinal adenopathy. Peripheral blood cell counts must be normal, and there may be no evidence of splenic or hepatic involvement. Finally, at laparotomy disease must be restricted to the primary tumor with mesenteric lymph node involvement.[26]

Multiple histologic variations of lymphoma exist, showing significant geographic variability. The majority of primary intestinal NHL are of the B-cell type with T-cell lymphoma comprising only 10% to 25% of cases. Further classifications of B-cell and T-cell tumors have been proposed but none has been uniformly adopted. A significant number of gastrointestinal lymphomas appear to be low-grade lymphomas derived from mucosal-associated lymphoid tissue. These lymphomas arise predominantly in the stomach but also occur in the small bowel. In the stomach they are associated with *Helicobacter pylori* infection and may regress with treatment of this infection.[27] In the small bowel these low-grade lymphomas should be resected. T-cell lymphomas tend to have a worse prognosis than B-cell tumors.

Clinical Presentation

Similar to other small bowel malignancies, the majority of patients present with abdominal pain that is nonspecific and unlocalized. Malabsorption, obstruction, and evidence of a palpable mass may be present. Although rare, perforation is a more common presentation for gastrointestinal NHL than for adenocarcinoma, possibly related to a lack of a vigorous desmoplastic response in lymphoma. Signs that are common in nodal lymphoma, such as adenopathy and splenomegaly, are unusual in primary gastrointestinal NHL.

Diagnosis

Most small bowel lymphomas will be demonstrable on CT scan. Lymphomas may grow to be quite large. CT scan will demonstrate the mass as well as marked luminal dilatation, bowel wall thickening, and displacement of neighboring loops. (Figs. 52.3 and 52.4) Short strictures are more suggestive of adenocarcinoma but may be seen in lymphoma at times. Small bowel follow-through will reveal multifocal lesions in 10% to 25% of patients. To make a tissue diagnosis, biopsies must be obtained from the submucosa, as the overlying mucosa often demonstrates no tumor infiltration. CT guided biopsy may be diagnostic, although proximal lesions are best diagnosed with endoscopic submucosal biopsy.

TABLE 52.5 STAGING

STAGING OF NON-HODGKIN LYMPHOMA OF THE GI TRACT

Stage	Extent of disease
I	Tumor confined to the gastrointestinal tract, either as single primary site or multiple noncontiguous lesions
II	Tumor extends from primary gastrointestinal site, either to lymph nodes or direct invasion. Confined to below the diaphragm
IIE	Tumor penetrates serosa to involve adjacent structures
II_1	Local nodal involvement
II_2	Distant nodal involvement
III	Evidence of supradiaphragmatic disease
IV	Disseminated disease above and below the diaphragm

Staging and Prognosis

Unlike other solid tumors of the gastrointestinal tract, the TNM system does not apply to staging of gastrointestinal NHL. Rather, staging is based on site involvement, outlined in Table 52.5. Like tumors elsewhere in the gastrointestinal tract, lymphomas are typically diagnosed late with almost half of patients presenting as stage III or IV disease. Fewer than 30% of patients have surgically respectable tumors. Patients with stage I tumors have a 40% to 60% five year survival, whereas those with stage II disease have a 20% five year survival. The long-term survival for stages III and IV remains negligible, despite the aggressive use of chemoradiation therapy.

Treatment

With no randomized series and small numbers of cases at single institutions, the optimal treatment of gastrointestinal NHL remains controversial. Most agree that surgical resection of isolated small bowel lymphoma is the cornerstone of treatment. Resection with lymphadenectomy is important for local control and prevents perforation and bleeding. Small bowel lymphoma is the only small intestinal malignancy that responds to currently available adjuvant therapy.[28] For more extensive gastrointestinal lymphoma, there is no evidence-based consensus on optimal management.

CARCINOID TUMORS

Carcinoids are indolent malignant neuroendocrine tumors that arise from the enterochromaffin cells at the base of the crypts of Lieberkuhn. These cells are part of the amine precursor uptake and decarboxylation system and can secrete peptides responsible for the carcinoid syndrome. Although 80% of carcinoids arise in the gastrointestinal tract, 10% of primary carcinoids occur in the bronchus or lung. Other sites, such as the ovaries, testicles, pancreas, and kidney are far less common. Within the gastrointestinal tract, carcinoids are most often identified in the appendix, followed by the small bowel, which harbors approximately 30% of all gastrointestinal carcinoids. Almost half of these arise in the distal 2 feet of ileum.

Accounting for 5% to 35% of small bowel neoplasms, carcinoids are found slightly more often in men than in women. Mean age of presentation is 60 years. The tumors are frequently asymptomatic; the autopsy rate in one study was over 2000 times that of the annual incidence rate, indicating the potential for longstanding slow growth. When symptomatic, carcinoids typically present with pain or obstructive symptoms. Because these tumors are typically slow growing, symptoms may be

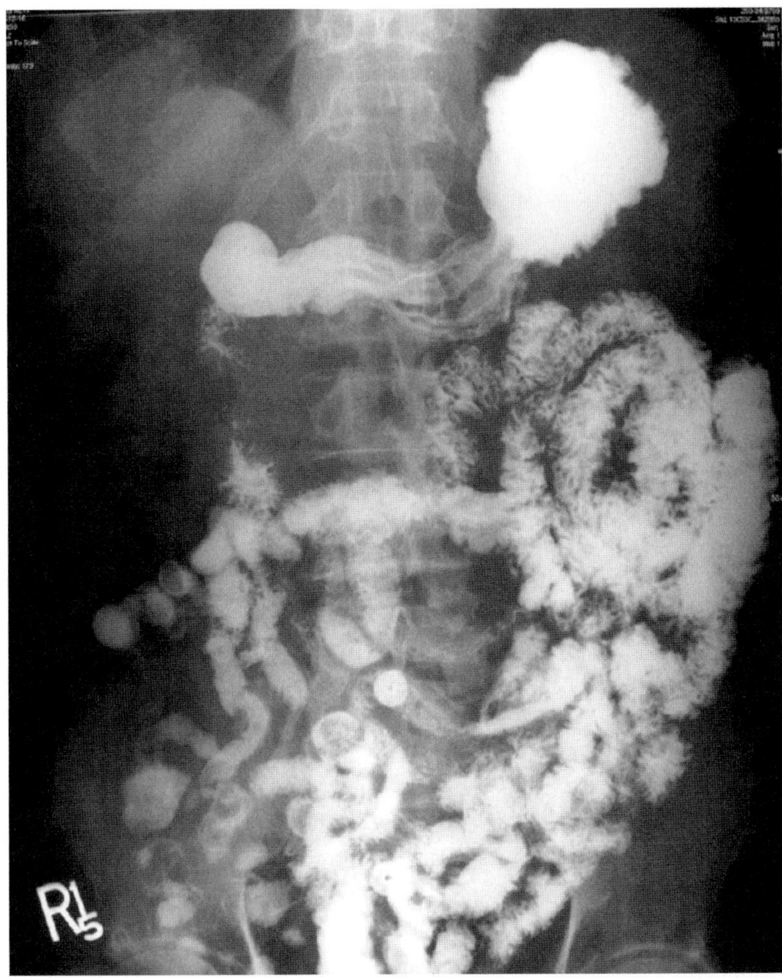

FIGURE 52.3 This small bowel-follow through was performed on a 71-year-old man with chronic symptoms of partial small bowel obstruction. It demonstrated a persistently dilated small bowel loop in the terminal ileum with a thickened wall. The computed tomography scan in the following figure was obtained.

present for 2 to 20 years prior to diagnosis. Ulceration is rare in carcinoids, so gastrointestinal bleeding is uncommon. Patients present with carcinoid syndrome in up to 40% of cases and only in the presence of symptoms of carcinoid syndrome is the diagnosis consistently made preoperatively.

There are five histologic patterns that correlate embryologically with the location of the tumor.[29] The foregut, or duodenal, lesions usually demonstrate a trabecular or ribbon pattern. An insular pattern predominates in the midgut or small bowel, and a mixed pattern is typical of the hindgut, or colorectum.

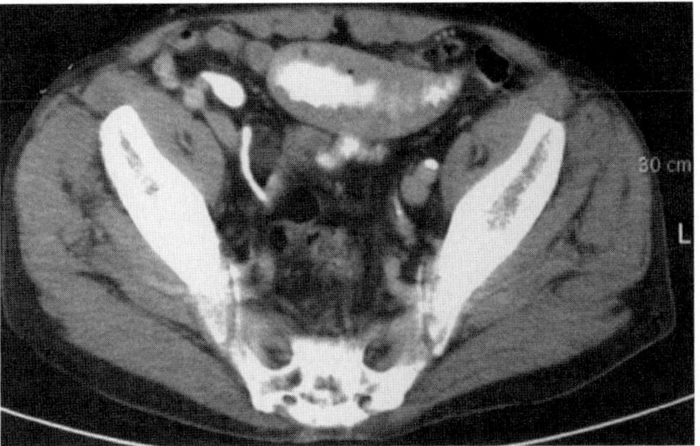

FIGURE 52.4 The computed tomography scan similarly demonstrated a thickened ileal loop with dilatation. No adenopathy was noted. At surgery, the patient was found to have a primary lymphoma of the small bowel.

The least common patterns are glandular or tubular and undifferentiated, both of which have a much poorer prognosis than the three more common variations. The histologic pattern does not affect treatment, but with other factors, appears to impact on long term survival.

Clinical Presentation and Diagnosis

The most common presenting symptom for patients with small bowel carcinoid is abdominal pain. As carcinoids grow, the polypoid lesions may serve as a lead point for intussusception. Intussusception is characterized by intermittent symptoms and signs of obstruction. Abdominal films often demonstrate a distal small bowel obstruction. The CT findings of intussusception are distinctive demonstrating a multilayer ringed structure in the ileocolic region (Figs. 52.5 and 52.6). If the patient does not have a complete small bowel obstruction, a contrast study may be helpful but yields a diagnosis in only 20% to 50%.

Unlike in the appendix where multicentricity is rare, carcinoids of the small bowel are multiple 30% to 40% of the time.[30] In addition, 30% to 50% of small bowel carcinoids are associated with second primary malignancies, most frequently of the breast and colon. Gastrointestinal carcinoids have the capacity to elicit a marked desmoplastic reaction. The mesentery of the small bowel becomes fibrotic and foreshortened, leading to kinking of the bowel or even intestinal ischemia as a result of sclerosis of the mesenteric blood vessels. The exact mechanism of this fibrosis, which is not only peritumoral but also distant in the heart and lungs, is still unknown.[31] This finding is readily identified on CT scan[32]

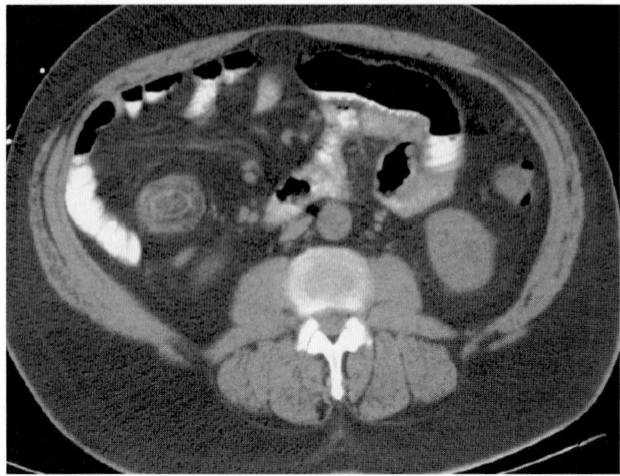

FIGURE 52.5 A 63-year-old man presented with a short history of abdominal pain that he described as similar to his pancreatitis pain. A computed tomography scan demonstrated an ileal carcinoid tumor as lead point for an intussusception into the cecum.

and is sometimes associated with calcifications while the small bowel appears fixed and angulated.

Stage and Prognosis

Tumor size is proportional to the risk for metastatic spread at initial diagnosis and must be considered in directing surgical strategies. In comparison to appendiceal carcinoids, which may cause appendicitis at a small size prior to lymph node metastasis, small bowel lesions often remain asymptomatic long enough to allow not only lymph node spread but also hepatic metastasis. For lesions smaller than 1 cm, there is a 20% to 30% incidence of nodal and hepatic spread. Tumors 1 to 2 cm in size have nodal spread in 60% to 80% and hepatic disease in 20%. The rate of nodal and hepatic metastasis for tumors larger than 2 cm is greater than 80% and 40% to 50% respectively.[33] These figures must guide the choice of operation. Whereas a small lesion less than 1 cm may be adequately treated with local excision, anything larger must be presumed to be metastatic and a wide resection with lymphadenectomy and careful examination of the liver is necessary.

Carcinoid Syndrome

Carcinoid syndrome refers to vasomotor, gastrointestinal, and cardiac manifestations induced by systemic circulation of a variety of peptides elaborated by carcinoid tumors. The amine precursor uptake and decarboxylation cells of carcinoid tumors can produce vasoactive products including serotonin, histamine, kallikrein, bradykinin, and prostaglandins, although the specific mediator or mediators of the syndrome remain unknown. Carcinoid syndrome is most reliably confirmed by finding elevated 24-hour 5-hydroxyindoleacetic acid urinary excretion, the primary stable metabolite of serotonin.

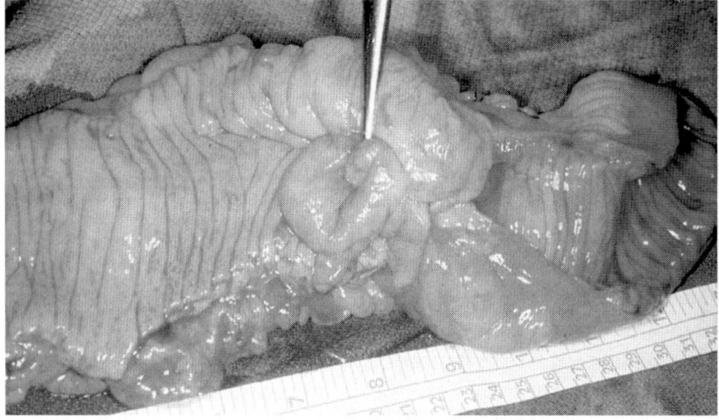

FIGURE 52.6 Resection of ileocolic segment of bowel in the patient shown in Fig. 52.5 to have an intussusception. Here carcinoid tumor can be seen as lead point for intussusception through ileocecal valve.

Attacks are initiated by stimuli including stress, alcohol, a large meal, or sexual intercourse, all of which manipulate the liver in some capacity. Flushing is the most common finding and affects approximately 80% of syndrome patients. The flush varies slightly by the location of the tumor, but in midgut carcinoids the flush is usually short-lived, lasting 5 to 10 minutes. Classically, the erythematous flush begins on the face and spreads to the trunk and limbs. Diarrhea, found in 75% of patients, seems to be caused by serotonin release. The diarrhea is intermittent, watery, and at times explosive. It may be associated with abdominal cramps and the patient may experience a certain degree of malabsorption. Although the diarrhea can be the most bothersome to a patient, the cardiac manifestations present in 60% to 70% of cases are the most serious. The tricuspid and pulmonary valves develop endocardial fibrosis, possibly secondary to high levels of 5-hydroxyindoleacetic acid. As the disease progresses, the fibrotic plaque stiffens, leading eventually to right heart failure.

Patients with gastrointestinal carcinoid tumors who present with carcinoid syndrome have metastatic disease in either the liver or retroperitoneum. The liver contains large amounts of monoamine oxidase which deactivates serotonin, one of the major effector hormones. Hence, to develop carcinoid syndrome, a patient must either have tumor in a location that does not primarily drain into the portal circulation, such as a bronchial carcinoid or retroperitoneal tumor, or have hepatic metastases of a magnitude that overwhelms the capacity of the monoamine oxidase to breakdown serotonin. The bioactive products from a small volume of hepatic metastases may be cleared by the hepatocytes, but larger tumor burden allows release of these products into the hepatic veins and the systemic circulation. It follows that patients with bronchial and ovarian carcinoids, or abdominal disease that has penetrated the retroperitoneum, which drains directly into the systemic circulation can manifest carcinoid syndrome from primary disease. Patients with gastrointestinal carcinoids, which drain into the portal circulation, must have metastatic disease prior to the development of the syndrome.

Management of patients with carcinoid syndrome may be approached surgically, radiologically, and medically, and often requires a combination of all three modalities. Surgical debulking of extensive hepatic disease or formal hepatic resection for resectable metastases may improve symptoms and prolong life. For patients with residual abdominal tumor and hepatic metastases, 5- and 10-year survival rates approached 60%, so although in general the initial surgery should involve attempts to debulk as much tumor as possible, it must also avoid catastrophic injuries such as those to the superior mesenteric vessels that may lead to short gut syndrome.[34] Hepatic artery embolization or radiofrequency ablation may be more appropriate for widespread hepatic metastases and in small series have been shown to give marked symptomatic relief and durable tumor control.[35,36] Medical therapy relies primarily on the use of a variety of somastatin analogues (octreotide) including short- and long-acting peptides for relief of carcinoid syndrome symptoms. Carcinoid tumors express somatostatin receptors and the somatostatin analogues inhibit vasoactive peptide release from carcinoid tumors. Efficacy of treatment can be documented by following excretion of the tumor marker 5-hydroxyindoleacetic acid. Palliation of symptoms is effective in 90% of patients with octreotide and some studies have even demonstrated a tumoristatic or tumor reduction effect after the administration of somatostatin, although these latter findings have not been consistently reproduced. Serotonin antagonists are useful in the management of gastrointestinal symptoms including rapid transit and diarrhea.

Potential chemotherapeutic agents for the treatment of metastatic carcinoid tumor have been used singly and in combination with each other in an effort to halt progression of disease as well as to promote regression. Common single agents include adriamycin, 5-fluorouracil, dacarbazine, and interferon-α, with response rates of approximately 20%. Combination protocols most often utilize streptozotocin and 5-fluorouracil. Preliminary reports on the use of targeted radiotherapeutics have been presented. Somatostatin analogues bind to somatostatin receptors on carcinoid tumors with high affinity. After binding, the ligand-receptor complex is internalized. This internalization has led to the development of "smart bombs" or radiolabeled somatostatin analogues that theoretically deliver radiation specifically to carcinoid cells. ^{111}-Indium-labeled pentetreotide demonstrated an enhanced tumor regression response compared with unlabeled analogue in one study.[37] Further investigations are ongoing.

GASTROINTESTINAL STROMAL TUMORS

Although GIST are the most common nonepithelial cell tumors of the small bowel, they are in fact rare tumors of the gastrointestinal tract representing only 0.2% of all gastrointestinal tumors. Approximately 25% of GIST arise in the small bowel, with 50% gastric, 15% rectal, and 10% colonic in origin.[38] GIST are diagnosed equally in men and women with a peak incidence in patients aged between 50 and 70 years. Arising from the interstitial cell of Cajal, the pacemaker cell of the gastrointestinal tract intercalated between the intramural neurons and the smooth muscle cells, GIST are characterized by the presence of activating c-kit mutations, a transmembrane receptor tyrosine kinase involved in the regulation of cellular proliferation, apoptosis, and differentiation. More than 95% of GIST express kit (CD117) mutations. This molecular marker allows for distinction of GIST from histologically similar mesenchymal tumors of the small bowel including leiomyomas, leiomyosarcoma, schwannomas and others. This molecular feature has lead to reclassification of up to 70% small bowel tumors as GIST that had previously been classified as a variety of mesenchymal tumors.[39] Those GIST that do not express c-kit mutations may express a mutation in another tyrosine kinase receptor, the platelet derived growth factor receptor alpha.[40] Present in approximately 5% to 7% of GIST, these activating mutations also result in abnormal cellular proliferation.

Like other primary small bowel tumors, GIST are characterized by indolent clinical symptoms including vague abdominal pain, weight loss and occult gastrointestinal bleeding. Although acute hemorrhage, perforation, or obstruction may lead to an emergency presentation, GIST may grow to a massive size prior to surgical presentation. Usually they grow insidiously as extraluminal masses from their submucosal origin in a noninvasive manner, characteristically pushing adjacent organs away from the expanding mass.

Diagnostic strategies are the same as for other tumors of the small bowel. Given the propensity of GIST to grow to a large size prior to diagnosis, CT scan is most likely to be the initial positive test. A characteristic finding is the presence of a large space-occupying mass, occasionally with calcification and hypervascularity and often with evidence of central necrosis and compression of adjacent organs (Fig. 52.7A).

All GIST should be considered to be malignant.[42] Malignant potential is based on two major criteria: size of the tumor and mitotic rate observed in the tumor (Table 52.6). Biologically aggressive tumors are large lesions with a high mitotic index, whereas tumors with benign features are small and exhibit a low mitotic index. Tumors are thus classified into very-low- to high-risk lesions for malignant potential, a classification that has prognostic significance.

Treatment

Surgery is the primary therapeutic option with the goal being complete resection. At operation, wide local excision of the primary tumor with in continuity resection of adherent organs is appropriate to attain curative resection (Fig. 52.7B). Lymph node metastasis is rare, negating the need for wide mesenteric resection.

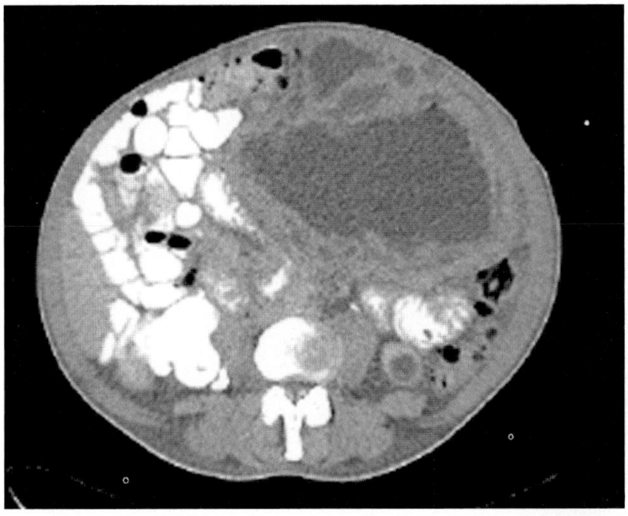

A

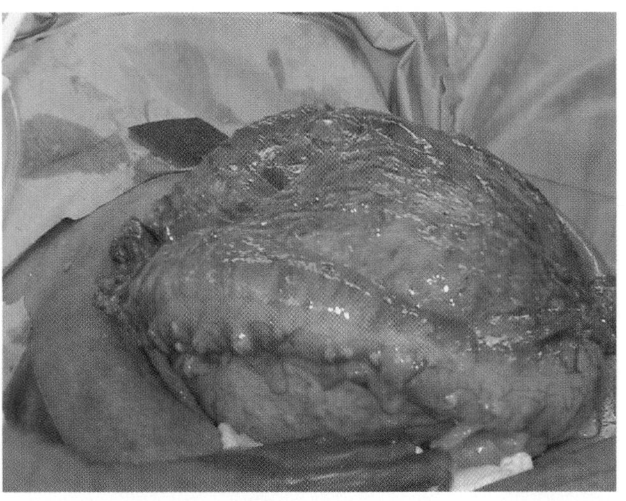

B

FIGURE 52.7 (*A*) Computed tomography image of a 76-year-old man with abdominal distention demonstrating a complex abdominal mass with varying degrees of thickness, central necrosis, and compression of adjacent organs. This was found to be a gastrointestinal stromal tumors with markedly increased mitotic activity. (*B*) Intraoperative photograph of the same patient, showing displacement of adjacent organs.

TABLE 52.6

MALIGNANT POTENTIAL AND PROGRESS OF GASTROINTESTINAL STROMAL TUMORS

Risk classification	Size	Mitotic rate	10-Year survival
High	Any size	>10/50 HPF	30%
	>10 cm	Any rate	
	>5 mm	>5/50 HPF	
Intermediate	5–10 cm	<5/50 HPF	60%
	<5 cm	6–10/50 HPF	
Low	2–5 cm	<5/50 HPF	75%
Very low	<2 cm	<5/50 HPF	80%
Normal population	—	—	80%

HPF, high power field.

Molecular Therapeutics and GIST

The discovery of activating mutations in the tyrosine kinases kit and more recently platelet-derived growth factor receptor alpha has stimulated development of therapeutic agents targeting these moieties. Activation of kit leads to phosphorylation of a receptor substrate protein initiating an intracellular phosphorylation cascade. This cytoplasmic cascade ultimately leads to nuclear activation of transcription events culminating in cell proliferation and survival. Imatinib mesylate is a small molecule that occupies the adenosine triphosphate binding pocket of the kit-kinase domain, blocking phosphorylation of the receptor and intracellular signaling. This binding arrests cellular proliferation and survival signaling.

Clinical use of imatinib is now routine in the management of GIST. This oral agent is well tolerated and highly effective for patients with metastatic GIST. Although complete regression of tumor is rare, partial regression of disease and arrest of progression of disease can be achieved for durable intervals with continuous treatment in up to 80% of patients. Efficacy of treatment can be predicted and followed using fluoro-D-glucose positron emission tomography scanning; these highly biologically active tumors will become metabolically silent with imatinib therapy in those patients with responsive tumors. With greater clinical experience with imatinib, resistant clones have been identified with eventual progression of disease. For these patients, a newer receptor tyrosine kinase inhibitor SU11248 has recently been introduced for clinical trials. This inhibitor has a broader spectrum of activity than imatinib and has shown early promise in patients with progression of disease on imatinib or in those relatively few patients who cannot tolerate imatinib.[42]

Use of imatinib in the neoadjuvant setting for unresectable or locally aggressive tumors is being currently being evaluated in cooperative group clinical trials. The efficacy of imatinib in the adjuvant setting for high risk or partially resected tumors is also being evaluated in ongoing trials. Given the favorable risk profile of the agent, such applications may prove useful in these settings as well, although definitive survival data are not yet available.

METASTATIC LESIONS TO THE SMALL BOWEL

The majority of malignant small bowel tumors are metastatic lesions from other primary sites rather than primary small bowel neoplasms. Metastatic spread can occur by direct invasion, hematogenous spread, or intraperitoneal seeding. Direct invasion from a colon or pancreatic cancer represents the most common mode of involvement. Hematogenous spread

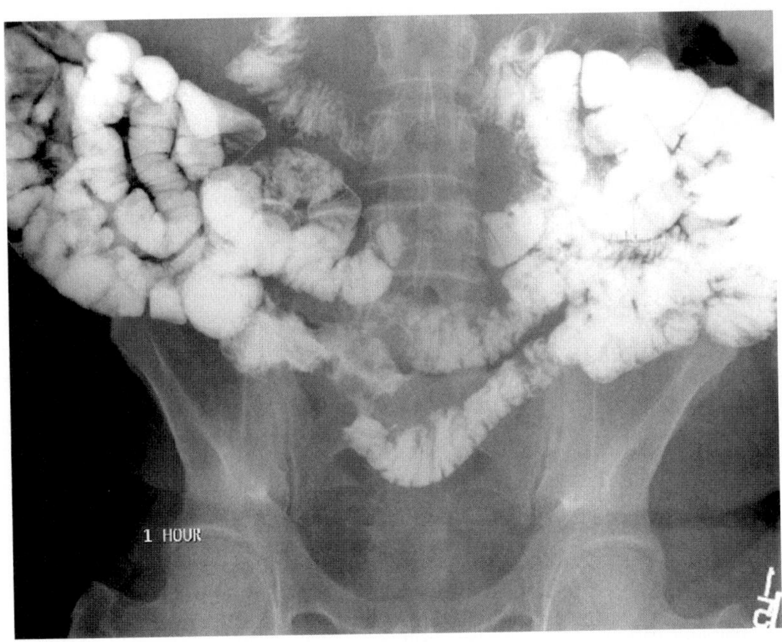

FIGURE 52.8 Small bowel follow-through in a 75-year-old man evaluated for significant weight loss and iron deficiency anemia. At exploration the above filling defect was found to be secondary to metastatic melanoma.

arises most frequently from bronchogenic or breast carcinoma or malignant melanoma. Peritoneal seeding has been documented from primary tumors of the stomach, liver ovary, appendix, and colon.

CT scan often demonstrates not only the degree of involvement of the small bowel but also the primary tumor. In metastatic small bowel tumors one may see bowel wall thickening as well as lesions in the mesentery or retroperitoneal fat. For small lesions, CT scan may be negative while small bowel follow through study may reveal an irregular luminal filling defect (Fig. 52.8) Carcinomatosis is frequently not specifically identifiable on imaging studies.

Optimal management is based on clinical criteria. Palliative intestinal resection or bypass to relieve hemorrhage, obstruction or pain is indicated except in the most terminal stages of disease. Case reports of prolonged survival after intestinal resection of solitary metastases have been reported, although progression of metastatic disease is more common.[43]

Management of patients with carcinomatosis, regardless of tumor origin, remains difficult. Palliative measures to maintain intestinal continuity and liberal use of decompressive gastrostomy tubes are indicated.

KEY POINTS

- **Although the small bowel accounts for 75% of the length and 90% of the mucosal surface of the gastrointestinal tract, it is the site of only 1% to 3% of gastrointestinal malignancies.**
- **As in the colon, small bowel adenomas may be histologically classified as tubular, tubulovillous, or villous. Adenomas occur predominantly in the duodenum with the majority found in the periampullary region.**
- **Like adenomas, adenocarcinomas have a predilection for the duodenum, with a marked decrease in frequency moving axially along the small bowel. Approximately 80% of tumors are located in the duodenum or proximal jejunum.**
- **The gastrointestinal tract is the site of 4% to 20% of all non-Hodgkin lymphomas, being the most common extranodal site. The stomach harbors the most lymphomas, followed by the small bowel, and then the colon.**
- **Carcinoids are indolent malignant neuroendocrine tumors that arise from the enterochromaffin cells at the base of the crypts of Lieberkühn.**

References

1. Ciresi DL, Scholten DJ. The continuing clinical dilemma of primary tumors of the small intestine. *Am Surg*. 1995;61:698–703.
2. Matsuo S, Eto T, Tsunoda T, et al. Small bowel tumors: an analysis of tumor-like lesions, benign and malignant neoplasms. *Eur J Surg Onc*. 1994;20:47–51.
3. Minardi AJ Jr, Zibari GB, Aultman DF, et al. Small-bowel tumors. *J Am Coll Surg*. 1998;186:664–668.
4. Johnson AM, Harman PK, Hanks JB. Primary small bowel malignancies. *Am Surg*. 1985;51:31–36.
5. Serour F, Dona G, Birkenfeld S, et al. Primary neoplasms of the small bowel. *J Surg Oncol*. 1992;49:29.
6. Sigel JE, Petras RE, Lashner BA, et al. Intestinal adenocarcinoma in Crohn's disease; a report of 30 cases with a focus on coexisting dysplasia. *Am J Surg Pathol*. 1999;23:651–655.
7. Abrahams NA, Halverson A, Fazio VW, et al. Adenocarcinoma of the small bowel: A study of 37 cases with emphasis on histologic prognostic factors. *Dis Colon Rectum* 2002;45:1496–1502.
8. **Howe JR, Karnell LH, Menck HR, et al. Adenocarcinoma of the small bowel: Review of the National Cancer Data Base, 1985-1995. *Cancer* 1999;86:2693–2706.**
9. O'Boyle CJ, Kerin MJ, Feeley K, et al. Primary small intestinal tumours: increased incidence of lymphoma and improved survival. *Ann R Coll Surg Engl*. 1998;80:332–334.
10. Green PH, Fleischauer AT, Bhagat G, et al. Risk of malignancy in patients with celiac disease. *Am J Med*. 2003;115:191–195.
11. Dong K, Li B. Peutz-Jeghers syndrome: case reports and update on diagnosis and treatment. *Chin J Dig Dis*. 2004;5:160–164.
12. Crump M, Gospodarowicz M, Shepherd FA. Lymphoma of the gastrointestinal tract. *Semin Oncol*. 1999;26:324–337.
13. Maglinte DDT, Reyes BL. Small bowel cancer: radiologic diagnosis. *Radiol Clin N Am*. 1997;35:361–380.
14. Buckley JA, Jones B, Fishman EK. Small bowel cancer; imaging features and staging. *Radiol Clin N Am*. 1997;35:381–402.
15. Waye JD: Small-bowel endoscopy. *Endoscopy* 2003;35:15–21.
16. Swain P. Wireless capsule endoscopy. *Gut* 2003;52 (suppl 4):48–50.
17. **Cave DR. Wireless video capsule endoscopy. *Clin Perspect Gastroenterol*. 2002;5:203–207.**
18. Adeonigbagbe O, Lee C, Karowe M, et al. A Brunner's gland adenomas as a cause of anemia. *J Clin Gastroenterol*. 1999;29:193–196.
19. Zangara J, Kushner H, Drachenberg C, et al. Iron deficiency anemia due to a Brunner's gland hamartoma. *J Clin Gastroenterol*. 1998;27:353–356.
20. Beger HG, Treitschke F, Gansange F, et al. Tumor of the ampulla of Vater. *Arch Surg*. 1999;134:526–532.
21. Sakorafas GH, Sarr MG, Tsiotos GG, et al. Villous tumors of the duodenum; reappraisal of local versus extended resection. *Gastroenterology* 1999;116:S0069.
22. Cunningham JD, Aleali R, Aleali M, et al. Malignant small bowel neoplasms; histopathologic determinants of recurrence and survival. *Ann Surg*. 1997;225:300–306.
23. Marcilla JAG, Bueno FS, Aquilar J, et al. Primary small bowel malignant tumors. *Eur J Surg Oncol*. 1994;20:630–634.
24. American Joint Committee on Cancer and TNM Committee of the International Union Against Cancer: Small intestine. In: Greene FL, Page DL, Fleming ID, et al., eds. *Handbook for the staging of cancer*. Philadelphia: JB Lippincott Co., 2002, pp.119–125.
25. Sohn TA, Lillemoe KD, Cameron JL, et al. Adenocarcinoma of the duodenum; factors influencing long-term survival. *J Gastrointest Surg*. 1998; 2:79–87.
26. Case 30-1999. Case Records of the Massachusetts General Hospital. *N Engl J Med*. 1999;341:1063–1071.
27. Cooper DL, Daria R, Salloum E. Primary gastrointestinal lymphomas. *Gastroenterologist* 1996;4:54–64.
28. Pandey M, Wadhwa MK, Patel HP, et al. Malignant lymphoma of the gastrointestinal tract. *Eur J Surg Oncol*. 1999;25:164–167.
29. Memon MA, Nelson H. Gastrointestinal carcinoid tumors; current management strategies. *Dis Colon Rectum* 1997;40:1101–1118.
30. Yantiss R. Odze R, Farraye F, et al. Solitary versus multiple carcinoid tumors of the ileum: a clinical and pathological review of 68 cases. *Am J Surg Pathol*. 2003;27:811–817.
31. Modlin IM, Shapiro MD, Kidd M. Carcinoid tumors and fibrosis: An association with no explanation. *Am J Gastroenterol*. 2004;99:2466–2478.
32. Sheth S, Horton K, Garland M, et al. Mesenteric neoplasms: CT appearance of primary and secondary tumors and differential diagnosis. *Radiographics* 2003;23:457–473.
33. Rothmund M, Kisker O. Surgical treatment of carcinoid tumors of the small bowel, appendix, colon and rectum. *Digestion* 1994;55:86–91.
34. **Soreide JA, van Heerden JA, Thompson GB, et al. Gastrointestinal carcinoid tumors: long-term prognosis for surgically treated patients. *World J Surg*. 2000;24:1431–1436.**
35. Schell S, Camp E, Caridi J, et al. Hepatic artery embolization for control of symptoms, octreotide requirements, and tumor progression in metastatic carcinoid tumors. *J Gastrointest Surg*. 2002;6:664–670.
36. Roche A, Girish B, de Baerre, et al. Trans-catheter arterial chemoembolization as first-line treatment for hepatic metastases from endocrine tumors. *Eur Radiol*. 2003;13:136–140.
37. Anthony L, et al. Indium-111-pentectreoctide prolongs survival in gastroenteropancreatic malignancies. *Semin Nucl Med*. 2002;32:123.
38. **Miettinen M, and Lasota J. Gastrointestinal stromal tumors—definition, clinical, histological, immunohistochemical, and molecular genetic features and differential diagnosis. *Virchows Arch*. 2001;438:1–12.**
39. Emory TS, Sobin LH, Lukes L, et al. Prognosis of gastrointestinal smooth-muscle (stromal) tumors: dependence on anatomic site. *Am J Surg Pathol*. 1999;23(1):82–87.
40. Heinrich MC, Corless CL, Duensing A.PDGFRA activating mutations in gastrointestinal stromal tumors. *Science*. 2003;299:708–710.
41. Fletcher CD, Berman JJ, Corless C, et al. Diagnosis of gastrointestinal stromal tumors: A consensus approach. *Hum Pathol*. 2002;33: 459–465.
42. **von Mehren M. New therapeutic strategies for soft tissue sarcomas. *Curr Treat Options Oncol*. 2003;4:441–451.**
43. Cipollone G, Santarelli G, Quitadamo S, et al. Small bowel metastases from lung cancer. *Chir Ital*. 2004;56:639–648.

SECTION G
PANCREAS

CHAPTER 53 ■ PANCREAS ANATOMY AND PHYSIOLOGY

SELWYN M. VICKERS, J. PABLO ARNOLETTI, AND F. CHARLES BRUNICARDI

The pancreas is a glandular structure located in the retroperitoneum that can have variable congenital abnormalities that often provide significant surgical insight. The normal development of the gland and its native location and anatomic boundaries, as well as its association with other structures, can often lead to insight into disease management and patient presentation as well as natural history of diseases.

Anteriorly, the pancreas is covered at the distal head and neck by the pylorus and the transverse mesocolon. The neck and body of the gland are covered anteriorly by the posterior gastric wall. The anterior surface of the pancreas is covered by a peritoneal leaf originating from the lesser sac. The gland lacks any formal capsule. Instead, it is covered by a tenuous layer of connective tissue that extends between the lobules of the gland. In the normal setting, the gland is extremely friable, with a texture that creates significant technical difficulties when it comes to suturing. In fact, normal pancreas has been found to be the key factor, determining either a leak or a fistula rate, when operative procedures are used to transect or reanastomose the gland. Thus, in its healthy state, it has the highest risk of having sutures pull out or cut through the gland.

The pancreas is routinely divided into the head (which usually includes the uncinate process), the neck, the body, and the tail (Fig. 53.1). The head is usually a flattened structure about 2 to 3 cm thick that is attached to the second and third portions of the duodenum to its right and to the left emerges into the neck. The border is determined by the insertion of the gastroduodenal artery (GDA). The neck of the pancreas is a narrow segment of the gland that straddles the superior mesenteric vein (SMV) and portal vein. At its inferior border, the superior mesenteric vessels emerge from this lower edge, and it is covered by the lesser sac in front. At its superior border, it is adjacent to the celiac axis with the hepatic artery to the right and the splenic artery just to its left. Just posterior to the neck, or the isthmus, lies the confluence of the splenic and SMVs, which form the portal vein. In this area, rarely are there any anterior branches to the body of the pancreas. Therefore, during a pancreaticoduodenectomy, this plane can be developed with limited risk of vessel perforation or tributaries interfering with the process.

The body of the pancreas is an elongated, flat structure with a sizable anterior and posterior surface encompassing, anteriorly, the splenic artery and, posteriorly, the splenic vein with its fascia. The lesser sac separates its anterior surface from the stomach, the posterior surface sits just above the aorta and anterior to the left adrenal gland, the left renal vessels, and the upper third of the left kidney. Again, the splenic vein runs firmly embedded in the posterior surface with some 10 to 12 short tributaries that drain directly into the posterior surface of the pancreas. There is a notable absence of any large vessels between the pancreatic body and its posterior surface in the retroperitoneum, creating a nearly avascular plane. The adrenal gland, however, lies just adjacent to the distal body of the pancreas and often may be involved in an oncologic resection. The inferior surface of the body is covered often by the transverse mesocolon. There are small branches of a finer nature from the epiploic veins to the greater omentum in this area. The only other major attachment is a middle colic artery and vein that often drain into the SMV, leaving the border of the neck and the body of the pancreas at its inferior surface. The tail of the pancreas lies at the level of the 12th thoracic vertebra. It is a short, mobile segment that ends within the splenic hilum. It may be injured during splenectomy, resulting in a postoperative fistula.

EMBRYOLOGY

The pancreas is of endodermal origin and develops from ventral and dorsal pancreatic buds. The ventral bud arises from the hepatic diverticulum, and the dorsal bud arises from the developing duodenum. During the fifth week of life, the dorsal bud appears first and grows rapidly. The ventral bud rotates clockwise behind the duodenum and fuses with the dorsal bud (Fig. 53.2). The ventral bud becomes the uncinate process and

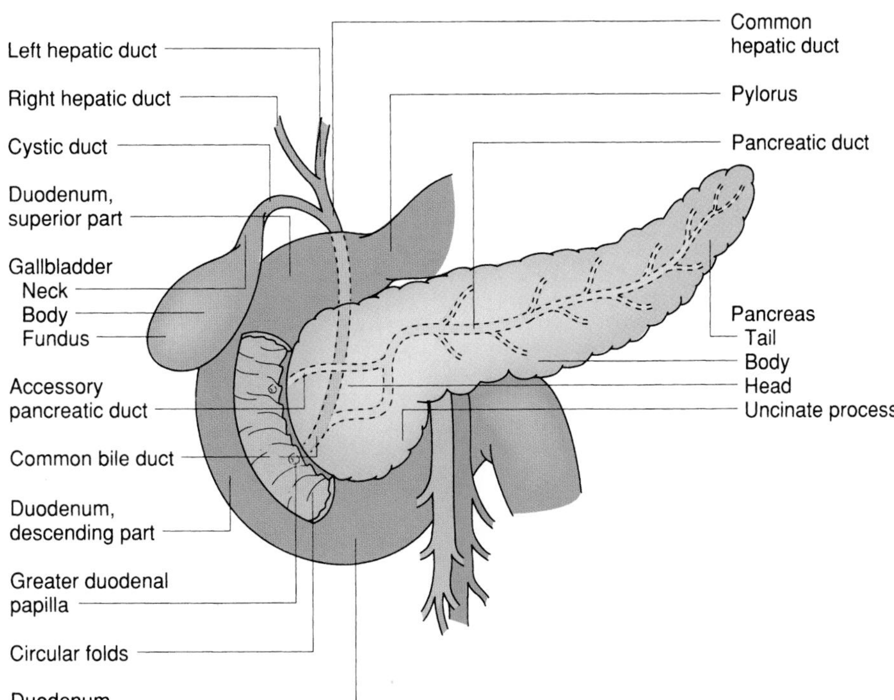

FIGURE 53.1 Relation of the pancreas to the duodenum and extrahepatic biliary system. (After Woodburne RT. *Essentials of human anatomy.* New York: Oxford University Press; 1973.)

inferior head of the pancreas; the dorsal bud becomes the neck, body and tail, and superior head of the pancreas. The ventral bud duct fuses with the dorsal bud to become the *main pancreatic duct*, or duct of Wirsung, which drains most of the pancreas. The proximal duct of the dorsal bud, known as the *lesser pancreatic duct*, or duct of Santorini, usually persists and drains into the duodenum through the lesser papilla. Abnormalities in the rotation or fusion of the developing pancreas can result in specific congenital disorders (Table 53.1; Figs. 53.3 and 53.4).

SURGICAL ANATOMY

Precise knowledge of pancreatic anatomy and physiology is critical for pancreatic surgeons. Pancreatic anatomy explains the unique presentation of patients with pancreatic disease. The pancreas is situated deep within the abdomen in the retroperitoneum at the level of the second lumbar vertebra. It extends in an oblique, transverse position from the duodenal C loop to the hilum of the spleen, at the level of the first and second lumbar vertebrae (Fig. 53.5). Its deep retroperitoneal location accounts for the late clinical manifestation and diagnosis of many pancreatic diseases. The pancreas is divided into four portions: the head; the uncinate process and neck, which extends from the duodenal C loop to the left flank of the superior mesenteric-portal vein confluence; the body, which lies behind the stomach and extends from the superior mesenteric-portal vein confluence to the left side of the abdominal aorta; and the tail, which includes the parenchyma located between the aorta and the hilum of the spleen. Resection of the head of the pancreas at the level of the neck results in a 60% to 70% reduction in pancreatic mass.

Relations to Other Structures

The pancreas is almost entirely retroperitoneal and has close relationships with numerous surrounding structures (see Fig. 53.5). The head of the pancreas fits closely into the curve of the duodenum and lies to the right of the superior mesenteric vessels. The head is crossed anteriorly by the root of the transverse mesocolon and is separated by the fusion fascia of Treitz from the adjacent inferior vena cava, renal veins, and right renal artery.

TABLE 53.1 ETIOLOGY

CONGENITAL DISORDERS RESULTING FROM DISORDERS AND ABNORMALTIES IN THE ROTATION OR FUSION OF THE DEVELOPING PANCREAS

Disorder	Description
Annular pancreas	Thin band of normal pancreatic parenchyma surrounds the second portion of the duodenum in continuity with the head of the pancreas causing variable degrees of duodenal stenosis. This thin band frequently carries a pancreatic duct remnant; thus, its division can often create an unwarranted fistula or pancreatitis due to ductal obstruction (see Fig. 53.4).
Pancreas divisum	Results from an incomplete fusion of the ventral pancreatic duct with the dorsal duct during fetal development and is present in 10%–12% of patients. In this anomaly, the lesser duct drains the entire pancreas; inadequacy of this pattern of drainage can result in pancreatitis and chronic pain (see Fig. 53.3).
Ectopic pancreatic tissue	Functional pancreatic tissue may be found in different ectopic locations such as stomach, duodenal wall, ileum, umbilicus, and even colon, appendix, or gallbladder.

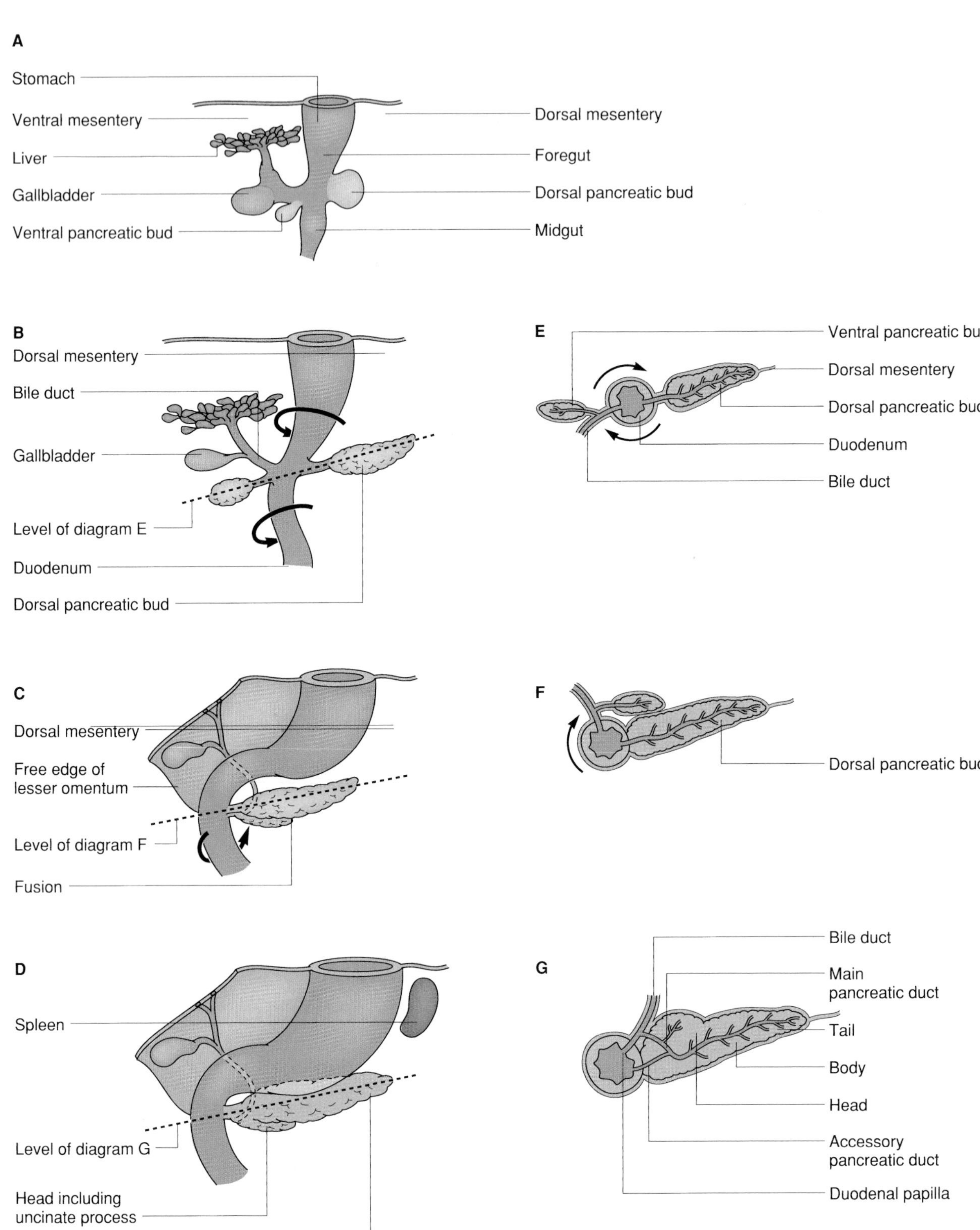

FIGURE 53.2 (*A–D*) Schematic drawings of the successive stages in the development of the pancreas from the fifth through the eighth weeks. (*E–G*) Diagrammatic transverse sections through the duodenum and the developing pancreas. Growth and rotation (*arrows*) of the duodenum bring the ventral pancreatic bud toward the dorsal bud, and they subsequently fuse. The bile duct initially attaches to the ventral aspect of the duodenum and is carried around to the dorsal aspect as the duodenum rotates. The main pancreatic duct is formed by the union of the distal part of the dorsal pancreatic duct and the entire ventral pancreatic duct. (After Moore KL. *The developing human,* 3rd ed. Philadelphia: WB Saunders; 1982.)

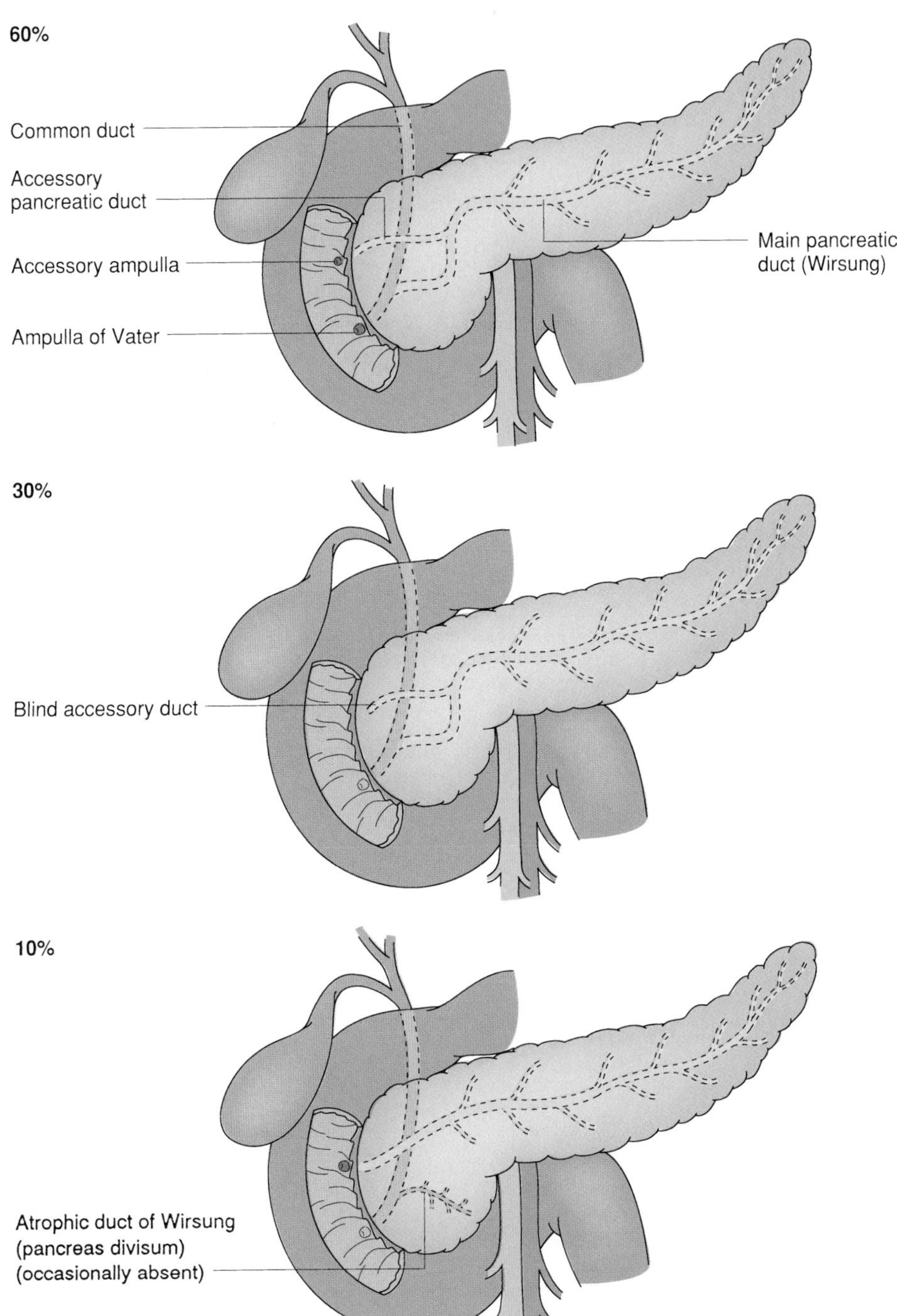

FIGURE 53.3 Anatomic configuration of the intrapancreatic ductal system. A lack of communication between the two ducts, which occurs in 10% of cases, is referred to as *pancreas divisum*. (After Silen W. Surgical anatomy of the pancreas. *Surg Clin North Am.* 1964;44:1253.)

These relationships must be taken into account when mobilizing the head of the pancreas and duodenum from the retroperitoneum (Kocher maneuver). The uncinate process, which is part of the head, wraps around and extends posteriorly to the superior mesenteric vessels. The intrapancreatic portion of the common bile duct descends in the posterior surface of the pancreatic head to join the main pancreatic duct at the ampulla of Vater. This structure has a significant degree variability as it enters the pancreatic head and ampulla—knowledge of its course is critical in Frey procedures and resection of choledochal cysts (Fig. 53.6).

The neck is defined as that portion of the pancreas overlying the superior mesenteric vessels and is identifiable from the head of the pancreas by a notch that contains the superior mesenteric vessels. This part of the pancreas is sometimes referred to as the *incisura pancreatis*. Usually, no anterior venous tributaries of the superior mesenteric or portal vein extend from the pancreatic neck. A plane can be developed between these vessels and the pancreas during pancreatic resection. In certain cases (10% to 20%), however, anterior venous collaterals may be present, almost always located on the superior border of the pancreas extending from the portal vein to the posterior surface of the bile duct or draining the inferior border of the bile duct or superior pancreas.

The body begins to the left of the neck. Its anterior surface is covered with peritoneum that forms the posterior floor of the lesser sac. The transverse mesocolon attaches to its inferior margin. The body lies behind the posterior wall of the stomach and overlies the aorta, celiac plexus nerve bundles, and the origin of the superior mesenteric artery (SMA). These anatomic relationships explain why an inflammatory process such as pancreatitis is frequently contained within the lesser sac.

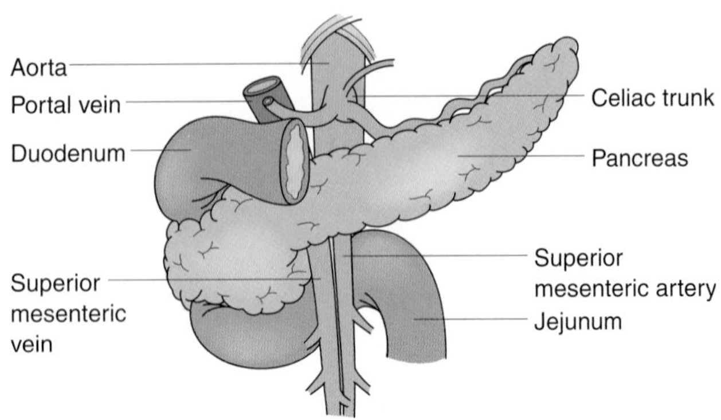

FIGURE 53.4 The ring of pancreatic tissue contains a large duct and may be heavily fixed to the duodenal musculature. The duodenum beneath the annulus is often stenosed. Thus, cutting the ring may not provide relief from symptoms of obstruction. There is also the danger of creating a pancreatic fistula or duodenal perforation. Duodenojejunostomy bypassing the annulus, is the accepted procedure. Annular pancreas usually produces symptoms in the first year of life, but where the stenosis is mild or absent, it may remain silent for many years. (After Gray SW, Skandalakis, JE. *Atlas of surgical anatomy for general surgeons.* Baltimore: Williams & Wilkins; 1985.)

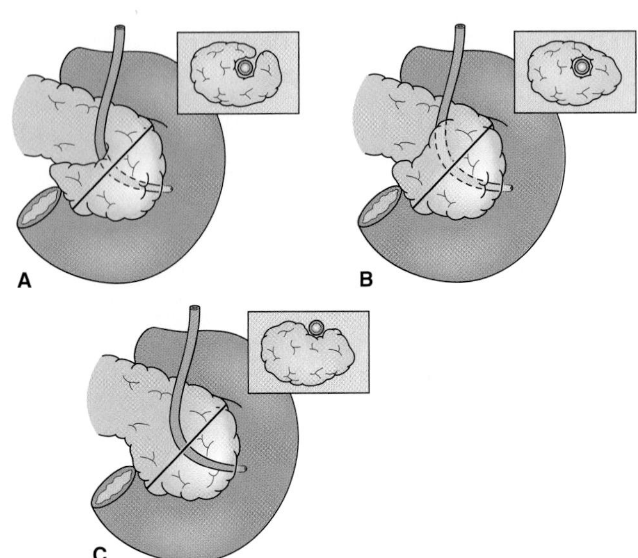

FIGURE 53.6 Variations of the retropancreatic segment of the common bile duct. (*A*) The duct is partially covered by pancreatic tissue. (*B*) The duct is completely covered by pancreas. (*C*) The duct runs freely behind the pancreas. (After Trede M. *Embryology and surgical anatomy of the pancreas.* New York: Churchill Livingstone; 1997.)

The small portion of the pancreas anterior to the left kidney is referred to as the *tail.* The tail of the pancreas lies close to the spleen, left colic flexure, left adrenal, and left kidney. The body and tail of the pancreas may be mobilized *en bloc* with the spleen, separating them from the rest of the retroperitoneum, by incising the retropancreatic fusion fascia of Toldt. An understanding of these complex relations can help avoid injury during surgery performed on the pancreas or any of its adjacent organs and structures.

Pancreatic Ducts

The main pancreatic duct, or duct of Wirsung, runs the entire length of the pancreas and joins the common bile duct to empty into the duodenum at the ampulla of Vater. The ampulla of Vater is usually located in the posterior aspect of the medial wall of the second portion of the duodenum, at approximately 7 to 10 cm from the pylorus. The ampulla of Vater represents the intersection of the biliary, pancreatic, and digestive tracts and has great functional and pathologic significance from both the endoscopic and surgical standpoints. The pancreatic duct usually runs midway between the superior and inferior borders and is usually closer to the posterior than to the anterior surface. The normal duct is only 2 to 4 mm in diameter and contains 20 secondary branches, which drain the tail, body, head, and uncinate process. Pancreatic ductal pressure is 15 to 30 mm Hg, whereas that in the common bile duct

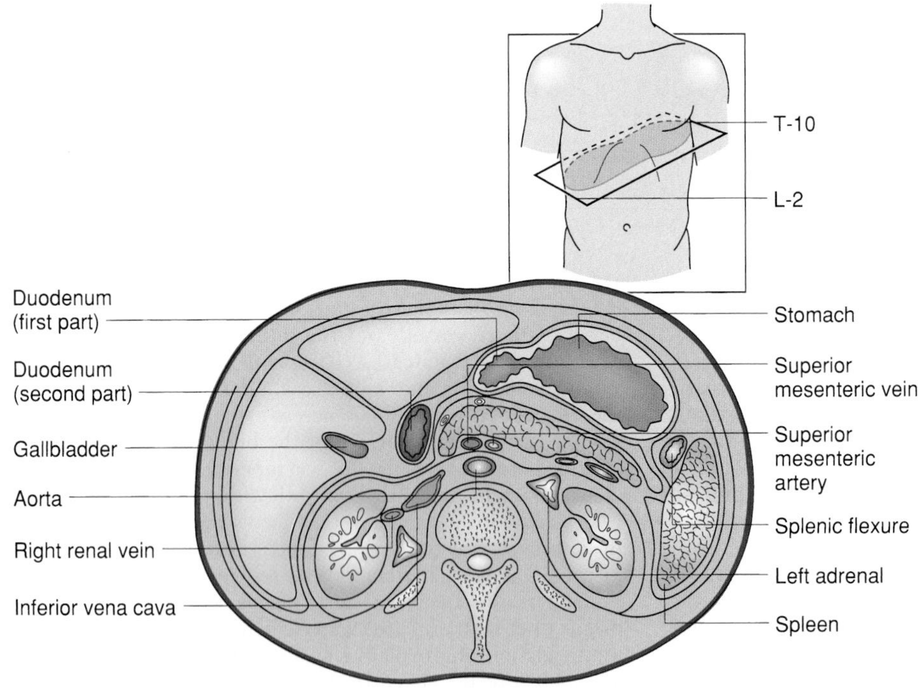

FIGURE 53.5 Cross-sectional relation of the pancreas to other abdominal structures in an oblique plane through the long axis of the pancreas extending from the level of L2 on the right to T10 on the left. (After Mackie CR, Moossa AR. Surgical anatomy of the pancreas. In: Moossa AR, ed. *Tumors of the pancreas.* Baltimore: Williams & Wilkins; 1980.)

is only 7 to 17 mm Hg. This normal pressure differential is thought to prevent damage to the pancreatic duct by reflux of bile. The drainage of the lesser duct, or duct of Santorini, is variable. The lesser duct commonly drains the superior portion of the head of the pancreas. It empties separately into the second portion of the duodenum through the minor papilla, which is 2 cm proximal to the ampulla of Vater. Eighty percent to 90% of the time, the lesser duct patently communicates with the main duct. Several variations in the ductal system may result from differences in embryologic development and can be of clinical significance as mentioned previously. Autopsy series demonstrate a 10% to 13% incidence of incomplete fusion of the dorsal and ventral buds of the pancreatic remnant. This condition of pancreas divisum may be associated with recurrent attacks of pancreatitis. The main pancreatic duct joins with the terminal common bile duct (with a normal diameter of approximately 6 mm at this level) to empty at the ampulla of Vater. At the level of the ampulla, the pancreatic duct opening is typically anterior and inferior to that of the terminal bile duct. A short *common channel,* containing flow from both secretory systems, is seen in a significant number of patients (Fig. 53.7). The surrounding sphincter of Oddi controls pancreatic and biliary secretions into the duodenal lumen. This sphincter, which is a complex set of muscular fibers surrounding the common bile duct and pancreatic duct, is regulated by neural and hormonal factors. The sphincter prevents reflux of duodenal contents into the ducts and can prevent reflux of bile into the pancreatic duct because of the differential in pancreatic and biliary ductular pressures.

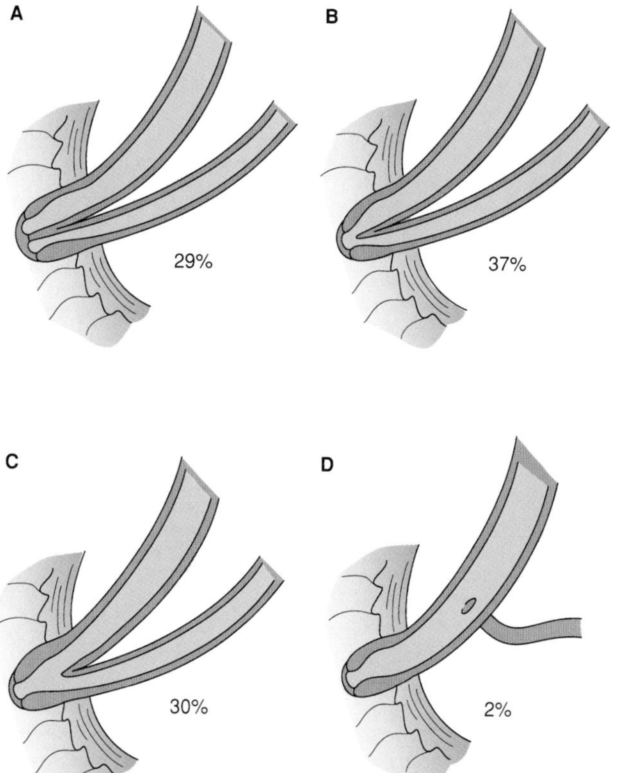

FIGURE 53.7 Variations in the relation between the intrapancreatic portion of the common bile duct and the main pancreatic duct at the ampulla of Vater. A common channel (C) is found in almost one third of subjects. (After Rienhoff WF Jr, Pickrell KL. Pancreatitis: anatomic study of pancreatic and extrahepatic biliary systems. *Arch Surg.* 1945;51:205.)

Arterial Supply

The unique arterial supply to the pancreas must be considered during pancreatic resection. The pancreas receives its blood supply from a variety of major arterial sources. The celiac and superior mesenteric arteries supply blood to the pancreas through their major branches (Fig. 53.8A and B). Collateral vessels generally form between arcades in the anterior and posterior surfaces of the head of the pancreas. These arcades arise from branches of the gastroduodenal and superior mesenteric arteries. The GDA is the first branch of the common hepatic artery and is divided when a pancreaticoduodenectomy is performed. Just distal to the first portion of the duodenum, the GDA becomes the superior pancreaticoduodenal artery, which divides into anterior and posterior branches. The inferior pancreaticoduodenal artery is the first branch of the SMA and divides into anterior and posterior branches. The anterosuperior pancreaticoduodenal artery lies in the anterior head of the pancreas, and collateral vessels usually extend between this artery and the anteroinferior pancreaticoduodenal artery. The posterosuperior pancreaticoduodenal artery crosses the common bile duct and forms the posterior arcade with the posteroinferior pancreaticoduodenal artery. These arcades provide a rich vascular supply shared by the head and second and third portions of the duodenum. Anomalies in the vascular supply to the head of the pancreas are found in 20% to 30% of patients and they mainly consist of the common hepatic, right hepatic, or GDA arising from the SMA. The most common anomaly (20% of the time) occurs with the relocation of the right hepatic artery originating from the superior border of the SMA traversing the upper edge of the uncinate process and traveling posterolateral to the portal vein, often becoming the most lateral structure in the hepatoduodenal ligament. Less often, the common hepatic originates from the SMA. In this setting the artery traverses the upper border of the uncinate, but lies anterior to the portal vein and posterior to the bile. This anomalous anatomy forces the GDA to enter the head of the pancreas directly posterior to the bile duct. Care must be taken to avoid confusing the common hepatic trunk for the GDA. Knowledge of these variations and careful attention to detail help the pancreatic surgeon avoid serious intraoperative mishaps.

Vascularization of the Duodenal Papilla

The duodenal papilla derives its blood supply from three main sources. A posterior pedicle, usually located at the 11 o'clock position, arises from the posterior and superior pancreaticoduodenal artery. A ventral commissural pedicle is situated at the 1 o'clock position and has branches from both pancreaticoduodenal arcades. An inferior pedicle (6 o'clock position) arises from the anterior and inferior pancreaticoduodenal artery.

The body and tail of the pancreas are supplied by the splenic artery. The splenic artery arises from the celiac trunk, is incorporated in the peripancreatic fascia, and courses along the posterosuperior surface of the pancreas to the spleen. About 10 branches of the splenic artery supply the body and tail of the pancreas. Three of the larger branches are the dorsal pancreatic artery, which lies close to the celiac trunk; the great pancreatic artery, or pancreatica magna, which supplies the midportion of the body; and the caudal pancreatic artery, which supplies the tail. Knowledge of these arteries is critical for performing central pancreatectomies and for splenic preservation during distal pancreatectomy. These three arteries course through the length of the pancreas and form collateral vessels with the inferior pancreaticoduodenal artery, which arises from the SMA.

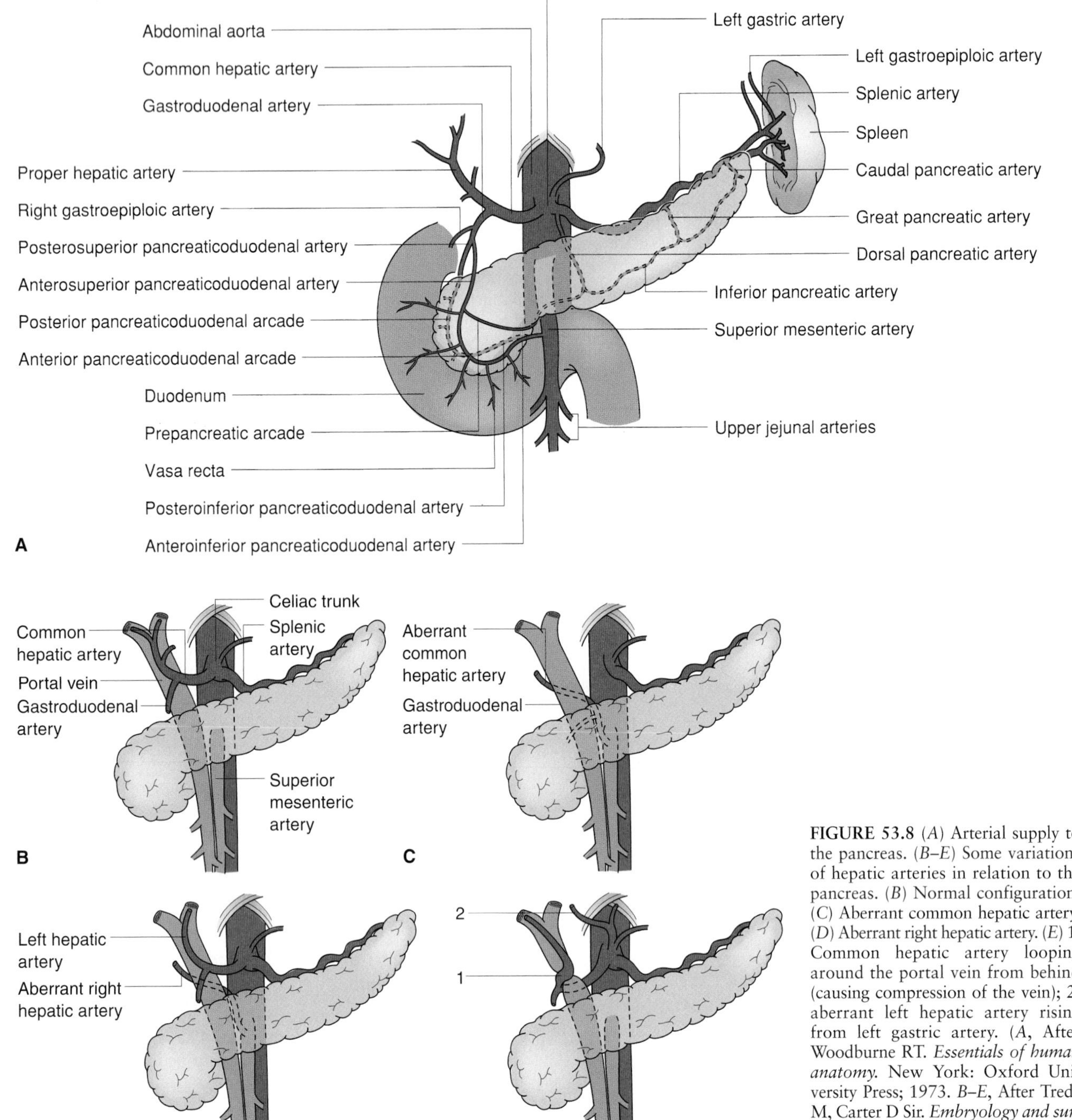

FIGURE 53.8 (*A*) Arterial supply to the pancreas. (*B–E*) Some variations of hepatic arteries in relation to the pancreas. (*B*) Normal configuration. (*C*) Aberrant common hepatic artery. (*D*) Aberrant right hepatic artery. (*E*) 1, Common hepatic artery looping around the portal vein from behind (causing compression of the vein); 2, aberrant left hepatic artery rising from left gastric artery. (*A*, After Woodburne RT. *Essentials of human anatomy.* New York: Oxford University Press; 1973. *B–E*, After Trede M, Carter D Sir. *Embryology and surgical anatomy of the pancreas.* New York: Churchill Livingstone; 1997.)

Venous Drainage

The venous drainage of the pancreas and duodenum follows the arterial supply (Fig. 53.9). The veins are usually superficial to the arteries, and the frequency of anomalies is similar. The anterior and posterior venous arcades drain the head, and the body and tail drain into the splenic vein. All venous effluent from the pancreas ultimately drains into the portal vein. The major venous drainage areas are the suprapancreatic portal vein, retropancreatic portal vein, splenic veins, and infrapancreatic SMV. The anterior and posterior venous arcades in the head of the pancreas drain directly into the suprapancreatic portal vein. The anteroinferior pancreaticoduodenal arcades drain with the right gastroepiploic vein to form a common venous trunk with the right colic vein. This trunk, known as Henle's *gastrocolic trunk,* enters the SMV just at the inferior border of the neck of the pancreas. Its location and identification is often critical to a successful and eventful dissection of the neck of the pancreas at the SMV notch. This drainage system forms a common trunk at its entrance into the SMV, but a centimeter above this point is a trifurcation of veins creating a difficult repair if injury or attempt division occurs at this point. The posteroinferior venous arcade empties directly into

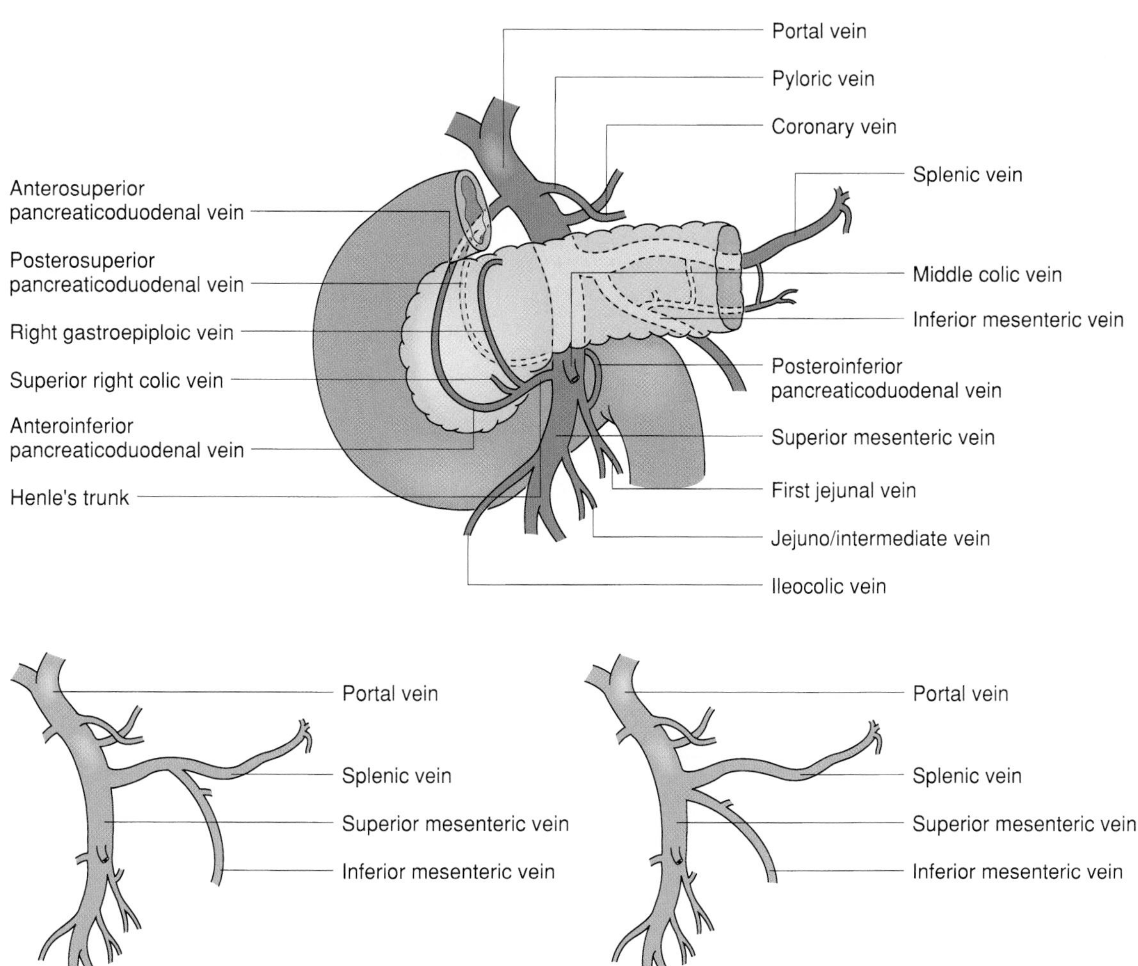

FIGURE 53.9 Venous drainage of pancreas. Variations in the relation of the portal, splenic, superior mesenteric, and inferior mesenteric veins are shown at the bottom. (After Mackie CR, Moossa AR. Surgical anatomy of the pancreas. In: Moossa AR, ed. *Tumors of the pancreas.* Baltimore: Williams & Wilkins, 1980.)

the SMV. The veins of the head drain laterally into the superior mesenteric and portal veins. For this reason, it is usually safe to "tunnel" and dissect the neck of the pancreas directly anterior to the portal vein during a pancreaticoduodenectomy. In some patients, however, the superior pancreaticoduodenal vein and the gastrocolic vein may enter the portal vein anteriorly.

Three major venous branches drain the body and tail of the pancreas. These are the inferior pancreatic vein, the caudal pancreatic vein, and the great pancreatic vein. All these branches drain into the splenic vein. The inferior mesenteric vein (IMV) courses behind the pancreas and joins either with the splenic vein or directly with the SMV. This variable insertion of the IMV must be noted in distal pancreatectomies or midbody resections to avoid injury to this structure.

Lymphatic Drainage

The abundant and ubiquitous lymphatic drainage of the pancreas provides a strong anatomic correlation to the high incidence of metastases associated with pancreatic cancer (Fig. 53.10). The lymphatic vessels of the pancreas arise from a rich periacinar network, which is followed by lymphatic trunks that drain into five main nodal groups. The superior nodes are located along the superior border of the pancreas and celiac trunk, and they drain the upper half of the head of the pancreas. The anterior lymphatics drain to the prepyloric and infrapyloric nodes. The inferior group of nodes is located along the inferior border of the pancreatic head and body and in turn drain to the superior mesenteric and periaortic nodes. The posterior pancreaticoduodenal lymph nodes include the distal common bile duct and ampullary lymphatics and drain into right periaortic nodes. Finally, the splenic group of nodes drains the tail of the pancreas along the splenic vessels and into the interceliomesenteric lymph nodes.[1] The absence of a peritoneal barrier on the posterior surface of the pancreas results in a direct communication of the intrapancreatic lymphatics with the retroperitoneal tissues, and this probably contributes to the high incidence of recurrence after presumably curative resections of pancreatic cancer.

Innervation

The exocrine and endocrine secretion of the pancreas is regulated by a rich neural supply that includes sympathetic fibers from the splanchnic nerves, parasympathetic fibers from the vagus, and peptidergic neurons that secrete amines and peptides.[2] The sympathetic and parasympathetic fibers give rise to intrapancreatic periacinar plexuses, which send neural fibers to the bases of acinar cell groups (Fig. 53.11). The pancreatic islets are innervated by similar plexuses that communicate

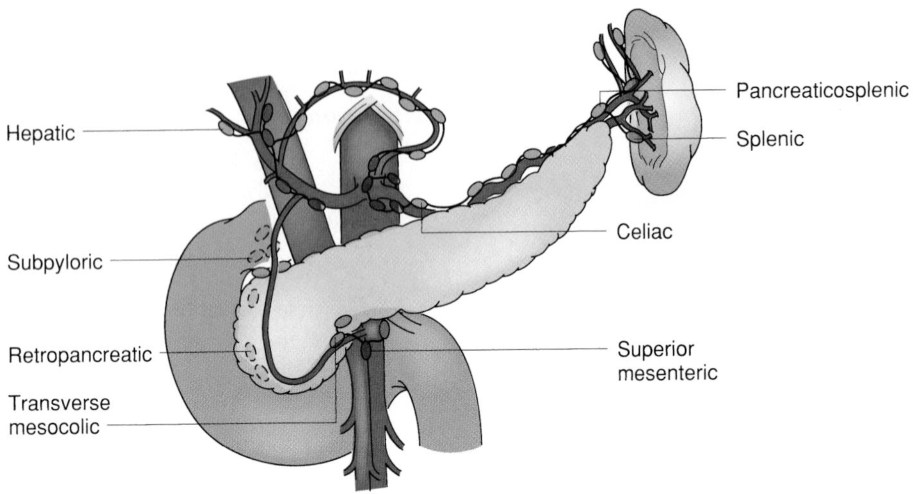

FIGURE 53.10 Lymph node groups receiving drainage from the pancreas.

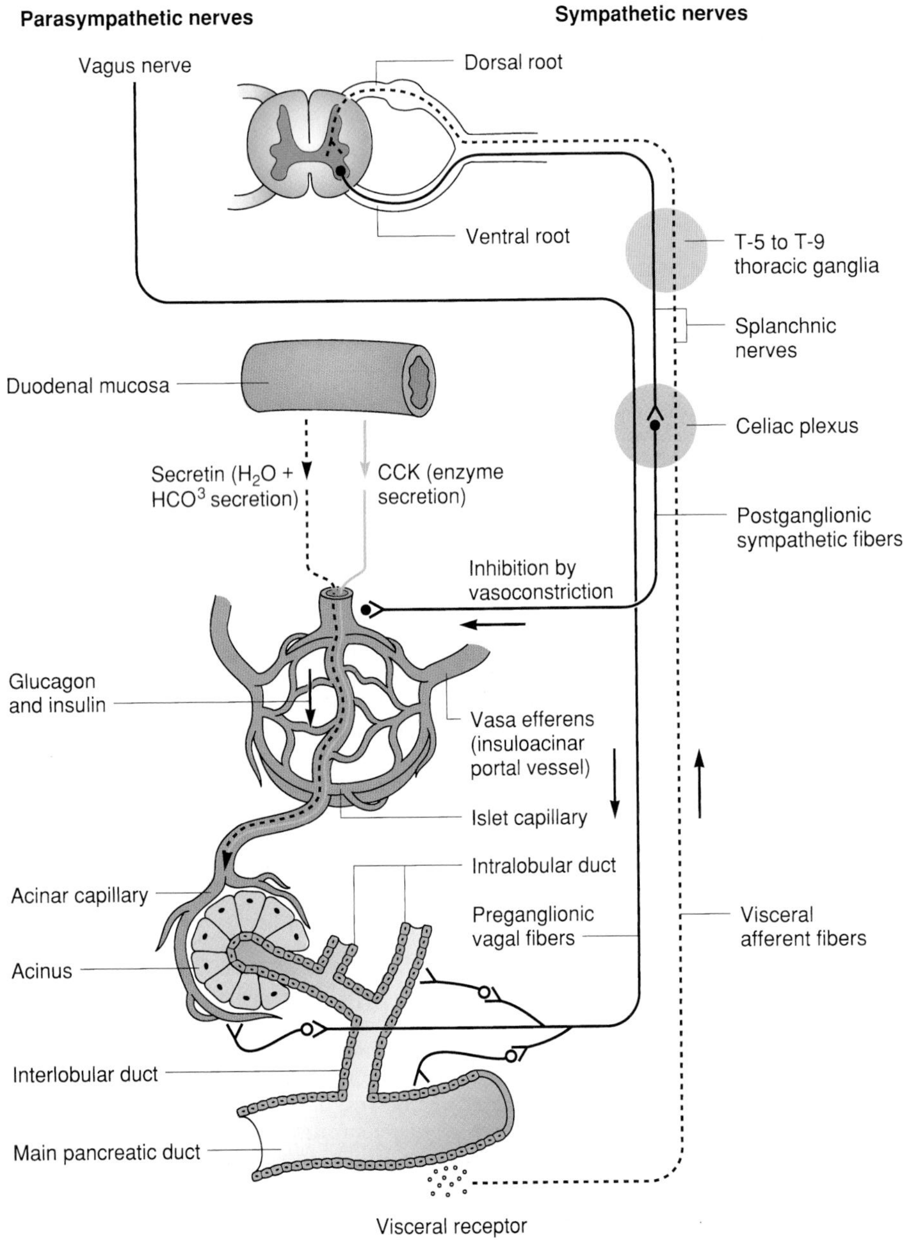

Parasympathetic nerves
Sympathetic nerves
Vagus nerve
Dorsal root
Ventral root
T-5 to T-9 thoracic ganglia
Splanchnic nerves
Duodenal mucosa
Celiac plexus
Secretin (H_2O + HCO^3 secretion)
CCK (enzyme secretion)
Postganglionic sympathetic fibers
Inhibition by vasoconstriction
Glucagon and insulin
Vasa efferens (insuloacinar portal vessel)
Islet capillary
Intralobular duct
Acinar capillary
Preganglionic vagal fibers
Visceral afferent fibers
Acinus
Interlobular duct
Main pancreatic duct
Visceral receptor

FIGURE 53.11 Schematic diagram of the neurohormonal control of the exocrine cells. Visceral receptors line the ductule system and carry the sensation of pain to the spinal cord. Sympathetic fibers first synapse in the celiac plexus after traveling through the thoracic ganglia and splanchnic nerves. Postganglionic fibers then synapse on intrapancreatic arterioles. Parasympathetic preganglionic fibers travel through the celiac plexus after leaving the vagus nerves and course with vessels and ducts to synapse on postganglionic fibers near acinar cells, islet cells, and the smooth muscle of major ducts. Stimulation of these parasympathetic fibers results in an immediate release of pancreatic enzymes. Secretin and cholecystokinin (CCK) first enter the pancreas through the capillary network of the islet cells, then enter the separate capillary network of the acinar tissue through the insuloacinar portal vessels. Glucagon, somatostatin, pancreatic polypeptide, and insulin from the islet cells reach the acinar tissue immediately after release. In this way, the islet cells can influence the acinar tissue responses to CCK and secretin. (After Tompkins RK, Traverso LW. The exocrine cells. In: Keynes WM, Keith RG, eds. *The pancreas.* New York: Appleton-Century-Crofts; 1981.)

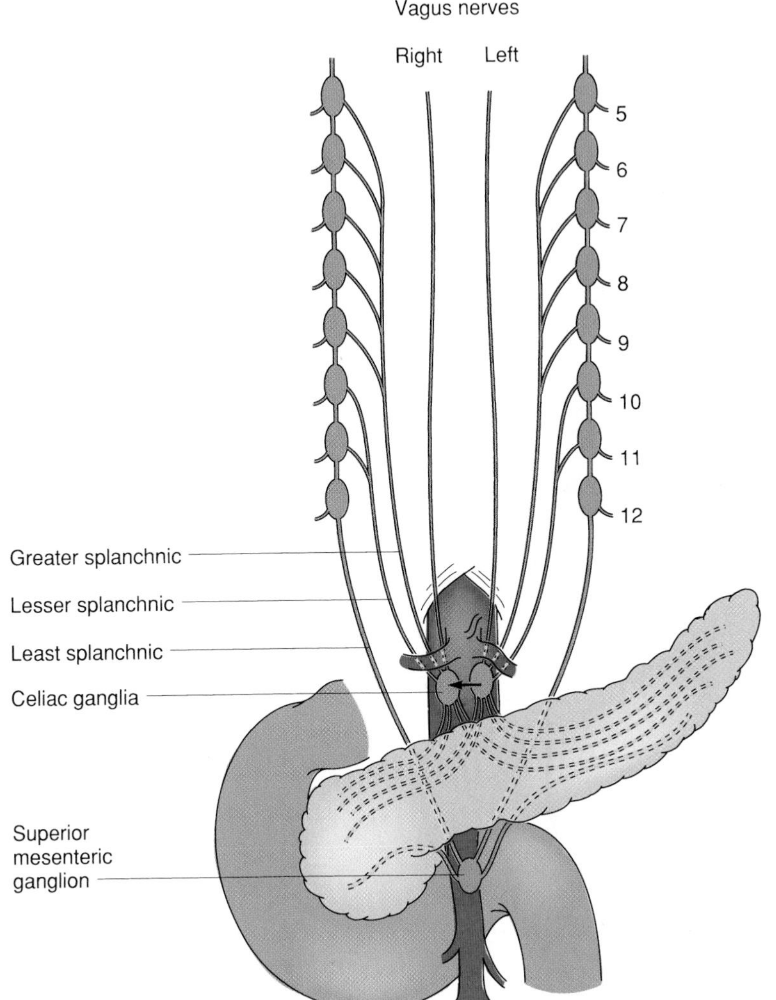

FIGURE 53.12 Diagram of the autonomic nerve supply to the pancreas. (After Skandalakis JE, Gray SW, Rowe JS Jr, et al. Anatomical complications of pancreatic surgery. *Contemp Surg.* 1979;15:17.)

with both the islet vasculature and the islet cells. In general, parasympathetic fibers stimulate both exocrine and endocrine secretion, whereas sympathetic fibers have a predominantly inhibitory effect.[3] The peptidergic neurons that innervate the pancreas secrete hormones such as somatostatin, vasoactive intestinal peptide (VIP), calcitonin gene-related peptide (CGRP), and galanin. Although the peptidergic neurons influence exocrine and endocrine function, their precise physiologic role is unknown. The pancreas also has a rich afferent sensory fiber network, which probably contributes to the severe intrinsic pancreatic pain often associated with pancreatic cancer and chronic pancreatitis (Fig. 53.12). Although results have been equivocal, ganglionectomy or celiac ganglion blockade (intraoperative or via endoscopic ultrasound) can be performed in an effort to interrupt these somatic fibers.[4]

STRUCTURE AND HISTOLOGY

Exocrine Structure

The two major components of the exocrine pancreas are the acinar cells and the ductular network. Together, they constitute 80% to 90% of the pancreatic mass. The acinar cells secrete the enzymes responsible for digestion. The cells are pyramidal and have an apex that faces the lumen of the duct. Within the apex of the cell are numerous zymogen granules, which contain the digestive enzymes. Twenty to 40 acinar cells coalesce into a unit called the *acinus* (Fig. 53.13). A second cell type in the acinus is the centroacinar cell, which is responsible for fluid and electrolyte secretion by the pancreas. These cells contain carbonic anhydrase and other enzymes necessary for bicarbonate and electrolyte transport.[5]

The ductular system is composed of a network of conduits that carry the exocrine secretions into the duodenum. The acinus drains into small, intercalated ducts. Several small, intercalated ducts join to form an interlobular duct. The interlobular ducts contribute to fluid and electrolyte secretion along with the centroacinar cells. The interlobular ducts form secondary ducts that empty into the main duct. Progressive destruction of the ductular network during recurrent episodes of pancreatitis contributes in part to exocrine insufficiency and pain. Research is under way to identify the precursor cell that gives rise to pancreatic ductal adenocarcinoma. Many assume that this cancer arises from ductal cells simply because the tumors exhibit a ductal structure. Some investigators believe pancreatic cancer arises from transdifferentiated acinar cells.[6] Others are convinced that pancreatic cancer arises more frequently from islets, most probably from reserve stem cells.[7] These cells are thought to be progenitor cells that can differentiate into endocrine or exocrine cells. The genetic mechanisms involved in this normal differentiation process and abnormal transformation into pancreatic cancer cells is under investigation.

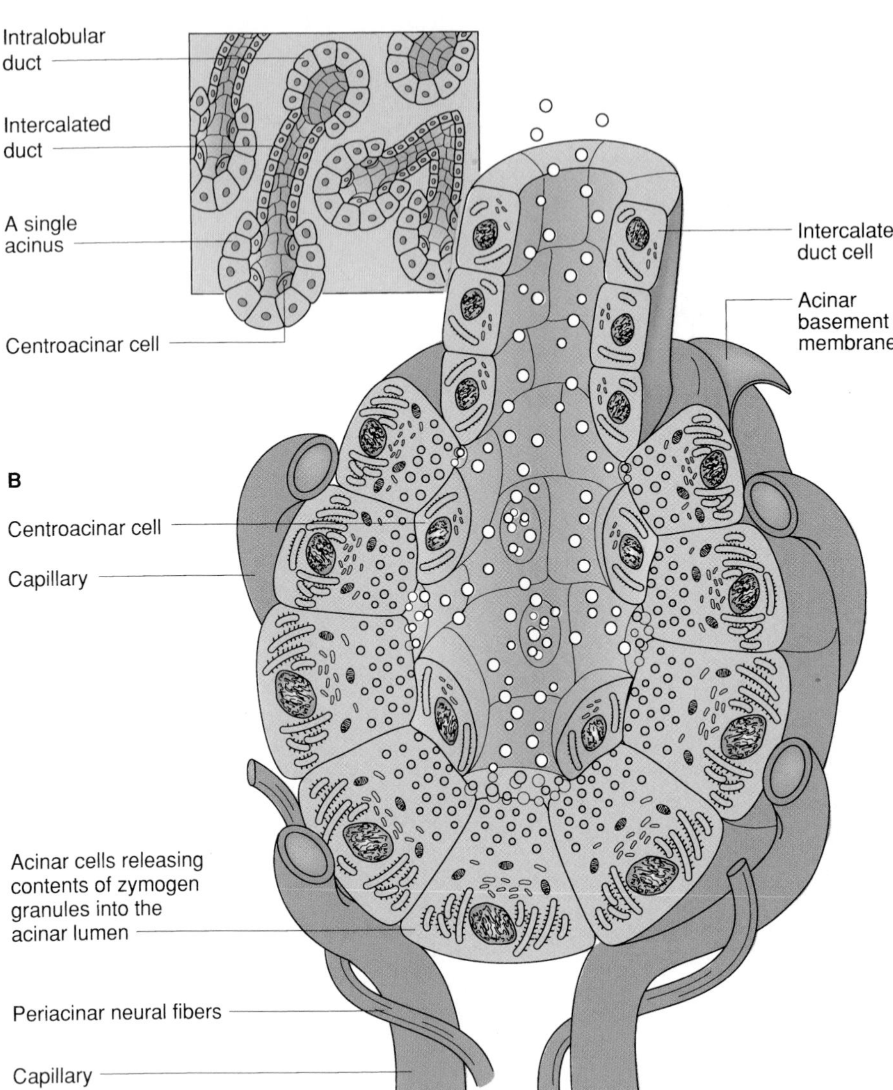

FIGURE 53.13 Histologic anatomy of the acinus. (*A*) Low-magnification view of a portion of the pancreas. (*B*) High-magnification view of a single acinus. (After Krstic RV. *Die Gewebes des Menschen und der Saugetiere*. Berlin: Springer-Verlag, 1978, with permission.)

Endocrine Structure

Within the pancreas are small nests of cells responsible for the secretion of hormones that control glucose homeostasis. These nests are called islets of Langerhans. In contrast to the exocrine cells, the endocrine pancreas accounts for only 2% of the pancreatic mass; the remaining portion of the gland consists of extracellular matrix, blood vessels, and major ducts. The islets contain an average of 3,000 cells and range in diameter from 40 to 900 mm. The islets are composed of four major cell types—alpha (A), beta (B), delta (D), and pancreatic polypeptide (PP) or F cells, which secrete glucagon, insulin, somatostatin, and PP, respectively. The B cells are centrally located within the islet and constitute 70% of the islet mass, whereas the PP, A, and D cells are located at the periphery of the islet. D cells have also been shown to be located within the core of human islets.[8] The PP, A, and D cells constitute roughly 15%, 10%, and 5% of the islet cell mass, respectively. Islet cells can secrete more than one hormone. For example, in addition to insulin, the B cells secrete amylin, which can also regulate glucose metabolism.[9] The cellular composition of the islets varies throughout the pancreas. Islets in the uncinate process are rich in PP cells and poor in A cells, whereas the islets in the body and tail are rich in A cells and poor in PP cells (Fig. 53.14). The B cells and D cells are evenly distributed throughout the pancreas.[10] The physiologic significance of this distribution remains largely unknown. As a consequence, certain operations can remove a specific islet population. For example, removal of 95% of the functioning PP cell mass during pancreaticoduodenectomy can contribute to subsequent glucose intolerance.[11]

Islets contain small numbers of additional cells that secrete hormones such as VIP, serotonin, and pancreastatin. The islets also secrete numerous neuropeptides, such as CGRP, neuropeptide Y, gastrin-releasing peptide, and somatostatin, which probably exert local regulatory effects on endocrine and exocrine secretion. Islet cells are physiologically and chemically distinct and are related to other neuroendocrine cells derived from the neural crest of the embryo. These groups of cells share the capacity of amine precursor uptake and decarboxylation and can give rise to tumors called APUDomas.

Intravascular Pattern

The blood flow to the pancreas has a distinctive pattern. The islets represent 2% of the pancreatic tissue but receive 20% to

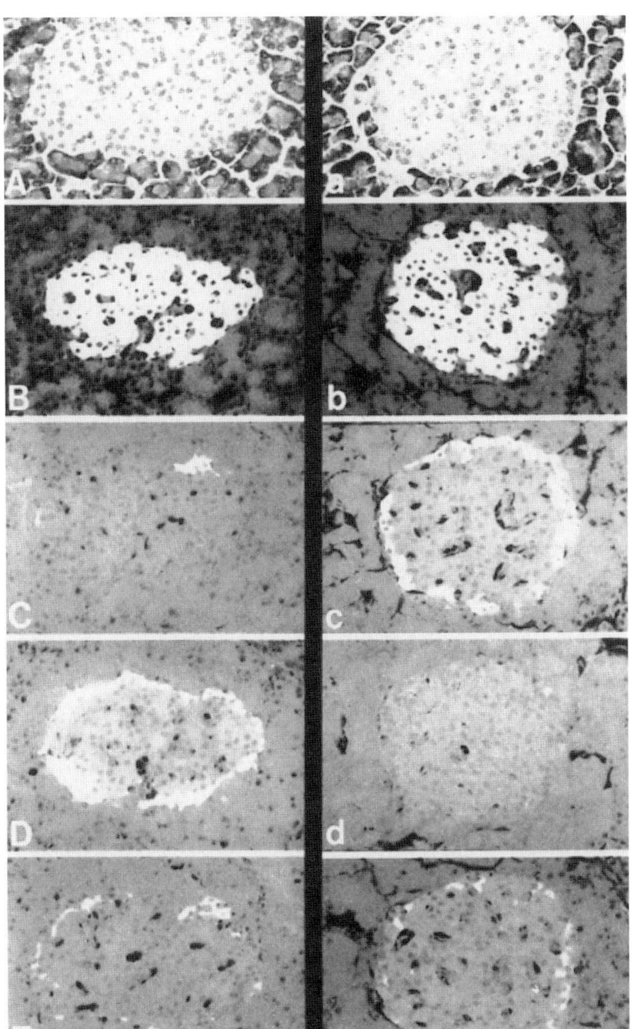

FIGURE 53.14 Histologic anatomy of the islet. Serial sections of a representative islet found in the ventral (*A–E*) and dorsal (*a–e*) portions of the pancreas. (A,a) Cells stained with hematoxylin and eosin. (B,b) B cells immunohistochemically stained with antiinsulin antisera. (C,c) A cells stained with antiglucagon antisera. (D,d) Pancreatic polypeptide cells stained with antipancreatic polypeptide antisera. (E,e) D cells stained with antisomatostatin antisera. (From Orci L. Macro- and micro-domains in the endocrine pancreas. *Diabetes* 1982;31:538.)

30% of the pancreatic arteriolar flow. The distribution of blood flow can change after a meal, when blood flow to different parts of the pancreas is redirected.[12]

Research is under way to determine the possible existence of different microvascular patterns within the islets depending on location (periductular or intralobular). In one pattern, the arteriole of the islet penetrates the islet and first perfuses the center, where the B cells are located.[13] The blood then flows toward the periphery, or mantle, of the islet, where the non-B cells are located, so that high concentrations of insulin modulate secretion of the non-B cells through a paracrine action (Fig. 53.15). In another pattern, the arteriole perfuses the mantle, then the core.[14,15] The collecting vessels drain the islets and then perfuse the acinar tissue. Perfusion of the acinar tissue with venous blood from the islet, known as the *insuloacinar portal system,* permits endocrine regulation of the exocrine pancreas. This regulation is principally effected by insulin, but the other islet hormones, such as PP and somatostatin, are also known to influence exocrine secretion.[16] Much of the acinar tissue is perfused directly by pancreatic arterial blood that bypasses the endocrine tissue.

PHYSIOLOGY

Exocrine Function

Early discoveries related to the exocrine pancreas were entirely separate from those involving the endocrine pancreas, as if the exocrine and endocrine pancreas were two separate organs.[17] Only recently has the intimate relation between exocrine and endocrine function been recognized. Islet peptide products are now known to influence the function of the exocrine pancreas. The final secretory product of the exocrine pancreas derives from the combination of ductal and acinar cell functions. The secretion of water and electrolytes originates in the centroacinar and intercalated duct cells. Pancreatic enzymes originate in the acinar cells. The final product is an alkaline fluid (or juice) that contains digestive enzymes; 500 to 800 mL of the fluid is secreted daily. The alkaline pH results from secreted bicarbonate, which serves to neutralize gastric acid and regulate the pH of the intestine, where the enzymes digest carbohydrates, proteins, and fats. Pancreatic fluid is colorless, odorless, and isosmotic. It contains 0.2% protein, mostly enzymes such as amylase, lipase, and trypsinogen.

Bicarbonate Secretion

The centroacinar cells and ductular epithelium secrete fluid containing 20 mmol of bicarbonate per liter in the basal state and up to 150 mmol of bicarbonate per liter under maximal stimulation. The fluid, with a pH that varies from 7.6 to 9.0, acts as a vehicle to carry inactive proteolytic enzymes to the duodenal lumen. Sodium and potassium concentrations are constant and equal those of plasma. Chloride secretion varies inversely with bicarbonate secretion, and the sum of these two cations remains constant and equal to that of plasma[18] (Fig. 53.16).

Bicarbonate is formed from carbonic acid by the enzyme carbonic anhydrase. Secretin, the major stimulant for bicarbonate secretion, is released from the duodenal mucosa in response to a duodenal luminal pH of less than 3.0. Cholecystokinin (CCK) only weakly stimulates bicarbonate secretion but potentiates secretin-stimulated bicarbonate secretion. Gastrin and acetylcholine are also weak stimulants of bicarbonate secretion.[19] Although cholinergic innervation appears to play a permissive role, bicarbonate secretion is inhibited by atropine and can be reduced 50% by a truncal vagotomy.[20] Islet peptide products such as somatostatin, PP, and glucagon are all thought to inhibit exocrine secretion.

Enzyme Secretion

The acinar cells secrete isozymes that fall into three major enzyme groups—amylases, lipases, and proteases. These enzymes include amylase, lipase, trypsinogen, chymotrypsinogen, procarboxypeptidases A and B, ribonuclease, deoxyribonuclease, proelastase, and trypsin inhibitor. The enzyme groups are not secreted in a fixed ratio, and stimulation by specific nutrients can result in a relative increase of one enzyme over another. Dietary alterations can also result in changes in the relative amounts of amylases, lipases, and proteases secreted. When enzyme secretion is absent or impaired, malabsorption or incomplete digestion occurs, resulting in fecal losses of fat and protein.

Enzyme secretion is regulated primarily through hormonal and neural factors. The enteric hormone CCK is the predominant regulator and stimulates acinar cells through specific

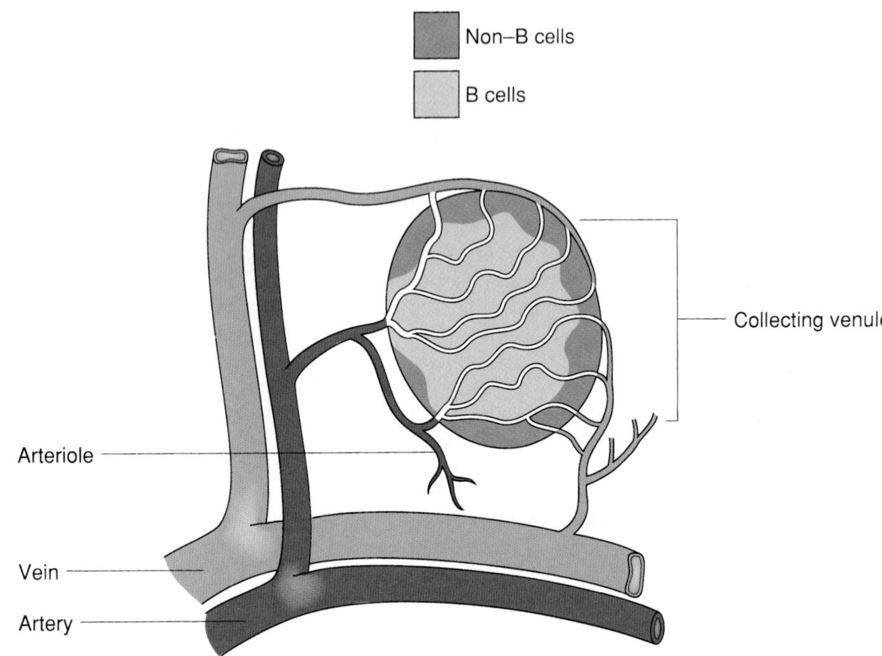

FIGURE 53.15 Diagram of a typical islet. Afferent arterioles enter the islet through discontinuities of the mantle of non-B cells and break into capillaries, most of which traverse the B-cell mass and pass through the mantle as efferent vessels. Occasionally, a capillary passes at the interface of the B cells and non-B cells and never enters the B-cell core. In the larger islets, the efferent capillaries coalesce at the edge of the islet and pass along the mantle as collecting venules before draining into a vein. (After Bonner-Weir S, Orci L. New perspectives on the microvasculature of the islets of Langerhans in the rat. *Diabetes* 1982;31:883.)

membrane-bound receptors. The intracellular effectors or second messengers are calcium and diacylglycerol. Acetylcholine strongly stimulates acinar cells when released from postganglionic fibers of the pancreatic plexus and acts in synergy with CCK to potentiate enzyme secretion (Fig. 53.17). Secretin and VIP weakly stimulate acinar cell secretion, but they potentiate the effect of CCK on the acinar cells. Acinar cell secretion also is influenced by islet hormones in the insuloacinar portal system. The enzymes are synthesized in the endoplasmic reticulum of the acinar cells and are packaged in the zymogen granules. These are released from the apical portion of the acinar cells into the lumen of the acinus and are then transported into the duodenal lumen, where the enzymes are activated.

Enzyme Groups

Amylase is secreted within the human body from both pancreatic and salivary tissue. Pancreatic amylase represents isoamylase type P. A pancreatic source of excess levels of amylase, as in pancreatitis, can be determined by the results of isoamylase studies. Amylase hydrolyzes starch and glycogen to glucose, maltose, maltotriose, and dextrins. Amylase is the only digestive enzyme secreted by the pancreas in an active form, although it functions optimally at a pH of 7.0.

Lipases emulsify and hydrolyze fat in the presence of bile salts. They hydrolyze insoluble esters of glycerol, alcohol esters, and water-soluble esters. Lipases function optimally at a pH of 7.0 to 9.0, and steatorrhea can result from excessive acidification of the duodenum and jejunum, as in gastric hypersecretory states. There are two phospholipases, A and B. Phospholipase A cleaves the fatty acid off lecithin or cephalin to form lysolecithin or lysocephalin. Phospholipase B cleaves the fatty acid off lysolecithin to form glycerol phosphatidylcholine.

The proteolytic enzymes are essential for protein digestion. These enzymes are secreted as proenzymes and require activation for proteolytic activity. The proenzymes of trypsin and chymotrypsin are trypsinogen and chymotrypsinogen. They are activated primarily by a duodenal enzyme, enterokinase, which converts trypsinogen to trypsin. Trypsin, in turn, activates chymotrypsin, elastase, carboxypeptidase, and phospholipase. Trypsinogen can also be activated by a fall in pH below 7.0. Within the pancreas, enzyme activation is prevented by an antiproteolytic enzyme secreted by the acinar cells. This enzyme inactivates trypsin by direct binding and thereby protects the pancreatic tissue from autodigestion.

Trypsinogen is a 229-amino-acid polypeptide that hydrolyzes proteins and also acts as a thrombokinase, accelerating

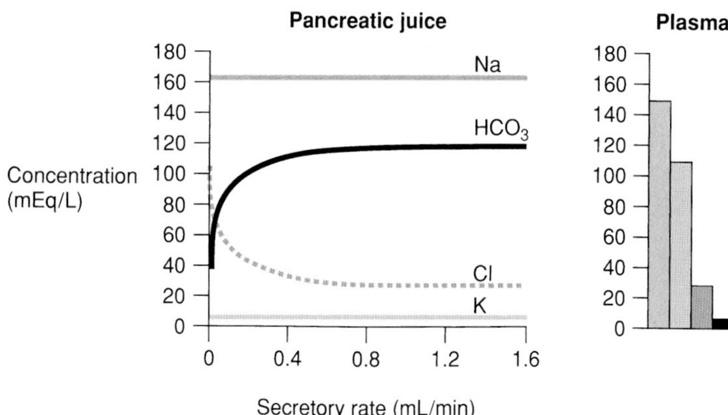

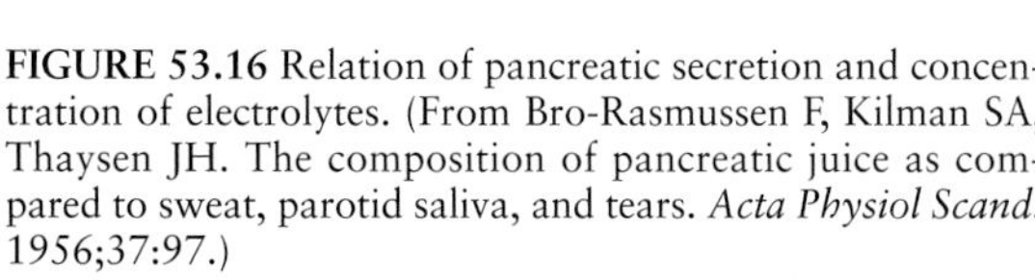

FIGURE 53.16 Relation of pancreatic secretion and concentration of electrolytes. (From Bro-Rasmussen F, Kilman SA, Thaysen JH. The composition of pancreatic juice as compared to sweat, parotid saliva, and tears. *Acta Physiol Scand.* 1956;37:97.)

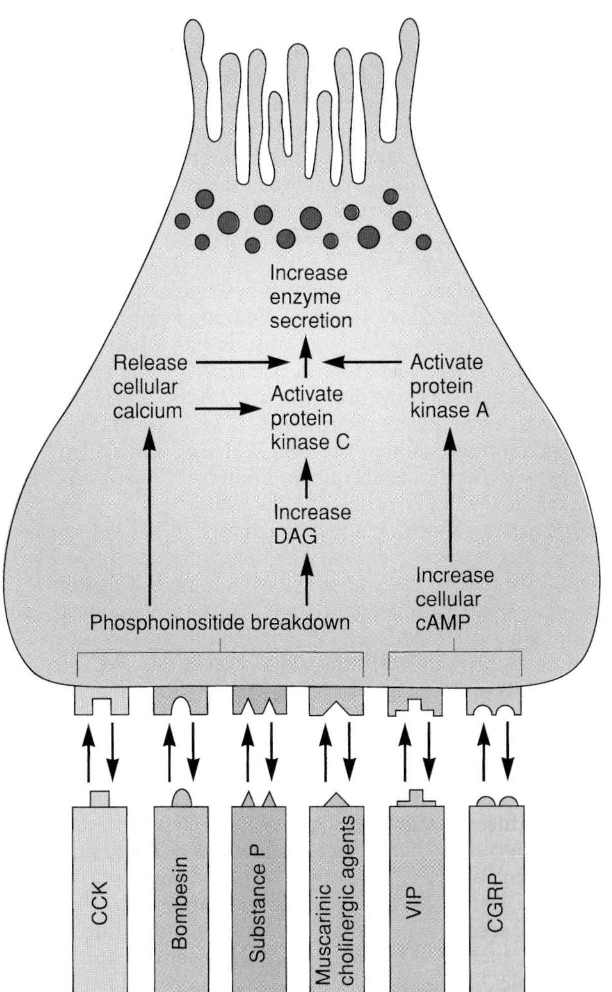

FIGURE 53.17 Schematic diagram of an acinar cell, demonstrating receptors for exocrine secretagogues and their intracellular bases of action. Six distinct classes of receptors are known, with principal ligands shown. CCK, cholecystokinin; VIP, vasoactive intestinal polypeptide; CRGP, calcitonin gene-related peptide; DAG, diacylglycerol.

coagulation of the blood. Trypsinogen can convert spontaneously to trypsin, but the change is accelerated by enterokinase, by acid, or by active trypsin itself. Chymotrypsinogen is a 246-amino-acid polypeptide. Chymotrypsinogen is converted to the active form, chymotrypsin, by trypsin or, indirectly, by enterokinase. The enzyme hydrolyzes proteins by a mechanism similar to that of trypsin but cleaves the proteins at a different site. The optimal activity of chymotrypsin and trypsin occurs at a pH of 8.0 to 9.0. Other proteolytic enzymes, such as carboxypeptidases A and B, further digest proteins that have been digested by trypsin and chymotrypsin. The nucleolytic enzymes, ribonuclease and deoxyribonuclease, hydrolyze nucleic acids into mononucleotides. Thus, through the secretion of the three classes of enzymes, the pancreas regulates the complete digestion of fats, carbohydrates, and proteins.

Endocrine Function

Insulin Synthesis, Secretion, and Action

Insulin is a 56-amino-acid polypeptide with a molecular weight of 6 kd. It consists of two polypeptide chains, an A and a B chain, joined by two disulfide bridges. Although species variation occurs in the amino acid sequence, the positions of the disulfide bridges are constant and important for biologic activity. Insulin is synthesized in the B cells of the islets of Langerhans. Destruction of the B cells in type I, or insulin-dependent, diabetes results in an absolute insulin deficiency. A considerable capacity exists for secretory reserves of insulin; 80% of the islet cell mass must be surgically removed before diabetes becomes clinically apparent.[21]

When the B cell is stimulated, a newly synthesized single-chain peptide, proinsulin, is transported from the endoplasmic reticulum to the Golgi complex. At this site, proinsulin is packaged into granules and cleaved into insulin and a residual connecting peptide, or C peptide (Fig. 53.18). The granules then move toward the outer membrane by way of microtubules and are released into the intervascular space through emiocytosis. Defects in the synthesis and cleavage of insulin can lead to rare forms of diabetes mellitus, such as Wakayama syndrome and the proinsulin syndromes.[22]

Insulin is secreted in two phases. The first phase consists of a burst of stored insulin that lasts 4 to 6 minutes. This is followed by a second phase of sustained secretion, attributed to an ongoing synthesis of insulin. The secretion of insulin is regulated by nutrient, neural, and hormonal factors. Glucose is the predominant nutrient regulator. The B cell is exquisitely sensitive to small changes in glucose concentration, with the maximal stimulation of insulin secretion occurring at a glucose concentration of 400 to 500 mg/dL.

Glucose is transported actively across cell membranes throughout the body by 55-kd membrane-bound facilitator peptides called *glucose transporters* (Fig. 53.19). Several classes of glucose transporters have been identified. The type of glucose transporter located on the B cell (GLUT-2) has a low affinity (or high K_m) for glucose, which results in a modest

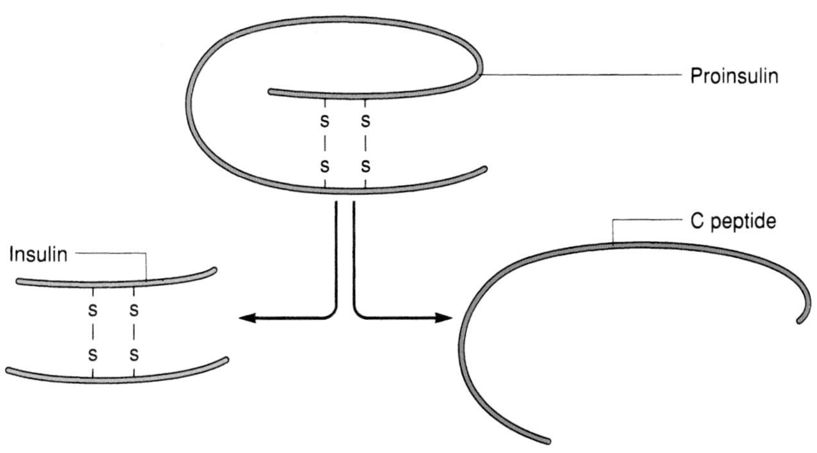

FIGURE 53.18 Synthesis of insulin. Proinsulin is synthesized by the endoplasmic reticulum and packaged within secretory granules of the B cell, where it is cleaved into insulin and C peptide. Equimolar amounts of insulin and C peptide are secreted into the bloodstream.

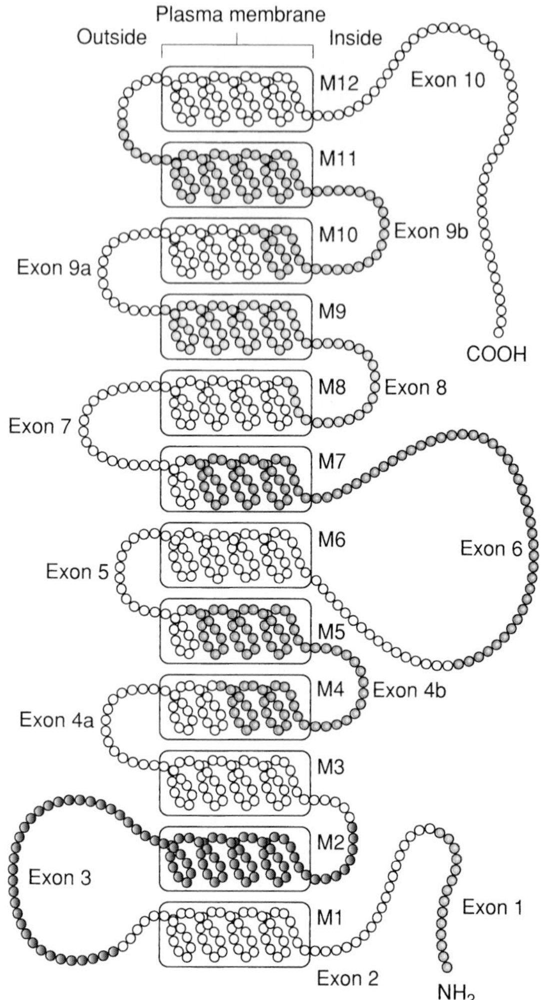

FIGURE 53.19 Model of the basic structure of a membrane-bound glucose transporter peptide, encoded by a gene divided into 10 exon regions. Membrane-spanning ß-helical peptide chains are numbered M1 through M12. Mutations of the promoter region of the gene or the synthesis of an abnormal form of the protein could result in altered transport of glucose. For the B-cell GLUT-2 transporter, this could cause reduced sensitivity to glucose. For the muscle and fat cell GLUT-4 transporter, this could result in decreased peripheral uptake of glucose. (After Bell GI, Kayano T, Buse JB, et al. Molecular biology of mammalian glucose transporters. *Diabetes Care* 1990;86:1615.)

rate of glucose transport at lower physiologic concentrations but an increased rate of transport and therefore an increase in subsequent insulin secretion at higher concentrations of glucose.[23] Studies suggest that a loss of B-cell GLUT-2 glucose transporters can precede, and therefore contribute to, the development of diabetes.[24]

Orally administered glucose stimulates a greater insulin response than an equivalent amount of glucose administered intravenously because of the release of enteric hormones that potentiate insulin secretion. This effect is known as the *enteroinsular axis.* Gastric inhibitory polypeptide (GIP) appears to be an important regulator of this incretion effect,[25] although other gut peptides, such as glucagon-like peptide-1, also contribute. Additional nutrients that regulate insulin secretion are amino acids, such as arginine, lysine, and leucine, and free fatty acids. Hormones that stimulate insulin secretion include glucagon, GIP, and CCK, whereas somatostatin, amylin, and pancreastatin are inhibitory. Insulin secretion is also stimulated by sulfonylurea compounds, which act independently of the glucose concentration and form the basis of treatment of type II, or non–insulin-dependent, diabetes.

The B cell is neurally regulated by cholinergic fibers that stimulate insulin secretion. b-Sympathetic fibers are also stimulatory, whereas a-sympathetic fibers strongly inhibit insulin secretion. A loss of pancreatic innervation, as after pancreatic transplantation, results in changes in the pattern or quantity of insulin secretion. Research is under way to define the role of neuropeptides such as CGRP and galanin in the regulation of insulin secretion.

Insulin is released in an oscillatory or pulsatile pattern, and release is controlled by an internal pacemaker, present even in isolated islets.[26] Once secreted, insulin has a half-life of 7 to 10 minutes and is metabolized primarily by the liver. Of the insulin secreted into the portal vein, 40% to 70% is cleared by the hepatocytes during the first pass. The brain and red blood cells take up no insulin. The liver, kidneys, and skeletal muscles slowly metabolize insulin and remove it from the circulation. Little insulin is excreted in the urine.

Insulin promotes glucose transport in all cells, except B cells, hepatocytes, and cells of the central nervous system. Insulin-stimulated glucose transport in muscle and adipose tissue can also result from insulin regulation of membrane-bound glucose transporters. Insulin inhibits glycogenolysis but stimulates protein synthesis. Insulin also inhibits fatty acid breakdown and therefore inhibits ketone formation.

Like all endocrine hormones, insulin binds to specific receptors. These receptors have been isolated and characterized. The insulin receptor is a glycoprotein with a molecular weight of 300 kd. Stimulation of the receptor depends on the insulin concentration. Insulin resistance can be the result of either a decreased number of receptors or a decreased affinity for insulin, whereas excessive receptors can result in hypoglycemia. Defects in insulin receptors can lead to the insulin resistance seen in type II diabetes mellitus and in rare forms of diabetes, such as the type A syndrome, leprechaunism, and lipotrophic diabetes.[27]

Glucagon Synthesis, Secretion, and Action

Glucagon is a single-chain, 29-amino-acid polypeptide with a molecular weight of 3.5 kd. Glucagon is secreted by the A cells of the islet and promotes hepatic glycogenolysis. Other forms of glucagon are released from the gut, including gastric glucagon, enteroglucagon, and glucagon-like peptides. Their physiologic role remains unclear.

Pancreatic glucagon secretion is controlled by neural, hormonal, and nutrient factors. Glucose is the primary regulator and has a potent suppressive effect on glucagon secretion. Glucagon and insulin respond in reciprocal fashion to changes in glucose concentrations; therefore, glucagon is considered a counterregulatory hormone to insulin. In a balance of actions, the two hormones work together to maintain basal glucose levels. Exaggerated or excess glucagon secretion can contribute to hyperglycemia, whereas a failure of glucagon secretion or an absence of glucagon-rich portions of the pancreas can contribute to profound hypoglycemia. Glucagon is stimulated by the amino acids arginine and alanine. Hormones such as GIP have been shown to have a stimulatory effect on glucagon secretion *in vitro* but not *in vivo*. Insulin and somatostatin have a potent suppressive effect on glucagon secretion and can regulate glucagon secretion through paracrine effects within the islet.

The neural regulation of glucagon is similar to that of insulin.[28] Cholinergic fibers have a strong stimulatory effect. a-Sympathetic fibers inhibit glucagon secretion, and b-sympathetic fibers are weakly stimulatory. The role of neuropeptides in glucagon secretion is unknown. Glucagon elevates blood glucose levels through the stimulation of glycogenolysis and gluconeogenesis. Along with epinephrine, cortisol, and growth hormone, glucagon is considered a stress hormone because it provides metabolic fuel during stress. The peptide is metabolized by the kidney and, to a lesser extent, by the liver.

Some authors consider dysfunctional A-cell secretion to play a major role in the elevation of blood sugar in diabetes. In the bidysfunctional theory of diabetes, absent or impaired insulin secretion and deranged glucagon secretion result in hyperglycemia, ketoacidosis, and accelerated lipolysis.[29] Suppression of glucagon secretion with somatostatin has resulted in improved glucose homeostasis in insulin-dependent, type I diabetes.[30]

Somatostatin Synthesis, Secretion, and Action

In 1973, Brazeau et al.[31] reported the isolation of a hypothalamic peptide that inhibits the release of growth hormone (somatotropin) and named it *somatostatin*. Somatostatin is a 14-amino-acid polypeptide that inhibits the release of almost all peptide hormones; it also inhibits gastric, pancreatic, and biliary secretion. Found in the D cell of the islet, the role of the hormone within the pancreas remains unclear. Although exogenous infusion of somatostatin has been shown to inhibit the release of insulin, glucagon, and PP, endogenous somatostatin has not been proved to influence the secretion of the adjacent islet cells directly. Therefore, the D cell is probably responsible for the paracrine regulation of islet cell hormone secretion.[32] Some researchers have suggested that the D cells regulate exocrine secretion as part of the insuloacinar portal system. Somatostatin has also been found in the neurons of the islet and can act as an inhibitory neuropeptide. The potent inhibitory effect of the peptide has been used to treat both endocrine and exocrine disorders.[33]

Pancreatic Polypeptide Synthesis, Secretion, and Action

Pancreatic polypeptide (PP) is a 36-amino-acid peptide that is secreted by the F cells of the islet. The F cells are located predominantly in the uncinate process of the pancreas and represent 5% to 15% of the islet cell mass. The physiologic role of PP remains unclear. The peptide has been shown to inhibit exocrine secretion in addition to choleresis and gallbladder emptying. The release of PP is regulated predominantly by cholinergic innervation. The rise in PP levels after a meal is ablated by vagotomy, and the ablation of this rise can be used as a marker of completion of vagotomy. Circulating PP levels are increased in diabetes and in normal aging because of increased secretion. Other studies suggest that PP is involved in glucose homeostasis and that a deficiency of PP in chronic pancreatitis or after pancreaticoduodenectomy contributes to glucose intolerance, so that PP deficiency has been linked to pancreatogenic diabetes.[34]

Many of the pathophysiologic responses observed in chronic pancreatitis are thought to be partly a consequence of either a disruption of the insuloacinar axis, destruction of islet cell mass, or both. Each of the four types of hormone-secreting islet cells is affected by the destructive process of chronic pancreatitis. The insulin-secreting B cells appear to be affected both qualitatively and quantitatively. Directly related to the changes in the B cells are the physiologic responses of the glucagon-secreting A cells. Their physiologic response in chronic pancreatitis appears to be related to the residual B-cell function. Recently, PP has been implicated as a contributor to abnormal glucose metabolism in pancreatogenic diabetes. The deficiency of this peptide appears to influence the expression of hepatocyte insulin receptors in chronic pancreatitis. In addition, PP deficiency and pancreatic exocrine insufficiency appear to be closely correlated. Although somatostatin appears to have a significant role within the insuloacinar axis, the effects of chronic pancreatitis on the role of somatostatin in the insuloacinar axis are still poorly understood. Further exploration of the relationship between the endocrine and exocrine pancreas is needed so that better methods can be developed to manage the alterations in glucose metabolism related to chronic pancreatitis.[35]

Other Peptide Products

Other peptides have been found to be secreted within the islet. These include neuropeptides, such as VIP, galanin, and serotonin, which are believed to play a role in the regulation of islet cell secretion. Amylin is a 36-amino-acid polypeptide that was discovered in 1988. It is secreted by the B cell but not in equimolar amounts to C peptide and insulin. Amylin inhibits insulin secretion and insulin uptake peripherally. It has been found in amyloid deposits within the pancreas of patients with type II diabetes and has been implicated in the development of type II diabetes mellitus. Furthermore, the peptide is absent in type I diabetes mellitus because the B cells are ablated in this disease. The significance of amylin deficiency is unknown.

Pancreastatin is another peptide found in large amounts in the pancreas. It is a derivative of a larger, ubiquitous endocrine tissue-related peptide, chromogranin A, and has been shown to inhibit insulin secretion. Its physiologic role is unknown.

Regulation of Hormone Secretion within the Islet

Because exogenous infusions of insulin, glucagon, and somatostatin have profound effects on islet hormone secretion, the paracrine regulation of islet hormone secretion has been an area of intense investigation. In 1982, it was demonstrated that the blood flow of the islet is centripetal—that is, a central artery penetrates into the islet and perfuses the centrally located B-cell mass first. The blood then flows outward toward the peripherally located A, D, and F cells, allowing a paracrine cascade. By using antibodies specific for each hormone, it has been possible to demonstrate that insulin secretion within the islet regulates the secretion of glucagon and somatostatin. This observation suggests that the suppression of glucagon during hyperglycemia is not regulated by glucose but rather by an increase in insulin secretion (Fig. 53.20). Intra-islet somatostatin is known to regulate insulin secretion.[32] The overall physiologic significance of the paracrine cascade is unknown, but it can result in the hyperglucagonemia and hypersomatostatinemia seen in insulin-dependent, type I diabetes.

Recent observations made during *in vivo* microscopic studies of the isolated perfused human pancreas have contributed to our understanding of the physiology of the endocrine pancreas.[36] The human endocrine pancreas is composed of approximately 1 million islets that act as end neurons of the central nervous system to secrete the appropriate hormonal milieu for glucose homeokinesis. To accomplish this, the endocrine pancreas secretes a hormonal milieu regulated by the microcirculation, nitric oxide, and neural and hormonal mechanisms. Changes in the arterial concentrations of nutrients and hormones are recognized simultaneously by all islets of the endocrine pancreas and by the central nervous system. Responses occur at two levels. At one level, the central nervous system sends neural signals to the endocrine pancreas to alter the microcirculation, which is regulated by internal and external gates. One of the final regulators of the gates is nitric oxide. Blood flow to the endocrine pancreas and within the islets is optimized to expose the appropriate cell type required to respond to the changes in the arterial milieu. The other level of response is within the islet. The islet cells respond directly to changes in the arterial concentrations of nutrients and hormones. Considerable communication between the cells within the islet is regulated by hormonal feedback loops and nitric oxide. These two levels of response result in secretion of the hormonal milieu necessary for glucose homeokinesis into the portal vein.

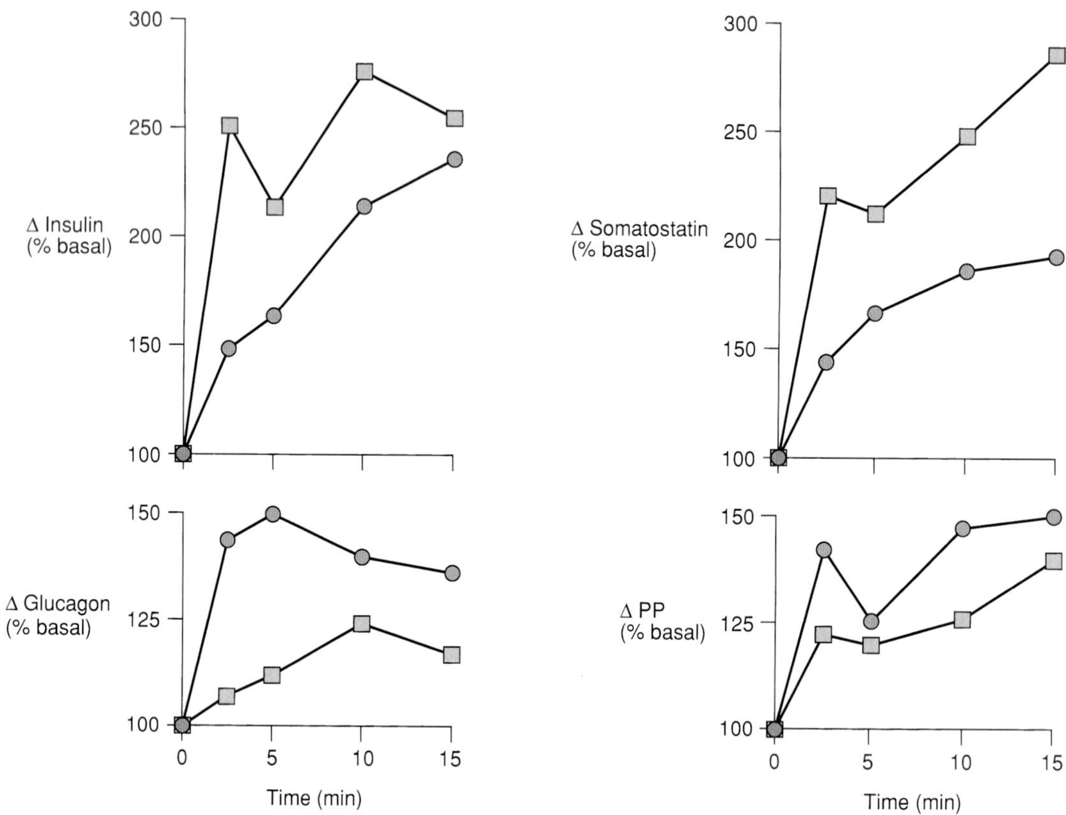

FIGURE 53.20 Paracrine modulation of islet secretion by insulin. The islet cell response to combined glucose (16 mmol) and gastric inhibitory polypeptide (1 nmol) perfusion in the isolated human pancreas is shown with (circles) and without (squares) the addition of 20 mU of insulin per milliliter to the arterial circuit. Venous insulin concentrations ranged from 1,500 to 3,000 mU/mL. Insulin and somatostatin secretion are inhibited, whereas glucagon and pancreatic polypeptide secretion are enhanced. These data suggest that insulin exerts negative feedback on insulin secretion from the islet and that insulin released from the B-cell core of the islet enhances somatostatin release from the D cells in the perimeter of the islet. (After Brunicardi FC, Druck P, Sun YS, et al. Regulation of pancreatic polypeptide secretion in the isolated perfused human pancreas. *Am J Surg.* 1988;155:63.)

For example, when an increase in arterial glucose is sensed by the endocrine pancreas and the brain, a two-tiered response occurs. The central nervous system sends a cholinergic signal to the endocrine pancreas that is mediated by nitric oxide. Both external gates, which shunt blood flow to the entire endocrine pancreas, and internal gates, which shunt flow to B cells in the core of the islet and away from A cells in the mantle, are opened. In addition, B cells and A cells respond directly to the increase in capillary glucose, and these responses are locally modified by hormonal feedback loops and nitric oxide. The two-tiered response results in two-phase insulin secretion and a decrease in glucagon secretion. Alterations in the hormonal milieu secreted from the endocrine pancreas into the portal circulation ultimately result in glucose homeokinesis. In this theoretical model of the endocrine pancreas, an effective physiologic response is possible to a wide variety of changes in the arterial milieu, and the appropriate portal venous hormonal milieu required for glucose homeokinesis is maintained.

TESTS OF PANCREATIC FUNCTION

Exocrine Function

The secretin test is the classic test for pancreatic exocrine function.[37] After the patient has fasted overnight, a double-lumen tube is placed in the duodenum. After 20-minute basal collections have been obtained, an intravenous bolus of 2 U of highly purified secretin per kilogram is administered, and four 20-minute collections of duodenal fluid are aspirated and analyzed for total volume, bicarbonate output, and enzyme secretion. The lower limits of normal for this study are 1.8 mL of pancreatic fluid per kilogram per hour, 6.2 mEq of bicarbonate output per hour, and 82 mEq of maximal bicarbonate content per hour. Amylase secretion normally ranges from 6 to 18 IU/kg. The test result is considered positive when abnormal values indicate pancreatic exocrine insufficiency (Table 53.2). In chronic pancreatitis, bicarbonate secretion is decreased because of stasis in the ducts. In pancreatic malignancy, volume is decreased because of replacement of normal pancreatic tissue with cancerous tissue. After cholecystectomy, the pancreatic juice can be diluted by bile, and results must be cautiously interpreted.

The fecal fat test is used to distinguish between pancreatic dysfunction and malabsorption secondary to enteric disease. Steatorrhea secondary to pancreatic disease is the result of lipase deficiency and is usually not present until lipase secretion is reduced by 90%. With a marked reduction of lipase secretion, the 24-hour fecal fat content is elevated to more than 20 g. Conversely, steatorrhea in the presence of low levels of fecal fat indicates intestinal dysfunction. A reduction in fecal fat indicates efficacy of pancreatic enzyme replacement in patients with exocrine insufficiency.

TABLE 53.2 DIAGNOSIS

CHARACTERISTIC RESULTS OF SECRETIN TESTING: FLOW BICARBONATE, AND ENZYME CHANGES OBSERVED IN PATIENTS WITH VARIOUS PANCREATIC AND OTHER DISORDERS

Disorder	Pattern	Flow rate	Maximum bicarbonate concentration	Enzyme secretion
End-stage pancreatitis, advanced pancreatic cancer	Total insufficiency	Decreased	Decreased	Decreased
Chronic pancreatitis	Qualitative insufficiency	Normal	Decreased	Normal
Pancreatic cancer	Quantitative insufficiency	Decreased	Normal	Normal
Malnutrition[a]	Isolated enzyme deficiency	Normal	Normal	Decreased
Hemochromatosis, Zollinger-Ellison syndrome, various cirrhoses	Hypersecretion	Increased	Normal	Normal

[a]Sprue, ulcerative colitis, and regional enteritis.
From Dreiling DA, Wolfson P. New insights into pancreatic disease revealed by the secretion test. In: Berk JE, ed. *Developments in digestive diseases*, vol 2. Philadelphia: Lea & Febiger; 1979: 155.

The dimethadione (DMO) test is based on the observation that the pancreas degrades trimethadione (Tridione), an anticonvulsant drug, and secretes its metabolite, DMO. The measurement of secreted DMO can be used as an assessment of exocrine function. Trimethadione is given to the patient orally; the dosage is 0.45 g three times a day for 3 days. A double-lumen tube is placed in the duodenum, and the secretin test is performed. The duodenal output of DMO correlates well with exocrine function and is impaired in patients with exocrine insufficiency.[38]

The Lundh test measures pancreatic enzyme secretion in response to a meal of carbohydrate, fat, and protein. The test relies on endogenous secretion of secretin and CCK in addition to pancreatic secretion; therefore, the test result can be abnormal in diseases involving the gastrointestinal mucosa. After an overnight fast, a double-lumen tube is placed in the duodenum and a basal collection of duodenal fluid is taken. The patient is given a mixed meal of 18 g of corn oil, 15 g of casein, and 40 g of glucose in 300 mL of water. Thirty-minute collections of the duodenal fluid are taken for 2 hours and are analyzed for trypsin, amylase, and lipase. The result of this test is abnormal in patients with chronic pancreatitis and diminished pancreatic reserve. Like the secretin and DMO tests, the Lundh test is limited by the need for duodenal intubation.

The triolein breath test is a noninvasive test of exocrine insufficiency.[39] Radiolabeled triglycerides are given orally, and the metabolite, 14C-carbon dioxide, can be measured in the breath. Twenty-five grams of corn oil containing 5 mCi of [14C]triolein is given orally, and breath samples are obtained 4 hours later. The radioactivity of the breath samples is then measured. Patients with disorders of fat digestion or absorption exhale less than 3% of the [14C]triolein dose per hour. The test is repeated after oral pancreatic enzyme replacement. Patients with exocrine insufficiency achieve a normal rate of excretion of 14C–carbon dioxide, whereas patients with enteric disorders show no improvement.

The paraaminobenzoic acid test is another noninvasive test of pancreatic insufficiency.[40] N-benzoyl-l-tyrosyl-paraaminobenzoic acid (BT-PABA) is cleaved by chymotrypsin to form PABA. PABA is excreted in the urine after being absorbed from the small intestine. One gram of BT-PABA in 300 mL of water is given orally, and urine collections are obtained for 6 hours. Patients with chronic pancreatitis excrete less than 60% of the ingested dose of BT-PABA. This test is useful in cases of moderate or severe pancreatic insufficiency.

The PP response to a test meal allows suspected pancreatic disease to be confirmed based on plasma levels of the islet hormone PP. Although no circulating peptide or compound changes specifically with pancreatic exocrine insufficiency, basal and meal-stimulated levels of plasma PP are reduced in severe chronic pancreatitis or after extensive pancreatic resection. After an overnight fast, a test meal consisting of 20% protein, 40% fat, and 40% carbohydrate is ingested. Basal levels of immunoreactive PP (normal, 100 to 250 pg/mL) are frequently less than 50 pg/mL in severe chronic pancreatitis.[41] PP levels normally rise to 700 to 1,000 pg/mL for 2 to 3 hours after the meal, but they are reduced to 250 pg/mL or less in severe disease. Because PP release depends on intact pancreatic innervation, the PP response can be depressed in cases of diabetic autonomic neuropathy or after truncal vagotomy or antrectomy (Table 53.3).

Endocrine Function

The oral glucose tolerance test, which is the most widely used test of pancreatic endocrine function, is an indirect assessment of the insulin response to an oral glucose load. After the patient has fasted overnight, two basal blood samples are drawn for glucose determination. An oral glucose load of 40 g/m^2 is given over 10 minutes. Blood samples are drawn every 30 minutes for 2 hours (Table 53.4). This test is used to help confirm the diagnosis of diabetes.[42] Caution must be used in interpreting the results because the oral glucose tolerance test measures the glucose profile and not the actual insulin response. The insulin response to oral glucose is affected by enteric factors, especially those hormones involved in the enteroinsular axis (e.g., GIP, glucagon-like peptide-1, CCK). The test result can also be affected by antecedent diet, drug use, exercise, and the age of the patient. Although a diagnosis of diabetes can be based on the result of the oral glucose tolerance test, insulin secretion per se is but one factor that affects the test result.

The intravenous glucose tolerance test reflects the pancreatic endocrine response to a bolus of intravenous glucose.[43] The test measures the disappearance of plasma glucose after administration of the glucose bolus, which indirectly reflects both the secretion and action of insulin. With this test, the gastrointestinal influences on glucose metabolism that affect the oral glucose tolerance test result are eliminated. After an overnight fast, two basal samples of blood are drawn. The patient is then

TABLE 53.3 DIAGNOSIS

DIFFERENTIAL DIAGNOSIS OF INTESTINAL AND PANCREATIC STEATORRHEA

Parameter	Intestinal steatorrhea	Pancreatitis
Fecal fat	<20 g monoglycerides and diglycerides; soapy consistency	>20 g tnglycendes; only seepage
D-Xylose	Low	Normal
Secretion test	Normal	Abnormal
Small-bowel series	Abnormal	Normal
Small-bowel biopsy	Abnormal	Normal
Lunch meal	Normal	Abnormal
PABA test	Normal	Abnormal
PP response to test meal	Normal	Low
Vitamin B_{12} and folate	Low	Normal
Treatment with pancreatic enzymes	No change	Improvement

PABA, paraaminobenzoic acid; PP, pancreatic polypeptide.
Modified from Brandt LJ. *Gastrointestinal disorders of the elderly.* New York: Raven Press; 1984:470.

given an intravenous bolus of 0.5 g of glucose per kilogram over 2 to 5 minutes. Blood samples are drawn every 10 minutes for 1 hour. The decline in glucose concentration (percentage of disappearance per minute) is called the *K value.* A K value of 1.5 or higher is normal. The intravenous glucose tolerance test response decreases with age, and results should be evaluated with age-adjusted criteria.

The intravenous arginine test is useful for the diagnosis of hormone-secreting tumors. The amino acid arginine stimulates the secretion of islet hormones. After an overnight fast, the patient is given a 30-minute infusion of 0.5 g of arginine per kilogram. Blood samples are taken every 10 minutes, and radioimmunoassays are performed for the specific hormones in question. This test is particularly useful for the diagnosis of glucagon-secreting tumors; elevations of plasma glucagon to above 400 pg/mL usually indicate a glucagonoma.

The tolbutamide response test is also useful in detecting hormone-secreting tumors. Tolbutamide is a sulfonylurea that stimulates insulin secretion. After the patient has fasted overnight, basal blood samples are drawn. One gram of sodium tolbutamide is given intravenously, and the blood glucose level is monitored for 1 hour. Blood samples are also drawn for radioimmunoassay of insulin or other suspected hormones, such as somatostatin. In normal patients, the blood glucose level falls to 50% of basal values after 30 minutes. Sustained hypoglycemia with hypersecretion of insulin is consistent with an insulinoma. In the case of a somatostatinoma, somatostatin levels are more than twice as high as the prevailing normal values for the particular somatostatin radioimmunoassay used.

KEY POINTS

- **Annular pancreas results when a thin band of pancreatic parenchyma surrounds the duodenum, causing variable degrees of duodenal stenosis.**
- **Pancreas divisum results from an incomplete fusion of the ventral pancreatic duct with the dorsal duct during fetal development, which may lead to inadequate drainage of the gland and result in pancreatitis.**
- **The tail of the pancreas is a short mobile segment of the gland, which ends within the splenic hilum making it susceptible to injury during splenectomy.**
- **Progressive destruction of the pancreatic ductular network occurs during recurrent episodes of pancreatitis, which contributes in part to exocrine insufficiency and chronic pain.**
- **The two major components of the exocrine pancreas, the acinar cells and the ductular network, constitute 80% to 90% of the pancreatic mass, whereas the endocrine pancreas accounts for only 2% of pancreatic mass.**
- **The pancreatic islet of Langerhans are composed of four major cell types—alpha (A), beta (B), delta (D), and pancreatic polypeptide (PP) or F cells, which secrete glucagon, insulin, somatostatin, and PP, respectively.**

TABLE 53.4 DIAGNOSIS

INTERPRETATION OF ORAL GLUCOSE TOLERANCE TEST RESULTS

Interpretation	Fasting glucose value (mg/dL)		Intermediate glucose value (mg/dL)		2-Hour glucose value (mg/dL)
Normal	<115	and	All values <200	and	140
Impaired glucose tolerance	<140	and	Any value ≥200	and	140–199
Diabetic	≥140 or <140		(Glucose tolerance test not necessary)		
		and	Any value ≥200	and	≥200
Nondiagnostic	Any combination of glucose values that does not fit into another category				

Modified from National Diabetes Data Group. Classification and diagnosis of diabetes mellitus and other categories of glucose intolerance. *Diabetes* 1979;28:1039.

- **Beta cells (or B cells) constitute 70% of islet cell mass.**
- **Approximately 500 to 800 mL of pancreatic juice is excreted daily and consists of a colorless, odorless, and isosmotic liquid that contains bicarbonate and pancreatic enzymes.**
- **Secretin is the major stimulant for pancreatic bicarbonate secretion, whereas pancreatic enzyme secretion is regulated through hormonal (CCK) and neural factors.**
- **Tests of pancreatic exocrine function include the secretin test, fecal fat determination, dimethadione (DMO) test, the Lundh test meal, the triolein breath test, and the para-aminobenzoic acid test.**

References

1. **Cubilla AC, Fortner JC, Fitzgerald PJ. Lymph node involvement in carcinoma of the head of the pancreas area. *Cancer* 1978;41:880.**
2. Ahren B, Taborsky GJ Jr, Porte D Jr. Neuropeptidergic versus cholinergic and adrenergic regulation of islet hormone secretion. *Diabetologia* 1986;29:827.
3. Havel PJ, Taborsky GJ Jr. The contribution of the autonomic nervous system to changes in glucagon and insulin secretion during hypoglycemic stress. *Endocr Rev.* 1989;10:332.
4. Sadar ES, Cooperman AM. Bilateral thoracic sympathectomy-splanchnicectomy in the treatment of intractable pain due to pancreatic carcinoma. *Cleve Clin Q.* 1974;41:185.
5. Gorelick FS, Jamieson JD. Structure–function relationship of the pancreas. In: Johnson LR, ed. *Physiology of the gastrointestinal tract.* New York: Raven Press; 1981:773.
6. Longnecker DS, Shinozuka H, Dekker A. Focal acinar cell dysplasia in human pancreas. *Cancer* 1980;45:534.
7. Pour PM, Schmied B. The link between exocrine pancreatic cancer and the endocrine pancreas. *Int J Pancreatol.* 1999;25:77.
8. Kleinman R, Gingerich R, Wong H, et al. The use of the Fab fragment for immunoneutralization of somatostatin in the isolated perfused pancreas. *Am J Surg.* 1994;167:114.
9. Cooper GJ, Day AJ, Willis AC, et al. Amylin and the amylin gene: structure, function, and relationship to islet amyloid and to diabetes mellitus. *Biochem Biophys Acta* 1989;1014:247.
10. Stefan Y, Orci L, Malaisse-Legae F, et al. Quantitation of endocrine cell content in the pancreas of non-diabetic and diabetic humans. *Diabetes* 1982;31:694.
11. Seymour NE, Brunicardi FC, Chaiken RL, et al. Reversal of abnormal glucose production after pancreatic resection by pancreatic polypeptide administration in man. *Surgery* 1988;104:119.
12. Jansson L, Hellerstrom C. Glucose-induced changes in pancreatic islet blood flow mediated by central nervous system. *Am J Physiol.* 1986;25:E644.
13. Bonner-Weir S, Orci L. New perspectives on the microvasculature of the islets of Langerhans in the rat. *Diabetes* 1982;31:883.
14. Murakami T, Fujita T, Ohtsuka A, et al. The insulino-acinar portal and insulino-venous drainage systems in the pancreas of the mouse, dog, monkey, and certain other animals: a scanning electron microscopic study of corrosion casts. *Arch Histol Cytol.* 1993;56:127.
15. Liu Y, Guth PH, Kaneko K, et al. Dynamic *in vivo* observation of rat islet microcirculation. *Pancreas* 1993;8:15.
16. Lee W, Kazunori M, Funakoshi A. Effects of somatostatin and pancreatic polypeptide on exocrine and endocrine pancreas in the rats. *Gastroenterol Jpn.* 1988;23:49.
17. **Busnardo AC, Didio L, Tidrick R, et al. History of the pancreas. *Am J Surg.* 1983;146:539.**
18. Davenport HW. Pancreatic secretion. In: Davenport HN, ed. *Physiology of the digestive tract,* 5th ed. Chicago: Year Book Medical Publishers; 1982:143.
19. Valenzuela JE, Weiner K, Saad C. Cholinergic stimulation of human pancreatic secretion. *Dig Dis Sci.* 1986;31:615.
20. Konturek SJ, Becker HD, Thompson JC. Effect of vagotomy on hormones stimulating pancreatic secretion. *Arch Surg.* 1974;108:704.
21. Leahy JL, Bonner-Weir S, Weir GC. Abnormal glucose regulation of insulin secretion in models of reduced B-cell mass. *Diabetes* 1984;33:667.
22. Nanjo K, Sanke T, Mujano M, et al. Diabetes due to secretion of a structurally abnormal insulin (insulin Wakayama): clinical and functional characteristics of Leu-A3 insulin. *J Clin Invest.* 1986;77:514.
23. Bell GI, Kayano T, Buse JB, et al. Molecular biology of mammalian glucose transporters. *Diabetes Care* 1990;13:198.
24. Orci L, Unger RH, Ravazzola M, et al. Reduced beta-cell glucose transporter in new onset diabetic BB rats. *J Clin Invest.* 1990;86:1615.
25. Ebert R, Creutzfeldt W. Gastrointestinal peptides and insulin secretion. *Diabetes Metab Rev.* 1987;3:1.
26. **Opara EC, Atwater I, Go VLM. Characterization and control of pulsatile secretion of insulin and glucagon. *Pancreas* 1988;3:484.**
27. Eisenbarth GS. Type I diabetes mellitus: a chronic autoimmune disease. *N Engl J Med.* 1986;314:1360.
28. **Brunicardi FC, Sun YS, Druck P, et al. Splanchnic neural regulation of insulin and glucagon secretion in the isolated perfused human pancreas. *Am J Surg.* 1987;153:34.**
29. Unger RH, Dobbs RE. Insulin, glucagon, and somatostatin in the regulation of metabolism. *Ann Rev Physiol.* 1978;40:307.
30. Gerich JE. Somatostatin and diabetes. *Am J Med.* 1981;70:619.
31. Brazeau P, Vale N, Burgus R, et al. Hypothalamic polypeptide that inhibits the secretion of immunoreactive pituitary growth hormone. *Science* 1973;179:77.
32. Kleinman R, Watt P, Ohning G, et al. The regulatory role of intraislet somatostatin on insulin secretion in the isolated perfused human pancreas. *Pancreas* 1993;9:172.
33. Mulvihill SJ, Pappas TN, Passaro E, et al. The use of somatostatin and its analogs in the treatment of surgical disorders. *Surgery* 1986;100:467.
34. Kennedy FP. Pathophysiology of pancreatic polypeptide secretion in human diabetes mellitus. *Diabetes Nutr Metab.* 1990;2:155.
35. Fagan SP, Anderson DK, Brunicardi FC. Islet cell hormones and chronic pancreatitis. *Probl Gen Surg.* 1998;15:7.
36. Moldovan S, Brunicardi FC. The endocrine pancreas: a summary of observations generated by surgical fellows. *World J Surg.* 2001;25:468.
37. Dreiling DA, Wolfson P. New insights into pancreatic disease revealed by the secretin test. In: Berk JE, ed. *Developments in digestive diseases,* Vol 2. Philadelphia: Lea & Febiger; 1979:155.
38. Noda A, Hayakowa T, Kondo T, et al. Clinical evaluation of pancreatic excretion test with dimethadione and oral BT-PABA test in chronic pancreatitis. *Dig Dis Sci.* 1983;30:230.
39. Goff JS. Two-stage triolein breath test differentiates pancreatic insufficiency from other causes of malabsorption. *Gastroenterology* 1982;83:44.
40. Arvanitakis C, Greenberger NJ. Diagnosis of pancreatic disease by a synthetic peptide: a new test of exocrine pancreatic function. *Lancet* 1976; 1:663.
41. **Nealon WH, Beauchamp RD, Townsend CM, et al. Diagnostic role of gastrointestinal hormones in patients with chronic pancreatitis. *Ann Surg.* 1986;204:430.**
42. National Diabetes Data Group. Classification and diagnosis of diabetes mellitus and other categories of glucose intolerance. *Diabetes* 1979;30:1039.
43. Andres R, Tobin JD. Endocrine systems. In: Finch CE, Hayflick L, eds. *Handbook of the biology of aging.* New York: Van Nostrand Reinhold; 1977:357.

CHAPTER 54 ■ ACUTE PANCREATITIS

EDWARD E. WHANG

Acute pancreatitis is an acute inflammatory process of the pancreas with variable involvement of other regional tissues or remote organ systems.[1] In the United States, more than 300,000 patients are hospitalized annually with acute pancreatitis as the primary diagnosis.[2] It is the principal cause of approximately 3,200 deaths per year and a contributing factor in an additional 4,000 deaths. The direct cost attributable to acute pancreatitis exceeds $2 billion per year in the United States.

Considerable investigation has focused on identifying strategies for reducing the formidable burden imposed by this disorder. These investigations have increased our understanding of the pathogenesis of acute pancreatitis and its complications. They have also led to an evolution in diagnostic and management algorithms. Although these advances have greatly improved outcomes associated with acute pancreatitis, the subset of patients with severe disease continue to pose some of the most difficult challenges in clinical surgery.

CLASSIFICATION AND DEFINITIONS

A useful and widely accepted classification system for describing the clinical spectrum of acute pancreatitis was developed during a multidisciplinary symposium held in 1992.[1] Consensus was reached on the definitions in Table 54.1.

PATHOLOGY AND PATHOPHYSIOLOGY

The typical pathologic correlate of mild acute pancreatitis is *interstitial (edematous) pancreatitis*, in which the pancreatic parenchyma is edematous and infiltrated with inflammatory cells. Gross architectural features are preserved. In contrast, severe acute pancreatitis (SAP) can be associated with *necrotizing pancreatitis*, in which variable amounts of pancreatic parenchyma and peripancreatic fat have undergone tissue necrosis, with vascular inflammation and thrombosis being prominent features.

Studies using experimental models suggest that prototypical molecular and cellular derangements lead to pancreatic injury, regardless of the specific etiology or inciting event that triggers an episode of acute pancreatitis. Among the earliest of these derangements appears to be abnormal activation of proteolytic enzymes within pancreatic acinar cells.[3] Under normal conditions, trypsinogen and other digestive zymogens are segregated from lysosomal enzymes (e.g., cathepsin B) within the acinar cell. Early in the course of acute pancreatitis these enzymes are hypothesized to become colocalized, allowing cathepsin B to hydrolyze trypsinogen, yielding active trypsin and trypsinogen activation peptide (TAP). In experimental pancreatitis induced by administration of the cholecystokinin (CCK) analogue cerulein, for example, trypsinogen activation occurs within minutes following administration of cerulein, precedes biochemical or morphologic evidence of acinar cell injury, and is prevented by inhibition of cathepsin B activity.[4]

Acinar cell injury induced by active trypsin allows it to be released into the pancreatic parenchyma (Fig 54.1) where it activates more trypsin and other digestive enzymes (e.g., chymotrypsin, phospholipase, and elastase). Trypsin can also activate the complement, kallikrein-kinin, coagulation, and fibrinolysis cascades within the pancreatic parenchyma. Activation of these enzymes is believed to initiate a vicious cycle in which activated enzymes cause cellular injury, an event that leads to the release of even more destructive enzymes. This cycle can overwhelm defense mechanisms that normally serve to limit the injurious consequences of premature trypsin activation within the pancreas (e.g., pancreatic secretory trypsin inhibitor-mediated inhibition of trypsin activity).

As injury progresses, the pancreatic parenchyma becomes infiltrated with macrophages and polymorphonuclear

TABLE 54.1 ■ CLASSIFICATION

CLASSIFICATION OF ACUTE PANCREATITIS

Term	Definition
Mild acute pancreatitis	Acute inflammation of the pancreas with minimal distant organ dysfunction and an uneventful recovery
Severe acute pancreatitis	Acute pancreatitis associated with pancreatic necrosis, distant organ failure, and/or the development of local complications, such as hemorrhage, abscess, or pseudocyst
Acute fluid collections	Fluid collections that occur early in the course of acute pancreatitis, are located in or near the pancreas, and lack a wall of granulation or fibrous tissue
Pancreatic necrosis	Diffuse or focal areas of nonviable pancreatic parenchyma, typically associated with peripancreatic fat necrosis
Pseudocyst	Collection of pancreatic secretions enclosed by a wall of fibrous or granulation tissue arising as a consequence of acute pancreatitis, chronic pancreatitis, or trauma to the pancreas
Pancreatic abscess	Collection of pus, usually near the pancreas, containing little or no pancreatic necrosis; arises as a consequence of acute pancreatitis or trauma to the pancreas

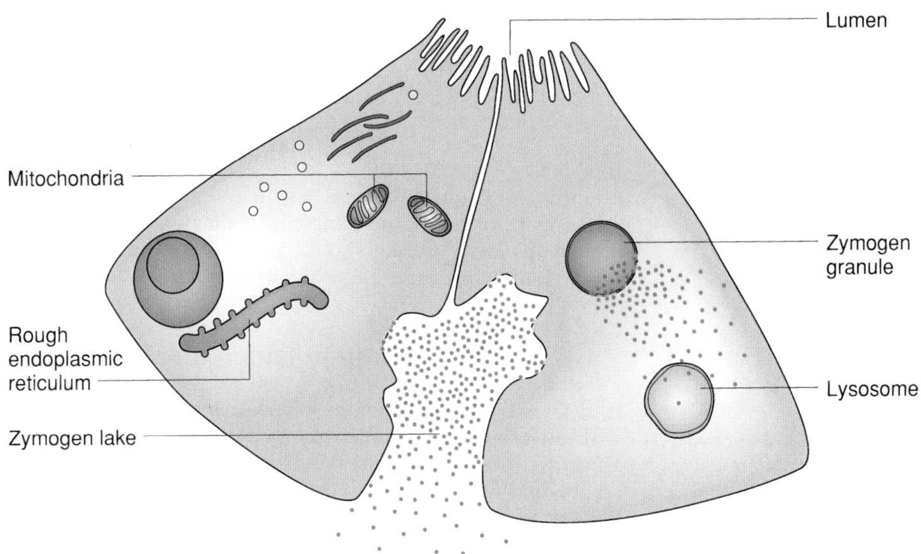

FIGURE 54.1 Schematic diagram depicting colocalization of the contents of zymogen granules and lysosomes within the pancreatic acinar cell. Lysosomal enzymes are hypothesized to induce premature activation of trypsin. Activated trypsin undergoes disordered basolateral discharge from the acinar cell into the pancreatic parenchyma.

leukocytes, resulting in the release of a broad range of proinflammatory mediators (e.g., tumor necrosis factor; interleukins 1, 6, and 8; prostaglandins; platelet-activating factor; leukotrienes; and reactive oxygen species). The result of these events is pancreatic autodigestion, with injury to the vascular endothelium, interstitium, and acinar cells. Increases in vascular permeability lead to interstitial edema. Vasoconstriction, thrombosis, and capillary stasis can lead to ischemic (and perhaps ischemia-reperfusion) injury and the development of pancreatic necrosis. The specific factors that determine whether an episode of acute pancreatitis is limited to interstitial pancreatitis or progresses to necrotizing pancreatitis are unknown.

With severe pancreatic injury, the systemic inflammatory response syndrome (SIRS) and distant organ failure can occur. The systemic complications are believed to be mediated by digestive enzymes and inflammatory mediators released from the injured pancreas. For example, activated phospholipase A-induced digestion of lecithin (an important component of pulmonary surfactant) may play a role in pathogenesis of acute respiratory distress syndrome (ARDS) that occurs in the setting of acute pancreatitis. In addition, the circulatory and inflammatory effects induced by acute pancreatitis are postulated to impair intestinal epithelial barrier function, allowing for the translocation of bacteria from the intestinal lumen into the systemic circulation. This phenomenon has been demonstrated to occur in animal models and may account for the pathogenesis of pancreatic and peripancreatic infection that can complicate necrotizing pancreatitis.

ETIOLOGY

A wide range of etiologies of acute pancreatitis has been identified (Table 54.2). In the United States, more than 75% of cases are attributable to either gallstones or alcohol. Patients for whom no etiology can be identified despite thorough evaluation are classified as having *idiopathic pancreatitis.*

Gallstones

Gallstones cause approximately 35% of episodes of acute pancreatitis in the United States. In a mechanistic model proposed over a century ago, a gallstone lodged at the papilla of Vater occludes the ampullary orifice, leading to retrograde reflux of bile into the pancreatic duct through a common channel shared by the common bile duct and the pancreatic duct (Fig. 54.2). Although elements of this model have been challenged, the prevailing view is that transient or persistent obstruction of the ampullary orifice by a gallstone or edema induced by stone passage is the inciting factor in the pathogenesis of gallstone-induced pancreatitis. *Microlithiasis* refers

TABLE 54.2 ETIOLOGY

ETIOLOGY OF ACUTE PANCREATITIS

- Gallstones
- Ethanol
- Iatrogenic causes
  - ERCP
  - Abdominal and nonabdominal operations
  - Cardiopulmonary bypass
- Trauma
- Neoplasms (e.g., pancreatic cancer)
- Pancreas divisum
- Sphincter of Oddi spasm
- Medications (see Table 54.3)
- Toxins
  - Parathion
  - Scorpion venom
- Hyperlipidemia
- Hypercalcemia
- Infectious agents
  - Viruses (e.g., mumps and Coxsackie B viruses; HIV)
  - Bacteria (e.g., *Salmonella* and *Shigella* species; hemorrhagic *Escherichia coli*)
  - Biliary parasites (e.g., *Ascaris lumbricoides*)
- Genetic causes
  - Hereditary pancreatitis
  - Cystic fibrosis
- Vasculitis (e.g., systemic lupus erythematosus and polyarteritis nodosa)
- Ischemia
- Pregnancy

ERCP, endoscopic retrograde cholangiopancreatography.

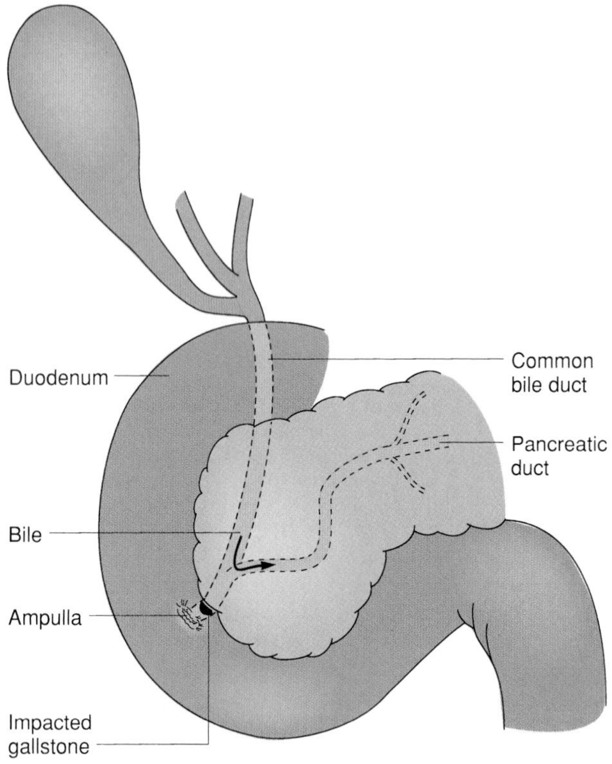

FIGURE 54.2 Illustration of the common channel concept. A gallstone lodged at the ampulla of Vater can cause reflux of bile into the pancreatic duct.

to aggregates (<5 mm in diameter) of cholesterol monohydrate crystals or calcium bilirubinate granules detected as "sludge" within the gallbladder on ultrasonography or on examination of bile obtained during endoscopic retrograde cholangiopancreatography (ERCP). An etiologic role for microlithiasis in acute pancreatitis remains unproved; however, data derived from case-control studies suggest that cholecystectomy or endoscopic sphincterotomy can reduce the risk of recurrent acute pancreatitis in patients with microlithiasis.

Alcohol

Ethanol causes approximately 40% of cases of acute pancreatitis in the United States. Most patients with alcohol-induced acute pancreatitis also have underlying chronic pancreatitis. Potential mechanisms by which alcohol induces pancreatitis include sphincter of Oddi spasm, obstruction of small pancreatic ductules by proteinaceous plugs, alcohol-induced metabolic abnormalities (e.g., hyperlipidemia), and direct toxic effects induced by alcohol and its metabolites (e.g., acetaldehyde, acetate, and nonesterified fatty acids).

Iatrogenic Causes and Trauma

Acute pancreatitis occurs following 1% to 5% of ERCP procedures. There is an increased incidence of both clinically overt acute pancreatitis and hyperamylasemia during the postoperative period. Potential mechanisms leading to postoperative pancreatitis include direct trauma to the pancreas and adjacent structures (in the case of abdominal operations), hypotension and ischemic pancreatic injury, and medication-induced pancreatic toxicity. Both penetrating and blunt trauma can cause pancreatitis. The body of the pancreas as it crosses anterior to the L2 vertebral body is susceptible to fracture in blunt trauma.

Neoplasms

Primary and metastatic neoplasms of the pancreas can cause acute pancreatitis. Acute pancreatitis diagnosed for the first time in an elderly patient should prompt thorough evaluation to rule out the presence of an underlying pancreatic cancer.

Autoimmune Pancreatitis

Also known as *sclerosing pancreatitis*, this condition presents with diffuse enlargement of the pancreas and characteristic abnormalities in laboratory tests, including elevations in serum immunoglobulin E (IgE) and IgG4 concentrations. Because obstructive jaundice and findings on cross-sectional imaging tests suggestive of focal pancreatic masses can accompany autoimmune pancreatitis, this condition can be misdiagnosed as pancreatic cancer. This form of pancreatitis resolves with corticosteroid therapy.

Pancreas Divisum

Based on autopsy series, this anatomic variant, in which there is incomplete or absent fusion between the ventral (Wirsung) and dorsal (Santorini) pancreatic ducts, occurs in approximately 7% of the population. The relationship between the presence of pancreas divisum and acute pancreatitis remains controversial. It is hypothesized that in some patients, resistance to flow of secretions from the dorsal duct caused by a diminutive orifice of the minor papilla leads to ductal hypertension-related pancreatitis. However, in most patients with pancreas divisum who develop acute pancreatitis, the pancreas divisum itself is not the cause of pancreatitis.

Medications

A wide range of drugs has been implicated in causing acute pancreatitis (Table 54.3). In most cases, the relationship between the agent and the development of pancreatitis is unclear, and the underlying mechanisms are unknown.

Hyperlipidemia and Hypercalcemia

Hyperlipidemia can be both a consequence and a cause of acute pancreatitis. Triglyceride levels of greater than 1,000 mg/dL are usually required to cause acute pancreatitis. The mechanism by which hyperlipidemia causes pancreatitis is likely related to the toxic effects of triglyceride metabolites (e.g., free fatty acids) within the pancreas. Hypercalcemia can induce increases in pancreatic duct permeability and trypsinogen activation within the pancreatic parenchyma. These effects may lead to either hyperamylasemia in the absence of overt pancreatitis or the development of clinical pancreatitis.

Genetic Causes

Hereditary pancreatitis is an autosomal dominant disorder with a nearly 80% penetrance. Affected individuals have attacks of pancreatitis that begin in childhood; they are also at high risk for developing chronic pancreatitis and pancreatic

TABLE 54.3

MEDICATIONS CAUSING ACUTE PANCREATITIS

Antiinflammatory drugs
Sulfasalazine
Sulindac
Salicylates
Antimicrobial agents
Didanosine
Metronidazole
Tetracycline
Nitrofurantoin
Pentamidine
Trimethoprim-sulfamethoxazole
Diuretics
Diazoxide
Ethacrynic acid
Furosemide
Thiazides
Immunosuppressive agents
Azathioprine
6-Mercaptopurine
Miscellaneous
ACE inhibitors
Calcium
Estrogen
Valproic acid

ACE, angiotensin-converting enzyme.

cancer. This form of pancreatitis is caused by mutations in the cationic trypsinogen gene (e.g., mutations in codons 29 and 122) that result in the synthesis of an abnormal form of trypsin that is resistant to proteolytic degradation. Other mutations have been identified that are associated with disorders of lower penetrance.

The relationship between pancreatitis and mutations in the cystic fibrosis transmembrane regulator (*CFTR*) gene remains incompletely understood. Most patients with cystic fibrosis develop pulmonary disease and pancreatic insufficiency but not pancreatitis. A distinct subset of patients with CFTR mutations, however, develops acute and chronic pancreatitis but not pulmonary disease. These patients are not homozygous for CFTR mutations that result in cystic fibrosis.

CLINICAL PRESENTATION

Abdominal pain, nausea, and vomiting are the most prevalent symptoms associated with acute pancreatitis. The pain is visceral in quality, is localized to the epigastrium, often radiates to the back, and may be alleviated with the patient leaning forward. Abdominal tenderness is the most prevalent sign of acute pancreatitis. Tachycardia and hypotension may result from intravascular hypovolemia. Low-grade fevers are common, but high-grade fevers are unusual in the absence of intra- or extrapancreatic infection. Jaundice may be evident in the presence of cholangitis (e.g., with gallstone-induced pancreatitis and persistent choledocholithiasis) or liver disease (alcohol-induced pancreatitis in a patient with cirrhosis). Evidence of retroperitoneal hemorrhage may be become apparent if blood dissects into the subcutaneous tissues of the flanks (Grey Turner's sign), umbilicus (Cullen's sign), or inguinal region (Fox's sign); however, these findings are unusual.

Approximately 80% of cases of acute pancreatitis are mild, associated with minimal systemic derangements, and generally resolve within 5 to 7 days, even with minimal therapy. The mortality rate associated with mild acute pancreatitis is less than 1%.

Approximately 20% of cases are classified as *severe acute pancreatitis*, defined as acute pancreatitis associated with one or more of the following: (a) necrosis of greater than one third of the pancreas; (b) distant organ failure (indicated by systolic blood pressure ≤90 mm Hg, serum creatinine >2.9 mg/dL, gastrointestinal blood loss exceeding 500 mL in volume within a 24-hour period, and/or PaO_2 ≤60 mm Hg); and/or (c) the development of local complications, such as hemorrhage, abscess, or pseudocyst.[1] The mortality rate associated with SAP ranges from 10% to 20% in contemporary series.[5,6] One half of deaths occur within the first 2 weeks after the onset of symptoms; these deaths are primarily the result of SIRS-induced multisystem organ failure. Most of the remaining deaths occur 2 to 3 weeks after presentation and result from complications of pancreatic necrosis, especially infection.

PANCREAS/LIVER

DIAGNOSIS

The differential diagnosis of acute pancreatitis includes other conditions causing acute upper abdominal pain, such as biliary colic and cholecystitis, acute mesenteric ischemia, small bowel obstruction, visceral perforation, and ruptured aortic aneurysm. Acute exacerbations of chronic pancreatitis can also be associated with clinical features resembling those of acute pancreatitis. The diagnosis of acute pancreatitis usually can be made by confirming biochemical evidence of pancreatic injury. Imaging tests should be used selectively, to rule out other diagnoses and for the indications discussed later.

Laboratory Tests

With pancreatic injury, a variety of digestive enzymes escape from acinar cells and enter the systemic circulation. Of these enzymes, amylase is the most widely assayed to confirm the diagnosis of acute pancreatitis. Amylase levels rise within several hours after onset of symptoms and typically remain elevated for 3 to 5 days during uncomplicated episodes of mild acute pancreatitis. Because of the short serum half-life of amylase (10 hours), levels can normalize as soon as 24 hours after disease onset. The sensitivity of this test depends on what threshold value is used to define a positive result (90% sensitivity with a threshold value just above the normal range vs. 60% sensitivity with a threshold value at three times the upper limit of normal). Specificity (which also varies with the threshold values selected) is limited because a wide range of disorders can cause elevations in serum amylase concentration (Table 54.4). Assays that detect increases in the serum concentration of amylase of pancreatic origin (P-isoamylase) alone are associated with greater specificity. Increased urinary amylase concentrations and amylase-to-creatinine clearance ratios occur with acute pancreatitis; however, these parameters offer no advantage over serum amylase concentrations, except in the evaluation of macroamylasemia (in which urinary amylase excretion is not increased despite elevations in serum amylase concentration).

Serum lipase concentrations increase with kinetics similar to those of amylase. It has a longer serum half-life than amylase, however, and may be useful for diagnosing acute pancreatitis late in the course of an episode (at which time serum amylase concentrations may have already normalized).

TABLE 54.4 ETIOLOGY

CONDITIONS CAUSING INCREASED SERUM AMYLASE LEVELS

Pancreatic disorders
Acute pancreatitis
Acute exacerbations of chronic pancreatitis
Pancreatic neoplasms and cysts
Nonpancreatic acute abdominal conditions
Acute appendicitis
Acute cholecystitis
Acute salpingitis
Common bile duct obstruction
Intestinal ischemia
Intestinal obstruction
Ruptured ectopic pregnancy
Visceral perforation
Salivary gland disorders
Mumps
Sialadenitis
Ethanol-induced secretion of salivary amylase
Extrapancreatic neoplasms
Ovarian neoplasms and cysts
Lung cancer
Renal insufficiency
Miscellaneous
AIDS
Anorexia nervosa
Diabetic ketoacidosis
Intracranial hemorrhage
Macroamylasemia

AIDS, acquired immunodeficiency syndrome.

Although lipase is more specific than amylase in the diagnosis of acute pancreatitis, note that lipase is produced at a range of nonpancreatic sites, including the intestine, liver, biliary tract, and stomach, and tongue.

The magnitude of the increases in amylase or lipase concentrations has no correlation with severity of pancreatitis. In general, the magnitude of increases in amylase concentrations tends to be greater in patients with gallstone pancreatitis than in those with alcohol-induced pancreatitis; however, this finding is unreliable in distinguishing between these two etiologies.

Imaging Tests

Findings on plain radiographs associated with acute pancreatitis are nonspecific and include ileus that may be generalized or localized to a segment of small intestine ("sentinel loop") or transverse colon ("colon cut-off sign"), psoas muscle margins that are obscured by retroperitoneal edema, an elevated hemidiaphragm, pleural effusions, and basilar atelectasis.

Ultrasonography may reveal a diffusely enlarged, hypoechoic pancreas. However, overlying bowel gas (particularly prominent with ileus) limits visualization of the pancreas in a large percentage of cases. Although ultrasonography has poor sensitivity in the diagnosis of acute pancreatitis, it plays an important role in the identification of the etiology of pancreatitis (i.e., the detection of gallstones).

Computed tomography (CT) scanning is the most important imaging test in the evaluation of acute pancreatitis. Specific applications of CT scanning are listed in Table 54.5. CT findings of mild acute pancreatitis include pancreatic enlargement and edema, effacement of the normal lobulated contour of the pancreas, and stranding of peripancreatic fat (Fig. 54.3). In addition, dynamic CT scanning performed after the bolus administration of intravenous contrast can demonstrate regions of pancreas that have poor or no perfusion, as seen with pancreatic necrosis (Fig. 54.4). Detection of necrosis plays an important role in assessment of disease severity, as discussed further later.

Magnetic resonance imaging (MRI) and magnetic resonance cholangiopancreatography (MRCP) are being used with increasing frequency in patients with acute pancreatitis. These examinations have the potential to offer better definition of pancreatic and biliary ductal abnormalities than CT scanning,

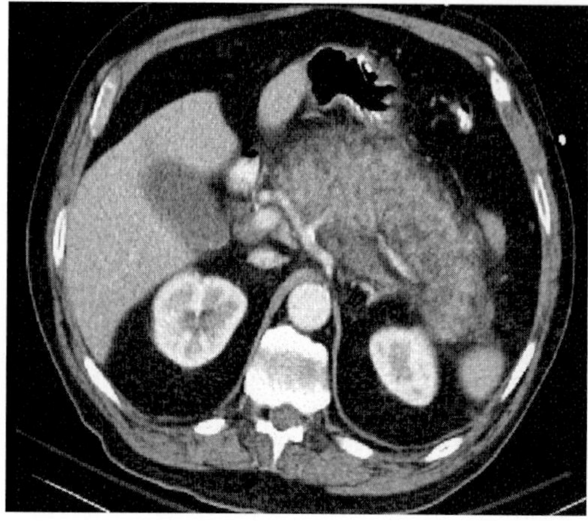

FIGURE 54.3 Computed tomography scan of acute interstitial pancreatitis.

TABLE 54.5 DIAGNOSIS

SPECIFIC APPLICATIONS OF COMPUTED TOMOGRAPHY SCANNING

Diagnosis confirmation in patients for whom diagnostic uncertainty exists despite completion of clinical assessment and laboratory testing
Assessment of disease severity
Detection of complications
Providing image guidance for interventional procedures

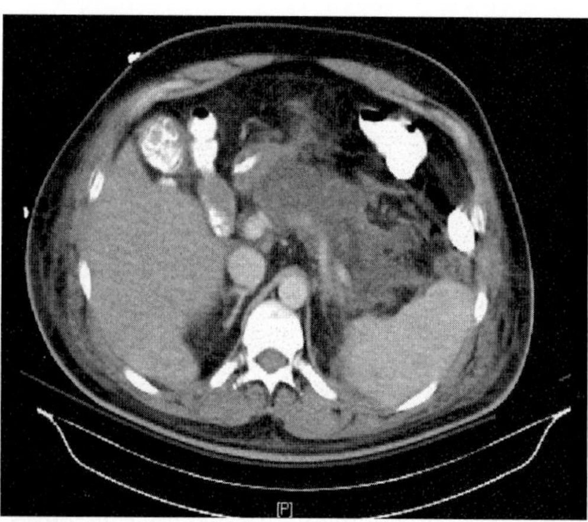

FIGURE 54.4 Computed tomography scan of acute necrotizing pancreatitis.

and they are applicable in patients for whom ionizing radiation or iodinated intravenous contrast agents used in CT scanning are contraindicated. Disadvantages of MRI include high cost, limited availability, and the long duration of examinations.

ASSESSMENT OF DISEASE SEVERITY

Accurate prediction of severity early in the course of disease offers potential benefits in that complications can be anticipated and detected early through the use of intensive monitoring and frequent clinical assessment, and early and aggressive therapies can be instituted to attempt to prevent these complications. Routine clinical assessment at the time of admission is associated with low sensitivities (<50%) in identifying patients with SAP.[7] Therefore, alternative methods for assessing disease severity based on scoring systems, CT scanning, and serum markers have been widely studied. In addition to these methods, hemoconcentration and obesity have been reported to be predictive of severe disease.[8]

Scoring Systems

The Ranson criteria (Table 54.6) are easily tabulated, and the resulting scores are well correlated with morbidity and mortality rates.[9] The presence of three or more of these criteria is indicative of SAP. An important limitation of the Ranson criteria is that the predictive score cannot be determined prior to 48 hours following admission and that it can only be used once. Furthermore, because these criteria were developed using a cohort of patients for whom alcohol was the predominant etiology of pancreatitis, their generalizability may be limited. A similar predictive scoring system (Table 54.7) developed using a cohort of patients for whom gallstones were the predominant etiology of pancreatitis is available.[7]

Acute Physiology and Chronic Health Evaluation (APACHE) II scores, which are based on patient age, indices of chronic health, and physiologic parameters, can be determined at any time after admission, can be updated continuously during the course of disease and may have greater predictive power than Ranson or Glasgow scores.[10] However, the complexity of calculating APACHE II scores limits its application in routine clinical practice. An even more complex scoring system (APACHE III) offers no advantage over APACHE II scoring in patients with acute pancreatitis. In contrast, the APACHE O score, which includes body mass index in addition to APACHE II variables, has been reported to have greater positive predictive value (up to 74%) for severe disease than standard APACHE II scoring.[11]

TABLE 54.6

RANSON CRITERIA FOR ASSESSING SEVERITY OF PANCREATITIS

AT ADMISSION	
Age	>55 yr
WBC count	>16,000/mm^3
Glucose	>200 mg/dL
LDH	>350 IU/L
AST	>250 IU/L
WITHIN 48 HOURS	
Hematocrit decrease	>10 pt
BUN increase	>5 mg/dL
Calcium	<8 mg/dL
PaO_2	<60 mm Hg
Base deficit	>4 mEq/L
Fluid requirement	>6 L

WBC, white blood cell; LDH, lactate dehydrogenase; AST, aspartate aminotransferase; BUN, blood urea nitrogen; PaO_2, arterial oxygen pressure.

TABLE 54.7

GLASGOW SYSTEM FOR ASSESSING SEVERITY OF PANCREATITIS

WBC count	>15,000/mm^3
Glucose	>180 mg/dL with no history of diabetes
BUN	>45 mg/dL
Pao_2	<60 mm Hg
Calcium	<8 mg/dL
Albumin	<3.2 g/dL
LDH	>600 IU/L
AST	>200 IU/L

WBC, white blood cell; BUN, blood urea nitrogen, Pao_2, arterial oxygen pressure, LDH, lactate dehydrogenase; AST, aspartate aminotransferase.

PANCREAS/LIVER

Computed Tomography Scanning

The diagnostic application of CT scanning was discussed previously. For assessment of disease severity, dynamic intravenous contrast-enhanced CT scanning should be obtained. This technique is associated with greater than 90% sensitivities in the detection of pancreatic necrosis, a finding that is predictive of severe disease, and is indicated if clinical deterioration occurs or if one the scoring systems discussed above suggests severe disease (e.g., presence of three or more Ranson criteria or APACHE II score ≥8). A CT severity index based on features identified on CT scanning (Table 54.8) has been developed.[12] Patients with a CT severity index greater than 5 have been reported to have a mortality rate eightfold greater than patients with a score less than 5. Because necrosis takes time to develop, a contrast-enhanced CT scan obtained too early in the disease course (e.g., at the time of admission) is unlikely to have predictive value. In addition, concerns that early administration of iodinated intravenous contrast agents used in CT scanning may exacerbate pancreatic injury have been raised, although these agents have not been shown to cause or exacerbate pancreatitis in humans.[13]

Serum and Urinary Markers

C-reactive protein (CRP) is an easily assayed marker for which serum concentrations are well correlated with disease severity. However, CRP levels do not become significantly elevated until 48 hours after onset of disease; therefore, this marker is not useful for early prediction of disease severity. Serum concentrations of neutrophil elastase and interleukin-6 and urinary concentrations of TAP (a product of trypsinogen activation) are also correlated with disease severity. Because these markers become elevated within 24 hours of disease onset, they may be relevant to early prediction strategies in the

TABLE 54.8

COMPUTED TOMOGRAPHY (CT) SEVERITY INDEX

GRADE BASED ON FINDINGS ON UNENHANCED CT

Grade	Findings	Score
A	Normal appearing pancreas	0
B	Focal or diffuse enlargement of pancreas No peripancreatic inflammation	1
C	Peripancreatic inflammation present	2
D	Intrapancreatic or extrapancreatic fluid collections present	3
E	Two or more collections of gas present in pancreas or retroperitoneum	4

NECROSIS SCORE BASED ON CONTRAST-ENHANCED CT

Percent of pancreas that is necrosed	Score
0	0
<33	2
33%–50	4
>50	6

CT severity index, unenhanced CT score + necrosis score.

future. Currently, however, assays for these markers are not widely available.

MANAGEMENT

The goals of management for patients with acute pancreatitis are given in Table 54.9.

Correcting Pathophysiologic Derangements and Ameliorating Symptoms

The most important component of initial management is fluid resuscitation. Third-space fluid losses can be large, with up to one third of plasma volume being sequestered. An indwelling urinary catheter should be placed, intravascular volume should be frequently assessed, and aggressive fluid and electrolyte replacement should be ensured.

Patients with SAP, as well as those for whom initial resuscitation fails, are best managed in a dedicated intensive care unit (ICU). Central venous monitoring will facilitate fluid management. Patients with severe cardiovascular derangements should have a Swan-Ganz catheter inserted for monitoring of pulmonary artery wedge pressure, cardiac output, and systemic vascular resistance. Patients should be closely monitored for development of distant organ failure, particularly respiratory, cardiovascular, and renal failure, so that supportive management of these conditions (positive-pressure ventilation, administration of vasopressor agents, and hemodialysis, respectively) can be instituted without delay.

Abdominal pain is usually ameliorated with intravenous narcotics. In the past, morphine was avoided because of concerns that morphine-induced increases in sphincter of Oddi pressure might exacerbate an episode of pancreatitis. However, there is no clinical evidence that morphine can induce or exacerbate acute pancreatitis. Other analgesic agents commonly used in patients with acute pancreatitis include meperidine and fentanyl. Evacuation of gastric contents using a nasogastric tube should be instituted if vomiting is a prominent symptom; otherwise, it is unnecessary.

TABLE 54.9 **TREATMENT**

GOAL OF TREATMENT FOR PATIENTS WITH ACUTE PANCREATITIS

Providing supportive care to correct pathophysiologic derangements (including those induced by distant organ failure) and to ameliorate symptoms
Minimizing the progression of pancreatic inflammation and injury
Treating the underlying etiologic factor responsible for causing pancreatitis
Managing complications of pancreatitis

Minimizing Progression of Pancreatic Inflammation and Injury

Identification of strategies for interrupting the inflammatory cascades that induce pancreatic injury and distant organ failure is an area of active investigation. Currently, the only method used in routine clinical practice is bowel rest (nothing by mouth). The rationale underlying this approach is that avoidance of oral nutrient intake may limit stimulation of pancreatic exocrine secretion induced by the presence of nutrients in the intestine, particularly the duodenum.

Patients with mild acute pancreatitis generally need no nutritional support, as their disease typically resolves within 1 week. In contrast, patients with SAP usually have a more prolonged disease course and should begin to receive nutritional support as early as feasible. Although these patients traditionally have been administered total parenteral nutrition (TPN), accumulating evidence suggests that enteral nutrition delivered to the jejunum is safe, is less costly, and may be associated with a lower complication rate than TPN in patients with acute pancreatitis.[14] Enteral nutrients delivered to the jejunum through nasojejunal tubes appear to have minimal stimulatory effects on pancreatic exocrine secretion. Administration of enteral nutrition is also associated with the theoretical advantage of helping to maintain the integrity of the intestinal mucosal barrier, thus potentially limiting or preventing bacterial translocation. However, TPN is still required in patients with severe ileus who do not tolerate enteral nutrition.

Clinical trials of agents that inhibit activated pancreatic enzymes, inhibit pancreatic secretion, or interrupt the inflammatory cascade have yielded disappointing results. Meta-analyses of clinical trials of gabexate mesylate (a proteinase inhibitor), somatostatin, and octreotide suggest these agents have limited, if any, efficacy in improving outcomes in acute pancreatitis.[15,16] A platelet-activating factor antagonist, lexipafant, showed promise in an initial study but not in a subsequent larger trial and is not currently recommended.[17,18] Other adjuncts for which clinical trials have failed to demonstrate efficacy in limiting pancreatic injury in patients with acute pancreatitis include glucagon, anticholinergics, fresh frozen plasma, and peritoneal lavage.

Treating the Underlying Cause

This discussion is particularly relevant to patients with gallstone pancreatitis. There is both theoretical and experimental rationale to believe that removal of gallstones impacted at the ampulla of Vater early in the course of an episode of acute gallstone pancreatitis might limit disease severity. The efficacy of early ERCP to accomplish this goal has been subjected to prospective, randomized clinical trials.[19,20] These studies show that early ERCP with stone extraction and sphincterotomy benefits the subset of patients with gallstone pancreatitis who have obstructive jaundice or cholangitis. In the absence of these features, early ERCP is associated with high complication rates but no apparent benefits and is therefore not recommended.

There is a 25% incidence of recurrent pancreatitis or other gallstone-related complications during the 6-week period following an episode of gallstone pancreatitis in patients who do not undergo cholecystectomy. Therefore, cholecystectomy should be performed in most patients once an episode of gallstone pancreatitis resolves. Endoscopic sphincterotomy is another option that is applicable in patients with comorbidities that preclude safe surgery.

Examples of other measures directed at correcting the underlying cause of pancreatitis include cessation of drugs known to cause pancreatitis and treatment of hypercalcemia or hyperlipidemia.

Preventing and Treating Complications

Complications of acute pancreatitis include pancreatic abscesses and infected necrosis, acute fluid collections and pseudocysts, pancreatic ascites and fistulas, splenic vein thrombosis, and arterial pseudoaneurysms. Infected necrosis and pseudoaneurysms are discussed in more detail later.

Infected Necrosis

Infection of pancreatic and peripancreatic necrosis complicates 30% to 70% of cases of acute necrotizing pancreatitis and most commonly becomes established during the second to third weeks after onset of disease. Historical data suggest that mortality rates associated with untreated infected necrosis approach 100%. The diagnosis of infected necrosis is made based on cultures of aspirates of fluid or necrotic tissue obtained during CT-guided fine needle aspiration (FNA) or specimens collected during surgery. The concordance rate between bacteriologic results of FNA and those of surgical specimens is greater than 95%.[21] In addition, the visualization of air bubbles within necrotic tissue on CT scans is highly suggestive of infection. Because presence or absence of infection has a strong impact on surgical decision making, FNA should be obtained in patients with acute necrotizing pancreatitis who exhibit clinical features of sepsis or whose clinical course deteriorates beyond 1 to 2 weeks after onset of disease.

If FNA indicates the presence of infected necrosis, surgical intervention is indicated. Unlike pancreatic abscesses, which are typically amenable to percutaneous drainage, infected necrosis consists of thick and tenacious material that must be mechanically débrided. The abdomen is entered through a vertical midline or bilateral subcostal incision. The anterior surface of the pancreas can be exposed by dividing the gastrocolic ligament (greater omentum) and entering the lesser sac. If inflammatory changes have obliterated the lesser sac, this approach may be hazardous. In such cases, an alternative route to the pancreas is achieved by dividing avascular portions of the transverse mesocolon, with care taken to preserve the middle colic vessels. Clearly nonviable tissue should be débrided bluntly. Anatomic resections should be avoided to minimize potential for removing viable pancreatic parenchyma. The débridement field is irrigated with several liters of sterile saline, after which large-bore drains are placed. Postoperatively, the drains are left in place at least 7 days and until the effluent becomes clear. If more prolonged drainage is necessary because a pancreatic fistula develops, the surgically placed drains should be replaced with soft, smaller-bore drains to minimize potential for bowel erosion.

The procedure described previously is known as *necrosectomy with closed drainage*. In a variant of this procedure, both gauze packing and drains are placed at the time of surgery and gradually withdrawn postoperatively. Other procedures include *necrosectomy with open packing* and *necrosectomy with planned, staged relaparotomy* in which the initial operation is followed by repeat laparotomies, during which gauze packing is changed or additional debridement is performed, every 2 days until all necrotic tissues have been removed. Another option is *necrosectomy with continuous lavage* in which high-volume lavage of the lesser sac is performed, using drains placed at the time of surgery, until the effluent becomes clear and the patients clinical course improves. These latter procedures are resource-intensive but may be necessary if necrosectomy is performed early in the course of disease, before clear demarcation between necrotic and viable tissues has occurred. Modern mortality rates associated with necrosectomy performed for infected necrosis range from 10% to 20%.[5,6] On long-term follow-up, approximately 25% of survivors develop exocrine insufficiency, and 30% develop endocrine insufficiency. Recently, laparoscopic and nonsurgical approaches to necrosectomy, such as endoscopic transgastric necrosectomy and percutaneous necrosectomy, have been reported. Complete débridement of all necrotic tissues is difficult to achieve using these methods; they should be considered investigational until improved outcomes are achievable.

Although surgical débridement is clearly indicated for infected necrosis, its role in sterile necrosis has undergone evolution.[22,23] In the past, early necrosectomy was recommended for patients with necrotizing pancreatitis, even in the absence of documented infection. The rationale for this approach was to prevent infection from developing and to remove the source of toxins and inflammatory mediators. Today, most authors recommend avoiding surgery in patients without documentation of infected necrosis, based on favorable outcomes reported using this conservative approach.[5,6] However, there remains a subset of patients with sterile necrosis who, despite prolonged supportive care, have persistent problems, including pain, malaise, and gastric outlet obstruction. If necrosectomy is performed to provide symptomatic palliation, it should be delayed until at least 4 weeks after onset of disease, to maximize the probability of clear-cut demarcation between viable and nonviable tissues.

Because of the high morbidity and mortality rates associated with infected necrosis, there has been much investigation into the use of antibiotics as prophylaxis against infection. Initial clinical trials failed to demonstrate a benefit of prophylactic antibiotics; however, these studies were flawed by the inclusion of patients with mild disease who were at low risk for developing infected necrosis and the use of antibiotics with poor penetration into the pancreas. Of the clinical trials reported in the past decade, five have shown a significant reduction in the incidence of pancreatic infection and one has shown a significant reduction in mortality among patients receiving antibiotic prophylaxis.[24] Based on this evidence, the use of antibiotic prophylaxis in patients documented to have necrotizing pancreatitis has become a widespread practice. Antibiotics demonstrated to have adequate penetration in pancreatic tissue (imipenem, third-generation cephalosporins, piperacillin, mezlocillin, fluoroquinolones, and metronidazole) should be used. The role of antibiotic prophylaxis in pancreatitis remains controversial, however, given the risks of fungal superinfection and the selection of resistant organisms. Further, studies that show no benefit of antibiotic prophylaxis continue to be reported.[25]

Pseudocysts

Acute fluid collections develop in up to 30% to 50% of patients with acute pancreatitis. As most resolve spontaneously, no specific treatment directed at acute fluid collections is necessary in the absence of evidence that the fluid is infected. However, in up to 10% of patients with acute pancreatitis, these fluid collections progress to develop a wall of fibrous granulation tissue, at which point they are classified as *pseudocysts.* The walls of pseudocysts generally require at least 4 weeks from the onset of pancreatitis to develop. Pseudocysts are distinguished from true pancreatic cysts, which have epithelium-lined walls.

Most pseudocysts are asymptomatic; however, they can cause upper abdominal pain, gastric outlet obstruction, and obstructive jaundice. They also have the potential to rupture, to bleed, and to become infected.

Pseudocysts are usually diagnosed on ultrasonography or CT scanning (Fig. 54.5). It is important to distinguish pseudocysts from neoplastic cysts of the pancreas, as some of these are malignant or have malignant potential and therefore may need to be managed aggressively. Neoplastic cysts should be suspected under the following circumstances: (a) there is no history of or other clinical evidence that suggests the presence of antecedent pancreatitis or pancreatic trauma and (b) the presence of internal septa within the cyst as detected on imaging studies. Aspiration and examination of cyst fluid may be required if a neoplastic cyst is suspected. Most pseudocysts communicate with the pancreatic duct; hence, pseudocysts usually contain fluid with high amylase concentrations. In contrast, most neoplastic cysts do not communicate with the pancreatic duct and contain fluid with low amylase concentrations. Because these criteria lack absolute predictive power, a high degree of suspicion for the presence of neoplastic cysts should be maintained if warranted by clinical findings.

The management of pseudocysts continues to evolve. In the past, surgical drainage of pseudocysts was recommended for pseudocysts (even if asymptomatic) that persisted beyond a 6-week period of observation. This recommendation was based on a widely quoted report that suggested that pseudocysts that persist more than 6 weeks rarely resolve spontaneously and are associated with high complication rates.[26] However, more recent reports suggest that the natural history of asymptomatic pseudocysts follows a more benign course, with most pseudocysts less than 6 cm in diameter resolving spontaneously without complications.[27,28]

Current well-accepted indications for intervention include the presence of symptoms attributable to the pseudocyst and growth during a period of observation. Whether large (>6 cm in diameter), asymptomatic pseudocysts that remain stable in size should undergo drainage is controversial.

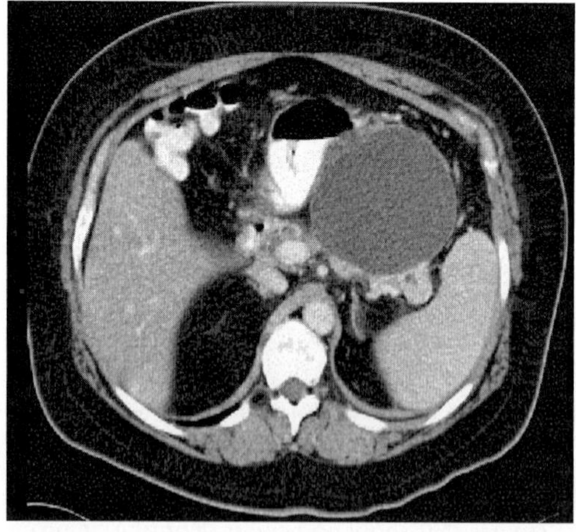

FIGURE 54.5 Computed tomography scan of pancreatic pseudocyst.

Treatment options include percutaneous aspiration, percutaneous drainage, internal drainage (performed surgically or endoscopically), and resection. These methods have yet to be compared in a controlled trial; however, available evidence suggests that surgical therapy is associated with the highest efficacy and lowest recurrence rates. Percutaneous aspiration alone is associated with high recurrence rates; even prolonged drainage is likely to fail in the presence of a pancreatic ductal stricture. Endoscopic cystgastrostomy is an option for patients in whom the pseudocyst is intimately adherent to the posterior wall of the stomach; however, high rates of bleeding-related complications have been reported in some series.

The most commonly performed surgical procedures used to treat pseudocysts include cystgastrostomy or cystoduodenostomy, applicable if a portion of the pseudocyst wall is adherent to the stomach or duodenum, respectively. Otherwise, the cyst wall can be anastomosed to a Roux limb of jejunum. These procedures, which can be performed as open or laparoscopic operations, should be delayed until pseudocyst wall maturation occurs. Mortality rates associated with surgical drainage procedures average less than 5%, with pseudocyst recurrence rates averaging 10%.

KEY POINTS

- **Severe acute pancreatitis accounts for about 20% of cases and is defined as acute pancreatitis associated with one or more of the following: pancreatic necrosis, distant organ failure, and the development of local complications such as hemorrhage, abscess, or pseudocyst.**
- **In the United States, more than 75% of cases of acute pancreatitis are attributable to either gallstones or alcohol.**
- **Approximately 80% of cases of acute pancreatitis are mild associated with minimal systemic derangements and generally resolve within 5 to 7 days, even with minimal therapy.**
- **The mortality rate associated with severe acute pancreatitis ranges from 10% to 20% with half of the deaths in the first 2 weeks as the result of SIRS-induced multisystem organ failure and the remaining occurring later as the result of pancreatic necrosis/infection.**
- **CT scanning is the most important imaging test for acute pancreatitis and is useful in confirming the diagnosis, assessing disease severity, and detecting complications.**
- **The most important component of initial management of acute pancreatitis is fluid resuscitation.**
- **Early ERCP with sphincterotomy and stone extraction has been shown in randomized controlled trials to benefit the subset of patients with gallstone pancreatitis and associated obstructive jaundice and cholangitis.**
- **Infection of pancreatic and peripancreatic necrosis complicates 30% to 70% of cases of acute necrotizing pancreatitis and most commonly becomes established during the second to third weeks after onset of disease.**
- **Treatment options for pancreatic pseudocysts include percutaneous aspiration, percutaneous drainage, internal drainage (performed surgically or endoscopically), or resection; surgical therapy is associated with the highest efficacy and lowest recurrence rates.**

References

1. Bradley EL III. A clinically based classification system for acute pancreatitis. Summary of the International Symposium on Acute Pancreatitis, Atlanta, GA, September 11 through 13, 1992. *Arch Surg.* 1993;128:586.

2. **Swaroop VS, Chari ST, Clain JE. Severe acute pancreatitis. *JAMA* 2004;291:2865.**
3. Steer ML. Pathogenesis of acute pancreatitis. *Digestion* 1997;58[suppl 1]: 46.
4. Saluja AK, Donovan EA, Yamanaka K, et al. Cerulein-induced in vitro activation of trypsinogen in rat pancreatic acini is mediated by cathepsin B. *Gastroenterology* 1997;113:304.
5. Ashley SW, Perez A, Pierce EA, et al. Necrotizing pancreatitis: contemporary analysis of 99 consecutive cases. *Ann Surg.* 2001;234:572.
6. Buchler MW, Gloor B, Muller CA, et al. Acute necrotizing pancreatitis: treatment strategy according to the status of infection. *Ann Surg.* 2000; 232:619.
7. Corfield AP, Cooper MJ, Williamson RC, et al. Prediction of severity in acute pancreatitis: prospective comparison of three prognostic indices. *Lancet* 1985;2:403.
8. Banks PA. Epidemiology, natural history, and predictors of disease outcome in acute and chronic pancreatitis. *Gastrointest Endosc.* 2002;56[6 suppl]: S226.
9. Ranson JHC, Rifkind KM, Roses DF, et al. Prognostic signs and the role of operative management in acute pancreatitis. *Surg Gynecol Obstet.* 1974; 139:69.
10. **Larvin M, McMahon MJ. Apache II score for assessment and monitoring of acute pancreatitis. *Lancet* 1989;334:201.**
11. Williams M, Simms HH. Prognostic usefulness of scoring systems in critically ill patients with severe acute pancreatitis. *Crit Care Med.* 1999; 27:901.
12. **Balthazar EJ, Robinson DL, Megibow AJ, et al. Acute pancreatitis: value of CT in establishing prognosis. *Radiology* 1990;174:331.**
13. Johnson CD, Stephens DH, Sarr MG. CT of acute pancreatitis: Correlation between lack of contrast enhancement and pancreatic necrosis. *Am J Radiol.* 1991;156:93.
14. Marik PE, Zaloga GP. Meta-analysis of parenteral nutrition versus enteral nutrition in patients with acute pancreatitis. *BMJ* 2004;328:1407. Epub 2004 Jun 02.
15. Messori A, Rampazzo R, Scroccaro G, et al. Effectiveness of gabexate mesylate in acute pancreatitis. A metaanalysis. *Dig Dis Sci.* 1995;40:734.
16. Andriulli A, Leandro G, Clemente R, et al. Meta-analysis of somatostatin, octreotide and gabexate mesylate in the therapy of acute pancreatitis. *Aliment Pharmacol Ther.* 1998;12:237.
17. Kingsnorth AN, Galloway SW, Formela LJ. Randomized, double-blind phase II trial of Lexipafant, a platelet-activating factor antagonist, in human acute pancreatitis. *Br J Surg.* 1995;82:1414.
18. Johnson CD, Kingsnorth AN, Imrie CW, et al. Double blind, randomised, placebo controlled study of a platelet activating factor antagonist, lexipafant, in the treatment and prevention of organ failure in predicted severe acute pancreatitis. *Gut* 2001;48:62.
19. Fan ST, Lai EC, Mok FP, et al. Early treatment of acute biliary pancreatitis by endoscopic papillotomy. *N Engl J Med.* 1993;328:228.
20. Bolsch UR, Nitsche R, Ludtke R, et al. German Study Group on Acute Biliary Pancreatitis: early ERCP and papillotomy compared with conservative treatment for acute biliary pancreatitis. *N Engl J Med.* 1997;336:237.
21. Gerzof SG, Banks PA, Robbins AH, et al. Early diagnosis of pancreatic infection by computer tomography-guided aspiration. *Gastroenterology* 1987;93:1315.
22. Warshaw AL. Pancreatic necrosis: to débride or not to débride—that is the question. *Ann Surg.* 2000;232:627.
23. **Connor S, Neoptolomos JP. Surgery for pancreatic necrosis: "whom, when, and what." *World J Gastroenterol.* 2004;10:1697.**
24. Golub R, Siddiqi F, Pohl D. Role of antibiotics in acute pancreatitis: A meta-analysis. *J Gastrointest Surg.* 1998;2:496.
25. Isenmann R, Runzi M, Kron M, et al, for the German Antibiotics in Severe Acute Pancreatitis Study Group. Prophylactic antibiotic treatment in patients with predicted severe acute pancreatitis: a placebo-controlled, double-blind trial. *Gastroenterology* 2004;126:997.
26. Bradley EL III, Clements JL Jr, Gonzales AC. The natural history of pancreatic pseudocysts: a unified concept of management. *Am J Surg.* 1979;137: 135.
27. Vitas GJ, Sarr MG. Selected management of pancreatic pseudocysts: operative versus expectant management. *Surgery* 1992;111:123.
28. Yeo CJ, Bastidas JA, Lynch-Nyhan A, et al. The natural history of pancreatic pseudocysts documented by computed tomography. *Surg Gynecol Obstet.* 1990;170:411.

CHAPTER 55 ■ CHRONIC PANCREATITIS

ISAAC SAMUEL AND RAYMOND J. JOEHL

DEFINITION

Chronic pancreatitis is a chronic inflammatory condition of the pancreas characterized by severe upper abdominal pain that often progresses to pancreatic exocrine (malabsorption) and endocrine (diabetes mellitus) insufficiency.

EPIDEMIOLOGY

North American and Danish studies indicate an incidence of chronic pancreatitis of 4 cases per 100,000 people per year and a prevalence of 13 cases per 100,000 inhabitants.[1,2] Although alcohol consumption is the most important predisposing factor for chronic pancreatitis, environmental and hereditary factors also possibly play a role as evidenced by the a greater per capita incidence of chronic pancreatitis in Denmark than in Sweden even though per capita alcohol consumption is greater in Sweden.

ETIOLOGY AND CLASSIFICATION

The etiologic factors of chronic pancreatitis are similar to acute pancreatitis, but chronic alcoholism is responsible for up to 80% of cases of chronic pancreatitis in developed countries. Although gallstones account for the majority of acute pancreatitis cases worldwide, gallstone-induced acute pancreatitis only occasionally results in chronic pancreatitis.

Most classification systems of chronic pancreatitis have placed undue dependence on the effects of chronic pancreatitis, resulting in the disproportionate inclusion of patients with end-stage and alcoholic chronic pancreatitis.[1,3] With a better understanding of the etiologic and pathobiologic aspects of the disease, and with the advent of improved imaging techniques, a new etiology-based classification system has been proposed.[1,3] The *TIGAR-O system* (Toxic-metabolic, Idiopathic, Genetic, Autoimmune, Recurrent severe acute pancreatitis, and Obstructive) for the classification of chronic pancreatitis has the potential to provide an approach in which earlier diagnosis and more timely preventive intervention are emphasized.[1,3]

Because chronic pancreatitis may be multifactorial in etiology, the TIGAR-O classification system inherently allows overlap between the groups, in which one disease entity appears under more than one classification group.

Toxic-Metabolic Chronic Pancreatitis

The toxic and metabolic factors implicated in the development of chronic pancreatitis include chronic alcohol abuse, tobacco smoking, hypercalcemia and hyperparathyroidism, certain toxins (e.g., organotin compounds), and probably also hyperlipidemia and chronic renal failure.

Idiopathic Chronic Pancreatitis

Most cases of nonalcoholic chronic pancreatitis in North America and Europe are idiopathic and show a bimodal age distribution. In the juvenile type, the predominant presenting symptom is pain. In the senile type, the disease is often painless presenting with exocrine insufficiency.[4] *Tropical chronic pancreatitis (nutritional pancreatitis),* for a long time thought to be related to chronic malnutrition, is also included under the idiopathic group because dietary factors could not be implicated in a pathogenic role.[1]

Genetic Factors in Chronic Pancreatitis

Several genes have been associated with the development of chronic pancreatitis.[1] In *hereditary chronic pancreatitis,* mutation of the cationic trypsinogen gene *PRSS1* (autosomal dominant, 80% penetrance) spontaneously incites a chronic inflammatory process due to premature trypsinogen activation within the pancreas and chronic pancreatitis begins in childhood (average age 10 to 12 years). On the other hand, certain genetic defects—such as mutations of the pancreatic secretory trypsin inhibitor (*SPINK1*) and cystic fibrosis transmembrane conductance regulator (*CFTR*) genes—do not cause chronic pancreatitis on their own but are associated with a greater risk of developing chronic pancreatitis.

Autoimmune Chronic Pancreatitis

Autoimmune chronic pancreatitis is distinct from other forms of chronic pancreatitis from the point of view of pathogenesis, clinical features, histologic findings, treatment, and prognosis.[1,3] It is most often primary (isolated) but may also be secondary to other immunologic disorders such as inflammatory bowel disease, primary biliary cirrhosis, primary sclerosing cholangitis, or Sjögren syndrome. The characteristic histologic feature of autoimmune pancreatitis is the prominent lymphocytic infiltration of the pancreatic parenchyma and the condition responds well to steroid therapy.

Recurrent Severe Acute Pancreatitis-induced Chronic Pancreatitis

Although a distinguishing feature between acute pancreatitis and chronic pancreatitis is that the pancreatic morphologic changes in acute pancreatitis typically reverse when the inciting event is overcome, recurrent attacks of severe acute pancreatitis can progress to the development of chronic pancreatitis with persistent and progressive changes in the pancreas.[1] Examples include alcoholic pancreatitis, hereditary pancreatitis, and hyperlipidemia-induced pancreatitis.

Obstructive Chronic Pancreatitis

Conditions causing mechanical obstruction of the pancreatic duct can result in the development of chronic pancreatitis.[1] Tumors, strictures, posttraumatic scarring, pancreatic pseudocysts, pancreas divisum, and sphincter of Oddi dysfunction cause a pathologically distinct form of chronic pancreatitis characterized by pancreatic ductal dilatation and parenchymal atrophy and fibrosis. In contrast to alcohol-induced chronic pancreatitis, obstruction-induced pancreatitis is rarely associated with the formation of intraductal stones, and parenchymal changes most often regress with relief of the obstruction. Additionally, the pancreatic duct is diffusely dilated in contrast to the segmental stricture and dilation of the duct seen in other forms of chronic pancreatitis.

PATHOLOGY

In individual cases of chronic pancreatitis the underlying cause is probably multifactorial involving interactions between two or more etiologies or risk factors. This may explain why only the minority (about 10%) of patients with long-term alcohol abuse actually develop chronic pancreatitis. For instance, there is a subgroup of patients that die of alcoholic hepatic cirrhosis without developing chronic pancreatitis. On the other hand, African-American alcoholics are more prone to develop chronic pancreatitis than cirrhosis.

In contrast to acute pancreatitis that is characterized by clinical and histologic improvement after the underlying cause has been treated or removed, the changes of alcoholic chronic pancreatitis are typically persistent and progressive. Destruction of the pancreatic parenchyma and fibrosis of the gland are characteristic, and these lead to strictures of the pancreatic duct, dilatations, and calcifications. On the other hand, obstructive chronic pancreatitis is most often reversed when the obstruction is relieved, and autoimmune chronic pancreatitis shows dramatic reversal when steroid therapy is instituted.[3] In obstructive pancreatitis pancreatic calculi and intraductal protein plugs are not observed and ductal epithelium is preserved. In autoimmune pancreatitis, the glandular enlargement and ductal stenosis are secondary to intense lymphocytic infiltration and not associated with duct epithelial destruction and thus respond to steroid treatment with reversal of structural and functional changes. Therefore, injury to the duct epithelium and basement membrane may contribute substantially to the progressive and irreversible nature of alcohol-induced chronic pancreatitis.

Although alcohol is the major cause of chronic pancreatitis, the mechanism of injury is not known. The type of alcohol and the manner of consumption do not seem to correlate with disease severity, but the severity of chronic pancreatitis does appear to increase with the amount and duration of alcohol consumption.[5] Additionally, susceptibility and disease severity appear to vary significantly between individual people, and chronic pancreatitis can progress even after the cessation of alcohol consumption. Chronic pancreatitis develops in only 10% of alcoholics, but autopsy series reveal an incidence of chronic pancreatitis that is 50 times greater in alcoholics than in nondrinking controls. The mechanisms of alcohol-induced cellular injury are unknown, but inferences can be drawn by examining the effects of alcohol on pancreatic secretion. It appears that long-term alcohol intake causes changes in the composition of pancreatic juice, including increased protein concentration, decreased flow, and decreased bicarbonate concentration.[6] These changes produce a juice with increased viscosity that is prone to forming stones and protein plugs. Ductal obstruction produces progressive injury and destruction of parenchyma, with a deterioration of both exocrine and endocrine function.

Pancreatitis develops in approximately 10% to 15% of patients with hyperparathyroidism, and if inadequately treated, it becomes chronic, presumably as a result of the effects of persistent hypercalcemia.[7] Calcium is a potent stimulator of pancreatic exocrine secretion. An increase in the concentration of calcium in pancreatic juice leads to intraductal precipitation.

Pancreas divisum, the most common congenital abnormality of the pancreas, results from incomplete or absent fusion of the ducts of the ventral and dorsal pancreas in embryologic development. It is postulated that the minor papilla is inadequate to handle all the exocrine secretion from the main body of the gland, so that the main duct becomes relatively obstructed. Whether or not pancreas divisum can cause chronic pancreatitis remains controversial. In an early report by Cotton,[8] the incidence of pancreas divisum on endoscopic retrograde cholangiopancreatography (ERCP) was 25.6% in patients with idiopathic pancreatitis and only 3.6% in patients undergoing ERCP for biliary tract disease. More recently, however, several studies have found the incidence of pancreas divisum to be similar in patients with and without pancreatitis.[9]

Blunt and penetrating trauma to the pancreas can lead to pancreatic injury. Parenchymal injury with duct disruption can lead to the formation of pseudocysts, pancreatic ascites, and pancreatic fistulae. Additionally, injury to the blood supply of the pancreas may result in ischemia and stricture of the pancreatic duct. Inadequate or delayed treatment can lead to persistent injury and ultimately chronic pancreatitis.

CLINICAL PRESENTATION

Pain

The intractable pain recalcitrant to various treatment modalities, repeated hospital admissions, narcotic dependence, malabsorption, diabetes mellitus and its attending complications, and the increased risk of pancreatic cancer, altogether make chronic pancreatitis an ominous disease entity. Upper abdominal pain that is aggravated by meals and radiates to the back (Fig. 55.1) is the earliest symptom of chronic pancreatitis and, as the condition progresses, the manifestations of exocrine and endocrine pancreatic insufficiency become apparent. However, morphologic changes of chronic pancreatitis can exist for long periods before symptoms develop. Conversely, a symptomatic patient can show a completely negative workup. Frequently, sitting upright and tilting the torso forward or lying prone alleviates the pain, whereas the supine position tends to aggravate the pain. The pain usually worsens but may even decrease and disappear completely ("pancreatic burnout") as the disease progresses.[10,11] Continued or recurrent inflammation of the head of the pancreas may result in duodenal narrowing and, more commonly, stenosis and obstruction of the distal common bile duct, both of which can be associated with abdominal pain.

Malabsorption

It takes almost a 90% loss of functional pancreas for symptoms such as diarrhea, steatorrhea, and azotorrhea to develop.[12] Pancreatic insufficiency resulting from alcohol-induced chronic pancreatitis usually takes 10 to 20 years to develop. The secretion of lipase is usually diminished earlier than the secretion of the proteolytic enzymes, and as a result, steatorrhea generally precedes proteinaceous diarrhea. Patients with fat malabsorption report loose, greasy, and foul-smelling stools associated with crampy abdominal pain and excessive flatus. Weight loss almost always occurs with malabsorption, and occasionally significant deficiencies of the fat-soluble vitamins develop. Postprandial pancreatic bicarbonate secretion is similarly diminished in long-standing, severe chronic pancreatitis. The duodenal pH may decrease (pH <4) within 90 minutes after ingestion of a meal, and when the bicarbonate concentration is inadequate, an acidic milieu with precipitation of bile salts and inactivation of pancreatic enzymes results in a further decrease in lipid and protein digestion.

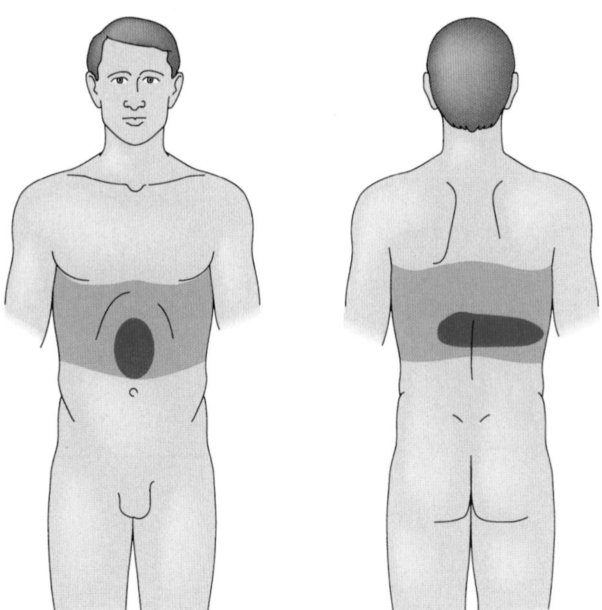

FIGURE 55.1 Topographic locations of pancreatic pain.

Endocrine Insufficiency

Although the derangement of pancreatic exocrine function is the most common clinical concern in chronic pancreatitis, glucose intolerance frequently develops early in the course of chronic pancreatitis, and clinically evident diabetes occurs later. Altered insulin secretion is observed in these patients, as is a blunted insulin and C-peptide response to oral or intravenous glucose. Endocrine insufficiency develops in up to 60% of patients, but in general not until after the diagnosis of chronic pancreatitis has been made. Diabetic ketoacidosis and nephropathy are rare, but diabetic neuropathy and retinopathy can occur.

DIAGNOSIS

Diagnostic investigations include imaging studies, pancreatic function tests, and histologic evaluation. Because obtaining a tissue sample of the pancreas is not easy, histologic studies are not performed on a routine basis. Imaging studies and pancreatic function tests used in a complementary fashion will reduce the possibility of missing the diagnosis in a significant number of patients. Serum amylase and lipase levels are often not elevated. Frequently, a typical history combined with a

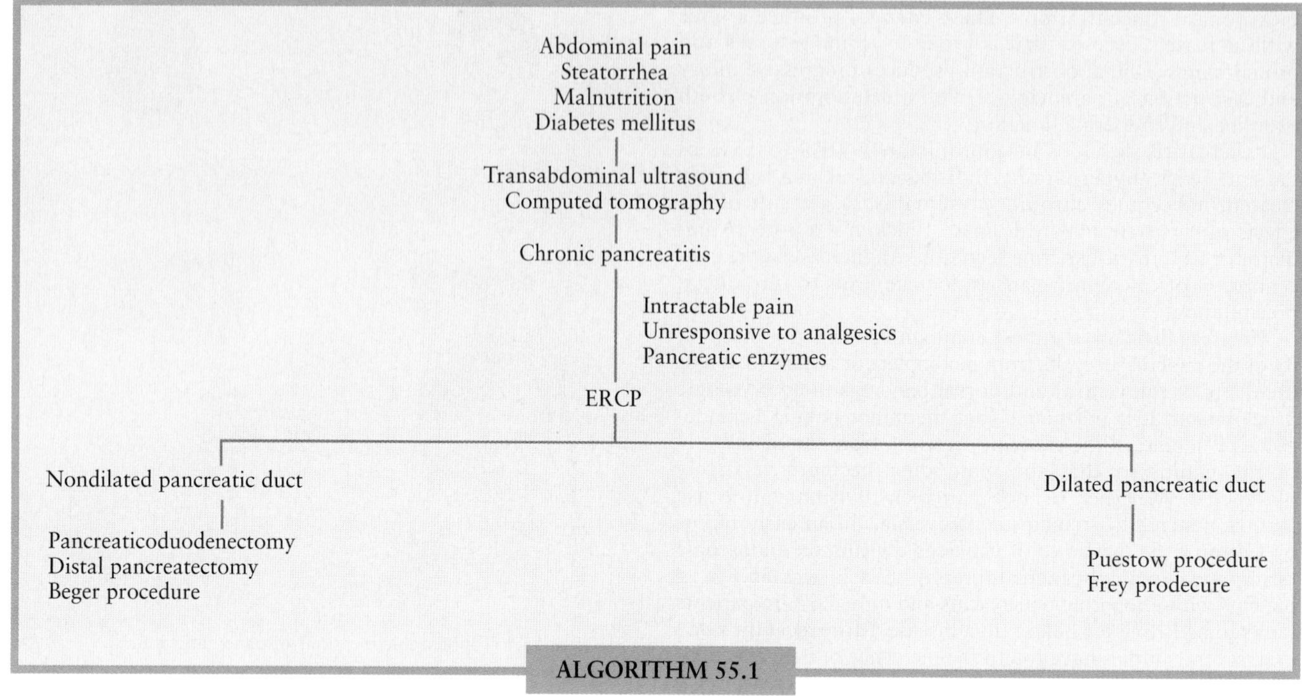

ALGORITHM 55.1 Diagnosis and treatment of chronic pancreatitis.

plain radiograph of the abdomen showing the classic findings of speckled calcification of the pancreas is sufficient to clinch the diagnosis. On the other hand, mild cases of symptomatic chronic pancreatitis may elude diagnosis due to a completely negative workup. In most instances the sensitivity and specificity of diagnostic modalities increase in parallel with increases in the severity of the disease.[1,3]

The diagnostic algorithm described here can be employed in all cases irrespective of the etiology[1,3] (Algorithm 55.1). First, noninvasive tests such as transabdominal ultrasound, computed tomography (CT), magnetic resonance imaging (MRI), and pancreatic function tests can be used. Measurement of fecal human specific elastase-1 concentration has been found to be more convenient, specific and sensitive than several other tests of pancreatic exocrine function. If the diagnosis is not apparent, then endoscopic tests such as ERCP and endoscopic high-resolution ultrasound are available. The secretin test is considered a gold standard but is performed only in some centers. Finally, histopathologic examination of pancreatic biopsies, obtained percutaneously or surgically, may be ultimately required to make a diagnosis.

Imaging Studies

Transabdominal ultrasonography has a sensitivity of 60% to 70% and a specificity of 80% to 90%. Ultrasonographic findings of a dilated main pancreatic duct (>4 mm), large cavitary dilatations (>1 cm), and calcifications correlate well with changes seen on ERCP and support the diagnosis of chronic pancreatitis.[13] *Computed tomography* is more sensitive than ultrasonography for identifying pancreatic calcifications and making the diagnosis of chronic pancreatitis. The most common findings include duct dilatation (Fig. 55.2), a shrunken calcified pancreas, and cystic lesions (Fig. 55.3). *Magnetic resonance imaging* is capable of detecting changes of chronic pancreatitis at an earlier stage than that possible by CT.[3] *Magnetic resonance cholangiopancreatography (MRCP)* is less sensitive than ERCP as it can evaluate main pancreatic duct abnormalities but not ductal branches; however, ionizing radiation and radiopaque contrast are avoided, and it can be used even if the papilla is inaccessible to ERCP such as after Roux-en-Y gastric bypass for morbid obesity.[1,3] *ERCP* has become the "gold standard" for making the diagnosis of chronic pancreatitis (Fig. 55.4) especially when tissue diagnosis is not available.[1,3] It is widely recognized as the most sensitive (90%) diagnostic test with an equally good specificity (90%). In moderate to severe chronic pancreatitis, the degree of ductal distortion (Figs. 55.5 and 55.6) correlates strongly with functional pancreatic reserve and histologic grade.[14] The specificity of ERCP is extremely high in advanced chronic pancreatitis, but with less severe disease, the peripheral ductal abnormalities (stricture, ectasia, and dilatation) associated with

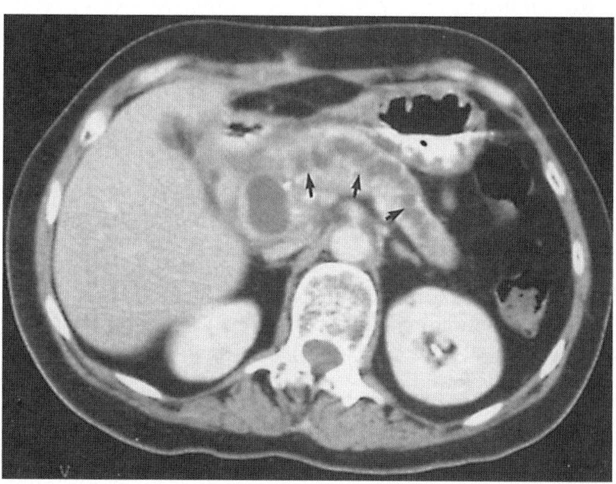

FIGURE 55.2 Abdominal computed tomography in a patient with chronic pancreatitis shows dilatation of the main pancreatic duct (*arrows*).

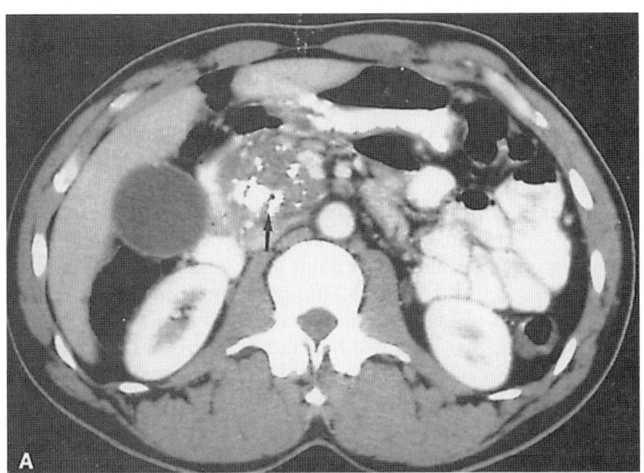

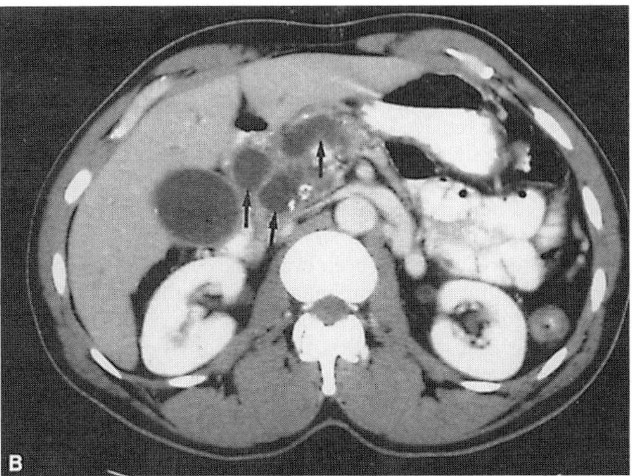

FIGURE 55.3 Abdominal computed tomography demonstrates pancreatic calcifications (*arrow, A*) and associated cystic lesions (*arrows, B*).

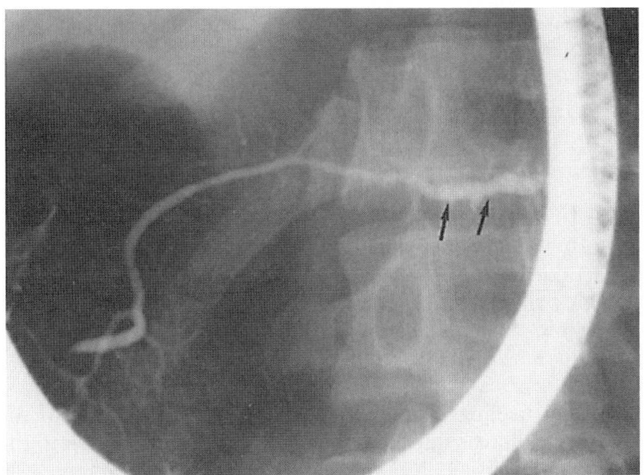

FIGURE 55.4 Endoscopic retrograde cholangiopancreatography (ERCP) illustrates early changes of chronic pancreatitis, with ductal ectasia confined to the pancreatic tail (*arrows*).

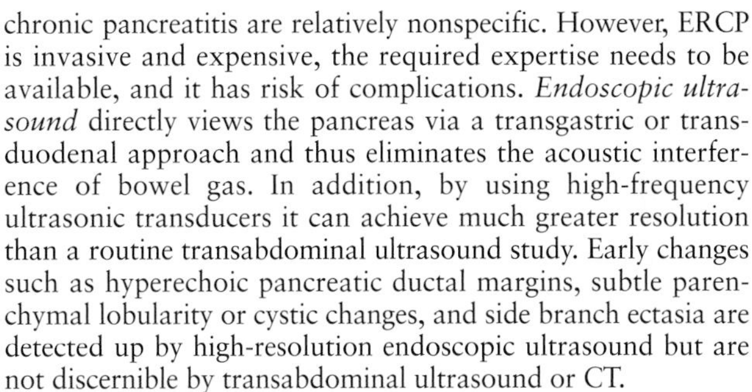

chronic pancreatitis are relatively nonspecific. However, ERCP is invasive and expensive, the required expertise needs to be available, and it has risk of complications. *Endoscopic ultrasound* directly views the pancreas via a transgastric or transduodenal approach and thus eliminates the acoustic interference of bowel gas. In addition, by using high-frequency ultrasonic transducers it can achieve much greater resolution than a routine transabdominal ultrasound study. Early changes such as hyperechoic pancreatic ductal margins, subtle parenchymal lobularity or cystic changes, and side branch ectasia are detected up by high-resolution endoscopic ultrasound but are not discernible by transabdominal ultrasound or CT.

Tests of Pancreatic Exocrine Function

Tests of pancreatic exocrine function either directly measure exocrine function or evaluate the secondary effects of impaired enzyme secretion. They can also be divided into invasive and noninvasive tests based on whether endoscopy is required or not. The secretin test is the gold standard but is performed only in a

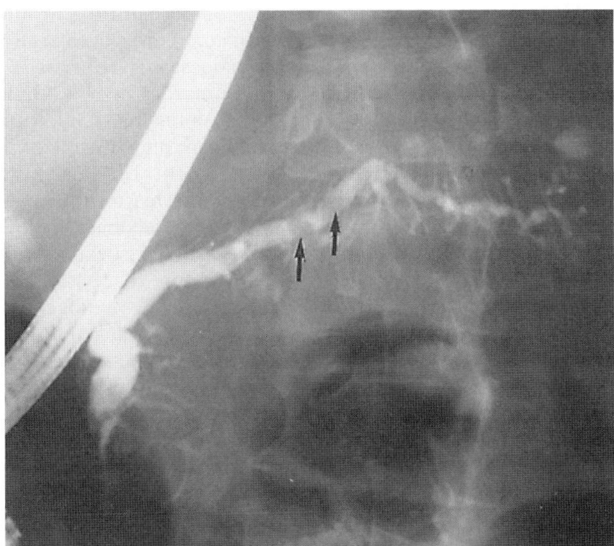

FIGURE 55.5 Endoscopic retrograde cholangiopancreatography (ERCP) illustrates moderate dilation of the main pancreatic duct and ectasia of the secondary ducts associated with moderately advanced chronic pancreatitis. Arrows indicate intraductal pancreatic stones.

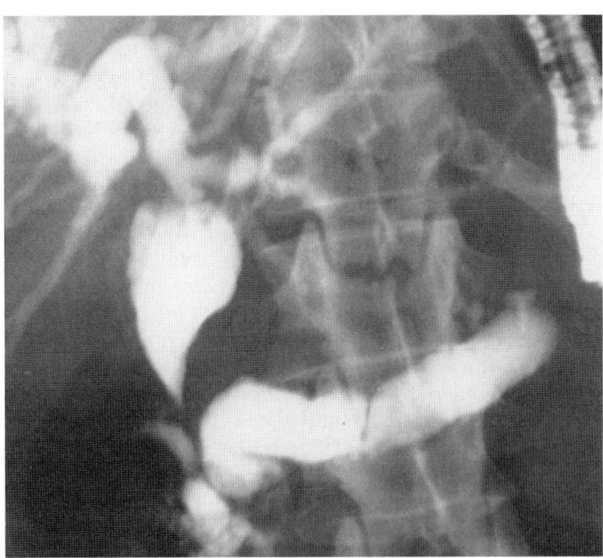

FIGURE 55.6 Endoscopic retrograde cholangiopancreatography demonstrates florid pancreatic ductal dilatation associated with end-stage chronic pancreatitis.

few specialized centers. Measurement of human specific elastase-1 concentration in feces is simple and accurate, has reasonable sensitivity when exocrine insufficiency is present, is useful even when patients are on pancreatic enzyme replacement therapy, and has therefore replaced other tests such as fecal chymotrypsin measurement, the bentiromide test, and the pancreolauryl test.

Direct measurements of pancreatic exocrine function require endoscopic cannulation of the pancreatic duct and assay of one or more components of pancreatic juice. A number of pancreatic juice components have been evaluated, but studies suggest that all pancreatic juice components are equally depressed in chronic pancreatitis. Moreover, not one of the components differentiates chronic pancreatitis from pancreatic cancer. The basal secretory rate of the exocrine pancreas is extremely variable in humans; thus, meaningful measurement of exocrine function requires some form of pancreatic stimulation. The most common method to stimulate the pancreas directly is the administration of secretin. Indirect stimulation can be achieved by feeding a standard meal (Lundh test), although this method is thought to be inferior to direct stimulation. Measurement of pancreatic juice components is most accurate only in the presence of severe disease. Direct measurement of exocrine pancreatic function is not commonly performed because of the inability to diagnose early disease consistently, the paucity of centers performing the studies, and the discomfort of an endoscopic procedure. Additionally, the direct measurement of pancreatic exocrine function is unreliable in patients with concomitant diabetes mellitus or cirrhosis.

Most of the indirect tests of pancreatic exocrine function measure the absorption of a compound that first must be digested by pancreatic enzymes. Unfortunately, malabsorption does not become detectable until pancreatic secretion has diminished to less than 10% of normal; therefore, the indirect tests of pancreatic exocrine function cannot detect early chronic pancreatitis. Interestingly, most of the indirect tests were first evaluated in patients with severe chronic pancreatitis and normal controls. The tests appeared promising until they were performed in patients with less severe disease, in whom the results were found to be much less sensitive and specific than originally thought.

In the *bentiromide test,* the patient ingests *N*-benzoyl-L-tyrosyl-*p*-aminobenzoic acid (NBT-PABA), which is digested by chymotrypsin to release PABA. Free PABA is absorbed in the small intestine and is excreted by the kidney. The quantity of excreted PABA is a measure of pancreatic exocrine function. The sensitivity of the bentiromide test is directly related to disease severity. In patients with end-stage disease the test can be almost 100% sensitive, whereas in patients with mild disease the test may only be 40% to 50% sensitive. In addition, the test can be inaccurate in the presence of coexistent diabetes mellitus, renal insufficiency, liver disease, or malabsorption states. The bentiromide test may be most useful in determining the severity of the chronic pancreatitis not in making the diagnosis.

Malabsorption of fat occurs in patients with significant chronic pancreatitis, and several tests have been directed at detecting this defect. Most of them involve ingestion of the triglyceride [^{14}C]olein. Subsequently, the [^{14}C]olein is hydrolyzed, and the breakdown product, [^{14}C]oleate, is absorbed, with resultant production and pulmonary excretion of carbon dioxide C-14. The level of carbon dioxide C-14 in the exhaled gas is a simple measure of triglyceride digestion.

DIFFERENTIAL DIAGNOSIS AND COMPLICATIONS

The most important condition to exclude during evaluation of a patient with chronic pancreatitis is pancreatic cancer. Even after histopathologic examination, a mass in the head of the pancreas associated with chronic pancreatitis can be difficult to distinguish from pancreatic cancer. In patients with localized calcification and chronic pancreatitis in the tail of the pancreas, the possibility of a tumor causing obstructive chronic pancreatitis must be entertained. Finally, there is an increased risk of developing pancreatic cancer in patients with chronic pancreatitis.

Other complications of chronic pancreatitis include obstructive jaundice, pseudocysts, pancreatic ascites and fistulae, vascular complications such as splenic artery aneurysm and splenic vein thrombosis, and gastrointestinal obstruction. Abnormalities of liver function, manifested by elevations in the liver enzymes, may be a result of either coexistent liver disease or obstruction of the common bile duct. Obstruction of the common bile duct in chronic pancreatitis may be secondary to the fibrotic process or may result from extrinsic compression by a pseudocyst or mass in the head of the pancreas. Although liver disease is frequently associated with alcoholism, the pattern of liver enzyme elevations is usually different from that seen with obstruction of the common duct. The presence of an obstructive pattern of the liver enzyme abnormalities warrants further investigation to identify the cause, primarily to exclude a concomitant pancreatic malignancy and determine the best method for bile duct decompression.

TREATMENT

Abdominal Pain

Intractable abdominal pain is the most frequent symptom of chronic pancreatitis that makes the patient seek help. The pain of chronic pancreatitis may be due to multiple factors such as parenchymal inflammation, inflammatory injury to neural sheaths, sensory nerve encasement, elevated intraductal pressures, and feedback neurohormonal hyperstimulation of the exocrine pancreas due to diminished trypsin secretion into the bowel lumen. If alcohol abuse is the cause of chronic pancreatitis, the treatment of pain should begin with abstinence. Although some report that up to 75% of alcoholic patients with chronic pancreatitis experience at least partial relief with abstinence,[15] others report no greater likelihood of pain relief.[16]

The mainstay of medical therapy for the pain of chronic pancreatitis is the administration of *analgesics.* Generally, treatment begins with nonnarcotic analgesics, such as acetaminophen and nonsteroidal antiinflammatory agents. Once narcotics become necessary, addiction is almost inevitable, and the evaluation of subsequent treatment is extremely difficult.

Oral replacement therapy in the form of pancreatic enzymes is currently being evaluated for the treatment of pain by inhibiting the pancreas through negative feedback. In the diseased state, a reduction of luminal trypsin is associated with a duodenal neurohormonal feedback response that stimulates the exocrine pancreas.[17,18] The administration of exogenous pancreatic enzymes can blunt the feedback exocrine pancreatic hyperstimulation and thus potentially relieve the pain of chronic pancreatitis. Six prospective, randomized trials have been published in which the benefit of exogenous oral enzyme replacement was examined.[19] Unfortunately, because of the heterogeneous population of patients and the significant placebo effect in the studies, it is difficult to draw conclusions about the benefits of this form of therapy.

Celiac plexus blockade can be performed endoscopically, under CT guidance, and either by open or laparoscopic surgery. However, pain relief after celiac plexus blockade has been found to be merely temporary and repeated treatments are even less effective.[20]

Endoscopic dilation and stent placement may be used to treat chronic pancreatitis secondary to pancreatic duct obstruction from stones, strictures, or papillary stenosis[21] but not without risk of injury caused by the stent itself.[19,22] Relief of pain after short-term stent drainage can be used to identify patients who will benefit from surgical drainage of the pancreatic duct.

Patients being considered for surgery must have failed medical management of their pain and their pancreatic anatomy must be completely delineated. Operations to relieve the pain of chronic pancreatitis can be divided into two categories: *drainage procedures* for patients with ductal dilatation and obstruction, and *resective procedures* for patients with a diseased pancreas but normal ductal size. The long-term postoperative relief of pain is the standard by which all operations for chronic pancreatitis are measured.

Drainage Procedures

Longitudinal Pancreaticojejunostomy (Puestow Procedure). In the presence of a dilated main pancreatic duct (>7 mm), longitudinal pancreaticojejunostomy is the most commonly performed operation. The gastrocolic ligament is divided to access the lesser sac, and the entire anterior surface of the pancreas is exposed (Fig. 55.7). The main pancreatic duct is identified by palpation, intraoperative ultrasonography or aspiration with a 25-gauge needle. Duct size is important because pain will be relieved in 65% to 80% of patients after longitudinal pancreaticojejunostomy if the duct is wider than 7 mm. If the operation is performed with a smaller duct, the long-term patency rate of the anastomosis is decreased. The main pancreatic duct is opened longitudinally (Fig. 55.8) preferably to within 1 cm of the duodenum to ensure that segments of the duct do not remain undrained and pancreatic duct stones are removed. A standard Roux-en-Y loop of jejunum is created, and an anastomosis is made between the Roux limb and the length of the opened pancreatic duct (Fig. 55.9). Immediate pain relief with the longitudinal pancreaticojejunostomy can be expected in more than 80% of patients. Operative mortality is less than 5%. Unfortunately, pain recurs in 25% to 50% of patients within 5 years (Fig. 55.10). The remaining pancreatic exocrine and endocrine function can be preserved because no pancreatic tissue is resected.

Local Resection of the Pancreatic Head with Longitudinal Pancreaticojejunostomy (Frey Procedure). This procedure was developed to facilitate ductal drainage in the head and uncinate process of the pancreas as a standard longitudinal pancreaticojejunostomy may provide inadequate drainage at the confluence of the ducts of Wirsung and Santorini.[23] In the Frey procedure, the head and uncinate process of the pancreas are "shelled out," and the resultant cavity is connected to the main pancreatic duct followed by longitudinal pancreaticojejunostomy with

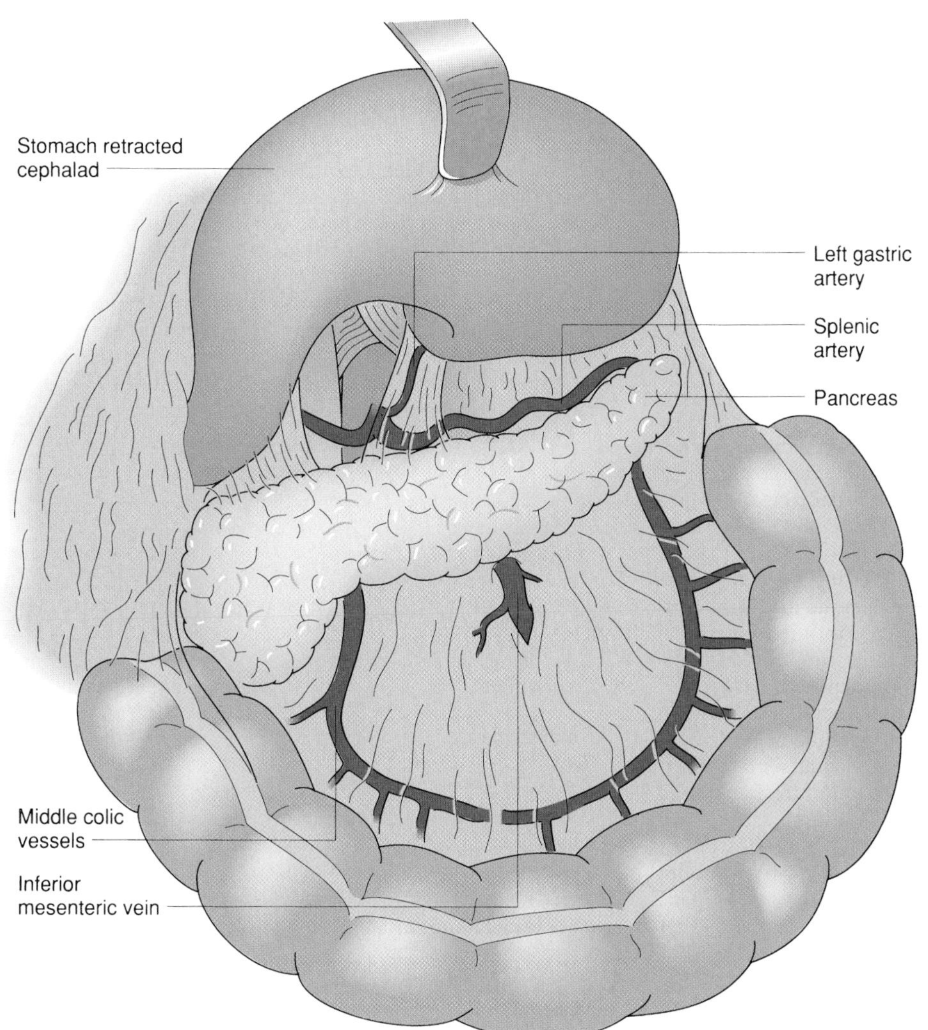

FIGURE 55.7 Exposure of the anterior surface of the pancreas through the lesser sac.

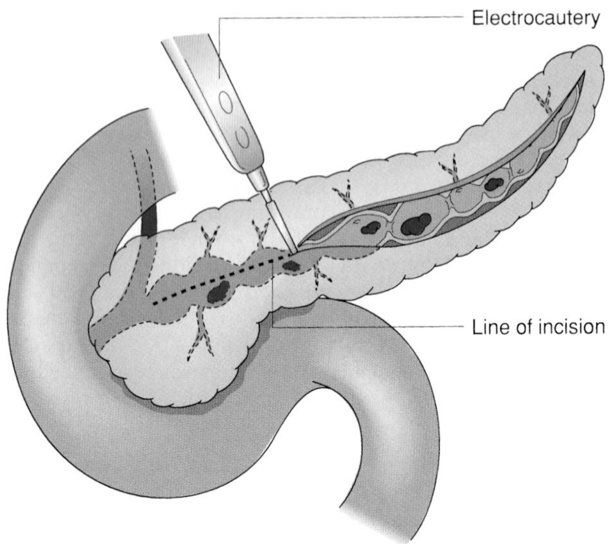

FIGURE 55.8 Longitudinal incision of the main pancreatic duct in preparation for lateral pancreaticojejunostomy.

a jejunal Roux limb. Frey reported excellent pain relief in 75% of patients after 3 years. Therefore, this modification may be preferable to the standard Puestow-type pancreaticojejunostomy in selected patients.

Resection Procedures

Patients with chronic pancreatitis whose duct size is too small are uniformly considered poor candidates for drainage procedures and then pancreatic resection would be the surgical option. Pancreatic resection is most beneficial if the disease is confined to one portion of the gland.

Distal Pancreatectomy. If changes of chronic pancreatitis are confined to the tail and body of the pancreas, a distal pancreatectomy may provide relief. If resection occurs at the level of the superior mesenteric vessels, approximately 50% of the gland is removed (Fig. 55.11). A spleen-preserving distal pancreatectomy is usually not practical in view of the chronic inflammatory changes. Thus, the preoperative administration of vaccines is indicated to prevent overwhelming postsplenectomy infections caused by encapsulated organisms (pneumococci, *Haemophilus influenzae*, meningococci).

Pancreaticoduodenectomy (Whipple Procedure). Resection of the pancreatic head may be indicated when the disease is confined predominantly to this region. Appropriate indications include a chronic inflammatory mass that cannot be differentiated from a malignancy, chronic inflammation associated with duodenal narrowing, multiple pseudocysts confined to the head of the gland, and failure of a pancreaticojejunostomy to drain the head and uncinate process adequately. Standard pancreaticoduodenectomy involves resection of the pancreatic head, duodenum, gallbladder, distal common duct, and antrum (Fig. 55.12). In the pylorus-preserving modification of the procedure, the antrum and proximal 1 to 2 cm of duodenum are preserved (Fig. 55.13). Regardless of the type of pancreaticoduodenectomy, the reported success rate for pain relief is between 60% to 80% after 5 years. If a mass in the head of the pancreas is identified and malignancy cannot be excluded, pancreaticoduodenectomy is indicated, and frequently an occult malignancy is identified on histologic examination.[24]

Ninety-five Percent Distal Pancreatectomy. The 95% distal pancreatectomy involves removal of the entire pancreas (and spleen) except for a small rim of gland adjacent to the duodenum. Although pain relief can be achieved in up to 80% of patients undergoing this procedure, the high incidence of insulin-dependent diabetes mellitus is a limitation.

Total Pancreatectomy. Total pancreatectomy is rarely performed for chronic pancreatitis in view of the morbid sequelae. In general, the procedure is reserved for patients who have undergone one resective procedure and have either persistent symptoms or a complication requiring further resection. Postoperatively, all patients develop insulin-dependent diabetes mellitus and also require pancreatic enzyme replacement therapy. Even with all the pancreatic tissue removed, pain relief is not uniform.

Duodenum-Preserving Resection of Pancreatic Head (Beger Procedure). Candidates for this procedure are the same as those who are candidates for a standard pancreaticoduodenectomy except when duodenal stenosis is present. The operation requires transection of the pancreas at its neck and removal of the head and uncinate process except for a rim of parenchyma between the common bile duct and the duodenum. A Roux-en-Y loop of jejunum is created and sewn to the open end of the body of the pancreas and the portion of pancreas adjacent to the duodenum. Although Beger reports pain relief in approximately 80% of patients, the operation is technically challenging and may offer little advantage in comparison with standard pancreaticoduodenectomy.[25]

Malabsorption

Two major consequences of pancreatic insufficiency include steatorrhea and azotorrhea, and on initial consideration, both would seem easy to treat with the administration of commercially available oral pancreatic enzyme supplements. Unfortunately, for a variety of reasons, complete correction of steatorrhea is infrequently achieved. Oral enzyme supplements (Table 55.1) must contain adequate amounts of lipase, with sufficient lipase activity delivered to the proximal small intestine. Fat absorption is adequate if 25,000 IU of lipase activity can be provided during the 4-hour postprandial period. Acid pepsin inactivates pancreatic enzymes, and

TABLE 55.1

COMMERCIALLY AVAILABLE PANCREATIC ENZYME PREPARATIONS

Preparation[a]	Lipase content (IU per pill)
Donnazyme	8,000
Ilozyme	3,600
Ku-Zyme HP	2,300
Cotazym-S	2,000
Pancrease	4,500
Viokase	3,800

[a]Each in capsule formulation.

Adapted from Owyang C, Levitt M. Chronic pancreatitis. In: Yamada T, Alpers DH, Powell DW, et al., eds. *Textbook of gastroenterology.* Philadelphia: JB Lippincott; 1991:1888.

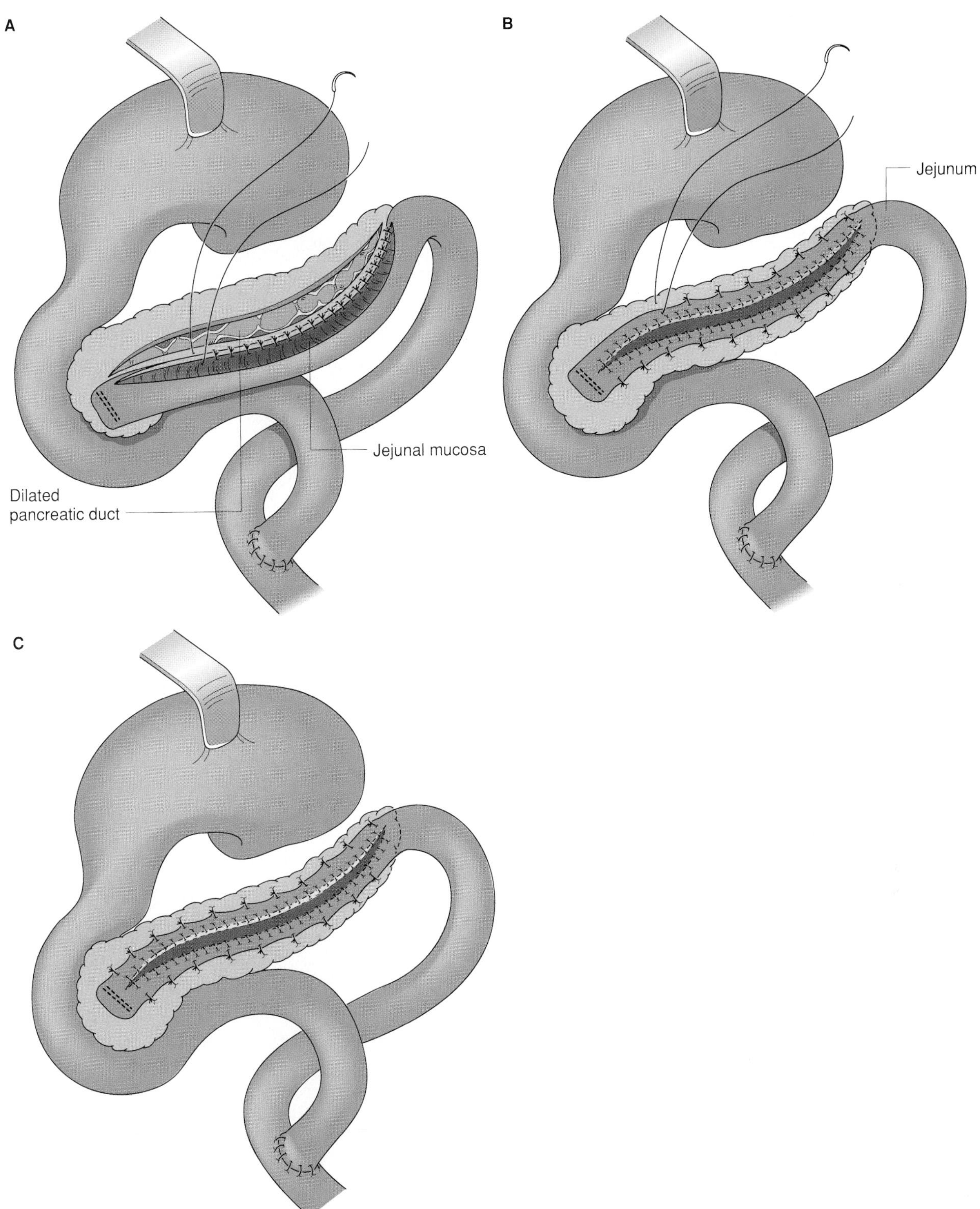

FIGURE 55.9 Lateral pancreaticojejunostomy.

gastric acidity is a major impediment to the delivery of active enzymes to the duodenum. Duodenal samples demonstrate recovery of less than 8% of ingested lipase and less than 22% of ingested trypsin. Pancreatic lipase is irreversibly denatured at a pH <4, and attempts to circumvent this problem have included the administration of large amounts of enzyme with meals and the inhibition of acid secretion with histamine (H_2) receptor antagonists. Enteric coating of pancreatic enzyme supplements is effective if the supplements are delivered to the duodenum with food and if sufficient intraduodenal dissolution occurs.

In general, the administration of adequate numbers of enzyme tablets to eliminate azotorrhea and decrease steatorrhea is ideal. This requires that multiple tablets be taken

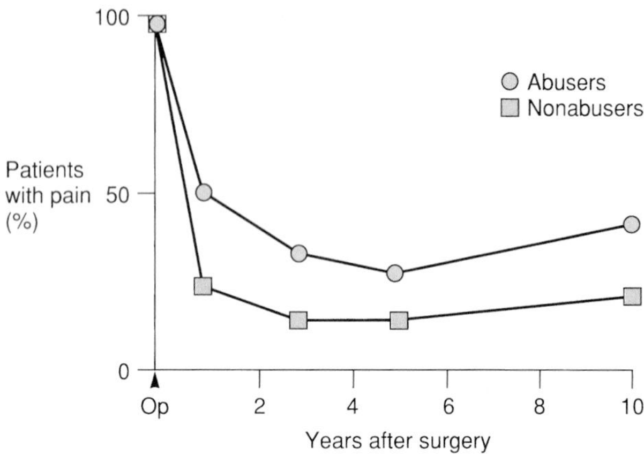

FIGURE 55.10 Long-term pain relief after pancreaticojejunostomy. (After Ihse I, Borch K, Larsson J. Chronic pancreatitis: results of operations for relief of pain. *World J Surg*. 1990;14:53.)

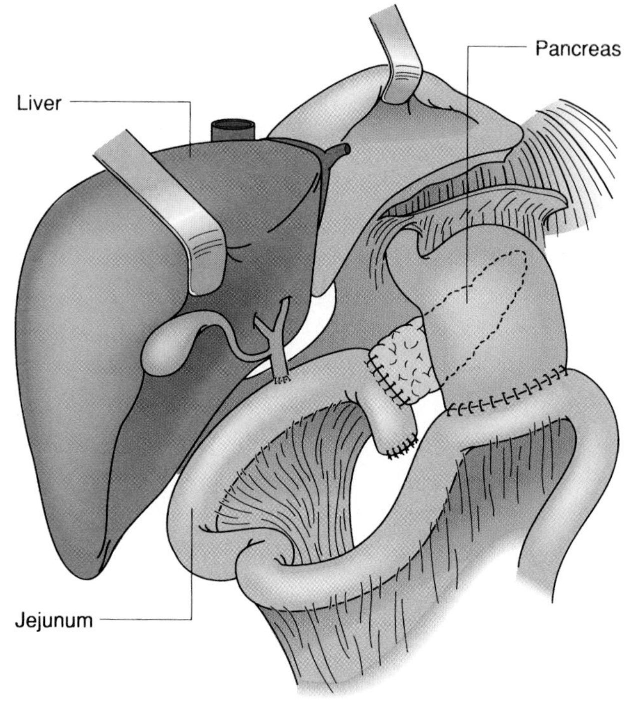

FIGURE 55.12 Reconstruction after standard pancreaticoduodenectomy.

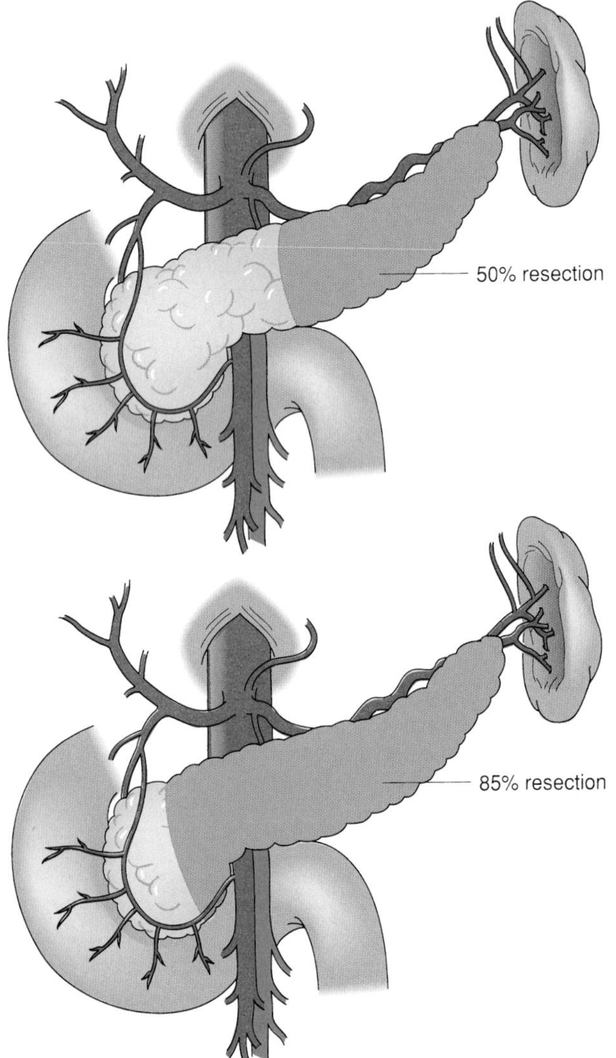

FIGURE 55.11 Points of parenchymal transection for 50% and 85% distal pancreatectomies.

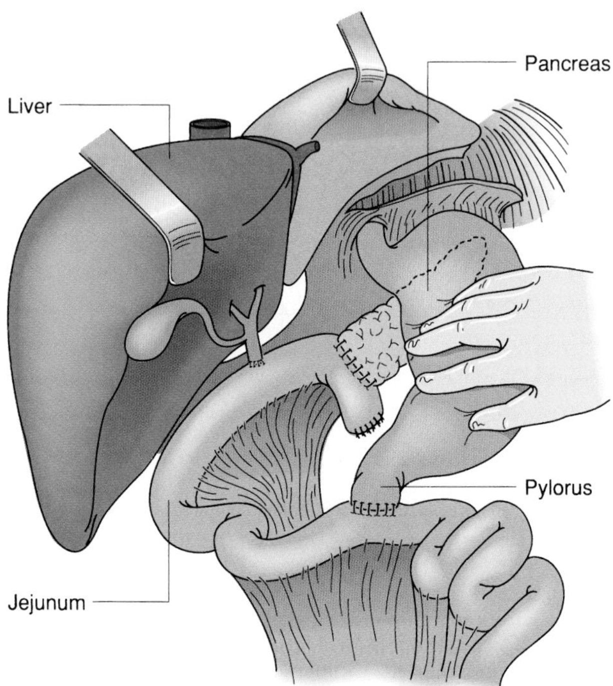

FIGURE 55.13 Reconstruction after pylorus-preserving pancreaticoduodenectomy.

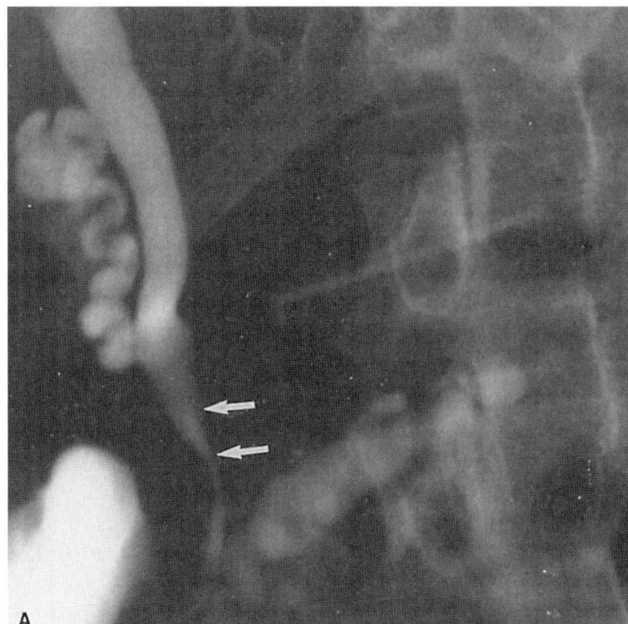

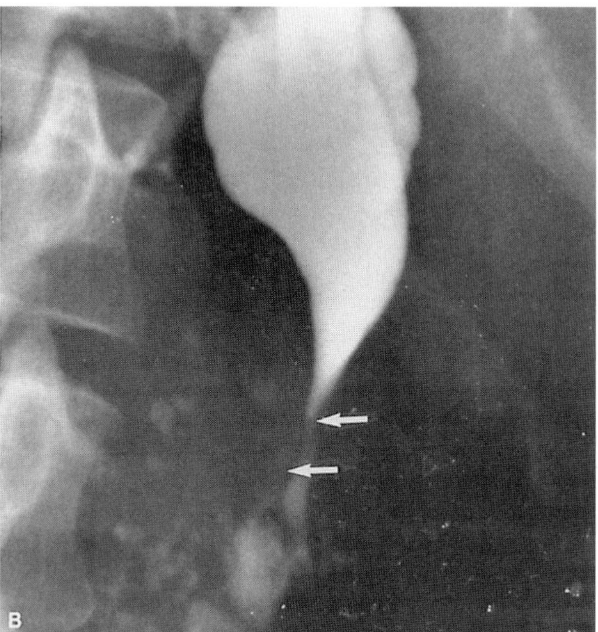

FIGURE 55.14 Endoscopic cholangiograms of early (*A*) and advanced (*B*) biliary stricture accompanying chronic pancreatitis. Smooth, tapering strictures (*arrows*) can be seen confined to the intrapancreatic portion of the bile duct.

with meals and snacks; if symptoms persist, the number of tablets should be increased or the fat content of meals decreased. With this regimen, most patients can achieve adequate nutritional status and maintain their weight. The addition of H_2 receptor antagonists or proton pump inhibitors should be reserved for patients who are relatively resistant to this regimen or who have documented acidic duodenal contents.

Pseudocysts

Pancreatic pseudocysts associated with chronic pancreatitis, when compared to those associated with acute pancreatitis, are less likely to resolve spontaneously due to underlying pancreatic duct abnormalities. Asymptomatic cysts less than 5 cm in size do not require therapy. Percutaneous drainage can be used to decompress symptomatic pseudocysts rapidly, but recurrence rates are as high as 25% once the drain is removed—especially if the pseudocyst remains in communication with the pancreatic ductal system and there is an element of ductal obstruction that maintains the fistulous communication with the pseudocyst. If pseudocysts recur after removal of a percutaneous drain, internal surgical drainage is indicated. Pseudocyst drainage rarely results in alleviation of pain from chronic pancreatitis. In addition to bowel or biliary tract compression, complications of pancreatic pseudocysts include infection, bleeding, and rupture.

Biliary Tract Complications

Significant fibrosis of the pancreatic head can lead to stenosis of the distal common bile duct and an elevation of serum alkaline phosphatase usually occurs before the appearance of jaundice. Although ultrasonography, CT, and percutaneous transhepatic cholangiography can provide valuable information, ERCP is commonly used to define the anatomy of the common duct (Fig. 55.14) and can also provide a tissue diagnosis. Bile duct stenosis associated with pancreatic head fibrosis is characterized by a long segment of narrowing, whereas a malignant stricture is characterized by abrupt termination of the bile duct lumen. Treatment options for bile duct stenosis caused by chronic pancreatitis include endoscopic stent placement and surgical drainage of the bile duct. Although the long-term use of stents to alleviate common duct obstruction has been reported, emphasis must be placed on ensuring that no malignancy is present. With the associated risk for malignancy, stent placement should be reserved for those patients who have cholangitis requiring immediate duct drainage or who are poor risks for surgical drainage. Either choledochoduodenostomy or choledochojejunostomy (Fig. 55.15) is an excellent choice for long-term surgical drainage of benign strictures of the common bile duct. At the time of surgery, if malignancy has not been sufficiently excluded, histologic samples should be taken or a pancreaticoduodenectomy should be performed as pancreatic cancer occurs in 4% of patients with chronic pancreatitis of 20 years duration.

PROGNOSIS

Patients with chronic pancreatitis have an excess mortality of 36% during 20 years and a decreased life expectancy in comparison with the general population. Fewer than 20% of patients with chronic pancreatitis die of direct complications of their disease. The majority of patients die of complications of tobacco or alcohol overuse. In addition, aerodigestive cancers, diabetic complications, and cirrhosis are frequent causes of death in patients with chronic pancreatitis.

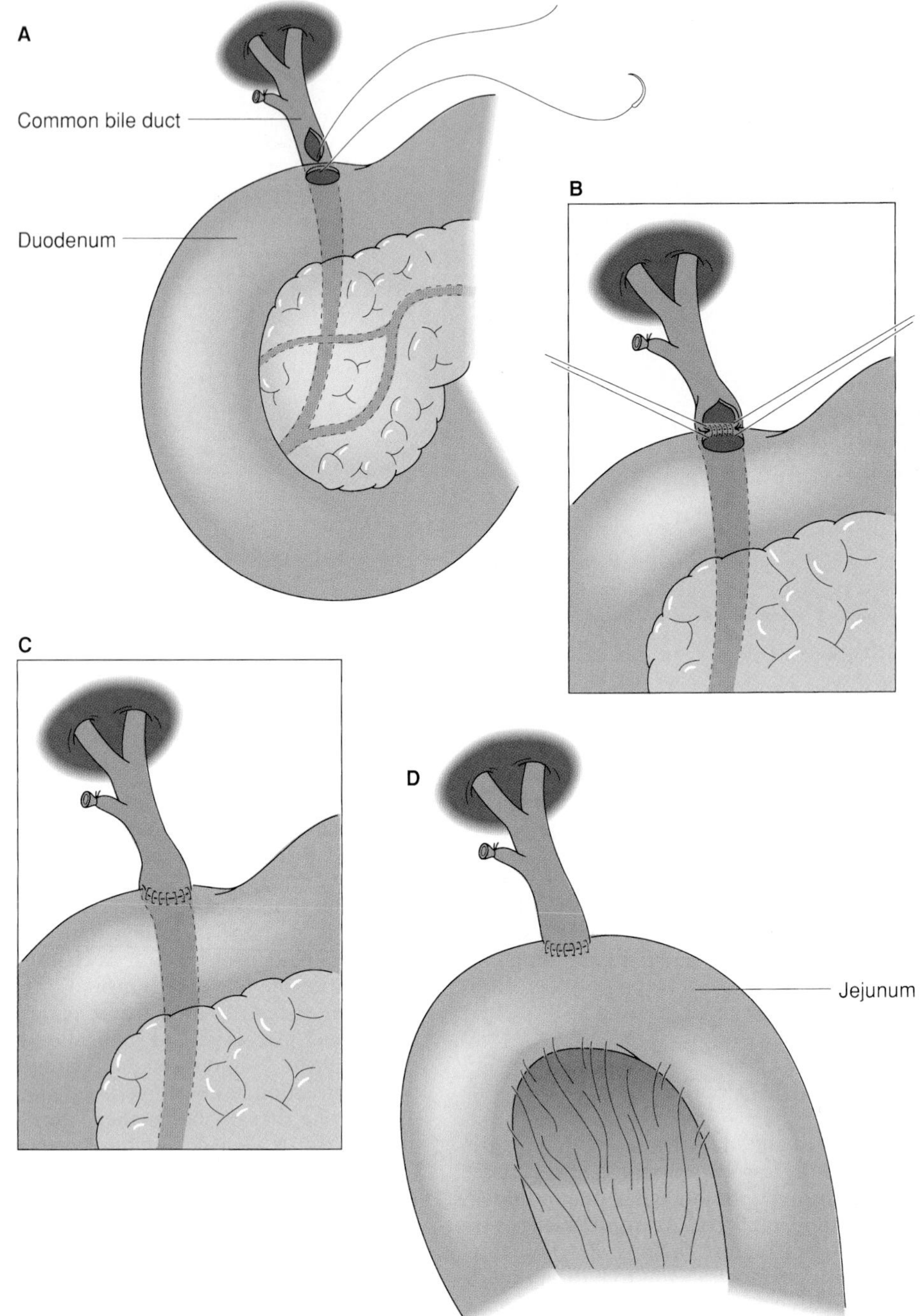

FIGURE 55.15 Operative construction of choledochoduodenostomy (*A–C*) and choledochojejunostomy (*D*).

KEY POINTS

- Chronic alcoholism is responsible for up to 80% of cases of chronic pancreatitis.
- The type of alcohol and the manner of consumption do not correlate with disease severity, but the severity of chronic pancreatitis does appear to increase with the amount and duration of alcohol consumption.
- It takes almost a 90% loss of functional pancreas for symptoms of malabsorption (diarrhea, steatorrhea) to develop.
- Although imaging studies such as transabdominal ultrasound and CT may be used to diagnose chronic pancreatitis, ERCP is the gold standard for diagnosis.
- Patients with chronic pancreatitis have an increased risk of pancreatic cancer.
- Analgesics and oral pancreatic enzymes are the first-line treatment for chronic pancreatitis.
- In the presence of a dilated pancreatic duct (>7 mm), longitudinal pancreaticojejunostomy (Puestow procedure) can provide pain relief in more than 80% of patients.
- Resection therapy is indicated for chronic pancreatitis in the absence of a dilated pancreatic duct.

- **Pancreaticoduodenectomy has a success rate of between 60% and 80% in patients with disease confirmed predominately to the head of the pancreas.**
- **Patients with chronic pancreatitis have a decreased life expectancy in comparison to the general population.**

References

1. **Etemad B, Whitcomb DC. Chronic pancreatitis: diagnosis, classification, and new genetic developments. *Gastroenterology* 2001;120:682.**
2. Copenhagen Pancreatitis Study. An interim report from a prospective epidemiological multicenter study. *Scand J Gastroenterol.* 1981;16:305.
3. **Otsuki M. Chronic pancreatitis. The problems of diagnostic criteria. *Pancreatology* 2004;4:28.**
4. Layer P, Kalthoff L, Clain JE, et al. Nonalcoholic chronic pancreatitis: two diseases? *Dig Dis Sci.* 1985;30:980.
5. Gastard J, Jobaud F, Farbos T, et al. Etiology and course of primary chronic pancreatitis in western France. *Digestion* 1973;9:416.
6. Sahel J, Sarles H. Modifications of pure human pancreatic juice induced by chronic alcohol consumption. *Dig Dis Sci.* 1979;24:897.
7. Bess MA, Edis AJ, van Heerden JA. Hyperparathyroidism and pancreatitis. *JAMA* 1980;243:246.
8. Cotton PB. Congenital anomaly of pancreas divisum as cause of obstructive pain and pancreatitis. *Gut* 1980;21:105.
9. Burtin P, Person B, Charneau J, et al. Pancreas divisum and pancreatitis: a coincidental association. *Endoscopy* 1991;23:55.
10. **Amman RW, Akovbiantz A, Largiader F, et al. Course and outcome of chronic pancreatitis: longitudinal study of a mixed medical—surgical series of 245 patients. *Gastroenterology* 1984;86:820.**
11. Gridwood AH. Does progressive pancreatic insufficiency limit pain in calcific pancreatitis with duct stricture or continued alcohol insult? *J Clin Gastroenterol.* 1981;3:241.
12. **DiMagno EP, Go VLW, Summerskill WHJ. Relations between pancreatic enzyme outputs and malabsorption in severe pancreatic insufficiency. *N Engl J Med.* 1973;288:813.**
13. Jones SN, Lees WR, Frost RA. Diagnosis and grading of chronic pancreatitis by morphological criteria derived by ultrasound and pancreatography. *Clin Radiol.* 1988;39:43.
14. Braganza JM, Hunt LP, Warwick R. Relationship between exocrine function and ductal morphology in chronic pancreatitis. *Gastroenterology* 1982;82:1341.
15. Trapnell JE. Chronic relapsing pancreatitis: a review of 64 cases. *Br J Surg.* 1979;66:471.
16. Lankisch PG, Lohr-happe A, Otto J, et al. Natural course in chronic pancreatitis: pain, exocrine and endocrine pancreatic insufficiency, and prognosis of the disease. *Digestion* 1993;54:148.
17. Samuel I, Joehl RJ. Enteral bile-pancreatic juice replacement-not cholinergic and cholecystokinin-receptor blockade-reverses acinar cell hyperstimulation after bile-pancreatic duct ligation. *Am J Surg.* 1996;171:207.
18. Samuel I, Joehl RJ. Bile and pancreatic enzyme exclusion from gut influences pathogenesis of early ligation-induced acute pancreatitis in opossums. *Dig Surg.* 1995;12:330.
19. **Warshaw AL, Banks PA, Fernandez-Del Castillo C. AGA technical review: treatment of pain in chronic pancreatitis. *Gastroenterology* 1998; 115:765.**
20. Leung JWC, Bowen-Wright M, Aveling W, et al. Celiac plexus block for pain control in pancreatic cancer and chronic pancreatitis. *Br J Surg.* 1983;70:730.
21. Geenen JE, Rolny P. Endoscopic therapy of acute and chronic pancreatitis. *Gastrointest Endosc.* 1991;37:377.
22. Smith MT, Sherman S, Ikenberry SO, et al. Alterations in pancreatic ductal morphology following polyethylene pancreatic stent therapy. *Gastrointest Endosc.* 1996;44:268.
23. **Frey CF, Mayer KL. Comparison of local resection of the head of the pancreas combined with longitudinal pancreaticojejunostomy (Frey procedure) and duodenum-preserving resection of the pancreatic head (Beger procedure). *World J Surg.* 2003;27:1217.**
24. **Thuluvath PJ, Imperio D, Nair S, et al. Chronic pancreatitis. Long-term pain relief with and without surgery, cancer risk, and mortality. *J Clin Gastroenterol.* 2003;36:98.**
25. **Beger HG, Buchler M. Duodenum-preserving resection of the head of the pancreas in chronic pancreatitis with inflammatory mass in the head. *World J Surg.* 1990;14:83.**

CHAPTER 56 ■ NEOPLASMS OF THE EXOCRINE PANCREAS

ATTILA NAKEEB, KEITH D. LILLEMOE, CHARLES J. YEO, AND JOHN L. CAMERON

In the United States it is estimated that nearly 33,000 new cases of pancreas cancer will be diagnosed with almost 32,000 people dying of the disease in 2005. Pancreatic cancer is the fourth leading cause of cancer death in this country.[1] The nonspecific symptoms associated with early pancreatic cancer, the inaccessibility of the pancreas to examination, the aggressiveness of the tumors, and the technical difficulties associated with pancreatic surgery make pancreatic cancer one of the most challenging diseases treated by general surgeons. In recent years, significant advances have been made in our understanding of the pathogenesis and clinical management of pancreatic cancer. This chapter reviews the epidemiology and risk factors associated with pancreatic cancer, discusses recent developments in the field of molecular genetics, and provides an update on the current management of pancreatic cancer.

EPIDEMIOLOGY AND RISK FACTORS

In the United States, approximately 11 new cases of pancreatic cancer are diagnosed per 100,000 population annually.[1] Although the incidence rate of pancreatic cancer has been relatively stable during the last two decades, it has increased nearly threefold since the beginning of the last century (Fig. 56.1). It has been argued that the apparent increase in the incidence of pancreatic cancer may represent a misclassification of pancreatic cancer as other types of upper gastrointestinal cancer, particularly gastric cancer, in the past. However, several analyses indicate that a portion of the threefold increase in the incidence of pancreatic cancer has been real.

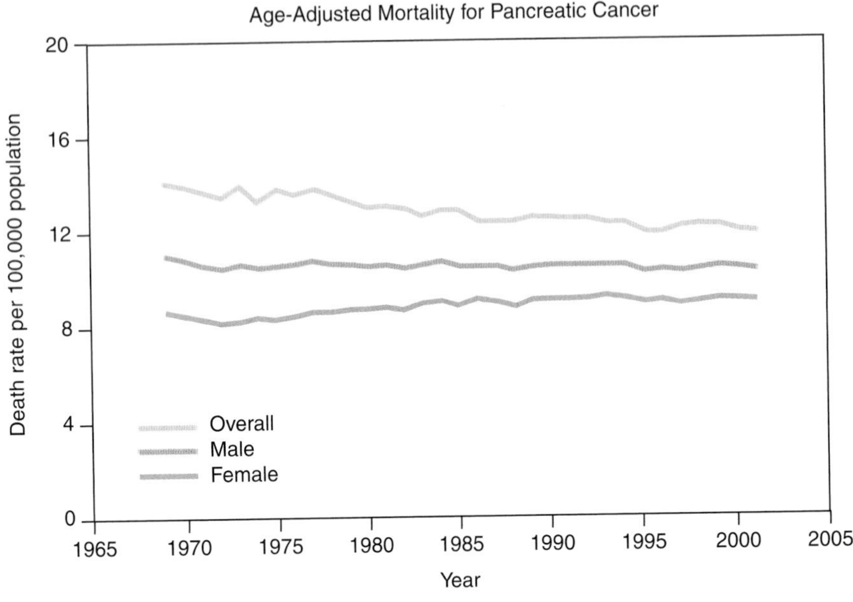

FIGURE 56.1 U.S. age-adjusted death rates for pancreatic carcinoma.

The risk for the development of pancreatic cancer is related to age, race, sex, tobacco use, diet, and specific genetic syndromes (Table 56.1). The incidence increases with advancing age. More than 80% of cases occur in persons between the ages of 60 and 80 years, and pancreatic cancer is rare in people younger than 40 years. The incidence and mortality rates for pancreatic cancer in African Americans of both sexes are higher than those in whites. The gender differences in pancreatic cancer have been equalizing during recent years. Pancreatic cancer is still more common in men than in women, but the incidence and mortality rates have increased in women while they have stabilized or slightly decreased in men.

Environmental and dietary factors have also been implicated as risk factors for the development of pancreatic cancer. The most consistently observed environmental risk for the development of pancreatic cancer is cigarette smoking. It has been estimated that cigarette smoking can increase the risk for pancreatic cancer between one and a half and five times. The mechanism is unknown, but carcinogens in cigarette smoke have been shown to produce pancreatic cancers in laboratory animals. In addition, autopsy studies have documented hyperplastic changes in pancreatic ductal cells with atypical nuclear patterns in smokers. Alcohol consumption does not seem to be a risk factor for pancreatic cancer despite conflicting past reports. Recent studies suggest that past studies linking pancreatic cancer to alcohol use may have been confounded by tobacco use. Similarly, coffee consumption and exposure to ionizing radiation have been shown not to be associated with an increased pancreatic cancer risk.

Several epidemiologic investigations have suggested that diet may play an important role in the development of pancreatic cancer. An apparent association has been noted between pancreatic cancer and an increased consumption of total calories, carbohydrate, cholesterol, meat, salt, dehydrated food, fried food, refined sugar, soy beans, and nitrosamines. The risks are unproved for the ingestion of fat, beta-carotene, and coffee. A protective effect has been reported for dietary fiber, vitamin C, fruits, and vegetables.[2]

TABLE 56.1

RISK FACTORS FOR PANCREATIC CANCER

	Increased risk	Possible risk	Unproved risk
Demographic factors	Advancing age Male sex Black race	Geography	Socioeconomic status Migrant status
Host factors	Hereditary nonpolyposis colorectal cancer Familial breast cancer Peutz-Jeghers syndrome Ataxia—telangiectasia Familial atypical multiple-mole melanoma Hereditary pancreatitis		Peptic ulcer surgery
Environmental factors	Tobacco	Diet Occupation	Alcohol Coffee Radiation

Modified from Gold EB, Goldin SB. Epidemiology of and risk factors for pancreatic cancer. *Surg Oncol Clin North Am.* 1998;7:67.

TABLE 56.2

GENETIC SYNDROMES ASSOCIATED WITH HEREDITARY PANCREATIC CANCER

Syndrome	Mode of inheritance	Gene	Fold increase in risk	Manifestation of pancreatic cancer
Peutz-Jeghers	AD	*STKll*	140×	Hamartomatous polyps of the gastrointestinal tract; mucocutaneous melanin macules
Hereditary pancreatitis	AD	*PRSSl*	60×	Recurrent episodes of severe pancreatitis starting at a young age
Familial pancreatic cancer	Unknown	Unknown	18×	At least one pair of first-degree relatives with pancreatic cancer
FAMMM	AD	p16	20×	Multiple nevi, atypical nevi, melanomas
Familial breast cancer 2	AD	*BRCA2*	10×	Breast, ovarian, and pancreatic cancer
HNPCC	AD	*MSH2* *HLHl*	Unknown	Colonic, endometrial, and gastric cancers; mutator phenotype

AD, autosomal dominant; FAMMM, familial atypical multiple mole melanoma; HNPCC, hereditary nonpolyposis colorectal cancer.

In addition to well-defined genetic syndromes, a number of common conditions have been thought to be etiologic factors in the development of pancreatic cancer. An apparent association between diabetes and pancreatic cancer has been suggested. Although the data are somewhat inconsistent, mostly they suggest that long-standing diabetes is not a risk factor for pancreatic cancer. Diabetes may actually be an early symptom of pancreatic cancer and not a causative factor. Chronic pancreatitis of any cause has been associated with a 25-year cumulative risk for the development of pancreatic cancer of approximately 4%. Other conditions for which a possible association with pancreatic cancer has been demonstrated include thyroid and other benign endocrine tumors, cystic fibrosis, and pernicious anemia.

Most cases of pancreatic cancer have no obvious predisposing factors. However, it is believed that between 5% to 10% of pancreatic cancers arise because of a familial predisposition.[3] Six genetic syndromes have been associated with an increased risk for the development of pancreatic cancer (Table 56.2). These include hereditary nonpolyposis colon cancer, familial breast cancer associated with the *BRCA2* mutation, Peutz-Jeghers syndrome, ataxia–telangiectasia syndrome, familial atypical multiple mole–melanoma syndrome, and hereditary pancreatitis.

MOLECULAR GENETICS

Tremendous advances have been made in understanding the molecular genetics of pancreatic cancer in recent years. In general, the genes involved in the pathogenesis of pancreatic cancer can be divided into three categories: tumor-suppressor genes, oncogenes, and DNA mismatch-repair genes (Table 56.3).

Tumor-suppressor genes normally function to control cellular proliferation. When these genes are inactivated by genetic events such as mutation, deletion, chromosome rearrangements, or mitotic recombination, their function as growth suppressors can be lost, and abnormal growth regulation is the result. The tumor-suppressor genes *p53*, *p16*, *DPC4*, and *BRCA2* are frequently inactivated in sporadic adenocarcinoma of the pancreas. The function of *p53* appears to be inactivated in up to 75% of all pancreatic cancers. The *p53* gene product is a DNA-binding protein that acts as both a cell cycle checkpoint and an inducer of apoptosis. Inactivation of the *p53* gene in pancreatic cancer leads to the loss of two important controls of cell growth: regulation of cellular proliferation and induction of cell death. The *p16* gene encodes a protein that binds cyclin to cyclin D–Cdk4 complexes. When the *p16* gene product binds to these complexes, it inhibits the phosphorylation of a number of growth and regulatory proteins. Inactivation of *p16* leads to the loss of an important cell cycle checkpoint and therefore relatively unchecked proliferation. *DPC4* is a tumor-suppressor gene that has been identified on chromosome 18q. This chromosome has been shown to be missing in nearly 90% of pancreatic cancers. The *DPC4* gene is inactive in almost 50% of pancreatic carcinomas. The mutation appears to be a homozygous deletion in 30% of pancreatic cancers, and a point mutation in another 20% of tumors. *DPC4* mutations are more specific than *p53* or *p16* mutations for pancreatic cancer. The function of *BRCA2* has not been established, but the gene product appears to be a tumor suppressor participating in DNA damage repair. Mutations in *BRCA2* have been linked to hereditary breast and ovarian

TABLE 56.3

GENETIC ALTERATIONS IN PANCREATIC ADENOCARCINOMAS

Gene	Chromosome locus	Frequency (%)
Oncogenes		
K-*ras*	12	90
Tumor suppressor genes		
p16	9p	95
p53	17p	50–75
DPC4	18q	55
BRCA2	13q	7
LKB1	17p	4
MKK4	19p	5
ALK4	12q	2
Genome maintenance genes *bMSH2, bMLH1*	2P, 3P	4

From Hruban RH. Pancreatic cancer: From genes to patient care. *J Gastrointest Surg.* 2001;5:583, with permission.

cancers. Recent studies also suggest a significantly increased risk of pancreatic cancer development in patients with germline *BRCA2* mutations.

Oncogenes are derived from normal cellular genes called *protooncogenes*. When overexpressed or activated by mutation, oncogenes encode proteins with transforming properties. Activating point mutations in the K-*ras* oncogene is the most common genetic alteration in pancreatic cancer. Point mutations in codons 12, 13, or 61 of the K-*ras* oncogene impair the intrinsic guanosine triphosphatase activity of its gene product; the result is a protein that is constitutively active in signal transduction. Mutations of K-*ras* have been found in 80% to 100% of pancreatic cancers and therefore may prove useful in the development of a molecular screening test for pancreatic cancer.

Mismatch-repair genes function to ensure the accuracy of DNA replication, and when these genes are mutated, errors in DNA replication are not repaired. The human mismatch-repair genes are *hMSH2, hMLH1, hPMS1, hPMS2, hMSH6/GTBP*, and *hMSH3*. The enzymes encoded by these genes repair single base pair changes and small insertions and deletions that occur during DNA replication. Approximately 4% of pancreatic cancers can be characterized by disorders of DNA mismatch-repair genes.[4]

PATHOLOGY

Tumors of the exocrine pancreas can be classified based on their cell of origin (Table 56.4). The most common neoplasms of the exocrine pancreas are ductal adenocarcinomas. Approximately 65% of pancreatic ductal cancers arise in the head, neck, or uncinate process of the pancreas; 15% originate in the body or the tail of the gland; and 20% diffusely involve the whole gland.

TABLE 56.4 CLASSIFICATION

HISTOLOGIC CLASSIFICATION OF 645 CASES OF PRIMARY NONENDOCRINE CANCER OF THE PANCREAS

Classification	Number
Duct cell origin	572 (89%)
Duct cell adenocarcinoma	494
Giant cell carcinoma	28
Adenosquamous carcinoma	20
Microadenocarcinoma	16
Mucinous carcinoma	9
Mucinous cystadenocarcinoma	5
Acinar cell origin	8 (1%)
Acinar cell carcinoma	7
Cystadenoma	1
Uncertain histogenesis	61 (9%)
Pancreaticoblastoma	1
Papillary and cystic neoplasm	1
Mixed type—duct and islet cells	1
Unclassified	58
Connective tissue origin	4 (1%)

Bell RH. Neoplasms of the exocrine pancreas. In: Greenfield LJ, Mulholland MW, Oldham KT, eds. *Surgery: scientific principles and practice,* 2nd ed. Philadelphia: Lippincott–Raven; 1997:901, with permission.

Solid Epithelial Tumors

Ductal Adenocarcinomas

Ductal adenocarcinomas account for more than 75% of all nonendocrine pancreatic cancers. Grossly, they are white–yellow, poorly defined, hard masses that often obstruct the distal common bile duct or main pancreatic duct. They are often associated with a desmoplastic reaction that causes fibrosis and chronic pancreatitis. Microscopically, they contain infiltrating glands of varying size and shape surrounded by dense, reactive fibrous tissue (Fig. 56.2). The epithelial cells sometimes form papillae and cribriform structures, and they frequently contain mucin. The nuclei of the cells can show marked pleomorphism, hyperchromasia, loss of polarity, and prominent nucleoli.

Ductal adenocarcinomas tend to infiltrate into vascular, lymphatic, and perineural spaces. At the time of resection, most ductal carcinomas have already metastasized to regional lymph nodes. In addition to the lymph nodes, pancreatic ductal adenocarcinoma frequently metastasize to the liver (80%), peritoneum (60%), lungs and pleurae (50% to 70%), and adrenal glands (25%). They also can directly invade the duodenum, stomach, transverse mesocolon, colon, spleen, and adrenal glands.

The histologic examination of a pancreas resected for cancer frequently reveals the presence of precursor lesions in the pancreatic ducts and ductules adjacent to the cancers.[5] This suggests that much like colon cancer, which arises from benign adenomas, pancreatic cancer may also demonstrate progression to malignant from benign precursor lesions. These precursor lesions are referred to as pancreatic intraepithelial neoplasia (PanIN). Briefly, PanIN-1A and PanIN-1B are proliferative lesions without remarkable nuclear abnormality that have a flat and papillary architecture, respectively. PanIN-3 is associated with severe architectural and cytonuclear abnormalities, but invasion through the basement membrane is absent. The older term for PanIN-3 includes carcinoma in situ (CIS). PanIN-2 is an intermediate category between PanIN-1 and PanIN-3 and is associated with a moderate degree of architectural and cytonuclear abnormality.[6] Several lines of evidence suggest that PanINs are precursors of infiltrating pancreatic cancer: PanINs are often found in association with ductal adenocarcinomas, three-dimensional mapping techniques that demonstrated a stepwise transformation from mild dysplasia to severe dysplasia in pancreatic duct lesions, and PanINs demonstrate some of the same genetic changes seen in infiltrating adenocarcinomas, most notably activating point mutations in codon 12 of K-*ras* and mutations in the *p16* and *p53* tumor-suppressor genes.

Adenoaquamous Carcinomas

Adenosquamous carcinoma is a rare variant of ductal adenocarcinoma that shows both glandular and squamous differentiation. This variant appears to be more common in patients who have undergone previous chemoradiation therapy. The biologic behavior of adenosquamous carcinoma appears to be similar to that of ductal adenocarcinoma, with similar rates of perineural invasion, lymph node metastases, and dissemination.

Acinar Cell Carcinomas

Acinar cell carcinomas account for only 1% of pancreatic exocrine tumors. Acinar tumors are typically smooth, fleshy, lobulated, hemorrhagic, or necrotic. Histologically, they form

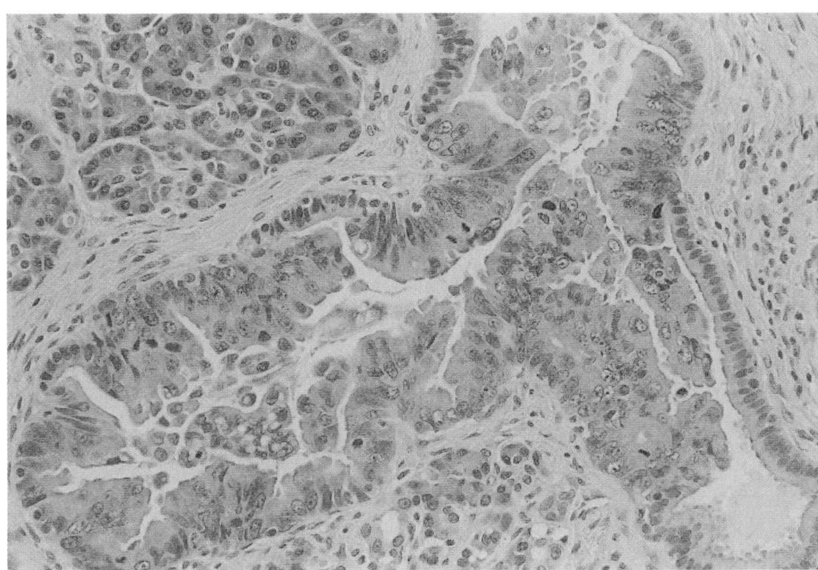

FIGURE 56.2 Microscopic appearance of ductal adenocarcinoma of the head of the pancreas demonstrating glands from an adenocarcinoma embedded in a fibrous matrix.

acini, and the cells display an eosinophilic, granular cytoplasm. Immunohistochemical staining demonstrates expression of trypsin, lipase, chymotrypsin, or amylase. These tumors are more common in males with a male-to-female predominance of approximately 2:1. The age of diagnosis is usually in the fifth to seventh decades. These tumors tend to be larger than ductal adenocarcinomas, often being larger than 10 cm. Although data are limited, it appears that patients with acinar cell carcinoma have a slightly better prognosis than patients with ductal carcinoma. Therefore, surgical resection is the treatment of choice.

Giant Cell Carcinomas

Giant cell carcinomas account for fewer than 5% of nonendocrine pancreatic cancers. They tend to be large, with average diameters greater than 15 cm. Microscopically, they contain large, uninucleated or multinucleated tumor cells, many of which are pleomorphic. The nuclei contain prominent nucleoli and numerous mitotic figures. Giant cell carcinomas are associated with a poorer prognosis than ductal adenocarcinomas. There is a variant of giant cell carcinoma termed *giant cell carcinoma with osteoclast-like giant cells*. These lesions tend to be well circumscribed with nonpleomorphic giant cells and are less aggressive than standard giant cell carcinomas.

Pancreatoblastoma

Pancreatoblastomas occur primarily in children ages 1 to 15 years. Pancreatoblastomas contain both epithelial and mesenchymal elements. The epithelial component appears to arise from acinar cells. The tumors are typically larger than 10 cm and often contain areas of degeneration and hemorrhage. The prognosis appears to be more favorable than that for typical ductal adenocarcinoma if the tumor can be resected.

Cystic Epithelial Tumors

Cystic neoplasms also arise from the exocrine pancreas. Cystic neoplasms are less common than ductal adenocarcinomas, tend to occur in women, and are evenly distributed throughout the gland. The vast majority of pancreatic and peripancreatic cysts are benign pseudocysts. However, it is important to recognize cystic neoplasms because their management is very different from that for nonneoplastic cysts. With advancements in imaging technology, cystic lesions of the pancreas are being detected with increased frequency. Although many of these lesions are small and asymptomatic, they can have malignant potential. Therefore, the management of these patients is complex, and knowledge of pancreatic cyst natural history and predictors of neoplasia are important.

Serous Cystic Neoplasms

Serous cysts are epithelial neoplasms composed of uniform cuboidal glycogen-rich cells that usually form numerous small cysts containing serous fluid. Serous cystadenomas or microcystic adenomas are more common in women than in men (2:1 preponderance). These tumors can vary from a few centimeters to more than 10 cm in size. Twenty-five percent to 30% of patients are asymptomatic; however, most patients present with symptoms such as abdominal or epigastric pain, dyspepsia, nausea, or vomiting. Serous cystadenomas can be located anywhere in the pancreas—head, body, or tail—and usually do not communicate with the pancreatic ducts. Plain computed tomography (CT) shows a honeycomb pattern of microlacunae, with thin septa separating different segments. Serous cystic neoplasms can have a sunburst pattern of central calcification, which is seen in 10% to 30% of cases. Grossly, they appear as spongy, well-circumscribed, multiloculated cysts. Microscopically, they consist of a layer of simple cuboidal cells separated by dense fibrous bands. Most serous cystic neoplasms are benign, although malignant behavior has been reported rarely (i.e., metastases to the liver or peripancreatic lymph nodes). Symptomatic cysts or cysts that cannot be differentiated from other potentially malignant cysts should undergo surgical excision.

Mucinous Cystic Neoplasms

Mucinous cystic neoplasms (MCNs) are neoplasms composed of mucin-producing epithelial cells associated with an ovarian-type of stroma. These cysts usually do not communicate with the larger pancreatic ducts. Invasive mucinous cystadenocarcinomas are MCNs associated with an invasive carcinoma, whereas non-invasive mucinous neoplasms can be categorized into adenomas, borderline neoplasms, and CIS based on the degree of architectural and cytologic atypia of the epithelial cells.

MCNs are relatively uncommon but account for almost 30% of all cystic neoplasms. The mean age at diagnosis is between 40 to 50 years. MCNs are more common in women with a female-to-male ratio of 9:1. Patients with mucinous cystadenocarcinomas tend to be 5 to 10 years older than patients with benign MCNs. Most patients with MCNs present with vague abdominal symptoms that include epigastric pain or a sense of abdominal fullness. The majority (70% to 90%) of MCNs arise in the body or tail of the pancreas, and only a minority (10% to 30%) involve the head of the gland. Microscopically, the cysts are lined by tall columnar mucin-producing epithelium. These columnar cells have basal nuclei and abundant intracytoplasmic apical mucin and can form flat sheets or papillae. The walls of the cysts contain a very distinctive "ovarian-type" stroma. This stroma is composed of densely packed spindle cells with sparse cytoplasm and uniform elongated nuclei.

Approximately, one third of all MCNs are associated with invasive carcinoma. The invasive and in situ carcinomas in MCNs can be very focal. Therefore, a benign diagnosis cannot be established on biopsy alone and the lesions should be completely resected. In addition, benign MCNs are considered to be premalignant lesions and should be completely resected to prevent progression to malignancy. The prognosis for patients with resected benign or borderline tumors is excellent. Patients with mucinous cystadenocarcinoma tend to do better than patients with ductal adenocarcinoma, with a 5-year survival of approximately 50%.

Intraductal Papillary-Mucinous Neoplasms

Intraductal papillary-mucinous neoplasms (IPMNs) are intraductal mucin-producing neoplasms with tall, columnar, mucin-containing epithelium with or without papillary projections. These neoplasms extensively involve the main pancreatic ducts and/or major side branches. In addition, IPMNs lack the ovarian stroma characteristic of MCNs. Similar to the well-defined adenoma-carcinoma sequence in pancreatic ductal adenocarcinoma (PanIN to invasive ductal carcinoma), IPMNs seem to follow a similar pattern progressing from IPMN adenoma, to borderline IPMN with dysplasia, to IPMN with CIS, and eventually to invasive carcinoma. Microscopically, they consist of papillary projections lined by columnar mucin-secreting cells. They show varying degrees of cellular atypia. The mean age of patients with invasive carcinoma is approximately 5 years older than patients with noninvasive IPMNs suggesting an approximately 5-year lag period for progression to malignancy.

IPMNs are usually found in individuals in their 60s to 80s. Some patients may experience symptoms that include: abdominal pain, steatorrhea, weight loss, jaundice, diabetes, and chronic pancreatitis. IPMNs appear to be more common in the head, neck, and uncinate process of the pancreas but can be found diffusely throughout the whole gland. CT scans will typically reveal a cystic mass in the head of the pancreas that appear to communicate with the pancreatic ductal system. On endoscopy, mucin can be seen oozing from the ampulla of Vater. Endoscopic retrograde cholangiopancreatography (ERCP) can be used to confirm that the cysts communicate with the pancreatic ducts.

MCNs are the main entity to consider in the differential diagnosis of IPMNs (Table 56.5). Two morphologic features distinguish IPMNs from MCNs: IPMNs communicate with ducts, mucinous cysts do not; IPMNs also lack an ovarian stroma that is present in mucinous cysts. In addition, mucinous cysts are usually seen in the tail of the pancreas and occur in middle-aged women, whereas IPMNs are found in the head of the pancreas and occur in older individuals of either sex.

TABLE 56.5

COMPARISON BETWEEN MUCINOUS CYSTIC NEOPLASM (MCN) AND INTRADUCTAL PAPILLARY MUCINOUS NEOPLASM (IPMN)

	MCN	IPMN
Age (years)	40 to 50	60 to 80
Gender	More common in females	More common in males
Location	Body/tail	Head
Communicates with pancreatic duct	No	Yes
Mucin at ampulla	No	Yes
Ovarian like stroma	Yes	No

As noted IPMNs represent a continuum of disease from benign to malignant. In a large series of resected IPMNs from the Johns Hopkins Hospital,[7] the prognosis for the benign forms of the disease appears to be significantly better than for invasive IPMNs with 1-, 2-, and 5-year actuarial survivals of 97%, 94%, and 77%, respectively. Although invasive IPMNs are associated with disease progression and death, the prognosis remains markedly better than for invasive ductal carcinoma of the pancreas with survivals of 72%, 58%, and 43% at 1, 2, and 5 years, respectively. The goal of surgical therapy for IPMNs should be a complete surgical resection yielding negative margins for all invasive and non-invasive disease. Unlike those patients with completely resected noninvasive MCNs (who are routinely cured), patients with completely resected noninvasive IPMNs should undergo careful follow-up and surveillance for the development of recurrent disease. Furthermore, patients with resected invasive IPMNs should also undergo careful follow-up and surveillance as they, too, remain at risk for the development of recurrent disease.

Solid and Cystic Papillary Neoplasms

Solid and cystic papillary neoplasms, also termed *Hamoudi tumors,* occur primarily in women in their third to fourth decade of life. Grossly, the masses range from 5 to 15 cm in diameter. The tumors show solid, cystic, and papillary components. Although most patients are cured after resection, metastases have been reported.

CLINICOPATHOLOGIC STAGING

Accurate pathologic staging of pancreatic cancer is important for providing prognostic information to patients and for comparing the results of various therapeutic trials. The American Joint Committee on Cancer (AJCC) staging for pancreatic cancer is shown in Table 56.6. This system, based on the TNM classification, takes into account the extent of the primary tumor (T), the presence of absence of regional lymph node involvement (N), and the presence or absence of distant metastatic disease (M).

TABLE 56.6 STAGING

AMERICAN JOINT COMMITTEE ON CANCER STAGING OF PANCREATIC CANCER

Stage	T	N	M	5-Year survival (%)
IA	T1	N0	M0	20–30
IB	T2	N0	M0	20–30
IIA	T3	N0	M0	10–25
IIB	T1, T2, T3	N1	M0	10–15
III	T4	Any N	M0	0–5
IV	Any T	Any N	M1	—

TUMOR (T)
TX: Primary tumor cannot be assessed
T0: No evidence of primary tumor
Tis: Carcinoma in situ
T1: Tumor limited to the pancreas, 2 cm or less in greatest dimension
T2: Tumor limited to the pancreas, more than 2 cm in greatest dimension
T3: Tumor extends beyond the pancreas but without involvement of the celiac axis or the superior mesenteric artery
T4: Tumor involves the celiac axis or the superior mesenteric artery (unresectable primary tumor)

REGIONAL LYMPH NODES (N)
NX: regional lymph nodes cannot be assessed
N0: no regional lymph node metastasis
N1: regional lymph node metastasis

DISTANT METASTASIS (M)
MX: distant metastasis cannot be assessed
M0: no distant metastasis
M1: distant metastasis

Adapted from American Joint Committee on Cancer. Exocrine pancreas. In: *AJCC cancer staging manual,* 6th ed. New York: Springer; 2002:157.

DIAGNOSIS

Clinical Presentation

Many of the difficulties associated with the management of pancreatic cancer result from our inability to make the diagnosis at an early stage. The early symptoms of pancreatic cancer include anorexia, weight loss, abdominal discomfort, and nausea. Unfortunately, the nonspecific nature of these symptoms often leads to a delay in the diagnosis. Specific symptoms usually develop only after invasion or obstruction of nearby structures has occurred. Most pancreatic cancers arise in the head of the pancreas, and obstruction of the intrapancreatic portion of the common bile duct leads to progressive jaundice, acholic stools, darkening of the urine, and pruritus. Pain is a common symptom of pancreatic cancer. The pain usually starts as vague upper abdominal or back pain that is often ignored by the patient or attributed to some other cause. It is usually worse in the supine position and is often relieved by leaning forward. Pain may be caused by invasion of the tumor into the splanchnic plexus and retroperitoneum, and by obstruction of the pancreatic duct. Other digestive symptoms are also common in pancreatic cancer (Table 56.7).

Occasionally, pancreatic cancer may be discovered in an unusual manner. The onset of diabetes may be the first clinical feature in 10% to 15% of patients. An episode of acute pancreatitis may also be the initial presentation of pancreatic cancer if the tumor partially obstructs the pancreatic duct. It is important to consider a pancreatic cancer in patients presenting with acute pancreatitis, especially those without an obvious cause for their pancreatitis (alcohol or gallstones).

The most common physical finding at the initial presentation is jaundice (Table 56.8). Hepatomegaly and a palpable gallbladder may be present in some patients. In cases of advanced disease, cachexia, muscle wasting, or a nodular liver, consistent with metastatic disease, may be evident. Other physical findings in patients with disseminated cancer include left supraclavicular adenopathy (Virchow's node), periumbilical adenopathy (Sister Mary Joseph's node), and pelvic drop metastases (Blumer's shelf). Ascites can be present in 15% of patients.

Laboratory Studies

In patients with cancer of the head of the pancreas, laboratory studies usually reveal a significant increase in serum total bilirubin, alkaline phosphatase, and γ-glutamyl transferase indicating bile duct obstruction. The transaminases can also be elevated but usually not to the same extent as the alkaline phosphatase. In patients with localized cancer of the body and tail of the pancreas, laboratory values are frequently normal early in the course. Patients with pancreatic cancer may also demonstrate a normochromic anemia and hypoalbuminemia secondary to the nutritional consequences of the disease. In patients with jaundice, the prothrombin time can be abnormally prolonged. This usually is an indication of biliary obstruction, which prevents bile from entering the gastrointestinal tract and leads to malabsorption of fat-soluble vitamins and

TABLE 56.7 DIAGNOSIS

SYMPTOMS OF PANCREATIC CANCER

Symptom	Patients (%)
HEAD	
Weight loss	92
Jaundice	82
Pain	72
Anorexia	64
Dark urine	63
Light stools	62
Nausea	45
Vomiting	37
Weakness	35
Pruritus	24
Diarrhea	18
Melena	12
Constipation	11
Fever	11
Hematemesis	8
BODY AND TAIL	
Weight loss	100
Pain	87
Weakness	43
Nausea	43
Vomiting	37
Anorexia	33
Constipation	27
Hematemesis	17
Melena	17
Jaundice	7
Fever	7
Diarrhea	3

decreased hepatic production of vitamin K–dependent clotting factors. The prothrombin time can usually be normalized by the administration of parenteral vitamin K. Serum amylase and lipase levels are usually normal in patients with pancreatic cancer.

A wide variety of serum tumor markers have been proposed for use in the diagnosis and follow-up of patients with pancreatic cancer. The most extensively studied of these is CA 19-9, a Lewis blood group-related mucin glycoprotein. Approximately 5% of the population lacks the Lewis gene and therefore cannot produce CA 19-9. When a normal upper limit of 37 U/mL is used, the accuracy of the CA 19-9 level in identifying patients with pancreatic adenocarcinoma is only about 80%. When a higher cutoff value of more than 90 U/mL is used, the accuracy improves to 85%, and increasing the cutoff value to 200 U/mL increases the accuracy to 95%.[8] The combined use of CA 19-9 and ultrasonography, CT, or ERCP can improve the accuracy of the individual tests, so that the combined accuracy approaches 100% for the diagnosis of pancreatic cancer. Levels of CA 19-9 have also been correlated with prognosis and tumor recurrence. In general, higher CA 19-9 values before surgery indicate an increased size of the primary tumor and increased rate of unresectability. In addition, the CA 19-9 level has been used to monitor the results of neoadjuvant and adjuvant chemoradiation therapy in patients. Increasing CA 19-9 levels usually indicate recurrence or progression of disease, whereas stable or declining levels indicate a stable tumor burden, absence of recurrence on imaging studies, and an improved prognosis.

TABLE 56.8 DIAGNOSIS

SIGNS OF PANCREATIC CANCER

Sign	Patients (%)
Head	
Jaundice	87
Palpable liver	83
Palpable gallbladder	29
Tenderness	26
Ascites	14
Abdominal mass	13
Body and tail	
Palpable liver	33
Tenderness	27
Abdominal mass	23
Ascites	20
Jaundice	13
Diarrhea	3

Radiologic Investigations

The early diagnosis of pancreatic cancer requires a high index of suspicion and appropriate aggressiveness in pursuing the diagnosis. Ultrasonography, CT, and magnetic resonance imaging (MRI) are all useful noninvasive tests in the patient suspected of having a pancreatic cancer.

Transabdominal ultrasonography is the most sensitive test for detecting gallstones, an ever-present issue in the elderly patient who is jaundiced. Ultrasonography is operator-dependent but can demonstrate dilated intrahepatic and extrahepatic bile ducts, liver metastases, pancreatic masses, ascites, and enlarged peripancreatic lymph nodes. Pancreatic cancer typically appears as a hypoechoic mass on ultrasonography. Ultrasonography will reveal a pancreatic mass in 60% to 70% of patients with cancer. Because helical CT is just as sensitive as ultrasonography and provides more complete information about surrounding structures and the local and distant extent of the disease, ultrasonography has been largely replaced by CT.

Helical or spiral CT is currently the preferred noninvasive imaging test for the diagnosis of pancreatic cancer. Pancreatic cancer usually appears as an area of pancreatic enlargement with a localized hypodense lesion (Fig. 56.3). For pancreatic lesions, a dual-phase intravenous contrast study is ideal. Thin cuts are obtained through the pancreas and liver during both an arterial phase and portal venous phase after the administration of intravenous contrast. In addition to determining the primary tumor size, CT is used to evaluate invasion into local structures or metastatic disease.

In general, MRI offers no significant advantages over CT because of a low signal-to-noise ratio, motion artifacts, lack of bowel opacification, and low spatial resolution. More recently, however, the introduction of magnetic resonance cholangiopancreatography (MRCP) has offered a promising noninvasive technique that can visualize both the bile duct and the pancreatic duct; images are similar to those obtained with ERCP.

Traditionally, the next step in the evaluation of the jaundiced patient has been cholangiography, either by the endoscopic or by the percutaneous route. If the endoscopic approach is used, the duodenum and ampulla can be visualized and biopsy specimens obtained if necessary. In addition, ERCP allows for direct imaging of the pancreatic duct.

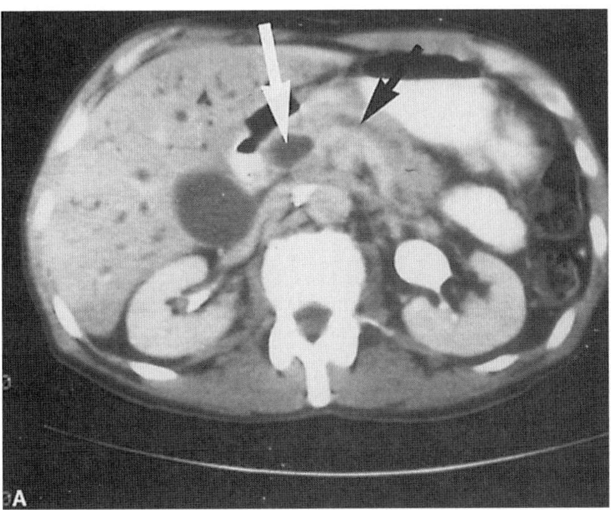

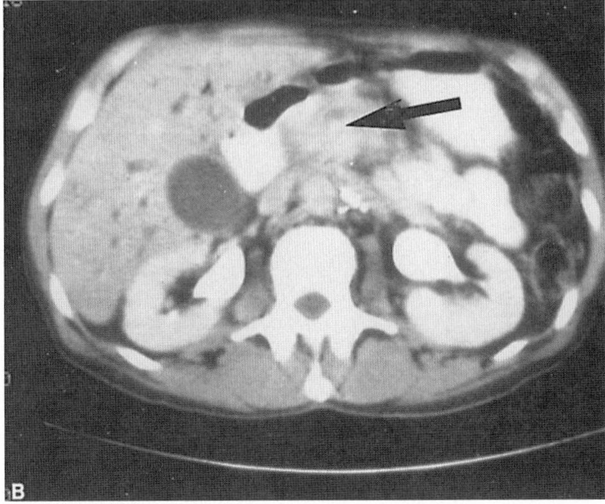

FIGURE 56.3 Computed tomogram of the abdomen of a patient with adenocarcinoma of the pancreas. (*A*) The obstructed and dilated common bile duct (*light arrow*) and pancreatic duct (*dark arrow*) can be seen. In the adjacent cross section (*B*), a large mass is present in the head of the pancreas (*arrow*).

The sensitivity of ERCP for the diagnosis of pancreatic cancer approaches 90%. The finding of a long, irregular stricture in an otherwise normal pancreatic duct is highly suggestive of a pancreatic cancer (Fig. 56.4). Often, the pancreatic duct will be obstructed with no distal filling. Although ERCP is reliable in confirming the presence of a clinically suspected pancreatic cancer, it should not be used routinely. Diagnostic ERCP should be reserved for patients with presumed pancreatic cancer and obstructive jaundice in whom no mass is demonstrated on CT, symptomatic but nonjaundiced patients without an obvious pancreatic mass, and patients with chronic pancreatitis in whom the development of a pancreatic mass is suspected based on clinical evidence or the development of jaundice.

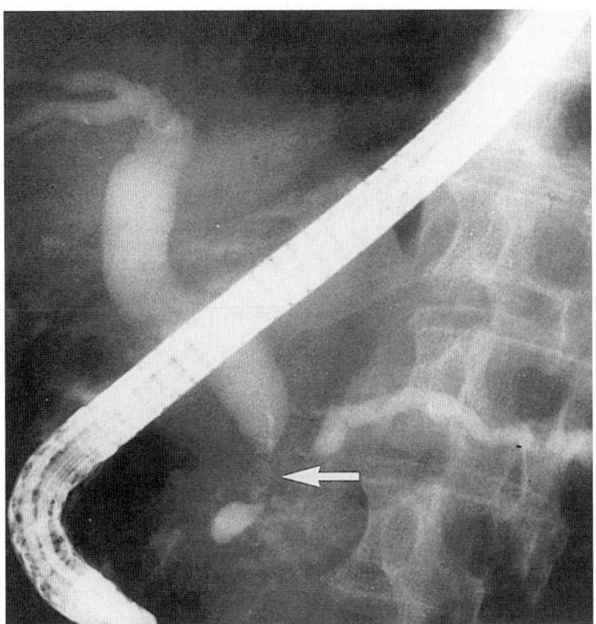

FIGURE 56.4 Endoscopic retrograde cholangiopancreatography in a patient with adenocarcinoma of the pancreas demonstrates a stricture of both the distal common bile duct and the pancreatic duct (*arrow*).

PREOPERATIVE STAGING

The goal of preoperative staging of pancreatic cancer is to determine the feasibility of surgery and the optimal treatment for each individual patient. In many cases, dynamic CT with oral and intravenous contrast may provide all the information necessary. Using objective, specific anatomy-based CT criteria that demonstrates the absence of extrapancreatic disease, a patent superior mesenteric vein (SMV)-portal vein confluence, and no evidence of direct tumor extension to the celiac axis or superior mesenteric artery, the accuracy of high-quality helical CT scanning to identify potentially resectable pancreatic cancer approaches 85%.[9] For tumors of the head, neck, or uncinate process of the pancreas, occlusion of the SMV or portal vein along with the presence of periportal collateral vessels is a sign of unresectability and typically precludes resection for cure. In contrast, for tumors of the body and tail of the pancreas, occlusion of the splenic vein with perigastric collaterals does not always preclude resection and should not be considered a sign of unresectability.

The extent of further staging to be performed depends on the individual patient and the surgeon's preference. If the surgeon's philosophy is to pursue a surgical treatment for all patients, either to attempt resection or to provide palliation, then further staging is not necessary. However, if the findings of staging could preclude an operation and lead to nonoperative palliation, then these efforts are worthwhile.

Endoscopic ultrasonography (EUS) is a minimally invasive technique in which a high-frequency ultrasonographic probe is placed into the stomach and duodenum endoscopically and the pancreas is imaged. Tumors appear as hypoechoic areas in the pancreatic substance (Fig. 56.5). The strengths of EUS techniques for pancreatic cancer are the clarification of small lesions (<2 cm) when CT findings are questionable or negative, detection of malignant lymphadenopathy, detection of vascular involvement, and the ability to perform EUS-guided fine needle aspiration (FNA) for definitive diagnosis and staging. EUS is not effective in assessing metastatic disease to the liver. In patients for whom a tissue diagnosis is required (poor operative candidates or undergoing neoadjuvant therapy), EUS-guided fine needle aspiration (FNA) has been used to acquire tissue samples for cytologic analysis. This approach

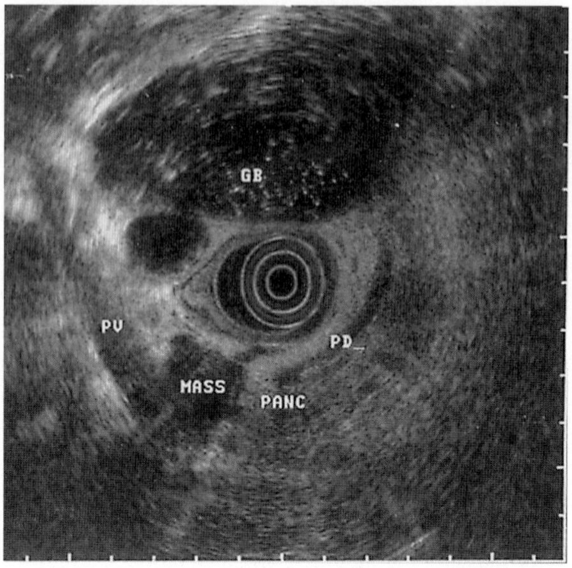

FIGURE 56.5 Endoscopic ultrasonogram of a 2.2-cm mass in the head of the pancreas. The transducer tip is located in the duodenum. The dilated common bile duct and gallbladder (GB) can be seen at the top of the image. The pancreatic duct (PD) is also dilated. The mass involves the portal vein (PV).

may avoid the risks of tumor seeding. The accuracy of EUS without FNA averages 85% for determining T stage and 70% for determining N stage disease. The combination of EUS and FNA has a sensitivity of 93% and a specificity of 100% for T stage and an accuracy of 88% for N stage.[10]

At the time of diagnosis, only 10% of patients have tumors confined to the pancreas, 40% have locally advanced disease, and more than 50% have distant spread. Unfortunately, only 10% to 20% of all patients are candidates for pancreatic resection. Therefore, accurate preoperative staging is important to determine which patients are candidates for curative resection and to avoid a nontherapeutic laparotomy in patients with unresectable disease. The use of diagnostic laparoscopy in pancreatic cancer remains controversial. Proponents believe that laparoscopy can identify a substantial number of unresectable patients with advanced disease and, therefore, should be uniformly applied to all patients with potentially resectable tumors.[11] On the other hand, opponents believe that the inherent cost of such a practice far outweighs the benefit to the small number of patients in whom diagnostic laparoscopy is useful. The liver and peritoneum are the most common sites of distant spread of pancreatic carcinoma. Once distant metastases have developed, survival is so limited that a conservative approach is usually indicated. Liver metastases larger than 1 cm in diameter can usually be detected by CT, but approximately 30% of these metastases are smaller and therefore may not be routinely detected. Moreover, peritoneal and omental metastases are usually only 1 to 2 mm in size and frequently can be detected only by direct visualization. With the recent improvements in CT imaging, the rate of positive peritoneal findings approaches 20% to 25% for all patients with pancreatic cancer and is significantly higher for patients with cancers of the body and tail. For example, patients presenting with obstructive jaundice secondary to tumors in the head of the pancreas typically have only a 15% to 20% incidence of unexpected intraperitoneal metastasis after routine staging studies. In contrast, unexpected peritoneal metastasis is found in up to 50% of patients with cancer of the body and tail of the pancreas.[12] Selective use of staging laparoscopy should be considered for patients at high risk of occult metastatic disease (Table 56.9). Percutaneous

TABLE 56.9 DIAGNOSIS

SIGNS OF HIGH RISK OF OCCULT METASTASTIC DISEASE

Large primary tumors
Lesions in the neck, body, or tail of the pancreas
Equivocal radiographic findings suggestive of occult distant metastatic disease
Low-volume ascites
CT findings indicating possible carcinomatosis
Small hypodense regions in the hepatic parenchyma that suggest hepatic metastases that are not amenable to percutaneous biopsy
Subtle clinical and laboratory findings suggesting more advanced disease (e.g., marked hypoalbuminemia and/or weight loss, significant increases in CA19-9 level, and relatively severe pain requiring narcotic analgesia)

CT, computed tomography.

FNA of pancreatic masses is helpful in selected patients. The technique is safe and generally reliable but is of limited use in patients in whom surgical exploration for attempted resection or palliation is planned. The reasons for not using FNA or percutaneous biopsy in potentially resectable lesions are twofold. First, even after repeated sampling, a negative result does not exclude malignancy; in fact, it is the smaller and likely more curable tumors that are likely to be missed by the needle. The second concern is the potential for seeding of the tumor, either along the needle tract or with intraperitoneal spread. Percutaneous biopsy is primarily indicated in patients with unresectable cancers based on preoperative staging to direct palliative chemoradiation therapy or in patients with cancer in the head of the pancreas for whom neoadjuvant protocols are being considered. Currently, however, EUS is the preferred technique when possible in either situation.

The information gained from preoperative staging provides the basis for planning therapy for each individual patient. If the results of preoperative staging with CT, angiography, and laparoscopy show localized disease, resectability rates may approach 80% for tumors in the head of the pancreas. A decision tree for the clinical staging of suspected pancreatic cancer is shown in Algorithm 56.1.

RESECTION OF PANCREATIC CARCINOMA

Carcinoma of the Head, Neck, or Uncinate Process

In 1912, Kaush[13] reported the first successful resection of the duodenum and a portion of the pancreas for an ampullary cancer. In 1935, Whipple et al.[14] described a technique for radical excision of a periampullary carcinoma. The operation was originally performed in two stages. A cholecystogastrostomy to decompress the obstructed biliary tree and a gastrojejunostomy to relieve gastric outlet obstruction comprised the first stage. The second stage was performed several weeks later when the jaundice had resolved and the nutritional status had improved. During the second stage, an *en bloc* resection of the second portion of the duodenum and head of the pancreas was performed without reestablishing pancreatic–enteric continuity. Although earlier contributions had been made, the

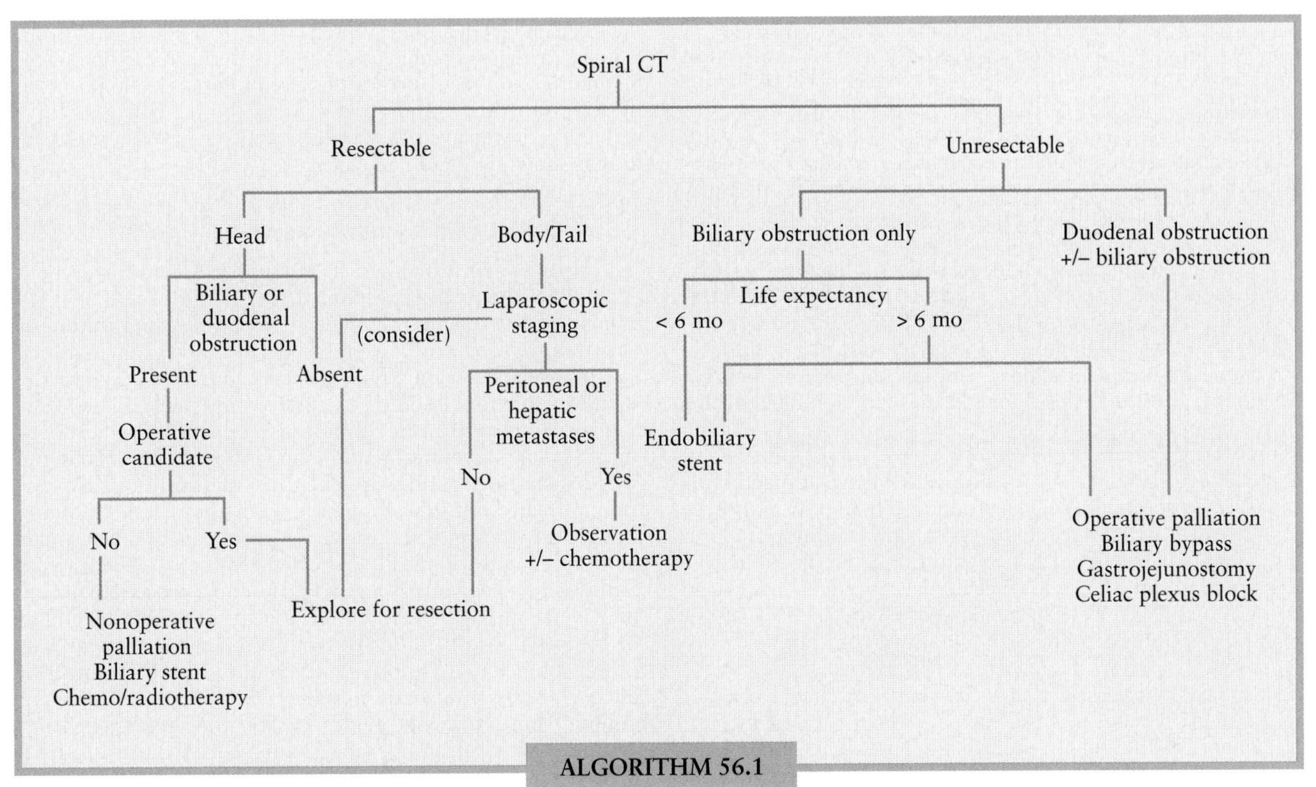

ALGORITHM 56.1 Diagnosis and management of pancreatic cancer. (After Tsiotis GG, Sarr MG. Diagnosis and clinical staging of pancreatic cancer. In: Howard JM, Idezuki Y, Ihse I, et al., eds. *Surgical disease of the pancreas,* 3rd ed. Baltimore: Williams & Wilkins; 1998:510, with permission.)

report by Whipple et al. began the modern-day approach to the treatment of pancreatic carcinoma.

Since Whipple's original description, pancreaticoduodenal resection has undergone numerous modifications and technical refinements. Unfortunately, during most of the first 50 years when the procedure was performed, the reported morbidity and mortality rates were unacceptably high, and long-term survival rates were disappointing. During the late 1960s and 1970s, the high operative morbidity and mortality and poor long-term survival rates led some surgeons to suggest that the Whipple procedure be abandoned. However, during the last two decades, a number of reports have documented improved operative results and long-term survival rates for patients with periampullary tumors following the Whipple procedure, so that a resurgence in its popularity has occurred.

The operative management of pancreatic cancer consists of two phases: first, assessing tumor resectability and then, if the tumor is resectable, completing a pancreaticoduodenectomy and restoring gastrointestinal continuity. After the abdomen has been opened through an upper midline or bilateral subcostal incision, a careful search for tumor outside the limits of a pancreaticoduodenal resection should be carried out. The liver, omentum, and peritoneal surfaces are inspected and palpated, and suspect lesions are sampled and specimens submitted for frozen section analysis. Next, regional lymph nodes are evaluated for tumor involvement. The presence of tumor in the periaortic lymph nodes of the celiac axis indicates that the tumor is beyond the limits of normal resection. However, the presence of tumor-bearing lymph nodes that normally would be incorporated within the resection specimen do not constitute a contraindication to resection.

Once distant metastases have been excluded, the primary tumor is assessed in regard to resectability. Local factors that preclude pancreaticoduodenal resection include retroperitoneal extension of the tumor to involve the inferior vena cava or aorta or direct involvement or encasement of the superior mesenteric artery, SMV, or portal vein. The technical aspects of determining local resectability begin with a Kocher maneuver and mobilization of the duodenum and head of the pancreas from the underlying inferior vena cava and aorta. Once the duodenum and head of the pancreas are mobilized sufficiently, the surgeon's hand can be placed under the duodenum and head of the pancreas to palpate the relationship of the tumor mass to the superior mesenteric artery. Inability of the surgeon to identify a plane of normal tissue between the mass and the arterial pulsation indicates direct tumor involvement of the superior mesenteric artery, and the possibility of complete tumor resection is eliminated.

The final step to determine resectability involves dissection of the superior mesenteric and portal veins to rule out tumor invasion. Identification of the portal vein can be simplified greatly if the common hepatic duct is divided and reflected early in the dissection. Once the hepatic duct has been divided, the posteriorly located portal vein can be identified easily. After the anterior surface of the portal vein is dissected posterior to the neck of the pancreas, the next step is to identify the SMV and dissect its anterior surface. This is done most easily by extending the Kocher maneuver past the second portion of the duodenum to include the third and fourth portions of the duodenum. During this extensive kocherization, the first structure that one encounters anterior to the third portion of the duodenum is the SMV. The anterior surface of the vein then can be cleaned rapidly and dissected under direct vision by retracting the neck of the pancreas anteriorly. The dissection is continued until it connects to the portal vein dissection from above.

Most experienced pancreatic surgeons, at this point, proceed with a pancreaticoduodenectomy without obtaining a tissue diagnosis. The clinical presentation, results of preoperative CT and cholangiography, and operative findings of a palpable mass in the head of the pancreas surpass the ability of an intraoperative biopsy to define the diagnosis of malignancy.

Having excluded regional and distant metastases and demonstrated no tumor involvement in major vascular structures, the surgeon can proceed with pancreaticoduodenectomy with a high degree of certainty that the tumor is resectable. In the pylorus-preserving modification of pancreaticoduodenectomy, the duodenum is first mobilized and divided approximately 2 cm distal to the pylorus. If a classic Whipple procedure is to be performed, the stomach is divided to include approximately 40% to 50% of the stomach with the resected specimen. The gastroduodenal artery is exposed, ligated, and divided near its origin at the common hepatic artery. It is always important to confirm, before ligation, that the structure to be ligated is indeed the gastroduodenal artery and not a replaced right hepatic artery. Next, the neck of the pancreas is divided, with care taken to avoid injury to the underlying superior mesenteric and portal veins. The portal and superior mesenteric veins are then dissected from the uncinate process and head of the pancreas. At this point, the fourth portion of the duodenum and the proximal jejunum are mobilized, with the proximal jejunum divided approximately 10 cm distal to the ligament of Treitz. The proximal jejunum and fourth portion of the duodenum are passed under the superior mesenteric vessels to the right, and the uncinate process is dissected from the superior mesenteric artery. The course of the superior mesenteric artery should be clearly identified to avoid injury to this structure. At this point, the specimen consisting of the gallbladder and common bile duct; the head, neck, and uncinate process of the pancreas; the entire duodenum; and the proximal jejunum (and the distal stomach for a traditional Whipple procedure) is freed completely and removed from the operative field (Fig. 56.6).

There are a number of techniques for restoring gastrointestinal continuity after a pancreaticoduodenal resection. Our preferred technique is to bring the end of the divided jejunum through the transverse mesocolon in a retrocolic fashion and perform an end to side pancreaticojejunostomy. The anastomosis is begun by placing a series of interrupted 3-0 silk sutures between the side of the jejunum and the posterior capsule of the end of the pancreas. A small enterotomy is then made in the jejunum to match the size of the pancreatic duct and an inner layer of interrupted 5-0 absorbable monofilament sutures are used to create a duct-to-mucosa anastomosis. A short segment of a pediatric feeding tube is often placed across the anastomosis to be used as a temporary indwelling stent. The anastomosis is completed with an outer layer of 3-0 silk sutures placed between the anterior pancreatic capsule and the jejunum. An alternative to this duct-to-mucosa technique is to create an enterotomy approximately the same size as the pancreatic neck and to complete a running anastomosis circumferentially around the entire gland. This technique then allows invagination of the neck 1 to 2 cm into the lumen of the bowel by the outer anterior layer of the anastomosis. The biliary-enteric anastomosis is performed 10 cm distal to the pancreaticojejunostomy. An end-to-side hepaticojejunostomy is performed with a single interrupted layer of 4-0 absorbable synthetic suture material. No T-tube or stent is generally necessary. Approximately 15 cm distal to the biliary-enteric anastomosis, an end-to-side duodenojejunostomy is performed with an inner continuous layer of 3-0 absorbable synthetic suture material and an outer interrupted layer of 3-0 silk. Alternatively, some experienced pancreatic surgeons perform the duodenal-jejunal anastomosis further distally in an antecolic position, feeling that this technique decreases the incidence of early postoperative delayed gastric emptying. The final reconstruction is shown in Figure 56.6C.

Extent of Resection

The classic pancreaticoduodenectomy performed for decades included a distal gastrectomy. In 1978, Traverso and Longmire[15] described the pylorus-preserving modification of the Whipple procedure. By preserving the antrum and pylorus, the pylorus-preserving Whipple procedure may reduce the incidence of troublesome postgastrectomy problems, including marginal ulceration. A number of studies have documented that gastrointestinal function is better preserved in the pylorus-sparing modification than in the traditional operation.[16,17] In addition, compared with the classic Whipple operation, the pylorus-preserving procedure is less time-consuming and technically easier to perform. Concerns exist in the use of the pylorus-preserving Whipple procedure for the management of pancreatic tumors because of the possibility of compromising the already small proximal surgical margin of resection. This question has been addressed by a number of authors, and no difference appears to be found in survival among those patients treated with the pylorus-sparing Whipple procedure and those managed by the traditional Whipple resection.[18,19]

An extension of the Whipple procedure to include a total pancreatectomy with removal of the spleen and more extensive regional lymph nodes has been advocated by some surgeons. The overall poor long-term survival following the standard Whipple operation was the impetus for the concept of extending resection to a total pancreatectomy. Advocates also cite the advantages of eliminating multicentric disease and preventing the spread of disease to the distal pancreas by direct extension, intraductal seeding, or lymphatic spread. In addition, it is felt that this is a better cancer operation, including a wider *en bloc* resection of the pancreas in addition to regional lymph nodes. Another advantage is elimination of the pancreaticojejunal anastomosis, which is a major cause of morbidity and mortality following the Whipple operation. Despite these rational arguments, no evidence has accumulated that a total pancreatectomy offers any survival advantage for patients with carcinoma of the head of the pancreas who are undergoing the procedure. Furthermore, no reduction in morbidity and mortality has been noted for those patients managed by a total pancreatectomy. The major disadvantage of the total pancreatectomy is the inevitable complete loss of pancreatic endocrine function, resulting in the development of diabetes that can be difficult to control. Total pancreatectomy should be reserved for those patients with histologic evidence of tumor at the margin of resection or those with gross multicentric disease. It also may be indicated in a subset of patients with IPMNs that have diffuse involvement of the pancreatic duct.

The concept of an even wider resection, or radical pancreatectomy, has also been suggested. These procedures include resection of the portal vein with reconstruction and an extensive regional lymph node dissection. Reports from Japanese centers have suggested a potential improvement in long-term survival with extended lymphadenectomy. However, these results have been uncontrolled and do not appear significantly better than those in recent Western reports.[20] One prospective randomized Italian trial[21] suggested a survival advantage to extended retroperitoneal lymph node dissection in patients with positive lymph nodes. Eighty-one patients with pancreatic adenocarcinoma were randomized to either standard or radical lymphadenectomy over 3 years at six different institutions. Although the two groups were similar with respect to preoperative parameters, operative morbidity, and overall survival, a subgroup analysis of the 48 patients with positive lymph nodes showed a statistically significant survival advantage for patients undergoing the extended lymph node dissection. However, a large prospective randomized trial from the Johns Hopkins Hospital failed to demonstrate a survival advantage for a radical resection as compared with a classic pancreaticoduodenectomy.[18] Two hundred and ninety-four patients undergoing resection for periampullary adenocarcinoma were randomized between a standard resection (pylorus preserving pancreaticoduodenectomy with *en bloc* resection of the anterior and posterior pancreaticoduodenal lymph nodes, lower hepatoduodenal lymph nodes, and nodes along the right lateral aspect of the superior artery and vein) and a radical resection (standard resection plus distal gastrectomy and retroperitoneal lymph node dissection extending from the right renal hilum to the left lateral border of the aorta and from the portal vein to the inferior mesenteric artery). The groups did not differ with respect to age, gender, site of primary tumor, lymph node status, or margin status. There were no significant differences in 1-, 3-, or 5-year and median survival when comparing the standard and radical groups (Fig. 56.7). However, the radical group had a higher overall morbidity (43% vs. 29%) with significantly higher

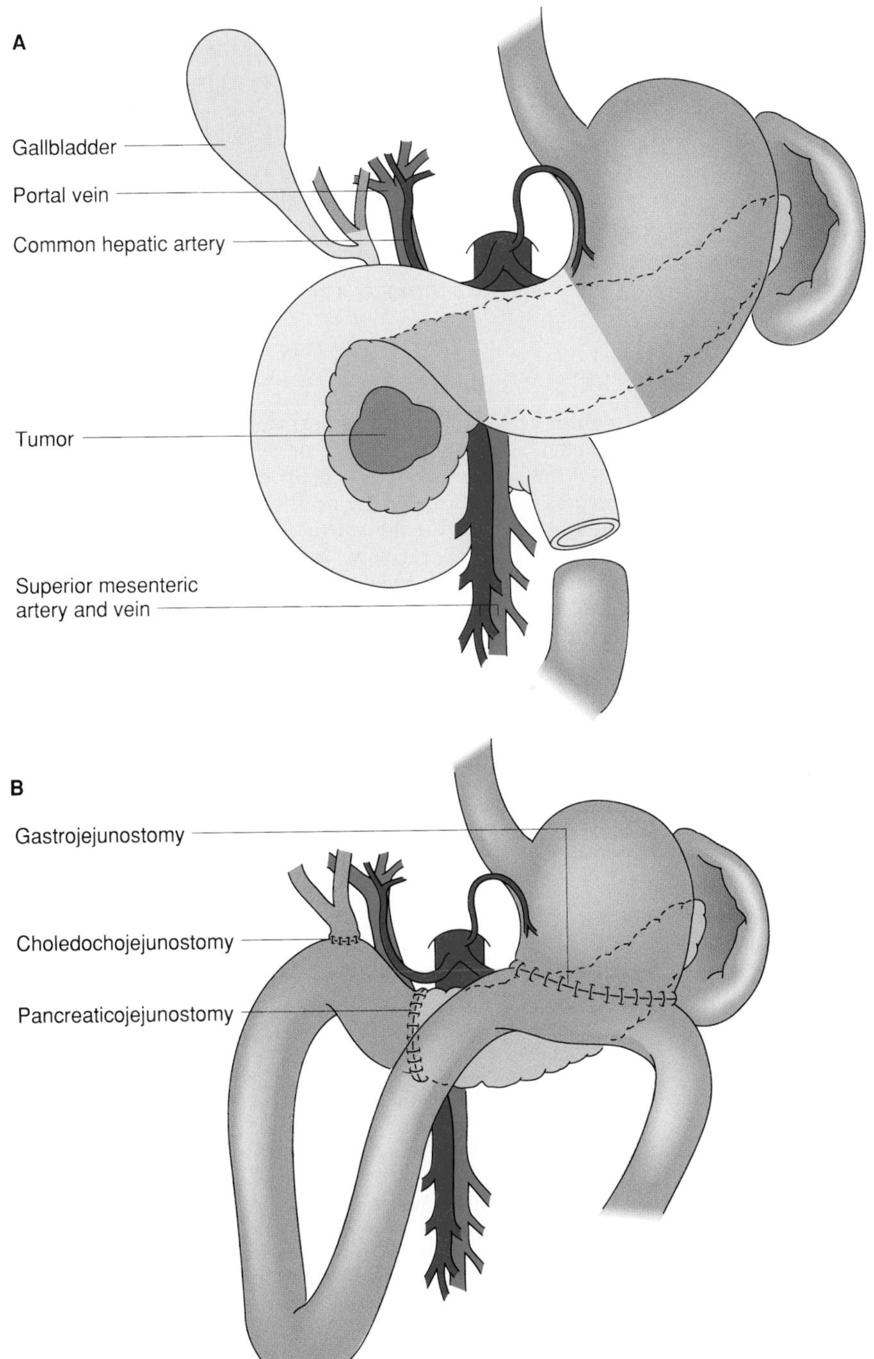

FIGURE 56.6 Pancreaticoduodenectomy. (*A*) The tissue to be resected in a standard pancreaticoduodenectomy. (*B*) Reconstruction after a standard pancreaticoduodenectomy. (*C*) Reconstruction after the pylorus-sparing variation.

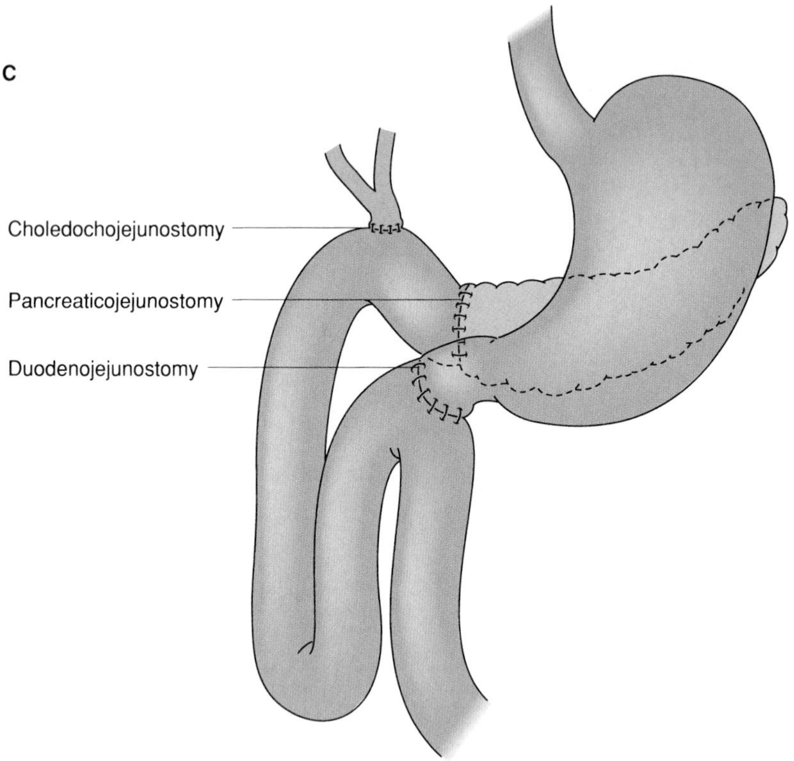

FIGURE 56.6 (*Continued*)

rates of delayed gastric emptying and pancreatic fistula in addition to a longer postoperative hospital stay.

Carcinoma of the Body and Tail

The surgical management of adenocarcinoma of the body and tail of the pancreas is much more limited than that of the head of the pancreas because of the extent of the disease usually present at the time of symptomatic presentation. Most patients are unable to undergo resection, based on findings of major vascular involvement on CT or peritoneal or liver metastases on laparoscopy. If an attempt at open exploration for possible cure is undertaken, the exploration should be started with a search for evidence of either metastatic disease to the liver or peritoneal implants. If this is not the case, the lesser sac is opened, and the SMV is identified as it passes under the neck of the pancreas. If this vessel is normal, and if the splenic vein does not appear to be obstructed preoperatively, a distal pancreatectomy with splenectomy is performed. The spleen is mobilized, as is the distal pancreas, and an *en bloc* resection of the structure, including the mass, is obtained. The resection should be extended as proximally as possible, with the transected pancreas simply oversewn. The tumor bed should be marked with the placement of clips for postoperative radiation therapy. If, as in most cases, the tumor cannot be resected, a tissue biopsy should be performed, in addition to a chemical

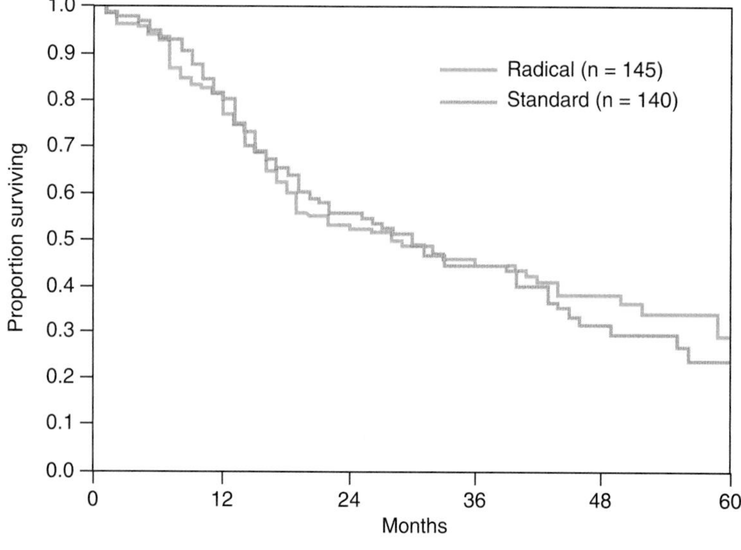

FIGURE 56.7 Actuarial survival for standard versus radical pancreaticoduodenectomy. (From Yeo CJ, Cameron JL, Lillemoe KD, et al. Pancreaticoduodenectomy with or without distal gastrectomy and extended retroperitoneal lymphadenectomy for periampullary adenocarcinoma, part 2: randomized controlled trial evaluating survival, morbidity, and mortality. *Ann Surg.* 2002;236:355, with permission.)

splanchnicectomy with alcohol for pain management. In some cases, a prophylactic gastrojejunostomy may be indicated because of the potential for obstruction by tumor at the ligament of Treitz.

Postoperative Results

During the 1960s and 1970s, many centers reported operative mortality following pancreaticoduodenectomy in the range of 20% to 40%, with postoperative morbidity rates as high as 40% to 60%. During the last two decades, a dramatic decline in operative morbidity and mortality following pancreaticoduodenectomy has been reported at a number of centers, with operative mortality rates in the range of 2% to 3%.[22–25] The reasons behind this decline appear to be the following: (a) fewer, more experienced surgeons are performing the operation on a more frequent basis, (b) preoperative and postoperative care has improved, (c) anesthetic management has improved, and (d) large numbers of patients are being treated at high-volume centers.[26]

Although the operative mortality rates for pancreatic cancer have been reduced significantly, the complication rates remain high (approximately 30%) (Table 56.10). Pancreatic fistula remains the most frequent serious complication following pancreaticoduodenectomy, with an incidence ranging from 5% to 15%. In the past, the development of pancreatic fistula after pancreaticoduodenectomy was associated with mortality rates of 10% to 40%. Although the incidence of pancreatic fistula following pancreaticoduodenectomy remains stable, the overall associated mortality rate has diminished owing to improved management. Important supportive measures include careful maintenance of fluid and electrolyte balance, parenteral nutrition, and controlling the pancreatic leak with percutaneous or intraoperative drainage.

Long-term Survival

Historically, 5-year survival rates for patients undergoing resection for adenocarcinoma of the head of the pancreas were reported to be in the range of 5%. However, a number of recent studies have suggested an improved survival for patients following pancreaticoduodenectomy.[23,24] In 2000, Sohn et al.[22] reported on 616 patients with of the pancreas managed by resection. The actuarial 5-year survival for these patients was 17%, with a median survival of 17 months (Fig. 56.8). In this study, factors found to be important predictors of survival included tumor diameter (<3 cm), negative resection margin status, well/moderate tumor differentiation, and postoperative chemoradiation treatment. Patients who underwent resection with negative margins had a median survival of 19 months and a 5-year survival of 21%, whereas those with positive margins fared significantly worse, with a median survival of 12 months and a 5-year survival of 6%.

TABLE 56.10 COMPLICATIONS

COMPLICATIONS AFTER PANCREATICODUODENECTOMY

COMMON
- Delayed gastric emptying
- Pancreatic fistula
- Intraabdominal abscess
- Hemorrhage
- Wound infection
- Metabolic
  - Diabetes
  - Pancreatic exocrine insufficiency

UNCOMMON
- Fistula
  - Biliary
  - Duodenal
  - Gastric
- Organ failure
  - Cardiac
  - Hepatic
  - Pulmonary
  - Renal
- Pancreatitis
- Marginal ulceration

From Yeo CJ, Cameron JL. Pancreatic cancer. *Curr Probl Surg.* 1999;36:61, with permission.

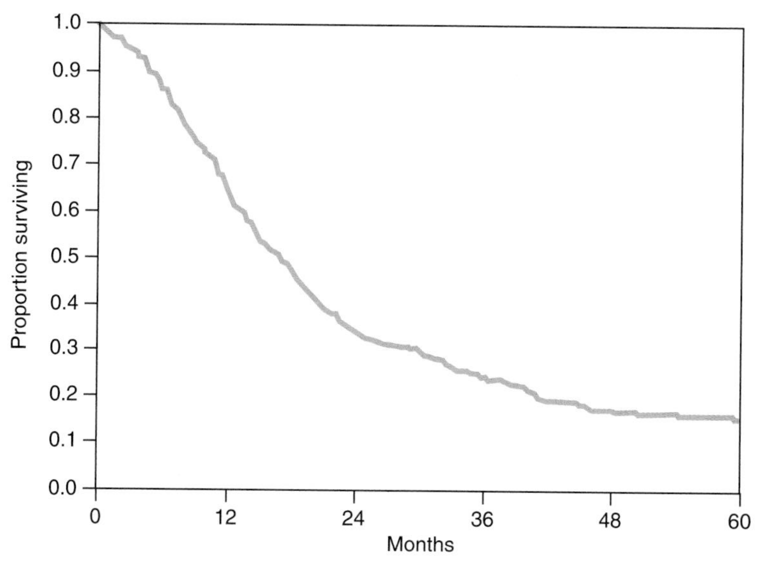

FIGURE 56.8 Kaplan-Meier actuarial survival for 616 patients with resected pancreatic adenocarcinoma. (From Sohn TA, Yeo CJ, Cameron JL, et al. Resected adenocarcinoma of the pancreas 616 patients: results, outcomes, and prognostic indicators. *J Gastrointest Surg.* 2000;4:567, with permission.)

The outcome was particularly favorable in the subgroup of patients with small tumors (<3 cm) who underwent margin-negative, node-negative resections; the median survival was 33 months and the 5-year survival was 31%.

ADJUVANT AND NEOADJUVANT THERAPY

At present, the general consensus of most surgeons treating patients with pancreatic carcinoma is that any future improvement in the management of this disease will involve improvements in adjuvant therapy. The role of adjuvant radiation therapy is emphasized by the pattern of relapse after surgical resection, as more than half of the patients undergoing resection experience local regional recurrence without evidence of distant metastases.[27]

In 1985, the Gastrointestinal Tumor Study Group reported encouraging results from a prospective, randomized trial to evaluate the efficacy of adjuvant radiation and chemotherapy following curative resection for adenocarcinoma of the head of the pancreas.[28] Forty-three patients were randomized to either adjuvant therapy with radiation and 5-fluorouracil (5-FU) or no adjuvant therapy. The median survival for the 21 patients who received adjuvant therapy was 20 months, and three (14%) survived 5 years or longer. For the 22 patients who received no adjuvant therapy, the median survival was 11 months, and only one patient (4.5%) survived 5 years. This finding was replicated in a randomized trial conducted by the European Organization for Research and Treatment of Cancer (EORTC), which also found an increase in median survival from 13 to 17 months.[29] In a single-institution nonrandomized study from Johns Hopkins,[30] 174 patients with resected pancreatic adenocarcinoma of the head, neck, or uncinate process of the pancreas were offered three options for postoperative treatment after pancreaticoduodenectomy: (a) standard therapy that consisted of external beam radiation to the pancreatic bed (4,000 to 4,500 cGy) given with two 3-day courses of 5-FU followed weekly by a bolus of 5-FU for an additional 4 months, (b) intensive therapy that consisted of external beam radiation to the pancreatic bed (5,040 to 5,760 cGy) with prophylactic hepatic irradiation (2,340 to 2,700 cGy) followed by infusional 5-FU plus leucovorin for 5 of 7 days/week for 4 months, (c) no therapy. In the 4-year period of this study, 174 patients underwent pancreaticoduodenectomy for pancreatic carcinoma. Patients who received either type of adjuvant therapy had a median survival of 19.5 months and a 2-year survival of 39%, significantly better than the survival rate of the patients who received no therapy (13.5 months and 30%) (Fig. 56.9). These results have been subsequently confirmed and provide strong support for the concept of postoperative combined adjuvant therapy.

Recently, however a report from the European Study Group for Pancreatic Cancer found that patients receiving adjuvant chemotherapy with 5-FU had a significant increase in survival, but those receiving chemoradiation with 20 Gray plus 5-FU had a significant decrease in survival.[31] Thus, the survival benefit of adjuvant chemoradiation for pancreatic cancer patients remains unclear, and the optimal regimen has yet to be determined.

A promising interferon-based adjuvant chemoradiation protocol for resected pancreatic adenocarcinoma has been proposed by the group at the Virginia Mason Medical Center.[32] This protocol consists of external-beam irradiation at a dose of 4,500 to 5,400 cGy (25 fractions over 5 weeks) and three-drug chemotherapy: continuous infusion 5-FU, weekly intravenous bolus cisplatin, and subcutaneus alpha-interferon. This chemoradiation is followed by continuous infusion 5-FU therapy. In the 43 patients studied the 1-, 2-, and 5-year actuarial survival was 95%, 64%, and 55%, respectively. Further investigations of this promising regimen are underway.

At present, a number of clinical trials are underway that are utilizing preoperative chemoradiation protocols for the treatment of pancreatic cancer. Preliminary results suggest that neoadjuvant therapy can be completed without increasing the subsequent morbidity and mortality of surgical resection. The group from the M.D. Anderson Cancer Center has reported on the multimodality treatment of 142 consecutive patients with localized adenocarcinoma of the pancreatic head.[33] A subset of 41 patients treated by preoperative chemoradiation and pancreaticoduodenectomy were compared with 19 patients receiving pancreaticoduodenectomy and postoperative adjuvant chemoradiation. Surgery did not have to be delayed for any patient who received preoperative chemoradiation because of chemoradiation toxicity, but 24% of the eligible patients did not receive their intended postoperative chemoradiation because of delayed recovery following pancreaticoduodenectomy. The patients treated with rapid fractionation were reported to have a significantly shorter duration of treatment (median, 62.5 days) than patients who received postoperative chemoradiation (median, 98.5 days). In early follow-up, no patient who received preoperative chemoradiation experienced a local recurrence, and peritoneal recurrence developed in only 10% of these patients. Local or regional recurrence developed in 21% of patients who

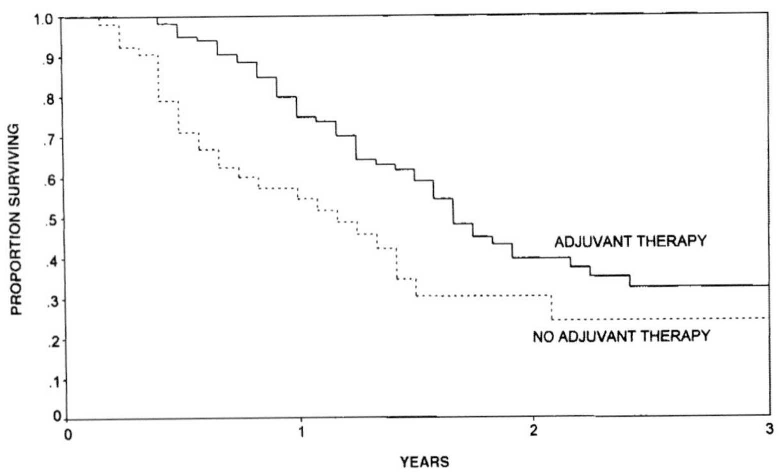

FIGURE 56.9 Actuarial survival curves for 173 patients who underwent pancreaticoduodenectomy. Patients who received adjuvant therapy (n = 120) are compared with those who declined adjuvant therapy (n = 53). (From Yeo CJ, Abrams RA, Grochow LB, et al. Pancreaticoduodenectomy for pancreatic adenocarcinoma: postoperative adjuvant chemoradiation improves survival: a prospective, single-institution experience. *Ann Surg.* 1997;225:621, with permission.)

received postoperative chemoradiation. The overall survival curves were similar for both cohorts. The use of neoadjuvant therapy remains controversial, with some groups reserving neoadjuvant therapy only for patients with evidence of locally unresectable tumors (as defined by imaging studies or laparotomy).

PALLIATION

Unfortunately, it has been the experience nationwide that only a minority of patients with carcinoma of the pancreas can undergo resection for possible cure at the time diagnosis is made. The overall median survival from the time of diagnosis is less than 5 months with a 1-year survival rate of 10% and a 5-year survival rate of only 3%. Therefore, the optimal palliation of symptoms to maximize quality of life is of primary importance in most patients with pancreatic cancer. Both operative and nonoperative options are available for the palliation of pancreatic cancer.

Jaundice

Obstructive jaundice is present in most patients who have pancreatic cancer. If left untreated, it can result in progressive liver dysfunction, hepatic failure, and early death. In addition, the pruritus associated with obstructive jaundice can be debilitating and usually does not respond to medication. When patients undergo exploration for possible cure and are found to have unresectable disease, a biliary bypass should be performed.

Traditionally, surgeons have performed either choledochojejunostomy or cholecystojejunostomy for the relief of malignant biliary obstruction. Both procedures are effective in relieving jaundice, but it appears that the rate of recurrent jaundice after cholecystojejunostomy is approximately 10%. Therefore, our preference for the palliation of obstructive jaundice is a hepaticojejunostomy or choledochojejunostomy reconstructed with a Roux-en-Y limb of jejunum. The surgical palliation of jaundice can be accomplished safely, with a mortality rate of less than 3% and an overall morbidity rate of 30% to 40%.[34] The gallbladder is usually removed at the time of choledochojejunostomy to prevent the development of late cholecystitis if the cystic duct becomes obstructed by tumor. In certain circumstances, however, it may be appropriate to use the gallbladder as a conduit for palliation. These include the presence of large bulky tumors that have invaded the porta hepatis or of large periductal varices that have developed as a result of portal vein thrombosis. If the gallbladder is to be used, the patency of the cystic duct should be confirmed, and the cystic duct should enter the common bile duct at least 2 cm away from any tumor.

In recent years, nonoperative palliation has become available as an option for managing patients who are deemed unresectable by preop staging. Plastic or metal stents can be placed across the biliary obstruction by either an endoscopic or a percutaneous technique. For pancreatic cancer, the endoscopic approach is usually preferred. The overall morbidity rate for endoscopic stenting ranges up to 35%, but the rate of major procedure-related morbidity is less than 10%. Early complications include cholangitis, pancreatitis, and bile duct or duodenal perforation. The major late complications of stent placement are cholecystitis, duodenal perforation, and stent migration. Stent occlusion can result in episodes of cholangitis and recurrent jaundice. For most patients, an exchange of stents is required every 3 to 6 months. The newer metal stents appear to remain patent for longer periods.

Nonoperative palliation appears to be associated with lower complication rates, lower procedure-related mortality rates, and shorter initial periods of hospitalization in comparison with surgical palliation. However, the rate of recurrent jaundice is higher. No advantage with respect to long-term survival has been noted for either approach. Therefore, nonoperative palliation should be offered to patients with advanced disease or poor performance status. Surgical palliation should be considered for patients with an anticipated life expectancy of at least 6 months.

Duodenal Obstruction

At the time that pancreatic cancer is diagnosed, approximately one third of patients have symptoms of nausea or vomiting. Although true mechanical obstruction of the duodenum seen by radiologic or endoscopic examination is much less frequent, duodenal obstruction develops in almost 20% of patients before they die as the disease progresses.[35] Duodenal obstruction can be caused in the C-loop by cancers of the head or at the ligament of Trietz by cancers of the body and tail. In patients with evidence of duodenal obstruction or impending obstruction, a gastrojejunostomy is indicated for palliation. This is typically performed as a retrocolic, isoperistaltic loop gastrojejunostomy with a loop of jejunum 20 to 30 cm distal to the ligament of Trietz.

In patients with unresectable pancreatic cancer who do not have symptoms of gastric outlet obstruction, whether or not to perform a prophylactic gastric bypass at the time of biliary bypass is a matter of debate. Surgeons who do not perform a prophylactic bypass feel that it needlessly increases the postoperative length of stay and can be associated with delayed gastric emptying and increased morbidity and mortality. However, data from a prospective, randomized trial of prophylactic gastrojejunostomy in patients with unresectable cancer do not support this view.[36] In this study, 44 patients were randomized to a gastrojejunostomy, and 43 did not undergo gastric bypass. No mortality occurred in either group. No difference was observed in either the complication rate or the postoperative length of stay (Table 56.11). However, late duodenal obstruction developed in 19% of the patients who did not undergo bypass. A recent multicenter prospective randomized controlled trial has confirmed these results.[37] Therefore, we believe that a prophylactic gastrojejunostomy should be performed in patients undergoing surgical palliation for unresectable pancreatic carcinoma.

Pain

Tumor-associated pain can be incapacitating in patients with unresectable pancreatic cancer. The postulated causes of tumor-associated pain are many and include tumor infiltration into the celiac plexus, increased parenchymal pressure caused by pancreatic duct obstruction, pancreatic inflammation, gallbladder distention resulting from biliary obstruction, and gastroduodenal obstruction. The management of pain in patients dying of carcinoma of the pancreas is one of the most important aspects of their care. The appropriate use of oral agents can be successful in most patients. Patients with significant pain should receive their medication on a regular schedule and not an "as-needed" basis. The use of long-acting morphine derivative compounds appears to be best suited for such treatment.

TABLE 56.11

PROSPECTIVE RANDOMIZED TRIAL OF PROPHYLACTIC GASTROJEJUNOSTOMY IN PATIENTS WITH UNRESECTABLE PERIAMPULLARY CANCER

	Patients (no.)	Morbidity (%)	Mortality (%)	Postoperative length of stay (d)	Late gastric outlet obstruction (%)
Gastrojejunostomy	44	32	0	8.5	0
No gastrojejunostomy	43	33	0	8.0	19

Adapted from Lillemoe KD, Cameron JL, Hardacre JM, et al. Is prophylactic gastrojejunostomy indicated for unresectable periampullary cancer? *Ann Surg*. 1999;230:322–330.

Percutaneous neurolytic block of the celiac axis, performed under either fluoroscopic or CT guidance, is also successful in the majority of patients at eliminating pain. Patients with unresectable cancer at the time of surgical exploration should receive a chemical splanchnicectomy, with 20 mL of 50% alcohol injected on either side of the aorta at the level of the celiac axis.[38]

Summary

The decision to perform nonoperative versus surgical palliation for pancreatic cancer is influenced by a number of factors, including the patient's symptoms, overall health status, predicted procedure-related morbidity and mortality, and projected survival. Surgical palliation can be completed with acceptable perioperative morbidity and mortality and postoperative length of stay. The avoidance of late complications of recurrent jaundice, duodenal obstruction, and disabling pain would strengthen the argument in favor of surgical palliation in those patients expected to survive 6 months or more. Nonoperative methods of palliation should be considered for patients in whom preoperative staging suggests distant metastatic disease or a locally unresectable tumor, patients who are not candidates for operative intervention, and those not expected to survive more than 3 months.

Radiation and Chemotherapy for Unresectable Pancreatic Carcinoma

Specific antitumor therapies in patients with advanced pancreatic carcinoma have been studied for years, with limited success. Trials evaluating the use of chemotherapy and radiation therapy both alone and in combination have shown a marginal improvement in survival, often with relatively high toxicity rates and some negative impact on quality of life. Recently gemcitabine, a deoxycytidine analogue capable of inhibiting DNA replication and repair, has become increasingly popular. When gemcitabine was compared with bolus 5-FU in a randomized phase III trial, it was shown to confer a significant survival benefit in advanced pancreatic cancer, increasing median survival from 4.4 months to 5.7 months and increasing 1-year survival from 2% to 18%, respectively.[39] A key end point in this study was "clinical benefit response," based on reducing pain, improving performance status, and inducing weight gain, which was attained in 24% of patients receiving gemcitabine compared with 5% for those receiving 5-FU. In patients with metastatic pancreatic cancer that had progressed with 5-FU and then been treated with gemcitabine, the median survival (in 63 of 74 patients enrolled) was 3.9 months.[40] Seventeen patients (27%) attained a clinical benefit response with a median duration of 14 weeks. Gemcitabine is generally well-tolerated with a low incidence of significant toxicity and therefore seems to be a reasonable choice for palliative therapy.

In addition to gemcitabine, other agents are currently being studied for a role in the palliation of patients with pancreatic adenocarcinoma. Examples of such agents are paclitaxel (Taxol), matrix metalloproteinase inhibitors (e.g., marimastat, perillyl alcohol), and inhibitors of angiogenesis, such as TNP-470. The results of such studies are eagerly awaited.

KEY POINTS

- **Approximately 65% of the pancreatic ductal cancers arise in the head, neck, or uncinate process of the pancreas, 15% originate in the body or the tail of the gland, and 20% diffusely involve the entire gland.**
- **There is increasing evidence that ductal pancreatic cancer arises from precursor lesions referred to as pancreatic intraepithelial neoplasia (PanIN) with progression from proliferative lesions without nuclear abnormality to carcinoma *in situ*, known as PanIn-3.**
- **Intraductal papillary mucinous neoplasm (IPMNs) are intraductal mucin-producing tumors that range from benign adenomas to invasive carcinoma and should be resected as all must be considered to have malignant potential.**
- **Spiral CT scan is the preferred noninvasive imaging test for the diagnosis and staging of pancreatic cancer demonstrating the primary lesion and its relationship to adjacent visceral vessels as well as metastatic disease to the liver and peritoneum.**
- **At the time of diagnosis only 10% of patients have tumors confined to the pancreas, 40% have locally advanced disease, and more than 50% have distant spread leaving only 10% to 20% as candidates for pancreatic resection.**
- **Perioperative mortality rates following pancreaticoduodenectomy have fallen to the range of 2% to 5% although perioperative complications occur in approximately 30% of patients.**
- **Although pancreatic fistula remains the most frequent serious complication following pancreaticoduodenectomy, occurring in 5% to 15% of patients, the mortality rate associated with the complication has been markedly diminished due to improved management.**
- **The survival rate after pancreaticoduodenectomy for pancreatic cancer is approximately 20% with factors influencing survival including tumors size, margin status, and node status.**

- **Although some controversy exists, most data support the role for adjuvant therapy, either chemotherapy or chemoradiation, for patients following resection of a pancreatic cancer.**
- **Surgical palliation of patients with pancreatic cancer located in the head found to be unresectable at laparotomy includes biliary bypass, gastrojejunostomy, and chemical splanchnicectomy to palliate the symptoms of jaundice, duodenal obstruction, and pain, respectively.**

References

1. Surveillance, Epidemiology, and End Results (SEER) Program (www.seer.cancer.gov) SEER*Stat Database.
2. Yeo CJ, Cameron JL. Pancreatic cancer. *Curr Probl Surg.* 1999;36:61.
3. Hruban RH. Pancreatic cancer: from genes to patient care. *J Gastrointest Surg.* 2001;5:583.
4. Goggins M, Oferhaus GJA, Hilgers W, et al. Adenocarcinoma of the pancreas with DNA replication errors (RER+) are associated with a characteristic histopathology: poor differentiation, a syncytial growth pattern, and pushing borders suggest RER+. *Am J Pathol.* 1998;152:1501.
5. **Wilentz RE, Hruban RH. Pathology of cancer of the pancreas. *Surg Oncol Clin North Am.* 1998;7:43.**
6. Takaori K, Hruban RH, Maitra A, Tanigawa M. Pancreatic intraepithelial neoplasia. *Pancreas* 2004;28:257.
7. **Sohn TA, Yeo CJ, Cameron JL, et al. Intraductal papillary mucinous neoplasms of the pancreas an updated experience. *Ann Surg.* 2004;239:788.**
8. Ritts RE, Pitt HA. CA 19-9 in pancreatic cancer. *Surg Oncol Clin North Am.* 1998;7:93.
9. Pisters PWT, Lee JE, Vauthey, et al. Laparoscopy in the staging of pancreatic cancer. *Br J Surg.* 2001;88:325.
10. Dye CE, Waxman I. Endoscopic ultrasound. *Gastroenterol Clin North Am.* 2002;31:863.
11. Conlon KC, Dougherty E, Klimstra DS, et al. The value of minimal access surgery in the staging of patients with potentially resectable peripancreatic malignancy. *Ann Surg.* 1996;223:134.
12. Barreiro CJ, Lillemoe KD, Koniaris LG, et al. Diagnostic laparoscopy for periampullary and pancreatic cancer: what is the true benefit? *J Gastrointest Surg.* 2002;6:75.
13. Kausch W. Das Carcinom der Papilla Duodeni and seine radikale Entfeinung. *Beitrage zur Klinische Chirurgie* 1912;78:439.
14. Whipple AO, Parsons WB, Mullins CR. Treatment of carcinoma of the ampulla of Vater. *Ann Surg.* 1935;102:763.
15. Traverso LW, Longmire WP Jr. Preservation of the pylorus in pancreaticoduodenectomy. *Surg Gynecol Obstet.* 1978;146:959.
16. Kozuschek W, Reith HB, Waleczek H, et al. A comparison of long term results of the standard Whipple procedure and the pylorus preserving pancreatoduodenectomy. *J Am Coll Surg.* 1994;178:443.
17. Takada T, Yasuda H, Amano H, et al. Results of a pylorus-preserving pancreatoduodenectomy for pancreatic cancer: a comparison with results of the Whipple procedure. *Hepatogastroenterology* 1997;44:1536.
18. Yeo CJ, Cameron JL, Lillemoe KD, et al. Pancreaticoduodenectomy with or without distal gastrectomy and extended retroperitoneal lymphadenectomy for periampullary adenocarcinoma, part 2: randomized controlled trial evaluating survival, morbidity, and mortality. *Ann Surg.* 2002; 236:355.
19. Tran KT, Smeenk HG, van Eijck CH, et al. Pylorus-preserving pancreaticoduodenectomy versus standard Whipple procedure a prospective randomized multicenter analysis of 170 patients with pancreatic and periampullary tumors. *Ann Surg.* 2004;240:738.
20. Yeo CJ, Cameron JL, Lillemoe KD, et al. Pancreaticoduodenectomy for cancer of the head of the pancreas: 201 patients. Ann Surg 1995;221:721–733.
21. Pedrazzoli S, DiCarlo V, Dionigi R, et al. Standard versus extended lymphadenectomy associated with pancreatoduodenectomy in the surgical treatment of adenocarcinoma of the head of the pancreas: a multicenter, prospective, randomized study. Lymphadenectomy Study Group. *Ann Surg.* 1998;228:508.
22. **Sohn TA, Yeo CJ, Cameron JL, et al. Resected adenocarcinoma of the pancreas 616 patients: results, outcomes, and prognostic indicators. *J Gastrointest Surg.* 2000;4:567.**
23. Richter A, Neidergethmann, Sturm JW, et al. Long-term results of partial pancreaticoduodenectomy for ductal adenocarcinoma of the pancreatic head: 25-year experience. *World J Surg.* 2003;27:324.
24. Fernandez-del Castillo, Rattner DW, Warshaw AL. Standards for pancreatic resection in the 1990s. *Arch Surg.* 1995;130:295.
25. Schmidt CM. Powell ES. Yiannoutsos CT, et al. Pancreaticoduodenectomy: a 20-year experience in 516 patients. *Arch Surg.* 2004;139:718.
26. **Sosa JA, Bowman HM, Gordon TA, et al. Importance of hospital volume in the overall management of pancreatic cancer. *Ann Surg.* 1998;228:320.**
27. Tepper J, Nardi G, Suit H. Carcinoma of the pancreas: review of MGH experience from 1963–1973: analysis of surgical failure and implications for radiation therapy. *Cancer* 1977;37:1519.
28. Kaiser MH, Ellenberg SS. Pancreatic cancer: adjuvant combined radiation and chemotherapy following curative resection. *Arch Surg.* 1985;97:28.
29. Kinkenbijl JH, Jeekel J, Sahmoud T, et al. Adjuvant radiotherapy and 5-fluorouracil after curative resection of cancer of the pancreas and periampullar region. *Ann Surg.* 1999;230:776.
30. Yeo CJ, Abrams RA, Grochow LB, et al. Pancreaticoduodenectomy for pancreatic adenocarcinoma: postoperative adjuvant chemoradiation improves survival: a prospective, single-institution experience. *Ann Surg.* 1997;225:621.
31. Neoptolemos JP, Stocken DD, Freiss H, et al. A randomized trial of chemoradiotherapy and chemotherapy after resection of pancreatic cancer. *N Engl J Med.* 2004;350:1200.
32. Picozzi VJ, Kozarek RA, Traverso LW. Interferon-based adjuvant chemoradiation therapy after pancreaticoduodenectomy for pancreatic adenocarcinoma. *Am J Surg.* 2003;185:476.
33. Spitz FR, Abbruzzese JL, Lee JE, et al. Preoperative and postoperative chemoradiation strategies in patients treated with pancreaticoduodenectomy for adenocarcinoma of the pancreas. *J Clin Oncol.* 1997; 15:928.
34. **Sohn TA, Lillemoe KD, Cameron JL, et al. Surgical palliation of unresectable periampullary carcinoma in the 1990s. *J Am Coll Surg.* 1999; 188:658.**
35. Sarr MG, Cameron JL. Surgical management of unresectable carcinoma of the pancreas. *Surgery* 1982;91:123.
36. Lillemoe KD, Cameron JL, Hardacre JM, et al. Is prophylactic gastrojejunostomy indicated for unresectable periampullary cancer? *Ann Surg.* 1999;230:322.
37. Van Heek NT, De Castro SM, van Eijck CH, et al. The need for a prophylactic gastrojejunostomy for unresectable periampullary cancer: a prospective randomized multicenter trial with special focus on assessment of quality of life. *Ann Surg.* 2003;238:894.
38. Lillemoe KD, Cameron JL, Kaufman HS, et al. Chemical splanchnicectomy in patients with unresectable pancreatic cancer: a prospective randomized trial. *Ann Surg.* 1993;217:447.
39. Burris HA, Moore MJ, Anderson J, et al. Improvements in survival and clinical benefit with gemcitabine as first-line therapy for patients with advanced pancreas cancer: a randomized trial. *J Clin Oncol.* 1997;15:2403.
40. Rothenberg ML, Moore MJ, Cripps MC, et al. A phase II trial of gemcitabine in patients with 5-FU refractory pancreas cancer. *Ann Oncol.* 1996;7:347.

CHAPTER 57 ■ NEOPLASMS OF THE ENDOCRINE PANCREAS

TAYLOR SOHN RIALL AND CHARLES J. YEO

The cells of the pancreatic islets are presumed to originate from neural crest cells, although some evidence suggests that they may have an endodermal origin.[1] Cells of this origin are called *amine precursor uptake and decarboxylation* (APUD) cells because they have a high amine content, are capable of amine precursor uptake, and contain and amino acid decarboxylase enzyme. A generalized derangement of the APUD system can cause abnormalities of multiple endocrine cells, as is observed in the multiple endocrine neoplasia (MEN) syndromes.

Neoplasms of the endocrine pancreas are rare, with an annual clinically recognized incidence in the United States of about five cases per million persons. These neoplasms are actually more common but clinically insignificant, with a prevalence in autopsy series of approximately 1 per 100 persons, in whom they are typically noted as incidental findings. These neoplasms can classified as *functional* or *nonfunctional* depending on whether or not they release one or more hormonal products into the bloodstream. The majority of pancreatic endocrine neoplasms discovered are functional, because the release of hormonal products lead to a clinically recognizable syndrome (Table 57.1). Patients with endocrine tumors of the pancreas but no recognizable clinical syndrome and normal serum levels (excluding pancreatic polypeptide and chromogranin) are considered to have nonfunctional pancreatic endocrine neoplasms. Patients with MEN-1 syndrome and von Hippel-Lindau disease have an inherited predisposition to pancreatic endocrine neoplasia.[2]

All neoplasms of the endocrine pancreas have a similar appearance under the light microscope. Routine histologic examination does not predict the biologic behavior or the endocrine manifestations of these neoplasms. Immunofluorescence techniques and the peroxidase—antiperoxidase procedure allow the demonstration of specific hormones within neoplastic cells. Malignancy is typically determined by the presence of local invasion that has spread to regional lymph nodes or by the existence of hepatic or distant metastases. A recent study on 82 resected tumors has shown that a low intramural microvascular density correlates with increased risk of metastases and shorter postresection survival.[3]

Three general principles apply to the treatment of patients with suspected functional neoplasms of the endocrine pancreas. One must *first* recognize the abnormal physiology or characteristic syndrome. Characteristic clinical syndromes are well described for insulinoma, gastrinoma, VIPoma, and glucagonoma. The somatostatinoma syndrome is nonspecific, much more difficult to recognize, and exceedingly rare. *Second* is the detection of hormone elevations in the serum by radioimmunoassay. Such assays are readily available for measuring insulin, gastrin, vasoactive intestinal peptide (VIP), and glucagon. Assays for somatostatin, pancreatic polypeptide (PP), prostaglandins, and other hormonal markers are less commonly available but can be obtained from certain laboratories. The *third* step involves localizing and staging the tumor in preparation for possible operative intervention (Algorithm 57.1).

LOCALIZATION AND STAGING

The initial imaging technique used to localize a pancreatic endocrine neoplasm and stage the disease is a high-quality spiral or multidetector three-dimensional computed tomography (CT) scan.[4–7] The accuracy of CT in detecting primary pancreatic endocrine neoplasms varies widely from 35% to 85% but has been significantly improved by modern techniques and focused scanning through the pancreas at 3- to 5-mm intervals.

TABLE 57.1 ■ CLASSIFICATION

CLASSIFICATION OF FUNCTIONAL PANCREATIC ENDOCRINE TUMORS

Tumor (syndrome)	Clinical features	Extrapancreatic location	Malignancy rate
Insulinoma	Hypoglycemia	Rare	10%
Gastrinoma (Zollinger-Ellison)	Peptic ulcer Diarrhea	Frequent	50%
VIPoma (Verner-Morrison; WDHA; pancreatic cholera)	Watery diarrhea Hypokalemia Achlorhydria/acidosis	10%	Most
Glucagonoma	Hyperglycemia Dermatitis	Rare	Most
Somatostatinoma	Hyperglycemia Steatorrhea Gallstones	Rare	Most

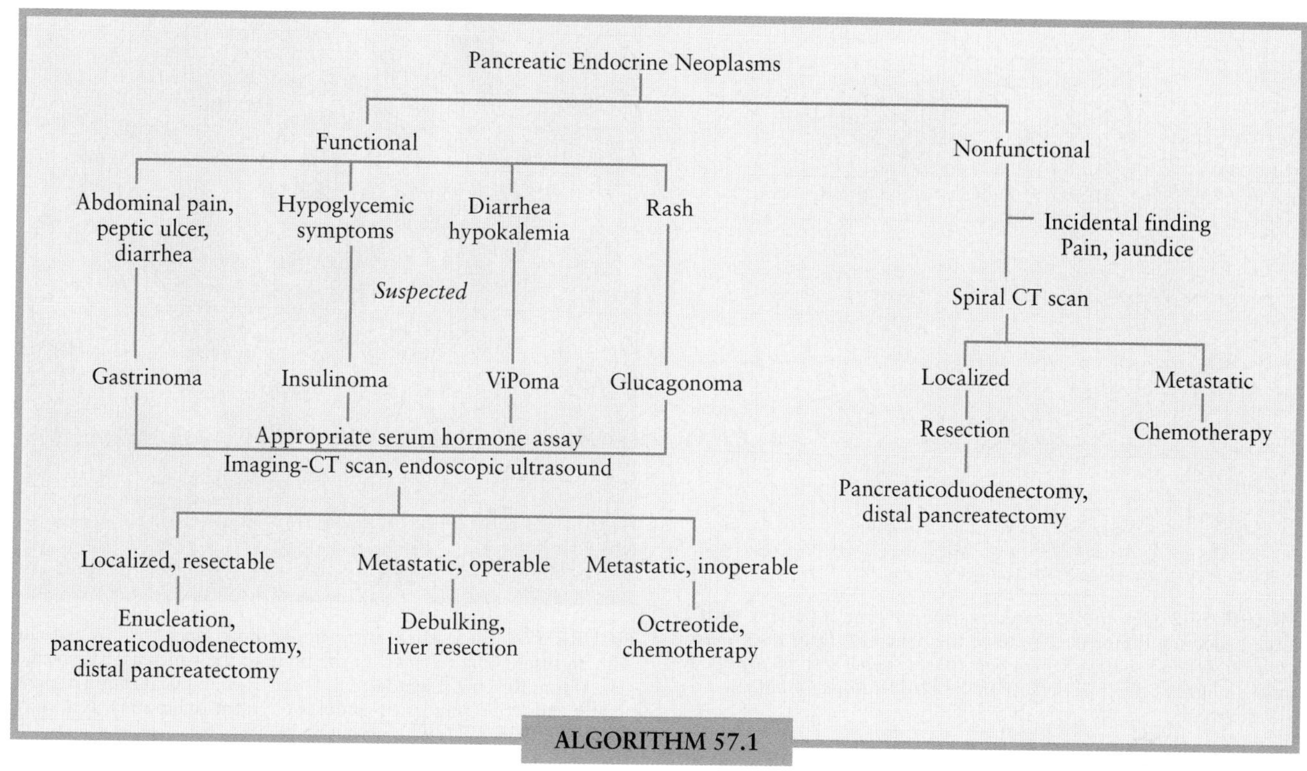

ALGORITHM 57.1 Diagnosis and management of pancreatic endocrine neoplasms.

CT is useful in assessing size and location of the primary tumor, peripancreatic lymph node involvement, and the presence or absence of liver metastases (Fig. 57.1).

Somatostatin receptor scintigraphy (SRS) also plays an important role in imaging patients with pancreatic endocrine tumors.[8–14] In this technique, the octapeptide analogue of somatostatin (Octreotide) labeled with indium-111 is administered intravenously to patients in whom a pancreatic endocrine neoplasm is suspected. Because neuroendocrine tumors often express large numbers of somatostatin receptors on their cell surfaces (Fig. 57.2), the tracer preferentially identifies tumors. Meko at al.[9] reported the overall sensitivity of SRS to be 74% for detecting local disease and 67% for detecting distant disease. They also reported a significant false-negative rate, indicating that negative SRS findings in patients with pancreatic endocrine neoplasms should be viewed with caution. Nonfunctional tumors and insulinomas seem to be localized less frequently by SRS than by CT or

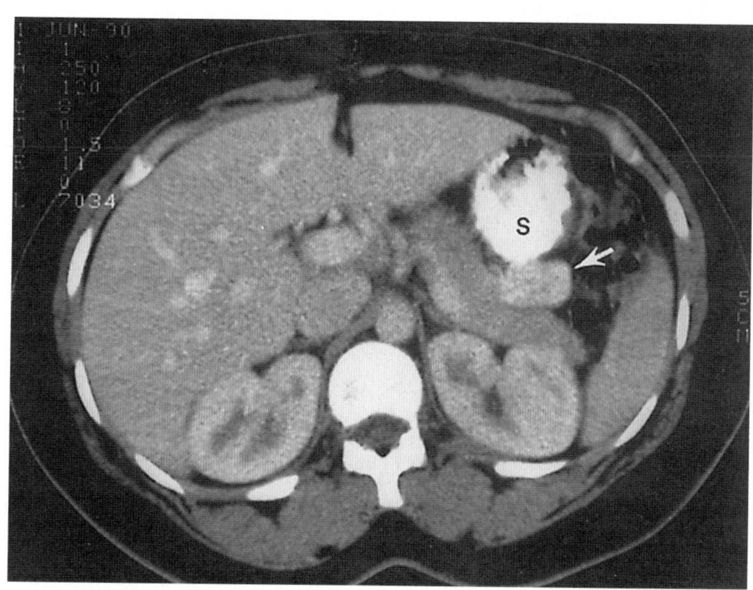

FIGURE 57.1 Computed tomography with oral and intravenous contrast in a patient with biochemical evidence of insulinoma. The neoplasm (*arrow*) is seen as a contrast-enhancing structure, 3 cm in diameter, in the tail of the pancreas posterior to the stomach (S). (From Yeo CJ. Islet cell tumors of the pancreas. In: Niederhuber JE, ed. *Current therapy in oncology*. St. Louis: Mosby; 1993:272, with permission.)

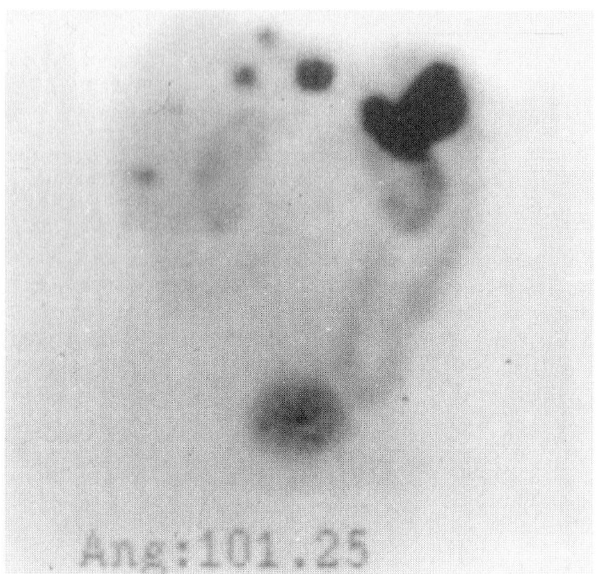

FIGURE 57.2 Octreotide scan (*anterior view*) in a patient with a large endocrine tumor in the tail of the pancreas (*large dark mass, upper right*) and several hepatic metastases (*upper left quadrant*). A small amount of the tracer is seen in the bladder (*lower midline*).

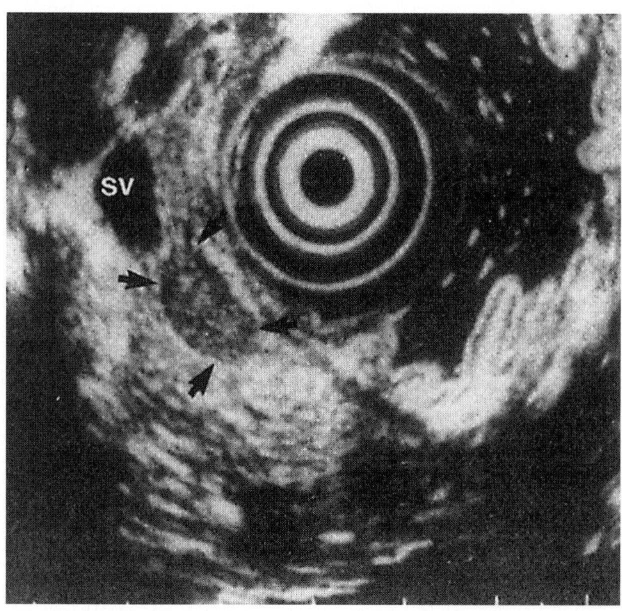

FIGURE 57.3 Endoscopic ultrasonographic image from a patient with an insulinoma (*arrows*) in the body of the pancreas. SV, splenic vein. (From Rosch T, Lightdale CJ, Botet JF, et al. Localization of pancreatic endocrine tumors by endoscopic ultrasonography. *N Engl J Med.* 1992;326:1721, with permission.)

ultrasonography, whereas SRS seemed superior for gastrinoma.[10] Most evidence suggests that SRS should play an important role in the preoperative localization and staging of gastrinoma, but the role of SRS in other pancreatic endocrine neoplasms is not as clear. In addition, SRS appears to play a role in the evaluation of patients with metastatic pancreatic endocrine tumors, especially in identifying extrahepatic tumor spread. In a study by Frilling et al.,[14] 54% of patients with liver metastases had extrahepatic tumor spread detected by SRS that was not detected by alternate imaging techniques.

Endoscopic ultrasonography (EUS) has also shown utility in localizing pancreatic endocrine neoplasms.[15–17] Rosch et al.[16] were able to localize 32 of 39 tumors (82%) correctly with EUS after CT had failed to locate the tumor (Fig. 57.3). In their experience, EUS was more sensitive than the combination of CT and visceral angiography. A more recent study, by Proye et al.,[18] evaluated preoperative EUS and SRS in 41 patients with insulinoma and gastrinoma. The sensitivity and positive predictive value of EUS were 77% and 94%, respectively, for pancreatic tumors; 40% and 100%, respectively, for duodenal gastrinomas; and 58% and 78%, respectively, for metastatic lymph nodes. These results have been duplicated by others and have led some to suggest that EUS should serve as the initial localization procedure in patients with insulinoma and gastrinoma. Of note, the drawback to EUS is that it does not evaluate for hepatic metastatic disease; rather, it is more sensitive than CT for imaging the duodenal wall, pancreatic parenchyma, and peripancreatic lymph nodes.

Visceral angiography has been used for selective visualization of the arterial supply to the pancreas and peripancreatic regions.[19] The accuracy of angiography has ranged from 45% to 85%. With the advent of SRS and EUS, this test is much less commonly utilized.

In a small number of cases, CT, SRS, and EUS are unsuccessful at localizing the pancreatic endocrine neoplasm. This happens most commonly with insulinomas and gastrinomas. Selective transhepatic portal venous hormone sampling may help in localizing the occult neoplasm.[20–24] The overall accuracy of this test ranges from 70% to greater than 95% depending on the number of samples obtained, the persistence of autonomous hormone production by the tumor, and the careful handling and assaying of all samples. This invasive test is designed to demonstrate an increase in hormone concentration at the site where its hormonal product drains into the portal system (Fig. 57.4).

A newer technique for the localization of occult functional pancreatic endocrine neoplasms is selective arterial secretin or calcium stimulation test. This technique involves the selective visceral arterial injection of secretin or calcium and concurrent

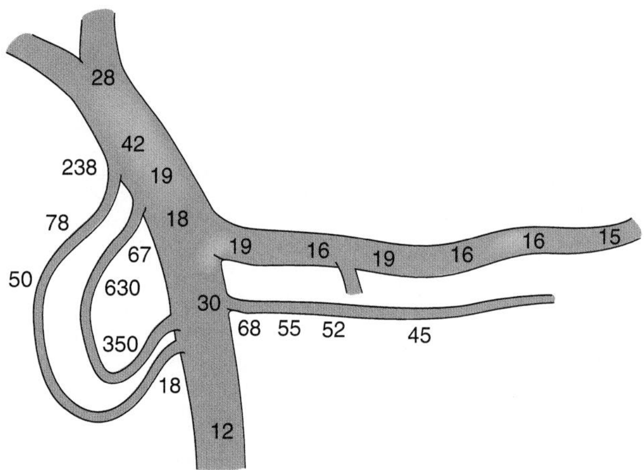

FIGURE 57.4 Schematic depiction of data from transhepatic portal venous insulin sampling in a patient with an insulinoma. Insulin levels are given in microunits per milliliter. These data localize the neoplasm to the head of the pancreas. (After Norton JA, Sigel B, Baker AR, et al. Localization of an occult insulinoma by intraoperative ultrasonography. *Surgery* 1985;97:381, with permission.)

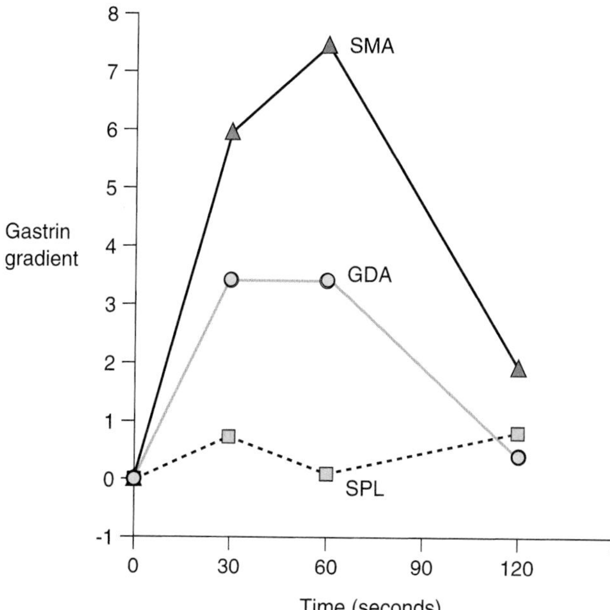

FIGURE 57.5 Graphic depiction of the results of a selective arterial secretin stimulation test in a patient with gastrinoma. The rise in hepatic vein gastrin concentration (gastrin gradient) is plotted on the y-axis, and basal values are plotted on the x-axis: 1, 100% rise; 2, 200% rise; and so forth. A rise in the hepatic vein gastrin concentration observed after the injection of secretin into the superior mesenteric artery (SMA) and gastroduodenal artery (GDA) localizes the neoplasm to the head of the pancreas or duodenum. SPL, splenic artery. (After Thom AK, Norton JA, Doppman JL, et al. Prospective study of the use of intraarterial secretin injection and portal venous sampling to localize duodenal gastrinomas. *Surgery* 1992;112:1002, with permission.)

hepatic venous sampling for either gastrin or insulin.[25,26] Gastrinoma cells are known to respond to secretin by releasing gastrin,[27,28] and insulinoma cells are known to respond to calcium by releasing insulin. The provocative secretogogue is serially injected through an arterial catheter into at least three sites—the splenic, gastroduodenal, and inferior pancreaticoduodenal arteries. Samples are subsequently drawn from an hepatic vein catheter before and immediately after each injection. The arterial supply to the occult tumor can then be deduced based on which selective secretogogue injection is followed by a large increase in hepatic vein hormone concentration (Fig. 57.5).

MOLECULAR GENETICS

Recent observations in the fields of classic and molecular genetics have added to our knowledge of pancreatic endocrine neoplasms. For example, up to half of malignant pancreatic endocrine tumors have been found to have clonal chromosomal abnormalities,[29] whereas *k-ras* oncogene mutations are absent in most of these tumors.[30] Gastrinoma has been shown to be associated with amplification of the *HER-2/neu* protooncogene,[31] and a high level of expression of mRNA for the alpha subunit of G_s protein has been demonstrated in insulinoma.[32] MAGE1, a protein identified in a number of neoplastic cell types including testicular germ cell cancer, breast cancer, and melanoma was found to be present in 86% of primary pancreatic endocrine neoplasms as well as in lymph node metastases. It may serve as a useful marker and potential therapeutic target for these neoplasms.[33] Aberrant hypermethylation of tumor suppressor genes in pancreatic endocrine neoplasms has been shown to be associated with advanced tumor stage.[34] In addition, hypermethylation of hMLH1 in pancreatic endocrine neoplasms leads to microsatellite instability and is associated with an improved prognosis.[35] Furthermore, sporadic pancreatic endocrine tumors and tumors arising as a manifestation of MEN-1 have both been shown to have mutations leading to genetic loss on chromosome 11 that inactivates a tumor-suppressor gene (menin) on that chromosome.[36]

Much progress has been made in the genetic understanding of MEN-1.[37] Chromosomal linkage studies have localized the genetic defect to the 11q13 locus, and studies of DNA markers have localized the MEN-1 gene between PYGM and D11S97. The gene contains 10 exons that code for a 610-amino acid protein called *menin*, whose function is unknown. Menin is expressed in diverse tissues and is highly conserved evolutionarily. Menin is predominately a nuclear protein, which binds to JunD and may repress JunD-mediated transcription. Studies in patients with MEN-1 have shown allelic deletions at chromosome 11q13 in nearly 100% of parathyroid tumors, 85% of nongastrinoma islet cell tumors, and up to 40% of gastrinomas. In patients with sporadic tumors (without MEN-1), the 11q13 deletions are seen in about 25%, 20%, and almost 50% of parathyroid, nongastrinoma islet cell tumors, and gastrinomas, respectively. Recently it has been shown that a comprehensive genetic testing program for patients at risk for MEN-1 can identify patients harboring an MEN-1 mutation almost 10 years before the development of clinical signs or symptoms of disease.[38]

Global expression analyses of pancreatic endocrine neoplasm tissue arrays have identified overexpression of putative oncogenes, growth factors, cell adhesion and migration molecules, and endothelial elements, as well as underexpression of some cell cycle checkpoint molecules. Such global expression analyses may help to identify potential therapeutic markers for these uncommon neoplasms.[39]

SURGICAL EXPLORATION

At the time of surgical exploration for pancreatic endocrine neoplasm, a complete evaluation of the pancreas and peripancreatic regions is performed. The body and tail of the pancreas are exposed by dividing the gastrocolic ligament. This portion of the pancreas can be partially elevated out of the retroperitoneum by dividing the inferior retroperitoneal attachments to the gland. After the second portion of the duodenum has been elevated out of the retroperitoneum by means of the Kocher maneuver, the pancreatic head and uncinate process are palpated bimanually. The liver is carefully assessed for evidence of metastatic disease. Potential extrapancreatic sites of tumor are evaluated in all cases, with particular attention paid to the duodenum, splenic hilum, small intestine and its mesentery, peripancreatic lymph nodes, and the reproductive tract in women. One technique that provides additional information in the operating room is intraoperative real-time ultrasonography, which can assist in tumor identification. The goals of surgical therapy for pancreatic endocrine neoplasms include controlling the symptoms of hormone excess, safely resecting maximal tumor mass, and preserving maximal pancreatic parenchyma. Management strategies, including preoperative, intraoperative, and postoperative considerations, vary for the different types of endocrine neoplasms of the pancreas. There have been scattered reports of laparoscopic resection of pancreatic endocrine tumors.

INSULINOMA

Insulinoma is the most common neoplasm of the endocrine pancreas (Table 57.2). The insulinoma syndrome is associated with the following features, known as *Whipple's triad:*[40]

1. Symptoms of hypoglycemia during fasting
2. Documentation of hypoglycemia, with a serum glucose level below 50 mg/dL
3. Relief of hypoglycemic symptoms following administration of exogenous glucose

Autonomous insulin secretion in insulinomas leads to spontaneous hypoglycemia, with symptoms that can be classified into two groups (see Table 57.2). Neuroglycopenic symptoms include confusion, seizure, obtundation, personality change, and coma. Hypoglycemia-induced symptoms, related to a surge in catecholamine levels, include palpitations, trembling, diaphoresis, and tachycardia. In most cases, patients consume carbohydrate-rich meals and snacks to relieve or prevent these symptoms.

Whipple's triad is not specific for insulinoma. The differential diagnosis of adult hypoglycemia is extensive and includes the following: reactive hypoglycemia, functional hypoglycemia associated with gastrectomy or gastroenterostomy, nonpancreatic tumors, pleural mesothelioma, sarcoma, adrenal carcinoma, hepatocellular carcinoma, carcinoid, hypopituitarism, chronic adrenal insufficiency, extensive hepatic insufficiency, and surreptitious self-administration of insulin or ingestion of oral hypoglycemic agents.

A common error made in evaluating a patient with suspected insulinoma is to begin with an oral glucose tolerance test. Instead, insulinoma is most reliably diagnosed by means of a monitored fast. During a monitored fast, blood is sampled for glucose and insulin determinations every 4 to 6 hours and when symptoms appear. Hypoglycemic symptoms typically occur when glucose levels are below 50 mg/dL, with concurrent serum insulin levels often exceeding 25 microunits/mL. Additional support for the diagnosis of insulinoma comes from the calculation of the insulin-to-glucose ratio at different times during the monitored fast. Normal persons have insulin-to-glucose ratios below 0.3, whereas patients with insulinoma typically demonstrate insulin-to-glucose ratios above 0.4 after a prolonged fast. Other measurable beta-cell products synthesized in excess in patients with insulinoma include C peptide and proinsulin.

TABLE 57.2 CLASSIFICATION

INSULINOMA

Parameter	Description
Symptoms	Neuroglycopenia causes confusion, personality change, coma Catecholamine surge causes trembling, diaphoresis, tachycardia
Diagnostic tests	Monitored fast Insulin-to-glucose ratio
Anatomic localization	Evenly distributed throughout pancreas

Elevated levels of both are typically found in the peripheral blood of patients with insulinoma.

The possibility of the surreptitious administration of insulin or oral hypoglycemic agents should be considered in all patients with suspected insulinoma. Levels of C peptide and proinsulin are not elevated in patients who self-administer insulin. Additionally, patients self-administering either bovine or porcine insulin may demonstrate antiinsulin antibodies in circulating blood. The ingestion of oral hypoglycemic agents, such as sulfonylureas, can be assessed by means of standard toxicologic screening.

Insulinomas are evenly distributed throughout the pancreas, with one third found in the head and uncinate process, one third in the body, and one third in the tail of the gland.[41] Ninety percent are found to be benign solitary nodules amenable to surgical cure. Ninety percent of insulinomas are sporadic, with approximately 10% being associated with the MEN-1 syndrome. In patients with MEN-1, the possibility of multiple insulinomas must be considered, and recurrence rates are higher. In approximately 10% of patients, insulinoma is metastatic to the peripancreatic lymph nodes, making the diagnosis of malignant insulinoma.

After the diagnosis of insulinoma has been confirmed biochemically, the appropriate localization and staging studies described earlier are performed (typically CT and EUS). Once the lesion has been localized,[42] patients undergo surgical exploration, where the pancreas is assessed not only by operative palpation but also by intraoperative ultrasonography. This allows for confirmation of preoperative localization and evaluates for the presence or absence of multiple primary tumors. Small, benign tumors that are not close to the main pancreatic duct can be removed by enucleation[43] (Fig. 57.6), regardless of their location in the gland. Larger tumors in the neck or proximal body may be resected via central pancreatectomy.[44–46] In the body and tail of the pancreas, insulinomas more than 2 cm in diameter and those close to the pancreatic duct are most commonly removed via distal pancreatectomy. Large lesions in the head or uncinate process of the gland may not be amenable to local resection and may occasionally require pancreaticoduodenectomy for complete excision.[47,48] In recent years, successful experience with laparoscopic resection of selected insulinomas has been reported.[49]

In rare instances, preoperative localization studies and intraoperative ultrasound fail to identify the tumor. Some authors have recommended a "blind" distal pancreatic resection to the level of the superior mesenteric vein (60% to 70% pancreatectomy), in the hope of excising an unidentified insulinoma in the body and tail. Others have suggested blind pancreaticoduodenectomy, because the thickness of the gland in this region makes it more likely to harbor an occult neoplasm. The favored approach at the current time is to defer any blind resection and to perform postoperative selective arterial calcium stimulation with hepatic venous insulin sampling to allow for specific tumor localization and directed surgical excision at a second operation.[50]

Approximately 10% of insulinomas are malignant, presenting with lymph node or liver metastases. In the presence of hepatic metastases, resection of the primary tumor and accessible metastases should be considered if it can be performed safely.[51–53] Such tumor debulking can be helpful in reducing hypoglycemic symptoms and improving long-term survival. In patients with unresectable disease, medications such as diazoxide and octreotide can be used to reduce insulin secretion from the tumor, minimizing hypoglycemia. Dietary manipulations including judicious spacing of carbohydrate-rich meals and the consumption of nighttime snacks, can also reduce the number of hypoglycemic

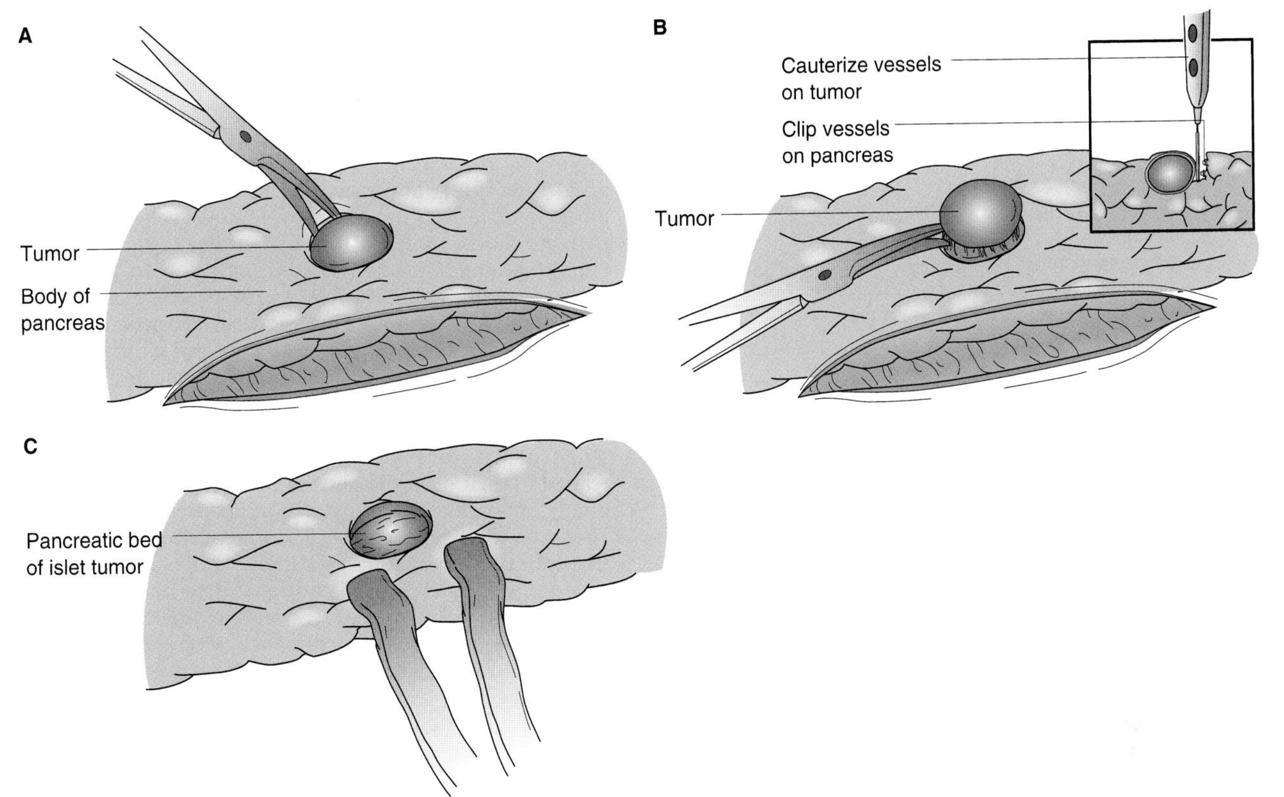

FIGURE 57.6 The technique for enucleating a benign pancreatic endocrine neoplasm with scissors (*A*) or electrocautery (*B*). (*C*) After enucleation, the site of excision is drained. (After Cameron JL. *Atlas of surgery,* vol 1. Philadelphia: BC Decker/Mosby; 1990:441, with permission.)

episodes. Multiple chemotherapeutic regimens have been used including streptozocin, dacarbazine, doxorubicin, and 5-fluorouracil.[54–56] Combination chemotherapy has yielded the highest response rates but has not been shown to be curative.

GASTRINOMA (ZOLLINGER-ELLISON SYNDROME)

In 1955, Zollinger and Ellison described two patients with severe peptic ulcer disease and pancreatic endocrine tumors and postulated that an ulcerogenic agent originated from the pancreatic tumor.[57,58] It is estimated that approximately 1 in 1,000 patients with primary duodenal ulcer disease and 2 in 100 patients with recurrent ulcer after ulcer surgery harbor gastrinomas.[59] Seventy-five percent of gastrinomas occur sporadically, and 25% are associated with the MEN-1 syndrome. Historically, the majority of gastrinomas were found to be malignant, with metastatic disease present at the time of initial workup. With increased awareness and screening for hypergastrinemia, the diagnosis of gastrinoma is made earlier and higher of percentage of patients present with benign and potentially curable neoplasms.[60]

The clinical symptoms of patients with gastrinoma are a direct result of increased levels of circulating gastrin (Table 57.3). Abdominal pain and peptic ulceration of the upper gastrointestinal (UGI) tract are seen in up to 90% of patients. Diarrhea is seen in 50% of patients, with 10% having diarrhea as their only symptom. Esophageal symptoms or endoscopic abnormalities resulting from gastroesophageal reflux are seen in up to half of patients. The diagnosis of gastrinoma should be suspected in several clinical settings including: the initial diagnosis of peptic ulcer disease, recurrent ulcer after medical or surgical therapy, postbulbar ulcer, family history of ulcer disease, ulcer with diarrhea, prolonged undiagnosed diarrhea, MEN-1 kindred, nongastrinoma pancreatic endocrine tumors (high association of secondary hormone elevations), and prominent gastric rugal folds on UGI examination. Serum gastrin levels should be obtained in all of these settings.

In most patients with gastrinoma, the fasting serum gastrin level is greater than 200 pg/mL. Gastrin levels greater than 1,000 pg/mL in the setting of hyperacidity and ulcer

TABLE 57.3 DIAGNOSIS

GASTRINOMA

Parameter	Description
Symptoms	Peptic ulcer disease Diarrhea Esophagitis
Diagnostic tests	Serum gastrin measurement Gastric acid analysis (or pH testing) Secretin stimulation test
Anatomic localization	Duodenum and head of pancreas (gastrinoma triangle)

TABLE 57.4 ETIOLOGY

DISEASE STATES ASSOCIATED WITH HYPERGASTRINEMIA

Nonulcerogenic causes (normal to low gastric acid secretion)
Atrophic gastritis
Pernicious anemia
Previous vagotomy
Renal failure
Short-gut syndrome
Ulcerogenic causes (excess gastric acid secretion)
Antral G-cell hyperplasia or hyperfunction
Gastric outlet obstruction
Retained excluded gastric antrum
Zollinger-Ellison syndrome

disease are virtually pathognomonic for gastrinoma. Because hypergastrinemia can occur in other pathophysiologic states (Table 57.4), fasting hypergastrinemia alone is not sufficient for the diagnosis of gastrinoma. Gastric acid analysis (or at least gastric pH testing) is critical in differentiating between ulcerogenic (high levels of acid) and nonulcerogenic (low levels of acid) causes of hypergastrinemia. To obtain an accurate gastric acid analysis, patients must not be taking antisecretory medications including histamine (H_2) receptor antagonists or proton pump inhibitors (PPIs). The diagnosis of gastrinoma is supported by a basal acid output above 15 mEq/hour in nonoperated patients, a basal acid output exceeding 5 mEq/hour in patients with previous vagotomy or ulcer operations, or a ratio of basal acid output to maximal acid output exceeding 0.6.

After documenting that hypergastrinemia and excessive acid secretion exist, provocative testing with secretin should be performed to differentiate between gastrinoma, antral G-cell hyperplasia or hyperfunction, and the other causes of ulcerogenic hypergastrinemia. This is achieved with a secretin stimulation test (Fig. 57.7). A baseline gastrin level is drawn. The patient is then stimulated with 2 units per kilogram of secretin as an intravenous bolus and subsequent gastrin samples are collected at 5 minute intervals for 30 minutes. An increase in the gastrin level by more than 200 pg/mL above the basal level supports the diagnosis of gastrinoma.

After the biochemical diagnosis of gastrinoma has been made, the gastric acid secretion should be pharmacologically controlled. The PPIs are now considered the drugs of choice for doing so.[61,62] The dose is adjusted to achieve a nonacidic pH during the hour immediately before the next dose of the drug. Typically, PPI doses needed for acid control exceed usual dosing levels. After the initiation of antisecretory therapy, all patients should undergo imaging studies to localize the primary tumor and to assess for metastatic disease.

If localization studies reveal *unresectable* hepatic metastases, the patient should undergo percutaneous or laparoscopic directed liver biopsy to obtain a definitive histologic diagnosis. These patients should be maintained on long-term PPI therapy. Virtually all patients can be rendered achlorhydric with an appropriate dose of PPI. Patients noncompliant with antisecretory therapy who experience complications related to their ulcer diathesis may require removal of the end organ (total gastrectomy) if tumor resection is not possible. However, total gastrectomy, once the operation of choice for gastrinoma, is now only rarely used.

If unresectable disease is not identified by staging studies, patients should be offered surgical exploration with curative intent. On exploration, the entire abdomen should be assessed for areas of extrapancreatic and extraduodenal gastrinoma. Most gastrinomas are found in the *gastrinoma triangle*[41,63] (Fig. 57.8), the area to the right of the superior mesenteric vessels, in the head of the pancreas or duodenum. Both intraoperative ultrasound and intraoperative upper endoscopy may be helpful in tumor localization. Transillumination of the duodenum may help identify small duodenal gastrinomas.[64,65] Well-encapsulated tumors less than 2 cm in size and distant from the pancreatic duct can be enucleated. Those situated deep in the parenchyma may require partial resection by pancreaticoduodenectomy or distal pancreatectomy. If no pancreatic tumor is identified, a longitudinal duodenotomy should be performed at the level of the second portion of the duodenum in search of duodenal microgastrinomas.[66,67] Small gastrinomas in the duodenal wall can be locally resected with primary

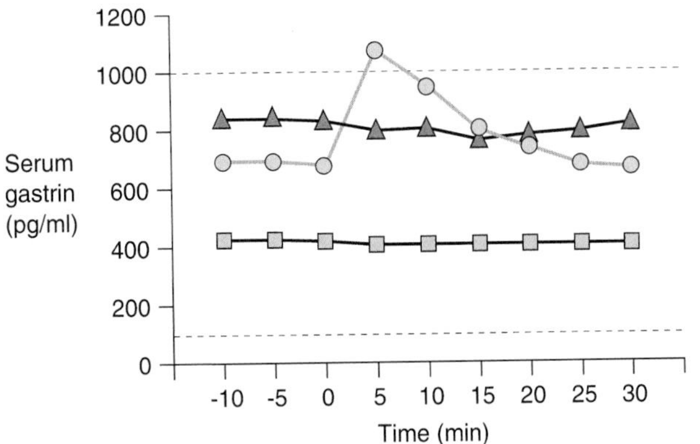

FIGURE 57.7 Results of intravenous secretin stimulation tests in patients with atrophic gastritis (triangles), gastric outlet obstruction (squares), and gastrinoma (circles). A positive test result, consistent with the presence of gastrinoma, is indicated by an increase over basal serum gastrin levels of at least 200 pg/mL. (After Wolfe MM, Jensen RT. Zollinger-Ellison syndrome: current concepts in diagnosis and management. *N Engl J Med.* 1987;317:1200, with permission.)

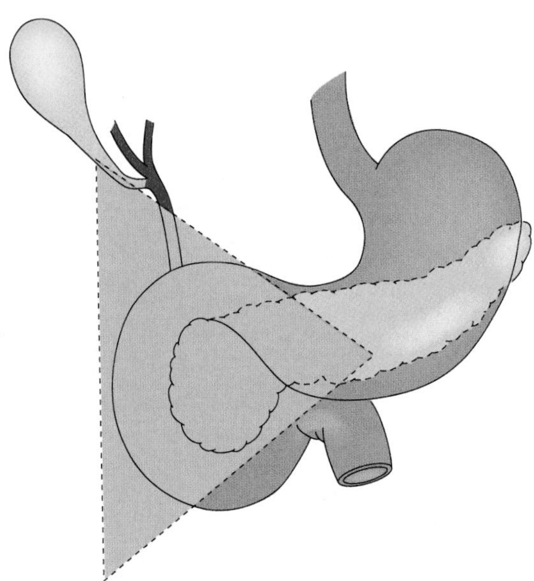

FIGURE 57.8 Most gastrinomas are found within the gastrinoma triangle. (After Stabile BE, Morrow DJ, Passaro E. The gastrinoma triangle: operative implications. *Am J Surg.* 1984;147:26, with permission.)

closure of the duodenal defect. A recent publication demonstrates that routine use of duodenotomy increases the short- and long-term cure rates in patients with sporadic gastrinoma, because such a duodenotomy allows detection of more duodenal gastrinomas.[68] Duodenotomy did not impact the occurrence of hepatic metastases or disease-related mortality. In a small percentage of patients, gastrinoma is found only in peripancreatic lymph nodes, with these lymph nodes harboring the apparent primary tumor. Resection of these apparent lymph node primary gastrinomas has been associated with long-term eugastrinemia and biochemical cure in up to half of cases.[69] A recent review from the National Institutes of Health identified likely primary lymph node gastrinomas in 26 of 176 gastrinoma patients (14.7%), with 69% being eugastrinemic at a mean of 10 years after resection.[70]

Occasionally, preoperative localization studies may identify the tumor in the gastrinoma triangle, but at the time of exploration, the tumor is not demonstrable. Several surgical options are available at this point. First, a parietal cell vagotomy has been proposed as a way to reduce antisecretory drug dose requirements in patients on high-dose antisecretory drug therapy but without prior life-threatening complications.[71] However, this approach leaves behind potentially resectable gastrinoma and has lost favor as an option. A second option is total gastrectomy; however, the availability of PPIs has drastically reduced the need to perform this operation for gastrinoma. It may have a limited role in patients whose tumors cannot be localized, if they cannot or will not take their PPIs. Like parietal cell vagotomy, this leaves tumor behind. A third, controversial option in patients with localization to the gastrinoma triangle is blind pancreaticoduodenectomy. Some argue this should include distal gastrectomy, as duodenal gastrinomas may arise close to the pylorus and be left behind during a pylorus-preserving resection.

Patients with sporadic gastrinomas tend to fare better following resection than those with MEN-1. In a series of 151 patients reported by Norton et al.,[72] 123 had sporadic gastrinoma and 28 had MEN-1 associated gastrinoma. Of those with sporadic gastrinoma, 34% were free of disease 10 years following resection. None of the MEN-1 patients were free of disease at 10 years. These data provide compelling evidence that patients with sporadic gastrinoma benefit from surgical exploration and complete tumor resection. The management of gastrinoma in MEN-1 is not as clear. The surgical treatment of hypercalcemia caused by parathyroid hyperplasia should precede any surgery for hypergastrinemia in patients with MEN-1. In these patients, gastrin-secreting tumors are often multicentric and associated with lymph node metastases. Although some groups have favored exploration only when MEN-1 gastrinoma tumors exceed 3 cm, it seems that earlier intervention may be warranted.[73,74] Unfortunately, more data from an appropriate clinical trial are needed to better define the timing of surgery for MEN-1 gastrinoma.

In the 1950s and 1960s, most gastrinomas were diagnosed late in the course of the disease, when the tumor burden was already significant. At that time, effective medical therapy did not exist, nor did sophisticated radiographic localization and staging techniques. Patients often suffered multiple ulcer complications, required total gastrectomy to control the ulcer diathesis, and typically succumbed to continued tumor growth following gastrectomy. Recent reviews of patients with surgically treated gastrinoma provide room for optimism.[75–78] Currently, up to 35% of patients who undergo resection with curative intent have been rendered eugastrinemic at follow-up. Cure rates approach 60% to 70% when the extent of disease allows a complete resection.

Most patients with incurable metastatic disease eventually die of tumor growth and dissemination. Multiple modalities have been used to treat such patients. Chemotherapy including streptozocin, 5-fluorouracil, and doxorubicin provides response rates of less than 50%.[79] Hormonal therapy with octreotide may relieve symptoms, reduce hypergastrinemia, and diminish hyperchlorhydria.[80,81] In patients with hepatic metastases, aggressive resection for debulking,[82–85] hepatic transplantation,[86] hepatic artery embolization, and interferon therapy have all been used, with variable favorable results.

VIPOMA (VERNER-MORRISON SYNDROME)

Synonyms for VIPoma include *WDHA syndrome* (watery diarrhea, hypokalemia, and either achlorhydria or acidosis) and *pancreatic cholera* syndrome (Table 57.5). Verner and Morrison[87] characterized this secretory diarrheal syndrome in a 1958 report. Patients characteristically present with intermittent, severe, watery diarrhea averaging up to 5 L/day. Hypokalemia results from fecal loss of large amounts of potassium. Low serum potassium levels lead to lethargy, muscle weakness, and nausea. A metabolic acidosis may be present, due to loss of bicarbonate in the diarrhea. Half of the patients may have hyperglycemia or hypercalcemia, and cutaneous flushing can be observed in a minority. The diagnosis of VIPoma is made after other common causes of diarrhea have been excluded (Table 57.6[88]) and an elevated serum VIP level is documented.

VIP secretion can be episodic, so repeated fasting levels should be measured if there is a strong clinical suspicion. Preoperative tumor localization is critical, because 10% of patients may have extrapancreatic tumors located in the retroperitoneum or chest. Most tumors are located in the distal pancreas where they are amenable to resection via distal pancreatectomy (Fig. 57.9). In most cases, hepatic metastases accompany the primary tumor. Therapies directed at debulking these metastases such as resection or ablative strategies are appropriate.

Surgical excision is appropriate in nearly all patients with the Verner-Morrison syndrome. Prior to surgery, fluid and electrolyte imbalances must be corrected. Octreotide can serve as a treatment adjunct, reducing the levels of circulating VIP, with a resultant decrease in the volume of diarrhea. Octreotide is also useful for symptom control in the setting of unresectable disease. Chemotherapy specific for this disease has not been well studied.

TABLE 57.5 DIAGNOSIS

VIPOMA

Parameter	Description
Symptoms	Watery diarrhea Weakness Lethargy Nausea
Diagnostic tests	Hypokalemia Achlorhydria Metabolic acidosis Serum VIP levels elevated
Anatomic localization	Most in body and tail of pancreas, with liver metastases

VIP, vasoactive intestinal peptide.

TABLE 57.6 DIAGNOSIS

DIFFERENTIAL DIAGNOSIS OF VERNER-MORRISON SYNDROME

Entity	Workup
Villous adenoma	Lower GI endoscopy
Laxative abuse	Stool examination for phenolphthalein
Celiac disease	Fecal fat measurement D-xylose tolerance test Small bowel biopsy
Parasitic and infectious diseases	Stool culture Ovum and parasite analysis *Clostridium difficile* toxin assay
Inflammatory bowel disease	Lower GI endoscopy Upper GI and small bowel series
Carcinoid syndrome	Urinary 5′-HIAA Upper GI and small bowel series Abdominal CT Serum serotonin measurement
Gastrinoma	Serum gastrin measurement Gastric acid analysis Secretin stimulation test

CT, computed tomography; GI, gastrointestinal; 5′-HIAA, 5′-hydroxyindoleacetic acid.

TABLE 57.7 DIAGNOSIS

GLUCAGONOMA

Parameter	Description
Symptoms	Dermatitis manifested as necrolytic migratory erythema Stomatitis Weight loss
Diagnostic tests	Hyperglycemia Hypoproteinemia Serum glucagon measurement Serum amino acid profile
Anatomic localization	Most in body and tail of pancreas, with liver metastases

GLUCAGONOMA

The most common findings in the glucagonoma syndrome are severe dermatitis, mild diabetes, stomatitis, anemia, and weight loss (Table 57.7). The dermatitis manifests as a characteristic skin rash termed *necrolytic migratory erythema.* This rash exhibits cyclic migrations, and it has been theorized that the hypoaminoacidemia accompanying glucagonoma is the cause.

The diagnosis of glucagonoma is suggested by the clinical presentation and biopsy of the skin lesions but is secured by the documentation of high fasting levels of serum glucagon. Most glucagonomas are located in the body and tail of the gland. These tumors are typically large and bulky, and surgical resection requires distal pancreatectomy (Fig. 57.10). Metastases are found in most patients and safe debulking of these

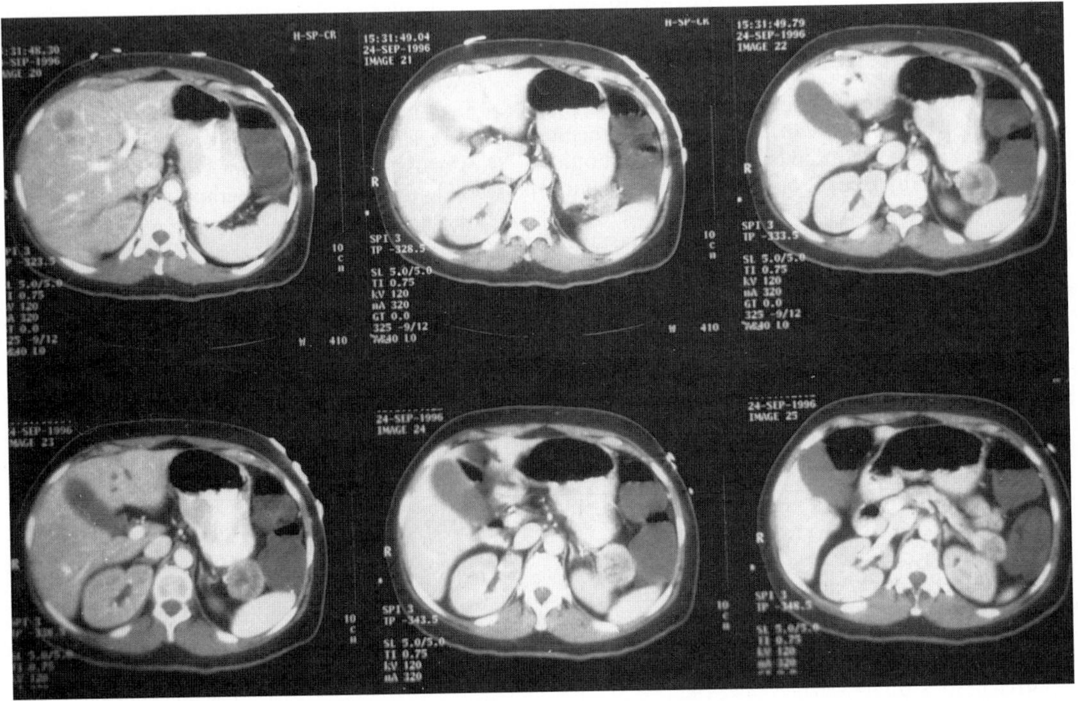

FIGURE 57.9 Several computed tomographic images from a patient with a primary VIPoma in the tail of the pancreas. The tumor is nearly spherical. Its location is posterior to the stomach and adjacent to the spleen.

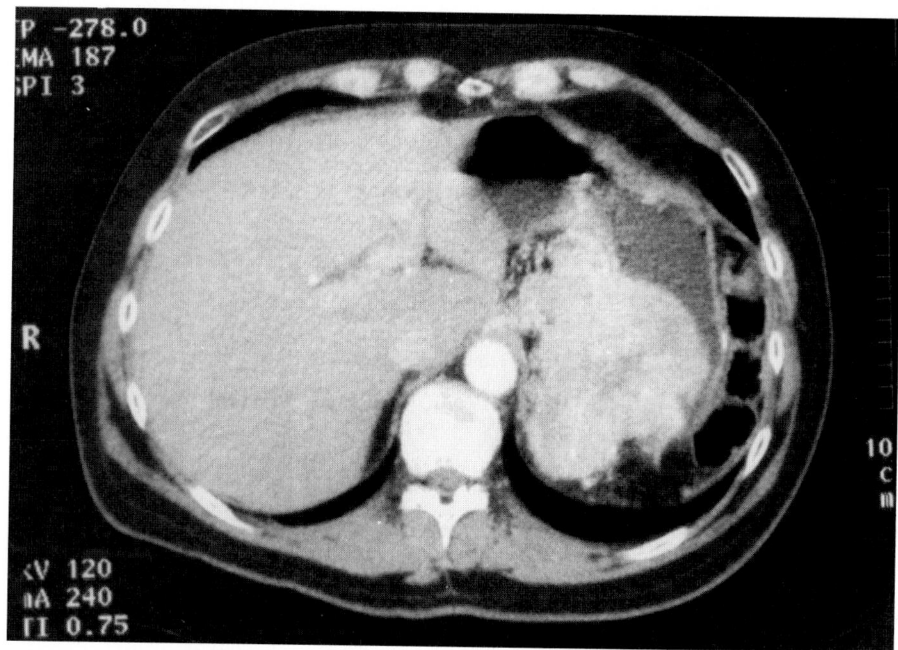

FIGURE 57.10 Computed tomography with oral and intravenous contrast in a patient with a glucagonoma. The large tumor appears to be posterior to the stomach and to the right of the aorta from the viewer's perspective.

should be considered.[89] As in patients with VIPoma and insulinoma, octreotide can be useful in controlling the signs and symptoms (hyperglycemia and dermatitis) associated with incurable glucagonoma.

SOMATOSTATINOMA

The somatostatinoma syndrome is the least common of the five generally accepted functional pancreatic endocrine neoplasia syndromes, occurring in less than 1 in 40 million people. The clinical features are nonspecific including steatorrhea, diabetes, hypochlorhydria, and cholelithiasis (Table 57.8). Fasting plasma somatostatin levels of greater than 100 pg/mL can be used to confirm the diagnosis.

Most somatostatinomas are located in the pancreatic head or periampullary region.[90] Tumors are of variable size and are often easily localized. Metastatic disease may be present at the time of diagnosis. Safe resection of the primary tumor and careful debulking of hepatic metastases are indicated.

TABLE 57.8 DIAGNOSIS

SOMATOSTATINOMA

Parameter	Description
Symptoms	Steatorrhea Right upper quadrant pain
Diagnostic tests	Hyperglycemia Hypochlorhydria Gallstones Serum somatostatin level
Anatomic localization	Most in head or uncinate process of pancreas; often periampullary

RARE CANDIDATE FUNCTIONAL PANCREATIC ENDOCRINE NEOPLASMS

Several rare clinical syndromes have been proposed as candidate functional pancreatic endocrine neoplasms. These include calcitoninoma,[91,92] parathyrinoma,[93] GRFoma, ACTHoma,[94] and neurotensinoma.[95] Calcitonin-secreting pancreatic neoplasms are associated with diarrhea. Parathyrinomas secrete parathyroid hormone-related protein (PTH-rp) and patients manifest the clinical features of hypercalcemia. GRFoma is marked by elevations of serum growth-hormone releasing factor and clinical features of acromegaly. ACTHoma is associated with features of Cushing's syndrome and elevated serum levels of adrenocorticotropic hormone (ACTH). Patients with neurotensinomas have tachycardia, hypotension, and malabsorption, with elevated serum levels of neurotensin.

NONFUNCTIONAL ISLET CELL TUMORS

Approximately one third to one half of patients with neoplasms of the endocrine pancreas have no defined clinical syndrome and no elevated hormone levels. The one hormone that may be elevated in these patients is PP, but this is not associated with a clinical syndrome. Another elevated serum marker may be chromogranin A. A study by Mutch et al.[96] determined a relationship between fasting plasma PP levels in patients with MEN-1 and the presence of radiographically detectable pancreatic endocrine tumor. A PP level that is more than three times the age-specific normal value is 95% sensitive and 88% specific for an islet cell tumor that can be imaged. Patients with nonfunctional endocrine tumors typically present with abdominal pain, weight loss, and jaundice, caused by the space-occupying nature of the mass in the pancreas. They are most commonly, located in the head, neck, or uncinate process of the gland and 50% to 90% are malignant. Occasionally, nonfunctional islet cell neoplasms may have a cystic appearance.[97] Overall, nonfunctional tumors tend to grow more slowly and have a much more indolent course and a better survival than pancreatic ductal adenocarcinoma.

Patients with resectable disease should undergo resection for potential cure via pancreaticoduodenectomy or distal pancreatectomy, depending on tumor location. Those with unresectable disease have shown partial responses to chemotherapy. In a study by Moertel et al.,[54] 105 patients with advanced nonfunctional endocrine tumors were randomly assigned to one of three groups. The lowest response rate (30%) was seen in patients receiving chlorozotocin alone, an intermediate response rate (45%) was seen in patients receiving the combination of streptozotocin plus 5-fluorouracil, and the highest response rate (69%) was noted in patients receiving streptozotocin plus doxorubicin. The last regimen also showed significant survival advantage in comparison with the other two treatments.

KEY POINTS

- **The majority of clinically recognized pancreatic endocrine neoplasms are functional, producing hormonal products leading to clinically recognizable syndromes.**
- **Malignant pancreatic endocrine neoplasms are determined by the presence of local invasion and lymph node or hepatic metastases not based on histologic examination.**
- **The initial imaging technique for a pancreatic endocrine neoplasm is a high-quality spiral CT scan.**
- **Endoscopic ultrasonography is particularly useful in localization of patients with gastrinoma and insulinoma.**
- **Insulinomas may present with either neuroglycopenic symptoms (confusion, seizure, obtundation, coma) or hypoglycemic-induced symptoms (palpitations, diaphoresis, tachycardia).**
- **Ninety percent of insulinomas are solitary, 90% are sporadic, and 90% are benign with location evenly distributed throughout the pancreas.**
- **Seventy-five percent of gastrinomas are sporadic (25% are associated with MEN-1 syndrome), and all should be considered to be of malignant potential.**
- **Most gastrinomas are located in the "gastrinoma triangle" and may be intrapancreatic, within the wall of the duodenum, or present only in a peripancreatic lymph node, and in all cases local resection (enucleation) may be adequate therapy.**
- **Glucagonomas usually present with a characteristic severe dermatitis (termed *necrolytic migratory erythema*) and are typically large and bulky and often with metastatic disease.**
- **Nonfunctional islet cell tumors of the pancreas, although often quite large at diagnosis, tend to grow slowly with a more indolent course than pancreatic ductal cancer.**

References

1. Andrew A. Further evidence that enterochromaffin cells are not derived from the neural crest. *J Embryol Exp Morphol.* 1974;31:589.
2. Lonser RR, Glenn GM, Walter M, et al. von Hippel-Landau disease. *Lancet* 2003;361:2059.
3. Marion-Audibert AM, Barel C, Gouysse G, et al. Low microvessel density is an unfavorable histoprognostic factor in pancreatic endocrine tumors. *Gastroenterology* 2003;125:1094.
4. Fedorak IJ, Ko TC, Gordon D, et al. Localization of islet cell tumors of the pancreas: a review of current techniques. *Surgery* 1993;113:242.
5. Frucht H, Doppman JL, Norton JA, et al. Gastrinomas: comparison of MR imaging with CT, angiography, and US. *Radiology* 1989;171:713.
6. Wank SA, Doppman JL, Miller DL, et al. Prospective study of the ability of computed axial tomography to localize gastrinomas in patients with Zollinger-Ellison syndrome. *Gastroenterology* 1987;92:905.
7. Yeo CJ, Wang BH, Anthone GJ, et al. Surgical experience with pancreatic islet-cell tumors. *Arch Surg.* 1993;128:1143.
8. Termanini B, Gibril F, Reynolds JC, et al. Value of somatostatin receptor scintigraphy: a prospective study in gastrinoma of its effect on clinical management. *Gastroenterology* 1997;112:335.
9. Meko JB, Doherty GM, Siegel BA, et al. Evaluation of somatostatin-receptor scintigraphy for detecting neuroendocrine tumors. *Surgery* 1996;120:975.
10. Kisker O, Bartsch D, Weinel RJ, et al. The value of somatostatin-receptor scintigraphy in newly diagnosed endocrine gastroenteropancreatic tumors. *J Am Coll Surg.* 1997;184:487.
11. Schirmer WJ, O'Dorisio TM, Schirmer TP, et al. Intraoperative localization of neuroendocrine tumors with ^{125}I-tyr^{3}-octreotide and a hand-held gamma-detecting probe. *Surgery* 1993;114:745.
12. Modlin IM, Tang LH. Approaches to the diagnosis of gut neuroendocrine tumors: the last word (today). *Gastroenterology* 1997;112:583.
13. Krausz Y, Bar-Ziv J, deJong RBJ, et al. Somatostatin-receptor scintigraphy in the management of gastroenteropancreatic tumors. *Am J Gastroenterol.* 1998;93:66.
14. Frilling A, Malago M, Martin H, et al. Use of somatostatin receptor scintigraphy to image extrahepatic metastases of neuroendocrine tumors. *Surgery* 1998;124:1000.
15. Glover JR, Shorvon PJ, Lees WR. Endoscopic ultrasound for localisation of islet cell tumours. *Gut* 1992;33:108.
16. Rosch T, Lightdale CJ, Botet JF, et al. Localization of pancreatic endocrine tumors by endoscopic ultrasonography. *N Engl J Med.* 1992;326:1721.
17. Thompson NW, Czako PF, Fritts LL, et al. Role of endoscopic ultrasonography in the localization of insulinomas and gastrinomas. *Surgery* 1994; 116:1131.
18. Proye C, Malvaux P, Patton F, et al. Noninvasive imaging of insulinomas and gastrinomas with endoscopic ultrasonography and somatostatin receptor scintigraphy. *Surgery* 1998;124:1134.
19. Maton PN, Miller DL, Doppman JL, et al. Role of selective angiography in the management of patients with Zollinger-Ellison syndrome. *Gastroenterology* 1987;92:913.
20. Norton JA, Shawker TH, Doppman JL, et al. Localization and surgical treatment of occult insulinomas. *Ann Surg.* 1990;212:615.
21. Vinik AI, Moattari AR, Cho K, et al. Transhepatic portal vein catheterization for localization of sporadic and MEN gastrinomas: a ten-year experience. *Surgery* 1990;107:246.
22. Pedrazzoli S, Pasquale C, Miotto D, et al. Transhepatic portal sampling for preoperative localization of insulinomas. *Surg Gynecol Obstet.* 1987; 165:101.
23. Vinik AI, Delbridge L, Moattari R, et al. Transhepatic portal vein catheterization for localization of insulinomas: a ten-year experience. *Surgery* 1991;109:1.
24. Fraker DL, Norton JA. Localization and resection of insulinomas and gastrinomas. *JAMA* 1988;259:3601.
25. Imamura M, Minematsu S, Suzuki T, et al. Usefulness of selective arterial secretin injection test for localization of gastrinoma in the Zollinger-Ellison syndrome. *Ann Surg.* 1987;205:230.
26. Rosato FE, Bonn J, Shapiro M, et al. Selective arterial stimulation of secretin in localization of gastrinomas. *Surg Gynecol Obstet.* 1990;171:196.
27. Gower WR Jr, Buzogany JA, Ellison EC, et al. Control of gastrin release in cultured gastrinoma-derived G cells. *Surgery* 1988;104:424.
28. Chiba T, Yamatani T, Yamaguchi A, et al. Mechanism for increase of gastrin release by secretin in Zollinger-Ellison syndrome. *Gastroenterology* 1989;96:1439.
29. Long PP, Hruban RH, Lo R, et al. Chromosome analysis of nine endocrine neoplasms of the pancreas. *Cancer Genet Cytogenet.* 1994;77:55.
30. Yashiro T, Fulton N, Hara H, et al. Comparisons of mutations of *ras* oncogene in human pancreatic exocrine and endocrine tumors. *Surgery* 1993;114:758.
31. Evers BM, Rady PL, Sandoval K, et al. Gastrinomas demonstrate amplification of the *HER-2/neu* protooncogene. *Ann Surg.* 1994;219:596.
32. Zeiger MA, Norton JA. Gs alpha: identification of a gene highly expressed by insulinoma and other endocrine tumors. *Surgery* 1993;114:458.
33. Hansel DE, House MG, Ashfaq R, et al. MAGE1 is expressed by a subset of pancreatic endocrine neoplasms and associated lymph node and liver metastases. *Int J Gastrointest Cancer* 2003;33:141.
34. House MG, Herman JG, Guo MZ, et al. Aberrant hypermethylation of tumor suppressor genes in pancreatic endocrine neoplasms. *Ann Surg.* 2003;238:423.
35. House MG, Herman JG, Guo MZ, et al. Prognostic value of hMLH1 methylation and microsatellite instability in pancreatic endocrine neoplasms. *Surgery* 2003;134:902.
36. Eubanks PJ, Sawicki MP, Samara GJ, et al. Putative tumor-suppressor gene on chromosome 11 is important in sporadic endocrine tumor formation. *Am J Surg.* 1994;167:180.
37. Marx S, Spiegel AM, Skarulis MC, et al. Multiple endocrine neoplasia type 1: clinical and genetic topics. *Ann Intern Med.* 1998;129:484.
38. **Lairmore TC, Piersall LD, DeBenedetti MK, et al. Clinical genetic testing and early surgical intervention in patients with multiple endocrine neoplasia Type 1 (MEN-1). *Ann Surg.* 2004;239:637.**
39. Maitra A, Hansel DE, Argani P, et al. Global expression analysis of well-differentiated pancreatic endocrine neoplasms using oligonucleotide microarrays. *Clin Cancer Res.* 2003;9:5988.

40. Whipple AO, Frantz VK. Adenoma of islet cells with hyperinsulinism: a review. *Ann Surg.* 1935;101:1299.
41. Howard TJ, Stabile BE, Zinner MJ, et al. Anatomic distribution of pancreatic endocrine tumors. *Am J Surg.* 1990;159:258.
42. Richards ML, Gauger PG, Thompson NW et al. Pitfalls in the surgical treatment of insulinoma. *Surgery* 2002;132:1040.
43. Menegaux F, Schmitt G, Mercadier M, et al. Pancreatic insulinomas. *Am J Surg.* 1993;165:243.
44. Sauvanet A, Partensky C, Sastre B et al. Medial pancreatectomy: A multi-institutional retrospective study of 53 patients by the French Pancreas Club. *Surgery* 2002;132:836.
45. Efron DT, Lillemoe KD, Cameron JL, Yeo CJ. Central pancreatectomy with pancreaticogastrostomy for benign pancreatic pathology. *J Gastrointest Surg.* 2004;8:532.
46. Goldstein MJ, Toman J, Chabot JA. Pancreaticogastrostomy: a novel application after central pancreatectomy. *J Am Coll Surg.* 2004;198:871.
47. Udelsman R, Yeo CJ, Hruban RH, et al. Pancreaticoduodenectomy for selected pancreatic endocrine tumors. *Surg Gynecol Obstet.* 1993;177:269.
48. Phan GQ, Yeo CJ, Cameron JL, et al. Pancreaticoduodenectomy for selected periampullary neuroendocrine tumors: fifty patients. *Surgery* 1997;122:989.
49. Jaroszewski DE, Schlinkert RT, Thompson GB, Schlinkert DK. Laparoscopic localization and resection of insulinomas. *Arch Surg.* 2004; 139:270.
50. Thompson GB, Service FJ, van Heerden JA, et al. Reoperative insulinomas, 1927 to 1992: an institutional experience. *Surgery* 1993;114:1196.
51. Carty SE, Jensen RT, Norton JA. Prospective study of aggressive resection of metastatic pancreatic endocrine tumors. *Surgery* 1992;112:1024.
52. Modlin IM, Lewis JJ, Ahlman H, et al. Management of unresectable malignant endocrine tumors of the pancreas. *Surg Gynecol Obstet.* 1993; 176:507.
53. McEntee GP, Nagorney DM, Kvols LK, et al. Cytoreductive hepatic surgery for neuroendocrine tumors. *Surgery* 1990;108:1091.
54. Moertel CG, Lefkopoulo M, Lipsitz S, et al. Streptozocin-doxorubicin, streptozocin-fluorouracil, or chlorozotocin in the treatment of advanced islet-cell carcinoma. *N Engl J Med.* 1992;326:519.
55. Moertel CG, Hanley JA, Johnson LA. Streptozocin alone compared with streptozocin plus fluorouracil in the treatment of advanced islet-cell carcinoma. *N Engl J Med.* 1980;303:1189.
56. Altimari AF, Badrinath K, Reisel HJ, et al. DTIC therapy in patients with malignant intra-abdominal neuroendocrine tumors. *Surgery* 1987;102: 1009.
57. Zollinger RM, Ellison EH. Primary peptic ulcerations of the jejunum associated with islet cell tumors of the pancreas. *Ann Surg.* 1955;142:709.
58. Zollinger RM, Ellison EC, Fabri PJ, et al. Primary peptic ulcerations of the jejunum associated with islet cell tumors: twenty-five-year appraisal. *Ann Surg.* 1980;192:422.
59. Wolfe MM, Jensen RT. Zollinger-Ellison syndrome: current concepts in diagnosis and management. *N Engl J Med.* 1987;317:1200.
60. Andersen DK. Current diagnosis and management of Zollinger-Ellison syndrome. *Ann Surg.* 1989;210:685.
61. Maton PN, Vinayek R, Frucht H, et al. Long-term efficacy and safety of omeprazole in patients with Zollinger-Ellison syndrome: a prospective study. *Gastroenterology* 1989;97:827.
62. Metz DC, Pisegna JR, Fishbeyn VA, et al. Currently used doses of omeprazole in Zollinger-Ellison syndrome are too high. *Gastroenterology* 1992;103:1498.
63. Stabile BE, Morrow DJ, Passaro E Jr. The gastrinoma triangle: operative implications. *Am J Surg.* 1984;147:25.
64. Sugg SL, Norton JA, Fraker DL, et al. A prospective study of intraoperative methods to diagnose and resect duodenal gastrinomas. *Ann Surg.* 1993;218:138.
65. Frucht H, Norton JA, London JF, et al. Detection of duodenal gastrinomas by operative endoscopic transillumination: a prospective study. *Gastroenterology* 1990;99:1622.
66. Farley DR, van Heerden JA, Grant CS, et al. Extrapancreatic gastrinomas: surgical experience. *Arch Surg.* 1994;129:506.
67. Chiarugi M, Pucciarelli M, Goletti O, et al. Outcome of surgical treatment for extrapancreatic gastrinomas. *Surg Gynecol Obstet.* 1993;177:153.
68. **Norton JA, Alexander HR, Fraker DL, et al. Does the use of routine duodenotomy (DUODX) affect rate of cure, development of liver metastases, or survival in patients with Zollinger-Ellison syndrome? *Ann Surg.* 2004; 239:617.**
69. Arnold WS, Fraker DL, Alexander HR, et al. Apparent lymph node primary gastrinoma. *Surgery* 1994;116:1123.
70. **Norton JA, Alexander HR, Fraker DL, et al. Possible primary lymph node gastrinoma: Occurrence, natural history, and predictive factors. A prospective study. *Ann Surg.* 2003;237:650.**
71. Richardson CT, Peters MN, Feldman M, et al. Treatment of Zollinger-Ellison syndrome with exploratory laparotomy, proximal gastric vagotomy, and H_2-receptor antagonists: a prospective study. *Gastroenterology* 1985;89:357.
72. Norton JA, Fraker DL, Alexander HR, et al. Surgery to cure the Zollinger-Ellison syndrome. *N Engl J Med.* 1999;341:635.
73. Cadiot G, Vuagnat A, Doukhan I, et al. Prognostic factors in patients with Zollinger-Ellison syndrome and multiple endocrine neoplasia type 1. *Gastroenterology* 1999;116:286.
74. Lowney JK, Frisella MM, Lairmore TC, et al. Pancreatic islet cell tumor metastasis in multiple endocrine neoplasia type 1: correlation with primary tumor size. *Surgery* 1999;125:1043.
75. Norton JA, Doppman JL, Jensen RT. Curative resection in Zollinger-Ellison syndrome: results of a 10-year prospective study. *Ann Surg.* 1992;215:8.
76. Fraker DL, Norton JA, Alexander HR, et al. Surgery in Zollinger-Ellison syndrome alters the natural history of gastrinoma. *Ann Surg.* 1994;220:320.
77. Delcore R, Friesen SR. The place for curative surgical procedures in the treatment of sporadic and familial Zollinger-Ellison syndrome. *Curr Opin Gen Surg.* 1994;2:69.
78. Zogakis TG, Gibril F, Libutti SK, et al. Management and outcome of patients with sporadic gastrinoma arising in the duodenum. *Ann Surg.* 2003;238:42.
79. von Schrenck T, Howard JM, Doppman JL, et al. Prospective study of chemotherapy in patients with metastatic gastrinoma. *Gastroenterology* 1988;94:1326.
80. Mozell E, Woltering EA, O'Dorisio TM, et al. Effect of somatostatin analog on peptide release and tumor growth in the Zollinger-Ellison syndrome. *Surg Gynecol Obstet.* 1990;170:476.
81. Mozell E, Cramer AJ, O'Dorisio TM, et al. Long-term efficacy of octreotide in the treatment of Zollinger-Ellison syndrome. *Arch Surg.* 1992;127:1019.
82. Elias D, Lasser P, Ducreux M, et al. Liver resection (and associated extra-hepatic resections) for metastatic well-differentiated endocrine tumors: a 15-year single center prospective study. *Surgery* 2003;133:375.
83. Sarmiento JM, Heywood G, Rubin J, et al. Surgical treatment of neuroendocrine metastases to the liver: a plea for resection to increase survival. *J Am Coll Surg.* 2003;197:29.
84. Sarmiento JM, Que FG, Grant CS, et al. Concurrent resections of pancreatic islet cell cancers with synchronous hepatic metastases: outcomes of an aggressive approach. *Surgery* 2002;132:976.
85. Norton JA, Kivlen M, Li M, et al. Morbidity and mortality of aggressive resection in patients with advanced neuroendocrine tumors. *Arch Surg.* 2003;138:859.
86. Florman S, Toure B, Kim L, et al. Liver transplantation for neuroendocrine tumors. *J Gastrointest Surg.* 2004;8:208.
87. Verner JV, Morrison AB. Islet cell tumor and a syndrome of refractory watery diarrhea and hypokalemia. *Am J Med.* 1958;25:374–380.
88. Schiller LR. Chronic diarrhea. *Gastroenterology* 2004;127:287.
89. Chu QD, Al-kasspooles MF, Smith JL, et al. Is glucagonoma of the pancreas a curable disease? *Int J Pancreatol.* 2001;29:155.
90. House MG, Yeo CJ, Schulick RD. Periampullary pancreatic somatostatinoma. *Ann Surg Oncol.* 2002;9:869.
91. McLeod MK, Vinik AI. Calcitonin immunoreactivity and hypercalcitoninemia in two patients with sporadic, nonfamilial, gastroenteropancreatic neuroendocrine tumors. *Surgery* 1992;111:484.
92. Howard JM, Gohara AF, Cardwell RJ. Malignant islet cell tumor of the pancreas associated with high plasma calcitonin and somatostatin levels. *Surgery* 1989;105:227.
93. Mao C, Carter P, Schaefer P, et al. Malignant islet cell tumor associated with hypercalcemia. *Surgery* 1995;117:37.
94. Aniszewski JP, Young WF Jr, Thompson GB et al. Cushing syndrome due to ectopic adrenocorticotropic hormone secretion. *World J Surg.* 2001;25:934.
95. Meko JB, Norton JA. Endocrine tumors of the pancreas. *Curr Opin Gen Surg.* 1994;2:186.
96. Mutch MG, Frisella MM, DeBenedetti MK, et al. Pancreatic polypeptide is a useful plasma marker for radiographically evident pancreatic islet cell tumors in patients with multiple endocrine neoplasia type 1. *Surgery* 1997;122:1012.
97. Ahrendt SA, Komorowski RA, Demeure MJ, et al. Cystic pancreatic neuroendocrine tumors: Is preoperative diagnosis possible? *J Gastrointest Surg.* 2002;6:66.

SECTION H
HEPATOBILIARY AND PORTAL VENOUS SYSTEM

CHAPTER 58 ■ HEPATOBILIARY ANATOMY

RICHARD D. SCHULICK

A precise knowledge of the anatomy of the liver and biliary tract, and their relationship to associated blood vessels are essential for the performance of hepatobiliary surgery. Every surgeon caring for a patient with a hepatobiliary problem should have a thorough understanding of the general anatomy and an absolute understanding of each individual patient's anatomy, because variations are common.

TOPOGRAPHIC ANATOMY

The normal adult liver is a large, wedge-shaped organ that occupies much of the right upper quadrant of the abdomen. Most of the liver bulk lays to the right of the midline where it molds to the undersurface of the right diaphragm, and where the lower border coincides with the right costal margin. The liver extends as a wedge to the left of the midline between the anterior surface of the stomach and the left dome of the diaphragm. The anterior surface of the liver is invested by visceral peritoneum that extends to the anterior abdominal wall in the midline from the ligamentum teres, or round ligament (the obliterated umbilical vessels), and by an obliquely oriented fusion of peritoneum known as the falciform ligament. Posteriorly, the investing peritoneum is contiguous with the peritoneum of the diaphragm and covers the liver, except for a *bare area* bounded by the *right and left triangular ligaments* (Fig. 58.1). Glisson's capsule is a thin, fibrous covering that envelops the liver deep to the peritoneum sending fibrous septa into the hepatic parenchyma investing the portal structures.

Ordinarily, the liver can be separated from adjacent organs and structures by simply moving it or dividing loose areolar tissue (Fig. 58.2). Neoplastic or inflammatory conditions may obliterate these planes. Superiorly and anteriorly, the diaphragm or abdominal wall and liver may jointly be involved in a pathologic process. Posteriorly, the right adrenal gland or upper pole of the right kidney may involve or be involved by the liver. Inferiorly, the gallbladder, colon, duodenum, or periportal lymphatics may be involved. Cancers of the stomach or gastroesophageal junction may involve the left liver or vice versa.

MORPHOLOGIC AND FUNCTIONAL ANATOMY

The description and definition of the anatomic divisions of the liver have been revised and written about numerous times in the past 100 years.[1–8] At present, there is still confusion between the various hepatic anatomic nomenclatures in the English and French literature. Based only on morphologic criteria and surface anatomy, the liver can be divided into right and left halves by forming a plane through the gallbladder fossa (Cantlie's line) and inferior vena cava (IVC) (Fig. 58.3). As will be shown later, this plane approximates the true division between the right and left halves using the more strict definition of a plane through the middle hepatic vein and IVC, but the middle hepatic vein is not obvious based solely on morphology and without ultrasound. Further subdivisions of the right half of the liver into a right anterior section and a right posterior section are not possible based only on surface anatomy. The left half of the liver can be further subdivided into a left medial section and left lateral section based on the umbilical fissure and falciform ligament. The caudate lobe of the liver is identified as lying posterior to the gastrohepatic ligament and emanating from a process of liver situated posterior to the main portal pedicle and anterior to the IVC.

The most widely accepted nomenclature is based on Couinaud's description of the discrete anatomic segments of the liver (Fig. 58.4).[6] The eight segments of a liver can be determined using surface anatomy, and location of the three main hepatic veins, the portal pedicle bifurcation into right and left, and the umbilical fissure and falciform ligament.

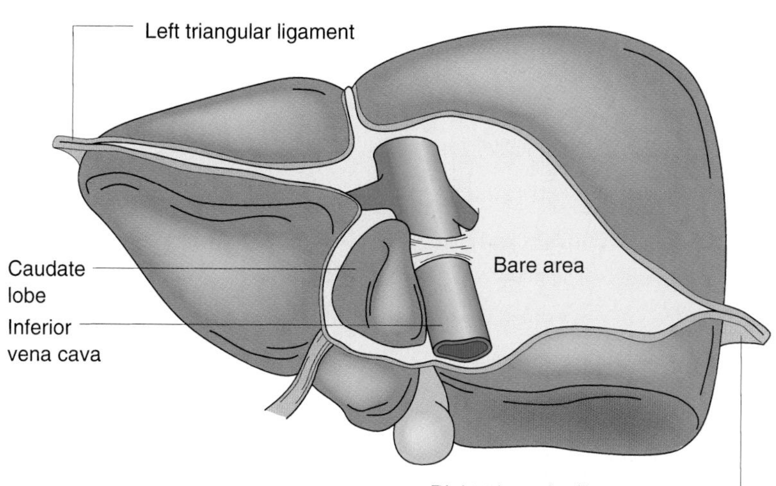

FIGURE 58.1 Posterior view of liver, showing the level of peritoneal reflections.

As described, the right and left halves of the liver are delineated by a plane through the middle hepatic vein and IVC. Segments II, III, and IV lie to the left of this plane and form the left half of the liver. Segments V, VI, VII, and VIII lie to the right of this plane and form the right half of the liver. Segment I, or the caudate lobe, is morphologically distinct from the two halves of the liver and emanates from a process of liver lying posterior to the portal pedicle and anterior to the IVC. Whereas the right and left halves of the liver derive blood supply from the corresponding right and left portal veins and hepatic arteries, segment I derives blood supply from both. Additionally, the right half of the liver has venous drainage through the right and middle hepatic veins, and the left half of the liver through the left and middle hepatic veins. Segment I, however, drains directly via small branches into the IVC.

The right half of the liver can be further subdivided using a plane through the right hepatic vein and the IVC. Liver anterior to this plane forms its right anterior section, and liver posterior to this plane forms the right posterior section. The right anterior section of the liver comprises segment V (inferior to the portal bifurcation) and segment VIII (superior to the portal bifurcation). The right posterior section of the liver comprises segment VI (inferior to the portal bifurcation) and segment VII (superior to the portal bifurcation).

The left half of the liver can be further subdivided using a plane through the umbilical fissure and falciform ligament. Liver medial to this plane forms the left medial section of the liver or segment IV, and liver lateral to this plane forms the left lateral section of the liver. The left lateral section of the liver is further subdivided into segment II (which is superior to the left hepatic vein) and segment III (which is inferior to the left hepatic vein).

Hepatic Veins

Three major hepatic veins carry blood from the liver to the IVC. Most patients have a single, large right hepatic vein that joins the right anterior wall of the IVC and a middle and left hepatic vein that converge into a common trunk 1 to 2 cm from the IVC and enter the left anterior wall of the IVC (Fig. 58.5). In approximately a third of patients, the three main hepatic veins join the IVC via three distinct trunks. These hepatic veins usually lie within the hepatic parenchyma. Sometimes a

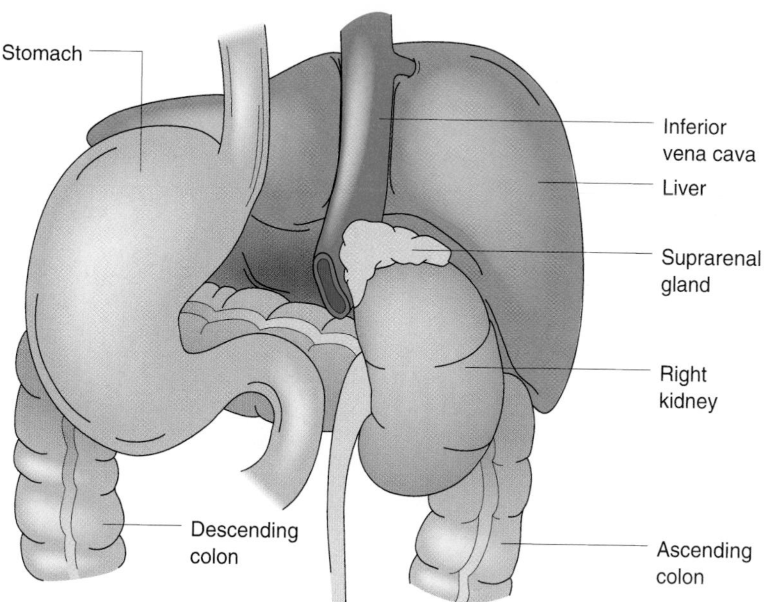

FIGURE 58.2 Posterior view of the liver, showing organs that produce impressions on its inferior surface.

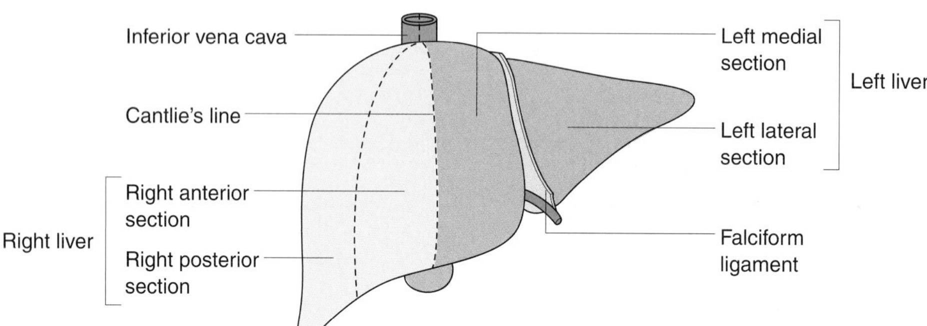

FIGURE 58.3 Anatomic division of the liver into right and left halves by a line extending from the gallbladder fossa posteriorly to the inferior vena cava.

definable extraparenchymal segment of the hepatic veins, especially the right, can be dissected out before it empties into the IVC, which makes outflow control safer and easier. Usually, multiple accessory right hepatic veins empty from the right half of the liver directly into the IVC as it courses posterior to the liver (Fig. 58.6). On occasion, these accessory right hepatic veins are sizable and may even support venous outflow should the native right hepatic vein need to be taken. Additionally, sometimes an umbilical vein can be appreciated running beneath the falciform ligament between the middle and left hepatic veins and emptying into the terminal portion of the left hepatic vein.

Portal Veins

The superior mesenteric and splenic veins join posterior to the neck of the pancreas to form the main portal vein. It receives pyloric and coronary vein branches as it courses cephalad and obliquely to the right to form the most posterior structure within the hepatoduodenal ligament (portal triad). In the hilus of the liver, the main portal vein bifurcates into a short oblique right portal vein and a longer, more transverse, and more superficial left portal vein (Fig. 58.7). These branches then enter the parenchyma and become invested along with the other components of the portal triad by extensions of Glisson's capsule. Both the right and left portal veins give off small branches to dually supply segment I. The right portal vein usually enters the hepatic parenchyma immediately and is quick to divide into a right anterior portal vein supplying segments V and VIII and a right posterior portal vein supplying segments VI and VII. The left portal vein may remain near the surface of the left half of the liver in the hilar plate for a significant distance as it courses to the umbilical fissure to give off medial branches to segment IV and lateral branches to segments II and III.

Hepatic Arteries

There is much variability in the hepatic arterial supply to the liver. The most common anatomy is a common hepatic artery that arises from the celiac trunk and courses near the superior border of the neck of the pancreas. After the origins of the gastroduodenal, supraduodenal, and right gastric arteries, the proper hepatic artery courses in the left anterior aspect of the hepatoduodenal ligament in front of the portal vein and to the left of the common hepatic duct. The proper hepatic artery usually bifurcates into right and left hepatic arteries outside the liver (Fig. 58.8). The right hepatic artery usually courses posterior to the common hepatic duct but anterior to the right portal vein to supply the right liver. The left hepatic artery usually remains extrahepatic until near the base of the umbilical fissure where it enters the liver to give off branches to segments

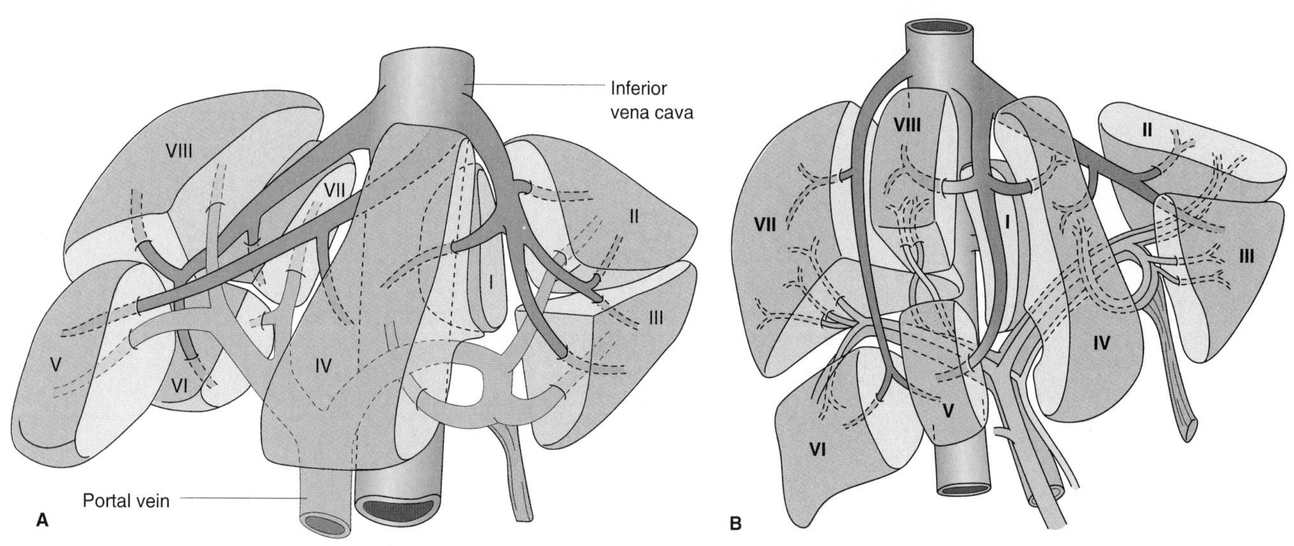

FIGURE 58.4 Functional divisions of the liver and liver segments according to Couinaud's nomenclature.

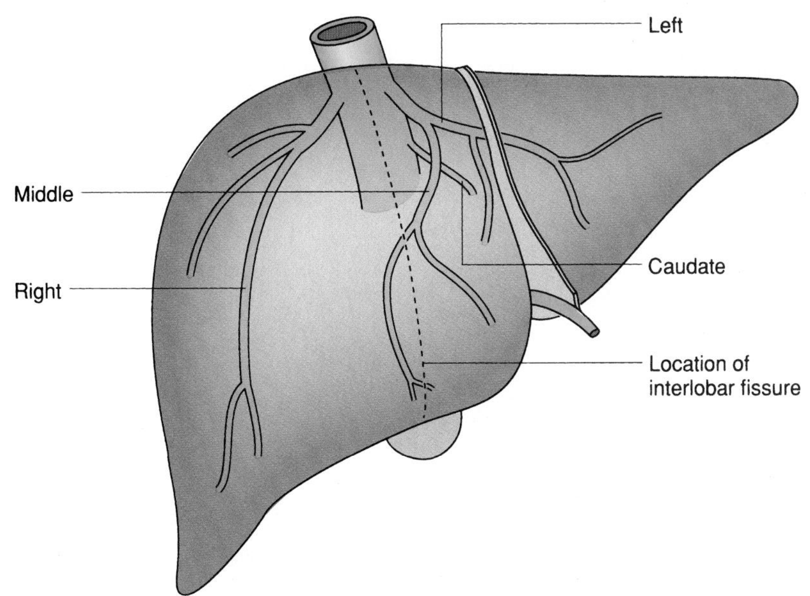

FIGURE 58.5 Three major hepatic veins drain the liver. The caudate segment of the liver usually drains directly into the inferior vena cava.

II, III, and IV. Small branches from near the bifurcation of the proper hepatic artery also supply segment I. A middle hepatic artery branch may arise from either the right or left hepatic arteries after bifurcation. Although this anatomy is described as normal, it is found only in approximately 50% to 60% of patients. A replaced or accessory right hepatic artery may arise off of the superior mesenteric artery near its origin, course posteriorly or through the head of the pancreas to lie along the right posterior border of the hepatoduodenal ligament. A replaced or accessory left hepatic artery may arise off of the left gastric artery and course transversely toward the base of the umbilical fissure in the lesser omentum. In general, within the hepatic parenchyma, the hepatic arterial branches course closely with bile duct branches and fairly closely with portal venous branches, but not always, and anatomic variations should be suspected. The descriptions and frequency of hepatic arterial variants have been well characterized by Michels.[9]

Intrahepatic Biliary Tree

The right and left livers are respectively drained by the right and left hepatic ducts, whereas the caudate (Segment I) is drained by several small ducts joining the bifurcation and the first several centimeters of both hepatic ducts. The intrahepatic ducts are tributaries of the corresponding hepatic ducts, which penetrate the liver invaginating Glisson's capsule at the hilus. Bile ducts are usually located above the corresponding portal branches, whereas hepatic arterial branches run inferiorly to the veins. The left hepatic duct directly drains the bile ducts to segments II, III, and IV, which constitute the left liver. The right hepatic duct drains the bile ducts from segments V, VI, VII, and VIII, which constitute the right liver. Usually, the bile ducts from segments V and VIII join to first form the anterior sectoral duct and the bile ducts from segments VI and VII join to first form the posterior sectoral duct prior to forming the right hepatic duct.

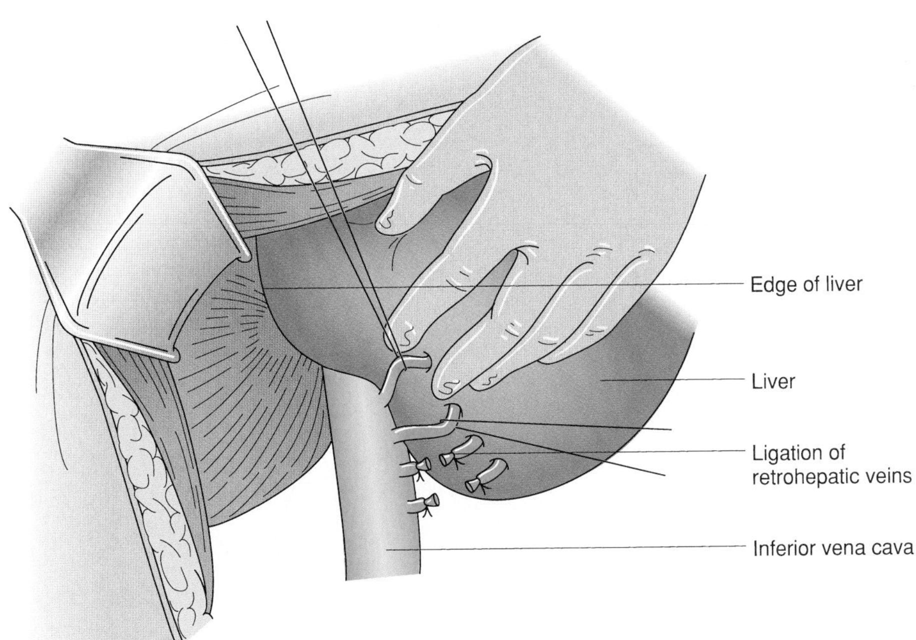

FIGURE 58.6 Retraction of right liver medially exposes small venous tributaries that drain the right liver directly into the retrohepatic vena cava. Several branches are ligated.

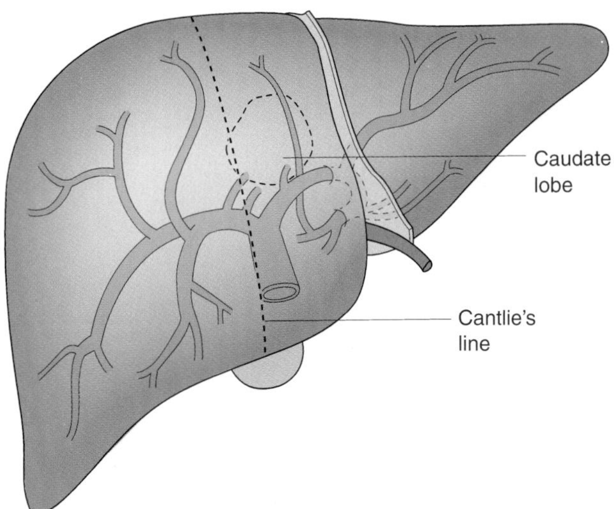

FIGURE 58.7 Intrahepatic divisions of the portal vein.

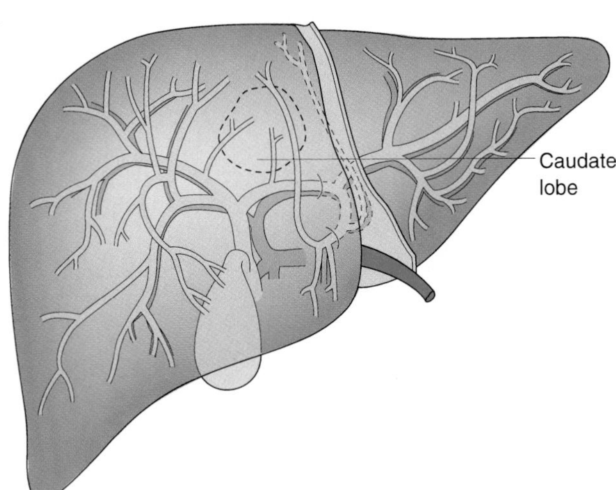

FIGURE 58.8 Intrahepatic divisions of bile ducts and hepatic arteries.

Gallbladder

The gallbladder is a reservoir for bile located on the undersurface of the liver at the confluence of the right and left halves of the liver. It is separated from the hepatic parenchyma by a cystic plate, which is constituted of connective tissue applied to Glisson's capsule. The gallbladder may be deeply imbedded into the liver or occasionally presents on a mesenteric attachment, but usually lays in a gallbladder fossa. The gallbladder varies in size and consists of a fundus, a body, and an infundibulum. The tip of the fundus usually reaches the free edge of the liver and is closely applied to the cystic plate. The infundibulum of the gallbladder makes an angle with the body and may obscure the common hepatic duct constituting a danger point during cholecystectomy. The cystic duct arises from the infundibulum of the gallbladder and extends to join the common hepatic duct. The lumen measures between 1 and 3 mm in diameter, and its length varies depending on the type of union with the common hepatic duct (Fig. 58.9). Callot's

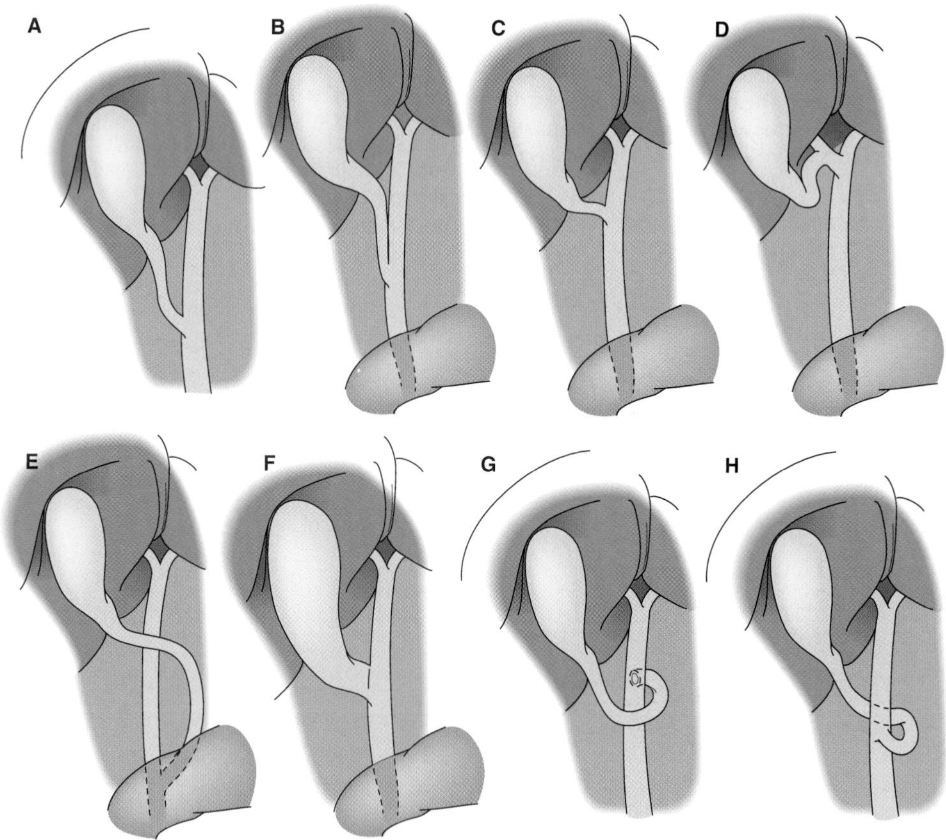

FIGURE 58.9 Variations in the junction of the cystic duct and common hepatic duct.

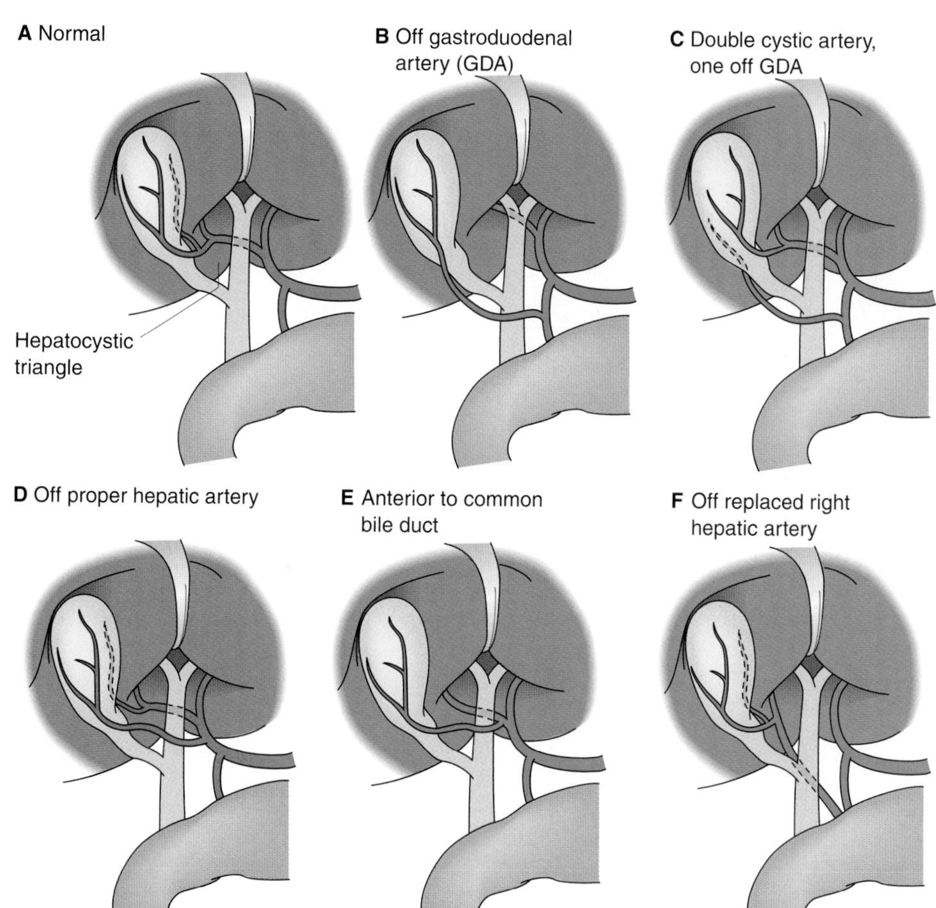

FIGURE 58.10 Variations in the origin and course of the cystic artery.

triangle is bounded by the common hepatic duct on the left, the cystic duct inferiorly, and the cystic artery superiorly. Arterial blood reaches the gallbladder via the cystic artery, which usually originates from the right hepatic artery. Several known variations in the origin and course of the cystic artery are illustrated in Figure 58.10. The venous drainage of the gallbladder is directly into the liver parenchyma or into the common bile duct plexus.

Common Bile Duct

The cystic and common hepatic ducts join to form the common bile duct. The common bile duct is approximately 8 to 10 cm in length and 0.4 to 0.8 cm in diameter. The common bile duct can be divided into three anatomic segments: supraduodenal, retroduodenal, and intrapancreatic (Fig. 58.11). The supraduodenal

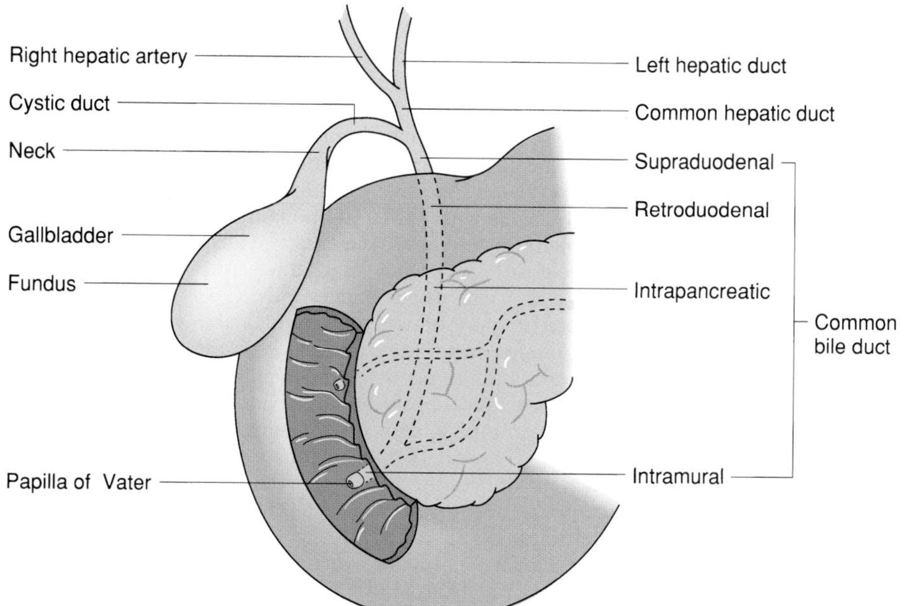

FIGURE 58.11 Anatomic divisions of the common bile duct.

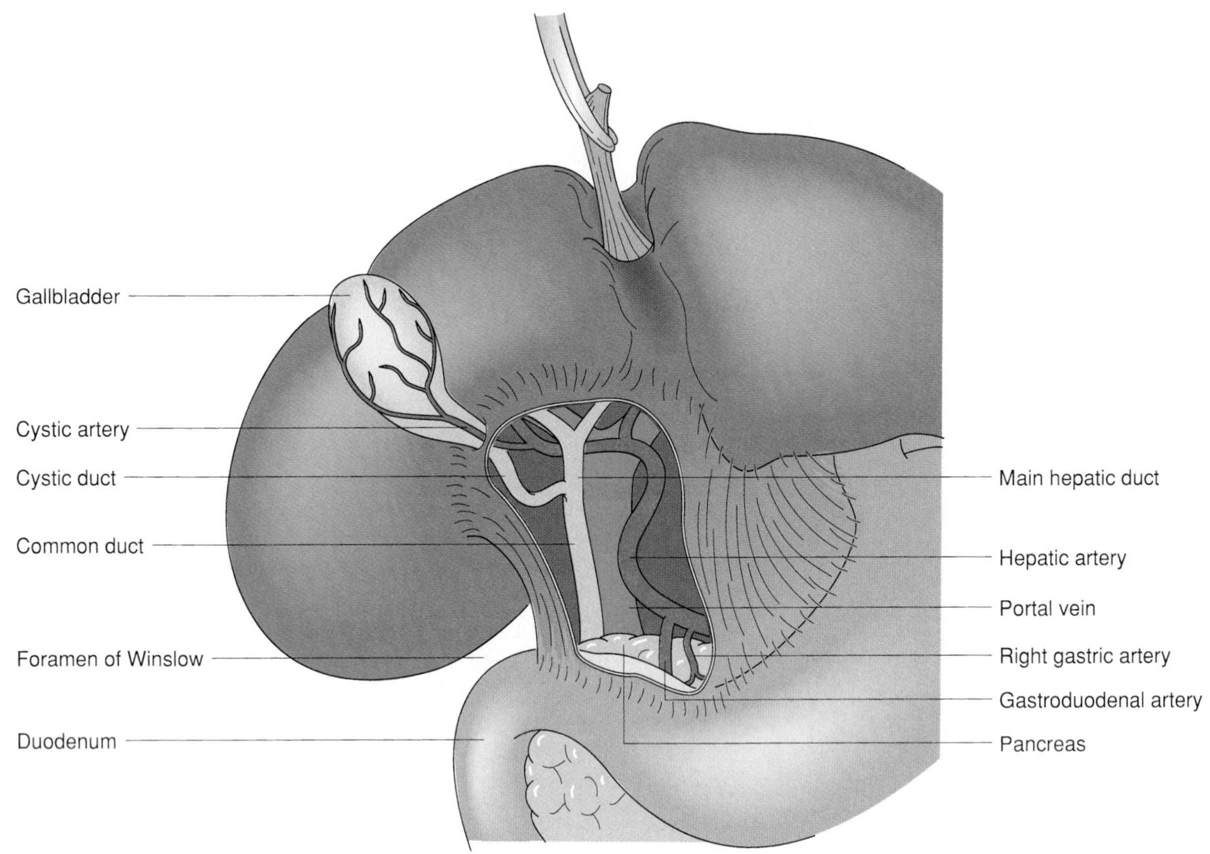

FIGURE 58.12 Relationship of structures within the hepatoduodenal ligament.

segment resides in the hepatoduodenal ligament lateral to the hepatic artery and anterior to the portal vein (Fig. 58.12). The anatomy of the hepatic artery is variable and should be familiar to surgeons operating in this area (Fig. 58.13). Approximately 45% of people have variant hepatic arterial anatomy.[9] The course of the retroduodenal segment is posterior to the first portion of the duodenum, anterior to the inferior vena cava, and lateral to the portal vein. The pancreatic portion of the duct lies within a tunnel or groove on the posterior aspect of the pancreas. The common bile duct then enters the medial wall of the duodenum, courses tangentially through the submucosal layer for 1 to 2 cm, and terminates in the major papilla in the second portion of the duodenum (Fig. 58.11). The distal portion of the duct is encircled by smooth muscle that forms the sphincter of Oddi. The common bile duct may enter the duodenum directly (25%) or join the pancreatic duct (75%) to form a common channel, termed the ampulla of Vater.

The blood supply of the common bile duct is segmental in nature and consists of branches from the cystic, hepatic, and gastroduodenal arteries. These meet to form collateral vessels that run in the 3 and 9 o'clock positions. The venous drainage forms a plexus on the anterior surface of the common bile duct that enters the portal system. The lymphatic drainage follows the course of the hepatic artery to the celiac nodes.

LIVER IMAGING

Computed Tomography

Computed tomography (CT) is widely available and quick and has become the main modality to initiate the assessment of hepatic processes. It also has the advantage of being able to quickly assess other organs within the abdominal cavity and chest. With the introduction of multidetector spiral CT, the resolution of hepatic lesions is quite good. This scanning technique allows total hepatic imaging in arterial, portal venous, and delayed phases after a rapid intravenous contrast bolus during a single breath hold by the patient (Fig. 58.14). In addition, three-dimensional reconstructions can be obtained to construct hepatic arteriograms that approach the quality of invasive angiography.

Magnetic Resonance Imaging

Magnetic resonance imaging (MRI) of the liver with gadolinium as a contrast agent is commonly used to help further characterize hepatic lesions. Resolution of some lesions may be slightly better with MRI. Additionally, certain lesions, such as hemangiomas and cysts, can easily be identified based on MRI characteristics when the CT characteristics are indeterminate (Fig. 58.15). The disadvantages of MRI are its increased cost, increased amount of time to perform, inability to quickly screen other organs and body cavities within the same session, and wide variability in quality from one imaging center to another.

Magnetic resonance cholangiopancreatography (MRCP) is becoming more widely used to noninvasively view biliary anatomy (Fig. 58.16). The scans are heavily T2-weighted, which maximizes the signal from the biliary tree. No injection of contrast agent is needed, and under optimal conditions the resulting imaging can rival that of formal cholangiography. Three-dimensional reconstructions can be performed to view the biliary tree from multiple angles and can be helpful in distinguishing between stones, strictures, and neoplasms.

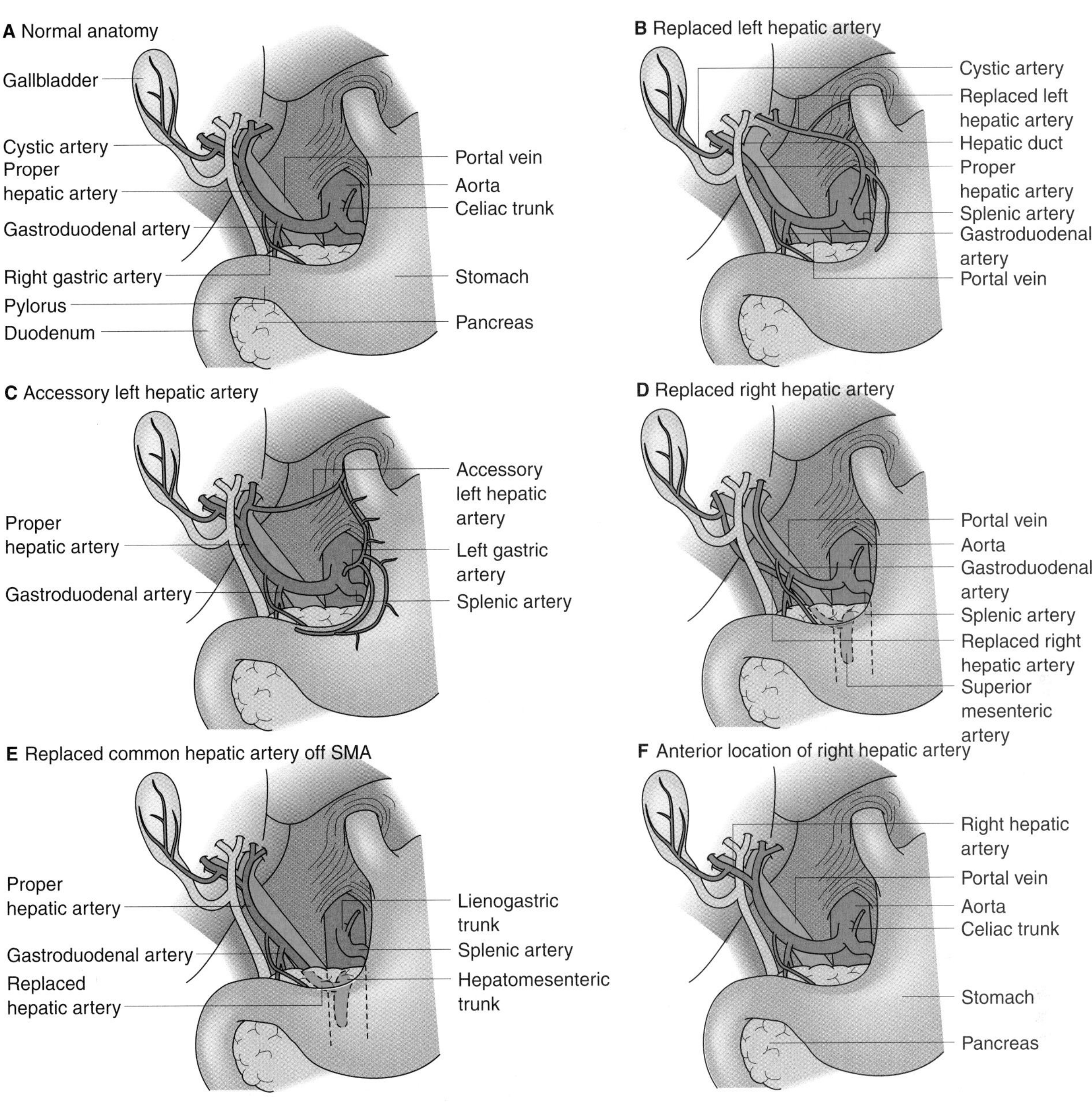

FIGURE 58.13 Variations in the origin and course of the hepatic artery and its relationship to the bile ducts.

Ultrasonography

Hepatic ultrasonography can be applied transcutaneously or intraoperatively via open surgery and laparoscopic surgery. It can be useful in identifying lesions within the hepatic parenchyma, to describe the consistency (i.e., fatty or cirrhotic) and identify dilatation of the biliary tree and any abnormalities or stones within the gallbladder. In many centers, intraoperative ultrasonography is used routinely to assess the anatomy of the pedicles (portal vein, hepatic artery, bile duct), the hepatic veins, and the hepatic parenchyma. It is useful both to further identify and characterize lesions within the hepatic parenchyma and to delineate their relationships within the eight anatomic segments of the liver. Additionally, it is often helpful to delineate proximity of lesions to major vascular structures and to survey for abnormal anatomy in planning a resection.

With ablational therapies more commonly employed, ultrasound has become indispensable in directing the use of radiofrequency ablation. This ablational therapy can be performed percutaneously, laparoscopically, and during open surgery.

Typically intraoperative assessment of the liver involves examining the portal pedicles. The main portal pedicle is identified within the hepatoduodenal ligament. It is followed superiorly to the portal bifurcation into the main right and left pedicle. The portal pedicles are invested with Glisson's capsule and have a very echogenic covering to them in contrast to hepatic vein branches. The main right portal pedicle is followed toward the right where it gives off an anterior and posterior branch (Fig. 58.17A,B). The right anterior branch gives off separate pedicles to segment V (inferiorly) and to segment VIII (superiorly). The right posterior branch gives off separate pedicles to segment VI (inferiorly) and to segment VII (superiorly). The main left pedicle is usually much longer and courses intact to the base of the umbilical fissure before branching into various segmental pedicles. At the base of the umbilical fissure, the main left pedicle courses anteriorly toward the

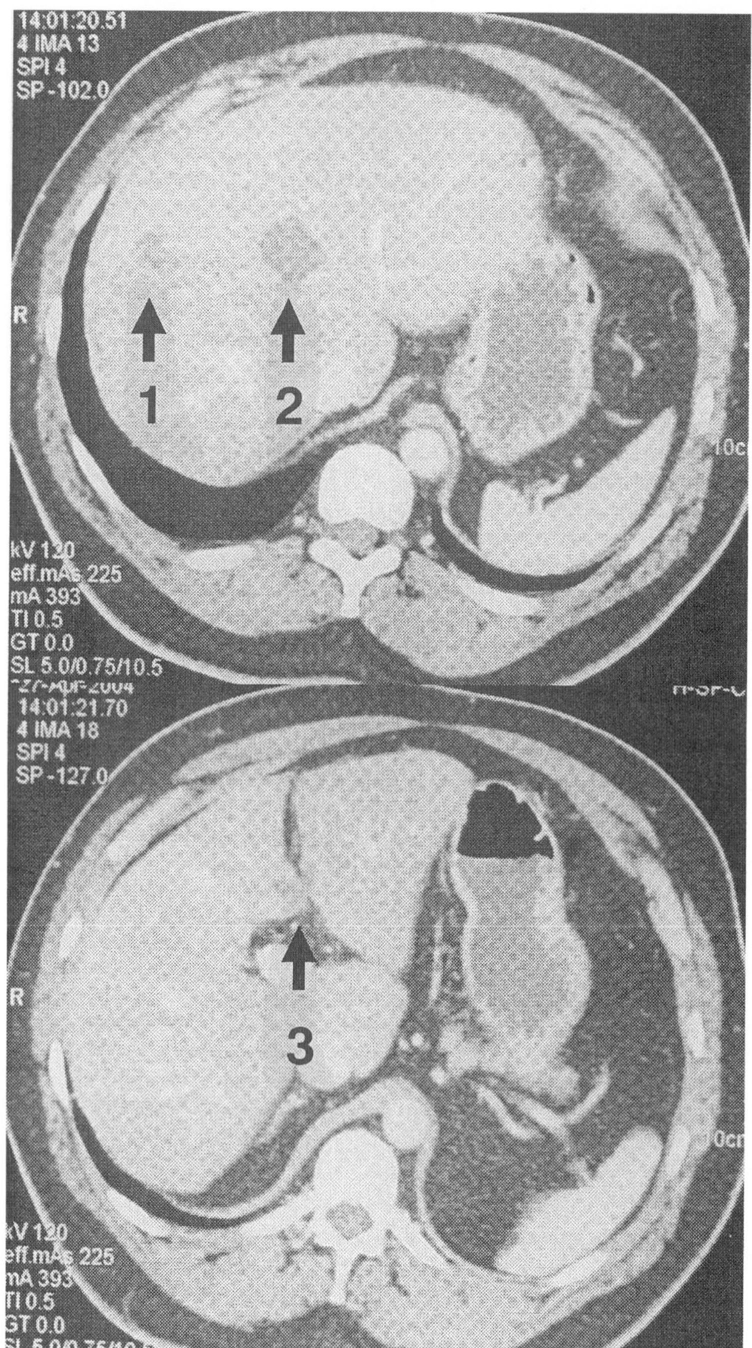

FIGURE 58.14 Portal venous phase of computed tomography (CT) scan from a patient with a history of colorectal cancer and three lesions in the liver. Lesion 1 in segment VIII is irregular and rim enhancing and was a colorectal cancer metastasis. Lesion 2 straddling segments IV and VIII has smooth borders, is not rim enhancing, and was found to be a cyst. Lesion 3 straddling segments IV and III across the umbilical fissure is irregular and rim enhancing and was a colorectal cancer metastasis.

round ligament and gives off a pedicle to segment IV medially and pedicles to segments II and III laterally. Next, if the bare area around the junction of the hepatic veins and IVC has been well mobilized, the hepatic veins can easily be visualized using intraoperative ultrasonography (Fig. 58.17C,D). As described previously, usually a larger right hepatic vein can be delineated and smaller left and middle hepatic veins joining into a common trunk before emptying into the IVC are seen. Commonly, an umbilical hepatic vein branch can be identified coursing between the middle and left hepatic veins and running under the falciform ligament. Not uncommonly, significant accessory right hepatic veins can be seen emptying from the posterior surface of the right liver directly into the IVC as it courses posterior to the liver. The identification of these accessory right hepatic veins is important for both vascular control and preservation of outflow from the liver. Lastly, the hepatic parenchyma is systematically scanned to identify lesions within the liver. It is sometimes useful to adjust the ultrasound settings on a known lesion defined preoperatively to maximize the echogenicity in the hopes of identifying other occult lesions not identified preoperatively.

Positron Emission Tomography

Positron emission tomography (PET), especially when combined with CT (PET—CT), has become a valuable tool in helping to select patients who will most benefit from aggressive liver resection. This technique is based on the increased metabolism of glucose in neoplastic tissues. A glucose analogue, fluorodeoxyglucose, that is tagged with fluorine 18 is

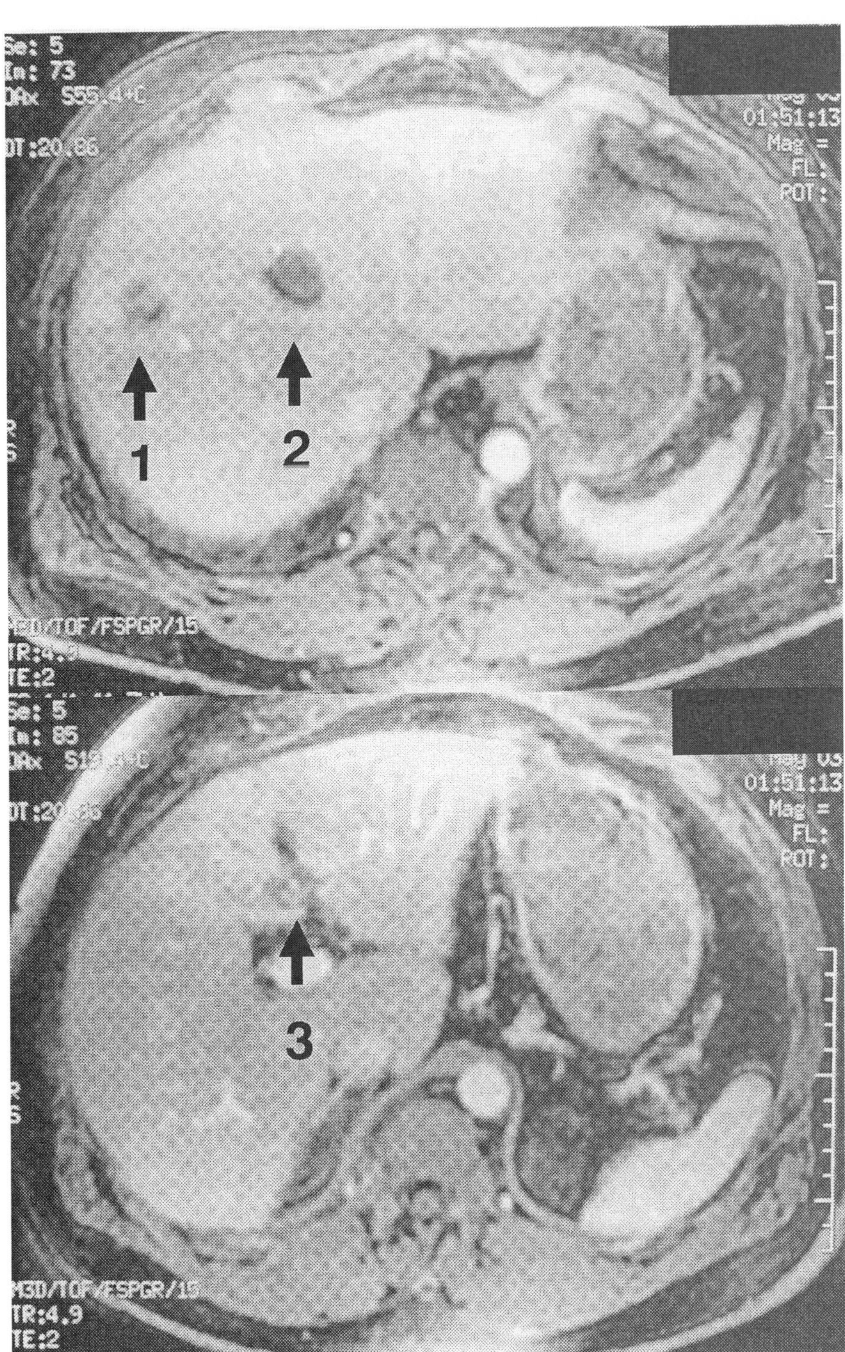

FIGURE 58.15 (*A*) and (*B*) T1-weighted magnetic resonance imaging (MRI) with gadolinium from the same patient as in Fig. 58.14 with history of colorectal cancer and three lesions in the liver. Lesion 1 in segment VIII is irregular and rim enhancing and was a colorectal cancer metastasis. Lesion 2 straddling segments IV and VIII has smooth borders, is not rim enhancing, and was found to be a cyst. Lesion 3 straddling segments IV and III across the umbilical fissure is irregular, rim enhancing, and was a colorectal cancer metastasis.

injected intravenously before scanning and is retained preferentially in metabolically active tumors over normal tissue. Sometimes PET scans will identify areas of occult disease within the liver, but more importantly, it can identify areas of extrahepatic occult disease previously unsuspected. When combined with a CT scanner within the same machine and the ability to fuse images, the areas of increased activity can be more precisely anatomically identified (Fig. 58.18).

Correlation of Computed Tomographic Images with Segmental Anatomy

Preoperative CT remains the primary imaging modality used by most surgeons before hepatic resection. Figure 58.14 is provided to help correlate CT images to the segmental anatomy defined previously. The segments of the liver are defined using identifiable structures on the CT (Fig. 58.19).

PREOPERATIVE EVALUATION OF HEPATIC RESERVE

Whenever a surgical resection is planned, an important consideration is whether the remnant liver will be sufficient to regenerate and sustain the patient long term. In patients with relatively normal hepatic parenchyma (without active hepatitis, cirrhosis, or metabolic defects), up to 70% to 75% of the hepatic volume can be resected with good recovery as long as the remnant liver has adequate portal venous and hepatic arterial inflow, adequate hepatic venous outflow, and adequate biliary drainage. Many groups around the world have used various strategies to predict hepatic reserve (Tables 58.1 and 58.2). None of these tests or

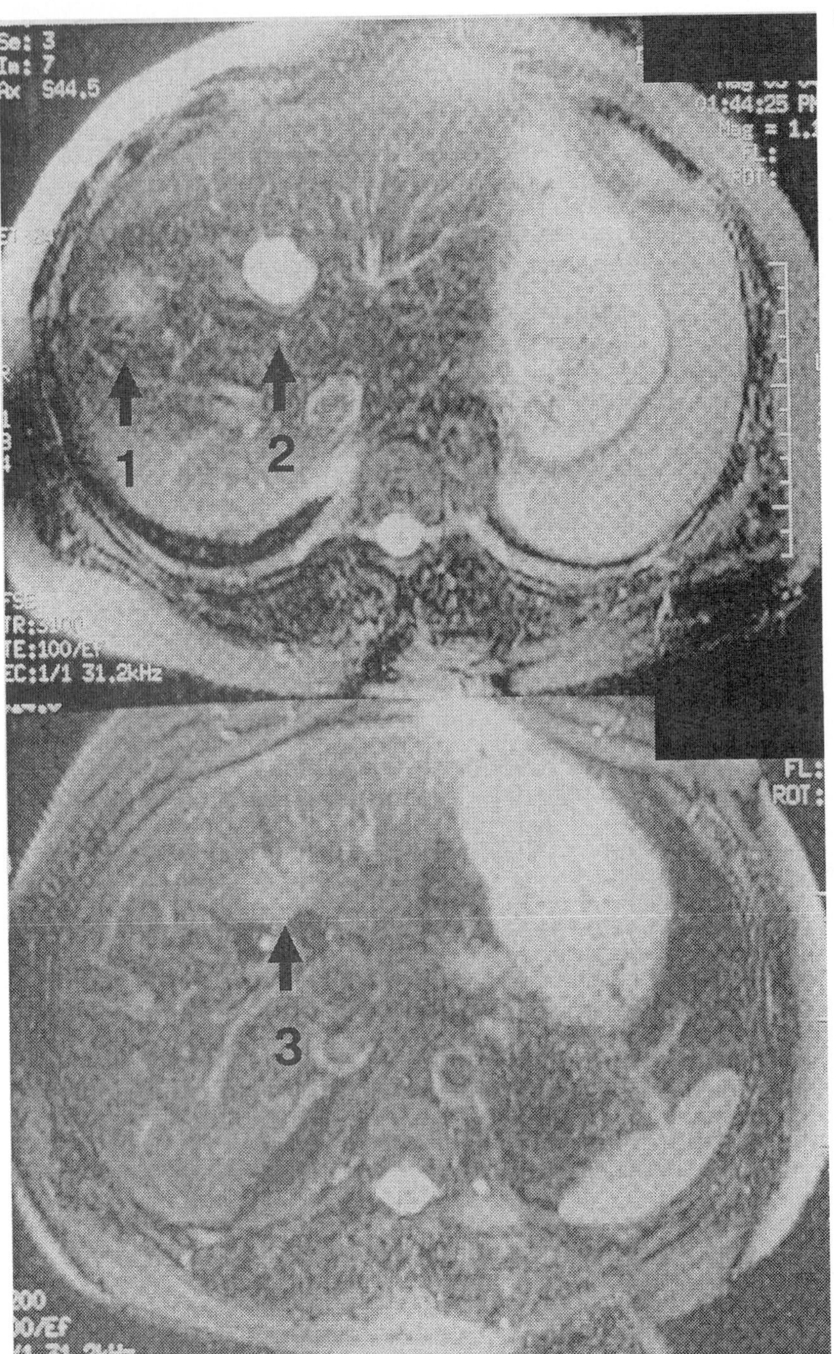

FIGURE 58.15 (*Continued*)
(*C*) and (*D*) T2-weighted MRI from same patient with history of colorectal cancer and three lesions in liver. Lesion 1 in segment VIII is irregular and mildly bright and was a colorectal cancer metastasis. Lesion 2 straddling segments IV and VIII has smooth borders, is very bright, and was found to be a cyst. Lesion 3 straddling segments IV and III across the umbilical fissure is mildly bright and was a colorectal cancer metastasis. Colorectal metastases and many tumors are mildly bright on T2-weighted MRI, whereas cysts and hemangiomas are typically very bright.

TABLE 58.1

STRATEGIES TO PREDICT HEPATIC RESERVE

- Child—Pugh score (Table 58.2) to assess synthetic ability (albumin, prothrombin time, and ascites), bile excretory function (total bilirubin), and metabolic function (changes in mental status from ammonia retention)
- Clearance of galactose or organic anionic dyes, such as indocyanine green
- Tests of microsomal function such as caffeine clearance, lidocaine clearance, or aminopyrine breath tests
- Volumetric measurements of the liver and prediction of liver remnant after resection based on three-dimensional reconstructions from computed tomography and magnetic resonance imaging

TABLE 58.2 CLASSIFICATION

CHILD—PUGH CLASSIFICATION

	1 Point	2 Points	3 Points
Bilirubin (mg/dL)	<2	2–3	>3
Albumin (g/dL)	>3.5	2.8–3.5	<2.8
Ascites	Absent	Moderate	Severe
Encephalopathy	Absent	Moderate	Severe
Prothrombin time			
Seconds prolonged	<4	4–6	>6
INR	<1.7	1.7–2.3	>2.3

INR, international normalized ratio.
A: 5–6 points; B: 7–9 points; C: 10–15 points.

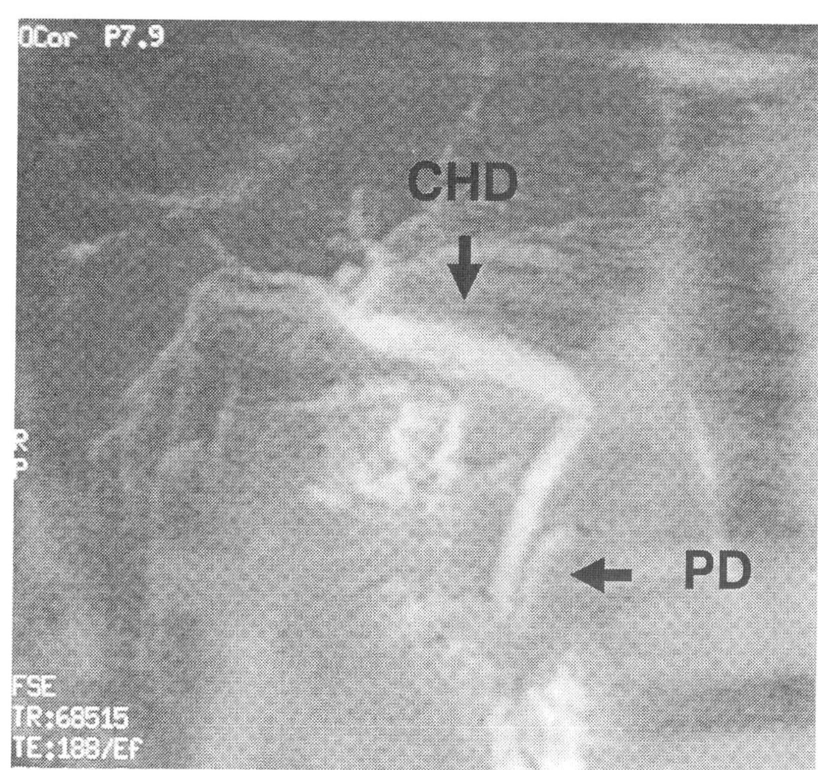

FIGURE 58.16 Magnetic resonance cholangiopancreatography (MRCP) of a patient after cholecystectomy with mild dilation of common hepatic duct (*CHD*). The pancreatic duct (*PD*) is also visible.

strategies has been demonstrated to clearly better predict outcome than another. Many centers in the United States rely simply on the Child—Pugh score and the prediction of adequate liver remnant volume after resection. In very select circumstances, it may be of benefit to perform portal vein embolization to the right or left half of the liver in the hopes of obtaining compensatory hypertrophy of the other side before resection. This is especially useful when the predicted liver remnant after resection is small or if the patient has an underlying hepatic dysfunction that may not allow the remnant to fully regenerate and sustain the patient long term. The disadvantages of portal vein embolization include the need to wait 4 to 6 weeks before resection to allow the compensatory hypertrophy to occur and, for more central lesions, the need to commit to taking out one or the other side with an extended hepatectomy without the benefit of intraoperative evaluation.

ONCOLOGIC CONSIDERATIONS IN HEPATIC RESECTION

The decision of when and whether to operate is often just as important as the technical details of successfully removing a liver lesion(s) identified in a patient. It is very important to consider the diagnosis in making the decision of whether to operate. For example, a solitary liver lesion presenting in an elderly patient, with a rising carcinoembryonic antigen (CEA), and a recent history of a resected colon cancer should be treated differently from a young woman with a solitary lesion, with radiologic characteristics of a focal nodular hyperplasia lesion. It is important to consider the biology of the tumor within the patient. For example, a patient who re-presents with a solitary hepatic colorectal cancer metastasis 4 years after resection of the primary tumor will more likely benefit from hepatic resection than another patient who presents with eight synchronous lesions in the liver at the time of diagnosis of the primary tumor. It is important to consider if the goal of resection is curative or palliative. For example, patients with neuroendocrine tumor metastases of the liver may be debulked of hepatic metastases, but they are rarely totally eradicated of disease. If the tumor is functional and difficult to control medically, then there may be a benefit to debulking. Even if the tumor is not functional, some evidence indicates that surgical debulking of liver metastases in carefully selected patients may benefit long-term survival. It is important to exclude other distant extrahepatic disease with a reasonable number of preoperative tests. For example, before performing hepatic resection for colorectal cancer metastases, it is often helpful to obtain a PET scan to exclude extrahepatic metastases. This will allow better selection of patients most likely to benefit from hepatic resection and will allow patients with previously unsuspected systemic disease to get systemic therapy sooner.

The comorbid status of the patient is also important. Extended hepatic resections with or without biliary reconstruction can exert a toll on even very fit patients. It is important to identify patients who may have difficulties with hepatic regeneration (e.g., those with a history of hepatitis, cirrhosis, or metabolic disorders). Patients with suspected cardiopulmonary disease should undergo appropriate preoperative evaluation and treatment before hepatic resection. Lastly, other effective treatments and the optimal sequence of treatments should be considered. For example, in the treatment of hepatocellular carcinoma the possibilities include liver transplantation, liver resection, liver ablation (radiofrequency, cryotherapy, or ethanol), embolization, and systemic chemotherapies. A patient with very poor hepatic reserve because of chronic liver disease and a single small hepatocellular carcinoma may be best treated with liver transplantation, whereas, a patient with normal liver parenchyma and a resectable lesion may be best treated with liver resection. Additionally, some patients may best be treated with ablative

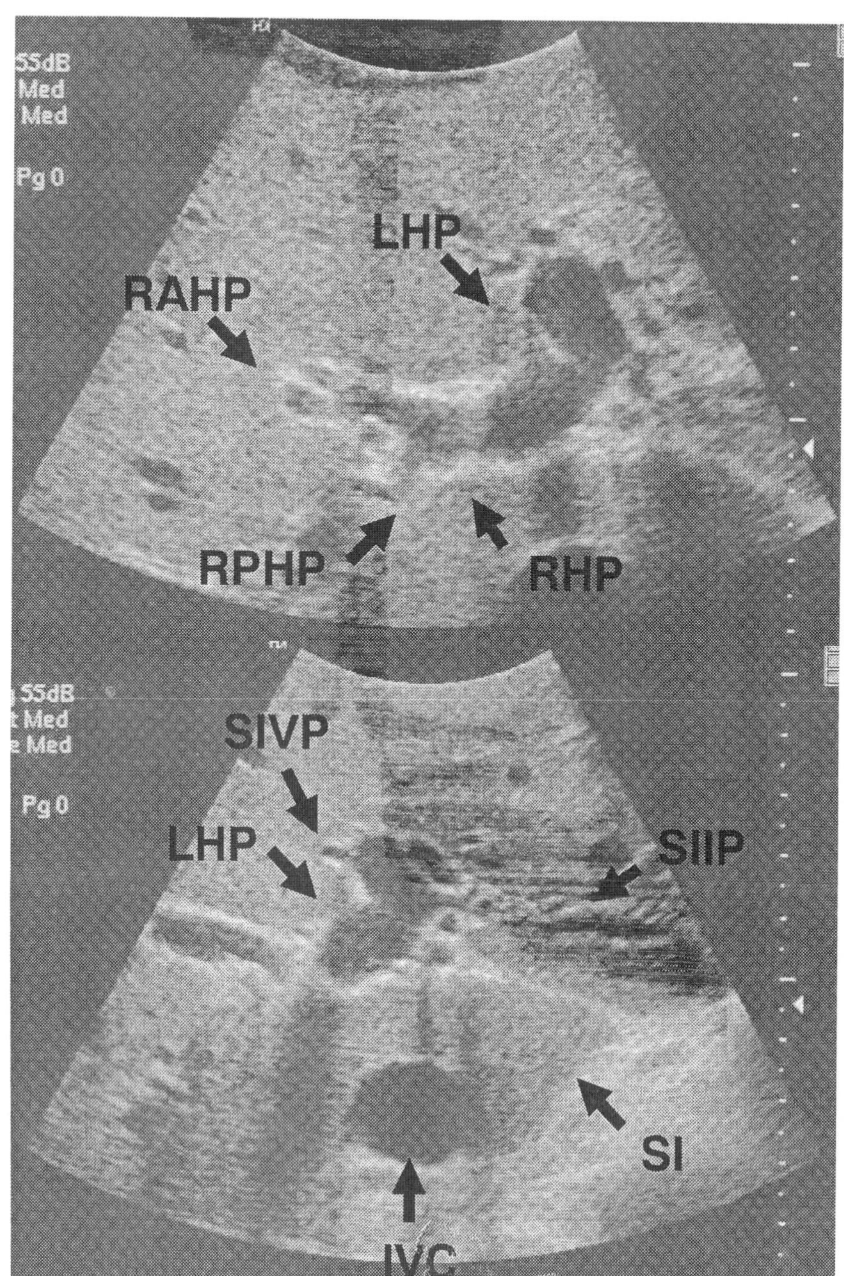

FIGURE 58.17 (A,B) Intraoperative ultrasound images of liver demonstrating right hepatic pedicle (*RHP*), right anterior section pedicle (*RASP*), right posterior section pedicle (*RPSP*), left hepatic pedicle (*LHP*), segment II pedicle (*SIIP*), segment IV pedicle (*SIVP*), segment I (*SI*), and inferior vena cava (*IVC*). (C,D) Intraoperative ultrasound images of liver demonstrating inferior vena cava (IVC), right hepatic vein (RHV), middle hepatic vein (*MHV*), left hepatic vein (LHV), segment I (SI), and a metastatic gastrointestinal stromal tumor lesion straddling segments IV and V of the liver.

techniques, especially if they have very small lesions that are easily approached percutaneously. Some patients are treated with a combination of these modalities. For example some centers will first treat patients with ethanol ablation and embolization before liver transplantation or resection for hepatocellular carcinoma.

INTRAOPERATIVE ASSESSMENT

Incisions for hepatic resections usually involve a right subcostal incision. Significant exposure can be obtained with a trifurcated incision as shown in Figure 58.20. In the majority of cases, however, all that is needed is an extended right subcostal incision with a vertical extension to the base of the xiphoid. The xiphoid can be resected for better exposure. For bulky lesions on the left or if the left half of the liver extends significantly to the left upper quadrant, a left subcostal component can be added. In rare circumstances, especially for lesions high on the dome, an intercostal extension or even median sternotomy may improve exposure. This is especially true for lesions involving the hepatic vein and IVC confluences.

Several versions of self-retaining costal margin retractors or ringed retractors are available that provide good access to the subdiaphragmatic surface. For complete intraoperative ultrasonography and for major resections, complete mobilization of the liver is required. The round ligament is divided and the falciform ligament divided close to the liver parenchyma. The right and left triangular ligaments are then divided to expose the bare areas of the liver. During exposure of the bare areas of the liver, care should be taken to avoid entering the right or left chest through the ligamentous portions of the diaphragm because this will cause excessive bellowing of the diaphragm

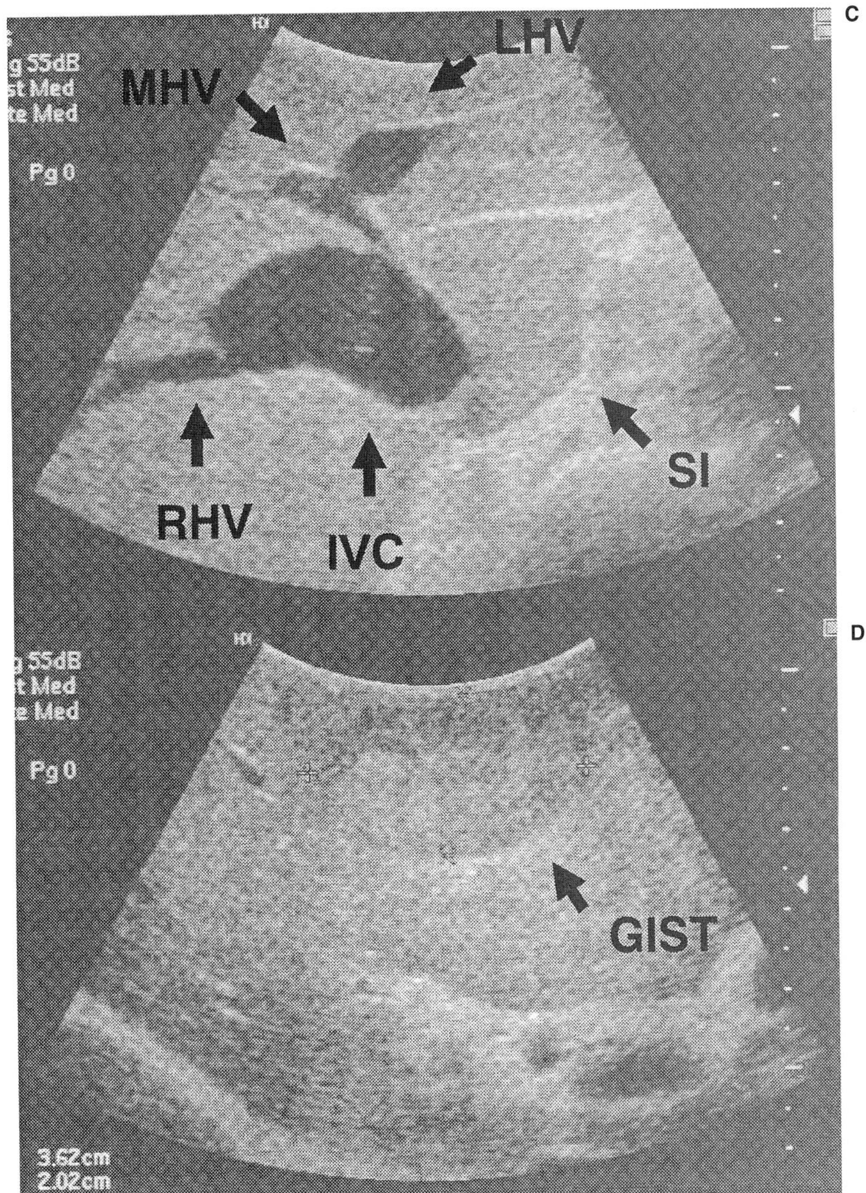

FIGURE 58.17 (*Continued*)

and poor exposure until a chest tube is placed on that side. Additionally, the right and left phrenic veins are very superficial on the hemidiaphragms and are prone to injury. The right colon can be mobilized out of the field by dividing Gerota's fascia over the right kidney and pulling the hepatic flexure inferiorly. To completely assess the caudate lobe, the overlying lesser omentum should be divided. Care should be taken to avoid inadvertently dividing a replaced or accessory left hepatic artery running in this space. After mobilization, a thorough bimanual examination should be performed and intraoperative ultrasonography used as previously described.

The porta hepatis is often dissected to identify the main bifurcations of the hepatic artery, bile duct, and portal vein. This allows individual ligation of the branches of these structures supplying one side of the liver while preserving the branches to the other side. Ligation of the hepatic artery and portal vein to one side also allows the liver parenchyma to demarcate a line of resection between the right and left liver. Greater exposure of the superior aspect of the hepatic hilum and exposure of a high or intraparenchymal bifurcation of a portal triad structure may be aided by exposing the hilar plate (Fig. 58.21) and dividing Glisson's capsule at the most inferior border of segment IV. Inflow control to the liver can also be obtained by pedicle ligations in which small hepatotomies are made around the main right pedicle, main left pedicle, the right anterior pedicle, or right posterior pedicle after identification with ultrasound (Fig. 58.22).[10] The pedicle of interest can be dissected out bluntly with a right angle or by palpation. The pedicle can then be clamped to confirm that it does indeed supply the area of liver of interest (i.e., right half, left half, right anterior section, or right posterior section). Once confirmed, the pedicle can be divided. Alternatively, the inflow pedicles can be divided as they are encountered while transecting hepatic parenchyma. With this technique, hemorrhage can be minimized by intermittent portal inflow occlusion, which is accomplished by gently clamping the main portal triad within the hepatoduodenal ligament.

Outflow control of the hepatic veins can be obtained before or after hepatic transaction and should be decided on a case-by-case basis. When there is a significant extraparenchymal

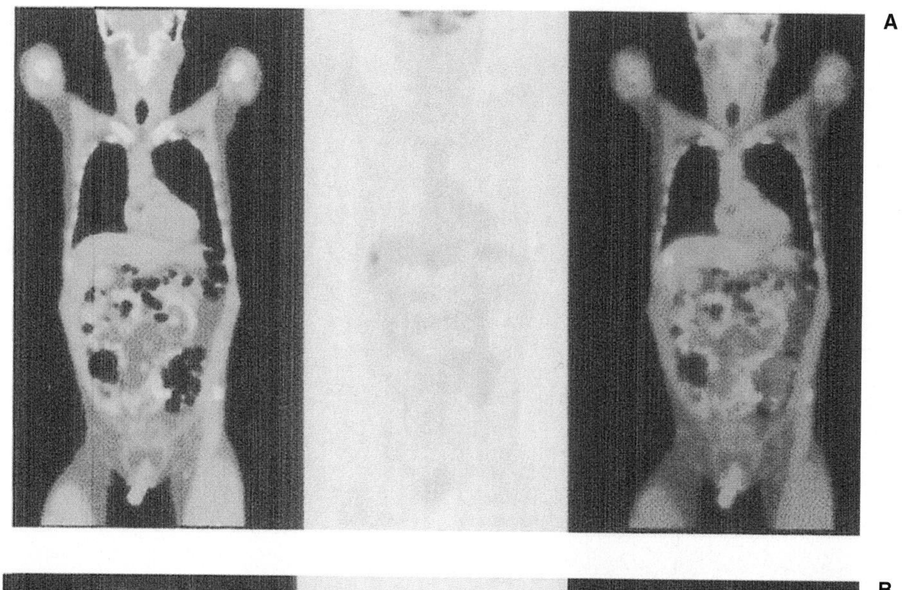

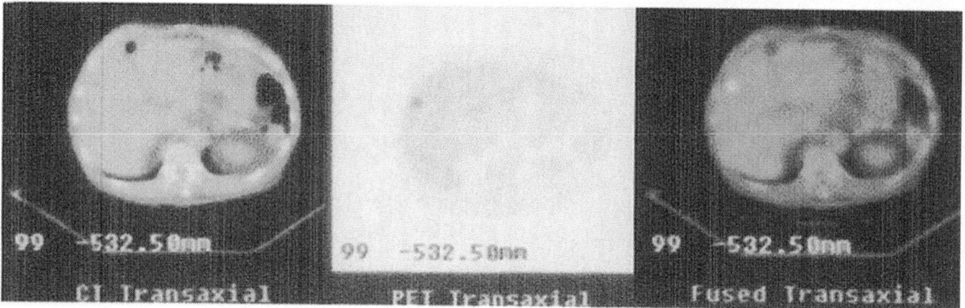

FIGURE 58.18 Positron emission tomography and computed tomography (PET—CT) scan images of patient in Figure 58.17B and C with solitary gastrointestinal stromal tumor metastasis straddling segments IV and V. Noncontrast CT images (*left*). PET images (*center*). Fusion images (*right*).

component to the hepatic vein(s) that need to be controlled, often it is easier to divide the hepatic vein(s) early and before parenchymal transection (but after inflow control) (Fig. 58.23). When the extraparenchymal component to the hepatic vein(s) is very short or absent and when the tumor margin is not near the junction of the hepatic vein(s) and IVC, it may be easier and safer to divide the hepatic vein(s) within the hepatic parenchyma after most of the parenchymal transection has been performed. The use of endoscopic vascular stapling devices has made the ligation of hepatic veins, whether extra- or intraparenchymally, much quicker and safer.[10] (Fig. 58.24) It is often useful to keep the central venous pressure (CVP) of the patient low (<5 mm Hg) until after parenchymal transection as this will decrease bleeding from the IVC and hepatic vein branches.[11]

MAJOR HEPATECTOMIES

To develop a uniform nomenclature understood by all, the American and International Hepato Pancreato Biliary Association (AHPBA and IHPBA) have adopted the Brisbane 2000 terminology of hepatic anatomy and resections. Right hepatectomy or right hemihepatectomy involves the resection of segments V through VIII. Left hepatectomy or hemihepatectomy involves the resection of segments II through IV. Either of these resections may or may not include resection of segment I, which should be stipulated. Extended right hepatectomy or hemihepatectomy involves the resection of segments IV through VIII. Extended left hepatectomy or hemihepatectomy involves the resection of segments II through V plus VIII. Again, either of these extended resections may or may not include resection of segment I, which should be stipulated.

Right anterior sectionectomy includes segments V and VIII. Right posterior sectionectomy includes segments VI and VII. Left medial sectionectomy removes segment IV. Left lateral sectionectomy includes segments II and III. A segmentectomy involves the resection of a single segment and a bisegmentectomy involves the resection of two contiguous segments.

The steps involved in each of these major hepatectomies include optimal exposure, vascular inflow control, vascular outflow control, and parenchymal transection. Vascular inflow control can be obtained by directly ligating the main right or left branches of the hepatic artery and portal vein in the hilum or by intermittent 10- to 20-minute intervals of a Pringle maneuver with 3 minutes in between to reestablish blood flow. It is the author's preference to encircle the hepatoduodenal ligament twice with a quarter inch Penrose drain that is tightened and clamped for a Pringle maneuver. Alternatively, pedicle ligations can be performed, as described previously, or the pedicles can be controlled as they are encountered during parenchymal transection. It is the author's preference to obtain vascular inflow by ligating the appropriate vessels in the hilum or by pedicle ligations, and to supplement this with intermittent Pringle maneuvers, as necessary, during parenchymal transection for hemihepatectomies. Vascular outflow to the right or left liver can be obtained by exposing and ligating the hepatic veins, as previously described, or by ligating the vessels intraparenchymally during transection of the liver tissue. Parenchymal transection can be performed using a multitude of techniques from finger fracture, using a Kelly clamp to fracture, Cavitron Ultrasonic Surgical Aspirator (CUSA), harmonic scalpel, stapling devices, electrocautery devices with or without saline perfusion, and high-pressure water jets. The superiority of any one of these techniques has not been established, and all are used. With these techniques, individual blood vessels and bile ducts are cauterized, clipped,

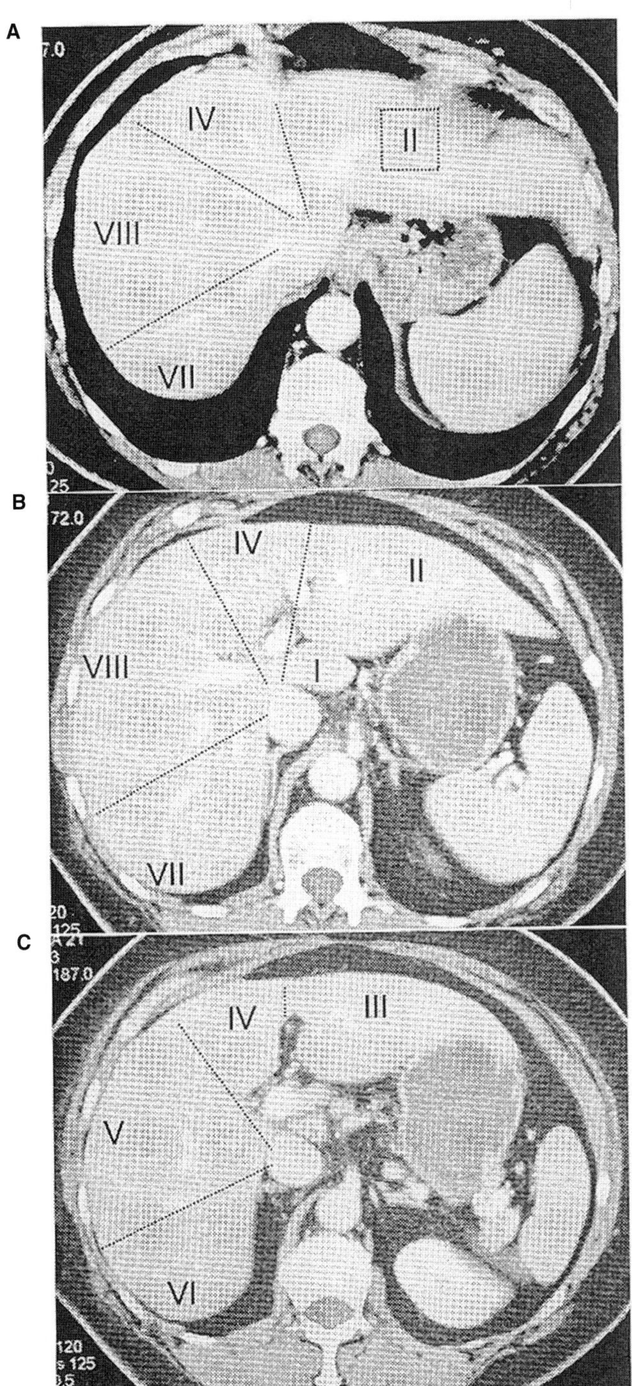

FIGURE 58.19 Computed tomography scan demonstrating segmental anatomy of the liver with cuts through the dome (*A*), just above the portal bifurcation (*B*), and below the portal bifurcation (*C*).

or sutured in rapid succession as they are encountered. Constant reevaluation of the direction of transection is important both to not injure vital structures to the remnant liver and to maintain a negative margin. After parenchymal transection and removal of the specimen, the raw surface of the liver is carefully inspected for bleeding and bile leakage, which can then be controlled by suture ligation, argon beam coagulation, or fibrin glue. It is the author's preference to place closed suction drains near resected liver surfaces to monitor and drain unrecognized postoperative bile leaks, but some centers will not routinely place drains.

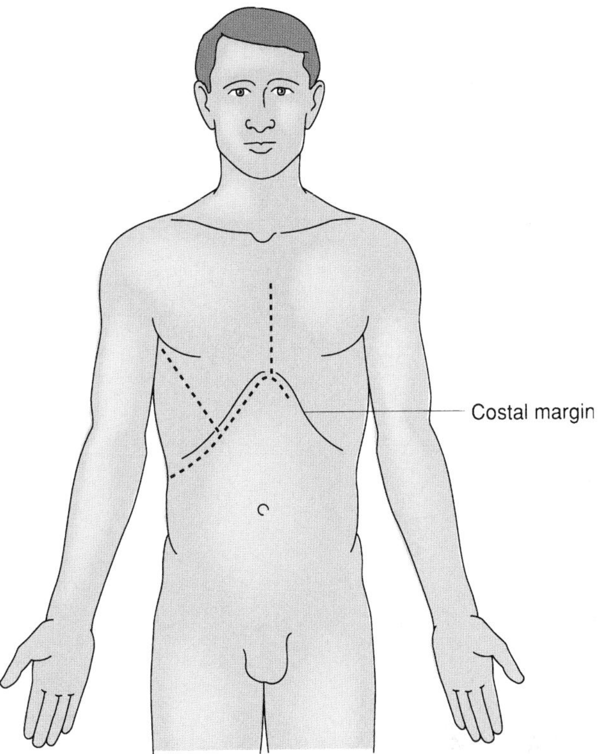

FIGURE 58.20 Incisions commonly used for hepatic resection.

SEGMENTAL RESECTIONS

To maximize functional reserve, (multi)segmental or subsegmental (or nonanatomic) hepatectomies can be performed. For example, left lateral sectionectomy (segments II and III), central hepatectomy to remove the right anterior section (segments V and VIII) and left medial section (segment IV),

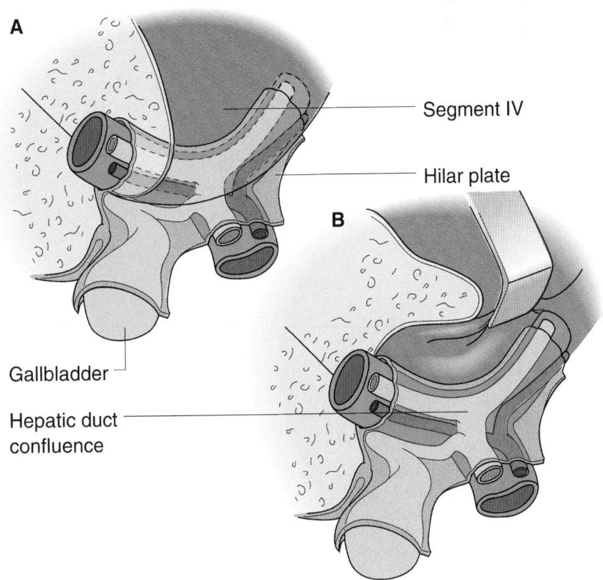

FIGURE 58.21 Lowering the hilar plate. (*A*) The inferior border of segment IV (quadrate lobe) overlies the hepatic duct confluence. (*B*) Division of the connective tissue investment allows elevation of segment IV, which results in a "lower" hilar plate and surgical exposure to the hepatic duct confluence. (From Blumgart LH, ed. *Surgery of the Liver and Biliary Tract*. New York: Churchill Livingstone, 1994, with permission.)

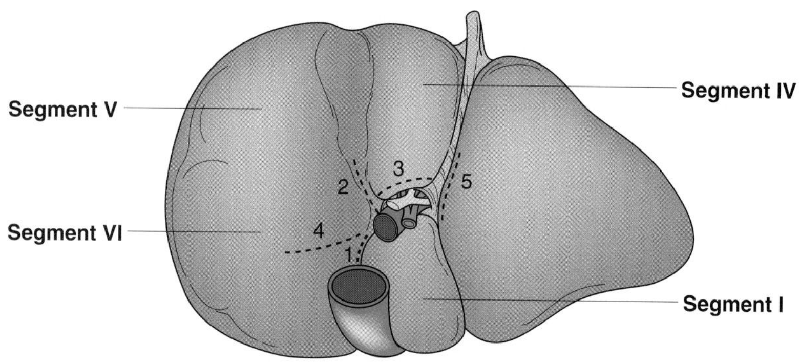

FIGURE 58.22 Hepatotomies to access pedicles for ligation: right hepatectomy, 1 and 4; left hepatectomy, 3 and 5; right anterior sectionectomy, 2 and 4; and right posterior sectionectomy, 1 and 4. (From Fong Y, Blumgart LH. Useful stapling techniques in liver surgery. *J Am Coll Surg.* 1997;185:93–100, with permission.)

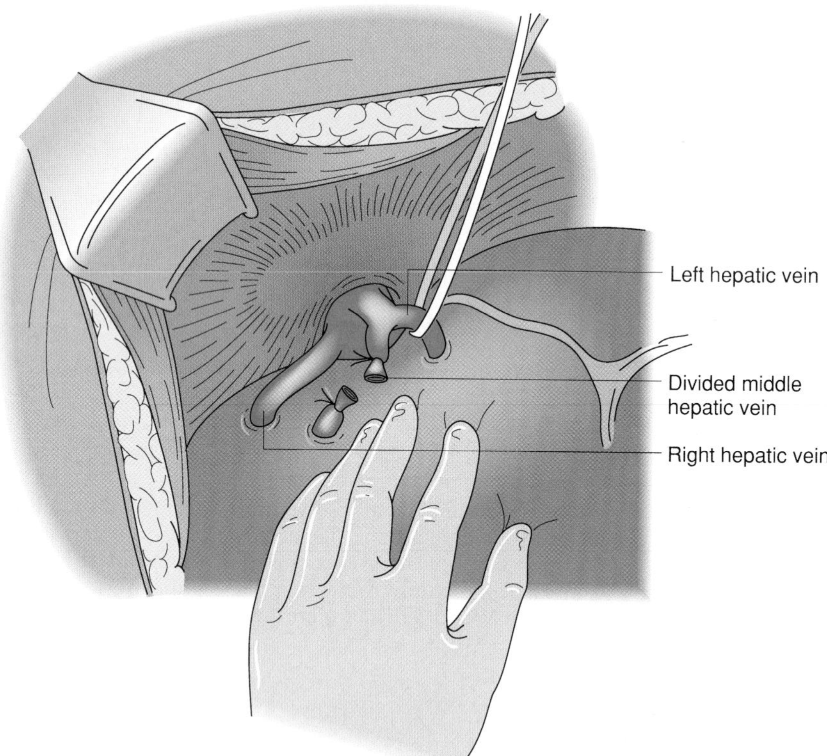

FIGURE 58.23 Caudal retraction of the left hepatic lobe with division of middle and left hepatic veins during left hepatic lobectomy.

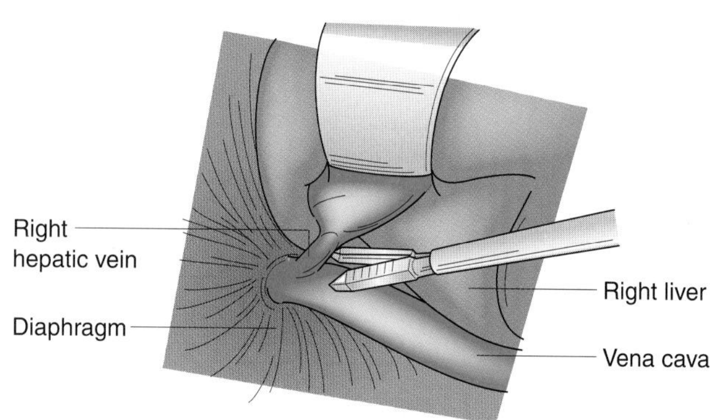

FIGURE 58.24 A vascular endoscopic stapling device is used to divide the right hepatic vein after the right side of the liver has been mobilized. (From Fong Y, Blumgart LH. Useful stapling techniques in liver surgery. *J Am Coll Surg.* 1997;185:93–100, with permission.)

right posterior sectionectomy (segments VI and VII), or caudate resection (segment I) are examples in which one, two, or three contiguous segments are removed to eradicate tumors within those regions of the liver. These resections are often done with intermittent Pringle maneuver until the specific pedicles supplying these areas are controlled.

KEY POINTS

- **The most widely accepted nomenclature for liver anatomy is based on Couinaud's description of eight anatomic segments of the liver.**
- **There are three major hepatic veins, with most patients having a single, large hepatic vein that joins the right anterior wall of the IVC and a middle and left hepatic vein that converge into a common trunk 1 to 2 cm from the IVC.**
- **Classic hepatic arterial anatomy exists in only approximately 50% to 60% of patients with a replaced right hepatic artery arising from the SMA and a replaced left hepatic artery arising from the left gastric artery being the most common variants each seen in 15% to 20% of patients.**

- Callot's triangle is bounded by the common hepatic duct on the left, the cystic duct inferiorly, and the cystic artery superiorly.
- The blood supply of the common bile duct is segmental in nature and consists of branches from the cystic, hepatic, and gastroduodenal arteries, which meet to form collateral vessels that run in the 3 o'clock and 9 o'clock positions.
- Magnetic resonance imaging of the liver with gadolinium as a contrast agent is commonly used to characterize hepatic lesions.
- Magnetic resonance cholangiopancreatography is widely used to view biliary anatomy as it involves no contrast agent and optimally can provide images that rival formal cholangiography.
- Intraoperative ultrasonography is used routinely to assess the anatomy of the hepatic pedicles (portal vein, hepatic artery, bile duct), hepatic veins, and to identify and characterize hepatic lesions within the parenchyma and their relationships within the eight anatomic segments.
- The portal pedicles are invested with Glisson's capsule and have a very echogenic covering to them on ultrasound in contrast to hepatic vein branches.
- The steps involved in major hepatectomy include optimal exposure, vascular inflow control, vascular outflow control, and parenchymal transection.

References

1. McIndoe AH, Counseller VX. A report on the bilaterality of the liver. *Arch Surg.* 1927;15:589.
2. Hjörtsjö CH. The topography of the intrahepatic duct systems. *Acta Anat.* 1931;11:599–615.
3. Tung TT. La vascularixation veineuse du foie et ses applications aux resections hepatiques. *Thèse Hanoi*, 1939.
4. Healy JE, Schroy PC. Anatomy of the biliary ducts within the human liver. Analysis of the prevailing pattern of branchings and the major variations of the biliary ducts. *American Medical Association Archives of Surgery* 1953;66:599–616.
5. Goldsmith NA, Woodvurne RT. Surgical anatomy pertaining to liver resection. *Surg Gynecol Obstet* 1957;195:310–318.
6. Couinaud C Le Foi. *Etudes anatomogiques et chirurgicales.* Paris: Masson, 1957.
7. Bismuth J, Houssin D, Castaing D. Major and minor segmentectomies–réglées–in liver surgery. *World J Surg.* 1982;6:10–24.
8. Blumgart LH, Hann LE. Surgical and radiologic anatomy of the liver and biliary tract. In Blumgart LH, Fong Y, eds. *Surgery of the Liver and Biliary Tract,* 3rd ed. Blumgart LH, Fong Y, eds. New York: WB Saunders, 2000.
9. Michels NA. Newer anatomy of the liver and its variant blood supply and collateral circulation. *Am J Surg.* 1966;112:337.
10. Fong Y, Blumgart LH. Useful stapling techniques in liver surgery. *J Am Coll Surg.* 1997;185:93–100.
11. Melendez JA, Arslan V, Fischer ME, et al. Perioperative outcomes of major hepatic resections under low central venous pressure anesthesia: blood loss, blood transfusion, and the risk of postoperative renal dysfunction. *J Am Coll Surg.* 1998. 187:620–625.

CHAPTER 59 ■ HEPATIC INFECTION AND ACUTE HEPATIC FAILURE

ERNESTO P. MOLMENTI AND ANDREW S. KLEIN

PYOGENIC LIVER ABSCESS

Pyogenic liver abscesses are of bacterial origin and constitute one of the two main types of liver abscesses, the other being amebic (caused by *Entamoeba histolytica*). Pyogenic liver abscesses, although infrequent, are potentially lethal. Outcome correlates directly with prompt diagnosis and rapid intervention. Over the past century, the pathogenesis of liver abscesses has changed. A classic study by Ochsner in the 1930s, prior to the introduction of antibiotics, reported that appendicitis and other intraabdominal infections were the most frequent cause of pyogenic liver abscess. The route of infection was attributable to the portal vein in 43% of instances, whereas the biliary tree was the source of infection in only 14% of cases. Over the past 20 years, invasive procedures involving the liver, biliary tree, and pancreas have resulted in an increased incidence of pyogenic liver abscesses. Currently, obstructive biliary malignancies and stone disease are the most common cause of liver abscesses. The use of stents to treat both malignant and nonmalignant strictures is a contributing factor. The portal vein serves as the conduit for infection from intraperitoneal sources in a minority of cases, and appendicitis has been replaced as the most frequent intraperitoneal source by infections associated with diverticulitis, perforated cancers, perforated ulcers, and inflammatory bowel disease. Hepatic abscesses that occur following liver transplantation should raise concern for the presence of hepatic artery thrombosis (Fig. 59.1) Most pyogenic abscesses are solitary and polymicrobial and involve the right lobe of the liver. Abscesses in liver metastases usually result from superinfection of a central area of necrosis. Hepatic abscesses may be further complicated by rupture into the peritoneum or retroperitoneum, pleuropulmonary fistulas, rupture into the pericardial cavity, rupture into the gastrointestinal tract, and involvement of surrounding blood vessels.[1–3]

Individuals over 50 years of age, males, liver transplant patients, diabetics, and those with malignancies are at highest risk for pyogenic liver abscesses. Fever is the most frequent presenting symptom. Right upper quadrant pain, chills, anorexia, weight loss, malaise, jaundice, and weakness are usually present. Hepatomegaly is less frequent than in amebic abscesses.[1,3,4]

Laboratory studies show leukocytosis in approximately 70% of patients. Elevated serum bilirubin, elevated alkaline phosphatase, elevated transaminases, or low albumin levels are observed in approximately 50% of all cases.[1,2]

Chest radiographs are abnormal in half of patients with pyogenic liver abscesses, reflecting an underlying inflammatory process. The most frequent findings include a right pleural effusion, elevation of the right hemidiaphragm, and atelectasis

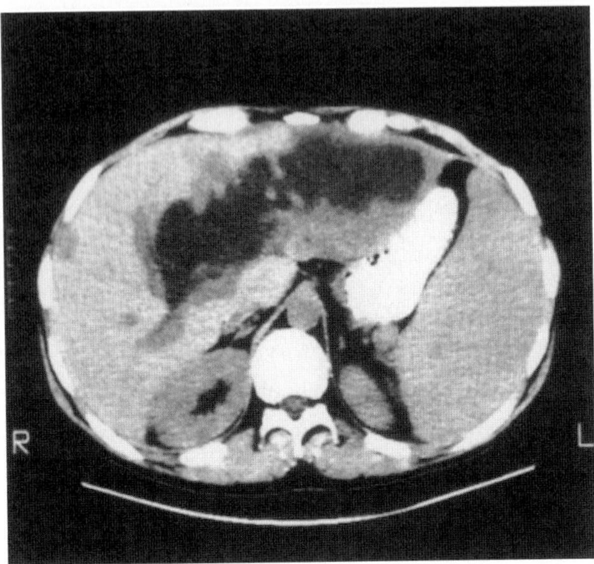

FIGURE 59.1 Computed tomogram of a pyogenic hepatic abscess in a liver transplant recipient with occlusion of the hepatic artery.

of the base of the right lung. Gas within the abscess may be seen in 10% to 20% of patients. Ultrasound evaluation is diagnostic in over 90% of cases. It is also quick, is radiation-free, can differentiate solid from cystic structures, is easy to perform, and can guide percutaneous drainage. It is, however, operator dependent and has a degree of resolution inferior to that of other imaging techniques. Computed tomography (CT) scanning is probably the most reliable diagnostic modality. In contrast—enhanced CT imaging, small abscesses appear as hypoattenuated areas with faint rim enhancement and surrounding edema that distinguishes them from hepatic cysts. Magnetic resonance (MR) imaging is frequently used but somewhat limited by its cost and the technical difficulties associated with the scanning process. Due to varying protein content, pyogenic abscesses exhibit variable signal intensity on T1- and T2-weighted images. T2-weighted images show slightly increased signal intensity associated with perilesional edema. Cholangiography (percutaneous or endoscopic) can define the anatomy of both biliary tree and hepatic abscess in about two thirds of cases. It is associated, however, with potential septic flares despite the administration of antibiotics due to disturbance of the bacterial flora.[1,5,6]

Gram-negative aerobes are encountered in two thirds of patients. Among these pathogens, *Escherichia coli*, *Klebsiella pneumoniae*, and *Proteus* species are the ones most frequently isolated. Anaerobes (such as *Bacteroides fragilis*) are found in 30% of cases. Streptococci, including aerobic and anaerobic forms, are present in approximately one third of patients. Approximately 60% of patients have concordant results of blood and abscess cultures. Broad-spectrum antibiotics aimed at gram-negative aerobes, streptococci, and anaerobes are indicated until bacterial sensitivities have been clearly identified. A frequently used antibiotic combination is ampicillin, an aminoglycoside, and either metronidazole or clindamycin. The aminoglycoside can be replaced with a third-generation cephalosporin (e.g., ceftriaxone) in patients at risk for renal toxicity. In instances of mixed pyogenic and fungal abscesses, antimycotic agents should be considered early, prior to the onset of fungemia. The duration of the treatment should be based on clinical response, toxicity of the regimen, and characteristics of the abscesses. Intravenous antibiotics are usually administered for 14 days, followed by oral agents for a total of 6 weeks.[1,2,7–9]

In the past, surgical drainage was the treatment of choice. Currently percutaneous drainage is considered the standard therapy. Its use, however, may be limited or contraindicated by the presence of ascites, multiple abscesses, a transpleural drainage route, large size of the abscess, and the presence of an intraabdominal source requiring an open approach. Unless appropriate therapy is started as soon as the diagnosis is made, death is the usual outcome. Reported mortality ranges from 2.5% to over 30% and is highest in patients with multiple abscesses, with non–*Klebsiella pneumonia* pathogens, with mixed bacterial and fungal abscesses, with respiratory symptoms, and with abscesses 5 cm or greater in diameter.[1,2,7,10,11]

AMEBIC LIVER ABSCESS

Amebic liver abscesses are caused by *Entamoeba histolytica,* a nonflagellated pseudopod-forming protozoan. Amebiasis is most prevalent in tropical and subtropical regions with poor sanitation, where up to 50% of the population may be infected. In the United States, the highest incidence of infection is encountered in the South, in areas with prominent concentrations of immigrants from areas such as Mexico and Southeast Asia. The incidence in these regions ranges from 7% to 10%. Hepatic abscesses, however, occur in only 3% to 7% of individuals with amebiasis. Especially at risk are patients confined to mental institutions, native Americans in reservations, some military personnel, travelers to endemic areas, and homosexual men. The peak incidence of amebic abscesses is observed in patients in their third or fourth decade of life. Men are affected more frequently than women.[1,12]

Fecal-oral transmission is the most frequent route of infection. Ingested cysts, containing four nuclei, pass unaltered through the stomach and reach the intestine. Once in the intestine, the cyst wall is degraded by trypsin and eight trophozoites are released. These infective forms multiply in the colonic lumen, especially in the cecum. While living within the colonic lumen, *Entamoeba histolytica* may become tissue invasive. Invasion may range from superficial mucosal ulceration to perforation. Amebic trophozoites that enter the mesenteric veins or lymphatics reach other organs. The portal vein is the route via which they reach the liver, the most frequent site of extraintestinal involvement. Amebic trophozoites cause obstruction of venules, thrombosis and infarction of the corresponding areas of hepatic parenchyma, and eventually abscesses (Fig. 59.2). In the distal colon they become cystic, undergo two consecutive divisions, are excreted in the feces as tetranucleate cysts, and remain viable for 8 to 30 days after being shed. Cysts are susceptible to acetic acid, iodine, chlorine, and temperatures greater than 68°C.[1,6,12]

Liver abscesses range in size from several millimeters to gigantic masses (Fig. 59.3). Differential diagnosis is with pyogenic abscess and malignancies. Homosexual men are particularly at risk because of their frequency of *E. histolytica* bowel carriage and a higher-than average risk for AIDS. Abscesses are encountered more frequently in the right lobe and tend to be single lesions. Amebic abscesses show slight inflammation on the periphery, and many times contain a dark hemorrhagic fluid known as "anchovy paste" (Fig. 59.4). Patients most frequently present with fever and abdominal pain. Other findings include hepatomegaly, weight loss, diarrhea, chills, and afternoon and night sweats. Jaundice is less frequent than in pyogenic abscesses. Abscesses have been classified into acute or chronic and benign or aggressive. The most feared complication is rupture into surrounding tissues or spaces. Bacterial superinfection of initially amebic abscesses may occur.[1,3,4,6,12–14]

Most patients with amebic abscesses have elevated white blood cell counts with no eosinophilia. Serum alkaline phosphatase is elevated in approximately 75% of cases.

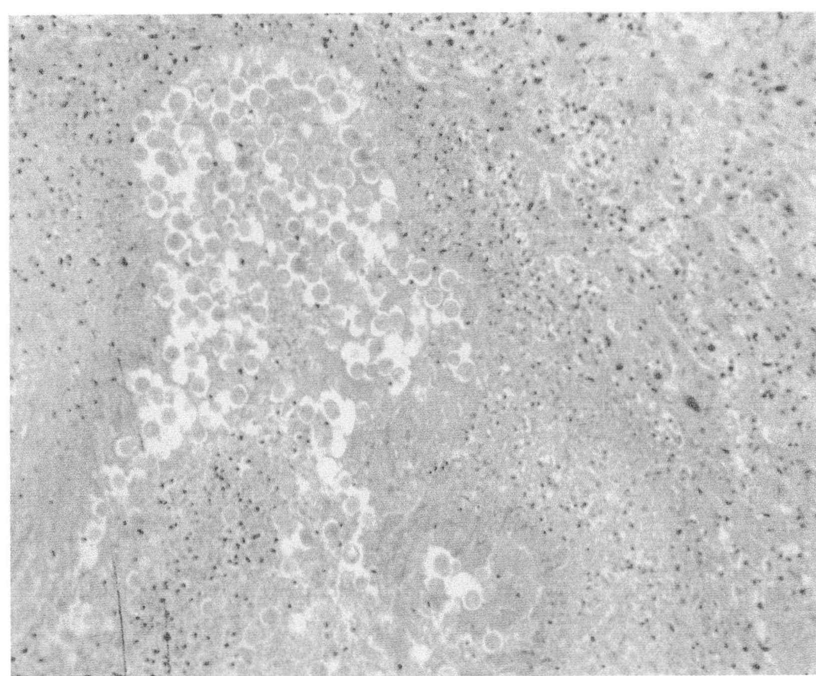

FIGURE 59.2 Amebic abscess of the liver. A photomicrograph of the margin of an amebic abscess shows fibroblastic proliferation surrounding the cavity and amebic trophozoites in the lumen. (From Rubin E, Farber JL. *Pathology*, 3rd ed. Philadelphia: Lippincott Williams & Wilkins, 1999.)

Hypoalbuminemia is also encountered. Serum bilirubin and transaminase levels are slightly elevated. *E. histolytica* is not found in fecal specimens of most patients with hepatic abscesses. Antibodies in serum are encountered in 90% to 100% of patients with amebic liver abscesses and are detectable 1 week to 10 days after the appearance of symptoms. Indirect hemagglutination and enzyme-linked immunosorbent assay have reported sensitivities of 99% and 97.9% and specificities of 99.8% and 94.8%, respectively. Other available diagnostic tests include indirect immunofluorescence, latex agglutination, complement fixation, gel diffusion, and counterimmunoelectrophoresis. Gel diffusion and counterimmunoelectrophoresis remain positive for only 6 to 12 months after infection and are used to distinguish acute from chronic infection.[1,12,15]

Chest radiographs are abnormal in the majority of patients with amebic hepatic abscesses. Findings include elevation of the right hemidiaphragm, right pleural effusion, atelectasis in the region of the base of the right lung, and a right pleural effusion. CT scanning is probably the imaging technique of choice, given the detailed information it provides. An enhancing wall and surrounding edema are usually observed in contrast-enhanced CT scans. Ultrasonography is very useful as well, but its accuracy is associated with the skills of the operator, is influenced by physiologic changes such as hepatic steatosis, and has a resolution inferior to that of CT scans. Amebic abscesses usually lack wall echoes by ultrasound. MR imaging shows homogeneous low signal intensity on T1 and high signal intensity on T2-weighted images. Technetium Tc99m nuclear scanning displays a photopenic area. Gallium scanning shows amebic abscesses as cold spots, because they do not contain leukocytes, which may aid in differentiating them from pyogenic abscesses.[1,6,12]

Treatment of hepatic amebic abscesses is based on amebicidal drugs. Metronidazole is the drug of choice. Standard dosing is 750 mg orally three times daily or 500 mg intravenously

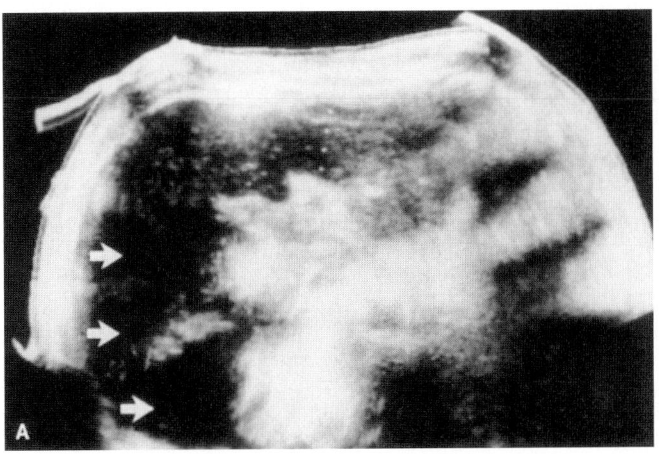

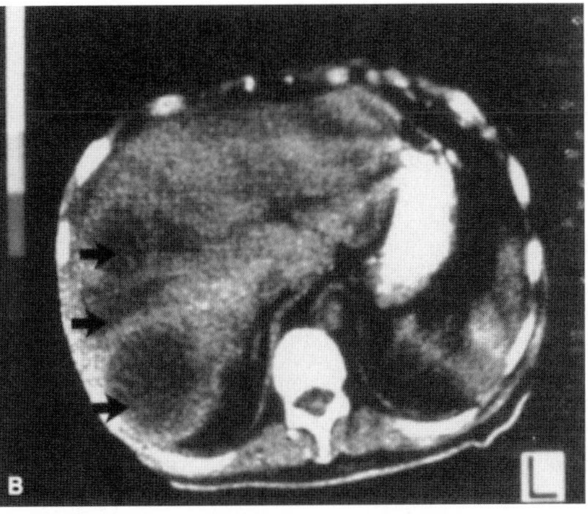

FIGURE 59.3 Sonogram (*A*) and computed tomogram (*B*) in a patient with multiple amebic abscesses (*arrows*).

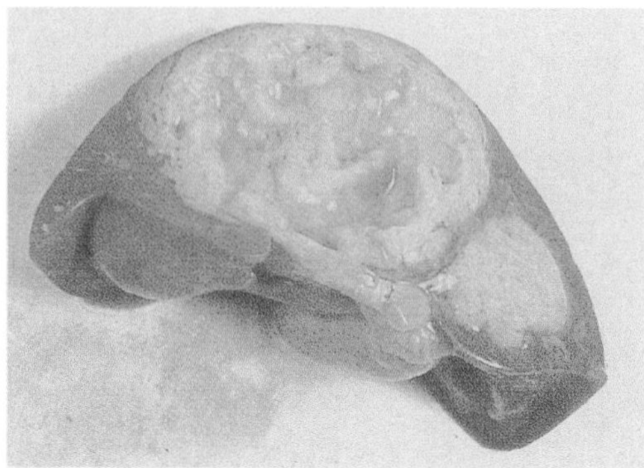

FIGURE 59.4 Amebic abscesses of the liver. The cut surface of the liver shows multiple abscesses containing "anchovy paste" material. (From Rubin E, Farber JL. *Pathology*, 3rd ed. Philadelphia: Lippincott Williams & Wilkins, 1999.)

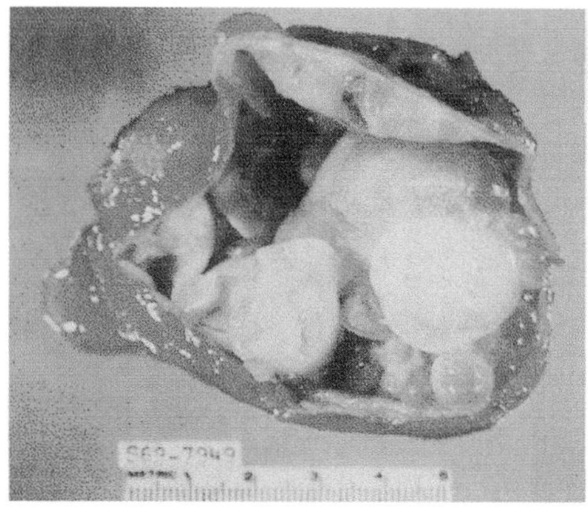

FIGURE 59.5 A partly opened hepatic hydatid cyst. Brood capsule and daughter cysts are visible in the cavity. (From Kean BH, Sun T, Ellsworth RM. *Color atlas/text of ophthalmic parasitology*. New York: Igaku-Shoin, 1991:188.)

every 6 hours for 7 to 10 days, with oral administration being the preferred route. Metronidazole has been shown to effectively treat both intestinal and extraintestinal sites. In cases resistant to metronidazole, chloroquine or chloroquine together with emetine or dehydroemetine is recommended. Glucose-6-phosphate dehydrogenase activity should be checked before chloroquine therapy is initiated. Percutaneous drainage is considered in cases of poor response to antiamebic agents, when superinfection is suspected, or when there is a risk of rupture. Open surgical drainage is almost never required and is recommended only in severe, complicated cases.[1,12,13]

ECHINOCOCCUS (HYDATID DISEASE)

Hydatid disease, caused by *Echinococcus granulosus, E. multilocularis*, and *E. vogeli*, is endemic in the Mediterranean basin and other regions with sheep-rearing economies but rare in the United States. *Echinococcus granulosus* is the species that most frequently results in liver involvement. Dogs are the definitive host, although the disease is endemic in sheep and cattle farming regions. The life cycle of the organism is complete when the definitive host ingests infected viscera, and scoleces released in the intestine develop into adult worms. Humans are intermediate hosts, and acquire echinococcal eggs by either ingestion of contaminated foods or contact with infected animals. The egg is digested in the duodenum and yields an embryo. Embryos invade the intestinal wall and reach the liver via the portal vessels. Although many embryos are destroyed in the liver, those that survive lodged in capillaries develop into hydatid cysts. The most frequent site of hydatid cysts is the liver (50% to 77% of cases), followed by the lungs (10% to 40% of cases).[6,16–18]

E. granulosus and *E. vogeli* cause liver cysts while *E. multilocularis* is associated with tumorlike lesions or alveolar disease. Liver involvement may lead to venous obstruction, portal hypertension, sepsis, and cholangitis. Hydatid cysts are fluid-filled and round and contain three layers of host tissue: an outer 2 to 4 mm thick fibrous *pericyst* composed of compressed and fibrotic liver tissue, a 2 mm thick middle anuclear hyaline layer or *ectocyst*, and an *internal germinal layer* or *endocyst* derived from the parasite. As the cyst matures, invagination of the germinal layer leads to development of daughter cysts in the periphery (Fig. 59.5). Calcifications may be observed in both viable and nonviable cysts.[6,17,18]

Cysts have an annual growth rate of 1 to 3 cm in diameter. Symptoms are caused by enlarging cysts that lead to abdominal pain (the most common presenting symptom), biliary obstruction, jaundice, and, rarely, portal hypertension. The only typical clinical finding of hepatic hydatid cyst is a palpable hepatic mass. Involvement of the biliary tree is seen in 12% to 80% of cases. Biliary findings may occur either as a result of communication between the pericyst and the biliary ducts or due to rupture of the cyst into the biliary tract. Fistulous communication of the cyst and bile ducts may be associated with secondary bacterial infection of the cyst, cholangitis, or biliary obstruction. Bacterial contamination occurs in 10% to 35% of cases. Occasionally, cysts spontaneously rupture into the peritoneal cavity and cause abdominal pain and anaphylaxis. Multiple intraabdominal cysts may develop as a result of intraperitoneal leakage. Hepatic hydatid cysts may perforate the diaphragm and lead to empyema, pulmonary cysts, biliary-bronchial fistulas, or pericardial collections.[19]

Routine laboratory tests in patients with hydatid cysts may be normal or nonspecifically abnormal (e.g., showing features of obstructive jaundice). Eosinophilia is frequently present. Serologic screening tests (e.g., indirect hemagglutination, latex agglutination, ELISA) based on crude antigens are associated with high rates of false-positive and false-negative results. However, ELISA detection of specific antigens and immune complexes of the cyst is associated with positive results in over 90% of cases. ELISA and RAST (radioallergosorbent test) detect specific IgE antibodies. Antigen 5 (arc-5) and antigen B8 are the parasitic antigens of major diagnostic value. Confirmatory arc-5 immunoelectrophoresis has a reported positive rate of over 90%. Purified fractions enriched in antigens 5 and B8 and glycoproteins from hydatid fluid are reported to have sensitivity and specificity rates of 95% and 100%, respectively.[6,16]

Hydatid cysts have a typical appearance on imaging studies. Furthermore, imaging studies are useful in detecting associated complications. Ultrasound images may show daughter cysts, peripheral calcifications, or the so-called water lily sign of curved bands of delaminated endocyst. On CT scans, hydatid cysts are usually seen as hypoattenuating lesions. Daughter cysts are visualized in approximately 75% of cases and calcifications within the surrounding cyst wall in 50% of cases. MR imaging is the technique that best demonstrates pericyst, matrix or "hydatid sand" (free scoleces), and daughter cysts. The fibrous and calcified pericyst appears as a hypointense ring on both T1- and T2-weighted images. The hydatid matrix is hyperintense on T2-weighted images and hypointense on

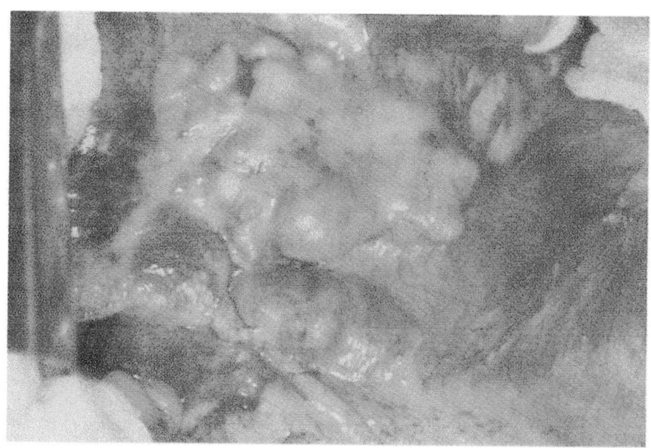

FIGURE 59.6 The external surface of the liver of a patient with echinococcosis before operation. (From Sun T. Parasitic Disorders: *Pathology, diagnosis, and management*, 2nd ed. Baltimore: Lippincott Williams & Wilkins, 1999.)

T1-weighted images. Daughter cysts are hypointense on both T1- and T2-weighted images. ERCP (endoscopic retrograde cholangiopancreatography) is especially useful in cases involving the bile ducts.[6,16]

Open surgical resection is classically the treatment of choice in cases of symptomatic or complicated hepatic cysts (Fig. 59.6). The goal is to remove the cyst intact. Alternative methods have been developed, however. One of them is to aspirate the cyst contents after the operative field has been protected to prevent any potential contamination should spillage of the cyst contents occur. In cases in which the aspirate is clear, ethyl alcohol or 20% sterile saline solution is injected to kill remaining scoleces. The cyst contents and pericystic wall are subsequently removed. In cases in which the aspirate is bilious and a communication with the biliary tree is suspected, the cyst is resected without injecting alcohol to prevent sclerosing cholangitis. Laparoscopic resections have also been reported. A percutaneous technique referred to as PAIR (*p*uncture, *a*spiration, *i*njection, *r*easpiration) simultaneously with albendazole therapy has been employed successfully and found to have several advantages over surgical resection. In this modality, after ultrasound-guided percutaneous puncture and aspiration of the hydatid cyst, 20% sodium chloride solution or 95% ethanol is injected into the cavity and subsequently reaspirated. Therapy with albendazole and/or mebendazole is not usually a curative approach by itself but should precede and follow the resection whenever possible. Recent studies report postoperative morbidity and mortality rates of 3% to 24% and 0% to 4%, respectively. Recurrence rates after surgery or invasive procedures range from 0% to 15% and are usually associated with residual vesicles or spillage of hydatid cyst contents.[16–23]

SCHISTOSOMA

Schistosomiasis constitutes a health risk for inhabitants of endemic regions as well as for visitors to these sites. *Schistosoma mansoni, S. japonicum,* and *S. hematobium* are the species of this trematode fluke that most frequently infect humans. Liver disease, although encountered with all species, is especially severe with *S. mansoni* and *S. japonicum*. Endemic areas where these trematodes are encountered are also frequently associated with a high prevalence of hepatitis B and C. The life cycle of Schistosoma species alternates between sexual reproduction in humans and asexual multiplication in water snails. Cercariae enter the human host by penetrating the skin. An irritating maculopapular rash that lasts for several days is one of the early manifestations. Schistosomes live in the intestinal lumen. Eggs reach the liver via the portal circulation and cause an inflammatory reaction.[17,18,24]

Infection is characterized by the presence of inflammatory granulomata surrounding schistosomal eggs. Acute schistosomiasis is seen most frequently in nonimmune visitors to endemic areas. Occasionally, it can lead to widespread granulomatous necrosis of the liver and even death. In contrast, chronic schistosomiasis is usually asymptomatic until variceal hemorrhage occurs as a result of presinusoidal portal hypertension. These patients exhibit hepatosplenomegaly, no ascites, and relatively normal hepatic synthetic function. Hepatomegaly involves mainly the left lobe. Severe decompensation tends to be observed in cases where schistosomal infections and viral hepatitis coexist. Hepatocellular carcinoma, colon cancer, and follicular lymphoma of the spleen have been reported in association with hepatic schistosomiasis.[6,17,18,25,26]

Active infection is usually diagnosed by the presence of schistosomal eggs in the stool (Kato-Katz smears), epidemiologic data, biochemical, or serologic findings. Laboratory features include eosinophilia, hypoalbuminemia, hypergammaglobulinemia, and elevated serum alkaline phosphatase. Serum transaminase levels are usually normal. ELISA serum antibody tests are highly sensitive but may not correlate with activity of the infection. Histologically, heavy infection can lead to prominent granulomata formation, normal liver architecture, and severe portal fibrosis (Symmers' pipestem fibrosis). In mild infections small white granulomata, each with a schistosomal egg at its center, are observed throughout the liver (Fig. 59.7). The hepatic parenchyma is darker than usual as a result of regurgitated heme-derived pigments from the schistosome gut.[6,17,18,26]

Imaging studies are not useful in the diagnosis of acute infection. Ultrasound examination in chronic *S. mansoni* infection shows echogenic thickening of the wall of the portal vein and its branches, in a bull's-eye pattern. Hypertrophy of the left hepatic lobe, splenomegaly, and engorged venous collaterals are also observed. On noncontrast CT scan the fibrosis around the portal vein branches presents as low-attenuation rings throughout the liver. Administration of intravenous contrast material leads to marked enhancement of the lesions. The periportal bands appear isointense on MR T1-weighted images and hyperintense on T2-weighted images.[6]

The preferred treatment of schistosomiasis is administration of praziquantel. The reported cure efficacy is approximately 90%. Oxamniquine has also been used to treat *S. mansoni*.[17,18]

VIRAL HEPATITIDES

Viral hepatitides represent a principal cause of chronic liver disease, cirrhosis, and hepatocellular carcinoma. Table 59.1 summarizes the characteristics of the five viruses most commonly associated with clinical hepatitis, their modes of transmission, and the consequences of infection. Hepatitis G virus (HGV) does not appear to be injurious to the liver and will not be considered further. Other viral infections can produce acute hepatitis in a fraction of patients (e.g., Epstein-Barr virus, cytomegalovirus [CMV], herpes simplex virus, and varicella virus). In some cases the hepatitis caused by these viruses generally associated with more systemic illness may be severe, and in fact liver involvement may be the dominant component of the infected patient's illness.

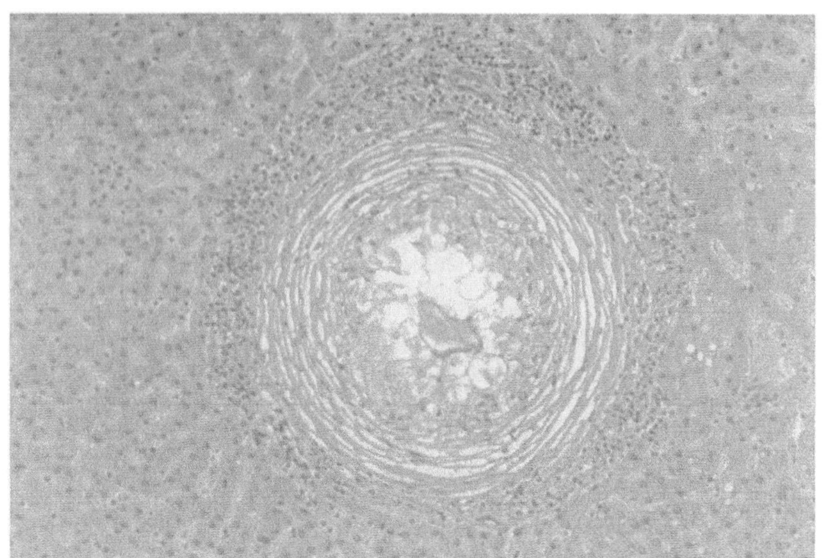

FIGURE 59.7 Hepatic schistosomiasis. A hepatic granuloma surrounds a degenerating egg of *S. mansoni*. (From Rubin E, Farber JL. *Pathology*, 3rd ed. Philadelphia: Lippincott Williams & Wilkins, 1999.)

HEPATITIS A VIRUS (HAV)

HAV (Table 59.1) is a nonenveloped single-stranded RNA virus, 27 nm in diameter and 7.5 kilobases in size that replicates in the cytoplasm of hepatocytes. It belongs to the Picornaviridae family, genus Hepatovirus. Only one serotype is known.[13,27,28]

The major mode of transmission is by fecal-oral spread. Humans are probably the only host for HAV infection, and the only organ injured seems to be the liver. The precise mechanism of injury is not completely understood. HAV infection can produce either icteric or anicteric syndromes. The incubation period is about 28 days. The anicteric prodrome lasts from 2 days to 3 weeks, and the diagnosis of hepatitis may be missed when it does not progress to jaundice. In cases where jaundice becomes manifest, it persists for 1 to 6 weeks. Acholia and choluria may precede the onset of jaundice. HAV infection leads to fulminant liver failure in 0.01% to 0.35% of cases of acute hepatitis A. The risk is higher in people over 40 years of age, IV drug users, homosexual men, habitants of endemic areas, and those with alcoholic, HBV, or HCV liver disease.[13,27,28]

Transaminase values are usually above 1,000 IU/mL. Serum IgM antibodies are detected in 95% of patients and strongly indicate the diagnosis. IgG antibodies become elevated as jaundice subsides and may persist for years (Fig. 59.8).[13,28]

A formalin-inactivated HAV vaccine was found to be safe and to induce an immune response in almost all recipients after two doses. Vaccination as recommended by the Advisory Committee on Immunization Practices of the CDC includes children 2 years of age or older in states or counties with high rates of infection (20 or more cases per 100,000 population from 1987 to 1997) as well as high-risk persons 2 years of age or older. Immune globulin, administered intramuscularly at a dose of 0.02 mL per kilogram of body weight within the first 14 days after exposure, prevents disease in more than 85% of cases. Close contacts of patients with recent onset of the illness, people exposed to contaminated foods, and selected travelers to endemic areas benefit the most.[29]

Most patients with HAV infection recover with simple nursing care and nutritional support. Hygiene should be a top priority to prevent spread of the virus, because fecal shedding of the virus occurs prior to the onset of symptoms and jaundice. Spontaneous survival in cases of acute liver failure may be as high as 40% to 60%. Liver transplantation is indicated in cases in which recovery is unlikely. Recurrence of HAV infection in the allograft may occasionally be encountered. This has led some to recommend administration of immunoglobulin in such instances.[28,30]

HEPATITIS B VIRUS (HBV)

HBV (see Table 59.1) is a DNA virus that belongs to the *hepadnavirus* (hepatotropic DNA virus) family. It is the smallest DNA virus with the ability to infect humans. HBV virions are 40- to 42 nm in diameter, with a double shell and an outer lipoprotein envelope. The viral nucleocapsid, or core, containing a 3.2-kb partially duplex DNA (Fig. 59.9) and a polymerase, lies within the envelope. Replication resembles that of retroviruses, in which viral DNA polymerase acts as a reverse transcriptase. The HBV polymerase lacks proofreading activity. This finding is associated with an estimated frequency of 10^5 to 10^6 mutations per nucleotide per year and the resultant development of mutant forms of the virus.[31–33]

It is estimated that 5 billion people are infected with HBV. Transmission is usually via nonsterile needles, intimate contacts, and blood transfusions. Infection by vertical transmission from mother to child is a serious problem in the developing world. There are no known animal reservoirs or evidence that insects could be involved in transmission of the disease.[31,34]

The hepatitis B virus replicates mainly in hepatocytes but is not itself cytotoxic. Hepatocyte injury seems to be due to the associated immune response. The incubation period in cases of acute infection is approximately 8 weeks. The presence of serum hepatitis B surface antigen (HBsAg) may precede the clinical onset of jaundice (Fig. 59.10). Acute infection is associated with serum HBV DNA, HBV DNA polymerase, hepatitis B early antigen (HBeAg), and liver HBV DNA and HBcAg. HBeAg is a useful marker of viral replication, except in individuals infected with mutant viruses where it may be absent despite active viral replication. In such circumstances, serum HBV DNA is detected by hybridization techniques. Serum anti-HBc IgM becomes detectable with the onset of jaundice. In most individuals, when HBV does not develop into chronic hepatitis, anti-HBc IgM becomes undetectable beyond 6 months. On occasion, however, it may persists for years after the acute infection or may recur as an amnestic phenomenon in reactivating chronic hepatitis B, thus limiting its usefulness as a marker of acute hepatitis B infection.[13,28]

TABLE 59.1

CHARACTERISTICS OF VIRUSES

Virus	Genus	Genome	Genome length (kb)	Mode of transmission	Incubation* (d)		Consequence of infection				Post-transplantation infection	
					Mean	Range	Acute hepatitis	Fulminant hepatic failure	Chronic hepatitis	Hepatoma	Recipient to allograft	New acquisition
Hepatitis A	Picornavirus	RNA	7.5	Fecal–oral Parenteral	28	15–50	Yes	Yes	No	No	No	No
Hepatitis B	Hepadnavirus	DNA	3.2	Parenteral Venereal ? Fecal–oral	84	28–160	Yes	Yes	Yes	Yes	Yes	Yes
Hepatitis C	Flavivirus	RNA	10.2	Parenteral ? Venereal ? Fecal–oral	56	14–160	Yes	Probable	Yes	Yes	Yes	Yes
Hepatitis D	Viroid	RNA	1.67	Parenteral	—	—	Yes	Yes	Yes	No	Yes	Uncertain
Hepatitis E	Probably calicivirus	RNA	7.6	Fecal–oral	40	22–60	Yes	Yes†	No	No	Uncertain	No

*Time from exposure to clinical hepatitis.
†Especially in pregnant women in third trimester.

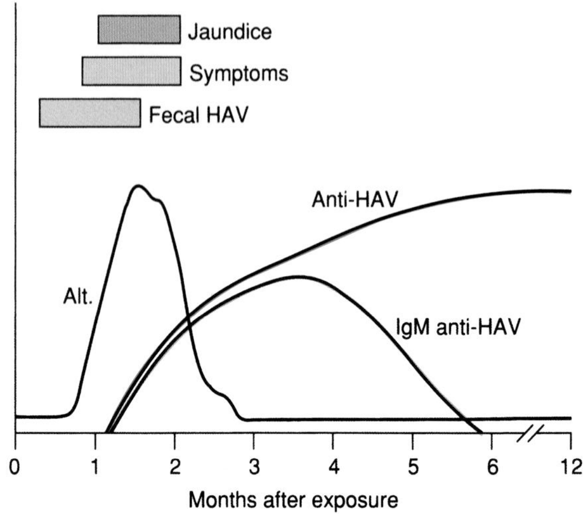

FIGURE 59.8 Clinical course of hepatitis A infection.

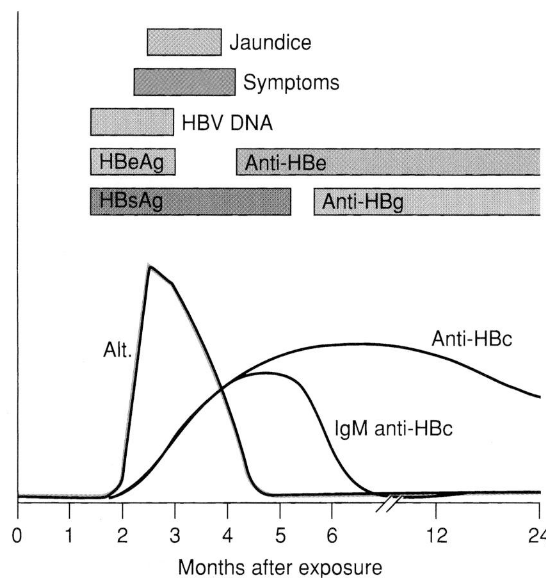

FIGURE 59.10 Clinical course of acute hepatitis B infection.

Although HBV accounts for 30% to 50% of cases of acute liver failure in developing countries, it is estimated that the incidence in the United States is approximately 10%. Hepatitis B becomes fulminant in approximately 1% of acute cases. Women, elderly individuals, HBV carriers, and those who sustain superinfection with another virus (such as HCV) seem to be at greater risk. Furthermore, the risk of acute liver failure is directly proportional to the antibody titers to HBc-Ag and HBs-Ag. Some cases of acute liver failure may be due to reactivation of HBV in patients with chronic infection. In cases of reactivation, reappearance of HBc-IgM Abs aids in the diagnosis. Spontaneous survival after HBV acute liver failure ranges from 15% to 36%.[27,28,35,36]

Most patients with acute HBV infection in the Western world (low carrier rates) recover completely (Fig. 59.11). Approximately 25% of adult cases in the Western world develop clinical jaundice but do not become HBV carriers. They usually retain HBcAb and HBsAb markers with no detectable HBsAg or HBV DNA. Approximately 10% of Western adults with acute HBV infection become chronic carriers, as determined by the presence of HBsAg in serum for more than 6 months. Most HBV carriers have a benign state (Figs. 59.11 and 59.12), with HBV DNA sequences integrating into their native genome. Histologically, these individuals show hepatocytes with ground-glass appearance resulting from cytoplasmic accumulation of HBsAg proteins (Fig. 59.13). Portal triad inflammation may or may not be present. The remainder of HBV carriers develop ongoing liver injury (see Figs. 59.11 and 59.12) usually have detectable HBeAg or HBV DNA and have free episomal HBV sequences in addition to the ones integrated into their native genomes. Histologically, there is evidence of active inflammation.[13]

About 350 million people have chronic HBV infection. In sub-Saharan Africa, most of Asia, and the Pacific, where 8% to 10% of the population is chronically infected, infection usually occurs during childhood. High rates of chronic infection

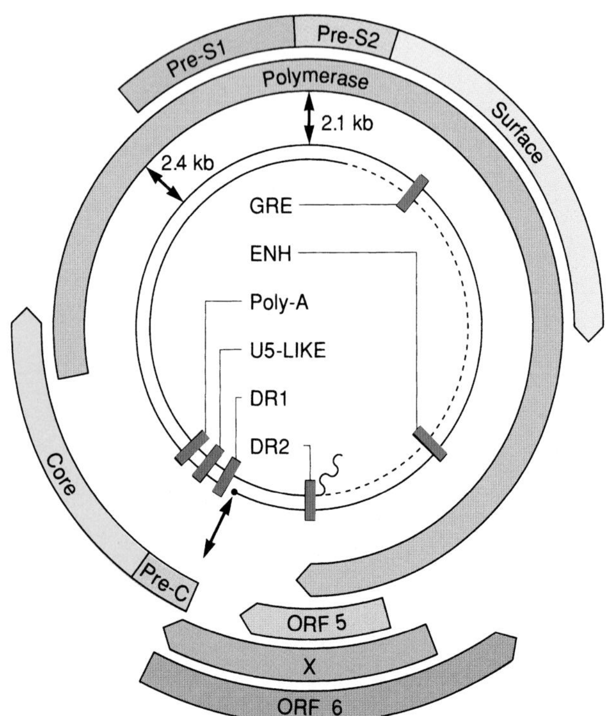

FIGURE 59.9 Hepatitis B viral genome.

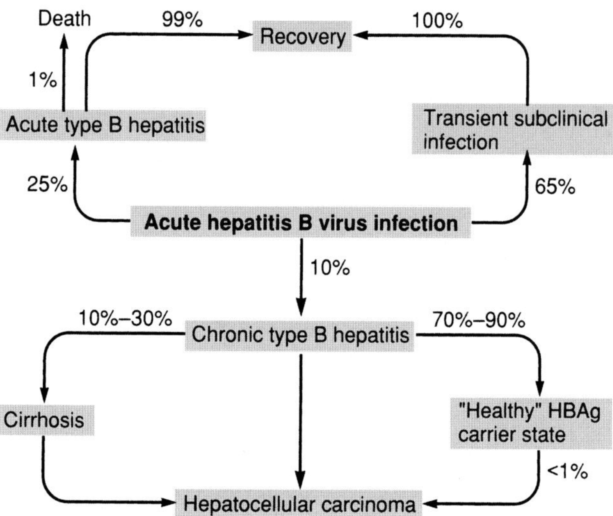

FIGURE 59.11 Common outcomes of acute hepatitis B.

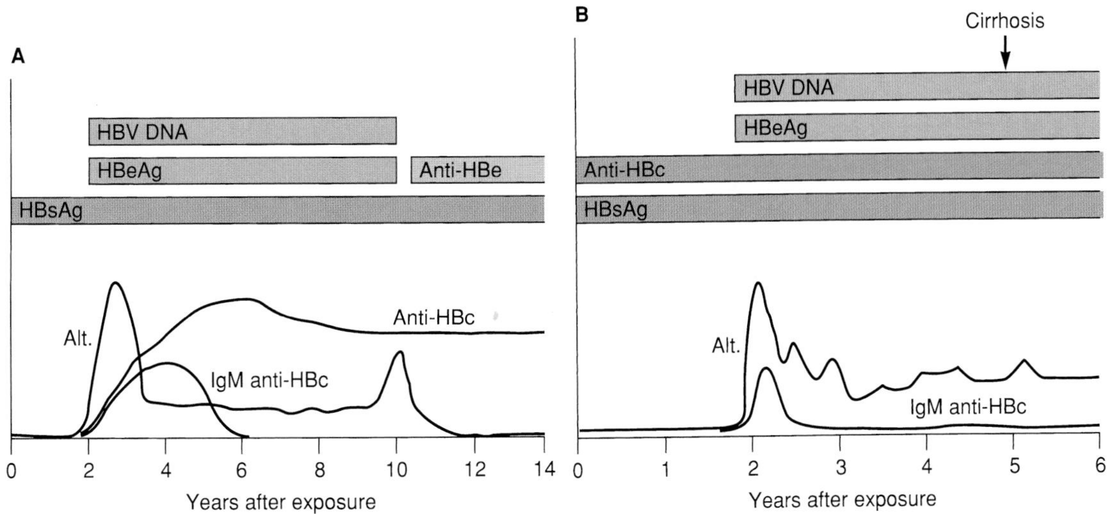

FIGURE 59.12 Clinical course of chronic hepatitis B. (*A*) A benign chronic carrier has continued production of hepatitis B surface antigen but an absence of serum markers of viral replication. (*B*) A pattern of continuing liver injury and serum markers of active viral replication.

are also observed in the Amazon and southern parts of Eastern and Central Europe. The incidence of chronic infection is approximately 5% in the Middle East and the Indian subcontinent. In Western Europe and North America, the overall incidence of chronic infection is less than 1%. It is estimated that there are 1 million deaths each year as a result of cirrhosis and hepatocellular carcinoma associated with chronic hepatitis B. Cirrhosis develops in 10% to 30% of individuals with evidence of active viral replication (Fig. 59.14) within 5 years and is especially high in patients infected early in life, with persistent seropositivity for HBeAg or with increased serum alanine aminotransferase levels after HBeAg seroconversion. Although imperfect, twice a year screening with hepatic ultrasound and/or α-fetoprotein levels is recommended for chronically infected patients.[13,31,32,34,37]

Primary prevention by means of vaccination constitutes the best treatment approach for HBV infection. Individuals at high risk include health-care workers, visitors to highly endemic areas, sexual contacts of chronic carriers or acutely infected people, and household contacts of those at high risk of infection (intravenous drug users, hemophiliacs, patients with thalassemia). The hepatitis B vaccine is given as a series

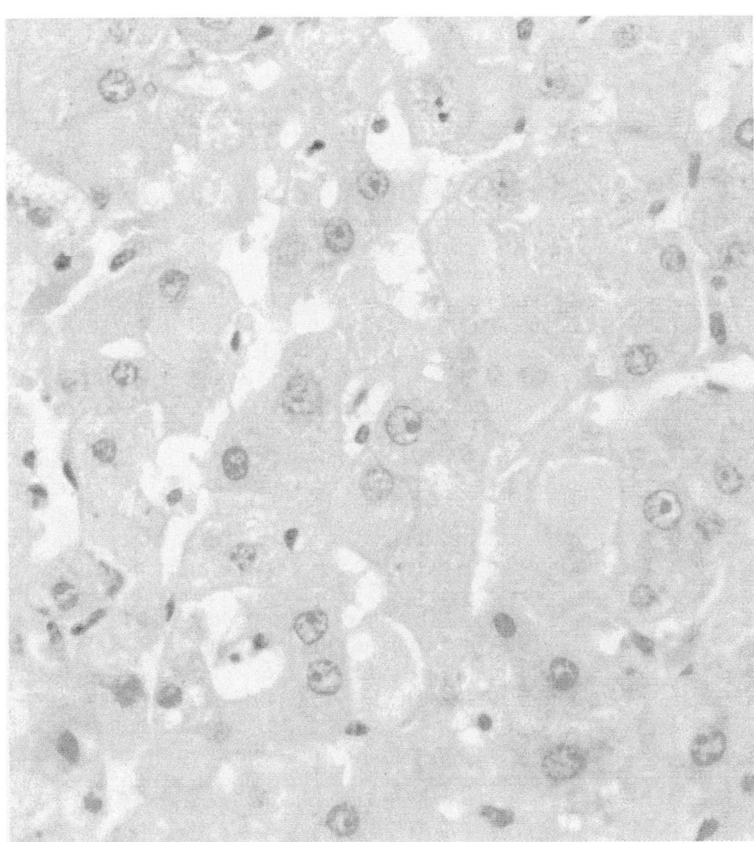

FIGURE 59.13 "Ground-glass" hepatocytes. A photomicrograph of a case of chronic persistent hepatitis B shows scattered hepatocytes with an abundant granular cytoplasm containing HBsAg. (From Rubin E, Farber JL. *Pathology*, 3rd ed. Philadelphia: Lippincott Williams & Wilkins, 1999.)

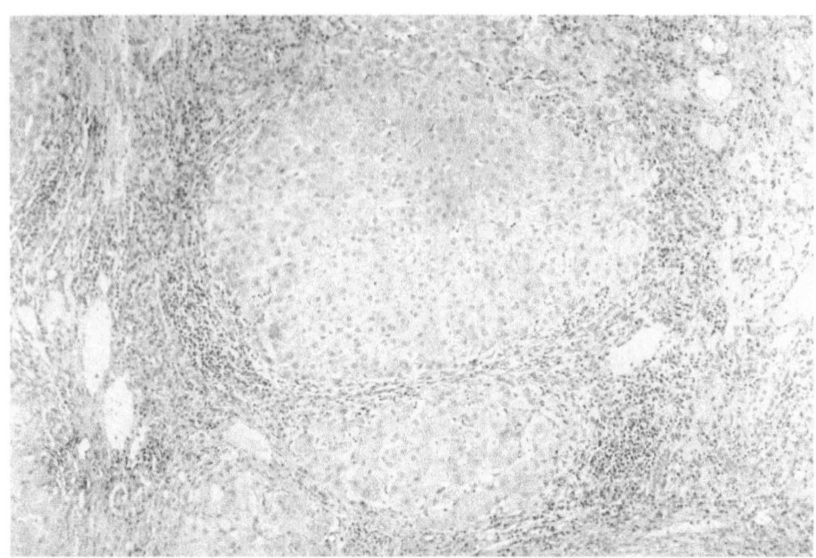

FIGURE 59.14 Chronic hepatitis B with cirrhosis. A photomicrograph of the liver from a patient with long-standing chronic active hepatitis B shows hepatocellular nodules and chronically inflamed fibrous septa. (From Rubin E, Farber JL. *Pathology*, 3rd ed. Philadelphia: Lippincott Williams & Wilkins, 1999.)

of three intramuscular doses and has an almost 100% efficacy among immunocompetent persons with antibody levels of at least 10 mIU per milliliter. Since the World Health Organization in 1991 called for all children to receive the vaccine, 116 countries have adopted it as a routine immunization. Hepatitis B immune globulin has a reported efficacy of 85% to 95% in the prevention of newborn infections and approximately 75% in cases of needle sticks or sexual infections in people exposed to the virus with no previous HBV immunity. It should be administered as soon as possible after exposure (for perinatal cases within 24 hours after birth, for needle-sticks within 7 days, and for sexual exposures within 14 days) together with the first dose of the hepatitis B vaccine series. Additional doses of the vaccine should follow according to the regular schedule. Testing for HBsAg is warranted in pregnant women to reduce the risk of vertical transmission.[13,31,34]

Therapy is usually directed at HBeAg-positive cases that have an increased risk of cirrhosis and hepatocellular carcinoma. It seems that HBeAg-negative patients with viremias of greater than 10^5 molecules per milliliter and liver dysfunction may also benefit from antiviral therapy. At present, antiviral therapy is not offered to asymptomatic HBeAg-negative chronic carriers with viral loads under 10^5 molecules per milliliter and normal alanine aminotransferase values. Therapeutic success in HBeAg-positive cases is determined by seroconversion to HBeAb and reduction of viral loads. Cure of infection as determined by loss of HBsAg and absent viremia by polymerase chain reaction (PCR) analysis in achieved in only 1% to 5% of cases. Patients with chronic hepatitis B and cirrhosis or advanced fibrosis showed a reduction in the incidence of hepatic decompensation and the risk of hepatocellular carcinoma after continuous treatment with lamivudine.[32,37]

Interferon alfa (5 million to 10 million units subcutaneously three times per week, for at least 3 months) used to constitute the main therapy in cases of HBV, achieving a successful response in approximately 30% of cases. However, its multiple side effects (fever, myalgias, bone marrow suppression, and depression, among others) made it difficult to tolerate. Furthermore, the potential for overt liver failure made it a risky treatment in people with advanced liver disease. Lamivudine is an orally effective antiviral agent that competitively inhibits the viral DNA polymerase. Its administration is associated with a more rapid seroconversion to HBeAg-positive status, a more rapid loss of HBeAg, improved aminotransferase levels, and a 3- to 4-log reduction in circulating levels of HBV DNA in the first 3 months of therapy. It is also associated with improved liver histologic findings in cases of chronic hepatitis. Lamivudine tends to be tolerated well. Its major limitation is development of drug resistance. Adefovir is an orally effective nucleotide analogue approved by the Food and Drug Administration (FDA) for the treatment of HBV infection. It has shown promising results by inhibiting replication of lamivudine-resistant HBV mutants.[32,33,38–40]

Liver transplantation is the treatment of choice in patients with hepatic failure. Recurrence of viral infection in the allograft can be as high as 80% in HBeAg-positive cases where no postoperative prophylaxis is administered. The combination of lamivudine and hepatitis B immune globulin posttransplantation reduced the reinfection rate to approximately 10%, and increased the 5-year HBV-free survival rate to approximately 80%.[32]

HEPATITIS C VIRUS (HCV)

HCV (see Table 59.1) is a lipid-enveloped, 9.4 kilobase, single-stranded RNA virus of the family *Flaviviridae*, genus hepacivirus. Six major genotypes and at least 15 subtypes have been identified so far. Over 70% of U.S. cases are due to genotype 1 virus. Worldwide, there are approximately 200 million carriers of the hepatitis C virus. The most commonly identified factors responsible for infection are exposure to blood or blood products and intravenous drug use. Other risk factors include occupational exposure, nosocomial spread, sexual contacts, workplace and household exposures, body piercing, tattooing, cocaine snorting, and vertical transmission. Approximately 30% of patients with HIV infection are also infected with HCV.

The usual incubation period is 5 to 10 weeks. Initial findings after infection include hepatitis characterized by elevated ALT levels (500 to 1,000 IU/mL) and very high HCV RNA titers (Fig. 59.15). Other clinical findings may be minimal or absent. HCV was found to clear spontaneously in 15% to 45% of individuals during primary infection. Hepatitis C infection by itself is only rarely associated with acute liver failure in the United States and Europe. Liver damage is presumably due to immune mechanisms rather than to viral hepatotoxicity. Hepatic injury leads to progressive fibrosis and cirrhosis (Fig. 59.16), in many cases undetected until the appearance of overt liver failure years or decades after the initial

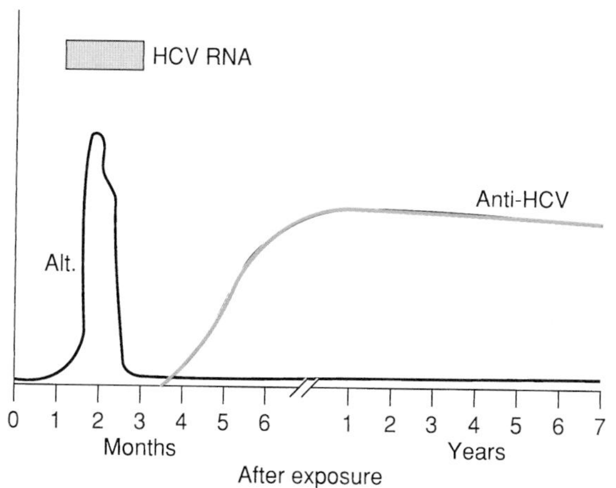

FIGURE 59.15 Clinical course in acute posttransfusion non-A, non-B hepatitis (hepatitis C).

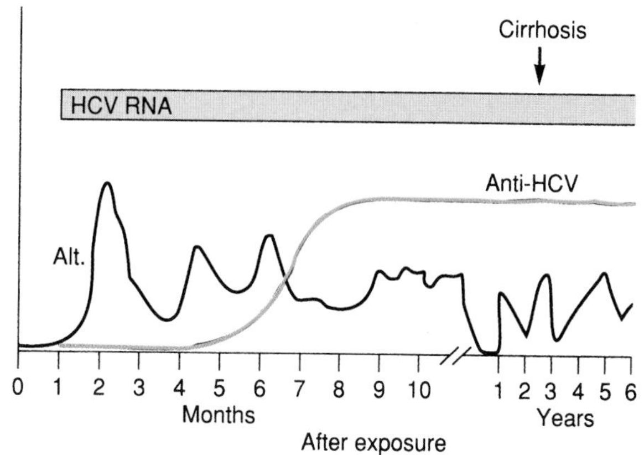

FIGURE 59.17 Clinical course in chronic posttransfusion non-A, non-B hepatitis (hepatitis C).

infection. Chronic infection develops in 55% to 70% of individuals. The 5-year incidence of hepatic decompensation (variceal hemorrhage, ascites, jaundice, encephalopathy) in the setting of cirrhosis is approximately 20%. Hepatitis C cirrhosis is strongly associated with the development of hepatocellular carcinoma. Some have also reported an association with cholangiocarcinomas. The risk of developing a hepatocellular carcinoma in the setting of HCV infection is further increased by the use of alcohol and dramatically increased by coinfection with the hepatitis B virus. Extrahepatic manifestations of hepatitis C include membranoproliferative glomerulonephritis, cryoglobulinemia, porphyria cutanea tarda, lichen planus, vitiligo, and non-Hodgkin's lymphoma.[13,27,28,33,41–52]

The diagnosis of hepatitis C is based on clinical and/or biochemical findings in association with serological demonstration of HCV RNA and/or antibodies. HCV RNA can be detected weeks earlier than antibodies, which are not observed until approximately 18 weeks after the initial illness. Chronic HCV infection tends to be characterized by transaminase levels ranging from normal to 200 to 400 IU/L. Viral replication is usually detectable in serum by PCR amplification (Fig. 59.17). However, quantitative levels of HCV RNA vary and may become transiently undetectable for brief periods of time.[13,27,28,41]

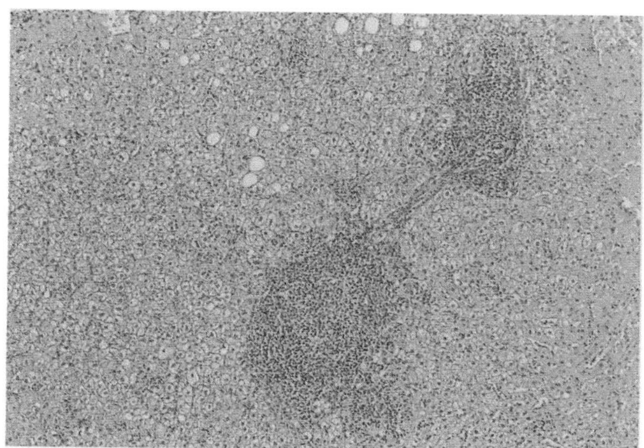

FIGURE 59.16 Chronic hepatitis C. A photomicrograph of the liver from a patient with long-standing hepatitis C exhibits two portal tracts connected by a fibrous bridge containing nodular aggregates of lymphoid cells. (From Rubin E, Farber JL. *Pathology*, 3rd ed. Philadelphia: Lippincott Williams & Wilkins, 1999.)

Therapy is indicated in cases of chronic hepatitis C with elevated serum aminotransferase concentrations, HCV antibodies in serum, and chronic hepatitis on liver biopsy. The current treatment of chronic hepatitis C is with a combination of pegylated interferon alfa and ribavirin. Pegylation of interferon alfa optimizes its pharmacodynamics and pharmacokinetics by providing sustained concentrations after single weekly injections. Its principal mechanism of action seems to be the immune clearance of infected cells. Ribavirin is a synthetic guanosine analogue that prevents relapses during and after therapy in patients who exhibit an initial response. Approximately 20% of patients with genotype 2 or 3 infection and 50% of patients with genotype 1 infection show failure to eradicate the virus. Male sex, race, advanced age, chronic infection, fibrosis, and high body weight are associated with diminished rates of sustained virologic response. Transplantation is the treatment of choice in terminal cases of hepatitis C where hepatic recovery is not expected. Transplantation does not ensure cure, because infection of the allograft is seen in the vast majority of cases.[38,42,51,53]

HEPATITIS D VIRUS (HDV)

The HDV (see Table 59.1), or delta agent, is an incomplete RNA virus that requires the concomitant presence of HBV for viral assembly and propagation. The only enzymatic activity of HDV is a ribozyme that autocleaves the circular RNA and makes it linear. It is estimated that the HDV virus is found in approximately 5% of HBV carriers. Transmission is similar to that of HBV, via parenteral or sexual exposure to blood or body fluids. HDV hepatitis occurs only in HBsAg-positive patients. Acute liver failure is seen with both coinfection (HDV and HBV simultaneously infect the host) (Fig. 59.18) and superinfection (HDV infects a host already infected with HBV) (Fig. 59.19). Superinfection seems to be associated with a higher mortality rate. Chronic HDV and HBV infection may coexist (Fig. 59.20). Cirrhosis is observed in at least two thirds of patients and occurs at a younger age than in patients infected with HBV alone.[13,28,54,55]

Acute infection is diagnosed by the presence of anti-HDV IgM. Anti-HBc IgM distinguishes coinfection from superinfection. The diagnosis in patients with chronic liver disease is made by the presence of HBsAg and antibodies against HDV in the serum and confirmed by the presence of HDV antigen in the liver or HDV RNA in the serum.[28,38]

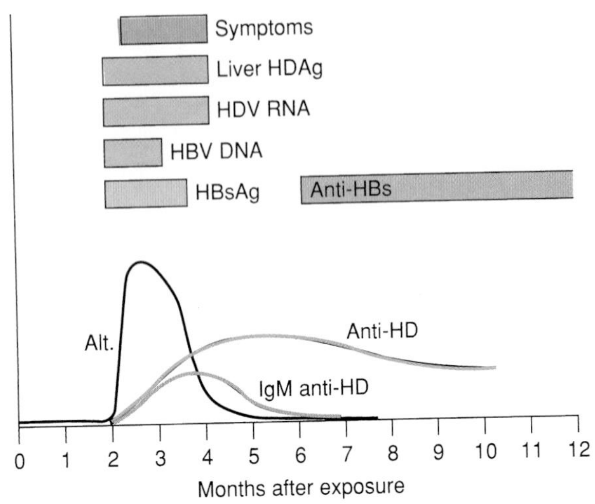

FIGURE 59.18 Synchronous infection with hepatitis B virus and hepatitis D virus.

Treatment and prevention of HDV are associated with that of hepatitis B, with which it always coexists. Vaccination with the hepatitis B vaccine is contributing to the decline in the incidence of HDV. α-Interferon (IFN) is the only currently available treatment for chronic HDV. Response rates correlate directly with dosage, and relapses are frequent after dose reduction. Sustained responses associated with clearance of HBsAg, improvement of liver histologic appearance, and conversion to HBsAb are unusual and relapses common. Treatment is complicated by the side effects of IFN, which include depression, weight loss, myalgias, fatigue, flu-like symptoms, and liver decompensation, among others. Pegylated IFN could be a potentially useful long-term therapy. IFN in combination with ribavirin for chronic cases was not found to be superior to IFN monotherapy. Liver transplantation is the only option in cases of end-stage liver disease. Allograft reinfection rates with long-term administration of hyperimmune serum against HBsAg seem to be lower for HDV than for HBV.[54,55]

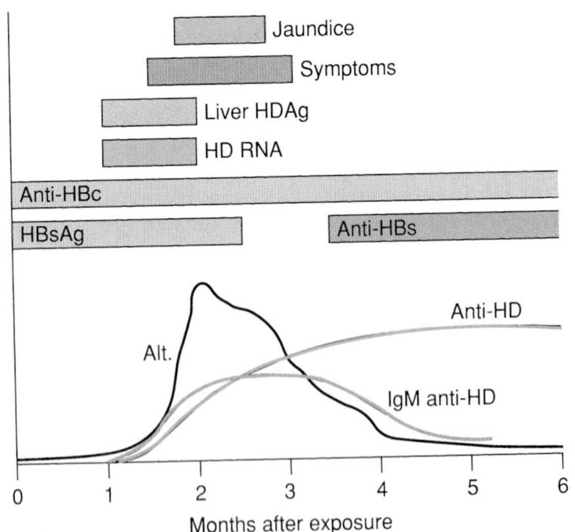

FIGURE 59.19 Superinfection of chronic hepatitis B carrier with hepatitis D.

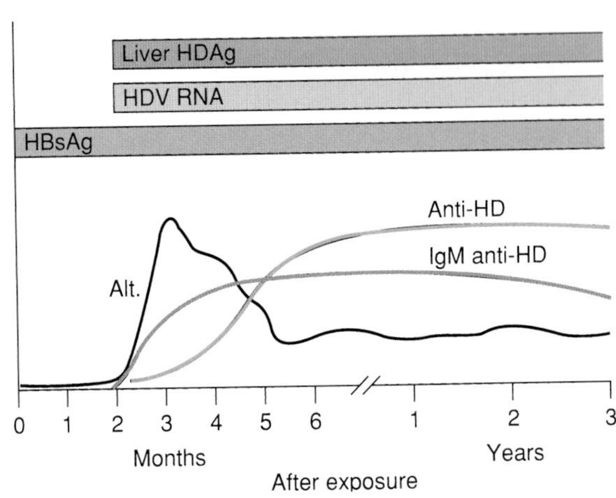

FIGURE 59.20 Clinical course of chronic hepatitis D infection.

HEPATITIS E VIRUS (HEV)

HEV (see Table 59.1) is an RNA virus, probably a calicivirus or similar to the calicivirus, of enteric transmission. Infection has been prominently observed in Asia and in regions of Sudan and Iraq. The incubation period usually lasts 3 to 8 weeks, and most individuals recover without chronic findings after a transient cholestatic jaundice. However, young adults and women in late stages of pregnancy may develop fulminant cases of hepatitis E. Mortality from HEV is 0.5% to 4% in the general population but up to 20% in pregnant women. Diagnosis is aided by amplification of serum and fecal viral genomes during the acute phase. The presence of anti-HEV IgM or follow up demonstration of IgG may be required. There is currently no specific treatment for HEV infection, and a vaccine has just undergone clinical trials. Improving sanitation and purifying or boiling water can reduce the incidence of this disease.[27,28,34,56]

CYTOMEGALOVIRUS

Cytomegalovirus (CMV) is a member of the β Herpesviridae family. It is usually associated with mild hepatitis but may occasionally cause acute liver failure. Transmission can be intrauterine, perinatal or postnatal, via infected fluids such as blood, or through transplanted organs. Infection is life-long and can be detected in up to 70% of individuals in U.S. urban cities. Organ injury can occur as a result of primary infection or reactivation of a latent infection. In the neonatal period, congenital infection is usually generalized and frequently fatal. In immunocompetent adults, liver dysfunction tends to be found in association with CMV mononucleosis. In immunosuppressed adults, infection leads to liver dysfunction with jaundice and at times liver failure. Acalculous gangrenous cholecystitis may also be encountered.[28,57,58]

Shell vial assay is the most sensitive and rapid method to detect infection. PCR assays increase the sensitivity. Detection of IgG is helpful in primary infection. Liver biopsy is of importance to establish the diagnosis of hepatitis. Microscopic examination shows inflammation and injury ranging from fatty changes to necrosis to fibrosis. Giant multinucleated cells and large nuclear inclusions can be encountered in hepatocytes and bile duct epithelial cells.[28,57,58]

Currently approved drugs for the treatment of CMV include ganciclovir, valacyclovir, valganciclovir, foscarnet, cidofovir, and fomivirsen.[39]

EPSTEIN-BARR VIRUS

Epstein-Barr virus (EBV) is a DNA virus and member of the *Herpesviridae* family. Infection persists for life and is usually transmitted in the course of close personal or intimate contact via oral secretions. Some degree of liver involvement is encountered in almost all cases of EBV mononucleosis. It is usually mild, with no major clinical manifestations, and resolves spontaneously. The presence of jaundice may reflect either more severe hepatitis or an associated hemolytic anemia. Occasional cases of fatal acute liver failure have been reported in both immunocompromised and immunocompetent patients. Leukocytosis is usually present, with lymphocytosis and monocytosis. The monospot test is sensitive but not specific. Diagnosis is by detection of nucleic acids with *in situ* hybridization, Southern blot analysis, and PCR of involved organ biopsies. Detection of IgG and IgM antibodies improves sensitivity and specificity. No antiviral agent has so far proved effective in EBV hepatitis. Liver transplantation has been reported in life-threatening situations.[39,57,59–60]

HERPES SIMPLEX VIRUS

The prevalence of antibodies to herpes simplex virus 1 (HSV-1) and to herpes simplex virus 2 (HSV-2) in the populations of industrialized nations is 50% and 20%, respectively. Liver involvement may be seen in neonates and immunocompromised, malnourished, and pregnant adults and is usually associated with multiorgan involvement. The course is usually fulminant, with a high mortality rate. Liver biopsy is of prime importance to establish the diagnosis, especially in pregnant women. Microscopic examination shows diffuse eosinophilic intranuclear inclusion bodies, multinucleated cells, widespread necrosis, and slight inflammation. Cowdry A type intranuclear inclusions are typical. Confirmation is by means of HSV DNA detection by PCR. Approved antivirals include acyclovir, famciclovir, and valaciclovir. Treatment should be started prior to confirmation of the etiology, because otherwise progression of the disease is extremely rapid and lethal. Liver transplantation can be considered even in selected cases of disseminated disease.[39,57,58]

VARICELLA ZOSTER VIRUS (VZV)

Herpesvirus varicellae is usually associated with mild hepatitis but may occasionally cause acute liver failure. Up to one fourth of children with varicella (chickenpox) may exhibit temporary mild biochemical liver abnormalities. Reye's syndrome may be encountered during the convalescence period, especially in those who receive aspirin. In such cases, mortality can be as high as 30%. Fulminant fatal hepatic failure can also be encountered in adults. Immunocompromised patients are at especially high risk. Confirmation of the diagnosis can be achieved by isolation of the virus from involved tissues. Any exposure to the virus in immunocompromised patients should be treated with antiviral therapy while awaiting diagnostic confirmation. Current therapies for VZV infection in immunocompetent and immunocompromised hosts include acyclovir, valacyclovir, penciclovir, and famciclovir. CDC guidelines should be followed for infection control.[28,39,57]

ACUTE LIVER FAILURE

Definition

Acute hepatic injury refers to a sudden loss of hepatocyte mass, most usually caused by a toxin, ischemia, or an inflammatory reaction in the liver. Acute liver failure (ALF) is manifested by a sudden increase in previously normal levels of liver transaminases. Typically, the serum level of ALT is more than 10 to 25 times the upper limits of the normal range. Fulminant liver failure is a term used to encompass various types of liver failure characterized by the presence of encephalopathy within 8 weeks of the onset of symptoms in previously healthy subjects or in subjects with previously compensated subclinical conditions. Identifying the etiology of ALF is not only of prognostic value but also may be vital for timely treatment. Worldwide, HBV infection is responsible for the majority of ALF cases. In Western nations, 30% to 40% of ALF cases have no identified etiology. In the United States and the U.K., acetaminophen toxicity is the most frequent cause of ALF, followed by other drug toxicities and cryptogenic causes. Submassive hepatic necrosis is similar to fulminant hepatic failure except that it is slower in onset. Submassive hepatic necrosis (also known as subfulminant hepatic failure and subacute hepatic failure) is defined as the development of acute hepatic encephalopathy within 9 to 24 weeks after the onset of symptomatic hepatocellular disease in a previously healthy person.[13,28,44]

Clinical Features

Acute hepatic injury in the absence of hepatic encephalopathy always resolves, except when it is caused by another ongoing systemic disease or when the elevated transaminase levels represent the first manifestation of previously covert chronic liver disease. The incidence of acute hepatic injury is unknown. It is estimated that 2,000 cases of fulminant hepatic failure and submassive hepatic necrosis occur in the United States annually and that 80% of these patients die. Outcome is determined by the course of encephalopathy, which is classified according to four grades (Table 59.2). In general, the deeper the coma, the worse will be the outcome. For example, patients in whom a grade III or IV coma develops have a higher mortality rate than patients with hepatic failure in whom encephalopathy never progresses beyond grade II. Paradoxically, the rapid onset of encephalopathy is a *favorable* prognostic sign. Consequently, most patients with acetaminophen-induced fulminant hepatic failure who experience grade III coma recover spontaneously. Delay in the onset of encephalopathy after the onset of jaundice indicates a lack of spontaneous recovery and is an unfavorable prognostic factor. For this reason, submassive hepatic necrosis has a particularly poor outcome. Cerebral edema, leading to increased intracranial pressure, is a common feature of severe fulminant hepatic failure and may cause permanent cerebral injury and death. Fulminant hepatic failure and submassive hepatic necrosis are always accompanied by severe coagulopathy.[13]

Causes of fulminant hepatic failure are listed in Table 59.3. Wilson's disease is usually included among the causes of fulminant hepatic failure despite the fact that it is a covert chronic disorder. A history of heavy alcohol use also suggests chronic injury, even though alcoholics are at particular risk for acetaminophen-induced hepatic failure. A characteristic clinical scenario is the development of hepatic failure when an alcohol abuser stops drinking and 24 to 48 hours later has abdominal pain from gastritis or pancreatitis or headache from a hangover. This person then takes a standard dose of acetaminophen to soothe the symptoms and unwittingly produces acute hepatic injury. When presented with an apparent case of acute hepatic injury, the physician must always answer two questions: Is this really an acute illness or rather the first presentation of a previously unrecognized chronic disorder? Are single or multiple factors contributing to the acute hepatic injury?[13]

TABLE 59.2 CLASSIFICATION

CLINICAL GRADES OF ACUTE HEPATIC ENCEPHALOPATHY

Grade	Mental state	Asterixus	Electroencephalogram result
I	Altered affect, subtle loss of mental acuity, slurred speech	Slight or none	Normal
II	Accentuation of stage I, confusion, drowsiness, inappropriate behavior, loss of sphincter control	Easily elicited	Abnormal, generalized slowing
III	Sleepy but rousable, marked confusion, can answer simple questions only	Present when patient can cooperate	Always abnormal
IV	Coma IVa—responds to pain IVb—no response to pain	Cannot cooperate	Always abnormal

Management and Treatment

Patients with hepatic failure who have ingested acetaminophen should receive a full course of *N*-acetylcysteine. Unconfirmed evidence suggests that *N*-acetylcysteine may be beneficial even in hepatic failure that is unrelated to acetaminophen.[13]

TABLE 59.3 ETIOLOGY

CAUSES OF FULMINANT HEPATIC FAILURE

VIRAL INFECTION
Hepatitis A
Hepatitis B
Hepatitis D
Other viruses (less common)
- Cytomegalovirus
- Epstein-Barr virus
- Varicella virus
- Herpesvirus

POISONS, CHEMICALS, AND DRUGS
Amanita phalloides
Acetaminophen
Tetracycline
Phosphorus
Halogenated volatile anesthetics (especially halothane)
Isoniazid
Methyldopa
Valproate
Monoamine oxidase inhibitors

ISCHEMIA AND HYPOXIA
Hepatic vascular occlusion
Acute circulatory stroke
Heat stroke
Gram-negative sepsis

MISCELLANEOUS
Acute fatty liver of pregnancy
Reye's syndrome
Wilson's disease
Hodgkin's disease and other lymphomas
Hereditary fructose intolerance
Galactosemia, tyrosinemia
Idiopathic (also called non-A non-B)

Liver biopsies are especially useful to identify the extent of hepatic injury as well as to identify unexpected etiologies where treatments may differ, such as in the case of hepatic lymphomas. Transjugular biopsies are probably the safest approach. Most viral infections lead to a disseminated panlobular injury similar to that seen with drug-induced idiosyncratic reactions. There is usually little portal tract inflammation.[27,28]

Before the advent of liver transplantation, ALF had a mortality rate of 40% to 95%. Cases of hyperacute liver failure have a spontaneous survival rate of approximately 35%. Cryptogenic cases, frequently associated with subacute findings, have reported survival rates of approximately 15%. In a recent series, 34% of patients with ALF died without liver transplantation, 25% survived with medical treatment, and 41% underwent transplantation. Death is usually associated with cerebral edema and sepsis. There have been many attempts to propose treatment guidelines and predict mortality. The King's College criteria (Table 59.4) predict the need for liver transplantation in cases of acetaminophen-induced and non–acetaminophen-induced fulminant hepatic failure. The Clichy criteria apply specifically to patients with viral hepatitis. According to the Clichy criteria, factor V levels less than 20% in patients under age 30 or factor V levels less than 30% in patients over 30 years of age, in the setting of stage 3 or 4 hepatic encephalopathy, are associated with a mortality of 90% or higher and are indicative for liver transplantation whenever possible. Lee observed that unbound serum Gc protein (≥ 34 μg/mL) was predictive of survival. Necrosis of greater than 70% of liver parenchyma on biopsy specimens was found to be of prognostic value in some studies. Other publications have identified α-fetoprotein as a marker of liver regeneration and correlate its levels with spontaneous recovery.[13,27,28,35,44,61–66]

Patients with any sign of compromise or instability should be admitted to an intensive care unit of a transplant center for close monitoring and potential transplantation. Clinical deterioration in cases of ALF can be very rapid. Rapid assessment and diagnosis are essential, given the wide variation in treatments associated with specific etiologies and the potential contraindication to transplantation as is seen in cases of malignancies. Medical management of patients with ALF requires a multidisciplinary dynamic approach to maintain the best homeostasis possible. Based on a thorough medical history and physical examination, a preliminary determination regarding the candidate's suitability for liver transplantation is made. Given the uncertainties of waiting time and the competition for transplantable organs it has proved prudent to place patients with ALF on the national organ transplant waiting list *before* a comprehensive assessment is complete. However, it should be emphasized that the *final* decision to actually perform a transplant is not made until a suitable organ from a

TABLE 59.4

PROGNOSTIC CRITERIA FOR PREDICTING REQUIRED LIVER TRANSPLANTATION IN PATIENTS WITH FULMINANT HEPATIC FAILURE

Cause of liver failure	Criteria
Acetaminophen toxicity	pH <7.3 (irrespective of grade of encephalopathy) or Prothrombin time >50 s and serum creatinine >3.4 mg/dL (300 μmol/L) in patients with grade III or IV encephalopathy
All other causes	Prothrombin time >50 s (irrespective of grade of encephalopathy) or Any three of the following variables (irrespective of grade of encephalopathy): Age <10 y or >40 y Liver failure from halothane or other drug idiosyncrasy or idiopathic hepatitis Duration of jaundice before encephalopathy >7 d Prothrombin time >25 s Serum bilirubin >17.5 mg/dL (300 mmol/L)

Adapted from O'Grady JG, Alexander GJM, Hayllar KM, et al. Early indicators of prognosis in fulminant hepatic failure. *Gastroenterology* 1989;97:439.

deceased (or live) donor becomes available. At this time there should be sufficient data for the transplant team to determine whether the risk/benefit ratio favors transplantation or nontransplant therapy. The hyperdynamic state typical of ALF can lead to hypoperfusion, diminished oxygenation, and eventually terminal cardiovascular collapse. Maintaining homeostasis under these adverse conditions requires careful management of all organ systems, including but not limited to fluids, electrolytes, acid–base status, cardiac rhythm, blood pressure, pulmonary status, infections, renal function, and neurological status. Acid–base status should be monitored frequently. During the initial stages, patients tend to present with respiratory alkalosis. As liver failure evolves, metabolic acidosis with elevated lactate and an increased anion gap emerge. Fluid and electrolyte management requires special attention. Hyponatremia, hypocalcemia, and hypomagnesemia are frequently encountered. Hypophosphatemia may be encountered in the early stages. Hyperphosphatemia develops in the presence of renal failure.[28,67]

Fresh frozen plasma (FFP) is classically administered in an attempt to correct the coagulopathy that occurs frequently in patients with ALF, especially in the setting of overt bleeding or impending invasive procedures. Plasmapheresis and vitamin K have also been used as corrective measures. However, in the absence of hemorrhage little data suggest that prophylactic administration of FFP or platelets is beneficial. In fact, the salt load associated with FFP administration may potentiate cerebral edema.

Pulmonary complications in the setting of ALF range from atelectasis to florid ARDS. Intubation and ventilation should be instituted to prevent ventilatory compromise, for airway protection, or to address intracranial hypertension. As the encephalopathy progresses, it may be difficult to determine whether the patient has lost his or her ability to protect the airway. There should be a low threshold for semielective intubation, which certainly should be considered in patients with grade III or IV encephalopathy.

Infectious complications constitute an ever-present potential catastrophe in ALF. Prevention and monitoring are vital steps in the care of these patients. Infections have been demonstrated in up to 80% of cases. The most frequent type was pneumonia, followed by bacteremia and urinary infections. Fungal infections were reported in up to slightly over 30% of cases and are also an important contributor to mortality. Surveillance cultures should be obtained. Administration of prophylactic antibiotics is probably of value.[28,68]

Factors that cause or could potentially cause renal insufficiency should be evaluated and avoided whenever possible. In the setting of renal insufficiency, continuous hemofiltration is preferred over hemodialysis because of the less pronounced blood pressure and fluid shifts. Variceal bleeding is unusual in ALF, except in venoocclusive diseases. Gastrointestinal bleeding tends to be associated with stress ulcers and gastric erosions. Maintaining the gastric pH above 4 to 5 is recommended. The value of nutritional support in ALF has not been carefully evaluated. It has been recommended that nutritional support may aid in the catabolic state associated with ALF. Encephalopathy and intracranial hypertension are classic findings of ALF and can lead to life-threatening complications. The effectiveness of lactulose in acute hepatic encephalopathy has been questioned, especially in the face of its potential detrimental side effects. Agitation may require pharmacologic sedation, although the reduced metabolism of the sedative drugs must be considered in dosing. No current effective therapy is available for prophylaxis of cerebral edema. Periodic electroencephalograms in comatose patients should be performed to rule out clinically inapparent seizure. Imaging studies such as CT or MRI should be performed as a baseline assessment and when there are significant changes in the neurologic examination. In experienced hands, placement of an extradural intracranial pressure monitoring device and assessment of cerebral perfusion pressure (CPP) may be helpful in management as well as the ultimate decision to proceed with liver transplantation. Prolonged periods of low CPP portend a dismal prognosis even with liver transplantation because irreversible brain damage or brain death may already be present.[28]

Liver transplantation remains the only effective therapy in cases of ALF without spontaneous recovery. The timing for liver transplantation is crucial. However, the decision concerning when to proceed with liver replacement is a very difficult one. As previously mentioned under the medical management section, several guidelines have been considered to predict outcome in ALF. They include the King's College criteria, the Clichy criteria, APACHE scores, liver biopsies, and unbound serum Gc protein levels, among others. Survival after liver transplantation has been reported to be approximately 65% and seems to be similar in the adult and pediatric populations. Outcome is associated, at least in part, with etiology of ALF, renal function, degree of encephalopathy, and quality of the allograft. Survival after liver transplantation for ALF is lower than that expected for chronic lever diseases. Both deceased and live donor liver transplantation have been employed in ALF. Auxiliary heterotopic liver transplantation, auxiliary partial orthotopic liver transplantation, and isolated hepatocyte transplantation have all been used with varying success. Bioartificial liver devices of various types have shown promising results as bridging therapies from the time of acute liver failure to either liver transplantation or liver regeneration. Further assessment of their safety and efficacy with controlled clinical trials is currently under way.[28,69–74]

KEY POINTS

- During the past several decades, the route of infection for pyogenic liver abscesses has changed from portal bacteremia due to intraabdominal infection to a biliary etiology.
- Gram-negative anaerobes account for two thirds of the cases of pyogenic liver abscesses with anaerobes isolated in 30% of cases.
- First-line treatment of hepatic amebic abscesses is oral metronidazole with percutaneous drainage considered with poor response to therapy or when superinfection is suspected.
- The treatment of choice for hydatid cysts is surgical resection of the intact cyst, often preceded by injection of ethyl chloride, 95% ethanol, or 20% sterile saline solution.
- Viral hepatitis, especially hepatitis B and C, represents a principal cause of chronic liver disease, cirrhosis, and hepatocellular carcinoma.
- Liver transplantation is the treatment of choice for patients with liver failure resulting from hepatitis, although recurrence of viral infection in the allograft can be as high as 80% in HBeAg-positive patients.
- Chronic infection develops in 55% to 70% of patient with hepatitis C, with a significant risk of development of both hepatic decompensation and hepatocellular carcinoma.
- Worldwide hepatitis B infection is the leading cause of acute liver failure, although in Western nations acetaminophen toxicity is the most frequent cause, followed by other drug toxicity and cryptogenic causes.
- Outcome for acute fulminant hepatic failure is determined by the course of encephalopathy with the deeper the coma, the worse will be the outcome.
- In recent series, 34% of patients with acute liver failure die without liver transplant, usually secondary to cerebral edema and sepsis, with 25% of patients surviving with medical treatment and 41% undergoing transplantation.

References

1. **Webb TH, Lillemoe KD, Pitt HA. Liver abscess. *Hosp Phys.* 1989:46–59.**
2. Rahimian J, Wilson T, Oram V, et al. Pyogenic liver abscess: recent trends in etiology and mortality. *Clin Infect Dis.* 2004;39:1654–1659. Epub 2004 Nov 9.
3. Yang DM, Kim HN, Kang JH, et al. Complications of pyogenic hepatic abscess: computed tomography and clinical features. *J Comput Assist Tomogr.* 2004;28:311–317.
4. Kaplan GG, Gregson DB, Laupland KB. Population-based study of the epidemiology of and the risk factors for pyogenic liver abscess. *Clin Gastroenterol Hepatol.* 2004;2:1032–1038.
5. Hanbidge AE, Buckler PM, O'Malley ME, et al. From the RSNA refresher courses: imaging evaluation for acute pain in the right upper quadrant. *Radiographics* 2004;24:1117–1135.
6. **Mortele KJ, Segatto E, Ros PR. The infected liver: radiologic-pathologic correlation. *Radiographics* 2004;24:937–955.**
7. Zibari GB, Maguire S, Aultman DF, et al. Pyogenic liver abscess. *Surg Infect (Larchmt).* 2000;1:15–21.
8. Lipsett PA, Huang CJ, Lillemoe KD, et al. Fungal hepatic abscesses: characterization and management. *J Gastrointest Surg.* 1997;1:78–84
9. Sharara AI, Rockey DC. Pyogenic liver abscess. *Curr Treat Options Gastroenterol.* 2002;5:437–442.
10. Tan YM, Chung AY, Chow PK, et al. An appraisal of surgical and percutaneous drainage for pyogenic liver abscesses larger than 5 cm. *Ann Surg.* 2005;241:485–490.
11. Yang CC, Yen CH, Ho MW, et al. Comparison of pyogenic liver abscess caused by non-Klebsiella pneumoniae and Klebsiella pneumoniae. *J Microbiol Immunol Infect.* 2004;37:176–184.
12. **Wells CD, Arguedas M. Amebic liver abscess. *South Med J.* 2004;97:673–682.**
13. Lucey MR. Hepatic infection and acute hepatic failure. In LJ Greenfield, MW Mulholland, KT Oldham, et al, eds. *Surgery: scientific principles and practice*, 3rd ed. Philadelphia: Lippincott Williams & Wilkins, 2001.
14. Lodhi S, Sarwari AR, Muzammil M, et al. Features distinguishing amoebic from pyogenic liver abscess: a review of 577 adult cases. *Trop Med Int Health* 2004;9:718–723.
15. Ahsan T, Jehangir MU, Mahmood T, et al. Amoebic versus pyogenic liver abscess. *J Pak Med Assoc.* 2002;52:497–501.
16. Sayek I, Tirnaksiz MB, Dogan R. Cystic hydatid disease: current trends in diagnosis and management. *Surg Today* 2004;34:987–996.
17. DiazGranados CA, Duffus WA, Albrecht H. Parasitic diseases of the liver. In D Zakim and TD Boyer, eds. *Hepatology. A textbook of liver disease*, 4th ed. Philadelphia: WB Saunders, 2003, pp. 1073–1107.
18. Dunn MA. Parasitic diseases. In: ER Shiff, MF Sorrell, Willis C. Maddrey, eds. *Schiff's diseases of the liver,* 8th ed.. Philadelphia: Lippincott Williams & Wilkins, 1999, pp. 1533–1548.
19. Kjossev KT, Losanoff JE. Classification of hydatid liver cysts. *J Gastroenterol Hepatol.* 2005;20:352–359.
20. Bastid C, Ayela P, Sahel J. Percutaneous treatment of a complex hydatid cyst of the liver under sonographic control. Report of the first case. *Gastroenterol Clin Biol.* 2005;29:191–192.
21. Chautems R, Buhler LH, Gold B, et al. Surgical management and long-term outcome of complicated liver hydatid cysts caused by *Echinococcus granulosus. Surgery* 2005r;137:312–316.
22. Gollackner B, Längle F, Auer H, et al. Radical surgical therapy of abdominal cystic hydatid disease: factors of recurrence. *World J Surg* 2000;24:717–721
23. Smego RA Jr, Sebanego P. Treatment options for hepatic cystic echinococcosis. *Int J Infect Dis.* 2005;9:69–76.
24. Godyn JJ, Siderits R, Hazra A. Schistosoma mansoni in colon and liver. *Arch Pathol Lab Med.* 2005;129:544–545.
25. Qiu DC, Hubbard AE, Zhong B, et al. A matched, case-control study of the association between *Schistosoma japonicum* and liver and colon cancers, in rural China. *Ann Trop Med Parasitol.* 2005;99:47–52.
26. El-Zayadi AR. Curse of schistosomiasis on Egyptian liver. *World J Gastroenterol.* 2004;10:1079–1081.
27. Lee WM, Shiodt FV. Fulminant hepatic failure. In: ER Shiff, MF Sorrell, and Willis C. Maddrey, eds. *Schiff's diseases of the liver,* 8th ed. Philadelphia: Lippincott Williams & Wilkins, 1999, pp. 879–893.
28. Sanyal AJ, Stravitz RT. Acute liver failure. In D Zakim and TD Boyer, eds. *Hepatology. A textbook of liver disease*, 4th ed. Philadelphia: WB Saunders, 2003, pp. 445–496.
29. Craig AS, Schaffner W. Prevention of hepatitis A with the hepatitis A vaccine. *N Engl J Med.* 2004;350:476–481.
30. Gane E, Sallie R, Saleh M, et al. Clinical recurrence of hepatitis A following liver transplantation for acute liver failure. *J Med Virol.* 1995;45:35–39.
31. Poland GA, Jacobson RM. Clinical practice: prevention of hepatitis B with the hepatitis B vaccine. *N Engl J Med.* 2004;351:2832–2838.
32. **Ganem D, Prince AM. Hepatitis B virus infection–natural history and clinical consequences. *N Engl J Med.* 2004;350:1118–1129.**
33. Wands JR. Prevention of hepatocellular carcinoma. *N Engl J Med.* 2004;351:1567–1570.
34. http://www.who.int/mediacentre/factsheets/fs204/en/
35. Schiodt FV, Atillasoy E, Shakil AO, et al. Etiology and outcome for 295 patients with acute liver failure in the United States. *Liver Transpl Surg.* 1999;5:29–34.
36. Lee WM. Hepatitis B virus infection. *N Engl J Med.* 1997;337:1733–1745.
37. Liaw YF, Sung JJ, Chow WC, et al., for the Cirrhosis Asian Lamivudine Multicentre Study Group. Lamivudine for patients with chronic hepatitis B and advanced liver disease. *N Engl J Med.* 2004 Oct 7;351:1521–1531.
38. **Hoofnagle JH, di Bisceglie AM. The treatment of chronic viral hepatitis. *N Engl J Med.* 1997;336:347–356.**
39. Hewlett G, Hallenberger S, Rubsamen-Waigmann H. Antivirals against DNA viruses (hepatitis B and the herpes viruses). *Curr Opin Pharmacol.* 2004;4:453–464.
40. Marcellin P, Lau GK, Bonino F, et al., for the Peginterferon Alfa-2a HBeAg-Negative Chronic Hepatitis B Study Group. Peginterferon alfa-2a alone, lamivudine alone, and the two in combination in patients with HBeAg-negative chronic hepatitis B. *N Engl J Med.* 2004;351:1206–1217.
41. Hoofnagle JH and Heller T. Hepatitis C. In D Zakim and TD Boyer, eds. *Hepatology. A textbook of liver disease,* 4th dd. Philadelphia: WB Saunders, 2003, pp. 1017–1062.
42. Pawlotsky JM. Treating hepatitis C in "difficult-to-treat" patients. *N Engl J Med.* 2004;351:422–423.
43. Piasecki BA, Lewis JD, Reddy KR, et al. Influence of alcohol use, race, and viral coinfections on spontaneous HCV clearance in a US veteran population. *Hepatology* 2004;40:892–899.
44. **Lee WM. Acute liver failure. N Engl J Med. 1993;329:1862–1872. Erratum in: *N Engl J Med.* 1994;330:584.**
45. Kuwada SK, Patel VM, Hollinger FB, et al. Non-A, non-B fulminant hepatitis is also non-E and non-C. *Am J Gastroenterol.* 1994;89:57–61.
46. Puoti M, Bruno R, Soriano V, et al, for the HIV HCC Cooperative Italian-Spanish Group. Hepatocellular carcinoma in HIV-infected patients: epidemiological features, clinical presentation and outcome. *AIDS* 2004;18:2285–2293.
47. Shaib YH, El-Serag HB, Davila JA, et al. Risk factors of intrahepatic cholangiocarcinoma in the United States: a case-control study. *Gastroenterology* 2005;128:620–626.
48. Morgan TR, Mandayam S, Jamal MM. Alcohol and hepatocellular carcinoma. *Gastroenterology* 2004;127(5 suppl 1):S87–S96.
49. Corrao G, Zambon A, Bagnardi V, et al., for the Collaborative SIDECIR Group. Nutrient intakes, nutritional patterns and the risk of liver cirrhosis: an explorative case-control study.*Eur J Epidemiol.* 2004;19:861–869.
50. Sulkowski MS, Thomas DL. Hepatitis C in the HIV-infected person. *Ann Intern Med.* 2003;138:197–207.
51. Pawlotsky JM. Mechanisms of antiviral treatment efficacy and failure in chronic hepatitis C. *Antiviral Res.* 2003;59:1–11.

52. El-Serag HB, Hampel H, Yeh C, et al. Extrahepatic manifestations of hepatitis C among United States male veterans. *Hepatology* 2002;36:1439–1445.
53. Pawlotsky JM. The nature of interferon-alpha resistance in hepatitis C virus infection. *Curr Opin Infect Dis.* 2003;16:587–592.
54. Niro GA, Rosina F, Rizzetto M. Treatment of hepatitis D. *J Viral Hepat.* 2005;12:2–9.
55. Kaymakoglu S, Karaca C, Demir K, et al. Alpha interferon and ribavirin combination therapy of chronic hepatitis D. *Antimicrob Agents Chemother.* 2005 49:1135–1138.
56. Emerson SU, Purcell RH. Running like water–the omnipresence of hepatitis E. *N Engl J Med.* 2004;351:2367–2368.
57. Yousfi MM, Douglas DD, Rakela J. Other hepatitis viruses. In D Zakim and TD Boyer, eds. *Hepatology. A textbook of liver disease*, 4th ed. Philadelphia: WB Saunders, 2003, pp. 1063–1072.
58. Schiff GM. Hepatitis caused by other viruses. In: ER Shiff, MF Sorrell, and Willis C. Maddrey, eds. *Schiff's diseases of the liver*, 8th ed. Philadelphia: Lippincott Williams & Wilkins, 1999, pp. 869–877.
59. Hinedi TB, Koff RS. Cholestatic hepatitis induced by Epstein-Barr virus infection in an adult. *Dig Dis Sci.* 2003;48:539–541.
60. Feranchak AP, Tyson RW, Narkewicz MR, et al. Fulminant Epstein-Barr viral hepatitis: orthotopic liver transplantation and review of the literature. *Liver Transpl Surg.* 1998;4:469–476.
61. O'Grady JG, Schalm SW, Williams R. Acute liver failure: redefining the syndromes. *Lancet* 1993;342:273.
62. O'Grady JG, Alexander GJ, Hayllar KM, et al. Early indicators of prognosis in fulminant hepatic failure. *Gastroenterology* 1989;97:439–445.
63. Bernuau J, Samuel D, Durand F. Criteria for emergency liver transplantation in patients with acute viral hepatitis and factor V below 50% of normal: a prospective study. *Hepatology* 1991;14:49A.
64. Lee WM, Galbraith RM, Watt GH, et al. Predicting survival in fulminant hepatic failure using serum Gc protein concentrations. *Hepatology* 1995;21:101–105. Erratum in: *Hepatology* 1995;21:1213.
65. Donaldson BW, Gopinath R, Wanless IR, et al. The role of transjugular liver biopsy in fulminant liver failure: relation to other prognostic indicators. *Hepatology* 1993;18:1370–1376.
66. Karvountzis GG, Redeker AG. Relation of alpha-fetoprotein in acute hepatitis to severity and prognosis. *Ann Intern Med.* 1974;80:156–160.
67. Ostapowicz G, Fontana RJ, Schiodt FV, et al., for the U.S. Acute Liver Failure Study Group. Results of a prospective study of acute liver failure at 17 tertiary care centers in the United States. *Ann Intern Med.* 2002;137:947–954.
68. Rolando N, Wade JJ, Stangou A, et al. Prospective study comparing the efficacy of prophylactic parenteral antimicrobials, with or without enteral decontamination, in patients with acute liver failure. *Liver Transpl Surg.* 1996;2:8–13.
69. Molmenti EP: Hepatic failure. In: Lillemoe K and Schulick R, eds. *Pocket general surgery* PocketMedicine.com, Inc, 2001.
70. Molmenti EP and Klintmalm GB. *Atlas of liver transplantation.* Philadelphia: WB Saunders, 2002.
71. Bismuth H, Samuel D, Castaing D, et al. Orthotopic liver transplantation in fulminant and subfulminant hepatitis. The Paul Brousse experience. *Ann Surg.* 1995;222:109–119.
72. Emre S, Schwartz ME, Shneider B, et al. Living related liver transplantation for acute liver failure in children. *Liver Transpl Surg.* 1999;5:161–165.
73. Molmenti EP and Scheel PJ. Clinical management of the necrotic liver during transplantation. In: RW Busuttil and GB Klintmalm, eds. 2nd ed. Philadelphia: Elsevier, In press.
74. van de Kerkhove MP, Hoekstra R, et al. Clinical application of bioartificial liver support systems. *Ann Surg.* 2004;240:216–230.

CHAPTER 60 ■ CIRRHOSIS AND PORTAL HYPERTENSION

MICHAEL R. MARVIN AND JEAN C. EMOND

CIRRHOSIS

BACKGROUND AND DEFINITION

The term *cirrhosis*, derived from the Greek word *kirrhos* (orange-yellow), was first coined by Laennec in 1826. In 1911, Mallory described the disease as a "progressive, destructive lesion with reparative activity and contraction of the connective tissue, resulting in obstruction of the bile ducts and interference of portal blood flow."[1] Multiple definitions of cirrhosis can be found in the literature, but all reflect the underlying pathology of injury, repair, regeneration, and scarring. Cirrhosis is not a localized process but one that, by definition, involves the entire liver. Cirrhosis is the end result of multiple, varied, repeated or chronic pathologic insults to the liver with subsequent repair that cause an irreversible derangement in the hepatic architecture; the primary histologic features are marked fibrosis, destruction of vascular and biliary elements, regeneration, and nodule formation.

Pathophysiology

Cirrhosis can be caused by a wide range of pathologic entities, including the viral hepatitides, alcohol, metabolic disorders, drug toxicity, and biliary obstruction, among others (Table 60.1). Regardless of the cause, the primary event that leads to cirrhosis is injury to hepatocellular elements, which leads to architectural destruction if the damage exceeds the regenerative capacity of the organ. Both acute and chronic injury initiate an inflammatory response with associated cytokine release; elaboration of toxic substances; destruction of hepatocytes, bile duct cells, and vascular endothelial cells; repair through cellular proliferation and regeneration; and formation of fibrous scar (Fig. 60.1). Understanding the deviation from successful regeneration with restoration of hepatocyte mass and normal architecture, to the path leading to fibrogenesis and cirrhosis, remains a central question in liver biology.

The primary cell implicated in the formation of fibrosis is the stellate cell (Ito cell, lipocyte, perisinusoidal cell), located in the perisinusoidal space of Disse (Fig. 60.2).[2] In the normal liver, these cells are primarily responsible for the storage of vitamin A.[3] In response to various stimuli, they become activated, as evidenced by cellular enlargement and proliferation, an increase in rough endoplasmic reticulum, loss of vitamin A droplets, expression of actin filaments, and increased expression of "fibril-forming" collagen types I, III, and V.[4,5] They also express components of the extracellular matrix, including heparan sulfate, dermatan, chondroitin sulfate,[6] laminin,[7] and fibronectin.[8]

The activation process may be influenced by Kupffer cells within the liver, which have been shown to enhance the activation

TABLE 60.1 CLASSIFICATION

CLASSIFICATION OF CIRRHOSIS

Alcohol
Viral hepatitis
Biliary obstruction
Primary
Secondary
Venoocclusive disease
Hemochromatosis
Wilson's disease
Autoimmune
Syphilis
Drugs and toxins
α_1 = Antitrypsin deficiency
Cystic fibrosis
Glycogen storage disease
Other metabolic diseases
Sarcoidosis
Copper
Small-bowel bypass
Idiopathic

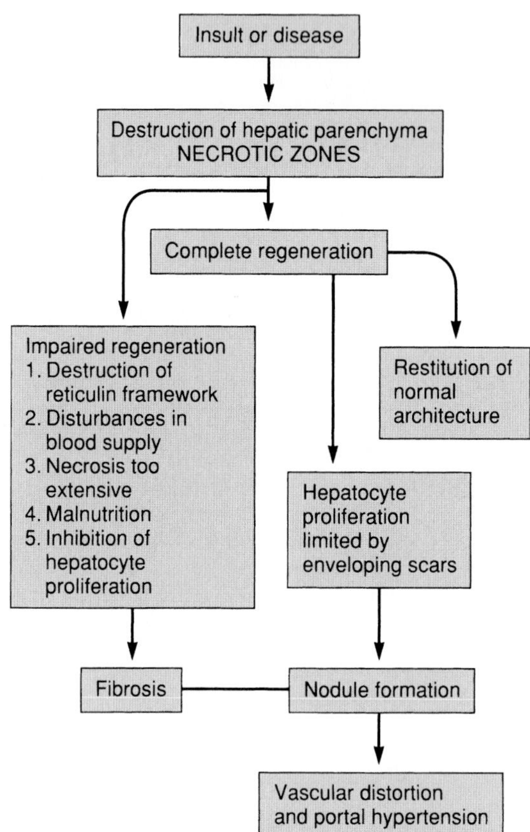

FIGURE 60.1 Evolution of cirrhosis. Fibrosis develops in nonregenerative necrotic areas, producing scars. The pattern of nodularity and scars reflects the type of response to injury (e.g., uniform vs. nonuniform necrosis) and the extent of injury.

of stellate cells *in vitro*,[9] perhaps by eliciting the production of cytokines such as transforming growth factor-β (TGF-β), platelet-derived growth factor (PDGF), tumor necrosis factor-α (TNF-α), interleukin-1 (IL-1), interleukin-6 (IL-6), and epidermal growth factor, in addition to their cellular receptors.[9–12] Both TGF-β and PDGF have been shown to enhance proliferation and fibrogenesis in animal models,[9,10] with TGF-β being the primary stimulator of collagen synthesis and fibrosis. Further evidence implicating TGF-β in the production of hepatic fibrosis is the observation that levels of TGF-β are reduced by therapy with interferon-α in patients who are positive for hepatitis C. This reduction has been correlated with a

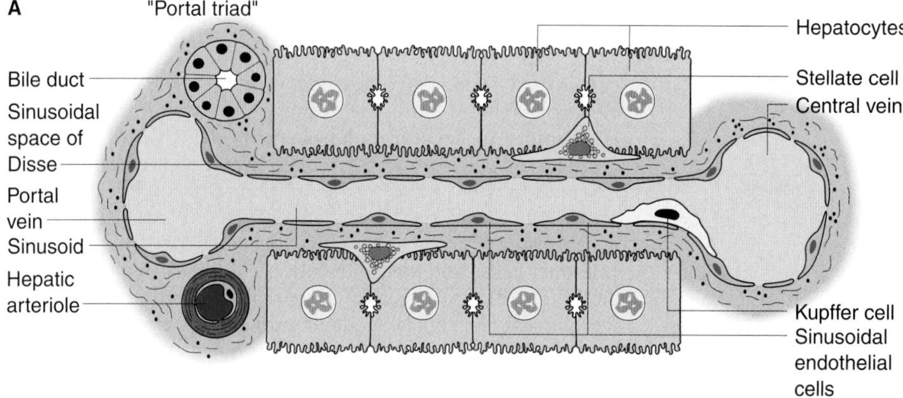

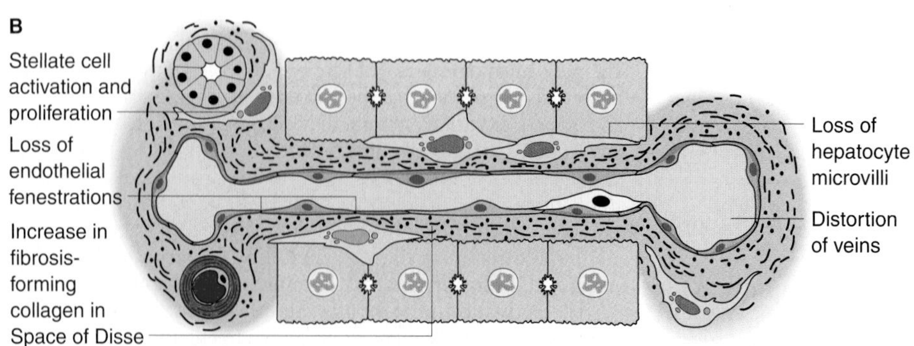

FIGURE 60.2 Matrix and cellular alterations in hepatic fibrosis. (*A*) In normal liver, a modest amount of low-density matrix is present in the subendothelial space of Disse. (*B*) In the fibrotic liver, the accumulation of fibril-forming matrix in this region leads to "capillarization" of the sinusoid and functional changes in all neighboring cell types. (From Friedman SL, Arthur MJP, Millward-Sadler. Cirrhosis and hepatic fibrosis. In: Wright R, et al., eds. *Liver and Biliary Disease*, 3rd ed. London: Bailliere Tindall, 1992: 822–881, with permission.)

regression of hepatic fibrosis.[13] As a result of the activation of stellate cells and a subsequent enhancement in collagen and extracellular matrix synthesis, the space of Disse becomes thickened, so that "capillarization" develops and the normal fenestrated architecture of the sinusoidal endothelium is lost.[14] Obliteration of sinusoidal fenestrations may be the essential component of fibrosis-induced hepatocellular dysfunction in cirrhosis, preventing the normal flow of nutrients to hepatocytes and increasing vascular resistance.[15] In addition, production of endothelin-1, a potent vasoconstrictor, by endothelial or stellate cells can cause contraction of the myofilaments within the stellate cell, influencing blood flow to injured areas and contributing to portal hypertension. Initially, fibrosis may be reversible if the inciting agents are removed. With sustained injury, the process of fibrosis becomes irreversible and leads to cirrhosis.

Classification Systems

Morphology

In 1977, the World Health Organization divided cirrhosis into three categories based on the morphologic characteristics of hepatic nodules (Fig. 60.3).[16]

Micronodular Pattern. Nodules are almost always less than 3 mm in diameter, are relatively uniform in size, are regularly distributed throughout the liver, and rarely contain portal tracts or efferent veins. Micronodular livers are usually of normal size or are mildly enlarged, and the fibrous septa vary in thickness. These changes reflect relatively early disease and are characteristic of a wide range of disease processes, including alcoholism, biliary obstruction, venous outflow obstruction, hemochromatosis, and Indian childhood cirrhosis.

Macronodular Pattern. In this category, nodules vary considerably in size and are larger than 3 mm in diameter, with some nodules measuring several centimeters. Portal structures and efferent veins are present but display architectural distortion. These livers are usually coarsely scarred with variably thick and thin septa and may be either normal or reduced in size. Two separate subcategories are recognized based on the nature of the fibrous septa. In the first one, characteristic of "posthepatitis" pathology and found in Wilson's disease, fine, sometimes incomplete septa link portal tracts; these are difficult to see on gross inspection of the liver. The second is characteristic of "postnecrotic" disease, commonly found in patients with viral hepatitis, and is characterized by coarse, thick septa that are readily apparent on gross examination. Because of the relatively large size of the nodules relative to the size of biopsy specimens, diagnosis by biopsy may be difficult in macronodular cirrhosis.

Mixed Pattern. This description is applied to livers in which both micronodules and macronodules are present in approximately equal proportions.

Etiology

Another commonly used method for classifying cirrhosis is by etiology. The causes of cirrhosis and the morphologic and histologic characteristics of the liver, however, overlap significantly. Oxidative stress leading to chronic injury and inflammation appears to be a common theme of these disorders, which leads to both scar formation and an increased risk of liver cancer.

Alcohol. The relationship between alcohol and liver disease has been well established. In 1849, Rokitansky, referring to the association of alcohol intake and liver disease, coined the term *Laennec's cirrhosis*.[17] More than 50% of alcoholics with cirrhosis and two thirds of patients with alcoholic hepatitis and cirrhosis die within 4 years of diagnosis.[18] Cirrhosis, however, develops in only 10% to 30% of heavy drinkers.[19] The reasons why cirrhosis develops in some alcoholics but not

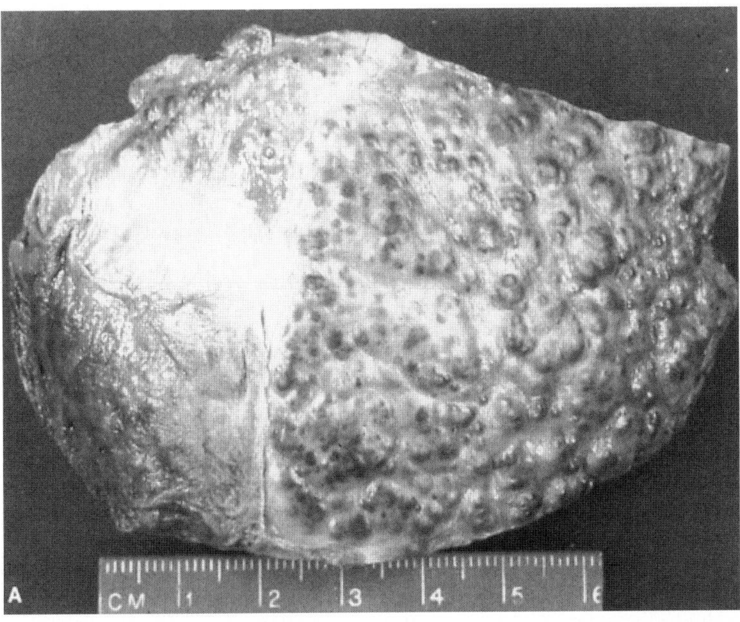

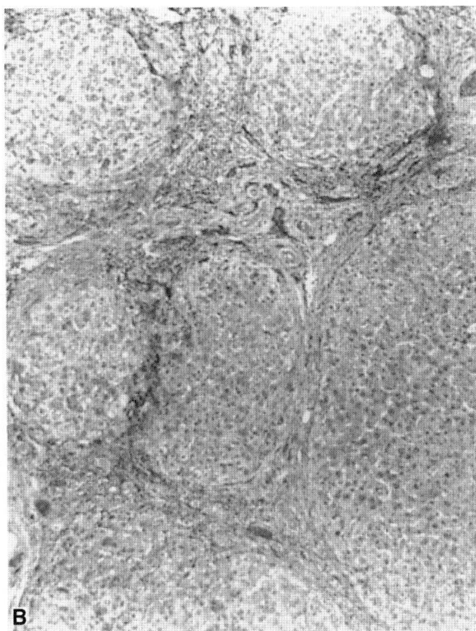

FIGURE 60.3 Small, shrunken liver and a fairly regular pattern of nodularity. This appearance is rather typical of end-stage cirrhosis, regardless of the cause. (*B*) Photomicrograph of cirrhotic liver tissue, showing irregular nodules of regenerating hepatocytes surrounded by scar. Trichrome stain.[60]

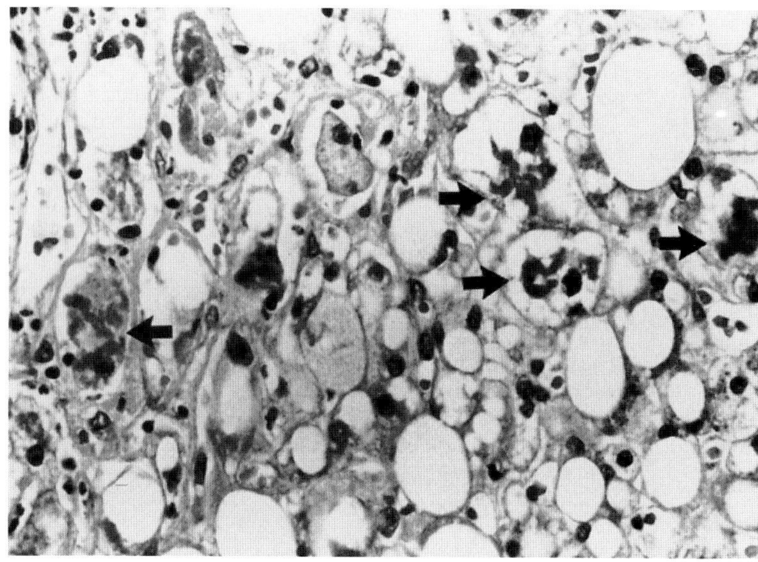

FIGURE 60.4 Alcoholic hepatitis. Mallory bodies (*arrows*) are evident within the swollen, clear cytoplasm of several hepatocytes. This hyaline material is chemotactic for leukocytes, many of which are seen within the field. Hematoxylin and eosin (H&E) stain.[470]

in others are not clear and may depend on a variety of factors, such as genetic predisposition, nutritional effects, concomitant drug use, and viral infection.

Alcoholic liver disease usually begins with a transition of normal architecture to fatty liver and alcoholic hepatitis, indicated histologically by the presence of megamitochondria, Mallory bodies (eosinophilic accumulations of intermediate filaments with cytokeratin proteins), inflammation and necrosis, and ultimately fibrosis (Fig. 60.4). Classically, the morphology of alcoholic cirrhosis is a micronodular pattern.

Although alcohol may directly activate stellate cells to produce collagen independently of inflammation and necrosis,[5] the key mediator in alcohol-induced liver disease is acetaldehyde, the product of alcohol metabolism by the enzyme alcohol dehydrogenase. Acetaldehyde (ADH) produces numerous deleterious effects on the liver, including the following: direct activation of stellate cells;[20] inhibition of DNA repair;[21] depletion of glutathione, which impairs mitochondrial function and the ability to handle free radical production;[19] damage to microtubules, which causes protein and water sequestration;[21] and formation of reduced nicotinamide adenine dinucleotide (NADH), which opposes gluconeogenesis and inhibits fatty acid oxidation, so that steatosis and hyperlipidemia develop.[21] ADH is most active in the perivenular/centrilobular zone 3 of the hepatic lobule; as a result, relatively high concentrations of acetaldehyde are found in this area of the liver. In addition, zone 3 is hypoxic because of its distance from portal venous and hepatic arterial inflow. These two factors are presumably responsible for the characteristic initial perivenular location of alcohol-induced liver disease.

Other effects of ADH include induction of lipid peroxidation with subsequent loss of integrity of cell membranes, which causes the characteristic "ballooning degeneration" of alcohol-induced liver disease.[22] Necrosis and inflammation in the perivenular region activate the stellate cells in the space of Disse, so that fibrosis develops. With continued ingestion of alcohol and hepatic injury, expansion of the areas of fibrosis toward the periportal regions leads to bridging fibrosis and ultimately cirrhosis.

Nonalcoholic Fatty Liver Disease (NAFLD)/Nonalcoholic Statohepatitis (NASH). This entity is becoming a more common cause of liver disease than in the past. Nonalcoholic steatohepatitis (NASH), as this disease was previously called, is only one stage in the NAFLD disease process.[23] It is characterized by infiltration of the liver with fat, with or without inflammation (hepatitis), that appears pathologically like alcohol-induced liver injury but in patients who do not abuse alcohol. It is associated with obesity, hyperlipidemia, and non–insulin-dependent diabetes. Most patients who are diagnosed with cryptogenic cirrhosis have NAFLD,[24] which is the most common cause of abnormal liver test results in the United States.[25]

Hepatitis. Viral hepatitis is the most common cause of cirrhosis worldwide, accounting for at least 50% of cases. Hepatitis A, B, C, D, and E have all been proved to cause acute hepatitis, characterized histologically by lymphocytic parenchymal and portal inflammation, focal necrosis, ballooning degeneration, cholestasis, Kupffer cell and macrophage hypertrophy and hyperplasia, and lobular disarray. Only hepatitis B, C, and D have been shown to progress to chronic hepatitis, defined by persistent liver cell necrosis and inflammation lasting longer than 6 months.

Chronic infection with hepatitis B virus (HBV) develops in less than 5% of patients who experience acute HBV infection. The development of cirrhosis in approximately 10% to 20% of chronically infected persons produces an overall rate of cirrhosis of approximately 1%. Of patients with hepatitis C virus (HCV), 90% become chronically infected, and chronic hepatitis develops in 60% of these. Of these patients with chronic hepatitis, 30% progress to cirrhosis,[17] so that the incidence of cirrhosis in patients initially infected with hepatitis C is approximately 10%.

Treatment of HCV hepatitis with interferon-α can completely eradicate infection in a small portion of patients (15% to 30%).[26] In patients who respond to interferon therapy, progression to cirrhosis is eliminated and hepatocellular carcinoma does not develop. In patients who do not respond to interferon therapy, cirrhosis develops in approximately 40%, and hepatocellular carcinoma develops in 16% of these.[27] Combination therapy with interferon and ribavirin has improved response rates, producing sustained remissions in 30% to 40% of patients.[28] Recently, pegylation of interferon has resulted in new drug formulations that have allowed for once weekly drug administration and improved sustained response rates to greater than 50%.[29] It should be noted that hepatitis C occurs naturally in multiple genotypes, of which, types 2 and 3, respond well to treatment with sustained viral suppression in 70% to 80% of patients.[29]

Hepatitis D virus (HDV) is an RNA virus that requires the presence of HBV to be pathogenic. Superinfection of HBV-positive patients with HDV leads to a more rapid clinical course, with progression to cirrhosis in 70% to 80% of patients.[30]

Among patients with compensated cirrhosis of viral origin, hepatocellular carcinoma developed in approximately 20% with HCV, 9% with HBV, and 41% with both HBV and HCV.[17]

Cholestasis. Cholestasis, defined as a decrease or absence of bile flow into the duodenum, may be caused by intrahepatic or extrahepatic biliary obstruction or defects in the ability of hepatocytes to excrete bile. Causes of cholestasis are presented in Table 60.2. Prolonged biliary obstruction leads to proliferation of bile ducts, formation of bile lakes caused by disruption of bile ducts, fibrosis, and ultimately secondary biliary cirrhosis as a result of the direct toxic effects of bile salts on hepatobiliary elements.

Immune or inflammatory cirrhosis. Although cholestasis is a generically toxic insult to the liver that can cause cirrhosis, several diseases that are characterized by cholestasis seem to be caused by underlying immune or inflammatory disorders affecting either small (primary biliary cirrhosis [PBC]) or large (primary sclerosing cholangitis [PSC]) bile ducts. Primary biliary cirrhosis is a chronic, slowly progressive disease that most commonly affects middle-aged women; it is characterized by portal inflammation, destruction of intrahepatic bile ducts, and progression to cirrhosis Approximately 95% of patients are women, and 95% of these women express antimitochondrial antibodies in serum.[31] The autoimmune inflammatory process damages both the bile ducts and, eventually, the hepatocytes as a result of leakage of bile acids into surrounding parenchyma.[32] Patients present with fatigue, jaundice, and pruritus, but as many as 50% to 60% of patients may be asymptomatic.[33] PBC progresses in the majority of patients; median survival times are approximately 10 to 15 years in asymptomatic and 7 years in symptomatic patients.[34,35] Poor prognostic factors include hyperbilirubinemia, advanced age, hepatosplenomegaly, and symptomatic disease. Treatment options include cholestyramine, colchicine and methotrexate for pruritus and fatigue, and ursodiol for slowing progression of the disease and delaying the need for transplant.[35,36] Orthotopic liver transplantation is the only known curative treatment.

Primary sclerosing cholangitis is a chronic, progressive cholestatic liver disease of unknown cause characterized by diffuse segmental intrahepatic or extrahepatic biliary ductular strictures with associated fibrosis and inflammation. The disease has no cure and often leads to secondary biliary cirrhosis, portal hypertension, hepatic failure, and cholangiocarcinoma if hepatic transplantation is not performed. PSC is strongly associated with inflammatory bowel diseases, most commonly ulcerative colitis, and probably shares an underlying disturbance related to disturbed mucosal immunity of the gastrointestinal tract.[37] Approximately 70% of patients with PSC also have ulcerative colitis.[38] Conversely, approximately 5% of patients with ulcerative colitis have PSC, though subtler forms of the disease may be present but clinically asymptomatic. PSC is thought to be autoimmune in nature; elevated levels of autoantibodies and an increased expression of HLA antigen class II molecules on biliary epithelial cells have been observed.[39,40] Approximately two thirds of patients are male and less than 45 years of age at the time of diagnosis.[41,42] Patients with PSC may be completely asymptomatic (up to 50%) or have signs of advanced disease at the time of diagnosis.[43] Commonly, the diagnosis is made in symptomatic patients after endoscopic retrograde cholangiopancreatography (ERCP) has been performed to evaluate elevated liver enzymes, including alkaline phosphatase and γ-glutamyltransferase. Symptomatic patients have a waxing and waning course and may present with complaints of fatigue (75%), pruritus (25% to 70%), jaundice (30% to 69%), abdominal pain (16% to 37%), and weight loss (10% to 34%).[38,44] Complications secondary to progression to cirrhosis are less common and include ascites, variceal bleeding, and acute cholangitis.

The diagnosis is suggested by a history of inflammatory bowel disease in the setting of elevated liver enzymes and is

TABLE 60.2 ETIOLOGY

CAUSES OF CHOLESTASIS

EXTRAHEPATIC
Common bile duct stones
Cancers
Pancreas
Ampulla of Vater
Bile duct
Cysts
Pancreatic
Choledochal
Infections
Parasites
AIDS
Chronic pancreatitis
Bile duct strictures
Benign
Ischemic
Hodgkin's disease
Biliary atresia
INTRAHEPATIC
Primary biliary cirrhosis
Space-occupying lesions
Primary or metastatic hepatic tumors
Lymphoma
Amyloidosis
Vanishing bile duct syndrome
Allograft rejection
Graft-vs.-host disease
Alagille's syndrome
Idiopathic adult ductopenia
Primary sclerosing cholangitis
Hodgkin's disease
Cystic fibrosis
HEPATOCELLULAR CHOLESTASIS
Genetic
α-Antitrypsin deficiency
Benign recurrent intrahepatic cholestasis
Blyer's syndrome
Cholestasis of pregnancy
Abnormal bile acid synthesis
Porphyrias
Acquired
Viral hepatitis
Drugs
Alcoholic hepatitis
Bacterial infections
Total parenteral nutrition
Renal carcinoma
Hodgkin's disease
Postoperative cholestasis

established by cholangiography. The disease process may range from a single dominant stricture to, more commonly, diffuse multifocal sclerosis of the intrahepatic and extrahepatic bile ducts. Pathologically, bile ductular proliferation, periductal fibrosis and inflammation, ductopenia, and, less commonly, obliterative fibrous cholangitis may be present. PSC may be considered a premalignant condition. Like ulcerative colitis, PSC confers a significant risk of malignant transformation of the biliary mucosa, which is one of the considerations in considering patients for transplantation. Natural history studies suggest that cholangiocarcinoma occurs in up to one third of patients, although the risk increases with the duration of disease and the degree of cholestasis.[45] Screening for premalignant changes with ERCP and cytologic examination and serum testing of CA19-9 have been helpful, though both have limited specificity and sensitivity. Transplantation should be performed before cancer develops and, generally, the discovery of cancer has been considered an absolute contraindication to transplantation because of poor outcomes. A recent aggressive protocol that includes neoadjuvant chemotherapy, radiotherapy, and brachytherapy followed by abdominal exploration before transplantation, however, has shown promising results with graft survival rates at 1 year of approximately 90%.[46]

Metabolic and Genetic Disorders. Some of these diseases are listed in Table 60.1. A description of all the metabolic disorders causing liver disease is beyond the scope of this chapter.

In hemochromatosis of the liver, an inborn error of metabolism causes an increased absorption of iron from the gastrointestinal tract. The pathophysiology of iron-induced hepatotoxicity is related to lipid peroxidation induced by iron in periportal regions of the liver. Activation of stellate cells by cytokines released from Kupffer cells that have phagocytosed necrotic hepatocytes injured by iron toxicity is also contributory.[47] Over time, the reaction progresses to bridging fibrosis and eventually to a mixed micronodular–macronodular cirrhosis. Treatment includes reduction of iron intake, repeated phlebotomy, and orthotopic liver transplantation.

Wilson's disease is an autosomal, recessively inherited disease caused by a deficiency in hepatocyte transport of copper into the bile. The disease is characterized biochemically by low serum ceruloplasmin levels and, clinically, by corneal pigmentation (Kayser-Fleischer rings), neuropsychiatric disease, and hepatic cirrhosis.[48] As copper accumulates in the liver, periportal inflammation develops that leads to piecemeal and lobular necrosis, bridging fibrosis, and a mixed micronodular–macronodular cirrhosis.[49] Treatment options include chelating penicillamine, trientine, zinc salts, and orthotopic liver transplantation.

Venous Outflow Obstruction. Cirrhosis may also result from obstruction of the hepatic veins. Causes include chronic right-sided heart failure as a result of severe tricuspid regurgitation, constrictive pericarditis, and the Budd-Chiari syndrome.

Hepatic dysfunction secondary to passive vascular congestion in the setting of right-sided heart failure and increased right-sided heart pressures is caused by the transmission of increased pressure to the hepatic venous system. This increased pressure leads to sinusoidal congestion, perivenular atrophy, hemorrhagic necrosis, and distortion and enlargement of sinusoidal fenestrations.[50] Increased pressure also causes perisinusoidal edema that eventually exceeds the clearance capabilities of hepatic lymphatics, so that ascites develops.[51] Grossly, the liver is described as having a "nutmeg" appearance in which areas of hemorrhage are interspersed with relatively normal yellowish parenchyma.[51] Histologically, perivenular fibrosis progresses to bridging fibrosis that spares the portal regions. Portal sparing is characteristic of "cardiac cirrhosis." In addition to causing ascites, chronic vascular congestion can lead to fibrosis in the space of Disse, which compromises nutrient delivery and contributes to portal hypertension and zone 3 hepatocellular injury.[52]

TABLE 60.3 ETIOLOGY

ETIOLOGIC FACTORS IN BUDD-CHIARI SYNDROME

- Idiopathic
- Hematologic disorders
  - Polycythemia vera
  - Paroxysmal nocturnal hemoglobinuria
  - Myeloproliferative disorders
  - Antithrombin III deficiency
  - Circulating lupus anticoagulants
- Oral contraceptives
- Pregnancy and postpartum
- Tumors
  - Hepatocellular carcinoma
  - Renal cell carcinoma
  - Adrenal carcinoma
  - Leiomyosarcoma of the inferior vena cava
- Vena caval webs
- Infections
  - Amebic abscess
  - Aspergillosis
  - Hydatid cyst
- Phlebitis
- Trauma
- Venoocclusive disease

Budd-Chiari syndrome is a rare disease caused by mechanical obstruction of the hepatic veins (Table 60.3). Obstruction may occur at the level of the terminal hepatic veins, the major hepatic veins, or the vena cava and may be caused by obstructing webs or membranes (most commonly in Africa and Asia) or thrombosis secondary to hypercoagulable states and neoplasms (most commonly in the West).

The range of presentations is wide; some patients are completely asymptomatic, whereas acute hepatic failure or cirrhosis develops in others.[53] These variations in symptoms are related to the degree and rate of progression of hepatic outflow obstruction. Patients classically present with abdominal pain, hepatomegaly, and ascites. The diagnosis can be made by duplex Doppler ultrasonography, which has a sensitivity of 85% to 95%.[54] Computed tomography (CT) is another diagnostic option.

Diagnosis

Although cirrhosis can be asymptomatic for decades, significant information can be obtained by performing a thorough history and physical examination. A history of alcohol abuse, hepatitis, toxin or drug exposure, upper gastrointestinal bleeding, enlarging hemorrhoids, infections, and alteration in mental status suggest the possibility of liver disease. Physical findings associated with cirrhosis are listed in Table 60.4. In addition to these findings, fetor hepaticus, purpura and bruising, decreased body hair, and white nails are common.

Laboratory tests of liver function are indicated if liver disease is suggested by the history and physical examination. Although levels of bilirubin, aspartate aminotransferase, alanine aminotransferase, and alkaline phosphatase are elevated in hepatic disease, the increases are not specific for liver pathology, and levels may be normal even in the setting of significant

TABLE 60.4 DIAGNOSIS

PHYSICAL FINDINGS IN CIRRHOSIS

Physical findings	Incidence [%]
Palpable liver	96
Jaundice	68
Ascites	66
Spider angiomas	49
Dilated abdominal wall veins	47
Palpable spleen	46
Testicular atrophy	45
Palmar erythema	24
Noninfectious fever	22
Hepatic coma	18
Gynecomastia	15
Dupuytren's contractures	5

disease. A very common finding in patients with cirrhosis is thrombocytopenia, caused by hypersplenism and portal hypertension. The platelet growth factor thrombopoietin, which is produced by the liver, has been shown to be decreased in patients with cirrhosis, and this deficit may contribute to the thrombocytopenia associated with hepatic disease.[55]

The definitive diagnosis of cirrhosis usually requires biopsy, either percutaneous or operative, or gross inspection during laparoscopy or laparotomy. Noninvasive methods to diagnose cirrhosis include ultrasonography, CT, and magnetic resonance imaging (MRI), which generally reveal an atrophic, nodular liver and an enlarged spleen. Ultrasonographic criteria for cirrhosis include the demonstration of multiple nodular irregularities on the ventral liver surface that are clearly separate from the anterior abdominal wall. Parenchymal texture is altered in the setting of fibrosis, though this feature can be subtle. When these criteria are used, ultrasonography has been shown to have a sensitivity, specificity, and accuracy of approximately 90% in the diagnosis of cirrhosis.[56] Indirect evidence of cirrhosis includes endoscopically discovered varices of the esophagus, and the presence of splenomegaly detected by CT or MRI.

Manifestations

Renal

Although *hepatorenal* syndrome is the most dramatic renal complication of liver failure, renal dysfunction in this setting is generally multifactorial. Renal insufficiency may develop in a patient with cirrhosis as a direct consequence of the underlying condition (i.e., primary biliary cirrhosis, amyloidosis), as a consequence of excessive diuretic use in the treatment of ascites and fluid overload, or as a secondary reaction to the release of cytokines or hormones by the liver that alter renal function. Renal dysfunction is characterized by avid sodium retention despite normovolemia or hypervolemia, dilutional hyponatremia secondary to free water overload, ascites, and ultimately renal failure and the hepatorenal syndrome.

An unresolved question is which of the above problems is a primary pathologic entity and which are the secondary consequences of circulatory dysfunction. Observations that support a secondary effect theory include the lack of anatomic renal abnormalities in patients with cirrhosis-related renal dysfunction, the normal function of previously dysfunctional kidneys transplanted into otherwise healthy recipients, and resolution of renal abnormalities after successful hepatic transplantation. The exact pathophysiology behind this process remains to be defined.

Sodium Retention. Patients with cirrhosis who do not have ascites have relatively normal sodium handling capabilities. Patients in whom ascites develops have a marked inability to excrete sodium. Because of this deficit, sodium intake in excess of renal excretion contributes to fluid overload. Three potential mechanisms have been invoked to explain the cause of sodium retention and the development of ascites in cirrhotic patients. The first is the "underfill" theory, whereby portal hypertension causes an increase in pressure in the splanchnic circulation. Ascites occurs when hepatic lymph production exceeds lymphatic return, with subsequent contraction of the blood volume and renal sodium retention. The second is the "overflow" theory, which suggests that the primary defect is inherent to the kidney. Abnormal renal retention of sodium leads to concomitant water retention, expansion of plasma volume, and subsequently edema and ascites.[57] The third explanation is the "arterial vasodilation hypothesis," which suggests that the responsible defect lies within the vascular system, with arterial hypotension as the primary event.[58] Arterial vasodilation in the splanchnic circulation leads to relative peripheral hypovolemia and activation of the renin–angiotensin–aldosterone and sympathetic nervous systems. The effects, in turn, are a release of antidiuretic hormone (arginine vasopressin), enhancement of sodium and water conservation, an increase in effective circulating volume, and edema and ascites.[59] Most evidence supports the latter hypothesis.

The cause of the splanchnic vasodilation is unclear. Some evidence suggests that nitric oxide may be the key mediator. Elevations in portal venous nitric oxide have been reported in both animal and human studies,[60,61] and inhibitors of nitric oxide production have been shown to reduce the activity of vasoconstrictor systems and enhance renal hemodynamics.[60] The exact role of nitric oxide activity in the pathophysiology of renal disease in cirrhosis remains to be determined.

Water Retention. Patients with cirrhosis and ascites may have a marked inability to handle free water. An increased production of antidiuretic hormone, decreased delivery of fluid to the diluting segments of the nephron, and reduced renal production of prostaglandins all may contribute.[38] Retention of water leads to dilutional hyponatremia (serum sodium 130 mEq/L), which can cause nausea, vomiting, lethargy, and seizures.

Hepatorenal Syndrome. Hepatorenal syndrome is a complication of cirrhosis, most often with ascites, characterized by progressive renal failure in the absence of intrinsic renal disease. This syndrome occurs in 10% of hospitalized patients with cirrhosis and ascites.[62] Manifestations of the disease include progressive oliguria, with urine outputs of 400 to 800 mL/d, a rising serum creatinine level, increased cardiac output, and decreased arterial pressure. The disease process is highly variable and is associated with marked renal cortical vasoconstriction induced by activity of the renin—angiotensin—aldosterone and sympathetic nervous systems. In addition, the powerful endothelium-derived vasoconstrictor endothelin-1, combined with decreased renal production of vasodilator prostaglandins, may play a role.

Hepatorenal syndrome may develop as a result of infection, use of nonsteroidal antiinflammatory drugs, variceal hemorrhage, or excessive diuretic use in patients who were previously well compensated. The differentiation of hepatorenal syndrome from acute renal failure is possible by the laboratory evaluation of urine and serum samples. Hepatorenal syndrome, however, is virtually indistinguishable by laboratory testing from prerenal azotemia. Both prerenal azotemia and hepatorenal syndrome are characterized by extremely low sodium concentrations in the urine, high urine osmolality, high urine-to-plasma ratios of creatinine, and normal urinary sediment (Table 60.5). Criteria for the diagnosis of hepatorenal syndrome are listed in Table 60.6.

TABLE 60.5 DIAGNOSIS

DIFFERENTIAL DIAGNOSIS OF ACUTE AZOTEMIA IN PATIENTS WITH LIVER DISEASE

	Prerenal azotemia	Hepatorenal syndrome	Acute renal failure
Urinary sodium	<10 mEq/L	<10 mEq/L	>30 mEq/L
Urine/plasma creatinine ratio	>30:1	>30:1	<20:1
Urine osmolality	100 mOsm, or more than plasma osmolality	100 mOsm, or more than plasma osmolality	Equal to plasma osmolality
Urine sediment	Normal	Normal	Casts: cellular debris

The treatment of ascites in patients with cirrhosis requires sodium and water restriction in addition to the use of diuretics. Excessive use of these treatment modalities may lead to increases in serum creatinine that can be difficult to distinguish from those of hepatorenal syndrome. A failure to respond to cessation of diuretics and fluid challenge suggests hepatorenal syndrome. If liver transplantation cannot be performed, patients with hepatorenal syndrome usually die within months of the development of severe disease, defined as a serum creatinine level above 2 mg/dL.[63] Recent studies, however, have shown improvement in renal function in patients with hepatorenal syndrome after treatment with vasopressors and albumin. Noradrenalin, terlipressin (an analogue of vasopressin) and midodrine have been effective as reflected by decreased creatinine, increased creatinine clearance, and increased urine output.[64,65] Although these preliminary results are encouraging, the only truly effective treatment for hepatorenal syndrome is orthotopic liver transplantation, after which the kidneys usually revert to normal function.

TABLE 60.6 DIAGNOSIS

DIAGNOSTIC CRITERIA FOR HEPATORENAL SYNDROME[a]

MAJOR CRITERIA

1. Low glomerular filtration rate, as indicated by serum creatinine >1.5 mg/dL or 24-hour creatinine clearance <40 mL/min.
2. Absence of shock, ongoing bacterial infection, fluid losses, and current treatment with nephrotoxic drugs.
3. No sustained improvement in renal function (decrease in serum creatinine to ≤1.5 mg/dL or increase in creatinine clearance to 340 mL/min) following diuretic withdrawal and expansion of plasma volume with 1.5 L of a plasma expander.
4. Proteinuria <500 mg/d and no ultrasonographic evidence of obstructive uropathy or parenchymal renal disease.

ADDITIONAL CRITERIA

1. Urine volume <500 mL/d.
2. Urine sodium <10 mEq/L.
3. Urine osmolality greater than plasma osmolality.
4. Urine red blood cells <50 per high-power field.
5. Serum sodium concentration <130 mEq/L.

[a]All major criteria must be present for the diagnosis of hepatorenal syndrome. Additional criteria are not necessary for the diagnosis but provide supportive evidence.

From Arroyo V, Gines Ginés P, Gerbes A, et al. Definition and diagnostic criteria of refractory ascites and hepatorenal syndrome in cirrhosis. Hepatology 1996;23:164.

Pulmonary

Many pathologic processes in patients with cirrhosis affect pulmonary function. Some reflect an underlying condition that causes both hepatic and pulmonary disease (i.e., cystic fibrosis, a_1-antitrypsin deficiency); others are primary pulmonary processes, such as interstitial lung disease, primary pulmonary hypertension (portopulmonary hypertension), and obstructive airway disease. Three main pulmonary manifestations of cirrhosis are discussed here; one is related to increased intraabdominal pressure secondary to ascites, one is caused by intrapulmonary shunting, and is known as the hepatopulmonary syndrome, and the last is portopulmonary hypertension.

The presence of copious ascitic fluid can lead to pulmonary dysfunction by compromising diaphragmatic excursion secondary to increases in intraabdominal and intrapleural pressures. Ascites may also induce large pleural effusions because of the presence of lymphatic transdiaphragmatic communications between the abdomen and thorax.[66] Effusions can compress the pulmonary parenchyma and impair gas exchange, so that ventilation–perfusion mismatch and hypoxemia develop. Patients present with worsening pulmonary symptoms in the setting of increasing abdominal girth. Pulmonary function testing reveals decreases in functional residual capacity and total lung capacity.[67] Marked improvement in pulmonary function results from large-volume paracentesis.[68] This intervention decreases the work of breathing and relieves symptoms. With control of ascites, even in the presence of pleural effusions, no other interventions may be necessary.

Hepatopulmonary syndrome occurs in patients with mild to severe hepatic disease and in approximately 10% to 50% of patients with hepatic dysfunction.[69,70] The criteria for diagnosis include hepatic dysfunction; an oxygen tension below 70 mm Hg or a diffusion gradient above 20 mm Hg, or both; and the presence of pulmonary vascular dilation in patients with structurally normal lungs.[71] Other manifestations include platypnea (increased shortness of breath with movement from a supine to an erect position) and orthodeoxia (decreased oxygen tension on moving from a supine to an erect position). These two positional deficits in pulmonary function are related to the increased number of dilated capillaries in the basal areas of the lung; flow is increased in these vessels while the subject is standing, so that shunting is increased. Physical findings include clubbing and cyanosis of the nail beds and spider nevi.

Although the underlying cause of hypoxemia in these patients is right-to-left intrapulmonary shunting, ventilation–perfusion mismatch and impaired hypoxic vasoconstriction also play a role. Patients usually present with dyspnea and worsening hypoxemia without evidence of a primary pulmonary process. Initial diagnostic tools include pulse oximetry and arterial blood gas analysis. When significant hypoxemia is found, pulmonary function testing is useful to rule out obstructive or restrictive airway disease. A definitive diagnosis can be obtained by the use of contrast-enhanced echocardiography (bubble study), spiral CT, or angiography, which will confirm the presence of a shunt. The only effective therapy for this disease is orthotopic liver transplantation.

Portopulmonary hypertension is defined as a mean pulmonary arterial pressure of greater than 25 mm Hg in the setting of liver disease. It is a relatively rare (<10%) complication of cirrhosis that, when severe, carries a substantial risk of mortality and is a relative contraindication to liver transplantation.[72] Screening of patients with cirrhosis by Doppler echocardiography will reveal evidence of elevated right heart pressures, which need to be confirmed by right heart catheterization. Although the high flow state of cirrhosis can elevate right-sided pressures, fixed obstruction of the pulmonary microcirculation is highly lethal and is not likely to improve with liver transplantation. The exact pathophysiology behind portopulmonary hypertension is not known, but portal hypertension is a necessary component of the disease process. The hyperdynamic state in portal hypertension may be the main contributory factor. Treatment with prolonged intravenous infusion of prostaglandins has been shown to be effective in improving pulmonary hemodynamics but does not prolong survival.[73]

Hepatic Encephalopathy

Etiology. Hepatic encephalopathy is a neuropsychiatric syndrome that occurs in the setting of hepatic disease. It is characterized by variable alterations in mental status, ranging from deficits detectable only by detailed psychometric tests to confusion, lethargy, and ultimately frank coma. The disease may present in association with acute hepatic failure, as a consequence of progression of chronic liver disease, or after the creation of a surgical portosystemic shunt. Usually, a precipitating cause, such as an acute variceal hemorrhage or infection, can be found.

The causative agent in hepatic encephalopathy has been the subject of much debate. Most evidence implicates ammonia in the development of this condition. Ammonia is produced during the bacterial digestion of proteins in the gut, is absorbed into the portal circulation, and usually undergoes extensive degradation in the liver.[74] Most researchers believe that encephalopathy is caused by products, such as ammonia, derived from the gastrointestinal tract that are usually metabolized by the liver. These agents reach the peripheral circulation as a result of poor hepatic metabolism or through portosystemic shunts that may be physiologic or the result of surgical procedures. In patients with cirrhosis, in addition to the accumulation of ammonia in the blood, the permeability of the brain to ammonia appears to be increased.[75] Other suggested etiologic agents for hepatic encephalopathy include γ-aminobutyric acid,[76] endogenous benzodiazepines,[77] branched-chain amino acids (e.g., tryptophan),[78] neurotoxic short-chain fatty acids, mercaptans, phenols,[79] and endogenous opiates.[80]

The following observations suggest that ammonia is the key mediator in hepatic encephalopathy: (a) Ammonia levels are increased in 80% to 90% of patients with the condition[81]; (b) factors that precipitate hepatic encephalopathy cause increases in ammonia levels; and (c) treatments that relieve hepatic encephalopathy lower ammonia levels.[82] Arguments against this hypothesis include the following: (a) Levels of ammonia correlate poorly with the severity of hepatic encephalopathy; (b) high ammonia levels alone do not cause encephalopathy;[83] (c) administration of ammonia to patients with cirrhosis but not hepatic encephalopathy does not cause encephalopathy;[840] and (d) treatments that reduce ammonia levels also reduce the levels of other putative toxins.[85]

Clinical Features. A wide range of neurologic symptoms may occur in patients with hepatic dysfunction. Subtle deficits may include changes in personality, memory loss, alterations in sleep patterns, and minor decreases in intellectual function. Defects may be detectable only by detailed psychometric testing. If no known underlying liver disease is suspected, establishing the cause of an alteration in mental status may be difficult.

With progression of disease, asterixis, a rapid repetitive flexion–extension of the wrist that occurs in response to sustained extension of the forearm and fingers, may occur. In addition, stigmata of liver disease are usually evident, including fetor hepaticus and spider angiomas. The combination of asterixis, elevated ammonia levels, and altered mental status in a patient with known liver disease strongly suggests the diagnosis. Electroencephalographic changes are nonspecific and may occur in patients with a variety of other conditions.

Factors that commonly precipitate hepatic encephalopathy include impaired renal function, variceal hemorrhage, constipation, infection, excessive dietary protein, and drugs, especially benzodiazepines and barbiturates.

Treatment. Treatment options for hepatic encephalopathy include correction of the precipitating factors, alterations in diet, bowel cleansing, medications that reduce ammonia production and neutralize its effects, and medications to treat possible neurotransmitter and nutrient deficiencies.

A search for precipitating factors is imperative and includes cultures of urine, sputum, and ascitic fluid; determination of electrolyte abnormalities; screening for viral infection; assessment of overall volume status; drug history; and endoscopy (Table 60.7).

Therapy begins with a trial of volume expansion via intravenous hydration to relieve azotemia and reduce concentrations of toxic substances by dilution. The mainstays of treatment are directed at the removal of nitrogenous compounds from the gut. Most ammonia is produced within the small and large bowel by bacterial metabolism of dietary and endogenous protein.[86] Orally administered cathartics and enemas are the

TABLE 60.7 TREATMENT

TREATMENT OF HEPATIC ENCEPHALOPATHY

Identify precipitating factors
- Disordered carbohydrate metabolism
- Narcotics
- Infection
- Hypotension
- Hypoxia
- Excess exogenous protein
- Gastrointestinal bleeding
- Electrolyte abnormalities
- Alkalosis

Supportive therapy
- Eliminate dietary nitrogen
- Purge gastrointestinal tract to remove blood and other nitrogenous compounds
- Nonabsorbable antibiotics (neomycin or metronidazole)
- Lactulose or lactitol

Dopamine receptor agonists
- L-Dopa and bromocriptine[a]

Branched-chain amino acid[b]

Temporary liver support

Orthotopic liver transplantation

[a]Arousal effect in selected patients may be secondary to enhanced renal function.
[b]High cost and equivocal benefits of intravenous amino acid mixtures make it difficult to justify routine use.

PANCREAS/LIVER

best methods to achieve bowel cleansing,[87] and these are combined with marked dietary restriction of protein.

The cathartic of choice is lactulose, a nonabsorbable disaccharide that reaches the distal ileum and colon essentially unmetabolized. Many theories regarding the mechanism of action of lactulose have been proposed. Initially, the presumed mechanism of action was that on reaching the colon, lactulose is metabolized by colonic bacteria to acidic products that lower the pH of the colon. Lowering the pH inhibits the growth of ammonia- and urea-producing bacteria and promotes the growth of *Lactobacillus,* a bacterium with little proteolytic activity.[88] The validity of this theory has been questioned.[89] It appears now that lactulose alters the metabolism of intestinal bacteria by providing carbohydrate, which enhances the bacterial uptake of ammonia. Combined with the osmotic diarrhea caused by the cathartic activities of lactulose, this effect leads to an increased excretion of ammonia.[82,90–92]

The dosage of lactulose, 45 to 90 g/day, is administered orally, divided into three or four doses. The dosage can be adjusted to produce two or three soft stools daily. Hourly doses of 30 to 45 mL can be used to induce more rapid improvement during the initial phase of therapy. Symptoms usually abate within 24 hours, but more than 48 hours may be required. Doses can be adjusted if side effects such as flatulence, diarrhea, and electrolyte abnormalities occur.

Nonabsorbable antibiotics have also been used to decrease the number and concentration of ammonia-forming bacteria in the gut. Most experience has accrued for neomycin and metronidazole. These antibiotics are active against gram-negative anaerobes such as *Bacteroides,* which are considered to be a major source of ammonia production.[93] The dosage of neomycin, 2 to 8 g/day, is divided into four doses and is continued for 4 to 10 days. Multiple double-blinded, randomized trials have determined the efficacy of antibiotics alone or in combination with lactulose. (For a complete review, see Chapman et al.[82]) For acute hepatic encephalopathy, studies have shown that neomycin for 4 days is equally as effective as lactulose,[94] and metronidazole for 7 days is as effective as neomycin.[95] In addition, for chronic hepatic encephalopathy, neomycin for 10 days was equal to lactulose.[96] Although only small amounts (1% to 3%) of neomycin are absorbed, a risk for nephrotoxicity and ototoxicity still exists.[97,98] Rifaximin, a macrolide antibiotic not approved for use in the United States, has similar efficacy when compared with lactulose and neomycin.[99–101]

PORTAL HYPERTENSION

Portal hypertension is defined as a portal vein pressure above the normal range of 5 to 8 mm Hg.[102] Portal hypertension may also be defined by the hepatic vein–portal vein pressure gradient, which is greater than 5 mm Hg in portal hypertensive states. Pressures in the portal venous system are usually measured indirectly via the wedged hepatic venous pressure. The technique is similar to that used to determine pulmonary capillary wedge pressure by pulmonary arterial (Swan-Ganz) catheterization.

Anatomy

The venous anatomy of the portal system is relatively constant, with the "usual" anatomy present in 98% of the population (Fig. 60.5). The portal vein is formed by the confluence of the superior mesenteric and splenic veins behind the neck of the pancreas. The inferior mesenteric vein most often joins the splenic vein before the portal vein is formed, but approximately one third of the time the inferior mesenteric vein joins the superior mesenteric vein. The superior mesenteric vein may not be present, and the portal vein may be formed by multiple small branches from the mesenteric system that join the splenic vein.

Many branches of the portal venous system are affected when portal pressure rises. As pressure increases, blood flow decreases and the pressure in the portal system is transmitted to its branches. This transmission of pressure through branches of the portal system is beneficial in that it decreases overall portal pressure. It also is responsible for many of the complications of portal hypertension, however, because of the resulting dilation of venous tributaries.

The coronary or left gastric vein becomes highly significant in portal hypertension, by diverting portal blood to the veins of the lesser curve of the stomach and the esophagus, leading to the formation of varices. Other important collaterals include the inferior mesenteric vein which connects with its rectal branches which, when distended, form hemorrhoids; the umbilical vein in the ligamentum teres of the falciform ligament, which joins the left portal vein and causes abdominal wall veins around the paraumbilical plexus to dilate (caput medusae); the short gastric veins, branches of the splenic vein, which communicate with gastric veins and contribute to gastric varices; and the retroperitoneal veins of Retzius, which communicate with the gastrointestinal veins through the bare areas of the liver where no peritoneal layer separates the abdominal viscera from the retroperitoneum. The retroperitoneal collaterals can also form large splenorenal shunts that may decompress the portal system but are associated with severe encephalopathy.

Physiology

Portal hypertension is caused by increased resistance to portal blood flow secondary to cirrhosis, portal vein thrombosis, or hepatic venous obstruction. Normally, the liver offers little resistance to portal flow because of the porous nature of the hepatic sinusoids. Moreover, the liver has no intrinsic control over portal blood flow; it is merely a passive recipient of splanchnic flow, the primary regulation of which occurs at the level of the splanchnic arterioles.[103] As discussed earlier, the deposition of collagen in the space of Disse (capillarization), in addition to the contractile properties of stellate cells, cause an increased resistance to portal blood flow in cirrhosis. In addition, various cytokines and hormones contribute to elevated portal pressures by inducing splanchnic vasodilation and an increase in splanchnic flow.

The increased blood flow through collateral vessels and subsequently increased venous return cause the characteristic hemodynamic features of portal hypertension, which include an increase in cardiac output and total blood volume[104] and a decrease in systemic vascular resistance. Arteriovenous shunts within the liver, stomach, and small intestine contribute to the augmented venous return and decreased peripheral vascular resistance. Early in the course of portal hypertension, blood pressure may be normal, but with progression of disease, blood pressure usually falls.[105]

The portal venous concentration of nitric oxide, a potent vasodilator, has been shown to be elevated in patients with cirrhosis and portal hypertension.[106] In addition to nitric oxide, many other vasodilators are elevated in portal hypertension, including prostacyclin, endotoxin, and glucagon.[107]

Etiology

Many pathologic processes can cause portal hypertension (Table 60.8). These are usually classified as prehepatic,

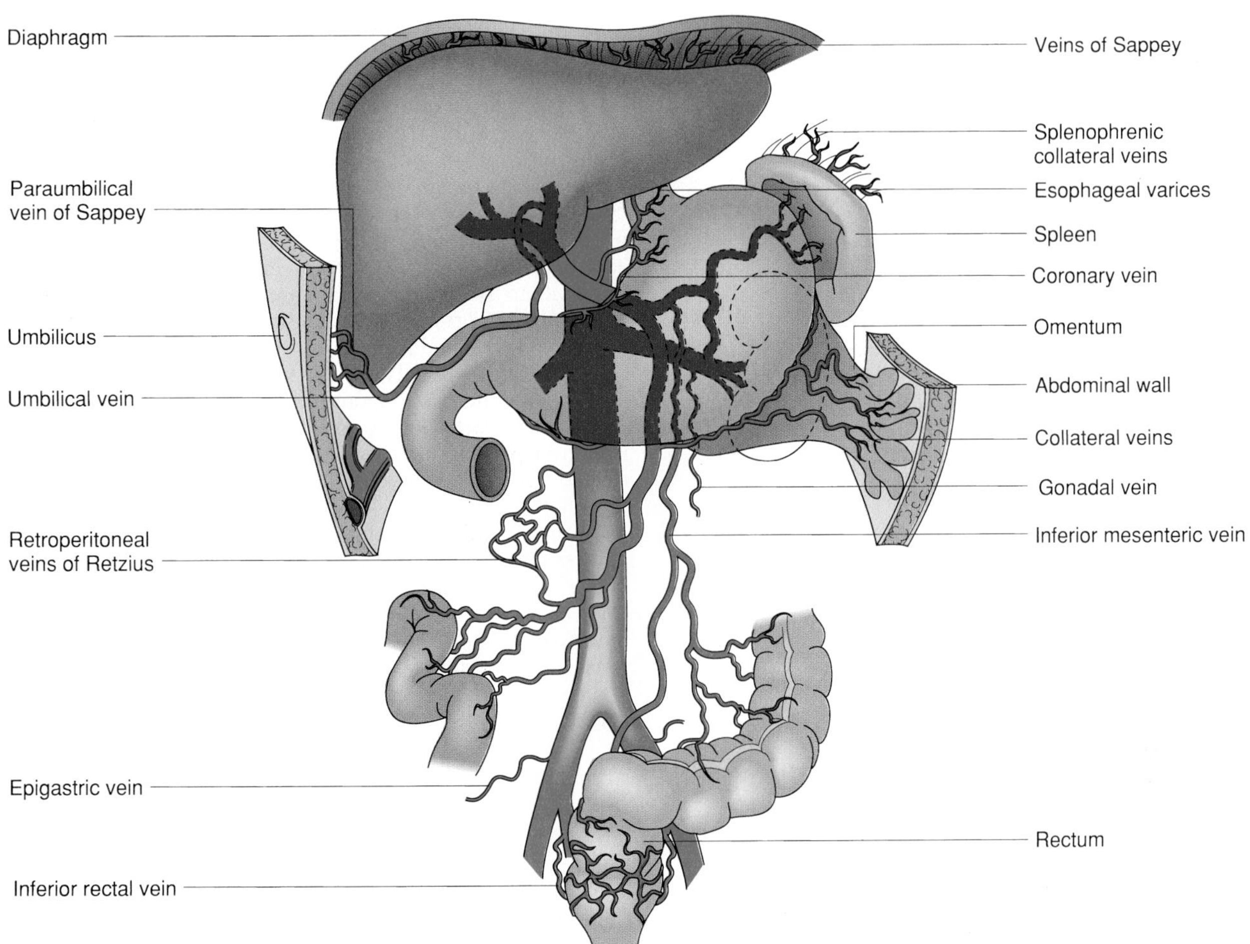

FIGURE 60.5 Potential venous collaterals that develop with portal hypertension. The veins of Sappey drain portal blood through the bare areas of the diaphragm and through paraumbilical vein collaterals to the umbilicus. The veins of Retzius form in the retroperitoneum and shunt portal blood from the bowel and other organs to the vena cava.

hepatic, or posthepatic (presinusoidal, sinusoidal, or postsinusoidal) conditions. In prehepatic and posthepatic conditions, portal hypertension is the result of mechanical venous obstruction at the level of the portal or hepatic veins, respectively, whereas cirrhosis is the main cause of hepatic portal hypertension.[108]

Budd-Chiari Syndrome and Venoocclusive Disease

The Budd-Chiari syndrome is caused by hepatic venous obstruction. The name of the syndrome is derived from two investigators, the first of whom (Budd)[109] described the classic presentation of abdominal pain, ascites, and hepatomegaly, and the second of whom (Chiari)[110] described the pathologic characteristics of the liver. The obstruction may occur at the level of the inferior vena cava, the hepatic veins, or the central veins within the liver itself and may be the result of congenital webs (most common in Africa and Asia), acute or chronic thrombosis (most common in the West), and malignancy. With occlusion of the hepatic veins, pressure increases in the central veins. As a result, centrilobular congestion, necrosis, and, with chronic disease, fibrosis and cirrhosis with portal hypertension develop.

In the West, the most common causes of this syndrome are hypercoagulable states associated with polycythemia vera, myeloproliferative disorders, paroxysmal nocturnal hemoglobinuria, and defects in the coagulation cascade, as in conditions associated with high estrogen levels (e.g., pregnancy, use of birth control pills).[111–114] Neoplasms may cause hepatic venous obstruction by direct invasion and occlusion of the vessels; or by establishment of a prothrombotic milieu secondary to the malignancy itself. In the East, the major causes of obstruction of the vena cava and hepatic veins are membranous webs that directly occlude the vessels. The etiology of vena cava webs is unknown.

Venoocclusive disease is characterized by obliterative endophlebitis of the intrahepatic veins (see Table 60.3). Causes of venoocclusive disease include medications, toxins, and pyrrolizidine alkaloids.

Budd-Chiari syndrome may present with acute, subacute, or chronic symptoms and is often misdiagnosed. This is unfortunate, because early treatment will prevent the development of hepatic fibrosis, which can lead to end-stage liver disease. Nearly 50% of patients have had symptoms for more than 3 months.[115] Acute symptoms include hepatomegaly, right upper quadrant abdominal pain, nausea, vomiting, and ascites. In the chronic form of the disease, patients may present with the sequelae of cirrhosis and portal hypertension, including variceal bleeding, ascites, spontaneous bacterial peritonitis, fatigue, and encephalopathy. In the chronic form, the entire liver atrophies except for the caudate lobe which may hypertrophy because its hepatic vein(s) enters the vena cava separately, so that venous outflow is not impeded.[116]

TABLE 60.8 ETIOLOGY

COMMON CAUSES OF PORTAL HYPERTENSION

DISORDERS THAT PRIMARILY INCREASE RESISTANCE TO FLOW
Prehepatic
Congenital atresia
Extrinsic compression
Schistosomiasis
Portal, superior mesenteric, or splenic vein thrombosis
Hepatic
CHRONIC–CIRRHOTIC
Hepatitis B, C
α_1-Antitrypsin deficiency
Cryptogenic
Cystic fibrosis
Hemochromatosis
Nutritional (alcoholic)
Wilson's disease
CHRONIC–NONCIRRHOTIC
Congenital hepatic fibrosis
Focal regenerative hyperplasia
Hepatic venoocclusive disease
Idiopathic
Metastatic carcinoma
Sarcoidosis
Toxin and drug injuries
ACUTE DISEASE
Acute fatty liver
Alcoholic hepatitis
Fulminant hepatic failure
Posthepatic
Budd-Chiari syndrome
Chronic heart failure
Constrictive pericarditis
Vena cava webs
DISORDERS THAT PRIMARILY INCREASE FLOW
Hepatocellular carcinoma
Mesenteric arteriosclerotic or aneurysmal vascular disease
Osler-Weber-Rendu syndrome
Splenomegaly

The hypertrophy of the caudate lobe creates a longitudinal narrowing of the retrohepatic vena cava which is surrounded by parenchyma, leading to secondary obstruction of the caval flow in the abdomen.

The diagnosis is most often made by ultrasonographic evaluation of the liver and its vasculature, which has a sensitivity of 85% to 95%.[117] Duplex scanning may reveal the location of the obstruction and characterize the flow within the vena cava and hepatic, portal, mesenteric, and splenic veins. Cross-sectional imaging using contrast-enhanced CT or MR is helpful in defining the entire abdominal venous circulation and assessing the status of the liver and its individual lobes, which is essential in planning therapy. Traditionally, the gold standard for the diagnosis has been angiography, which provides detailed information on the location and degree of obstruction.

The management of patients with this syndrome has traditionally been surgical intervention. Liver biopsies are usually performed preoperatively. The response rates to medical therapy, which does not relieve the obstruction to portal outflow, are poor,[118] and survival rates without surgical intervention are approximately 10%. Antithrombotic agents may be used in the rare patient who presents early with acute venous occlusion. The mainstay of therapy is surgical decompression with a side-to-side portosystemic shunt (see later). After shunt placement, the pressure on the vena cava by the caudate lobe is gradually relieved, leading to restoration of liver function.

A more direct solution, which is necessary in the face of complete caval obstruction, is the creation of a mesoatrial shunt which was popularized by Cameron and Maddrey.[119] This radical procedure has been largely supplanted by percutaneous portocaval shunting (transjugular intrahepatic portosystemic shunt [TIPS]). The rates of postprocedural encephalopathy are usually not increased in patients with Budd-Chiari syndrome, as they are in patients with cirrhosis who undergo portosystemic shunting for esophageal bleeding. In patients with end-stage liver disease, liver transplantation may be performed.[120] The 5-year survival rate for patients with good hepatic function before the shunt procedure is approximately 60%, with a 34% to 88% survival for patients after liver transplantation.[115,121–123] Postoperatively, patients are treated with long-term anticoagulation to prevent recurrent thrombosis.[121]

As noted, minimally invasive treatment using TIPS may be first-line therapy, and it has supplanted surgical shunting in our practice. Case reports and small series have suggested efficacy for this technique,[124] and a recent larger study has indicated 1- and 5-year survival rates of 93% and 74%, respectively.[125] Many patients develop shunt occlusion, however, and further angiographic manipulation is required to maintain patency.

Portal Vein Thrombosis

Portal vein thrombosis is the cause of portal hypertension in fewer than 10% of adult patients but is the most common cause in children.[126] In contrast to patients with cirrhosis-induced portal hypertension, these patients have normal liver function and are not as susceptible to the development of complications, such as encephalopathy. Causes of portal vein thrombosis include umbilical vein infection (the most common cause in children), coagulopathies (protein C and antithrombin III deficiency), hepatic malignancy, myeloproliferative disorders, inflammatory bowel disease, pancreatitis, trauma, and previous splenorenal shunt.[127,128] Most cases in adults are idiopathic.

The diagnosis can be made by sonography, which reveals an echogenic lesion in the lumen of the portal vein and an absence of portal venous flow on duplex examination.[129] With time, cavernous transformation of the portal vein may occur, in which channels develop within the clotted portal vein.[130] CT and MRI are also useful in establishing the diagnosis. Often, the initial manifestation of portal vein thrombosis is variceal bleeding in a noncirrhotic patient with normal liver function. Splenomegaly is another common finding.

Therapeutic options for the control of hemorrhage caused by portal vein thrombosis are esophageal variceal ligation and sclerotherapy. If unsuccessful, the distal splenorenal shunt is the preferred surgical treatment for patients with isolated portal vein thrombosis. In patients whose intrahepatic portal vein is patent (most commonly children), however, a shunt created by placing an internal jugular vein graft between the superior mesenteric vein and the patent left portal vein within the parenchyma of the liver (Rex shunt) may be the optimal therapeutic procedure for reestablishing physiologic portal flow.[130] This is the most elegant solution for portal obstruction because the portal pressure is reduced by restoring blood flow to the liver, preventing chronic hepatic atrophy and dysfunction, which can occur in a patient with long-standing portal decompression. In fact, in our practice, the Rex shunt is the first-line treatment and we reserve splenorenal shunting for patients who have no remnant intrahepatic portal system to receive the shunted blood.

Splenic Vein Thrombosis

Splenic vein thrombosis is most often caused by disorders of the pancreas, including acute and chronic pancreatitis, trauma, pancreatic malignancy, and pseudocysts. This association is related to the location of the splenic vein behind and close to the pancreas. Other causes include retroperitoneal masses, abscesses, and inflammatory bowel disease; the remaining cases are idiopathic. Gastric varices are present in approximately 80% of patients, and esophageal varices in 30% to 40%.[131] Isolated "sinistral" or left-sided portal hypertension occurs in the setting of normal liver function, and patients are readily cured with splenectomy, although observation for asymptomatic patients is acceptable.[131] The main indication for splenectomy is variceal hemorrhage.

Complications of Portal Hypertension

The most important complications of portal hypertension are gastrointestinal bleeding secondary to esophageal and gastric varices, ascites, and hepatic encephalopathy. The severity of portal hypertension and its complications and how amenable these conditions are to treatment with surgical intervention have been graded by a scoring scale initially called the *Child-Turcotte score* and subsequently modified to the *Child-Turcotte-Pugh score* (Table 60.9). These indices incorporate clinical and laboratory data as a means to assess the functional status of the liver, estimate hepatic reserve, and predict morbidity and mortality.[132] They have been adopted by the United Network for Organ Sharing (UNOS) as a tool for determining the need for liver transplantation. Child A patients have adequate hepatic reserve and survival rates similar to those of noncirrhotic patients, whereas Child C patients have mortality rates in excess of 50% and may not tolerate any intervention short of hepatic transplantation. Although initially used to determine the potential success of surgical interventions, these scores are now used globally to assess the prognosis for all patients with hepatic dysfunction.

Varices

One of the most life-threatening complications of portal hypertension is bleeding from esophageal varices. Esophageal varices are dilated veins found most commonly in the distal 5 cm of the esophagus. In the normal esophagus, a venous plexus is located in the submucosa; it becomes more superficially located to the lamina propria in the distal esophagus.[133,134] This more superficial location in the distal esophagus is consistent with the known increased occurrence of bleeding varices in that location. In addition, 10% to 15% of patients with esophageal varices have gastric varices.

The pressure in the portal system is an important determinant of the likelihood for varices to develop. Varices do not develop in persons with hepatic vein–portal vein gradients below 12 mm Hg. Pressure gradients above 12 mm Hg are invariably present in patients with varices, but this pressure does not necessarily produce varices in all patients. Other, undetermined factors must play a role. The prevalence of varices in patients with cirrhosis varies from 25% to 70%, depending on the severity of their liver disease.[135]

In approximately 10% of all patients presenting with acute upper gastrointestinal bleeding, esophageal varices are the cause of bleeding. Rates of bleeding from varices vary among studies. In a study of the natural history of varices in which patients were prospectively followed for 6 years, esophageal varices developed in approximately 8% of patients with cirrhosis each year during the first 2 years of observation; the percentage increased to 30% by 6 years. Of the patients who had small varices detected at initial endoscopy, large varices developed in 25%.[136] Other studies show an incidence of varices of up to 90% for patients with cirrhosis.[137,138] Once varices are present, bleeding occurs in 25% to 35% of cases, with the highest risk occurring within the first year after diagnosis.[139,140] Of patients who survive an episode of bleeding, 30% experience rebleeding within 6 weeks, and 70% at 1 year.[141,142] Mortality rates from bleeding varices range from 5% to 50%, with rates of 5%, less than 25%, and more than 50% for Child A, B, and C patients, respectively.[135,141]

TABLE 60.9 CLASSIFICATION

CHILD-TURCOTTE CRITERIA FOR HEPATIC FUNCTIONAL RESERVE

Criterion	Class A	Class B	Class C
Encephalopathy	None	Minimal	Advanced
Ascites	None	Easily controlled	Poorly controlled
Bilirubin (mg/dL)	<2	2–3	>3
Albumin (g/gL)	>3.5	3–3.5	<3
Nutrition	Excellent	Good	Poor, "wasting"

CHILD-TURCOTTE-PUGH GRADING OF SEVERITY OF LIVER DISEASE

Score	1	2	3
Encephalopathy	None	1 or 2	3 or 4
Ascites	None	Mild	Moderate
Bilirubin (mg/dL)	1–2	2.1–3	≥3.1
Albumin (g/dL)	≥3.5	2.8–3.5	≦2.7
Protime (s)	1–4	4.1–6	≥6.1
or INR	<1.7	1.7–2.3	>2.3
Grade A, 5–6; grade B, 7–9; grade C, 10–15.			

INR, international normalized ratio.

From Wantz GE, Payne MA. Experience with portacaval shunt for portal hypertension. *N Engl J Med* 1961;265:721, with permission.

TABLE 60.10

ENDOSCOPIC SIGNS THAT CORRELATE WITH RISK FOR VARICEAL RUPTURE

Basic color
White varices
Blue varices
Signs
Red color sign
Red wale marking
Cherry red spot
Hematocystic spot
Diffuse redness
Form
Linear
Tortuous
Large

Adapted from Japanese Research Society for Portal Hypertension.

The propensity for varices to bleed has been extensively studied. When combined with clinical data, certain endoscopic characteristics of varices have been correlated with initial episodes of bleeding (Table 60.10). These factors include variceal size, Child-Pugh class, and the presence of red wale markings (longitudinal dilated venules that resemble whip marks),[139] in addition to active alcohol consumption. Direct and indirect measurements of portal pressure have been used to predict the likelihood of bleeding, with hemorrhage occurring only in patients with portal—hepatic venous gradients above 12 mm Hg.[144,145]

Prevention of Initial Variceal Bleeding. Because of the severe consequences of variceal bleeding, methods to prevent first (primary prophylaxis) and recurrent (secondary prophylaxis) episodes of bleeding have been developed. These include control of the underlying cause of cirrhosis (i.e., alcohol consumption) and pharmacologic and surgical interventions to lower portal pressure. The next section discusses methods of primary prophylaxis to prevent initial episodes of bleeding (Table 60.11).

Beta blockade. Use of nonspecific β-adrenergic blockade has been studied extensively in randomized, controlled trials of the primary prophylaxis of variceal bleeding. The mechanism of action of these drugs (propranolol, nadolol) involves effects of both β_1-adrenergic and β_2-adrenergic blockade, including decreased cardiac output and increased splanchnic arteriolar vasoconstriction as a result of the loss of opposing β_2-adrenergic dilation.[145,146] The combined effects decrease portal blood flow and subsequently portal pressure.

These drugs are effective in portal hypertension associated with prehepatic, intrahepatic, and posthepatic conditions,[147,148] regardless of whether ascites is present.[149] Not all patients respond to therapy, however. Two meta-analyses have evaluated seven randomized, controlled trials comparing propranolol or nadolol with placebo in the prevention of initial variceal bleeding. Both analyses concluded that beta blockade is significantly correlated with a reduced incidence of bleeding. A reduction of 40% was noted overall after all trial results were combined, with bleeding developing in approximately 16% of treated and 27% of untreated patients. The goal of therapy is to reduce the hepatic vein–portal vein gradient to below 12 mm Hg or to more than 20% below baseline.[150]

In addition to reducing the number of first episodes of bleeding, beta blockade therapy has been shown to reduce

TABLE 60.11 TREATMENT

PREVENTION/TREATMENT OPTIONS FOR VARICEAL BLEEDING

Drug	Dose
Propranolol	10–20 mg bid titrated weekly maximum of 160 mg bid
Nadolol	20 mg orally qd, titrated to reduction of HR by 20%–25%, absolute HR of 55–60, symptoms
Isosorbide-5-mononitrate	20 mg orally tid
Vasopressin with nitroglycerin	0.4 U/min to maximum of 1.0 U/min, titrated to maintain SBP at approximately 100 mm Hg
Octreotide	50 mg bolus, followed by 50 mg/h for 5 days or until definitive treatment

HR, heart rate; SBP, systolic blood pressure.

Adapted from Rikkers LF. Variceal hemorrhage: surgical therapy. Gastroenterol Clin North Am 1993;22(4):821–842.

mortality in most clinical trials.[151–155] However, the differences were significant in only one study.[154] A meta-analysis of these studies concluded that mortality from bleeding is reduced in patients with large varices.[156]

Nitrates. Organic nitrates such as isosorbide-5-mononitrate, a vasodilator, have been used to reduce portal pressures. The possible mechanisms of action may include the following: (a) reflex splanchnic vasoconstriction secondary to peripheral venodilation and venous pooling; (b) decreased collateral resistance by arterial vasodilation; and (c) decreased intrahepatic resistance, possibly as a result of inhibition of stellate cell contractility.[157] These agents may be used alone in patients with contraindications to beta-blocker therapy, such as chronic obstructive pulmonary disease and congestive heart failure, or in combination with beta blockade in patients who do not have contraindications but respond inadequately to beta blocker therapy alone. Studies have indicated an enhanced reduction of portal pressure and a decreased incidence of bleeding in patients who receive combination therapy.[158,159] In the only study that compared combination therapy with beta blocker therapy alone, approximately 8% of patients treated with the combined regimen experienced bleeding, compared with 18% of patients treated with beta blocker therapy alone.[160] Thus, combination therapy may become the mainstay for prevention of bleeding in cirrhotic patients with varices.

Surgical intervention. In the 1950s and 1960s, surgeons created prophylactic portosystemic shunts in an attempt to prevent variceal bleeding. These procedures were studied in a randomized, controlled fashion and, although effective in preventing variceal bleeding, they caused an increased incidence of hepatic failure and encephalopathy and had no effect on overall survival.[161,162] Therefore, they are no longer performed for this indication.

Endoscopic sclerotherapy and variceal ligation. In the past, prophylactic sclerotherapy to prevent variceal bleeding was an accepted practice. An increased mortality in alcoholic patients treated with sclerotherapy, however, has been seen.[163] This therapeutic option is no longer used for the primary prevention of variceal bleeding. Investigations of the effectiveness of variceal ligation as a method of primary prophylaxis to prevent initial bleeding in high-risk patients with esophageal varices have reported mixed results.[164,165] In one study, no statistically significant differences in the incidence of initial bleeding and mortality were found in a comparison of patients after variceal ligation with controls.[164] A subgroup analysis revealed a significant decrease in the incidence of initial bleeding for Child-Pugh class B patients. In another report, a comparison of patients undergoing sclerotherapy or ligation with controls demonstrated a significant difference between both the sclerotherapy group and the ligation group versus the controls. Variceal ligation may be most appropriately indicated in primary prophylaxis in patients who do not tolerate beta-blocker therapy.

Treatment of Esophageal Variceal Bleeding

Initial management. Initial management of the patient with acute variceal includes the following: (a) establishment and maintenance of an airway; (b) hemodynamic monitoring; (c) placement of large-bore intravenous lines; (d) full laboratory investigation, including measurement of hemoglobin and hematocrit, coagulation profile, liver function tests, measurement of electrolytes, and assessment of renal function; (e) administration of blood products as needed, including packed red cells, platelets, and fresh frozen plasma; and (f) intensive care unit monitoring.

Pharmacologic therapy. Administration of vasoactive medications can be commenced almost immediately after patient presentation if the history and physical findings suggest variceal bleeding. This practice decreases the rate of bleeding and enhances the endoscopic ability to visualize the site(s) of bleeding.

Vasopressin (antidiuretic hormone) has potent splanchnic vasoconstrictive properties that decrease portal venous and collateral flow and reduce portal pressure. In randomized, prospective trials, as well as in a meta-analysis, continuous intravenous administration of vasopressin has proved to reduce variceal bleeding. When vasopressin was compared with placebo, bleeding stopped in an average of 52% of patients who received vasopressin and 18% of patients who received placebo.[166–168] Rates of rebleeding as high as 45% were noted, however. Because of coronary vasoconstrictive effects, vasopressin is often used in combination with a vasodilator, such as nitroglycerin.[169] The combination provides protection from adverse cardiac events and increases the effectiveness of vasopressin by decreasing intrahepatic and collateral resistance.[170,171] A meta-analysis of three randomized, controlled trials[172–174] confirmed the increased effectiveness of vasopressin and nitroglycerin in comparison with vasopressin alone. A derivative of vasopressin, terlipressin, has similar efficacy with fewer side effects,[172] but this drug is not available in the United States.

Somatostatin and octreotide, its longer acting eight-amino acid derivative, have been used extensively for the treatment of variceal bleeding. These agents decrease splanchnic blood flow indirectly by reducing the levels of other factors, such as glucagon, vasoactive intestinal peptide, and substance P, rather than by direct vasoconstriction.[175,176] The effects of somatostatin are limited to the splanchnic circulation, so that side effects are minimized.[177] A somatostatin and octreotide combination has proved to be as effective as vasopressin, sclerotherapy, and balloon tamponade in multiple studies.[178–184] Because of the lack of complications related to somatostatin therapy, octreotide is the initial drug of choice for the treatment of acute variceal hemorrhage.

Endoscopic interventions. The two main nonpharmacologic interventions for the treatment of variceal bleeding are endoscopic sclerotherapy and endoscopic variceal ligation. Both can be performed at the bedside. The technique of sclerotherapy (Fig. 60.6) entails performing upper gastrointestinal endoscopy with a flexible endoscope, visualizing the varices, and injecting 1 to 5 mL of sclerosing agent into or in close proximity to each varix. Sclerosing agents include sodium morrhuate, ethanolamine, polidocanol, and sodium tetradecyl sulfate. Total injection volume is 20 to 30 mL. The injections are begun at the distal esophagus and are continued circumferentially and proximally until all clinically relevant varices have been injected. Complications of sclerotherapy occur in 10% to 30% of patients and include fever, retrosternal chest pain (most common), dysphagia, and, more significantly, perforation with mediastinitis, bleeding from sclerosant-induced ulcers, esophageal stenosis, and sepsis. Overall, the treatment-related mortality rate is less than 2%. In the approximately 1% of patients in whom perforation occurs, the mortality rate

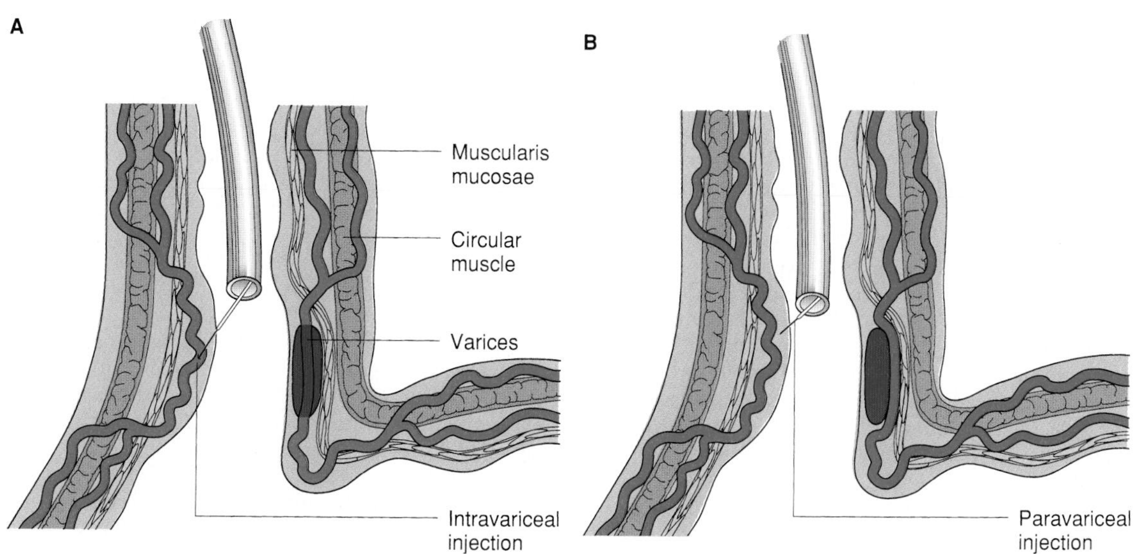

FIGURE 60.6 Techniques of intravariceal (*A*) and paravariceal (*B*) injection of esophageal varices.

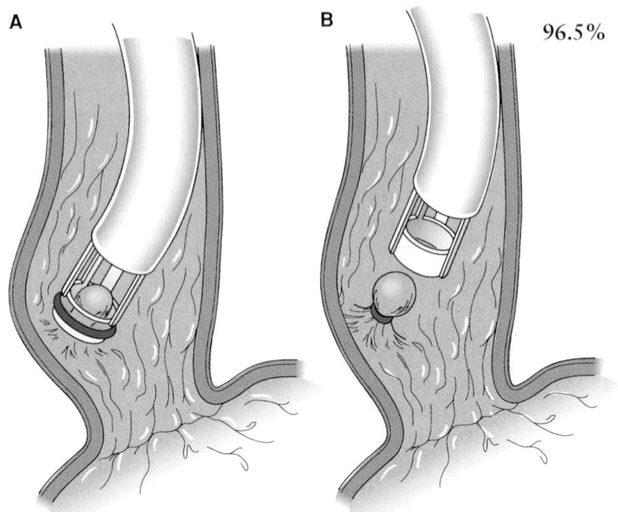

FIGURE 60.7 Endoscopic ligation of esophageal varices. The device used for ligation is based on the standard Barron-type ligator for the treatment of anal hemorrhoids. The esophageal varix is drawn up into the ligating device with suction (*A*), and the base of the varix is ligated with an O-ring (*B*). Up to six varices can be treated at a single session.

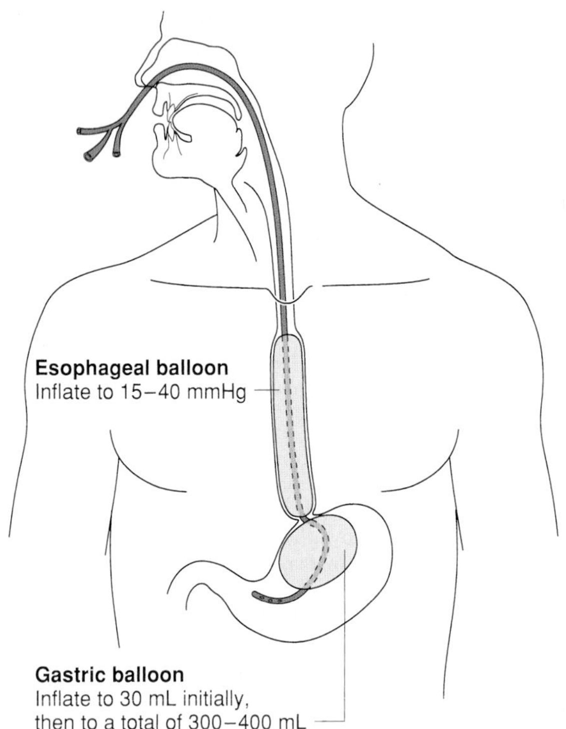

FIGURE 60.8 The Sengstaken-Blakemore tube is used to tamponade acutely bleeding gastroesophageal varices. The tube has three lumina—one to aspirate the stomach, another to inflate the gastric balloon, and a third to inflate the esophageal balloon. Patients treated with balloon tamponade should be in an intensive care unit, and endotracheal tubes should be placed in almost all to prevent aspiration.

may be as high as 50%. Success rates for initial control of variceal bleeding by sclerotherapy range from 60% to 90%,[185] but more than one session is required to stop bleeding completely in up to 95% of cases.

Although sclerotherapy has been the initial intervention of choice, it has been supplanted by endoscopic variceal ligation. The technique of ligation (Fig. 60.7) includes placing an endoscope over a sheath (which allows multiple insertions and removal of the endoscope), suctioning of a varix into the lumen of a plastic channel, and then placing a rubber band around the tissue. The procedure is similar to the ligation of hemorrhoids. The tissue then sloughs in 1 to 3 days, leaving a shallow ulcer. Up to six bands can be placed at each session. Newer endoscopes allow for the placement of multiple bands without removal of the endoscope. The placement of bands follows the same pattern as in sclerotherapy.

Success rates for variceal ligation range from 80% to 100%, in comparison with 77% to 94% for sclerotherapy, in controlled trials.[186–190] A meta-analysis[191] that examined these data and compared the results of seven randomized, controlled trials[186–190,192,193] indicated an equal or better success rate for variceal ligation than for sclerotherapy in eliminating esophageal variceal bleeding, with fewer complications. When patients who underwent ligation therapy were compared with patients who underwent sclerotherapy, a reduction of approximately 50% in the incidence of rebleeding (50% vs. 25%) and death from bleeding (17% vs. 10%) and a reduction of 30% in overall mortality (32% vs. 24%) were noted in the ligation group. In addition, the incidence of esophageal stricture, bleeding from treatment-related ulceration, and the number of treatment sessions were decreased with ligation. In patients with profuse bleeding, the type of endoscope used for variceal ligation may make visualization of the bleeding varices difficult. Some investigators choose to perform sclerotherapy in these patients and use variceal ligation once bleeding is somewhat controlled.

Balloon tamponade. The vast majority of patients (75% to 90%) with bleeding esophageal varices respond to endoscopic or pharmacologic therapy. For patients who fail these interventions, balloon tamponade (Fig. 60.8) is an alternative therapy with a high success rate in controlling bleeding. It entails the placement of a specialized nasogastric tube with two balloons that can be inflated separately and to different pressures. The most commonly used tubes are the Sengstaken-Blakemore tube and the Minnesota tube. The former consists of a gastric balloon and an esophageal balloon with a sump port for gastric suctioning. The latter tube has an additional port above the esophageal balloon for the aspiration of saliva and other material from the esophagus and pharynx.

Placement of these tubes begins with the establishment of a safe airway by endotracheal intubation. The tube is then passed through the nose and into the stomach. Radiographic confirmation that the tip of the tube is in the stomach is required before balloon inflation to prevent inadvertent intraesophageal inflation of the gastric balloon and resultant perforation. The gastric balloon is inflated with 200 mL of air and firmly pulled backward against the gastroesophageal junction to tamponade any proximal gastric bleeding. The esophageal balloon is then inflated to a pressure of 30 to 40 mm Hg, and the tube is secured to the patient by means of a face mask or helmet to ensure adequate stability of the tube and prevent inadvertent removal.

Because of the possible complications of balloon tamponade (e.g., aspiration, esophageal and gastric perforation, necrosis), which occur in 10% to 20% of patients, its use is restricted to approximately 24 hours. Success rates for cessation of bleeding are 70% to 80%, but more than half of all patients rebleed when the balloons are deflated. Although this method is highly effective in the initial control of bleeding, with an efficacy similar to that of pharmacologic agents, because of its transient effects it can be used only as a temporizing measure in anticipation of a more definitive procedure (e.g., TIPS, placement of a surgical shunt, or transplantation) and is used only after endoscopic and pharmacologic therapies have failed.

Transjugular intrahepatic portasystemic shunt. In the 10% to 20% of patients who continue to bleed or who have early rebleeding, a shunt procedure (to bypass the high-pressure hepatic vascular bed) may be indicated. The mortality rate associated with failure to control bleeding can be as high as 90%,[194] and surgically created shunts in this setting are associated with a high morbidity and mortality rate.

The transjugular intrahepatic portosystemic shunt (Fig. 60.9) has become first-line treatment for bleeding esophageal varices when the above-mentioned attempts fail. After ultrasonographic confirmation of patency of the portal vein, the procedure is performed in the interventional radiology suite, where a wire-guided stent (8 to 12 mm in diameter) is placed

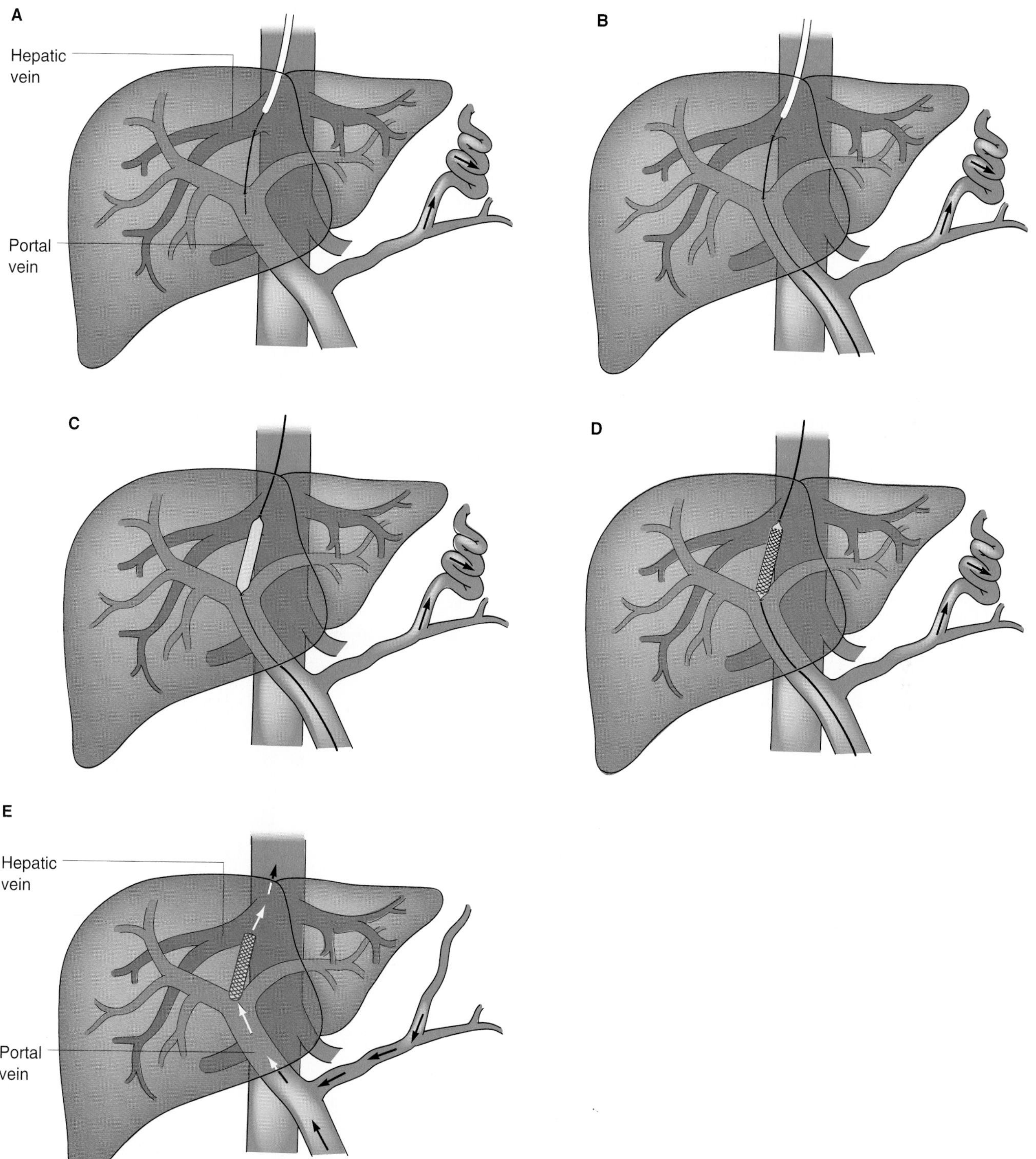

FIGURE 60.9 Schematic representation of the steps used to create a transjugular intrahepatic portosystemic shunt. (From Zemel G, Katzen BT, Becker GJ, et al. Percutaneous transjugular portosystemic shunt. *JAMA* 1991;266:390, with permission.)

percutaneously into the jugular vein. The wire is then guided through the superior vena cava, right atrium, and inferior vena cava into a hepatic vein, after which the catheter traverses the hepatic parenchyma and joins the hepatic vein to a portal vein. This connection effectively creates a side-to-side portacaval shunt. Success rates in the cessation of variceal bleeding are as high as 90% to 100%, with an incidence of recurrent bleeding of approximately 10%.[195,196]

The therapeutic goal is to reduce the hepatic–portal venous pressure gradient to below 12 mm Hg. TIPS reduces the portosystemic pressure gradient to a mean of approximately 9 to 15 mm Hg (average, 10 mm Hg) or to 40% to 62% below baseline.[197,198] Mortality rates are high (40% to 60% at 6 to 7 weeks) despite the relative noninvasiveness of the procedure and reflect the gravity of the clinical condition of most patients requiring this intervention.[195,196] One potential cause of the high mortality is a delay in instituting the TIPS until multiple unsuccessful attempts at sclerotherapy or banding have been made. This delay allows the patient's hepatic function and overall stability to deteriorate.

As with all portosystemic shunts, a significant complication of TIPS is the development of hepatic encephalopathy. After placement of a TIPS, the incidence of hepatic encephalopathy rises from 10% before treatment to 25%,[199] and the incidence of progression to accelerated liver failure is approximately 3% to 5%.[194]

Although in early series, stenoses or occlusion of the stent developed in up to 50% to 60% of patients in the first year, long-term patency can be maintained by ongoing surveillance of the shunt with redilatation, as needed. Shunt stenosis is managed angiographically with thrombolytic therapy, dilation, or replacement of the stent. The newest shunts are lined with polytetrafluoroethylene (PTFE) and seem to have a much higher patency than the original permeable Wallstents.[200] Patients are usually followed at 3-month intervals by ultrasonography to assess the patency of the shunt. At 6 months of follow-up, 92% of patients had had no episodes of rebleeding, and 82% were free of hemorrhage at 1 year.[124] It is safe to assert that the TIPS is now the standard procedure used to halt bleeding in patients who fail medical therapy. The ability to effectively decompress the portal circulation without open surgery in these critically ill patients has transformed clinical hepatology. Patients become medically stable and can be evaluated for transplantation electively. Patients with reversible liver disease (e.g., abstinent alcoholics) may recover fully without further intervention because the TIPS will slowly close as the liver heals.

Surgical Decompression

Background. Surgeons have been performing shunt procedures since the 1800s. The first was an end-to-side portacaval shunt with ligation of the distal portal vein, performed by Nicolai Eck (Eck fistula) in dogs. In 1945, Whipple and Blakemore at the Columbia-Presbyterian Medical Center in New York performed this shunt for the first time for the indication of variceal bleeding.[201] This group was also responsible for the development of the tube for the tamponade of bleeding esophageal varices, which adopted the name of Blakemore, as discussed previously.

Surgical interventions for the treatment of bleeding varices are divided into three main types: (a) liver transplantation, (b) shunt procedures, and (c) devascularization procedures. The only definitive procedure for the treatment of portal hypertension caused by cirrhosis is orthotopic liver transplantation, and the success of this option during the past two decades has revolutionized the treatment of portal hypertension and its complications in patients with end-stage liver disease. However, for the treatment of portal hypertension in patients without cirrhosis or in those whose liver function does not warrant a transplant (e.g., patients with portal vein thrombosis), decompressive surgically created shunts or devascularization procedures may be performed.

Shunts. Surgical shunts can be divided into three categories: (a) totally diverting shunts, (b) partially diverting shunts, and (c) selective shunts. Total shunts are created by completely bypassing the flow of blood away from the liver. Examples include the end-to-side portacaval shunt (Eck fistula) (Fig. 60.10) and the large-diameter (>10 mm) side-to-side portacaval (Fig 60.11), mesocaval, and central splenorenal shunts. These large side-to-side shunts divert all blood flow through the path of least resistance, so that flow in the portal vein, which becomes the outflow tract for portal blood flow, is reversed. One of the causes of ascites in patients with portal hypertension is high pressure at the level of the hepatic sinusoids. The main difference between end-to-side and side-to-side shunts is that maintenance of high pressure with end-to-side shunts may worsen ascites, whereas side-to-side procedures effectively relieve this problem by reducing sinusoidal pressure. Complete portal blood flow diversion lowers portal pressure and is highly effective in the treatment of bleeding esophageal varices.

The main complications of totally diverting shunts are a worsening of liver function and hepatic encephalopathy as a result of decreased flow through the liver and loss of hepatotropic factors from the mesenteric venous system. Another disadvantage of portocaval shunts is that the porta hepatis

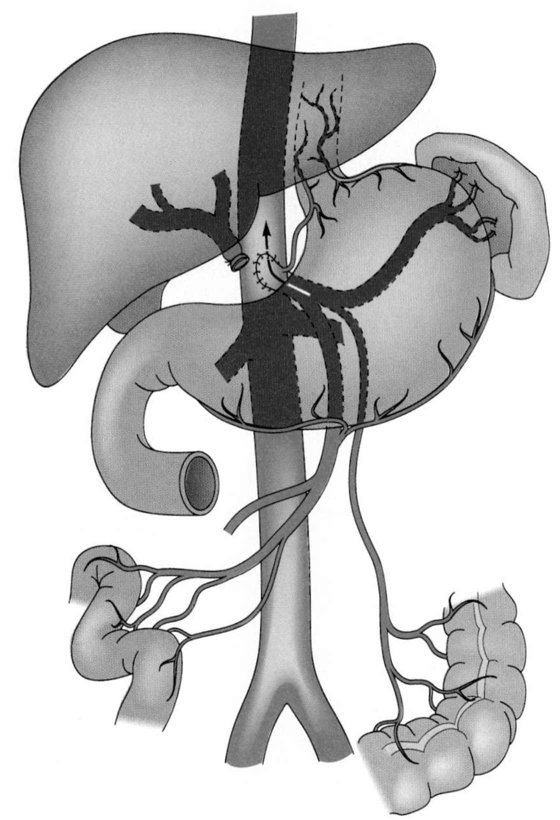

FIGURE 60.10 End-to-side portacaval shunt, also referred to as an Eck fistula. The portal vein is divided, the hepatic limb of the portal vein is ligated, and the splanchnic end of the portal vein is anastomosed end-to-side to the vena cava. All portal blood is necessarily diverted into the vena cava, and the hepatic limb of the portal vein cannot serve as an outflow tract.

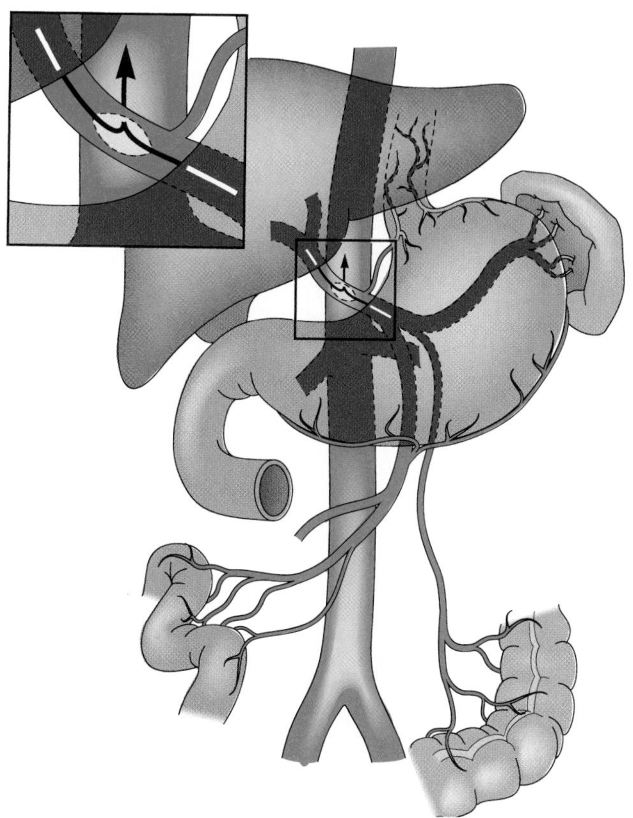

FIGURE 60.11 Side-to-side portacaval shunt. An anastomosis is made between the side of the portal vein and the side of the inferior vena cava. With a shunt of standard diameter, almost all splanchnic blood is diverted around the liver into the low-pressure vena cava. The hepatic limb of the portal vein serves as an outflow tract from the liver toward the low-pressure vena cava.

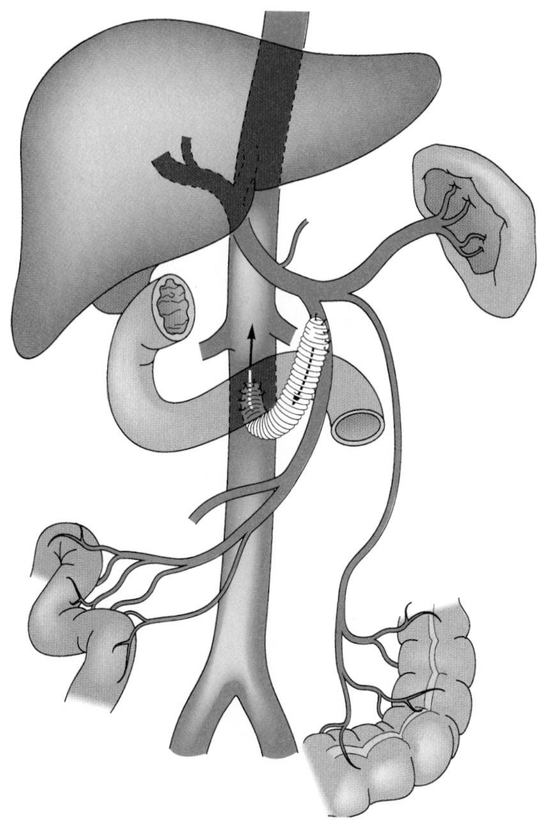

FIGURE 60.12 Interposition mesocaval shunt. A plastic prosthesis or an autogenous internal jugular vein is used for the shunt. One end is anastomosed to the inferior vena cava, and the other end is anastomosed to the trunk of the superior mesenteric vein. The shunt curves around the lower edge of the third portion of the duodenum and is sometimes called a C-shunt.

must be dissected, so that future surgical procedures in the area (e.g., liver transplantation) are more difficult.

Partially diverting shunts allow for the maintenance of hepatopetal flow while decompressing the high pressures in the portal system. The original shunts were larger than 10 mm in diameter and were able to create a gradient between the portal vein and vena cava that maintained some prograde hepatic flow. All these shunts, however, dilated over time and became complete shunts in that the portal vein-to-inferior vena cava pressure gradient disappeared. The small-diameter (8 mm) side-to-side mesocaval (Fig. 60.12) and portacaval (Sarfeh) (Fig. 60.13) shunts are performed with an interposition graft made of either expanded PTFE or Dacron. A significant component of the Sarfeh procedure is ligation of the coronary (left gastric), gastroepiploic, and other collateral veins. Bleeding from varices resolves in more than 90% of patients.[202,203] This smaller-diameter shunt has a higher resistance than the larger shunt, is synthetic and therefore does not dilate, can maintain hepatic perfusion and is associated with a lower incidence of hepatic encephalopathy. With these shunts, portal pressure gradients can be reduced to the critical 12 mm Hg while hepatopetal flow is maintained in up to 80% to 90% of patients.[204] In addition, the maintenance of mesenteric pressure at or relatively close to normal levels may prevent the hyperammonemia associated with total shunts.[205] One relatively common complication is graft thrombosis, which occurs in up to 16% of patients.[202] Shunt thrombosis can usually be treated angiographically. Dissection at the porta hepatis leads to the formation of adhesions, which may compromise later liver transplantation.

Selective shunts are designed to create two separate drainage systems within the portal venous network. A high pressure is maintained within the mesenteric system and a low pressure is created in the esophagogastric system by shunting blood from the latter into the systemic circulation without decompressing the mesenteric network. The most frequently used selective shunt is the distal splenorenal shunt (Fig. 60.14).[206] Another rarely used selective shunt is the coronary–caval shunt.[203] The distal splenorenal shunt selectively decompresses the gastroesophageal venous system through an anastomosis between the distal end of the splenic vein and the side of the renal vein. Decompression occurs through the short gastric veins, which are in continuity with the splenic vein. In addition, as in the small side-to-side shunts described above, collateral veins must be ligated.

Advantages to this procedure are the following: (a) Control of bleeding is excellent in more than 90% of patients; (b) no dissection of the porta hepatis is required; (c) hepatopetal flow is maintained; and (d) the incidence of encephalopathy (5% to 24%) and progressive liver failure is lower.[207–210] Experience with this shunt has revealed that most patients have hepatopetal flow, with 84% of alcoholic and 90% of nonalcoholic patients having prograde flow at 4 years after surgery.[211,212] Some loss of prograde portal flow does occur as a result of either portal vein thrombosis (approximately 10% of patients) or increased flow through collaterals located along the pancreas. This latter mechanism can be prevented by complete dissection of the splenic vein from the posterior aspect of the pancreas (splenopancreatic disconnection),[212] but this additional technique adds to the complexity of the operative procedure and to the incidence of complications.

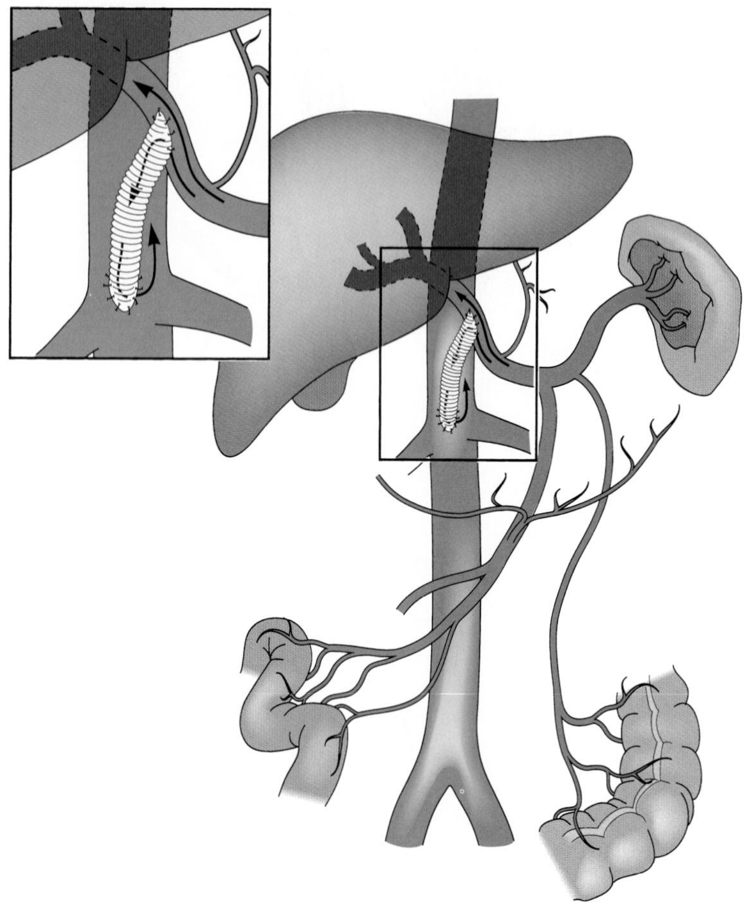

FIGURE 60.13 Small-diameter interposition portacaval Sarfeh shunt. A vascular prosthesis measuring 8 to 10 mm in diameter is interposed between the side of the vena cava and the side of the portal vein. The goal is to reduce portal pressure partially and thereby prevent variceal hemorrhage but still maintain sufficient pressure to permit the prograde flow of portal blood to the liver. This procedure is simpler to perform than that for the Warren shunt and theoretically avoids the problem of diversion of an increasing proportion of portal blood away from the liver over time, as occurs with the Warren shunt.

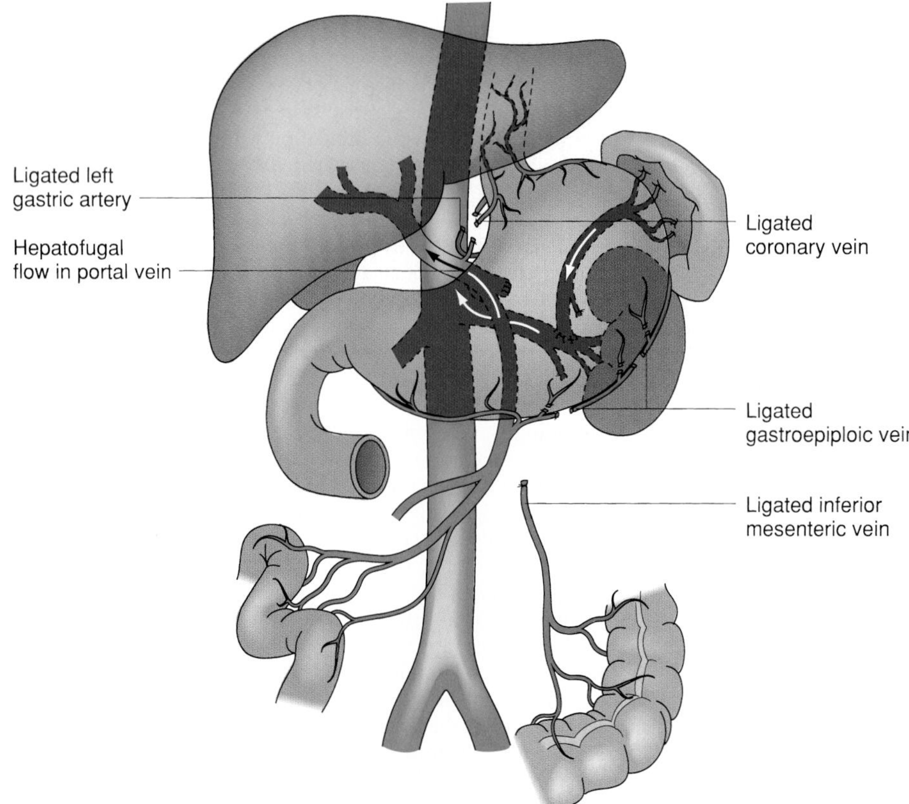

FIGURE 60.14 Distal splenorenal Warren shunt. The splenic vein is divided near its junction with the superior mesenteric vein. The distal end of the splenic vein is anastomosed to the renal vein. Varices are selectively decompressed through the stomach and short gastric veins into the splenic vein and then into the vena cava through the renal vein. Portal hypertension is maintained in the portal and superior mesenteric veins to provide enough pressure to drive portal blood through the diseased liver.

The distal splenorenal shunt is relatively contraindicated in patients with significant ascites. Because no portal venous decompression occurs, ascites may increase after a distal splenorenal shunt is created. In addition, ligation of collateral vessels and lymphatics during the procedure contributes to increased portal pressures and subsequent increase in ascites. Patients with small splenic veins (<8 mm) have a relatively high incidence of shunt thrombosis.[213]

Several trials comparing side-to-side total shunts with the distal splenorenal shunt found that they are equally effective (>90%) in stopping variceal hemorrhage.[214] The incidence of hepatic encephalopathy is lower after the distal splenorenal shunt, with rates of 36% and 15% for the total and selective shunts, respectively. Rates of rebleeding were similar and ranged from zero to 30%, with no survival advantage for either procedure.

Investigators have also used the side-to-side nonselective total shunt for the emergency treatment of bleeding varices.[215] Bleeding stopped in more than 90% of patients with medical therapy alone, although bleeding often restarted shortly thereafter. Bleeding stopped in all patients after surgery, and 99% of patients were completely free of episodes of rebleeding. The 5-year survival was approximately 80%, with the majority of deaths occurring during the first year after surgery as a result of progressive hepatic failure. Hepatic encephalopathy requiring recurrent intervention, including dietary restriction and lactulose or neomycin therapy, occurred in 8% of patients. These data support an aggressive, systematic approach to caring for these patients before, during, and after surgery.

Devascularization procedures. Devascularization procedures are nonshunting techniques in which the venous drainage of the stomach and esophagus is disconnected from the liver and intestinal vessels. These procedures are relatively less technically demanding than shunting procedures and can be performed in patients with extensive portal thromboses that preclude other options. They do not interfere with hepatopetal blood flow and therefore do not increase the incidence of hepatic encephalopathy.

The procedures range in complexity from simple esophageal transection and reanastomosis with an end-to-end anastomosis (EEA) stapler combined with ligation of the coronary vein (Fig. 60.15) to the Sugiura procedure (Fig. 60.16). The Sugiura procedure requires both abdominal and thoracic incisions, through which a splenectomy, devascularization of the proximal stomach and esophagus, transection of the esophagus with reanastomosis, and ligation of all gastroesophageal collaterals are performed.[216] The latter procedure can also be performed via a single abdominal incision.[217] Bleeding recurs in fewer than 5% of patients in Japan, but rates of rebleeding range from 10% to 54% in other countries.[216,218] Operative mortality rates range from 10% to 35%.[218]

Four controlled trials have compared devascularization procedures with sclerotherapy.[214,219–221] Although esophageal transection appeared to be associated with a lower incidence of rebleeding, the mortality rates were higher.

Hepatic transplantation. Liver transplantation is the definitive therapy for portal hypertension and cirrhosis and the complications thereof. The limited number of organs and the potential complications of this procedure make it one of last resort. Only patients with end-stage liver disease (Child C patients with cirrhosis) are candidates for transplantation. When successful, transplantation treats both the underlying disease and any acute complication.

Algorithm for the treatment of variceal bleeding. Treatment recommendations assume the following: (a) adequate expertise in all aspects of caring for cirrhotic patients, including expert endoscopy and interventional radiology; (b) the availability of trained surgeons capable of performing the indicated surgical procedures; and (c) the availability of hepatic transplantation or transfer to a center where it is available (Algorithm 60.1).

Resuscitation and primary control. At presentation, patients should immediately undergo resuscitation and hemodynamic monitoring, followed by establishment of the diagnosis of variceal bleeding. A pharmacologic agent should be commenced immediately in the emergency department, consisting of octreotide or beta blockade, or both. Second-tier agents include vasopressin and nitroglycerin. Upper gastrointestinal endoscopy should be performed expeditiously in the appropriate setting to attempt variceal ligation. Sclerotherapy is a second choice. Rapid triage is imperative, and repeated attempts at endoscopic therapy in the setting of continued bleeding may lead to worsening of the patient's overall status and increased morbidity and mortality. For the majority of patients (75% to 90%), these interventions will be effective in controlling the hemorrhage. If rebleeding occurs, another attempt at endoscopic therapy is warranted while preparations are made for decompressive therapy in the event of treatment failure. In the relatively small number of patients in whom primary control is not achieved, balloon tamponade is usually the next

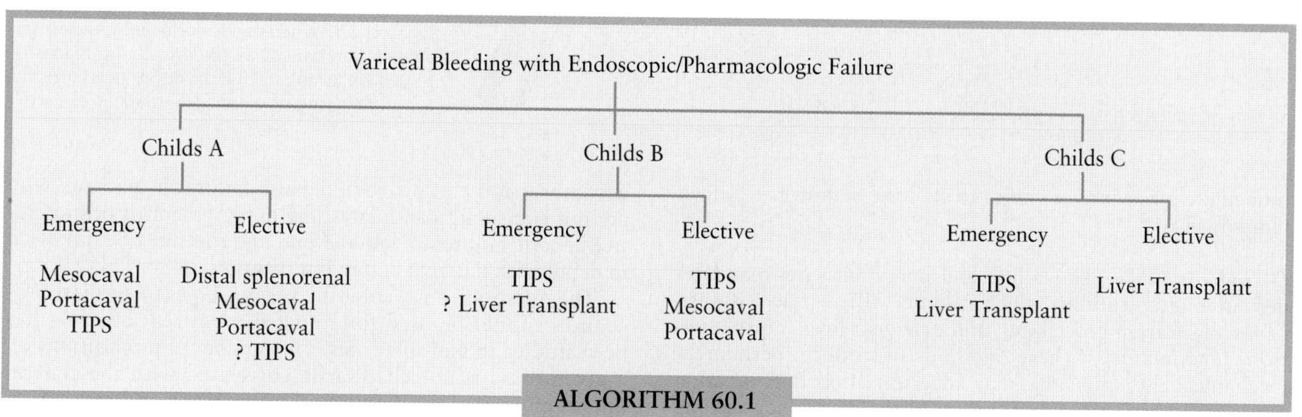

ALGORITHM 60.1 Suggested treatment options, in order of preference, for patients who fail medical management for variceal bleeding.

PANCREAS/LIVER

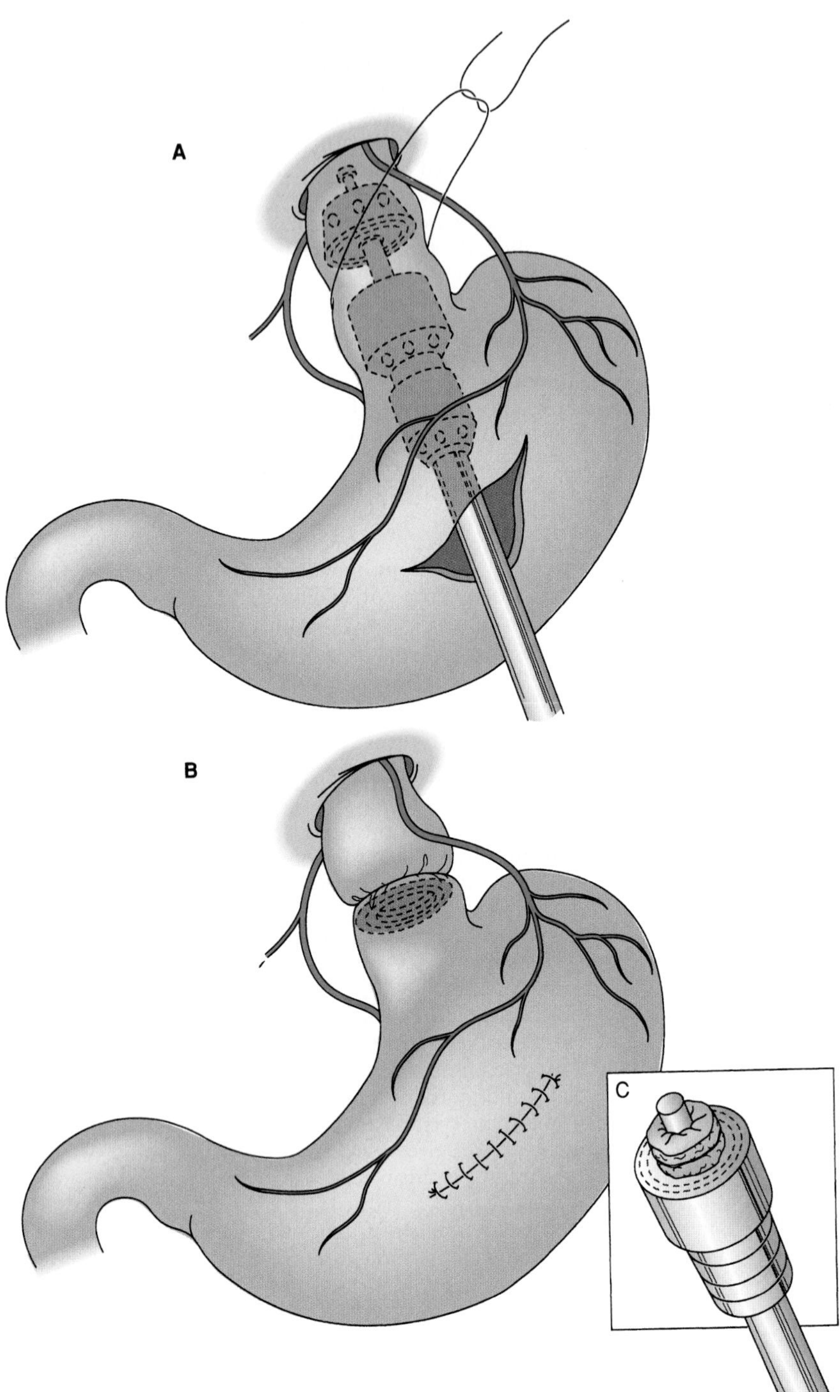

FIGURE 60.15 Transection and reanastomosis of the distal esophagus with the stapling device to control variceal hemorrhage. (*A*) A stapling device is inserted through a small gastrotomy incision. (*B*) When the device is fired, the esophagus is simultaneously transected and reanastomosed with staples. (*C*) If the device fires correctly, a complete ring of esophageal tissue is excised.

immediate procedure of choice to stop the hemorrhage, albeit temporarily.

Definitive control. The failure of primary measures mandates definitive interventions, which include TIPS, surgical shunts, devascularization procedures, and emergent liver transplantation (uncommon). These methods introduce permanent mechanical alterations that may adversely affect liver function and are of varying practical utility in the emergency setting. Proper decision making requires primary stratification based on hepatic function and secondary stratification according to treatment setting (emergent vs. elective). It is critical that the issue of eligibility for hepatic transplantation be addressed before these interventions are undertaken because portal decompression can provoke hepatic failure. In patients who are not transplant candidates, the development of postoperative hepatic failure is a lethal event, and this must be discussed in detail with patients before intervention.

The question of which of the various types of surgical procedures should be used for emergency variceal bleeding has been studied in multiple trials. The number of publications on a given topic is not necessarily correlated with the general applicability of a specific surgical intervention and may reflect the referral pattern or hospital system in which the studies were performed. As in all complex operative procedures, the technical ability of an individual surgeon to perform a given procedure is crucial to its success and is correlated with complications. The following recommendations are based on the

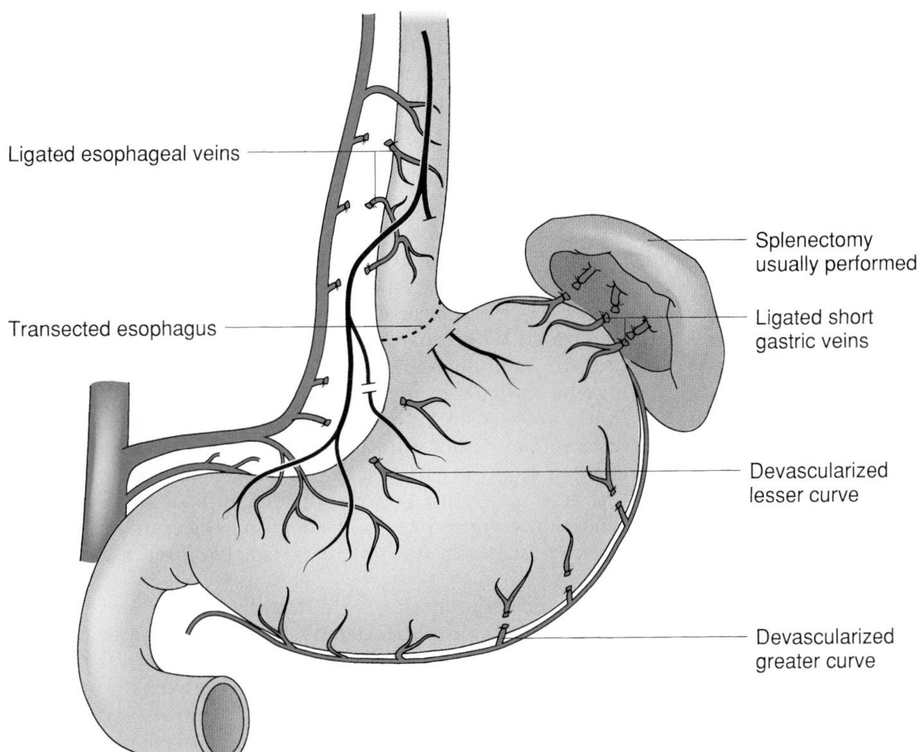

FIGURE 60.16 Sugiura esophageal transection and devascularization operation.

assumption that well-trained surgeons are performing these procedures.

Patients with well-compensated liver function (Child's A) rarely fail to respond to pharmacologic and endoscopic therapy. Patients who continue to bleed should undergo TIPS, particularly if they are potential transplant candidates. TIPS does not disturb surgical anatomy and avoids the technical difficulty associated with transplantation in patients with previous shunts of any type. The rare patients with anticipated long-term survival without a transplant may be candidates for a distal splenorenal shunt. Excellent results have also been reported in this setting with small-diameter portacaval H-graft shunts. The arguments for the H-graft are that it is technically easier to perform and provides excellent control of bleeding. In addition, it is associated with high rates of long-term maintenance of prograde portal flow and patency and low rates of hepatic encephalopathy and mortality. Similar arguments can be made for the small-diameter mesocaval H-graft shunts. Mesocaval shunts have the added advantage of eliminating the need for portal dissection and subsequent adhesion formation.

In the hemodynamically unstable Child A cirrhotic patient, a TIPS is the procedure of choice. If this is not an option, nonselective side-to-side portacaval or mesocaval shunt can be performed for immediate control of bleeding. For patients who are noncompliant or live far from tertiary care medical centers capable of performing and maintaining the TIPS, a simple operation such as the side-to-side shunt, which requires comparatively little follow-up, may be more appropriate.

Hemodynamically stable Child B patients with cirrhosis without medically untreatable ascites who are transplant candidates can be treated with a TIPS or with a distal splenorenal or mesocaval shunt to avoid dissection in the porta hepatis. Unstable patients may undergo the same procedures, with the caveat that the distal splenorenal shunt should be avoided. If the patient has medically uncontrollable ascites, a TIPS is the procedure of choice. Small-diameter shunts are less effective for patients with ascites.

For Child C patients with cirrhosis, the options are much more limited. These patients should undergo TIPS, with the expectation that liver function will deteriorate and hepatic encephalopathy may worsen unless urgent transplant can be performed. In nontransplant candidates who fail nonoperative therapy and continue to bleed, TIPS may be life saving in the short term, but many patients will die of progressive liver failure.

Currently, the only indication for devascularization procedures is the presence of extensive thrombosis in the portal vessels, which precludes the use of a shunt.

In conclusion, open surgical intervention for patients with portal hypertension is becoming a rarity. With the advent of TIPS, the indications for surgically created shunts are dwindling. Child A patient with cirrhosis may become the only true candidates for surgically created shunts in the setting of esophageal variceal bleeding, with most Child B patients undergoing the TIPS procedure. Although some studies have shown an increased need for reintervention in patients who have undergone TIPS for variceal bleeding,[222] the overwhelming efficacy and safety of TIPS has essentially settled the issue and today, even in large liver centers, open portal decompressive procedures are rarely performed.

Prevention of recurrent variceal bleeding. The risk for rebleeding in untreated patients with a history of prior variceal bleeding ranges from 47% to 70%, with an associated mortality rate of 20% to 70%.[163] The risk factors for subsequent bleeding from esophageal varices are the same as those for initial bleeding and include continued alcohol abuse, size of varices, Child class, and the presence of red markings on endoscopic evaluation.

Multiple randomized trials,[223–232] including a meta-analysis,[163] have shown a reduction in rebleeding rates with the use of beta-blocker therapy in comparison with placebo. Mortality rates were reduced in most of those trials. All patients without a contraindication to beta-blocker therapy should be treated with one of these agents. In addition, combination therapy with beta blockade and nitrates reduces rates of rebleeding in comparison with either agent alone.[233]

As indicated in the section on treatment of bleeding varices, endoscopic variceal ligation has surpassed sclerotherapy in stopping bleeding. Moreover, in preventing rebleeding, variceal ligation has proved to be at least as effective as sclerotherapy, with fewer complications, and has become the endoscopic intervention of choice.[234]

Almost 10 randomized trials have been performed to compare endoscopic intervention with TIPS.[235–243] The vast majority of data support the use of TIPS, which is associated with significantly decreased rates of rebleeding (approximately 25% less) and no increase in mortality. Because the incidence of significant encephalopathy is doubled, however, TIPS should be reserved for patients who fail other means of therapy.

Many randomized trials have compared endoscopic sclerotherapy with elective shunt surgery to prevent recurrent bleeding from esophageal varices.[244–248] The majority used the distal splenorenal shunt. Rates of rebleeding varied from 3% to 17% for shunts and from 35% to 60% for sclerotherapy, with no difference in overall survival. For good-risk patients without medically intractable ascites, the distal splenorenal shunt appears to be a better option to prevent recurrent variceal bleeding than repetitive sclerotherapy.

Gastropathy and Gastric Varices. Approximately 10% of patients with esophageal varices also have gastric varices. Conversely, about 90% of patients with gastric varices have esophageal varices.[249–252] Bleeding from gastric varices occurs in approximately 25% of affected patients, is usually more severe than bleeding from esophageal varices, and is poorly controlled by sclerotherapy. Rebleeding occurs in up to 30% of patients after an initial bleed.[252] The same pharmacologic interventions used for esophageal varices are used to treat gastric varices. Balloon tamponade may also be used. The surgical procedure of choice for bleeding gastric varices is the distal splenorenal shunt.

Portal hypertensive gastropathy is a condition characterized by dilation of the venules and capillaries of the gastric mucosa without associated inflammation.[253,254] The major complication of gastropathy is bleeding; gastropathy accounts for 4% to 38% of all episodes of acute bleeding in patients with cirrhosis.[255,256]

Ascites

One of the most important consequences of hepatic dysfunction in cirrhosis and portal hypertension is ascites. This development portends a significant worsening of the patient's condition, with markedly decreased survival rates. Ascites is defined as the accumulation of free fluid within the abdominal cavity (normally <150 mL). Causes of ascites are listed in Table 60.12. In cirrhosis, the fluid is derived from a combination of hepatic (high in protein) and splanchnic (low in protein) lymph that cannot be absorbed as a result of the increased hydrostatic pressures within the liver and splanchnic systems secondary to cirrhosis and capillarization of the space of Disse. Because of the loss of sinusoidal fenestrations and a subsequent decrease in their permeability, splanchnic lymph is more abundant than hepatic lymph in patients with advancing cirrhosis,, so that the protein content of ascitic fluid is relatively low.[257] The main underlying pathophysiology in the development of ascites is renal sodium retention and associated water retention, which lead to fluid overload. Peripheral vasodilation and lower pressures are thought to be secondary to the dilator effects of nitric oxide, glucagon, and prostaglandins[136] on nascent arteriovenous shunts present throughout the splanchnic vascular system, as well as in muscle, skin, and brain.[258] The severity of liver disease is not uniformly correlated with the presence or absence of ascites.

Clinical and Laboratory Features. Ascites may be present in patients with cirrhosis who have no other overt signs or symptoms. Patients may present with subtle signs of weight gain and an inability to fit into clothes. Physical examination reveals shifting dullness to percussion (1.5 L of ascitic fluid), fluid waves (10 L), and bulging flanks.[258] With progression of disease and massive ascites, respiratory status may be compromised secondary to increased intraabdominal pressure and pleural effusions, which are often present and usually located on the right side. The progression may be slow or more rapid after an inciting event, such as a variceal bleed or infection.

Stigmata of poor liver function include peripheral muscle wasting, palmar erythema, spider angiomas, peripheral edema, a palpable liver, and caput medusae (dilated periumbilical veins). With progressive ascites and increased abdominal pressure, umbilical and inguinal hernias often develop and may be difficult to manage. Abdominal distention may be caused by gastrointestinal gas rather than ascites. Gas can be differentiated from fluid by eliciting hyperresonance to percussion, secondary to gas, as opposed to dullness with fluid. The most widely used test for the diagnosis of ascites is ultrasonography, which can also be helpful in determining the best location for therapeutic and diagnostic paracentesis.

Diagnostic Paracentesis. The differential diagnosis of ascites is presented in Table 60.12. Determination of the character of the ascitic fluid is helpful in establishing the diagnosis. Paracentesis may be performed in the midline, midway between the umbilicus and the pubic symphysis. The fluid from patients with cirrhosis is usually straw-colored and clear; measurements of protein (usually <2 g/dL), quantitative cell counts, and microbiologic culture and determination of pH, amylase, glucose, and albumin levels should be obtained. The serum-to-ascitic fluid albumin-gradient (SAG) is calculated by subtracting the albumin concentration in ascites from the level found in serum. This gradient is helpful in determining the cause of ascites; high values (>1.1 g/dL) are generally associated with portal hypertension,

TABLE 60.12 DIAGNOSIS

DIFFERENTIAL DIAGNOSIS OF ASCITES

PORTAL HYPERTENSION
Cirrhosis and other intrahepatic diseases
Hepatic congestion
  Congestive heart failure
  Constrictive pericarditis
  Inferior vena cava obstruction
  Budd-Chiari syndrome
Portal vein occlusion

HYPOALBUMINEMIA
Nephrotic syndrome
Protein-losing enteropathy
Malnutrition

MISCELLANEOUS DISORDERS
Myxedema
Ovarian disease (Meigs' syndrome, struma ovarii)
Peritoneal carcinomatosis
End-stage renal disease
Chylous ascites
Bile ascites
Urine ascites

From Sleisenger MH, Fordran JS. *Gastrointestinal disease: pathophysiology, diagnosis and management*, 4th ed. Philadelphia: WB Saunders, 1989:433.

TABLE 60.13 TREATMENT

TREATMENT OF ASCITES

Bed rest
Sodium restriction
1–2 g/d (45–90 mEq/d)
Fluid restriction
1–1.5 L/d
Diuretics
Spironolactone
50 mg po q8h
maximum of 100 mg q6h
Furosemide
40–370 mg/d
Antibiotics
Cefotaxime
2 q IV q12h
Ofloxacin
400 mg po q12h
Prophylaxis
Norfloxacin
400 mg/d while hospitalized
Ciprofloxacin
750 mg po weekly
Norfloxacin
400 mg/d for 6 mo
Trimethoprim/sulfamethoxazole
One double-strength table 5 times a week

whereas lower levels may be associated with other disorders, including malignancy.

Treatment. Initial therapy is usually directed at control of renal sodium and water retention, with bed rest and dietary manipulation. The upright position exacerbates sodium retention as a result of venous pooling and relative hypovolemia. Up to 15% of patients respond to this therapy alone with a natriuresis. A low-sodium diet is a critical part of the management of patients with cirrhosis (1 to 2 g of sodium per day or 45 to 90 mEq/d). A major problem with a strict low-sodium diet is lack of palatability and poor compliance. Fluid restriction is also an essential component of therapy in patients in whom hyponatremia develops (sodium concentration <125 mEq/L), with only 1,000 to 1,500 mL of fluid allowed each day.

For the 85% to 95% of patients who do not respond to bed rest and fluid and salt restriction, the mainstay of treatment is diuresis (Table 60.13). The loop diuretic furosemide and the potassium-sparing diuretic spironolactone are the two most widely used agents, and they can be combined to minimize side effects and maximize effectiveness. A diuresis of approximately 500 mL/day is the goal for patients with mild ascites and of up to 1 to 2 L/day for patients with both ascites and peripheral edema. More than 90% of patients respond to the combination of dietary manipulation and diuretics.[259]

Complications of the use of spironolactone include painful breast enlargement in males, hyperkalemia, and metabolic acidosis. Complications of the more potent furosemide include prerenal azotemia, which occurs in approximately 20% of patients as a result of excessive diuresis and hypovolemia.[258] Additional complications include hyponatremia and encephalopathy.

Large-volume paracentesis (removal of 4 to 6 L of ascitic fluid per day) and total paracentesis are techniques that can be used for patients with large amounts of fluid who are experiencing symptoms and are not responding to the above-mentioned therapeutic endeavors. Patients requiring paracentesis usually have severe underlying liver disease and a 1-year survival rate of 25%.[260] The technique of paracentesis involves placing a catheter into the abdominal cavity, either in the lower midline or in one of the lower quadrants. Care is taken to enter lateral to the rectus muscle and avoid the inferior epigastric artery. More than 30 L of fluid can be removed by means of total paracentesis, with 6 to 10 g of albumin infused for each liter of ascitic fluid removed.[258] The albumin commonly is administered in the form of 25% albumin (12.5 g/50 mL). Controversy exists regarding the need for albumin replacement therapy in patients undergoing total paracentesis and repetitive large-volume paracentesis. Patients who have less than 5 L of ascitic fluid removed do not require albumin replacement.[261]

The efficacy of paracentesis in the treatment of tense ascites has been studied extensively. Repetitive large-volume paracentesis has been shown to be as effective as diuretics in the treatment of moderate to severe ascites, with fewer systemic complications. A decreased length of hospital stay with no increase in the incidence of spontaneous bacterial peritonitis has been noted.[262–264] Paracentesis has become the therapy of choice for severe ascites.

Peritoneovenous shunts are surgically placed tubes that connect the peritoneal cavity with the superior vena cava via the internal jugular vein (Fig. 60.17). The two main types are the LeVeen shunt and the Denver shunt, both of which have a one-way valve that allows unidirectional movement of ascitic

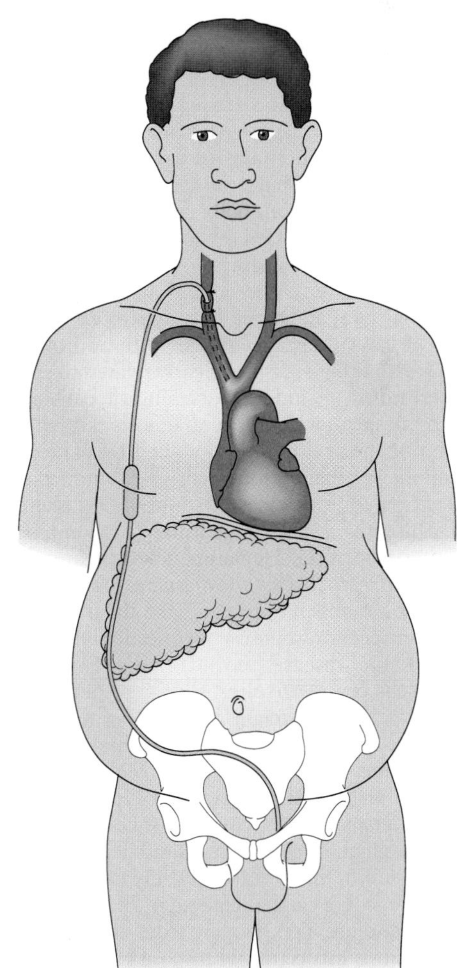

FIGURE 60.17 LeVeen peritoneovenous shunt used for routing ascitic fluid into the systemic circulation. The shunt consists of fenestrated tubing for insertion into the peritoneal cavity, a one-way valve, and a length of venous tubing for insertion into the superior vena cava.

fluid from the peritoneal cavity into the systemic circulation. Although these shunts are effective in decreasing the volume of ascitic fluid, a significant number of major complications have been noted, including disseminated intravascular coagulation, heart failure, and sepsis,[260,265] and associated mortality rates are high (approximately 20%).[266] The shunt is occluded in approximately 50% of patients at 1 year, and no improvement in survival is noted.[260] The use of these shunts has drastically decreased with the development of the TIPS procedure.

Surgically created portosystemic shunts have been used in the past for the treatment of ascites. Because of high morbidity and mortality rates, an increase in encephalopathy and progression to liver failure, and the addition of the TIPS procedure to treatment options, surgically created shunts are now used infrequently for this indication alone. As discussed earlier, the TIPS is a total nonselective shunt that decompresses the portal system and reduces pressure at the hepatic sinusoids, thereby eliminating the drive for the production of ascitic fluid. In a study evaluating the use of TIPS for the treatment of medically refractory ascites, the ascites resolved completely in almost 75% of patients, and a partial response was noted in an additional 20%.[267] In addition, renal function improved during the 6 months of follow-up. TIPS in this group of patients, however, was associated with an increase in the number of cases of encephalopathy. Although survival appears to be unaffected by a TIPS procedure when compared with large volume paracentesis,[268] the requirement for repeated paracentesis after TIPS may be justification for enhanced placement on the liver transplant waiting list, thus shortening waiting time for a transplant.

Spontaneous bacterial peritonitis is a potentially lethal complication of portal hypertension with ascites that occurs in up to 10% of patients. The cause of spontaneous bacterial peritonitis is unknown. Antecedent gastrointestinal hemorrhage is common, and spontaneous bacterial peritonitis in this setting may be related to bacterial translocation from the gut. Deficits in immune function, both systemically and within the abdomen, including depressed reticuloendothelial function,[268] low ascitic protein concentration,[269] and deficient ascitic opsonic activity,[270] may play a role. Patients often present with abdominal pain and fever, but 10% to 20% of cases are discovered on routine paracentesis.[265] In addition, patients may present with other signs not clearly related to spontaneous bacterial peritonitis, including worsening encephalopathy and deteriorating renal function. The diagnosis is easily made by examination of the ascitic fluid obtained by paracentesis. An elevated number of white blood cells ($>250/mm^3$) is diagnostic. The vast majority of cases of spontaneous bacterial peritonitis are caused by a single organism, most commonly gram-negative enteric bacteria. Hematogenous spread may lead to infection with *Streptococcus pneumoniae.* (Table 60.14).[265] If more than one organism is present, the diagnosis of spontaneous bacterial peritonitis must be questioned, and a search for intraabdominal disease (secondary peritonitis), such as a perforated viscus or diverticulitis, should be performed.

The treatment of spontaneous bacterial peritonitis consists of supportive care and broad-spectrum antibiotics, most commonly cefotaxime, a third-generation cephalosporin. Other antibiotics with proved efficacy include ofloxacin, a quinolone. This antibiotic has potent activity against gram-negative organisms and reaches high levels in ascitic fluid. For patients who are clinically stable and able to take oral medications, this is the drug of choice.[272] Cure can be achieved in 75% to 90% of cases, but mortality rates are high, ranging from 20% to 40%.[272–276] The poor prognosis associated with spontaneous bacterial peritonitis warrants consideration of liver transplantation.

Prophylactic oral or intravenous antibiotics are indicated for two distinct groups of patients with cirrhosis with ascites: (a) those with gastrointestinal hemorrhage, and (b) those with low protein counts in the ascitic fluid (<10 to 15 g/L).[273]

TABLE 60.14

BACTERIOLOGY OF SPONTANEOUS BACTERIAL PERITONITIS

Organisms	Percentage of total
Escherichia coli	40
Pneumococci	15
Streptococci	14
Klebsiella	7
Pseudomonas	3
Proteus	3
Staphylococci	3
Anaerobes	5
Other	20
Multiple isolates	10

Adapted from Targan S, Chow A, Gluze L. Role of anaerobic bacteria in spontaneous peritonitis of cirrhosis. *Am J Med* 1977;62:397.

The antibiotics used in patients with hemorrhage are neomycin, colistin, and nystatin in combination, and ofloxacin alone.[277,278] These antibiotics reduce the incidence of spontaneous bacterial peritonitis from approximately 15% to 20% to 3% to 9% and cause few side effects. A meta-analysis evaluating the use of prophylactic antibiotics in patients with gastrointestinal hemorrhage confirmed the utility of prophylaxis, with an approximately 30% decrease in the incidence of infection, a 20% decrease in the incidence of spontaneous bacterial peritonitis and bacteremia, and a 10% improvement in overall survival.[279] In patients with low protein levels in the ascitic fluid, multiple regimens have proved effective in reducing the incidence of spontaneous bacterial peritonitis, from approximately 20% to less than 5%.[280–283]

Hernias and Ascites

Hernias of the anterior abdominal wall occur in up to 20% of patients with cirrhosis. The causes include increased intraabdominal pressure and nutritional deficits, with muscular wasting and thinning of the fascia. If the hernias are left untreated, complications include incarceration, rupture, strangulation, and leakage. Hernias should be treated electively, with preoperative paracentesis to decrease intraabdominal pressure. No increase in complication rates was noted in a study comparing the outcome of umbilical hernia repair in patients with and without ascites. A longer hospital stay and a significantly higher recurrence rate (73% vs. 14%) was noted, however, in the group of patients with ascites.[284] We favor the use of abdominal drains to remove the ascites until the incision is healed, thereby preventing ascites from leaking through the wound. Meticulous fluid management is essential during the postoperative period to prevent early reaccumulation of ascites. In patients with severe ascites, TIPS should be performed before hernia repair to ensure a good result. Emergency repair of hernias complicated by skin breakdown with ascites leak or incarceration or strangulation are managed in a similar fashion with preoperative large volume paracentesis, and aggressive control of ascites postoperatively.

KEY POINTS

- **Although the causes of cirrhosis and the morphologic and histologic changes seen in the liver overlap significantly, oxidative stress leading to chronic injury and inflammation appears to be a common theme.**

- The key mediator in alcohol-induced liver disease is acetaldehyde, which produces numerous deleterious effects on the liver.
- Nonalcoholic fatty liver disease or nonalcoholic steatohepatitis (NASH) is characterized by infiltration of the liver with fat and is associated with obesity, hyperlipidemia, and non–insulin-dependent diabetes.
- Viral hepatitis is the most common cause of cirrhosis worldwide, accounting for at least 50% of cases.
- Budd-Chiari syndrome is a rare disease caused by mechanical obstruction of the hepatic veins owing to obstructing webs or membranes (most commonly in Asia and Africa) or thrombosis secondary to hyper coagulable states and neoplasms (most commonly in the West).
- Hepatorenal syndrome is a complication of cirrhosis, usually associated with ascites, characterized by progressive renal failure in the absence of intrinsic renal disease.
- Hepatic encephalopathy is a neuropsychiatric syndrome that occurs in the setting of hepatic disease and is characterized by variable alterations in mental status ranging from deficits detectable only by detailed psychometric tests to confusion, lethargy, and ultimately coma.
- Portal hypertension is defined as a portal pressure above the normal range of 5 to 8 mm Hg and can be secondary to cirrhosis (hepatic), portal vein thrombosis (presinusoidal) or hepatic venous obstruction (postsinusoidal).
- The use of transjugular intrahepatic portosystemic shunts (TIPS) has become the first-line therapy for bleeding esophageal varies with 6-month and 1-year patency rates and prevention of rebleeding in a 92% and 82% of patients, respectively.
- The Child-Turcotte-Pugh score is a scoring scale that incorporates clinical and laboratory data as a means to assess the functional status of the liver, estimate hepatic reserve, and predict morbidity and mortality of liver disease. It is used as a tool for determining the need for liver transplantation.
- Although the surgical interventions for treatment of bleeding varices are divided into three main types; (a) liver transplantation, (b) shunt procedures, and (c) devascularization procedures, the only definitive procedure in patients with cirrhosis is orthotopic liver transplant.
- Spontaneous bacterial peritonitis is a potentially lethal complication of unknown etiology associated with portal hypertension with ascites that occurs in up to 10% of patients.

References

1. Mallory FB. Cirrhosis of the liver: five different types of lesions from which it may arise. *Bull Johns Hopkins Hosp* 1911;22:69–75.
2. Friedman SL, Roll FJ, Boyles J, et al. Hepatic lipocytes: the principle collagen-producing cells of normal rat liver. *Proc Natl Acad Sci USA* 1985;82:8681–8685.
3. Wake K. "Sternzellen" in the liver: perisinusoidal cells with special reference to storage of vitamin A. *Am J Anat* 1971;132:429–462.
4. Takahara T, Kojima T, Miyabayashi C. Collagen production in fat-storing cells after carbon tetrachloride intoxication in the rat: immunoelectron microscopic observation of type I, type III collagens, and prolyl hydroxylase. *Lab Invest* 1988;59:509–521.
5. Friedman SL. The cellular basis of hepatic fibrosis. *N Engl J Med* 1993;328:1828–1835.
6. Gressner AM, Bachem MG. Cellular sources of noncollagenous matrix proteins: role of fat-storing cells in fibrogenesis. *Semin Liver Dis* 1990;10:30–46.
7. Loreal O, Levasseur F, Rescan PY, et al. Differential expression of laminin chains in hepatic lipocytes. *FEBS Lett* 1991;290:9–12.
8. Ramadori G, Knittel T, Odenthal M, et al. Synthesis of cellular fibronectin by rat liver fat-storing (Ito) cells: regulation by cytokines. *Gastroenterology* 1992;103:1313–1321.
9. Friedman SL, Arthur MJP. Activation of cultured rat hepatic lipocytes by Kupffer cell conditioned medium: direct enhancement of matrix synthesis and stimulation of cell proliferation via induction of platelet-derived growth factor receptors. *J Clin Invest* 1989;84:1780–1785.
10. Pinzani M, Gesualdo L, Sabbah GM, et al. Effects of platelet-derived growth factor and other polypeptide mitogens on DNA synthesis and growth of cultured rat liver fat-storing cells. *J Clin Invest* 1989;84:1786–1793.
11. Matsuoka M, Pham N-T, Tsukamoto H. Differential effects of interleukin-1 alpha, tumor necrosis factor alpha, and transforming growth factor beta-1 on cell proliferation and collagen formation by cultured fat-storing cells. *Liver* 1989;9:71–78.
12. Gressner AM. Cytokines and cellular crosstalk involved in the activation of fat-storing cells. *J Hepatol* 1995;22:28–36.
13. Tsushima H, Kawata S, Tamura S. Reduced plasma transforming growth factor-b_1 levels in patients with chronic hepatitis C after interferon-a therapy: association with regression of hepatic fibrosis. *J Hepatol* 1999; 30:1–7.
14. Schaffner F, Popper H. Capillarization of hepatic sinusoids in man. *Gastroenterology* 1963;44:239–242.
15. Friedman SL. Hepatic fibrosis. In: Schiff ER, Sorrell MF, Maddrey WC, eds. *Diseases of the Liver,* 8th ed. Philadelphia: JB Lippincott, 1999: 371–386.
16. Anthony PP, Ishak KG, Nayak NC, et al. The morphology of cirrhosis: definition, nomenclature, and classification. *Bull World Health Organ* 1977;55:521–540.
17. Chiaramonte M, Stroffolini T, Vian A, et al. Rate of incidence of hepatocellular carcinoma in patients with compensated viral cirrhosis. *Cancer* 1999;85:2132–2137.
18. Chedid A, Mendenhall CL, Garside P, et al. Prognostic factors in alcoholic liver disese. *Am J Gastroenterol* 1991;86:210–216.
19. Lieber CS. Medical disorders of alcoholism. *N Engl J Med* 1995;333: 1058–1065.
20. Moshage H, Casini A, Lieber CS. Acetaldehyde selectively stimulates collagen production in cultured rat liver fat-storing cells but not in hepatocytes. *Hepatology* 1990;12:511–518.
21. Lieber CS, ed. *Medical and Nutritional Complications of Alcoholism: Mechanisms and Management*. New York: Plenum, 1992.
22. Flier JS, Underhill LH. Medical disorders of alcoholism. *N Engl J Med* 1995;333:1058–1065.
23. **Angulo P. Nonalcoholic fatty liver disease. *N Engl J Med* 2002;346(16).**
24. Browning JD, Kumar KS, Saboorian MH, Thiele DL. Ethnic differences in the prevalence of cryptogenic cirrhosis. *Am J Gastroenterol* 2004;99(2):292–298.
25. Angulo, Clark JM, Brancati FL, Diegl AME. Nonalcoholic fatty liver disease: the most common cause of abnormal liver enzymes in the U.S. population. Gastroenterololgy 2001;120:Suppl:A-65(abst).
26. Di Bisceglie AM, Martin P, Kassianides C, et al. Recombinant interferon alpha therapy for chronic hepatitis C: a randomized, double-blind, placebo-controlled trial. *N Engl J Med* 1989;321:1506–1510.
27. Shindo M, Ken A, Okuno T. Varying incidence of cirrhosis and hepatocellular carcinoma in patients with chronic hepatitis C responding differently to interferon therapy. *Cancer* 1999;85:1943–1950.
28. **Fried MW, Shiffman ML, Reddy R, et al. Peginterferon alfa-2a plus ribavirin for chronic hepatitis C virus infection. *N Engl J Med* 2002;347:975-982.**
29. Davis GL. Treatment of chronic hepatitis C: combination treatment with interferon and ribavirin for chronic hepatitis C. *Clin Liver Dis* 1999;3: 811–826.
30. Szakacs JG, Szakacs JE. Progress in diagnosis of hepatitis and the cirrhotic liver. *Ann Clin Lab Sci* 1999;29:87–103.
31. Kaplan MM. Primary biliary cirrhosis. *N Engl J Med* 1996; 335: 1570–1580.
32. Portmann B, Popper H, Neuberger J, et al. Sequential and diagnostic features in primary biliary cirrhosis based on serial histologic study in 209 patients. *Gastroenterology* 1985;88:1777–1790.
33. Tornay AS Jr. Primary biliary cirrhosis: natural history. *Am J Gastroenterol* 1980;73:223–226.
34. Balasubramaniam K, Grambasch PM, Wiesner RH, et al. Diminished survival in asymptomatic primary biliary cirrhosis: a prospective study. *Gastroenterology* 1990;98:1567–1571.
35. Mahl TC, Shockcor W, Boyer JL. Primary biliary cirrhosis: survival of a large cohort of symptomatic and asymptomatic patients followed for 24 years. *J Hepatol* 1994;20:707–713.
36. Heathcote EJ, Lindor KD, Poupon R, et al. Combined analysis of French, American, and Canadian randomized controlled trials of ursodeoxycholic acid therapy in primary biliary cirrhosis. *Gastroenterology* 1995;108[Suppl]: A1082(abst).
37. Chapman RW, Varghese Z, Gaul R, et. al. Association of primary sclerosing cholangitis with HLA-B8. *Gut* 1983;24:38–41.
38. Angulo P, Lindor KD. Primary biliary cirrhosis and primary sclerosing cholangitis. *Clin Liver Dis* 1999;3:529–570.
39. Broome U, Glaumann H, Hultcrantz R, et al. Distribution of HLA-DR, HLA-DP, HLA-DQ antigens in liver tissue from patients with primary sclerosing cholangitis. *Scand J Gastroenterol* 1990;25:54.
40. Zauli D, Schrumpf E, Crespi C, et al. An autoantibody profile in primary sclerosing cholangitis. *J Hepatol* 1987;5:14.
41. Wiesner RH. Current concepts in primary sclerosing cholangitis. *Mayo Clin Proc* 1994;69:969.

42. Martin FM, Braasch JW. Primary sclerosing cholangitis. *Curr Probl Surg* 1992;29:133.
43. Okolicsanyi L, Fabris L, Viaggi S, et al. Primary sclerosing cholangitis: clinical presentation, natural history, and prognostic variables—an Italian multicenter study. *Eur J Gastroenterol Hepatol* 1996;8:685.
44. Bergquist A, Broome U. Primary biliary cirrhosis, primary sclerosing cholangitis, and adult cholangiopathies. *Clin Liver Dis* 1998;2:283–301.
45. Broome U, Lofberg R, Veress R, et al. Primary sclerosing cholangitis and ulcerative colitis: indicator of increased neoplastic potential. *Hepatology* 1995;22:1404.
46. De Vreede I, Steers JL, Burch PA. Prolonged disease-free survival after orthotopic liver transplantation plus adjuvant chemoirradiation for cholangiocarcinoma. *Liver Transpl* 2000;6:309–316.
47. Stal P, Broome U, Scheynius A. Kuppfer cell iron overload induced intercellular adhesion molecule-1 expression on hepatocytes in genetic hemochromatosis. *Hepatology* 1995;21:1301–1316.
48. Schilsky ML, Tavill AS. Wilson's disease. In: Schiff ER, Sorrell MF, Maddrey WC, eds. *Diseases of the Liver,* 8th ed. Philadelphia: JB Lippincott, 1999:1091.
49. Leggett BA, Halliday JW, Brown NN, et al. Prevalence of haemochromatosis amongst asymptomatic Australians. *Br J Haematol* 1990;74: 525–530.
50. Safran AP, Schaffner F. Chronic passive congestion of the liver in man: electron microscopic study of cell atrophy and intralobular fibrosis. *Am J Pathol* 1967;50:447–463.
51. Dunn GD, Hayes P, Breen KJ, et al. The liver in congestive heart failure: a review. *Am J Med Sci* 1973;265:174–189.
52. Rosenberg PM, Friedman LS. The liver in circulatory failure. In: Schiff ER, Sorrell MF, Maddrey WC, eds. *Diseases of the Liver*, 8th ed. Philadelphia: JB Lippincott, 1999:1217.
53. Tilanus HW. Budd-Chiari syndrome. *Br J Surg* 1995;82:1023–1030.
54. Gupta S, Barter S, Pillips GW, et al. Comparison of ultrasonography, computed tomography, and ^{99m}Tc liver scan in diagnosis of Budd-Chiari syndrome. *Gut* 1987;28:242–247.
55. Ishikawa T, Ichida T, Matsuda Y, et al. Reduced expression of thrombopoietin is involved in thrombocytopenia in human and rat liver cirrhosis. *J Gastroenterol Hepatol* 1998;13:907–913.
56. Simonovsky V. The diagnosis of cirrhosis by high-resolution ultrasound of the liver surface. *Br J Radiol* 1999;72:29–34.
57. Lieberman FL, Denison EK, Reynolds TB. The relationship of plasma volume, portal hypertension, ascites, and renal sodium retention in cirrhosis: the overflow theory of ascites formation. *Ann N Y Acad Sci* 1970;170:202.
58. Schrier RW, Arroyo V, Bernardi M, et al. Peripheral arterial vasodilation hypothesis: a proposal for the initiation of renal sodium and water retention in cirrhosis. *Hepatology* 1988;8:1151.
59. Ginès P, Arroyo V, Rodes J. Renal complications. In: Schiff ER, Sorrell MF, Maddrey WC, eds. *Diseases of the Liver,* 8th ed. Philadelphia: JB Lippincott, 1999:453.
60. Martin PY, Ginès P, Schrier RW. Nitric oxide as a mediator of hemodynamic abnormalities and sodium and water retention in cirrhosis. *N Engl J Med* 1998;339:533–541.
61. Sarela AI, Mihaimeed FMA, Batten JJ, et al. Hepatic and splanchnic nitric oxide activity in patients with cirrhosis. *Gut* 1999;44:749–753.
62. Rodes J, Bosch J, Arroyo V. Clinical types and drug therapy of renal impairment in cirrhosis. *Postgrad Med J* 1975;55:492.
63. Gines A, Escorsell A, Ginès P, et al. Incidence, predictive factors, and prognosis of the hepatorenal syndrome in cirrhosis with ascites. *Gastroenterology* 1993;105:229.
64. Ortega R, Gines P, Uriz J, et al. Terlipressin therapy with and without albumin for patients with hepatorenal syndrome: results of a prospective, nonrandomized study. *Hepatology* 2002;36:941–948.
65. Angeli P, Volpin R, Gerunda G, et al. Reversal of type 1 hepatorenal syndrome with the administration of midodrine and octreotide. *Hepatology* 1999;29:1690–1697.
66. Singer JA, Kaplan MM, Katz RL. Cirrhotic pleural effusion in the absence of ascites. *Gastroenterology* 1977;73:575.
67. Fitz G. Systemic complications of liver disease. In: Feldman M, ed. *Sleisenger and Fordtran's Gastrointestinal and Liver Disease,* 6th ed. Philadelphia: WB Saunders, 1998:1340–1342.
68. Berkowitz KA, Butensky MS, Smith RL. Pulmonary function changes after large volume paracentesis. *Am J Gastroenterol* 1993;88:905.
69. Hopkins WE, Waggoner AD, Brazilai B. Frequency and significance of intrapulmonary right-to-left shunting in end-stage hepatic disease. *Am J Cardiol* 1992;70:516–519.
70. Hourani JM, Bellamy PE, Tashkin DP, et al. Pulmonary dysfunction in advanced liver disease: frequent occurrence of an abnormal diffusing capacity. *Am J Med* 1991;90:693–700.
71. Scott VL, Dodson SF, Kang Y. The hepatopulmonary syndrome. *Surg Clin North Am* 1999;79:23–41.
72. De Wolf AM, Begliomini B, Gasior TA, et al. Right ventricular function during orthotopic liver transplantation. Anesth Analg 1993;76: 562–568.
73. Swanson KL, McGoon MD, Krowka MJ. Survival in patients with portopulmonary hypertension. Am J Respir Crit Care Med 2003; 167:A693.
74. Nomura F, Ohnishi K, Terabayashi J, et al. Effect of intrahepatic portal-systemic shunting on hepatic ammonia extraction in patients with cirrhosis. *Hepatology* 1994;20:1478–1481.
75. Lockwood AH, Yap EW, Wong WH. Cerebral ammonia metabolism in patients with severe liver disease and minimal hepatic encephalopathy. *J Cereb Blood Flow Metab* 1991;11:337–341.
76. Schafer DF, Jones EA. Hepatic encephalopathy and the g-aminobutyric acid neurotransmitter system. *Lancet* 1982;1:18–19.
77. Mullen KD, Martin JV, Mendelson WB, et al. Could an endogenous benzodiazepine ligand contribute to hepatic encephalopathy? *Lancet* 1988;1: 457–459.
78. Bengtsson F, Gage FH, Jeppson B, et al. Brain monoamine metabolism and behavior in portacaval shunted rats. *Exp Neurol* 1985;70:21–35.
79. Zieve L, Doizaki WM, Zieve J. Synergism between mercaptans and ammonia or fatty acids in the production of coma: a possible role for mercaptans in the pathogenesis of hepatic coma. *J Lab Clin Med* 1974; 83:16–28.
80. Yurdaydin C, Li Y, Ha JH, et al. Brain and plasma levels of opioid peptides are altered in rats with thioacetamide-induced fulminant hepatic failure: implications for the treatment of hepatic encephalopathy with opioid antagonists. *J Pharmacol Exp Ther* 1995;273:185–192.
81. Schenker S, Bay MK. Portal systemic encephalopathy. *Clin Liver Dis* 1997;1:157–184.
82. Mullen KD, Dasarathy S. Hepatic encephalopathy. In: Schiff ER, Sorrell MF, Maddrey WC, eds. *Diseases of the Liver,* 8th ed. Philadelphia: JB Lippincott, 1999:545.
83. Flannery DB, Hsia YE, Wolf B. Current status of hyperammonemia syndrome. *Hepatology* 1982;2:495–506.
84. Eichler M, Bessman SP. A double-blind study of the effects of ammonium infusion on psychological functioning in cirrhotic patients. *J Nerv Ment Dis* 1962;134:539–542.
85. Zeneroli ML, Venturini I, Stefanilli S, et al. Antibacterial activity of rifaximin reduces the levels of benzodiazepine-like compounds in patients with liver cirrhosis. *Pharmacol Res* 1997;35:537–560.
86. Lockwood AH. Ammonia. In: Lockwood AH, ed. *Hepatic Encephalopathy.* Boston: Butterworth-Heineman, 1992:65–72.
87. Conn HO, Lieberthal MM. Management of acute portal systemic encephalopathy. In: Conn HO, Lieberthal MM, eds. *The Hepatic Coma Syndrome and Lactulose.* Baltimore: Williams & Wilkins, 1978:189–219.
88. Conn HO, Floch MH. Effects of lactulose and *Lactobacillus acidophilus* on the fecal flora. *Am J Clin Nutr* 1970;23:1588–1594.
89. Price JB, Sawoda M, Voorhees AB. Clinical significance of intraluminal pH in intestinal ammonia transport. *Am J Surg* 1970;119:595–598.
90. Fessel JM, Conn HO. Lactulose in the treatment of acute hepatic encephalopathy. *Am J Med Sci* 1973;266:103–110.
91. Mortensen PB. The effect of orally administered lactulose on colonic nitrogen metabolism and excretion. *Hepatology* 1992;16:1350–1356.
92. Weber FL Jr, Banwell JG, Fresard KM, et al. Nitrogen in fecal bacteria, fiber, and soluble fractions of cirrhotic patients: effects of lactulose and lactulose plus neomycin. *J Lab Clin Med* 1987;110:259–263.
93. Vince AJ, Burridge SM. Ammonia production by intestinal bacteria: effects of lactose, lactulose, and glucose. *J Med Microbiol* 1980;13: 177–191.
94. Atterbury CE, Maddrey WC, Conn HO. Neomycin, sorbitol, and lactulose in the treatment of acute portal systemic encephalopathy: a controlled double-blind clinical trial. *Am J Dig Dis* 1978;23:398–406.
95. Morgan M, Read AE, Speller PCE. Treatment of hepatic encephalopathy with metronidazole. *Gut* 1982;23:1–7.
96. Conn HO, Leevy CM, Vlahcevic ZR, et al. Comparison of lactulose and neomycin in the treatment of chronic portal systemic encephalopathy. *Gastroenterology* 1977;72:573–583.
97. Kunin CM, Chalmers TC, Leevy CM, et al. Absorption of orally administered neomycin and kanamycin with special reference to patients with severe hepatic and renal disease. *N Engl J Med* 1960;262:380–385.
98. Berk DP, Chalmers T. Deafness complicating antibiotic therapy of hepatic encephalopathy. *Ann Intern Med* 1970;73:393–396.
99. DiPiazza S, Filippazzp MC, Valenza LM, et al. Rifaximin vs. neomycin in the treatment of portosystemic encephalopathy. *Ital J Gastroenterol* 1991;23:403–407.
100. Pedretti G, Calzetti C, Missale C, et al. Rifaximin versus neomycin on hyperammonemia in chronic portal systemic encephalopathy of cirrhosis: a double-blind randomized trial. *Ital J Gastroenterol* 1991;23:175–178.
101. Fera G, Agostinacchio F, Nigro M, et al. Rifaximin in the treatment of hepatic encephalopathy. *Eur J Clin Res* 1992;4:57–66.
102. Reynolds TB, Redecker AG, Geller HM. Wedged hepatic vein pressure. *Am J Med* 1957;22:341.
103. Vorobioff J, Bredfeldt JE, Groszmann RJ. Increased blood flow through the portal system in cirrhotic rats. *Gastroenterology* 1984;87:1120–1126.
104. Moller S, Christensen E, Henriksen JH. Continuous blood pressure monitoring in cirrhosis: relations to splanchnic and systemic haemodynamics. *J Hepatol* 1997;27:284–294.
105. Battista S, Bar F, Mengozzi G, et al. Hyperdynamic circulation in patients with cirrhosis: direct measurement of nitric oxide levels in hepatic and portal veins. *J Hepatol* 1997;26:75–80.
106. Jaffe DL, Chung RT, Friedman LS. Management of portal hypertension and its complications. *Med Clin North Am* 1996;80:1021–1034.

107. Gupta TK, Chen L, Groszmann RJ. Pathophysiology of portal hypertension. *Clin Liver Dis* 1997;1:1–12.
108. Budd G. *On Diseases of the Liver*. London: John Churchill, 1845:146.
109. Chiari H. Über die selbstandige phlebitis obliterans der hauptstamme der venae hepaticae als todesursache. *Beitr Z Pathol Anat* 1899;26:1–18.
110. Tilanus HW. Budd-Chiari syndrome. *Br J Surg* 1995;82:1023–1030.
111. Gordon SC, Polson DJ, Shirkoda A. Budd-Chiari syndrome complicating preeclampsia: diagnosis by magnetic resonance imaging. *J Clin Gastroenterol* 1991;13:460–462.
112. Ilan Y, Oren R, Shouval D. Postpartum Budd-Chiari syndrome with prolonged hypercoagulability state. *Am J Obstet Gynecol* 1990;162: 1164–1165.
113. Valla D, Le MG, Poynard T, et al. Risk of hepatic vein thrombosis in relation to recent use of oral contraceptives: a case-control study. *Gastroenterology* 1986;90:807–811.
114. Mitchell MC, Boitnott JK, Kaufman S, et al. Budd-Chiari syndrome: etiology, diagnosis, and management. *Medicine* 1982;61:199–218.
115. Faust TW, Sorrell MF. Budd-Chiari syndrome. In: Schiff ER, Sorrell MF, Maddrey WC, eds. *Diseases of the Liver,* 8th ed. Philadelphia: JB Lippincott, 1999:1207–1214.
116. Gupta S, Barter S, Phillips GW, et al. Comparison of ultrasonography, computed tomography, and ^{99m}Tc liver scan in diagnosis of Budd-Chiari syndrome. *Gut* 1987;28:242–247.
117. McCarthy PM, vanHeerden JA, Adson MA, et al. The Budd-Chiari syndrome: medical and surgical management of 30 patients. *Arch Surg* 1985;120:657–662.
118. Cameron JL, Maddrey WC. Mesoatrial shunt: a new treatment for the Budd–Chiari syndrome. *Ann Surg* 1978; 187: 402–406
119. Halff G, Todo S, Tzakis AG, et al. Liver transplantation for the Budd-Chiari syndrome. *Ann Surg* 1990;211:43–49.
120. Hemming AW, Langer B, Greig P, et al. Treatment of Budd-Chiari syndrome with portosystemic shunt or liver transplantation. *Am J Surg* 1996;171:176–181.
121. Campbell DA, Rolles K, Jamieson N, et al. Hepatic transplantation with perioperative and long-term anticoagulation as treatment for Budd-Chiari syndrome. *Surgery Gynecology Obstetrics* 1988;166:511–518.
122. Shaked A, Goldstein RM, Klintmalm GB, et al. Portosystemic shunt versus orthotopic liver transplantation for the Budd-Chiari syndrome. *Surgery Gynecology Obstetrics* 1992;174:453.
123. Uhl MD, Roth DB, Reily CA. Transjugular intrahepatic portosystemic shunt (TIPS) for Budd-Chiari syndrome. *Dig Dis Sci* 1996;41:1494–1499.
124. Rossle M, Olschewski M, Siegerstetter V. The Budd-Chiari syndrome: outcome after treatment with the transjugular intrahepatic portosystemic shunt. *Surgery* 2004;135:394–403.
125. Belli L, Romani F, Riolo F, et al. Thrombosis of portal vein in absence of hepatic disease. *Surgery Gynecology Obstetrics* 1989;169:46.
126. Orozco H, Takahashi T, Mercado MA, et al. Surgical management of extrahepatic portal hypertension and variceal bleeding. *World J Surg* 1994;18:246–250.
127. Choen J, Edelman RR, Chopra S. Portal vein thrombosis: a review. *Am J Med* 1992;92:173–182.
128. Parvey HR, Raval B, Sandler CM. Portal vein thrombosis: imaging findings. *AJR Am J Roentgenol* 1994;152:77–81.
129. de Ville de Goyet J, Alberti D, Clapuyt P, et al. Direct bypassing of extrahepatic portal venous obstruction in children: a new technique for combined hepatic portal revascularization and treatment of extrahepatic portal hypertension. *J Pediatr Surg* 1998;33:597–601.
130. Loftus FP, Nagorney DM, Ilstrup D, et al. Sinistral portal hypertension: splenectomy or expectant management. *Ann Surg* 1993;217:35–40.
131. Child CG, Turcotte JG. Surgery and portal hypertension. In: Child CG II, ed. *Major Problems in Clinical Surgery: The Liver and Portal Hypertension,* Vol 1. Philadelphia: WB Saunders, 1964:1.
132. Spence R. The venous anatomy of the lower esophagus in normal subjects and patients with varices: an image analysis study. *Br J Surg* 1984;71:739.
133. Noda T. Angioarchitectural study of esophageal varices with special reference to variceal rupture. *Virchows Arch [A]* 1984;404:381.
134. Roberts LR, Kamath PS. Pathophysiology and treatment of variceal hemorrhage. *Mayo Clin Proc* 1996;71:973–983.
135. Pagliaro L, D'Amico G, Pasta L, et al. Portal hypertension in cirrhosis: natural history. In: Bosch J, Groszmann R, eds. *Portal Hypertension: Pathophysiology and Treatment.* Oxford: Blackwell Science, 1994:72–92.
136. Cales P, Desmorat H, Vinel J, et al. Incidence of large esophageal varices in patients with cirrhosis: application to prophylaxis of first bleeding. *Gut* 1990;31:1298–1302.
137. Christensen E, Fauerholdt L, Schlichting P, et al. Aspects of the natural history of gastrointestinal bleeding in cirrhosis and the effects of prednisone. *Gastroenterology* 1981;81:944–952.
138. North Italian Endoscopic Club. Prediction of the first variceal hemorrhage in patients with cirrhosis of the liver and esophageal varices. *N Engl J Med* 1988;319:983.
139. Graham D, Smith J. The course of patients after variceal hemorrhage. *Gastroenterology* 1981;80:800–809.
140. Grace ND, Bhattacharya K. Pharmacologic therapy of portal hypertension and variceal hemorrhage. *Clin Liver Dis* 1997;1:59–75.
141. Polio J, Groszmann RJ. Hemodynamic factor in the development and rupture of esophageal varices: a pathophysiologic approach to treatment. *Semin Liver Dis* 1986;6:318.
142. Garcia-Tsao G, Groszmann RJ, Fisher RL, et al. Portal pressure, presence of gastroesophageal varices, and variceal bleeding. *Hepatology* 1985;5:419.
143. Boyer TD. The natural history of portal hypertension. *Clin Liver Dis* 1997;1:31.
144. Kroeger R, Groszmann R. The effect of selective blockade of b_2-adrenergic receptors on portal and systemic hemodynamics in a portal hypertensive model. *Gastroenterology* 1985;88:896.
145. Price H, Cooperman L, Warden J. Control of the splanchnic circulation in man: role of beta-adrenergic receptors. *Circ Res* 1967;1(21):333.
146. Braillon A, Moreau R, Hadengue A, et al. Hyperkinetic circulatory syndrome in patients with presinusoidal portal hypertension: effect of propranolol. *J Hepatol* 1989;9:312.
147. Kiire C. Controlled trial of propranolol to prevent recurrent variceal bleeding in patients with non-cirrhotic portal fibrosis. *BMJ* 1989; 298:1363.
148. Poynard T, Cales P, Pasta L, et al. Beta-adrenergic-antagonist drugs in the prevention of gastrointestinal bleeding in patients with cirrhosis and esophageal varices: an analysis of data and prognostic factors in 589 patients from four randomized clinical trials. *N Engl J Med* 1991;324: 1532–1538.
149. Feu F, Garcia-Pagan J, Bosch J, et al. Relation between portal pressure response to pharmacotherapy and risk of recurrent variceal haemorrhage in patients with cirrhosis. *Lancet* 1995;346:1056–1059.
150. Conn H, Grace N, Bosch J, et al. Propranolol in the prevention of the first hemorrhage from esophagogastric varices: a multicenter, randomized clinical trial. *Hepatology* 1991;13:902.
151. Andreani T, Poupon R, Balkau B, et al. Preventive therapy of first gastrointestinal bleeding in patients with cirrhosis: results of a controlled trial comparing propranolol, endoscopic sclerotherapy, and placebo. *Hepatology* 1990;12:1413.
152. Ideo G, Bellati G, Fesce E, et al. Nadolol can prevent the first gastrointestinal bleeding in cirrhotics: a prospective, randomized study. *Hepatology* 1988;8:6.
153. Pascal J, Cales P, Multicenter Study Group. Propranolol in the prevention of first upper gastrointestinal tract hemorrhage in patients with cirrhosis of the liver and esophageal varices. *N Engl J Med* 1987;317:856.
154. PROVA. Prophylaxis of first hemorrhage from esophageal varices by sclerotherapy, propranolol or both in cirrhotic patients: a randomized multicenter trial. *Hepatology* 1991;14:1016–1024.
155. Poynard T, Cales P, Pasta L, et al. b-Adrenergic antagonists in the prevention of first gastrointestinal bleeding in patients with cirrhosis and esophageal varices: an analysis of data and prognostic factors in 589 patients from four randomized clinical trials. *N Engl J Med* 1991;324: 1532–1538.
156. Groszmann RJ, de Franchis R. Portal hypertension. In: Schiff ER, Sorrell MF, Maddrey WC, eds. *Diseases of the Liver*, 8th ed. Philadelphia: JB Lippincott, 1999:387–442.
157. Angelica M, Carli R, Piat C, et al. Isosorbide-5-mononitrate versus propranolol in the prevention of first bleeding in cirrhosis. *Gastroenterology* 1993;104:1460–1465.
158. Vorobioff J, Picabea E, Gamen M. Propranolol compared with propranolol plus isosorbide dinitrate in portal-hypertensive patients: long-term hemodynamics and renal effects. *Hepatology* 1993;18:477–484.
159. Merkel C, Marin R, Enzo E, et al. Randomized trial of nadolol alone or with isosorbide mononitrate for primary prophylaxis of variceal bleeding in cirrhosis. *Lancet* 1996;348:1677–1681.
160. Conn HO. The rational evaluation and management of portal hypertension. In Schaffner F, Sherlock S, Leevey CM, eds. *The Liver and Its Diseases*. New York: Intercontinental, 1974:289–306.
161. Grace ND, Muench H, Chalmers TC. The present status of shunts for portal hypertension in cirrhosis. *Gastroenterology* 1966;50:684–691.
162. D'Amico G, Pagliaro L, Bosch J. The treatment of portal hypertension: a meta-analytic review. *Hepatology* 1995;22:332.
163. Lo GH, Lai KH, Cheng JS, et al. Prophylactic banding ligation of high-risk esophageal varices in patients with cirrhosis: a prospective, randomized trial. *J Hepatol* 1999;31:451–456.
164. Svoboda P, Kantorova I, Ochmann J, et al. A prospective randomized controlled trial of sclerotherapy vs. ligation in the prophylactic treatment of high-risk esophageal varices. *Surg Endosc* 1999;13:580–584.
165. Fogel M, Knauer C, Andres L, et al. Continuous intravenous vasopressin in active upper gastrointestinal bleeding. *Ann Intern Med* 1982;96:565.
166. Chojkier M, Groszmann R, Atterbury C, et al. A controlled comparison of continuous intra-arterial and intravenous infusions of vasopressin in hemorrhage from esophageal varices. *Gastroenterology* 1979;77:540.
167. Merigan TP, Plotkin GR, Davidson CS. Effect of intravenously administered posterior pituitary extract on hemorrhage from bleeding esophageal varices. *N Engl J Med* 1962;266:134.
168. Zito RA, Diez AR, Groszmann RJ. Comparative effects of nitroglycerin and nitroprusside on vasopressin-induced cardiac dysfunction in the dog. *J Cardiovasc Pharmacol* 1983;5:586.
169. Groszmann R, Kravetz D, Bosch J, et al. Nitroglycerin improves the hemodynamic response to vasopressin in portal hypertension. *Hepatology* 1982;2:757.
170. Iwao T, Toyonaga A, Ikegami M, et al. Portohepatic pressures, hepatic function, and blood gases in the combination of nitroglycerin and

vasopressin: search for additive effects in cirrhotic portal hypertension. *Am J Gastroenterol* 1992;87:719–724.
171. Gimson A, Westaby D, Hegarty J, et al. A randomized trial of vasopressin and vasopressin plus nitroglycerin in the control of acute variceal hemorrhage. *Hepatology* 1986;6:410.
172. Bosch J, Groszmann R, Garcia-Pagan J, et al. Association of transdermal nitroglycerin to vasopressin infusion in the treatment of variceal hemorrhage: a placebo-controlled clinical trial. *Hepatology* 1989;10:962.
173. Tsai Y, Lay C, Lai K, et al. Controlled trial of vasopressin plus nitroglycerin vs. vasopressin alone in the treatment of bleeding esophageal varices. *Hepatology* 1986;6:406–409.
174. Sonneburg G, Keller U, Perruchoud A, et al. Effect of somatostatin on splanchnic hemodynamics in patients with cirrhosis of the liver and in normal subjects. *Gastroenterology* 1981;80:526–532.
175. Sieber C, Mosca P, Groszmann R. Effect of somatostatin on mesenteric vascular resistance in normal and portal hypertensive rats. *Am J Physiol* 1992;262:274–277.
176. Bosch J, Kravetz D, Rodes J. Effects of somatostatin on hepatic and systemic hemodynamics in patients with cirrhosis of the liver: comparison with vasopressin. *Gastroenterology* 1981;80:518–525.
177. Jenkins S, Baxter J, Corbett W, et al. A prospective randomized controlled clinical trial comparing somatostatin and vasopressin in controlling acute variceal hemorrhage. *BMJ* 1985;290:275.
178. Burroughs A, McCormick P, Hughes M, et al. Randomized, double-blind, placebo-controlled trial of somatostatin for variceal bleeding: emergency control and prevention of early variceal rebleeding. *Gastroenterology* 1990;99:1388.
179. Kravetz D, Bosch J, Teres J, et al. Comparisons of intravenous somatostatin and vasopressin infusions in the treatment of acute variceal hemorrhage. *Hepatology* 1984;4:442.
180. Saari A, Klvilaakso E, Inberg M, et al. Comparison of somatostatin and vasopressin in bleeding esophageal varices. *Am J Gastroenterol* 1990;85:804.
181. Hsia H, Lee F, Tsai Y, et al. Comparison of somatostatin and vasopressin in the control of acute esophageal variceal hemorrhage: a randomized, controlled study. *Chin J Gastroenterol* 1990;7:71–78.
182. Jaramillo J, de la Mata M, Mino G, et al. Somatostatin versus Sengstaken balloon tamponade for primary haemostasis of bleeding esophageal varices. *J Hepatol* 1991;12:100–105.
183. Avgerinos A, Klonis C, Rekoumis G, et al. Controlled trial of somatostatin and balloon tamponade in bleeding esophageal varices. *J Hepatol* 1991;13:78–83.
184. Burroughs AK, Hamilton G, Phillips A, et al. A comparison of sclerotherapy with staple transection of the esophagus for the emergency control of bleeding from esophageal varices. *N Engl J Med* 1989;321:857–862.
185. Stiegmann G, Goff J, Michaletz-Onody P, et al. Endoscopic sclerotherapy as compared with endoscopic ligation for bleeding esophageal varices. *N Engl J Med* 1992;326:1527–1532.
186. Young M, Sanowski R, Rasche R. Comparison and characterization of ulcerations induced by endoscopic ligation of esophageal varices versus endoscopic sclerotherapy. *Gastrointest Endosc* 1993;39:119–122.
187. Mundo F, Mitrani C, Rodriquez G, et al. Endoscopic variceal treatment: is band ligation taking over sclerotherapy? *Am J Gastroenterol* 1993;88: 1493(abst).
188. Laine L, El-Newihi H, Migikowsky B, et al. Endoscopic ligation compared with sclerotherapy for the treatment of bleeding esophageal varices. *Ann Intern Med* 1993;119:1–7.
189. Gimson A, Ramage J, Panos M, et al. Randomized trial of variceal banding ligation versus injection sclerotherapy for bleeding esophageal varices. *Lancet* 1993;342:391–394.
190. Laine L, Cook D. Endoscopic ligation compared with sclerotherapy for treatment of esophageal variceal bleeding: a meta-analysis. *Ann Intern Med* 1995;123:280–287.
191. Jensen D, Kovacs T, Randall G, et al. Initial results of a randomized prospective study of emergency banding vs. sclerotherapy for bleeding gastric or esophageal varices. *Gastrointest Endosc* 1993;39:279(abst).
192. Lo G, Lai K, Cheng J, et al. A prospective, randomised trial of injection sclerotherapy versus banding ligation in the management of bleeding esophageal varices. *Hepatology* 1995;22:466–471.
193. McCormick PA, Dick R, Panagou EB, et al. Emergency trans-jugular intrahepatic portasystemic stent shunting as salvage treatment for uncontrolled variceal bleeding. *Br J Surg* 1994;81:1324–1327.
194. LaGerge JM, Ring EJ, Gordon RL, et al. Creation of transjugular intrahepatic portosystemic shunts with the Wallstent endoprosthesis: results in 100 patients. *Radiology* 1993;187:413–420.
195. Sanyal A, Freedman A, Luketic V, et al. Transjugular intrahepatic portosystemic shunts for patients with active variceal hemorrhage unresponsive to sclerotherapy. *Gastroenterology* 1996;111:138–146.
196. Miller-Catchpole R. Transjugular intrahepatic portosystemic shunt (TIPS): diagnostic and therapeutic technology assessment (DATTA). *JAMA* 1995; 21:1824–1830.
197. Kerlan RK Jr, LaBerge JM, Gordon RL, et al. Transjugular intrahepatic portosystemic shunts: current status. *AJR Am J Roentgenol* 1995;164: 1059–1066.
198. Rossle M, Haag K, Ochs A, et al. The transjugular intrahepatic portosystemic stent–shunt procedure for variceal bleeding. *N Engl J Med* 1994;330:165–171.
199. Hernandez-Guerra M, Turnes J, Rubinstein P, et al. PTFE-covered stents improve TIPS patency in Budd—Chiari syndrome. *Hepatology*. 2004;40(5): 1197–202
200. Whipple AO. The problem of portal hypertension in relation to the hepatosplenopathies. *Ann Surg* 1945;122:449–475.
201. Sarfeh IJ, Rypins EB. Partial versus total portacaval shunt in alcoholic cirrhosis: results of a prospective, randomized clinical trial. *Ann Surg* 1994;219:353–361.
202. Rosemurgy AS, Goode SE, Zwiebel BR, et al. A prospective trial of transjugular intrahepatic portasystemic stent shunts versus small-diameter prosthetic H-graft portacaval shunts in the treatment of bleeding varices. *Ann Surg* 1996;224:378–384.
203. Sarfeh IJ, Rypins EB, Mason GR. A systemic appraisal of portocaval H-graft diameters: clinical and hemodynamic perspectives. *Am Surg* 1986; 204:356–363.
204. Johansen KH, Girod C, Lee SS, et al. Mesenteric venous stenosis reduces hyperammonemia in the portacaval-shunted rat. *Eur Surg Res* 1990;22:170–174.
205. Inokuchi K. A selective portacaval shunt. *Lancet* 1968;2:51–52.
206. Hermann RE, Henderson JM, Vogt DP, et al. Fifty years of surgery for portal hypertension at the Cleveland Clinic Foundation: lessons and prospects. *Ann Surg* 1995;221:459–466.
207. Henderson JM, Gilmore GT, Hooks MA, et al. Selective shunt in the management of variceal bleeding in the era of liver transplantation. *Ann Surg* 1992;216:248–254.
208. Rikkers LF. Is the distal splenorenal shunt better? *Hepatology* 1988; 8:1705–1707.
209. Orozco H, Mercado MA, Garcia JG, et al. Selective shunts for portal hypertension: current role of a 21-year experience. *Liver Transpl Surg* 1997;3:475–480.
210. Warren WD, Millikan WJ Jr, Henderson JM, et al. Ten years' portal hypertensive surgery at Emory. *Ann Surg* 1982;195:530.
211. Henderson JM, Warren WD, Millikan WJ, et al. Distal splenorenal shunt with splenopancreatic disconnection: a 4-year assessment. *Ann Surg* 1989;210:332–339.
212. Jin G, Rikkers LF. Etiology and management of upper gastrointestinal bleeding after distal splenorenal shunt. *Surgery* 1990;112:719.
213. Henderson JM. Variceal bleeding: which shunt? *Gastroenterology* 1986;91:1021–1023.
214. Orloff MJ, Orloff MS, Orloff SL, et al. Three decades of experience with emergency portacaval shunt for acutely bleeding esophageal varices in 400 unselected patients with cirrhosis of the liver. *J Am Coll Surg* 1995; 180:257–272.
215. Sugiura M, Futagawa S. Esophageal transection with paraesophagogastric devascularizations (the Sugiura procedure) in the treatment of esophageal varices. *World J Surg* 1984;8:673–679.
216. Yamamoto S, Hidemura R, Sanada M, et al. The late results of terminal esophago-proximal gastrectomy (TEPG) with extensive devascularization and splenectomy for bleeding esophageal varices in cirrhosis. *Surgery* 1976;80:106.
217. Wexler MJ, Stein BL. Nonshunting operations for variceal hemorrhage. *Surg Clin North Am* 1990;70:425.
218. Cello JP, Crass R, Trunkey DD. Endoscopic sclerotherapy versus esophageal transection in Child's class C patients with variceal hemorrhage: comparison with results of portacaval shunt—preliminary report. *Surgery* 1982;91:333.
219. Hamilton G, Burroughs AK, McIntyre N, et al. The final report on prospective randomized trial of endoscopic sclerotherapy versus esophageal stapled transection in uncontrolled variceal bleeding. Presented at the Second World Congress on Hepato-pancreato-biliary Surgery, Amsterdam, May 29–April 3, 1988.
220. Huizinga WKJ, Angorn IB, Baker LW. Esophageal transection versus injection sclerotherapy in the management of bleeding esophageal varices in patients of high risk. *Surg Gynecol Obstet* 1985;160:539.
221. Helton WS, Maves R, Wicks K, et al. Transjugular intrahepatic portosystemic shunt vs. surgical shunt in good-risk cirrhotic patients. *Arch Surg* 2001;136:17–20.
222. Villeneuve J, Pomier-Layrargues G, Infante-Rivard C, et al. Propranolol for the prevention of recurrent variceal hemorrhage: a controlled trial. *Hepatology* 1986;6:1239.
223. Lebrec D, Poynard T, Berneau J, et al. A randomized controlled study of propranolol for prevention of recurrent gastrointestinal bleeding in patients with cirrhosis: a final report. *Hepatology* 1984;4:355.
224. Burroughs A, Jenkins W, Sherlock S, et al. Controlled trial of propranolol for the prevention of recurrent variceal hemorrhage: a controlled trial. *N Engl J Med* 1983;309:1539.
225. Queuniet A, Czernichow P, Lerebours E, et al. Étude controlée du propranolol dans la prévention des récidives hémorragiques chez les patients cirrhotiques. *Gastroenterol Clin Biol* 1987;11:41.
226. Gatta A, Merkel C, Sacerdoti D, et al. Nadolol for prevention of variceal rebleeding in cirrhosis: a controlled clinical trial. *Digestion* 1987;37:22.
227. Ink O, Servent L, Attali P, et al. Propranolol prevention of hemorrhagic recurrence caused by rupture of esophageal varices: worsened prognosis in ascites and jaundice. *Gastroenterologie Clinique et Biologique* 1985; 9:819–823.

228. Garden O, Mills P, Birnie G, et al. Propranolol in the prevention of recurrent variceal hemorrhage in cirrhotic patients. *Gastroenterology* 1990;98:185.
229. Sheen I, Chen T, Liaw Y. Randomized controlled study of propranolol for prevention of recurrent esophageal bleeding in patients with cirrhosis. *Liver* 1989;9:1.
230. Rossi V, Cales P, Pascal B, et al. Prevention of recurrent variceal bleeding in alcoholic cirrhotic patients: prospective controlled trial of propranolol and sclerotherapy. *J Hepatol* 1991;12:283–289.
231. Colman J, Jones P, Finch C, et al. Propranolol in the prevention of variceal hemorrhage in alcoholic cirrhotic patients. *Hepatology* 1990;12:851(abst).
232. Villanueva C, Balanzo J, Novella M, et al. Nadolol plus isosorbide mononitrate compared with sclerotherapy for the prevention of variceal rebleeding. *N Engl J Med* 1996;334:1624–1629.
233. Westaby D, Binmoller K, de Franchis R, et al. Baveno II consensus statements: the endoscopic management of variceal bleeding. In: de Franchis R, ed. *Portal hypertension II. Proceedings of the Second International Consensus Workshop on Definitions, Methodology, and Therapeutic Strategies*. Oxford: Blackwell Science, 1996:126.
234. Sauer P, Theilmann L, Benz T, et al. Transjugular intrahepatic portosystemic stent shunt (TIPS) vs. sclerotherapy in the prevention of variceal rebleeding: a randomized study. *Gastroenterology* 1996;110:A1313(abst).
235. Sanyal A, Freedman A, Luketic V, et al. Transjugular intrahepatic portosystemic shunts compared with endoscopic sclerotherapy for the prevention of recurrent variceal hemorrhage: a randomized controlled trial. *Ann Intern Med* 1997;126:849–857.
236. Cabera J, Maynar M, Granados R, et al. Transjugular intrahepatic portosystemic shunt (TIPS) vs. sclerotherapy in the elective treatment of variceal bleeding. *Gastroenterology* 1996;110:832–839.
237. Cello J, Ring E, Elcott E, et al. Transjugular intrahepatic portosystemic shunt vs. sclerotherapy for variceal hemorrhage. *Gastroenterology* 1995;108:A1045(abst).
238. Jalan R, Forrest E, Stanley A, et al. TIPS vs. variceal band ligation for the prevention of variceal rebleeding in cirrhosis: a randomized controlled study. *Hepatology* 1996;24:247A(abst).
239. Rossle M, Deibert P, Haag K, et al. TIPS versus sclerotherapy and b-blockage: preliminary results of a randomized study in patients with recurrent variceal hemorrhage. *Hepatology* 1994;20:107A(abst).
240. Garcia-Villarreal L, Martinez-Lagares F, Sierra A, et al. TIPS vs. sclerotherapy for the prevention of variceal rebleeding: preliminary results of a randomized study. *Hepatology* 1996;24:208A(abst).
241. Groupe d'Étude des Anastomoses Intra-Hepatiques. TIPS vs. sclerotherapy + propranolol in the prevention of variceal rebleeding: preliminary results of a multicenter randomized trial. *Hepatology* 1995;22:297A(abst).
242. Merli M, Riggio O, Capocaccia L, et al. Transjugular intrahepatic portosystemic shunt (TIPS) vs. endoscopic sclerotherapy (ES) in preventing variceal rebleeding: preliminary results of a randomized controlled trial. *Hepatology* 1994;20:107A(abst).
243. Henderson J, Kutner M, Millikan WJ, et al. Endoscopic variceal sclerosis compared with distal splenorenal shunt to prevent recurrent variceal bleeding in cirrhosis: a prospective, randomized trial. *Ann Intern Med* 1990;112:262.
244. Planas R, Boix J, Broggi M, et al. Portacaval shunt versus endoscopic sclerotherapy in the elective treatment of variceal hemorrhage. *Gastroenterology* 1991;100:1078–1086.
245. Rikkers L, Burnett D, Valentine G, et al. Shunt surgery versus endoscopic sclerotherapy for long-term treatment of variceal bleeding: early results of a randomized trial. *Ann Surg* 1987;206:261.
246. Spina G, Santambrogio R, Opocher E, et al. Distal splenorenal shunt vs. endoscopic sclerotherapy in the prevention of variceal rebleeding: first stage of a randomized controlled trial. *Ann Surg* 1990;211:178.
247. Teres J, Bordax J, Rodes J. Sclerotherapy versus distal splenorenal shunt in the elective treatment of variceal hemorrhage: a randomized controlled trial. *Hepatology* 1987;7:430.
248. Watanabe K, Kimura K, Matsutani S, et al. Portal hemodynamics in patients with gastric varices: a study in 230 patients with esophageal or gastric varices using portal vein catheterization. *Gastroenterology* 1988;95:434–440.
249. Sarin S, Lahoti D, Saxena S, et al. Prevalence, classification, and natural history of gastric varices: long-term follow-up study in 568 patients with portal hypertension. *Hepatology* 1992;16:1343–1349.
250. Sarin S, Kumar A. Gastric varices: profile, classification, and management. *Am J Gastroenterol* 1989;84:1244.
251. Kim T, Shijo H, Kokawa H, et al. Risk factors for hemorrhage from gastric fundal varices. *Hepatology* 1997;25:307–312.
252. Quintero F, Pique J, Bombi J, et al. Gastric mucosal vascular ectasias causing bleeding in cirrhosis. *Gastroenterology* 1987;93:1054–1061.
253. Sarfeh I, Tarnawsky A. Gastric mucosal vasculopathy in portal hypertension. *Gastroenterology* 1987;93:1129–1131.
254. D'Amico G, Montalbano L, Pagliaro L, et al. Natural history of congestive gastropathy in cirrhosis. *Gastroenterology* 1990;99:1558.
255. McCormack T, Sims J, Eyre-Brook I, et al. Gastric lesions in portal hypertension: inflammatory gastritis or congestive gastropathy? *Gut* 1985;26:1226.
256. Huet P-M, Goresky CA, Villeneuve J-P, et al. Assessment of liver microcirculation in human cirrhosis. *J Clin Invest* 1982;70:1234–1244.
257. Roberts LR, Kamath PS. Ascites and hepatorenal syndrome: pathophysiology and management. *Mayo Clin Proc* 1996;73:874–881.
258. Stanley MM, Ochi S, Lee KK, et al. Peritoneovenous shunting as compared with medical treatment in patients with alcoholic cirrhosis and massive ascites. *N Engl J Med* 1989;321:1632–1638.
259. Bories P, Compean DG, Michel H, et al. The treatment of refractory ascites by the LeVeen shunt: a multi-centre controlled trial (57 patients). *J Hepatol* 1986;2:212–218.
260. Aiza I, Perez GO, Schiff ER. Management of ascites in patients with chronic liver disease. *Am J Gastroenterol* 1994;89:1949–1956.
261. Ginès P, Arroyo V, Quintero E, et al. Comparison of paracentesis and diuretics in the treatment of cirrhotics with tense ascites. *Gastroenterology* 1987;93:234–241.
262. Salerno F, Badalamenti S, Incerti P, et al. Repeated paracentesis and i.v. albumin infusion to treat "tense" ascites in cirrhotic patients: a safe alternative therapy. *J Hepatol* 1987;5:102–108.
263. Sola R, Andreu M, Coll S, et al. Spontaneous bacterial peritonitis in cirrhotic patients treated using paracentesis or diuretics: results of a randomized study. *Hepatology* 1995;21:340.
264. Olafsson S, Blei AT. Diagnosis and management of ascites in the age of TIPS. *AJR Am J Roentgenol* 1995;165:9–15.
265. Greig PD, Langer B, Blendis LM, et al. Complications after peritoneovenous shunting for ascites. *Am J Surg* 1980;139:125–131.
266. Ochs A, Rossle M, Haag K, et al. The transjugular intrahepatic portosystemic stent—shunt procedure for refractory ascites. *N Engl J Med* 1995; 332:1192–1197.
267. Sanyal AJ, Genning C, Reddy KR, et al. The North American Study for the Treatment of Refractory Ascites. *Gastroenterology* 2003;124:634-641
268. Rimola A, Soto R, Bory F, et al. Reticuloendothelial system phagocytic activity in cirrhosis and its relation to bacterial infections and prognosis. *Hepatology* 1984;4:53–58.
269. Runyon BA. Low-protein-concentration ascitic fluid is predisposed to spontaneous bacterial peritonitis. *Gastroenterology* 1986;91:1343–1346.
270. Almdal TP, Skinhoj RG, Craxi A, et al. Spontaneous bacterial peritonitis in cirrhosis: incidence, diagnosis, and prognosis. *Scand J Gastroenterol* 1987;22:295–300.
271. Rimola A, Salmeron JM, Clemente G, et al. Two different dosages of cefotaxime in the treatment of spontaneous bacterial peritonitis in cirrhosis: results of a prospective, randomized, multicenter study. *Hepatology* 1995;21:674–679.
272. Felisart J, Rimola A, Arroyo V, et al. Cefotaxime is more effective than is ampicillin-tobramycin in cirrhotics with severe infections. *Hepatology* 1985;5:457–462.
273. Runyon BA, McHutchison JG, Antillon MR, et al. Short-course versus long-course antibiotic treatment of spontaneous bacterial peritonitis. *Gastroenterology* 1991;100:1737–1742.
274. Runyon BA. Patients with deficient ascitic fluid opsonic activity are predisposed to spontaneous bacterial peritonitis. *Hepatology* 1988;8:632–635.
275. Toledo C, Salmeron JM, Rimola A, et al. Spontaneous bacterial peritonitis in cirrhosis: predictive factors of infection resolution and survival in patients treated with cefotaxime. *Hepatology* 1993;17:251–257.
276. Rimola A, Bory F, Teres J, et al. Oral, nonabsorbable antibiotics prevent infection in cirrhotics with gastrointestinal hemorrhage. *Hepatology* 1985;5:463–467.
277. Soriano G, Guarner C, Tomas A, et al. Norfloxacin prevents bacterial infection in cirrhotics with gastrointestinal hemorrhage. *Gastroenterology* 1992;103:1267–1272.
278. Bernard B, Grange JD, Khac EN, et al. Antibiotic prophylaxis for the prevention of bacterial infections in cirrhotic patients with gastrointestinal bleeding: a meta-analysis. *Hepatology* 1999;29:1655–1661.
279. Grange JD, Roulot D, Pelletier G. Primary prophylaxis of bacterial infections with norfloxacin in cirrhotic patients with ascites: results of a double-blind, placebo-controlled trial. *Gastroenterology* 1994;106:901A.
280. Rolachon A, Cordier L, Bacq Y, et al. Ciprofloxacin and long-term prevention of spontaneous bacterial peritonitis: results of a prospective controlled trial. *Hepatology* 1995;22:1171–1174.
281. Singh N, Gayowski T, Yu VL, et al. Trimethoprim-sulfamethoxazole for the prevention of spontaneous bacterial peritonitis in cirrhosis: a randomized trial. *Ann Intern Med* 1995;122:595–598.
282. Soriano G, Guarner C, Teixido M, et al. Selective intestinal decontamination prevents spontaneous bacterial peritonitis. *Gastroenterology* 1991;100:477–481.
283. Runyon BA, Juler GL. *Am J Gastroenterology* 1985;80:38–39.

CHAPTER 61 ■ HEPATIC NEOPLASMS

KEITH A. DELMAN AND STEVEN A. CURLEY

ANATOMY AND PHYSIOLOGY

Because the details of hepatic anatomy and physiology are specifically discussed in other chapters of this book, we will repeat only a brief overview in this chapter. The liver lies in the right upper quadrant, nestled underneath the rib cage. It is completely surrounded by a peritoneal membrane, known as Glisson's capsule. This investing sheath also envelopes the portal vascular structures as they enter the liver. In contrast, hepatic veins are not covered by Glisson's capsule. The liver receives a dual blood supply from both the hepatic artery and portal vein. The portal vein supplies approximately 75% of the blood supply with the hepatic artery providing the remainder. The liver is drained predominantly by three major veins: the left, right, and middle hepatic veins, with the balance of drainage occurring through several small vessels directly entering the vena cava from the posterior aspect of the liver.

For surgical approaches to hepatic neoplasms, it is important to recognize the variability of the extrahepatic arterial anatomy.[1,2] In the majority of patients, the common hepatic artery arises from the celiac trunk giving off the gastroduodenal artery, followed by a right gastric artery. The proper hepatic artery gives rise to the cystic artery followed by the right and left hepatic arteries. The cystic artery, however, frequently arises from the right hepatic artery, and rarely may arise from the left hepatic artery. Anatomic variants include a replaced right hepatic artery (right hepatic artery arising from the superior mesenteric artery) and a replaced left hepatic artery (left hepatic artery arising from the left gastric artery). The importance of these variants in hepatic surgery is in recognizing their presence so as to prevent inadvertent injury. Other anatomic variants exist, including accessory vessels (a vessel that exists in conjunction with a vessel with a more standard origin) and variations in the cystic artery anatomy.

Although also discussed elsewhere, an understanding of biliary anatomy is paramount to the successful performance of surgery for hepatic neoplasms. The proximal right hepatic duct is largely intrahepatic, whereas the proximal left hepatic duct is extrahepatic and runs perpendicular to the common hepatic duct to the level of the round ligament. At the round ligament, the left hepatic duct is formed by confluence of ducts from segment IV and segments II and III. The confluence of the left and right hepatic ducts is cephalad and ventral to the portal vein bifurcation. The hepatic bile duct confluence gives rise to the common hepatic duct, the portion of the duct between the confluence and the cystic duct entrance. The common bile duct extends from the cystic duct to the ampulla of Vater. The blood supply to the extrahepatic bile duct arises from the right hepatic artery superiorly and from the gastroduodenal artery inferiorly and runs longitudinally along its course.

One of the greatest advances in hepatic surgery is the understanding of the segmental anatomy of the liver. The Couinaud system for liver segmental nomenclature is widely accepted (Fig. 61.1).[3,4] The liver is divided into longitudinal planes drawn through each hepatic vein to the vena cava and a transverse plane at the level of the main portal bifurcation. The plane of the middle hepatic vein and the primary bifurcation of the portal vein, which divide the liver into a right and left lobe, runs from the inferior vena cava to the tip of the gallbladder fossa (also know as "Cantlie's line" or the portal fissure). The secondary portal bifurcations on the right and left give rise to four sectors (or sections). On the right side, this produces the anterior and posterior sectors that are split by the plane of the right hepatic vein. The tertiary branches on the right supply four segments, two in each sector. On the left, the ascending branch gives off recurrent branches to the medial sector,[5] whereas the left lateral sector is supplied by separate branches supplying segments II and III. Segment I, the caudate lobe, receives blood supply from both the left and right portal pedicles; bile ducts from segment I also drain into the right and left hepatic ducts.

The translation of understanding surgical segmental anatomy to axial radiologic imaging is important in evaluating diagnostic computer tomographic (CT) or magnetic resonance imaging (MRI) studies. Reading axial studies should begin with the identification of the hepatic vein insertions into the vena cava and the plane of the portal bifurcation. Any segments cephalad to the portal vein bifurcation are VII, VIII, IVA, or II. Those caudal to the portal vein bifurcation are VI, V, IVB, and III.

DIAGNOSIS

History, Physical, and Laboratory Examination

The majority of patients who present with liver tumors are diagnosed through imaging performed for some other indication, as part of a screening protocol, or during follow-up for a known primary malignancy of another organ site. If symptomatic, patients complain variably of dull right upper quadrant pain, fullness or bloating, and in some instances nausea or vomiting, depending on the size and location of the tumor.[6] Some patients may present with systemic complaints such as malaise, fever, weight loss, or increasing abdominal girth. Specific questioning regarding high-risk behaviors or known hepatitis virus infection, travel to areas where hepatitis B or C is endemic, alcohol use, exposure to hepatotoxins, use of oral contraceptives or hormone replacement therapy, or a history of hereditary liver diseases is important for patients suspected of having primary liver tumors such as hepatocellular carcinoma (HCC) or hepatic adenoma. For patients presenting with suspected metastatic lesions, diagnosis often occurs during follow-up and the patient's history of prior malignancy will make the evaluation more focused.

Depending on the stage of the lesion, physical examination may or may not reveal a palpable mass. Some patients may present with liver tenderness, which can be formidable.[6] Attention to characteristic abnormalities seen in patients with

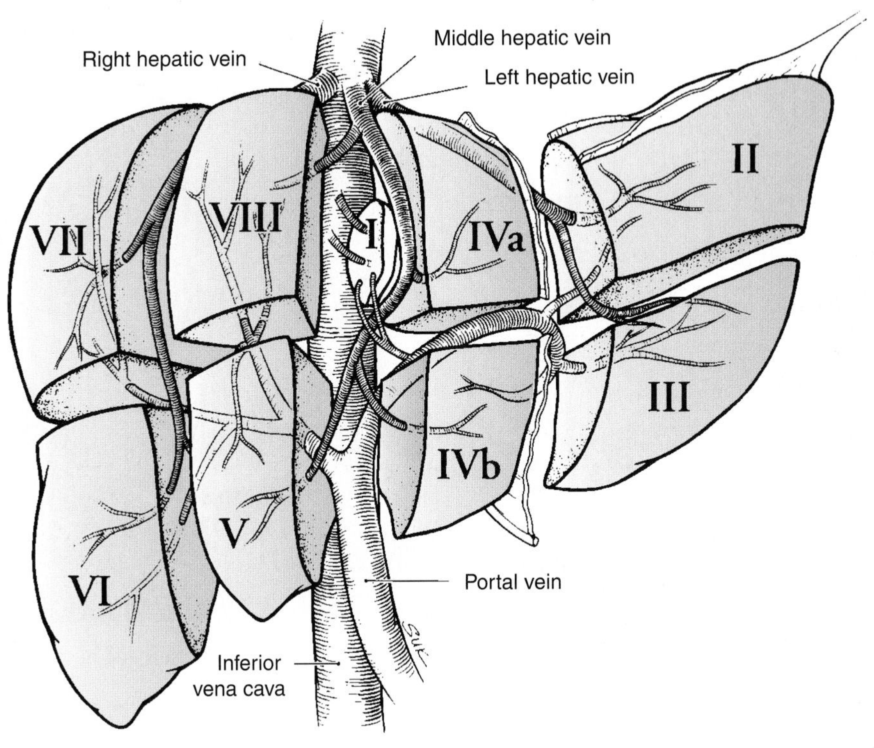

FIGURE 61.1 Couinaud's segmental anatomy of the liver. Segments II to IV make up the left lobe and segments V to VIII constitute the right lobe.

advanced cirrhosis is appropriate; for example, splenomegaly and ascites are frequently seen in patients with portal hypertension.[6] A history of easy bruising or signs of ecchymoses can serve as indicators of liver dysfunction with associated platelet and coagulation abnormalities.

Laboratory evaluation should include liver function studies, coagulation parameters, and measurement of hematologic parameters, including hemoglobin, hematocrit, and platelet counts. In patients with suspected metastatic disease, appropriate tumor markers should be obtained. In most patients with benign liver lesions, liver function tests will be normal, whereas in 97% of patients with HCC at least one liver function assay will be abnormal.[7] In patients with underlying liver disease, many of the laboratory studies may also be abnormal even without the presence of a hepatic tumor; however, in patients with HCC the serum α-fetoprotein (AFP) level is the most useful laboratory test to suggest its diagnosis.[8] Other laboratory tests have also been shown to play a role in diagnosis and prognosis of HCC. Specifically, protein induced by vitamin K absence or antagonist-II (PIVKA-II), also known as des-γ-carboxy prothrombin (DCP), has been shown to be elevated in some patients with HCC. New assays for this protein have enhanced its clinical utility, allowing it to aid in diagnosis and to serve as a prognostic factor, predictive of poor outcome and vascular invasion in patients with HCC. Its presence in the serum of patients with HCC is independent of the presence of AFP and therefore the two tests are complementary.[9,10]

Radiographic Evaluation and Imaging Techniques

Computed Tomography Scanning

Modern computed tomography scans are helical and are highly sensitive at spatial discrimination and quantification of lesions in the liver.[11–13] Lesions can be characterized as solid or cystic, and the enhancement characteristics can be evaluated during the arterial, portal, and delayed phases. The smallest detectable lesion size is approximately 1 cm. Current generation CT scanners allow for rapid acquisition and multidetector technologies can generate three-dimensional reconstructions. These reconstructions are useful in preoperative planning, assessment of hepatic inflow and outflow blood vessels, and measurement of liver volume, which is useful for planning both resection and transplantation.[14] CT scans utilizing arterial, portal, and delayed phase bolus intravenous contrast (Fig. 61.2) are more accurate than standard CT or portal venous phase CT in detecting colorectal liver metastases, although the overall detection rate is still 85%, with a false—positive rate of up to 5%.[15,16] CT scan is not as effective in detecting small HCC as it is in detecting metastatic lesions. The small HCC detection rate ranges from 40% to 60% and is complicated by the limited ability of the CT scan to differentiate between macronodular regenerating nodules arising in a cirrhotic liver and HCC.[17,18] CT is still the preferred method for evaluating the

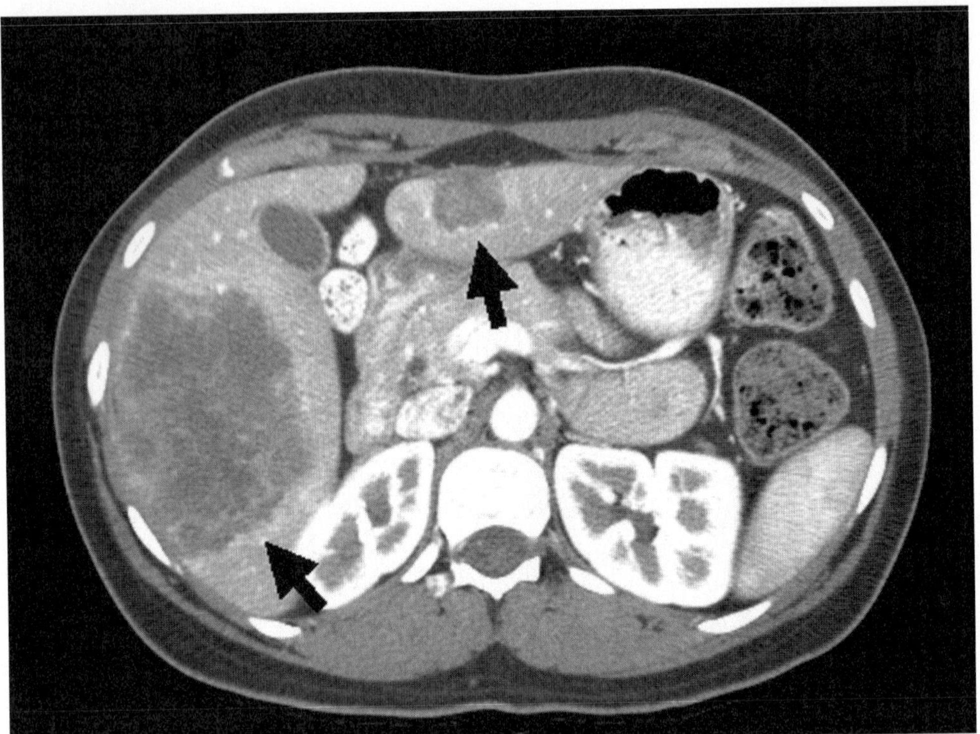

FIGURE 61.2 Arterial phase of a three-phase computed tomography scan of hepatic metastases from colorectal carcinoma. *Black arrows* mark the lesions.

remainder of the abdomen to exclude the presence of extrahepatic malignant disease. In patients with liver metastases, the CT is used to evaluate for peritoneal disease, portal lymphadenopathy, and other remote lesions.

Magnetic Resonance Imaging

Magnetic resonance imaging scans are more sensitive than helical CT in detecting early HCC and in distinguishing between HCC and macroregenerative nodules (Fig. 61.3). The application of liver-specific contrast agents has improved the diagnostic accuracy of MRI for both primary and metastatic liver malignancies, and can also be useful in differentiating between a benign and a malignant liver tumor.[17,18] MR-cholangiography is an excellent study for the evaluation of the biliary tree and is critical to the operative planning for hilar bile duct malignancies requiring liver resection. MR-venography is another useful adaptation of this technology that can be used for the noninvasive study of the extrahepatic portal system and that is particularly adept in identifying extrahepatic portal venous occlusion.

Ultrasound

Transcutaneous ultrasonography has been used to detect the presence of liver tumors, to guide percutaneous biopsies of liver tumors, and to guide therapy for selected tumors with direct injection or ablation techniques. Like CT and MRI, ultrasonographic technology continues to improve. Ultrasonography is rarely used as a screening or follow-up evaluation tool in patients with metastatic liver tumors, but because it is a readily available and relatively inexpensive technology, ultrasonography is commonly used in programs that screen high-risk populations for the development of HCC. In studies from Western centers, ultrasonography has been shown to be superior to serum AFP measurement for early detection of HCC in chronic viral hepatitis patients.[19,20]

The development of new ultrasound technologies, including microbubble contrast agents and multidimensional imaging, may increase the utility of ultrasound in the evaluation of benign or malignant solid tumors. Initial studies of these agents suggest that the sensitivity of ultrasound to detect metastatic disease can be improved as much as 20%, and the mean size of the smallest lesions detected is reduced to less than 1 cm.[21] Doppler ultrasound, even in the absence of contrast agents, is effective in determining the patency and flow direction of all major hepatic blood vessels and also in evaluating tumor vascularity.

Despite the advances in transcutaneous ultrasound techniques, perhaps the most significant application of ultrasound technology in the management of patients with hepatic neoplasms is in its use as an intraoperative tool. Intraoperative ultrasonography (IOUS) has become the gold standard against which all other diagnostic imaging modalities are compared to detect the number, extent, and association of tumors with intrahepatic blood vessels in both primary and metastatic liver tumors. IOUS can be performed laparoscopically or during an open procedure.[22] All patients undergoing liver resection for tumor should undergo an IOUS evaluation to rule out smaller undetected lesions before proceeding with resection. IOUS can also be used to guide resection, specifically with respect to how the line of parenchymal transection relates to relevant vascular structures. IOUS is also necessary for intraoperative image-guided procedures such as biopsy and radiofrequency ablation.

Positron Emission Tomography

Positron emission tomography (PET) is a nuclear medicine study that is being widely evaluated in patients with malignant disease. PET does not provide the anatomic detail and definition of modern CT or MRI, but offers the potential advantages of whole body imaging and ability to detect subclinical disease in the liver and at extrahepatic sites. PET scanning is a whole-body, multiaxial imaging technique where ^{18}F-flurodeoxyglucose (FDG) is injected systemically through an intravenous catheter

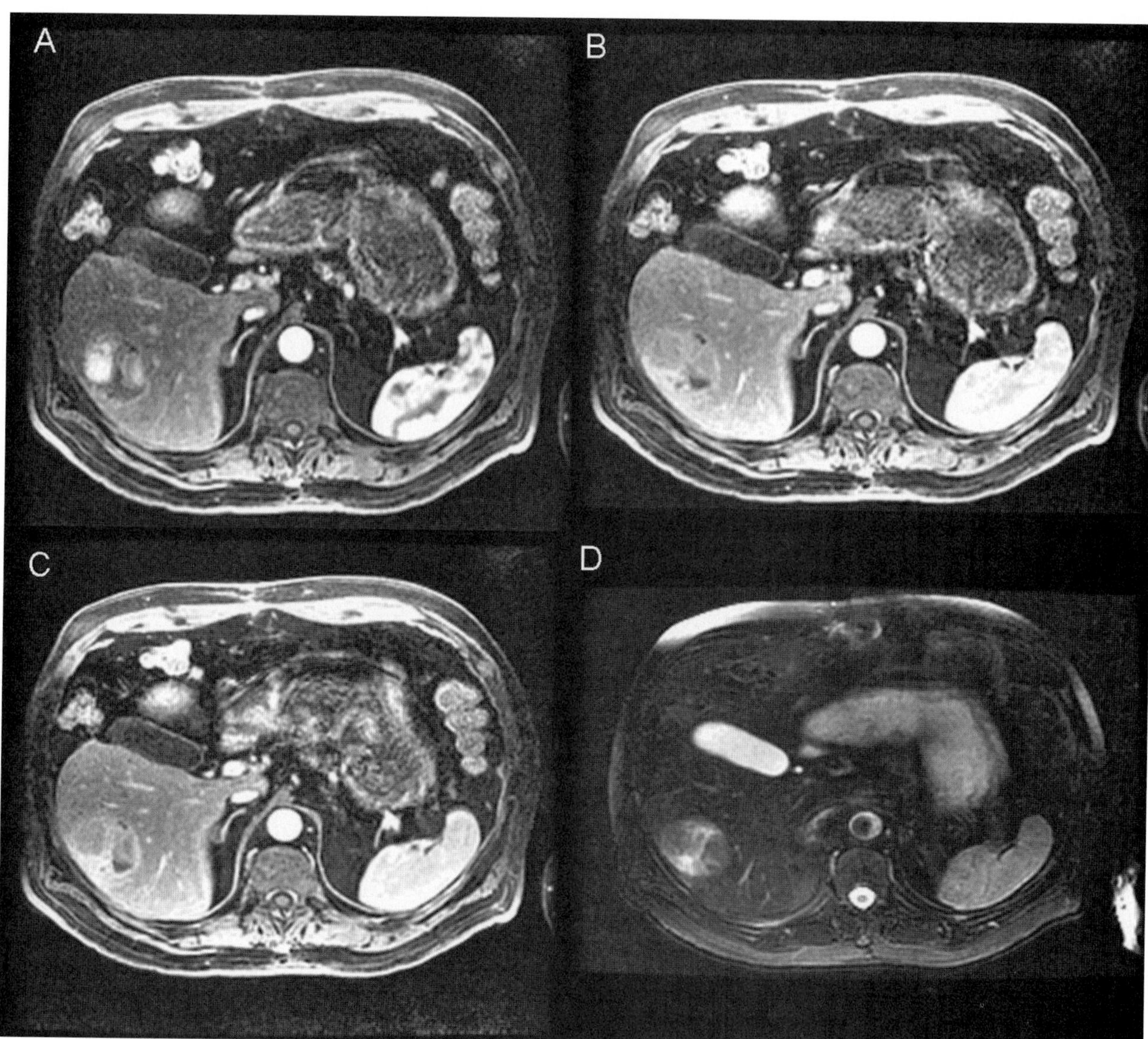

FIGURE 61.3 Magnetic resonance image (MRI) of hepatocellular carcinoma. The heterogeneity is characteristic of the lesion, which is both hypervascular and fibrotic. (*A*) The arterial phase of a T1 weighted scan. The bright area is a result of the marked arterial vascularity of the lesion. (*B*) The portal phase of the MRI, which shows considerable washout of the lesion but with persistent heterogeneity indicative of the underlying fibrosis, similarly seen in (*C*), the venous phase of the study. (*D*) is a T2-weighted study contrasting the lesion against normal hepatic parenchyma.

and glucose avid (metabolically active) tissue (e.g., the brain or neoplastic cells) absorbs and traps the radiotracer. A detector and processor is then used to interpret and quantify the uptake as it is distributed throughout the body.[23]

A significant survival benefit has been shown in some studies of patients undergoing PET scan screening before potentially curative liver resection.[24,25] In one study from the authors' institution, PET was shown to have a sensitivity, specificity, and accuracy of 84%, 89%, and 85%, respectively, in identifying colorectal liver metastases. When used in conjunction with CT scan, the sensitivity, specificity, and accuracy increased to 96%, 88%, and 95%, respectively.[26] In up to 11% of patients being considered for liver resection, PET can be used to exclude patients from surgical consideration because of the presence of extrahepatic disease (Fig. 61.4).[27,28] PET does have a false–negative rate of 7% to 10%, but, in contrast, the false–positive rate appears to be significantly lower. PET has been less useful in the evaluation of patients with HCC because many of these tumors do not have a significantly higher uptake of the radioisotope when compared with the surrounding hepatic parenchyma.[29] Current advances in PET scanning include "fusion" scans applying simultaneous CT and PET scan evaluations. This technology allows for the synchronous assessment of lesions for both their anatomic characteristics and their metabolic activity. The use of fusion scans is presently still in its infancy.

Angiography

Angiography is becoming less important in the evaluation of liver tumors. The present generation CT and MRI scans are capable of defining vascular anatomy and characterizing tumors in the majority of circumstances. Rarely, atypical hemangiomas will be undiagnosed and in these situations angiography may be diagnostic. Planned angiography for hepatic arterial chemoembolization is a potential therapy for

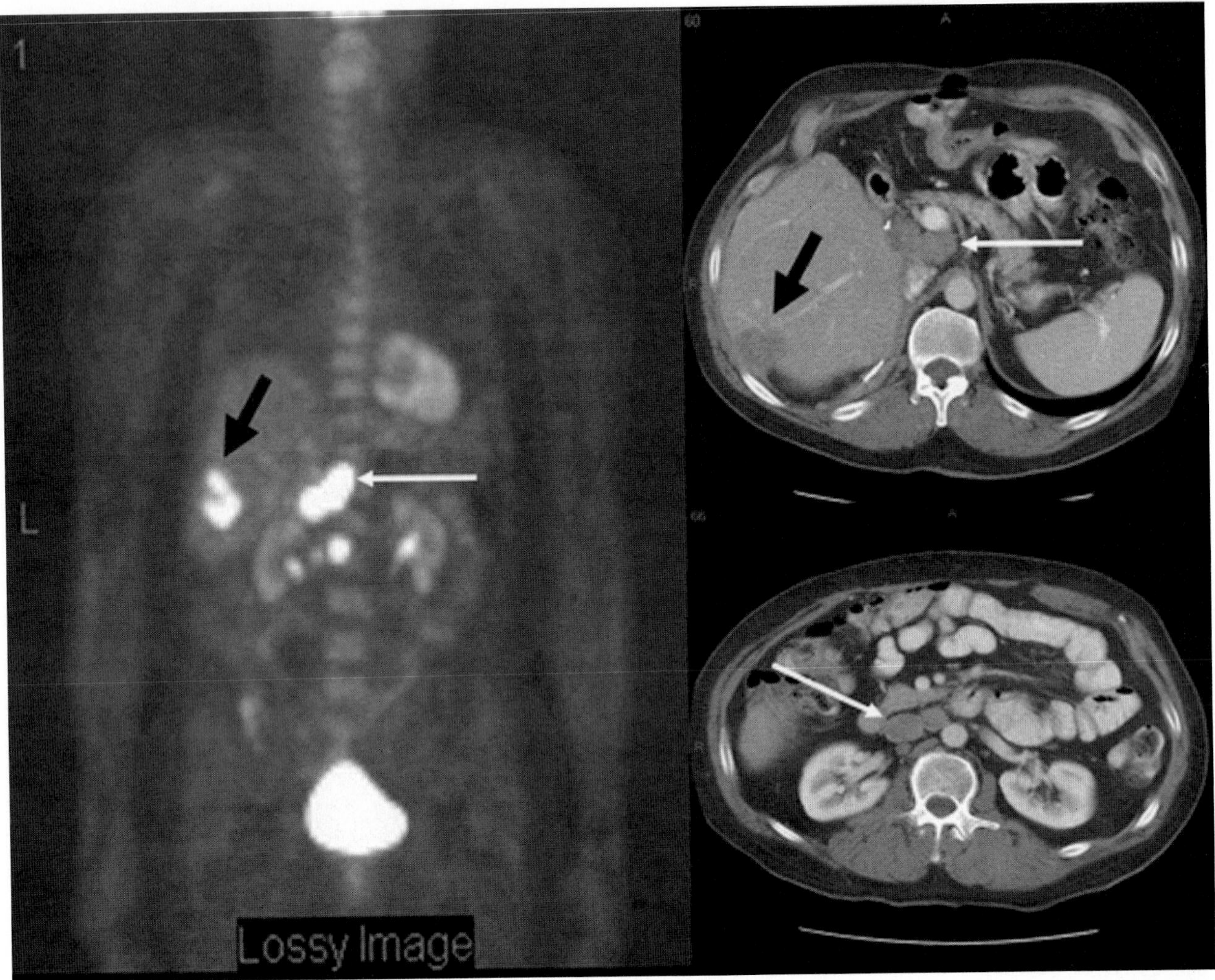

FIGURE 61.4 Positron emission tomography scan confirming hypermetabolic activity of lesions identified on corresponding computed tomography scans. *Black arrows* indicate hepatic metastases, and the *white arrows* demonstrate portal and para-aortic lymph node metastases.

unresectable malignant tumors, including HCC and neuroendocrine tumors.

Diagnostic Laparoscopy

Although technically not an imaging technique, laparoscopy is a minimally invasive method of obtaining a direct view of the liver and peritoneum. Diagnostic laparoscopy can be considered the final step in evaluation of a hepatic neoplasm for resectability before resection.[30] The goal of the preoperative evaluation in hepatic neoplasms is to detect surgically treatable disease. In most malignancies, contraindications to resection or ablation include such findings as extrahepatic disease, extensive intrahepatic disease, and severe portal hypertension. Although some controversy exists as to the utility of diagnostic laparoscopy, its ability to evaluate the entire abdomen, including the parietal and visceral peritoneal surfaces, perform intraoperative laparoscopic ultrasound, and evaluate the porta hepatis in a minimally invasive manner is compelling. A number of centers have published results indicating that in up to 20% of patients undergoing exploration for liver malignancy the tumors will be deemed unresectable.[31] Identification of patients whose tumors are unresectable in a minimally invasive manner avoids a laparotomy, decreasing morbidity and reducing hospital stay in patients who ultimately are not candidates for curative surgery.

Screening

Screening programs for patients with chronic hepatitis B or C virus infection who are at high risk to develop HCC may be able to increase the number of patients diagnosed with early stage disease. As previously mentioned, in conjunction with AFP determination, ultrasound has been shown to be a highly effective tool for screening high-risk populations.[19,20,32–34] Importantly, these studies have shown that up to 60% of patients who develop tumors have either normal AFP levels or their levels fluctuate between normal and abnormal. Furthermore, these studies uniformly show that ultrasound is more sensitive at detecting tumors less than 3 cm than AFP determination alone.[33–35] The goal of these programs is to increase the proportion of patients with HCC who can be treated surgically, especially if preoperative evaluation indicates that they will tolerate the proposed resection. Screening programs that combine transcutaneous ultrasonography and serum AFP measurement have been shown to detect between one third and one half of patients at a stage when their tumors are resectable. Although definitive evidence for a survival benefit in patients detected via screening is lacking, the quality of life of patients treated with resection of HCC has been shown to be significantly better than that of patients treated nonsurgically.[36] It is currently recommended that high- and moderate-risk chronic hepatitis B or C virus-infected populations undergo screened and that surgical therapy be considered in patients with potentially resectable lesions.

BENIGN TUMORS

Cystic Lesions

Cystic lesions of the liver include congenital cysts, cysts associated with polycystic liver disease, neoplastic cysts, and lesions secondary to parasitic infections (e.g., hydatid and amebic cysts). Infectious, polycystic, and congenital cysts fall outside of the scope of this chapter and will not be discussed further. Neoplastic cysts are discussed in the section on malignant tumors; however, simple cysts warrant further elaboration.

Simple cysts are the most common tumor found in the liver and result from excluded hyperplastic bile duct rests (Fig. 61.5). They are distributed across all age groups and do not demonstrate a gender predilection. Although the vast majority of patients with these lesions are asymptomatic, when the cysts are very large they can produce pain, epigastric fullness, or early satiety.[37] If patients are symptomatic, treatment may include initial attempts via a percutaneous approach. Percutaneous aspiration, installation of absolute alcohol, and reaspiration has a success rate as high as 80%.[37,38] If percutaneous therapy fails or the lesion is anatomically not amenable to this approach, surgical therapy is an alternative. If technically feasible, laparoscopic wide fenestration is the surgical procedure of choice.[39,40] At the time of surgery, a portion of the cyst wall should be biopsied and the remaining cyst inspected for evidence of gross neoplastic changes. Recurrence after fenestration is rare (<5%) and it is extremely unusual for simple cysts to require resection in the form of enucleation or hepatectomy.

Solid Lesions

Benign solid lesions of the liver should be discernible based on imaging and clinical presentation. These lesions can usually be differentiated from malignant lesions without the need for percutaneous biopsy, which is important because many of these lesions can be managed conservatively.[41–43]

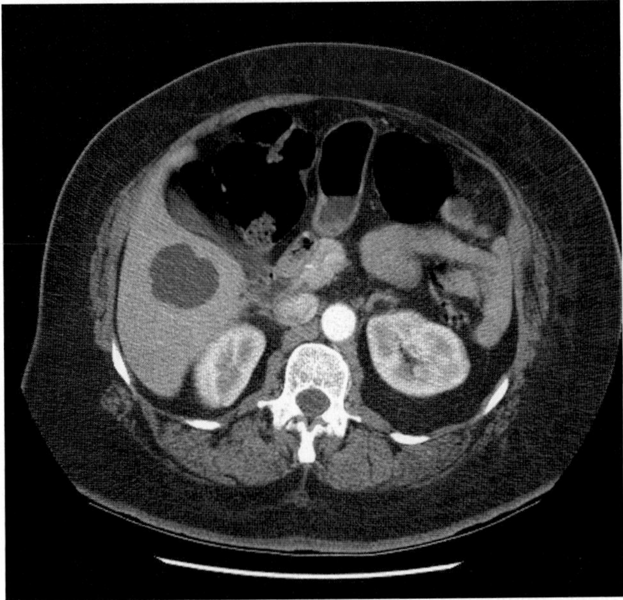

FIGURE 61.5 Computed tomography scan demonstrating a simple hepatic cyst.

Hepatic Adenoma

Hepatic adenomas occur in women of reproductive age, more commonly in individuals using oral contraceptives.[44,45] Up to 75% of adenomas may be symptomatic at presentation, with up to one quarter presenting after rupture and an episode of acute hemorrhage. The most common presenting symptom in patients with hepatic adenomas is abdominal or flank pain.

The radiographic distinction of hepatic adenomas from focal nodular hyperplasia (FNH) poses a common diagnostic dilemma.[46,47] Multiphase CT scan is often a good first study (Fig. 61.6). Although both lesions demonstrate rapid contrast enhancement followed by rapid washout, adenomas do not have a central scar and FNH is often found to have an overt feeding artery.[44,48,49] MRI has also been shown to be useful in that some adenomas demonstrate an increased fat signal intensity on MRI when compared with FNH.[50] If the diagnosis remains ambiguous after CT or MRI, a technetium marcoaggregated albumin liver scan should be considered. Typically, adenomas will not demonstrate uptake, whereas FNH will, because the latter tumor contains Kupffer cells and the former does not.

Once the diagnosis of adenoma is confirmed, management is segregated by size. In patients with lesions less than 4 cm, cessation of oral contraceptive use is an appropriate initial intervention. If regression is noted, as is commonly seen, observation without further intervention may be appropriate.[43] Surgical resection is indicated for patients with lesions larger than 4 cm, those who cannot medically cease hormonal therapy, those whose lesions do not shrink after cessation of hormonal therapy, and those who plan to become pregnant.[43,51] Although radiofrequency ablation is another potential therapeutic option, particularly in individuals with multiple adenomas, until further follow-up data are available, resection remains the standard of care. Finally, a number of large, resected adenomas harbored foci of well-differentiated HCC, although no studies have demonstrated a strong association between oral contraceptive use and an increased risk to develop HCC.[52]

Focal Nodular Hyperplasia

Focal nodular hyperplasia differs from hepatic adenoma in that it does not typically present with symptoms nor pose the risk of rupture or malignant degeneration.[46] A majority of these lesions will demonstrate a central scar on axial imaging and many will demonstrate a feeding artery (Fig. 61.7).[48,49,53] These lesions are often peripherally located and, therefore, lend themselves to laparoscopic approaches for resection if indicated by symptomatology.[43,54] Although resection with a thin margin of normal tissue is an acceptable approach in patients with FNH, formal segmental resection is associated with a lower morbidity and therefore should be considered, either by a laparoscopic or an open approach.

Hemangioma

Hemangiomas are also termed cavernous hemangiomas. They are common lesions that are characteristically diagnosed by CT scan or MRI. Radiographic findings include peripheral enhancement followed by gradual centripetal enhancement and subsequently washout on delayed films (Fig. 61.8). On T2 weighted MRI, hemangiomas will be bright. If any ambiguity remains surrounding the identification of a lesion as a hemangioma, a tagged red cell scan using technetium may be confirmatory.

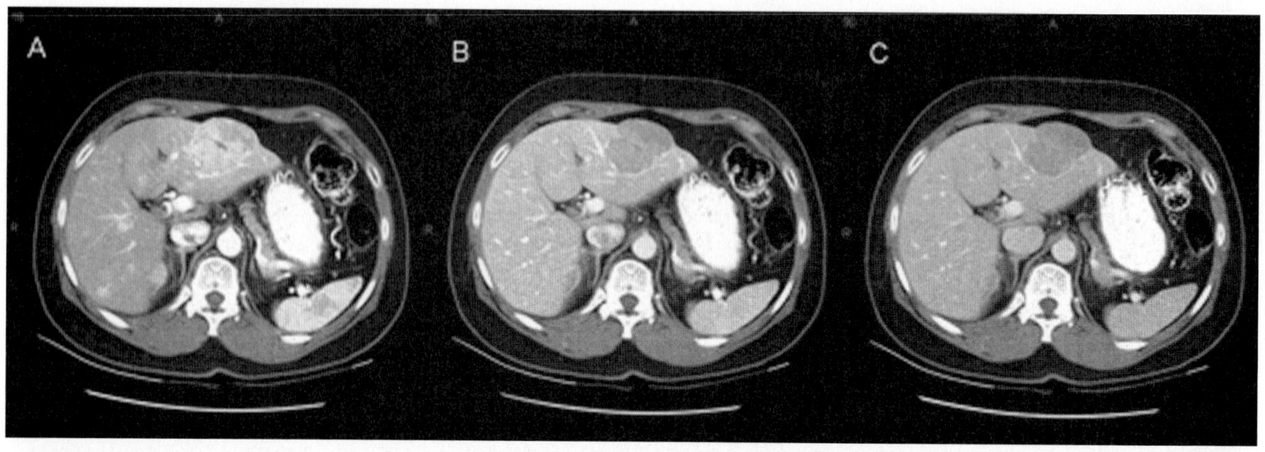

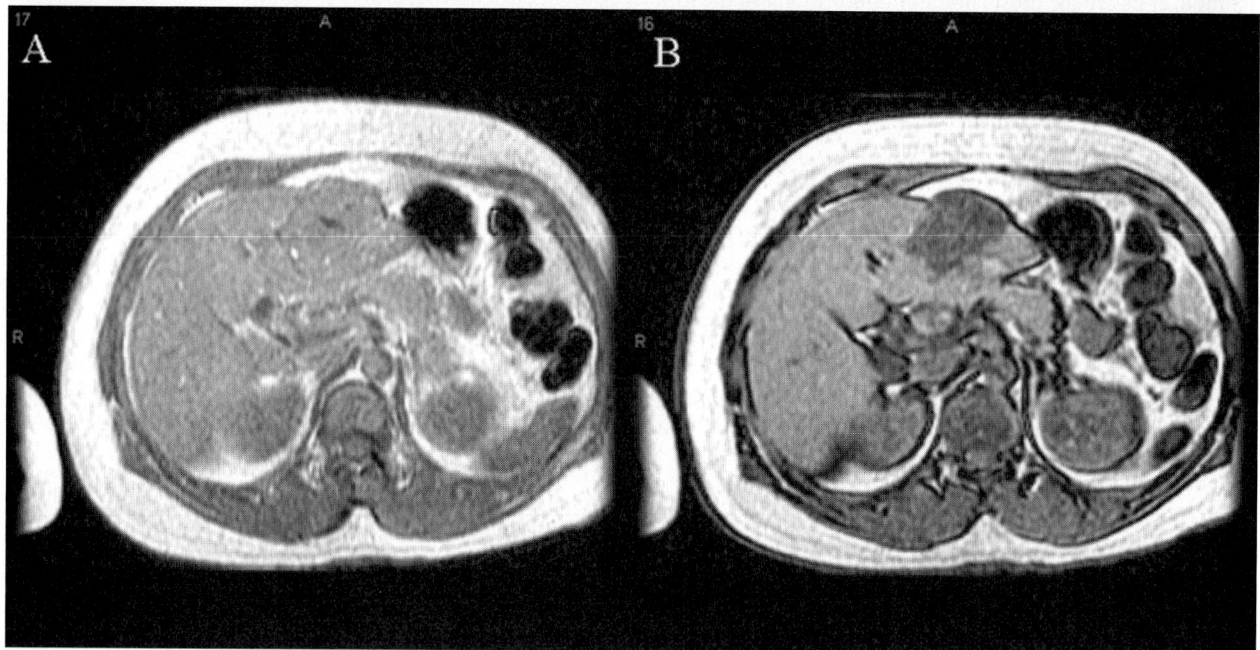

FIGURE 61.6 (*A*) Three-phase computed tomography scan of a hepatic adenoma. *Left*: arterial phase; *center*: portal phase; *right*: venous phase. (*A*) In-phase (*left*) and out-of-phase (*right*) magnetic resonance image of the same hepatic adenoma. As a result of the high fat content of the lesion, the signal cancels out on the out-of-phase image. The lesion, therefore, appears to be nonenhancing.

Generally, hemangiomas may present with chronic, mild, right upper quadrant abdominal pain if they are symptomatic at all.[55] If symptomatic, they can be treated by enucleation or a formal segmental or lobar resection.[56,56]

Bile Duct Hamartomas

Bile duct hamartomas are the most common liver lesions identified incidentally at laparotomy. They are peripherally located, firm, smooth and white in appearance, and are generally less than 1 cm in diameter. They are often difficult to distinguish from miliary metastases from colorectal carcinoma or bile duct cancers and, therefore, biopsy is often necessary to clarify the diagnosis.

MALIGNANT TUMORS

Overview

The goal of surgical therapy for solid tumors is complete extirpation of all malignant tissue. To achieve this end in tumors of the liver, a multitude of therapeutic modalities have been used, ranging from percutaneous, minimally invasive approaches to open resections of up to 80% of the hepatic parenchyma in patients without underlying liver disease. Before undertaking a review of specific malignant hepatic lesions, it is beneficial to have an understanding of the options available to treat these lesions and the planning required to optimize the outcome from major hepatic resections.

Until Couinaud's[3] seminal treatise on the segmental liver anatomy was published in 1957 most surgeons were selective about the patients in whom they attempted liver resection, if they attempted resection at all. Couinaud's description, based on portal venous inflow and hepatic venous outflow, was paramount in the evolution of safe, anatomically based hepatic resections. With this foundation, elective operations for liver surgery are performed with increasing frequency and with marked reduction in morbidity and mortality rates. Currently, when undertaken at major centers by experienced hepatobiliary surgeons, hepatic resection can be performed with an operative mortality of less than 3%.[58–60]

The size, number, and location of liver tumors generally dictate the selection of therapies to be applied to a particular clinical

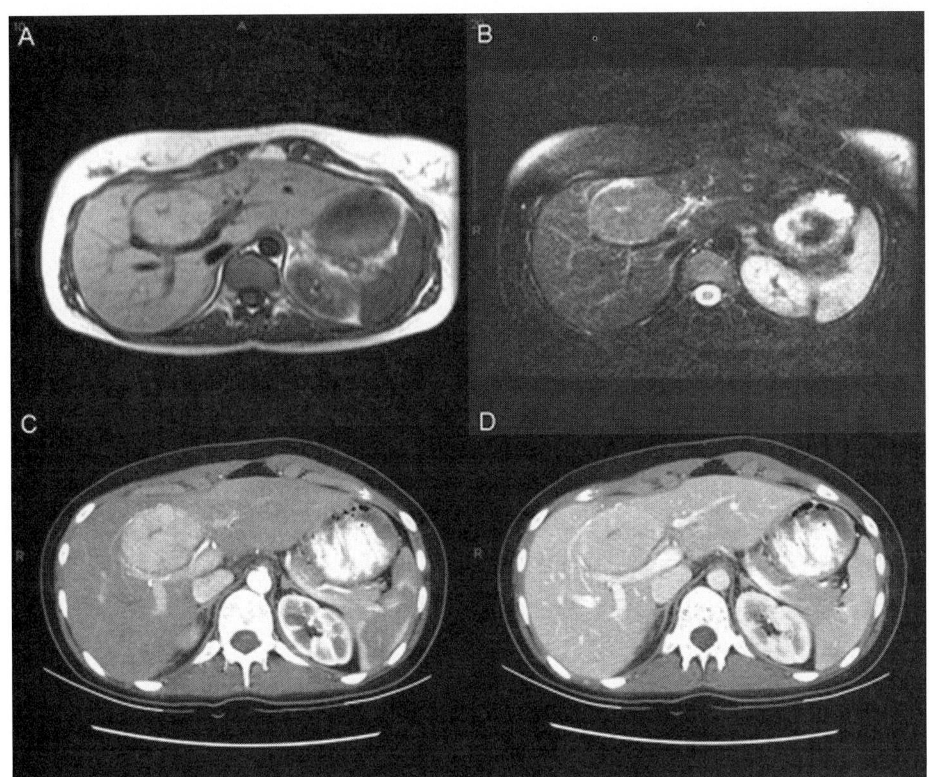

FIGURE 61.7 Focal nodular hyperplasia on cross-sectional T1-weighted (*A*) and T2-weighted (*B*) magnetic resonance imaging. Both scans were made using manganese-based contrast, an agent taken up by hepatocytes generating a hyperintense appearance in the lesion with a high concentration of hepatocytes. Note also, the obvious peripheral vessel on the T2 weighted image. (*C*) Arterial phase computed tomography scan of the same lesion, again hyperintense compared with background liver parenchyma. (*D*) The lesion washes out during the portal phase, demonstrating the importance of three-phase imaging in characterizing and detecting lesions within the liver.

scenario, specifically, in patients with resectable tumors, the amount of hepatic parenchyma that needs to be removed. In patients with normal hepatic parenchyma and normal serum liver function tests, resection of 80% of the liver volume is possible because the remaining 20% of normal, perfused liver can meet metabolic demands while undergoing regeneration. In contrast, patients with abnormal liver function related to steatosis or underlying cirrhosis may not tolerate a significant hepatic resection and are at risk of postoperative liver insufficiency, failure, or even death. Evaluation of functional hepatic reserve is therefore paramount in patients with underlying liver disease or anatomic constraints to resection.

Evaluation of Functional Hepatic Reserve

Typically, individuals whose hepatic reserve is assessed are those with cirrhosis who develop HCC. Assessing the risk of postoperative liver failure based on a clinical classification schema, such as the Child-Turcotte classification, alone is inadequate; the postresection mortality rate from liver failure for Child-Turcotte class A or B patients ranges from 8% to 25%.[61] For patients with cirrhosis who are being considered for resection of malignant liver disease, quantitative or functional hepatic studies can improve patient selection, determine the extent of hepatic parenchymal resection that will be tolerated, and reduce the postoperative mortality rate from liver failure to between 0% and 5%.[62]

A number of functional tests are used to assess hepatic reserve. The most commonly used test is the indocyanine green (ICG) clearance rate. ICG is a dye bound by plasma lipoproteins and cleared by the liver.[63] There are disadvantages to this test, however. Principally, it is not a true measure of hepatocyte function (ICG delivery may be limited by the rate of hepatic blood flow) and, for patients whose clearance values fall in the middle of the ICG risk assessment range, the test does not accurately predict risk for postoperative liver failure and death. Several other tests are not dependent on hepatic

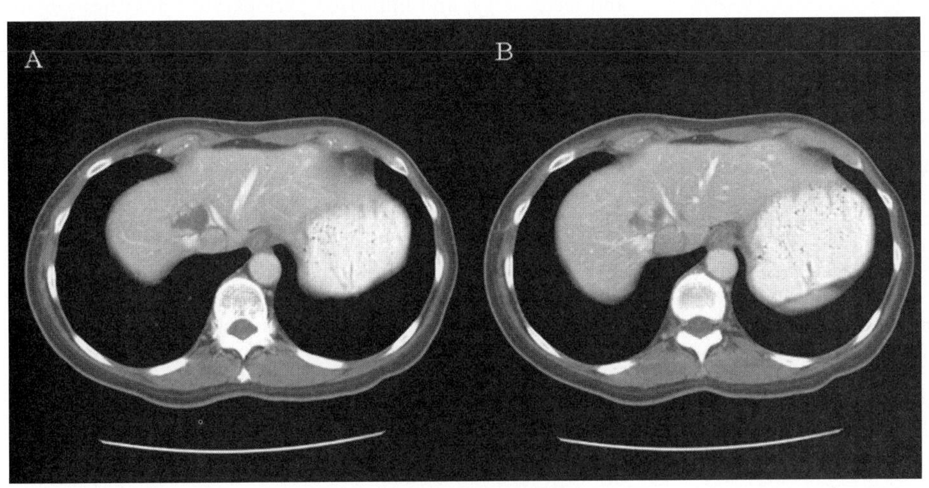

FIGURE 61.8 Cavernous hemangioma. Note the contrast collecting within the lesion. Called "puddling" or alternatively a "globular pattern" of enhancement, it is indicative of contrast pooling within a lesion filled with blood and is characteristic of hemangioma. (*A* and *B*) Different cuts through the same lesion.

blood flow and therefore may provide a more accurate measure of hepatic function. These include the aminopyrine and phenylalanine breath tests in which a patient is injected with either radiolabeled aminopyrine or phenylalanine. The amount of exhaled radioactive CO_2 from hepatic microsomal metabolism of the parent molecules is collected and measured over 2 hours.[61,63,64] Other tests include the measurement of the conversion rate of lidocaine to its metabolite monoethylgylinexylidide (MEGX), and a recently reported application of the hippurate ratio, a novel measurement of glycine conjugation of paraaminobenzoic acid. The MEGX test may be limited by the fact that it measures only particular enzymatic reactions and, therefore, may not be reflective of global hepatic reserve. In contrast, the hippurate ratio was compared to ICG clearance in a study of 61 patients and was shown to be a better predictor of postoperative liver failure.[65]

Assessment of functional hepatic reserve is also another role for nuclear medicine studies. Dynamic single photon emission computed tomography (SPECT) imaging after intravenous administration of ^{99m}Tc-galactosyl-serum albumin has been used to assess functional reserve in patients with liver disease before and after hepatectomy.[66] Positron emission tomography (PET) scanning using radiolabeled water has also been shown to be a noninvasive approach to the measurement of portal venous and hepatic blood flow,[67,68] but this test is still undergoing evaluation as a prognostic indicator in patients with cirrhosis who are intended for liver resection.

Finally, there has been considerable interest in the application of CT volumetry in patients planned for extended hepatic resection with a future liver remnant calculated to be less than 20% of functional liver volume.[69] Although first reported in a small group of patients with HCC,[70] this process is often applied in patients intended to undergo an extended hepatic resection who have normal hepatic parenchyma but an anatomically small future liver remnant. CT volumetry is used in conjunction with preoperative portal vein embolization, which will be discussed subsequently. In brief, the procedure involves a rapid sequence, thin-section helical CT scan that directly measures specific liver volumes.[71] The segments of liver remaining after resection are then considered the future liver remnant and this volume is then divided by the total estimated liver volume to obtain a percent future liver remnant. Recent studies have indicated this percentage to be more than 20% in patients with normal hepatic parenchyma[69] and more than 40% in patients with underlying cirrhosis or severe steatosis.[72] If the future liver remnants are not adequate, then portal vein embolization is considered to induce hypertrophy of those residual or remaining segments after the planned resection.

Portal Vein Embolization

Portal vein embolization (PVE) was first reported as a method for inducing hypertrophy in the liver in a small group of patients with HCC.[70] Since that time, PVE has garnered greater interest because extended hepatectomy has become a safe and appropriate treatment option in patients with a variety of primary and secondary hepatic malignancies. Despite the overall safety of extended hepatectomy, complications related to postoperative liver insufficiency such as cholestasis, coagulopathy, fluid retention, and impaired hepatic synthetic function, persist and can often prolong recovery and hospital stay.[73] PVE provides the additional benefit of offering some patients with prohibitively small anticipated liver remnants the possibility of resection if they undergo an adequate hypertrophic response.

At the authors' institution, PVE is generally offered to patients with a future liver remnant calculated to be less than 20% of the total liver volume. This is based on a recent study demonstrating that the incidence of complications in patients with a future liver remnant less than 20% was significantly higher (50% vs. 13%) than in those with future liver remnants greater than 20% of total liver volume (Fig. 61.9).[69] CT volumetry is performed as described previously in the section on the assessment of effective hepatic reserve. Another method of estimating the total liver volume is based on the association between body surface area (BSA) and total liver volume (TLV) using the following equation:[74]

$$TLV = 706.2 \times BSA + 2.4$$

There is some concern over the reliability of this formula, however, particularly in patients with multiple tumors and those with bile duct cancers.[72,75]

The PVE technique involves a percutaneous transhepatic approach.[76] This technique allows direct access to the lobar and segmental branches to be embolized and minimizes the risk of main trunk thrombosis or injury to the vessels supplying the future liver remnant. The side effects are minimal and include transient mild pain and low-grade fever. If an extended right hepatectomy (segments IV, V, VI, VII, and VIII to be resected) is planned, it is important to embolize the branches to segment IV to restrict potential segment IV tumor growth.[77]

A number of studies have documented changes in future liver remnant ranging from 18% to 36% of TLV preembolization to 31% to 59% post-PVE.[71,76,78–83] Complications are infrequent and there have been no reported deaths with the procedure. One caveat remains, however, because not all patients ultimately undergo surgery after PVE: some fail to respond to the intervention, whereas others suffer from rapid progression of their malignant disease.

Treatment Options

Hepatic Resection

Surgical resection remains the optimal choice for the treatment of solid tumors of the liver. If nodal metastases are excluded, the liver is the most common site of metastasis from solid tumors of other sites.[84] Furthermore, HCC is one of the most common solid tumors worldwide, with an estimated 1 million new patients affected annually.[85,86] Surgical resection of HCC and metastatic lesions from a variety of solid tumors has demonstrated a significant survival benefit in appropriately selected patients.[59,87–90] Improved preoperative imaging studies, routine use of intraoperative ultrasonography, a thorough understanding of the vascular and segmental anatomy of the liver, application of new surgical instruments and technology, and improved perioperative anesthesia management have resulted in an increase in the number of patients who successfully undergo hepatic resection.

Candidacy for operative resection of solid hepatic lesions differs somewhat based on the status of the underlying hepatic parenchyma. Patients with HCC often have a diseased liver, in contrast to those with liver metastases. Therefore, the two groups must be approached with different surgical mindsets. Patients with metastatic disease may tolerate up to 80% of their liver being removed, whereas patients with HCC will tolerate a much smaller volume of resection and still have a higher morbidity rate from the procedure.

With a considerable volume of evidence demonstrating the benefit of resection in treating hepatic tumors, interest has increased in expanding the group of patients who are candidates for this approach. This interest has led to novel approaches to patients with hepatic tumors. One such approach, PVE, has been discussed previously. Others, however, include the

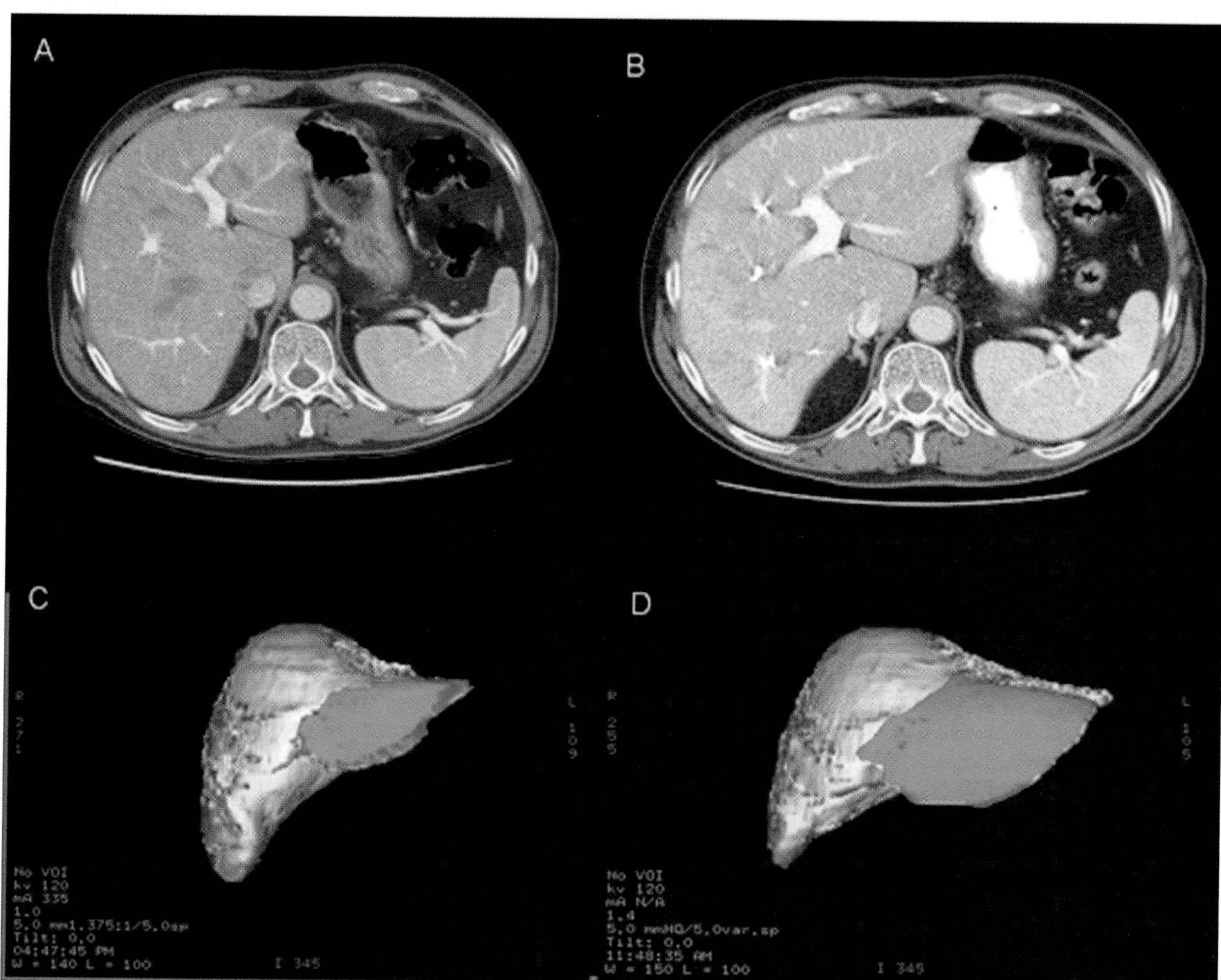

FIGURE 61.9 Images before and after portal venous embolization. (*A*) The cross-sectional and (*C*) the three-dimensional reconstruction of the liver before portal vein embolization of segments IV-XIII with the future liver remnant highlighted. (*B*) The corresponding cross-sectional image after portal vein embolization. (*D*) The reconstructed image, again with the future liver remnant highlighted. The increase in size in segments II and III is readily apparent in *B* and *D*.

application of a two-stage hepatectomy and the use of neoadjuvant chemotherapy in select patients. Two-stage hepatectomy has been advocated by some authors and essentially entails two planned hepatic resections.[91,92] Initially described, the procedure includes a first operation wherein as many tumors as possible are resected. This is followed by an interval of recovery and hepatic regeneration during which the patient receives systemic chemotherapy. The second operation is then approached as though the patient presented *de novo* and, presuming the patient remains a candidate for resection, the second operation is performed with a curative intent.[92] Another approach to this technique uses an open ligation of the right portal vein and simultaneous resection of all left-sided disease at the initial operation to allow for hypertrophy to occur in the subsequently disease-free future liver remnant. Right hepatectomy is then performed as a second procedure after hypertrophy is complete.[91]

Another effort to expand the indications for surgical resection involves the use of neoadjuvant chemotherapy. A number of studies have demonstrated the applicability and safety of this approach in patients with multiple metastatic lesions.[60,93–96] A large single-institution study demonstrated in 330 patients with initially deemed unresectable tumors that a reduction in tumor burden to permit resectability was achievable in 15% of those individuals.[96] Follow-up from the same group analyzing a total of more than 700 patients confirmed the finding that nearly 15% of patients who presented initially with unresectable disease were able to have their disease resected after neoadjuvant chemotherapy and, with subsequent resection, had an overall 5-year survival rate similar to that seen in patients who undergo resection alone.[94] Currently, interest lies in evaluating the benefit of neoadjuvant protocols in patients regardless of the resectability of their disease at presentation. A potential survival benefit in patients utilizing this approach has been observed,[97] but investigation is ongoing.

The application of certain devices not primarily used for hepatic surgery has also led to changes in the approach to hepatic surgery. In particular, stapling devices have led to a reduction in operative time and intraoperative blood loss (Figs. 61.10 to 61.13).[98]

The use of a stapling device does not obviate the need for mobilization, as a key point in the safe application of a stapler as an adjunct to hepatic resection is the complete mobilization of the lobe to be resected.[99] These techniques should be applied judiciously and the surgeon should refrain from their use if the tumor sits near a vascular pedicle because there is a negative prognostic impact if a positive resection margin is obtained. When tumor is near the main portal vein branches,

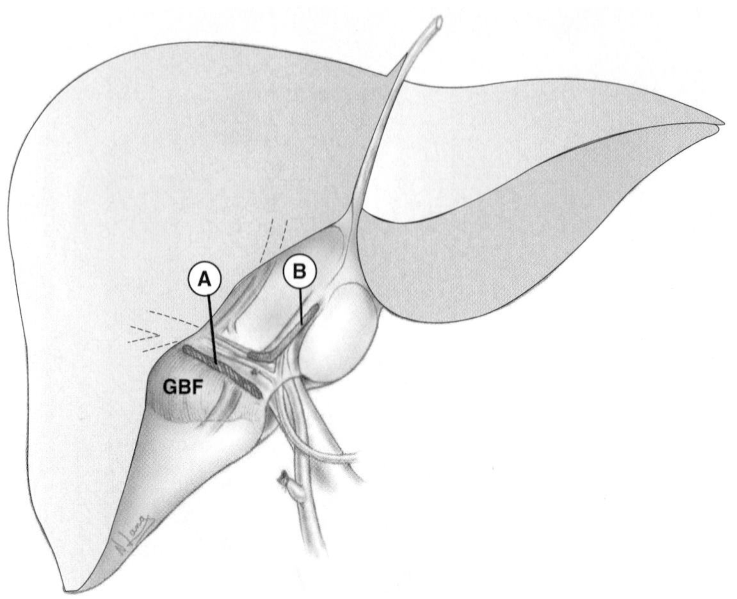

FIGURE 61.10 Technical aspects of hepatic resection. Approach to the inflow. *A* indicates the right main portal triad, and *B* indicates the left main portal triad, which generally has a longer extrahepatic segment than the right. *GBF*, gallbladder fossa. (Copyright ©2003, the University of Texas M.D. Anderson Cancer Center.)

RHV

IVC

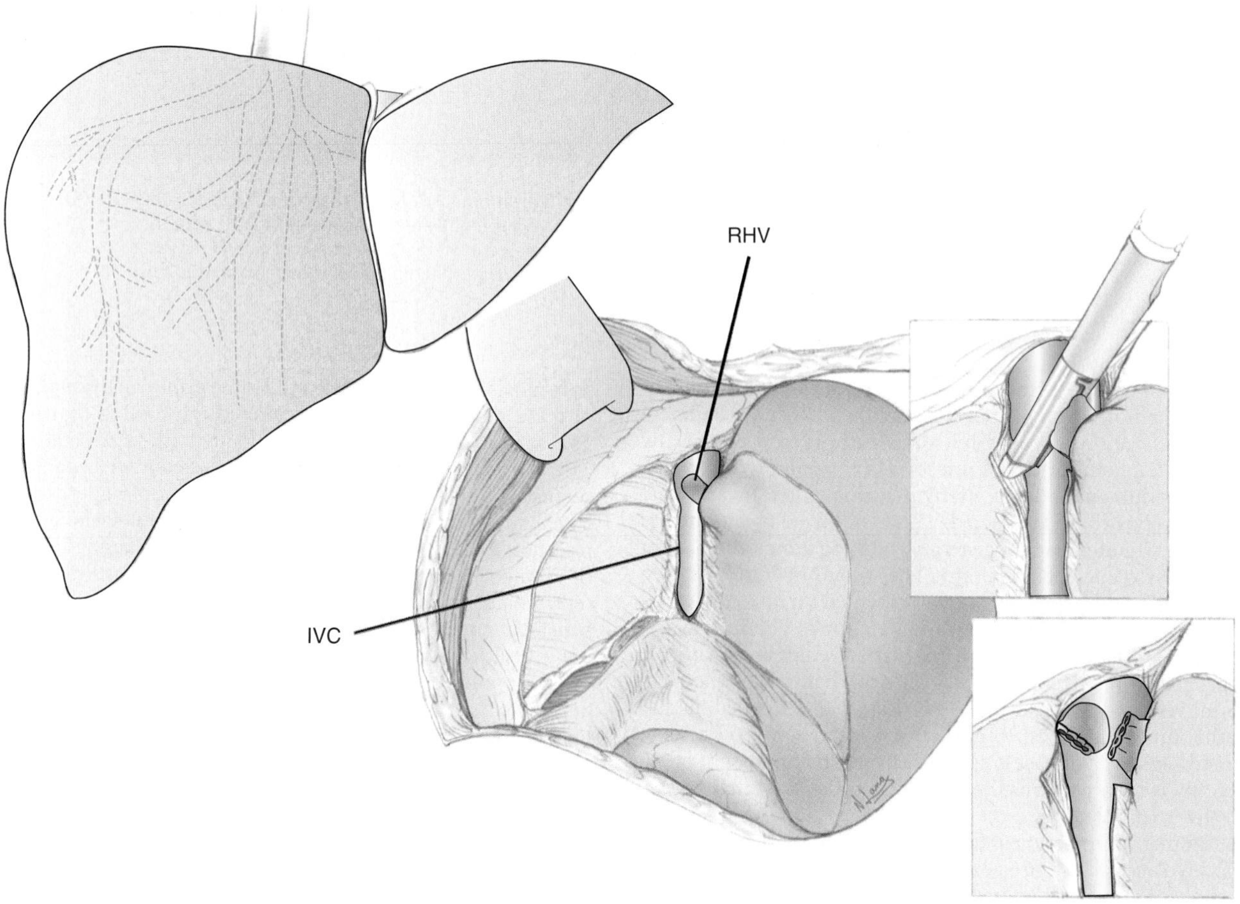

FIGURE 61.11 Approach to the outflow tract for a planned right hepatectomy. Note the application of the endoscopic linear stapler to ligate and divide the right hepatic vein (*RHV*). The liver is retracted medially and anteriorly after mobilization. (Copyright ©2003, the University of Texas M.D. Anderson Cancer Center.)

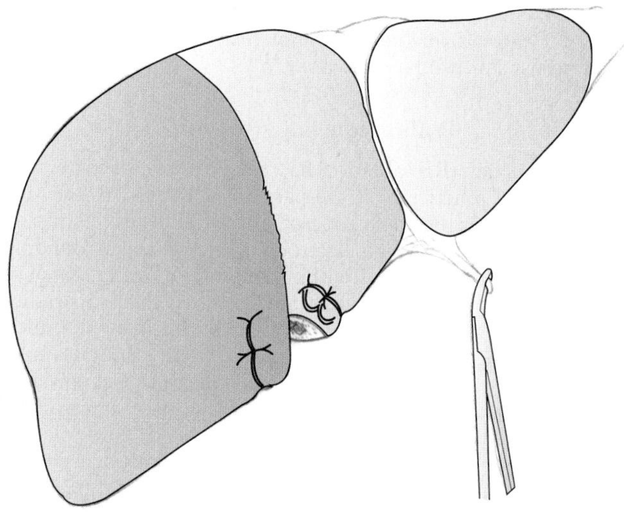

FIGURE 61.12 The specimen is dusky and demarcated after vascular isolation and the parenchymal transection is begun. Note the two sutures placed in the peripheral edge of the liver for both traction and some minor additional hemostasis. (Copyright ©2003, the University of Texas M.D. Anderson Cancer Center.)

the standard approach of extrahepatic dissection and ligation of the portal vein, hepatic artery, and bile duct branch is advocated. The physical attributes of a laparoscopic linear vascular stapler make it an excellent instrument for control of venous outflow through ligation and division of hepatic veins. This technique is most commonly used with the right hepatic vein but, with proper mobilization, the middle and left hepatic veins can also be divided with this device.[99]

Laparoscopic approaches to hepatic resection have evolved to play a definite role in the diagnosis and staging of liver tumors. Although a therapeutic role for laparoscopic liver resection has yet to be established, the development of endoscopic vascular staplers and the harmonic scalpel have spurred interest in applying this technique in cases of benign and malignant lesions. At present, a multitude of anecdotal studies have demonstrated the applicability and safety of this modality in a variety of hepatic tumors.[54,100–102]

Repeat hepatic resection has also become feasible. Because of improvements in technology and anesthesia, selected patients can undergo resection of isolated intrahepatic recurrences for both metastatic and primary tumors. Because disease-free survival rates are 40% or lower, for most resected malignant hepatic tumors, this scenario is becoming more common. Criteria for re-resection are similar to those with initial hepatic resections (i.e., recurrent tumors must be located in anatomic sites amenable to removal and patients must have undergone sufficient regeneration for the future liver remnant to provide adequate functional reserve). The patients most frequently considered for repeat hepatectomy are those with recurrent colorectal metastases.[103,104] Of patients who have undergone resection for colorectal metastases, only 10% to 15% of patients will be candidates for repeat hepatectomy. The experience at The University of Texas M.D. Anderson Cancer Center with repeat hepatectomy consisted of 23 patients with colorectal metastases. There were no perioperative deaths and a 22% complication rate. The median survival was 39 months, with a 5-year survival rate of only 13%.[103] In contrast, other authors report 5-year survival rates as high as 35%.[104]

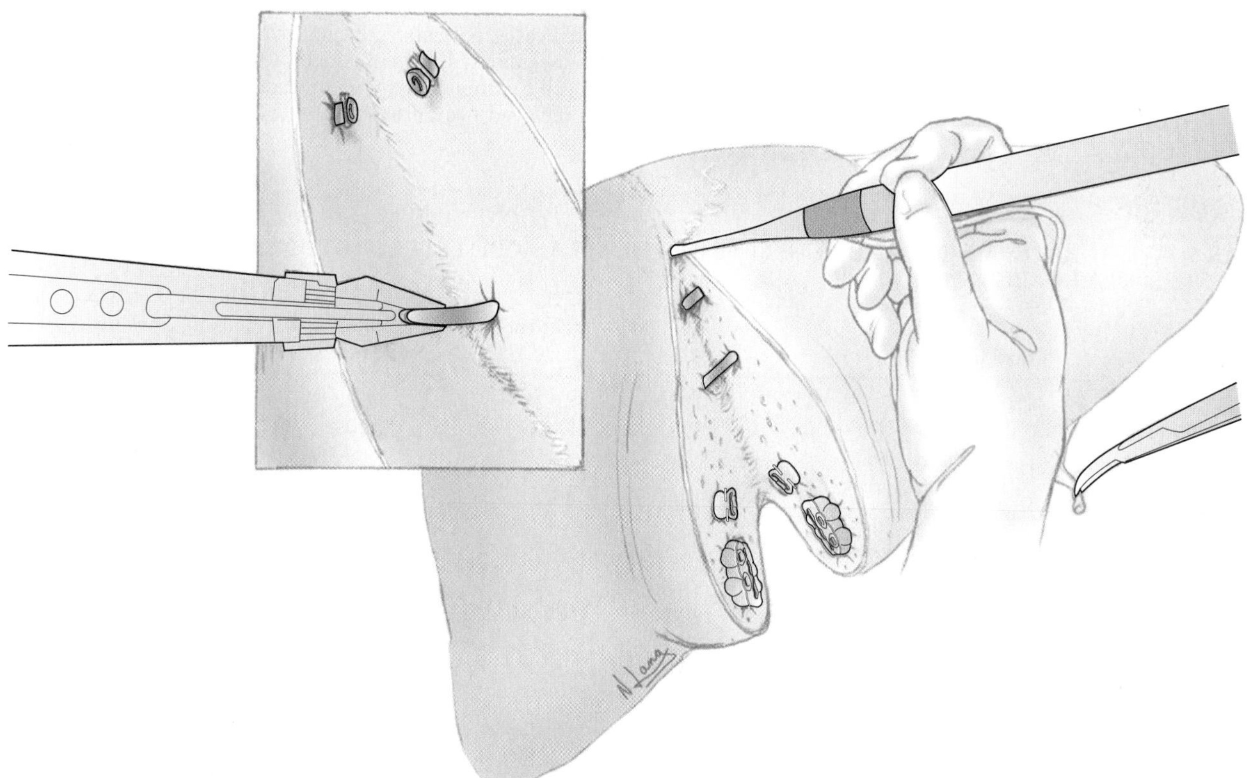

FIGURE 61.13 Parenchymal transection is carried out along the plane identified after vascular isolation. Parenchymal division can be performed by a number of different techniques, including coagulation dissecting devices or ultrasonic dissection. Large crossing ducts and vessels can be ligated with suture or clips, whereas smaller vessels are often readily coagulated with a variety of electrosurgical techniques. (Copyright ©2003, the University of Texas M.D. Anderson Cancer Center.)

Although repeat hepatectomy for colorectal metastases is more common, repeat hepatic resection can be used in selected patients with HCC. Isolated intrahepatic recurrence is actually more common in patients with HCC than in those with metastatic disease, but the number of patients who have sufficient hepatic function to tolerate repeat resection is lower. In selected patients, repeat resection for HCC can lead to long-term survival rates of up to 30%.[105,106] The incidence of postresection liver failure in these patients is no higher than in those undergoing an initial resection, an indication of the important role careful selection plays in these procedures.

Transplantation

Attitudes regarding the use of orthotopic liver transplantation as a therapeutic option for HCC have undergone a remarkable evolution in recent years. Prior to the adoption of strict criteria for candidacy for transplantation, results using this modality were dismal.[107,108] In 1996, Mazzaferro et al. published their data demonstrating a 75% 4-year survival in a small cohort of patients meeting strict criteria regarding tumor size and number.[109] Now uniformly identified as the Milan Criteria, candidates for transplantation in this study had solitary tumors 5 cm or less in diameter or three or fewer tumors all 3 cm or less in greatest diameter. Subsequent studies have demonstrated that in patients meeting these criteria, resection and transplantation afford similar 5-year overall survival rates (Table 61.1).[110]

Considerable interest in outcomes after transplantation has identified predictors of tumor recurrence, in addition to size and number: specifically, vascular invasion, high tumor grade, and high preoperative serum AFP values.[111–114] Since the adoption of these criteria by the United Network for Organ Sharing (UNOS), further changes have been made in the manner in which organs are distributed. In February 2002, UNOS adopted the model for end-stage liver disease (MELD) as a mechanism for prioritizing patients to receive organs. Since the initial adoption of these policies using the Milan Criteria as a guideline, UNOS has amended the MELD criteria to give weight to patients with HCC who are otherwise not candidates for surgical resection.[115] As a result of these changes, dropout rates from the transplant list have decreased and waiting-list survival has increased.[116]

Radiofrequency Ablation

Radiofrequency (RF) ablation has been a focus of increasing research and practice over the past several years. Briefly, RF ablation involves the application of a high-frequency alternating current from the tip of an electrode to the tissue surrounding that electrode. As the ions within the tissue move in response to this current, frictional heat is generated. As the temperature in the tissue increases above 60°C, cells begin to die, ultimately leading to coagulative necrosis.[117] RF electrodes may be applied via a percutaneous, laparoscopic, or open approach. Generally, ultrasound is used to guide the placement of the needle and ensure a complete therapeutic field. Once placed, RF energy is then applied across the needle electrode using an established protocol specific for the instrument (Figs. 61.14 and 61.15).[118] Smaller tumors can often be treated with one application, whereas larger tumors (>2.5 cm) will require more than one deployment of the electrode to ensure complete destruction of the lesion. Overlapping zones of coagulative necrosis are a key element in the use of RF ablative techniques requiring more than one deployment. To mimic a surgical margin of resectability, the electrode array is positioned so as to obtain a field of thermal necrosis including, when possible, a 1-cm perimeter of normal hepatic parenchyma surrounding each ablated lesion. After RF ablation CT scans demonstrate cystic areas ideally larger than the original tumors. These ablation zones decrease in size over time.

Candidates for RF ablation of hepatic tumors are generally patients who do not meet criteria for resection of their disease but do not have evidence of extrahepatic disease.[118,119] In selected cases, patients with tumors that are usually associated with disseminated, systemic metastatic disease (e.g., breast or renal cell carcinoma) may be considered for RF ablation if they have received 6 months or more of effective chemotherapy

TABLE 61.1 RESULTS

5-YEAR SURVIVAL RATES BEFORE AND AFTER USE OF THE MILAN CRITERIA FOR TRANSPLANTATION FOR HEPATOCELLULAR CARCINOMA

Author	Institution	Year	Patients (N)	5-Year overall survival (%)	5-Year disease-free survival (%)
Olthoff et al.	UCLA	1990	28	31	NR
Ringe et al.	Klinik for Abdominal and Transplant Surgery	1989	95	20.4	NR
O'Grady et al.	Kings College Hospital	1988	50	NR[b]	NR[b]
Penn	U of Cincinnati	1991	365[c]	18	NR
Mazzaferro et al.	U of Milan	1996	48	75[d,e]	83[d,e]
Llovet et al.	U of Barcelona	1998	58	74	NR
Shetty et al.	U of Penn	2004	109	65	65
Yedibela et al.	U of Erlangen-Nuremberg	2004	45	64[e]	73[e]

NR, Not reported.
[a]Number of patients reflects patients treated with hepatocellular carcinoma, if reported. Earlier studies frequently included all patients undergoing transplant for malignancy regardless of etiology.
[b]This report does not specify 5-year overall survival rates or disease-free survival rate, however only 3 patients of those reported lived beyond 5-years.
[c]This report includes 637 patients of which 365 were documented hepatocellular carcinoma.
[d]The 4-year actuarial survival rates were reported rather than 5-year in this study.
[e]Reported disease-free survival rates can be higher than overall survival rates in patients treated for HCC because many patients die of their underlying liver disease without evidence of recurrence of malignancy.

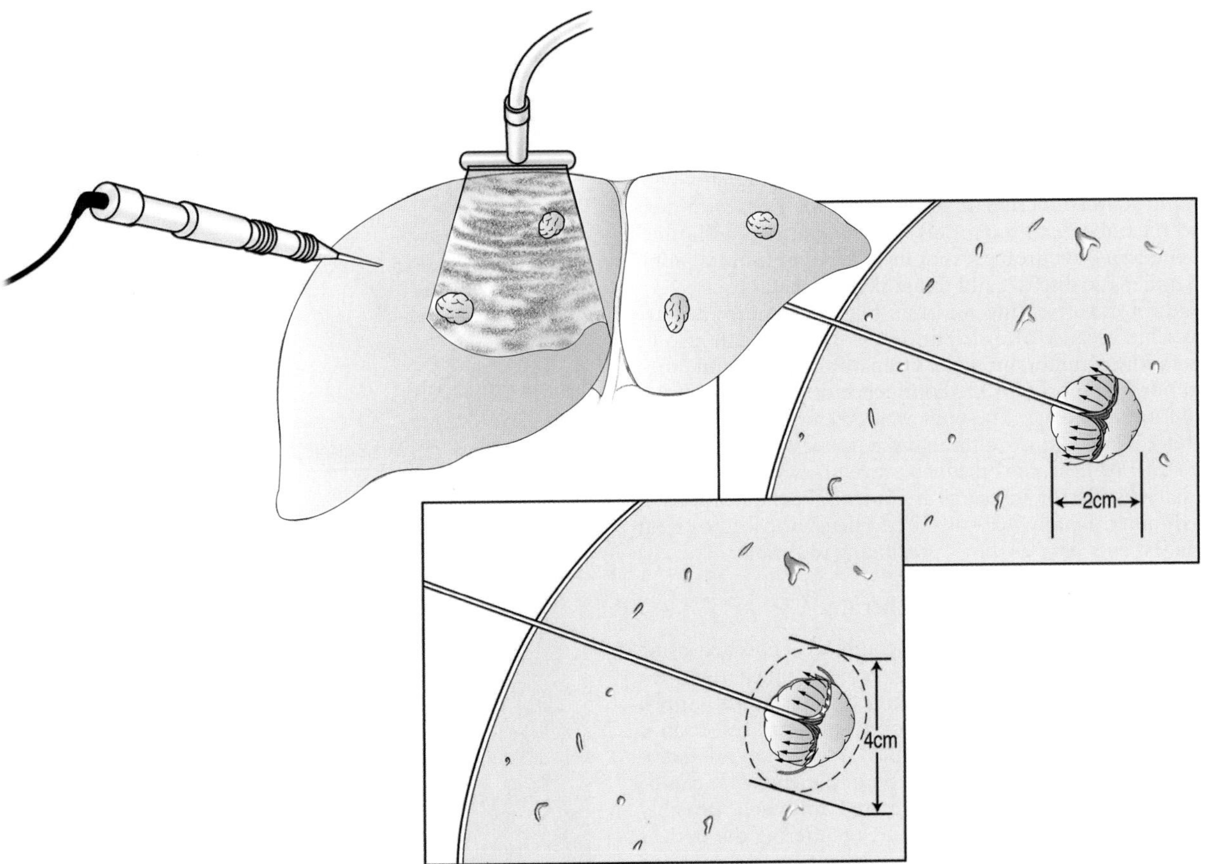

FIGURE 61.14 Technique for radiofrequency ablation. Using ultrasound guidance, the probe is inserted into a lesion and the array is opened so that it encompasses the entire lesion.

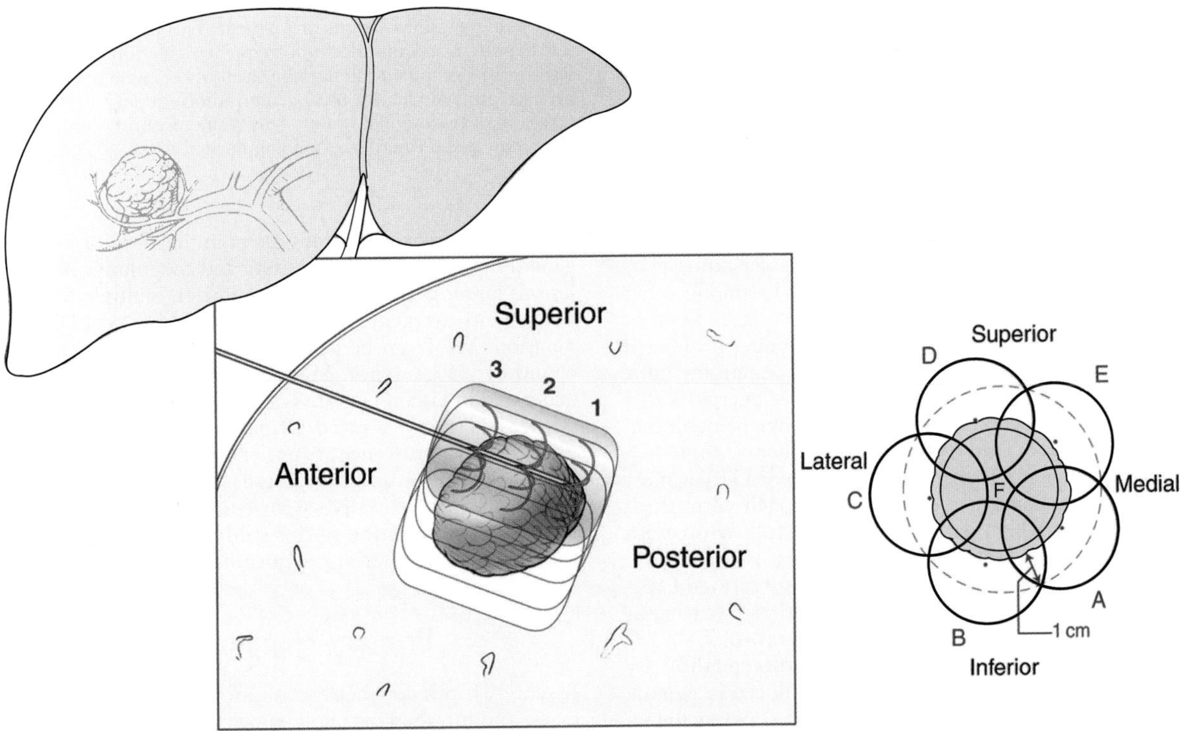

FIGURE 61.15 Technique for larger lesions. Overlapping ablations are performed so that the entire lesion, along with a margin of normal tissue, is submitted to the ablative current.

and have evidence of metastases isolated to the liver. This group of patients is small, and only a few will derive long-term benefit from aggressive liver-directed interventions.[120] As a result, RF ablation should be used only in patients with no preoperative or intraoperative evidence of extrahepatic disease and only for tumors with a reasonable probability of metastases restricted to the liver. Because some patients with metastatic neuroendocrine tumors can live for years with their disease, the only exception to this rule is in patients with functional endocrine syndromes from these types of tumors, minimal extrahepatic disease, and treatable liver metastases.

In addition to treating multiple bilobar tumors that are unresectable because of distribution, RF ablation can also be used to address tumors in areas of anatomic constraint, such as a tumor juxtaposed to the confluence of the hepatic veins and inferior vena cava. The only area precluding RF ablation is the hilar plate because, although the portal vein and hepatic arteries tolerate heat, the bile ducts traveling with them do not and biliary fistulae or strictures are potential complications of thermal injury. Finally, RFA is an excellent modality to treat HCC in patients with cirrhosis precluding resection.[119]

Combination Therapy

Some patients are candidates for a combined approach using both resection and RF ablation. When considering patients for this approach, standard surgical considerations apply. Although the addition of RF ablation to standard resection is not a replacement for complete surgical resection of all identified disease, it expands the population of patients who can be treated with an aggressive, liver-directed approach, possibly improving survival and quality of life, or offering the patient palliative treatment (Fig. 61.16). Two recent studies analyzed the outcome of this combined approach and although complete surgical extirpation remained the optimal therapeutic choice, these studies indicated that some long-term survival benefit may be derived from a regimen us RF ablation combined with liver resection over one using chemotherapy alone.[121,122]

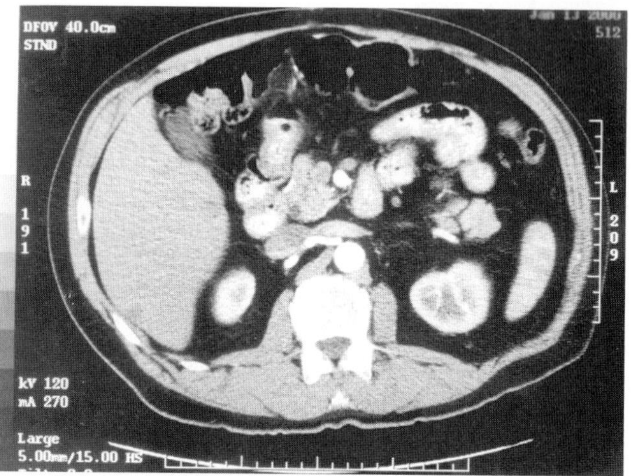

A

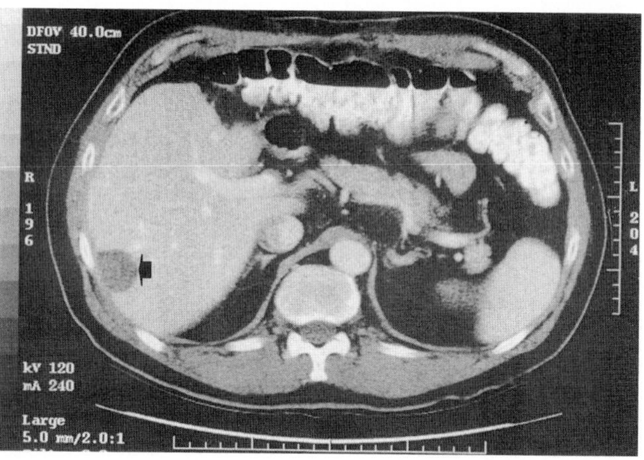

B

FIGURE 61.16 (*A*) Computed tomography scan demonstrating one of several metastatic lesions in a patient. This patient had a combined left hepatic resection and radiofrequency ablation of the right lobe lesion. (*B*) Computed tomography scan of the same patient 6 months after treatment, demonstrating the radiofrequency cavity, which is larger than the original lesion. This results from the need to destroy the tumor and a rim of surrounding normal tissue.

Alternative Ablative Techniques

In addition to RF ablation, other ablative techniques are used to treat hepatic tumors. These include interstitial laser hyperthermic ablation and microwave coagulation therapy (MCT). Both of these approaches are similar to RF ablation in that they induce a thermal injury and coagulative necrosis to the tumor and a rim of surrounding normal hepatic parenchyma.

Interstitial laser hyperthermic ablation, also known as laser-induced interstitial thermotherapy (LITT) among other acronyms, is performed by the insertion of a laser fiber or fibers into a tumor. This fiber is then used to induce prolonged heating of the target tissue in a progressively enlarging zone of radiant and conductive heating. The laser energy is dispersed to naturally occurring chromophores like hemoglobin, myoglobin, bilirubin, and cytochrome pigments, that then produce exothermic photochemical reactions.[123] LITT is most often performed using a percutaneous approach with ultrasonographic or MRI guidance. Currently, follow-up with LITT, as with other novel ablative techniques, is short term, limiting the value of outcome data. The largest reported experience with LITT consists of 705 patients with a 3-year actuarial survival rate of 50% and a complication rate of 7.5%.[124]

Microwave coagulation therapy is another method by which thermal coagulative necrosis can be induced in hepatic tumors and a surrounding rim of normal hepatic parenchyma. Although initially developed as a method of achieving hemostasis,[125] it has since found a better application as an ablative instrument. MCT works by inducing agitation of water molecules within cells and tissues from direct application of microwaves, generating rapid frictional heating and coagulative necrosis. For lesions larger than 2 to 3 cm in diameter, multiple MCT needle placements are generally necessary. Similar to LITT and RF ablation, MCT can be performed percutaneously, using ultrasound or CT guidance. Most data regarding MCT have been generated in Japan. One study of 19 patients with HCC treated with MCT demonstrated 10 patients without radiographic evidence of recurrence, 6 patients who died from progression of either underlying liver disease or HCC, and 3 patients who were alive with evidence of new HCC nodules.[126] The limitation of this study, however, is that patients received hepatic arterial chemoembolization as well.

Primary Hepatic Tumors

Essentially, primary hepatic tumors include HCC, neoplastic cysts, and intrahepatic cholangiocarcinoma. Because the management of cholangiocarcinoma is discussed elsewhere in this book, this discussion is limited to HCC and, briefly, neoplastic cystic lesions. HCC is one of the most common solid human

TABLE 61.2 ETIOLOGY

FACTORS ASSOCIATED WITH AN INCREASED RISK OF DEVELOPING HEPATOCELLULAR CARCINOMA

Hepatitis B virus infection
Hepatitis C virus infection
Aflatoxin B_1 ingestion
Cirrhosis
Ethanol ingestion
Primary biliary cirrhosis
Exogenous hormone intake
Hemochromatosis
α_1-Antitrypsin deficiency
Glycogen storage diseases
Hypercitrullinemia
Porphyrias
Hereditary tyrosinemia
Wilson's disease
Hepatotoxin exposure (thorotrast, polyvinyl chloride, carbon chloride)

cancers with an annual incidence of approximately 1 million new patients.[85] Its incidence increases with age and is greatest between the third and fifth decades of life.[86] There is a marked geographic disparity, with parts of Asia and Africa considered to be high-incidence and much of Europe and North America considered low incidence.[127] As a result of this significant disparity in the geographic incidence of this disease, environmental factors have always been suspect as causative agents. In fact, there are several risk factors for HCC, but essentially the common pathway for each is that they lead to or are a marker of chronic hepatocellular injury. These risk factors include chronic hepatitis B and C virus infection (simultaneous infection portends a greater risk than either individually), cirrhosis, ethanol ingestion, exogenous hormone intake, genetic diseases, and toxin exposure. The complete list is enumerated in Table 61.2. Patients who are at high risk for the development of HCC may be followed with a screening protocol using ultrasonography and serum AFP; however, the frequency and duration of follow-up is not established. Diagnosis is dependent on histologic examination of a biopsy or FNA specimen, although in high-risk populations, serum AFP and imaging alone are adequate for a presumptive diagnosis.

Of note, a histologic variant of HCC has been recognized. Fibrolamellar HCC, also known as eosinophilic HCC with lamellar fibrosis, comprises less than 10% of all cases. Significantly, however, this variant differs from more common histologic subtypes in that the patients are usually younger (median age of onset 25 years), it is less frequently associated with cirrhosis, and it occurs equally in women and in men.[128–130] Importantly, patients with fibrolamellar HCC more frequently present with resectable lesions and are thought to have a higher cure rate after resection and transplantation.[131–133]

The natural history of untreated HCC is bleak, with a median survival between 6 and 20 months.[134–136] Systemic chemotherapy and radiation have yet to yield worthwhile improvements in survival and therefore treatment of this disease relies on surgical extirpation, by resection, transplantation, or ablative techniques. Currently, resection remains the gold standard of therapy, with transplantation reserved for individuals prohibited from resection by their underlying liver disease and ablation used either as an adjunct or in patients who are otherwise not candidates for either of the other approaches.

For all patients with HCC who undergo resection, current 5-year survival rates have been reported as high as 25% to 49%.[137] In patients who meet criteria for transplantation, the 5-year overall survival rate after resection or transplantation is on the order of 70%. Interestingly, transplantation offers a 5-year, disease-free survival rate as high as 65%,[114] whereas resection affords a 5-year disease-free survival rate on the order of 48%,[110] a disparity largely thought to result from the fact that transplantation addresses and treats the underlying liver disease, whereas resection does not. Finally, RF ablation of HCC has been the subject of recent review. One study of 110 patients with a median follow-up of 19 months demonstrated a local recurrence rate of 3.6% (all had lesions >4.0 cm) and all of those whose disease recurred locally developed disease in other areas of the liver as well. In this study, 50% of the patients had no evidence of disease at the time of last follow-up.[119] In a follow-up to this study, the authors report long-term results on the cohort now totaling 194 patients treated with RF ablation. At a median follow-up of 34.8 months, there was a 5-year survival rate of 55.4% with a complication rate of only 12%.[138]

Neoplastic cysts are more common in women and in those individuals older than 40 years. These lesions are symptomatic and have a characteristic appearance on ultrasound and other axial imaging studies.[139] The surgical management of neoplastic cysts relies on the initial differentiation between biliary cystadenoma and biliary cystadenocarcinoma.[140] Biliary cystadenocarcinoma is uncommon and is associated with marked thickening of the cyst wall and vascular enhancement on axial imaging studies. Biliary cystadenomas can be either enucleated or resected as dictated by the anatomy.[141] If there is any concern of biliary cystadenocarcinoma based on the axial imaging studies, a formal liver resection with adequate tumor-free parenchymal margins should be planned.

Metastatic Lesions

A number of solid tumors metastasize to the liver, but the most common that merit surgical attention are metastases from colorectal carcinoma. Without treatment, patients with metastatic colorectal cancer have a median survival of approximately 9 months, depending on the volume of disease.[142] Most patients are not candidates for surgical resection because of extent or distribution of disease. Patient selection resulting from a better understanding of tumor biology and prognostic factors has improved, however, leading to improved outcomes after hepatic metastasectomy. As such, the boundaries of surgical therapy for hepatic metastases have expanded and more patients with a wider variety of histologic findings are being considered for resection.

Resection of metastatic lesions of the liver has been thoroughly investigated. Historical analyses of patients with hepatic metastases focus on colorectal carcinoma and originally advocated offering hepatic resection to patients with fewer than four metastases, in whom the primary tumor was stage I or II and in individuals in whom at least a 1-cm negative margin of resection could be achieved.[143] Recent studies using the entire armamentarium of tools available to the hepatic surgeon have demonstrated a survival benefit in patients undergoing resection of four or more lesions, with overall 5-year survival rates greater than 23%.[144,145] In one analysis, only positive resection margin and increasing number of metastases were independent prognostic factors.[144]

In analyzing all patients undergoing resection, several reviews have identified a 5-year survival rate of more than 30% after hepatic resection.[58,146] One group analyzed trends in survival and noted that in patients having surgery after 1992, the 5-year survival rate was 58% compared with those having surgery during the period 1984 to 1992, who were found to only have a 31% 5-year survival.[59] A recent study from M.D. Anderson Cancer Center confirmed this improved long-term outcome with patients undergoing resection since 1995 having a 58% 5-year survival rate.[122] Another study reported a 10-year survival of nearly 25%.[147] Despite increasingly aggressive approaches to hepatic colorectal metastases, these recent analyses also demonstrate improved perioperative morbidity and mortality, with highly specialized centers reporting operative mortality rates as low as 0%[59,60] and perioperative morbidity as low as 23%.[59] It is clear from these examples that surgical resection for hepatic colorectal metastases is both efficacious and safe.

Most colorectal metastases are found either at the time the primary lesion was identified (in up to 25% of patients) or in follow-up after treatment of a primary lesion (in an additional 20%) using CT scan.[147] Three-phase helical CT scan is the most useful nonoperative tool in detecting liver lesions, although the overall detection rate, as mentioned previously, is 85% with a false—positive rate of up to 5%.[15,16] As a result, no patient should undergo hepatic resection for metastatic disease without the benefit of intraoperative ultrasound, which remains the gold standard for identifying liver lesions. Intraoperative ultrasonography, whether via a laparoscopic or open technique, detects small liver tumors not visualized on preoperative CT or MRI studies in up to 27% of patients.[148–150]

Metastases other than those from colorectal carcinoma can be grouped into two broad categories: those that arise from a neuroendocrine primary and those that are classified as "non-neuroendocrine, noncolorectal" and encompass lesions arising from other histologic primary tumors (e.g., breast cancer, sarcoma, ovarian cancer). In addressing lesions of either category, standard surgical principles apply. Criteria for technical resectability remain based on anatomic and volume of disease concerns, but the ultimate question regarding the role of surgery lies in the benefit to the patient. With the low morbidity and mortality currently observed after major hepatic resection, a greater number of patients with disease that fall into these categories are undergoing surgical treatment.

Neuroendocrine tumors pose a unique management problem because hepatic tumor burden can lead to endocrine syndromes that can produce debilitating symptoms in patients. These individuals are candidates for surgical extirpation and should undergo either resection or ablation, if possible. In a study of 74 patients undergoing hepatic resection for metastatic neuroendocrine tumors, resection was shown to improve symptoms in up to 90% of patients.[151] This study also demonstrated that, when compared with surgery for a curative intent, debulking afforded a similar short-term (2-year) survival rate. Because of the relatively indolent nature of most neuroendocrine tumors, a 5-year survival rate for patients who are untreated is relatively good. Despite this, results after surgery have shown survival rates as high as 73% at 4 years, compared with 30% to 40% in those untreated. In a follow-up to this study, the same group reported on 170 patients. Although 84% of these patients had recurrence within 5 years of resection, the study noted a 61% 5-year and 35% 10-year survival rate, with symptom improvement in 96% of patients.[90] Although surgery for neuroendocrine metastases is infrequently curative, patients often are relieved of symptoms and enjoy prolonged survival after resection; therefore, an aggressive liver-directed approach is appropriate in this group, when feasible.

Non-neuroendocrine, noncolorectal hepatic metastases encompass a wide variety of histologies. Included in this group are lesions arising from breast, sarcoma, ovarian, and melanoma primary lesions, as well as many others. Because of this wide array of histologic findings, patients must be approached on a case-by-case basis with only a select few considered for aggressive liver-directed therapy. Not surprisingly, outcome after resection varies widely based on the histology of the primary tumor: Some patients who undergo resection of sarcoma metastases have a 30% 5-year survival rate, according to one report,[89] whereas patients who undergoing resection for metastatic melanoma are noted to have a dismal outcome, with only anecdotal reports of long-term survival.[152] In one single-institution review of 96 patients with a variety of histologic findings, an overall 37% 5-year survival rate was observed, with the authors noting that histology and completion of resection were predictors of outcome.[153] One histologic type that has gained recent attention is breast cancer. With improvements in systemic therapy for this disease, aggressive approaches to isolated liver metastases have become more commonplace. Two recent reports identify 5-year survivals of 46% and 50% in patients undergoing R0 resections.[154,155] Of the more than 50% of patients with breast cancer who develop liver metastases, however, in only 5% will that disease be confined to their liver. As a result, despite evidence of a potential survival benefit from surgery, only a small, select group of patients are candidates for resection.

Last, gastrointestinal stromal tumors (GIST) warrant special mention in this category as the management of these tumors is rapidly evolving with the development of Gleevec (Fig. 61.17). Most studies reporting survival after resection for sarcomas metastatic to the liver include GIST and may reflect a disparate group, because these tumors may carry a different prognosis with the advent of targeted therapy. Although the safety and efficacy of Gleevec for metastatic GIST has been demonstrated, its role in treating patients continues to be a focus of active investigation. Most patients with liver metastases from GIST are considered inoperable based on diffuse tumor distribution. With the advent of Gleevec, however, the treatment of these patients is likely to include an approach utilizing combination therapy and therefore resection and thermal ablation may become feasible in a larger number of patients.

Adjuvant and Neoadjuvant Therapy

There currently is no uniformly accepted, superior, single combination of agents for use as an adjuvant to hepatic resection for colorectal metastases or HCC. One thing that has become evident, however, is that chemotherapy in either the adjuvant or the neoadjuvant setting is safe in conjunction with major hepatic surgery.[60,156,157] As mentioned previously, some authors have documented the conversion of patients from an unresectable to resectable status with chemotherapy,[93–96] whereas others have shown a potential survival benefit with the application of neoadjuvant chemotherapy in patients who initially present with resectable disease.[97] Currently, neoadjuvant chemotherapy is an area of ongoing investigation. In contrast, adjuvant chemotherapy, either via systemic or hepatic arterial infusion, has undergone a more rigorous evaluation.

Adjuvant chemotherapy for isolated hepatic metastases from colorectal carcinoma can be delivered either via a systemic route or via direct hepatic arterial infusion. A randomized, prospective trial assigned 156 patients undergoing resection of colorectal cancer liver metastases to one of two adjuvant treatment arms.[158] The patients received either six monthly cycles of systemic intravenous fluorouracil (5-FU) and folinic acid or hepatic arterial infusion chemotherapy with floxuridine (FUDR) and dexamethasone plus systemic intravenous 5-FU, with or without folinic acid. This study identified a significant improvement in actuarial overall 2-year survival in the group treated with regional arterial combined with systemic chemotherapy (86% 2-year actuarial survival) compared with the group treated with adjuvant systemic chemotherapy alone (72% 2-year actuarial survival). The rate of hepatic recurrence was significantly lower in the patients treated with regional chemotherapy combined with systemic chemotherapy. With a median follow-up of 63 months, the median survival in

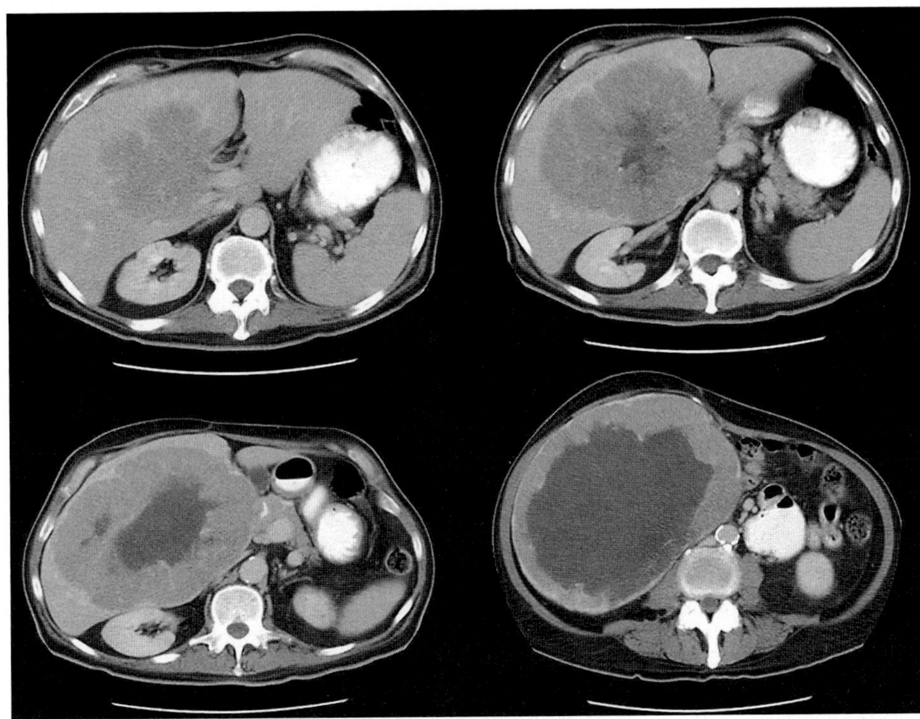

FIGURE 61.17 Computed tomography scan of a massive metastatic gastrointestinal stromal tumor. This lesion was successfully resected and the patient receive adjuvant therapy later.

the combined regional and systemic chemotherapy group was 72 months versus 59 months in the patients who received adjuvant systemic therapy only. Chemotherapy-related side effects occurred with equal frequency in the two treatment arms, but the rate of diarrhea and abnormalities in serum liver function tests was higher in patients in the combined regional and systemic chemotherapy arm. Many of the patients in the combined regional and systemic therapy arm were unable to complete the planned 6 months of adjuvant therapy because of chemotherapy-induced elevations in serum liver function tests. This article served as an important publication in the adjuvant therapy of colorectal hepatic metastases and spurred considerable interest in hepatic artery infusion (HAI) pumps.

Since that article's publication, little progress has been made in agents for use in HAI therapy, whereas new agents have been developed for use in systemic treatments. These newer systemic agents have been used in a variety of combinations, some of which have demonstrated response rates of almost 55%.[159] These successes, in concert with some of the problems associated with HAI therapy (e.g., biliary sclerosis, gastritis, and ulcer)[160] have left HAI therapy with an ambiguous role in the current therapeutic approach to colorectal liver metastases.

A recent prospective, randomized intergroup study investigating the benefits of combined modality (HAI and systemic) adjuvant therapy found that combination therapy provides a 4-year recurrence-free and 4-year liver recurrence-free rate of 46% and 67%, respectively compared with 25% and 43% without chemotherapy.[161] This study, however, did not utilize some of the newer chemotherapeutic combination regimens for its chemotherapy arm, and therefore it may not reflect response rates attainable with current systemic regimens.

Adjuvant therapy for HCC has also been investigated. This is primarily performed through the technique of hepatic artery chemoembolization. This modality arose from initial studies of hepatic artery ligation, which resulted in significant morbidity and mortality. Currently, selective embolization of tumor-feeding vessels has evolved as a safer, more tumor-specific approach. Arterial chemoembolization involves the administration of a variety of chemotherapeutic agents that are infused in conjunction with compounds that prolong the duration of contact between tumor tissue and the treatment drug. Chemotherapeutic agents currently in use include FUDR, mitomycin C, epirubicin, cisplatin, and styrene maleic acid neocarzinostatin. Two compounds such as lipiodol and ethiodol (contrast media) are administered with the drugs to prolong their contact with tumor. In some instances, these compounds are labeled with radioactive iodine and deliver therapy primarily.

A randomized, prospective trial assigned patients with HCC to a single postoperative dose via hepatic artery infusion of ^{131}I-lipiodol or no further treatment.[162] With a median follow-up of 35 months, recurrent HCC developed in 6 of 21 patients (28.5%) who received adjuvant ^{131}I-lipiodol compared with 13 of 22 (59%) control patients. A significant improvement was seen in median disease-free survival in the treatment group (57.2 months) compared with the surgery alone group (13.6 months). Additionally, the 3-year overall survival was significantly improved in the treatment versus control group, 86.4% versus 46.3%, respectively. There was no significant toxicity related to the infusion of ^{131}I-lipiodol.

Another approach for transarterial therapy in HCC utilizes biodegradable microspheres that are either radiolabeled or that contain chemotherapeutic agents. These spheres transiently occlude hepatic arterial flow, but within 48 to 72 hours are degraded and resorbed. Currently, this remains a palliative approach, but adjuvant studies are ongoing and some results are encouraging.

Novel and Experimental Therapy

Despite advances in surgical resection for hepatic malignancies, the results from this approach are still poor. As a result, treatment of these entities is an area of active investigation and a multitude of novel agents and experimental approaches are currently being studied. Although these entities are the subject of numerous chapters and publications on their own, many at least warrant mention in this chapter. These agents can be grouped into broad categories for their reference here: antiangiogenic agents, chemosensitizing agents that manipulate the apoptotic pathways, and oncolytic viral agents.

Presently, antiangiogenic agents may be the most significant of these novel therapies because they have recently been approved by the U.S. Food and Drug Administration for use in the treatment of metastatic colorectal carcinoma. The two presently approved agents in this class target vascular endothelial growth factor and the epidermal growth factor receptor.[163,164] Because angiogenesis plays a role in both pathologic and homeostatic processes, the efficacy of antiangiogenic therapy must be tightly balanced between inhibition of tumor angiogenesis and permission of physiologic angiogenesis. One particular concern in surgical patients is the role these agents have on wound healing. This issue remains unclear, but a presumptive attitude that these agents do inhibit wound healing is likely appropriate at the present time.[165–168] Studies involving both approved agents have shown marginal benefit in patients with metastatic colorectal cancer refractory to other treatment modalities; however, their mild side-effect profile has fostered their usage.[169–171]

Apoptosis and apoptotic pathways are an area of intense investigation in the field of gene therapy for cancer. Genetic aberrations, either as a result of a spontaneous mutation or genetic insult, lead to the abnormalities that permit the expression of a malignant phenotype. These abnormalities appear to alter not only the rate of cell replication but the rate of cell death as well. In HCC in particular, a down-regulation of apoptosis appears to be critical to early tumor development.[172] This, along with increasing evidence that a significant mechanism by which oncogenes induce tumorigenesis is at least in part mediated through effects on apoptotic pathways, has spurred interest in this field. Particular genes of interest are the p53 tumor suppressor gene and the *Bcl-2* family of genes. P53 mutations have been noted in as many as 60% to 80% of colorectal cancers[173] and as many as 25% to 50% of HCC.[174–175] These genetic aberrations provide targets for experimental therapeutics that can potentially serve to enhance the response to standard chemotherapeutic regimens.

Oncolytic viral therapy is another area of active experimental investigation. A variety of different viral agents have been used to selectively infect and subsequently lyse tumor cells within the liver. Additionally, several of these agents have been genetically modified so as to transcribe and ultimately produce a variety of proteins, such as cytokines, intended to enhance their anti-tumor efficacy. Finally, these agents are often modified to induce non-specific and specific antitumor immunity and in this role, genetic manipulation of the viral vectors to produce immunomodulatory proteins is frequently performed as well. Some viral vectors are currently undergoing clinical trials and therefore warrant specific mention. ONYX-15 is an adenovirus under investigation in the treatment of p53-deficient hepatic malignancies (among others) and has undergone phase I and II trials. To date, the safety of this agent when administered to patients has been documented, but its therapeutic role has yet to be defined.[176] The replication-defective herpes simplex virus type 1 (HSV-1) is another viral agent that has been proved safe in limited human trials and primate studies and is the focus of an ongoing phase I trial. The advantage HSV-1 offers is the potential for a large area of its genome to be replaced with a variety of different transgenes, allowing for combination approaches to antitumor therapy. These approaches have been validated in experimental models but have yet to evolve to clinical use.[177,178] Although it is still early to characterize the clinical applicability of oncolytic viral agents, experimental models and limited human studies provide encouraging data supporting their potential.

Lastly, another agent of note is a compound used exclusively in primary hepatic malignancies, recently reported in a combined phase I and II clinical trial of 19 patients.[179] Pegylated arginine deiminase is a form of therapy that takes advantage of the fact that HCC do not express the enzyme argininosuccinate synthase and, therefore, do not maintain the salvage pathway to produce arginine that normal hepatocytes do. Monopolizing on this disparity, investigators demonstrated that the administration of this agent leads to a depletion of systemic arginine in patients with minimal side effects and encouraging disease responses. This recent report supports further investigation of this novel approach.

SUMMARY

Hepatic tumors range from benign to malignant and include both primary and metastatic lesions. Advances in technology and perioperative care, combined with improvements in systemic therapy, have led to a considerable increase in the number of patients who are candidates for aggressive, liver-directed therapy. For the vast majority of malignant hepatic tumors, complete surgical extirpation remains the only chance at long-term cure. Current areas of active investigation pursue new forms of adjuvant and neoadjuvant treatment modalities that may improve outcomes from surgical therapy alone.

KEY POINTS

- **Modern helical computed tomography scans are highly sensitive at spatial discrimination and quantification of lesions (of at least 1 cm in size) and can characterize lesions as solid or cystic and define enhancement characteristics during arterial, portal, and delayed phases.**
- **CT scanning with intravenous contrast has an overall detection rate of 85% with a false—positive rate of 5% for colorectal liver metastases, but can detect only 40% to 60% of small hepatocellular carcinomas because of the limited ability to differentiate between macronodular regenerating nodules in a cirrhotic liver versus tumors. Intraoperative ultrasonography has become the gold standard against which all other modalities are compared to detect the number, extent, and association of tumors with intrahepatic vessels in both primary and metastatic liver tumors.**
- **Positive emission tomography scanning used in conjunction with CT scan increases the sensitivity (96%), specificity (88%), and accuracy (95%) in detecting colorectal metastatic disease and may exclude up to 11% of patients being considered for liver resection because of extrahepatic disease.**
- **Up to 75% of hepatic adenomas, which also may harbor malignancy, are symptomatic at presentation with one quarter presenting after rupture or an episode of acute hemorrhage; therefore, lesions more than 4 cm in size should be treated with surgical resection.**
- **In patients with cirrhosis being considered for resection of malignant liver disease, addition of quantitative or functional hepatic studies can improve patient selection, determine the extent of hepatic parenchymal resecting that will be tolerated, and reduce the postoperative mortality from liver failure to between 0 and 5%.**
- **Patients with metastatic disease to the liver can tolerate up to 80% of the liver being removed, whereas patients with HCC will tolerate a much smaller volume of resection and still have a higher mortality rate from the procedure.**
- **Primary solitary liver tumors 5 cm or smaller in diameter of (the Milan Criteria) who undergo hepatic transplantation can expect 5-year overall survival rates in excess of 65%, whereas resection affords a lower survival (48%), in large part because of the problems related to the underlying liver disease.**
- **The natural history of untreated HCC is bleak, with a median survival between 6 and 20 months; therefore, as nonsurgical therapies yield little improvement, treatment consists of surgical extirpation, either by resection, transplantation, or ablative techniques.**

- **Recent studies using the combined techniques of liver resection and RF ablation report 5-year survival rates in excess of 50%, often with operative mortality rates as low as 0 and perioperative morbidity as low as 25%.**

References

1. Gruttadauria S, Foglieni CS, Luca A, et al. Hepatic artery anomalies: anatomy review. *Liver Transpl* 2002;8:981.
2. Jones RM, Hardy KJ. The hepatic artery: a reminder of surgical anatomy. *J R Coll Surg Edinb* 2001;46:168–170.
3. Couinaud C. Etudes anatomiques et chirurgales. Paris: Mason, 1957.
4. Strasberg SM, Belghiti J, Clavien P-A, et al. The Brisbane 2000 terminology of liver anatomy and resections. *HPB* 2000;2:333–339.
5. Botero AC, Strasberg SM. Division of the left hemiliver in man—segments, sectors, or sections. *Liver Transplantation Surg* 1998;4:226–231.
6. Kassianides C, Kew MC. The clinical manifestations and natural history of hepatocellular carcinoma. *Gastroenterol Clin North Am* 1987;16:553–562.
7. Chlebowski RT, Tong M, Weissman J, et al. Hepatocellular carcinoma. Diagnostic and prognostic features in North American patients. *Cancer* 1984;53:2701–2706.
8. Nomura F, Ohnishi K, Tanabe Y. Clinical features and prognosis of hepatocellular carcinoma with reference to serum alpha-fetoprotein levels. Analysis of 606 patients. *Cancer* 1989;64:1700–1707.
9. Fujiyama S, Tanaka M, Maeda S, et al. Tumor markers in early diagnosis, follow-up and management of patients with hepatocellular carcinoma. *Oncology* 2002;62[Suppl 1]:57–63.
10. Nagaoka S, Yatsuhashi H, Hamada H, et al. The des-gamma-carboxy prothrombin index is a new prognostic indicator for hepatocellular carcinoma. *Cancer* 2003;98:2671–2677.
11. **Vauthey JN, Rousseau DL, Jr.. Liver imaging. A surgeon's perspective. *Clin Liver Dis* 2002;6:271–295.**
12. Harisinghani MG, Hahn PF. Computed tomography and magnetic resonance imaging evaluation of liver cancer. *Gastroenterol Clin North Am* 2002;31:759–776, vi.
13. Fenchel S, Fleiter TR, Merkle EM. Multislice helical CT of the abdomen. *Eur Radiol* 2002;12[Suppl 2]:S5–10.
14. Mortele KJ, McTavish J, Ros PR. Current techniques of computed tomography. Helical CT, multidetector CT, and 3D reconstruction. *Clin Liver Dis* 2002;6:29–52.
15. Valls C, Andia E, Sanchez A, et al. Hepatic metastases from colorectal cancer: preoperative detection and assessment of resectability with helical CT. *Radiology* 2001;218:55–60.
16. Scott DJ, Guthrie JA, Arnold P, et al. Dual phase helical CT versus portal venous phase CT for the detection of colorectal liver metastases: correlation with intra-operative sonography, surgical and pathological findings. *Clin Radiol* 2001;56:235–242.
17. Rode A, Bancel B, Douek P, et al. Small nodule detection in cirrhotic livers: evaluation with US, spiral CT, and MRI and correlation with pathologic examination of explanted liver. *J Comput Assist Tomogr* 2001;25:327–336.
18. Peterson MS, Baron RL. Radiologic diagnosis of hepatocellular carcinoma. *Clin Liver Dis* 2001;5:123–144.
19. Tong MJ, Blatt LM, Kao VW. Surveillance for hepatocellular carcinoma in patients with chronic viral hepatitis in the United States of America. *J Gastroenterol Hepatol* 2001;16:553–559.
20. Izzo F, Cremona F, Ruffolo F, et al. Outcome of 67 patients with hepatocellular cancer detected during screening of 1125 patients with chronic hepatitis. *Ann Surg* 1998;227:513–518.
21. Blomley MJ, Cooke JC, Unger EC, et al. Microbubble contrast agents: a new era in ultrasound. *BMJ* 2001;322:1222–1225.
22. John TG, Greig JD, Crosbie JL, et al. Superior staging of liver tumors with laparoscopy and laparoscopic ultrasound [comments]. *Ann Surg* 1994;220:711–719.
23. Akhurst T, Fong Y. Positron emission tomography in surgical oncology. *Adv Surg* 2002;36:309–331.
24. Strasberg SM, Dehdashti F, Siegel BA, et al. Survival of patients evaluated by FDG-PET before hepatic resection for metastatic colorectal carcinoma. a prospective database study [comment]. *Ann Surg* 2001;233:293–299.
25. Strasberg SM, Siegal BA. Survival of patients staged by FDG-PET before resection of hepatic metastases from colorectal cancer [comment]. *Ann Surg* 2002;235:308; discussion 310.
26. Bauer TW, Curley S, Macapinlac HA, et al. The impact on patient management of whole-body FDG-PET scanning in patients with liver metastases from colorectal carcinoma. Proceedings ASCW 2004, New Orleans, Louisiana, *J Clin Oncol* 2004;22(145):3569.
27. Johnson K, Bakhsh A, Young D, et al. Correlating computed tomography and positron emission tomography scan with operative findings in metastatic colorectal cancer. *Dis Colon Rectum* 2001;44:354–357.
28. Topal B, Flamen P, Aerts R, et al. Clinical value of whole-body emission tomography in potentially curable colorectal liver metastases. *Eur J Surg Oncol* 2001;27:175–179.
29. Shiomi S, Nishiguchi S, Ishizu H, et al. Usefulness of positron emission tomography with fluorine-18-fluorodeoxyglucose for predicting outcome in patients with hepatocellular carcinoma. *Am J Gastroenterol* 2001;96:1877–1880.
30. Giger U, Schafer M, Krahenbuhl L. Technique and value of staging laparoscopy. *Dig Surg* 2002;19:473–478.
31. D'Angelica M, Fong Y, Weber S, et al. The role of staging laparoscopy in hepatobiliary malignancy: prospective analysis of 401 cases. *Ann Surg Oncol* 2003;10:183–189.
32. Cottone M, Turri M, Caltagirone M, et al. Early detection of hepatocellular carcinoma associated with cirrhosis by ultrasound and alfafetoprotein: a prospective study. *Hepatogastroenterology* 1988;35:101–103.
33. Liaw YF, Tai DI, Chu CM, et al. Early detection of hepatocellular carcinoma in patients with chronic type B hepatitis. A prospective study. *Gastroenterology* 1986;90:263–267.
34. Maringhini A, Cottone M, Sciarrino E, et al. Ultrasonography and alphafetoprotein in diagnosis of hepatocellular carcinoma in cirrhosis. *Dig Dis Sci* 1988;33:47–51.
35. Colombo M, de Franchis R, Del Ninno E, et al. Hepatocellular carcinoma in Italian patients with cirrhosis. *N Engl J Med* 1991;325:675–680.
36. Poon RT, Fan ST, Yu WC, et al. A prospective longitudinal study of quality of life after resection of hepatocellular carcinoma. *Arch Surg* 2001;136:693–699.
37. Regev A, Reddy KR, Berho M, et al. Large cystic lesions of the liver in adults: a 15-year experience in a tertiary center. *J Am Coll Surg* 2001;193:36–45.
38. Ammori BJ, Jenkins BL, Lim PC, et al. Surgical strategy for cystic diseases of the liver in a western hepatobiliary center. *World J Surg* 2002;26:462–469.
39. Katkhouda N, Hurwitz M, Gugenheim J, et al. Laparoscopic management of benign solid and cystic lesions of the liver. *Ann Surg* 1999;229:460–466.
40. Gigot JF, Metairie S, Etienne J, et al. The surgical management of congenital liver cysts. *Surg Endosc* 2001;15:357–363.
41. Semelka R, DR DM, C CB, et al. Focal liver lesions: comparison of dual-phase CT and multisequence multiplanar MR imaging including dynamic gadolinium enhancement. *J Magn Reson Imaging* 2001;13:397–401.
42. Horton KM, Bluemke DA, Hruban RH, et al. CT and MR imaging of benign hepatic and biliary tumors. *Radiographics* 1999;19:431–451.
43. Charny CK, Jarnagin WR, Schwartz LH, et al. Management of 155 patients with benign liver tumours. *Br J Surg* 2001;88:808–813.
44. Trotter JF, Everson GT. Benign focal lesions of the liver. *Clin Liver Dis* 2001;5:17–42, v.
45. Reddy KR, Kligerman S, Levi J, et al. Benign and solid tumors of the liver: relationship to sex, age, size of tumors, and outcome. *Am Surg* 2001;67:173–178.
46. De Carlis L, Pirotta V, Rondinara GF, et al. Hepatic adenoma and focal nodular hyperplasia: diagnosis and criteria for treatment. *Liver Transpl Surg* 1997;3:160–165.
47. Kim J, Ahmad SA, Lowy AM, et al. An algorithm for the accurate identification of benign liver lesions. *Am J Surg* 2004;187:274–279.
48. Buetow PC, Pantongrag-Brown L, Buck JL, et al. Focal nodular hyperplasia of the liver: radiologic-pathologic correlation [erratum appears in *Radiographics* 1997;(Mar–Apr)17(2):524]. *Radiographics* 1996;16:369–388.
49. Ruppert-Kohlmayr AJ, Uggowitzer MM, Kugler C, et al. Focal nodular hyperplasia and hepatocellular adenoma of the liver: differentiation with multiphasic helical CT. *AJR Am J Roentgenol* 2001;176:1493–1498.
50. Mortele KJ, Praet M, Van Vlierberghe H, et al. Focal nodular hyperplasia of the liver: detection and characterization with plain and dynamic-enhanced MRI. *Abdom Imaging* 2002;27:700–707.
51. Ribeiro A, Burgart LJ, Nagorney DM, et al. Management of liver adenomatosis: results with a conservative surgical approach. *Liver Transpl Surg* 1998;4:388–398.
52. Foster JH, Berman MM. The malignant transformation of liver cell adenomas. *Arch Surg* 1994;129:712–717.
53. Brancatelli G, Federle MP, Grazioli L, et al. Focal nodular hyperplasia. CT findings with emphasis on multiphasic helical CT in 78 patients. *Radiology* 2001;219:61–68.
54. Descottes B, Glineur D, Lachachi F, et al. Laparoscopic liver resection of benign liver tumors [erratum appears in *Surg Endosc* 2003 Apr;17(4):668]. *Surg Endosc* 2003;17:23–30.
55. Baer HU, Dennison AR, Mouton W, et al. Enucleation of giant hemangiomas of the liver. Technical and pathologic aspects of a neglected procedure. *Ann Surg* 1992;216:673–676.
56. Gedaly R, Pomposelli JJ, Pomfret EA, et al. Cavernous hemangioma of the liver: anatomic resection vs. enucleation. *Arch Surg* 1999;134:407–411.
57. Terkivatan T, Vrijland WW, Den Hoed PT, et al. Size of lesion is not a criterion for resection during management of giant liver haemangioma. *Br J Surg* 2002;89:1240–1244.
58. Fong Y, Fortner J, Sun RL, et al. Clinical score for predicting recurrence after hepatic resection for metastatic colorectal cancer: analysis of 1001 consecutive cases. *Ann Surg* 1999;230:309–318; discussion 318–321.
59. **Choti MA, Sitzmann JV, Tiburi MF, et al. Trends in long-term survival following liver resection for hepatic colorectal metastases. *Ann Surg* 2002;235:759–766.**
60. Parikh AA, Gentner B, Wu TT, et al. Perioperative complications in patients undergoing major liver resection with or without neoadjuvant chemotherapy. *J Gastrointest Surg* 2003;7:1082–1088.

61. Curley SA. Surgical management of hepatocellular carcinoma. In: Curley SA, ed. *Liver Cancer*. New York: Springer-Verlag, 1998:28–52.
62. Noguchi T, Imai T, Mizumoto R. Preoperative estimation of surgical risk of hepatectomy in cirrhotic patients. *Hepato-Gastroenterology* 1990;37: 165–171.
63. Lau H, Man K, Fan ST, et al. Evaluation of preoperative hepatic function in patients with hepatocellular carcinoma undergoing hepatectomy. *Br J Surg* 1997;84:1255–1259.
64. Kobayashi T, Kubota K, Imamura H, et al. Hepatic phenylalanine metabolism measured by the [13C] phenylalanine breath test. *Eur J Clin Invest* 2001;31:356–361.
65. Hamming AW, Gallinger S, Greig PD, et al. The hippurate ratio as an indicator of functional hepatic reserve for resection of hepatocellular carcinoma in cirrhotic patients. *J Gastrointest Surg* 2001;5:316–321.
66. Hwang EH, Taki J, Shuke N, et al. Preoperative assessment of residual hepatic functional reserve using 99mTc-DTPA-galactosyl-human serum albumin dynamic SPECT. *J Nucl Med* 1999;40:1644–1651.
67. Shiomi S, Iwata Y, Sasaki N, et al. Assessment of hepatic blood flow by PET with 15O water: correlation between per-rectal portal scintigraphy with 99Tc(m)-pertechnetate and scintigraphy with 99Tc(m)-GSA. *Nucl Med Commun* 2000;21:533–538.
68. Taniguchi H, Kunishima S, Koh T. The reproducibility of independently measuring human regional hepatic arterial, portal and total hepatic blood flow using [15O] water and positron emission tomography. *Nucl Med Commun* 2003;24:497–501.
69. **Abdalla EK, Barnett CC, Doherty D, et al. Extended hepatectomy in patients with hepatobiliary malignancies with and without preoperative portal vein embolization. *Arch Surg* 2002;137:675–680; discussion 680–671.**
70. Kinoshita H, Sakai K, Hirohashi K, et al. Preoperative portal vein embolization for hepatocellular carcinoma. *World J Surg* 1986;10:803–808.
71. Vauthey JN, Chaoui A, Do KA, et al. Standardized measurement of the future liver remnant prior to extended liver resection: methodology and clinical associations. *Surgery* 2000;127:512–519.
72. Kubota K, Makuuchi M, Kusaka K, et al. Measurement of liver volume and hepatic functional reserve as a guide to decision-making in resectional surgery for hepatic tumors. *Hepatology* 1997;26:1176–1181.
73. Melendez J, Ferri E, Zwillman M, et al. Extended hepatic resection: a 6-year retrospective study of risk factors for perioperative mortality. *J Am Coll Surg* 2001;192:47–53.
74. Urata K, Kawasaki S, Matsunami H, et al. Calculation of child and adult standard liver volume for liver transplantation. *Hepatology* 1995;21:1317–1321.
75. Ogasawara K, Une Y, Nakajima Y, et al. The significance of measuring liver volume using computed tomographic images before and after hepatectomy. *Surg Today* 1995;25:43–48.
76. Nagino M, Kamiya J, Kanai M, et al. Right trisegment portal vein embolization for biliary tract carcinoma: technique and clinical utility. *Surgery* 2000;127:155–160.
77. Elias D, De Baere T, Roche A, et al. During liver regeneration following right portal embolization the growth rate of liver metastases is more rapid than that of the liver parenchyma [comments]. *Br J Surg* 1999;86: 784–788.
78. Azoulay D, Castaing D, Smail A, et al. Resection of nonresectable liver metastases from colorectal cancer after percutaneous portal vein embolization. *Ann Surg* 2000;231:480–486.
79. de Baere T, Roche A, Elias D, et al. Preoperative portal vein embolization for extension of hepatectomy indications. *Hepatology* 1996;24:1386–1391.
80. Imamura H, Shimada R, Kubota M, et al. Preoperative portal vein embolization: an audit of 84 patients. *Hepatology* 1999;29:1099–1105.
81. Shimamura T, Nakajima Y, Une Y, et al. Efficacy and safety of preoperative percutaneous transhepatic portal embolization with absolute ethanol: a clinical study. *Surgery* 1997;121:135–141.
82. Wakabayashi H, Okada S, Maeba T, et al. Effect of preoperative portal vein embolization on major hepatectomy for advanced-stage hepatocellular carcinomas in injured livers: a preliminary report. *Surg Today* 1997;27:403–410.
83. Elias D, Cavalcanti A, De Baere T, et al. Resultats carcinologiques a long terme des hepatectomies realisee apres embolisation portal selective. *Ann Chir* 1999;53:559–564.
84. Weiss L, Grundmann E, Torhorst J, et al. Haematogenous metastatic patterns in colonic carcinoma: an analysis of 1541 necropsies. *J Pathol* 1986;150:195–203.
85. Di Bisceglie AM, Carithers RL, Jr., Gores GJ. Hepatocellular carcinoma. *Hepatology* 1998;28:1161–1165.
86. Anthony PP. Hepatocellular carcinoma: an overview. *Histopathology* 2001;39:109–118.
87. Bilimoria MM, Lauwers GY, Doherty DA, et al. Underlying liver disease, not tumor factors, predicts long-term survival after resection of hepatocellular carcinoma. *Arch Surg* 2001;136:528–535.
88. Fong Y, Cohen AM, Fortner JG, et al. Liver resection for colorectal metastases. *J Clin Oncol* 1997;15:938–946.
89. DeMatteo RP, Shah A, Fong Y, et al. Results of hepatic resection for sarcoma metastatic to liver. *Ann Surg* 2001;234:540–547; discussion 547–548.
90. Sarmiento JM, Heywood G, Rubin J, et al. Surgical treatment of neuroendocrine metastases to the liver: a plea for resection to increase survival. *J Am Coll Surg* 2003;197:29–37.
91. Kianmanesh R, Farges O, Abdalla EK, et al. Right portal vein ligation: a new planned two-step all-surgical approach for complete resection of primary gastrointestinal tumors with multiple bilateral liver metastases. *J Am Coll Surg* 2003;197:164–170.
92. Adam R, Laurent A, Azoulay D, et al. Two-stage hepatectomy. A planned strategy to treat irresectable liver tumors. *Ann Surg* 2000;232:777–785.
93. **Adam R. Chemotherapy and surgery: new perspectives on the treatment of unresectable liver metastases. *Ann Oncol* 2003;14[Suppl 2]:ii13–16.**
94. Adam R, Avisar E, Ariche A, et al. Five-year survival following hepatic resection after neoadjuvant therapy for nonresectable colorectal. *Ann Surg Oncol* 2001;8:347–353.
95. Adam R, Huguet E, Azoulay D, et al. Hepatic resection after down-staging of unresectable hepatic colorectal metastases. *Surg Oncol Clin N Am* 2003;12:211–220.
96. Bismuth H, Adam R, Levi F, et al. Resection of nonresectable liver metastases from colorectal cancer after neoadjuvant chemotherapy. *Ann Surg* 1996;224:509–520; discussion 520–502.
97. Tanaka K, Adam R, Shimada H, et al. Role of neoadjuvant chemotherapy in the treatment of multiple colorectal metastases to the liver. *Br J Surg* 2003;90:963–969.
98. Yanaga K, Nishizaki T, Yamamoto K, et al. Simplified inflow control using stapling devices for major hepatic resection. *Arch Surg* 1996; 131:104–106.
99. Ramacciato G, Balesh AM, Fornasari V. Vascular endostapler as aid to hepatic vein control during hepatic resections. *Am J Surg* 1996;172: 358–362.
100. Cherqui D, Husson E, Hammoud R, et al. Laparoscopic liver resections: a feasibility study in 30 patients. *Ann Surg* 2000;232:753–762.
101. Morino M, Morra I, Rosso E, et al. Laparoscopic vs open hepatic resection: a comparative study. *Surg Endosc* 2003;17:1914–1918.
102. O'Rourke N, Fielding G. Laparoscopic right hepatectomy: surgical technique. *J Gastrointest Surg* 2004;8:213–216.
103. Tuttle TM, Curley SA, Roh MS. Repeat hepatic resection as effective treatment for recurrent colorectal liver metastases. *Ann Surg Oncol* 1996;4:125–130.
104. Imamura H, Kawasaki S, Miyagawa S, et al. Aggressive surgical approach to recurrent tumors after hepatectomy for metastatic spread of colorectal cancer to the liver. *Surgery* 2000;127:528–535.
105. Nakajima Y, Ko S, Kanamura T, et al. Repeat liver resection for hepatocellular carcinoma. *J Am Coll Surg* 2001;192:339–344.
106. Matsuda M, Fujii H, Kono H, et al. Surgical treatment of recurrent hepatocellular carcinoma based on the mode of recurrence: repeat hepatic resection or ablation are good choices for patients with recurrent multicentric cancer. *J Hepatobiliary Pancreat Surg* 2001;8:353–359.
107. Iwatsuki S, Gordon RD, Shaw BW, Jr., et al. Role of liver transplantation in cancer therapy. *Ann Surg* 1985;202:401–407.
108. O'Grady JG, Polson RJ, Rolles K, et al. Liver transplantation for malignant disease. Results in 93 consecutive patients. *Ann Surg* 1988; 207:373–379.
109. **Mazzaferro V, Regalia E, Doci R, et al. Liver transplantation for the treatment of small hepatocellular carcinomas in patients with cirrhosis. *N Engl J Med* 1996;334:693–699.**
110. Cha CH, Ruo L, Fong Y, et al. Resection of hepatocellular carcinoma in patients otherwise eligible for transplantation. *Ann Surg* 2003;238:315–321; discussion 321–313.
111. **Vauthey JN, Lauwers GY, Esnaola NF, et al. Simplified staging for hepatocellular carcinoma. *J Clin Oncol* 2002;20:1527–1536.**
112. Tsai TJ, Chau GY, Lui WY, et al. Clinical significance of microscopic tumor venous invasion in patients with resectable hepatocellular carcinoma. *Surgery* 2000;127:603–608.
113. Jonas S, Bechstein WO, Steinmuller T, et al. Vascular invasion and histopathologic grading determine outcome after liver transplantation for hepatocellular carcinoma in cirrhosis. *Hepatology* 2001;33:1080–1086.
114. Shetty K, Timmins K, Brensinger C, et al. Liver transplantation for hepatocellular carcinoma validation of present selection criteria in predicting outcome. *Liver Transpl* 2004;10:911–918.
115. Organ Procurement and Transplantation Network. Organ Procurement and Distribution Policies, Richmond, VA. United Network for Organ Sharing, 2004.
116. Sharma P, Balan V, Hernandez JL, et al. Liver transplantation for hepatocellular carcinoma: the MELD impact. *Liver Transpl* 2004;10:36–41.
117. McGahan JP, Brock JM, Tesluk H, et al. Hepatic ablation with use of radio-frequency electrocautery in the animal model. *J Vasc Interv Radiol* 1992;3:291–297.
118. Curley SA, Izzo F, Delrio P, et al. Radiofrequency ablation of unresectable primary and metastatic hepatic malignancies: results in 123 patients. *Ann Surg* 1999;230:1–8.
119. Curley SA, Izzo F, Ellis LM, et al. Radiofrequency ablation of hepatocellular cancer in 110 patients with cirrhosis. *Ann Surg* 2000;232:381–391.
120. **Curley SA. Radiofrequency ablation of malignant liver tumors. *The Oncologist* 2001;6:14–23.**
121. Pawlik TM, Izzo F, Cohen DS, et al. Combined resection and radiofrequency ablation for advanced hepatic malignancies: results in 172 patients. *Ann Surg Oncol* 2003;10:1059–1069.
122. **Abdalla EK, Vauthey JN, Ellis LM, et al. Recurrence and outcomes following hepatic resection, radiofrequency ablation, and combined resection/ablation for colorectal liver metastases. 2004;239:818–825; discussion 825–817.**

123. Germer CT, Albrecht D, Roggan A, et al. Technology for in situ ablation by laparoscopic and image-guided interstitial laser hyperthermia. *Semin Laparosc Surg* 1998;5:195–203.
124. Mack MG, Straub R, Eichler K, et al. Percutaneous MR imaging-guided laser-induced thermotherapy metastases. *Abdom Imaging* 2001;26: 369–374.
125. Tabuse K, Katsumi M, Kobayashi Y, et al. Microwave surgery: hepatectomy using a microwave tissue coagulator. *World J Surg* 1985;9:136–143.
126. Sato M, Watanabe Y, Ueda S, et al. Microwave coagulation therapy for hepatocellular carcinoma. *Gastroenterology* 1996;110:1507–1514.
127. Falk H. Liver. In: DS, Fraumeni JF, Jr., eds. *Cancer Epidemiology and Prevention*. Philadelphia: WB Saunders, 1982:668.
128. Cooke C, Mooy N, Matz LR, et al. Test and teach. Number fifty-three. Diagnosis. Fibrolamellar carcinoma of the liver. *Pathology* 1986;18:281–282, 357.
129. Berman MM, Libbey NP, Foster JH. Hepatocellular carcinoma. Polygonal cell type with fibrous stroma—an atypical variant with a favorable prognosis. *Cancer* 1980;46:1448–1455.
130. Craig JR, Peters RL, Edmondson HA, et al. Fibrolamellar carcinoma of the liver: a tumor of adolescents and young adults with distinctive clinicopathologic features. *Cancer*1980;46:372–379.
131. Berman MA, Burnham JA, Sheahan DG. Fibrolamellar carcinoma of the liver: an immunohistochemical study of nineteen cases and a review of the literature. *Hum Pathol* 1988;19:784–794.
132. Ihde DC, Matthews MJ, Makuch RW, et al. Prognostic factors in patients with hepatocellular carcinoma receiving systemic chemotherapy. Identification of two groups of patients with prospects for prolonged survival. *Am J Med* 1985;78:399–406.
133. Soreide O, Czerniak A, Bradpiece H, et al. Characteristics of fibrolamellar hepatocellular carcinoma. A study of nine cases and a review of the literature. *Am J Surg* 1986;151:518–523.
134. Barbara L, Benzi G, Gaiani S, et al. Natural history of small untreated hepatocellular carcinoma in cirrhosis: a multivariate analysis of prognostic factors of tumor growth rate and patient survival. *Hepatology* 1992;16: 132–137.
135. Pawarode A, Voravud N, Sriuranpong V, et al. Natural history of untreated primary hepatocellular carcinoma: a retrospective study of 157 patients. *Am J Clin Oncol* 1998;21:386–391.
136. Okuda K. Natural history of hepatocellular carcinoma including fibrolamellar and hepato-cholangiocarcinoma variants. *J Gastroenterol Hepatol* 2002;17:401–405.
137. Poon RT, Fan ST, Lo CM, et al. Improving survival results after resection of hepatocellular carcinoma: a prospective study of 377 patients over 10 years. *Ann Surg* 2001;234:63–70.
138. Raut CP, Izzo F, Marra P, et al. Significant long-term survival following radiofrequency ablation of unresectable hepatocellular carcinoma in cirrhotic patients. *Ann Surg Oncol* 2005;12:616–628.
139. Mortele KJ, Ros PR. Cystic focal liver lesions in the adult: differential CT and MR imaging features. *Radiographics* 2001;21:895–910.
140. Lauffer JM, Baer HU, Maurer CA, et al. Biliary cystadenocarcinoma of the liver: the need for complete resection. *Eur J Cancer* 1998;34:1845–1851.
141. Kim K, Choi J, Park Y, et al. Biliary cystadenoma of the liver. *J Hepatobiliary Pancreat Surg* 1998;5:348–352.
142. Stangl R, Altendorf-Hofmann A, Charnley RM, et al. Factors influencing the natural history of colorectal liver metastases. *Lancet* 1994;343:1405–1410.
143. Multiple. Resection of the liver for colorectal carcinoma metastases: a multi-institutional study of indications for resection. Registry of Hepatic Metastases. *Surgery* 1988;103:278–288.
144. Weber SM, Jarnagin WR, DeMatteo RP, et al. Survival after resection of multiple hepatic colorectal metastases. *Ann Surg Oncol* 2000;7:643–650.
145. Minagawa M, Makuuchi M, Torzilli G, et al. Extension of the frontiers of surgical indications in the treatment of liver metastases from colorectal cancer: long-term results. *Ann Surg* 2000;231:487–499.
146. Scheele J, Altendorf-Hofmann A, Grube T, et al. [Resection of colorectal liver metastases. What prognostic factors determine patient selection?]. *Chirurg* 2001;72:547–560.
147. Altendorf-Hofmann A, Scheele J. A critical review of the major indicators of prognosis after resection of hepatic metastases from colorectal carcinoma. *Surg Oncol Clin N Am* 2003;12:165–192, xi.
148. Jarnagin WR, Bach AM, Winston CB, et al. What is the yield of intraoperative ultrasonography during partial hepatectomy for malignant disease? *J Am Coll Surg* 2001;192:577–583.
149. Fuhrman GM, Curley SA, Hohn DC, et al. Improved survival after resection of colorectal liver metastases. *Ann Surg Oncol* 1995;2:537–541.
150. Scaife CL, Chaan CS, Ellis LM, et al. The accuracy of preoperative imaging of hepatic tumors with helical computed tomography. *Ann Surg Oncol* 2005 (*in press*).
151. Que FG, Nagorney DM, Batts KP, et al. Hepatic resection for metastatic neuroendocrine carcinomas. *Am J Surg* 1995;169:36–42; discussion 42–33.
152. Feldman ED, Pingpank JF, Alexander HR, Jr.. Regional treatment options for patients with ocular melanoma metastatic to the liver. *Ann Surg Oncol* 2004;11:290–297.
153. Harrison LE, Brennan MF, Newman E, et al. Hepatic resection for noncolorectal, non-neuroendocrine metastases: a fifteen-year experience with ninety-six patients. *Surgery* 1997;121:625–632.
154. Elias D, Maisonnette F, Druet-Cabanac M, et al. An attempt to clarify indications for hepatectomy for liver metastases from breast cancer. *Am J Surg* 2003;185:158–164.
155. Carlini M, Lonardo MT, Carboni F, et al. Liver metastases from breast cancer. Results of surgical resection. *Hepatogastroenterology* 2002; 49:1597–1601.
156. Figueras J, Valls C, Rafecas A, et al. Resection rate and effect of postoperative chemotherapy on survival after surgery for colorectal liver metastases. *Br J Surg* 2001;88:980–985.
157. Carlo WF, Hummer AJ, Schwartz L, et al. Extent of hepatic resection does not correlate with toxicity following adjuvant chemotherapy. *J Surg Oncol* 2004;87:85–90.
158. Kemeny N, Huang Y, Cohen AM, et al. Hepatic arterial infusion of chemotherapy after resection of hepatic metastases from colorectal cancer [comments]. *N Engl J Med* 1999;341:2039–2048.
159. Tournigand C, Andre T, Achille E, et al. FOLFIRI followed by FOLFOX6 or the reverse sequence in advanced colorectal cancer. a randomized GERCOR study. *J Clin Oncol* 2004;22:229–237.
160. Vauthey JN, Marsh Rde W, Cendan JC, et al. Arterial therapy of hepatic colorectal metastases. *Br J Surg* 1996;83:447–455.
161. Kemeny MM, Adak S, Gray B, et al. Combined-modality treatment for resectable metastatic colorectal carcinoma to the liver: surgical resection of hepatic metastases in combination with continuous infusion of chemotherapy—an intergroup study. *J Clin Oncol* 2002;20:1499–1505.
162. Lau WY, Leung TW, Ho SK, et al. Adjuvant intra-arterial iodine-131-labelled lipiodol for resectable hepatocellular carcinoma: a prospective randomised trial [comments]. *Lancet* 1999;353:797–801.
163. Ellis LM, Takahashi Y, Liu W, et al. Vascular endothelial growth factor in human colon cancer: biology and therapeutic implications. *Oncologist* 2000;5[Suppl 1]:11–15.
164. Hoff PM, Ellis LM, Abbruzzese JL. Monoclonal antibodies: the foundation of therapy for colorectal cancer in the 21st century? *Oncology (Huntingt)* 2004;18:736–741; discussion 742, 745–736.
165. Abramovitch R, Dafni H, Neeman M, et al. Inhibition of neovascularization and tumor growth, and facilitation of wound repair, by halofuginone, an inhibitor of collagen type I synthesis. *Neoplasia (New York)* 1999;1: 321–329.
166. Klein SA, Bond SJ, Gupta SC, et al. Angiogenesis inhibitor TNP-470 inhibits murine cutaneous wound healing. *J Surg Res* 1999;82:268–274.
167. Bloch W, Huggel K, Sasaki T, et al. The angiogenesis inhibitor endostatin impairs blood vessel maturation during wound healing. *FASEB J* 2000;14:2373–2376.
168. Berger AC, Feldman AL, Gnant MF, et al. The angiogenesis inhibitor, endostatin, does not affect murine cutaneous wound healing. *J Surg Res* 2000;91:26–31.
169. Fernando NH, Hurwitz HI. Targeted therapy of colorectal cancer: clinical experience with bevacizumab. *Oncologist* 2004;9[Suppl 1]:11–18.
170. Hurwitz H, Fehrenbacher L, Novotny W, et al. Bevacizumab plus irinotecan, fluorouracil, and leucovorin for metastatic colorectal cancer. *N Engl J Med* 2004;350:2335–2342.
171. Cunningham D, Humblet Y, Siena S, et al. Cetuximab monotherapy and cetuximab plus irinotecan in irinotecan-refractory metastatic colorectal cancer. *N Engl J Med* 2004;351:337–345.
172. Grasl-Kraupp B, Ruttkay-Nedecky B, Mullauer L, et al. Inherent increase of apoptosis in liver tumors: implications for carcinogenesis and tumor regression. *Hepatology* 1997;25:906–912.
173. Fearon ER, Vogelstein B. A genetic model for colorectal tumorigenesis. *Cell* 1990;61:759–767.
174. Bellamy CO, Clarke AR, Wyllie AH, et al. p53 Deficiency in liver reduces local control of survival and proliferation, but does not affect apoptosis after DNA damage. *FASEB J* 1997;11:591–599.
175. Soini Y, Virkajarvi N, Lehto VP, et al. Hepatocellular carcinomas with a high proliferation index and a low degree of apoptosis and necrosis are associated with a shortened survival. *Br J Cancer* 1996;73: 1025–1030.
176. Hecht JR, Bedford R, Abbruzzese JL, et al. A phase I/II trial of intratumoral endoscopic ultrasound injection of ONYX-015 with intravenous gemcitabine in unresectable pancreatic carcinoma. *Clin Cancer Res* 2003;9:555–561.
177. Cozzi PJ, Malhotra S, McAuliffe P, et al. Intravesical oncolytic viral therapy using attenuated, replication-competent herpes simplex viruses G207 and Nv1020 is effective in the treatment of bladder cancer in an orthotopic syngeneic model. *FASEB J* 2001;15:1306–1308.
178. McAuliffe PF, Jarnagin WR, Johnson P, et al. Effective treatment of pancreatic tumors with two multimutated herpes simplex oncolytic viruses. *J Gastrointest Surg* 2000;4:580–588.
179. Izzo F, Marra P, Beneduce G, et al. Pegylated arginine deiminase treatment of patients with unresectable hepatocellular carcinoma: results from phase I/II studies. *J Clin Oncol* 2004;22:1815–1822.

CHAPTER 62 ■ CALCULOUS BILIARY DISEASE

ATTILA NAKEEB, STEVEN A. AHRENDT, AND HENRY A. PITT

Calculus biliary disease is a major health-care problem in developed countries as well as in many underdeveloped countries. In the United States, approximately 12% of the population or more than 30,000 Americans have gallstones. Currently more than 750,000 cholecystectomies are performed annually in the United States, and the cost of caring for these patients is estimated to be between 7 and 10 million dollars per year.[1] To properly manage these patients, surgeons should understand biliary physiology and gallstone pathogenesis, incidence, risk factors, and natural history as reviewed in the following discussion. In addition, this chapter reviews the diagnostic options, clinical manifestations, management options, and expected outcomes for calculus biliary disease.

BILIARY PHYSIOLOGY

Bile Flow

The bile ducts, gallbladder, and sphincter of Oddi act in concert to modify, store, and regulate the flow of bile. Approximately 600 to 750 mL of bile is produced daily. During its passage through the bile ductules, canalicular bile is modified by the absorption and secretion of electrolytes and water. The gastrointestinal hormone, secretin, increases bile flow primarily by increasing the active secretion of chloride-rich fluid by the bile ducts. Bile ductular secretion is also stimulated by other hormones such as cholecystokinin and gastrin. The bile duct epithelium is also capable of water and electrolyte absorption, which may be of primary importance in the storage of bile during fasting in patients who have previously undergone cholecystectomy. The main functions of the gallbladder are to concentrate and store hepatic bile during the fasting state and deliver bile into the duodenum in response to a meal. The usual capacity of the human gallbladder is approximately 40 to 50 mL. Only a small fraction of the 600 to 750 mL of bile produced each day would be stored were it not for its remarkable absorptive capacity. The gallbladder mucosa has the greatest absorptive capacity per unit of any structure in the body.

Bile Composition

Bile is usually concentrated fivefold to 10-fold by the absorption of water and electrolytes leading to a marked change in bile composition (Table 62.1).[2] Active sodium chloride transport by the gallbladder epithelium is the driving force for the concentration of bile. Water is passively absorbed in response to the osmotic force generated by solute absorption. The concentration of bile may affect the solubilities of two important components of gallstones, cholesterol and calcium. Although the gallbladder mucosa does absorb calcium, this process is not nearly as efficient as the absorption of sodium or water, leading to a greater relative increase in calcium concentration. As the gallbladder bile becomes concentrated, several changes occur in the capacity of bile to solubilize cholesterol. The solubility in the micellar fraction is increased, but the stability of phospholipid-cholesterol vesicles is greatly decreased. Because cholesterol crystal precipitation occurs preferentially by vesicular rather than micellar mechanisms, the net effect of concentrating bile is an increased tendency to form cholesterol crystals.[2]

Bile facilitates the intestinal absorption of lipids and fat-soluble vitamins and represents the route of excretion for certain organic solids such as bilirubin and cholesterol. The major organic solutes in bile are bilirubin, bile salts, phospholipids, and cholesterol. Bilirubin is the breakdown product of spent red blood cells and is conjugated with glucuronic acid prior to being excreted. Bile salts solubilize lipids and facilitate their absorption. Phospholipids are synthesized in the liver in conjunction with bile salt synthesis. The final major solute of bile is cholesterol, which is also produced primarily by the liver with little contribution from dietary sources. Cholesterol is highly nonpolar and insoluble in water and thus in bile as well.

Gallbladder Function

As a result of active absorption, the gallbladder stores concentrated bile that reenters the distal bile duct and is secreted into the duodenum in response to a meal. In addition to absorption and concentration, the gallbladder's mucosa actively secretes glycoproteins and hydrogen ions. Secretion of mucus glycoproteins occurs primarily from the glands of the

TABLE 62.1

COMPOSITION OF HEPATIC AND GALLBLADDER BILE

Characteristic	Hepatic	Gallbladder
Sodium (mEq/L)	160	270
Potassium (mEq/L)	5	10
Chloride (mEq/L)	90	15
Bicarbonate (mEq/L)	45	10
Calcium (mEq/L)	4	25
Magnesium (mEq/L)	2	—
Bilirubin (mEq/L)	1.5	15
Protein (mEq/L)	150	—
Bile acids (mEq/L)	50	150
Phospholipids (mEq/L)	8	40
Cholesterol (mEq/L)	4	18
Total solids (mEq/L)	—	125
pH	7.8	7.2

gallbladder neck and cystic duct. The resultant mucin gel is believed to constitute an important part of the unstirred layer (diffusion-resistant barrier) that separates the gallbladder cell membrane from the luminal bile. This mucus barrier may be very important in protecting the gallbladder epithelium from the strong detergent effect of the highly concentrated bile salts found in the gallbladder. However, considerable evidence also suggests that mucin glycoproteins play a role as a pronucleating agent for cholesterol crystallization. The transport of hydrogen ions by the gallbladder epithelium leads to a decrease in gallbladder bile pH through a sodium-exchange mechanism. Acidification of bile promotes calcium solubility, thereby preventing its precipitation as calcium salts. The gallbladder's normal acidification process lowers the pH of entering hepatic bile from 7.5 to 7.8 down to 7.1 to 7.3.[2]

Biliary Motility

Gallbladder

Gallbladder filling is facilitated by tonic contraction of the ampullary sphincter, which maintains a constant pressure in the common bile duct (CBD) (10 to 15 mm Hg). However, the gallbladder does not simply fill passively and continuously during fasting. Rather, periods of filling are punctuated by brief periods of partial emptying (10% to 15% of its volume) of concentrated gallbladder bile. Emptying periods are coordinated with each passage through the duodenum of phase III of the migrating myoelectric complex (MMC). This process is mediated, at least in part, by the hormone motilin. Following a meal, the release of stored bile from the gallbladder requires a coordinated motor response of gallbladder contraction and sphincter of Oddi relaxation. One of the main stimuli to gallbladder emptying is the hormone, cholecystokinin, which is released from the duodenal mucosa in response to a meal. When stimulated by eating, the gallbladder empties 50% to 70% of its contents within 30 to 40 minutes. Gallbladder refilling then occurs gradually over the next 60 to 90 minutes. Many other hormonal and neural pathways are also necessary for the coordinated action of the gallbladder and sphincter of Oddi. Defects in gallbladder motility, which increase the residence time of bile in the gallbladder, play a central role in the pathogenesis of gallstones.[2]

Sphincter of Oddi

The human sphincter of Oddi is a complex structure that is functionally independent from the duodenal musculature. Endoscopic manometric studies have demonstrated that the human sphincter of Oddi creates a high-pressure zone between the bile duct and the duodenum. The sphincter regulates the flow of bile and pancreatic juice into the duodenum and also prevents the regurgitation of duodenal contents into the biliary tract. These functions are achieved by keeping pressure within the bile and pancreatic ducts higher than duodenal pressure. The sphincter of Oddi also has very high-pressure phasic contractions, which may play a role in preventing the regurgitation of duodenal contents into the biliary tract.

Both neural and hormonal factors influence the sphincter of Oddi. In humans, sphincter of Oddi pressure and phasic wave activity diminish in response to cholecystokinin. Thus, sphincter pressure relaxes after a meal, allowing the passive flow of bile into the duodenum. During fasting, high-pressure phasic contractions of the sphincter of Oddi persist through all phases of the MMC. However, recent animal studies suggest that sphincter of Oddi phasic waves do vary to some degree in concert with the MMC. Thus, sphincter of Oddi activity is undoubtedly coordinated with the partial gallbladder emptying and increases in bile flow that occur during phase III of the MMC. This activity may be a preventative mechanism against the accumulation of biliary crystals during fasting.[2]

Neurally mediated reflexes link the sphincter of Oddi with the gallbladder and stomach to coordinate the flow of bile and pancreatic juice into the duodenum. The cholecystosphincter of Oddi reflex allows the human sphincter to relax as the gallbladder contracts. Similarly, antral distension causes both gallbladder contraction and sphincter relaxation.

GALLSTONE PATHOGENESIS

Gallstone Types

Gallstones represent a failure to maintain certain biliary solutes, primarily cholesterol. and calcium salts in a solubilized state. Gallstones are classified by their cholesterol content as either cholesterol or pigment stones. Pigment stones are further classified as either black or brown (Fig. 62.1). Pure cholesterol gallstones are uncommon (10%) with most cholesterol stones containing calcium salts in their center, or nidus. In most American populations, 70% to 80% of gallstones are cholesterol, and black pigment stones account for most of the remaining 20% to 30%.

An important biliary precipitate in gallstone pathogenesis is biliary "sludge," which refers to a mixture of cholesterol crystals, calcium bilirubinate granules, and a mucin gel matrix. Biliary sludge has been observed clinically in prolonged fasting states or with the use of long-term total parenteral nutrition (TPN). Both of these conditions are also associated with gallstone formation. The finding of macromolecular complexes of mucin and bilirubin, similar to biliary sludge in the central core of most cholesterol gallstones, suggests that sludge may serve as the nidus for gallstone growth.

Cholesterol Gallstones

The pathogenesis of cholesterol gallstones is clearly multifactorial but essentially involves four factors: (a) cholesterol supersaturation in bile, (b) crystal nucleation, (c) gallbladder dysmotility, and (d) gallbladder absorption. For many years, gallstones were thought to result primarily from a defect in the hepatic secretion of biliary lipids. More recently, it has become increasingly clear that gallbladder mucosal and motor function also play key roles in gallstone formation.

Biliary Lipids. The key to maintaining cholesterol in solution is the formation of both micelles, a bile salt-phospholipid-cholesterol complex, and cholesterol-phospholipid vesicles (Fig. 62.2). Present theory suggests that in states of excess cholesterol production, these large vesicles may also exceed their capability to transport cholesterol, and crystal precipitation may occur. Cholesterol solubility depends on the relative concentration of cholesterol, bile salts, and phospholipid. By plotting the percentages of each component on triangular coordinates, the micellar zone in which cholesterol is completely soluble can be demonstrated (Fig. 62.3). In the area above the curve, bile is supersaturated with cholesterol, and precipitation of cholesterol crystals can occur.

Cholesterol Crystallization. Cholesterol supersaturation is present in many normal humans without gallstones. As bile is concentrated in the gallbladder, a net transfer of phospholipids and cholesterol from vesicles to micelles occurs. The phospholipids are transferred more efficiently than cholesterol,

A

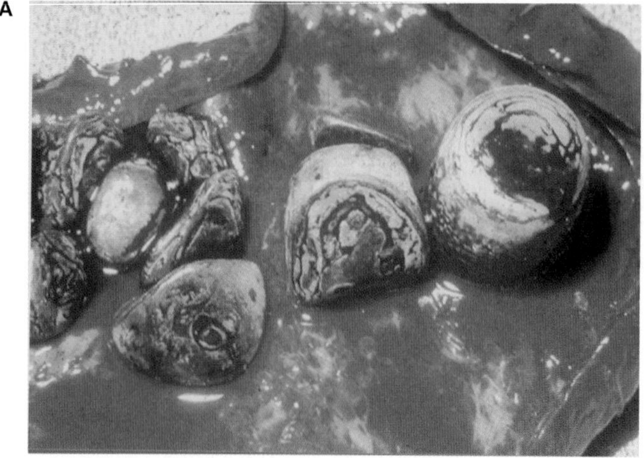

B

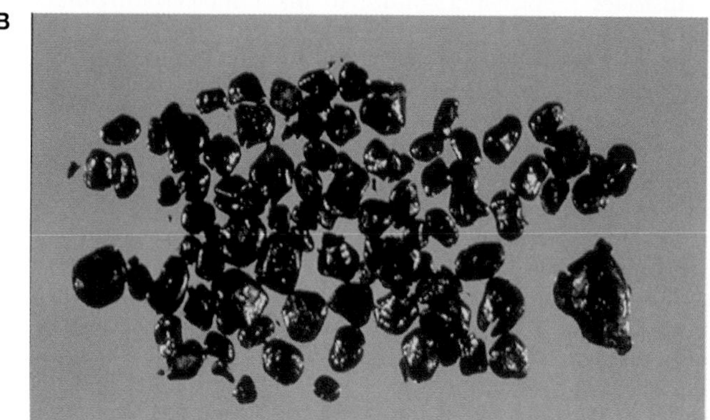

C

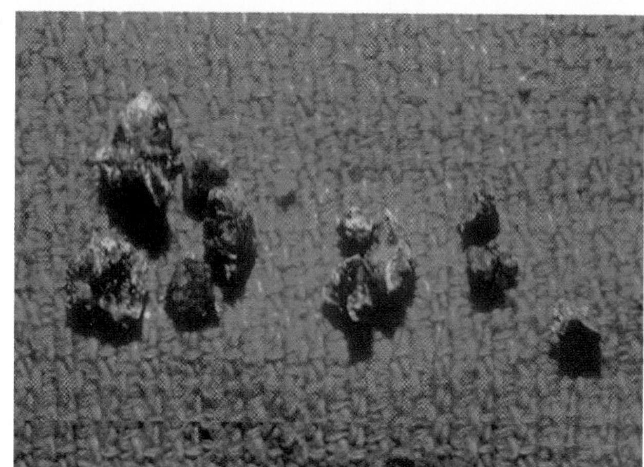

FIGURE 62.1 (*A*) Cholesterol gallstones. (*B*) Black pigment gallstones. (C) Brown pigment gallstone.

leading to cholesterol enrichment of the remaining vesicles. These cholesterol-rich vesicles aggregate to form large multilamellar liquid vesicles that then precipitate cholesterol monohydrate crystals. Several pronucleating factors including mucin glycoproteins, immunoglobulins, and transferrin accelerate the precipitation of cholesterol in bile.

Gallbladder Motility. For gallstones to cause clinical symptoms, they must obtain a size sufficient to produce mechanical injury to the gallbladder or obstruction of the biliary tree. Growth of stones may occur in two ways: (a) progressive enlargement of individual crystals or stones by deposition of additional insoluble precipitate at the bile-stone interface, or

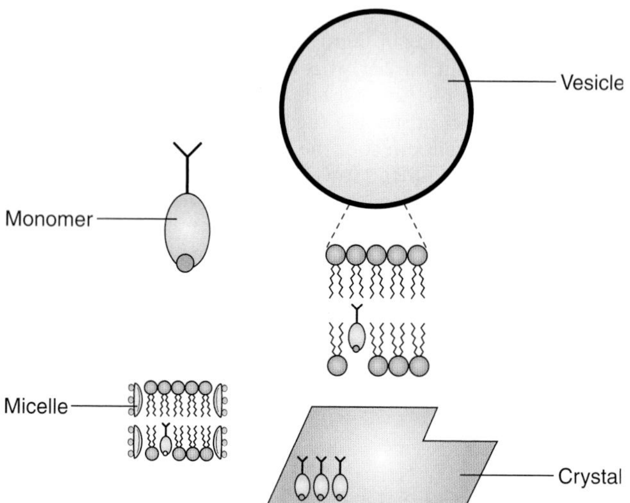

FIGURE 62.2 Phases of cholesterol in bile.

(b) fusion of individual crystals or stones to form a larger conglomerate. In addition, defects in gallbladder motility increase the residence time of bile in the gallbladder thereby playing a role in stone formation. Gallstone formation occurs in clinical states with gallbladder stasis, as seen with prolonged fasting, the use of long-term parenteral nutrition, after vagotomy, in diabetic patients, and in patients with somatostatin-producing tumors or in those receiving long-term somatostatin therapy.[2]

Gallbladder Absorption. As noted previously, the gallbladder is a very effective absorptive organ, and a normal function of the gallbladder is to concentrate and acidify bile. For many years, three factors have been thought to be key in cholesterol gallstone pathogenesis: cholesterol supersaturation, cholesterol crystallization, and biliary motility. However, a fourth factor, gallbladder absorption/secretion, also may be key to gallstone formation. Alterations in sodium, chloride, bicarbonate, and water absorption may alter the milieu for cholesterol saturation and crystal formation as well as for calcium precipitation.

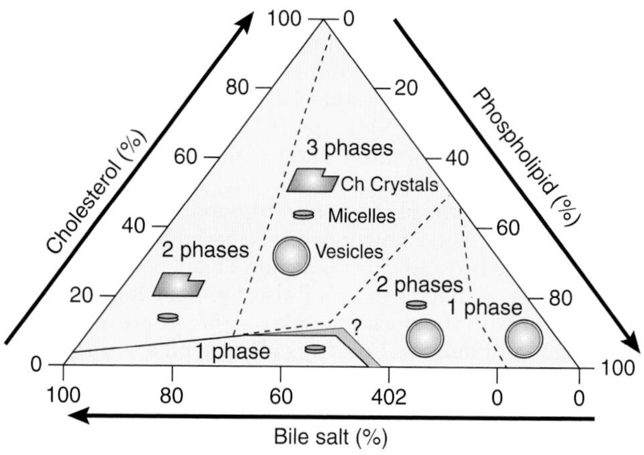

FIGURE 62.3 Equilibrium phase diagram for bile salt–lecithin–cholesterol–water at a concentration of 10% solids, 90% water. The monomeric phase is not depicted as a phase because it exists at the same concentration throughout. The one-phase zone contains only micelles. Several other zones exist, but only the two on the left above the one-phase zone apply to human gallbladder bile, and both contain cholesterol monohydrate crystals at equilibrium.

Pigment Gallstones

Black Pigment Stones. With the recognition that calcium salts are present in most, if not all, cholesterol gallstones, renewed interest has developed in the events leading to the precipitation of calcium with the anions, bilirubin, carbonate, phosphate, or palmitate. Precipitation of these anions as insoluble calcium salts serves as a nidus for cholesterol stone formation. Furthermore, calcium bilirubinate and calcium palmitate also form major components of pigment gallstones. Pigment gallstones are classified as either black or brown pigment stones. Black pigment stones are typically tarry and frequently are associated with hemolytic conditions or cirrhosis. In hemolytic states, the bilirubin load and concentration of unconjugated bilirubin increases. These stones are usually not associated with infected bile and are located almost exclusively in the gallbladder.

Brown Pigment Stones. In contrast to black pigment stones, brown pigment stones are earthy in texture and are typically found in the bile ducts, especially in Asian populations. Brown stones often contain more cholesterol and calcium palmitate than black stones and occur as primary common duct stones in Western patients with disorders of biliary motility and associated bacterial infection. In these settings, bacteria-producing slime and bacteria containing the enzyme glucuronidase cause enzymatic hydrolysis of soluble conjugated bilirubin glucuronide to form free bilirubin, which then precipitates with calcium.[2]

GALLSTONE INCIDENCE AND RISK FACTORS

Incidence

Cholesterol gallstones account for 70% to 80% of all stones in Western industrialized countries. Their prevalence increases with patient age. Stones are uncommon in patients younger than age 20 years, but a sharp increase is noted, especially in women, with each decade to approximately age 70 years (Fig. 62.4). The disease is epidemic, with about 20% of women and 10% of men having stones by age 60 years. Recent studies have shown that approximately 14 million American women and 6 million American men harbor gallstones.[3] In certain populations, such as American Indians, the incidence is extremely high, especially in women. In Chileans and Bolivians of Indian ancestry, the incidence of gallstones is also very high and is associated with a high incidence of gallbladder cancer. In fact, gallbladder cancer is the most common gastrointestinal cancer in these countries. In the United States, the prevalence of stones is highest in Mexican American women (26%), and the prevalence in white women (17%) is higher than in black women (14%).[3]

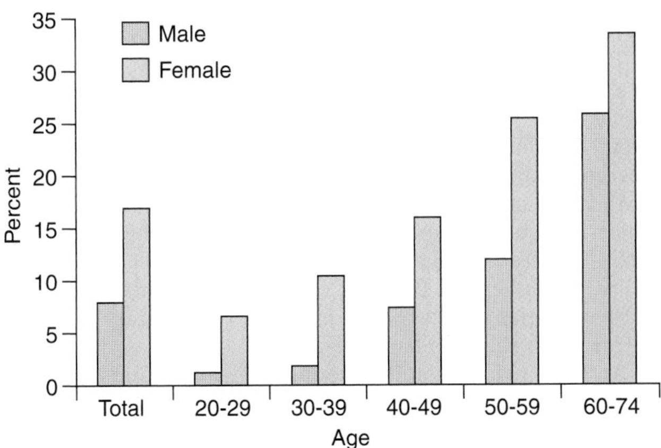

FIGURE 62.4 Influence of age and gender on gallstone incidence. (After the National Health and Nutrition Examination and Survey III (1988–1994). The National Center for Health Statistics, Division of Health Examination Studies, Center for Disease Control and Prevention, October 1996.

Risk Factors

Gallstones are more common in women, especially those who have had multiple pregnancies, are taking birth control pills, are obese, are undergoing rapid weight loss, or who have elevated serum triglyceride levels. Diet plays an important role in cholesterol supersaturation. Cholesterol gallstones do not form in vegetarians. Cholesterol gallstones are common in populations consuming a Western diet, which is relatively high in animal fat. The incidence of cholesterol gallstones rises in a population as it shifts to a higher consumption of dietary fat. Diabetic patients also have an increased incidence of gallstones, which may be caused, in part by alterations in gallbladder motor function and/or absorption. Gallstones also are known to occur more frequently in certain families. However, the genetic factors underlying this phenomenon have not been elucidated. Nevertheless, current data suggest that approximately 30% of the risk for gallstone formation is hereditary whereas 70% is environmental, with diet being the primary environmental factor.[4]

As mentioned previously, prolonged fasting, TPN, ileal resection, vagotomy, hemolytic states and cirrhosis are additional risk factors, and many of these factors lead to black pigment stone formation. Finally, bile duct stasis, as occurs with biliary strictures, congenital cysts, chronic pancreatitis, sclerosing cholangitis, and perivaterian duodenal diverticula, is the primary risk factor for brown pigment stone formation.

NATURAL HISTORY OF GALLSTONES

An understanding of the natural history of gallstone disease is necessary for the appropriate management of patients with cholelithiasis. The presence or absence of symptoms remains the most important factor in the determination of the natural history of gallstones. Gallstone disease can be considered as a spectrum of clinical entities that includes asymptomatic gallstones, symptomatic gallstones and complicated gallstone disease. The complications of gallstone disease include (a) acute cholecystitis, (b) choledocholithiasis with or without cholangitis, (c) gallstone pancreatitis, (d) gallstone ileus, and (e) gallbladder carcinoma.

Asymptomatic Gallstones

Asymptomatic gallstones are often discovered at the time of laparotomy or during abdominal imaging for nonbiliary disease. The vast majority of patients with gallstones are asymptomatic. The stones remain in the gallbladder and do not obstruct the cystic duct. As a result, the gallbladder fills and empties normally, and the gallstones remain silent. Over time, asymptomatic gallstones can progress to symptomatic disease. Symptomatic gallstones usually present with what is termed *biliary colic*, describing right upper quadrant or epigastric abdominal pain that typically develops postprandially and may be associated with nausea and vomiting. The pain results from the impaction of a gallstone at the neck of the gallbladder or cystic duct. Studies that have followed asymptomatic patients have shown that 20% to 30% of patients become

TABLE 62.2

NATURAL HISTORY OF GALLSTONES

Degree of symptoms	Symptoms requiring cholecystectomy	Complications of gallstones
Asymptomatic	1% to 2%/yr	1% to 2%/yr
Mild symptoms	6% to 8%/yr	1% to 3%/yr
Symptomatic	5% to 30%/yr	7%/yr

symptomatic within 20 years.[5,6] Approximately 1% to 2% of asymptomatic individuals with gallstones per year develop serious symptoms or complications related to their gallstones (Table 62.2). The longer stones remain silent, the less likely symptoms are to develop. In addition, almost all patients will develop symptomatic disease before developing one of the complications of gallstones. Therefore, prophylactic cholecystectomy is not generally indicated in patients with asymptomatic gallstones.

In select groups of patients, however, prophylactic cholecystectomy should be considered (Table 62.3). Children with gallstones almost always develop symptoms and should be considered for early cholecystectomy. In patients with sickle cell disease, cholecystitis can precipitate a crisis with substantial operative risks. Therefore, these patients are best treated with elective cholecystectomy. A nonfunctioning gallbladder usually indicates advanced disease with more than 25% of these patients developing symptoms that require cholecystectomy. Large gallstones (>2.5 cm) are more frequently associated with acute cholecystitis and gallbladder carcinoma, and prophylactic cholecystectomy may also be indicated in these patients. In the past, the presence of a porcelain gallbladder (calcified gallbladder wall) was thought to be associated with a 25% risk of malignant transformation,[7] and prophylactic cholecystectomy has been recommended. More recent data suggest that the true risk may be less than 5%,[8,9] but is still high enough to justify cholecystectomy. Patients with a long common channel between the bile and pancreatic ducts also are at significant risk for gallbladder cancer and should undergo prophylactic cholecystectomy.

In obese patients in whom gallstones have already developed and who undergo bariatric surgery, cholecystectomy is indicated because in a large number of these patients symptoms develop that are difficult to distinguish from symptoms caused by complications of their primary operation. Moreover, in 36% of patients who require gastric bypass operations for morbid obesity who did not have gallstones previously, gallstones developed within 6 months of their operation during the period of rapid weight loss. Even more remarkable is that symptoms develop in 40% of these patients and 28% require cholecystectomy during the first year after operation. Prophylactic cholecystectomy adds minimal morbidity and mortality risks to most bariatric operations and is clearly indicated in patients with gallstones. Finally, acute cholecystitis is a potentially life-threatening condition in immunosuppressed patients. For this reason, prophylactic cholecystectomy has been recommended prior to major organ transplantation.

Prophylactic cholecystectomy is not indicated in patients with diabetes and asymptomatic gallstones. Although diabetic patients have an increased risk of surgery with emergent cholecystectomy, recent studies have shown that they also have an increased risk with elective cholecystectomy. This increased risk is related to comorbid conditions not to the diabetes itself. Furthermore, no evidence suggests that asymptomatic diabetics are at increased risk to develop complications of gallstone disease.

TABLE 62.3 INDICATIONS/CONTRAINDICATIONS

INDICATIONS FOR PROPHYLACTIC CHOLECYSTECTOMY

Pediatric gallstones
Congenital hemolytic anemia
Gallstones >2.5 cm in diameter
Calcified (porcelain) gallbladder
Bariatric surgery
Incidental gallstones found during intraabdominal surgery
Long common channel of bile and pancreatic ducts
No access to medical care

Symptomatic Gallstones

Patients with mild symptoms (intermittent biliary colic) are at higher risk for developing gallstone-related complications or requiring cholecystectomy than asymptomatic patients who have gallstones. Approximately 1 to 3% of mildly symptomatic patients per year will develop gallstone-related complications, and at least 6 to 8% per year will require a cholecystectomy to manage their gallbladder symptoms. The diagnosis of symptomatic gallstones requires the presence of characteristic symptoms and the documentation of gallstones on diagnostic imaging.

The primary symptom associated with chronic cholecystitis or symptomatic cholelithiasis is pain. This pain is often referred to as *biliary colic*, a term that is inaccurate and suggests that the pain related to gallstones is intermittent and spasmodic like other colicky pain. In fact, obstruction of the cystic duct results in a progressive increase in tension in the gallbladder wall, leading to constant pain in the majority of patients. The pain is usually located in the right upper quadrant and/or epigastrium and frequently radiates to the back and right scapula. The intensity of the pain is often severe enough that patients often seek immediate medical attention with the first episode. Classically, the pain of biliary colic occurs following fatty meals, although this situation does not occur in most cases. An association with meals is present in only 50% of patients, and in these patients, the pain often develops more than 1 hour after eating. In the remaining patients, the pain is not temporally related to meals and often begins at nighttime waking the patient from sleep.

The duration of pain is typically 1 to 5 hours. The attacks rarely persist for more than 24 hours and are rarely shorter than 1 hour. Pain lasting beyond 24 hours suggests that acute inflammation or cholecystitis is present. The attacks are often discrete and severe enough that the patient can accurately recall and number them. The episodes of biliary colic are usually less frequent than one episode per week. Other symptoms such as nausea and vomiting often accompany each episode (60 to 70% of cases). Bloating and belching are also present in 50% of patients. Fever and jaundice occur much less frequently with simple biliary colic.

Atypical pain is common. Sometimes the pain is continuous rather than episodic. The pain may be located predominantly in the back or the left upper or right lower quadrant. Not all attacks are necessarily severe, and some patients do not relate their pain to meals or time of day. The less typical the pain, the more carefully the clinician should search for another cause, even in the presence of stones—causes such as renal colic, peptic ulcer disease, hiatal hernia, abdominal wall hernia, liver disease, and disease of the small and large intestine. Treatment of atypical biliary colic is appropriate when other causes of pain have been eliminated.

Complicated Gallstones

Acute cholecystitis occurs in approximately 10% to 20% of patients with symptomatic gallstones and results from occlusion of the cystic duct by one or more gallstones. Obstruction of the cystic duct incites an inflammatory response in the gallbladder and can lead to significant complications, including gangrene, empyema, emphysematous cholecystitis, perforation, or cholecystenteric fistula. Choledocholithiasis (CBD stones) is present in 8% to 15% of patients with symptomatic gallstones. The incidence varies with age and is about 5% in younger patients and more than 20% in older patients with gallstones. CBD stones typically develop in the gallbladder and subsequently enter the CBD via the cystic duct. CBD stones may result in cirrhosis, cholangitis, and pancreatitis.

DIAGNOSTIC IMAGING

Abdominal Plain Films

In general, abdominal plain films have a low yield in diagnosing biliary tract problems. They are most useful in diagnosing other causes of acute abdominal pain such as a perforated viscus or a bowel obstruction. Only approximately 15% of gallstones contain sufficient calcium to appear radiopaque on a plain X-ray. Rarely, abdominal films may show a calcified gallbladder wall or pneumobilia that may aid in the diagnosis of biliary disease.

Ultrasound

Transabdominal ultrasound is the radiologic procedure of choice for identifying gallstones and bile duct dilation. Ultrasound is noninvasive, inexpensive, and widely available. Patients should receive nothing by mouth for several hours prior to performing an ultrasound examination so that the gallbladder is fully distended. Gallstones create echoes that are reflected back to the ultrasound probe. The ultrasound waves cannot penetrate the stones; and therefore, acoustic shadowing is seen posterior to the stones (Fig. 62.5). In addition, gallstones that are free-floating in the gallbladder will move to a dependent position when the patient is repositioned during scanning. When these two features are present, the accuracy of ultrasound at diagnosing gallstones approaches 100%. Echoes without shadows may be caused by gallbladder polyps.

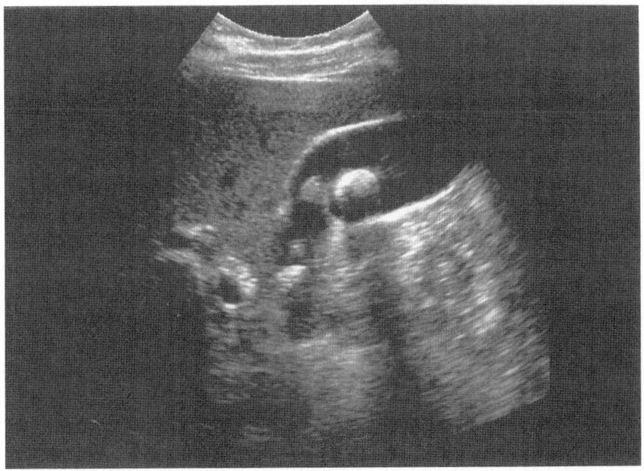

FIGURE 62.5 Abdominal ultrasound of gallbladder with multiple echogenic gallstones.

Several features lower the diagnostic accuracy of ultrasound in detecting gallstones. Small gallstones may not demonstrate an acoustic shadow. Furthermore, a lack of fluid (bile) around the gallstones (stone impacted in cystic duct, gallbladder filled with gallstones) also impairs their detection. In addition, an ileus with increased abdominal gas as occurs with acute cholecystitis may hamper gallbladder visualization. Overall, the false negative rate for ultrasound in detecting gallstones is approximately 5% but may increase to 15% with acute cholecystitis.

Ultrasound can also demonstrate dilatation of the intrahepatic or proximal extrahepatic bile ducts with at least an 80% accuracy rate.[10,11] The normal extrahepatic bile duct diameter is less than 10 mm, and normal intrahepatic duct diameter is less than 4 mm. Dilated ducts may signify the presence of stones in the CBD.

Cholescintigraphy

Cholescintigraphy provides a noninvasive evaluation of the liver, gallbladder, bile duct, and duodenum with both anatomic and functional information. ^{99m}Technetium–labeled iminodiacetic acid derivatives (hepatic 2,6-dimethyl-iminodiacetic acid [HIDA], diisopropyl-acetanilido-iminodiacetic acid, P-isopropylacetanilido imidodiacetic acid) are injected intravenously, rapidly extracted from the blood, and excreted into the bile. These radionuclide scans provide functional information about the liver's ability to excrete radiolabeled substances into a nonobstructed biliary tree. Uptake by the liver, gallbladder, CBD, and duodenum should all be present after 1 hour. Slow uptake of the tracer by the liver suggests hepatic parenchymal disease. Filling of the gallbladder and CBD with delayed or absent filling of the intestine suggests an obstruction at the ampulla.

The primary use of cholescintigraphy is in the diagnosis of acute cholecystitis. Although used less frequently for this indication than in the past because of the availability and accuracy of ultrasound, cholescintigraphy demonstrates the presence of cystic duct obstruction, which is invariably present in acute cholecystitis. Nonvisualization of the gallbladder 1 hour after the injection of the radioisotope with filling of the CBD and duodenum is consistent with total or partial cystic duct obstruction and acute cholecystitis. The sensitivity and specificity of cholescintigraphy for diagnosing acute cholecystitis are each about 95%. False positive results are increased in the setting of gallbladder stasis as in critically ill patients or in patients on parenteral nutrition.

Computerized Tomography/Magnetic Resonance Imaging

Abdominal computed tomography (CT) is less sensitive in diagnosing gallstones than ultrasound. Calcified gallstones are visualized in approximately 50% of patients. The role of CT scanning is primarily limited to the diagnosis of complications of gallstone disease such as acute cholecystitis (gallbladder wall thickening, pericholecystic fluid), choledocholithiasis (intrahepatic and extrahepatic bile duct dilation), pancreatitis (pancreatic edema and inflammation), and gallbladder cancer. More recently, magnetic resonance imaging has been shown to be highly sensitive in the diagnosis of both gallstones and common duct stones when heavily weighted T2-weighted images are obtained.

TREATMENT

Nonoperative Therapy

The nonsurgical options for the treatment of gallstone disease include oral dissolution therapy with the bile acids, ursodeoxycholic acid and chenodeoxycholic acid; contact dissolution therapy with organic solvents (methyl tert-butyl ether); and extracorporeal shock wave biliary lithotripsy. These treatments are rarely used today. Oral dissolution therapy is indicated in symptomatic patients with cholesterol gallstones and a functioning gallbladder. These agents are effective in the dissolution of cholesterol gallstones only and therefore are not indicated if stones are radiopaque or if calcifications can be detected on CT scan. In carefully selected series, complete stone dissolution can be achieved in 40% of patients; however, the recurrence rate is 50% within 5 years if therapy is stopped. Contact dissolution with organic solvents requires cannulation of the gallbladder with direct infusion of the agent into the gallbladder. Again, only cholesterol gallstones are amenable to contact dissolution, and the recurrence rate is similar to that of oral dissolution therapy. Extracorporeal shock wave lithotripsy was originally thought to be a promising nonoperative alternative for the management of symptomatic gallstones. Extracorporeal shock wave lithotripsy is a reasonable therapy for patients with single stones 0.5 to 2 cm in diameter, which have a lower recurrence rate of about 20%. Again, only a small percentage of patients with stones fit these criteria. Moreover, extracorporeal shock wave biliary lithotripsy has never been approved for gallstone dissolution by the U.S. Food and Drug Administration. Finally, the widespread application of laparoscopic cholecystectomy has greatly limited the role of all nonoperative techniques to a very select group of patients.

Operative Therapy

The operative management of gallstones has been the standard of care over the past 140 years. Cholecystectomy is the most common gastrointestinal operation performed in the United States. Since the introduction of laparoscopic cholecystectomy, the number of cholecystectomies performed in the United States has increased from approximately 500,000 per year to 700,000 per year. John Stough Bobb of Indianapolis is credited with performing the first operation on the biliary tract. In 1867, Bobb explored a 32-year-old woman with a large abdominal mass and discovered a massive gallbladder hydrops. A cholecystotomy was made, the gallstones removed, and the gallbladder sutured closed. Fifteen years later, in 1882, Carl Langenbuch of Berlin is credited with performing the first cholecystectomy in a 43-year-old man with a 16-year history of biliary colic. In the late 1980s, German and French surgeons described the first laparoscopic cholecystectomies. Currently, most cholecystectomies are performed laparoscopically.

Laparoscopic Cholecystectomy

Symptomatic cholelithiasis is the main indication for laparoscopic cholecystectomy. As experience with advanced laparoscopy has increased, however, many surgeons will attempt a laparoscopic cholecystectomy in situations of complicated gallstone disease. Contraindications to laparoscopic cholecystectomy include the inability of the patient to withstand a general anesthetic, intractable bleeding disorders, and end-stage liver disease. In addition, patients with severe chronic obstructive pulmonary disease or congestive heart failure may not tolerate the pneumoperitoneum required for performing laparoscopic surgery. The technical difficulty of laparoscopic cholecystectomy is increased in several clinical settings. Laparoscopic cholecystectomy can be performed safely in acute cholecystitis albeit with a higher conversion rate and operative time than in the elective setting. Morbid obesity, once thought to be a relative contraindication to the laparoscopic approach, is not associated with a higher conversion rate. Longer trocars and instruments and an increase in intraabdominal pressure may be helpful in these patients. Prior upper abdominal surgery may increase the difficulty of or preclude laparoscopic cholecystectomy. Elective laparoscopic cholecystectomy has also been completed safely in patients with well-compensated cirrhosis (Child's class A and B) although difficulty retracting the firm liver and increased bleeding from collaterals have been noted.

Patients undergoing laparoscopic cholecystectomy are prepared and draped in a similar fashion to open cholecystectomy. Conversion to an open operation is necessary in up to 5% of patients undergoing elective cholecystectomy and up to 30% of patients undergoing laparoscopic cholecystectomy for acute cholecystitis. A Foley catheter and orogastric tube are inserted to avoid inadvertent injury and improve exposure. Either an open or closed technique can be used to establish a pneumoperitoneum. With the open technique, a small incision is made at the umbilicus, and a blunt cannula (Hasson cannula) is inserted into the peritoneal cavity and anchored to the fascia. In the closed technique a Veress needle is inserted into the peritoneal cavity through a supraumbilical incision and used for insufflation. An 11-mm trocar is inserted through the supraumbilical incision once a pneumoperitoneum is established. A 30°-laparoscope is then inserted through the umbilical port, and an examination of the peritoneal cavity is performed. An 11-mm operating port is placed subxiphoid, and two additional 5-mm trocars are positioned subcostally in the right upper quadrant in the midclavicular and anterior axillary lines.

The two 5-mm ports are used for grasping the gallbladder and exposing the gallbladder and cystic duct (Fig. 62.6). The

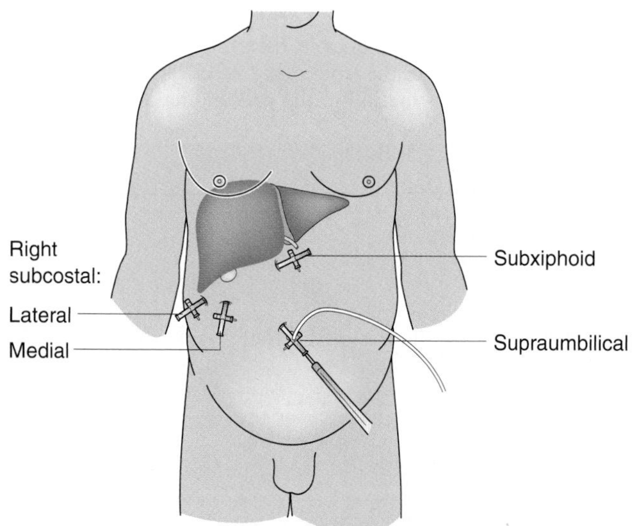

FIGURE 62.6 Trocar placement for laparoscopic cholecystectomy. The laparoscope is placed through a 10-mm port just above the umbilicus. Additional ports are placed in the epigastrium, subcostally in the mid clavicular, and near the anterior axillary lines.

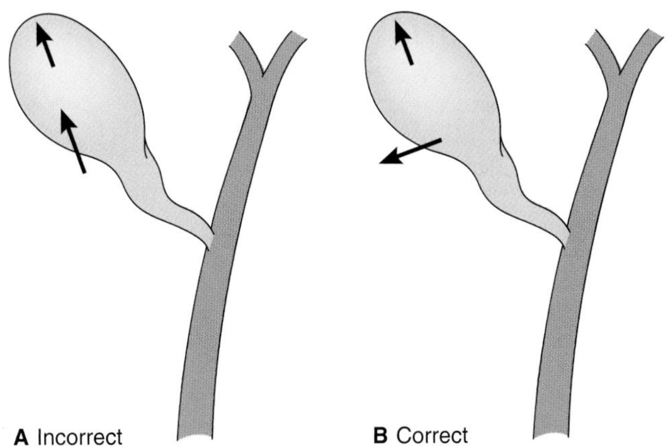

FIGURE 62.7 Incorrect (*A*) and correct (*B*) methods of retracting the gallbladder brings the cystic and common ducts into alignment and makes them appear as one.

medial 5-mm cannula is used to grasp the gallbladder infundibulum and retract it laterally to further expose the triangle of Calot. Traction on the fundus should be upward and to the right, and traction on the pouch of Hartmann laterally to the right. This combination "disaligns" the common duct and cystic duct so that they appear as distinct structures. Incorrect traction aligns the ducts so that they appear as a continuous structure and as a consequence the chance of biliary injury is increased (Fig. 62.7). The junction of the gallbladder and cystic duct is identified by stripping the peritoneum off the gallbladder neck and removing any tissue surrounding the gallbladder neck and proximal cystic duct. This dissection is continued until the triangle of Calot is cleared of all fatty and lymphatic tissue and the gallbladder infundibulum is elevated off of the liver bed (Fig. 62.8). At this point two structures (cystic artery and cystic duct) should be seen entering the gallbladder. Once the cystic duct is identified, an intraoperative cholangiogram may be performed by

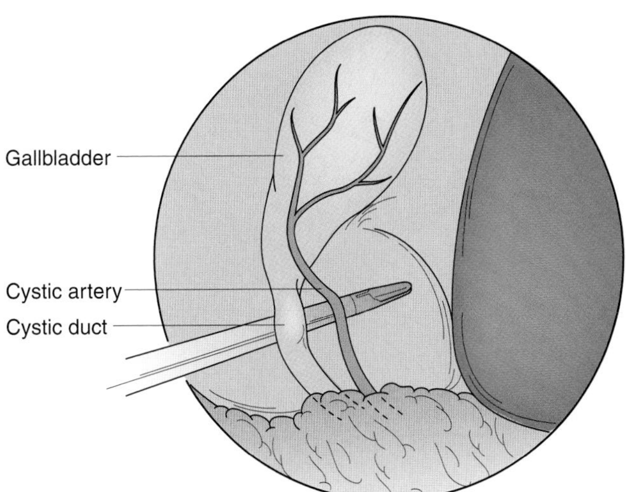

FIGURE 62.8 The "critical view of safety." The triangle of Calot is dissected free of all tissue except for the cystic duct and artery, and the base of the liver bed is exposed. When this view is achieved, the two structures entering the gallbladder can only be the cystic duct and artery. Visualization of the common bile duct is not necessary. (After Strasberg SM, Hertl M, Soper NJ. An analysis of the problem of biliary injury during laparoscopic cholecystectomy. *J Am Coll Surg.* 1995;180:101.)

placing a ligating clip proximally on the cystic duct, incising the anterior surface of the duct, and passing a cholangiogram catheter into the cystic duct. Once the cholangiogram is completed, two clips are placed distally on the cystic duct, which is then divided (Fig. 62.9). Alternatively, the CBD may be evaluated for stones using laparoscopic ultrasound. The sensitivity of laparoscopic ultrasound for detecting CBD stones is comparable to intraoperative cholangiography (80% to 96% versus 75% to 99%).

The next step is the division of the cystic artery. The artery is usually encountered running parallel to and behind the cystic duct. Once identified and isolated, clips are placed proximally and distally, and the artery is divided. The peritoneum overlying the gallbladder is placed on tension using the two grasping forceps, and the peritoneum and adventitia between the gallbladder and liver are divided with the cautery, and the gallbladder is dissected out of the gallbladder fossa. (Fig. 62.9). Prior to removing the gallbladder from the liver, the operative field is carefully searched for hemostasis and adequate placement of the cystic duct and artery clips is confirmed. The gallbladder is then dissected off the liver and is usually removed through the umbilical port. The fascial defect and skin incision may need to be enlarged to remove the gallbladder and contained gallstones. If the gallbladder has been entered during the dissection or if it is acutely inflamed or gangrenous, the gallbladder should be placed in a plastic specimen retrieval bag prior to removing it from the peritoneal cavity.[12,13]

Elective laparoscopic cholecystectomy can be safely performed as an outpatient procedure.[14] Among patients selected for outpatient management, 77% to 97% of patients can be successfully discharged the same day. Factors contributing to overnight admission include uncontrolled pain, nausea and vomiting, operative duration greater than 60 minutes, and cases completed late in the day.

Routine operative cholangiography has been advocated to avoid ductal injury. Opinion on the subject is sharply divided. Biliary injuries appear to be less frequent in the hands of surgeons who perform operative cholangiography routinely. However, in about 50% of ductal injuries, a cholangiogram fails to prevent the injury although abnormal anatomy is present (i.e., cholangiograms are often incorrectly interpreted). The indications for intraoperative cholangiography, when it is performed selectively, are known choledocholithiasis, a history of jaundice, a history of pancreatitis, a large cystic duct and small gallstones, any abnormality in preoperative liver function tests, and dilated biliary ducts on preoperative sonography. Provided these indications are carefully followed, selective cholangiography is as effective in detecting clinically relevant stones as routine cholangiography.

Serious complications of laparoscopic cholecystectomy are rare, the mortality rate being less than 0.1%. As cholecystectomy rates have risen, however, the total number of deaths has not decreased.[15] The single greatest problem in laparoscopic cholecystectomy is biliary injury. The incidence of major bile duct injury following laparoscopic cholecystectomy is between 0.3% and 0.6%; but if all bile leaks are considered, the injury rate in these reports ranges from 0.6% to 1.5%, which is three to four times the injury rate at open surgery.[16] Major vascular injuries to the hepatic arteries, especially the right hepatic artery, may occur in association with biliary injuries and sometimes lead to intraoperative blood loss. Isolated vascular injuries to hepatic vessels are rare. Although the increase in cholecystectomy rates means that the total number of deaths from cholecystectomy has not decreased, an individual patient's risk for death is smaller.

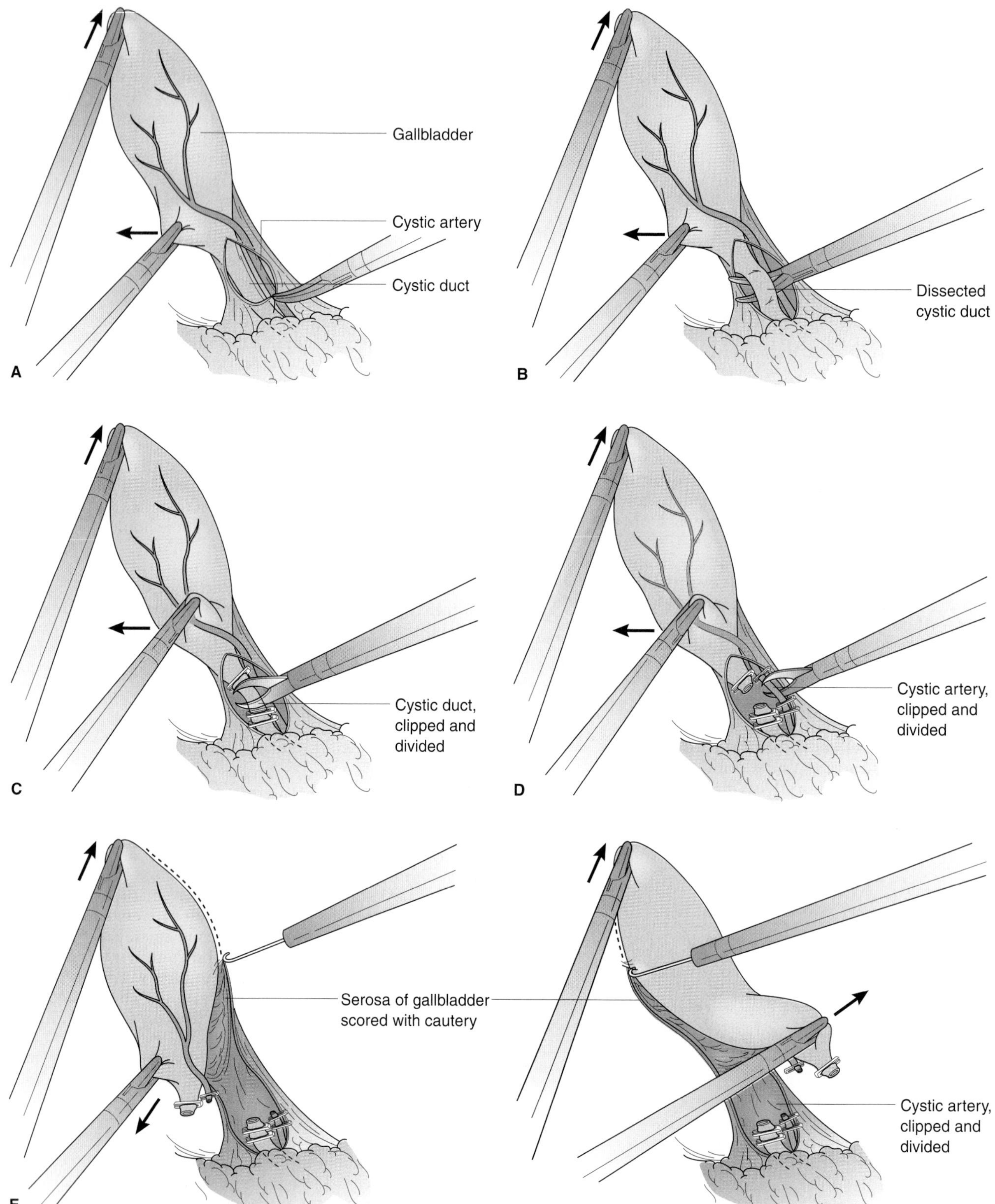

FIGURE 62.9 (*A*) The peritoneum overlying the cystic duct gallbladder junction is opened with blunt dissection. (*B*) The cystic duct is isolated. (*C*) The cystic duct is clipped proximal and distal and divided with the hook scissors. (*D*) The cystic artery is dissected, clipped and divided. (*E*) The gallbladder is dissected from the liver by scoring the serosa with electrocautery.

Spillage of stones into the peritoneal cavity during laparoscopic cholecystectomy occurs in 10% or more of cases. Leaving stones in the peritoneal cavity may not be innocuous.[17] Intraabdominal abscess, subcutaneous abscess, and later discharge of stones through the abdominal wall or through the lung and trachea have all been described. Every attempt should be made to remove spilled stones by picking and irrigating them out. Clearance is usually quite successful with the use of retractors to lift the liver and the 30-degree laparoscope, which allows the depths of the recess between liver and kidney to be visualized. Laparoscopic ultrasonography may be useful to detect stones. Large stones or massive spills should be cleaned up by laparotomy if necessary. If concern exists that stones have been left behind, the patient should be informed.

As in open cholecystectomy, a gallbladder containing an unsuspected cancer is excised one to three times per 1,000 laparoscopic cholecystectomies. Therefore, a good practice is to open the gallbladder and inspect it and obtain frozen sections if a suspect lesion is observed. If cancer is suspected, the gallbladder should be extracted in an impermeable bag. If a cancer is discovered, further surgery may be indicated.

Open Cholecystectomy

Open cholecystectomy can be performed through either an upper midline or right subcostal (Kocher) incision. Identification and division of the cystic duct and artery initially limits bleeding from the gallbladder for the remainder of the dissection. With lateral traction on the gallbladder neck, the peritoneum overlying the triangle of Calot is incised, and the cystic duct is identified and ligated distally. A cholangiogram is performed at this time if indicated. The cystic duct is then ligated proximally and divided. Similarly, the cystic artery is ligated and divided after carefully tracing it onto the gallbladder. If the anatomy cannot be clearly identified, the gallbladder should be dissected from the fundus downward towards the gallbladder neck, making the ductal and vascular anatomy easier to identify. The gallbladder is dissected out of the gallbladder bed by incising the overlying peritoneum with cautery.

CLINICAL MANIFESTATIONS

Chronic Calculous Cholecystitis

Pathogenesis

The term *chronic cholecystitis* implies an ongoing or recurrent inflammatory process involving the gallbladder. In most patients (more than 90%), gallstones are the causative factor and lead to recurrent episodes of cystic duct obstruction manifest as biliary pain or colic. Over time, these recurrent attacks can lead to scarring and a nonfunctioning gallbladder. Histopathologically, chronic cholecystitis is characterized by an increase in subepithelial and subserosal fibrosis and a mononuclear cell infiltrate.

Clinical Presentation

The primary symptom associated with chronic cholecystitis or symptomatic cholelithiasis is pain, often labeled *biliary colic*. The pain is usually located in the right upper quadrant and/or epigastrium and frequently radiates to the right upper back, right scapula, or between the scapulae (as noted in the previous discussion of symptomatic gallstones). Other symptoms such as nausea and vomiting often accompany each episode (60% to 70% of cases). The physical examination is usually completely normal in patients with chronic cholecystitis, particularly if they are pain free. During an episode of biliary colic, mild right upper quadrant tenderness may be present. Laboratory values such as serum bilirubin, transaminases, and alkaline phosphatase are also usually normal in patients with uncomplicated gallstones.

Diagnosis

The diagnosis of chronic calculous cholecystitis requires two findings: abdominal pain consistent with biliary colic and the presence of gallstones. The presence of symptoms (usually pain) attributable to the gallbladder is necessary to consider any treatment for gallstones. Patients without symptoms (approximately two thirds of patients with gallstones) develop symptoms at a low rate and complications of gallstones at an even lower rate (as noted in the previous discussion of natural history). In most cases treatment is not necessary in these asymptomatic patients. The presence of gallstones should also be documented. Ultrasound is sensitive (95% to 98%) for documenting the presence of gallstones and also provides additional anatomical information, including the presence of polyps, the diameter of the CBD, and any hepatic parenchymal abnormalities. Gallstones are occasionally identified on abdominal radiographs (15%) or CT scans (50%) because gallstones contain enough calcium to be visualized.

Management

The treatment of choice for patients with symptomatic gallstones is elective laparoscopic cholecystectomy. The mortality of laparoscopic cholecystectomy is approximately 0.1% with cardiovascular complications being the most frequent cause of death. The most significant complication following laparoscopic cholecystectomy is injury to the biliary tract. Overall, complications occur in fewer than 10% of patients. Conversion to an open cholecystectomy is necessary in less than 5% of patients undergoing laparoscopic cholecystectomy for chronic cholecystitis. Conversion rates are increased in elderly, obese, and male patients.

The long-term results of laparoscopic cholecystectomy in appropriately selected patients with chronic cholecystitis are excellent. More than 90% of patients with typical biliary pain and gallstones are symptom-free following cholecystectomy. For patients with atypical symptoms or painless dyspepsia (fatty food intolerance, flatulence, belching, or bloating), the percentage of patients experiencing relief of symptoms decreases.

Acute Calculous Cholecystitis

Pathophysiology

Acute cholecystitis is the most common complication of gallstones occurring in 20% to 30% of patients with symptomatic disease. As in biliary colic, acute cholecystitis results from a stone impaction at the gallbladder-cystic duct junction (Fig. 62.10). The extent of inflammation and the progression of acute cholecystitis is related to the duration and degree of obstruction. In the most severe cases (5% to 18%), this process can lead to ischemia and necrosis of the gallbladder wall. More frequently, the gallstone is dislodged, and the inflammation gradually resolves. Acute cholecystitis is primarily an inflammation and not an infectious process with bacterial infection appearing as a secondary event. Approximately 50% of patients with acute cholecystitis will have positive bile cultures, with *Escherichia coli* being the most common organism.

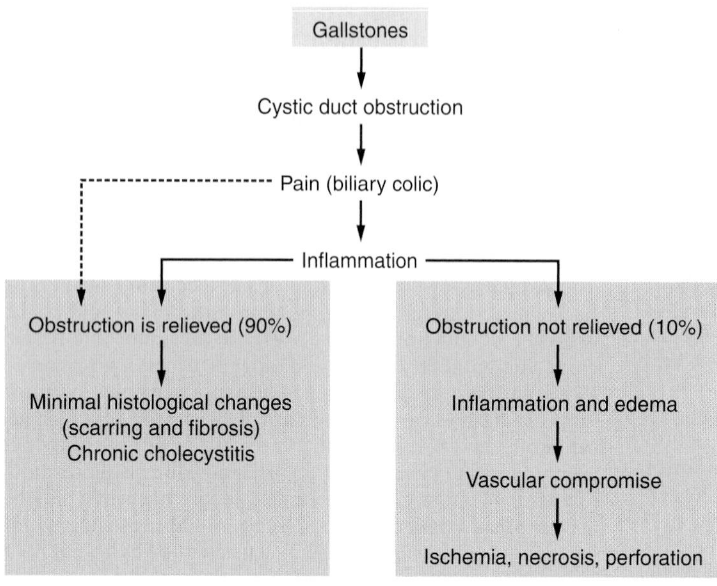

FIGURE 62.10 Pathophysiology of acute cholecystitis.

Clinical Presentation

Patients with acute cholecystitis typically present with right upper quadrant pain that is similar to that of biliary colic. In acute cholecystitis, however, the pain is usually unremitting, may last several days, and is often associated with nausea, emesis, anorexia, and fever. On physical examination, patients with acute cholecystitis usually have a low-grade fever, and exhibit localized right upper quadrant tenderness and guarding which distinguishes the episode from simple biliary colic. The presence of Murphy's sign, an inspiratory arrest during deep palpation of the right upper quadrant, is the classic physical finding of acute cholecystitis. A palpable right upper quadrant mass is appreciated in one third of patients and usually represents omentum that has migrated to the area around the gallbladder in response to the inflammation. Severe jaundice is rare, but mild jaundice may be present—up to 6 mg/dL. Severe jaundice suggests the presence of CBD stones, cholangitis, or obstruction of the common hepatic duct by severe pericholecystic inflammation resulting from impaction of a large stone in Hartmann's pouch, which mechanically obstructs the bile duct (Mirizzi's syndrome). Acute cholecystitis may coexist with choledocholithiasis or it complications (acute cholangitis and gallstone pancreatitis). The coexistence of two of these conditions often explains an unusual or atypical clinical presentation.

Laboratory evaluation can show a mild leukocytosis (white blood cell count [WBC] 12,000 to 15,000 cells/mm^3). However, many patients have a normal WBC. A white cell count greater than 20,000 should suggest further complications of cholecystitis, such as gangrene, perforation, or cholangitis. Mild elevations in serum bilirubin (<4 mg/dL), alkaline phosphatase, the transaminases, and amylase may also be seen with acute cholecystitis.

Diagnosis

Ultrasound is the most useful radiologic examination in the patient with suspected cholecystitis. First, in the patient without known gallstones, ultrasound is a sensitive test for establishing the presence or absence of gallstones. Additional findings suggestive of acute cholecystitis include thickening of the gallbladder wall (>4 mm) and pericholecystic fluid. Focal tenderness directly over the gallbladder (sonographic Murphy's sign) is also suggestive of acute cholecystitis. Ultrasound has a sensitivity and specificity of 85% and 95%, respectively, for diagnosing acute cholecystitis.

Radionuclide scanning is used less frequently for the diagnosis of acute cholecystitis but may provide additional information in the atypical case. Nonfilling of the gallbladder with the radiotracer (^{99}Tc-HIDA) indicates an obstructed cystic duct, and in the right clinical setting is highly sensitive (95%) and specific (95%) for acute cholecystitis. Computed tomography (Fig. 62.11) occasionally is performed in evaluating the patient with abdominal pain and acute illness. CT may demonstrate evidence of acute cholecystitis, including gallbladder wall thickening, pericholecystic fluid and edema, gallstones, and air in the gallbladder or gallbladder wall (emphysematous cholecystitis), although it is less sensitive for these conditions than ultrasonography.

Management

Once the diagnosis of acute cholecystitis is made, the patient should be given nothing by mouth, and intravenous hydration should begin. A nasogastric tube is placed if there is persistent nausea and vomiting or abdominal distention. In almost all cases, broad-spectrum antibiotics, such as a broad-spectrum

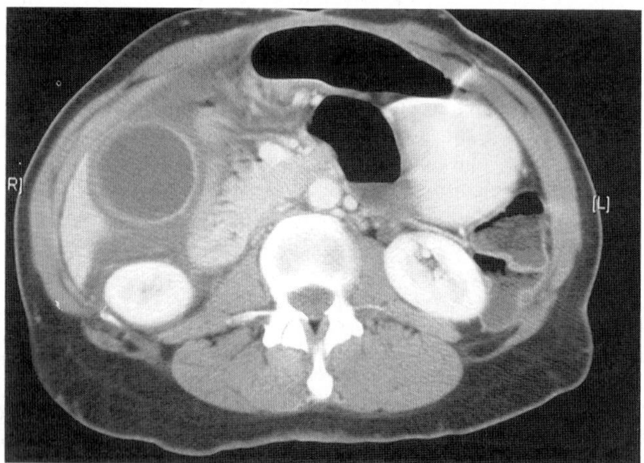

FIGURE 62.11 Computed tomography of a patient with acute cholecystitis showing gallbladder wall thickening and pericholecystic fluid.

TABLE 62.4 RESULTS

RANDOMIZED PROSPECTIVE TRIALS OF EARLY VERSUS DELAYED LAPAROSCOPIC CHOLECYSTECTOMY FOR ACUTE CHOLECYSTITIS

	Queen Mary hospital[19]		Prince of Wales hospital[20]	
	Early	Late	Early	Late
Number of patients	45	41	53	46
Operative time	135 min	105 min	123 min	106 min
Conversion	11%	23%	21%	24%
Morbidity	13%	29%	21%	24%
Total LOS	6 days	11 days	7.6 days	11.6 days
Recurrent symptoms	—	36%	—	17%

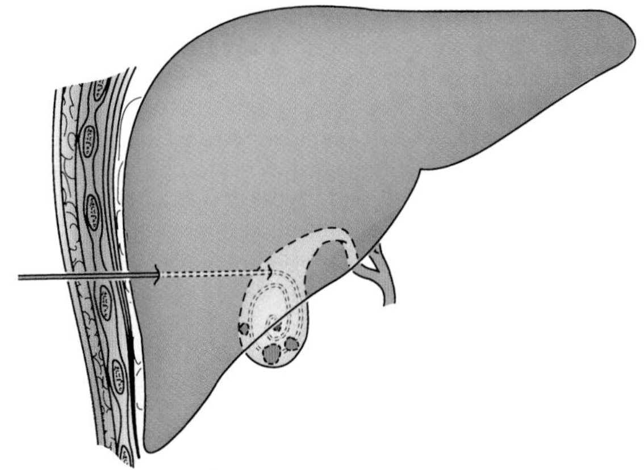

FIGURE 62.12 Schematic demonstration of the technique of percutaneous placement of a pigtail catheter into the gallbladder.

penicillin should be started and maintained into the immediate postoperative period. Parenteral analgesia should also be administered. Unfortunately, narcotics increase biliary pressure whereas nonsteroidal analgesics, which inhibit prostaglandin synthesis, reduce gallbladder mucin production, and, therefore, reduce pressure and pain.

The treatment of choice for acute cholecystitis is cholecystectomy. Open cholecystectomy had been the standard treatment for acute cholecystitis for many years. Initially, acute cholecystitis was felt to be a contraindication to laparoscopic cholecystectomy. As experience has increased, however, it has become clear that laparoscopic cholecystectomy can be performed safely in the setting of acute cholecystitis. In prospective, randomized trials, the morbidity rate, length of hospital stay, and time to return to work have all been lower in patients undergoing laparoscopic cholecystectomy than open cholecystectomy.[18] However, the conversion rate in the setting of acute cholecystitis (10% to 35%) is higher than with chronic cholecystitis.

The timing of cholecystectomy for acute cholecystitis has been studied for several decades. In the distant past, delayed cholecystectomy was preferred in the setting of acute cholecystitis. Patients were initially managed nonoperatively and discharged home after their symptoms resolved. Elective cholecystectomy was then performed 6 weeks later after the acute inflammation had resolved. Recent prospective randomized trials have shown that early laparoscopic cholecystectomy (within 3 days of symptom onset) can be accomplished with a similar morbidity and mortality rate as delayed cholecystectomy (Table 62.4).[19,20] No significant differences were observed in the conversion rate to open cholecystectomy among patients undergoing early cholecystectomy versus those managed with delayed surgery. Hospital stay, and therefore cost, however, were significantly reduced in both trials in the early laparoscopic cholecystectomy group. In addition, approximately 20% of patients in the delayed surgery arm failed initial medical therapy and required operation during the initial admission or before the end of the planned cooling-off period.

Laparoscopic cholecystectomy should be performed within 24 to 72 hours of diagnosis. Early conversion to an open procedure should be considered if dissection is difficult or clear progress cannot be made by the laparoscopic technique. In certain high-risk patients whose medical conditions precludes cholecystectomy, a cholecystostomy can be performed for acute cholecystitis. Although previously performed operatively and under local anesthesia, percutaneous drainage techniques can usually be accomplished (Fig. 62.12). In most cases, prompt improvement is seen after gallbladder drainage and appropriate antibiotics. These patients must be observed closely, however, and if improvement does not occur within 24 hours, laparotomy is indicated. Failure to improve after percutaneous cholecystostomy is usually caused by gangrene of the gallbladder or perforation. After the acute episode resolves, the patient can undergo either cholecystectomy or percutaneous stone extraction and removal of the cholecystostomy tube. The latter is an option in elderly or debilitated patients for whom a general anesthetic is contraindicated.

Complications of Acute Cholecystitis

Several complications of acute cholecystitis are recognized in clinical practice. These complications include empyema of the gallbladder, emphysematous cholecystitis, perforation, and cholecystenteric fistula. All of these complications can be associated with significant morbidity and mortality and, therefore, require prompt surgical intervention.

Empyema. Gallbladder empyema represents an advanced stage of cholecystitis with bacterial invasion of the gallbladder and actual pus in the lumen. Patients present with severe right upper quadrant pain, high-grade fever, rigors, and significant leukocytosis. Sepsis including cardiovascular collapse may be seen. Treatment consists of broad-spectrum antibiotics, including anaerobic coverage, and emergent cholecystectomy or cholecystostomy; however, cholecystostomy may not be adequate to relieve sepsis in patients with empyema of the gallbladder.

Emphysematous Cholecystitis. Emphysematous cholecystitis develops more commonly in males and patients with diabetes mellitus. Severe right upper quadrant pain and generalized sepsis are frequently present. Abdominal films or CT scans may demonstrate air within the gallbladder wall or lumen. Prompt antibiotic therapy to cover the common biliary pathogens including *E. coli, enterococcus, Klebsiella*, as well as *Clostridia* species and emergency cholecystectomy are appropriate treatments.

Gangrene/Perforation. Gangrene of the gallbladder occurs when the wall becomes ischemic and leads to perforation. Gallbladder perforation can be categorized as being either localized or free. The incidence of perforation in acute cholecystitis is approximately 10%. Localized perforation generally results in the formation of a pericholecystic abscess as the omentum walls of the perforation and limits it to the right upper quadrant. Free perforation is less frequent (1%

of cases) and occurs if the omentum is unable to wall off the inflammatory process. Free perforation results in the spilling of bile into the peritoneal cavity and a generalized peritonitis. Perforation should be suspected if the patient's clinical course deteriorates. Evidence for perforation includes an increase in pain and tenderness, fever and chills, elevation in white blood cell count, and hypotension. These patients require aggressive fluid resuscitation, antibiotics, and emergent operative exploration. Cholecystostomy will usually not be adequate therapy for patients with gangrene or perforation of the gallbladder.

Cholecystoenteric Fistula. In 1% to 2% of patients with acute cholecystitis, the gallbladder will perforate into an adjacent hollow viscus. The duodenum (79%) and the hepatic flexure of the colon (17%) are the most common sites. Generally, after the fistula forms, the episode of acute cholecystitis resolves as the gallbladder spontaneously decompresses. If a large gallstone passes from the gallbladder into the small intestine, a mechanical bowel obstruction may result which is termed gallstone ileus. Gallstone ileus occurs in 10% to 15% of patients with a cholecystoenteric fistula. Patients with gallstone ileus present with signs and symptoms of intestinal obstruction–nausea, vomiting, and abdominal pain. The pain may be episodic and recurrent as the impacted stone temporarily impacts in the gut lumen and then dislodges and moves distally (tumbling obstruction). A history of gallstone-related symptoms (right upper quadrant pain) may only be present in 50% of these patients. Abdominal films will demonstrate small bowel distension and air-fluid levels and may give additional clues to the source of the obstruction (pneumobilia or a calcified gallstone distant from the gallbladder). The site of obstruction is most frequently in the narrowest part of the small intestine (ileum) or large intestine (sigmoid colon).

The initial management of gallstone ileus includes relieving the obstruction. Most frequently, this goal can be achieved by removing the gallstone through an enterotomy (Fig. 62.13). Additional gallstones should be sought as recurrent obstruction has been reported in up to 10% of patients with gallstone ileus. Takedown of the biliary-enteric fistula and cholecystectomy may be warranted as recurrent cholecystitis and cholangitis are common in patients with a biliary-enteric fistula, and gallbladder cancer has been reported in 15% of these patients. However, in patients with a significant inflammatory process in the right upper quadrant or who are too unstable to withstand a prolonged operative procedure, the fistula can be addressed at a second laparotomy.

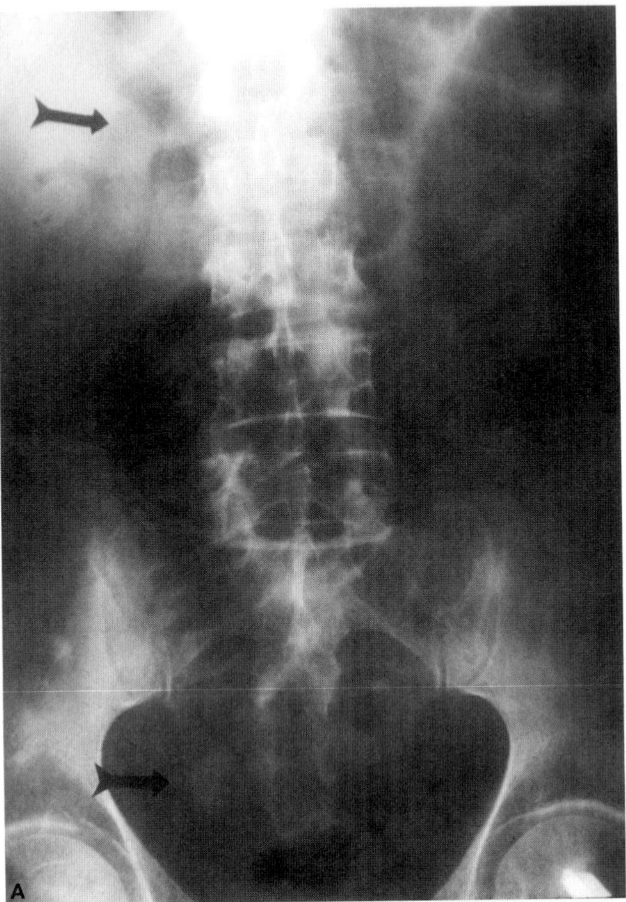

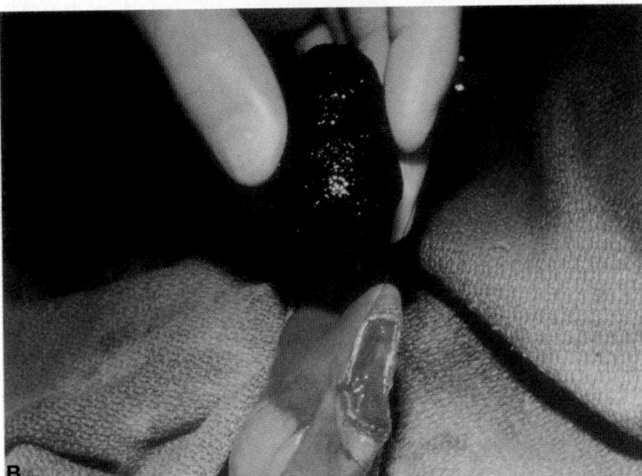

FIGURE 62.13 (*A*) Abdominal plain film demonstrating small bowel obstruction secondary to gallstone ileus. *Arrows* show a gallstone in the right lower quadrant and air in the biliary tree. (*B*) Operative photograph demonstrating removal of a large gallstone from the ileum.

Acute Acalculous Cholecystitis

Acute acalculous cholecystitis accounts for 5% to 10% of all patients with acute cholecystitis. The disease often has a more fulminant course than acute calculous cholecystitis and frequently progresses to gangrene, empyema, or perforation. Acute acalculous cholecystitis usually occurs in the critically ill patient following trauma, burns, long-term parenteral nutrition, and major nonbiliary operations such as abdominal aneurysm repair and cardiopulmonary bypass. The etiology of acute acalculous cholecystitis remains unclear although gallbladder stasis and ischemia have been most often implicated as causative factors. Stasis is common in critically ill patients not being fed enterally and may lead to colonization of the gallbladder with bacteria. Visceral ischemia is also a common denominator in patients with acute acalculous cholecystitis and may explain the high incidence of gallbladder gangrene. Decreased arteriolar and capillary filling is present in acute acalculous cholecystitis in contrast to the dilation of these vessels observed in acute calculous cholecystitis.

The symptoms and signs of acute acalculous cholecystitis are similar to acute calculous cholecystitis with right upper quadrant pain and tenderness, fever, and leukocytosis most frequently present. CT scan and ultrasound findings are similar to calculous cholecystitis and include gallbladder wall thickening and pericholecystic fluid in the absence of gallstones. Cholescintigraphy demonstrates absent gallbladder filling in acute acalculous cholecystitis; however, the false positive rate (absent gallbladder filling without acute acalculous cholecystitis) may be as high as 40%.

Emergency cholecystectomy is the appropriate treatment once the diagnosis is established or the suspicion is high. The incidence of gangrene, perforation, and empyema exceeds 50%; and therefore, cholecystectomy rather than cholecystostomy is usually required in this setting. The mortality rate for acute acalculous cholecystitis in recent series remains high (40%) in large part because of the concomitant illnesses in patients who develop this disease.

Chronic Acalculous Cholecystitis

A subgroup of patients presenting with typical symptoms of biliary colic (postprandial right upper quadrant pain, fatty food intolerance, and nausea) do not have any evidence of gallstones on ultrasound examination. Further investigations have usually been performed in these patients to exclude any other pathology. This workup often includes an abdominal CT scan, esophagogastroduodenoscopy, or even an endoscopic retrograde cholangiogram. In these patients, the diagnosis of biliary dyskinesia or chronic acalculous cholecystitis should be considered. The cholecystokinin-Tc-HIDA scan has been useful in identifying patients with this disorder. Cholecystokinin (CCK) is infused intravenously after the gallbladder has filled with the ^{99}Tc-labeled radionuclide. Twenty minutes after the administration of CCK, a gallbladder ejection fraction is calculated. An ejection fraction less than 35% at 20 minutes is considered abnormal.

Patients with symptoms of biliary colic and an abnormal gallbladder ejection fraction should be managed with a laparoscopic cholecystectomy. Between 85% and 94% of patients with a low gallbladder ejection fraction and symptoms of biliary colic will be asymptomatic or improved by cholecystectomy. Most of these patients have histopathologic evidence of chronic cholecystitis.

Sphincter of Oddi Dysfunction

Sphincter of Oddi dysfunction may be caused by either a structural or functional abnormality involving the sphincter. Fibrosis of the sphincter from gallstone migration, operative or endoscopic trauma, pancreatitis, or other nonspecific inflammatory processes can lead to elevated sphincter pressures. Elevated sphincter pressures may also present in the absence of a structural abnormality, and these cases of sphincter of Oddi dyskinesia or spasm are often associated with more diffuse abnormalities of gastrointestinal motility.[21]

Sphincter of Oddi dysfunction should be suspected in patients with typical episodic biliary-type pain without an obvious organic cause. Approximately 1% of patients undergoing cholecystectomy are estimated to have sphincter of Oddi dysfunction. Numerous diagnostic tests have been used to diagnose sphincter of Oddi dysfunction, but none are sensitive or specific. Elevated serum amylase or transaminases may be present in patients with sphincter of Oddi dysfunction. Ultrasound evidence of sphincter of Oddi dysfunction includes a dilated (>12 mm) CBD, an increase in CBD diameter in response to cholecystokinin, or an increase in pancreatic duct diameter in response to secretin. Delayed emptying of contrast from the CBD after endoscopic retrograde cholangiopancreatography is also indicative of abnormal sphincter function. Endoscopic manometry has also been used to evaluate the sphincter of Oddi, and an elevated basal sphincter pressure (>40 mm Hg) has been correlated with successful response to sphincter ablation.

Both endoscopic sphincterotomy and transduodenal sphincteroplasty with transampullary septotomy have been used to manage patients with sphincter of Oddi dysfunction. Results of both treatments appear to be similar and are more dependent on the presence of objective signs of sphincter dysfunction than on the procedure performed. The surgical approach (transduodenal sphincteroplasty with transampullary septotomy) has the advantage of including division of the transampullary septum, which can impede pancreatic duct drainage when chronically inflamed and fibrotic. A further advantage is that mucosa to mucosa apposition can be achieved minimizing the risk of scarring and restenosis. When objective evidence of sphincter dysfunction is present (elevated transaminases, delayed biliary emptying, dilated CBD, elevated basal sphincter pressure), 60% to 80% of patients will be pain-free or improved following sphincterotomy or sphincteroplasty.[21]

Acute Cholangitis

Acute cholangitis is a bacterial infection of the biliary ductal system, which varies in severity from mild and self-limited to severe and life threatening. The clinical triad of fever, jaundice, and pain associated with cholangitis was first described in 1877 by Charcot. He postulated that stagnant bile associated with obstructive biliary pathology was a significant factor in the pathogenesis of this disease.

Pathophysiology

Clinical cholangitis results from a combination of two factors: significant bacterial concentrations in the bile and biliary obstruction. Although cultures of the gallbladder and bile ducts are usually sterile, in the presence of CBD stones or other obstructing pathology the incidence of positive bile duct cultures increases. The most common organisms recovered from the bile in patients with cholangitis include *E. coli, Klebsiella pneumonia*, the enterococci, and *Bacteroides fragilis*.[22] Nevertheless, even in the presence of high biliary bacterial concentrations, clinical cholangitis and bacteremia do not develop unless obstruction causes elevated intraductal pressures.

Normal biliary pressures range from 7 to 14 cm H_2O. In the presence of bactibilia and normal biliary pressures, hepatic vein blood and perihepatic lymph are sterile. In cases of partial or complete biliary obstruction, however, intrabiliary pressures rise to 18 to 29 cm H_2O, and organisms rapidly appear in both the blood and lymph. The fever and chills associated with cholangitis are the result of systemic bacteremia caused by cholangiovenous and cholangiolymphatic reflux (Fig. 62.14).

Etiology. The most common causes of biliary obstruction are choledocholithiasis, benign strictures, biliary enteric anastomotic strictures, and cholangiocarcinoma or periampullary cancer. Prior to 1980, choledocholithiasis was the cause of approximately 80% of the reported cases of cholangitis. In recent years, malignant strictures have become a frequent cause of cholangitis particularly at tertiary referral centers. Endoscopic cholangiography, percutaneous transhepatic cholangiography, and stent placement via either the endoscopic or percutaneous route are all known to cause bacteremia. These procedures are frequently performed in patients with unresectable malignant obstruction.

Clinical Presentation. Cholangitis may present with a wide spectrum of disease. Patients may have a self-limited illness and never seek attention. At the other end of the spectrum, patients with toxic cholangitis present with a severe illness, including jaundice, fever, abdominal pain, mental obtundation, and hypotension (Reynolds' pentad). Fever is the most common presenting symptom and is often accompanied by

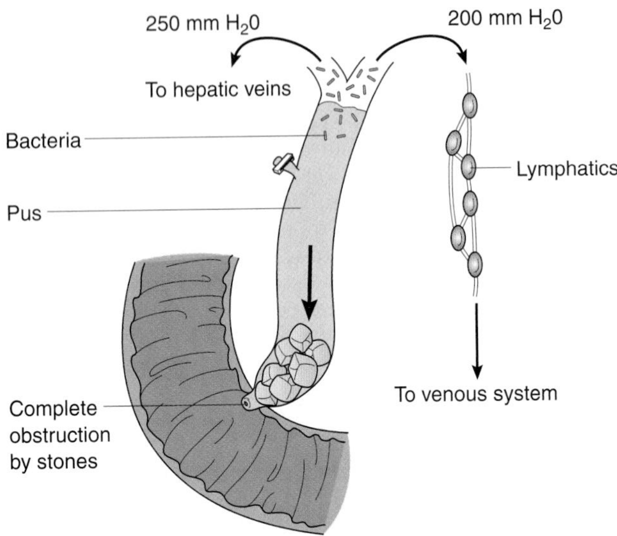

FIGURE 62.14 Cholangitis is caused by the combination of biliary obstruction and bactibilia. Bacteria then reflux into the hepatic veins and perihepatic lymphatics, resulting in systemic bacteremia.

chills. Jaundice is a frequent physical finding but may be absent, especially in patients with an indwelling endoprosthesis or biliary stent. Pain is also commonly present but is often mild. Severe pain or marked tenderness should prompt consideration of an alternate diagnosis such as acute cholecystitis. Up to 33% of East Asian patients with choledocholithiasis present with toxic cholangitis characterized by septic shock.[23]

Diagnosis. Although cholangitis is a clinical diagnosis, laboratory tests can support evidence of biliary obstruction. Leukocytosis, hyperbilirubinemia, and elevations of alkaline phosphatase and transaminases are all common in patients with cholangitis. Radiological studies are also helpful in confirming the diagnosis. CT, ultrasound, and magnetic resonance image scanning can provide noninvasive evidence of biliary ductal dilation, pancreatic masses, and occasionally CBD stones. Cholangiography is usually required prior to or as part of therapy. Both endoscopic and percutaneous transhepatic cholangiography are associated with a 4% to 7% incidence of cholangitis, and systemic antibiotics should be administered prior to these procedures.

Management. The initial treatment of the patient with cholangitis includes antibiotics. Some patients are only mildly ill and can be managed as outpatients with oral antibiotics. Patients with toxic cholangitis may require intensive care unit monitoring and vasopressors to support blood pressure. Most patients will require intravenous fluids and antibiotics. The antibacterial regimen should cover the common pathogens isolated from the biliary tract or be based on current or prior bile cultures.

Most patients with cholangitis respond to antibiotic therapy alone with clinical improvement; however, emergency biliary decompression may be necessary, in the 15% of patients who do not respond to antibiotics within 12 to 24 hours or in patients with toxic cholangitis. Biliary decompression may be performed endoscopically or via the percutaneous transhepatic route. The selection of which procedure to perform should be based on the level and nature of the biliary obstruction. In patients with a proximal perihilar obstruction or a biliary-enteric anastomotic stricture, percutaneous drainage may be the preferred route of decompression. Choledocholithiasis and cholangitis associated with periampullary malignancies are best approached endoscopically. Endoscopic biliary drainage may include endoscopic sphincterotomy and stone extraction or simply placement of an endoscopic biliary stent in the hemodynamically unstable patient. In experienced hands, successful endoscopic CBD stone clearance can be achieved in more than 90% of patients.[23] In settings in which either endoscopic or percutaneous biliary drainage is not possible, CBD exploration and placement of a T-tube remains a life-saving procedure for seriously ill patients with toxic cholangitis. However, the mortality for patients treated surgically is considerably higher than for patients successfully managed endoscopically.

Overall, the mortality rate associated with an episode of gallstone cholangitis is approximately 2% but is higher in patients with toxic cholangitis (5%). Renal failure, hepatic abscess, and malignancy are all associated with higher morbidity and mortality. The success of the initial antibiotic therapy and biliary drainage is significantly lower in patients with malignant biliary obstruction, and these patients frequently require changes in antibiotic therapy and repeat biliary manipulations to adequately decompress the biliary tract.[22] Hepatic abscesses are frequently observed in patients with biliary pathology and should be considered in patients who do not respond to therapy. Patients with gallstone cholangitis should undergo interval laparoscopic cholecystectomy within 6 to 12 weeks. The incidence of recurrent biliary symptoms is significantly higher if the gallbladder is left in situ (6% versus 25%).[23]

CHOLEDOCHOLITHIASIS

Classification and Etiology

CBD stones can be classified as either primary or secondary. Primary duct stones develop *de novo* within the bile ducts, whereas secondary stones develop in the gallbladder and subsequently fall into the CBD. In the United States more than 85% of all bile duct stones are secondary. Primary duct stones typically occur in patients with benign biliary strictures, sclerosing cholangitis, choledochal cyst disease, or sphincter of Oddi dysfunction. These conditions are associated with bile stasis, which promotes the overgrowth of bacteria in bile with subsequent deconjugation of bilirubin and the breakdown of biliary lipids, resulting in the formation of brown pigment stones. Secondary bile duct stones have a composition similar to gallbladder stones. Approximately 75% are cholesterol stones, and 25% are black pigment stones. The classification of CBD stones into primary or secondary is of therapeutic importance because primary stones require removal of the stones and a drainage procedure (choledochoenterostomy or sphicteroplasty) whereas secondary stones can be treated by removal of the stones and cholecystectomy.

Clinical Presentation

Common duct stones are often asymptomatic and only discovered during cholangiography at the time of cholecystectomy. CBD stones are present in 8% to 15% of patients with symptomatic gallstones. The incidence varies with age and is approximately 5% in younger patients and more than 20% in older patients with gallstones. Patients with symptomatic choledocholithiasis will present with biliary colic, extrahepatic biliary obstruction, cholangitis, or pancreatitis. Clinical features suspicious for biliary obstruction caused by CBD stones include biliary colic, jaundice, lightening of the stools, and darkening of the urine. Typically, the pain and jaundice associated with CBD stones are more intermittent and transient than when the biliary obstruction is caused by a malignancy. In addition, fever and chills may be present in patients with choledocholithiasis and cholangitis. Gallstone pancreatitis can develop from the obstruction of the ampulla of Vater by common duct stones. CBD stones are responsible for up to 50% of all cases of pancreatitis. Most patients with gallstone pancreatitis experience a mild self-limited attack from which they recover within a few days; however, some patients will progress to develop severe pancreatitis with peripancreatic necrosis, infection, or pseudocyst formation.

Predictors of Common Bile Duct Stones

No single clinical variable is completely accurate in predicting the presence of choledocholithiasis. Therefore, the results of a detailed history and physical examination, laboratory evaluations, and diagnostic imaging tests must be taken together when assessing the likelihood that a patient has CBD stones. Serum liver function tests (bilirubin, alkaline phosphatase, and transaminases) can be useful in predicting common duct stones. If any one value of the liver profile is elevated, the risk for CBD stones approaches 20%. With two elevated values the risk increases to nearly 40%, and with three or more elevated values the risk for CBD stones is nearly 50%. However, between 5% and 7% of patients with no liver function abnormalities have CBD stones identified by cholangiography at the time of cholecystectomy. A recent meta-analysis has shown that the presence of cholangitis, CBD stones identified on ultrasound and jaundice to be the strongest indicators of CBD stones.[24] A patient with any one of these indicators has at least ten times the risk of having CBD stones compared with a patient without the risk factor (Table 62.5).

Diagnostic Studies

Ultrasonography

Ultrasound is very sensitive for the diagnosis of gallstones within the gallbladder. Unfortunately, its sensitivity for the detection of CBD stones is only 15% to 30%. Ultrasound can identify CBD dilation, which can suggest choledocholithiasis. If the extrahepatic bile duct diameter is less than 3 mm, CBD stones are exceedingly rare, whereas a diameter greater than 10 mm in a jaundiced patient predicts CBD stones in more than 90% of cases. Ultrasound successfully identifies the presence of CBD stones in only 70% of patients because the distal end of the bile duct is frequently obscured by duodenal or colonic gas.

Magnetic Resonance Imaging

Magnetic resonance cholangiopancreatography (MRCP) has recently been developed as another noninvasive means of imaging the biliary tract (Fig. 62.15). Several studies have shown that MRCP can diagnose CBD stones with a sensitivity of 90%, a specificity of 100%, and an overall diagnostic accuracy of 97%. The main advantage of MRCP is that it allows for the direct imaging of the biliary tract without the need for contrast or an invasive procedure. Disadvantages include its high cost, lack of availability, and lack of therapeutic capacity. Magnetic resonance cholangiography has been used to screen patients at low and moderate risk of having common duct stones prior to endoscopic cholangiography. A normal magnetic resonance cholangiogram can avoid the need for an invasive endoscopic cholangiogram. MRCP may become more popular as costs are reduced and surgeons become more skilled with laparoscopic techniques for managing CBD stones.

Endoscopic Ultrasound

Endoscopic ultrasound (EUS) is a semiinvasive test that can be performed with a very low rate of complications (<0.1%).[25] The sensitivity and specificity for the diagnosis of CBD stones by EUS ranges from 92% to 100% and 95% to 100%, respectively. The negative predictive value for EUS is more than 97%.[26] Therefore, when EUS is negative for common duct stones, ERCP or intraoperative cholangiography can be avoided.

Preoperative Cholangiography

Endoscopic cholangiography is the gold standard for the diagnosis of CBD stones. Both endoscopic retrograde cholangiography (ERC) and percutaneous transhepatic cholangiography (PTC) techniques can be used to directly visualize the biliary tree. A comparison of endoscopic retrograde cholangiography and percutaneous transhepatic cholangiography techniques is noted in Table 62.6. Endoscopic cholangiography (Fig. 62.16) has the advantage of providing a therapeutic option at the time CBD stones are identified and is therefore the preferred approach for patients with suspected CBD stones. Skilled endoscopists can successfully cannulate the CBD in approximately 90% to 95% of patients. Complications of diagnostic

TABLE 62.5 DIAGNOSIS

PREDICTIVE VALUES OF PREOPERATIVE INDICATORS OF COMMON BILE DUCT STONES

Indicator	Positive likelihood ratio	Negative likelihood ratio	Sensitivity	Specificity
Cholangitis	18.3	0.93	0.11	0.99
Common bile duct stones on ultrasound	13.6	0.70	0.38	1.00
Preoperative jaundice	10.1	0.69	0.36	0.97
Elevated bilirubin	4.8	0.77	0.69	0.88
Elevated alkaline phosphatase	2.6	0.65	0.57	0.86
Pancreatitis	2.1	0.96	0.10	0.95
Cholecystitis	1.6	0.94	0.50	0.76
Amylase	1.5	0.99	0.11	0.95

Adapted with permission from Abboud BA, Malet PF, Berlin JA, et al. Predictors of common bile duct stones prior to cholecystectomy: a meta-analysis. *Gastrointest Endosc.* 1996;44:450.

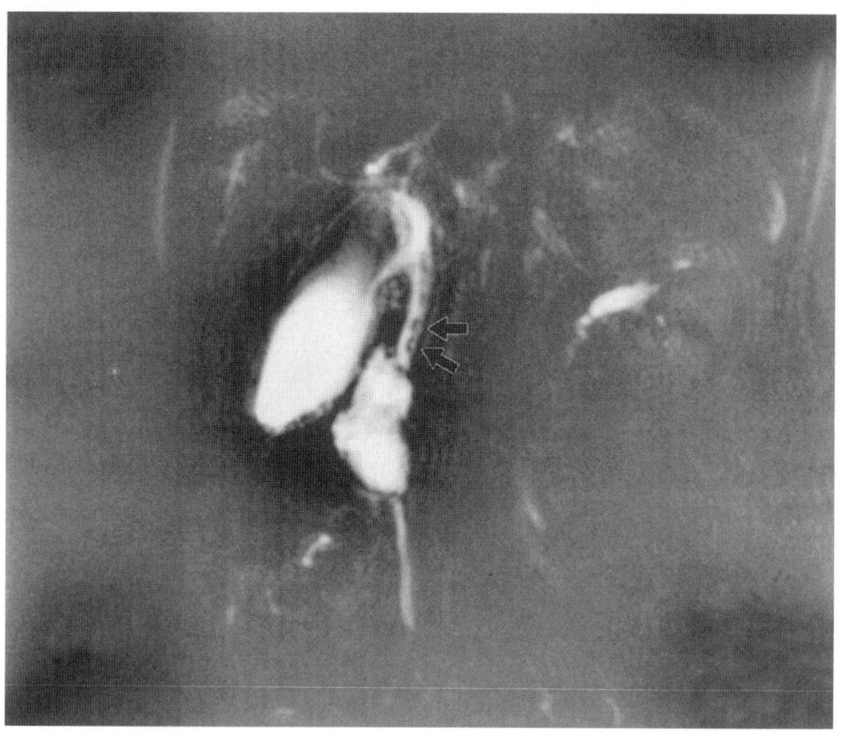

FIGURE 62.15 Magnetic resonance cholangiogram showing common bile duct stones (*arrows*).

cholangiography include pancreatitis and cholangitis and occur in up to 5% of patients. ERC may be unsuccessful in patients with previous gastric surgery (Bilroth II reconstruction), periampullary diverticula, or tortuous biliary ducts. Percutaneous transhepatic cholangiography may be used to image the bile ducts if ERC is unsuccessful.

Intraoperative Cholangiography

Intraoperative cholangiography (IOC) can be successfully accomplished in more than 95% of cases. The cholangiogram should be carefully evaluated for filling defects within the ducts, presence of contrast in the duodenum, and the intrahepatic biliary anatomy. Debate continues over the need to perform routine intraoperative cholangiography at the time of cholecystectomy. Advocates of routine IOC argue that asymptomatic CBD stones can be identified and biliary injuries prevented by performing routine IOC. Critics of this approach suggest that the incidence of retained stones is no greater when cholangiography is performed selectively based on clinical and laboratory criteria. The indications for performing cholangiography during cholecystectomy include: (a) a dilated CBD, (b) a wide cystic duct, (c) palpable CBD stones, (d) elevated serum liver function tests or bilirubin, and (e) a history of pancreatitis. If these criteria are strictly followed, approximately 30% of patients will require IOC at the time of cholecystectomy. IOC can identify the size, number, and location of CBD stones in addition to defining biliary anatomy. This information is critical in choosing the most appropriate treatment for CBD stones.

Intraoperative Ultrasonography

Intraoperative ultrasonography can also be used to identify CBD stones at the time of cholecystectomy. In experienced hands, intraoperative ultrasonography has been shown to be comparable to intraoperative cholangiography for the diagnosis of CBD stones. Laparoscopic ultrasonography is

TABLE 62.6 TREATMENT

COMPARISON OF PERCUTANEOUS TRANSHEPATIC CHOLANGIOGRAPHY AND ENDOSCOPIC RETROGRADE CHOLANGIOGRAPHY

Criterion	Transhepatic cholangiography	Endoscopic cholangiography
Success rate	>90% with dilated ducts, 70% with nondilated ducts	80 to 90% with either dilated or non-dilated ducts
Identification of cause of obstruction	90% to 100%	75% to 90%
Complications	5%, (range, 3% to 10%)	5% (range, 2% to 7%)
Mortality	0.2% to 0.9%	0.1% to 0.2%
Expense	Less	More
Skill required	Less	More
Patient selection	Proximal lesions, altered gastroduodenal anatomy, failed endoscopic cholangiography	Distal lesions, pancreatic pathology, coagulopathy, ascites, failed transhepatic cholangiography

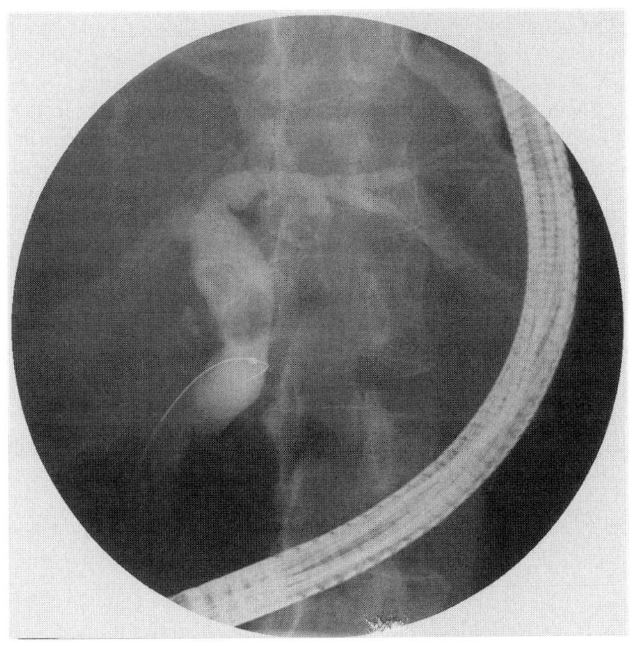

FIGURE 62.16 Endoscopic retrograde cholangiogram showing common bile duct stones.

performed with a high frequency (7.5- to 10-mHZ) probe, and the bile duct is imaged in the transverse and longitudinal planes. The distal bile duct can be visualized in more than 95% of cases.

The choice of radiologic studies used to evaluate a patient with suspected choledocholithiasis should be based on the probability of this diagnosis. Patients at highest risk for choledocholithiasis should undergo endoscopic cholangiography. Patients at intermediate risk may be screened with magnetic resonance cholangiography or endoscopic ultrasound and proceed to laparoscopic cholecystectomy if no stones are identified. Those patients at low risk of harboring common duct stones may be evaluated with intraoperative cholangiography at the time of laparoscopic cholecystectomy with laparoscopic CBD exploration or postoperative endoscopic stone extraction reserved for the few patients with a positive study.[27]

Management

Currently, several options are available to the surgeon for the treatment of CBD stones. In choosing the most appropriate approach for an individual patient, factors such as the local endoscopic expertise, the surgeon's laparoscopic skill, and the patient's clinical condition must be considered. A potential approach to the management of CBD stones is shown in Algorithm 62.1.

Endoscopic

Endoscopic retrograde cholangiography (ERC) with endoscopic sphincterotomy permits CBD stones to be removed without the need for conventional surgery. Stones can be successfully removed from the CBD in 85% to 95% of cases. The endoscopic approach is particularly useful for patients prior to cholecystectomy in whom a high suspicion exists for CBD

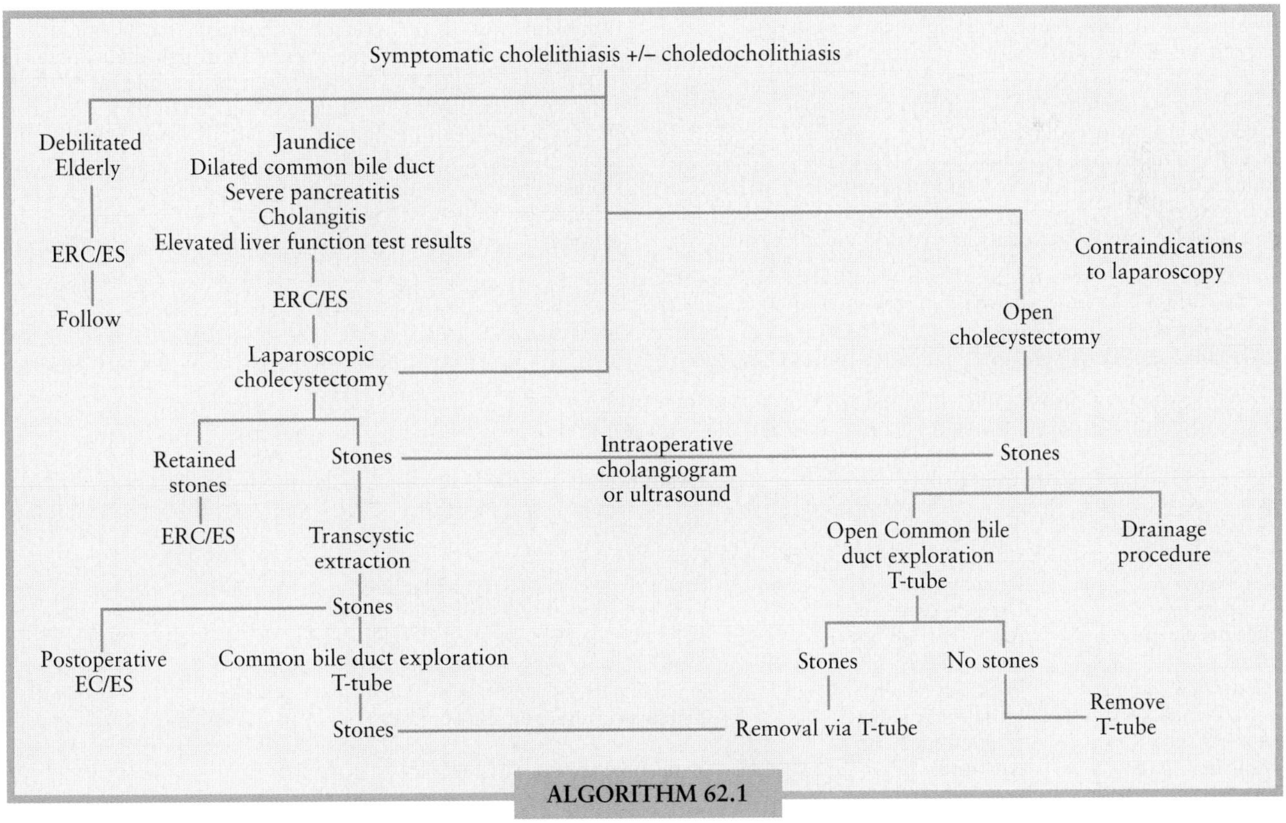

Symptomatic cholelithiasis +/– choledocholithiasis

Debilitated
Elderly
ERC/ES
Follow

Jaundice
Dilated common bile duct
Severe pancreatitis
Cholangitis
Elevated liver function test results
ERC/ES
Laparoscopic cholecystectomy

Contraindications to laparoscopy
Open cholecystectomy

Retained stones
ERC/ES

Stones
Transcystic extraction
Stones

Intraoperative cholangiogram or ultrasound

Stones
Open Common bile duct exploration T-tube
Drainage procedure

Postoperative EC/ES
Common bile duct exploration T-tube
Stones

Stones
No stones
Removal via T-tube
Remove T-tube

ALGORITHM 62.1

ALGORITHM 62.1 Algorithm for the management of common bile duct stones.

calculi, particularly if laparoscopic CBD exploration is not available. Endoscopic clearance of stones from the CBD precholecystectomy can avoid the need for an open operation. Furthermore, if endoscopic stone extraction is not possible because of multiple gallstones, intrahepatic stones, large gallstones, impacted stones, duodenal diverticula, prior gastrectomy, or bile duct stricture, this information is known before cholecystectomy, and an open CBD exploration or drainage procedure can be performed. After sphincterotomy, most stones smaller than 1 cm in diameter pass spontaneously. A balloon catheter or stone basket can also be used to retrieve stones if needed. If endoscopic clearance is incomplete, an endoscopic stent can be placed into the CBD to maintain drainage and prevent cholangitis.

Endoscopic sphincterotomy and stone extraction is well tolerated in most patients. Complications occur in 5% to 8% of patients and include cholangitis, pancreatitis, perforation, and bleeding. The overall mortality rate is 0.2% to 0.5%. Complete clearance of all common duct stones is achieved endoscopically in 71% to 75% of patients at the first procedure and in 84% to 95% of patients after multiple endoscopic procedures.[28]

Preoperative ERC plus endoscopic sphincterotomy is the preferred management option for CBD stones in several conditions. In the setting of acute suppurative cholangitis morbidity and mortality are significantly decreased if preoperative biliary decompression and stone removal are accomplished before cholecystectomy. Patients with severe gallstone pancreatitis or a significant deterioration of their clinical condition have also been shown to benefit from early ERC and stone clearance. Cholecystectomy can then be performed after the pancreatitis has resolved. In patients with a dilated CBD (>8 mm) on ultrasound and jaundice an ERC should also be performed to rule out a malignancy or biliary stricture that would alter the surgical management. In patients who are high operative risks ERC plus endoscopic sphincterotomy can be performed to remove CBD stones and the gallbladder left in place.

Following endoscopic sphincterotomy and stone extraction, patients with a stone-filled gallbladder remain at high risk of developing future biliary symptoms. A recent prospective, randomized trial demonstrated a significantly greater incidence of recurrent biliary symptoms among patients managed with a wait and see approach versus laparoscopic cholecystectomy (47% versus 2%, $P<0.0001$) following endoscopic stone extraction. A large percentage (37%) of patients managed expectantly later required cholecystectomy.[29]

Laparoscopic

Laparoscopic exploration of the CBD for choledocholithiasis enables appropriate patients to undergo complete management of their calculous biliary tract disease with one invasive procedure. The laparoscopic approach is ideal for patients with CBD stones identified during intraoperative cholangiography or ultrasound or in patients with suspected choledocholithiasis managed at centers where laparoscopic CBD exploration is routinely performed. Intraoperative cholangiography is accomplished via the cystic duct prior to duct exploration.

The two approaches for laparoscopic bile duct exploration are laparoscopic transcystic duct bile duct exploration (LTCBDE) or laparoscopic choledochotomy (Table 62.7). The indications for transcystic duct exploration are filling defects noted on cholangiography (CBD stones), stones less than 9 mm in diameter, stones below the cystic duct entrance to the bile duct, and less than six stones. Contraindications to LTCBDE are a small friable cystic duct, more than 8 stones in the CBD, common hepatic duct stones, and stones larger than 1 cm. Laparoscopic choledochotomy can be performed if LTCBDE fails or is contraindicated, if stones are present above the cystic duct, or when multiple stones are present. The only contraindication to laparoscopic choledochotomy is a small common duct (<6 mm) that might be narrowed during its closure.

***Laparoscopic* Transcystic Duct Bile Duct Exploration.** The technique of LTCBDE involves the blunt dissection of the cystic duct down to its junction with the CBD. A cystic ductotomy is then made and a guide wire inserted into the bile duct. A cholangiocatheter can then be advanced over the guide wire into the bile duct and saline irrigated through the catheter in an attempt to flush small stones out of the bile duct. If the stones in the CBD are larger than the lumen of the cystic duct, the cystic duct can be dilated with a balloon catheter. Stone retrieval baskets can be inserted over the guide wire and stones extracted under fluoroscopic guidance (Fig. 62.17). Flexible choledochoscopy via the cystic duct can also be performed and stones extracted under direct vision. Success rates

TABLE 62.7 TREATMENT

FACTORS IN LAPAROSCOPIC TRANSCYSTIC COMMON BILE DUCT EXPLORATION VERSUS LAPAROSCOPIC CHOLEDOCHOTOMY

	Transcystic	Choledochotomy
Stone characteristics		
Number	<8	Any
Size	>9 mm	Any
Location	Distal to cystic duct	Entire duct
Bile duct size	Any	>6 mm
Drain	Optional cystic duct tube	T-tube
Contraindications	Friable cystic duct Intrahepatic stones Multiple large stones	Small diameter duct Inability to suture laparoscopically
Advantages	No T-tube Short hospital stay	T-tube for postoperative access

Adapted with permission from Phillips EH, Korman JE. Laparoscopic management of common bile duct stones. In: Cameron JL, ed. *Current Surgical Therapy.* 6th ed.; St. Louis, MO: Mosby, 1998.

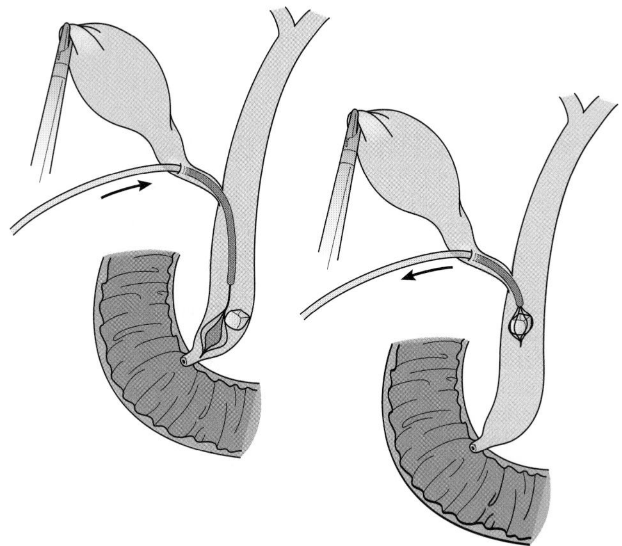

FIGURE 62.17 Laparoscopic transcystic bile duct exploration.

greater than 95% have been reported for bile duct clearance using choledochoscopy. To document stone clearance a completion cholangiogram should be performed. A cystic duct drainage tube can be left in place if there are equivocal findings on the cholangiogram. This tube can be used postoperatively for cholangiography and radiographic treatment of retained stones if necessary.

Laparoscopic Choledochotomy. Laparoscopic choledochotomy is another excellent approach to CBD stones when the CBD diameter is 6 mm or greater. The anterior wall of the CBD is bluntly dissected and a longitudinal choledochotomy made in the anterior wall below the cystic duct. The choledochotomy should be made as long as the diameter of the largest stone. Two stay sutures can be placed in the common duct and used to tent the anterior wall up to facilitate the incision. A larger choledochoscope (3.3 mm, 2.4 mm-working channel) can then be placed into the bile duct and stones extracted with baskets or balloon catheters. The choledochotomy is then closed over a T-tube with a 4-0 absorbable suture.

Advantages of laparoscopic choledochotomy to LTCBDE include the ability to remove larger stones (>1 cm), to remove stones from the proximal hepatic ducts, to remove multiple stones, and to use biliary lithotripsy to fragment impacted stones. The disadvantages of laparoscopic choledochotomy are that it requires a T-tube and that it requires considerable laparoscopic suturing skill to close the choledochotomy.

Clearance of all CBD stones is achieved in 75% to 95% of patients with laparoscopic CBD exploration.[30] The morbidity and mortality of laparoscopic CBD exploration are similar to laparoscopic cholecystectomy alone. In a recent prospective randomized trial comparing laparoscopic CBD exploration at the time of laparoscopic cholecystectomy with postoperative endoscopic stone extraction following laparoscopic cholecystectomy, the complication rate and retained stone rate were similar between the two groups. The median hospital stay was significantly shorter for patients managed with the single invasive procedure (1 day versus 3.5 days).

Open Common Bile Duct Exploration. Open CBD exploration is performed much less frequently with the increased use of endoscopic, percutaneous, and laparoscopic techniques to remove CBD stones. Occasionally, when these methods fail, are not available, are not possible because of prior surgery, or when open operation is otherwise necessary, open CBD exploration becomes necessary. The technique will be described briefly because open CBD exploration is not commonly performed in the era of laparoscopic cholecystectomy. The first step is to perform a full Kocher maneuver in the duodenum so that a hand can be placed behind the head of the pancreas and the distal CBD palpated. Any impacted stones may be milked more proximally. The supraduodenal bile duct is then exposed and two stay sutures placed in the CBD just below the cystic duct. The anterior wall of the bile duct is then elevated with the stay sutures and a longitudinal choledochotomy made. The bile duct can then be explored for stones. Rigid instruments should not be used to extract stones because they can injure the delicate ductal epithelium. A soft rubber irrigating catheter can be used to gently flush out any stones or debris. Balloon-tipped catheters can then be passed proximally and distally into the ducts to retrieve stones. Adequate clearance of the duct should be confirmed visually with flexible choledochoscopy. Remaining stones can be removed by irrigation or the use of instruments such as stone forceps, wire baskets, or balloon catheters. A T-tube should be placed in the bile duct and the choledochotomy closed with 4-0 absorbable suture. Completion cholangiography is performed before closing the abdomen to rule out the presence of retained stones or a bile leak around the T-tube. Postoperatively, a T-tube cholangiogram is performed 3 to 7 days after the exploration. If the cholangiogram is normal, the tube can be clamped and the tube pulled 3 to 6 weeks later. If retained stones are detected, the tract is allowed to mature, and percutaneous extraction can be performed by a radiologist in 4 to 6 weeks. Open CBD exploration can be accomplished with almost no mortality in patients younger than age 60 years, but can have a mortality of up to 4% in septic patients.

Drainage Procedures

Patients with an impacted stone at the ampulla that cannot be removed with a CBD exploration or with multiple stones in a nondilated system duct may require a transduodenal sphincteroplasty. A sphincteroplasty is also indicated in the presence of an ampullary stenosis or a choledochocele. The first step in a sphincteroplasty is to perform a Kocher maneuver. A small longitudinal duodenotomy is made over the ampulla and two stay sutures placed on each side of the ampulla to elevate it. A small incision is made at the 11-o'clock position in the sphincter taking care to avoid the pancreatic duct, which is usually found at the 5-o'clock position. The sphincterotomy is extended through the sphincter (approximately 1.5 cm) and the impacted stone removed. The bile duct and duodenal mucosa are then reapproximated with interrupted 4-0 absorbable sutures. The duodenotomy should be closed transversely to prevent narrowing of the lumen.

Patients with grossly dilated bile ducts (>2 cm), multiple stones (>5), intrahepatic stones, primary duct stones, or a distal biliary stricture should be considered for a biliary drainage procedure. The two options are a choledochoduodenostomy or a Roux-en-Y choledochojejunostomy. The choledochoduodenostomy can be performed in either a side-to-side or an end-to-side fashion. Advantages of a choledochoduodenostomy are that it can be performed rapidly, requires only one anastamosis, and the bile duct can still be accessed endoscopically. However, a side-to-side anastamosis leaves the distal CBD in continuity and can lead to the sump syndrome. In this situation, food debris from the duodenum can enter the distal limb of the duct and obstruct the anastamosis or the pancreatic duct orifice leading to cholangitis or pancreatitis. Roux-en-Y choledochojejunostomy is also an excellent option for biliary drainage. This operation is performed by dividing the common duct and doing an end-to-end anastamosis to a 60-cm Roux limb. Development of the sump syndrome is not a concern because a choledochojejunostomy is completely diverting.

Intrahepatic Stones

Intrahepatic stones are relatively uncommon in Western countries. These stones are more prevalent in Asia and represent a difficult management problem. Intrahepatic stones are primarily brown pigment stones. They typically occur in association with diseases characterized by prolonged partial bile duct obstruction, such as sclerosing cholangitis, benign and malignant biliary strictures, choledochal cysts, and biliary parasites.

Cholangiography, either endoscopic or percutaneous, is the most valuable technique in the evaluation of patients with intrahepatic stones. The transhepatic percutaneous approach is preferable in most patients because it allows for direct access to the intrahepatic bile ducts for therapeutic interventions. Transhepatic biliary drainage catheters can be inserted and gradually upsized to a 16-Fr size. The tract is then allowed to mature for 5 to 6 weeks, and stones are removed by using steerable stone retrieval baskets under fluoroscopic guidance, or with percutaneous choledochoscopy.

Although some patients with intrahepatic stone disease can be managed nonoperatively, many patients will require surgical intervention. A Roux-en-Y hepaticojejunostomy is usually constructed and intraoperative choledochoscopy used to clear the bile ducts of stones. Large bore transhepatic stents can be placed intraoperatively to provide access to the biliary tree for percutaneous stone extraction or the treatment of strictures postoperatively. Using this approach, a stone clearance rate of greater than 90% can be expected (Table 62.8).[31] Another option for management of intrahepatic stones is the creation of a hepaticocutaneous jejunostomy. This technique involves creating a Roux-en-Y hepaticojejunostomy with a longer than usual Roux limb and extending the Roux limb beyond the anastamosis up to the anterior abdominal wall. The limb is then marked with metal wire or clips, which allows percutaneous access to the biliary system if needed. If the intrahepatic stone disease is isolated to a single lobe or segment of liver and is associated with significant intrahepatic biliary strictures or atrophy a hepatic resection may be indicated to treat the stone disease.

TABLE 62.8 RESULTS

SUMMARY OF TREATMENT AND OUTCOMES FOR INTRAHEPATIC STONE DISEASE AT THE JOHNS HOPKINS HOSPITAL

Patient, *n*	54
Percutaneous treatment only	26% of patients
Surgical treatment	74% of patients
Postoperative percutaneous treatment	33% of patients
Mean follow-up	60 months
Successful stone clearance	94% of patients
Symptom-free state	87% of patients
Recurrent stones or stricture	20% of patients

Adapted with permission from Pitt HA, Venbrux AC, Coleman JA, et al. Intrahepatic Stones: the transhepatic team approach. *Ann Surg.* 1994;219:527.

KEY POINTS

- **Gallstones are classified by their cholesterol content as either cholesterol (70% to 80%) or pigment (20% to 30%) with pigment stones further classified as black or brown.**
- **Biliary sludge refers to a mixture of cholesterol crystals, calcium bilirubinate granules, and a mucin gel matrix and is thought to serve as the nidus for gallstone growth.**
- **The pathogenesis of cholesterol gallstones is clearly multifactorial but essentially involves four factors: a) cholesterol supersaturation in bile, b) crystal nucleation, c) gallbladder dysmotility, and d) gallbladder absorption.**
- **Prophylactic cholecystectomy is generally not indicated in patients with asymptomatic gallstones, because studies show that only 20% to 30% will become symptomatic within 20 years and only 1% to 2% will develop serious complication per year.**
- **Elective laparoscopic cholecystectomy is associated with a mortality rate of less than 0.1% and an overall complication rate of 10% with less than 5% of patients requiring conversion to an open procedure.**
- **Randomized trials have shown that laparoscopic cholecystectomy performed for acute cholecystitis can result in a lower morbidity rate, shorter hospital stay and quicker return to work than open cholecystectomy.**
- **Chronic acalculous cholecystitis is associated with typical symptoms of biliary colic without evidence of gallstones and is diagnosed by cholecystokinin–Tc-hepatic 2,6-dimethyl-iminodiacetic acid scan ejection fraction of less than 35% at 20 minutes.**
- **Acute cholangitis results from the combination of significant bacterial concentration in bile and increased biliary pressure associated with biliary obstruction.**
- **The strongest clinical indications for a common bile duct stone include the presence of cholangitis, common bile duct stones identified on ultrasound, and jaundice; with a patient having one of these indicators having at least a 10 times increased risk of common bile duct stones.**
- **Endoscopic cholangiography is the gold standard for the diagnosis of common bile duct stones being successful in 90% to 95% of patients although associated with complications of cholangitis or pancreatitis in up to 5% of patients.**

References

1. National Center for Health Statistics. *Health, United States, 2004 With Chartbook on Trends in the Health of Americans.* Hyattsville, MD, 2004.
2. Klein A, Lillemoe K, Yeo C, et al. Liver, biliary tract, and pancreas. In: O'Leary J, ed. *Physiologic basis of surgery*. Baltimore: Williams and Wilkins, 1996, pp. 441–78.
3. Everhart JE, Khare M, Hill M, et al. Prevalence and ethnic differences in gallbladder disease in the United States. *Gastroenterology* 1999;117:632.
4. **Nakeeb A. Comuzzie AG. Martin L, et al. Gallstones: genetics versus environment. *Ann Surg.* 2002;235:842.**
5. Friedman GD, Raviola CA, Fireman B. Prognosis of gallstones with mild or no symptoms: 25 years of follow-up in a health maintenance organization. *J Clin Epidemiol.* 1989;42:127.
6. Ransohoff DF, Gracie WA, Wolfenson LB, et al. Prophylactic cholecystectomy or expectant management for silent gallstones: a decision analysis to assess survival. *Ann Intern Med.* 1983;99:199.
7. Berk RN, Armbuster TG, Saltzstein SL. Carcinoma in the porcelain gallbladder. *Radiology* 1973;106:29.
8. Towfigh S, McFadden DW, Cortina GR, et al. Porcelain gallbladder is not associated with gallbladder carcinoma. *Am Surgeon.* 2001;67:7.

9. Stephen AE, Berger DL. Carcinoma in the porcelain gallbladder: a relationship revisited. *Surgery* 2001;129:699.
10. Thomas MJ, Pellegrini CA, Way LW. Usefulness of diagnostic tests for biliary obstruction. *Am J Surg*. 1982;144:102.
11. Baron RL, Stanley RJ, Lee JK, et al. A prospective comparison of the evaluation of biliary obstruction using computed tomography and ultrasonography. *Radiology* 1982;145:91.
12. Cameron JL. *Atlas of surgery, Vol. 2*. Philadelphia: BC Decker, Inc., 1994.
13. Curet M, Zucker K. Laparoscopic surgery of the biliary tract and liver. In: Zuidema G, ed. *Shackelford's surgery of the alimentary tract*. Philadelphia: WB Saunders, 1996.
14. Calland J, Tanaka K, Foley E, et al. Outpatient laparoscopic cholecystectomy: patient outcomes after implementation of a clinical pathway. *Ann Surg*. 2001; 233:704.
15. **Steiner CA, Bass EB, Talamini MA, et al. Surgical rates and operative mortality for open and laparoscopic cholecystectomy in Maryland. *N Engl J Med*. 1994;330:403.**
16. Strasberg SM, Hertl M, Soper NJ. An analysis of the problem of biliary injury during laparoscopic cholecystectomy. *J Am Coll Surg*. 1995;180:101.
17. Leslie KA, Rankin RN, Duff JH. Lost gallstones during laparoscopic cholecystectomy: are they really benign? *Can J Surg*. 1994;37:240.
18. Kiviluoto T, Siren J, Luukonen P, et al. Randomized trial of laparoscopic versus open cholecystectomy for acute and gangrenous cholecystitis. *Lancet* 1998;351:321.
19. **Lo CM, Liu CL, Fan ST, et al. Prospective randomized study of early versus delayed laparoscopic cholecystectomy for acute cholecystitis. *Ann Surg*. 1998;227:461.**
20. Lai P, Kwong K, Leung K, et al. Randomized trial of early versus delayed laparoscopic cholecystectomy for acute cholecystitis. *Br J Surg*. 1998;85:764.
21. Tzovaras G, Rowlands B. Diagnosis and treatment of sphincter of Oddi dysfunction. *Br J Surg*. 1998; 85:588.
22. Thompson JE, Pitt HA, Doty JE, et al. Broad spectrum penicillin as an adequate therapy for acute cholangitis. *Surg Gynecol Obstet*. 1990; 171:275.
23. Poon RT, Liu CL, Lo CM. Management of gallstone cholangitis in the era of laparoscopic cholecystectomy. *Arch Surg*. 2001;136:11.
24. **Abboud BA, Malet PF, Berlin JA, et al. Predictors of common bile duct stones prior to cholecystectomy: a meta-analysis. *Gastrointest Endosc*. 1996;44:450.**
25. Rosch T, Dittler HJ, Fockens P, et al. Major complications of endoscopic ultrasonography: results of a survey of 42105 cases. *Gastrointest Endosc*, 1993;39:341.
26. Vilgrain V, Palazzo L. Choledocholithiasis: role of US and endoscopic ultrasound. *Abdom Imaging*. 2001;26:7.
27. Liu T, Consorti E, Kawashima A, et al. Patient evaluation and management with selective use of magnetic resonance cholangiography and endoscopic retrograde cholangiopancreatography before laparoscopic cholecystectomy. *Ann Surg*. 2001;234:.
28. **Freeman M, Nelson D, Sherman S, et al. Complications of endoscopic biliary sphincterotomy. *N Engl J Med*. 1996;335:909.**
29. Boerma D, Rauws W, Keulemans Y, et al. Wait-and-see policy or laparoscopic cholecystectomy after endoscopic cholecystectomy for bile-duct stones: a randomized trial. *Lancet* 2002;360:761.
30. **Rhodes M, Sussman L, Cohen L, et al. Randomized trial of laparoscopic exploration of common bile duct versus postoperative endoscopic retrograde cholangiography for common bile duct stones. *Lancet* 1998; 351:159.**
31. **Pitt HA, Venbrux AC, Coleman J, et al. Intrahepatic stones: the transhepatic team approach. *Ann Surg*. 1994;219:527.**

CHAPTER 63 ■ BILIARY INJURIES AND STRICTURES AND SCLEROSING CHOLANGITIS

KEITH D. LILLEMOE

Benign strictures of the biliary tree are among the most difficult challenges that a surgeon faces. Although numerous technologic developments have facilitated diagnosis and management, bile duct strictures remain a significant clinical problem. If they go unrecognized or are managed improperly, life-threatening complications, such as biliary cirrhosis, portal hypertension, and cholangitis, can develop. To avoid these complications, virtually every patient with a bile duct stricture should undergo evaluation and treatment with the goal of relieving the obstruction to bile flow and its associated hepatic injury.

Benign bile duct strictures can have numerous causes (Table 63.1). Most biliary strictures occur after primary operations on the gallbladder or biliary tree. With the introduction of laparoscopic cholecystectomy, bile duct injuries and associated strictures have been seen with increased frequency. Operative injury to the bile ducts can also occur during nonbiliary operations on the gallbladder or biliary tree or as a result of external penetrating or blunt abdominal trauma. Inflammatory conditions and fibrosis caused by chronic pancreatitis, gallstones in the gallbladder or the bile duct, stenosis of the sphincter of Oddi, or biliary tract infections can also cause benign bile duct strictures. Finally, primary sclerosing cholangitis, a rare disease of unknown cause, can result in multiple strictures of the intrahepatic and extrahepatic bile ducts. This chapter focuses primarily on postoperative bile duct strictures and primary sclerosing cholangitis.

POSTOPERATIVE BILE DUCT STRICTURES

Pathogenesis

Most benign bile duct strictures result from operations in or near the right upper quadrant. More than 80% of strictures occur after injury to the bile ducts during cholecystectomy. The exact incidence of bile duct injury is unknown because many cases may go unreported in the literature. Data suggest that the incidence of bile duct injury during open cholecystectomy is one in 500 to 1,000 cases. The incidence of bile duct injury during laparoscopic cholecystectomy is clearly higher. Although a wide range in the incidence of injury can be found in reported series, the most accurate data most likely come from surveys encompassing thousands of patients. These

TABLE 63.1 ETIOLOGY

CAUSES OF BENIGN BILE DUCT STRICTURES

POSTOPERATIVE STRICTURES
Injury at primary biliary operations
■ Laparoscopic cholecystectomy
■ Open cholecystectomy
■ Common bile duct exploration
INJURY AT OTHER OPERATIVE PROCEDURES
■ Gastrectomy
■ Hepatic resection
■ Portacaval shunt
Stricture of a biliary-enteric anastomosis
Blunt or penetrating trauma
Strictures caused by inflammatory conditions
Chronic pancreatitis
Cholelithiasis and choledocholithiasis
Primary sclerosing cholangitis
Stenosis of the sphincter of Oddi
Duodenal ulcer
Crohn's disease
Viral infections
Toxic drugs

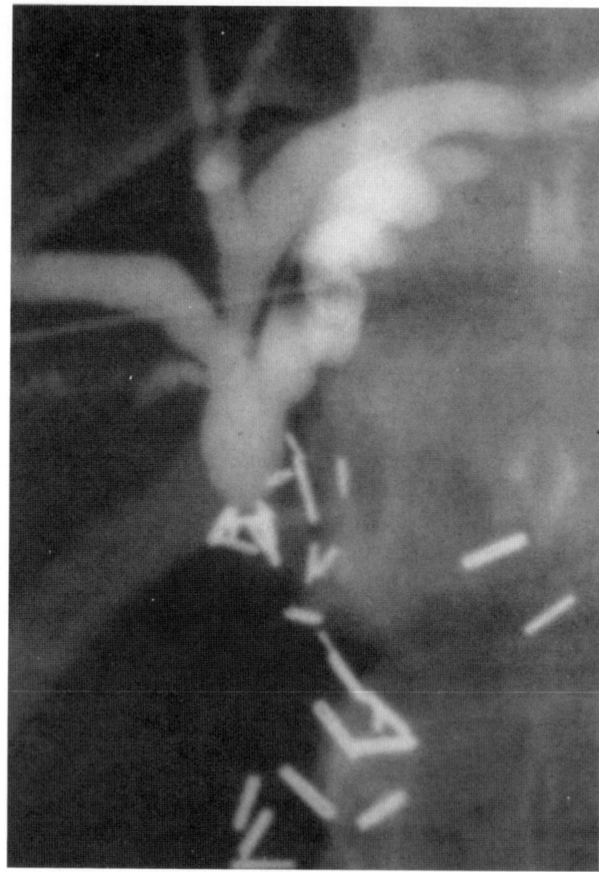

FIGURE 63.1 Percutaneous transhepatic cholangiogram in a patient with a bile duct stricture secondary to iatrogenic injury during cholecystectomy. Numerous surgical clips can be seen in the area of the stricture. (From Lillemoe KD, Pitt HA, Cameron JL. Postoperative bile duct strictures. *Surg Clin North Am.* 1990;70:1356.)

reports reflect the results from a large number of surgeons in both community and teaching hospitals. The results of such series suggest an incidence of bile duct injury during laparoscopic cholecystectomy ranging from 0.3% to 0.7%.[1] Furthermore, the incidence of bile duct injury associated with laparoscopic cholecystectomy does not appear to have diminished in more recent surveys, suggesting that the previously observed increase is not simply the result of a learning curve associated with the laparoscopic technique.

A number of factors are associated with bile duct injury during either open or laparoscopic cholecystectomy, including acute or chronic inflammation, inadequate exposure, patient obesity, and failure to identify structures before clamping, ligating, or dividing them. More specific causes of bile duct injury also exist. Bleeding from the cystic or hepatic arteries can lead to bile duct injury during attempts to gain hemostasis. The generous application of Liga clips at either open or laparoscopic cholecystectomy to hilar areas not well visualized can result in placing a clip on or across a bile duct, with resultant injury (Fig. 63.1). Failure to recognize congenital anatomic anomalies of the bile ducts, such as insertion of the right hepatic duct into the cystic duct or a long common wall between the cystic duct and the common bile duct, can also lead to injury (Fig. 63.2). A number of technical factors are associated with laparoscopic cholecystectomy that can also increase the risk of bile duct injury compared with the open procedure. These factors include the use of an end-viewing laparoscope, which alters the surgeon's perspective of the operative field. Excessive cephalad retraction of the gallbladder fundus can cause the cystic duct and common bile duct to become aligned in the same plane. This distortion often results in the classic laparoscopic injury, in which the common bile duct is mistaken for the cystic duct and clipped and divided (Fig. 63.3).[2] The role of intraoperative cholangiography in preventing bile duct injury during laparoscopic cholecystectomy is controversial. Based on a number of published series advocating either routine or selective cholangiography, it appears that cholangiography does not prevent bile duct injury. The procedure can, however, minimize the extent of injury. Finally, ample evidence exists to support the conclusion that the experience of the surgeon in performing laparoscopic cholecystectomy can be correlated with the risk of bile duct injury.

In recent years there has been a growing understanding of surgeon cognitive factors associated with bile duct injury during laparoscopic cholecystectomy. An analysis examining 252 biliary injuries during laparoscopic cholecystectomy using human error factor and cognitive science techniques found that 97% of injuries were caused by visual-perceptual illusion or inadequate visualization.[3] Further work from the same group has determined a major explanation for the surgeon's frequent inability to recognize bile duct injury. These bile duct injuries appear to be associated with confirmation bias, which is a propensity to seek cues to confirm a belief and to discount cues that might discount the belief. Although cognitive factors are important for the understanding of the psychological issues associated with bile duct injuries, surgeons must continue to have the appropriate corrective mechanisms in place to minimize the chance of these injuries, including knowledge of anatomy, typical mechanisms of injury, and an appropriate level of suspicion and logic.

The importance of ischemia of the bile duct in the formation of postoperative strictures has been emphasized. Unnecessary dissection around the bile duct during cholecystectomy or bile duct anastomosis can divide or injure the major arteries of the bile duct that run in the 3-o'clock and 9-o'clock positions. Another important factor contributing to the formation of biliary strictures is the intense connective tissue response with fibrosis and scarring that can occur after bile duct injury.

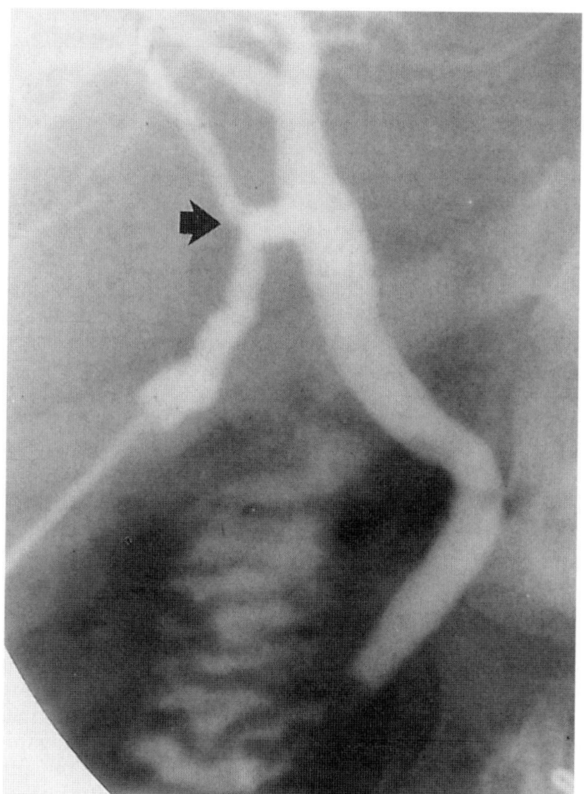

FIGURE 63.2 Operative cholangiogram demonstrating a right lobe segmental bile duct entering the cystic duct (*arrow*). Division of the cystic duct proximal to this insertion can result in a bile leak or obstruction of bile flow from a significant segment of the liver.

Experimental studies of bile duct ligation in a canine model have demonstrated immediate and sustained elevation of bile duct pressure and progressive increase in bile duct diameter. Histologic changes at 1 month after ligation have shown that the bile duct wall is thickened, with a reduction of mucosal folds and loss of surface microvilli, associated with a well-defined epithelial degeneration. Biochemical analysis of connective tissue response to ligation showed that collagen synthesis and prolene hydroxylase activity is increased within 2 weeks in the obstructed bile duct and is sustained throughout the period of observation. Finally, a marked local inflammatory response can develop in the adjacent tissue in association with bile leakage, which occurs with many bile duct injuries. This inflammation can be further intensified in the face of infection. This inflammation results in fibrosis and scarring in the periductal tissue, further contributing to stricture formation. These factors can be of major importance in bile duct injuries during laparoscopic cholecystectomy, which are frequently associated with bile leaks.

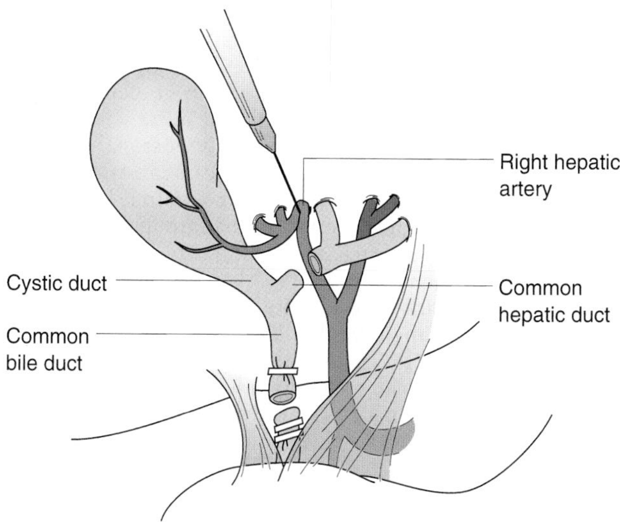

FIGURE 63.3 Classic laparoscopic bile duct injury. The common bile duct is mistaken for the cystic duct and transected. A variable extent of the extrahepatic biliary tree is resected with the gallbladder. The right hepatic artery, in background, is also often injured. (After Branum G, Schmidt C, Baillie J, et al. Management of major biliary complications after laparoscopic cholecystectomy. *Ann Surg.* 1993;217:532.)

After cholecystectomy and common bile duct exploration, the two most common operations associated with bile duct injury are gastrectomy and hepatic resection. The most common situation resulting in bile duct injury during gastrectomy involves dissection of the pyloric region and the first portion of the duodenum in the face of inflammation from peptic ulcer disease. The injury occurs during mobilization of the duodenum either for creation of a Billroth I gastroduodenostomy or for closure of the duodenal stump. Biliary injury during liver resection is most likely to occur during dissection of the hepatic hilum.

In addition to iatrogenic bile duct injury occurring during cholecystectomy or other operations, bile duct strictures can also occur at biliary anastomoses. Such strictures can occur at a biliary-enteric anastomosis performed for reconstruction after resection for benign or malignant disease of the pancreaticobiliary system, or after end-to-end bile duct anastomosis performed for hepatic transplantation or for repair of traumatic injury. Ischemia of the anastomosis caused by excessive skeletonization of the duct in preparation for the anastomosis is an important factor in many such strictures.

Unfortunately, the recurrence of bile duct strictures after an initial attempt at repair is not uncommon and can also account for a number of anastomotic strictures.[4,5] A number of other factors have been evaluated in patients who have a recurrent bile duct stricture, including the location of the stricture, the length of follow-up, the influence of previous operations, the type of operation performed, the type of sutures used, and the use and duration of postoperative stenting.[4] Previous attempts at repair and performance of a procedure other than choledochojejunostomy or hepaticojejunostomy and stricture location higher in the biliary tree appear to be associated with a higher incidence of recurrent stricture. The type of suture material used for repair does not influence the outcome. When postoperative biliary stents are used, a longer period of stenting appears to be favorable. Finally, long-term follow-up of a bile duct anastomosis is important because strictures can develop years after the original anastomosis.

Clinical Presentation

Most patients with benign postoperative bile duct strictures present early after their initial operation (Fig. 63.4). After open cholecystectomy, only approximately 10% of postoperative strictures are actually suspected within the first week, but nearly 70% are diagnosed within the first 6 months, and more than 80% are diagnosed within 1 year of surgery.[4] In series reporting bile duct injuries during laparoscopic cholecystectomy, the injury is usually recognized either during the procedure (25% to 30%) or, more commonly, in the early postoperative period.

Patients suspected of having a postoperative bile duct injury within days to weeks of initial operation usually

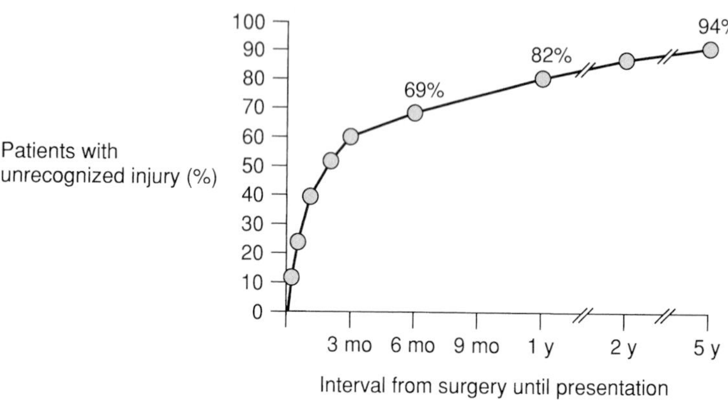

FIGURE 63.4 The cumulative percentage of patients in whom symptoms develop is shown with respect to the time from the procedure during which the injury occurred until the presentation of the symptoms. (After Pitt HA, Miyamoto T, Parapatis SK, et al. Factors influencing outcome in patients with postoperative biliary strictures. *Am J Surg.* 1982;144:14–21.)

present in one of two ways. One presentation is the progressive elevation of liver function test results, particularly total bilirubin and alkaline phosphatase levels. These changes can often be seen as early as the second or third postoperative day. The second mode of early presentation is with leakage of bile from the injured bile duct. This presentation appears to occur most often in patients presenting with bile duct injuries after laparoscopic cholecystectomy. Bilious drainage from operatively placed drains or through the wound after cholecystectomy is abnormal and represents some form of biliary injury. In patients without drains (including patients in whom the drains have been removed), the bile can leak freely into the peritoneal cavity or it can loculate as a collection. Free accumulation of bile into the peritoneal cavity results in either biliary ascites or bile peritonitis. Similarly, a loculated bile collection can result in sterile biloma (Fig. 63.5) or in an infected subhepatic or subdiaphragmatic abscess.

Patients with postoperative bile duct strictures who present months to years after the initial operation frequently have evidence of cholangitis. The episodes of cholangitis are often mild and respond to antibiotic therapy. Repetitive episodes usually occur before the definitive diagnosis. Less commonly, patients may present with painless jaundice and no evidence of sepsis. Finally, patients with markedly delayed diagnoses may present with advanced biliary cirrhosis and its complications.

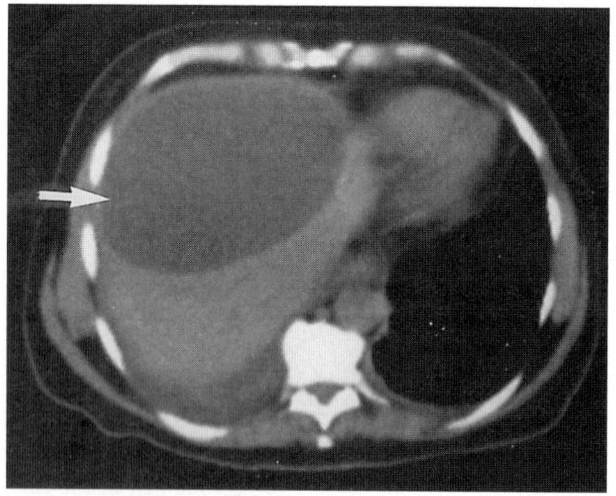

FIGURE 63.5 Large bile duct collection (biloma; *arrow*) occurring after bile duct injury. (From Lillemoe KD, Pitt HA, Cameron JL. Postoperative bile duct strictures. *Surg Clin North Am.* 1990;70:1362.)

Laboratory Investigation

Liver function tests usually show evidence of cholestasis. The serum bilirubin can fluctuate; occasionally, this value is normal. In patients with bile leakage, the bilirubin can be normal or minimally elevated because of absorption from the peritoneal cavity. When elevated, serum bilirubin usually ranges from 2 to 6 mg/dL, unless secondary biliary cirrhosis has developed. Serum alkaline phosphatase is usually elevated. Serum aminotransferase levels can be normal or minimally elevated except during episodes of cholangitis. If advanced liver disease exists, hepatic synthetic function can be impaired, with lowered serum albumin and a prolongation of prothrombin time. Serum electrolytes and complete blood count are typically normal unless there is associated biliary sepsis.

Radiologic Examination

The imaging techniques of abdominal ultrasound and computed tomography (CT) play an important initial role in the evaluation of patients with benign postoperative biliary strictures. In patients who present in the early postoperative period with evidence of a bile leak or biliary sepsis, these studies are useful to rule out the presence of intraabdominal collections that might require drainage (Fig. 63.5). CT and ultrasound are also important in the initial evaluation of the patient presenting with a bile duct stricture months to years after initial operation. Both studies can confirm biliary obstruction by demonstrating a dilated biliary tree. CT is especially useful in identifying the level of obstruction of the extrahepatic bile duct.

In patients suspected of having early postoperative bile duct injury, a radionucleotide biliary scan can confirm bile leakage. In patients with postoperative external bile fistula, injection of water-soluble contrast media through the drainage tract (sinography) can often define the site of leakage and the anatomy of the biliary tree.

The gold standard for evaluation of patients with bile duct strictures is cholangiography. Percutaneous transhepatic cholangiography (PTC) is usually more valuable than endoscopic retrograde cholangiography (ERC). PTC is more useful in that it defines the anatomy of the proximal biliary tree that is to be used in the surgical reconstruction (Fig. 63.6). Furthermore, PTC can be followed by placement of percutaneous transhepatic catheters, which can be useful in decompressing the biliary system either to treat or prevent cholangitis and to control an ongoing bile leak. These catheters can also be of assistance in surgical reconstruction and provide access to the biliary tree for nonoperative dilation. ERC is often less useful than PTC because the discontinuity of the extrahepatic bile duct usually prevents adequate filling of the proximal biliary tree (Fig. 63.7). Often, ERC can demonstrate a normal-sized

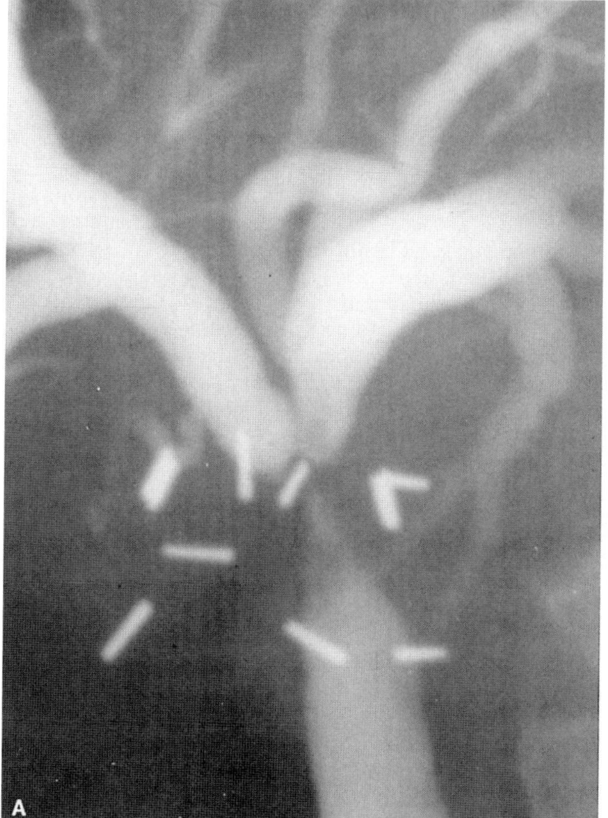

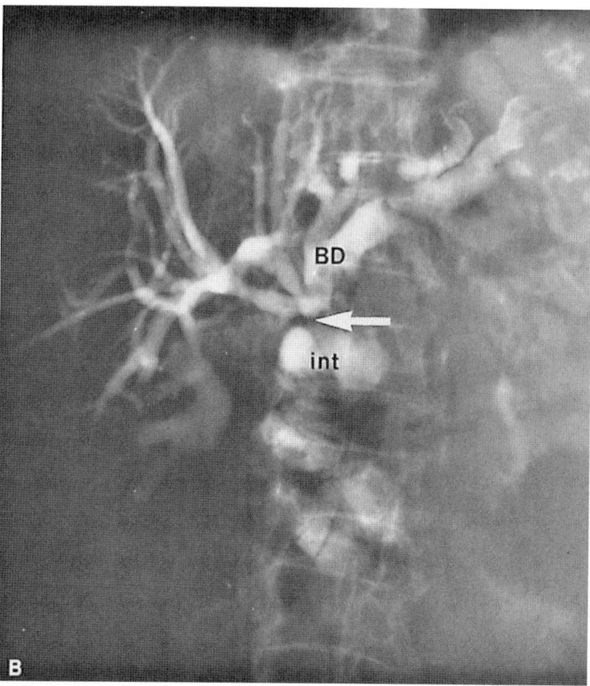

FIGURE 63.6 (*A*) Percutaneous transhepatic cholangiogram demonstrating bile duct stricture at hepatic duct bifurcation with proximal duct dilatation. (*B*) Percutaneous transhepatic cholangiogram demonstrating stricture (*arrow*) at a hepaticojejunostomy anastomosis. BD, bile duct; int, intestine.

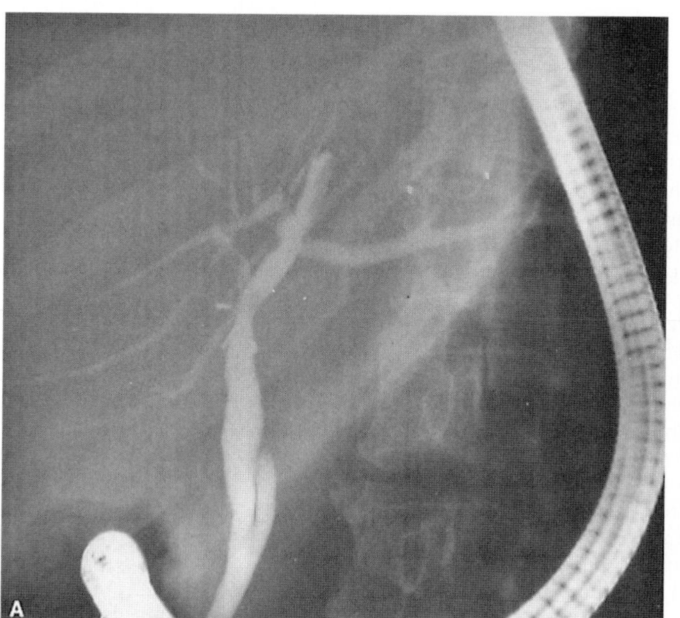

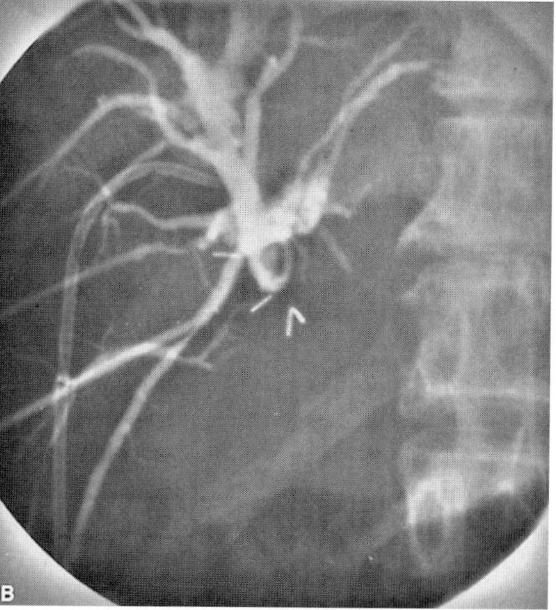

FIGURE 63.7 (*A*) Endoscopic retrograde cholangiogram showing a relatively normal biliary tree in a patient with a postoperative bile collection (see Fig. 63.5). (*B*) Percutaneous transhepatic cholangiogram of same patient, showing entire right hepatic posterior lobe segment obstructed as the result of ligation of the segmental duct. The patient had an unrecognized anatomic variant similar to that shown in Fig. 63.2.

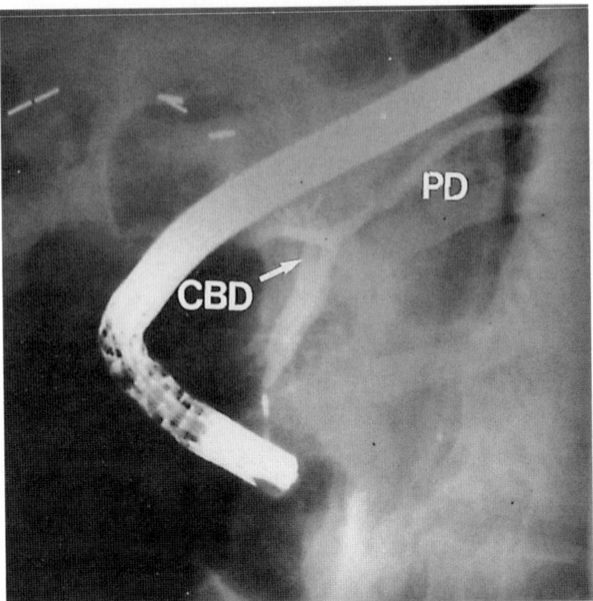

FIGURE 63.8 Endoscopic retrograde pancreaticocholangiogram showing filling of a normal pancreatic duct (PD). The common bile duct (CBD), however, does not fill beyond the large clip that appears to be placed across the duct. (Adapted with permission from Lillemoe KD, Pitt HA, Cameron JL. Postoperative bile duct strictures. *Surg Clin North Am* 1990;70:1363.)

distal bile duct up to the site of the stricture without visualization of the proximal biliary system (Fig. 63.8). This finding is frequently the case in patients with injury during laparoscopic cholecystectomy, when the distal bile duct is often clipped and divided. The development of magnetic resonance cholangiopancreatography has provided a noninvasive technique that provides excellent delineation of the biliary anatomy. The quality of these images has led some surgeons to advocate this technique as the initial step in the evaluation of patients with suspected bile duct injuries and may eliminate the need for a diagnostic ERC in many patients.

Preoperative Management

The preoperative management of a patient with a postoperative bile duct stricture depends primarily on the timing of the presentation. Patients presenting in the early postoperative period can be septic with either cholangitis or intraabdominal bile collections. Sepsis must be controlled first with broad-spectrum parenteral antibiotics, percutaneous biliary drainage, and percutaneous or operative drainage of biliary leaks. Once sepsis is controlled, there is no hurry in proceeding with surgical reconstruction of the bile duct stricture. The combination of proximal biliary decompression and external drainage allows most biliary fistulae to be controlled or even to close. The patient can then be discharged home to allow several weeks to elapse for resolution of the inflammation in the periportal region and recovery of overall health.

The management of a suspected bile duct injury after laparoscopic cholecystectomy presenting with a bile leak deserves special mention. Often, when bile leakage is suspected, the surgeon believes that urgent surgical exploration is necessary. Unfortunately, at laparotomy, the marked inflammation associated with bile spillage and the small decompressed biliary tree that appears retracted high into the porta hepatis make recognition of the injury and repair virtually impossible. In such cases, every attempt should be made to define the biliary anatomy by preoperative cholangiography and to control the bile leak with percutaneous stents. In many cases, early operative intervention is not required because the bile either can be drained percutaneously or simply is absorbed from the peritoneal cavity. Delayed reconstruction, aided by percutaneous biliary catheters, then allows optimal surgical results.[6]

In patients who present with a biliary stricture remote from the initial operation, symptoms of cholangitis can necessitate urgent cholangiography and biliary decompression. Biliary drainage is best accomplished by the transhepatic method, although successful endoscopic stent placement can also be accomplished. Parenteral antibiotics and biliary drainage should be continued until sepsis is controlled. In patients who present with jaundice but without cholangitis, cholangiography should be performed to define the anatomy. Preoperative biliary decompression in patients without cholangitis has not been demonstrated to improve outcome.

Surgical Management

The goal of operative management of bile duct stricture is the establishment of bile flow into the proximal gastrointestinal tract in a manner that prevents cholangitis, sludge or stone formation, restricture, and biliary cirrhosis. This goal is best accomplished with a tension-free anastomosis between healthy tissues. A number of surgical alternatives exist for primary repair of bile duct strictures, including end-to-end repair, Roux-en-Y hepaticojejunostomy or choledochojejunostomy, choledochoduodenostomy, and mucosal grafting. The choice of repair depends on a number of factors, including the extent and location of the strictures, the experience of the surgeon, and the timing of the repair.

Immediate Repair of Intraoperative Bile Duct Injury

In many cases, initial proper management of bile duct injury recognized at the time of cholecystectomy can avoid the development of a bile duct stricture. Unfortunately, recognition of a bile duct injury is uncommon during either open or laparoscopic cholecystectomy. If bile leakage is observed or atypical anatomy is encountered during laparoscopic cholecystectomy, early conversion to an open technique and prompt cholangiography are imperative. If a segmental or accessory duct less than 3 mm has been injured and cholangiography demonstrates segmental or subsegmental drainage of the injured ductal system, simple ligation of the injured duct is adequate. If the injured duct is 4 mm or larger, however, it is likely to drain multiple hepatic segments or the entire right or left lobe and thus requires operative repair.

If the injury involves the common hepatic duct or the common bile duct, repair should also be carried out at the time of injury. The aims of any repair should be to maintain ductal length and not to sacrifice tissue as well as to effect a repair that will not result in postoperative bile leakage. To accomplish these goals, all repairs at the time of initial operation should involve some sort of external drainage. If the injured segment of the bile duct is short (<1 cm) and the two ends can be opposed without tension, an end-to-end anastomosis can be performed with placement of a T-tube through a separate choledochotomy either above or below the anastomosis. (Fig. 63.9A) Generous mobilization of the duodenum out of the retroperitoneum (Kocher maneuver) can be useful to help approximate the injured ends of the bile duct. An end-to-end repair, however, should be avoided if the ductal injury is near the hepatic duct bifurcation.

For proximal injuries or if the injured segment of bile duct is greater than 1 cm in length, an end-to-end bile duct anastomosis should be avoided because of the excessive tension that usually exists in these situations. In these circumstances, the distal bile duct should be oversewn, and the proximal bile duct should be débrided of injured tissue and anastomosed in

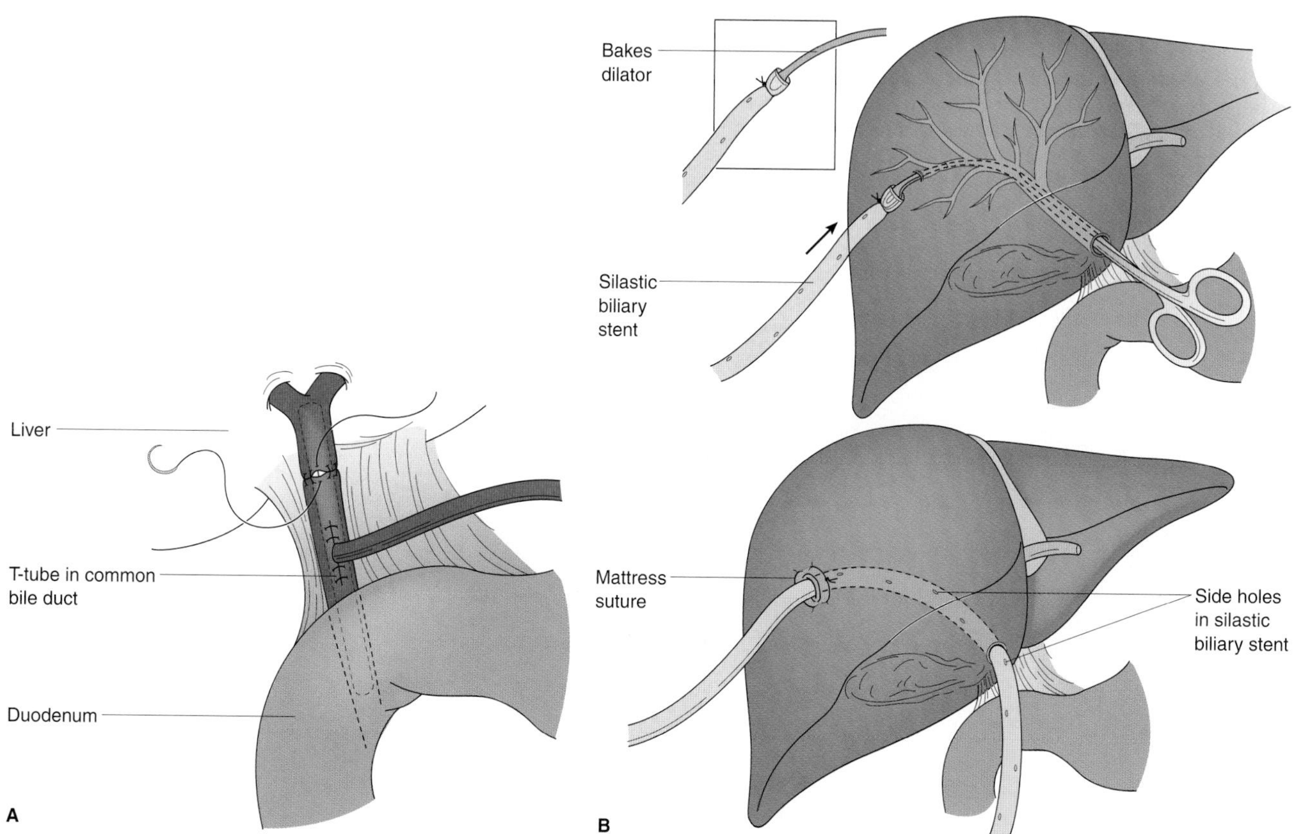

FIGURE 63.9 All biliary anastomosis performed for the reconstruction of acute bile duct injury should have external drainage. (*A*) If the injured segment of bile duct is short (<1 cm), and the two ends can be opposed without tension, and end-to-end anastomosis can be performed with placement of a T-tube through a separate choledochotomy either above or below the anastomosis. The T-tube should not be brought out directly through the anastomosis. (*B*) With more proximal injuries or if the segment of injured bile duct is greater than 1 cm, an end-to-end bile duct anastomosis should be avoided and a Roux-en-Y hepaticojejunostomy should be constructed. A transanastomotic stent can be placed retrograde through the transected duct and exited to the hepatic paraenchyma to allow postoperative external drainage. (After Cameron JL. Resection of benign bile duct stricture with reconstruction utilizing Silastic transhepatic biliary stents and hepaticojejunostomy. *Atlas of Surgery.* Vol 1. Ontario: BC Decker; 1990;47.)

an end-to-side fashion to a Roux-en-Y jejunal limb. The use of a Roux-en-Y jejunal limb is preferable to anastomosis to the duodenum because, in the latter case, an anastomotic leak results in a duodenal fistula. A transanastomotic Silastic stent can be placed retrograde through the transected duct and exiting the hepatic parenchyma, (Fig. 63.9B) to allow for postoperative external drainage.

The long-term results of immediate repair of common bile duct injuries is uncertain. Most injuries occur away from major centers, and therefore even the successes are unlikely to be reported in the literature. In a Swedish report, early primary repair with end-to-end anastomosis resulted in good results in only 22% of patients. Anastomotic leak requiring reoperation occurred in 32% of patients, and late stricture occurred in another 37% of patients. In patients undergoing immediate repair with a biliary-enteric anastomosis, good results were seen in 54% of patients, with strictures occurring in only 12% of patients. Similar poor late results were observed in another series in which 29 of 36 patients with primary end-to-end repair had postoperative strictures within 4 years.

Elective Repair of Bile Duct Injuries and Established Strictures

Several principles are associated with successful repair of a biliary injury or stricture: exposure of healthy proximal bile ducts that provide drainage of the entire liver; preparation of a suitable segment of intestine that can be brought to the area of the stricture without tension, most frequently a Roux-en-Y jejunal limb; and creation of a direct biliary-enteric mucosal-to-mucosal anastomosis. A number of alternatives for elective repair of bile duct strictures exist. The choice of procedure is dictated by the location of the stricture, the history of previous unsuccessful attempts at repair, and the surgeon's personal preference. Simple excision of a bile duct stricture and end-to-end bile duct anastomosis or repair of the damaged duct can rarely be accomplished because of the invariable loss of duct length as a result of fibrosis associated with the injury. Similarly, anastomosis of the proximal bile duct to the duodenum as a choledochoduodenostomy is not suitable for most postcholecystectomy strictures because an adequate length of bile duct for creating a tension-free anastomosis to the duodenum usually cannot be obtained. Thus, in almost all cases, hepaticojejunostomy constructed to a Roux-en-Y limb of jejunum is the preferred procedure.

Many surgeons believe that a transanastomotic stent is helpful in almost all cases. In the early postoperative period, a stent is used to decompress the biliary tree and provide access for cholangiography. If the injury involves the common bile duct or the common hepatic duct at least 2 cm distal to the hepatic duct bifurcation, and adequate proximal bile duct mucosa can be defined, the use of long-term biliary stents is not necessary. In these situations, the preoperatively placed percutaneous transhepatic catheter or operatively placed T-tube is used to decompress the biliary-enteric anastomosis for 4 to 6 weeks after surgery. When adequate proximal bile duct is not available for a good mucosa-to-mucosa anastomosis, long-term stenting of the biliary-enteric anastomosis with a Silastic transhepatic stent is recommended. For strictures involving the hepatic duct bifurcation, both the right and left main hepatic ducts should be individually stented.

An operative technique for biliary reconstruction with transhepatic stents using the preoperatively placed percutaneous transhepatic catheters begins with dissection of the porta hepatis, which usually involves separating adhesions of the duodenum and hepatic flexure of the colon to Glisson's capsule and the gallbladder fossa.[7] Identification of the proximal biliary segment can be difficult and can be aided by the presence of the transhepatic biliary catheter. This is particularly true for bile duct transections that will retract high into the porta. If a primary duct

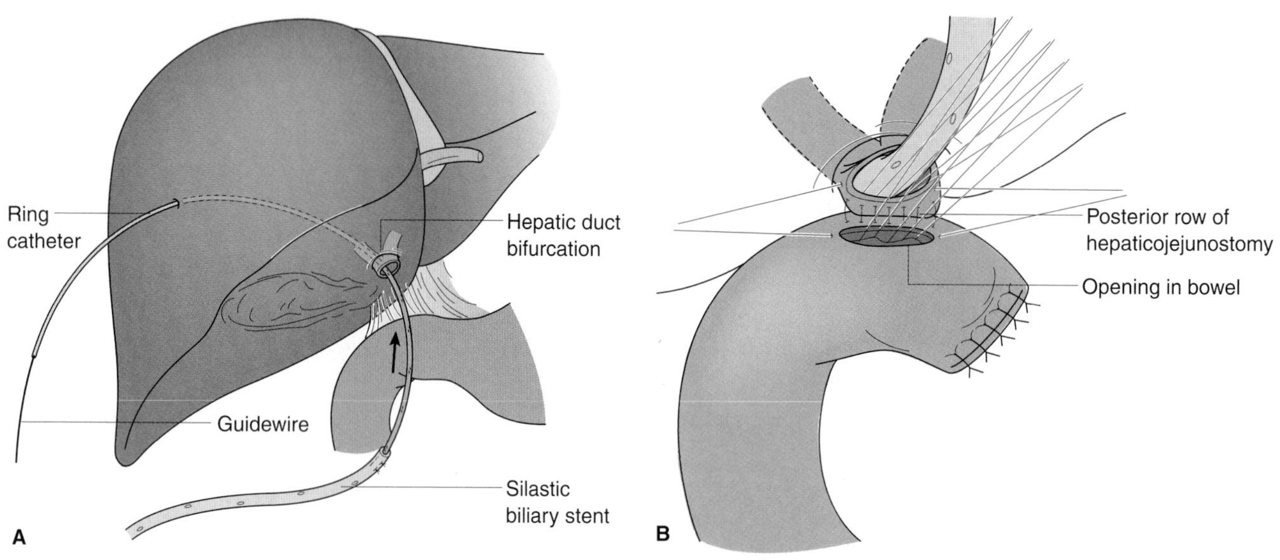

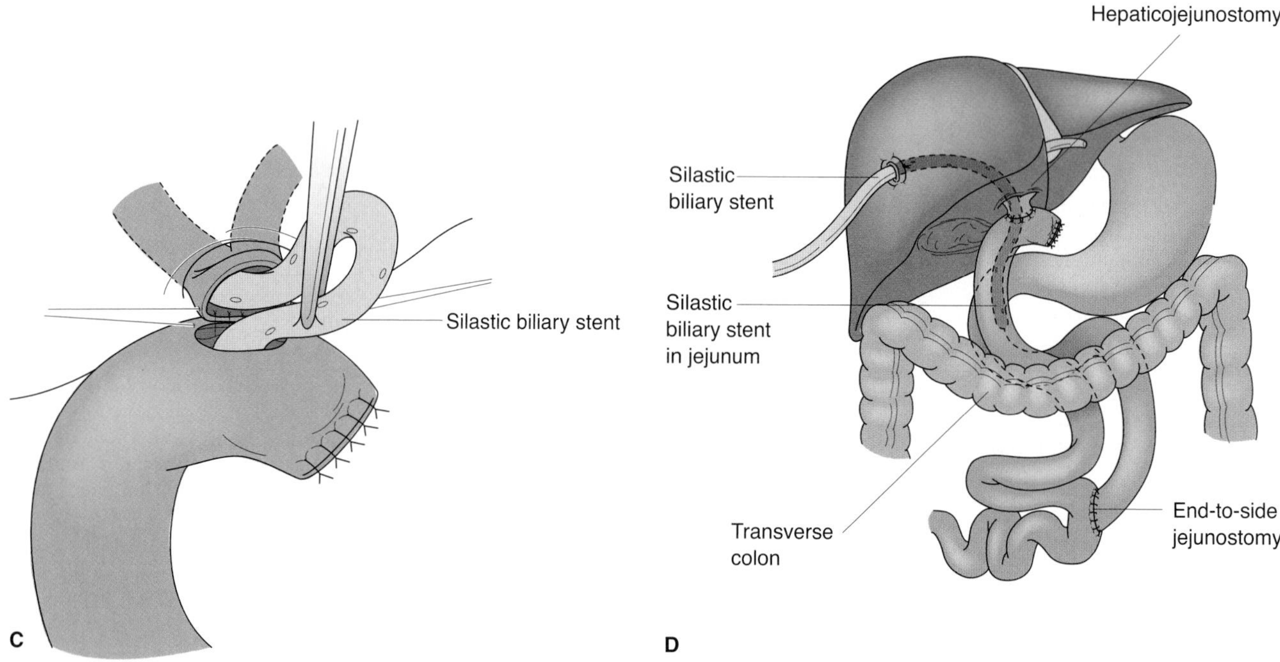

FIGURE 63.10 Technique of biliary reconstruction. (*A*) A Silastic stent is sutured to the preoperatively placed transhepatic catheter, which protrudes through the transected hepatic duct and through the catheter tract in the hepatic parenchyma. (*B*) A Roux-en-Y jejunal loop is then anastomosed to the hepatic duct and (C) the silastic stent is placed through the anastomosis. (*D*) A completed Roux-en-Y hepaticojejunostomy with a transanastomotic stent. (After Cameron JL. Resection of benign bile duct stricture with reconstruction utilizing silastic transhepatic biliary stents and hepaticojejunostomy. *Atlas of Surgery*, Vol 1, BC Decker; 1990;45, 55, 57.)

stricture exists the bile duct is then divided at the lowest extent of the stricture and dissected proximally. A segment of the strictured duct should be resected and submitted for pathologic examination. The distal duct is then oversewn, and the bile duct proximal to the stricture is carefully dissected circumferentially in a cephalad direction for a distance not to exceed 5 mm. Excessive dissection should be avoided to prevent vascular compromise of this segment of duct, which will be used for the anastomosis. After mobilization and division of the bile duct, the biliary catheters protrude through the proximal end (Fig. 63.10A). A radiologic guide wire is then placed through these catheters. The preoperatively placed catheter can then be exchanged over the wire for a properly sized Silastic stent. These stents are 70 cm long and range from 12 Fr to 22 Fr. Multiple side holes are present along 40% of the length of the stent. These side holes are left to reside within the intrahepatic biliary tree and the portion of the Roux-en-Y jejunal limb used for the biliary anastomosis. The end of the stent without the side holes exits through the hepatic parenchyma and is brought out through a stab wound in the upper anterior abdomen. After stent placement, a Roux-en-Y jejunal limb is prepared, and the anastomosis is then performed as an end-to-side hepaticojejunostomy (Fig. 63.10B–D).

An alternative technique has been described for management of bile duct strictures involving the bifurcation and one or both of the hepatic ducts in which a side-to-side anastomosis of the left hepatic duct to the Roux-en-Y limb is constructed. A long opening along the anterior surface of the left hepatic duct is anastomosed to the side of the Roux-en-Y limb. Because it is possible to dissect the anterior surface of the left hepatic duct high up into the hepatic parenchyma, this procedure permits anastomosis to normal mucosa, even though there can be fibrosis and stricture at the bifurcation of the ducts and in the distal portion of the hepatic duct. This technique can avoid the need for postoperative stenting.

Surgical Outcome

Morbidity and Mortality

Repairs of bile duct strictures are performed primarily in major medical centers by experienced surgeons, yet these operations are still associated with significant morbidity and mortality. In 1982, a review of 38 series published since 1900 that included more than 7,643 procedures performed on 5,586 patients reported an overall operative mortality rate of 8.3%.[8] More recently the incidence of operative mortality has decreased markedly with improved technology and a multidisciplinary approach as well as improved surgical experience. A recent series of 200 consecutive patients managed at the Johns Hopkins Hospital reported three deaths in patients who did not undergo an attempt at repair who were referred with sepsis secondary to an uncontrolled biliary leak for a mortality rate of 1.5%. Definitive surgical reconstruction was performed in 175 patients with a perioperative mortality of only 1.7%.[9] In this series the timing of repair, the mode of presentation, previous attempts of repair and the level of injury did not influence outcome. Chronic liver disease can be an important factor for operative mortality and morbidity with advanced biliary cirrhosis and portal hypertension leading to mortality rates approaching 30%. Fortunately in the modern era, such advanced disease is uncommon. In most series postoperative mortality rates are in the range of 20% to 40%. In the recent Hopkins series, complications occurred in 41% of patients. Most of the complications were minor and could be managed with either interventional radiology techniques or conservative management. No patient required reoperation for postoperative complications. The median length of stay in this series was 8 days.

TABLE 63.2 RESULTS

RESULTS OF SURGICAL MANAGEMENT OF BILE DUCT STRICTURES

Investigators	Patients	Success (%)	Follow-up (mo)
Pitt et al., 1982[4]	66	86	60
Pelligrini et al., 1984[9]	60	78	102
Genest, 1986	105	82	60
Innes, 1988	22	95	72
Pain, 1988	163	72	133
Pitt et al., 1989[17]	25	88	57
David et al., 1993[15]	35	83	50
Lillemoe et al., 2000[11]	142	91	58

Long-term Results

Historically, excellent long-term results were achieved in 70% to 90% of patients who underwent repair of bile duct strictures (Table 63.2). The definition of satisfactory results in most series requires that patients have no symptoms, jaundice, or cholangitis. Length of follow-up is important in analyzing final results because recurrent strictures can occur up to 20 years after the initial procedure (Fig. 63.11).[4,5] Approximately two thirds of restrictures are evident within 2 years, and 90% are seen within 7 years. The percentage of patients with good results is inversely related to the number of previous repairs. Other factors that favor a good outcome include young age at the time of stricture repair, use of a Roux-en-Y biliary-enteric anastomosis, absence of infection and hepatic fibrosis, and use of transhepatic stents.

As illustrated above, in the era before laparoscopic cholecystectomy, excellent long-term results were obtainable in

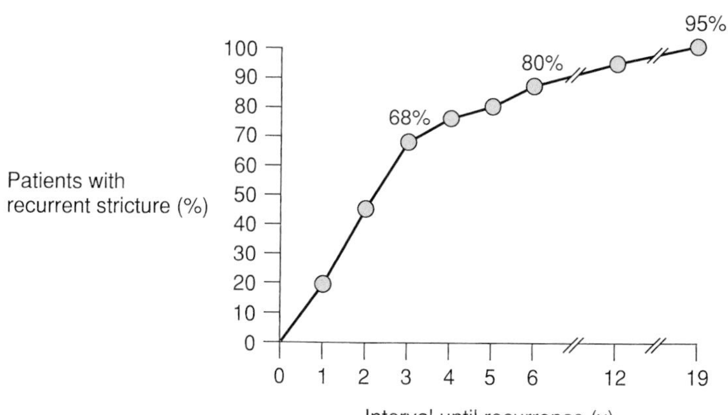

FIGURE 63.11 The cumulative percentage of recurrent strictures with respect to the time from the initial repair until the next repair. (After Pitt HA, Miyamoto T, Parapatis SK, et al. Factors influencing outcome in patients with postoperative biliary strictures. *Am J Surg.* 1982;144:14.)

tertiary care centers, specializing in the management of these problems. Questions had arisen as to whether the excellent results of bile duct strictures after open cholecystectomy could be directly transferred to patients sustaining laparoscopic bile duct injuries. Some researchers had suggested that the mechanism of bile duct injury during laparoscopic cholecystectomy, the complex nature of many of these injuries, and the frequent association of significant inflammation and fibrosis secondary to sustained, unrecognized bile leakage might result in poor long-term results. Furthermore, the high percentage of these patients who have undergone unsuccessful operations, often performed by the primary laparoscopic surgeon, might also lead to a poor long-term outcome. Evidence for the latter hypothesis was provided by a review of the records of 85 patients who underwent a total of 112 biliary repairs.[10] Four factors determined the success or failure of treatment in this series. These factors included performance of preoperative cholangiography, the choice of surgical repair, details of the operative repair, and experience of the surgeon performing the repair. The importance of preoperative delineation of anatomy was clear, in that 96% of procedures in which cholangiograms were not obtained before repair were unsuccessful, and 69% of repairs were not successful when the cholangiographic data were incomplete. When cholangiographic data were complete, the initial repair was successful in 84% of patients. The type of repair was also of significance in influencing outcome. A primary end-to-end ductal repair over a T-tube was unsuccessful in all patients in whom a complete transection of the bile duct had taken place, whereas 63% of Roux-en-Y hepaticojejunostomies were successful. Attempts at repair by the primary surgeon were successful only in 17% of cases, and in no case was a secondary repair by the primary surgeon successful. In those cases in which the first repair was performed by a tertiary care biliary surgeon, a 94% success rate was obtained.

The outcome of management of 142 patients with major bile duct injuries treated during the 1990s has been reported.[11] Laparoscopic cholecystectomy was the initial operation in 75% of these patients, and 41% had undergone a previous attempt or attempts at surgical repair before referral. In this series with a median follow-up of 58 months (range, 11 to 119 months), a successful outcome was obtained in 91% of patients. In this series the level of injury, clinical presentation, history of prior repair, and length of biliary stenting did not influence outcome. These results suggest that surgical reconstruction of major bile duct injuries after laparoscopic cholecystectomy can still result in excellent long-term results.

Despite the overall high levels of success in surgical management of laparoscopic bile duct injuries associated with laparoscopic cholecystectomy, there is an impression that patients may have an impaired quality of life even after successful repair of their bile duct injury. Quality of life assessments after laparoscopic cholecystectomy bile duct injury have been addressed in several recent reports. These results have generally reported either comparable or mildly diminished quality of life compared with matched controls. In one such study, patients following successful surgical repair reported overall quality of life scores comparable to controls in the physical and social domains of a standardized health–related quality-of-life assessment.[12] Only in the psychological domain were patients following bile duct injury repair found to have significantly worse scores as compared to controls. Interestingly patients that reported pursuing a law suit following their injury has significantly worse quality of life scores in all domains when compared to those who did not entertain legal action.

Nonoperative Management

Operative management of bile duct strictures is technically difficult and continues to be associated with significant postoperative morbidity and mortality. Moreover, in all series, recurrent strictures develop in a proportion of patients. These factors, in addition to technical advances in the fields of therapeutic radiology and endoscopy, have led to the development of nonoperative techniques for management of bile duct strictures.

Percutaneous Balloon Dilation

The largest nonoperative experience in the management of benign bile duct strictures is using the percutaneous transhepatic route. The procedure in many cases can be performed with a combination of local anesthesia and intravenous sedation. In this technique, access to the proximal biliary tree is gained and the stricture is traversed with a guide wire under fluoroscopic guidance. At this point, the stricture is dilated using angioplasty-type balloon catheters, chosen on the basis of the location of the stricture and the diameter of the normal duct (Fig. 63.12). After the procedure, a transhepatic stent is left in place across the stricture to allow access to the biliary tree for follow-up cholangiography, repeat dilation, and maintenance of a lumen during the healing process. In most series, numerous dilations are required.

The results from a number of series have been encouraging (Table 63.3). In a multicenter review of bile duct strictures treated in the open cholecystectomy era, 3-year follow-up showed a 67% patency rate for anastomotic and a 76% patency rate for iatrogenic primary bile duct strictures, yielding an overall 70% success rate.[13] A report of 51 patients with bile duct strictures after laparoscopic cholecystectomy managed with percutaneous dilation showed a success rate of 58% with a mean follow-up of 76 months.[14]

Complications of balloon dilation are frequent. Cholangitis, hemobilia, and bile leaks can occur in up to 20% of patients. Bleeding, usually from the hepatic parenchyma, has been reported, with transfusions often necessary. Sepsis due to cholangitis can occur despite antibiotic prophylaxis. Sepsis and significant bleeding seldom occur in patients dilated by a T-tube tract, suggesting that much of the morbidity is the result of traversing the hepatic parenchyma by the large percutaneously placed catheters.

Endoscopic Balloon Dilation

The experience with endoscopic balloon dilation is more limited. This technique is technically possible only in patients with primary bile duct strictures or with strictures at a choledochoduodenal anastomosis. This technique begins with ERC and endoscopic sphincterotomy. The stricture is traversed retrograde with an atraumatic guide wire, and sequential balloon dilation is used. Reevaluation with cholangiography is performed every 3 to 6 months. Redilation is performed as necessary. In most cases, an endoprosthesis is left in place after dilation for at least 6 months.

The reported experience with endoscopic dilation of benign bile duct strictures is shown in Table 63.4. The largest experience

TABLE 63.3 RESULTS

RESULTS OF TRANSHEPATIC BALLOON DILATION OF BILE DUCT STRICTURES

Investigators	Patients	Success (%)	Follow-up (mo)
Mueller et al., 1986[13]	61	70	36
Williams, 1987	64	78	28
Moore, 1987	18	83	33
Pitt et al., 1989[17]	20	55	59
Citron et al., 1991	28	93	38
Misra et al., 2004	51	58	76

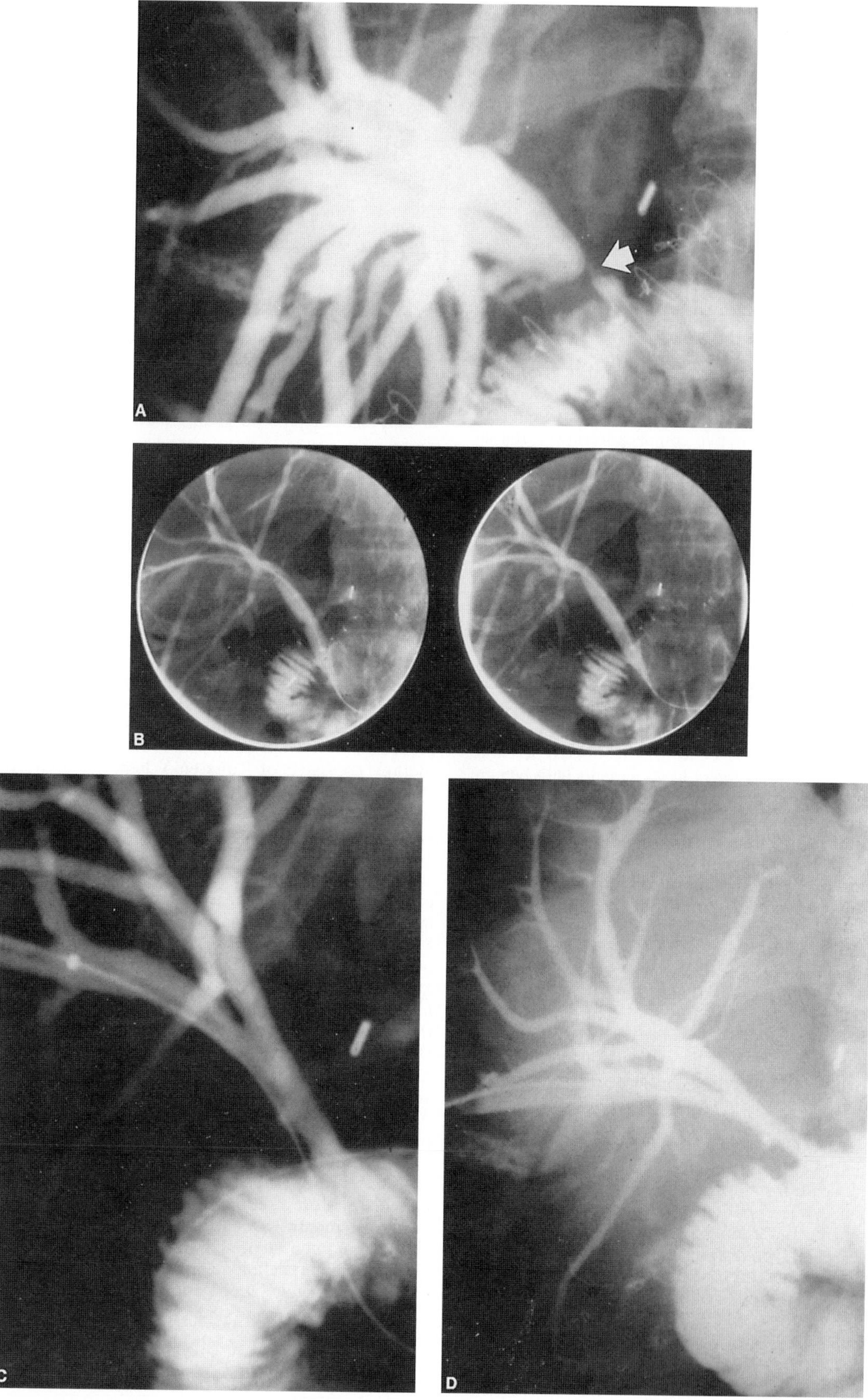

FIGURE 63.12 (*A*) Transhepatic cholangiogram demonstrating stricture (*arrow*) at a previous choledochojejunostomy. (*B*) Progressive dilation of the strictured anastomosis with an angioplasty balloon catheter. (*C*) Postdilation stenting of the anastomotic stricture for prolonged periods. (*D*) Subsequent cholangiogram demonstrating resolution of the anastomotic stricture. (From Pitt HA, Kaufman SL, Coleman J, et al. Benign postoperative biliary strictures: operate or dilate? *Ann Surg*. 1989;210:417.)

TABLE 63.4 RESULTS

RESULTS OF ENDOSCOPIC BALLOON DILATATION OF BILE DUCT STRICTURES

Investigators	Patients	Success (%)	Follow-up (mo)
Foutsch, 1985	9	55	6
Geenen et al., 1989[16]	25	88	48
David et al., 1993[15]	46	83	48

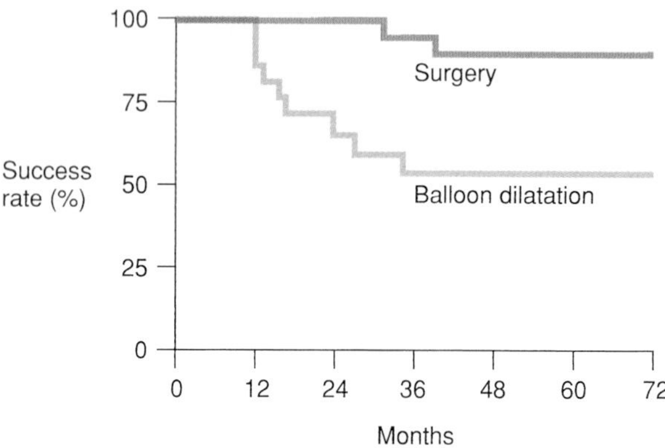

FIGURE 63.13 Actuarial success rates over 72 months for surgery (89%) and balloon dilation (52%). The difference is statistically significant (P <.01). (After Pitt HA, Kaufman SL, Coleman J, et al. Benign postoperative biliary strictures: operate or dilate? *Ann Surg.* 1989;210:417.)

comes from the group in The Netherlands and is discussed in the following section, Comparative Data.[15] A similar experience was reported in the United States.[16] In this series, 18 of 25 strictures were postoperative. Strictures were located at the cystic duct junction in 17 patients and in the distal bile duct in the remaining 8 patients. Of 25 patients, 22 (88%) had significant clinical benefit from the therapy. Only two complications occurred in this series—one case each of pancreatitis and cholangitis.

Comparative Data

Comparison of results of nonoperative dilation with those of surgery have been difficult. Few centers have a significant experience with both operative and nonoperative management. Furthermore, the definition of a successful procedure, the reporting of complications, and the length of follow-up have not been consistent in the literature. There are no prospective, randomized studies to compare these techniques; however, two retrospective comparative studies exist. In the first study, a retrospective review of the results at the Johns Hopkins Hospital between 1979 and 1987 compared percutaneous balloon dilation and surgery in 43 patients with benign postoperative bile duct strictures.[17] Twenty-five patients underwent surgical repair with Roux-en-Y hepaticojejunostomy with postoperative transhepatic stenting for a mean of 13 ± 1.3 months. Twenty patients had percutaneous balloon dilation, a mean of 3.9 times, and were stented transhepatically for a mean of 13.3 ± 2 months. Three patients were managed with both surgery and balloon dilation. The two groups were similar with respect to multiple parameters that might have influenced outcome, including age, sex, associated medical problems, and presentation with either obstructive jaundice or biliary fistulas. No patients died after any of the procedures. Procedure-related morbidity occurred in 20% of surgical patients and in 35% of the patients undergoing balloon dilation. For both groups, a successful outcome was defined as no evidence of cholangitis or jaundice requiring another procedure more than 12 months from the onset of treatment. A failed treatment was defined as the need for crossover to the other treatment modality, either operation or dilation, or late death from liver failure, biliary sepsis, or portal hypertension. A successful repair was achieved in 89% of the surgical patients and in only 52% of the balloon dilation patients (Fig. 63.13). The overall late mortality rate in this series was 10%. One late death occurred in the surgical group, whereas three late deaths followed balloon dilation (4% versus 15%, respectively). No deaths, however, were attributed to liver failure, biliary sepsis, or portal hypertension associated with the bile duct stricture.

To define further the relative benefits of the two procedures, total hospital stay and total procedural costs were determined. As expected, initial hospitalization was longer for surgery than for balloon dilation. When rehospitalization for further dilation, complications, or recurrences were considered, total hospital stay did not differ significantly between the two groups. Cost data paralleled hospitalization data and did not differ significantly between the groups. Thus, the authors concluded that until properly designed, randomized, prospective, controlled trials can be performed, surgical repair for benign postoperative strictures appears to be associated with fewer problems and a greater success rate.

In the second comparative study, the group from The Netherlands compared endoscopic versus surgical treatment of benign bile duct strictures.[15] Thirty-five patients were treated surgically, and 66 were treated by endoscopic stenting. Patient characteristics, initial injury, previous repairs, and the level of obstruction were comparable in both groups. Surgical therapy consisted of Roux-en-Y hepaticojejunostomy, and endoscopic therapy consisted of placement of an endoprosthesis with trimonthly elective exchange for 1 year. Successful stent placement was accomplished in 94% of patients managed endoscopically. Six of the 66 endoscopic patients, however, underwent surgical reconstruction either for failed stent placement or for other reasons. Early complications occurred more frequently in the surgically treated group (26% versus 8%; $P < 0.03$). However, the only procedure-related death occurred in a patient in whom severe pancreatitis developed after endoscopic stent placement. Late complications, which included primarily episodes of cholangitis, occurred only in the endoscopic group (27%). The overall complication rates, therefore, were similar at 26% for surgical patients and 35% for endoscopic patients. The mean follow-up and definition of success were similar to those in the aforementioned study. After surgery, excellent results were observed in 83% of patients, with a recurrent stricture developing in 6 patients at a mean of 40 months after the initial operation. After endoscopic stenting, excellent results were observed in 72% of patients, with restricture developing in 18% of patients at a mean of 3 months after stent removal. The investigators concluded that endoscopic stenting should be considered for the initial attempt at definitive management in suitable patients in the hope of avoiding reoperation.

PRIMARY SCLEROSING CHOLANGITIS

Primary sclerosing cholangitis is an idiopathic disease characterized by intrahepatic and extrahepatic inflammatory strictures of the bile ducts that cannot be attributed to other specific causes. The cause of primary sclerosing cholangitis is unknown.

TABLE 63.5

DISEASES ASSOCIATED WITH PRIMARY SCLEROSING CHOLANGITIS

Disease	Frequency (%)
Ulcerative colitis	40–60
Pancreatitis	12–25
Diabetes mellitus	5–10
Retroperitoneal fibrosis	Rare
Riedel's thyroiditis	Rare
Crohn's disease	Rare
Histiocytosis X	Rare
Sicca complex	Rare
Rheumatoid arthritis	Rare
Hypertrophic osteoarthropathy	Rare
Sarcoidosis	Rare
Angioimmunoblastic lymphadenopathy	Rare
Acquired immunodeficiency syndrome	Rare

Many experts consider primary sclerosing cholangitis to be an autoimmune reaction because it is associated with other autoimmune diseases, such as ulcerative colitis, retroperitoneal fibrosis, and Riedel's thyroiditis (Table 63.5). It is likely that a number of causes, including viral or bacterial infections, toxic drug reactions, and congenital anomalies, can all result in the same end-stage injury that is recognized as primary sclerosing cholangitis.

The usual clinical presentation of patients with primary sclerosing cholangitis involves intermittent jaundice, which begins insidiously in the fourth or fifth decade of life. Right upper quadrant pain, pruritus, fever, weight loss, and fatigue can also occur. The disease is characterized by cyclic remissions and exacerbations. Despite the nomenclature, acute cholangitis is uncommon without previous biliary manipulation or surgery. The diagnosis is suggested by clinical presentation associated with cholestatic liver function test abnormalities. The levels of bilirubin often fluctuate with respect to the remissions and exacerbations of the disease and the extent of hepatic injury. Alkaline phosphatase is usually elevated out of proportion to the serum bilirubin, and is a more persistent finding. The diagnosis, however, usually is confirmed by cholangiography, which reveals multiple dilatations and strictures (beading) of the intrahepatic and extrahepatic bile ducts (Fig. 63.14). ERC is the preferred procedure because of difficulties in cannulation of the intrahepatic ducts by the percutaneous transhepatic route, because the ducts are usually nondilated and fibrotic. The disease should be followed closely by cholangiography and liver biopsy to provide appropriate management before the development of biliary cirrhosis.

No known specific medical therapy is effective for primary sclerosing cholangitis. The most encouraging results, from a prospective, randomized, placebo-controlled trial, suggest that ursodeoxycholic acid significantly improves serum liver function tests and liver histologic appearance. Unfortunately, there were no significant differences in clinical outcome between the two groups at up to 6 years of follow-up.[15] Nonoperative dilation therapy (discussed earlier), by either the transhepatic or endoscopic route, has been used for dominant strictures. In a multicenter review of percutaneous balloon dilation, only 43% of patients with primary sclerosing cholangitis had successful long-term results.[12] The results of endoscopic dilation and stenting may be more favorable.

An aggressive surgical approach is advocated for most symptomatic patients with primary sclerosing cholangitis

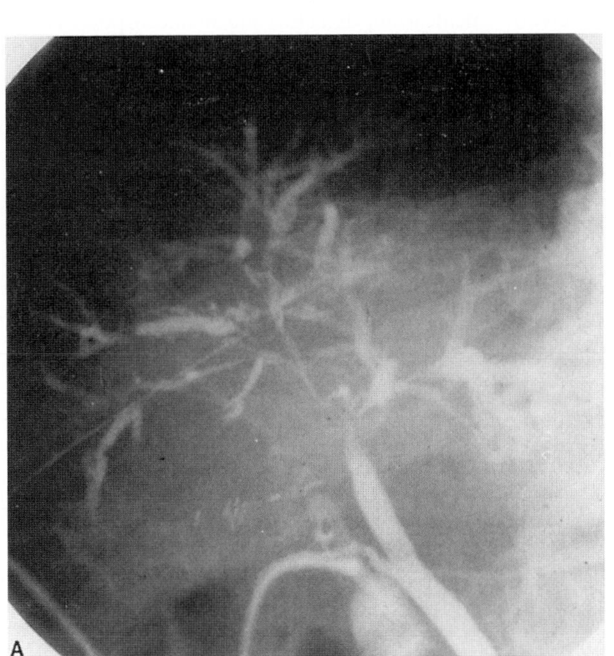

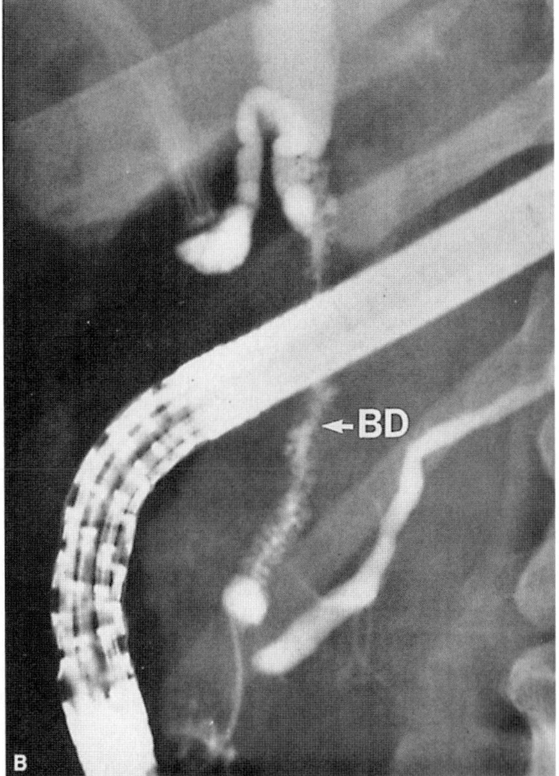

FIGURE 63.14 (*A*) Cholangiogram of a patient with primary sclerosing cholangitis. Multiple irregular strictures and dilatation (beading) of intrahepatic bile ducts can be seen. (*B*) Endoscopic retrograde cholangiogram showing extensive involvement of extrahepatic bile duct (BD) with primary sclerosing cholangitis. (*B* from Lillemoe KD, Pitt HA, Cameron JL. Primary sclerosing cholangitis. *Surg Clin North Am.* 1990;70:1390.)

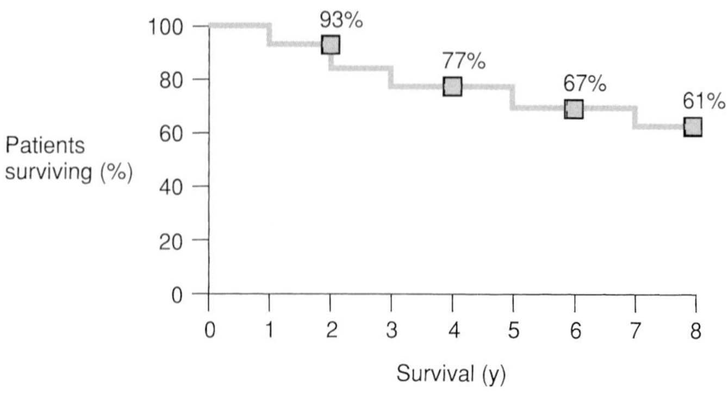

FIGURE 63.15 Actuarial survival rates among 31 noncirrhotic patients with primary sclerosing cholangitis who underwent resection of the hepatic bifurcation and longterm transhepatic stenting. (From Lillemoe KD, Pitt HA, Cameron JL. Primary sclerosing cholangitis. *Surg Clin North Am.* 1990;70:1397.)

because of the lack of effective medical therapy. One surgical approach, in patients with a dominant stricture at the hepatic duct bifurcation, uses resection of the bifurcation and long-term transhepatic stenting with Silastic(r) stents. This mode of therapy was reported in 31 patients.[19] Indications for operation included persistent jaundice in 29 patients and recurrent cholangitis in 2 patients. Five of the 31 patients had secondary biliary cirrhosis before surgery, with the remaining 26 patients having varying degrees of fibrosis without cirrhosis. The 1- and 5-year actuarial survival rates for patients with fibrosis were 92% and 71%, respectively, whereas the actuarial survival rate at 1 and 5 years was 20% in patients with established biliary cirrhosis (Fig. 63.15). Four patients have undergone hepatic transplantation for progressive disease. A more recent report of this form of surgical therapy has demonstrated a greater and longer biochemical improvement, improved survival until death or liver transplantation, and a lower incidence of cholangiocarcinoma than was observed in patients treated medically or with endoscopic or percutaneous dilation.[20]

The role of biliary surgery in primary sclerosing cholangitis, however, has decreased considerably with the growing success of liver transplantation. Primary sclerosing cholangitis has become one of the most common indications for liver transplantation in the United States, with 5-year actuarial survival and graft survival rates of 85% and 72%, respectively.[21] Liver transplantation should be considered before the disease is too advanced. The development of a poor quality of life as a result of disabling fatigue, intractable pruritus, severe muscle wasting, and chronic or recurrent bacterial cholangitis or persistent elevations in serum bilirubin are primary indications for referral for liver transplantation.

Preoperative recognition of cholangiocarcinoma is extremely important in this population in that the development of this complication significantly worsens the result after liver transplantation. The presence of known malignancy results in patients being refused transplantation. The microscopic identification of intrahepatic cholangiocarcinoma in the absence of lymph node involvement, often demonstrated in the explanted liver specimen, however, does not usually portend a poor prognosis.

Patients with primary sclerosing cholangitis have a significantly higher rate of development of nonanastomotic biliary strictures after liver transplantation, with histologic features on posttransplantation biopsy consistent with recurrence of the disease. Other causes of stricture, such as hepatic artery thrombosis, preservation-related ischemia, cytomegalovirus infection, and chronic ductopenic rejection, can cause similar lesions. Recurrent primary sclerosing cholangitis usually does not have an aggressive course.

Resection of the hepatic duct bifurcation and long-term transanastomotic stenting in selected patients can preclude or delay the need for hepatic transplantation. Moreover, this operation does not eliminate or influence the results of hepatic transplantation. Resection of the hepatic bifurcation and long-term transhepatic stenting can be recommended for selected patients with primary sclerosing cholangitis with severe strictures at or distal to the hepatic duct bifurcation but without established biliary cirrhosis. In patients with biliary cirrhosis, hepatic transplantation is recommended.

BILE DUCT STRICTURES SECONDARY TO CHRONIC PANCREATITIS

Chronic pancreatitis is an uncommon cause of benign bile duct strictures, resulting in less than 10% of such cases. Transient partial obstruction of the distal common bile duct caused by inflammation and edema frequently occurs in patients with acute pancreatitis. With chronic pancreatitis, however, the clinical problem is distal bile duct obstruction caused by inflammation and parenchymal fibrosis of the gland. These strictures classically involve the entire intrapancreatic segment of the common bile duct and are associated with dilatation of the entire proximal biliary tree (Fig. 63.16). In most cases, the cause of the chronic pancreatitis is alcoholism. Often, advanced disease is present in that the incidence of pancreatic calcification, diabetes, and malabsorption is increased at the time of presentation with jaundice compared with patients with chronic pancreatitis without jaundice. Common bile duct strictures have been reported to occur in 3% to 29% of patients with chronic alcoholic pancreatitis. In a review of a number of clinical series, the overall incidence of common bile duct strictures in patients with chronic pancreatitis was 5.7%.[22] The exact incidence of common bile duct strictures is not known, however, because cholangiography is not routinely performed in patients with chronic pancreatitis.

The clinical presentation of patients with common bile duct strictures secondary to chronic pancreatitis is variable. Some patients have no symptoms, with the diagnosis of bile duct strictures suggested only by abnormal liver function test results. The serum alkaline phosphatase appears to be the most sensitive laboratory finding and is elevated in more than 80% of patients. Abdominal pain with or without jaundice is another common presentation. In some cases, the abdominal pain can be difficult to distinguish from the pain associated with chronic pancreatitis. Failure to recognize and address a bile duct stricture, however, can lead to ultimate failure of operative procedures performed for chronic pain in patients with chronic pancreatitis. Finally, the development of jaundice in patients with chronic pancreatitis must be differentiated from underlying periampullary malignancy.

The definitive evaluation of patients with a bile duct stricture caused by chronic pancreatitis is cholangiography. Either endoscopic retrograde cholangiopancreatography (ERCP) or PTC can be useful. ERCP offers the advantage of demonstrating

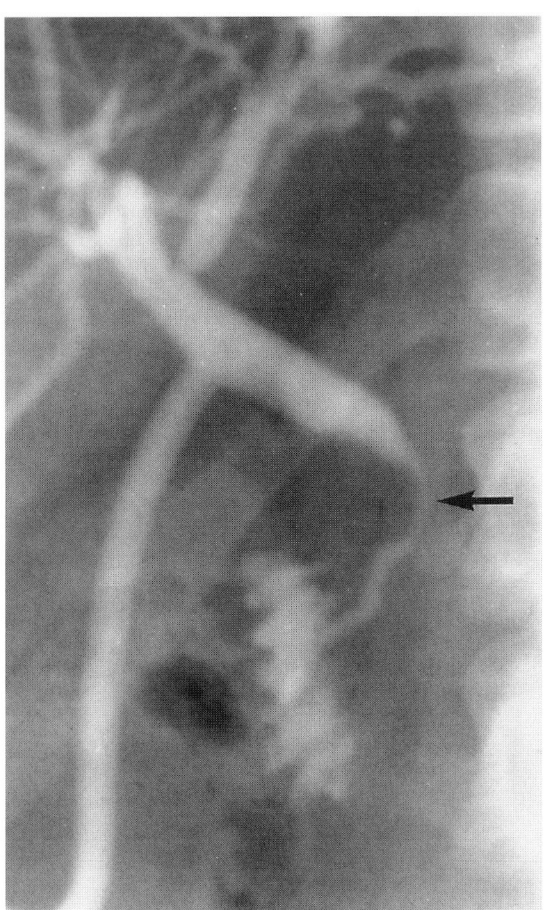

FIGURE 63.16 Cholangiogram of a patient with a long distal common bile duct stricture (*arrow*) caused by chronic pancreatitis.

pancreatic ductal anatomy and possible abnormality, which is essential in optimal surgical management of chronic pancreatitis. Both techniques allow decompression of the obstructed biliary tree if necessary for cholangitis or severe jaundice. A long (usually 2 to 4 cm), smooth, gradual tapering of the common bile duct is most compatible with a benign stricture due to chronic pancreatitis (Fig. 63.16).

The indications for surgical management of common bile duct strictures due to chronic pancreatitis are clear in patients with significant pain, jaundice, or cholangitis. Controversy exists, however, concerning the necessity of biliary decompression in patients with an asymptomatic elevation of serum alkaline phosphatase. In general, biliary bypass is indicated because changes from obstructive biliary cirrhosis have been observed in liver biopsy specimens obtained from patients with longstanding, functionally significant biliary obstruction due to chronic pancreatitis.[23,24]

Choledochoduodenostomy and Roux-en-Y choledochojejunostomy are acceptable methods of biliary bypass in patients with bile duct strictures caused by chronic pancreatitis. Choledochoduodenostomy is preferred by many surgeons because it does not divert bile from the duodenum, is technically easier to perform, and leaves the jejunum intact for any associated procedures required for decompression of an obstructed gastrointestinal tract or pancreatic duct. Finally, in patients in whom periampullary malignancy cannot be completely ruled out by the clinical course or imaging studies, or in patients with significant chronic pain thought secondary to proximal pancreatic duct disease, pancreaticoduodenectomy offers an excellent treatment option. The results of surgical management of distal bile duct structures due to chronic pancreatitis are usually excellent, with a low rate of perioperative complications and excellent long-term results.

Transduodenal sphincteroplasty is not recommended for the management of common bile duct strictures caused by chronic pancreatitis because the stricture is too long to be managed adequately by this technique. Similarly, endoscopic sphincterotomy has no role in the management of biliary obstruction due to chronic pancreatitis. Limited experience has been reported with balloon dilation of distal bile duct strictures secondary to pancreatitis, with little long-term follow-up.

MISCELLANEOUS CAUSES OF BILE DUCT STRICTURES

Benign strictures of the bile duct can result from the chronic inflammation associated with gallstones in either the gallbladder or common bile duct. This cause of bile duct strictures is uncommon and is a rare complication of gallstone disease. Bile duct strictures caused by cholelithiasis are usually associated with a narrowing at the level of the common hepatic duct caused by a stone impacted in the infundibulum of the gallbladder. The narrowing can be caused by two means. First, simple compression can occur from a large stone lying adjacent to the common hepatic duct. Second, chronic or acute inflammation arising from the gallbladder or cystic duct can extend to the contiguous bile duct, resulting in stricture formation. The biliary obstruction associated with either of these conditions is known as *Mirizzi's syndrome*.

The clinical presentation of a bile duct stricture caused by cholelithiasis is often associated with acute cholecystitis and hyperbilirubinemia. In some long-standing cases, these findings exist in the face of chronic gallbladder symptoms. If hyperbilirubinemia is present and urgent cholecystectomy is not indicated, ERCP or PTC can help to delineate the preoperative biliary anatomy. Most cases that are associated with acute cholecystitis, however, are recognized at the time of cholecystectomy and operative cholangiography. When the duct compression is associated with acute inflammation, the common hepatic duct almost always returns to normal after the offending stone has been removed by cholecystectomy and the inflammatory process has resolved. Care must be taken during the dissection to avoid creation of a defect in the common hepatic duct. Rarely, after the acute episode has resolved, a well-established stricture presents months to years after the acute episode. In such cases, management by Roux-en-Y hepaticojejunostomy is appropriate.

Strictures due to choledocholithiasis are also rare. The presumed mechanism is erosion of the epithelium of the distal duct, creating inflammation with subsequent fibrosis and stricture. Because of the anatomic tapering of the common bile duct, nearly all stones are entrapped in the intrapancreatic portion of the duct and are often difficult to remove by the supraduodenal route.

Excessive intraoperative manipulation at the time of bile duct exploration with forceps, scoops, and catheters can often create additional trauma to an already friable distal duct. After the stone has been removed, the distal bile duct should be gently sized with a soft rubber catheter to be sure that no stricture exists. If a stricture persists after stone removal, it may not be recognized until the time of postoperative T-tube cholangiography. If recognized in the postoperative period, time should be allowed for resolution of inflammation before considering stricture repair. If a distal bile duct stricture does persist, a biliary-enteric anastomosis with either Roux-en-Y choledochojejunostomy or a choledochoduodenostomy is indicated. If the proximal duct is adequately dilated (>2 cm in diameter) to allow a large choledochoduodenal anastomosis, this procedure is usually preferable because of its technical ease and excellent results.

Stenosis of the sphincter of Oddi, or papillitis, is a benign intrinsic obstruction of the outlet of the common bile duct, usually associated with inflammation, fibrosis, or muscular hypertrophy. Sphincter stenosis can result in any of three clinical conditions: (a) common bile duct obstruction due to fibrotic stenosis of the papilla, (b) recurrent pancreatitis, or (c) recurrent right upper quadrant pain without jaundice or pancreatitis. The pathogenesis of the inflammation of sphincter stenosis is unclear. In many cases, it is thought to result from the trauma of the passage of multiple small stones from the common duct through the ampulla. This trauma results in inflammation, scarring, and stricture formation. Many patients with papillary stenosis have no gallstones. Other potential mechanisms include primary sphincter motility disorders and congenital anomalies. The clinical presentation is usually either jaundice or cholangitis. In some cases, an impacted common bile duct stone may be present. The diagnosis can be supported with either PTC or ERC. This condition can be managed by sphincterotomy performed either endoscopically or operatively. If a cholecystectomy was performed previously, endoscopic papillotomy is the initial procedure of choice.

Cholangiohepatitis is an unusual infection of the biliary tree frequently associated with *Clonorchis sinensis* and other parasites. These infections are most commonly seen in natives of Asia. Most patients present with recurrent episodes of cholangitis. Cholangiography can demonstrate multiple strictures of both the intrahepatic and extrahepatic biliary tree, with the bile ducts filled with sludge and stones (Fig. 63.17). Surgical management consists of cholecystectomy and improved biliary drainage with either Roux-en-Y choledochojejunostomy or choledochoduodenostomy. Access to the biliary tree for postoperative management of intrahepatic stones or sludge should be maintained with either transhepatic biliary stents or a choledochojejunocutaneous or subcutaneous fistula. No specific medical management is available for this condition.

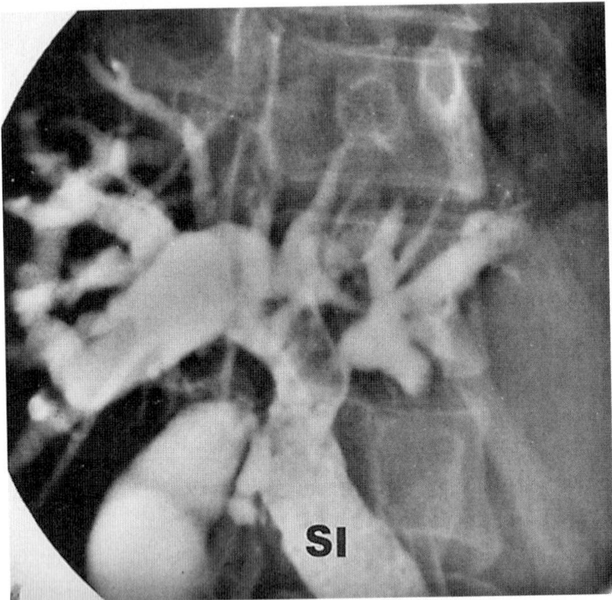

FIGURE 63.17 Cholangiogram of a patient with cholangiohepatitis with diffuse bile duct dilatation. The biliary tree is filled with sludge (Sl) and stones.

Finally, rare causes of benign intrahepatic and extrahepatic bile duct strictures have been reported secondary to intrahepatic arterial infusion of 5-fluorouracil used in the treatment of hepatic metastases of colorectal carcinoma. The clinical picture closely resembles primary sclerosing cholangitis but usually can be managed by simple discontinuation of infusion and, in some cases, percutaneous transhepatic drainage. Surgery should be reserved for patients with persistent evidence of biliary obstruction. A similar cholangiographic appearance has been reported in patients with acquired immunodeficiency syndrome. The pathogenesis of this injury is believed to be viral and related to cytomegalovirus infection. No experience in the surgical management of this condition has been reported.

References

1. **Hall JG, Pappas TN. Current management of biliary strictures. *J Gastrointest Surg.* 2004;8:1098.**
2. **Branum G, Schmitt C, Baillie J, et al. Management of major biliary complications after laparoscopic cholecystectomy. *Ann Surg.* 1993;17:532.**
3. Way LW, Stewart L, Gantert W, et al. Causes and prevention of laparoscopic bile duct injuries: analysis of 252 cases from a human factors and cognitive psychology perspective. *Ann Surg.* 2003;273:460.
4. Pitt HA, Miyamoto T, Parapatis SK, et al. Factors influencing outcome in patients with postoperative biliary strictures. *Am J Surg.* 1982;144:14.
5. Pellegrini CA, Thomas MJ, Way LW. Recurrent biliary stricture: patterns of recurrent and outcome of surgical therapy. *Am J Surg.* 1984;147:175.
6. Lillemoe KD, Martin SA, Cameron JL, et al. Major bile duct injuries during laparoscopic cholecystectomy: follow-up after combined surgical and radiologic management. *Ann Surg.* 1977;225:459–71.
7. Lillemoe KD. Treatment of laparoscopic bile duct injuries. *Curr Tech Gen Surg.* 1997;6:1.
8. Warren KW, Christophi C, Armendari ZR. The evolution and current perspectives of the treatment of benign bile duct strictures: a review. *Surg Gastroenterol.* 1982;1:141.
9. Sicklick JK, Camp MS, Lillemoe KD, et al. Surgical management of bile duct injuries sustained during laparoscopic cholecystectomy: Perioperative results in 200 patients. *Ann Surg.* 2005. In press.
10. **Stewart L, Way LW. Bile duct injuries during laparoscopic cholecystectomy. *Arch Surg.* 1995;130:1123.**
11. **Lillemoe KD, Melton GB, Cameron JL, et al. Postoperative bile duct strictures: management and outcome in the 1990s. *Ann Surg.* 2000;232:430.**
12. Melton GB, Lillemoe KD, Cameron JL, et al. Major bile duct injuries associated with laparoscopic cholecystectomy: Effect on quality of life. *Ann Surg.* 2002;235:888.
13. Mueller PR, van Sonnenberg E, Ferrucci JT Jr, et al. Biliary stricture dilatation: multicenter review of clinical management in 73 patients. *Radiology* 1986;160:17.
14. Misra S, Melton GB, Geschwind JF, et al. Percutaneous management of bile duct strictures and injuries associated with laparoscopic cholecystectomy: A decade of experience. *J Am Coll Surg.* 2004;198:218.
15. David PHP, Tanka AKF, Rauws EAJ, et al. Benign biliary strictures: surgery or endoscopy? *Ann Surg.* 1993;217:237.
16. Geenen DJ, Geenen JE, Hogan WJ, et al. Endoscopic therapy for benign bile duct strictures. *Gastrointest Endosc.* 1989;35:367.
17. Pitt HA, Kaufman SL, Coleman J, et al. Benign postoperative biliary strictures: operate or dilate? *Ann Surg.* 1989;210:417.
18. Lindor KD. Ursodiol for primary sclerosing cholangitis. Mayo Primary Sclerosing Cholangitis-Ursodeoxycholic Acid Study Group. *N Engl J Med.* 1997;336:691.
19. Lillemoe KD, Pitt HA, Cameron JL. Primary sclerosing cholangitis. *Surg Clin North Am.* 1990;70:1381.
20. **Ahrendt SA, Pitt HA, Kalloo AN, et al. Primary sclerosing cholangitis: resect, dilate, or transplant. *Ann Surg.* 1998;227:412.**
21. Gross JA, Shackelton CR, Farmer DG, et al. Orthotopic liver transplantation for primary sclerosing cholangitis: a 12-year single center experience. *Ann Surg.* 1997;225:472.
22. **Stahl TJ, Allen MO, Ansel M, et al. Partial biliary obstruction caused by chronic pancreatitis: an appraisal of indications for surgical biliary drainage. *Ann Surg.* 1988;207:26.**
23. Warshaw AL, Schapiro RH, Ferrucci JT Jr, et al. Persistent obstructive jaundice, cholangitis, and biliary cirrhosis due to common bile duct stenosis in chronic pancreatitis. *Gastroenterology* 1976;70:562.
24. Afroudakis A, Kaplowitz N. Liver histopathology in chronic bile duct stenosis due to chronic alcoholic pancreatitis. *Hepatology* 1981;1:65.

CHAPTER 64 ■ BILIARY NEOPLASMS

SHARON WEBER AND YUMAN FONG

Tumors arising in the gallbladder and biliary tree are often asymptomatic until late in the course of the disease. Consequently, these tumors commonly present in an advanced, often unresectable, stage. Surgery remains the only curative option for biliary malignancies. Resection of biliary neoplasms, however, often requires radical resections and complex biliary reconstructions that have only recently become safe in routine practice. Surgery also offers effective palliation for these cancers, including biliary bypasses for jaundiced patients with unresectable tumors. Both the late diagnosis and the complex operative techniques required for potentially curative resection contribute to the challenge of these cases. In addition, there are no proven effective options for adjuvant treatment. This chapter reviews the incidence, diagnosis, and therapy of these malignancies as well as the outcome of treatment.

GALLBLADDER CARCINOMA

Gallbladder cancer is a rare malignancy with a dismal outlook because of its insidious onset, propensity for local invasion, and rapid disease progression. Overall, most series report a 5-year survival of less than 5%. Extent of surgical resection remains ill defined because of the rarity of this lesion and its poor prognosis.

Incidence

Only 6,000 to 7,000 new cases of gallbladder cancer are diagnosed nationally each year.[1] Attesting to the rarity of this lesion, after routine screening abdominal ultrasounds in asymptomatic patients in Japan, only 19/194,767 (0.01%) were found to have gallbladder cancer.[2] This tumor occurs more frequently in women (female-to-male ratio = 3:1) and peak incidence is in the seventh decade.[1] There is an increased risk of gallbladder cancer in Native American populations of the United States and Mexico.[3] The increased risk of gallbladder cancer with cholelithiasis is well established; 70% to 90% of all patients with carcinoma also have gallstones. However, less than 0.5% of patients with gallstones are found to have gallbladder cancer.[3] After elective cholecystectomy for gallstones, gallbladder cancer is found incidentally in 1% of patients.[4] The association of gallstones with carcinoma is probably related to chronic inflammation. Larger stones (>3 cm) are associated with a 10-fold increased risk of cancer.[5]

The association of gallbladder cancer with gallstone disease has led some investigators to question whether all patients with gallstones should undergo cholecystectomy. The argument against this approach is that the use of cholecystectomy only for symptomatic patients, thus leaving the gallbladder in place in patients with asymptomatic gallstones, has not led to an increase in the prevalence of gallbladder cancer over time. Also, epidemiologic studies have found that the 20-year risk of developing cancer in patients with gallstones is less than 0.5% for the overall population and 1.5% for high-risk groups.[3] Thus, routine cholecystectomy for asymptomatic gallstones because of concern for gallbladder cancer does not appear to be warranted.

In the past, the finding of a calcified gallbladder wall, called "porcelain gallbladder" (Fig. 64.1), was associated with a high risk of cancer, in some series ranging from 25% to 60%.[6] Thus, the recommendation was for all patients with porcelain gallbladder to undergo open cholecystectomy, even if asymptomatic. Recent series evaluating this issue, however, suggest that the risk of gallbladder cancer in patients with porcelain gallbladder has likely been greatly overestimated.[7,8] In fact, although patients with limited areas of calcification of the wall may have a higher incidence of gallbladder cancer (7%), patients with diffuse calcification of the gallbladder wall, the classic presentation for porcelain gallbladder, do not appear to have an increased risk of gallbladder cancer.[7,8]

Patients with choledochal cysts have an increased risk of carcinoma developing anywhere in the biliary tree, but the incidence is highest in the gallbladder. This risk increases with age.[9] Therefore, complete surgical resection is recommended for all patients with choledochal cysts at the time of diagnosis.

Pathology and Staging

More than 80% of gallbladder cancers are adenocarcinomas; there are several histologic subtypes, including papillary, nodular, and tubular. Papillary tumors, which grow predominately into the gallbladder lumen, have an improved prognosis compared with the other subtypes.[10] Poor prognostic signs in gallbladder cancer include grade[10,11] and vascular invasion.[10] The most important prognostic sign may be lymph node status,[12] although 5-year survivors with nodal involvement have been documented.[13] Less than 5% of cases are squamous cell carcinomas, with the remaining 10% being anaplastic lesions.

Gallbladder cancer spreads via the lymphatic and venous drainage. Because of drainage of the cholecystic veins directly into the adjacent liver, these tumors often involve hepatic parenchyma, most often portions of segments IV and V. Lymphatic spread is first to the cystic duct (Calot's) node, then to pericholedochal and hilar nodes, and finally to peripancreatic, duodenal, periportal, celiac, and superior mesenteric artery nodes. Nodal disease in the porta hepatis often causes common bile duct obstruction and resultant jaundice, which is the first clinical symptom in 30% of patients. Jaundice may also be caused by tumors arising in the infundibulum, which may spread directly to the cystic duct and common hepatic duct. Although peritoneal metastases are frequent, distant extraperitoneal metastases are not.

Limited information exists regarding the genetic changes in gallbladder cancer. The most widely reported gene abnormalities associated with gallbladder cancer include p53,[14] K-ras,[14,15] and CDKN2 (9p21) mutations.[15,16] The finding that patients with an anomalous pancreaticobiliary junction have a greater frequency of K-ras mutations has led investigators to believe that reflux of pancreatic enzymes into the biliary tree may contribute to the development of cancer.[15] Because of our limited knowledge of the sequence of molecular changes, there are no known

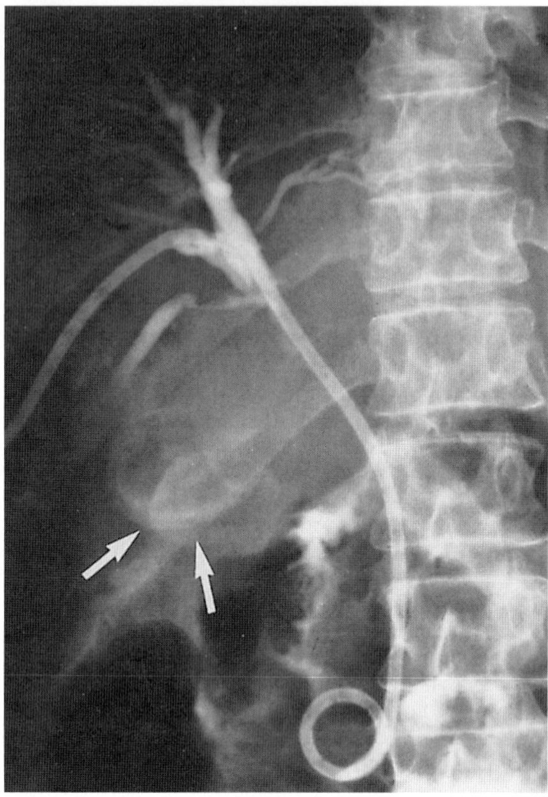

FIGURE 64.1 Unresectable gallbladder cancer demonstrating palliative transhepatic percutaneous stent placed to relieve jaundice. Porcelain gallbladder is present (*arrows*).

detectors of early disease or of risk assessment. Clearly, this is an area that needs improvement, particularly in endemic areas.

The American Joint Committee on Cancer's (AJCC, 6th edition, 2002) tumor, node, metastasis (TNM) Staging System (Table 64.1) reflects prognostic characteristics of tumor depth, regional nodal disease, or distant spread. The gallbladder differs histologically from the rest of the gastrointestinal tract in that it lacks a muscularis mucosa and submucosa. The gallbladder wall is composed of (a) a single layer of columnar cells, the mucosa, and lamina propria; (b) a fibromuscular layer; (c) a perimuscular, subserosal layer containing lymphatics and neurovascular structures; and (d) a serosal surface, except where the gallbladder is embedded in the liver.[17] Because lymphatics are present in the subserosal layer only, tumors invading less than the full thickness of the muscular layer have minimal risk of nodal spread. Thus, disease invading into, but not through, the muscular layer of the gallbladder is stage IA disease, whereas invasion into the perimuscular connective tissue is stage IB. Stage IIA disease includes tumors that have perforated the serosa or have directly invaded the liver or other surrounding structures, which are clearly more advanced but still potentially resectable. Lymph node metastasis is now classified as stage IIB. In line with other pancreaticobiliary malignancies, the stage III grouping refers to locally advanced, unresectable disease and stage IV indicates metastatic disease.

Clinical Findings and Diagnosis

The majority of patients are found to have gallbladder cancer during workup or treatment of cholelithiasis or choledocholithiasis. In patients with symptoms, abdominal pain consistent with biliary colic or acute cholecystitis is most common. Patients also present with jaundice, weight loss, anorexia, or an increase in abdominal girth secondary to ascites. Physical findings include right upper quadrant tenderness or a palpable mass, hepatomegaly, and ascites. Laboratory investigation, if abnormal, is most often consistent with biliary obstruction. Because of its nonspecific presentation and the lack of reliable screening tests, gallbladder cancer is not diagnosed preoperatively in over half the cases.

Imaging evaluation often reveals a thickened gallbladder wall or a mass within or replacing the gallbladder on ultrasound examination. Because polyps and carcinoma can have an echogenicity similar to the gallbladder wall, these lesions are often difficult to distinguish. This is even more difficult when inflammation is present from gallstones. At times, ultrasound can visualize invasion of the liver, adjacent adenopathy, and a dilated biliary tree. The ability of ultrasound to differentiate benign from neoplastic disease is enhanced using endoscopic ultrasound, and may be more specific than computed tomography (CT) or magnetic resonance imaging (MRI).[18,19]

A dynamic contrast-enhanced CT scan may identify a gallbladder mass or invasion into the liver parenchyma or adjacent organs. The classic finding in a patient with gallbladder cancer is asymmetric thickening of the gallbladder wall. The sensitivity and specificity of contrast-enhanced CT in diagnosing neoplastic lesions is close to 90%.[6] Staging of gallbladder carcinoma using CT, however, is limited by poor sensitivity in identifying nodal spread.[20]

In patients who are jaundiced, direct cholangiography may be useful to delineate extent of biliary involvement as well as to palliate symptoms of biliary obstruction. A midbile duct obstruction not caused by gallstones is gallbladder cancer until proved otherwise (Fig. 64.2). More recently, with improvements in MRI technology, magnetic resonance cholangiopancreatography (MRCP) has evolved into a single, noninvasive imaging modality that allows complete assessment of biliary, vascular, hepatic parenchymal, and nodal involvement, as well as involvement of adjacent organs (Fig. 64.3).[21–23]

Surgery

It is clear that the only curative option in patients with gallbladder cancer is complete surgical resection. It is essential for optimal patient care that patients with gallbladder cancer be recognized before laparoscopic cholecystectomy is performed, because of the risk of port site seeding and bile spillage, with its potential for subsequent carcinomatosis.[24]

Role of Staging Laparoscopy

Because a large percentage of patients with gallbladder cancer are found to have occult, unresectable disease at the time of surgical exploration, several authors have investigated the use of initial staging laparoscopy for this disease.[25–28] Because gallbladder cancer has such a propensity to spread intraabdominally, this tumor is ideal for detection of intraabdominal metastases with laparoscopy. This is demonstrated by the fact that up to 50% of patients are found to have unresectable disease at the time of laparoscopy.[25,29] Patients who are found to have unresectable disease at laparoscopy can begin other forms of systemic therapy earlier and may undergo the procedure as an outpatient. Particularly because patients with unresectable disease have a median survival of only 6 months, the impact on quality of life, including decreased length of stay in the hospital, cannot be overemphasized.

Cholecystectomy with or without Partial Hepatectomy

Gallbladder cancer, if not completely surgically removed, results in rapid local progression and death. In a collected

TABLE 64.1 STAGING

AMERICAN JOINT COMMITTEE ON CANCER 6TH EDITION STAGING SYSTEM FOR GALLBLADDER CARCINOMA

Stage	Tumor	Nodes	Metastasis
0	Tis	N0	M0
IA	T1	N0	M0
IB	T2	N0	M0
IIA	T3	N0	M0
IIB	T1	N1	M0
	T2	N1	M0
	T3	N1	M0
III	T4	Any N	M0
IV	Any T	Any N	M1

DEFINITION OF TNM

Primary tumor (T)

TX Primary tumor cannot be assessed
T0 No evidence of primary tumor
Tis Carcinoma *in situ*
T1 Tumor invades the lamina propria or muscle layer
  T1a Tumor invades the lamina propria
  T1b Tumor invades the muscle layer
T2 Tumor invades the perimuscular connective tissue; no extension beyond the serosa or into the liver
T3 Tumor perforates the serosa (visceral peritoneum) or directly invades the liver or one other adjacent organ or structure (e.g., stomach, duodenum, colon, pancreas, omentum, or extrahepatic bile ducts)
T4 Tumor invades main portal vein or hepatic artery or invades multiple extrahepatic organs or structures

Regional lymph nodes (N)

NX Regional lymph nodes cannot be assessed
N0 No regional lymph node metastasis
N1 Regional lymph node metastasis

Distant metastasis (M)

MX Presence of distant metastasis cannot be assessed
M0 No distant metastasis
M1 Distant metastasis

review of 5,836 patients with gallbladder cancer, the overall mean survival was between 2 and 5 months, whereas the 5-year survival was 4%.[3] The 5-year survival of patients undergoing resection with curative intent was 17%. Of the 2,115 patients with unresectable disease, only a single survivor was found at 5 years.[3] Although surgical resection represents the treatment of choice and the only potentially curative therapy available, resection is possible in only 25% of patients at presentation because of the advanced nature of the disease.[3]

There is little doubt that the results of treatment, as well as the scope of operation, are related to depth of tumor penetration (Table 64.2). For tumors limited to the muscular layer of the gallbladder (T1), there is near-universal agreement that simple cholecystectomy is adequate.[30–33] T1 tumors have not yet invaded the subserosal layer, which contains lymphatics, and therefore lymphadenectomy is not required. Attesting to the fact that early gallbladder carcinoma is completely curable, simple cholecystectomy has resulted in nearly 100% survival when early cancer is an incidental finding after elective cholecystectomy.[33,34]

Difficulty can arise at the time of surgery in evaluating polypoid lesions of the gallbladder as either benign or early gallbladder cancer. Although it appears that frozen section diagnosis is fairly reliable in distinguishing whether lesions are malignant or benign (95% accurate), the accuracy in correctly assessing depth of invasion is only 70%.[35] Thus, it may be difficult at the time of surgery to determine the extent of resection. Because of this, pursuing a more aggressive resection if the depth of invasion is in doubt is important for adequate tumor clearance.[36]

The extent of surgical resection for T2 or greater tumors is controversial, with recommendations ranging from simple cholecystectomy to radical excision, including hepatectomy. For advanced local disease, some groups have advocated radical resections, including hepatectomy and pancreatectomy. Whereas it is clear that major hepatic resection can be performed safely with a mortality less than 5% (Table 64.3)[31–34,37,38] it has not been universally accepted that more aggressive resections improve survival. To understand the rationale for extensive resections, it is also important to understand the pattern of spread of gallbladder cancer. Direct extension to the adjacent liver parenchyma often occurs first, followed by adjacent organ involvement, including duodenum, colon, and stomach (see Fig. 64.2). Lymphatic spread of gallbladder cancer is routine, often involving nodes in the porta hepatis, peripancreatic region, celiac axis, and the aortocaval nodal basins.

Because the gallbladder is not surrounded by serosa where it is attached to the liver in the gallbladder fossa, even T2 tumors (full thickness invasion of the muscular layer into the perimuscular connective tissue, no extension beyond serosa or into liver) can invade the normal plane of dissection in the gallbladder fossa during simple cholecystectomy. Therefore, T2 tumors cannot be completely removed with cholecystectomy alone and a radical cholecystectomy, with resection of a 1- to 2-cm rim of normal liver around the gallbladder fossa, is the minimal resection that is required. Many authors, however, have found that segmental resection of segments 4b and 5 of the liver, which abut the gallbladder fossa, results in a more anatomically controlled dissection with less blood loss.[39] An additional part of

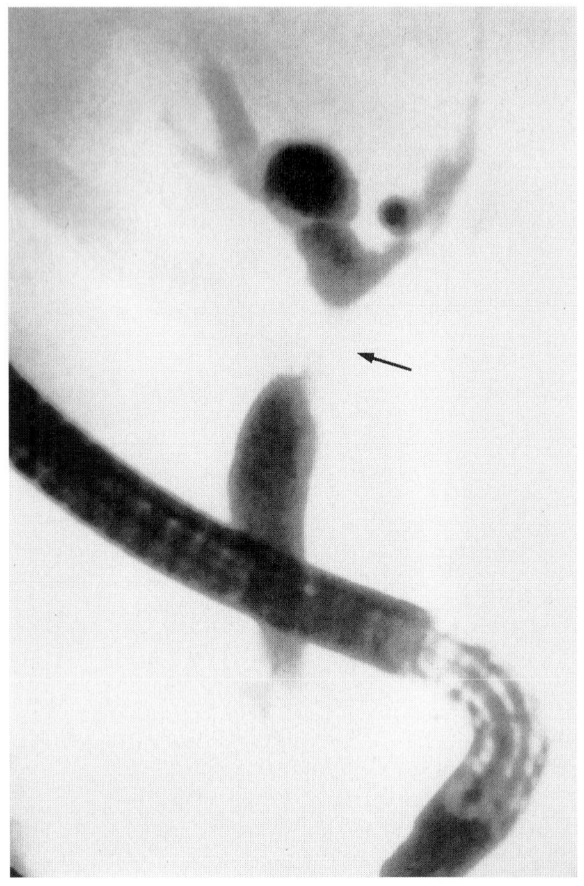

FIGURE 64.2 Endoscopic retrograde cholangiopancreatogram obtained from a patient with gallbladder cancer. Midbile duct obstruction (*arrow*) is caused by direct extension of tumor to the cystic and common hepatic duct.

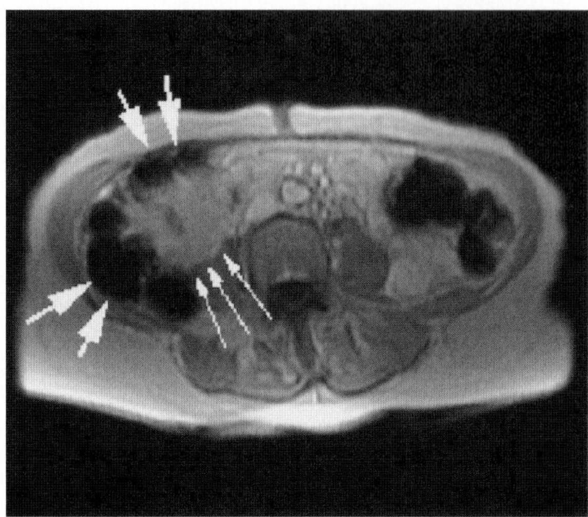

FIGURE 64.3 T_1-weighted magnetic resonance imaging scan of a patient with gallbladder cancer (*small arrows*) with extension into the duodenum and the hepatic flexure of colon (*large arrows*).

the definitive surgical treatment is regional lymphadenectomy, because about half the patients with T2 tumors are found to have nodal spread after resection.[12] Dissection of lymph nodes should include all tissue from the bifurcation of the hepatic ducts to the distal common bile duct. Proponents of this approach advocate liver resection on the basis that it is the only way to obtain an adequate margin on the hepatic side of the gallbladder and resection of the regional nodes allows the best chance for complete tumor clearance. For all of these reasons, simple cholecystectomy is inadequate for T2 or greater tumors. When larger anatomic hepatic resections have been performed in patients with T2 tumors, it has increased the 5-year survival from 25% to 40% after simple cholecystectomy to 70% to 100% after radical resection.[30–32,37,40,41]

For T3 and T4 lesions, there is a high likelihood of intraperitoneal and hematogenous spread and significant morbidity from the radical procedures that are often necessary for excision of local disease. Recent series, however, support an aggressive approach to resection of these large tumors, particularly if no indication of nodal involvement is found (see Table 64.3). For T3 and resectable T4 tumors, a minimal resection includes segments 4b and 5, and in many cases an extended right hepatectomy (segments 4, 5, 6, 7, and 8) may be necessary to obtain complete resection. With aggressive

TABLE 64.2 RESULTS

FIVE-YEAR SURVIVAL AFTER RESECTION FOR GALLBLADDER CANCER

	T1 or T2 tumors		T3 or T4 tumors	
Author	**Simple cholecystectomy (%)**	**Radical cholecystectomy or segmental resection (%)**	**Simple cholecystectomy (%)**	**Radical cholecystectomy or segmental resection (%)**
Wanebo et al., 1982[41]	33	—	3	13
Ouchi et al., 1987[30]	57	100	0	23
Nakamura et al., 1989[38]	—	100	—	15
Donohue et al., 1990[31]	—	—	0	29
Shirai et al., 1992[33]	—	72	—	37
Fong et al., 2000[47]	—	58 (T2)	—	25%
Wakai et al., 2001[117]	100* (10-year survival, T1b only)	75* (10-year survival, T1b only)	—	—

*No significant difference.

TABLE 64.3 RESULTS

RESULTS AFTER RADICAL RESECTION FOR GALLBLADDER CANCER

Author	Number resected	Mortality (%)	Five-year survival (%)
Nakamura et al., 1989[38]	15	0	25
Donohue et al., 1990[31]	42	2	33
Ogura et al., 1991[32]	1686	5	51
Shirai et al., 1992[33]	40	0	65
Bartlett et al., 1996[37] and Fong et al., 2000[47]	102	4	58
Taner et al., 2004[118]	131	2	13

resection, long-term survival can be achieved even for patients with these more advanced tumors.[31–33,37,38,42]

Surgical exploration should be performed for all patients without medical contraindications. If a T1 tumor is suspected, a cholecystectomy and biopsy of regional nodes should be performed after thorough examination of the abdominal cavity for any signs of tumor dissemination. The pathology and depth of penetration should be confirmed by frozen section, and the procedure terminated if a T1 tumor with negative margins is confirmed. For T2 lesions, either a radical cholecystectomy (wedge resection of the hepatic bed) or a segment 4b and 5 resection with lymphadenectomy should be performed.[37] For T3 lesions, a segment 4b and 5 resection or extended right hepatectomy is performed. Finally, for T4 lesions, a more radical excision of the liver, such as extended right hepatectomy, usually must be performed for adequate tumor clearance.

Tumor location may be important in determining the extent of resection. If the tumor arises in the gallbladder infundibulum, the common bile duct is often involved with tumor, either by direct extension or external invasion of the hepatoduodenal ligament. In this case, an extended liver resection and removal of a portion of the common bile duct (CBD) should be performed. Reconstruction is then performed by Roux-en-Y hepaticojejunostomy. Tumor arising in the fundus of the gallbladder, however, can be treated with limited hepatic resection without excision of the CBD. To clear the lymph nodes in the porta hepatis, complete lymphadenectomy should be performed skeletonizing the CBD, hepatic artery, and portal vein.

Incidentally or Laparoscopically Discovered Gallbladder Cancer

Gallbladder cancer is often discovered during pathologic examination after cholecystectomy for presumed benign gallstone disease. Because of the popularization of laparoscopic cholecystectomy in the past decade, an increasing number of patients with gallbladder cancer are found incidentally. Patients with T2 or greater tumors and no signs of distant disease should be offered radical resection to eradicate all disease. Even if grossly normal, excision of laparoscopic port sites should also be performed because of the well-documented history of port-site seeding.[40,43–45]

Patients presenting with gallbladder cancers after a recent cholecystectomy pose additional technical challenges. Often postoperative inflammation occurs in the right upper quadrant that hinders distinction of tumor from normal tissue. Bile spillage at the time of the initial operation may result in carcinomatosis.[46] Determination of ductal or nodal involvement by tumor is always difficult at the time of reoperation. In addition, postoperative fibrosis often encases the right hepatic artery, which crosses behind the bile duct in most patients. Because of this, during a second operation for incidentally discovered gallbladder cancer, an extended right hepatectomy along with excision of the extrahepatic biliary tree and portal lymphadenectomy is often necessary. This resection allows adequate exposure for lymphadenectomy, greater confidence of a negative margin on the bile duct, and permits biliary reconstruction to only one side of the liver. The disadvantage is that a large portion of normal liver parenchyma is sacrificed and, consequently, transient postoperative liver dysfunction is common. Although it may be more difficult to curatively resect disease in patients with incidentally discovered gallbladder cancer after laparoscopic cholecystectomy, there is no difference in overall survival between patients with incidentally discovered gallbladder cancer who are submitted to curative resection and those patients who undergo initial curative resection.[47]

When a patient presents with T1 gallbladder cancer discovered after simple cholecystectomy, the pathology should be reviewed to determine if the entire gallbladder has been removed and if the cystic duct margin is clear of tumor. If the cystic duct margin is positive, the patient requires bile duct excision. If all margins are negative, no further therapy is warranted. If the tumor is proved to be T2 or greater, the patient should undergo reexcision to attempt complete resection if the extent of disease evaluation is negative. Patients with a known or suspected early gallbladder carcinoma should not undergo laparoscopic cholecystectomy. Rather, open exploration and cholecystectomy should be performed.

Adjuvant Therapy

Adjuvant therapy for gallbladder cancer remains a controversial and unproved consideration. Very few randomized trials have been conducted, and those that have are limited because of the number of patients included. Given the relative rarity of these malignancies in the United States, large-scale, randomized trials are feasible only in the context of a multi-institutional or cooperative group setting.

One recent prospective, randomized phase III trial of adjuvant chemotherapy with 5-flurouracil and mitomycin C versus surgery alone for patients with pancreaticobiliary malignancies having resection found that in the subset of patients with gallbladder cancer (n = 112), the 5-year survival rate was significantly better in the adjuvant group (26%) versus the control group (14%).[48] Similarly, the 5-year. disease-free survival rate was 20.3% versus 11.6%, clearly favoring the adjuvantly treated group. This trial suggests that adjuvant chemotherapy may offer benefit for patients with resected gallbladder cancer; however, replication in a larger scale setting is required before definitive conclusions can be drawn.

Prognosis

The 5-year survival rate for all patients with gallbladder cancer is less than 5% in most series, with a median survival of 6 months. This is primarily because most patients present with unresectable disease. Of those patients undergoing resection, survival is dependent on depth of penetration and nodal status. Nearly 100% survival is reported after simple cholecystectomy for T1 disease, whereas patients with T2 and T3 tumors without nodal disease have a 5-year survival greater than 50%.[33,37,38,40] Node positivity is an ominous finding, with few series reporting 5-year survivors.

Follow-up after Resection for Gallbladder Cancer

The most common sites of recurrence after resection of gallbladder cancer include carcinomatosis, intrahepatic metastases, or nodal recurrence in the retroperitoneum. Jaundice is a common sign, but patients with recurrence may also present with ascites caused by carcinomatosis. For most tumors, local recurrence is found synchronously with diffuse intraabdominal spread. Therefore, surgical treatment of recurrence has little potential for cure. If recurrent disease is found after resection, prognosis is exceedingly poor, with death occurring secondary to biliary sepsis or liver failure within months of diagnosis.

The main goal of follow-up after resection of gallbladder cancer is to provide palliation for symptomatic recurrences. The main symptoms associated with recurrence requiring palliation are pruritus or cholangitis associated with jaundice, or bowel obstruction associated with carcinomatosis. Additional goals of follow-up are to detect benign complications of surgical treatment such as biliary stricture. When jaundice or cholangitis is the presenting symptom of possible recurrence, a nonsurgical palliative approach using percutaneous transhepatic cholangiogram (PTC) and stenting is usually favored unless a benign postsurgical stricture is suspected. Because of the rapid growth of tumor in patients with recurrence, the hospitalization and recovery time from a surgical bypass is usually not justified for recurrences resulting in biliary obstruction.

The routine follow-up of a patient after resection of gallbladder cancer includes office visits every 3 months with physical examination and measurement of liver function tests. Although CA19-9 may be elevated in patients with gallbladder cancer, the sensitivity and specificity are poor[49] and, thus, should not be used for screening patients for recurrence. Because an asymptomatic recurrence of gallbladder cancer has only limited treatment options, overaggressive use of imaging studies is not warranted. Therefore, the use of imaging studies should be individualized.

Issues for the Future

Clearly, improving our ability to recognize early gallbladder cancer in high-risk geographic areas would have an important impact on outcome in these patients. This will likely require improvements in understanding the sequential molecular changes associated with gallbladder cancer. Other improvements in screening programs in high-risk areas, which could result in prophylactic cholecystectomy, would likely be beneficial.[50]

BILE DUCT CARCINOMA

One of the most technically difficult surgical resections occurs in patients with bile duct tumors arising in the hepatic hilus, named Klatskin tumors, or hilar cholangiocarcinoma. Bile duct cancers can arise at other sites, including within the liver (intrahepatic cholangiocarcinoma) and below the biliary bifurcation but above the pancreas (midbile duct cholangiocarcinoma). Distal cholangiocarcinoma involves that portion of the bile duct within the pancreas, which requires pancreaticoduodenectomy. The location of the tumor affects prognosis as well as the potential for curative resection.

Resection of biliary neoplasms, particularly hilar cholangiocarcinoma, often requires radical resections and complex biliary reconstructions that have only recently become safe in routine practice. Surgery may also offer effective palliation for these cancers by providing biliary bypass for jaundiced patients with unresectable tumors. Because disease is often diagnosed late in the course and because complex operative techniques are required for potentially curative resection, these tumors represent one of the greatest challenges for definitive treatment. Adding to this is that there are no proved effective options for adjuvant treatment.

Incidence

The overall incidence of hilar cholangiocarcinoma in the United States is 1.0/100,000 per year, although other geographic regions such as Israel and Japan have higher rates.[51] The incidence of intrahepatic cholangiocarcinoma in the United States is approximately 0.7/100,000 with a similar mortality. During the last 30 years, it appears that both the incidence and mortality in the United States are increasing.[52] Cholangiocarcinomas arise slightly more often in males,[53] with a male-to-female ratio of 1.3:1 and an average age of 50 to 70 years.

Risk factors for this disease include primary sclerosing cholangitis, ulcerative colitis, choledochal cysts, and biliary tract infection, either with *Clonorchis* or in chronic typhoid carriers.[54] Treating patients with cholangiocarcinoma arising from one of these underlying conditions is challenging.[55] Some industrial chemicals (e.g., nitrosamines, dioxin, asbestos, and polychlorinated biphenyls) have also been implicated in the pathogenesis of cholangiocarcinoma.[51] Although there has been some suggestion of an increased risk of cholangiocarcinoma arising after transduodenal sphincteroplasty,[56] it is difficult to determine if this is caused by the surgical intervention or the underlying disease leading to sphincteroplasty.

Pathology and Staging

Similar to gallbladder cancer, bile duct tumors tend to invade locally. Over 95% of these tumors are adenocarcinomas. They are morphologically described as nodular, which is the most common, scirrhous, diffusely infiltrating, or papillary. Histologic subtypes include acinar, ductular, trabecular, alveolar, and papillary. Papillary tumors appear to have an improved outcome. Much less common types of bile duct tumors include cystadenocarcinomas, hemangioendotheliomas, and mucoepidermoid carcinomas. Perineural invasion is clearly a poor prognostic sign.[57]

In patients with intrahepatic cholangiocarcinoma, negative prognostic signs include vascular invasion, multiple tumors, positive margin, large size, and lymph node metastases.[58] These tumors can be either sclerotic, masslike lesions, or cystic lesions.

Historically, cholangiocarcinomas have been classified according to their location in the upper (60%), middle (15% to 20%), or lower third (15% to 20%) of the bile duct. Middle-third lesions arise between the cystic duct and the superior border of the duodenum. Lower-third lesions are found below the superior border of the duodenum, but above the ampulla. The problem with this classification is that the anatomic landmarks are somewhat arbitrary and not clinically useful. Most midbile duct malignant obstructions are caused by gallbladder cancer. Even when it is truly a midbile duct cholangiocarcinoma, very few of these tumors are amenable to treatment by local excision of the bile duct.

A more useful classification is to divide these lesions into upper half or lower half tumors, based on the location of the cystic duct as it enters the common duct (in the case of normal anatomy). The usefulness of this classification scheme is that it allows the surgeon to delineate whether a hepatic or pancreatic resection will be required for clearance of tumor. The AJCC TNM Staging System (6th edition) for bile duct cancers is described in Table 64.4.

Other staging systems have been created that attempt to incorporate clinically important indicators of resectability for hilar cholangiocarcinoma that are defined preoperatively, including hepatic lobe atrophy or portal vein involvement.[59] With the increasing acceptance of major hepatic resection for these tumors, this preoperative staging system attempts to define whether there is ipsilateral involvement alone, because tumors with bilateral extension past the primary biliary radicles are not resectable.

Clinical Findings and Diagnosis

The vast majority of patients with cholangiocarcinoma present with painless jaundice, though mild right upper quadrant pain, pruritus, anorexia, malaise, and weight loss may also be reported. Cholangitis is the presenting symptom in 10% to 30% of patients. Some patients have cancer discovered on evaluation for otherwise asymptomatic elevations of alkaline phosphatase and gamma glutamyl transferase.

Patients with intrahepatic cholangiocarcinoma are usually asymptomatic. Many patients are found to have a liver tumor present on cross-sectional imaging obtained for other reasons. Many of these patients will present to the surgeon with a biopsy showing adenocarcinoma without a known primary tumor. The standard evaluation in these patients should include tumor markers to rule out an elevated carcinoembryonic antigen (CEA) or α-fetoprotein (AFP), upper and lower endoscopy to evaluate for a gastrointestinal source; CT scan to assess for a primary tumor in the gastrointestinal tract or pancreas; and, in women, a mammogram. If no site of primary disease is found, in the majority of patients, the diagnosis is intrahepatic cholangiocarcinoma.

A variety of imaging tests are available to assess patients with hilar cholangiocarcinoma. Abdominal ultrasound is noninvasive, easily available, and inexpensive, and thus is commonly used as a first imaging modality. It can establish the level of biliary obstruction and rule out cholelithiasis or choledocholithiasis as the etiology. CT scans frequently reveal dilated intrahepatic biliary ducts with a normal, collapsed gallbladder, and, depending on the level of the tumor, a nondilated or partially dilated extrahepatic biliary tree (Fig. 64.4). In addition, the presence of hilar adenopathy can be assessed. Portal vein patency can be determined with ultrasound or helical CT. In addition, signs of hepatic lobar atrophy should be sought, because this is associated with a high incidence of ipsilateral portal vein involvement by tumor. MRCP offers the potential of evaluating parenchymal, vascular, biliary, and nodal involvement with a single noninvasive examination.[21–23] Frequently, it is possible to visualize the tumor itself with MRI (Figs. 64.5, 64.6).

In most centers, direct cholangiography is used to evaluate the extent of biliary involvement and provide palliation for

TABLE 64.4 STAGING

AMERICAN JOINT COMMITTEE ON CANCER, 6TH EDITION, STAGING SYSTEM FOR EXTRAHEPATIC BILE DUCT CARCINOMA

Stage	Tumor	Nodes	Metastasis
0	Tis	N0	M0
IA	T1	N0	M0
IB	T2	N0	M0
IIA	T3	N0	M0
IIB	T1	N1	M0
	T2	N1	M0
	T3	N1	M0
III	T4	Any N	M0
IV	Any T	Any N	M1

DEFINITION OF TNM

Primary tumor (T)

TX Primary tumor cannot be assessed
T0 No evidence of primary tumor
Tis Carcinoma *in situ*
T1 Tumor confined to bile duct histologically
T2 Tumor invades beyond the wall of the bile duct
T3 Tumor invades the liver, gallbladder, pancreas, or unilateral branches of the portal vein or hepatic artery
T4 Tumor invades any of the following: main portal vein or its branches, common hepatic artery, or other adjacent structures (e.g., colon, stomach, duodenum, abdominal wall).

Regional lymph nodes (N)

NX Regional lymph nodes cannot be assessed
N0 No regional lymph node metastasis
N1 Regional lymph node metastasis

Distant metastasis (M)

MX Presence of distant metastasis cannot be assessed
M0 No distant metastasis
M1 Distant metastasis

jaundice. Endoscopic retrograde cholangiopancreatography (ERCP) has little role to play in high biliary obstruction because opacification of the proximal biliary tree is difficult. ERCP, however, can be effectively used to image more distal lesions. At the time cholangiography is performed, some authors advocate the routine preoperative placement of biliary drainage catheters to aid in intraoperative identification of the bile ducts.[60,61] Others have found a higher incidence of infectious complications[62] and mortality,[63] and a longer hospital stay[64] after preoperative placement of biliary drainage catheters. The difficulty in making the decision regarding preoperative stenting is that many patients are severely symptomatic because of jaundice and pruritus and require palliation, thus with a delay in operative intervention many patients require palliation.

In many cases, it is difficult to obtain pathologic confirmation of cholangiocarcinoma except in very advanced cases, even with the use of biliary brushings and cytology obtained at the time of direct cholangiography. In most cases, patients are offered surgical therapy based on clinical suspicion and radiographic appearance. In patients with intrahepatic cholangiocarcinoma, cross-sectional imaging with CT scan is usually sufficient. Tumors may be masslike or may have cystic areas.

Surgery

Proximal Cholangiocarcinomas

Untreated, most patients with bile duct cancers die within a year of diagnosis.[64,65] Surgical excision is the treatment of choice, with no other potentially curative therapy. The immediate causes of death are most commonly hepatic failure or cholangitis related to tumor growth and inadequate drainage of the biliary tree.[66] Therefore, the objectives of management for patients with cholangiocarcinoma include both complete removal of tumor and adequate biliary drainage. It has become clear over the last three decades that curative treatment for patients with tumors involving the upper half of the bile duct depends on aggressive excision that often requires a major liver resection. Until as recently as one decade ago, treatment of hilar cholangiocarcinomas was associated with mortality as high as 30%.[67–71] Recently, major improvements in the safety of these operations has been demonstrated, and resection of hilar tumors now results in mortality of less than 10%, even when liver resections are required.[67,68,70,72]

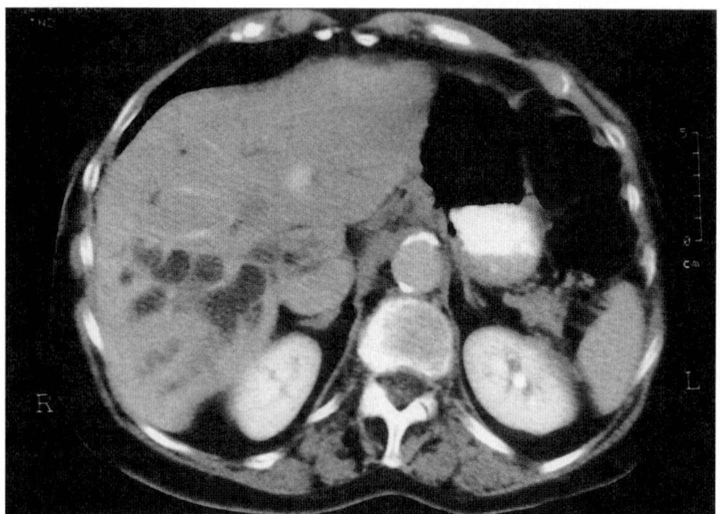

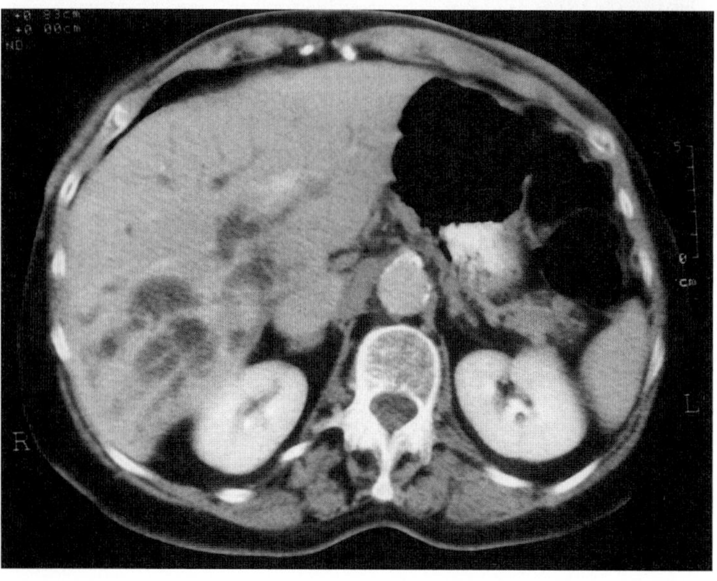

FIGURE 64.4 Computed tomography scan in a patient with hilar cholangiocarcinoma, demonstrating dilated intrahepatic ducts in the right lobe but inability to directly visualize tumor.

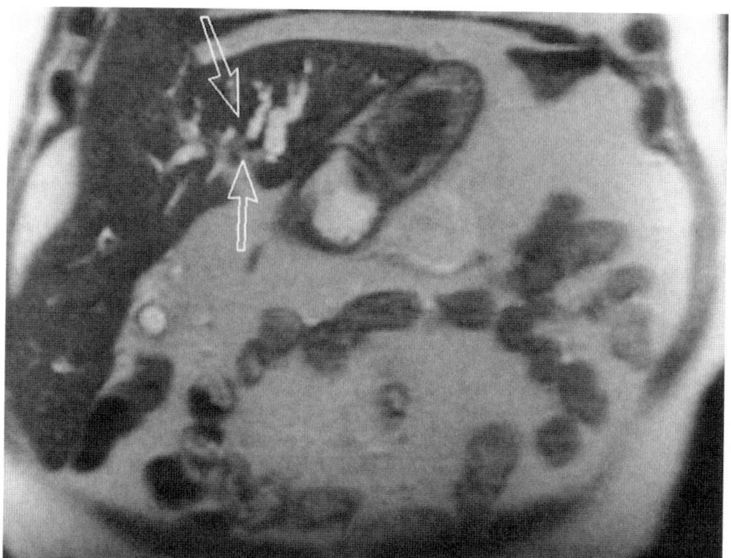

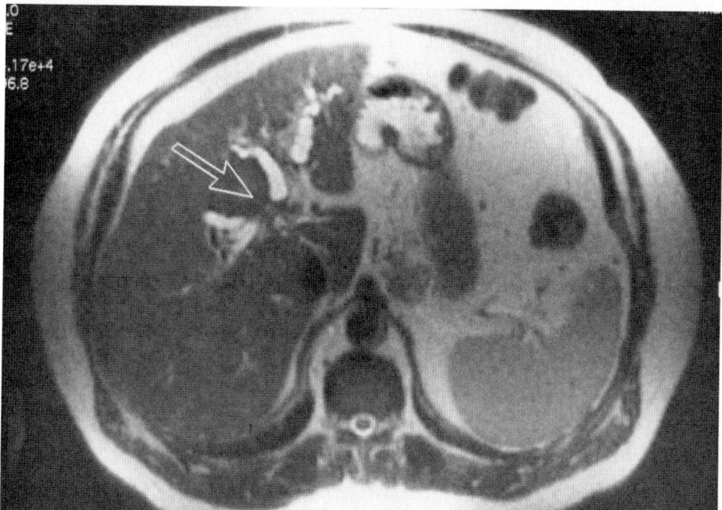

FIGURE 64.5 Coronal (*A*) and axial (*B*) magnetic resonance imaging in a patient with hilar cholangiocarcinoma. Dilated intrahepatic ducts are present with a soft tissue density consistent with tumor (*arrows*).

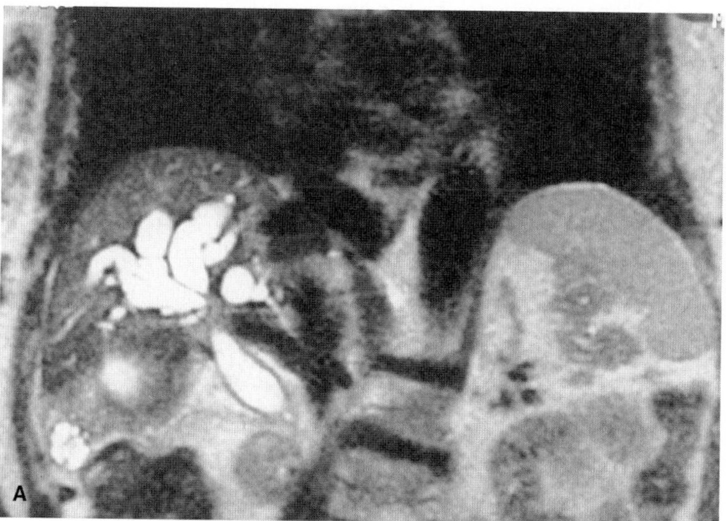

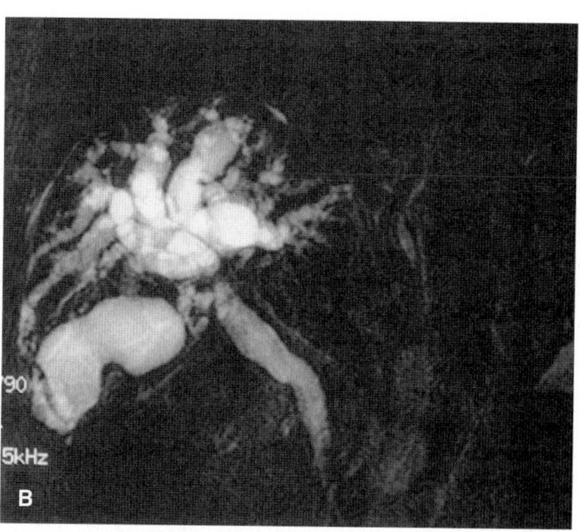

FIGURE 64.6 Coronal (*A*) magnetic resonance imaging and magnetic resonance cholangiopancreatography (*B*) in a patient with hilar cholangiocarcinoma, demonstrating dilated intrahepatic ducts narrowing at the area of obstruction.

Assessment of Resectability and Surgical Procedure

Surgical exploration is often the only means of assessing resectability. Because of the potential morbidity of a laparotomy that has no therapeutic benefit, staging laparoscopy has been advocated to save patients from unnecessary laparotomy. In patients with hilar cholangiocarcinoma, up to 25% will benefit from staging laparoscopy because of detection of occult extrahepatic disease.[25,29] Laparoscopy is a very sensitive means to detect peritoneal metastases or additional intrahepatic disease through the use of laparoscopic ultrasound, but is less sensitive in detecting nodal metastases or locally invasive tumors.[25]

Hilar cholangiocarcinoma is considered unresectable because of both local factors and metastatic spread. Clearly, patients with disease outside the liver, including most commonly peritoneal and intrahepatic metastases, are not amenable to curative resection. Local factors that make these tumors unresectable include invasion of the main portal vein or both the right and left portal vein and hepatic arteries and tumor extension into second-order biliary radicals of both right and left hepatic lobes. By contrast, tumors extending into second- or third-order biliary radicles on one side of the liver without vascular involvement can be resected with curative outcome.

The goals of surgical management for cholangiocarcinomas are both eradication of tumor and establishment of adequate biliary drainage. Tumors of the biliary confluence are particularly difficult to treat because symptoms often appear late in the course of disease when the lesion has already involved adjacent structures including the portal vein or adjacent hepatic parenchyma. Complete resection, therefore, requires biliary and hepatic resection and often major vascular reconstruction. It is not surprising, therefore, that in the past the surgical therapy for proximal biliary malignancies consisted mainly of biliary-enteric bypass as palliation for jaundice and cholangitis. The therapeutic approach to hilar cholangiocarcinoma was largely nihilistic, because of difficulty in delineating the extent of disease and the technical challenge of complete resection for such lesions.

Over the last decade, surgical approaches have become more aggressive, as demonstrated by the increasing number of hepatic resections that have been performed for bile duct cancers.[67–71] Recent improvements in ultrasound, CT, MRI, and angiography have greatly facilitated preoperative diagnoses and staging of cholangiocarcinoma. This has allowed improved patient selection and surgical planning. The location and local extension of tumor dictates the extent of resection, with most lesions requiring an extended right or left hepatectomy for complete excision. Caudate resection is often required because of direct extension into caudate biliary radicles or parenchyma.[59,70,71] CBD excision and portal lymphadenectomy are also essential for tumor clearance.

Prognosis after Resection

Results of major studies on resection of hilar cholangiocarcinoma are summarized in Table 64.5. In patients amenable to curative resection, the median survival is 35 months with a 5-year survival rate of 10% to 30%.[60,67,68,71,73–80] Surgical resection provides both improved survival and improved quality of life.[81] The greatest risk factors for recurrence include the presence of positive margins[81] and node-positive tumors.[82]

Prognosis after Resection for Intrahepatic or Distal Cholangiocarcinoma

In patients with intrahepatic cholangiocarcinoma, expected 3-year survival rates as high as 60% have been reported,[25,83] with 5-year survival rates of 30% to 45%.[84] Patients with unresectable disease have a median survival of 12 months.[85,86] Thus, completely resected intrahepatic cholangiocarcinoma appears to have an improved prognosis over proximal (hilar) cholangiocarcinoma.

Most patients with distal cholangiocarcinomas are definitively managed with pancreaticoduodenectomy (Whipple procedure) to obtain adequate clearance of tumor, because of the intrapancreatic location of the distal CBD. Patients with cholangiocarcinomas arising in the distal bile duct have both an increased resectability rate and improved prognosis over those with hilar cholangiocarcinomas.[72] Patients with resectable distal bile duct cancer have a 5-year survival rate of 30% to 50%,[84,87] with a decreased survival if nodes are involved with tumor.[87]

Surgical Treatment of Unresectable Cholangiocarcinoma

For patients with unresectable hilar cholangiocarcinomas, significant improvement in quality of life can occur with surgical bypass. Palliative bypass can be performed in several ways. A partial excision of the left lateral segment and biliary-enteric anastomosis to the left hepatic duct (Longmire procedure)

TABLE 64.5 RESULTS

RESULTS AFTER RESECTION FOR HILAR CHOLANGIOCARCINOMA

Author	N	Percent resected	Postoperative mortality (%)	Five-year survival (%)	Survival (months)	
					Mean	Median
Cameron et al., 1990[60]	96	55	2	8		18
Hadjis et al., 1990[71]	131	21	7	12	25	
Altaee et al., 1991[67]	70	21		19		12
Baer et al., 1993[68]	48	44	4	23	34	
McMasters et al., 1997[75]	91	44	0	26		22
Klempnauer et al., 1997[78]	151		10	28		24
Nagino et al., 1999[76]	173	80	10	26		
Nakeeb et al., 2002[77]	72	57		34		
Jarnagin et al., 2001[79]	225	71	10	27		35
Rea et al., 2004[80]	46		9	26		28

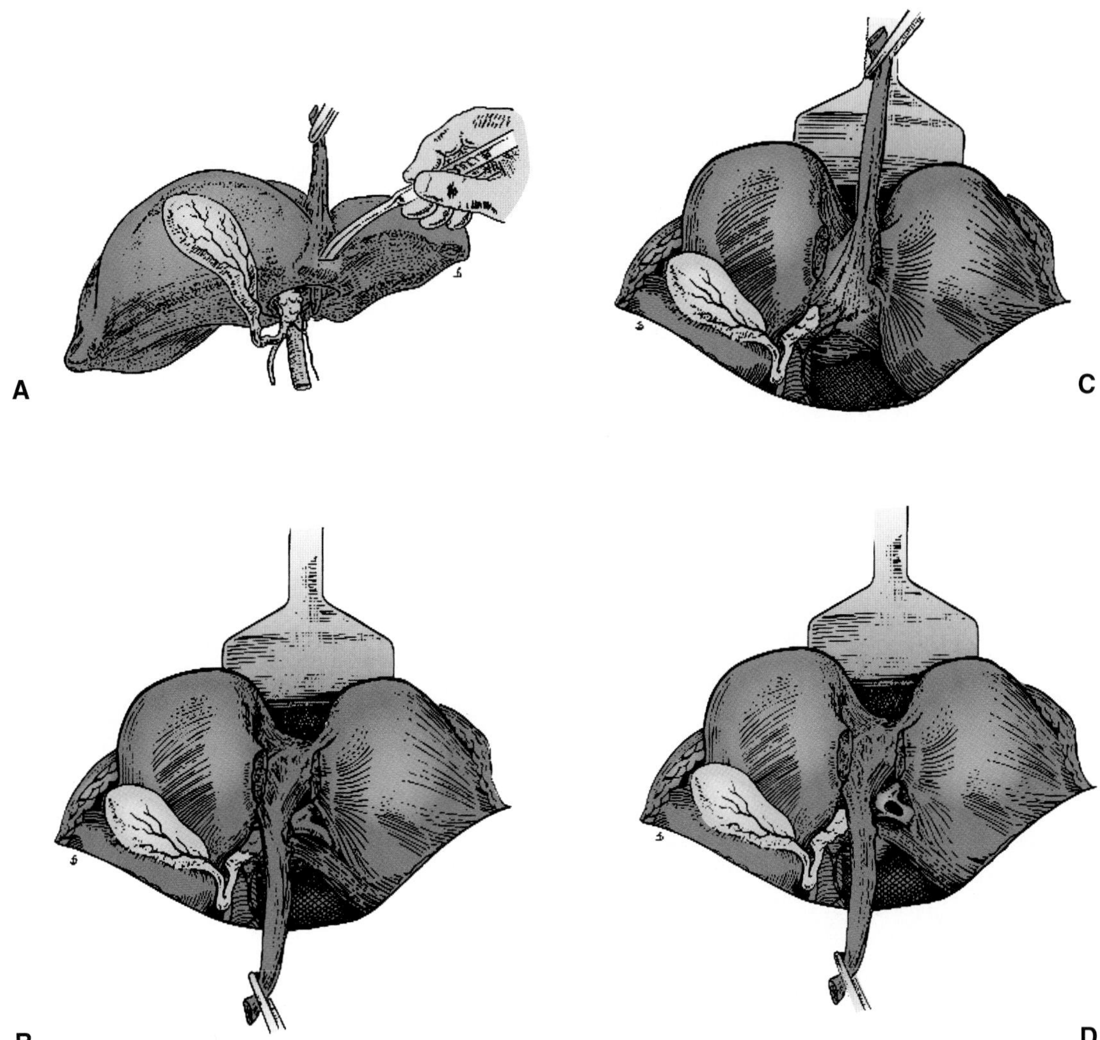

FIGURE 64.7 Surgical approach to segment III duct. (*A*) The bridge of tissue present at the base of the liver is divided. (*B*) The ligamentum teres is held superiorly to expose the tissue overlying the segment III duct. (*C*) The segment III duct is exposed. (*D*) The duct is opened in preparation for anastomosis with a Roux-en-Y jejunal limb. (Courtesy of Dr. L. H. Blumgart.)

was used commonly in the past, but more recently surgical techniques have become less complicated and do not require hepatic parenchymal transection. One technique involves biliary decompression through the left duct, approached through the round ligament, a segment III bypass (Fig. 64.7). Opening the bridge of tissue just beneath the ligamentum teres allows access to the duct. In this position, a long anastomosis can be performed from the segment III duct to a jejunal limb because of the horizontal course of the duct in this location. Although less commonly used, the right hepatic duct can be approached at the base of the gallbladder fossa. This is technically more difficult and results in a higher rate of late bypass failure.[88]

Nonoperative palliative biliary decompression can be accomplished with percutaneous or endoscopic stenting, depending on the level of obstruction. Proximal lesions are usually approached percutaneously with placement of expandable stents or drainage catheters (Fig. 64.8). Internal stents result in fewer electrolyte abnormalities and improvement in patient comfort, although morbidity and mortality occurs in up to 30% of patients and stent occlusion is common.[89–91] There is a significant risk of cholangitis with external and internal drainage, occurring in over 90% of patients with metallic expandable internal stents in one series.[90] Bleeding and bile leaks are also frequent complications. More recent techniques (e.g., photodynamic therapy) have been used to palliate patients with biliary obstruction and may hold some promise for the future.[92]

Because patients with unresectable disease have a short median survival, those whose disease is clearly unresectable on preoperative imaging should undergo percutaneous internal or external drainage. In patients who undergo exploratory surgery and whose disease is found to be unresectable, surgical bypass offers fewer episodes of cholangitis, with an improved quality of life. In some series, surgical bypass for patients with unresectable disease is the only biliary drainage procedure ever required by the patient.

In patients with unresectable distal cholangiocarcinomas, palliation can be achieved with surgical bypass, percutaneous biliary drains, or ERCP-placed stents. The simplest and most effective way to relieve jaundice is usually with an ERCP stent. Although surgical bypass offers improved patency and fewer episodes of cholangitis, the morbidity of the procedure is not warranted in patients with these aggressive tumors.

A

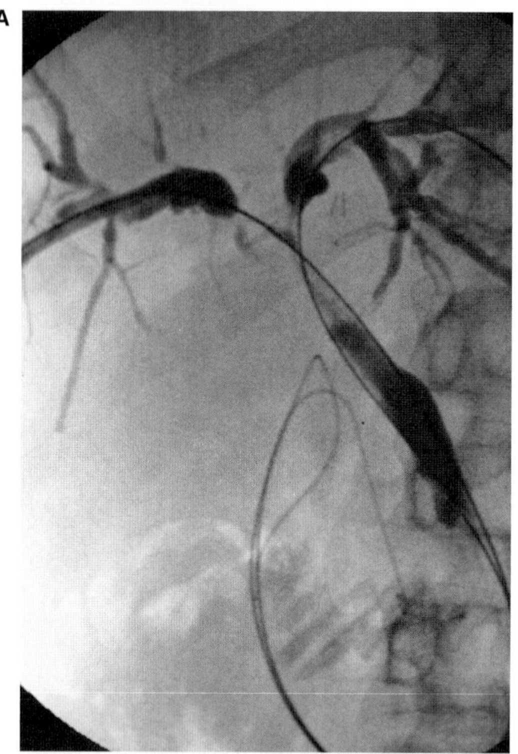

B

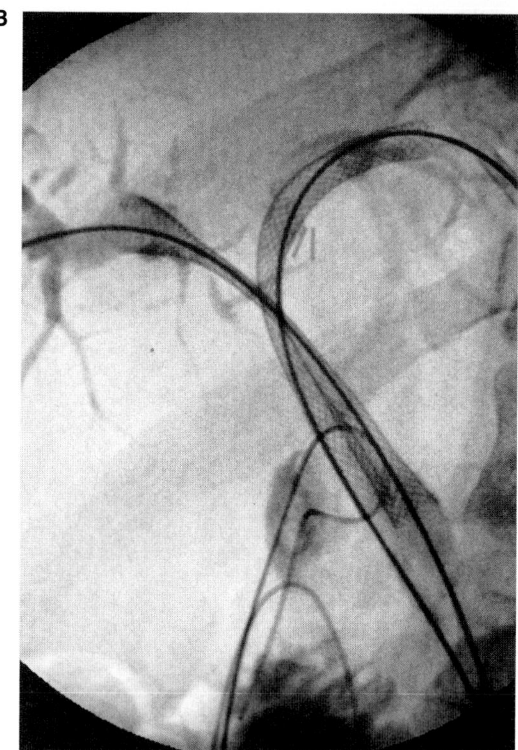

C

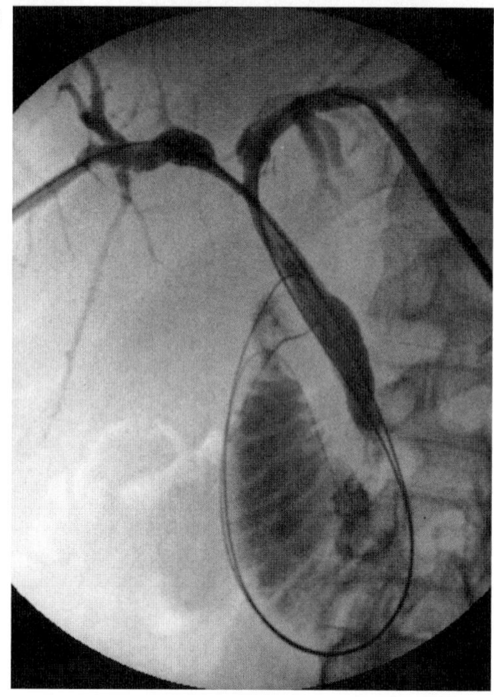

FIGURE 64.8 (*A*) Percutaneous transhepatic cholangiogram in a patient with hilar cholangiocarcinoma, demonstrating biliary obstruction at the confluence. The patient has previously had placement of internal/external stents for biliary drainage. (*B*) Film demonstrates appearance of wall stents after deployment into the left and right biliary ducts. (*C*) After stenting, the cholangiogram demonstrates adequate biliary drainage, with contrast filling the duodenum.

INTRAHEPATIC CHOLANGIOCARCINOMA

Patients with intrahepatic cholangiocarcinoma typically present with single liver lesions. The procedure of choice is anatomically based hepatic resection. Because these tumors are frequently asymptomatic, there are fewer issues with palliative management.

Adjuvant Therapy

To date, no chemotherapeutic regimen has consistently shown activity against cholangiocarcinoma. Many of the issues that pertain to chemotherapy trials in gallbladder cancer are directly relevant to the interpretation of trials for cholangiocarcinomas. Studies performed to date have typically been small, single institution trials, including patients with both gallbladder and bile duct cancers.[93]

Although 5-fluorouracil (5-FU)–based chemotherapy is often offered to patients with unresectable disease, the likelihood of response is less than 10%. Capecitabine as a single agent may have some modest activity in cholangiocarcinomas.[94] The use of mitomycin C and doxorubicin (Adriamycin), in combination with 5-FU, has resulted in combined response rates of less than 30%, with higher toxicity than 5-FU alone.[95] There is no proved role for adjuvant chemotherapy in the treatment of cholangiocarcinoma.

In cases of unresectable cholangiocarcinoma, the use of external beam radiation therapy has been explored.[96–99] To date, no study has clearly demonstrated efficacy for this modality. Anecdotal reports of long-term survivors after external beam radiotherapy show that some individuals may benefit from such treatment, but this must be weighed against the potential complications (e.g., duodenal or bile duct stenosis and duodenitis). The most encouraging results involve use of intraoperative[97,100] or interstitial radiation.[90,98,101] Our current practice is to use combined interstitial radiation and external beam radiation in unresectable cases after palliative bypass. In patients whose disease is resected, adjuvant radiotherapy has not been shown to increase quality of life or survival.[102]

Follow-up after Resection of Cholangiocarcinoma

The most likely site of recurrence after resection of a hilar cholangiocarcinoma is locally within the bile duct, regional lymph nodes, or liver. Therapy for recurrence is palliative. Surgical re-excision is usually impossible because of the challenging anatomic location and the radical procedures that are required for resection of the primary tumor. Therefore, the goal of follow-up is diagnosis of symptomatic recurrences to direct palliative therapy and diagnosis of benign complications of surgical treatment (e.g., biliary strictures). The main symptoms of recurrence that demand palliation are pruritus or cholangitis associated with jaundice. For biliary drainage to relieve jaundice or cholangitis, either surgical drainage[90] or drainage by PTC can be effective.[103] Endoscopic drainage has little role in the relief of jaundice in patients who have had Roux-en-Y biliary reconstruction. For limited recurrences, intraluminal brachytherapy[104] or external beam radiotherapy[105] may improve palliation and, potentially, survival.

Routine follow-up consists of office visits every 3 months with physical examination and measurement of liver function tests. Although a rising alkaline phosphatase level is a good indicator of evolving biliary obstruction, patients recovering from liver resection and biliary obstruction can have persistent elevations of alkaline phosphatase. Up to 10% of patients with biliary surgical reconstruction, however, may develop a benign anastomotic stricture. Most patients with recurrence or a benign stricture will present with jaundice or cholangitis. Because there is a low likelihood of effective therapy for recurrences, the routine use of tumor markers is not recommended, although a fair percentage of biliary malignancies will express CEA or CA 19-9. The routine use of imaging studies to follow patients with cholangiocarcinoma after resection should be limited for the same reasons. When patients become symptomatic with jaundice, an abdominal ultrasound should be obtained. Other imaging will usually be dictated by the sonographic findings.

Issues for the Future

The only known curative therapy for intra- and extrahepatic bile duct cancers is surgery. No proven role is seen for adjuvant chemotherapy alone or adjuvant combined chemoradiation, although further studies are needed to fully define the role of these therapies. Continued assessment of new drugs, novel radiosensitizers, and biologic agents is warranted. A better understanding of the molecular pathogenesis and genetics of bile duct cancers may lead to new therapeutic and ultimately preventive strategies for high-risk populations.

BENIGN GALLBLADDER NEOPLASMS

Incidence

Benign tumors of the biliary tract are rare, but have been reported more frequently as imaging modalities (e.g., ultrasound and CT scan) have come into widespread and frequent use. In patients undergoing cholecystectomy, the reported incidence of benign gallbladder tumors is less than 3%.

Pathology

Polyps and Pseudotumors

Benign gallbladder tumors are most frequently polyps or polypoid lesions. The incidence of polyps in asymptomatic patients is about 5%.[2] Cholesterol polyps (cholesterolosis), accounting for half of all gallbladder polypoid lesions,[106] result from epithelium-covered, cholesterol-laden macrophages in the lamina propria. These lesions are likely a result of an error in cholesterol metabolism. They extend from the mucosa on a narrow stalk, grossly appearing as yellow spots on the mucosal surface. Nearly all are multiple and most are less than 10 mm in size.[6,106,107] When a polyp is pedunculated, it is benign in most cases; alternatively, sessile "polyps" are more often malignant (Fig. 64.9).[107] Inflammatory polyps result from chronic inflammation, and extend by a narrow vascularized stalk into the gallbladder lumen. None of these lesions are considered premalignant, although isolated cases of cholesterolosis associated with *in situ* carcinoma have been reported.[108]

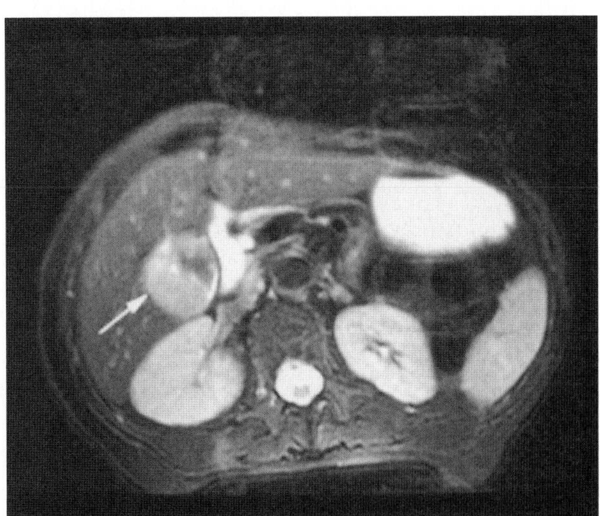

FIGURE 64.9 T_2-weighted magnetic resonance imaging scan showing a sessile polyp within the gallbladder (*arrow*) that was malignant on histologic examination.

Adenomas

Gallbladder adenomas are found infrequently. They may be tubular or papillary, both arising from the epithelial layer of the gallbladder. Multiple papillary adenomas, or papillomas, are called *papillomatosis*. A direct association between benign adenoma, adenoma containing carcinoma *in situ*, and invasive carcinoma has been demonstrated, thus these lesions are considered premalignant.[109] Malignant transformation, however, has only rarely been reported, primarily from large adenomas. In one series, all benign adenomas were less than 12 mm in diameter, whereas the adenomas with cancerous foci were greater than 12 mm.[110]

Adenomyomatosis

Adenomyomatosis of the gallbladder is characterized by localized or diffuse hyperplastic extensions of the mucosa into, and often beyond, a hypertrophied gallbladder muscular layer. Hyperplasia occurs at outpouchings of the mucosa of the gallbladder through the wall (Rokitansky–Aschoff sinuses) and through the crypts of Luschka. This can result in focal thickening of the gallbladder wall, resembling gallbladder adenocarcinoma. The etiology is unknown. This lesion may be premalignant, because cases of adenocarcinoma arising in or near adenomyomatosis have been reported,[110,111] but this relationship is unclear.

Other Benign Gallbladder Tumors

Other benign lesions include tumors arising from the tissue of the gallbladder wall, such as leiomyomas, lipomas, hemangiomas, and granular cell tumors, and heterotopic tissue, including gastric, pancreatic, or intestinal epithelium.

Clinical Findings

Patients with benign gallbladder tumors typically present with symptoms consistent with choledocholithiasis, including right upper quadrant pain, fatty food intolerance, and nausea. Many benign gallbladder lesions are also discovered incidentally after elective cholecystectomy. Therefore, symptoms caused by benign lesions are difficult to separate from those caused by gallstones. Most lesions, however, are asymptomatic and are discovered incidentally during imaging for other abdominal conditions.

Diagnosis

Diagnosis of benign gallbladder polyps is usually made when an ultrasound study is obtained to evaluate a patient for symptoms consistent with gallstones. On ultrasound, a filling defect that does not change with position is likely a polyp or carcinoma and not a gallstone. Cholesterol polyps are typically small, submucosal, multiple, and hyperechoic on ultrasound because of their high cholesterol content. Other than this typical appearance and the fact that malignant polyps are usually more than1 cm in size,[6,106,107] it is difficult to differentiate benign from malignant polyps.

Both intravenous-contrast enhanced and unenhanced CT may be important in distinguishing benign from malignant polyps. In a recent series examining 31 polypoid lesions of the gallbladder, contrast-enhanced CT detected all of the lesions. Benign polyps were not visualized with unenhanced CT, unlike neoplastic tumors, thus improving the ability to distinguish these lesions when both enhanced and unenhanced CT scans were obtained.[6] Endoscopic ultrasound has also been used to image these lesions, and may be more accurate than transabdominal ultrasound in differentiating benign from malignant tumors.[18]

Treatment

Large polyps, greater than 10 mm, have the greatest malignant potential.[6,106,107] Without evidence of invasion or metastatic disease, however, no radiologic test can reliably differentiate benign from malignant lesions. Therefore, if large (>1 cm) polyps are present, even in asymptomatic patients without stones, cholecystectomy is warranted.[104] Smaller pedunculated lesions with the gross characteristics of a benign cholesterol polyp may be observed and resected only if symptomatic. Although these lesions have routinely been followed with ultrasound, a recent prospective study suggested that polyps smaller than 1 cm do not progress to carcinoma.[112] Cholecystectomy, however, is still considered the standard of care if there is any increase in size.

BENIGN BILE DUCT NEOPLASMS

Incidence

Benign bile duct tumors, at times clinically resembling hilar cholangiocarcinoma, are less common, occurring in less than 1% of patients.[1]

Pathology

Attesting to the rarity of these lesions, only two cases of benign extrahepatic bile duct disease occurred in 4,200 biliary tract operations in one institution.[113] The most common benign tumors of the extrahepatic biliary tree arise from the glandular epithelium lining the ducts; about two thirds of benign tumors are polyps, adenomatous papilloma, or bile duct adenomas. Most are found in the periampullary region, but can be distributed throughout the entire biliary tree (Fig. 64.10). Multiple papilloma also have been reported throughout the intra- and extrahepatic biliary tree, termed *multiple biliary papillomatosis*. Although local recurrence and progression to death from

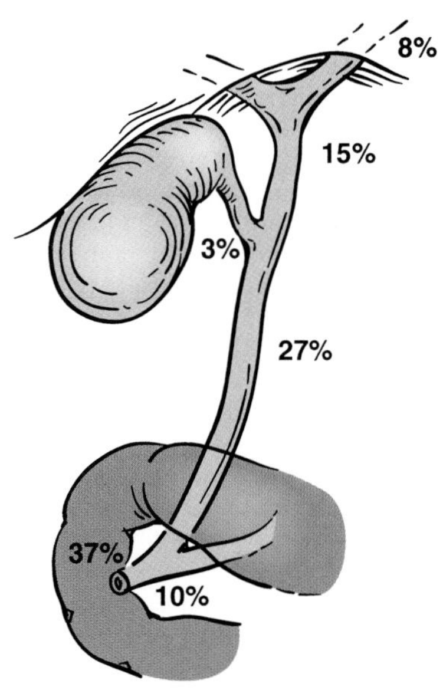

FIGURE 64.10 Distribution of papillomas and adenomas of the biliary tree. The ampulla and common bile duct are the most frequent sites.

obstructive jaundice and cholangitis occur frequently in these rare cases, these tumors have little, if any, malignant potential. Other benign tumors (e.g., cystadenoma, granular cell myoblastoma, leiomyoma, and heterotopic tissue) have also been reported.

One condition that deserves consideration is the case of "malignant masquerade," an inflammatory, fibrotic lesion clinically resembling hilar cholangiocarcinoma, but pathologically consisting only of extensive fibrosis and inflammatory cells without evidence of dysplasia or preneoplastic change.[114–116] In patients being considered for palliative treatment alone with presumed hilar cholangiocarcinoma, it is essential to obtain a tissue diagnosis. It is inappropriate to treat benign lesions by percutaneous stenting because of the excellent outcome after resection of these lesions.

Clinical Findings

Biliary obstruction, with resultant jaundice or cholangitis, is frequently the presenting symptom in patients with benign bile duct tumors. Symptoms may also include epigastric pain or nausea. Because these tumors are indolent, symptoms may be intermittent or gradually progressive.

Diagnosis

Because of the presence of jaundice, benign bile duct tumors are usually initially evaluated with ultrasound. Many patients then undergo ERCP or PTC and CT scan. A diagnosis of malignant masquerade should be suspected in patients with mass lesions that resemble hilar cholangiocarcinomas, but without lobar atrophy or portal vein involvement.

Treatment

Resection and reconstruction are performed to relieve jaundice and cholangitis. The preferred reconstruction is a Roux-en-Y choledochojejunostomy to decrease the risk of postoperative biliary stricture or recurrent cholangitis.

KEY POINTS

- **Gallbladder cancer is a rare malignancy with a dismal outlook because of its insidious onset, propensity for local invasion, and rapid disease progression.**
- **The only curative option in patients with gallbladder cancer is complete surgical resection.**
- **Risk factors for this disease include primary sclerosing cholangitis, ulcerative colitis, choledochal cysts, and biliary tract infection, either with *Clonorchis* or in chronic typhoid carriers.**
- **Most patients with cholangiocarcinoma present with painless jaundice.**
- **Because patients with unresectable disease have a short median survival, those whose disease is clearly unresectable on preoperative imaging should undergo percutaneous internal or external drainage.**
- **There is no proved role for adjuvant chemotherapy alone or adjuvant combined chemoradiation.**

References

1. Diehl AK. Epidemiology of gallbladder cancer: a synthesis of recent data. *J Natl Cancer Inst* 1980;65:1209–1214.
2. Okamoto M, Okamoto H, Kitahara F, et al. Ultrasonographic evidence of association of polyps and stones with gallbladder cancer. *Am J Gastroenterol* 1999;94:446.
3. Piehler JM, Crichlow RW. Primary carcinoma of the gallbladder. *Surgery, Gynecology and Obstetrics* 1978;147:929.
4. Anderson JH, Cooper WJ WC. Adenocarcinoma of the extrahepatic biliary tree. *J R Coll Surg* 1985;67:130.
5. Diehl AK. Gallstone size and the risk of gallbladder cancer. *JAMA* 1983;250:2323–2326.
6. Shinkai H, Kimura W, Muto T. Surgical indications for small polypoid lesions of the gallbladder. *Am J Surg* 1998;175:114.
7. Towfigh S, McFadden DW, Cortina GR, et al. Porcelain gallbladder is not associated with gallbladder carcinoma. *Am Surg* 2001;67:7.
8. Stephen AE, Berger DL. Carcinoma in the porcelain gallbladder: a relationship revisited. *Surgery* 2001;129:699.
9. Aoki H, Sugaya H, et al. A clinical study on cancer of the bile duct associated with anomalous arrangements of the pancreaticobiliary ductal system: analysis of 569 cases collected in Japan. 1987;8:1539.
10. Henson DE, Albores-Saavedra J, Corle D. Carcinoma of the gallbladder. Histologic types, stage of disease, grade, and survival rates. *Cancer* 1992;70:1493.
11. Yamamoto M, Nakajo S, Tahara E. Carcinoma of the gallbladder: the correlation between histogenesis and prognosis. *Virchows Arch* 1989;414:83.
12. **Bartlett DL, Fong Y, Fortner JG, et al. Long-term results after resection for gallbladder cancer. Implications for staging and management. *Ann Surg* 1996;224:639.**
13. Shirai Y, Yoshida K, Tsukada K, et al. Radical surgery for gallbladder carcinoma. Long-term results. *Ann Surg* 1992;216:565.
14. Wistuba II, Sugio K, Hung J, et al. Allele-specific mutations involved in the pathogenesis of endemic gallbladder carcinoma in Chile. *Cancer Res* 1995;55:2511.
15. Matsubara T, Sakurai Y, Sasayama Y, et al. K-ras point mutations in cancerous and noncancerous biliary epithelium in patients with pancreaticobiliary maljunction. *Cancer* 1996;77:1752.
16. Wistuba II, Albores-Saavedra J. Genetic abnormalities involved in the pathogenesis of gallbladder carcinoma. *J Hepatobiliary Pancreat Surg* 1999;6:237.
17. Cotran RS KVRS. *Robbins pathological basis of disease*, 1989.
18. Sugiyama M, Xie XY, Atomi Y, Saito M. Differential diagnosis of small polypoid lesions of the gallbladder: the value of endoscopic ultrasonography. *Ann Surg* 1999;229:498.
19. Mizuguchi M, Kudo S, Fukahori T, et al. Endoscopic ultrasonography for demonstrating loss of multiple-layer pattern of the thickened gallbladder wall in the preoperative diagnosis of gallbladder cancer. *Eur Radiol* 1997;7:1323.
20. Ohtani T, Shirai Y, Tsukada K, et al. Spread of gallbladder carcinoma: CT evaluation with pathologic correlation. *Abdom Imaging* 1996;21:195.
21. Soto JA, Barish MA, Yucel EK, et al. Magnetic resonance cholangiography: comparison with endoscopic retrograde cholangiopancreatography. *Gastroenterology* 1996;110:589.
22. Demachi H, Matsui O, Hoshiba K, et al. Dynamic MRI using a surface coil in chronic cholecystitis and gallbladder carcinoma: radiologic and histopathologic correlation. *J Comput Assist Tomogr* 1997;21:643.
23. Schwartz LH, Coakley FV, Sun Y, et al. Neoplastic pancreaticobiliary duct obstruction: evaluation with breath-hold MR cholangiopancreatography. *AJR American Journal of Roentgenology* 1998;170:1491.
24. Fong Y, Brennan MF, Turnbull A, et al. Gallbladder cancer discovered during laparoscopic surgery. Potential for iatrogenic tumor dissemination. *Arch Surg* 1993;128:1054.
25. **Weber SM, DeMatteo RP, Fong Y, et al. Staging laparoscopy in patients with extrahepatic biliary carcinoma. Analysis of 100 patients. *Ann Surg* 2002;235:392.**
26. Barbot DJ, Marks JH, Feld RI, et al. Improved staging of liver tumors using laparoscopic intraoperative ultrasound. *J Surg Oncol* 1997;64:63.
27. Bhargava DK, Sarin S, Verma K, Kapur BM. Laparoscopy in carcinoma of the gallbladder. *Gastrointest Endosc* 1983;29:21.
28. Dagnini G, Marin G, Patella M, Zotti S. Laparoscopy in the diagnosis of primary carcinoma of the gallbladder. A study of 98 cases. *Gastrointest Endosc* 1984;30:289.
29. **Vollmer CM, Drebin JA, Middleton WD, et al. Utility of staging laparoscopy in subsets of peripancreatic and biliary malignancies. *Ann Surg* 2002;235:1.**
30. Ouchi K, Owada Y, Matsuno S, Sato T. Prognostic factors in the surgical treatment of gallbladder carcinoma. *Surgery* 1987;101:731.
31. Donohue JH, Nagorney DM, Grant CS, et al. Carcinoma of the gallbladder. Does radical resection improve outcome? *Arch Surg* 1990;125:237.
32. Ogura Y, Mizumoto R, Isaji S, et al. Radical operations for carcinoma of the gallbladder: present status in Japan. *World J Surg* 1991;15:337.
33. Shirai Y, Yoshida K, Tsukada K, et al. Radical surgery for gallbladder carcinoma. Long-term results. *Ann Surg* 1992;216:565.
34. Yamaguchi K, Tsuneyoshi M. Subclinical gallbladder carcinoma. *Am J Surg* 1992;163:382.
35. Yamaguchi K, Chijiiwa K, Saiki S, et al. Reliability of frozen section diagnosis of gallbladder tumor for detecting carcinoma and depth of its invasion. *J Surg Oncol* 1997;65:132.
36. Yamaguchi K, Tsuneyoshi M. Subclinical gallbladder carcinoma. *Am J Surg* 1992;163:382.
37. Bartlett DL, Fong Y, Fortner JG, et al. Long-term results after resection for gallbladder cancer. Implications for staging and management. *Ann Surg* 1996;224:639.

38. Nakamura S, Sakaguchi S, Suzuki S, Muro H. Aggressive surgery for carcinoma of the gallbladder. *Surgery* 1989;106:467.
39. Billingsley KG, Jarnagin WR, Fong Y, Blumgart LH. Segment-oriented hepatic resection in the management of malignant neoplasms of the liver. *J Am Coll Surg* 1998;187:471.
40. Shirai Y, Yoshida K, Tsukada K, Muto T. Inapparent carcinoma of the gallbladder. An appraisal of a radical second operation after simple cholecystectomy. *Ann Surg* 1992;215:326.
41. Wanebo HJ, Castle WN, Fechner RE. Is carcinoma of the gallbladder a curable lesion? *Ann Surg* 1982;195:624.
42. Chijiiwa K, Tanaka M. Carcinoma of the gallbladder: an appraisal of surgical resection. *Surgery* 1994;115:751.
43. Fong Y, Brennan MF, Turnbull A, et al. Gallbladder cancer discovered during laparoscopic surgery. Potential for iatrogenic tumor dissemination. *Arch Surg* 1993;128:1054.
44. Drouard F, Delamarre J, Capron JP. Cutaneous seeding of gallbladder cancer after laparoscopic cholecystectomy. *N Engl J Med* 1991;325:1316.
45. Pezet D, Fondrinier E, Rotman N, et al. Parietal seeding of carcinoma of the gallbladder after laparoscopic cholecystectomy. *Br J Surg* 1992;79:230.
46. Weiland ST, Mahvi DM, Niederhuber JE, et al. Should suspected early gallbladder cancer be treated laparoscopically? *J Gastrointest Surg* 2002;6:50.
47. Fong Y, Jarnagin W, Blumgart LH. Gallbladder cancer: comparison of patients presenting initially for definitive operation with those presenting after prior noncurative intervention. *Ann Surg* 2000;232:557.
48. Takada T, Amano H, Yasuda H, et al. Is postoperative adjuvant chemotherapy useful for gallbladder carcinoma? A phase III multicenter prospective randomized controlled trial in patients with resected pancreaticobiliary carcinoma. *Cancer* 2002;95:1685.
49. Kim HJ, Kim MH, Myung SJ, et al. A new strategy for the application of CA19-9 in the differentiation of pancreaticobiliary cancer: analysis using a receiver operating characteristic curve. *Am J Gastroenterol* 1999;94:1941.
50. Lazcano-Ponce EC, Miquel JF, Munoz N, et al. Epidemiology and molecular pathology of gallbladder cancer. *CA Cancer J Clin* 2001;51:349.
51. Pitt HA, Dooley WC, et al. Malignancies of the biliary tree. *Curr Probl Surg* 1995;32:1.
52. Patel T. Increasing incidence and mortality of primary intrahepatic cholangiocarcinoma in the United States. *Hepatology* 2001;33:1353.
53. Henson DE, Albores-Saavedra J, Corle D. Carcinoma of the extrahepatic bile ducts. Histologic types, stage of disease, grade, and survival rates. *Cancer* 1992;70:1498.
54. **de Groen PC, Gores GJ, LaRusso NF, et al. Biliary tract cancers. *N Engl J Med* 1999;341:1368.**
55. Kaya M, de Groen PC, Angulo P, et al. Treatment of cholangiocarcinoma complicating primary sclerosing cholangitis: the Mayo Clinic experience. *Am J Gastroenterol* 2001;96:1164.
56. Hakamada K, Sasaki M, Endoh M, et al. Late development of bile duct cancer after sphincteroplasty: a ten- to twenty-two-year follow-up study. *Surgery* 1997;121:488.
57. Bhuiya MR, Nimura Y, Kamiya J, et al. Clinicopathologic studies on perineural invasion of bile duct carcinoma. *Ann Surg* 1992;215:344.
58. Yamamoto M, Takasaki K, Yoshikawa T. Lymph node metastasis in intrahepatic cholangiocarcinoma. *Jpn J Clin Oncol* 1999;29:147.
59. Burke EC, Jarnagin WR, Hochwald SN, et al. Hilar Cholangiocarcinoma: patterns of spread, the importance of hepatic resection for curative operation, and a presurgical clinical staging system. *Ann Surg* 1998; 228:385.
60. Cameron JL, Pitt HA, Zinner MJ, et al. Management of proximal cholangiocarcinomas by surgical resection and radiotherapy. *Am J Surg* 1990;159:91.
61. Nakayama T, Ikeda A, Okuda K. Percutaneous transhepatic drainage of the biliary tract: technique and results in 104 cases. *Gastroenterology* 1978;74:554.
62. Hochwald SN, Burke EC, Jarnagin WR, et al. Association of preoperative biliary stenting with increased postoperative infectious complications in proximal cholangiocarcinoma. *Arch Surg* 1999;134:261.
63. McPherson GA, Benjamin IS, Hodgson HJ, et al. Pre-operative percutaneous transhepatic biliary drainage: the results of a controlled trial. *Br J Surg* 1984;71:371.
64. Pitt HA, Gomes AS, Lois JF, et al. Does preoperative percutaneous biliary drainage reduce operative risk or increase hospital cost? *Ann Surg* 1985;201:545.
65. Okuda K, Kubo Y, Okazaki N, et al. Clinical aspects of intrahepatic bile duct carcinoma including hilar carcinoma: a study of 57 autopsy-proven cases. *Cancer* 1977;39:232.
66. Ottow RT, August DA, Sugarbaker PH. Treatment of proximal biliary tract carcinoma: an overview of techniques and results. *Surgery* 1985;97:251.
67. Altaee MY, Johnson PJ, Farrant JM, Williams R. Etiologic and clinical characteristics of peripheral and hilar cholangiocarcinoma. *Cancer* 1991;68:2051.
68. Baer HU, Stain SC, Dennison AR, et al. Improvements in survival by aggressive resections of hilar cholangiocarcinoma. *Ann Surg* 1993;217:20.
69. Bengmark S, Ekberg H, Evander A, et al. Major liver resection for hilar cholangiocarcinoma. *Ann Surg* 1988;207:120.
70. Bismuth H, Nakache R, Diamond T. Management strategies in resection for hilar cholangiocarcinoma. *Ann Surg* 1992;215:31.
71. Hadjis NS, Blenkharn JI, Alexander N, et al. Outcome of radical surgery in hilar cholangiocarcinoma. *Surgery* 1990;107:597.
72. Nagorney DM, Donohue JH, Farnell MB, et al. Outcomes after curative resections of cholangiocarcinoma. *Arch Surg* 1993;128:871.
73. Iwasaki Y, Okamura T, Ozaki A, et al. Surgical treatment for carcinoma at the confluence of the major hepatic ducts. *Surgery, Gynecology and Obstetrics* 1986;162:457–464.
74. Iida S, Tsuzuki T, Ogata Y, et al. The long-term survival of patients with carcinoma of the main hepatic duct junction. *Cancer* 1987;60:1612.
75. McMasters KM, Tuttle TM, Leach SD, et al. Neoadjuvant chemoradiation for extrahepatic cholangiocarcinoma. *Am J Surg* 1997;174:605.
76. Nagino M, Nimura Y, Kamiya J, et al. Segmental liver resections for hilar cholangiocarcinoma. *Hepatogastroenterology* 1998;45:7.
77. Nakeeb A, Tran KQ, Black MJ, et al. Improved survival in resected biliary malignancies. *Surgery* 2002;132:555.
78. Klempnauer J, Ridder GJ, von Wasielewski R, et al. Resectional surgery of hilar cholangiocarcinoma: a multivariate analysis of prognostic factors. *J Clin Oncol* 1997;15:947.
79. **Jarnagin WR, Fong Y, DeMatteo RP, et al. Staging, resectability, and outcome in 225 patients with hilar cholangiocarcinoma. *Ann Surg* 2001;234:507.**
80. Rea DJ, Munoz-Juarez M, Farnell MB, et al. Major hepatic resection for hilar cholangiocarcinoma: analysis of 46 patients. *Arch Surg* 2004;139:514.
81. Blumgart LH, Hadjis NS, Benjamin IS, Beazley R. Surgical approaches to cholangiocarcinoma at confluence of hepatic ducts. *Lancet* 1984;1:66.
82. Reding R, Buard JL, Lebeau G, Launois B. Surgical management of 552 carcinomas of the extrahepatic bile ducts (gallbladder and periampullary tumors excluded). Results of the French Surgical Association Survey. *Ann Surg* 1991;213:236.
83. Lieser MJ, Barry MK, Rowland C, et al. Surgical management of intrahepatic cholangiocarcinoma: a 31-year experience. *J Hepatobiliary Pancreat Surg* 1998;5:41.
84. Nakeeb A, Pitt HA, Sohn TA, et al. Cholangiocarcinoma. A spectrum of intrahepatic, perihilar, and distal tumors. *Ann Surg* 1996;224:463.
85. **Weber SM, Jarnagin WR, Klimstra D, et al. Intrahepatic cholangiocarcinoma: resectability, recurrence pattern, and outcomes. *J Am Coll Surg* 2001;193:384.**
86. Berdah SV, Delpero JR, Garcia S, Hardwigsen J, Le Treut YP. A western surgical experience of peripheral cholangiocarcinoma. *Br J Surg* 1996;83:1517.
87. Fong Y, Blumgart LH, Lin E, et al. Outcome of treatment for distal bile duct cancer. *Br J Surg* 1996;83:1712.
88. Jarnagin WR, Burke E, Powers C, et al. Intrahepatic biliary enteric bypass provides effective palliation in selected patients with malignant obstruction at the hepatic duct confluence. *Am J Surg* 1998;175:453.
89. Glattli A, Stain SC, Baer HU, et al. Unresectable malignant biliary obstruction: treatment by self-expandable biliary endoprostheses. *J Hepatobiliary Pancreat Surg* 1993;6:175.
90. Kuvshinoff BW, Armstrong JG, Fong Y, et al. Palliation of irresectable hilar cholangiocarcinoma with biliary drainage and radiotherapy. *Br J Surg* 1995;82:1522.
91. Lee BH, Choe DH, Lee JH, et al. Metallic stents in malignant biliary obstruction: prospective long-term clinical results. *AJR American Journal of Roentgenology* 1997;168:741.
92. Rumalla A, Baron TH, Wang KK, et al. Endoscopic application of photodynamic therapy for cholangiocarcinoma. *Gastrointest Endosc* 2001;53:500.
93. Yee K, Sheppard BC, Domreis J, et al. Cancers of the gallbladder and biliary ducts. *Oncology (Huntingt)* 2002;16:939.
94. Stemmler J, Heinemann V, Schalhorn A. Capecitabine as second-line treatment for metastatic cholangiocarcinoma: a report of two cases. *Onkologie* 2002;25:182.
95. Oberfield RA, Rossi RL. The role of chemotherapy in the treatment of bile duct cancer. *World J Surg* 1988;12:105.
96. Cameron JL, Broe P, Zuidema GD. Proximal bile duct tumors: surgical management with silastic transhepatic biliary stents. *Ann Surg* 1982;196:412.
97. Iwasaki Y, Ohto M, Todoroki T, et al. Treatment of carcinoma of the biliary system. *Surgery, Gynecology and Obstetrics* 1977;144:219.
98. Fletcher MS, Brinkley D, Dawson JL, et al. Treatment of high bile duct carcinoma by internal radiotherapy with iridium-192 wire. *Lancet* 1981;2:172.
99. Kopelson G, Gunderson LL. Primary and adjuvant radiation therapy in gallbladder and extrahepatic biliary tract carcinoma. *J Clin Gastroenterol* 1983;5:43.
100. Todoroki T, Iwasaki Y, Okamura T, et al. Intraoperative radiotherapy for advanced carcinoma of the biliary system. *Cancer* 1980;46:2179.
101. Ikeda H, Kuroda C, Uchida H, et al. Intraluminal irradiation with iridium-192 wires for extrahepatic bile duct carcinoma—a preliminary report. [Japanese]. *Nippon Igaku Hoshasen Gakkai Zasshi—Nippon Acta Radiologica* 1979;39:1356.
102. Pitt HA, Nakeeb A, Abrams RA, et al. Perihilar cholangiocarcinoma. Postoperative radiotherapy does not improve survival. *Ann Surg* 1995;221:788.
103. Polydorou AA, Cairns SR, Dowsett JF, et al. Palliation of proximal malignant biliary obstruction by endoscopic endoprosthesis insertion. *Gut* 1991;32:685.
104. Aldridge MC, Bismuth H. Gallbladder cancer: the polyp-cancer sequence. *Br J Surg* 1990;77:363.

105. Shiina T, Mikuriya S, Uno T, et al. Radiotherapy of cholangiocarcinoma: the roles for primary and adjuvant therapies. *Cancer Chemother Pharmacol* 1992;31:[suppl 8].
106. Koga A, Watanabe K, Fukuyama T, et al. Diagnosis and operative indications for polypoid lesions of the gallbladder. *Arch Surg* 1988;123:26.
107. Furukawa H, Kosuge T, Shimada K, et al. Small polypoid lesions of the gallbladder: differential diagnosis and surgical indications by helical computed tomography. *Arch Surg* 1998;133:735.
108. Akiyama T, Sahara H, Seto K, et al. Gallbladder cancer associated with cholesterosis. *J Gastroenterol* 1996;31:470.
109. Kozuka S, Tsubone N, Yasui A, et al. Relation of adenoma to carcinoma in the gallbladder. *Cancer* 1982;50:2226.
110. Aldridge MC, Gruffaz F, Castaing D, et al. Adenomyomatosis of the gallbladder. A premalignant lesion? *Surgery* 1991;109:107.
111. Kurihara K, Mizuseki K, Ninomiya T, et al. Carcinoma of the gall-bladder arising in adenomyomatosis. *Acta Pathologica Japonica* 1993;43:82.
112. Csendes A, Burgos AM, Csendes P, et al. Late follow-up of polypoid lesions of the gallbladder smaller than 10 mm. *Ann Surg* 2001;234:657.
113. Farris KB, Faust BF. Granular cell tumors of biliary ducts. Report of two cases and review of the literature. *Arch Pathol Lab Med* 1979;103:510.
114. Hadjis NS, Collier NA, Blumgart LH. Malignant masquerade at the hilum of the liver. *Br J Surg* 1985;72:659.
115. Standfield NJ, Salisbury JR, Howard ER. Benign non-traumatic inflammatory strictures of the extrahepatic biliary system. *Br J Surg* 1989; 76:849.
116. Verbeek PCM, Vanleeuwen DJ, Dewit LT, et al. Benign fibrosing disease at the hepatic confluence mimicking Klatskin tumors. *Surgery* 1992; 112:866.
117. Wakai T, Shirai Y, Yokoyama N, et al. Early gallbladder carcinoma does not warrant radical resection. *Br J Surg* 2001;88:675.
118. Taner CB, Nagorney DM, Donohue JH. Surgical treatment of gallbladder cancer. *J Gastrointest Surg* 2004;8:83.

SECTION I
COLON, RECTUM, AND ANUS

CHAPTER 65 ■ COLONIC ANATOMY AND PHYSIOLOGY

JOHN F. SWEENEY

EMBRYOLOGY

The primitive gut begins to form during the fourth week of gestation. For descriptive purposes, it is divided into the foregut, midgut, and hindgut. In this chapter, the discussion will focus only on the midgut and hindgut.

Midgut derivatives include the entire small intestine distal to the ampulla of Vater, the cecum and appendix, the ascending colon, and the right half to two-thirds of the transverse colon. These structures receive their blood supply from branches of the superior mesenteric artery. At the beginning of the sixth week of gestation, the midgut loop undergoes a physiologic umbilical herniation and migrates into the extraembryonic coelom. During the next 4 weeks the midgut loop elongates considerably and also undergoes a series of counterclockwise rotations around the axis of the superior mesenteric artery. During the tenth week of gestation, the midgut structures return into the abdomen, having undergone a total counterclockwise rotation of 270 degrees. During the final months of gestation, the cecum grows down into the right iliac fossa.

The hindgut structures include the left one-third to one-half of the transverse colon, the descending colon, the sigmoid colon, the rectum, and the superior portion of the anal canal. Branches of the inferior mesenteric artery supply all these hindgut structures.

ANATOMY OF THE COLON

The colon begins in the right lower quadrant of the abdomen where the distal ileum empties into posteromedial aspect of the cecum at the ileocecal valve (Fig. 65.1). The colon extends from the ileocecal valve to the anal canal and can range between 3 to 6 feet in total length. The approximately 7.5- to 8.5-cm diameter of the cecum makes it the widest portion of the colon. The appendix projects from the lowest portion of the cecum. From the cecum, the colon ascends along the right side of the abdomen for a distance of approximately 20 to 30 cm to a level overlying the inferior pole of the right kidney. At this point, the colon forms a medial, anterior, and downward angulation, the hepatic flexure, which is the portion of the ascending colon that joins the transverse colon. During mobilization of the hepatic flexure in a right hemicolectomy, it is important to stay in the plane close to the colon to avoid injury to the right kidney and duodenum.

The transverse colon extends from the hepatic flexure to the splenic flexure and is the longest segment of colon, ranging between 30 and 60 cm. The transverse colon is suspended by the transverse mesocolon and is considered to be completely intraperitoneal. It is the most mobile portion of the colon and can be located anywhere from the upper abdomen to the pelvis. The greater omentum descends from the greater curve of the stomach in front of the transverse colon and then ascends to attach to the transverse colon on its anterosuperior edge. The splenic flexure is the angle between the distal transverse colon and the descending colon. The splenic flexure is situated high in the left upper quadrant, more cephalad than the hepatic flexure. The flexure lies anterior to the midportion of the left kidney and also closely abuts the lower pole of the spleen. The attachments to the diaphragm and spleen (phrenocolic and splenocolic ligaments) should be carefully identified and divided during mobilization of the splenic flexure to avoid injuring the spleen.

The descending colon is approximately 20 to 30 cm in length and courses from the splenic flexure to its junction with the sigmoid colon at the pelvic brim. The anterior, lateral, and medial portions of the descending colon are covered by peritoneum, but the posterior surface is adherent to the posterior abdominal wall and frequently lies in close contact with the left ureter. The sigmoid colon extends from the pelvic brim to the sacral promontory, where it continues as the rectum. The sigmoid colon can vary from 15 to 50 cm in length. The sigmoid colon is extremely mobile and has a generous mesentery

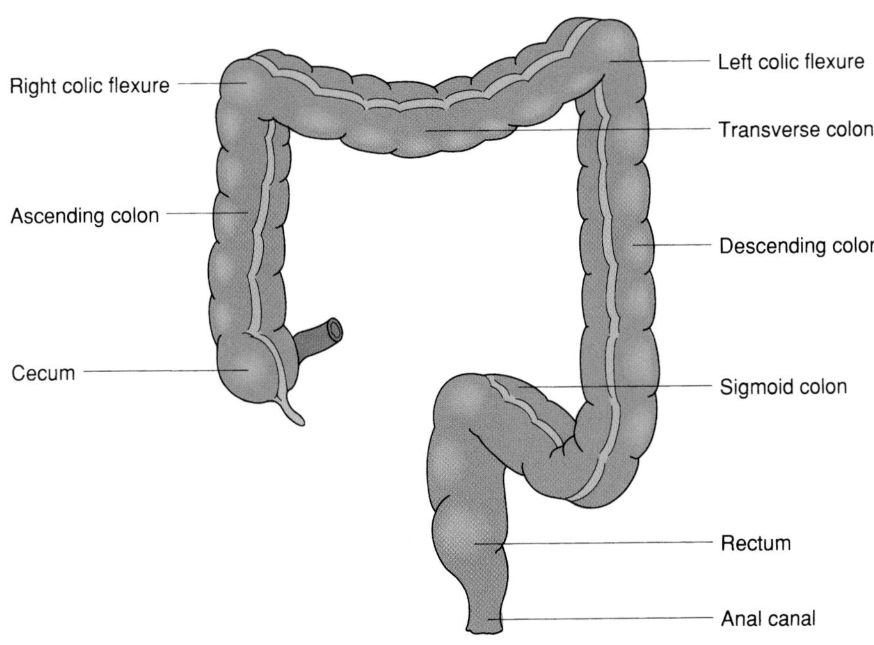

FIGURE 65.1 General anatomic components of the colon.

that extends along the pelvic brim from the iliac fossa across the sacroiliac joint to the second or third sacral segment. When the sigmoid colon is mobilized, care should be taken to identify the left ureter as it runs in the intersigmoid fossa and crosses anterior to the point where the common iliac artery bifurcates into the internal and external iliac arteries.

Anatomists have classically described the beginning of the rectum at the level of the third sacral vertebra. Surgeons often consider the rectum to begin at the level of the sacral promontory. From here, the rectum proceeds posteriorly and caudally along the curvature of the sacrum and coccyx and ends by passing through the levator ani muscles, at which point it turns abruptly caudal and posterior becoming the anal canal.

The four layers of the colonic wall include the mucosa, submucosa, circular muscle layer, and longitudinal muscle layer (Fig. 65.2). The mucosal surface of the colon consists of columnar epithelium made up of regularly arranged crypts and numerous goblet cells. Unlike that of the small intestine, the columnar epithelium of the colon does not possess villi. The muscularis propria of the colon consists of an inner circular layer and an outer longitudinal layer. The thick circular muscle forms a continuous layer around the entire circumference of the colon. In contrast, the outer longitudinal muscle layer is grouped into three bands known as *taeniae*. These bands are positioned approximately 120 degrees apart about the circumference of the colon, with one taenia along the mesenteric border and the other two found on the antimesenteric border of the colon. The taeniae begin proximally at the appendix and disappear as distinct bands at the level of the upper rectum. At this point, the longitudinal muscle layer coalesces to form a continuous layer around the circumference of the rectum. The sacculations seen between the taeniae are called the *haustra coli*.

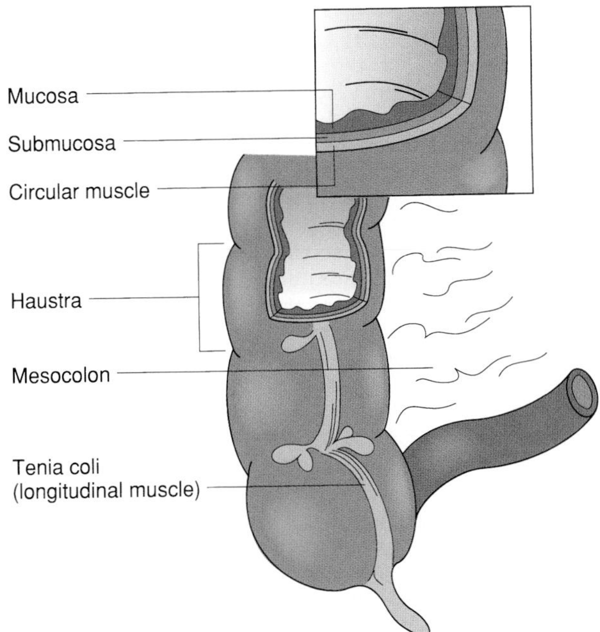

FIGURE 65.2 Layers of the colonic wall.

Arterial Blood Supply

The superior mesenteric artery arises from the aorta, runs posterior to the pancreas, and passes anterior to the third portion of the duodenum (Fig. 65.3). The superior mesenteric artery gives rise to the ileocolic and middle colic branches that supply the cecum, ascending colon, and proximal transverse colon. The right colic artery, which also supplies the ascending colon, can originate as a branch of the ileocolic artery or may arise directly from the superior mesenteric artery. The inferior mesenteric artery arises from the infrarenal aorta and supplies the distal transverse colon, descending colon, sigmoid colon, and upper rectum via its left colic, sigmoid, and superior hemorrhoidal branches. The middle and inferior hemorrhoidal arteries arise from the hypogastric arteries and supply the distal two-thirds of the rectum. A series of arterial arcades along the mesenteric border of the entire colon, known as the marginal *artery of Drummond,* connect the superior mesenteric and inferior mesenteric arterial systems. This important collateral circulation allows the left colon to remain viable while the inferior mesenteric artery is ligated during an extended sigmoid resection.

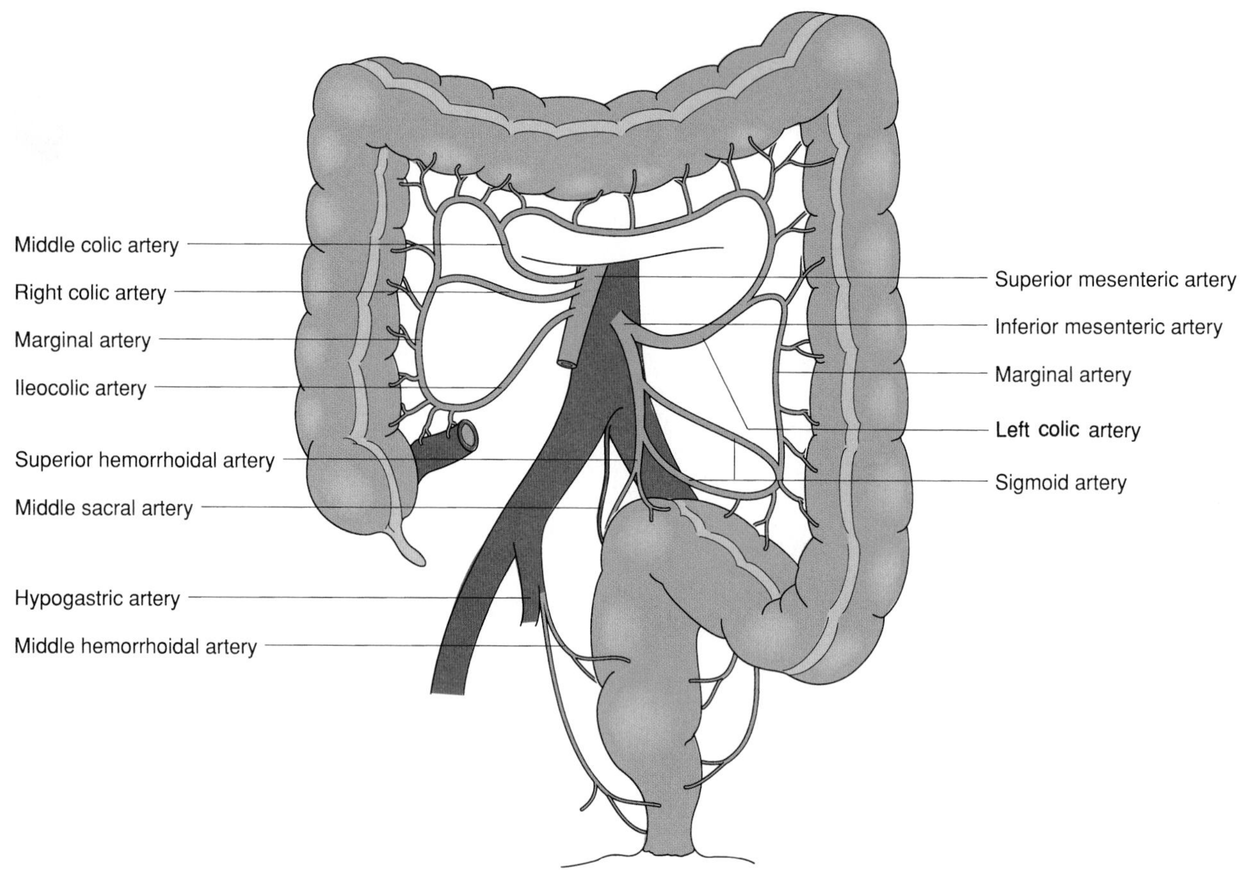

FIGURE 65.3 Arterial blood supply of the colon.

Venous Drainage

The veins that drain the large intestine bear the same terminology and follow a course similar to that of their corresponding arteries (Fig. 65.4). The veins from the right colon and transverse colon, along with the veins draining the small intestine, drain into the superior mesenteric vein. The superior mesenteric vein runs slightly anterior to and to the right of the superior mesenteric artery. The superior mesenteric vein courses beneath the neck of the pancreas, where it joins with the splenic vein to form the portal vein. The inferior mesenteric vein drains blood from the left colon, sigmoid colon, rectum, and superior anal canal. The inferior mesenteric vein ascends over the psoas muscle in a retroperitoneal plane. The vein courses under the body of the pancreas to drain into the splenic vein. The superior hemorrhoidal veins drain blood from the rectum into the portal system via the inferior mesenteric vein. The middle and inferior hemorrhoidal veins drain blood from the lower rectum and anal canal into the systemic venous circulation via the internal iliac veins. In the setting of portal hypertension, the superior, middle, and inferior hemorrhoidal veins interact to shunt venous blood from the portal system into the systemic circulation.

Lymphatic Drainage

Lymphatic drainage generally follows the arterial blood supply of the colon and rectum (Fig. 65.5). In the anal canal, lesions above the dentate line ultimately drain into inferior mesenteric lymph nodes. Lesions below the dentate line drain into the internal iliac nodes.

Neural Components

The colon possesses extrinsic and intrinsic (enteric) neuronal systems. The extrinsic system consists of sympathetic and parasympathetic nerves that generally inhibit or stimulate colonic peristalsis, respectively. The sympathetic innervation to the right colon originates from the lower thoracic segments of the spinal cord and travel in the thoracic splanchnic nerves to the celiac and superior mesenteric plexuses. Postganglionic fibers emerge from here and course along the superior mesenteric artery and its branches to the right side of the colon. The parasympathetic innervation originates from the right vagus nerve and travels along with the sympathic nerves to the right side of the colon. The left side of the colon and the rectum receive sympathetic fibers that arise from L1 through L3. The parasympathetic supply to the left side of the colon and the rectum arises from S2 through S4.

The intrinsic, or enteric, nervous system consists of two groups of plexuses that are identified by their location within the wall of the colon. Meissner's plexus is located in the submucosa between the muscularis mucosae and the circular muscle of the muscularis propria. The myenteric plexus, also known as *Auerbach's plexus*, is located between the inner circular muscle and outer longitudinal muscle layers of the colon.

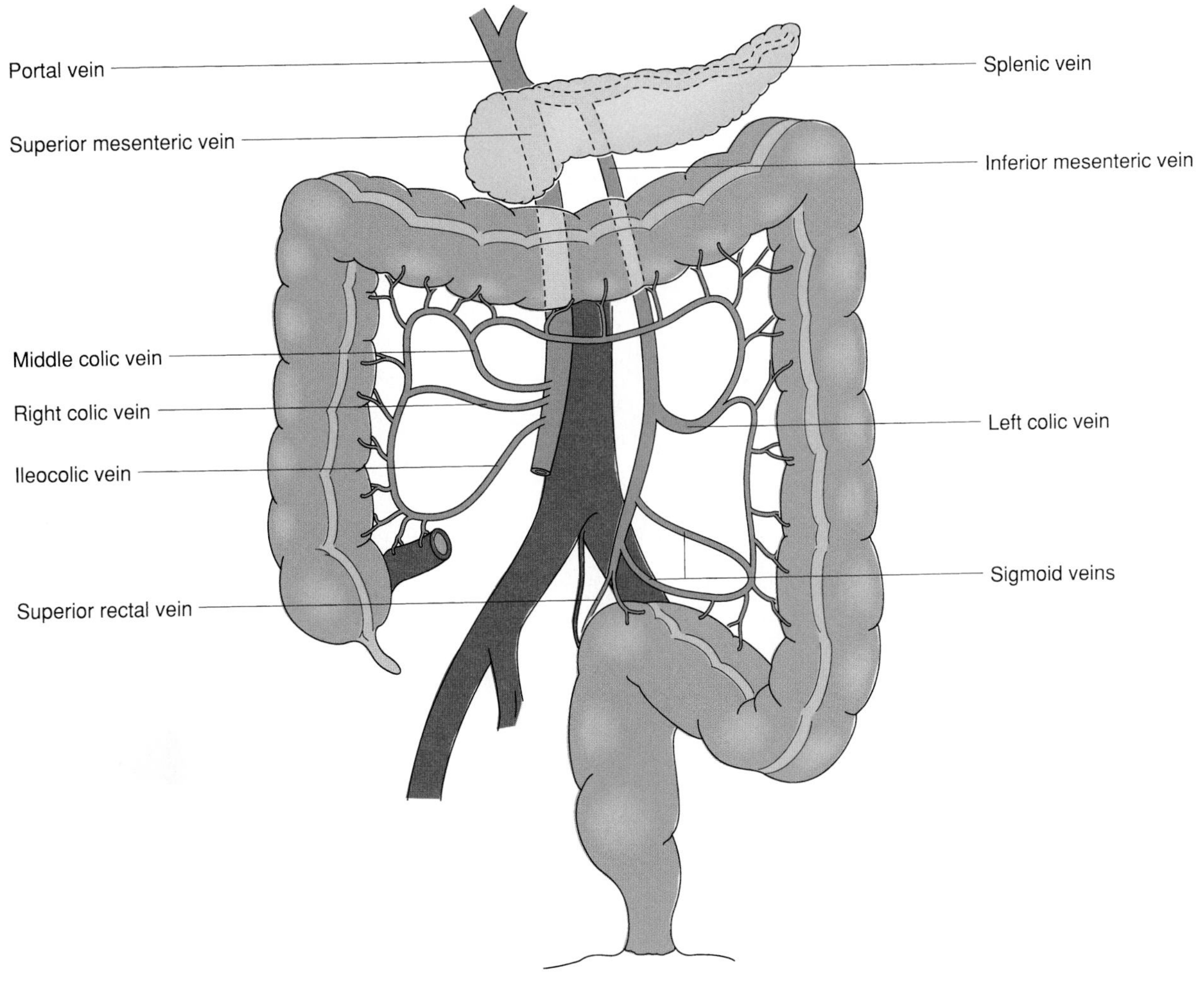

FIGURE 65.4 Venous drainage of the colon by the portal vein.

COLORECTAL

PHYSIOLOGY

Absorption

The colon absorbs water, sodium, and chloride while it secretes potassium and bicarbonate. The physiologic control of colonic water and electrolyte transport requires careful integration of neural, endocrine, and paracrine components. Although colonic epithelium does not actively absorb glucose or amino acids, as the small-intestinal epithelium does, the colon does absorb short-chain fatty acids and vitamins that are produced by bacterial breakdown of nonabsorbed sugars and amino acids. These short-chain fatty acids, which include acetate, butyrate, and propionate, are absorbed in a concentration-dependent fashion. They are a major energy substrate for colonic epithelial cells and are the major fecal anions.[1,2]

Approximately 1,500 mL of ileal effluent reaches the cecum in a 24-hour period, of which 90% is water. Of this amount, only 100 to 150 mL of water remains in the stool. The colon has a tremendous capacity that allows it to absorb as much as 5 to 6 L of water within a 24-hour period.[3] Normally formed feces consist of 70% water and 30% solid material. Almost half of the solid material is made up of bacteria and the other half is composed of undigested food material and desquamated epithelium. Water absorption in the colon is a passive process that depends primarily on the osmotic gradient established by the active transport of sodium across the colonic epithelium. The composition of ileal effluent and luminal flow rates also play an important role in water absorption. Upsetting the balance of these three factors results in diarrhea. The absorptive capacity is not the same throughout each segment of the colon. Salt and water absorption is greatest in the right colon. Patients undergoing a right hemicolectomy should therefore be counseled preoperatively that they may experience loose bowel movements or frank diarrhea in the early postoperative period. Patients should also be reassured that this will resolve with time as the remaining colon adapts.

Sodium absorption by colonic epithelium is an active cellular transport process similar to that seen in small intestinal and renal epithelial cells.[4] Initially, sodium absorption involves the passive movement of sodium across the apical membrane into the mucosal cell down an electrochemical gradient. To maintain an adequate electrochemical gradient, intracellular sodium is removed from the cell into the interstitial space in exchange for potassium. This is an energy-dependent process that is controlled by Na^+-K^+-adenosine triphosphatase (ATPase). Mineralocorticoids (aldosterone) and glucocorticoids accelerate sodium absorption and potassium excretion in the colon by increasing Na^+-K^+-ATPase activity.[5] Potassium movement into the colonic lumen is primarily a passive process

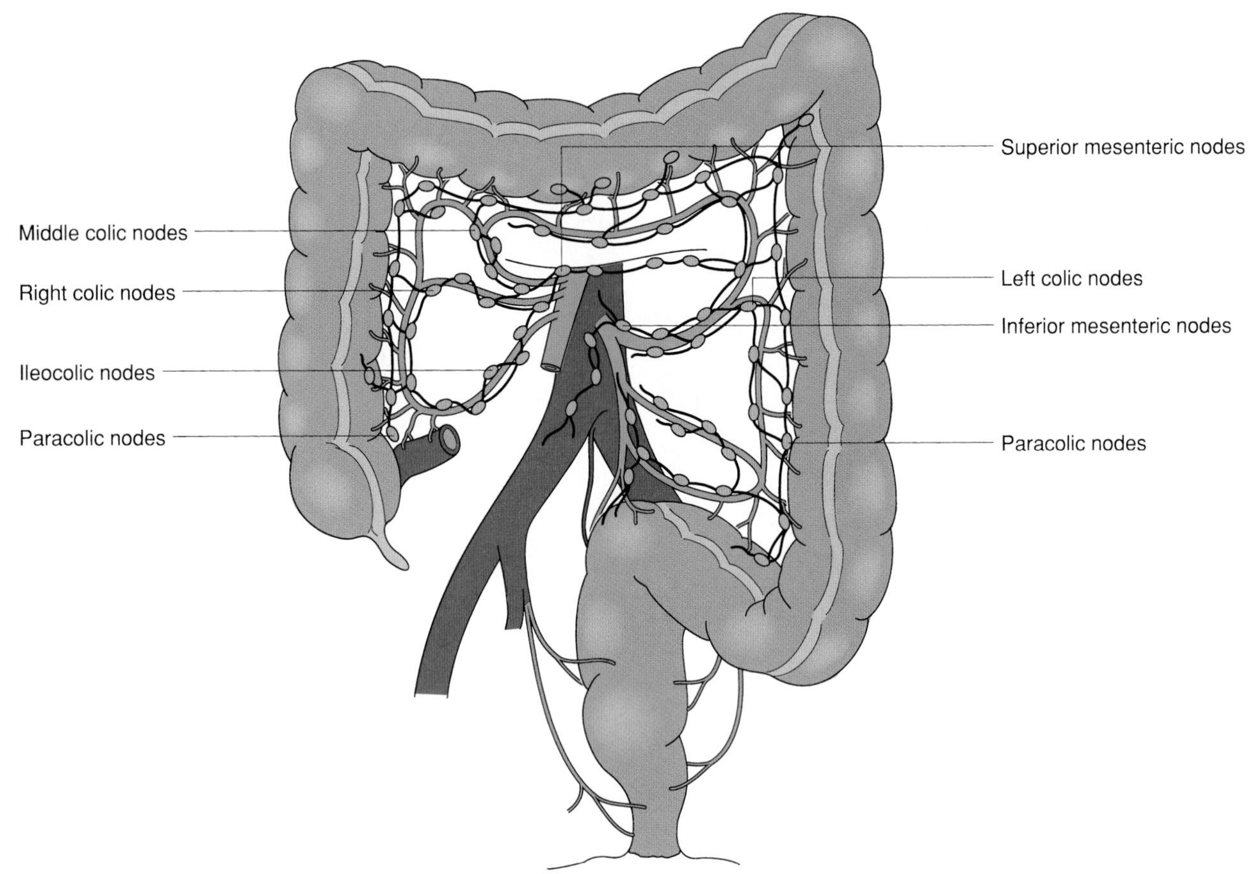

FIGURE 65.5 Lymphatic drainage of the colon.

that depends on the electrochemical gradient generated by the active transport of sodium across colonic epithelial cells. Chloride absorption in the colon is generally thought to be an energy-independent process that is associated with reciprocal exchange for bicarbonate at the luminal border of the mucosal cell.[6]

Colonic Flora

The bacterial flora of the colon is established soon after birth and depends in large part on dietary and environmental factors. Approximately 400 different species of bacteria have been identified in the human colon. Bacteria constitute between 40% to 55% of fecal solids in a person who consumes a normal Western diet. The vast majority of the normal colonic flora consists of anaerobic bacteria, with *Bacteroides* species, especially *B. fragilis*, the most prevalent.[7] Other anaerobic bacteria include *Lactobacillus bifidus, Clostridium* species, and *Eubacterium* species. Aerobic colonic bacteria are mainly coliforms and enterococci. *Escherichia coli* is the predominant coliform. Other aerobic coliforms include *Klebsiella, Proteus,* and *Enterobacter*. The principal enterococcus is *Streptococcus faecali*.

Fecal flora plays an important role in many physiologic processes. The host absorbs vitamin K, which is produced by many colonic microorganisms. The enterohepatic circulation of bilirubin and bile acids depends greatly on bacterial enzymes produced by fecal flora, and the degradation of bile pigments by colonic bacteria gives stool its characteristic brown color. Colonic bacteria also influence colonic motility and absorption, generate intestinal gases, and play an important role in the prevention of infection by keeping the growth of pathogenic bacteria such as *C. difficile* in check.

Colonic Motility

Motor activity varies greatly throughout the colon. Three patterns of colonic smooth-muscle contraction are known to exist: retrograde movement, segmental contractions, and mass movements. *Retrograde movements* are a unique pattern of antiperistaltic contractions that originate in the distal right side of the colon and travel toward the cecum, slowing the movement of the luminal contents.[8,9] These contractions facilitate a thorough mixing of the ileal effluent and prolong exposure of the luminal contents to the mucosa of the right colon, thereby promoting microbial metabolism and water and electrolyte absorption.[10] *Segmental contractions* are intermittent contractions of the longitudinal and circular muscles that result in the segmented appearance of the colon.[11] Segmental contractions are most commonly seen in the transverse and descending colon. These contractions propel luminal contents in a back-and-forth pattern over short distances to cause further mixing of fecal matter. The final type of colonic activity, termed *mass movement*, consists of strong, propulsive contractions of the smooth muscle that involve a long segment of colon.[12] The contractions move the luminal contents forward at a rate of 0.5 to 1.0 cm/s and typically last for 20 to 30 seconds.[13] Mass movement contractions occur three to four times per day, primarily after awakening and after meals.

The orderly progression of colonic luminal contents from cecum to anus requires the coordination of smooth-muscle contractions. Calcium-dependent cyclic depolarization and repolarization of the colonic smooth-muscle cell membrane generates a basic electrical pattern of slow-wave activity. This activity allows each smooth-muscle cell to control its own contraction and to couple with adjacent smooth-muscle cells.[14] The extrinsic (autonomic) and intrinsic (enteric) neuronal systems also interact to influence colonic motility.

Defecation

As the fecal mass enters the rectum, the internal anal sphincter relaxes while the external anal sphincter contracts to maintain continence. Distention of the rectum in this setting is the primary stimulus for the initiation of defecation. At this point, the urge to defecate may be suppressed by conscious contraction of the external anal sphincter. Receptive relaxation of the rectal ampulla accommodates the fecal mass and the urge to defecate passes unless the volume of feces is extremely large or the sphincter mechanism is impaired. If the subject voluntarily accedes to the urge to defecate, a squatting position is assumed, which straightens the anorectal angle. A Valsalva's maneuver is then performed, which increases the intraabdominal and intrathoracic pressure and overcomes the resistance of the external anal sphincter. Relaxation of the pelvic muscles causes the pelvic floor to descend and the anorectal angle to straighten further. Conscious inhibition of the external anal sphincter then allows passage of the feces. On completion, the pelvic floor returns to its resting position and the anal sphincter muscles return to their resting activity, closing the anal canal. Under normal circumstances, this process occurs once every 24 hours; however, the interval between bowel movements may vary between 8 and 12 hours and 2 to 3 days in normal subjects. The frequency of defecation is influenced by multiple environmental and dietary factors.

DISORDERS OF COLONIC MOTILITY

Constipation

To the layperson, constipation means infrequent stools or difficulty in passing stools. The Rome definition,[15] however, requires specific criteria to be present before a diagnosis of constipation can be assigned (Table 65.1). The causes of constipation are numerous and include faulty dietary and life-style habits; structural/functional, neurologic, and endocrine/metabolic disorders; and iatrogenic causes/medication (Table 65.2). The recent onset of constipation in an otherwise healthy adult is a warning sign and should prompt a search to exclude an obstructing anatomic lesion.

TABLE 65.1 DIAGNOSIS

ROME CRITERIA FOR THE DIAGNOSIS OF CONSTIPATION

Two or more of the following:
Straining on >25% of bowel movements
Incomplete evacuation of the rectum on >25% of bowel movements
Hard stool consistency on >25% of bowel movements
Three or fewer bowel movements weekly

TABLE 65.2 ETIOLOGY

CAUSES OF CONSTIPATION

Faulty Dietary and Lifestyle Habits
Inadequate dietary fiber
Inadequate fluids
Lack of exercise
Environmental changes (e.g., travel, hospitalization)
Structural/Functional
Slow transit
Pelvic floor dysfunction (e.g., rectocele, procidentia)
Immobilization
Depression
Irritable bowel syndrome
Diverticulosis
Colonic obstruction (e.g., neoplasm, volvulus, inflammation)
Scleroderma
Amyloidosis
Neurologic Disorders
Central nervous system (e.g., stroke, Parkinson's disease, Alzheimer's disease)
Spinal cord (e.g., multiple sclerosis, tumor, herniated disk, trauma)
Nervi erigentes damage
Aganglionosis (Hirschsprung's disease, Chagas' disease)
Iatrogenic/Medication
Narcotics
Anticholinergics
Antacids
Antihypertensives
Antidepressants
Iron
Barium
Endocrine/Metabolic
Hypothyroidism
Hypercalcemia
Pheochromocytoma
Diabetes
Pregnancy
Uremia
Dehydration

The standard initial treatment for patients with constipation involves dietary manipulation with bulk-forming agents to increase dietary fiber. Patients should also be encouraged to increase their fluid intake. Patients who fail an initial trial of bulk-forming agents may respond to stool softeners such as docusate (Colace). These agents increase the stool water content by inhibiting the normal water-absorptive capacity of the colon. Although they soften the stool, they do not promote defecation. If bulk-forming agents and stool softeners do not successfully treat the constipation, the next preferred therapy involves osmotic laxatives. These agents (which include magnesium citrate, sodium sulfate, phosphate, and potassium tartrate) are poorly absorbed chemicals that increase the stool water content through an osmotic effect. Caution should be exercised in prescribing them for patients with significant underlying cardiac, renal, or hepatic disease. Polysaccharides such as lactulose or sorbitol are also poorly absorbed substances that have an osmotic effect and increase stool water. They may cause excess cramping, bloating, flatulence, and fluid loss. Stimulant laxatives act on the mucosa to reduce water and electrolyte secretion; they also increase colonic motility. Examples include diphenylmethane derivatives (e.g., bisacodyl) and anthraquinone cathartics (senna, cascara sagrada).

Treatment of constipation should result in a normal frequency and consistency of stools and freedom from associated discomfort. This goal is achieved in most patients simply by increasing dietary fiber and water intake. Additional agents should be added in a graded fashion at the lowest effective dose. Long-term laxative abuse should be avoided. Surgical treatment should be reserved for patients with new onset of constipation and an underlying anatomic cause (e.g., diverticular stricture or obstructing colon carcinoma). The surgical treatment of chronic constipation is poorly defined and should not be considered until a complete workup has been completed.

Postoperative Ileus

Postoperative ileus is most commonly seen in patients who have undergone intraabdominal operative procedures, but it can also occur after major extraabdominal (e.g., cardiothoracic or orthopedic) surgical procedures. The colon appears to be most profoundly affected by postoperative ileus, with the stomach and small intestine recovering function earlier. The cause of this phenomenon is unclear and is likely multifactorial. Bowel manipulation is one factor that has often been cited.[16] The observation that postoperative ileus is less severe after minimally invasive surgery adds credence to this theory.[17] Anesthetic agents utilized intraoperatively and postoperative analgesia can also influence the duration of postoperative ileus.[18] Electrolyte abnormalities, including deficits in potassium, magnesium, and calcium, are also known to alter intestinal motility following surgery.

Irritable Bowel Syndrome

Irritable bowel syndrome is defined as abdominal pain that is not associated with an anatomic abnormality and may or may not be associated with alterations in bowel habits. The causes of this disorder are uncertain. Emotional stress and psychiatric illness have been implicated in the pathogenesis and may exacerbate symptoms.[19] Physiologic abnormalities have also been demonstrated in patients with irritable bowel syndrome.[20,21] Abnormal colonic motility in response to an ingested meal has been demonstrated in some patients with irritable bowel syndrome. Other studies have cited altered myoelectric activity and abnormal gut hormone secretion as causes.

Because no one clear cause of irritable bowel syndrome has been demonstrated, no specific treatment regimen has been defined for this disorder. Most patients have asymptomatic periods interrupted by intervals of symptoms. The approach to treatment begins with an evaluation of the factors associated with irritable bowel syndrome. Diagnosis and treatment of an underlying psychiatric problem may resolve the patient's symptoms. A careful dietary history should also be taken, and factors that contribute to constipation or diarrhea should be adjusted appropriately. If these management strategies are not successful, a gradual introduction of anticholinergic medications may be helpful. Anticholinergic agents can reduce the rate of myoelectric activity and decrease tonic contractions in the colon, thereby relieving the cramping and bloating that many patients experience. Low doses of tricyclic antidepressants, including imipramine, amitriptyline, and nortriptyline, often decrease or eliminate abdominal symptoms. Constipation is known to be one major side effect of these agents, which may be helpful in patients with irritable bowel syndrome and underlying diarrhea but a problem in patients with preexisting constipation. The myriad of treatment options described for irritable bowel syndrome underscores the poor understanding of this clinical entity.

Colonic Pseudoobstruction

Colonic pseudoobstruction, also known as *Ogilvie syndrome*, is a clinical entity in which signs and symptoms of bowel obstruction are present without an actual mechanical obstruction. Pseudoobstruction is usually observed in patients with serious underlying medical conditions who have undergone a major (usually extraabdominal) surgical procedure. The most frequent presenting symptoms include abdominal pain and distention. Constipation/obstipation or diarrhea may be present. Nausea and vomiting may also be seen. Physical examination usually demonstrates tympany to percussion and mild tenderness on palpation. Abdominal radiographic findings are significant for marked colonic distention that is typically localized to the right side of the colon (Fig. 65.6). The management of colonic pseudoobstruction is initially nonoperative and consists of nasogastric decompression, correction of fluid and electrolyte imbalances, gentle enemas, rectal tube placement, and avoidance of narcotics and anticholinergics. With these conservative measures, colonic pseudoobstruction usually resolves in more than 75% of cases.[22] In cases in which conservative measures fail or the luminal diameter of the cecum reaches 10 to 12 cm, a more aggressive approach is warranted because of the risk for cecal perforation. Decompressive colonoscopy has historically been the method of choice in this setting.[23] More recently, the intravenous administration of 2.5 mg of neostigmine during 2 to 3 minutes has been found to decompress the colon promptly in nearly all patients.[24] Surgery is reserved for patients with obvious peritoneal signs or who

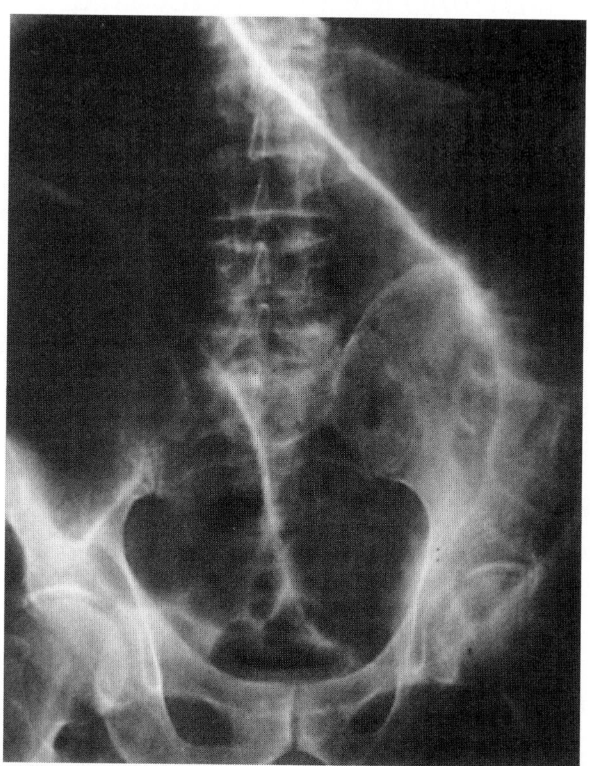

FIGURE 65.6 Pseudoobstruction of the colon (Ogilvie syndrome).

fail all forms of nonoperative therapy. In the latter setting, when the possibility of cecal perforation is high, a cecostomy is warranted.

KEY POINTS

- **The colon receives arterieal blood supply from both the superior and inferior mesenteric arteries.**
- **The veins that drain the large intestine bear the same terminology and follow a course similar to that of their corresponding arteries.**
- **The colon absorbs water, sodium, and chloride while it secretes potassium and bicarbonate.**
- **The bacterial flora of the colon is established soon after birth and depends in large part on dietary and environmental factors. Approximately 400 different species of bacteria have been identified in the human colon.**
- **Colonic pseudoobstruction, also known as Ogilvie syndrome, is a clinical entity in which signs and symptoms of bowel obstruction are present without an actual mechanical obstruction.**

References

1. Cummings JH, Macfarlane GT. The control and consequences of bacterial fermentation in the colon. *J Appl Bacteriol.* 1991;70:443–459.
2. **Latella G, Caprilli R. Metabolism of the large bowel mucosa in health and disease. *Int J Colorectal Dis.* 1991;6:127–132.**
3. Pemberton JH, Phillips SF. Colonic absorption. *Perspect Colon Rectal Surg.* 1988;1:89–103.
4. Grady GF, Duhamel RC, Moore EW. Active transport of sodium by human colon in vitro. *Gastroenterology* 1970;59:583–588.
5. Giller J, Phillips SF. Electrolyte absorption and secretion in the human colon. *Am J Dig Dis.* 1972;17:1003–1011.
6. Powell DW. Transport in the large intestine. In: Giebisch G, Tosteson DC, Ussing HH, eds. *Membrane transport in biology*. New York: Springer-Verlag, 1978, pp. 318–327.
7. Dunn DL. Autochthonous microflora of the gastrointestinal tract. *Perspect Colon Rectal Surg.* 1989;2:105–119.
8. Cannon WB. The movements of the intestine studied by means of roentgen rays. *Am J Physiol.* 1902;6:251–277.
9. Elliott TR, Barclay-Smith E. Antiperistalsis and other muscular activities of the colon. *J Physiol.* 1904;31:272–304.
10. Cohen S, Snape WJ. Movement of the small and large intestine. In: Fordtran J, Sleisinger M, eds. *Gastrointestinal disease*, 3rd ed. New York: McGraw-Hill, 1983, pp. 56–71.
11. Ritchie JA. Movements of segmental constrictions in the human colon. *Gut* 1971;6:251–277.
12. Herz AF. The passage of food along the human alimentary canal. *Guy's Hosp Rep.* 1907;61:389–427.
13. Ritchie JA. Mass peristalsis in the human colon after contact with oxyphenisatin. *Gut* 1972;13:211–219.
14. Daniel EE. Electrophysiology of the colon. *Gut* 1975;16:298–329.
15. Drossman DA, Thompson WG, Talley NJ, et al. Identification of sub-groups of functional gastrointestinal disorders. *Gastroenterol Int.* 1990;3:159–172.
16. **Benson MJ, Roberts JP, Wingate DL, et al. Small bowel motility following major intra-abdominal surgery: the effects of opiates and rectal cisapride. *Gastroenterology* 1994;106:924–936.**
17. Bohm B, Milsom JW, Fazio VW. Postoperative intestinal motility following conventional and laparoscopic intestinal surgery. *Arch Surg.* 1995;130: 415–419.
18. Olgilvy AJ, Smith G. The gastrointestinal tract after anaesthesia. *Eur J Anaesthesiol.* 1995;12(suppl 10):35–42.
19. Walker EA, Byrnne PP, Katon WJ. Irritable bowel syndrome and psychiatric illness. *Am J Psychiatry* 1990;147:565–572.
20. **Munakata J, Naliboff B, Harraf F, et al. Repetitive sigmoid stimulation induces rectal hyperalgesia in patients with irritable bowel syndrome. *Gastroenterology* 1997;112:55–63.**
21. Snape WJ Jr, Carlson GM, Cohen S. Colonic myoelectrical activity in the irritable bowel syndrome. *Gastroenterology* 1976;70:326–330.
22. Sloyer A, Panella V, Demas B. Ogilvie's syndrome: successful management with colonoscopy. *Dig Dis Sci.* 1988;33:1391–1396.
23. Nakhgevany KB. Colonoscopic decompression of the colon in patients with Olgivie's syndrome. *Am J Surg.* 1984;148:317–320.
24. **Hutchinson R, Griffiths C. Acute colonic pseudo-obstruction: a pharmacological approach. *Ann R Coll Surg Engl.* 1992;74:364–367.**

CHAPTER 66 ■ GASTROINTESTINAL MOTILITY DISORDERS

GEORGE A. SAROSI, JR. AND MASSIMO ASOLATI

Orderly progression of a swallowed food bolus from the mouth though the entire digestive system and expulsion of the residual material remaining after digestion is the normal function of gastrointestinal motility. Loss of normal gastrointestinal motor activity causes failure of major gastrointestinal functions, including absorption of nutrients and fluid and secretion of waste products. Although many acute surgical diseases result in secondary failure of gastrointestinal motor function, the majority of diseases causing primary gastrointestinal motor dysfunction are not surgically treated. Because many primary motility disorders can present in a similar fashion to common surgical diseases, and a few primary motility disorders are surgically treated diseases, surgeons must be familiar with gastrointestinal motility disorders. This chapter provides a broad overview of gastrointestinal motility disorders with a focus on the pathophysiology of motility disturbances.

DISORDERS AFFECTING THE ENTIRE DIGESTIVE TRACT

Ileus

Ileus is defined as impairment in the aboral passage of intestinal contents secondary to a failure of normal intestinal motility in the absence of an obstructing lesion. Ileus is the most common gastrointestinal motility disorder encountered by surgeons. Broadly defined, there are two major categories of ileus: postoperative ileus and ileus related to metabolic abnormalities, drugs, inflammation or ischemia (Table 66.1). The most common etiology of ileus is the postsurgical state, as some component of postoperative ileus is associated with essentially all major intraabdominal procedures and many nonabdominal procedures.[1]

TABLE 66.1 ETIOLOGY

CAUSES OF ILEUS

Abdominal surgery
Electrolyte abnormalities
Drugs
Intraabdominal inflammation
Retroperitoneal trauma or inflammation
Intestinal ischemia
Systemic sepsis

Although the pathophysiology of ileus remains incompletely understood, in recent years the basic mechanisms of postoperative ileus have been elucidated. In the immediate postoperative period all three functional segments of the gastrointestinal tract, the stomach, small intestine and the colon, display impaired motility characterized by disorganized electrical activity and a lack of coordinated propulsion.[2] Although all segments of the gastrointestinal tract are affected by ileus in the postoperative period, the duration of the dysmotility varies by segment. Small bowel motility normalizes first, often within a few hours.[3] Gastric motility usually returns to normal within 24 to 48 hours, but colonic motility takes 2 to 5 days to normalize and it is this functional segment that contributes most to the clinical effects of postoperative ileus.[4,5]

The pathophysiologic mechanisms underlying postoperative ileus are multifactorial. Three major contributing factors are spinal and local sympathetic reflexes, local and systemic inflammatory mediators, and exogenous factors including opioid analgesics and electrolyte disturbances. The role of spinal and sympathetic reflexes in ileus has been investigated in animal models, in which interventions such as spinal cord transection or pharmacologic neuronal depletion have been shown to decrease the duration of postoperative ileus.[6] These animal observations have been confirmed in human studies which demonstrate that interruption of gastrointestinal tract spinal reflexes with epidural local anesthetics significantly reduce the duration of postoperative ileus.[7] Multiple neurotransmitters intrinsic to the enteric nervous system may play a role in regulating gastrointestinal motility in the postoperative period. Nitric oxide, vasoactive intestinal polypeptide (VIP), and substance P reduce intestinal motility and have been linked to postoperative ileus in animal studies.[8,9] In contrast, both motilin and ghrelin promote motility during the resolution of postoperative ileus in both humans and animals.[10,11]

Local inflammation and systemic inflammatory mediators play an important role in postoperative ileus. Animal studies have demonstrated that surgical manipulation results in the accumulation of inflammatory cells in the muscular layer of the small intestine and that the degree of inflammation correlates with the degree of manipulation. In elegant animal studies, investigators have demonstrated that this infiltrate results in muscular dysfunction and jejunal dysmotility and that inhibition of leukocyte infiltration reduces ileus.[12] The correlation between intestinal inflammatory cell infiltration and degree of bowel manipulation may help explain the reduction in postoperative ileus observed with laparoscopic surgical approaches. Elevated serum levels of inflammatory cytokines such as interleukin-1 (Il-1) and Il-6 are seen in the postoperative period and may also be associated with decreased gastrointestinal function.[13]

Opioid analgesics are the mainstay of postoperative pain control and have a powerful influence on gastrointestinal motility through actions on peripheral opioid receptors found throughout the gastrointestinal tract.[14] Opioid analgesics have been shown to directly inhibit gastric, small bowel, and colonic motility, and limited narcotic use reduces postoperative colonic dysmotility in humans.[15,16] Electrolyte abnormalities are common in patients dependent on intravenous fluids for hydration, and one study has linked hypokalemia with prolonged postoperative ileus and demonstrated resolution of ileus with potassium therapy.[17]

Preventing ileus or reducing its duration has enormous potential to reduce health care expenditures and improve patient comfort in the perioperative period. Although no single treatment exists that can eliminate postoperative ileus, there are several interventions that may shorten the duration of this motility disorder. The two most effective interventions are thoracic epidural analgesia with local anesthetics and minimally invasive surgical approaches. Six of eight randomized trials comparing the effects of epidural analgesia to systemic opiates on postoperative ileus demonstrate a statistically significant reduction in the duration of ileus with epidural analgesia, with a typical effect size of 1 to 2 fewer days of ileus.[7] This effect is observed with epidural local anesthetics but not with epidural narcotics. Laparoscopic surgery appears to reduce the duration of postoperative ileus by reducing the amount of bowel manipulation and intraperitoneal inflammatory response. Four of six randomized trials comparing laparoscopic with open colectomy have shown a significant decrease in postoperative ileus with a typical effect size of 24 hours.[7]

Multiple pharmacologic interventions have been studied including promotility agents such as metoclopramide, erythromycin and cisapride, adrenergic blockade, parasympathomimetic agents, and opiate antagonists. Of these agents, only cisapride, which is no longer available in the United States, and the peripheral opiate antagonist ADL8-2698, have been shown to reduce the duration of postoperative ileus.[18] Nonpharmacologic measures that show promise in reducing postoperative ileus include early enteral feeding, sham feeding, and gum chewing. These interventions have not been proven to have benefit in large randomized trials. Standard interventions such as early ambulation and nasogastric decompression have no effect or prolong postoperative ileus when careful studies are performed, despite being considered standard of care.[19] Multimodality therapy, combining several interventions shows promise in reducing postoperative ileus, but systematic studies have not yet been performed.

Irritable Bowel Syndrome

Irritable bowel syndrome (IBS) is a chronic gastrointestinal illness characterized by frequent unexplained abdominal pain associated with bloating and disturbance in normal bowel function. Although in the strictest sense not a gastrointestinal motility disorder, IBS is associated with many of the symptoms of gastrointestinal motility disorders and patients with IBS have alterations in gastrointestinal motor function. IBS is an illness, a condition of gastrointestinal and mental disharmony, versus a specific medical disease. IBS is a common disorder with an estimated prevalence of 12% in adults in the United States. The peak incidence of the disease is in the second through fifth decades of life, and it is rare in patients older than age 50 years. There is a 2:1 female to male predominance.[20] The combination of abdominal pain in association with constipation, diarrhea, or alternating constipation and diarrhea that does not fit the pattern of a conventional gastrointestinal disorder should lead to consideration of the diagnosis of IBS. No single test can diagnose IBS, rather the condition is diagnosed by the presence of specific symptoms known as the Rome II criteria (Table 66.2), in the absence of other organic diseases.[21]

IBS is characterized by abnormal patterns of small bowel and colon electrical activity known as *discrete clusters of contractions*.[22] Rather than representing a true gastrointestinal motility disorder, these patterns are thought to be an exaggeration of the normal intestinal stress response.[23]

TABLE 66.2 DIAGNOSIS

ROME II DIAGNOSTIC CRITERIA FOR IRRITABLE BOWEL SYNDROME

At least 12 weeks or more, which need not be consecutive, in the preceding 12 months of abdominal discomfort or pain that has two of the following three features:
Relief by defecation Onset is associated with a change in stool frequency Onset is associated with a change in stool appearance
Symptoms that cumulatively support the diagnosis of irritable bowel syndrome
Abnormal stool frequency (>3/day or <3/week) Abnormal stool form (lumpy/hard or loose/watery) Abnormal stool passage (straining, urgency or incomplete evacuation) Passage of mucus Bloating/abdominal distention

Patients with IBS also have increased visceral sensitivity to bowel distention, and are more likely to perceive this distention as a noxious stimulus than normal controls.[24] This combination of heightened sensitivity associated with an exaggerated intestinal motility response to stress is thought to explain the symptoms of IBS. The cause of the heightened sensitivity to visceral stimulation is not clear, but inflammation triggered by infection, the postoperative state, or perhaps food allergies may play a role.[25]

The treatment of IBS is directed at symptomatic control. Importantly for surgeons, patients with IBS appear to have higher rates of common surgical procedures such as cholecystectomy, hysterectomy, and appendectomy than patients without the diagnosis of IBS.[26] The reasons for this observation are not clear. Three possible explanations include the overlap of IBS symptoms with the symptoms of surgically treated diseases, increased health-seeking behavior in IBS patients, and the ability of postsurgical inflammation to create visceral sensitization. For these reasons, rigorous attention to surgical indications in patients with IBS symptoms is critical.

Dietary modification and teaching patients to more effectively manage stressful life events that trigger symptoms are the usual starting points of therapy. Psychotherapy, including cognitive behavioral therapy has been shown to be beneficial. Management of constipation with fiber therapy and diarrhea with anti-diarrheal agents is helpful. Antispasmodic agents may reduce pain symptoms, although they do not appear to affect motility disturbances.[20] Tricyclic antidepressants appear to control motility disturbances in selected patients. This effect is independent from antidepressant actions, as serotonin re-uptake inhibitors have not been shown to be effective.[27] Two serotonin axis agents, the serotonin-3 receptor antagonist alosetron and the serotonin-4 agonist tegaserod, have been shown to be beneficial in diarrhea-predominant and constipation-predominant IBS, respectively.[28,29]

DISORDERS AFFECTING SPECIFIC ORGANS

Esophagus

Achalasia. The term *achalasia* is derived from the ancient Greek *chalasis*, or relaxation; thus *achalasis*, failure to relax. This word describes the characteristic motility disorder of achalasia: failure of the lower esophageal sphincter (LES) to relax.[30,31] Hypermotility of the body of the esophagus is usually the initial response to the functional obstruction of the LES, eventually resulting in hypomotility and aperistalsis. When the esophageal body becomes aperistaltic, the viscus becomes a large pouch in which food remains for days with minimal transit to the stomach.

TABLE 66.3 DIAGNOSIS

CLINICAL MANIFESTATIONS OF ACHALASIA

Dysphagia Chest pain Regurgitation Pulmonary symptoms

Achalasia is a rare disorder, with an incidence in the Western world of 0.5 to 1.1/100,000.[32] Achalasia can occur at any age, and both sexes are equally affected. Symptoms are the hallmarks of the disease; dysphagia is the predominant symptom with dysphagia for solid food present in the majority of the patients, and dysphagia for liquids present in two-thirds of cases (Table 66.3). The combination of dysphagia to both liquids and solids is more suggestive of functional disease rather than anatomical obstruction such as a stricture or tumor. The symptoms of dysphagia typically plateau over time, as patients learn to alleviate symptoms and improve esophageal function with postural maneuvers or other strategies that increase intra-esophageal pressure and promote esophageal emptying.

Approximately 50% of achalasia patients complain of chest pain. The relationship of pain to esophageal function is unclear as improvement of esophageal emptying does not necessarily ameliorate pain. Regurgitation occurs in 90% of patients and is associated with aspiration of esophageal contents and pulmonary complications in 10%. Weight loss usually occurs late in the course of achalasia. The clinical presentation of achalasia is often subtle in early stage disease but may be dramatic in the decompensated phases of the disease.

A barium swallow study is an appropriate initial test in a patient with suspected achalasia. Abnormal or absent clearance of the barium bolus is seen, particularly in the recumbent position. In achalasia, relaxation of the LES fails to occur with swallowing, causing radiographic findings resembling a "bird's beak." In the late phases of the disease a dilated esophagus is commonly present. Videofluoroscopy may help to establish the correct diagnosis in the early phases of the disease when the body of the esophagus may not be dilated. An epiphrenic diverticulum proximal to the LES is often seen in this disease. Its size may vary, and its presence may make diagnostic tests difficult.

The etiology of primary achalasia is not understood; several mechanisms have been postulated including immunologic, infectious, and genetic causes.[33] Dysfunction of inhibitory neurons containing nitric oxide and VIP innervating the LES and proximal portion of the stomach is postulated to be the major mechanism underlying the motor dysfunction of achalasia. Neural degeneration with resultant denervation of the smooth muscle segment of the esophagus has been demonstrated in patients with achalasia.[34] An autoimmune or inflammatory mechanism is suggested by the presence of T-lymphocytes infiltrating degenerating nervous fibers.[35] Whether lymphocyte infiltration is a primary or secondary event is unclear.[36] Patients with achalasia exhibit exaggerated LES contractions in response to acetylcholine and cholecystokinin (CCK), a classic deinnervation response, suggesting that lack of inhibitory neurons is the primary defect.[36] Loss of regulatory inhibition of the sphincter tone results in failure of the LES to relax.

Failure of the LES to relax and high resting LES pressure create a functional esophageal obstruction. Over time, this obstruction results in failure of the muscles of the esophageal body with esophageal dilation and aperistalsis. Muscle from the LES in patients with achalasia does not relax compared to muscle from normal individuals.[37]

Restoration of normal motility in the damaged esophagus is not possible and normal peristalsis and LES relaxation are not achievable with any therapeutic modality. All treatment options are targeted at reducing pressure across the LES, which will facilitate esophageal transit by gravity. Reduction of pressure across the LES can be achieved by surgical myotomy, pneumatic dilation, or pharmacologic agents; the choice of treatment depends on comorbid medical conditions. Because surgical myotomy is the most effective method to provide long-term pressure reduction across the LES, this treatment modality should be offered to patients who are good surgical candidates.[38] Anterior esophageal myotomy is carried out across the esophageal sphincter and should be extended a few centimeters along the anterior gastric wall. Because myotomy destroys the LES in the setting of hypomotility of the esophageal body, inadequate esophageal acid clearance is a potential source of uncontrolled gastroesophageal reflux. Whether an antireflux procedure should be combined with esophageal myotomy remains controversial.[39] Myotomy and fundoplication (Dor, Toupet or loose Nissen techniques) is usually done laparoscopically through the abdomen. Residual gastroesophageal reflux has been reported in 10% of patients treated in this way and overall results are satisfactory in 80% to 100% of the patients.

The most effective non-surgical treatment of achalasia is pneumatic dilation. The goal of this treatment is to "rupture" the LES. This result is obtained with inflation of a balloon across the LES tearing the muscle fibers of the sphincter. The balloons have different sizes (3.0, 3.5, and 4.0 cm) and clinical response is directly proportional to the size of the balloon used for dilation. The procedure can be done on an outpatient basis with minimum discomfort to the patient. About 25% to 30% of patients require multiple dilations. Esophageal perforation is the main complication with an incidence of about 2%.

Muscle relaxants such as calcium channel blockers or sublingual isosorbide dinitrate can be used before meals or to relieve symptoms. The efficacy of these medications is variable and usually decreases with prolonged use. Injection of botulinum toxin into the LES is a relatively new non-surgical approach for the treatment of achalasia. Botulinum toxin inhibits the release of acetylcholine from nerve terminals, counteracting the effect of loss of the inhibitory neurotransmitters. This treatment has an initial reported efficacy rate of about 80% to 85%. Unfortunately, symptom recurrence can be as high as 50% within 6 months. Receptor regeneration has been postulated as the main cause of failure after botulinum toxin injection. Some authors reported that myotomy can be more difficult and less effective after botulinum toxin injection.[40] Patient selection is extremely important when considering this type of treatment for achalasia (Algorithm 66.1). Patients with vigorous achalasia and older patients have been reported to have a prolonged response.

Improvement of symptoms is clinically used to evaluate the efficacy of pneumatic dilation or surgical myotomy. Symptom scores are not necessarily correlated with improvement in esophageal emptying; one-third of patients have poor esophageal emptying despite symptomatic improvement. Long-term patient follow-up has shown that good esophageal emptying is associated with better long-term results. Manometric or radiological studies may help to define objective improvement in esophageal body motility and transit through the manipulated LES.

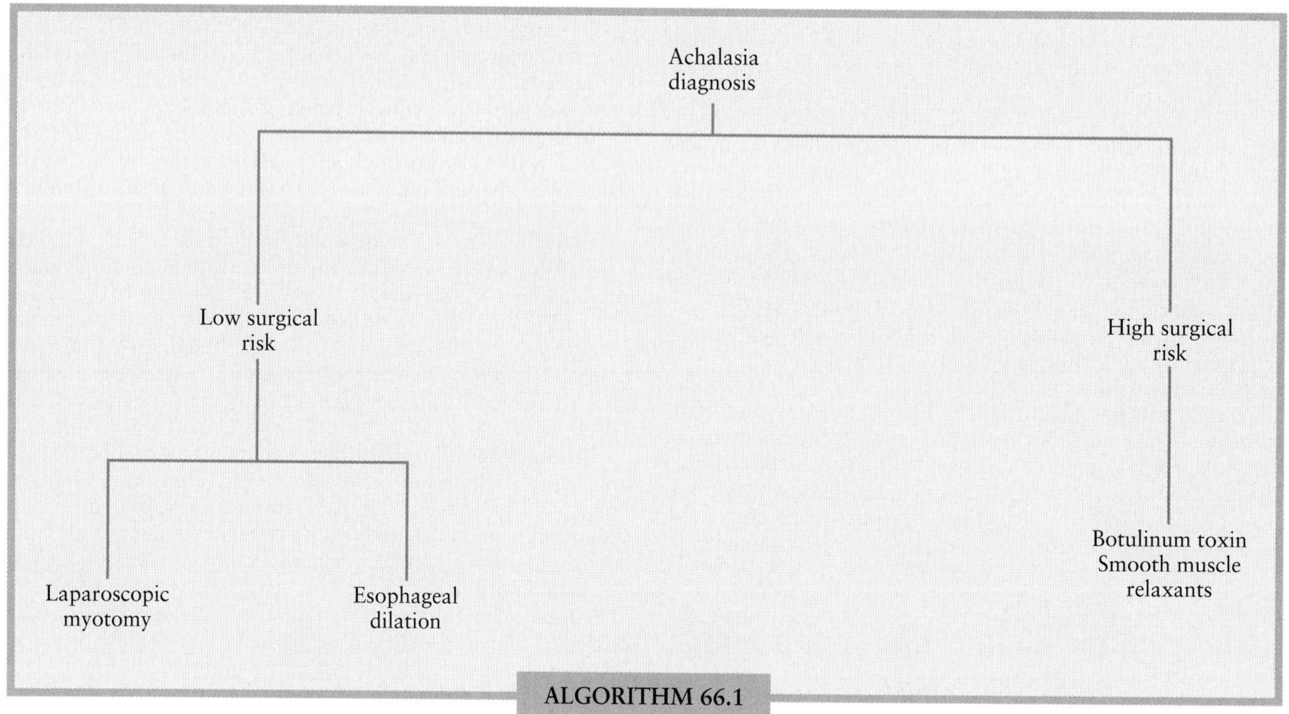

ALGORITHM 66.1 A proposed approach to the patient with achalasia. (Adapted with permission from Richter JE. Oesophageal motility disorders. *Lancet.* 2001;358: 823–828.)

Diffuse Esophageal Spasm. Normal esophageal peristalsis interrupted by simultaneous contractions is the hallmark of diffuse esophageal spasm. Roughly 3% to 5% of patients assessed for esophageal motility disorders have diffuse esophageal spasm. Diffuse esophageal spasm can affect patients at any age but is more common in those older than 50 years. The typical symptoms of diffuse esophageal spasm are chest pain and dysphagia. The chest pain of diffuse esophageal spasm is similar to cardiac angina and may respond to nitrites; however, this symptom is usually not related to exertion and is often associated with meals. Intermittent, nonprogressive dysphagia to liquids and solids that can be precipitated by rapid eating, extreme food temperatures, and stress is also commonly noted with diffuse esophageal spasm. An association of diffuse esophageal spasm with IBS, urinary disturbances, and sexual dysfunction has been reported.[41] Manometry is the diagnostic test of choice for the diagnosis of diffuse esophageal spasm.[42] The manometric findings are consistent, intermittent simultaneous contractions mixed with normal peristalsis and the presence of simultaneous contractions after 20% or more of wet swallows.[41]

The pathophysiology of diffuse esophageal spasm is unclear, but neural dysfunction has been suggested. Patients with diffuse esophageal spasm are more sensitive to hormonal and cholinergic stimulations, which cause esophageal contractions. Defects in inhibitory neural circuits have been implicated with a possible decrease in nitric oxide synthesis.[43] Gastroesophageal reflux and stress can produce diffuse esophageal spasm and some patients with diffuse esophageal spasm develop achalasia, suggesting that dysfunction of inhibitory motor circuits may be a common pathogenetic mechanism to both disorders.

Diffuse esophageal spasm is a nonprogressive disorder, and treatment is predominately directed at symptomatic control. Because there are many nonesophageal causes of chest pain, and the relationship between esophageal dysmotility and chest pain can be difficult to confirm, it is critical to exclude these problems before embarking on a course of therapy for dysmotility induced chest pain. Two pharmacologic approaches have been utilized, smooth muscle relaxants such as nitrates and calcium channel blockers, and chronic pain control with antidepressant medication. No randomized trials support the use of nitrates, although uncontrolled studies suggest they help with chest pain symptoms. Three small, randomized trials of calcium channel blockers have shown that despite significant manometric changes, calcium channel blockers were no more effective than placebo in reducing chest pain.[44] Both tricyclic antidepressants and trazodone have shown benefits in symptom relief without improvements in manometric findings in randomized controlled trials.[45] Despite these disappointing results, long-term follow-up of pharmacologically treated patients suggests that most patients improve with reassurance. For patients with refractory symptoms, nonrandomized case series suggest that thoracoscopic esophageal myotomy can result in good long-term symptom control when performed by experienced esophageal surgeons.[46]

Esophageal Hypermotility. High-pressure contractions in the esophageal body have been described as "nutcracker esophagus." High resting pressure in the LES is labeled as *hypertensive LES*. The entities have been grouped as a syndrome of spastic esophagus or esophageal hypermotility. Other causes of high-pressure contractions (e.g., gastroesophageal reflux) must be excluded prior to the diagnosis of esophageal hypermotility. The main symptom is chest pain, which is typically retrosternal and may radiate to the back. Dysphagia is an associated symptom in 50% of patients. Esophageal manometry is the most useful diagnostic test, with more than 40% of patients meeting manometric criteria. Manometry is characterized by mean distal esophageal peristaltic amplitude more than 180 mm Hg or mean distal duration greater than 6 seconds.[47] Treatment options are the same as those for diffuse esophageal spasm. Response to treatment is not always predictable.

Esophageal Hypomotility. Low-amplitude peristaltic contractions, simultaneous contractions, or failed contraction in the distal esophagus have been grouped as hypocontracting esophagus or as ineffective esophageal motility. Peristaltic waves with amplitude of less than 30 mm Hg do not provide effective esophageal transport and clearance. Two major groups of patients with esophageal hypomotility exist, those with hypomotility secondary to systemic diseases and those with idiopathic hypomotility. Connective tissue disorders are the most common causes of ineffective esophageal motility, including scleroderma, rheumatoid arthritis, and systemic lupus erythematosus. Up to 80% of patients with scleroderma have esophageal motility disorders.[48] This autoimmune disease causes diffuse vasculitis. In the esophagus and gastroesophageal junction vasculitis affects both smooth muscles and innervation resulting in low amplitude peristalsis of the distal esophagus and LES pressures below 10 mm Hg. Other causes of ineffective esophageal motility include autonomic neuropathy, amyloidosis, mixedema, multiple sclerosis, and alcoholism.

Gastroesophageal reflux is present in most patients with ineffective esophageal motility. Acid damage in the distal esophagus may contribute to dysmotility and diminished esophageal acid clearance is responsible for increased acid exposure with ineffective esophageal motility.[49] The close relationship between esophageal hypomotility and gastroesophageal reflux disease (GERD) is emphasized by the fact that patients with esophageal hypomotility typically present with reflux symptoms rather than dysphagia.

Many patients with reflux disease have similar manometric findings to patients with primary or secondary esophageal hypomotility. Whether gastroesophageal reflux is cause or result of these abnormal manometric findings is a subject of debate. Some patients with esophageal hypomotility in the setting of GERD obtain marked improvement in esophageal contractility with antireflux surgery.[50] There is currently no specific treatment available to improve esophageal contractility and symptomatic control of the gastroesophageal reflux is the only option for these patients.

Stomach

Diabetic Gastroparesis. Diabetic autonomic neuropathy is one of the major complications of diabetes mellitus and is most common in patients with long-term diabetes, poor glycemic control, and peripheral neuropathy. Autonomic neuropathy may affect the entire gastrointestinal tract producing constipation, abdominal pain, nausea, vomiting, dysphagia, diarrhea, and fecal incontinence. Diabetic gastroparesis may affect 50% of diabetic patients. Symptoms of diabetic gastroparesis include nausea, vomiting, and early satiety. In addition, impaired gastric motility predisposes to bezoar formation that can result in a vicious cycle of worsened gastric motility and early satiety. Delayed gastric emptying secondary to diabetic gastroparesis can make glucose homeostasis challenging, with resultant diabetic ketoacidosis or hypoglycemia. The diagnosis is usually suspected in a patient with symptoms of nausea, vomiting and early satiety in the setting of diabetes. An upper endoscopy should be performed in all patients suspected of diabetic gastroparesis to exclude other organic causes of their symptoms. A nuclear medicine gastric emptying study is the most accepted diagnostic test for gastroparesis and can also be used in follow-up to assess response to treatment.

The pathophysiology of diabetic gastroparesis is complicated, incompletely understood and multifactorial. Vagal nerve dysfunction can cause multiple changes in the normal physiology of gastric emptying. Vagal dysfunction can result in abnormal receptive relaxation of the stomach, decreased gastric antral contractility with failure of the antral pump, and prolonged contraction of the pylorus resulting in pylorospasm.[51] Neuropathy of the gastric enteric nervous system can exacerbate vagal dysfunction and may contribute to gastric myoelectric dysrythmias.[52] Hyperglycemia itself can disrupt normal gastric motility and delay gastric emptying.[53]

There is no single, specific treatment for diabetic gastroparesis. Aggressive glycemic control may prevent progressive neuropathy. Prokinetic agents such as metoclopramide and domperidone and dopamine antagonists promote gastric tone and improve gastric emptying. In addition, these drugs act as central nervous system–mediated antiemetic agents, reducing symptoms of nausea. The motilin agonist, erythromycin, has also been shown to be effective in patients with diabetic gastroparesis.[54] Erythromycin use has been limited by long-term tachyphylaxis. Pancreatic transplantation, by restoring glycemic control, has been reported to improve gastric motility as documented by gastric-emptying studies. Gastric electrical pacing using gastric pacemaker leads placed directly on the stomach has shown promise, but remains experimental.

Postsurgical Gastroparesis. Postsurgical gastroparesis is a syndrome characterized by gastric hypomotility in the absence of mechanical obstruction. The incidence of this disorder has been estimated at 2% to 3% after partial gastrectomy and vagotomy.[55] Postsurgical gastroparesis appears to occur more commonly after operations for gastric outlet obstruction and in diabetic patients. Patients with postsurgical gastroparesis develop symptoms of abdominal pain, postprandial nausea, vomiting, and weight loss months after gastric resection. The diagnosis is one of exclusion, and careful evaluation with endoscopy and barium studies are required to exclude mechanical gastric outlet obstruction. A solid phase gastric emptying study is necessary and is the only abnormal test in 45% of patients with this motility disorder.[56]

The pathogenic mechanism of this syndrome is related to loss of vagal innervation of the stomach, coupled with loss of antral pump function after antrectomy. Underlying gastric motor dysfunction in diabetic patients may also contribute to postsurgical gastroparesis. Treatment of postsurgical gastroparesis consists of prokinetic agents such as metoclopramide and erythromycin or revisional gastric surgery. Most authors recommend a 6- to 12-month trial of medical therapy prior to revisional surgery. Success rates of medical therapy have been disappointing, with response rates in the 20% to 30% range.[56] Surgical therapy is directed at eliminating the gastric reservoir with a near completion gastrectomy and Roux-en Y gastrojejunostomy. In selected patient series, symptomatic success rates of 70% to 80% have been reported.[57]

Dumping Syndrome. Dumping syndrome is a clinically defined spectrum of symptoms observed after gastric surgery thought to be a consequence of accelerated gastric emptying following vagotomy and bypass or destruction of the pylorus. Symptoms occur after the ingestion of food; they are absent in the fasting state. The incidence of dumping syndrome after gastric surgery is variable and depends on the operation performed. Overall, about 10% of patients will have clinically significant symptoms.[58] A diagnosis of dumping is made on clinical grounds and hinges on the presence of typical symptoms in a postoperative patient. Dumping occurs in the postprandial period and is classified into two forms. Early dumping occurs within 30 to 60 minutes of eating and typically presents with both gastrointestinal and vasomotor symptoms. Late dumping occurs 2 to 3 hours after eating and usually presents with only vasomotor symptoms. Gastrointestinal symptoms include postprandial fullness, crampy abdominal pain, nausea, vomiting, and explosive diarrhea. Vasomotor symptoms include diaphoresis, weakness, dizziness, flushing, palpitations, and an intense urge to lie down. In patients with severe dumping symptoms, weight loss and food fear may also be present.

Radioisotopic gastric emptying studies demonstrate rapid gastric emptying. Investigators have suggested a simple provocative test to confirm the diagnosis of dumping. After ingestion of 50 g of oral glucose a heart rate rise of greater than 10 beats per minute in the first hour is a sensitive predictor of early dumping.[59] Late dumping is confirmed with this test by documenting typical vasomotor symptoms in the postchallenge period.

The pathophysiologies of early and late dumping are different. In early dumping, rapid delivery of hyperosmolar chyme into the small intestine secondary to rapid gastric emptying results in several maladaptive responses. The presence of hyperosmolar proximal small intestinal contents leads to fluid shifts into the intestinal lumen causing intestinal distention and precipitating gastrointestinal symptoms. Rapid delivery of glucose to the proximal small bowel leads to both peripheral and splanchnic vasodilatation and blood pooling, which results in the vasomotor symptoms of early dumping. In addition, gastrointestinal hormone release is enhanced in patients with early dumping including secretion of enterglucogon, VIP, peptide YY, pancreatic polypeptide, and neurotensin.[60] Rapid delivery of glucose to the small bowel followed by rapid glucose absorption causes late dumping symptoms by producing an exaggerated serum insulin release. Exaggerated insulin secretion, combined with rapid gastric emptying, results in an excess insulin state 2 to 3 hours after eating with subsequent hypoglycemia and vasomotor symptoms. The cause of the excess insulin secretion is unclear, but the enteric hormone glucagon-like peptide 1 may play a role in late dumping.[61]

Most cases of dumping syndrome fade with time.[62] The initial mainstay therapy for dumping syndrome is dietary modification, which will effectively control dumping symptoms in most patients. An antidumping diet consists of: (1) frequent small meals, ideally six or more per day, (2) a diet low in simple sugars with a moderate amount of fat and high in complicated carbohydrates, protein, and fiber, and (3) dry meals with liquid ingestion delayed at least 30 minutes after solid intake. Dietary fiber supplementation has been shown to help with late dumping. Acarbose, a competitive inhibitor of carbohydrate absorption has also been shown to improve late dumping although long-term use can cause malabsorption.[60] In patients with severe dumping, or those whose symptoms fail to respond to dietary modification, the next step should be the use of octreotide, the long-acting somatostatin analog. Octreotide acts to delay intestinal transit time, cause splanchnic vasoconstriction, and suppress the release of a variety of enteral hormones including insulin.[58] For patients with debilitating dumping symptoms that are refractory to dietary modification and octreotide, remedial surgery may be considered. A cautious approach is appropriate, as most cases of dumping will improve with time and no remedial operation has a 100% success rate. Reconstruction of the pylorus and conversion to Roux-en Y gastrojejunostomy have both been used successfully to correct intractable dumping.[62]

Gallbladder and Biliary Tract

Gallbladder Dyskinesia. The term *biliary dyskinesia* indicates a poorly characterized motility disorder of the gallbladder and the sphincter of Oddi. Gallbladder dyskinesia has been recognized as a cause of biliary symptoms, and may be a manifestation of generalized dysmotility of the gastrointestinal tract.[63] The most common presenting symptom of gallbladder dyskinesia is abdominal pain in the absence of gallstones or other structural cause of right upper quadrant pain. The prevalence of biliary pain without gallstones has been estimated to be 6 % to21% with a three-to-one female to male predominance. The diagnosis of gallbladder dyskinesia is usually made by CCK cholescintigraphy obtained after an ultrasound negative for gallstones. During CCK cholescintigraphy, a gallbladder ejection fraction less than 35% is considered diagnostic by most authors.

Defects in the function and distribution of CCK receptors on cells within the gallbladder wall with resultant abnormal responses to endogenous CCK have been implicated as causes of this disorder. In addition to an intrinsic motility disorder, inflammation and anatomical abnormalities have also been reported. Inflammatory bowel disease is associated with abnormal gallbladder contractility and patients with slow–transit constipation have been reported to have decreased gallbladder ejection fraction.[64,65]

There is no effective medical therapy for this disorder. Laparoscopic cholecystectomy is the major treatment option for patients with gallbladder dyskinesia, with symptomatic improvement noted in 90% of selected patients. Because of the frequent association of gallbladder dyskinesia with other motility disorders of the gastrointestinal tract, symptoms related to gastrointestinal dysmotility may not be relieved. Although 81% of the patients with gallstones become asymptomatic after laparoscopic cholecystectomy, only 47% of patients with gallbladder dyskinesia are asymptomatic postoperatively.[66]

Sphincter of Oddi Dysfunction. Sphincter of Oddi dysfunction describes a clinical syndrome arising from abnormalities of sphincter of Oddi contractility. The disorder can be caused by fibrosis and stenosis or by functional obstruction of the pancreaticobiliary junction. Ductal hypertension, hypersensitivity of the papilla and possible ischemia from spastic contraction have been postulated as causes of pain, pancreatitis and severe liver enzyme abnormalities.[67] The disorder can occur at any age and affects females more frequently than males. Estimates of the incidence of sphincter of Oddi dysfunction in patients with elevation of liver enzymes or biliary symptoms range between 40% and 53%. Fewer than 50% of patients with active symptoms have liver enzyme abnormalities.

Abdominal pain, usually in the epigastrium or right upper quadrant, is the most common symptom. The pain is often associated with oral intake and use of narcotics and does not respond to acid reducing or prokinetic medical therapy. Jaundice and fever are uncommon. There are no characteristic findings on physical examination aside from nonspecific abdominal tenderness. Because of the absence of a classic symptom or finding, patients with the diagnosis of sphincter of Oddi dysfunction are sometimes difficult to distinguish from patients with other organic or dysmotility disorders. Rome II criteria for the diagnosis of sphincter of Oddi dysfunction are listed in Table 66.4.

TABLE 66.4 DIAGNOSIS

ROME II CRITERIA FOR SPHINCTER OF ODDI DYSFUNCTION

Criteria
Epigastric or right upper quadrant pain
Symptoms at least 30 minutes with pain-free intervals
Symptoms of 12 months duration
Pain requires medical attention and affects daily activities
No evidence of structural abnormalities

(Adapted with permission from Sherman S, Lehman GA. Sphincter of Oddi dysfunction: diagnosis and treatment. *J Panc.* 2001;2:382–400.)

Initial diagnostic tests include complete blood count, liver function tests, and determination of serum amylase and lipase. Imaging studies include abdominal computed tomography scan and ultrasonography. All of these tests are most sensitive when performed during active symptoms. Endoscopic retrograde pancreatography (ERCP) is conventionally used to exclude other pathologies that may cause symptoms similar to sphincter of Oddi dysfunction and provides visual evaluation of the peripapillary area. Sphincter of Oddi manometry is considered the standard for the diagnosis of sphincter of Oddi dysfunction and is the only method to measure the activity of the sphincter directly. Manometry is usually performed during ERCP with selective cannulation of the pancreatic duct and biliary duct. Although a variety of invasive and noninvasive tests have been used in the diagnosis of sphincter of Oddi dysfunction, noninvasive testing cannot be recommended for general clinical use due to low sensitivity and specificity.[67] Invasive tests such as ERCP and manometry have a relatively high complication rate and are indicated only if definitive therapy is planned in the presence of abnormal results. Because of the difficulty in establishing the diagnosis of sphincter of Oddi dysfunction, and predicting the response to therapy, the Hogan-Geenen classification system was developed in an effort to correlate symptoms and diagnostic tests with abnormal manometric findings and predict the response to sphincterotomy (Tables 66.5 and 66.6). Abnormal liver tests in biliary type II disease may predict symptomatic response to endoscopic sphincterotomy.[68]

The aim of therapy is to decrease the resistance to the flow of bile and pancreatic juice. Medical therapy is based on smooth muscle relaxants. Nifedipine has been shown to reduce pain in sphincter of Oddi dysfunction in 75% of the patients in the short term.[69] Long-term outcomes have not been reported. Despite the lack of long-term data, medical approaches should be considered when patients are not severely symptomatic (class III and II sphincter of Oddi dysfunction).

Reduction of resistance at the sphincter of Oddi via endoscopic means by stenting or sphincterotomy is the mainstay of therapy for sphincter of Oddi dysfunction.[70] According to Hogan-Geenen classification, manometry may predict outcome from sphincter ablation in patients with biliary-type pain. The use of stents in sphincter of Oddi dysfunction is controversial, with a reported high incidence of pancreatitis (38%). Stenting may predict outcome from sphincterotomy when stenting provides resolution of pain for at least 12 weeks. Currently, endoscopic sphincteroplasty is standard therapy for sphincter of Oddi dysfunction, with clinical

TABLE 66.5 CLASSIFICATION

HOGAN-GEENEN CLASSIFICATION: SYMPTOMS

Biliary type	Description
I	Patient with biliary-type pain, abnormal AST or alkaline phosphatase (2 times normal) on two or more occasions, delayed drainage from ERCP contrast >45 minutes, and dilated CBD more than 12 mm diameter.
II	Patient with biliary-type of pain but only one of two of the above criteria.
III	Biliary-type pain only

AST, aspartate aminotransferase; ERCP, endoscopic retrograde pancreatography; CBD, common bile duct. (Adapted with permission from Sherman S, Lehman GA. Sphincter of Oddi dysfunction: diagnosis and treatment. *J Panc.* 2001;2:382–400.)

TABLE 66.6 CLASSIFICATION

HOGAN-GEENEN CLASSIFICATION: BILIARY SYMPTOMS AND RESPONSE TO TREATMENT

Patient characteristics	Abnormal manometry (%)	Sphincterotomy efficacy		Indication for manometry: prior sphincterotomy
		Normal (%)	Abnormal (%)	
Biliary I	75–95	90–95	90–95	Unnecessary
Biliary II	55–65	35%	85	Highly recommended
Biliary III	25–60	<10%	55–65	Mandatory

(Adapted with permission from Sherman S, Lehman GA. Sphincter of Oddi dysfunction: diagnosis and treatment. *J Panc.* 2001;2:382–400.)

improvement reported in 55% to 95% of cases.[71] The role of sphincter ablation is evolving; complication rates remain higher than in patients with ductal stones. Surgical approaches such as transduodenal sphincteroplasty with pancreatic septoplasty have been largely replaced by endoscopic therapy.

Patient selection is paramount considering the high complication rate for endoscopic therapy.[71] Evolving manometric techniques are improving knowledge of sphincter of Oddi dysfunction. Patient selection is also important to tailor medical therapy.

Small Intestine

Chronic Intestinal Pseudoobstruction. Chronic intestinal pseudoobstruction is a clinical syndrome caused by ineffective intestinal propulsion and characterized by signs and symptoms of intestinal obstruction in the absence of mechanical cause.[72] The disorder is a rare clinical syndrome, caused by a variety of pathogenic mechanisms. Although sophisticated clinicopathologic classification systems exist for chronic intestinal pseudoobstruction, important etiologies include visceral myopathies, visceral neuropathies, systemic disorders involving smooth muscle such a systemic sclerosis, developmental abnormalities of the myenteric plexus, and systemic neurodegenerative disorders.[73] Although small intestinal dysmotility is the prominent finding in most cases, the syndrome can involve all portions of the gastrointestinal tract from esophagus to colon.

Patients with intestinal pseudoobstruction present with variable amounts of abdominal pain, distention and vomiting. The vomitus often consists of partially digested food and can be feculent in character. Patients with small bowel involvement can develop bacterial overgrowth and may have symptoms of diarrhea and steatorrhea. In patients with significant colonic dysmotility, constipation symptoms may predominate. A family history of similar problems may be present in up to one third of cases, and many patients have a history of abdominal surgery.

On physical examination, patients may exhibit wasting with marked abdominal distention and visible bowel loops against the abdominal wall. Although tenderness is often present peritonitis is unusual. In most ways it will be impossible to distinguish chronic intestinal pseudoobstruction from true mechanical bowel obstruction, except for the chronic nature of symptoms and a history of prior episodes with waxing and waning severity. It is imperative for surgeons evaluating patients with chronic intestinal pseudoobstruction to avoid mistaking this syndrome for simple bowel obstruction, because once a patient with chronic intestinal pseudoobstruction has undergone abdominal surgery the potential exists for both pseudoobstruction and adhesive bowel obstruction to coexist. The best way to confirm a suspected diagnosis of chronic intestinal pseudoobstruction is through barium contrast studies of the entire gastrointestinal tract. The identification of multiple sites of abnormality on such studies in the absence of a clear mechanical transition point is most consistent with the diagnosis. The finding of a single area of dilation isolated to the small intestine should raise suspicion of mechanical small bowel obstruction.

There is no definitive treatment for this motility disorder; no pharmacologic therapy or surgical procedure will correct the underlying motility disorder. Therapy is therefore directed at palliating symptoms and ensuring that patients receive adequate nutrition. A variety of promotility agents have been used. Metoclopramide and domperidone have not been found to be effective.[73] Erythromycin has shown benefit in some patients for up to 1 year, but tachyphylaxis appears to limit its long-term value.[72] Cisapride, although no longer available in the United States, improves symptoms in the majority of patients in noncontrolled trials.[74] Low-dose (50µg) octreotide may be of benefit in patients with systemic sclerosis, but has not been shown to be useful in other patients.[75]

In patients with suspected pseudoobstruction, avoiding operation is critical because a nontherapeutic operation for bowel obstruction will predispose the patient to adhesive mechanical bowel obstruction in the future. In patients with confirmed chronic intestinal pseudoobstruction, surgical therapy can be important in palliating specific symptoms of the syndrome such as bloating and malnutrition, or in managing failures of medical management. For patients with localized dysfunctional bowel, bypass or segmental resection of the involved bowel can result in satisfactory long-term results.[76] In patients with diffuse intestinal involvement, venting enterostomy and intravenous access for long-term parenteral nutrition may represent the only surgical options. Small intestinal transplant has been reported in small series with good functional results.[77]

Acquired Jejunoileal Diverticular Disease. Acquired jejunoileal diverticulosis appears to occur as a consequence of a small bowel motility disorder. This rare finding has a prevalence of between 0.1% and 2.3%, depending on whether autopsy or radiological data are used.[78,79] These lesions are usually found in patients in the seventh decade of life. There is no apparent sex predilection. These acquired lesions are pseudodiverticula whose wall includes only the mucosal and submucosal layers of the bowel. They are found on the mesenteric surface of the bowel and commonly lie within the mesentery. Eighty percent of patients have the diverticula localized to the jejunum; in 15% of patients, lesions are found in the ileum, and 5% have diverticula distributed throughout the small intestine. Eighty percent of patients, particularly those with jejunal diverticula, have multiple lesions.[80]

It has been postulated that these acquired lesions are caused by a motility disturbance of the involved intestine. Poorly coordinated neuromuscular function with ineffective peristalsis and resultant high intraluminal pressures cause protrusion of the mucosa through the muscular layers of the bowel wall at the point that the vasa recta enter the bowel wall. Abnormalities of both intestinal smooth muscle and the myenteric plexus found in patients with jejunoileal diverticulosis support this hypothesis.[81] Mild variants of the same disorders may lead to the development of acquired small bowel diverticulosis. Pseudodiverticula are found in the colon and duodenum in 40% to 50% of patients with jejunoileal diverticulosis, supporting the role of a diffuse intestinal motility disorder in pathogenesis.

The role of surgical therapy in this motility disorder lies in the management of complications and in palliating symptoms secondary to the diverticula. The majority of patients (50% to 60%) have asymptomatic diverticula noted on radiological study or found incidentally at laparotomy.[78] Because these patients are likely to remain symptom-free there is no indication for resection in these instances. Twenty to 40% of patients will present with a nonspecific constellation of chronic abdominal complaints including pain, postprandial bloating, diarrhea, malabsorption, and vitamin B_{12} deficiency.[80] In these patients, symptoms are related to bacterial overgrowth and malabsorption. Most of these patients respond to a regimen of a high protein, low residue diet coupled with vitamin B_{12} supplementation and intermittent broad-spectrum antibiotic treatment. Only when this approach fails should resection be contemplated. Only 10% to 15% of patients will present with acute complications, either bleeding, diverticulitis or perforation, requiring urgent surgical intervention.[82] In emergent cases, resection of the involved segment of small bowel with anastomosis is the best surgical approach.

Colon

Colonic Inertia. Constipation is a common complaint, affecting up to 20% of the population.[83] Although the overwhelming majority of cases of constipation do not require surgical attention, one disorder, idiopathic slow transit constipation is both a motility disorder and amenable to surgical therapy. Idiopathic slow transit constipation or colonic inertia is caused by a variety pathogenic mechanisms including abnormalities of myenteric plexus formation, disorders of extrinsic enervation of the colon and disorders of colonic neuromuscular transmission. From a diagnostic and therapeutic standpoint these disorders may be considered a single syndrome.[84]

The diagnosis of colonic inertia is established in a chronically constipated patient with markedly prolonged colonic transit time in the absence of anorectal dysfunction. Colonic transit time is assessed either with radiopaque markers or by scintigraphic colonic transit studies. Radiopaque marker study involves ingestion of three capsule markers on 3 consecutive days followed by abdominal radiographs on days 4 and 7. In patients with normal motility, the mean transit time of markers is 36 hours, and transit is considered pathologic when it exceeds 72 hours.[85] Scintigraphic colonic transit studies are less widely available, but require only 24 hours to obtain accurate segmental transit times.[86]

After establishing a diagnosis of slow colonic transit, anorectal function must be assessed, as disorders of anorectal function will slow colonic transit. Fluoroscopic defecography and anorectal manometry are used to exclude anorectal dysfunction. Normal findings on these evaluations are required to establish a diagnosis of idiopathic slow transit constipation.[87]

The initial management of chronic constipation is medical, including behavior modification, dietary changes, fiber supplementation, and use of oral low volume polyethylene glycol electrolyte solution.[88]

In the few patients with intractable constipation found to have isolated colonic inertia, total abdominal colectomy with ileorectal anastomosis results in excellent functional outcomes in 90% of patients. The key to good results with surgical therapy for constipation is careful preoperative evaluation of colonic function. In series without complete evaluation, acceptable outcome rates of as low as 67% have been reported.[87]

Acute Colonic Pseudoobstruction (Ogilvie Syndrome). Acute colonic pseudoobstruction is a clinical syndrome characterized by massive dilation of the colon in the absence of mechanical obstruction. The disorder is characterized by the loss of effective colonic peristalsis and subsequent distention of the proximal colon. This syndrome generally develops in ill patients, hospitalized initially for other significant medical problems, and is also observed in surgical patients after a variety of non-gastrointestinal operations.[89] If left untreated, massive colonic dilation can result in ischemia of the right colon and cecum with associated perforation. The overall mortality rate of acute colonic pseudoobstruction is quite variable, ranging between 0 and 32%, and appears to depend on the underlying cause of the pseudoobstruction.[90] With the development of ischemia and perforation, mortality rises to 30% to 50%.

The pathophysiology of acute colonic pseudoobstruction remains unclear. A current hypothesis invokes an imbalance in neural input to the colon distal to the splenic flexure with an excess of sympathetic stimulation and a paucity of parasympathetic input, resulting in a spastic contraction of the distal colon and functional obstruction.[91] Multiple independent circumstantial lines of evidence support this hypothesis, including the finding of colonic dilation in only the right and transverse colon in the majority of cases, the observation that epidural anesthesia improves the condition in a majority of cases, and the effective use of parasympathomimetic agents to treat the syndrome. The role of inhibitory neurotransmitters such as nitric oxide in the pathogenesis of acute colonic pseudoobstruction has been suggested in vitro, but not yet confirmed in human studies.

Acute colonic pseudoobstruction should be suspected in a hospitalized patient who develops marked abdominal distention over a period of 1 to 2 days. Obstipation is seen in the majority of patients, but up to 40% of cases will present with diarrhea or passage of flatus. Abdominal discomfort is present in the majority of patients, and tenderness on physical examination raises the concern for bowel ischemia.[89]

Plain films of the abdomen, with the finding of proximal dilation of the colon associated with a decompressed distal colon with some gas in the rectosigmoid region, are highly suggestive of acute colonic pseudoobstruction. The diagnostic challenge initially is to exclude mechanical colonic obstruction, and early performance of a water soluble contrast enema is critical if mechanical obstruction cannot be ruled out on clinical grounds. The diameter of the cecum on plain film is important in directing the therapeutic approach to acute colonic pseudoobstruction. Both animal studies and large retrospective human series suggest that the risk of cecal ischemia and perforation exists with cecal diameters greater than 12 cm, and rises dramatically with cecal diameters greater than 14 cm.[89]

For patients with a cecal diameter less than 14 cm, an initial trial of conservative therapy is indicated. Conservative therapy includes correction of electrolyte disorders, avoidance of narcotic and anticholinergic agents, hydration, mobilization, tap water enemas and placement of a nasogastric tube.[92] During this course of conservative therapy patients should receive frequent abdominal evaluation and serial abdominal radiographs to assess cecal diameter. Several small cases series suggest that resolution rates of acute colonic pseudoobstruction approximating 90% can be achieved with a conservative regimen. Roughly 70% of the cases that resolve with conservative therapy do so within 2 days, suggesting that a 48-hr trial in stable patients is warranted.[93] However, postponing colon decompression beyond 4 days increases the mortality rate in patients with acute colonic pseudoobstruction.[89]

Patients who fail conservative therapy for more than 48 hours should be considered for active intervention with the first line treatment consisting of intravenous administration of the cholinesterase inhibitor neostigmine. More than five non-controlled trials and one randomized controlled trial have shown that intravenous neostigmine at a dose of 2 to 2.5 mg given over 3 to 5 minutes results in immediate colonic decompression in 80% to 90% of patients, and sustained colon decompression is achieved in more than 60%.[91,94] Because symptomatic bradycardia is a serious side effect of neostigmine, all patients being treated with the drug require cardiac monitoring. Neostigmine is contraindicated in patients with significant bradycardia. In patients with a contraindication to neostigmine and for those who fail to respond to the drug, decompressive colonoscopy is the next line of therapy. Colonoscopy to the cecum with evacuation of the contents of the proximal colon and placement of a long tube for decompression results in resolution of acute colonic pseudoobstruction in 70% to-80% of cases. Roughly 40% of cases require multiple colonscopies.[95]

Colonoscopy in this setting is associated with a 2% to 3% perforation rate and the case fatality rate of acute colonic pseudoobstruction in patients requiring colonoscopy is up to 30%.[96] In patients who develop findings suggestive of colonic ischemia or those who fail colonoscopic decompression, surgical therapy with either resection, or a stoma is necessary although it is associated with a 30% to 50% mortality rate.[89] Laparoscopic approaches have been reported for stoma creation and may avoid laparotomy in an elderly or frail patient.

KEY POINTS

- **Ileus is defined as impairment in the aboral passage of intestinal contents secondary to a failure of normal intestinal motility in the absence of an obstructing lesion. Ileus is the most common gastrointestinal motility disorder encountered by surgeons.**
- **Irritable bowel syndrome is a chronic gastrointestinal illness characterized by frequent unexplained abdominal pain associated with bloating and disturbance in normal bowel function.**
- **Normal esophageal peristalsis interrupted by simultaneous contractions is the hallmark of diffuse esophageal spasm.**
- **Diabetic gastroparesis may affect 50% of diabetic patients.**
- **Dumping syndrome is a clinically defined spectrum of symptoms observed after gastric surgery thought to be a consequence of accelerated gastric emptying following vagotomy and bypass or destruction of the pylorus.**
- **The most common presenting symptom of gallbladder dyskinesia is abdominal pain in the absence of gallstones or other structural cause of right upper quadrant pain.**
- **The diagnosis of colonic inertia is established in a chronically constipated patient with markedly prolonged colonic transit time in the absence of anorectal dysfunction.**
- **Acute colonic pseudoobstruction is a clinical syndrome characterized by massive dilation of the colon in the absence of mechanical obstruction. The syndrome generally develops in ill patients, hospitalized initially for other significant medical problems.**

References

1. **Baig MK, Wexner SD. Postoperative ileus: a review. *Dis Colon Rectum.* 2004;47:516–526.**
2. Livingston EH, Passaro EP Jr. Postoperative ileus. *Dig Dis Sci.* 1990;35:121–132.
3. Miedema BW, Schillie S, Simmons JW, et al. Small bowel motility and transit after aortic surgery. *J Vasc Surg.* 2002;36:19–24.
4. Waldhausen JH, Shaffrey ME, Skenderis BS II, et al. Gastrointestinal myoelectric and clinical patterns of recovery after laparotomy. *Ann Surg.* 1990;211:777–784; discussion 785.
5. Behm B, Stollman N. Postoperative ileus: etiologies and interventions. *Clin Gastroenterol Hepatol.* 2003;1:71–80.
6. Holzer P, Lippe IT, Holzer-Petsche U. Inhibition of gastrointestinal transit due to surgical trauma or peritoneal irritation is reduced in capsaicin-treated rats. *Gastroenterology* 1986;91:360–363.
7. Holte K, Kehlet H. Postoperative ileus: a preventable event. *Br J Surg.* 2000;87:1480–1493.
8. De Winter BY, Robberecht P, Boeckxstaens GE, et al. Role of VIP1/PACAP receptors in postoperative ileus in rats. *Br J Pharmacol.* 1998;124:1181–1186.
9. Espat NJ, Cheng G, Kelley MC, et al. Vasoactive intestinal peptide and substance P receptor antagonists improve postoperative ileus. *J Surg Res.* 1995;58:719–723.
10. Trudel L, Tomasetto C, Rio MC, et al. Ghrelin/motilin-related peptide is a potent prokinetic to reverse gastric postoperative ileus in rat. *Am J Physiol Gastrointest Liver Physiol.* 2002;282:G948–952.
11. Rennie JA, Christofides ND, Mitchenere P, et al. Neural and humoral factors in postoperative ileus. *Br J Surg.* 1980;67:694–698.
12. Kalff JC, Schraut WH, Simmons RL, et al. Surgical manipulation of the gut elicits an intestinal muscularis inflammatory response resulting in postsurgical ileus. *Ann Surg.* 1998;228:652–663.
13. Bellon JM, Manzano L, Larrad A, et al. Endocrine and immune response to injury after open and laparoscopic cholecystectomy. *Int Surg.* 1998;83:24–27.
14. Kaufman PN, Krevsky B, Malmud LS, et al. Role of opiate receptors in the regulation of colonic transit. *Gastroenterology* 1988;94:1351–1356.
15. Yee MK, Evans WD, Facey PE, et al. Gastric emptying and small bowel transit in male volunteers after i.m. ketorolac and morphine. *Br J Anaesth.* 1991;67:426–431.
16. Ferraz AA, Cowles VE, Condon RE, et al. Nonopioid analgesics shorten the duration of postoperative ileus. *Am Surg.* 1995;61:1079–1083.
17. Lowman RM. The potassium depletion states and postoperative ileus. The role of the potassium ion. *Radiology* 1971;98:691–694.
18. Brown TA, McDonald J, Williard W. A prospective, randomized, double-blinded, placebo-controlled trial of cisapride after colorectal surgery. *Am J Surg.* 1999;177:399–401.
19. Cheadle WG, Vitale GC, Mackie CR, et al. Prophylactic postoperative nasogastric decompression. A prospective study of its requirement and the influence of cimetidine in 200 patients. *Ann Surg.* 1985;202:361–366.
20. Mertz HR. Irritable bowel syndrome. *N Engl J Med.* 2003;349:2136–2146.
21. Thompson WG, Longstreth GF, Drossman DA, et al. Functional bowel disorders and functional abdominal pain. *Gut* 1999;45(suppl 2):II43–47.
22. Kellow JE, Gill RC, Wingate DL. Prolonged ambulant recordings of small bowel motility demonstrate abnormalities in the irritable bowel syndrome. *Gastroenterology* 1990;98(5 Pt 1):1208–1218.
23. Kellow JE, Phillips SF, Miller LJ, et al. Dysmotility of the small intestine in irritable bowel syndrome. *Gut* 1988;29:1236–1243.
24. Mertz H, Naliboff B, Munakata J, et al. Altered rectal perception is a biological marker of patients with irritable bowel syndrome. *Gastroenterology* 1995;109:40–52.
25. Collins SM, Vallance B, Barbara G, et al. Putative inflammatory and immunological mechanisms in functional bowel disorders. *Baillieres Best Pract Res Clin Gastroenterol.* 1999;13:429–436.
26. Longstreth GF, Yao JF. Irritable bowel syndrome and surgery: a multivariable analysis. *Gastroenterology* 2004;126:1665–1673.
27. Jackson JL, O'Malley PG, Tomkins G, et al. Treatment of functional gastrointestinal disorders with antidepressant medications: a meta-analysis. *Am J Med.* 2000;108:65–72.
28. Novick J, Miner P, Krause R, et al. A randomized, double-blind, placebo-controlled trial of tegaserod in female patients suffering from irritable bowel syndrome with constipation. *Aliment Pharmacol Ther.* 2002;16:1877–1888.
29. Camilleri M, Northcutt AR, Kong S, et al. Efficacy and safety of alosetron in women with irritable bowel syndrome: a randomised, placebo-controlled trial. *Lancet* 2000;355:1035–1040.
30. **Richter JE. Oesophageal motility disorders. *Lancet.* 2001;358:823–828.**
31. Wong RHK, Maydonovich CL. Achalasia. In: Castell DO, Richter JE, eds. *The Esophagus.* Philadelphia: Lippincott Williams and Wilkins, 1999, p. 185.
32. Podas T, Eaden J, Mayberry M, et al. Achalasia: a critical review of epidemiological studies. *Am J Gastroenterol.* 1998;93:2345–2347.
33. Goldblum JR, Whyte RI, Orringer MB, et al. Achalasia. A morphologic study of 42 resected specimens. *Am J Surg Pathol.* 1994;18:327–337.
34. Cassella RR, Ellis FH Jr, Brown AL Jr. Fine-structure changes in achalasia of the esophagus. I. Vagus Nerves. *Am J Pathol.* 1965;46:279–288.
35. Raymond L, Lach B, Shamji FM. Inflammatory aetiology of primary oesophageal achalasia: an immunohistochemical and ultrastructural study of Auerbach's plexus. *Histopathology* 1999;35:445–453.
36. Clark SB, Rice TW, Tubbs RR, et al. The nature of the myenteric infiltrate in achalasia: an immunohistochemical analysis. *Am J Surg Pathol.* 2000;24:1153–1158.
37. Misiewicz JJ, Waller SL, Anthony PP, et al. Achalasia of the cardia: pharmacology and histopathology of isolated cardiac sphincteric muscle from patients with and without achalasia. *Q J Med.* 1969;38:17–30.
38. Vaezi MF. Achalasia: diagnosis and management. *Semin Gastrointest Dis.* 1999;10:103–112.

39. Donahue PE, Horgan S, Liu KJ, et al. Floppy Dor fundoplication after esophagocardiomyotomy for achalasia. *Surgery* 2002;132:716–722; discussion 722–723.
40. Horgan S, Hudda K, Eubanks T, et al. Does botulinum toxin injection make esophagomyotomy a more difficult operation? *Surg Endosc.* 1999;13:576–579.
41. Richter JE, Castell DO. Diffuse esophageal spasm: a reappraisal. *Ann Intern Med.* 1984; 100:242–245.
42. Peters L, Maas L, Petty D, et al. Spontaneous noncardiac chest pain. Evaluation by 24-hour ambulatory esophageal motility and pH monitoring. *Gastroenterology.* 1988;94:878–886.
43. Behar J, Biancani P. Pathogenesis of simultaneous esophageal contractions in patients with motility disorders. *Gastroenterology* 1993;105:111–118.
44. Richter JE, Dalton CB, Bradley LA, et al. Oral nifedipine in the treatment of noncardiac chest pain in patients with the nutcracker esophagus. *Gastroenterology* 1987;93:21–28.
45. Storr M, Allescher HD, Classen M. Current concepts on pathophysiology, diagnosis and treatment of diffuse oesophageal spasm. *Drugs* 2001;61: 579–591.
46. Patti MG, Pellegrini CA, Arcerito M, et al. Comparison of medical and minimally invasive surgical therapy for primary esophageal motility disorders. *Arch Surg.* 1995;130:609–615; discussion 615–616.
47. Spechler SJ, Castell DO. Classification of oesophageal motility abnormalities. *Gut* 2001;49:145–151.
48. Bassotti G, Battaglia E, Debernardi V, et al. Esophageal dysfunction in scleroderma: relationship with disease subsets. *Arthritis Rheum.* 1997;40: 2252–2259.
49. Fouad YM, Katz PO, Hatlebakk JG, et al. Ineffective esophageal motility: the most common motility abnormality in patients with GERD-associated respiratory symptoms. *Am J Gastroenterol.* 1999;94:1464–1467.
50. Rydberg L, Ruth M, Lundell L. Does oesophageal motor function improve with time after successful antireflux surgery? Results of a prospective, randomised clinical study. *Gut.* 1997;41:82–86.
51. Horowitz M, Edelbroek M, Fraser R, et al. Disordered gastric motor function in diabetes mellitus. Recent insights into prevalence, pathophysiology, clinical relevance, and treatment. *Scand J Gastroenterol.* 1991;26:673–684.
52. Quigley EM. The pathophysiology of diabetic gastroenteropathy: more vague than vagal. *Gastroenterology* 1997;113:1790–1794.
53. Kong MF, Horowitz M. Gastric emptying in diabetes mellitus: relationship to blood-glucose control. *Clin Geriatr Med.* 1999;15:321–338.
54. Janssens J, Peeters TL, Vantrappen G, et al. Improvement of gastric emptying in diabetic gastroparesis by erythromycin. Preliminary studies. *N Engl J Med.* 1990;322:1028–1031.
55. **Eagon JC, Miedema BW, Kelly KA. Postgastrectomy syndromes. *Surg Clin North Am.* 1992;72:445–465.**
56. Pellegrini CA, Broderick WC, Van Dyke D, et al. Diagnosis and treatment of gastric emptying disorders. Clinical usefulness of radionuclide measurements of gastric emptying. *Am J Surg.* 1983;145:143–151.
57. Eckhauser FE, Conrad M, Knol JA, et al. Safety and long-term durability of completion gastrectomy in 81 patients with postsurgical gastroparesis syndrome. *Am Surg.* 1998;64:711–716; discussion 716–717.
58. Li-Ling J, Irving M. Therapeutic value of octreotide for patients with severe dumping syndrome—a review of randomised controlled trials. *Postgrad Med J.* 2001;77:441–442.
59. van der Kleij FG, Vecht J, Lamers CB, et al. Diagnostic value of dumping provocation in patients after gastric surgery. *Scand J Gastroenterol.* 1996;31:1162–1166.
60. Vecht J, Masclee AA, Lamers CB. The dumping syndrome. Current insights into pathophysiology, diagnosis and treatment. *Scand J Gastroenterol Suppl.* 1997;223:21–27.
61. Andreasen JJ, Orskov C, Holst JJ. Secretion of glucagon-like peptide-1 and reactive hypoglycemia after partial gastrectomy. *Digestion* 1994;55:221–228.
62. Carvajal SH, Mulvihill SJ. Postgastrectomy syndromes: dumping and diarrhea. *Gastroenterol Clin North Am.* 1994;23:261–279.
63. Moriarty KJ, Dawson AM. Functional abdominal pain: further evidence that whole gut is affected. *Br Med J (Clin Res Ed).* 1982;284:1670–1672.
64. Kellow JE, Miller LJ, Phillips SF, et al. Altered sensitivity of the gallbladder to cholecystokinin octapeptide in irritable bowel syndrome. *Am J Physiol.* 1987;253(5 Pt 1):G650–655.
65. Kamath PS, Gaisano HY, Phillips SF, et al. Abnormal gallbladder motility in irritable bowel syndrome: evidence for target-organ defect. *Am J Physiol.* 1991;260(6 Pt 1):G815–819.
66. Tabet J, Anvari M. Laparoscopic cholecystectomy for gallbladder dyskinesia: clinical outcome and patient satisfaction. *Surg Laparosc Endosc Percutan Tech.* 1999;9:382–386.
67. Sherman S, Lehman GA. Sphincter of Oddi dysfunction: diagnosis and treatment. *J Panc.* 2001;2:382-400.
68. Lin OS, Soetikno RM, Young HS. The utility of liver function test abnormalities concomitant with biliary symptoms in predicting a favorable response to endoscopic sphincterotomy in patients with presumed sphincter of Oddi dysfunction. *Am J Gastroenterol.* 1998;93:1833–1836.
69. Khuroo MS, Zargar SA, Yattoo GN. Efficacy of nifedipine therapy in patients with sphincter of Oddi dysfunction: a prospective, double-blind, randomized, placebo-controlled, cross over trial. *Br J Clin Pharmacol.* 1992;33:477–485.
70. Rolny P, Geenen JE, Hogan WJ. Post-cholecystectomy patients with "objective signs" of partial bile outflow obstruction: clinical characteristics, sphincter of Oddi manometry findings, and results of therapy. *Gastrointest Endosc.* 1993;39:778–781.
71. Toouli J, Roberts-Thomson IC, Kellow J, et al. Manometry based randomised trial of endoscopic sphincterotomy for sphincter of Oddi dysfunction. *Gut.* 2000;46:98–102.
72. Verne GN, Sninsky CA. Chronic intestinal pseudo-obstruction. *Dig Dis Sci.* 1995;13:163–181.
73. Schuffler MD. Chronic Intestinal Pseudo-obstruction. In: Feldman MF, L; Schleisenger, M, ed. *Schleisenger & Fordtrans gastrointestinal and liver disease*, vol. 2. Philadelphia: WB Saunders, 2002, pp. 2140–2150.
74. Reyntjens A, Verlinden M, Schuermans V. Cisapride in the treatment of chronic intestinal pseudo-obstruction. *Z Gastroenterol.* 1990;28 (suppl 1):79–84; discussion 92–93.
75. Verne GN, Eaker EY, Hardy E, et al. Effect of octreotide and erythromycin on idiopathic and scleroderma-associated intestinal pseudoobstruction. *Dig Dis Sci.* 1995;40:1892–1901.
76. Murr MM, Sarr MG, Camilleri M. The surgeon's role in the treatment of chronic intestinal pseudoobstruction. *Am J Gastroenterol.* 1995;90:2147–2151.
77. Iyer K, Kaufman S, Sudan D, et al. Long-term results of intestinal transplantation for pseudo-obstruction in children. *J Pediatr Surg.* 2001 Jan:174–177.
78. Maglinte DD, Chernish SM, DeWeese R, et al. Acquired jejunoileal diverticular disease: subject review. *Radiology* 1986;158:577–580.
79. Altemeier WA, Bryant LR, Wulsin JH. The surgical significance of jejunal diverticulosis. *Arch Surg.* 1963;86:732–745.
80. Palder SB, Frey CB. Jejunal diverticulosis. *Arch Surg.* 1988;123:889–894.
81. Krishnamurthy S, Kelly MM, Rohrmann CA, et al. Jejunal diverticulosis. A heterogeneous disorder caused by a variety of abnormalities of smooth muscle or myenteric plexus. *Gastroenterology* 1983;85:538–547.
82. Kouraklis G, Glinavou A, Mantas D, et al. Clinical implications of small bowel diverticula. *Isr Med Assoc J.* 2002;4:431–433.
83. Higgins PD, Johanson JF. Epidemiology of constipation in North America: a systematic review. *Am J Gastroenterol.* 2004;99:750–759.
84. Bassotti G, Iantorno G, Fiorella S, et al. Colonic motility in man: features in normal subjects and in patients with chronic idiopathic constipation. *Am J Gastroenterol.* 1999;94:1760–1770.
85. Metcalf AM, Phillips SF, Zinsmeister AR, et al. Simplified assessment of segmental colonic transit. *Gastroenterology* 1987;92:40–47.
86. Camilleri M, Zinsmeister AR. Towards a relatively inexpensive, noninvasive, accurate test for colonic motility disorders. *Gastroenterology.* 1992;103:36–42.
87. Knowles CH, Scott M, Lunniss PJ. Outcome of colectomy for slow transit constipation. *Ann Surg.* 1999;230:627–638.
88. Camilleri M, Thompson WG, Fleshman JW, et al. Clinical management of intractable constipation. *Ann Intern Med.* 1994;121:520–528.
89. Vanek VW, Al-Salti M. Acute pseudo-obstruction of the colon (Ogilvie's syndrome). An analysis of 400 cases. *Dis Colon Rectum.* 1986;29:203–210.
90. Delgado-Aros S, Camilleri M. Pseudo-obstruction in the critically ill. Pseudo-obstruction in the critically ill, 2003;17:427–444.
91. De Giorgio R, Barbara G, Stanghellini V, et al. Review article: the pharmacological treatment of acute colonic pseudo-obstruction. *Aliment Pharmacol Ther.* 2001;15:1717–1727.
92. Eisen GM, Baron TH, Dominitz JA, et al. Acute colonic pseudo-obstruction. *Gastrointest Endosc.* 2002;56:789–792.
93. Sloyer AF, Panella VS, Demas BE, et al. Ogilvie's syndrome. Successful management without colonoscopy. *Dig Dis Sci.* 1988;33:1391–1396.
94. **Ponec RJ, Saunders MD, Kimmey MB. Neostigmine for the treatment of acute colonic pseudo-obstruction. *N Engl J Med.* 1999;341:137–141.**
95. Geller A, Petersen BT, Gostout CJ. Endoscopic decompression for acute colonic pseudo-obstruction. *Gastrointest Endosc.* 1996;44:144–150.
96. Rex DK. Colonoscopy and acute colonic pseudo-obstruction. *Gastrointest Endosc Clin N Am.* 1997 July:499–508.

CHAPTER 67 ■ ACUTE GASTROINTESTINAL HEMORRHAGE

LAWRENCE T. KIM, MAUREEN HELDMANN, AND RICHARD H. TURNAGE

Acute gastrointestinal (GI) hemorrhage is categorized as upper or lower depending upon the location of the bleeding relative to the ligament of Treitz. Upper GI (UGI) hemorrhage (i.e., bleeding from the esophagus, stomach, or duodenum) accounts for about 80% of cases of acute GI blood loss, with nearly all the remaining cases in the colon. The small intestine is the site of hemorrhage in about 1% of cases.[1] The incidence of UGI bleeding is estimated to be about 37 to 150 episodes per 100,000 individuals depending upon the population sampled,[2–4] whereas the incidence of lower GI bleeding is about 20 cases per 100,000 individuals.[5]

The differential diagnosis of overt upper and lower GI hemorrhage and the relative frequency of the most common causes of GI bleeding are shown in Tables 67.1 and 67.2 and Fig. 67.1, respectively. The most common causes of acute UGI hemorrhage are peptic ulcer disease (31% to 58%), gastritis (9% to 30%), and gastroesophageal varices (3% to 23%),[1,2] whereas diverticulosis (24% to 47%), colitis (6% to 26%), neoplasms (9% to 17%), and angiodysplasia (2% to 12%) account for most instances of lower GI hemorrhage.[1,5–9]

PATIENT CHARACTERISTICS

Patients who have significant GI hemorrhage are more commonly older and male than are individuals without GI bleeding. Affected individuals are more likely to use alcohol, tobacco, aspirin, nonsteroidal antiinflammatory drugs (NSAIDs) and anticoagulants.[1,10] Predictors of risk for acute GI bleeding are shown in Table 67.3.

Both UGI and lower GI hemorrhage are more common in elderly than in younger individuals. In a study from the Netherlands, van Leerdam et al.[11] found that 71% of patients presenting with acute UGI bleeding were more than 60 years of age and 24% were older than age 80 years. In this population, the average age of patients suffering an UGI hemorrhage was 71 years.[2]

Lower GI bleeding is also more common in the elderly. Peura et al.[1] found that the average age of patients with a lower GI bleed was about 60 years and was not different than that of patients presenting with UGI bleeding. Longstreth reported that the frequency of lower GI hemorrhage increased more than 200-fold from the third to the ninth decade of life.[8]

Coexisting chronic illnesses are common in patients suffering either an upper or lower GI hemorrhage. Various studies have suggested a relationship between GI bleeding and correlates of poor health such as the use of multiple medications, reduced levels of physical activity, and inability to complete basic self-care tasks.[10,12] Vreeburg et al.[2] found that 85% of patients with an UGI bleed had concomitant chronic illnesses. Cardiovascular disease and renal disease are independent risk factors for acute GI bleeding.[10,13] The presence of these chronic illnesses, as well as chronic obstructive pulmonary disease and cirrhosis, also greatly increases the risk of rebleeding after endoscopic control.[14]

TABLE 67.1 ■ DIAGNOSIS

DIFFERENTIAL DIAGNOSIS OF ACUTE UPPER GASTROINTESTINAL HEMORRHAGE BY ANATOMIC SITE

Esophagus
Esophagitis
- Reflux
- Infectious (fungal, viral)

Esophageal varices
Neoplasms

Stomach
Peptic ulcer disease
- Gastric ulcer

Gastroesophageal varices
- Portal gastropathy

Dieulafoy ulcer
Arteriovenous malformation
Neoplasms
- GI stroma tumors
- Lymphoma
- Adenocarcinoma
- Carcinoid tumors

Mallory-Weiss tear
Stress gastritis

Duodenum
Peptic ulcer disease
- Duodenal ulcer

Arteriovenous malformation
Neoplasms
- Duodenal adenocarcinoma
- Pancreatic adenocarcinoma
- Carcinoid tumors

Dieulafoy ulcers
Aortoduodenal fistula
Diverticula

Hepatopancreatic-biliary
Hemobilia
Pancreatitis-induced pseudoaneurysm

Many studies have related the use of NSAIDs and aspirin to significant GI bleeding, particularly UGI bleeding. In Vreeburg's review of 951 patients with UGI hemorrhage, 41% used NSAIDs or aspirin. In this study, the odds ratio for UGI bleeding for patients taking NSAIDs was 2.33 (95% confidence interval [CI] = 1.76, 3.07).[2] van Leerdam et al.[11] reported that more than half of the patients bleeding from ulcers were actively taking NSAIDs or acetylsalicylic acid (aspirin). Mellemkjaer et al.[15] found that the

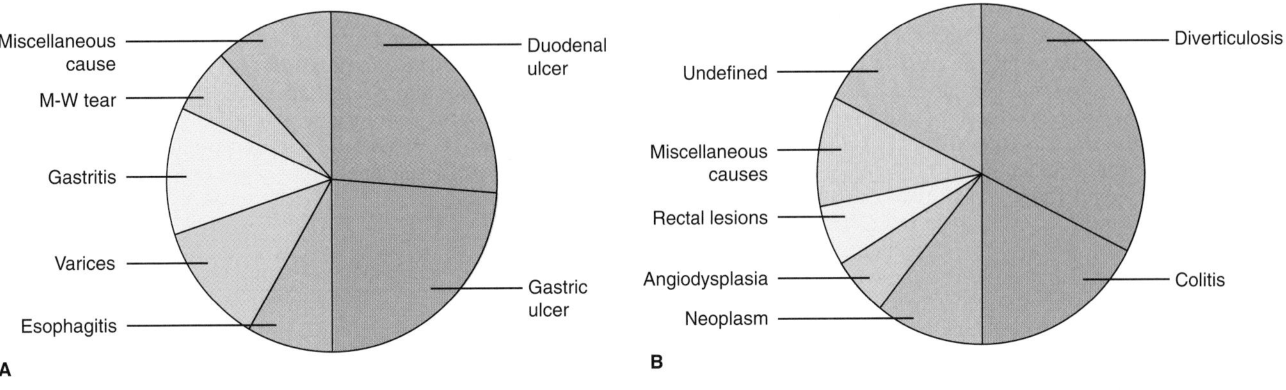

FIGURE 67.1 (*A*) The relative frequency of the most common causes of upper gastrointestinal hemorrhage in the United States. These data represent the percentage of patients with each of these causes of UGI hemorrhage for of 482 patients in a survey of the members of the American College of Gastroenterology published by Peura et al.[1] in 1997. These data are very similar to that reported by Vreeburg et al.[2] in a multi-institutional study of 951 patients sustaining an UGI hemorrhage in the hospital in and surrounding Amsterdam. M-W = Mallory Weiss. (*B*) The relative frequency of the most common causes of lower gastrointestinal hemorrhage. These data, reported by Lingenfelser and Ell[5] are the percentage of patients with each of these causes of lower GI hemorrhage in 912 patients collected in five studies from Europe, Asia, and the United States.[1,6–9]

TABLE 67.2 DIAGNOSIS

DIFFERENTIAL DIAGNOSIS OF ACUTE LOWER GASTROINTESTINAL HEMORRHAGE BY ANATOMIC SITE

Small Intestine
NSAID-induced ulcers
Diverticula
- Meckel's diverticula
- Pseudodiverticula

Neoplasms
- Lymphoma
- GI Stroma tumors
- Adenocarcinoma
- Carcinoid tumor

Inflammation
- Crohn disease
- Radiation enteritis
- Ischemic enteritis
- Infectious enteritis

Arteriovenous malformations
Aortoenteric fistula

Colon and Rectum
Diverticulosis
Colitis
- Crohn disease
- Ulcerative colitis
- Radiation colitis
- Infectious colitis
- Ischemic colitis

Neoplasms
- Adenocarcinoma
- GI Stromal tumors
- Lymphoma
- Carcinoid tumors

Arteriovenous malformation
Iatrogenic
- Polypectomy sites

Benign rectal diseases
- Hemorrhoids
- Rectal ulcers

NSAID, nonsteroidal antiinflammatory drug.

observed to expected ratio of UGI hemorrhage in a cohort of 156,138 users of NSAIDs was 4.1 (95% CI = 3.8, 4.5).

The use of anticoagulants is also an important risk factor for acute GI bleeding. Kaplan et al[10] found the age- and sex-adjusted hazard ratio for GI bleeding in patients taking oral anticoagulants was 2.59 (95% CI = 1.71, 3.93). Vreeburg et al.[2] reported that 17% of study patients with UGI hemorrhage were taking coumarins and the international normal ratio (INR) was greater than 4 in more than half of these patients. Tobacco is also associated with a higher rate of significant GI hemorrhage. A prospective cohort study of 5888 men and women found that the multivariate-adjusted hazard ratio for subjects who smoked more than half a pack per day was 2.14 (95% CI = 1.22, 3.75) for UGI bleeding.[10]

CLINICAL PRESENTATION

Usually patients with overt GI bleeding present to the hospital after observing the passage of blood from the GI tract as hematemesis (the vomiting of blood), melena, or hematochezia.

TABLE 67.3

CHARACTERISTICS OF INDIVIDUALS AT AN INCREASED RISK OF DEVELOPING ACUTE GASTROINTESTINAL BLEEDING

Increased age
Male sex
Unmarried (vs. married)
Perceived fair or poor health status
Cardiovascular disease
Diabetes mellitus
Renal disease
Difficulty with activities of daily living
Low level of physical activity
Increased numbers of medications
Oral anticoagulant use

(From Kaplan RC, Heckbert SR, Koepsell TD, et al. Risk factors for hospitalized gastrointestinal bleeding among older persons. Cardiovascular Health Study Investigators. *J Am Geriatr Soc.* 2001; 49:126–133.)

Melena is a black, tarry stool resulting from the degradation of blood by enteric bacteria. It may occur with the loss of as little as 50 to 200 mL of blood.[16,17] Bleeding from the small intestine or right colon may also appear black if the blood has remained in the GI tract for more than 12 to14 hours.[18] Hematochezia is the passage of bright red blood from the rectum and is usually indicative of a lower GI source, although massive UGI hemorrhage may also cause hematochezia. Patients with acute GI bleeding may present with the hemodynamic consequences of hemorrhage including lightheadedness, dizziness, orthostatic syncope or near-syncope, shortness of breath, or palpitations from tachycardia.

The medical history and physical examination provide important clues of the etiology of the patient's hemorrhage and the potential risk to the patient's life. The occurrence of melena after several days of worsening epigastric or upper abdominal pain suggests peptic ulcer disease, whereas hematemesis or melena following vomiting or retching strongly suggests a Mallory-Weiss tear. Massive, painless UGI hemorrhage in a patient with cirrhosis suggests bleeding from gastroesophageal varices, although other etiologies including peptic ulcer disease or a Mallory-Weiss tear must also be considered. Taking the medical history should elicit the presence of risk factors for GI hemorrhage as previously discussed (see Table 67.3).

A systematic physical examination will document the magnitude of bleeding and the patient's ability to compensate. Massive hemorrhage is associated with signs and symptoms of hypovolemic shock, including cool, clammy, mottled skin, tachycardia, tachypnea, flat jugular veins, oliguria, and perhaps hypotension. These responses may be altered by advanced age, concomitant medical problems, and particular medications. Physical examination should also document evidence of cirrhosis and portal hypertension (i.e., ascites, spider angiomas, hepatosplenomegaly, palmar erythema, large hemorrhoidal veins). A rectal examination may demonstrate bright red blood or melena.

PROGNOSTIC FACTORS

Most patients (about 80%) who have GI hemorrhage will stop bleeding spontaneously, and those who don't, or those who rebleed are at particularly high risk to suffer an inhospital complication, require operative control of their hemorrhage, or die. Several classification systems have been developed to separate low-risk from high-risk patients with acute UGI and lower GI hemorrhage. These systems have also been used to stratify those patients who may be safely managed as an outpatient from those requiring inhospital care.[19] The BLEED classification system consists of the following parameters: ongoing bleeding, low systolic blood pressure, elevated prothrombin time, erratic mental status, and unstable co-morbid disease. Patients with at least one BLEED criterion are more likely to suffer in-hospital complications from UGI bleeding (31% versus 4%) or lower GI bleeding (38% versus 12%) than are patients with no criteria.[20] The importance of age and comorbid disease as independent risk factors is expressed in the

TABLE 67.4

ROCKALL RISK SCORING SYSTEM AND RATES OF REBLEEDING AND MORTALITY

SCORING SYSTEM

Variable	Score 0	Score 1	Score 2	Score 3
Age	<60 years	60–79 years	≥80 years	
Shock	"No shock" Systolic blood pressure ≥100 Heart rate <100	"Tachycardia" Systolic blood pressure ≥100 Heart rate ≥100	"Hypotension" Systolic blood pressure <100	
Comorbidity	None	None	Cardiac failure Ischemic heart disease Any major comorbidity	Renal failure Liver failure Disseminated malignancy
Diagnosis	Mallory-Weiss tear No lesion identified No stigmata of recent hemorrhage	All other diagnosis	Malignancy of the UGI tract	
Major stigmata of recent hemorrhage	None or dark spot only		Blood in UGI tract Adherent clot Visible or spurting vessel	

SCORE-RELATED MORTALITY

Score	0	1	2	3	4	5	6	7	8+
Mortality (%)	0	0	0.2	2.9	5.3	10.8	17.3	27	41

UGI, upper gastrointestinal.
(From Rockall TA, Logan RF, Devlin HB, et al. Risk assessment after acute upper gastrointestinal haemorrhage. *Gut* 1996;38:316–321.)

Rockall score for assessing the risk of death and re-bleeding in patients with UGI hemorrhage (Table 67.4). Using this model, Rockall et al.[21] found that rebleeding occurred in less than 5% of patients and mortality was virtually 0 (0 to 0.2) in patients with scores of 0 to 2. In contrast, one-fourth to nearly one-half of patients with a Rockall score of 5 to 8+ rebled; the mortality rates for these patients was 11% to 41%. In this study, rebleeding significantly affected the likelihood of death, particularly for patients with intermediate scores of 3 or 4 and 5 to 7 in which there was a three- to five-fold increase in mortality rates. Clinical and endoscopic factors that have been associated with an increased risk of rebleeding and death are shown in Tables 67.5 and 67.6, respectively.[22]

TABLE 67.5

PREDICTORS OF PERSISTENT OR RECURRENT BLEEDING IN PATIENTS WITH NONVARICEAL UPPER GASTROINTESTINAL HEMORRHAGE

Clinical factors	Range of odds ratios for increased risk
Age >65 years	1.3
>70 years	2.30
Shock (systolic blood pressure <100 mm Hg)	1.2–3.65
Health status (ASA class 1 versus 2–5)	1.94–7.63
Comorbid illness	1.6–7.63
Erratic mental status	3.21 (95% CI = 1.53, 6.74)
Ongoing bleeding	3.14 (95% CI = 2.40–4.12)
Laboratory factors	
Initial hemoglobin <10 g/dL or hematocrit <0.30	0.8–2.99
Coagulopathy (prolonged partial thromboplastin time)	1.96 (95% CI:1.46,2.64
Presentation of bleeding	
Melena	1.6 (95% CI = 1.1, 2.4)
Red blood on rectal examination	3.76 (95% CI = 2.26, 6.26)
Blood in gastric aspirate or stomach	1.1–11.5
Hematemesis	1.2–5.7
Endoscopic factors	
Active bleeding on endoscopy	2.5–6.48
Endoscopic high-risk stigmata	1.91–4.81
Clot	1.72–1.9
Ulcer size ≥2 cm	2.29–3.54
Diagnosis of gastric or duodenal ulcer	2.7 (95% CI= 1.2, 4.9)
Ulcer location	
High on lesser curvature	2.79
Superior wall	13.9
Posterior wall	9.2

ASA, American Society of Anesthesiologists.
(From Barkun A, Bardou M, Marshall JK. Nonvariceal Upper GI Bleeding Consensus Conference Group. Consensus recommendations for managing patients with nonvariceal upper gastrointestinal bleeding. *Ann Intern Med.* 2003;139:843–857.)

TABLE 67.6

PREDICTORS OF MORTALITY IN PATIENTS WITH NONVARICEAL UPPER GASTROINTESTINAL HEMORRHAGE

Clinical factors	Range of odds ratios for increased risk
Age	
60–69 years	3.5 (95% CI 5 = 1.5, 4.7)
≥70 years	4.5–12.7
>80 years	5.7 (95% CI = 2.9, 10.2)
Shock (systolic blood pressure <100 mm Hg)	1.18–6.4
Health status (ASA Class 1 vs. 2–5)	2.6–9.52
Comorbid illness	1.19–12.1
Continued or rebleeding	5.29–76.23
Sepsis	5.4 (95% CI =1.5,19.6)
Presentation of bleeding	
Red blood on rectal examination	2.95 (95% CI = 1.29, 6.76)
Blood in gastric aspirate or stomach	0.43–18.9
Hematemesis	2.0 (95% CI = 1.1,3.5)
Onset of bleeding while hospitalized for other causes	2.77 (95% CI = 1.64, 4.66)
Laboratory factors	
Elevated blood urea nitrogen level	5.5–18
Elevated serum creatinine level	14.8 (95% CI = 2.6,83.5)
Elevated serum aminotransferase levels	4.2–20.2

ASA, American Society of Anesthesiologists.
(From Barkun A, Bardou M, Marshall JK. Nonvariceal Upper GI Bleeding Consensus Conference Group. Consensus recommendations for managing patients with nonvariceal upper gastrointestinal bleeding. *Ann Intern Med.* 2003;139:843–857.)

INITIAL EVALUATION AND RESUSCITATION

On presentation, two large-bore intravenous lines should be placed in peripheral veins and intravascular volume resuscitation begun with an isotonic saline solution. Most patients stop bleeding spontaneously, and crystalloid volume resuscitation is all that is required. Blood is drawn for type and cross-match, complete blood count with platelet count, electrolyte determination, liver function tests, and coagulation profiles. It is important to emphasize that on presentation, the hematocrit or hemoglobin level does not accurately reflect the magnitude of acute blood loss. Estimates of the severity of hemorrhage must be based on clinical parameters.

The massively bleeding patient should receive packed red blood cells to restore intravascular volume and oxygen-carrying capacity. The decision to transfuse blood or blood products depends on the individual needs of the patient and the cause of the bleeding. The risks of the blood products (i.e., infection and allergic reactions) must be weighed against the risks of withholding transfusion (i.e., anemia, decreased oxygen-carrying capacity, coagulopathy). In general, blood products are used early in the management of patients with limited cardiac and pulmonary reserve (who are unable to withstand or compensate for an acute reduction in their systemic oxygen delivery) and those with lesions that are at particular

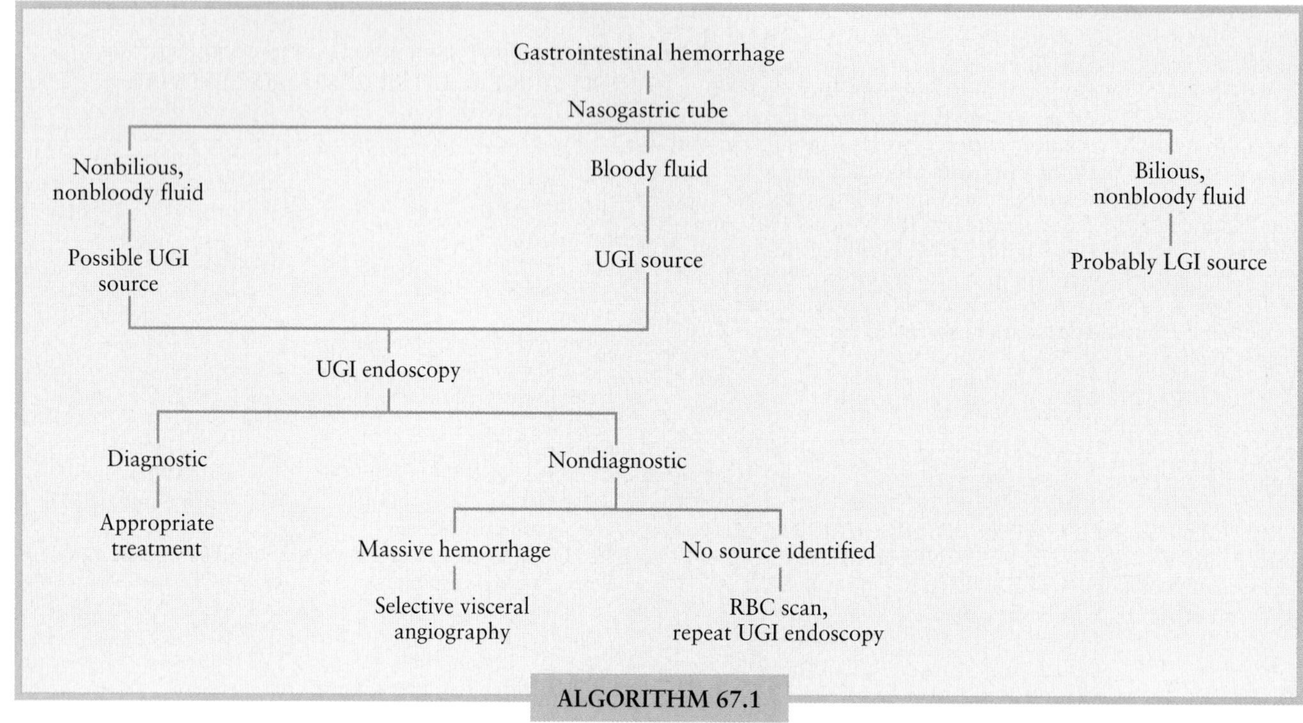

ALGORITHM 67.1 Diagnostic steps in the evaluation of acute upper gastrointestinal hemorrhage.

high risk for continued or recurrent hemorrhage (e.g., gastroesophageal varices).

Careful hemodynamic monitoring of these potentially critically ill patients is vital to successful management. Patients who are actively bleeding and those who have recently sustained significant hemorrhage should be admitted to an intensive care unit for close monitoring of hemodynamic parameters and evidence of continued or recurring hemorrhage. The presence of significant underlying illnesses, such as cardiac, renal, hepatic, or pulmonary insufficiency, may necessitate invasive cardiac monitoring with cardiac and arterial catheters. The information gained from these devices allows cardiac performance to be optimized during intravascular volume replacement. Central venous catheterization should be performed only after initial volume resuscitation through peripheral sites. The placement of a urinary catheter and frequent monitoring of heart rate, blood pressure, gastric aspirate, urine output and mental status are the minimum necessary to monitor patients who have suffered GI hemorrhage. The importance of prompt, adequate resuscitation and diligent observation cannot be overemphasized as the cornerstone for managing these potentially mortally ill patients.

DIAGNOSTIC APPROACH

After the restoration of circulating blood volume, the next step is to identify the source of bleeding so definitive therapy may be instituted. If the patient presents with hematemesis, localization of the bleeding to the esophagus, stomach, or duodenum is relatively straightforward and esophagogastroduodenoscopy (EGD) should be performed promptly to identify the source of bleeding. When blood or coffee-ground guiac-positive material is present in the gastric aspirate, EGD will define the site of bleeding. Bright red blood per rectum strongly suggests a lower GI source of bleeding unless the patient is hemodynamically unstable, in which case the hemorrhage may originate from a source proximal to the ligament of Treitz. General algorithms for evaluating patients with acute upper and lower GI hemorrhage is presented in Algorithms 67.1 and 67.2, respectively.

Gastric Aspiration

In the absence of hematemesis, aspiration of gastric fluid after the placement of a nasogastric tube has been used to distinguish between an upper and lower GI source of bleeding. Two recent studies with more than 700 patients found that the presence of blood in the gastric aspirate was a good indicator of an UGI source; however, its absence was unreliable in predicting the presence or absence of an UGI source.[23,24] In one study of 220 patients with UGI sources of bleeding, the sensitivity, specificity and accuracy of the nasogastric aspirate was 42% (95% CI = 32, 51%), 91% (95% CI = 83, 95%), and 66% (95% CI = 59, 72%), respectively.[24] Bloody fluid in the gastric aspirate was associated with lesions at high risk for continued or recurrent bleeding with an odds ratio of 4.82 (95% CI = 2.3, 10.1). The odds ratio for high risk lesions in patients with clear or bilious fluid was 2.8 (95% CI = 1.8, 4.3).[23]

Endoscopy

Esophagogastroduodenoscopy

EGD will identify the site of bleeding in about 95% of cases of UGI bleeding and is the initial diagnostic study for patients suspected of bleeding from the esophagus, stomach, or duodenum.[25,26] The sensitivity of the procedure is significantly enhanced when performed within the first 24 hours of presentation.[2] A systematic review of the literature found that early endoscopy (i.e., performed within 24 hours of admission) was associated with a decreased transfusion requirement and

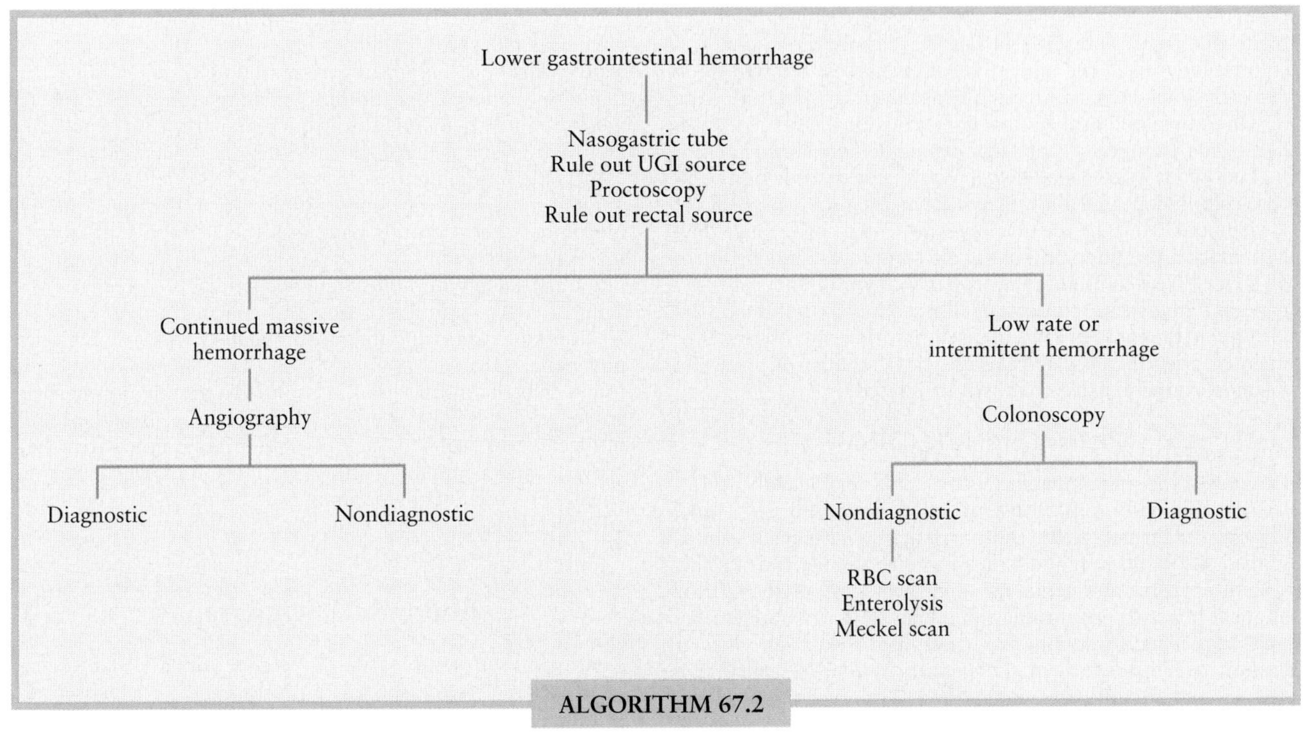

ALGORITHM 67.2 Diagnostic steps in the evaluation of acute lower gastrointestinal hemorrhage.

decreased length of stay.[27] A prospective, randomized trial found that early endoscopy allowed the triaging of 46% of patients to outpatient care without any adverse effects.[28] Previous consensus guidelines and several cohort studies have related various endoscopic stigmata of recent or active hemorrhage to a heightened risk of rebleeding or continued bleeding.[22,29–34] Laine and Peterson[29] analyzed data from 37 prospective trials in which patients with bleeding ulcers did not receive endoscopic therapy; they found that the rate of further bleeding was less than 5% for those patients with a clean ulcer base and increased to 10% for patients with a flat spot, 22% for those with an adherent clot, 43% for those with a non-bleeding visible vessel, and 55% for those with active bleeding. Endoscopic features predictive of persistent or recurrent bleeding and mortality are shown in Tables 67.5, 67.6, and 67.7. In addition to these ulcer-specific factors, endoscopy allows identification of lesions with a high risk of continued hemorrhage and mortality (i.e., gastroesophageal varices) and those with a low risk (e.g., Mallory-Weiss tears). The efficacy of endoscopy-based modalities to control UGI hemorrhage is discussed in subsequent sections.

TABLE 67.7

FORREST CLASSIFICATION OF ENDOSCOPIC APPEARANCE OF BLEEDING ULCERS

Type	Description
Ia	Spurting, bleeding
Ib	Nonspurting, active bleeding
IIa	Visible vessel
IIb	Nonbleeding ulcer with overlying clot
IIc	Ulcer with hematin-covered (black) base
III	Clean ulcer base

(From Pilotto A, Leandro G, Di Mario F, et al. Role of *Helicobacter pylori* infection on upper gastrointestinal bleeding in the elderly: a case-control study. *Dig Dis Sci.* 1997;42:586–591.)

Colonoscopy

Although the efficacy of colonoscopy in determining the cause of occult GI bleeding is undisputed, its role in the evaluation of patients with acute lower GI bleeding is less well agreed upon. The procedure is best suited for patients who are actively bleeding at the time of the study, but not massively bleeding. Colonic lavage with a polyethylene glycol solution will clear the lumen of clot and stool providing adequate visualization of the mucosa. Others have reported good visualization of the mucosa even in the absence of mechanical bowel preparation.[35]

A meta-analysis examined the role of colonoscopy as the primary diagnostic modality for patients with acute lower GI bleeding and found that 69% (range 48% to 90%) of urgent colonoscopies identified a source or a presumptive source of bleeding.[36] Even in the setting of unprepped bowel, urgent colonoscopy has been shown to identify bleeding colon and distal ileal lesions in 82 of 85 patients (97%).[35] Stigmata of recent hemorrhage for lower GI bleeding are similar to those of UGI lesions and include an actively bleeding site, a nonbleeding visible vessel, and an adherent clot; these findings have been associated with continued hemorrhage and the need for urgent colectomy.[6,37] Jensen et al.[38] reported that 25% to 50% of patients with *any* of these three factors continued to bleed, or rebled, and required urgent colectomy. Others have found colonoscopy to be less accurate in the diagnosis of lower GI bleeding. For example, Al Qahtani et al.[39] reported a series of 136 patients in which colonoscopy identified only 45% of the sources of bleeding.

Enteroscopy

For patients who present with hematochezia in whom the initial EGD and colonoscopy are nondiagnostic, repeating these studies before evaluating the small intestine is warranted given the very small frequency in which the bleeding originates from the small intestine (1%). Repeating the EGD and colonoscopy when the patient is better resuscitated will often detect lesions such as ulcers or vascular ectasias that were obscured by blood at the initial endoscopy or the vasoconstriction of the GI mucosa that accompanies hemorrhagic shock.

Endoscopy of the small bowel with an enteroscope or a pediatric colonoscope will allow inspection of the proximal 60 cm of the jejunum[40] and the use of a long videoenteroscope may allow visualization of 100 to 150 cm of intestine beyond the ligament of Treitz.[41] Jensen et al., in an experience with more than 200 patients with obscure sources of GI bleeding, reported success in identifying the cause in 79% of instances using enteroscopy.[42] In their experience, vascular ectasias and postbulbar ulcers were the most common causes of obscure GI bleeding.

Wireless Capsule Endoscopy

Imaging of the small intestine is also now possible with a wireless capsule endoscope consisting of a battery, light source, imaging-capturing system and transmitter. This capsule endoscope is 11 × 30 mm and is moved solely by peristalsis. This system captures and sends up to two images per second for about 5 hours to an ultrahigh frequency band radiotelemetry unit worn by the patient. The location of the capsule is suggested by the strength of the signal. Two large series have shown high diagnostic yields (>90% in overtly bleeding patients) using this technique in selected patients.[43,44] Several recent prospective studies have compared wireless capsule enteroscopy and push enteroscopy in patients with obscure GI bleeding and found that wireless capsule enteroscopy may increase the diagnostic yield in these very difficult patients.[45–49]

Selective Visceral Arteriography

Selective visceral arteriography is primarily useful in patients with upper or lower GI bleeding in whom endoscopy cannot be performed or has been unsuccessful in determining the site of ongoing, rapid hemorrhage. Successful angiographic identification of the source of bleeding occurs in 27% to 86% of instances and depends primarily upon the presence of active arterial bleeding at the time of the study.[39,50,51] (Fig. 67.2). The extravasation of contrast may be detected if the patient is bleeding at rates greater than 0.5 to 1 milliliters per minute;[52] this correlates clinically with the requirement for continuous volume infusion to maintain hemodynamic stability. Pennoyer et al.,[53] however, were unable to identify any clinical parameter (including tachycardia, numbers of transfusions, or orthostatic hypotension) that could increase the diagnostic yield of selective angiography, including scintigraphy demonstrating ongoing bleeding. Several groups have used heparin, vasodilators or thrombolytics to improve the diagnostic yield of arteriography in patients with non-diagnostic studies. Mernagh et al.[54] found that the administration of heparin intravenously for 24 hours increased the diagnostic yield of visceral angiography from 33% (6 of 18) to 67% (12 of 18). Others have found that the intraarterial infusion of a vasodilator, heparin, and/or urokinase (a thrombolytic) failed to identify the source of bleeding in 5 of 7 patients.[55] It should be noted that these provocative techniques are not commonly employed. The therapeutic potential of angiography is described in detail in subsequent sections.

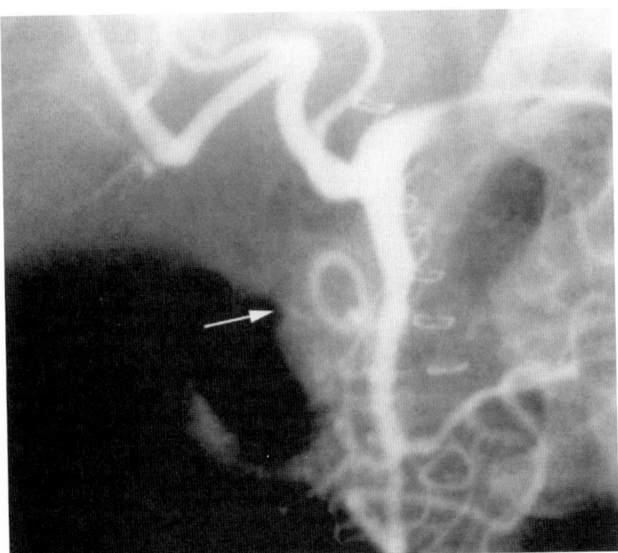

FIGURE 67.2 Selective celiac arteriography with injection into the common hepatic artery in a patient bleeding from a duodenal diverticulum. Extravasation of contrast from a branch of the gastroduodenal artery can be seen (*arrow*).

Abdominal Scintigraphy

Abdominal scintigraphy with ^{99m}technetium (Tc)-labeled red blood cells lacks the spatial resolution and diagnostic precision of angiography and endoscopy; however, it is of most value in detecting intermittently bleeding lesions or those with very low rates of hemorrhage, such as vascular malformations. Abdominal scintigraphy utilizing ^{99m}Tc-RBCs has been shown to detect bleeding rates as low as 0.04 to 0.1 mL per minute[56,57] In a review of seven retrospective studies with nearly 400 patients the median diagnostic accuracy of scintigraphy was 82% (range, 52% to 95%); in this review, ^{99m}Tc-RBCs was incorrect in 5% to 48% of instances (median 18%).[51] Suzman et al.[58] summarized 20 retrospective studies containing 804 positive studies and reported a false-positive rate of 19%. Precise localization of the site of bleeding may be complicated by the rapid distribution of isotope throughout the intestine by peristalsis or by accumulation in the right colon. More recent techniques of cinescintigraphy may improve the diagnostic accuracy (Fig. 67.3).[59] One area where radionuclide scanning has a clear role is in the diagnosis of Meckel's diverticulum. ^{99}Tc-pertechnate is secreted by ectopic gastric mucosa in Meckel's diverticula.[60] This study should be considered early in the evaluation of young individuals with lower GI bleeding.

COMMON CAUSES OF GASTROINTESTINAL HEMORRHAGE AND TREATMENT

Upper Gastrointestinal Hemorrhage

Peptic Ulcer Disease

Peptic ulcer disease is the most common cause of acute UGI hemorrhage, accounting for nearly 40% of cases in most series although this proportion may be decreasing.[61] About 15% to 20% of patients with peptic ulcer disease experience bleeding during the course of their disease and as many as 20% of these patients will have bleeding as the initial manifestation. Hemorrhage is the principal cause of death from peptic ulcer disease and has replaced intractable pain as the most frequent indication for surgery. Complications of peptic ulcer disease occur more commonly in older patients who often have medical

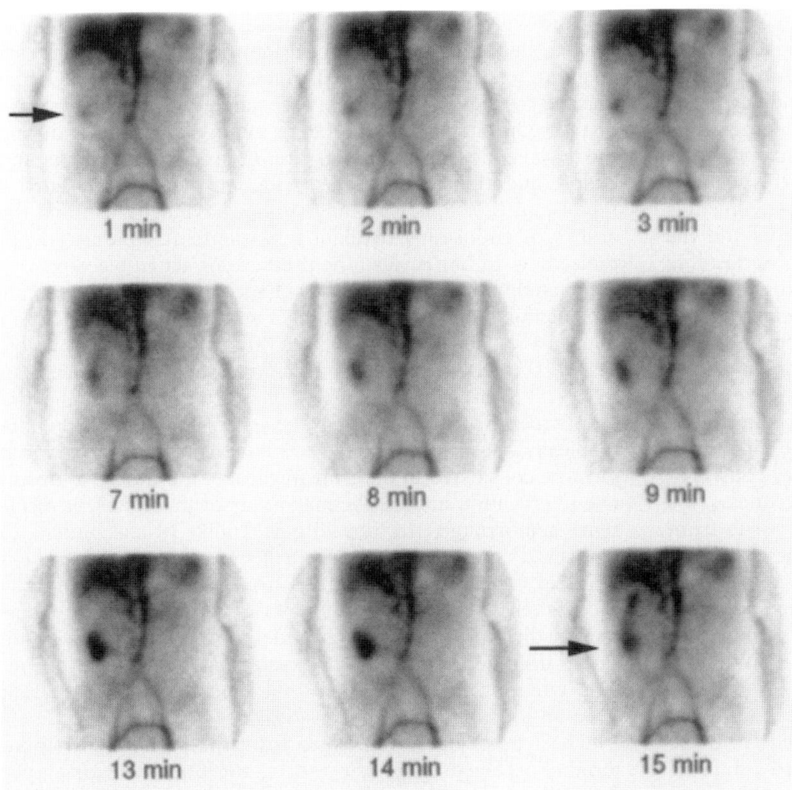

FIGURE 67.3 Cine-^{99}Tc erythrocyte scintigraphy showing extravasation of isotope in the right colon. Only a small portion of the image set is shown. *Arrows* point to accumulation of isotope in right colon. Bleeding was due to delayed hemorrhage following endoscopic polypectomy.

problems that profoundly influence their risk of morbidity and mortality.

Duodenal ulcers occur slightly more frequently than gastric ulcers. Penetration of the ulcer through the posterior wall of the duodenal bulb is associated with erosion into the gastroduodenal artery or one of its branches, resulting in brisk hemorrhage. Patients may present with hematemesis of bright red blood and clots or with melena alone. Between 80% and 90% of patients stop bleeding spontaneously during the initial stages of therapy with volume resuscitation and gastric lavage.

In general, patients with gastric ulcers tend to be older and have coexisting medical problems that increase morbidity and mortality compared with duodenal ulcers. Bleeding may occur from any site in the stomach, although ulcers occurring at the incisura are most common. At this site, involvement of the branches of the left gastric artery may result in brisk, if not torrential, hemorrhage. The clinical presentation of patients bleeding from gastric ulcers is similar to that of duodenal ulcers, with hematemesis, melena, and hematochezia.

An important risk factor for the development of GI hemorrhage and gastroduodenal ulcer formation is the use of NSAIDs. NSAID use has been associated with a continuum of mucosal injury ranging from small acute mucosal hemorrhages to large chronic ulcers. It has been estimated that 10% to 15% of regular NSAID users have chronic gastric ulcers.[62] Symptoms correlate poorly with the degree of mucosal injury since as many as 20% of ulcers penetrating the muscularis are asymptomatic.[63] Case control and cohort studies have suggested that NSAIDs are associated with a relative risk of GI hemorrhage and ulceration ranging from about 2 to 9.1.[64] Ketorolac, in particular, has been associated with a high risk of GI bleeding (relative risk approaches 25).[65,66] The risk of NSAID-associated complications is highest in patients with a history of UGI bleeding, the elderly, those patients taking oral anticoagulants or corticosteroids.[67] Patients with a prior history of peptic ulcer disease also appear to be at increased risk of NSAID-associated GI hemorrhage and tend to have a significantly worse outcome compared with individuals not using NSAIDs.[68,69]

The tremendous frequency with which the elderly use NSAIDs underscores the magnitude of this problem. Individuals with a history of NSAID-induced hemorrhage may benefit from the prostaglandin E_1 analogue, misoprostol, which has been shown to prevent NSAID-induced gastric erosions and ulcers.[70] Histamine (H_2)-receptor blockers (ranitidine and cimetidine) are effective in preventing NSAID-induced duodenal ulcers, but appear to have little effect on the occurrence of gastric lesions.[63,71,72] Proton pump inhibitors (PPI) have also been shown to be protective in patients on NSAIDs, with greater efficacy than H_2 blockers[73] NSAIDs are also associated with lower GI bleeding, including lesions not generally considered related to NSAID-induced ulcers, such as diverticulosis.[74–76] Selective COX-2 inhibitors have been widely marketed as being safer than nonselective NSAIDs. Most studies confirm a reduced risk of GI hemorrhage compared with nonselective NSAIDs, but not to baseline risk.[66,77,78]

Medical Treatment. Once bleeding has stopped, either spontaneously or through an intervention, treatment with a PPI should be initiated. Acute use of a PPI has been shown in several studies to decrease rebleeding.[22,79] An 80-mg intravenous bolus of omeprazole or pantoprazole followed by an infusion at 8 mg/hr produces the most reliable acid suppression.[80] All patients should be tested for *Helicobacter pylori* infection and treated if found. Treatment of the infection significantly reduces the recurrence of hemorrhage compared with no treatment or chronic antisecretory treatment alone.[81,82] Interestingly *H. pylori* infection may be less common in patients with bleeding ulcers than in those with non-bleeding ulcers.[83]

Endoscopic Treatment. The endoscopic appearance of a bleeding ulcer has important prognostic and therefore therapeutic implications, as alluded to in Tables 67.5 and 67.6. A modification of the system employed by Forrest et al.[84] is shown in Table 67.7. In this system category I findings are indicative of active bleeding whereas category II findings provide evidence of recent hemorrhage. In general, only actively bleeding ulcers (i.e., Forrest category I lesions) are treated endoscopically. A variety of endoscopic techniques are available to arrest hemorrhage from bleeding ulcers. The precise method of treatment is less important than the correct selection of patients and the experience of the endoscopist. Mechanical ligation of bleeding vessels can be achieved with endoscopic ligation (banding) or endoscopic clipping or endoloop ligation.[85,86] Heater probes and monopolar and bipolar electrocoagulation probes also can effectively control UGI hemorrhage. Monopolar probes apply high-frequency electrical current to the tissue, resulting in localized heating to 100°C and sealing of the bleeding vessel by coagulation necrosis of the surrounding tissue and vessel wall. Multipolar electrocoagulation (bicap) probes consist of three equally spaced pairs of bipolar microelectrodes. This orientation of electrodes allows coagulation of tissue from tangential approaches and eliminates some of the disadvantages of the monopolar probe, such as the unpredictable depth of thermal injury, adherence of tissue, and clot dislodgement. Direct thermal coagulation of a bleeding point can also be produced by applying a heater probe, consisting of an aluminum tip coated with Teflon. The tip is rapidly heated to 250°C by an inner coil. The tip can be irrigated with a water jet to prevent accumulation of debris and clot. Heat conducted from the probe produces tissue coagulation to a depth of 1 to 5 mm.

Injection of epinephrine to induce vasoconstriction has been used successfully to control acutely bleeding ulcers, particularly as an adjunct to electrocautery. One study comparing epinephrine injection alone, bipolar coagulation, and injection plus coagulation found that although epinephrine injection alone was as effective as the other treatments in initial control of bleeding, it was associated with a higher frequency of rebleeding.[87] Another group reported no difference in outcomes between acutely bleeding patients treated with epinephrine injection versus epinephrine plus heater probe except in a small subgroup of patients with spurting hemorrhage.[88]

The injection of sclerosants has been well described as a method of treating esophageal varices and has recently been popular for controlling nonvariceal bleeding. Sodium morrhuate and ethanolamine oleate are most commonly used to treat esophageal varices, whereas ethanol and polidocanol are most commonly used for nonvariceal sites. These agents act by thrombosing bleeding vessels and causing necrosis and subsequent fibrosis of surrounding tissue. Clinical experience with sclerosants has been similar to that obtained with electrocoagulation. In one large multicenter study of 332 actively bleeding patients or patients with stigmata of recent hemorrhage who underwent injection of 98% alcohol around the lesions, less than 1% continued to bleed, 6% rebled, and only 3% required emergency operative intervention.[89]

A meta-analysis of 25 randomized trials of endoscopic therapy for bleeding ulcers concluded that endoscopic treatment methods have a beneficial effect on survival by reducing the rate of recurrent hemorrhage. This analysis suggested that endoscopic therapy results in a relative reduction of 69% in recurrent bleeding, 62% in emergent surgery, and 30% in mortality rate, with the greatest benefit seen in actively bleeding ulcers and ulcers with nonbleeding visible vessels.[90] The effectiveness of early aggressive endoscopic diagnosis and treatment is further supported by a report of 562 patients bleeding from a variety of causes of whom only 2.5% required emergency operations to control hemorrhage.[91]

Operative Treatment. The successful use of endoscopic therapies has relegated operative procedures to a rescue role for those cases in which endoscopy is unsuccessful in arresting hemorrhage. Numerous studies have attempted to identify patients at greatest risk of continued or recurrent bleeding. Of the many factors examined, those associated with the highest risk of rebleeding included patients in hypovolemic shock during the initial endoscopy, ulcers greater than 2 cm in diameter and endoscopic stigmata of recent or ongoing hemorrhage (Forrest type I and II lesions).[92] Many studies have demonstrated the ability of endoscopy to identify patients at greatest risk of rebleeding. In one review, the presence of active bleeding was associated with a 90% to 100% chance of continued or recurrent hemorrhage. A nonbleeding visible vessel had a 40% to 50% chance, adherent clot 20% to 30%, oozing without visible vessel 10%, flat spot 5% to 10%, and clean-based ulcer 1% to 2%.[93] Even in patients who rebleed following initial endoscopic therapy, two-thirds may be successfully retreated endoscopically, thus avoiding operative intervention.[62] Factors that must be considered in decisions regarding the timing of operative intervention include the magnitude of the initial (or recurrent) hemorrhage, the physiologic ability of the patient to withstand continued or recurrent hemorrhage, and the likelihood of recurrent or continued hemorrhage. It is generally accepted that elderly patients and those with significant concurrent medical problems should undergo operative intervention earlier during the course of the hemorrhage since these individuals will poorly tolerate continued hemorrhage, recurrent hypotension, and repeated transfusions.

The type of operation depends on the pathology encountered. For bleeding gastric ulcers, the operation of choice depends on the patient's condition and location of the ulcer. For favorably located ulcers in stable patients, the preferred procedure is gastric resection (to include the ulcer in the resected specimen) with or without vagotomy, depending on the ulcer type. In those patients who are hemodynamically unstable, excision of the ulcer with closure of the gastrotomy will provide hemostasis and tissue for histologic evaluation without the need for a more formal gastric resection. If the ulcer is unfavorably located, for example near the gastroesophageal junction, simple undersewing of the bleeding ulcer may adequately control bleeding.[94] Subsequent endoscopic biopsy may allow the exclusion of a neoplastic etiology. Extensive gastric resections such as subtotal or total gastrectomies are generally unwise in these unstable patients.

For patients bleeding from duodenal ulcers, truncal vagotomy, pyloroplasty, and oversewing of the bleeding vessel is the most widely used operation. Highly selective vagotomy with duodenotomy and oversewing of the bleeding vessel has also been recommended. Direct ligation of the bleeding vessel through the duodenotomy should incorporate the gastroduodenal artery proximal and distal to the ulcer as well as the transverse pancreatic artery.

Stress Gastritis

Although studies in the 1960s and 1970s demonstrated acute erosions of the gastric mucosa in as many as 60% to 100% of critically ill patients, the incidence has markedly decreased over the past two decades. Factors postulated to have been important in this phenomenon include: (1) the widespread use of prophylactic gastric alkalinization; (2) improvements in the ability to detect and treat sepsis; (3) improvements in the ability to monitor and correct hemodynamic instability; and (4) the ability to provide adequate nutritional support of critically ill patients.

In general, stress gastritis is characterized by the appearance of multiple superficial gastric ulcerations within 12 to 14 hours of an acute injury. These lesions, initially localized to the fundus and body of the stomach, later involve the entire gastric surface. Patients at greatest risk include those with sepsis, major burns, or severe trauma. Critically ill patients with a coagulopathy and respiratory insufficiency appear to be at highest risk of developing stress gastritis.[95,96] In this setting, the disease appears to represent the gastric component of the multiorgan failure syndrome.

The primary defect is in the protective processes that maintain the integrity of the gastric mucosal barrier. Although some gastric acid secretion is required for the development of stress gastritis, it is clear that the hypersecretion of acid is not the cause of mucosal injury. Altered gastric mucosal blood flow and impaired clearance of hydrogen ions from the mucosa appear to be of particular importance. Stress gastritis should be differentiated from the deep, often solitary ulcerations occurring in patients with severe central nervous system lesions (Cushing ulcers).

Generally hemorrhage is the only symptom that patients with stress gastritis experience. Overt bleeding is often heralded by the appearance of flecks of blood in the gastric aspirate. The superficial nature of the lesions makes perforation unlikely.

Prophylactic therapy is directed toward preventing hemorrhage, primarily by neutralizing gastric acid, augmenting mucosal defenses, and removing or preventing physiologic stress. Antacids, H_2-receptor antagonists, and sucralfate have all been used successfully to prevent stress gastritis. Alkalinization of the gastric contents is associated with oral and fecal flora colonization of the stomach and has raised concerns about an increased risk of nosocomial pneumonia. This concern has prompted the use of sucralfate as a preferred prophylactic agent instead of antacids or cimetidine.[97] However a prospective, randomized trial of 1200 critically ill patients receiving either ranitidine or sucralfate for stress ulcer prophylaxis found that those patients receiving ranitidine had a lower bleeding rate (1.7%) than the sucralfate group (3.8%). There was no difference in mortality or incidence of ventilator-assisted pneumonia.[98]

The success of these prophylactic measures has led to a dearth of recent experience in managing patients bleeding from stress gastritis. Based on early reports, attention to blood replacement, intravascular volume restoration, and correction of coagulation defects are associated with the cessation of hemorrhage in nearly 80% of cases and as such are the principal means of initial treatment. A variety of nonoperative techniques have been employed with variable success in arresting hemorrhage from stress gastritis including endoscopic and embolization techniques and the selective catheterization of the left gastric artery with continuous infusion of vasopressin.[99]

Based on these same early experiences, very few patients bleeding from erosive gastritis require operative intervention to arrest hemorrhage. A variety of surgical treatment options have been reported including vagotomy and pyloroplasty with oversewing of bleeding sites, vagotomy and hemigastrectomy, total gastrectomy, and gastric devascularization. The dilemma facing the surgeon is that these critically ill patients poorly tolerate extensive procedures, yet lesser operations often fail to control hemorrhage. Regardless of the operation performed, mortality risk depends on the underlying illness, particularly in the presence of multiple organ failure. Mortality rates between 30% and 60% are commonly quoted, with as many as one-fourth of the deaths resulting from continued hemorrhage. Rebleeding rates ranging from 25% to 61% have been reported. The combination of vagotomy, hemigastrectomy, and oversewing of bleeding points has been touted as more successful in these patients; however, rebleeding rates of 11% to 44% and operative mortality rates ranging from 33% to 63% have been associated with this procedure.[100] More extensive operations, such as near total gastrectomy or total gastrectomy are associated with significant mortality although they successfully stop hemorrhage.

Gastroesophageal Varices

Cirrhosis is a leading cause of death in the United States and variceal hemorrhage is a common mode of death for these patients. About 30% of people with cirrhosis develop gastroesophageal varices, and of these individuals, about 30% bleed as a result, usually within 1 to 2 years of diagnosis. Gastroesophageal varices are a significant cause of UGI hemorrhage, accounting for about 20% of such cases. Patients with bleeding gastroesophageal varices tend to have much higher rebleeding rates, transfusion requirements, lengths of hospitalization, and risk of death than do patients bleeding from nonvariceal causes.[91,101,102]

Although the basic tenets of resuscitation for massive variceal hemorrhage are similar to those for any source of massive hemorrhage, intravenous volume resuscitation should be particularly judicious. The hyperaldosteronemic state of cirrhosis promotes sodium and water retention with aggravation of ascites and peripheral edema. Accurate blood replacement is imperative since over-transfusion may worsen portal hypertension and exacerbate hemorrhage. Invasive cardiac monitoring with Swan-Ganz catheterization may be particularly useful for guiding volume replacement. Coagulation deficits should be aggressively corrected by administering fresh frozen plasma. Thrombocytopenia, secondary to hypersplenism or dilution, should be treated promptly with pooled platelet transfusions. Sedatives are best avoided or used sparingly because cirrhosis impairs the liver's ability to metabolize many of these drugs. Adequate prophylaxis for delirium tremens should be administered to alcoholic patients.

As with other sources of UGI hemorrhage, early endoscopy is imperative for successful diagnosis and therapy. The identification of varices alone is not adequate to incriminate them as the source of the hemorrhage since up to half of patients with cirrhosis bleed from a source other than varices. Furthermore, endoscopy may identify factors associated with a heightened risk of variceal hemorrhage such as the size and number of varices and the presence of red, blue, or other colored spots on the varix. The presence of gastric and duodenal varices and portal hypertensive changes in the gastric mucosa (portal gastropathy) will influence therapeutic decisions and prognosis.

Although vasopressin has commonly been used in the management of variceal hemorrhage, recent reports suggest the superiority of somatostatin or its synthetic analogue, octreotide. Meta-analyses have shown that the infusion of somatostatin is more effective and safer than vasopressin in the pharmacologic control of variceal hemorrhage.[103,104] Other studies have shown that somatostatin or octreotide can improve the results of sclerotherapy or endoscopic variceal ligation.[105–107] In addition to the enhanced efficacy in controlling hemorrhage, the use of octreotide eliminates the cardiac risks of vasopressin infusion (i.e., coronary artery vasoconstriction, myocardial ischemia, and infarction). Although neither somatostatin nor vasopressin plus nitroglycerin definitively treat the bleeding esophageal varices, these modalities may provide initial control of hemorrhage, reducing transfusion requirements and providing time for resuscitation before definitive treatment.

Another temporizing method used for massively bleeding patients is balloon tamponade using a Sengstaken-Blakemore or a Minnesota tube. These devices consist of a gastric tube with esophageal and gastric balloons. In the case of a Minnesota tube, a proximal esophageal lumen allows for the aspiration of swallowed secretions. Inflation of the gastric (and if required esophageal) balloons tamponade the bleeding varices, controlling hemorrhage in more than 80% of cases. Hemorrhage recurs in 25% to 50% of patients on deflation of the balloons, thus limiting this technique to a temporizing role.[108] The greatest value of these tubes is for arresting massive hemorrhage that has been unresponsive to other measures, allowing time for resuscitation and angiographic definition of the portal system before definitive treatment.

When used inappropriately, these tubes can be associated with significant morbidity and mortality. Complications occur in 4% to 9% of patients with the most frequent being aspiration pneumonitis. Measures to prevent pulmonary complications include endotracheal intubation before tube insertion and the placement of an esophageal tube to remove swallowed salivary secretions. Other significant complications include esophageal rupture or necrosis and airway occlusion during the attempted removal of an incompletely deflated gastric balloon.

Endoscopic sclerotherapy, endoscopic clipping, and endoscopic variceal ligation (banding) have become the most widely used modalities for the initial definitive control of bleeding esophageal varices. Several studies have confirmed that these techniques arrest acute variceal hemorrhage in 90% to 95% of patients. In general a patient bleeding from esophageal varices should undergo urgent sclerotherapy or banding of the varices at the time of the first emergency endoscopy. A single treatment controls variceal bleeding in more than 70% of patients, and a second treatment increases the rate of control to 90% to 95%. Continued or recurrent hemorrhage after endoscopic treatment requires temporary control with balloon tamponade and somatostatin, usually followed by emergency portal decompression either with transjugular intrahepatic portosystemic shunting (TIPS) or with surgery.[109,110] Following an initial episode of variceal hemorrhage several options are available for the prevention of further episodes of hemorrhage.

Mallory-Weiss Tears

The Mallory-Weiss syndrome is acute UGI hemorrhage that occurs after retching or vomiting. Mallory and Weiss[111] described the laceration of the gastric cardia and postulated that violent emesis against an unrelaxed cardia was the mechanism of injury. They were able to produce similar mucosal tears in cadavers by forcing gastric contents against an occluded gastroesophageal junction. The typical patient is an alcoholic who begins to retch and vomit after an alcohol binge, although this syndrome may also be found in nonalcoholic patients with bouts of emesis. Initially the vomitus consists of gastric contents without blood and subsequently the patient develops hematemesis and/or melena. Overall, these lesions account for about 5% to 10% of patients with UGI bleeding.[91,101,102]

The initial management of these patients is similar to that of patients bleeding from other sources of UGI hemorrhage and includes volume resuscitation, gastric lavage, and decompression. Most patients with Mallory-Weiss tears stop bleeding spontaneously, either before treatment or after these early measures. Once bleeding has stopped, rebleeding is rare.

In patients who continue to bleed despite these maneuvers, nonoperative and operative therapeutic options are available. Nonoperative management, consisting of endoscopic electrocoagulation, banding or injection therapy, has been successfully applied to these lesions.[112] In cases not amenable to endoscopic therapy, operative management consists of oversewing the laceration through an anterior longitudinal gastrotomy in the middle third of the stomach.

LOWER GASTROINTESTINAL HEMORRHAGE

Although the passage of maroon or bright red blood per rectum may occur in the presence of a massive UGI hemorrhage, this finding most commonly indicates a source distal to the ligament of Treitz. The absence of blood in bilious nasogastric lavagate further supports a distal location of hemorrhage. Although numerous potential causes of lower GI hemorrhage are possible (see Table 67.2), colonic diverticulosis and colitis are by far the most common. Small bowel sources and other colonic pathology such as colon cancer are relatively unusual causes of acute GI hemorrhage.

Colonic Diverticulosis

In Western society, the prevalence of colonic diverticula increases with age such that about 60% of people in their seventh decade of life are affected and the incidence increases roughly 1% per year. Only about 20% of patients with diverticulosis have symptoms attributable to these lesions, and less than 5% experience hemorrhage.[113] Hemorrhage from diverticular disease is most often massive, associated with hematochezia and varying degrees of hemorrhagic shock. Classically, patients present with a sudden occurrence of mild lower abdominal discomfort, rectal urgency, and the subsequent passage of a large maroon or melanic stool. Because the colon can contain large volumes of blood, neither the volume nor the frequency of bloody stools is a reliable guide to the rate of hemorrhage. Despite the massive nature of hemorrhage, most patients with diverticular disease stop bleeding spontaneously. In one series, 76% of patients initially stopped bleeding spontaneously, though 38% of these rebled. Of those who rebled, less than one fourth required surgery.[114]

Bleeding associated with diverticular disease comes from a perforated vasa recta located at the neck or apex of a diverticulum. The vasa recta penetrates the colonic wall from the serosa to the submucosa through obliquely oriented connective tissue septa. Protrusion of colonic mucosa through this connective tissue plane causes apposition of the diverticulum and the vasa recta (Fig. 67.4). Ulceration of the mucosa within the neck of the diverticulum and disruption of the arterial wall produces hemorrhage into the lumen of the bowel. Although diverticular

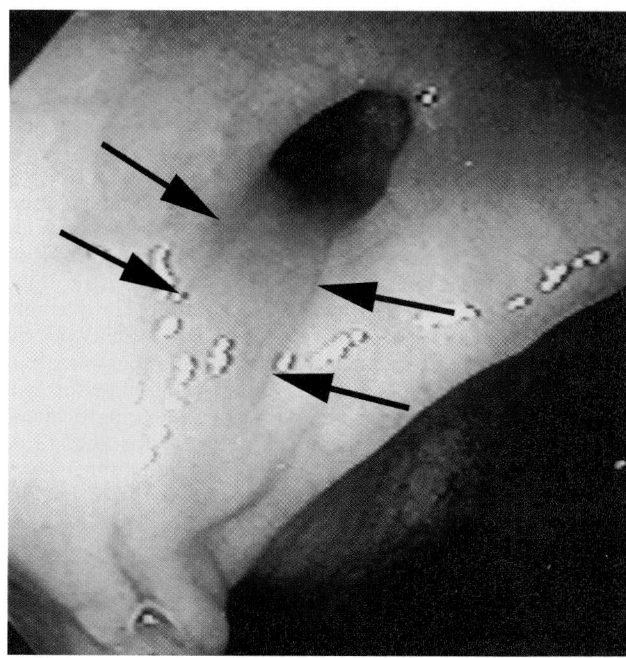

FIGURE 67.4 Colonoscopic view of a colonic diverticulum. A vasum rectum is seen entering the diverticulum and forming one of the walls.

disease is more prevalent in the left colon, right-sided lesions account for half or more episodes of bleeding.[114,115]

The massive nature of the bleeding caused by colonic diverticula limits the diagnostic usefulness of colonoscopy. Rarely is a bleeding vessel seen within a diverticulum and the presence of blood or clot within diverticula is of no diagnostic benefit. Selective mesenteric arteriography may demonstrate the luminal extravasation of contrast; however, in one study of patients bleeding from diverticulosis, angiographic localization was effective in less than 20% of patients.[116] Failure to visualize a bleeding point is usually due to cessation of active bleeding at the time of angiography.

Given the relatively low risk of recurrent hemorrhage, patients who stop bleeding should be treated expectantly. About 10% of patients bleeding from colonic diverticula continue to bleed and ultimately require operative intervention. Embolization of bleeding vessels in the colon has been reported to be safe and effective in the majority of patients; however there is a definite risk of ischemic complications.[117–120] The rapid nature of the hemorrhage and the difficulty in defining the site of bleeding through the endoscope have largely thwarted endoscopic attempts at control of diverticular hemorrhage.

Patients who continue to bleed from diverticular disease should undergo resection of the colon segment that contains the site of bleeding. Even after successful localization of a bleeding source, the least operation that can usually be contemplated is a hemicolectomy or wide segmental colectomy. Tagged red blood cell scanning, though sensitive, cannot pinpoint a bleeding site with great accuracy. Although angiography usually gives more precise localization, correlation between the vascular pattern and the anatomic location is sufficiently imprecise to warrant at least a segmental resection. Lastly, measurement with colonoscopy is notoriously misleading with even experienced endoscopists making mistakes about the precise site of a lesion.

Although a subtotal colectomy for nonlocalized ongoing colonic hemorrhage may occasionally be necessary, it should be performed only after exhaustive attempts to localize the site of bleeding. Subtotal colectomy is associated with greater perioperative morbidity rates than is segmental resection and postoperative diarrhea may present a significant problem to elderly patients. However, if the patient continues to bleed massively from the colon and all attempts at preoperative and intraoperative localization are unsuccessful, subtotal colectomy with ileoproctostomy may be required.

Colonic Angiodysplasia

Sometimes called *vascular ectasias* or *arteriovenous malformations*, these lesions are believed to arise from the age-related degeneration of previously normal intestinal submucosal veins and overlying mucosal capillaries. Angiodysplasia is located most frequently in the cecum and ascending colon, although it may be found more distally in 20% to 30% of cases. Multiple lesions may be present in as many as 40% to 75% of all cases.[121] Microscopically, angiodysplasia consists of dilated, thin-walled vessels that appear to be ectatic veins and venules localized within the submucosa. A dilated submucosal vein is often found and occasionally an enlarged artery. Smooth muscle is usually absent. Angiodysplasia is generally thought to be an acquired lesion associated with aging, but the exact etiology is unknown.

The prevalence of colonic angiodysplasia in the general population appears to be less than 1%.[122] These lesions may present with hematochezia, melena, occult blood loss, or iron deficiency anemia. Bleeding lesions are most commonly found in the right colon. As compared to diverticular bleeding, episodes of hemorrhage from vascular ectasias are usually less severe, and are somewhat more likely to recur. After the initial episode of hemorrhage, the majority of patients will stop bleeding spontaneously.[123]

Vascular ectasias may be diagnosed by either colonoscopy or by selective mesenteric angiography. Colonoscopy has been reported to have a sensitivity of 80% in demonstrating vascular ectasias.[124] However, colonoscopic diagnosis of these lesions in actively bleeding patients may be confounded by the presence of other incidental lesions including traumatic and suction artifacts produced during the examination. In addition, after significant bleeding and hypovolemia, the shunting of blood flow away from the intestinal mucosa may obscure these lesions in inadequately resuscitated patients. Colonoscopy can be used effectively to treat vascular ectasias either by coagulation or injection of sclerosants.[125,126]

Selective mesenteric angiography may also demonstrate these lesions and compliment colonoscopy, particularly in patients who are massively bleeding or in whom colonoscopy was unrevealing or incomplete. Characteristic angiographic findings include a densely opacified and slowly emptying, dilated, tortuous vein (found in 90% of patients), a vascular tuft (seen in 66% to 75% of patients), and an early-filling vein (usually a segmental vein in the cecum or right colon, although at times it may be the ileocolic vein).

The natural history of these lesions was revealed by the clinical course of 101 patients with colonic vascular ectasias.[124] Of the 15 asymptomatic individuals without a history of bleeding, none bled during a period of follow-up to 68 months (mean, 23 months). For 31 patients with overt bleeding or anemia who were treated only with blood transfusion, the rebleeding rate at 1 and 3 years was 26% and 46%, respectively. This study suggests that the risk of bleeding for incidentally discovered lesions is minimal, whereas the risk of recurrent hemorrhage for most symptomatic patients is substantial and may increase with time.

Patients bleeding from colonic vascular ectasias can be treated endoscopically. Nonrandomized investigations with vascular ectasias managed with monopolar electrocoagulation, endoscopic injection sclerotherapy, contact probes and lasers have been published with good results. All methods appear to be effective for treating bleeding vascular ectasias and all are associated with procedure-related morbidity rates of 2% to 10%. Perforation has been reported in all of these experiences with rates of 2% to 3%.

Patients bleeding from vascular ectasias in whom endoscopic hemostatic methods are unsuccessful or unavailable can be treated with resection of the colon following preoperative localization of the bleeding site. For the usual patient bleeding from a vascular ectasia in the cecum or ascending colon, a right colectomy with ileotransverse colostomy is the treatment of choice. The value of preoperative localization of the bleeding site cannot be overstated, and every effort should be made to determine the site of hemorrhage prior to laparotomy.

Ischemic Colitis

Ischemic colitis is a common cause of lower GI hemorrhage especially in the elderly. Its exact incidence is unknown, but is thought to be underdiagnosed. Bleeding is a common presenting manifestation of ischemic colitis occurring in approximately one-half to three-fourths of patients.[127,128] The etiology of ischemic colitis is unknown. Although it may occur with occlusion of a major artery, such as ligation of the inferior mesenteric artery during abdominal aortic aneurysm repair, in most cases major vascular occlusion cannot be demonstrated. Ischemic colitis usually occurs in the elderly and debilitated with significant comorbidities. Renal failure requiring hemodialysis, hypertension, cardiovascular disease, vasoactive medications, and a variety of other risk factors have been associated with the disease. Any segment of the colon may be involved. Profound ischemia may lead to full-thickness necrosis, peritonitis, and perforation. Lesser degrees of ischemia may result in vague abdominal pain, diarrhea, and mild to moderate bleeding. Life-threatening hemorrhage is uncommon.

The diagnosis of ischemic colitis is usually made by colonoscopy. Angiography is only occasionally helpful.[128] Surgical treatment is often required, usually due to peritonitis or other signs of full-thickness necrosis. Mortality is common though a large number of patients, the majority in some series, will recover uneventfully with supportive care alone.

UNUSUAL CAUSES OF ACUTE GASTROINTESTINAL HEMORRHAGE

As outlined in Tables 67.1 and 67.2, a wide variety of other pathologic processes may present with acute GI hemorrhage. Although these lesions generally comprise a relatively small percentage of the total number of cases of overt GI hemorrhage, they can present vexing problems to the clinician faced with a bleeding patient in whom the usual causes have been excluded. There are a number of case reports in the literature of extremely rare causes of GI bleeding that will not be discussed here. The following lesions occur commonly enough that an individual clinician is likely to encounter them.

Dieulafoy Vascular Malformation

Dieulafoy vascular malformation is an unusual cause of recurrent hematemesis, in which bleeding originates from an unusually large (1- to 3mm diameter) artery running through the gastric submucosa for variable distances. Erosion of the gastric mucosa overlying the vessel results in necrosis of the arterial wall and brisk hemorrhage. The size of the mucosal defect is usually small (2 to 5 mm) and without evidence of chronic inflammation. Other anatomic locations of these lesions including the colon have been described.[129–131]

Painless hematemesis and melena are typical. Recurrent bleeding with spontaneous cessation are also common. In a collective review of 101 cases, the mean age of the patients was 52 years, and the lesion occurred twice as frequently in men as women. There was no significant association with alcohol abuse or antecedent symptoms.[132]

The diagnosis is most frequently made endoscopically by demonstrating arterial bleeding from a pinpoint mucosal defect. Occasionally, a small arterial vessel may be seen protruding from the gastric mucosa. Characteristically, the lesions are located within 6 cm of the esophagogastric junction along the lesser curvature although they may occur in other sites as well.

Most patients can be managed endoscopically by injection of epinephrine, sclerotherapy, banding, clipping, or coagulation.[133–135] A subset of patients will require retreatment or surgical excision for control of hemorrhage. After cessation of hemorrhage few patients rebleed from these lesions even when treated only be endoscopic methods.[136]

Angiodysplasia of the Stomach and Small Intestine

Angiodysplastic lesions may occur throughout the GI tract. Similar to colonic lesions they appear as minute, flat or slightly raised red lesions with round or stellate shapes. The margins are characteristically sharp with a pale mucosal halo surrounding the lesion. The lesions are frequently multiple and are found most commonly in the stomach and duodenum, although esophageal and small intestinal involvement has also been described.

In general these lesions may be diagnosed by endoscopy although their minute size and sessile nature may complicate their detection. The lesions may also be readily mistaken for submucosal hemorrhage associated with acute gastritis or trauma artifact from a nasogastric tube or the endoscope. The lesions may also be demonstrated arteriographically since they have many of the features described for colonic vascular ectasia.

Endoscopic injection of sclerosants, electrocoagulation, and laser photocoagulation have all been used to treat gastroduodenal angiodysplasia with good results. The multiplicity of lesions often necessitates several courses of therapy to eliminate recurring hemorrhage. Surgical resection of the gastric or intestinal wall containing the lesion as well as oversewing of the bleeding lesion have been reported to successfully control hemorrhage.

Aortoenteric Fistula

Although communication between the aorta and the intestine may occur as a result of aneurysmal disease or infectious aortitis *(primary aortoenteric fistula)*, most of those encountered currently are due to the erosion of an aortic vascular prosthesis through the wall of the distal duodenum *(secondary aortoenteric fistula)*. The incidence of aortoenteric fistula following aortic reconstructive surgery is about 1% with most of these fistulas arising from the proximal graft anastamosis. Secondary aortoenteric fistulas are believed to develop after prolonged contact of a prosthetic graft with a fixed segment of intestine. Ultimately, erosion of the graft through the bowel wall results in a low-grade infection around the graft; involvement of the infection with the suture line leads to dehiscence of the anastomosis and massive hemorrhage.

The interval between aortic reconstructive surgery and the onset of GI hemorrhage may range from a few days to many years; the median interval is about 3 years.[137] Most patients have an initial episode of GI bleeding (i.e., herald bleed) that is followed in hours, days, or weeks by catastrophic hemorrhage. Patients may also complain of back or abdominal pain and less commonly have fever or signs of sepsis from infection of the graft.

The diagnosis of an aortoenteric fistula must be considered in any patient with an aortic prosthesis or an abdominal aortic aneurysm who presents with GI hemorrhage. Endoscopy should be urgently performed following resuscitation to disclose evidence of an aortoenteric fistula or another cause of bleeding (e.g., peptic ulcer disease with stigmata of recent hemorrhage). If endoscopy fails to demonstrate an aortoenteric fistula or another convincing source of bleeding and the patient is not massively bleeding, computed tomography may be helpful in detecting perigraft infection or other evidence of an aortoenteric fistula. In patients who are actively bleeding, exploratory laparotomy with exposure of the proximal graft should be undertaken. Identification of an aortoenteric fistula or erosion requires resection of the graft with extraanatomical bypass and repair of the duodenal wall.

Meckel's Diverticulum

Bleeding from a Meckel's diverticulum is a common cause of lower GI hemorrhage in children but is rare in older adults.

Meckel's diverticula are present in approximately 2% of the population. The lifetime risk of a complication from a Meckel's diverticulum is about 4%.[138] About 25% of patients with symptomatic Meckel's diverticula present with hemorrhage.[139] In a series of 17 patients who bled from Meckel's diverticula, 11 experienced frank hemorrhage, whereas 6 had chronic occult blood loss. The incidence of GI hemorrhage is greatest in the first decade of life and steadily decreases from that point. In one series, no patient older than 40 years , and only one patient older than age 31 years, bled from a Meckel's diverticulum,[139] although it has been reported in the very elderly.[140] The pathogenesis of this bleeding involves the occurrence of ectopic gastric mucosa with peptic ulceration of adjacent bowel wall. Although these lesions may be demonstrated by enteroclysis, abdominal scintigraphy following the intravenous injection of ^{99}technetium pertechnetate demonstrates the ectopic gastric mucosa within the diverticulum suggesting the correct diagnosis. Treatment consists of resecting the diverticulum with a cuff of adjacent bowel. Diverticulectomy alone will be associated with persistence of the ulcer and the possibility of recurrent hemorrhage.

Small Intestinal Diverticulum

Diverticular disease of the small intestine is another uncommon cause of either UGI hemorrhage (duodenal) or lower GI hemorrhage (jejunoileal diverticula).[141] The pathogenesis is similar to that of colonic diverticula with erosion of a vasa recta through the diverticular wall and the acute onset of massive hemorrhage. Depending on the location of the diverticulum, patients may present with either hemetemesis, melena, or hematochezia. Hemorrhage from this source can be a vexing diagnostic problem because jejunoileal lesions are beyond the reach of the gastroscope and bleeding from duodenal diverticula may be difficult to discern. Mesenteric angiography or intraoperative enteroscopy may localize the site of hemorrhage in actively bleeding patients. Segmental resection of the involved intestine is the treatment of choice.

Hemorrhage Following Endoscopic Procedures

Significant hemorrhage can occur following endoscopic biopsy, sphincterotomy, and other traumatic procedures. Fortunately these complications are uncommon. Hemorrhage following endoscopic biliary sphincterotomy occurs in approximately 2% of patients.[142–144] Mild immediate bleeding is common and is usually self-limited. Late hemorrhage usually occurs within 48 hours of the procedure but can occur many days after sphincterotomy.[145] More severe hemorrhage can usually be controlled by epinephrine injection making the need for operative treatment uncommon.[145,146]

Biopsy of lesions in the GI tract may also cause bleeding. Usually this bleeding is minor and self-limited. Clinically significant hemorrhage after colonic polypectomy is seen in approximately 0.2% of biopsies and may occur up to 12 days after the procedure.[147] The bleeding site can be confirmed by tagged red cell scanning, arteriography, or colonoscopy. Arteriography and colonoscopy can be used therapeutically as described previously. Endoscopically placed bands such as those used for esophageal varices have also been reported to be successful in arresting hemorrhage.[73] Surgical treatment is rarely required.

KEY POINTS

- **Patients with overt GI bleeding present after observing the passage of blood from the GI tract as hematemesis (the vomiting of blood), melena, or hematochezia.**
- **Melena is a black, tarry stool resulting from the degradation of blood by enteric bacteria. Bleeding from the small intestine or right colon may also appear black if the blood has remained in the GI tract for more than 12 to14 hours.**
- **Hematochezia is the passage of bright red blood from the rectum and is usually indicative of a lower GI source.**
- **Esophagogastroduodenoscopy will identify the site of bleeding in about 95% of cases of UGI bleeding and is the initial diagnostic study for patients suspected of bleeding from the esophagus, stomach or duodenum.**
- **Peptic ulcer disease is the most common cause of acute upper GI hemorrhage, accounting for nearly 40% of cases in most series.**
- **Cirrhosis is a leading cause of death in the United States and variceal hemorrhage is a common mode of death for these patients. About 30% of people with cirrhosis develop gastroesophageal varices, and of these individuals, about 30% bleed as a result.**
- **The Mallory-Weiss syndrome is acute UGI hemorrhage that occurs after retching or vomiting.**
- **Colonic angiodysplasia may cause hematochezia, melena, occult blood loss, or iron deficiency anemia. Bleeding lesions are most commonly found in the right colon.**

References

1. Peura DA, Lanza FL, Gostout CJ, et al. The American College of Gastroenterology Bleeding Registry: preliminary findings. *Am J Gastroenterol.* 1997;92:924–928.
2. Vreeburg EM, Snel P, de Bruijne JW, et al. Acute upper gastrointestinal bleeding in the Amsterdam area: incidence, diagnosis, and clinical outcome. *Am J Gastroenterol.* 1997;92:236–243.
3. Cutler JA, Mendeloff AI. Upper gastrointestinal bleeding. Nature and magnitude of the problem in the U.S. *Dig Dis Sci.* 1981;26(suppl):90S–6S.
4. Yavorski RT, Wong RK, Maydonovitch C, et al. Analysis of 3,294 cases of upper gastrointestinal bleeding in military medical facilities. *Am J Gastroenterol.* 1995;90:568–573.
5. Lingenfelser T, Ell C. Lower intestinal bleeding. *Baillieres Best Pract Res Clin Gastroenterol.* 2001;15:135–153.
6. Richter JM, Christensen MR, Kaplan LM, et al. Effectiveness of current technology in the diagnosis and management of lower gastrointestinal hemorrhage. *Gastrointest Endosc.* 1995;41:93–98.
7. Bramley PN, Masson JW, McKnight G, et al. The role of an open-access bleeding unit in the management of colonic haemorrhage. A 2-year prospective study. *Scand J Gastroenterol.* 1996;31:764–769.
8. Longstreth GF. Epidemiology and outcome of patients hospitalized with acute lower gastrointestinal hemorrhage: a population-based study. *Am J Gastroenterol.* 1997;92:419–424.
9. Kok KY, Kum CK, Goh PM. Colonoscopic evaluation of severe hematochezia in an Oriental population. *Endoscopy* 1998;30:675–680.
10. Kaplan RC, Heckbert SR, Koepsell TD, et al. Risk factors for hospitalized gastrointestinal bleeding among older persons. Cardiovascular Health Study Investigators. *J Am Geriatr Soc.* 2001;49:126–133.
11. van Leerdam ME, Vreeburg EM, Rauws EA, et al. Acute upper GI bleeding: did anything change? Time trend analysis of incidence and outcome of acute upper GI bleeding between 1993/1994 and 2000. *Am J Gastroenterol.* 2003;98:1494–1499.
12. Pahor M, Guralnik JM, Salive ME, et al. Disability and severe gastrointestinal hemorrhage. A prospective study of community-dwelling older persons. *J Am Geriatr Soc.* 1994;42:816–825.
13. Fiaccadori E, Maggiore U, Clima B, et al. Incidence, risk factors, and prognosis of gastrointestinal hemorrhage complicating acute renal failure. *Kidney Int.* 2001;59:1510–1519.
14. Cheng HC, Chuang SA, Kao YH, et al. Increased risk of rebleeding of peptic ulcer bleeding in patients with comorbid illness receiving omeprazole infusion. *Hepato Gastroenterology* 2003;50:2270–2273.
15. Mellemkjaer L, Blot WJ, Sorensen HT, et al. Upper gastrointestinal bleeding among users of NSAIDs: a population-based cohort study in Denmark. *Br J Clin Pharmacol.* 2002;53:173–181.
16. Daniel WA Jr, Egan S. The Quantity of Blood Required to Produce a Tarry Stool. *JAMA* 1939;113:2232.

17. Schiff L, Stevens RJ, Shapiro N, et al. Observations on the oral administration of citrated blood in man. II. The effect on the stools. *Am J Med Sci.* 1942;203:409–412.
18. Hilsman JH. The color of blood-containing feces following the instillation of citrated blood at various levels of the small intestine. *Gastroenterology* 1999;15:131–134.
19. Longstreth GF, Feitelberg SP. Outpatient care of selected patients with acute non-variceal upper gastrointestinal haemorrhage . *Lancet* 1995;345: 108–111.
20. **Kollef MH, O'Brien JD, Zuckerman GR, et al. BLEED: a classification tool to predict outcomes in patients with acute upper and lower gastrointestinal hemorrhage. *Crit Care Med.* 1997;25:1125–1132.**
21. Rockall TA, Logan RF, Devlin HB, et al. Risk assessment after acute upper gastrointestinal haemorrhage. *Gut* 1996;38:316–321.
22. **Barkun A, Bardou M, Marshall JK. Nonvariceal Upper GI Bleeding Consensus Conference Group. Consensus recommendations for managing patients with nonvariceal upper gastrointestinal bleeding. *Ann Intern Med.* 2003;139:843–857.**
23. Aljebreen AM, Fallone CA, Barkun AN. Nasogastric aspirate predicts high-risk endoscopic lesions in patients with acute upper-GI bleeding. *Gastrointest Endosc.* 2004;59:172–178.
24. Witting MD, Magder L, Heins AE, et al. Usefulness and validity of diagnostic nasogastric aspiration in patients without hematemesis. *Ann Emerg Med.* 2004;43:525–532.
25. Kovacs TO, Jensen DM. Endoscopic control of gastroduodenal hemorrhage. *Annu Rev Med.* 1987;38:267–277.
26. Chung YF, Wong WK, Soo KC. Diagnostic failures in endoscopy for acute upper gastrointestinal haemorrhage. *Br J Surg.* 2000;87:614–617.
27. Spiegel BM, Vakil NB, Ofman JJ. Endoscopy for acute nonvariceal upper gastrointestinal tract hemorrhage: is sooner better? A systematic review. *Arch Intern Med.* 2001;161:1393–1404.
28. Lee JG, Turnipseed S, Romano PS, et al. Endoscopy-based triage significantly reduces hospitalization rates and costs of treating upper GI bleeding: a randomized controlled trial. *Gastrointest Endosc.* 1999;50: 755–761.
29. Laine L, Peterson WL. Bleeding peptic ulcer. *N Engl J Med.* 1994;331: 717–727.
30. Anonymous. Consensus conference: Therapeutic endoscopy and bleeding ulcers. *JAMA* 1989;262:1369–1372.
31. Hsu PI, Lin XZ, Chan SH, et al. Bleeding peptic ulcer—risk factors for rebleeding and sequential changes in endoscopic findings. *Gut* 1994;35: 746–749.
32. Villanueva C, Balanzo J, Espinos JC, et al. Prediction of therapeutic failure in patients with bleeding peptic ulcer treated with endoscopic injection. *Dig Dis Sci.* 1993;38:2062–2070.
33. Chung IK, Kim EJ, Lee MS, et al. Endoscopic factors predisposing to rebleeding following endoscopic hemostasis in bleeding peptic ulcers. *Endoscopy* 2001;33:969–975.
34. Terdiman JP, Ostroff JW. Risk of persistent or recurrent and intractable upper gastrointestinal bleeding in the era of therapeutic endoscopy. *Am J Gastroenterol.* 1997;92:1805–1811.
35. Chaudhry V, Hyser MJ, Gracias VH, et al. Colonoscopy: the initial test for acute lower gastrointestinal bleeding. *Am Surg.* 1998;64:723–728.
36. Zuckerman GR, Prakash C. Acute lower intestinal bleeding. Part II: etiology, therapy, and outcomes. *Gastrointest Endosc.* 1999;49:228–238.
37. Foutch PG. Diverticular bleeding: are nonsteroidal anti-inflammatory drugs risk factors for hemorrhage and can colonoscopy predict outcome for patients? *Am J Gastroenterol.* 1995;90:1779–1784.
38. Jensen DM, Machicado GA, Jutabha R, et al. Urgent colonoscopy for the diagnosis and treatment of severe diverticular hemorrhage. *N Engl J Med.* 2000;342:78–82.
39. Al Qahtani AR, Satin R, Stern J, Gordon PH. Investigative modalities for massive lower gastrointestinal bleeding. *World J Surg.* 2002;26: 620–625.
40. Rossini FP, Pennazio M. Small-bowel endoscopy. *Endoscopy* 2000;32: 138–145.
41. Kovacs TO, Jensen DM. Recent advances in the endoscopic diagnosis and therapy of upper gastrointestinal, small intestinal, and colonic bleeding. *Med Clin North Am.* 2002;86:1319–1356.
42. Jensen DM, Kovacs TO, Jutabha R. Gastrointestinal bleeding (GIB) of obscure origin in an era of managed care and push enteroscopy. *Gastrointest Endosc.* 1997;45:AB92.
43. Pennazio M, Santucci R, Rondonotti E, et al. Outcome of patients with obscure gastrointestinal bleeding after capsule endoscopy: report of 100 consecutive cases. *Gastroenterology* 2004;126:643–653.
44. Fireman Z, Eliakim R, Adler S, et al. Capsule endoscopy in real life: a four-centre experience of 160 consecutive patients in Israel. *Eur J Gastroenterol Hepatol.* 2004;16:927–931.
45. Adler DG, Knipschield M, Gostout C. A prospective comparison of capsule endoscopy and push enteroscopy in patients with GI bleeding of obscure origin. *Gastrointest Endosc.* 2004;59:492–498.
46. Saurin JC, Delvaux M, Gaudin JL, et al. Diagnostic value of endoscopic capsule in patients with obscure digestive bleeding: blinded comparison with video push-enteroscopy. *Endoscopy* 2003;35:576–584.
47. Ell C, Remke S, May A, et al. The first prospective controlled trial comparing wireless capsule endoscopy with push enteroscopy in chronic gastrointestinal bleeding. *Endoscopy* 2002;34:685–689.
48. Mylonaki M, Fritscher-Ravens A, Swain P. Wireless capsule endoscopy: a comparison with push enteroscopy in patients with gastroscopy and colonoscopy negative gastrointestinal bleeding. *Gut* 2003;52:1122–1126.
49. Mata A, Bordas JM, Feu F, et al. Wireless capsule endoscopy in patients with obscure gastrointestinal bleeding: a comparative study with push enteroscopy. *Aliment Pharmacol Ther.* 2004;20:189–194.
50. Zuckerman GR, Prakash C. Acute lower intestinal bleeding: part I: clinical presentation and diagnosis. *Gastrointest Endosc.* 1998;48:606–617.
51. Vernava AM III, Moore BA, Longo WE, et al. Lower gastrointestinal bleeding. *Dis Colon Rectum.* 1997;40:846–858.
52. Nusbaum M, Baum S. Radiographic demonstration of unknown sites of GI bleeding. *Surg Forum* 1963;14:374.
53. Pennoyer WP, Vignati PV, Cohen JL. Mesenteric angiography for lower gastrointestinal hemorrhage: are there predictors for a positive study? *Dis Colon Rectum.* 1997;40:1014–1018.
54. Mernagh JR, O'Donovan N, Somers S, et al. Use of heparin in the investigation of obscure gastrointestinal bleeding. *Can Assoc Radiol J.* 2001;52:232–235.
55. Bloomfeld RS, Smith TP, Schneider AM, et al. Provocative angiography in patients with gastrointestinal hemorrhage of obscure origin. *Am J Gastroenterol.* 2000;95:2807–2812.
56. Smith R, Copely DJ, Bolen FH. 99mTc RBC scintigraphy: correlation of gastrointestinal bleeding rates with scintigraphic findings. *AJR Am J Roentgenol.* 1987;148:869–874.
57. Thorne DA, Datz FL, Remley K, et al. Bleeding rates necessary for detecting acute gastrointestinal bleeding with technetium-99m-labeled red blood cells in an experimental model. *J Nucl Med.* 1987;28:514520.
58. Suzman MS, Talmor M, Jennis R, et al. Accurate localization and surgical management of active lower gastrointestinal hemorrhage with technetium-labeled erythrocyte scintigraphy. *Ann Surg.* 1996;224:29–36.
59. Maurer AH, Rodman MS, Vitti RA, et al. Gastrointestinal bleeding: improved localization with cine scintigraphy. *Radiology* 1992;185:187–192.
60. Singh PR, Russell CD, Dubovsky EV, et al. Technique of scanning for Meckel's diverticulum. *Clin Nucl Med.* 1978;3:188–192.
61. Boonpongmanee S, Fleischer DE, Pezzullo JC, et al. The frequency of peptic ulcer as a cause of upper-GI bleeding is exaggerated. *Gastrointest Endosc.* 2004;59:788–794.
62. Hirschowitz BI, Lanas A. NSAID association with gastrointestinal bleeding and peptic ulcer. *Agents Actions Suppl.* 1991;35:93–101.
63. Ehsanullah RS, Page MC, Tildesley G, et al. Prevention of gastroduodenal damage induced by non-steroidal anti-inflammatory drugs: controlled trial of ranitidine. *BMJ.* 1988;297:1017–1021.
64. Strom BL, Taragin MI, Carson JL. Gastrointestinal bleeding from the non-steroidal anti-inflammatory drugs. *Agents Actions Suppl.* 1990;29: 27–38.
65. Garcia RL, Cattaruzzi C, Troncon MG, et al. Risk of hospitalization for upper gastrointestinal tract bleeding associated with ketorolac, other non-steroidal anti-inflammatory drugs, calcium antagonists, and other antihypertensive drugs. *Arch Intern Med.* 1998;158:33–39.
66. Laporte JR, Ibanez L, Vidal X, et al. Upper gastrointestinal bleeding associated with the use of NSAIDs: newer versus older agents. *Drug Safety* 2004;27:411–420.
67. Shorr RI, Ray WA, Daugherty JR, et al. Concurrent use of nonsteroidal anti-inflammatory drugs and oral anticoagulants places elderly persons at high risk for hemorrhagic peptic ulcer disease. *Arch Intern Med.* 1993;153:1665–1670.
68. Armstrong CP, Blower AL. Non-steroidal anti-inflammatory drugs and life threatening complications of peptic ulceration. *Gut* 1987;28:527–532.
69. Klein WA, Krevsky B, Klepper L, et al. Nonsteroidal antiinflammatory drugs and upper gastrointestinal hemorrhage in an urban hospital. *Dig Dis Sci.* 1993;38:2049–2055.
70. Lanza FL, Fakouhi D, Rubin A, et al. A double-blind placebo-controlled comparison of the efficacy and safety of 50, 100, and 200 micrograms of misoprostol QID in the prevention of ibuprofen-induced gastric and duodenal mucosal lesions and symptoms. *Am J Gastroenterol.* 1989;84: 633–636.
71. Robinson MG, Griffin JWJ, Bowers J, et al. Effect of ranitidine on gastroduodenal mucosal damage induced by nonsteroidal antiinflammatory drugs. *Dig Dis Sci.* 1989;34:424–428.
72. Roth SH, Bennett RE, Mitchell CS, Hartman RJ. Cimetidine therapy in nonsteroidal anti-inflammatory drug gastropathy. Double-blind long-term evaluation. *Arch Intern Med.* 1987;147:1798–1801.
73. Pfaffenbach B, Adamek RJ, Wegener M. Endoscopic band ligation for treatment of post-polypectomy bleeding. *Z Gastroenterol.* 1996;34: 241–242.
74. Wilcox CM, Alexander LN, Cotsonis GA, et al. Nonsteroidal antiinflammatory drugs are associated with both upper and lower gastrointestinal bleeding. *Dig Dis Sci.* 1997;42:990–997.
75. Lanas A, Sekar MC, Hirschowitz BI. Objective evidence of aspirin use in both ulcer and nonulcer upper and lower gastrointestinal bleeding. *Gastroenterology* 1992;103:862–869.

76. Holt S, Rigoglioso V, Sidhu M, et al. Nonsteroidal antiinflammatory drugs and lower gastrointestinal bleeding. *Dig Dis Sci.* 1993;38: 1619–1623.
77. Hunt RH, Harper S, Watson DJ, et al. The gastrointestinal safety of the COX-2 selective inhibitor etoricoxib assessed by both endoscopy and analysis of upper gastrointestinal events. *Am J Gastroenterol.* 2003;98: 1725–1733.
78. Norgard B, Pedersen L, Johnsen SP, et al. COX-2-selective inhibitors and the risk of upper gastrointestinal bleeding in high-risk patients with previous gastrointestinal diseases: a population-based case-control study. *Aliment Pharmacol Ther.* 2004;19:817–825.
79. Barkun A, Sabbah S, Enns R, et al. The Canadian Registry on Nonvariceal Upper Gastrointestinal Bleeding and Endoscopy (RUGBE): Endoscopic hemostasis and proton pump inhibition are associated with improved outcomes in a real-life setting. *Am J Gastroenterol.* 2004;99:1238–1246.
80. Dore MP, Graham DY. Ulcers and gastritis. *Endoscopy.* 2004;36:42–47.
81. Laine LA. *Helicobacter pylori* and complicated ulcer disease. *Am J Med.* 1996;100(5A):52S–7S.
82. Vergara M, Casellas F, Saperas E, et al. *Helicobacter pylori* eradication prevents recurrence from peptic ulcer haemorrhage. *Eur J Gastroenterol Hepatol.* 2000;12:733–737.
83. Pilotto A, Leandro G, Di Mario F, et al. Role of *Helicobacter pylori* infection on upper gastrointestinal bleeding in the elderly: a case-control study. *Dig Dis Sci.* 1997;42:586–591.
84. Forrest JA, Finlayson ND, Shearman DJ. Endoscopy in gastrointestinal bleeding. *Lancet* 1974;2:394–397.
85. Raju GS, Gajula L. Endoclips for GI endoscopy. *Gastrointest Endosc.* 2004;59:267–279.
86. Naga MI, Okasha HH, Foda AR, et al. Detachable endoloop vs. elastic band ligation for bleeding esophageal varices. *Gastrointest Endosc.* 2004;59:804–809.
87. Lin HJ, Lo WC, Lee FY, et al. A prospective randomized comparative trial showing that omeprazole prevents rebleeding in patients with bleeding peptic ulcer after successful endoscopic therapy. *Arch Intern Med.* 1998;158: 54–58.
88. Chung SS, Lau JY, Sung JJ, et al. Randomised comparison between adrenaline injection alone and adrenaline injection plus heat probe treatment for actively bleeding ulcers. *BMJ* 1997;314:1307–1311.
89. Asaki S. Endoscopic haemostasis by local absolute alcohol injection for UGI tract bleeding: a multicentre study. In: Okabe H, Honda T, Ohshiba S, eds. *Endoscopic surgery.* New York: Elsevier, 1999, p. 105.
90. Sacks HS, Chalmers TC, Blum AL, et al. Endoscopic hemostasis. An effective therapy for bleeding peptic ulcers. *JAMA* 1990;264:494–499.
91. Sugawa C, Steffes CP, Nakamura R, et al. Upper GI bleeding in an urban hospital. Etiology, recurrence, and prognosis. *Ann Surg.* 1990;212:521–526.
92. Lau JY, Sung JJ, Lam YH, et al. Endoscopic retreatment compared with surgery in patients with recurrent bleeding after initial endoscopic control of bleeding ulcers. *N Engl J Med.* 1999;340:751–756.
93. Gupta PK, Fleischer DE. Nonvariceal upper gastrointestinal bleeding. *Med Clin North Am.* 1993;77:973–992.
94. Teenan RP, Murray WR. Late outcome of undersewing alone for gastric ulcer haemorrhage. *Br J Surg.* 1990;77:811–812.
95. Schuster DP, Rowley H, Feinstein S, et al. Prospective evaluation of the risk of upper gastrointestinal bleeding after admission to a medical intensive care unit. *Am J Med.* 1984;76:623–630.
96. Cook DJ, Fuller HD, Guyatt GH, et al. Risk factors for gastrointestinal bleeding in critically ill patients. Canadian Critical Care Trials Group. *N Engl J Med.* 1994;330:377–381.
97. Driks MR, Craven DE, Celli BR, et al. Nosocomial pneumonia in intubated patients given sucralfate as compared with antacids or histamine type 2 blockers. The role of gastric colonization. *N Engl J Med.* 1987;317:1376–1382.
98. Cook D, Guyatt G, Marshall J, et al. A comparison of sucralfate and ranitidine for the prevention of upper gastrointestinal bleeding in patients requiring mechanical ventilation. Canadian Critical Care Trials Group. *N Engl J Med.* 1998;338:791–797.
99. Athanasoulis CA. Therapeutic applications of angiography (first of two parts). *N Engl J Med.* 1980;302:1117–1125.
100. Robert A, Kauffman GL Jr. Stress ulcers, erosions and gastric mucosal injury. In: Sleisenger and Fordtran's gastrointestinal and liver disease: pathophysiology, diagnosis, management, 4 ed. Philadelphia: WB Saunders; 1999, p. 772.
101. Silverstein FE, Gilbert DA, Tedesco FJ, et al. The national ASGE survey on upper gastrointestinal bleeding. II. Clinical prognostic factors. *Gastrointest Endosc.* 1981;27:80–93.
102. Wilcox CM, Clark WS. Causes and outcome of upper and lower gastrointestinal bleeding: the Grady Hospital experience. *South Med J.* 1999;92: 44–50.
103. Imperiale TF, Teran JC, McCullough AJ. A meta-analysis of somatostatin versus vasopressin in the management of acute esophageal variceal hemorrhage. *Gastroenterology* 1995;109:1289–1294.
104. Burroughs AK. Octreotide in variceal bleeding. *Gut* 1994;35(3 suppl): S23–S27.
105. Avgerinos A, Nevens F, Raptis S, et al. Early administration of somatostatin and efficacy of sclerotherapy in acute oesophageal variceal bleeds: the European Acute Bleeding Oesophageal Variceal Episodes (ABOVE) randomised trial . *Lancet* 1997;350:1495–1499.
106. Besson I, Ingrand P, Person B, et al. Sclerotherapy with or without octreotide for acute variceal bleeding. *N Engl J Med.* 1995;333:555–560.
107. Sung JJ, Chung SC, Yung MY, et al. Prospective randomised study of effect of octreotide on rebleeding from oesophageal varices after endoscopic ligation. *Lancet* 1995;346(8991–8992):1666–1669.
108. Hermann RE, Traul D. Experience with the Sengstaken-Blakemore tube for bleeding esophageal varices. *Surg Gynecol Obstet.* 1970;130: 879–885.
109. Monescillo A, Martinez-Lagares F, Ruiz-del-Arbol L, et al. Influence of portal hypertension and its early decompression by TIPS placement on the outcome of variceal bleeding. *Hepatology* 2004;40:793–801.
110. Orloff MJ, Orloff MS, Orloff SL, et al. Three decades of experience with emergency portacaval shunt for acutely bleeding esophageal varices in 400 unselected patients with cirrhosis of the liver. *J Am Coll Surg.* 1995;180:257–272.
111. Mallory GK, Weiss S. Hemorrhages from lacerations of the cardiac orifice of the stomach due to vomiting. *Am J Med Sci.* 1929;178:506–515.
112. Park CH, Min SW, Sohn YH, et al. A prospective, randomized trial of endoscopic band ligation vs. epinephrine injection for actively bleeding Mallory-Weiss syndrome. *Gastrointest Endosc.* 2004;60:22–27.
113. McGuire HHJ, Haynes BW Jr. Massive hemorrhage for diverticulosis of the colon: guidelines for therapy based on bleeding patterns observed in fifty cases. *Ann Surg.* 1972;175:847–855.
114. McGuire HH, Jr. Bleeding colonic diverticula. A reappraisal of natural history and management. *Ann Surg.* 1994;220:653–656.
115. Casarella WJ, Kanter IE, Seaman WB. Right-sided colonic diverticula as a cause of acute rectal hemorrhage. *N Engl J Med.* 1972;286:450–453.
116. Boley SJ, DiBiase A, Brandt LJ, et al. Lower intestinal bleeding in the elderly. *Am J Surg.* 1979;137:57–64.
117. Nicholson AA, Ettles DF, Hartley JE, et al. Transcatheter coil embolotherapy: a safe and effective option for major colonic haemorrhage. *Gut* 1998;43:79–84.
118. Kuo WT, Lee DE, Saad WE, et al. Superselective microcoil embolization for the treatment of lower gastrointestinal hemorrhage. *J Vasc Interv Radiol.* 2003;14:1503–1509.
119. Gady JS, Reynolds H, Blum A. Selective arterial embolization for control of lower gastrointestinal bleeding: recommendations for a clinical management pathway. *Current Surgery* 2003;60:344–347.
120. Gordon RL, Ahl KL, Kerlan RK, et al. Selective arterial embolization for the control of lower gastrointestinal bleeding. *Am J Surg.* 1997;174: 24–28.
121. Foutch PG. Angiodysplasia of the gastrointestinal tract. *Am J Gastroenterol.* 1993;88:807–818.
122. Foutch PG, Rex DK, Lieberman DA. Prevalence and natural history of colonic angiodysplasia among healthy asymptomatic people. *Am J Gastroenterol.* 1995;90:564–567.
123. Sharma R, Gorbien MJ. Angiodysplasia and lower gastrointestinal tract bleeding in elderly patients. *Arch Intern Med.* 1995;155:807–812.
124. Richter JM, Hedberg SE, Athanasoulis CA, et al. Angiodysplasia. Clinical presentation and colonoscopic diagnosis. *Dig Dis Sci.* 1984;29:481–485.
125. Gupta N, Longo WE, Vernava AM. Angiodysplasia of the lower gastrointestinal tract: an entity readily diagnosed by colonoscopy and primarily managed nonoperatively. *Dis Colon Rectum* 1995;38:979–982.
126. Bemvenuti GA, Julich MM. Ethanolamine injection for sclerotherapy of angiodysplasia of the colon. *Endoscopy* 1998;30:564–569.
127. Medina C, Vilaseca J, Videla S, et al. Outcome of patients with ischemic colitis: review of fifty-three cases. *Dis Colon Rectum* 2004;47:180–184.
128. Scharff JR, Longo WE, Vartanian SM, et al. Ischemic colitis: spectrum of disease and outcome. *Surgery* 2003;134:624–629.
129. Chaer RA, Helton WS. Dieulafoy's disease. *J Am Coll Surg.* 2003;196: 290–296.
130. Lee YT, Walmsley RS, Leong RW, et al. Dieulafoy's lesion. *Gastrointest Endosc.* 2003;58:236–243.
131. Gimeno-Garcia AZ, Parra-Blanco A, Nicolas-Perez D, et al. Management of colonic Dieulafoy lesions with endoscopic mechanical techniques: report of two cases. *Dis Colon Rectum* 2004;47:1539–1543.
132. Veldhuyzen vZS, Bartelsman JF, Schipper ME, et al. Recurrent massive haematemesis from Dieulafoy vascular malformations—a review of 101 cases. *Gut.* 1986;27:213–222.
133. Baettig B, Haecki W, Lammer F, et al. Dieulafoy's disease: endoscopic treatment and follow up. *Gut* 1993;34:1418–1421.
134. Park CH, Sohn YH, Lee WS, et al. The usefulness of endoscopic hemoclipping for bleeding Dieulafoy lesions. *Endoscopy* 2003;35:388–392.
135. Cheng CL, Liu NJ, Lee CS, et al. Endoscopic management of Dieulafoy lesions in acute nonvariceal upper gastrointestinal bleeding. *Dig Dis Sci.* 2004;49(7–8):1139–1144.
136. Romaozinho JM, Pontes JM, Lerias C, et al. Dieulafoy's lesion: management and long-term outcome. *Endoscopy* 2004;36:416–420.
137. Nagy SW, Marshall JB. Aortoenteric fistulas. Recognizing a potentially catastrophic cause of gastrointestinal bleeding. *Postgrad Med.* 1921;93:211–212.

138. Yahchouchy EK, Marano AF, Etienne JC, et al. Meckel's diverticulum. *J Am Coll Surg*. 2001;192:658–662.
139. Mackey WC, Dineen P. A fifty year experience with Meckel's diverticulum. Surg *Gynecol Obstet*. 1983;156:56–64.
140. Lichtstein DM, Herskowitz B. Massive gastrointestinal bleeding from Meckel's diverticulum in a 91-year-old man. *South Med J*. 1998;91:753–754.
141. El-Haddawi F, Civil ID. Acquired jejuno-ileal diverticular disease: a diagnostic and management challenge. *ANZ Journal of Surgery* 2003;73:584–589.
142. Halme L, Doepel M, von Numers H, et al. Complications of diagnostic and therapeutic ERCP. *Ann Chir Gynaecol*. 1999;88:127–131.
143. Freeman ML, Nelson DB, Sherman S, et al. Complications of endoscopic biliary sphincterotomy. *N Engl J Med*. 1996;335:909–918.
144. Gholson CF, Favrot D, Vickers B, et al. Delayed hemorrhage following endoscopic retrograde sphincterotomy for choledocholithiasis. *Dig Dis Sci*. 1996;41:831–834.
145. Vasconez C, Llach J, Bordas JM, et al. Injection treatment of hemorrhage induced by endoscopic sphincterotomy. *Endoscopy* 1998;30:37–39.
146. Leung JW, Chan FK, Sung JJ, Chung S. Endoscopic sphincterotomy-induced hemorrhage: a study of risk factors and the role of epinephrine injection. *Gastrointest Endosc*. 1995;42:550–554.
147. Gibbs DH, Opelka FG, Beck DE, et al. Postpolypectomy colonic hemorrhage. *Dis Colon Rectum* 1996;39:806–810.

CHAPTER 68 ■ ULCERATIVE COLITIS

EMINA HUANG

Ulcerative colitis is a nonspecific inflammatory bowel disease (IBD) of unknown etiology that affects the mucosa of the colon and rectum. The disease presents in both genders, with onset principally in the second to fourth decades. Because ulcerative colitis affects the mucosa, clinical features include diarrhea and bleeding per rectum. Although current medical treatment may temporarily improve the symptoms, allowing long periods of quiescence, this therapy does not provide cure. Currently, the only definitive treatment is surgical, involving resection of the colon and rectum.

EPIDEMIOLOGY

Broadly speaking, epidemiology is the study of occurrence of illness. More specifically, epidemiology studies the distribution of factors important in determining the nature of the disease. Initially, ulcerative colitis and Crohn disease were believed to be different manifestations of the same disease. Despite more than 50 years of investigation, efforts to understand the underlying biologic mechanisms have failed to reveal an inciting event or process.[1]

IBD is not an entity discovered in the 20th century. Case series of ulcerative colitis have been documented in the 19th century.[2] After World War II, the incidence of both ulcerative colitis and Crohn disease increased, with an incidence of approximately 2.2 to 14.3 cases per 100,000 person-years for ulcerative colitis in North America.[3–5] Regional differences do exist; the highest incidence rates are in northern Europe, the United Kingdom, and North America, with rising incidences on the continents of Asia, Africa, and South America.[6] When these numbers are extrapolated to the combined 320 million persons of North America, between 7,000 and 46,000 new cases of ulcerative colitis occur per year.[7]

Although ulcerative colitis typically begins in the teen years or early adulthood, a second and perhaps a third peak of incidence are noted. Secondary peaks of disease activity occur in the 40- to 60-year age range, with a smaller third peak after the age of 70 years,[8] The male gender exhibits mild predominance. Some studies reveal gender-related differences in late onset disease, in that men are more likely than women to be diagnosed in the fifth and sixth decades of life.[8]

Risk Factors for Ulcerative Colitis

Many risk factors have been examined for this enigmatic disease. Though diet, oral contraceptive use, perinatal factors (breastfeeding), measles infection/vaccination, and other infections have all been implicated, the data connecting these factors to ulcerative colitis are weak. Presented below are factors with multiple lines of association.

Cigarette Smoking

For more than 20 years, a decreased incidence of ulcerative colitis has been noted in individuals who smoke.[9] In 1989, meta-analytical studies revealed that smokers were 40% as likely as nonsmokers to develop ulcerative colitis.[10] The mechanisms underlying this protective effect are unclear; however, the related conditions of primary sclerosing cholangitis and pouchitis are both decreased in those who smoke, suggesting, at least in the case of primary sclerosing cholangitis, a systemic protective effect.[11,12] Equally fascinating is the observation that those who have ceased smoking are at increased risk.[13] Indeed, smoking has been associated with the course of ulcerative colitis. Active smokers are half as likely to be hospitalized as nonsmokers, and former smokers are 50% more likely to be hospitalized and twice as likely as current smokers or those who have never smoked to require colectomy[14] One French study revealed that those patients with ulcerative colitis who ceased smoking had more active disease, more hospitalizations, and greater need for immunosuppressants that those who continued to smoke[15]

Appendectomy

Large meta-analyses reveal a protective effect of nearly 70% of appendectomy for the development of ulcerative colitis.[16] Two large studies in the Netherlands, one Swedish investigation[17] and another Danish cohort study.[18,19] have provided conflicting results. In the former, the cohorts were followed for 5 million person-years, and observed for a subsequent diagnosis of ulcerative colitis. Those having had an appendectomy had only three-quarters the incidence of ulcerative colitis compared with controls. However the Danish study only revealed a 13% decreased likelihood for the development of ulcerative colitis.

Like smoking, appendectomy may also influence the course of ulcerative colitis. At least two studies, one Japanese and one Australian, corroborate this possibility. In the Japanese study, those who developed ulcerative colitis after appendectomy were less likely to develop recurrent symptoms than colitis patients with an intact appendix [20] In the Australian study, ulcerative colitis patients who had undergone appendectomy prior to the diagnosis were significantly less likely to require colectomy.[21]

Genetics

IBD has been shown to cluster within families, implicating genetics in determining susceptibility. Twin studies reveal a concordance rate of 10% in monozygotic twins, and 3% in dizygotic twins.[22] Population based studies report that 5% to 10% of those affected have a positive family history.[23] Cohort studies reveal a population relative risk of 10 for relatives of patients with ulcerative colitis.[24] In 75% of those multiply affected families, there is concordance for disease type, that is, one member with ulcerative colitis, then all members have ulcerative colitis; whereas 25% of the families are mixed,[25] suggesting multiple susceptibility genes.

Expression of antibodies also segregates with disease processes. The expression of perinuclear antineutrophil cytoplasmic antibodies versus antibodies to the cell wall of mannan polysaccharide (anti-*Saccharomyces cerevisiae* antibodies [ASCA]) segregates such that antineutrophil cytoplasmic antibodies correlate with ulcerative colitis, whereas ASCA is a marker for Crohn disease. Unfortunately, neither antibody is sensitive enough to serve as a sole screening test because up to 64% of patients with Crohn disease have ASCA.[26] Nevertheless, these antibodies are part of the Prometheus panel, which helps to determine if a patient may have IBD and which type of disease may be present.

Genome-wide scans are used to type genetic markers in families containing more than one affected member and to identify chromosomal regions shared in excess of statistical expectation. These genetic linkage studies have revealed that the IBD2 locus (12q13) may be associated with ulcerative colitis. Unfortunately, several important genes in this region, including the $\beta 7$ integrin family and signal transducer and activator of transcription 6 have not been found to correlate with this disease.[27] The most intensively studied region has been the chromosome 6 region (IBD3), especially regions associated with major histocompatibility complex class II genes. Meta-analysis combining results from 29 studies from 1966 to 1998 reveal positive associations to DR2, DR9, and DRB1*0103.[28]

PATHOLOGY

Macroscopic Appearance

Ulcerative colitis is a disease largely limited to the mucosa and submucosa of the colorectum. The rectum is always involved, and the disease presents in a continuous fashion from this point proximally. The proximal extent of disease and the severity may vary from patient to patient. When the entire colon is involved, termed *pancolitis*, a phenomenon called *backwash ileitis* may occur, characterized by a dilated, mildly inflamed terminal ileum. The typical presentation may be less

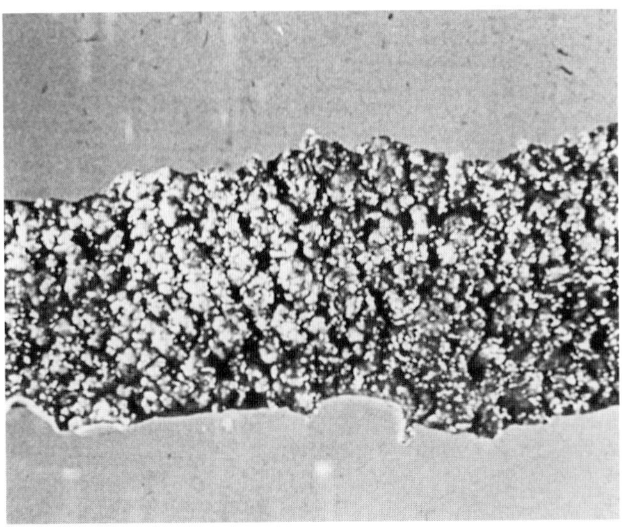

FIGURE 68.1 Pseudopolyps (colonoscopic photo). (From Corman ML, ed. *Colon and rectal surgery*, 5th ed. Philadelphia: Lippincott Williams & Wilkins, 2005, p. 1337.)

clear if a patient develops toxic megacolon initially. In this case, a constellation of septic clinical symptoms associated with dilation of the colon may cloud the inciting disease process, and may cause diffuse colonic thickening,[29] gangrene and perforation.

Gross inspection of the colon reveals confluence of numerous ulcers with areas of heaped up, regenerating mucosa, called *pseudopolyps* (Fig. 68.1). This process is continuous, beginning at the rectum, and extending proximally for variable distances. Superficial fissures, consisting of linear coalescence of ulcerating lesions, are seen. In contradistinction to Crohn disease, ulcerative colitis is not transmural, and therefore lacks thickening, fibrosis, and chronic inflammation. The loss of the mucosa eventually leads to the loss of the normally visualized endoscopic vascular pattern (Fig. 68.2).

Microscopic Appearance

Early in the inflammatory process, the disease involves acute inflammatory cells, predominantly neutrophils, infiltrating into the crypts of Lieberkühn at the base of the mucosa to form crypt abscesses (Fig. 68.3). As the process continues, crypt abscesses coalesce, and superficial desquamation of overlying epithelium leads to the formation of ulcers. Cryptitis undermines the adjacent mucosa, which becomes edematous. If this inflammation is severe, the muscularis propria may undergo myocytolysis, resulting in hyperemia and wall thinning during severe attacks. Granulation tissue is formed as the ulcerated areas heal, which extends to, but rarely through, the submucosa.

CLINICAL FEATURES/COURSE

The usual presentation of ulcerative colitis includes bloody diarrhea, abdominal pain, and fever. The majority of patients present with a mild attack of predominantly distal disease (80%) and a minority (20%) develop pancolitis[30] In 40%, the initial presentation is proctitis. The next most common presentation is left-sided colitis (35%), with disease distal to the splenic flexure. In those patients whose initial presentation is

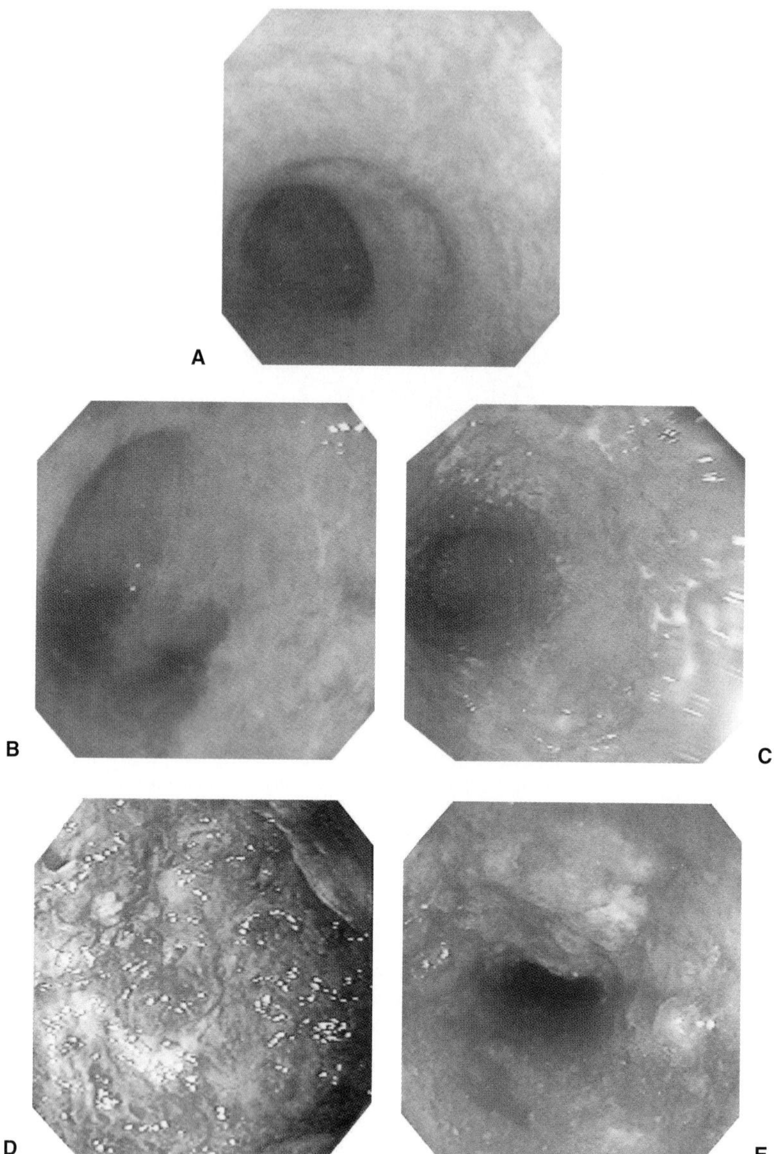

FIGURE 68.2 (*A*) Loss of normal vascular pattern (colonoscopic photo) (*B*) Contact bleeding (*C*) Granularity (*D*) Ulceration and friability (*E*) Colonic stricture. (From Corman ML. Colon and rectal surgery. 5th ed. Philadelphia: Lippincott Williams & Wilkins, 2005.)

distal disease, 10% will progress to pancolitis.[30] In 10% to 20% of patients, an initial attack will rapidly progress to fulminant colitis, characterized by frequent, bloody bowel movements, fever, and abdominal tenderness.

The severity, duration, and location of disease dictate the physical findings. In patients with proctitis, or proctosigmoiditis, urgency and bloody, mucoid diarrhea dominate the clinical picture. Patients complain of urgency, frequency and tenesmus. Though abdominal examination may be unremarkable, rectal examination will reveal a friable mucosa with blood and mucous on the gloved finger. Anoproctoscopy will demonstrate an inflamed mucosa.

In patients with total colitis, anemia, anergia, fatigue, and anorexia may be present. These patients may exhibit weight

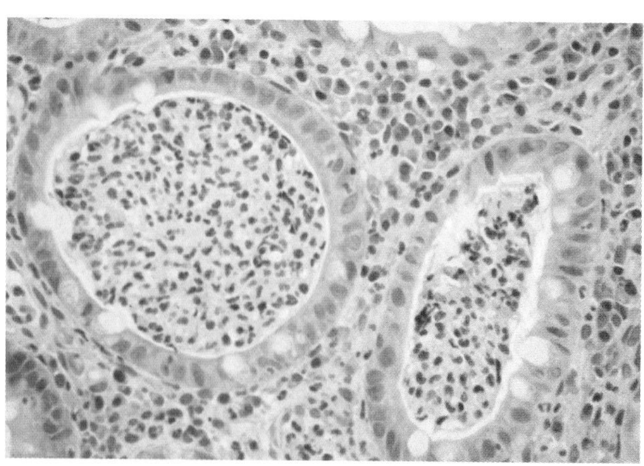

FIGURE 68.3 Histograph of crypt abscess. (Courtesy of Henry Appelman, University of Michigan, Ann Arbor, MI.)

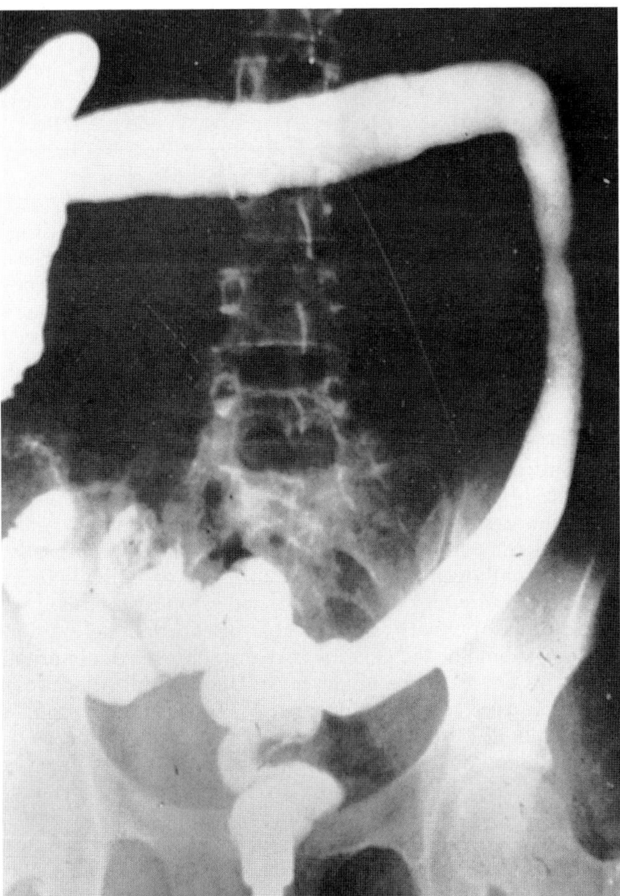

FIGURE 68.4 Lead-pipe colon radiograph. (From Corman ML. *Colon and Rectal Surgery*. 5th ed. Philadelphia: Lippincott Williams & Wilkins, 2005, color plate)

loss due to decreased oral intake during attacks, increased metabolism, and protein loss during chronic or recurrent episodes. Patients with chronic colitis have loss of mucosal folds and haustra. The walls of the colon undergo fibrosis and shortening, leading to a "lead pipe" on contrast radiography (Fig. 68.4). With the loss of functional mucosa, the colon may be unable to absorb fluid, leading to diarrhea.

Extraintestinal manifestations involve dermatologic, ocular, articular, and hepatic tissues (Table 68.1). These manifestations complicate 25% to 30% of cases,[31] and may become the impetus for surgical treatment. With treatment, dermatologic and ocular manifestations may resolve. Unfortunately, hepatic and articular manifestations do not resolve, and primary sclerosing cholangitis may require liver transplantation for management.

Of dermatologic manifestations, erythema nodosum and pyoderma gangrenosum are the most common. Erythema nodosum, found in approximately 9% of patients with ulcerative colitis,[32] is a rash consisting of tender, symmetric, raised erythematous papules, dominantly found on the extensor surfaces of the arms and legs (Fig. 68.5A). These lesions are named descriptively; they appear erythematous but palpate as nodules. Skin disease commonly parallels the activity, but not the severity or extent of bowel disease, and may rarely precede the diagnosis of IBD. The uncommon condition of pyoderma gangrenosum, is associated with IBD in 50% of cases.[33] Pyoderma gangrenosum begins as an erythematous plaque, papule, or bleb, usually in the pretibial region, but may progress to an ulcerated, necrotizing, tender wound with ill-defined, purple-red margins (Fig. 68.5B). In both diseases, treatment of the underlying bowel disease process is key to management.

TABLE 68.1 DIAGNOSIS

EXTRAINTESTINAL MANIFESTATIONS OF ULCERATIVE COLITIS

DERMATOLOGIC
Pyoderma gangrenosum
Erythema nodosum
Clubbing
OCULAR
Iritis
Uveitis
Scleritis
RHEUMATOLOGIC
Ankylosing spondylitis
Sacroiliitis
Peripheral arthritis
HEPATOBILIARY
Sclerosing cholangitis
Fatty liver
Cirrhosis
VASCULAR
Thromboembolism
Coagulopathy

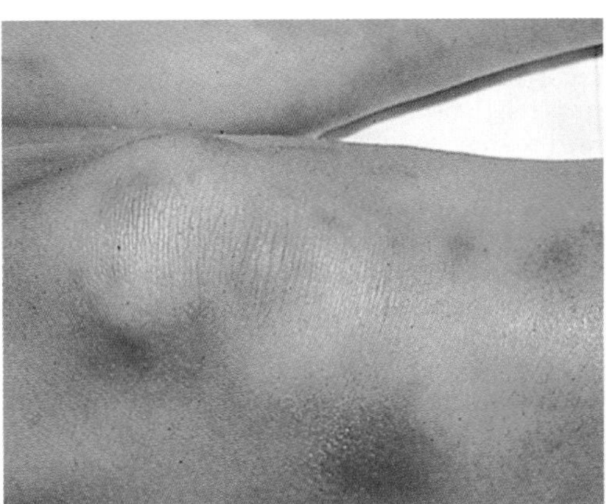

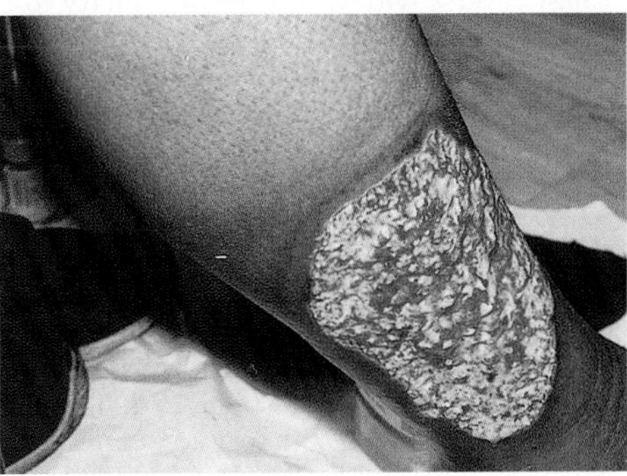

FIGURE 68.5 (*A*) Erythema nodosum. (*B*) Pyoderma gangrenosum. (*A* from Goodheart HP. *A photoguide of common skin disorders: diagnosis and management*. Baltimore: Lippincott Williams & Wilkins, 1999.)

The ocular manifestations of ulcerative colitis are commonly episcleritis, and less commonly, but more seriously, iritis and uveitis. Episcleritis is characterized by the development of eye redness without visual disturbance, whereas scleritis and iritis/uveitis may be associated with blindness if left untreated. Episcleritis is associated with pain or tenderness to palpation, but is not associated with loss of vision, photophobia, or loss of a normal pupillary response to light. Episcleritis is related to active IBD. Episcleritis may be confused with conjunctivitis; however, the latter is not associated with discomfort. Scleritis is a more severe ocular disorder, which may result in impaired vision. Scleritis differs from episcleritis in that with episcleritis the sclera remain white, as opposed to pink in scleritis. Scleritis may lead to retinal detachment or optic nerve swelling[34] Uveitis and iritis are often associated with joint and skin extraintestinal manifestations. The inflammation includes the iris, ciliary body, and posteriorly, the vitreous, choroids, or retina. These complications are characterized by the acute onset of painful eyes, blurred vision, and headache, and may herald the diagnosis of ulcerative colitis. Slit lamp examination establishes the diagnosis. Treatment of uveitis involves cycloplegics and topical steroids, but may require systemic steroids and immunosuppression.

The musculoskeletal manifestations of ulcerative colitis are the most common extraintestinal complications.[35] The arthritic component is believed to be associated with loss of intestinal integrity associated with colitis, and the release of bacteria, lipopolysaccharide, and cytokines. A generalized inflammatory response is revealed by arthritic discomfort. Acute synovitis may occur in up to 20% of patients, reported as sudden joint pain with effusion and tenderness, synovitis usually associated with increased disease activity.[35] Medical therapy targeted at improving mucosal integrity or altering bacterial flora relieves symptoms.

Ankylosing spondylitis occurs in a small percentage of patients with ulcerative colitis (3% to 5%), with the highest risk patients possessing the human leukocyte antigen (HLA) B27 haplotype.[35] Unfortunately, sacroiliitis/spondylitis does not bear a relationship to clinically active bowel disease and thus may progress unnoticed. On examination, these patients have tenderness of the sacroiliac joint, loss of truncal motion, and, later, will have decreased chest expansion with cervical fusion. In longstanding disease, pain may dissipate as the spinal ligaments or joints ossify. Neither medical nor surgical therapy has an effect on these manifestations, and thus treatment is geared towards slowing disability and minimizing deformity.

Asymptomatic abnormalities of hepatic enzymes are the most common manifestation of hepatobiliary disturbances in ulcerative colitis. At least 50% of patients have fatty infiltration of the liver, with cirrhosis present in 3% to 5%.[36] Though fatty liver may reverse with treatment of primary disease, cirrhosis will not.

The most severe extraintestinal manifestation of ulcerative colitis is primary sclerosing cholangitis. This chronic cholestatic syndrome is characterized by fibrosing obliteration of the bile ducts. Best diagnosed by endoscopic retrograde cholangiopancreatography or magnetic resonance cholangiopancreatography, primary sclerosing cholangitis demonstrates bead-like extrahepatic and intrahepatic bile ducts. Primary sclerosing cholangitis present in a minority of patients with ulcerative colitis, but of those patients with primary sclerosing cholangitis, 50% have ulcerative colitis.[37] Not only may primary sclerosing cholangitis eventuate into in failure necessitating a liver transplant, but in patients with ulcerative colitis, the relative risk of development of cholangiocarcinoma also is 31 times greater than those without ulcerative colitis.[38] In general, primary sclerosing cholangitis is a chronic, progressive disease with the rate of progression being variable. Current medical treatment involves the use of ursodeoxycholic acid and endoscopic dilation of the bile duct strictures until transplantation is necessary.

DIAGNOSIS

The diagnosis of ulcerative requires a combination of history and endoscopic/radiologic findings (Algorithm 68.1). Diarrhea, often with blood or mucus, is a dominant symptom. Urgency of bowel movements may be disabling, with tenesmus due to an inflamed rectum. If the disease is more severe, associated systemic symptoms, including fever, arthritis, skin manifestations, and weight loss, may ensue. On a chronic basis, the disease causes fatigue and malaise.

At first presentation, the disease must be differentiated from infectious causes. Stool may be collected seeking the presence of fecal leukocytes, to verify an inflammatory source. Stool cultures should be obtained to rule out common infectious colonic pathogens, such as *Campylobacter, Salmonella, Shigella*, pathogenic *Escherichia coli*, and in individuals at risk, *Clostridium difficile*, *Giardia*, and cytomegalovirus.

Colonoscopy with ileal intubation or flexible sigmoidoscopy should be the next invasive test. Biopsies of abnormal and quiescent areas are of key importance, with the locations of the biopsies carefully documented. Because the rectum is involved in 90% to 95% of cases with ulcerative colitis, flexible sigmoidoscopy may establish the initial diagnosis. In early cases, findings include a granular texture, resembling small bowel, and mucosal friability. With moderately active disease, spontaneous hemorrhage occurs, whereas in severe cases, the mucosa is ulcerated with copious bleeding and a purulent exudate. Over time, the mucosa regenerates, with multiple areas of raised granulation tissue and mucosa (pseudopolyps).

Examination at initial presentation accompanying symptoms and histologic examination of biopsies may help to differentiate ulcerative colitis from Crohn disease (Table 68.2). Distinguishing features include the clinical presentation, which for Crohn disease may include cramping abdominal pain, suggestive of small bowel involvement. At colonoscopy, the presence of discontinuous disease or "skip areas" suggests Crohn disease, and, if possible, ileal intubation with biopsies should be attempted. Edema of the interhaustral septa with thickening and blunting suggests ulcerative colitis. In both diseases, grossly normal appearing mucosa should also be biopsied, as histopathologic abnormalities are frequently present, and may lend further clues regarding the diagnosis. If severe acute inflammation exists, a limited flexible sigmoidoscopy may be all that is necessary to initiate treatment, whereas a more aggressive examination may predispose to colonic perforation.

Radiologic examination may be helpful to determine the extent of disease and to distinguish from Crohn disease. Rarely, the initial presentation is one of toxicity, and a dilated transverse colon, with a diameter of 5 to 7 cm, may herald progressive disease. Mild cases of ulcerative colitis may be seen on air contrast barium enema with spiculation and collar button ulcers. When contrast studies are used to visualize longstanding ulcerative colitis, the loss of haustra with a flat mucosa and narrowed caliber (lead-pipe colon) (see Figure 68.4), will be seen. Additionally, in Crohn disease, the small bowel is often involved and should be investigated with a small bowel follow-through or enteroclysis or the more contemporary imaging techniques of video-capsule endoscopy or computed tomography enterography.[39]

The presentation of ulcerative colitis and Crohn disease may overlap sufficiently in the initial presentation that discrimination of the two entities is not possible. In the 8% to

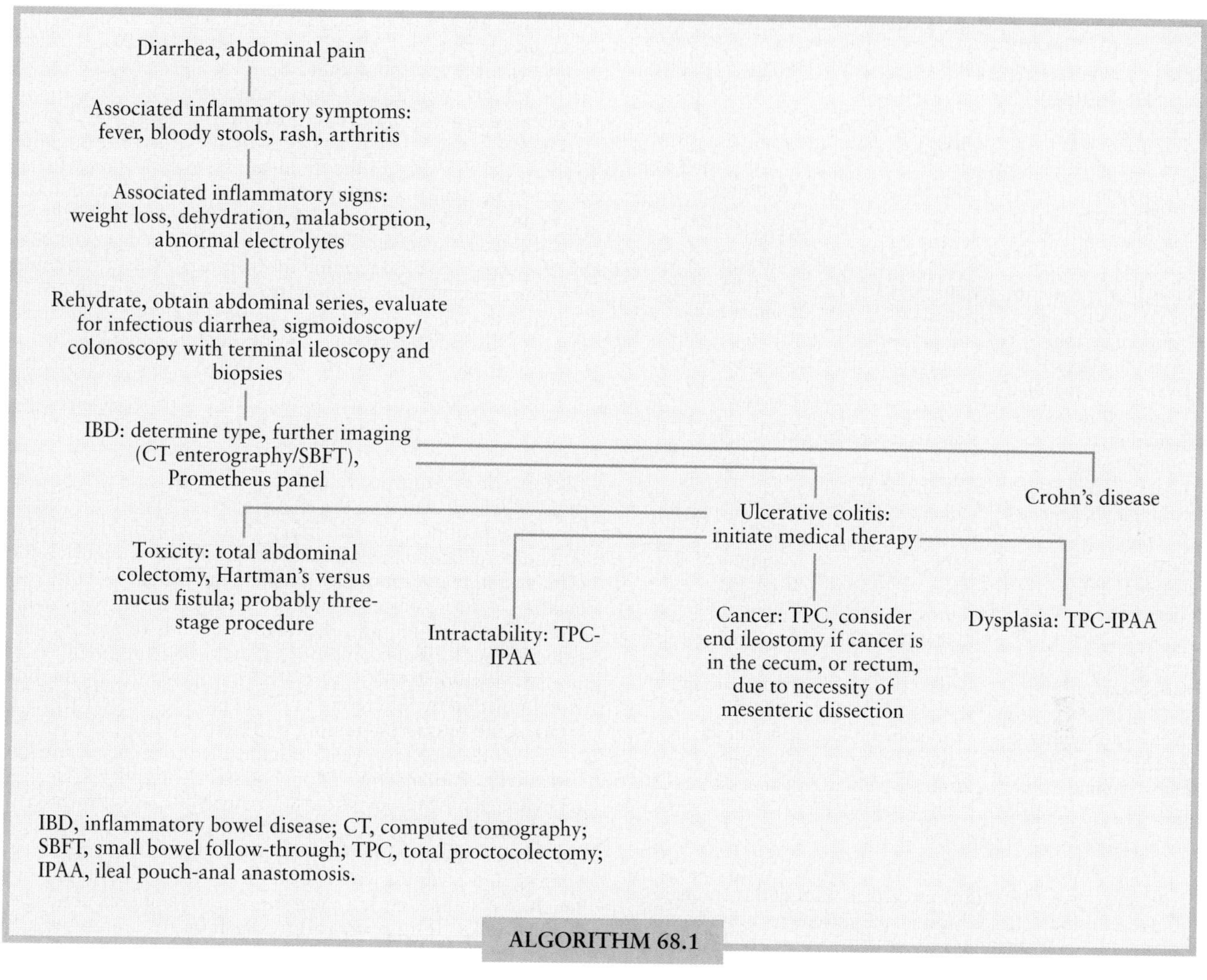

ALGORITHM 68.1 Diagnosis and management of ulcerative colitis.

10% of cases in which this occurs, the colitis is labeled "indeterminate." Because the natural history of these two diseases is different, diagnosis is paramount. However, most surgeons treat cases of indeterminate colitis as ulcerative colitis, offering these patients standard treatment for ulcerative colitis, counseling that should the patient develop sequelae of Crohn disease occur, the diagnosis will then be changed.

MEDICAL MANAGEMENT

Table 68.3 summarizes the medical management for ulcerative colitis. The natural history of ulcerative colitis involves disease flares followed by remission. Approximately 10% of patients with proctitis or proctosigmoiditis will have proximal extension of disease.[40] Of those presenting with pancolitis, 50% will require colectomy at 5 years.

Steroids

Corticosteroids remain the mainstay of therapy for moderate to severe ulcerative colitis or for patients who have failed aminosalicylate treatment. The use of corticosteroids is designed to control symptoms, not to maintain long-term remission. *In vivo* effects of steroids are multiple because they act via pluripotent, ubiquitous steroid receptors. Both immunologic and anti-inflammatory effects are noted because the steroids affect the NFκB and AP-1 cytokine cascades and also have effects on prostaglandin production and leukocyte function.[41,42]

Of patients with ulcerative colitis, a fraction does not respond to systemic steroids. Attempts to identify this fraction have indicated higher levels of glucocorticoid receptors.[43] Additionally, proinflammatory cytokines have been noted to permit accrual of the β isoform of the glucocorticoid receptor, which inhibits the α isoform, thus increasing inflammatory cytokine transcription.[44]

A contemporary formulation of budesonide shows promise regarding effectiveness, with decreased side effects. Budesonide is believed to have greater potency due to high affinity for the glucocorticoid receptor and low systemic bioavailability due to extensive first-pass hepatic metabolism.[45] Budesonide capsules delay the release of the active component until the ileum and ascending colon, where the pH is greater than 5.5.

TABLE 68.2 DIAGNOSIS

CLINICOPATHOLOGIC FEATURES OF ULCERATIVE COLITIS VERSUS CROHN DISEASE

Manifestation	Ulcerative colitis	Crohn disease
Transmural inflammation	Seldom	Common
Granulomas	Seldom	>50%
Fissuring	Rare	Common
Fibrosis	Rare	Common
Submucosal inflammation	Rare	Common
Crypt abscesses	Common	Uncommon
Dysplasia associated lesion or mass		
Small bowel involvement	Rare (backwash ileitis)	Common
Anatomic location	Continuous	Skip
Rectal involvement	Common	May be spared
Bleeding	Common	Absent
Fistulas	Rare	Common
Perianal disease	Rare	Common
Ulcers	Rare	Common
Surrounding mucosa	Pseudopolyps	Relatively normal
Cobblestoning of mucosa	None	Longstanding disease
Mucosal friability	Common	Uncommon
Vascular pattern	Absent	Normal
Fat wrapping	Rare	Common

In severe cases, prednisone, 40 to 60 mg/day, is used to induce remission. If a hospitalized patient exhibits toxicity, intravenous steroids, in a dose equivalent to 300 mg of hydrocortisone or 60 mg of methylprednisolone, should be administered.

Aminosalicylic Acid Compounds

Aminosalicylates are the dominant medical treatment modality for mild to moderate ulcerative colitis to both induce remission and prevent relapse. Sulfasalazine, composed of 5 aminosalicylic acid (ASA) linked to sulfapyridine by a diazo-bond, was the first compound in this family identified. The active component is 5-ASA, and formulations have been created to release the active moiety at different pH level. Mesalamine (Asacol) is released at pH greater than 7; for Pentasa, controlled release begins in the duodenum. Rowasa is released at pH greater than 6, thus facilitating distal ileal and colonic exposure. Rowawa may be compounded into suppositories or enemas. Colonic bacteria contain azo-reductase enzymes that are able to split sulfasalazaine to liberate 5-ASA in the colon where it is believed to act topically. Although multiple formulations exist, each with touted benefits, several studies have failed to show differential benefit of these formulations.[46]

Immunomodulators

Cyclosporine therapy for refractory colitis is effective in 40% of patients who have failed steroids alone.[47,48] Cyclosporine is a lipophilic peptide with inhibitory effects on both the cellular and humoral immune systems. Cyclosporine down-regulates the cellular immune response by blocking the production of interleukin (IL)-2 by T-helper lymphocytes. Molecularly, cyclosporine binds to cyclophilin, and this complex binds to and inhibits calcineurin, a cytoplasmic phosphatase enzyme involved in the activation of T-cells.[49] Cyclosporine also indirectly inhibits B-cell function by interfering with the production of activation factors, and interferon-gamma by T-helper cells.[50]

The dose of cyclosporine recommended to induce remission is 4 mg/kg. Patients with hypocholesterolemia, hypokalemia, or hypomagnesemia must have a reduced dose of 2 mg/kg to avoid seizures. Long-term therapy is avoided due to the associated side effects of hypertension, renal insufficiency, paresthesias, and seizures, with transition to either salicylates or to an antimetabolite, such as azathioprine, or 6-mercaptopurine. Additionally, long-term follow-up fails to demonstrate a decreased incidence of colectomy, with 60% to 80% of these patients requiring operation within 1 year.[51] This delay may allow an elective operation instead of an emergency situation.

Another calcineurin inhibitor, tacrolimus, a member of the macrolide antibiotic family, may be useful adjunctive therapy for steroid-refractory ulcerative colitis. Tacrolimus has improved absorption compared to cyclosporine. The fact that tacrolimus is a member of the macrolide antibiotic family contributes to a promotility effect.[52]

TABLE 68.3 MANAGEMENT

MEDICAL TREATMENT FOR ULCERATIVE COLITIS

Disease type	Extent	Treatment
INDUCTION THERAPY		
Mild disease	Distal	Oral/rectal aminosalicylate [mesalamine (Asacol 1.6–4.8 g/d po; Rowasa enemas)]
	Extensive	Oral aminosalicylate
Severe disease	Distal	Oral/rectal corticosteroid [prednisone 40–60 mg/d; cortenemas]
	Extensive	Oral corticosteroid
Fulminant disease	Extensive	Parenteral corticosteroid/Intravenous cyclosporine
MAINTENANCE THERAPY		
	Distal	Oral/rectal aminosalicylate
		Azathiaprine (2.5 mg/kg) or 6-mercaptopurine (1.5 mg/kg)
	Extensive	Oral aminosalicylate
		Azathiaprine or 6-mercaptopurine

The purine antimetabolites, azathioprine and its metabolite, 6-mercaptopurine, may also be used to achieve steroid-sparing remission. These agents are used to facilitate a remission induced by cyclosporine. These agents act via inhibition of purine biosynthesis, nucleotide interconversions, DNA and RNA synthesis and chromosomal replication.[53] A prolonged interval of 3 to 6 months may be necessary for these agents to demonstrate their full suppressive potential. Approximately 60% of patients achieve long-term remission.[54] Measurement of the activity of the thiopurine-methyltransferase, as well as 6-thioguanine levels allow for dose adjustment. Toxicities induced by this family include bone marrow suppression, especially leukopenia, which is dose dependent. Additionally, liver toxicity and allergic reactions, manifested as a combination of fever, rash, myalgias or arthralgias, may limit utilization. Pancreatitis occurs as another manifestation of hypersensitivity in 2% of patients.[55]

Biological Agents

Anti-Tumor Necrosis Factor

The success of anti-tumor necrosis factor (TNF) therapy achieved by Infliximab for Crohn disease has not been replicated for ulcerative colitis though clinical trials are continuing. Although TNF is present in the mucosa, TNF does not seem responsible for the inflammatory response. Although one small trial revealed benefit in 88% of steroid-refractory patients,[56] a multiple other trials have failed to corroborate these findings.[57–59]

Two other humanized antibodies against TNF are currently undergoing evaluation: CDP571 and RDP58. The former has had limited success. The latter has a novel molecular mechanism, targeted at interfering with TNF production at the posttranscriptional level, also inhibiting the production of interferon-gamma, IL-2, and IL-12.[60,61] In a phase II study, dose-dependent improvement has been noted, and this agent may become more prominent in the future.[62]

Anti-Interleukin-2R

As cyclosporine inhibits IL-2, antibodies targeted at the IL-2 receptor may also have benefit in ulcerative colitis. Daclizumab, a recombinant humanized immunoglobulin monoclonal antibody to IL-2R(, recently was reported to induce clinical response in 8 of 10 patients after 2 weeks, with remission achieved in 5 of 10 of these patients.[63] Similarly, basiliximab, a chimeric monoclonal antibody to IL-2R was evaluated in another small pilot study; a single dose resulted in 9 of 10 patients achieving clinical remission in 8 weeks.[64] Though the majority of these patients relapsed, remission was easily reestablished.

Anti-CD3

Apoptosis of activated T-cells has been reported with visilizumab, a humanized antibody directed at the CD3e chain of the T-cell receptor complex. This agent was recently used in a trial of seven patients with steroid-refractory ulcerative colitis, resulting in five of seven remissions, persisting for several months and permitting steroid withdrawal.[65]

Growth Factors

Experimentally, growth factors aid in restoration of mucosa. Epidermal growth factor has been used topically for the healing of skin wounds, and systemically for the treatment of necrotizing enterocolitis in neonates. Epidermal growth factor was recently reported, in conjunction with mesalamine enemas to treat 12 patients with mild to moderate colitis. Of the 12 patients, 10 experienced remission early on, with 8 sustaining remission at 12 weeks.[66]

INDICATIONS FOR SURGICAL INTERVENTION

The acute indications for surgical intervention are: bleeding, perforation, infection, and malignancy. Failure of medical management associated extraintestinal manifestations, and dysplasia are also indications for operation.

The most common indication for elective proctocolectomy is intractability. These patients often have longstanding colitis and have failed aggressive outpatient medical regimens with significant side effects due to medications or have extraintestinal manifestations not well controlled despite adequate management of colitis. Many of these patients have delayed surgery due to concerns about difficulties with adaptation to a temporary or permanent ileostomy. Many patients and their referring physicians are not aware of reconstructive options.

Many extraintestinal manifestations are quiescent when colitis is well controlled, but two extraintestinal manifestations are not reversible, even with excellent disease management. Irreversible changes include cirrhosis, in patients with associated primary sclerosing cholangitis, and ankylosing spondylitis. Epidemiologic studies have shown that nearly 70% of patients with primary sclerosing cholangitis have ulcerative colitis, whereas the incidence of primary sclerosing cholangitis in patients with ulcerative colitis is only 2% to 7%.[37,67] This disease is characterized by a progressive, inflammatory fibrosis which may affect the entire biliary tree. Currently, the only known curative treatment for primary sclerosing cholangitis is orthotopic liver transplantation. Whether the addition of the immunosuppression to maintain the transplanted organ ameliorates colitic symptoms and affects the advent of colonic malignant degeneration is not clear.[68,69]

Cancer prophylaxis is sometimes a motive for elective colectomy. Most investigators believe that oncogenesis is related to the severity and duration of disease. Though the risk is low during the first 8 to 10 years of ulcerative colitis, cancer incidence increases at a rate of 1% to 2% per year following this interval.[70–72] Malignancy may be present in up to 18% of patients with an intact colon having sustained 30 years of disease,[73] and reflects an increase in relative risk of 2.6- to 5.4-fold relative to the general population. The cancer develops in the flat mucosa, not in inflammatory regions. Colitis-associated cancer appears to undergo a different pathogenesis than conventional colorectal cancer.[74–76]

Surveillance colonoscopy has been advocated. Notably, at the first colonoscopy for surveillance, approximately 10% of patients will already have dysplasia,[77] with a rate of 3% for the development of dysplasia if the first colonoscopy is unrevealing.[78] Current recommendations include a minimum of 18 biopsies to have 95% sensitivity for any type of dysplasia, and most recommend four biopsies from at least nine sites with at least four sites in the rectosigmoid.[79] When low-grade dysplasia is found, 20% of patients already have cancer present, and low-grade dysplasia progresses to high-grade dysplasia in up to 50% of patients in 5 years.[80] Thus, a diagnosis of dysplasia of any type warrants surgical intervention.

Surgical Emergencies

Hemorrhage is an unusual indication for surgery in ulcerative colitis because the disease is limited to the mucosa. Usually, bleeding is controlled with medical treatment of the disease. Total abdominal colectomy may not be sufficient to arrest hemorrhage because the disease begins with the rectum, and proctectomy, which may complicate later reconstruction, may be a necessary life-saving maneuver.

Failure of medical management for severe (fulminant) colitis forms another indication for acute surgical intervention. Severe colitis is defined as the passage of more than six bloody stools per day with a temperature higher than 37.5°C, tachycardia, hemoglobin less than 75% of normal, and an increased sedimentation rate. Affected patients are hospitalized, resuscitated, and placed on intravenous steroids. At times, fulminant or severe colitis may constitute the initial presentation of colonic infectious etiologies. If these patients fail to resolve with intravenous steroids, a trial of cyclosporine may be warranted.

Toxic megacolon is the most feared presentation, and is defined by severe systemic signs of illness, such as fever, abdominal pain and tenderness, tachycardia, leukocytosis, and dilation of the colon (more than 6 cm transverse colon on abdominal radiograph).[29] When either toxic megacolon or severe colitis occurs perforation is a possible sequelae associated with a 20% increase in mortality.[81,82] Perforation may be present without radiologic evidence in 25% of patients.

Emergency Surgery for Ulcerative Colitis

The indications for emergency surgery for ulcerative colitis are summarized in Table 68.4. Perforation and bleeding are among these indications, and toxic colitis and toxic megacolon are also motivations for operation.

Acute, severe, fulminant, or toxic colitis requires hospital admission and intensive treatment. Supportive care, including repletion of fluids, electrolytes, transfusion for anemia, nutritional support, and anti-inflammatory treatment with high-dose steroids, is required. The findings of fever, defecation greater than 8 to10 times per 24-hour period, frequent bloody movements, hypoalbuminemia, and abdominal tenderness all herald surgical intervention. Barium enema, narcotics, anticholinergics drugs, and antidiarrheal agents should be avoided because these agents may precipitate toxic megacolon.

Likewise, toxic dilation of the colon, or toxic megacolon, is an indication for urgent surgery (see Table 68.4). A plain abdominal film will reveal a colonic diameter of greater than 6 cm. This finding may presage perforation, which was historically associated with an increased mortality rate.[83] Recent advances in medical and surgical intervention have decreased mortality to less than 3%.[84]

Emergency surgery for ulcerative colitis consists of total abdominal colectomy, with management of the rectal stump. The rectum is preserved to minimize the chance of presacral bleeding in a systemically ill patient and to facilitate future pelvic procedures, including the creation of a pelvic reservoir. The rectal stump may be managed by either suturing or stapling the proximal end. If disease in this area precludes such management due to inflammation or edema, the stump may be left with enough sigmoid to create a mucous fistula to the anterior abdominal wall. Formerly, blowhole colostomy and ileostomy had been advocated for management of toxic megacolon, in which a dilated, edematous, thin-walled colon might lead to intraoperative spillage with subsequent septic complications.[85] With improved medical management and earlier surgical intervention, fewer patients with advanced disease and perforation are currently forced to surgery, and therefore this procedure is rarely used.

Total abdominal colectomy with end ileostomy is the most common and safest procedure for patients who require emergency intervention for ulcerative colitis. This procedure is rapid, removes the greatest source of the patient's symptoms, facilitates subsequent pelvic procedures, allows withdrawal of steroids, and improves nutrition. However, this management may mandate a second procedure (completion proctectomy, pouch formation, and diverting loop ileostomy), and perhaps a third procedure (ileostomy closure). During performance of this procedure, the patient is placed in the supine position. In the planning for subsequent procedures, preservation of the ileocolic trunk and superior mesenteric vessels for possible pouch construction is desirable. The ileum is mobilized only enough to reach the anterior abdominal wall, with length maximally preserved by dividing the bowel close to the cecum. The inferior mesenteric vessels are maintained; to remove the sigmoid colon, the vessels are ligated individually. This approach facilitates mobilization of sigmoid colon to the anterior abdominal wall, and minimizes pelvic scarring and damage to pelvic autonomic nerves.

The rectal stump may be managed by three different techniques. Simple suture or stapled closure is the easiest. If the stump is very friable, it may be mobilized as a mucus fistula and matured to the skin. If the end will not reach the skin or if an immediate mucus fistula is not desirable, the end may be brought through the fascia and sutured in the subcutaneous space. A third possibility is to place a large catheter intraanally to stent the sphincters open, facilitating dependent drainage.

TABLE 68.4 INDICATIONS/CONTRAINDICATIONS

INDICATIONS FOR URGENT SURGERY IN ULCERATIVE COLITIS

Acute severe colitis (70%)
Toxic colonic dilatation (20%)
Perforation (<10%)
Hemorrhage (<5%)

(From Nicholls, RJ. Review article: ulcerative colitis—surgical indications and treatment. *Aliment Pharmacol Ther.* 2002;16(suppl. 4): 25–28.

Elective Surgery

The advantages, disadvantages, indications, and contraindications for elective surgical options are summarized in Table 68.5.

Total Proctocolectomy

The manifestations of ulcerative colitis are cured by removal of the colon and rectum. Therefore, the disease is cured by total proctocolectomy. In the early 1950s, the technique of the Brooke ileostomy was described.[86] Prior to this description, ileostomies were matured in such a fashion that stricturing occurred, causing high ileostomy outputs. With Brooke's description, this problem was alleviated. Still, patients were left with the constant need to wear an appliance. Professor Nils Kock developed the continent ileostomy in 1969.[87] Though initially received by patients and surgeons with great enthusiasm, this procedure has largely been replaced. The procedure is technically difficult with a significant complication of valve slippage and a need for reoperation in more than 50% of patients.

Parks[88] and Utsonomiya[89] independently reported the development of a technique that adapted Kock's ileal pouch and, instead of connecting the pouch to the abdominal wall, anastomosed it to the anus. This type of reconstruction avoids a permanent ileostomy, and the route of evacuation is sustained. Options for reconstruction were limited until this adaptation of a pediatric surgery technique, which facilitated restoration of intestinal continuity. This technique is now commonly referred to as the *ileal pouch—analanastomosis, restorative proctocolectomy*, or *pelvic pouch*.[90]

TABLE 68.5 INDICATIONS/CONTRAINDICATIONS

ADVANTAGES/DISADVANTAGES AND INDICATIONS/CONTRAINDICATIONS FOR ELECTIVE SURGICAL OPTIONS FOR ULCERATIVE COLITIS

Procedure	Advantage	Disadvantage	Contraindications
Total proctocolectomy/ Ileostomy	Single operation	Permanent ileostomy	
Kock pouch	Continent abdominal Reconstruction	Frequent complications requires multiple procedures, Permanent ileostomy	Crohn disease
Total abdominal colectomy Ileorectal anastomosis	Single operation, preserves native continence	Maintains rectum, which is usually diseased	
Total proctocolectomy/Ileal pouch Anal anastomosis	Removes nearly all disease continent reconstruction	In addition to complications due to proctectomy, anastomotic leak, pouchitis, and, if used, complications related to the ileostomy Frequent bowel movements/leakage	Crohn disease, incontinence distal rectal cancer

Colectomy with Ileorectal Anastomosis

In this procedure the entire abdominal colon is removed, and the ileum is anastomosed to the rectum at approximately the level of the sacral promontory. The postoperative leak rate is very low, around 2%,[91] and the procedure is technically easy to perform with either a hand-sewn or stapled end-to-side anastomosis. The procedure spares the anus. Bowel movements are more numerous and looser than before operation, but with the addition of bulking agents or antidiarrheal agents, the number of movements may be minimized. The morbidity associated with a pelvic dissection is avoided.

Unfortunately, for most patients with ulcerative colitis, this procedure is not an optimal long-term solution because the disease always involves the rectum and the possibility of neoplastic degeneration mandates surveillance. Indeed, the incidence of carcinoma in the rectal stump at 20 years is approximately 5% to 17%.[92] At least 10% of patients require subsequent proctectomy for refractory proctitis, and another 10% require proctectomy for poor function. This procedure is a compromise for patients with minimal rectal disease, wishing intermediate-term preservation of parasympathetic nerve function with continence.

Total Proctocolectomy with Brooke Ileostomy

This procedure is one of the earliest for ulcerative colitis, and is still considered the standard against which other procedures must be compared. In this procedure, the entire colon and rectum are removed, thus eliminating all of the disease and the possibility of neoplastic transformation. An intersphincteric perineal dissection creates a smaller perineal wound than that traditionally completed for an abdominoperineal dissection. Morbidity is low, associated with the perineal wound and a permanent ileostomy.

Kock Pouch

The Kock pouch is designed to create a reservoir formed from the ileum with a valve that prevents spontaneous emptying. A catheter is inserted into the valve, allowing ileal contents to be emptied. This construction is created so that motivated patients who did not wish to maintain a permanent, spontaneously emptying ileostomy would be able to intubate the pouch. The nipple valve forms the major source for either a successful or on unsuccessful pouch. The pouch is created from two to three limbs of ileum to form a reservoir, whereas the valve is formed by a portion of the efferent limb intussuscepted into the pouch. This procedure is now rarely performed because of the greater than 50% need for revision due to valve failure and incompetence, technical difficulties with intubation, fistula formation and because of the advent of the restorative proctocolectomy.

Restorative Proctocolectomy

This procedure has increased in utilization over the past 25 years and is now the most commonly used operation in the elective management of ulcerative colitis.[93] Contraindications include Crohn disease, fulminant colitis, low rectal neoplasia, disseminated carcinoma, incontinence, and the inability to withstand a long anesthetic period (usually 4 to 6 hours). Relative contraindications include obesity because a thick mesentery will preclude mobilization of the bowel into the distal pelvis. A patient with an android-shaped pelvis or a tall patient may have similar difficulties.

The restorative proctocolectomy is usually performed in two stages: (1) total or completion proctocolectomy, pouch formation and pouch-anal anastomosis, diverting loop ileostomy, and (2) closure of loop ileostomy. The procedure may be performed with laparoscopic assistance. The patient is prepared for the operation and is placed in the modified lithotomy position, permitting access to the perineum for dissection and anastomosis. The entire colon is mobilized. Most surgeons preserve the major ileocolic trunks by staying close to the cecum, maintaining the vessels that may provide blood supply to the future pouch. The small bowel mesentery is then mobilized, and an estimate that a created pouch will reach into the anastomosis is made by grasping the most dependent portion of the bowel, and measuring that it will reach 3 to 6 cm beyond the bony symphysis pubis.

If it is not clear that the pouch will reach the anal region, a number of maneuvers may increase length. The small bowel mesentery may be mobilized to the third part of the duodenum. Peritoneal windows may be over the vessel causing tension to the apical portion of the pouch. These windows may be repeated on both sides of the mesentery. Transillumination will identify vascular arcades that must be preserved, but will also identify vessels that may be ligated to increased length.

A vessel clamp with either palpation or Doppler confirmation of adequate blood flow prior to ligation is recommended. Ileocolic vessels may be ligated near their origin to create greater length, and the superior mesenteric artery is able to provide adequate blood supply. The right branch of the middle colic artery may be preserved, which may facilitate blood supply to the ileum in the absence of both the ileocolic and the superior mesenteric artery.

Multiple pouch constructions have been suggested. Though initially the S- and W-pouches were favored for their increased reservoir capacity, and possible length, the J-pouch is now the most popular construction, probably due to the ease of construction, fit into the pelvis, reservoir capacity, and emptying. The J-pouch is constructed by stapling two 15- to 20-cm limbs of ileum together, via an enterotomy created at the apex of the J-pouch (Fig. 68.6A). To complete the common wall, another firing of the GIA stapler is necessary, with the distal pouch accordioned onto the forks of the stapler. Other constructions include the S-pouch and W-pouch (Figs. 68.6B, 68.6C). An ileoanal anastomosis may be performed by double stapling or, following mucosectomy, via a hand-sewn anastomosis. Stapling preserves the anal transition zone, and this preservation seems to enhance function[94] by retaining neorectal sensation and continence. However, this approach does retain a small area of potentially neoplastic tissue, and some investigators have favored mucosectomy. To facilitate mucosectomy, the perineal operator uses a retractor to expose the dentate line. Dilute epinephrine is injected submucosally to raise the mucosa and to prevent bleeding. A needle tip cautery is helpful to precisely excise the mucosa for a length of several centimeters. The pouch is then lowered into pelvis and pulled down endoanally for a hand-sewn anastomosis with absorbable sutures.

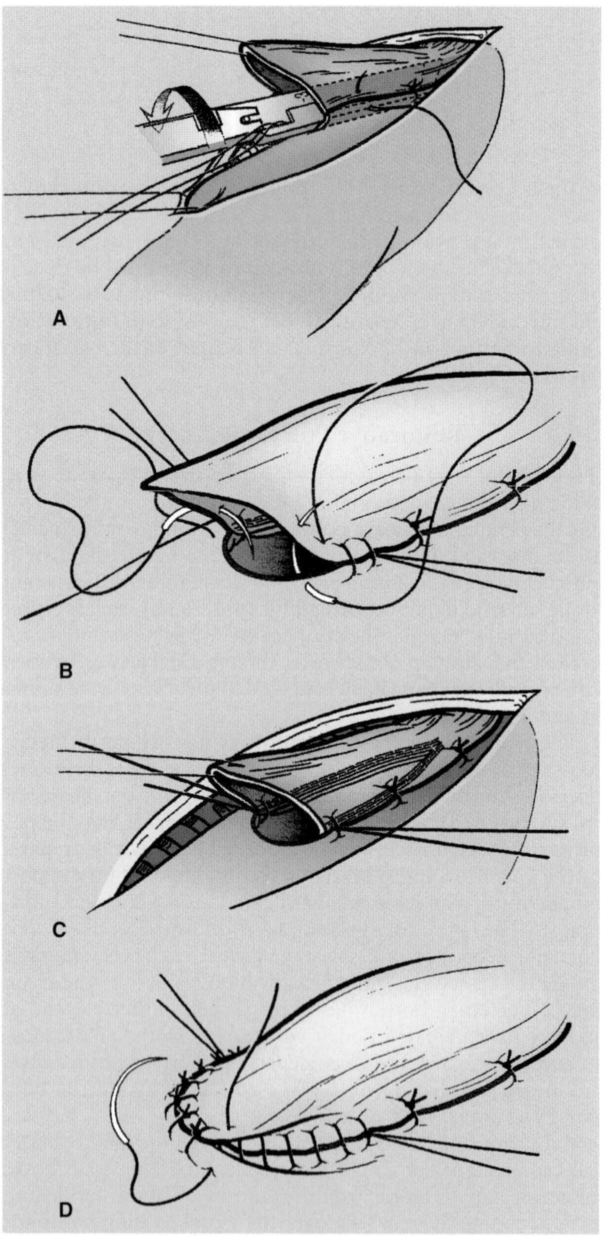

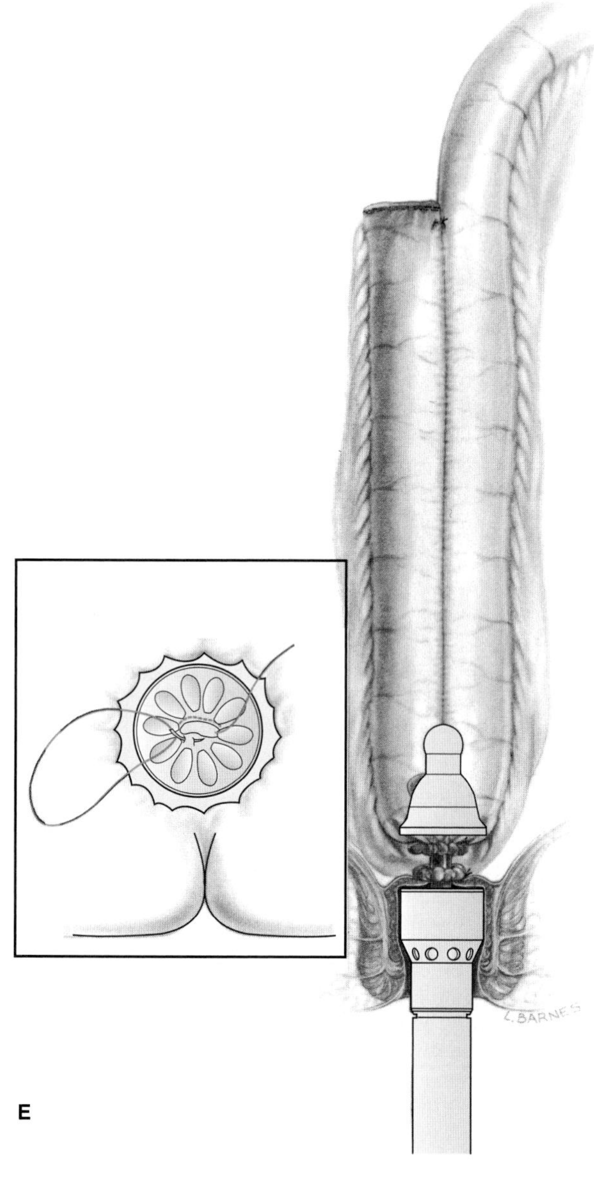

FIGURE 68.6 Ileal pouch construction. (*A*) An electrocautery is used to create an enterotomy at the apex of the 15-cm loop of terminal ileum. (*B*) The forks of an intestinal anastomosing stapler are pressed into the intestinal limbs, and the instrument is fired. (*C*) This is repeated once or twice while the limbs are telescoped onto the stapler, until a 15-cm side-to-side anastomosis is completed. (*D*) The apical enterotomy is closed with a simple purse string stitch. E: The stapled construction of the J-pouch. (*E* From Corman ML. Colon and Rectal Surgery, 5th ed. Philadelphia: Lippincott Williams & Wilkins, 2005, p. 1418.)

Postoperative Complications

The most common early postoperative complications are small bowel obstruction and sepsis. Small bowel obstruction complicates 11% to 26% of ileal pouch procedures.[95,96] The loop ileostomy increases this risk significantly.[97] A series of 1,005 patients reported in 1995 revealed 25% of patients had small bowel obstruction, with two thirds of the patients having the temporary loop ileostomy as the cause.[98] Of this 25%, 7.5% had early obstructions and 18% had later obstruction. Overall, of the 254 patients with a small bowel obstruction, 28% required reoperation. The most common site of obstruction was the ileostomy,[99] which has led some surgeons to perform the procedure without ileostomy. Others have implemented the use of Seprafilm (Genzyme Corporation, Cambridge, MA; modified sodium hyaluronic acid and carboxymethylcellulose), which has been found in a randomized, prospective trial, to decreased adhesions by 50%.[100] Causes of small bowel obstruction include adhesions, internal hernia, stenosis, and volvulus around the ileostomy. Though many of the patients resolve obstruction nonoperatively, approximately one-quarter require operative intervention.[101] If the obstruction occurs prior to planned ileostomy closure, then pre-closure evaluation, including pouch studies, should be expedited and the ileostomy closed.

The second most common early complication is sepsis, either in the form of pelvic abscess or leak. Sepsis complicates 3% to 37% of cases.[95,98,102–104] As in all bowel anastomoses, the abscess may be an expression of leak. Leakage of the pouch or the pouch-anal anastomosis occurs in 2% to 15% of cases.[98,105,106] This serious complication may be revealed radiologically, clinically as an abscess, or as a fistula to either another intraabdominal structure or to the perineum or vagina. The rate of leakage is increased in patients with ulcerative colitis compared to those with familial adenomatous polyposis.[105] The incidence of leak is only 9% for polyposis relative to 24% for those with ulcerative colitis. The most common location for the leak is at the pouch-anal anastomosis. The most commonly cited association for leak is ingestion of greater than 40 mg of daily prednisone. The use of steroids may influence the choice of procedure, that is, patients who are more ill are likely to be on higher dose steroids. Some centers have performed routine pouch procedures without a defunctioning ileostomy.[109]

A defunctioning loop ileostomy does not prevent leakage, but the ileostomy may decrease the morbidity associated with the leak. The leak may be adequately managed with diversion and drainage while allowing time and support for healing. However, the most common cause of eventual pouch excision is an anastomotic leak, usually due to poor long-term functional results. In one series, 58 patients required pouch excision: 39% due to a leak from the ileoanal anastomosis and 12% due to leak from the pouch. Others have reported an association of leak with pouch failure in up to 24% of patients requiring pouch excision.[108]

Fistula is another expression of sepsis, which may extend to another organ, the perineum or vagina. Fistula may occur in the early postoperative period, but may also present months or years later. Pouch fistulas occur with a frequency of 2.8% to 12%.[95,98,99,104,109] Fistulas are complex to manage, and regardless of whether a local or abdominal technique is used, only half of attempted repairs will be successful.[110] Contributing factors include pouch ischemia, anastomotic leak, vaginal inclusion in the anastomotic suture line, cryptoglandular infection, and Crohn disease. Abscess drainage, prolonged diversion with loop ileostomy, antibiotics, and local therapy may lead to closure, but variable success has been noted with seton placement, fibrin glue instillation, ileoanal flaps, and vaginal flaps.[110]

TABLE 68.6 ETIOLOGY

POUCHITIS DISEASE ACTIVITY INDEX

Criteria	Score[a]
CLINICAL CRITERIA	
Stool frequency	
Usual stool frequency	0
1–2 stool/day > postoperative usual	1
3 or more stools/day > postoperative usual	2
Rectal bleeding	
None or rare	0
Present daily	1
Fecal urgency	
None	0
Occasional	1
Usual	2
Fever (temperature >100°F)	
Absent	0
Present	1
ENDOSCOPIC CRITERIA	
Edema	1
Granularity	1
Friability	1
Loss of vascular pattern	1
Mucus exudates	1
Ulcerations	1
ACUTE HISTOLOGIC CRITERIA	
Polymorphonuclear infiltration	
Mild	1
Moderate—crypt abscess	2
Severe + crypt abscess	3
Ulcerations per low-power field (mean)	
<25%	1
25% to 50%	2
>50%	3

[a]Pouchitis is defined as total score of ≥ 7 points.
(From Sandborn WJ, Tremaine WJ, Batts KP, Pemberton JH, Phillips SF. Pouchitis after ileal pouch-anal anastomosis: a pouchitis disease activity index. *Mayo Clin Proc.* 1994;69:409–415.)

Long-term Sequelae

Pouchitis

This complication is unique to patients with an ileal pouch, and is increased in patients with IBD.[111] The syndrome is manifested as inflammation in the pouch, increased stool frequency, urgency, incontinence, bleeding, crampy abdominal pain, with malaise and a low-grade fever. Pouchitis occurs in 30% to 50% of patients.[107] The cumulative probability of suffering a second episode after an initial attack within 2 years of an restorative proctocolectomy is 64%; interestingly, after single episode, only 15% experience chronic symptoms[112] On pouchoscopy, the mucosa is inflamed, with friability, ulceration and discharge. Histology must confirm the diagnosis. The Pouchitis Activity Index quantifies severity of symptoms (Table 68.6).

The cause of pouchitis is unknown, though mechanical factors such as a poorly emptying pouch or an anastomotic stricture have been invoked. In most of those affected, no etiology is documented. Pouchitis may be due to bacterial stasis, with toxins causing ulceration of the mucosa, or due to ischemia, leading to

COLORECTAL

the production of free radicals. The syndrome is associated with pancolitis and extraintestinal manifestations, including primary sclerosing cholangitis. Luckily, the initial treatment with antimicrobial agents, including metronidazole or a fluoroquinolone, leads to remission in the majority of cases. In refractory cases, a 5-ASA compound is added. Newer data suggest that probiotics may be beneficial in preventing pouchitis and in maintaining remission.[113,114] Chronic or disabling pouchitis leads to pouch excision in up to 12% of those affected.[115]

Anastomotic Stricture

A small degree of narrowing is often present, particularly during the period of fecal diversion, and is not problematic. This complication involves 7% to 15% of cases.[95,98,116] This narrowing may be associated with disuse and usually yields to digital or balloon dilation prior to ileostomy closure, but may herald more complex difficulties, such as a healed leak, tension, ischemia, fistula formation, or cuffitis. If nonoperative approaches fail to manage the complication, pouch revision may be necessary to manage the complication, as the stricture will adversely affect pouch emptying.

Cuffitis

The stapled pouch and anastomosis retains a small remnant of the anal transition zone. This area retains the possibility of symptomatic inflammation or "cuffitis." These patients may present with symptoms similar to those of pouchitis, including diarrhea, abdominal pain, urgency, perianal pain and bloody movements.[117] The majority of these patients may be treated with topical 5-ASA suppositories.[118]

Cancer

Reports of cancer in patients having undergone the restorative proctocolectomy have been rare. Both the retained cuff of rectum and the pouch are at risk. The residual rectum has been documented to develop cancer. These cases have occurred in patients in whom a mucosectomy was performed as well as in patients in whom a mucosectomy was not performed. Patients at increased risk are those who had either dysplasia or cancer in the original proctocolectomy. Additionally, patients with primary sclerosing cholangitis are at increased risk. Therefore, continued screening for patients with prolonged disease duration, dysplasia or cancer in the excised specimen, and primary sclerosing cholangitis is recommended.

Pouch Failure

A failure rate of 5% to 10% has been reported at most high-volume centers. Risk factors include hand sewn anastomosis, tension on the ileoanal anastomosis, use of an ileostomy, Crohn disease, and leak.[119] One series reported a failure rate of 10%, due mostly to poor function (28%), unsuspected Crohn disease (5%), and sepsis.[108] The failure rate may increase over time, and other series report fistula as predictive of failure.[120]

Sexual Dysfunction

Though dissection in a plane close to the rectum has been recommended for this otherwise benign disease, men are still at risk for injury to the parasympathetic nerve trunks. The morbidity from this injury includes difficulty with bladder emptying, impotence, and retrograde ejaculation. These symptoms may be transient or permanent, occurring in 1% to 3% of patients.[111]

Women may also suffer from dyspareunia (7%), and leaking during intercourse (2%).[121] Fertility following restorative proctocolectomy may be reduced.[122] Infertility may be due to adhesion formation.

Quality of Life

Quality of life incorporates not only physical or functional outcomes, but also includes psychosocial aspects regarding the well being of patients. Patients who have had any of the procedures to manage their disease express happiness and satisfaction, even with a conventional ileostomy, probably linked to their physical status.[123] The pelvic pouch patients may exhibit imperfect functional results, with an average of six bowel movements per day, seepage of stool in 20% of patients during the day and in 50% at night. Despite these results, 95% of patients exhibit satisfaction with postoperative outcomes.[123–125]

KEY POINTS

- **Ulcerative colitis is a disease largely limited to the mucosa and submucosa of the colorectum.**
- **Gross inspection of the colon reveals confluence of numerous ulcers with areas of heaped up, regenerating mucosa, or so-called pseudopolyps. This process is continuous, beginning at the rectum, and extending proximally for variable distances.**
- **The usual presentation of ulcerative colitis includes bloody diarrhea, abdominal pain, and fever.**
- **The acute indications for surgical intervention are bleeding, perforation, infection, and malignancy. Failure of medical management associated extraintestinal manifestations, and dysplasia are also indications for operation.**
- **The manifestations of ulcerative colitis are cured by removal of the colon and rectum; the disease is cured by total proctocolectomy.**

References

1. Ekbom A. The epidemiology of IBD: a lot of data but little knowledge. How shall we proceed? *Inflamm Bowel Dis.* 2004;10(suppl 1):S32–34.
2. Wilks S, Moxon W. *Lectures on pathological anatomy*. 2nd ed. London: J & A Churchill; 1875.
3. Stowe SP, Redmond SR, Stormont JM, et al. An epidemiologic study of inflammatory bowel disease in Rochester, New York. Hospital incidence. *Gastroenterology* 1990;98(1):104–110.
4. Loftus EV Jr, Silverstein MD, Sandborn WJ, et al. Ulcerative colitis in Olmsted County, Minnesota, 1940–1993: incidence, prevalence, and survival. *Gut* 2000;46(3):336–343.
5. Bernstein CN, Blanchard JF, Rawsthorne P, et al. Epidemiology of Crohn's disease and ulcerative colitis in a central Canadian province: a population-based study. *Am J Epidemiol.* 1999;149(10):916–924.
6. Langholz E, Munkholm P, Nielsen OH, et al. Incidence and prevalence of ulcerative colitis in Copenhagen county from 1962 to 1987. *Scand J Gastroenterol.* 1991;26(12):1247–1256.
7. **Loftus EV Jr. Clinical epidemiology of inflammatory bowel disease: Incidence, prevalence, and environmental influences. *Gastroenterology* 2004;126(6):1504–1517.**
8. Stonnington CM, Phillips SF, Melton LJ 3rd, et al. Chronic ulcerative colitis: incidence and prevalence in a community. *Gut* 1987;28(4):402–409.
9. Harries AD, Jones L, Heatley RV, et al. Smoking habits and inflammatory bowel disease: effect on nutrition. *Br Med J (Clin Res Ed).* 1982; 284(6323):1161.
10. Calkins BM. A meta-analysis of the role of smoking in inflammatory bowel disease. *Dig Dis Sci.* 1989;34(12):1841–1854.
11. Loftus EV Jr, Sandborn WJ, Tremaine WJ, et al. Primary sclerosing cholangitis is associated with nonsmoking: a case-control study. *Gastroenterology* 1996;110(5):1496–1502.
12. van Erpecum KJ, Smits SJ, van de Meeberg PC, et al. Risk of primary sclerosing cholangitis is associated with nonsmoking behavior. *Gastroenterology.* 1996;110(5):1503–1506.
13. Boyko EJ, Koepsell TD, Perera DR, et al. Risk of ulcerative colitis among former and current cigarette smokers. *N Engl J Med.* 1987;316(12): 707–710.
14. Boyko EJ, Perera DR, Koepsell TD, et al. Effects of cigarette smoking on the clinical course of ulcerative colitis. *Scand J Gastroenterol.* 1988;23(9): 1147–1152.
15. Beaugerie L, Massot N, Carbonnel F, et al. Impact of cessation of smoking on the course of ulcerative colitis. *Am J Gastroenterol.* 2001;96(7): 2113–2116.
16. Koutroubakis IE, Vlachonikolis IG, Kouroumalis EA. Role of appendicitis and appendectomy in the pathogenesis of ulcerative colitis: a critical review. *Inflamm Bowel Dis.* 2002;8(4):277–286.
17. Andersson RE, Olaison G, Tysk C, et al. Appendectomy and protection against ulcerative colitis. *N Engl J Med.* 2001;344(11):808–814.
18. Frisch M, Biggar RJ. Appendectomy and protection against ulcerative colitis. *N Engl J Med.* 2001;345(3):222–223; author reply 223–234.

19. Frisch M, Johansen C, Mellemkjaer L, et al. Appendectomy and subsequent risk of inflammatory bowel diseases. *Surgery* 2001;130(1):36–43.
20. Naganuma M, Iizuka B, Torii A, et al. Appendectomy protects against the development of ulcerative colitis and reduces its recurrence: results of a multicenter case-controlled study in Japan. *Am J Gastroenterol.* 2001; 96(4):1123–1126.
21. Radford-Smith GL, Edwards JE, Purdie DM, et al. Protective role of appendicectomy on onset and severity of ulcerative colitis and Crohn's disease. *Gut.* 2002;51(6):808–813.
22. Watts DA, Satsangi J. The genetic jigsaw of inflammatory bowel disease. *Gut* 2002;50 (suppl 3):III31–36.
23. Farmer RG, Michener WM, Mortimer EA. Studies of family history among patients with inflammatory bowel disease. *Clin Gastroenterol.* 1980;9(2):271–277.
24. **Orholm M, Munkholm P, Langholz E, et al. Familial occurrence of inflammatory bowel disease. *N Engl J Med.* 1991;324(2):84–88.**
25. Binder V. Genetic epidemiology in inflammatory bowel disease. *Dig Dis.* 1998;16(6):351–355.
26. Nakamura RM, Matsutani M, Barry M. Advances in clinical laboratory tests for inflammatory bowel disease. *Clin Chim Acta.* 2003;335(1–2):9–20.
27. Satsangi J, Parkes M, Louis E, et al. Two stage genome-wide search in inflammatory bowel disease provides evidence for susceptibility loci on chromosomes 3, 7 and 12. *Nat Genet.* 1996;14(2):199–202.
28. Stokkers PC, Reitsma PH, Tytgat GN, et al. HLA-DR and -DQ phenotypes in inflammatory bowel disease: a meta-analysis. *Gut* 1999;45(3):395–401.
29. Gan SI, Beck PL. A new look at toxic megacolon: an update and review of incidence, etiology, pathogenesis, and management. *Am J Gastroenterol.* 2003;98(11):2363–2371.
30. Holtmann MH, Galle PR. Current concept of pathophysiological understanding and natural course of ulcerative colitis. *Langenbecks Arch Surg.* 2004;389(5):341–349.
31. Bernstein CN. Extraintestinal manifestations of inflammatory bowel disease. *Curr Gastroenterol Rep.* 2001;3(6):477–483.
32. Apgar JT. Newer aspects of inflammatory bowel disease and its cutaneous manifestations: a selective review. *Semin Dermatol.* 1991;10(3):138–147.
33. Danzi T. Extraintestinal manifestation of idiopathic inflammatory bowel disease. *Arch Intern Med.* 1988;148:297–302.
34. Mintz R, Feller ER, Bahr RL, et al. Ocular manifestations of inflammatory bowel disease. *Inflamm Bowel Dis.* 2004;10(2):135–139.
35. Levine JB, Lukawski-Trubish D. Extraintestinal considerations in inflammatory bowel disease. *Gastroenterol Clin North Am.* 1995;24(3):633–646.
36. Raj V, Lichtenstein DR. Hepatobiliary manifestations of inflammatory bowel disease. *Gastroenterol Clin North Am.* 1999;28(2):491–513.
37. Olsson R, Danielsson A, Jarnerot G, et al. Prevalence of primary sclerosing cholangitis in patients with ulcerative colitis. *Gastroenterology* 1991;100(5 Pt 1):1319–1323.
38. Mir-Madjlessi SH, Farmer RG, Sivak MV Jr. Bile duct carcinoma in patients with ulcerative colitis. Relationship to sclerosing cholangitis: report of six cases and review of the literature. *Dig Dis Sci.* 1987;32(2): 145–154.
39. Wold PB, Fletcher JG, Johnson CD, et al. Assessment of small bowel Crohn disease: noninvasive peroral CT enterography compared with other imaging methods and endoscopy—feasibility study. *Radiology* 2003;229(1):275–281.
40. Hendriksen C, Kreiner S, Binder V. Long term prognosis in ulcerative colitis—based on results from a regional patient group from the county of Copenhagen. *Gut.* 1985;26(2):158–163.
41. Refojo D, Liberman AC, Holsboer F, et al. Transcription factor-mediated molecular mechanisms involved in the functional cross-talk between cytokines and glucocorticoids. *Immunol Cell Biol.* 2001;79(4):385–394.
42. Yamamoto Y, Gaynor RB. Therapeutic potential of inhibition of the NF-kappaB pathway in the treatment of inflammation and cancer. *J Clin Invest.* 2001;107(2):135–142.
43. Schottelius A, Wedel S, Weltrich R, et al. Higher expression of glucocorticoid receptor in peripheral mononuclear cells in inflammatory bowel disease. *Am J Gastroenterol.* 2000;95(8):1994–1999.
44. Honda M, Orii F, Ayabe T, et al. Expression of glucocorticoid receptor beta in lymphocytes of patients with glucocorticoid-resistant ulcerative colitis. *Gastroenterology* 2000;118(5):859–866.
45. Thalen A, Brattsand R, Andersson PH. Development of glucocorticosteroids with enhanced ratio between topical and systemic effects. *Acta Derm Venereol Suppl (Stockh).* 1989;151:11–19, 47–52.
46. Sandborn WJ, Hanauer SB. Systematic review: the pharmacokinetic profiles of oral mesalazine formulations and mesalazine pro-drugs used in the management of ulcerative colitis. *Aliment Pharmacol Ther.* 2003; 17(1): 29–42.
47. Lichtiger S, Present DH. Preliminary report: cyclosporin in treatment of severe active ulcerative colitis. *Lancet* 1990;336(8706):16–19.
48. Lichtiger S, Present DH, Kornbluth A, et al. Cyclosporine in severe ulcerative colitis refractory to steroid therapy. *N Engl J Med.* 1994;330(26): 1841–1845.
49. Liu J, Farmer JD Jr, Lane WS, et al. Calcineurin is a common target of cyclophilin-cyclosporin A and FKBP-FK506 complexes. *Cell* 1991;66(4): 807–815.
50. Reed JC, Prystowsky MB, Nowell PC. Regulation of gene expression in lectin-stimulated or lymphokine-stimulated T lymphocytes. Effects of cyclosporine. *Transplantation* 1988;46(2 (suppl):85S–89S.
51. Hyde GM, Thillainayagam AV, Jewell DP. Intravenous cyclosporin as rescue therapy in severe ulcerative colitis: time for a reappraisal? *Eur J Gastroenterol Hepatol.* 1998;10(5):411–413.
52. Loftus CG, Egan LJ, Sandborn WJ. Cyclosporine, tacrolimus, and mycophenolate mofetil in the treatment of inflammatory bowel disease. *Gastroenterol Clin North Am.* 2004;33(2):141–169, vii.
53. Lennard L. The clinical pharmacology of 6-mercaptopurine. *Eur J Clin Pharmacol.* 1992;43(4):329–339.
54. Hawthorne AB, Logan RF, Hawkey CJ, et al. Randomised controlled trial of azathioprine withdrawal in ulcerative colitis. *BMJ.*1992;305(6844): 20–22.
55. Present DH, Meltzer SJ, Krumholz MP, et al. 6-Mercaptopurine in the management of inflammatory bowel disease: short- and long-term toxicity. *Ann Intern Med.* 1989;111(8):641–649.
56. Chey WY, Hussain A, Ryan C, et al. Infliximab for refractory ulcerative colitis. *Am J Gastroenterol.* 2001;96(8):2373–8231.
57. Actis GC, Bruno M, Pinna-Pintor M, et al. Infliximab for treatment of steroid-refractory ulcerative colitis. *Dig Liver Dis.* 2002;34(9): 631–634.
58. Gornet JM, Couve S, Hassani Z, et al. Infliximab for refractory ulcerative colitis or indeterminate colitis: an open-label multicentre study. *Aliment Pharmacol Ther.* 2003;18(2):175–181.
59. Probert CS, Hearing SD, Schreiber S, et al. Infliximab in moderately severe glucocorticoid resistant ulcerative colitis: a randomised controlled trial. *Gut* 2003;52(7):998–1002.
60. Iyer S, Kontoyiannis D, Chevrier D, et al. Inhibition of tumor necrosis factor mRNA translation by a rationally designed immunomodulatory peptide. *J Biol Chem.* 2000;275(22):17051–17057.
61. Iyer S, Lahana R, Buelow R. Rational design and development of RDP58. *Curr Pharm Des.* 2002;8(24):2217–2229.
62. Travis S, Yap L, CJ H. Novel and effective therapy for ulcerative colitis: results of a parallel, prospective, placebo-contrials [N2](abstr). *Am J Gastroenterol.* 2003;98:S239.
63. Van Assche G, Dalle I, Noman M, et al. A pilot study on the use of the humanized anti-interleukin-2 receptor antibody daclizumab in active ulcerative colitis. *Am J Gastroenterol.* 2003;98(2):369–376.
64. Creed TJ, Norman MR, Probert CS, et al. Basiliximab (anti-CD25) in combination with steroids may be an effective new treatment for steroid-resistant ulcerative colitis. *Aliment Pharmacol Ther.* 2003;18(1):65–75.
65. Plevy S, Salzberg B, Reguiro M. A humanized anti-CD3 monoclonal antibody, visilizumab, for treatment of severe steroid-refractory ulcerative colitis: preliminary results of a phase I study [abstract]. *Gastroenterology.* 2003;124:A7.
66. Lim WC, Hanauer SB. Emerging biologic therapies in inflammatory bowel disease. *Rev Gastroenterol Disord.* 2004;4(2):66–85.
67. Wiesner RH, Grambsch PM, Dickson ER, et al. Primary sclerosing cholangitis: natural history, prognostic factors and survival analysis. *Hepatology* 1989;10(4):430–436.
68. MacLean AR, Lilly L, Cohen Z, et al. Outcome of patients undergoing liver transplantation for primary sclerosing cholangitis. *Dis Colon Rectum* 2003;46(8):1124–1128.
69. Kelly DM, Emre S, Guy SR, et al. Liver transplant recipients are not at increased risk for nonlymphoid solid organ tumors. *Cancer.* 1998;83(6): 1237–1243.
70. Collins RH Jr, Feldman M, Fordtran JS. Colon cancer, dysplasia, and surveillance in patients with ulcerative colitis. A critical review. *N Engl J Med.* 1987;316(26):1654–1658.
71. Ekbom A, Helmick C, Zack M, et al. Ulcerative colitis and colorectal cancer. A population-based study. *N Engl J Med.* 1990;323(18):1228–1233.
72. Ekbom A. Risk of cancer in ulcerative colitis. *J Gastrointest Surg.* 1998;2(4):312–313.
73. **Eaden JA, Abrams KR, Mayberry JF. The risk of colorectal cancer in ulcerative colitis: a meta-analysis. *Gut* 2001;48(4):526–535.**
74. Fearon ER, Vogelstein B. A genetic model for colorectal tumorigenesis. *Cell* 1990;61(5):759–767.
75. Brentnall TA, Crispin DA, Rabinovitch PS, et al. Mutations in the p53 gene: an early marker of neoplastic progression in ulcerative colitis. *Gastroenterology* 1994;107(2):369–378.
76. Yin J, Harpaz N, Tong Y, et al. p53 Point mutations in dysplastic and cancerous ulcerative colitis lesions. *Gastroenterology* 1993;104(6): 1633–1639.
77. Bernstein CN, Shanahan F, Weinstein WM. Are we telling patients the truth about surveillance colonoscopy in ulcerative colitis? *Lancet* 1994;343(8889):71–74.
78. Connell WR, Lennard-Jones JE, Williams CB, et al. Factors affecting the outcome of endoscopic surveillance for cancer in ulcerative colitis. *Gastroenterology* 1994;107(4):934–944.
79. Bernstein CN. Ulcerative colitis with low-grade dysplasia. *Gastroenterology* 2004;127(3):950–956.
80. Ullman T, Croog V, Harpaz N, et al. Progression of flat low-grade dysplasia to advanced neoplasia in patients with ulcerative colitis. *Gastroenterology* 2003;125(5):1311–1319.
81. Strauss RJ, Flint GW, Platt N, et al. The surgical management of toxic dilatation of the colon: a report of 28 cases and review of the literature. *Ann Surg.* 1976;184(6):682–688.
82. Greenstein AJ, Sachar DB, Gibas A, et al. Outcome of toxic dilatation in ulcerative and Crohn's colitis. *J Clin Gastroenterol.* 1985;7(2):137–143.
83. Nicholls RJ. Review article: ulcerative colitis—surgical indications and treatment. *Aliment Pharmacol Ther.* 2002;16(suppl 4):25–28.
84. Hawley PR. Emergency surgery for ulcerative colitis. *World J Surg.* 1988;12(2):169–173.

85. Turnbull RB Jr, Hawk WA, Weakley FL. Surgical treatment of toxic megacolon. Ileostomy and colostomy to prepare patients for colectomy. *Am J Surg*. 1971;122(3):325–331.
86. Brooke BN. The management of an ileostomy, including its complications. *Lancet* 1952;2(3):102–104.
87. Kock NG. Intra-abdominal "reservoir" in patients with permanent ileostomy. Preliminary observations on a procedure resulting in fecal "continence" in five ileostomy patients. *Arch Surg*. 1969;99(2):223–231.
88. **Parks AG, Nicholls RJ, Belliveau P. Proctocolectomy with ileal reservoir and anal anastomosis. *Br J Surg*. 1980;67(8):533–538.**
89. **Utsunomiya J, Iwama T, Imajo M, et al. Total colectomy, mucosal proctectomy, and ileoanal anastomosis. *Dis Colon Rectum* 1980;23(7): 459–466.**
90. Martin LW, LeCoultre C, Schubert WK. Total colectomy and mucosal proctectomy with preservation of continence in ulcerative colitis. *Ann Surg*. 1977;186(4):477–480.
91. Oakley JR, Jagelman DG, Fazio VW, et al. Complications and quality of life after ileorectal anastomosis for ulcerative colitis. *Am J Surg*. 1985;149(1): 23–30.
92. Baker WN, Glass RE, Ritchie JK, et al. Cancer of the rectum following colectomy and ileorectal anastomosis for ulcerative colitis. *Br J Surg*. 1978;65(12):862–868.
93. Melville DM, Ritchie JK, Nicholls RJ, et al. Surgery for ulcerative colitis in the era of the pouch: the St Mark's Hospital experience. *Gut* 1994;35(8):1076–1080.
94. Sugerman HJ, Newsome HH. Stapled ileoanal anastomosis without a temporary ileostomy. *Am J Surg*. 1994;167(1):58–65; discussion 65–66.
95. Fleshman JW, Cohen Z, McLeod RS, et al. The ileal reservoir and ileoanal anastomosis procedure. Factors affecting technical and functional outcome. *Dis Colon Rectum* 1988;31(1):10–16.
96. Wexner SD, Rosen L, Lowry A, et al. Practice parameters for the treatment of mucosal ulcerative colitis—supporting documentation. The Standards Practice Task Force. The American Society of Colon and Rectal Surgeons. *Dis Colon Rectum* 1997;40(11):1277–1285.
97. Sagar PM, Lewis W, Holdsworth PJ, et al. One-stage restorative proctocolectomy without temporary defunctioning ileostomy. *Dis Colon Rectum* 1992;35(6):582–588.
98. **Fazio VW, Ziv Y, Church JM, et al. Ileal pouch-anal anastomoses complications and function in 1005 patients. *Ann Surg*. 1995;222(2):120–127.**
99. Marcello PW, Roberts PL, Schoetz DJ Jr, et al. Obstruction after ileal pouch-anal anastomosis: a preventable complication? *Dis Colon Rectum* 1993;36(12):1105–1111.
100. Becker JM, Dayton MT, Fazio VW, et al. Prevention of postoperative abdominal adhesions by a sodium hyaluronate-based bioresorbable membrane: a prospective, randomized, double-blind multicenter study. *J Am Coll Surg*. 1996;183(4):297–306.
101. Senapati A, Nicholls RJ, Ritchie JK, et al. Temporary loop ileostomy for restorative proctocolectomy. *Br J Surg*. 1993;80(5):628–630.
102. Mikkola K, Luukkonen P, Jarvinen HJ. Long-term results of restorative proctocolectomy for ulcerative colitis. *Int J Colorectal Dis*. 1995;10(1): 10–14.
103. Tan HT, Connolly AB, Morton D, et al. Results of restorative proctocolectomy in the elderly. *Int J Colorectal Dis*. 1997;12(6):319–322.
104. Blumberg D, Opelka FG, Hicks TC, et al. Restorative proctocolectomy: Ochsner Clinic experience. *South Med J*. 2001;94(5):467–471.
105. Heuschen UA, Hinz U, Allemeyer EH, et al. Risk factors for ileoanal J pouch-related septic complications in ulcerative colitis and familial adenomatous polyposis. *Ann Surg*. 2002;235(2):207–216.
106. Heuschen UA, Allemeyer EH, Hinz U, et al. Outcome after septic complications in J pouch procedures. *Br J Surg*. 2002;89(2):194–200.
107. McLeod RS. Surgery for inflammatory bowel diseases. *Dig Dis*. 2003; 21(2):168–179.
108. Gemlo BT, Wong WD, Rothenberger DA, et al. Ileal pouch-anal anastomosis. Patterns of failure. *Arch Surg*. 1992;127(7):784–786; discussion 787.
109. Wexner SD, Wong WD, Rothenberger DA, et al. The ileoanal reservoir. *Am J Surg*. 1990;159(1):178–183; discussion 183–185.
110. Shah NS, Remzi F, Massmann A, et al. Management and treatment outcome of pouch-vaginal fistulas following restorative proctocolectomy. *Dis Colon Rectum* 2003;46(7):911–917.
111. Dozois RR, Kelly KA, Welling DR, et al. Ileal pouch-anal anastomosis: comparison of results in familial adenomatous polyposis and chronic ulcerative colitis. Ann Surg. 1989;210(3):268-71; discussion 272–273.
112. Stocchi L, Pemberton JH. Pouch and pouchitis. *Gastroenterol Clin North Am*. 2001;30(1):223–421.
113. Gionchetti P, Amadini C, Rizzello F, et al. Probiotics for the treatment of postoperative complications following intestinal surgery. *Best Pract Res Clin Gastroenterol*. 2003;17(5):821–831.
114. Gionchetti P, Rizzello F, Helwig U, et al. Prophylaxis of pouchitis onset with probiotic therapy: a double-blind, placebo-controlled trial. *Gastroenterology* 2003;124(5):1202–1209.
115. Yantiss RK, Sapp HL, Farraye FA, et al. Histologic predictors of pouchitis in patients with chronic ulcerative colitis. *Am J Surg Pathol*. 2004;28(8): 999–1006.
116. Kelly KA. Anal sphincter-saving operations for chronic ulcerative colitis. *Am J Surg*. 1992;163(1):5–11.
117. Lavery IC, Sirimarco MT, Ziv Y, et al. Anal canal inflammation after ileal pouch-anal anastomosis. The need for treatment. *Dis Colon Rectum* 1995;38(8):803–806.
118. Shen B, Lashner BA, Bennett AE, et al. Treatment of rectal cuff inflammation (cuffitis) in patients with ulcerative colitis following restorative proctocolectomy and ileal pouch-anal anastomosis. *Am J Gastroenterol*. 2004; 99(8):1527–1531.
119. MacRae HM, McLeod RS, Cohen Z, et al. Risk factors for pelvic pouch failure. *Dis Colon Rectum* 1997;40(3):257–262.
120. Lepisto A, Luukkonen P, Jarvinen HJ. Cumulative failure rate of ileal pouch-anal anastomosis and quality of life after failure. *Dis Colon Rectum*. 2002;45(10):1289–1294.
121. Damgaard B, Wettergren A, Kirkegaard P. Social and sexual function following ileal pouch-anal anastomosis. *Dis Colon Rectum*. 1995; 38(3):286–289.
122. Gorgun E, Remzi FH, Goldberg JM, et al. Fertility is reduced after restorative proctocolectomy with ileal pouch anal anastomosis: a study of 300 patients. *Surgery* 2004;136(4):795–803.
123. McLeod RS, Baxter NN. Quality of life of patients with inflammatory bowel disease after surgery. *World J Surg*. 1998;22(4):375–381.
124. Pemberton JH, Phillips SF, Ready RR, et al. Quality of life after Brooke ileostomy and ileal pouch-anal anastomosis. Comparison of performance status. *Ann Surg*. 1989;209(5):620–626; discussion 626–628.
125. Kohler LW, Pemberton JH, Zinsmeister AR, et al. Quality of life after proctocolectomy. A comparison of Brooke ileostomy, Kock pouch, and ileal pouch-anal anastomosis. *Gastroenterology* 1991;101(3):679–684.

CHAPTER 69 ■ COLONIC POLYPS AND POLYPOSIS SYNDROMES

C. RICHARD BOLAND AND ROBERT S. BRESALIER

COLORECTAL POLYPS

The gastrointestinal tract accounts for more neoplastic disease than any other organ system in the body. In North America, neoplasms of the colon and rectum have attracted the greatest interest because of their relatively high incidence and because appropriate intervention can dramatically modify the morbidity and mortality associated with them. The adenoma is the most common precursor of colorectal cancer, and early removal of adenomatous polyps can interrupt the natural history of the disease and prevent death.

Colorectal cancers can develop through one of at least three molecular pathways, and each variety appears to have some unique clinical and pathologic features. The adenoma–carcinoma sequence is virtually canonical at this time and describes the common pathway taken by neoplasms that have "chromosomal instability." It has subsequently been proposed that "serrated" polyps may be precursors of colon cancers with the microsatellite instability (MSI) phenotype. These polyps are a pathologic hybrid, showing features of both hyperplastic and adenomatous polyps. It is becoming increasingly important to understand the clinical behavior of colorectal neoplasms in the context of the genetic and molecular bases of these lesions.

Classification of Colorectal Polyps

The term *polyp* (from the Greek *polypous*, "morbid excrescence") refers to a macroscopic protrusion of the colonic mucosa into the bowel lumen. This can result from abnormal growth of the mucosa or from a submucosal process that causes the mucosa to protrude into the lumen. Mucosal polyps can be *sessile*, protruding directly from the colonic wall, or *pedunculated*, extending from the mucosa through a fibrovascular stalk.

Mucosal polyps in the colon can be categorized as *neoplastic*, with malignant potential, or *non-neoplastic*, with no malignant potential (Table 69.1). Neoplastic polyps include benign adenomatous polyps that may evolve to carcinoma, adenomatous polyps that contain foci of intramucosal carcinoma (carcinoma in situ), and adenomatous polyps in which carcinoma has penetrated the muscularis mucosae (invasive carcinoma). A serrated polyp contains adenomatous features admixed with features of a hyperplastic polyp. Serrated adenomas appear to originate in a manner unique from typical adenomas, but are premalignant lesions. Sometimes a polyp is found in which carcinoma has completely obliterated the adenomatous tissue from which it arose (polypoid carcinoma).

TABLE 69.1 CLASSIFICATION

CLASSIFICATION OF COLORECTAL POLYPS

Mucosal polyps
NEOPLASTIC
Benign
Adenomatous polyps
Tubular adenoma
Tubulovillous adenoma
Villous adenoma
Serrated polyp
Malignant
Carcinoma in situ
Invasive carcinoma
Polypoid carcinoma
NONNEOPLASTIC
Hyperplastic polyps
Juvenile polyps
Peutz-Jeghers polyps
Inflammatory polyps
Normal epithelium
Submucosal polyps
Lipomas
Leiomyomas
Colitis cystica profunda
Pneumatosis cystoides intestinalis
Lymphoid aggregates
Lymphoma (primary or secondary)
Carcinoids
Metastatic neoplasms

Nonneoplastic mucosal polyps include hyperplastic polyps, juvenile polyps, Peutz-Jeghers hamartomas, and a variety of inflammatory polyps, including those associated with inflammatory bowel disease. Any submucosal lesion can expand to push the mucosa into the bowel lumen and thus appear as a polypoid lesion. Examples include lipomas, leiomyomas, colitis cystica profunda, pneumatosis cystoides intestinalis, lymphoid aggregates, primary or secondary lymphomas, carcinoid tumors, and other metastatic neoplasms.

Neoplastic Mucosal Polyps

Most colorectal cancers arise in preexisting adenomatous polyps. Neoplastic mucosal epithelium evolves through a series of progressive, cumulative molecular and cellular steps that lead to altered proliferation, cellular accumulation, and glandular disarray. In some instances, the polyp also achieves the ability to invade and metastasize through the adenoma-to-carcinoma sequence.

Several lines of evidence support the assumption that colorectal adenocarcinomas arise from adenomatous polyps. The descriptive epidemiology of colonic adenomas parallels that of carcinomas, but the benign lesions occur earlier. Adenomas are rare in geographic regions with a low prevalence of colon cancer, and the distribution of adenomas in the colon parallels that of carcinomas. Adenomas often occur in anatomic proximity to colon cancers, and cancer risk is proportional to the number of adenomas present synchronously or metachronously in a patient. Cancer is often present in polyps removed endoscopically or surgically, and the risk for cancer is proportional to the degree of dysplasia or atypia in the polyp. Conversely, histologically evident residual adenomatous tissue may be found surrounding carcinomas. Most important, results from several studies indicate that the systematic removal of adenomatous polyps during screening proctosigmoidoscopy or surveillance colonoscopy decreases the risk for the development of colorectal cancers and death from this disease.

Pathogenesis

Molecular Biology

Genetic changes that lead to the development of adenomas (and carcinomas) can be loosely organized into three major classes: alterations in protooncogenes, loss of tumor-suppressor gene activity, and abnormalities of genes involved in DNA repair (Fig. 69.1). Several different mechanisms are involved in altering these genes. Typically, oncogenes become overactive by mutation or amplification. Tumor suppressor genes become inactivated by mutation, deletion, or by silencing through promoter methylation. Tumor suppressor genes require inactivation of both copies and alleles, making this process more complex. It is now clear, however, that the development of adenoma and carcinoma is always associated with the progressive accumulation of genetic changes.[1]

In familial adenomatous polyposis (FAP), Lynch syndrome (also called *hereditary nonpolyposis colorectal cancer*), and other familial syndromes, the first genetic alteration is inherited in the germline. Environmental factors are then required for the additional genetic mutations that lead to malignant transformation. The phenotype for the inherited predispositions to gastrointestinal cancer is initially normal; such individuals might be thought of as having an exceptional susceptibility to environmental stress. The germline mutation provides the first "hit," which greatly increases the likelihood of neoplasia and greatly increases the likelihood that the disease will occur at a young age.[2]

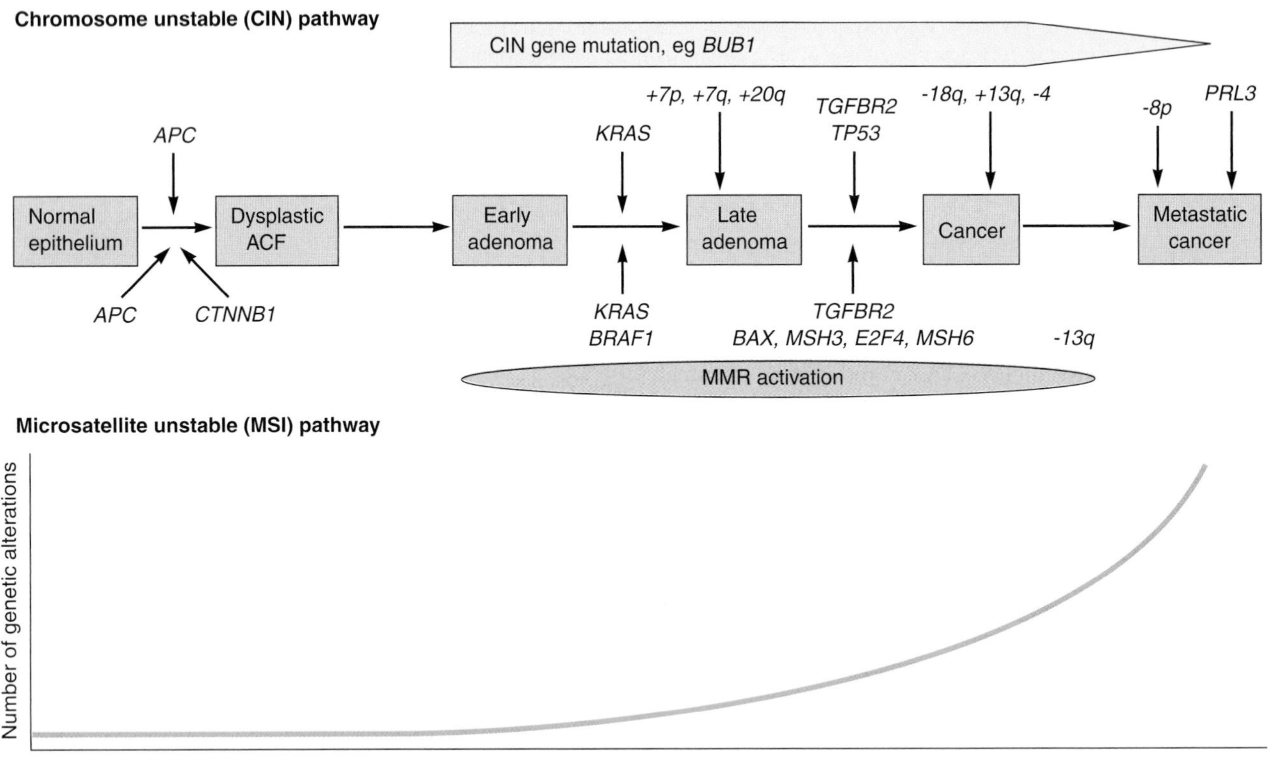

FIGURE 69.1 Proposed sequence of molecular genetic events in the evolution of colon cancer. Carcinomas arise from an accumulation of events whose sequence has been defined for two of the carcinogenesis pathways. As illustrated here, tumors progress through the adenoma-to-carcinoma sequence along pathways marked by chromosomal instability (CIN) or microsatellite instability (MSI). At least one more pathway, characterized by promoter methylation of tumor suppressor genes, serrated polyps, and cancers with variable degrees of microsatellite instability, is incompletely understood, and not shown here. ACF, aberrant crypt focus; TGF, transforming growth factor. (After Grady WM. Genomic instability and colon cancer. *Cancer Metastasis Rev.* 2004;23:11.)

"Sporadic" polyps and cancers are associated with multiple somatic mutations, all of which are caused by spontaneous decay or environmental insults. Adenomas and cancers that develop in both cases arise in the context of genomic instability, a process that increases the likelihood that epithelial cells will acquire the number of mutations needed to attain a neoplastic state.[3] Destabilization of the genome is a prerequisite to carcinogenesis and most commonly involves chromosomal instability with widespread chromosomal deletions, duplications, and rearrangements that produces aneuploidy. Alternatively, increased rates of mutations, often in tandemly repeated DNA sequences known as *microsatellites* (microsatellite instability) or a form of epigenetic instability called the *CpG island methylator phenotype* (or, CIMP), in which genes are inappropriately silenced by promoter methylation,[4] are mechanisms that can lead to progressive multistep carcinogenesis. Genomic (or epigenetic) instability generates a large number of random alterations, and the successive accumulation of those changes that are advantageous to the cell will eventually facilitate the evolution of the neoplastic cell.

Cellular protooncogenes are a group of evolutionarily conserved genes that play a role in signal transduction and the normal regulation of cell growth. Inappropriate activation of these genes, usually through mutation, leads to abnormal transmission of growth regulatory signals, which produce excessive cellular proliferation. Mutations of the K-*ras* oncogene, for example, can be found in about half of sporadic colorectal neoplasms and appear to play a role in accelerating the growth potential of the early adenoma. Only 9% of small adenomas have *K-ras* mutations, whereas 58% of adenomas >1 cm have altered *K-ras* genes. *K-ras* mutations are more common in pedunculated than flat adenomas. However, by themselves, K-ras mutations are not sufficient either for the neoplastic phenotype or for tumor progression. This mutation provides one mechanism for an epithelial cell to grow and achieve autonomous growth, which increases the likelihood that additional genetic alterations will occur.

The tumor suppressor gene *APC* on chromosome 5q is critical to the evolution of the colorectal adenoma. Allelic losses of chromosome 5q occur early during carcinogenesis in the colon.[5] A combination of mutation of one allele, and loss of the other allele of *APC*, occurs in the majority of colorectal adenomas. *APC* acts as the "gatekeeper" of colonic epithelial proliferation, and inactivation of this gene will lead to net cellular proliferation and initiation of neoplasia in the colon.[6] The protein produced by the *APC* gene plays a central role in regulating the intracellular concentrations of the intracellular protein β-catenin. This protein is highly expressed in actively proliferating cells at the base of the colonic crypt, where it stimulates cell proliferation in its role as a transactivating protein.[7] As the cell commits to terminal differentiation, the *APC* gene is turned on, which down-regulates b-catenin by phosphorylation, targeting its subsequent degradation.

Other genetic changes occur later in the adenoma-to-carcinoma sequence. Stepwise tumor progression is associated in more than 75% of cases with loss of one or more tumor-suppressor genes located on chromosome 18q. Several candidate genes are present in this location, and loss of chromosome 18 in the tumor is associated with a poor prognosis. Loss of the *SMAD 4* gene on 18q probably contributes the most to the progressively aggressive nature of neoplasms that advance through this pathway. Deletions of chromosome 17p involve the *p53* tumor-suppressor gene, whose product normally prevents cells with damaged DNA from progressing from the G_1 to the S phase in the cell cycle. Inactivation of the *p53* gene mediates the conversion from adenoma to carcinoma.[8]

Alterations in genes that mediate DNA mismatch repair during replication cause Lynch syndrome, which has also been called hereditary nonpolyposis colorectal cancer, or HNPCC.[9] The genes responsible for Lynch syndrome are *hMSH2, hMLH1, hMSH6*, and *hPMS2*. In the hereditary disease, germline mutations inactivate one copy of the gene, and the other allele is inactivated by a "somatic" event that occurs locally in an individual colonic epithelial cell. This inactivation creates an inability to repair DNA mismatches and results in a diffuse mutational signature in the tumor, called *microsatellite instability* (MSI) as previously described. This defect leads to the mutational inactivation of several key genes important for maintaining normal cellular behavior. The type II receptor for transforming growth factor-beta (TGF-beta RII), for example, is mutated in 85% of MSI colorectal cancers. The MSI multistep carcinogenesis pathway to tumor development is seen in about 12% of all colorectal cancers,[10] and progression from adenoma to carcinoma occurs in a shorter time period than occurs the chromosomal instability pathway seen in most colorectal cancers, which is thought to require a period of at least 10 to 20 years. MSI colorectal neoplasms appear to account for two clinical observations. First, the MSI pathway may account for the occurrence of cancers 1 or 2 years after a negative colonoscopic exam. Second, it may account for the relatively small number of adenomatous polyps found with MSI because they may not exist for a prolonged period.

Histopathology and Malignant Potential

Adenomatous polyps are characterized according to their physical features, size, glandular structure, and degree of dysplasia, which all have important implications for clinical management. Polyps may be sessile, with a broad-based attachment to the colonic wall, or pedunculated, attached to the colonic wall by way of a fibrovascular stalk (Fig. 69.2). Whether a polyp is sessile or pedunculated typically determines whether the endoscopist can remove the polyp completely by snare polypectomy. Diminutive polyps that measure 5 mm or less in diameter are not likely to contain high-grade dysplasia or invasive carcinoma. Malignant potential increases with polyp size in all histologic groups of adenoma.

Adenomas are classified histologically according to their glandular structure. Aberrant (dysplastic) crypts and microadenomas may be the earliest lesions detected in the flat mucosa of patients at risk. These microadenomas enlarge and progress to macroscopic adenomatous polyps. Tubular adenomas are characterized by a complex network of branching adenomatous glands, whereas villous adenomas contain fronds or folds of mucosa that have overgrown their underlying stroma, and project toward the colonic lumen (Fig. 69.3). Often, both histologic types coexist in a mixed tubulovillous adenoma.

All adenomas, by definition, consist of dysplastic mucosa. The term *dysplasia* refers to abnormalities in crypt architecture (such as irregular branching or crowded "back-to-back" glands) and cytologic detail (enlarged pleomorphic and hyperchromatic nuclei with multiple mitoses and pseudostratification [Fig. 69.4]). Dysplasia may be mild, moderate, or severe, depending on the degree to which these characteristics are present. Severe, or high-grade, dysplasia represents carcinoma-in-situ when the basement membrane is intact. Extension into the lamina propria denotes intramucosal carcinoma. Invasion into the muscularis mucosae defines invasive carcinoma, and the malignant polyp. The degree of dysplasia usually correlates with polyp size and the extent of villous architecture.

Even though nearly all adenocarcinomas of the colon and rectum arise in adenomatous polyps, not all polyps evolve into carcinoma; in fact, most do not. The malignant potential of adenomatous polyps is related to polyp size and the histologic characteristics. Large polyps and those with predominantly villous architecture are more likely to contain coincident carcinoma (Fig. 69.5). These features are interdependent, however, because large polyps are more likely to be villous and dysplastic. Adenomas that measure 0.5 cm or less are most often tubular adenomas and rarely contain severe dysplasia or carcinoma (<0.5% in autopsy series). Likewise, only 1% to 2% of adenomatous polyps smaller than 1 cm contain carcinoma, but autopsy studies suggest that as many as 40% of adenomas larger than 2 cm contain cancer. Data derived from the examination of colonoscopic polypectomy specimens indicate similar trends but suggest a lower incidence of cancer-containing polyps.

Epidemiology

Prevalence

The descriptive epidemiology of adenomatous polyps of the colon and rectum parallels that of colorectal carcinoma with relation to geographic distribution, age, prevalence, and genetic susceptibility. Like colorectal cancer, adenomas are common in Western countries such as the United States, but their prevalence is low in parts of Asia, South America, and sub-Saharan Africa. Estimates of adenoma prevalence in the United States vary depending on the mode of data collection. Data from older studies were collected from autopsies and sometimes grouped all polyps together, whereas more recent studies have examined adenoma prevalence in the context of endoscopic screening. Studies using colonoscopy suggest an adenoma prevalence in patients without symptoms who are older than 50 years that ranges between 20% and 40%. Prevalence rates from autopsy studies are 50% higher. Based on autopsy studies, one half to two thirds of people older than 65 years have colonic adenomas. Adenoma prevalence increases with age in all populations. Age-associated prevalence rates suggest that adenomas precede carcinomas in a given population by at least 5 to 10 years; this time period may be much longer because polyps do not produce symptoms and, unlike cancers, dating the onset can only be estimated. Advancing age also correlates with multiplicity of polyps, polyp size, and higher degrees of dysplasia. In addition, 30% to 50% of patients with one adenoma have a synchronous adenoma elsewhere in the colon.[11]

Heredity

Heredity plays a role not only in FAP and Lynch syndrome, but also in the development of sporadic adenomas. Sporadic (nonsyndromic) adenomatous polyps and colon cancers represent more than 90% of colorectal neoplasms. Clinical studies, including case-control and prospective analyses, indicate a two fold to three fold increased risk for colon cancer among first-degree relatives of patients with a history of colonic adenoma or carcinoma.[12] The relative risk increases with the number of affected relatives and when adenomas and carcinomas occur in relatives at a younger age.[13] The impact of family history becomes insignificant in patients whose polyps are discovered after age 60. In most families, it is not possible to

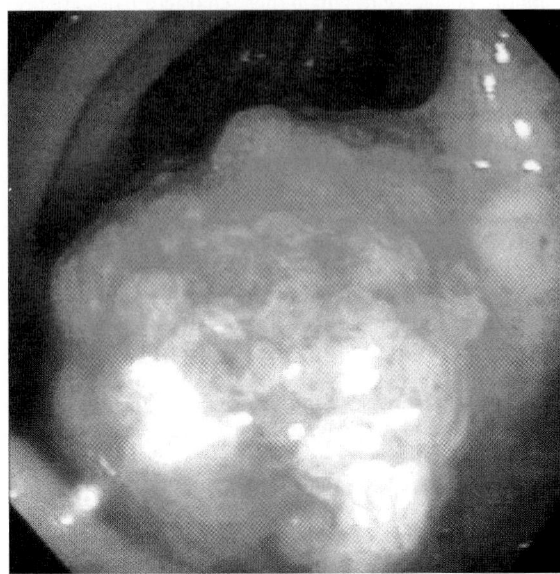

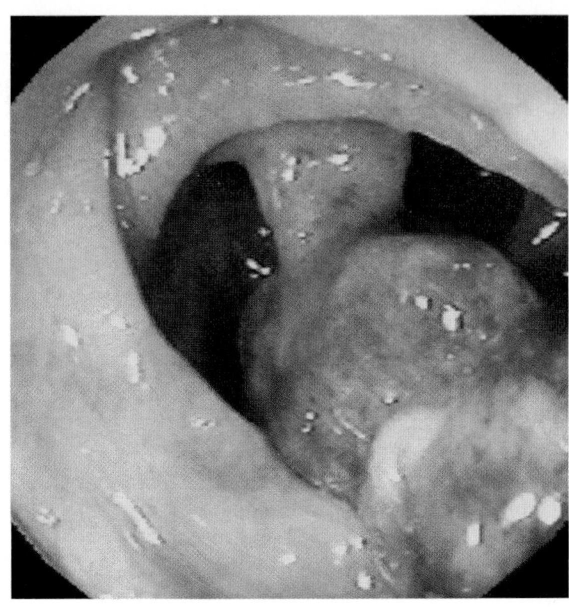

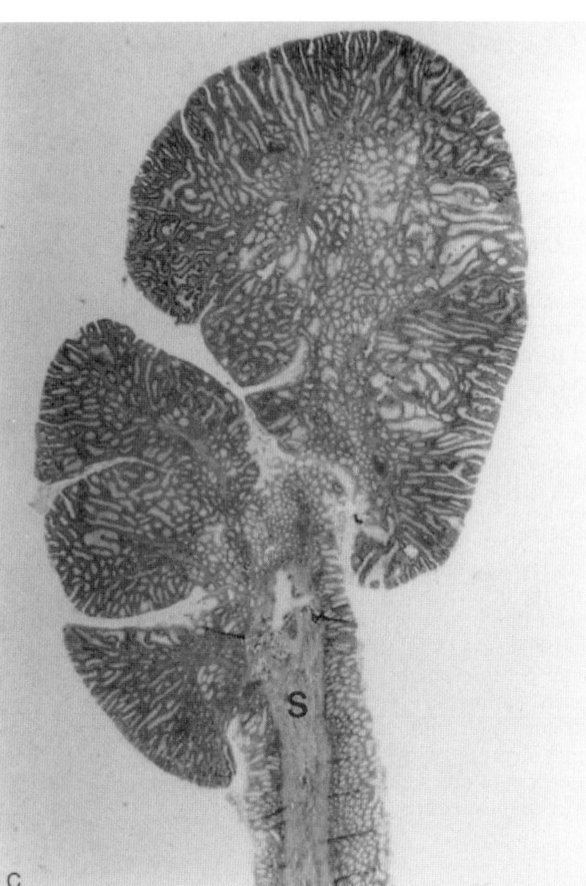

FIGURE 69.2 Mucosal polyps of the colon may be sessile, protruding directly from the colonic wall, or pedunculated, extending from the mucosa through a fibrovascular stalk. (*A*) Large sessile polyp seen at colonoscopy. The polyp has a broad-based attachment to the mucosa. (*B*) Pedunculated polyp seen at colonoscopy. The polyp is attached to the mucosa through a distinct stalk. (*C*) Low-power photomicrograph of a pedunculated polyp (a tubular adenoma) cut in cross section to demonstrate its fibrovascular stalk (S).

separate the impact of commonly shared genes from the impact of shared environmental exposures.

Anatomic Distribution

Autopsy series and colonoscopic examination of patients who do not have symptoms suggest that although adenomas are uniformly distributed throughout the colon, the distribution of clinically important larger adenomas is more similar to that of carcinomas, with a left-sided predominance.

Natural History

Adenomas are common in people older than 50 years, and although most carcinomas arise in adenomatous polyps, relatively few adenomas progress to carcinoma. Little precise information is available regarding what percentage of adenomas evolves to carcinomas. In Norway, an example of a high-risk Western population, it has been estimated that colorectal adenomas are present in 29% of the population older than 35 years. The conversion rate from adenoma to carcinoma in this

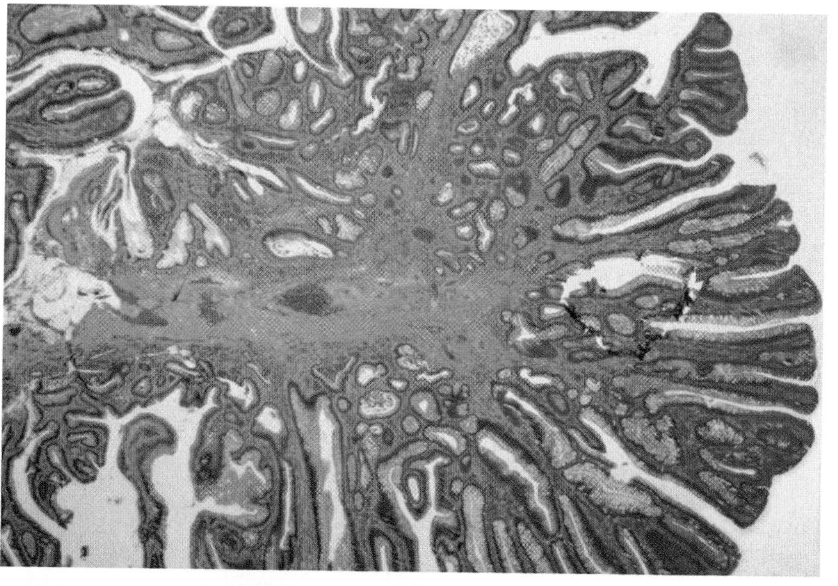

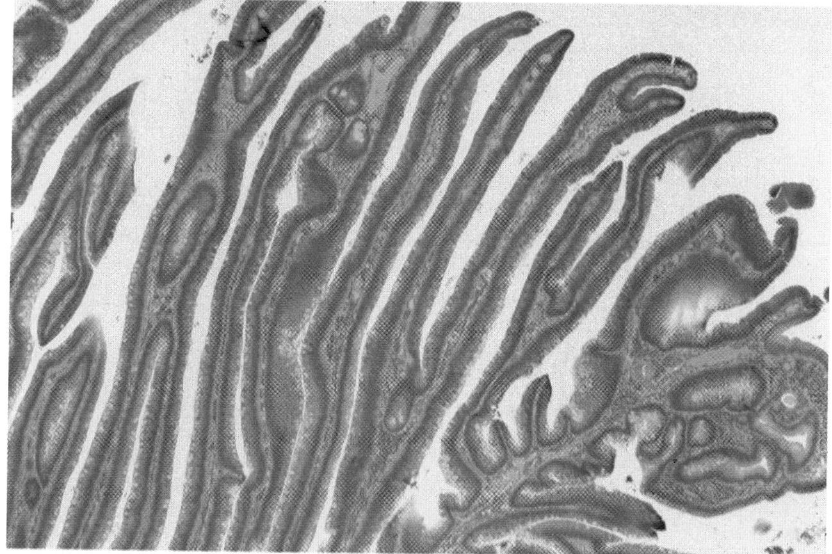

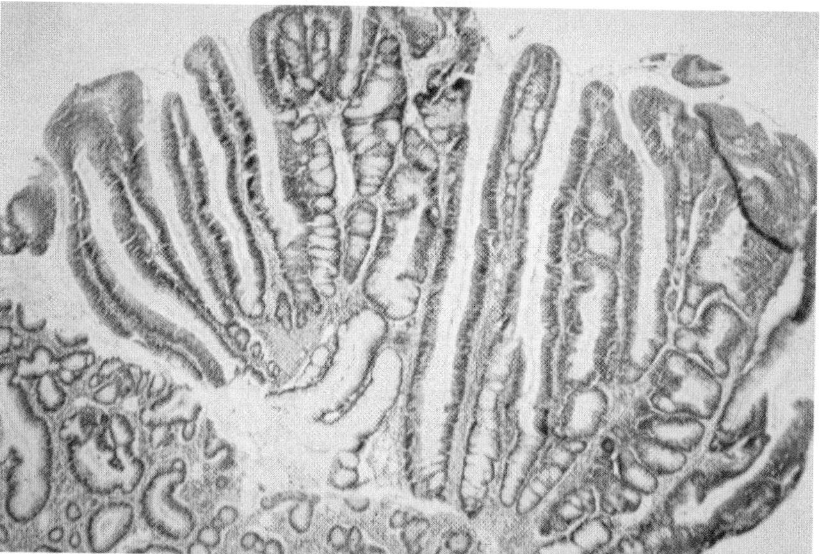

FIGURE 69.3 Histology of adenomatous polyps. (*A*) Tubular adenomas are characterized by a complex network of branching adenomatous glands (see also *C*). (*B*) Villous adenomas consist of glands that extend straight down from the surface to the base as fingerlike projections; this pattern may be suggested by the gross appearance of these polyps. (*C*) Tubulovillous adenoma.

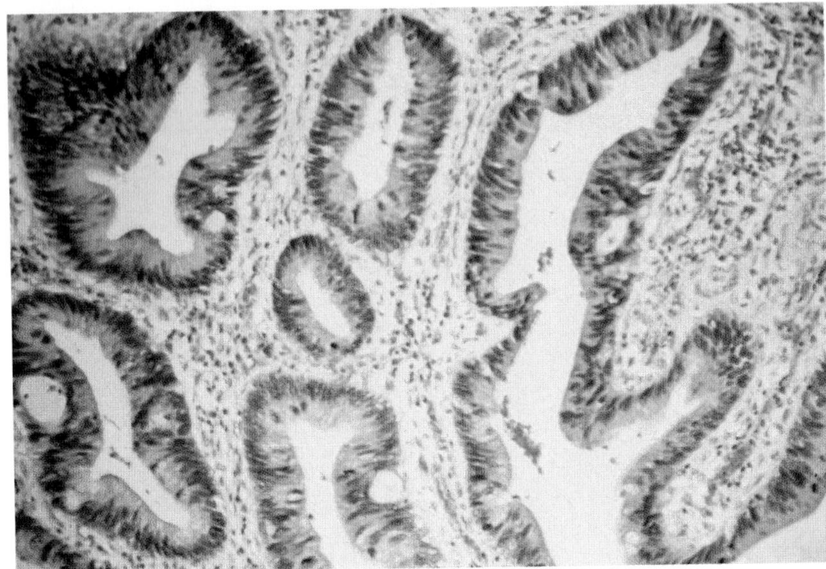

FIGURE 69.4 Moderate dysplasia. Dysplastic mucosa is characterized by crowded, irregular glands and cells with enlarged, hyperchromatic nuclei of varied size and shape that do not line up uniformly on the basement membrane (pseudopalisading). Adenomas are composed of dysplastic mucosa in which the degree of atypia may vary. These changes precede the development of invasive carcinoma.

group (based on cancer incidence from multiple tumor registries) has been calculated to be 0.25% per year. In other words, the risk that a colorectal cancer will develop in a polyp-bearing person within 10 years is 2.5%. The annual conversion rates to invasive cancer for people with adenomas larger than 1 cm, villous components, and severe dysplasia have been estimated to be 3%, 17%, and 37%, respectively, based on these inferences.

Both longitudinal follow-up of a small number of people with unresected adenomas and studies of age distribution provide indirect evidence that the evolution from adenoma to carcinoma takes at least 5 to 10 years. Age prevalence data from the National Polyp Study, for example, suggest that it may take as long as 5 to 10 years for normal-appearing mucosa to develop into a macroscopically visible adenomatous polyp, and an additional 3 to 5 years for invasive carcinoma to develop, in most instances. Case-control studies also support

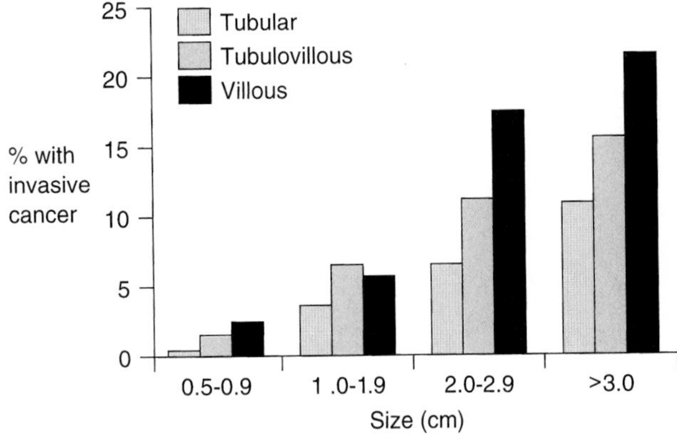

FIGURE 69.5 The relation of adenoma size and histology to malignant potential based on an analysis of 7,000 endoscopically removed polyps. The incident of polyp-associated carcinoma determined from examination of polypectomy specimens is lower than that derived from early autopsy studies. (Data derived from Shinya H, Wolff WI. Morphology, anatomic distribution, and cancer potential of colonic polyps. *Ann Surg* 1979;1990:675, with permission.)

that the development of adenomas in the colon and the evolution to carcinoma occurs slowly. Several studies have estimated that the protective effect of screening sigmoidoscopy may last at least 10 years.[14]

Associated Disease States

A number of clinical situations have been associated with a greater than average risk for adenoma development, but the evidence in most cases is tenuous. Although adenomas and carcinomas develop frequently in patients who have undergone urinary diversion by way of ureterosigmoidoscopy, this finding is largely of historical interest. Nonetheless, patients who have undergone this procedure require periodic colonoscopic surveillance for adenoma and carcinoma development. An increased prevalence of colonic adenomas and carcinomas has been reported in patients with acromegaly, and patients with elevated gastrin levels have been reported to be at risk for neoplasia. Alleged associations between colorectal adenomas and a history of prior cholecystectomy, atherosclerosis, acrochordons (skin tags), and hyperplastic polyps remain unproven.

Clinical Features

Adenomatous polyps of the colon and rectum are highly prevalent in Western societies, but most patients with colonic adenomas do not have symptoms directly referable to these lesions. Overt bleeding manifesting as hematochezia may occur with larger polyps, which may be evident when the polyps are located distally in the rectum. Adenomas typically lose less than 1 mL of blood daily unless they are 2 cm or greater in size. Although colorectal polyps are the most common lesions detected in patients without symptoms undergoing colonoscopy because of the presence of fecal occult blood, the polyps are probably not responsible for the bleeding. Very large colonic polyps may be associated with obstructive symptoms, such as lower abdominal cramping or alterations in bowel habits, but this finding is unusual. Secretory diarrhea with accompanying hypokalemia and hypochlorhydria has been associated with very large villous adenomas of the distal colon and rectum. This is a rare syndrome, and the search for secretagogues such as vasoactive intestinal polypeptide or prostaglandins in patients with polyps and diarrhea is infrequently productive.

Adenomas Associated with Lynch Syndrome and Its Variants

Lynch syndrome is a disease of autosomal dominant inheritance in which cancers arise in discrete adenomas, but polyposis (i.e., dozens or hundreds of polyps) does not occur. This entity is most narrowly defined by the Amsterdam criteria: families must have at least three relatives with colorectal cancer, one of whom is a first-degree relative of the other two; colorectal cancer must involve at least two generations, and at least one cancer case must occur before 50 years of age. Broader definitions of Lynch syndrome take into account the occurrence of extracolonic tumors and smaller kindreds.[15] Adenomas and carcinomas in Lynch syndrome arise at an early age (adenomas may occur in patients in their 20s and 30s, with a mean age for carcinoma development of 40 to 45 years), and the polyps are often proximal in location and multiple. Some families with Lynch syndrome are prone to cancers of the female genital tract (endometrium and ovary) and other sites in addition to colorectal neoplasms. The frequency of Lynch syndrome in the general population is difficult to determine, but Lynch syndrome accounts for about 3% to 5% of all colorectal cancer cases; this suggests that Lynch syndrome may occur in about 2 per 1,000 of the population.

Turcot syndrome is a term of historical significance, in which there is a concurrence of primary brain tumors and multiple colorectal adenomas or cancer in young people. With the advent of accurate genetic characterization, these families are categorized as either FAP or Lynch syndrome, as brain tumors are an occasional complication of both diseases.[16]

Diagnosis

Most colorectal adenomas are asymptomatic and are often detected in the setting of an evaluation for unrelated colonic symptoms or occult blood in the stool. Similarly, adenomatous polyps are frequently detected when patients without symptoms are screened for colorectal neoplasia. Nevertheless, data strongly suggest that the detection and removal of adenomatous polyps are important in reducing colorectal cancer-related mortality.

Fecal Occult Blood Tests

Screening studies from both Europe and the United States indicate that a polyp is detected in about 30% of patients without symptoms who are 50 years of age or older and undergo colonoscopy for follow-up of a positive fecal occult blood test result. Blood loss from polyps is related to polyp size, and positive fecal occult blood test results are related to polyp size and proximity to the rectum. In one study in which rehydrated Hemoccult slides were used (rehydration results in greater sensitivity but also increases the number of false-positive findings), only 15% of polyps smaller than 1 cm were associated with a positive Hemoccult test result, whereas 80% of polyps larger than 2 cm were associated with a positive result. In another study, standard testing with Hemoccult cards detected 17% of adenomas smaller than 1 cm and 42% of adenomas larger than 1 cm. A prospective, randomized study of fecal occult blood tests in which rehydrated Hemoccult cards were used indicated that annual testing reduces colorectal cancer-related deaths by 33% through 18 years of follow-up.[17] This study, in addition to two European trials, have also demonstrated a 15% to 21% reduction in colon cancer-related death from biennial fecal occult blood testing.[18] Thus, unless one rigorously performs the fecal occult blood test on an annual basis, the reduction in colorectal cancer mortality will be disappointing.

Results from the National Polyp Study strongly indicate that the removal of index polyps detected by fecal occult blood testing and other methods, together with subsequent colonoscopic surveillance, results in a very substantial reduction in colorectal cancer mortality; in fact, the reduction may be as high as 76% to 90% (see later).[19]

Sigmoidoscopy

The National Cancer Institute, the American Cancer Society, the American College of Physicians, the American Gastroenterological Association, and the World Health Organization Collaborating Center for Prevention of Colorectal Cancer all advocate screening sigmoidoscopy every 5 years in conjunction with yearly fecal occult blood tests beginning at 50 years of age.[20] The benefit of sigmoidoscopy in interrupting the adenoma-to-carcinoma sequence is suggested by a number of studies. Investigators compared the use of rigid sigmoidoscopy in 261 members of the Kaiser Permanente Medical Care Program who died of cancer of the rectum or distal colon versus that in 868 matched controls.[14] Only 8.8% of those with cancer had undergone screening sigmoidoscopy, compared with 24.2% of controls. The impact of sigmoidoscopy was limited to the development of fatal colon cancer within reach of the sigmoidoscope and was long-standing (at least 10 years). Other investigators determined the long-term risk of colorectal cancer development after rigid sigmoidoscopy and polypectomy in 1,618 patients with rectosigmoid adenomas. The overall risk for subsequent rectal cancer in these patients was similar to that in the general population, but subject analysis revealed that risk depended on histologic type, size, and number of adenomas removed.[21] Based on existing data, the Health Care Financing Administration decided to provide coverage for colon cancer screening procedures to Medicare beneficiaries beginning in 1998. This includes yearly fecal occult blood testing and flexible sigmoidoscopy every 4 years in persons at average risk.

The 60-cm flexible sigmoidoscope has supplanted the rigid scope because it causes less discomfort to the patient, visualizes 2.5 times more surface area, and detects two to three times more adenomas. Flexible sigmoidoscopy can be mastered by paramedical personnel and has been successfully used in screening programs by nurse-practitioners.[22]

Other Screening Modalities

Given the high cost of repeated screening of average-risk, asymptomatic patients for adenomas and carcinomas and the long natural history of the adenoma-to-carcinoma sequence, some have advocated a single air-contrast barium enema or colonoscopy at 50 years of age, with no further screening in patients without symptoms who have negative examination results. However, the American Cancer Society and other groups consider colonoscopy every 10 years or barium enema every 5 to 10 years beginning at age 50 as a screening option in average-risk individuals.[23]

A nonendoscopic screening approach is desirable to reach patients who do not have access to colonoscopy or will not accept this procedure. Computed tomographic (CT) colography, also known as *virtual colonoscopy*, uses thin-section helical CT of an air-distended, prepped colon to generate high-resolution images. Several studies have demonstrated that experienced radiologists using optimized hardware, software, and bowel prep can detect more than 90% of polyps greater than 6 mm in size with an acceptably low false positive rate.[24] However, the failure to optimize the technical aspects of the examination reduces the results to an unacceptable level.[25]

Detection of adenoma-associated antigens or mutated genes in stool is possible, but this approach is currently insufficiently sensitive, and the technical aspects of fecal DNA testing is still in evolution.[26] Technical improvements in this approach could lead to a replacement of the fecal occult blood test.

Management

Management of Adenomas

Index Polypectomy. Once detected, adenomas should be completely removed, preferably by endoscopic snare polypectomy (Fig. 69.6). Polypectomy is relatively safe and easily performed when adenomas are small or pedunculated but is more difficult when polyps are large or sessile. Potential complications include bleeding and perforation of the polypectomy site. Large sessile villous adenomas (larger than 2 cm) have a great potential for malignant degeneration. If such lesions cannot be completely removed by snare polypectomy, and when there is uncertainty about the polypectomy margin in the case of pathologically advanced lesions, segmental surgical resection may be necessary. Diminutive polyps, in contrast, have little malignant potential. If they are too small for snare polypectomy, ablation with a hot biopsy forceps is a reasonable approach. Because 30% to 50% of patients with one adenoma have a synchronous adenoma elsewhere in the colon, the entire colon should be "cleared" by colonoscopy in polyp-bearing patients.

Follow-Up. Much of our current practice has come from information gained through the National Polyp Study (NPS), first organized in 1978. Additional metachronous adenomas are likely to develop in patients who have had adenomas removed. Colonoscopic surveillance studies have provided estimates of the frequency and time course of recurrence in these patients. Data from the NPS suggested a recurrence rate of 32% to 42% by 3 years after index polypectomy. A prospective colonoscopic analysis also demonstrated a cumulative recurrence rate at 3 years of 42%. Most adenomas detected at this 3-year interval were small tubular adenomas. Age older than 60 years, multiple adenomas at index polypectomy, and large size of the index adenoma predicted polyp recurrence in the NPS, but only multiplicity predicted recurrence of polyps with advanced pathologic features (i.e., >1 cm, high-grade dysplasia or invasive cancer) at follow-up. The 3-year recurrence rate in patients with a known history of adenoma (42%) was higher than the incidence rate of adenoma appearance *de novo* during this period in patients who had no adenomas detected on index colonoscopy (16%).[19] The high recurrence rate of adenomas after index polypectomy supports the use of postpolypectomy surveillance in patients with known histories of adenoma. Colonoscopy is the preferred means of follow-up in these patients. Air-contrast barium enemas are inadequate for surveillance examinations; they will miss a substantial number of large lesions and most small polyps. This approach will be supplanted by the use of CT, as discussed previously. Colonoscopy is the most accurate means of evaluating the colonic mucosa, and most importantly, allows biopsy and removal of polyps.

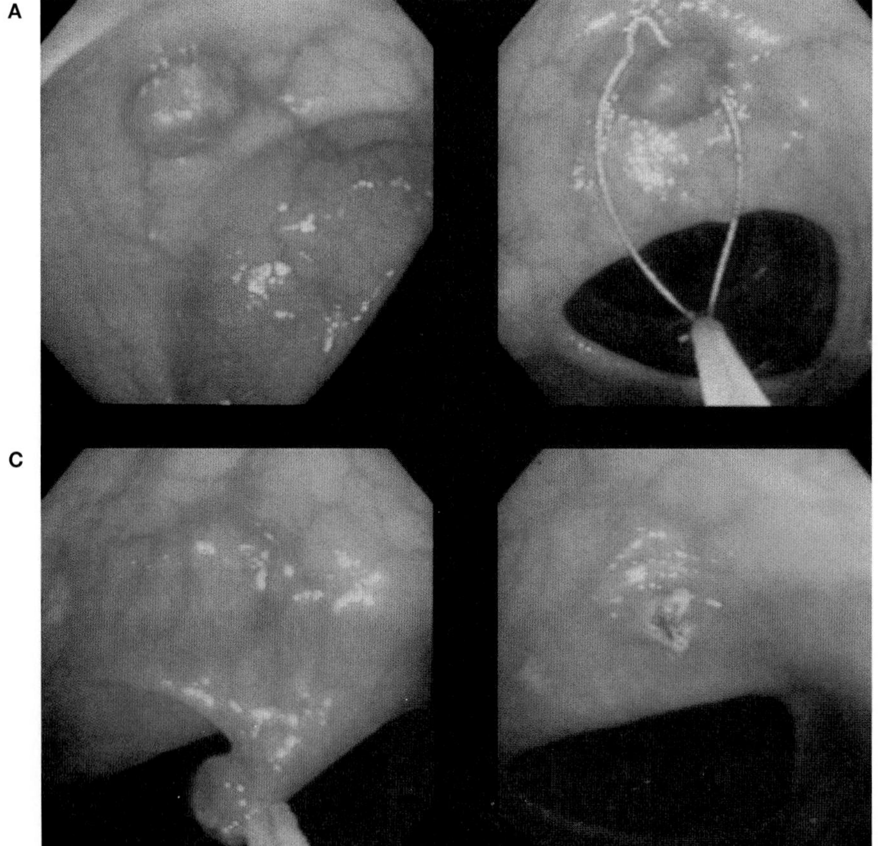

FIGURE 69.6 Endoscopic snare polypectomy. (*A*) A small colonic polyp. (*B*) The polypectomy snare is placed around the polyp. (*C*) The snare is closed around the base of the polyp, and the head of the polyp is gently pulled away from the wall and into the lumen. Current is applied to cut the stalk and cauterize the site. (*D*) The site after completion of polypectomy.

Data from the NPS indicate that colonoscopy need not be repeated at intervals shorter than 3 years in patients whose index polyp demonstrates no evidence of high-grade dysplasia or carcinoma. Although patients undergoing postpolypectomy surveillance at both 1 and 3 years after index polypectomy had a greater number of polyps detected in this study than did those undergoing colonoscopy at 3 years only, the percentage of patients whose adenomas had advanced pathologic features was similarly low in both groups (3.3%). Subsequent studies have confirmed the low incidence of recurrent advanced adenomas 3 to 5 years after polypectomy. Recent recommendations suggest an initial follow-up interval of 3 years after polypectomy. If the result of this colonoscopy is negative, the interval can be extended to every 5 years (Algorithm 69.1).[20]

The NPS has demonstrated that colonoscopic polypectomy and surveillance result in a 76% to 90% reduction in colorectal cancer incidence in comparison with historical reference groups. This study and others have demonstrated, however, that in patients with no family history of colorectal cancer, most adenomas detected at interval follow-up are small tubular adenomas. In addition, when the index polyp is a small tubular adenoma, the risk for the subsequent development of a histologically important lesion is low. This finding is especially true of the diminutive polyp (less than 6 mm in diameter). Given the high cost of repeated colonoscopy procedures, it will be necessary to establish better who may benefit most from colonoscopic surveillance and who may require less rigorous follow-up. A reasonable guideline would be to follow-up polyps with high-grade dysplasia or cancer at 1 year, large (1 cm or larger) adenomas or tubulovillous adenomas in 5 years, and small solitary adenomas in 10 years. Data are not yet available to know what proportion of patients will develop invasive cancers in spite of this approach.

Management of Malignant Polyps

Endoscopic polypectomy is adequate treatment for an adenomatous polyp containing cancer if it can be demonstrated that the cancer is confined to the head of the polyp (i.e., carcinoma in situ or intramucosal carcinoma (Fig. 69.7). The adequacy of simple polypectomy has been controversial in cases in which malignant cells have invaded the polyp stalk (Fig. 69.8), but most studies indicate that polypectomy is adequate treatment provided that a margin of more than 2 mm is present, the cancer is not poorly differentiated, and no vascular or lymphatic invasion is noted. The presence of cancer at or near

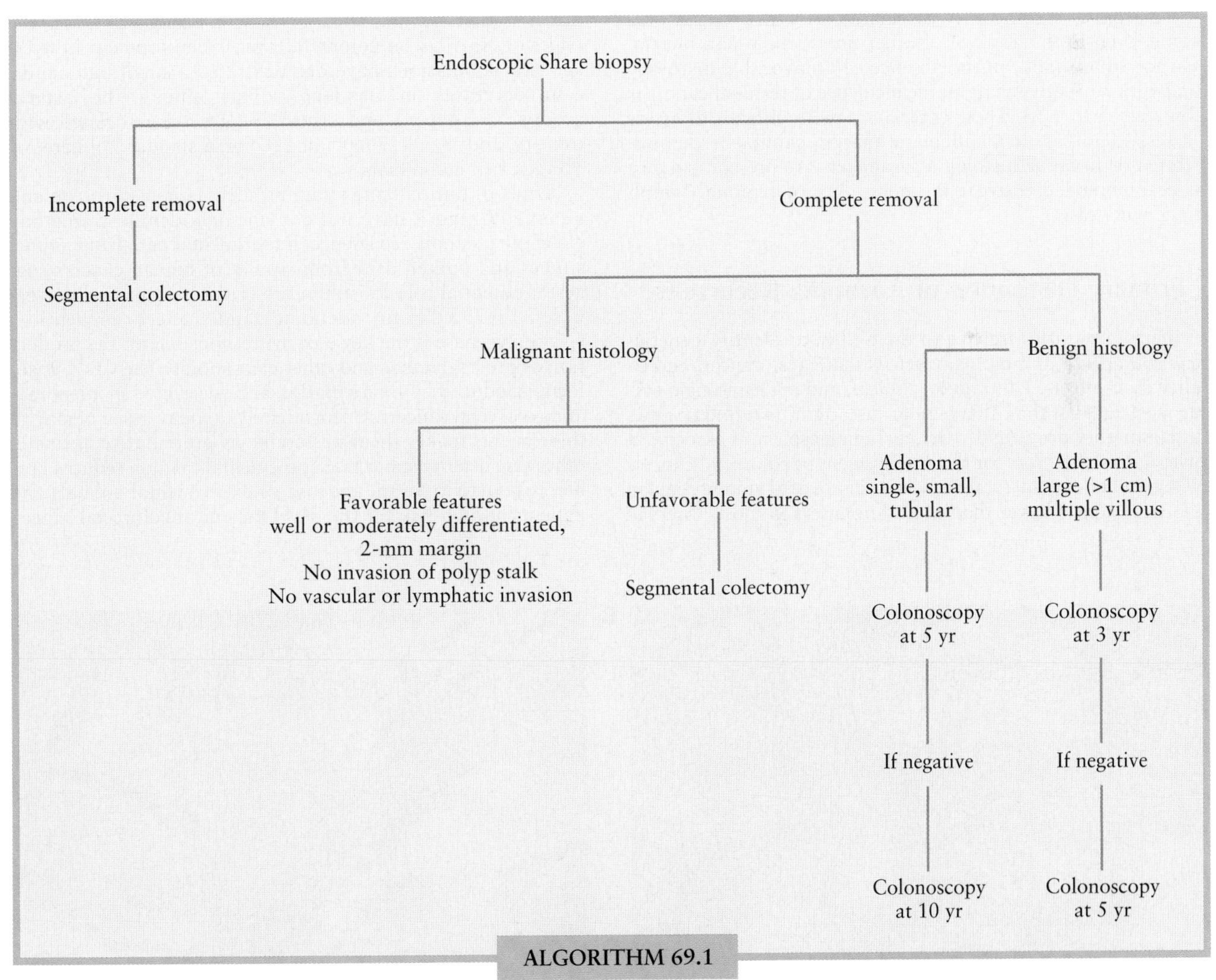

ALGORITHM 69.1 Management of colonic adenoma.

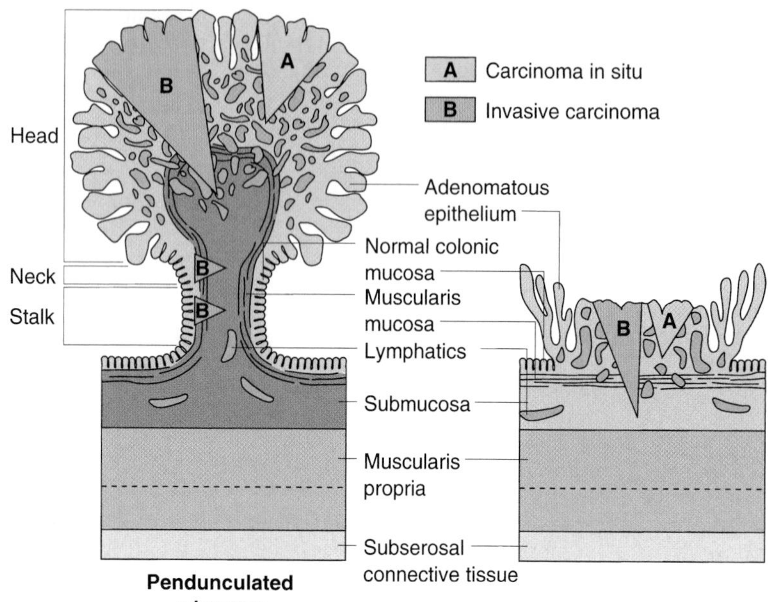

FIGURE 69.7 Diagram representation of cancer-containing polyps. Pedunculated adenoma is described on the left and a sessile adenoma of the right. In carcinoma is situ, malignant cells are confined to the mucosa. These lesions are adequately treated by endoscopic polypectomy. Polypectomy is adequate treatment for invasive carcinoma only if the margin is sufficient (2 mm), the carcinoma is not poorly differentiated, and no evidence of venous or lymphatic invasion is found. (After Haggitt RC, Glotzbach RE, Soffen EE, et al. Prognostic factors in colorectal carcinomas arising in adenomas: implications for lesions removed by endoscopic polypectomy. *Gastroenterology* 1985;89:328.)

the margin is significantly associated with an adverse outcome, even in the absence of other unfavorable parameters. On the other hand, in the absence of unfavorable histology and with a negative margin, the incidence of residual cancer is low (less than 1%). These criteria are more difficult to assess in sessile polyps. If an adequate margin cannot be demonstrated or negative histologic parameters are present, surgery is recommended to treat the possibility of regional lymph node metastases.

Primary Prevention of Adenoma Recurrence

Primary prevention relates to the ability to identify genetic, environmental, and biologic factors that cause cancer, and to alter their effects. Laboratory, clinical, and epidemiologic evidence suggests that the regular use of nonsteroidal anti-inflammatory drugs (NSAIDs), including aspirin, is associated with a decreased risk for the development of colorectal cancer. The number of colorectal adenomas discovered among regular NSAID users is lower than that in nonusers in most observational studies. Several trials of varying designs to assess the effect of NSAIDs on colorectal cancer development in average-risk populations have demonstrated a small but significant decreases in incident polyps among the aspirin groups.[27,28] Aspirin and other NSAIDs are associated with toxicity, and their use has not become a standard of care for average-risk individuals.

Trials of antioxidant vitamins such as beta-carotene and vitamins C and E have not convincingly demonstrated any effect on adenoma recurrence. Experimental data from animal studies and limited data from studies of human cancers suggest a potential role for inhibitors of the enzyme cyclooxygenase-2 (COX-2) in adenoma and cancer prevention. Cyclooxygenase is the key enzyme responsible for the production of prostaglandins and other eicosanoids. The COX-2 isoform is induced by inflammation and is elevated in adenomas and colorectal cancers. Unfortunately, toxicity associated with these agents makes them unsuitable as preventative agents in otherwise healthy subjects. Supplemental calcium reduces proliferative activity in the mucosa of experimental animals and patients at high-risk for the development of colorectal cancer.

A
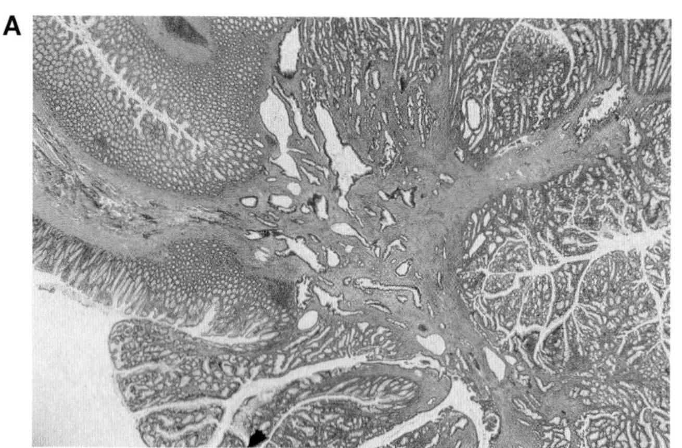
B
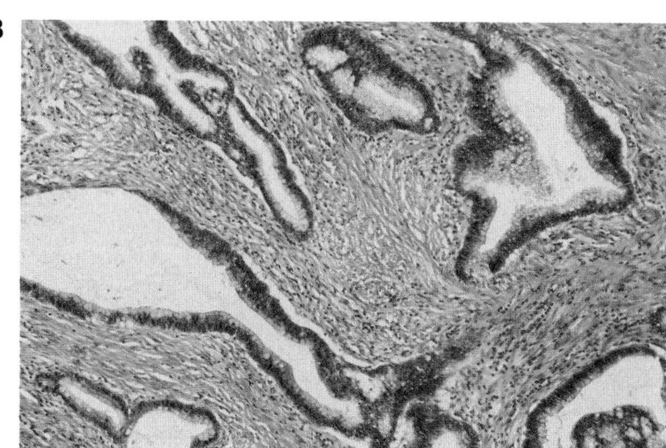

FIGURE 69.8 Invasive carcinoma in the stalk of an adenomatous polyp. (*A*) Low power view. Malignant glands can be seen invading fibrovascular stalk. (*B*) High power magnification of malignant glands in stalk. Nuclei are large, hyperpigmented, and crowded.

Clinical evidence suggests a modest reduction in polyp recurrence in patients taking supplemental daily calcium.[29] Little harm, and little impact on polyp incidence or progression will result from calcium supplements alone.

NONNEOPLASTIC MUCOSAL POLYPS

Hyperplastic Polyps

Hyperplastic polyps are small, usually sessile lesions most frequently encountered in the distal colon and rectum (Figure 69.9A). Although grossly indistinguishable from small adenomas, they carry no significant potential for malignant degeneration. Microscopically, hyperplastic polyps are characterized by a serrated epithelial pattern representing micropapillary luminal infoldings of columnar absorptive cells and mature, frequently hyperdistended goblet cells (Fig. 69.9B). Elongation and subsequent in-folding of the epithelium may be caused by an expanded, but otherwise normally located, replication zone in the crypt. The cytologic atypia found in adenomatous polyps is not seen in these lesions.

Hyperplastic polyps are common age-related lesions found in about one third of the population older than 50 years. Although they often coexist with adenomas in polyp-bearing patients, no convincing evidence has been found that hyperplastic polyps are harbingers of adenoma development. These polyps are most common in the distal colon and rectum and are usually diminutive. Because hyperplastic polyps are asymptomatic and carry no malignant potential, no specific treatment is required for these lesions. If a hyperplastic polyp is the only lesion detected on index flexible sigmoidoscopy or colonoscopy, no further evaluation is indicated.

In contrast, serrated polyps have the dysplastic cytological features of the adenoma, and the serrated surface features of the hyperplastic polyp. These may create difficult diagnostic decisions for non-experienced pathologists. There is evidence

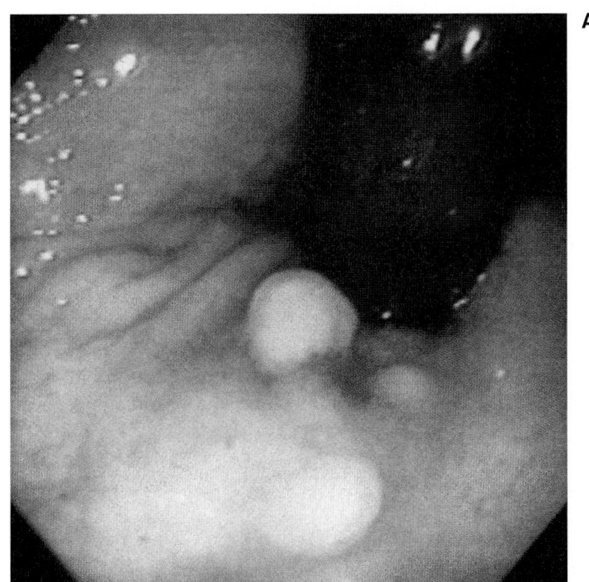

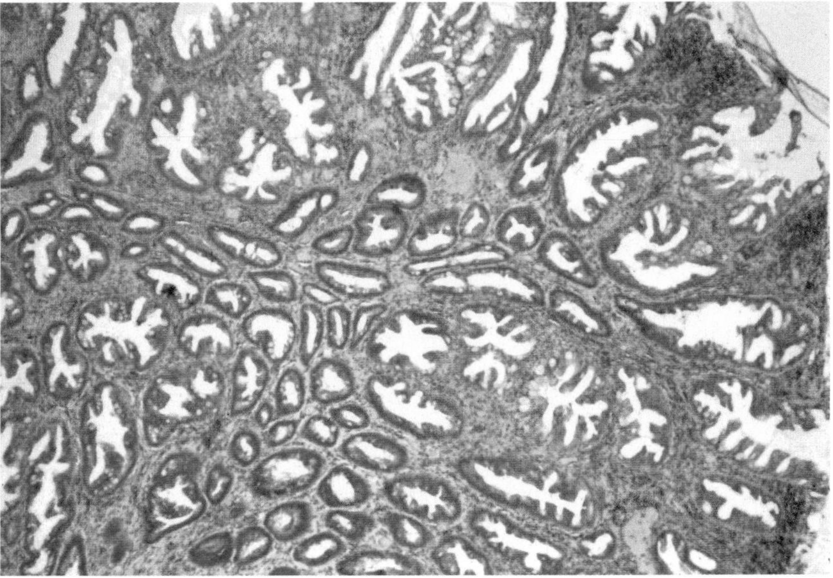

FIGURE 69.9 Hyperplastic polyps. (*A*) Several diminutive hyperplastic polyps seen in the rectum during flexible sigmoidoscopy. (*B*) Photomicrograph of a hyperplastic polyp, characterized by elongated glands with papillary infoldings that have a typical serrated epithelial pattern.

that large, serrated polyps in the proximal colon may be the precursors to colorectal cancers of the MSI phenotype. Thus, good clinical judgment would suggest that the small hyperplastic polyps commonly seen in the distal colon should not be a trigger for colonoscopic surveillance, but that larger "serrated polyps" in the proximal colon should raise clinical concerns, and be followed up like an advanced adenoma.[30]

Juvenile Polyps

Juvenile polyps, also known as *retention polyps,* can occur sporadically or as part of a familial polyposis syndrome. These mucosal polyps consist of dilated cystic mucus-filled glands, and abundant lamina propria with an inflammatory infiltrate. Seventy-five percent of these occur in children younger than 10 years of age, often appearing as single pedunculated cherry-red polyps with a smooth surface and contour. The exact prevalence of such lesions has not been determined, but they are thought to be acquired lesions detectable in about 2% of children who do not have symptoms. Juvenile polyps often present in the form of hematochezia because they are highly vascularized lesions. Rectal prolapse and autoamputation may occur with distal lesions, whereas intussusception may be precipitated by proximal juvenile polyps found in the context of familial syndromes. Individually, these polyps have no malignant potential, but symptomatic polyps should be removed to prevent further complications. Juvenile polyposis, in contrast, is associated with an increased risk for the early development of cancer.

Inflammatory Polyps

Inflammatory mucosal polyps are common in the setting of idiopathic inflammatory bowel disease. Marked inflammation and ulceration coexist with granulation tissue in a distorted mucosal architecture that appears polypoid because of confluent areas of ulceration, leaving behind islands of intact epithelium (Fig. 69.10A). Subsequent healing leads to the appearance of polypoid, nonneoplastic excrescences covered by normal colonic epithelium, so-called *pseudopolyps* (Fig. 69.10B). They need not be removed and are important largely because they make it difficult to recognize subtle, early neoplastic lesions in these high-risk patients. Severe chronic inflammation of any kind, including a variety of infectious diseases (tuberculosis, amebiasis, schistosomiasis, amebic colitis), may result in inflammatory polyps that resemble those found in idiopathic inflammatory bowel disease.

Submucosal Polyps

Submucosal masses can expand to push the colonic mucosa into the bowel lumen and thus appear as polypoid lesions. Many submucosal lesions (e.g., lipomas, leiomyomas) are clinically asymptomatic and must be differentiated from neoplastic lesions. Others are malignant lesions that require early detection, such as lymphomas and metastatic tumors. Many submucosal lesions are not detected on endoscopic mucosal biopsy because standard biopsy forceps do not reach beyond the mucosa. If a submucosal lesion is suspected, multiple biopsy specimens of the same site sometimes provides tissue for diagnosis.

Lipomas are benign fatty tumors that occur throughout the gastrointestinal tract but are most commonly found in the cecum near the ileocecal valve (Fig. 69.11). They appear endoscopically as soft, smooth polyps that are pliable and deformable. The overlying mucosa is intact but may be light yellow in appearance. These are benign lesions that have little clinical significance, and are commonly seen in obese patients.

Isolated *lymphoid nodules* consisting of benign lymphoid tissue may appear as sessile smooth polyps of various sizes, with a predilection for the distal colon and rectum. These are usually asymptomatic. Diffuse nodular lymphoid hyperplasia

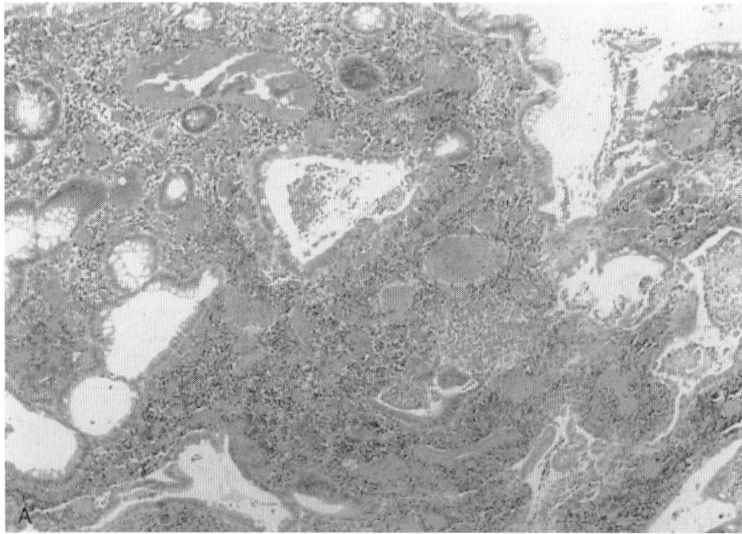

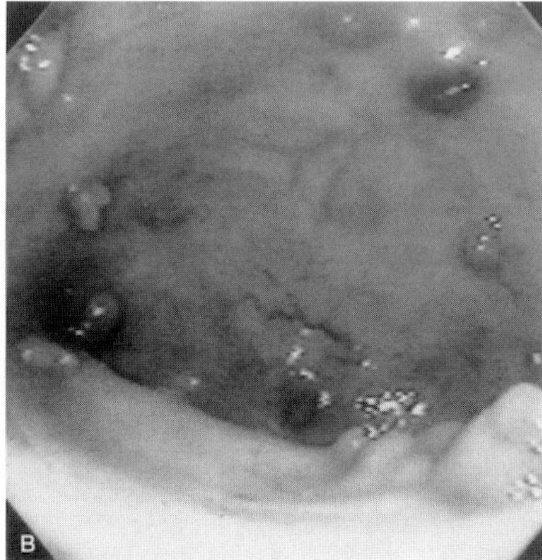

FIGURE 69.10 Inflammatory polyps. (*A*) Severe mucosal inflammation with infiltrates and granulation tissue shown here microscopically can appear clinically with a polypoid configuration. (*B*) Resolution of inflammation can leave exuberant polyps covered by normal epithelium, which are called *pseudopolyps*, a misnomer. These are truly polyps, but are not neoplastic.

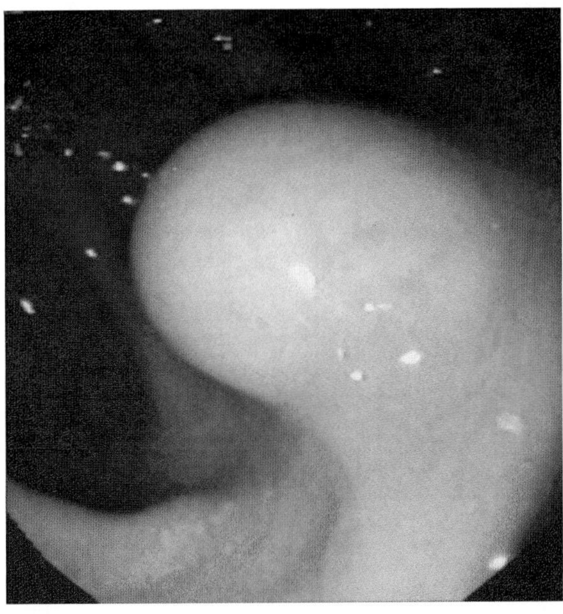

A

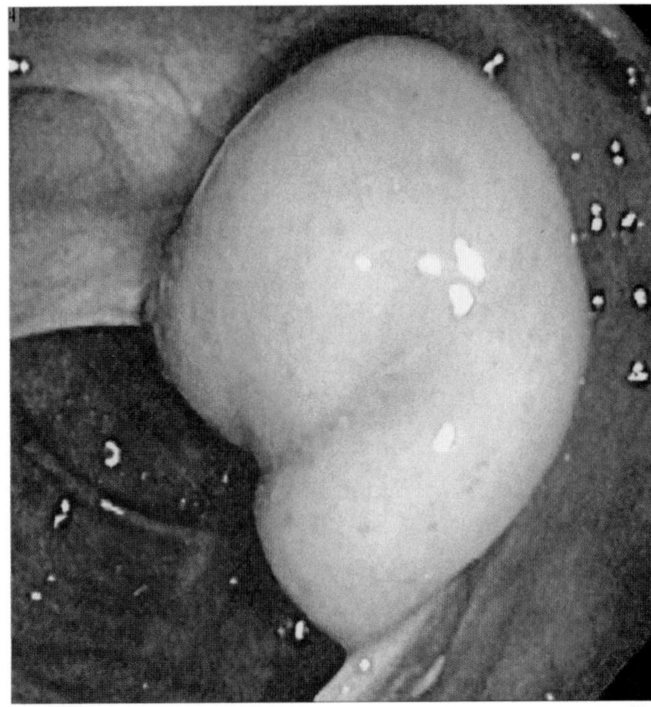

B

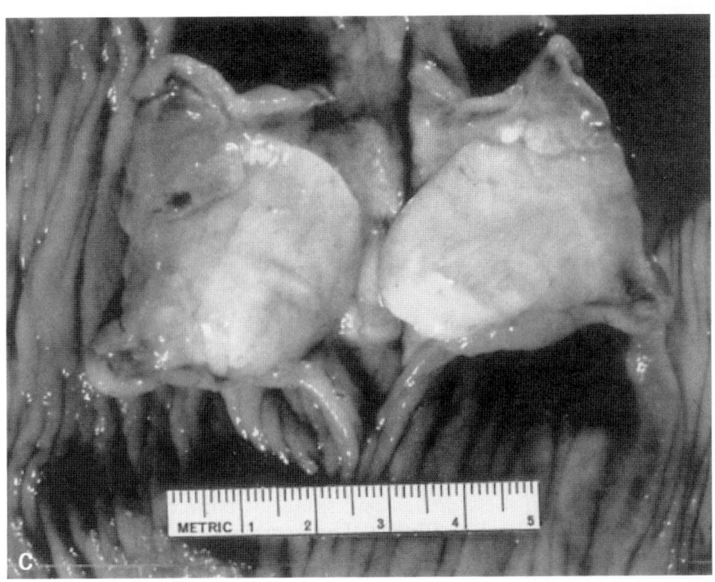

C

FIGURE 69.11 Submucosal lipomas. (*A*) Lipoma seen at colonoscopy. Submucosal fatty tissue causes the mucosa to protrude into the lumen; such protrusion appears as a polyp. Overlying mucosa is smooth. (*B*) Lipomatous infiltration of ileocecal valve seen at colonoscopy. (*C*) Colectomy specimen showing a large submucosal lipoma cut in cross section.

also occurs in children as an incidental finding. The nodules must be distinguished from primary or secondary lymphoma of the large intestine, which may present as mucosal nodularity resembling the pseudopolyposis of inflammatory bowel disease or even polyposis (Fig. 69.12).

Pneumatosis cystoides intestinalis consists of multiple air-filled cysts within the submucosa. This may be an incidental finding in patients with chronic obstructive pulmonary disease, scleroderma, or asymptomatic pneumoperitoneum secondary to recent surgery or instrumentation, in which air or colonic gas diffuses into the cysts. These cysts sometimes resolve with administration of oxygen. A far more virulent form of pneumatosis is associated with fulminant mucosal inflammation, ischemia, or necrotizing enterocolitis in children. These cysts are thought to result from mucosal invasion by gas-producing bacteria.

Colitis cystica profunda is a rare condition in which the intestinal wall is thickened by submucosal mucus-filled cysts of various sizes and an accumulation of fibroblasts in the lamina propria. It can present as an ulcerating or mass lesion in the rectosigmoid in association with the solitary rectal ulcer syndrome. Although the pathogenesis of this condition is unknown, it may result from the downward displacement of colonic glands during trauma or chronic inflammation followed by healing. The appearance of aberrant submucosal glandular epithelium and acellular mucous lakes must be distinguished from a colloid carcinoma, because this lesion has no malignant potential.

Carcinoid tumors of the rectum appear as isolated, small, yellow-gray submucosal nodules. These findings are often incidental during sigmoidoscopy. Most carcinoid tumors of the rectum are smaller than 1 cm, have little malignant

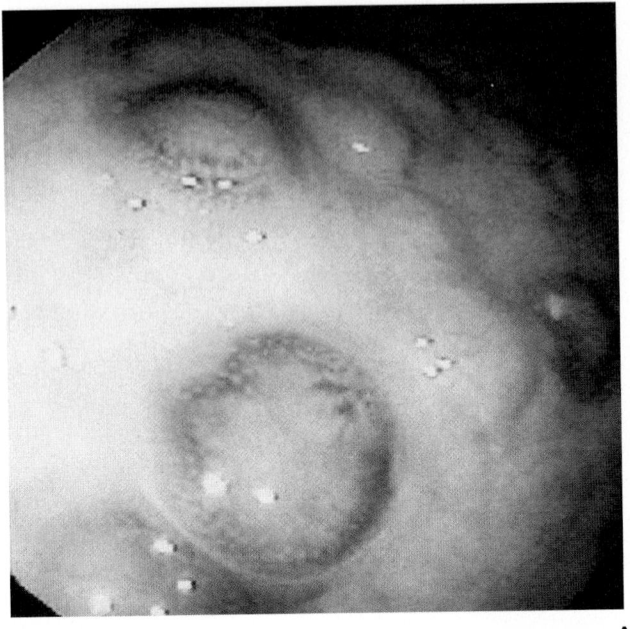

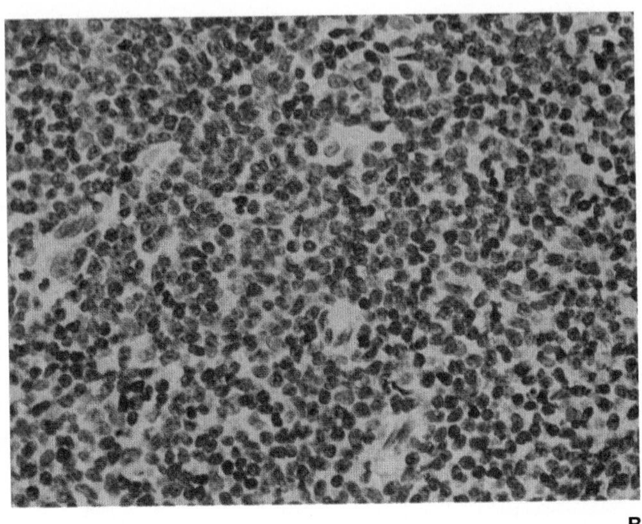

FIGURE 69.12 Lymphomatous polyposis of the colon. (*A*) Colonoscopic view of B-cell lymphoma presenting as multiple colonic polyps. (*B*) Histology of lymphoma is one of the polyps.

potential, and are amenable to local excision. Lesions larger than 2 cm are more likely to be malignant, but seldom give rise to metastases. These lesions should be treated aggressively with complete excision. Rectal carcinoid tumors are usually asymptomatic but may present with hematochezia. They are not associated with the carcinoid syndrome. Carcinoid tumors in the proximal colon may be locally invasive or metastasize to the liver, liberating vasoactive peptides into the systemic circulation and producing the carcinoid syndrome.

Other lesions that can present as submucosal polyps include *metastatic tumors*, such as malignant melanoma, and benign lesions, such as *leiomyomas*, *fibromas*, *lymphangiomas*, *hemangiomas*, and *endometriosis*.

GASTROINTESTINAL POLYPOSIS SYNDROMES

Gastrointestinal polyposis indicates the presence of a systemic process that promotes the development of multiple polyps throughout the gastrointestinal tract. In some instances, the polyps are located predominantly in the colon; however, in others, polyps may be found in the stomach, small intestine, colon, and rectum. The classification of the polyposis syndromes has traditionally been based on the histologic characteristics of the polyps, but gradually an awareness of the genetic basis for the most important of these syndromes has permitted more precise diagnosis and rational approaches to treatment.

Familial Adenomatous Polyposis

FAP is an autosomal dominant, genetic disease characterized by the development of multiple adenomatous polyps throughout the colon and rectum (Fig. 69.13). The polyps first appear in adolescence, with the median age of onset being about 16 years. The number of polyps in each patient is variable, and they increase in number and size with advancing age. The genetic basis for this disease is a germline mutation in the *APC* gene located on chromosome 5q. In part, the age of onset, number of polyps, and age at which cancer develops are determined by the location of the mutation in the *APC* gene. More than 5,000 polyps eventually develop in patients with the most severe types of mutation, and cancer develops in these patients at a mean age of 35 years. Other mutations in the APC gene can give rise to attenuated forms of the disease in which only a few (i.e., 20 to 100) polyps are likely, and the median age for cancer development may be in the 50s or 60s. Additional factors not related to the mutation on the *APC* gene, some genetic and some environmental, also modify the clinical characteristics of the disease.[31,32]

Gastrointestinal Features

Polyps in the stomach and small intestine develop in about 90% of patients with FAP. The gastric polyps primarily consist of fundic gland hyperplasia, which is not a premalignant lesion. Occasionally, gastric adenomas are found, but stomach cancer is only rarely reported as a complication of FAP in North America, where the incidence of gastric cancer is low.

Small-intestinal neoplasia is not rare in FAP and principally occurs in the periampullary region of the duodenum. Duodenal adenomatous polyps, which typically appear later than the colonic lesions, may be multiple but tend not to carpet the proximal small intestine. The ampulla of Vater is a particular target for neoplastic development. With time, carcinoma develops in up to 5% to10% of these patients, so that duodenal surveillance is required. Adenomas and carcinomas occur in the jejunum and ileum, but these are rare. Polyps in the terminal ileum are more likely to represent lymphoid aggregates than adenomas and should be sampled for diagnostic purposes.

Classically, it has been stated that the natural history of FAP is for cancer to develop at a median age of 40 to 45 years. As mentioned, the development of cancer is variable and again is based in part on the location of the germline mutation in the *APC* gene. Colon cancer is rare before age 30 years, and cancer may not develop in patients with the attenuated form of

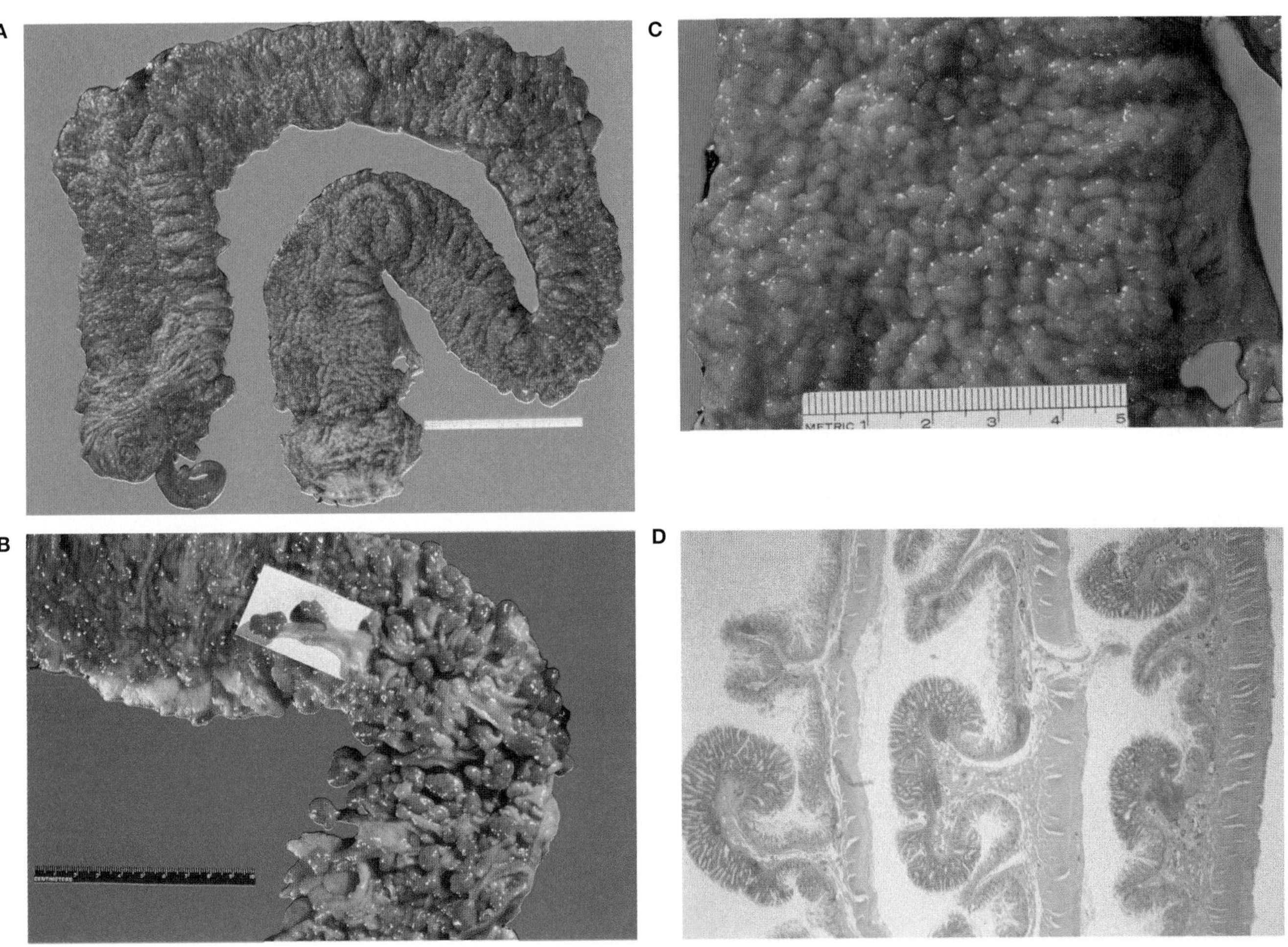

FIGURE 69.13 Familial adenomatous polyposis (FAP). (*A*) Gross specimen of a resected colon from a patient with FAP. (*B*) Sessile and pedunculated adenomatous polyps in the colon of a patient with FAP. (*C*) Close-up view of a profuse type of FAP, in which the mucosa is carpeted with innumerable polyps. (*D*) Photomicrograph demonstrating profuse FAP with both sessile and pedunculated adenomatous polyps.

FAP until they are in their 50s or 60s. Cancer occurring in the teenage years has been reported as a result of a patient who had both FAP and Lynch syndrome.[33] Thus, the treatment of these patients relies increasingly on a genetic characterization of the disease.

Extraintestinal Features

Traditionally, patients with manifestations of FAP together with extraintestinal manifestations were considered to have Gardner syndrome. It is now appreciated that families with FAP all have extraintestinal manifestations and that no distinction can be made between families with Gardner's syndrome and other families with FAP.[34] FAP is characterized by osteomas of the mandible, skull, and long bones and a variety of other benign soft-tissue tumors, such as fibromas and lipomas (Fig. 69.14). Osteomas are commonly found in the skull and may be multiple. Some of these lesions have been reported to regress and later reappear. Osteomas may also be found in the mandible, and radiographs of the mouth may reveal impacted or supernumerary teeth. Congenital hypertrophy of the retinal pigmented epithelium (CHRPE) is present in some families with FAP, depending on the location of the mutation in the *APC* gene. CHRPE lesions may be seen in the general population but are small and usually single. Multiple, bilateral, and large CHRPE lesions are essentially diagnostic of FAP.

Malignant tumors in the colon are considered to be nearly inevitable, and they may occur occasionally in the duodenum or (less commonly) elsewhere in the gastrointestinal tract. Patients with FAP are also at increased risk for brain tumors (particularly medulloblastomas), thyroid tumors, adrenal tumors, and malignant tumors of the hepatobiliary tree. The occurrence of a malignant brain tumor in conjunction with intestinal polyposis was traditionally referred to as *Turcot syndrome*, although this is not a distinctive disease process. Medulloblastomas are a rare complication of FAP, and the risk for this tumor is increased 99-fold in FAP families. Interestingly, one of the index families initially reported by Turcot in 1959 (and several others characterized as Turcot syndrome) did not have FAP, but actually had Lynch syndrome complicated by astrocytomas.[16]

Desmoid Tumors

Desmoid tumors are currently the major cause of mortality and morbidity in FAP (after colorectal cancer), and develop in 10% to 15% of such patients, often as a complication of laparotomy, but sometimes spontaneously. These are benign

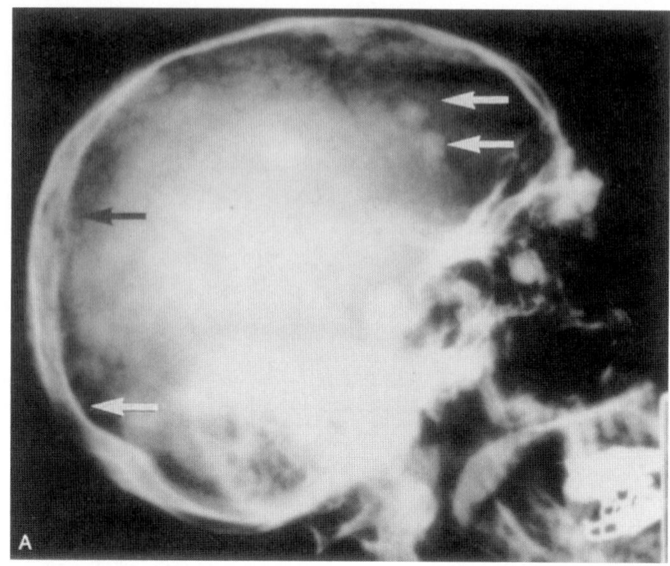

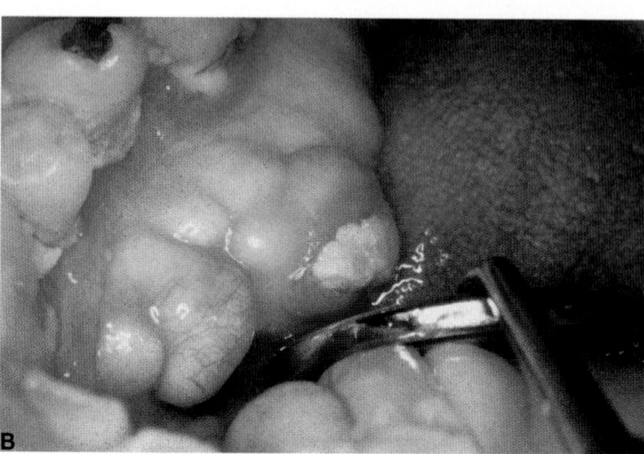

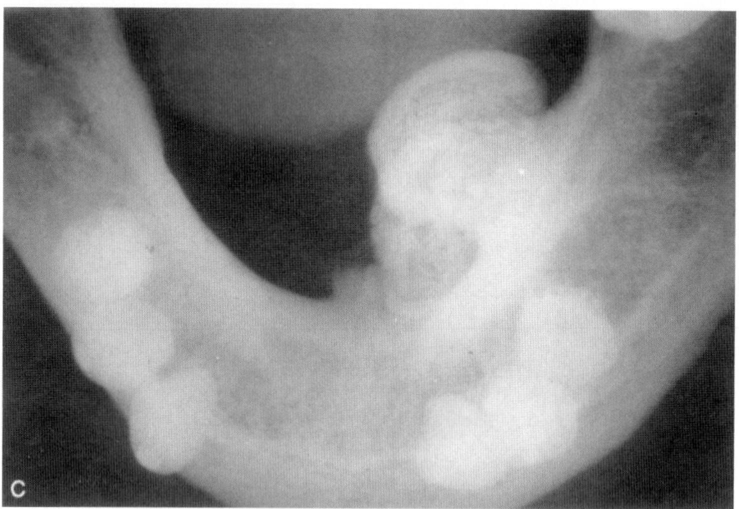

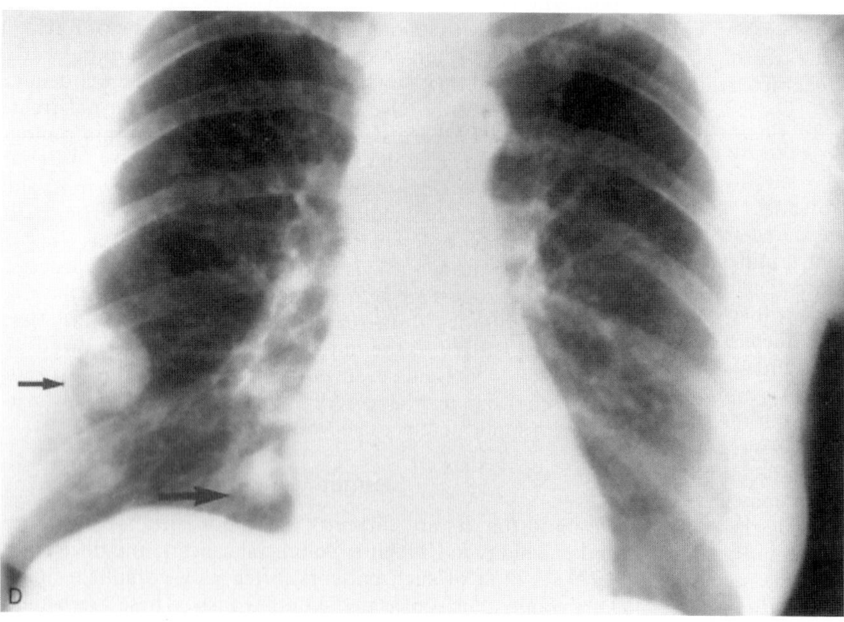

FIGURE 69.14 Extraintestinal manifestations of familial adenomatous polyposis (FAP). (*A*) Skull film demonstrating osteomas of the calvarium (*arrows*). (*B*) Photograph of the mandible demonstrating protuberant mandibular osteomas. (*C*) Mandibular radiograph demonstrating a large osteoma of the mandible. (*D*) Chest radiograph demonstrating multiple fibromas (*arrows*) in a patient with FAP.

but aggressive tumors of mesenteric fibroblasts that can envelop and obstruct the gastrointestinal tract, arteries, veins, or ureters. They frequently occur in the abdominal wall. In some instances, desmoid tumors can become quite large, may virtually fill the abdominal cavity, and can be lethal.

Genetic Basis

FAP occurs when a germline mutation in the *APC* gene inactivates the function of the *APC* gene product. In most instances, the genetic lesion creates a premature stop codon in the *APC* gene, which in turn leads to the translation of a truncated APC protein. The *APC* gene encodes a large protein (311 kd) that binds to other intracellular proteins—namely the catenins and E-cadherin.[5] Depending on the location of the premature stop codon, the mutant protein is of variable length. The *APC* gene encodes 2843 codons (i.e., one for each amino acid) and is broken into 15 translated exons. The structure of the *APC* gene is unique in that the 15th exon makes up about 75% of the coding sequences of the gene. Because it is unusually large, this long, open reading frame is a natural target for the types of mutations that result in premature stop codons.

The location of the germline mutation is of some clinical significance (Fig. 69.15). For example, mutations that occur at the 5-prime end of the gene, particularly in the first three exons, result in a clinically mild or "attenuated" form of FAP, in which the number of polyps is smaller and the onset of disease about 10 years later, with cancer developing in the sixth or seventh decade.[35] This occurs because the APC gene has a ribosomal reentry site downstream of the mutation, which permits the cell to bypass and ignore the premature stop codon. To complicate the situation, family members with the same mutation may have variable manifestations of the disease. Indeed, some members who inherit this mutation have few polyps and no cancer, yet can pass an increased risk for cancer to their progeny.

In contrast, mutations that occur in the "mutation cluster region" of the 15th exon, in a segment between codons 1250 and 1464, are associated with a particularly virulent form of the disease, in which the number of polyps is greater than 5,000 and the average age for the development of colorectal cancer at significantly earlier (median age, 34 years). A majority of the acquired mutations that occur in sporadic cancers are also located in this region. For reasons that are not entirely clear, mutations at the extreme 3-prime end of the gene are also associated with a milder phenotype, with fewer polyps, and later onset of cancer.

In families who have FAP with CHRPE lesions, the mutations are almost always in exons 9 to 15, and rarely in families whose mutations are in the first eight exons. Thus, a detailed knowledge of the location of the germline mutation can be used to predict the clinical manifestations and guide therapy.

Diagnosis

The clinical diagnosis of FAP is usually obvious clinically, but the availability of a genetic diagnosis has changed the approach to this disease. Currently, optimal practice is to obtain a germline diagnosis in an individual who is definitely affected, in order to characterize and counsel the family. A mutation in *APC* can be found in most approximately 80%) of these individuals using commercially available reference laboratories. This test will assist in the early and definitive identification of family members who carry the disease-causing mutation and will alleviate anxiety for those who do not. The risk to inherit the mutated gene from an affected parent is 50%, and there is no gender preference.

In some instances, the phenotype indicates FAP, but no mutation can be found in the *APC* gene. In this instance, the relatives at risk should undergo surveillance sigmoidoscopy on an annual basis beginning in their middle teens. The entire colon is at risk for the development of neoplasia, so sigmoidoscopy is sufficient to detect carriers of the abnormal gene. If a single adenoma appears in a teenager at risk, the disease is strongly suspected, and the individual should be managed as if he or she is a mutation carrier. Almost no other disease produces multiple adenomatous polyps in young patients.

About 25% of patients have FAP that does not appear to be present in either parent. This can represent a new mutation, an autosomal recessive form of the disease (*MYH*-associated polyposis, as discussed later), misattribution of paternity, or phenotypic variation in which a parent actually has a milder form of the disease.

Genetic testing can be fraught with misunderstandings. The genetic results are sometimes ambiguous and difficult for the physician to interpret.[36] Additionally, some patients mistake the germline test as a test for cancer. Issues of guilt and denial are prominent in genetic disorders. It is strongly recommended that physicians enlist the involvement of genetic counselors when performing genetic testing and counseling in such patients.

Management

Surgery is the only reasonable management option in FAP, and the clinical decision involves the selection and timing of the operation. The diagnosis of FAP is often made in adolescence, but the development of cancer may not be anticipated for 20 to 30 years after the first polyp appears, depending upon the location of the mutation in the *APC* gene. When an child is found to have a germline mutation in *APC*, sigmoidoscopy should begin in the early teenage years, particularly if the mutation is in the "mutation cluster region," or the family's phenotype is known to be associated with thousands of polyps. Ideally, one would like a patient to reach adulthood prior to the colectomy, as the pelvis is larger, and the individual is better able to cope with the disease psychologically. The safest surgical approach is a total proctocolectomy with an ileoanal pouch anastomosis. No rectal mucosa should be left behind because it is at risk for the development of neoplasia. Even with careful endoscopic surveillance of the rectal segment, invasive carcinomas may develop.

The fact that small adenomatous polyps of the rectum can spontaneously regress after a subtotal colectomy and ileorectal anastomosis underscores the reversible nature of the benign adenoma. Additionally, it has been found that adenomas can regress in FAP in response to treatment with sulindac (Clinoril). Several reports have confirmed that even large numbers of polyps regress in patients on 150 to 200 mg of sulindac twice per day.[37] Unfortunately, the polyps reappear when the drug is stopped, and development of cancer despite treatment with sulindac has been reported. Medical treatment is therefore not a safe or reliable first-line treatment for FAP, but it may be of some benefit in patients who delay operative intervention. Although no data are available to support this approach, sulindac may be a useful adjunct in patients with milder forms of FAP (i.e., smaller numbers of polyps with relative rectal sparing) and in circumstances in which residual rectal tissue must be left behind. Sulindac is not effective in the management of upper gastrointestinal tract neoplasia.

Management of Extracolonic Disease. In addition to the risks for colorectal neoplasia, patients with FAP are at risk for the development of osteomas, lipomas, fibromas, and a variety of other lesions. Although the these mesenchymal tumors can degenerate into sarcomas, this is a sufficiently rare event that prophylactic surveillance and surgery are not indicated. Likewise, the CHRPE lesions do not require ther-

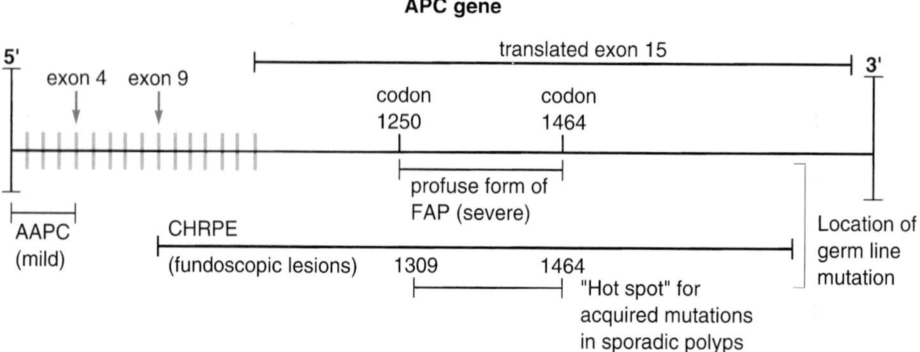

FIGURE 69.15 This scheme of the *APC* (*adenomatous polyposis coli*) gene illustrates the genotype-phenotype correlations. Most mutations of *APC* result in premature stop codons; therefore, the site of the mutation usually indicates the relative length of the mutant protein product. Mutations at the 5′ end of the gene produce "attenuated" FAP, a milder form of the disease. The retinal lesions (congenital hypertrophy of retinal pigmented epithelium, or CHRPE) occur when the mutations are between exons 9 and 15. The portion of the *APC* gene that binds to other cytoskeletal elements in the cell (β-catenins) is represented at the 3′ end of the 15th exon. Mutations in a hot spot immediately downstream from the β-catenin-binding site (between codons 1250 and 1464) result in a more virulent, profuse form of familial adenomatous polyposis. This site is also the location of most of the acquired mutations in sporadic colorectal neoplasms.

apy. Gastric carcinoma is distinctly uncommon in North American populations, and it is not necessary to provide endoscopic surveillance of the stomach. The risk for this disease is about 1%.

The two major management issues after removal of the colon and rectum are periampullary neoplasia and desmoid tumors. One or more adenomas are found in the duodenum in 90% of patients with FAP, usually close to the ampulla of Vater. These lesions should be excised for biopsy and destroyed by electrocautery, laser, or other ablative approaches. Although no data are available to indicate the optimal intervals for safe surveillance, it seems prudent to examine the duodenum about every 2 years. Complex neoplasms, including adenomas with varying degrees of dysplasia, may require individualized management, including the use of biliary stents while extensive ablative therapy of the periampullary region is performed. Surgical approaches may be required for advanced neoplasms (i.e., carcinoma in situ or invasive carcinoma), but therapeutic endoscopy remains the first option. Duodenotomy with local surgical excision is an option for these lesions; rarely, a Whipple's procedure is required for difficult lesions in this region.

Desmoid tumors are aggressive benign tumors of fibroblasts that can cause multiple clinical complications; they are a significant cause of morbidity and mortality in FAP. They typically grow slowly and can surround or compress vascular structures, nerves, or the abdominal viscera. They are more commonly seen in women and may be hormonally responsive, so estrogen administration (oral contraceptives or hormone replacement therapy) should be avoided in these patients. Surgical management is generally avoided unless simple local excision of an abdominal wall lesion is possible, and postoperative recurrences are common. Radiotherapy has been used to control the growth of some of these tumors but is generally reserved for superficial lesions of the abdominal wall. No medical approach to this disease has been uniformly successful. A combination of sulindac plus tamoxifen may be tried for intraabdominal tumors and has been successful in some patients. Cytotoxic chemotherapy with doxorubicin was successful in a patient whose tumor was refractory to other treatment. Anecdotally, some of these lesions may have *c-kit* mutations, and are responsive to imatinib (Gleevec).

Familial Adenomatous Polyposis Variants

A number of names, especially *Gardner syndrome,* have been attached to variations of FAP to emphasize the presence of particular extracolonic findings. Actually, Gardner syndrome is the same entity as FAP; all families with Gardner syndrome have mutations in the *APC* gene, and virtually all families with FAP have the stigmata previously attributed to Gardner syndrome. A few families with prominent sebaceous cysts were formerly said to have Oldfield syndrome, and families with brain tumors were said to have Turcot syndrome. All these syndromes represent the variable expression of germline mutations in the *APC* gene and are largely of historical interest. The current mode of classifying FAP families is based on the *APC* gene mutation.

MYH-Associated Polyposis

An autosomal recessive form of polyposis has been linked to inheritance of germline mutations in the base excision repair gene *MYH*, a DNA glycolase.[38] This association should be considered when multiple adenomatous polyps occur in siblings or in a person who has no family history of polyposis and in which is no detectable germline mutation in the *APC* gene. These patients have a relatively mild (attenuated) form of adenomatous polyposis, will develop 20 to 500 adenomas, and the polyposis is typically detected in patients 35 to 65 years old. These patients are at very high risk for colorectal cancer, and the disease may present with cancer. The extraintestinal manifestations of FAP, such as duodenal adenomas or CHRPE lesions occur, but are less common in this condition. The pathogenesis of this disease is that the germline mutations in *MYH* permit an excess number of acquired mutations in the *APC* gene to occur in the colon; these mutations are typically G:C (T:A transversions), which is a consequence of losing the DNA base excision repair system. More than 1.3% of the Caucasian population carries single Y165C, G382D, or E466X mutations, and these carriers have a slight increase in colon cancer risk.[39] Many reference laboratories are currently testing for the three commonest *MYH* mutations on DNA sent from patients with a diagnosis of FAP if there is no detectable germline mutation (or deletion) in *APC*.

Peutz-Jeghers Syndrome

Peutz-Jeghers syndrome is an autosomal dominant familial syndrome associated with multiple gastrointestinal polyps and characteristic skin pigmentation. The gene responsible for this disease is on chromosome 19p3.3, and encodes a serine/threonine kinase called *LKB1* or *STK11* (Table 69.2); carriers of the gene are predisposed to a number of early-onset cancers.

Gastrointestinal Features

The gastrointestinal polyps in Peutz-Jeghers syndrome are non-neoplastic hamartomas consisting of a supportive framework of smooth muscle tissue covered by somewhat hyperplastic epithelium (Fig. 69.16). These are histologically distinct from juvenile polyps and show no inflammatory cell infiltrate. Polyps may be found in the stomach, small intestine, or colon, and in each instance they have a distinctive appearance. Peutz-Jeghers polyps can usually be identified as such by the pathologist, and the characteristic cutaneous pigmentation makes this syndrome readily recognizable.

Skin Lesions

The cutaneous manifestations of Peutz-Jeghers syndrome may be found early in life and consist of dark, macular lesions on the mouth (both on the skin and in the buccal mucosa), nose, lips, hands, feet, genitalia, and anus. These lesions tend to become less obvious by the time of puberty. Unlike ordinary freckles, the cutaneous lesions of Peutz-Jeghers syndrome are present from birth. Moreover, ordinary freckles typically do not extend beyond the vermilion border of the lips, nor is the buccal mucosa involved, as it is in Peutz-Jeghers syndrome.

Clinical Complications

The principal complication of Peutz-Jeghers syndrome is intestinal obstruction, which may develop in infancy or childhood. This complication is most prominent in the small intestine because of its narrower diameter. Gastrointestinal bleeding may also be seen in this disease.

Cancer in the small intestine or colon can occur in Peutz-Jeghers syndrome; however, this is an uncommon complication.[40] It is thought that neoplasia may arise from foci of adenomatous epithelium found in some Peutz-Jeghers polyps. The risk for cancer is such that prophylactic surgery is not recommended.

Patients with Peutz-Jeghers syndrome are at increased risk for cancers within and outside the gastrointestinal tract. Cancer developed in about half of the patients in one large study at a median age of about 50 years. At risk are the stomach, small intestine, colorectum, gonads, breasts, pancreas, and biliary tree. Ovarian cysts and sex cord tumors are seen in 5% to 12% of female patients, and boys are at risk for endocrinologically active Sertoli's cell testicular tumors that may produce feminizing features before puberty. No internal organ is individually at sufficiently high risk for cancer that a specific screening regimen or prophylactic surgery is indicated. The clinician should be aware of these risks, however, and should be particularly alert to gonadal tumors (which are otherwise rare) and breast cancer (for which screening should start at an early age, and bilateral disease should be suspected).

Management

The management of Peutz-Jeghers syndrome is limited to the removal of polyps; endoscopic techniques should be used when possible. Surgery may be required for intussusception caused by small-intestinal polyps. The risk for neoplastic development should be kept in mind, but these patients are not candidates for prophylactic removal of any section of the gastrointestinal tract. As mentioned earlier, gonadal neoplasms and breast cancer are potential complications that may require surgery.

Juvenile Polyposis

Juvenile polyps are pathologically characteristic lesions that can be solitary or part of a polyposis syndrome. Juvenile polyps are most commonly solitary lesions found in the rectum during childhood. The lesions may be large and are made up of an edematous, mildly inflamed lamina propria covered by normal colonic epithelium (Fig. 69.17). If multiple polyps are found, a familial juvenile polyposis syndrome should be suspected. Three different syndromic presentations have been reported; it is not known, however, whether these are truly distinctive syndromes. They may consist of familial juvenile polyposis limited to the colon, familial juvenile polyposis throughout the gastrointestinal tract, and familial juvenile polyposis limited to the stomach. The genetic basis of this syndrome is not understood, but germline mutations in the *SMAD4* (also called the *MADH4* gene) and *BMPR1A* genes each account for about 20% of juvenile polyposis cases in which the genetic cause can be found.[41,42] Both these genes are involved in the TGF-beta signaling pathway (Table 69.2). Although alterations the *PTEN* gene had initially been linked to juvenile polyposis, germline mutations in this gene are only found in the rare Bannayan-Riley-Ruvalcaba variant, a childhood disorder characterized by macrocephaly, intestinal polyps and unique pigmented macules of the penis;[43] this disorder shares features with Cowden's syndrome, which is also caused by *PTEN* mutations.[44] Juvenile polyposis is a topic in need of additional clarification at the genetic and clinical levels.

The manifestations of juvenile polyposis can vary but are largely limited to bleeding, intussusception, obstruction, and the passage of autoamputated lesions. In some children, a life-threatening protein-losing enteropathy may develop that requires surgical resection of the affected segment of intestine. Patients with familial juvenile polyposis are at some increased risk for the development of colorectal cancer. It has been suggested that the presence of mixed juvenile and adenomatous polyps indicates which lesions are premalignant. It is important that the pathologist examine lesions carefully for the presence of adenomatous tissue in such polyps. When mixed lesions are found, patients in these families should be subjected to colonoscopic surveillance, perhaps as often as every 2 years.

TABLE 69.2

GENETIC ALTERATIONS IN COLONIC POLYPOSIS SYNDROMES

Polyposis syndrome	Chromosome	Gene
Familial adenomatous polyposis	5q21	*APC* (dominant) *MYH* (recessive)
Peutz-Jeghers syndrome	19p13.3	LKB1/STK11
Juvenile polyposis coli	18q21.1	SMAD4/MADH4 BMPR1A
Bannayan-Riley-Ruvalcaba	10q23	PTEN
Cowden disease	10q23	PTEN
Hereditary mixed polyposis	6q (?)	Unknown

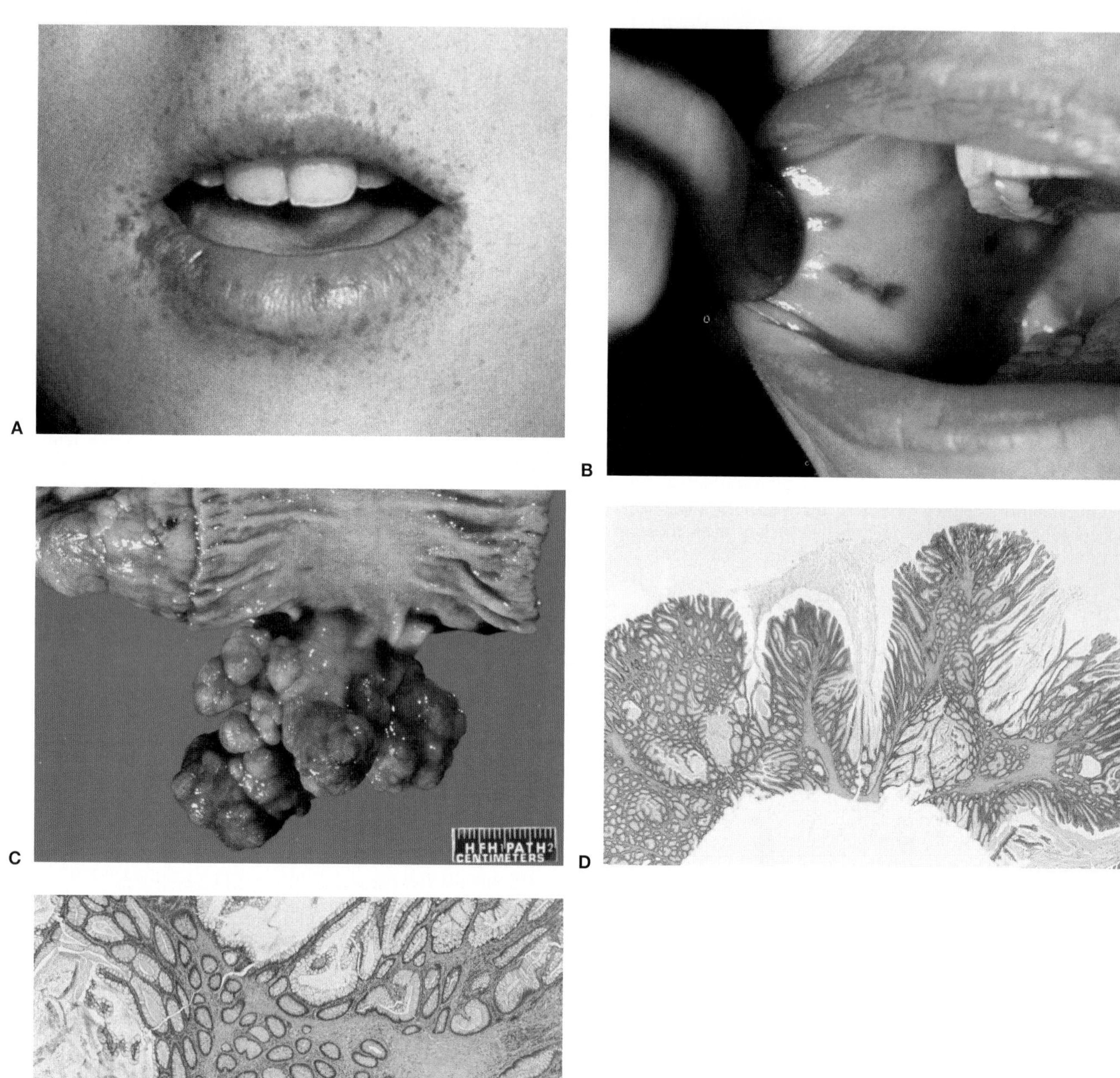

FIGURE 69.16 Peutz-Jeghers syndrome. (*A*) Perioral hyperpigmentation (*B*) Hyperpigmented buccal mucosa (*C*) Gross specimen of a Peutz-Jeghers polyp illustrating a large, multilobular lesion. (*D*) Low-power photomicrograph of a Peutz-Jeghers polyp of the colon revealing smooth-muscle stroma covered by non-neoplastic colonic epithelium. (*E*) photomicrograph of the Peutz-Jeghers polyp at higher power indicates that the stroma contains arborizing bands of smooth muscle.

Other Familial Polyposis Syndromes

A variety of other rare syndromes may give rise to multiple gastrointestinal polyps. Cowden syndrome consists of multiple gastrointestinal hamartomas and may be complicated by multiple lesions of the face that arise from follicular epithelium and are pathologically trichilemmomas.[45] The diagnosis of Cowden syndrome should be considered for patients with multiple trichilemmomas. Gastrointestinal polyps, which are usually asymptomatic, may develop in these patients. The polyps include a variety of nonspecific hamartomas and may include hyperplastic polyps and ganglioneuromas of the colon. Glycogenic acanthosis of the esophagus may also occur and usually is found incidentally as multiple, diminutive, flat polyps of the esophagus. These patients are at increased risk for the development of breast cancer and benign and malignant complications of the thyroid gland. No specific therapy need be directed toward the gastrointestinal tract. Germline mutations of the *PTEN* gene can be identified in most families with Cowden syndrome.[46]

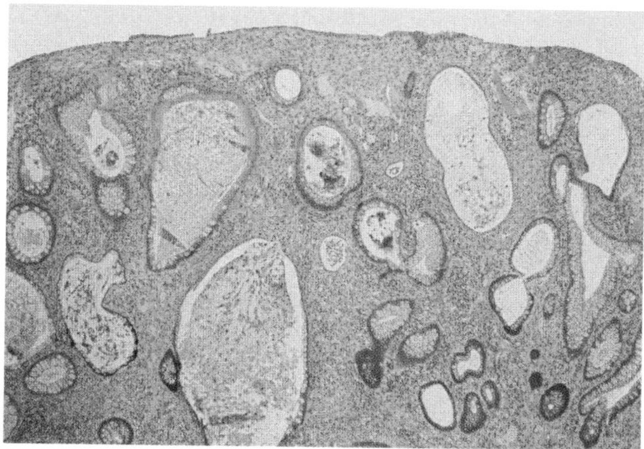

FIGURE 69.17 Photomicrograph of a juvenile polyp reveals an attenuated surface epithelium overlying an edematous lamina propria with fluid-and mucus-filled cystic structures.

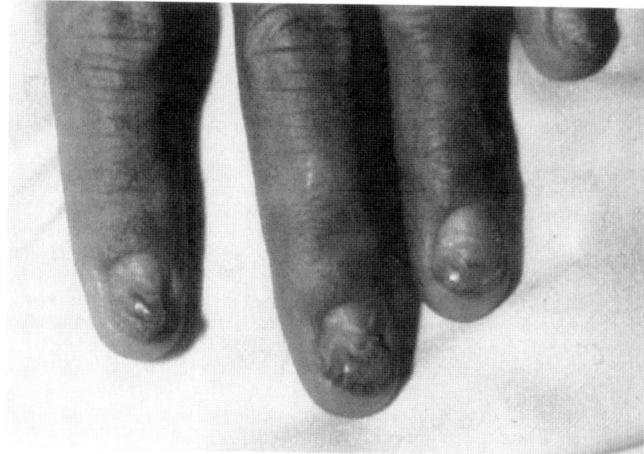

FIGURE 69.18 Cronkhite-Canada syndrome. Onycholysis and hyperpigmentation are characteristic cutaneous manifestations of Cronkhite-Canada syndrome, a nonfamilial, poorly understood, and acquired condition in which multiple juvenile, inflammatory-type gastrointestinal polyps and characteristic cutaneous features are found.

Other diseases, such as neurofibromatosis (von Recklinghausen syndrome) and the basal cell nevus syndrome, may be associated with multiple gastrointestinal polyps; however, symptomatic complications of these polyps are uncommon. Bannayan-Riley-Ruvalcaba syndrome is a generalized hamartoma syndrome inherited in an autosomal dominant manner that is characterized by ileal and colonic polyps and lingual lesions. Other characteristics include ocular abnormalities, delayed motor development, lipid storage myopathy, and Hashimoto disease. This disease is also linked to germline mutations in the *PTEN* gene and appears to be a variant of familial juvenile polyposis.

NONFAMILIAL GASTROINTESTINAL POLYPOSIS SYNDROMES

Multiple gastrointestinal polyps are occasionally seen in nonfamilial syndromes. The Cronkhite-Canada syndrome is an acquired, nonfamilial syndrome characterized by cutaneous lesions (Fig. 69.18), chronic diarrhea, protein-losing enteropathy, and gastrointestinal polyps. The enteropathy may produce progressive inanition that can result in death. The diarrhea is attributable to diffuse mucosal injury of the small intestine but may be complicated by bacterial overgrowth. Gastrointestinal polyps are present in most patients and occur in the stomach, small intestine, colon, and rectum. These polyps are pathologically similar to juvenile retention-type polyps. The lamina propria is edematous and contains an inflammatory infiltrate. As has been reported in juvenile polyps, the lesions in this syndrome may contain adenomatous epithelium, and occasionally carcinomas have complicated this disease. A variety of medical and surgical measures have been used as treatment, and primary attention should be drawn to the treatment of the diarrhea and maintenance of the nutritional status. The cutaneous lesions consist of onycholysis, alopecia, and hyperpigmentation. In a number of cases, treatment of the bacterial overgrowth with antibiotics and maintenance of the nutritional status have resulted in complete resolution of the cutaneous features. Curiously, the cutaneous features may resolve despite persistence of the gastrointestinal polyps.

Other acquired lesions that may present with multiple gastrointestinal polyps include inflammatory pseudopolyps in the setting of inflammatory bowel disease, lymphoma, pneumatosis cystoides intestinalis, and multiple lipomas or hyperplastic polyps. None of these syndromes requires specific surgical treatment.

KEY POINTS

- **Non-neoplastic mucosal polyps include hyperplastic polyps, juvenile polyps, Peutz-Jeghers hamartomas, and a variety of inflammatory polyps, including those associated with inflammatory bowel disease.**
- **Most colorectal cancers arise in preexisting adenomatous polyps.**
- **Neoplastic mucosal epithelium evolves through a series of progressive, cumulative molecular and cellular steps that lead to altered proliferation, cellular accumulation, and glandular disarray.**
- **The malignant potential of adenomatous polyps is related to polyp size and the histologic characteristics.**
- **Lynch syndrome is a disease of autosomal dominant inheritance in which cancers arise in discrete adenomas, but polyposis does not occur.**
- **Familial adenomatous polyposis is an autosomal dominant, genetic disease characterized by the development of multiple adenomatous polyps throughout the colon and rectum.**
- **Peutz-Jeghers syndrome is an autosomal dominant familial syndrome associated with multiple gastrointestinal polyps and characteristic skin pigmentation.**

References

1. Vogelstein B, Kinzler KW. Cancer genes and the pathways they control. *Nat Med*. 2004;10:789–799.
2. Kinzler KW, Vogelstein B. Lessons from hereditary colorectal cancer. *Cell* 1996;87:159–170.
3. Boland CR, Ricciardiello L. How many mutations does it take to make a tumor? *Proc Natl Acad Sci USA*. 1999;96:14675–14677.
4. **Herman JG, Baylin SB. Gene silencing in cancer in association with promoter hypermethylation. *N Engl J Med*. 2003;349:2042–2054.**
5. Powell SM, Zilz N, Beazer-Barclay Y, et al. APC mutations occur early during colorectal tumorigenesis. *Nature* 1992;359:235–237.

6. **Kinzler KW, Vogelstein B. Cancer-susceptibility genes. Gatekeepers and caretakers. *Nature* 1997;386:761, 763.**
7. Su LK, Vogelstein B, Kinzler KW. Association of the APC tumor suppressor protein with catenins. *Science* 1993;262:1734–1737.
8. Boland CR, Sato J, Appelman HD, et al. Microallelotyping defines the sequence and tempo of allelic losses at tumour suppressor gene loci during colorectal cancer progression. *Nat Med.* 1995;1:902–909.
9. **Boland CR. Hereditary non-polyposis colorectal cancer (HNPCC). In: Scriver CR, Beaudet AL, Sly AL, et al., eds. *The molecular and metabolic bases of inherited diseases.* 8th ed. New York: McGraw-Hill; 2001, pp. 769–783.**
10. **Umar A, Boland CR, Terdiman JP, et al. Revised Bethesda guidelines for hereditary nonpolyposis colorectal cancer (Lynch syndrome) and microsatellite instability. *J Natl Cancer Inst.* 2004;96:261–268.**
11. O'Brien MJ, Winawer SJ, Zauber AG, et al. The National Polyp Study. Patient and polyp characteristics associated with high-grade dysplasia in colorectal adenomas. *Gastroenterology* 1990;98:371–379.
12. Fuchs CS, Giovannucci EL, Colditz GA, et al. A prospective study of family history and the risk of colorectal cancer. *N Engl J Med.* 1994;331:1669–1674.
13. Winawer SJ, Zauber AG, Gerdes H, et al. Risk of colorectal cancer in the families of patients with adenomatous polyps. National Polyp Study Workgroup. *N Engl J Med.* 1996;334:82–87.
14. Selby JV, Friedman GD, Quesenberry CP Jr, et al. A case-control study of screening sigmoidoscopy and mortality from colorectal cancer. *N Engl J Med.* 1992;326:653–657.
15. Boland CR, Thibodeau SN, Hamilton SR, et al. A National Cancer Institute Workshop on Microsatellite Instability for cancer detection and familial predisposition: development of international criteria for the determination of microsatellite instability in colorectal cancer. *Cancer Res.* 1998;58:5248–5257.
16. Hamilton SR, Liu B, Parsons RE, et al. The molecular basis of Turcot's syndrome. *N Engl J Med.* 1995;332:839–847.
17. Mandel JS, Bond JH, Church TR, et al. Reducing mortality from colorectal cancer by screening for fecal occult blood. Minnesota Colon Cancer Control Study. *N Engl J Med.* 1993;328:1365–1371.
18. Mandel JS. Screening of patients at average risk for colon cancer. *Med Clin North Am.* 2005;89:43–59, vii.
19. Winawer SJ, Zauber AG, Ho MN, et al. Prevention of colorectal cancer by colonoscopic polypectomy. The National Polyp Study Workgroup. *N Engl J Med.* 1993;329:1977–1981.
20. **Winawer S, Fletcher R, Rex D, et al. Colorectal cancer screening and surveillance: clinical guidelines and rationale-Update based on new evidence. *Gastroenterology* 2003;124:544–560.**
21. Atkin WS, Morson BC, Cuzick J. Long-term risk of colorectal cancer after excision of rectosigmoid adenomas. *N Engl J Med.* 1992;326:658–662.
22. Schoenfeld PS, Cash B, Kita J, et al. Effectiveness and patient satisfaction with screening flexible sigmoidoscopy performed by registered nurses. *Gastrointest Endosc.* 1999;49:158–162.
23. Byers T, Levin B, Rothenberger D, et al. American Cancer Society guidelines for screening and surveillance for early detection of colorectal polyps and cancer: update 1997. American Cancer Society Detection and Treatment Advisory Group on Colorectal Cancer. *CA Cancer J Clin.* 1997;47:154–160.
24. Pickhardt PJ, Choi JR, Hwang I, et al. Computed tomographic virtual colonoscopy to screen for colorectal neoplasia in asymptomatic adults. *N Engl J Med.* 2003;349:2191–2200.
25. Cotton PB, Durkalski VL, Pineau BC, et al. Computed tomographic colonography (virtual colonoscopy): a multicenter comparison with standard colonoscopy for detection of colorectal neoplasia. *JAMA* 2004; 291:1713–1719.
26. Imperiale TF, Ransohoff DF, Itzkowitz SH, et al. Fecal DNA versus fecal occult blood for colorectal-cancer screening in an average-risk population. *N Engl J Med.* 2004;351:2704–2714.
27. Chan AT, Giovannucci EL, Schernhammer ES, et al. A prospective study of aspirin use and the risk for colorectal adenoma. *Ann Intern Med.* 2004;140:157–166.
28. Baron JA, Cole BF, Sandler RS, et al. A randomized trial of aspirin to prevent colorectal adenomas. *N Engl J Med.* 2003;348:891–899.
29. Baron JA, Beach M, Mandel JS, et al. Calcium supplements for the prevention of colorectal adenomas. Calcium Polyp Prevention Study Group. *N Engl J Med.* 1999;340:101–107.
30. **Jass JR, Whitehall VL, Young J, et al. Emerging concepts in colorectal neoplasia. *Gastroenterology* 2002;123:862–876.**
31. Powell SM, Petersen GM, Krush AJ, et al. Molecular diagnosis of familial adenomatous polyposis. *N Engl J Med.* 1993;329:1982–1987.
32. Giardiello FM, Krush AJ, Petersen GM, et al. Phenotypic variability of familial adenomatous polyposis in 11 unrelated families with identical APC gene mutation. *Gastroenterology* 1994;106:1542–1547.
33. Scheenstra R, Rijcken FE, Koornstra JJ, et al. Rapidly progressive adenomatous polyposis in a patient with germline mutations in both the APC and MLH1 genes: the worst of two worlds. *Gut* 2003;52:898–899.
34. Giardiello FM, Petersen GM, Piantadosi S, et al. APC gene mutations and extraintestinal phenotype of familial adenomatous polyposis. *Gut* 1997;40: 521–525.
35. Giardiello FM, Brensinger JD, Luce MC, et al. Phenotypic expression of disease in families that have mutations in the 5′ region of the adenomatous polyposis coli gene. *Ann Intern Med.* 1997;126:514–519.
36. Giardiello FM, Brensinger JD, Petersen GM, et al. The use and interpretation of commercial APC gene testing for familial adenomatous polyposis. *N Engl J Med.* 1997;336:823–827.
37. Giardiello FM, Hamilton SR, Krush AJ, et al. Treatment of colonic and rectal adenomas with sulindac in familial adenomatous polyposis. *N Engl J Med.* 1993;328:1313–1316.
38. **Sieber OM, Lipton L, Crabtree M, et al. Multiple colorectal adenomas, classic adenomatous polyposis, and germ-line mutations in MYH. *N Engl J Med.* 2003;348:791–799.**
39. Wang L, Baudhuin LM, Boardman LA, et al. MYH mutations in patients with attenuated and classic polyposis and with young-onset colorectal cancer without polyps. *Gastroenterology* 2004;127:9–16.
40. Giardiello FM, Welsh SB, Hamilton SR, et al. Increased risk of cancer in the Peutz-Jeghers syndrome. *N Engl J Med.* 1987;316:1511–1514.
41. Howe JR, Sayed MG, Ahmed AF, et al. The prevalence of MADH4 and BMPR1A mutations in juvenile polyposis and absence of BMPR2, BMPR1B, and ACVR1 mutations. *J Med Genet.* 2004;41:484–491.
42. Howe JR, Shellnut J, Wagner B, et al. Common deletion of SMAD4 in juvenile polyposis is a mutational hotspot. *Am J Hum Genet.* 2002;70: 1357–1362.
43. Marsh DJ, Coulon V, Lunetta KL, et al. Mutation spectrum and genotype-phenotype analyses in Cowden disease and Bannayan-Zonana syndrome, two hamartoma syndromes with germline PTEN mutation. *Hum Mol Genet.* 1998;7:507–515.
44. Chi SG, Kim HJ, Park BJ, et al. Mutational abrogation of the PTEN/MMAC1 gene in gastrointestinal polyps in patients with Cowden disease. *Gastroenterology* 1998;115:1084–1089.
45. Marra G, Armelao F, Vecchio FM, et al. Cowden's disease with extensive gastrointestinal polyposis. *J Clin Gastroenterol.* 1994;18:42–47.
46. Eng C. PTEN: one gene, many syndromes. *Hum Mutat.* 2003;22:183–198.

CHAPTER 70 ■ COLORECTAL CANCER

ALFRED E. CHANG AND ARDEN M. MORRIS

Adenocarcinoma of the large intestine is the fourth most common malignancy in the United States, with approximately 146,000 new cases diagnosed annually.[1] Malignancies more prevalent than colorectal cancer are those of the prostate, breast, and lung, in decreasing order (Fig. 70.1). Nevertheless, colorectal carcinoma is the second leading cause of all cancer-related deaths after lung cancer. Approximately 56,000 persons die each year in the United States of colorectal cancer. If diagnosed in its early stages, however, this malignancy is curable by surgical treatment with minimal morbidity and mortality.

Because of the potential for cure of early-stage disease, the definition of populations at risk and screening of asymptomatic patients are important considerations. Controlled clinical trials have demonstrated that the multidisciplinary approach to the treatment of localized colorectal cancer has decreased the morbidity and mortality associated with this disease (Fig. 70.2).[2] For recurrent disease, various therapeutic approaches are reviewed. Other colorectal tumors, such as lymphomas, sarcomas, gastrointestinal stromal tumors, and carcinoid tumors, are distinct from adenocarcinoma and are discussed separately at the end of the chapter.

EPIDEMIOLOGY

Worldwide, colorectal cancer ties with breast cancer as the third most frequent cancer, after gastric and lung cancers.[3] An important feature of colorectal cancer is the wide variation in incidence (as much as 30-fold) noted between population groups according to geographic region (Fig. 70.3). These differences do not appear to be solely the result of genetic factors because populations migrating from low- to high-incidence regions experience an increase in the rate of colorectal cancer. Such data provide indirect evidence that environmental factors are involved in the pathogenesis of this disease. Industrialized countries have the highest incidence rates, and numerous studies have linked dietary factors to the development of colorectal cancer. Evidence suggests that this disease may be responsive to dietary manipulations and that its incidence may therefore be reducible.

In the United States, the incidence of colorectal cancer overall has been in decline since 1992, a phenomenon largely attributed to screening. This advantageous trend has been statistically significant only for white males,[4] possibly associated

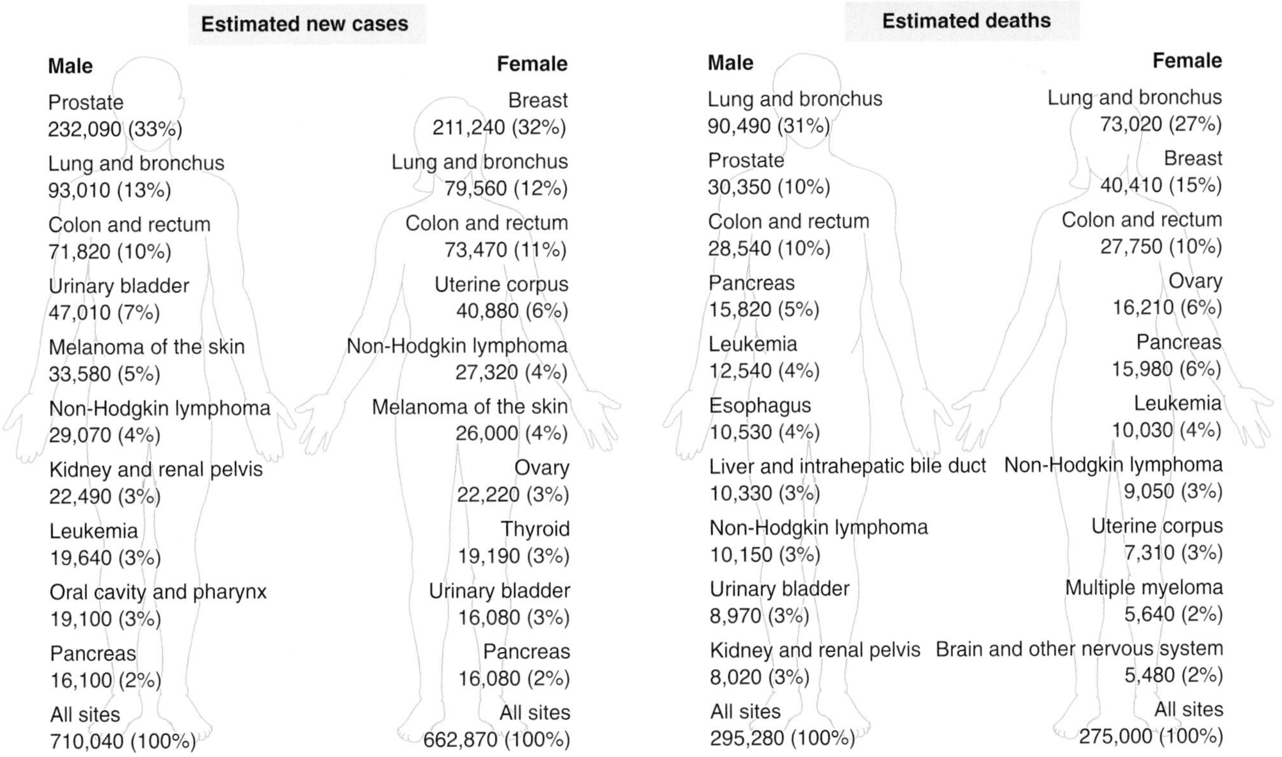

Estimated new cases		Estimated deaths	
Male	**Female**	**Male**	**Female**
Prostate 232,090 (33%)	Breast 211,240 (32%)	Lung and bronchus 90,490 (31%)	Lung and bronchus 73,020 (27%)
Lung and bronchus 93,010 (13%)	Lung and bronchus 79,560 (12%)	Prostate 30,350 (10%)	Breast 40,410 (15%)
Colon and rectum 71,820 (10%)	Colon and rectum 73,470 (11%)	Colon and rectum 28,540 (10%)	Colon and rectum 27,750 (10%)
Urinary bladder 47,010 (7%)	Uterine corpus 40,880 (6%)	Pancreas 15,820 (5%)	Ovary 16,210 (6%)
Melanoma of the skin 33,580 (5%)	Non-Hodgkin lymphoma 27,320 (4%)	Leukemia 12,540 (4%)	Pancreas 15,980 (6%)
Non-Hodgkin lymphoma 29,070 (4%)	Melanoma of the skin 26,000 (4%)	Esophagus 10,530 (4%)	Leukemia 10,030 (4%)
Kidney and renal pelvis 22,490 (3%)	Ovary 22,220 (3%)	Liver and intrahepatic bile duct 10,330 (3%)	Non-Hodgkin lymphoma 9,050 (3%)
Leukemia 19,640 (3%)	Thyroid 19,190 (3%)	Non-Hodgkin lymphoma 10,150 (3%)	Uterine corpus 7,310 (3%)
Oral cavity and pharynx 19,100 (3%)	Urinary bladder 16,080 (3%)	Urinary bladder 8,970 (3%)	Multiple myeloma 5,640 (2%)
Pancreas 16,100 (2%)	Pancreas 16,080 (2%)	Kidney and renal pelvis 8,020 (3%)	Brain and other nervous system 5,480 (2%)
All sites 710,040 (100%)	All sites 662,870 (100%)	All sites 295,280 (100%)	All sites 275,000 (100%)

FIGURE 70.1 Leading sites of new cancer cases and deaths in the United States, 2005. (American Cancer Society. [website], Cancer Facts and Figures 2005. Available at: http://www.cancer.org. Accessed January 2005.)

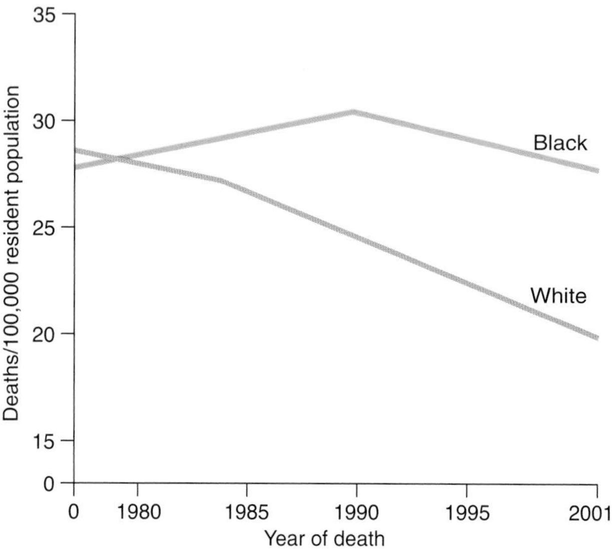

FIGURE 70.2 Mortality trends (1977–2001) for colorectal cancer in the United States for white and black populations. (National Cancer Institute [website], Cancer Statistics. Available at: http://www.nci.nih.gov/statistics/. Accessed January 2005.)

with a greater likelihood of polyp and tumor formation in the rectosigmoid area compared with other demographic groups.[5] Incidence of colon and rectal cancer among white females and black persons has been stable, without a significant annual decline.

In North America, the pattern of geographic regions with a substantially increased risk does not suggest the presence of an important carcinogenic agent, although the incidence of colorectal cancers tends to be greater in urban populations and people of higher socioeconomic status. In addition, no high-risk occupations have been found consistently, and smoking does not play an etiologic role.[6]

ETIOLOGY

Dietary Factors

Evidence from epidemiologic studies suggests that dietary factors play important causative and protective roles in the development of large-bowel cancers. Fat intake has been the most consistently positive association and fiber intake the most consistently inverse association noted in the incidence of colorectal cancer.

In comparisons between countries, the rates of colon cancer are strongly associated with the intake of animal fat and meat (Fig. 70.4).[7] The associations between per capita consumption of total fat, saturated fat, and cholesterol and the national incidence rates of colon cancer are strongly positive.[8] The proposed mechanism by which dietary fat increases the risk for colonic cancer is its interaction with bile acids, discussed in more detail later. In industrialized countries, red meat intake has consistently been associated with elevated long-term risk of cancer in the distal but not the proximal colon.[9–11] The site-specific nature of fat- and meat-associated tumorigenesis may be a result of prolonged toxin exposure in the distal colon, given its relatively slower transit time and narrowed lumen. The relation between fiber intake and colon cancer was initially noted by Burkitt,[12] who reported low rates of colon cancer in areas of Africa where fiber consumption and stool bulk are high. In general, epidemiologic studies have demonstrated that fiber intake is higher in nonindustrialized countries with lower incidence rates of colon cancer. However, in countries where fiber intake is high, the intake of fat and frequently the life expectancy also tend to be lower, so that confounding variables are introduced. The role of fiber was originally seen simply as the provision of bulk to dilute potential carcinogens and speed their transit through the colon. Data now suggest that this is an oversimplification and that the relation between fiber intake and colon cancer is more complex. Certain fibers can bind mutagens, reducing their contact with colonic epithelium; others can favorably change the fecal pH or participate in other complex interactions.

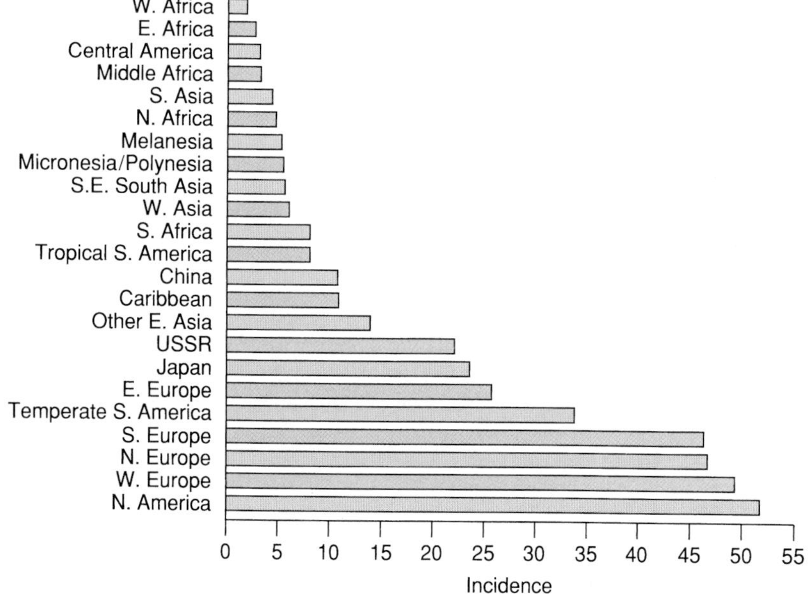

FIGURE 70.3 Incidence of colorectal cancer per 100,000 persons in 23 geographic regions during 1980. (After Parkin DM, Laara E, Muir CS. Estimates of the worldwide frequency of sixteen major cancers in 1980. *Int J Cancer* 1988;41:184.)

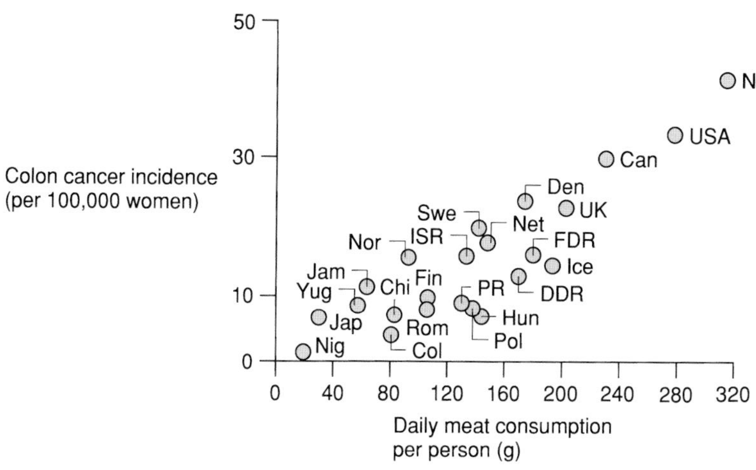

FIGURE 70.4 Correlation between meat intake and the incidence of colon cancer among women in 23 countries. (After Willett W. The search for the causes of breast and colon cancer. *Nature* 1989;338:389.)

The difficulty in sorting out the association of fiber intake with risk for colon cancer reflects the heterogeneous nature of fiber, the nondigestible component of carbohydrates. Fiber is derived from cereal products, vegetables, and fruit. Dietary fiber comprises a diverse collection of carbohydrates that are unlikely to have identical physiologic effects. Although the protective role of fiber is incompletely defined, recent evidence indicates a potential 20% to 50% risk reduction, particularly noted among frequent consumers of dark green vegetables.[9]

Mutagenesis

Carcinogenesis in the colon and rectum has been described in terms of an initiation–promotion model based on experimental observations in laboratory animals. According to this model, the first step involves initiating factors that directly interact with cellular DNA to induce mutations in the genome. Afterward, the process is driven by promotional factors, which are not mutagenic by themselves but enhance cellular proliferation of previously mutated cells. Although this concept represents an oversimplification of a complex, multiple-step process, it serves as a useful framework to understand data generated from animal models examining the pathogenesis of large-bowel cancer. One can enhance or reduce tumorigenesis in experimental animals both by maneuvers that modify the generation of a mutagen (or carcinogen) and by those that alter promotional factors long after the administration of an initiating agent.

The human diet contains a myriad of naturally occurring mutagens or substances that can be metabolized into mutagens. A wide range of such substances are generated from interactions between the diet, microbial flora, and colonic mucosal enzymes. In addition, protective mechanisms are present throughout the mucosa to detoxify these compounds. The action of carcinogens on DNA appears not to be an entirely random process. Mutagens typically alkylate DNA at specific carbon residues and cause nucleotide misreading during the next cycle of DNA replication. A mutation commonly seen early in colonic carcinogenesis results in activation of the *ras* protooncogene, one of several genetic events presumed to occur during malignant transformation.[13] The activation of *ras* may be involved in the initiation or promotion of carcinogenesis. Because of the ubiquitous presence of mutagens in the gut, many strategies that aim to reduce colon cancer attempt to interfere with the interaction between mutagens and the target colonic cells.

In animal studies, the role of fat in the pathogenesis of colon cancer appears to be that of a promotional factor. With increasing fat intake, total fecal bile acid increases significantly. Available data suggest that bile acids stimulate the generation of reactive oxygen metabolites that enhance the conversion of unsaturated fatty acids to compounds that promote cellular proliferation. Theoretically, this would facilitate the emergence of a mutated clone of neoplastic cells. Enhanced proliferation of these transformed cells can either compress the time required for carcinogenesis or, perhaps, make the process more efficient. An extension of this concept is the observation that increased dietary calcium has been associated with a decreased risk for colorectal cancer. Experimental data demonstrate that an increase in dietary calcium tends to inhibit colonic proliferative indices.

Molecular Genetics

The molecular genetic events that lead to colorectal cancer have served as a paradigm for the multiple-step process of tumorigenesis. This concept arose from frequent clinical and pathologic observations of an orderly progression of cellular transformation from normal colonic or rectal epithelium to small adenoma, then to large adenoma, and finally to carcinoma. These rather distinct stages have allowed scientists to elucidate the genetic alterations that may be responsible for the progression of the neoplastic process. Coincident with this line of investigation was the discovery of the genetic basis of several familial cancer syndromes in which colorectal cancer is a prominent feature of the phenotype. When taken together, the evidence suggests that colorectal cancers result from a series of genetic alterations leading to progressive disordering of the normal mechanisms that control cellular growth and differentiation (Fig. 70.5). It should be recognized that not every colorectal tumor will acquire each of the mutations described. Furthermore, other genetic events are likely to be necessary for cancer formation, and each tumor may have a unique genetic profile. Such a model of multiple-step tumorigenesis, however, helps us to understand better the complex molecular genetics of cancer. Within this paradigm, mutations in three distinct types of genes are known to contribute to colorectal cancer formation: oncogenes, tumor-suppressor genes, and DNA mismatch repair genes. The former two mechanisms, comprising the *loss of heterozygosity* or *chromosomal instability* pathway, account for about 85% of colon and rectal tumors. Mutations in mismatch repair genes, termed the *replication error* or *microsatellite instability* (MSI) *pathway*, account for about 15% of large bowel tumors.

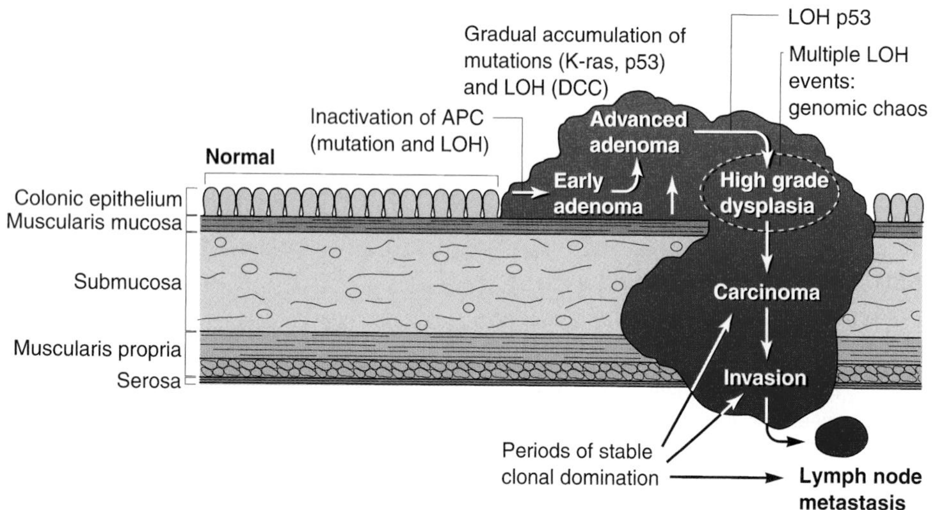

FIGURE 70.5 Model of genetic events mediating neoplastic progression in the colon. LOH, loss of heterozygosity.

In colon cancer, an important genetic alteration that has been demonstrated is a mutation of the K-*ras* protooncogene. The *ras* protooncogenes are a family of normal genes (N-*ras*, H-*ras*, and K-*ras*) that are highly conserved in nature and encode the production of guanosine triphosphate-binding proteins (G proteins), which are important for signal transduction. G proteins are involved in the transduction of proliferative signals induced by growth factors or factors involved in cell differentiation. The product of a mutated *ras* gene is an abnormal G protein that becomes constitutively activated and continuously stimulates autonomous cell growth. Experimentally, transfection of normal fibroblasts by mutated *ras* genes confers neoplastic properties to those cells.

About half of colorectal carcinomas and a similar percentage of adenomas larger than 1 cm in diameter have been found to have the *ras* gene mutation.[13,14] By contrast, fewer than 10% of adenomas smaller than 1 cm have this mutation. The *ras* gene mutation may be the initiating event in some colorectal carcinomas or, alternatively, may promote the clonal expansion of a mutated cell population. It appears that the *ras* gene mutation alone is not responsible for tumorigenesis. Other molecular events are required in addition to *ras* gene mutations.

The concept of tumor-suppressor genes arose from several observations. Cytogenetic studies demonstrated that tumor cells often have losses of specific chromosomal regions and suggested that loss of a particular gene or genes could contribute to tumor formation and progression. Conversely, experimental evidence documented that replacement of specific chromosomes or portions of chromosomes in tumor cells could result in inhibition of growth. It was thus deduced that genes exist that function to keep cellular growth and proliferation in check, and that their loss results in unregulated growth and neoplastic transformation. One such tumor-suppressor gene associated with colon cancer is the adenomatous polyposis coli (APC) gene, mutations in which result in the familial cancer syndrome, familial adenomatous polyposis (FAP). In persons affected with FAP, hundreds to thousands of colorectal adenomatous polyps develop, all of which have the potential to progress to a cancer. The lifetime risk for the development of colon cancer is virtually 100%.[15] When linkage analysis was performed in families with FAP, the *APC* gene was mapped to chromosome 5q21 and was subsequently cloned by several groups.[16,17] The *APC* gene encodes a large protein of 2,843 amino acids that contains a number of functional domains. A key function of the protein is to bind and thereby decrease intracellular levels of beta-catenin. Mutations of the *APC* gene that result in loss of this binding function lead to an increase in free beta-catenin, which then activates the expression of other genes involved in cellular growth.[18,19]

Mutations of the *APC* gene are also commonly found in sporadic cases of colorectal cancer. Approximately 70% of all sporadic cases of colorectal cancer have such mutations. Among those cancers in which *APC* is not mutated, a number have mutations in beta-catenin that disrupt its ability to bind to the APC protein, and as such, they are phenotypically similar to those in which *APC* is mutated.[19,20] Mutations in the *APC* gene appear to be an early or initiating event in sporadic colorectal cancer, as mutations in the gene have been identified in aberrant crypt foci, one of the earliest events in the neoplastic proliferation of colonic mucosa.[21]

Mutation or loss of the *p53* tumor-suppressor gene, located on chromosome 17p, is another common genetic event in colorectal cancer. Although *p53* mutations have been found in 75% of sporadic colorectal cancers, they are seen infrequently in earlier lesions, which suggests that inactivation of *p53* is an important event in the transition from adenoma to carcinoma. The *p53* gene codes for a 393-amino acid phosphoprotein that has the ability to bind to DNA in a sequence-specific manner. When bound to DNA, the p53 protein can activate the expression of certain genes that are presumed to participate in growth inhibition. Mutations that disrupt this ability to bind DNA result in a decrease in the expression of growth-inhibitory genes and an increase in cellular proliferation.[22] Germline mutations in *p53* are responsible for the Li-Fraumeni syndrome. Interestingly, colorectal cancer is not a prominent feature of the phenotype.

Chromosome 18q21 appears to have an important role in the development of colorectal cancer, as allelic loss of this region is observed in many cases. The clinical importance of such a loss is controversial; one report has identified 18q21 allelic loss as an independent negative prognostic factor in patients with stage II tumors, whereas others have failed to identify such an association.[23,24] Several candidate tumor-suppressor genes have been identified on chromosome 18q21, including deleted in colon cancer *(DCC)*, deleted in pancreatic cancer locus 4 *(DPC4)* and mad-related *(smad2)* genes. The role of these genes and others in the 18q21 region in colorectal tumorigenesis is not well defined. Investigation has been hampered by the inability to identify a significant number of mutations in any of these genes in sporadic colon cancers and by the lack of any familial syndromes in which germline mutations can be identified.

A third mechanism that has been implicated in colorectal tumorigenesis, the MSI pathway, involves disruption of the normal surveillance for and repair of DNA damage. Maintaining the fidelity of the genome during DNA replication and cell division is of paramount importance for the normal growth and development of an organism. Ordinarily, cells have numerous mechanisms that constantly survey DNA for damage or replication errors and, if present, repair them. In this manner, the integrity of the genome is ensured, and the accumulation and propagation of mutations is minimized. If these survey and repair mechanisms are defective, genetic instability and accelerated rates of mutation follow. If such mutations result in the activation of oncogenes or the inactivation of tumor-suppressor genes, affected cells gain a growth advantage.

In the early 1990s, several investigators observed that a subset of colorectal tumors have widespread instability in microsatellite repeats in tumor DNA, and that such instability is present in the tumors of many patients affected by familial nonpolyposis colorectal cancer, also called hereditary nonpolyposis colorectal cancer (HNPCC).[25–27] Simultaneously, bacterial and yeast geneticists described a set of DNA repair enzymes, termed *DNA mismatch repair enzymes,* that function to excise and repair nucleotide base mismatches that occur during DNA replication. The connection between DNA mismatch repair enzymes and HNPCC was solidified when it was found that tumor cells from patients with HNPCC lack DNA mismatch repair activity in vitro.[28] Subsequently, the first human mismatch repair homologue, *hMSH2,* was cloned and was found to be mutated in many patients with HNPCC.[29,30] Soon thereafter, a second human homologue of a mismatch repair enzyme, *hMLH1,* was cloned and demonstrated to be altered in a subset of patients with HNPCC who had normal *hMSH2*.[31,32]

It is now understood that DNA mismatch repair in the eukaryotic cell requires the participation of at least four other enzymes, *hPMS1, hPMS2, hMSH6* (formerly called *GTBP*), and *hMSH3*.[33] Together, these enzymes form two complexes that perform the many aspects of the DNA mismatch repair process. Single base pair insertions or errors are recognized by a MSH2-MSH6 heteroduplex, which then binds a MLH1-PMS2 heteroduplex to initiate DNA excision. Similarly, larger DNA insertion or deletion loops are recognized by a MSH2-MSH3 heteroduplex, which again binds a MLH1-PMS2 heteroduplex and initiates DNA excision.[34,35] It follows that *hMSH2* or *hMLH1* mutator phenotypes result in the highest MSI and account for more than 60% of the mutations found in HNPCC kindreds. In addition to the germ-line inactivation of mismatch repair genes seen in HNPCC, spontaneous development of MSI-high tumors results from hypermethylation of the promoter region of MLH1.

Delineation of the molecular genetic alterations responsible for colorectal tumor development has defined much of our current understanding of the multiple-step process of tumorigenesis. Yet despite these discoveries, an even greater number of questions remain to be answered. For example, among individuals who carry mutations in the *APC* gene, there is a wide variability in the phenotype; those affected with mutations that preserve the beta-catenin binding domain may manifest a much more attenuated, or even absent, polyposis phenotype with substantially later and less aggressive tumor presentation. Similarly, although MSI high tumors are associated with some unfavorable features (poor differentiation, larger size, mucinous subtype) compared with chromosomal unstable tumors, MSI high status confers a marked survival advantage. What accounts for such variability, and how will this impact on clinical management? Clearly, there are a myriad of interacting and modifying factors that contribute to the ultimate phenotype, with each being expressed to varying degrees in affected individuals. It is the elucidation of these interacting pathways that will be paramount to the understanding of colorectal cancer and to the design of more specific treatment or prevention strategies.

CLINICAL RISK FACTORS

Familial Cancer Syndromes

The vast majority of colorectal cancer cases have no apparent familial association and, as such, are considered truly sporadic. Epidemiologic studies have suggested that at least 15% of all colorectal cancers occur in a dominantly inherited pattern, and that an inherited susceptibility to polyps and cancer could account for up to 90% of the total number of colorectal cancers in the population.[36,37] The two best-described familial colorectal cancer syndromes are FAP and HNPCC. Currently, it is estimated that 3% to 5% of all colorectal cancers occur in persons affected with one of these two syndromes (Table 70.1).

FAP is an autosomal, dominantly inherited disease caused by mutations in the *APC* gene. In affected subjects, hundreds to thousands of adenomatous polyps typically develop throughout the colon and rectum, each of which has the potential to progress to an invasive cancer. The average age for the diagnosis of colorectal cancer is 42 years, markedly earlier than the average age of 63 years in sporadic cases. Cancer develops in virtually all affected persons by age 55 years. Polyps are also found in other regions of the gastrointestinal tract in patients with FAP, the most common locations being the duodenum and stomach. Polyps of the stomach have little propensity to progress to cancer. The duodenal and periampullary polyps, however, are associated with an increased risk for the development of cancer.[38,39] Additionally, a number of extraintestinal manifestations of FAP have been described, including congenital hypertrophy of the retinal pigment

TABLE 70.1 ETIOLOGY

CLINICAL RISK FACTORS FOR COLORECTAL CANCER

Genetic
POLYPOSIS SYNDROMES
Familial polyposis coli
Gardner syndrome
Turcot syndrome (central nervous system tumors)
Oldfield syndrome (sebaceous cysts)
Peutz-Jeghers syndrome (hamartomas)
NONPOLYPOSIS SYNDROMES
Lynch syndrome I
Lynch syndrome II (associated extracolonic cancers)
PREEXISTING DISEASE
Ulcerative colitis
Crohn disease
Prior colorectal cancer
Neoplastic polyps
Pelvic irradiation
Breast or genital tract cancer
General
Age >40 years
Family history of colorectal cancer

epithelium (CHRPE), osteomas, and desmoid tumors. These and other polyposis syndromes are discussed in more detail in Chapter 69. The first description of HNPCC kindreds was made by Aldred Warthin, a pathologist at the University of Michigan, in 1913.[40] One of these kindreds, referred to as *family G*, has been followed extensively through the years and represents a classic example of the HNPCC syndrome.[41] A more systematic collection of families and analysis of their pedigrees was performed by Henry Lynch et al. at Creighton University. It was recognized that although colorectal cancer is the most predominant cancer in the syndrome and these tumors derive from adenomatous polyps, an associated polyposis phenotype is not seen, in contrast to patients with FAP. For this reason, the syndrome was given the "nonpolyposis" designation. Two phenotypic variants of HNPCC have been described: Lynch syndromes I and II. Lynch syndrome I families manifest only colon cancer. Lynch syndrome II families manifest colon cancer in addition to a number of others, including endometrial, ovarian, gastric, small-bowel, liver and biliary tract, upper urologic tract, and central nervous system cancers. The median age for the development of either colorectal or endometrial cancer in HNPCC patients is 39 to 46 years.[42] The penetrance of HNPCC is not accurately known, but is estimated at 70% to 90% for colon cancer. An unusual clinical variant of HNPCC is the Muir-Torre syndrome, in which affected members have sebaceous tumors (both benign and malignant) and keratoacanthomas in addition to the spectrum of tumors found in Lynch syndrome II.

The clinical criteria necessary for identifying a family as an HNPCC kindred were established by an international collaborative group meeting in Amsterdam in 1990. These criteria, termed the *Amsterdam criteria,* include the following: (a) exclusion of FAP; (b) at least three relatives with histologically verified colorectal cancer, with at least one being a first-degree relative of the other two; (c) at least two successive generations affected; and (d) diagnosis of colorectal cancer in one of the relatives before the age of 50 years.[43] With further study of HNPCC kindreds, the Amsterdam criteria have been revised as *Amsterdam II*, to include at least three relatives with *HNPCC-associated* cancers in lieu of colorectal cancers only.[44] However, a proportion of individuals at risk for HNPCC still do not satisfy the Amsterdam II criteria. To better guide recommendations for genetic evaluation, the *Bethesda criteria* were developed and recently revised as an alternative system for identifying HNPCC kindreds (Table 70.2).[45,46] Although these criteria schemes provide acceptable capture of patients, test characteristics and ease of use differ. The tumors of patients in families that satisfy Amsterdam II or the revised Bethesda criteria should be tested for MSI (positive two of five mononucleotide markers including BAT25, BAT26, D2S123, D5S346, D17S250), and potentially undergo further germline analysis for MSH2/MLH1 abnormalities.

Recently, a novel type of mutation was described that by itself does not result in a tumor phenotype but indirectly confers a predisposition for the development of colorectal cancer. A single base pair alteration was identified in the *APC* gene that results in the substitution of a lysine for an isoleucine at codon 1,307. This mutation does not alter the function of the encoded protein but does produce an extended mononucleotide tract that becomes a hypermutable region of the gene. It was hypothesized that this unstable region of the gene leads to a higher rate of detrimental somatic mutations and cancer. The 1,307 mutation has been found in 6% of Ashkenazi Jews and in 28% of Ashkenazim with a family history of colorectal cancer.[47]

In the future, more and more patients with cancer will be determined to have a responsible hereditary defect in either a specific tumor gene or in a modifying gene that imparts a predisposition to cancer. Obtaining a thorough family history is now a necessity in the workup of any patient with cancer, especially one with onset at a young age or with multiple tumors. The easy availability of genetic testing by many commercial laboratories has been problematic, as most physicians are not prepared to interpret the results or to counsel patients regarding their cancer risk and treatment. In a study of patients undergoing genetic testing for familial polyposis by a commercial company, it was found that only 19% of patients received genetic counseling before the test, and in 32% of cases, the physician ordering the test misinterpreted the results.[48] Although most problems with misinterpretation are encountered with negative results, the interpretation of a positive result also can be difficult. It must be emphasized that a negative result can provide reassurance only if the predisposing mutation in the family is already known. Otherwise, a negative result may mean that the mutation was missed, that it occurred in a promoter or intronic sequence not evaluated, or that a cancer predisposition still exists because of a mutation in another known or unknown disease gene.[49] In the case of a positive result, one must be sure that the mutation does in fact confer a cancer risk and that it is not merely a benign polymorphism. Therefore, when identified, patients suspected of having an inherited cancer syndrome should be offered counseling by a cancer geneticist or experienced genetic counselor, both before the test is ordered and after the results are known.

Inflammatory Bowel Disease

A strong association exists between inflammatory bowel disease and bowel cancer. For patients with ulcerative colitis, the incidence of malignancy is proportional to the extent of colonic involvement, age at onset, and severity and duration of disease. The duration of inflammatory bowel disease is a critical factor in predicting the likelihood of adenocarcinoma. Cancer develops in about 3% of patients during the first 10 years after the onset of colitis, and in an additional 20% during each of the next two decades. The cure rate in patients with ulcerative colitis who are treated for cancer is similar to that in noncolitic patients treated for cancer.[50]

Patients with Crohn disease are also at increased risk for colon cancer in addition to small-bowel cancer. The risk for malignancy is lower than that reported for ulcerative colitis. Like the cancers associated with ulcerative colitis, the cancers associated with Crohn disease tend to occur at an earlier age than those in patients without inflammatory bowel disease.

Polyps

Traditionally, colorectal polyps have been divided into two broad categories: neoplastic and nonneoplastic. Nonneoplastic polyps included hyperplastic, inflammatory, juvenile, and hamartomatous polyps, none of which were considered precursors to colorectal cancer. Neoplastic polyps were adenomas and had the potential to develop into malignant cancers. The incidence of colorectal malignancy is two to five times higher in patients with adenomatous polyps than in those without them. Carcinoma is twice as likely to develop in patients with multiple polyps as in patients with a single polyp. Evidence suggests the existence of a common inherited susceptibility toward both sporadic colonic adenomatous polyps and colorectal cancer.[36]

Adenoma histology can be classified as tubular (75% to 100% tubular components), tubulovillous (25% to 75% villous components), or villous (75% to 100% villous components). Tubular adenomas, or adenomatous polyps, are the most common type and constitute about 75% of neoplastic

TABLE 70.2 DIAGNOSIS

COMPARISON OF CLINICAL CRITERIA FOR HEREDITARY NONPOLYPOSIS COLORECTAL CANCER (HNPCC)[a]

	Criteria	Sensitivity[109]	Specificity[109]	Strengths	Weaknesses
AMSTERDAM[43]	Three relatives with colorectal cancer, meeting all of the following criteria: (i) One of whom is a first-degree relative of the other two; (ii) colorectal cancer in at least two generations; (iii) one or more colorectal cancer cases diagnosed before age 50 years	61%	67%	Easy to remember and apply; good specificity	Limited sensitivity
AMSTERDAM II[44]	Three relatives with HNPCC-associated cancer,[b] meeting all of the following criteria: (i) One of whom is a first-degree relative of the other two; (ii) colorectal cancer in at least two generations; (iii) one or more colorectal cancer cases diagnosed before age 50 years	78%	61%	Easy to remember and apply	Improved but limited sensitivity
BETHESDA GUIDELINES[45]	Meeting any of the following criteria:[c] (i) Subjects with cancer in families that fulfill Amsterdam criteria; (ii) subjects with two HNPCC-related cancers; (iii) subjects with colorectal cancer and a first-degree relative with HNPCC-related cancer and/or colorectal adenoma; one of the cancers diagnosed at age <45 years and the adenoma diagnosed at age <40 years	94%	49%	Increased sensitivity	Complexity in the clinic setting
REVISED BETHESDA GUIDELINES[46]	Meeting any of the following criteria: (i) Colorectal cancer diagnosed in a patient younger than age 50 years; (ii) presence of synchronous or metachronous HNPCC-associated tumors, regardless of age; (iii) colorectal cancer with microsatellite instability high histology in a patient younger than age 60 years; (iv) colorectal cancer in one or more first-degree relatives with an HNPCC-related tumor, with one of the cancers diagnosed at age younger than 50 years; or (v) colorectal cancer diagnosed in two or more first- or second-degree relatives with HNPCC-associated tumors, regardless of age			Easier to apply in the clinical setting	Due to recent development, limited data regarding test

[a]After exclusion of familial adenomatous polyposis.
[b]HNPCC-associated cancers are colorectal, endometrial, ovarian, stomach, small intestine, biliary tract, ureter, renal pelvis, and brain cancers, and sebaceous gland adenomas and keratoacanthomas in Muir-Torre syndrome.
[c]Three additional original Bethesda criteria did not increase the sensitivity, but their inclusion decreased the specificity to 25%: (iv) Subjects with colorectal cancer or endometrial cancer at age <45 years; (v) subjects with right-sided colorectal cancer with an undifferentiated histopathologic pattern diagnosed at age <45 years; (vi) subjects with signet-ring cell type colorectal cancer diagnosed at age <45 years; (vii) subjects with adenomas diagnosed at age <40 years.

polyps.[51] (Table 70.3). Tubulovillous adenomas account for 15% and purely villous adenomas for 10% of neoplastic polyps. All adenomas contain some degree of dysplasia or cellular atypia, which can be graded from mild to severe. Carcinoma in situ and severe dysplasia have been grouped together under the classification of high-grade dysplasia. In contrast to invasive carcinoma, carcinoma in situ has not invaded the muscularis mucosae (Fig. 70.6). The incidence of invasive malignancy differs markedly for the three histologic subtypes. In general, malignancies are seen in 5% of adenomatous polyps, in 22%

TABLE 70.3

NEOPLASTIC COLORECTAL POLYPS

Type	Histologic features	Incidence (%)	Invasive malignancy (%)
Adenomatous (tabular adenoma)	Branching tubules embedded in lamina propria	75	5
Villous (villous adenoma)	Finger-like projections of epithelium over lamina propria	10	40
Intermediate (tubulovillous adenoma)	Mixture of adenomatous and villous patterns	15	22

of tubulovillous adenomas, and in 40% of villous lesions. Although villous lesions are much less common, they are more likely to harbor a malignancy.

Polyp size is also directly correlated with the presence of dysplasia or malignancy.[52] Polyps that are 10 mm in diameter or larger have long been considered "high risk," harboring invasive carcinoma in about 3% of cases. Polyps 5 mm or less in diameter are considered to be diminutive, with 0 to 0.05% frequency of carcinoma based on extremely large cohort studies.[53,54] Polyps 6 to 9 mm in diameter may harbor dysplasia or malignancy but there is no definitive agreement regarding the benefit to risk ratio associated with their removal. Recent reviews have demonstrated 3% of such polyps to have severe dysplasia but only 0.05 to 0.15% contain invasive cancer.[54,55]

Recently, an additional histologic family of neoplastic polyps has been proposed, the *serrated polyps*. Serrated polyps include hyperplastic-like polyps, mixed polyps (part hyperplastic, part dysplastic), and serrated adenomas. The serrated polyps appear to be susceptible to or initiated by inactivation of MLH1 by methylation, which in turn is thought to initiate rapid acquisition of microsatellite DNA instability. In contrast to most hyperplastic polyps, which are seen in the distal colon, the serrated hyperplastic-like polyps are found in the proximal colon. Other clinical features include higher prevalence among women and older patients, rapid growth, and large size at diagnosis, all of which are also associated with proximal colon cancer. Although this alternative pathway to colorectal cancer is not universally accepted, supportive data include (a) the frequency of sporadic MSI high cancers but paucity of MSI-high adenomatous polyps (except in HNPCC), (b) loss of expression of MLH1 but not MSH2 among both serrated polyps and sporadic MSI high cancers, and (c) the natural history of hyperplastic polyposis and associated prevalence of right-sided colon cancer.[56–59]

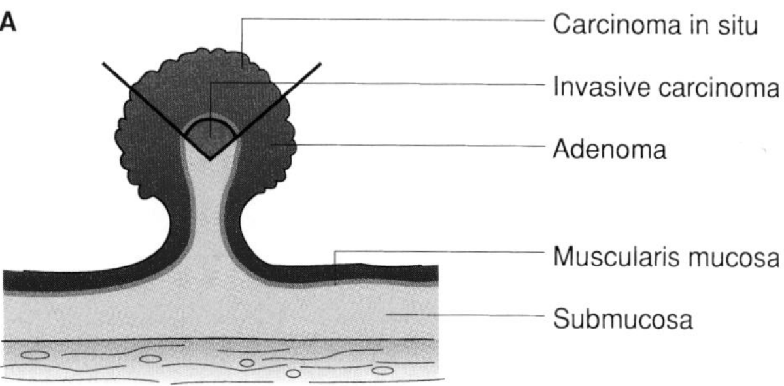

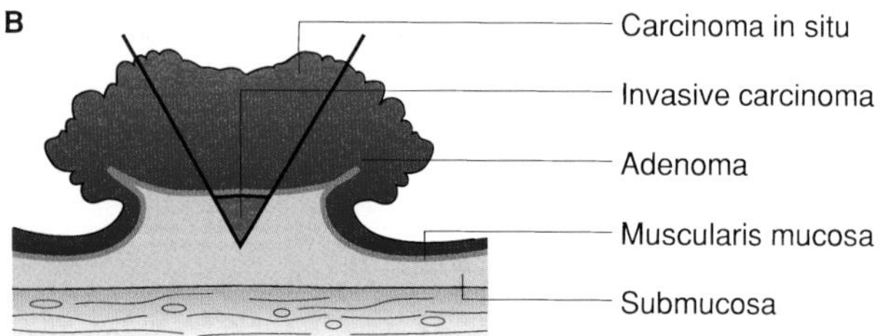

FIGURE 70.6 Anatomic distinction between carcinoma *in situ* and invasive malignancy in a pedunculated (*A*) and a sessile (*B*) adenomatous polyp. Carcinoma *in situ* is characterized by the absence of invasion into the muscularis mucosae.

Other Risk Factors

People older than 40 years have an increased risk for colorectal cancer, and this risk increases proportionally to the eighth decade. Patients who have received irradiation for gynecologic cancer have a twofold to threefold increased risk for the development of colorectal cancer. Patients with previously resected colorectal cancer have a threefold increased risk for the development of a second primary large-bowel cancer. Women with breast or genital tract cancer also are at increased risk for large-bowel cancer.

DIAGNOSIS

Symptoms

The diagnosis of colorectal cancer can be based on the evaluation of a symptomatic patient or on the results of screening or surveillance programs for asymptomatic patients. The symptoms of colorectal cancer can be nonspecific, such as intermittent pain, bleeding, nausea, and vomiting. Bleeding may present as melena, which is more commonly associated with right-sided colon cancers, or as gross red blood, associated with left-sided colon and rectal cancers. Lesser amounts of bleeding may be detected on a fecal occult blood test. Iron-deficiency anemia associated with fatigue may develop in patients with chronic blood loss.

Malignant obstruction can result in abdominal pain with nausea and vomiting. In the presence of obstruction, a perforation may develop either at the site of the tumor or through the proximal uninvolved intestine. With rectal tumors, compromise of the rectal reservoir can cause a change in bowel habits, such as constipation, decreased stool caliber, or even diarrhea and changes in continence. With locally advanced rectal cancers, symptoms of tenesmus, urgency, and perineal pain can occur.

Screening and Diagnostic Tests

Screening refers to testing that is applied to an asymptomatic group without prior disease, in order to identify those at greater risk for disease. Screening tests should demonstrate simplicity, accuracy and reliability, safety, cost-effectiveness, and good compliance. A broad range of screening and diagnostic studies can be employed in the evaluation of a suspected large-bowel cancer. The least expensive and potentially most informative study for rectal tumors is the digital examination. This permits the localization of distal rectal and anal neoplasms. In addition, stool can be obtained for the evaluation of occult bleeding.

The fecal occult blood test is most commonly employed screening test for colorectal cancer. Stool samples are placed on guaiac-impregnated paper slides that change color in the presence of peroxidase activity from hemoglobin. Patients are instructed to test two samples from three consecutive bowel movements. Several factors affect the utility of this test. First, not all colonic cancers or polyps are associated with bleeding, and even in those that are, bleeding is often intermittent. Second, patients must be instructed to remain on diets low in peroxidase (no rare beef or horseradish) before testing to avoid false-positive results. Third, certain medications, such as iron, cimetidine, antacids, and ascorbic acid, may interfere with the peroxidase reaction and lead to a false-negative result. The experience with annual, unrehydrated fecal occult blood testing in asymptomatic populations has shown that about 2.5% of tested patients have positive results. Among these, only 10% to 15% have colorectal cancer.[60] Thus, a positive screening fecal occult blood test would necessarily lead to a more specific diagnostic test, colonoscopy, which would lead in turn to the opportunity for biopsy or polypectomy. After 18 years of follow-up, the Minnesota Colon Cancer Control Study [61] has determined that, even with 50% to 75% compliance, annual fecal occult blood test use decreased the incidence of colorectal cancer by about 20%. Table 70.4 compares test characteristics of fecal occult blood testing and other screening and diagnostic examinations described later in this section.

Rigid sigmoidoscopy with a 25-cm instrument is comparatively inexpensive but is limited by the length of intestine that can be examined and by patient compliance. Flexible fiberoptic sigmoidoscopy has gained more acceptance. Instruments measuring 35 and 65 cm are available, and an examination of the sigmoid colon and rectum can usually be performed after cleansing enemas have been administered. Patient comfort is much higher than with rigid sigmoidoscopy. In addition, the ability to perform this test adequately without a total bowel cathartic and without sedation have a positive influence on patient compliance. Because of the risk of retained methane gas, electrocautery-assisted biopsy is unsafe.

Colonoscopy with the 180-cm fiberoptic instrument is the most widely used diagnostic study to evaluate the colon. A valuable aspect of this procedure is the ability to obtain mucosal biopsy specimens and perform polypectomies. Thus colonoscopy provides both diagnostic and therapeutic benefit, making it the accepted criterion standard for assessing other screening and diagnostic tests. Data from the National Polyp Study[62] indicate a lower rate of cancer among patients who have undergone colonoscopic polypectomy, implying that colonoscopy is the only screening test that can potentially prevent cancer development. Unfortunately, colonoscopy is also the only cancer screening test that has an associated mortality rate. The incidence of severe complications that require surgical intervention (e.g., hemorrhage, perforation) is 0.1% to 0.3%.

The barium enema is the traditional study for the diagnosis of colonic polyps and cancers. The double-contrast technique in which air insufflation is used is superior to the standard single-contrast barium enema to detect early polyps or cancers. The classic apple core defect has been described for colonic cancers (Fig. 70.7). Colonoscopy has largely supplanted use of barium enema but the examination is still useful in the setting of strictures or adhesions that cannot be negotiated with a flexible scope. Another advantage of barium enema over colonoscopy is the routine visualization of the right side of the colon, which is not possible in 5% to 10% of colonoscopic examinations.

Two emerging screening tests under active investigation are virtual colonoscopy and fecal DNA screening. Virtual colonoscopy, also termed *CT colonography*, was introduced in 1994 and has gradually captured public appeal due to its potential to improve patient comfort, minimize risk, and eradicate the need for sedation.[63] After air insufflation of the prepared colon, thin-cut axial images are gathered by a high speed helical CT scanner; both prone and supine scans are obtained in minutes. Based on both image sets, the two dimensional axial images are reconstituted into three dimensional replications of the entire colon (Fig. 70.8). Another advantage of this technique is good visualization of the entire colon, including antegrade and retrograde views of haustral folds that sometimes elude the traditional colonoscopist.

It must be noted that virtual colonoscopy is not diagnostic; that is, patients with positive findings must undergo a traditional

TABLE 70.4 DIAGNOSIS

COMPARISON OF COLORECTAL CANCER SCREENING TEST CHARACTERISTICS

	Unrehydrated FOBT[61,110]	Flexible sigmoidoscopy[82,111]	Colonoscopy[86,111]	Double-contrast barium enema[112–114]
ACCURACY				
Sensitivity	33%–40%	70%	97.5%	70%–85%
Specificity	97%		100%	86%–97%
COST, 2000 $US[115,116]	$3.50	$400	$695	$296
CONSEQUENCES [117,80,118]	Negligible	Perforation = 0 to 0.011%	Hemorrhage = 0.15 to 4% Perforation = 0.2 to 3% Mortality =0.006%	Negligible
COMPLIANCE	60%–86%	47%–74%	28%–38%	
EFFECTIVENESS (REDUCTION in CRC mortality)[116]	18%–55%	34%–66%	64%–90%	33%–47%

FOBT, fecal occult blood test, unrehydrated. CRC, colorectal cancer.

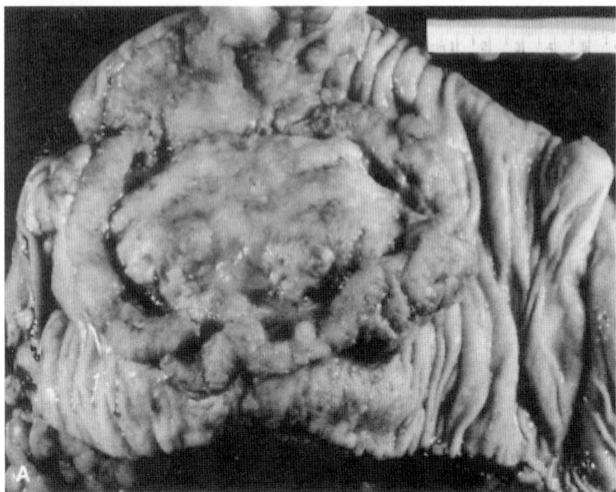

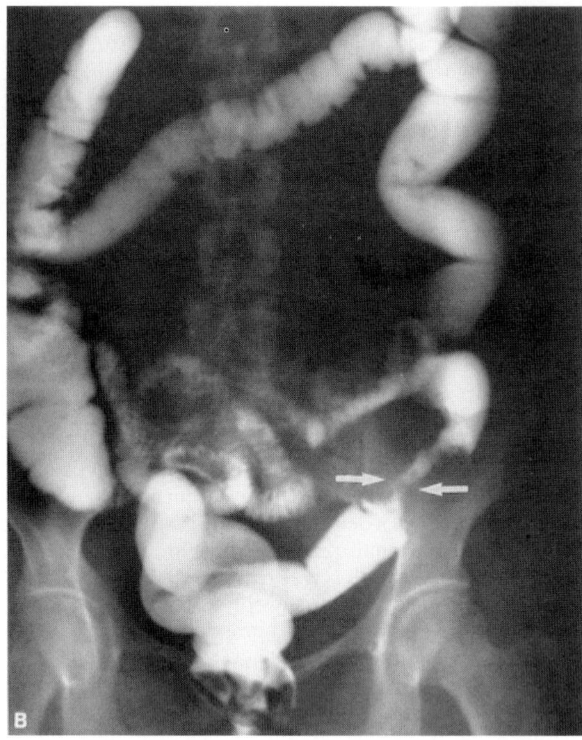

FIGURE 70.7 Surgical specimen with correlating barium enema examination of an invasive sigmoid carcinoma. (*A*) The tumor is a circumferential lesion. (*B*) The barium enema study demonstrates features of the apple core defect (*arrows*).

colonoscopy for biopsy or polypectomy. Among high-risk patients, per-patient sensitivity and specificity as high as 92% and 94% for patients with polyps or lesions 6 mm or larger have been reported from a single center.[64] To better assess generalizability of the technique, a multicenter trial examined high risk patients in nine different institutions and reported a combined sensitivity of only 39% for lesions 6 mm or larger with high interobserver variation.[65] This study has been criticized for its reliance on older technology and high interobserver variation. However, such issues may more accurately reflect broad-scale generalizability.

As a rule, accuracy improves as lesions increase in size, but the accuracy of screening tests generally declines with decreasing prevalence of disease. It follows that virtual colonoscopy test characteristics may be less positive among the *average-risk* population. A recent prospective, blinded study subjected a combination of high and average risk patients to virtual colonoscopy followed by conventional colonoscopy.[66] Sensitivity and specificity were 84% and 83% for polyps or lesions 6 mm or larger. More important, using a 6-mm lesion cutoff, the per-patient negative predictive value was 95%. A strong negative predictive value indicates that a negative test result reliably reflects a lesion-free state; that is, patients with a negative test result may safely forego invasive conventional colonoscopy. False-negative and false-positive results are primarily a result of retained stool, which can be minimized by a full bowel cathartic. Stool-tagging techniques can also help to distinguish small lesions from fecaliths that adhere to the mucosa despite repositioning.[67] A recent three-center study of virtual colonoscopy among 1201 average-risk patients revealed a sensitivity and specificity of 88.7% and 79.6% for adenomas larger than 6 mm.[68] The authors attributed their excellent results to preprocedural stool tagging, extensive interpreter experience, and primary reliance on three dimensional reconstituted images over the two dimensional axial images. When similar results can be widely replicated and definitive test characteristics are known for average-risk individuals, virtual colonoscopy will become part of the screening armamentarium.

Stool DNA screening refers to polymerase chain reaction analysis of sloughed mucosal cells in stool, seeking genetic alterations associated with colorectal cancer. Despite technically challenging contaminants, stool is a useful medium for development of such tests because it reflects mucosal cells from the entire colon. Although the sequence of genetic changes in colorectal cancer is well documented, screening for any of these markers individually may be a painstaking process with no better accuracy than the well entrenched fecal occult blood test. Conversely, a screening method for some optimal combination of genetic markers could be very useful. Among specimens from known cancer patients, small early feasibility studies demonstrated 71% to 91% sensitivity and more than 93% specificity searching for a combination of *K-ras*, p53, *APC* gene, BAT-26, and long-segment DNA indicating extinguished apoptosis.[69,70] A recent multicenter cohort study of more than 4400 average risk patients compared fecal DNA screening to fecal occult blood testing, using follow-up colonoscopy as a standard.[71] Sensitivity for invasive cancer was 51.6% versus 12.9%, respectively; specificity was 94.4% versus 95.2%. Compared with no testing, fecal DNA testing is cost effective.[72] However, the substantially higher cost and essentially identical specificity render the fecal DNA test less advantageous than fecal occult blood testing followed by diagnostic colonoscopy as indicated.

Screening and Surveillance Recommendations

The previous section described goals and characteristics of screening tests. Screening regimens, that is the periodic application of these tests, should be undertaken for diseases that are serious, prevalent, and curable with early diagnosis. Colorectal cancer is clearly a serious health issue, resulting in

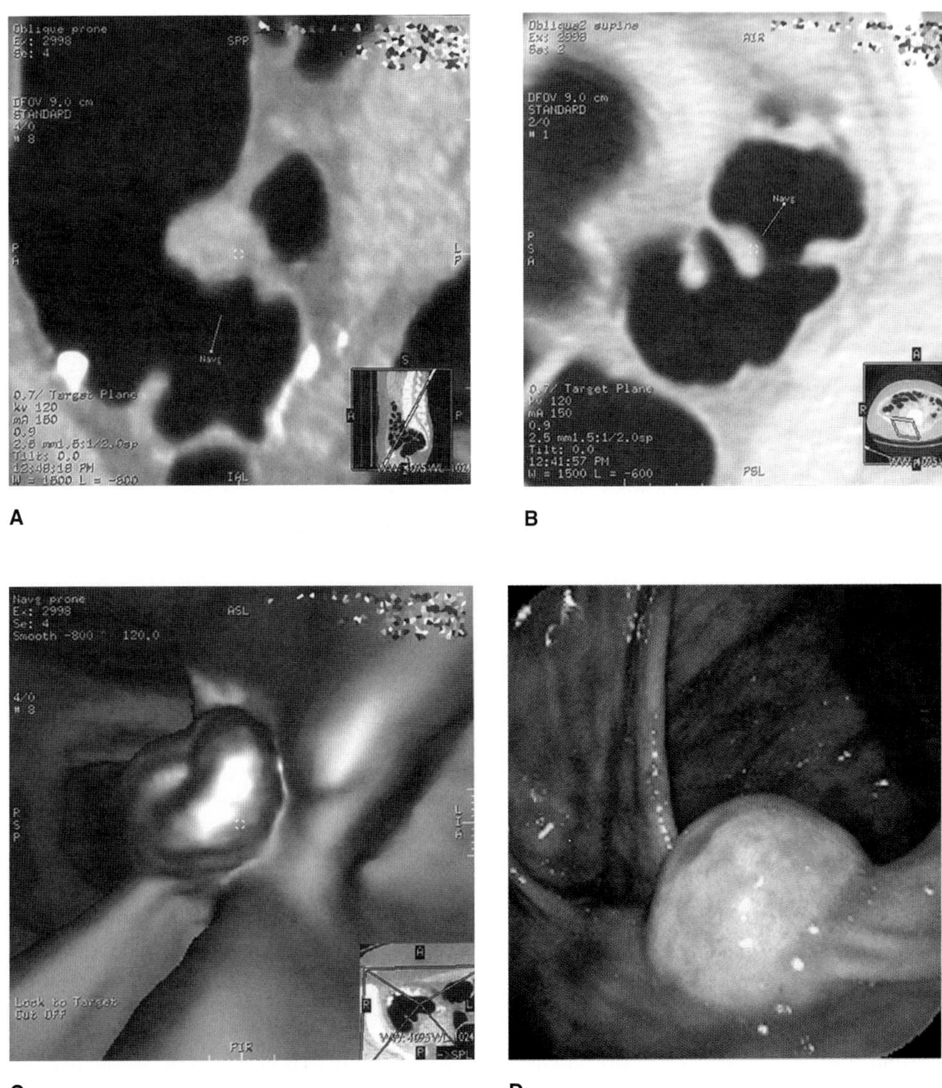

FIGURE 70.8 Prominent ileocecal valve with an associated tumor. (*A*) Identified on two-dimensional axial computed tomography image, sagittal view. (*B*) Identified on two-dimensional axial computed tomography image, coronal view. (*C*) Identified on reconstituted three-dimensional virtual colonoscopy image. (*D*) As pictured on colonoscopy performed for biopsy.

more than 57,000 deaths per year. The increased prevalence among individuals older than 60 years justifies recommendations to begin screening at age 50 years for average-risk individuals. Last, effective treatment is available and earlier stage at diagnosis is associated with better outcome, implying that screening that results in early diagnosis and initiation of treatment confers a survival benefit.

Screening for colorectal cancer begins with risk stratification in order to determine the appropriate timing of initiation and follow-up. Table 70.5 delineates different risk categories, including average risk, moderate risk, and high risk. For average-risk individuals, no one strategy currently dominates the others in combined cost-effectiveness, patient safety, and compliance.[73] Therefore, the U.S. Multisociety Task Force on Colorectal Cancer (USMSTF) has endorsed a variety of cost-effective screening regimens for asymptomatic, average-risk individuals beginning at age 50 years.[74]

The annual or biennial fecal occult blood test is the only screening regimen that has been shown to directly reduce colorectal cancer mortality.[61,75–78] Table 70.6 summarizes the results of four separate trials comprising more than 400,000 persons. Follow-up was substantial, ranging from 8 to 18 years. All these studies reported a higher percentage of earlier-stage (i.e., stage I) cancers detected in the screened group than in the control group. Based on intention to treat (screen), annual fecal occult blood testing was associated with a 33% decrease in colorectal cancer mortality. If noncompliant patients from the Minnesota study are excluded, it is estimated that a 50% reduction in colorectal cancer mortality would be observed. Clearly, improving compliance would have a major impact on colorectal cancer mortality. Eliminating dietary restrictions may improve patient compliance, as with the newer guaiac-based fecal immunochemical tests.[79] The updated recommendations for the fecal occult blood testing regimen among average-risk adults from the USMSTF includes (a) annual, unrehydrated fecal occult blood testing with dietary restriction or fecal immunochemical test without restriction (b) testing of two samples from three consecutive bowel movements, and (cv) following a positive screening test result with diagnostic colonoscopy.

Although data from randomized, controlled trials of screening endoscopy are not yet mature,[80,81] three large case-control

TABLE 70.5

RISK STRATIFICATION FOR COLORECTAL CANCER SCREENING

Average Risk for Colorectal Cancer
(must fulfill all criteria below)
Age 50 years or older
No personal history of polyps or colorectal cancer
No first-degree relatives with polyps or colorectal cancer
Fewer than two second-degree relatives with colorectal cancer

Moderate Risk for Colorectal Cancer
(any criteria below)
First-degree relative with colorectal cancer or polyp at age younger than 60 years
First-degree relative with colorectal cancer or polyp at age 60 years or older
Two or more second-degree relatives with colorectal cancer

Increased Risk for Colorectal Cancer
(any criteria below)
Gene carrier or at risk for familial adenomatous polyposis
Gene carrier or at risk for hereditary nonpolyposis colorectal cancer

Surveillance (any criteria below)
Personal history of colorectal polyps
Personal history of colorectal cancer
Personal history of inflammatory bowel disease

studies demonstrated that periodic screening sigmoidoscopy reduced the mortality from distal colorectal cancers between 60% to 80%.[82–84] Approximately 70% of all large-bowel polyps and cancers should be within reach of a flexible sigmoidoscope. A study of 3121 veterans demonstrated that flexible sigmoidoscopy, followed by full colonoscopy if a distal polyp were found, would identify 70% to 80% of patients with proximal neoplasia.[85] Current recommendations for average-risk individuals include flexible sigmoidoscopy once every 5 years. An alternative recommendation combines fecal occult blood testing (to be performed first) yearly with flexible sigmoidoscopy every 5 years, which increases the detection rate from 70% to 76%.[86]

Data from studies of colonoscopy suggest that this procedure can be an effective screening tool. In the National Polyp Study, patients who underwent colonoscopy and subsequent removal of benign polyps were followed with periodic colonoscopy for an average duration of 6 years.[62] A 90% decrease in colorectal cancer in patients participating in the National Polyp Study was noted in comparison with a general population registry. These data indicate that colonoscopy can be a very effective tool in reducing the incidence of colorectal cancer. The USMSTF recommends screening every 10 years, the estimated time for transformation from an adenoma to invasive malignancy. Recent changes in Medicare to include coverage of screening colonoscopy have encouraged the use of this modality.

Double-contrast barium enema is used less commonly but remains an option among screening regimens. The double-contrast barium enema provides a structural examination of the entire colon, and is associated with fewer than 0.0001% complication rate. The accuracy of this examination is markedly poorer than that for conventional colonoscopy and therefore recommended examination intervals have been shortened to every 5 years.

Table 70.7 outlines screening regimen options detailed above for average-risk patients.[74] Currently, less than half of Americans older than age 50 years have undergone any colorectal cancer screening.[87] It is hoped that choosing a screening regimen based on patient and provider preferences and resources will enhance screening compliance. Although colorectal cancer mortality is decreased with screening, it is unclear whether the overall mortality of the screened populations is different from that of the control groups. Mortality may be shifted to other causes (e.g., cardiovascular deaths) in the screened population. Cost-effective analyses do indicate that all of the recommended colorectal cancer screening strategies cost between $10,000 and $25,000 per year of life saved,

TABLE 70.6

SUMMARY OF PROSPECTIVE RANDOMIZED TRIALS OF FECAL OCCULT BLOOD TESTING

Study	No. of patients	Randomized groups	Type of FOBT	Cancers follow-up period (y)	Detected by FOBT (%)	RR of CRC Dukes A cancers (%)	Death with screening (95% CI)
Mandel et al. (47, 48) Minnesota, US	46,551	Annual Biennial Control	Rehydrated	18	Annual 50 Biennial 39	Annual 33 Biennial 29 Control 25	Annual 0.67 (0.51–0.89) Biennial 0.79 (0.62–0.97)
Hardcastle et al. (49) Nottingham, U.K.	152,850	Biennial Control	Unhydrated	7.5 (median)	27	Screen 21 Control 12	0.85 (0.74–0.98)
Kronburg et al (50) Funen. Denmark	140,000	Biennial Control	Unhydrated	10	25	Screen 23 Control 12	0.82 (0.68–0.99)
Kewenter et al. (51)	63,308	Two, screens, 16–22 mo. apart	Rehydrated	8.2 (median)	28	Screen 26	0.88 (0.69–1.12)
Gothenburg, Sweden		Control				Control 9	

FOBT, fecal occult blood testing; CRC, colorectal cancer; CI, confidence interval; RP, relative risk.

TABLE 70.7

GUIDELINES FOR COLORECTAL CANCER SCREENING[a]

Individuals at Average Risk, Age >50 years		
Test[b]	**Interval**	**Comment**
Fecal occult blood test	Annually	No rehydration
Flexible sigmoidoscopy	Every 5 years	
Fecal occult blood test and flexible sigmoidoscopy	Fecal occult blood test annually, flexible sigmoidoscopy every 5 years	Fecal occult blood test first; if positive, skip sigmoidoscopy and follow with colonoscopy
Colonoscopy	Every 10 years	
Double contrast barium enema	Every 5 years	
Individuals at moderate risk		
Risk	**Initiate screening**	**Comments**
First-degree relative with colorectal cancer or polyp at age ≥60 years OR ≥two or more second-degree relatives with colorectal cancer	Age 40 years	Same screening regimens and intervals as average risk.
First-degree relative with colorectal cancer or polyp at age <60 years OR >two or more first-degree relatives with colorectal cancer	Age 40 years or 10 years younger than youngest family member at the time of diagnosis, whichever comes first	Colonoscopy every 5 years
Individuals at increased risk, colonoscopy only		
Familial risk	**Initiate surveillance**	**Interval if normal colonoscopy result**
Familial adenomatous polyposis; consider genetic counseling and testing; colectomy if genetic testing is positive.	Age 10–12 years	Annual sigmoidoscopy, stopping at age 40 years if normal
Attenuated adenomatous polyposis coli	Late teens	Annual colonoscopy, no stopping at age 40 years
Hereditary nonpolyposis colon cancer	Age 20–25 years or 10 years younger than earliest family diagnosis	Biennial colonoscopy to age 40 years, then annual

[a]Endorsed by the American Cancer Society, American College of Gastroenterology, American Society of Colon and Rectal Surgeons, American Society for Gastrointestinal Endoscopy, Oncology Nursing Society, and Society of American Gastrointestinal Endoscopic Surgeons.
[b]Diagnostic evaluation with colonoscopy should be performed for any patients with either positive findings on screening with fecal occult blood testing or symptoms suggestive of colorectal cancer or polyps.

which is substantially less than the cost for other currently recommended screening measures (i.e., mammography).[73]

Patients with known disease or a personal history of polyps or cancer are in a separate surveillance category. Surveillance is defined as routine collection of data from a population known to be at high risk for disease. For the purposes of colorectal cancer, this population includes patients with inflammatory bowel disease or a personal history of polyps or cancer. The USMSTF Surveillance Guidelines recommend periodic endoscopy as outlined in Table 70.8.[74]

STAGING

Pathology

Of all large bowel cancers, 90% to 95% are adenocarcinomas, with the remaining histologic types being squamous cell carcinomas, adenosquamous carcinomas, lymphomas, sarcomas, and carcinoid tumors. Most colonic adenocarcinomas are moderately differentiated or well differentiated tumors. About 20% of adenocarcinomas are poorly differentiated or undifferentiated, and these are associated with a poorer prognosis. Another commonly described characteristic of adenocarcinomas is the relative amount of mucin that is produced. Ten percent to 20% of tumors are described as mucinous or colloid carcinomas based on the abundant production of mucin. These tumors are associated with a poorer 5-year survival rate in comparison with nonmucinous tumors. Other histologic features associated with a poorer prognosis include blood vessel invasion, lymphatic vessel invasion, and the absence of a lymphocytic response to the tumor.

Dukes Classification

The most important prognostic factor in colorectal cancer is the depth of invasion of the primary tumor. The first practical staging system to incorporate this observation was described by Dukes, who classified the depth of invasion of rectal tumors in stages from A to C. In his original classification, stage A indicated penetration through the muscularis propria but not through the intestinal wall (Fig. 70.9). Stage B represented penetration through the muscularis propria into the perirectal fat. Stage C represented metastasis to lymph nodes regardless

TABLE 70.8

GUIDELINES FOR COLORECTAL CANCER ENDOSCOPIC SURVEILLANCE[a]

Personal history risk	Initiate surveillance	Interval
Following resection of single <1 cm adenoma	5 years postpolypectomy	If first colonoscopy is normal, resume average-risk recommendations
Following resection of ≥1 cm or high-risk adenoma	3 years postpolypectomy	Repeat colonoscopy in 3 years; if normal, return to average-risk recommendations
Following curative resection for colorectal cancer	Within 1 year postoperatively	Repeat in 3 years, then every 5 years
Inflammatory bowel disease	Within 8 years of diagnosis	Survey for dysplasia Every 1–2 years

[a]Endorsed by the American Cancer Society, American College of Gastroenterology, American Society of Colon and Rectal Surgeons, American Society for Gastrointestinal Endoscopy, Oncology Nursing Society, and Society of American Gastrointestinal Endoscopic Surgeons.

of the extent of intestinal wall penetration. This application of this classification was strictly confined to rectal tumors lying beneath the peritoneal reflection, and therefore the concept of serosal involvement was not relevant.

Since Dukes' original description, various modifications of this system have been described to stage tumors in the rectum and throughout the colon. One of the more commonly used staging systems is the modified Astler-Coller system (Fig. 70.9). According to this system, stage A represents tumors that invade into the mucosa only. Stage B1 tumors invade into but not through the muscularis propria. Stage B2 lesions invade through the intestinal wall without involving adjacent organs, whereas stage B3 tumors involve adjacent organs. Stage C tumors involve regional lymph nodes and are subgrouped into stages C1, C2, and C3 according to the depth of intestinal wall penetration. Stage D represents evidence of distant organ involvement.

TNM Classification

The American Joint Committee on Cancer and the International Union Against Cancer (AJCC/UICC) have proposed an alternative staging system based on the extent of the primary tumor (T), regional node involvement (N), and metastasis (M). The TNM system is correlated with equivalent Dukes and modified Astler-Coller stages in Table 70.9. The TNM method has been generally adopted in the field of oncology as the universal colorectal cancer staging system, and is subjected to continuous, data-driven quality improvement reviews. In contrast to the modified Astler-Coller system, the TNM system includes carcinoma *in situ* (Tis) and stratifies

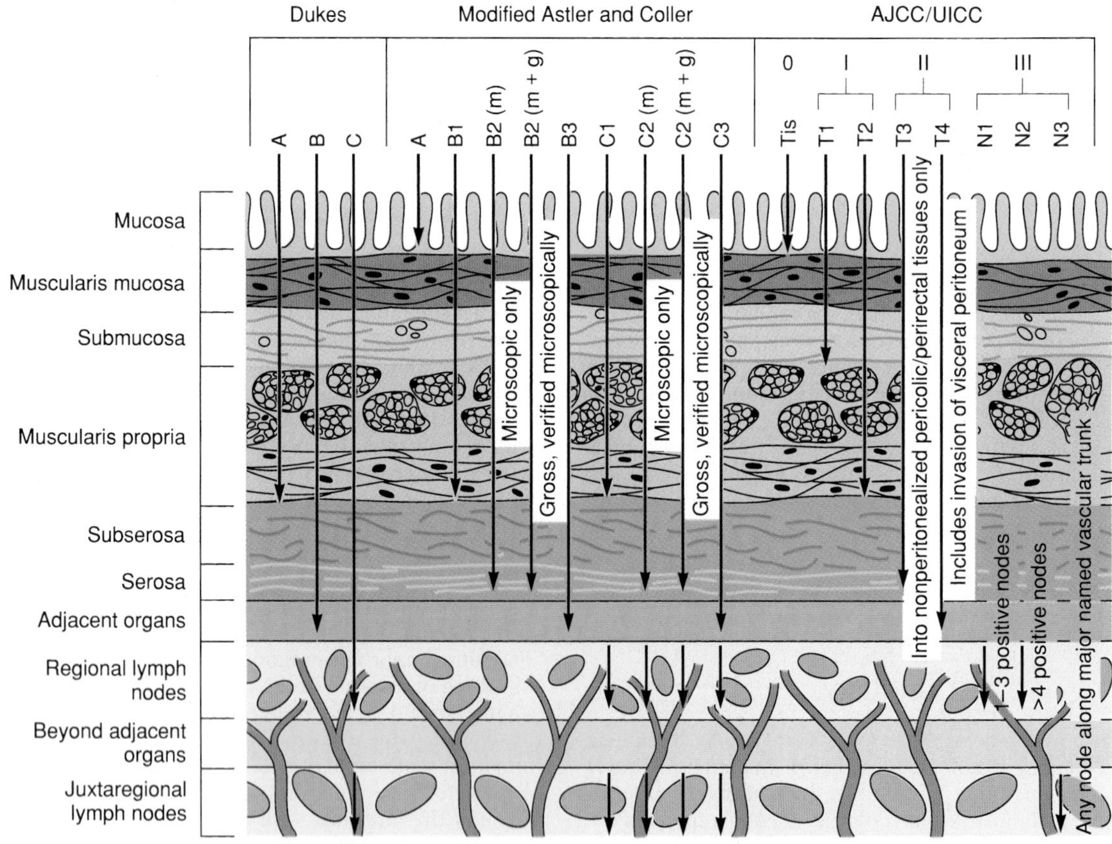

FIGURE 70.9 Schematic description of the staging systems with respect to depth of invasion.

according to number of positive nodes (Fig. 70.9). Stage 0 represents Tis tumors that do not metastasize, stage I includes T1 and T2 tumors, stage II includes T3 and T4 tumors, and stage III includes any tumors with nodal involvement (N1 to N3). Stage IV includes any cancer with distant metastases.

In 2002, the TNM staging system for colorectal cancer was updated to better reflect the impact of depth of penetration and number of involved lymph nodes.[88] National Cancer Database evidence of significantly different survival times among more than 50,000 patients with node positive cancer led to expansion into subcategories A, B, and C. Stage IIA indicates a T1,2 N0 lesions; stage IIB indicates T3,4 N0 disease; stage IIIA indicates a T1,2 N1 lesion; stage IIB indicates T2,3 N1 disease; and stage IIIC indicates any N2 disease. The prognostic validity of this subclassification has been demonstrated using the Surveillance, Epidemiology, and End Results (SEER) national cancer registry.[89] When applied to more than 100,000 patients in the SEER registry, the AJCC 5th edition TNM system revealed overall 5-year colon cancer survival rates of 93.2% for stage I, 82.5% for stage II, 59.5% for stage III, and 8.1% for stage IV. The AJCC 6th edition revised TNM system revealed 5-year colon cancer survival rates of 93.2% for stage I, 84.7% for stage IIA, 72.2% for stage IIB, 83.4% for stage IIIA, 64.1% for stage IIIB, 44.3% for stage IIIC, and 8.1% for stage IV.[89]

Survival of stage IIIA is notably better than that of stage IIB. Two immediate hypotheses may explain this prognostic discrepancy. First, the poorer survival rate among stage IIB patients may reflect the lack of accepted recommendations for adjuvant treatment of these patients. Second, an accurate staging system is predicated on adequate node retrieval. Stage designation may be inaccurate because of an inadequate number of nodes retrieved intraoperatively. A minimum number of 12 lymph nodes must be examined for reliable designation of node negative status. However, a review of more than 100,000 stage I to III colorectal cancer patients found that only 41% of specimens from stage II patients had an adequate lymph node evaluation.[90]

NATURAL HISTORY

The natural progression of colorectal cancer comprises three processes: local invasion, lymphatic spread, and hematogenous spread. Studies described by Dukes in the 1930s led to the theory of an orderly progression from local tumor invasion to subsequent lymphatic and hematogenous spread after the tumor had penetrated the intestinal wall. Today, we know that these observations are not entirely correct because in some subsets of patients with tumors that do not invade through the intestinal wall, lymphatic metastases or distant disease develops nonetheless. In this regard, even patients who undergo curative resection of apparently localized colorectal cancers should be viewed as harboring blood-borne metastases. The risk for the development of disseminated disease can be predicted by the depth of tumor invasion into the intestinal wall and the involvement of draining lymph nodes. Therapies designed to reduce the development of recurrent disease after surgical resection are discussed in later sections of this chapter.

Local growth of an adenocarcinoma is initially characterized by intramural expansion of the tumor into the bowel lumen. Subsequent lateral invasion into the intestinal wall usually progresses in a transverse direction rather than longitudinally and thereby leads to circumferential involvement of the intestine. The incidence of lymphatic metastasis increases with extent of local invasion through the intestinal wall; however, 10% to 20% of patients with cancer limited to the intestinal wall are found to have positive lymph nodes.

TABLE 70.9

STAGING OF COLORECTAL CANCER*

Stage	Description
TUMOR-NODE-METASTASIS (TNM) SYSTEM	
Primary Tumor	
TX	Primary tumor cannot be assessed
T0	No evidence of tumor in resected specimen (prior polypectomy or fulguration)
Tis	Carcinoma in situ
T1	Invades into submucosa
T2	Invades into muscularis propria
T3/T4	Depends on whether serosa is present
Serosa Present	
T3	Invades through muscularis propria into subserosa Invades serosa (but not through) Invades pericolic fat within the leaves of the mesentery
T4	Invades through serosa into free peritoneal cavity or through serosa into a continguous organ
NP Serosa (distal two thirds of rectum, posterior left or right colon)	
T3	Invades through muscularis propria
T4	Invades other organs (vagina, prostate, ureter, kidney)
Regional Lymph Node Involvement	
NX	Nodes cannot be assessed (e.g., local excision only)
N0	No regional node metastases
N1	1–3 positive nodes
N2	4 or more positive nodes
N3	Central nodes positive
Distant Metastasis	
MX	Presence of distant metastases cannot be assessed
M0	No distant metastases
M1	Distant metastases present

Stage	Description		
0	Tis	N0	M0
I	T1,2	N0	M0
IIA	T3	N0	M0
IIB	T4	N0	M0
IIIA	T1,2	N1	M0
IIIB	T3,4	N1	M0
IIIC	Any T	N2	M0
IV	Any T	Any N	M1

DUKES STAGING SYSTEM CORRELATED WITH TNM SYSTEM

Dukes A	T1, N0, M0 (stage I) T2, N0, M0 (stage I)
Dukes B	T3, N0, M0 (stage II) T4, N0, M0 (stage II)
Dukes C	T (any), N1, M0; T (any), N2, M0 (stage III)
Dukes D	T (any), N (any), M1 (stage IV)

MODIFIED ASTLER-COLLER (MAC) SYSTEM CORRELATED WITH TNM SYSTEM

MAC A	T1, N0, M0 (stage I)
MAC B1	T2, N0, M0 (stage I)
MAC B2	T3, N0, M0 (stage II)
MAC B3	T4, N0, M0 (stage II)
MAC C1	T2, N1, M0; T2, N2, M0 (stage III)
MAC C2	T3, N1, M0; T3, N2, M0 (stage III) T4, N1, M0; T4, N2, M0 (stage III)
MAC C3	T4, N1, M0; T4, N2, M0 (stage III)

*In all pathologic staging systems, particularly those applied to rectal cancer, the abbreviations m and g may be used; m denotes microscopic transmural penetration; g or m + g denotes transmural penetration visible on gross inspection and confirmed microscopically.

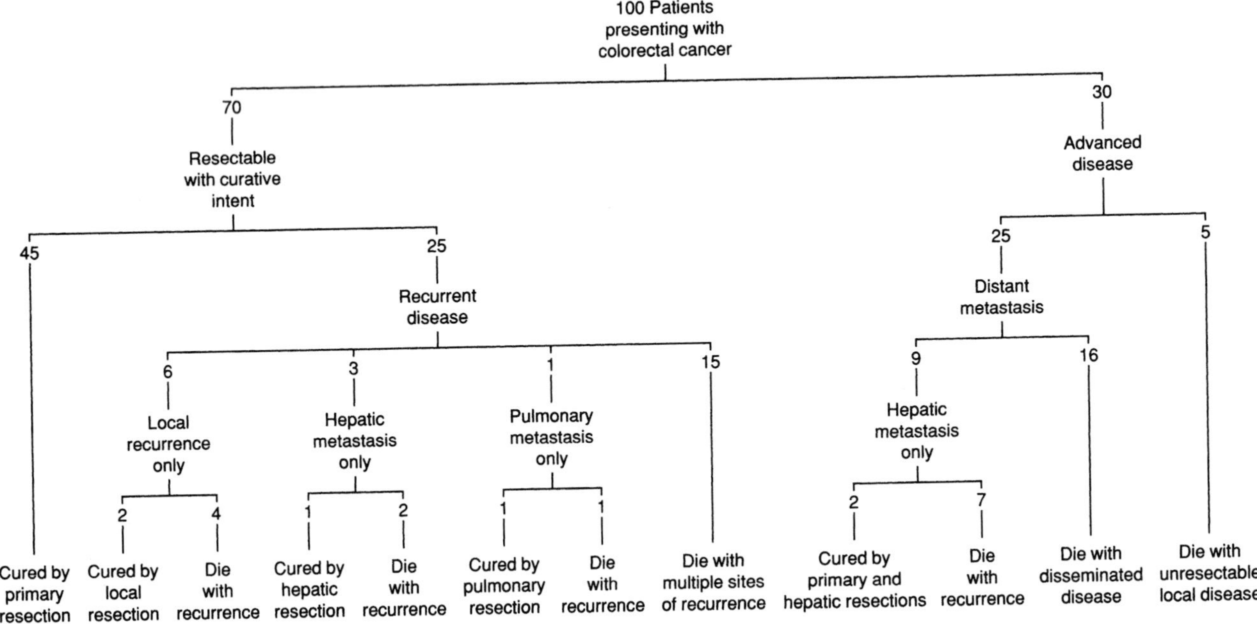

FIGURE 70.10 The natural history of colorectal cancer.

The liver is the most common site of hematogenous spread of colorectal cancer; liver metastasis occurs in about half of all cases.[91] The liver is the first capillary network exposed to tumor emboli traveling through the portal system and represents the major site of venous drainage of the colon and upper rectum. The liver can be the sole site of tumor metastasis, as evidenced by the successful resection of liver metastases for cure in selected patients. By contrast, the lower rectum has a dual drainage system, draining into the portal system and the vena cava by way of the middle and inferior hemorrhoidal veins, respectively. Some think that isolated lung metastases can develop from lower rectal tumors when tumor emboli travel through the systemic venous drainage system. The lung is the second most common site of metastasis from colorectal tumors. Tumor involvement of other sites in the absence of liver and lung metastases is unusual. In certain circumstances, isolated bone metastases to the sacrum or vertebral bodies can arise when tumor emboli travel through portal–vertebral venous communications known as *Batson's plexus*.

Another potential mode of spread is by intraluminal or extraluminal exfoliation of tumor cells with subsequent implantation. Tumor implantation may occur during surgical resection; spillage of tumor cells can cause recurrences in bowel anastomoses, abdominal incisions, or other intraabdominal sites. When tumors penetrate the intestinal wall, shed tumor cells can be implanted intraperitoneally and cause peritoneal carcinomatosis.

Figure 70.10 depicts a summary of the natural history of patients who present with colorectal cancer.[91] For every 100 patients initially evaluated, 30 have clinically evident distant spread, and the remaining 70 undergo resection for localized disease. Among these 70 patients, 45 are cured and disease recurs in the remainder. Extrapolation of these data to the approximately 146,000 patients in whom colorectal cancer is diagnosed each year in the United States implies that 65,700 patients can be cured with surgical resection alone; disease recurs in the remaining 80,300 patients after resection, or they have disseminated tumor at the time of diagnosis. Table 70.10 lists prognostic factors.

TREATMENT OF PRIMARY COLORECTAL TUMORS

Neoplastic Polyps

With the availability of colonoscopy, endoscopic polypectomy has become the standard approach for the treatment of neoplastic polyps unless it is medically contraindicated. The

TABLE 70.10

PROGNOSTIC FACTORS FOR PRIMARY COLORECTAL CANCER

Factor	Association
Age	Patients <40 y old often present with more advanced stage of disease
Symptoms	Symptomatic patients tend to have more advanced stage of disease
Obstruction and perforation	Poorer prognosis when present
Location of primary	Rectosigmoid and rectal cancers have lower cure rates compared with cancers elsewhere in the colon
Tumor configuration	Exophytic tumors are associated with less advanced stage of cancer compared with ulcerative tumors
Blood vessel invasion	Poorer prognosis when present
Lymphatic vessel invasion	Poorer prognosis when present
Perineural invasion	Poorer prognosis when present
Lymphocytic infiltration	Improved prognosis when present
Carcinoembryonic antigen study	Poorer prognosis when elevated before primary tumor resection
Aneuploidy	Poorer prognosis when present

risk of this procedure is extremely low, with a complication rate of less than 1%. Almost all pedunculated polyps can be removed endoscopically with a snare. Sessile lesions can frequently be removed piecemeal, but several sessions may be required. A dilemma in treating colonic polyps occurs if a resected lesion contains a malignant focus. A decision must then be made about the need for a colectomy. If the lesion does not penetrate the muscularis mucosae, it should be considered a malignancy in situ that does not have the propensity to metastasize and therefore does not require further surgery. If the lesion penetrates the muscularis mucosae, it is an invasive cancer and may require surgery. In general, if evidence of invasion is found, colectomy with resection of paracolonic lymph nodes is indicated. In selected cases of pedunculated polyps, conservative management without colectomy may be undertaken if the lesion does not contain poorly differentiated tumor cells or show evidence of vascular invasion and if a negative resection margin has been obtained at the level of the stalk. Lesions that are poorly differentiated or have evidence of vascular invasion, regardless of a negative surgical margin, should be treated by colectomy.

Large villous tumors of the rectum can pose a challenge. Total excision is required to assess the presence of invasive cancer accurately. A full thickness transanal excision with sphincteric muscle and mucosal approximation is preferred; however, other approaches, such as low anterior resection, coloanal procedures, or abdominoperineal resection, may have to be employed to excise extensive benign rectal lesions totally.

Invasive Colorectal Cancers

Surgery

The surgical options for colorectal cancer depend on the location of the primary tumor. Table 70.11 summarizes these surgical procedures.

Before surgical resection, evaluation for sites of metastatic disease is important. A careful physical examination determines the presence of hepatomegaly, ascites, or adenopathy. For rectal tumors, the distance of the tumor from the anal verge and its mobility are important in assessing resectability and the type of operation required. Rectal ultrasonography is currently the most accurate method for preoperatively assessing the extent of local invasion, sphincter involvement, and the presence of enlarged lymph nodes within the mesorectum (Fig. 70.11). Laboratory studies should include a complete blood cell count, determination of serum liver enzymes, and a carcinoembryonic antigen (CEA) assay. Determination of a baseline CEA level can be useful in subsequent follow-up of the patient (see later). Abnormal results of liver function studies may indicate the need to perform abdominal computed tomography (CT) to assess the presence of liver metastases. It is not unreasonable to perform preoperative abdominal CT in all patients with colorectal cancer. The presence of metastatic disease may alter the planned surgical procedure—that is, a low rectal cancer with evidence of hepatic metastases may be better palliated with fulguration than with abdominoperineal resection. A full colonoscopy or air-contrast barium enema should be performed to rule out the presence of other primary colorectal polyps or cancers.

TABLE 70.11 TREATMENT

SURGICAL OPTIONS FOR COLORECTAL CANCER

INTRAPERITONEAL COLON AND UPPER THIRD OF THE RECTUM
Resection and anastomosis
MIDDLE THIRD OF THE RECTUM
Abdominoperineal resection
Low anterior resection
Abdominosacral resection
Coloanal resection
Local excision or fulguration
Primary radiation therapy
LOWER THIRD OF THE RECTUM
Abdominoperineal resection
Local excision or fulguration
Primary radiation therapy

The surgical goals in the resection of a primary colorectal cancer are to achieve an *en bloc* resection that encompasses an adequate amount of normal colon proximal and distal to the tumor, to obtain adequate lateral margins if the tumor is adherent to contiguous structures, and to remove regional lymph nodes. Accomplishment of these goals optimizes the chance of preventing locoregional recurrence of the disease. The extent of bowel resection has been the subject of numerous debates. In pathologic studies, tumor rarely extends intramurally more than 2 cm beyond the area of gross involvement. Traditionally, 5 cm of normal large intestine proximal and distal to the tumor has been advocated as a margin that is adequate to encompass intramural spread completely. The actual margin of intestine removed is often determined by the extent of the lymphadenectomy. The paracolic and intermediate draining lymph nodes should be removed as part of a curative resection (Fig. 70.12). Extensive resections of bowel along with more central or retroperitoneal lymph nodes are not indicated because they add minimal oncologic benefit and substantially increase operative complications. At the time of surgical resection, the abdominal viscera, particularly the liver and peritoneal surfaces, should be thoroughly investigated. If evidence of disseminated disease is apparent, a less extensive resection of the primary lesion for palliation to avoid complications of obstruction or bleeding may be indicated.

Intraperitoneal colon and upper third of the rectum. The surgical resection of cancers in different sites in the colorectum requires attention to specific anatomic details. Resection plus primary anastomosis is the surgical procedure of choice for cancers of the colon and upper third of the rectum. Whenever possible, a mechanical bowel preparation, along with oral antibiotics, should be instituted preoperatively to reduce infectious complications. The choice of anastomotic technique (i.e., stapling versus hand sewing) depends on the surgeon's preference.

Tumors of the cecum and ascending colon should be resected by a right hemicolectomy. Ligation of the ileocolic, right colic, and right branches from the middle colic artery is required (Fig. 70.12). For tumors in the hepatic flexure, an extension of a right hemicolectomy is performed with ligation of the middle colic artery near its origin. Care must be taken during the mobilization of the ascending colon and hepatic flexure because the right ureter and testicular or ovarian vessels, inferior vena cava, superior mesenteric vein, and duodenum are all close together.

For lesions of the transverse colon, a transverse colectomy is accomplished by proximal ligation of the middle colic artery (Fig. 70.12). Cancer of the splenic flexure can be treated with a segmental resection in which the middle transverse colon is anastomosed to the middle descending colon. For this procedure, the left colic artery is divided and the middle colic artery is preserved. Mobilization of the splenic flexure requires care to avoid injury to the spleen.

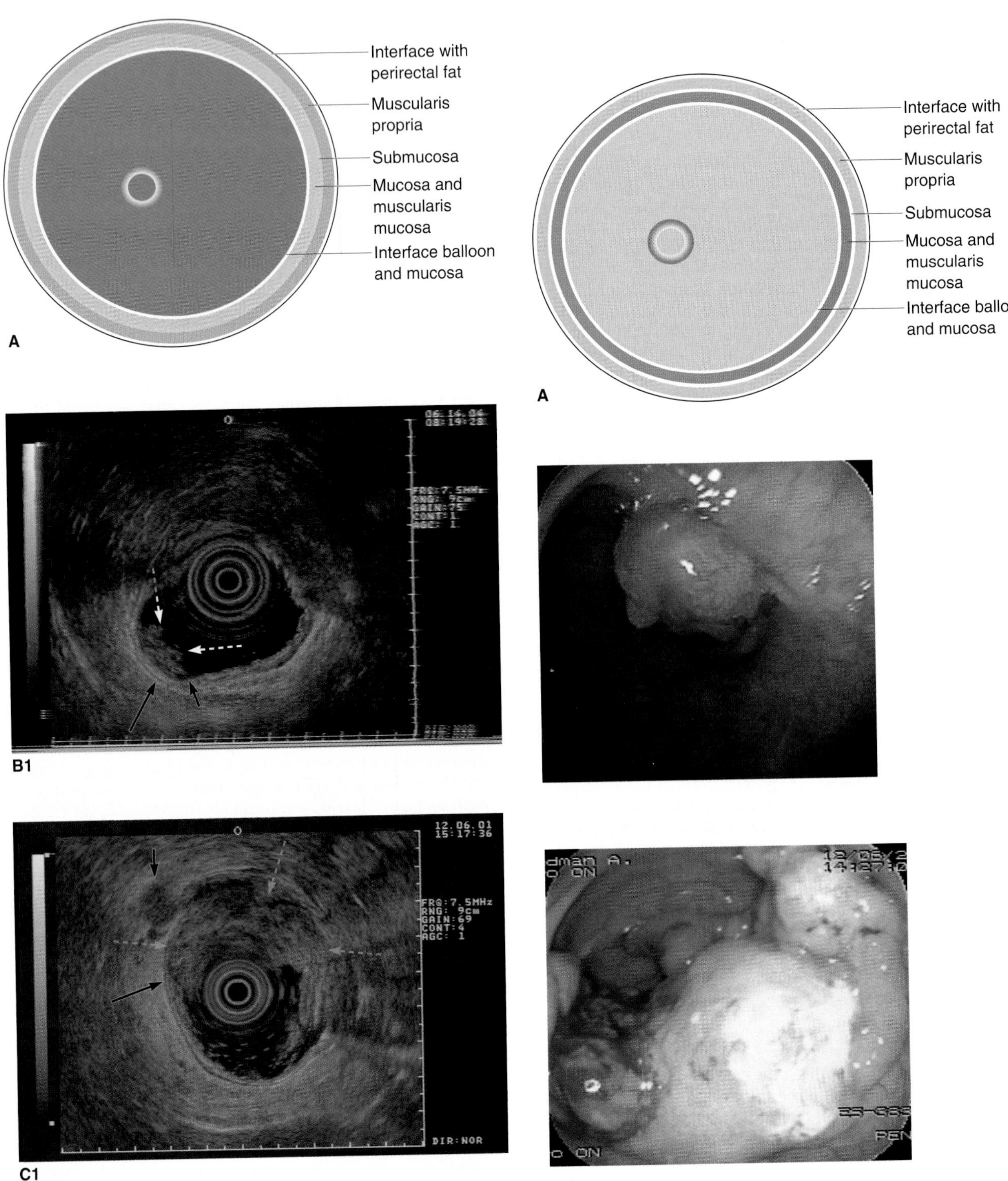

FIGURE 70.11 Endoscopic ultrasound for rectal cancer staging. (*A*) Schematic view of wall structures. (*B* and *C*) Rectal polyp (no mucosal invasion). (*D* and *E*) Stage X tumor (invasion of the XXX).

A left hemicolectomy with removal of intestine from the middle transverse to the distal sigmoid colon can be used for tumors of the descending colon (Fig. 70.12). High ligation of the inferior mesenteric artery is necessary in this operation. For cancers of the sigmoid colon, a segmental resection can be performed with ligation of the sigmoid artery near its origin. Rectosigmoid cancers and tumors confined to the upper third of the rectum are removed by an anterior resection. The upper third of the rectum is about 12 to 16 cm from the anal verge and is located above the peritoneal reflection ending proximally where the tenia flare (Fig. 70.13). The pelvic peritoneum is incised circumferentially around the rectum, and the intestine is mobilized from the presacral fascia. Laterally, the middle hemorrhoidal vessels are ligated, and anteriorly, the rectum is mobilized from the seminal vesicles and prostate or the vagina. The mesenteric vessels are divided at the origin of the

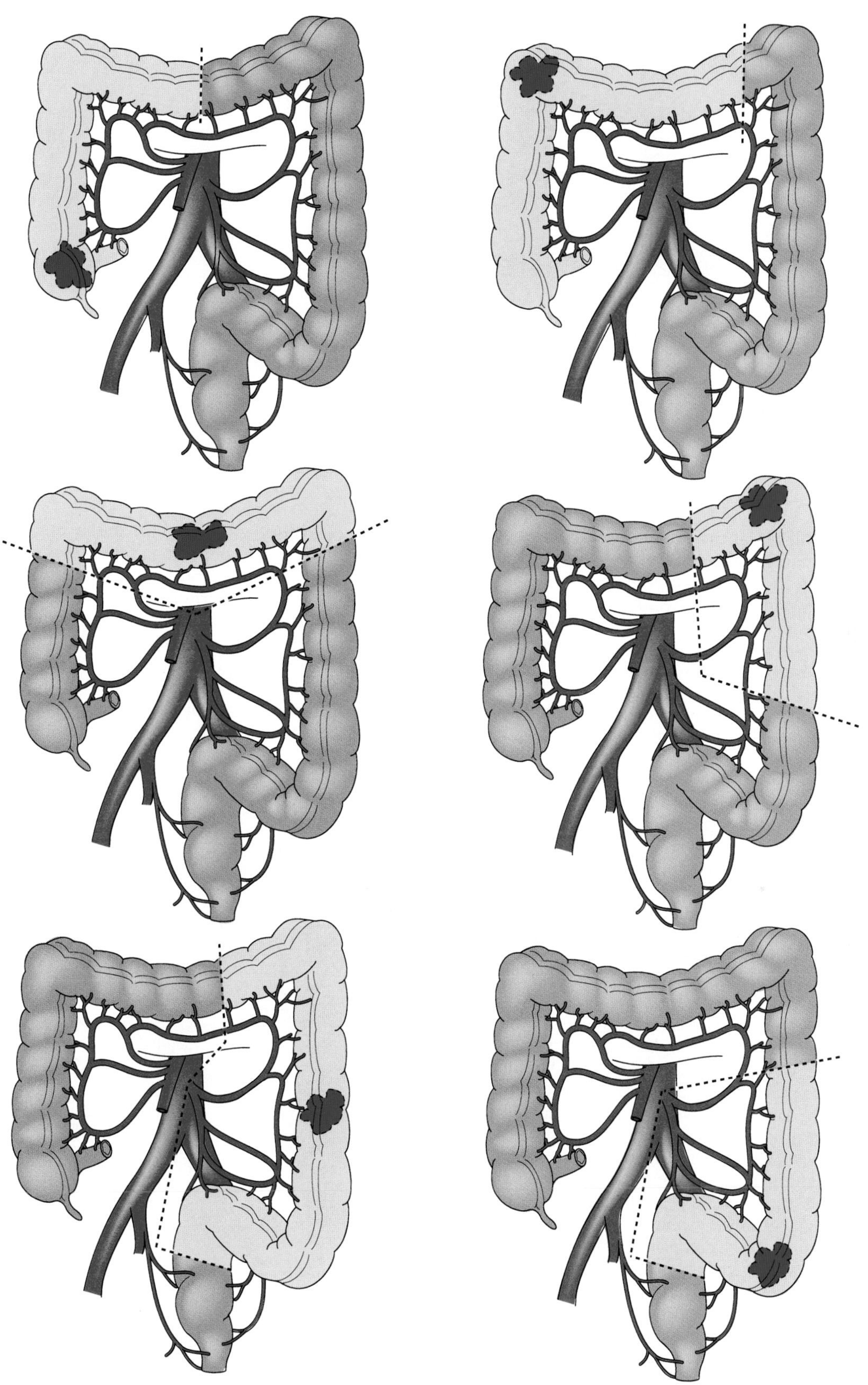

FIGURE 70.12 Segmental resections for cancers of the colon and upper third of the rectum.

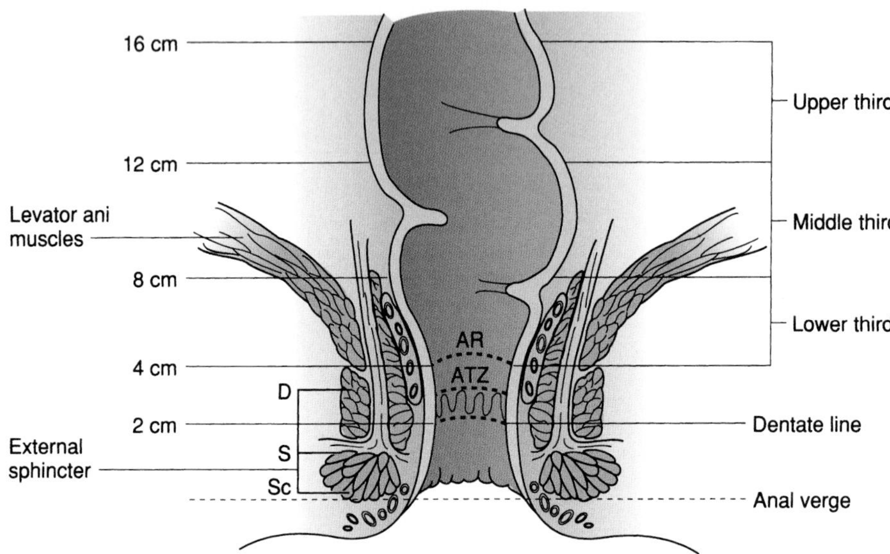

FIGURE 70.13 Anorectal anatomy with important landmarks. Approximate measurements are relative to the anal verge. D, deep; S, superficial; Sc, subcutaneous; AR, anorectal ring; ATZ, anal transition zone.

sigmoid artery or higher, at the origin of the inferior mesenteric artery, if further mobilization of the splenic flexure is required to obtain a tension-free anastomosis.

Laparoscopy provides a new technique for resection of colon and upper rectal cancers. Although the operative steps and surgical principles are identical, laparoscopic resection for colorectal cancer was met initially with skepticism. Critics questioned potential for port-site metastases, possible inadequacy of resection, compromise of patient safety, and increased cost and time investment for questionable gain. The Clinical Outcomes and Surgical Therapy (COST) Study Group recently reported mid-term data from a multicenter trial of 872 colon cancer patients randomized to undergo laparoscopic versus conventional cancer resection.[92] With 3 years of follow-up, there was no difference in recurrence rate, wound recurrence, overall survival, perioperative complications, readmission, and reoperation. The laparoscopic group had a slightly shorter median hospital stay and briefer use of analgesics. This noninferiority trial suggests that laparoscopic resection for appropriate patients is a viable alternative to conventional open surgery.

Middle and Lower Third of the Rectum. Cancers located in the lower third of the rectum, between the anorectal ring and 7 to 8 cm from the anal verge, are reliably treated by abdominoperineal resection. The procedure involves wide excision of the rectum to include the lateral attachments and pelvic mesocolon and establishment of a colostomy. The extent of surgery for an abdominoperineal resection is illustrated in Figure 70.14. With the patient in a modified lithotomy position, the abdominal and perineal procedures can be performed simultaneously by two teams or sequentially by one team. Alternatively, the abdominal procedure can be completed with the patient in the supine position, and the perineal portion completed afterward, with the patient turned in the lateral position. On opening of the abdomen, evidence of intraabdominal spread is ascertained. The discovery of extensive disseminated disease may eliminate the need for an abdominoperineal resection because a local excision or fulguration to preserve anal function may be more appropriate for palliation. If an abdominoperineal resection is performed, ligation of the superior hemorrhoidal vessels at their origin from the left colic artery is required. Occasionally, if extensive nodal disease is present, higher arterial ligation may be necessary. The rectum is mobilized in a fashion similar to that described for an anterior resection, but the dissection is carried down to the pelvic floor muscles, which are excised *en bloc* with the anus. An end-sigmoid colostomy is brought out through the rectus sheath. Efforts to exclude small intestine from a future radiation field by use of the uterus, omentum, peritoneum, or absorbable mesh should be considered. Primary closure of the perineal wound over drains can usually be accomplished without complications.

Cancer of the middle third of the rectum, between 8 and 12 cm from the anal verge (Fig. 70.13), can be managed by a variety of techniques. For these tumors, abdominoperineal resection does not yield results superior to those of other pro-

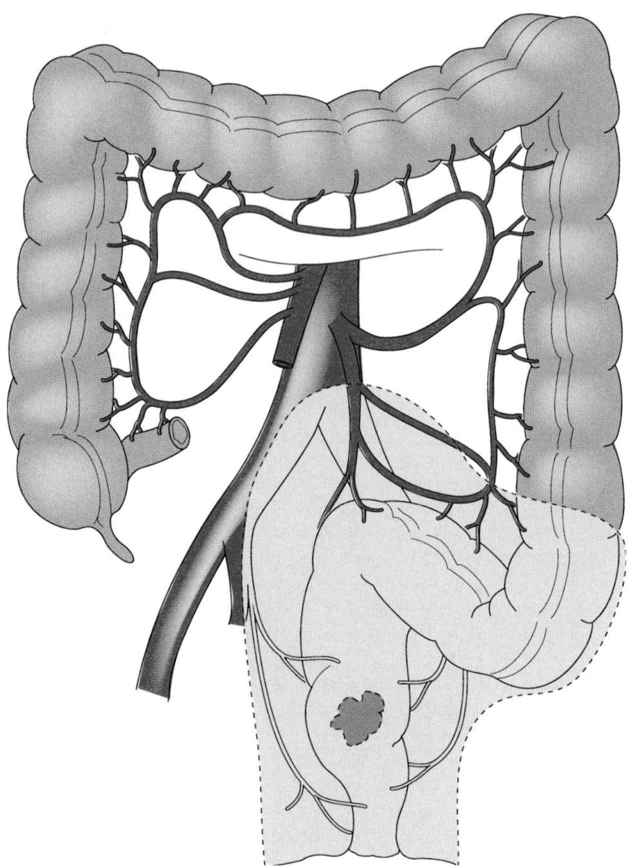

FIGURE 70.14 Extent of surgery in abdominoperineal resection.

cedures that spare the anal sphincter. Therefore, an effort should be made to maintain intestinal continuity. Low anterior resection is a commonly used technique that involves resection of the middle rectum with primary anastomosis. The introduction of the end-to-end anastomosis stapler has increased the use of this sphincter-saving procedure (Fig. 70.15A). If a transanal reconstruction with a stapler is contemplated, the patient should be placed in the lithotomy position. The initial stages of the operation, with complete mobilization of the rectum to the level of the pelvic floor, are identical to those for an abdominoperineal resection. After removal of the tumor, the anastomosis, which can be end-to-end or end-to-side, is joined with sutures or staples (Fig. 70.15B,C). A temporary transverse colostomy or loop ileostomy should be employed if the integrity of the anastomosis is a concern.

Other sphincter-saving approaches have been described for middle rectal cancers.[93] Coloanal anastomosis involves restoring bowel continuity by bringing the colon to the level of the anus and dentate line (Fig. 70.15D). A straight coloanal anastomosis commonly results in stool frequency, urgency, and incontinence, which can be tempered by a side-to-end anastomosis or a formation of a colonic J-pouch (Fig. 70.15E). Creation of an adequate but not overlarge reservoir is an important technical point in order to avoid future difficulty with evacuation. Abdominosacral resections were described in the 1940s and allowed surgeons more direct visualization of low, hand-sewn anastomoses. The rectum is mobilized through an abdominal approach, and a second incision is made above the anus, with resection of the coccyx for visualization into the pelvis. A hand-sewn anastomosis is completed through the transsacral incision (Fig. 70.15F). This procedure has largely been supplanted by the use of stapling devices.

One of the controversies concerning sphincter-saving procedures for rectal tumors concerns the length of an adequate distal mucosal margin. The traditional dictum of 5 cm for a margin is not substantiated by any studies. Only 2.5% of patients have intramural spread beyond 2 cm from the palpable tumor, and these patients usually have dissemination of tumor despite aggressive local therapy. No correlation has been found between local recurrence and extent of the distal margin when it is greater than 2 cm. Ideally, a surgical margin of 3 cm, measured on the fresh specimen, should be achieved. If the end-to-end anastomosis stapler is used, then a margin of 2 cm plus the additional "doughnut" specimen obtained by the stapler should be adequate. If, in the surgeon's judgment, this length of margin cannot be obtained, then abdominoperineal resection should be performed. The segment of rectum located between the tumor and the pelvic floor, determined preoperatively, can be lengthened as much as 4 cm after the rectum is mobilized from its pelvic attachments (Fig. 70.16).

Radial margins are more relevant than longitudinal margins for local control of mid to low rectal cancers. The practical importance of lateral spread is demonstrated by results of total mesorectal excision (TME) *en bloc* with the rectal specimen. By means of TME, the Basingstoke group initially reported a dramatic reduction in local recurrence from the norm of 30% to 40% to 3.7% over a 4 year follow-up period. [94] Subsequent studies consistently showed a decline in local recurrence of 15% to 40% using conventional techniques to 4% to 11% using TME. [95–98] The technique of TME includes sharp dissection posteriorly in the presacral avascular plane from the superior hemorrhoidal vessels to the levator ani, laterally encompassing the entire peritoneal reflection, and anteriorly including Denonvilliers fascia in the specimen (Fig. 70.17).

As with many oncologic surgical procedures, increased interest has been shown in less radical types of surgery to manage cancers of the middle and lower third of the rectum in an effort to preserve the anal sphincters and avoid an abdominoperineal resection. Initially, these local procedures, such as excision, ablation, and irradiation, were reserved for patients with advanced disease or with medical contraindications to radical surgery. Evidence is increasing, however, that for selected patients with low rectal cancers local excision is an acceptable treatment option that is associated with rates of local recurrence and survival similar to those seen after radical surgery. A multicenter, prospective study addressing this question was recently published.[99] To be eligible, patients had to have an adenocarcinoma of the rectum that was 10 cm or less from the dentate line and 4 cm or less in diameter, and that involved 40% or less of the rectal lumen. All patients registered underwent local excision of their tumor. Those determined to have T1 tumors with negative surgical margins received no further treatment, and those with T2 tumors underwent postoperative radiation and chemotherapy. The 6-year disease-free survival rates were 83% and 87%, respectively, and the overall survival rates were 71% and 85%for T1 and T2 tumors, respectively. Two of 59 patients with T1 tumors and 7 of 51 patients with T2 tumors experienced an isolated local recurrence and underwent salvage abdominoperineal resection. Four of these patients died of recurrent local or distal disease. Data from the remaining patients were not mature enough to comment on whether salvage abdominoperineal resection performed for local recurrences provides the same chance for survival as abdominoperineal resection performed at the time of primary cancer treatment.[99] A case control study from the Minnesota group examining transanal excision versus radical surgery without adjuvant therapy found a significantly higher local recurrence rate of 47% versus 6%, respectively.[100] More importantly, T2 patients undergoing local versus radical initial excision experienced a respective 5-year survival difference of 65% versus 81% among patients with T2 tumors, in spite of salvage abdominoperineal resection. Until more detailed prospective data are available, a radical excision should be strongly considered for clinical stage T2 tumors. If a local excision is performed and the tumor is upstaged pathologically to T2, the patient and surgeon should consider an abdominoperineal resection depending on the patient's health and functional status.

Other forms of local treatment for low rectal cancers should still be reserved for patients who are not candidates for abdominoperineal resection or local excision. Ablation by transanal electric fulguration of the tumor in multiple stages has been reported to be an acceptable treatment in patients who are poor surgical candidates; however, this procedure cannot be used for circumferential tumors.[101] Endocavitary irradiation as a primary curative therapy for early cancers has been reported with some success. The neodymium:yttrium-aluminum garnet laser has been found to be effective in palliating obstructive or bleeding lesions of locally advanced colorectal tumors.

Adjuvant Radiation Therapy

Radiation therapy combined with surgical resection for colorectal cancer has been demonstrated to reduce the incidence of local tumor recurrence. In general, the use of radiation therapy has been limited to rectal tumors in which the incidence of local recurrence is significant, including those extending through the intestinal wall or with lymph node involvement. Overall, for stage IIA (T3, N0) rectal tumors, the incidence of local recurrence is about 30% to 35% but can be reduced to 5% with adjuvant radiation therapy. For stage III (any T, N1-2) rectal cancers, the use of adjuvant radiation therapy decreases local recurrences from the range of 45% to 65% down to 10%. Multiple phase III studies of adjuvant and neoadjuvant radiation have demonstrated improved local control.[102] Although no survival advantage has been shown at 2 years follow-up, one randomized controlled trial revealed an overall 5-year survival

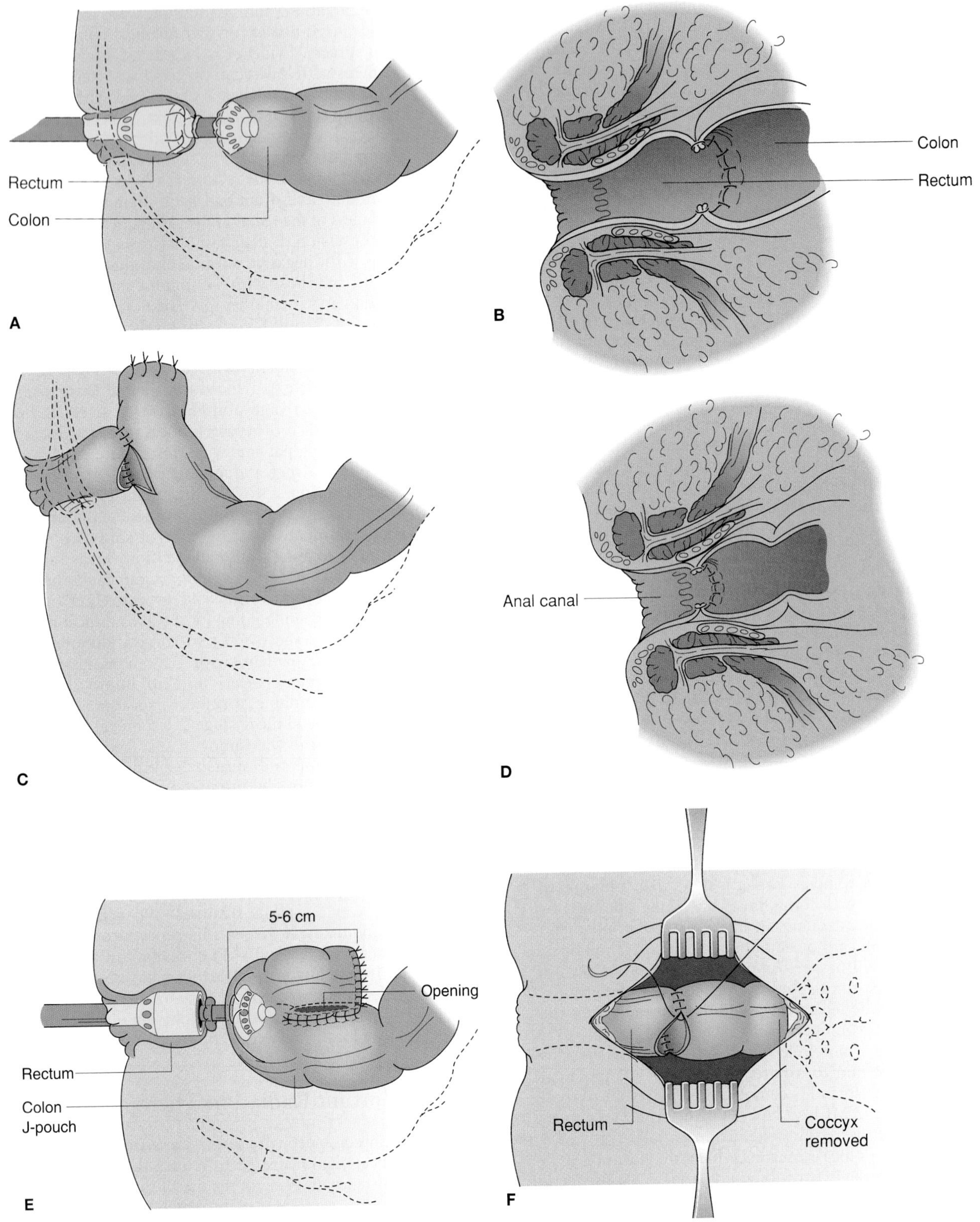

FIGURE 70.15 Techniques for low anterior resections. (*A*) End-to-end stapler. (*B*) Single layer with sutures. (*C*) Side-to-end anastomosis. (*D*) Pull-through. (*E*) Colon J-pouch (5- to 6-cm pouch). (*F*) Transsacral resection.

rate of 58% for radiation plus surgery versus 48% for the surgery alone group.[103]

The technical aspects of radiation therapy relate to dose and timing. The effectiveness of radiation therapy is directly proportional to the total dose. It appears that the most effective dose of radiation to eradicate microscopic disease is at least 5,000 cGy. Adjuvant radiation therapy can be delivered preoperatively, postoperatively, or in a combined "sandwich" approach, in which small doses of preoperative treatment are followed by postoperative treatment to a high total cumulative dose. Recent

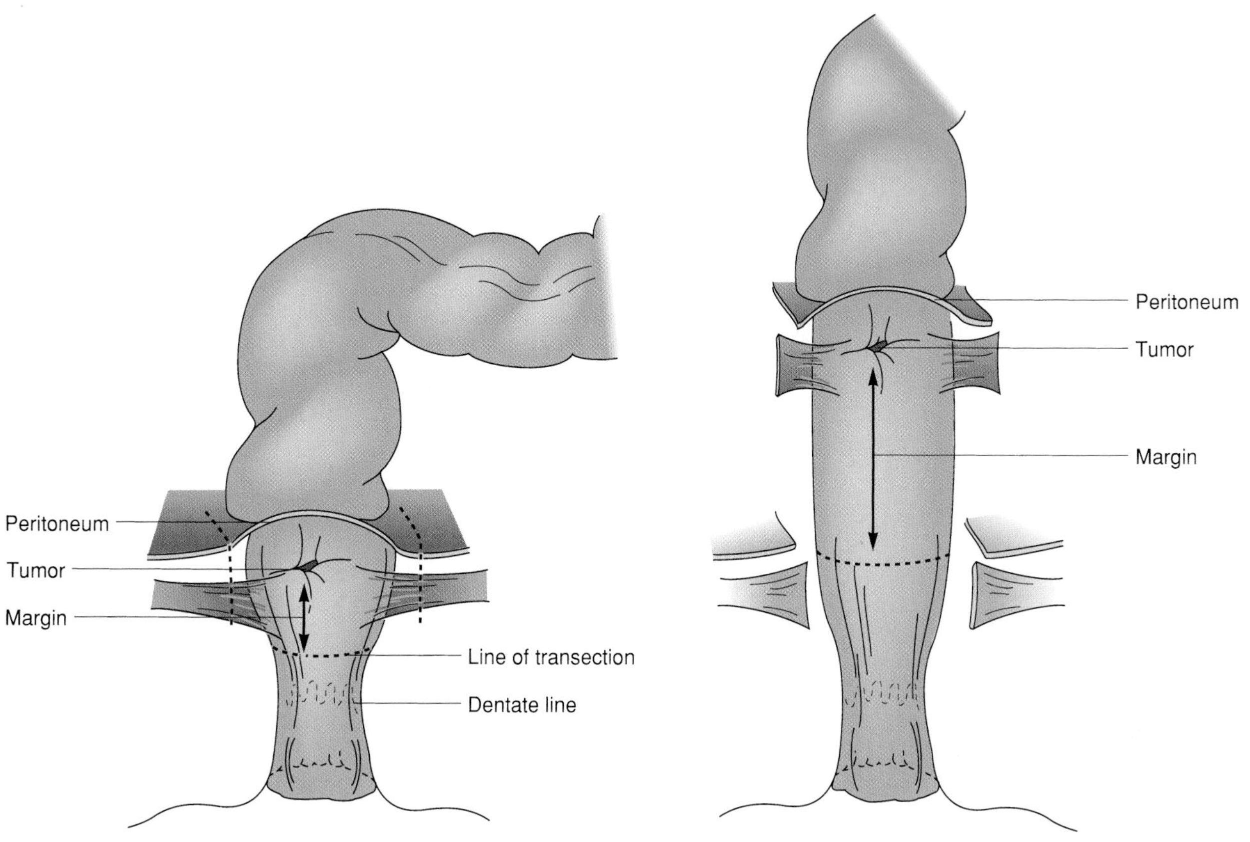

FIGURE 70.16 Dissection of the rectum from pelvic attachments lengthens distal tumor-free margins and may permit a sphincter-saving procedure.

data from a randomized trial of preoperative versus postoperative therapy for stage II and III patients indicate no overall survival superiority. However, patients who received preoperative therapy experienced only a 6% rate of local recurrence and significantly fewer toxic effects than the postoperative radiotherapy group who had a 12% rate of local recurrence.[104]

Less experience has been reported for adjuvant radiation therapy of resected colon cancer. Adjuvant radiation therapy for colon cancer is associated with special problems of toxicity because of the large amount of small intestine that may lie within the treatment field. Nevertheless, several reports indicate that in high-risk cases, such as tumors involving adjacent viscera or perforated lesions, adjuvant radiation therapy can decrease local and regional recurrences.

Adjuvant Chemotherapy

Even if local tumor control is adequate, patients with colorectal cancer die of disseminated disease. In about 25% of patients with stage II tumors, and 50% of those with stage III tumors, the growth of micrometastatic disease present at the time of primary tumor resection eventually causes death. Several randomized, prospective studies have demonstrated that postoperative adjuvant systemic chemotherapy benefits certain subgroups of patients.

The National Comprehensive Cancer Network (NCCN) is a consortium of major cancer centers in the United States that have established practice guidelines for a variety of cancers.[105] The guidelines have been established based upon the best evidence available. For node positive colon cancer (associated with any T stage), adjuvant chemotherapy is recommended. The standard chemotherapy regimen is currently 5-fluorouracil (5-FU) and leuocovorin. Capecitabine appears to be equivalent to 5-FU/leucovorin in recent studies. Also, the combination of 5-FU/leucovorin/oxaliplatin (FOLFOX) is being evaluated as a better alternative to the standard 5-FU/leucovorin regimen. For node negative colon cancers, adjuvant chemotherapy may be considered for high risk lesions (i.e., T3, grade 3-4, lymphovascular invasion or bowel obstruction) as opposed to participation in a clinical trial or observation. Any T4 colon lesion should also be considered for adjuvant radiotherapy.

In colon cancer, local recurrence is infrequent; in rectal cancer, the use of adjuvant chemotherapy combined with radiation has proved effective in improving local control and increasing the survival rate. In rectal cancer, it is almost as important to prevent local failure and ensuing symptoms as it is to prevent death from distant metastasis. As noted in the previous section, radiation therapy is routinely recommended for patients with stage IIA (T3, N0) or III (any T, N1-2) rectal cancers. In addition, the NCCN guidelines recommend adjuvant chemotherapy (either 5-FU or FOLFOX) for these stages of rectal cancer.

TREATMENT OF RECURRENT COLORECTAL CANCER

A subset of patients with recurrent colorectal cancer can be cured, so that a comprehensive follow-up program in patients who have undergone resection of their primary tumor is appropriate (Table 70.12). Of cancers that recur, 50% do so within 18 months after surgery, and 90% of recurrences are evident by 3 years. Therefore, careful follow-up is important during the 3-year period after primary tumor resection.

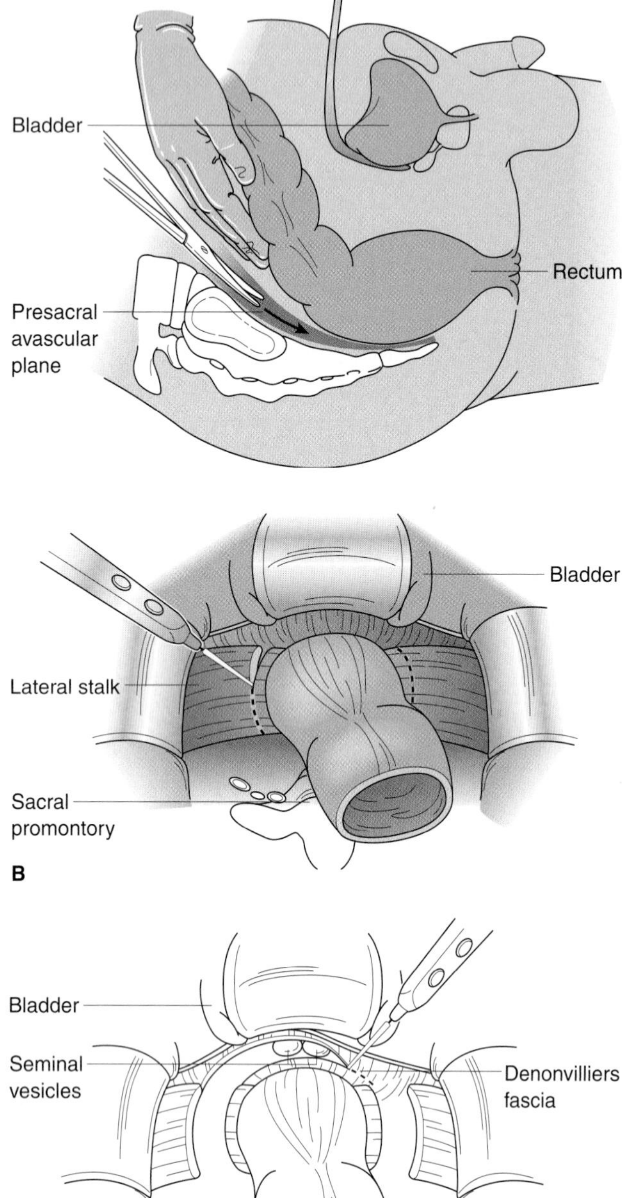

FIGURE 70.17 Technique of total mesorectal excision. (*A*) Posterior sharp dissection in the presacral avascular plane. (*B*) lateral dissection encompassing the peritoneal reflection. (*C*) Anterior dissection including Denonvilliers fascia in the specimen.

Besides identifying recurrences, a careful follow-up program also identifies the 5% of patients in whom a metachronous primary tumor of the large intestine develops.

The CEA assay is a sensitive serologic test in the diagnosis of recurrent colorectal cancer. CEA is a glycoprotein that was originally described as a tumor-specific antigen derived from neoplasms of the gastrointestinal tract. It is now known that CEA is not tumor-specific because its concentration can be elevated in a variety of malignancies from different sites and in some benign conditions. CEA is an oncofetal antigen that is also expressed by early embryonic or fetal cells. CEA is not useful as a screening or diagnostic test but is useful as a tumor marker. The CEA concentration is elevated in more than 90% of patients with disseminated colorectal cancer and in about 20% of patients with localized disease. Serum levels usually are elevated in proportion to the mass of the tumor present and often correlate with response to therapy. CEA measurement provides useful information when elevated levels fall to normal after curative resection. In about two thirds of patients with recurrent disease, an increased CEA level is the first indicator of tumor recurrence; therefore, serial CEA testing, combined with regular physical examinations, is one of the most useful means for detecting recurrent colorectal cancer. In fact, the CEA determination, along with the history and physical examination, is the only surveillance test recommended for patients after curative resection of stage II or III disease. The NCCN guidelines recommend CEA testing along with history and physical examinations every 3 months for 2 years, then every 6 months for a total of 5 years. Colonoscopy is recommended 1 year after resection and then every 2 to 3 years thereafter if negative.

TABLE 70.12

GUIDELINES FOR SURVEILLANCE STUDIES AFTER RESECTION OF STAGE II OR III COLORECTAL CANCER*

Test	Recommendations
Carcinoembryonic antigen	If patient is medically fit to undergo liver resection for liver metastases, evaluate every 2–3 mo for 2 y or more; an elevated result warrants further evaluation for metastatic disease but does not justify systemic therapy for presumed disease
History and physical examination	Every 3–6 mo for first 3 y and yearly thereafter
Colonoscopy	Every 3–5 y to detect new cancers and polyps
Computed tomography	Not indicated
Chest roentgenography	Not indicated
Complete blood cell count	Not indicated
Liver chemistries	Not indicated
Fecal occult blood	Not indicated

*Endorsed by the American Society of Clinical Oncology.

Hepatic Metastases

The liver is the most frequent site of blood-borne metastases from primary colorectal cancers. In a subgroup of patients, the liver is the only site of recurrent disease, and surgical excision of the metastases is the only curative option for these patients. Overall, surgical resection is associated with a 5-year survival rate of 25% to 30% (Fig. 70.18).[106] Patients eligible for hepatic resection of metastatic disease are those who have no evidence of extrahepatic tumor, no medical contraindications to surgery, and a limited number of lesions that are amenable to resection with negative surgical margins.

Patients who have unresectable hepatic metastases that appear to be confined to that organ have been treated with regional chemotherapy through the hepatic artery (e.g., fluorodeoxyuridine). Several studies have demonstrated significantly higher tumor response rates with regional chemotherapy than with systemic chemotherapy. A meta-analysis has demonstrated that regional chemotherapy of unresectable liver metastases can confer improved survival of several months.

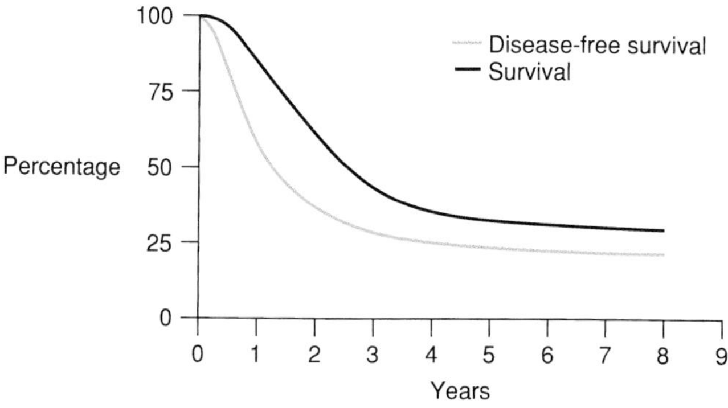

FIGURE 70.18 Disease-free and overall survival in patients who underwent hepatic resection for colorectal carcinoma metastases to the liver. (After Hughes KS, Simon R, Songhorabodi S, et al. Registry of hepatic metastases: resection of the liver for colorectal carcinoma metastases: A multiinstitutional study of indications for resection. *Surgery* 1988;103:278.)

Pulmonary Metastases

Pulmonary metastases develop in about 10% of all patients with colorectal cancer, usually in association with widespread metastatic disease. Because the colon is drained solely by the portal system, one would not expect metastases to the lung without evidence of tumor in the liver. In contrast, rectal cancers may spread through the portal or systemic venous systems and can theoretically give rise to isolated pulmonary metastases. In select patients, particularly those with rectal cancers, resection of pulmonary recurrences can result in a 5-year survival rate of 20%.[107]

Local/Regional Recurrence

Colon cancer recurs locally in about 20% of cases, and the local lesion is the only site of recurrence in about one third of these cases. If the recurrent tumor is isolated to the suture line, resection of such recurrence can be curative. Locoregional failure occurs in 30% to 65% of patients with transmural or node-positive rectal cancers. Often, pelvic recurrences of rectal cancer after a low anterior or abdominoperineal resection are diffuse and associated with disseminated disease. If pelvic recurrences are localized, they should be resected if negative surgical margins can be achieved. Surgical procedures necessary to accomplish this include *en bloc* partial sacrectomy or total pelvic exenteration.

Disseminated Disease

Recurrent colorectal cancer is not usually localized to one site that is amenable to surgical resection. More commonly, colorectal cancer recurs in multiple sites. In these cases, systemic therapy may be considered. No studies have clearly documented that systemic therapies for disseminated colorectal cancer improve the survival rate; however, systemic treatment is commonly used for palliation.

The current management of disseminated colorectal cancer employs a variety of active agents, both in combination and as single agents: 5-FU/leucovorin, irinotecan, oxaliplatin, and capecitabine and bevacizumab. The choice of therapy is based on the performance status of the patient (i.e., whether the patient can tolerate or not tolerate intensive therapy), prior therapies, and patient preference. Patients with poor performance characteristics should receive supportive care only.

OTHER COLORECTAL TUMORS

Carcinoid Tumors

Carcinoid tumors are neoplasms derived from cells that are capable of synthesizing a wide variety of hormones. Most gastrointestinal tract carcinoids occur in the ileum and the appendix. The rectum is the next most common site, and occasionally carcinoid tumors occur in the colon. Tumor size is an extremely important prognostic factor. About 60% of rectal carcinoids present as asymptomatic submucosal nodules measuring less than 2 cm in diameter. Transanal local excision suffices for definitive therapy because small tumors rarely metastasize. Malignant potential is seen almost exclusively in tumors larger than 2 cm. More radical excisions of larger rectal lesions may be required for local control; however, the results of radical excisions for large rectal carcinoids are poor because these tumors are prone to metastasize. In contrast to rectal carcinoids, colon carcinoids should be treated by standard curative operation. Among carcinoid tumors of the colon smaller than 2 cm , 22% have metastasized to regional lymph nodes, whereas 79% of tumors larger than 2 cm have positive nodes.[108]

Lymphomas

Colorectal lymphomas are rare and account for fewer than 0.5% of all colorectal malignancies. The documentation of widespread dissemination of lymphoma in most cases underscores the concept that lymphoma of the gastrointestinal tract is a systemic disease in which tumor cells are present in other organ sites. Because this disease is highly responsive to chemotherapy and radiation, surgery is not the primary mode of therapy. If the clinical workup reveals a focal site of disease in the large intestine, surgical resection may be considered. Usually, for localized, low-grade colorectal lymphomas, radiation therapy is considered first-line therapy. For intermediate- and high-grade lymphomas, chemotherapy combined with radiation therapy should be the primary treatment modality. Surgery for colorectal lymphomas has been primarily for diagnostic and staging purposes and for the management of treatment-related complications (i.e., perforation or bleeding).

Sarcomas

Colorectal sarcomas are extremely rare and account for fewer than 0.1% of all large bowel malignancies. The most common histologic sarcoma subtype is leiomyosarcoma. With these tumors, the most significant prognostic indicator is the tumor grade. Patients with high-grade tumors do poorly. These tumors usually metastasize to the liver and peritoneal surfaces. If the tumors are clinically localized at initial presentation, a radical *en bloc* excision should be performed to obtain a margin of uninvolved normal tissue. Because of the rarity of this tumor, no studies have addressed whether adjuvant radiation therapy or chemotherapy is beneficial.

Gastrointestinal Stromal Tumors

Gastrointestinal stromal tumors (GISTs) are a more recently identified tumor subtype, previously often mislabeled as "sarcoma." GISTs originate from the pluripotential interstitial cells of Cajal, the gastrointestinal pacemaker cell, and can occur anywhere in the gut. These are submucosal, slow-growing tumors that can reach immense sizes before becoming symptomatic. Frozen section histology is often consistent with a spindle cell appearance; immunohistochemical staining nearly always reveals a positive kit receptor. The metastatic potential is assessed by size and mitotic index. These mesenchymal tumors spread hematogenously, generally recurring locally, in the peritoneum, or in the liver. The mainstay of treatment is complete surgical resection. GISTs are not responsive to traditional chemotherapy or to radiation. For metastatic disease, a tyrosine kinase inhibitor, iminitab mesylate, is extremely effective at controlling tumor growth and spread.

KEY POINTS

- **Mutations in three distinct types of genes are known to contribute to colorectal cancer formation: oncogenes, tumor-suppressor genes, and DNA mismatch repair genes. The former two mechanisms, comprising the *loss of heterozygosity* or *chromosomal instability pathway*, account for about 85% of colon and rectal tumors. Mutations in mismatch repair genes, termed the *replication error* or *microsatellite instability pathway*, account for about 15% of large bowel tumors.**
- **Epidemiologic studies have suggested that 15% of colorectal cancers occur in a dominantly inherited pattern. The two best-described familial colorectal cancer syndromes are familial adenomatous polyposis (FAP) and hereditary nonpolyposis colorectal cancer (HNPCC). Currently, it is estimated that 3% to 5% of all colorectal cancers occur in persons affected with one of these two syndromes.**
- **A strong association exists between inflammatory bowel disease and bowel cancer.**
- **The incidence of invasive malignancy differs markedly for the three histologic subtypes of colon polyps, being lowest in adenomatous polyps, intermediate in tubulovillous adenomas, and highest in villous lesions. Polyp size is also directly correlated with the presence of dysplasia or malignancy.**
- **The most important prognostic factor in colorectal cancer is the depth of invasion of the primary tumor.**
- **The surgical goals in the resection of a primary colorectal cancer are to achieve an *en bloc* resection that encompasses an adequate amount of normal colon proximal and distal to the tumor, to obtain adequate lateral margins if the tumor is adherent to contiguous structures, and to remove regional lymph nodes.**
- **The liver is the most frequent site of blood-borne metastases from primary colorectal cancers.**

References

1. American Cancer Society. Statistics for 2004. Available at: http://www.cancer.org. Accessed January, 2005.
2. National Cancer Institute. Colon cancer treatment. Available at: http://www.cancer.gov/. Accessed January 2005.
3. Parkin DM, Laara E, Muir CS. Estimates of the worldwide frequency of sixteen major cancers in 1980. *Int J Cancer* 1988;41:184–197.
4. Jemal A, Clegg LX, Ward E, et al. Annual report to the nation on the status of cancer, 1975–2001, with a special feature regarding survival. *Cancer* 2004;101:3–27.
5. Dominitz JA, Samsa GP, Landsman P, et al. Race, treatment, and survival among colorectal carcinoma patients in an equal-access medical system. *Cancer* 1998;82:2312–2320.
6. Nyren O, Bergstrom R, Nystrom L, et al. Smoking and colorectal cancer: a 20 year follow-up study of Swedish construction workers. *J Natl Cancer Inst.* 1996;88:1302–1307.
7. Willett W. The search for the causes of breast and colon cancer. *Nature* 1989;338:389–394.
8. Willett WC, MacMahon B. Diet and cancer—an overview (second of two parts). *N Engl J Med.* 1984;310:697–703.
9. Satia-Abouta J, Galanko JA, Martin CF, et al. Food groups and colon cancer risk in African-Americans and Caucasians. *Int J Cancer* 2004; 109:728–736.
10. Chao A, Thun MJ, Connell CJ, et al. Meat consumption and risk of colorectal cancer. *JAMA* 2005;293:172–182.
11. Larsson SC, Rafter J, Holmberg L, et al. Red meat consumption and risk of cancers in the proximal colon, distal colon, and rectum: The Swedish Mammography Cohort. *Int J Cancer* 2005;113:829–834.
12. Burkitt DP. Epidemiology of cancer of the colon and rectum. *Dis Colon Rectum* 1993;36:1071–1082.
13. Bos JL, Fearon ER, Hamilton SR, et al. Prevalence of ras gene mutations in human colorectal cancers. *Nature* 1987;327:293–297.
14. Fearon ER, Vogelstein B. A genetic model for colorectal tumorigenesis. *Cell.* 1990;61:759–767.
15. Arvanitis ML, Jagelman DG, Fazio VW, et al. Mortality in patients with familial adenomatous polyposis. *Dis Colon Rectum* 1990;33:639–642.
16. Kinzler KW, Nilbert MC, Su LK, et al. Identification of FAP locus genes from chromosome 5q21. *Science* 1991;253:661–665.
17. Groden J, Thliveris A, Samowitz W, et al. Identification and characterization of the familial adenomatous polyposis coli gene. *Cell* 1991; 66:589–600.
18. Korinek V, Barker N, Morin PJ, et al. Constitutive transcriptional activation by a beta-catenin-Tcf complex in APC-/- colon carcinoma. *Science* 1997; 275:1784–1787.
19. Morin PJ, Sparks AB, Korinek V, et al. Activation of beta-catenin-Tcf signaling in colon cancer by mutations in beta-catenin or APC. *Science* 1997;275:1787–1790.
20. Powell SM, Zilz N, Beazer-Barclay Y, et al. APC mutations occur early during colorectal tumorigenesis. *Nature* 1992;359:235–237.
21. Smith AJ, Stern HS, Penner M, et al. Somatic APC and K-ras codon 12 mutations in aberrant crypt foci from human colons. *Cancer Res.* 1994;54:5527–5530.
22. Vogelstein B, Kinzler KW. p53 function and dysfunction. *Cell* 1992; 70:523–526.
23. Jen J, Kim H, Piantadosi S, et al. Allelic loss of chromosome 18q and prognosis in colorectal cancer. *N Engl J Med.* 1994;331:213–221.
24. Carethers JM, Hawn MT, Greenson JK, et al. Prognostic significance of allelic lost at chromosome 18q21 for stage II colorectal cancer. *Gastroenterology* 1998;114:1188–1195.
25. Thibodeau SN, Bren G, Schaid D. Microsatellite instability in cancer of the proximal colon. *Science* 1993;260:816–819.
26. Ionov Y, Peinado MA, Malkhosyan S, et al. Ubiquitous somatic mutations in simple repeated sequences reveal a new mechanism for colonic carcinogenesis. *Nature* 1993;363:558–561.
27. Aaltonen LA, Peltomaki P, Leach FS, et al. Clues to the pathogenesis of familial colorectal cancer. *Science* 1993;260:812–816.
28. Parsons R, Li GM, Longley MJ, et al. Hypermutability and mismatch repair deficiency in RER+ tumor cells. *Cell* 1993;75:1227–1236.
29. Leach FS, Nicolaides NC, Papadopoulos N, et al. Mutations of a mutS homolog in hereditary nonpolyposis colorectal cancer. *Cell* 1993; 75: 1215–1225.
30. Fishel R, Lescoe MK, Rao MR, et al. The human mutator gene homolog MSH2 and its association with hereditary nonpolyposis colon cancer. *Cell* 1993;75:1027–1038.
31. Papadopoulos N, Nicolaides NC, Wei YF, et al. Mutation of a mutL homolog in hereditary colon cancer. *Science* 1994;263:1625–1629.
32. Bronner CE, Baker SM, Morrison PT, et al. Mutation in the DNA mismatch repair gene homologue hMLH1 is associated with hereditary nonpolyposis colon cancer. *Nature* 1994;368:258–261.
33. Kolodner R. Biochemistry and genetics of eukaryotic mismatch repair. *Genes Dev.* 1996;10:1433–1442.
34. Marsischky GT, Filosi N, Kane MF, et al. Redundancy of Saccharomyces cerevisiae MSH3 and MSH6 in MSH2-dependent mismatch repair. *Genes Dev.* 1996;10:407–420.
35. Umar A, Risinger JI, Glaab WE, et al. Functional overlap in mismatch repair by human MSH3 and MSH6. *Genetics* 1998;148:1637–1646.
36. Cannon-Albright LA, Skolnick MH, Bishop DT, et al. Common inheritance of susceptibility to colonic adenomatous polyps and associated colorectal cancers. *N Engl J Med.* 1988;319:533–537.
37. Houlston RS, Collins A, Slack J, et al. Dominant genes for colorectal cancer are not rare. *Ann Hum Genet.* 1992;56:99–103.
38. Offerhaus GJ, Giardiello FM, Krush AJ, et al. The risk of upper gastrointestinal cancer in familial adenomatous polyposis. *Gastroenterology* 1992;102:1980–1982.
39. Tonelli F, Nardi F, Bechi P, et al. Extracolonic polyps in familial polyposis coli and Gardner's syndrome. *Dis Colon Rectum* 1985;28:664–668.
40. Classics in oncology. Heredity with reference to carcinoma as shown by the study of the cases examined in the pathological laboratory of the University of Michigan, 1895–1913. By Aldred Scott Warthin. 1913. *CA Cancer J Clin* 1985;35:348–359.
41. Lynch HT, Krush AJ. Cancer family "G" revisited: 1895-1970. *Cancer* 1971;27:1505–1511.
42. Watson P, Lynch HT. Extracolonic cancer in hereditary nonpolyposis colorectal cancer. *Cancer* 1993;71:677–685.
43. Vasen HF, Mecklin JP, Khan PM, et al. The International Collaborative Group on Hereditary Non-Polyposis Colorectal Cancer (ICG-HNPCC). *Dis Colon Rectum* 1991;34:424–425.
44. Vasen HF, Watson P, Mecklin JP, et al. New clinical criteria for hereditary nonpolyposis colorectal cancer (HNPCC, Lynch syndrome) proposed by the International Collaborative group on HNPCC. *Gastroenterology* 1999;116:1453–1456.
45. Rodriguez-Bigas MA, Boland CR, Hamilton SR, et al. A National Cancer Institute Workshop on Hereditary Nonpolyposis Colorectal Cancer Syndrome: meeting highlights and Bethesda guidelines. *J Natl Cancer Inst.* 1997;89:1758–1762.

46. Umar A, Boland CR, Terdiman JP, et al. Revised Bethesda Guidelines for hereditary nonpolyposis colorectal cancer (Lynch syndrome) and microsatellite instability.. *J Natl Cancer Inst.* 2004;96:261–268.
47. Laken SJ, Petersen GM, Gruber SB, et al. Familial colorectal cancer in Ashkenazim due to a hypermutable tract in APC. *Nat Genet.* 1997; 17:79–83.
48. Giardiello FM, Brensinger JD, Petersen GM, et al. The use and interpretation of commercial APC gene testing for familial adenomatous polyposis. *N Engl J Med.* 1997;336:823–827.
49. Ponder B. Genetic testing for cancer risk. *Science* 1997;278:1050–1054.
50. Gyde SN, Prior P, Thompson H, et al. Survival of patients with colorectal cancer complicating ulcerative colitis. *Gut* 1984;25:228–231.
51. Muto T, Bussey HJ, Morson BC. The evolution of cancer of the colon and rectum. *Cancer* 1975;36:2251–2270.
52. O'Brien MJ, Winawer SJ, Zauber AG, et al. The National Polyp Study. Patient and polyp characteristics associated with high-grade dysplasia in colorectal adenomas. *Gastroenterology* 1990;98:371–379.
53. Nusko G, Mansmann U, Altendorf-Hofmann A, et al. Risk of invasive carcinoma in colorectal adenomas assessed by size and site. *Int J Colorectal Dis.* 1997;12:267–271.
54. Church JM. Clinical significance of small colorectal polyps. *Dis Colon Rectum* 2004;47:481–485.
55. Aldridge AJ, Simson JN. Histological assessment of colorectal adenomas by size. Are polyps less than 10 mm in size clinically important? *Eur J Surg.* 2001;167:777–781.
56. Goldstein NS, Bhanot P, Odish E, et al. Hyperplastic-like colon polyps that preceded microsatellite-unstable adenocarcinomas. *Am J Clin Pathol.* 2003;119:778–796.
57. Wynter CV, Walsh MD, Higuchi T, et al. Methylation patterns define two types of hyperplastic polyp associated with colorectal cancer. *Gut* 2004;53:573–580.
58. Hyman NH, Anderson P, Blasyk H. Hyperplastic polyposis and the risk of colorectal cancer. *Dis Colon Rectum* 2004;47:2101–2104.
59. Jass JR, Young J, Leggett BA. Hyperplastic polyps and DNA microsatellite unstable cancers of the colorectum. *Histopathology* 2000;37:295–301.
60. Hardcastle JD, Armitage NC, Chamberlain J, et al. Fecal occult blood screening for colorectal cancer in the general population. Results of a controlled trial. *Cancer* 1986;58:397–403.
61. Mandel JS, Church TR, Bond JH, et al. The effect of fecal occult-blood screening on the incidence of colorectal cancer. *N Engl J Med.* 2000; 343:1603–1607.
62. Winawer SJ, Zauber AG, Ho MN, et al. Prevention of colorectal cancer by colonoscopic polypectomy. The National Polyp Study Workgroup. *N Engl J Med.* 1993;329:1977–1981.
63. Vining D, Gelfand D, Bechtold R, et al. Technical feasibility of colon imaging with helical CT and virtual reality. *AJR Am J Roentgenol.* 1994;162(suppl):104.
64. Fenlon HM, Nunes DP, Schroy PC III, et al. A comparison of virtual and conventional colonoscopy for the detection of colorectal polyps. *N Engl J Med.* 1999;341:1496–1503.
65. Cotton PB, Durkalski VL, Pineau BC, et al. Computed tomographic colonography (virtual colonoscopy): a multicenter comparison with standard colonoscopy for detection of colorectal neoplasia. *JAMA.* 2004;291:1713–1719.
66. Pineau BC, Paskett ED, Chen GJ, et al. Virtual colonoscopy using oral contrast compared with colonoscopy for the detection of patients with colorectal polyps. *Gastroenterology* 2003;125:304–310.
67. Iannaccone R, Laghi A, Catalano C. Computed tomographic colonography without cathartic preparation for the detection of colorectal polyps. *Gastroenterology* 2004;127:1300–1311.
68. Pickhardt PJ, Choi JR, Hwang I, et al. Computed tomographic virtual colonoscopy to screen for colorectal neoplasia in asymptomatic adults. *N Engl J Med.* 2003;349:2191–2200.
69. Ahlquist DA, Skoletsky JE, Boynton KA, et al. Colorectal cancer screening by detection of altered human DNA in stool: feasibility of a multitarget assay panel. *Gastroenterology* 2000;119:1219–1227.
70. Dong SM, Traverso G, Johnson C, et al. Detecting colorectal cancer in stool with the use of multiple genetic targets. *J Natl Cancer Inst.* 2001;93:858–865.
71. Imperiale TF, Ransohoff DF, Itzkowitz SH, et al. Fecal DNA versus fecal occult blood for colorectal-cancer screening in an average-risk population. *N Engl J Med.* 2004;351:2704–2714.
72. Song K, Fendrick AM, Ladabaum U. Fecal DNA testing compared with conventional colorectal cancer screening methods: a decision analysis. *Gastroenterology* 2004;126:1270–1279.
73. Pignone M, Saha S, Hoerger T, et al. Cost-effectiveness analyses of colorectal cancer screening: a systematic review for the U.S. Preventive Services Task Force. *Ann Intern Med.* 2002;137:96–104.
74. Winawer S, Fletcher R, Rex D, et al. Colorectal cancer screening and surveillance: clinical guidelines and rationale-Update based on new evidence. *Gastroenterology* 2003;124:544–560.
75. Mandel JS, Bond JH, Church TR, et al. Reducing mortality from colorectal cancer by screening for fecal occult blood. Minnesota Colon Cancer Control Study. *N Engl J Med.* 1993;328:1365–1371.
76. Hardcastle JD, Chamberlain JO, Robinson MH, et al. Randomised controlled trial of faecal-occult-blood screening for colorectal cancer. *Lancet* 1996;348:1472–1477.
77. Kronborg O, Fenger C, Olsen J, et al. Randomised study of screening for colorectal cancer with faecal-occult-blood test. *Lancet* 1996;348:1467–1471.
78. Kewenter J, Brevinge H, Engaras B, et al. Results of screening, rescreening, and follow-up in a prospective randomized study for detection of colorectal cancer by fecal occult blood testing. Results for 68,308 subjects. *Scand J Gastroenterol.* 1994;29:468–473.
79. Young G, St. John J, Winawer S, Rozen P. Choice of fecal occult blood tests for colorectal cancer screening: recommendations based on performance characteristics in population studies. A WHO and OMED Report. *Am J Gastroenterol.* 2002;97:2499–2507.
80. Single flexible sigmoidoscopy screening to prevent colorectal cancer: baseline findings of a UK multicentre randomised trial. *Lancet* 2002;359:1291–1300.
81. Segnan N, Senore C, Andreoni B, et al. Baseline findings of the Italian multicenter randomized controlled trial of "once-only sigmoidoscopy"—SCORE. *J Natl Cancer Inst.* 2002;94:1763–1772.
82. Selby JV, Friedman GD, Quesenberry CP Jr, et al. A case-control study of screening sigmoidoscopy and mortality from colorectal cancer. *N Engl J Med.* 1992;326:653–657.
83. Muller AD, Sonnenberg A. Protection by endoscopy against death from colorectal cancer. A case-control study among veterans. *Arch Intern Med.* 1995;155:1741–1748.
84. Newcomb PA, Norfleet RG, Storer BE, et al. Screening sigmoidoscopy and colorectal cancer mortality. *J Natl Cancer Inst.* 1992;84:1 572–1575.
85. Lieberman DA, Weiss DG, Bond JH, et al. Use of colonoscopy to screen asymptomatic adults for colorectal cancer. Veterans Affairs Cooperative Study Group 380. *N Engl J Med.* 2000;343:162–168.
86. Lieberman DA, Weiss DG. One-time screening for colorectal cancer with combined fecal occult-blood testing and examination of the distal colon. *N Engl J Med.* 2001;345:555–560.
87. Seeff LC, Nadel MR, Klabunde CN, et al. Patterns and predictors of colorectal cancer test use in the adult U.S. population. *Cancer*2004;100:2093–2103.
88. Greene F, Page D, Fleming I, eds. *AJCC cancer staging manual,* 6th ed. New York: Springer-Verlag, 2002.
89. O'Connell J, Maggard M, Ko C. Colon cancer survival rates with the New American Joint Committee on Cancer Sixth Edition Staging. *J Natl Cancer Inst.* 2004;96:1420–1425.
90. Baxter N, Virnig DJ, Rothenberger D, et al. Lymph node evaluation in colorectal cancer patients: a population-based study. *J Natl Cancer Inst.* 2005;97:219–225.
91. August DA, Ottow RT, Sugarbaker PH. Clinical perspective of human colorectal cancer metastasis. *Cancer Metastasis Rev.* 1984;3:303–324.
92. Laparoscopically assisted colectomy is as safe and effective as open colectomy in people with colon cancer. Abstracted from: Nelson H, Sargent D, Wieand HS, et al.; for the Clinical Outcomes of Surgical Therapy Study Group. A comparison of laparoscopically assisted and open colectomy for colon cancer. *N Engl J Med.* 2004;350:2050–2059. *Cancer Treat Rev.* 2004;30:707–709.
93. Yeatman TJ, Bland KI. Sphincter-saving procedures for distal carcinoma of the rectum. *Ann Surg.* 1989;209:1–18.
94. Heald RJ, Ryall RD. Recurrence and survival after total mesorectal excision for rectal cancer. *Lancet* 1986;1:1479–1482.
95. Bulow S, Christensen IJ, Harling H, et al. Recurrence and survival after mesorectal excision for rectal cancer. *Br J Surg.* 2003;90:974–980.
96. Heald RJ, Moran BJ, Ryall RD, et al. Rectal cancer: the Basingstoke experience of total mesorectal excision, 1978–1997. *Arch Surg.* 1998;133:894–899.
97. Wibe A, Moller B, Norstein J, et al. A national strategic change in treatment policy for rectal cancer—implementation of total mesorectal excision as routine treatment in Norway. A national audit. *Dis Colon Rectum* 2002;45:857–866.
98. Martling A, Holm T, Rutqvist LE, et al. Impact of a surgical training programme on rectal cancer outcomes in Stockholm. *Br J Surg.* 2004; 92:225–229.
99. Steele GD Jr, Herndon JE, Bleday R, et al. Sphincter-sparing treatment for distal rectal adenocarcinoma. *Ann Surg Oncol.* 1999;6:433–441.
100. Mellgren A, Sirivongs P, Rothenberger DA, et al. Is local excision adequate therapy for early rectal cancer? *Dis Colon Rectum* 2000;43: 1064–1071.
101. Madden JL, Kandalaft SI. Electrocoagulation as a primary curative method in the treatment of carcinoma of the rectum. *Surg Gynecol Obstet.* 1983;157:164–179.
102. Adjuvant radiotherapy for rectal cancer: a systematic overview of 8,507 patients from 22 randomised trials. *Lancet* 20 2001;358:1291–1304.
103. Improved survival with preoperative radiotherapy in resectable rectal cancer. Swedish Rectal Cancer Trial. *N Engl J Med.* 3 1997;336:980–987.
104. Sauer R, Becker H, Hohenberger W, et al. Preoperative versus postoperative chemoradiotherapy for rectal cancer. *N Engl J Med.* 2004;351: 1731–1740.
105. The National Comprehensive Cancer Network. The NCCN Clinical Practice Guidelines in Oncology. Available at: http://www.nccn.org/. Accessed January 2005.
106. Resection of the liver for colorectal carcinoma metastases: a multi-institutional study of indications for resection. Registry of Hepatic Metastases. *Surgery* 1988;103:278–288.
107. Kern KA PH, Roth JA. Surgical treatment of pulmonary metastases. In: SA Rosenberg, ed. *Surgical treatment of metastatic cancer,* vol 69. Philadelphia: JB Lippincott, 1987.
108. Stinner B, Kisker O, Zielke A, et al. Surgical management for carcinoid tumors of small bowel, appendix, colon, and rectum. *World J Surg.* 1996;20:183–188.

CHAPTER 71 ■ DIVERTICULAR DISEASE

MARY F. OTTERSON AND GARY B. KORUS

Diverticular disease of the colon includes both diverticulosis and diverticulitis. In *diverticulosis,* noninflamed diverticula are present with or without symptoms. *Diverticulitis* occurs with inflammation of one or more diverticula. The spectrum of inflammation can range from pericolic infection (*peridiverticulitis*) or abscess formation, to free perforation with peritonitis, fistula formation, or obstruction. Hinchey et al.[1] devised a classification for the extent of inflammation encountered in diverticulitis. Stage I is a small confined pericolonic abscess, stage II is a larger collection, stage III is suppurative peritonitis, and stage IV refers to fecal peritonitis.

Before 1940, diverticulosis of the colon was recognized infrequently. Retrospective reviews of colon radiographs and pathologic specimens from this period recorded an incidence of diverticulosis of 5% to 10%.[2] Currently, the incidence of diverticulosis is age-specific and varies from less than 2% in patients younger than 30 years old to 30% to 50% in patients older than 50 years.[3] Although most patients with diverticulosis of the colon are asymptomatic or have only mild symptoms, complications of hemorrhage or infection occur in 15% to 30% of affected patients and about 30% of these patients require operative treatment.

PATHOLOGIC ANATOMY

True diverticula are rare and involve all layers of the bowel wall: mucosa, submucosa, and muscularis externa. False diverticula (pseudo diverticula) are much more common and involve herniation of mucosa and submucosa through the muscularis externa. These false diverticula emanate from weak points in the colonic wall where mesenteric blood vessels penetrate the circular muscle layer (Fig. 71.1) Pseudo diverticula can also occur along the antimesenteric border in the intertaenial area.[4]

Most diverticula are found in the sigmoid colon, although they can be scattered throughout the intraabdominal colon.[2–4] In up to 65% of patients, diverticulosis is limited to the sigmoid colon. In about 35% of patients, at least one other area of the colon is involved. Diverticular disease spares the sigmoid colon in only 1% to 4% of patients.

PATHOPHYSIOLOGY

Diverticulosis is a disease of affluent society and refined food products. As the people of Western nations have decreased their intake of dietary fiber, the incidence of diverticulosis has increased. Decrease in fiber is the most consistent factor associated with the high incidence of diverticulosis in Western populations.[4] In contrast, diverticulosis is rare in less affluent, nonindustrialized countries. Interestingly, diverticulosis is unusual in Japan, where, although society is industrialized, the population continues to eat a diet high in fiber. It will be interesting to see if the new fad of extremely low carbohydrate dieting alters the incidence or natural history of diverticulosis in the future.

There is epidemiologic evidence that a low fiber diet is associated with the formation of diverticula.[5] A current hypothesis of the etiology of diverticula is that circular muscle contracts the colonic lumen until total occlusion. This effect may be worse with the smaller stool volume of patients consuming low fiber diets. When two such contractions occur close together, the lumen of the intervening segment of colon is isolated from the remainder of the colon, and high pressure is generated in that segment. Theoretically, diverticula formation is a function of increased intraluminal pressure and decreased tensile strength of the colonic wall, particularly at sites of penetrating blood vessels. Pressure–volume curves in patients with diverticulosis demonstrate decreased colon wall tension compared with controls. The combination of colonic segmentation and decreased wall tension may be more important than either factor in isolation.[6]

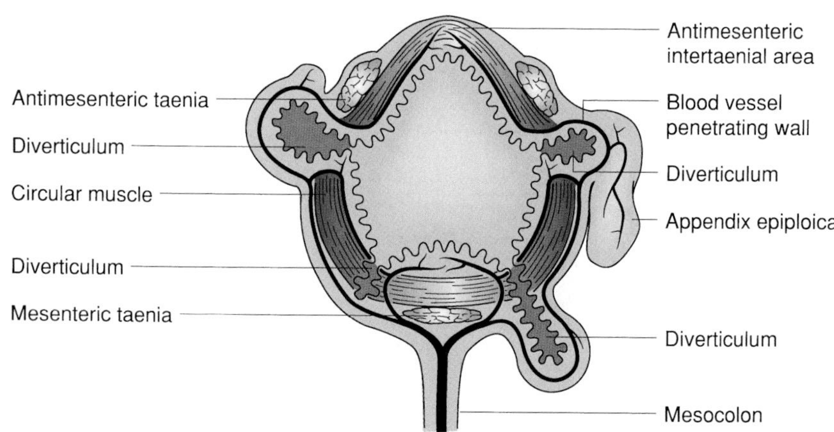

FIGURE 71.1 Cross section of the colon illustrating the relation of diverticula to the blood vessels penetrating the circular muscle layer, the taeniae, and the appendices epiploicae.

CLINICAL PRESENTATION AND DIFFERENTIAL DIAGNOSES

Diverticulosis

Most patients with evidence of colonic diverticula on barium enema have mild or no symptoms. In patients with abdominal pain and evidence of noninflamed diverticula on barium enema, the diverticula are not usually the cause of symptoms (Fig. 71.2). Rather, the excessive pressure exerted by segmentation of the colon may be the source of abdominal discomfort. Although diverticulosis should be considered in the differential diagnosis of a patient with intermittent, mild to moderate lower abdominal pain, other causes of the pain need to be considered. Other diagnoses that should be eliminated include chronic constipation, diverticulitis, irritable bowel syndrome, and adenocarcinoma of the colon. If pain is severe and constant, diverticulitis should be considered. Irritable bowel syndrome is thought by some to be a prediverticular condition and a diagnosis made by exclusion. In patients in whom barium enema does not demonstrate diverticula, a diagnosis of irritable bowel or chronic constipation should not be made until colonoscopy has eliminated carcinoma or inflammatory bowel disease.

Diverticulitis

Symptoms of diverticulitis include fever, lower abdominal pain, and lower abdominal tenderness. Nausea, vomiting, constipation, diarrhea, dysuria, and urinary frequency are less common symptoms. A lower abdominal mass, tachycardia, and an elevated white blood cell count with a left shift may be noted. Abdominal pain and tenderness can vary depending on the location of the inflamed colonic segment and whether there is free perforation into the abdominal cavity. When there is free perforation and generalized peritonitis, it is often difficult to differentiate diverticulitis from other causes of peritonitis. Suspicion of diverticular complications is heightened when the process is localized to the left lower quadrant and there is a palpable, tender mass. The differential diagnosis for diverticulitis without free perforation includes perforated, yet contained colon cancer, acute appendicitis, perforated peptic ulcer, acute-onset ischemic colitis, Crohn disease, infections, and ulcerative colitis.

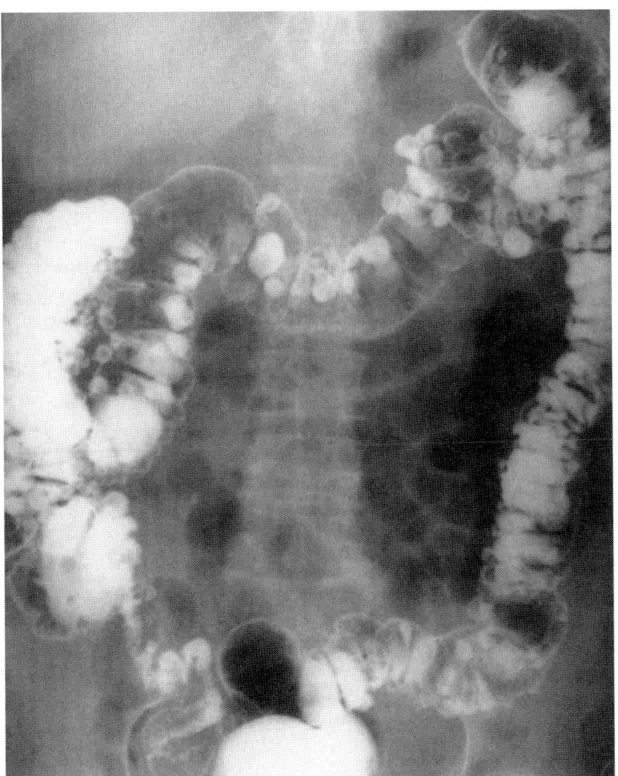

FIGURE 71.2 Barium enema showing multiple diverticula of the colon.

Perforated colon cancer is difficult to differentiate from diverticulitis. Both diseases frequently involve the sigmoid colon, and can produce a tender, left lower quadrant mass. Patient histories are frequently similar with vague, poorly defined lower abdominal pain. Although helpful, colonoscopy is not always diagnostic. The inflammation can make colonoscopy difficult, and it may be impossible to visualize the involved area. Therefore, if carcinoma cannot be eliminated preoperatively, a thorough examination must be performed intraoperatively. Computed tomography (CT) scan evidence of pericolic lymphadenopathy is more frequent in patients with colonic cancer than in patients with diverticulitis. Detection of pericolic lymph nodes in patients suspected of having diverticulitis should raise the suspicion of underlying colonic cancer.[7] The patient's history is usually helpful in differentiating appendicitis from diverticulitis unless the diverticula are right-sided in origin. Inflammatory bowel disease and ischemic colitis can be diagnosed by colonoscopy or flexible sigmoidoscopy. Diverticulitis may be difficult to distinguish from ulcerative colitis or Crohn disease when the onset of symptoms is acute unless the patient's history includes a diagnosis of inflammatory bowel disease. Caution should be exercised in diagnosing Crohn disease in the presence of diverticular disease.[8]

Hemorrhage can occur as a result of diverticular disease (Fig. 71.3). It is important to distinguish hemorrhage as a complication of diverticulosis from colonic angiodysplasia.[9] Similar to diverticulosis, patients who bleed from angiodysplasia are usually asymptomatic before hemorrhage and the blood loss can be massive. Carcinoma of the colon is seldom a cause of acute massive bleeding. Patients who develop massive bleeding secondary to inflammatory bowel disease usually have a history of colitis. Occasionally, a patient with colitis presents with a fulminant course and no history of the disease. Ischemic colitis is usually accompanied by a history of abdominal pain, diarrhea, and vascular occlusive disease. The differential diagnosis of lower gastrointestinal bleeding must always include the various causes of massive upper gastrointestinal bleeding.

Obstruction

Diverticulitis and its complications account for about 13% of cases of large bowel obstruction. Significant problems in evaluating patients with sigmoid colon obstruction include the relatively high incidence (7%) of carcinoma in patients with symptomatic sigmoid diverticular disease and the relative difficulty of making the diagnosis of carcinoma of the colon when a large phlegmonous mass is present.[7] Colonoscopy is helpful only when the endoscope can pass the area of obstruction and biopsy specimens can be obtained because colonoscopy distal to the obstruction does not exclude carcinoma.

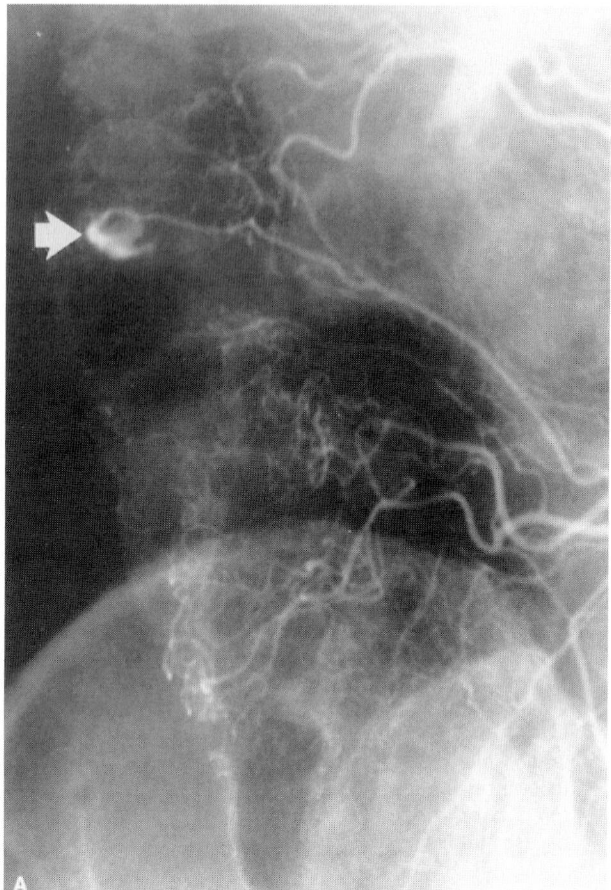

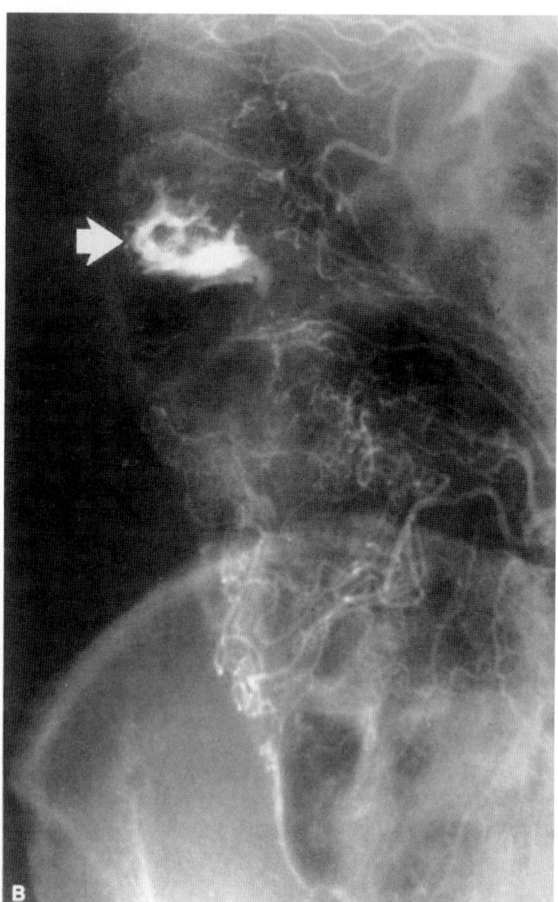

FIGURE 71.3 Superior mesenteric arteriogram from a patient with bleeding from a right colon diverticulum. (*A*) Early radiograph with contrast material outlining the diverticulum (*arrow*). (*B*) Late radiograph demonstrating overflow of contrast material into the colonic lumen.

DIAGNOSIS AND THERAPY

Diverticulosis

Patients with a combination of chronic, intermittent, lower abdominal pain and diverticula on barium enema should be treated symptomatically. The diverticula are not considered to be the cause of the pain, and surgical therapy is not indicated. Colectomy should be reserved for treatment of complications of diverticular disease.

Population studies have demonstrated that consuming a diet high in fiber can prevent diverticula, and such a diet has been widely prescribed for the treatment of symptomatic diverticulosis. No study, however, has shown that a diet high in fiber prevents the complications of diverticulosis. Likewise, the efficacy of fiber supplements or bulk laxatives to treat the pain associated with diverticula is controversial. Studies have demonstrated that an increase in dietary fiber can improve symptoms related to constipation.

In more than 70% of patients with diverticular hemorrhage, bleeding stops spontaneously, and 75% of these patients do not have recurrent bleeding. Most patients who bleed are taking aspirin or nonsteroidal antiinflammatory drug (NSAID) therapy.[10] In the 25% of patients whose bleeding recurs, even if the bleeding is managed successfully by nonoperative means, segmental colectomy should be performed because most of these patients have subsequent hemorrhage. The management of diverticular hemorrhage is discussed in more detail in Chapter 44. Reports suggest that angiodysplasia of the right colon is a more common cause of massive lower gastrointestinal bleeding than previously appreciated. In one series, half the patients with angiodysplasia had diverticula, which is not surprising because both diseases occur predominately in the elderly. All the bleeding angiodysplastic lesions were in the right colon, which explains why massive colonic hemorrhage tends to be right-sided in origin.

Diverticulitis is a complication of diverticulosis. One theory is that diverticulitis occurs when impaction of feces in a single diverticulum causes obstruction of the neck of the diverticulum or abrasion of the thin-walled diverticulum, resulting in invasive infection. Another theory states that microperforation occurs as a result of increased intraluminal pressure, leading to spillage of colonic contents. Either event could result in infection of the surrounding pericolic tissues or free perforation. The process, once initiated, could result in a self-limiting infection without clinical symptoms or could cause progression to clinically significant infection, requiring hospitalization and surgical intervention. When the infection is progressive, other complications can occur.

If a clinical diagnosis of mild diverticulitis is made, therapy should be initiated immediately (Algorithm 71.1). Treatment for mild distress in a patient tolerating oral hydration should include 7 to 10 days of oral broad-spectrum antimicrobral therapy, which includes anaerobic coverage.[11,12] Most patients with diverticulitis severe enough to require hospitalization can

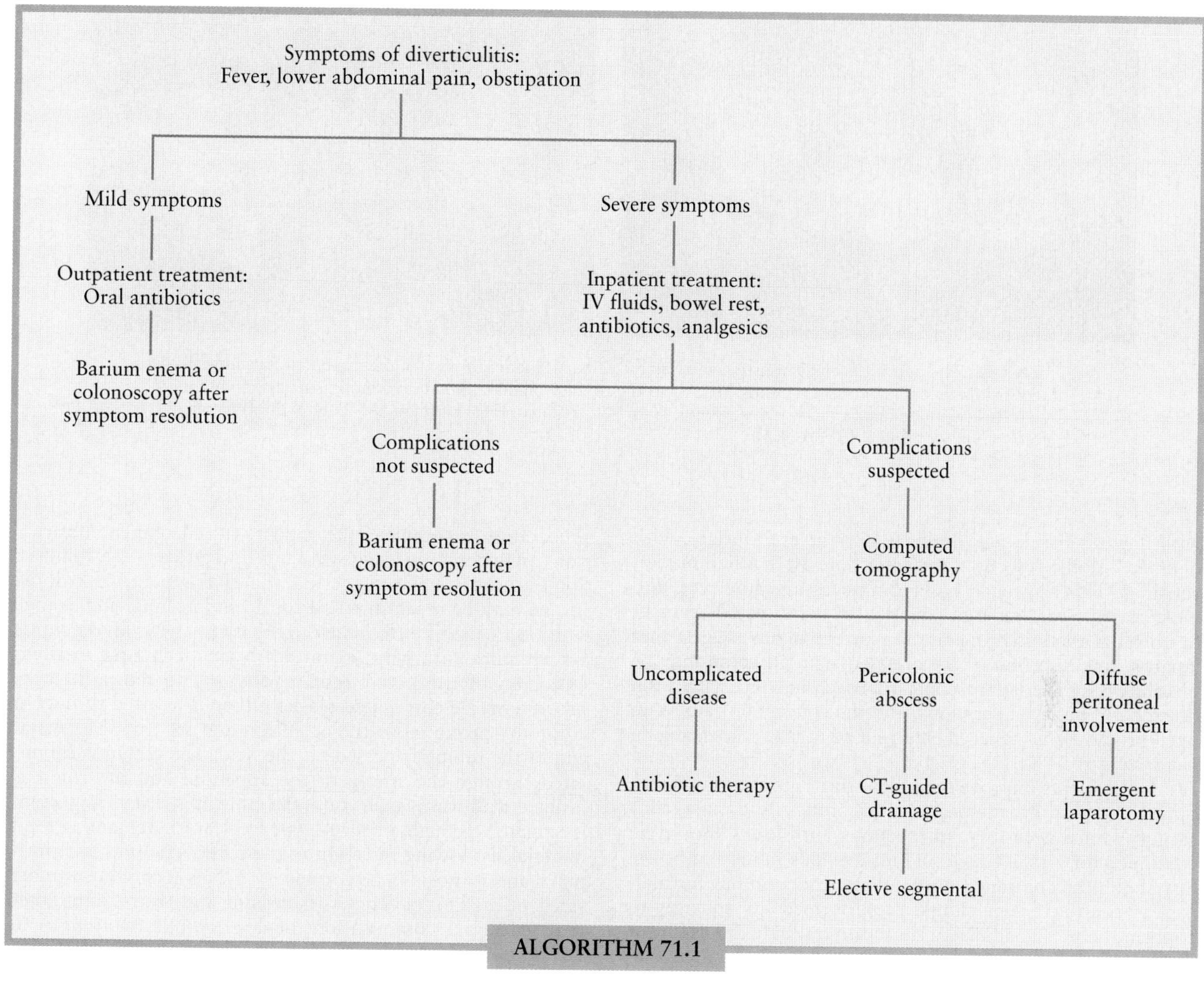

ALGORITHM 71.1 Management of acute diverticulitis. IV, intravenous; CT, computed tomography.

be treated with intravenous fluids, bowel rest, broad-spectrum antibiotics, and analgesics.[2] Signs and symptoms of severe diverticulitis include fever, tachycardia, leukocytosis with left shift of the differential count, abdominal pain (usually in the left lower quadrant) severe enough to require analgesics, abdominal tenderness, and a lower abdominal mass. If nausea, vomiting, or abdominal distention develops, nasogastric suction and acid suppression should be instituted. The patient should be reexamined frequently for progression of disease. If despite maximal therapy the patient does not improve within 48 hours, complications of diverticulitis probably exist and further therapy is necessary. Only about 20% of patients develop complications with their first episode of diverticulitis; this incidence rises to 60% with recurrent episodes. Although a water-soluble contrast enema radiograph frequently provides the diagnosis of diverticulitis, CT has become the preferred diagnostic test in patients who do not improve within 48 hours, who are assumed to have a complication of diverticulitis (Fig. 71.4).[11,13,14] CT is the safest and most cost effective method and has the additional potential benefits of percutaneous drainage for the treatment of abscess.[9] Radiologically guided percutaneous drainage is recommended as the initial therapeutic maneuver in patients with diverticular abscesses greater than 5 cm in diameter. Most smaller abscess will regress with antibiotics and do not require radiologic drainage. After CT drainage of an abscess, 50% to 90% of patients undergo a successful one-stage procedure of segmented colectomy and primary anastomosis.[14] If percutaneous drainage is not feasible or an abscess is not identified, surgical intervention is recommended.

At the time of exploratory laparotomy, if the disease is localized, a segmental colectomy should be performed. The distal extent of the resection should always extend to the proximal rectum to decrease the chance of recurrence. The proximal extent of resection should include the segment involved with the acute disease plus any additional colon with signs of chronic disease or many diverticula. With this approach, the recurrence rate after surgical resection is less than 10%. The only absolute contraindications to primary anastomosis are free perforation with generalized peritonitis, obstruction with unprepared bowel, and intraoperative conditions that do not warrant primary anastomosis, such as septic shock, ureteral injury, and other medical conditions that make a prolonged operation inadvisable. If resection is thought to be unsafe in the presence of a massive phlegmon or the patient is too unstable to undergo a resection, a diverting end colostomy

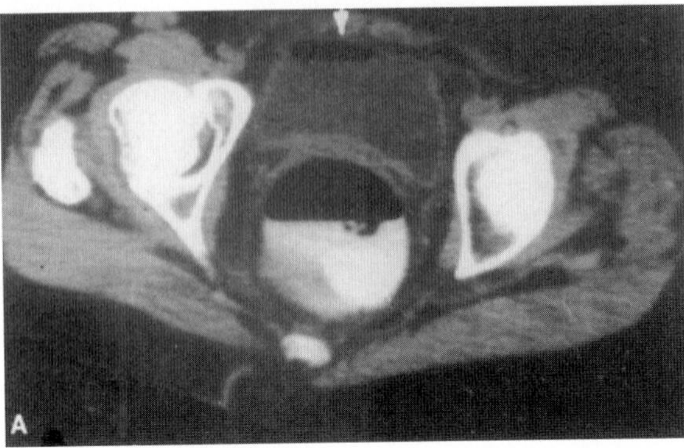

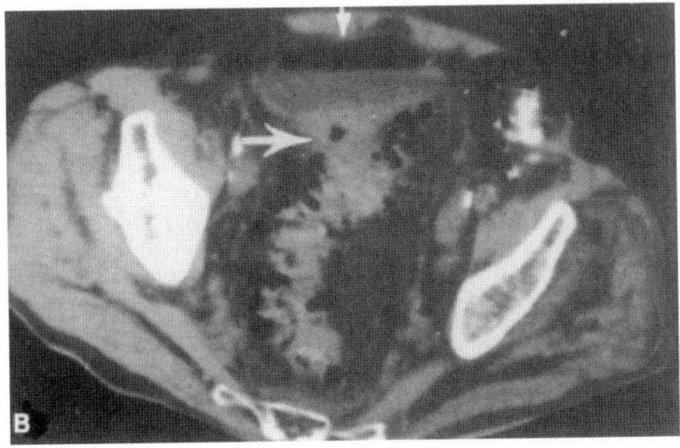

FIGURE 71.4 (*A*) CT scan demonstrating air in the urinary bladder (*arrow*) in the presence of a colovesical fistula secondary to diverticulitis. (*B*) Air in the urinary bladder (*small arrow*) in association with a paravesical inflammatory mass (*large arrow*). (Sarr MG, Fishman EK, Goldman SM. Enterovesical fistula. *Surg Gynecol Obstet*. 1987;164:2.)

with mucous fistula and drainage may be appropriate, with planned colonic resection at a later date after inflammation subsides. This approach is seldom necessary, however, and most patients can undergo resection of the diseased segment of bowel at the initial operation. Current trends suggest that laparoscopic resection of the diseased sigmoid colon may be possible.[15–18] The laparoscopic approach has primarily been utilized for elective operations, and the conversion rate to an open procedure is higher in emergent or urgent cases (ranging from 10% to 53%).

Most patients improve on a regimen of intravenous fluids, bowel rest, and broad-spectrum antibiotics, and emergency surgery is not necessary. Intravenous antibiotics should be continued for 7 to 10 days, and intravenous fluids and bowel rest should be continued until colonic function has normalized. A contrast enema should be performed subsequently to confirm the presumed diagnosis and to evaluate the extent of disease. If there is minimal disease and no sign of obstruction, fistula formation, or abscess, the patient can be discharged and followed as an outpatient. If any of these complications are present, a segmental resection should be performed. After a second episode of diverticulitis, a resection should be performed because the risk of further episodes of diverticulitis increases with each episode.

Obstruction

Patients who have experienced one or more episodes of diverticulitis can develop a fibrotic colonic stricture and large bowel obstruction. When obstruction is diagnosed, it is important to differentiate between diverticulitis, colon carcinoma or colonic volvulus. All patients should undergo sigmoidoscopy or colonoscopy to allow biopsy of any masses. Water-soluble contrast radiographs of the colon should be obtained to define completeness of obstruction. The extent of the workup depends on the condition of the patient and the degree of obstruction. Patients with an incomplete obstruction should be given a thorough but rapid preoperative evaluation in an attempt to secure an exact diagnosis. Because patients with complete obstructions require urgent operation, it is not always feasible to complete all tests before surgery.

If the obstruction is partial, complete preoperative bowel preparation should be carried out, including oral antibiotics. Patients with high-grade colonic obstructions do not tolerate rapid bowel preparation with laxatives or polyethylene glycol. Such patients should be prepared slowly, with extra time allowed for completion of the bowel cleansing. Once bowel preparation is complete, the patient with incomplete obstruction can undergo one-stage resection and primary anastomosis. Some authors have suggested that intraoperative colonic lavage may be a safe method for accomplishing single stage resection of the colon in selected patients with diverticulitis who require an urgent operation.[19] This technique involves occlusion of the bowel lumen proximal to the pathologic process. Sterile corrugated plastic tubing is inserted through a colotomy proximal to the occlusion and secured. The distal end of the tubing is passed off the field. The cecum is cannulated through the stump of the appendix and the colon is lavaged with warm saline until the effluent is clear. The rectum is irrigated through a proctoscope to clear the remaining fecal material. Following resection of the pathologic process, a primary anastomosis is performed.[20,21] This technique is most safely utilized for patients with bleeding and obstruction rather than infectious complications of diverticulitis. Only 35% to 75% of patients who undergo colostomy for diverticular disease go on to have colostomy closure, probably because of the debilitated condition of many of these patients. In spite of this, a staged procedure is virtually mandated in the presence of generalized peritonitis. Unless colon carcinoma has been eliminated as a possible diagnosis, a cancer operation should be performed for this circumstance.

Patients with complete obstruction that cannot undergo bowel preparation, and in whom a one-stage operation is not feasible, should undergo an urgent diverting colostomy to relieve the obstruction. Resection of the diseased, obstructed segment of bowel can be performed during this operation or can be delayed until additional workup is complete. The workup to differentiate between carcinoma and diverticulitis should be completed after the patient has recovered from the initial surgery.

After recovery, the next procedure may be performed. Depending on placement of the colostomy, the second operation can be resection of the colostomy and the diseased segment of colon and reestablishment of bowel continuity by colocolostomy. When the diseased segment of bowel was removed during the first operation, the secondary procedure is colostomy closure.

Fistula Formation

Diverticular disease can also be complicated by the development of fistulas from the diseased colon to other viscera or to skin. Colovesical fistulas account for about half of the fistulas due to diverticulitis. Most patients with colovesical fistulas present with urinary tract symptoms, including urgency, dysuria, pneumaturia, and fecaluria. Despite what in retrospect often appear to be obvious symptoms, the diagnosis of colovesical fistula can be difficult to establish conclusively. Recurrent urinary tract infections in an elderly man should increase suspicion. Barium enema usually demonstrates diverticula and occasionally shows sigmoid narrowing. Only rarely is the fistulous tract actually filled. Cystoscopy demonstrates hyperemia and inflammation, but the fistulous opening is seldom seen. CT with intraluminal contrast material has emerged as the most sensitive test for the presence of a colovesical fistula. In addition, after the rectal administration of barium, the patient's urine sediment should be checked for barium by radiograph of a spun urine sample. The presence of barium in the urine is diagnostic of a colovesical fistula. In more than 90% of patients, air is in the urinary bladder and an indurated segment of sigmoid colon is observed adjacent to a locally thickened bladder wall.[22]

Most patients with colovesical fistulas are treated effectively with a one-stage procedure consisting of segmental colectomy and closure of the fistulous opening in the bladder. The proximal margin of resection should include the entire segment of thickened, contracted colon and any additional colon that is involved in the acute inflammation. As stated earlier, although it is not necessary to resect the entire colon involved with diverticulosis, the resection should include sufficient colon to allow the anastomosis to be performed in an area of colon relatively free of diverticula. The distal resection margin should be the proximal rectum. If the fistulous opening is not identifiable, indicating that it is small in diameter, nothing needs to be done to identify the bladder fistula. Urinary catheter drainage for 7 to 10 days, followed by cystographic verification of closure of the fistula, is sufficient therapy. Depending on the severity of the related complications of diverticulitis (obstruction, inflammation, abscess, sepsis, other fistulas), it may occasionally be necessary to perform a two-stage procedure, the first stage being segmental colectomy and colostomy formation and the second stage consisting of closure of the colostomy. Either the one- or two-stage procedure can be done with low morbidity and mortality and with less than a 5% recurrence rate. An alternate to the standard two-stage procedure is primary anastomosis with a diverting loop ileostomy. The colon must be relatively prepped to allow this procedure. The diverting loop ileostomy is completely diverting and does not interfere with the blood supply of the colon as is possible with a loop colostomy. In addition, closure of a loop ileostomy rather than repeat exploratory laparotomy is a much smaller surgical procedure. The three-stage approach of diverting colostomy, then resection, and finally colostomy closure is not recommended because the inflammatory process and the fistula are not removed at the first operation, leaving potential sources of sepsis.

Although rare in the past, recent reports indicate an increase in the occurrence of colovaginal fistulas. Almost all patients with colovaginal fistulas have had hysterectomies. The only consistent symptom is feculent vaginal discharge. About 40% of patients have intermittent abdominal pain and distention. A mass may be felt on pelvic examination; on vaginal speculum examination, the fistula opening is visible in 85% of cases. The diagnosis is confirmed in 50% of cases by barium enema. Vaginal contrast studies may also be helpful. Unless other complications of diverticulitis are present, a one-stage procedure is appropriate. The involved colon is resected and a primary anastomosis performed. The vaginal defect is closed if this can be easily accomplished, but such a defect usually closes spontaneously if left open.

Diarrhea, abdominal pain, and constitutional symptoms are frequently observed in patients with diverticular coloenteric fistulas. The usual signs of coloenteric fistula are abdominal tenderness, abdominal distention, and pelvic mass. Barium enema is diagnostic in 40% to 100% of patients. The preferred operative management of an uncomplicated coloenteric fistula is en bloc resection of the involved segment of small intestine, the fistula, and the diseased segment of colon. Primary anastomoses of both the small intestine and colon are then performed. If there are complicating factors, such as other fistulas, intraabdominal abscess, or inadequate bowel preparation secondary to obstruction, primary anastomosis of the small intestine, combined with colostomy formation, is performed as the first stage of a two-stage procedure.

DIVERTICULITIS OF THE CECUM AND ASCENDING COLON

The actual incidence of right-sided diverticula is not known; estimates based on barium enema examinations are between 5% and 10%.[23] The incidence of true diverticula is higher in the cecum and ascending colon than in the remainder of the colon, but false diverticula still predominate. True diverticula tend to be solitary and to originate in the anterior cecum close to the ileocecal valve. They occur in only 1% to 2% of the population. Most are asymptomatic, and the diagnosis is usually made by pathologic examination. Seven to 30% of people with left-sided diverticulosis will have right-sided diverticula.[23] In a study of more than 250 patients with right colonic diverticulitis, 81% had a solitary diverticulum whereas 19% had multiple diverticula.[24] There is an increased incidence of right colonic diverticula and diverticulitis and a lower than expected incidence of left-sided diverticulitis in Asian patients.[25]

When patients with right-sided diverticula develop diverticulitis, the symptom complex is similar to that in acute appendicitis, and misdiagnosis is frequent.[24,26] Patients with right-sided diverticulitis are generally younger than patients with left-sided disease and are older than most patients with appendicitis.[26] Patients with right-sided diverticulitis are usually in their late 30s or 40s; patients with left-sided diverticulitis are usually more than 50 years of age.[26] Patients with right-sided diverticulitis have a longer duration of illness than patients with appendicitis, infrequently vomit, and feel pain initially in the right lower quadrant rather than the mid abdomen. Despite these dissimilarities, misdiagnosis of acute appendicitis is made in more than 60% of patients who are later found to have right-sided diverticulitis.[24,26] In only 20% of cases is the correct diagnosis made preoperatively. CT scanning may improve diagnosis of right-sided diverticulitis. CT findings include thickening of the colonic wall, extraluminal mass involving the cecum or ascending colon, and signs of pericolic inflammation. CT scanning is recommended in patients with atypical appendicitis who are elderly and in who right-sided diverticulitis is being considered as a diagnosis. Barium enema examination is seldom helpful because many patients have a single diverticulum that is not visible on barium examination. Associated findings, such as compression of the colon, are nonspecific and usually nondiagnostic.

At the time of operation, it may be difficult to establish a diagnosis of diverticulitis of the cecum or ascending colon. Most series report a correct intraoperative diagnosis in fewer than 60% of cases.[26] The presence of an intact, normal appendix eliminates appendicitis as the diagnosis in almost all circumstances. Usually, a large inflammatory mass involves the cecum and ascending colon. In many cases, however, it is difficult to distinguish the mass from a perforated carcinoma, and a right hemicolectomy should be performed. If the resection can be accomplished without contamination of the peritoneal cavity and a mechanical bowel preparation had been accomplished preoperatively, a primary anastomosis is acceptable.

If there is spillage of abscess contents or bowel preparation was not feasible, an end ileostomy and mucous fistula can be performed. When the only abnormality noted at laparotomy is an inflamed diverticulum, a few authors propose leaving the diverticulum *in situ* and treating the patient with broad-spectrum antibiotics. If this therapy is undertaken, an appendectomy should be performed to avoid confusion if right lower quadrant symptoms recur. Most patients treated in this manner do not develop recurrent diverticulitis.

If the diagnosis of right-sided diverticulitis is made before operation, the patient should be treated as with sigmoid diverticulitis. If improvement is noted with intravenous fluids, broad-spectrum antibiotics, bowel rest, and analgesics, therapy should be continued and further testing performed when the patient recovers. If the patient does not improve or deteriorates, laparotomy is recommended.

GIANT COLONIC DIVERTICULUM

Although uncommon, giant colonic diverticulum is a well-described clinical entity. Giant diverticula usually occur in the sigmoid colon, although they have been described in other areas of the left colon. Giant diverticula almost always arise from the antimesenteric border of the colon, unlike most left-sided diverticula, which develop where the vascular supply passes through the muscularis externa. Most are gas filled and therefore visible on plain abdominal radiographs. They range in size from 3 to 35 cm, with an average of 13.5 cm.

The pathogenesis of giant diverticula is not understood; they are assumed to be a complication of diverticulosis and not a separate entity. One explanation is that inflammation of a diverticulum causes narrowing of its neck and results in a ball-valve mechanism that entraps gases that pass into the diverticulum from the colon. The predominant symptoms are abdominal pain, bloating, nausea, vomiting, and diarrhea. Physical findings include abdominal tenderness and a movable, lower abdominal mass. Perforation causes abdominal pain, leukocytosis, fever, and signs of localized or generalized peritonitis. Although the diagnosis can be suspected based on plain radiographs of the abdomen, barium enema and CT scanning confirm the diagnosis. On barium enema, the diverticula fills with barium in 50% to 70% of cases, and frequently, other diverticula are demonstrated (Fig. 71.5). CT scanning of giant diverticula performed with intraluminal contrast usually demonstrates apposition of the colon and the giant diverticulum as well as the presence of barium in the diverticulum. On CT scan, wall thickness is variable and not diagnostic.

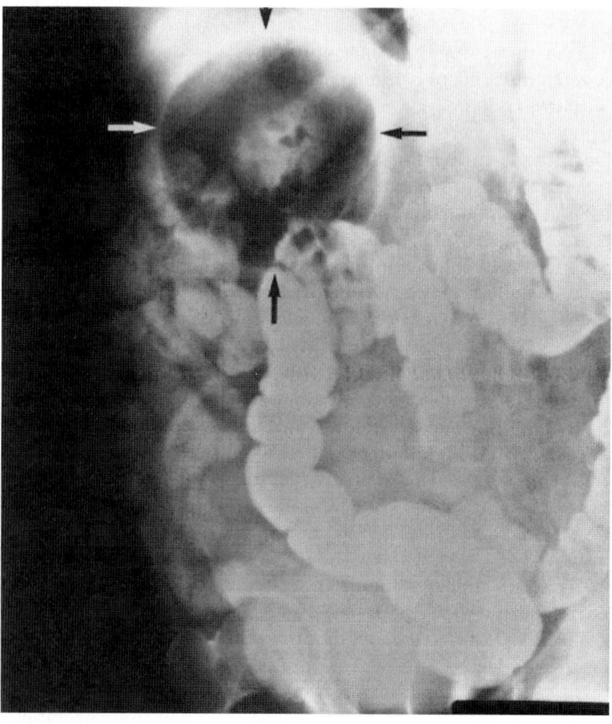

FIGURE 71.5 Postevacuation film of barium enema, demonstrating a giant colonic diverticulum (*arrows*) partially filled with barium. (McNutt R, Schmitt D, Schulte W. Giant colonic diverticula. *Dis Colon* 1988;31:625.)

Giant colonic diverticula are managed surgically. The patient should undergo standard mechanical bowel preparation, and the diverticulum and adjacent colon should be resected.

KEY POINTS

- **Colonic diverticuli are actually pseudodiverticuli, involving herniation of mucosa and submucosa through the muscularis externa. These false diverticula emanate from weak points in the colonic wall where mesenteric blood vessels penetrate the circular muscle layer.**
- **Diverticulosis is a disease of affluent societies and refined food products. With decreased intake of dietary fiber, the incidence of diverticulosis has increased.**
- **Most patients with diverticulosis have mild or no symptoms. Symptoms of diverticulitis include fever, lower abdominal pain, and lower abdominal tenderness.**
- **Most patients with diverticulitis severe enough to require hospitalization should be treated with intravenous fluids, bowel rest, broad-spectrum antibiotics, and analgesics.**
- **Computed tomography is the preferred diagnostic test in patients who do not improve within 48 hours, who are assumed to have a complication of diverticulitis.**
- **At the time of laparotomy, a segmental colectomy should be performed. The distal extent of the resection should extend to the proximal rectum to decrease the chance of recurrence. The proximal extent of resection should include the segment involved with the acute disease plus additional colon with signs of chronic disease or many diverticula.**
- **Diverticular disease can be complicated by the development of fistulas from the diseased colon to other viscera or to skin.**

References

1. Hinchey EJ, Schaal PGH, Richards GK. Treatment of perforated diverticular disease of the colon. *Adv Surg.* 1978;12:85–109.
2. Spriggs EI, Marxer OA. Intestinal diverticula. *Q J Med.* 1925;19:1.
3. Hughes LE. Postmortem survey of diverticular disease of the colon. *Gut* 1969;10:336–344.
4. Slack WW. The anatomy, pathology and some clinical features of diverticulitis of the colon. *Br J Surg.* 1962;50:185–190.
5. **Aldoori WH, Giovannuci EL, Rockett HR, et al. A prospective study of dietary fiber types and symptomatic diverticular disease in men. *J Nutr.* 1998;128:714–719.**
6. **Floch MH, Bina I. The natural history of diverticulitis: fact and theory. *J Clin Gastroenterol.* 2004;38(suppl):S3.**
7. Chintapalli KN, Esola CC, Chopra S, et al. Pericolic mesenteric lymph nodes: An aid in distinguishing diverticulitis from cancer of the colon. *AJR.* 1997;169:1253–1255.
8. Gledhill A, Dixon MF. Crohn's-like reaction in diverticular disease. *Gut* 1998;42:392–395.

9. Welch CE, Athanasoulis CA, Galdabini JJ. Hemorrhage from the large bowel with special reference to angiodysplasia and diverticular disease. *World J Surg*. 1978;2:73–83.
10. Holt S, Rigoglioso V, Sidhu M, et al. Nonsteroidal antiinflammatory drugs and lower gastrointestinal bleeding. *Dig Dis Sci*. 1993;38(9):1619–1623.
11. **Ferzoco LB, Raptopoulos V, Silen W. Acute Diverticulitis. *New Engl J Med*. 1998;338:1521–1526.**
12. Freeman SR, McNally PR. Diverticulitis. *Med Clin North Am*. 1993;77:1149–1167.
13. Stabile BE, Puccio E, Van Sonnenberg E, et al. Preoperative percutaneous drainage of diverticular abscesses. *Am J Surg*. 1990;159:99–104.
14. Spivak H, Weinrauch S, Harvey JC, et al. Acute colonic diverticulitis in the young. *Dis Colon Rectum* 1997;49:570–574.
15. Memon MA, Fitztgibbons RJ. The role of minimal access surgery in the acute abdomen. *Surgical Clin North Am*. 1997;77:1333–1353.
16. Bruce CJ, Coller JA, Murray JJ, et al. Laparoscopic resection for diverticular disease. *Dis Colon Rectum* 1996;39(suppl):S1–S6.
17. **Eijsbouts QA, Cuesta MA, deBrauw LM, et al. Elective laparoscopic-assisted sigmoid resection for diverticular disease. *Surg Endosc*. 1997;11: 750–753.**
18. Sher ME, Agachan F, Bortul M, et al. Laparoscopic surgery for diverticulitis. *Surg Endosc*. 1997;11:264–267.
19. Lee EC, Murray JJ, Coller JA, et al. Intraoperative colonic lavage in nonelective surgery for diverticular disease. *Dis Colon Rectum* 1997;40:669–674.
20. Murray JJ, Schoetz DJ, Coller JA, et al. Intraoperative colonic lavage and primary anastomosis in nonelective colon resection. *Dis Colon Rectum* 1991;34:527–531.
21. Scott HJ, Lane IF, Glynn MJ. Colonic hemorrhage: a technique for rapid intraoperative bowel preparation and colonoscopy. *Br J Surg*. 1986;73:390–391.
22. Woods RJ, Lavery IC, Fazio VW, et al. Internal fistulas in diverticular disease. *Dis Colon Rectum* 1988;31:591–596.
23. Beranbaum SL, Zausner J, Lane B. Diverticular disease of the right colon. *Radiology* 1972; 115:334–348.
24. Graham SM, Ballantyne GH. Cecal diverticulitis: a review of the American experience. *Dis Colon Rectum* 1987;30:821–826.
25. Katz DS, Lane MJ, Ross BA, et al. Diverticulitis of the right colon revisited. *AJR*. 1998; 171:151–156.
26. Gouge TH, Coppa GF, Eng K, et al. Management of diverticulitis of the ascending colon: 10 years' experience. *Am J Surg*. 1983;145:387–391.

CHAPTER 72 ■ ANORECTAL DISORDERS

ARDEN M. MORRIS, ROBERT MADOFF, AND SANTHAT NIVATVONGS

ANATOMY AND PHYSIOLOGY

The Rectum

The rectum extends from the level of the promontory of the sacrum to the level of the levator ani muscle and varies in length from 12 to 15 cm. The rectum differs from the colon in that the outer layer is covered circumferentially by longitudinal muscle rather than the three taeniae bands. The rectum has two or three lateral curves that form submucosal folds in the lumen, known as the *valves of Houston*. The posterior part of the rectum is devoid of peritoneum and is covered with the endopelvic fascia. The presacral fascia is a strong, endopelvic fascia that covers the entire anterior surface of the sacrum and also covers the underlying vessels and nerves. At about the level of S4, the presacral fascia runs forward and downward and attaches to the rectum, an area known as the *rectosacral fascia* or *Waldeyer's ring* (Fig. 72.1).[1] This fascia must be incised for full mobilization of the rectum during abdominoperineal resection or low anterior resection. Peritoneum covers the upper two thirds of the rectum anteriorly and the upper one third of the rectum laterally; the lower third of the rectum is entirely devoid of peritoneum. In general, the anterior peritoneal reflection is about 6 to 8 cm from the anal verge. The extraperitoneal portion of the rectum is covered by the endopelvic fascia. On the anterior surface, this is called *Denonvilliers fascia* and lies just posterior to the seminal vesicles in males. The lateral endopelvic fascia, called the *lateral rectal stalks*, also require division for full rectal mobilization.

The Anal Canal and Sphincters

The anal canal, about 4 cm in length, is the terminal portion of the large bowel that passes through the levator ani muscle and opens to the anal verge. The muscular wall of the anal canal, derived from the circular smooth muscular layer of the rectum, is thickened and forms the internal anal sphincter. The anal canal is wrapped by the striated external anal sphincter muscle and the puborectalis muscle, which are arranged in three U-shaped loops.[2] Although the possibility of puborectalis inclusion in the external sphincter was previously debated,[3] recent sophisticated imaging studies indicate that the top loop, or deep external anal sphincter, is separated from the puborectalis by a layer of fat which can be appreciated on magnetic resonance imaging (MRI) coronal views.[4] The intermediate loop is the superficial external sphincter muscle; the origin of this loop at the tip of the coccyx is known as the *anococcygeal ligament*. The basal loop is composed of the subcutaneous portion of the external sphincter muscle (Fig. 72.2).

At the upper portion of the anal canal, called the *anorectal ring*, the internal sphincter muscle thickens and the puborectalis muscle can be palpated digitally. From the level of the anorectal ring distally and between the internal and external anal sphincter muscles, the longitudinal muscle coat of the rectum is joined by fibers of the levator ani and puborectalis to form the conjoined longitudinal muscle (Fig. 72.3). These muscle fibers traverse the lower portion of the distal external sphincter to insert in the perianal skin, causing wrinkling of the anal verge known as the corrugator cutis ani.

At about the midpoint of the anal canal, 2 cm from the anal verge, there is an undulating demarcation called the *dentate or pectinate line*. Longitudinal folds of the mucosa above the dentate line are known as the *columns of Morgagni*. For a distance of about 1 cm above the dentate line, the epithelial lining may be columnar, transitional, or stratified squamous epithelium; this area is referred to as the *transitional or cloacogenic zone*. The internal hemorrhoidal plexus lies deep to the mucosa at this location. The area above the transitional zone is lined by columnar epithelium and the area below the dentate line is lined by squamous epithelium (see Fig. 72.3).

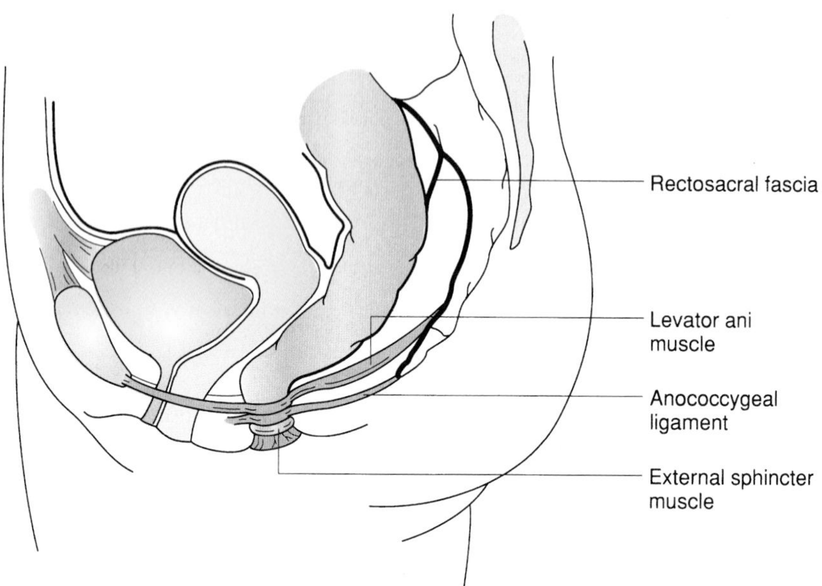

FIGURE 72.1 Fascial attachments of the rectum.

Pelvic Floor Muscles

The pelvic floor muscles consist of the levator ani muscle and the iliococcygeal muscle. The levator ani muscle is a broad, thin muscle that forms the floor of the pelvic cavity and is innervated by the fourth sacral nerve. This muscle has traditionally been considered to consist of three muscles—the iliococcygeal, the pubococcygeal, and the puborectalis.[5]

The iliococcygeal muscle arises from the ischial spine and posterior part of the obturator fascia, passes downward, backward, and medially, and becomes inserted on the last two segments of the sacrum and the anococcygeal raphe as described later (Fig. 72.4). The pubococcygeal muscle arises from the anterior half of the obturator fascia and the back of the pubis. The fibers of the pubococcygeal muscle are directed backward, downward, and medially, where they decussate with fibers of the opposite side. The line of decussation is called the *anococcygeal raphe* (see Fig. 72.4). Some fibers that lie more posteriorly are attached directly to the tip of the coccyx and the last segment of the sacrum. This muscle also sends fibers to share in the formation of the conjoined longitudinal muscle. The puborectalis and levator ani muscles have a reciprocal action: as one contracts, the other relaxes. In the upright standing position, the puborectalis is contracted, creating an anorectal angle while the levator ani muscle supports the viscera. During defecation, the puborectalis relaxes while the levator ani contracts, effectively widening the hiatus, straightening the anorectal angle, and elevating the lower rectum and anal canal to create a straight path for evacuation.

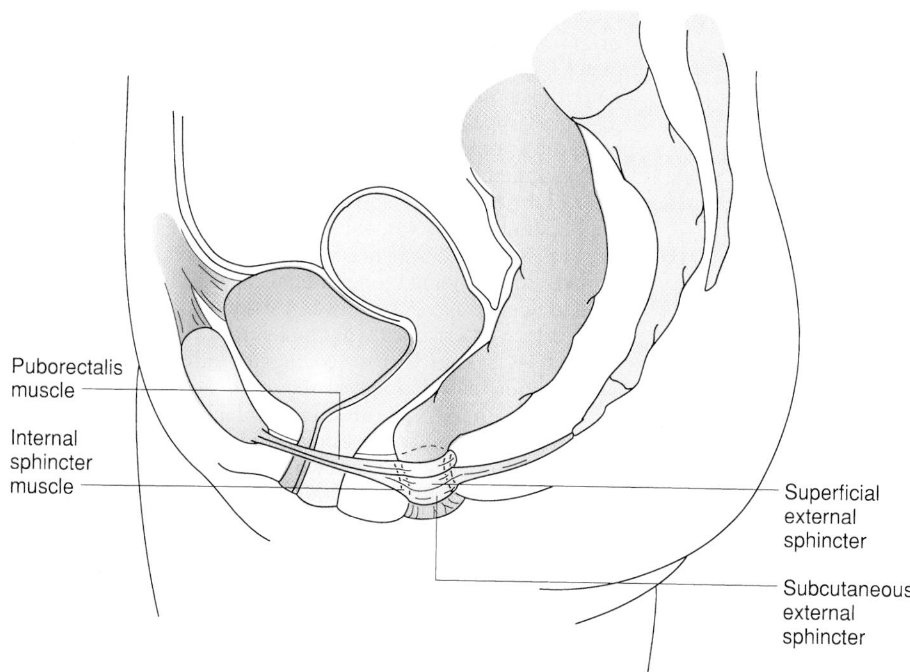

FIGURE 72.2 Arrangement of the external sphincter muscles.

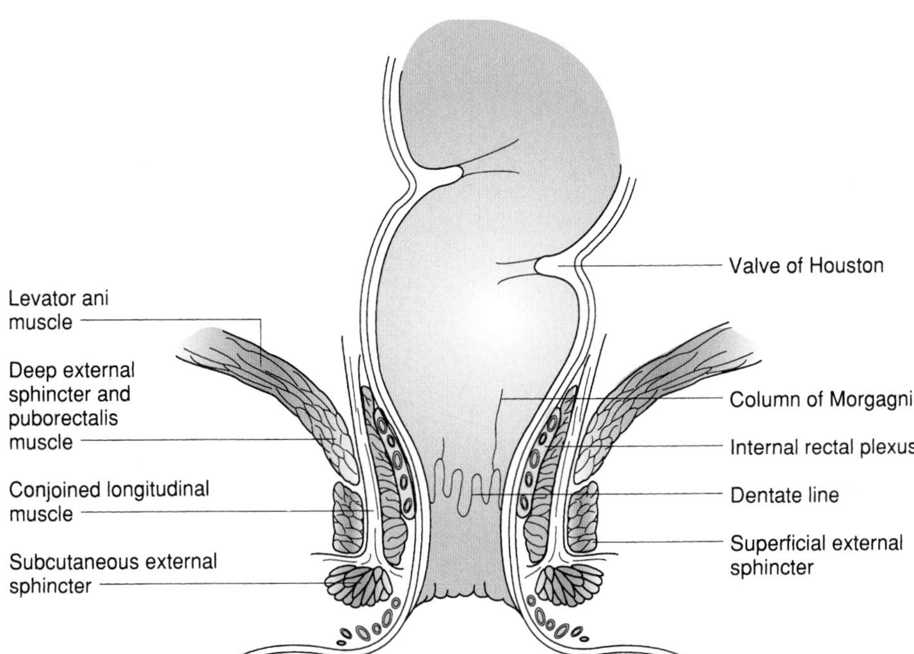

FIGURE 72.3 Anatomy of the anal canal.

Perianal and Perirectal Spaces

Surrounding the anorectum are several potential spaces that are normally filled with areolar tissues or fat. These spaces are clinically important because they are sites where abscesses can form. The perianal space immediately surrounds the anus. Laterally, the perianal space is contiguous with the subcutaneous fat of the buttocks. Medially, it is bound by the anoderm to the level of the dentate line. The ischioanal space is a triangular-shaped region below the levator ani muscle, bound medially by the external sphincter muscle, laterally by the ischium, and inferiorly by the transverse septum of the ischiorectal fossa (Fig. 72.5). The ischioanal space on each side is filled with fat and contains the inferior rectal vessels and lymphatics. The deep postanal space or space of Courtney connects the ischioanal space on each side posteriorly and lies between the levator ani muscle above and the anococcygeal ligament below (Fig. 72.6). The deep postanal space is an important pathway in the formation of abscess; spread from one ischiorectal fossa to the other may result in a so-called *horseshoe abscess*. The intersphincteric space lies between the internal and external sphincter muscles. It is continuous with the perianal space below and extends above into the wall of the rectum. The supralevator spaces are situated on each side of the rectum above the levator ani muscle (see Fig. 72.5). The supralevator spaces communicate posteriorly and may allow spread of infection cephalad into the retroperitoneum (see Fig. 72.6).

Arterial Supply of the Rectum and Anal Canal

The superior rectal (hemorrhoidal) artery is the continuation of the inferior mesenteric artery and descends posterior to the rectum, where it bifurcates to supply the rectum and the upper portion of the anal canal (Fig. 72.7). The middle rectal (hemorrhoidal) arteries arise from the internal iliac artery on each side and enter the lower portion of the rectum anterolaterally at variable points but usually in the lower third of rectum. The middle rectal arteries are inconsistent and cannot be relied on after ligation of the superior rectal artery. The inferior rectal arteries (hemorrhoidal) arise from the internal pudendal artery, a branch of the internal iliac artery, and traverse the ischioanal fossa on each side to supply the anal

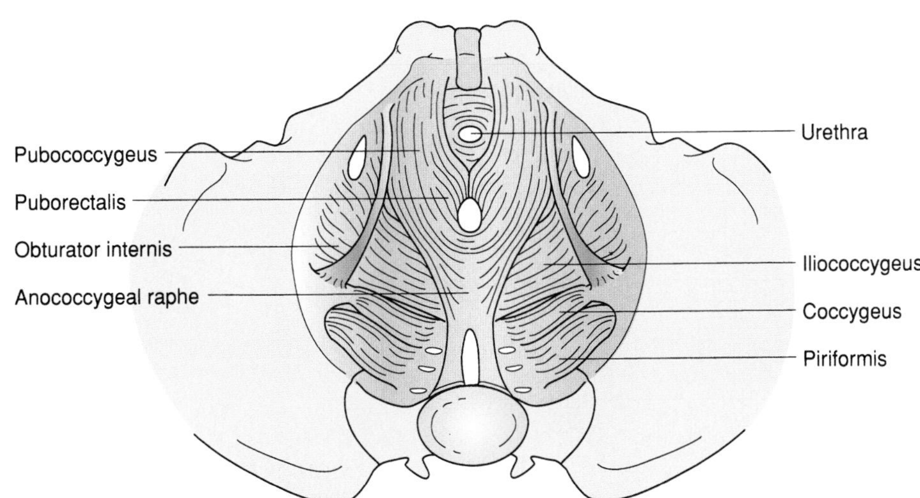

FIGURE 72.4 Muscles of the pelvic floor.

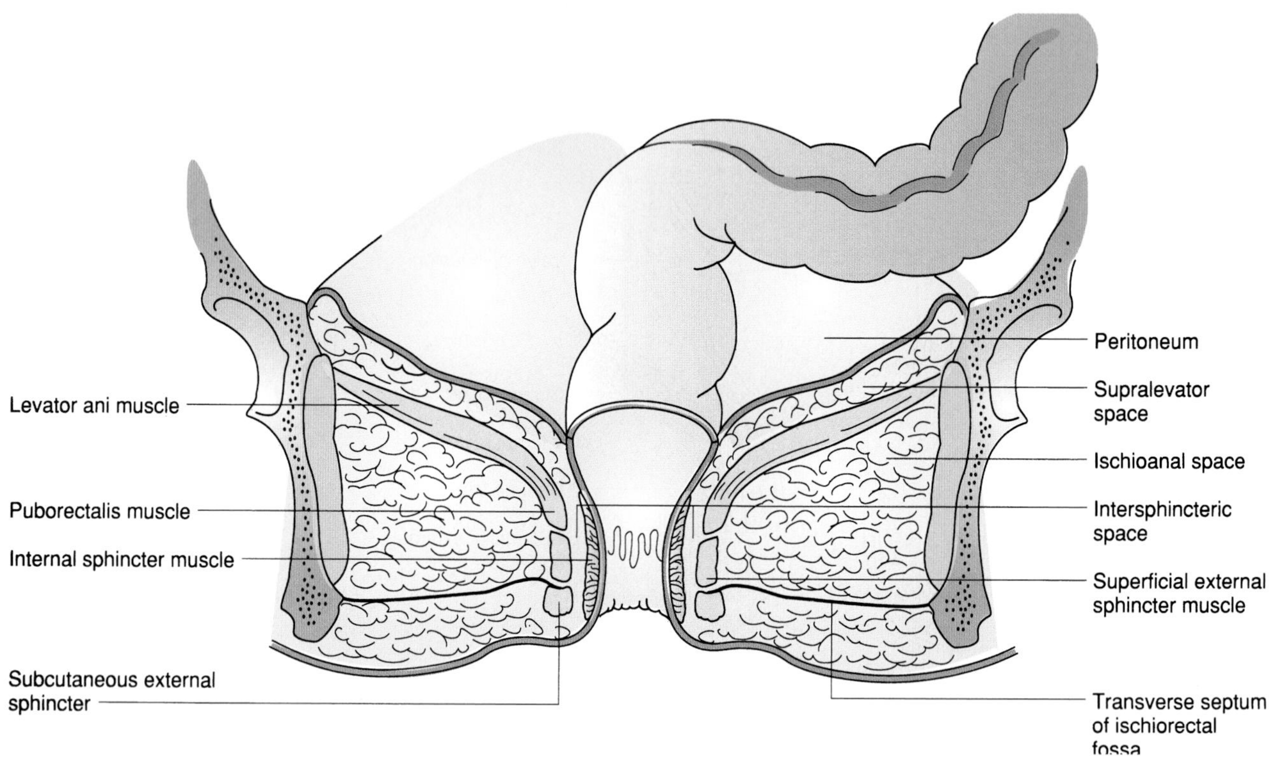

FIGURE 72.5 Anatomy of the perianorectal spaces (anteroposterior view).

sphincter muscles. Although there is no extramural anastomosis among the superior, middle, and inferior rectal arteries on cadaver dissection, arteriography shows abundant intramural anastomoses, thus rectal ischemia is an exceedingly rare event even after substantial devascularization.

Venous Drainage of the Rectum and Anal Canal

The return of blood from the rectum and anal canal occurs by two systems—portal and systemic (Fig. 72.8). The superior rectal (hemorrhoidal) vein drains the rectum and upper part of the anal canal into the portal system through the inferior mesenteric vein. The middle rectal veins drain the lower part of the rectum and the upper part of the anal canal; they accompany the middle rectal arteries and terminate in the internal iliac veins. The inferior rectal veins, following the corresponding arteries, drain the lower part of the anal canal by way of the internal pudendal veins, which empty into the internal iliac veins.

Lymphatic Drainage of the Rectum and Anal Canal

Lymph from the upper and middle portions of the rectum ascends along the superior rectal artery and subsequently to the inferior mesenteric lymph nodes. The lower part of the rectum

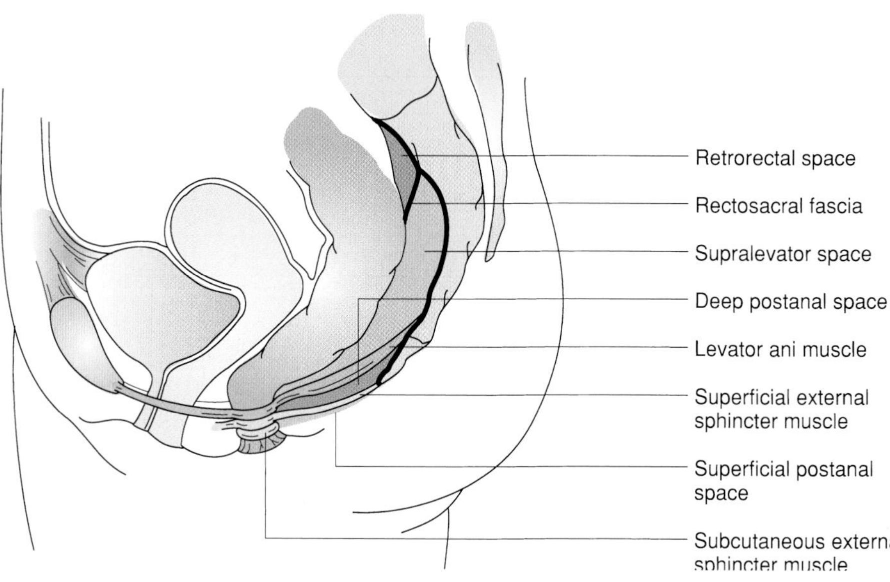

FIGURE 72.6 Anatomy of the perianorectal spaces (lateral view).

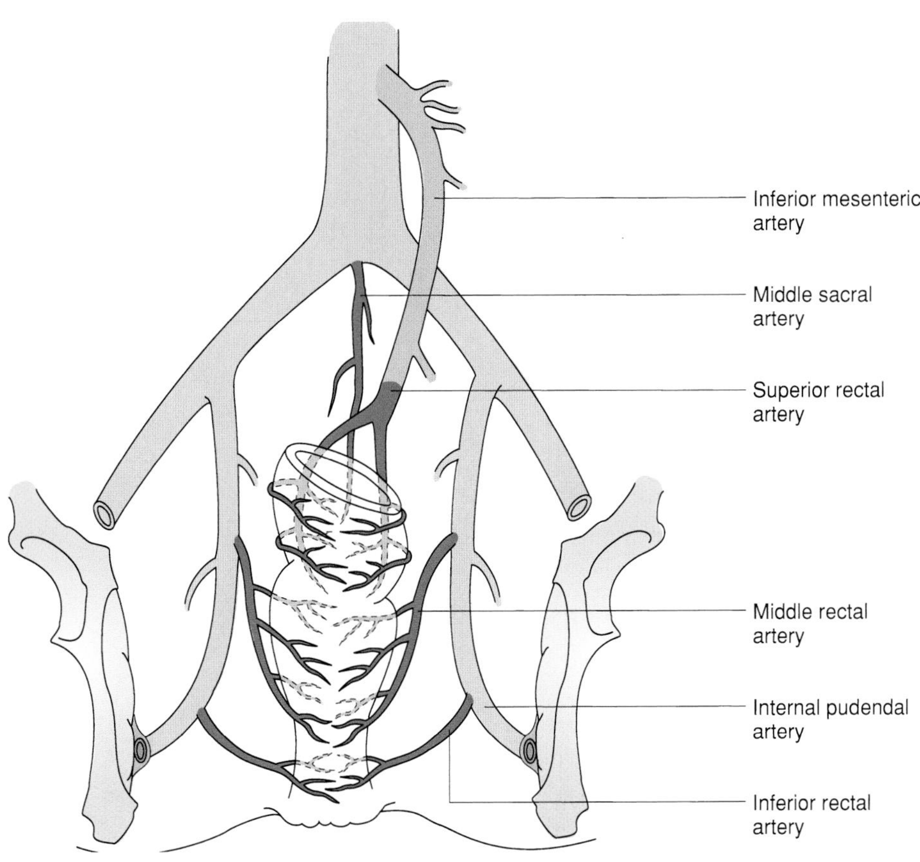

FIGURE 72.7 Arterial supply of the rectum and anal canal.

drains cephalad by way of the superior rectal lymphatics to the inferior mesenteric nodes, and laterally by way of the middle rectal lymphatics to the internal iliac nodes (Fig. 72.9). Lymphatics from the anal canal above the dentate line drain cephalad through the superior rectal lymphatics to the inferior mesenteric nodes, and laterally along both middle rectal vessels and inferior rectal vessels through the ischioanal fossa to the internal iliac nodes. Lymph from the anal canal below the dentate line usually drains to the inguinal nodes, although it can also drain to the superior rectal lymph nodes or along the inferior rectal lymphatics to the ischioanal fossa, if obstruction occurs in the primary drainage (Fig. 72.10).

Nerve Supply of the Rectum and Urogenital Organs

Sympathetic and parasympathetic nerves of the autonomic nervous system supply the anorectum and also send branches to the adjacent urogenital organs. Nerve trunks are close to the rectum and are prone to injury during mobilization of the rectum unless specific precautions are taken.

Sympathetic nerve fibers to the rectum are derived from the first three lumbar segments of the spinal cord. Sympathetic fibers pass through ganglionated sympathetic chains before forming the preaortic plexus. Preaortic fibers extend below the bifurcation of the aorta to form the hypogastric plexus or the presacral nerve (Fig. 72.11). The plexus thus formed divides into left and right branches on each side of the pelvis, where they are joined by the parasympathetic nerves.

The pelvic parasympathetic nerve supply is from the nervi erigentes, which originate from the second, third, and fourth sacral nerve roots. The fibers pass inward and forward to join the sympathetic nerve fibers to form the pelvic plexus. The pelvic plexus on each side is encased in the mid portion of the lateral stalk, which is located just above the levator ani muscle (see Fig. 72.11). From the pelvic plexuses, both types of nerve fibers are distributed to urinary and genital organs.

In women, the sympathetic nerve fibers from the hypogastric plexus are directed toward the uterosacral ligament close to the rectum. In men, the nerve fibers from the hypogastric plexus pass immediately adjacent to the anterolateral wall of the rectum in the retroperitoneal tissue.

The pelvic plexus gives rise to the periprostatic plexus, an important subdivision that is essential to sexual function in men. The periprostatic plexus distributes fibers to the prostate, seminal vesicles, corpora cavernosum, terminal part of the vas deferens, prostatic and membranous urethra, ejaculatory ducts, and bulbourethral glands. Both parasympathetic and sympathetic nervous systems are involved in erection. Nerve impulses from the parasympathetic nerves, which lead to erection, produce vasodilation and increase blood flow in the cavernous spaces of the penis. Activity of the sympathetic system adds to vascular engorgement and sustained erection. Moreover, sympathetic activity causes contraction of the ejaculatory ducts, seminal vesicles, and prostate, with subsequent expulsion of semen into the posterior urethra. Depending on which nerves have been damaged, deficiencies may include incomplete erection, lack of ejaculation, retrograde ejaculation, or total impotence.[6] Table 72.1 lists precautions to help avoid nerve injury during low rectal operations.[7]

The pudendal nerve arises from the sacral plexus (S2 to S4). It leaves the pelvis through the greater sciatic foramen, crosses the ischial spine, and then continues in the pudendal canal toward the ischial tuberosity in the lateral wall of the ischioanal fossa on each side. Three of its important branches are the inferior rectal, perineal, and dorsal nerves of the penis or clitoris. The pudendal nerve is anatomically protected from injury during mobilization of the rectum. Sensory stimuli from the penis and clitoris are mediated by a branch of the pudendal nerve and thus are preserved after proctectomy.

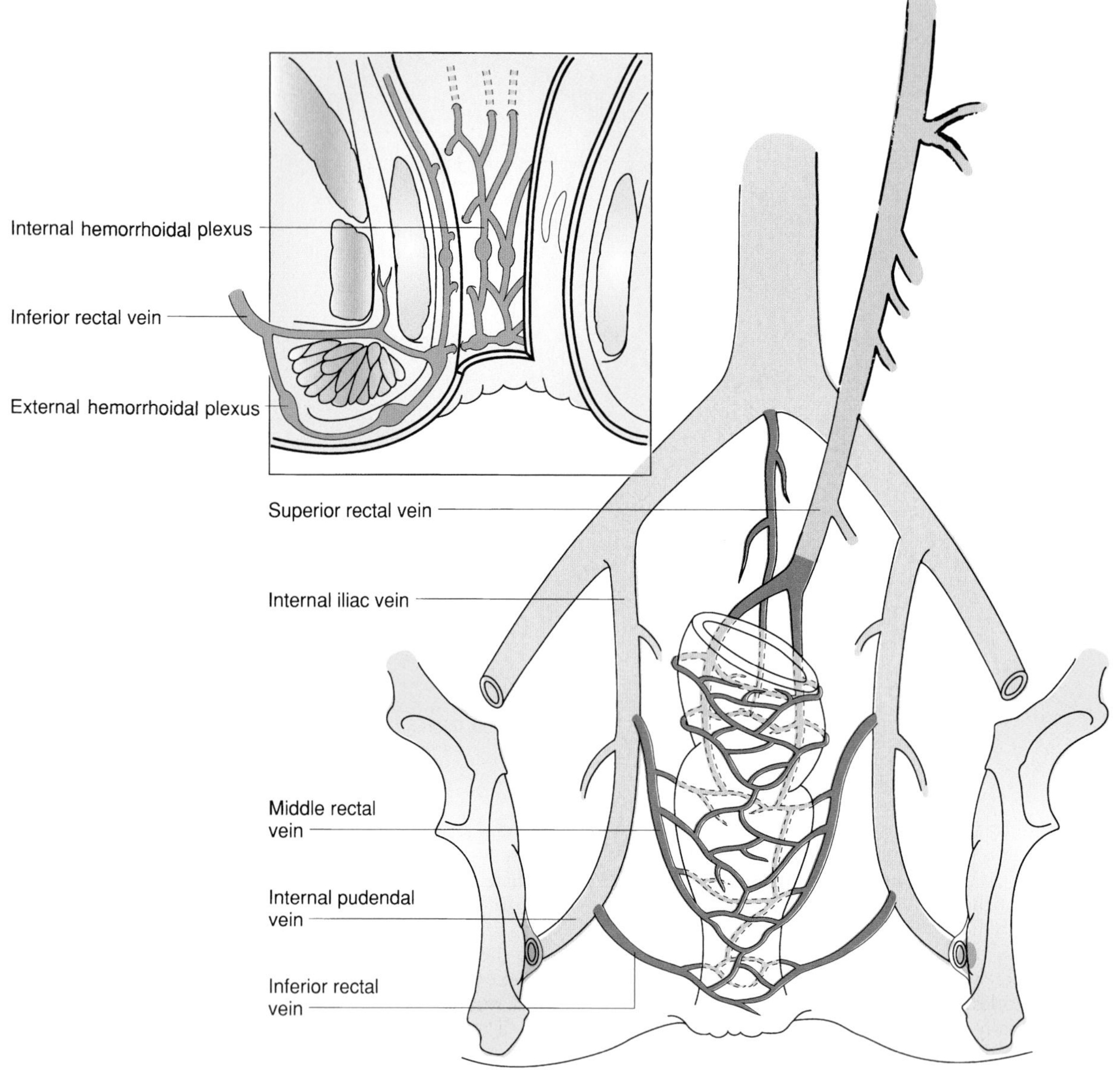

FIGURE 72.8 Venous drainage of the rectum and anal canal.

Nerve Supply of the Anal Canal

Motor Innervation

Both sympathetic and parasympathetic nerves supply the internal sphincter. The sympathetic and parasympathetic nerves are inhibitory to the internal anal sphincter. The external sphincter is supplied by the inferior rectal branch of the internal pudendal nerve and the perineal branch of the fourth sacral nerve. The levator ani is supplied not only by the pudendal nerve but also by direct branches of the third, fourth, and often the fifth sacral nerves, the fifth lying above the pelvic floor.

Sensory Innervation

The sensory nerve supply of the anal canal comes from the inferior rectal nerve, a branch of the pudendal nerve. The epithelium of the anal canal is profusely innervated with sensory nerve endings, especially in the vicinity of the dentate line. Painful sensations in the anal canal can be felt up to 1.5 cm proximal to the dentate line.

Physiology of the Anorectum

Sensation of the Anorectum

Complete anal continence cannot be achieved unless the subject can sense the presence of material in the rectum and can discriminate the quality of the substances (feces or gas). The receptors responsible for the appreciation of rectal fullness and impending evacuation lie outside the anorectal wall, probably within the levator ani muscle. The epithelium of the anal canal is rich with sensory nerve endings, and, although this sensitive area plays an important role in discriminating between flatus and feces, it is not a critical factor in preserving anal continence. When the anoderm is anesthetized with a topical anesthetic, the ability to differentiate between air and water is impaired, but the continence of rectally infused saline is maintained.[8]

Mechanism of Anal Continence

Stool can accumulate in the rectum for a variable period of time before the urge to defecate is experienced. The ability of

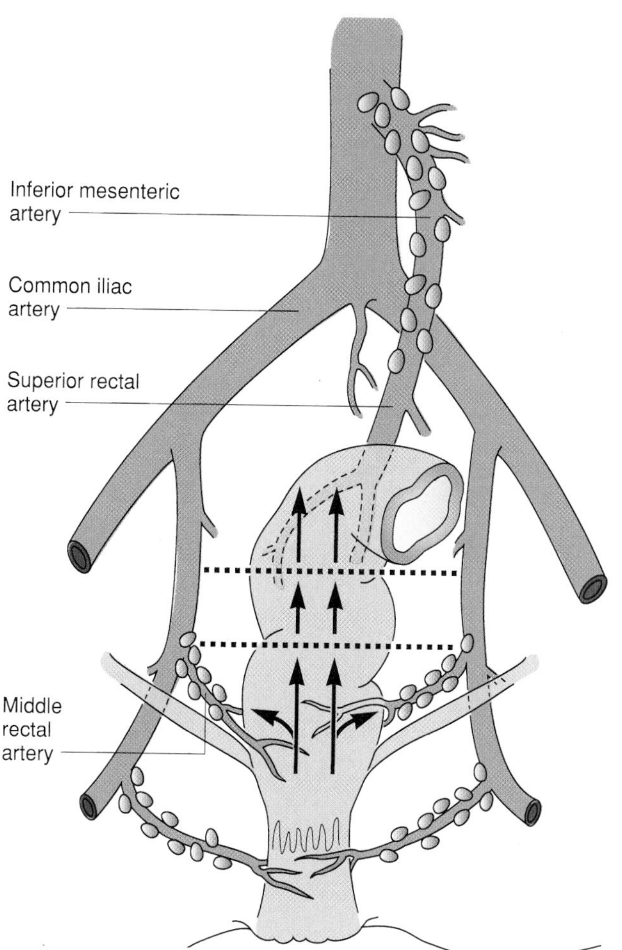

FIGURE 72.9 Lymphatic drainage of the rectum.

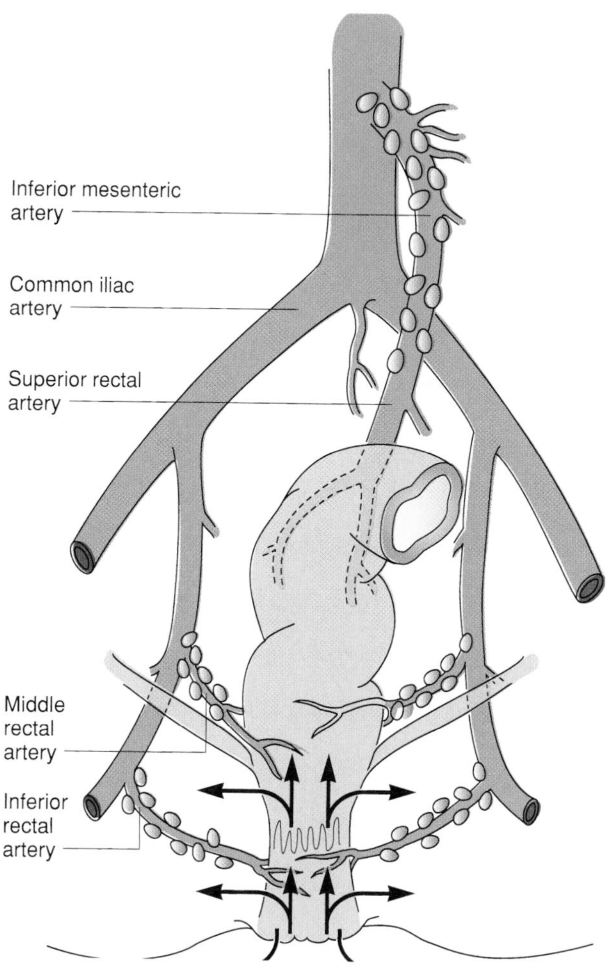

FIGURE 72.10 Lymphatic drainage of the anal canal.

the rectum to retain stool is known as *reservoir continence*. Continence is favored by the influence of pelvic muscles on rectal shape. The anal canal is pulled forward by the puborectalis muscle, which, as a U-shaped sling, creates an angle of 80 to 90 degrees to the rectum. This anorectal angle, maintained by the continuous tonic activity of the puborectal muscle, is effective in preventing stool in the rectum from entering the anal canal. Although it has been postulated that the mucosa of the anterior wall of the lower rectum is pressed firmly into the anal canal, creating a flap valve effect, recent studies have suggested that continence is maintained by sphincteric action rather than such a valvular mechanism. In the upper part of the anal canal, the hemorrhoidal pillars function as submucosal anal cushions, which contribute to continence by engorging during brisk involuntary Valsalva, such as coughing or sneezing.

Due to innervation by the autonomic nervous system, the internal sphincter is not considered subject to voluntary control. This powerful muscle exists in a continuously tonic state, maintaining approximately 85% of the anal canal resting pressure in a "high-pressure zone." The external sphincter contributes to anal pressure when a bolus of stool is present within the anal canal. The increase in pressure during voluntary contraction (squeeze pressure) is exclusively caused by the activity of the external sphincter. The high resting pressure in the anal canal acts as a barrier to prevent leakage of mucus and gas.

When the rectum is distended, the increased volume stimulates pressure receptors located on the puborectalis and pelvic floor muscles, which in turn stimulate the rectoanal inhibitory reflex. The rectoanal inhibitory reflex consists of internal anal sphincter relaxation and external anal sphincter contraction, allowing sampling of anal canal contents without leakage. This contact allows the sensory epithelium of the anal canal to sense and discriminate the nature of the material. If rectal distention is maintained, that is defecation is deferred, the rectal ampulla adapts to decrease the rectal pressure, called the *accommodation response*. Incontinence may occur with an abrupt and marked distention of the rectum (approximately 400 mL), which inhibits external sphincter contraction. Although volitional contraction of the external sphincter can be sustained only for short periods, it is the most important mechanism of voluntary continence.

Mechanism of Defecation

Defecation, the act of evacuating fecal material from the rectum, is a complex process that involves both a reflex response and voluntary performance (Fig. 72.12). When the anal canal is deemed to have solid contents and a decision to defecate is made, the subject assumes a squatting or sitting position to help straighten the anorectal angle and perform a Valsalva maneuver. With Valsalva, the glottis closes, pelvic floor muscles contract, and diaphragm and abdominal wall muscles contract, all increasing abdominal pressure. The puborectalis muscle relaxes, resulting in further straightening of the anorectal angle, and the pelvic floor descends slightly. The external anal sphincter relaxes and anal canal contents are evacuated. On normal complete evacuation, the pelvic floor rises and sphincters contract once more in a "closing reflex." After defecation is completed, voluntary sphincters contract actively, and the normal postural tone is restored.

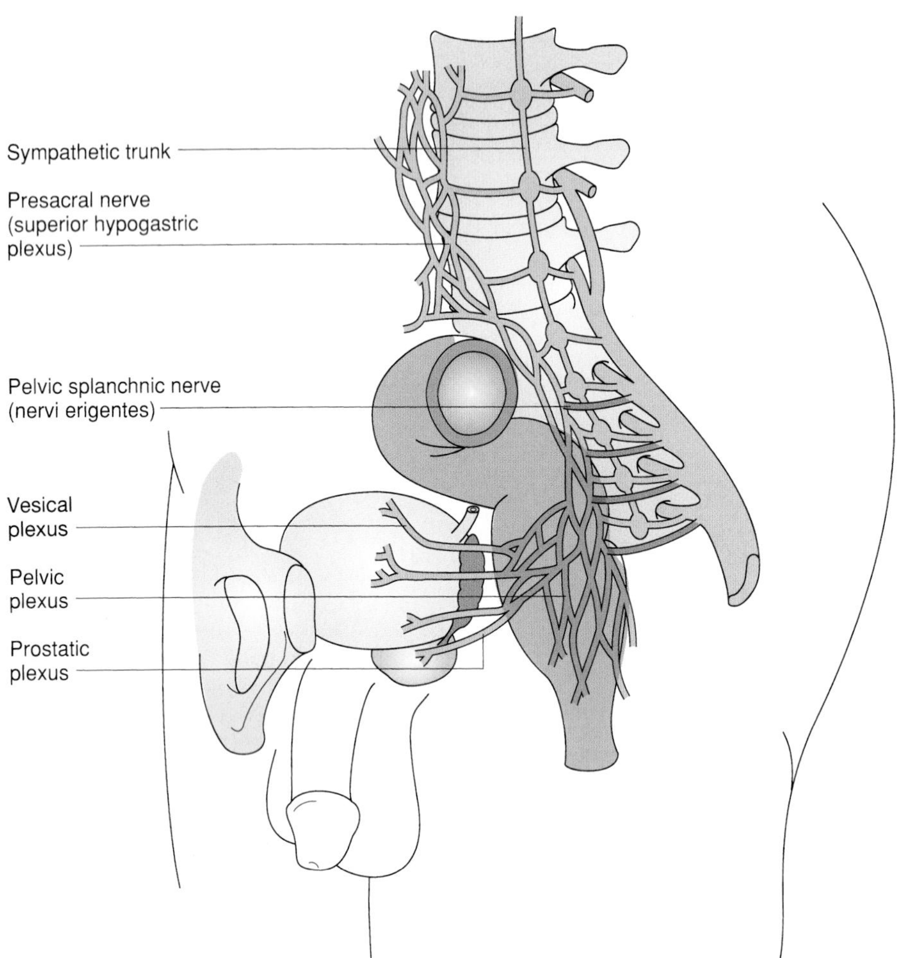

FIGURE 72.11 Sympathetic and parasympathetic nerve supply of the rectum.

BENIGN ANORECTAL DISEASE

Hemorrhoids

In the upper anal canal, the hemorrhoidal cushions are composed of three submucosal pillars of sinusoids within connective tissue, generally in the left lateral, right anterior, and right posterior. During the act of defecation, the hemorrhoidal cushions become engorged with blood, cushioning the anal canal and supporting the anal canal lining. The pathologic term *hemorrhoid* is used to describe the downward displacement of the cushion along with dilation of the contained sinusoids and sometimes bleeding from the arteriole, venule, or sinusoidal portion.[9,10] Hence, hemorrhoids develop when the supporting tissues of the anal cushion deteriorate or with extensive downward pressure, as in prolonged straining at stool or pregnancy.[11]

TABLE 72.1

AVOIDING NERVE INJURY DURING LOW RECTAL OPERATIONS

- When mobilizing the upper rectum for nonmalignant disease, dissect close to the bowel wall posteriorly and do not disturb the retroperitoneal tissue, to avoid injury to the hypogastric plexus.
- Incise the lateral peritoneum close to the rectum and brush the retroperitoneal tissue laterally to avoid injury to the left and right branches of the hypogastric plexus.
- Divide the lateral stalks close to the rectum to avoid injury to the nervi erigentes and the pelvic plexus.
- Note that the bulk of the pelvic plexus is located lateral and posterior to the seminal vesicles.[7] Separation of the rectum from Denonvilliers fascia should start at the midline and continue laterally to the edge of the seminal vesicle, then curve inferiorly to avoid injury to the neurovascular bundle.

Classification

External hemorrhoids are defined by their location below the dentate line. Thrombosed external hemorrhoids are intravascular clots in the sinusoids or venules of the external hemorrhoids. Internal hemorrhoids are the anal cushions located above the dentate line that have become prolapsed. The appearance and symptoms of internal hemorrhoids depend on the severity. For practical purposes, internal hemorrhoids are graded according to the degree of prolapse (Table 72.2).

Clinical Manifestations

The most common complaints of burning, itching, swelling, and pain usually are not from hemorrhoids but result from pruritus ani, anal abrasion, anal fissure, thrombosed external hemorrhoids, or prolapsed anal papilla. Symptoms are aggravated by constipation and diarrhea. The most common manifestation of hemorrhoids is painless, bright red rectal bleeding associated with bowel movement. With severe hemorrhoids,

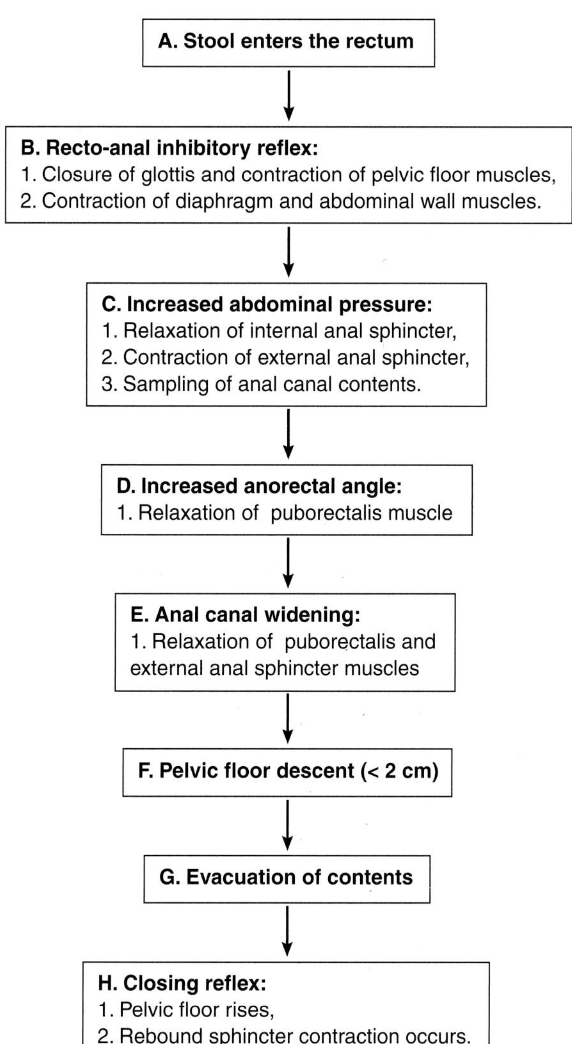

FIGURE 72.12 Mechanics of defecation.

the patient commonly describes the bleeding episode as blood dripping into the toilet bowl. A feeling of incomplete evacuation is also common. In chronic prolapse, exposed rectal mucosa often causes perianal irritation and mucus staining on the underwear. Congestion of external hemorrhoids or skin tags can cause discomfort. Except in the presence of thrombosis, pain is rarely an early symptom of hemorrhoidal disease and other diagnoses should be excluded.

TABLE 72.2 CLASSIFICATION

GRADING OF INTERNAL HEMORRHOIDS

Degree	Description
First	Hemorrhoids prolapse beyond the dentate line on straining
Second	Hemorrhoids prolapse through the anus on straining but reduce spontaneously
Third	Hemorrhoids prolapse through the anus and require manual reduction
Fourth	Prolapsed hemorrhoids cannot be manually reduced

Examination

Because many benign and malignant pathologic conditions are initially misdiagnosed as hemorrhoids, a thorough examination is critical for accurate diagnosis (Table 72.3). Although the examination can be performed in prone jackknife position, the left lateral or Sims position is usually less stressful and embarrassing to patients. The physician's discretion, sensitivity, and communication, for example warning the patient of pressure to the perineum or anus, makes a complete inspection easier and more thorough. Careful record of a thorough examination can be helpful with operative planning and future assessment of refractory pathology.

Anal skin tags, an external fistula opening, perianal excoriation from anal discharge, and anal fissure can be easily detected. The most accurate method of diagnosis for hemorrhoids is to ask the patient to sit on the toilet and strain and to watch for the prolapse.

Internal hemorrhoids cannot be palpated. Digital examination may detect anal stenosis or an anal scar. The anal sphincter tone and sphincter squeeze can be subjectively evaluated. A mass in the anal canal can be detected, and, in male patients, prostatic hypertrophy can be diagnosed.

After the visual inspection and digital examination, anoscopy is ideal for completing the anorectal exam. For patients in the prone jackknife position, the table should not be tilted during the examination. The patient is asked to strain to estimate the

TABLE 72.3

THE COMPLETE DIGITAL RECTAL EXAMINATION

Preparation
Enema
Left lateral decubitus position
Lighting, gloves, lubrication, anoscope

Visualization
Distract the buttocks
Inspect for:
- Soiling
- Excoriation or abrasion
- Scarring
- Patulous anus, deformity or flattening of folds
- Fissure
- External fistula opening
- Anal wink reflex
- Prolapse through anus with strain
- External hemorrhoids

Palpation
Slow insertion of gloved, lubricated finger
Pain with exam
Palpable sphincter defect
Perineal body scarring
Anal stenosis
Relaxed or increased tone
Prostate abnormalities (men) or anterior rectocele (women)
Gross blood present
Muscle function: squeeze
- Adequate
- Accessory muscle use

Strain
- Adequate
- Puborectalis relaxation
- Prolapsing tissue
- Other organ prolapse

degree of prolapse of the hemorrhoids. During anoscopy, one must exclude a coexisting anal fissure or fistula. Proctoscopy or flexible sigmoidoscopy should be used in all cases to rule out coexisting rectal abnormalities, particularly carcinoma and inflammatory bowel disease, both of which can cause symptoms similar to hemorrhoidal complaints. In young patients, if the rectal bleeding is obviously from the hemorrhoids, a complete colonic examination is not indicated, although follow-up is warranted. In patients older than age 49 years or in patients with a family history of epithelial cancers, a complete colonoscopy should be performed.

Treatment

According to modern concepts, prolapse of anal cushions is initiated by the shearing effect of the passage of a hard stool or by excessive downward pressure as with constipation, pregnancy, or childbirth, or by the precipitous act of defecation as in urgent diarrhea. If prolapse of the vascular cushions can be prevented or if the congesting effect of a tight anal canal can be abolished, the anal cushions return to their normal state and symptoms are ameliorated without necessitating removal of the cushions themselves. Therefore, the rationale of giving bulk in the diet is to eliminate straining at defecation by producing soft, bulky stool. A high-fiber diet usually reduces symptoms of hemorrhoids and is ideal for first- and second-degree hemorrhoids.

Rubber Band Ligation. Rubber band ligation is suitable for symptomatic first-, second-, and some third-degree internal hemorrhoids that do not respond to bulk-forming agents. Aspirin, nonsteroidal anti-inflammatory drugs, and anticoagulants should be discontinued at least 1 week before and 2 weeks after the procedure. After preparation with an enema, the procedure may be performed in the office through an anoscope. The band should be placed on the rectal mucosa just above the internal hemorrhoid (Fig. 72.13). Ligation of up to two or three hemorrhoids at one setting has been practiced with good results, and additional ligation can be performed 4 to 6 weeks later.

Rubber band ligation is not painless. The patient should be warned of anal discomfort or even pain, usually from anal sphincter spasm. Warm sitz baths reduce the pain, and an appropriate analgesic should be prescribed. Increasing fruits and vegetables in the diet or a bulk-forming agent with plenty of water should be taken for at least 6 to 8 weeks. Immediate severe or progressive pain is an indication of misplaced rubber band ligation, too close to the dentate line, and requires immediate removal of the rubber band with a number 11 blade. Symptoms of delayed anal pain, urinary retention, and fever are clues to the development of perianal infection. Prompt and aggressive treatment should include antibiotics, drainage of abscesses, and excision of necrotic tissues. Severe infection after rubber band ligation is rare, but deaths caused by acute perianal sepsis have been reported. A recent large retrospective review indicated a cumulative success rate of 80% for eradication of all grades of internal hemorrhoids, with a 29.5% recurrence rate after the first banding episode.[12] The postbanding complication rate was 2.8% for bleeding, 1.5% for thrombosis, 0.09% for bacteremia. Because of these potentially severe complications, rubber band ligation should be applied considered carefully for patients with immune deficiencies.

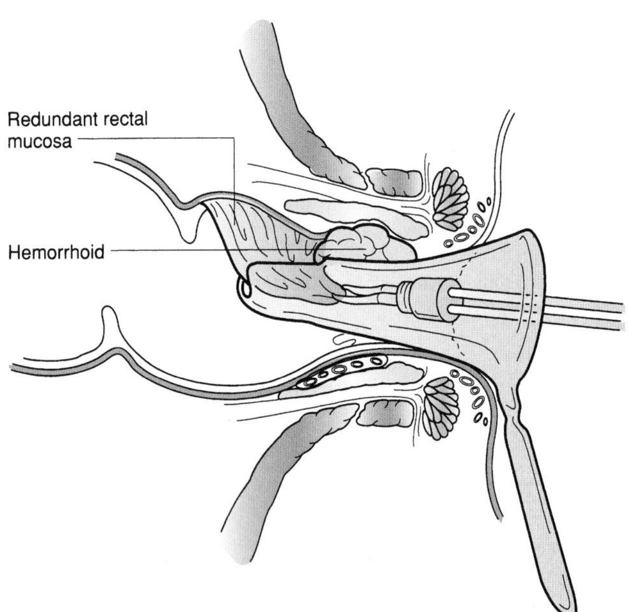

FIGURE 72.13 Rubber band ligation of an internal hemorrhoid.

Sclerotherapy. Sclerotherapy with a variety of substances (phenol, olive oil, sodium tetradecyl sulfate) can be performed in the office setting for first- or second-degree hemorrhoids in conjunction with banding or hemorrhoids that are too small to band. Using an anoscope, a small gauge needle is used to inject 1- to 2-mL sclerosant in the submucosal space just proximal to the hemorrhoidal bundle.

Infrared Photocoagulation. Infrared photocoagulation coagulates tissue protein or evaporates water in the cells, depending on the intensity and duration of application. As for sclerotherapy, an infrared probe is applied just proximal to the internal hemorrhoids through an anoscope. Infrared photocoagulation results for first- and second-degree hemorrhoids are comparable with those of rubber band ligation. Pain and complications occur infrequently. A regular electrocautery unit with a flat or ball tip works as well or even better.

Hemorrhoidectomy. Hemorrhoidectomy should be considered when the hemorrhoids are mixed internal and external, are severely prolapsed through the anus, or are complicated by associated pathology, such as ulceration, fissures, fistulas, large hypertrophied anal papillae, or extensive skin tags. Beginning a bowel regimen with fiber and a stool softener several days before operative intervention can help to prevent painful postoperative constipation. In many cases, hemorrhoidectomy can be performed using local anesthesia with mild sedation. In muscular or obese individuals, general or regional block anesthesia may be preferred. The patient is placed in the prone jackknife position with buttocks taped apart for visualization. An elliptic excision starts at the anoderm, includes external and internal hemorrhoids, and ends at the anorectal ring. The mucosa and submucosa are dissected off of the underlying internal sphincter muscle through the alveolar plane (Fig. 72.14). Excessive bleeding indicates that the hemorrhoidal bundle is being violated and can make visualization difficult. Alternatively, excising too deeply damages the internal sphincter fibers. Unless there is an associated anal stenosis or chronic anal fissure, internal sphincterotomy is not performed. The entire wound is closed with running absorbable sutures, and dressed with antibiotic ointment, fluff dressing to the perineum, and mesh shorts.

Urinary retention is a common complication of hemorrhoidectomy, unless intravenous fluids are restricted during the procedure and minimized for the next 6 to 8 hours.[13] Warm sitz baths are started the next morning, and patients are encouraged to use a gentle laxative as necessary.

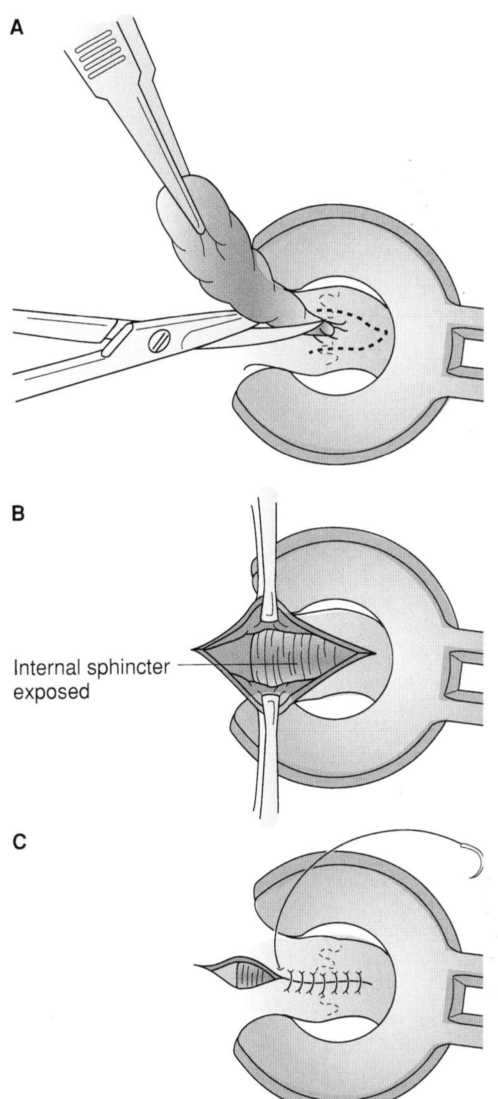

FIGURE 72.14 Technique of interanal closed hemorrhoidectomy. (*A*) Exposure of hemorrhoid with elliptic excision starting at perianal skin and extending to anorectal ring. (*B*) Submucosal hemorrhoidal plexus dissected from the internal sphincter, anoderm, and mucosa. (*C*) Wound closed with a running suture.

Procedure for Prolapsed Hemorrhoids. The procedure for prolapsed hemorrhoids or circular stapled procedure has been a relatively dramatic innovation in treatment for prolapsing internal hemorrhoids.[14] After placing the patient in prone jackknife position and administering local anesthesia, a dilator and obturator are inserted transanally into the distal rectum (Fig. 72.15). The dilator is secured to the perianal skin and a purse string suture is placed in the submucosa 4 to 5 cm proximal to the dentate line. The pursestring is gently tightened as the open stapler is inserted above it into the rectum. After the anvil passes proximal to the pursestring, the suture ends are pulled through designated channels in the stapler to use as stay sutures and manipulate the redundant rectal mucosa. The stapler is closed, advanced into the rectum, and pressure is held to aid in hemostasis. In female patients, a digital vaginal examination is performed to ascertain no incorporated vaginal tissue is in the staple line before firing. After firing the stapler, pressure is held for an additional minute. Frequently after stapler withdrawal, additional sutures are required across the anastomosis to assist with hemostasis.

A randomized trial comparing the procedure for prolapsed hemorrhoids with rubber band ligation found significantly increased pain and morbidity using the stapler but significantly increased recurrent bleeding with bands.[15] A recent systematic review of 15 randomized trials of the procedure for prolapsed hemorrhoids versus excisional hemorrhoidectomy, demonstrated significantly shorter operative time (weighted mean difference, –12.82 minutes), return to work (–4.03 days), and significantly decreased subjective pain, promoted as the main advantage of the procedure for prolapsed hemorrhoids.[16] At 6 months postoperatively, odds of recurrence using this technique were calculated at 3.64 compared with conventional excision. A recent report of long-term (1 year) results from a randomized trial of the stapled technique versus Ferguson hemorrhoidectomy reported similar significant short-term benefits, along with a significantly decreased number of patients requiring further anorectal surgery in the first postoperative year.[17]

Management of special cases. The following discussion reviews management for several other types of hemorrhoids, including thrombosed external hemorrhoids, strangulated hemorrhoids, hemorrhoids in pregnant and postpartum women, acute hemorrhoidal bleeding caused by portal hypertension, and hemorrhoids in inflammatory bowel disease.

Thrombosed external hemorrhoids. Thrombosis is a fairly common complication of hemorrhoidal disease. Most patients give no history of straining or physical exertion and do not have histories of hemorrhoidal disease. The complication develops with an abrupt onset of anal mass and pain that peaks within 48 hours. Usually, the pain becomes minimal after the fourth day. Occasionally, the skin overlying the hematoma becomes necrotic, causing bleeding and discharge or infection, which causes further necrosis and more pain. Treatment should be aimed at relief of severe pain, prevention of recurrent clot, and prevention of residual skin tags. If the patient is experiencing severe pain at the time of examination, excision should be performed. Conversely, if the pain is already subsiding and the clot is starting to shrink, thrombosis may be managed conservatively with warm sitz baths for comfort, proper anal hygiene, and bulk-producing agents such as bran or psyllium seed. The procedure can often be performed with the use of local anesthesia, and the wound can be left open without packing. Relief of pain is usually immediate. Postoperative care is simple and is aimed at keeping the wound clean with warm sitz baths and washing. An analgesic drug may be required during the first 24 hours. Patients must be warned of a relatively high recurrence rate: 6% after excision and 25% with noninvasive treatment.[18]

Strangulated hemorrhoids. Strangulation results from prolapsed third or fourth degree hemorrhoids that have become irreducible. History reveals a long-standing hemorrhoidal prolapse on straining. On examination, one may observe marked edema of both external and internal hemorrhoids everting through the anus. Untreated, strangulation may progress to ulceration and necrosis. Pain is usually severe and urinary retention is common. Proper treatment requires an urgent or emergent hemorrhoidectomy. The operation should be performed in the operating room or ambulatory surgical center and can usually be done under local anesthesia. Antibiotics are not indicated. The wound can be closed as in other hemorrhoidectomy.

Hemorrhoids in pregnant and postpartum women. Hemorrhoids can occur as the result of downward pressure from a gravid uterus or from prolonged labor, and may be exacerbated by hormonal changes. The problem may manifest as

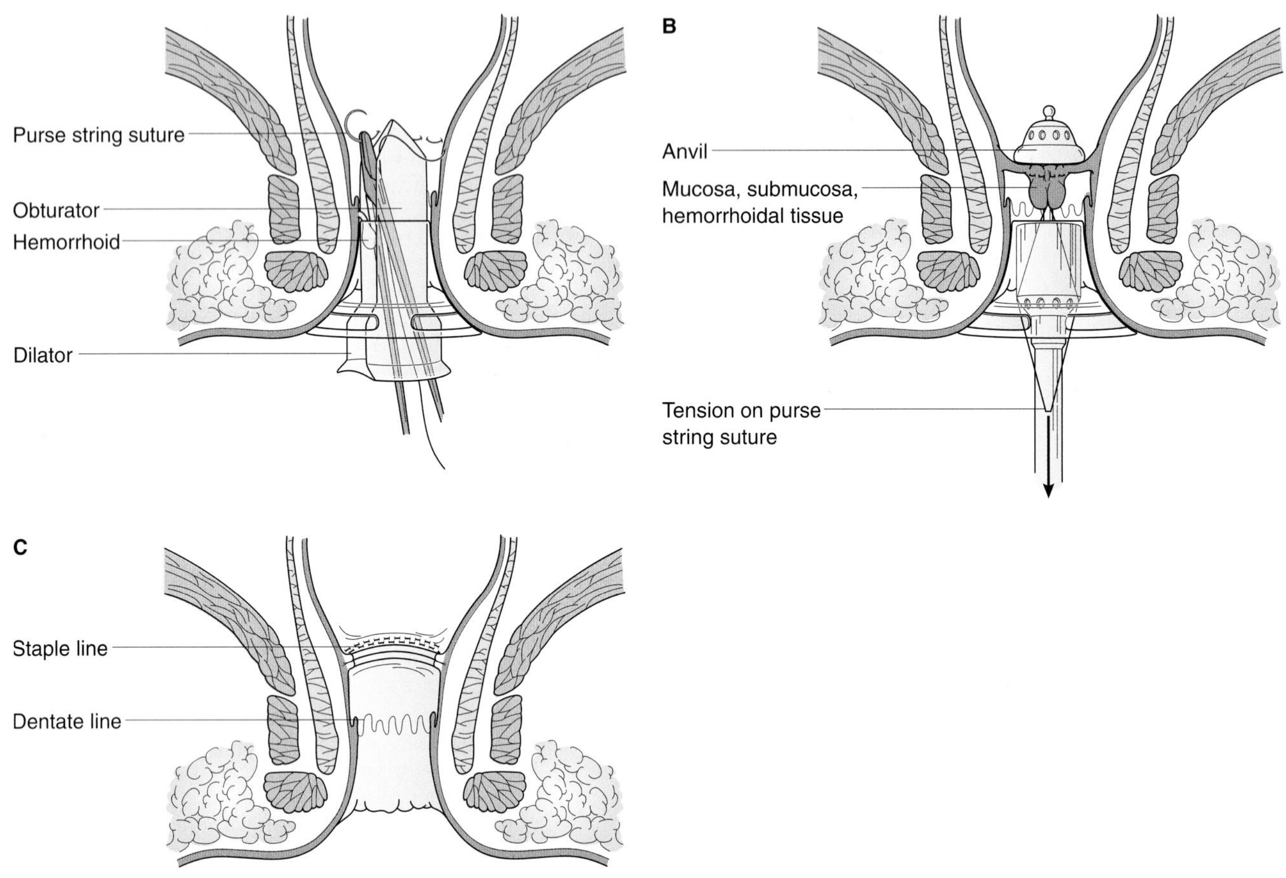

FIGURE 72.15 Stapled circular hemorrhoidectomy or procedure for prolapsing hemorrhoids. (*A*) A purse string suture is placed in the rectal mucosa proximal to hemorrhoids. (*B*) The stapler anvil is placed proximal to the purse string and purse string is tied down to draw hemorrhoidal tissue into the staple line. (*C*) The stapler is fired and removed, effectively excising hemorrhoidal tissue and creating a stapled anastomosis.

thrombosed external and internal hemorrhoids or strangulated hemorrhoids; treatment should be directed accordingly. Positioning in a left lateral decubitus position with additional retraction assistance is recommended for patients in later trimester pregnancy.

Acute hemorrhoidal bleeding caused by portal hypertension. Despite the communication between external and portal systems in the anal canal, the incidence of hemorrhoidal disease in portal hypertension is no greater than in the normal population. Although uncommon, massive bleeding from hemorrhoids in patients with portal hypertension can be life-threatening. Anoscopic examination is essential to identify the site of bleeding; proctoscopy or flexible sigmoidoscopy may miss the bleeding point entirely.

Suture of the bleeding site must incorporate the mucosa, submucosa, and internal sphincter. It is essential to correct any coexisting coagulopathy. Hemorrhoidectomy should be reserved for the rare situation when the stick-tie method fails to control the bleeding.

Hemorrhoids in inflammatory bowel disease. Hemorrhoidal problems in inflammatory bowel disease are uncommon. Most anal problems are the result of diarrhea causing perianal irritation and swelling, rather than the result of hemorrhoids themselves. The frontline treatment is anal hygiene and symptomatic relief of pain. If noninvasive therapy is ineffective, hemorrhoidectomy can be safely performed for patients with ulcerative colitis, but should be avoided in patients with Crohn disease because of the high incidence of nonhealing in these patients.

Rectal Prolapse

Prolapse of the rectum (procidentia) is an uncommon condition in which the full thickness of the rectal wall prolapses through the anal canal. Typically, the extruded rectum can be identified by concentric rings of mucosa, in contrast to prolapsing hemorrhoids, which display radially oriented folds.

Pathophysiology

Although the cause of rectal prolapse is poorly understood, the disorder is best considered an extension of intussusception. The intussusception usually starts in the lower rectum anteriorly, at a level about 8 cm from the anal verge, although the starting point may be at the rectosigmoid junction. Many patients with rectal prolapse have a history of straining associated with intractable constipation or, less commonly, chronic diarrhea. Studies of anorectal function and defecation dynamics in patients with rectal prolapse reveal that these patients have impaired resting and voluntary sphincter activity, decreased functional rectal capacity, impaired continence and puborectalis dyssynergy during defecation. Perhaps associated with difficult bowel habits or with effects of medication, rectal prolapse is disproportionately seen among patients with dementia, mental retardation, or schizophrenia.

Anatomic Abnormalities

Prolapse of the rectum predominates in female patients, with a female/male ratio of 5:1 or 6:1. Several anatomic defects or abnormalities are consistently demonstrated in patients with

TABLE 72.4 ETIOLOGY

ANATOMIC DEFECTS OR ABNORMALITIES IN PATIENTS WITH CHRONIC RECTAL PROLAPSE

- Abnormally deep rectovaginal or rectovesical pouch
- Lax and atonic musculature of the pelvic floor
- Lack of normal fixation of the rectum and an elongated mesorectum
- Unusually redundant sigmoid colon
- Lax and atonic anal sphincter

chronic rectal prolapse (Table 72.4). These defects are seen concurrently with long-standing prolapse, making the distinction between cause and effect difficult.

Classification

Although prolapse is generally classified informally as intussusception or frank prolapse, traditional classification is given in Table 72.5.[19]

Clinical Manifestations

One of the early symptoms of rectal prolapse is anorectal discomfort during defecation. Difficulty in initiating bowel movements, sensation of obstructed bowel movements, and the feeling of incomplete evacuation are common. Some patients require digital evacuation of the stool in the rectum. In many patients, difficulty with evacuating because of a nonrelaxing puborectalis muscle or rectocele, can lead to increased straining. A self-feeding cycle develops as the prolapse causes obstruction and further straining. Occult prolapse or solitary rectal ulcer syndrome is a vexing constellation of bleeding because of mucosal sheer stress, tenesmus, and sometimes a nonhealing ulcer. In an overt prolapse, initially the protrusion occurs only during or after defecation. As the problem becomes more pronounced, the protrusion may be precipitated by coughing, exertion, or walking.

Fecal and urinary incontinence are associated symptoms in prolapse of long duration. Loss of continence is caused by eversion of rectal mucosa resulting in decreased sensation, and by mechanical stretching of the sphincters and the pudendal nerves.[20]

Evaluation

Physical examination reveals a patulous anus with decreased sphincter tone. Anoscopy or rigid proctoscopy may demonstrate associated conditions, such as erythema on the anterior rectal wall. Anal manometry is helpful to establish baseline function among patients preoperatively but does not help to predict the outcome of surgery. Cinedefecography is extremely useful to confirm the diagnosis of intussusception (Fig. 72.16) and other potential anatomic or functional abnormalities, such as nonrelaxing puborectalis muscle or enterocele. Although minimally useful for the diagnosis of prolapse, colonoscopy is indicated to rule out an associated lesion, particularly among patients who have had family history of colorectal cancer. Colonoscopy can also identify occult prolapse or solitary rectal ulcer syndrome by revealing friable rectal mucosa 6 to 8 cm from the verge, generally on the anterior side. Diagnosis is confirmed by a characteristic histologic appearance of submucosal glands on biopsy. Surgical intervention for solitary rectal ulcer syndrome is generally ineffective at relieving symptoms of pain and tenesmus; patients are counseled to change dietary and bowel habits and referred for biofeedback physical therapy.

TABLE 72.5 CLASSIFICATION

CLASSIFICATION OF RECTAL PROLAPSE

Prolapse	Description
Incomplete (partial)	Prolapse of rectal mucosa only
Complete	Involving all layers
First degree	Occult prolapse or solitary rectal ulcer syndrome
Second degree	Prolapse to, but not through, the anus or intussusception
Third degree	Protrusion through the anus for a variable distance or frank prolapse

Treatment

Acute prolapse should be reduced with steady manual pressure to prevent incarceration and strangulation. Incarcerated prolapse is often reducible after application of granulated table sugar. For nonacute prolapse, strategies of surgical care include removal of the intussusception and measures to prevent recurrence. Most methods of repair use a transabdominal approach, although in male patients who are concerned regarding a risk to sexual function or in unfit patients a transperineal approach may be more appropriate initially.

The rectal sling operation introduced by Ripstein has been a common technique for prolapse repair in the United States. The operation consists of the construction of a sling of Teflon or Marlex to wrap the fully mobilized rectum anteriorly and attach it to the presacral fascia. The anterior rectal wrap was plagued with problems of obstructed defecation, therefore Ripstein later changed to posterior wrap,[21] in a technique described by Wells in 1959 (Fig. 72.17). Although mechanical obstruction has been eliminated, the constipation problems persist.[22] Additionally, patients are subjected to the risk of mesh erosion into the bowel, chronic pain associated with mesh, and the potential for smoldering infection.

Transabdominal rectosigmoid resection and suture rectopexy, described in detail by Frykman and Goldberg, is a composite surgical procedure with a full mobilization of the rectum to the level of the pelvic floor musculature. The redundant sigmoid and the rectum are resected with primary anastomosis, and the endorectal tissue and peritoneum on each side of the midrectum are sutured to the presacral fascia (Fig. 72.18). The recurrence rate has been reported to be 6% to 9% with up to 10-year follow-up.[23,24] Similar to mesh wrap, suture rectopexy is associated with constipation in about 50% of cases.[24,25]

A recently published multicenter cohort study compared abdominal approaches to prolapse repair and found pooled 5- and 10-year recurrence rates of 7% and 29%, respectively. No recurrence difference was identified based on performance of mobilization, resection, or rectopexy; that is, mobilization-only had the same recurrence rate as mobilization-resection-rectopexy, nor was a recurrence difference identified between suture and mesh rectopexy or between laparoscopic and open approaches.[26] Although there was substantial heterogeneity between centers and the study was likely underpowered, these findings support the notion that prolapse is probably alleviated by formation of presacral adhesions during the postoperative period.

Perineal rectosigmoidectomy is a transanal approach in which the prolapsed rectum and redundant sigmoid colon are excised endorectally. The prolapse must protrude at least 3 cm through the anus. The operation is performed with the patient in the lithotomy (Fig. 72.19) or prone jackknife position. The

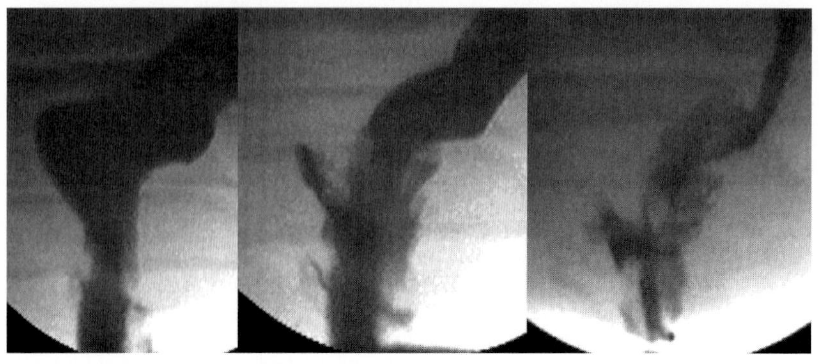

FIGURE 72.16 Cinedefecography demonstrating internal rectal prolapse, or intussusception. (Figure courtesy of Susan Congilosi Parker, MD.)

operation is well tolerated by patients, and the postoperative pain is minimal. Among patients with fecal incontinence, an anterior levatoroplasty can be performed simultaneously without an additional incision and may help to recreate the anorectal angle. Several series report a recurrence rate of about 16% with a relatively short-term follow-up.[24,27] Major long-term postoperative complications include recurrence, increased urgency with the smaller sigmoid reservoir after rectal excision, increased tenesmus, and anastomotic stricture.

The modified Delorme procedure is another transperineal approach. This technique is used for rectal prolapse that comes down to but not through the anus or for overt prolapse that protrudes less than 3 cm through the anus. The procedure is conducted with the patient in the prone jackknife position. The submucosa from the dentate line is stripped circumferentially with the use of electrocautery, continuing proximally until it is taut. At this point, the submucosal tube is transected. The proximal cut end is then brought down and anastomosed to the dentate line. The denuded rectal wall is incorporated into the stitches to eliminate the dead space (Fig. 72.20). Similar to perineal rectosigmoidectomy, it is well tolerated by patients and causes little postoperative pain, but is associated with a high rate of recurrence.

About 50% of patients with fecal incontinence from rectal prolapse improve after repair of the prolapse. Because the return of continence takes as long as 6 to 12 months, operative treatment for incontinence should be postponed for a year after a successful prolapse repair.

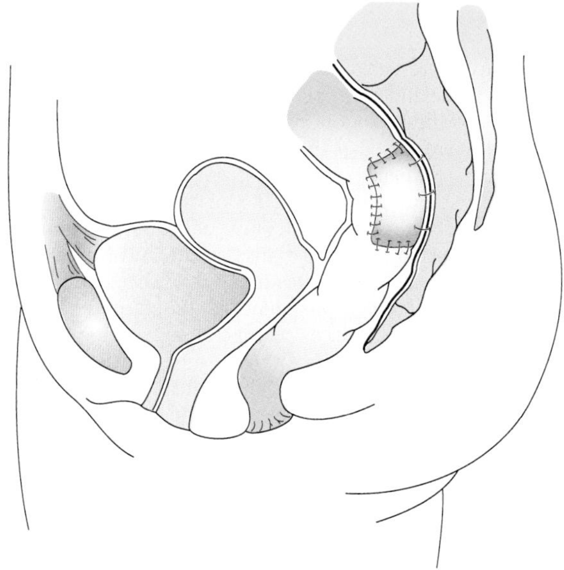

FIGURE 72.17 Marlex or Teflon mesh sutured to the presacral fascia, then wrapped the rectum posteriorly to three fourths of circumference.

Anal Incontinence

Definition and Etiology

The term *anal incontinence* describes a broad spectrum of anorectal functional impairment, ranging from simple involuntary passage of flatus to complete loss of sphincteric tone with involuntary passage of formed stool. Anal incontinence results when there is loss or disturbance of normal anorectal anatomy or physiology. A contracted rectum, poor rectal compliance, or a resection of the rectum with loss of normal rectal reservoir function may result in incontinence. A neurologic disturbance of anorectal sensation may prevent awareness of stool in the anorectum or even leakage from the anal canal. A large volume of diarrheal stool emptying rapidly into the anorectum may overcome the continent mechanism, even in healthy persons. Direct mechanical injuries to the sphincter muscles include obstetric tear, fistulotomy, hemorrhoidectomy, internal sphincterotomy, anal stretching, and perianal trauma. Age and female gender are the two major risk factors for incontinence and appear to have an important but poorly understood interaction; incontinence often does not manifest for 2 to 4 decades after obstetrical injury.

Evaluation

The previously outlined physical examination (Table 72.3) can help to differentiate the presence of a neurologic or muscular issue. For example, a patulous or lax anus may indicate neurogenic dysfunction of the sphincter muscles. Flattening of the corrugator cutis ani anteriorly may indicate a rectocele, essentially a tear in the rectovaginal fascia with intact overlying rectal and vaginal mucosa. A scar or defect in the anal region may indicate surgical injuries to the sphincter muscle.

In addition to history and physical examination, a number of anorectal anatomic and physiologic tests are available. Perhaps the most useful, endoanal ultrasonography has revolutionized investigation of the anal sphincter by providing a circumferential anatomic image of the internal and external sphincter. Endoanal ultrasonography can clarify presence of a large sphincter defect, indicating a need for sphincteroplasty and provide a map of the sphincter defect, or conversely can reveal the presence of an intact sphincter, thus preventing a futile attempt at sphincteroplasty. An intact but thinned area of sphincter may be due to denervation, which a pudendal nerve terminal motor latency test can help to confirm. Anal manometry is useful to establish baseline resting and exertional pressures, although results do not necessarily correlate with outcome of operative intervention. Defecography is a

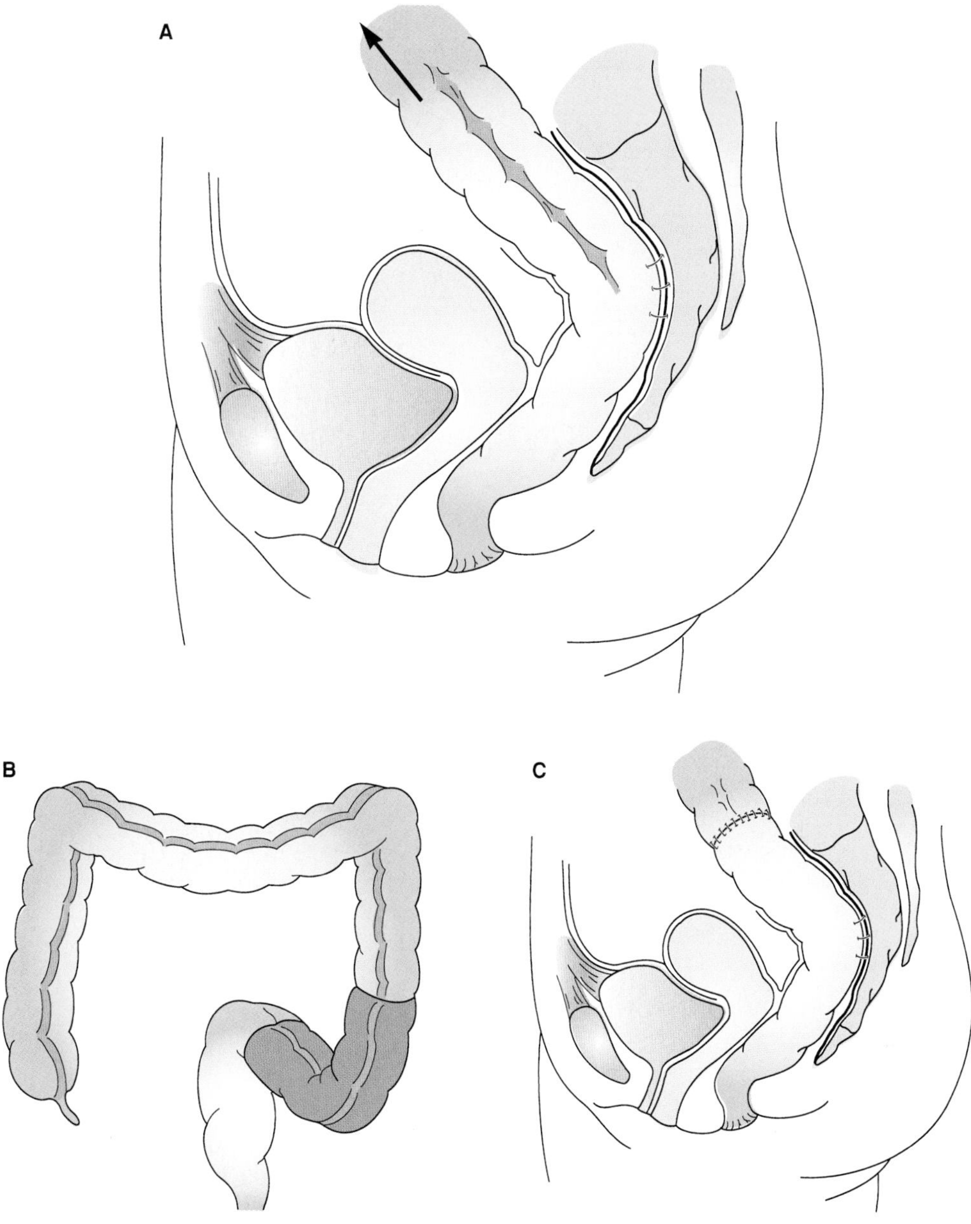

FIGURE 72.18 Transabdominal proctopexy. (*A*) After full mobilization of the rectum, the endorectal fascia and peritoneum on each side is sutured to presacral fascia, below the promontory of the sacrum. (*B*) Resection of redundant rectosigmoid colon. (*C*) Completed colonic anastomosis.

dynamic radiologic test that demonstrates the anatomic relationships of the pelvic floor organs during rectal evacuation. Although its uses are limited for defining the etiology of incontinence, defecography can be an invaluable aid to planning operative therapy in the presence of other previously unrecognized disorders, such as rectocele or internal prolapse. It is important to note that none of these tests individually correlates with incontinence. For example, fully continent control subjects also may display sphincter defects or manometric abnormalities. Anorectal physiology tests are most useful as complementary parts of the etiologic picture. Understanding the etiology underlying incontinence is an important first step to treatment planning.

The clinical evaluation of fecal incontinence is incomplete without a patient-centered assessment of symptom severity and quality of life. The subjective experience of these symptoms may be surprisingly different among patients. For example, one patient may be housebound because of fear of minor soiling, whereas another patient may make little change in daily activities despite occasional episodes of complete incontinence. Because anal incontinence is more an issue of quality of life than one of increasing mortality risk, determination of a need for intervention lies with the patient. Although a formal assessment is not generally necessary, it can be helpful in establishing a preoperative baseline score for postoperative comparison. Several validated severity and quality of life scores are available and have been reviewed in detail.[28]

Management

One of the most important first steps in treatment is medical regulation of bowel habits, with the goal of decreasing the bowel movement to once a day or once every other day. Sometimes this simple intervention resolves chronic and difficult symptoms. A high-fiber diet enhances stool bulk, easing evacuation of the rectum. Antidiarrheal drugs may be prescribed, such as

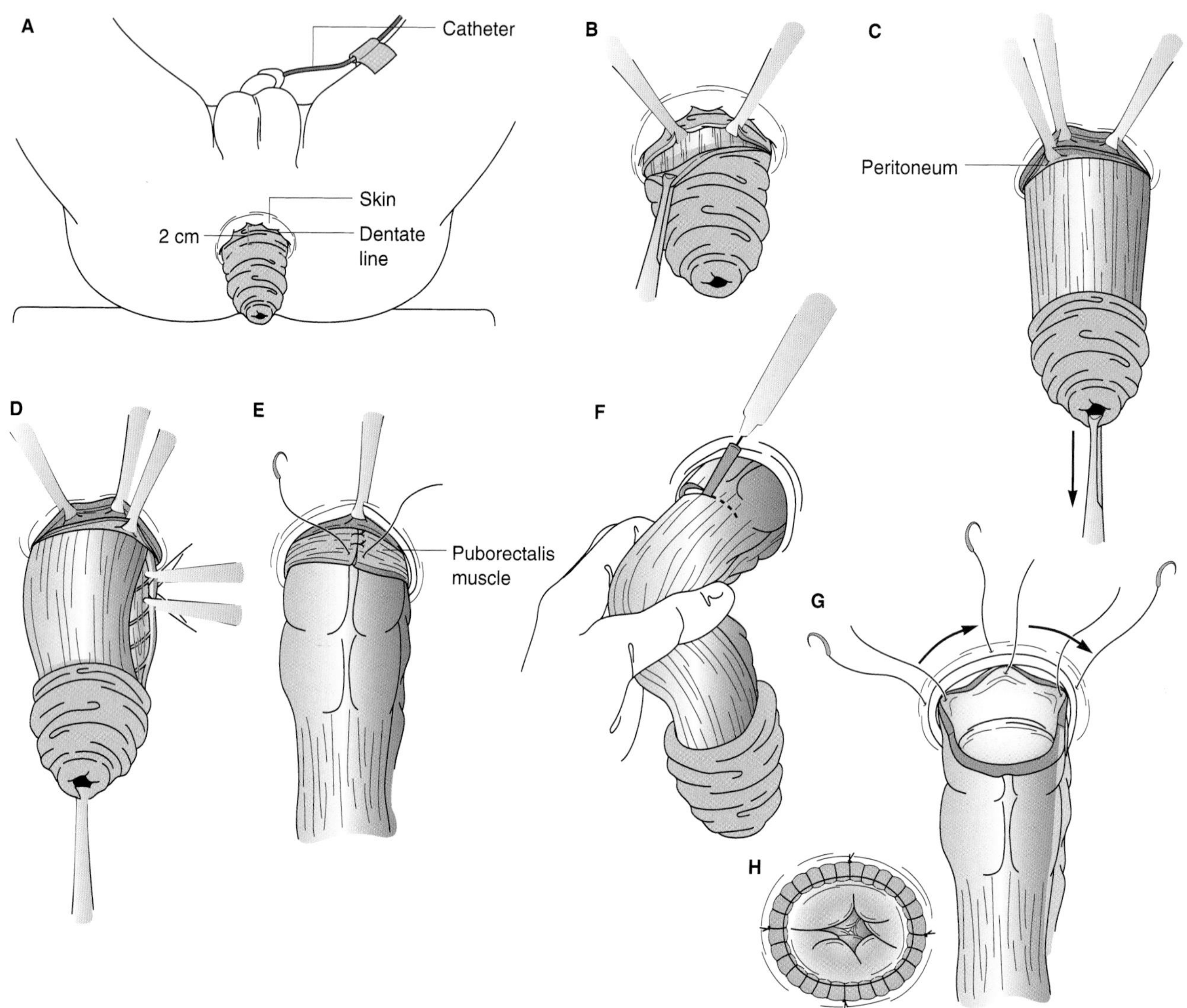

FIGURE 72.19 Perineal rectosigmoidectomy. The patient is placed in the lithotomy position with both legs in gynecologic stirrups. (*A* and *B*) A circular incision is made on the prolapsed rectum 2 cm proximal to the dentate line. (*C*) The peritoneal attachment is dissected from the anterior rectal wall, thus opening into the peritoneal cavity. (*D*) The mesorectum or mesosigmoid is clamped and divided laterally and posteriorly. (*E*) The previously opened peritoneum is sutured to the anterior wall of the rectum or sigmoid colon as high as possible. This is followed by approximation of the puborectalis (optional). (*F*) The anterior wall of the protruding rectum is cut 1 cm distal to the anal verge. (*G*) Stay sutures of 3-0 synthetic absorbable material are placed in four quadrants. (*H*) Anastomosis with running stitches.

loperamide, diphenoxylate, and bile acid binders to alter bowel consistency. Loperamide decreases intestinal motility and secretion, and may also increase sphincter pressure.

Biofeedback physical therapy can be used to regain anorectal sensation and to retrain coordinated contraction/relaxation of the pelvic floor and sphincter muscles. Biofeedback training helps about 85% of patients with various causes of anal incontinence.[29] The most common system consists of a triple-balloon catheter attached to a pressure transducer. With the patient watching the rectal manometer tracings, the balloon is inflated, and the patient is coached to contract the sphincter muscle to elevate the sphincter tracing. Several sessions may be required before the patient is aware of the sensation in the rectum and can specifically contract the anal sphincter. Eventually the patient can learn to contract the sphincter muscle without the instrument. A small, portable anorectal biofeedback system can be used to practice at home.

Operative treatment is reserved for incontinence that is refractory to conservative management. Sphincteroplasty is most suitable for incontinence secondary to obstetric injury or injury after previous anorectal surgery, but requires preoperative documentation of a sphincter defect. The procedure begins with a curved incision overlying the sphincter disruption and parallel to the anal verge. The sphincters are mobilized laterally to allow an overlapping plication with mattress suture. The buttock tape must be released from under the surgical drapes to allow modest tension of the overlap, and the anus should still permit digitation (Fig. 72.21). A simultaneous levatorplasty can help to support the repair and recreate the anorectal angle, but may contribute to postoperative dyspareunia. The overlapping sphincteroplasty achieves short-term success in about 85% of patients.[30] A recent review of long-term results in 191 consecutive patients found that only 40% maintained continence over a median interval of 10 years.[31] The only identified predictor of recurrence was patient age. Still, 74% of patients studied at 10 years postoperatively stated they were satisfied with their treatment.

Gracilis muscle transposition has been used in the presence of significant loss of the anal sphincter muscle mass. These

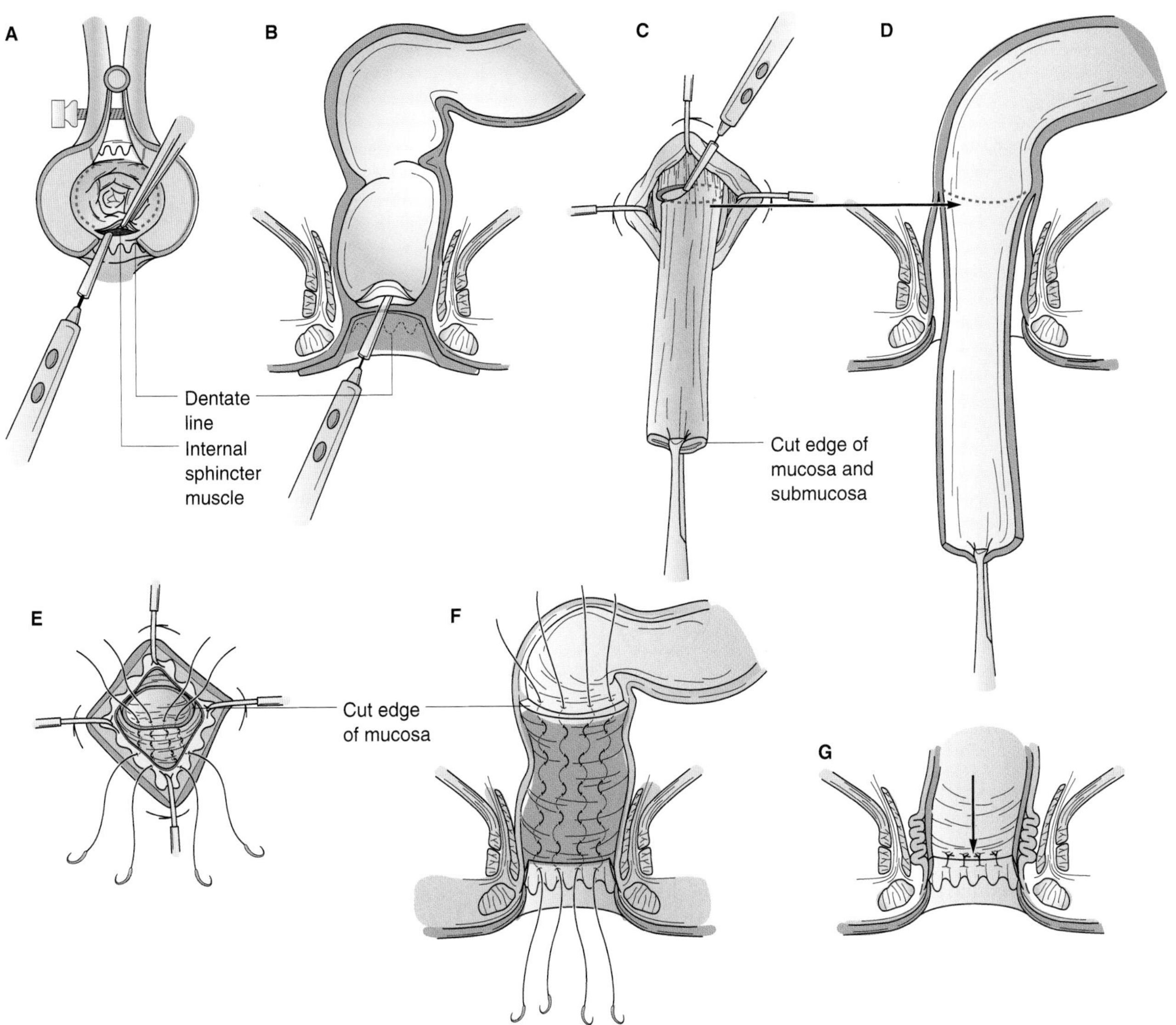

FIGURE 72.20 Modified Delorme procedure. Patient is placed in the prone position. (*A* and *B*) With a Pratt speculum used for exposure, a circumferential incision is made 1 cm proximal to the dentate line. The submucosa is dissected from the underlying internal sphincter. At the level of the anorectal ring, the Pratt speculum is replaced by Gelpi retractors placed at a right angle to the dentate line. (*C* and *D*) Proximal to the anorectal ring, the dissection continues in the mucosal plane until the mucosa resists being pulled down. The mucosal tube is then cut. (*E* and *F*) With 3-0 synthetic absorbable sutures, the mucosa at the upper cut end is brought down to the mucosa at the lower cut end, taking along the denuded anorectal wall. Eight such sutures are placed all around. (*G*) At completion of the anastomosis, the anorectum is plicated.

striated muscles are capable of producing a voluntary contraction to occlude the anal canal. However, the gracilis muscles are unable to preserve a closed lumen at all times because of a lack of an inherent tone, unlike the resting anal tone generated by the internal sphincter muscle. Traditional gracilis transposition has fallen out of favor because of unsatisfactory short-term successes of about 50%.[32,33] Gluteal muscle transposition yields similar results.[34]

The dynamic graciloplasty, in which an implanted electrical stimulating device stimulates the gracilis muscle, yields short-term success of 75%.[35] The chronic low-frequency electrical stimulation of skeletal muscle converts a fast-twitch muscle into a slow-twitch muscle capable of sustained activity. Although this operation has been received with enthusiasm in Europe, it is not approved for clinical applications by the U.S. Food and Drug Administration.

A recent development with promising results is the artificial anal sphincter (Acticon Neosphincter, American Medical Systems, Minnetonka, MN; Fig. 72.22), now approved by the U.S. Food and Drug Administration. The sphincter consists of an inflatable cuff of silicone rubber placed around the upper anal canal via two small perianal incisions. The pressure-regulating balloon is placed extraperitoneally to the left or right of the bladder, and the pump by which the patient can inflate and deflate the cuff is placed in the labia majora or in the scrotum. A multicenter trial of the artificial anal sphincter revealed results similar to those for dynamic graciloplasty.[36] Reoperation was required in 46% of patients, primarily because of infection; 37% required device explantation, 20% of whom were reimplanted with a new device. In patients with a functioning device, 85% achieved continence. Long-term (more than 2 years) results of artificial sphincter placement have recently been published.[37] About 50% of patients required explantation for infection or other problems, and about half of those were successfully reimplanted. Approximately 25% of patients in the cohort ultimately required an end colostomy.

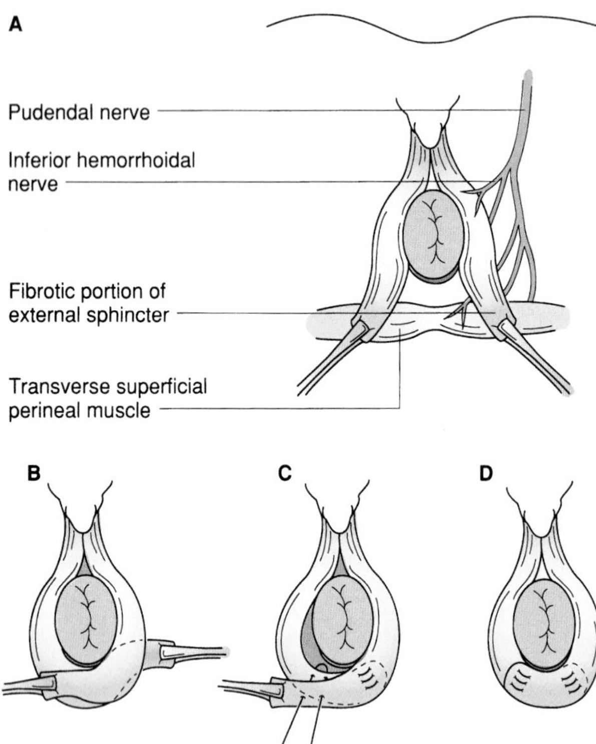

FIGURE 72.21 Overlapping anal sphincteroplasty.

A number of novel therapeutic interventions for anal incontinence are emerging.[38] Sacral nerve stimulation, or neuromodulation, does not attempt to repair a defect but instead augments physiologic functioning through stimulation of S2, S3, and S4 nerves exiting the sacral foramina. The mechanism is incompletely understood but likely associated with some combination of electrical recruitment of striated muscle, increased sensation, enhanced anal resting tone, and improvement in local reflexes. At a median of 2 years follow-up, Kenefick et al.[39] reported about 73% full return of continence among a cohort of women with various etiologies of liquid and solid stool incontinence. The Secca procedure (Curon Medical, Fremont, CA) consists of radiofrequency energy delivery to the submucosa through a transanally placed, heat-controlled probe. Although the mechanism of action is poorly understood, improvement in continence may be a result of collagen contraction after heating. Shorter term results indicate about 80% at least partial response among patients undergoing the Secca procedure.[40]

For patients with refractory incontinence or who are unable to tolerate extensive intervention, other options such as anal plug devices and anal bulking agents have also been described. Among patients with incapacitating fecal incontinence who have failed other forms of treatment, a permanent end-sigmoid colostomy is the best choice.

Anal Fissure

Definition

Anal fissure is an ulcer in the lower portion of the anal canal. Fissures can be classified as acute or chronic and further subdivided as either primary or secondary. A primary fissure occurs without association with other local or systemic diseases. Secondary fissure develops in association with other systemic diseases, such as Crohn disease, leukemia, aplastic anemia, or agranulocytosis.

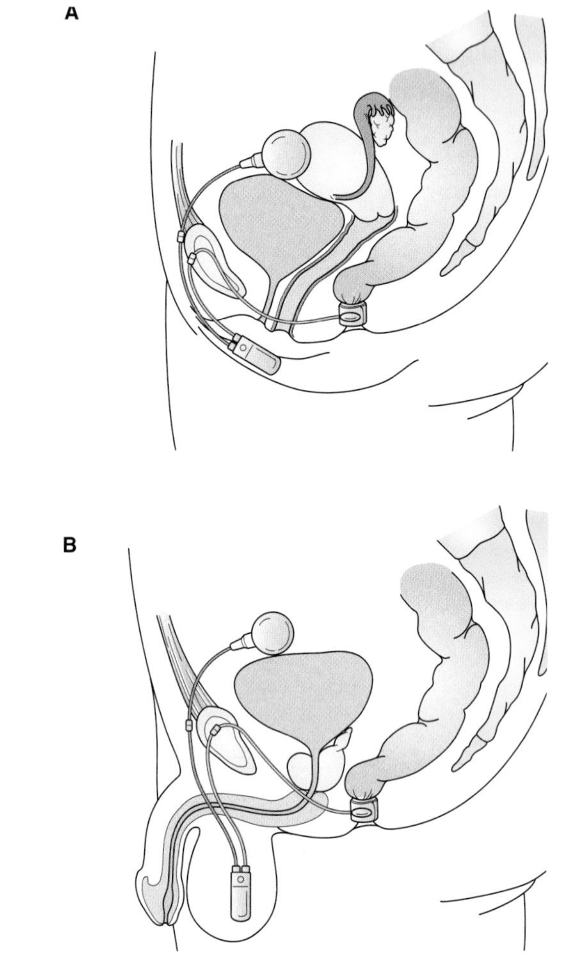

FIGURE 72.22 Implanted silicone neosphincter. (*A*) Female. (*B*) Male.

Pathophysiology

Most tears of the anal canal can be traced to the passage of a large, hard stool or explosive diarrhea, trauma to the anus, or tearing during vaginal delivery. In men, almost all fissures are located in the posterior midline, whereas 10% of fissures in women are in the anterior midline. Numerous studies on anal sphincteric function reveal that the resting anal pressure (internal sphincter) in patients with anal fissure is significantly higher than normal, whereas the squeeze pressure (external sphincter) is normal. Increased anal pressure is caused by increased internal sphincter tone. Doppler flowmetry has demonstrated perfusion of the anal canal to be poorest posteriorly and has also demonstrated reduced anodermal blood flow at fissure sites, suggesting that chronic nonhealing fissures are caused by ischemia. Reduction of anal pressure by sphincterotomy improves anodermal blood flow, resulting in fissure healing.[41]

Clinical Manifestations

Anal pain, particularly during and after bowel movement, is the most prominent symptom, followed by bleeding with defecation. The pain is described as sharp, burning, throbbing, or dull aching. In acute anal fissure, the pain can be severe and incapacitating and may last for many hours. If there is fever, fissure may mimic an anorectal abscess, especially intersphincteric abscess. Constipation is a common association, both as a precipitating event and subsequent to fissure development due to pain associated with defecation.

Diagnosis

Although pain and bleeding are typical of anal fissure, the diagnosis is confirmed by examination. When performed gently, inspection of the anus by spreading the buttocks will reveal the fissure in most cases. On digital examination, the fissure can be appreciated as a small fibrotic defect. Digital examination can also detect hypertonicity of the anal canal, another clue indicating an anal fissure. A small anoscope is useful to visualize the fissure, if the patient can tolerate it. Occasionally, the examination must be performed under anesthesia because of severe pain.

Management

Initial treatment of acute anal fissure is pain relief, with proper anal hygiene and warm sitz baths to relax the anal canal. Application of a topical anesthetic jelly directly to the fissure before bowel movement is helpful. Bulking and softening the stool with oral bran or psyllium seed will usually relieve constipation. Acute anal fissures should heal within 6 weeks. Surgery is not usually required unless the fissure is an exacerbation of a chronic anal fissure.

Chronic anal fissures are usually deep, exposing the internal anal sphincter, and are often accompanied by a sentinel skin tag, and hypertrophied anal papilla. The sentinel tag is the fibrotic or edematous skin adjacent to the fissure. A reasonable first conservative treatment for chronic anal fissure is the application of 0.2% to 0.4% nitroglycerin ointment on a cotton swab applied directly to the anal fissure twice a day. Nitroglycerin reduces the anal resting pressure and increases the anodermal blood flow. Patients should be warned of associated headaches, which tend to subside in severity over the 6-week therapeutic period. Fissure resolution after 6 weeks of therapy has been reported at 50% to 75%, but about half of these will recur. Topical diltiazem or nifedipine have been reported to yield better than 50% resolution at 6 weeks, but again are associated with headache side effects and frequent fissure recurrence. Botulinum toxin A injection into the internal sphincter to reduce hypertonicity may enhance fissure healing, although technique, dose, and success rates have varied widely. A long-term cohort study of fissure patients treated with botulinum injection demonstrated 42% recurrence at a median of 42 months.[42] Potential side effects of botulinum injection include transitory incontinence (generally lasting no more than 3 months), hematoma, thrombosis, and infection.

Lateral internal sphincterotomy has become the treatment of choice for the unhealed chronic anal fissure refractory to medical therapy (Fig. 72.23).[43] The procedure can be performed under local, regional, or general anesthesia. Most patients can return home on the same day of the surgery. In the closed method, the left or right lateral quadrant of the anal canal is exposed with an anal speculum. The speculum is gently and gradually opened to its maximum. The stretched internal sphincter can be easily felt, like a bow string. A knife blade is passed through the skin at the lateral border of the internal sphincter muscle, in the subcutaneous plane, with the blade in the horizontal position. The knife blade is then advanced to the level of the dentate line. At this point, the blade is turned 90 degrees, with the cutting edge on the muscle. The internal sphincter muscle is then cut to its full thickness by gentle pressure on the blade while it is withdrawn. The stab wound is left open (Fig. 72.24). The fissure in the posterior or anterior midline is left undisturbed, but the redundant skin or the hypertrophied anal papilla can be excised as appropriate. With the open technique, the skin and subcutaneous tissue from the dentate line to the anal verge are incised; an anal speculum is used to expose the left or right lateral quadrant. The internal sphincter muscle is identified and incised to its full thickness. The wound is closed with running sutures (Fig. 72.24). A recent cohort study of 35 male patients who had failed nonoperative management reported 94% fissure healing after open sphincterotomy.[44] Three patients had a decreased fecal continence score but only one patient had a decreased quality of life score postoperatively. A recent

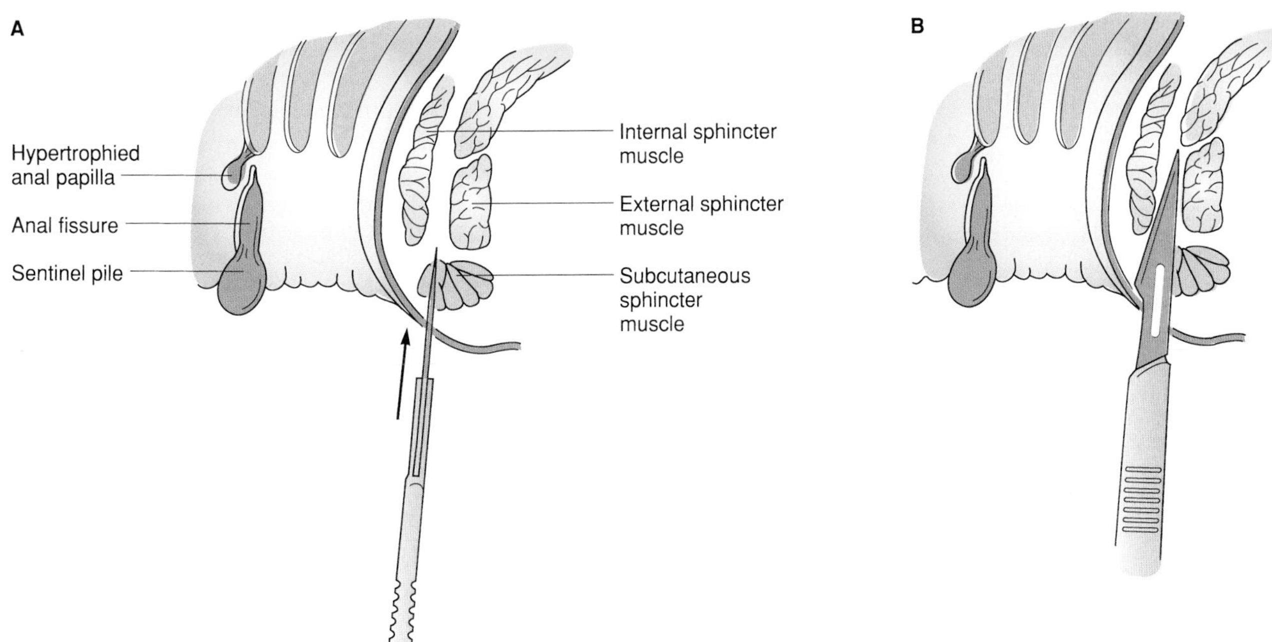

FIGURE 72.23 Lateral internal sphincterotomy (closed technique). (*A*) Triad of fissure, sentinel pile, and hypertrophied anal papilla. With an anal speculum used for exposure of the lateral quadrant, a no. 11 scalpel blade stabs into the subcutaneous tissue from the anal verge to the dentate line, with the knife in the horizontal position. (*B*) The knife is turned 90 degrees and the internal sphincter muscle is cut while the anal canal is stretched open.

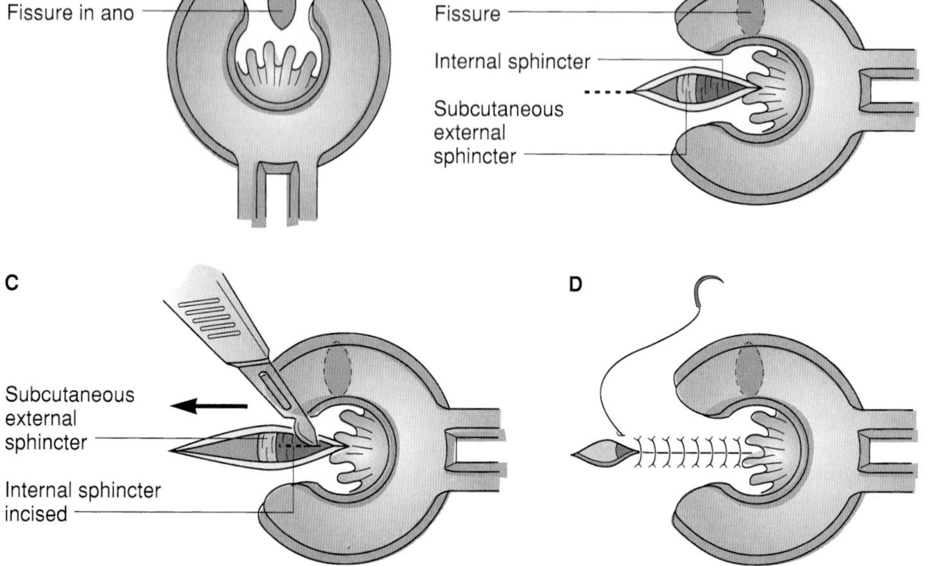

FIGURE 72.24 Lateral internal sphincterotomy (open method). (*A*) The fissure in the midline is left alone. (*B*) With a speculum used to expose the left lateral quadrant, an incision is made through the subcutaneous tissue to expose both the subcutaneous external sphincter and the internal sphincter. (*C*) The internal sphincter is incised to its full thickness; care is taken not to cut the external sphincter. (*D*) The wound is closed.

Cochrane review of surgical interventions indicated that stretch therapy and posterior sphincterotomy are less effective and more likely to result in incontinence.[45] No difference was found between open and closed lateral internal sphincterotomy techniques.

Secondary Anal Fissure

Fissures or ulcers that develop as a result of underlying disease, such as Crohn disease, tend to be larger and deeper than primary anal fissures and less likely to be found in the posterior midline. The skin around the ulcer is edematous, macerated, and erythematous. As a rule, pain is not as severe as that associated with idiopathic primary fissure; severe pain from a fissure in Crohn disease may be a sign of abscess formation. The treatment of fissure associated with Crohn disease is proper anal hygiene, local care of the lesion, and control of constipation or diarrhea. Surgery should be avoided and is contraindicated in the presence of active Crohn disease.

A non-midline or otherwise abnormal appearing fissure should undergo margin biopsy, to assist in diagnosis of the underlying disorder and to rule out malignancy. Anal fissure or ulcer may occur in patients with leukemia, aplastic anemia, and agranulocytosis. The fissure usually follows a bout of diarrhea or constipation at a time when the patient is neutropenic. The ulcer is extremely painful and often necrotic at its base. Fever or septicemia is common; if present, broad-spectrum antibiotics should be given. Treatment is directed at perineal hygiene and relief of pain with a non-constipating analgesic drug. The ulcer usually heals when the white blood cell count rises above 1,000/mL. Surgery should be avoided.

Anorectal Abscesses

Pathogenesis

In the wall of the anal canal, a variable number of anal glands (4 to 10) lined by stratified columnar epithelium have direct openings into the anal crypts at the dentate line. Infection of the anal glands is the most common origin of perianal abscesses. Because the anal glands lie between the internal and external sphincter muscles, an intersphincteric abscess is formed. The infection may then spread to different spaces (Fig. 72.25). Abscess locations, in order of frequency, are perianal, ischioanal, intersphincteric, and supralevator.

Clinical Manifestations

The initial symptom of most anorectal abscesses is severe pain in the anal region. The pain is throbbing or dully aching in character and is aggravated by walking, straining, coughing, and sneezing. Depending on the location of the abscess, a swollen mass may be felt. Fever or even septicemia may be present. In some patients, urinary retention occurs.

Management

Like an abscess in any other part of the body, an anorectal abscess must be drained as soon as possible. In general, antibiotics are not necessary after the abscess is adequately drained, but in patients with immune deficiencies and in those with prostheses or cardiac valvular abnormalities, appropriate antibiotics should be considered. Additionally, among patients with Crohn disease, oral metronidazole or ciprofloxacin seems to have a mitigating effect. Packing of a perianal or perirectal abscess is generally discouraged because it can help to maintain the potential space.

Perianal abscesses are the most superficial and the easiest to treat. The abscess is usually small and can be drained under local anesthesia. An elliptical or cruciate incision is made on the most prominent part of the skin and subcutaneous tissue overlying the abscess cavity. Redundant skin edges are excised to prevent premature closure of the abscess. The abscess cavity is thoroughly curetted and irrigated. No packing is necessary.

An ischioanal abscess causes a diffuse swelling of the ischioanal fossa. Drainage is similar to perianal abscess. Bilateral ischioanal or horseshoe abscess has its origin in the deep postanal space, with spreads to both sides of the ischioanal space. A horseshoe abscess should be drained

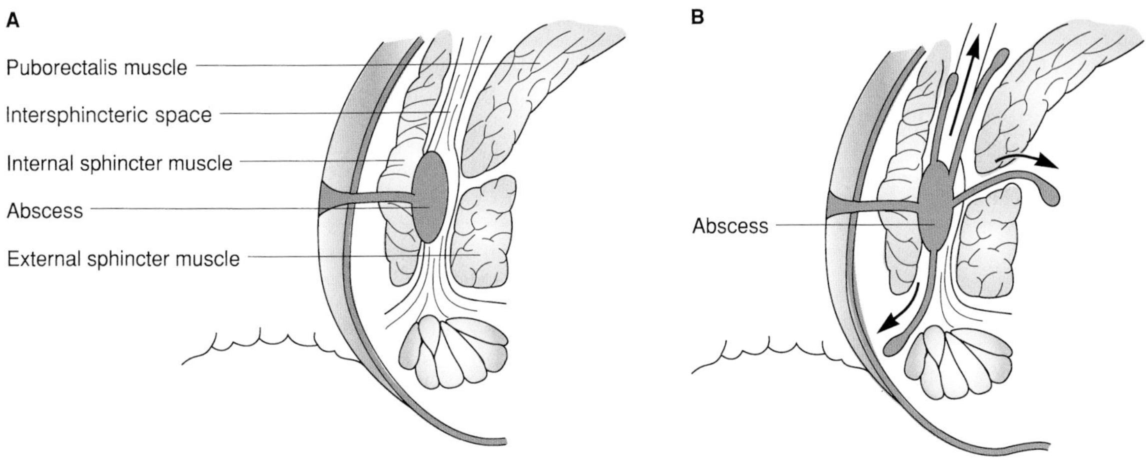

FIGURE 72.25 Pathways of infection start in the intersphincteric space (*A*) and then spread to perianal spaces, forming perianal abscesses (*B*).

through the deep postanal space. A longitudinal incision is made in the skin between the tip of the coccyx and the anus to expose the anococcygeal ligament. The anococcygeal ligament is incised along its fibers, and the deep postanal space is entered. After the abscess cavity is drained, curetted, and irrigated, a counterdrainage incision is made on one or both limbs of the ischioanal space. No packing is needed.

Unlike perianal and ischioanal abscesses, there are no apparent signs of swelling or induration in the perianal area in intersphincteric abscesses. The diagnosis is suspected when anorectal pain is so severe that rectal examination is impossible. A deep-seated tenderness is present when circumanal pressure is applied. Most intersphincteric abscesses are located in the posterior quadrant. An indurated or bulging mass can be felt in the anal wall above the dentate line and can extend into the rectum to a variable distance. Intersphincteric abscesses are drained by incising the anal canal lining and incising through the internal sphincter muscle. The abscess cavity is curetted and irrigated with saline solution until clean. No packing is placed. Postoperative care consists of warm sitz baths for comfort. A bulk-producing agent is started the next day.

Supralevator abscess is uncommon and can be difficult to diagnose. Because of its proximity to the abdominal cavity, a supralevator abscess can mimic acute intraabdominal conditions. Digital examination reveals an indurated or bulging tender mass on either side of the lower rectum or posteriorly above the level of the anorectal ring. The supralevator abscess may arise in one of three ways: through upward extension of an intersphincteric abscess, by upward extension of an ischioanal abscess, or from intraabdominal processes such as diverticular abscess, appendiceal abscess, or abscess from Crohn disease. It is essential to determine the origin of the abscess before treatment. If the abscess is secondary to upward extension of an intersphincteric abscess, it should be drained into the rectum. If such an abscess is drained through the ischioanal fossa, a complicated suprasphincteric fistula can be formed. If a supralevator abscess arises from the upward extension of an ischiorectal abscess, it should be drained through the ischioanal fossa. Attempts at draining this kind of abscess into the rectum may result in an extrasphincteric fistula. If the abscess is secondary to an intraabdominal disease, the primary disease is treated and the supralevator abscess is drained into the rectum, through the ischioanal fossa, or through the abdominal wall.

Fistula-in-ano

Fistula-in-ano is a chronic form of perianal abscess that is spontaneously or surgically drained but in which the abscess cavity does not heal completely, becoming instead an inflammatory track with a primary opening (internal opening) in the anal crypt at the dentate line and a secondary opening (external opening) in the perianal skin.

Classification

There are four main forms of fistula-in-ano, based on the relation of the fistula to the sphincter muscles (Fig. 72.26).[46]

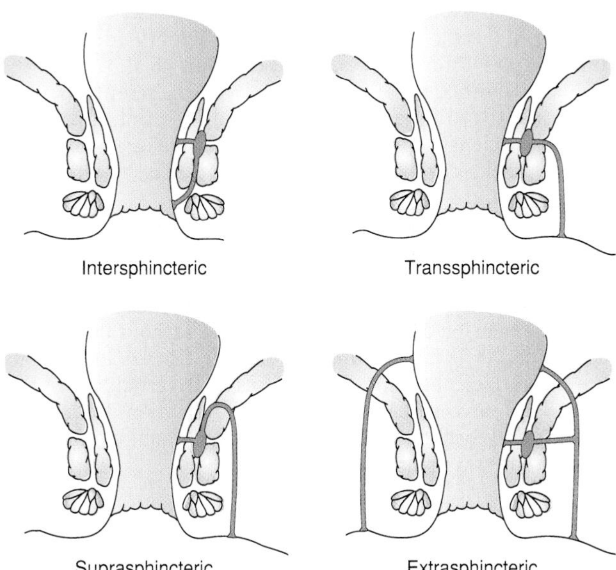

FIGURE 72.26 The four main anatomic types of fistula.

Intersphincteric Fistula. The fistulous track is in the intersphincteric plane. The external opening is usually in the perianal skin close to the anal verge.

Transsphincteric Fistula. The fistula starts in the intersphincteric plane or in the deep postanal space. The fistulous track traverses the external sphincter, with the external opening at the ischioanal fossa. Horseshoe fistulas are also in this category.

Suprasphincteric Fistula. The fistula starts in the intersphincteric plane in the midanal canal and then passes upward to a point above the puborectal muscle. The fistula passes laterally over this muscle and downward between the puborectal muscle and the levator ani muscle into the ischioanal fossa.

Extrasphincteric Fistula. The fistula passes from the perineal skin through the ischioanal fossa and the levator ani muscle and finally penetrates the rectal wall. Extrasphincteric fistulas may arise from a cryptoglandular origin, trauma, a foreign body, or a pelvic abscess, such as diverticular or appendiceal abscess.

Clinical Manifestations

Most patients have a previous history of anorectal abscess subsequently associated with intermittent drainage. Recurrence of a perianal abscess suggests the presence of a fistula-in-ano. The external opening is usually visible as a red elevation of granulation tissue with purulent or serosanguineous drainage on compression. In the simple or superficial fistula, the track can be palpated as an indurated cord. Deeper fistulas usually are not palpable.

Anoscopy should be done to identify the internal opening. Proctoscopy or flexible sigmoidoscopy is performed to rule out other lesions and inflammatory bowel disease. A fistula probe can be introduced into the fistulous track to determine its direction, although it is not always possible to pass the probe through the internal opening. Occasionally the internal fistula opening or fistula pathway may be hard to discern based on physical examination. Injection of the external opening with hydrogen peroxide while performing endoanal ultrasound can demonstrate a track, effectively creating a fistula map, and can also help to identify an unrecognized internal opening. Buchanan et al.[47] recently studied a cohort of 108 patients with recurrent fistulae using digital examination, endoanal ultrasound, and MRI on each patient Digital examination correctly identified 61% of tracks compared with 81% of tracks by endoanal ultrasound and 90% by MRI.

Several disorders must be considered in the differential diagnosis of a fistula-in-ano. Hidradenitis suppurativa is differentiated by the presence of multiple perianal skin openings with the surrounding leather-like skin. A pilonidal sinus with perianal extension and infected perianal sebaceous cysts must be considered. It is important to exclude fistulas associated with ulcerative colitis and Crohn disease. Diverticulitis of the sigmoid colon, with perforation and fistulization to the perineum, rarely occurs. Low rectal and anal canal carcinomas may present as a fistula in the perineum.

Management

The principles of fistula surgery include unroofing the fistula, eliminating the internal opening (infective source), and establishing adequate drainage. Failure to open the entire track may lead to recurrence. In most fistulas, the treatment of choice involves opening the entire fistulous track, with a fistulous probe in place. Granulation tissues are curetted and the edges of the wound marsupialized. Fistulectomy, the excision of the fistulous track, has no advantages over fistulotomy, which is lay open of the track. Horseshoe fistula, an uncommon form of fistula-in-ano, is a direct extension of an intersphincteric abscess and usually starts in the deep postanal space. Radical unroofing results in a large wound and is not necessary. Incision of the deep postanal space combined with excision or curettage of the lateral tracks is the procedure of choice.

In young patients, transection of the internal and external sphincter muscle in the posterior half, when performed in the course of a fistulotomy, does not always jeopardize anal continence. In older patients and in women, however, transection of the external sphincter muscle, particularly in the anterior half, risks incontinence. When sphincter transection appears likely, a staged procedure with the use of a seton, or cord made of nonreactive material drawn through the fistula, is recommended. Setons are tied loosely around the muscles covering the fistula to allow drainage of infection. Tight seton application, designed to slowly cut through the sphincter and create fibrosis, was commonly performed in the past but has been associated with incontinence and is no longer encouraged. In the second stage (average interval, 6 to 8 weeks), seton removal and fistulotomy or curettage of epithelialized tissue, closure of the internal opening and fibrin glue application to the fistula track may be performed. Fibrin glue application has the distinct advantage of few to no side effects; however, this technique has overall less than a 50% long-term success rate. Fibrin glue can be applied multiple times, potentially with subsequent fistula healing and has shown a small success rate among patients with complex fistulae among whom fistulotomy would likely result in incontinence.[47]

After draining the fistula and resolving infection with use of a seton, an anal advancement flap is another interventional option for patients who fail less invasive therapy. With the patient in prone jackknife position and well anesthetized, the fistula track is curetted. A U-shaped flap of mucosa is created, encompassing the internal fistula opening adjacent to the distal edge. The flap is advanced and the distal strip with the internal opening is excised. The flap is affixed with simple absorbable suture to eradicate the internal opening.

Anal Fistula Associated With Crohn Disease

Fistulas associated with Crohn disease are often asymptomatic. They resemble the ordinary fistulas seen in patients without Crohn disease in that there is an indurated opening in the skin that exudes pus and a palpable track passing toward the anal canal. The fistulas can be simple and superficial, complex with multiple tracks, or deep with the origin in the upper anal canal or lower rectum.

The most important part of treatment is adequate and aggressive medical therapy, including medications for active Crohn disease. Metronidazole and ciprofloxacin have been found to be useful in some patients. Methotrexate and azathioprine have met with very limited success. Infliximab, a monoclonal antibody directed against tumor necrosis factor, has shown promising efficacy for Crohn disease fistulas. In a placebo-controlled trial of patients with fistulizing Crohn disease in which 90% of patients also had perianal disease, 62% experienced at least 50% reduction in the number of draining fistulas compared with 26% of the placebo group.[48] Nearly half of patients treated with infliximab experienced complete closure of all fistulas with short- to mid-term follow-up.

Aggressive surgical intervention is discouraged because of extremely poor healing among these patients. The basic principle of surgery is to locally curette the granulation tissue in the fistulous tracks, lay open the superficial tracks, open and clean the abscess cavity. Long-term indwelling setons are an acceptable alternative in this patient population.

Rectovaginal Fistula

A rectovaginal fistula is a communication between the anterior wall of the anal canal or rectum and the posterior wall of the vagina. There are many possible causes (Table 72.6), but obstetric injury accounts for the majority. Rectovaginal fistulas are considered low if a repair can be done from a perineal approach and high if repair can be accomplished only transabdominally (Fig. 72.27). Simple or complex classification is based on location, size, and cause (Table 72.7).

Clinical Manifestations

Symptoms of rectovaginal fistulas depend on location, size, and cause. In low or small fistulas, the most common complaint is passage of gas per vagina. In large fistulas, symptoms include vaginal discharge with fecal odor, passage of flatus and stool per vagina, and painful vaginitis. Some patients have fecal incontinence as well.

Diagnosis

Definitive diagnosis is made by examination. In low fistula, digital examination of the anal canal reveals scar and a defect in the anterior wall. Bimanual examination with one finger in the rectum and a finger of the other hand in the vagina is also helpful. Anoscopy can also detect the opening in the anal canal. Middle and high fistulas require proctoscopy. If the fistula cannot be seen, a tampon is placed in the vaginal canal and 100 mL of diluted methylene blue is instilled into the anorectum. After a time, the tampon is removed and checked for evidence of blue staining. Barium enema is usually not helpful but may be indicated in certain patients with inflammatory bowel disease or previous irradiation.

TABLE 72.6 ETIOLOGY

CAUSES OF RECTOVAGINAL FISTULA

Congenital maldevelopment
Trauma
Obstetric
Operative
Blunt and penetrating injury
Foreign body
Infection of anal canal or vaginal septum
Pelvic irradiation
Neoplasm

Management

Spontaneous or nonoperative healing of a rectovaginal fistula depends primarily on its cause and, to a lesser extent, on its size. About one half of small rectovaginal fistulas secondary to obstetric trauma heal spontaneously.

Healing often follows removal of a foreign body. Similarly, proper treatment of an infectious process may allow the fistula to heal. Fistula caused by Crohn disease or irradiation rarely heals spontaneously. For a low, simple fistula and some midrectovaginal fistulas, endorectal advancement of an anorectal flap technique gives the best results. The rectal flap, which consists of mucosa, submucosa, internal sphincter, and the circular muscle of the lower rectum, is outlined lateral and distal to the fistula. It is important to base the flap at least 4 cm cephalad to the fistula, and the base should be about twice the length of the flap to ensure adequate blood supply. After the flap is raised from the apex to the base, the underlying fistula and the excess flap are excised. The cut edges of the internal sphincter and the circular muscle of the lower rectum are approximated, thus obliterating the opening of the fistula in

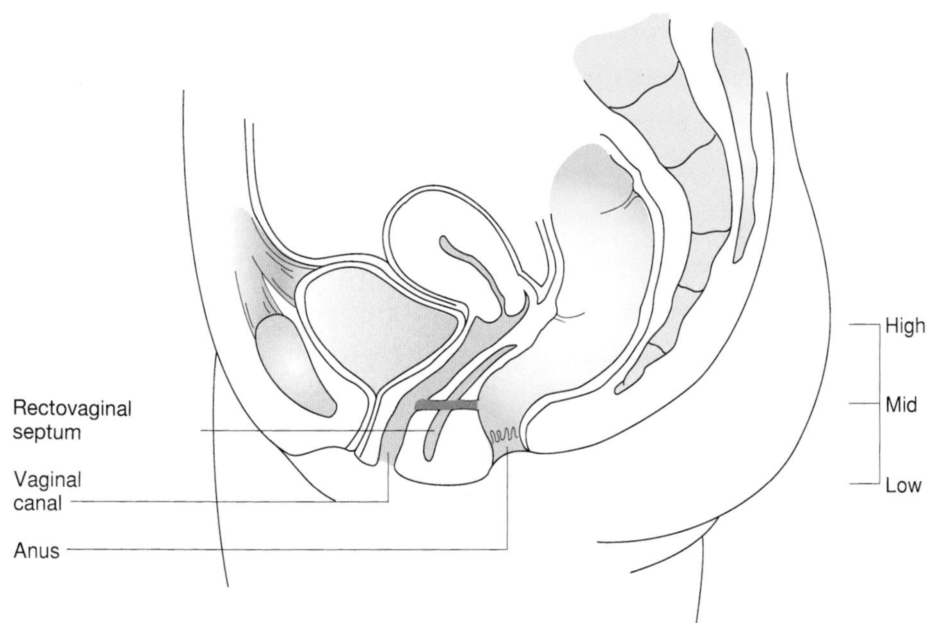

FIGURE 72.27 Rectovaginal fistula classified by location. Fistulas are low when located at or just cephalad to the dentate line, high when near the cervix, and mid when located in between.

TABLE 72.7 CLASSIFICATION

CLASSIFICATION OF RECTOVAGINAL FISTULA

Characteristic	Simple	Complex
Location	Low to mid-vaginal septum	High vaginal septum
Size	2.5 cm or less in diameter	2.5 cm or more in diameter
Cause	Traumatic or infectious cause	Inflammatory bowel disease, irradiation, neoplastic cause

the anal canal. The opening in the vagina is left open for drainage. The anorectal flap is then advanced over the repaired area and sutured (Fig. 72.28). If the rectovaginal fistula is associated with incontinence resulting from injury to the external sphincter, a sphincteroplasty is also performed. In this technique, the ends of the transected muscle are identified and mobilized. The fistula is excised, and the muscle ends are then overlapped and sutured. The results of endorectal advance-

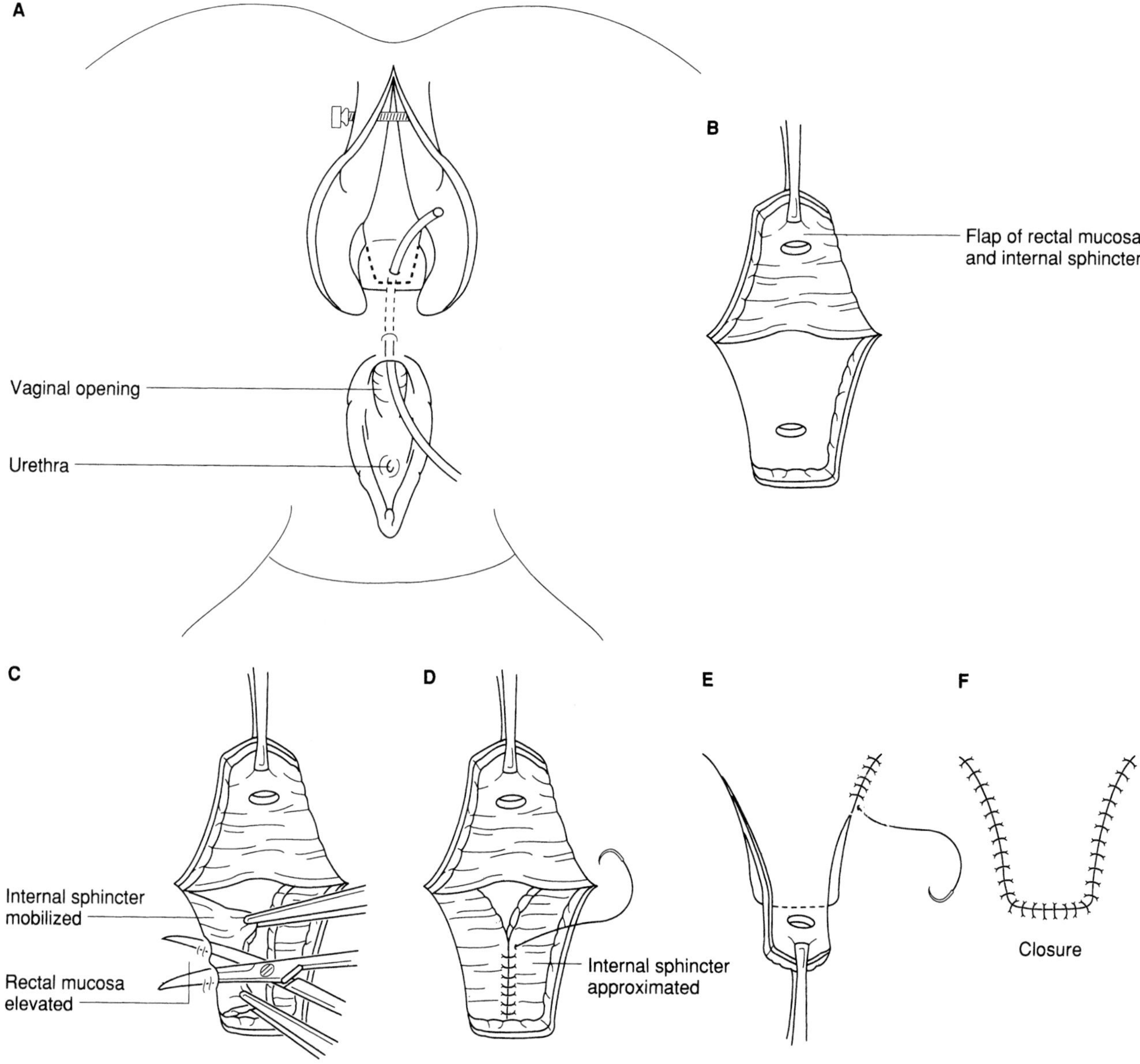

FIGURE 72.28 Endorectal advancement of anorectal flap. (*A*) Exposure is gained by an anal speculum, and the fistula is identified. Outline of endorectal flap, extending proximally to 7 cm from the anal verge. (*B*) The full-thickness flap is created to include the internal sphincter muscle.(C) Lateral mobilization is made on each side in the submucosal plane. (*D*) Anorectal wall on each side is approximated. (*E* and *F*): The endorectal flap is pulled down to cover the wound and sutured. The fistula is excised. The aperture in the vagina is not sutured but is left open for drainage.

ment flap for treatment of simple rectovaginal fistula are good, with 83% of treated patients achieving primary healing of the fistula.[49] It is important to wait, usually 3 to 6 months, until the inflammation has subsided before considering a surgical repair. An alternative repair is to lay open the rectovaginal fistula and convert it to fourth degree perineal tear. A layered closure of the anal and vaginal defect is performed using synthetic absorbable sutures.

High fistulas and some midrectovaginal fistulas require a transabdominal approach. Simple fistulas with healthy surrounding tissues can be repaired by mobilization of the rectovaginal septum, division of the fistula, and layer closure of the rectal defect without bowel resection. If the local tissues are damaged by irradiation, infection, or inflammatory diseases, an extended low anterior resection with coloanal anastomosis should be performed.

Although most simple rectovaginal fistulas do not require a diverting colostomy, complex rectovaginal fistulas are best managed by a preliminary colostomy. For elderly or unfit patients, for most radiation-induced fistulas, and for rectovaginal fistulas associated with Crohn disease, a permanent colostomy may be the procedure of choice.

Pilonidal Sinus

Most authors now accept the fact that pilonidal sinuses start with infection of the hair follicle in the sacrococcygeal area. Reports that pilonidal sinus occurs in unusual positions such as the umbilicus, healed amputation stumps, and interdigital clefts all support the acquired etiology of this disease. Pilonidal sinuses are more likely to occur in the hirsute patient.

Clinical Manifestations

The average patient with pilonidal disease is a hirsute, moderately obese man in his second or third decade. Pilonidal disease is rare in people younger than age 15 years, rises sharply to peak between ages 16 and 20 years, and remains high until age 25 years, when the incidence declines quickly. Pilonidal disease occurs less frequently in women, almost always in teenagers or young adults. Pilonidal disease may present as an acute abscess at the sacrococcygeal area that ruptures spontaneously, leaving unhealed sinuses with chronic drainage. When sinuses develop, pain is usually minimal.

Diagnosis

A painful and fluctuant mass is the most common presentation of the acute process. In its earliest stage, only cellulitis may be present, whereas in the chronic state the diagnosis is confirmed by the sinus opening in the intergluteal fold, about 5 cm above the anus. Most sinus tracks run cephalad (93%); the rest run caudad (7%) and may be confused with fistula-in-ano or suppurative hidradenitis. On careful examination, one can always find a pit or pits in the midline, representing infected hair follicles. The differential diagnoses include furuncles of the skin, anal fistula, syphilitic or tuberculous granulomas, and osteomyelitis with multiple draining sinuses in the skin. Actinomycosis in the sacral region has been described as virtually indistinguishable from pilonidal disease.

Treatment

Drainage of a pilonidal abscess can almost always be accomplished under local anesthesia. A longitudinal incision is made lateral to the midline in the coccygeal area. The incision is deepened into the subcutaneous tissue, entering the abscess cavity. All the hairs in the abscess cavity, if present, must be removed, and the wound is lightly packed with fine gauze. The patient is instructed to clean the wound at least once a day and to apply light packing. An antibiotic is not usually indicated.

For chronic pilonidal sinuses, the chronic infected cavity is open lateral to the midline. The sinus tracks to the midline pits are probed and laid open. The granulation tissue in the cavity is curetted and the wound packed. Healing is rapid and usually the wound is completely closed within 4 weeks.[50] This is the technique of choice for most primary pilonidal sinuses with or without abscess. Excision of pilonidal sinuses in the midline with marsupialization, primary closure, or Z-plasty is plagued by delayed healing, nonhealing or recurrence.

Postoperative Care

The postoperative care is as important as the operation. The wound should be washed in the bathtub or shower at least once a day. If the cavity is large, it should be packed with fine gauze. If it is small, it should be swabbed to remove any foreign body, especially hair, at least once a day. The patient should return for follow-up at 1- to 2-week intervals until the wound is completely healed.

Pilonidal Sinus Complicated by Carcinoma

Carcinoma arising from chronic pilonidal sinus is rare; 44 cases had been reported in the world literature up to 1994.[51] Almost all are well-differentiated squamous cell carcinomas. The average duration of pilonidal disease in these patients was 23 years. The appearance of the wound should alert one to suspect carcinoma. There is usually an ulcer with a friable, bleeding, and fungating margin. Wide excision is the treatment of choice. When inguinal node metastasis is present, the prognosis is poor.

SEXUALLY TRANSMITTED DISEASES OF THE ANORECTUM

Anal Condylomata Acuminata

Anal condylomata acuminata are caused by human papilloma virus (HPV), primarily HPV-6 and HPV-11. In most patients, the warts involve the perianal skin, anal verge, and anoderm. Occasionally, the lesions also involve the mucosa of the upper anal canal and the lower rectum. The extent of the disease varies from a few small warts to an extensive mass occluding the anus. The diagnosis is usually obvious by the characteristic papillary appearance. Anoscopic examination is essential to detect intra-anal involvement. Because most cases are transmitted by sexual contact after a 1- to 3-month incubation period, other coexisting venereal diseases should be excluded.

Small perianal warts can be destroyed by applying podophyllin solution or bichloracetic acid. Both podophyllin and bichloracetic acid are caustic; therefore, the uninvolved skin should be protected with petroleum jelly before these agents are applied so that caustic injury can be prevented. Extensive warts in the perianal area or in the anal canal are best treated by excision and fulguration with electrocautery.

Frequent postoperative follow-up is necessary because the recurrence rate is higher than 65%. The follow-up should be done every 3 months until at least 6 months have passed with no disease recurrence. Immunotherapy (with the use of autogenous wart tissue vaccine) in conjunction with excision of the lesions has been found to be effective, but the role of immune mechanisms in recurrent wart formation has yet to be determined. Preliminary enthusiasm for HPV vaccine use against anal condylomata has waned.

Malignant transformation of condylomata acuminata is rare and is usually associated with the more aggressive serotypes 16 and 18, although serotypes 30, 42, 44, 51, and 54 also have malignant potential. Other risks for malignant transformation include longstanding condylomata and patient immunosuppression, such as posttransplant state or HIV positivity. The microscopic picture includes squamous dysplasia with proliferation and disorganization of epidermal cells, individual cell keratinization, keratin pearl formation, an increased number of normal and abnormal mitoses, and, most importantly, invasion into the underlying tissue. Treatment of anal condylomata acuminata with invasive carcinoma should follow the treatment of squamous cell carcinoma of the anus.

Gonococcal Proctitis and Syphilis

Patients with gonococcal proctitis are generally asymptomatic but may have mild anal burning, pain, discharge, or bleeding in the acute phase. Proctoscopic examination reveals hyperemic and edematous anorectal mucosa with purulent discharge in the anal crypts at the dentate line. In the chronic phase, the anorectum may appear normal. Diagnosis is confirmed by observing *Neisseria gonorrhoeae* on stained smears of the discharge and by plating the exudate immediately onto Thayer-Martin culture medium. In the United States, antimicrobial resistance in the gonococcus continues to evolve, and coinfection with *Chlamydia trachomatis* is a serious problem. Chlamydial infection may be documented in up to 45% of gonorrhea cases when adequate chlamydial cultures are performed.

The recommended treatment is ceftriaxone, 250 mg intramuscularly once, plus doxycycline, 100 mg orally twice a day for 7 days.[52] For those patients who cannot take ceftriaxone, ciprofloxacin, 500 mg orally once, plus doxycycline, 100 mg orally twice a day for 7 days, is a good alternative.[53] Doxycycline or tetracycline alone is not adequate, but these drugs can be added to counter possible coexisting chlamydial infection.

All patients treated for gonorrhea should have a serologic test for syphilis. *Treponema pallidum* is still sensitive to penicillin. Benzathine penicillin G, 2.4 million units given intramuscularly, maintains treponemicidal levels for 2 weeks. For latent syphilis, 2.4 million units weekly for 3 weeks is given. Patients who are allergic to penicillin may be treated with tetracycline or erythromycin, 500 mg four times a day for 30 days.[52]

Follow-up cultures should be obtained from the anorectum 3 to 7 days after completion of treatment. Recurrent gonococcal infections after treatment with recommended schedules are commonly caused by reinfection rather than treatment failure and indicate a need for improved sex partner tracing and patient education. Because antimicrobial resistance is a cause of treatment failure, all posttreatment isolates should be tested for antimicrobial susceptibility.

Chlamydial Proctitis

Chlamydia trachomatis is the most common cause of sexually transmitted disease in the United States, affecting 4 million Americans each year. Although most chlamydial infections affect the urethra, anorectal involvement among male homosexuals is common. Proctoscopy reveals a picture of nonspecific proctitis with friable, granular, and edematous mucosa. Immunofluorescent microscopy provides an accurate and rapid diagnosis. The specimen should be collected by swabbing the anorectal mucosa.

Treatment includes tetracycline hydrochloride, 500 mg by mouth four times daily for 7 days, or doxycycline, 100 mg by mouth twice daily for 7 days. For patients in whom tetracyclines are contraindicated, erythromycin base or stearate, 500 mg by mouth four times daily for 7 days, or erythromycin ethylsuccinate, 800 mg by mouth four times daily for 7 days, may be used. When taken as directed, the tetracycline and erythromycin regimens described previously are highly effective (more than 95% cure rate). Therefore, posttreatment *C. trachomatis* test-of-cure cultures may be omitted if laboratory resources are limited. Although cultures may not become positive until 3 to 6 weeks after treatment, when they are positive, patients should be retreated with one of the previously described regimens, and any interim sex partners should also be contacted.

Two new drugs have been approved by the U.S. Food and Drug Administration for the treatment of *Chlamydia*—azithromycin, 1 g orally in a single dose, and ofloxacin, 300 mg orally two times a day for 7 days. A substantial advantage of azithromycin, compared with all other therapies, is that a single dose is effective; this antimicrobial may prove most useful for situations in which compliance with a 7-day regimen of another antimicrobial cannot be ensured. In view of the high efficacy of tetracycline and doxycycline, cost should also be considered when selecting a treatment regimen.[54]

Herpes Simplex Viral Proctitis

Anorectal herpes is caused by herpesvirus hominis type II, the same organism implicated in genital herpes. The usually severe anorectal pain is associated with fever, inguinal adenopathy, tenesmus, constipation, anorectal discharge, and bleeding. Neurologic symptoms in the distribution of the sacral roots are noted in some patients. These may include urinary retention, dyspareunia, and impotence. Examination reveals erythematous areas with small groups of vesicles that rupture and become ulcerated. Proctoscopic examination may reveal a nonspecific proctitis.[55,56]

The diagnosis can be made by staining the exudate with the Papanicolaou or Giemsa method. A finding of multinucleated giant cells is diagnostic. One may also use immunofluorescence or immunoperoxidase staining of lesion scrapings to detect the herpes simplex virus (HSV) antigens. Both techniques are rapid and useful when positive but are less sensitive than viral isolation in tissue culture from the vesicles or ulcers.

For the first episode, acyclovir, 200 mg by mouth five times daily for 7 to 10 days, is effective if initiated within 6 days of the onset of lesions. This treatment shortens the median duration of first-episode eruptions by 3 to 5 days and may reduce systemic symptoms in primary episodes. For patients with severe symptoms or complications that necessitate hospitalization, acyclovir, 5 mg/kg intravenously every 8 hours for 5 to 7 days, is recommended. This treatment shortens the median course of first episodes by about 7 days. Topical acyclovir ointment has a marginal benefit in decreasing virus shedding but has no significant effect on symptoms or healing time.

For recurrent anorectal herpes, because benefit may be minimal, treatment should be limited to those patients who typically have severe symptoms and who are able to begin therapy at the beginning of the prodrome or within 2 days of the onset of lesions. Acyclovir, 200 mg orally five times a day for 5 days, is used. This drug shortens the mean clinical course by about 1 day. Intravenous or topical acyclovir is not indicated for recurrences.

ANORECTAL DISEASES IN PATIENTS WITH AIDS AND HIV POSITIVITY

Kaposi Sarcoma

Kaposi sarcoma, normally a rare tumor of the skin, is one of the most common malignant tumors in AIDS patients. Most Kaposi sarcoma tumors of the colon and rectum are asymptomatic, but bleeding, diarrhea, and obstruction may occur. The lesion has a characteristic red, round, submucosal nodule with central umbilication. A deep biopsy is required to yield an accurate result. The diagnosis is useful as a prognostication because there is no effective medical treatment. Surgery is indicated only to control massive bleeding, perforation, or obstruction.

Cytomegalovirus

Although cytomegalovirus (CMV) has been found in virtually every human organ system, its presence is not uniformly associated with pathologic changes. Symptomatic CMV proctocolitis occurs in at least 10% of AIDS patients. CMV in immunocompromised patients, however, leads to serious complications. In about 50% of the patients with AIDS who harbor the virus, the infection is serious. Disseminated CMV has been identified at postmortem examination in 90% of patients with AIDS, with 30% having CMV in the gastrointestinal tract. CMV enteroproctocolitis occurs in 5% to 10% of patients with AIDS but is responsible for 70% of all deaths in these patients who undergo major abdominal surgery on an emergency basis.[27,57] Symptoms of CMV enterocolitis are diarrhea, fever, right lower quadrant abdominal pain, and weight loss. Not uncommon are coinfection with one or more opportunistic agents such as *Salmonella, Shigella, Campylobacter, Clostridium difficile, Cryptosporidium, Microsporida, Entamoeba,* and *Giardia.*

The morphologic hallmarks of CMV enteroproctocolitis are sharply demarcated areas of shallow ulcers, frequently covered with fibrin. Biopsy gives an accurate diagnosis. The pathognomonic histopathologic features include large basophilic intranuclear CMV inclusions. The problems that most commonly necessitate emergency or urgent surgical intervention are bleeding and perforation of the CMV ulcers. These complications occur in 60% to 100% of emergency exploratory celiotomies performed in patients with AIDS. Medical treatment consists of ganciclovir.[27]

Lymphoma

There is an increased incidence of non-Hodgkin's lymphoma in patients with HIV positivity and AIDS. In the United States, about 3% of AIDS cases present with lymphoma. When the gastrointestinal tract is the primary site, the stomach is affected more than the colon. Identification of anorectal lymphoma is difficult because the disease is extraluminal in most cases. Most patients are brought to the operating room with perianal abscesses as a preoperative diagnosis.[27] The diagnosis relies on microscopic identification of B-cell immunoblastic configuration of extranodular lymphoma. A consideration in the treatment of AIDS-related lymphoma is that radiation and chemotherapy may actually accelerate the demise of the patient through further immunosuppression. It is worthwhile, in patients with resectable tumors, to excise the lesion.[58]

Anal Carcinoma

Although anal carcinoma is uncommon in general population, anal carcinoma and its precursor lesion, anal intraepithelial neoplasia (AIN) are increased in homosexual men. The association of these lesions with HPV is clear. There has been a good deal of evidence suggesting that there has been a rise in the incidence of invasive anal carcinoma since the onset of the HIV epidemic but little published data on the morbidity or mortality associated with anal carcinoma among HIV-infected men. It is likely that as the life span of HIV-infected individuals is prolonged by highly active antiretroviral therapy, anal carcinoma will become a more common complication of HIV infection with considerable morbidity and mortality.[59]

Relatively little is known about the prevalence of AIN among patients with AIDS, primarily because until recently there has never been any screening for what are generally subclinical, asymptomatic lesions. AIN can be detected using cytologic smears (Papanicolaou staining). Using this approach, it has become apparent that such pathology is exceedingly common. Low-grade AIN regresses and can simply be followed. High-grade AIN is the counterpart of carcinoma in situ, ablation of visible lesions is recommended.[58]

Anorectal Ulcers

Individuals practicing anoreceptive intercourse have an increased proclivity for various viral, bacterial, and parasitic diseases of the anorectum. Anal ulcers are common among HIV-positive patients. About half of the anal ulcers are idiopathic. Most ulcers are in the posterior midline of the anus, somewhat closer to the dentate line than the ordinary anal fissure. Idiopathic ulcers in HIV-positive patients are extremely erosive, dissecting along the submucosal and intersphincteric planes and many times skeletonizing the internal sphincter muscle. These erosions create pockets in which stool and pus collect, causing severe pain, especially on defecation.[60]

Examination of the anorectum under general anesthesia is usually necessary. Biopsy specimens should be taken and sent for viral culture and dark-field examination if indicated. If lymphoma is suspected, the tissue should be sent for typing. Pocketing of the ulcers should be corrected by division of a portion of the internal sphincter muscle along with débridement. In patients with intolerable pain from anal ulcers, a sigmoid colostomy gives symptomatic relief. Specific ulcers in HIV-positive patients are usually from syphilis, tuberculosis, HSV, cytomegalovirus, and other bacterial infections.

ANAL CANCERS

Anal cancers—cancers of the perianal skin and the anal canal—are uncommon. Although the literature is replete with reports on this subject, the use of terminology and classification has not been uniform; consequently, interpreting the results of treatment is difficult because the malignant neoplasms at different locations with different behaviors were grouped together. To overcome this confusion, the World Health Organization (WHO) and the American Joint Committee on Cancer have developed a universally agreed-on description terminology for the histologic typing of neoplasms of the anal region.[61,62]

Anatomic Landmarks

The anal canal extends from the anorectal ring to the anal verge, or the "surgical" anal canal. The mucosal lining is divided into three zones: upper or rectal, middle or transitional, and lower or squamous. The transitional zone extends proximally from the dentate line for a distance of approximately 1 cm.[61,62] This definition is in contrast to many series in the literature that use the dentate line as the dividing line describing the anal canal as the area above the dentate line and the anal margin as the area below the dentate line.[63,64] Numerous other reports never define the landmarks. The perianal skin[65,66] starts from the lateral border of the anal verge. The lateral or distal extent of the perianal skin is defined as 5 to 6 cm from the anal verge.[66,67]

The area above the dentate line up to the anorectal ring (the first 6 to 10 mm referred to as the transitional zone) has primarily cephalad lymphatic drainage via the superior rectal lymphatics to the inferior mesenteric nodes. It also has lesser drainage laterally along both the middle rectal vessels and inferior rectal vessels through the ischioanal fossa to the internal iliac nodes. Lymphatic drainage from the anal canal below the dentate line drains to the inguinal nodes. However, secondary drainage can follow the inferior rectal lymphatics to the ischioanal nodes and internal iliac nodes, and along the superior rectal nodes. Lymphatic drainage of the perianal skin is entirely to the inguinal nodes.

Perianal Neoplasms

Anal Intraepithelial Neoplasia

Anal intraepithelial neoplasia (AIN) is classified as AIN I (low-grade) or AIN II or III (high grade) (Fig. 72.29). High-grade AIN has many euphemisms, including *anal atypia* or *dysplasia*, *squamous cell carcinoma in situ*, and *Bowen disease*. HPV infection has been shown to cause an increased risk of anal AIN in a manner that closely parallels the role of HPV infection in the genesis of cervical carcinoma. HPV 16 and 18 are integrated into host DNA, explaining the different propensity to initiate the development of carcinoma.[68] HPV 16 and 18 also have a predilection for the less stable epithelium of the upper anal canal (transitional zone) rather than the modified skin of the lower anal canal (anoderm), but can still be identified in the anal margin area.[69] Increased risks of anal carcinoma are found in immunosuppressed patients such as renal transplant and cardiac allograft recipients, and in patients with carcinomas after chemotherapy.

High-grade AIN is rare, slow growing, and can occur in any age group.[3,70] The lesions appear as a discrete scaly or crusted plaque, sometimes exhibiting a moist surface, and are often pigmented. The patient may report itching, burning, or spotty bleeding. Although symptoms and gross appearance are suggestive, only a biopsy can confirm the diagnosis. The disease is considered a precursor to invasive squamous cell carcinoma.[70] Widespread AIN III has been treated by laser (with about 80% recurrence), by local excision (with about 50% recurrence), and by wide local excision, the traditional treatment of choice.[3,70] The recurrence rate even with wide local excision is discouraging at 25% to 50%. Mapping the extent of involvement by obtaining multiple biopsies 1 cm from the lesion all around the perianal area, including the dentate line, the anal verge, and the perineum can assist with operative planning and with establishing a baseline for future surveillance. Extensive long-term surveillance is essential, with recurrences reported as late as 9 years postoperatively. The value of coloposcopy for surveillance continues to be debated.

Squamous Cell Carcinoma

Squamous cell carcinomas of the perianal area resemble those occurring in skin elsewhere. They grow slowly and typically have rolled, everted edges with central ulceration. Any chronic unhealed or indurated ulceration in the perianal area should be considered squamous cell carcinoma until biopsy proves otherwise. Squamous cell carcinomas are usually well differentiated histologically, with well-developed patterns

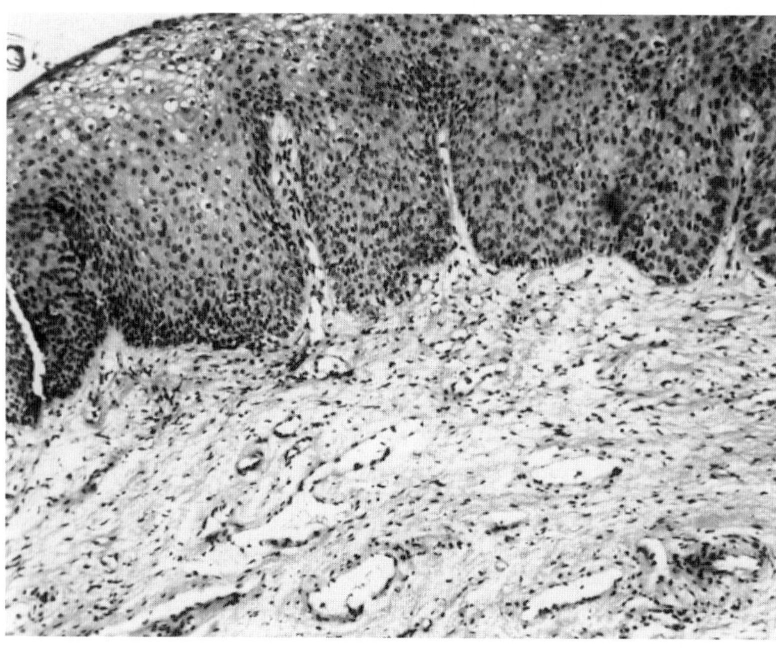

FIGURE 72.29 Bowen disease. Atypical epithelial cells involve the full thickness of the epidermis (carcinoma *in situ*).

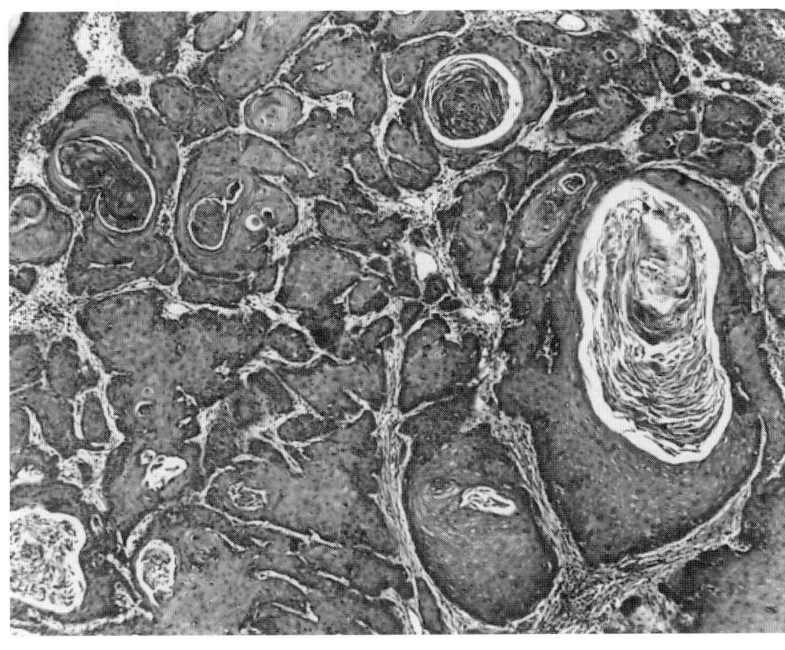

FIGURE 72.30 Photomicrograph of squamous cell carcinoma of the perianal skin. Note the presence of keratin.

of keratinization (Fig. 72.30). Lymphatic spread from squamous carcinomas of the perianal area is mainly to inguinal lymph nodes. Despite their superficial location, most lesions are usually diagnosed late, with half of the cases detected more than 22 months after the onset of symptoms, and the carcinoma is often discovered as a late stage measuring 5 cm or larger in diameter.[71]

Wide local excision has remained the cornerstone of the treatment of perianal squamous cell carcinoma, but only in properly selected cases. For in situ or microinvasive carcinoma, local excision has a 100% cure rate.[65,72] For other less favorable lesions, chemoradiation should be used.[66] Abdominoperineal resection is reserved for patients who cannot tolerate chemoradiation or in patients with anal incontinence. The size of the carcinoma determines the patient survival. The 5- and 10-year survival rates for T_1 lesions are 100% and 100%, respectively, compared with 60% and 40% for T_2 lesions, respectively.[67]

Perianal Paget Disease

In 1874, Sir James Paget first described this disease in relationship to the nipple of the breast in females. Extramammary Paget disease can be found in the axilla and the anogenital region (labia majora, penis, scrotum, groin, pubic area, perineum, perianal region, thigh, and buttock). The histogenesis of perianal Paget disease is not fully understood, but ultrastructural and immunohistochemical studies have helped to clarify the debate. Most authors agree that Paget cells are of glandular and probably of apocrine origin.[73,74] An alternative hypothesis implicating pluripotential intraepidermal cells cannot be excluded, but the evidence for such a histogenesis is lacking.[73] In contrast to Paget disease of the nipple, which is invariably associated with an underlying invasive or *in situ* ductal adenocarcinoma, perianal Paget disease starts out as a benign neoplasm. It may eventually become invasive and gives rise to an adenocarcinoma.

Perianal Paget disease occurs mostly in elderly people at an average age of 68 years.[75] The lesions appear as a slowly enlarging pruritic, erythematous, eczematous, and often sharply demarcated perianal rash that may ooze or scale. Because of its similarity to other perianal conditions such as idiopathic pruritus ani, hidradenitis suppurativa, condyloma acuminatum, Crohn disease, AIN III, and squamous cell carcinoma, the diagnosis of perianal Paget disease is often delayed by clinical diagnostic error. In almost one third of the cases, the lesion involves the entire circumference of the perianal skin and the anus.[76]

The diagnosis must be confirmed by biopsy and by identification of the characteristic Paget cells—large, pale, vacuolated cells with hyperchromatic eccentric nuclei (Fig. 72.31). The cells invariably contain acid mucosubstances, an important feature in distinguishing this lesion from AIN III and melanoma. True Paget disease of the perianal skin must be distinguished from downward intraepidermal spread of a signet-ring cell carcinoma of the rectum. A complete large bowel investigation with emphasis on thorough examination of the rectum and anal canal should be performed. The coexistence of visceral carcinomas has been documented in up to 50% of patients.[77]

In the absence of invasive carcinoma, wide excision is the treatment of choice. Obtaining an adequate microscopically clear margin is important. Because perianal Paget disease may extend beyond the gross margin of the lesion, mapping the extent of involvement by obtaining multiple biopsies 1 cm from the edge of the lesion all around the perianal area, including the dentate line, the anal verge, and the perineum is performed. The large wound defect of the perianal area and the anal canal can be reconstructed with sliding V-Y subcutaneous skin flaps. Successful radiation therapy has been reported for perianal Paget disease.[76,78] If necessary, such treatment is an option.

For more advanced lesions with an underlying invasive carcinoma, an abdominoperineal resection along with inguinal lymph node dissection is recommended. Sentinel node dissection has not been explored for this rare disease. Whether preoperative chemoradiation is helpful remains to be seen. Because of the commonly delayed diagnosis (average 4 years), approximately 25% of patients with invasive adenocarcinoma in Paget disease already have metastasis. The sites of the metastasis in order of frequency are the inguinal and pelvic lymph nodes, liver, bone, lung, brain, bladder, prostate, and adrenal gland.[79]

Long-term follow-up is essential to detect local recurrence and development of invasive Paget disease or intercurrent

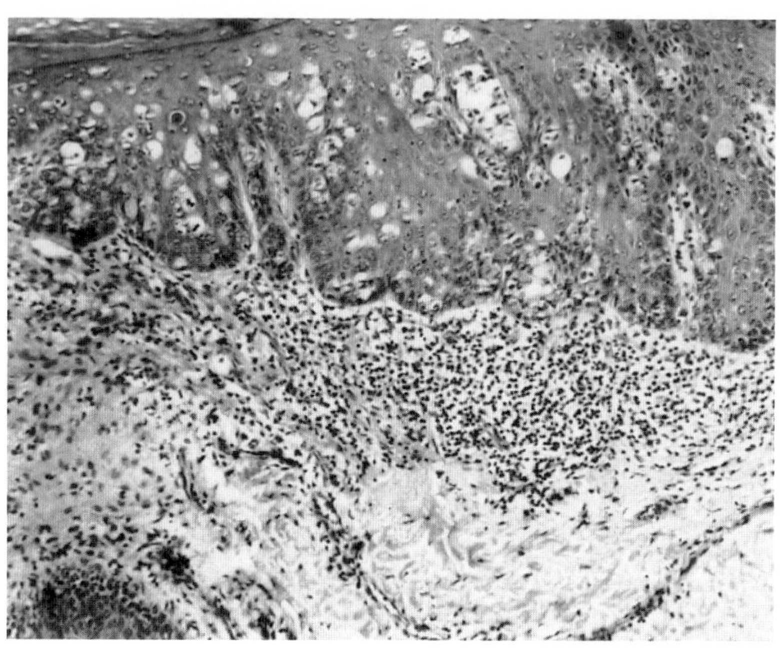

FIGURE 72.31 Perianal Paget's disease. Paget's cells are above the basal layer.

invasive carcinoma of the rectum and anal canal. A patient with invasive perianal Paget disease has a poor prognosis despite abdominoperineal resection, since in most cases distant metastasis has already occurred at the time of diagnosis.

Verrucous Carcinoma

Although there is no universal agreement, there is a growing consensus that the entity that has been termed a *giant condyloma acuminatum* or a *Buschke-Löwenstein tumor* represents a verrucous carcinoma. These lesions typically present as large (8 × 8 cm), slow-growing, painful, wart-like growths that are relatively soft and have a cauliflower-like appearance. The lesions may arise in the perianal skin, anal canal, or distal rectum and are frequently indistinguishable from condylomata acuminata. Although they are histologically benign, their behavior is clinically malignant.

The clinical course of these lesions is one of relentless progression and expansion of the neoplasm by extensive erosion and pressure necrosis of surrounding tissues with invasion of the ischioanal fossa, perirectal tissues, and even the pelvic cavity. The invasive nature of these lesions may cause multiple sinuses and fistulous tracts, which may invade the fascia, muscle, the rectum, the uterus, and may cause inflammation, infection, and hemorrhage. The extent of involvement can be precisely determined by computed tomography examination.

Microscopically, the lesion bears a marked resemblance to condylomata acuminata with papillary proliferation, keratinization, acanthosis, parakeratosis, and vacuolization of superficial layers. Metastasis from these tumors has not been reported to date.

The basic treatment is wide local excision. If the carcinoma involves the anal sphincters, an abdominoperineal resection should be performed. At the present time, there have been no reports regarding the use of multimodality therapy in the treatment of verrucous carcinoma, but such consideration may obviate the need for radical extirpation surgery.[80,81]

Basal Cell Carcinoma

Basal cell carcinoma of the perianal area is rare and occurs more frequently in men than in women, usually appearing in the sixth decade. The lesions are characterized by central ulceration and irregular, raised edges. Basal cell carcinomas are usually superficial, are not fixed to deeper structures, and rarely metastasize. Inguinal lymphadenopathy develops frequently from reactive inflammation. The patient most frequently presents with complaints of mild discomfort, itching, or bleeding.

A wide local excision is the treatment of choice. Local recurrence after excision is common, however, and occurs in almost one third of patients. Reexcision is indicated. Abdominoperineal resection is reserved for large lesions and for uncontrollable local recurrence or in patients with anal incontinence. The 5-year survival is around 70%.[82]

Neoplasms of the Anal Canal

Squamous Cell or Epidermoid Carcinoma

Squamous cell carcinoma of the anus is rare, with an incidence of about 3,500 cases per year in the United States general population, but this disease is increasing in frequency. The anal canal accounts for about 85% of cases and has a radically different treatment and prognosis than anal margin cancer. Squamous cell or epidermoid cancer encompasses a number of different microscopic appearances, including large-cell keratinizing, large-cell nonkeratinizing (transitional), and basaloid. The term *cloacogenic carcinoma* has been used especially for the basaloid and large-cell nonkeratinizing (transitional) forms of squamous carcinoma. Most squamous cell carcinomas of the anal canal above the dentate line are nonkeratinizing (Fig. 72.32). Mucoepidermoid carcinoma is extremely rare.

The presentation of squamous cell carcinomas generally follows a long history of minor perianal problems, such as bleeding, pruritus, discharge, pain, and an indurated anal mass. Almost one third of the patients with anal canal squamous cell carcinoma are initially incorrectly diagnosed as having benign or inflammatory disease.

The most important part of diagnosis is digital examination of the anal canal. The size, consistency, and fixation of the primary lesion and the presence or absence of pararectal lymph nodes should be recorded. Proctoscopy can confirm the digital findings and allow for biopsy. A colonoscopy examination is indicated to rule out more proximal associated lesions.

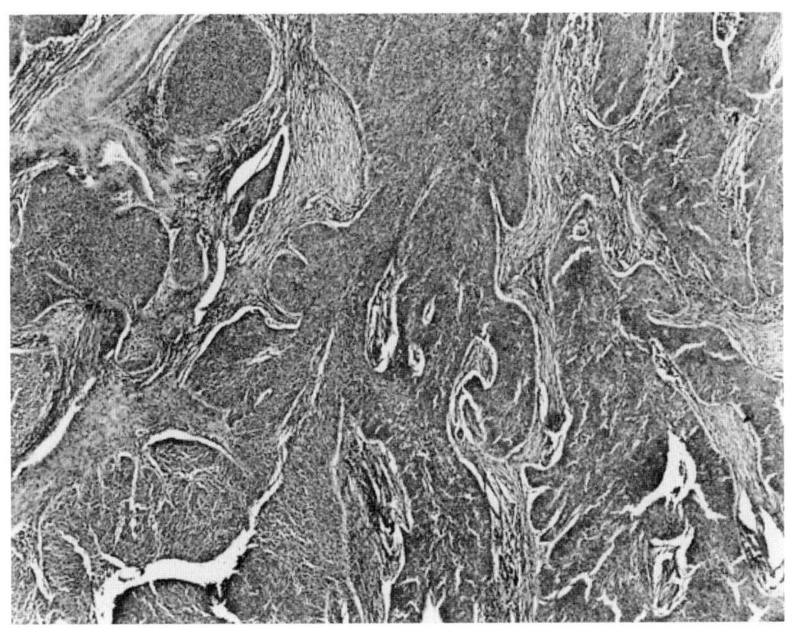

FIGURE 72.32 Squamous cell carcinoma of the anal canal. Note the absence of keratin.

Endorectal ultrasonography is useful in evaluating the depth of invasion and detection of lymph node metastasis. Both groins must be examined carefully to detect any enlargement of lymph nodes. Enlarged or suspicious lymph nodes in the groin area should be assessed by excision or biopsy because reactive lymphadenopathy is common.

The anal canal has extensive lymphatic pathways. If the carcinoma is situated above the dentate line, metastasis are found along the superior rectal vessels; if the carcinoma is at the dentate line, the lymphatic drainage is towards the internal pudendal, hypogastric, and obturator nodes; and if the carcinoma is below the dentate line, the lymphatic drainage is via the inguinal nodes. About 40% of lymph node metastasis are in lymph nodes less than 5 mm in diameter,[83] indicating potential value in sentinel node investigation.

Inguinal metastasis is found in 15% to 20% of patients at the time of diagnosis and become apparent later in an additional 10% to 25%.[84] The risk of lymphatic metastasis is correlated with the depth of the invasion, the size, and the histologic grade. Nodal metastasis is present in 30% of patients when the smooth muscle is infiltrated and in 58% when the infiltration is beyond the external sphincter. When carcinoma is less than 2 cm in diameter, only 3% of patients are found to have lymph node metastasis.[85] Although distant metastasis is uncommon at presentation, subsequent metastasis is common: 40% of carcinoma-related deaths occur from disease identified outside the pelvis. Appropriate staging is important for treatment planning and prognostication. The tumor, node, metastases (TNM) classification system has recently been updated by the American Joint Committee on Cancer, as detailed in Table 72.8.[86]

The treatment of squamous cell carcinoma of the anal canal represents a remarkable success story for nonsurgical therapy. The combination of fluorouracil, mitomycin C, and pelvic radiation therapy was pioneered by Nigro[87] in 1972. Neoadjuvant therapy was originally attempted because of high recurrence rates after radical resection. Nigro found that after neoadjuvant therapy, many patients had no residual disease in the resection specimen. Ultimately, clinicians eschewed radical resection and began to simply biopsy the scar 6 weeks after completion of chemoradiation to rule out residual disease. Five-year survival rates increased from about 35% to 70% after surgical treatment to 65% to 90% after combined chemoradiotherapy. Subsequently, three large prospective randomized trials established the most effective combination of chemoradiation for local control, avoidance of colostomy, and overall survival.[88–90] The modified Nigro regimen is summarized in Table 72.9.

Other therapy combinations, such as cisplatin in place of mitomycin, continue to be investigated in hopes of identifying effective but less toxic regimens. Late adverse effects associated with radiation include proctitis, diarrhea, incontinence, anal ulcers and stenosis, leading to a need for permanent colostomy in about 10% of patients.

Although abdominoperineal resection is no longer the primary treatment for invasive squamous cell carcinoma of the anal canal, it continues to play a role for residual or recurrent local disease. A recently published review of such patients demonstrated crude 5-year survival rates of 60% to 70%, although only 31% to 48% of patients were disease free at 5 years.[91] A larger cohort study demonstrated about 31% actuarial 5-year survival for patients with residual disease and 51% 5-year survival for patients with recurrent disease.[92]

Adenocarcinoma

Adenocarcinomas of the anus are rare, constituting 3% to 9% of all anal carcinomas.[93,94] WHO classifies these malignancies into rectal type, anal gland type, and anorectal fistula type.[61]

Rectal Type. Rectal type adenocarcinoma arises within the upper zone lined by colorectal-type mucosa. Histology is that of an adenocarcinoma of the large intestine. It may be difficult or impossible to separate adenocarcinoma of the anal canal from adenocarcinoma of lower rectum.

Anal Gland Type. The ducts of the anal glands are lined by stratified columnar epithelium with mucin-secreting or goblet cells. The histologic picture of these lesions, therefore, may be one of adenocarcinoma or mucoepidermoid carcinoma. The most characteristic feature of anal duct carcinoma is its extramucosal adenocarcinoma without involvement of the surface epithelium, except when the lesion has become advanced.

Anorectal Fistula Type. Well-differentiated mucinous adenocarcinomas within an anorectal fistula may be developmental or acquired.[61] Most often these carcinomas arise in patients

TABLE 72.8 STAGING AND CLASSIFICATION

AMERICAN JOINT COMMITTEE ON CANCER STAGING CLASSIFICATION FOR SQUAMOUS CELL CARCINOMA OF THE ANAL CANAL

Primary Tumor (T)
Tx: Primary tumor cannot be assessed
T0: No evidence of primary tumor
Tis: Carcinoma *in situ*
T1: Tumor 2 cm or less in greatest dimension
T2: Tumor more than 2 cm but not more than 5 cm in greatest dimension
T3: Tumor more then 5 cm in greatest dimension
T4: Tumor of any size invades adjacent organ(s), e.g., vagina, urethra, bladder (involvement of the sphincter muscle[s] alone is not classified as T4)

Regional Lymph Nodes (N)
Nx: Regional lymph nodes cannot be assessed
N0: No regional lymph node metastasis
N1: Metastasis in perirectal lymph node(s)
N2: Metastasis in unilateral internal iliac and/or inguinal lymph nodes
N3: Metastasis in perirectal and inguinal lymph nodes and/or bilateral internal iliac and/or inguinal lymph nodes

Distant Metastasis (M)
Mx: Distant metastasis cannot be assessed
M0: No distant metastasis
M1: Distant metastasis

Stage Grouping
Stage 0
Tis, N0, M0

Stage I
T1, N0, M0

Stage II
T2, N0, M0
T3, N0, M0

Stage IIIA
T1, N1, M0
T2, N1, M0
T3, N1, M0
T4, N0, M0

Stage IIIB
T4, N1, M0
Any T, N2, M0
Any T, N3, M0

Stage IV
Any T, Any N, M

TABLE 72.9 TREATMENT

MODIFIED NIGRO REGIMEN FOR SQUAMOUS CELL CARCINOMA OF THE ANAL CANAL

Treatment	Dose	Schedule
External radiation	50 Gy, to the primary carcinoma and 35-45 Gy to pelvic inguinal nodes	Start day 1 (2 Gy/day, 5 days a week for 5 weeks)
Systemic chemotherapy	Fluorouracil, 1,000 mg/m^2/24 hr as a continuous infusion for 4 days	Start day 1; repeat 4-day infusion starting day 28
Mitomycin C	10-15 mg/m^2 as intravenous bolus	Day 1 only

with longstanding perianal fistula disease.[95] Some authors believe that they originate in the anal glands and ducts.[96,97]

As treatment for rectal-type adenocarcinoma, a wide local excision can be performed for small and well-differentiated carcinomas that have not invaded the muscular layer of the anorectum; otherwise, an abdominoperineal resection is indicated. An abdominoperineal resection is indicated for adenocarcinomas of the anal gland or an anal fistula. The role of adjuvant therapy is not yet defined due to uncommon disease. The Nigro chemoradiation regimen has been successfully used; among nine patients who were treated with this protocol, six patients were free of disease on follow-up of 2 to 4 years.[98]

Small Cell Carcinoma

This very rare carcinoma may arise in the anorectal region. It is similar in histology, behavior, and histochemistry to small-cell (oat cell) carcinoma of the lung. Small cell carcinoma is often widely disseminated at the time of discovery. The term *neuroendocrine* has been applied to this carcinoma but implies an embryologic derivation that is as yet unproved[61] The treatment of these carcinomas is the same as for adenocarcinomas. The prognosis can be expected to be poor.

Undifferentiated Carcinoma

Undifferentiated carcinoma is also very rare. This type of malignant lesion has no glandular structure or other features to indicate definite differentiation. The treatment is the same as for adenocarcinomas. The prognosis can be expected to be poor.

Melanoma

Melanoma accounts for less than 1% of all malignancies of the anal canal. The anal canal, nevertheless, represents the third most common site for melanomas, exceeded only by skin and eyes. Almost all anal melanomas arise from the epidermoid lining of the anal canal. Most melanomas occur adjacent to the dentate line, although a few reports have been made of these tumors arising in the rectum. The female-to-male ratio is approximately 2:1, and the average age at presentation is approximately 63 years.[99]

Rectal bleeding is the most common symptom. Melanoma is suspected when a deeply pigmented lesion is seen. Most tumors, however, are pigmented lightly or are nonpigmented, and they are often misdiagnosed as polyps or squamous cell carcinomas. In amelanotic melanomas, tissue biopsy can be misinterpreted as a poorly differentiated or undifferentiated squamous cell carcinoma.

Anal canal melanomas have a marked tendency to spread submucosally into the rectum, but rarely invade adjacent organs, possibly because most patients die before this occurs. Lymphatic spread to the mesenteric nodes is seen in about one third of patients at the time of diagnosis; spread to the inguinal nodes is less common. Hematogenous spread to the liver and lung is early and rapid, accounting for most of the deaths.[100]

Melanomas of the anal canal are radioresistant and do not respond to chemotherapy or immunotherapy. The surgical approach to this malignant neoplasm is controversial. Abdominoperineal resection confers no survival benefit compared with wide local excision. Postoperative 5-year survival rates are about 15% to 20%,[99,101,102] and distant metastases are the most common cause of death. A reasonable approach is to perform wide local excision if this can be accomplished without causing fecal incontinence. Sentinel node excision has not been systematically explored in this population because of the paucity of subjects.

KEY POINTS

- **The most common manifestation of hemorrhoids is painless, bright-red rectal bleeding associated with bowel movement.**
- **A high-fiber diet usually reduces symptoms of hemorrhoids and is ideal for first- and second-degree hemorrhoids.**
- **Rubber band ligation is suitable for symptomatic first- and second- and some third-degree internal hemorrhoids that do not respond to bulk-forming agents.**
- **Hemorrhoidectomy should be considered when the hemorrhoids are mixed internal and external, are severely prolapsed through the anus, or are complicated by associated pathology, such as ulceration, fissures, fistulas, large hypertrophied anal papillae, or extensive skin tags.**
- **Rectal prolapse is best considered a form of rectal intussusception.**
- **Anal fissure is an ulcer in the lower portion of the anal canal.**
- **Infection of the anal glands is the most common origin of perianal abscesses.**
- **Fistula-in-ano is a chronic form of perianal abscess that is spontaneously or surgically drained but in which the abscess cavity does not heal completely, becoming instead an inflammatory track with a primary opening (internal opening) in the anal crypt at the dentate line and a secondary opening (external opening) in the perianal skin.**
- **Anal condylomata acuminata are caused by human papillomavirus.**

References

1. Crapp AR, Cuthbertson AM. William Waldeyer and the rectosacral fascia. *Surg Gynecol Obstet.* 1974;138:252–256.
2. Shafik A. A new concept of the anatomy of the anal sphincter mechanism and the physiology of defecation. The external anal sphincter: a triple-loop system. *Invest Urol.* 1975;12:412–419.
3. Marchesa P, Fazio VW, Oliart S, et al. Perianal Bowen's disease: a clinicopathologic study of 47 patients. *Dis Colon Rectum* 1997;40:1286–1293.
4. Kashyap P, Bates N. Magnetic resonance imaging anatomy of the anal canal. *Australas Radiol.* 2004;48:443–449.
5. Shafik A. New concept of the anatomy of the anal sphincter mechanism and the physiology of defecation. II. Anatomy of the levator ani muscle with special reference to puborectalis. *Invest Urol.* 1975;13:175–182.
6. Bauer JJ, Gelernt IM, Salky B, et al. Sexual dysfunction following proctocolectomy for benign disease of the colon and rectum. *Ann Surg.* 1983;197:363–367.
7. Lepor H, Gregerman M, Crosby R, et al. Precise localization of the autonomic nerves from the pelvic plexus to the corpora cavernosa: a detailed anatomical study of the adult male pelvis. *J Urol.* 1985;133:207–212.
8. Cherry DA, Rothenberger DA. Pelvic floor physiology. *Surg Clin North Am.* 1988;68:1217–1230.
9. Thomson WH. The nature of haemorrhoids. *Br J Surg.* 1975;62:542–552.
10. **Loder PB, Kamm MA, Nicholls RJ, et al. Haemorrhoids: pathology, pathophysiology and aetiology. *Br J Surg.* 1994;81:946–954.**
11. Bernstein WC, What are hemorrhoids and what is their relationship to the portal venous system? *Dis Colon Rectum* 1983;26:829–834.
12. Iyer, VS, Shrier I, Gordon PH. Long-term outcome of rubber band ligation for symptomatic primary and recurrent internal hemorrhoids. *Dis Colon Rectum* 2004;47:1364–1370.
13. Buls JG, Goldberg SM. Modern management of hemorrhoids. *Surg Clin North Am.* 1978;58:469–478.
14. Longo A. Treatment of hemorrhoidal disease by reduction of mucosa and hemorrhoidal prolapse with a circular suturing device: a new procedure. In: The 6th World Congress of Endoscopic Surgery. Rome, Italy.
15. Peng BC, Jayne DG, Ho YH. Randomized trial of rubber band ligation vs. stapled hemorrhoidectomy for prolapsed piles. *Dis Colon Rectum* 2003;46:291–297.
16. Nisar PJ, Acheson AG, Neal KR, et al. Stapled hemorrhoidopexy compared with conventional hemorrhoidectomy: systematic review of randomized, controlled trials. *Dis Colon Rectum* 2004;47:1837–1845.
17. **Senagore AJ, Singer M, Abcarian H, et al. A prospective, randomized, controlled multicenter trial comparing stapled hemorrhoidopexy and Ferguson hemorrhoidectomy: perioperative and one-year results. *Dis Colon Rectum* 2004;47:1824–1836.**
18. Greenspon J, Williams SB, Young HA, et al. Thrombosed external hemorrhoids: outcome after conservative or surgical management. *Dis Colon Rectum.* 2004;47:1493–1498.

19. Beahrs OH, Theuerkauf FJ Jr, Hill JR. Procidentia: surgical treatment. *Dis Colon Rectum* 1972;15:337–346.
20. Parks AG, Swash M, Urich H. Sphincter denervation in anorectal incontinence and rectal prolapse. *Gut* 1977;18:656–665.
21. McMahan JD, Ripstein CB. Rectal prolapse. An update on the rectal sling procedure. *Am Surg*. 1987;53:37–40.
22. Aitola PT, Hiltunen KM, Matikainen MJ. Functional results of operative treatment of rectal prolapse over an 11-year period: emphasis on transabdominal approach. *Dis Colon Rectum* 1999;42:655–660.
23. Wolff B, Dietzen C. Abdominal resectional procedures for rectal prolapse. *Semin Colon Rectal Surg*. 1991;2:184–186.
24. Kim DS, Tsang CB, Wong WD. Complete rectal prolapse: evolution of management and results. *Dis Colon Rectum* 1999;42:460–469.
25. Huber FT, Stein H, Siewert JR. Functional results after treatment of rectal prolapse with rectopexy and sigmoid resection. *World J Surg*. 1995;19: 138–143.
26. Raftopoulos Y, Senagore AJ, Di Giuro G, et al. Recurrence rates after abdominal surgery for complete rectal prolapse: a multicenter pooled analysis of 643 individual patient data. *Dis Colon Rectum* 2005;48(March).
27. Agachan F, Reissman P, Pfeifer J, et al. Comparison of three perineal procedures for the treatment of rectal prolapse. *South Med J*. 1997;90:925–932.
28. Baxter NN, Rothenberger DA, Lowry AC., Measuring fecal incontinence. *Dis Colon Rectum* 2003;46:1591–1605.
29. Patankar SK, Ferrara A, Levy JR, et al. Biofeedback in colorectal practice: a multicenter, statewide, three-year experience. *Dis Colon Rectum* 1997;40:827–831.
30. Wijnen JT, Vasen HF, Khan PM, et al. Clinical findings with implications for genetic testing in families with clustering of colorectal cancer. *N Engl J Med*. 1998;339:511–518.
31. Baxter N, et al. Long-term results of sphincteroplasty for acquired fecal incontinence. In: *American Society of Colon and Rectal Surgeons Annual Meeting*. New Orleans; 2003.
32. Christiansen J, Sorensen M, Rasmussen MM. Gracilis muscle transposition for faecal incontinence. *Br J Surg*. 1990;77:1039–1040.
33. Faucheron JL, Hannoun L, Thome C, et al. Is fecal continence improved by nonstimulated gracilis muscle transposition? *Dis Colon Rectum* 1994;37:979–983.
34. Devesa JM, Madrid JM, Gallego BR, et al. Bilateral gluteoplasty for fecal incontinence. *Dis Colon Rectum* 1997;40:883–888.
35. Baeten CG, Geerdes BP, Adang EM, et al. Anal dynamic graciloplasty in the treatment of intractable fecal incontinence. *N Engl J Med*. 1995;332: 1600–1605.
36. Wong WD, Congliosi SM, Spencer MP, et al. The safety and efficacy of the artificial bowel sphincter for fecal incontinence: results from a multicenter cohort study. *Dis Colon Rectum* 2002;45:1139–1153.
37. Parker SC, Spencer MP, Madoff RD, et al. Artificial bowel sphincter: long-term experience at a single institution. *Dis Colon Rectum* 2003;46:722–729.
38. Parker S, Morris A, Thorson A: New developments in anal surgery: incontinence. *Semin Colon Rectal Surg*. 2003;14:82–92.
39. Kenefick NJ, Vaizey CJ, Cohen RC, et al. Medium-term results of permanent sacral nerve stimulation for faecal incontinence. *Br J Surg*. 2002;89:896–901.
40. Takahashi T, Garcia-Osogobio S, Valdovinos MA, et al. Radio frequency energy delivery to the anal canal for the treatment of fecal incontinence. *Dis Colon Rectum* 2002;45:915–922.
41. Schouten WR, Briel JW, Auwerda JJ, et al. Ischaemic nature of anal fissure. *Br J Surg*. 1996;83:63–65.
42. Minguez M, Herreros B, Espi A, et al. Long-term follow-up (42 months) of chronic anal fissure after healing with botulinum toxin. *Gastroenterology* 2002;123:112–117.
43. Gordon PH, Vasilevsky CA. Symposium on outpatient anorectal procedures. Lateral internal sphincterotomy: rationale, technique and anesthesia. *Can J Surg*. 1985;28:228–230.
44. **Hyman N. Incontinence after lateral internal sphincterotomy: a prospective study and quality of life assessment. *Dis Colon Rectum* 2004;47:35–38.**
45. **Nelson R. Operative procedures for fissure in ano. In: *2005, The Cochrane Database of Systematic Reviews*. 2005: Issue 2. Art. No.: CD002199. Pub2. DOI: 10.1002/14651858.CD002199.pub2.**
46. Parks AG, Gordon PH, Hardcastle JD. A classification of fistula-in-ano. *Br J Surg*. 1976;63:1–12.
47. Buchanan GN, Halligan S, Bartram CI, et al. Clinical examination, endosonography, and MR imaging in preoperative assessment of fistula in ano: comparison with outcome-based reference standard. *Radiology* 2004;233:674–681.
48. Present DH, Rutgeerts P, Targan S, et al. Infliximab for the treatment of fistulas in patients with Crohn's disease. *N Engl J Med*. 1999;340: 1398–1405.
49. Lowry AC, Thorson AG, Rothenberger DA, et al. Repair of simple rectovaginal fistulas. Influence of previous repairs. *Dis Colon Rectum* 1988;31:676–678.
50. Bascom, J. Pilonidal disease: long-term results of follicle removal. *Dis Colon Rectum*1983;26:800–807.
51. Davis KA, Mock CN, Versaci A, et al. Malignant degeneration of pilonidal cysts. *Am Surg*. 1994;60:200–204.
52. Centers for Disease Control and Prevention. 1998 guidelines for treatment of sexually transmitted diseases. *MMWR Recomm Rep*. 1998;47:1–111.
53. Echols RM, Heyd A, O'Keeffe BJ, et al. Single-dose ciprofloxacin for the treatment of uncomplicated gonorrhea: a worldwide summary. *Sex Transm Dis*. 1994;21:345–352.
54. Minnesota Department of Health. *Disease Control Newsletter* 1994;22:1–8.
55. Jacobs E. Sexually transmitted diseases of the anorectum and intestine. *Perspect Colon Rectal Surg*. 1989;2:27–43.
56. Milsom J. Herpes simplex infections of the anorectum. *Semin Colon Rectal Surg*. 1992;3:222–226.
57. Soderlund C, Bratt GA, Engstrom L, et al. Surgical treatment of cytomegalovirus enterocolitis in severe human immunodeficiency virus infection. Report of eight cases. *Dis Colon Rectum* 1994;37:63–72.
58. Surawicz C, Kiviat N. A rational approach to anal intraepithelial neoplasia. *Semin Colon Rectal Surg*. 1998;9:99–106.
59. Stadler RF, Gregorcyk SG, Euhus DM, et al. Outcome of HIV-infected patients with invasive squamous-cell carcinoma of the anal canal in the era of highly active antiretroviral therapy. *Dis Colon Rectum* 2004;47: 1305–1309.
60. Bernstein M. Benign human immunodeficiency virus/acquired immune deficiency syndrome-specific anorectal conditions. *Semin Colon Rectal Surg*. 1998;9:94–98.
61. Jass JR, Sobin LH. *Histologic Typing of Intestinal Tumors*. 2nd ed. New York: Springer-Verlag, 1989, pp. 32–3, 41–6.
62. Fleming ID, Cooper JS, Henson DE. *American Joint Committee on Cancer*. 5th ed. Philadelphia: Lippincott-Raven, 1997, pp. 91–95, 157–161.
63. Brown DK Oglesby AB, Scott DH, et al. Squamous cell carcinoma of the anus: a twenty-five year retrospective. *Am Surg*. 1988;54:337–342.
64. **Nigro ND. Multidisciplinary management of cancer of the anus. *World J Surg*. 1987;11:446–451.**
65. Beahrs OH Wilson SM. Carcinoma of the anus. *Ann Surg*. 1976;184:422–8.
66. Cummings BJ. Editorial. *Oncology* 1996;10:1853–1854.
67. Jensen SL, Hagen K, Shokouh-Amiri MH, et al. Does an erroneous diagnosis of squamous-cell carcinoma of the anal canal and anal margin at first physician visit influence prognosis? *Dis Colon Rectum* 1987;30:345–351.
68. Saclarides T, Klem D. Genetic alterations and virology of anal cancer. *Semin Colon Rectal Surg*. 1995;6:131–134.
69. Deans GT, McAleer JJ, Spence RA. Malignant anal tumours. *Br J Surg*. 1994;81:500–508.
70. Sarmiento JM, Wolff BG, Burgart LJ, et al. Perianal Bowen's disease: associated tumors, human papillomavirus, surgery, and other controversies. *Dis Colon Rectum* 1997;40:912–918.
71. Papillon J, Chassard JL. Respective roles of radiotherapy and surgery in the management of epidermoid carcinoma of the anal margin. Series of 57 patients. *Dis Colon Rectum* 1992;35:422–429.
72. Schraut WH, Wang CH, Dawson PJ, et al. Depth of invasion, location, and size of cancer of the anus dictate operative treatment. *Cancer* 1983;51:1291–1296.
73. Day D, Jass D. *Morson and Dawson's gastrointestinal pathology*. London: Blackwell Scientific 1990:673–675.
74. Rosai J, Ackerman LV. *Ackerman's surgical pathology*, 8th ed. St. Louis: Mosby, 1996, pp. 808–809.
75. Sarmiento JM, Wolff BG, Burgart LJ, et al. Paget's disease of the perianal region—an aggressive disease? *Dis Colon Rectum* 1997;40:1187–1194.
76. Jensen SL, Sjolin KE, Shokouh-Amiri MH, et al. Paget's disease of the anal margin. *Br J Surg*. 1988;75:1089–1092.
77. Beck DE. Paget's disease and Bowen's disease of the anus. *Semin Colon Rectal Surg*. 1995;6:143–149.
78. Brown RS, Spittle MF. Radiotherapy for perianal Paget's disease. *J R Soc Med*. 1998;91:114–115.
79. Helwig EB, Graham JH. Anogenital (extramammary) Paget's disease. A clinicopathological study. *Cancer* 1963;16:387–403.
80. Cintron J. Buschke-Loewenstein tumor of the perianal and anorectal region. *Semin Colon Rectal Surg*. 1995;6:135–139.
81. Gordon PH. Current status—perianal and anal canal neoplasms. *Dis Colon Rectum* 1990;33:799–808.
82. Nielsen OV, Jensen SL. Basal cell carcinoma of the anus—a clinical study of 34 cases. *Br J Surg*. 1981;68:856–857.
83. Wade DS, Herrera L, Castillo NB, et al., Metastases to the lymph nodes in epidermoid carcinoma of the anal canal studied by a clearing technique. *Surg Gynecol Obstet*. 1989;169:238–242.
84. Greenall MJ, Quan SH, Urmacher C, et al. Treatment of epidermoid carcinoma of the anal canal. *Surg Gynecol Obstet*. 1985;161:509–517.
85. Boman BM, Moertel CG, O'Connell MJ, et al. Carcinoma of the anal canal. A clinical and pathologic study of 188 cases. *Cancer* 1984;54:114–125.
86. Greene F, Page D, Fleming I, eds. *AJCC Cancer Staging Manual*, 6th ed. Springer: New York, 2002.
87. Nigro ND. An evaluation of combined therapy for squamous cell cancer of the anal canal. *Dis Colon Rectum*. 1984;27:763–766.
88. **Flam M, John M, Pajak TF, et al. Role of mitomycin in combination with fluorouracil and radiotherapy, and of salvage chemoradiation in the definitive nonsurgical treatment of epidermoid carcinoma of the anal canal: results of a phase III randomised intergroup study. *J Clin Oncol*. 1996;14:2527–2529.**

89. **UKCCCR Anal Cancer Trial Working Party. Epidermoid anal cancer: results from the UKCCCR randomised trial of radiotherapy alone versus radiotherapy, 5-fluorouracil, and mitomycin C. *Lancet* 1996;348:1049–1054.**
90. Bartelink H, Roelofsen F, Eschwege F, et al. Concomitant radiotherapy and chemotherapy is superior to radiotherapy alone in the treatment of locally advanced anal cancer: results of a phase III randomized trial of the European Organization for Research and Treatment of Cancer Radiotherapy and Gastrointestinal Cooperative Groups. *J Clin Oncol.* 1997;15:2040–2049.
91. Ghouti L, Houvenaeghel G, Moutardier V, et al. Salvage abdominoperineal resection after failure of conservative treatment in anal epidermoid cancer. *Dis Colon Rectum* 2005;48:16–22.
92. Akbari RP, Paty PB, Guillem JG, et al. Oncologic outcomes of salvage surgery for epidermoid carcinoma of the anus initially managed with combined modality therapy. *Dis Colon Rectum* 2004;47:1136–1144.
93. Basik M, Rodriguez-Bigas MA, Penetrante R, et al. Prognosis and recurrence patterns of anal adenocarcinoma. *Am J Surg* 1995;169:233–237.
94. Tarazi R, Nelson R. Adenocarcinoma of the Anus. *Semin Colon Rectal Surg.* 1995;6:169–173.
95. Jensen SL, Shokouh-Amiri MH, Hagen K, et al., Adenocarcinoma of the anal ducts. A series of 21 cases. *Dis Colon Rectum* 1988;31:268–272.
96. Fenger C, Morson BC. Anal duct carcinoma. *Dis Colon Rectum* 1989;32: 355–357.
97. Getz SB Jr, Ough YD, Patterson RB, et al. Mucinous adenocarcinoma developing in chronic anal fistula: report of two cases and review of the literature. *Dis Colon Rectum* 1981;24:562–566.
98. Tarazi R, Nelson RL. Anal adenocarcinoma: a comprehensive review. *Semin Surg Oncol.* 1994;10:235–240.
99. Thibault C, Sagar P, Nivatvongs S, et al. Anorectal melanoma—an incurable disease? *Dis Colon Rectum* 1997;40:661–668.
100. Cooper PH, Mills SE, Allen MS Jr. Malignant melanoma of the anus: report of 12 patients and analysis of 255 additional cases. *Dis Colon Rectum* 1982;25:693–703.
101. Brady MS, Kavolius JP, Quan SH. Anorectal melanoma. A 64-year experience at Memorial Sloan-Kettering Cancer Center. *Dis Colon Rectum* 1995;38:146–151.
102. Pessaux P, Pocard M, Elias D, et al. Surgical management of primary anorectal melanoma. *Br J Surg.* 2004;91:1183–1187.

SECTION J
HERNIA, ACUTE ABDOMEN, AND SPLEEN

CHAPTER 73 ■ ABDOMINAL WALL HERNIAS

ALAN T. RICHARDS, THOMAS H. QUINN, AND ROBERT J. FITZGIBBONS, JR.

One of the most frequently performed operations by general surgeons worldwide is the repair of an abdominal wall hernia. In the United States, approximately 1 million hernia operations are performed each year.[1] Because hernias are far less age-dependent than other conditions are, a large proportion of the patients undergoing hernia repair are relatively young.

ANATOMY OF THE ABDOMINAL WALL AND GROIN

The anatomy of the abdominal wall and the inguinal region are presented, first from the viewpoint of the surgeon using open techniques and subsequently from the perspective of the surgeon utilizing the laparoscope. Anatomic terms for which synonyms and eponyms are commonly used are listed in Table 73.1. Specific anatomic nomenclature can now be found in *Terminologia Anatomica,* the successor to *Nomina Anatomica.*

The abdominal wall spans the gap between the lower ribs and the pelvis; the lowest ribs, pelvic brim, and lumbar spine comprise its only skeletal support. The muscular and aponeurotic structures that provide much of the integrity of the wall must not only compress and contain abdominal viscera but also contribute to the support and movement of the spine and pelvis.

The sheets of relatively thin muscles and aponeuroses that make up the abdominal wall would, individually, seem to predispose to visceral eventration. The lamination of most of the wall precludes this in most cases. The most common sites of hernia formation are found between laminations, where only peritoneum and fascia are found between the viscera and skin. These weak areas are most important to the hernia surgeon and are described in detail in the subsequent sections dealing with the anterior and posterolateral abdominal wall and the inguinal region.

Anterior Abdominal Wall

Superficial Fascia, Vessels, and Nerves

The anterior abdominal wall does not consist solely of muscle and aponeurosis; it can also be the repository for copious amounts of adipose tissue (panniculus adiposus) in its superficial

TABLE 73.1

ANATOMIC TERMS WITH COMMON SYNONYMS AND EPONYMS

FASCIAL STRUCTURES/SPACES
Fatty layer of superficial fascia; panniculus adiposus; Camper's fascia
Investing fascia of external abdominal oblique; fascia innominata
Membranous layer of superficial fascia; Scarpa's fascia
Retroinguinal space; space of Bogros
Retropubic space; space of Retzius
LIGAMENTOUS STRUCTURES
Iliopectineal ligament; iliopectineal arch
Iliopubic tract; Thompson's ligament (band)
Inguinal ligament; Poupart's ligament
Lacunar ligament; Gimbernat's ligament
Pectineal ligament; Cooper's ligament
APONEUROSIS-DERIVED STRUCTURES
Arcuate line; semicircular line; linea semicirculars; line of Douglas
Falx inguinalis (often incorrectly referred to as *conjoined tendon*)
Reflected inguinal ligament; reflex ligament; Colles' ligament
Semilunar line; linea semilunaris; Spigelius' line

fascial layer, often called *Camper's fascia*. This layer, which is continuous inferiorly with the outer layer of fascia covering the perineum and genitalia, also contains the dartos muscle fibers of the scrotum. The major blood vessels of the superficial fatty layer are the superficial epigastric vessels and superficial circumflex iliac vessels, which are tributaries of the femoral vessels. The superficial fascia is also replete with lymphatic vessels that drain into the inguinal lymph nodes inferior to the umbilicus. The lymphatic structures cross the inguinal ligament, so that they are potentially placed in the surgical field during open herniorrhaphy.[2–6]

A second fascial layer in the superficial abdominal wall is the deep fascia of Scarpa. Although most commonly considered a distinct anatomic layer, Scarpa's fascia actually consists of compressed fibrous components of the superficial fascia.[7] The deeper fibrous tissue of the superficial fascia forms the fundiform ligament of the penis (suspensory ligament of the female clitoris), continues onto the penis and scrotum, and ultimately fuses with the superficial fascia of the perineum.

The superficial fascia also fuses with the layer of fascia (fascia innominata) investing the external abdominal oblique muscle. This fascia is bound inferiorly to the inguinal ligament and pubis before continuing onto the thigh, where it blends with the fascia lata to seal the space beneath and inferior to the inguinal ligament, which is the inferior portion of the myopectineal orifice (Fig. 73.1). This portion of the inguinal region includes Hesselbach's (inguinal) triangle superiorly and therefore constitutes the weakest aspect of the groin.

The skin of the anterior abdominal wall is segmentally innervated in the familiar dermatome pattern. The nerve branches to this area are derived from the anterior and lateral cutaneous branches of the ventral rami of the seventh to 12th intercostal nerves and from the ventral rami of the first and second lumbar nerves. Disruption of one of these nerves is rarely noted by the postoperative patient because the dermatome fields overlap significantly. The anterior and lateral cutaneous branches reach the subcutaneous layer by coursing between the flat lateral muscles and by piercing the sheath of the rectus abdominis.

Anterior Musculature and Ligaments

The division of the wall into anterior and posterior segments is somewhat artificial because the anterior muscles, with the exception of the rectus abdominis, arise posteriorly and also form part of the posterior wall.

The three muscles of the lateral aspect of the anterior abdominal wall (Fig. 73.2) are composed of a variable amount of muscle with a large aponeurosis. The aponeurosis is the tendon of insertion for the lateral muscles, and it also forms the sheath of the rectus abdominis. The midline decussation of the three aponeuroses forms the linea alba. Fibrous tissue layers are of great importance to the hernia surgeon because of their ability to support sutures. Fascia and aponeurosis are terms commonly used to describe these fibrous structures but are often confused and used interchangeably. In this chapter, an aponeurosis is defined as the nonmuscle fiber containing portion of a muscle usually present at insertion points. Muscle fibers are said to "give way" to the corresponding aponeurosis. Fascia on the other hand is the fibrous tissue that lines or envelops muscles.

External Abdominal Oblique Muscle and Associated Ligaments

The external abdominal oblique muscle (Figs. 73.2 and 73.3A and B) is the most superficial of the three lateral abdominal muscles. The external abdominal oblique arises from the posterior aspects of the lower eight ribs and interdigitates with both the serratus anterior and the latissimus dorsi at its origin. The direction of the muscle fibers varies from nearly horizontal in its upper portion to oblique in the middle and lower portions. The mostly horizontal fibers, which originate posteriorly, insert onto the anterior portion of the iliac crest. The obliquely arranged anteroinferior fibers of insertion fold on themselves to form the inguinal ligament. The remaining portion of the aponeurosis inserts into the linea alba after contributing to the anterior portion of the rectus abdominis sheath. Some fibers cross the linea alba to reinforce further the anterior rectus sheath of the opposite side.

The more medial fibers of the aponeurosis of the external oblique divide into a medial and a lateral crus to form the external or superficial inguinal ring. The spermatic cord (or round ligament) and branches of the ilioinguinal and genitofemoral nerves pass through this opening. The *inguinal ligament* (Fig. 73.4) is worthy of special consideration because of its important role as both a landmark and an integral component of many groin hernia repairs. The inguinal ligament is formed by obliquely oriented anteroinferior aponeurotic fibers of the external abdominal oblique. The ligament is formed when the aponeurosis folds beneath itself. Its lateral

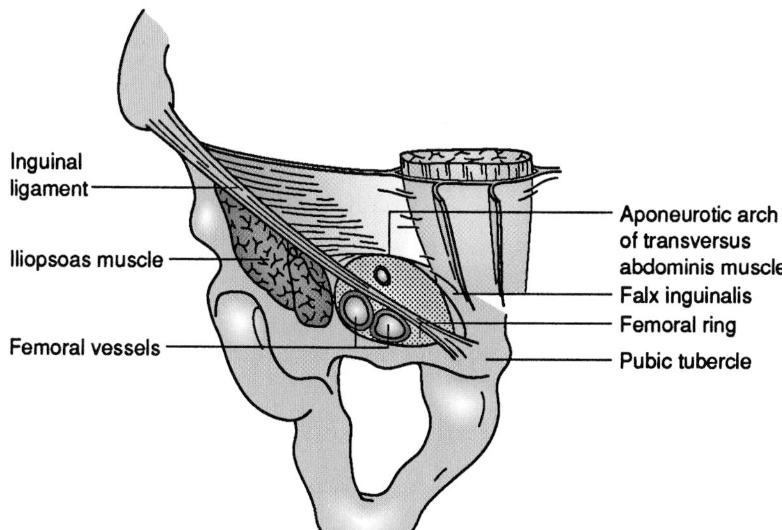

FIGURE 73.1 The myopectineal orifice. Superior to the inguinal ligament, this area includes the inguinal (Hesselbach's) triangle. Inferior to the ligament, the orifice transmits the iliopsoas muscle, the femoral nerve and vessels, and the femoral canal and sheath. (From Wantz GE. *Atlas of hernia surgery*. New York: Raven Press; 1991:4, with permission.)

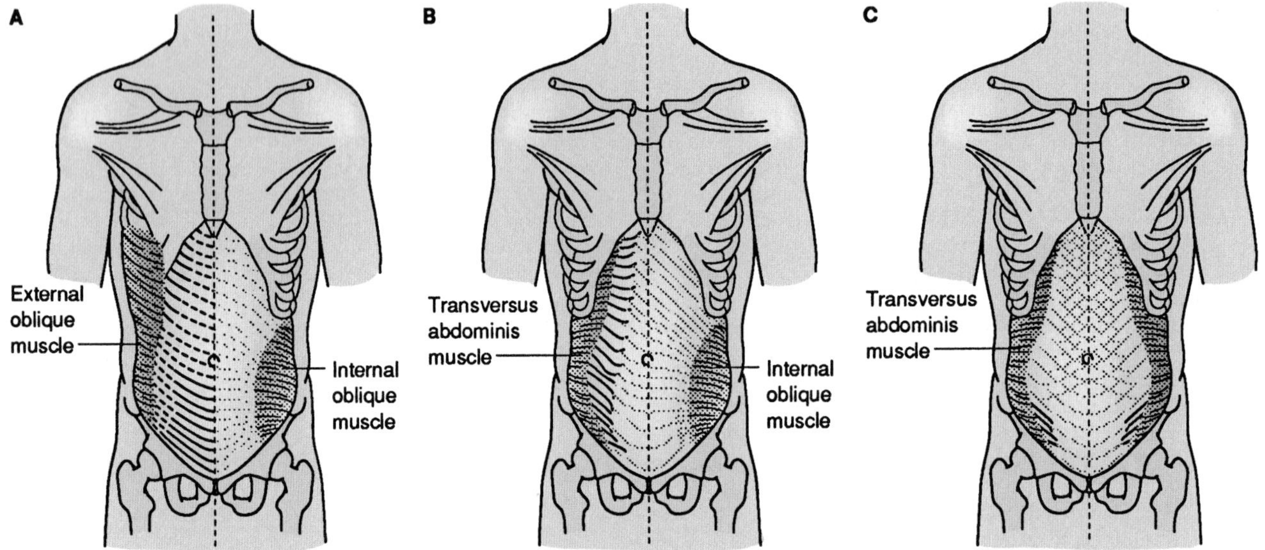

FIGURE 73.2 Pattern of crossing of the aponeurotic fascicles of the abdominal wall musculature. (*A*) Fascicles from the right external oblique and anterior lamina of the left internal oblique. (*B*) Fascicles from the right transversus abdominis and posterior lamina of the left internal oblique. (*C*) Fascicles between the right and left transversus abdominis muscles.

attachment is to the anterior superior iliac crest; its medial insertion is primarily on the pubic tubercle.

The medial insertion of the inguinal ligament in most persons is dual. One portion runs along the superior surface of the pubic tubercle and symphysis to form (or at least reinforce) the superior pubic ligament. The other portion is fan-shaped and spans the distance between the inguinal ligament proper and the pectineal line of the pubis. This fan-shaped portion of the ligament is called the *lacunar ligament* (see Fig. 73.4). It blends laterally with the pectineal (Cooper's) ligament.

Internal Abdominal Oblique Muscle and Aponeurosis

The middle layer of the lateral abdominal group is the internal abdominal oblique muscle (see Figs. 73.2 and 73.3B and C). This muscle primarily arises from the iliac fascia along the iliac crest and forms a band of iliac fascia fused with the inguinal ligament. The uppermost fibers course obliquely toward the distal ends of the lower three or four ("floating") ribs. The muscle fibers of the internal oblique fan out following the shape of the iliac crest, so that the lowermost fibers are directed inferiorly. These fibers arch over the round ligament, or spermatic cord. Some of the lower muscle bundles in the male join fibers of the transversus abdominis to form the cremaster muscle. The aponeurosis of the internal oblique (Fig. 73.5A) above the level of the umbilicus splits to envelop the rectus abdominis, re-forming in the midline to join and interweave with the fibers of the linea alba. Below the level of the umbilicus (see Fig. 73.5B), the aponeurosis does not split but rather runs anterior to the rectus muscle, continues medially as a single sheet, joins the anterior rectus sheath, and finally contributes to the linea alba. The aponeurotic portion of the internal oblique is widest at the level of the umbilicus.

Transversus Abdominis Muscle and Aponeurosis

The transversus abdominis muscle (see Figs. 73.2 and 73.3C) arises from the fascia along the iliac crest and inguinal ligament and from the lower six costal cartilages and ribs, where it interdigitates with the lateral diaphragmatic fibers. The muscle bundles of the transversus abdominis for the most part run horizontally. The lower medial fibers, however, may continue in a more inferomedial course toward the site of insertion on the crest and pecten of the pubis.

The aponeurosis of the transversus abdominis joins the posterior lamina of the internal abdominal oblique, forming above the umbilicus a portion of the posterior rectus sheath. Below the umbilicus, the transversus abdominis aponeurosis is a component of the anterior rectus sheath. The gradual termination of aponeurotic tissue on the posterior aspect of the rectus abdominis forms the arcuate line (of Douglas) (Fig. 73.6). The medial aponeurotic fibers of the transversus abdominis insert on the pecten pubis and the crest of the pubis to form the falx inguinalis. These fibers infrequently are joined by a portion of the internal oblique aponeurosis; only then is a true conjoined tendon formed.[8]

The arch formed by the termination of the aponeurotic fibers of the transversus abdominis is called the *aponeurotic arch* (see Fig. 73.6). The area beneath the arch varies. A high arch may be a predisposing factor in direct inguinal hernia. Contraction of the transversus abdominis causes the arch to move down toward the inguinal ligament in a kind of shutter mechanism, which reinforces the weakest area of the groin when intraabdominal pressure is raised.

Rectus Abdominis

The rectus abdominis (see Figs. 73.3D and 73.5) forms the central and anchoring muscle mass of the anterior abdomen. The rectus muscle arises from the fifth to the seventh costal cartilages and inserts on the pubic symphysis and pubic crest. Each rectus muscle is segmented by tendinous intersections at the levels of the xiphoid process and the umbilicus and at a point midway between these two. The principal blood supply reaches the muscle from the superior and inferior epigastric arteries (see Fig. 73.5), which anastomose just superior to the umbilicus. Other vessels are anterior branches of the intercostal arteries; these reach the muscle by entering the lateral aspect of the rectus sheath. The

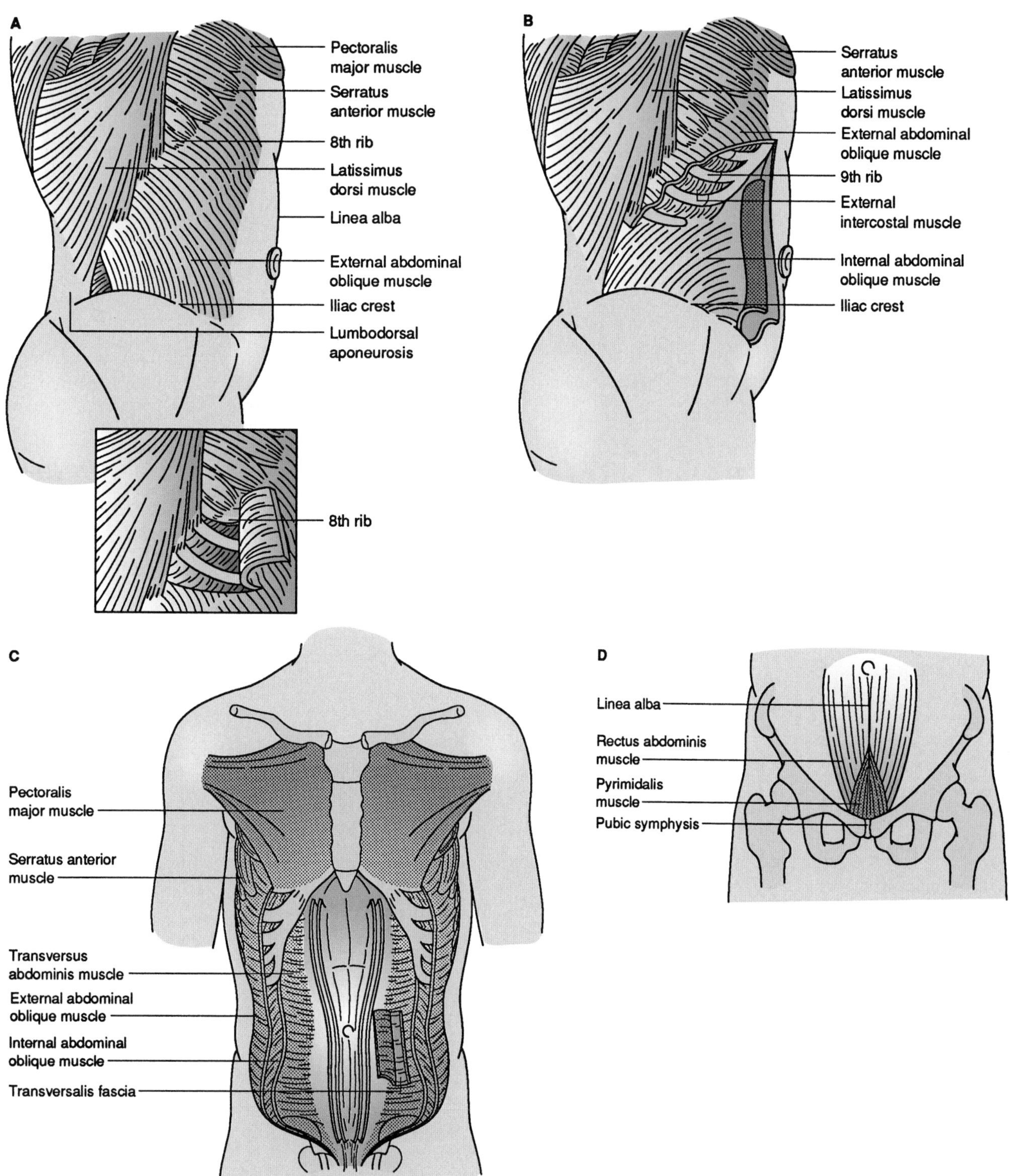

FIGURE 73.3 (*A*) External oblique muscle and aponeurosis. (*B*) Internal oblique muscle and aponeurosis. (C) Transversus abdominis muscle and aponeurosis. (*D*) Lower rectus abdominis and pyramidalis muscle. The linea alba is formed by the intermeshed fibers of the aponeuroses of the lateral muscle layers; it is tensed by the pyramidalis, which inserts into it.

innervation of the muscle is from the seventh to the 12th intercostal nerves, which laterally pierce the aponeurotic sheath of the muscle. The lateral edge of the muscle is demarcated by a slight depression in the aponeurotic fibers coursing toward the muscle; this depression is the *semilunar line*.

The small pyramidalis muscle (see Fig. 73.3D) accompanies the rectus abdominis at its origin in a minority of people. The pyramidalis arises from the pubic symphysis. It lies within the rectus sheath and tapers to attach to the linea alba, the conjunction of the two rectus sheaths and the major site of insertion of three aponeuroses from all three lateral muscle layers.

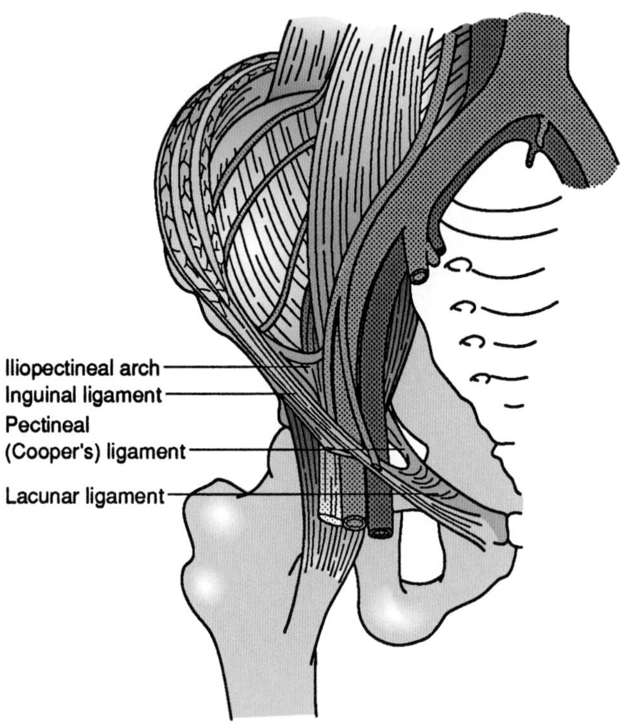

FIGURE 73.4 Ligamentous structures of the inguinal region. The iliopubic tract is not seen in this view because it is obscured by the inguinal ligament. The lacunar ligament is the expanded medial end of the inguinal ligament; on the pecten pubis, it blends with the inguinal (Cooper's) ligament.

Rectus Sheath

Although the components of the rectus sheath individually have been discussed in relation to the three lateral abdominal muscles, it should also be considered as a distinct entity. Three features of the rectus muscle and its sheath can be observed even topographically in well-muscled or very thin subjects:

1. The semilunar line is a slight depression in the aponeurotic fibers corresponding to the lateral edge of the rectus muscle. It marks the site of initial lateral insertion of the aponeurotic tendons of the lateral abdominal muscles.
2. The tendinous inscriptions divide each muscle into three parts.[9] These are the basis of the expression "six pack," popularized by bodybuilders.
3. The linea alba is the midline confluence of the aponeuroses of the rectus muscles and also the internal and external oblique muscles.

The composition of the rectus sheath varies depending on the level sampled. The anterior sheath superior to the umbilicus is composed of the aponeurosis of the external abdominal oblique and the anterior lamina of the internal abdominal oblique. The transversalis aponeurosis does not participate in the formation of the anterior sheath at this level. At a variable level inferior to the umbilicus, the anterior sheath is a composite of all the aponeurotic layers.

The posterior sheath of the rectus muscle superior to the umbilicus is a lamination of the posterior lamina of the aponeurosis of the internal abdominal oblique and the transversus abdominis aponeurosis. The external abdominal oblique does not participate in the formation of the posterior portion of the rectus sheath. At a highly variable site inferior to the umbilicus, all the aponeurotic tendons pass anteriorly to form the anterior rectus sheath. The fibers of the posterior sheath are seen to attenuate gradually. The aponeurotic fibers do not end abruptly at the arcuate line. This transfer of connective tissue away from the posterior rectus sheath causes the arcuate line (of Douglas) to form on the posterior surface of the muscle (see Fig. 73.6). The tissue covering the deep surface of the rectus muscle inferior to the arcuate line is primarily the transversalis fascia.

Some have questioned this traditional scheme of rectus sheath composition, contending that each of the aponeurotic layers superior to the umbilicus is actually bifid, with both contributing to the anterior and posterior sheaths.[10] The fibers of the posterior sheath are seen to attenuate gradually. The concept of rectus sheath composition favored by most is shown in Figure 73.7.[11]

Innervation and Blood Supply of the Anterior Abdominal Wall

The innervation of the anterior wall muscles is multiple. The lower intercostal and upper lumbar nerves (T7 to T12, L1, L2) contribute most of the innervation to the lateral muscles and to the rectus abdominis and overlying skin. The nerves pass anteriorly in a plane between the internal abdominal oblique and the transversus abdominis, eventually piercing the lateral aspect of the rectus sheath to innervate the muscle therein. The external oblique muscle receives branches of the intercostal nerves, which penetrate the internal oblique. The anterior ends of the nerves form part of the cutaneous innervation of the abdominal wall. The first lumbar nerve divides

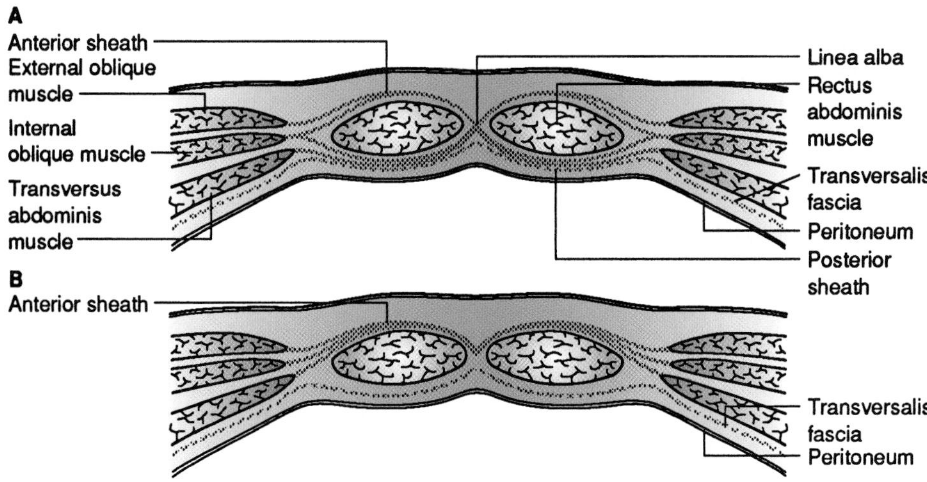

FIGURE 73.5 (*A*) Immediately superior to the umbilicus, the rectus sheath consists of anterior and posterior components. The anterior sheath is composed of the aponeuroses of the external and internal abdominal oblique muscles, and the posterior sheath consists of the posterior aponeurotic lamina of the internal oblique and the aponeurosis of the transversus abdominis muscle. (*B*) The rectus sheath inferior to the arcuate line (of Douglas) consists of an anterior portion made up of fibers from all aponeurotic layers; the posterior portion at this point comprises only transversalis fascia covered internally by peritoneum.

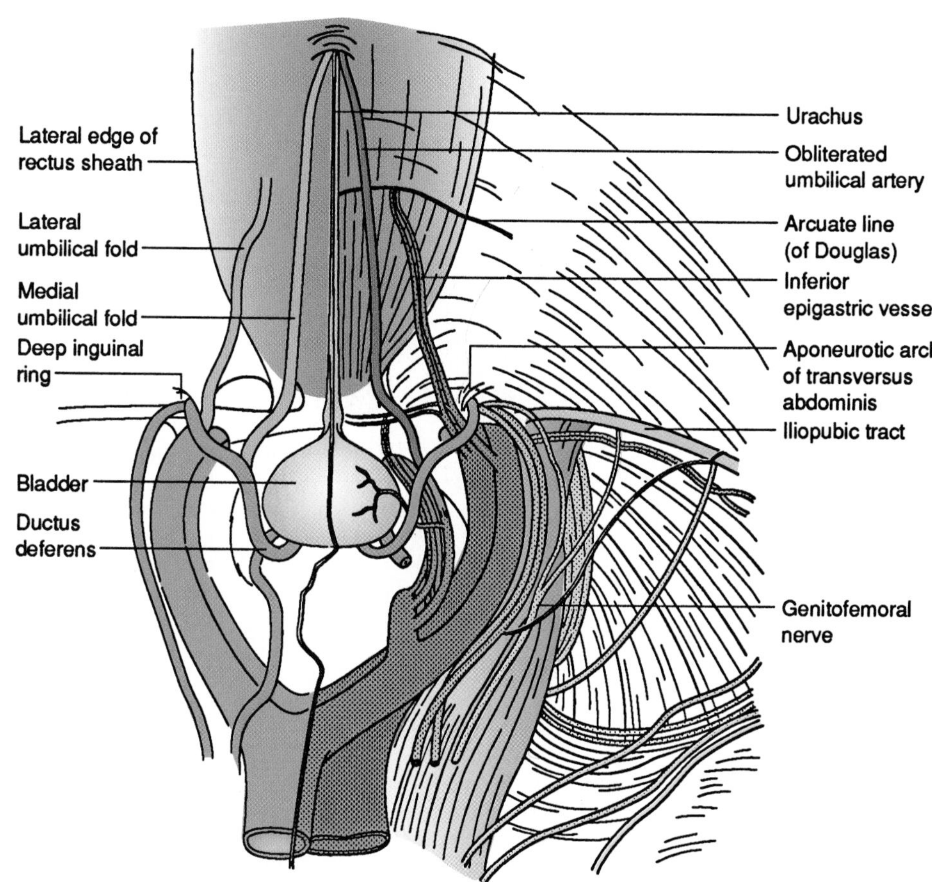

FIGURE 73.6 The deep inguinal region, pelvis, and anterior abdominal wall from the viewpoint of a surgeon using a laparoscopic technique. The anterior wall folds upward approximately at the iliopubic tract in this illustration.

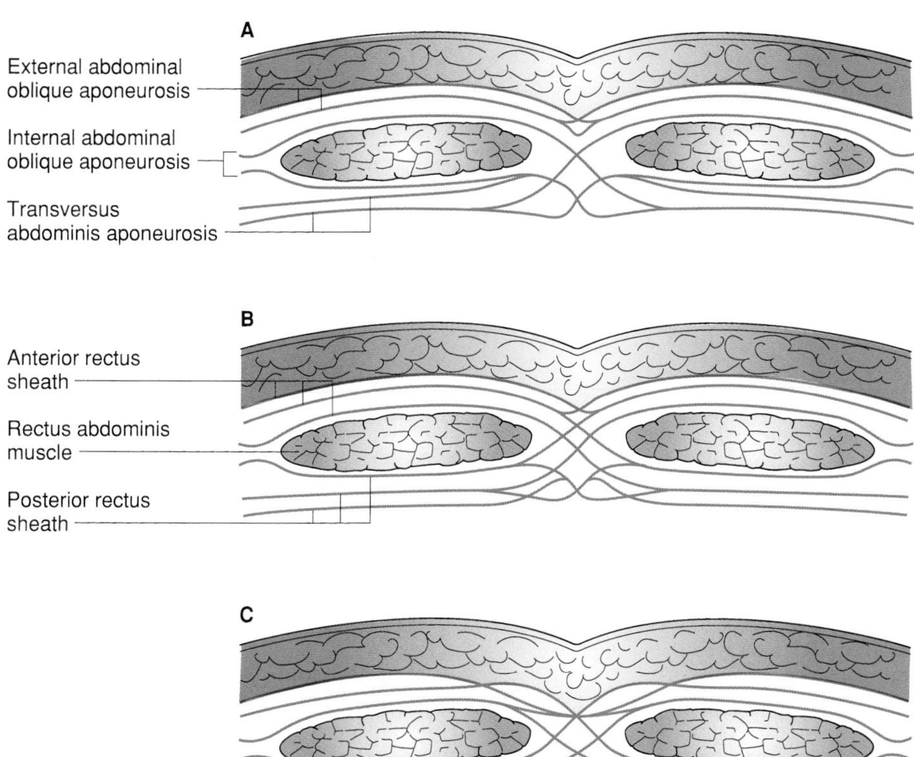

FIGURE 73.7 Patterns of midline decussation of the aponeuroses. (*A*) Single anterior and posterior lines of decussation. (*B*) Single anterior and triple posterior lines of decussation. (*C*) Triple anterior and posterior lines of decussation. (After Askar O. Surgical anatomy of the aponeurotic expansions of the anterior abdominal wall. *Ann R Coll Surg Engl*. 1977;59: 313, with permission.)

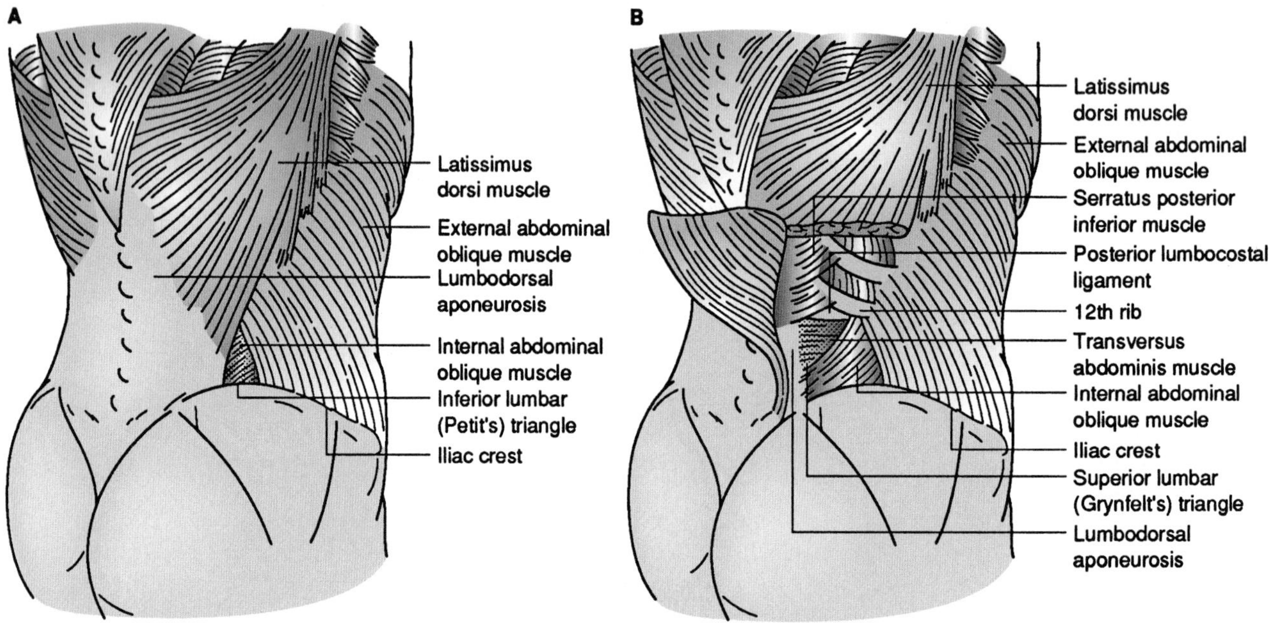

FIGURE 73.8 The lumbar abdominal wall with the inferior lumbar triangle (*A*) and the superior lumbar triangle (*B*).

into the ilioinguinal and iliohypogastric nerves. These may divide within the psoas major muscle or between the internal oblique and transversus abdominis muscles. The ilioinguinal nerve may communicate with the iliohypogastric nerve before innervating the internal oblique. The ilioinguinal nerve then passes through the external inguinal ring to run with the spermatic cord, whereas the iliohypogastric nerve pierces the external oblique to innervate the skin above the pubis. The cremaster muscle fibers, which are derived from the internal oblique muscle, are innervated by the genitofemoral nerve (L1, L2).

The blood supply of the lateral muscles of the anterior wall is primarily from the lower three or four intercostal arteries, the deep circumflex iliac artery, and the lumbar arteries. The rectus abdominis has a complicated blood supply derived from the superior epigastric artery (a terminal branch of the internal thoracic, or internal mammary, artery), the inferior epigastric artery (a branch of the external iliac artery), and the lower intercostal arteries. The latter arteries enter the sides of the muscle after traveling between the oblique muscles. The superior and inferior epigastric arteries enter the rectus sheath and anastomose near the umbilicus.

Posterolateral (Lumbar) Abdominal Wall

The posterolateral or lumbar portion of the abdominal wall (Fig. 73.8) often is overlooked in discussions of abdominal hernia, perhaps because of the much more common occurrence of groin and femoral hernias. The configuration of the muscle layers in the lumbar area also predisposes to hernia formation. For the purposes of this discussion, the lumbar portion of the abdominal wall is defined as the area bounded superiorly by the 12th rib, inferiorly by the iliac crest, and medially by the erector spinae group. Eight muscles arrayed in three layers constitute the posterolateral or lumbar portion of the abdominal wall.

The most superficial layer is composed of the external abdominal oblique muscle, which arises from the posteroinferior portion of the lower ribs and inserts in part along the posterior iliac crest. Closely associated with the external oblique in this area is the latissimus dorsi, which arises from the posterior iliac crest, the spinous processes of the sacrum and lumbar vertebrae, and the lumbodorsal fascia. The muscle courses obliquely toward its insertion on the medial aspect of the intertubercular groove of the humerus. The triangular space formed by the two muscles just described and the iliac crest is called the *inferior lumbar (Petit's) triangle* (see Fig. 73.8A).

The middle layer of lumbar abdominal muscles consists of the erector spinae, the internal abdominal oblique, and the extremely thin insignificant serratus posterior inferior. The erector spinae forms a significant portion of the abdominal wall in the lumbar region, with fibers extending nearly the length of the spinal column. The internal abdominal oblique muscle forms the remainder of the layer. The serratus posterior inferior arises from the lumbodorsal fascia and inserts on the lower four ribs. The middle layer of lumbar muscle is associated with the superior lumbar triangle, a more common site of hernia than the inferior lumbar triangle described previously. The superior triangle (see Fig. 73.8B) is formed superiorly by the 12th rib, the serratus posterior inferior, and the superior lumbocostal ligament; inferiorly by the upper border of the internal abdominal oblique; and medially by the erector spinae.

The deep layer of the lumbar abdominal wall includes three muscles: the quadratus lumborum, the psoas major, and the transversus abdominis. The quadratus lumborum primarily arises from the posterior iliac crest and inserts on the 12th rib. The psoas major arises from vertebrae T12 through L5 and passes beneath the inguinal ligament to insert on the lesser trochanter of the femur.

Deep Inguinal Region

Laparoscopic View

Deep Aspect of the Anterior Abdominal Wall, Peritoneal Folds, and Associated Structures. If one creates a space in the abdominal cavity by distending it with gas, an excellent view of the anterior wall can be obtained. The umbilical peritoneal

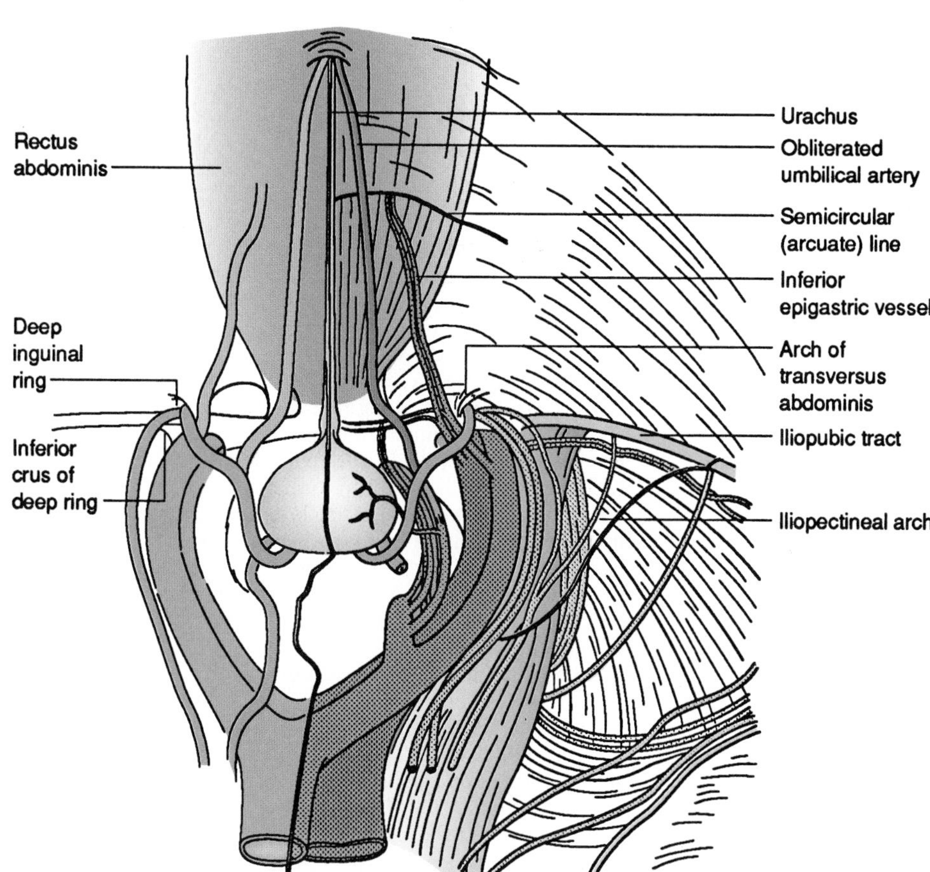

FIGURE 73.9 The deep inguinal region and the anterior abdominal wall seen from within the abdomen. The urachus, the obliterated portion of the umbilical artery, and the inferior epigastric vessels are covered by peritoneal folds, respectively called the median, medial, and lateral umbilical folds.

folds (Fig. 73.9) in most subjects are very prominent and provide easily identified landmarks. The folds (ligaments) primarily exist because the peritoneum covers underlying structures.

The single median umbilical fold extends from the umbilicus to the urinary bladder and covers the urachus, the fibrous remnant of the fetal allantois. The urachus may be patent for a short distance in adults or may open into the umbilical scar in newborns. The medial umbilical fold is formed by the underlying obliterated portion of the fetal umbilical artery. This normally cordlike structure, like the urachus, may be patent for a portion of its length. Indeed, the proximal, patent portion of the artery normally supplies the superior vesicular arteries to the bladder. The lateral fold covers the inferior epigastric arteries as they course toward the posterior rectus sheath, which they enter approximately at the level of the arcuate line.

Between the median and the medial ligaments, a depression is usually found that is called the *supravesical fossa*. This is the site of hernias of the same name. The fossa formed between the medial and lateral ligaments is the medial fossa; this is the site of direct inguinal hernias. The lateral fossa is less well delineated than the others. The medial border of the fossa is formed by the lateral umbilical ligament and the rectus abdominis. This fossa does not have a lateral border; rather the concavity slowly attenuates. The deep inguinal ring is located in the lateral fossa and therefore is the site of the congenital or indirect inguinal hernia.

Transversalis Fascia

The transversalis fascia (endoabdominal fascia) is perhaps the most commonly misunderstood structure in the literature devoted to groin hernia. Confusion results because surgeons may actually be referring to very different anatomic structures when discussing various hernia repairs; however, each may use the same anatomic term or eponym. Indeed, perhaps the biggest reservation among surgeons intent on performing a Shouldice repair is a precise definition of what is being sewn to what.

The transversalis fascia proper is a continuous sheet that extends throughout the extraperitoneal space. The term *transversalis fascia* generally is defined as the deep or endoabdominal fascia covering the internal surface of the transversus abdominis, the iliacus, the psoas muscles, and the obturator internus and portions of the periosteum. One variant of this convention is the use of terms specific to the muscle covered by the fascia (e.g., iliac fascia).

Most authors feel that only one layer of transversalis fascia exists, whereas others maintain that the transversalis fascia comprises two layers, or laminae.[12–16] The posterior lamina is a layer of fibrous connective tissue that widely varies in density and continuity and is interspersed with adipose tissue, as seen in Figure 73.10. This layer is often referred to simply as the *preperitoneal fascia*. The anterior lamina is more uniform and is adherent to the deep surface of the transversus abdominis and the rectus abdominis. The posterior lamina is contained within the preperitoneal space, which is defined as the space between the peritoneum and the anterior lamina of the transversalis fascia. The inferior epigastric vessels are enclosed by, or interspersed with, the adipose tissue and the fibrous tissue of the posterior lamina of the transversalis fascia. The vessels are in contact anteriorly with the anterior lamina of the transversalis fascia as they course upward to enter the rectus abdominis sheath.

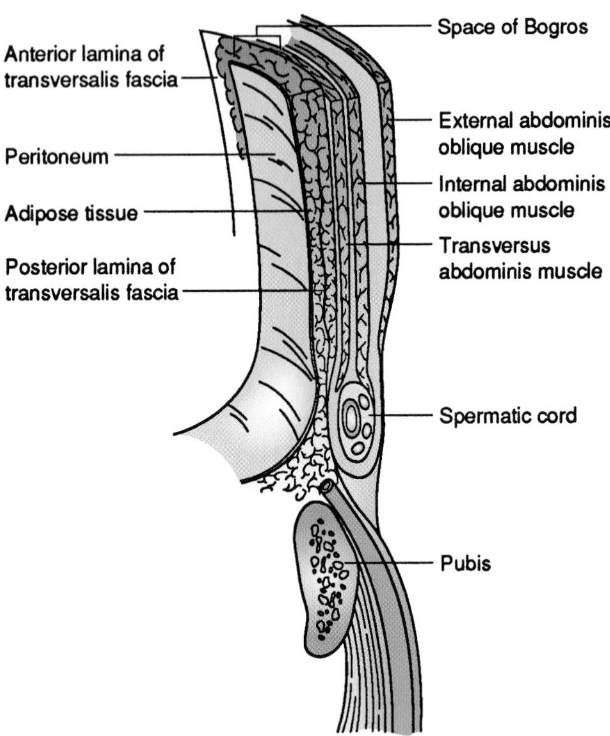

FIGURE 73.10 A parasagittal section through the layers of the anterior abdominal wall and groin. Observe that the transversalis fascia is depicted as a bilaminar structure.

Transversalis Fascia Derivatives

The transversalis fascia analogues or derivatives are the iliopectineal arch, iliopubic tract, and crura of the deep inguinal ring. The superior and inferior crura form a transversalis fascia sling, a structure shaped like a "monk's hood," around the deep inguinal ring (see Fig. 73.9). The transversalis fascia also contributes the internal spermatic fascia to the spermatic cord at this point. This "sling" has functional significance; when the transversus abdominis contracts, the crura of the ring are pulled upward and laterally, which results in a valvular action that helps to prevent the indirect formation of a hernia.

The iliopubic tract (Figs. 73.9 and 73.11) has become an increasingly important landmark for surgeons as the use of laparoscopic technology has increased.[17,18] The iliopubic tract is the thickened band of transversalis fascia formed at the zone of transition between the deep surfaces of the iliac and transversus abdominis muscles. The structure courses parallel to the more superficially located inguinal ligament, is attached to the iliac crest laterally, and inserts on the pubic tubercle medially. The tract forms along its course a portion of the inferior crus of the deep inguinal ring and then contributes to the anterior and medial walls of the femoral sheath. The tract fuses with the inguinal ligament to form a component of the inferior wall of the inguinal canal. At its insertion on the pubic tubercle, it curves backward slightly to blend with Cooper's pectineal ligament. The pectineal ligament actually is a condensation of periosteum and is not a true analogue of the transversalis fascia, but it is reinforced by fibers from the iliopubic tract and inguinal ligament.

The iliopubic tract contains not only fibrous connective tissue but also some elastic fibers.[19] In one series, the iliopubic tract was a substantial structure, suitable for use in hernia repairs, in 42% of the specimens examined. The tract, whether substantial or not, can be used as a readily identified landmark.

The iliopubic tract has particular significance because of its importance as a landmark to the laparoscopic surgeon. Many of the branches of the lumbar plexus run inferior to the tract, and damage to these nerves may be the result of aggressive dissection or the placement of tacks or staples to affix a prosthesis below this structure. The tract is not obviously visible in every patient from a laparoscopic view, but its location should always be immediately known to the surgeon because of its constant relationship to the other landmarks in this area.

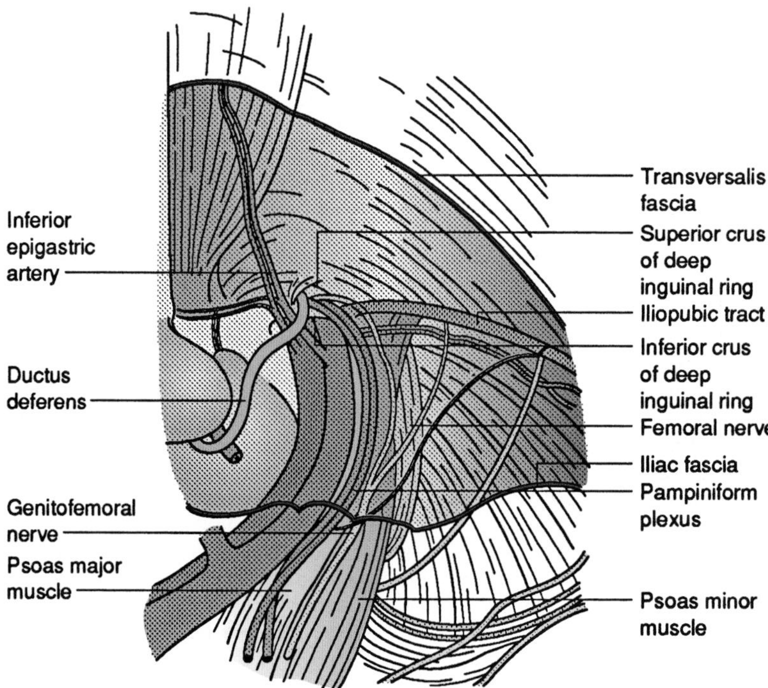

FIGURE 73.11 A schematic representation of the deep inguinal region. The iliopubic tract is shown as a thickening of the transversalis fascia, inferior to which many of the branches of the lumbar plexus exit the pelvis.

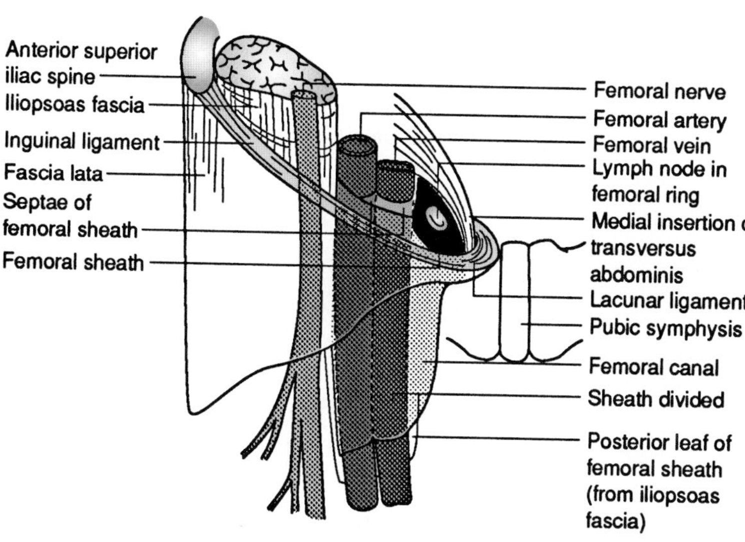

FIGURE 73.12 Schematic view of the femoral sheath, ring, and canal. The transversalis fascia forms the anterior portion of the sheath, and the iliopsoas fascia forms the posterior portion. Septa separate the vessels from each other and the vein from the femoral canal. The femoral ring contains a lymph node. The ring is formed medially by the aponeurosis of the transversus abdominis aponeurosis, anteriorly by the inguinal ligament, posteriorly by the pubic bone, and laterally by the femoral sheath.

The iliopectineal arch (see Fig. 73.9) is also a condensation of the transversalis fascia. The iliopectineal arch commences at the medial border of the iliacus muscle, where it is continuous with the iliac fascia, itself a portion of the transversalis (endoabdominal) fascia. The arch separates the vascular compartment containing the femoral vessels from the neuromuscular compartment containing the iliopsoas muscle, femoral nerve, and lateral femoral cutaneous nerve. The iliopectineal arch also contributes to the proximal portion of the femoral sheath, thereby joining the iliopubic tract in the formation of the femoral sheath.

Femoral Sheath, Canal, and Ring

The femoral sheath (Fig. 73.12) is composed primarily of extensions of the transversalis fascia. The sheath is best understood in terms of the structures contained within. As the external iliac artery and vein pass beneath the inguinal ligament to become the femoral vessels, they are covered anteriorly by the transversalis fascia proper. This fascial layer is posteriorly and laterally joined by portions of the iliopsoas fascia, which are themselves continuations of the transversalis fascia. At the inguinal ligament, the iliopsoas fascia forms the iliopectineal arch. This arch divides the vascular compartment (lacuna vasorum), containing the femoral vessels, from the muscular portion (lacuna musculorum), which contains the iliopsoas muscle, femoral nerve, and lateral femoral cutaneous nerve. The vascular lacuna is further divided by septa into compartments for the vessels and the femoral branch of the genitofemoral nerve.

The medial border of the femoral sheath follows the transversus abdominis aponeurosis to its insertion just lateral to that of the lacunar ligament and extends inferiorly to fuse eventually with the medial septum and adventitia of the femoral vein. The resultant cone-shaped cul-de-sac is the femoral canal. The canal normally contains only wisps of connective tissue and small lymphatic nodes. The wider proximal part of the canal, the femoral ring, contains a large node, which is often referred to as *Cloquet's node.*

The femoral ring is the extraperitoneal opening of the canal. The boundaries of the ring are formed medially by the curved edge of the transversus abdominis aponeurosis, not the lacunar ligament, which inserts more medially.[20] Laterally, the ring is bounded by the connective tissue septum and the adventitia that is interposed between it and the femoral vein. The anterior boundary is the inguinal ligament; posteriorly, the ring is reinforced by the iliopubic tract and iliopectineal ligament. The canal is not in direct communication with the pelvic cavity. The transversalis fascia is not a component of the roof of the canal because it is diverted at this point to form the femoral sheath. This weakened area is therefore quite prone to hernia formation, especially in female subjects.

Inguinal (Hesselbach's) Triangle

The inguinal triangle is the site of direct inguinal hernias. This triangle is most often described from the anterior aspect (Fig. 73.13), in which case the inguinal ligament forms the base of the triangle, the rectus abdominis the medial border, and the inferior epigastric vessels the superolateral border. The triangle as originally described by Hesselbach had the pectineal ligament as its base. The latter description is quite useful to the surgeon viewing the abdomen from within because the inguinal ligament cannot be seen from this viewpoint. When the inguinal

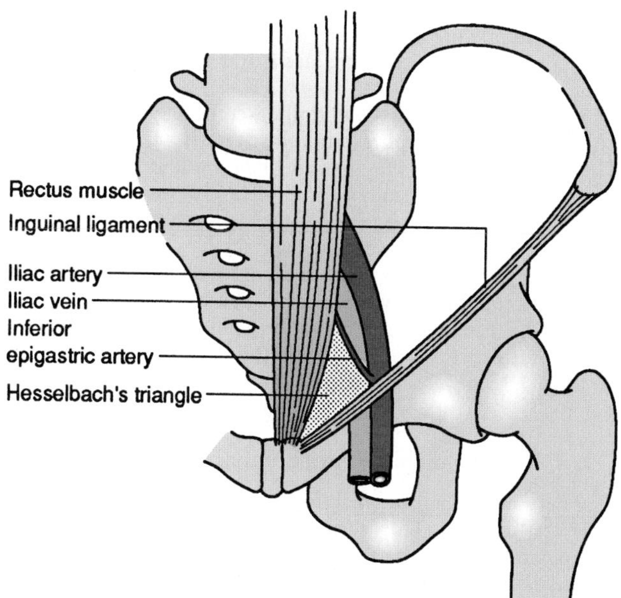

FIGURE 73.13 The inguinal (Hesselbach's) triangle.

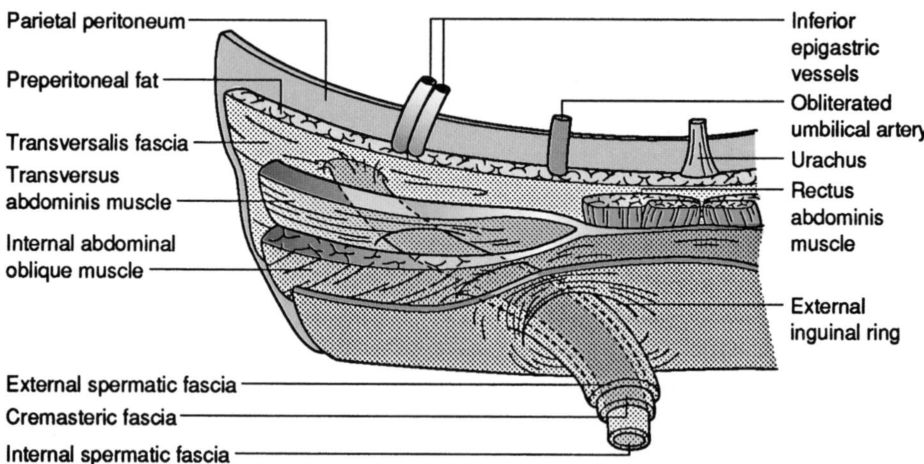

FIGURE 73.14 The component layers covering the contents of the spermatic cord.

triangle is transilluminated, the thinness and translucency of the area of abdominal wall within the triangle underscores its importance in hernia development and repair. In the most translucent area, little or no muscle is present. Only the peritoneum and the transversalis fascia cover the triangle here. The aponeurotic arch of the transversus abdominis crosses the triangle just below the apex in most people. A high aponeurotic arch affords less reinforcement to the triangle and may therefore predispose a person to the formation of a direct inguinal hernia.

Components of the Spermatic Cord

The spermatic cord (Figs. 73.11 and 73.14) is closely associated with the deep inguinal ring. The spermatic cord is most appropriately described at this point because the deep ring itself is formed by derivatives of transversalis fascia, as is the innermost covering layer of the spermatic cord, the internal spermatic fascia. The middle covering layer is called the *cremasteric fascia* and contains the cremasteric muscle bundles; both are derived from the internal abdominal oblique muscle and fascia. The outermost covering of the spermatic cord is the external spermatic fascia, which is continuous with the investing fascia of the external abdominal oblique muscle.

The tunica vaginalis is initially a component of the cord, but normally it atrophies and closes early in neonatal life. This structure is an evagination of peritoneum. The testicle descends retroperitoneally in fetal life and is merely in contact with the posterior aspect of the tunica. An indirect congenital hernia enters the patent tunica vaginalis.

The cord structures enclosed by the coverings described above are the ductus (vas) deferens, the pampiniform venous plexus, the testicular artery, and the genital branch of the genitofemoral nerve, a branch of the lumbar plexus (Figs. 73.9, 73.11, 73.15).

Branches of the Lumbar Plexus

The nerves crossing the iliac fossa are some of the most variable in the body. This variability may be the cause of frequent intraoperative injury to the fragile nerves. The lumbar plexus is formed by roots from the 12th thoracic nerve and the first through fourth lumbar nerves. Cutaneous territories innervated by branches of the lumbar plexus are seen in Figure 73.15A. The five terminal branches commonly encountered in laparoscopic herniorrhaphy can be discerned in many people as they course across the iliacus muscle covered by peritoneum and the iliac fascia (a portion of the transversalis–endopelvic fascia). The nerves form within or deep to the psoas major muscle (Fig. 73.15B), often ramifying with other nerves within or close to the muscle. The nerve branches initially lie within the so-called triangle of pain,[21] bordered medially by the psoas muscle, anteriorly and inferiorly by the iliopubic tract, and laterally by the iliac crest. With the exception of the genital branch of the genitofemoral nerve, the branches of the lumbar plexus destined for the thigh run beneath the iliopubic tract.

The most anterior of the nerves encountered, the genitofemoral nerve, is also the most variable.[22] This nerve may occur as a single trunk lying deep to the peritoneum and fascia on the anterior surface of the psoas muscle. The nerve may also divide into its component genital and femoral branches within the muscle. The genital branch travels with the spermatic cord, entering at the deep inguinal ring; it ultimately innervates the cremaster muscle and the lateral scrotum. The femoral branch of the nerve innervates the skin of the proximal midthigh.

The lumbar plexus branch encountered immediately deep to the lateral aspect of the psoas muscle is the large femoral nerve. Although not routinely encountered during laparoscopy, the femoral nerve has been injured in some cases.[23] The lateral femoral cutaneous nerve crosses the iliac fossa under the iliac fascia to run deep to the iliopubic tract and the inguinal ligament, which it pierces to enter the thigh.

The iliohypogastric nerve typically arises with the ilioinguinal by a common trunk from the first lumbar nerve. They may exchange fibers within the muscle, but they usually diverge immediately to form individual nerves. The iliohypogastric nerve crosses the iliac fossa just inferior to the kidney and pierces the transversus abdominis. The subsequent course of the nerve carries it between the transversus and the internal abdominal oblique until it pierces the aponeuroses of both obliques just above the external inguinal ring.

The ilioinguinal nerve normally crosses the iliac fossa just inferior to the iliohypogastric nerve. In its typical further course, the nerve pierces the transversus abdominis and internal abdominal oblique above the iliac crest and eventually enters the inguinal canal. The nerve may run more diagonally through the iliac fossa and then pierce the iliopubic tract to reach the inguinal canal.[24] This path "can obviously render the nerve more vulnerable to iatrogenic injury."[24]

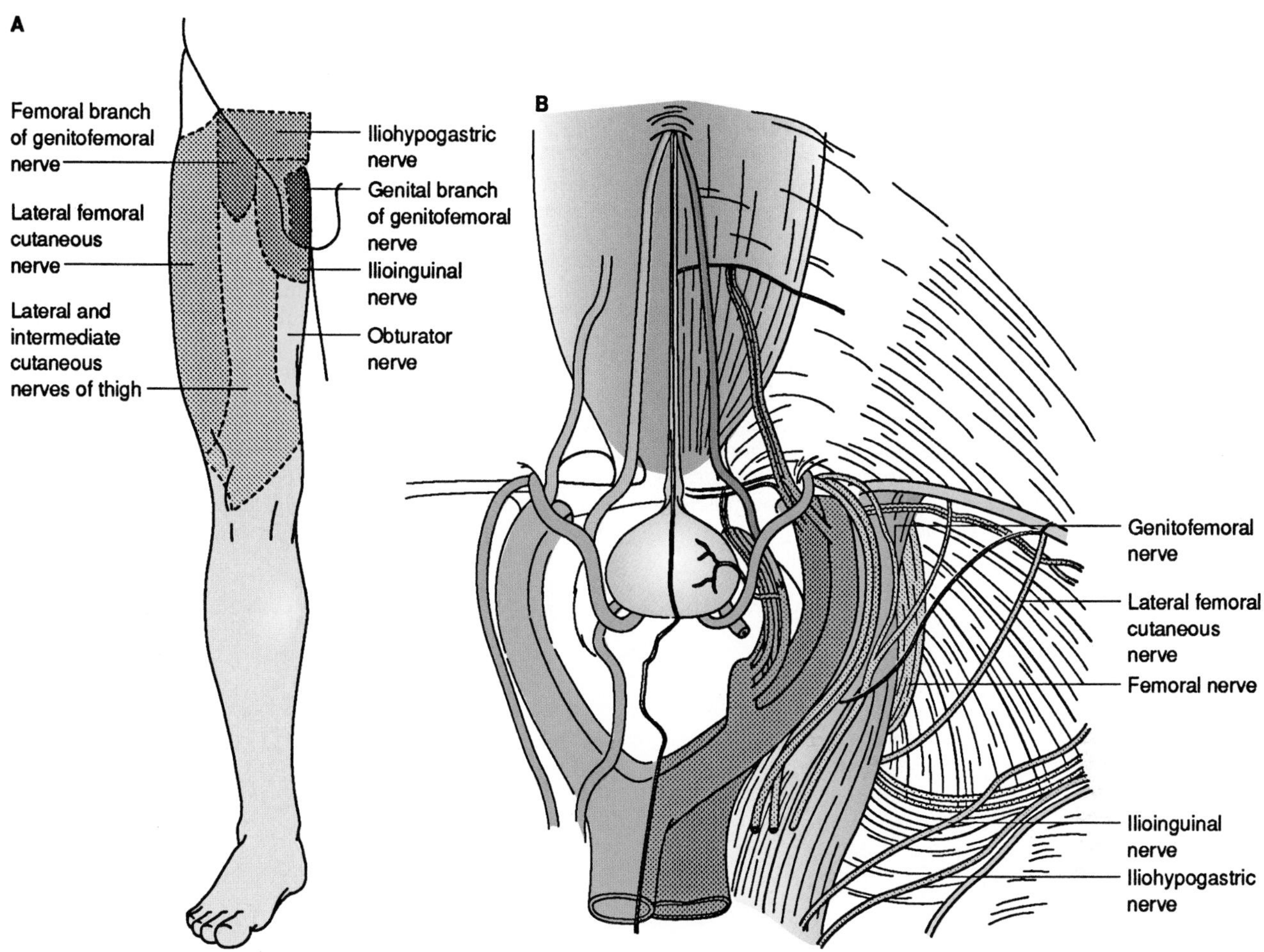

FIGURE 73.15 (*A*) The cutaneous territories innervated by several branches of the lumbar plexus. (*B*) Some of the branches of the lumbar plexus seen from within the abdomen.

Vasculature of the Abdominal Wall and Deep Inguinal Region

The vasculature of the deep inguinal region and anterior abdominal wall has been analyzed by surgeons for well over 100 years. The importance and variability of these vessels has been underscored by the ominous mnemonics used to refer to them—"crown of death" (*corona mortis*) and "triangle of doom." The primary blood supply to the deep anterior wall is from the inferior epigastric artery. This artery is a branch of the external iliac artery. In many cases, an artery called the "aberrant" obturator artery arises from the inferior epigastric, which joins the "normal" obturator artery and thereby forms a circle—the corona mortis—before entering the obturator foramen. Injury to the circle, usually sustained while the surgeon is working in the area of Cooper's ligament, causes copious bleeding. Recent studies have indicated that aberrant obturator vessels are present in between 60% and 90% of whole pelves studied.[25,26]

The veins in this area also are prone to injury because many, especially the iliopubic veins and obturator veins and their tributaries, may be much larger than their accompanying arteries. One network of veins in the area is situated on the inferior deep surface of the rectus muscles. The veins of this network, which anastomose with the pubic branches discussed above, have been called the *rectusial veins*.[27]

The vessels in the vascular compartment of the deep inguinal region are the external iliac artery and vein. They arise within a triangular area bordered laterally by the gonadal vessels and medially by the ductus deferens. The primary continuations of the external iliac vessels are the femoral artery and vein. The inferior epigastric artery is a branch of the external iliac. The obturator artery may arise from either of these arteries as a replacement or accessory to the obturator branch of the internal iliac artery.

A final vessel to consider in this review is the deep circumflex iliac artery (see Fig. 73.10). The origin of this artery is extremely variable, but its course is predictable along the iliopubic tract. It pierces the transversalis fascia and runs along the iliac fossa to anastomose eventually with a deep lumbar artery. Because the deep circumflex artery runs along the iliopubic tract, it can inadvertently be stapled or otherwise injured during laparoscopic herniorrhaphy.

Pelvic Floor and Obturator Muscles

The pelvic musculature normally affords remarkable support to the structures within the true pelvis. Although a myoaponeurotic hammock-like sheet forms the pelvic diaphragm, obturator muscles and membrane, and urogenital diaphragm, herniation of fat or viscera through or around any of these layers occurs. The potential for hernia formation is increased because of the openings through which many structures exit or enter the pelvis.

The Latin term *obturator* is translated as "stopper for a bottle." The aptly named obturator internus, along with its membrane and the obturator externus, closes off nearly all the large obturator foramen. The small superolateral aperture through which the obturator vessels and nerve pass is the site where obturator hernias form. The obturator internus arises from the deep surface of parts of all three pelvic bones. The muscle fibers converge on a tendon, which leaves the pelvis through the lesser sciatic foramen to insert on the greater trochanter. The dense internal obturator fascia covers the muscle and is thickened to form the arcuate ligament, from which the levator ani muscles (the pelvic diaphragm) are in part suspended. The obturator internus fascia splits to enclose the pudendal vessels in the pudendal canal. The external obturator muscle arises from the pelvic bones surrounding the obturator foramen and from the anterior portion of the obturator membrane. The external obturator muscle is supplied by the obturator nerve and vessels.

The component muscles of the bowl-shaped pelvic diaphragm, the pubococcygeus, iliococcygeus, and puborectalis, along with the coccygeus form the floor of the pelvis. The pubococcygeus arises from the posterior aspect of the pubis and the thickened portion of the internal obturator fascia, called the *tendinous arch* (Fig. 73.16), that spans the distance between the pubis and ischial spine. The puborectalis, the midportion of the diaphragm, arises from the pubis and loops around the rectum as the puborectal sling. The iliococcygeus is suspended at its origin from the tendinous arch and inserts on the coccyx. The coccygeus muscle completes the diaphragm posteriorly, arising from the ischial spine and inserting on the sides of the coccyx.

The area remaining between the sacrum and the greater sciatic foramen is filled for the most part by the piriformis muscle. The piriformis arises from the anterior surface of the second through fourth sacral vertebrae and the sacrotuberous ligament. This muscle exits the pelvis through the greater sciatic foramen, which is thereby divided into suprapiriform and infrapiriform portions (Figs. 73.16 and 73.17). The superior

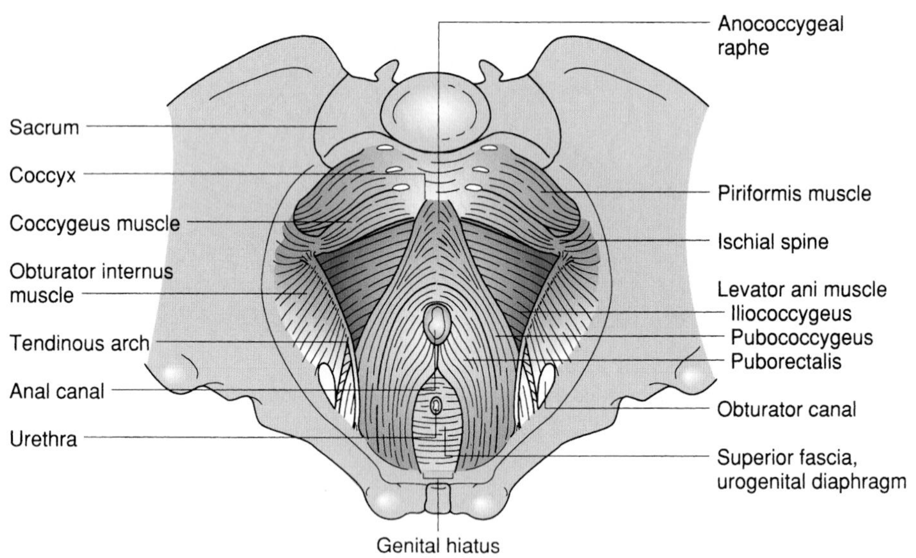

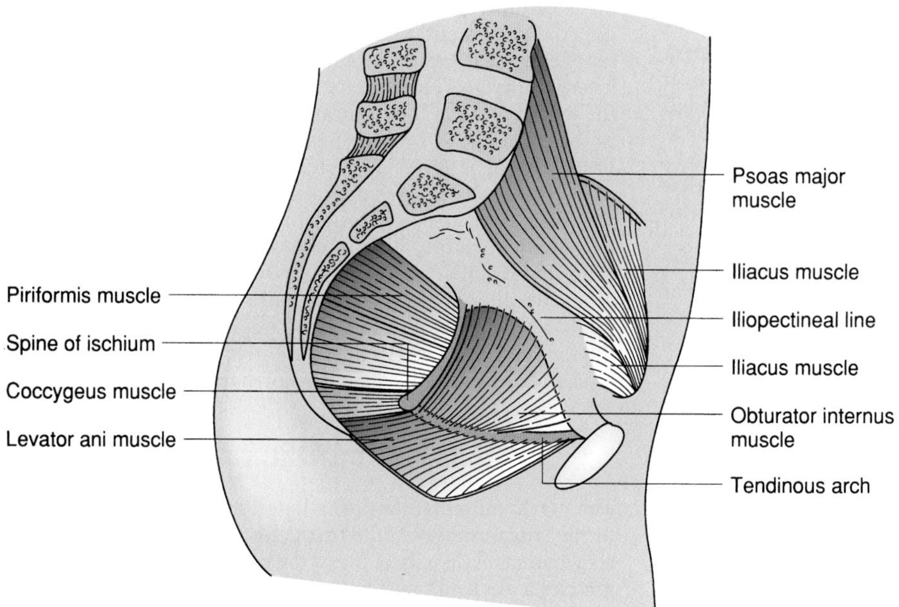

FIGURE 73.16 (*A*) The pelvic diaphragm (levator ani and the piriformis) and the urogenital diaphragm viewed from within the pelvis. (*B*) Hemisection of the pelvis revealing the levator ani, piriformis, obturator internus, and psoas muscles.

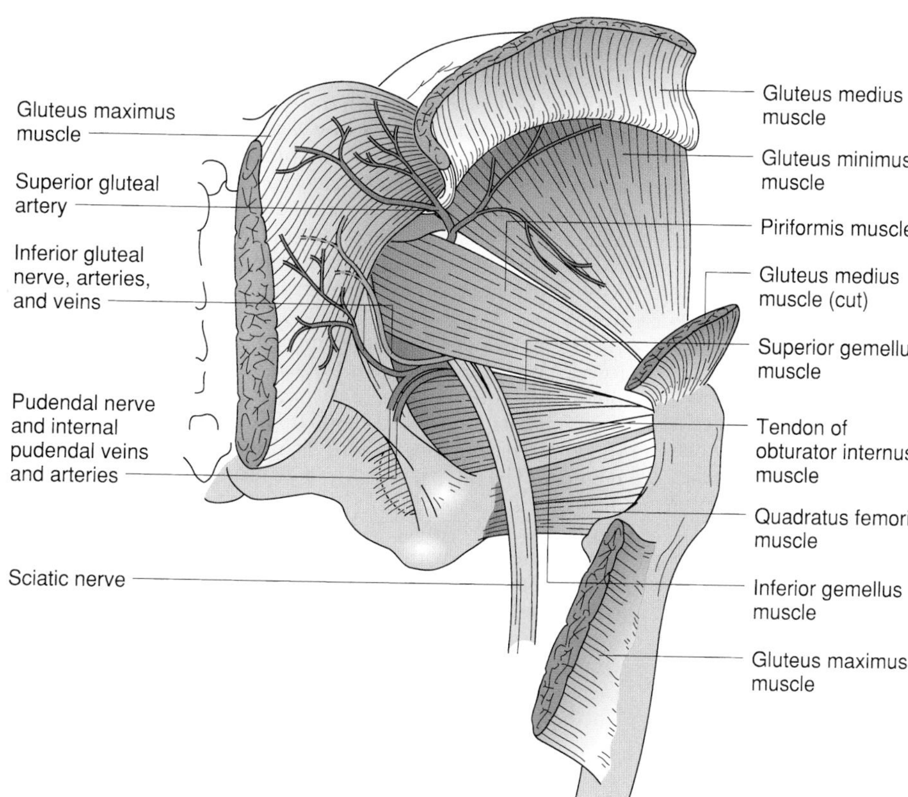

FIGURE 73.17 The gluteal muscles and lateral rotators of the hip. External relations of the sciatic foramen are also evident.

gluteal nerves and vessels pass through the suprapiriform foramen, whereas the inferior gluteal nerves and vessels in company with the sciatic nerve pass through the infrapiriform foramen.

The most pronounced deficit in the pelvic diaphragm is situated anteriorly, where an aperture must allow the urogenital structures to pass out of the pelvis. This area is reinforced by the urogenital diaphragm, a structure primarily consisting of the superficial and deep transverse perineal muscles. The deep transverse perineal muscle is enclosed by a weak superior fascia and a sturdier inferior perineal fascia. The urogenital diaphragm recently has been shown to be more funnel-shaped than sandwich-like, as previously depicted in many atlases.[28] The urogenital diaphragm exists only in humans because the human pelvic outlet faces inferiorly, unlike that of quadrupeds.[29]

CLINICAL FEATURES OF HERNIAS

Inguinal hernias occur in persons of all ages, from the neonate to the elderly. The incidence of inguinal hernias in premature babies is approximately 10%. The duration of symptoms varies from individual to individual; some patients have had a hernia for many years at the time of presentation, whereas in others the development of a strangulated hernia is the initial presentation. The patient may give a history of a lump or swelling that develops on straining. This may be painful if it occurs suddenly after straining, with stretching of a preexisting processus vaginalis.

On clinical examination, a swelling is noted that has a cough impulse. An uncomplicated hernia reduces spontaneously when the patient relaxes or lies down. When the upright position is assumed, the hernia becomes more prominent because the abdominal viscera fall forward. With hernias about the umbilicus or incisional hernias, the edges of the defect in the abdominal wall can be palpated easily, and the size of the neck of the hernia can be assessed accurately. When the hernia is reduced, a gurgle of the intestinal contents in the abdomen can be heard and felt by the examiner. Auscultation of the hernia elicits bowel sounds. A hernia does not transmit light, as opposed to a hydrocele, which usually transilluminates brilliantly. After the hernia is reduced, if the hand is placed over the defect and the patient strains or coughs, the hernia does not protrude.

COMPLICATIONS OF HERNIAS

Incarceration

Incarcerated means "trapped" or "imprisoned." Clinically, an incarcerated hernia is an irreducible hernia. Incarceration does not denote obstruction. The contents of the hernia may be omentum, nonobstructed bowel, or ovary, and its irreducibility is associated with adhesions to the hernial sac.

The hernia itself is not necessarily tense to palpation, and the overlying skin appears normal. Normal bowel sounds may be heard within the hernia. It is important to differentiate an incarcerated hernia from a hydrocele of the cord. One can get above the hydrocele with the examining fingers. One cannot get above a hernia, however, as it communicates with the abdominal cavity. A hydrocele will transilluminate clearly, but a hernia will not.

The recommended treatment of an incarcerated hernia is surgical, but the need for treatment is not urgent because no life-threatening complications are present. This routine recommendation is currently being tested in a multicenter, randomized trial of watchful waiting versus operation that is being sponsored by the Unites States government's Agency for Health Research and Quality.

Intestinal Obstruction

One hundred years ago, the most common cause of intestinal obstruction was a hernia. At the present time, hernia is third, after adhesive obstructions and cancer. Hernia is an important cause of obstruction that is not infrequently missed on clinical examination. When a patient with an intestinal obstruction is examined, great emphasis should be placed on adequate exposure of the entire abdominal wall and groin area (from nipples to knees). Proper lighting is essential because previous scars can fade with time and become barely perceptible. The patient with intestinal obstruction as a result of a hernia will have a tense hernia that is irreducible. The abdomen itself will be distended, and high-pitched bowel sounds with frequent rushes will be heard. If the process continues to the complication of strangulation, these signs will disappear. Unlike adhesive small-bowel obstructions, partial small-bowel obstructions secondary to hernia are rare. Most patients will have had vomiting and obstipation.

A plain roentgenogram of the abdomen will reveal the signs of an intestinal obstruction—dilated loops of bowel with air–fluid levels and no bowel gas distal to the obstruction. Frequently on a plain roentgenogram, one can see bowel shadows in the region of the hernia. A lateral view is often useful to demonstrate this feature more clearly. Contrast studies are not usually necessary in this instance. Computed tomography (CT) reliably demonstrates the hernia with characteristic features of obstruction and should be considered if the clinical diagnosis is not certain (Fig. 73.18) because a distal intestinal obstruction secondary to another cause (e.g., adhesions) may result in significant distention of a coincidental nonobstructing hernia of the abdominal wall. Should the examiner focus attention exclusively on the hernia, the real cause of the obstruction may be missed when the hernia is repaired.

The patient is sedated and placed in bed. The Trendelenburg position should facilitate reduction of a groin hernia. An attempt should be made at the initial examination to reduce the hernia. The maneuver of taxis entails grasping the neck of the hernia with the fingers of one hand and then applying intermittent pressure on the most distal part of the hernia with the other hand. Taxis has the effect of elongating the neck of the hernia so that the contents of the hernia may be guided through this area back into the abdominal cavity with a rocking movement. Mere pressure on the most distal part of the hernia causes bulging of the hernial sac around the neck, which can occlude the neck and prevent it from being reduced (Fig. 73.19). The maneuver of taxis should not be performed with excessive pressure or too vigorously. If the hernia is strangulated, gangrenous bowel might be reduced into the abdomen or perforated in the process. One or two gentle attempts should be made at taxis. If they are unsuccessful, this procedure should be abandoned. Rarely, the hernia together with its peritoneal sac and constricting neck may be reduced into the abdomen (reduction *en masse*). The patient would then have persistent obstruction after reduction of the hernia.

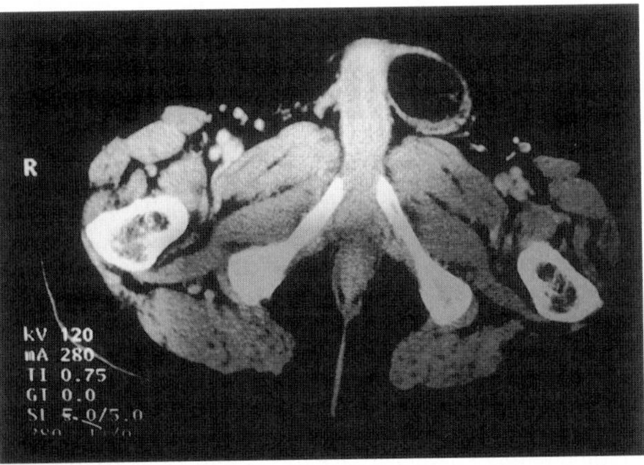

FIGURE 73.18 Computed tomogram showing a left-sided inguinal hernia.

The next steps in management include resuscitation followed by urgent surgery. At surgery, an approach directly over the hernia is used. In all patients, the entire gastrointestinal tract must be assessed to eliminate causes of obstruction other than the hernia itself. This is done before the hernia is repaired. The bowel, if viable, is reduced into the abdomen. If difficulty is encountered in reducing the hernia, the neck of the hernia can be widened. In the case of an inguinal hernia, division of the neck with or without ligation and division of the inferior epigastric vessels, is safe, and the hernia contents can be reduced into the abdomen. In the case of a femoral hernia, the inguinal ligament can be split anteriorly and the hernia contents reduced into the abdomen. If the bowel is nonviable, then a bowel resection can be performed with anastomosis. The hernia is then repaired.

Strangulation

Strangulation of a hernia is a serious and life-threatening condition in which the hernial contents become ischemic and nonviable. The pathogenesis of this condition involves bowel within the hernia sac. Straining may push more bowel into the sac, and the tense sac then causes pressure at the neck. This pressure initially produces venous congestion, as a result of which the bowel becomes edematous. Eventually, the pressure is so great that the arterial supply is obstructed and the bowel becomes gangrenous.

In addition to having an irreducible hernia and intestinal obstruction, the patient is toxic, dehydrated, and febrile. Examination of the abdomen reveals the signs of an intestinal obstruction, with distention and increased bowel sounds. Absolute constipation and vomiting are other manifestations. The hernia itself is tense, irreducible, and very tender, and the overlying skin may be discolored with a reddish or bluish tinge. No bowel sounds are heard within the hernia itself. The patient commonly manifests a leukocytosis with a predominance of polymorphonuclear leukocytes. Blood gases may reveal metabolic acidosis.

Management of these patients requires urgent attention to detail. No attempt should be made to reduce the hernia. Rapid resuscitation should commence immediately, with nasogastric suction and replacement of fluids and electrolytes. The patient should be given antibiotics. Once the patient is resuscitated, urgent surgery commences to expose the hernia, open the sac, and assess the viability of the bowel. More bowel can be pulled into the hernia so that viable bowel can be transected and the gangrenous portion removed. An end-to-end anastomosis should be performed and the bowel then reduced into the abdominal cavity. The hernia is then repaired.

Richter's Hernia

In this interesting complication, part of the bowel wall herniates through the defect and may become ischemic and gangrenous.

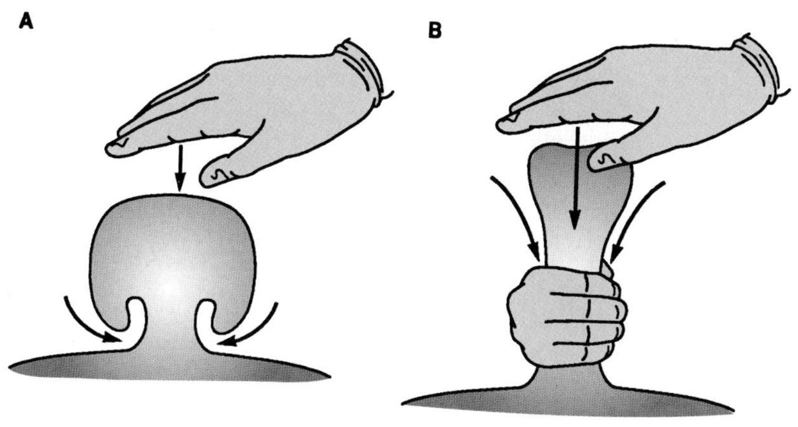

FIGURE 73.19 Reduction of a hernia by taxis. (*A*) Applying pressure on the hernia directly occludes the neck. (*B*) Elongating the neck of the hernia while applying pressure allows reduction.

However, intestinal obstruction does not occur (Fig. 73.20). The overlying skin may be discolored.

The herniated bowel wall is exposed by opening the sac. The neck of the sac is enlarged to allow delivery of the bowel into the wound. The gangrenous patch is excised and the bowel wall reconstituted. The hernia is then repaired.

Massive Hernia

In these defects, a large portion of the abdominal contents is situated within the hernia. These hernias have usually been present for many years, and because of chronicity, the contents of the hernia have lost their "right of domain" within the abdomen. Reduction of the hernia with replacement of contents into the abdominal cavity and repair of the hernia can increase the intraabdominal tension tremendously, resulting in an abdominal compartment syndrome. Problems often affect the skin overlying a massive hernia. The skin can become edematous and cellulitis can develop.[28] It is imperative that the skin over the hernia be in healthy condition before the hernia is repaired.

Some authors recommend the use of pneumoperitoneum when returning contents to the abdominal cavity is likely to be difficult.[29] The maneuver involves injecting 500 to 1,500 mL of air every 1 to 3 days for about 3 weeks before the repair. This technique is designed to stretch the abdominal wall so that it can accommodate the bowel that has lost its right of domain. However, the injected gas can enter the hernial sac, distending the sac and stretching the abdominal cavity but little.

The repair of these hernias requires opening the sac and reducing the contents into the abdomen. Because the defect is usually large, a prosthetic repair is most appropriate.

GROIN HERNIAS

Edoardo Bassini[30] described the principle of reinforcement of the posterior wall of the inguinal canal in 1887. It is generally agreed that Bassini ushered in the modern era of inguinal hernia repair. His scientific approach to the problem led to the development of several distinct steps essential for the procedure (Table 73.2).

The desire to reduce recurrence rates led to the development of numerous variations of Bassini's operation that have undergone phases of popularity. The fact that so many types of repair have been described attests to the frequency of the major complication of the surgical procedure, recurrence of the hernia. In the mid-20th century, a variety of repairs were developed; strengthening of the endoabdominal fascia was claimed to be an integral component of all of them. As noted in the section on anatomy, a consistent definition of the endoabdominal fascia was then and is now still lacking. Nevertheless, McVay (Cooper's ligament) and Shouldice repairs became especially popular and were until recently the most commonly used and most successful (lowest rate of recurrence) techniques. Although it is true that the Bassini repair and its modifications were associated with a much lower incidence of recurrence than historical controls, surgeons realized that the results were far from perfect, particularly when performed outside specialty centers. Indeed,

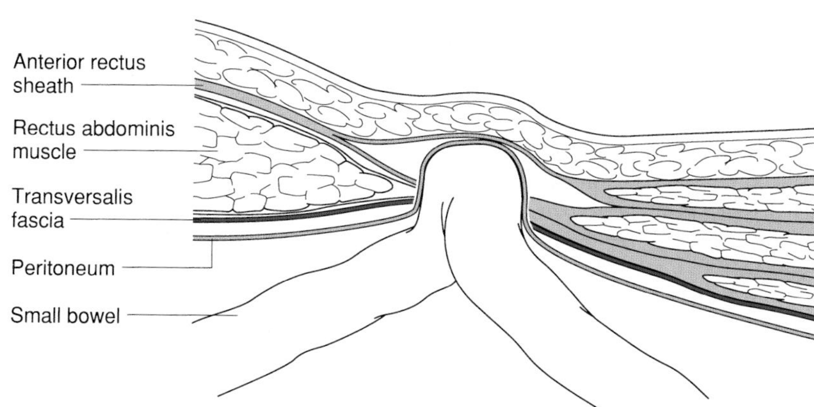

FIGURE 73.20 Richter's hernia. Part of the bowel wall herniates through the defect in the abdominal wall.

TABLE 73.2 TREATMENT

ESSENTIAL STEPS FOR THE INGUINAL HERNIA REPAIR

1. Complete division of the external oblique aponeurosis and the transversalis fascia
2. Differentiation between indirect and direct defects
3. Isolation of the spermatic cord
4. Ligation and removal of the sac at the deep inguinal ring flush with the peritoneum
5. Oblique reconstruction of the inguinal canal with an anterior and posterior wall and an internal and external ring

population-based studies, such as those conducted by the Rand Corporation, confirmed recurrence rates to be in the 10% to 30% range, with the lesser figure applying to the repair of simple, small hernias and the higher rate to the repair of recurrent hernias.[31]

The excessive recurrence rate is not surprising because the Bassini repair and its modifications all create tension at the suture line when muscle and fascia are sutured to close the defect. The tension thus created has been considered the root cause of late failure (recurrence), pain, and disability.

Four developments in the latter half of the 20th century significantly decreased morbidity and favorably influenced the recurrence rate to the currently accepted level of less than 5%: routine use of prosthetic materials, widespread acceptance of the "tension-free" concept, realization that the preperitoneal space can be used for hernia repair, and therapeutic laparoscopy.

Prosthetic materials: The use of prostheses for many medical applications increased during the 20th century. The development of a wide variety of materials that can be used for abdominal wall reconstruction now makes it possible to individualize the selection of a prosthesis so that they can be used in almost all clinical situations.[32] The materials that have emerged as suitable for routine use in hernia surgery include polypropylene, either monofilament (Marlex, Prolene) or polyfilament (Surgipro); Dacron (Mersilene); and expanded polytetrafluoroethylene (e-PTFE) (Gore-Tex). Absorbable prosthesis such as polyglactin are not durable and have no place in groin hernia surgery. The newer biologic prostheses made of human cadaver skin, porcine cross-linked dermal collagen or porcine small-intestinal submucosa are more expensive and have no advantage over synthetic material for an uncomplicated hernia repair. However, they can be useful in infected groin wounds.[33]

Widespread acceptance of the "tension-free" concept: For a consistently successful inguinal hernia repair to be achieved, the reconstruction of the posterior wall of the inguinal canal is necessary in addition to closure of the defect through which the hernia protrudes. Techniques, both conventional and laparoscopic, have been developed that avoid the creation of tension by using a nonabsorbable prosthesis to reconstruct the inguinal floor, with or without closure of the defect itself. Reported rates of recurrence are lower than those with previous techniques that include tension at muscle and fascia suture lines. In their series of 4,000 patients, Lichtenstein et al.,[35] recorded a recurrence rate of 0.1%, including procedures for recurrent hernias; other complications occurred only rarely. Studies in which this technique was used by surgeons outside Lichtenstein's clinic have confirmed a low recurrence rate, which indicates that the good results were not necessarily related to the fact that the operation was performed by an enthusiastic proponent in a highly specialized hernia unit.[36–38]

Use of the preperitoneal space: The key to the preperitoneal hernia repair is the placement of a large prosthesis in the preperitoneal space on the abdominal side of the defect in the transversalis fascia rather than on the external oblique aponeurosis. The preperitoneal space can be entered through a variety of incisions (lower midline, paramedian, Pfannenstiel, groin and laparoscopic). The hernia defect itself may or may not be closed, depending on the preference of the surgeon. Unlike the extraperitoneal repair, in which abdominal pressure is a major contributing factor in recurrence, the preperitoneal repair makes use of the abdominal pressure to help fix the mesh material against the abdominal wall, which adds strength to the repair.[39,40] A variety of sutured and nonsutured repairs have been introduced that are based on the theory that ". . . by covering the hernia defect and adjacent areas far beyond the limits of the defect with the mesh, the intraabdominal pressure becomes an efficient means of fixation of the mesh over the site of the hernia rather than a factor in recurrence."[42–44]

Laparoscopic techniques: At about the same time that surgeons were beginning to accept the routine use of a prosthetic mesh for repair of an inguinal hernia, laparoscopic cholecystectomy was introduced. With laparoscopy, the intraabdominal space can be accessed with minimal perioperative discomfort—hence the interest in intraabdominal herniorrhaphy under laparoscopic guidance. The advantage of laparoscopic herniorrhaphy over a conventional, open procedure is a matter of intense study at present.

Etiology, Epidemiology, and Natural History

Spontaneous abdominal hernias occur in about 5% of the world population over a lifetime. The prevalence may be as high as 10%.[33] Inguinal hernias are the most common of all the abdominal wall hernias and constitute about 80% of cases, with 800,000 inguinal hernia repairs in the United States in 2003.[45] Femoral hernias occur in about 5% of instances. Incisional, umbilical, epigastric, and a host of miscellaneous hernia types make up the other 15%. The majority of inguinal hernias occur in male subjects, with a male-to-female ratio of 7:1. With femoral hernias, a female predominance of about 1.8:1 is seen.

The prime cause of an indirect inguinal hernia is a patent processus vaginalis. The processus vaginalis is the direct result of the migration of the testis from its abdominal location to the scrotum, which is completed by about 28 weeks of gestation. Normally, the processus becomes obliterated in the first few months of life. If all or part of the processus remains patent, the defect can give rise to an indirect inguinal hernia, a scrotal hydrocele, or an encysted hydrocele of the cord or hydrocele of the canal of Nuck in a female patient. The congenital etiology of indirect inguinal hernias has resulted in controversy over the incidence of bilaterality of groin hernias. In a 38-year follow-up of 1,944 patients, investigators found a contralateral lesion in 15.8%.[46] In a large series of patients with hernias occurring in childhood, others reported that the patent processus vaginalis closed over a period of time in most cases.[47] In premature babies, both sides were patent. In the neonatal period, the contralateral side was patent in 60% of cases, but by the age of 2 years, only 40% of the children had a patent processus vaginalis. This 40% rate persists into adult life, but in only 20% of these cases does symptomatic hernia develop; the other 20% have a lifelong patent processus that does not produce any symptoms.[46,47]

The myopectineal orifice of Fruchaud (see Fig. 73.1) is an area of transversalis fascia that is not protected by the posterior rectus sheath or by muscle. This is an area of potential weakness through which all groin hernias emerge. Some degree of protection is afforded by the shutter mechanism, whereby with increased intraabdominal pressure the curved fibers of the internal oblique and the falx inguinalis flatten and move toward the inguinal ligament. Contraction of the transversus abdominis muscle also pulls up and tenses the crura of the internal ring.

Hernias are also caused by a mechanical disparity between visceral pressure and resistance of the abdominal musculature. Causes of increased abdominal pressure include coughing, constipation, prostatism, pregnancy, and unusual exertion (especially lifting heavy weights). Under these circumstances, when a patent processus vaginalis is present or the endoabdominal fascia is attenuated, hernia results. The sudden onset of a painful hernia in a young person after lifting a heavy weight is usually associated with a patent processus vaginalis. This potential space expands suddenly like a collapsed balloon, giving rise to the notion the patient "ruptured" himself. In older persons, the abdominal muscles and fascia weaken with the aging process, so even moderate effort may be sufficient to produce a hernia. Although obesity has traditionally been regarded as a causative factor, this is probably not as true for inguinal hernias as it is for other abdominal hernias.

The fascia transversalis, like other fascial tissue, derives its strength from collagen fibers that are continually being produced and reabsorbed. A disturbance of this balance results in attenuation of the fascia. Congenital defects, such as occur in Marfan, Ehlers-Danlos, and Hunter-Hurler syndromes, can predispose to hernia formation. It appears that certain lifestyles can lead to defective collagen production, including the now rare condition of lathyrism, in which a patient ingests large quantities of foods, particularly peas, that contain e_1-aminopropionitrile.[48] This substance prevents covalent cross-linking between and within forming collagen molecules, so that collagen is produced that is reduced in tensile strength. An association between cigarette smoking and groin hernias has also been demonstrated.[49] Levels of circulating serum elastolytic activity have been shown to be significantly greater in patients who smoke.

The natural history of an untreated inguinal hernia is poorly understood, with almost no modern data available. This lack of information is a consequence of the commonly held opinion that all inguinal hernias should be repaired when diagnosed to prevent complications. In fact, the risk of a major complication, such as incarceration, obstruction, or strangulation, is very low. It has been estimated that an 18-year-old man has a 0.272 lifetime risk of strangulation and that the risk for a 75-year-old is 0.034.[50] This extremely low incidence of major complications may offset the ninefold to 10-fold increase in mortality in patients presenting with intestinal obstruction in comparison with nonobstructed patients. Other investigators have reported the annual risk of a major complication to be 0.002 to 0.0037.[51] Based on this incidence, coupled with the life expectancy in 1971 and the operative mortality rates for uncomplicated and complicated hernia repair in the Medicare population in 1971, elective operation was associated with a greater loss of life than no operation was. A randomized, prospective trial is currently accruing patients to compare operative management versus careful observation for minimally symptomatic patients with inguinal hernias. This study will provide the data needed to understand the natural history of an inguinal hernia, so that the indications for elective repair can be better defined.

Classification

Groin hernias may be primary or recurrent. Hernias are classified as inguinal and femoral, the inguinal hernias being further subdivided into direct and indirect hernias (Fig. 73.21)

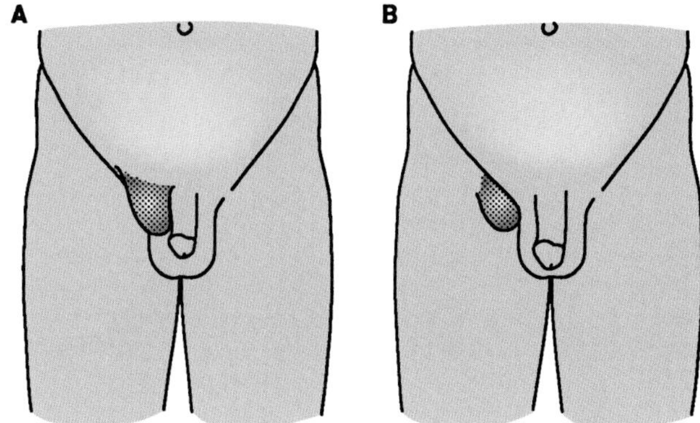

FIGURE 73.21 (*A*) Inguinal hernia. This presents above the inguinal ligament and extends below it. (*B*) Femoral hernia. This presents below the inguinal ligament.

(Table 73.3). An indirect hernia occurs as a protrusion of abdominal contents through the internal ring, lateral to the inferior epigastric vessels, into the inguinal canal. Indirect inguinal hernias are situated within the spermatic cord and therefore may extend into the scrotum. In female patients, the hernia follows the round ligament and may present as a swelling in the labium. A direct hernia is a protrusion through the triangle of Hesselbach medial to the inferior epigastric vessels. These hernias develop through an area where the endoabdominal fascia is not protected by overlying muscle. Direct hernias do not usually involve the cord, as they tend to protrude forward. However, they occasionally track alongside the cord down the entire length of the inguinal canal and even enter the scrotum. For this reason, the only absolute distinction between a direct and an indirect hernia is the relationship to the inferior epigastric vessels. A femoral hernia protrudes through the femoral canal, which is bordered by the inguinal ligament superiorly, the pubic ramus medially and inferiorly, and the femoral vein laterally. This hernia presents below the

TABLE 73.3 CLASSIFICATION

NYHUS CLASSIFICATION OF GROIN HERNIAS

Type	Description
I	Indirect hernia Normal-size internal ring Typically in infants, children, small adults
II	Indirect hernia Dilated internal ring Posterior wall intact Inferior epigastric vessels not displaced Does not extend to the scrotum
III	Posterior wall defect
IIIA	Direct hernia Size not taken into account
IIIB	Indirect hernia Dilated internal ring encroaching on Hesselbach's triangle (massive scrotal, sliding, or pantaloon type)
IIIC	Femoral hernia
IV	Recurrent hernia
IVA	Direct
IVB	Indirect
IVC	Femoral
IVD	Combined

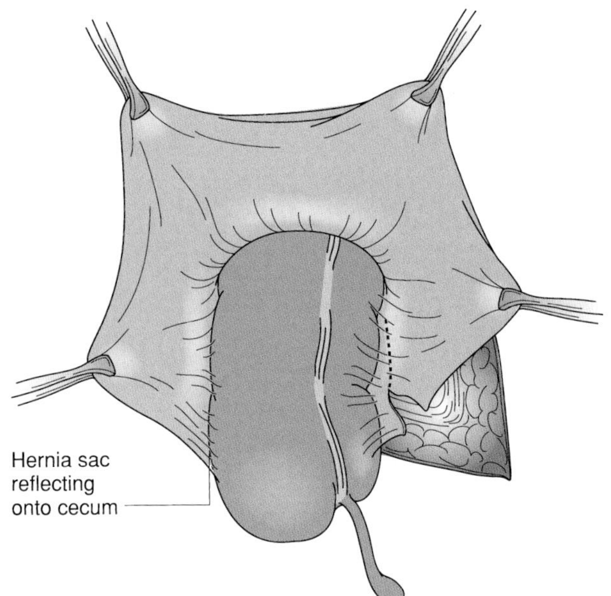

FIGURE 73.22 Sliding hernia (right indirect inguinal).

inguinal ligament. In a sliding hernia, part of the sac is formed by the viscera, on the left side the sigmoid colon or bladder and on the right side the cecum or bladder[52] (Fig. 73.22).

The previous description is regarded as the traditional classification. A more modern classification brings in size and recurrence for a more practical approach.[53]

Clinical Diagnosis

Groin hernias present with a swelling that has a cough impulse. With indirect hernias, the swelling may extend down into the scrotum. The swelling reduces when the patient lies down. Sometimes, the hernia does not reduce easily and the patient has to reduce it manually. Applying pressure over the midinguinal point (midway between the anterior superior iliac spine and the pubic tubercle and just above the inguinal ligament) with the fingertip will control an indirect hernia and prevent it from protruding when the patient strains. A direct hernia will not be controlled with this maneuver. Similarly, if the scrotum is invaginated with the index finger and the tip of the finger is placed through the external inguinal ring into the canal, and the patient is then asked to strain, an indirect hernia will push against the fingertip, whereas a direct hernia will push against the pulp of the finger. It should be noted that the accuracy of this clinical assessment is questioned by many authorities. A femoral hernia presents as a swelling below the inguinal ligament and just lateral to the pubic tubercle (see Fig. 73.21).

Differential Diagnosis

The clinical presentation of a groin hernia, especially when large, is frequently obvious to the examiner. Smaller hernias and recurrent hernias can be confused with a number of different conditions that can be mistaken for a hernia (Table 73.4).

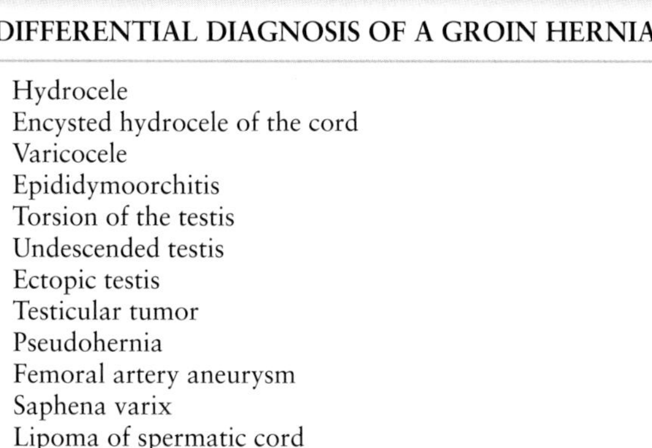
TABLE 73.4 DIAGNOSIS

DIFFERENTIAL DIAGNOSIS OF A GROIN HERNIA

Hydrocele
Encysted hydrocele of the cord
Varicocele
Epididymoorchitis
Torsion of the testis
Undescended testis
Ectopic testis
Testicular tumor
Pseudohernia
Femoral artery aneurysm
Saphena varix
Lipoma of spermatic cord
Inguinal lymphadenopathy
Psoas abscess
Cutaneous lesions (e.g., sebaceous cyst, skin tumor)

A hydrocele extending into the scrotum or an encysted hydrocele of the cord can involve the groin area. The distinguishing features are that the examining hand can get above a hydrocele but not above a hernia and that a hydrocele transilluminates very clearly. A varicocele does not transilluminate, has the characteristic feel of a "bag of worms," and is more tubelike in conformation. Lesions of the testicle may sometimes mimic a hernia, particularly in inflammatory conditions, such as epididymoorchitis. The distinguishing features are intense pain extending down into the scrotum. The testicle itself is enlarged and tender, as is the epididymis. On rectal examination, the seminal vesicles are tender. This condition may be bilateral. Torsion of the testicle is distinguished by the fact that the testicle is absent from the scrotum and the swelling in the groin feels firm. A sonogram reveals a solid mass in the testicle, which has been pulled up because of the torsion. Testicular tumors, if large enough, may extend up to the groin area, but they have a solid feel and sonography can distinguish them.

Pseudohernia is a condition that occurs in patients with denervation of the abdominal wall musculature (e.g., after polio). The abdominal wall muscles bulge forward on straining and have the appearance of a hernia. An aneurysm of the femoral artery may present as a groin swelling but with an expansile impulse and sometimes a bruit. If thrombosis develops in the aneurysm, pulsation may be lost. In this instance, the aneurysm becomes tender. Femoral aneurysms move from side to side but not up and down. A saphena varix usually presents below the inguinal ligament and represents a varicosity of one of the branches of the long saphenous vein as it emerges from the hiatus. Like a hernia, the varix has a cough impulse and becomes more prominent when the patient is standing. Compression over the femoral hiatus obliterates this lesion. The varix is sometimes associated with varicose veins farther down the lower limb. The overlying skin has an associated bluish discoloration.

A lipoma within the spermatic cord is a very common condition and, from anatomic studies and surgical dissection, is now regarded as a hernia of the extraperitoneal fat.[54,55] If found at surgery, the lipoma is removed to avoid a persistent bulge in the inguinal region despite a successful hernia repair.

Enlargement of inguinal lymph nodes may also be mistaken for herniation. Inflammatory nodes are usually tender; metastatic lymphadenopathy is usually not tender. If inguinal lymph nodes are replaced by metastasis, a primary lesion should be looked for in the skin in any part of the lower limb. The perineum and anal canal should also be examined. Lymphadenopathy can also be caused by lymphoma, and groin nodes may be the only site. Lymphadenopathy characteristically appears as a well-circumscribed mass below the inguinal ligament that one can get above with the examining hand. Lymph nodes are solid on ultrasonography, and for this reason, it may be difficult to differentiate nodes from a femoral hernia containing omentum.

Treatment

The current surgical literature suggests that all inguinal hernias should be repaired unless specific contraindications are present. This recommendation is based on the presumption that complications of incarceration, obstruction, and strangulation are greater threats than are the risks of operation. The operative mortality, especially in the elderly, is increased at least ninefold to 10-fold when obstruction occurs.[56–62] However, because of the low incidence of life-threatening complications of groin hernias and the possibility of the development of chronic groin pain in 10% to 12% of patients after herniorrhaphy, the notion that the presence of an inguinal hernia is an indication for repair has come under scrutiny. Until more data are available, the treatment of a groin hernia is surgical unless a serious medical condition precludes repair. Because of the ease with which groin hernias can be repaired under local anesthesia, very few conditions preclude surgery. If it is impossible for the patient to undergo surgery, a truss can be worn. This is a type of belt with an appliance that compresses the area through which the hernia protrudes. Trusses are successful in controlling symptoms in a certain percentage of patients, but complications can develop despite their use.

Open Approach

In the first of the three basic types of hernia repair, the *herniotomy*, the patent processus vaginalis is ligated at its origin at the internal ring and divided, so-called high ligation of the sac. This procedure is used for Nyhus type I hernias, such as those that occur in children. The skin incision starts at the pubic tubercle and is extended laterally. The external oblique aponeurosis is opened in the line of its fibers through the external ring and the lower leaf is freed from the spermatic cord. The spermatic cord is freed from the floor of the inguinal canal and the pubic bone. The genital branch of the genitofemoral nerve and the spermatic vessels are included with the cord. The ilioinguinal and iliohypogastric nerves are usually preserved. The cremasteric fibers are separated, and the hernia sac is dissected from the cord structures to a point proximal to the internal ring. Ligation can be performed at this point (high ligation), followed by division of the neck of the sac. Prior to this the sac can be opened to allow a digital examination of the abdominal cavity and femoral ring. No form of repair is necessary, and an excellent result can be expected.

The second type of hernia operation is the *herniorrhaphy*, which is used to repair Nyhus type II or III hernias. The sac is ligated at its origin. Large scrotal hernias are transected at the midpoint of the canal, and the distal sac is left *in situ*. The area of weakness in the posterior wall is then reinforced with the patient's own tissues. The Bassini, Shouldice, and McVay repairs are good examples of this type of operation.

In the Bassini repair, the transversus abdominis aponeurosis together with the transversalis fascia is sutured to the shelving edge of the inguinal ligament with nonabsorbable interrupted sutures (Fig. 73.23). In the Shouldice repair, the transversalis fascia is divided from the internal ring to the pubic tubercle and lifted from the peritoneum. The fascia is then overlapped with two rows of running sutures (Fig. 73.24). Two further rows of sutures are applied to bring the transversus abdominis muscle to the shelving edge of the inguinal ligament. Although the suture material originally used for this repair was stainless steel wire, other nonabsorbable materials, such as Prolene, are now used. The McVay repair (Fig. 73.25) addresses both inguinal and femoral hernias. The central attenuated portion of the inguinal floor is excised. Cooper's ligament must be clearly identified. The inguinal floor is then repaired by approximating the transversus abdominis aponeurosis and transversalis fascia to Cooper's ligament between the pubic tubercle and the femoral vein. More laterally, the transversus abdominis muscle and transversalis fascia are approximated to the iliopubic tract and femoral sheath up to the internal ring.

A relaxing incision is necessary for repairs of large indirect hernias and whenever the McVay repair is used. Failure to make a relaxing incision has been implicated in a greater incidence of recurrence. The relaxing incision is made in the internal lamina of the anterior rectus sheath in a vertical direction and is extended 1 to 2 cm above the pubis to a level opposite the internal ring (see Fig. 73.25). The resulting defect in the sheath is protected posteriorly by the body of the rectus muscle, which prevents herniation at that site.

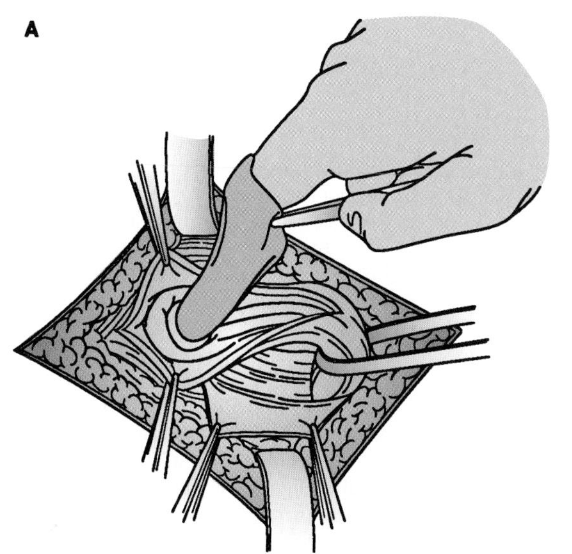

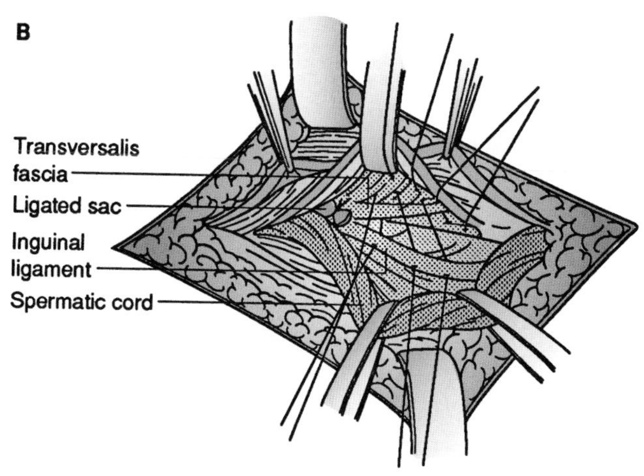

FIGURE 73.23 Bassini repair.

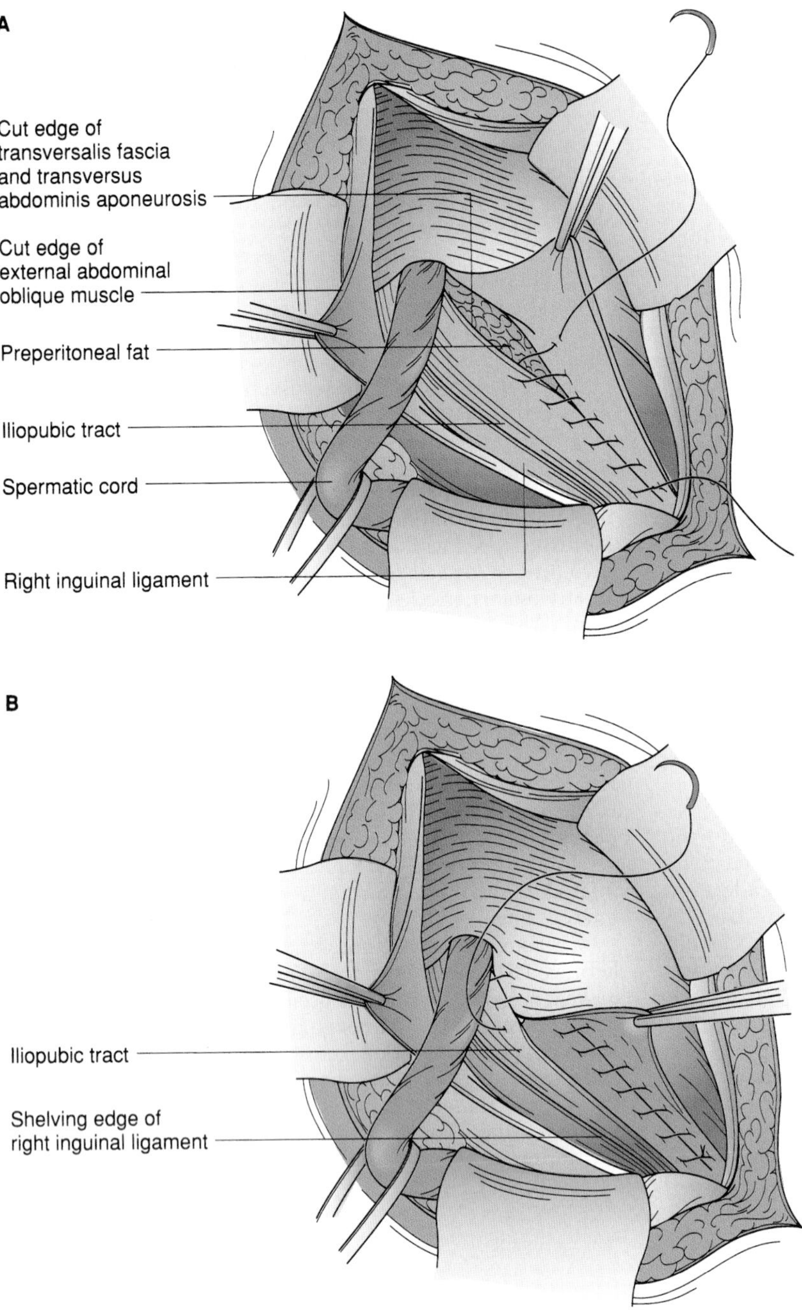

FIGURE 73.24 Shouldice repair.

In the third type of repair, *hernioplasty*, the hernial sac is ligated at the neck, as described previously. Alternatively, the sac may be simply inverted. The proponents of not opening the sac feel that with this method the patient experiences less pain because the highly innervated peritoneum has not been violated.[63] The repair then consists of reinforcement of the posterior abdominal wall defect with synthetic material. The prosthesis can be placed either as a plug to invert the hernial sac or as a patch, which may be an underlay, overlay, or a combined type (Fig. 73.26). The overlay patch technique is currently the most popular.[34,37,63–65]

In the Lichtenstein operation[34] (Fig. 73.27), the incision starts at the pubic tubercle and is extended laterally for about 10 cm. The exposure of the cord is as described previously. The hernial sac is dealt with and then the defect is repaired with synthetic mesh. The upper leaf of the external oblique aponeurosis is separated from the underlying internal oblique muscle and anterior rectus sheath so that the mesh will be able to overlap 2 to 3 cm above the upper border of Hesselbach's triangle. A 15 × 11-cm sheet of polypropylene mesh is used, the medial end of which is rounded to the shape of the medial corner of the inguinal canal. This medial end is sutured to the aponeurotic tissue over the pubic bone with a 2-0 polypropylene suture so that it overlaps the pubic bone by 2 cm. The periosteum of the bone is avoided. The suture is continued to attach the lower edge of the prosthesis to the shelving edge of the inguinal ligament up to a point just lateral to the internal ring. If a femoral hernia is present, the posterior surface of the mesh is sutured to Cooper's ligament after the inferior edge has been attached to the inguinal ligament. This closes the femoral canal. The repair is then continued by securing the superior border of the mesh to the internal oblique aponeurosis and the anterior rectus sheath. A slit is cut in the lateral end of the mesh to produce a narrow (one third-width) tail below and a wider

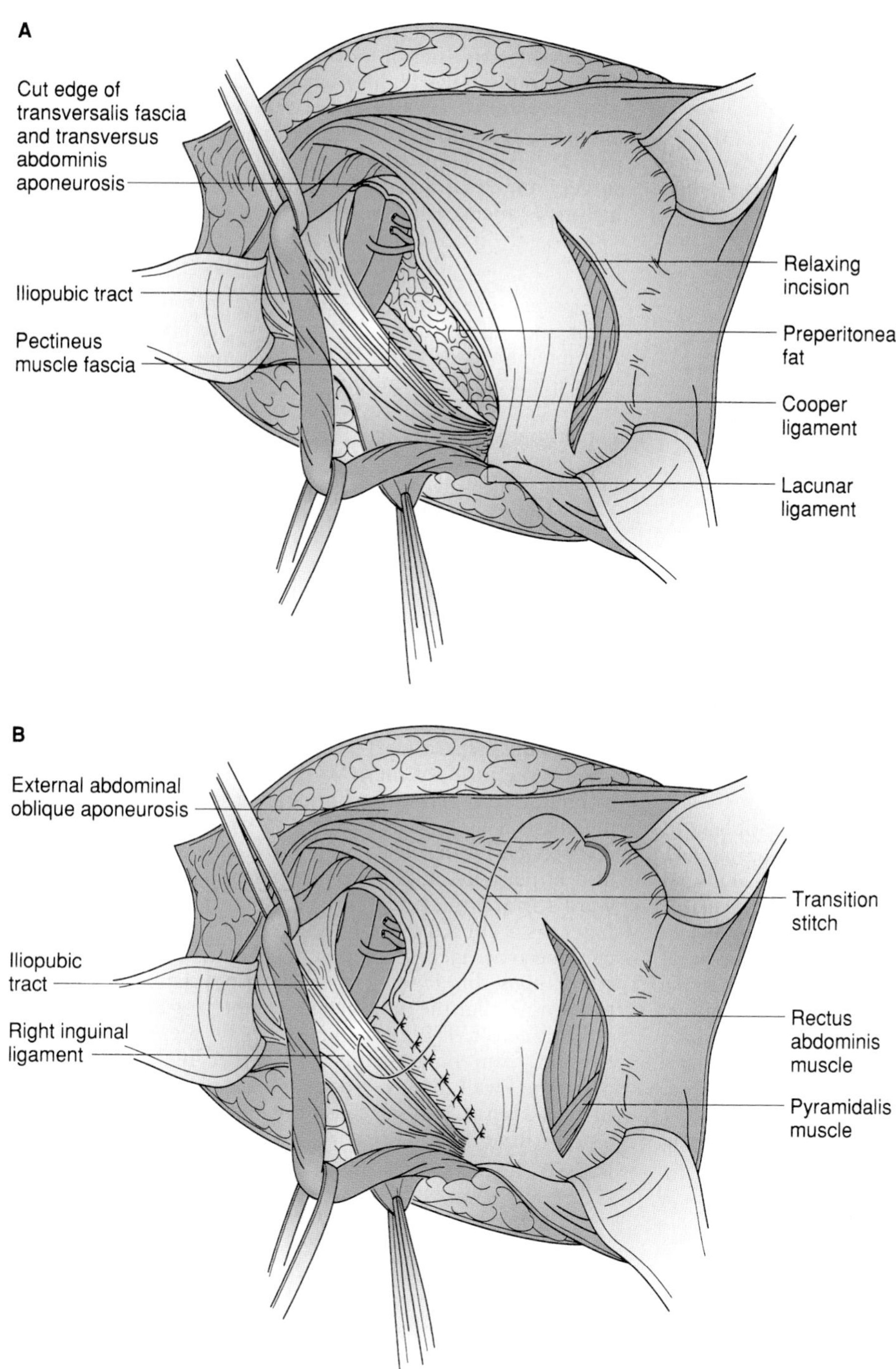

FIGURE 73.25 McVay (Cooper's ligament) repair.

(two thirds-width) tail above. The spermatic cord is positioned between the two tails. The wider tail is placed over the narrow one and held there with a hemostat. The cord is retracted downward and the upper edge of the patch is sutured to the internal oblique muscle and anterior rectus sheath, with care taken to avoid injury to the iliohypogastric nerve. This part of the repair is performed with upward retraction of the internal oblique, so that when it is released, there will be no tension on the repair. With a single polypropylene suture, the lower edges of the two tails are now fixed to the shelving margin of the inguinal ligament, so that a new, snug-fitting internal ring is created. Any excess prosthesis is trimmed, with 4 to 5 cm left lateral to the internal ring. The external oblique aponeurosis is closed to re-create the external ring. The wound is closed in layers.

During a 25-year period, investigators used the tension-free method to repair bilateral hernias in 2,953 patients.[66] Postoperative pain was mild and the recovery period short. The recurrence rate was 0.1%. Repair of bilateral hernias via the laparoscopic approach has also yielded excellent results.

Femoral hernias can be repaired from a lower approach, in which a vertical incision is made over the femoral triangle in the upper thigh. The hernia is approached from below the inguinal ligament and reduced, and then the defect is closed by suturing the inguinal ligament to Cooper's ligament from below. With the Lichtenstein technique, a rolled plug of mesh

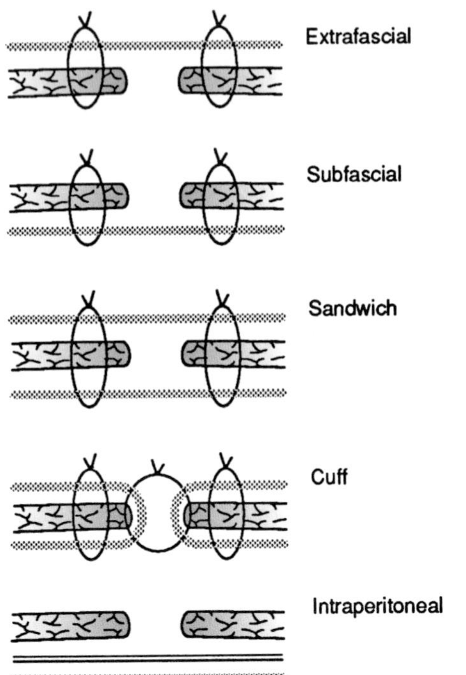

FIGURE 73.26 Various techniques for placing an abdominal wall prosthesis.

can be inserted into the defect and sutured to the periphery of the inguinal ligament and Cooper's ligament.[67] Alternatively, the repair can be carried out from above via an inguinal approach, as in the McVay repair. The posterior floor of the inguinal canal is dissected out, and Cooper's ligament is repaired after the hernia has been reduced. A third type of femoral hernia repair is the preperitoneal repair. Access to the preperitoneal space is gained through a midline abdominal incision. Femoral hernias are more common in women and often present with an acute episode of incarceration, intestinal obstruction, or strangulation, so that emergency surgery is necessary. It can be difficult to reduce the hernia at surgery, and is not uncommon to have to divide the inguinal ligament to obtain greater freedom to perform this reduction.

Another important factor contributing to the well-being of the patient after hernia is the use of local anesthesia.[68,69] Throughout the world, local anesthesia has become the standard method of anesthesia for this operation. When local anesthesia is used, the procedure can be carried out on an outpatient basis. The patient can walk immediately after the surgery and return to normal activities in a day. Hernias in high-risk patients can be safely repaired under local anesthesia.

Preperitoneal Approach

The preperitoneal space is situated between the transversalis fascia and the peritoneum. The transversus abdominis muscle and its aponeurosis and fascial coverings are probably the most important layer in the groin. The aim of hernia repairs should be to return this layer to normal. By strengthening the preperitoneal area, this goal can be achieved.

An operation may be performed through a lower midline incision, which gives one access to the preperitoneal space.[40] The peritoneum can be dissected away from the undersurface of the transversalis fascia to expose the defect through which the hernia protrudes. Alternatively, a lateral rectus approach via a transverse incision can be used to expose the defect. A few centimeters above the pubic tubercle, the rectus sheath can be opened and the rectus muscle retracted medially.[70] Access is then gained to the preperitoneal space, through which the repair is performed.

In 1983, investigators developed the concept of reinforcement of the preperitoneal layer in the lower abdomen by placing a large piece of mesh in this area.[71] This can be done through a transverse lower abdominal incision.[72–76] A large prosthesis is used that extends far beyond the margins of the myopectineal orifice and envelops the visceral sac. The mesh is held in place by intraabdominal pressure, which pushes outward toward the undersurface of the transversalis fascia. Later, as a consequence of connective tissue ingrowth, the mesh becomes incorporated in the body tissues, which further strengthens this layer. The mesh also adheres to the peritoneum, so that the peritoneum cannot protrude through the parietal defect. This technique works by preventing the peritoneum from bulging outward rather than by repairing abdominal wall defects. No sutures are placed in this method of hernia repair, and it is tension-free. Because the incision for a preperitoneal hernia repair is away from the groin area and directly accesses the preperitoneal space, dissection of the

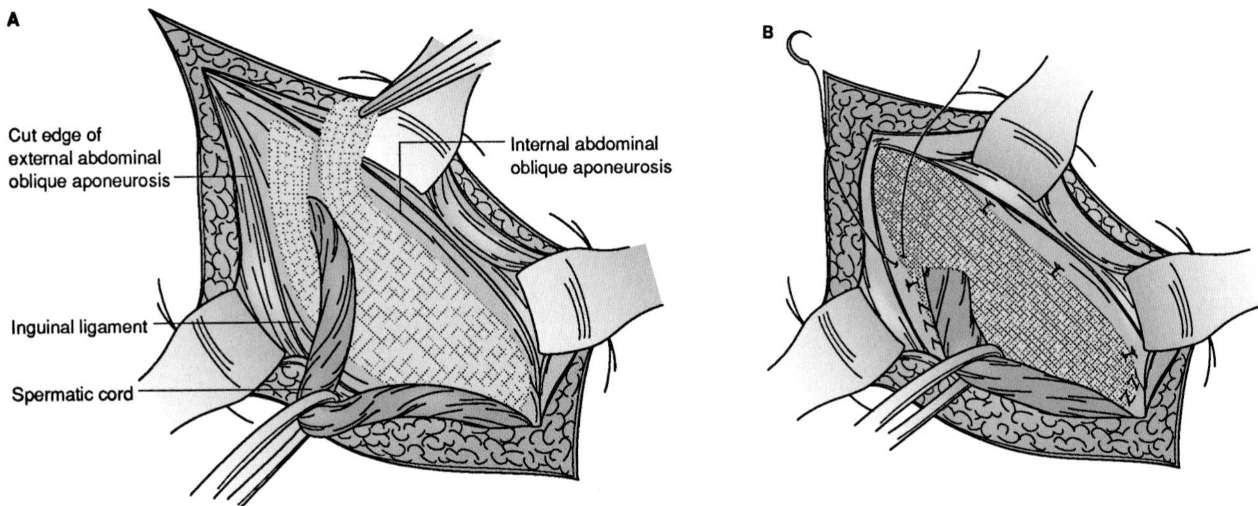

FIGURE 73.27 The Lichtenstein hernioplasty, showing placement of the mesh.

inguinal canal, spermatic cord, or sensory nerves of the groin is not performed. The complications involving these structures that occur with other hernia repairs are very rare with the preperitoneal repair. If the hernial sac is large, it is amputated or inverted beneath a pursestring suture to smooth the external surface of the visceral sac. The distal peritoneal sac is left in place, undissected and attached to the cord. With a sliding indirect hernia, the sac would have to be dissected away from the cord. The mesh is composed of multifilament fibers of Dacron, which is soft, elastic, supple, and rapidly integrated into tissue. Other meshes are not suitable because they are semirigid and buckle when bent in two directions.

In a bilateral repair, the chevron-shaped mesh is usually measured to be transversely 2 cm less than the distance between the anterior superior iliac spines and vertically the distance between the umbilicus and the symphysis pubis. The mesh is placed in the preperitoneal space so that it underlies the rectus muscle for a width of about 2 to 3 cm and extends this same distance above the level of the myopectineal orifice in all directions. The mesh is held in place by sutures attaching it to the undersurface of the abdominal wall.

The preperitoneal or posterior approach for the repair of groin hernias is particularly useful with very large or recurrent hernias.[70] Laparoscopic hernioplasty is an extension of the preperitoneal concept. In many of the laparoscopic repairs, the prosthesis is placed in the preperitoneal space.

Three newer less invasive techniques have been developed to place a mesh in the preperitoneal space. A preperitoneal plug is placed via a conventional groin incision and its edges sutured to the edges of the defect in the transversalis fascia.[42] In the second method, also approached via a groin incision, a bilayered mesh is placed with one layer in the preperitoneal space, and the other in the inguinal canal.[43] In the third procedure, which is done via a small incision over the deep inguinal ring, a bilayered mesh with a reinforcing ring that holds the shape of the mesh is placed entirely within the preperitoneal space.[44] All three of these methods give a recurrence rate of less than 1%. Currently, the Lichtenstein repair is used for 40%, the Mesh plug repair for 25%, the Kugel ring for 8%, the double mesh for 2% and laparoscopic repairs for 15% of all groin hernia repairs in the United States. Traditional sutured repairs now account for less than 10%.[45]

Laparoscopic Approach

The laparoscopic method was introduced into general surgery in the late 1980s for the treatment of gallbladder disease and immediately became popular among patients because it was perceived to be less invasive than conventional open surgery. Many commonly performed open general surgical operations were adapted to be performed laparoscopically and inguinal hernia repair was no exception. The terminology to describe a laparoscopic inguinal herniorrhaphy can be confusing.[77] A laparoscopic preperitoneal hernia repair, in which a laparoscopy is performed and the preperitoneal space is entered with a second incision in the peritoneum, is called a *transabdominal preperitoneal repair,* or TAPP repair. An inguinal hernia repair in which prosthetic material is placed intraperitoneally over the defect under laparoscopic guidance is referred to as an *intraperitoneal onlay mesh repair,* or IPOM repair. The third general type of laparoscopic approach is the *totally extraperitoneal laparoscopic repair,* or TEP repair. Laparoscopy, by definition, implies that the peritoneal cavity has been entered. To refer to this technique as *extraperitoneal* therefore represents a contradiction in terms. However, because a laparoscope and related instruments are used, it is fitting to discuss the extraperitoneal approach along with the other laparoscopic inguinal herniorrhaphies.

The TAPP and the TEP laparoscopic inguinal herniorrhaphies are the most popular. Both are modeled after the conventional preperitoneal operations. The major difference is that the preperitoneal space is entered through three trocar sites rather than through a large conventional incision. The ensuing radical dissection of the preperitoneal space with placement of a large prosthesis is similar to the conventional preperitoneal operation.

Laparoscopic Versus Conventional Herniorrhaphy. Randomized controlled trials as well as meta-analysis of pooled data from these trials have shown that on average patients undergoing laparoscopic herniorrhaphy have less pain initially than open, tension-free herniorrhaphy and return to normal activities sooner.[78–80] The difference is even greater when the comparison is made to non prosthetic repairs. However, the potential advantages of laparoscopic herniorrhaphy must be interpreted in light of the disadvantages, which include complications related to the laparoscopy such as bowel perforation or major vascular injury, potential adhesive complications at sites where the peritoneum has been breached or prosthetic material has been placed, the need for a general anesthetic, and increased cost because of the expensive equipment. On the other hand, the conventional operation can be performed under local anesthesia on an outpatient basis, with minimal risk of intraabdominal injury, and the cost is less. The majority of randomized trials, most of which come from single centers with an interest in laparoscopic herniorrhaphy, demonstrate a recurrence rate similar to a conventional tension-free operation. The notable exception is the highly publicized multicenter trial conducted in the Veterans Administration (VA) comparing a laparoscopic preperitoneal inguinal herniorrhaphy (mostly TEP) with a standardized Lichtenstein approach.[81] Recurrences were more common in the laparoscopic group (87 of 862 patients or 10.1%) than in the open group (41 of 834 patients or 4.9% and this was statistically significant. The significance of the VA may be that it is a better indicator of the "real world" and has caused many to suggest that the operation should be confined to specialty centers. Complication rates have been similar in most series but the severity in the laparoscopic group can be much greater.

Patient Selection. Perhaps the most important element in patient selection has nothing to do with the patient but has to do with the surgeon's skill. Laparoscopic inguinal herniorrhaphy is more challenging technically than a conventional open tension-free procedure. Assuming equivalence for recurrence and complication rates between laparoscopic inguinal herniorrhaphy and a tension-free herniorrhaphy for a given surgeon, all adult patients with inguinal hernias who are candidates for general anesthesia can be considered candidates for laparoscopic inguinal hernia repair. Certain hernia types, such as those that are recurrent, bilateral, or otherwise complicated, are particularly suited for the laparoscopic approach.

Contraindications include intraabdominal infection and coagulopathy. Relative contraindications include intraabdominal adhesions from previous surgery, ascites, or previous retropubic space surgery, because of the increased risk for bladder injury. Severe underlying medical illness is also a relative contraindication because of the added risk of general anesthesia. These patients are better suited for a conventional operation under local anesthesia. An incarcerated sliding scrotal hernia is a relative contraindication, especially when it involves the sigmoid colon, because of the high risk for perforation during the dissection.

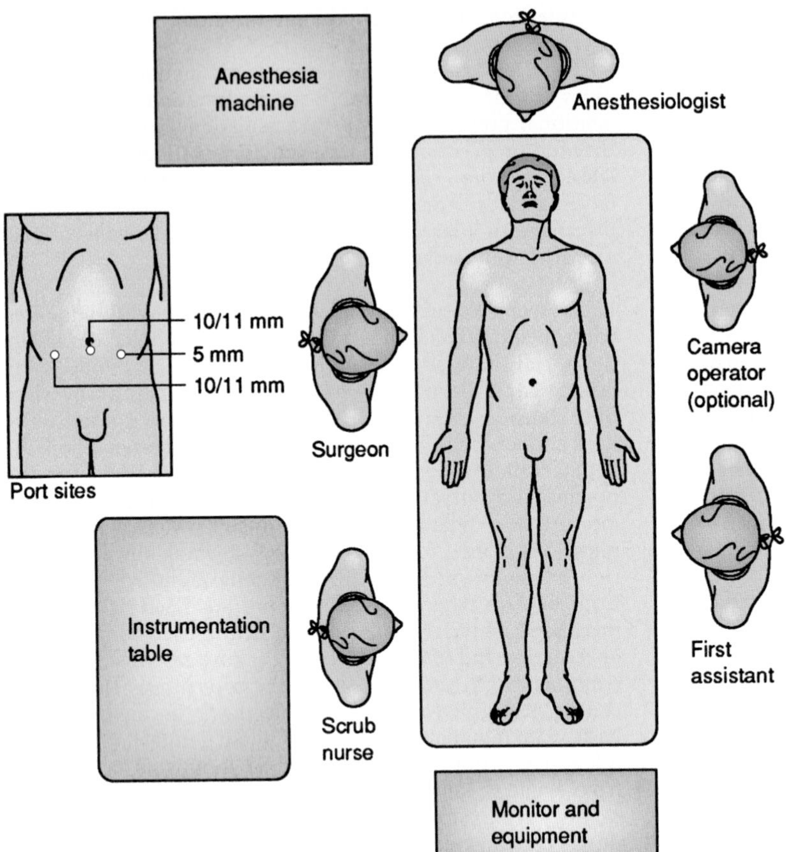

FIGURE 73.28 Typical operative setup and cannula site selection for a transabdominal preperitoneal (TAPP) laparoscopic inguinal herniorrhaphy.

Operative Techniques

TAPP. The procedure is begun with a thorough diagnostic laparoscopy to rule out unrelated pathology and carefully inspect both myopectineal orifices. Two additional cannulae are placed just lateral to the rectus sheath on either side of the umbilicus (Fig. 73.28). For a unilateral hernia, a transverse incision is begun at the lateral side of the medial umbilical ligament and extended to open its lateral leaf to the anterior superior iliac spine. If the medial umbilical ligament appears to compromise exposure, it can be divided. Electrocautery is used to minimize bleeding from the remnants of the embryologic umbilical artery. A radical dissection of the preperitoneal space is then performed with mostly blunt dissection and generous use of electrocautery, as bleeding in this area is particularly troublesome if it interferes with illumination. The ipsilateral and contralateral pubic tubercles, the inferior epigastric vessels, Cooper's ligament, and the iliopubic tract are identified (Fig. 73.29). The cord structures are mobilized, and the peritoneal flap is dissected several centimeters proximal to the bifurcation of the vas deferens and the internal spermatic vessels. Recurrences have been attributed to inadequate mobilization of the peritoneal flap, which does not allow the prosthesis to lie flat in this area. If small, an indirect sac is mobilized away from the cord structures and reduced. If large, the sac is divided at a convenient point distal to the internal ring and only the proximal portion is mobilized. A direct sac readily reduces during the preperitoneal dissection. An easily visible layer of fatty tissue separates the thinned out transversalis fascia lining the defect and the peritoneum.

A large piece of polypropylene mesh (at least 14 × 8 cm) is placed in the preperitoneal space to cover the contralateral pubic tubercle medially and extending onto the anterior abdominal wall superiorly at least 2 cm above the hernia defect, to the anterior superior iliac spine laterally, and over Cooper's ligament inferiorly. Most surgeons prefer to fasten the prosthesis with staples or tacks, but some feel this is not necessary when a large prosthesis is used that widely overlaps the entire myopectineal orifice. Staples or tacks are never placed below the iliopubic tract when lateral to the internal spermatic vessel because of the danger of damage to the important nerves in this area. The last step is to cover the prosthesis with the inferior peritoneal flap. Sutures, tacks, staples, or glue can be used for this. The goal is to isolate the prosthesis from the abdominal viscera rather than to always achieve precise approximation of the peritoneal edges. This is because gaps can form if the peritoneum is closed under tension allowing bowel to migrate into the preperitoneal space. A better option is to secure the inferior peritoneal flap to the transversalis fascia above the prosthesis and leave the superior flap alone.

For bilateral inguinal hernias, the same peritoneal incision and preperitoneal dissections are used. The symphysis pubis is completely exposed so that both preperitoneal dissections communicate with each other. This exposure allows the placement of one large prosthesis (at least 25 × 8 cm) that essentially covers the entire lower pelvis. By not incising the peritoneum between the two medial umbilical ligaments, one avoids the theoretical complication of dividing a patent urachus.

TEP. An incision is made at the umbilicus, as if one were planning to perform open laparoscopy. The rectus sheath is opened on one side and the rectus muscle is retracted laterally. Blunt dissection is then begun in the space between the rectus muscle and the posterior rectus sheath. Once the space is large enough, two additional cannulae are placed in the midline, one approximately 5 cm above the symphysis pubis and the other midway between the umbilicus and the symphysis pubis.

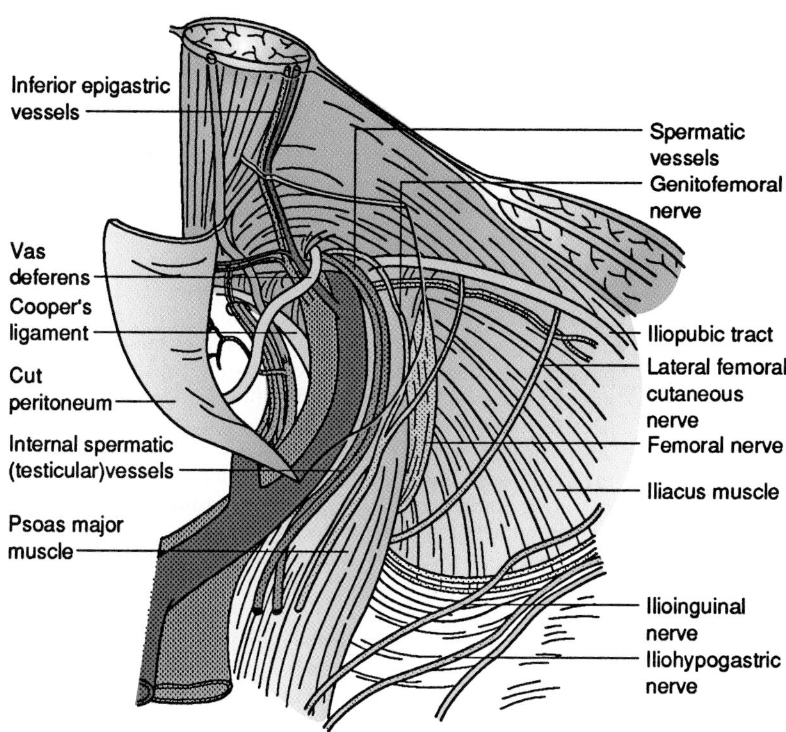

FIGURE 73.29 Important structures that must be identified after a preperitoneal dissection: inferior epigastric vessels, Cooper's ligament, spermatic vessels, vas deferens, iliopubic tract, genitofemoral nerve, femoral nerve, lateral femoral cutaneous nerve, ilioinguinal nerve, iliacus muscle, psoas major muscle.

The dissection of the preperitoneal space is completed under direct vision. The rest of the operation is identical to the TAPP procedure, described previously except that peritoneal closure is not necessary. Popular alternatives are to use a water- or air-filled balloon dissector to perform the preperitoneal dissection and to place the two accessory cannulae on either side of the umbilicus, as in the TAPP procedure, instead of in the midline.

The presumed advantages of the TEP procedure are that the inherent complications of entering the peritoneal cavity, such as intraabdominal organ injury or postoperative bowel obstruction secondary to adhesions or trocar site herniation, are avoided. However, the operative space is limited, and considerable experience is required to become familiar with the anatomy from this perspective. In addition, it is not yet clear whether inadvertent breaches in the peritoneal cavity that are difficult to visualize because of the direction of the optics might negate the potential benefits of this approach.

IPOM. The TAPP and the TEP herniorrhaphies are better considered minimal access procedures rather than minimally invasives because of the extensive dissection required in the preperitoneal space. The IPOM procedure was developed to be a truly minimally operation. By placing the prosthesis one layer deep to the preperitoneal space directly onto the peritoneum, one can eliminate the need for a radical preperitoneal dissection. Initial laparoscopy and accessory cannula placement are the same as in the TAPP procedure. A large piece of prosthetic material is introduced into the peritoneal cavity and secured in place with staples, tacks, or sutures. An attempt is made to use the same landmarks described previously for the TAPP procedure. The main concern is development of the complications of intraperitoneal placement of a prosthesis in contact with intraabdominal organs. For this reason, it should be considered an experimental operation suitable for use in controlled trials only. However, should a completely inert prosthesis be developed it may assume a more important place especially for indirect inguinal hernia for which it seems to be particularly effective.

Complications of Repair

The complications of groin hernia repair are many and varied (Table 73.5), but fortunately uncommon. The complications of inguinal herniorrhaphy can be categorized according to whether they are related to the laparoscopy, the patient, or the herniorrhaphy. Except for the complications unique to laparoscopy, complications occur at similar rates in both laparoscopic and conventional procedures.

Complications Related to Laparoscopy

Vascular Injury. The most serious injuries occur to vessels that reside in the retroperitoneum.[82,83] For all laparoscopic procedures, the risk for major vascular injury that requires operative intervention is 0.05%.[84] The vessels most at risk are the distal aorta, common iliac arteries and veins, and inferior vena cava. Injuries to the renal vessels have also been reported. These vessels are fixed and may be penetrated even if the safety mechanisms of the needle or trocar are working properly. The mesenteric and omental vessels are also at risk, especially in the presence of adhesions. The epigastric arteries may be injured with secondary cannula placement.

The insufflation needle is the most common cause of vascular injury but may be self-limiting; On the other hand, injuries caused by a trocar are usually more obvious and catastrophic. The mortality associated with retroperitoneal injury secondary to trocar insertion ranges from 9% to 36%, even with rapid identification and repair. When suspected, immediate conventional laparotomy is almost always indicated. Most abdominal wall vascular complications occur during the placement of secondary cannulae. Usually, pressure can be applied to bleeding at the trocar site with the cannula. Occasionally, suture ligation is required, which has been simplified by the development of disposable "exit devices" designed to facilitate the placement of fascial sutures. Most of

TABLE 73.5 COMPLICATIONS

COMPLICATIONS OF LAPAROSCOPIC HERNIORRHAPHY

RELATED TO LAPAROSCOPY
- Vascular injury
  - Intraabdominal
  - Retroperitoneal
  - Abdominal wall
  - Gas embolism
- Visceral injury
  - Bowel perforation
  - Bladder perforation
- Trocar site complications
  - Hematoma
  - Hernia
  - Wound infection
  - Keloid
- Bowel obstruction
  - Trocar or peritoneal closure site hernia
  - Adhesions
- Diaphragmatic dysfunction
- Hypercapnia

RELATED TO PATIENT
- Urinary infection
- Ileus
- Nausea and vomiting
- Aspiration pneumonia
- Cardiovascular and respiratory insufficiency

RELATED TO HERNIORRHAPHY
- Recurrence
- Neurologic
  - Iliohypogastric
  - Ilioinguinal
  - Genitofemoral
  - Lateral cutaneous
- Cord and testicular problems
- Wound infection
- Seroma
- Hydrocele
- Hematoma
  - Wound
  - Scrotal
  - Retroperitoneal
- Osteitis pubis
- Prosthetic complications
  - Contraction
  - Erosion
  - Infection
  - Rejection
  - Pain

these complications can be avoided by placing the secondary trocars under direct vision.

Gas Embolism. This is caused by intravascular insufflation.[82,85] It is an uncommon complication, unique to the needle insufflation technique, with an incidence of 0.003%. Careful attention to tests confirming proper peritoneal needle placement will keep the incidence of this complication low.

Visceral Injury. Visceral injuries are uncommon, occurring in 0.05% to 0.4% of all laparoscopic procedures, but they have a mortality rate of 5%. The most common means of injury is the insufflation needle. Simple repair laparoscopically is usually possible as most are self-limiting. If the injury is caused by a trocar, formal repair of the injury will be needed. The injury can be repaired laparoscopically if the skill of the laparoscopic surgeon is sufficient. Otherwise laparotomy is mandatory. Quite often, these injuries goes unnoticed at the time of insult, so that visceral injury is the most common cause of late morbidity and mortality associated with laparoscopic access. Patients typically present with peritonitis and sepsis 2 days to 1 week after surgery.

Bladder Injury. This complication is possible during peritoneal access but is rare, usually the result of failure to decompress a distended bladder. Less commonly, injury is associated with a congenital bladder abnormality. Bladder injury has not been reported with the open access technique. When bladder injury occurs, it is usually obvious. Urine is withdrawn into the syringe, or blood and gas are noticed in the urine if the patient is catheterized. A minor injury can be treated conservatively with postoperative decompression via an indwelling catheter. When the injury is caused by a trocar, formal bladder repair is usually necessary.

Bowel Obstruction. This problem plagued the developmental stages of laparoscopic inguinal herniorrhaphy for two reasons. First, the importance of closing trocar sites at the fascial level if greater than 5 mm was not appreciated resulting in the occasional patient with an incarcerated or strangulated ventral hernia at the trocar site resulting in the clinical presentation of a bowel obstruction.[86,87] There are now several different types of reusable and disposable appliances designed to facilitate trocar site fascial closure which should minimize the incidence of these hernias (Fig. 73.30). The second is inadequate peritoneal closure over the prosthesis, which allows bowel to migrate into the preperitoneal space also resulting in intestinal obstruction. Steps taking to avoid tension at the peritoneal closure site (see TAPP technique section) have decreased this problem. Theoretically the TEP procedure eliminates the possibility of this complication because the abdomen is not entered. However, inadvertent breaches of the peritoneum during a TEP herniorrhaphy are common especially in patients with thin peritoneum or those that have scar tissue associated with previous lower abdominal surgery. These peritoneal lacerations can be difficult to recognize because they are not in the visual field of the limited working space and indeed intestinal obstruction has been reported.[88]

Diaphragmatic Dysfunction. Phrenic nerve palsy has been reported with a variety of laparoscopic procedures; it is usually transient but has been known to require a short period of mechanical ventilation. Stretching during the pneumoperitoneum probably causes this complication.

Hypercapnia. This is the result of inadequate compensatory ventilation, given the fact that, in the vast majority of laparoscopic procedures, carbon dioxide is used as the insufflating agent.

Complications Related to the Patient

Urinary Retention. This occurs in a significant number of patients after herniorrhaphy. Older age and a history of urinary symptoms are often associated. General anesthesia, overhydration with intravenous fluid, and opiates has also been implicated as predisposing factors. Treatment consists of repeated bladder catheterization until normal voiding resumes.[89]

Ileus. Ileus can be seen with either the conventional or the laparoscopic procedure but is more common with the latter.

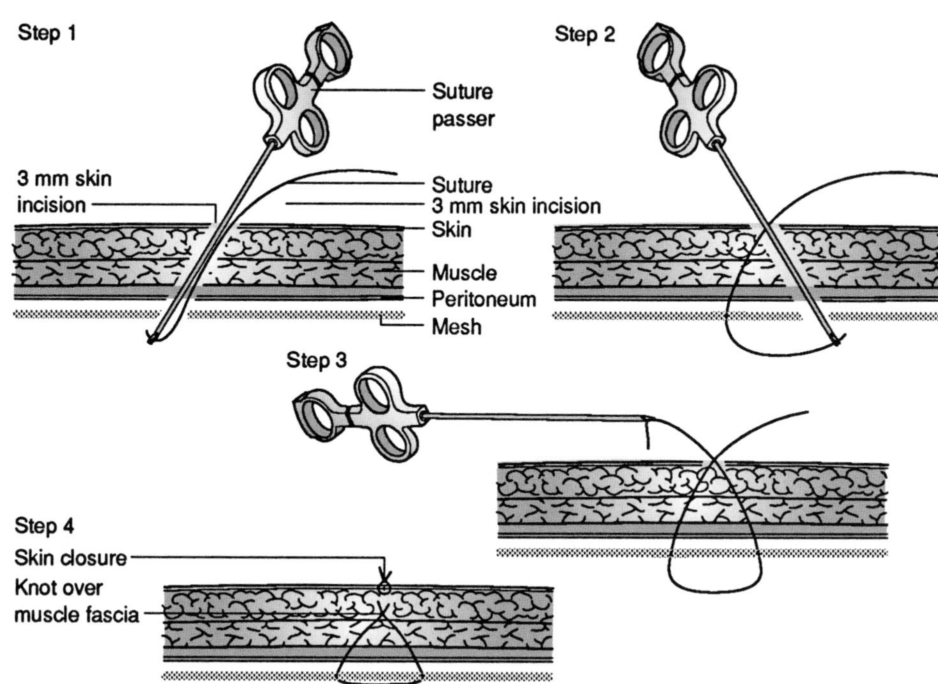

FIGURE 73.30 Fixation of prosthesis to the peritoneal surface of the abdominal wall with use of a suture passer. Step 1: The suture passer device with a heavy nonabsorbable suture is passed through a 3-mm stab incision in the skin at an oblique angle. The device and suture traverse the entire abdominal wall and then the prosthesis. Once the peritoneal cavity is entered, the suture is released and the passer is withdrawn back into the subcutaneous tissue. Step 2: The device is redirected at a different angle through the abdominal wall and prosthesis and the suture is grasped. Step 3: The suture is pulled out of the abdominal cavity so that the two free ends are extracorporeal. Step 4: The suture is tied with the knot resting on the fascia. The skin is then closed.

Treatment is symptomatic, and spontaneous resolution is the rule. Nasogastric decompression is occasionally needed.

Complications Related to the Herniorrhaphy

Recurrence. The shift from the routine use of non prosthetic techniques for the repair of an inguinal hernia to the acceptance of the tension-free concept observed in the last part of the twentieth century resulted in a marked decrease in the recurrence rate.[90] Recurrence rates of 2% or less are now routinely reported from specialty centers performing either laparoscopic or conventional tension-free repairs.[91] Although the recurrence rate for hernia repairs is less than 1% at the Shouldice Clinic, others have not been able to duplicate this outstanding record with this or any of the other nonprosthetic repairs.[92] A recent study from the VA reported a higher recurrence rate at 2 years (4% for Lichtenstein and 10% for laparoscopy) and may be more reflective of the general population outside of specialty centers.[81]

A consistent definition of a recurrent hernia does not exist because of the difficulty in differentiating a lipoma of the cord, seroma, or an expansile bulge of the internal oblique muscle from a true hernia recurrence. A hernia should not be classified recurrent unless there is a visible bulge or there is unequivocal evidence of a hernia by an imaging modality such as ultrasound, CT or magnetic resonance imaging (MRI). This is especially important for patients who present with pain after their hernia repair because their pain is likely due to a preoperative condition or a postinguinal herniorrhaphy pain syndrome and might be exacerbated by further groin surgery. Femoral recurrences are occasionally seen after a Lichtenstein repair because the femoral canal is not routinely closed with the classic technique.

The general principle for managing recurrent hernias depends on the original repair. The logical approach is to perform the herniorrhaphy in the space that has not been dissected. If the patient had a previous conventional repair then a preperitoneal repair is best chosen. On the other hand, if the index operation was a preperitoneal one, then a repair that is performed in the conventional inguinal space is best. The dissection of the preperitoneal space after a failed herniorrhaphy has been performed there is particularly challenging with significant risk for vascular, neurologic, and bladder injury. It is not for the uninitiated.

Postherniorrhaphy Groin Pain. Now that the recurrence rate has been brought down to a minimum using modern hernioplasty techniques, chronic postoperative groin pain syndromes have emerged as the biggest issue facing inguinal hernia surgeons. Poobalan et al.[93] published a critical review of inguinal herniorrhaphy studies between 1987 and 2000. The frequency of at least some long-term groin pain was as high as 53% at 1 year (range: 0% to 53%). On average, moderate or severe postinguinal herniorrhaphy groin pain probably occurs in about 10%.[94] Perhaps the most important single determination for the postherniorrhaphy patient is to decide if the pain is the same or different from that which brought the hernia to the attention of the physician in the first place. There are varieties of conditions that cause groin pain (Table 73.6). CT, ultrasonography, herniography, laparoscopy, and MRI all have their place in the evaluation of these patients. MRI is perhaps the most beneficial because of its ability to differentiate between muscle tear, osteitis pubis, bursitis, and stress fracture. Strain of the adductor muscle complex (adductor longus, brevis, and magnus and gracilis muscles) is commonly overlooked in this group.

True postherniorrhaphy groin pain should be divided into two types: (a) nociceptive pain, which is caused by tissue damage and is further subdivided into somatic and visceral and (b) neuropathic pain, which means direct nerve damage. Somatic pain is the most common and is usually caused by damage to ligaments, tendons, and muscles. Visceral pain refers to that which is related to a specific visceral function such as urination or ejaculation (see dysejaculation syndrome later). Neuropathic pain is much less common but is important to recognize because surgical treatment is possible if the cause is incorporation of a nerve in staples or suture material. The nerves that are usually involved are the ilioinguinal nerve, the iliohypogastric nerve, both the genital and femoral branches of the genitofemoral nerve, and the lateral cutaneous nerve of the thigh. The former two are especially prone to injury during a

TABLE 73.6 DIAGNOSIS

CONDITIONS OTHER THAN A HERNIA ASSOCIATED WITH GROIN PAIN

Muscle injury
Adductor strains
Tendon injury
Iliopsoas bursitis
Osteitis pubis
Pelvic stress fractures
Snapping hip syndrome
Lumbosacral disorders
Connective tissue disease
Nerve entrapment
Hip disorders
- Synovitis
- Avascular necrosis
- Osteoarthritis
- Legg-Calvé-Perthes disease
- Slipped femoral capital epiphysis
- Osteochondritis dissecans or avascular necrosis of the femoral head
- Acetabular labral tears

Prostatitis
Epididymitis
Nephrolithiasis
Urinary tract infection
Lymphadenitis

conventional herniorrhaphy, whereas the latter are most likely damaged during laparoscopy. A femoral nerve injury is extremely rare and is usually the result of a gross technical misadventure. Pain and/or paraesthesia in their distribution characterize patient's symptoms for the more common nerves. There is significant overlap of these nerves and therefore it is commonly difficult to sort out exactly which nerve is damaged. Both nociceptive and neuropathic pain is best treated initially with reassurance and conservative treatment with antiinflammatory medications and local nerve blocks because commonly these will resolve spontaneously. The only exception might be the patient who complains of severe pain immediately (i.e., in the recovery room). This patient may be best treated by immediate reexploration before scar tissue develops. When groin exploration is required, neurectomy and neuroma excision, adhesiolysis, and foreign body removal (i.e., mesh) are all possibilities. The results are often less than satisfying.

Cord and Testicles

Infertility. The cause of infertility can be related to either the vas deferens or the testicle. The incidence of injury to the vas deferens during inguinal herniorrhaphy has been estimated at 0.3% for adults and between 0.8% to 2.0% for children.[95] Injuries to the vas that may present as an obstruction include division, ligation, clipping, stapling, electrocauterization, devascularization, and scarification. Obstruction is not the only reason why an injury to the vas deferens may lead to infertility. For example, traction injuries during normal cord mobilization may damage the muscular layer of the vas deferens, which then interferes with rapid sperm transfer during ejaculation.[96] Sperm antibodies may develop as a result of extravasation of sperm at an injury site, which is why a unilateral injury can also result in infertility.[97]

Ischemic orchitis. Damage to the blood supply of the testicle can cause ischemic orchitis and testicular atrophy.[98] Ischemic orchitis occurs in about 1% of primary hernioplasties but is much more common with operations performed for recurrent hernias.[99] It manifests as postoperative inflammation of the testicle developing within 1 to 2 days after surgery. The patient has a painfully enlarged testicle that is hard in consistency and associated with low-grade fever. Pain is severe and may last several weeks. Ischemic orchitis is caused by thrombosis of the veins draining the testicle after extensive dissection of the spermatic cord. It is generally accepted that the incidence can be decreased by division of large inguinal-scrotal sacs leaving the distal sac open *in situ* rather than excising it.[100] The majority of patients with testicular swelling as an immediate complication of herniorrhaphy recover without testicular atrophy. In one recent report, testicular atrophy developed in 19 patients among 52,583 primary inguinal hernia repairs (0.036%) and 33 patients among 7,169 recurrent inguinal hernia repairs (0.46%).[99] A substantial number of patients who develop testicular atrophy after inguinal herniorrhaphy have no history of a testicular problem at the time of the index operation. The management of a patient with ischemic orchitis is usually conservative with elevation and antiinflammatory medication. Antibiotics and steroids have been used but their value is unproved.

Miscellaneous. Hydroceles occasionally develop after inguinal herniorrhaphy but the cause is not known and therefore a preventative measure is not possible. The urologic literature suggests that the practice of leaving the distal aspect of an indirect inguinal sac *in situ* rather than removing it should be incriminated but this is not accepted by most experienced hernia surgeons. The treatment is the same as for any other hydrocele. Testicular descent is a complication felt to be related to complete division of the cremasteric muscle but the occurrence is variable. The cord structures loose their tethering effect allowing the testicle to descend into the most dependent portion of the scrotum. Due to the elasticity of the scrotum, with time gravity causes the scrotum to elongate. Patients complain their testicle "drops into the toilet" and can be quite unhappy. Few hernia surgeons now routinely completely divide the cremasteric muscle so it is hoped that this will become a rare phenomena. The dysejaculation syndrome is characterized by searing, burning, painful sensations throughout the groin around the time of ejaculation. The incidence is approximately 0.04%.[99]

Wound Infection. This is a surprisingly rare complication of groin herniorrhaphy (less than 5%) and the reason for the "protected" status especially when compared to prosthetic ventral herniorrhaphy is not known.[101]

Seromas. Seromas are common with the use of synthetic mesh in laparoscopic hernia repairs and are possibly related to the size of the mesh used. The fluid eventually resorbs spontaneously. Aspiration is performed for symptomatic relief only.

Bleeding. Hemorrhage can occur from the cremasteric, internal spermatic, or inferior epigastric vessels.[89] Conservative treatment with reassurance is preferred. Evacuation is rarely required. Injuries to the deep circumflex artery, the corona mortis, or the external iliac vessels may result in a large retroperitoneal hematoma.

Prosthetic Complications. Shrinkage of polypropylene as well other meshes should be considered by surgeons when performing prosthetic repairs. Sufficient overlap anticipating a 20% contracture is accepted by most.[102] The decrease in size is felt to be due to scarification of the recipient's tissue. Intestinal obstruction or fistulization is possible by erosion especially if there is physical contact between intestine and the prosthesis. Intraabdominal placement of a mesh prosthesis should be avoided in favor of ePTFE or perhaps a biologic prosthesis whenever possible. Rejection because of an allergic response is possible but extremely rare. What patients call rejection in their histories usually is the result of infection. Local erosion into the cord structures has also been reported.[103]

PERIUMBILICAL HERNIAS

Umbilical and periumbilical hernias are caused by improper healing of the umbilical scar, which results in a defect in the fascia covered by skin. In infants, the fascial defect varies in size but is most commonly 1 to 2 cm. A large proportion of pediatric umbilical hernias heal spontaneously, and 80% of them close by the time the patient is 2 years old. Persistent umbilical hernias require surgery. In older patients, the onset is usually sudden and the defect is relatively small. An underlying cause of increased intraabdominal pressure, such as ascites or intraabdominal tumors, should be sought.

The differential diagnosis of umbilical hernia includes the varicosities that extend radially from the umbilicus in persons with portal hypertension, the so-called caput medusae (Fig. 73.31). The varicosities have a bluish discoloration and fill when the patient is straining. A metastatic deposit of intraabdominal cancer at the umbilicus may mimic umbilical herniation. Cancer cells reach this area via lymphatics in the falciform ligament. Metastasis presents as a hard nodule, and biopsy is diagnostic. Other periumbilical masses that can be confused with an umbilical hernia include umbilical granulomas, omphalomesenteric duct remnant cysts, and urachal cysts.

The management of umbilical hernias is conservative in children up to the age of 2 years. In those who require surgery,

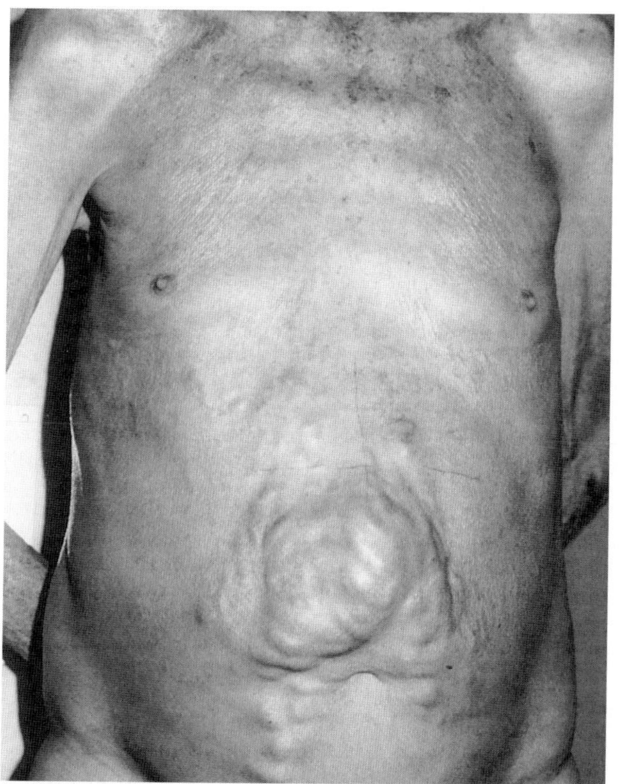

FIGURE 73.31 Caput medusae. Large periumbilical collaterals in a patient with portal hypertension.

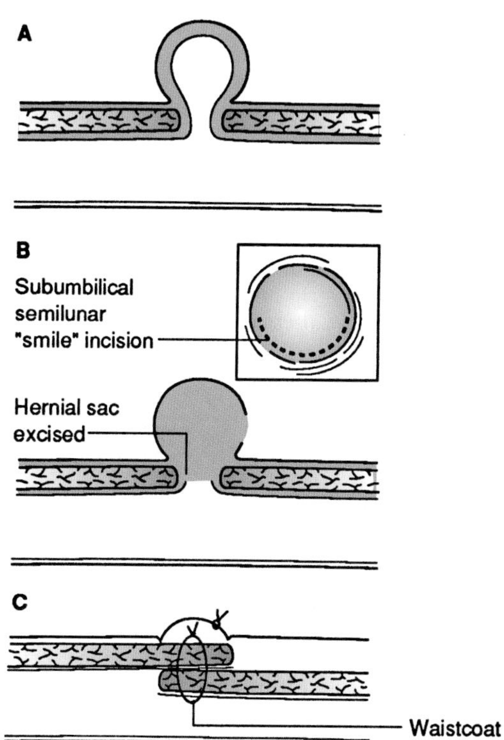

FIGURE 73.32 Repair of an umbilical hernia. (*A*) Diagram of longitudinal section through the hernia. (*B*) Subumbilical "smile" incision. The hernial sac is excised. (*C*) Waistcoat type of closure.

the repair depends on the size of the hernia. The majority are small, and the defect can be closed by simple suture. A subumbilical semilunar incision is made. The sac of the hernia is opened and the contents reduced into the abdomen. The sac is then excised. An overlapping or waistcoat technique is used in which the upper edge of the linea alba overlaps the lower edge. Nonabsorbable sutures are used (Fig. 73.32). For larger hernias, particularly in adults, the sac may be dissected away from the undersurface of the skin of the umbilicus and reduced into the preperitoneal space. A prosthesis can then be used to bridge the fascial defect without contact with the intraabdominal viscera. The prosthesis is sutured circumferentially to the defect or to the undersurface of the posterior rectus sheath and the linea alba above the peritoneal closure. If it is not possible to keep the peritoneum intact beneath the defect, omentum should be tacked to the peritoneum circumferentially to isolate the abdominal viscera from the prosthesis.

EPIGASTRIC HERNIAS

Epigastric hernias occur through a defect in the linea alba. In the majority of patients, only a single decussation of the fibers of the linea alba is present rather than the usual triple decussation (see Fig. 73.6). The incidence of epigastric herniation reported varies from less than 1% to as high as 5%. Epigastric hernias are two to three times more common in men than in women. Twenty percent are multiple. Most are less than 1 cm and contain only incarcerated preperitoneal fat without a peritoneal sac. For this reason, epigastric hernias cannot be visualized with laparoscopy. Patients complain of a painful nodule in the upper midline. Repair by reduction of the preperitoneal fat and simple closure of the defect is curative. These hernias are prone to recur, with rates as high as 10%. Left untreated, an epigastric hernia can become large enough for a peritoneal sac to form, into which the intraabdominal contents can protrude. The sac is usually wide, and serious complications are not common.

In *diastasis recti,* the two rectus muscles are separated widely. The area of the linea alba is stretched and protrudes like a fin. Although diastasis recti is easily reducible and almost never produces complications, many patients find the defect unsightly and request treatment. Surgical therapy involves removal of a strip of the weakened linea alba and reapproximation. The alternative is a mesh repair done laparoscopically.

INCISIONAL HERNIAS

Incisional hernias occur as a complication of prior surgery. These hernias can follow any type of abdominal surgery, regardless of the type of incision. The highest incidence is with midline and transverse incisions,[104,105] but hernias are well documented following paramedian, subcostal, appendectomy gridiron, and Pfannenstiel incisions. Poor surgical technique, rough handling of tissues, use of rapidly degraded absorbable suture materials, closure of the abdomen under tension, and infection of the wound are important causes of incisional hernias. Morbid obesity, cigarette smoking, pulmonary disease, and hypoalbuminemia have been incriminated as associated predisposing conditions. Many authorities believe that incisional hernias can be prevented by closing abdominal wounds with continuous running sutures and monofilament suture material. Sutures are placed 1 cm away from the edge and 1 cm apart from each other. The length of the suture should be four times the length of the wound to avoid excessive tension[106] (Fig. 73.33).

Repair of an incisional hernia depends on the size of the hernia. If the defect is solitary and 3 cm or less in size, primary closure with nonabsorbable suture material can be performed. For larger hernias or hernias with multiple small defects, primary closure results in unacceptably high recurrence rates. With large defects, the recurrence rate has been significantly reduced by using a tension-free mesh repair.[107–111] When a hernia defect is bridged with mesh, attempts should be made to isolate the material from the intraabdominal viscera to prevent erosion with fistula formation or adhesive bowel obstruction. This can be accomplished with a peritoneal flap or omentum. When contact with intraabdominal organs cannot be avoided, e-PTFE should be considered.

Laparoscopic surgeons performing an incisional herniorrhaphy prefer e-PTFE. In this procedure, the abdominal contents are reduced from the hernia defect under direct laparoscopic guidance. The number and location of the sites of trocar placement vary depending on the size and location of the hernia. The prosthesis is introduced through the largest cannula and positioned onto the peritoneum so that it widely overlaps the hernia defect. The prosthesis is secured to the anterior abdominal wall with staples, tacks, or sutures. A suture passer introduced through circumferentially located stab incisions is particularly useful for laparoscopic herniorrhaphy because it allows sutures to be placed through the prosthesis and the full thickness of the musculofascial elements of the abdominal wall. The sutures can be tied extracorporeally and then allowed to retract back into the subcutaneous tissue of the stab incisions. The skin is then closed over them[112,113] (see Fig. 73.30). Recent reports of using a bioactive material made from porcine submucosa have demonstrated its safety in repair of infected or contaminated hernias.[113–115]

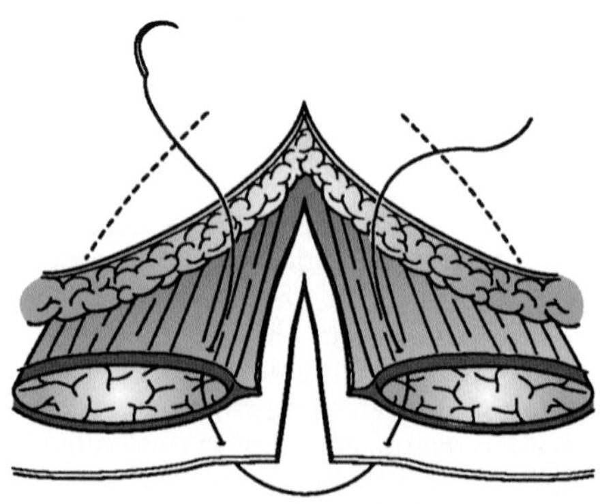

FIGURE 73.33 Mass closure of abdominal wall surgical wound.

Alternatively, the posterior rectus sheath can be opened on each edge of the hernia defect and dissected away from the undersurface of the rectus muscles for a distance of 10 to 15 cm. The posterior rectus sheaths are then approximated to each other primarily. A large mesh prosthesis (e-PTFE if the approximation of the posterior rectus sheath is inadequate) is then placed in this pocket outside the repaired posterior sheath but beneath the rectus muscles. The mesh is secured in this position with several sutures placed through small stab incisions at the periphery of the prosthesis with a suture passer and then tied in the subcutaneous tissue above the fascia.[116–118]

Infection remains a major problem with prosthetic incisional hernia repairs. The incidence of infection is about 5%, and when infection occurs, healing can be delayed for a prolonged period. Factors leading to infection are preexisting infection or ulceration of the skin over the hernia, obesity, incarcerated or obstructed bowel within the hernia, and perforation of the bowel at the time of hernia repair. Seromas are common when a large prosthesis is required or flap dissection of the subcutaneous layer from the fascia has been extensive. Untreated seromas can become secondarily infected. Suction drains can be useful, but if left in place too long, they also result in infection of the prosthesis. Strategies to prevent and manage seromas are largely based on empiricism and personal opinion, as objective data are nearly absent. It is not always necessary to remove the mesh prosthesis in the presence of infection. A trial of local wound care after opening of the incision and débridement is warranted.

Several other factors contribute to the poor results obtained in repairing incisional hernias. These include preexisting comorbid conditions. Debilitation from cancer, morbid obesity, the use of steroids, and chemotherapy all influence results. In the past, incisional hernia repair was associated with a 30% to 40% recurrence rate; with modern tension-free repairs, the recurrence rate has been dramatically reduced.[107–110,120,121]

PARASTOMAL HERNIAS

This incisional hernia is one of the most common complications of stoma formation. Studies designed with very careful follow-up suggest that a paracolostomy hernia develops in more than 50% of patients followed for longer than 5 years.[121] The rate of herniation with small-bowel stomas is less than for colon stomas. Poor site selection or technical errors, such as making the fascial opening too large or placing a stoma in an incision, account for some of these hernias. Placing a stoma

TABLE 73.7 INDICATIONS/CONTRAINDICATIONS

INDICATIONS FOR REPAIR OF A PARASTOMAL HERNIA

ABSOLUTE
Obstruction
Incarceration with strangulation
RELATIVE
Incarceration
Prolapse
Stenosis
Intractable dermatitis
Difficulty with appliance management
Large size
Cosmesis
Pain

lateral to the rectus sheath is widely touted as a cause. Obesity, malnutrition, advanced age, collagen abnormalities, postoperative sepsis, abdominal distention, constipation, obstructive uropathy, steroid use, and chronic lung disease also contribute.[122] Novel techniques for stomal reconstruction, such as extraperitoneal tunneling, have had little impact.

Fortunately, patients tolerate these hernias well, and life-threatening complications, such as bowel obstruction or strangulation, are rare. Fewer than 20% of patients with parastomal hernias have a complication that mandates repair.[122] Routine repair is therefore not recommended. Table 73.7 lists possible indications.

The three general types of stomal hernia repair are fascial repair, stomal relocation, and prosthetic repair. Fascial repair involves a local exploration around the stoma site, with primary closure of the defect. This approach should be considered of historical interest only. Stomal relocation produces better results than simple fascial repair. This approach is especially indicated in patients with other stomal problems, such as skin excoriation or suboptimal stomal construction. The use of a prosthesis with stomal relocation is not recommended because of the inherent danger of contamination.

Prosthetic repair is associated with the complications inherent in using a foreign body. Care must be taken to isolate the exit of the stoma from the abdominal wall from the surgical field to avoid infection of the prosthesis. The prosthesis can be placed extraperitoneally by making an incision around the stoma that is usually outside the periphery of the stomal appliance. Some surgeons make the incision underneath the appliance. Once the subcutaneous tissue is divided, dissection proceeds along the fascia until the hernia sac is identified and removed. The defect can be closed and an overlying prosthesis buttress sutured in place (Fig. 73.34). Alternatively, the fascial defect can be bridged with the prosthesis for a tension-free repair. The extraperitoneal approach seems logical but can actually be technically demanding, because it is sometimes difficult to define the entire extent of the hernia defect. In addition, the undermining of subcutaneous tissue leads to seroma formation and eventual infection. An intraabdominal prosthetic repair has also been described, which enlists the mechanical advantage of placing the prosthesis on the peritoneal side of the abdominal wall.[123,124] Intraabdominal pressure becomes a force that serves to fuse the prosthetic material to the abdominal wall instead of a factor in recurrence. The intraabdominal approach is particularly suited for laparoscopy, and several techniques have been described.[125,126]

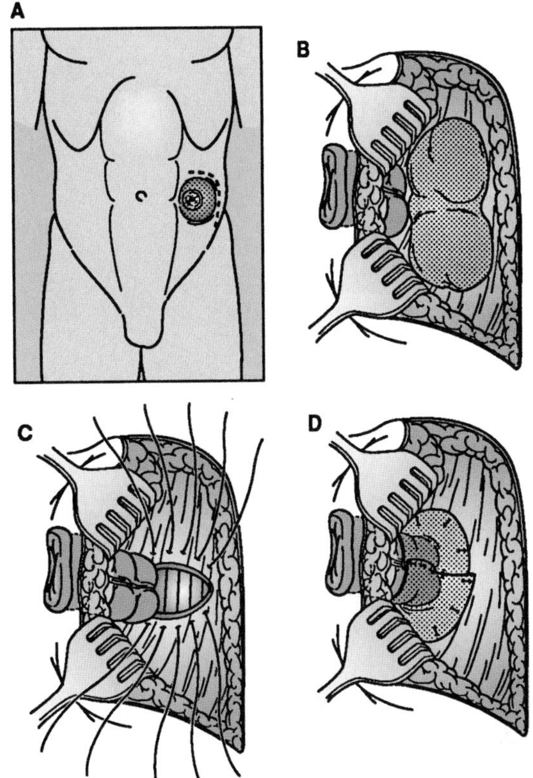

FIGURE 73.34 Repair of a parastomal hernia. (*A*) Incision around hernia. (*B*) Hernial sac is identified, the contents are reduced, and the peritoneum is closed. (*C*) The edges of the fascial defect are reapproximated. (*D*) The fascial repair is reinforced with polypropylene mesh, which is wrapped around the subcutaneous portion of the colon and sutured in place. (After Pearl RK. Para-stomal hernias. *World J Surg.* 1989;13:569, with permission.)

UNUSUAL HERNIAS

Spigelian Hernia

A Flemish anatomist, Adriaan van der Spieghel, first described the semilunar line, which is the lower limit of the posterior rectus sheath. A spigelian hernia protrudes through an area of weakness just lateral to the rectus sheath and just below this line (Fig. 73.35). The hernia is usually interparietal, rarely penetrating the external oblique fascia, and therefore can be difficult to appreciate. This is an unusual hernia; only 744 cases have been described in the literature, although the number may increase because this form of herniation is so easily diagnosed at laparoscopy. The usual presentation is a lower abdominal swelling just lateral to the border of the rectus muscle. Spigelian hernias often occur in elderly female patients. They are usually small, about 1 to 2 cm in diameter, although large hernias up to 14 cm in diameter have been described. Omentum and small or large bowel may enter the sac. Incarceration and strangulation are common complications of this hernia. Because the hernia is deep to the external oblique fascia, the clinical presentation may not be obvious. Pain and tenderness may be the only signs. Plain roentgenograms may show a bowel shadow in this area, and CT can demonstrate the defect well. Treatment is operative repair. A transverse incision is centered over the mass. The external oblique aponeurosis is split to reveal the protrusion.

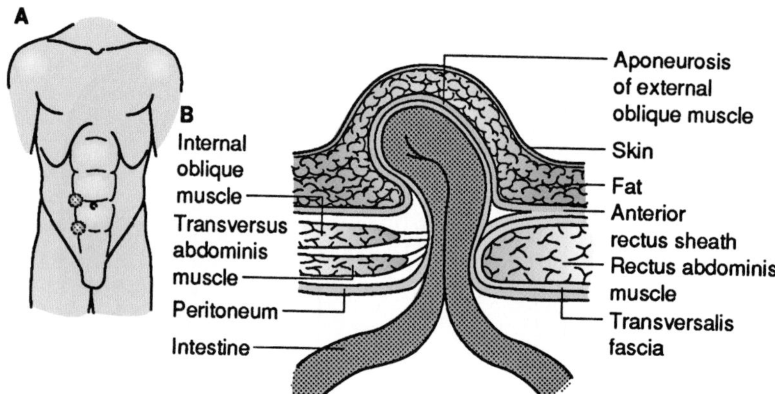

FIGURE 73.35 Spigelian hernia. (*A*) Usual site of occurrence. (*B*) Transverse section of abdominal wall showing site of defect.

If a large sac is present, it is divided and sutured. The aponeurotic defect is triangular, with its base at or near the lateral border of the rectus muscle. The defect is closed by joining the separated transversus and internal oblique layers. Recurrence is uncommon.

Lumbar Hernia

The lumbar region is the area bounded inferiorly by the iliac crest and superiorly by the 12th rib. Posteriorly, the boundary is the erector spinae group of muscles, and anteriorly, it is the posterior border of the external oblique muscle as it extends from the 12th rib to the iliac crest. The three varieties of lumbar hernia are given in Table 73.8 (Fig. 73.36). These hernias require repair if they are large, and because of the size of the defect, synthetic mesh is used. For the inferior lumbar hernia, a rotation flap of fascia lata can be used (Fig. 73.37).

Obturator Hernia

Obturator hernia occurs through the obturator canal accompanied by the obturator vessels and nerves. Obturator herniation is seen mostly in women and is associated with a laxity

TABLE 73.8 CLASSIFICATION

TYPES OF LUMBAR HERNIA

Type	Description
Superior lumbar hernia of Grynfeltt	Occurs through a space between the latissimus dorsi, the serratus posterior inferior, and the posterior border of the internal oblique muscle
Inferior lumbar hernia of Petit	Occurs through a defect in the space bounded by the latissimus dorsi posteriorly, the iliac crest inferiorly, and the posterior border of the external oblique anteriorly
Secondary lumbar hernia	Develops as a result of trauma, mostly surgical (e.g., renal surgery), or infection; lumbar hernias were encountered relatively frequently in the past in cases of spinal tuberculosis with paraspinal abscesses

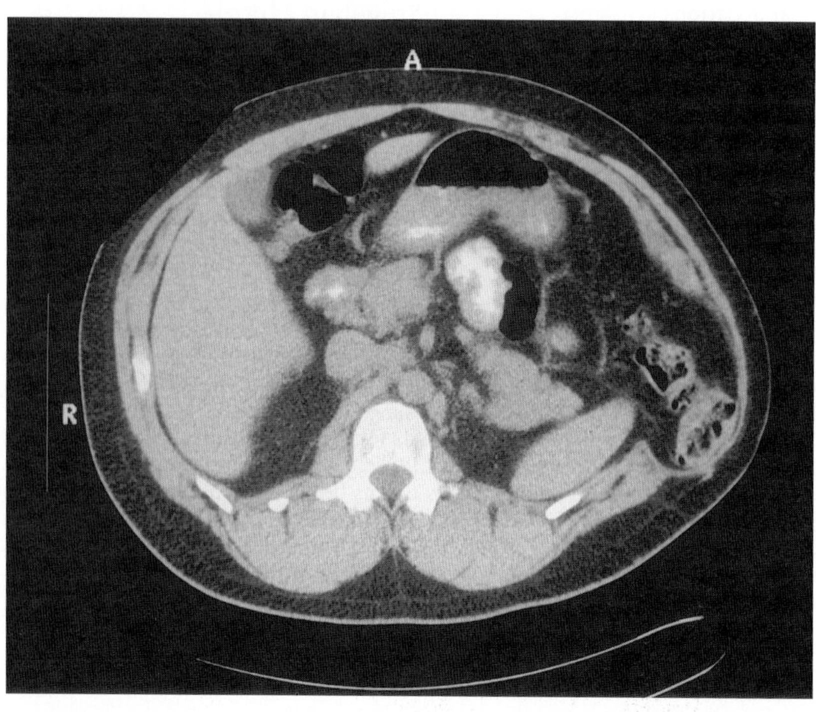

FIGURE 73.36 Computed tomogram of a left-sided lumbar hernia following nephrectomy for renal cell cancer.

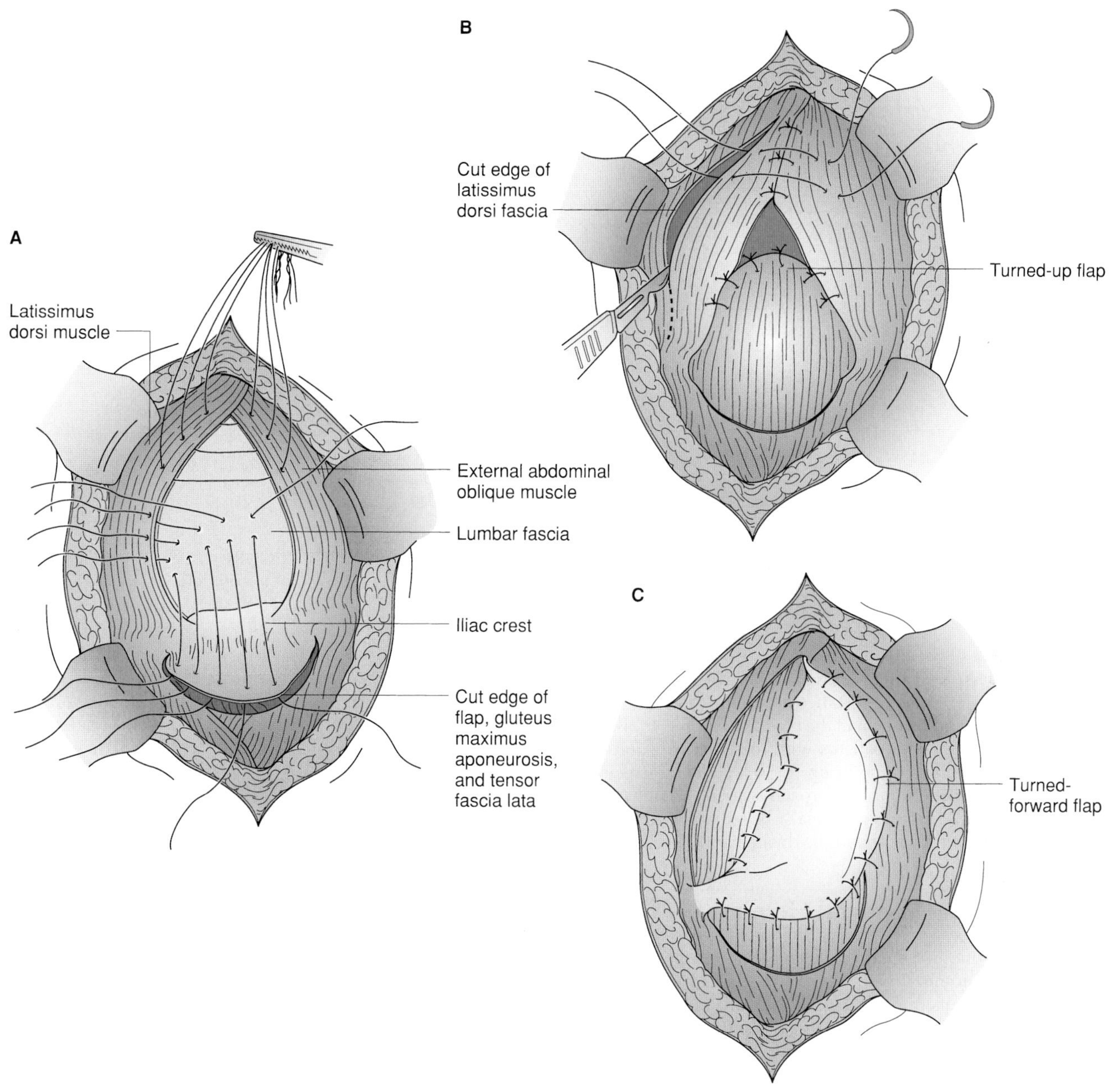

FIGURE 73.37 Sciatic hernias. (*A*) Suprapiriform. (*B*) Infrapiriform. (*C*) Subspinous.

of the pelvic floor. The main symptom is intermittent pain. Occasionally, a mass can be palpated in the upper medial thigh, especially with the hip flexed and externally rotated and abducted. A mass can sometimes be palpated on vaginal examination. The defect is approached transperitoneally; the hernia is reduced and mesh placed over the defect.

Sciatic Hernia

A sciatic hernia is a protrusion of a peritoneal sac through the major or minor sciatic foramen (Fig. 73.38). These very rare hernias present with a swelling on the buttock. The sciatic nerve may be involved. A ureter can become obstructed if it is included with the herniated tissues. The treatment of these hernias is surgical. Both transperitoneal and transgluteal approaches have been described. A combination of the two is sometimes used. The defect usually requires a prosthetic mesh repair.

Supravesical Hernia

This hernia is anterior to the urinary bladder and forms when the integrity of the transversus abdominis muscle and the transversalis fascia fail, both of which insert into Cooper's ligament. The preperitoneal space is continuous with the retropubic space of Retzius, and the hernial sac protrudes into this area. The sac of the hernia is directed laterally, emerges at the lateral border of the rectus muscle, and presents in the inguinal, femoral, or obturator region. It can also be associated with an inguinal, femoral, or obturator hernia. Treatment of this hernia depends on recognizing it at the time of groin exploration and reinforcing the defect.

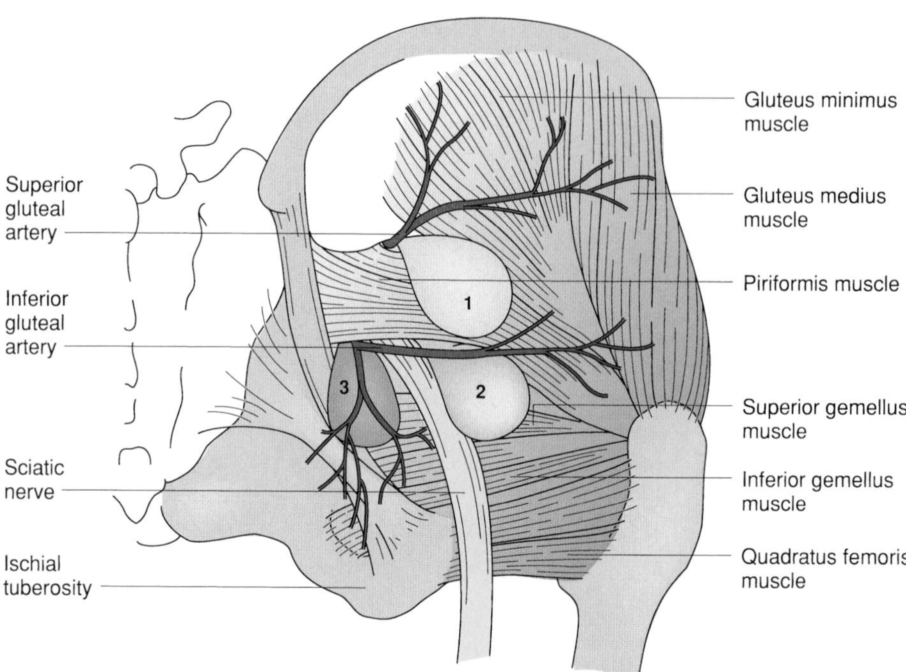

FIGURE 73.38 Technique of repair of inferior lumbar hernia.

A second variety of these hernias is known as an internal supravesical hernia. They are classified according to whether they cross in front of, beside, or behind the bladder (Fig. 73.39). Bowel symptoms predominate in patients with these hernias, and urinary tract symptoms develop in up to 30%. The treatment is surgical, and a transperitoneal approach is used through a low midline incision. The hernias can usually be reduced without difficulty. The neck of the sac should be divided and closed.

Interparietal Hernia

This hernia is one in which the hernial sac lies between the layers of the abdominal wall. It may be either *preperitoneal* (between the peritoneum and the transversalis fascia) or *interstitial* (between the muscle layers of the abdominal wall). The majority are inguinal, in which case they are designated *inguinal interstitial* hernias. An *inguinal crural* hernia occurs when the sac passes behind the inguinal ligament in the region of the femoral ring.

The cause of these hernias appears to be related to congenital abnormalities; they have been associated with failure of the testis to descend, congenital pouches, and other abnormalities, such as absence of the cremaster and absence of the external abdominal ring.

The diagnosis of these hernias is difficult because no swelling of the abdominal wall is obvious unless the hernia is large. Pain is commonly the only symptom, and it is not unusual for patients to present with intestinal obstruction secondary to incarceration. CT, ultrasonography, and laparoscopy can be helpful in making the diagnosis. Not infrequently, the correct diagnosis is made only at operation. The defect is repaired according to the principles described for inguinal and incisional hernias.

Littre's Hernia

Littre's hernia is a groin hernia containing a Meckel's diverticulum. These hernias sometimes also contain the appendix.

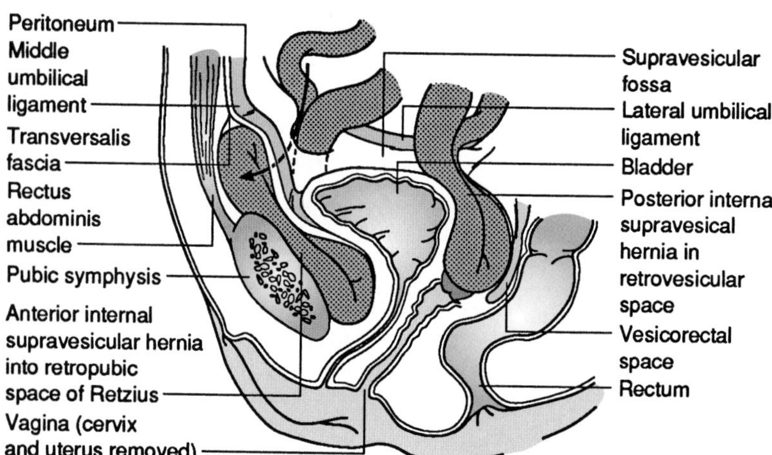

FIGURE 73.39 Internal supravesical hernias. (After Skandalakis JE. Internal and external supravesical hernia. *Am Surg.* 1976;42:142, with permission.)

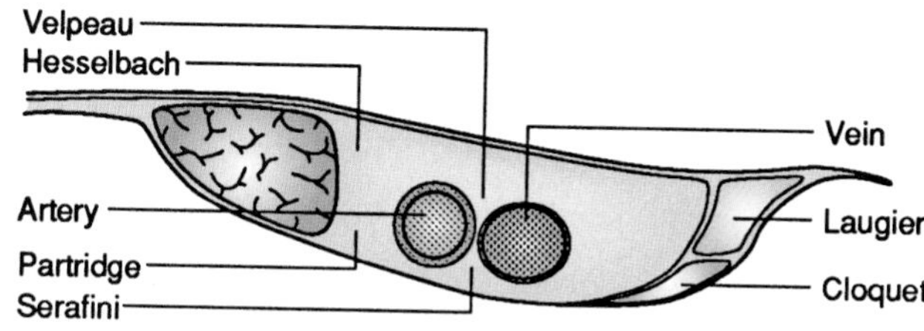

FIGURE 73.40 Perivascular hernias and their eponyms.

If the diverticulum is symptomatic or strangulated, then it is mandatory to resect it at the time of the hernia repair.

Perineal Hernia

These hernias are more common in older female patients and are related to a lax pelvic floor. They are termed *anterior* or *posterior* according to their relationship to the transversus perinei muscle. The anterior hernias usually present as a swelling in the labium or lateral vaginal wall. The posterior hernias present between the rectum and the ischial tuberosity. Surgical repair requires a transperitoneal approach, and, if the opening is large, a prosthetic mesh repair is required.

Perivascular Hernia

These hernias present through defects between the inguinal ligament and the iliopubic bone. They are known by various eponyms according to their position. The hernia protruding through a defect in the lacunar ligament is *Laugier's hernia.* The hernia protruding through the pectineal fascia is *Cloquet's hernia.* The hernia extending anterior to the femoral vessels but behind the inguinal ligament is *Velpeau's hernia.* The hernia behind the vessels is *Serafini's hernia.* Lateral to the femoral artery are two hernias, the anterior one being *Hesselbach's hernia* and the more posterior one *Partridge's hernia* (Fig. 73.40).

KEY POINTS

- **Currently hernias are the third most common cause of intestinal obstruction after adhesive obstructions and cancer.**
- **The performance of a "tension-free" inguinal hernia repair dramatically reduces the risk of recurrent hernia to a rate generally reported to be less than 2%.**
- **Inguinal hernias constitute approximately 80% of abdominal hernias with femoral hernia accounting for 5% and incisional, umbilical, and epigastric making up the other 15%.**
- **Inguinal hernias occur with a 7:1 male-to-female ratio, whereas femoral hernias have a female predominance of 1.8:1.**
- **The risk of a major complication, such as incarceration, obstruction, or strangulation, is very low with the annual risk estimated from 0.002 to 0.0037.**
- **The most popular laparoscopic techniques for repair of an inguinal hernia are the transabdominal preperitoneal repair (TAPP) or the totally extraperitoneal laparoscopic repair (TEP).**
- **A recent major prospective randomized multicenter trial showed that laparoscopic repair was associated with a significantly increased risk of recurrent hernia than open repair (10.1% vs. 4.9%).**
- **The frequency of at least some long term groin pain may be as high as 50% at 1 year following inguinal hernia repair with moderate to severe pain in up to 10% of patients.**
- **Ischemic orchitis occurs in about 1% of primary hernia repairs but is more common following repair of a recurrent hernia.**
- **Historical recurrence rates of 30% to 40% following ventral hernia repair have been dramatically reduced by modern tension-free repairs.**

References

1. **Rutkow IM. Epidemiologic, economic, and sociologic aspects of hernia surgery in the United States in the 1990s. *Surg Clin North Am.* 1998;78:941.**
2. Whitely MS, Laws SA, Wise MH. Use of a hand-held Doppler to avoid abdominal wall vessels in laparoscopic surgery. *Ann R Coll Surg Engl.* 1994;76:348.
3. Hurd WW, Bude RO, DeLancy OL, et al. The location of abdominal wall blood vessels in relationship to abdominal landmarks apparent at laparoscopy. *Am J Obstet Gynecol.* 1994;171:642.
4. Chatzipappas IK, Magos AL. A simple technique of securing inferior epigastric vessels and repairing the rectus sheath at laparoscopic surgery. *Obstet Gynecol.* 1997;90:304.
5. Green LS, Loughlin KR, Kavousi L. Management of epigastric vessel injury during laparoscopy. *J Endourol.* 1992;6:99.
6. Hurd WW, Pearl ML, DeLancey OL, et al. Laparoscopic injury of abdominal wall blood vessels: a report of three cases. *Obstet Gynecol.* 1993;82:673.
7. Hollingshead HW. The abdominal wall and inguinal region. *Anatomy for surgeons,* vol 2. New York: Hoeber-Harper, 1961, p. 224.
8. **Condon RE. The anatomy of the inguinal region and its relation to groin hernia. In: Nyhus LM, Condon RE, eds. *Hernia.* Philadelphia: JB Lippincott, 1995, p. 31.**
9. Milloy FJ, Anson BJ, McCaffee DK. The rectus abdominis muscle and the epigastric arteries. *Surg Gynecol Obstet.* 1960;110;293.
10. Rizk NN. A new description of the anterior abdominal wall in man and mammals. *J Anat.* 1980;131:373.
11. Askar O. Patterns of midline decussation of the aponeurosis. *Ann R Coll Surg Engl.* 1977;59:313.
12. Cooper A. *The anatomy and surgical treatment of abdominal hernia.* Philadelphia: Lee and Blanchard, 1804, p. 26.
13. Zimmerman LM, Anson BJ. *Anatomy and surgery of hernia.* Baltimore: Williams & Wilkins,1953, p. 85.
14. Condon RE. Surgical anatomy of the transversus abdominis and transversalis fascia. *Ann Surg.* 1971;173:1.
15. Read RC. Cooper's posterior lamina of transversalis fascia. *Surg Gynecol Obstet.* 1992;174:426.
16. Colborn GL, Skandalakis JE. Laparoscopic inguinal anatomy. *Hernia* 1998;2:179.
17. **Quinn TH, Ryberg A, Annibali R, et al. Anatomy of the anterior abdominal wall and deep inguinal region from the laparoscopic surgeon's perspective. In: Lansafame RJ, ed. *Prevention and management of complications in minimally invasive surgery.* New York: Igaku Shoin, 1996, p. 107.**
18. Page DW, Gilroy A, Marks SC Jr. The iliopubic tract: an essential guide in teaching and performing groin hernia repairs. *Contemp Surg.* 1996; 49:219.
19. Gilroy A, Marks SC Jr, Quinfang L, et al. Anatomical characteristics of the iliopubic tract: implications for repair of inguinal hernias. *Clin Anat.* 1992;5:255.
20. McVay CB, Anson BJ. Aponeurotic and fascial continuities in the abdomen, pelvis, and thigh. *Anat Rec.* 1940;76:213.
21. Annibali R, Quinn TH, Fitzgibbons RJ Jr. Anatomy of the inguinal region from the laparoscopic perspective: critical areas for laparoscopic hernia repair. In: Bendavid R, ed. *Prostheses and abdominal wall hernias.* Austin, TX: Landes, 1994, p. 82.
22. Urbanowicz Z. External structure of the genitofemoral nerve in postfetal life in man. *Folia Morphol (Warsz).* 1975;34:425.
23. Annibali R, Quinn TH, Fitzgibbons RJ Jr. Avoiding nerve injury during laparoscopic hernia repair: critical areas for staple placement. In: Arregui ME, Nagan RF, eds. *Inguinal hernia: advances or controversies?* Oxford: Radcliffe Medical, 1994, p. 41.
24. Colborn GL, Skandalakis JE. Laparoscopic inguinal anatomy. *Hernia* 1998;2:179.
25. Gilroy AM, Hermey DC, Dibenedetto LM, et al. Variability of the obturator vessels. *Clin Anat.* 1997;10:328.
26. Missankov AA, Asvat R, Maoba KI. Variation of the pubic vascular anastomoses in black South Africans. *Acta Anat.* 1996;155:212.
27. Bendavid R. The space of Bogros and the deep inguinal venous circulation. *Surg Gynecol Obstet.* 1992;174:356.
28. Flament JB, Visse CA, Palot JP. Tropic ulcers in giant incisional hernias—pathogenesis and treatment: a report of 33 cases. *Hernia* 1997;1:71.
29. Raynor RW, Deguercio LRM. The place of pneumoperitoneum in the repair of massive hernia. *World J Surg.* 1989;13:581.

30. Bassini E. Nuovo metodo per la crura radicale dell'emia. *Atti Congr Ass Med Ital.* 1889;2:179.
31. Rand Corporation. *Conceptualization and measurement of physiologic health of adults.* Santa Monica, CA: Rand Corporation, 1983, p. 15.
32. Jansen PL, Mertens Pr P, Klinge U, Schumpelick V. The biology of hernia formation. *Surgery* 2004;136:1.
33. Franklin ME Jr, Gonzalez JJ Jr, Michaelson RP, et al. Preliminary experience with new bioactive prosthetic material for repair of hernias in infected fields. *Hernia* 2002;6:171 (Epub Oct 19, 2002).
34. **Amid PK, Shulman AG, Lichtenstein IL. Open "tension-free" repair of inguinal hernias: the Lichtenstein technique. *Eur J Surg.* 1996;162:447.**
35. Amid PK, Shulman AG, Lichtenstein IL. Critical scrutiny of the open "tension-free" hernio-plasty. *Am J Surg.* 1993;165:369.
36. Amid PK. Lichtenstein tension-free hernioplasty: its inception, evolution, and principles. *Hernia* 2004;8:1 (Epub September 20, 2003).
37. Wantz GE. Experience with the tension-free hernioplasty for primary inguinal hernias in men. *J Am Coll Surg.* 1996;182:351.
38. Shulman AG, Amid PK, Lichtenstein IL. A survey of non-expert surgeons using the open tension-free mesh repair for primary inguinal hernias. *Int Surg.* 1995;80:35.
39. Cheatle GL. An operation for the radical cure of inguinal and femoral hernia. *Br Med J.* 1920;2:68.
40. Henry AK. Operation for femoral hernia by a midline extraperitoneal approach, with a preliminary note on the use of this route for reducible inguinal hernia. *Lancet* 1936;1:531.
41. Rignault DP. Preperitoneal prosthetic inguinal hernioplasty through a Pfannenstiel approach. *Surg Gynecol Obstet.* 1986;163:465.
42. **Robbins AW, Rutkow IM. Mesh plug repair and groin hernia surgery. *Surg Clin North Am.* 1998;78:1007.**
43. Gilbert AI, Graham MF, Voight WJ. A bilayer patch for inguinal hernia repair. *Hernia* 1999;3:161.
44. Kugel RD. Minimally invasive, non-laparoscopic, preperitoneal and sutureless inguinal hernia repair. *Am J Surg.* 1999;178:298.
45. Rutkow IM. Demographic and socioeconomic aspects of hernia repair in the United States in 2003. *Surg Clin North Am.* 2003;83:1045.
46. Sparkman RS. Bilateral exploration in inguinal hernia in juvenile patients. *Surgery* 1962;51:393.
47. Rowe MI, Clatworthy HW. The other side of the pediatric hernia. *Surg Clin North Am.* 1971;51:6.
48. Abrahamson J. Factors and mechanisms leading to recurrence. In: Bendavid R, ed. *Prostheses and abdominal wall hernias.* Austin, TX: Landes, 1994, p. 138.
49. Read RC. The role of protease—antiprotease in the pathogenesis of hernia and abdominal aortic aneurysm in certain smokers. *Post Grad Gen Surg.* 1992;14:161.
50. Metropolitan Life Insurance Company. Expectation of life and mortality rates at single years of age, by race and sex: United States, 1991. *Stat Bull Metrop Insur Co.* 1996;75:16.
51. Neuhauser D. Elective inguinal herniorrhaphy versus truss in the elderly. In: Bunker JP, Barnes BA, Mosteller F, eds. *Costs, risks, and benefits of surgery.* New York: Oxford University Press, 1977, p. 223.
52. Ponka JL. Surgical management of large bilateral indirect sliding inguinal hernias. *Am J Surg.* 1966;112:52.
53. Zollinger RM. Classification systems for groin hernias. *Surg Clin North Am.* 2003;83:1053.
54. Heller CA, Marucci DD, Dunn T, et al. Inguinal canal lipoma. *Clin Anat.* 2002;15:280.
55. Read RC, Schaefer RF. Lipoma of the spermatic cord, fatty herniation and liposarcoma. *Hernia* 2000;4:149.
56. Williams JS, Hale HW. The advisability of inguinal herniorrhaphy in the elderly. *Surg Gynecol Obstet.* 1966;122:100.
57. Nehme AE. Groin hernias in elderly patients: management and prognosis. *Am J Surg.* 1983;146:257.
58. Tingwald GR, Cooperman M. Inguinal and femoral hernia repair in geriatric patients. *Surg Gynecol Obstet.* 1982;154:704.
59. Rorbaek-Madsen M. Herniorrhaphy in patients aged 80 years or more: a prospective analysis of morbidity and mortality. *Eur J Surg.* 1992; 158:591.
60. Primatesta P, Goldacre MJ. Inguinal hernia repair: incidence of elective and emergency surgery, readmission, and mortality. *Int J Epidemiol.* 1996;25:835.
61. Nilsson E, Kald A, Anderberg B, et al. Hernia surgery in a defined population: a prospective three-year audit. *Eur J Surg.* 1997;163:823.
62. Cook TM, Britton DC, Craft TM, et al. An audit of hospital mortality after urgent and emergency surgery in the elderly. *Ann R Coll Surg Engl.* 1997;79:361.
63. Rutkow IM, Robbins AW. Mesh plug hernia repair: a follow-up report. *Surgery* 1995;117:597.
64. Lichtenstein IL, Shulman AG, Amid PK, et al. The tension-free hernioplasty. *Am J Surg.* 1989;157:188.
65. Amid PK, Shulman AG, Lichtenstein IL. The Lichtenstein open "tension-free" mesh repair of inguinal hernias. *Jpn J Surg.* 1995;25:619.
66. **Amid PK, Shulman AG, Lichtenstein IL. Simultaneous repair of bilateral inguinal hernias under local anesthesia. *Ann Surg.* 1996;223:249.**
67. Amid PK, Shulman AG, Lichtenstein IL. Femoral hernia resulting from inguinal herniorrhaphy: the "plug" repair. *Contemp Surg.* 1991;39:19.
68. Amid PK, Shulman AG, Lichtenstein IL. Local anesthesia for inguinal hernia repair step-by-step procedure. *Ann Surg.* 1994;220:735.
69. Kark AE, Kurzer MN, Belsham PA. Three thousand one hundred seventy-five primary inguinal hernia repairs: advantages of ambulatory open mesh repair using local anesthesia. *J Am Coll Surg.* 1998;186:447.
70. Nyhus LM, Pollak R, Bombeck CT, et al. The preperitoneal approach and prosthetic buttress repair for recurrent hernia. *Ann Surg.* 1988; 208:733.
71. Wantz GE. The technique of giant prosthetic reinforcement of the visceral sac performed through an anterior groin incision. *Surg Gynecol Obstet.* 1993;177:497.
72. Wantz GE. Giant prosthetic reinforcement of the visceral sac: the Stoppa groin hernia repair. *Surg Clin North Am.* 1998;78:6 1075.
73. Mathonnet M, Cubertafond P, Gainant A. Bilateral inguinal hernias: giant prosthetic reinforcement of the visceral sac. *Hernia* 1997;1:93.
74. Munshi IA, Wantz GE. Management of recurrent and perivascular femoral hernias by giant prosthetic reinforcement of the visceral sac. *J Am Coll Surg.* 1996;182:417.
75. Hoffman HC, Vinton Traverso AL. Preperitoneal prosthetic herniorrhaphy: one surgeon's successful technique. *Arch Surg.* 1993;128:964.
76. Champault G, Rizk N, Catheline JM, et al. Inguinal hernia repair: totally pre-peritoneal laparoscopic approach versus Stoppa operation—randomized trial: 100 cases. *Hernia* 1997;1:31.
77. Fitzgibbons RJ Jr, Camps J, Cornet DA, et al. Laparoscopic inguinal herniorrhaphy: results of a multicenter trial . *Ann Surg.* 1995;221:3.
78. **Memon MA, Cooper NJ, Memon B, et al. Meta-analysis of randomized clinical trials comparing open and laparoscopic inguinal hernia repair. *Br J Surg.* 2003;90:1479.**
79. Collaboration EH. Laparoscopic compared with open methods of groin hernia repair: systematic review of randomized controlled trials. *Br J Surg.* 2000;87:860.
80. McCormack K, Scott NW, Go PM, et al., for the EU Hernia Trialists Collaboration. Laparoscopic techniques versus open techniques for inguinal hernia repair. *Cochrane Database Syst Rev.* 2003;CD001785.
81. **Neumayer L, Giobbie-Hurder A, Jonasson O, et al., for the Veterans Affairs Cooperative Studies Program 456 Investigators. *N Engl J Med.* 2004;350:1819.**
82. Crist DW, Gadacz TR. Complications of laparoscopic surgery. *Surg Clin North Am.* 1993;73:265.
83. Baadsgaard SE, Bille S, Egeblad K. Major vascular injury during gynecologic laparoscopy. *Acta Obstet Gynecol Scand.* 1989;68:283.
84. Mintz M. Risks and prophylaxis in laparoscopy: a survey of 100,000 cases. *J Reprod Med.* 1977;18:269.
85. McMahon AJ, Baxter JN, O'Dwyer PJ. Preventing complications of laparoscopy. *Br J Surg.* 1993;80:1592.
86. Boughey JC, Nottingham JM, Walls AC. Richter's hernia in the laparoscopic era: four case reports and review of the literature. *Surg Laparosc Endosc Percutan Tech.* 2003;13:55.
87. Patterson M, Walters D, Browder W. Postoperative bowel obstruction following laparoscopic surgery. *Am Surg.* 1993;59:656.
88. Rink J, Ali A. Intestinal obstruction after totally extraperitoneal laparoscopic inguinal hernia repair. *JSLS* 2004;8:89.
89. Condon RE, Nyhus LM. Complications of groin hernia. In: Condon RE, Nyhus LM, eds. *Hernia,* 4th ed. Philadelphia: JB Lippincott; 1995:269.
90. Nathan JD, Pappas TN. Inguinal hernia: an old condition with new solutions. *Ann Surg.* 2003;238(suppl):S148.
91. EU Hernia Trialists Collaboration. Repair of groin hernia with synthetic mesh: meta-analysis of randomized controlled trials. *Ann Surg.* 2002; 235:322.
92. Bendavid R. The Shouldice technique: a cannon in hernia repair. *Can J Surg.* 1997;40:199, 207.
93. Poobalan AS, Bruce J, Smith WC, et al. A review of chronic pain after inguinal herniorrhaphy. *Clin J Pain* 2003;19:48.
94. Cunningham J, Temple WJ, Mitchell P, et al. Cooperative hernia study: pain in the postrepair patient. *Ann Surg.* 1996;224:598.
95. Sheynkin YR, Hendin BN, Schlegel PN, Goldstein M. Microsurgical repair of iatrogenic injury to the vas deferens. *J Urol.* 1998;159:139.
96. Ceylan H, Karakok M, Guldur E, et al. Temporary stretch of the testicular pedicle may damage the vas deferens and the testis. *J Pediatr Surg.* 2003;38:1530.
97. Matsuda T, Muguruma K, Horii Y, et al. Serum antisperm antibodies in men with vas deferens obstruction caused by childhood inguinal herniorrhaphy. *Fertil Steril.* 1993;59:1095.
98. Wantz GE. Testicular atrophy and chronic residual neuralgia as risks of inguinal hernioplasty. *Surg Clin North Am.* 1993;73:571.
99. **Bendavid R. Complications of groin hernia surgery. *Surg Clin North Am.* 1998;78:1089.**
100. Wantz GE. Testicular atrophy as a risk inguinal hernioplasty. *Surg Gynecol Obstet.* 1982;154:570.
101. Sanchez-Manuel FJ, Seco-Gil JL. Antibiotic prophylaxis for hernia repair. *Cochrane Database Syst Rev.* 2003;(2):CD003769.
102. Amid PK. How to avoid recurrence in Lichtenstein tension-free hernioplasty. *Am J Surg.* 2002;184:259.
103. Silich RC, McSherry CK. Spermatic granuloma: an uncommon complication of the tension-free hernia repair. *Surg Endosc.* 1996;10:537.

104. Ellis H, Bucknall TE. Abdominal incisions and their closure. *Curr Probl Surg*. 1985;22:1.
105. Bucknall TE, Cox PJ, Ellis H. Burst abdomen and incisional hernia: a prospective study of 1,129 major laparotomies. *Br Med J*. 1982;284:931.
106. Israelsson LA, Jonsson T, Knutsson A. Suture technique and wound healing in midline laparotomy incisions. *Eur J Surg*. 1996;162:605.
107. Santora TA, Roslyn JJ. Incisional hernia. *Surg Clin North Am*. 1993; 73:557.
108. Makela JT, Kiviniemi H, Juvonen T, et al. Factors influencing dehiscence after midline laparotomy. *Am J Surg*. 1995;170:387.
109. Temudon T, Saidati M, Sarr MG. Repair of complex giant or recurrent ventral hernias by using tension-free intraparietal prosthetic mesh (Stoppa technique): lessons learned from our initial experience (50 patients). *Surgery* 1996;120:738.
110. Bebawi MA, Moqtaderi F, Vijay V. Giant incisional hernia: staged repair using pneumoperitoneum and expanded polytetrafluoroethylene. *Am Surg*. 1997;63:375.
111. Liujendijk RN, Hop WCJ, van den Tol MP, et al. A comparison of suture repair with mesh repair for incisional hernia. *N Engl J Med*. 2000;343:392.
112. Heniford BT, Ramshaw BJ. Laparoscopic ventral hernia repair. A report of 100 consecutive cases. *Surg Endosc*. 2000;14:419.
113. Franklin ME, Gonzalez JJ, Glass JL. Laparoscopic ventral and incisional hernia repair; an 11 year experience. *Hernia* 2004;8:23.
114. Franklin ME, Gonzalez JJ, Michalson RP. Preliminary experience with new bioactive prosthetic material for repair of hernias in infected fields. *Hernia* 2002;6:171.
115. Edelman DS. Laparoscopic herniorrhaphy with porcine small intestinal submucosa. A preliminary study. *J Soc Laparoendosc Surg*. 2002;6:203.
116. de Vries Reilingh TS, van Geldere D, Langenhorst BLAM, et al. Repair of large midline incisional hernias with polypropylene mesh: comparison of 3 operative techniques. *Hernia* 2004;8:56.
117. Heniford BT, Park A, Ramshaw BJ, Voeller G. Laparoscopic ventral and incisional hernia repair in 407 patients. *J Am Coll Surg*. 2000;196:645.
118. Knight R, Fenoglio M. The use of the Kugel mesh in ventral hernia repairs. *Am J Surg*. 2002;183:642.
119. Sugerman HJ, Kellum JM, Reines HD, et al. Greater risk of incisional hernia with morbidly obese than steroid-dependent patients and low recurrence with prefascial polypropylene mesh. *Am J Surg*. 1996;171: 80.
120. Anthony T, Bergen PC, Lawrence TK. Factors affecting recurrence following incisional herniorrhaphy. *World J Surg*. 2000;24:95.
121. Rubin MS, Schoetz DJ Jr, Matthews JB. Parastomal hernia: is stoma relocation superior to fascial repair? *Arch Surg*. 1994;129:413; discussion 418.
122. Pearl RK. Parastomal hernias. *World J Surg*. 1989;13:569.
123. Byers JM, Steinberg JB, Postier RG. Repair of parastomal hernias using polypropylene mesh. *Arch Surg*. 1992;127:1246.
124. Sugarbaker PH. Peritoneal approach to prosthetic mesh repair of paraostomy hernias. *Ann Surg*. 1985;201:344.
125. Bickel A, Shinkarevsky E, Eitan A. Laparoscopic repair of paracolostomy hernia. *J Laparoendosc Adv Surg Tech A*. 1999;9:353.
126. Porcheron J, Payan B, Balique JG. Mesh repair of paracolostomy hernia by laparoscopy. *Surg Endosc*. 1998;12:1281.

CHAPTER 74 ■ ACUTE ABDOMEN AND APPENDIX

JEFFREY B. MATTHEWS AND RICHARD A. HODIN

APPROACH TO THE PATIENT WITH ACUTE ABDOMINAL PAIN

Abdominal pain is one of the most frequent reasons for visits to physician offices and hospital emergency rooms and is a leading cause for hospital admission in the United States. Although most patients will be found to suffer from self-limited conditions of little consequence, a subset of patients with acute abdominal pain will harbor serious intraabdominal or retroperitoneal pathology that requires major surgical or medical intervention. It is this latter population to whom the term "acute abdomen" is commonly applied, although "abdominal emergency" might be more descriptive. The experienced clinician understands that the severity of the pain does not always correlate with the gravity of the situation, nor do all patients with the so-called acute abdomen require surgical intervention. Early diagnosis, and particularly the early distinction of conditions that require urgent operation from those best managed nonsurgically, must be the paramount principle that outweighs all other concerns. Evaluation by a surgical consultant and performance of appropriate radiologic studies must proceed promptly regardless of time of day or disruption of normal routines and schedules.[1]

In the vast majority of cases, a thorough history and physical examination will reveal the cause of the abdominal pain or at least sufficiently narrow down the possibilities to allow initial treatment decisions to be made.[2] Important features to be elicited include the time and mode of onset of the illness, the location of the pain, the character of the pain, and the presence of associated symptoms and their relation to the pain (Table 74.1). Examination of the patient includes an assessment of general appearance and attitude in bed in addition to the abdominal examination itself (Table 74.2). The ability to group the symptoms and signs of acute abdominal pain and to weigh their relative importance ("pattern recognition") perhaps best distinguishes the novice from the expert diagnostician in this setting. Blood tests may be complementary but are

TABLE 74.1 DIAGNOSIS

KEY HISTORICAL FEATURES IN ACUTE ABDOMINAL PAIN

Age
Time and mode of onset of pain
Duration of symptoms
Character of pain
Location of pain and site(s) of radiation
Associated symptoms and their relation to pain
Nausea or anorexia
Vomiting
Diarrhea or constipation
Menstrual history

TABLE 74.2 DIAGNOSIS

EXAMINATION OF THE PATIENT WITH ACUTE ABDOMINAL PAIN

General observations
General appearance
Attitude in bed
Vital signs, including temperature
Chest
Auscultation
Abdomen
Inspection (distention, localized swelling, hernia)
Percussion (tympany or dullness, tenderness, referred tenderness)
Palpation (muscle rigidity, tenderness, [rebound pain], hyperesthesia)
[Auscultation]
Pelvis
Rectal examination (tenderness, presence of stool, occult blood, mass)
Bimanual examination (cervical motion tenderness, adnexal masses)
Obturator sign
Back and flanks
Percussion (costovertebral angle tenderness)
Iliopsoas sign

only occasionally of major importance in the initial evaluation. The same is generally true for radiologic studies, although in some circumstances, newer techniques of abdominal imaging do appear to enhance diagnostic accuracy. However, it cannot be overstated that an excessive reliance on tests can lead to unnecessary delay and must be avoided.

Most patients with acute abdominal pain evaluated in the emergency room setting will not require either hospital admission or surgical intervention.[3] The most common causes of abdominal pain requiring admission include acute appendicitis, nonspecific abdominal pain, pain of urologic origin, intestinal obstruction, and biliary tract disease, depending on the population and geographic region considered.[4] With improvements in diagnostic imaging over the past few decades, more patients with acute abdominal pain are able to be assigned a specific diagnosis and there are fewer instances of missed surgical disease.[5] The proportion of all patients evaluated for abdominal pain that are admitted to hospital may also be declining.

EMBRYOLOGIC AND PHYSIOLOGIC CONSIDERATIONS

The developing gastrointestinal (GI) tract is divided into three regions based on blood supply and innervation, relationships that are maintained from embryonic to adult life. The foregut consists of oropharynx, esophagus, stomach, proximal duodenum, pancreas, liver, biliary tract, and spleen. The midgut runs from distal duodenum (ligament of Treitz) and includes the small intestine, appendix, cecum, ascending colon, and proximal two thirds of the transverse colon. The remainder of the colon and rectum make up the hindgut.

The intestinal tract itself, from the stomach to the distal sigmoid colon (with the exception of the duodenum), is lined by a layer of mesodermally derived visceral peritoneum. The liver, spleen, and gallbladder are largely covered by visceral peritoneum; the pancreas is located within the retroperitoneum. Although continuous with the parietal peritoneum that lines the abdominal cavity, the visceral peritoneum is supplied by autonomic (sympathetic and parasympathetic) nerves. In contrast, the parietal peritoneal layer has an entirely somatic innervation derived from spinal nerves. This difference accounts for the distinct character of the pain associated with irritation or inflammation of the parietal peritoneum (which is generally perceived as sharp, severe, and persistent) compared to painful stimuli involving the visceral peritoneum (perceived as dull, cramping or aching, poorly localized, and often associated with nausea and/or diaphoresis). The visceral peritoneum and its associated organs are insensitive to touching, pinching, cutting, burning, and electrical stimulation, but the sensation of pain from these sites can be induced by stretching, distention, or vigorous contraction against resistance. Additional painful stimuli to visceral organs include certain chemicals, ischemia, and inflammation. Visceral pain usually indicates the presence of significant intraabdominal disease but is not in itself an indication for surgical therapy. A transition from visceral to somatic pain implies extension of the underlying disease process to include the parietal peritoneum and often heralds the need for urgent operative intervention (e.g., acute appendicitis, intestinal obstruction with strangulation). However, somatic pain of intraabdominal origin should not be equated with the invariable need for operation (e.g., acute diverticulitis). In this regard, it is important to distinguish between localized somatic pain and diffuse somatic pain. Although conditions associated with localized peritonitis may require operation, the degree of urgency is far less than in diffuse peritonitis, which generally indicates a surgical emergency.

The central gut tube is invested with bilateral nerve supply, accounting for the midline location of the visceral pain originating from these organs. Pain of foregut origin is usually perceived in the epigastrium, midgut pain in the periumbilical region, and hindgut pain in the hypogastrium. In contrast, pain deriving from the bladder, prostate, uterus, ovaries, and fallopian tubes may be localized as pelvic or, occasionally, perineal. Pain originating from the abdominal wall musculature or parietal peritoneum is usually perceived in precise relation to the anatomic location of the stimulus because somatic pain nerve fibers enter the spinal cord ipsilaterally. The anterior and lateral abdominal wall is innervated from vertebral segments T7 to L1, whereas the posterior abdominal wall is from L2 to L5.

In addition to pain of the somatic and visceral categories, a third form of pain related to acute abdominal disorders is referred pain. Referred pain is perceived at a site removed from the anatomic location of the pathology but in a region that shares a common embryonic origin. The most common example is the radiation of pain of biliary origin to the right subscapular region or right shoulder. This phenomenon reflects the fact that the phrenic nerve is derived from the fourth cervical nerve. Thus, irritation of the undersurface of the right hemidiaphragm, such as by an inflamed gallbladder or hepatic abscess, may induce pain or hyperesthesia in the skin distribution of the fourth cervical nerve. Similarly, splenic pathology (e.g., rupture) may be perceived as pain in the left shoulder (Kehr's sign). Other examples of referred pain are listed in Table 74.3.

Inflammation of the parietal peritoneum leads to rigidity and tenderness of the overlying muscle groups, a phenomenon of great clinical significance in the diagnosis of acute abdominal pain. These include not only the muscles of the anterior abdominal wall such as the rectus abdominus but also the diaphragm, psoas, quadratus lumborum, erector spinae, pyriformis, and obturator internus. Thus, an inflamed retrocecal appendix overlying the right psoas muscle may produce spasm reflected by the preference of the patient to maintain the right

TABLE 74.3 DIAGNOSIS

SITES OF REFERRED PAIN

Site	Organ(s)	Common examples
Right subscapular or shoulder	Diaphragm, gallbladder, liver	Biliary colic, perforated ulcer, pneumoperitoneum
Left subscapular or shoulder	Diaphragm, spleen, stomach, tail of pancreas, splenic flexure	Splenic rupture, pancreatitis
Back	Pancreas, duodenum, aorta	Pancreatitis, ruptured AAA
Coccyx	Uterus, rectum	Uterine colic
Groin or genitalia	Kidney, ureter, iliac arteries	Ureterolithiasis

AAA, abdominal aortic aneurysm.

thigh in flexed position; similarly, placing the patient on the left side and fully extending the right thigh may produce pain (psoas sign). Similarly, the presence of an inflamed appendix or periappendiceal abscess may be deduced by a positive finding in the so-called obturator test (pain on internal rotation of the right thigh). In contrast, irritation of the deep pelvic peritoneum is generally not associated with any overlying muscle group, accounting for the striking lack of abdominal wall rigidity in cases of pelvic abscess from appendicitis or diverticulitis.

DIFFERENTIAL DIAGNOSIS

The sheer number of conditions that produce acute abdominal pain is overwhelming. However, the differential diagnosis may be narrowed substantially by anatomic considerations and an understanding of the general characteristics of the episode of the pain.

It is useful to subdivide the abdomen into four quadrants and consider the conditions that cause abdominal pain localized to each region (Table 74.4). Pain that does not lateralize in this fashion can be characterized as epigastric, periumbilical, or hypogastric, and a relatively limited differential diagnosis can also be generated for each midline location (Table 74.5). Diffuse abdominal pain (Table 74.6) can be mild and without significant physical findings, as in early acute appendicitis, or it can be severe and associated with generalized abdominal muscle rigidity, as in diffuse peritonitis.

There are a limited number of pathologic processes affecting abdominal viscera that produce abdominal pain, and each is associated with a characteristic evolution of clinical symptoms and signs (Table 74.7). *Obstruction* of a hollow viscus results in a form of pain termed colic, consisting of a deep, nauseating ache that may be cyclical, as in intestinal colic, or steady, as in biliary colic. *Inflammation* can be the result of bacterial infection and generally produces only mild pain until the process becomes transmural, at which point the resultant peritoneal irritation can cause localized somatic pain. *Perforation* or rupture of a hollow viscus or other structure (e.g., an ovarian cyst or a hepatic adenoma) typically results in a pain of sudden onset that builds to maximum intensity over minutes to hours, producing signs of peritoneal irritation that are initially localized but may soon become generalized. *Torsion* may also produce a severe pain of sudden onset but usually physical findings in the initial phase are limited to the site of torsion and do not generalize. Finally, *ischemia* of a solid or hollow viscus produces a severe pain frequently described as out of proportion to physical findings.

As a first step in differential diagnosis, it is useful to tentatively assign the abdominal pain episode to one of these pathologic processes and to one of the previously mentioned locations. These categories are of course not absolute, because overlapping presentations are seen in a variety of conditions. For example, sigmoid volvulus simultaneously represents torsion and obstruction, whereas acute cholecystitis is initially due to obstruction (of the cystic duct) but then progresses to transmural inflammation. It is not unusual for a pain that is initially due to one process to evolve into another (e.g., intestinal ischemia and infarction developing as a consequence of untreated adhesive obstruction).

EVALUATION OF THE PATIENT WITH ABDOMINAL PAIN

It has been said that the most important diagnostic instrument available to the clinician is a chair, and this is perhaps nowhere more true than in the setting of the evaluation of a patient with acute abdominal pain. While eliciting the history, the clinician should take the opportunity to observe the patient's attitude in bed, the facial expression particularly during paroxysms of pain, and the contour of the abdomen.[2]

The course of the episode of illness should be retraced, beginning with the exact time and mode of onset of the pain as well as any prodromic events occurring in the hours or days from the point at which the patient was subjectively at baseline health. The location and character of the pain, the direction of radiation of the pain, and changes in intensity or shifts in location over time are elicited. The presence of associated symptoms, in particular anorexia and vomiting, and their relation to the onset and evolution of pain is determined. Nausea and vomiting are usually due either to severe irritation of the peritoneal or mesenteric nerves or to obstruction of a hollow viscus. The character and time of the most recent bowel movement or the occurrence of diarrhea is noted. The relevant past medical history is then documented in detail, with particular attention to prior episodes of similar pain, the presence of major digestive or other systemic disorders, and previous abdominal operations. Current medications are documented. Corticosteroid use or other conditions associated with immunosuppression may diminish the symptoms produced by inflammation and obscure a serious degree of intraabdominal disease. The presence of familial disorders or concurrent illness in family or other contacts should be noted.

The age of the patient should be taken into account, as the differential diagnosis shifts considerably when dealing with the pediatric versus the geriatric population. In women, a recent menstrual history is obtained and prior pregnancies noted. Gynecologic causes of acute abdominal pain to be considered include mittelschmerz or ruptured ovarian cyst, pelvic inflammatory disease, ectopic pregnancy, tubo-ovarian abscess (with or without rupture), and ovarian torsion.

As indicated previously, the physical examination should begin with inspection of the general appearance, attitude in bed, and facial expression. Unwillingness to change position

TABLE 74.4 DIAGNOSIS

PAIN LOCALIZING TO AN ABDOMINAL QUADRANT

RIGHT UPPER QUADRANT PAIN
- Biliary colic/cholecystitis
- Cholangitis
- Hepatic abscess
- Hepatitis (toxic or viral)
- Perihepatitis (Fitzhugh-Curtis syndrome)
- Hepatic congestion
- Budd-Chiari syndrome
- Hepatic tumor (primary or secondary)
- Appendicitis
- Perforated peptic ulcer
- Perinephritis
- Pneumonia (right lower lobe)
- Pulmonary infarction
- Pleuritis
- Myocardial ischemia
- Empyema
- Rib fracture
- Herpes zoster

LEFT UPPER QUADRANT PAIN
- Splenic rupture
- Splenic infarction
- Splenomegaly
- Ruptured splenic artery aneurysm
- Gastritis
- Perforated gastric ulcer (phlegmonous gastritis)
- Jejunal diverticulitis
- Pancreatitis
- Diverticulitis (splenic flexure)
- Perinephritis
- Pneumonia (left lower lobe)
- Pulmonary infarction
- Pleuritis
- Pericarditis
- Myocardial ischemia
- Empyema
- Rib fracture
- Herpes zoster

RIGHT LOWER QUADRANT PAIN
- Appendicitis
- Acute enterocolitis (viral or bacterial)
- Crohn's disease (ileitis)
- Foreign body perforation
- Right-sided diverticulitis
- Cecal diverticulitis
- Meckel's diverticulitis
- Torsion of appendix epiploica
- Mesenteric adenitis
- Intestinal obstruction
- Perforated peptic ulcer
- Pancreatitis
- Ruptured ovarian cyst (including Mittelschmerz)
- Ovarian torsion
- Endometriosis
- Salpingitis (pelvic inflammatory disease)
- Ectopic pregnancy
- Cholecystitis
- Ruptured iliac artery aneurysm
- Renal or ureteral calculi
- Pyelonephritis
- Psoas abscess
- Seminal vesiculitis
- Rectus sheath hematoma
- Herpes zoster

LEFT LOWER QUADRANT PAIN
- Diverticulitis
- Appendicitis
- Perforated colon cancer
- Intestinal obstruction
- Crohn's colitis
- Ischemic colitis
- Ruptured iliac artery aneurysm
- Ruptured ovarian cyst (including Mittelschmerz)
- Ovarian torsion
- Endometriosis
- Salpingitis (pelvic inflammatory disease)
- Ectopic pregnancy
- Renal or ureteral calculi
- Pyelonephritis
- Psoas abscess
- Seminal vesiculitis
- Rectus sheath hematoma
- Herpes zoster

TABLE 74.5 ETIOLOGY

CAUSES OF MIDLINE ABDOMINAL PAIN

EPIGASTRIC
- Peptic ulcer
- Pancreatitis
- Gastritis
- Esophagitis
- Mesenteric ischemia
- Appendicitis (early)
- Myocardial ischemia
- Pericarditis
- Cholecystitis

PERIUMBILICAL
- Small intestinal obstruction
- Appendicitis
- Pancreatitis
- Mesenteric ischemia
- Acute glaucoma

HYPOGASTRIC
- Large intestinal obstruction
- Intussusception
- Appendicitis
- Diverticulitis
- Enterocolitis
- Ovarian torsion
- Testicular torsion
- Degeneration or torsion of uterine fibroid
- Cystitis

may indicate underlying peritonitis; conversely, an inability to find a comfortable position may be seen with ureteral colic due to nephrolithiasis. A patient with acute pancreatitis or mesenteric ischemia may prefer to lean forward. Intermittent grimacing may be observed in a patient with intestinal obstruction. Vital signs are measured. The presence of cool, clammy skin or of jaundice may be observed at this time.

Inspection of the abdomen will reveal generalized distention or focal swelling. The presence of a hernia must be specifically excluded by direct examination of all hernial orifices and abdominal incisions. Auscultation of the abdomen may be performed next, although this only rarely provides valuable information. Auscultation of the chest, particularly the basilar regions, may reveal pneumonic consolidation that can simulate an acute abdominal process or may reveal a pleuritic rub.

TABLE 74.6 ETIOLOGY

CAUSES OF DIFFUSE ABDOMINAL PAIN

- Early appendicitis
- Perforated appendicitis
- Perforated peptic ulcer
- Perforated diverticulitis
- Stercoral perforation of colon
- Peritonitis (primary or secondary)
- Pancreatitis
- Mesenteric adenitis
- Mesenteric ischemia
- Ruptured abdominal aortic aneurysm
- Diabetic coma
- Tuberculous peritonitis
- Food poisoning
- Heavy metal poisoning
- Acute porphyria
- Sickle cell crisis
- Acute leukemia

TABLE 74.7 ETIOLOGY

PATHOLOGIC PROCESSES UNDERLYING ABDOMINAL PAIN

Process	Common examples
Obstruction	Intestinal colic, renal calculi, biliary colic
Inflammation	Enterocolitis, mesenteric adenitis
Perforation	Perforated peptic ulcer
Torsion	Ovarian torsion, sigmoid volvulus
Ischemia	Mesenteric artery thrombosis, splenic infarction

Gentle percussion of the abdomen will help distinguish gaseous distention from ascites; loss of dullness over the liver may indicate free intraperitoneal air, as in perforated duodenal ulcer. Tenderness to percussion, either localized or across the abdomen, suggests focal or diffuse peritonitis. Referred tenderness to percussion (pain perceived away from the site of percussion) is an extremely important finding that is essentially pathognomonic for peritonitis.

Palpation of the abdomen must be gentle. Rough or sudden deep palpation will frighten the patient, cause voluntary guarding, and hamper subsequent attempts to palpate the abdomen. The presence of subtle muscle rigidity (involuntary guarding) or of an intraabdominal mass is more likely to be detected by a gentle approach. It may be useful to ask the patient to flex the thighs during this phase of the examination. Areas of skin hyperesthesia may be noted during gentle palpation. Elicitation of rebound tenderness rarely provides additional information beyond that obtained by careful percussion and palpation and is not recommended. The psoas and obturator tests may be performed next. In patients with a colostomy or ileostomy, direct examination of the stoma along with digitalization is important. The back is examined with attention to the presence of spinal tenderness or tenderness in the costovertebral angle or flanks.

Examination of the pelvis is extremely important in most patients with abdominal pain. Suprapubic palpation may reveal an enlarged bladder or tenderness indicative of deeper disease. Digital rectal examination may reveal focal tenderness due to a periappendiceal or peridiverticular pelvic abscess. Anterior palpation may reveal the only evidence of pelvic peritonitis, particularly in males. A bimanual vaginoabdominal examination in females will reveal pathology in the pouch of Douglas or involving the uterus, tubes, or ovaries.

Whether it is prudent to administer analgesics to the patient undergoing evaluation for acute abdominal pain has remained a controversial question. Certainly, once the diagnosis is established or a definitive plan of action has been made, it is not justifiable to withhold such treatment. There is a considerable literature to suggest that administration of morphine can provide substantial pain relief without changing important physical signs (in particular, the presence of peritoneal irritation), although there is limited high-quality prospective, randomized data.[6–8]

Laboratory and Radiologic Examination

The common practice of ordering a "routine" panel of tests, even prior to evaluation by a physician, is wasteful of resources and may lead to unnecessary delays in diagnosis and treatment, particularly when normal values lull caregivers into a false sense of security. For example, the white blood cell count is notoriously normal in a substantial fraction of patients with serious intraabdominal pathology and is frequently elevated in cases of nonsurgical disease.[9] However, a hematocrit and serum electrolytes and blood urea nitrogen may be useful to guide fluid resuscitation. A serum amylase and liver chemistries are usually indicated in patients with upper abdominal pain but only rarely so in lower abdominal pain. Although liberal use of human chorionic gonadotrophin testing may avoid a missed tubal pregnancy, its routine use in females with abdominal pain is not likely to be cost-effective. A urinalysis is frequently of value to screen for urologic causes of abdominal pain, but routine urine culture is unnecessary.

Plain radiographs of the abdomen are ordered far in excess of their usefulness in the evaluation of abdominal pain.[10,11] Despite occasional positive findings (e.g., air-fluid levels, a fecalith, gallstones), plain films tend to be relatively nonspecific, complementing what is already obvious on history and examination, and rarely redirect therapeutic thinking. They are most helpful in patients with suspected ureteral calculus or intestinal obstruction. It is important to remember that abdominal films are frequently normal or nondiagnostic in patients with strangulating obstruction. An upright chest film is the least expensive and perhaps best test to identify free intraperitoneal air.

Upper GI series performed with water-soluble contrast is occasionally helpful in detecting ulcer perforation and determining whether such perforation is free or contained. A water-soluble contrast enema may be useful in cases of suspected large bowel obstruction. Intravenous pyelography may be used to identify ureteral stones. All of these studies, however, have been supplanted in many centers by computed tomography (CT), which, although somewhat more expensive, yields considerably more information of practical importance.[12] CT is quite useful in patients with abdominal pain who do not require emergency surgery, particularly in delineating the cause and suggesting therapeutic strategy in patients with no prior history of abdominal disease.[13] Arteriography may be useful in patients with suspected mesenteric ischemia, although CT angiography and magnetic resonance imaging are increasingly applied to this situation. Ultrasound examination of the right upper quadrant may reveal gallstones, but it is important to remember that ultrasonographic signs of acute cholecystitis may be no more accurate than clinical examination. Ultrasonography for lower abdominal pain may improve diagnostic accuracy beyond clinical impression alone but is highly experience- and operator-dependent.[14] A guiding principle in ordering radiologic tests is that the result should substantially influence plans for further testing or therapy. Redundant tests should be avoided.

Diagnostic laparoscopy may be appropriate in certain circumstances, especially the evaluation of acute lower abdominal pain in females. This has become a more attractive option as techniques of therapeutic laparoscopy (e.g., appendectomy) have been refined.[15–17] Nevertheless, laparoscopy requires a general anesthetic and should not be used without due consideration.

Conditions Mimicking the Acute Abdomen

A variety of nonsurgical conditions may be associated with acute abdominal pain, including a variety of cardiovascular, respiratory, metabolic, and toxic conditions. For example, myocardial ischemia may produce epigastric pain, nausea, and vomiting that simulates acute cholecystitis; conversely, and perhaps more frequently, acute cholecystitis is mistaken for pain of cardiac origin. Abdominal wall injury, radiculopathy, and rectus sheath hematoma (the latter particularly in patients on anticoagulant therapy) may cause acute abdominal pain. Abdominal pain and vomiting may accompany influenza. Diabetic ketoacidosis and, rarely, blood dyscrasias such as acute porphyria or sickle cell hemolytic crisis may produce severe abdominal pain. Urologic disorders such as pyelonephritis or obstruction of the ureter, renal pelvis, or bladder outlet may be mistaken for intraabdominal pathology. Urinalysis and renal ultrasound may confirm the diagnosis. Testicular torsion can also be associated with severe abdominal pain.

Abdominal Pain in Special Circumstances

The pediatric population represents a particularly difficult subset in which to evaluate acute abdominal pain. In neonates and infants, congenital causes such as midgut volvulus or pyloric stenosis must be considered, and entities such as intussusception and Meckel's diverticulitis are far more common than in adults. It may be impossible to obtain key historical information, and physical examination may be difficult.[18] Evaluation of older children is generally easier. It should be noted that anorexia may be absent in children with appendicitis or other important abdominal pathology. Diarrhea as a manifestation of appendicitis is also frequent and may simulate acute infectious enterocolitis. Abdominal films may be more informative in pediatric than adult patients. In certain instances, it may be appropriate to consider whether child abuse has occurred. The geriatric population can also present diagnostic difficulty and if dementia is present, it may be impossible to elicit a meaningful history. In such patients, serious intraabdominal pathology may present with few or subtle signs, and there may be only minimal tenderness on examination despite diffuse peritonitis. Laboratory values are frequently normal despite the presence of serious pathology in this population.[19] The majority of geriatric patients evaluated in the emergency setting will be found to have significant disease requiring hospitalization.[20]

Acute abdominal pain in immunosuppressed patients represents a particular diagnostic challenge, for example, in the setting of organ transplantation, immunosuppressive therapy for autoimmune disorders, chemotherapy, and acquired immune deficiency syndrome (AIDS). Unusual infectious causes of acute abdominal pain, including cytomegalovirus (CMV), mycobacteria, protozoal species, and fungi should be considered; these may affect the GI tract, gallbladder, liver, and pancreas. Perforation of the GI tract due to CMV, *Mycobacterium tuberculosis* or *Mycobacterium avium-intracellulare,* lymphoma, or Kaposi sarcoma or associated with corticosteroid use are seen in immunosuppressed patients. Acalculous cholecystitis should be considered in patients with AIDS and is often associated with *Cryptosporidia* or CMV. Splenic abscess due to *Candida* or *Salmonella* may be a cause of left upper quadrant pain. Neutropenic enterocolitis is a common cause of abdominal pain and fever in patients with bone marrow suppression due to chemotherapy. In the transplant population, acute graft-versus-host disease should be considered. Although abdominal pain in immunosuppressed patients is often treated nonoperatively, vigilance must be maintained lest serious surgical pathology be overlooked.

Acute abdominal pain after cardiac or major abdominal vascular surgery merits special mention because of the frequency of serious diagnoses that carry particularly high mortality in this setting. Mesenteric or segmental colonic ischemia is commonly reported, as are acute colitis and cholecystitis (often acalculous). Acute pancreatitis associated with extracorporeal cardiopulmonary bypass occurs in about 2% of cases.[21] Severe acute abdominal pain in hemodialysis patients is most commonly due to mesenteric ischemia.[22]

The diagnosis of abdominal pain in patients with spinal cord injury is particularly challenging. Mortality in this setting is high (about 10%), usually due to delayed diagnosis.[23] Classical signs such as tenderness, guarding, and even fever are unreliable; more helpful are the presence of shoulder pain, abdominal distention, nausea, vomiting, and autonomic dysreflexia.[24]

Finally, evaluation of abdominal pain occurring during pregnancy carries additional considerations.[25] Anatomic relationships may be distorted by the gravid uterus; in particular, the appendix is often displaced upward into the right upper quadrant. Nonsurgical causes of abdominal and pelvic pain are common. Interpretation of blood work should recognize physiologic alterations; leukocytosis is frequently present during normal pregnancy. Although one should not hesitate to obtain radiologic tests when essential, unnecessary exposure to x-rays must be avoided. Ultrasound is a particularly valuable diagnostic modality in these patients.

APPENDIX

The clinical entity of appendiceal inflammation followed by perforation, abscess formation, and peritonitis was first described in 1889 by Reginald Fitz.[26] Since that time, appendectomy has remained among the most common abdominal operations and, in fact, is the most common surgical procedure performed on an emergency basis in Western countries. Appendectomy remains the mainstay of treatment, but with the development of modern antibiotics and percutaneous drainage techniques, some cases are best managed nonoperatively. The morbidity and mortality associated with acute appendicitis has diminished over time, although because it usually affects young, healthy people, the overall effect on our work force remains significant. When not treated appropriately, appendicitis remains a potentially lethal condition. A case in point is that of the famous magician, Harry Houdini, who would occasionally entertain by withstanding punches to the abdomen delivered by members of his audience. Unfortunately, Mr. Houdini once performed this "act" while suffering from an appendiceal abscess, only to die several days later from diffuse peritonitis and sepsis, the abscess having been ruptured from one of the assaults.[27]

Anatomy and Pathophysiology

The appendix is considered a vestigial organ with no known function in human beings. However, examination of the phylogenetic tree reveals that the appendix is absent from a number of carnivores, such as the dog, tiger, and lion, and, surprisingly, there is progressive development of the appendix in apes and as one ascends the primate scale.[28] The appendix contains large amounts of lymphoid aggregates, similar to those within the Peyer patches of gut-associated lymphoid tissue. Lymphoid nodules containing both B and T cells within its lamina propria differentiate the appendix from the adjacent colon.[29] Because of this prominence of lymphoid tissue, some have hypothesized that the appendix may have an immune function similar to that of the thymus or bursa of Fabricius, although no actual function has ever been documented. The appendiceal mucosa produces minimal amounts of fluid and digestive juices, suggesting that it has no important exocrine function. There have been some associations made between the lack of an appendix and various disease states (inflammatory bowel disease), but a causal relationship remains unproved.

The appendix develops as an antimesenteric outpouching from the cecum and is first delineated during the fifth month of gestation. The position of the appendix can vary greatly. The appendix, in almost two thirds of the population, is located in a retrocecal position, whereas in others it is located over the pelvic brim, occasionally descending low down in the pelvis. When the appendix occupies an unusual location, the diagnosis of appendicitis may be more difficult and contribute to delays in either presentation and/or diagnosis. The three taeniae coli of the ascending colon meet at the base of the appendix, with the anterior taenia serving as an important landmark. Following the taeniae can be a useful maneuver in identifying a difficult appendix at the time of operation. The appendix can vary in length from 2 to 20 cm, averaging approximately 9 cm. The blood supply of the appendix is from the appendicular artery, which is a branch of the ileocolic. Similarly, the lymphatic drainage follows that of the ileocolic nodes, and these are often hyperplastic in cases of acute appendicitis. The neural innervation of the appendix is derived from the autonomic nervous system. As with other visceral organs, there are no somatic pain fibers within the appendix. As such, early inflammation leads to poorly localizable pain and is referred to the periumbilical region because the autonomic nerves follow the midgut embryologic origin. As inflammation of appendicitis progresses, irritation of the surrounding parietal peritoneum results in the activation of somatic pain fibers and localization of symptoms and signs to the right lower quadrant.

In cross-section, the appendix contains the same layers as those of the adjacent colon, including the mucosa, submucosa with prominent lymphoid tissue, circular and longitudinal muscle layers, and the overlying serosa. Neurosecretory cells are located within the subepithelial layer and are the presumed source of carcinoid tumors, which are often found within the appendix.

The etiology of appendicitis remains somewhat unclear. In most patients, there is probably luminal obstruction that leads to bacterial overgrowth and increased luminal pressure, leading to obstruction of venous outflow and then arterial inflow, resulting in gangrene and eventual perforation. The cause for the luminal obstruction that initiates the process of appendicitis is postulated to involve lymphoid hyperplasia, a condition that is especially common in the teenage years which correlates with the high incidence of appendicitis in this age group. It is felt that either viral or bacterial infections such as *Shigella, Salmonella,* infectious mononucleosis, and so forth can precede the episode of appendicitis, presumably by initiating the lymphoid hyperplasia and subsequent luminal obstruction.

In addition to lymphoid hyperplasia, fecaliths can also lead to appendiceal obstruction and subsequent appendicitis. It is thought that approximately 30% of cases of acute appendicitis in adults are linked to fecaliths. Fecaliths are thought to occur following entrapment of vegetable matter with subsequent mucus deposition and eventual calcification. The "obstructive" model for appendicitis does not appear to explain the etiology in all cases, however, because some patients with appendicitis appear to have a patent lumen by radiologic, gross, and histologic examination. The pathophysiology of these cases remains unclear.

Diagnosis

Early diagnosis remains the most important clinical goal in patients with suspected appendicitis. Although mortality rates in modern series are well under 1%,[30,31] the morbidity of perforated appendicitis is much higher than in nonperforated cases and is related to increased rates of wound infection, intraabdominal abscess formation, lengths of hospital stay, and delayed return to full activity.[32]

TABLE 74.8 — DIAGNOSIS

TYPICAL SEQUENCE OF SYMPTOMS AND SIGNS OF ACUTE APPENDICITIS

Periumbilical pain—vague, visceral, poorly localized
Anorexia, nausea, and/or vomiting
Right lower quadrant pain and tenderness—localized
Fever
Leukocytosis

By a thorough history and physical examination, experienced clinicians can accurately diagnose acute appendicitis in the majority of cases.[2] A typical presentation (Table 74.8) is that of vague periumbilical pain (sometimes located more superiorly in the epigastric region) followed by anorexia, nausea, or even frank vomiting. When vomiting occurs in appendicitis, it is usually of a limited nature, as opposed to patients with viral gastroenteritis who generally have more severe vomiting. The pain then shifts to the right lower quadrant region as the inflammatory process progresses and involves the localized overlying peritoneum. Eventually, fever ensues and this is followed by the development of leukocytosis. These clinical features are not entirely reliable, however. For example, not all patients will complain of anorexia, so that the fact that a given patient expresses hunger should not necessarily deter one from surgical intervention for presumed acute appendicitis. Occasionally, patients will complain of urinary symptoms, perhaps because of some inflammation adjacent to the ureter and/or bladder. Microscopic hematuria is quite common, and the clinician should not mistake the primary problem as residing in the urinary tract. Intestinal function is usually unaffected in appendicitis, but some patients will note diarrhea, perhaps related to the inflammation adjacent to the rectum and/or colon. Appendicitis can also be associated with adynamic ileus, leading to the complaint of constipation.

Physical examination is generally the most reliable indicator of appendicitis. Aside from the young child, very elderly, or otherwise neurologically impaired, patients with appendicitis will have at least some degree of tenderness on palpation of the abdomen. In cases of an appendix located entirely in the pelvis, the tenderness on abdominal examination may be minimal, but on rectal examination the tenderness will be evident as the pelvic peritoneum is manipulated. Pelvic examination with cervical motion will also manipulate the pelvic peritoneum and elicit tenderness when there is an inflamed appendix in that region. Therefore, the finding of cervical motion tenderness does not necessarily indicate gynecologic pathology but rather is a nonspecific sign of inflammation in the pelvis.

Peritoneal irritation can be elicited on physical examination with the findings of percussion and/or rebound tenderness. Any movement including coughing (Dunphy sign) may cause increased pain. The most reliable indicator of peritoneal irritation, however, is involuntary guarding, a reflex contraction of the abdominal wall musculature overlying the inflamed peritoneum. The involuntary nature of this response is less dependent on the individual variation seen in response to external stimuli. Other physical signs (Table 74.9) associated with appendicitis include the occurrence of pain in the right lower quadrant during palpation of the left lower quadrant (Rovsing's sign), pain on internal rotation of the hip (obturator sign, suggesting a pelvic appendix), and pain on right hip extension (iliopsoas sign, typical of a retrocecal appendix).

TABLE 74.9 DIAGNOSIS

SIGNS ON PHYSICAL EXAMINATION SUGGESTIVE OF ACUTE APPENDICITIS

Sign	What it indicates	Description
Dunphy	Inflammation involving the partial peritoneum	Increased pain with coughing or other movement
Rovsing	Localized peritoneal inflammation in the right lower quadrant	Lower left quadrant palpation induces right lower quadrant pain
Obturator	Pelvic appendicitis	Pain on internal rotation of the right hip
Iliopsoas	Retrocecal appendicitis	Pain on extension of right hip

In addition to the history and physical examination, a white blood cell count is usually obtained and in most patients will be elevated, although it may be in the normal range during the early stages. A very high white blood cell count (>20,000 white blood cells per mL) suggests complicated appendicitis with either gangrene or perforation. A urinalysis can also be helpful to rule out pyelonephritis or nephrolithiasis. However, in patients with pyelonephritis, the fever and white blood cell count will generally be much higher than that seen in appendicitis, symptoms of dysuria will be present, and the tenderness is centered more in the flank or costovertebral angle region. Minimal pyuria, frequently seen in elderly women, should not deter one from the correct diagnosis of appendicitis. Although microscopic hematuria is common in appendicitis, gross hematuria is uncommon and may indicate the presence of a kidney stone. As a kidney stone passes down the urinary tract through the distal ureter, pain can often be referred to the right lower quadrant region and occasionally down into the testicle. The pain is quite severe and entirely visceral in nature. Therefore, the signs of peritoneal irritation should not exist in the patient with nephrolithiasis. Other blood tests are generally not helpful nor indicated in the patient with suspected appendicitis.

Plain abdominal radiographs are of little use in the patient with suspected appendicitis. Occasionally, a calcified appendicolith may be evident, but this is a rare event (~17%) and, in any case, does not really establish the diagnosis even if present.[33] Plain abdominal films can show indications of mechanical bowel obstruction or the presence of free intraperitoneal air, but such conditions should rarely be confused with appendicitis.

Given the inherent limitations in establishing the diagnosis of acute appendicitis and a concern that a delay may result in perforation with increased associated morbidity and possible mortality, a false appendectomy rate of approximately 20% has been considered acceptable. Certainly, if the negative appendectomy rate were much higher, one could question the diagnostic acumen and experience of the clinicians involved. On the other hand, in some centers a negative appendectomy rate of less than 10% has been accomplished,[31] and it is likely that the addition of newer imaging modalities to evaluate acute abdominal pain has improved accuracy to the point where the modern standard-of-care should be substantially better than the historical target of 20%. Clearly, clinical experience and expertise is an important factor in establishing a correct diagnosis. In addition, in-hospital observation has been touted as an excellent way to closely follow patients and quickly intervene for worsening abdominal pain, peritoneal irritation, or fever. Using this approach, White et al.[34] reported a negative appendectomy rate of 6%. Cost-effectiveness of in-hospital observation strategies has not been determined. Of course, with a low negative appendectomy rate, one must ensure that there are few patients who develop perforated appendicitis while being observed in the hospital or after being sent home from an emergency room visit.

To improve diagnostic accuracy in patients with suspected appendicitis, other radiologic tests have been used. Ultrasonography has been reported to aid in the diagnosis of acute appendicitis[35,36] by the demonstration of a so-called target lesion (i.e., a thick walled, noncompressible, luminal structure in the right lower quadrant). In more advanced cases, peritoneal fluid and even a frank abscess may be found. However, a number of large series[37,38] have shown ultrasound to be unreliable, both in terms of sensitivity and specificity, such that it probably should not be used in the routine diagnosis of acute appendicitis. Ultrasound may be helpful if it suggests a diagnosis other than appendicitis, especially gynecologic pathology in women of menstrual age. It must be cautioned, however, that simple cysts of the ovary are common and usually nonpathologic. As such, the presence of an ovarian cyst does not weigh against the diagnosis of acute appendicitis. On the other hand, if ultrasonographic signs of a tubo-ovarian abscess, ovarian torsion, or even rare complications related to uterine fibroids are present, then the diagnosis of appendicitis may be excluded (Fig. 74.1).

More recently, abdominal and pelvic CT scan has been used in the setting of suspected acute appendicitis[39,40] and appears to be more accurate than ultrasound.[41] Rao et al.[42] suggested that CT scan can lead to significant cost savings, because a normal study virtually excludes the diagnosis and obviates the need (and costs) of in-hospital observation. CT scan should include thin cuts through the area of the appendix and the use of rectal contrast to distend the cecum and make the adjacent inflammatory changes more evident. The role of CT scan in the diagnosis of appendicitis, however, remains controversial, because in most patients an accurate diagnosis can be reached simply by history and physical examination. In the setting of early acute appendicitis, pathologic changes in the gross appearance of the appendix may be minimal even with direct observation at the time of surgery and may well be missed by all radiologic techniques. One advantage of CT scan, similar to that of ultrasound, may be the detection of pathology other than acute appendicitis.[43]

Barium enema has also been used in the past in an attempt to diagnose appendicitis.[44] Failure to fill the appendix has been associated with appendicitis, but up to 20% of normal appendices do not fill and therefore the diagnosis cannot be accurately established using this criterion. Occasionally, in more advanced cases, with abscess formation, a mass effect will be seen compressing the adjacent cecum. However, such a finding would probably be better visualized by CT, which also provides the opportunity for percutaneous drainage. On occasion, barium enema can detect a colonic mucosal lesion such as a neoplasm or terminal ileal abnormalities related to Crohn's disease, thereby establishing a diagnosis other than appendicitis. Overall, however, barium enema has little role in the modern management of suspected acute appendicitis.

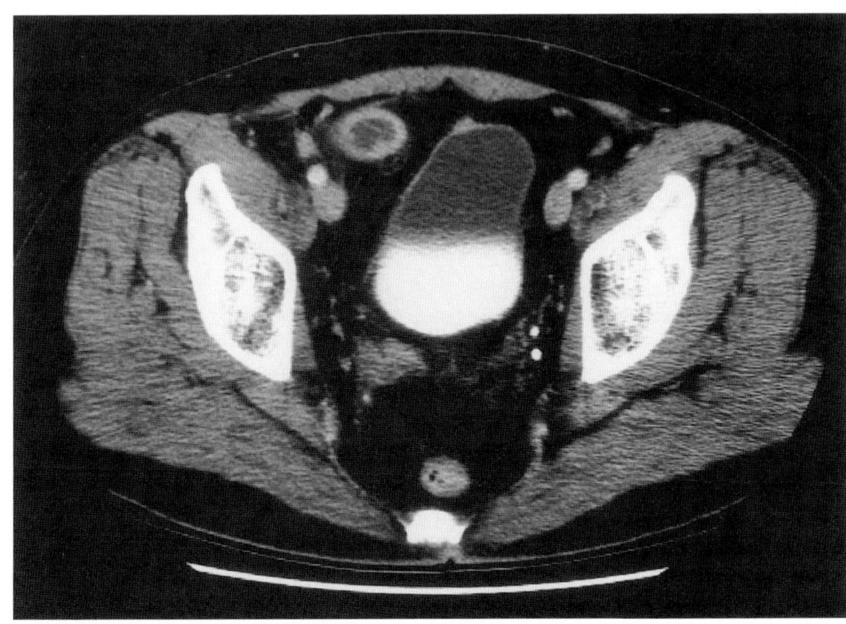

FIGURE 74.1 Acute appendicitis in a 53-year-old woman with fever and right lower quadrant pain and tenderness. Note the thick-walled, fluid-filled appendix with surrounding inflammation. A gangrenous appendix was found at operation.

Treatment

The standard treatment for suspected appendicitis is appendectomy via a right lower quadrant incision (Algorithm 74.1). The classical McBurney incision employs an oblique approach, incising each of the three abdominal wall muscle layers lateral to the rectus sheath. Ideally, the incision should follow Langer's skin lines to provide an optimal cosmetic result. The aponeurosis overlying the external oblique can be sharply incised, and the remaining muscle layers split by retraction. The peritoneum is opened, the appendix is identified, and its blood supply is then ligated, usually from tip to base. Depending on the degree of surrounding inflammation and the length of time of the illness, mobilization of the appendix may be difficult and may require division of the lateral attachments of the cecum. The appendix itself is usually ligated with an absorbable suture and then inverted into the cecal wall through the use of a purse-string or Z-stitch. Inversion of the appendiceal stump has been advocated to prevent leakage and fistulization, but numerous reports have shown no difference in complication rates between inversion and simple ligation of the appendiceal stump.[45] Following appendectomy, irrigation of the peritoneal cavity should be carried out and then the peritoneum and muscles should be closed in layered fashion, usually with absorbable sutures. The skin incision can generally be safely closed, although in grossly contaminated cases, one may consider delayed primary closure or simply healing by secondary intention. Intraperitoneal drains have not proven to be useful even in cases of perforated appendicitis.[46]

If a normal appendix is found at the time of laparotomy, other causes for the abdominal pain should be sought. The cecum and proximal ascending colon should be examined for right-sided diverticulitis, neoplasms, or other pathology. The terminal ileum should be examined for Crohn's disease or acute ileitis and the ileum should be inspected for at least two feet proximal to the ileocecal valve for the presence of a Meckel's diverticulum. If Crohn's disease is encountered, the appendix may be safely removed as long as the cecum and particularly the base of the appendix is not involved with the inflammatory process. If uncomplicated Crohn's inflammation is detected, ileal resection is not indicated, but in the case of a gross perforation or advanced Crohn's disease with obstruction, resection should be performed. Occasionally, sigmoid diverticulitis may be mistaken for acute appendicitis, especially when a redundant sigmoid colon reaches the right side of the abdomen. Finally, the fallopian tubes, ovaries, and uterus should be carefully examined in female patients.

Laparoscopy

The role of laparoscopy and laparoscopic appendectomy remains to be established. Many surgeons advocate diagnostic laparoscopy especially for young women. Laparoscopy allows easy visualization of the pelvic organs as well as the appendix and can establish the diagnosis of appendicitis or other processes.[47,48] Laparoscopic appendectomy has gained substantial popularity. Generally, the laparoscope is inserted through a periumbilical incision and then additional trocars are placed, one in the right lower quadrant to grasp the appendix, and another on the left side to perform dissection, ligation, and, ultimately, removal of the appendix. Endoscopic stapling devices have simplified transection and closure of the appendiceal stump at its base as well as hemostatic division of the mesoappendix. Numerous series have compared laparoscopic to open appendectomy.[49,50] As in many other minimally invasive procedures, a learning curve clearly exists and may explain the longer operative times in initial reports. With experience, however, operative times for the laparoscopic approach probably equal and may be superior to open appendectomy. Complication rates appear to be low and are probably no different between the laparoscopic and open techniques, although postoperative infections may be less common with laparoscopy. Laparoscopy may also be of benefit in regard to hospital stay and overall recovery. Most reports in the literature indicate that length of stay is significantly shorter using the laparoscopic route, as is narcotic usage and other parameters associated with postoperative morbidity.[51] In a large retrospective series,[31] laparoscopic appendectomy was found to be particularly valuable in cases of gangrenous and/or perforated appendicitis. For simple acute appendicitis, hospital stay and recovery periods were short, regardless of operative approach. However, in the more advanced cases, laparoscopy was associated with shorter hospital stays and faster recovery.

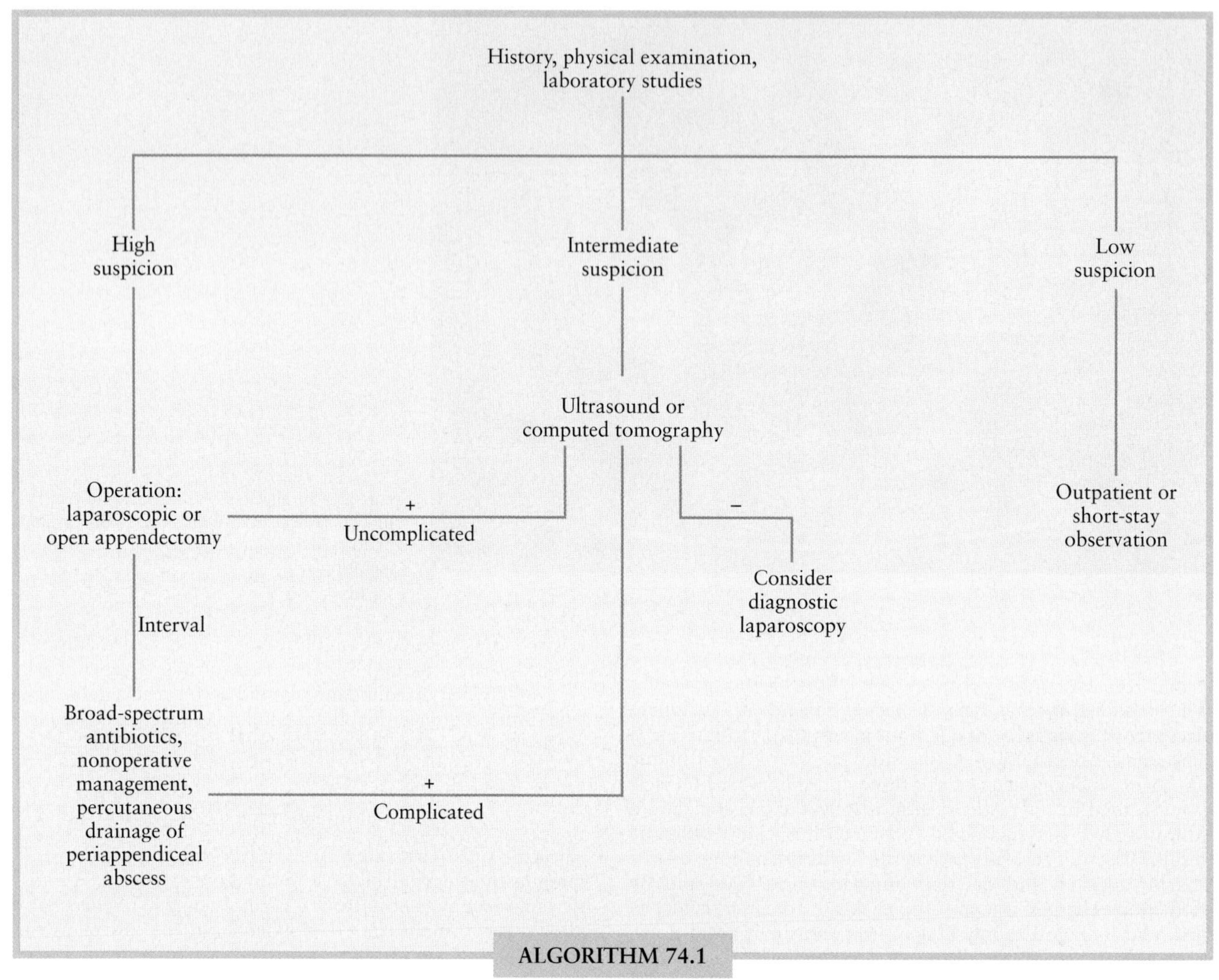

ALGORITHM 74.1 Management of suspected appendicitis.

Appendiceal Mass

Some patients with appendicitis will present at a relatively late stage (greater than about 5 days). Although, in most cases, acute appendicitis progresses to perforation and diffuse peritonitis within the first few days of the illness, virtually forcing the patient to seek medical attention, occasionally an appendiceal perforation is contained by surrounding structures including the omentum and adjacent bowel. Instead of developing diffuse peritonitis, these patients develop a localized inflammatory mass or phlegmon with or without a discrete abscess. The associated pain and other systemic signs are limited by this process, which may explain the delayed presentation. Such patients usually have right lower quadrant abdominal pain, tenderness on examination, with a palpable mass or fullness, although overlying guarding of the abdominal wall musculature may obscure the mass. The key diagnostic feature to be recognized in these patients is the length of time of the illness, because a walled-off appendiceal mass generally requires a minimum of 5 days to form. In such cases, CT scan may establish the diagnosis and allow for percutaneous abscess drainage (Fig. 74.2). In the acute setting, these patients are best treated nonoperatively, because, although the appendix can be removed, there is added risk of injury to adjacent structures, including the small bowel. The overall morbidity in these patients appears to be decreased by the nonoperative approach, with or without percutaneous drainage.[52] Intravenous antibiotics are administered initially, and most of these patients will respond within a 24- to 48-hour period with a decrease in pain and fever. The patients can then be safely discharged on a course of oral antibiotics and a normal diet. The appendiceal inflammation generally subsides within 1 to 2 weeks. Antibiotics should continue for a total of approximately 2 weeks.

It should be noted that patients who have undergone percutaneous or open drainage of a periappendiceal abscess rarely develop fistulization from the cecum. Similarly, patients with perforated appendicitis almost always have pus within the peritoneal cavity, rather than actual enteric contents. These observations support the concept that most cases of appendicitis are associated with some obstruction of the lumen of the appendix. Following the successful nonoperative treatment of an appendiceal mass, consideration should be given to interval appendectomy. A period of approximately 8 weeks will allow resolution of the inflammatory changes

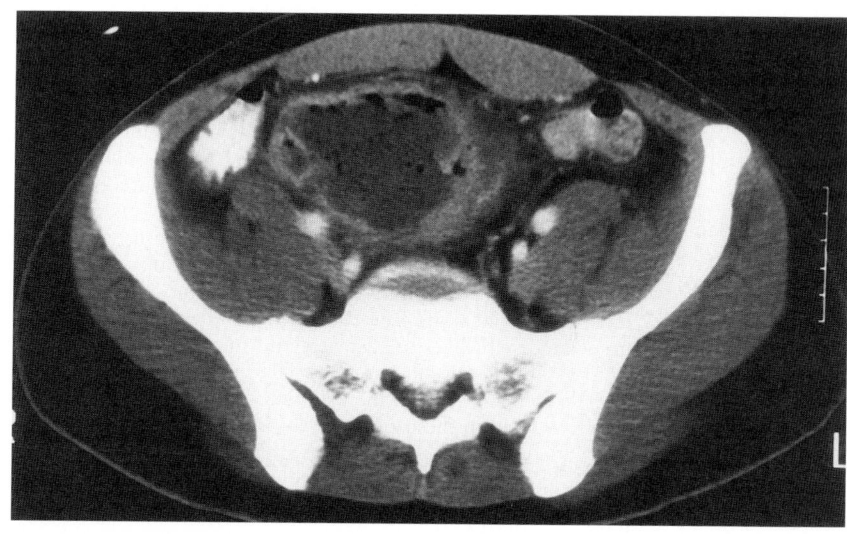

FIGURE 74.2 A 23-year-old man with 2 weeks of right lower quadrant pain, fever, and leukocytosis. Note the large periappendiceal abscess containing gas. The patient was successfully treated with percutaneous drainage and antibiotics.

surrounding the appendix. Removal of the appendix after such a time period is generally safe and simple, although in rare circumstances, a significant amount of periappendiceal scar tissue and inflammation will persist. Whether or not to perform an interval appendectomy remains controversial. A number of investigators have examined the incidence of recurrent appendicitis following presentation with an appendiceal mass and successful nonoperative treatment. Based on a recurrence rate of approximately 10% (6-month to 13-year follow-up), Ein and Shandling[53] suggested that interval appendectomy is not indicated in all patients. The incidence of recurrence may be higher in younger patients and therefore the decision to perform the interval appendectomy should probably be individualized by patient age. One must remember, however, especially in the elderly patient, that the original diagnosis of appendicitis may have been mistaken and it is important to rule out a cecal neoplasm in such patients if interval appendectomy is not performed.

More recently, interval laparoscopic appendectomy has been shown to be a safe and simple procedure with a high degree of patient acceptance. The operation can generally be performed on an outpatient basis with minimal morbidity.[54] Laparoscopy, therefore, may have shifted the risk/benefit ratio in favor of interval appendectomy.

Antibiotic Therapy

Patients with acute appendicitis should be treated with perioperative broad-spectrum antibiotics directed against colonic flora, including gram-positive, gram-negative, and anaerobic organisms. Peritoneal cultures are generally not clinically helpful in the selection of the type of antibiotics.[55] The optimal length of antibiotic therapy is not known. In simple cases of acute appendicitis, 24 hours or less is generally sufficient. However, in cases of perforated appendicitis, longer courses of antibiotics are generally used, approximately 5 to 7 days.

Recurrent Appendicitis

Rarely, a patient will present with recurrent episodes of presumed acute appendicitis. At each presentation, spontaneous resolution may occur, with or without the use of antibiotics. Such patients may eventually come to appendectomy, and it is only in retrospect that the previous episodes are recognized to have been due to acute appendicitis. Recurrent appendicitis is occasionally termed chronic appendicitis, but this is probably a misnomer because the appendix is almost certainly uninflamed in the interval between episodes. Some patients will present in the outpatient setting for evaluation of chronic or intermittent right lower quadrant pain raising the question of recurrent and/or chronic appendicitis. This difficult scenario requires clinical expertise to rule out etiologies other than appendicitis and to determine whether surgery is indicated. In general, discrete episodes of right lower quadrant pain, especially associated with fever and/or leukocytosis, are the best indicators of pathology within the appendix, and these patients respond most favorably to appendectomy. In contrast, patients with chronic right lower quadrant pain recurring frequently or even daily, in the absence of associated fever, are unlikely to benefit from appendectomy.

Appendicitis in Special Patient Populations

Children

The diagnosis of acute appendicitis is generally more difficult in young children compared to adults.[56] An accurate history may be difficult to obtain, and some of the signs of appendicitis such as nausea, vomiting, abdominal pain, and tenderness are often associated with extraabdominal processes (e.g., pneumonia, meningitis, otitis media). The difficulty in establishing an accurate diagnosis in children is the presumed reason for a higher perforation rate in this population, reported to be as high as 50%. As such, the use of radiologic studies such as CT scan may be of particular benefit in children with suspected appendicitis. Recent data suggest a negative appendectomy rate as low as 4% can be achieved with routine use of ultrasound or CT.[57] However, this has not been the experience of all groups, and there is concern about the potential increase in lifetime risk of cancer in children who have undergone radiation exposure due to a single CT scan.[58]

Elderly Patients

As in a number of other disease entities, elderly patients tend to present later in their course of appendicitis and clearly have higher associated rates of morbidity and mortality.[59] Perforation rates in elderly patients with appendicitis are quite high (>50%). Elderly patients tend to have less subjective pain, have decreased findings of peritonitis on examination, and may have a delayed leukocytosis. Therefore, the index of suspicion for an intraabdominal inflammatory/infectious process, including acute appendicitis, must be higher in elderly patients compared to the general population.

Immunocompromised Patients

The patient with an impaired immune system who complains of abdominal pain represents a particularly challenging problem for the clinician.[60] Patients with AIDS or those who have been exposed to high-dose chemotherapy are susceptible to specific disease entities, including CMV-related bowel perforations and typhlitis (neutropenic colitis). Because these disease processes most commonly effect the terminal ileum and cecum, they can often be confused with acute appendicitis. CT scan can be particularly helpful in this setting in order to establish a definitive diagnosis, although in some cases the findings of pericecal inflammation are nonspecific. In general, regardless of the underlying disease process, surgery is indicated in the patient with spreading peritonitis or with systemic signs of sepsis related to an intraabdominal infection.

Pregnancy

Appendicitis is the most frequent nonobstetric indication for laparotomy during pregnancy. Pregnant women will often present with abdominal pain, particularly in the lower abdomen, raising the suspicion of appendicitis. A diagnosis can be difficult to establish, especially because abdominal pain, nausea, and vomiting are quite common in early pregnancy. The white blood cell count is slightly elevated in normal pregnancy, adding further difficulties to establishing the diagnosis of appendicitis. In addition, as the uterus enlarges, the anatomic location of the appendix will be shifted upward, and the uterus may cover the appendix, thereby diminishing the signs of peritoneal inflammation. Because of these complicating factors, the perforation rate of appendicitis during pregnancy is probably higher than in the general population.[61,62] Unfortunately, perforated appendicitis is also associated with high fetal mortality (>30%), whereas simple acute appendicitis has a risk of fetal loss in the range of 10%, and poses negligible risk to the mother. As such, it is best to be aggressive in recommending surgical exploration in pregnant women with suspected appendicitis, especially because a "negative" appendectomy is well tolerated with minimal morbidity to mother and fetus. Numerous reports have indicated the safety of laparoscopy in the setting of pregnancy.[63] However, in the third trimester, the enlarged uterus may limit the exposure and preclude a laparoscopic approach.

Appendiceal Neoplasms

Approximately 1% of all appendectomy specimens will contain a neoplasm.[64] The most common tumor is the carcinoid. Rare tumors of the appendix include benign and malignant mucoceles, adenocarcinoma, and adenocarcinoids.

Carcinoids

Approximately one third to two thirds of all appendiceal neoplasms are carcinoids, tumors of neural crest origin and derived from enteroendocrine cells. Of all carcinoid tumors within the GI tract, approximately half arise within the appendix. Carcinoid tumors of the appendix are usually found incidentally on pathologic examination of the inflamed appendix. These tumors have a characteristic firm yellow appearance and are often associated with a surrounding desmoplastic reaction. In regard to treatment and prognosis, the key feature is the size of the tumor. Most carcinoids are less than 1.5 cm in diameter, and these tumors are adequately treated by simple appendectomy. The chance of lymphatic or distant metastasis is essentially zero and the prognosis for cure should be excellent. On the other hand, tumors that are 2 cm in size or greater begin to show metastatic potential. In such cases, a formal right hemicolectomy is generally indicated, and the prognosis remains quite good. Other indications for right colectomy include high-grade malignant lesions with high mitotic index, mesoappendiceal invasion, tumors located at the base of the appendix with positive margins, and goblet cell adenocarcinoid tumors.[65] Rarely, appendiceal carcinoids are associated with liver metastases, and in these cases the carcinoid syndrome may be present. The number and location of liver lesions, as well as the associated symptoms, would dictate treatment in these cases.[66,67]

Mucoceles

Mucoceles of the appendix can be due to both benign and malignant disease, either cystadenomas or cystadenocarcinomas. These tumors obstruct the appendiceal lumen, leading to a large mucin-filled structure, often with calcification in the wall. Such tumors can generally be diagnosed by CT scan.

Appendectomy is curative for benign cystadenomas, even if rupture has occurred with mucinous ascites. However, with rupture of a cystadenocarcinoma, peritoneal tumor implantation can occur, leading to mucin secretion and a condition known as pseudomyxoma peritonei. The presence of mucin-secreting cellular elements in the peritoneal cavity distinguishes this malignant condition from the benign cystadenoma rupture with simple mucinous ascites. There is no effective treatment for pseudomyxoma peritonei, and these patients can develop secondary complications including bowel obstruction and perforation. The neoplastic process tends to be fairly indolent (5-year 50% survival), and repeated debulking procedures may be indicated.[68]

Adenocarcinoma

Adenocarcinoma of the appendix is extremely rare and like other appendiceal neoplasms is generally found unexpectedly at the time of appendectomy. Unfortunately, up to one half of the patients have metastatic disease at the time of diagnosis, usually with peritoneal spread presumably from rupture of the associated inflammatory process. Staging and treatment for appendiceal adenocarcinoma is similar to that for the more common colon carcinoma. Early lesions confined to the mucosa or submucosa (Dukes A) may be treated by simple appendectomy, as long as clear surgical margins are present. Dukes B and C lesions require formal right hemicolectomy, with adjuvant therapy indicated similar to colon carcinoma. Interestingly, appendiceal adenocarcinomas are associated with secondary tumors in up to 35% of patients, most often involving other areas of the GI tract.[69]

KEY POINTS

- **Pathologic processes affecting abdominal viscera that produce abdominal pain with characteristic symptoms and signs include obstruction, inflammation, perforation, torsion, and ischemia.**
- **Acute abdominal pain in immunosuppressed patients presents a particular diagnostic challenge both in making the diagnosis and due to the unusual infectious causes of abdominal pain that may be present.**
- **The cause of acute appendicitis in most patients is luminal obstruction that leads to bacterial overgrowth and increased luminal pressure leading to obstruction of venous**

outflow and then arterial inflow, resulting in gangrene and eventual perforation.

- Ultrasonographic findings of acute appendicitis include demonstration of a so-called target lesion (i.e., a thick-walled noncompressible, luminal structure in the right lower quadrant with peritoneal fluid and even frank abscess in advanced cases).
- A number of studies suggest that laparoscopic appendectomy is associated with a benefit in regard to shorter hospital stay, narcotic use, and overall recovery with a perioperative complication rate comparable to open appendectomy.
- A patient presenting late with appendicitis and an appendiceal mass should undergo initial percutaneous drainage and intravenous antibiotics followed by interval appendectomy in about 8 weeks.
- The diagnosis of acute appendicitis in children is difficult leading to a perforation rate as high as 50%.
- The diagnosis of acute appendicitis in the elderly is difficult leading to a perforation rate as high as 50% and higher associated rates of morbidity and mortality.
- Appendicitis is the most frequent nonobstructive indication for laparotomy during pregnancy and the difficulty in diagnosis leads to a high perforation rate and associated high fetal mortality.
- Carcinoid tumors less than 1.5 cm are adequately treated by appendectomy, whereas tumors 2 cm in size or greater have metastatic potential and a right hemicolectomy is indicated.

References

1. **Gill BD JJ. Cost-effective evaluation and management of the acute abdomen. *Surg Clin North Am.* 1996;76:71.**
2. Silen W. *Cope's early diagnosis of the acute abdomen,* 19th ed. New York: Oxford University Press, 1996.
3. Brewer BJ, Golden GT, Hitch DC, et al. Abdominal pain. An analysis of 1,000 consecutive cases in a University Hospital emergency room. *Am J Surg.* 1976;131:219.
4. Hawthorn IE. Abdominal pain as a cause of acute admission to hospital [see comments]. *J Royal Coll Surg Edinb.* 1992;37:389.
5. **Powers RD, Guertler AT. Abdominal pain in the ED: stability and change over 20 years. *Am J Emerg Med.* 1995;13:301.**
6. Wolfe JM, Smithline HA, Phipen S, et al. Does morphine change the physical examination in patients with acute appendicitis? *Am J Emerg Med.* 2004;22:280.
7. Thomas SH, Silen W. Effect on diagnostic efficiency of analgesia for undifferentiated abdominal pain. *Br J Surg.* 2003;90:5.
8. Thomas SH, Silen W, Cheema F, et al. Effects of morphine analgesia on diagnostic accuracy in emergency department patients with abdominal pain: a prospective, randomized trial. *J Am Coll Surg.* 2003;196:18.
9. Nauta RJ, Magnant C. Observation versus operation for abdominal pain in the right lower quadrant. Roles of the clinical examination and the leukocyte count. *Am J Surg.* 1986;151:746.
10. McCook TA, Ravin CE, Rice RP. Abdominal radiography in the emergency department: a prospective analysis. *Ann Emerg Med.* 1982;11:7.
11. Anyanwu AC, Moalypour SM. Are abdominal radiographs still overutilized in the assessment of acute abdominal pain? A district general hospital audit. *J R Coll Surg Edinb.* 1998;43:267.
12. **Gupta H, Dupuy DE. Advances in imaging of the acute abdomen. *Surg Clin North Am.* 1997;77:1245.**
13. Siewert B, Raptopoulos V, Mueller MF, et al. Impact of CT on diagnosis and management of acute abdomen in patients initially treated without surgery. *AJR Am J Roentgenol.* 1997;168:173.
14. Carrico CW, Fenton LZ, Taylor GA, et al. Impact of sonography on the diagnosis and treatment of acute lower abdominal pain in children and young adults. *AJR Am J Roentgenol.* 1999;172:513.
15. Mutter D, Navez B, Gury JF, et al. Value of microlaparoscopy in the diagnosis of right iliac fossa pain. *Am J Surg.* 1998;176:370.
16. Memon MA, Fitzgibbons RJ Jr. The role of minimal access surgery in the acute abdomen. *Surg Clin North Am.* 1997;77:1333.
17. Chung RS, Diaz JJ, Chari V. Efficacy of routine laparoscopy for the acute abdomen. *Surg Endosc.* 1998;12:219.
18. Neblett WW, Pietsch JB, Holcomb GW Jr. Acute abdominal conditions in children and adolescents. *Surg Clin North Am.* 1988;68:415.
19. Potts FE, Vukov LF. Utility of fever and leukocytosis in acute surgical abdomens in octogenarians and beyond. *J Gerontol A Biol Sci Med Sci.* 1999;54:M55.
20. Marco CA, Schoenfeld CN, Keyl PM, et al. Abdominal pain in geriatric emergency patients: variables associated with adverse outcomes. *Acad Emerg Med.* 1998;5:1163.
21. Simic O, Strathausen S, Hess W, et al. Incidence and prognosis of abdominal complications after cardiopulmonary bypass. *Cardiovasc Surg.* 1999;7:419.
22. Bender JS, Ratner LE, Magnuson TH, et al. Acute abdomen in the hemodialysis patient population. *Surgery* 1995;117:494.
23. Sheridan R. Diagnosis of the acute abdomen in the neurologically stable spinal cord-injured patient. A case study. *J Clin Gastroenterol.* 1992;15:325.
24. Bar-On Z, Ohry A. The acute abdomen in spinal cord injury individuals. *Paraplegia* 1995;33:704.
25. **Tarraza HM, Moore RD. Gynecologic causes of the acute abdomen and the acute abdomen in pregnancy. *Surg Clin North Am.* 1997;77:1371.**
26. Fitz R. Perforating inflammation of the vermiform appendix: with special reference to its early diagnosis and treatment. *Trans Assoc Am Physicians* 1886;1:107.
27. Silverman K. *Houdini: the career of Ehrich Weiss.* New York: HarperCollins; 1996.
28. Scott G. The primate caecum and appendix vermiformis: a comparative study. *J Anat.* 1980;131:549.
29. Gray H. *Gray's anatomy,* 29th ed. Philadelphia: Lea & Febiger, 1973.
30. **Styrud J, Eriksson S, Segelman J, et al. Diagnostic accuracy in 2,351 patients undergoing appendicectomy for suspected acute appendicitis: a retrospective study 1986–1993. *Dig Surg.* 1999;16:39.**
31. **Nguyen DB, Silen W, Hodin RA. Appendectomy in the pre- and post-laparoscopic eras. *J Gastrointest Surg.* 1999;3:67.**
32. **Hale DA, Molloy M, Pearl RH, et al. Appendectomy: a contemporary appraisal. *Ann Surg.* 1997;225:252.**
33. Olutola PS. Plain film radiographic diagnosis of acute appendicitis: an evaluation of the signs. *Can Assoc Radiol J.* 1988;39:254.
34. White JJ, Santillana M, Haller JA Jr. Intensive in-hospital observation: a safe way to decrease unnecessary appendectomy. *Am Surg.* 1975;41:793.
35. Zielke A, Hasse C, Sitter H, et al. Influence of ultrasound on clinical decision making in acute appendicitis: a prospective study. *Eur J Surg.* 1998;164:201.
36. Ooms HW, Koumans RK, Ho Kang You PJ, et al. Ultrasonography in the diagnosis of acute appendicitis. *Br J Surg.* 1991;78:315.
37. Franke C, Bohner H, Yang Q, et al. Ultrasonography for diagnosis of acute appendicitis: results of a prospective multicenter trial. Acute Abdominal Pain Study Group. *World J Surg.* 1999;23:141.
38. Wade DS, Marrow SE, Balsara ZN, et al. Accuracy of ultrasound in the diagnosis of acute appendicitis compared with the surgeon's clinical impression. *Arch Surg.* 1993;128:1039.
39. Choi YH, Fischer E, Hoda SA, et al. Appendiceal CT in 140 cases. Diagnostic criteria for acute and necrotizing appendicitis. *Clin Imaging* 1998;22:252.
40. Lane MJ, Katz DS, Ross BA, et al. Unenhanced helical CT for suspected acute appendicitis. *AJR Am J Roentgenol.* 1997;168:405.
41. Balthazar EJ, Birnbaum BA, Yee J, et al. Acute appendicitis: CT and US correlation in 100 patients. *Radiology* 1994;190:31.
42. **Rao PM, Rhea JT, Novelline RA, et al. Effect of computed tomography of the appendix on treatment of patients and use of hospital resources [see comments]. *N Engl J Med.* 1998;338:141.**
43. Shaff MI, Tarr RW, Partain CL, et al. Computed tomography and magnetic resonance imaging of the acute abdomen. *Surg Clin North Am.* 1988; 68:233.
44. Smith DE, Kirchmer NA, Stewart DR. Use of the barium enema in the diagnosis of acute appendicitis and its complications. *Am J Surg.* 1979;138:829.
45. Street D, Bodai BI, Owens LJ, et al. Simple ligation vs. stump inversion in appendectomy. *Arch Surg.* 1988;123:689.
46. Greenall MJ, Evans M, Pollack AV. Should you drain a perforated appendix? *Br J Surg.* 1978;65:880.
47. Tytgat SH, Bakker XR, Butzelaar RM. Laparoscopic evaluation of patients with suspected acute appendicitis. *Surg Endosc.* 1998;12:918.
48. Thorell A, Grondal S, Schedvins K, et al. Value of diagnostic laparoscopy in fertile women with suspected appendicitis. *Eur J Surg.* 1999;165:751.
49. Chiarugi M, Buccianti P, Celona G, et al. Laparoscopic compared with open appendicectomy for acute appendicitis: a prospective study. *Eur J Surg.* 1996;162:385.
50. **Chung RS, Rowland DY, Li P, et al. A meta-analysis of randomized controlled trials of laparoscopic versus conventional appendectomy. *Am J Surg.* 1999;177:250.**
51. Sackier JM. Laparoscopy for acute appendicitis. *Semin Laparosc Surg.* 1996;3:185.
52. Brown CV, Abrishami M, Muller M, et al. Appendiceal abscess: immediate operation or percutaneous drainage? *Am Surg.* 2003;69:829.
53. Ein S, Schandling B. Is interval appendectomy necessary after rupture of an appendiceal mass? *J Pediatr Surg.* 1996;31:849.
54. **Nguyen DB, Silen W, Hodin RA. Interval appendectomy in the laparoscopic era. *J Gastrointest Surg.* 1999;3:189.**
55. Mosdell DM, Morris DM, Fry DE. Peritoneal cultures and antibiotic therapy in pediatric perforated appendicitis. *Am J Surg.* 1994;167:313.
56. Neblett WW, Pietsch JB, Holcomb GW Jr. Acute abdominal conditions in children and adolescents. *Surg Clin North Am.* 1988;68:415.

57. Kaiser S, Mesas-Burgos C, Söderman E, et al. Appendicitis in children: impact of US and CT on the negative appendectomy rate. *Eur J Pediatr Surg*. 2004;14:260.
58. Martin AE, Vollman D, Adler B, et al. CT scans may not reduce the negative appendectomy rate in children. *J Pediatr Surg*. 2004;39:886.
59. Horattas MC, Guyton DP, Wu D. A reappraisal of appendicitis in the elderly. *Am J Surg*. 1990;160:291.
60. Nylander WA Jr. The acute abdomen in the immunocompromised host. *Surg Clin North Am*. 1988;68:457.
61. Tamir IL, Bongard FS, Klein SR. Acute appendicitis in the pregnant patient. *Am J Surg*. 1990;60:571.
62. Horowitz MD, Gomez GA, Santiesteban R, et al. Acute appendicitis during pregnancy. Diagnosis and management. *Arch Surg*. 1985;120:1362.
63. Nezhat FR, Tazuke S, Nezhat CH, et al. Laparoscopy during pregnancy: a literature review. *J Soc Laparoendosc Surg*. 1997;1:17.
64. Connor SJ, Hanna GB, Frizelle FA. Appendiceal tumors: retrospective clinicopathologic analysis of appendiceal tumors from 7,970 appendectomies. *Dis Colon Rectum* 1998;41:75.
65. **Goede AC, Caplin, ME, Winslet MC. Carcinoid tumour of the appendix. *Br J Surg*. 2003;90:1317.**
66. Moertal CG, Weiland LH, Nagorney DM, et al. Carcinoid tumor of the appendix: treatment and prognosis. *N Engl J Med*. 1987;317:1699.
67. **Sandor A, Modlin IM. A retrospective analysis of 1570 appendiceal carcinoids. *Am J Gastroenterol*. 1998;93:422.**
68. Smith JW, Kemeny N, Caldwell C, et al. Pseudomyxoma peritonei of appendiceal origin. The Memorial Sloan-Kettering Cancer Center experience. *Cancer* 1992;70:396.
69. Cortina R, McCormick J, Kolm P, et al. Management and prognosis of adenocarcinoma of the appendix. *Dis Colon Rectum* 1995;38:848.

CHAPTER 75 ■ SPLENIC DISORDERS

DOUGLAS L. FRAKER

The spleen has been a mysterious organ throughout surgical and medical history, with a clear understanding and appreciation of its function emerging only in the latter half of the 20th century. The reasons for this paucity of knowledge on the spleen are multifactorial. The spleen has no obvious function that can be discerned from its anatomical structures or features. There are no clear relationships of gross pathology of the spleen with many of the diseases for which it is important, and even today it is difficult to obtain a biopsy of the spleen, thereby limiting the amount of tissue available for pathologic study. The diseases (other than trauma) in which the spleen has importance are generally of a hematologic or immunologic nature. Understanding of the normal physiology and subsequent pathophysiology of the spleen is important for surgical decision making regarding when to recommend splenectomy and whether a partial splenectomy is possible. The only surgical procedure for the majority of the history of medicine applied to the spleen was splenectomy. Current variations on that procedure include laparoscopic splenectomy, partial splenectomy, and other splenic preservation procedures. The history of splenic surgery, its anatomy and physiology, and the disease processes as well as operative techniques involving the spleen are reviewed in this chapter.

HISTORY

The spleen has had a colorful history based on the function ascribed to this organ by many of the prominent scientists throughout the ages (Table 75.1).[1] Even the origin of the English word *spleen* is unclear. It is thought to come from the Greek *splen*, which may have derived from the Greek *splancknon*. "a viscus," or the Greek *spaw*, "to draw."[1] The dark purple-red color led ancients to believe that the spleen may draw spoiled or bad parts of the blood to itself, which predates one of the major roles of the spleen as a filtration device for senescent red blood cells. In ancient Greece, the spleen was thought to be the source of black bile, which was one of the four cardinal humors related to melancholy.[2] However, ancient authors wrote in the Talmud that the spleen was the seat for laughter and removal of the spleen would limit mirth in that person.[2] It was thought that the spleen was a source of discomfort sometimes felt as "a stitch in the side" for athletes and that by removal or ablation of the spleen an individual would run faster. Reports of the earliest procedures on the spleen indicate that runners in ancient Greece may have had their spleens ablated in an effort to improve their performance. This hypothesis was studied in an experimental model almost 2,000 years later at Johns Hopkins in which splenectomized mice versus control mice were evaluated for their ability to run a race, and the splenectomized mice were reported to be faster.[2]

During the Renaissance, scientists began to question the various roles ascribed to splenic function. Princelsus rejected the black bile theory and questioned in the early 16th century whether the spleen had any meaningful role at all. One of his students, named Zaccarella, reportedly performed the first splenectomy in the year 1549 in Palermo, Italy, removing the large spleen of a 24-year-old woman successfully (Table 75.1).[2] This organ was reportedly displayed in the town square after this landmark, but unsubstantiated, procedure. Versalius during that same era performed splenectomy in mice and other animals and determined that the spleen was not essential to life, because there was no clear difference following

TABLE 75.1

HISTORICAL MILESTONES IN SURGERY OF THE SPLEEN

1549	First reported splenectomy by Zaccarella in Italy
1826	First documented splenectomy by Quitterbaum in Germany
1865	First successful splenectomy by Paen in France
1892	First trauma splenectomy by Reigner in Germany
1911	Elective splenectomy for autoimmune hemolytic anemia
1916	Elective splenectomy for immune thrombocytopenia purpura
1952	First report of overwhelming postsplenectomy sepsis
1962	First report of splenic salvage procedure for trauma
1991	Laparoscopic splenectomy

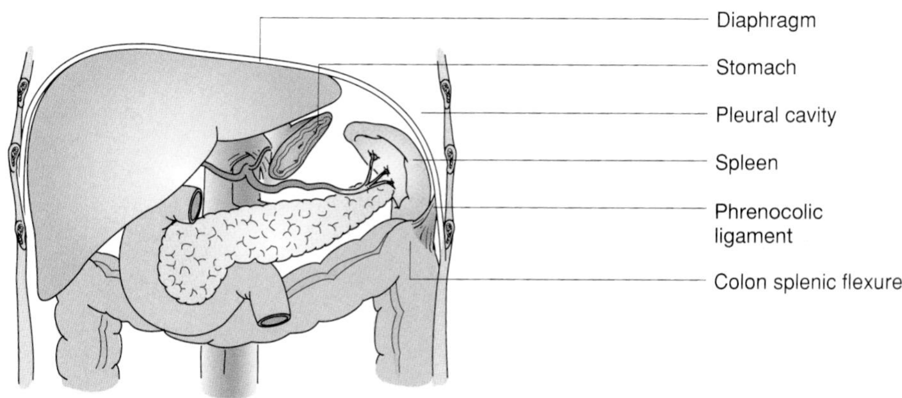

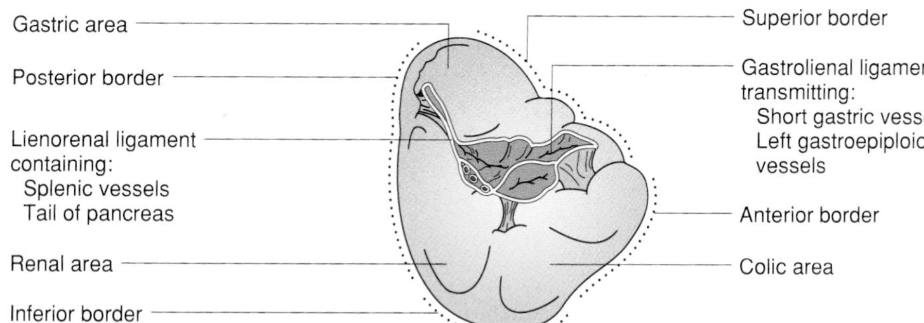

FIGURE 75.1 Anatomic relation of the spleen to the liver, diaphragm, pancreas, colon, and kidney. The stomach is sectioned to illustrate the anatomic relation *in situ*.

removal. Carl Frederick Quitterbaum performed the first authenticated splenectomy in Germany in 1826 in a patient with secondary hypersplenism due to cirrhosis. This high-risk patient succumbed 6 hours after the procedure. The first successful operation in which the patient survived was performed by Jules Pean in France in 1865 for a large splenic cyst. This patient underwent the procedure for what was thought to be an ovarian cystic mass. The mass was found to be arising from the inferior portion of the spleen and required splenectomy for removal; the patient survived. In this early period of splenic surgery, there was much pessimism because of the high operative mortality rate, primarily from hemorrhage. A collective series published in 1877 reported 50 splenectomies with a 70% overall mortality rate. By 1900, Bessel-Hagen reported 360 splenectomies with a 40% mortality rate.

The 20th century brought technical advances in the form of hemostasis and blood transfusion as well as an understanding of the pathophysiology of splenic function.[3] In 1911 Micheli identified the spleen as the site of red cell destruction in autoimmune hemolytic anemia. Paul Kaznelson, a Czech medical student, postulated in 1916 that the removal of the spleen in patients with idiopathic thrombocytopenic purpura would be beneficial, and he reported the successful treatment of a patient with that disease with splenectomy. Throughout the 20th century, as the understanding of the pathophysiology of hematologic and immune disorders associated with the spleen increased, the roles for splenectomy that are pertinent to modern-day practice became clearer.

EMBRYOLOGY AND ANATOMY

The spleen develops from the mesoderm as an outpouching from the mesogastrium during the 5th week of gestation.[4,5] Natural rotation of the gut during subsequent development places the spleen in its typical position in the left upper quadrant of the abdomen (Fig. 75.1). In that location, the spleen relates to the diaphragm both superiorly and laterally, and it generally spans the 9th, 10th, and 11th ribs along the left mid to posterior axillary line. The ventral surface of the spleen relates to the greater curvature of the stomach and the tail of the pancreas. The tail of the pancreas touches the splenic capsule in 30% of cases and is 1 cm away in 73% of cases. The inferior pole relates to the left kidney posteriorly and the splenic flexure of the colon anteriorly.

The normal size of the spleen is approximately 13 × 7 × 4 cm.[4] The typical weight of a spleen in a young adult is thought to be 150 to 200 g, and this decreases to approximately 100 g in the elderly population (Fig. 75.2).[6,7] It is thought that the spleen must double in size to the range of 300 to 400 g to project below the costal margin and thereby to allow palpation of the spleen tip on abdominal examination in a patient undergoing deep inspiration.[8] The weight assigned to the spleen in defining massive splenomegaly has been arbitrarily set at 1,500 grams or 10 times the average adult splenic weight. There can be a significant cleft in the capsule of the spleen, which may be confused with splenic disruption on computed tomography (CT) scan obtained for trauma.

The vascular anatomy of the spleen is straightforward.[9] The splenic artery is one of the three major trunks, along with the left gastric artery and common hepatic artery, branching off from the celiac axis (Fig. 75.3). This artery has a characteristic appearance on celiac arteriograms as a serpentine artery with loops extending both superiorly and inferiorly. There are several small pancreatic branches that supply blood to the body and tail of the pancreas along the length of this vessel. The first major splenic branch, called the superior polar artery, occurs approximately 2 to 3 cm from the hilum. The main artery then divides into between three and five segmental branches that enter along the trabecula of the spleen.

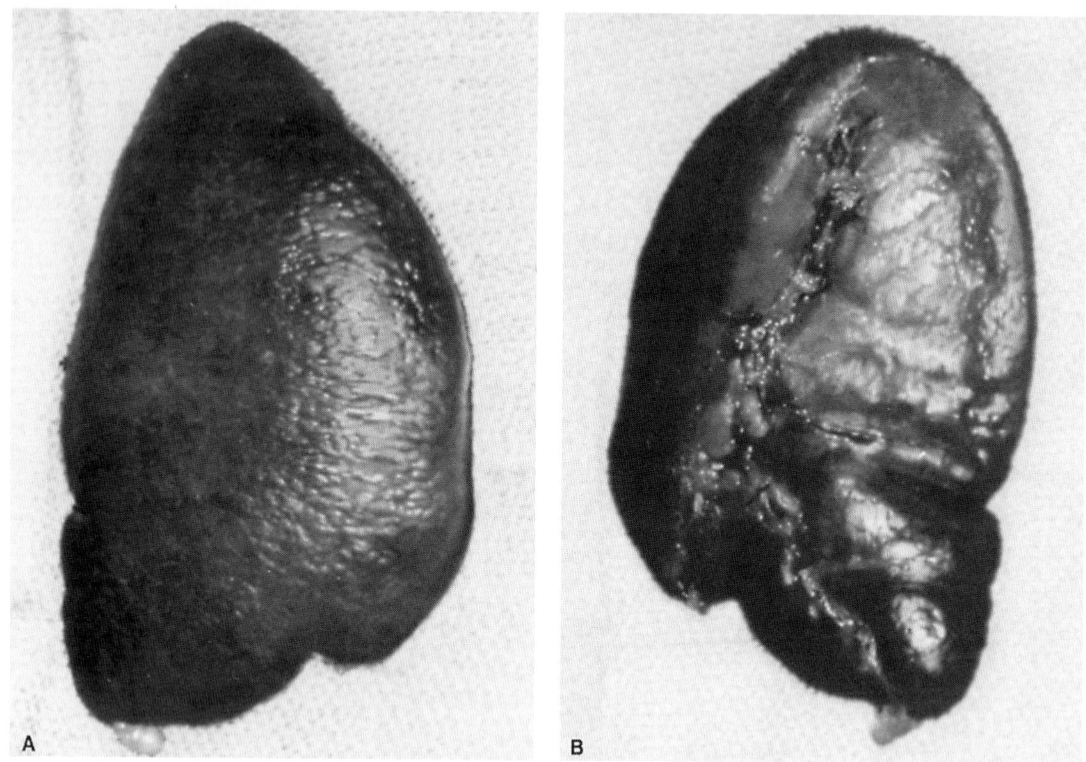

FIGURE 75.2 (*A*) The lateral or diaphragmatic surface of the spleen, showing the lobulated edge and the glistening capsule. (*B*) The hilar surface of the spleen, showing the ligatures on the cephalad short gastric vessels and the caudal hilar vessels.

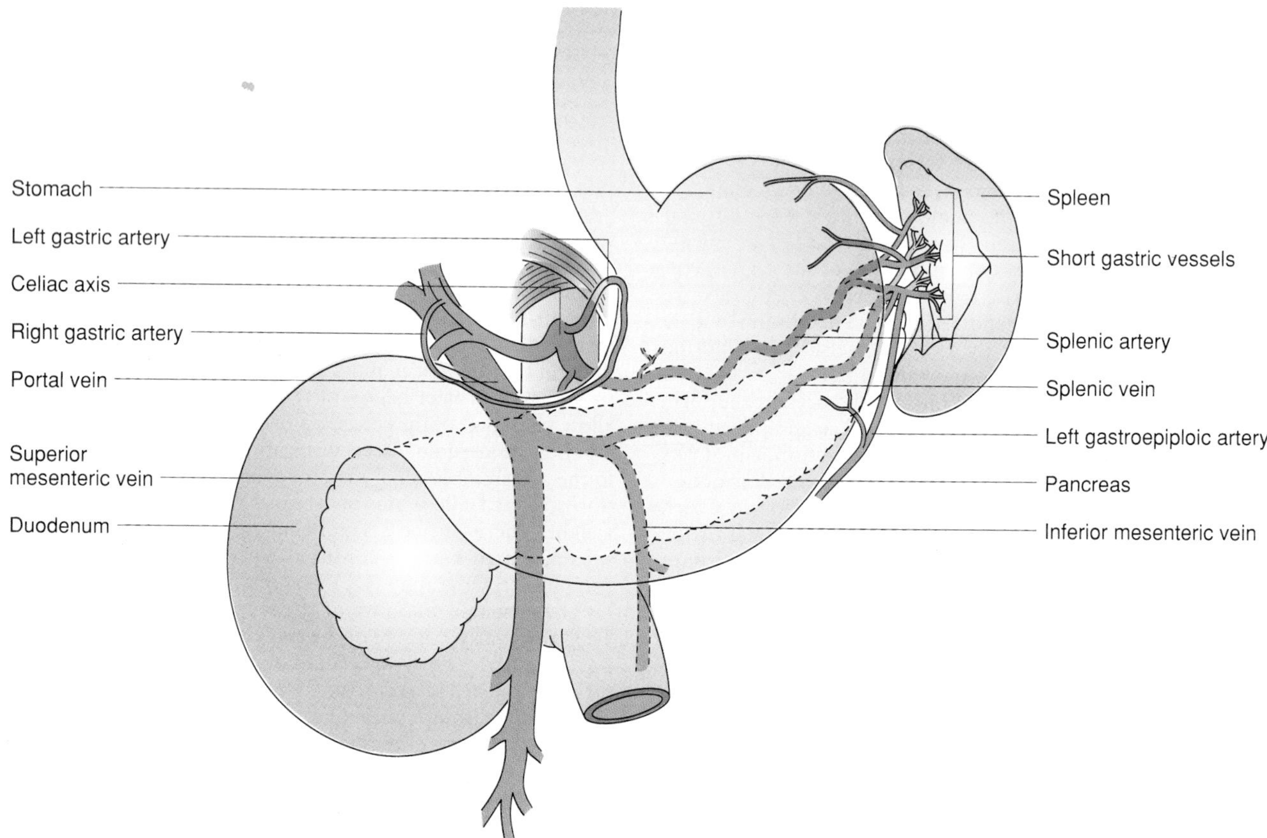

FIGURE 75.3 The arterial blood flow to the spleen is derived from the splenic artery, the left gastroepiploic artery, and the short gastric arteries (vasa brevia). The venous drainage into this portal vein is also shown.

Additional blood supply to the spleen comes from the left gastroepiploic artery via the short gastric vessels. When the spleen is massively enlarged, it may have direct vessels that are parasitized from the omentum, the diaphragm, or the mesentery of the splenic flexure of the colon. The splenic artery generally travels outside the parenchyma of the pancreas just at the superior border; loops that go inferiorly may be completely covered by the posterior surface of the pancreas, whereas superior loops may be well away from the pancreatic surface. These curves that lie more cranially are the optimal place to provide a ligature for control of the splenic artery during procedures in which there is significant thrombocytopenia or for enlarged spleens. These are generally areas that have few pancreatic branches and avoid proximity to the splenic which occurs when the artery loops inferiorly.

The splenic vein is formed by segmental venous branches that leave the trabecula and coalesce into the main splenic vein in the hilum of the spleen (Fig. 75.3). The splenic vein is intimately associated with the posterior surface of the tail and body of the pancreas to its junction with the superior mesenteric vein forming the portal vein. The inferior mesenteric vein may join the splenic vein directly at several areas along its course or may come together right at the junction of the superior mesenteric vein. There are again several pancreatic branches that directly enter this splenic vein. The blood flow to the spleen in the typical adult is estimated to be 200 to 300 mL/minute, or approximately 5% of the cardiac output.[9]

The lymph node drainage generally follows the vasculature. The primary lymph nodes are located in the hilum of the spleen and also along the splenic artery at the superior border of the pancreas and along the short gastric vessels.

Several ligaments maintain the spleen in its fixed position in the left upper quadrant (Fig. 75.4).[9] Three of these ligaments are virtually always present (except in the condition of the "wandering spleen"),[10] and two may be present to variable extents, depending on the individual patient and the disease process. The first ligament that is constant is the splenogastric ligament, which is a left-sided superior extension of the greater omentum along the proximal greater curvature of the stomach. Within this area supplied by the left gastroepiploic vessels are short gastric vessels that branch to the upper pole of the spleen and often provide the upper two thirds of the spleen with an alternative blood supply. The second and very important ligament is the splenorenal ligament, which runs parallel to the posterolateral border of the spleen and attaches to the superior pole of Gerota's fascia developing the left kidney. This ligament is divided when mobilizing the spleen during splenectomy and allows reflection of the spleen with or without the tail of the pancreas medially. The splenocolic ligament is short and may be avascular or have small blood vessels that go from the inferior tip of the spleen to the splenic flexure of the colon. This ligament may be divided by cautery or may have vessels that need to be controlled with ties or clips during mobilization of the splenic flexure of the colon.

Two ligaments that are variably present are the splenoomental attachments and the splenophrenic attachments (see Fig. 75.4). The free part of the greater omentum may have variable association with the splenic capsule along the inferior pole. There are often small vessels that can be controlled by electrocautery. This attachment may be absent or may be quite extensive over the lower pole of the spleen. It is this attachment to the omentum that often leads to disruption of the capsule along the inferior pole causing bleeding in other abdominal procedures and may even eventually result in splenectomy for control with an inadvertent injury. Before exerting inferior traction on the omentum, during any procedure the extent of attachments to the lower pole of the spleen should be investigated, and if present they should be divided prior to more vigorous mobilization. There may be direct ligaments connecting the spleen to the diaphragm, identified as splenophrenic ligaments. These typically are present to a greater degree when the spleen is diseased or enlarged. They may be avascular or may have branches of vessels parasitized from the diaphragm blood supply, especially with large spleens.

The anatomy of the spleen itself is segmental, being fed by arteries and drained by veins that leave via the trabecular.[11] The trabecula are fibrous bands that attach to the splenic capsule. The parenchyma of the spleen between these trabecula is divided into a small area of white pulp surrounding the arteries, a marginal zone, and the larger predominant area of red pulp that makes up 75% of the splenic parenchyma.[12] The capsule of the spleen is quite thin because it is only a few cell layers thick. The capsule consists of a single layer of mesothelium and several layers of fibroelastic tissue. In mammals other than humans, there may be variable amounts of smooth muscle in the capsule. This smooth muscle would allow contraction and mobilization of the circulating blood cells that are stored in the spleen.[13] The trabecula arteries that enter the spleen as continuations of the segmental arterial branches then give off perpendicular branches to form the central arteries (Fig. 75.5). Surrounding these central arteries is the periarterial lymphatic sheath (PALS), which comprises T-lymphocytes and follicles with B cells at various stages of development. During antigenic stimulation, this area greatly expands with more mature and secondary follicles. The marginal zone is the borderline between the white pulp and the red pulp and contains a mixture of lymphatics and macrophages. The structure

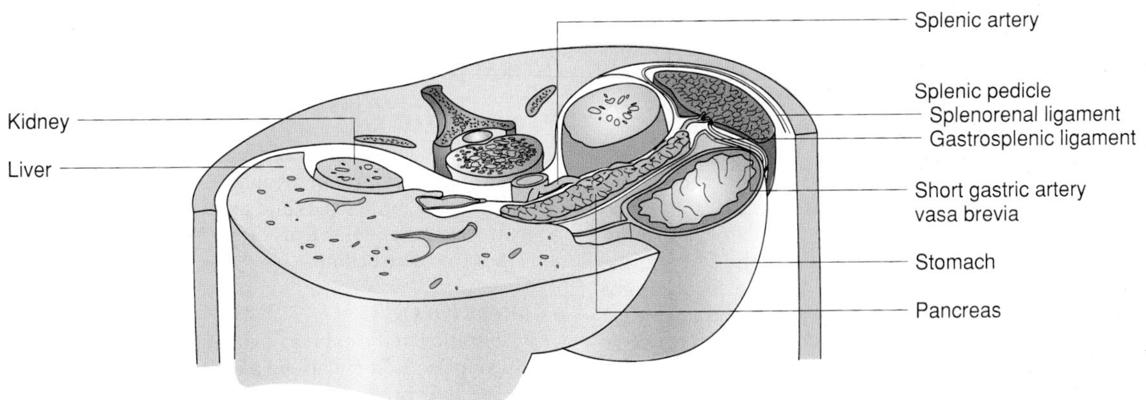

FIGURE 75.4 The relations of the spleen to the abdominal and retroperitoneal viscera are seen in a cross section of the left-facing torso.

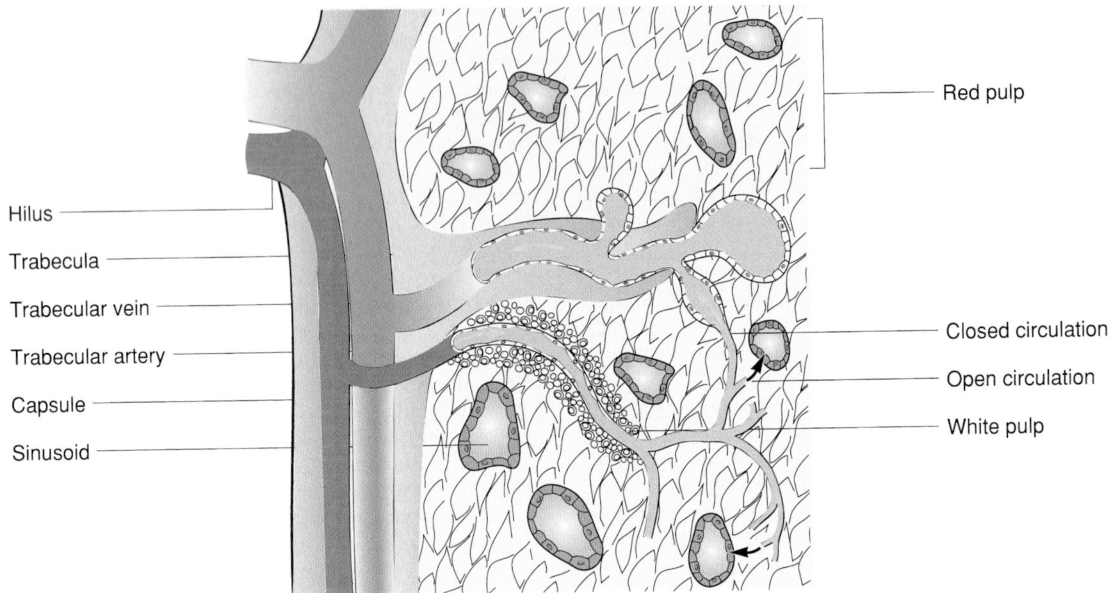

FIGURE 75.5 The splenic microanatomy is shown with depictions of both the open and closed circulations.

of the red pulp comprises splenic cords with an intervening area called *splenic sinuses*. The splenic cords, also known as the cords of Billroth, are a meshwork of fibroblasts and a large number of mature macrophages. The splenic sinuses are an interconnective meshwork of fairly random red cell spaces that are thin-walled and generally filled with large numbers of erythrocytes.[5]

Studies on blood flow show two alternative routes to the spleen being fast flow and slow flow.[14] A small proportion of the blood goes through the splenic arteries and returns rapidly to the splenic veins. This fast-flow pattern consists of a greater predominance of plasma and few erythrocytes because of streaming and accounts for only 10% of flow. A particularly large portion of the erythrocytes that enter the spleen travel through the highly fenestrated meshwork in the red pulp as part of the filtration process of the spleen. This slow path or slow flow makes up 90% of the splenic blood flow and relates to the role of the spleen in clearly senescent erythrocytes.

Accessory spleens are small nodules of splenic tissue that are completely separate from the main body of the spleen. They typically range in size from 0.5 cm to 3 or 4 cm. The incidence of accessory spleens ranges in reports between 10% and 20%. The most common locations for these small nodules of splenic tissue are in the splenic hilum; the omentum, most commonly between the stomach and transverse colon but also within the greater omentum; and the small bowel mesentery. However, they can occur anywhere in the abdomen, including the retroperitoneum behind the spleen and in the pelvis. Accessory spleens are important in disease processes in which a complete removal of all splenic tissue is mandatory for long-term cure, such as certain autoimmune disorders. The routine use of laparoscopic splenectomy to treat this disorder highlights the importance of the accessory spleens, because they are more difficult to identify with a minimally invasive approach rather than an open operation. However, several reports demonstrate that accessory spleens can be successfully removed laparoscopically, particularly with the aid of a nuclear medicine spleen scan if needed to identify sources of residual tissue.[15]

PHYSIOLOGY

The major functions of the spleen can be divided into two general categories: hematologic and immunologic (Table 75.2). For hematologic functions, the spleen primarily is an organ related to the destruction or clearance of the circulating blood cell elements as a normal physiologic mechanism.[16] This physiologic filtration function is increased in disease states that produce hypersplenism. The spleen may play a minor role in hematopoiesis and storage of blood cells that can be mobilized for the circulation, with the predominantly stored cell being platelets. In terms of the immunologic functions, the spleen relates to the vascular system in many of the same ways that lymph nodes relate to the lymphatic system. The white pulp and marginal zones are most important for the immunologic functions, whereas the red pulp is primarily related to the hematologic functions. However, the macrophages that line the cords or fill the cords in the red pulp are clearly also important for immunosurveillance for intravascular pathogens.

TABLE 75.2

NORMAL FUNCTIONS OF THE SPLEEN

HEMATOLOGIC
- Culling or destruction of senescent erythrocytes
- Pitting or removal of cytoplasm inclusive in erythrocytes
- Reservoir for platelets and granulocytes
- Hematopoiesis—as fetus or in conditions with bone marrow destruction

IMMUNOLOGIC
- Filtration and trapping of circulatory antigens
- Lymphocyte stimulation and proliferation
- Antibody production in germinal follicles
- Production of opsonin-tuftsin and properdin
- Opsonins: tuftsin and properdin

The primary hematologic function of the spleen is removal of senescent erythrocytes or remodeling of abnormal red blood cells with various deformities.[14] The average life span of a normal erythrocyte measured on clearance studies in humans is estimated to be approximately 120 days.[17] It is also estimated that the spleen destroys approximately 100 billion erythrocytes daily in the red pulp.[16] The process of removal or phagocytosis of erythrocytes or other blood cells is called culling (see Table 75.2). The blood flow patterns of the spleen lead to a hemoconcentrated erythrocyte-laden fluid that enters the sinuses of the red pulp. Here a slow flow through the sinusoid network with adjacent macrophage-filled cords leads to the environment in which erythrocytes may become trapped and then phagocytized by the macrophages. The precise mechanism by which senescent red cells are identified for destruction in normal physiology is unclear. One hypothesis is that over the course of the life span of an erythrocyte, there is loss of either membrane elements or total membrane material such that the red cells become less compliant and therefore become trapped in the mesh of the sinusoids. A second hypothesis is that specific cell surface marker molecules may become either more exposed or less available to allow identification of senescent cells targeted for destruction. Pathologic destruction of red cells occurs in diseases such as hereditary spherocytosis or elliptocytosis in which a genetic defect creates abnormal red cell pliability, limiting its passage through the red pulp. Similarly, in sickle cell anemia, the genetic defect in the hemoglobin alters red cell shape and creates destruction with clogging of the sinusoids. A second pathologic mechanism in which destruction of red cells is increased is disease processes that increase the spleen size and lead to increased removal of red cells not because of red blood cell or hemoglobin abnormalities but because of increased red pulp volume. This condition is known as hypersplenism.

The second physiologic process involving circulating erythrocytes is remodeling or pitting, which is partial removal of the cell membrane typically associated with the cytoplasmic inclusions. Erythrocytes with a remnant of the cell nucleus remaining pass more slowly through the splenic red pulp because of their larger size.[16] The nuclear remnant may be trapped passing through a small space in the spleen and this solid particle that does not allow deformation and gets pinched off in the process of pitting. Intracytoplasmic inclusions include Howell-Jolly bodies, which are nuclear remnants; Heinz bodies, which are denatured hemoglobin; and Pappenheimer bodies, which are iron granules.

The destruction of the other circulating cellular elements of the blood (platelets and leukocytes) is more in the realm of pathophysiology of the spleen than normal physiologic function. The disease processes in which these cells are removed are either related to autoantibodies to cell surface elements or related to hypersplenism. If either platelets or white blood cells become coated with antibodies, the Fc portion of the immunoglobulin will interact with the Fc receptors on the macrophages in the splenic cords leading to phagocytosis of these cell types. With splenic enlargement from various causes of hypersplenism, a similar process of destruction may occur even without any autoantibodies or defects in the cells just because of the increase in splenic mass.

The spleen serves as a potential source for hematopoiesis of all cell types during gestation. In normal humans, there is thought to be very little if any production of red cells, granulocytes, or platelets, which is not true in other mammals. In the white pulp of the spleen there are germinal centers with amplification and production of reactive lymphocytes. The cords of the spleen are filled with macrophages, and throughout normal adult life there may be production of lymphocytes and macrophages in the spleen. In certain disease states, the spleen may develop the capacity for erythropoiesis and myelopoiesis. The best example is agnogenic myeloid metaplasia. In this disease, the bone marrow is replaced with fibrotic scar and a portion of the hematopoietic function of the marrow is taken over by the spleen, which is typically quite enlarged.

The final hematologic function of the spleen may be as a reservoir of circulating cellular elements.[13] In man, the only significant cell type that is stored in the spleen is platelets, and it is estimated that 30% of all platelets may reside in the spleen. This function may be more important than in other mammals, particularly those with significant smooth muscle lining the capsule of the spleen that allows contracture with expulsion of large numbers of stored cells as a physiologic response to injury.

The immunologic function of the spleen is primarily to generate an immune response to antigens that are identified and cleared from the blood system (see Table 75.2). Opsonized antigens and specific encapsulated microorganisms are important examples of target antigens trapped by the spleen. The spleen is an ideal environment for generation of either a cellular or a humoral immune response. All of the necessary cells types for stimulation of the immune response are present, including phagocytic cells, dendritic cells, T-cells, and B-cells, which may form general follicles to generate specific antibody responses. These interactions primarily occur in the marginal zone in the white pulp, which may become quite enlarged and hypertrophied during antigen stimulation. These cellular components and the structure of the germinal follicles are essentially identical to those found in lymph node tissue, which becomes enlarged in a similar way with antigenic stimulation by microbes or antigens in the lymphatic system.

The spleen is also involved in nonspecific immune responses. It is the site of synthesis of both properdin and tuftsin which are opsonins. Tuftsin is a small peptide that binds to the surface of granulocytes and promotes phagocytic function by these cells.[18] Properdin can initiate the alternate pathway of complement activation, which may be important in destruction of abnormal cells or bacteria that are antibody bound. The spleen is not the only source of these nonspecific immune-enhancing proteins, and therefore splenectomy may lead to only a modest alteration in this function.

PATHOPHYSIOLOGY

Some characteristic responses share many common features under the broad category of hyposplenism and hypersplenism. These features highlight the normal physiologic functions of the spleen and provide guidelines and influence clinical decision making when managing patients after splenectomy or in deciding which patients should undergo splenectomy. By far the most common cause of hyposplenism is surgical removal.[19] Other explanations would be an unusual situation of a congenitally small or absent spleen or acquired destruction of splenic tissue, as occurs in sickle cell anemia. Hypersplenism is the most frequent indication for elective splenectomy. There are a variety of causes of hypersplenism that are typically neoplastic but may be related to primary blood cell dysfunction or abnormalities or other conditions such as portal hypertension due to cirrhosis or splenic vein thrombosis.

Hyposplenism

Hyposplenism or the changes seen after a splenectomy are predictable from the known functions of the spleen. Hematologic changes in the circulating cells can be predicted from the splenic functions of culling and pitting and because the spleen is a reservoir for platelets (Table 75.3). Changes in

TABLE 75.3

RESULTS OF SPLENECTOMY/HYPOSPLENIC CONDITION

ERYTHROCYTES
- Howell-Jolly bodies (nuclear fragments)
- Heinz bodies (hemoglobin deposits)
- Pappenheimer bodies (iron deposits)
- Target cells
- Spur cells (acanthocytes)

PLATELETS
- Transient thrombocytosis

LEUKOCYTES
- Transient leukocytosis
- Persistent lymphocytosis
- Persistent monocytosis

the immunologic responses are important primarily in infants or young children because they lead to the problem of overwhelming postsplenectomy sepsis.

The changes in circulating blood cells after splenectomy in cases of hyposplenism affect the erythrocytes, leukocytes, and platelets. Over time, the intracytoplasmic inclusions in the red cells that are normally cleared by the spleen accumulate, resulting in presence of Howell-Jolly bodies, Heinz bodies, and Pappenheimer bodies as well as target cells with excess red blood cell membrane and occasionally increases in the circulating nucleated red blood cells or reticulocytes. Because the spleen is the storage organ for a large proportion of the platelets, a splenectomy often results in thrombocytosis with postsplenectomy platelet counts ranging from 500,000 to one million in some cases. This increased platelet count tends to be transient and may reflect that the spleen, although a storage organ for platelets, may not be a primary area of platelet destruction after the typical half-life of 10 days. The immediate response after a splenectomy in white cells is leukocytosis, again reflecting storage of a large proportion of white cells in the spleen.[20] As with thrombocytosis, this effect is transient, but there may be long-term increases in the proportion of circulating lymphocytes and monocytes after splenectomy. Preserving even a small amount of spleen can preserve splenic function in clearing senescent blood cells.[21]

The changes seen with hyposplenism or after splenectomy in immune function are most importantly manifested by the phenomenon of overwhelming postsplenectomy sepsis.[22] This was initially recognized as an important epidemiologic phenomenon in the early 1950s, and multiple studies of splenectomized patients define key features of this increased susceptibility to infection. It is clear that the risk of postsplenectomy sepsis is inversely related to age.[23] The younger the patient is, the more impact and greater risk of developing overwhelming postsplenectomy sepsis.[24] This feature has clinical implications because elective splenectomies are not performed for patients with hereditary erythrocyte syndromes until after age 6 to 10 years. In adults, there is still between a 40% and 60% increased risk of sepsis compared to patients with normal splenic function. These postsplenectomy septic episodes typically occur within the first 2 years of splenectomy in 80% of cases. In adults, the reason for performing splenectomy also relates to the incidence of sepsis. In trauma, the instance of sepsis in a large series was 1.4%, whereas in thalassemia the incidence was 24.8%. Patients with any associated immunodeficiency such as malignancies or patients undergoing chemotherapy for treatment of Hodgkin disease are also at increased risk for sepsis. The mortality rate of postsplenectomy sepsis is between 50% and 60% in most series.

The types of organisms that account for infection are typically encapsulated organisms. These bacteria may have special features that allow them to be opsonized and cleared from the circulation by the spleen, making them more dangerous in hyposplenic or splenectomized patients. The most common organism causing postsplenectomy sepsis is *Streptococcus pneumoniae*, which accounts for 50% of septic episodes in most series. In decreasing order of frequency, other bacteria associated with postsplenectomy sepsis are *Haemophilus influenzae*, *Neisseria meningitidis*, β-hemolytic *Streptococcus*, *Staphylococcus aureus*, *Escherichia coli*, and *Pseudomonas* species.[23] The current recommendation for patients who are having elective splenectomy is to vaccinate susceptible individuals to pneumococcus strains (Table 75.4).[23] This is ideally done 2 weeks before surgery if possible but can be done at any time preoperatively or even postoperatively if the patient was not vaccinated. Recent studies have shown that administration of vaccine with the first postoperative visit does not lead to beneficial immune stimulation. Waiting for 14 days postoperatively is equivalent to waiting 1 month or longer.[25] Therefore, vaccination at 2 weeks after an unplanned splenectomy is ideal timing. There are choices of polyvalent vaccines including Pneumovax 23 and Pnu-Immune 23, both of which provide protection against virtually all common strains of pneumococcus.[25] For patients who are at particularly high risk because they may be immunosuppressed, there are also polyvalent vaccines against *Neisseria meningitides* and *Haemophilus influenzae* type B. Patients under the age of 2 years and patients receiving chemotherapy for malignant disease may not be able to generate an immune response to vaccines and should be vaccinated either after age 2 years or when not receiving chemotherapy, respectively. Finally, because of the risk of very rapid progression of sepsis in a postsplenectomy state, patients who have had splenectomy for any reason should be given a MedicAlert bracelet.

A recent survey of practicing surgeons indicated patterns of utilization of immunization for splenectomy patients. Of the practices, 99.2% of active surgeons said they do immunize patients they treat with splenectomy.[26] Virtually everyone administers vaccine to pneumococcus. Of practicing surgeons, 72.4% routinely use a *H. influenzae*-type vaccine, 62.8% give meningococcal vaccination, and 56.7% use all three vaccines. A small portion of practicing surgeons immunize their patients who have splenorrhaphy (15.7%), and a very small proportion immunize patients who have splenic injury but who are managed nonoperatively. Current guidelines are that all patients with elective splenectomies should have prophylactic immunization prior to surgery, whereas patients who have unexpected splenectomy should have immunization 14 days

TABLE 75.4

GUIDELINES FOR PREVENTION OF POSTSPLENIC SEPSIS

- Vaccinate with polyvalent pneumococcal vaccine at least 10–14 days prior to splenectomy, if possible.
- If splenectomy is urgent wait until at least 14 days post procedure to vaccinate
- For high-risk patients (immunosuppressed, children <10 years of age), meningococcal vaccine and *Haemophilus influenza* vaccine
- Antibiotic prophylaxis for children <5 years of age
- Early antibiotic treatment for initial signs of infection
- MedicAlert bracelet

TABLE 75.5

DEFINITION OF HYPERSPLENISM

Decrease in circulating cell count of erythrocytes and/or platelets and/or leukocytes
and
Normal compensatory hematopoietic responses present in bone marrow
and
Correction of cytopenia by splenectomy
with or without
Splenomegaly

after the procedure. All patients should get pneumococcal vaccines, and patients at high risk should have vaccination for *H. influenzae* and meningococcus.[26]

Hypersplenism

Hypersplenism is increased splenic function that is manifested clinically by the decrease in one or more of the circulating blood elements (Table 75.5). The specific criteria for hypersplenism are: (a) documented anemia, thrombocytopenia, or leukopenia; (b) normal compensatory response by the bone marrow to correct the cytopenia; and (c) correction of this cytopenia by splenectomy.[27] Some definitions of hypersplenism may also include the criteria for splenomegaly. If one states that an enlarged spleen is mandatory for a diagnosis of hypersplenism, then one would not classify diseases or disorders related to the abnormalities in circulating blood cells such as idiopathic thrombocytopenic purpura (ITP) or autoimmune hemolytic anemia in this category. The second approach to defining hypersplenism is to categorize disorders in which the spleen is normal anatomically and the disease is related to the circulating cells, with a second category in which the circulating cells are normal and there is a primary alteration in the spleen either anatomically or functionally (Table 75.6). For either situation the pathophysiology is that the spleen is the site of destruction for one or more circulating blood elements. In cases of significantly enlarged spleen, additional symptoms relate to mass effect from the spleen on adjacent organs. The most important symptom is early satiety and weight loss as the stomach is compressed between the liver and the enlarged spleen. Hypersplenism is the most important indication for elective isolated splenectomy, to reverse the cytopenia and often to relieve compressive symptoms from splenomegaly.

TABLE 75.6 ETIOLOGY

CAUSES OF HYPERSPLENISM

PRIMARY DISEASES OF BLOOD CELLS; NORMAL SPLEEN
Congenital
Erythrocyte abnormalities
Hereditary spherocytosis
Hereditary elliptocytosis
Glucose 6 phosphate dehydrogenase deficiency
Pyruvate kinase deficiency
Hemoglobin abnormalities
Thalassemia major
Sickle cell anemia (eventually results in splenic infarction and hyposplenism)
Platelet abnormalities
Wiskott-Aldrich syndrome
Acquired
Autoimmune hemolytic anemia
Autoimmune neutropenia—Felty's syndrome
Immune thrombocytopenia purpura
Thrombotic thrombocytopenia purpura
PRIMARY DISORDERS OF THE SPLEEN
Neoplastic
Hairy cell leukemia
Chronic lymphocytic leukemia
Chronic myelogenous leukemia
Non-Hodgkin lymphoma
Cellular infiltrative (Hematopoiesis)
Agnogenic myeloid metaplasia
Mastocytosis
Chediak-Higashi syndrome
Metabolic infiltration
Gaucher disease
Sarcoidosis
Vascular
Splenic vein thrombosis
Portal vein hypertension (cirrhosis)

SURGICAL TREATMENT

Until recently, the only pertinent operation to discuss in relationship to disease involving the spleen was splenectomy. Appreciation of the increased risk of infection in inpatients who are asplenic or hyposplenic in the late 1960s and the early 1970s led to two new surgical procedures. First, there was an interest in splenic preservation that resulted in procedures including splenorrhaphy and other ways to save damaged spleen. Second, procedures to do partial splenectomy were developed primarily for elective surgery for patients in whom hypersplenism existed but a complete splenectomy was not necessary and there were advantages to partial splenectomy. The most recent change in surgery of the spleen relates to the explosion in minimally invasive surgery that has happened over the past 15 years. The spleen is very susceptible to laparoscopic excision, and recent reports have utilized laparoscopic splenectomy for virtually all indications including removing massive spleens. In most major centers, laparoscopic splenectomy is now the procedure of choice for elective splenectomy.

To better describe and understand operative indications in surgery of the spleen, one could categorize the splenectomy or procedures of the spleen into eight general areas:

1. *Trauma or injury to the spleen.*
2. *Autoimmune/erythrocyte* disorders. In this category of disease, specific cytopenias are related to antibodies targeting platelets, erythrocytes, or neutrophils, and the second category of diseases is related to intrinsic structural changes within the erythrocyte. In these procedures, it is often important to obtain total splenectomy for complete cure.
3. *Hypersplenism* results in decreased circulating blood cells, often including all subtypes of platelets and red blood cells. Hypersplenism may be related to neoplastic infiltration of the spleen or infiltration with lipids and other stored products that links to massive spleen. Hypersplenism also may cause symptoms due to the splenic size.
4. *Incidental splenectomy.* The spleen may be removed as part of a standard operation to remove the distal pancreas most commonly and also for proximal gastric cancers resulting from direct or nodal involvement. Other enlarged tumors of the left upper quadrant and retroperitoneum, including sarcoma and adrenal tumor, and left nephrectomy may

require splenectomy because of association with the spleen or its vessels even though it is not a primary tumor of the spleen.

5. *Iatrogenic splenectomy.* This category may be underreported but relates to the splenectomy or splenic preservation procedures that result from incidental injury to the spleen during surgery within the general abdominal cavity or, specifically, the left upper quadrant.
6. *Diagnostic procedures.* This category of splenectomy occurs when the spleen is removed primarily to make a clinical diagnosis when none is available.[28] A subcategory would be staging laparotomy for Hodgkin disease, which is rapidly becoming more of a historical footnote because the treatment of this lymphoma now rarely requires splenectomy to make the diagnosis.
7. *Vascular procedures.* Splenectomy for vascular procedures includes patients with splenic vein thrombosis or, less commonly, splenic artery aneurysms.
8. *Miscellaneous procedures.* This category includes treatment of simple and neoplastic cysts, echinococcal cysts, and treatment of the wandering spleen when symptomatic as a congenital anomaly.

Two recent reports have been published describing 10-year experiences for all splenectomies done in their respective institutions. The first report is the combined series of 1,280 splenectomies over a 10-year interval from the Barnes Hospital in St. Louis and the Brigham and Women's Hospital in Boston.[28] The second report is a single institution over the identical time period from Vanderbilt University.[29] The Barnes/Brigham series included 1,280 splenectomies, and in the Vanderbilt series there were 896 splenectomies (Table 75.7). One can see that, dependent on the type of institution and referral patterns, the indications for splenectomy vary to some degree. In the Vanderbilt series, the majority of splenectomies were done for trauma, which accounts for 41.5% of all operations done in that institution. In the Barnes/Brigham series, the most common indication was incidental splenectomy in which the spleen was removed as part of an excision of another organ, typically large tumor somewhere in the left upper quadrant of the abdomen. The second most frequent indication for splenectomy was staging laparotomy for Hodgkin disease, which is likely to be different in the ensuing decade because both treatment indications and diagnostic techniques significantly eliminated this practice after 1990. The differences between these institutions highlight that in centers with a large trauma population, splenectomies are done for that indication, whereas in centers in which there may be significant association with major cancer referral bases, there are alternative indications. It also should be noted that if one eliminates the traumatic, incidental, and staging procedures, the most common indication in both series relates to autoimmune or erythrocyte disorder.

In the subsequent sections of this chapter, the details of the indications for splenectomy in each of these categories will be discussed. The specific indications for splenectomy, the alternative treatments that are available, and the results from surgical removal of the spleen will be discussed. The options to do partial splenectomy and the application of minimally invasive or laparoscopic splenectomy for these indications will also be described.

TABLE 75.7 INDICATIONS/CONTRAINDICATIONS

INDICATIONS FOR SPLENECTOMY IN TWO LARGE SERIES FROM ACADEMIC MEDICAL CENTERS

N	Barnes/Brigham and Women's[28] 1,280	Vanderbilt[29] 896
Dates	1986–1995	1986–1995
Trauma	167 (13.0%)	372 (41.5%)
Autoimmune/ erythrocyte disorders	219 (17.1%)	140 (15.6%)
Hyperplasia	99 (7.7%)	138 (15.4%)
Incidental	336 (26.3%)	110 (12.3%)
Iatrogenic	N.A.	33 (8.1%)
Diagnostic unknown	122 (9.5%)	18 (2.0%)
Diagnostic staging for Hodgkin disease	258 (20.2%)	N.A.
Vascular	74 (5.8%)	21 (2.3%)
Miscellaneous	5 (0.4%)	24 (2.7%)

Trauma of the Spleen

The spleen is the most common intraabdominal organ injured by blunt trauma in the United States, and in many institutions splenectomy remains the most common operative procedure performed on the spleen.[30] The history of splenic surgery mirrors the history of surgery for trauma. In the ancient medical literature, the spleen is described as often herniating through a flank wound and there are reports of either partial splenectomy of the herniated portions or total splenectomy.[31] The first documented splenectomy for penetrating trauma was performed in San Francisco by a British naval surgeon named O'Brien in 1816 when a spleen protruded from the side of a knife wound.[2] In the late 19th century, Theodor Billroth observed, during an autopsy of a patient who had died of head trauma 5 days earlier, that there was minimal blood in the peritoneum from the fracture of the splenic capsule and predicted that these injuries may be managed operatively. Although in the earlier part of the 20th century splenic trauma was uniformly managed by a complete splenectomy, Dr. Campos Christo of Brazil reported partial splenectomy and splenic salvage for both penetrating and blunt trauma in 1962 (see Table 75.1).[2,3] This initial report, combined with the ability to obtain repeated cross-sectional imaging and with the understanding of splenic function and the appreciation for overwhelming postsplenectomy sepsis, has led to the current management guidelines with nonoperative management of lower grade splenic injuries and operative management centered around splenic preservation when possible.[32,33]

The most common modes of blunt injuries leading to splenic rupture are motor vehicle accidents and bicycle accidents, in which upper abdominal trauma may occur. The signs and symptoms of isolated splenic injury include tenderness in the left upper quadrant of the abdomen. Attention must be directed toward the lower lateral left ribs, and focal tenderness over ribs 9 through 11 in that region should raise suspicion of possible splenic injury. Approximately 20% of cases of rib fracture can be demonstrated on radiographs. Patients may have referred pain to the left shoulder (Kehr's sign) particularly when placed in the Trendelenburg position with palpation of the upper abdomen. The spleen itself is rarely palpable, but a palpable left upper quadrant mass represents contained hematoma or a subcapsular hematoma and this is known as Ballance's sign. Depending on the severity of the injury, patients may have no hemodynamic instability or may be in frank hypovolemic shock. The staging system for splenic trauma is shown in Table 75.8.

The diagnostic studies associated with splenic rupture potentially include a decrease in hematocrit and hemoglobin, although initial assessment before volume resuscitation may show normal levels. After a short time there is often a leukocytosis in the range of 15,000 to 20,000. Plain abdominal radiographs, in addition to possibly showing left rib fractures,

TABLE 75.8 CLASSIFICATION

SPLEEN INJURY SEAL

Grade	Laceration	Hamartoma
I	<1 cm in depth	Subcapsular <10% of surface
II	1 to 3 cm in depth not involving a trabecular vessel	Subcapsular 10%–50% of surface area or 5 cm in diameter
III	>3 cm depth or any depth involving a trabecular vessel	Subcapsular >50% of surface area or intraparenchymal
IV	Segmental or hilar vessel involvement	
V	Shattered spleen or hilar vessel disruption	

may show displacement or a corrugated appearance along the greater curvature of the stomach because of a hematoma infiltrating the gastrosplenic ligament (Fig. 75.6). Peritoneal lavage will reveal the presence of blood in the abdomen. The most important current tool for diagnosis, particularly in patients who have enough hemodynamic stability to be managed conservatively, is the computed tomography (CT) scan. Contrast CT scan will show the splenic contour and will also show the amount of extrasplenic blood (Fig. 75.7).[34]

Overall, blunt injuries make up the majority of splenic trauma, but the spleen is susceptible to penetrating trauma in the retroperitoneum, lower thoracic penetrating trauma, or upper abdominal penetrating trauma. The management and diagnosis of penetrating trauma of the thorax and upper abdomen is less of a diagnostic dilemma because a majority of these patients undergo abdominal exploration because of associated injuries. In some series, there are additional injuries in 90% to 100% of patients with penetrating trauma to the spleen and 40% to 60% associated injuries for blunt trauma.

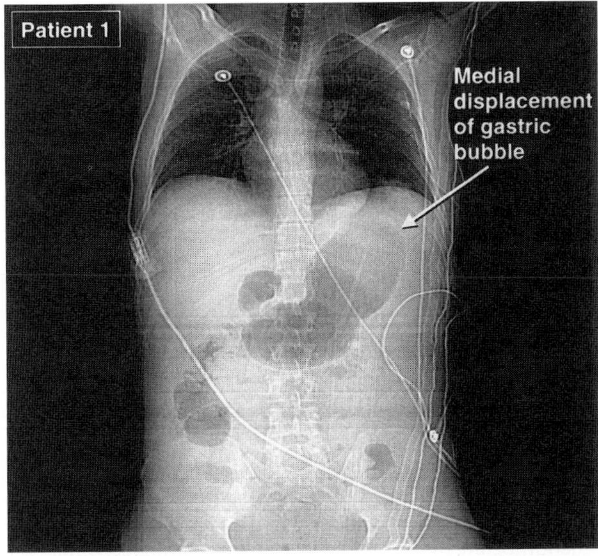

FIGURE 75.6 Abdominal film in a patient with a splenic rupture from blunt trauma with a perisplenic hematoma displacing the greater curvature of the stomach medially. The scalloped appearance is indicative of blood in the gastrosplenic ligament. (Courtesy of Dr. C. William Schwab.)

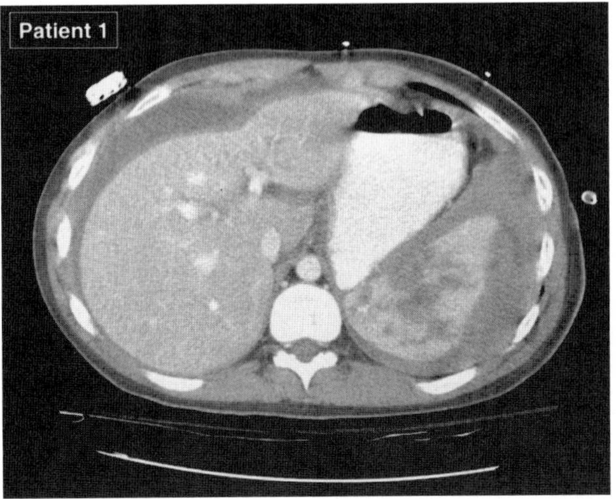

FIGURE 75.7 A contrast computed tomography scan of a patient with splenic rupture near the hilum. There is considerable blood in the perisplenic fossa as well as free blood in the peritoneal cavity around the liver. (Courtesy of Dr. C. William Schwab.)

Management of splenic injuries historically has been a laparotomy with splenectomy. Since Christo introduced the ability to do either partial splenectomy or splenorrhaphy, there has been an increased trend to try to repair or preserve part if not all of the spleen. The current trend in management is a nonoperative approach with observation in serial CT scans.[35] The presence of peritonitis, associated injuries requiring surgery, the overall injury severity, evidence of hypovolemic shock and ongoing bleeding, and the patient's age are the primary factors that are taken into consideration when deciding on nonoperative versus operative management of blunt splenic injuries.[36] When patients have diffuse peritonitis or have hypotension related to hypovolemic shock, urgent laparotomy is indicated. For patients who are hemodynamically stable and do not have other injuries that require surgical management, the recommendation is to attempt nonoperative observation of these patients. In some pediatric series, this comprises the vast majority of the patient population. In other recent series of adult patients, approximately 30% to 50% of patients require urgent splenectomy because of associated injuries and ongoing bleeding (Fig. 75.8). Of patients stable enough to obtain a CT scan, 50% to 80% may be candidates for observation. Between 3% and 15% of patients selected for observation will ultimately need an operation for continued or recurrent bleeding.

The standard nonoperative management protocol includes very close observation in an intensive care unit or other similar monitored environment. Patients have serial abdominal examinations as well as serial hemoglobin and hematocrit assessments. Any change in status in which patients remain somewhat stable is evaluated with a follow-up CT scan to see whether progressive or ongoing bleeding is demonstrated by increased hemoperitoneum or expansion of splenic hematoma. A recent report noted that routine follow-up CT scans did not alter management in patients treated nonoperatively.[37] Only patients with changes in hemodynamic parameters had a change in management. With this conservative management, the majority of patients avoid laparotomy for isolated splenic blunt trauma.[38] In the past, there was a concept of a delayed splenic rupture that was thought to be due to capsular hematoma that subsequently liquefied and led to rupture, typically with 75% of these cases occurring within 2 weeks of the date of injury. However, delayed rupture may occur a month or up to several years after the trauma.[37,39] The recent approach of nonoperative

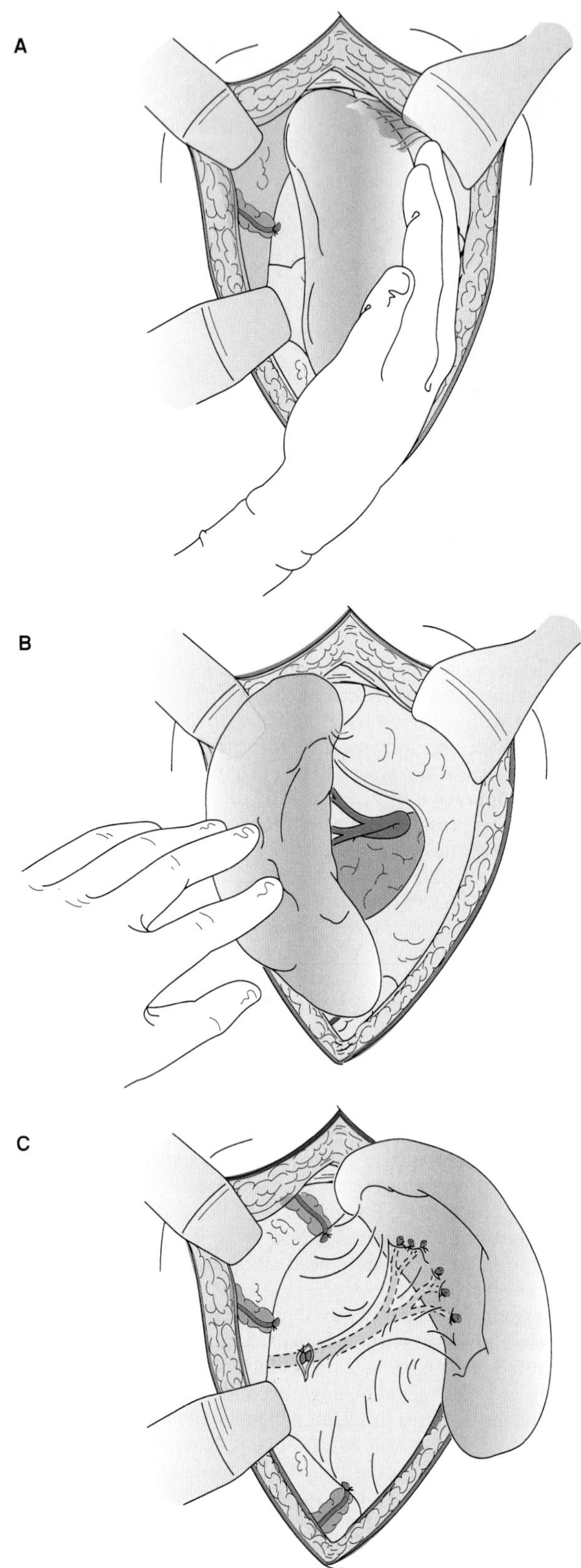

FIGURE 75.8 (*A* and *B*) Rapid mobilization of a bleeding spleen can be accomplished in most patients by blunt dissection of the lateral attachments. (C) The splenic hilum can then be quickly controlled.

management of splenic trauma supplemented by sequential CT imaging studies has defined this phenomenon with delayed rupture to be a relatively rare event when patients are followed prospectively.

A laparotomy is appropriate for blunt splenic trauma in patients who are older or in those who have associated injuries or who have ongoing blood loss.[31,40] Again, the nature of the splenic injury is graded relative to the degree of damage to the splenic parenchyma and the proximity to the splenic hilum and major blood vessels (Table 75.8). The principles of operative management include stopping ongoing hemorrhage while preserving the maximal amount of viable splenic parenchyma.[41] Nonviable or devascularized tissue must be débrided.[42] Partial splenectomy has been popularized based on the concept of segmental blood supply via the trabecular arteries. A variety of approaches can be taken to more minor peripheral splenic trauma, including primary repair or mesh repair (Fig. 75.9). Multiple materials that are available for hemostasis, including microfibrillar collagen, thrombins of Gelfoam, or fibrin glue sealants, have been used to obtain control of splenic hemorrhage. The argon beam coagulator is a very useful instrument for repair of capsular tear or evulsions.[43] Of note, all of these techniques that have been applied to the patient suffering from blunt trauma can be similarly applied to patients who have inadvertent trauma to the spleen during operations on the splenic flexure of the colon or the left kidney, adrenal gland, or stomach.

In a recent trauma registry of more than 1,480 patients with blunt splenic trauma, 54.8% were managed conservatively; 38.5% went immediately to the operating room because of the magnitude of the injury and hemodynamic instability. Of the 54.8% that had nonoperative management, 89.2% did not need surgery, whereas 10.8% went to the operating room. Of the conservative management failures, 60% happened within the first 24 hours.[44] The results with blunt trauma for the pediatric population show even a greater rate of splenic preservation. In the Pennsylvania Trauma Registry between 1993 and 1997, there were 754 pediatric patients with blunt splenic trauma. Of these, 77.5% were managed nonoperatively, 7.4% went to the operating room and had a splenorrhaphy, and only 15.1% had a splenectomy. The factors that increased the risk of splenectomy were the grade and magnitude of the injury and not dynamic instability. Also, patients who were seen at designated pediatric trauma centers had a much higher rate of splenic preservation compared with patients not cared for at trauma centers. Even in patients who do need a splenectomy because of the magnitude of the injury, there are attempts to preserve splenic function by either implanting spleens in the omentum or causing splenosis. In institutional series reported in 505 patients with splenic injury, 29% (145 patients) went to the operating room, whereas 71% were managed nonoperatively. Of those who had surgery, 23% had a splenectomy and 5% had a splenorrhaphy. A small subgroup of patients, based on the surgeons' preference, who underwent splenectomy had splenic implantation to the omentum.[35] Ten of the patients who had splenic implantation had follow-up CT scans, and virtually all of these were read as a postoperative abscess within the omentum, which corresponded to the splenic implant. Follow-up scans showed recovery of the splenic implant in the majority of cases.

Autoimmune/Erythrocyte Disorders

There are two categories of disease in which abnormalities do not originate in terms of the histology, pathology, or size of the spleen but rather are a result of either autoimmune phenomenon or intrinsic diseases within circulating cells that lead to their destruction. The most common and obvious example of this is immune thrombocytopenic purpura (ITP), in which antibodies to platelet antigens lead to destruction of platelets and thrombocytopenia, with the spleen being the primary source of platelet elimination. Related diseases affecting erythrocytes

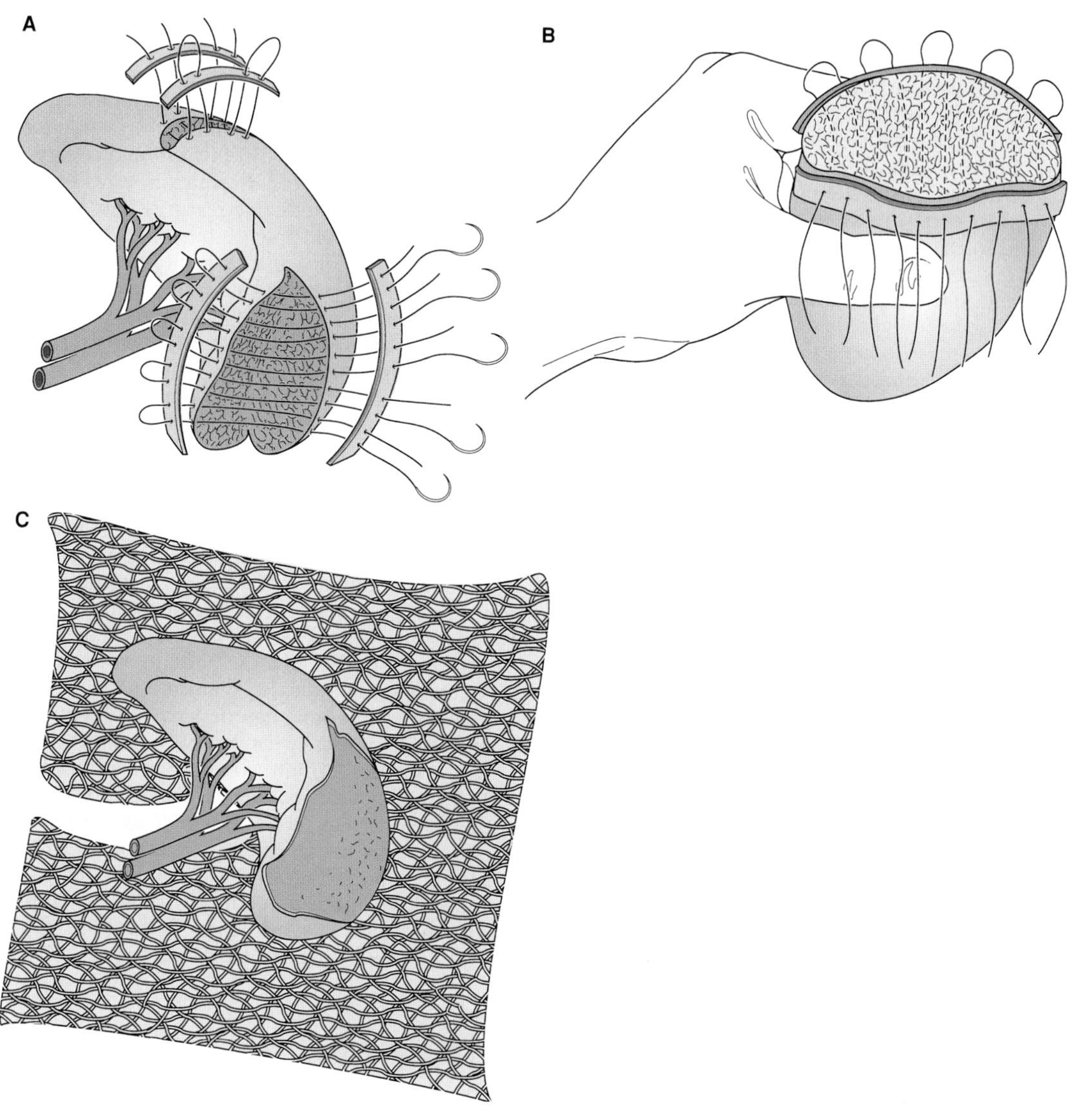

FIGURE 75.9 (*A*) Techniques to suture superficial splenic lacerations. (*B*) Technique to control bleeding after hemisplenectomy. The sutures can be interlocked. (*C*) Polyglycolic acid mesh sheets or mesh bags can be applied to spleens that have had the capsule stripped away.

and neutrophils with specific antibodies and splenic elimination occur to lesser degrees.

A second category of disease is not an autoimmune phenomenon but rather an intrinsic cellular defect that leads to a shortened half-life of this specific blood cell within the circulation primarily to elimination within the spleen. As discussed in the physiology section previously, a normal role of the spleen is to eliminate senescent erythrocytes, and the anatomic structures of splenic circulation are well suited to that task. Alteration in the structure of erythrocytes may lead to more rapid elimination. In other diseases, genetic differences in the hemoglobin may result in splenic changes, particularly in the setting of hypoxia, which occurs within the splenic sinusoids. The most obvious example of this condition is sickle cell anemia. Another example is an alteration in the cellular adhesion molecule that leads to increased interaction and thrombocytopenia in Wiskott-Aldrich syndrome.

Immune Thrombocytopenic Purpura

ITP is a disease characterized by autoimmune destruction of platelets with clinical manifestations of thrombocytopenia, which include susceptibility to easy or excessive bleeding.[45] ITP may be classified as either an acute form or a chronic form. Acute ITP generally occurs in children under age 8 years following a viral upper respiratory illness. Of children with acute ITP, 80% to 90% have spontaneous remissions.[46] Only 8% to 10% of adults who develop ITP have remission, and the majority develop chronic ITP. This disease is usually self-limited and requires surgical intervention only in the case of intracranial bleeding. Chronic ITP accounts for the vast majority of cases considered for splenectomy. Similar to autoimmune hemolytic anemia, this disease may be idiopathic or may be secondary to a lymphoproliferative disorder, a connective tissue disorder such as systemic lupus erythematosus, or drug or bacterial exposure. The average age at diagnosis is in the 4th decade of life, and it affects women more commonly than men. As HIV was identified in the mid-1980s, it was noted that patients with acquired immunodeficiency syndrome (AIDS) were developing disease virtually identical to ITP.[47] Clinical manifestations of the disease reflect low platelets. In women, this may be manifested by increased menstrual bleeding that is noted in an insidious manner. As platelet counts reach lower levels, petechiae and spontaneous bleeding or inability to clot following minor injury generally makes the diagnosis apparent.

The pathophysiology of ITP is development of an IgG antibody to a platelet antigen. This is thought to be most commonly directed against the fibrinogen receptor (glycoprotein IIb/IIIa).[48] The spleen plays a predominant role in this disease because it may be the site of initial antibody production,[49] it is almost certainly the site of continued antibody production, and in the majority of patients it is the primary site of platelet destruction. Because the targeted antigen is an intravascular cell, and because the spleen stores large numbers of platelets, it is thought that the initial reaction to the platelet cell antigen may occur in the spleen. Studies on antibody levels have indicated that overall IgG production in spleens from patients with ITP is markedly increased over that in individuals with normal spleens. Similarly, following splenectomy the amount of IgG antibody is somewhat decreased. The IgG antibody is not eliminated because helper T cells as well as plasma cells may be located or be redistributed in other areas, particularly the bone marrow after prolonged immune stimulation. The spleen is also the predominant site of platelet destruction. As noted previously, the macrophages located in the cords of Billroth have receptors for the Fc portion of the IgG and will bind and phagocytize the antibody-coated platelets.

For a patient to be considered to have ITP, the platelet count has to at least be less than 100,000, but typically patients do not become symptomatic unless platelet counts are less than 50,000. Platelet counts in this disorder may drop to very low levels, well below 10,000 on occasion. Assays are now available to identify the IgG antiglobulin on the platelet surface, verifying the disease. Bone marrow analysis shows increased megakaryocyte production as a compensatory mechanism to the thrombocytopenia. In this disorder, there is often no splenomegaly and the spleen may be somewhat smaller than typical. Only 2% of patients with ITP have palpable spleens. For this reason, there is virtually no leukopenia or anemia associated with ITP due to hypersplenism. There may be anemia secondary to chronic blood loss. The overall risk of a fatal hemorrhage in patients with ITP is 0.47/year and for patients with platelet counts less than 30,000 ranges between 1.6 and 6.9%.[46]

The treatment of ITP includes standard measures to treat any ongoing bleeding, medical therapies designed to increase platelet count, and splenectomy. Options for initial medical therapy include platelet transfusion, corticosteroids, gamma-immunoglobulin, and the recently approved Rho(d) immunoglobulin.[50] Platelet transfusions should be discouraged unless patients are actively bleeding because platelets will become rapidly coated with IgG and will be sequestered and destroyed in the spleen. High-dose corticosteroids produce an initial response in the majority of patients, but this response unfortunately is not sustained. Approximately 75% of the patients will have an increase in platelet count that is significant within 24 hours of starting high-dose steroids.[51] However, only 15% to 25% of patients will have a sustained remission with chronic ITP following steroid therapy.

A second-line treatment for chronic ITP has been administration of intravenous IgG immunoglobulin. This treatment takes only between 3 and 5 days to show an effect and generally does not put patients into complete remission. This IgG may be a useful treatment to try to boost platelet counts prior to elective splenectomy to decrease the chance of intraoperative bleeding. The mechanism of action of immune gamma globulin is thought to be saturation of the Fc receptors on the splenic macrophages.[52] The administered gamma globulin may coat red cells, and they may provide a competitive interference such that platelet destruction is decreased. The newest available drug is the recently approved Rho(d) immunoglobulin, which specifically targets the Fc receptors. Initial experience indicates significant benefit in ITP, but the long-term role of this agent remains to be seen.

In patients who have not achieved a sustained remission with medical therapy, which is the majority of patients with chronic ITP, an elective splenectomy is recommended. A recent series analyzed 135 institutional reports between 1966 and 2004[53] and reported results in terms of normalization of platelet counts, predictive features that would indicate who would benefit from splenectomy, and reported complications including morbidity and mortality (Table 75.9). The percentage of patients who normalized platelets achieved a normal platelet count of only splenectomy was 68.9% with over 5,000 patients reported. If one evaluated case series with adults only, this was only slightly lower at 66% and when adults and children were combined it was 72.1%. There was no analysis of pediatric patient populations only, although it is believed that children had to do better in terms of overall cure rate. These results seem to be durable because in the subset of this series, which is approximately 20% of all reported patents, there was 5-year follow-up and the cure rate at 5 years was 67.2% (see Table 75.9).[53] In assessing disease characteristics and demographic features such as age, sex, duration of illness, platelet count, and response to medical therapy, one tries to identify which patients would be in the subgroup that would respond versus the patients who would not respond. A recent study indicated that only patients with short disease duration at a young age (less than 16 years) had benefit on univaried analysis, whereas only the short duration of disease was a feature in multivaried analysis.[54] In the review of the 135 combined series, there was no predictive value of any of these features in terms of which patients would respond to therapy. The overall mortality rate from splenectomy in this patient population was 0.81% and tended to be lower in the subgroup of patients treated with laparoscopic splenectomy. This may reflect decreased risk with laparoscopic splenectomy, it also would in spite of the fact that all of the laparoscopic

TABLE 75.9 RESULTS

RESULTS FROM 135 COMBINED CASE SERIES EVALUATING SPLENECTOMY FOR ITP

CURE RATE		
% of patients with normalized platelet counts		
All reports	68.9%	(3,506/5,086)
Adult series only	66.0%	(1,731/2,623)
Adult pediatric combined	72.1%	(1,785/2,468)
% of patients with normalized platelet counts with 5 year follow-up	67.2%	(779/1,159)
COMPLICATIONS		
Perioperative mortality		
Total	0.81%	51/6,256
Laparotomy	0.96%	48/4,955
Laparoscopy	0.23%	3/1,301
Perioperative complications		
Total	12.0%	406/3,386
Laparotomy	12.9%	318/2,465
Laparoscopy	9.6%	88/921

ITP, idiopathic thrombocytopenic purpura.
(Adapted from Kojouri K, Vesely SK, Terrell DR, George JN. Splenectomy for adult patients with idiopathic thrombocytopenic purpura: a systematic review to assess long-term platelet count responses, prediction of response, and surgical complications. *Blood* 2003;104:2623–2634.)

procedures have been performed in the last 10 to 15 years of this 4-year analysis. This mortality rate, particularly with laparoscopic splenectomy, compares favorably to the risk of a fatal hemorrhage in patients who have significant thrombocytopenia with this disease. The overall complication rate was 12%.

A recent study evaluated the role of indium-labeled platelets as a predictor for response to splenectomy in ITP.[55,56] In this study, if the radiolabeled platelets predominantly tracked to the spleen, 96% of patients under the age of 30 had complete remission, and 91% of patients over the age of 30 had complete remission. If the radiolabeled platelets tracked to the liver or elsewhere, there was only an 8% success rate. If the spleen/liver ratio is less than one almost no patients achieve benefit.[57] This test, which has remarkably predictive results, contrasts with earlier studies using chromium-labeled platelets in a similar manner, which did not show correlation with outcome.

One cause for a failed splenectomy for ITP is residual splenic tissue, most commonly in the form of a missed accessory spleen but also in the form of splenosis.[15] Both problems of accessory spleens and splenosis are felt to have increased somewhat in the current era of laparoscopic splenectomy. Again, ITP spleens are predominantly small and are ideally suited for a laparoscopic approach. The incidence of accessory spleens identified with open procedures is in the range of 15% to 30%, whereas the incidence of accessory spleens reported with the laparoscopic approach is between 0% and 15%.[58] In a recent study, two of three patients who were failures after surgical splenectomy had accessory spleens that were missed at the time of the laparoscopic splenectomy. Reports have indicated that use of indium-labeled platelets, particularly with single photon emission computed tomography (SPECT) imaging techniques, precisely identified the location of accessory spleens and allowed removal with subsequent success. The second operation to remove the accessory spleen generally can be accomplished with a laparoscopic approach as well.[59,60]

Thrombotic Thrombocytopenia Purpura

Thrombotic thrombocytopenia purpura (TTP), or Moschcowitz syndrome, is a poorly understood, much more virulent syndrome than ITP, in which thrombocytopenic purpura is only one manifestation. This disease is characterized by widespread occlusion of arterioles and capillaries by hyalin membranes, which are composed of a combination of platelets and fibrinogen. The classic pentad of symptoms reflects various organ injuries with this microvascular process. This includes thrombocytopenic purpura, with microvascular disease in the skin; neurologic manifestations resulting from microvascular disease in the central nervous system; renal failure or hematuria caused by microvascular disease in the kidney; microvascular hemolytic anemia owing to destruction of red cells traveling to damaged small vessels; and fever. The precise etiology is unknown but may be related to an autoimmune response to small vessel endothelial cell antigen.

The therapeutic options for this disease include administration of fresh frozen plasma or plasmapheresis, or both; high-dose corticosteroids; and antiplatelet drugs.[61] The benefits seen with plasmapheresis indicate that there is a toxic substance that is contributing to the etiology of this disorder circulating in the plasma, whereas the benefit of administration of fresh frozen plasma indicates lack of some necessary substance that has yet to be identified. High-dose corticosteroids also lead to some benefit. Aspirin and dipyridamole block platelet agglutination. A combination of these therapies now leads to significant improvement of symptoms in 70% of patients. For patients failing to respond or patients who relapse, a splenectomy has been performed with some success.[62,63] The majority of the long-term survivors with TTP have undergone splenectomy, implying that this organ has some major role in the pathophysiology of this disease.[64] The precise mechanism of splenic contribution is unclear. Mortality rates in the past have been as high as 90% to 95% for this disorder, but are improving with aggressive treatment plans and a better understanding and diagnosis of this disorder.

Autoimmune Hemolytic Anemia

Autoimmune hemolytic anemia or acquired hemolytic anemia results from antibodies produced to red cell membrane proteins that lead to red cell destruction. This disease is more common in women than in men by a ratio of 2:1, and it typically presents after age 50 years. Patients present with acute symptoms consisting of anemia, jaundice, and occasional fever. The spleen is enlarged in approximately half of the patients. Laboratory diagnosis shows a positive direct Coombs test, indicating antibody coating the erythrocytes. There is also significant reticulocytosis and increased indirect bilirubin in the serum.

The disease is considered to be either idiopathic in 40% to 50% of the cases in which no drug or infectious cause is identified or secondary to infection or drug. Of the secondary causes, the most common infections are mycoplasmal pneumonia, viral infections, infectious mononucleosis, and AIDS and it can also occur with neoplastic diseases such as leukemia and lymphoma. The major drugs that cause secondary autoimmune hemolytic anemia are penicillin, quinidine, hydralazine, and methyldopa.

A second way in which autoimmune hemolytic anemia is categorized is by either cold or warm antibodies. Warm antibodies are predominantly IgG, whereas cold antibodies are predominantly IgM. This distinction is important when considering splenectomy as a treatment. The spleen contains macrophages that bind the Fc portion of IgG. For this reason, in patients with warm antibody hemolytic anemia the spleen is the primary source of destruction of the red cells by the red pulp macrophages. However, because the spleen does not contain receptors to bind IgM or the cold antibodies, there is no destruction of the red cells in this form of hemolytic anemia. Rather, IgM either causes complement fixation with destruction of red cells in the liver predominantly or there is agglutination of red cells in peripheral circulation, such as the distal extremities leading to peripheral red cell destruction with clinical manifestations similar to Raynaud's phenomenon. Splenectomy is not effective for patients with cold antibody or IgM hemolytic anemia.

The treatment of autoimmune hemolytic anemia initially consists of supportive therapy, such as blood transfusions. For patients who have disease secondary to an acute infection such as a mycoplasm pneumonia, the disease may be self-limited. For drug-induced hemolytic anemia, the offending agent is removed as quickly as possible. The initial form of treatment is typically high-dose corticosteroids, which cause a beneficial response in 75% of the patients. If patients again have drug-induced disease and the offending agent is removed or the acute infection resolves, this may lead to long-term resolution. In idiopathic autoimmune hemolytic anemia, only 25% of patients have sustained remission from steroid use. In patients who have relapse after steroid therapy or who are ineligible for steroid therapy and have warm antibodies, a splenectomy has a high likelihood of benefit. About 80% of patients show a good response in correcting the anemia by splenectomy.[65] This is thought to be almost certainly related to removal of the site of destruction of the erythrocytes but may be due to a decrease in production of the source of the antibodies.

Autoimmune Neutropenia (Felty Syndrome)

Approximately 1% of patients with chronic rheumatoid arthritis will develop splenomegaly and neutropenia. This triad of rheumatoid arthritis, neutropenia, and splenomegaly is known as Felty syndrome.[66] High levels of IgG have been identified on the surface of neutrophils with evidence of increased production of granulocytes in the bone marrow. Pathologic analysis of spleens removed in patients with Felty syndrome show a significant but proportional increase in the white pulp of the spleen as opposed to other conditions of splenomegaly.[67] Microscopically, there is evidence of excess accumulation of neutrophils in both the T-cell zone and the white pulp as well as the cords and sinuses of the red pulp.

Patients with this disease have recurrent infections due to neutropenia as well as dysfunction of the available neutrophils that are coated with antineutrophil IgG. Recurrent infections and chronic leg ulcers are the predominant symptoms. Symptomatic patients should undergo splenectomy, and the vast majority of patients will have resolution of their neutropenia within 2 to 3 days.[68] Even patients who do not have a significant increase in neutrophil count should get some benefit because of improved neutrophil function.[69]

Hereditary Spherocytosis

Hereditary spherocytosis, also known as congenital hemolytic jaundice or familial hemolytic anemia, is an autosomal dominant disease that is the most common of the congenital hemolytic anemias, affecting one in 5,000 individuals. There are a variety of genetic defects in this syndrome that primarily affect spectrin and ankyrin, which alter the binding of the cytoskeleton to the erythrocyte cellular membrane causing decreased cellular plasticity with membrane loss.[70] The normal shape of the erythrocyte is changed from a biconcave disc into a sphere, and the decreased membrane-to-volume cell ratio causes a lack of deformability that impacts the passage of erythrocytes through channels of the splenic red pulp. Because of this delay in cell transit, there is adenosine 5′-triphosphate (ATP) deprivation, resulting in increased cellular destruction. The condition is more frequent in whites and in African-Americans and is usually noted in childhood or adolescent ages. Because it is an autosomal dominant inheritance, patients may be screened and diagnosed at an early age.

The diagnosis is primarily made by evaluation of the red cell smear showing a large number of spherocytes. Spherocytes may also appear during autoimmune hemolytic anemias, but in hereditary spherocytosis the Coombs test is negative and an osmotic fragility test may be performed, which is diagnostic. Also contributing to the diagnosis is a positive family history.

Patients with hereditary spherocytosis have mild to moderate anemia, splenomegaly, and jaundice. The patients may have intermittent flares of disease, which cause significant increased rates of hemolysis causing jaundice. Between 30% and 60% of patients have been reported to have pigmented gallstones owing to the breakdown of hemoglobin.

The treatment for hereditary spherocytosis is splenectomy, and it is indicated in virtually all patients.[71] This treatment does not remove the spherocytes, but it relieves all symptoms.[72] The major question involving management of these patients is the timing of splenectomy. Because of the increased incidence of overwhelming postsplenectomy sepsis in very young children, it is usually recommended that patients wait until after the age of at least 4 years if not 6 before undergoing splenectomy. For younger patients who are very symptomatic and require splenectomy, partial splenectomies have been reported to be beneficial in relieving the abdominal symptoms as well as the anemia and may be a useful alternative procedure until patients reach an age at which total splenectomy is safer.[73,74,75] Patients with partial splenectomies had regrowth of tissue but with short-term did not have recurrent anemia.[65] Patients should be assessed for the presence of gallstones at the time of scheduling a splenectomy, and a laparoscopic cholecystectomy should be performed if stones are identified.

Hereditary Elliptocytosis

Hereditary elliptocytosis is a disease that is related to hereditary spherocytosis, although it is not as severe. For patients who are symptomatic, virtually all of the same comments regarding pathophysiology and treatment of hereditary spherocytosis can be made about hereditary elliptocytosis. This disease is also inherited in an autosomal dominant pattern, and the defect is thought to be present in spectrin. The predominant abnormality changes spectrin such that it exists as a dimer instead of tetramer, which is the normal structure. This change leads to an alteration in membrane plasticity that creates cells that are more elliptically shaped instead of a biconcave disc.

The signs and symptoms caused in this disease are much more mild than those of hereditary spherocytosis, in that only 10% of patients have clinical manifestations of anemia, splenomegaly, and in some cases jaundice. The treatment recommendation for symptomatic patients is again splenectomy, which may be performed with laparoscopic techniques, and also cholecystectomy if gallstones are present.

Hereditary Nonspherocytic Hemolytic Anemia

There is a heterogeneous group of rare hemolytic anemias caused by inherited defects, primarily of enzymes involved in glycolysis. It is thought that these genetic defects may decrease cellular energy production such that during their passage through the red pulp of the spleen some cells do not have the ability to produce ATP in this relatively hypoxic environment, leading to increased red cell destruction. The most common subtypes in this group of hemolytic anemias are pyruvate kinase deficiency and glucose 6-phosphate dehydrogenase (G6PD) deficiency. Patients present with anemia, jaundice, increased reticulocytes, and possibly cholelithiasis. The differential diagnosis can be made in that the shape of the cell does not typically show spherocytes and there is normal osmotic fragility.

The primary treatment for these diseases is blood transfusion. In G6PD deficiency, splenectomy is not believed to be beneficial, whereas it may reverse some of the symptoms associated with pyruvate kinase deficiency.

Thalassemia

Thalassemia is an autosomal dominant disease with a variety of structural defects in one of the globin chains. The disease is categorized as alpha, beta, gamma, or delta thalassemia, depending on which of the globin chains is defective. The vast majority of patients in North America have beta-thalassemia. Thalassemia major, otherwise known as Mediterranean anemia or Cooley anemia, is a homozygous expression of this genetic defect. Thalassemia minor is a heterozygous expression, and patients are only mildly symptomatic and are carriers for the more severe form of the disease.

The pathophysiology of thalassemia major or beta-thalassemia is the lack of production of normal beta-chain hemoglobin, leading to a surplus of alpha-chain hemoglobin in adult patients. These excess globin chains precipitate in the cytoplasm and attach to the inner surfaces of cytoplasmic membrane, leading to poor passage of these cells through the splenic sinusoids. This intracellular inclusion then leads to increased destruction and over time causes significant splenomegaly resulting from the increased clearance of red cells.

The diagnosis is made by identifying microcytic hypochromic anemia with target cells and an increase in reticulocytes on the peripheral smear. Protein electrophoresis shows very low levels of hemoglobin A, with predominant amounts of the fetal hemoglobin, or hemoglobin F. The clinical symptom of alpha-thalassemia major is severe anemia within the first year of life. Decreased growth rate, enlargement of the head, splenomegaly, and hepatomegaly are the typical clinical findings.[76]

The primary treatment for thalassemia major is frequent transfusions combined with iron chelation therapy. Some patients may develop significant splenomegaly because of overload or hypertrophy from excess trapping of red cells.[77] Patients with symptomatic splenomegaly or those with massive and frequent transfusion requirements may be referred for splenectomy. One report suggested that episodes of transfusion are decreased from 18 per year to four per year after splenectomy. In general, if there are symptoms of massive splenomegaly, they will be resolved with splenectomy as well. As with other hematologic disorders in children, there has been a recent trend toward partial splenectomy, particularly in children less than 4 to 5 years of age.[78] This will result in symptomatic improvement in 1 to 2 years, with recurrent disease caused by hypertrophy of the residual splenic remnant.[79]

Although splenectomy may be beneficial in terms of the transfusion requirements and local symptoms, the typical mode of death with this disease is myocardial failure as a result of hemosiderin accumulation. Splenectomy does not alter this cardiac problem to any great extent.

Sickle Cell Anemia

Sickle cell anemia is a hereditary hemolytic anemia that is due to a genetic alteration of a single amino acid substitution in the beta chain. This results in a change from glutamic acid to valine in the sixth amino acid position of the beta chain of hemoglobin molecule. Because of this substitution, patients who are homozygous for sickle cell defect have a characteristic stiffening or sickling of the red blood cells when they become hypoxic.[80] This change in red cell shape leads to blockage in hypoxic areas such as the red pulp of the spleen. There can occasionally be sequestration crises in which a portion of the blood volume gets actively trapped or sequestered to the spleen during the sickle cell crisis. This pattern of red cell shape change in relatively hypoxic areas can lead to tissue infarction with bone pain, hematuria, abdominal pain, and priapism.

The incidence of this disease, which occurs almost exclusively in the black population, is approximately 0.5% for homozygous disease, with approximately 8% of African-Americans being carriers for the sickle cell trait. Patients who have a combination of a sickle cell allele as well as a beta thalassemia allele manifest a similar disease process.

The clinical signs of the disease usually appear during the second 6 months of life; in early infancy the patient is asymptomatic because of the presence of fetal hemoglobin. The patients may have acute crises with abdominal pain and bone pain in conjunction with significant anemia. During acute crises of splenic sequestration there may be massive enlargement of the spleen, and an urgent decompressive splenectomy may be required. Patients who do not need splenectomy for splenic sequestration may be followed as this disease goes through a natural progression of ischemic necrosis of large areas of the spleen, with eventual hyposplenism and a shrunken organ by early adolescence. Splenectomy is reserved for very young patients who have massive splenomegaly in sequestration crises early in life.

Wiskott-Aldrich Syndrome

Wiskott-Aldrich syndrome is an X-linked disease characterized by thrombocytopenia, combined B- and T-cell deficiency, eczema, and a propensity to develop other malignancies. The genetic defect in this disease is thought to be related to an abnormal adhesion molecule affecting immune cell interaction as well as platelet adhesion. Thrombocytopenia is the major problem with this rare disease, and most patients present with manifestations of poor clotting, bloody diarrhea, epistaxis, and petechiae at a young age. The platelet count typically ranges between 20,000 and 40,000, the platelets that are present are dysfunctional because of their small size, and platelet volume is 25% to 50% of normal. In this disease, the spleen sequesters platelets and partially degrades them, releasing "microplatelets" back into the circulation.[81]

Splenectomy in the Wiskott-Aldrich syndrome was initially avoided because of its very problematic postoperative course, which is characterized by severe and fatal infections resulting from the underlying immunodeficiency combined with the potential for overwhelming postsplenectomy infection. However, splenectomy does increase the number, size, and function of platelets and can lead to amelioration of the bleeding problems in very symptomatic patients.[81] The combination of splenectomy with antibiotic suppression, particularly in younger patients, may be beneficial. The optimal treatment for Wiskott-Aldrich syndrome is a human leukocyte antigen (HLA)–match sibling bone marrow transplantation.[82] However, splenectomy with antibiotics results in better survival than unmatched bone marrow transplantation. Patients who do not undergo bone marrow transplantation or splenectomy typically do not survive past the age of 5 years. The pathology of spleens removed for Wiskott-Aldrich syndrome shows a near complete depletion of white pulp supporting the clinical immune deficiency seen in this syndrome.[83]

Hypersplenisim

Hypersplenism is a physical enlargement of the spleen that can be broadly categorized as the neoplastic disorders, hematopoietic disorders of the bone marrow, and metabolic or storage disorders. In the neoplastic disorders, the spleen is infiltrative and large, typically by leukemic or lymphoma cells. This enlargement often happens in the mid or late course of a patient's disease, but can be associated with isolated splenomegaly in which the splenectomy is performed not only to treat hypersplenism, but also to make the definitive diagnosis (see Diagnostic Splenectomy, later). Hypersplenism is associated with diseases of hematopoiesis related to myeloid metaplasia, in which the bone marrow is infiltrated with fibrotic material and the spleen becomes a site of secondary non–bone marrow hematopoiesis. Enlargement can lead to symptoms of hypersplenism because of the massive size of the spleen, and often the benefits of extramedullary hematopoiesis are outweighed by the sites of circulating blood cell destruction in the enlarged spleen. The final category is secondary hyposplenism, in which there may be deposition of lipid within the spleen, such as in Gaucher disease, leading to enlargement that can cause pancytopenia. Each of these areas of secondary hypersplenism is associated with pancytopenia and mass effect of the spleen, causing early satiety and weight loss. These disorders typically lead to spleen size of more than 1,500 g and can result in a spleen that essentially fills the entire left side of the abdomen.

Chronic Lymphocytic Leukemia

Chronic lymphocytic leukemia (CLL) is the most common of all chronic leukemias. It predominantly affects males more than females by 2:1 predominance and has a peak incidence in the 6th decade of life or older. This indolent disease presents with fatigue, lymphadenopathy, hepatosplenomegaly, and eventually anemia and thrombocytopenia. The disease may progress over a 5- to 10-year period.

Patients by definition in stage II or greater CLL will have splenomegaly and anemia and thrombocytopenia secondary to hypersplenism. Splenomegaly often reaches a very large size, and patients may have symptoms secondary to the compressive effects of the large spleen on the stomach with early satiety and pain (Fig. 75.10). Treatment for early stage disease is either observation or treatment with nontoxic doses of alkylating agents such as chlorambucil and cyclophosphamide. A newer agent that is becoming a standard therapy is fludarabine. Medical therapy is never curative, and eventually the predominant symptoms result from hypersplenism and splenomegaly. One strategy that has been employed in particular for patients who are nonoperative candidates is splenic radiation.[84] The splenic radiation has decreased the size of the spleen, improving symptoms due to mass effect, but it may have complications of further thrombocytopenia and leukopenia.

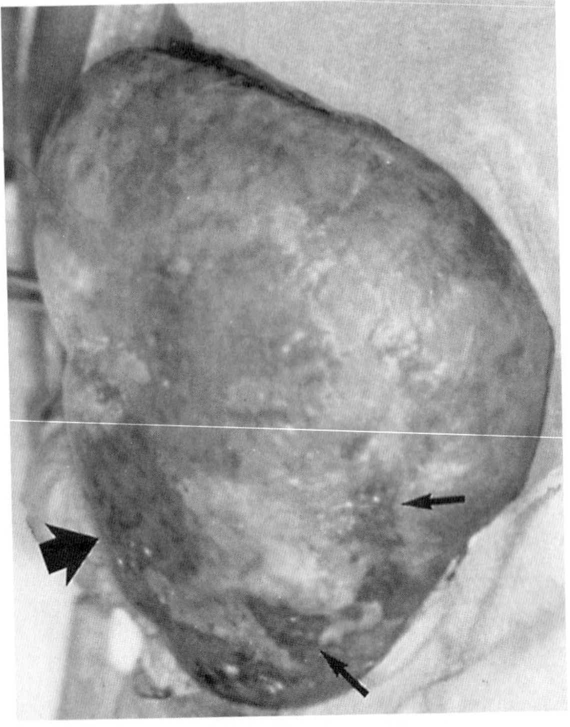

FIGURE 75.10. A massively enlarged, 2.2-kg spleen from a patient with chronic lymphocytic leukemia. Superficial areas of infarction are indicated by thin arrows and splenic infarction by the thick arrow.

Splenectomy is a highly successful treatment for both the pressure effects caused by splenomegaly and the cytopenias.[85,86,87] Reports of 85% resolution of thrombocytopenia and 100% resolution of anemia have been published.[88] The negative features of splenectomy in this patient population are that they are typically elderly and are typically debilitated from having gone through years of having CLL and potentially prior chemotherapy treatment. In one series in which a prospective comparison was made between splenectomy and fludarabine for later stage CLL, there was a 9% perioperative mortality in the splenectomy group primarily due to sepsis in this patient population.[89] However, in this same study, there were highly significant improvements in thrombocytopenia and anemia. The patient who is younger and has a larger spleen tends to do better. In this comparative study patients with Rai stage IV CLL had a 55% survival in the splenectomy arm and a 29% survival in the fludarabine arm. At present, splenectomy is recommended for patients who have failed medical therapy and have anemia with transfusion requirements or thrombocytopenia with bleeding or compressive symptoms such as splenomegaly.

CHRONIC MYELOGENOUS LEUKEMIA

Chronic myelogenous leukemia (CML) is a leukemia in which the cell of origin is a primitive hematopoietic cell. This primordial cell can differentiate into myeloid cell lines, erythroid cell lines, platelet cell lines, and possibly B lymphoid and T lymphoid cells. CML occurs preferentially in men to women at a 1.5:1 ratio, and like CLL typically occurs in the 6th decade of life or older. This disease varies from CLL in that it invariably progresses from a chronic stage to an accelerated and blastic stage, whereas CLL remains more indolent. The initial chronic phase may last between 1 and 5 years and is characterized by splenomegaly, constitutional symptoms of fatigue, abdominal fullness, and weight loss.[90] The accelerated phase is apparent with 15% of circulating cells being more immature blast cells, and then within 3 to 6 months this generally converts to the terminal blast phase in which the blastic cells fill the bone marrow and the circulating blood at greater than 30% of leukocytes and may cause destruction of other organs. Death due to infection or bleeding invariably results after the blast crisis begins.

The diagnosis of CML is made by the leukocytosis with myeloid differentiation and the presence of granulocytes filling the bone marrow space. Ninety percent of patients have the classic Philadelphia chromosome, which is a reciprocal translation between chromosomes 9 and 22. On the basis of randomized trials, there is no benefit in terms of delaying the accelerated and blast phases of the disease by doing a splenectomy during the chronic phase of the disease. Certain select patients who have significant hypersplenism or splenomegaly may benefit with symptomatic improvement during the chronic phase.[91,92]

A recent study from M. D. Anderson Cancer Center reports their experience of splenectomy during the accelerated or blast phase of disease.[93] Patients were referred for this procedure with symptoms of splenomegaly in 42% of cases and thrombocytopenia in 30% of cases, to potentially improve administration of chemotherapy by reducing the hypersplenism in 19% of cases and because of symptoms with both hypersplenism and thrombocytopenia in 9% of cases. The perioperative mortality in this series of 55 patients was 2% with one patient death.[93] There was universal benefit of symptoms related to splenomegaly, and there was a marked improvement of platelet count and requirement for platelet transfusions in patients with preoperative thrombocytopenia. The median 6-month transfusion requirements decreased from 21 to 1, combining both platelet and red cell transfusions. The median postsplenectomy survival was 19 months for patients in the accelerated phase and 6.5 months for patients in the blastic phase of their disease. This report concludes that for select patients who have severe transfusion requirements or severe symptoms of splenomegaly, or both, there is objective benefit with relatively low morbidity in patients with this later stage of CML.

Non-Hodgkin Lymphoma

Non-Hodgkin lymphoma is the most common cause of lymphoma, outnumbering Hodgkin disease by a ratio of almost 6:1 in the United States. Non-Hodgkin lymphoma is a much more heterogeneous disease, with a large range of histologic cell types defined by morphology and immunohistochemistry studies to differentiate subgroups of the disease. The clinical course of these different subgroups correlates with these microscopic findings. In general, diffuse or infiltrative non-Hodgkin lymphoma tends to have a worse prognosis than nodular NHL. The diffuse high-grade type occurs most commonly in the younger patient population (age less than 35 years) or in the very elderly. More aggressive non-Hodgkin lymphomas tend to be T-cell lymphomas with the low grade tending to be B cell. Non-Hodgkin lymphoma, as opposed to Hodgkin disease, occurs at presentation in approximately one third of cases in extranodal sites, with two thirds limited to lymphadenopathy.[94,95] In general, the disease is more diffuse at the time of presentation, mandating treatment by combination chemotherapy. It is for this reason that the staging laparotomy classically used in Hodgkin disease (see later) is not applicable in NHL.

Of patients dying of non-Hodgkin lymphoma, up to 80% will have significant splenic involvement with splenomegaly due to lymphatic infiltration.[96] As is true with other infiltrative neoplastic diseases, symptoms of pancytopenia and splenomegaly are common in patients with NHL. Patients who are operative candidates have significant benefit, with up to 80% having decreased transfusion requirements and the majority having relief of gastric oppression and pain symptoms due to splenomegaly.[97] In terms of the response of the pancytopenias, it is somewhat dependent on the bone marrow reserve, which may have been heavily pretreated with prior chemotherapy or radiation therapy. There is no differential test to identify adequate marrow reserve, and the only assessment in that situation is whether a patient has a response following splenectomy.

Hairy Cell Leukemia

Hairy cell leukemia is a low-grade lymphoproliferative disorder with characteristic "hairy cells" due to irregular filament projections from the cell surface that give an appearance of hair under light microscopy. This leukemia is a B-lymphocyte tumor that infiltrates the bone marrow and spleen with almost no peripheral lymphadenopathy. There may or may not be enlargement of the liver. The disease is much more common in males than females by a fourfold difference, and the onset of disease is typically in the 5th or 6th decade of life.

The initial symptoms most commonly relate to enlargement of the spleen either by direct effects of splenomegaly or by pancytopenia resulting from hypersplenism (Fig. 75.11).[98] Patients may have early satiety or upper quadrant pain with a large palpable spleen infiltrated with leukemic cells. The enlarged spleen often causes symptoms related to anemia with a transfusion requirement, bleeding caused by thrombocytopenia, and frequent infections because of leukopenia. In the past, splenectomy was recommended as the primary treatment because virtually all patients would have resolution of symptoms of splenomegaly, and 80% to 90% of patients had initial improvement in their cell counts. However, the vast majority of patients relapsed, some as early as 6 to 12 months later, and only 40% to 50% of patients received long-term benefit from the cytopenias due to bone marrow replacement with hairy cell infiltrates.

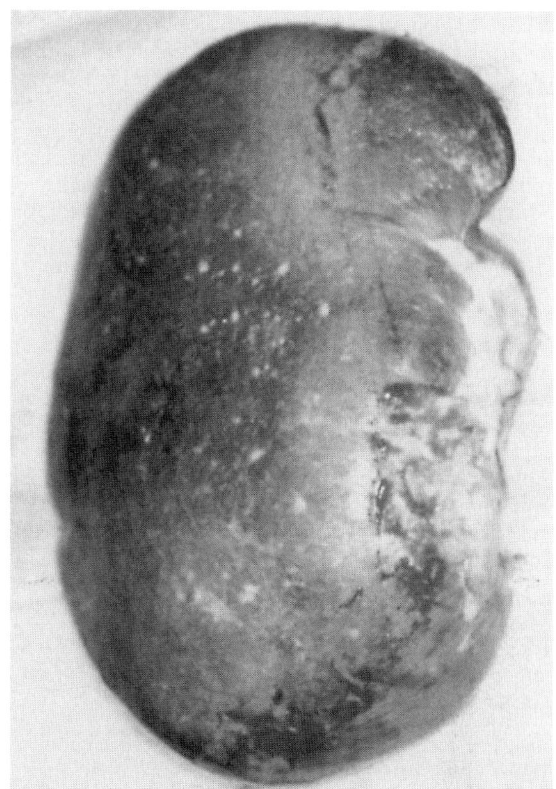

FIGURE 75.11 Spleen from a patient with hairy cell leukemia. Note the whitened anterior edge of the spleen and the white "sugar-coating" spots on the surface.

In the past 2 decades, medical therapy initially with recombinant α-interferon led to responses.[99] Newer trials with purine analogs such as pentostatin (2-doxycoformycin) and 2-chlorodoxydenosine provided a beneficial nonsurgical therapy.[100] A randomized trial comparing pentostatin with α-interferon showed a complete response rate of 78% with pentostatin versus 11% with α-interferon, and this has become a first-line therapy.[101] The majority of these patients will have sustained significant benefit and can avoid splenectomy. Of patients who are resistant to medical therapy, 5% to 10% may be offered splenectomy as a salvage therapy.

Myelodysplastic Syndrome

Agnogenic myeloid metaplasia (AMM) or myelodysplastic syndrome (MDS) with myeloid metaplasia is a poorly understood disorder characterized by a fibrotic replacement of the bone marrow compartment with extramedullary hematopoiesis and massive splenomegaly.[102] The pathophysiology of the disease is poorly understood but includes a nonclonal proliferation of fibroblasts making a dense fibrous stroma that fills the marrow space as well as contributes to hepatosplenomegaly and lymphadenopathy. This fibrous proliferation may be under control of secreted growth factors such as transformin growth factor beta.[103] Other myeloproliferative diseases include polycythemia vera and essential or idiopathic thrombocytosis.

The clinical symptoms and features of MDS relate to anemia and splenomegaly via direct mass effects or hypersplenism. Patients tend to be in the 5th decade of life or older. They present with constitutional symptoms including weight loss and fatigue as well as abdominal fullness and discomfort due to splenomegaly. There may be pain from splenic infarctions. Patients may present with bleeding due to thrombocytopenia. Hepatomegaly is present in 50% to 75% of patients, and splenomegaly is present in virtually all patients. The massively enlarged spleens in MDS are often some of the largest spleens by weight in most clinical series.

The combination of massive splenomegaly with increased blood flow via the enlarged spleen and hepatomegaly with fibrosis leading to relative portal hypertension creates a unique situation in which some of the clinical symptoms may be similar to those of portal hypertension from other cause as patients may present with varices and ascites. The diagnosis is made by evaluation of peripheral blood smear, which shows immature red cells with poikilocytes and tear-shaped cells. There can either be thrombocytopenia or thrombocytosis with platelet counts of greater than one million. Similarly, there may be leukopenia or there may be elevated white cell counts similar to those seen in CML. Bone marrow biopsy often produces a dry tap because of the fibrotic replacement of the marrows.

Treatment is generally targeted to palliate the symptoms that are present. Anemia and thrombocytopenia can be treated with transfusions. There is some role for alkylating agents and steroids, and in patients with thrombocytosis hydroxyurea is of benefit.[104] Splenectomy is indicated for relief of significant symptoms of hypersplenism or splenomegaly.[105] Hypersplenism is manifested by anemia and thrombocytopenia with increasing transfusion requirements of bleeding. Patients who have significant pain and early satiety with massively enlarged spleens may benefit from removal of mass effect. Finally, MDS is a unique situation in which splenectomy may treat portal hypertension because it will move a good bit of the increased blood flow through a fibrotic and enlarged liver, decreasing variceal bleeding and possibly ascites.[106]

It was initially debated whether the loss of the spleen as source of extramedullary hematopoiesis would be beneficial or harmful in this disease.[107] The success rate in terms of correction of cytopenias with MDS is less than with other causes of neoplastic secondary hypersplenism discussed earlier. A recent review of 223 patients with MDS from the Mayo Clinic showed indications for splenectomy in this disease were thought to be 45% due to transfusion-related anemia, 39% due to mass effects from splenomegaly, 11% due to portal hypertension, and 5% due to thrombocytopenia.[108] Correction of the anemia or a decrease in transfusion requirements occurred in only 23% of patients, and no patient had significant response of the thrombocytopenia in this disease. However, for the majority of patients the symptoms resulting from splenomegaly and 50% of patients with portal hypertension showed significant improvement. The operative mortality rate in this series was 9%.[108]

Two recent treatment strategies have been employed in MDS in the past 5 years. One is antiangiosyngenic therapy and the other is immunosuppressive treatment. It was recently identified that there was an increase in neovascularity of the bone marrow in patients with MDS and vascular endothelial cell growth factor (VEGF) appears to play a prominent role in pathophysiology. Specific antiangiogenic therapy to block VEGF, including the recently reported trial of thalidomide, led to independence from needing transfusions in a subgroup of patients with MDS. Interest in immunosuppressive therapy in MDS occurred because the subset of these patients with refractory anemia has autoimmune pathophysiology. Young patients or patients with HLA-DR 15 appear to have autoimmune etiology and have responded to immunosuppressive therapy.

Mastocytosis

Mastocytosis or systemic mast cell disease (SMCD) is a rare condition that is characterized by mast cell infiltration of a number of tissues, including the spleen.[109] Two categories of SMCD exist, one that is indolent and one that has an aggressive clinical course. In indolent SMCD, there is no need for consideration of splenectomy. Aggressive SMCD is a hematologic disease that has the characteristics of a malignant lymphoma. Splenomegaly may occur with subsequent hypersplenism, with the most predominant in this syndrome being thrombocytopenia. In this subgroup of patients with aggressive disease and symptomatic hypersplenism, splenectomy improves platelet counts and is associated with a longer median survival time than for patients with aggressive disease who do not undergo splenectomy.[110]

Chediak-Higashi Syndrome

Chediak-Higashi syndrome is a rare autosomal recessive disease characterized by immunodeficiency, which increases the susceptibility to bacterial and viral infections, recurrent fevers, nystagmus, and photophobia. The majority of patients experience widespread infiltration of tissues with histiocytes similar to that seen with lymphoma. Secondary hepatosplenomegaly with lymphadenopathy, leukopenia, and bleeding complications occur in the accelerated phase of Chediak-Higashi syndrome. Standard treatment includes chemotherapy, high-dose steroids, and ascorbic acid. These patients have a poor prognosis. Patients with hypersplenism who can tolerate a procedure have been shown to have beneficial results from a splenectomy.[111]

Metabolic or Infiltrative Diseases

Gaucher disease is an autosomal recessive disorder with a deficiency in the lysosomal hydrolase β-glucosidase, which is encoded by chromosome 1. Gaucher disease is the most common lysosomal storage disease. β-Glucosidase typically degrades sphingolipids such as glucocerebroside. There is a marked increase incidence of this disorder in Ashkenazi Jews. There are three types of this disease. Type I, the adult form, makes up 99% of cases and is the one in which splenectomy in the past was useful. The defect in the acid β-glucosidase causes an accumulation of undegraded glycolipids that are taken up by the reticuloendothelial cells and result in infiltration of the spleen, liver, and bone marrow. The most common symptoms of this disease relate to hypersplenism as well as direct effects on massive splenomegaly. Thrombocytopenia with bleeding problems and anemia causing fatigue are the most common effects of hypersplenism. Patients also may have such massive spleens that they have early satiety and weight loss due to gastric compression.

The diagnosis can be confirmed by the measurement of acid β-glucosidase activity in peripheral white blood cells or cultured fibroblasts. With the cloning of the gene, patients can be screened by molecular techniques to identify carriers. Prenatal diagnosis is also available by amniocentesis.

In the past, treatment has included supportive care with platelet transfusions as well as erythrocyte transfusions. Splenectomy was frequently performed for advanced cases, and in this disease a significant experience with partial splenectomy was developed in the early 1990s.[112,113,114] The goals of the subtotal splenectomy are partially to prevent the complications of overwhelming postsplenectomy sepsis and partially to protect the lipid and bone marrow by leaving a residual splenic fragment for continued deposition of lipid. In this disease, the techniques have worked out to safely perform partial splenectomy leaving a small residual upper pole fragment vascularized from the short gastric vessels.

Recently, it has been established that enzyme replacement with purified placental acid β-glucosidase is safe and has good efficacy. Patients are given between 30 and 60 units per kilogram of enzyme intravenously every other week, and the symptoms and signs are typically reversed. A recombinant β-glucosidase (alglucerase) is now available for therapy, and the role of splenectomy has been displaced by this medical management.

Sarcoidosis

Sarcoidosis is a granulomatous disease of unknown origin that can involve virtually any organ or area of the body.[115] Pulmonary disease is the most common, but autopsy studies have shown that the spleen is the second most common site of sarcoid deposits, with enlargement by noncaseating granulomas in 50% to 60% of patients. The majority of patients do not have splenomegaly, but when this does occur with significant deposits of granulomas, patients can suffer from hypersplenism. Also, patients with very bulky disease typically have the hypercalcemia of sarcoidosis.[116] In this subgroup of patients, splenectomy is indicated as a curative procedure.

INCIDENTAL SPLENECTOMY

In a large series evaluating reasons for splenectomy from the combined series from Barnes Hospital and Brigham and Women's Hospital, the single most common indication for removing the spleen is as an incidental procedure. This would be categorized as an operation primarily for an adjacent organ or tumor in which the spleen needs to be removed either for completeness of resection or because of removal or ligature of the splenic vasculature. In this large series, over 26% of the splenectomies performed over a 10-year period were incidental splenectomies (see Table 75.7).[28] The actual primary treatments of those various disease entities in adjacent organs are subjects of multiple other chapters within this textbook, but a few comments need to be made regarding the reasons for splenectomy and whether it is always appropriate.

The one common indication for an incidental splenectomy to remove tumors is during removal of the distal pancreas. For decades, the standard procedure when a distal pancreatectomy was performed was a splenectomy. The reason for splenectomy is that the splenic vein is intimately associated with the undersurface of the pancreas and has many direct branches to the pancreatic parenchyma. The splenic artery generally is superior to the pancreatic border and could be preserved, but because of removal of the splenic vein and for completeness of the resection, an *en bloc* resection of the distal pancreas and spleen is typically performed. Because of the interest in splenic preservation due to the incidence of postsplenectomy infection, two different approaches have been used to remove the distal pancreas without removing the spleen. The more technically challenging operation is a distal pancreatectomy with preservation of the splenic artery and vein. This can be performed only if there is a relatively small amount of invasive tumor or for benign neoplasia in which the splenic vein can be tediously dissected away from the pancreatic tissue, tying multiple side branches and then dividing the pancreatic parenchyma and leaving the splenic vessel intact. The second spleen-preserving distal pancreatectomy involves ligation of the splenic artery and vein but preservation of short gastric vessels and utilizing those vessels as collateral inflow and outflow to maintain splenic viability. Removal of the distal pancreas with splenic preservation has also recently been reported as a laparoscopic procedure as well.[117] For patients with tumors that mandate removal of the lymph nodes of the splenic hilum or with direct association of the tumor with splenic parenchyma, certainly it is more appropriate to do an operation based on neoplastic principles and perform a distal pancreatectomy/splenectomy. In other indications if the anatomy is appropriate and the completeness of tumor resection is not compromised, splenic preservation is certainly possible.

Another procedure in which it is common to perform a splenectomy is proximal gastric cancer resection. The importance of complete nodal dissection in terms of long-term results in gastric resections has been debated for several decades. A report from Japan noted that in 20% of proximal gastric cancers positive splenic hilum nodes were identified as level X lymph nodes.[118] These authors emphasize the need to perform associated splenectomy with grossly positive nodal disease in the splenic hilum. A long-term retrospective review from Memorial Sloan-Kettering Cancer Center noted that in 23% of gastrectomies in which complete resection of cancer was accomplished, adjacent organs had to be removed, most commonly the spleen.[119] There was long-term survival in this patient population, but it was emphasized that this aggressive surgery should be employed only when removal of all gross disease is achieved.[120]

Other tumors of the left upper quadrant and retroperitoneum may require splenectomy, including large renal cell carcinomas, left adrenal tumors, and retroperitoneal sarcomas that may infiltrate upward into the spleen. Often splenectomy is performed in these situations to provide adequate exposure to cleanly dissect bulky disease that lies posterior to the spleen. Although the asplenic state does make patients susceptible to infections (see Hyposplenism, earlier), the spleen should be viewed as an expendable organ if necessary to accomplish complete resection of malignancies, and there should be no hesitation to remove the spleen in those settings to achieve complete resection.

IATROGENIC SPLENECTOMY

A poorly reported and uncommonly discussed area of spleen surgery is removal or preservation of the iatrogenically traumatized spleen during unrelated abdominal operations. Procedures in which mobilization of the left upper quadrant such as reflection of the spleen and pancreas medially to expose retroperitoneal tissue, left adrenalectomy, and left nephrectomy put the spleen at risk.[121] Simple mobilization of the splenic flexure of the colon can lead to bleeding from the inferior pole of the spleen that may be difficult to control. The ligaments that go directly from the omentum to the capsule of the spleen may be the most common cause of iatrogenic splenic trauma, because it is a common practice to aggressively retract the omentum as needed for exposure. Direct branches, which sometimes may be sizable, from the omentum to the splenic capsule could lead to capsular disruption and troublesome bleeding. A national database on antireflux procedures of 86,411 patients reported an incidence of iatrogenic splenectomy of 2.3%, which translates into 1,987 iatrogenic splenectomies for that indication alone.[122]

Probably the best data for the incidence of iatrogenic splenectomy comes from the recently reported series from Vanderbilt, which listed 73 iatrogenic splenectomies over a 10-year period or an average of 7 per year.[29] This comprised 8.1% of all splenectomies performed during that time interval. There are probably several times that number of minor or moderate injuries to the spleen during unrelated surgeries in which the spleen was not removed but was repaired or salvaged. Just as in trauma to the spleen, the techniques of splenorrhaphy can be employed to preserve the spleen. A recent report indicates that use of a mesh wrap splenorrhaphy even in the setting of bowel surgery does not lead to an increased incidence of infection.[35] For minor capsular disruption, the use of the argon beam coagulator for surface cautery is a helpful technique.

The primary teaching point regarding iatrogenic injuries is that the best way to preserve the spleen is to not damage it in the first place. This requires caution when mobilizing tissue in and around the spleen as well as visual inspection of the attachments of the spleen prior to blunt mobilization. Whenever possible, an attempt should be made to preserve the spleen to decrease the risk of postsplenectomy sepsis.

DIAGNOSTIC SPLENECTOMY

One indication for splenectomy is for diagnosis in an otherwise asymptomatic patient. One situation in which splenectomy may be needed to make a diagnosis is when a dissecting mass lesion is seen within the spleen on CT scan, ultrasound, or magnetic resonance imaging (MRI) scan for which a definitive diagnosis cannot be made radiographically. Another example is for patients who have either palpable spleens on physical examination or enlarged spleens by scan but otherwise have no clear diagnostic disorder. Table 75.10 lists the final pathology diagnoses in spleens removed for these two indications over a 10-year period in two major academic medical centers.[28] In that series, a total of 121 diagnostic splenectomies were performed; 52 were for splenic mass and 41 were for splenomegaly with no other clear diagnosis. An additional 29 were done to further characterize a known hematologic malignancy.

For patients who had an isolated splenic mass, 60% turned out to be malignant lesions and 40% turned out to be benign lesions (Table 75.10).[28] The majority of the malignant lesions were lymphoma with another large group of metastatic carcinomas including some in which the primary diagnosis had not been made previously. Two patients had metastatic sarcoma to the spleen. In the benign diagnoses, more than half were cysts and there were also splenic hamartomas and splenic hemangiomas.

In terms of diagnosis of an isolated splenic mass, the majority of these lesions could have been diagnosed by doing a fine-needle aspiration biopsy. Certain of these lesions, such as the cystic lesions or the hemangiomas, would have classic appearance on gadolinium-enhanced MRI scan; this is another imaging modality that could be used to sort out mass lesions without the use of tissue biopsy. Although there may be some hesitation to do fine-needle aspiration biopsies on splenic lesions, because of the risk of bleeding, for most mass lesions this would have made the diagnosis and with the exception of splenic hemangiomas essentially all of these lesions could be aspirated without any significant consequence.

The second diagnostic indication for splenectomy is unexplained splenomegaly. In this series, over 10 years there were 41 cases, or 4 cases per year, at these two hospitals in which a massively enlarged spleen was removed purely for diagnosis.[28] The majority of these (58%) turned out to be lymphoma. The remaining 42% were split relatively evenly among benign lymphoid proliferation, benign vascular lesions, granulomatous disease, and splenic infarction and hemorrhage. The role of fine-needle aspiration and other percutaneous biopsies for splenomegaly is limited because there is considerable risk of bleeding in this indication and there would be very low yield in terms of being able to make that diagnosis with that form of biopsy.

Another type of diagnostic procedure is a staging laparotomy for Hodgkin disease. Discussion of this procedure is more of a historical note because it has limited use in today's current practice in treating this form of lymphoma. A standard practice for pathologic staging between 1960 and 1990 was performance of a staging laparotomy in most patients with Hodgkin disease. The reason to perform this invasive procedure was based on reports that laparotomy altered the clinical stage of disease in approximately 35% of patients. Approximately two thirds, or 20% to 25% of patients, were upstaged to a more advanced level by staging laparotomy and approximately one third, or 10% to 15%, were down-staged to a lower clinical level based on laparotomy results. If the treatment of Hodgkin disease depended on accurate staging (i.e., early stages were treated differently from more advanced stages), the staging laparotomy was essential in determining the proper therapeutic intervention for patients with Hodgkin disease.

Staging laparotomy was performed via an upper abdominal midline incision.[123] This included exploration of the entire abdomen for any abnormal lymph nodes, including nodes identified by lymphogram. Even if no abnormalities were found, multiple tissues were removed for pathologic

TABLE 75.10 DIAGNOSIS

FINAL PATHOLOGIC DIAGNOSES IN 122 SPLEENS REMOVED FOR DIAGNOSTIC PURPOSES

Indication	Diagnosis	No.
Splenic mass		52
	Lymphomas	17
	Metastatic cancer	14
	Carcinoma	12
	Sarcoma	2
	Benign	20
	Cysts	11
	Hamartoma	3
	Hemangioma	3
	Other	3
Splenomegaly		41
	Lymphoma	24
	Benign lymphoid proliferation	5
	Benign vascular	4
	Granulomatous disease	4
	Infarction/hemorrhage	4
Categorize lymphoma		29
	Malignant (successful)	28
	Benign	1

(Adapted from Kraus MD, Fleming MD, Vonderheide RH. The spleen as a diagnostic specimen: a review of 10 years' experience at two tertiary care institutions. *Cancer* 2001;91:2001–2009.)

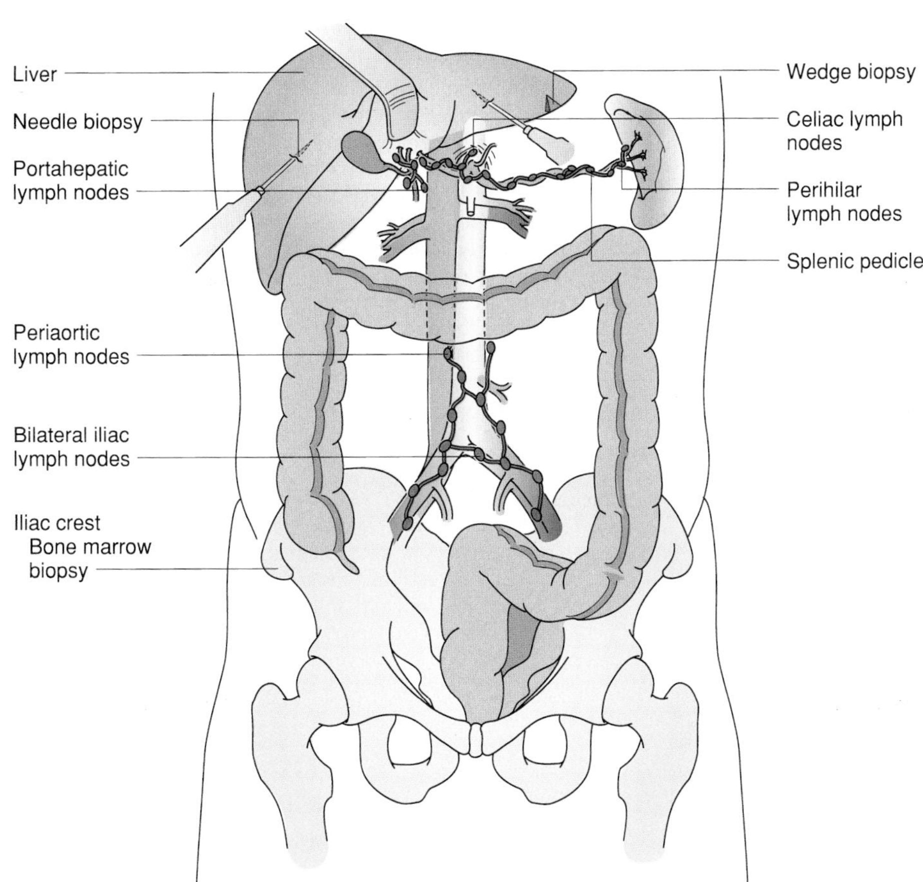

FIGURE 75.12 The tissues to be removed or to undergo biopsy in a staging laparotomy for Hodgkin disease. Splenectomy, liver biopsy, and lymph node sampling in the specific sites are shown. Bone marrow biopsy can be done if necessary.

assessment (Fig. 75.12). This included removal of the spleen, bilobar hepatic wedge resections, bilobar hepatic core biopsies, and multiple lymph nodes samplings. Lymph nodes were typically removed from the porta hepatis area, the celiac region, the splenic hilum, the periaortic region, and the bowel mesentery. If any iliac lymph nodes were palpated, they were removed as well. The spleen removed during a staging laparotomy for Hodgkin disease is bread-loafed in pathology at 3- to 4-mm thicknesses, and any suspicious nodule, particularly in the white pulp, will be examined microscopically for presence of Hodgkin disease.

There are several reasons the incidence of performing staging laparotomy has decreased over the past 10 to 15 years.[124] The primary reason is that it does not alter treatment of Hodgkin disease based on results of recent clinical series. The treatment of patients with stage IB, IIB, IIIB, IVB, IIIA, and IVA Hodgkin disease almost always involves systemic chemotherapy. Because systemic chemotherapy treats the whole patient, accurate pathologic staging makes no impact on the treatment outcome or treatment decisions. The only patients who may theoretically benefit from staging laparotomy at present are those with stage IA or IIA Hodgkin disease, who typically may receive treatment with radiation therapy. Even in this subgroup of patients there is a trend toward not performing staging laparotomy. First, many oncologists use combination chemotherapy even for early stage disease. Second, for patients who were treated with radiation therapy alone for stage IA and IIA disease, it has been demonstrated in several recent clinical series that ultimate outcome is equivalent whether these patients undergo staging laparotomy or whether they are treated up-front with radiation therapy.[125,126,127] The reason is that if these patients recur outside of the radiation field during long-term follow-up, they can be salvage obtained with systemic chemotherapy. Third, performance of staging laparotomy is obviously a major abdominal operation with potential for morbidity and also the reality that treatment for the Hodgkin disease will be delayed typically between 4 and 6 weeks. Finally, there are data showing that patients who survive Hodgkin disease and receive combination chemotherapy are at increased risk for the development of a secondary malignancy that is primarily acute, nonlymphocytic leukemia (ANLL).[128,129,130] In some series, the risk of developing ANLL is increased up to tenfold in patients who have undergone splenectomy as part of their staging workup for Hodgkin disease compared with patients undergoing similar chemotherapy regimens who did not undergo splenectomy. For all of these reasons, this procedure, which also accounted for a large number of the splenectomies performed in major tertiary referral centers and cancer centers, is rarely performed today.

VASCULAR DISORDERS OF THE SPLEEN

Vascular problems with the spleen that can lead to splenectomy include both venous and arterial problems. The most common situation would be splenic vein thrombosis, and splenectomy in this setting is very gratifying and curative for the patient. Splenic artery aneurysms are one of the more common visceral aneurysms and also can be an indication for splenectomy.

Splenic Vein Thrombosis

Splenic vein thrombosis is an unusual cause of upper gastrointestinal hemorrhage that can be cured by splenectomy. The pathophysiology of this disease is an isolated thrombosis of the splenic vein as it travels along the posterior pancreatic body and tail. The splenic venous outflow is then diverted to the short gastric vessels as collateral venous outflow channels. This increased flow via the short gastric veins leads to high pressure with a dilatation of the submucosal venous plexus primarily in the gastric cardia and fundus with eventual development of gastric varices.[131]

The cause of splenic vein thrombosis does not involve any pathology of the spleen, but rather typically pathology of the pancreas and possibly the stomach. Pancreatitis or pancreatic pseudocyst is the cause of splenic vein thrombosis in more than 50% of patients in most series. Pancreatic carcinoma with direct invasion and infiltration of the splenic vein is the second most common cause. Other unusual causes may be a penetrating gastric ulcer posteriorly or retroperitoneal fibrosis.

The diagnosis is made in patients who have upper gastrointestinal bleeding with only gastric varices on endoscopy. Because there is no portal vein hypertension and no cirrhosis of the liver, there are no esophageal varices. The spleen may or may not be enlarged, but again there are no other signs and symptoms of cirrhosis. Definitive diagnosis in the past has been made by a celiac angiogram, which demonstrates absence of the splenic vein with collateral flow via the gastric veins. MR angiograms/venograms as well as high-resolution ultrasound may also make the diagnosis.

Splenectomy is curative because it removes the blood flow via the splenic artery through this organ. This removes all the excess collateral flow that leads to the venous hypertension, and the associated symptoms resolve. Whenever splenic vein thrombosis is diagnosed, even if the patient has not had an episode of bleeding, elective splenectomy should be performed as a prophylactic measure.

Patients with portal hypertension and cirrhosis or partial vein thrombosis have a complex collection of symptoms that include hypersplenism with splenomegaly and thrombocytopenia and anemia. However, the operative risk associated with portal vein hypertension is excessive, and splenectomy is virtually never indicated in this setting.

Splenic Artery Aneurysm

Splenic artery aneurysm is uncommon even though it is the second most frequent abdominal artery to undergo aneurysmal changes.[132] Splenic aneurysms occur twice as often in women as in men. Patients can be divided into two distinct groups. First, there are elderly patients whose aneurysms are manifestations of atherosclerosis. Second, young women have apparent congenital predisposition to form splenic artery aneurysms. In these young women, there is an increased risk of rupture of these aneurysms during pregnancy. Inflammatory processes such as pancreatitis may involve the splenic artery and occasionally lead to aneurysm, but more frequently it leads to acute bleeding.

Splenic artery aneurysms are typically asymptomatic and may be initially identified as a widened rim of calcification in the left upper quadrant defining the aneurysm boundaries. They may also be discovered as incidental findings on CT scan. If symptomatic, patients experience left upper quadrant pain, nausea, and vomiting. The presence of symptoms suggesting pending aneurysmal rupture, and urgent splenectomy with ligation of the splenic arteries is indicated.

When a calcified atherosclerotic splenic artery aneurysm is discovered in a patient over age 60 years with no splenomegaly and no symptoms, surgical excision is not indicated and the aneurysm may be followed to look for signs of enlargement. In younger patients who have a symptomatic aneurysm identified, particularly young women of childbearing age, an elective splenectomy is recommended to prevent rupture. Nonsurgical approaches are to embolize the splenic artery in patients who are poor risks for open laparotomy.[132]

MISCELLANEOUS INDICATIONS FOR SPLENECTOMY

Splenectomy may be performed in relatively infrequent events for a miscellaneous collection of indications, including splenic cysts, infectious cysts, and splenic abscesses. Also included in discussion in this section is the frequently described wandering spleen, which is a normal spleen that lacks the normal ligamental attachments to keep it in the left upper quadrant. This can present in a variety of ways, from an undiagnosed mass to a torsion of the splenic hilum that causes acute pain.

Cysts

The splenectomy is performed as described often for hematologic malignancies, including multiple forms of leukemia and lymphoma, primarily for symptoms of hypersplenism or splenomegaly, or as a staging procedure. Splenectomy for primary neoplasms of the spleen is an infrequent indication. These primary neoplastic processes are listed in Table 75.11.

Hemangioma is the most common benign primary neoplasm of the spleen. It is often an incidental finding and may be solitary or multiple. During operation, it can be identified as a more intensely bluish-purple–colored lesion when seen from the surface compared with the reddish-purple color of the splenic parenchyma. Hemangiomas can be identified with excellent sensitivity and specificity by MRI characteristics. It is ill advised to perform a biopsy of a lesion that may be a splenic hemangioma.[133,134] Hemangiomas of the spleen rarely cause symptoms, but massive hemangiomas either rupture spontaneously or make the spleen more susceptible to a traumatic rupture. In cases of massive hemangioma with capsular distention with pain, either a splenectomy or partial splenectomy may be indicated.

Hemangioendothelioma is a neoplasm that is thought to be slightly more aggressive than the typical benign hemangioma. It is considered to be pathologically an intermediate benign hemangioma rather than a malignant angiosarcoma. It is not thought to have metastatic potential, and generally is an

TABLE 75.11

PRIMARY NEOPLASMS AND CYSTS OF SPLEEN

Hemangioma
Hemangioendothelioma
Lymphangioma
Pseudotumor
Mycobacterial pseudotumor
Hamartomas
Primary cyst
Echinococcal cyst

incidental finding. Larger lesions may cause symptoms or be noted for their size and rupture either spontaneously or with minor trauma is the typical circumstance in which patients with these lesions have splenectomy.

Lymphangiomas also occur in the spleen and are much less common than hemangiomas. They may be multiple or solitary and can be identified by a lighter color and compressibility when seen in surgery.

Two mass lesions that occur in the spleen that are not true neoplasms are hamartomas and inflammatory pseudotumors. Hamartomas are focal development of abnormalities that occur in the spleen and other solid organs such as the liver. Hamartomas contain normal cellular elements and are non-neoplastic but have a random fibrotic organization. The major significance of hamartomas is that they are identified either at laparotomy as incidental findings or they are seen as incidental lesions on CT scans done for other reasons.[135] Inflammatory pseudotumors are described throughout most organs and have been described in the spleen. These sometimes are quite large with a wide variety of reactive cells. A subcategory of inflammatory pseudotumors of the spleen is related to mycobacterial infection, particularly in HIV-positive patients. There have been reports of primary splenic pregnancy, which is considered the rarest site of ectopic pregnancies.

Cysts of the spleen are almost uniformly not related to parasitic infection. They are also relatively common lesions seen across all age groups and may be multifocal. The diagnosis of splenic cysts can be ascertained by ultrasound or CT scan. These benign lesions have no clinical significance unless they reach a large size. As discussed earlier in the history of splenic surgery, the first reported case of a successful elective splenectomy was done for a splenic cyst. This was an enormous cyst at the tip of the spleen and was felt to be likely an ovarian mass and found to be arising from the spleen at laparotomy (Fig. 75.13). Today there would be a tendency to do a cyst enucleation or partial splenectomy for peripheral cystic lesions that are large and symptomatic. An alternative approach is unroofing the cyst and leaving a portion of the cyst wall in place, which can be done laparoscopically.[136]

The only parasitic cyst involving the spleen is from *Echinococcus granulosus* or a hydatid cyst. The incidence of echinococcal cyst in the spleen compared to the liver is a ratio of approximately 30:1. However, the spleen is the third most common site of echinococcal cysts behind the liver and lung.[137] Diagnosis should be suspected in patients in areas where echinococcal disease is common, such as New Zealand, Australia, and parts of the western United States. The complement fixation test is the most reliable serologic study for this organism. The treatment for echinococcal cysts is splenectomy. As with echinococcal cysts of the liver, it is of utmost importance not to rupture the cyst and expose the patient to the scoleces. For large and peripheral cysts in which risk of rupture is high, the contents of the cyst should be carefully aspirated and replaced with hypertonic saline.[138] In a recent report from Greece, surgeons preserved 8 of 19 spleens with echinococcal cysts by doing partial splenectomy.[137]

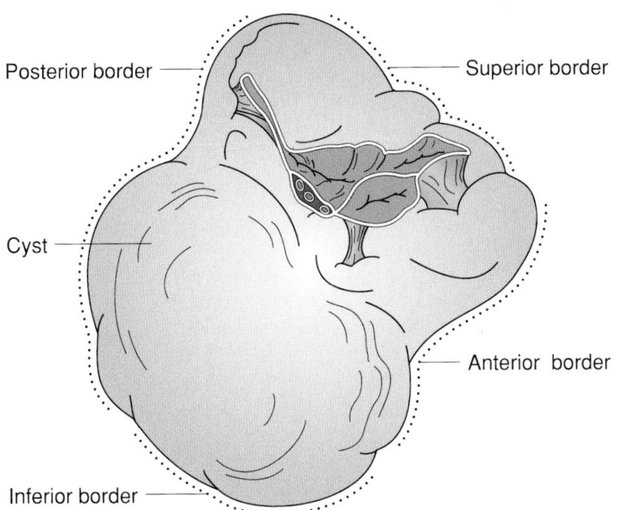

FIGURE 75.13 The visceral surface of a spleen with a true congenital splenic cyst.

Abscess

Splenic abscesses are uncommon, but this is an important disease because it is associated with a significant mortality rate and may be cured by splenectomy.[139] In most series, the mortality rate ranges between 40% and 100%.[140] The typical patient has hematogenous seeding of the spleen by bacteria from a remote source such as endocarditis or from intravenous drug abuse.[141] There may be, in some cases, direct spread of infection from adjacent intraabdominal sources. Finally, splenic trauma treated conservatively may eventually result in an infected splenic hematoma. In 80% of the cases, there is an additional source of infection other than the spleen, and in only 20% of cases is the splenic abscess the sole source of sepsis identified. Enteric organisms account for two thirds of the splenic abscesses and staphylococcus and streptococcus comprise the remainder of the cases.

The patients present with signs and symptoms of sepsis, including fever, malaise, and leukocytosis. When the spleen is the sole site of infection, patients will have significant left upper quadrant tenderness and guarding. Abdominal radiographs may show gas in the spleen, and an ultrasound and CT scan with contrast will be diagnostic to show an abscess with reactive rim.

The treatment of choice for patients who can undergo a laparotomy and have the splenic abscess as an isolated or prominent component of septic syndrome is splenectomy. If the spleen is the only source of infection, removal of the spleen should be curative and result in the recovery of the patient. If patients have multiple sites of infection or are too sick to undergo laparotomy, percutaneous drainage of splenic abscesses may be attempted, but this is not as successful because of frequent spillage and assimilation of bacteria in the left upper quadrant of the abdomen.

Ectopic Spleen (Wandering Spleen)

Ectopic spleens, or the so-called wandering spleens, occur because of either extreme laxity or absence of the normal ligaments that attach the spleen to the left upper quadrant. This allows the spleen to essentially drop to the lower abdomen in either the right or the left lower quadrant by the force of gravity attached by its vascular pedicle. Wandering spleen occurs 13 times more frequently in women than in men. Wandering spleen presents most commonly in adults but can cause symptoms in children.[142] The diagnosis may be made by palpable lower abdominal mass confirmed by CT scan or shown on a nuclear imaging scan to be splenic tissue. The ectopic spleen creates symptoms typically when there is torsion of the pedicle causing acute ischemia and acute pain. The treatment for a wandering spleen as an incidental finding at laparotomy or if the torsion can be corrected and the spleen appears to be viable is to do a splenopexy tacking the spleen to its native position in the left upper quadrant. If the spleen appears infarcted, then a splenectomy must be performed.[143] The wandering spleen is ideally suited for laparoscopic splenectomy because it is generally free from ligaments or attachments and other organs.[144]

SPLENECTOMY

The choices of operations available currently to approach the spleen in an elective manner are open splenectomy, laparoscopic splenectomy, or partial splenectomy. Table 75.12 lists indications for splenectomy and whether a partial splenectomy is indicated. Certain principles apply to all patients undergoing elective splenectomy. First, all patients should receive appropriate preoperative vaccination with Pneumovax and possibly also vaccination against *Haemophilus influenzae* and *Neisseria meningococcus* 10 to 14 days prior to the procedure if possible. Patients must have appropriate blood products ready because patients often are anemic and thrombocytopenic due to hypersplenism as described previously.

The operative technique for open splenectomy involves either a midline abdominal incision or a left subcostal incision. For patients with massive splenomegaly defined as greater than 1,500 g in adults and greater than 1,000 g in children, a long midline incision should be used.[145] The components of the splenectomy include division of the avascular lateral and posterior attachments to mobilize the spleen, ligation of the short gastric vessels separating the upper half of the spleen from the greater curvature of the stomach, and ligation of splenic hilar vessels in a controlled manner to avoid injury to the pancreatic tail. Although one approach particularly for small spleens that are mobile is to initially divide the lateral attachments and place packs in the left upper quadrant to elevate the spleen and then proceed with the vascular dissection (Fig. 75.14), this should be discouraged particularly in patients who are thrombocytopenic or patients with massive splenomegaly. In this situation, the splenectomy should start by obtaining vascular control before manipulating the spleen and leading to capsular rupture and significant blood loss.

The preferred operative approach in patients with splenomegaly[146] and hypersplenism is to first divide the attachments of the left lateral segment of the liver and retract this segment to the right side of the abdomen, exposing the greater curvature of the stomach. Then, starting at the midportion of the greater curvature of the stomach, the branches of the left gastroepiploic artery and vein including the short gastric vessels are ligated sequentially, completely dissociating the stomach from the superior portion of the spleen (Fig. 75.15). Through this window into the lesser sac created by dissecting the short gastric vessels, the splenic artery can be identified at variable locations along the superior border of the pancreas. A loop of this tortuous artery at its most superior or cranial portion is safest because at those points it is farthest away from the splenic vein as well as away from the pancreatic parenchyma. The artery may simply be ligated once or twice with heavy silk ties at that location and does not need to be divided. By dividing the short gastric arteries as well as ligating the main splenic artery, the vast majority if not all of the blood flow into the spleen is controlled prior to even touching the spleen to mobilize it. If capsular disruption occurs, the amount of blood loss is greatly minimized. Following vascular control, the lateral and posterior attachments are divided and the spleen is elevated to near the level of the abdominal wall musculature ventrally. The splenic hilum can then be dissected, tying vessels in a controlled manner.

TABLE 75.12 INDICATIONS/CONTRAINDICATIONS

OPERATIVE INDICATIONS FOR SPLENECTOMY AND WHETHER TOTAL OR PARTIAL SPLENECTOMY IS INDICATED

Disease	Need for splenectomy	Partial splenectomy
Hereditary spherocytosis	Always	Yes
Hereditary elliptocytosis	Sometimes	Yes
Thalassemia	Sometimes	Yes
Sickle cell anemia	Rarely	No
Wiskott-Aldrich syndrome	Sometimes	No
Autoimmune hemolytic anemia	Usually	No
Autoimmune neutropenia	Sometimes	No
Immune thrombocytopenia purpura	Usually	No
Thrombotic thrombocytopenia purpura	Sometimes	No
Hairy cell leukemia	Rarely[a]	No
Chronic lymphocytic leukemia	Sometimes	No
Chronic myelogenous leukemia	Sometimes	No
Non-Hodgkin lymphoma	Sometimes	No
Angiogenic myeloid metaplasia	Sometimes	Yes
Mastocytosis	Rarely	No
Gaucher disease	Rarely[a]	Yes
Hodgkin disease	Rarely[b]	No
Splenic vein thrombosis	Always	No
Splenic abscess	Usually	No
Splenic cyst	Rarely	Yes
Echinococcal cyst	Always	No

[a]Splenectomy rarely indicated in current practice because of effective medical therapy
[b]Splenectomy rarely indicated because of change in current therapy

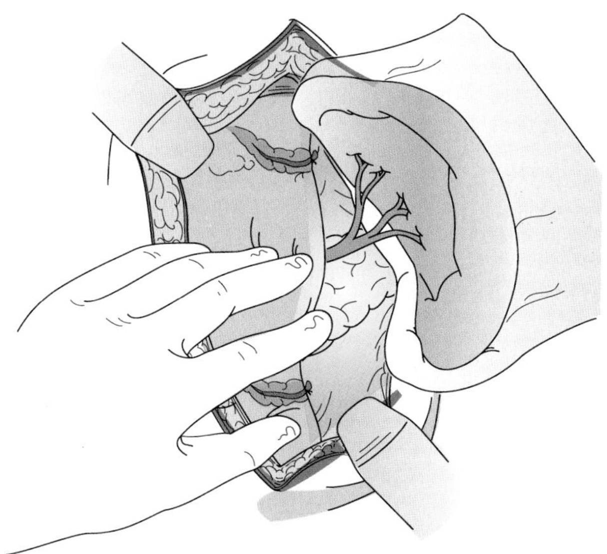

FIGURE 75.14 Lateral mobilization permits the spleen to reach the surface of a midline wound despite the presence of intact hilar vessels.

For patients with ITP, platelets should not be given until the spleen is either removed or at least until the arterial inflow is controlled because of clearance of transfused platelets by the spleen in this disease. Similarly, for this disease as well as other diseases in which the spleen is the site of platelet or blood cell destruction, it is important to identify and remove accessory spleens. The majority of the accessory spleens occur in the splenic hilum, and they can also occur in the omentum, along the superior border of the pancreas, in the bowel mesentery, and in the pelvis in some situations. The incidence of accessory spleens and open splenectomy ranges between 15% and 30%.

Partial splenectomy can be performed based on the segmental blood supply to the spleen. The spleen is mobilized with good visualization. The inferior segmental arteries are generally ligated, and the artery and veins are ligated as a predemarcation of blood flow to the spleen. The splenic parenchyma is then transected and the cut to the surface can be controlled using materials that induce coagulation or the argon beam coagulator.[147,148]

Over the past 5 to 10 years, the standard practice for an elective splenectomy in most large centers has become a laparoscopic approach. Even patients with massive splenomegaly are now being approached with a laparoscopic splenectomy with use of a hand port. In one recent series, there were no conversions in 16 consecutive patients with massive splenomegaly.[149] Another series noted a higher incidence of conversion to an open procedure when the spleen weighed more than 2,000 g.[150]

The technique of laparoscopic splenectomy can either treat patients supine with a roll under their hips to prop that portion of the abdomen up approximately 30 degrees, or it can be done with the patient in the lateral decubitus position. The omental, inferior attachments and the short gastric vessels are divided with a harmonic scalpel device. It has been reported that careful exposure of the splenic hilum with the direct ligation of the vessels is a much safer technique than the laparoscopic equivalent of a trauma splenectomy in which the hilum is stapled without precise vessel dissection.[151] Once the vessels are ligated, the spleen is placed into a large plastic bag and brought to the port and this allows careful morselization of the spleen without having to enlarge the incision and without fracture and spillage elsewhere in the abdomen.

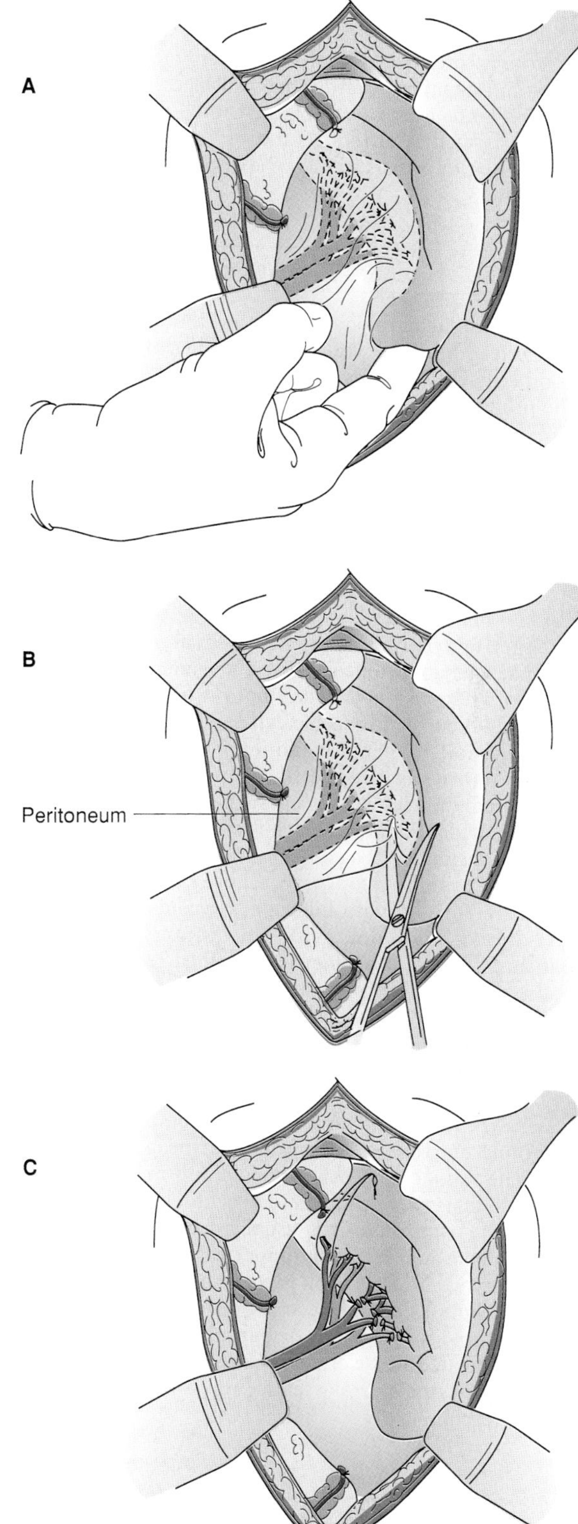

FIGURE 75.15 Technique for elective splenectomy. (*A*) The inferior pole is reflected laterally by the assistant's fingers, exposing the lower edge of the hilar peritoneal envelope. (*B*) The hilar peritoneum is opened, here shown progressing from inferior to superior. (*C*) Individual vessels are identified and suture ligated.

Virtually all indications for splenectomy can be approached laparoscopically.[152] Laparoscopic splenectomy has been reported for removal of a wandering spleen.[144] In this indication it is actually a much easier operation because the spleen is free and the hilum is very easily exposed. There has been a report that accessory spleens are identified to a lesser degree and consequently missed to a greater degree with a laparoscopic approach. The use of lymphoscintigrams after failed splenectomy can identify accessory spleens. Accessory spleens can be removed laparoscopically as well, and reports indicate that adding a hand port for palpation assists in this type of procedure.[153]

KEY POINTS

- The primary hematologic function of the spleen is removal of senescent erythrocytes or remodeling of abnormal red blood cells with various deformities.
- The primary immunologic function of the spleen is to generate an immune response to antigens that are identified and cleared from the blood stream.
- The most important immunologic change associated with hyposplenism or after splenectomy is overwhelming postsplenectomy sepsis resulting from increased susceptibility to infection with encapsulated organisms including *Streptococcus pneumoniae, Haemophilus influenzae,* and *Neisseria meningitis.*
- The specific criteria for hypersplenism are: (a) documented anemia, thrombocytopenia, or leukopenia; (b) normal compensatory response by the bone marrow to correct the cytopenia; and (c) correction of the cytopenia by splenectomy.
- The decision to perform nonoperative management of splenic injuries is affected by the presence of peritonitis, associated injuries requiring surgery, the overall injury severity, evidence of hypovolemic shock and ongoing bleeding, and the patient's age.
- Immune thrombocytopenia purpura is generally initially treated medically with high-dose steroids or intravenous IgG immunoglobulin, with splenectomy indicated for patients who do not achieve a sustained remission with an approximately 70% predictable chance of success.
- Patients with hereditary spherocytosis present with mild to moderate anemia, splenomegaly, and jaundice, with 30% to 60% of patients having pigment gallstones.
- Hypersplenism is the physical enlargement of the spleen because of neoplastic disorders, hematopoietic disorders of the bone marrow, or metabolic or storage disorders and can cause associated pancytopenia and mass effect symptoms, such as early satiety and weight loss.
- Splenic vein thrombosis is usually caused by pathology of the pancreas and results in upper gastrointestinal bleeding from gastric varices, which is cured by splenectomy.
- Surgical options for splenectomy include open splenectomy, laparoscopic splenectomy, or partial splenectomy, with the latter indicated for selected cases of hereditary spherocytosis, elliptocytosis, thalassemia, myeloid metaplasia, and splenic cysts.

References

1. McClusky DA III, Skandalakis LJ, Colborn GL, et al. Tribute to a triad: history of splenic anatomy, physiology, and surgery—part 1. *World J Surg.* 23:311–325, 1999.
2. Morgenstern L. A history of splenectomy. In: *Surgical diseases of the spleen.* Hiatt JR, Phillips EH, Morgenstern L, eds. Berlin: Springer-Verlag, 1997.
3. McClusky DA, Skandalakis LJ, Colborn GL, et al. Tribute to a triad: history of splenic anatomy, physiology, and surgery—part 2. *World J Surg.* 1999.
4. Patterson KD, Drysdale TA, Krieg PA. Embryonic origins of spleen asymmetry. *Development* 2000;127:167–175.
5. Chadburn A. The spleen: anatomy and anatomical function. *Semin Hematol.* 37:13–21, 2000.
6. Sprogoe-Jakobsen S, Sprogoe-Jakobsen U. The weight of the normal spleen. *Forensic Sci Int.* 1997;88:215–223.
7. Ravaglia G, Forti P, Biagi F, et al. Splenic function in old age. *Gerontology* 1998;44:91–94.
8. Hoefs JC, Wang FW, Lilien DL, et al. A novel, simple method of functional spleen volume calculation by liver-spleen scan. *J Nucl Med.* 1999;40;1745–1755.
9. Skandalakis PN, Colborn GL, Skandalakis LJ, et al. The surgical anatomy of the spleen. *Surg Clin N Am* 1993;73:747–768.
10. Desai DC, Hebra A, Davidoff AM, et al. Wandering spleen: a challenging diagnosis. *South Med J.* 1997;90:439–443.
11. Liu DL, Xia S, Xu W, et al. Anatomy of vasculature of 850 spleen specimens and its application in partial splenectomy. *Surgery* 1996;120:574.
12. Kraus MD. Pathology of the spleen. Introduction. *Semin Diagn Pathol.* 2003;20:83.
13. Espersen K, Frandsen H, Lorentzen T, et al. The human spleen as an erythrocyte reservoir in diving-related interventions. *J Appl Physiol.* 2002;92: 2071–2079.
14. Peters AM. Splenic blood flow and blood cell kinetics. *Clin Haematol.* 1983;12:421.
15. Phom H, Kumar A, Tripathi M, et al. Comparative evaluation of Tc-99m–heat-denatured RBC and Tc-99m—anti-D IgG opsonized RBC spleen planar and SPECT scintigraphy in the detection of accessory spleen in postsplenectomy patients with chronic idiopathic thrombocytopenic purpura. *Clin Nucl Med.* 2004;29:403–409.
16. Gielchinsky Y, Elstein D, Hadas-Halpern I, et al. Is there a correlation between degree of splenomegaly, symptoms and hypersplenism? A study of 218 patients with Gaucher's disease. *Br J Haematol* 1999;106:812–816.
17. Were JM, Willekens FL, Bosch FH, et al. The red cell revisited—matters of life and death. *Cell Mol Biol.* 2004;50:139–145.
18. Zoli G, Corazza GR, D'Amato G, et al. Splenic autotransplantation after splenectomy: tuftsin activity correlates with residual splenic function. *Br J Surg.* 1994;81:716–718.
19. Feder HM Jr, Pearson HA. Assessment of splenic function in familial asplenia. *N Engl J Med.* 1999;341:210–212.
20. Horowitz J, Leonard D, Smith J, et al. Postsplenectomy leukocytosis: physiologic or an indicator of infection? *Am Surg.* 1992;58:387.
21. Resende V, Petroianu A. Functions of the splenic remnant after subtotal splenectomy for treatment of severe splenic injuries. *Am J Surg.* 2003;185:311–315.
22. **Lutwick LI. Life threatening infections in the asplenic or hyposplenic individual. *Surg Clin Top Infect Dis* 2002;22:78–96.**
23. Hansen K, Singer DB. Asplenic-hyposplenic overwhelming sepsis: postsplenectomy sepsis revisited. *Pediatr Dev Pathol.* 2001;4:105–121.
24. Lane PA. The spleen in children. *Curr Opin Pediatr.* 1995;7:36–41.
25. Shatz DV, Romero-Steiner S, Elie CM, et al. Antibody responses in postsplenectomy trauma patients receiving the 23-valent pneumococcal polysaccharide vaccine at 14 versus 28 days postoperatively. *J Trauma Injury Infect Crit Care* 2002;53:1037–1042.
26. Shatz DV. Vaccination practices among North American trauma surgeons in splenectomy for trauma. *J Trauma Injury Infect Crit Care* 2002;53:950–956.
27. **Gielchinsky Y, Elstein D, Hadas-Halpern I, et al. Is there a correlation between degree of splenomegaly, symptoms and hypersplenism? A study of 218 patients with Gaucher's disease. *Br J Haematol.* 1999;106: 812–816.**
28. **Kraus MD, Fleming MD, Vonderheide RH. The spleen as a diagnostic specimen: a review of 10 years' experience at two tertiary care institutions. *Cancer* 2001;91:2001–2009.**
29. **Rose AT, Newman MI, Debelak J, et al. The incidence of splenectomy is decreasing: lessons learned from trauma experience. *Am Surg.* 2000;66: 481–486.**
30. Peitzman AB, Ford HR, Harbrecht BG, et al. Injury to the spleen. *Curr Probl Surg.* 2001;38:932–1008.
31. Upadhyaya P. Conservative management of splenic trauma: history and current trends. *Pediatr Surg Int.* 2003;19:617–627.
32. Morrell DG, Chang FC, Helmer SD. Changing trends in the management of splenic injury. *Am J Surg.* 1995;170:686–689.
33. Williams MK, Young DH, Schiller WR. Trend toward nonoperative management of splenic injuries. *Am J Surg.* 1990;160:588.
34. **Gavant ML, Schurr M, Flick PA, et al. Predicting clinical outcome of nonsurgical management of blunt splenic injury: using CT to reveal abnormalities of splenic vasculature. *Am J Roentgenol.* 1997; 168:207–212.**
35. Berry MF, Rosato EF, Williams NN. Dexon mesh splenorrhaphy for intraoperative splenic injuries. *Am Surg.* 2003;69:176–180.
36. Smith JS Jr, Cooney RN, Mucha P Jr. Nonoperative management of the ruptured spleen: a revalidation of criteria. *Surgery* 1996;120:745–750.
37. Uecker J, Pickett C, Dunn E. The role of follow-up radiographic studies in nonoperative management of spleen trauma. *Am Surg.* 2001;67:22–25.
38. Konstantakos AK, Barnoski AL, Plaisier BR, et al. Optimizing the management of blunt splenic injury in adults and children. *Surgery* 1999;126: 805–812.
39. Emery KH, Babcock DS, Borgman AS, et al. Splenic injury diagnosed with CT: US follow-up and healing rate in children and adolescents. *Radiology* 1999;212:515–518.

40. Gaunt WT, McCarthy MC, Lambert CS, et al. Traditional criteria for observation of splenic trauma should be challenged. *Am Surg.* 1999;65:689– 691.
41. Wisner DH, Blaisdell FW. When to save the ruptured spleen. *Surgery* 1992;111:121–122.
42. Khan ZA, Dikki PE. Return of a normal functioning spleen after traumatic splenectomy. *J R Soc Med.* 2004;97:391–392.
43. Chen HH, Yan NS, Hou KY, et al. Subtotal splenectomy with a microwave coagulator. *Br J Surg.* 1993;80:612–613.
44. Peitzman AB, Heil B, Rivera L. et al. Blunt splenic injury in adults: multi-institutional study of the Eastern Association for the Surgery of Trauma. *J Trauma Injury Infect Crit Care* 2000;49:177–187.
45. George JN, el-Harake MA, Raskob GE. Chronic idiopathic thrombocytopenic purpura. *N Engl J Med.* 1994;331:1207–1211.
46. Morris KT, Horvath KD, Jobe BA, Swanstrom LL. Laparoscopic management of accessory spleens in immune thrombocytopenic purpura. *Surg Endosc.* 1999;13:520–522.
47. Ballem PJ, Belzberg A, Devine DV, et al. Kinetic studies of the mechanism of thrombocytopenia in patients with human immunodeficiency virus infection. *N Engl J Med.* 1992;327:1779–1784,.
48. Beer JH, Rabaglio M, Berchtold P, et al. Autoantibodies against the platelet glycoproteins (GP) IIb/IIIa, Ia/IIa, and IV and partial deficiency in GPIV in a patient with a bleeding disorder and a defective platelet collagen interaction. *Blood* 1993;82:820–829.
49. Hoo M, Lv B, He Q, et al. Both splenic CD5(+) B and CD5(−) B cells produce platelet glycoprotein-specific autoantibodies in chronic ITP. Thromb Res. 2003;110:1–5.
50. Dan K, Gomi S, Kuramoto A, et al. A multicenter prospective study on the treatment of chronic idiopathic thrombocytopenic purpura. *Int J Hematol.* 1992;55:287–292.
51. Andersen JC. Response of resistant idiopathic thrombocytopenic purpura to pulsed high-dose dexamethasone therapy. *N Engl J Med.* 1994;330:1560–1564.
52. Sandler SG. The spleen and splenectomy in immune (idiopathic) thrombocytopenic purpura. *Semin Hematol.* 2000;37:10–12.
53. **Kojouri K, Vesely SK, Terrell DR, et al. Splenectomy for adult patients with idiopathic thrombocytopenic purpura: a systematic review to assess long-term platelet count responses, prediction of response, and surgical complications. *Blood* 2003;104:2623–2634.**
54. Tsereteli Z, Smith CD, Branum GD, et al. Are the favorable outcomes of splenectomy predictable in patients with idiopathic thrombocytopenic purpura (ITP)? *Surg Endosc.* 2001;15:1386–1389.
55. Najean Y, Rain JD, Billotey C. The site of destruction of autologous ^{111}In-labeled platelets and the efficiency of splenectomy in children and adults with idiopathic thrombocytopenic purpura: a study of 578 patients with 268 splenectomies. *Br J Haematol.* 1997;97:547–550.
56. Suga K, Nishigauchi K, Shimizu K, et al. SPECT with In-111 autologous platelets to detect residual splenic tissue in two patients with relapsed thrombocytopenia. *Clin Nucl Med.* 1997;22:141–146.
57. Kinuya K, Matano S, Nakashima H, et al. Scintigraphic prediction of therapeutic outcomes of splenectomy in patients with thrombocytopenia. *Ann Nucl Med.* 2003;17:161–164.
58. Targarona EM, Espert JJ, Balague C, et al. Residual splenic function after laparoscopic splenectomy: a clinical concern. *Arch Surg.* 1998;133:56–60.
59. Morris KT, Horvath KD, Jobe BA, et al. Laparoscopic management of accessory spleens in immune thrombocytopenic purpura. *Surg Endosc.* 1999;13:520–522.
60. Antevil J, Thoman D, Taller J, et al. Laparoscopic accessory splenectomy with intraoperative gamma probe localization for recurrent idiopathic thrombocytopenic purpura. *Surg Laparosc Endosc Percutan Tech.* 2002;12:371–374.
61. Onundarson PT, Rowe JM, Heal JM, et al. Response to plasma exchange and splenectomy in thrombotic thrombocytopenic purpura. A 10-year experience at a single institution. *Arch Intern Med.* 1992;152:791–796.
62. Wells AD, Majumdar G, Slater NG, et al. Role of splenectomy as a salvage procedure in thrombotic thrombocytopenic purpura. *Br J Surg.* 1991;78:1389–1390.
63. Aqui NA, Stein SH, Konkle BA, et al. Role of splenectomy in patients with refractory or relapsed thrombotic thrombocytopenic purpura. *J Clin Apheresis* 2003;18:51–54.
64. Modic M, Cernelc P, Zver S. Splenectomy: the last option of immunosuppressive therapy in patients with chronic or relapsing idiopathic thrombotic thrombocytopenic purpura? *Transplant Proc.* 2002;34:2953–2954.
65. Rice HE, Oldham KT, Hillery CA, et al. Clinical and hematologic benefits of partial splenectomy for congenital hemolytic anemias in children. *Ann Surg.* 2003;237:281–288.
66. Balint GP, Balint PV. Felty's syndrome. *Best Prac Res Clin Rheumatol.* 2004;18:631–645.
67. Van Krieken JH, Breedveld FC, te Velde J. The spleen in Felty's syndrome: a histological, morphometrical, and immunohistochemical study. *Eur J Haematol.* 1988;40:58.
68. Blumfelder TM, Logue GL, Shimm DS. Felty's syndrome: effects of splenectomy upon granulocyte count and granulocyte-associated IgG. *Ann Int Med.* 1981;94:623–628.
69. Logue GL, Huang AT, Shimm DS. Failure of splenectomy in Felty's syndrome. The role of antibodies supporting granulocyte lysis by lymphocytes. *N Engl J Med.* 1981;304:580–583.
70. Eber S, Lux SE. Hereditary spherocytosis—defects in proteins that connect the membrane skeleton to the lipid bilayer. *Semin Hematol.* 2004;41:118–141.
71. **Bolton-Maggs PH, Stevens RF, Dodd NJ, et al. Guidelines for the diagnosis and management of hereditary spherocytosis. *Br J Haematol.* 2004;126: 455–474.**
72. Reliene R, Mariana M, Zanella A, et al. Splenectomy prolongs in vivo survival of erythrocytes differently in spectrin/ankyrin- and band 3–deficient hereditary spherocytosis. *Blood* 2002;100:2208–2215.
73. Tchernia G, Gauthier F, Mielot F, et al. Initial assessment of the beneficial effect of partial splenectomy in hereditary spherocytosis. *Blood* 1993;81:2014–2020.
74. Tchernia G, Bader-Meunier B, Berterottier P, et al. Effectiveness of partial splenectomy in hereditary spherocytosis. *Curr Opin Hematol.* 1997;4:136–141.
75. Tsereteli Z, Smith CD, Branum GD, et al. Are the favorable outcomes of splenectomy predictable in patients with idiopathic thrombocytopenic purpura (ITP)? *Surg Endosc.* 2001;15:1386–1389.
76. Olivieri NF, Nathan DG, MacMillan JH, et al Survival in medically treated patients with homozygous beta-thalassemia. *N Engl J Med.* 1994;331:574–578.
77. Pinca A, DiPalma A, Soriani S, et al. Effectiveness of partial splenic embolization as treatment for hypersplenism in thalassemia major: a 7-year follow up. *Eur J Haematol.* 1992;49:49–52.
78. Idowu O, Hayes-Jordan A. Partial splenectomy in children under 4 years of age with hemoglobinopathy. *J Pediatr Surg.* 1998;33:1251–1253.
79. Al-Salem AH, al-Dabbous I, Bhamidibati P. The role of partial splenectomy in children with thalassemia. *Eur J Pediatr Surg.* 1998;8:334–338.
80. Levasseur DN, Ryan TM, Reilly MP, et al. A recombinant human hemoglobin with anti-sickling properties greater than fetal hemoglobin. *J Biol Chem.* 279:27518–27524,.
81. Corash L, Shafer B, Blaese RM. Platelet-associated immunoglobulin, platelet size, and the effect of splenectomy in the Wiskott-Aldrich syndrome. *Blood* 1985;65:1439–1443.
82. Muller CA, Anderson KD, Blaese RM. Splenectomy and/or bone marrow transplantation in the management of the Wiskott-Aldrich syndrome: long-term follow-up in 62 cases. *Blood* 1993;82:2961.
83. Verni W, Blanzuoli L, Kraus MD, et al. The spleen in the Wiskott-Aldrich syndrome: histopathologic abnormalities of the white pulp correlate with the clinical phenotype of the disease. *Am J Surg Pathol.* 1999;23:192–191.
84. Elliott MA, Tefferi A. Splenic irradiation in myelofibrosis with myeloid metaplasia: a review. *Blood Rev.* 1999;13:163–170.
85. Delpero JR, Houvenaeghel G, Gastaut JA, et al. Splenectomy for hypersplenism in chronic lymphocytic leukemia and malignant non-Hodgkin's lymphoma. *Br J Surg.* 1990;77:554–559.
86. Thiruvengadam R, Piedmonte M, Barcos M, et al. Splenectomy in advanced chronic lymphocytic leukemia. *Leukemia* 1990;4:758–760..
87. Delpero JR, Houvenaeghel G, Gastaut JA, et al. Splenectomy for hypersplenism in chronic lymphocytic leukemia and malignant non-Hodgkin's lymphoma. *Br J Surg.* 1990;77:443–449.
88. Neal TF Jr, Tefferi A, Witzig TE, et al. Splenectomy in advanced chronic lymphocytic leukemia: a single institution experience with 50 patients. *Am J Med.* 1992;93:435–440.
89. Seymour JF, Cusack JD, Lerner SA, et al. Case-control study of the role of splenectomy in chronic lymphocytic leukemia. *J Clin Oncol.* 1997;15:52–60.
90. Savage DG, Szydlo RM, Goldman JM. Clinical features at diagnosis in 430 patients with chronic myeloid leukemia seen at a referral centre over a 16-year period. *Br J Haematol.* 1997;96:111–116.
91. Hester JP, Waddell CC, Coltman CA, et al. Response of chronic myelogenous leukemia patients to COAP-splenectomy: a Southwest Oncology Group Study. *Cancer* 1984;54:1977–1982.
92. The Italian Cooperative Study on Chronic Myeloid Leukemia: results of a prospective randomized trial of early splenectomy in chronic myeloid leukemia. *Cancer* 1984;54:333–338..
93. Bouvet M, Babiera GV, Termuhlen PM, et al. Splenectomy in the accelerated or blastic phase of chronic myelogenous leukemia: a single-institution, 25-year experience. *Surgery* 1997;122:20–25.
94. Morel P, Dupriez B, Gosselin B, et al. Role of early splenectomy in malignant lymphomas with prominent splenic involvement (primary lymphomas of the spleen): a study of 59 cases. *Cancer* 1993;71:207–215.
95. Nair S, Shukla J, Chandy M. Non-Hodgkin's lymphoma presenting with prominent splenomegaly—clinicopathologic diversity in relationship to immunophenotype. *Acta Oncologica* 1997;36:725–727.
96. Lehne G, Hannisdal E, Langholm R, et al. A 10-year experience with splenectomy in patients with malignant non-Hodgkin's lymphoma at the Norwegian Radium Hospital. *Cancer* 1994;74:933–939.
97. Brodsky J, Abcar A, Styler M. Splenectomy for non-Hodgkin's lymphoma. *Am J Clin Oncol.* 1996;19:588–561.
98. Tallman MS, Hakimian D, Peterson L. Massive splenomegaly in hairy cell leukemia. *J Clin Oncol.* 1998;16:1232–1233.
99. Smalley RV, Connors J, Tuttle RL, et al. Splenectomy vs alpha interferon: a randomized study in patients with previously untreated hairy cell leukemia. *Am J Hematol.* 1992;41:13–18.
100. Saven A, Piro L. Newer purine analogues for the treatment of hairy-cell leukemia. *N Engl J Med.* 1994;330:691–697.
101. Grever M, Kopecky K, Foucar MK, et al. Randomized comparison of pentostatin versus interferon alpha-2a in previously untreated patients with hairy cell leukemia: an intergroup study. *J Clin Oncol.* 1995;13: 974–982.

102. Reilly JT. Pathogenesis of idiopathic myelofibrosis: present status and future directions. *Br J Haematol.* 1994;88:1–8.
103. Kraus MD, Bartlett NL, Fleming MD, et al. Splenic pathology in myelodysplasia: a report of 13 cases with clinical correlation. *Am J Surg Pathol.* 1998;22:1255–1266.
104. Benbassat J, Gion D, Penchas S. The choice between splenectomy and medical treatment in patients with advanced agnogenic myeloid metaplasia. *Am J Hematol.* 1990;33:128–135.
105. Barosi G, Ambrosetti A, Buratti A, et al. Splenectomy for patients with myelofibrosis with myeloid metaplasia: pretreatment variables and outcome prediction. *Leukemia* 1993;7:200–206.
106. Lopez-Guillermo A, Cervantes F, Bruguera M, et al. Liver dysfunction following splenectomy in idiopathic myelofibrosis: a study of 10 patients. *Acta Haematologica* 1991;85:184–188.
107. Towell BL, Levine SP. Massive hepatomegaly following splenectomy for myeloid metaplasia. Case report and review of the literature. *Am J Med.* 1987;82:371–375.
108. Tefferi A, Mesa RA, Nagorney DM, et al. Splenectomy in myelofibrosis with myeloid metaplasia: a single-institution experience with 223 patients. *Blood* 2000;95:2226–2233.
109. Austen KF. Systemic mastocytosis. *N Engl J Med.* 1992;326:639–640.
110. Friedman B, Darling G, Norton J, et al. Splenectomy in the management of systemic mast cell disease. *Surgery* 1990;107:94–100.
111. Harfi HA, Malik SA. Chediak-Higashi syndrome: clinical, hematologic, and immunologic improvement after splenectomy. *Ann Allergy* 1992;69: 147–150.
112. Cohen IJ, Katz K, Freud E, et al. Long-term follow-up of partial splenectomy in Gaucher's disease. *Am J Surg.* 1992;164:345–347.
113. Morgenstern L, Verham R, Weinstein I, et al. Subtotal splenectomy for Gaucher's disease: a follow-up study. *Am Surg.* 1993;59:860–855.
114. Zer M, Freud E. Subtotal splenectomy in Gaucher's disease: towards a definition of critical splenic mass. *Br J Surg.* 1992;79:742–744.
115. Haran MZ, Feldbewrg E, Miller G, et al. Sarcoidosis presenting as massive splenomegaly and bicytopenia. *Am J Hematol.* 2000;63:232–233.
116. Kruithoff KL, Gyetko MR, Scheiman JM. Giant splenomegaly and refractory hypercalcemia due to extrapulmonary sarcoidosis. Successful treatment by splenectomy. *Arch Intern Med.* 1993;153:2793–2796.
117. Fermandez-Cruz L, Martinez I, Gilabert R, et al. Laparoscopic distal pancreatectomy combined with preservation of the spleen for cystic neoplasms of the pancreas. *J Gastrointest Surg.* 2004;8:493–501.
118. Ikeguchi M, Kaibara N. Lymph node metastasis at the splenic hilum in proximal gastric cancer. *Am Surg.* 2004;70:645–648.
119. Martin RC, Jaques DP, Brennan MF, et al. Extended local resection for advanced gastric cancer: increased survival versus increased morbidity. *Ann Surg.* 2002;236:159–165.
120. Martin RC, Jaques DP, Brennan MF, et al. Achieving RO resection for locally advanced gastric cancer: is it worth the risk of multiorgan resection? *J Am Coll Surg.* 2002;194:568–577.
121. Cassar K, Munro A. Iatrogenic splenic injury. *J R Colle Surg Edinb.* 2002;47:731–741.
122. Flum DR, Koepsell T, Heagerty P, et al. The nationwide frequency of major adverse outcomes in antireflux surgery and the role of surgeon experience. *J Am Coll Surg.* 2002;195:611–618.
123. Muskat PC, Johnson RA, Bowers GJ. Staging laparotomy in Hodgkin's lymphoma. *Am J Surg.* 1991;162:603–606.
124. Mendenhall NP, Cantor AB, Williams JL, et al. With modern imaging techniques, is staging laparoscopy necessary in pediatric Hodgkin's disease? A Pediatric Oncology Group study. *J Clin Oncol.* 1993;11:2218–2225.
125. Blackwell EA, Joshua DE, McLaughlin AF, et al. Early supradiaphragmatic Hodgkin's disease. High dose gallium scanning obviates the need for staging laparotomy. *Cancer* 1986;58:883.
126. Gospodarowicz MK, Sutcliffe SB, Clark RM, et al. Analysis of supradiaphragmatic clinical stage I and II Hodgkin's disease treated with radiation alone. *Int J Radiat Oncol Biol Phys.* 1992;22:859.
127. Wasserman TH, Trenkner DA, Fineberg B, et al. Cure of early stage Hodgkin's disease with subtotal nodal irradiation. *Cancer* 1991;68:1208.
128. Swerdlow AJ, Douglas AJ, Vaughan Hudson G, et al. Risk of second primary cancer after Hodgkin's disease in patients in the British National Lymphoma Investigation: relationships to host factors, histology, and stage of Hodgkin's disease, and splenectomy. *Br J Cancer* 1993; 68:1006–1011.
129. Tura S, Fiacchini M, Zinzanni PL, et al. Splenectomy and the increasing risk of secondary acute leukemia in Hodgkin's disease. *J Clin Oncol.* 1993; 11:925–930.
130. Linet MS, Yren O, Gridley G, et al. Risk of cancer following splenectomy. *Int J Cancer* 1996;66:611–616.
131. Loftus JP, Nagorney DM, Ilstrup D, et al. Sinistra portal hypertension: splenectomy or expectant management. *Ann Surg.* 1993;217:35–40.
132. Lambert CJ Jr, Williamson JW. Splenic artery aneurysm: a rare cause of upper gastrointestinal bleeding. *Am Surg.* 1990;56:543–545.
133. Keagan MT, Freed KS, Parks EK, et al. Imaging-guided percutaneous biopsy of focal splenic lesions: update on safety and effectiveness. *Am J Roentgenol.* 1999;172:933–937.
134. Lishner M, Lang R, Hamlet Y, et al. Fine needle aspiration biopsy in patients with diffusely enlarged spleens. *Acta Cytologica* 1996;40:196– 198.
135. Yu RS, Zhang SZ, Hua JM. Imaging findings of splenic hamartoma. *World J Gastroentrol.* 2004;10:13–15.
136. Mackenzie RK, Youngson GG, Mahomed AA. Laparoscopic decapsulation of congenital splenic cysts: a step forward in splenic preservation. *J Ped Surg.* 2004;39:88–90.
137. Atmatzidis K, Papaziogas B, Mirelis C, et al. Splenectomy versus spleen-preserving surgery for splenic echinococcosis. *Dig Surg.* 2003;20: 527–531.
138. Manouras AJ, Nikolaou CC, Katergiannakis VA, et al. Spleen-sparing surgical treatment for echinococcosis of the spleen. *Br J Surg.* 1997;84:1162.
139. Cohen MAA, et al. Splenic abscess. *World J Surg.* 1990;14:513.
140. De Bree E, Tsiftsis D, Christodoulakis M, et al. Splenic abscess: a diagnostic and therapeutic challenge. *Acta Chirurgica Belgica* 1998;98:199–202.
141. Robinson SL, Saxe JM, Lucas CE, et al. Splenic abscess associated with endocarditis. *Surgery* 1992;112:781–786.
142. Flum DR, Koepsell T, Heagerty P, et al. The nationwide frequency of major adverse outcomes in antireflux surgery and the role of surgeon experience. *J Am Coll Surg.* 2002;195:611–618.
143. Haj M, Bickel A, Weiss M, et al. Laparoscopic splenopexy of a wandering spleen. *J Laparoendosc Adv Surg Tech A.* 1999;9:357–360.
144. Corcione F, Caiazzo P, Cuccurullo D, et al. Laparoscopic splenectomy for the treatment of wandering spleen. *Surg Endosc.* 2004;18:554–556.
145. Nelson EW, Mone MC. Splenectomy in high-risk patients with splenomegaly. *Am J Surg.* 1999;178:581–586.
146. Letoquart JP, LaGamma A, Kunin N, et al. Splenectomy for splenomegaly exceeding 1000 grams: analysis of 47 patients. *Br J Surg.* 1993;80:334– 335.
147. Petroianu A, da Silva RG, Simal CJ, et al. Late postoperative follow-up of patients submitted to subtotal splenectomy. *Am Surg.* 1997;63:735–740.
148. Targarona EM, Espert JJ, Balague C, et al. Splenomegaly should not be considered a contraindication for laparoscopic splenectomy. *Ann Surg.* 1998;228:35–39.
149. Borrazzo ED, Daly JM, Morrisey KP, et al. Hand-assistant laparoscopic splenectomy for giant spleen. *Surg Endosc.* 2003;17:918–920.
150. Terrosu G, Baccarani U. Bresadola V, et al. The impact of splenic weight on laparoscopic splenectomy for splenomegaly. *Surg Endosc.* 2002;16: 103–107.
151. Machado MA, Makdissi FF, Herman P, et al. Exposure of splenic hilum increases safety of laparoscopic splenectomy. *Surg Laparosc Endosc Percutan Tech.* 2004;14:23–25.
152. Tanoue K, Okita K, Akahoshi T, et al. Laparoscopic splenectomy for hematologic diseases. *Surgery* 2002;131:S318–323.
153. Kaban GK, Czerniach DR, Perugini RA, et al. Use of a laparoscopic hand-assist device for accessory splenectomy. *Surg Endosc.* 200418:1001.

SECTION K
SURGICAL ENDOCRINOLOGY

CHAPTER 76 ■ BREAST DISEASE

MONICA MORROW AND SEEMA KHAN

ANATOMY

The adult female breast lies between the second and sixth ribs and between the sternal edge and the midaxillary line (Fig. 76.1). Breast tissue frequently extends into the axilla as the axillary tail of Spence. Posteriorly, the upper portion of the breast rests on the fascia of the pectoralis major muscle; inferolaterally, it is bounded by the fascia of the serratus anterior. Bands of fibrous tissue, known as *Cooper's ligaments*, extend from the fascia to the fibrous tissue of the dermis and support the breast. The size of the adult female breast varies widely among individuals, and considerable discrepancy in breast size is seen between the breasts of an individual woman. This is rarely a sign of breast disease. The breast is composed of skin, subcutaneous tissue, and breast tissue. The breast tissue includes both epithelial parenchymal elements and stroma. The epithelial component comprises about 10% to 15% of the breast mass, with the remainder being stroma. Each breast consists of 15 to 20 lobes of glandular tissue that are supported by a framework of fibrous connective tissue. The space between lobes is filled by adipose tissue. Variations in breast size are accounted for by differences in the amount of adipose tissue in the breast rather than the epithelial elements. Much of the epithelial tissue of the breast is found in the upper outer quadrant, which is why this is the most frequent site of both benign and malignant breast disease.

The lobes of the breast are subdivided into lobules, which are made up of branched tubuloalveolar glands. Each lobe ends in a lactiferous duct, 2 to 4 mm in diameter. Beneath the areola, the lactiferous ducts dilate into lactiferous sinuses and then open through a constricted orifice onto the nipple (Fig. 76.2).

The nipple is located over the fourth intercostal space in the nonpendulous breast and is surrounded by a circular, pigmented areola. Beneath the nipple and areola are bundles of radially arranged smooth-muscle fibers that are responsible for the erection of the nipple in response to a variety of stimuli. The nipple and areola contain sebaceous glands and apocrine sweat glands, but no hair follicles. In addition, the tubercles of Morgagni are nodular elevations formed by the openings of the Montgomery glands at the periphery of the areola. These glands are capable of secreting milk and are believed to represent an intermediate stage between sweat and mammary glands. The nipple and areolar region, as well as the remainder of the breast, is richly supplied with sensory innervation.

The blood supply of the breast is derived from the internal mammary and lateral thoracic arteries. The medial and central portions of the breast receive their major blood supply from anterior perforating branches of the internal mammary artery, and the upper outer quadrant is primarily supplied by the lateral thoracic artery. In general, the venous drainage of the breast follows the arterial supply.

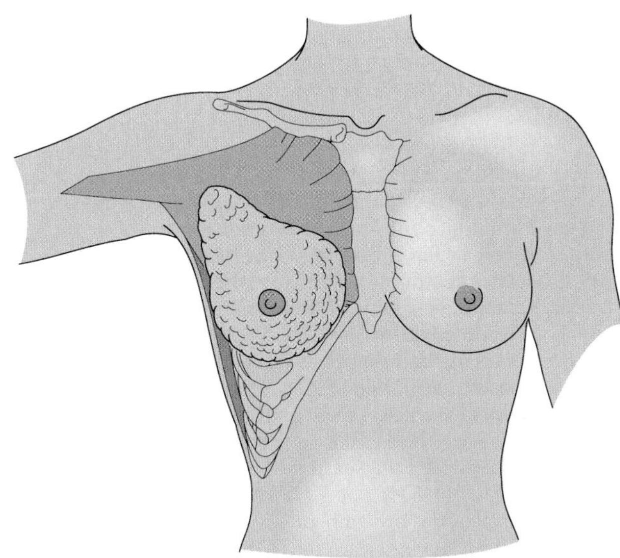

FIGURE 76.1 The adult female breast. The upper and medial portions of the breast rest on the pectoralis major muscle, and the inferolateral portion rests on the serratus anterior.

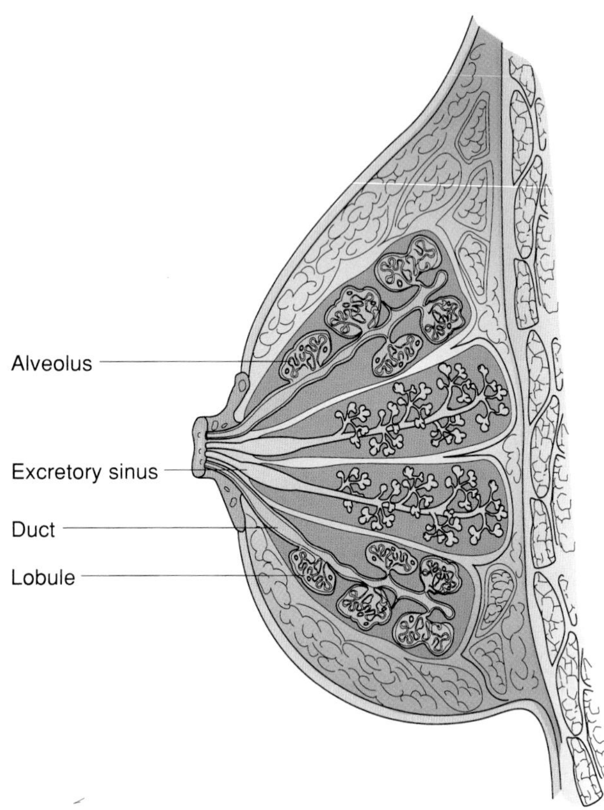

FIGURE 76.2 The breast consists of 15 to 20 lobes of glandular tissue. Within each lobe, the lobules are composed of branched tubuloalveolar glands. Each lobule ends in a lactiferous duct. These ducts dilate into lactiferous sinuses beneath the nipple.

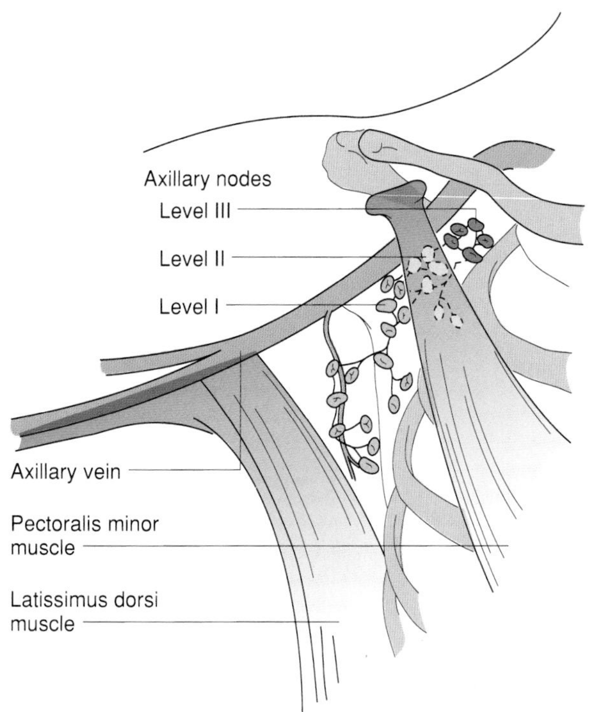

FIGURE 76.3 The axillary lymph nodes are divided into three levels by the pectoralis minor muscle. The level I nodes are inferior and lateral to the pectoralis minor, the level II nodes are below the axillary vein and behind the pectoralis minor, and the level III nodes are medial to the muscle against the chest wall.

LYMPHATIC DRAINAGE

The lymphatics of the breast are thin-walled, valveless vessels that drain unidirectionally except when obstructed by inflammatory or neoplastic disease. The superficial subareolar lymphatic plexus drains primarily the skin of the breast and the nipple and areola, in addition to some of the central portion of the gland. This plexus is interconnected with the deep lymphatic plexus, which drains most of the breast parenchyma. Injections of radioactively labeled colloid have demonstrated that about 97% of the lymphatic flow from the breast drains directly into the axillary lymph nodes, with the remaining 3% draining into the internal mammary nodes.[1] All quadrants of the breast drain into the internal mammary nodes.

The axillary space is bordered by the axillary vein superiorly, the latissimus dorsi laterally, and the serratus anterior medially (Fig. 76.3). The pectoralis major lies anterior to the axillary space, and the subscapularis comprises its posterior wall. Structures of clinical importance within this space include the long thoracic nerve, which innervates the serratus anterior; the thoracodorsal neurovascular bundle, which innervates and supplies blood to the latissimus dorsi; and the intercostobrachial nerves, which are sensory to the upper inner aspect of the arm.

The axillary nodes are embedded in fat and are variable in number. Surgeons have traditionally divided the axillary nodes into three levels: level I nodes, inferior and lateral to the pectoralis minor; level II nodes, behind the pectoralis minor and inferior to the axillary vein; and level III nodes, medial to the pectoralis minor and against the chest wall. The interpectoral (or Rotter's) nodes are located between the pectoralis major and minor muscles along the lateral pectoral nerve. Involvement of this node group in the absence of axillary metastases is extremely rare,[2] and thus they are of limited clinical significance. The supraclavicular nodes are contiguous with the apex of the axilla. Metastatic involvement of this nodal group in the absence of extensive axillary disease is also uncommon, although direct lymphatic drainage to this node group is occasionally seen.

The internal mammary nodes are located in the first six intercostal spaces within 3 cm of the edge of the sternum. The highest concentration of internal mammary nodes is found in the first three intercostal spaces.[3]

PHYSIOLOGY

Development of the Breast

Breast development is controlled by a large number of hormonal and biochemical factors. In the female, estrogens interact with the primordial breast bud to promote ductal development, whereas in the male, the interaction of androgen with the breast bud results in destruction of the epithelial component. In the female, ductal elongation and branching begin in puberty and are regulated by pituitary growth hormone, which may act through insulinlike growth factor I locally.[4] In addition, the presence of estrogen and progesterone is required to stimulate DNA synthesis. This effect is believed to occur through both receptor-mediated and paracrine pathways.

Changes in breast size and shape begin at puberty and are secondary to growth of both the glandular and stromal elements of the breast. Russo and Russo[5] have described three types of breast lobules, related to a woman's parity and menopausal status. The type 1 (or virginal) lobule consists of a cluster of 11 alveolar buds around a terminal duct; it is the predominant lobule seen in nulliparous and postmenopausal women. Type 2 lobules contain an average of 47 alveolar buds, and type 3 lobules have 80, at which time they are referred to as *ductules* or *alveoli*. In parous women, type 3 lobules predominate, with a peak frequency in the early reproductive years until they begin to decline in the fourth decade of life. Cells within these lobules have been shown to proliferate at different rates, the rate being 10 times higher in type 1 than in type 3 lobules, and three times higher in type 1 than in type 2 lobules. The presence of estrogen receptor-α and the progesterone receptor within these lobules is directly proportional to the rate of cell proliferation.[6] These differences in cell proliferation may explain some of the differences in breast cancer risk observed on the basis of parity and age at first birth (see section on breast cancer risk factors).

The cyclical increases in estrogen and progesterone that occur in the menstrual cycle also influence the gross and microscopic character of the breast. Many women experience increased breast fullness, nodularity, and sensitivity in the premenstrual period. During the follicular phase of the menstrual cycle (days 4 through 14), epithelial proliferation occurs, with epithelial sprouting and an increased mitotic rate. During the luteal phase of the cycle (days 15 through 28), when progestins predominate, proliferation is maximal, with ductal dilation and differentiation of the alveolar epithelial cells to secretory cells. This results in the formation of lipid droplets in the alveolar cells and some intraluminal secretion. With the onset of menstruation, secretory activity regresses secondary to epithelial apoptosis, or programmed cell death.

Pregnancy

Significant ductal, lobular, and alveolar growth occurs during pregnancy as a result of exposure to estrogen, progesterone, growth hormone, prolactin, and placental hormones. Clinically, this is manifested as breast enlargement, with associated dilation of the superficial veins and darkening of the nipple. At delivery, the breast may be three times the size of the nonlactating breast. Microscopically, lobular–alveolar differentiation to type 3 lobules begins in the first trimester, and the stromal elements of the breast are gradually replaced by the proliferating glandular epithelium. During the third trimester, terminal differentiation of the epithelium results in the development of secretory cells that are able to synthesize and secrete milk proteins. Oxytocin induces myoepithelial proliferation and differentiation.[6]

Lactation and Involution

After delivery, the sudden fall in estrogen and progesterone levels results in lactation. Prolactin, in conjunction with growth hormone and insulin, induces the production and secretion of milk. Initially, colostrum, a sticky serous fluid rich in growth factors, is secreted, followed by milk. Milk secretion is regulated by the pituitary production of oxytocin, which is released in response to neural reflexes activated by suckling.

Following weaning, the secretory activity of the lactogenic epithelium gradually decreases. Retained secretory products are removed by phagocytosis, although ruptured alveoli containing milk may be clinically manifested as galactoceles. Atrophy of glandular, ductal, and stromal elements results in a decrease in breast size. Withdrawal of the steroid hormones and growth factors of pregnancy and lactation results in apoptosis of the terminally differentiated secretory cells of the epithelial lumen. As previously noted, however, type 3 lobules persist.

Menopause

After menopause, the breast undergoes regression. Type 1 lobules predominate, as in the breasts of nulliparous women. Overall, involution of the ductal and glandular elements of the breast occurs, and the breast becomes predominantly fat and stroma. With aging, a progressive decrease in the fat content and supporting stroma results in breast shrinkage and loss of contour.

BREAST EXAMINATION

A careful history is the initial step in a breast examination. Regardless of the presenting complaint, baseline information regarding menstrual status and breast cancer risk factors should be obtained. The basic elements of a breast history are listed in Table 76.1. In premenopausal women, knowing the date of the last menstrual period and the regularity of the cycle is useful in evaluating breast nodularity, pain, and cysts. Postmenopausal women should be questioned about the use of hormone replacement therapy, given that many benign breast problems are uncommon after menopause in the absence of exogenous hormones. Specific information about the patient's presenting complaint is then elicited. A breast lump is most often the clinical problem that causes women to seek treatment and remains the most common presentation of breast carcinoma. Today, many women present for a breast examination after an abnormality has been identified on a screening mammogram. Although the majority of these lesions are not clinically evident, a careful physical examination is an important part of the evaluation of a patient with an abnormal mammogram. Breast pain, a change

TABLE 76.1 DIAGNOSIS

MEDICAL HISTORY OF A BREAST PROBLEM

GENERAL
Age at menarche
Number of pregnancies
Number of live births
Age at first birth
Family history of breast cancer, including affected relative, age of onset, and presence of bilateral disease
History of breast biopsies (and histologic diagnosis, if available)
Premenopausal women
- Date of last menstrual period
- Length and regularity of cycles
- Use of oral contraceptives

Postmenopausal women
- Date of menopause
- Use of hormone replacement therapy

SPECIFIC
Onset
Duration
Frequency
Severity
Relationship to menstrual cycle or use of hormone replacement therapy

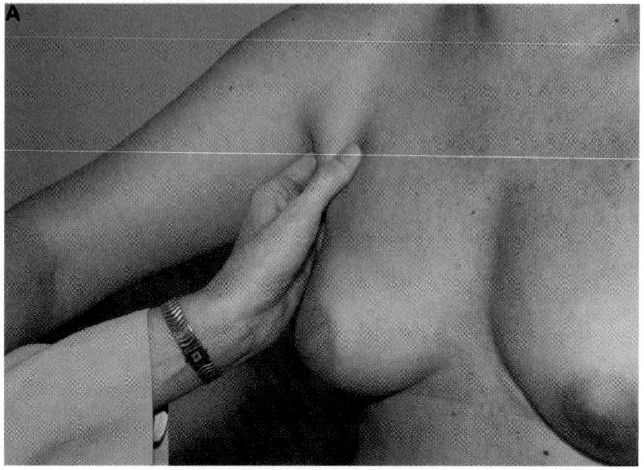

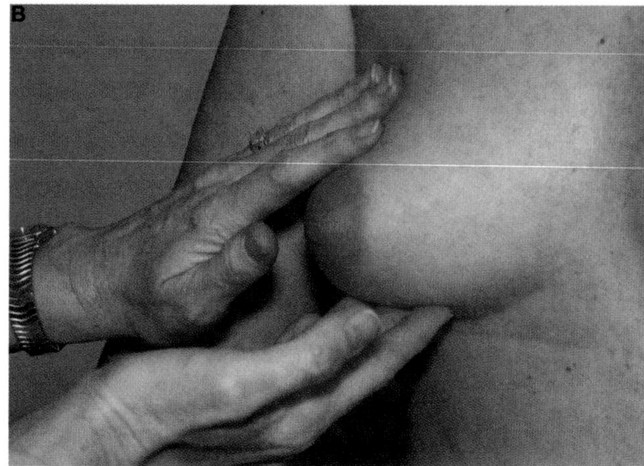

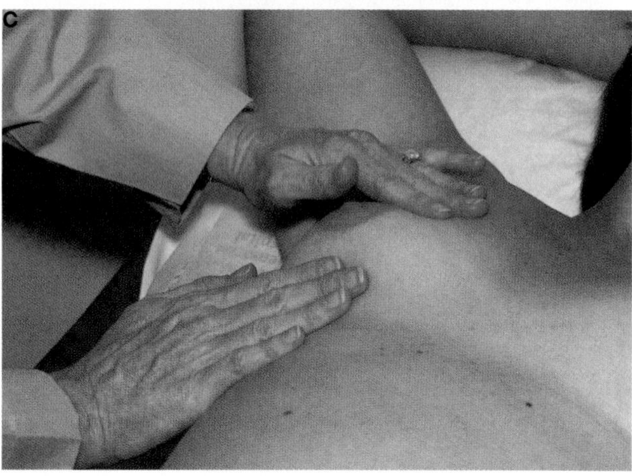

FIGURE 76.4 Breast examination. (*A*) The patient's ipsilateral arm is supported by the examiner to relax the pectoral muscle while the axillary nodes are examined. (*B*) Bimanual examination of the breast in the upright position. (*C*) Bimanual examination in the supine position with the arm raised over the head.

in the size and shape of the breast, nipple discharge, and changes in the appearance of the skin are infrequent symptoms of carcinoma. The evaluation and management of these conditions are described in the section on clinical breast problems. For any breast complaint, the duration of the symptoms, their persistence over time, and their fluctuation with the menstrual cycle or relationship to exogenous estrogen should be ascertained.

Technique

A woman must be disrobed from the waist up for a complete breast examination. Although attention to modesty is appropriate and a gown or drape should be provided, inspection is an important part of the examination, and subtle abnormalities are best appreciated by comparing the appearance of both breasts. The breast examination should be performed with the patient in both the sitting and supine positions, and care should be taken at all times to be gentle. The steps of a breast examination are illustrated in Figure 76.4.

The breasts are initially inspected while the patient is in the sitting position with the arms relaxed. The size and shape of the breasts should be compared. If a discrepancy in size is noted, determine its chronicity. In many women, the breasts are not identical in size, and the finding of small discrepancies in size is rarely a sign of malignancy. Differences in breast size of recent onset or progressive in nature, however, may be caused by both benign and malignant tumors and require further evaluation (Fig. 76.5). Alterations in breast shape, in the absence of previous surgery, are of more concern. Superficially located tumors can cause bulges in the breast contour or retraction of the overlying skin. The skin retraction seen with superficial tumors may be caused by direct extension of tumor or

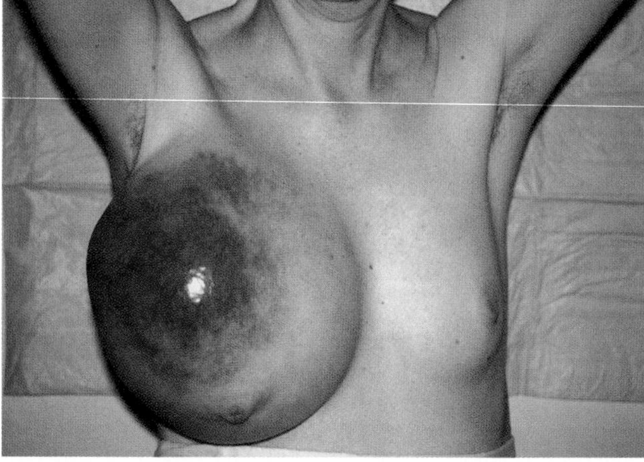

FIGURE 76.5 Breast asymmetry resulting from a benign phyllodes tumor. Skin changes are caused by pressure necrosis.

fibrosis. Tumors deep within the substance of the breast that involve the fibrous septa (Cooper's ligaments) can also cause retraction. Retraction is not itself a prognostic factor except when it is caused by the direct extension of tumor into the skin, and for this reason, it is not a part of the clinical staging of breast cancer.[7] Although retraction is usually a sign of malignancy, benign lesions of the breast, such as granular cell tumors and fat necrosis, also cause retraction. Other benign causes of retraction include surgical biopsy and thrombophlebitis of the thoracoepigastric vein (Mondor's disease).

The skin of the breast and the nipples should also be carefully inspected. Edema of the skin of the breast *(peau d'orange)*, when present, is usually extensive and readily apparent. Localized edema is frequently most prominent in the lower half of the breast and periareolar region and is most noticeable when the patient's arms are raised. Erythema is another sign of disease that is evident on inspection. It may be caused by cellulitis or abscess in the breast, but a diagnosis of inflammatory carcinoma should always be considered.

Examination of the nipples should include inspection for symmetry, retraction, and changes in the character of the skin. The new onset of nipple retraction should be regarded with a high index of suspicion, except when it occurs immediately after cessation of breast-feeding. Ulceration and eczematous changes of the nipple may be the first signs of Paget's disease.

After inspection with the arms relaxed, ask the patient to raise her arms to allow a more complete inspection of the lower half of the breasts. A final inspection is made with the hands on the hips and the pectoral muscles contracted.

The regional nodes are then examined with the patient upright. Assess the size, character (soft, tender, firm), and number, and note whether the nodes are matted. The axillary nodes are most readily examined with the ipsilateral arm supported to relax the pectoral muscle (Fig. 76.4A). Bimanual examination of the breast is also carried out with the patient upright (Fig. 76.4B).

Complete the breast examination with the patient in the supine position and the ipsilateral arm raised above the head (Fig. 76.4C). Then systematically examine the breast tissue. Whether the examination is performed with a radial or a concentric circular search pattern is unimportant, provided that the entire breast is examined. The examination should extend superiorly to the clavicle, inferiorly to the lower rib cage, medially to the sternal border, and laterally to the midaxillary line.

One of the most difficult aspects of breast examination relates to the nodular, irregular texture of normal breasts in premenopausal women. Normal breasts tend to be most nodular in the upper outer quadrants, where the glandular tissue is concentrated, in the inframammary ridge area, and in the subareolar region. Generalized lumpiness is not a pathologic finding. Comparing the breasts is often helpful in determining whether a questionable area requires further evaluation. When the patient notices a mass that is not evident to the examiner, she should be asked to indicate the area of concern. If uncertainty remains regarding the significance of an area of nodular breast tissue in a premenopausal woman, a repeated examination at a different time during the menstrual cycle may clarify the issue. If a dominant mass is identified, measure it and record its location, mobility, and character in the medical record. The evaluation of a breast mass is discussed in detail in the section on clinical breast problems.

Screening Mammography

A screening mammogram consists of two views of the breast (craniocaudal and mediolateral oblique), which are obtained in asymptomatic women in an effort to detect cancer in a preclinical state, when the likelihood of cure is higher. It is important that screening not be confused with a diagnostic workup, which is performed to evaluate a woman with a clinical breast complaint and is discussed in the section on diagnostic imaging.

The ultimate measure of the effectiveness of a screening test is its effect on mortality. Eight randomized clinical trials, beginning with the Health Insurance Plan of New York study in 1963, have compared breast cancer mortality in women undergoing screening mammography at 1- to 2-year intervals with mortality in control populations. A 20% to 30% decrease in mortality has been demonstrated for screened women age 50 and older.[8] The benefit of screening in women ages 40 to 49 has been controversial. Many of the trials were not designed to allow a separate analysis of women in this age group, and mortality benefits were often not apparent until after 8 years or more of follow-up. A meta-analysis of women ages 40 to 49 in the randomized trials, however, suggests a 29% mortality reduction with screening in this age group.[9]

The mortality reduction from screening is achieved by identifying abnormalities that cannot be detected on physical examination. These include microcalcifications and masses smaller than 1 cm in size, the usual clinical limit of detection. In addition to reducing breast cancer mortality, identifying smaller tumors increases the likelihood that a woman will be a candidate for breast-conserving surgery. In one study, only 10% of women with tumors 2 cm or less in size had contraindications to breast conservation, compared with 30% of women with tumors larger than 2 cm but less than 5 cm in size.[10] Current screening recommendations are for annual mammography for women age 40 and older.

Screening mammography is a sensitive but nonspecific test, and only 20% to 30% of mammographically detected abnormalities that are examined further are found to be malignant. Biopsies for clinically occult, benign lesions represent the major induced cost of screening. The positive predictive value of a mammographic lesion varies with its appearance. For spiculated or stellate masses, the likelihood of malignancy is 75%; this falls to 20% for lobulated masses with slightly irregular margins and to 5% for well-circumscribed masses (Fig. 76.6). The classification of calcifications has proved to be even more difficult. Calcifications are analyzed based on their size, number, distribution, and morphology; those that are irregular in size and shape, particularly when they have a branching pattern suggestive of a ductal distribution, are most likely to be malignant (Fig. 76.7).

In an effort to standardize the reporting of mammographic abnormalities, the American College of Radiology has created a breast imaging reporting and data system (BI-RADS).[11] The BI-RADS classification is listed in Table 76.2. Category 3 lesions are those with a less than 2% probability of malignancy, and short-interval follow-up usually consists of repeated imaging studies at 6 months. Category 4 lesions range in risk from 2% to 50%, and a decision regarding biopsy is based on the appearance of the lesion and the patient's level of risk.

The BI-RADS also includes a category 0, which is used when analysis is incomplete and additional studies, such as magnification views or ultrasonography, are needed before a final BI-RADS classification can be assigned. In practice, the majority of abnormalities detected on screening mammography should undergo a diagnostic workup before biopsy. With additional views, the need for biopsy of benign lesions is often avoided, as illustrated in Figure 76.8, where what appears to be a mass lesion resolves with spot compression and magnification views. Sickles[12] reported that of 302 cases of calcifications felt to be equivocal (i.e., BI-RADS category 4) after a screening examination, 61% were shown to be benign on additional views. Even with lesions that are clearly malignant on a screening examination, additional views allow a better definition of the extent of the lesion for treatment planning.

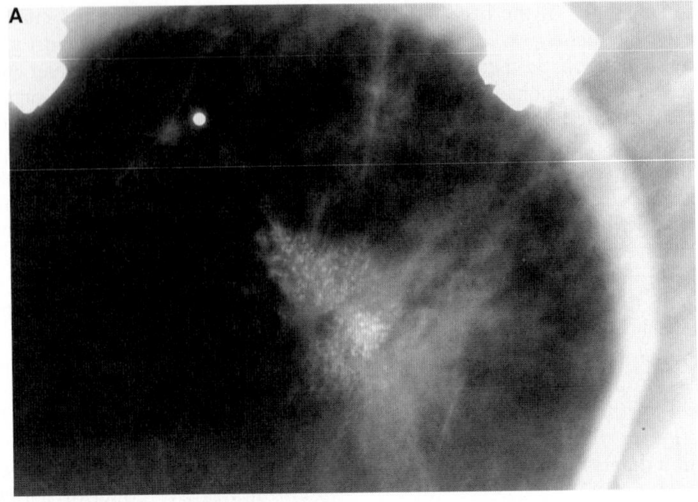

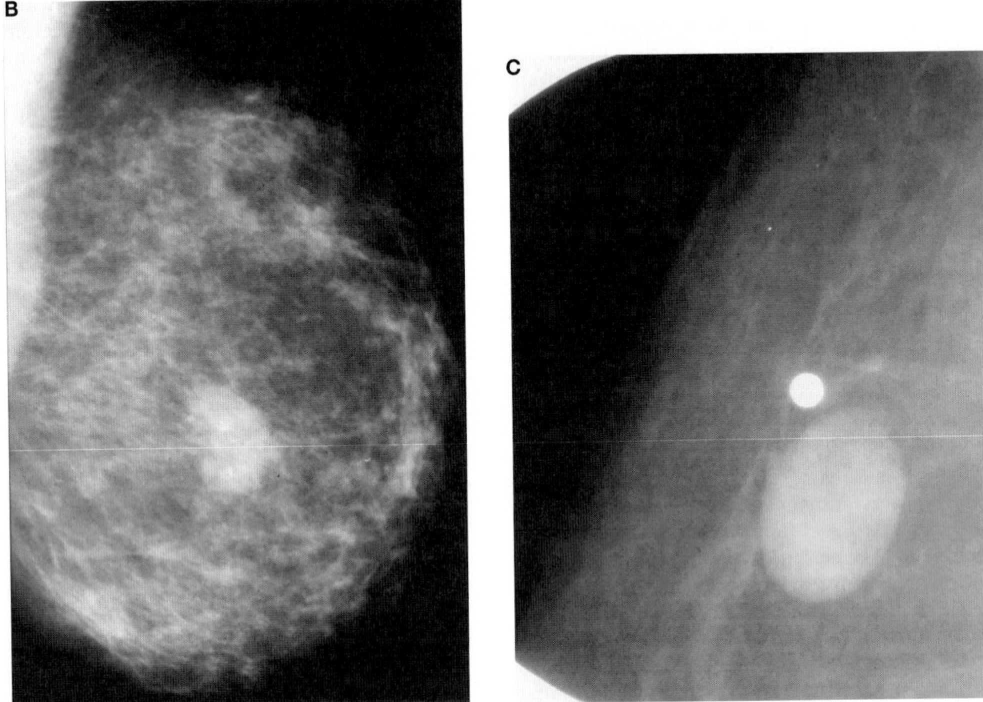

FIGURE 76.6 Mammographic masses. (*A*) Spiculated mass with calcifications. (*B*) Lobulated mass with indistinct posterior margin. (*C*) Well-circumscribed mass.

TABLE 76.2 CLASSIFICATION

BI-RADS CLASSIFICATION OF MAMMOGRAPHIC ABNORMALITIES

Category	Assessment	Recommendation
1	Negative	Routine screening.
2	Benign finding	Routine screening
3	Probably benign finding	Short-interval follow-up
4	Suspicious abnormality	Definite probability of malignancy; consider biopsy
5	Highly suggestive of malignancy	High probability of cancer; appropriate action should be taken.

BI-RADS, breast imaging reporting and data system.

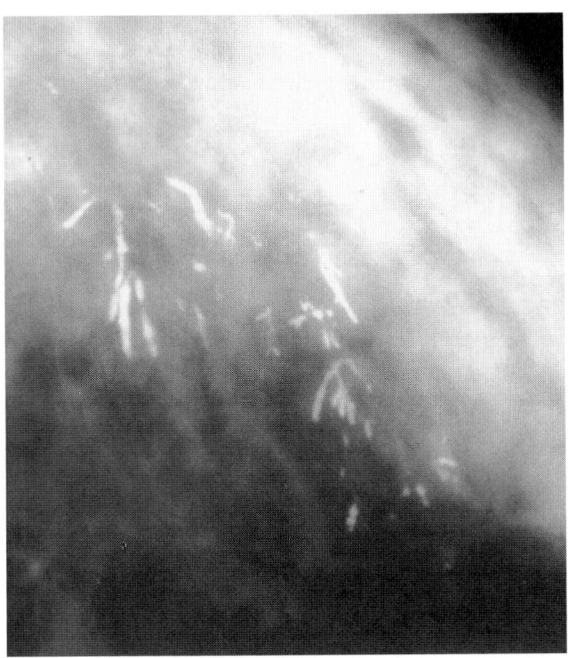

FIGURE 76.7 Microcalcifications. The branching, irregular appearance is classic for ductal carcinoma *in situ*.

Biopsy Techniques for Lesions Detected on Screening

After a physical examination has confirmed that a mammographically detected abnormality is not clinically evident, a histologic diagnosis can be obtained by needle localization and excision or an image-guided core biopsy. For many years, needle localization with excision was the gold standard for the diagnosis of mammographic abnormalities. Recognition that the majority of mammographic abnormalities are benign, however, has resulted in the replacement of surgical biopsy with image-guided needle biopsy techniques.

Mass lesions can be sampled under ultrasonographic or stereotactic guidance; calcifications generally require stereotactic guidance. A comparison of the results of stereotactic core biopsy and surgical biopsy demonstrates concordance rates of 71% to 99%.[13–15] Based on clinical experience, a number of circumstances in which a benign core biopsy should be followed by a surgical excision have been identified. These are listed in Table 76.3. The finding of atypical ductal hyperplasia on a core biopsy is associated with carcinoma in 18% to 50% of cases, even when large vacuum-assisted biopsy devices are used.[15–17] The majority of these are intraductal carcinomas, but approximately one third are invasive lesions. Similarly, radial scar has been found to be associated with coexistent carcinoma in 20% of cases. Lesions suspected of being radial scars are best approached initially with needle localization and excision.

Lack of concordance between the appearance of a mammographic abnormality and the histologic diagnosis obtained with core biopsy is an important indication for surgical biopsy. For example, the finding of a small amount of hyperplasia in a largely fatty specimen would not adequately explain a mass lesion seen on a mammogram. In addition, biopsies that reveal only fat, provide material insufficient for diagnosis, or lack calcifications on specimen radiography (if performed for that indication) must be repeated. An assessment of the cause of an insufficient sample (i.e., superficial location of the lesion, poor targeting, breast too thin after compression) will aid in determining if a repeated core biopsy is appropriate or if surgical excision is needed.

For most mammographic abnormalities, core biopsy is a more cost-effective, less morbid diagnostic technique than needle localization and excision and diagnosis by core biopsy increases the likelihood that local therapy will be completed with a single surgical procedure.[18,19] When needle localization and excision is indicated, the localizing

ENDOCRINE

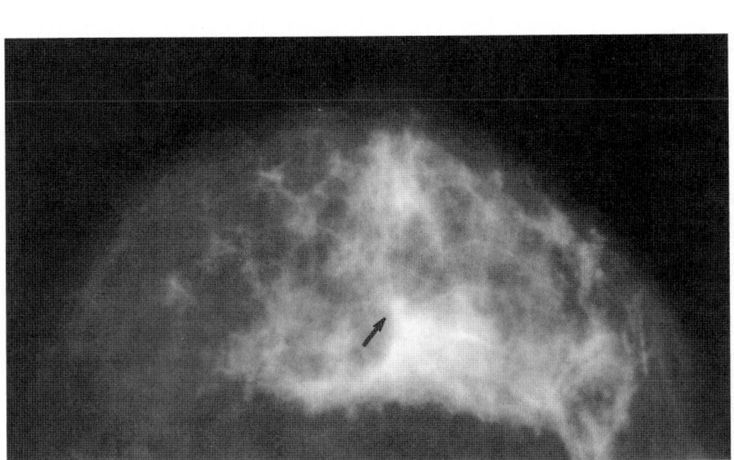

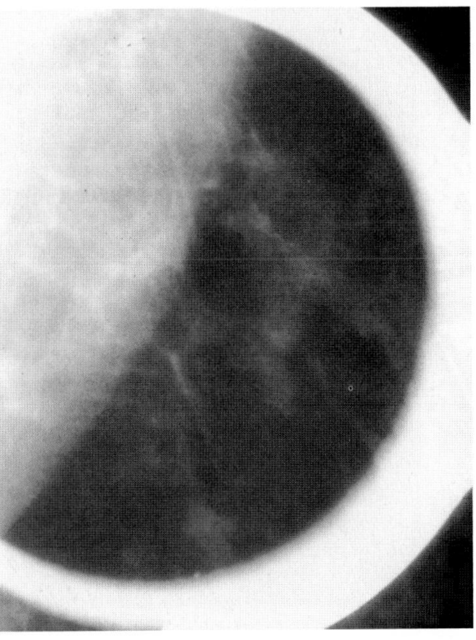

A B

FIGURE 76.8 Workup of abnormal screening mammogram. (*A*) Craniocaudal view showing an increased density with a slightly spiculated appearance (*arrow*). (*B*) Spot magnification view of the density demonstrating normal breast tissue.

TABLE 76.3 INDICATIONS/CONTRAINDICATIONS

INDICATIONS FOR SURGICAL BIOPSY AFTER CORE BIOPSY

- Atypical ductal hyperplasia
- Radial scar
- Lack of concordance between appearance of mammographic lesion and histologic diagnosis
- Nondiagnostic specimen (including absence of calcifications on specimen radiograph when biopsy is performed for calcifications)

wire should be placed within 1 cm of the lesion, and the incision should be placed over the abnormality (Fig.76.9). Incisions at the point of wire entry should be used only when the wire has a short course within the breast. Specimen radiography should be performed routinely to document removal of the target abnormality. The clinical approach to a patient with a mammographic abnormality is summarized in Algorithm 76.1.

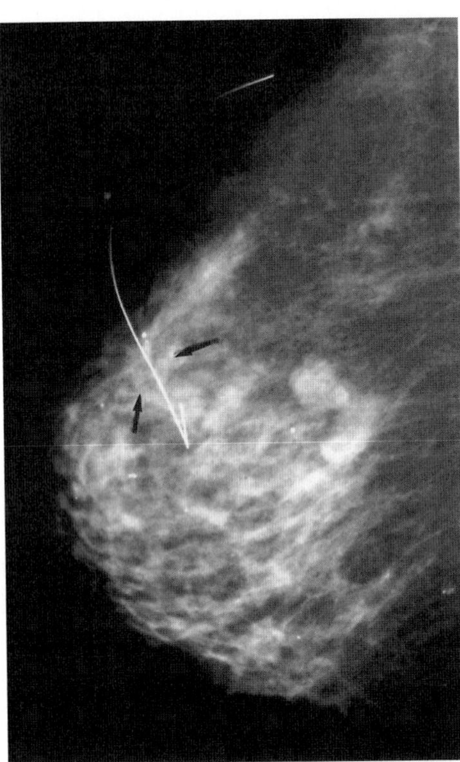

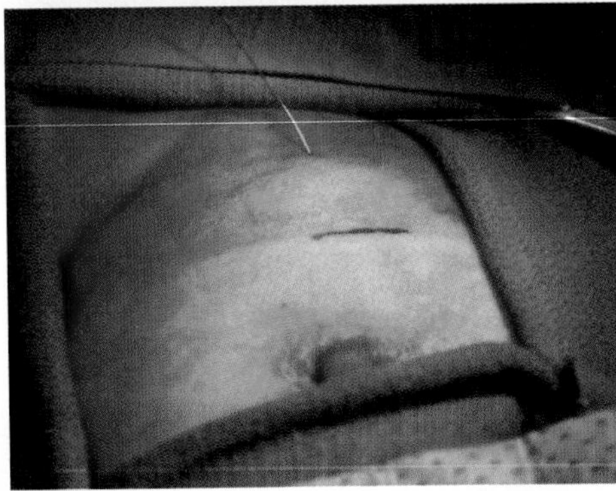

FIGURE 76.9 Incision placement for needle localization biopsy. (*A*) The mammogram demonstrates that the lesion (*arrow*) is inferior to the point of wire entry. (*B*) Incision placement inferior to wire entry to allow access to the lesion.

CLINICAL BREAST PROBLEMS

Most breast complaints that cause a woman to seek medical attention are benign. The purpose of the evaluation of any breast problem is first to determine if it is caused by a benign or malignant condition. If the process is malignant, a prompt diagnosis with sufficient information to plan treatment is the goal. If the process is benign, reassurance and relief of troublesome symptoms are the goals. Clinical breast problems can be divided into the general categories of breast pain, nipple discharge, breast masses, and breast infections. Each is associated with different causes and a different risk for malignancy, and each is considered separately.

Breast Pain

Breast pain is a common problem that is rarely a presenting sign of breast carcinoma. Breast pain may originate from the breast itself or may be referred from extramammary structures, such as the ribs, vertebrae, or occasionally the teeth. Clinically, breast pain can be divided into two categories, cyclic and noncyclic: cyclic breast pain waxes and wanes with the menstrual cycle, is frequently bilateral, and often involves the upper outer quadrants of the breasts with radiation to the axillae or down the arms. It tends to be most severe immediately before the menses, but may persist throughout the month. In contrast, noncyclic pain occurs in postmenopausal women or, when seen in premenopausal women, bears no relationship to the menstrual cycle.

No specific hormonal abnormalities or histologic correlates have been identified in women with breast pain, but the problem is clearly hormonally related, because it affects premenopausal women much more frequently than their postmenopausal counterparts. Breast pain is often precipitated by hormonal change, and a history of menstrual irregularity or a new medication should be sought. In the evaluation, it is important to ascertain whether fear of an underlying cancer or the need for pain relief is the patient's primary concern. In almost all cases, fear of cancer predominates. A careful physical examination should be performed to exclude a specific cause of the pain, particularly for focal, noncyclic mastalgia, which is occasionally secondary to the presence of a fibroadenoma or cyst and may be relieved by treatment of the underlying lesion. In women age 35 and older, a mammogram is usually part of the evaluation of breast pain unless one has been obtained within the preceding year. In the vast majority of women with breast pain, examination and mammography demonstrate no evidence of breast disease. In these cases, reassurance that a malignancy is not the cause of the pain and a discussion of the normal physiology of the breast are usually all that is necessary. In the patient with persistent, localized pain, physical examination should be accompanied by imaging studies, including ultrasound, to exclude the presence of carcinoma.

Approximately 5% of patients have disabling breast pain requiring further treatment. Several agents have been tested in randomized controlled trials; these include danazol (an antigonadotropin),[20] bromocriptine (a dopaminaergic agonist),[21] and tamoxifen (a selective estrogen receptor [ER]

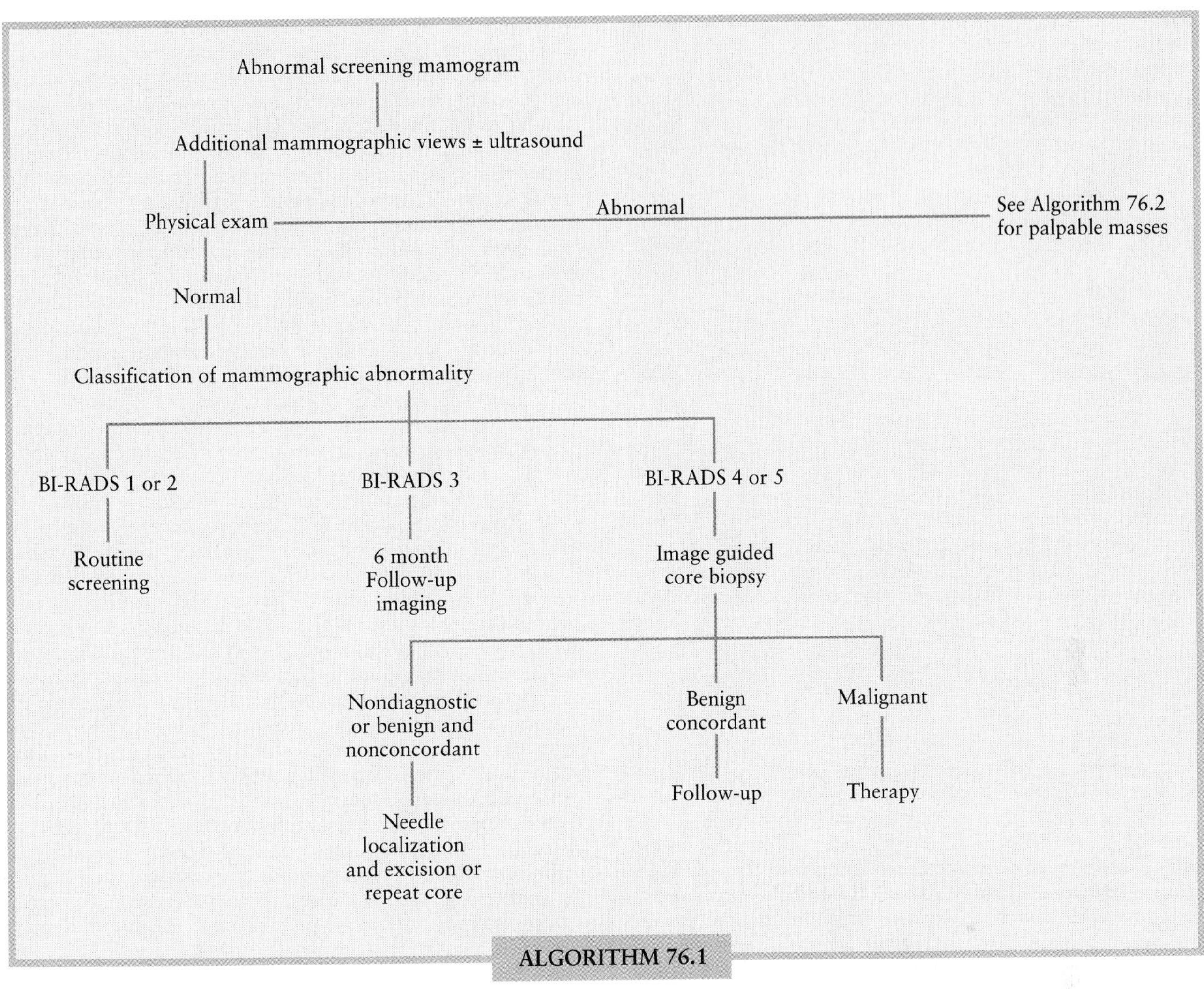

ALGORITHM 76.1 Diagnosis and management of mammographically detected breast lesions. A careful physical examination and a diagnostic imaging workup must be performed before a decision is made about the need for biopsy. *BI-RADS*, breast imaging, reporting, and data system.

modulator)[22] Danazol, which appears to be more effective than bromocriptine, has a response rate of approximately 50% for cyclical pain at doses of 100 to 400 mg, but is recommended only for severe, activity-limiting pain because of its side effects, which include menstrual irregularity, acne, weight gain, and hirsutism.[23] In addition, women starting therapy with danazol should be advised to use barrier contraception because of potential teratogenicity and possible interference with oral contraceptives. Tamoxifen appears to be effective at doses of 10 mg daily and has been used for 3- to 6-month intervals for the treatment of breast pain, but long-term use is not recommended because of its serious adverse effects (see later). Other agents, such as vitamins E and B_6, diuretics, and avoidance of caffeine have failed to demonstrate a reduction in symptoms in controlled clinical trials.[24–26] Evening primrose oil, which contains the long-chain fatty acid γ-linolenic acid, has also been proposed as therapy for cyclic breast pain, but clear evidence of its efficacy is lacking. Surgery should be avoided, even for apparently localized pain, because it rarely results in long-term pain relief.

Mondor disease, or thrombophlebitis of the lateral thoracic or superior thoracoepigastric vein, is an uncommon cause of breast pain that is readily identified clinically by the presence of a tender, subcutaneous cord in the lateral aspect of the breast. Skin retraction may be associated (Fig. 76.10), which raises concern about the presence of carcinoma.Mondor disease may develop secondary to trauma, surgical procedures on the breast, or breast irradiation. In approximately 50% of cases, no predisposing condition can be identified. Mondor disease is occasionally seen in women with a nonpalpable breast cancer,[27] and for this reason, a mammogram should be obtained in women age 35 and older who present with the condition. Mondor disease resolves spontaneously and requires no specific therapy, although antiinflammatory agents may be used for pain relief.

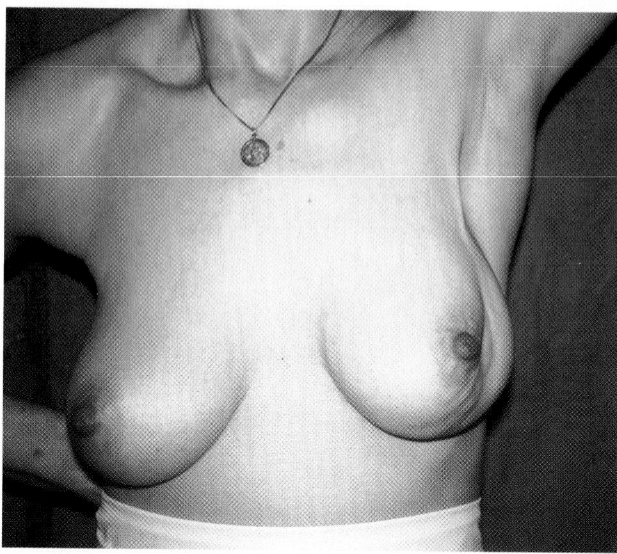

FIGURE 76.10 Mondor disease. Thrombophlebitis of the thoracoepigastric vein causes retraction of the lateral portion of the breast, which crosses to the midline at the inferior areolar margin and is accompanied by a palpable cord.

Nipple Discharge

Evaluation

Nipple discharge is a common complaint, particularly in premenopausal women, and has a benign cause in approximately 95% of women who present with it. The initial step in the evaluation of nipple discharge is to determine whether it is physiologic or pathologic. Discharges are considered pathologic if they are spontaneous and localized to one duct; they may be bloody or serous and are almost always unilateral. In one study, 32% of women over the age of 60 who presented with pathologic nipple discharge and no mass had carcinoma, compared with 7% of women under age 60 with the same presentation.[28] In contrast, physiologic discharges occur only with nipple compression, frequently originate from multiple ducts, and are often bilateral. If the remainder of the breast evaluation is normal, patients with physiologic discharge should be advised to stop squeezing their nipples and be assured that no further therapy is needed.

The clinical evaluation of a pathologic discharge should include testing the fluid for occult blood and identifying the quadrant of the breast from which the discharge originates. Although 70% to 85% of the discharges associated with carcinoma contain blood,[29] a nonbloody discharge that meets the other criteria of a pathologic discharge is an indication for further evaluation. Cytology is not usually useful in the evaluation of nipple discharge because the absence of malignant cells does not reliably exclude carcinoma, and false-positive cytologic findings are not rare.[30] Mammography and ultrasonography should be performed and may identify nonpalpable masses, calcifications, or dilated ducts. The presence of imaging abnormalities in women with a pathologic nipple discharge increases the likelihood of malignancy[31] and biopsy of the abnormality should be performed. The role of galactography in the management of nipple discharge is controversial. Although ductal lesions are visualized in many women (Fig. 76.11), biopsy is still required to determine whether they are benign or malignant, and a normal galactogram in a woman with a pathologic discharge does not reliably exclude the presence of significant ductal disease.[30,32] Galactography, or the recently introduced technique of ductoscopy (mammary endoscopy),[33] however, may be useful in identifying lesions in the periphery of the breast that would not be removed with a standard terminal duct excision, and in minimizing the portion of the ductal system that is removed in women of childbearing age.

Galactorrhea, defined as the nonpuerperal discharge of milky fluid from both nipples, is not a sign of primary breast pathology. It should prompt a workup to exclude an underlying endocrine disorder, particularly a variety of amenorrhea syndromes that result in hyperprolactinemia. In addition, it may be secondary to hypothyroidism, pituitary adenoma, or chest trauma (including thoracotomy). A variety of medications, including oral contraceptives, phenothiazines, tricyclic antidepressants, metoclopramide, and reserpine, also cause galactorrhea. Persistent galactorrhea in a patient not taking any of these medications should be evaluated with measurement of the prolactin level. A persistently elevated prolactin level should prompt a search for a pituitary adenoma, but if there is

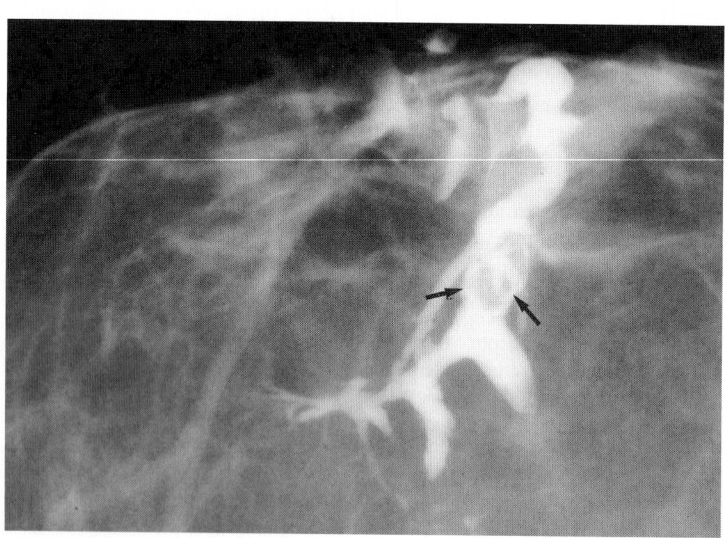

FIGURE 76.11 Ductogram. A large defect (*arrow*) represents an intraductal papilloma.

no evidence of an endocrine abnormality, these women may be followed without intervention.

Etiology

The most common cause of pathologic discharge identified in surgical specimens is a solitary papilloma (about 60% of cases); these lesions are most common in the major subareolar ducts. They consist of an epithelial layer covering a fibrovascular stroma. Peripheral papillomas are a distinctly different clinical entity, in which multiple papillomas develop in the peripheral ducts of the breast. These lesions are less likely to produce nipple discharge and tend to present as a palpable or image-detected mass.[34] Duct hyperplasia, typical or atypical, is found in 15% to 20% of women undergoing duct excision for spontaneous nipple discharge, whereas ductal carcinoma *in situ* is found in 5% to 20%.[29,31] Invasive carcinoma presenting as discharge alone is rare. Ductal ectasia may also cause nipple discharge, which is classically thick and opaque, and varies in color from pale yellow to blue-green. It may be accompanied by periductal mastitis, causing nipple inversion, and mimic carcinoma. The discharge of ductal ectasia is sometimes mistaken for an infectious process, but the ducts are usually sterile.[35]

Management

When a pathologic discharge has been identified, an attempt should be made to localize the source of the discharge within the ductal tree by galactography, or by ductoscopy. If the intraductal lesion is centrally located, terminal duct excision, also called *microdochectomy*, is the appropriate management. If the lesion is peripheral, it is necessary to localize it for excision, either by wire localization of the abnormal area on galactogram, or by ductoscopy immediately preceding the surgical excision. In a woman with clearly pathologic nipple discharge, it is reasonable to proceed with terminal duct excision even if radiologic investigations (including galactography) are normal.[30,32] Exceptions to this rule include women with a single, nonreproducible episode of discharge with normal imaging evaluation, and women with bloody nipple discharge during pregnancy.

Terminal duct excision is carried out through a circumareolar incision that includes a quarter to a third of the circumference of the areola. Duct removal should begin on the dermal surface of the nipple, as ductal disease often occurs in the proximal duct. The dilated duct is visualized after the subareolar space has been entered and excised to a depth of 2 to 3 cm in the breast parenchyma. Identification of the diseased duct can be aided by inserting a lacrimal probe into the discharging ductal orifice, or the instillation of blue dye. If ductoscopy is performed before the duct excision, the outer cannula of the endoscope can be left in place to guide resection of the appropriate segment of the duct. Patients should be warned that some nipple sensation may be lost after the procedure, in addition to the ability to breast-feed.

Breast Masses

Definition

The first step in the evaluation of a woman with a complaint of a breast mass is to verify that a dominant mass is actually present. Dominant masses may be cystic or solid and are characterized by their persistence throughout the menstrual cycle. They may be discrete or poorly defined, but they differ in character from the surrounding breast tissue and the corresponding area in the contralateral breast. Often, what the patient perceives as a breast mass is actually a normal variant of breast tissue. In premenopausal women, the normal glandular tissue of the breast is nodular, and patients often confuse such nodular glandular tissue with a dominant breast mass. Nodularity, particularly when it waxes and wanes during the menstrual cycle, is a physiologic process and not a predictor of breast disease. Morrow et al.[36] reviewed 605 women younger than 40 years of age who were referred for evaluation of a breast mass. Only 36% of the 484 masses detected by patient self-examination and 29% of the 121 masses detected by a primary care provider were confirmed surgically. The differential diagnosis of a palpable breast mass includes macrocyst, fibroadenoma, prominent areas of fibrocystic change, fat necrosis, and carcinoma.

Cysts

Cysts are a common cause of dominant breast masses, with a peak incidence in women in their 40s and perimenopausal years. Cysts are thought to result from cystic lobular involution; acini within the lobule distend to form microcysts, which in turn give rise to macrocysts. Clinically evident macrocysts are estimated to develop in 7% of Western women.

Cysts are usually well demarcated from the surrounding breast tissue, mobile, and firm. It is often difficult to distinguish a cystic from a solid lesion on physical examination, although cysts may fluctuate with the menstrual cycle, whereas solid lesions do not. Cystic lesions in postmenopausal women who are not on hormone replacement therapy are uncommon, and they should be regarded with a higher degree of suspicion than those found in premenopausal women because they may be secondary to ductal obstruction by a malignant lesion.

The initial step in the evaluation of a possible cyst is aspiration. If fluid is obtained that is not grossly bloody and the mass resolves completely, no further therapy other than a follow-up examination is needed. However, if the cystic fluid is bloody, the palpable abnormality does not resolve completely, or the same cyst recurs multiple times in a short time period, a biopsy to exclude the presence of a malignant lesion in the cyst wall is required. Cytologic examination of cyst fluid is of little value because intracystic carcinoma is rare and malignant cells are seen in fewer than 1% of cases.[37] The presence of atypical cells, an indication for surgical biopsy, is not uncommon when cyst fluid is examined, and it may pose a dilemma when a patient's cyst has resolved with aspiration and the examination and mammographic findings are now normal.

Many patients present to the surgeon with a palpable mass and an ultrasonographic examination demonstrating that the mass is a simple cyst. If the cyst is symptomatic or alarming to the patient, it can be aspirated. Otherwise, because the diagnosis has been made, it can be left alone. Nonpalpable lesions that are proved to be simple cysts by ultrasonography do not require aspiration. The management of cystic lesions is summarized in Algorithm 76.2. A dominant breast mass should not be dismissed as a cyst unless the diagnosis is confirmed by ultrasonography or cyst aspiration.

Solid Masses

Fibroadenomas. Fibroadenomas present most frequently in patients between the ages of 20 and 50 years. Their characteristic clinical presentation is that of a well-defined palpable mass that is rubbery in texture and mobile. Fibroadenomas

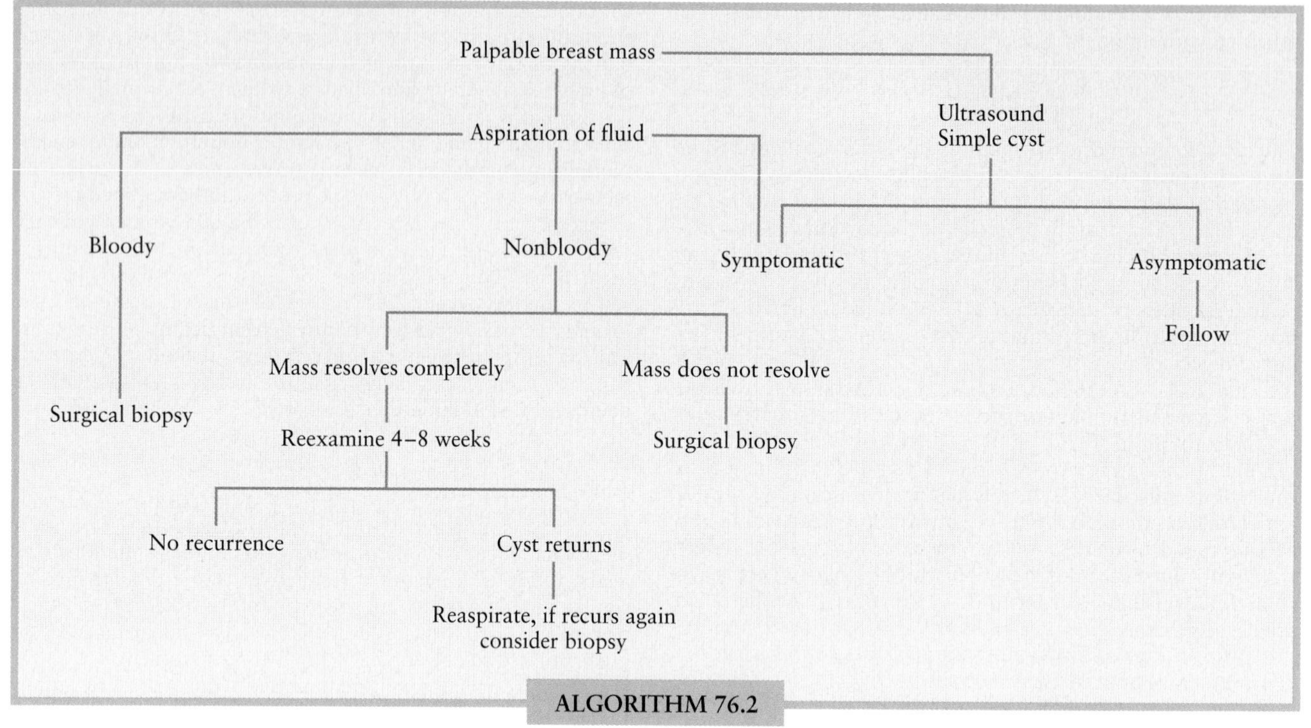

ALGORITHM 76.2 Diagnosis and management of cystic lesions. Bloody fluid on aspiration, failure of the mass to resolve completely, and prompt refilling of the same cyst are indications for surgical biopsy.

present as multiple lesions in 10% to 15% of cases. Although they have a characteristic clinical appearance, a clinical diagnosis of fibroadenoma is accurate in only one half to two thirds of cases.[38] In women younger than age 20, however, fibroadenomas account for 75% of breast biopsies.

Fibroadenomas are thought to be the result of a minor aberration in the normal process of lobular development. Hormonal factors appear to be important in their growth, as evidenced by the clinical observation of the involution of fibroadenomas after menopause and their dramatic increase in size during pregnancy. In postmenopausal women receiving estrogen alone, fibroadenomas may increase in size relative to the surrounding breast parenchyma.

Sonographic criteria for the diagnosis of fibroadenoma include a round or oval, well-circumscribed, solid mass with homogeneous, low-level internal echoes and intermediate acoustic attenuation. As many as 30% of fibroadenomas, however, lack these "classic" features.

In rare circumstances, fibroadenomas have been associated with carcinoma. More than 160 cases of associated cancers have been reported in the literature, including ductal carcinoma *in situ* and infiltrating lobular and ductal carcinomas. Historically, it has been widely accepted that fibroadenomas do not confer an increased breast cancer risk. However, four population-based retrospective studies have shown a small (relative risk of 1.3 to 1.9) but significant increased risk for breast cancer development that persists over time.[39–42] This slight increase in risk should have no impact on the clinical management of fibroadenomas. Although fibroadenomas can be suspected on the basis of their characteristic clinical presentation, a final diagnosis cannot be made without histologic or cytologic confirmation.

Fibrocystic Disease. *Fibrocystic disease* is a common term that is used to describe a variety of benign breast disorders. It is not a clinically meaningful term because it encompasses a heterogeneous group of processes, some pathologic and some physiologic, with widely varying cancer risks. The cancer risks associated with benign breast disease are discussed in the section on breast cancer risk factors. The term *fibrocystic change* is not a synonym for lumpy breasts, and if used at all, it should be reserved for women in whom a breast biopsy has demonstrated one of the histologic components of fibrocystic change. Frequently, when a breast biopsy is performed for vague areas of nodularity that lack mammographic or ultrasonographic correlates, a fibrocystic process is the diagnosis.

Fat Necrosis. Fat necrosis in the breast may occur secondary to trauma, breast surgery, infection, or radiation therapy, although in approximately 50% of cases, no antecedent cause can be identified. Fat necrosis is seen most commonly in women with pendulous breasts and those who are overweight. It is clinically significant in that on both physical examination and mammography, it may be indistinguishable from carcinoma. The lesions of fat necrosis are typically firm, painless, and poorly defined. Because fat necrosis usually occurs in the superficial breast tissue, it may be accompanied by skin thickening, dimpling, or retraction. The mammographic findings of fat necrosis include spiculated masses, microcalcifications, and architectural distortion. Only when the characteristic oil cyst, a circumscribed mass of mixed soft-tissue density and fat with a rim that is often calcified, is seen can an unequivocal diagnosis of fat necrosis be made radiographically (Fig. 76.12). In the absence of this finding or a clear history of trauma, biopsy is required to exclude the presence of malignancy.

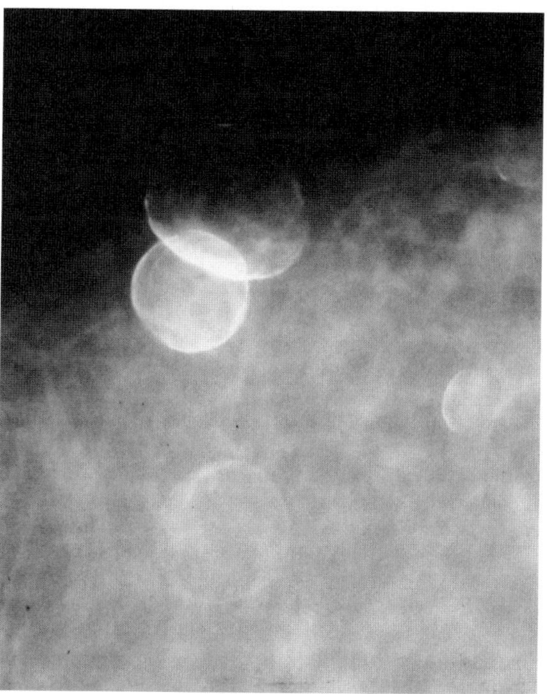

FIGURE 76.12 Oil cysts. The calcified rims of these cysts in a patient with a history of trauma are diagnostic.

Diagnostic Imaging. When a clinical abnormality has been identified in a woman over age 40, a diagnostic mammogram should be obtained before a histologic diagnosis is attempted. Imaging studies are used to define the extent of a potential malignancy and to identify nonpalpable masses or associated calcifications elsewhere in the ipsilateral or contralateral breast that might influence definitive therapy. The decision to perform a biopsy, however, is based on the clinical determination that a dominant mass is present, and nonvisualization of a mass on imaging studies should not dissuade the surgeon from performing a breast biopsy. In two reports, between 10% and 22% of patients with palpable breast cancer had tumors that were not visible by mammography.[43,44] Obtaining a diagnostic, rather than a screening, mammogram ensures that a marker will be placed on the area of palpable concern, so that the clinical and radiographic findings can be correlated. Identifying the site of a lesion also ensures that lesions at the periphery of the breast will be included on the film, which helps to eliminate one cause of false–negative mammograms. A diagnostic mammogram also includes magnification views of the lesion, which are useful in determining the extent of any associated calcifications.

The routine use of ultrasonography for the evaluation of solid palpable masses remains controversial. Studies of high-resolution ultrasonography have demonstrated that the technique is more accurate and sensitive and has a better negative predictive value than mammography alone.[45] If follow-up of a clinically benign lesion is being considered, ultrasonography is a useful adjunct to mammography, as discussed in the section on the clinical approach to the patient with a solid breast mass. In the patient with a clinically suspect mass who will undergo biopsy regardless of the results of imaging studies, ultrasonography has been shown to provide a more accurate estimate of lesion size than mammography,[46] and it may also identify satellite lesions not seen on mammography. Ultrasonography is also useful in the woman with a palpable mass that is not clearly seen on mammography; in such cases, it may help to define the extent of the lesion more completely than physical examination alone.

In women under age 40 presenting with a clinically unworrisome breast mass, the rationale for mammographic imaging is less compelling because carcinoma is uncommon and the density of the breasts often obscures mass lesions. Directed ultrasonography allows the presence of a true mass lesion to be confirmed when the significance of a physical finding is clinically uncertain.[36] The presence of benign characteristics on ultrasonography also supports the use of a follow-up approach. In younger women with clinically suspect masses, mammography should be performed.

Other Imaging Studies. Magnetic resonance imaging (MRI) of the breast is increasingly being used for clinical breast imaging, although the lack of standardization of the procedure, the difficulty in sampling lesions seen on MRI alone, the lack of specificity of the procedure, and the high cost of MRI have limited its application. There is great interest in the use of MRI in women with known breast cancer to improve selection for breast-conserving therapy (BCT). In a multicenter study of 426 patients with cancer, 24% were found to have additional abnormalities by MRI. Of the 78 who were biopsied, 56 were shown to be cancer.[47] Other studies of MRI in this setting report additional cancer in 10% to 34% of subjects. A major unanswered question is the clinical significance of these occult cancer foci. Pathology studies have documented the presence of additional microscopic areas of cancer in 32% to 63% of patients with clinically localized carcinoma.[48] The presence of these multifocal and multicentric areas of cancer was used to argue that mastectomy was the only appropriate surgical therapy for breast cancer. Extensive clinical experience has shown that radiotherapy controls the majority of these occult tumor foci. Although MRI is capable of identifying some of these occult tumor foci, before this is used as rationale for the routine use of MRI, improvement in clinical end points such as local recurrence of the number of surgeries needed to obtain negative margins must be demonstrated.

Other clinical applications of MRI are to detect an implant rupture and to look for a primary breast tumor in patients presenting with axillary adenopathy caused by metastatic tumor from an unknown primary site (see section on occult primary tumor presenting with nodal metastases). The role of MRI in assessing the response of a tumor to preoperative chemotherapy is also under study. The role of screening MRI in women at very high risk of breast cancer development is discussed in "Management of the High-Risk Woman."

Positron emission tomography (PET) with 18F fluorodeoxyglucose (FDG) can be used not only to image breast abnormalities but also to assess their metabolic activity for diagnostic and prognostic purposes. FDG uptake is increased in both primary and metastatic breast cancer. Whole-body PET scanning is currently used to evaluate undiagnosed lesions that could represent metastatic disease. Its use as a diagnostic technique for indeterminate breast masses and to monitor response to therapy is under study.[49]

Biopsy Techniques for Solid Breast Masses. A variety of biopsy techniques are available to obtain a pathologic diagnosis of clinically evident breast masses. Each has advantages and disadvantages, and no single technique is applicable to all clinical circumstances.

Fine-needle aspiration biopsy. Fine-needle aspiration (FNA) cytology has a very high diagnostic accuracy rate in the hands

TABLE 76.4 TREATMENT

MANAGEMENT OF BREAST MASSES BASED ON FINE-NEEDLE ASPIRATION (FNA) DIAGNOSIS

FNA diagnosis	Treatment
Malignant	Definitive therapy
Suspicious	Surgical biopsy
Atypia	Surgical biopsy
Benign	Possible observation[a]
Nondiagnostic	Repeated FNA or surgical biopsy

[a]See discussion in text on clinical approach to the patient with a solid breast mass.

of experienced clinicians and cytopathologists. In a review of 31,340 procedures,[50] its sensitivity ranged from 65% to 98%. In most series, false–positive rates are less than 1%, false—negative rates are below 10%, and the incidence of insufficient specimens ranges from 4% to 13%. Small tumor size, fibrotic tumors, and certain histologic tumor types, such as infiltrating lobular, tubular, and cribriform carcinoma, have been associated with a higher likelihood of false-negative results. Most false-negative results are the consequence of sampling errors rather than misinterpretation by the cytopathologist.

The advantages of FNA include its simplicity and quickness, low cost, low morbidity, and availability as an office procedure. Because an unequivocal diagnosis of malignancy by FNA is reliable, treatment options can be discussed with the patient and definitive surgery can be performed without the need for a surgical biopsy. It is imperative, however, that the surgeon be aware of the meaning of positive cytology at a particular institution, because the sensitivities of FNA at institutions that do not have access to an experienced cytopathologist may not be as high as those reported in the literature. Stratification of FNA diagnoses as described in Table 76.4 will help to minimize this problem. The management of breast lesions on the basis of FNA results is summarized in Table 76.4.

Core needle biopsy. Core needle biopsy is another office diagnostic technique that is rapid, inexpensive, and relatively painless. A core needle biopsy differs from FNA in that a core of tissue is obtained for histologic examination, so that a more detailed characterization of the lesion is possible and the adequacy of the specimen can be evaluated at the time of the biopsy. In addition, the material can be evaluated by any surgical pathologist. In one series in which the diagnostic accuracy of aspiration cytology was compared with core needle biopsy in 81 patients who had breast masses, aspiration cytology was diagnostic in 95% of cases, and core needle biopsy was diagnostic in 70% of the cases in which it was used.[51] False–negative results occur when the needle is deflected into the surrounding fat by a hard tumor mass. In practice, the selection of the type of needle biopsy (FNA or core) often depends on the availability of a cytopathologist and the surgeon's level of comfort with a cytologic diagnosis of malignancy without further histologic detail. The difference between an FNA specimen and a core needle specimen is illustrated in Figure 76.13.

Excisional biopsy. Excisional biopsy is the complete removal of a breast mass. It is definitive therapy for a benign breast mass and may also serve as a therapeutic lumpectomy if the specimen includes a margin of normal breast tissue around a malignant tumor. Kearney and Morrow[52] obtained negative margins with a conservative diagnostic lumpectomy in 161 of 173 (93.1%) consecutive patients. The adequacy of a biopsy specimen cannot be assessed unless the margins of the specimen are inked. The use of orienting sutures in two margins of the specimen makes it possible to identify which margin contains tumor should the excision be incomplete; as a result, less normal breast tissue has to be removed in a repeated excision. In this era of breast-conserving surgery, orientation and inking of excisional breast biopsy specimens should be routine practice.

Excisional biopsy is an outpatient procedure that can usually be carried out under local anesthesia with intravenous sedation, as needed. Excisional biopsy is usually planned as a two-step procedure, (i.e., excisional biopsy with additional therapy at a later date if required). This allows for a detailed review of the pathology and a discussion of treatment options

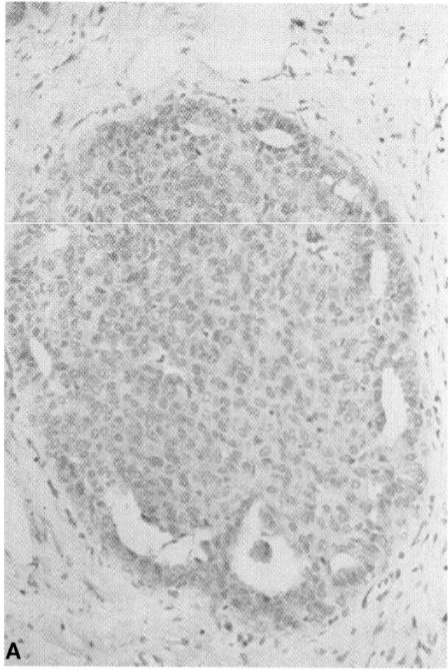

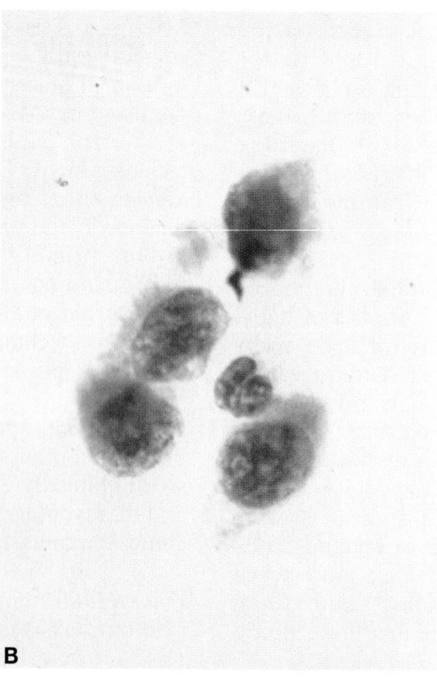

FIGURE 76.13 Comparison of core needle biopsy specimen (*A*) and fine-needle aspiration specimen (*B*). Architectural detail is seen only in the core specimen.

with the patient, in addition to consultation with a radiation oncologist or reconstructive surgeon as desired by the patient. Delays of up to 1 month from the time of diagnosis to definitive therapy have not been shown to affect prognosis[53]; therefore, the two-step procedure is the preferred method of management. However, diagnosis by needle biopsy techniques is reliable, more cost-effective than surgical biopsy, and avoids placement of an incision on the breast before definitive local therapy. For the vast majority of breast masses, needle biopsy is the preferred diagnostic technique.

Incisional biopsy. Incisional biopsy is a diagnostic procedure reserved for masses that are too large to be completely excised. Today, the indications for incisional biopsy are few, because FNA or core needle biopsy can be used to make a diagnosis of breast cancer with less morbidity and at lower cost. The widespread availability of immunohistochemistry allows hormone receptor status to be determined and tumor markers to be studied in core specimens or cytologic aspirates.

Clinical approach to the patient with a solid breast mass. The accuracy of physical examination alone to detect carcinoma is limited because the clinical characteristics of benign and malignant masses are not absolute, and a clinical diagnosis is correct in only 60% to 85% of cases.[51,54] The difficulty of distinguishing benign from malignant lesions is greatest in young women, and the use of other studies to confirm the clinical diagnosis of a benign breast mass is essential before the patient is returned to routine follow-up.

The extent of the workup necessary to exclude the presence of carcinoma varies with the degree of suspicion and the age of the patient. In the patient with a clinically suspect mass, regardless of age, diagnostic mammography and ultrasonography should be performed before a histologic diagnosis is sought. A needle biopsy (either aspiration cytology or core biopsy) is the preferred initial method of making a diagnosis, for the reasons discussed in the preceding sections on fine-needle aspiration biopsy and core needle biopsy. If a diagnosis of malignancy is obtained, treatment options are discussed with the patient. If a diagnosis of cancer is not obtained, excisional biopsy is undertaken because of the known false–negative rates of both FNA and core biopsy. This approach is summarized in Algorithm 76.3.

In the woman with a clinically benign mass, management varies somewhat with age (Algorithm 76.4). In women under age 40, the first step is to determine if the patient wants the mass to be excised, regardless of the likelihood of malignancy. If so, imaging studies are not indicated because of the low risk for carcinoma in this age group. For the patient who desires follow-up, ultrasonography and FNA or core biopsy should be performed. If both confirm that the lesion has benign features, clinical follow-up can be undertaken, with regular monitoring of the lesion for a period of 1 to 2 years to confirm that carcinoma is not present. The combination of clinical examination, FNA, and ultrasonography provides an accurate differentiation between benign and malignant lesions in 95% of cases.[55] For this reason, in addition to the low risk for malignancy in this age group, follow-up is a safe approach.

In patients over age 40, mammography and ultrasonography should be obtained before a decision about the need for excision or follow-up is made. If follow-up is chosen, needle biopsy is also performed. If the mass is visualized on

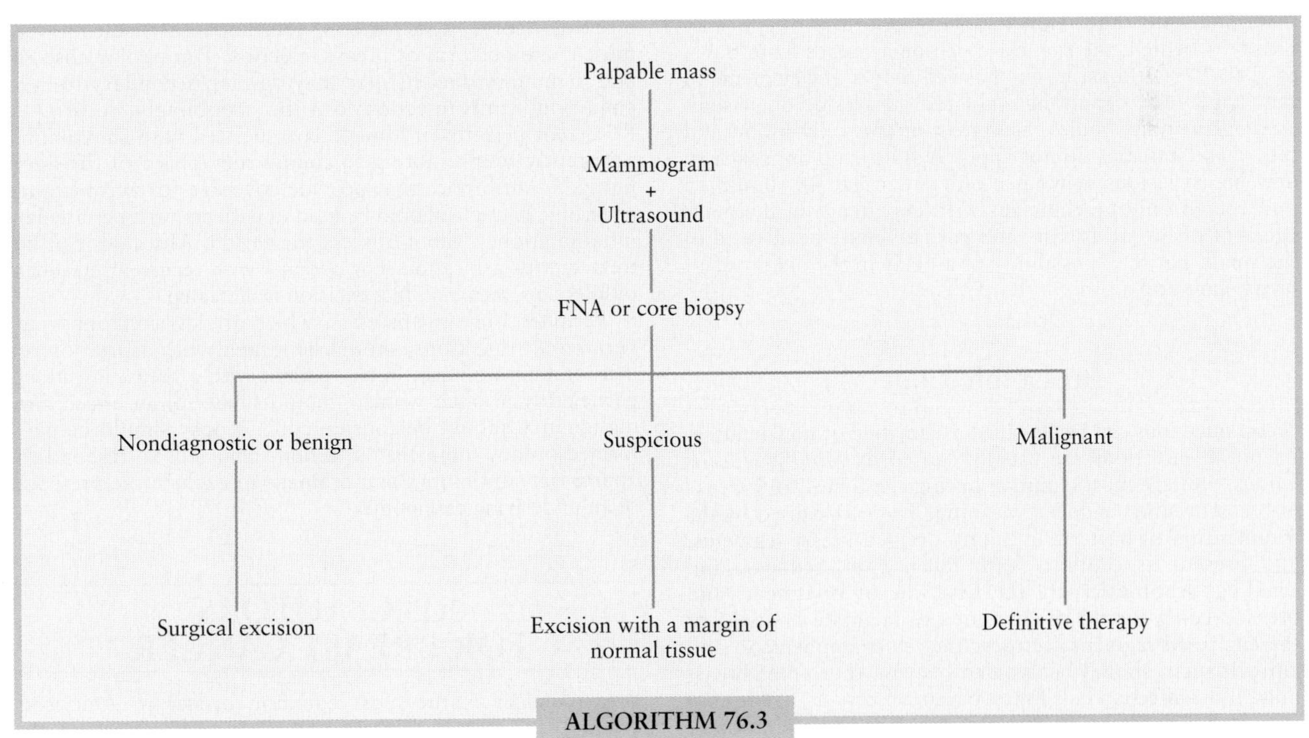

ALGORITHM 76.3 Diagnosis and management of the patient with a clinically indeterminate or suspect solid breast mass. In this circumstance, imaging studies are insufficient to exclude malignancy, and tissue sampling is required.

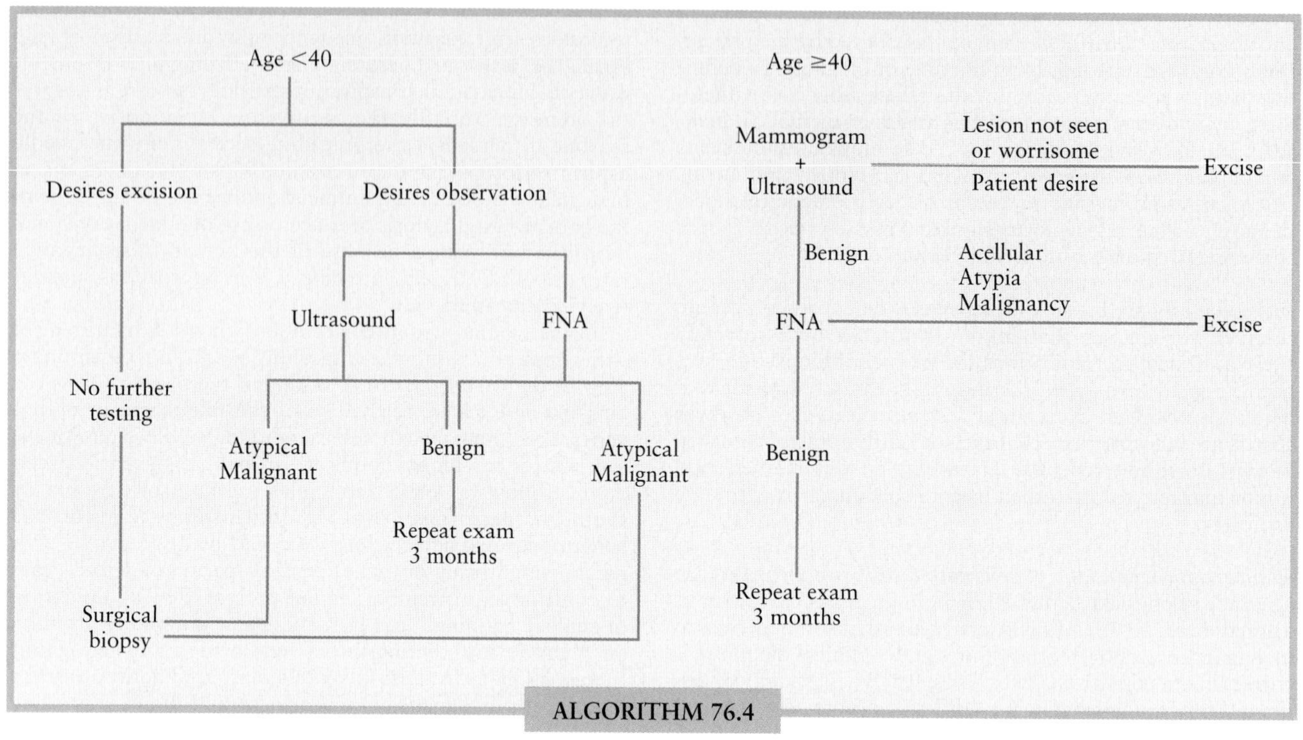

ALGORITHM 76.4 Diagnosis and the management of clinically benign breast masses. The use of imaging studies varies according to age because carcinoma is infrequent in women under age 40.

mammography and appears benign, and if the needle biopsy is benign, the risk for carcinoma ranges from 0.6% to 3.4%.[56,57] It must be emphasized that if any elements of the "triple test" cannot be evaluated (i.e., lesion not visualized on imaging studies, aspirate contains only blood and fat), these statistics do not apply. A follow-up approach to new breast lesions in women older than age 40 should be undertaken only by clinicians with experience in the management of breast disease, and patients must be advised of the small, but real, possibility of a delay in the diagnosis of breast carcinoma.

Breast Infections

Breast infections can be classified as lactating or nonlactating. Lactating infections are usually caused by *Staphylococcus aureus*, and are most common during the first 4 to 6 weeks of breast-feeding or during weaning. They are caused by the proliferation of bacteria in poorly drained breast segments, and present as cellulitis with fever, pain, redness, and swelling. Antibiotics are the first line of treatment, and breast-feeding should be continued to facilitate drainage of the engorged segment. Tetracycline, chloramphenicol, and ciprofloxacin should be avoided because they enter breast milk. If the infection fails to resolve, an abscess should be considered. When the breast skin is intact, repeated aspiration of the abscess combined with antibiotics is the preferred treatment.[58] When the skin is thinned, a small incision will facilitate drainage.

In nonlactating women, a syndrome characterized by periareolar inflammation, sometimes associated with a purulent nipple discharge, which affects premenopausal women, is the most common form of breast infection. Periareolar abscess and mammary duct fistulae may develop secondary to this condition, and infection can be troublingly recurrent. Recurrent periareolar abscess is associated with smoking,[59] apparently by promoting squamous metaplasia of the duct lining.[60] Antibiotics that provide coverage for aerobic and anaerobic bacteria should be used in patients with periareolar inflammation without abscess formation. Abscesses can be treated with aspiration. For patients with recurrent episodes of infection, terminal duct excision is indicated.

Peripheral breast abscesses, which are less common than periareolar infections, should be treated with aspiration or incision and drainage. In any patient with a breast infection, particularly in older women, the possibility of an underlying malignancy should be considered. A biopsy should be performed on any apparent "infection" that fails to respond to appropriate antibiotics and drainage to exclude the presence of an underlying carcinoma.

RISK FACTORS FOR BREAST CANCER

Breast cancer is the most common cancer in American women, the second most common cause of cancer death, and a major cause of cancer death in most industrialized nations. Approximately 192,000 cases of breast cancer and 44,000 breast cancer deaths occur annually in American women. Many factors that increase the risk for the development of breast cancer have been identified, and have become clinically important since the demonstration that tamoxifen use can protect high-risk women from breast cancer (see section on management of the high-risk woman). Risk can be described as the absolute risk for the development of breast cancer, either over the lifetime (usually to age 90) or within a given time interval (e.g., 2.5% during the next 5 years). Risk may also be expressed as a relative risk (RR), a comparison of the incidence of disease in a population having a particular risk factor with the incidence in a population lacking that risk factor. Understanding the clinical implications of RR requires a knowledge of the absolute risk of breast cancer in the index population and, although it is a useful measure for research purposes, it is not particularly useful for the discussion of risk clinically. Risk information is best provided to patients as absolute risk within a given time period.

Age

The most common breast cancer risk factor is age. Half of a woman's lifetime risk for breast cancer development occurs after age 65. Between the ages of 35 to 55, the risk for breast cancer development is only 2.5%, and the risk for breast cancer death is only about one third of that.[61] The incidence of breast cancer across age groups has been fairly stable, although an increase in the number of young women in the population has resulted in an increase in the number of cases seen in this group, without a change in incidence rate. Breast cancer at a young age is more common in black women than in white women. At age 40, the incidence curves cross, and the disease becomes more common in white women.

Family History

There are two distinct types of risk associated with a family history of breast carcinoma. Approximately 20% to 30% of women with breast cancer have a family history of the disease, but only 5% to 10% have an inherited mutation in a breast cancer susceptibility gene.[62,63] Distinguishing between familial and true hereditary breast cancer is important because the associated level of risk varies widely.

The majority of cases of genetic breast cancer are caused by mutations of *BRCA1* and *BRCA2*. Mutations of either of these genes carry a lifetime risk for breast cancer development of 37% to 85%,[64,65] a high risk of contralateral breast cancer, and an increased risk for ovarian cancer. Although the risk for ovarian cancer is elevated with mutations of both *BRCA1* and *BRCA2*, it is greater in carriers of the *BRCA1* mutation. In *BRCA2* families, the risk for male breast cancer, prostate cancer, and pancreatic cancer is increased.[66,67] These mutations can be inherited from both maternal and paternal relatives, and are summarized in Table 76.5. The carrier frequency of these mutations varies with the population under study. The frequency of *BRCA1* mutations is between 1/500 and 1/800, and the frequency of *BRCA2* mutations is lower in the general population. In persons of Ashkenazi Jewish descent, however, two specific mutations of *BRCA1* (185delAG and 5382insC) and one *BRCA2* mutation (6174delT) are seen with a background frequency of 2.3%.[64] These are known as *founder mutations*, thought to arise from common ancestry, and have been identified in other ethnic populations in Iceland, France, Russia, Holland, Sweden, and Belgium.

Features of the family history that suggest mutations in *BRCA1* or *BRCA2* include having two or more relatives affected with early-onset breast or ovarian cancer, or both, with involvement of two or more generations in a pattern consistent with autosomal dominant inheritance. This can be through maternal or paternal relatives. A typical pedigree is shown in Figure 76.14. The likelihood of a mutation also varies with ethnic ancestry. For example, in an Ashkenazi Jewish family with two cases of breast cancer and one case of ovarian cancer, the chance of a *BRCA1* mutation is 75%, but in a non-Ashkenazi family with the same history, the probability is only 33%.[68] Models have been developed and validated to assist clinicians in estimating the probability of a mutation.[69]

Genetic testing for mutations of *BRCA1* and *BRCA2* is now a commercially available option for women with a family history suggestive of a genetic mutation. Genetic testing should always be preceded by a counseling session in which the complexities of genetic testing and the potential emotional and financial ramifications of test results are discussed. The information obtained from testing will be maximized by first testing a family member affected with breast or ovarian cancer, or both. If the affected person does not carry a mutation, testing an unaffected relative is unlikely to be informative.

Other, infrequent genetic breast cancer syndromes include the Li-Fraumeni syndrome, Cowden's syndrome, and the Lynch syndromes. The Li-Fraumeni syndrome is associated with mutations in the tumor-suppressor gene *p53*, and is an autosomal dominant condition characterized by soft-tissue sarcomas, osteosarcomas, brain tumors, leukemia, adrenocortical malignancies, and early-onset breast cancer.[70]

For the majority of women with a family history of breast cancer that is not associated with an inherited mutation, the level of risk is much lower and rarely exceeds 30%.

TABLE 76.5

ESTIMATED LIFETIME CANCER RISKS FOR *BRCA1* AND *BRCA2* MUTATIONS (TO AGE 70)

Type of cancer	General population (%)	*BRCA1* carrier (%)	*BRCA2* carrier (%)
Breast cancer	8.0	40–85	40–85
Contralateral breast cancer	0.5–1/year	40–65	40–65
Male breast cancer	0.1	1–5	5–10
Ovarian cancer	1.4	30–45	10–20

(Modified from Isaacs C, Peshkin BN, Lerman C. Evaluation and management of women with a strong family history of breast cancer. In: Harris JR, Lippman ME, Morrow M, et al., eds. *Diseases of the breast*, 3rd ed. Philadelphia: Lippincott Williams & Wilkins, 2004, p. 316.)

Hormonal Factors

Numerous studies have linked breast cancer risk to the lifetime exposure to estrogens, as refected by age at menarche, menopause and first pregnancy, and postmenopausal obesity.[71] Conversely, women who undergo bilateral oophorectomy before menopause are at decreased risk, with the magnitude of benefit increasing as the age at oophorectomy decreases. In general, hormonal risk factors are associated with RR in

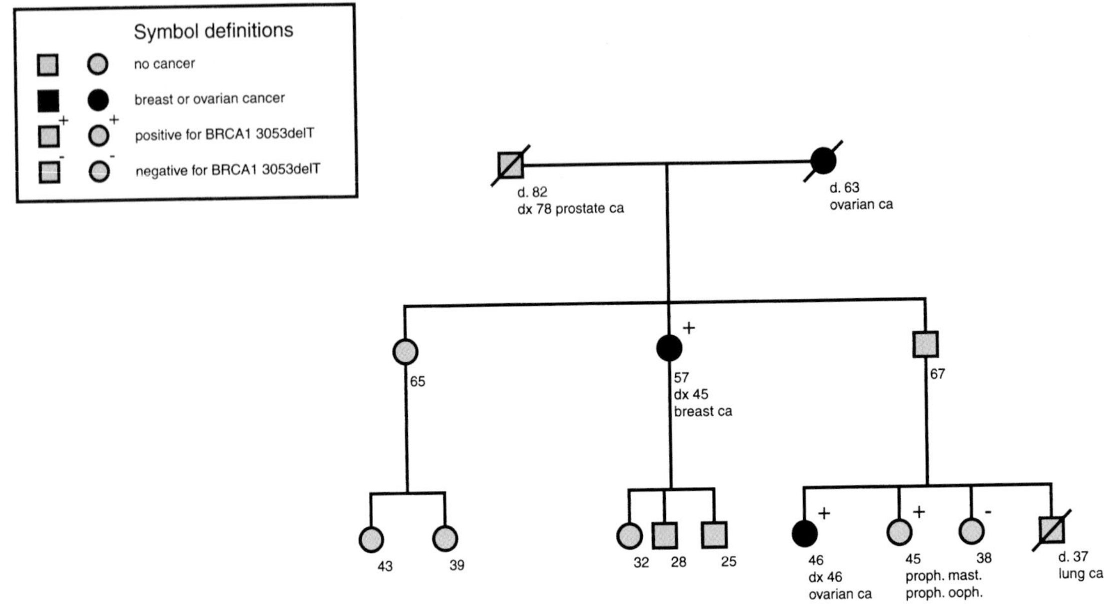

FIGURE 76.14 Pedigree of genetic breast cancer. The family illustrated in the pedigree carries a mutation of the *BRCA1* gene; multiple relatives are affected with breast and ovarian cancer.

the range of 1.5 to 2.0. Studies of the effect of lactation on breast cancer risk have been inconclusive, but a long duration of lactation appears to reduce risk in premenopausal women.[72]

There is no convincing evidence for an effect of oral contraceptive use on breast cancer risk, despite extensive study,[73] but use of combination postmenopausal hormone replacement therapy (estrogen plus progesterone), appears to be associated with a small increase in breast cancer risk.[74]

Environmental Factors and Diet

Exposure to ionizing radiation, whether from a nuclear explosion or medical procedure, increases breast cancer risk. The level of risk varies with age at exposure, being greatest for exposures in childhood and adolescence, and minimal for exposures after age 40. Patients who were treated with mantle irradiation for Hodgkin's lymphoma in their adolescent or childhood years are the group at risk on the basis of radiation exposure most commonly encountered today.[75]

Much attention has been devoted to the role of diet in breast cancer etiology, but prospective studies of diet and breast cancer risk within the context of American diets fail to confirm this relationship, at least for fat consumption within adult life.[76,77] Stronger evidence exists to support an association between alcohol intake and breast cancer risk.[78]

BENIGN BREAST DISEASE

Benign breast lesions are classified as nonproliferative, proliferative, or proliferative with atypia (Table 76.6). Nonproliferative lesions, which are not associated with an increased risk for breast cancer development, account for approximately 70% of palpable breast masses.[79] Proliferative lesions without atypia are associated with a small increase in breast cancer risk (RR, 1.5 to 2.0). Proliferative lesions with atypia are uncommon, comprising only 3.6% of palpable breast masses and 7% to 10% of nonpalpable abnormalities. Atypical lesions are associated with a RR of 4.0 to 5.0, which increases to 9.0 when they are found in a woman having a first-degree relative with breast cancer.[79]

TABLE 76.6 CLASSIFICATION

CLASSIFICATION OF BENIGN BREAST DISEASE

Nonproliferative: No Increase in Risk
Cysts: micro or macro
Ductal ectasia
Simple fibroadenoma
Mastitis
Fibrosis
Metaplasia: squamous or apocrine
Mild hyperplasia
Proliferative: RR 1.5–2.0
Complex fibroadenoma
Papilloma
Sclerosing adenosis
Hyperplasia; moderate or severe
Proliferative with Atypia: RR 4.5–5.0
Atypical ductal hyperplasia
Atypical lobular hyperplasia

RR, relative risk.

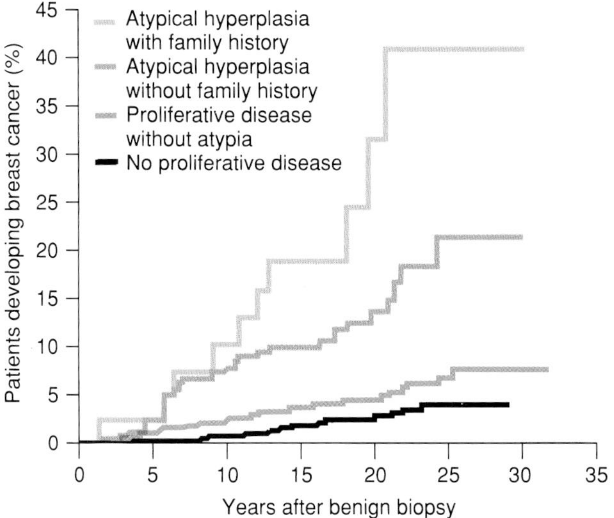

FIGURE 76.15 Cumulative risk for the development of invasive breast cancer after a biopsy for benign breast disease. Women with atypical hyperplasia (ductal or lobular type) are at a significantly increased risk for the development of breast cancer. (From Page DL, Dupont WD. Anatomic markers of human premalignancy and risk of breast cancer. *Cancer* 1990;66:1326, with permission.)

As illustrated in Figure 76.15, however, breast cancer will have developed at 15 years in only 10% of women with atypical hyperplasia alone.

Lobular Carcinoma *In Situ*

Lobular carcinoma *in situ* (LCIS) is now accepted as a breast cancer risk factor and is not thought to be a malignancy that progresses locally. Lobular proliferation is designated as lobular intraepithelial neoplasia (LIN) with lobular hyperplasia without atypia being described as grade1 LIN, atypical lobular hyperplasia as grade 2 LIN, and LCIS as grade 3 LIN, with the intention of clarifying its role as a high risk lesion rather than a malignancy. LIN occurs predominantly in premenopausal women; it generally does not form lumps or cause radiologic changes, and is usually identifed incidentally with other benign changes in women who require biopsy. Women diagnosed with grade 3 LIN have a RR for breast cancer development ranging from 5.4 to 12.[80–86] This translates in most studies to a risk for breast cancer development of about 1% per year (Table 76.7). The risk affects both breasts, and subsequest cancer may be infiltrating ductal carcinoma or infiltrating lobular carcinoma.[81–86] The increased risk for breast cancer development after a diagnosis of LCIS persists indefinitely.

TABLE 76.7

RISK FOR BREAST CANCER DEVELOPMENT AFTER LOBULAR CARCINOMA IN SITU

Study	No. patients	Invasive cancer (%)	Follow-up (y)	Relative risk
Haagensen.[80]	287	18	16.3	6.9
Rosen et al.[81]	99	12.5	24	9.0
Andersen[82]	47	26.4	15	12.0
Page et al.[83]	44	23	18	9.0
Salvadori et al.[84]	80	6.3	5	10.3
Ottesen et al.[85]	69	11.6	5	11.0
Bodian et al.[86]	236	26[a]	18	5.4
Fisher et al.[91]	182	33	5	—

[a]Includes intraductal and invasive cancer.

CLINICAL ASSESSMENT OF RISK

Many factors that increase breast cancer risk have been identified in studies of large populations and are summarized in Table 76.8, but are of uncertain benefit in counselling the individual woman. Several of these have been integrated into a model to allow calculation of risk for an individual woman by Gail and colleagues.[87] These include age, age at menarche, age at first live birth, number of first-degree relatives with breast cancer, number of prior breast biopsies, and whether or not any of the biopsies showed atypical hyperplasia. This model calculates risk over a defined time interval, allows comparison with age-specific incidence figures, and has been shown to predict risk accurately in groups of women undergoing annual mammographic screening. It is a useful tool for counseling women who are concerned about their level of risk. It is not an appropriate model, however, for women at risk because of a strong family history of breast cancer, particularly early onset breast cancer, or those with LCIS. A sample Gail model risk calculation is shown in Figure 76.16. A more appropriate risk model for women with strong family histories, which has not, however, been validated to the same extent as the Gail model, was described by Claus et al.,[88] and considers both the age at onset in affected relatives and the history of cancer in second-degree relatives.

TABLE 76.8

MAGNITUDE OF KNOWN BREAST CANCER RISK FACTORS

RELATIVE RISK <2
Early menarche
Late menopause
Nulliparity
Proliferative benign disease
Obesity
Alcohol use
Hormone replacement therapy

RELATIVE RISK 2–4
Age >35 first birth
First-degree relative with breast cancer
Radiation exposure
Prior breast cancer

RELATIVE RISK >4
Gene mutation
Lobular carcinoma in situ
Atypical hyperplasia

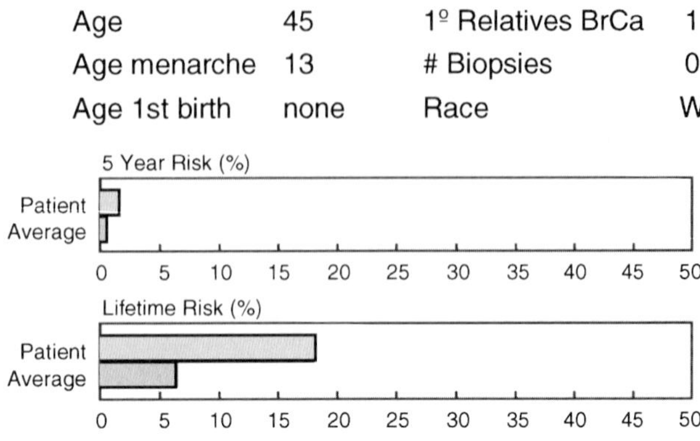

FIGURE 76.16 Breast cancer risk assessment according to the Gail model. This woman's 5-year risk for the development of breast cancer is 1.6%, and her lifetime risk is 18%.

MANAGEMENT OF THE HIGH-RISK WOMAN

Two strategies are available to reduce the risk for breast cancer development in women at increased risk—prophylactic mastectomy and tamoxifen. Prophylactic mastectomy does not provide 100% protection against breast cancer development. Both subcutaneous and total (simple) mastectomies have been used for prevention, and the development of carcinoma in residual breast tissue has been reported after both types of surgery. The efficacy of prophylactic mastectomy in a group of high-risk women was defined in a study of 639 women from the Mayo Clinic, of whom 90% underwent subcutaneous mastectomy and 10% received total mastectomy.[89] At a median of 14 years, prophylactic mastectomy reduced the risk for breast cancer by 90%. Prophylactic mastectomy is a radical prevention option that should be undertaken only after a complete risk assessment, consultation with a reconstructive surgeon, and a thorough discussion of management alternatives. Women should be advised of their level of risk and assisted in determining if that level of risk is unacceptable to them, rather than being told to undergo prophylactic surgery. When prophylactic mastectomy is performed, the procedure should be a total mastectomy with removal of the nipple–areola complex, extended to the same anatomic limits as a therapeutic mastectomy. Patients undergoing prophylactic mastectomy are ideal candidates for a skin-sparing approach to facilitate immediate breast reconstruction (Fig. 76.17).

An alternative strategy for breast cancer prevention is the selective ER modulator (SERM), tamoxifen. Tamoxifen has been used to treat breast cancer for more than 25 years. Data from treatment trials, most recently updated in the 2001 Oxford Overview Analysis,[90] demonstrated that women taking tamoxifen for 5 years had a 47% reduction in the incidence of contralateral breast cancer. Similar findings from earlier studies served as the impetus for the National Surgical Adjuvant Breast and Bowel Project (NSABP) P-1 prevention trial, in which 13,388 women at increased risk for breast cancer development were randomized to tamoxifen or placebo.[91] Risk was defined by the Gail model.[87] Eligible women included those who were age 60 or older, or those between the ages of 35 and 59 years with a predicted 5-year breast cancer risk of 1.66% or more. After a median follow-up of 54.6 months, a 49% reduction in the risk for invasive cancer and a 50% reduction in the risk for noninvasive cancer

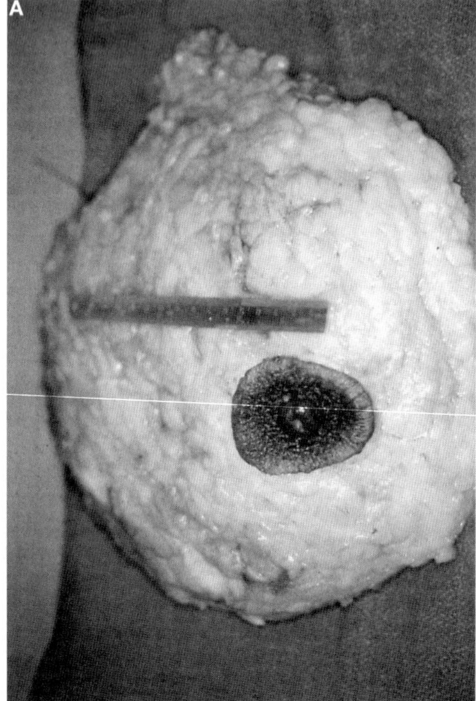

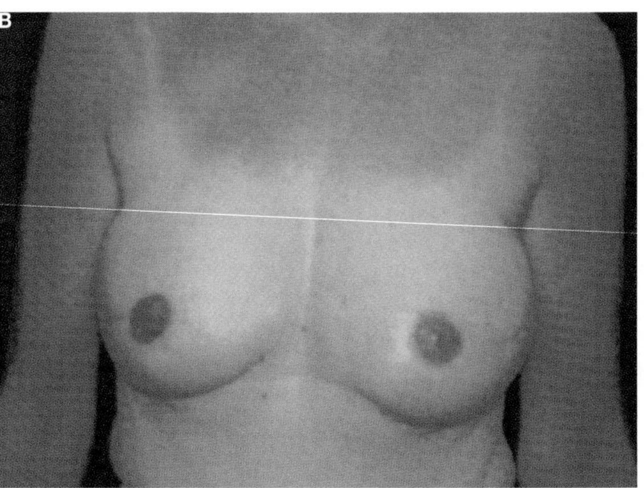

FIGURE 76.17 Skin-sparing mastectomy. (*A*) The only skin removed was the nipple–areola complex. (*B*) Cosmetic outcome after bilateral skin-sparing mastectomy and transverse rectus abdominis myocutaneous (TRAM) flap reconstruction.

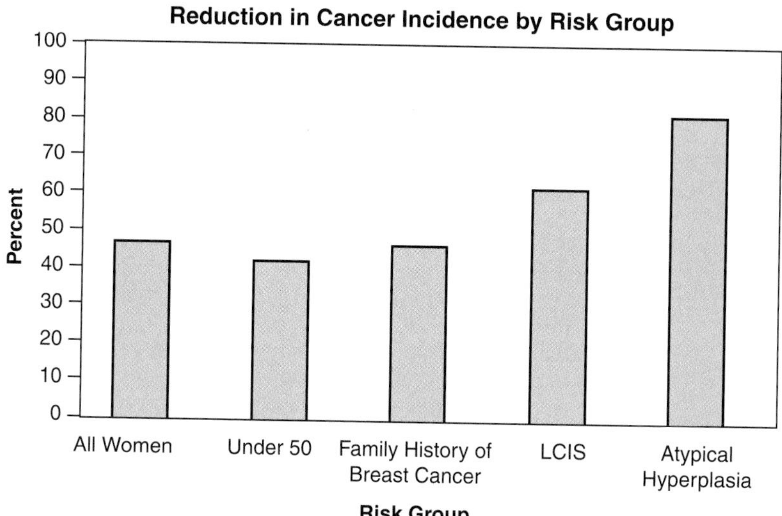

FIGURE 76.18 Tamoxifen for breast cancer prevention. Although tamoxifen was effective in all subgroups of high-risk women, particular benefit was seen in those at risk on the basis of lobular carcinoma *in situ* and atypical hyperplasia.

were seen in the tamoxifen group (Fig. 76.18). The reduction occurred only in ER-positive tumors, and the occurrence of ER-negative tumors was unchanged. Tamoxifen was of benefit in all age groups, in women at risk on the basis of a family history, as well as those eligible for the study on the basis of other risk factors. A particular benefit was observed in women at risk on the basis of LCIS and atypical hyperplasia, in whom risk reductions of 65% and 86%, respectively, were seen.[91] Postmenopausal women experienced a 19% reduction in the incidence of fractures, including a 45% reduction in hip fracture. This approached statistical significance.

The most common side effects of tamoxifen were hot flashes and vaginal discharge. Participants who took tamoxifen had a 2.5 times greater risk for endometrial carcinoma than those in the placebo group, and all the excess risk was seen in postmenopausal women. An increased risk for venous thrombosis, including pulmonary embolism, was also seen in the postmenopausal women taking tamoxifen. The rate of pulmonary embolism in these women, however, was 1/1,000 annually. The presence of these competing risks emphasizes the need for a complete assessment of a woman's health status before a decision is made regarding the use of tamoxifen for prevention.

Raloxifene is a newer SERM used for osteoporosis management that also may be effective in reducing breast cancer incidence. Initial trials in 7,705 postmenopausal women demonstrated that in addition to maintaining bone density, raloxifene reduced the incidence of invasive breast cancer by 66%.[92] As in the tamoxifen trial, this effect was observed on the incidence of ER-positive tumors only. These findings remain tentative because only 40 women developed breast cancer in this osteoporosis study. A prospective, randomized trial in 20,000 postmenopausal women at increased risk for breast cancer development (Study of Tamoxifen and Raloxifene [STAR]) has completed accrual and will directly compare the risks and benefits of tamoxifen and raloxifene for breast cancer prevention.

DUCTAL CARCINOMA IN SITU

Ductal carcinoma *in situ* (DCIS), also known as *intraductal carcinoma,* is a distinct entity from LCIS, the other lesion classified as noninvasive breast cancer, with differences in both clinical presentation and biologic potential. DCIS is characterized by a proliferation of abnormal, presumably malignant epithelial cells that are confined within the basement membrane of the mammary ductal–lobular system (Fig. 76.19).

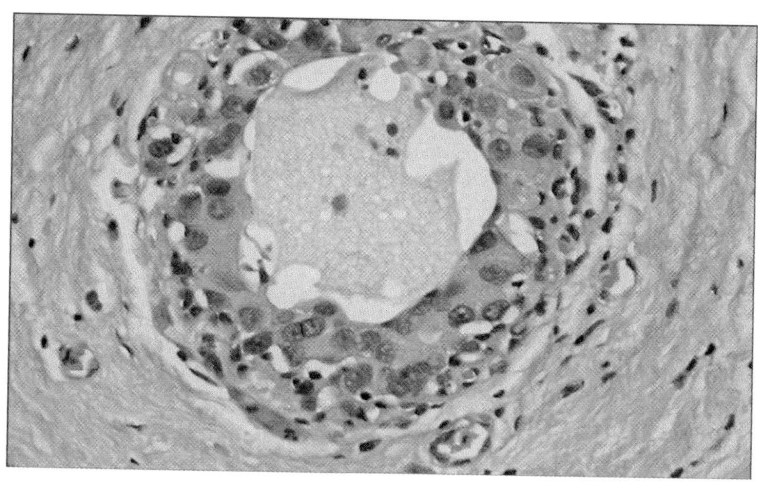

FIGURE 76.19 Photomicrograph of ductal carcinoma *in situ.* The abnormal cells do not cross the ductal basement membrane. The necrotic debris in the center of the duct is responsible for the calcification seen on mammography.

Presentation

Ductal carcinoma *in situ* has a variety of clinical presentations: palpable mass, pathologic nipple discharge, or Paget's disease of the nipple, all of which are relatively uncommon. The overwhelming majority of palpable breast cancers are invasive carcinoma; fewer than 2% are DCIS. Today, clustered microcalcifications on a mammogram are the most frequent presentation of DCIS, although approximately 10% of nonpalpable masses may also be DCIS. In many reports of biopsies performed for mammographic abnormalities, DCIS accounts for 30% to 50% of the malignancies identified. The number of cases of DCIS seen each year has increased dramatically as screening mammography has become more widely adopted. This increase has been observed in both white and African American women. DCIS may also lack both clinical and mammographic findings and be discovered incidentally in a biopsy done for other indications.

Pathology

Ductal carcinoma *in situ* has traditionally been classified on the basis of architectural pattern as comedo, cribriform, micropapillary, papillary, or solid. Because a mixed architectural pattern is seen in as many as 30% to 60% of DCIS lesions, however, the utility of this classification system is limited. Newer systems classify DCIS lesions on the basis of nuclear grade and necrosis and usually recognize three groups of lesions: high, intermediate, and low grade. Multiple systems have been proposed, but their reproducibility and ability to predict the behavior of DCIS remain to be proved.

Management

Mastectomy, excision and irradiation (radiation therapy [RT]), and excision alone have all been proposed as management strategies for DCIS because of uncertainty about the natural history of the disease. Mastectomy is a curative treatment for approximately 98% of patients with DCIS, regardless of lesion size or grade.[93,94] Treatment failure after mastectomy for DCIS is thought to be a consequence of unrecognized invasive carcinoma; as many as 26% of patients undergoing mastectomy for DCIS are found to have invasive carcinoma that was not identified preoperatively.[93,94] Invasive carcinoma is most frequently found in large, high-grade DCIS lesions.

Although mastectomy is an effective treatment for DCIS, it is a radical approach for a lesion that may not progress to invasive carcinoma during a patient's lifetime and is too small to be detected clinically. The use of BCT with excision and RT for invasive carcinoma (see section on local management of stages I and II breast cancer) has stimulated greater interest in the use of this approach for DCIS. No randomized trial has ever compared the treatment of DCIS by mastectomy with treatment by excision and RT. A large number of clinical studies have demonstrated that local recurrence after treatment with excision and RT is seen in 10% to 15% of cases after 10 years,[93–97] and that approximately half of the local recurrences are invasive carcinoma. Deaths from DCIS are rare; 14 breast cancer deaths occurred in 814 patients followed for 8 years after treatment with excision and RT.[96]

Because DCIS is a local problem in the breast and all DCIS does not progress to invasive carcinoma during a patient's lifetime, some authors have suggested that DCIS can be treated by wide excision alone. Three prospective, randomized trials have addressed this question and the results are summarized in Table 76.9. Despite differences in study design, the trial results are remarkably similar.[96,98,99] The studies demonstrate that the use of RT reduces ipsilateral breast tumor recurrence by 50% to 60%, and this reduction persists through 12 years of follow-up in the NSABP B17 study. The use of RT reduces both invasive and noninvasive recurrences; with the use of RT, the annual rate of invasive recurrence is 0.5% to 1.0%. In patients treated with excision alone or excision and RT, approximately 50% of recurrences are invasive and 50% are DCIS. No survival benefit for RT has been observed. In a more detailed pathologic analysis,[97] the greatest benefits of RT were seen in the patients at highest risk for recurrence (those with comedo necrosis and uncertain margins), but even in the most favorable subgroup (absent or slight comedo necrosis, clear margins), the use of RT reduced the absolute incidence of breast recurrence by 7% at 8 years. A retrospective study has suggested that excision of DCIS with a 1-cm margin of normal breast tissue eliminates the need for RT,[100] but an attempt to prospectively duplicate this observation was unsuccessful.[101]

Treatment selection for the patient with DCIS begins with a careful evaluation of the extent of the DCIS lesion by means of magnification mammography. Standard two-view mammography significantly underestimates the extent of well-differentiated DCIS.[102] If the extent of the DCIS is too large relative to the patient's breast size to allow a cosmetically acceptable breast-conserving approach, the patient should be counseled about the options of mastectomy alone or mastectomy with immediate breast reconstruction. In patients with localized DCIS suitable for a breast-conserving approach, the decision regarding the need for RT should be made based on the estimated risk for recurrence and the patient's attitude toward risk. Patients with larger tumors, high-grade lesions, and close margins

TABLE 76.9 RESULTS

RESULTS OF RANDOMIZED TRIALS OF RADIOTHERAPY IN DUCTAL CARCINOMA IN SITU

Study	Patients (No.)	Median follow-up (Mo)	IBTR (%)		Survival (%)	
			E	RT	E	RT
NSABP B17[96]	813	129	32	16	86	87
EORTC 10853[98]	1002	51	16	9	99	99
United Kingdom[99]	1,030	53	14	6	NA	NA

NSABP, National Surgical Adjuvant Breast Project; EORTC, European Organization for Research and Treatment of Cancer; IBTR, ipsilateral breast tumor recurrence; E, excision alone; RT, radiation therapy.

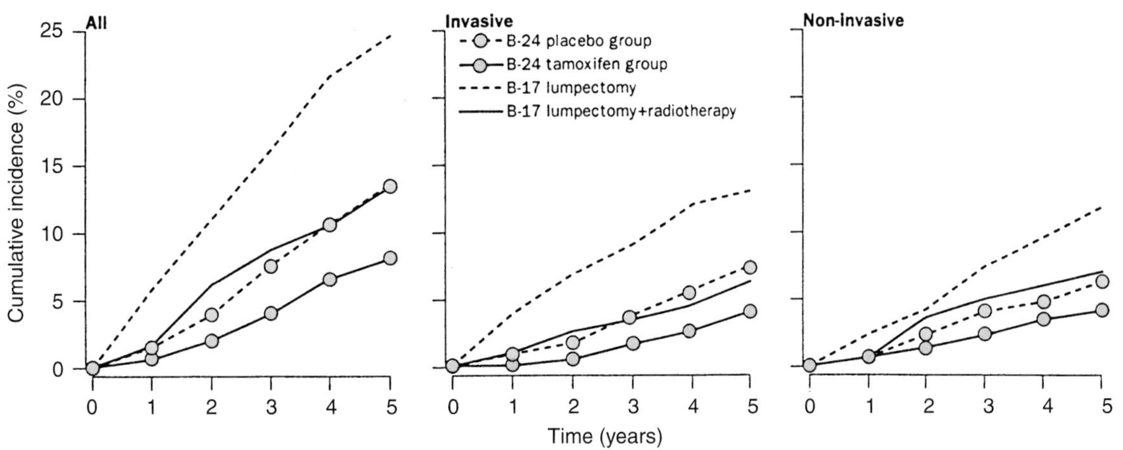

FIGURE 76.20 Benefits of radiation therapy and tamoxifen in ductal carcinoma *in situ*. The cumulative incidence of breast cancer events in the ipsilateral and contralateral breasts for patients treated in the National Surgical Adjuvant Breast and Bowel Project B-17 and B-24 trials is shown. The reduction in recurrence is greatest for patients receiving radiotherapy and tamoxifen.

appear to derive the greatest benefit from RT. It also appears that younger women are at higher risk for recurrence than their older counterparts.[98,103] However, even patients with small, low-grade lesions appear to benefit from RT,[97–99] and it is in this low-risk subgroup that the patient's attitude toward risk becomes important.

Tamoxifen has been shown to be of benefit in reducing the risk for subsequent invasive carcinoma in patients with DCIS. In NSABP B-24,[103] 1,804 women with DCIS treated by excision and RT were randomized to tamoxifen or placebo for 5 years. A reduction in the incidence of all breast cancer events from 17% to 10.0% was seen with tamoxifen ($P = .01$). The benefit of tamoxifen was observed in women over and under age 50 and in those with negative and positive margins. A benefit for tamoxifen was also observed whether or not comedo necrosis was present in the tumor. A subset analysis of 676 patients for whom estrogen receptor status could be determined was performed retrospectively. The benefit of adding tamoxifen to RT in reducing all breast cancer events was 59%, compared with 37% in the overall patient population. Little benefit for tamoxifen in ER-negative DCIS was seen, and its use is not warranted in these patients. The UK trial[99] compared treatment with excision alone with excision plus tamoxifen. After a median follow-up of 53 months, no differences in the rate of local recurrence were seen between groups. The findings of this study indicate that tamoxifen is not a replacement for RT. The effects of RT and tamoxifen in the NSABP B-17 and B-24 trials[96,103] are illustrated in Figure 76.20. The decision to use RT, tamoxifen, or both in the patient with DCIS will depend on the patient's personal level of risk and attitude toward small benefits from therapeutic intervention, but both should be considered. Identification of markers that predict which women with DCIS will develop an invasive recurrence is a research priority that will greatly improve our ability to tailor treatment to an individual's level of risk.

BIOLOGY AND NATURAL HISTORY OF BREAST CANCER

Breast cancer is a disease characterized by marked heterogeneity among patients and a long natural history. This is evident in the Middlesex Hospital series, in which Bloom et al.[104] reported the outcome of 250 patients with breast cancer observed without treatment between 1805 and 1933. Patients were generally admitted for advanced disease, with only 2% having stage II disease, 23% stage III, and 74% stage IV. Only 39% presented within 1 year of their first symptom. Despite this, 18% of patients receiving no treatment survived 5 years, and 4% survived 10 years. The mortality was constant over time, with approximately 25% of patients who were alive at the beginning of any given year dying during that year. In modern series, patients with varying annual hazards of death can also be identified, and these remain constant for at least 10 years after the diagnosis. For this reason, some have concluded that breast cancer is never cured, and that if death from other causes did not intervene, cancer eventually would recur in all patients. Although this may be true in the abstract, from a practical point of view, failures more than 20 years after treatment are rare, and many patients have a normal life expectancy after breast cancer treatment. The clinical variations in breast cancer are believed to reflect variable genetic changes that result in the disease.

The initial clinical understanding of breast cancer, as articulated by Halsted,[105] was one of orderly disease progression, suggesting that *en bloc* extirpation of the primary tumor with a wide margin of normal tissue (i.e., the breast) and the draining lymphatics was the most likely strategy to cure breast cancer. Over time, it became clear that the majority of women with breast cancer were not cured by radical mastectomy. Recognition of this fact initially led to larger operations, such as the extended radical mastectomy to remove more of the lymphatic drainage of the breast. When these procedures failed to improve survival, however, a dramatic shift in thinking occurred. In the new disease paradigm, championed by Bernard Fisher,[106] most breast cancer was considered to be systemic at the time of diagnosis, so that the extent of locoregional treatment would have little impact on survival from breast cancer. Acceptance of this concept led to the adoption of the modified radical mastectomy, and subsequently breast-conserving surgery, for the treatment of stages I and II breast cancer, in addition to the widespread use of adjuvant chemotherapy and hormonal therapy.

More recently, a spectrum hypothesis has been advanced suggesting that breast cancer exists in a local, a locoregional, and in a systemic form, and that metastasis can occur during the clinical course of the disease.[107] In this paradigm, effective locoregional treatment does contribute to survival. The potential for locoregional treatment to affect survival has been emphasized in the recent studies of postmastectomy radiation therapy in node-positive breast cancer, in which a survival benefit was noted when chest wall and nodal irradiation were given.[108–110] These studies are discussed in more detail in the section on postmastectomy radiotherapy. The spectrum theory suggests that treatment strategies should be tailored according to the characteristics of an individual patient's disease rather than based on the assumption that most breast cancers are systemic at the time of diagnosis. Traditonally, treatment strategies have been selected on the basis of clinically determined prognostic factors. Emerging data, discussed in the section on prognostic factors, suggest that genetic profiling may improve our ability to identify women with the metastatic phenotype. Ultimately, we may be able to identify those factors responsible for the locally invasive as well as the metastatic phenotype, and it will be possible to adjust the intensity of both local and systemic therapy according to the unique genetic profile of each tumor.

INVASIVE CARCINOMA

Pathology

Invasive carcinomas are defined as those in which tumor cells have crossed the basement membrane and have the biologic capability to metastasize. Any breast lesion that is surgically removed should be considered potentially malignant. Breast biopsy specimens should be oriented in the operating room and inked before sectioning so that the margin status can be assessed. The pathologic evaluation of a breast tumor should routinely include size, histologic type, grade, margin status, and hormone receptor status.

Histologic Type

Infiltrating ductal carcinoma is the most common type of breast carcinoma, accounting for 65% to 80% of all cases of breast cancer. Microscopically, they vary widely in appearance and often have features of other histologic subtypes of breast cancer, with areas of lobular, medullary, or tubular differentiation. For prognostic purposes, these mixed tumors are considered to be infiltrating ductal carcinomas.

Infiltrating lobular carcinoma is the second most frequently encountered subtype of invasive carcinoma. Approximately 10% of cancers are classified as lobular. Histologically, lobular cancers grow as a single file of malignant cells that tend to be arranged circumferentially around ducts and lobules. Because of this growth pattern, they are often difficult to recognize on clinical examination and mammography because they may not produce the distinctive mass lesions characteristic of infiltrating ductal carcinomas. Infiltrating lobular carcinoma has been said to have a rate of bilaterality as high as 30% to 50%. When patients with LCIS are excluded from consideration, however, the incidence of contralateral breast cancer in patients with infiltrating lobular carcinoma differs little from that in patients with ductal carcinoma. In one study of 4,748 patients, a contralateral cancer had developed after 5 years in 5.3% of patients with infiltrating lobular cancer, and in 4.0% of those with infiltrating ductal tumors.[111] Thus, the routine use of bilateral mastectomy for patients with tumors of lobular histology cannot be justified. Lobular carcinoma is more likely to metastasize to the intraabdominal viscera, uterus, ovaries, and peritoneal surfaces than other histologic types of breast carcinoma. Most studies have found no difference in survival between patients with infiltrating ductal and those with lobular carcinoma after stratification for appropriate prognostic factors.

Favorable histologic subtypes of breast carcinoma include pure tubular and mucinous carcinoma. Tubular carcinomas form normal-appearing breast ductules or tubules. At least 75% of a tumor must be tubular to be classified in this subtype. Tubular carcinomas are uncommon, accounting for 2% or fewer of all cancers, although they are more frequent in women undergoing screening mammography. Their significance lies in their excellent prognosis. Nodal metastases are extremely rare in tubular carcinomas smaller than 1 cm, and even when nodal metastases do occur, the prognosis is much better than that for ductal or lobular carcinoma at the same stage. Mucinous or colloid carcinomas are also uncommon. They are characterized by relative acellularity and large pools of extracellular mucus. The prognosis is similar to that for tubular carcinoma. Medullary carcinoma is another variant of infiltrating ductal carcinoma with a favorable prognosis, although this is less well recognized than in tubular and mucinous tumors, perhaps because of the aggressive microscopic appearance of medullary carcinoma. The tumor cells have large pleomorphic nuclei and a high mitotic rate and are associated with an intense lymphoplasmacytic infiltrate. Grossly, the tumors are well circumscribed and may be mistaken for benign lesions. Medullary carcinomas are less likely to be associated with axillary nodal metastases than ductal or lobular carcinomas of the same size, and survival is also better. Other histologic types of breast cancer account for fewer than 2% of all cancers.

Grading Systems

The grade of a carcinoma is an estimate of differentiation. It may be histologic or nuclear. Nuclear grading is a cytologic assessment of the similarity of tumor nuclei to the nuclei of normal cells. The nuclear grade is usually reported as well differentiated, intermediate, or poorly differentiated. The histologic grade considers not only the cytologic differentiation but also the growth pattern of the carcinoma. The extent of tubule formation, nuclear hyperchromasia, and the mitotic index are assessed. In one of the most widely used systems, the Elston modification of the Scharf-Bloom-Richardson classification, each of these three elements is scored on a scale of 1 to 3, with a resultant classification of grade 1 (score of 3 to 5), grade 2 (score of 6 or 7), or grade 3 (score of 8 or 9).[112] Approximately 19% of the 2,000 cases reviewed by Elston and Ellis[112] were grade 1, 34% were grade 2, and 47% were grade 3.

Hormone Receptors

The concept of an estrogen receptor was described by Jensen and Jacobsen in 1962,[113] based on the observation that estrogens tagged with radioactive isotopes are preferentially concentrated in the estrogen target organs of animals (i.e., breast, uterus, vagina) and in human breast cancers. Subsequently, a second hormone receptor, the progesterone receptor (PR), was identified. ERs and PRs belong to a superfamily of nuclear hormone receptors that function as transcription factors when bound to their respective ligands. Approximately 70% of breast carcinomas are hormone receptor-positive; well-differentiated tumors and those occurring in older postmenopausal women have the highest rates of receptor positivity. Approximately 60% of patients with ER-positive tumors respond to endocrine therapy, but only 5% to 10% of patients with ER-negative tumors do so, and responses probably result from false-negative receptor results.[114] It is now apparent that there are two receptors for estrogen, ERα (the classical receptor identified by Jensen) and ERβ, identified by Gustaffson's laboratory in 1996.[115] At present, the clincal significance of ERβ in breast cancer management is uncertain. Tumor ERα and PR content is measured by immunohistochemical techniques. Determination of hormone receptor status is a critical part of the pathologic analysis of breast tumors and is used to ascertain whether the patient is a candidate for hormonal therapy (see section on adjuvant systemic therapy).

Clinical Evaluation and Staging

The extent of the preoperative workup should be guided by the clinical stage of the disease and the patient's symptoms. Patients with DCIS do not require screening for metastatic disease. Bone scans are frequently used as a preoperative screening test for patients with invasive cancer, but in a large review, the incidence of occult bony metastases detected by scanning in patients with stage I or II disease was less than 5%.[116] False-positive results are frequent, especially in older women. In asymptomatic women with stage III disease, 8.3% had bony metastases. The yield of liver screening studies is less than 1%, even for women with stage III disease and the test is of little benefit in preoperative evaluation.

Serum tumor markers have not been shown to be of value preoperatively. Studies of carcinoembryonic antigen, CA15-3, CA27.29, and the shed extacellular domain of erbB2 do not demonstrate sufficient sensitivity or specificity to indicate or exclude the presence of occult metastatic disease.

Staging refers to the grouping of patients according to the extent of their disease. The stage is useful in (a) determining the choice of treatment for an individual patient, (b) estimating prognosis, and (c) comparing the results of different treatment programs. Staging can be based on either clinical or pathologic findings.

Currently, the staging of cancer is determined by the American Joint Committee on Cancer (AJCC). The AJCC system is a clinical and pathologic staging system based on the TNM (tumor, node, metastasis) system.[7]

The clinical stage is based on all the information available before the first definitive treatment is administered. This includes the findings from physical examination, imaging studies, operation, and pathologic examination of the breast or other tissues. The clinical stage is useful in selecting and evaluating therapy.

The pathologic stage (designated pTNM) is based on all the data used for clinical staging in addition to data derived from the pathologic examination of the primary carcinoma and axillary lymph nodes. A tumor cannot be evaluated for pathologic staging (pTX) if excision of the primary carcinoma reveals tumor in any margin of resection by gross pathologic examination. The pathologic stage provides the most precise data to estimate the prognosis and calculate the end result. The current staging system is given in Table 76.10.[7]

Local Management of Stage I and Stage II Breast Cancer

The goal of the local therapy of breast cancer is to eradicate all clinically evident tumor in the breast and axillary lymph nodes. This can be accomplished with a modified radical mastectomy, a modified radical mastectomy with immediate breast reconstruction, or BCT, which consists of removal of the primary tumor with a margin of normal tissue and RT. Six modern prospective, randomized trials have compared mastectomy with BCT and have demonstrated no survival differences, even after long-term follow-up (Table 76.11).[117–122] Mastectomy alone has never been compared with mastectomy and reconstruction in a randomized trial, but there is no reason to suspect that reconstruction would decrease survival. In the absence of survival differences, the role of the surgeon is to identify medical contraindications to the procedures and to counsel the patient regarding what is involved in each one.

Breast-conserving Therapy

For BCT to be successful, three conditions must be met: It must be possible to (a) reduce the tumor burden to a microscopic level likely to be controlled by irradiation, (b) safely deliver radiation therapy, and (c) promptly detect local recurrence. The contraindications to BCT arise logically from these conditions. In 1992, a joint committee of the American College of Surgeons, American College of Radiology, College of American Pathologists, and Society of Surgical Oncology developed guidelines for BCT. These were updated in 2002 and are listed in Table 76.12.[123]

The incidence of the contraindications to BCT in the breast cancer population determines the number of patients who are advised to undergo mastectomy for medical reasons. Morrow et al.[10] reported a study in which a multidisciplinary team of physicians prospectively evaluated 456 patients with DCIS, clinical stage I breast cancer, or clinical stage II breast cancer between 1988 and 1991. Medical contraindications to breast preservation were present in only 26% of the patients, and the incidence and type of contraindications varied significantly by stage, with only 10% of patients with stage I disease having contraindications to BCT.

In an effort to increase the number of patients eligible for breast conservation, the use of neoadjuvant chemotherapy to shrink the primary tumor before surgical therapy has been studied.[124] In a large randomized trial, NSABP protocol B-18, 1,523 patients with tumors of any size were randomized to receive four cycles of doxorubicin (A) and cyclophosphamide (C) either preoperatively or postoperatively.[125] All patients over age 50 received tamoxifen. A reduction in tumor diameter of 50% was noted clinically in 80% of the patients, and in 37%, no tumor could be felt after chemotherapy. Only one fourth of the patients thought to be complete responders, however, had no tumor identified microscopically after surgery. Significant axillary down-staging also was observed, with pathologically negative nodes seen in 60% of the neoadjuvant group and in 42% of the postoperative adjuvant group ($P < .001$). Despite these impressive response rates, the rate of breast conservation increased by only 8%, from 60% to 68%. In a subsequent study, the addition of docetaxel to AC treatment preoperatively increased the clinical complete response rate from 40.1% to 63.6% ($P < .001$) and the pathologic complete response rate from 13.7% to 26.1% ($P < .001$).[126] Despite this increase in response rate, the use of BCT did not differ between patients receiving preoperative AC and those receiving AC plus taxotere. This is probably because of the inability of the physical examination and imaging studies to reliably predict the degree of pathologic response. To date, neoadjuvant therapy has not been shown to improve survival in comparison with therapy given postoperatively.

In addition to the medical contraindications to BCT discussed earlier, patient desire is another indication for mastectomy. Not all women who are eligible for BCT opt for this therapy. In one study, 19% of eligible patients selected treatment with mastectomy, either alone or with immediate reconstruction.[10] This decision was independent of age or race.

TABLE 76.10 STAGING

TUMOR, NODE, METASTASIS (TNM) CLASSIFICATION FOR BREAST CANCER STAGING

TNM DEFINITIONS

Primary Tumor

Tx	Primary tumor cannot be assessed
T0	No evidence of primary tumor
Tis	Carcinoma *in situ*, ductal or lobular or Paget disease of the nipple with no tumor
T1	Tumor 2 cm or less in greatest dimension
T2	Tumor more than 2 cm but not more than 5 cm in greatest dimension
T3	Tumor more than 5 cm in greatest dimension
T4	Tumor of any size with direct extension to the chest wall (not including pectoralis muscle), skin edema, skin ulceration, satellite skin nodules or inflammatory carcinoma

Regional Lymph Nodes (pathologic)

Nx	Nodes cannot be assessed
N0	No regional node metastases histologically, no additional examination for isolated tumor cells (ITC)
N1	Metastasis to 1–3 axillary nodes or in internal mammary (IM) nodes with microscopic disease detected by sentinel node biopsy which is not clinically apparent
N2	Metastases in 4 to 9 axillary nodes or in clinically apparent IM nodes in the absence of axillary node metastasis
N3	Metastases in 10 or more axillary nodes; or in infraclavicular nodes, or in IM nodes in the presence of 1 or more positive axillary nodes; or in more than 3 axillary nodes with IM metastases, or in supraclavicular nodes

Distant Metastases

Mx	Distant metastasis cannot be assessed
M0	No distant metastasis
M1	Distant metastasis

STAGE GROUPING

Stage 0	Tis	N0	M0
Stage I	TI	N0	M0
Stage IIA	T0	N1	M0
	T1	N1	M0
	T2	N0	M0
Stage IIB	T2	N1	M0
	T3	N0	M0
Stage IIIA	T0	N2	M0
	T1	N2	M0
	T2	N2	M0
	T3	N1	M0
	T3	N2	M0
Stage IIIB	T4	N0	M0
	T4	N1	M0
	T4	N2	M0
Stage IIIC	Any T	N3	M0
Stage IV	Any T	Any N	M1

TABLE 76.11 RESULTS

SURVIVAL IN PROSPECTIVE RANDOMIZED TRIALS COMPARING BREAST-CONSERVING THERAPY WITH MASTECTOMY

		Overall survival		Local recurrence	
Trial	Follow-up (y)	BCT (%)	Mastectomy (%)	BCT (%)	Mastectomy (%)
Institut Gustave Roussy[117]	15	73	65	9	14
Milan I[118]	20	42	41	7	2
NSABP B06[119]	20	46	47	14	10
NCI[120]	18	59	58	22	6
EORTC[121]	10	65	66	20	12
Danish[122]	6	79	82	3	4

BCT, breast-conserving therapy; EORTC, European Organization for Research and Treatment of Cancer; NCI, National Cancer Institute; NSABP, National Surgical Adjuvant Breast and Bowel Project.

TABLE 76.12 INDICATIONS/CONTRAINDICATIONS

CONTRAINDICATIONS TO BREAST-CONSERVING THERAPY IN INVASIVE CARCINOMA

ABSOLUTE CONTRAINDICATIONS

- Two or more primary tumors in separate quadrants of the breast
- Persistent positive margins after reasonable surgical attempts
- Pregnancy is an absolute contraindication to the use of breast irradiation. When cancer is diagnosed in the third trimester, it may be possible to perform breast-conserving surgery and treat the patient with irradiation after delivery.
- A history of prior therapeutic irradiation to the breast region that would result in re-treatment to an excessively high radiation dose
- Diffuse malignant-appearing microcalcifications

RELATIVE CONTRAINDICATIONS

- A history of scleroderma or active systemic lupus erythematosus
- Extensive, gross, multifocal disease in the same quadrant. Studies in this area are not definitive.
- Large tumor in a small breast that would result in cosmesis unacceptable to the patient
- Very large or pendulous breasts if reproducibility of patient setup and adequate dose homogeneity cannot be ensured

The amount of breast tissue to be resected in a lumpectomy to minimize the risk for local recurrence while optimizing the cosmetic appearance remains a major issue. The goal of surgery is to reduce the tumor burden to a microscopic level that is likely to be controlled with RT. In a study of mastectomy specimens in 264 patients in which serial sectioning and radiography were used, only 39% of specimens had no additional tumor beyond the primary tumor site.[48] The likelihood of finding additional tumor was not related to the size of the primary tumor. Other studies have shown that the risk for residual tumor varies with the histology of the primary tumor, being lowest in pure infiltrating ductal carcinoma and highest in infiltrating ductal carcinoma with an extensive intraductal component (EIC); the risk in infiltrating lobular carcinoma falls between the other two.[127] These studies indicate that the ideal balance between cosmesis and local failure is unlikely to be achieved by resecting the same amount of breast tissue in all patients. Magnification mammography is essential to identify the extent of the tissue that must be resected, and it allows large "quadrantectomy"-type resections to be reserved for patients with multifocal disease. With the use of physical examination and magnification mammography, the patients who can undergo breast conservation can be identified with a success rate higher than 95%.[128] The extent of surgical resection is the major determinant of cosmetic outcome, and approximately 90% of patients treated with conservative resection rate their cosmetic outcome as excellent or good (Fig. 76.21).

Local recurrence of tumor in the breast after BCT has been the subject of many studies. Local recurrence may be a consequence of inappropriate patient selection, inadequate surgery or RT, or biologic characteristics of the tumor. The presence of tumor at the margin of resection significantly increases the risk for local recurrence, as does the use of radiation doses to the whole breast of less than 4,500 to 5,000 cGy. Six randomized trials have attempted to identify a subgroup of patients with invasive carcinoma who do not require RT. All have shown a large reduction (average, 75%) in the rate of local recurrence with RT,[129] and RT should be considered a standard part of BCT for invasive carcinoma. Studies are now ongoing to evaluate the efficacy of partial breast irradiation to the quadrant of the tumor on local control. Patient factors, such as young age, have also been associated with an increased risk for local failure after BCT. Young age, however, has also been shown to increase rates of local failure after mastectomy, which indicates that young age is a prognostic factor rather than one that can be used to select therapy. In contrast, a family history of breast cancer does not increase local failure rates. In women with mutations of *BRCA1* or *BRCA2*, the risk of new second primary cancers is increased in both breasts, but the risk of local failure does not seem to be elevated.[130] A number of tumor factors, such as size and involvement of axillary lymph nodes, that are strong predictors of the risk for distant recurrence are not associated with

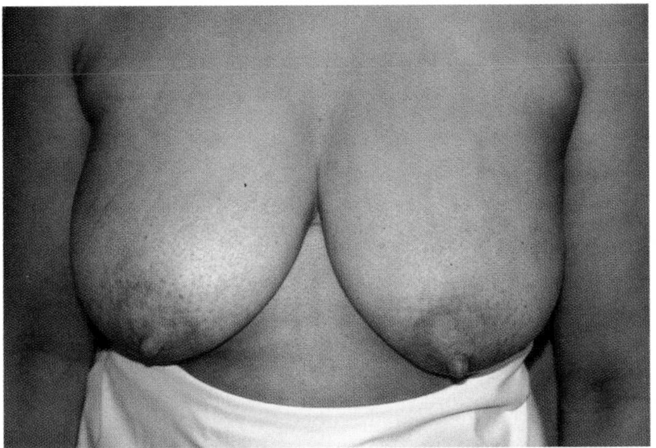

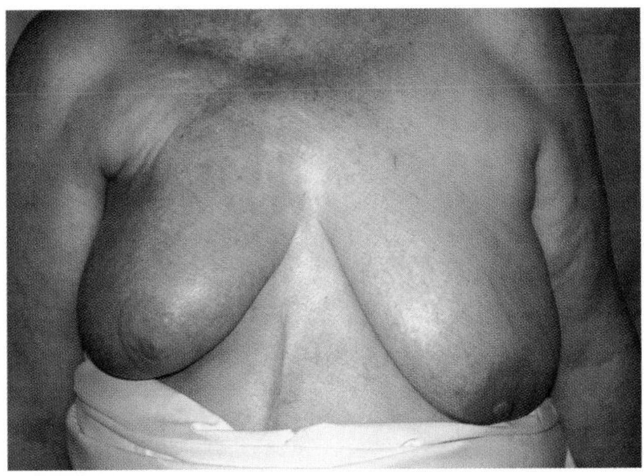

FIGURE 76.21 Cosmetic outcome after breast-conserving therapy with radiation. (*A*) Excellent cosmetic outcome. The treated breast (*left*) is identical to the untreated breast. (*B*) Fair cosmetic outcome. Significant shrinkage and loss of ptosis is evident in the treated right breast.

the risk for recurrence in the breast. Histologic tumor type also is not a risk factor, and studies have shown that recurrence rates after excision of infiltrating lobular carcinoma to negative margins do not differ from those after excision of infiltrating ductal tumors. Most studies also indicate that histologic grade is not predictive of recurrence. Some studies have identified lymphatic invasion at the primary tumor site as a risk factor, but this has also been shown to be a risk factor for local recurrence after mastectomy.

In the past, an EIC, defined as the presence of intraductal carcinoma both within an infiltrating ductal carcinoma and in adjacent grossly normal breast tissue, was thought to be associated with an increased risk for local, but not distant, recurrence. More recent studies indicate that when EIC-positive tumors are excised to negative margins, local failure rates are similar to those seen with EIC-negative tumors.[131] The use of adjuvant chemotherapy or tamoxifen in patients who have received breast RT reduces the risk for breast recurrence by approximately 50%. In modern series, local failure rates of 4% to 8% at 10 years are commonly reported in patients receiving RT plus systemic therapy. The information on factors associated with local recurrence suggests that two types of recurrences develop after BCT. One type of recurrence represents a heavy tumor burden in the breast that is not controlled by breast irradiation. This type of recurrence can be minimized by meticulous patient selection and attention to the technical details of surgery and irradiation. The other type of recurrence is a manifestation of a biologically aggressive tumor and represents a first site of metastatic disease. This type of recurrence is similar to the majority of chest wall recurrences seen after mastectomy.

Modified Radical Mastectomy

The term *modified radical mastectomy* encompasses several different operative procedures, depending on whether the pectoralis minor muscle is preserved, removed, or divided. In all the operations, the breast tissue and some of the axillary lymph nodes are removed. Modified radical mastectomy is performed through an elliptical incision that encompasses the nipple–areola complex and the biopsy scar, if an open biopsy has been performed, in addition to the excess skin of the breast (Fig. 76.22). If the skin is needed for reconstruction, it can be preserved and exposure obtained through incision rather than excision. Skin flaps are raised in the plane between the subcutaneous fat and the underlying breast tissue. To encompass all the breast tissue, the dissection should extend superiorly to the inferior border of the clavicle, medially to the lateral border of the sternum, inferiorly to the superior extent of the rectus sheath, and laterally to the latissimus dorsi. The fascia overlying the pectoralis major is the deep margin of resection, but it can be preserved when needed to facilitate reconstruction.

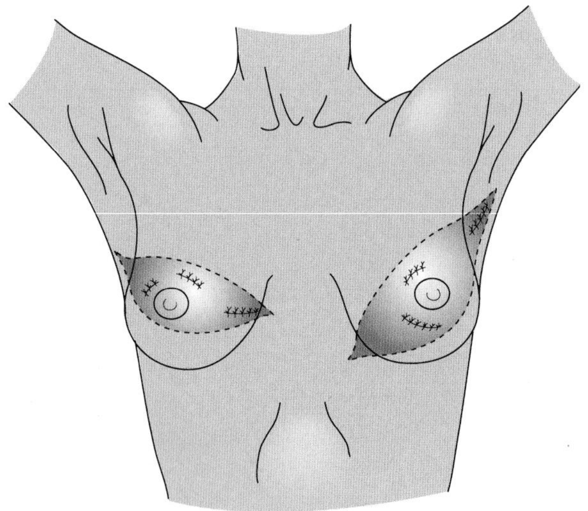

FIGURE 76.22 Incision placement for modified radical mastectomy. The incision should include the nipple–areola complex, biopsy scar, and excess skin of the breast.

Mastectomy is an extremely safe operation. A review of the Surveillance, Epidemiology, and End Results (SEER) from the National Center for Health Statistics data for 10,056 patients treated between 1960 and 1973 reports a 30-day operative mortality of 0.35%.[132] Early postoperative complications include wound infections, which tend to present as cellulitis and are seen in from 2% to 14% of cases.[133] Open surgical biopsy before mastectomy (as opposed to a needle biopsy technique) has been shown to increase the rate of infection. Skin flap necrosis is relatively uncommon today. Factors associated with flap necrosis include vertical incisions, technical error with denuding of the subcutaneous fat from the flap, and closure under tension. Seromas form in 100% of patients and should be considered a side effect and not a complication. Extensive axillary nodal involvement is the strongest predictor of prolonged lymphatic drainage after mastectomy. Seroma formation can be minimized by leaving suction drains in place until their output is less than 30 mL/24 hours rather than arbitrarily removing them on a predetermined day. Anesthesia of the chest wall is another side effect of mastectomy that patients should be informed of preoperatively.

Mastectomy and Immediate Reconstruction

The techniques of breast reconstruction have evolved dramatically during the past 30 years, and the switch from radical mastectomy to modified radical mastectomy has made immediate reconstruction an option for most women. Tissue expansion followed by removal of the expander and replacement with a permanent implant is the most common form of reconstruction in the United States. The advantage of this technique is that it adds little to the length of surgery or the time of recovery. Disadvantages include the need for a second surgical procedure routinely and the limitations in cosmetic outcome, particularly for women with large or pendulous breasts. These differences, however, are minimized when a bra is worn (Fig. 76.23).

The alternative to implant reconstruction is the use of autologous tissue flaps. Both the transverse rectus abdominis myocutaneous (TRAM) flap and a latissimus dorsi flap have been used for reconstruction. These flaps have the advantage of allowing a more natural look and feel to the breasts than can be achieved with implants (see Fig. 76.17B). The TRAM reconstruction has the added advantage of an abdominoplasty. Both, however, add significant time to the operative procedure, hospitalization, and recovery period, and they may not be suitable for patients with major comorbid conditions. In addition, in most women the latissimus flap does not provide enough tissue to create a breast mound, and an implant must be added.

The major oncologic issue in immediate reconstruction has been the incidence and detection of local recurrence. This has never been examined in a prospective randomized trial, but retrospective studies do not suggest an increase in the rate of local failure, even after skin-sparing mastectomies.[134] The detection of local failure also does not appear to be altered by the presence of a reconstruction because the majority of chest wall failures occur in the skin or subcutaneous fat. A second issue is the use of immediate reconstruction in patients who will require postoperative RT. The incidence of implant loss

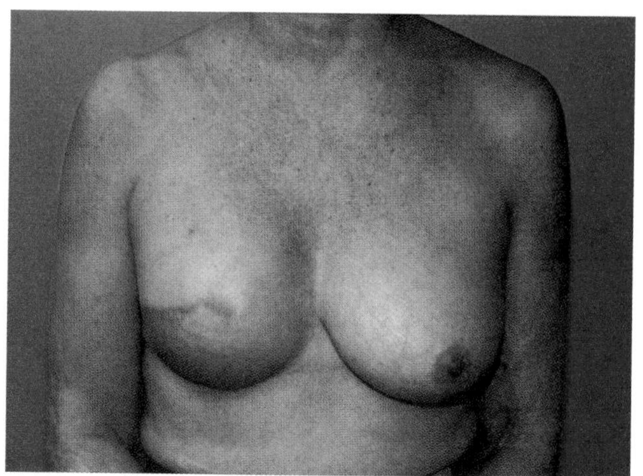

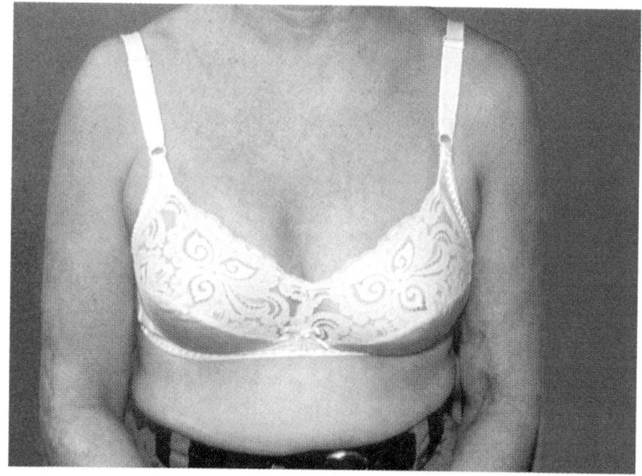

FIGURE 76.23 Breast reconstruction with tissue expanders. Although the breasts are not identical, this is not evident when a bra is worn.

and poor cosmetic outcome is clearly increased in patients who undergo postoperative RT, whereas flap necrosis, fibrosis, and shrinkage can occur in TRAM flaps after radiation. As the indications for postoperative RT are expanded (discussed later), the issue of the optimal method and timing of reconstruction assumes greater importance. One approach to the patient who is highly likely to require postoperative RT is to place an expander to allow skin preservation at the time of initial surgery.[135] Once postoperative RT is completed, a decision to continue with the expander and implant or to switch to a flap reconstruction can be made.

Management of the Axillary Nodes

Axillary dissection has been a part of the surgical management of breast cancer since the era of Halsted. Initially, axillary dissection was thought to be therapeutic, but came to be regarded as a staging procedure when it became evident that the majority of women with nodal metastases died of breast cancer after receiving local therapy alone. In the 1990s, the increasing use of adjuvant systemic therapy for node-positive and node-negative breast cancer, the more frequent detection of small cancers associated with a low risk for nodal metastases, and an increased awareness of the morbidity of axillary dissection resulted in attempts to identify subgroups of patients who would not benefit from the procedure. In most studies, tumor size was used to identify a low-risk subgroup. Even for tumors smaller than 5 mm, however, the incidence of nodal metastases ranges from 3% to 12%.[129] For the majority of patients with breast cancer, the axillary nodal status cannot be reliably predicted on the basis of the characteristics of the primary tumor. Today, sentinel node biopsy allows the reliable identification of patients with axillary metastases with a low morbidity staging procedure.

Sentinel Node Biopsy

A sentinel lymph node (SN) is defined as the first lymph node that receives drainage from a cancer. The procedure of lymphatic mapping and SN biopsy can be performed with lymphazurin blue dye, colloids labeled with radioactive isotopes (usually technetium), or a combination of the two agents. The SN technique was initially developed and validated in studies from single surgeons or institutions where SN biopsy was followed by axillary dissection.[136]

A number of multiinstitutional studies have examined the ability to identify an SN and the accuracy of the SN in predicting the status of the remaining axillary nodes.[137–142] These are summarized in Table 76.13. These studies indicate that regardless of the technique used, surgeons learning the procedure can identify a SN in approximately 90% of patients, which will predict the status of the remaining axillary nodes in about 90% of cases. It is apparent that SN biopsy can be performed in most patients with breast cancer.

TABLE 76.13 RESULTS

RESULTS OF MULTIINSTITUTIONAL STUDIES OF LYMPHATIC MAPPING AND SENTINEL NODE BIOPSY

Study	No. patients	%SN indentification	%false–negative
Krag et al.[141]	443	91	11
McMasters et al.[139]	1817	91.7	9
Shivers et al.[142]	560	85	4
Tafra et al.[137]	535	87	13
Bergkvist et al.[138]	498	90	11
Chua et al.[140]	547	88	22

SN, sentinel node.

TABLE 76.14 INDICATIONS/CONTRAINDICATIONS

CONTRAINDICATIONS TO SENTINEL NODE BIOPSY

- Clinically suspicious axillary adenopathy
- Inflammatory or other locally advanced breast cancer
- Pregnant or lactating patient
- Prior axillary surgery

Contraindications to SN biopsy are listed in Table 76.14. A randomized comparison has demonstrated that equal numbers of node-positive women are identified with SN biopsy and axillary dissection.[143] The morbidity of SN biopsy is significantly lower than that of axillary dissection, both 6 months and 2 years postoperatively, and the incidence of lymphedema is significantly lower.[143] After SN biopsy alone, isolated axillary recurrence occurs in fewer than 1% of patients, making it the axillary staging procedure of choice for most patients with breast cancer. Sentinel node biopsy also offers the pathologist the opportunity to perform a much more detailed study of the lymph node that is most likely to contain metastases than is possible when an entire axillary specimen containing 15 to 30 nodes is evaluated. With the use of multiple sections or immunohistochemistry, it is possible to identify tumor deposits in approximately 20% of nodes found to be "negative" with routine sectioning and hematoxylin and eosin staining. The prognostic significance of these micrometastases, however, is uncertain. Prospective clinical trials being performed by the American College of Surgeons Oncology Group and the NSABP will determine whether immunohistochemistry of the SN is a useful way to refine our ability to predict the risk for recurrence.

Axillary Dissection

Axillary dissection is indicated in patients found to have metastatic disease in the SN or those with contraindications to SN biopsy. The extent of axillary dissection has been defined on the basis of the number of nodes removed or their anatomic location. As discussed in the section on anatomy, the axilla is divided into three anatomic levels. Removal of the level I and II nodes accurately identifies metastases in 98% of patients because isolated metastases to level III are uncommon. A level I and II dissection is standard practice, with the removal of level III being reserved for patients with evidence of gross nodal involvement. Isolated axillary recurrence after a level I and II dissection is uncommon and is seen in fewer than 3% of patients undergoing BCT. With random node removal, a clear relationship is noted between the number of nodes removed and the incidence of axillary failure.

It has become increasingly apparent that axillary dissection is accompanied by significant morbidity. Major complications, such as injury to the axillary vein and motor nerves of the axilla, are rare, but numbness in the distribution of the intercostobrachial nerve is seen in 70% to 80% of patients unless the nerve is preserved and pain and weakness are seen in 20% to 30% of patients 1 year after surgery.[143] The risk of lymphedema after axillary surgery persists for the patient's lifetime, and the frequency of lymphedema increases as the time from surgery increases. In a review of reports published in the 1990s,[144] the incidence of lymphedema was found to range from 6% to 30%. The incidence of lymphedema is related to the extent of axillary dissection, being higher when level III is removed than when lesser dissections are performed. The radiation of an axillary field after surgical dissection significantly increases the risk for lymphedema. Beyond these two treatment-related factors, there is little agreement regarding which patient characteristics are associated with an increased risk for lymphedema.

Postmastectomy Radiotherapy

The reasons for irradiating the chest wall and draining lymph node basins after mastectomy are twofold: first, to reduce the risk for locoregional recurrence of tumor, and second, to improve survival by eradicating residual locoregional disease that may be resistant to systemic therapy. The risk for local failure after mastectomy is significant and is clearly related to the presence of axillary node metastases, and large (>5 cm) tumor size. Reported locoregional recurrence rates in randomized trials of mastectomy alone range from 4% to 26%.[145] In patients with negative axillary nodes, local failure rates are usually less than 4%. An overview analysis of 40 trials (19,582 women) of RT after both mastectomy and BCT demonstrated that RT reduces the risk for local recurrence by approximately two thirds.[146] A much smaller decrease in breast cancer mortality was also seen (proportional reduction 9%) but, in older studies, was offset by a significant increase in late cardiac mortality in women who underwent radiation for left-sided cancers.

Recent studies have examined the use of RT in patients receiving adjuvant systemic therapy and have reported an improvement in survival with the addition of RT. The Danish Breast Cancer Group reported a randomized study of 1,708 premenopausal women with stage II or III breast cancer who received eight cycles of cyclophosphamide, methotrexate, and fluorouracil and were randomized to locoregional RT or no further treatment.[108] After a median follow-up of 114 months, overall survival was 54% in the RT group versus 45% in the chemotherapy alone group ($P < .01$). A smaller trial of premenopausal women, from British Columbia, showed similar survival benefits.[109] Further support for this concept comes from the Danish trial in postmenopausal women receiving tamoxifen, in which RT improved overall survival from 36% to 45% ($P < .05$).[110] To date, postmastectomy RT has been used primarily in patients with involvement of four or more axillary nodes to reduce the risk for locoregional recurrence. These studies suggest that RT may be considered in patients with involvement of one to three nodes to improve survival.

PROGNOSTIC FACTORS

The clinical course of breast cancer varies from patient to patient. Prognostic factors can be used to predict the natural history of a tumor, usually in terms of disease-free or overall survival. Prognostic factors must be distinguished from predictive factors, which are associated with response to a particular therapy. Clinically, prognostic factors are used to determine which patients have such a favorable outcome after local therapy that adjuvant systemic therapy is not warranted. Although multiple prognostic factors have been described, those in standard use today include axillary lymph node status, tumor size, histologic subtype (discussed in the section on pathology), nuclear or histologic grade, and ER and PR status. Measurements of proliferation, such as S-phase fraction or Ki67, are more controversial but are used in many institutions. Newer factors under study include cyclins, growth factor receptors, plasminogen activators, and inhibitors and markers of cell death (e.g., BCL-2).

The presence of metastases to the axillary nodes is the single most important prognostic factor in breast cancer. Although clinical studies usually divide patients into groups with negative nodes, one to three positive nodes, and four or more positive nodes, the number of involved nodes indicates the prognosis as a continuous variable. Because patients with node-positive disease are uniformly recognized as requiring adjuvant systemic therapy, most studies have concentrated on prognostic factors in patients with node-negative disease. Tumor size is another strong predictor of outcome.[147,148] Only 10% or less patients with tumors 1 cm or less in size and negative axillary lymph nodes experience recurrence during long-term follow-up.[147]

Tumor grade has also been shown to predict outcome in breast cancer. However, the availability of multiple grading systems, poor reproducibility among different observers unless specific guidelines are provided, and the failure in the past of many pathologists to include a grade on the pathology report have limited its utility as a prognostic factor. Hormone receptor (ER and PR) status has long been recognized as a predictive factor for response to endocrine manipulations (e.g., tamoxifen or oophorectomy). In addition, studies have demonstrated that ER and PR are prognostic factors that are associated with increases in disease-free survival of about 10% at 5 years.[149] ER and PR levels are strongly correlated with histologic grade and patient age and inversely correlated with measures of proliferation.

Although many prognostic factors have been examined, relatively few have shown clinical utility. In addition, most studies of prognostic factors have examined one or two factors, making it difficult to predict the outcome of patients with a mixture of favorable and unfavorable prognostic features. Microarray technology has made it possible to examine the messenger RNA (mRNA) expression of thousands of genes simultaneously, producing a tumor fingerprint, which may be a more accurate predictor of prognosis. In a study of sporadic breast cancer, Perou et al.[150] demonstrated that patients could be separated into four major subgroups on the basis of gene clustering with those in the luminal subgroup having the best prognosis and those in the basal cell group a significantly worse prognosis. In a subsequent study, Van de Vijver et al.[151] used expression levels of 70 genes to classify 295 patients with breast cancer into good or poor prognosis groups. Interestingly, women with node-positive and node-negative disease were evenly distributed between the two groups, whereas other recognized poor prognostic factors (e.g., ER negativitiy, high histologic grade) were clustered in the poor prognosis group. The 10-year disease-free survival was 94.5% in the good prognosis group and 50.6% in the poor prognosis group. The gene expression profiling provided a significantly better prediction of outcome than currently used clinical criteria. These results are extremely promising, but additional work is needed to confirm these results before widespread clinical application.

ADJUVANT SYSTEMIC THERAPY

Adjuvant therapy is defined as the use of cytotoxic chemotherapy or endocrine therapy after the local treatment of breast cancer to eliminate clinically occult micrometastases, thereby preventing recurrence and increasing survival. Initially, adjuvant systemic therapy trials were carried out in patients with node-positive disease, who are at the highest risk of relapse. Subsequently, the recognition that breast cancer death occurs in up to 40% of patients with node-negative breast cancer led to trials of systemic treatment in that group.

The Early Breast Cancer Trialists Collaborative Group has conducted metaanalyses of the major prospective, randomized trials of chemotherapy, with the most recent analysis published in 1998 (Table 76.15).[152] After 15 years of follow-up, this analysis confirmed that adjuvant chemotherapy reduces the proportional risk of death equally in patients with node-positive and those with node-negative disease. A small benefit was seen for anthracycline-based treatment (e.g., doxorubicin) versus cytoxan, methotrexate, and fluorouracil. The benefit of

TABLE 76.15 RESULTS

OVERVIEW ANALYSIS OF CHEMOTHERAPY, 2000

	Reduction in annual odds	
Treatment	**Breast cancer recurrence (% ± SE)**	**Breast cancer death (% ± SE)**
Any multidrug chemotherapy	22 ± 2	15 ± 2
CMF vs. none	24 ± 2	16 ± 3
Anthracycline vs. none	24 ± 5	14 ± 5
Anthracycline vs. CMF	11 ± 3	16 ± 3
Anthracycline, age <50	33 ± 8	26 ± 9
Anthracycline, age 50–59	21 ± 4	17 ± 5

CMF, cytoxan, methotrexate, 5-fluorouracil; SE, standard error. (Modified from Stearns V, Davidson NE. Adjuvant chemotherapy and chemoendocrine therapy. In: Harris JR, Lippman ME, Morrow M, et al., eds. *Diseases of the breast*, 3rd ed. Philadelphia: Lippincott Williams & Wilkins, 2004, p. 895.)

chemotherapy was greatest in younger women, reducing the odds of death by 27% in those under 40 and by 8% in those ages 60 to 69. Recent studies have investigated the utility of adding a taxane (paclitaxel or docetaxel) to an anthracycline-based regimen in women with node-positive disease, and have demonstrated a small added benefit for this group of patients.[153] The utility of newer agents such as vinorelbine and herceptin (an antibody against the c-*HER2-neu* protein) as adjuvant therapy is currently being defined.

Tamoxifen is a nonsteroidal agent that exhibits site-specific estrogen agonist and antagonist properties.[154] It was the first drug identified in the class now referred to as SERMs (selective estrogen receptor modulators). Tamoxifen acts as an antiestrogen in the breast through competitive blockade of the ER. In bones and lipids, tamoxifen acts as an estrogen agonist, preserving bone density and lowering blood cholesterol. Tamoxifen also acts as an agonist in the uterus, increasing the incidence of endometrial carcinoma (see section on management of the high-risk woman). A metaanalysis, most recently updated in 2000, has been conducted of more than 42,000 patients in 63 trials of tamoxifen.[155] The use of tamoxifen reduces the annual odds of breast cancer recurrence by 47% and the annual odds of death by 26%. Tamoxifen is beneficial in women of all ages, and 5 years of therapy is superior to shorter durations of treatment. These benefits are limited to patients whose tumors express ER, PR, or both. A newer adjuvant therapy option for postmenopausal women consists of aromatase inhibitor therapy: these drugs function by inhibiting the peripheral conversion of androgens to estrogen, thereby lowering estrogen levels. One of these agents, anastrozole, was recently compared with tamoxifen alone or in combination with anastrozole in a large randomized clinical trial.[156] At 4 years follow-up, the anastrozole-alone arm showed a modest benefit compared with tamoxifen, with the combination arm being similar to tamoxifen. The tolerability profile of anastrozole was somewhat better than that for tamoxifen, with fewer hot flashes, no endometrial effects, and fewer thromboembolic events. Anastrozole is therefore a valid alternative to tamoxifen in postmenopausal women.

The overview analysis of randomized trials[152,155] also demonstrates that combined therapy with chemotherapy and tamoxifen is superior to treatment with either agent alone in both premenopausal and postmenopausal women. In postmenopausal women, however, the benefit from the addition of

TABLE 76.16 TREATMENT

RECOMMENDATIONS FOR ADJUVANT THERAPY

Patient group	Recommended treatment
NODE-NEGATIVE, LOW RISK	
Tumor <1 cm	No treatment or endocrine therapy if ER+
Special histologic types 1–2 cm, grade 1, ER+	
NODE-NEGATIVE, HIGHER RISK	
ER+	Endocrine therapy OR chemotherapy + endocrine therapy
ER−	Chemotherapy
NODE-POSITIVE	
ER+	
Premenopausal	Chemotherapy plus endocrine therapy
Postmenopausal	Chemotherapy + endocrine therapy or endocrine therapy alone
ER−	Chemotherapy

ER+, estrogen receptor-positive; ER−, estrogen receptor-negative.

chemotherapy is modest and must be weighed against the toxicity of the treatment in the context of the patient's overall health. General guidelines for the use of adjuvant therapy are shown in Table 76.16, but final treatment decisions are influenced by the individual attitudes of patients toward possibly small benefits and treatment toxicities. The proportional reduction in mortality must be translated into an absolute reduction to be meaningful for the individual patient. Thus, a 24% reduction in mortality for a patient with a 1-cm, node-negative tumor who has a 10% risk for death at 10 years corresponds to about a 2% benefit. The same proportional reduction in mortality for the patient with six positive nodes and a 75% risk for death at 10 years translates to a 30% absolute benefit.

SPECIAL PROBLEMS

Breast Cancer in the Elderly

Approximately 50% of breast cancers in the United States are diagnosed in women aged 65 and older. Therapy in the elderly should be based on physiologic, not chronologic, age. Mastectomy can be performed safely in the majority of older women, regardless of age, albeit with a slightly higher mortality (0.39% for all ages, and 0.9% for the subgroup of women age 75 and older).[132] Mastectomy is an excellent means of obtaining local control and may minimize outpatient visits, but many older women prefer BCT if offered this option. This is clearly a lesser operative procedure than a mastectomy, and several studies[157] suggest that local failure rates after BCT with RT are lower in women over age 65 than in their younger counterparts. Radiotherapy is generally well tolerated by older women, but daily visits for RT may be difficult for the elderly patient with limited mobility. In elderly women with tumors under 2 cm in size, the benefit of RT may be marginal and treatment with wide excision of the tumor and endocrine therapy is an option.[158,159] When omission of breast irradiation in the treatment of an elderly patient with larger tumors is considered, it is useful to remember that the majority of local failures occur in the first 6 postoperative years.

In the elderly woman with significant comorbid conditions, tamoxifen has been studied as an alternative to conventional surgical treatment. In three randomized trials comparing tamoxifen alone versus surgical therapy alone or with tamoxifen, no survival advantages were observed for surgical therapy.[158–160] Although wide resection with free surgical margins was not uniformily required in these studies, significant improvements in local control were noted in the surgically treated woman. Newer endocrine agents include the aromatase inhibitors; one of these (letrozole) has been compared with tamoxifen in a randomized trial of neoadjuvant therapy, with superior local response seen with letrozole. Response rates to primary endocrine therapy are high, but 12 months or more are often needed to achieve the best response. With long-term follow-up, the risk for disease progression may be significant. Because surgical treatment is well tolerated by the majority of older women, there is no reason to routinely substitute primary endocrine therapy. For the elderly woman with a limited life span who is a poor operative risk, however, endocrine therapy represents a viable alternative as a primary therapy.

Breast Cancer in Pregnancy

Breast cancer occurring during pregnancy is relatively uncommon when all cases of breast cancer are considered. If only patients with breast cancer in their childbearing years are evaluated, 7% to 14% are found to be pregnant at diagnosis.[161] If pregnant women are used as a denominator, approximately 2.2 breast cancers per 10,000 pregnancies can be anticipated.

The clinical presentation of breast cancer during pregnancy is the same as in the nonpregnant patient, and a palpable mass is the most common symptom. Mammography is not particularly helpful in the evaluation of breast masses in pregnant women because of the increased density of the breast. Ultrasonography is often useful in distinguishing a true mass from the normal nodularity of pregnancy, but ultimately the decision about the need for biopsy should be made on the basis of the physical examination. Delay in the diagnosis of breast cancer during pregnancy remains a major problem, and most of this delay is physician-induced. Core needle biopsy or breast biopsy under local anesthesia are safe at any time during pregnancy and should be performed for any suspicious mass.

The options for the local treatment of breast cancer during pregnancy are limited for the woman who wishes to continue her pregnancy. The use of irradiation during any trimester of pregnancy is contraindicated because of the inability to shield the fetus from internal radiation scatter. If breast cancer is diagnosed in the third trimester, lumpectomy can be performed and radiation delayed until after delivery. The effect of longer delays in radiation to allow breast preservation is unknown and may be detrimental. Immediate reconstruction with tissue flaps is also contraindicated during pregnancy because of the risk to the fetus of a more prolonged anesthesia and increased blood loss, in addition to the inability to obtain symmetry with the postpartum breast. Thus, mastectomy remains the mainstay of the surgical therapy of breast cancer during pregnancy. The radiocolloids and blue dyes used for SN biopsy are not known to be safe during pregnancy, so axillary staging is done with an axillary dissection. Therapeutic abortion does not appear to play a role in the treatment of nonmetastatic breast carcinoma. A number of small, nonrandomized studies have failed to show a survival advantage associated with termination of pregnancy. Some patients may opt to terminate a pregnancy because of concerns about the long-term prognosis or the risk for fetal damage, but patients should not be advised that this is of therapeutic benefit.

Breast cancer during pregnancy is often thought to be a particularly aggressive disease with a poor prognosis. Much of the poor prognosis, however, seems to be secondary to advanced disease at the time of diagnosis. These women are generally too young to undergo regular mammographic screening before pregnancy, and even in recent series, more than 60% of patients with pregnancy-associated breast cancer had positive axillary nodes. After correction for age and tumor stage, some studies suggest that survival in women treated during pregnancy is similar to that in nonpregnant patients. Populaton-based studies in Denmark, Sweden, and the United States indicate, however, that survival decreases significantly when breast cancer is diagnosed during pregnancy or shortly thereafter.[162–164]

Chemotherapy can be given to the pregnant patient with breast cancer but is generally delayed until after the first trimester. Fetal malformation is seen in approximately 20% of patients treated during the first trimester, and this risk falls to about 2% for exposure in the second and third trimesters. Some series, however, have reported low birth weight in as many of 40% of infants exposed to chemotherapy during pregnancy, and the long-term effects of chemotherapy exposure on growth, development, and cancer risk are largely unknown.[165] The decision to treat any woman with chemotherapy during pregnancy depends on her risk for relapse and the woman's desire for treatment after a thorough discussion of the risks and benefits, and these decisions must be resolved on a case-by-case basis. When breast cancer is diagnosed in the third trimester, chemotherapy can usually be delayed until fetal maturity, when delivery can be induced. The effects of longer delays on the efficacy of chemotherapy is unknown. Tamoxifen is contraindicated in pregnant women.

Male Breast Cancer

Cancer of the male breast is an uncommon disease. Risk factors include Klinefelter's syndrome, a family history of breast cancer, mutations of the *BRCA2* gene, hepatic disorders, and radiation exposure. With the exception of the gynecomastia seen with Klinefelter's disease, there is no clear association with gynecomastia. The mean age of patients at presentation with male breast cancer is approximately 10 years older than that of women with the disease.[166] The typical presentation is a mass beneath the nipple–areola complex, with retraction or ulceration of the nipple; nipple discharge is less frequent. Approximately 80% of male breast cancers are hormone receptor–positive.

The most common local treatment for male breast carcinoma is mastectomy. Radical mastectomy is no longer the standard therapy, and when the tumor is not fixed to the pectoral muscle, a total mastectomy can be performed. With limited muscle involvement, the portion of the pectoralis adherent to the tumor can be excised. When extensive pectoral muscle invasion is present, radical mastectomy may be necessary, although preoperative chemotherapy, as in female breast cancer, is also an option. BCT for male breast carcinoma is rarely feasible because of the small size of the breast and the central location of most tumors. Several small studies in men with breast cancer support the use of SN biopsy if the axilla is clinically negative; axillary dissection is indicated if suspicious axillary nodes are palpable.[167]

The survival rate of men with breast cancer is similar to that in women with disease of the same stage[168] and axillary nodal status is the major predictor of outcome. The benefit of adjuvant systemic therapy in male breast cancer has not been evaluated in randomized clinical trials, but the natural history and response to therapy of metastatic breast carcinoma in men is similar to that in postmenopausal women, leading to similar practice in the adjuvant setting. Because most male breast cancers contain hormone receptors, the largest adjuvant experience has been gained with hormonal therapy. The administration of tamoxifen to men with stage II or III disease resulted in a 55% 5-year survival, versus 28% in historical controls who received no systemic treatment.[169] Tamoxifen, however, may not be as well tolerated in men as in women, and frequently causes decreased libido. The use of aromatase inhibitors in men with breast cancer is being explored, but tamoxifen remains the mainstay of endocrine therapy. In general, the use of adjuvant systemic therapy should be based on prognosis and hormone receptor status, and the guidelines for postmenopausal women should be followed. Orchiectomy is an option as second-line hormonal manipulation in men with metastatic disease, with an 80% response rate to castration, in men with receptor-positive cancer.[170]

Occult Primary Tumor Presenting with Nodal Metastases

Breast cancer presenting as metastatic disease in the axillary nodes with no evident tumor in the breast is uncommon, accounting for fewer than 1% of cases in most large series. Metastatic adenocarcinoma in axillary nodes may be secondary to a variety of primary cancers, but in women, breast cancer is by far the most common type. In the patient without historical or clinical evidence suggesting a primary tumor at another site, the radiologic evaluation should be confined to breast imaging and a chest radiograph. Examination of the nodal tissue for hormone receptors helps to confirm a breast primary tumor if the tissue is hormone receptor–positive, but the breast cannot be excluded as the site of the primary tumor if the nodal tissue does not contain receptors.

Magnetic resonance imaging is often successful in identifying a primary tumor when mammography and ultrasound are normal. Olson et al.[171] identified a primary tumor in 28 of 40 (70%) patients presenting with axillary adenopathy and other small series report similar results. Identification of a primary tumor greatly facilitates BCT and, in this circumstance, the patient can be managed in the same way as any stage II cancer.

Historically, when a primary tumor has not been identified, most women with axillary node metastases secondary to a presumed breast cancer have been treated with mastectomy, and a breast carcinoma was identified during the pathologic evaluation in approximately 65% of these cases. In older reports, the size of the occult tumors varied widely, with lesions as large as 6 cm reported. In more recent studies of patients evaluated with modern imaging techniques, large tumors are uncommon, and this has stimulated interest in breast preservation even when the tumor cannot be identified. In the largest reported series from the Institute Curie, 54 patients received whole breast irradiation (median dose 59Gy). The 5- and 10-year rates of ipsilateral breast recurrence were 7.5% and 20%, supporting the idea that this is a reasonable approach.[172] In contrast, studies in which the breast was observed without treatment indicate that evident breast cancers develop in close to 50% of patients within 5 years.[173,174] Additional positive axillary nodes are frequent in this circumstance, so axillary dissection should be performed regardless of the method that is selected for managing the breast.

The prognosis for patients with occult primary tumors is similar to that for patients with clinically evident tumors matched for the number of involved nodes, and adjuvant systemic therapy should be administered according to established guidelines for patients with node-positive disease.

Locally Recurrent Breast Carcinoma

Local recurrence in the breast after BCT may be a consequence of inappropriate patient selection, poor surgical or radiotherapeutic technique, or tumor biology. When errors in technique and selection are excluded, local recurrence in the first two postoperative years is uncommon. From years 2 to 6, local recurrence develops at a constant rate, usually at or adjacent to the site of the original tumor. After year 6, most local recurrence develops in other quadrants of the breast, which suggests that these are new primary tumors rather than true local failures. This idea is supported by the observation that the risk for late recurrence in other quadrants of the breast, approximately 1% annually, is equal to the risk for development of a new contralateral breast carcinoma.

Most recurrences are in the breast parenchyma, with approximately 5% to 10% developing in the skin as diffuse inflammatory-type recurrences.[175] Before further local therapy, an evaluation to exclude metastatic disease is appropriate because concomitant distant metastases are present in 5% to 10% of cases. In the absence of distant metastases, complete mastectomy has been the mainstay of therapy. Five-year relapse-free survival rates range from 60% to 79% after the procedure, and further chest wall recurrences are uncommon. Small experiences with further attempts at breast preservation by using excision alone or repeated irradiation of small areas of the breast after surgical excision have been reported, but larger numbers of patients and longer follow-up periods are needed to determine the role of these therapies. The role of adjuvant systemic therapy in the management of recurrence is not well defined. In patients who have not received prior systemic therapy, we use the same criteria for treatment that are used for patients with newly diagnosed cancer. Treatment decisions for patients who received adjuvant systemic therapy at the time of diagnosis are made on a case-by-case basis.

Local recurrence after mastectomy develops in a different time frame, and the predictors and outcome are different than for local recurrence after BCT. Approximately 75% of cases of local recurrence after mastectomy develop in the first 3 postoperative years, and about half of these are associated with the development of distant metastases at the time of local recurrence or within a few years. The number of axillary nodes containing metastasis is the best predictor of the risk for chest wall recurrence.

An evaluation for distant metastases is an essential part of the workup of local recurrence after mastectomy. Small, localized recurrences are usually excised, but even with complete excision, RT should be administered to the chest wall because it is safe to assume that all the lymphatics are seeded with tumor. The supraclavicular space is usually included in the radiation field because these nodes are the second most frequent site of locoregional recurrence. The value of treating the axillary space and the internal mammary nodes is uncertain because clinical recurrence at these sites is uncommon. The value of additional systemic therapy for patients who have received postoperative adjuvant therapy is also uncertain.

Paget's Disease of the Nipple

Paget's disease of the nipple comprises 1% to 3% of all breast cancers. It is characterized by eczematoid changes of the nipple (Fig. 76.24), frequently present for 6 months or more before diagnosis, and often accompanied by itching, erythema, and nipple discharge. Paget's disease is diagnosed histologically by the presence of large cells with pale cytoplasm and prominent nucleoli (Paget's cells) involving the epidermis of the nipple. In 1874, Sir James Paget reported that this condition is invariably followed by cancer of the breast, usually within 1 year of diagnosis.[176] It is now recognized that the majority of women with Paget's disease have an associated infiltrating or intraductal carcinoma, which may manifest as a palpable mass, or as mammographic findings.

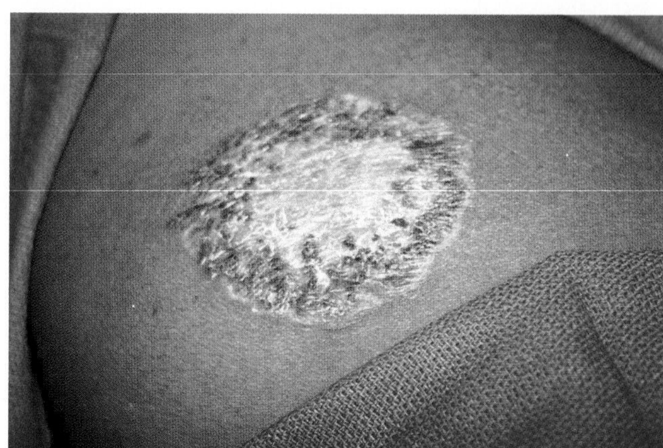

FIGURE 76.24 Paget disease of the nipple. Depigmentation and desquamation of the nipple and areola are evident.

Paget's disease has traditionally been treated with mastectomy. The reasons include the need to sacrifice the nipple–areola complex, the fact that subareolar ducts may be diffusely involved with tumor, and the observation that carcinoma may be found at a considerable distance from the nipple. A limited experience with breast-conserving procedures in the management of Paget's disease has been described. Because Paget's disease is a noninvasive carcinoma involving the nipple that usually is associated with intraductal or invasive carcinoma in the underlying breast parenchyma, the appropriateness of BCT is determined by the extent of the underlying involvement. A detailed mammographic evaluation (including magnification views of the subareolar region) and histologic evaluation with margin assessment are essential components of this assessment. For patients with evidence of diffuse involvement or disease at a distance from the nipple, mastectomy remains the standard therapy. In patients with disease localized to the subareolar area or the nipple–areola complex, BCT can be considered. This treatment requires removal of the entire nipple–areola complex and some of the underlying ductal region. In carefully selected patients, local failure rates with this approach appear to be similar to those reported for other breast carcinomas. Radiotherapy has been increasingly employed as part of BCT for Paget's disease, but no randomized trials have been performed, because of the rarity of the condition.[177] The prognosis in Paget's disease is related to the stage of the disease and appears to be similar to that of women with other types of breast carcinoma. If invasive breast cancer is found, adjuvant systemic therapy should be administered according to the same guidelines used for other patients with invasive cancer.

Phyllodes Tumor

The term *phyllodes tumor* denotes a group of lesions of varying malignant potential, ranging from completely benign tumors to fully malignant sarcomas. (The previous name, *cystosarcoma phyllodes*, is now reserved for fully malignant lesions.) A palpable mass is the most common clinical presentation, and rapid growth is often reported. On examination, phyllodes tumors are smooth, rounded, multinodular lesions that may be indistinguishable from fibroadenomas. Skin ulceration is seen with very large tumors, but this is usually caused by pressure necrosis rather than invasion of the skin by malignant cells (see Fig. 76.5). Histologically, phyllodes tumor, like fibroadenoma, is composed of epithelial elements and a connective tissue stroma.

Phyllodes tumors are classified as benign, borderline, or malignant, based on the nature of the tumor margins (pushing or infiltrative) and the presence of cellular atypia, mitotic activity, and overgrowth in the stroma. Which of these criteria is most important is a matter of disagreement, although most experts favor stromal overgrowth. The percentage of phyllodes tumors classified as malignant ranges from 23% to 50%.[178,179] Axillary metastases are reported in fewer than 5% of cases but are a poor prognostic sign when present. Metastases more commonly follow the pattern seen with sarcomas (with the lung as the most common site) and histologically resemble sarcomas. Approximately 20% of benign and malignant phyllodes tumors recur locally if excised with no margin or a margin of a few millimeters of normal breast tissue. A wide excision with a 1- to 2-cm margin of normal breast tissue is appropriate therapy for benign and borderline phyllodes tumors unless they are so large that this is not cosmetically feasible. In the past, many authors advocated mastectomy for the management of malignant phyllodes tumors. Because phyllodes tumors are not multicentric, there is no clear-cut biologic rationale for mastectomy, and the successful treatment of malignant phyllodes tumors with wide excision has been reported.[180] The use of systemic therapy for malignant phyllodes tumors is based on the guidelines for treating sarcomas.

OTHER CANCERS IN THE BREAST

Sarcomas, lymphomas, and melanomas may all present as breast masses and are generally managed as recommended when they develop in other sites. Angiosarcoma is reported to involve the breast more frequently than other sites in the body. The tumors frequently grow rapidly and may be associated with a bluish discoloration of the skin. Bilateral disease is not uncommon. Angiosarcoma has traditionally been treated with mastectomy to clear margins. Axillary metastases are rare, and axillary dissection is not routinely indicated. The prognosis appears to be related to the grade of the lesion. No advantage has been proved for adjuvant RT or chemotherapy. Other sarcomas occur infrequently in the breast. Surgery is the primary therapy, and the decision to perform mastectomy or wide local excision is based on tumor size.

Melanoma arising from the skin of the breast is a more frequent finding in men than women. The diagnosis, treatment, and prognosis of melanoma arising in the breast are the same as for melanoma arising in other parts of the body. Mastectomy is not necessary for treatment of this lesion.

Primary breast lymphomas are rare and account for fewer than 1% of breast malignancies. They are believed to arise from intramammary lymph nodes or periductal and perilobular lymphoid tissue. Bilateral disease is seen in as many as 25% of patients. The diagnosis is usually made only after a biopsy, as neither the clinical nor the mammographic appearance of these lesions is diagnostic. Once the diagnosis of lymphoma is established, treatment is with chemotherapy or RT, or both, according to the disease stage and histologic subtype.

LOCALLY ADVANCED BREAST CANCER

The designation of *locally advanced breast cancer* includes T3 and T4 tumors, those with extensive regional nodal involvement (N2 or N3), and inflammatory breast cancer (Fig. 76.25).

Historical studies have demonstrated that for inflammatory carcinoma and tumors with evidence of skin involvement, chest wall fixation, or extensive axillary nodal disease, initial surgical therapy is associated with a high rate of locoregional recurrence and very poor 5-year survival, with treatment failure usually occurring within 2 years of diagnosis.[181] For this reason, locally advanced breast cancer is now approached with a combination of chemotherapy, surgery, and RT. Anthracycline-based neoadjuvant chemotherapy results in partial (50% reduction in primary tumor volume) or complete clinical reponse (no clinically detectable residual tumor) in 60% to 80% of patients.[182] Response rates are further increased to 80% to 95% by the addition of taxanes to the neoadjuvant protocol, with a significant increase in clinical complete responses, and an increase in pathologic complete response (no residual tumor present on pathologic examination) from 15% to 31%.[183] Women who experience a pathologic complete response have significantly better long-term survival than those who do not.[184] Although induction chemotherapy is effective in reducing tumor burden and facilitates surgical therapy, no survival advantage has been demonstrated for the use of preoperative, as opposed to postoperative, chemotherapy in randomized trials.

For patients with stage IIIB carcinoma, induction chemotherapy is the standard initial approach. After three to four cycles of treatment or maximal response, mastectomy or lumpectomy is undertaken. Depending on the extent of residual tumor, additional chemotherapy may be given postoperatively, followed by chest wall RT to reduce the risk for local recurrence. For the patient with stage IIIA carcinoma that is operable by traditional criteria, the initial therapy can be surgery or chemotherapy. If the patient desires breast preservation, chemotherapy can shrink the tumor sufficiently to allow this in some women. If not, mastectomy can be performed, with chemotherapy and RT given postoperatively in the traditional sequence.[185] Women with HR-positive disease should receive endocrine therapy. Inflammatory breast cancer is a special subtype of locally advanced breast cancer that is characterized by erythema, edema, and peu d'orange and by diffuse thickening

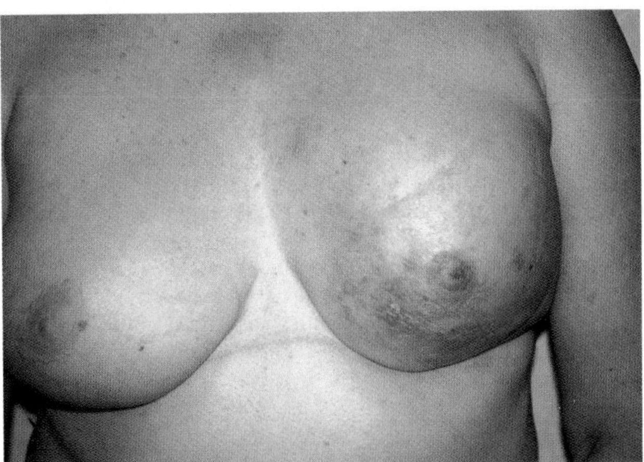

FIGURE 76.25 Locally advanced breast cancer. The breast is lifted and the upper half is bulging because of the large tumor. Distortion in the inferolateral contour is evident. The medial skin changes are caused by dermal tumor satellites.

of the breast tissue. This appearance is caused by obstruction of the dermal lymphatics with tumor cells. Inflammatory cancer is always treated with chemotherapy as the initial approach. If all inflammatory skin changes resolve, mastectomy is performed. Radiation to the chest wall is also part of therapy. With modern combined-modality therapy, locoregional control can be maintained in 80% of patients with locally advanced and inflammatory cancer, and 5-year survival rates of 50% to 80% have been reported.[183–186] However, 50% of patients eventually die of metastatic disease, which underscores the need for further research in this area.

KEY POINTS

- **Screening mammography appears to reduce breast cancer mortality by 20% to 30% as well as increasing the likelihood of breast-conserving surgery.**
- **Comparison of the results of stereotactic core biopsy and surgical biopsy demonstrates concordance rates of 71% to 99%. The diagnosis of atypical ductal hyperplasia and radial scar are circumstances of concern for a false-negative diagnosis.**
- **The most common cause of pathologic nipple discharge is a solitary papilloma (60%) duct hyperplasia (15% to 20%), followed by ductal carcinoma *in situ* in 5% to 20% of patients.**
- **If aspiration of a breast cyst yields nonbloody fluid and the masses resolve, no further therapy is needed, whereas if the fluid is bloody, the palpable abnormality does not resolve completely, or the same cyst recurs multiple times, biopsy to exclude malignancy is required.**
- **Approximately 20% to 30% of women with breast cancer have a family history of the disease, but only 5% to 10% have an inherited mutation in a breast cancer susceptibility gene, most commonly *BRCA1* and *BRCA2*.**
- **The use of tamoxifen in high-risk women results in approximately 50% reduction in risk for invasive and noninvasive breast cancer.**
- **For breast conserving therapy to be successful in the treatment of invasive breast cancer, three conditions must be met: It must be possible to (a) reduce the tumor burden to a microscopic level likely to be controlled by irradiation, (b) safely deliver radiation therapy, and (c) promptly detect local recurrence.**
- **Radiation therapy leads to approximately 75% reduction in local recurrence after breast conservation therapy with tumor at the margin of resection, young age, and whole breast radiation dose less than 4,500 to 5,000 cGy being risk factors for local recurrence.**
- **Regardless of the technique of sentinel node biopsy used, a sentinel node will be identified in 90% of cases, which will predict the status of the remaining axillary nodes in about 90% of cases.**
- **The use of tamoxifen reduces the annual odds of breast cancer recurrence by 47% and the annual odds of death by 20% in patients of all ages who express estrogen receptors or progesterone receptors, or both.**
- **Locally advanced breast cancer includes T3 and T4 tumors, those with extensive regional nodal involvement (N2 or N3), and inflammatory breast cancer and should be treated with a combination of induction chemotherapy, surgery, and postoperative radiation therapy.**

References

1. Turner-Warwick RT. The lymphatics of the breast. *Br J Surg.* 1959; 46:574.
2. Cody HS 3rd, Egeli RA, Urban JA. Rotter's node metastases. Therapeutic and prognostic considerations in early breast carcinoma. *Ann Surg.* 1984;199:266–270.
3. Sacre R. Modern thoughts on lymph nodes in breast cancer. *Semin Surg Oncol.* 1989;5:118–125.
4. Daniel C, Silberstein, GB. Development of the mammary gland. In: Neville M, Daniel, CW, eds. *The mammary gland.* New York: Plenum, 1987, pp. 3–10.
5. Russo J, Russo IH. Development of the human breast. In: Russo J, Russo IH, eds. *Encyclopedia of reproduction.* New York: Academic Press, 1998, pp. 71–76.
6. Dickson RB, Russo J. Biochemical control of breast development. In: Harris JR, Lippman ME, Morrow M, eds. *Diseases of the breast.* Philadelphia: Lippincott, Williams & Wilkins, 2000, pp. 303–318.
7. American Joint Committee on Cancer Staging. *Manual for staging of cancer*, 6th ed. New York: Springer, 2002.
8. Shapiro S. Screening: assessment of current studies. *Cancer* 1994;74: 231–238.
9. Hendrick RE, Smith RA, Rutledge JH 3rd, et al. Benefit of screening mammography in women aged 40–49: a new meta-analysis of randomized controlled trials. *J Natl Cancer Inst Monogr.* 1997:87–92.
10. Morrow M, Bucci C, Rademaker A. Medical contraindications are not a major factor in the underutilization of breast conserving therapy. *J Am Coll Surg.* 1998;186:269–274.
11. American College of Radiology. *Breast Imaging Reporting and Data System (BI-RADS)*, 2nd ed. Reston, VA, 1995.
12. Sickles EA. Further experience with microfocal spot magnification mammography in the assessment of clustered breast microcalcifications. *Radiology* 1980;137:9–14.
13. Dowlatshahi K, Yaremko, ML, Kluskens LF, et al. Nonpalpable breast lesions: findings of stereotactic needle-core biopsy and fine-needle aspiration cytology. *Radiology* 1991;183:745–750.
14. Parker SH, Burbank F, Jackman RJ, et al. Percutaneous large-core breast biopsy: a multi-institutional study. *Radiology* 1994;193:359–364.
15. Venta L. Image-guided breast biopsy. In: Harris J, Lippman ME, Morrow M, et al., eds. *Diseases of the Breast*, 3rd ed. Philadelphia: Lippincott, Williams & Wilkins, 2004, pp. 199–219.
16. Liberman L, Cohen MA, Dershaw DD, et al. Atypical ductal hyperplasia diagnosed at stereotaxic core biopsy of breast lesions: an indication for surgical biopsy. *AJR Am J Roentgenol* 1995;164:1111–1113.
17. Jackman RJ, Burbank F, Parker SH, et al. Atypical ductal hyperplasia diagnosed at stereotactic breast biopsy: improved reliability with 14-gauge, directional, vacuum-assisted biopsy. *Radiology* 1997;204:485–488.
18. Golub RM, Bennett CL, Stinson T, et al. Cost minimization study of image-guided core biopsy versus surgical excisional biopsy for women with abnormal mammograms. *J Clin Oncol.* 2004;22:2430–2437.
19. Morrow M, Venta L, Stinson T, et al. Prospective comparison of stereotactic core biopsy and surgical excision as diagnostic procedures for breast cancer patients. *Ann Surg.* 2001;233:537–541.
20. Mansel RE, Wisbey JR, Hughes LE. Controlled trial of the antigonadotropin danazol in painful nodular benign breast disease. *Lancet* 1982;1: 928–930.
21. Mansel RE, Dogliotti L. European multicentre trial of bromocriptine in cyclical mastalgia. *Lancet* 1990;335:190–193.
22. Fentiman IS, Caleffi M, Hamed H, et al. Dosage and duration of tamoxifen treatment for mastalgia: a controlled trial. *Br J Surg.* 1988;75:845–846.
23. Pye JK, Mansel RE, Hughes LE. Clinical experience of drug treatments for mastalgia. *Lancet* 1985;2:373–377.
24. London RS, Sundaram GS, Murphy L, et al. The effect of vitamin E on mammary dysplasia: a double-blind study. *Obstet Gynecol.* 1985;65: 104–106.
25. Allen SS, Froberg DG. The effect of decreased caffeine consumption on benign proliferative breast disease: a randomized clinical trial. *Surgery* 1987;101:720–730.
26. Smallwood J, Ah-Kye D, Taylor I. Vitamin B_6 in the treatment of pre-menstrual mastalgia. *Br J Clin Pract.* 1986;40:532–533.
27. Catania S, Zurrida S, Veronesi P, et al. Mondor's disease and breast cancer. *Cancer* 1992;69:2267–2270.
28. Seltzer MH, Perloff LJ, Kelley RI, et al. The significance of age in patients with nipple discharge. *Surg Gynecol Obstet.* 1970;131:519–522.
29. King TA, Carter KM, Bolton JS, et al. A simple approach to nipple discharge. *Am Surg.* 2000;66:960–965; discussion 965–966.
30. Simmons R, Adamovich T, Brennan M, et al. Nonsurgical evaluation of pathologic nipple discharge. *Ann Surg Oncol.* 2003;10:113–116.
31. Cabioglu N, Hunt KK, Singletary SE, et al. Surgical decision making and factors determining a diagnosis of breast carcinoma in women presenting with nipple discharge. *J Am Coll Surg.* 2003;196:354–364.
32. Dawes LG, Bowen C, Venta LA, et al. Ductography for nipple discharge: no replacement for ductal excision. *Surgery* 1998;124:685–691.
33. Dietz JR, Crowe JP, Grundfest S, et al. Directed duct excision by using mammary ductoscopy in patients with pathologic nipple discharge. *Surgery* 2002;132:582–587; discussion 587–588.
34. Schnitt S, Connelly, J. Pathology of benign breast disorders. In: Harris J, Lippman ME, Morrow M, et al., eds. *Diseases of the breast*, 2nd ed. Philadelphia: Lippincott Williams & Wilkins, 2000, pp. 75–94.
35. Aitken RJ, Hood J, Going JJ, et al. Bacteriology of mammary duct ectasia. *Br J Surg.* 1988;75:1040–1041.
36. Morrow M, Wong S, Venta L. The evaluation of breast masses in women younger than forty years of age. *Surgery* 1998;124:634–640; discussion 640–641.

37. Cowen PN, Benson EA. Cytological study of fluid from breast cysts. *Br J Surg.* 1979;66:209–211.
38. Wilkinson S, Anderson TJ, Rifkind E, et al. Fibroadenoma of the breast: a follow-up of conservative management. *Br J Surg.* 1989;76:390–391.
39. Dupont WD, Page DL, Parl FF, et al. Long-term risk of breast cancer in women with fibroadenoma. *N Engl J Med.* 1994;331:10–15.
40. Dupont WD, Parl FF, Hartmann WH, et al. Breast cancer risk associated with proliferative breast disease and atypical hyperplasia. *Cancer* 1993; 71:1258–1265.
41. London SJ, Connolly JL, Schnitt SJ, et al. A prospective study of benign breast disease and the risk of breast cancer. *JAMA* 1992;267:941–944.
42. McDivitt RW, Stevens JA, Lee NC, et al. Histologic types of benign breast disease and the risk for breast cancer. The Cancer and Steroid Hormone Study Group. *Cancer* 1992;69:1408–1414.
43. Shelty MK, Shah YP, Sharman RS. Prospective evaluation of the value of combined mammographic and sonographic assessment in patients with palpable abnormalities of the breast. *J Ultrasound Med.* 2003;22:263–268.
44. Morrow M, Schmidt RA, Bucci C. Breast conservation for mammographically occult carcinoma. *Ann Surg.* 1998;227:502–506.
45. Lister D, Evans AJ, Burrell HC, et al. The accuracy of breast ultrasound in the evaluation of clinically benign discrete, symptomatic breast lumps. *Clin Radiol.* 1998;53:490–492.
46. Yang WT, Lam WW, Cheung H, et al. Sonographic, magnetic resonance imaging, and mammographic assessments of preoperative size of breast cancer. *J Ultrasound Med.* 1997;16:791–797.
47. Schnall M, Blume, J, Bluemke D, et al. MRI detection of multifocal breast carcinoma: report from the International Breast MRI Consortium. *J Clin Oncol.* 2004;22(14s):4s (abst 504).
48. Holland R, Veling SH, Mravunac M, et al. Histologic multifocality of Tis, T1-2 breast carcinomas. Implications for clinical trials of breast-conserving surgery. *Cancer* 1985;56:979–990.
49. Schelling M, Avril N, Nahrig J, et al. Positron emission tomography using [(18)F]Fluorodeoxyglucose for monitoring primary chemotherapy in breast cancer. *J Clin Oncol.* 2000;18:1689–695.
50. Giard RW, Hermans J. The value of aspiration cytologic examination of the breast. A statistical review of the medical literature. *Cancer* 1992;69: 2104–2110.
51. Shabot MM, Goldberg IM, Schick P, et al. Aspiration cytology is superior to Tru-Cut needle biopsy in establishing the diagnosis of clinically suspicious breast masses. *Ann Surg.* 1982;196:122–126.
52. Kearney TJ, Morrow M. Effect of reexcision on the success of breast-conserving surgery. *Ann Surg Oncol.* 1995;2:303–307.
53. Fisher ER, Sass R, Fisher B. Biologic considerations regarding the one and two step procedures in the management of patients with invasive carcinoma of the breast. *Surg Gynecol Obstet.* 1985;161:245–249.
54. Layfield LJ, Glasgow BJ, Cramer H. Fine-needle aspiration in the management of breast masses. *Pathol Annu.* 1989;24 Pt 2:23–62.
55. Greenberg R, Skornick Y, Kaplan O. Management of breast fibroadenomas. *J Gen Intern Med.* 1998;13:640–645.
56. Bell DA, Hajdu SI, Urban JA, et al. Role of aspiration cytology in the diagnosis and management of mammary lesions in office practice. *Cancer* 1983;51:1182–1189.
57. Donegan WL. Evaluation of a palpable breast mass. *N Engl J Med.* 1992;327:937–942.
58. Dixon JM. Repeated aspiration of breast abscesses in lactating women. *BMJ* 1988;297:1517–1518.
59. Bundred NJ, Dover MS, Aluwihare N, et al. Smoking and periductal mastitis. *BMJ* 1993;307:772–773.
60. Meguid MM, Oler A, Numann PJ, et al. Pathogenesis-based treatment of recurring subareolar breast abscesses. *Surgery* 1995;118:775–782.
61. National Center for Health Statistics. *SEER Cancer Statistics Review, 1973–1995.* Bethesda, MD: National Cancer Institute, 1998.
62. Slattery ML, Kerber RA. A comprehensive evaluation of family history and breast cancer risk. The Utah Population Database. *JAMA* 1993; 270:1563–1568.
63. Claus EB, Risch NJ, Thompson WD. Age at onset as an indicator of familial risk of breast cancer. *Am J Epidemiol.* 1990;131:961–972.
64. Struewing JP, Hartge P, Wacholder S, et al. The risk of cancer associated with specific mutations of BRCA1 and BRCA2 among Ashkenazi Jews. *N Engl J Med.* 1997;336:1401–1408.
65. **King MC, Marks JH, Mandell JB. Breast and ovarian cancer risks due to inherited mutations in BRCA1 and BRCA2. *Science* 2003;302: 643–646.**
66. Kirchhoff T, Kauff ND, Mitra N, et al. BRCA mutations and risk of prostate cancer in Ashkenazi Jews. *Clin Cancer Res.* 2004;10:2918–2921.
67. Hahn SA, Greenhalf B, Ellis I, et al. BRCA2 germline mutations in familial pancreatic carcinoma. *J Natl Cancer Inst.* 2003;95:214–221.
68. Shattuck-Eidens D, Oliphant A, McClure M, et al. BRCA1 sequence analysis in women at high risk for susceptibility mutations. Risk factor analysis and implications for genetic testing. *JAMA* 1997;278: 1242–1250.
69. Euhus DM, Smith KC, Robinson L, et al. Pretest prediction of BRCA1 or BRCA2 mutation by risk counselors and the computer model BRCAPRO. *J Natl Cancer Inst.* 2002;94:844–851.
70. Hisada M, Garber JE, Fung CY, et al. Multiple primary cancers in families with Li-Fraumeni syndrome. *J Natl Cancer Inst.* 1998;90:606–611.
71. Colditz GA. Epidemiology of breast cancer. Findings from the nurses' health study. *Cancer* 1993;71:1480–1489.
72. Newcomb PA, Storer BE, Longnecker MP, et al. Lactation and a reduced risk of premenopausal breast cancer. *N Engl J Med.* 1994;330:81–87.
73. Collaborative Group on Hormonal Factors in Breast Cancer. Breast cancer and hormonal contraceptives: collaborative reanalysis of individual data on 53,297 women with breast cancer and 100,239 women without breast cancer from 54 epidemiological studies. *Lancet* 1996;347:1713–1727.
74. **Chlebowski RT, Hendrix SL, Langer RD, et al. Influence of estrogen plus progestin on breast cancer and mammography in healthy postmenopausal women: the Women's Health Initiative Randomized Trial. *JAMA* 2003; 289:3243–3253.**
75. Hancock SL, Tucker MA, Hoppe RT. Breast cancer after treatment of Hodgkin's disease. *J Natl Cancer Inst.* 1993;85:25–31.
76. Hunter DJ, Spiegelman D, Adami HO, et al. Cohort studies of fat intake and the risk of breast cancer—a pooled analysis. *N Engl J Med.* 1996;334:356–361.
77. Willett W, Hunter, DJ, Stampfer, MJ, et al. Dietary fat and fiber in relation to risk of breast cancer: an 8 year follow-up. *JAMA* 1992;268:2037–2044.
78. Hamajima N, Hirose K, Tajima K, et al. Alcohol, tobacco and breast cancer—collaborative reanalysis of individual data from 53 epidemiological studies, including 58,515 women with breast cancer and 95,067 women without the disease. *Br J Cancer* 2002;87:1234–1245.
79. Dupont WD, Page DL. Risk factors for breast cancer in women with proliferative breast disease. *N Engl J Med.* 1985;312:146–151.
80. Haagensen CD. Lobular neoplasia (lobular carcinoma in situ). In: Haagensen CD, Bodian C, Haagensen DE, eds. *Breast carcinoma: risk and detection.* Philadelphia: WB Saunders, 1981, pp. 238–291.
81. Rosen P, Kosloff, C, Lieberman, PH, et al. Lobular carcinoma in situ of the breast: detailed analysis of 99 patients with average follow-up of 24 years. *Am J Surg Pathol.* 1978;2:225–251.
82. Andersen JA. Lobular carcinoma in situ of the breast. An approach to rational treatment. *Cancer* 1977;39:2597–602.
83. Page DL, Kidd TE Jr, Dupont WD, et al. Lobular neoplasia of the breast: higher risk for subsequent invasive cancer predicted by more extensive disease. *Hum Pathol.* 1991;22:1232–1239.
84. Salvadori B, Bartoli C, Zurrida S, et al. Risk of invasive cancer in women with lobular carcinoma in situ of the breast. *Eur J Cancer* 1991;27:35–37.
85. Ottesen GL, Graversen HP, Blichert-Toft M, et al. Lobular carcinoma in situ of the female breast. Short-term results of a prospective nationwide study. The Danish Breast Cancer Cooperative Group. *Am J Surg Pathol.* 1993;17:14–21.
86. Bodian CA, Perzin KH, Lattes R. Lobular neoplasia. Long term risk of breast cancer and relation to other factors. *Cancer* 1996;78:1024–1034.
87. Gail MH, Brinton LA, Byar DP, et al. Projecting individualized probabilities of developing breast cancer for white females who are being examined annually. *J Natl Cancer Inst.* 1989;81:1879–1886.
88. Claus EB, Risch N, Thompson WD. Autosomal dominant inheritance of early-onset breast cancer. Implications for risk prediction. *Cancer* 1994; 73:643–651.
89. Hartmann LC, Schaid DJ, Woods JE, et al. Efficacy of bilateral prophylactic mastectomy in women with a family history of breast cancer. *N Engl J Med.* 1999;340:77–84.
90. Early Breast Cancer Trialists' Cooperative Group. Effects of chemotherapy and hormonal therapy for early breast cancer recurrence and 15 year survival. *Lancet* 2005;365:1687–1717.
91. **Fisher B, Costantino JP, Wickerham DL, et al. Tamoxifen for prevention of breast cancer: report of the National Surgical Adjuvant Breast and Bowel Project P-1 Study. *J Natl Cancer Inst.* 1998;90:1371–1388.**
92. Cummings SR, Eckert S, Krueger KA, et al. The effect of raloxifene on risk of breast cancer in postmenopausal women: results from the MORE randomized trial. Multiple outcomes of raloxifene evaluation. *JAMA* 1999;281:2189–2197.
93. Morrow M, Harris JR. Ductal carcinoma in situ and microinvasive carcinoma. In: Harris JR, Lippman ME, Morrow M, eds. *Diseases of the breast,* 3rd ed. Philadelphia: Lippincott Williams & Wilkins, 2004, pp. 521–540.
94. Silverstein M. Van Nuys/USC experience by treatment. In: Silverstein M, ed. *Ductal carcinoma in situ of the breast,* 2nd ed. Philadelphia: Lippincott Williams & Wilkins, 2002, pp. 337–342.
95. Solin LJ, Kurtz J, Fourquet A, et al. Fifteen-year results of breast-conserving surgery and definitive breast irradiation for the treatment of ductal carcinoma in situ of the breast. *J Clin Oncol.* 1996;14:754–763.
96. **Fisher B, Dignam J, Wolmark N, et al. Lumpectomy and radiation therapy for the treatment of intraductal breast cancer: findings from National Surgical Adjuvant Breast and Bowel Project B-17. *J Clin Oncol.* 1998; 16:441–452.**
97. Fisher ER, Dignam J, Tan-Chiu E, et al. Pathologic findings from the National Surgical Adjuvant Breast Project (NSABP) eight-year update of protocol B-17: intraductal carcinoma. *Cancer* 1999;86:429–438.
98. Julien JP, Bijker N, Fentiman IS, et al. Radiotherapy in breast-conserving treatment for ductal carcinoma in situ: first results of the EORTC randomised phase III trial 10853. EORTC Breast Cancer Cooperative Group and EORTC Radiotherapy Group. *Lancet* 2000;355:528–533.
99. UK Coordinating Committee on Cancer Research Ductal Carcinoma in Situ Working Party. Radiotherapy and tamoxifen in women with completely excised ductal carcinoma in situ of the breast in the UK, Australia, and New Zealand: randomized controlled trial. *Lancet* 2003;362:95–102.
100. Silverstein MJ, Lagios MD, Groshen S, et al. The influence of margin width on local control of ductal carcinoma in situ of the breast. *N Engl J Med.* 1999;340:1455–1461.

101. Wong J, Gadd M, Gelman R, et al. Wide excision alone for ductal carcinoma in situ (DCIS) of the breast. *Proc Am Soc Clin Oncol.* 2003;22:12 (abst).
102. Holland R, Hendriks JH, Vebeek AL, et al. Extent, distribution, and mammographic/histological correlations of breast ductal carcinoma in situ. *Lancet* 1990;335:519–522.
103. Fisher B, Dignam J, Wolmark N, et al. Tamoxifen in treatment of intraductal breast cancer: National Surgical Adjuvant Breast and Bowel Project B-24 randomised controlled trial. *Lancet* 1999;353:1993–2000.
104. Bloom HJ, Richardson WW, Harries EJ. Natural history of untreated breast cancer (1805–1933). Comparison of untreated and treated cases according to histological grade of malignancy. *BMJ* 1962;5299:213–221.
105. Halsted W. The results of radical operations for the cure of carcinoma of the breast. *Ann Surg.* 1907;66:1–19.
106. Fisher B. Laboratory and clinical research in breast cancer—a personal adventure: the David A. Karnofsky memorial lecture. *Cancer Res.* 1980; 40:3863–3874.
107. Hellman S. Karnofsky Memorial Lecture. Natural history of small breast cancers. *J Clin Oncol.* 1994;12:2229–2234.
108. Overgaard M, Hansen PS, Overgaard J, et al. Postoperative radiotherapy in high-risk premenopausal women with breast cancer who receive adjuvant chemotherapy. Danish Breast Cancer Cooperative Group 82b Trial. *N Engl J Med.* 1997;337:949–955.
109. Ragaz J, Jackson SM, Le N, et al. Adjuvant radiotherapy and chemotherapy in node-positive premenopausal women with breast cancer. *N Engl J Med.* 1997;337:956–962.
110. Overgaard M, Jensen MB, Overgaard J, et al. Postoperative radiotherapy in high-risk postmenopausal breast-cancer patients given adjuvant tamoxifen: Danish Breast Cancer Cooperative Group DBCG 82c randomised trial. *Lancet* 1999;353:1641–1648.
111. Broet P, de la Rochefordiere A, Scholl SM, et al. Contralateral breast cancer: annual incidence and risk parameters. *J Clin Oncol.* 1995;13:1578–1583.
112. Elston CW, Ellis IO. Pathological prognostic factors in breast cancer. I. The value of histological grade in breast cancer: experience from a large study with long-term follow-up. *Histopathology* 1991;19:403–410.
113. Jensen C, Jacobsen HI. Basic guides to the mechanism of estrogen action. *Recent Prog Horm Res.* 1962;18:387.
114. McGuire W, Carbone P, Sears M, et al. Estrogen receptors in human breast cancer: an overview. In: McGuire W, Vollmer E, Carbone P, eds. *Estrogen receptors in human breast cancer.* New York: Raven Press, 1975, pp. 1–7.
115. Kuiper G, Enmark E, Pelto-Huikko M, et al. Cloning of a novel receptor expressed in rat prostate and ovary. *Proc Natl Acad Sci USA* 1996;93: 5925–5930.
116. Myers RE, Johnston M, Pritchard K, et al. Baseline staging tests in primary breast cancer: a practice guideline. *CMAJ* 2001;164:1439–1444.
117. Arriagada R, Le MG, Rochard F, et al. Conservative treatment versus mastectomy in early breast cancer: patterns of failure with 15 years of follow-up data. Institut Gustave-Roussy Breast Cancer Group. *J Clin Oncol.* 1996;14:1558–1564.
118. Veronesi U, Cascinelli N, Mariani L, et al. Twenty-year follow-up of a randomized study comparing breast-conserving surgery with radical mastectomy for early breast cancer. *N Engl J Med.* 2002;347:1227–1232.
119. **Fisher B, Anderson S, Bryant J, et al. Twenty-year follow-up of a randomized trial comparing total mastectomy, lumpectomy, and lumpectomy plus irradiation for the treatment of invasive breast cancer. *N Engl J Med.* 2002;347:1233–1241.**
120. Poggi MM, Danforth DN, Sciuto LC, et al. Eighteen-year results in the treatment of early breast carcinoma with mastectomy versus breast conservation therapy: the National Cancer Institute Randomized Trial. *Cancer* 2003;98:697–702.
121. van Dongen JA, Voogd AC, Fentiman IS, et al. Long-term results of a randomized trial comparing breast-conserving therapy with mastectomy: European Organization for Research and Treatment of Cancer 10801 trial. *J Natl Cancer Inst.* 2000;92:1143–1150.
122. Blichert-Toft M, Rose C, Andersen JA, et al. Danish randomized trial comparing breast conservation therapy with mastectomy: six years of life-table analysis. Danish Breast Cancer Cooperative Group. *J Natl Cancer Inst Monogr.* 1992:19–25.
123. **Morrow M, Strom EA, Bassett LW, et al. Standard for breast conservation therapy in the management of invasive breast carcinoma. *CA Cancer J Clin.* 2002;52:277–300.**
124. Bonadonna G, Veronesi U, Brambilla C, et al. Primary chemotherapy to avoid mastectomy in tumors with diameters of three centimeters or more. *J Natl Cancer Inst.* 1990;82:1539–1545.
125. Fisher B, Bryant J, Wolmark N, et al. Effect of preoperative chemotherapy on the outcome of women with operable breast cancer. *J Clin Oncol.* 1998;16:2672–2685.
126. Bear H, Anderson, S, Brown, A, et al. The effect on tumor response of adding sequential preoperative docetaxel to preoperative doxorubicin and cyclophophamide: preliminary results from National Surgical Adjuvant Breast and Bowel Project B-27. *J Clin Oncol.* 2003;22:4165–4174.
127. Schmidt-Ullrich RK, Wazer DE, DiPetrillo T, et al. Breast conservation therapy for early stage breast carcinoma with outstanding 10-year locoregional control rates: a case for aggressive therapy to the tumor bearing quadrant. *Int J Radiat Oncol Biol Phys.* 1993;27:545–552.
128. Morrow M, Schmidt R, Hassett C. Patient selection for breast conservation therapy with magnification mammography. *Surgery* 1995;118:621–626.
129. Morrow M, Harris JR. Local management of invasive cancer: breast. In: Harris J, Lippman ME, Morrow M, et al., eds. *Diseases of the breast*, 3rd ed. Philadelphia: Lippincott Williams & Wilkins, 2004, pp. 719–744.
130. Haffty BG, Harrold E, Khan AJ, et al. Outcome of conservatively managed early-onset breast cancer by BRCA1/2 status. *Lancet* 2002;359: 1471–1477.
131. Schnitt SJ, Abner A, Gelman R, et al. The relationship between microscopic margins of resection and the risk of local recurrence in patients with breast cancer treated with breast-conserving surgery and radiation therapy. *Cancer* 1994;74:1746–1751.
132. Schneiderman M, Axtell LM. Deaths among female patients with carcinoma of the breast treated by surgical procedure alone. *Surg Gynecol Obstet.* 1979;148:193–196.
133. Platt R, Zucker JR, Zaleznik DF, et al. Prophylaxis against wound infection following herniorrhaphy or breast surgery. *J Infect Dis.* 1992;166: 556–560.
134. Chagpar AB. Skin-sparing and nipple-sparing mastectomy: preoperative, intraoperative, and postoperative considerations. *Am Surg.* 2004;70: 425–432.
135. Cordiero P, Pusic A, Disa JJ, et al. Irradiation after immediate tissue expander/implant breast reconstruction. *Plast Reconstr Surg.* 2004;113: 877–881.
136. Giuliano AE, Kirgan DM, Guenther JM, et al. Lymphatic mapping and sentinel lymphadenectomy for breast cancer. *Ann Surg.* 1994;220:391–398.
137. Tafra L, Lannin DR, Swanson MS, et al. Multicenter trial of sentinel node biopsy for breast cancer using both technetium sulfur colloid and isosulfan blue dye. *Ann Surg.* 2001;233:51–59.
138. Bergkvist L, Frisell J, Liljegren G, et al. Multicentre study of detection and false–negative rates in sentinel node biopsy for breast cancer. *Br J Surg.* 2001;88:1644–1648.
139. McMasters KM, Wong SL, Chao C, et al. Defining the optimal surgeon experience for breast cancer sentinel lymph node biopsy: a model for implementation of new surgical techniques. *Ann Surg.* 2001;234:292–299.
140. Chua B, Olivotto IA, Donald JC, et al. Outcomes of sentinel node biopsy for breast cancer in British Columbia, 1996 to 2001. *Am J Surg.* 2003; 185:118–126.
141. Krag D, Weaver D, Ashikaga T, et al. The sentinel node in breast cancer—a multicenter validation study. *N Engl J Med.* 1998;339:941–946.
142. Shivers S, Cox C, Leight G, et al. Final results of the Department of Defense multicenter breast lymphatic mapping trial. *Ann Surg Oncol.* 2002;9:248–255.
143. **Veronesi U, Paganelli G, Viale G, et al. A randomized comparison of sentinel-node biopsy with routine axillary dissection in breast cancer. *N Engl J Med.* 2003;349:546–553.**
144. Petrek JA, Heelan MC. Incidence of breast carcinoma-related lymphedema. *Cancer* 1998;83:2776–2781.
145. Morrow M. Postmastectomy radiation therapy: a surgical perspective. *Semin Radiat Oncol.* 1999;9:269–274.
146. **Early Breast Cancer Trialists' Collaborative Group. Favourable and unfavourable effects on long-term survival of radiotherapy for early breast cancer: an overview of the randomized trials. *Lancet* 2000;355: 1757–1770.**
147. Morrow M, Krontiras H. Who should not receive chemotherapy? Data from American databases and trials. *J Natl Cancer Inst Monogr.* 2001: 109–113.
148. Quiet CA, Ferguson DJ, Weichselbaum RR, et al. Natural history of node-positive breast cancer: the curability of small cancers with a limited number of positive nodes. *J Clin Oncol.* 1996;14:3105–3111.
149. Clark GM, McGuire WL. Steroid receptors and other prognostic factors in primary breast cancer. *Semin Oncol.* 1988;15:20–25.
150. Perou CM, Sorlie T, Eisen MB, et al. Molecular portraits of human breast tumours. *Nature* 2000;406:747–752.
151. van de Vijver MJ, He YD, van't Veer LJ, et al. A gene-expression signature as a predictor of survival in breast cancer. *N Engl J Med.* 2002;347:1999–2009.
152. **Early Breast Cancer Trialists' Collaborative Group. Polychemotherapy for early breast cancer: an overview of the randomized trials. *Lancet* 1998; 352:930–942.**
153. **Henderson IC, Berry DA, Demetri GD, et al. Improved outcomes from adding sequential Paclitaxel but not from escalating doxorubicin dose in an adjuvant chemotherapy regimen for patients with node-positive primary breast cancer. *J Clin Oncol.* 2003;21:976–983.**
154. Jordan VC, Morrow M. Tamoxifen, raloxifene, and the prevention of breast cancer. *Endocr Rev.* 1999;20:253–278.
155. Early Breast Cancer Trialists' Collaborative Group. Tamoxifen for early breast cancer: an overview of the randomized trials. *Lancet* 1998;351: 1451–1467.
156. Baum M, Buzdar A, Cuzick J, et al. Anastrozole alone or in combination with tamoxifen versus tamoxifen alone for adjuvant treatment of postmenopausal women with early-stage breast cancer: results of the ATAC (arimidex, tamoxifen alone or in combination) trial efficacy and safety update analyses. *Cancer* 2003;98:1802–1810.

157. Veronesi U, Salvadori B, Luini A, et al. Conservative treatment of early breast cancer. Long-term results of 1232 cases treated with quadrantectomy, axillary dissection, and radiotherapy. *Ann Surg.* 1990;211:250–259.
158. Bates T, Riley DL, Houghton J, et al. Breast cancer in elderly women: a Cancer Research Campaign trial comparing treatment with tamoxifen and optimal surgery with tamoxifen alone. The Elderly Breast Cancer Working Party. *Br J Surg.* 1991;78:591–594.
159. Mustacchi G, Milani S, Pluchinotta A, et al. Tamoxifen or surgery plus tamoxifen as primary treatment for elderly patients with operable breast cancer: The G.R.E.T.A. Trial. Group for Research on Endocrine Therapy in the Elderly. *Anticancer Res.* 1994;14:2197–2200.
160. Robertson JF, Ellis IO, Elston CW, et al. Mastectomy or tamoxifen as initial therapy for operable breast cancer in elderly patients: 5-year follow-up. *Eur J Cancer* 1992;28A:908–910.
161. Rugo HS. Management of breast cancer diagnosed during pregnancy. *Current Treatment Options in Oncology* 2003;4:165–173.
162. Kroman N, Wohlfahrt J, Andersen KW, et al. Time since childbirth and prognosis in primary breast cancer: population based study. *BMJ* 1997;315:851–855.
163. Rosenberg L, Thalib L, Adami HO, et al. Childbirth and breast cancer prognosis. *Int J Cancer* 2004;111:772–776.
164. Whiteman MK, Hillis SD, Curtis KM, et al. Reproductive history and mortality after breast cancer diagnosis. *Obstet Gynecol.* 2004;104:146–154.
165. Ebert U, Loffler H, Kirch W. Cytotoxic therapy and pregnancy. *Pharmacol Ther.* 1997;74:207–220.
166. Anderson WF, Althuis MD, Brinton LA, et al. Is male breast cancer similar or different than female breast cancer? *Breast Cancer Res Treat.* 2004;83:77–86.
167. Port ER, Fey JV, Cody HS 3rd, et al. Sentinel lymph node biopsy in patients with male breast carcinoma. *Cancer* 2001;91:319–323.
168. Giordano SH, Cohen DS, Buzdar AU, et al. Breast carcinoma in men: a population-based study. *Cancer* 2004;101:51–57.
169. Ribeiro G, Swindell R. Adjuvant tamoxifen for male breast cancer (MBC). *Br J Cancer* 1992;65:252–254.
170. Donegan WL, Redlich PN. Breast cancer in men. *Surg Clin North Am.* 1996;76:343–363.
171. Olson JA Jr, Morris EA, Van Zee KJ, et al. Magnetic resonance imaging facilitates breast conservation for occult breast cancer. *Ann Surg Oncol.* 2000;7:411–415.
172. Fourquet A, Melinier M, Campana F. Occult primary cancer with axillary metastases. In: Harris J, Lippman ME, Morrow M, et al., eds. *Diseases of the breast*, 3rd ed. Philadelphia: Lippincott Willliams & Wilkins, 2004.
173. Ellerbroek N, Holmes F, Singletary E, et al. Treatment of patients with isolated axillary nodal metastases from an occult primary carcinoma consistent with breast origin. *Cancer* 1990;66:1461–1467.
174. Merson M, Andreola S, Galimberti V, et al. Breast carcinoma presenting as axillary metastases without evidence of a primary tumor. *Cancer* 1992;70:504–508.
175. Gage I, Schnitt SJ, Recht A, et al. Skin recurrences after breast-conserving therapy for early-stage breast cancer. *J Clin Oncol.* 1998;16:480–486.
176. Paget J. Disease of the mammary areola preceding cancer of the mammary gland. *Saint Bartholomew's Hospital Journal.* 1874;10:79–89.
177. Bijker N, Rutgers EJ, Duchateau L, et al. Breast-conserving therapy for Paget disease of the nipple: a prospective European Organization for Research and Treatment of Cancer study of 61 patients. *Cancer* 2001;91: 472–477.
178. Salvadori B, Cusumano F, Del Bo R, et al. Surgical treatment of phyllodes tumors of the breast. *Cancer* 1989;63:2532–2536.
179. Kessinger A, Foley JF, Lemon HM, et al. Metastatic cystosarcoma phyllodes: a case report and review of the literature. *J Surg Oncol.* 1972;4:131–147.
180. Zissis C, Apostolikas N, Konstantinidou A, et al. The extent of surgery and prognosis of patients with phyllodes tumor of the breast. *Breast Cancer Res Treat.* 1998;48:205–210.
181. Haagensen CD, Stout AP. Carcinoma of the breast. II. Criteria of operability. *Ann Surg.* 1943;118:859–872.
182. Hortobagyi G, Singletary SE, Strom EA. Locally advanced breast cancer. In: Harris J, Lippman ME, Morrow M, et al., eds. *Diseases of the breast*, 3rd ed. Philadelphia: Lippincott Williams & Wilkins, 2004, pp. 951–969.
183. Smith IC, Heys SD, Hutcheon AW, et al. Neoadjuvant chemotherapy in breast cancer: significantly enhanced response with docetaxel. *J Clin Oncol.* 2002;20:1456–1466.
184. Thomas E, Holmes FA, Smith TL, et al. The use of alternate, non-cross-resistant adjuvant chemotherapy on the basis of pathologic response to a neoadjuvant doxorubicin-based regimen in women with operable breast cancer: long-term results from a prospective randomized trial. *J Clin Oncol.* 2004;22:2294–2302.
185. Chen AM, Meric-Bernstam F, Hunt KK, et al. Breast conservation after neoadjuvant chemotherapy: the MD Anderson Cancer Center experience. *J Clin Oncol.* 2004;22:2303–2312.
186. Low JA Berman AW, Steinberg SM, et al. Long-term follow-up for locally advanced and inflammatory breast cancer patients treated with multimodality therapy. *J Clin Oncol.* 2004;22:4067–4074.

CHAPTER 77 ■ THYROID GLAND

PAUL G. GAUGER

Largely as a function of disease prevalence, surgical treatment of thyroid disorders is relatively common. Excellent patient outcomes require a through understanding of embryology, anatomy, physiology, and relevant pharmacology. Delicate and deliberate surgical technique and careful attention to detail are required to prevent common complications of thyroid resections.

EMBRYOLOGY AND SURGICAL IMPLICATIONS

Developmental Embryology

As the first endocrine gland to develop, the thyroid is mostly of endodermal origin and originates from the ventral embryologic digestive tract. A midline diverticulum arises in the area of the foramen cecum at the base of the tongue at approximately 4 weeks of gestational age. The rudimentary thyroid tissue descends as the *median thyroid component* (or *anlage*), which ultimately becomes the isthmus (overlying the upper tracheal rings) and most of each lateral lobe. It reaches its final position by gestational week 7 and undergoes histologic differentiation into recognizable follicles between week 8 and 11.[1] The embryology of the median component is fairly well understood. Its initial appearance in evolution seems to be the endostyle, a groove in the pharyngeal floor of the ammocaete larva of sea urchins, which takes up iodine in a fashion similar to the human thyroid.[2] The portion associated with the foramen cecum ruptures and resorbs during week 6 of gestational age leaving behind a regressive fibrous tract, which becomes the thyroglossal duct tract (including the portion associated with the central hyoid bone). The distal end associated with the isthmus persists as a pyramidal thyroid lobe in about 30% to 50% of individuals. The *lateral thyroid component* (also known as the ultimobranchial body in some vertebrates) develops on each side from the caudal pharyngeal endoderm (with the contribution of the fourth and fifth branchial pouches).[1,3,4] They arise later in development than the median component. These fuse with the posterior portion of the median component on each side and, with this process, C cells (from neural crest origin) migrate into the superolateral portion of the lobes and eventually secrete calcitonin. The median and lateral thyroid components unite by a complicated mechanism in which the lateral components move anteriorly and cranially and the median component migrates posteriorly and cranially.[5] Only after this point does the unified thyroid begin to differentiate into thyroid follicles. Basic glandular function begins on a cellular level by the third month of gestation when iodine trapping occurs and thyroid hormones are first secreted. The control of descent and fusion of thyroid tissue appears to be influenced by multiple transcription factors such as TTF-1, TTF-2, and Pax-8.[6] The lateral components become increasingly removed from the pharynx leaving a tapering connection on each side, which eventually detaches and is replaced by mesenchyme.[7] The residual posterolateral projection from the lateral thyroid component toward the pharynx, when present, is known as the tubercle of Zuckerkandl [attributed to Viennese anatomist Emil Zuckerkandl (1849–1910)]. Because of its branchial pouch origin, the lateral thyroid component is closely associated with the superior parathyroid anlage (from fourth pouch).

Congenital Abnormalities

An uncommon developmental malformation is the lingual thyroid gland, which is most often associated with agenesis of thyroid tissue in the standard position. It represents a failure of the median thyroid component to descend from the region of the foramen cecum. The size of a lingual thyroid can often be decreased by using exogenous thyroid hormone to suppress thyroid-stimulating hormone (TSH) or, in some cases, by ^{131}I ablation. Surgical excision may be required if airway obstruction, obstructive dysphagia, or hemorrhage occurs. Ectopic thyroid tissue can be found in other areas of the central cervical compartment and the mediastinum. These can be sequestered nodules associated with multinodular goiters or they may be embryologic rests of thyroid tissue. Although the concept of *lateral aberrant thyroid* tissue was originally used to describe the findings of follicular tissue in the carotid sheath or the lateral compartments of the neck, it is now generally agreed that this cannot occur as an embryologic abnormality. If thyroid tissue is found in these areas, it most likely represents a regional nodal metastasis of an occult thyroid cancer—typically a follicular variant of papillary thyroid cancer, which may have follicular architecture that is similar to normal thyroid tissue.

Thyroglossal duct cysts occur in the midline of the neck along the path of descent of the median thyroid component. They may occur from the base of the tongue to the low central neck, although most are located just inferior to the hyoid bone. Although they are often discovered during infancy and childhood, it is not uncommon for them not to be evident until adulthood—discovered either because of complaints of mass or evidence of infection. Because the posterior wall of the cyst abuts the flexible anterior pharynx, enlargement of the cyst can cause dysphagia and choking. When examining the patient, elevation of the mass with protrusion of the tongue is very suggestive of a thyroglossal duct cyst. Resection of a thyroglossal duct cyst involves excision of the entire thyroglossal duct on either side of the cyst. The tract is often intimately associated with the central portion of the hyoid bone and, for that reason, excision of this segment of bone is critical to prevent recurrence (known as the Sistrunk procedure). The epithelial lining usually contains some thyroid cells and, thus, thyroid carcinomas (usually of papillary type) can arise primarily in thyroglossal duct cysts. Excision of the cyst and the thyroglossal duct may be sufficient for small, limited carcinomas, but if regional nodal metastases are present or if the tumor is of sufficient size, total thyroidectomy should be included to facilitate subsequent ^{131}I scanning and therapy.

ANATOMY AND SURGICAL IMPLICATIONS

A normal thyroid gland (especially in patients from iodine-sufficient regions) weighs between 15 and 20 g. The normal color is a dark shade of burgundy. Conditions such as chronic thyroiditis may change the color to a pink–gray, whereas nodular disease often adds a brown or tan discoloration. Fluid-filled cysts typically have a blue appearance. If the patient has previously been prescribed minocycline (often for acne), the thyroid adopts permanent black coloration.[8] The upper portion of the isthmus typically crosses at or below the level of the cricoid cartilage and overlies the second and third tracheal rings. The isthmus itself is approximately 1 to 2 cm in transverse and vertical dimensions and the lower margin of the lobe is normally near the fourth or fifth tracheal ring. The lateral lobes lie adjacent to the thyroid cartilage and cricothyroideus muscles as well as the lateral trachea and a portion of the lateral esophagus on each side. The two lateral lobes are roughly conical, approximately 5 cm long and 2 to 3 cm in transverse and anteroposterior dimensions. The pyramidal lobe may attach to the center of the isthmus but often is found on a slightly lateral aspect (often the left). It may be situated in front of the potential space that exists between the superior thyroid pole and the cricothyroideus muscle. In that case, it will need to be mobilized and divided to facilitate development of the cricothyroid space and, thus, safe mobilization of the superior pole during thyroidectomy. Occasionally the pyramidal lobe is accompanied by a small group of skeletal muscle fibers, which has been termed the "levator glandulae superioris."[9]

Muscular, Fascial, and Airway Relationships

The thyroid lies in the central compartment of the neck bordered by the contents of the carotid sheath on each side. The anterolateral surface is covered by the sternothyroid muscles, which do not completely meet in the midline above the level of the isthmus. The oblique upper muscular insertion into the thyroid cartilage is the limiting factor preventing the lobes from encroaching further toward the midline and onto the underlying thyrohyoid muscle. Superficial to that are the paired sternohyoid muscles that meet in the midline raphe marking the most common plane of dissection used to expose the thyroid gland. These muscles are innervated by the ansa cervicalis (ansa hypoglossi) formed from the descendens hypoglossi (containing fibers of C1), and the descendens cervicalis (containing fibers of C2 and C3) and contributory branches can be seen on the lateral aspects. The thyroid is invested in a thin layer of connective tissue that is an expansion of the pretracheal fascia (often called the "thyroid sheath"). The plane defined by this layer is usually easy to develop as the thyroid is mobilized away from surrounding structures. Especially near the superior portion of the thyroid, the sheath defines a coronal plane that, when opened, exposes the potential space between the pharynx and esophagus and the cervical vertebral bodies. The superior parathyroid gland may be found between the sheath and the thyroid capsule, within the sheath, or posterior to the sheath. The sheath is not to be confused with the thyroid capsule, which is more integral to the gland itself. The sheath is condensed as the anterior suspensory ligament above the isthmus. The sheath also suspends the inner surface of the thyroid gland to the trachea rings and cricoid cartilage. It is condensed posteromedially into the ligament of Berry on each side. The ligament of Berry is often a very firm attachment to the trachea near the cricothyroid interval, which means that it is often intimately associated with the recurrent laryngeal nerve (RLN). It is in the course of dividing these attachments that the RLN is most vulnerable to iatrogenic injury.

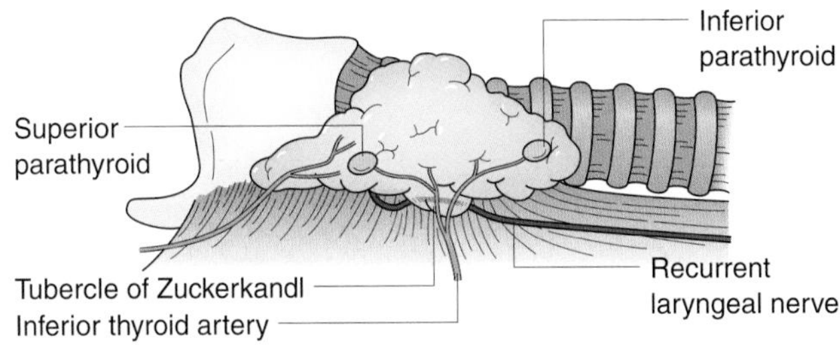

FIGURE 77.1 The standard anatomic relationship whereby the recurrent laryngeal nerve (RLN) passes medial to the tubercle of Zuckerkandl before its insertion into the cricothyroid interval.

Vascular Relationships

The thyroid gland has a very high blood flow index per tissue mass and receives its arterial supply from a paired system of superior thyroid arteries (originating from the external carotid arteries) and the inferior thyroid arteries (originating from the thyrocervical trunks). The superior artery courses along the inferior pharyngeal constrictor muscle group and branches near the tip of the superior pole of the thyroid, usually into at least the anterior and posterior branch. The inferior thyroid artery (ITA) courses upward behind the carotid artery and then crosses medially and often in a slightly downward course to serve the thyroid lobe. The ITA has multiple branches that course in a plane between the sheath and the capsule of the gland. The relationship of the ITA to the RLN is an important landmark. There is always an intersection (except in the case of a direct laryngeal nerve), but the specific relationship may be variable. Occasionally, the lowest thyroid artery (arteria thyroidea ima) arises from the aorta or innominate artery and directly serves the inferior portion of the thyroid gland. Venous drainage is by a widely anastomotic system that condenses into three main trunks: The superior thyroid veins course adjacent to the superior thyroid arteries but empty into the internal jugular vein at the level of the carotid bifurcation. The inferior thyroid veins form nearly all of the vascular connections found at the inferior poles of the thyroid lobes. The number and configuration of these veins can be quite variable, but in general they descend along the course of the thyrothymic tract to drain into the ipsilateral innominate or brachiocephalic veins. Middle thyroid veins are present in approximately half of patients. The number and course are highly variable as they drain laterally to the internal jugular vein. These veins are divided in the course of mobilizing the thyroid lobe. If a vessel is seen passing from the region of the carotid sheath to the thyroid and it is not immediately apparent whether it is ITA or middle thyroid vein, its identity can be confirmed by tracing it laterally. If it passes anterior to the carotid artery, it is a middle thyroid vein while if it passes deep to the carotid, it is the ITA.

Neurologic Relationships

Two nerves have critical importance during thyroidectomy: the RLN (also known as the inferior laryngeal nerve) and the external branch of the superior laryngeal nerve. The right recurrent laryngeal nerve arises from the vagus at the level of the subclavian artery and passes (recurs) around the posterior aspect of the artery before ascending into the central compartment. The nerve takes an oblique course in the central neck and may be 1 to 2 cm lateral to the trachea low in the central neck before traveling toward its entry into the larynx. The left RLN arises from the vagus nerve as it crosses the aortic arch. It passes inferior and medial to the arch and ascends to the larynx in the tracheoesophageal groove along a course that is typically linear and more vertical. The RLN often lays immediately posterolateral to the ligament of Berry, but it is not infrequent that it can be embedded in the fibrous connections of the ligament itself, especially the anterior branch if the nerve bifurcates outside the larynx. Although it may be tempting to describe this as the nerve "running through thyroid tissue," that cannot actually occur. Pelizzo has recently described the tubercle of Zuckerkandl as a constant anatomic landmark to facilitate identification of the recurrent laryngeal nerve during thyroid resection.[10] In the standard anatomic relationship, the tubercle of Zuckerkandl is lateral to the RLN (Fig. 77.1). An uncommon, but high-risk anatomic arrangement occurs when the RLN is lateral to the tubercle of Zuckerkandl (Fig. 77.2). As the thyroid lobe is retracted anteromedially during thyroidectomy, the RLN may seem to be anterolateral to the tubercle. If the surgeon is unaware of this possibility (which often exists when the tubercle has undergone nodular enlargement), the nerve is subject to iatrogenic injury. The nerve usually bifurcates extralaryngeally but often at a point less than 0.5 cm from the cricoid cartilage. Up to 58% of recurrent laryngeal nerves will bifurcate proximal to inferior border of the cricoid cartilage.[11] Extralaryngeal trifurcations exist in approximately 1% of RLNs.

It is critical to be aware of the occasional "direct" laryngeal nerve (also called the "nonrecurrent laryngeal nerve"). This anomaly results from abnormal embryonic development of the aortic arch. The anomaly is more common on the right (approximately 0.5% to 0.7%) than on the left (approximately 0.04%).[12] On the right, a direct nerve is the consequence of the formation of the *arteria lusoria* vascular abnormality, in which the innominate artery is absent and the right common carotid and right subclavian arteries originate directly from the arch. The subclavian artery takes a retroesophageal course. A "false" nonrecurrent inferior laryngeal nerve has been described as a communicating branch between the cervical sympathetic system and the RLN, which can mimic a nerve that appears to

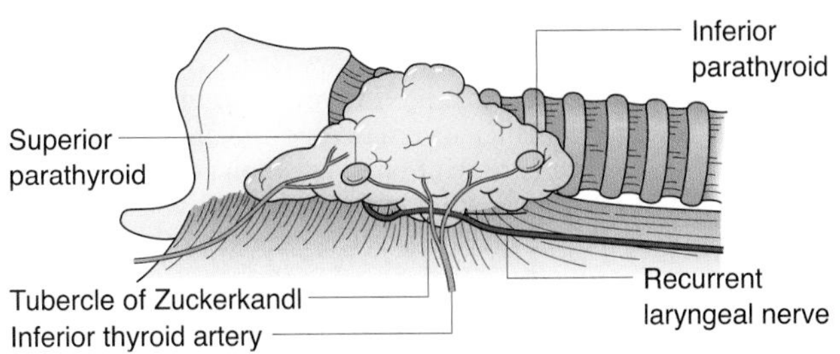

FIGURE 77.2 The uncommon, but high-risk anatomic variation where the recurrent laryngeal nerve (RLN) courses lateral to the tubercle of Zuckerkandl, which is often enlarged. The nerve is encountered much earlier in the dissection required for thyroidectomy and is at risk of being misidentified as a vascular structure.

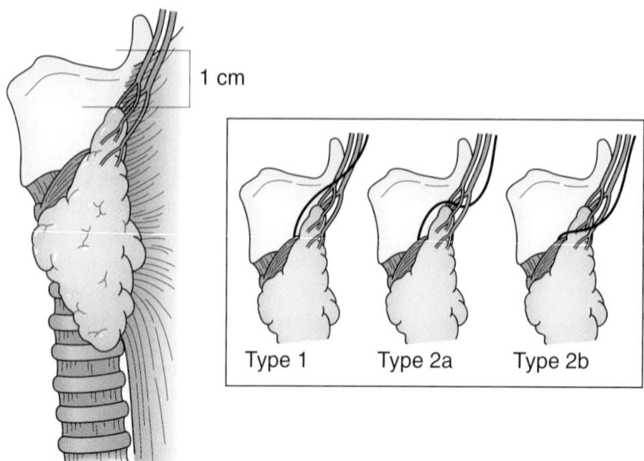

FIGURE 77.3 Cernea classification of the anatomic relationships between the external branch of the superior laryngeal nerve (EBSLN), the superior pole of the thyroid, and the superior thyroid artery. With type 1 anatomy, the nerve crosses the superior thyroid vessels 1 cm or more above the superior thyroid pole. With type 2 anatomy, the nerve crosses the vessels less than 1 cm above (type 2a) or even below (type 2b) the superior pole. Type 2 variants are the most vulnerable to iatrogenic injury.

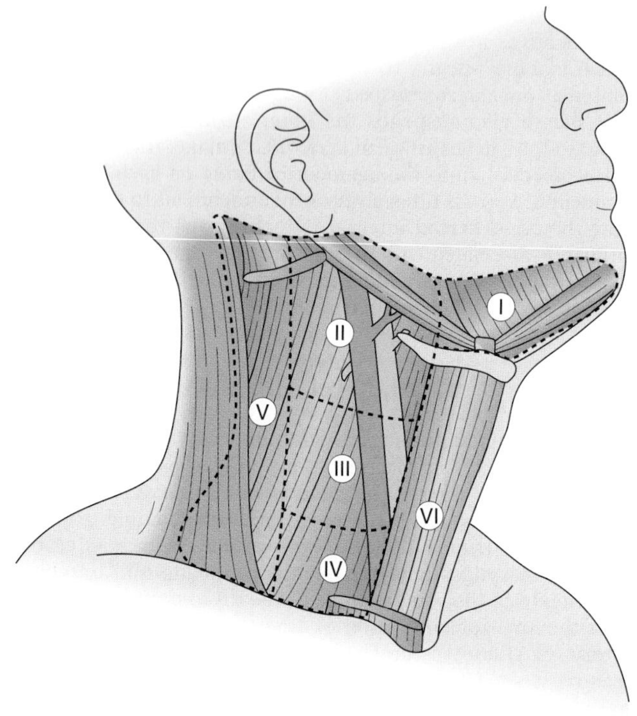

FIGURE 77.4 Classification scheme for regional lymph node basins in the neck.

emerge from the region of the vagus nerve as would be seen with a direct nerve.[13] To have a direct nerve on the left side, a number of other anomalies must exist. Specifically, the aortic arch must be right sided (as occurs in *situs inversus viscerum*), the origin of the left subclavian artery must be abnormally sited on the aortic arch, and the ligamentum arteriosum must be displaced to the right.

The superior laryngeal nerve arises from the vagus at the nodose ganglion near the base of the skull and descends with along the course of the internal carotid artery. At the level of the hyoid bone, it divides into the internal branch (which enters the larynx at the thyrohyoid membrane to provide sensory innervation to the superior larynx) and the external branch (which provides motor innervation to the cricothyroideus muscle). It has a variable course in relation to the inferior pharyngeal constrictor muscle and the branches of the superior thyroid artery. It is this fact that makes the external branch of the superior laryngeal nerve (EBSLN) vulnerable to iatrogenic injury. One classification of the anatomic variations is depicted in Figure 77.3.

Lymphatic Relationships

The thyroid gland has intracapsular lymph channels, which provide some communication from lobe to lobe across the isthmus. A rich plexus of lymphatics surrounds the region of the thyroid and, consequently, lymph flows in multiple directions from the gland. These factors are important to understand for treatment of thyroid malignancies. Within the anterior suspensory ligament is a small group of midline lymph nodes known as the Delphian nodes. Along with the pretracheal and paratracheal nodes and those along the recurrent laryngeal nerves, these central compartment lymph nodes are classified as level VI. The upper jugular (level II), midjugular (level III), and lower jugular (level IV) lymph nodes divide the central compartment from the lateral compartment of the neck, whereas the posterior triangle lymph nodes are level V (Fig. 77.4). The superior mediastinal lymph nodes (level VII) may also be involved by thyroid cancer. Thyroid cancers with regional lymph node metastases tend to involve level VI lymph node metastases before sequentially involving level III and level IV and ultimately level V. Level II and level VII involvement is less common but does occur. Level I involvement is rare. Rare documented cases of "skip" metastases directly to the lateral compartment with no level VI involvement have been reported.[14]

Parathyroid Relationships

Parathyroid glands in normal or typical location are encountered during thyroidectomy by virtue of their association with the thyroid gland. Parathyroid glands that develop in ectopic locations will typically not be encountered during thyroidectomy and are not discussed here. The superior parathyroid gland is typically located in a relatively constant area largely because of the embryologic association between the lateral thyroid component and the superior parathyroid anlage (both associated with branchial pouch IV). The tubercle of Zuckerkandl was noted by Gilmour to be anatomically associated with the position of the ipsilateral superior parathyroid gland as well as the recurrent laryngeal nerve.[15] In relation to the point at which the RLN intersects the inferior thyroid artery, a 2-cm circumscribed area on the cranial aspect will often contain the superior parathyroid gland. It may also be found tucked posterior to the inferior thyroid artery or even posteromedial to the superior thyroid pole. Superior parathyroid glands are nearly never found within the thyroid capsule. If a superior parathyroid gland is found on one side, the chance of the contralateral gland being in a similar position is approximately 80%.

The location of the normal inferior parathyroid gland may be more variable. It may be found on the anterior aspect of the inferior thyroid pole (especially with Hashimoto's disease or large multinodular goiter) but is often on the inferolateral aspect. It may also be in the triangular region caudal to the inferior thyroid artery and anterior to the RLN. If it is not in these locations, it is often embedded in fat and thymic tissue within the thyrothymic tract. It may also be located under the thyroid capsule in an intrathyroidal position. The symmetry of inferior parathyroid glands from side to side is approximately 70%.

THYROID PHYSIOLOGY

Production of Thyroid Hormones

The thyroid gland produces thyroxine (T_4), triiodothyronine (T_3), and calcitonin under complicated regulatory mechanisms. The regulation of thyroid hormone secretion is well understood, but it can be affected by many physiologic and pharmacologic factors. Approximately 100 to 150 μg of dietary iodide is required for normal thyroid hormone synthesis to occur. Daily intake from iodine-containing foods is usually far in excess of that in most developed regions of the world. The kidneys excrete the excess iodide not utilized by the thyroid. The availability of thyroid hormones to all tissues is conceptually divided into the process of hormone production within the thyroid gland (specifically within the follicular cells) and the delivery and metabolism of the hormones in peripheral tissues. The integration of these systems to maintain a euthyroid state is ultimately orchestrated by the anterior pituitary gland through its secretion of thyrotropin (TSH). The active uptake of iodide in the thyroid occurs on the basolateral aspect of the follicular cells and is performed by a $Na+/K+$ adenosine triphosphatase (ATPase)-mediated pump. This symporter system is influenced by both TSH and the circulating concentration of iodide. TSH secretion is increased in response to decreased circulating T_3 levels. TSH acts within the thyroid gland to regulate the synthesis of thyroglobulin (Tg), the active uptake of iodide, its incorporation with tyrosine (an oxidative reaction catalyzed by thyroid peroxidase [TPO]), and the subsequent production of T_4 and T_3 (and their storage bound to Tg in the colloid component of the gland), and ultimately the release of both T_4 and T_3 into the circulation. Hormone release is again an active process of micropinocytosis that involves resorption of the bound Tg into the follicular cell where enzymatic degradation releases the T_4 and T_3, which is released from the basal portion of the cell into the circulation. T_4 is produced in preference to T_3 in the thyroid gland by a ratio of approximately 13:1. This ratio can be altered to increase the relative fraction of T_3 in situations of iodine deficiency or by TSH hyperstimulation. T_4 has a relatively weak biologic action so a peripheral conversion to the more active T_3 hormone is required. Most of this takes place in the plasma and liver by type 1 deiodinase enzymes. All of the T_4 in the circulation is derived from the thyroid, whereas far less than 20% of T_3 in the circulation is from the thyroid, the majority being produced enzymatically from monodeiodination of T_4 in nonthyroidal tissues. In circulation, most thyroid hormone (>99% of both T_4 and T_3) is bound to proteins such as thyroxine-binding globulin (TBG), albumin, and thyroxine-binding prealbumin. Protein-bound thyroid hormones are considered biologically inert because they do not enter cells until they are released from proteins to circulate in the very small free fraction. The half-life of T_4 is approximately 7 days, whereas the half-life of T_3 is much shorter—on the order of 8 to 12 hours.

Action of Thyroid Hormones

Thyroid hormones have many broad effects on various body tissues. The peripheral conversion from T_4 to T_3 increases the binding affinity of thyroid hormone for the nuclear thyroid receptor protein at least tenfold. Specific T_3 receptors are present on the cell membrane to assist in transport into the cell. Triiodothyronine acts within the nucleus of peripheral tissues via the thyroid hormone receptor to activate T_3-regulated gene transcription. Four T_3 nuclear receptor subtypes have been identified with slightly different downstream actions. Ultimately, the physiologic actions of thyroid hormone relate to growth, differentiation, calorigenesis, and TSH suppression.

Calcitonin is physiologically effective in many other species, but in humans it is apparently less important. Although exogenous calcitonin may have a therapeutic effect, endogenous calcitonin secretion rarely results in an impact on serum calcium levels.

RELEVANT LABORATORY TESTS

An understanding of the normal relationship between free T_4 (FT_4) levels and TSH levels is critical for appropriate interpretation of thyroid function tests. Thyroid dysfunction can be determined directly, by measuring FT_4 levels or, indirectly, by measuring TSH. If TSH is to be used as the primary indicator of thyroid dysfunction, an intact hypothalamic—pituitary axis is required. Normally, a log/linear inverse relationship between TSH and FT_4 is defined by the negative feedback inhibition of TSH secretion by circulating thyroxine levels. Therefore, high TSH and low FT_4 levels are indicative of hypothyroidism and, conversely, low TSH and high FT_4 levels are characteristic of hyperthyroidism. It is likely that each individual has a genetically determined FT_4 set point. Early subtle deviation from that set point (via *in situ* conversion to FT_3 in the pituitary) will cause amplified changes in the TSH value, thus making TSH a very sensitive early indicator of incipient thyroid dysfunction.

Calcitonin

Calcitonin is a 32–amino acid polypeptide, which is currently measured by immunometric techniques using monoclonal antibodies (one each to C-terminal and N-terminal region). Calcitonin levels are generally less than 10 pg/mL for normal healthy people and for nearly all patients with thyroid disease, other than medullary thyroid carcinoma (MTC). Therefore, calcitonin serves as a very specific tumor marker for MTC. Basal calcitonin levels are useful for diagnosis and observation of these patients.

Free Thyroxine (FT_4) and Free Triiodothyronine (FT_3)

Technically, it is easier to measure the total (free + protein-bound) hormone levels (measured at nanomolar levels) as compared to the very small free hormone concentrations (measured at picomolar ranges). Because T_4 is more tightly protein bound than T_3, it is less bioavailable and, consequently, very difficult to measure directly. Measurement of free hormone levels in clinical laboratories involves index methods (requiring two separate tests), single-test ligand assays, or physical separation methods to isolate the free fraction before direct measurement. Ligand assays performed on automated immunoassay analyzers are fairly common in clinical use and are standardized against known hormone concentrations. Because this method does not rely on physical separation of the free and protein-bound hormone fractions, it is more accurately considered a free hormone estimate. The only reason to measure FT_4 or FT_3 in preference to total thyroxine (T_4) or total triiodothyronine (TT_3) is to improve the ability to detect thyroid dysfunction in the presence of thyroid hormone-binding abnormalities, which are relatively common. For example, some common drugs such as phenytoin, carbamazepine, furosemide, and aspirin may compete with thyroid hormone for binding to serum proteins.

Thyroglobulin

Serum thyroglobulin is reflective of three factors: the mass of thyroid tissue present, the presence of injury or inflammation of the gland, which allows leakage of Tg, and the degree of stimulation of the TSH receptor. The primary clinical use of Tg measurement is as a tumor marker, which serves as an index of the amount of differentiated thyroid cancer present (assuming that total thyroidectomy has been performed). Tg is measured in the serum by radioimmunoassay methods or increasingly, by immunometric assays. The latter is more susceptible to competitive interference by thyroglobulin autoantibodies (TgAb), which cause an artifactual decrease in the measured levels. The particular assay utilized must be very sensitive to detect Tg levels at the lower end of the reference range (1 to 3 μg/L) to be useful in monitoring for recurrence of differentiated thyroid carcinoma (DTC). It is critical to understand that the TSH level is a major influence on the level of Tg and, consequently, interpretation of any level requires an understanding of whether the patient was hypothyroid or not at the time of measurement.

Thyroid Autoantibodies

Thyroid peroxidase autoantibodies (TPOAb) were initially described as antimicrosomal antibodies because they were found to react with crude preparations of thyroid cell membranes. Currently, competitive and noncompetitive immunoassay methods are used to quantify TPOAb, but there is wide variability in the sensitivity and specificity of the available quantitative assays. It is the most sensitive test for detecting autoimmune thyroid disease and TPOAb is often the first abnormality to appear in Hashimoto's disease because hypothyroidism develops (present in >95% of such patients). A significant fraction (up to 12%) of people with no apparent thyroid disorder, however, may also have positive TPOAb titers.

During thyroid hormone synthesis and release, thyroglobulin is polymerized and degraded, creating a complex structure that consequently leads to the equally complex immunologic structure of thyroglobulin autoantibodies (TgAb). TgAb are measured by competitive and noncompetitive immunoassays. They may be present in approximately 3% to 10% of the general population and are even more common (20%) in patients with differentiated thyroid carcinoma. In fact, sensitive quantitative TgAb determination is a critical accompaniment to serum Tg measurement, which is common during management of thyroid carcinoma. TgAb measurements, however, are not as useful as TPOAb in evaluation of autoimmune thyroid disease.

Thyroid-stimulating hormone receptor autoantibodies (TRAb) are heterogeneous and may mimic the action of TSH to cause hyperthyroidism as seen in Graves' disease or, conversely, may block the action of TSH and cause hypothyroidism as seen in neonates of a mother with thyroid autoantibodies. The specific different types include thyroid-stimulating antibodies (TSAb), TSH receptor blocking antibodies (TBAb), Thyroid growth simulating antibodies (TGI), thyroid binding inhibiting immunoglobulins (TBII).

Thyroid-Stimulating Hormone (Thyrotropin)

Now that the sensitivity and specificity of TSH assays are very high, the indirect approach of measuring TSH levels is the most sensitive method for detecting thyroid dysfunction. The inverse relationship between TSH and FT_4 also dictates that small alterations in FT_4 will lead to a larger response in TSH, thus adding further support to this strategy. For many years, assays have easily detected the elevated TSH levels, which indicated hypothyroidism, but until the assays became ultrasensitive (thus able to detect very low TSH levels), the ability to diagnose hyperthyroidism by a TSH level alone was very limited. Modern methods are generally based on nonisotopic immunometric assays and are able to achieve a sensitivity of 0.02 mIU/L or less. At present, the upper limit of the normal range is considered to be approximately 5 mIU/L, but this is likely to be redefined at approximately 2.5 mIU/L in the future as it becomes more clear that many patients in the interval between these values progress to develop hypothyroidism, especially if thyroid autoantibodies are present. It is this range of 0.5 to 2.0 mIU/L that is generally considered the target range for TSH when patients are treated with levothyroxine (LT_4) for hypothyroidism because, consequently, most patients then have FT_4 levels in the upper third of the normal reference range.

Total Thyroxine (TT_4) and Total Triiodothyronine (TT_3)

Currently, TT_4 and TT_3 hormones are measured by competitive immunoassay methods (with enzymes, fluorescence, or chemiluminescence used for signaling). Total hormone assays require an inhibitor to block or displace the hormone from its binding proteins. This factor, along with large sample dilution, allows binding of the hormone to the antibody reagent. Because of the tenfold lower concentrations of T_3 in the serum, the TT_3 assay requires even greater sensitivity and precision. Because of variability in the quantity and the binding capacity of serum proteins, however, abnormal TT_4 and TT_3 measurements are more commonly caused by these factors instead of true thyroid dysfunction. Older free hormone indices (FT_4I or FT_3I) are basically derived from the mathematical relationship between the measured total hormone concentration and an "uptake" test (also called thyroid hormone binding ratio tests).

RELEVANT PHARMACOLOGY

Thionamide

The common antithyroid drugs propothiouracil (PTU), methimazole (Tapazole), and carbimazole (commonly used in the United Kingdom, but not in the United States) are examples of the thionamide drug class. PTU prevents oxidation iodide to iodine and the incorporation of iodine and tyrosine by inhibiting TPO. PTU also inhibits peripheral conversion of T_4 to T_3, whereas methimazole does not. For this reason, PTU is the preferred thionamide during treatment of thyroid storm. Because the half-life is only 2 to 3 hours, it requires multiple doses per day, whereas methimazole can be given just once or twice daily. Both drugs have significant side effect profiles. The most common is skin rash (3% with PTU, 7% with methimazole), whereas the most serious is agranulocytosis (0.44% with PTU, 0.12% with methimazole).[16] These drugs are effective in pregnancy but the minimal necessary dose should be used because the placental passage which will decrease thyroid hormone production in the fetus.

Ionic Inhibitor

Iodine, usually supplied in a preparation such as Lugol's iodine (KI), can function as a short-term antithyroid medication by inhibiting thyroglobulin proteolysis as well as blocking organification and inhibition of thyroid hormone release. When used in preparation for an operation to ameliorate hyperthyroidism, it can also decrease the vascularity of the gland as well, which can be beneficial. Its effect only lasts 10 to 14 days, after which an escape phenomenon can occur.

T_3 Production Inhibitors

Although PTU, glucocorticoids, and iopanoic acid (Telpaque) act to inhibit the peripheral conversion of T_4 to T_3, this is the major role for β-adrenergic blocking agents such as propranolol or metoprolol. Many hyperthyroid patients are prepared for operation using these drugs alone if the severity of symptoms is moderate.

Inhibitors of Peripheral Thyroid Action

β-Blockers also serve to ameliorate the peripheral effects of hyperthyroidism, such as palpitations, diaphoresis, nervousness, and tremor. These drugs will have an impact on symptoms within a couple of days when administered orally or even within hours if administered intravenously.

Radioactive Iodine

Radioiodine is usually administered in the form of ^{131}I. It is trapped by follicular cells, incorporated into the iodine–tyrosine complex, and deposited into colloid. Once accumulated within the cells, ^{131}I undergoes beta decay, releasing high-energy electrons for a short distance into the surrounding tissues. This cytotoxicity is focused (and essentially limited to tissues that possess the ability to concentrate iodine) and generally thought to affect tissues only within a 2-mm radius. Gamma rays are also released that allow for the use of the radioisotope for scanning procedures (usually requiring only a low dose). In moderate doses, it can be used to treat hyperthyroidism and, in higher doses, it is used to destroy differentiated thyroid carcinoma.

THYROID IMAGING TECHNIQUES

It is common for patients to present to the surgeon after having undergone multiple imaging tests. In general, only ultrasonography is routinely useful in evaluation of the patient with a thyroid nodule. In other specific circumstances, various other tests may be useful.

Nuclear Medicine Imaging

Radionuclide imaging provides functional imaging of the thyroid gland with limited anatomic detail. Therefore, it is unique when compared with other thyroid imaging techniques in that the image provided depends on the specific functional characteristics of the thyroid tissue.

Technetium Pertechnetate ^{99m}Tc Scintigraphy

^{99m}Tc is the radionuclide most commonly available for thyroid imaging. The ^{99m}Tc pertechnetate component is actively trapped by functional thyroid cells in a manner similar to iodine but is not organified or stored in the thyroid. The isotope emits gamma (γ) radiation (the mechanism of scintigraphic imaging) and very small amounts of other types of radiation. Because the thyroid rapidly absorbs the injected 99mTc pertechnetate, imaging can occur early after administration and an entire study may take only an hour. A normal result demonstrates equal distribution bilaterally. Abnormal results include either concentration of the tracer in the region of a known nodule indicating an area of hyperfunction or, conversely, an area of photopenia (the "cold nodule") indicating a region of hypofunction. Before the era of fine-needle aspiration (FNA) biopsy, this finding elevated the concern for potential malignancy.

^{123}Iodine Scintigraphy

Because ^{123}I is trapped and organified by the thyroid gland, it can better indicate the functional characteristics of thyroid tissue. It is produced in a cyclotron and has a short half-life (about 13 hours). These factors are responsible for the substantial cost associated with this test. ^{123}I emits x-rays, some β particles and γ rays. After administration of an oral dose, the thyroid absorbs sufficient isotope to allow imaging by 4 hours. Images are also obtained at 24 hours, and the total fraction of dose retained by the thyroid can then be calculated as the 24-hour radioactive iodine uptake (RAIU).

^{131}Iodine Scintigraphy

^{131}I concentrates in the thyroid by the same mechanism as ^{123}I, but it has a much longer half-life (about 8 days) and emits much more β radiation along with β radiation at a range that is suboptimal for clear image creation. Because of its long half-life and thorough clearance from background tissues, however, it remains the isotope of choice for imaging of patients with differentiated thyroid carcinoma. Ultimately, treatment or ablation of residual or metastatic carcinoma (largely by the effect of the ß irradiation) is accomplished with higher doses of the isotope than required for imaging.

Positron Emission Tomography

^{18}F fluorodeoxyglucose positron emission tomography (PET) scanning with 3-dimensional tomographic reconstruction can be very helpful in imaging thyroid carcinomas. Because of the expense and the inconsistent insurance coverage, usage is currently limited to unusual circumstances such as recurrent thyroid malignancy which is otherwise occult (Fig. 77.5). The sensitivity in thyroid carcinomas is approximately 60% to 70% and false-positive findings are very rare.[17] PET scanning is so frequently used in the evaluation of other solid malignancies that occult thyroid carcinomas are occasionally discovered.[18] All thyroid incidentalomas discovered by PET scanning are not malignant, however. In one series, just over 25% of such tumors were thyroid cancers and elevated standard uptake values (SUV) were often suggestive of this compared with those tumors ultimately proved to be benign.[19]

^{99m}Tc SestaMIBI Scintigraphy

Although ^{99m}Tc-SestaMIBI scintigraphy is commonly used in localization of parathyroid tumors, it has incidentally been noted to concentrate in follicular tumors, most notably those with Hürthle cell cytology. For this reason, it may have a role in localizing persistent disease in patients with Hürthle cell carcinoma. In contrast to radioactive iodine, however, it does not have therapeutic potential in ablating tissue. If a thyroid nodule is incidentally imaged on SestaMIBI scanning, there is no capability to predict whether it is a benign or malignant tumor.[20]

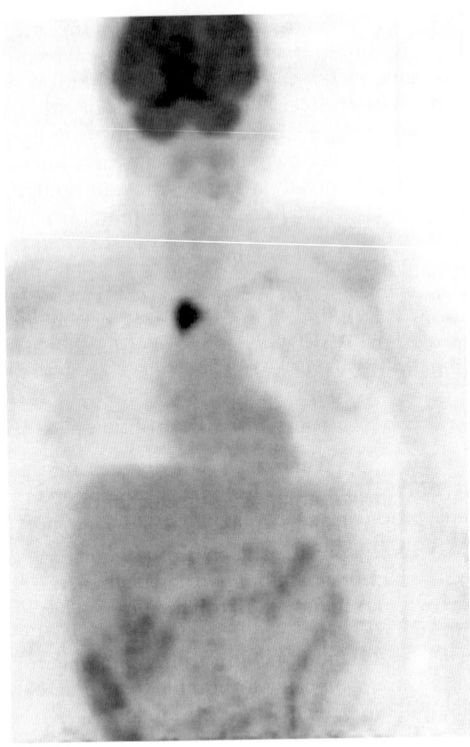

FIGURE 77.5 ^{18}F fluorodeoxyglucose (FDG) PET scan of a patient with late recurrence of differentiated thyroid carcinoma in the mediastinum. The tumor is the intensely FDG-avid mass superior to the cardiac activity.

^{111}Indium-Octreotide Scintigraphy

Octreotide scanning (somatostatin receptor scintigraphy) has been occasionally useful in imaging differentiated thyroid carcinoma, especially when radioiodine scintigraphy has failed to do so. Its therapeutic potential is undefined.

Ultrasonography

Ultrasound of the thyroid requires a high-frequency "small parts" probe (generally 7.5 to 10 mHz or higher). It is a very sensitive technique to determine the size, number, and distribution of thyroid nodules. Ultrasound often detects very small, subtle nodules that are not otherwise clinically evident. Studied prospectively, the prevalence of asymptomatic thyroid nodules (thyroid incidentalomas) detected by ultrasonography is 67%.[21] Because ultrasonography can detect nodules at a preclinical stage, it follows that proper perspective about the significance or insignificance of these nodules must be maintained. In practical terms, selective FNA biopsy should be limited to those nodules greater than 1 cm or those that have increased in size under serial ultrasound measurement. As with any imaging technique that depends on individual performance of the test, a user-dependent sensitivity range exists. Also, the specific measurement of the dimensions of the nodules can vary between examiners because of variable placement of both the transducer and the measurement cursor. Despite these factors, ultrasonography is a very valuable enhancement to the workup of the thyroid nodule or multinodular goiter. It can be especially useful when employed by the surgeon who will be performing the thyroid resection. Additionally, it has a rapidly developing role in the preoperative staging and the postoperative follow-up of patients with differentiated thyroid carcinoma. In experienced hands, it is a very sensitive technique for detecting abnormally enlarged lymph nodes or recurrence within the thyroid bed. Its utility is even further enhanced by ultrasound guidance of the subsequent FNA biopsy.[22]

Cross-sectional Imaging

Computed tomography (CT) scans and magnetic resonance imaging (MRI) scans are useful in certain circumstances. In large nodules firmly fixed to contiguous structures or accompanied by new vocal cord paralysis, the concern for an invasive thyroid cancer is raised. CT scan may suggest invasion of the laryngeal or tracheal cartilages, which may modify the operative approach. Large goiters that have an obvious substernal component on physical examination or that are accompanied by an upper airway obstructive component may warrant preoperative CT scan to define the extent of the goiter, not only to help plan the specific operative plan but also to facilitate anesthetic evaluation for difficult airway management techniques such as fiberoptic intubation (Fig. 77.6).

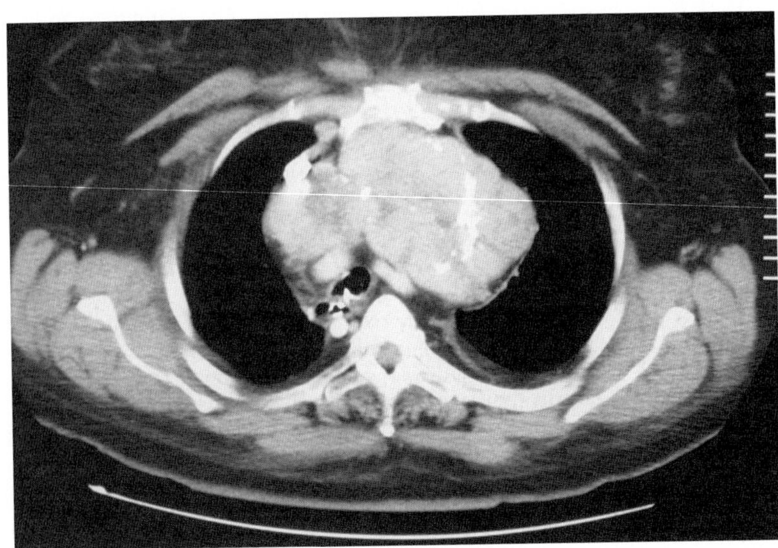

FIGURE 77.6 Example of a multinodular goiter with a large substernal component causing tracheal displacement and compression.

FUNCTIONAL DISORDERS AND GENERAL TREATMENT CONSIDERATIONS

Hyperthyroidism

Hyperthyroidism can be caused by diverse pathophysiology, such as Graves' disease, toxic multinodular goiter, and solitary toxic adenoma. Typical symptoms are heat intolerance, sweating, palpitations, tremor, hyperphagia, thirst, and sleep disturbances. Elderly patients can present with muscle wasting, atrial fibrillation, angina pectoris, or congestive heart failure. Regardless of specific cause, the need to control hyperthyroidism before operation is critical to prevent thyroid crisis (i.e., thyroid storm). Maximal safety is assured with thionamides combined with β-blockade, but many studies suggest that propranolol or metoprolol used without thionamides are as safe and effective.[23,24] β-Blockade alone is not universally accepted because of the occasional occurrence of postoperative thyroid crisis, tachycardia, hyperhydrosis, or anxiety.[25] Doses of β-blockers must continue until the morning of surgery and should not be stopped abruptly postoperatively. Lugol's solution (iodine plus potassium iodide, 6 mg per drop) can be administered as 5 to 10 drops three times daily for 2 weeks preoperatively to decrease vascularity. Henry S. Plummer at the Mayo Clinic was the first physician to define the role of iodine preoperatively in Graves' disease, which contributed to remarkable improvements in perioperative mortality.

Graves' Disease

Graves' disease, which was described by Dr. Robert Graves in the 1830s as a toxic diffuse goiter associated with exophthalmos and palpitations, is an autoimmune disorder with a genetic predisposition and a female predominance (five to seven times higher than the incidence in males). It is characterized by the presence of thyroid-stimulating antibodies (TSAb). These antibodies bind to the TSH receptor on follicular cells and stimulate thyroid hormone release. The autoimmune disease may also affect the eyes to cause exophthalmos and pretibial regions to cause myxedema. Graves' ophthalmopathy may be the first manifestation of disease, and it covers a wide spectrum from very mild changes in acuity or ocular dryness to obvious proptosis. It may be clinically so severe as to require aggressive ophthalmologic treatment in approximately 5% of patients. The pathophysiology is not entirely understood, but the ophthalmopathy appears to have some relationship to inflammation of the periorbital fibroblasts. Aside from the ophthalmopathic findings of proptosis and lid lag on physical examination, patients with Graves' disease have a diffuse goiter, which may be smooth or occasionally irregular. The gland is by nature very vascular and may occasionally have an audible bruit overlying it. T_4 and T_3 levels are increased and TSH levels are suppressed. The uptake of ^{131}I generally shows a symmetrically enlarged gland with increased 24-hour RAIU measurements.

Three main treatment modalities for Graves' disease are medical therapy, radioactive iodine treatment, and thyroidectomy. Selection of therapy depends on age, disease severity, goiter size, and patient preference. Practice patterns differ dramatically across the world, especially regarding the use of radioiodine (it is less common in Europe and especially Japan compared to the United States). The most common initial treatment involves thionamides and often β-blockade. In a small fraction of patients, antithyroid drugs may be the only therapy necessary, but in general, this strategy is considered an impermanent solution. Although the drugs may theoretically be used long term, they are associated with a small, but real risk of life-threatening agranulocytosis. Additionally, a number of less severe side effects make tolerance difficult for many, and the recurrence of thyrotoxicosis can be unpredictable. Ultimately, most patients pursue a permanent, or "ablative" therapy such as radioactive iodine (RAI) or surgery. Treatment with RAI is very effective and has not been associated with secondary risk of development of a new malignancy, yet there is still a practical hesitance to use this treatment in young children. RAI takes a full 1 to 2 months to provide definitive results and thus antithyroid medications must continue during this period. Although euthyroidism is the most common result of therapy, the effects are slowly progressive such that over 95% of patients become hypothyroid within 10 years following treatment. RAI therapy has been occasionally associated with exacerbation of Graves' ophthalmopathy, although the effect is ameliorated by corticosteroids and the early addition of LT_4 posttreatment.[26–28] Because of this concern, patients with severe ophthalmopathy should consider total thyroidectomy instead of RAI to prevent such an exacerbation; however, ultimate resolution of ophthalmopathy is no more likely with operation.

Surgery for Graves' disease has the advantage of rapid correction of the hyperthyroid state. The specific operation has typically been either bilateral subtotal thyroidectomy or total thyroidectomy. Subtotal thyroidectomy intends to remove enough tissue to resolve the hyperthyroidism but leave enough to maintain euthyroidism. Graves' disease is dynamic and, thus, remissions and exacerbations are common. This factor makes the determination of exactly how much tissue to leave as a remnant very challenging (typically estimated between 4 and 8 g of thyroid tissue). For these reasons, total thyroidectomy is becoming the preferred operation for treatment of Graves' disease with the intention of obviating the chance of recurrence but accepting hypothyroidism requiring LT_4 therapy. The transient hypocalcemia that can occur after total thyroidectomy (from the effect on the parathyroid glands) may be greatly worsened in the patient with Graves' disease because of the increased bone turnover observed with hyperthyroidism. With proper supportive treatment, however, recovery is common and the incidence of permanent hypoparathyroidism should be no higher than in other patients.

Toxic Multinodular Goiter

The term *toxic multinodular goiter* (MNG) refers to thyrotoxicosis that is caused by a multinodular goiter that may be of endemic or nonendemic etiology. H. S. Plummer first distinguished toxic adenomatous goiter from Graves' disease. Although the eponym "Plummer disease" now more commonly refers to the patient with a solitary toxic nodule (see below), many clinicians still include toxic MNG under that historical blanket. Thyrotoxicosis may occur as a progression from euthyroid multinodular goiter that was originally TSH dependent, which then progressed to a state of autonomy whereby it is not suppressible with LT_4. After that, it may progress to a toxic state in which distinct nodular areas are overproducing T_4 and T_3 with resultant TSH suppression. Although the cause is clearly distinct, it is possible that some patients included in this diagnostic category actually have Graves' disease with nodular degeneration of their diffuse goiter. Patients with toxic MNG, however, are often easily distinguished from those with Graves' disease. The typical patient is female and more than 50 years old with a previous history of multinodular goiter. Thyrotoxicosis may be precipitated in a MNG with or without areas of autonomy when an iodide load is provided (the Jod-Basedow phenomenon). Historically, this has been seen over a period of years following public health efforts to iodinate salt or flour in an iodine-deficient population. This is still seen after exposure to iodinated radiographic contrast media, expectorants, or iodide-containing drugs such as amiodarone.

Hyperthyroidism present in a patient with MNG can involve a wide spectrum of severity such that it is not uncommon for a patient having indications for thyroidectomy, for reasons such as continued nodular growth or substernal extension, to have a suppressed TSH in the absence of major functional symptoms. This subclinical thyrotoxicosis is another potential indication for thyroidectomy because it rarely resolves spontaneously and prolonged hyperthyroidism, even when mild, may have deleterious health effects. Thyroidectomy is a relatively common treatment for toxic MNG, with radioiodine treatment representing a less-common alternative because it often requires high doses or repeated treatments because of the large goiter size and low radioiodine uptake. Long-term remissions from antithyroid drug treatment are even less common or predictable than seen in treatment of Graves' disease.[29]

Solitary Toxic Adenoma

Patients with thyrotoxicosis and a new dominant thyroid nodule may have a toxic adenoma. Nodules must usually grow to at least 2 cm in size before hyperthyroidism is clinically evident. As expected, T_3or T_4, or both are elevated and TSH is suppressed. Thyroid scintigraphy will demonstrate a single "hot" area corresponding to the known nodule with suppression of the remainder of the thyroid substance. FNA is rarely helpful and the incidence of malignancy within these nodules is negligible. Treatment options include ^{131}I RAI therapy or resection. RAI is effective in controlling the hyperthyroidism, but depending on nodule size, may leave behind a palpable abnormality. In particular, younger patients with sizable nodules may choose operation. The resection is typically a hemithyroidectomy and isthmusectomy. The contralateral lobe is often normal and will maintain normal thyroid hormone production after the hyperthyroidism is remedied.

Hypothyroidism

Primary hypothyroidism can arise from intrinsic thyroid disease, iatrogenic thyroid removal or destruction, and antithyroid drug effects. Secondary hypothyroidism can also occur from failure of thyrotropic function (via TSH) of the pituitary gland because of disease, removal, or destruction of that gland as well. Rarely, tertiary hypothyroidism can occur with destructive disorders of the hypothalamus via decreased production of thyrotropin-releasing hormone. The most common cause of primary hypothyroidism in adult patients is Hashimoto's thyroiditis. In large part, hypothyroidism is straightforward to address with exogenous LT_4 therapy, with the exception of the patient with thyroid hormone resistance. As defined by hypothyroidism itself, the role for surgical therapy is limited. The structural thyroid disorder causing the hypothyroidism, however, may be an indication for thyroidectomy (e.g. goiter).

Thyroiditis

A summary of conditions causing a painful neck mass is delineated in Table 77.1. Inflammatory conditions of the thyroid are a disparate family of conditions that require surgical therapy in the minority of situations. However, they can be quite prevalent in patients undergoing evaluation for thyroid surgery and a thorough understanding is required to avoid diagnostic and therapeutic misadventures. The different types of thyroiditis are presented in descending order of clinical frequency.

TABLE 77.1 DIAGNOSIS

DIFFERENTIAL DIAGNOSIS OF THE PAINFUL NECK MASS

THYROIDAL CAUSES
Acute thyroiditis
Subacute thyroiditis
Acute thyroid cyst (hemorrhage into cyst or nodule)
Rapidly enlarging thyroid carcinoma
Painful Hashimoto's thyroiditis
Radiation thyroiditis
NONTHYROIDAL CAUSES
Infected thyroglossal duct cyst
Infected branchial cleft cyst
Infected cystic hygroma
Cervical adenitis
Globus hystericus (no mass palpable)

(Adapted from Farwall AP, Braverman LE. Thyroiditis. In Randolph GW, ed. *Surgery of the thyroid and parathyroid glands*. Philadelphia: WB Saunders, 2003, p. 49.)

Hashimoto's Thyroiditis

Also known as chronic thyroiditis, autoimmune thyroiditis, and lymphocytic thyroiditis, this condition was described by Hashimoto in 1912 as *struma lymphomatosa* based on the histologic findings. It affects perhaps up to 10% of the general population and is the most common cause of both goiter and hypothyroidism in the United States. Although it can occur at nearly any age, the peak is from age 30 to 60. Female to male preponderance is as high as 9:1. It is clearly an autoimmune condition and there is a moderate genetic predisposition, associated with HLA-DR3, -DR5, and -B8. The disease prevalence is increased in iodine-sufficient regions and this may be because immunogenicity of the thyroglobulin molecule increases with the degree of iodination. The histologic changes are characterized by lymphocytic infiltration with fibrosis and germinal centers. Some follicular cells may undergo metaplasia to Hürthle cells. The typical presentation is that of a painless diffuse goiter in a young woman discovered on physical examination or associated with hypothyroidism. Patients often note a sense of fullness in, or awareness of, the region of the thyroid. When the associated goiter is large, compressive symptoms of dysphagia or dyspnea may occur. The goiter is typically firm and rubbery and slightly "bumpy" with prominent lateral lobes. Nodular disease can and does occur in a gland affected by Hashimoto's disease and needs to be investigated with FNA to rule out coexisting malignancy, typically papillary cancer or, rarely, thyroid lymphoma. Thyroid autoantibody titers are elevated, primarily TPOAb and secondarily, TgAb, and erythrocyte sedimentation rate (ESR) is normal. A 24-hour RAIU is variable and can be elevated, normal, or often depressed. Patients are often hypothyroid but may be euthyroid at the time of presentation. If patients are euthyroid, approximately 5% per year will progress to hypothyroidism.[30] In approximately 5% of patients, a transient phase of hyperthyroidism, termed "Hashitoxicosis," may be seen at the onset of disease and, in fact, the subsequent pattern in thyroid function changes are nearly indistinguishable from that of silent thyroiditis. For the majority of patients, treatment of Hashimoto's thyroiditis is limited to LT_4 therapy in those with hypothyroidism, which is dosed for the goal of a TSH level in the lower portion of the normal range. Surgery is indicated in patients with large goiters, significant compressive symptoms, local symptoms refractory to LT_4 therapy, or the inability to rule out malignancy (typically in the nodular subtype).

Painless or Postpartum Thyroiditis

Sporadic silent (painless) thyroiditis and postpartum thyroiditis are known as destruction-induced thyroiditities and are probably variants of the same process, distinguished only by the relationship to pregnancy.[31] Along with subacute thyroiditis, these conditions are characterized by the onset of thyrotoxicosis, a goiter, and low 24-hour RAIU. Even excluding postpartum cases, there is a female predominance by 2:1 and the age range of affected patients is broad. The cause appears to be autoimmune, but the genetic predisposition is low. There is no fever or malaise and the goiter is painless, but persistent. Thyroid autoantibodies titers are often high, and the ESR is usually normal. Thyroid function is dynamic and follows a pattern similar to that of subacute thyroiditis with the abrupt onset of thyrotoxicosis followed by a period of euthyroidism, then hypothyroidism. Permanent hypothyroidism is fairly common, especially if the disease course was characterized by very limited hyperthyroidism with evident progressive hypothyroidism. A 24-hour RAIU is very low (usually <5%), consistent with leakage of preformed thyroid hormones from a thyroid gland that is damaged on the cellular level. At the histologic level, lymphocytic infiltration is seen along with destruction of follicular cells. If it is pregnancy associated, it is likely to relapse with future pregnancies. If symptoms of thyrotoxicosis are significant, β-adrenergic blocking drugs may be used, but antithyroid drugs are not appropriate because the gland is not hyperfunctioning at the follicular cell level. Rarely, severe thyrotoxicosis may be impacted by iopanoic acid, which markedly inhibits peripheral conversion of T_4 to T_3. If LT_4 therapy is instituted during the hypothyroid phase for symptomatic relief, it can be withdrawn after 6 to 9 months to determine if recovery has occurred.

Subacute Thyroiditis

Subacute thyroiditis is a common form of thyroiditis that affects women more often than men by a 5:1 ratio and often in the age group of 20 to 60. There are a number of synonymous terms, such as de Quervain's thyroiditis, giant cell thyroiditis, pseudogranulomatous thyroiditis, subacute painful thyroiditis, and subacute granulomatous thyroiditis. The cause is not entirely certain, but it appears to be virally related or mediated. There may be moderate genetic predisposition. A prodrome consistent with an upper respiratory viral infection is very common. The patient often has fever and malaise and an exquisitely painful and firm goiter that is also transient. The goiter is usually unilaterally dominant, and the patient may have pain that radiates to the ipsilateral ear. At a histologic level, giant cells (which may also be seen on FNA, thus supporting the diagnosis) and granulomas often infiltrate the thyroid. It is common to see a dynamic picture of thyroid function with subclinical or obvious thyrotoxicosis followed by hypothyroidism, which may occasionally be permanent. Consistent with follicular cell destruction, serum Tg levels may be elevated. Antithyroid antibodies may be present in low titers and the ESR is often high. A 24-hour RAIU is usually quite low (<5%). Management is similar to painless thyroiditis in that β-blockers may be used, but antithyroid medications are not useful. Salicylates or nonsteroidal anti-inflammatory drugs (NSAIDs) are adequate to control pain in most cases, with the occasional need for oral glucocorticoids. Although the course of disease can be protracted for weeks or months, relapse is rare and management is usually limited to management of symptoms.

Amiodarone-Induced Thyrotoxicosis or Thyroiditis

Although the significance of amiodarone-induced thyrotoxicosis or thyroiditis is usually related to the thyrotoxicosis induced by the Jod-Basedow mechanism, increased understanding of the condition has led to the realization that it often includes a component of destructive thyroiditis as well, especially when background iodine deficiency is not a factor.[32] The antiarrhythmic drug amiodarone is 37% iodine by weight and the iodine load can induce thyrotoxicosis. Amiodarone therapy results in thyrotoxicosis in 3% of patients in iodine-sufficient regions and up to 10% of patients in iodine-deficient regions.[33] In addition, the drug inhibits 5′ deiodinase. Secondary medical treatment of the hyperthyroidism is difficult because of both the long half-life of the drug and the decompensation in cardiac function related to underlying heart disease. Amiodarone-induced destructive thyroiditis is very common in the United States. Two types of amiodarone-induced hyperthyroidism can occur, but distinction between the types can be clinically difficult. Type I is iodine-induced and is more common in iodine-deficient areas (type Ia is often associated with preexisting multinodular goiter). In general, amiodarone should be stopped and thionamides may be variably effective. A 24-hour RAIU may be normal or elevated in iodine-deficient areas (opening that therapeutic possibility) but in iodine-sufficient areas (type Ib is often associated with Graves' disease), 24-hour RAIU is decreased. Type II, defined primarily by destructive thyroiditis, is usually seen in iodine-sufficient areas and can be self-limited. Decreased thyroid parenchymal blood flow on color flow Doppler imaging is typical. A 24-hour RAIU is typically very low and serum interleukin-6 may be elevated. Corticosteroids are used therapeutically and, if tolerated, β-blockers as well. If hyperthyroidism is severe in either type I or II, thyroidectomy may be required to resolve the thyrotoxicosis and allow continuation of amiodarone. Some recommend iopanoic acid before thyroidectomy. Because of the cardiac decompensation, thyroidectomy may need to be done under local anesthesia and sedation to avoid the risks of general anesthesia.

Acute Thyroiditis

Acute thyroiditis refers to a rare suppurative condition caused by bacterial organisms. It may occur in children or young adults (approximately age 20 to 40 years) with equal sex predisposition and no evidence of genetic predisposition. Patients with acquired immunodeficiency syndrome (AIDS) may be at risk for this condition. A clinical prodrome, usually a viral or bacterial upper respiratory infection, may occur and the patient is often affected by a significant fever and malaise and may have radiating pain to the region of the ipsilateral ear. *Staphylococcus aureus* and *Streptococcus pyogenes* are the most common pathogens, but many other possibilities exist. A painful, but ultimately transient goiter may be evident, which often is a thyroidal or perithyroidal abscess. The patient usually remains euthyroid and antithyroid antibody titers are normal. ESR may be elevated. If a 24-hour RAIU scan is performed, it is often normal but uptake may be focally decreased in the region of active infection. Bacterial infection of the thyroid may occur via hematologic spread from a distant site or local infiltration from other head and neck infections. If acute thyroiditis is related to a fistulous communication with the pyriform sinus, the condition may recur repeatedly. It is the potential for abscess formation or pyriform sinus fistula that makes this a disease that occasionally requires surgical intervention even if FNA is able to determine the causative organism and if appropriate parenteral antibiotics are instituted. In general, this condition is still associated with some risk of mortality and these patients should be admitted to the hospital for appropriately aggressive management.

Riedel's Thyroiditis

Also known as Riedel's struma or invasive fibrous thyroiditis, this rare disorder affects mainly women (by a ratio of 4:1) and usually occurs between the ages of 30 and 60. The cause is unknown and a genetic predisposition is not apparent. There is no prodrome and no fever or malaise. The patient presents with a painless but persistent, and often progressive, goiter. Patients are usually euthyroid at presentation but may eventually become hypothyroid. They may have detectable antithyroid antibody titers and a normal ESR. If obtained, the 24-hour RAIU is often normal or somewhat decreased. Physical examination reveals an exceptionally firm goiter often described as "woody." Most commonly, this is a diffuse, bilobar process. Histologically, the disease is characterized by extensive fibrosis, which may progress to a point of compression of adjacent structures such as the trachea and esophagus. Riedel's thyroiditis is often accompanied by other equally mysterious focally sclerotic conditions such as retroperitoneal fibrosis, mediastinal fibrosis, retroorbital fibrosis, and sclerosing cholangitis.[34] Because of its infiltrative nature, it is important to differentiate Riedel's thyroiditis from thyroid carcinoma. FNA is often inadequate and open biopsy may be required. If substantial compression exists, surgery is often required to relieve these symptoms. Extensive resection is often unsafe or impossible, and wedge resections, especially of the isthmus, may be very effective in relieving symptoms. Medical therapy, including corticosteroids, methotrexate, or tamoxifen, may have a positive impact in the chronic setting.[35]

NODULAR THYROID DISEASE AND GENERAL TREATMENT CONSIDERATIONS

Nontoxic Multinodular Goiter

From a world health perspective, endemic goiter is still a significant issue affecting up to 12% of the world's population. Endemic goiters are caused by dietary iodine deficiency, which ultimately is also responsible for endemic cretinism—another major world health issue. Goitrogenic substances found in diets may also be contributory. Iodine deficiency in a region is addressed over time by iodination of dietary components (e.g., salt, bread flour, or vegetable oil).

In endemic goiter, T_4 levels may be normal or decreased, whereas T_3 levels are normal or often increased. This reflects an adaptive regulatory mechanism by which the thyroid preferentially shifts production to the more biologically potent T_3. Exogenous thyroxine therapy will induce a decrease in goiter size in roughly 80% of patients treated. Resection may be indicated for large size, increase in size while on T_4, or compression of the trachea, esophagus, or superior vena cava.

In most developed countries, the term *goiter* generically refers to a group of diseases causing thyroid enlargement in patients not affected by iodine deficiency. Specifically, it can refer to conditions such as Graves' disease, nodular goiter, chronic lymphocytic thyroiditis, subacute thyroiditis, and Reidel's thyroiditis. In common usage, *goiter* typically refers to patients with nodular goiter, which may be uninodular or multinodular. Asymptomatic, multinodular goiter is common and if reasonable assurance that the goiter is not harboring a malignancy can be obtained by FNA, thyroidectomy is not usually indicated. Sometimes, because of the number of nodules if significant size (>1 cm), repeated FNA during longitudinal observation becomes impractical. Patients may grow frustrated with the prospects of multiple FNAs and elect thyroidectomy to simplify management. Compressive symptoms involving the airway or esophagus are also an indication for thyroidectomy. A multinodular goiter causing subclinical or obvious thyrotoxicosis (toxic multinodular goiter) should also be removed (see later). Options for removal include subtotal thyroidectomy or total thyroidectomy. Total thyroidectomy is the preferred option because of the significant chance for recurrent nodular degeneration of the thyroid remnant after subtotal thyroidectomy. If a goiter develops a substernal portion, thyroidectomy is warranted because of the inability to monitor continuing growth in the mediastinum. If tracheal compression develops gradually, it may be largely asymptomatic. The natural history of that situation is the unpredictable possibility of sudden respiratory obstructive crisis usually exacerbated by an upper respiratory infection. Because all of the important attachments to the thyroid parenchyma remain in the neck, even very large substernal goiters can be removed through a cervical incision. Less than 5% to 10% will require partial sternotomy for full removal.

Solitary or Dominant Thyroid Nodule

Thyroid nodular disease is very common, whereas thyroid malignancy is relatively rare. The prevalence of thyroid nodules is approximately 4% to 7% in the general population and, in fact, thyroid nodules are present in approximately 50% of autopsy specimens. In contrast, the incidence of thyroid cancer (in the absence of significant risk factors) is 4 per 100,000 per year. Therefore, a great deal of culling needs to occur to appropriately identify those patients who require operation and to avoid operation for a large fraction of patients who do not.

When assessing a patient with a solitary thyroid nodule, first assess factors in the history that may indicate the likelihood of benign or malignant disease. A new thyroid nodule that occurs at the extremes of age is more likely to be malignant than one that occurs in the third through seventh decade. The risk of a solitary thyroid nodule in a child under 14 being malignant may be as high as 50%.[36] Patient gender itself does not generally confer risk of malignancy, and the fact that thyroid cancer occurs in a greater number of women than men is related more to the increased prevalence of nodular thyroid disease in women. A new thyroid nodule that occurs after the age of 60, however, is more likely to be malignant in a man than in a woman.

Many factors apparent on physical examination or imaging can also be used to assess the potential for malignant disease in the patient with a thyroid nodule. The consideration that nodular disease is uninodular (e.g., solitary) instead of multinodular has traditionally implied that the former situation is more concerning for malignancy. Especially in the era of thyroid ultrasound, this distinction is inappropriately overemphasized because at least half of nodules considered solitary by clinical examination are actually just a dominant nodule in a multinodular goiter. It is mostly a practical consideration that the dominant nodule (largest or most apparent) of a multinodular gland is the one that dictates subsequent clinical decision-making. The physical characteristics of a nodule (size, firmness, texture) have a limited ability to predict malignancy. Significant fixation to surrounding tissues can greatly elevate the level of concern, but this is not entirely reliable. Associated lymphadenopathy in the central or lateral cervical compartments is certainly concerning for potential malignancy. Although many patients with benign thyroid disease describe hoarseness or a change in voice, this is often largely subjective and is of limited concern unless accompanied by objective hoarseness and ipsilateral recurrent laryngeal nerve paralysis. Thyroid functional status can be important in two ways. First, if the nodule is truly solitary and the patient is hyperthyroid, it may be a toxic autonomous nodule. If this is confirmed by nuclear scintigraphy, the risk of malignancy in this nodule is negligible. If the patient is chronically hypothyroid (likely from Hashimoto's disease), a firm, indistinct nodule raises the question of whether an extranodal lymphoma may be present.

Several hereditary environmental factors and hereditary conditions can increase the risk of developing thyroid cancer. A critical question in assessing any patient with a thyroid nodule is whether any history of radiation exposure exists. At least 90% of radiation-associated thyroid cancers are papillary thyroid carcinoma. Typical exposures have included external beam irradiation treatment for acne, tinea capitis, external otitis, recurrent tonsillitis, or neonatal thymic enlargement, treatments that were common in the 1940s and 1950s but that are no longer used. In the current era, excessive diagnostic radiation or too high-dose therapeutic irradiation (e.g., treatment of lymphoma or head and neck malignancies) is responsible for relevant exposures. The association is well documented and there appears to be a linear relationship between the dose of radiation and the risk for thyroid cancer with even a higher risk among those exposed at a young age.[37] The typical latent period between exposure and clinically evident cancer appears to be in the 3- to 8-year range. It is not clear, however, exactly when, if ever, the risk is no longer present. Cases appear to increase for up to three decades after exposure and then begin to tail off. Another source of radiation exposure to the thyroid gland is nuclear fallout, related to either atomic weapons or nuclear power plant accidents, such as Chernobyl in 1986, which exposed 1.5 million people in southern Belarus and northern Ukraine. This acute γ radiation exposure is likely the main risk factor, but longer term exposure to diverse radioisotopes of iodine that secondarily contaminate the regional water and food supplies may also be contributory.

Another critical question to investigate is whether a family history of thyroid cancer or associated conditions exists. The prototypical issue here is to uncover a family history of medullary thyroid cancer, which suggests the potential for an inherited syndrome such as familial medullary thyroid carcinoma or multiple endocrine neoplasia type 2. Papillary thyroid cancer, however, may have a familial association as well, either independently or, more commonly, associated with Cowden's syndrome or Gardner's syndrome (familial adenomatous polyposis).

In most situations, extensive thyroid function testing is not necessary and a TSH is all that is required. After initial clinical assessment, thyroid nodular disease is often assessed by ultrasound (USN). Relevant factors include the size of the nodule and other sonographic characteristics. Hyperechoic nodules are often benign, whereas thyroid malignancies, regardless of cell type, are often hypoechoic. Irregular margins between the nodule and surrounding tissues will raise the concern for malignancy. A sonolucent dark rim around the nodule is referred to as a "halo" and is much more likely to occur with a benign nodule, although it is occasionally seen with a malignancy as well. Significant calcification with acoustic shadowing (e.g., "eggshell") is usually indicative of chronicity and is more likely associated with a benign nodule, whereas subtle microcalcifications, which are too small to cause acoustic shadowing and which cause a "twinkling" effect when the transducer is moved, are highly correlated with malignancy. Also important is whether the nodule is truly solitary or whether there are additional nodules, especially in the contralateral lobe, that may affect the specific surgical recommendations. Although it is still common for patients to undergo thyroid scintigraphy, its utility is actually very limited and it should not be a routine investigation for a thyroid nodule. The only helpful role is to determine the specific nature of a nodule in a patient with hyperthyroidism. The additional diagnostic information provided by knowing the nodule is "cold" or "photopenic" is very limited, especially in the era of FNA, which can categorize the potential for malignancy to a much greater degree. Both USN and FNA are able to confirm if the nodule is cystic in character. Although smaller cysts may resolve with aspiration, recurrence is very likely if the cyst is 4 cm or greater and, consequently, these patients should consider resection.

FNA is the cornerstone of diagnostic evaluation of the thyroid nodule. It can reliably identify colloid nodules, benign nodular hyperplasia, thyroiditis, papillary thyroid carcinoma (PTC), medullary thyroid carcinoma, and anaplastic thyroid carcinoma. FNA may suggest an extranodal lymphoma. It can also classify nodules as follicular lesions or Hürthle cell lesions. These lesions currently require at least partial thyroidectomy (e.g., lobectomy) to determine whether it is a follicular (or Hürthle cell) adenoma or follicular (or Hürthle cell) carcinoma. That is because the determination of malignancy can be made only by the demonstration of capsular or vascular invasion. FNA should have a false-positive rate of 0 to 0.5% and a false-negative rate of 0 to 5%. The potential for a nondiagnostic interpretation is directly related to the number of follicular cells recovered for analysis. This is ultimately related to technique and the number of sampling needle passes performed. Ultrasound guidance can help ensure that the biopsy results are representative of the nodule of interest, but ultimately, it will not significantly change the possibility of a nondiagnostic result if inadequate technique is employed.

Standard disposable needles from 23- to 27-gauge size range and 10-mL syringes are used. The target nodule is fixed between two fingers on the nondominant hand while multiple passes through portions of the nodule are made without requiring a separate skin puncture for each. An average of three separate biopsy maneuvers is reasonable practice. The technique does not rely heavily on aspiration or suction as the name might imply. The ideal sample remains mostly in the needle hub and barrel before expelling it onto a slide or into fixative for cytologic preparation. Current limitations require that decisions based on FNA are contingent on the cytologic appearance. It is likely that in the near future, however, specific molecular markers or gene expression data will be identified that will allow specific testing of FNA specimens to indicate risk of malignancy.

THYROID MALIGNANCY AND GENERAL TREATMENT CONSIDERATIONS

General Considerations

Thyroid cancers exhibit a wide spectrum of behavior, from the inconsequential, occult, well-differentiated thyroid carcinomas to the nearly uniformly fatal course of undifferentiated anaplastic cancers. Fortunately, at least 98% of thyroid cancers are well differentiated. Although the general treatment strategy for thyroid carcinomas is familiar (surgical resection, staging of disease, appropriate application of adjuvant treatments, and secondary screening or follow-up), a number of unique points are emphasized below.

Tumor Classification

Differentiated thyroid cancers are of follicular cell origin (papillary thyroid carcinoma and its variants, follicular thyroid carcinoma, and Hürthle cell carcinoma) or parafollicular (C-cell) origin (medullary thyroid carcinoma). There is, then, a spectrum of dedifferentiation that exists between these tumors and undifferentiated cancers such as anaplastic carcinoma. Tumors such as insular carcinoma exist along this spectrum. In a general sense along this progression, prognosis is directly related to the degree of differentiation. A number of classification systems exist. Although the original systems were based on architectural characteristics noted during histopathologic analysis, most current systems include certain cytologic and biologic behavioral attributes as well. The American Thyroid Association (ATA), the Armed Forces Institute of Pathology (AFIP), and the World Health Organization (WHO) all consider papillary thyroid cancers, including classic papillary carcinoma, mixed papillary-follicular variants, and follicular variants, and follicular thyroid carcinomas (FTC) as DTC. Still some disagreement exists about the classification of Hürthle cell carcinomas (HCC). In general, the ATA and WHO consider HCC as a subtype of follicular thyroid carcinoma, although the AFIP does not. Support for considering HCC as a subtype of follicular thyroid carcinoma includes the histologic demonstration of the transition of follicular to Hürthle cells, in intact TSH receptor adenylate cyclase system in Hürthle cells, and the ability of Hürthle cells to produce thyroglobulin and thus maintain Tg positivity on immunohistochemical staining).[38] Other characteristics, however, such as higher oncogene expression in HCC than FTC and the general impression that HCC can display a more aggressive clinical course than FTC cause some to classify HCC tumors outside the FTC family.[39] Medullary thyroid carcinoma is also a differentiated thyroid carcinoma but is of parafollicular cell origin.

Papillary Thyroid Carcinoma

Papillary thyroid carcinoma (PTC) accounts for approximately 80% of thyroid carcinomas. Although it occurs across the spectrum of age from childhood to the elderly, the peak incidence begins in the third and fourth decades of life. It is more common in females than males. It is especially prevalent in iodine-sufficient regions of the world. Papillary carcinoma arises from the follicular cells, is characterized by papillary architecture, and is often associated with calcifications, psammoma bodies, squamous metaplasia, and fibrosis. Cytology is diagnostically important and typical findings include large, overlapping nuclei, which are optically clear (known as Orphan Annie nuclei), and intranuclear grooving. As a whole, the prognosis is excellent, especially in those patients with tumors that define a low risk for recurrence. Greater than 30% of PTC is multicentric throughout the thyroid. Although multifocality does not signify a worse prognosis, this characteristic, in part, influences the rationale for total thyroidectomy discussed below. The incidence of cervical lymph node metastases varies across series and is influenced by whether lymphadenectomy is performed for prophylactic or therapeutic reasons. In general, it approximates 30% to 40%. Distant metastases occur in 2% to 14% of patients with PTC.[38] At least 70% of PTC can take up radioiodine and thus, RAI scanning is an important part of the treatment strategy.

Variants. A follicular variant of papillary thyroid carcinoma essentially combines the histologic and architectural appearance of follicular tumors with the cytologic features of papillary carcinoma. In terms of treatment and biologic behavior, this variant behaves in the same manner as classic PTC. The dilemma caused by this variant is based on the fact that, in contrast to classic PTC, it is very difficult to diagnose on frozen section analysis. It is often interpreted as a follicular lesion with the final diagnosis deferred until formal histopathology when the cytologic features are more apparent. More aggressive variants of papillary carcinoma include tall cell and columnar types, which also exist on the spectrum of dedifferentiation toward anaplastic carcinoma.

Microcarcinoma. PTC less than 1 cm in size are considered microcarcinomas (occult or incidental tumors). They may be multifocal and are usually clinically unapparent until thyroidectomy is performed for another indication. Although they are by definition malignant, this group of tumors requires a different set of considerations based on "nonmalignant" biologic behavior and patient outcome. Prognosis is exceptionally good, with a 0.4% cause-specific mortality rate.[37] If such a microcarcinoma is found after lobectomy, adequate treatment has already been rendered and completion thyroidectomy or radioiodine scanning, or both, are not indicated. Somewhat in contrast, if these microcarcinomas are diagnosed preoperatively, which is difficult because of their size, thyroid resection is usually recommended. Some groups, however, have chosen to follow these patients closely with ultrasound. Approximately 70% do not increase in size significantly.[40] Nonetheless, these tumors cannot be completely discounted. It is not uncommon for PTC to be diagnosed by biopsy of a lateral compartment lymph node even if the associated primary tumor is not apparent. If these patients are treated with total thyroidectomy, very careful histologic sectioning will be required to find the associated primary tumor, which may be as small as 1 mm.

Follicular Carcinoma. Follicular thyroid carcinoma (FTC) accounts for approximately 10% to 20% of all thyroid cancers. Again there is a female-to-male predominance, and the incidence begins to increase in the 5th decade of life. Determination that a follicular neoplasm is a carcinoma is not contingent only on the specific cellular architecture, but instead is based on the findings of vascular invasion and capsular invasion. This determination is rarely able to be made on frozen section and the information is often not available until final histopathology results.[41] FTC is often more advanced at the time of diagnosis compared with PTC. For example, it is more common for FTC to be locally infiltrative of muscles and perithyroidal vascular structures. Because of this difference in stage at diagnosis, the overall 10-year survival for patients with FTC is slightly worse than for those with PTC, but when patients are matched for age and stage with PTC, this difference largely disappears.[42] In contrast to PTC, follicular cancers are usually solitary. Approximately one third of patients with FTC have distant metastases at the time of diagnosis and the pattern is consistent with a mechanism of hematogenous spread, with lung and bone most often being involved. Lymph node involvement is limited to only about 10% of patients. Importantly, at least 80% of FTC will take up radioiodine, opening up this therapeutic possibility.

Minimally Invasive Follicular Carcinoma. Follicular neoplasms with demonstrable capsular invasion but no vascular invasion are classified as minimally invasive follicular cancers. These patients have an excellent prognosis, conceptually equivalent to patients with incidental papillary microcarcinomas. If such a tumor is found after hemithyroidectomy, there is no reason for the patient to undergo completion thyroidectomy and radioiodine scanning as would be recommended for true FTC.[43]

Hürthle Cell Carcinoma. Malignant Hürthle cell neoplasms account for approximately 5% of thyroid carcinomas and, in general, occur in patients slightly older than those with PTC or FTC. Despite their relatively uncommon nature, HCC enters diagnostic consideration frequently because Hürthle cells are frequently seen on FNA cytology from thyroid nodules. Patients with Hashimoto's disease or colloid nodules may demonstrate Hürthle cells. It is the nodule that contains almost entirely Hürthle cells, however, that raises concern for HCC. If this is suggested on FNA, operation, which at minimum is a thyroid lobectomy, is appropriate to establish the nature of the tumor. Hürthle cell adenomas (neoplasms with no evidence of capsular or vascular invasion) certainly exist but, occasionally, a tumor that is otherwise histologically compatible with a Hürthle cell adenoma is found to be associated with lymph node or distant metastases. For these reasons and considering the perspective that HCC may behave more aggressively, many surgeons advocate total thyroidectomy for any Hürthle cell neoplasm.[44] Again, HCC is more prevalent in women than men and is more often associated with lymph node metastases and distant metastases than PTC and FTC in general. Although it is a DTC likely of follicular cell origin, very few HCC tumors will take up radioiodine (only approximately 10%). For this reason, and considering the concern of a more unpredictably aggressive biologic behavior for HCC, aggressive and complete surgical resection is especially important in this disease. Therefore, total thyroidectomy may often be combined with central compartment lymphadenectomy and perhaps modified radical neck dissection if lymph node involvement is evident.

Medullary Carcinoma. MTC arises from the parafollicular C cells and accounts for about 7% of all thyroid malignancies. Approximately 75% occur in a sporadic fashion and 20% to 25% may be familial (multiple endocrine neoplasia [MEN] types 2A and 2B, as well as familial medullary thyroid carcinoma). These are autosomal-dominant inherited endocrinopathies related to a group of specific mutations on chromosome 10q11.2 (RET proto-oncogene) (Table 77.2). The familial forms of MTC have different degrees of aggressiveness related to the specific syndrome. Familial MTC has the most indolent course, whereas MEN 2B has the most aggressive course, with MEN 2A intermediate to these. Most sporadic MTC is relatively slow growing and may be quite indolent. These patients typically do not present before approximately 30 years of age. A subset of patients with sporadic MTC have a much more aggressive course. This variability in biologic behavior accounts for the overall 10-year survival rate of approximately 50%. Overall, MTC is more aggressive than other DTC and is more likely to metastasize, first to the level VI lymph nodes and then to the lateral compartment nodes (e.g., level III, IV, and V). At least 50% to 75% of patients with sporadic MTC have nodal metastases already present at the time of diagnosis. Distant metastases may involve the liver, lungs, and bone. FNA can be diagnostic for medullary cancer, especially if the specimen is stained for calcitonin. MTC is unique in that a very specific tumor marker is used for diagnosis and to guide subsequent follow-up. Serum calcitonin is the most useful marker, but most MTC also makes carcinoembryonic antigen (CEA) as well.

Approximately 20% of patients thought to have sporadic MTC may in fact be index cases of familial MTC. Therefore, any patient with a new diagnosis of MTC should have direct genetic testing for the genetic abnormalities associated with MEN 2A (RET protooncogene analysis). Appropriate screening for pheochromocytoma (which would be treated before the cervical operation) and hyperparathyroidism are required.

The treatment strategy for MTC is distinct to that of DTC of follicular cell origin. Because of the high likelihood of lymph node metastases and the fact that there is no effective adjuvant therapy (MTC does not take up radioiodine), a more extensive initial surgical resection is warranted. The appropriate operation for MTC is a total thyroidectomy with central compartment lymphadenectomy (level VI nodes). Because intraoperative assessment of lymph node involvement is relatively inaccurate, consideration should be given to ipsilateral modified radical neck dissection as well. Some advocate bilateral modified radical neck dissection initially and others advocate very extensive "microdissection" designed to completely remove any lymph node-bearing tissue in these areas and more durably render the patient normocalcemic.[45] Because of technical issues and an unclear influence on prognosis, this approach has not met with widespread acceptance.

It is common for patients to have persistent hypercalcitoninemia even after an extensive initial operation. Most patients have a subsequent indolent course, although some patients will progress more rapidly. Experience with remedial neck dissections in an attempt to render the patient normocalcemic has generally been disappointing and requires an appropriate search for distant metastases. This may include extensive imaging tests such as CT scanning, ultrasound, octreotide scanning, selective venous sampling for calcitonin levels, and laparoscopy to investigate for hepatic metastases. For most patients, the strategy of observation by clinical examination, biochemical markers, and imaging tests is adopted with interval reassessment for resectable regional and metastatic disease. When this is detected, especially if it is in a location whereby ongoing growth could cause significant morbidity (e.g., tracheoesophageal groove), resection can be offered. Hepatic resections for diffuse metastatic disease are inappropriate, whereas such an operation may be considered for isolated bulky metastatic deposits. Chemotherapy has largely been ineffective, although trials with tyrosine kinase-inhibiting drugs are ongoing. External beam radiotherapy may be useful for locoregional tumor control, especially in those patients with evidence of locally aggressive tumor behavior. This should not be employed, however, until appropriate surgical options are exhausted.

Provocative testing (e.g., pentagastrin or calcium stimulated calcitonin levels) was until recently a standard screening maneuver to identify patients with heritable forms of MTC. Now, these familial forms of MTC, or at least the risk of developing the manifestations, may be diagnosed with the aid of genetic testing for mutations in the RET proto-oncogene. The best use of such testing is to identify the specific mutation in affected family members, which then guides testing of the progeny. When other kindred members with the mutation are identified, thyroidectomy may be performed before malignancy develops. In the setting of MEN 2A, MTC typically does not develop before 12 years of age but is nearly always present by age 30. Accordingly, children with MEN 2A should undergo total thyroidectomy, usually with central neck lymphadenectomy, at approximately 6 years of age. The thyroid resection must be absolutely complete because the region of

TABLE 77.2

DISEASE PHENOTYPES RELATED TO MUTATION OF THE RET PROTO-ONCOGENE

Phenotype	Clinical features	Prevalence (%)
MEN 2A (60%)	Medullary thyroid carcinoma	100
	Pheochromocytoma	10–60
	Hyperparathyroidism	5–20
MEN 2B (5%)	Medullary thyroid carcinoma	100
	Pheochromocytoma	50
	Marfanoid habitus	100
	Mucosal neuromas (gut) and ganglioneuromatosis	100
FMTC (35%)	Medullary thyroid carcinoma	100

MEN 2A, multiple endocrine neoplasia type 2A; MEN 2B, multiple endocrine neoplasia type 2B; FMTC, familial medullary thyroid carcinoma.

thyroid that remains after a near total or subtotal thyroidectomy is the region that is most densely populated with C-cells. If hyperparathyroidism is present and enlarged parathyroid glands are encountered at operation, they should be removed as well. A subtotal parathyroidectomy or total parathyroidectomy and autotransplantation (similar to that which would be considered for MEN 1) are excessive options for the parathyroid disease encountered in MEN 2A and, instead, resection may be guided by morphologic changes in the parathyroid glands. Children identified to have MEN 2B should undergo thyroidectomy and central neck lymphadenectomy as soon as the diagnosis is made, preferably by 2 years of age.[46] If MTC is already evident at the time of diagnosis (as opposed to only C-cell hyperplasia), patients should undergo ipsilateral neck dissection as well. There is no consensus about at which age patients confirmed to have the FMTC mutation should undergo thyroidectomy, although this decision may be guided by the specifics of the family history.

Anaplastic Carcinoma. Although it formerly accounted for a larger fraction of thyroid malignancies, undifferentiated or anaplastic cancer now accounts for just 1% to 2% of thyroid cancers. Most commonly, this occurs in elderly patients who have a long-standing goiter. There is significant evidence to infer that most anaplastic thyroid cancers of the spindle cell or giant cell type arise from transformation of DTC, especially follicular and papillary carcinoma. Because of the improved outcome of lymphoma compared with anaplastic cancer(see later), it is critical to further investigate a tumor classified as a small cell anaplastic carcinoma. Appropriate studies must determine if the tumor is actually a lymphoma or a poorly differentiated MTC. Anaplastic thyroid carcinoma is one of the most aggressive and rapidly lethal malignancies known. Nearly all are too far advanced at the time of diagnosis to be adequately treated by currently available therapies. The diagnosis may be made by appropriate clinical suspicion (rapidly growing firm thyroid mass) and needle biopsy (FNA or core). If not, excisional biopsy at operation may be required. If airway compromise is present or impending, operation may include debulking and tracheostomy. Occasionally, a small anaplastic cancer is found that is confined to the thyroid or is minimally extensive to surrounding tissues (e.g., trachea). Especially in a young patient, aggressive resection may be legitimately considered. The long-term prognosis for these patients, however, is usually limited by metastatic disease, which may not be apparent at diagnosis. Adjuvant or primary palliative therapy consisting of chemotherapy and external beam radiotherapy is still frequently employed. It is common to see a measurable response early in therapy, but eventual tumor progression is typical. Unfortunately, the overall impact is often very limited, so no single regimen has become a standardized approach. Although doxorubican, taxol, and other drugs have been tried, doxorubicin and cisplatin are more frequently used. Radiation therapy is often given in combination by using a hyperfractionated routine such as two daily fractions, 5 days per week, until a total of 40 Gy is delivered to the cervical compartments and superior mediastinum.[47] Most often, chemotherapy and radiotherapy follow an operation performed for diagnosis or airway control, but such a regimen may also be used occasionally as neoadjuvant therapy before an attempt at resection is undertaken.

Thyroid Lymphoma. Primary thyroid lymphomas are rare tumors that account for less than 5% of thyroid malignancies. The majority are classified as non-Hodgkin's lymphomas of B-cell origin. Nearly all arise within from a background of Hashimoto's thyroiditis. Thyroid lymphoma usually affects patients between 50 and 80 years of age and is more common in women than men. Most patients present with a rapidly enlarging thyroid mass with compressive symptoms (e.g., dyspnea, dysphagia, choking, pain) and most have a history of hypothyroidism (from Hashimoto's thyroiditis). The cornerstone of treatment is chemotherapy (e.g., cyclophosphamide, doxorubicin, vincristine, prednisone), often combined with radiotherapy. The diagnosis, however, must be firmly established. Modern immunophenotypic analysis often allows this to occur with a small amount of tissue obtained by FNA or core needle sampling. Operation is still occasionally required, however, to obtain adequate tissue samples for diagnosis. Substantial surgical resection is often not required, but there is a subset of patients with significant compressive symptoms who benefit from palliative total or subtotal thyroidectomy.[48]

Metastases to Thyroid Gland. Isolated metastases from other primary cancers can occur in the thyroid gland, although they are rare. The most common tumor type to do so is renal cell carcinoma, although it can occur from lung and gastrointestinal carcinomas as well as melanoma and sarcoma.[49]

Staging of Thyroid Malignancy

A number of patient factors have been investigated to predict risk and prognosis for patients with DTC, such as age, gender, tumor size, involvement of lymph nodes, extrathyroidal invasion, tumor grade or histologic features, and completeness of surgical removal. Many of these factors are included in the staging systems outlined later. Although there are differences in these systems, in general, they agree that younger patients with smaller tumors have an excellent prognosis with decreased risk of recurrence and death compared with older patients.

One early prognostic staging scheme proposed by investigators from the Mayo Clinic was the AGES system (*age*, histologic grade, extrathyroidal disease [invasion and distant metastases], and tumor size).[50] Although useful, the scheme was later modified to exclude histologic tumor grade because there was not uniform agreement on DTC grading by pathologists.

Another system from the Lahey Clinic is the AMES system (*a*ge, *m*etastases, *e*xtrathyroidal invasion, and tumor *s*ize), which was originally described for patients with DTC.[51] The main criticism of this scheme is that it was defined based on a patient population, which included both papillary and follicular thyroid carcinomas, and that there was no accounting for those patients with low-risk versus-high risk FTC (see previously).

Another useful prognostic system is the MACIS scoring system (*m*etastases, *a*ge, *c*ompleteness of resection, extrathyroidal *i*nvasion and distant metastases, and tumor *s*ize). This system calculates a composite score based on these factors, then stratifies prognosis in proportion to these scores (<6.00 is very low risk and >8.00 represents greatly increased risk).[52]

The European Organization for Research on Treatment of Cancer (EORTC) based their prognostic scoring system on a multivariate analysis of patients with all types of thyroid malignancies and found that patients with scores of less than 50 had a 5-year survival rate of 95%, whereas those with scores greater than 109 had a 5-year survival rate of 5%.[53] This system has not been universally adopted for use in DTC because the high-risk, poor prognostic group contained a large fraction of patients with anaplastic thyroid cancer. Although medullary thyroid carcinoma is considered a differentiated cancer, its biologic behavior differs sufficiently from DTC of follicular cell origin that their inclusion in this staging system also confounds the prognostic ability somewhat.

The familiar TNM system (*t*umor size, *n*odal status, distant *m*etastases) is also used to provide prognostic information for patients. When used for thyroid cancer, the TNM system has been modified to account for the risk-reducing influence of low

TABLE 77.3 STAGING

TUMOR, NODE, METASTASIS STAGING SYSTEM FOR DIFFERENTIATED THYROID CARCINOMA (PAPILLARY AND FOLLICULAR TYPES)

Stage	Age <45 years	Age >45 years
I	T_{any} N_{any} M0	T1 N0 M0
II	T_{any} N_{any} M1	T2 N0 M0
		T3 N0 M0
III		T4 N0 M0
		T_{any} N1 M0
IV		T_{any} N_{any} M1

T1, ±1 cm; T2, >1 cm, ±4 cm; T3, >4 cm; T4, extrathyroidal extension; N0, no nodal involvement; N1, regional nodal metastases; M0, no distant metastases; M1, distant metastases.

patient age (Table 77.3). This system can provide consistency when comparing patients across different series. This system, like all prognostic scoring systems, still has limited utility in guiding initial treatment decisions (e.g., extent of resection) because the important components are not known preoperatively.

Selection of Surgical Procedure

Although thyroidectomy as a primary treatment for DTC is well accepted to be both effective and safe, some controversy persists about the extent of thyroidectomy necessary, especially when the controversial questions are applied to individual patients who are likely to have low-risk tumors and an excellent prognosis regardless of the specifics of surgical treatment. The advantages of total thyroidectomy for all DTC of follicular cell origin include: (a) radioiodine can be used to localize and treat small amounts of residual normal thyroid tissue, and especially regional or distant metastases; and (b) serum thyroglobulin may then be used as a sensitive marker of persistent or recurrent disease. If only lobectomy is performed, radioiodine treatment is usually not possible because of the avidity of normal thyroid tissue for RAI, and thyroglobulin measurements also lose their utility. Total thyroidectomy also addresses multifocal tumors (especially PTC) even if they are not obvious at the time of operation. After treatment with lobectomy, recurrence develops in the contralateral lobe in about 7% of patients, and half go on to die of thyroid cancer.[38] The risk of recurrence is decreased somewhat in patients treated with bilobar resections (e.g., total thyroidectomy) compared with patients undergoing only unilateral lobectomy. Overall, the application of total thyroidectomy in patients with DTC also decreases the likelihood of requiring reoperation in the central compartment of the neck in the future.

Radioiodine Therapy

Radioiodine may be used in two ways after thyroidectomy: low doses are used to demonstrate remaining thyroid tissue or metastatic disease as part of a radioiodine thyroid scan, whereas higher doses are used for ablation or therapy. The timing of the initial postoperative scan is dictated by the physiology of T_4 and the fact that remnant thyroid or DTC tissue must be stimulated by elevated levels of TSH to take up RAI. Although no precise threshold has been established, a general consensus is held that the TSH should be at least 30 mIU/mL. The TSH rise is generally achieved by thyroxine withdrawal, although recombinant human TSH is available (Thyrogen, currently approved for diagnostic scanning only). The half-life of thyroxine is approximately 7 days, so TSH values are significantly elevated 4 to 5 weeks after total thyroidectomy or withdrawal from thyroxine treatment. To minimize the duration of hypothyroid symptoms, patients can be managed on T_3 (triiodothyronine, Cytomel) for the first 4 postoperative weeks. Because of the much shorter half-life of T_3 (8 to 12 hours), it is held for only 2 weeks before scanning. One shortcoming of this strategy is that the rise of TSH can be slightly unpredictable and the specific RAI scanning schedule may need to be adjusted.

Radioiodine therapy is well suited to DTC because most tumor cells retain the ability to concentrate radioiodine. Additionally, many studies have shown a decreased rate of recurrence and increased disease-specific and overall survival when ^{131}I is used. Mazzaferri[54] reported in 1997 a threefold decrease in the incidence of distant metastatic disease and local tumor recurrence in tumors treated with radioiodine.[54] In another study, the risk of cancer death was decreased by half (from 16% to 8%) when radioiodine was used after surgery compared with hormone replacement or external radiation alone.[55] Many clinicians agree that radioiodine is beneficial and well tolerated, but certainly this is not a unanimous conclusion.

There are no prospective, randomized trials with subgroup analysis to shed light on the dilemma of which patients should receive postoperative radioiodine. The argument is further complicated by the fact that because of the multiple staging and prognostic systems are used, comparisons across studies can be difficult. Postoperative RAI is commonly used, even for lower-risk cancers, and thyroid remnant ablation is generally accepted as part of the postoperative treatment of patients who have undergone total or near-total thyroid excision for DTC. It is also widely recognized that this approach may not be the final answer, and it is not entirely evident that using postoperative radioiodine to "clear" a whole-body scan will impact the patient's recurrence or survival. Perhaps the most appropriate approach is to select patients for postoperative radioiodine therapy based on individual risk assessment.

Several situations exist wherein it is generally agreed that ^{131}I is not beneficial. If the cancer is nondifferentiated and does not concentrate radioiodine, ablative or therapeutic efforts will be futile. Lesions smaller than 1 cm without evidence of metastatic disease are not treated with radioiodine because of their exceptionally low potential for local or distant recurrence. Finally, if only a lobectomy is performed, the radioiodine ablation is possible only 25% of the time because of the volume of residual tissue and its avidity for RAI.

Proponents of ^{131}I therapy advocate that all patients who meet the indications for total thyroidectomy should undergo postoperative radioiodine therapy because it should not be assumed that residual thyroid tissue in the neck is tumor-free. Importantly, less than 30% of well-differentiated thyroid cancers will be multifocal, multicentric, or microscopic. In these settings, postoperative remnant thyroid ablation after total thyroidectomy serves to destroy remaining thyroid tissue that may harbor occult microscopic carcinoma. There are additional compelling reasons to provide postoperative radioiodine ablation. In short, it is easier to manage and follow the patient without remaining thyroid tissue. Without competing normal tissue, visualization of local or distant recurrences on follow-up ^{131}I scanning is possible. If large amounts of thyroid tissue remained after the initial operation, the bright emission of ^{131}I from the residual thyroid will obscure any small areas of local recurrence. Additionally, remaining thyroid tissue will cause TSH suppression, which can decrease the uptake of ^{131}I during postoperative imaging. Finally, thyroglobulin measurements are the most specific tests for recurrent cancer when no normal thyroid tissue or Tg antibodies (Tg-Ab) are present and when Tg level is measured during a period of hypothyroidism—none of which is feasible when a remnant remains. It follows, therefore, that only patients with a small cancer (<1 cm) carrying an exceptionally low risk of recurrence should be routinely excluded from consideration of treatment with postoperative radioiodine therapy.

External Beam Radiotherapy

If gross residual disease remains after surgical resection, external radiotherapy may be considered to assist in local tumor control. This is most often a consideration with tumors that invade the tracheoesophageal axis. This occurrence is frequent with poorly differentiated tumors, but it certainly can complicate DTC as well. It has also been considered for patients with extensive lymph node involvement that is characterized by extranodal invasion of metastatic tumor. Bone metastases are rarely treated completely with ^{131}I and, thus, external beam radiotherapy may be effective.[56] Complications include skin erythema and desquamation, and tracheoesophageal mucositis.

Thyroid-Stimulating Hormone Suppression

Levothyroxine therapy to suppress TSH levels is commonly recommended for patients with differentiated thyroid carcinoma because TSH is considered a trophic factor for these cancers. The efficacy is inferred from uncontrolled retrospective studies. It is important to individualize the degree of suppression in patients, balancing the risk of recurrence with the risks of subclinical hyperthyroidism (e.g., osteoporosis, cardiac arrhythmias). Many physicians will suppress TSH to undetectable levels ($<$0.01 mIU/L) in high-risk cancers and less severely (TSH 0.05 to 0.1 mIU/L) in low-risk cancers. If a patient has no evidence of recurrence and has extremely low or undetectable thyroglobulin levels 5 to 10 years after treatment, it may be appropriate to lessen the degree of TSH suppression.

New Horizons and Future Directions

Adjunctive treatment of DTC is dependent on the uptake and concentration of radioiodine by cancerous thyroid tissue. Problematically, it has been reported that as many as 30% of advanced DTC will eventually de-differentiate, and a portion of these cancers will lose the ability to concentrate radioiodine. This may result from decreased expression of the human sodium iodide symporter (hNIS). Both *in vivo* and *in vitro* research has shown that follicular cancer cell lines have greater iodine uptake when stably transfected with hNIS.[57,58] Application of these gene therapy techniques to human subjects is not a current reality, but remains an exciting area of research. Certain therapies have been used in humans in effort to "re-differentiate" thyroid cancer cells such that they would regain the ability to concentrate radioiodine. In early pilot studies, retinoic acid has been shown to increase radioiodine uptake and decrease thyroglobulin levels in advanced thyroid carcinomas, and further studies hold promise for the treatment of de-differentiated tumors.[59]

There are no significantly effective medical therapies to offer patients with radioiodine-resistant thyroid cancers. In addition to the dedifferentiation therapies mentioned earlier, the past two decades of research into the molecular biology and genetics of thyroid cancer have identified potential targets for alternate therapies. Clinical trials have been established for a variety of drugs with wide-ranging targets and molecular mechanisms of actions, including drugs that target intracellular signaling molecules (ras and raf inhibition), receptor tyrosine kinases (anti-VEGF, anti-EGFR, anti Her2/neu, and VEGF/EGF receptor inhibitors), angiogenesis (thalidomide, combretastatins), apoptotic pathways (TNF-related apoptosis-inducing ligand [TRAIL]), and the effect of rapamycin on the mTOR gene (mammalian target of rapamycin). To ensure future progress in the treatment of patients with thyroid malignancies, all patients with radioiodine-resistant tumors should be considered as candidates for clinical trials.

THYROID SURGERY

The first recorded goiter excision was by Abdul Kasan Kelebis Abis in Baghdad in AD 500. The patient survived despite massive hemorrhage. Wilhelm Fabricus performed the first thyroidectomy using scalpels in 1646. The patient did not survive and the surgeon was subsequently imprisoned. By the mid-nineteenth century, the mortality associated with thyroid surgery was still as high as 40%. Substantial improvements began with the discovery of anesthesia, antisepsis, and improved hemostasis. It was with this background that Albert Theodor Billroth, Theodor Kocher, and William Halsted were able to make substantial technical contributions in making thyroidectomy safe and efficacious.

Technique

There is little if any place for odd thyroid resections (e.g., nodulectomy) and only an occasional role for isthmusectomy. Total thyroid lobectomy is the total extracapsular removal of the lobe and the isthmus while preserving both parathyroid glands, the recurrent laryngeal nerve, and the external branch of the superior laryngeal nerve. Total thyroidectomy is a matter of performing a total thyroid lobectomy on the contralateral side during the same operation. Near-total thyroidectomy and subtotal thyroidectomy will not be discussed here. For most thyroid procedures, the patient is placed in supine position or semi-Fowler position with the arms tucked to the side. A support is placed transversely under the shoulders to aid in extending the neck. This extension must not be too extreme or a significant amount of postoperative pain may occur in the occipitocervical region. After skin preparation, a curvilinear incision is made approximately one to two fingerbreadths above the clavicular heads and not any higher than the level of the cricoid cartilage (Fig. 77.7). If possible, it should be disguised in an existing skin crease. Subplatysmal skin flaps are

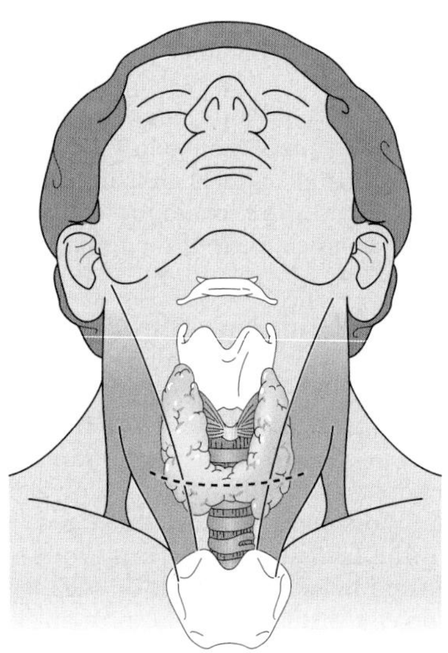

FIGURE 77.7 With the patient's neck extended, the line above indicates the appropriate site of incision for thyroid resection. Camouflage within an existing skin crease is often possible.

raised with an electrocautery to the level of the thyroid cartilage above and the sternal notch below. These are carried onto the sternocleidomastoid muscles laterally, taking care to avoid the anterior jugular veins. The plane of the midline raphe is developed to expose the anterior trachea and the isthmus. The sternohyoid is reflected off the sternothyroid and then the sternothyroid is bluntly dissected from the thyroid lobe. It is this maneuver that leads to division of the thyroid sheath layer as the paraesophageal space is entered. The middle thyroid veins are divided and ligated. Instead of lateral retraction of the strap muscles, it is occasionally useful to divide the strap muscles transversely, instead of in the midline raphe, in the case of exceptionally large goiters. This greatly improves exposure of the superior pole vessels and allows easier blunt mobilization of the enlarged lobes.

If a pyramidal lobe is present, it is mobilized and divided from the fibrous tissue in any remaining thyroglossal duct tract. The anterior suspensory ligament is divided to mobilize the superior aspect of the isthmus.

These procedures should be performed in a logical orderly sequence as follows: (a) exposure of the thyroid gland, (b) dissection of the superior pole of the thyroid with preservation of the external branch of the superior laryngeal nerve, (c) dissection of the inferior pole of the thyroid lobe with preservation of the inferior parathyroid gland, (d) dissection of the posterolateral aspect of the thyroid gland with preservation of the superior parathyroid gland and the recurrent laryngeal nerve, and (e) closure. Figure 77.8 indicates the plane of dissection relevant to tasks c and d.

Dissection of the superior pole of the thyroid must take place in the plane directly adjacent to the thyroid capsule after the largely avascular space between the pole and the cricothyroideus muscle is seen. To do so more proximally along the superior pole vessels imperils the EBSLN. This nerve is not always seen during thyroidectomy, but it can nearly always be preserved by utilizing the technique. Unequivocal identification of the recurrent laryngeal nerve is mandatory. This is done by many surgeons as direct dissection and exposure in the proximal portion of the RLN before its intersection with the ITA and the ligament of Berry. The safety provided by this maneuver, however, is contingent on continuing the exposure more distally along the nerve as it approaches the cricothyroid interval, because it is at this point of genu that the nerve is most vulnerable to iatrogenic injury. Another technique of nerve exposure is provided by the close capsular dissection that takes place when the lobe is retracted anteromedially and as the terminal branches of the ITA are divided. As the ligament of Berry is divided, the genu of the nerve is identified and protected. Although visual identification of the RLN remains the gold standard, palpation can aid in the process. The nerve is often easy to palpate because it is a slightly firm linear structure (similar to the feel of the vas deferens encountered during pediatric hernia repair) as the lobe is retracted anteromedially. Although helpful, this technique should not supplant visual confirmation.

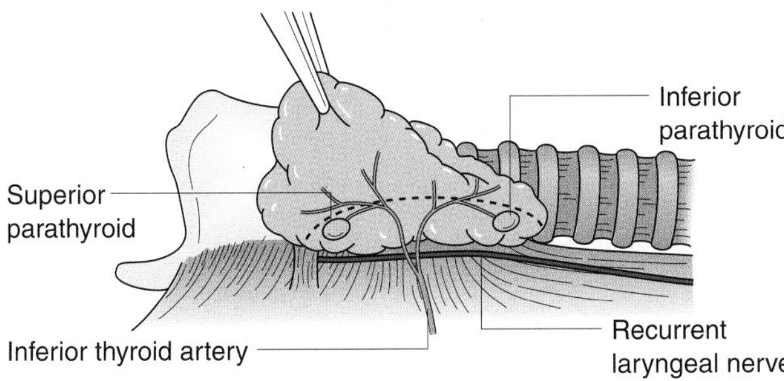

FIGURE 77.8 The capsular dissection necessary to preserve well-vascularized parathyroid tissue and a fully functional recurrent laryngeal nerve begins in the area outlined above.

The ability to routinely preserve well-vascularized parathyroid tissue during thyroidectomy is mandatory for surgeons performing these operations. Normal parathyroid tissue is subtle and may be difficult to identify. It can be distinguished from surrounding fat by slight color differences and a fine capillary vascular pattern that is not present in the adjacent fat or thymus.

Complications

The risk of death or major disability during thyroidectomy should be diminutive. The key outcomes by which to measure the quality of surgical care, especially relevant to total thyroidectomy, include recurrent laryngeal nerve paralysis and hypoparathyroidism. Although both complications can occur in a self-limited fashion, the persistence or permanence (defined at 6 months after operation) of these complications is a critical measure. The rate of unintended permanent recurrent laryngeal nerve dysfunction should be no greater than 1% and the rate of permanent hypoparathyroidism should be no greater than 1% to 2%.

Injury to a RLN results in paralysis of the vocal cord it innervates. Depending on the specific branch or combination of branches injured, the cord may remain in a paramedian position (also called cadaveric position) or may remain abducted. If the contralateral cord is able to adduct to the midline or beyond, the patient may have a voice that is not particularly hoarse, but is weak. If the cord is paralyzed in the abducted position, vocal quality is very poor because of the difficulty in approximating the cords during speaking. The patient's cough also has a bovine quality where there is a lack of a sharp, percussive initiation. If both vocal cords are paralyzed, the consideration of the specific cord positions is even more critical. If both cords are paralyzed in the abducted position, the patient may have essentially no ability to speak. In this situation, the patient may gradually develop some degree of airway obstruction as the cords gradually migrate toward the midline. If both cords are paralyzed in the paramedian position, the airway is critically narrowed. In this situation, stridor is usually apparent very soon after extubation and an emergent procedure (e.g., cricothyroidotomy or tracheostomy) may be required to establish the airway.

Functional monitoring of EBSLN integrity is feasible, but somewhat cumbersome and is not routinely employed. Recurrent laryngeal nerve monitoring has been much more evident in recent thyroid surgery practice. Although the technology has improved to a point that the technique is relatively easy to employ, large studies have failed to detect a major improvement in RLN injury rates (largely related to the low incidence of this complication in the proper hands despite specific technique employed).[60] Even so, RLN monitoring can be very helpful in facilitating nerve identification and protection during complex reoperations, or initial thyroidectomy for very large goiter or malignancy, even if it will not materially change the chance of injury.[61]

Injury to the EBSLN is both more common and more difficult to detect than injury to the RLN. Because of anatomic variations, the EBSLN is at risk for injury during thyroidectomy in 15% to 68% of cases.[62] The symptoms of injury may be only slightly evident to the patient or can be devastating in the case of the vocal professional. Symptoms typically include early vocal fatigue, decreased pitch range, and decreased projection ability. Findings on laryngoscopy are subtle and include bowing and inferior displacement of the affected vocal cord and rotation of the posterior glottis toward the injured side. Laryngeal videostroboscopy or percutaneous electromyography of the cricothyroideus muscle may be required to detect injury in subtle cases. Because there is no effective treatment for this condition, prevention is extremely important, usually by careful surgical technique to ligate the individual branches of the superior thyroid artery at the level of the thyroid capsule.

The parathyroid glands are at risk during thyroid resection by virtue of the fact that they are often firmly invested within the thyroid sheath or occasionally even within the thyroid capsule. Parathyroid glands are served by end arteries, most often only a single branch. Inferior parathyroid glands are served ultimately by the inferior thyroid artery. Superior parathyroid glands are often served by the inferior thyroid artery but may also have contributions from the superior thyroid artery distribution as well. Ligation of the trunk of the ITA must be avoided to preserve blood supply to the parathyroid glands. Every attempt should be made to mobilize the parathyroid glands away from the thyroid tissue being resected while preserving the blood supply. If at the end of mobilization, a parathyroid gland appears blue and congested, it may be to the result of constriction of the venous outflow. The capsule of the gland may be incised carefully and if mild arterial bleeding is seen and the congestion appears to resolve, the parathyroid gland can be left *in situ*. If the gland appears pale and devascularized, the arterial supply is probably compromised. Such a parathyroid gland is unlikely to survive after the operation and should be immediately autotransplanted. This may be done by mincing the gland and inserting or injecting the pieces into well-vascularized skeletal muscle (e.g., sternocleidomastoid or pectoralis).[63] Even during thyroid lobectomy, meticulous technique must be used to preserve parathyroid viability, even though permanent, or even temporary, hypoparathyroidism is unlikely. With total thyroidectomy, this is even more critical. Temporary hypoparathyroidism is relatively common from relative mild devascularization of parathyroid glands during mobilization. Approximately 20% to 40% of patients will have mild temporary hypocalcemia beginning about 12 to 36 hours after operation. This may not even be symptomatic and is usually easy to control with oral calcium or occasionally vitamin D supplements (calcitriol, Rocaltrol). Severe symptomatic hypocalcemia can be treated with intravenous calcium gluconate (calcium chloride is not safely administered through a peripheral intravenous site outside of emergency settings). Temporary hypoparathyroidism complicating thyroidectomy usually resolves over days to weeks, although occasionally it may take months to do so. Hypoparathyroidism that persists longer than 6 months is usually, but not always, destined to be permanent. The rate of permanent hypoparathyroidism after total thyroidectomy must be low (approximately 1% to 2%).

The central compartment of the neck contains level VI lymph nodes and is bordered by the hyoid bone above, the innominate vein below, and the carotid sheaths laterally. Removal of the central compartment lymph nodes is a critical component of an operation to treat medullary thyroid carcinoma. It is a reasonable consideration in the treatment of HCC and PTC because lymph node involvement is both common and difficult to treat with a remedial operation in the future. If central neck dissection is to be added to the routine performance of total thyroidectomy to treat low-risk PTC, however, it must be assured that the incidence of hypoparathyroidism is not increased, because it can be technically difficult to maintain parathyroid vascularization with a thorough level VI lymphadenectomy.

These complications can largely be avoided or ameliorated by delicate and deliberate surgical technique. A thorough understanding of the function and anatomy, both normal and abnormal, of the thyroid and of the rationale behind various treatment options are also critical to ensure the best outcomes for our patients.

KEY POINTS

- **The thyroid is mostly from endodermal origin and originates from the ventral embryologic digestive tract.**
- **The upper portion of the isthmus typically crosses the trachea at or below the level of the cricoid cartilage and overlies the second and third tracheal rings.**
- **The thyroid gland produces thyroxine (T_4), triiodothyronine (T_3), and calcitonin under complicated regulatory mechanisms.**
- **Ultrasonography is a very valuable enhancement to the workup of the thyroid nodule or multinodular goiter.**
- **Hyperthyroidism can be caused by diverse pathophysiology such as Graves' disease, toxic multinodular goiter, and solitary toxic adenoma, and can be treated by medications, radioiodine or operation.**
- **Differentiated thyroid cancers (DTC) are of follicular cell origin (papillary thyroid carcinoma and its variants, follicular thyroid carcinoma, and Hürthle cell carcinoma) or parafollicular (C-cell) origin (medullary thyroid carcinoma).**
- **The advantages of total thyroidectomy for all DTC of follicular cell origin include the fact that radioiodine can be used to localize and treat small amounts of residual normal thyroid tissue, and especially regional or distant metastases, and that serum thyroglobulin can then be used as a sensitive marker of persistent or recurrent disease.**
- **Anaplastic thyroid carcinoma is one of the most aggressive and rapidly lethal malignancies known.**

References

1. Moore KL. *The developing human: clinically oriented embryology*, 4th ed. Philadelphia: WB Saunders, 1993.
2. Brookes M, Zietman Z. *Clinical embryology. A color atlas and text.* Boca Raton, FL: CRC Press, 1998.
3. Larsen WJ. *Human embryology*. New York: Churchill Livingstone, 1997.
4. Merida-Velasco JA, Garcia-Garcia JD, Espin-Ferra J, et al. Origin of the ultimobranchial body and its colonizing cells in human embryos. *Acta Anat.* 1989;136:325–330.
5. Weller GL. *Development of the thyroid, parathyroid, and thymus glands in man.* Washington DC: Carnegie Institute of Washington, 1933.
6. Sackett WR, Reeve TS, Barraclough B, et al. Thyrothymic thyroid rests: incidence and relationship to the thyroid gland. *J Am Coll Surg.* 2002; 195:635–640.
7. Gauger PG, Delbridge LW, Thompson NW, et al. Incidence and importance of the tubercle of Zuckerkandl in thyroid surgery. *Eur J Surg.* 2001;167:249–254.
8. Tarjan G, Nayar R. Black thyroid syndrome. *Thyroid* 2002;12:343–344.
9. **Bliss RD, Gauger PG, Delbridge LW. Surgeon's approach to the thyroid gland: surgical anatomy and the importance of technique. *World J Surg.* 2000;2:891–897.**
10. Pelizzo MR, Toniato A, Gemo G. Zuckerkandl's tuberculum: an arrow pointing to the recurrent laryngeal nerve (constant anatomical landmark). *J Am Coll Surg.* 1998;187:333–336.
11. Katz AD. Extralaryngeal division of the recurrent laryngeal nerve. *Am J Surg.* 1986;152:407–410.
12. Henry JF, Audiffret J, Denizot A, et al. The nonrecurrent inferior laryngeal nerve: review of 33 cases, including two on the left side. *Surgery* 1988;104:977–984.
13. Raffaelli M, Iacobone M, Henry JF. The "false" nonrecurrent inferior laryngeal nerve. *Surgery* 2000;128:1082–1087.
14. **Machens A, Holzhausen HJ, Dralle H. Skip metastases in thyroid cancer leaping the central lymph node compartment. *Arch Surg.* 2004;139:43–45.**
15. Gilmour JR. The gross anatomy of the parathyroid glands. *J Pathol.* 1938;46:133.
16. Cooper DS, Goldminz D, Levin AA, et al. Agranulocytosis associated with antithyroid drugs. Effects of patient age and drug dose. *Ann Intern Med.* 1983;98:26–29.
17. Scanga DR, Martin WH, Delbeke D. Value of FDG PET imaging in the management of patients with thyroid, neuroendocrine, and neural crest tumors. *Clin Nucl Med.* 2004;29:86–90.

18. Davis PW, Perrier ND, Adler L, et al. Incidental thyroid carcinoma identified by positron emission tomography scanning obtained for metastatic evaluation. *Am Surg.* 2001;67:582–584.
19. Kang KW, Kim SK, Kang HS, et al. Prevalence and risk of cancer of focal thyroid incidentaloma identified by 18F-fluorodeoxyglucose positron emission tomography for metastasis evaluation and cancer screening in healthy subjects. *J Clin Endocrinol Metab.* 2003;88:4100–4104.
20. Boi F, Lai ML, Deias C, et al. The usefulness of 99mTc-SestaMIBI scan in the diagnostic evaluation of thyroid nodules with oncocytic cytology. *Eur J Endocrinol.* 2003;149:493–498.
21. Tan GH, Gharib H. Thyroid incidentalomas: management approaches to nonpalpable nodules discovered incidentally on thyroid imaging. *Ann Intern Med.* 1997;126:226–231.
22. **Rausch P, Nowels K, Jeffrey RB Jr. Ultrasonographically guided thyroid biopsy: a review with emphasis on technique. *J Ultrasound Med.* 2001;20:1261–1262.**
23. Lennquist S, Jortso E, Anderberg B, et al. Beta blockers compared with antithyroid drugs as preoperative treatment in hyperthyroidism: drug tolerance, complications, and postoperative thyroid function. *Surgery* 1985;98:1141–1146.
24. Alderberth A, Stenstrom G, Hasselgren P. The selective beta 1 blocking agent metoprolol compared with antithyroid drug and thyroxine as preoperative treatment of patients with hyperthyroidism. Results from a prospective randomized study. *Ann Surg.* 1987;205:182–188.
25. Eriksson M, Rubenfeld S, Garber A, et al. Propranolol does not prevent thyroid storm. *N Engl J Med.* 1977;296:263–264.
26. Tallstedt L, Lundell G, Blomgren H, et al. Does early administration of thyroxine reduce the development of Graves' ophthalmopathy after radioiodine treatment? *Eur J Endocrinol.* 1994;130:494–497.
27. Tallstedt L, Lundell G, Torring O, et al. Occurrence of ophthalmopathy after treatment for Graves' hyperthyroidism. The Thyroid Study Group. *N Engl J Med.* 1992;326:1733–1738.
28. Bartalena L, Marcocci C, Bogazzi F, et al. Use of corticosteroids to prevent progression of Graves' ophthalmopathy after radioiodine therapy for hyperthyroidism. *N Engl J Med.* 1989;321:1349–1352.
29. van Soestbergen M, van der Vijver J, Graafland A. Recurrence of hyperthyroidism in multinodular goiter after long-term drug therapy: a comparison with Graves' disease. *J Endocrinol Invest.* 1992;15:797–800.
30. Tunbridge WM, Brewis M, French JM, et al. Natural history of autoimmune thyroiditis. *Br Med J Clin Res.* 1981;282:258–262.
31. Smallridge RC, DeKeyser FM, VanHerle AJ, et al. Thyroid iodine content and serum thyroglobulin: cues to the natural history of destruction-induced thyroiditis. *J Clin Endocrinol Metab.* 1986;62:1213–1219.
32. Bartalena L, Grasso L, Brogioni S, et al. Serum interleukin-6 in amiodarone-induced thyrotoxicosis. *J Clin Endocrinol Metab.* 1994;78:423–427.
33. Harjai KJ, Licata AA. Effects of amiodarone on thyroid function. *Ann Intern Med.* 1997;126:63–73.
34. Violaris NS, Windle-Taylor PC. Idiopathic fibrosis of the upper aerodigestive tract. *J Laryngol Otol.* 1989;103:333–334.
35. Few J, Thompson NW, Angelos P, et al. Riedel's thyroiditis: treatment with tamoxifen. *Surgery* 1996;120:998–999.
36. Harness JK, Thompson NW, Nishiyama RH. Childhood thyroid carcinoma. *Arch Surg.* 1971;102:278–284.
37. DeGroot LJ, Kaplan EL, McCormick M, et al. Natural history, treatment, and course of papillary thyroid carcinoma. *J Clin Endocrinol Metab.* 1990;71:414–424.
38. **Kebebew E, Clark OH. Differentiated thyroid cancer: "complete" rational approach. *World J Surg.* 2000;24:942–951.**
39. Jossart GH, Clark OH. Well-differentiated thyroid cancer. *Curr Probl Surg.* 1994;31:933–1012.
40. Ito Y, Tomoda C, Uruno T, et al. Papillary microcarcinoma of the thyroid: how should it be treated? *World J Surg.* 2004;28:1115–1121.
41. Chen H, Nicol TL, Udelsman R. Follicular lesions of the thyroid. Does frozen section evaluation alter operative management? *Ann Surg.* 1995; 222:101–106.
42. Emerick GT, Duh QY, Siperstein AE, et al. Diagnosis, treatment, and outcome of follicular thyroid carcinoma. *Cancer* 1993;72:3287–3295.
43. van Heerden JA, Hay ID, Goellner JR, et al. Follicular thyroid carcinoma with capsular invasion alone: a non-threatening malignancy. *Surgery* 1992;112:1130–1138.
44. Thompson NW, Nishiyama RH, Harness JK. Thyroid carcinoma: current controversies. *Curr Probl Surg.* 1978;15:1–67.
45. **Tisell LE, Hansson G, Jansson S, et al. Reoperation in the treatment of asymptomatic metastasizing medullary carcinoma of the thyroid. *Surgery* 1986;99:60–66.**
46. Skinner MA, DeBenedetti MK, Moley JR, et al. Medullary thyroid carcinoma in children with multiple endocrine neoplasia types 2A and 2B. *J Pediatr Surg.* 1996;31:177–181.
47. Crevoisier RD, Baudin E, Bachelot A, et al. Combined treatment of anaplastic thyroid carcinoma with surgery, chemotherapy, and hyperfractionated accelerated external radiotherapy. *Int J Radiat Oncol Biol Phys.* 2004;60:1137–1143.
48. Sippel RS, Gauger PG, Angelos P, et al. Palliative thyroidectomy for malignant lymphoma of the thyroid. *Ann Surg Oncol.* 2002;9:907–911.
49. Mirallie E, Rigaud J, Mathonnet M, et al. Management and prognosis of metastases to the thyroid gland. *J Am Coll Surg.* 2005;200:203–207.
50. Hay ID, Grant CS, Taylor WF, et al. Ipsilateral lobectomy versus bilateral lobar resection in papillary thyroid carcinoma: a retrospective analysis of surgical outcome using a novel prognostic scoring system. *Surgery* 1987; 102:1088–1095.
51. Cady B, Rossi R. An expanded view of risk-group definition in differentiated thyroid carcinoma. *Surgery* 1988;104:947–953.
52. **Hay ID, Bergstralh EJ, Goellner JR, et al. Predicting outcome in papillary thyroid carcinoma: development of a reliable prognostic scoring system in a cohort of 1779 patients surgically treated at one institution during 1940 through 1989. *Surgery* 1993;114:1050–1057.**
53. Byar DP, Green SB, Dor P, et al. A prognostic index for thyroid carcinoma: a study of the E.O.R.T.C. thyroid cancer cooperative group. *Eur J Cancer* 1979;15:1033–1041.
54. Mazzaferri EL. Thyroid remnant ^{131}I ablation for papillary and follicular thyroid carcinoma. *Thyroid* 1997;7:265–271.
55. **Mazzaferri EL, Jhiang SM. Long-term impact of initial surgical and medical therapy on papillary and follicular thyroid cancer. *Am J Med.* 1994;97: 418–428.**
56. Brierley JD, Tsang RW. External-beam radiation therapy in the treatment of differentiated thyroid cancer. *Semin Surg Oncol.* 1999;16:42–49.
57. Smit JW, Shroder-van der Elst JP, Karperien M, et al. Reestablishment of in vitro and in vivo iodide uptake by transfection of the human sodium iodide symporter (hNIS) in a hNIS defective human thyroid carcinoma cell line. *Thyroid* 2000;10:939–943.
58. Spitzweg C, Morris JC. Gene therapy for thyroid cancer: current status and future prospects. *Thyroid* 2004;14:424–434.
59. Haugen BR. Redifferentiation therapy in advanced thyroid cancer. Current drug targets. *Immune, Endocrine, & Metabolic Disorders* 2004;4:175–180.
60. **Dralle H, Sekulla C, Haerting J, et al. Risk factors of paralysis and functional outcome after recurrent laryngeal nerve monitoring in thyroid surgery. *Surgery* 2004;136:1310–1322.**
61. **Yarbrough DE, Thompson GB, Kasperbauer JL, et al. Intraoperative electromyographic monitoring of the recurrent laryngeal nerve in reoperative thyroid and parathyroid surgery. *Surgery* 2004;136:1107–1115.**
62. Teitelbaum BJ, Wenig BL. Superior laryngeal nerve injury from thyroid surgery. *Head Neck* 1995;17:36–40.
63. Gauger PG, Reeve TS, Wilkinson M, et al. Routine parathyroid autotransplantation during total thyroidectomy: the influence of technique. *Eur J Surg* 2000;166:605–609.

CHAPTER 78 ■ PARATHYROID GLANDS

GERARD M. DOHERTY

ANATOMY

Typically, a person has four parathyroid glands—two superior and two inferior (Fig. 78.1).[1] The normal parathyroid glands are flat, ovoid, and red-brown to yellow. They are 5 to 7 mm × 3 to 4 mm × 0.5 to 2 mm and weigh between 30 and 50 mg each. The lower glands are usually larger than the upper glands. The superior glands are most often embedded in the fat on the posterior surface of the upper thyroid lobe near the site where the recurrent laryngeal nerve enters the larynx. The inferior glands are usually more ventral and lie close to or within the portion of the thymus gland that extends from the inferior pole of the thyroid gland into the chest. Although this anatomy is fairly consistent, substantial variations from the norm can occur, and it is essential that the surgeon have a thorough understanding of these anatomic variations.

Variations in parathyroid anatomy are primarily caused by differences in patterns of embryogenesis. During the fourth and fifth weeks of fetal development, a series of four pharyngeal pouches develop (Fig. 78.2). The superior parathyroid arises from the fourth pharyngeal pouch in conjunction with the lateral thyroid, and the inferior gland arises from the third pouch along with the thymus. The derivatives of each pouch then migrate together so that the superior parathyroid usually remains in close association with the upper pole of the thyroid, although it may occasionally be loosely attached by a long vascular pedicle, migrating caudad along the esophagus into the posterior mediastinum. Occasionally, a gland may be totally embedded in the thyroid parenchyma. The inferior parathyroid descends with the thymus, but this migration is extremely variable. Inferior glands can be found anywhere from the pharynx to the mediastinum. Regardless of their location, they usually adhere to the thymus or are within the thyrothymic ligament. Supernumerary glands can be identified in up to 15% of patients, most often in association with the thymus. Autopsy studies suggest that four parathyroid glands are virtually always present.

The arterial supply to both the superior and inferior parathyroid glands is usually from the inferior thyroid artery, although it may arise from the superior thyroid or thyroidea ima arteries or from the rich anastomosis of vessels supplying the larynx, trachea, and esophagus. It has been suggested that a mediastinal parathyroid gland that descended during embryonic development usually receives its blood supply from either the internal mammary artery or small arteries within the thymus. In adults, however, an enlarged parathyroid gland that migrates into the mediastinum usually carries with it the corresponding branch of the inferior thyroid artery. The inferior, middle, and superior thyroid veins, which drain the parathyroid glands, empty into the internal jugular vein or the innominate vein.

Histologically, the normal adult parathyroid is about half parenchyma and half stroma, including fat cells (Fig. 78.3). In children, the gland is almost entirely composed of parenchymal chief cells. Beginning at puberty, adipocytes appear and, with age, occupy an increasing proportion of the gland. Also with increasing age, acidophilic, mitochondria-rich oxyphil cells are present in increasing numbers and are intermixed with the glycogen-laden, polygonal, water-clear cells. The functional significance of the various cell types remains unclear, although the water-clear cells and oxyphil cells are probably derived from the chief cells and secrete parathyroid hormone (PTH).

PHYSIOLOGY

The primary physiologic role of the parathyroid gland is the endocrine regulation of calcium and phosphate metabolism. Average daily exchanges of these ions from the gastrointestinal tract, bone, and kidney are shown in Fig. 78.4.

Calcium

Calcium ion plays a critical role in all biologic systems. It participates in enzymatic reactions and is a mediator in hormone metabolism. Calcium is intimately involved in the physiology of neurotransmission, muscle contraction, and blood coagulation. It is the major cation in bone and teeth. It represents about 2% of the average body weight, and almost all calcium is contained in the skeleton. The normal range of serum calcium is 9 to 10.5 mg/dL (4.5 to 5.2 mEq/L), and the daily variation in a normal person is generally less than 10%. About half of the total serum calcium is in an ionized, biologically active form; 40% is bound to serum protein, mainly albumin, and 10% forms compounds with organic ions, such as citrate. The total serum calcium concentration is a function of the serum protein content, and because hydrogen ion competes with calcium for the same binding sites on albumin, the body fluid pH is important. In general, for every change of 1 g/dL in the serum albumin level, a direct alteration of 0.8 mg/dL occurs in the serum calcium concentration. Almost all the physiologically important activity of calcium is represented by the unbound, or free, fraction.

Calcium is absorbed in its inorganic form from the duodenum and proximal jejunum. The rate of absorption is precisely regulated according to body calcium status. The calcium in the extracellular fluid is constantly being exchanged with that in the intracellular fluid, the exchangeable bone, and the glomerular filtrate. Calcium reabsorption by the kidney is closely related to that of sodium, and about 99% of the filtered load is reabsorbed under normal conditions.

Phosphate

Phosphate anion is also an integral component of most biologic systems. It is critical to the pathways of glycolysis and is the functional group for a number of high-energy transfer compounds, including adenosine triphosphate. It is also the major anion in crystalline bone. Normal levels of plasma phosphate range from 2.5 to 4.3 mg/dL, and the level varies inversely with the serum level of calcium. The relation is such that the product of plasma calcium and phosphate is constant

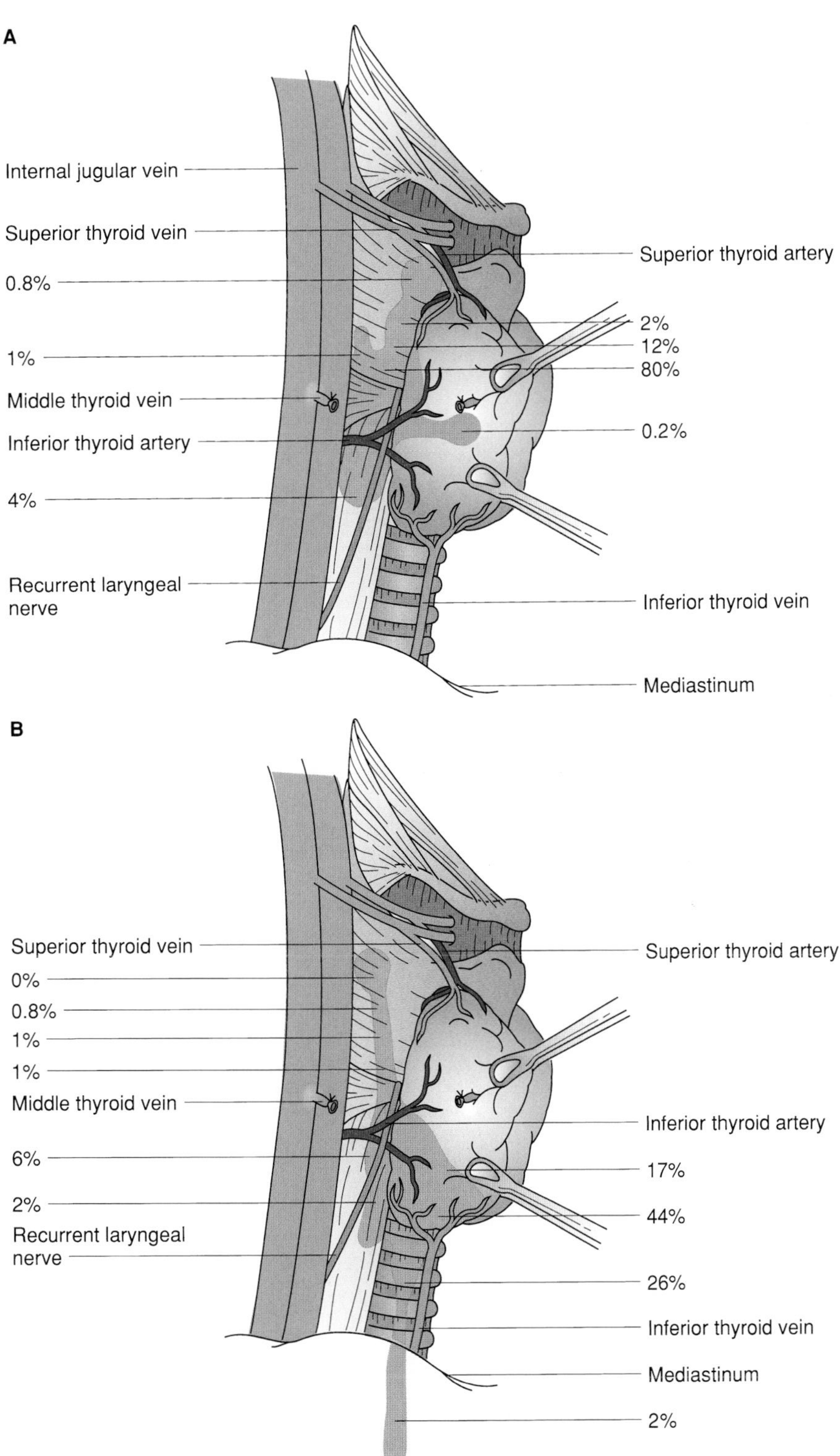

FIGURE 78.1 Schematic illustration of the location of the superior (*A*) and inferior (*B*) parathyroid glands from 503 autopsy studies. The more common locations are indicated by the shaded areas. The numbers represent the percentage of glands found at each location. Typically, the glands were posterolateral to the thyroid and above or below the junction of the inferior thyroid artery with the recurrent laryngeal nerve. (After Akerstrom G, Malmaers J, Bergstrom R. Surgical anatomy of human parathyroid glands. *Surgery* 1984;95:14.)

and ranges between 30 and 40 mg/dL. When it increases above this level, a potential develops for the precipitation of calcium phosphate in body tissues.

In contrast to the percentage of calcium absorbed, the percentage of phosphate absorbed from the diet is relatively constant, and excretion usually provides the major mechanisms for regulating phosphate balance (Fig. 78.4). Unlike stores of calcium, the readily exchangeable soft-tissue stores of phosphate, such as those in muscle, are large.

Regulation of Calcium and Phosphate Metabolism

The maintenance of calcium and phosphate homeostasis depends on major contributions from three organ systems—the gastrointestinal tract, the skeleton, and the kidneys—with minor contributions from the skin and liver.[2] The primary hormonal regulators of this metabolism are PTH, vitamin D,

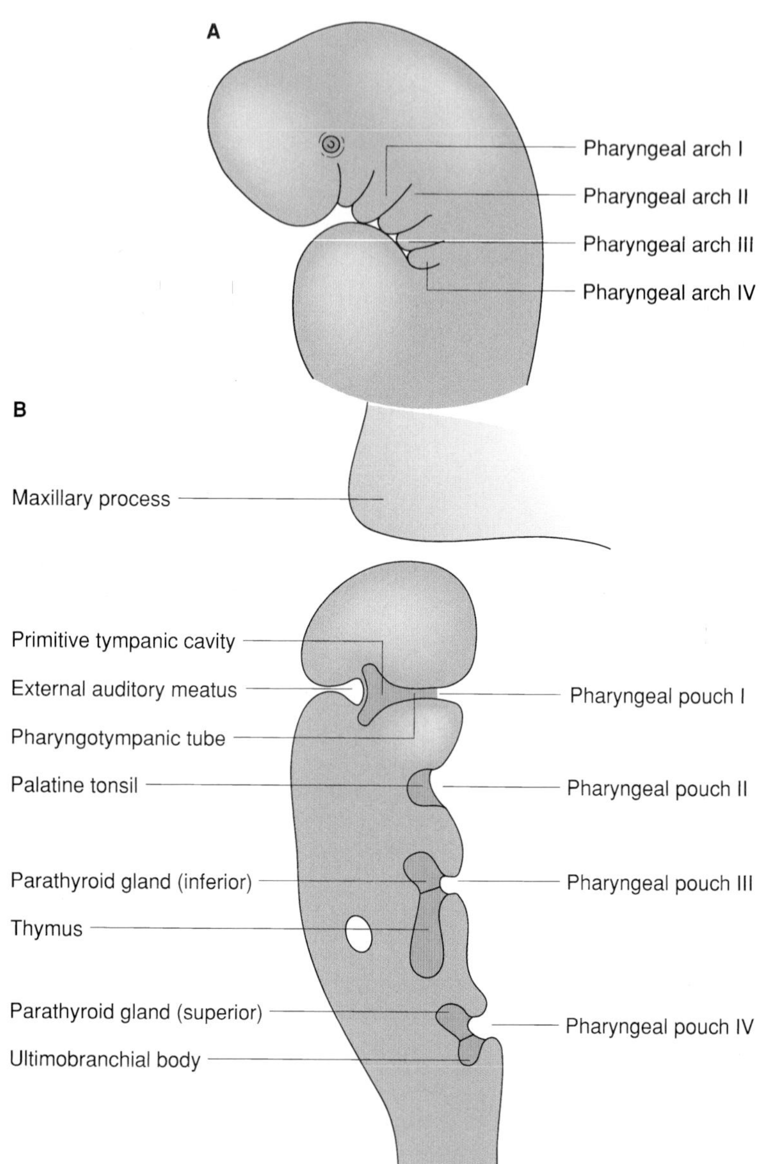

FIGURE 78.2 (*A*) pharyngeal arches in a 5-week embryo. The corresponding pouches extend from within the pharynx into each arch. (*B*) Schematic representation of the differentiating epithelium of the respective pharyngeal pouches. (After Langman J. *Medical embryology and human development: normal and abnormal.* Baltimore: Williams & Wilkins, 1975, p. 262.)

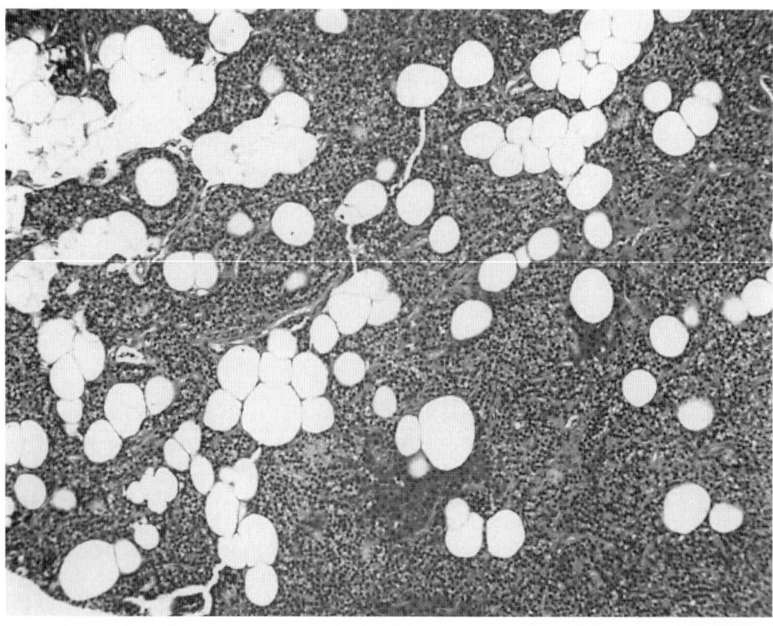

FIGURE 78.3 A normal adult parathyroid is composed of about half parenchyma and half fat (×150).

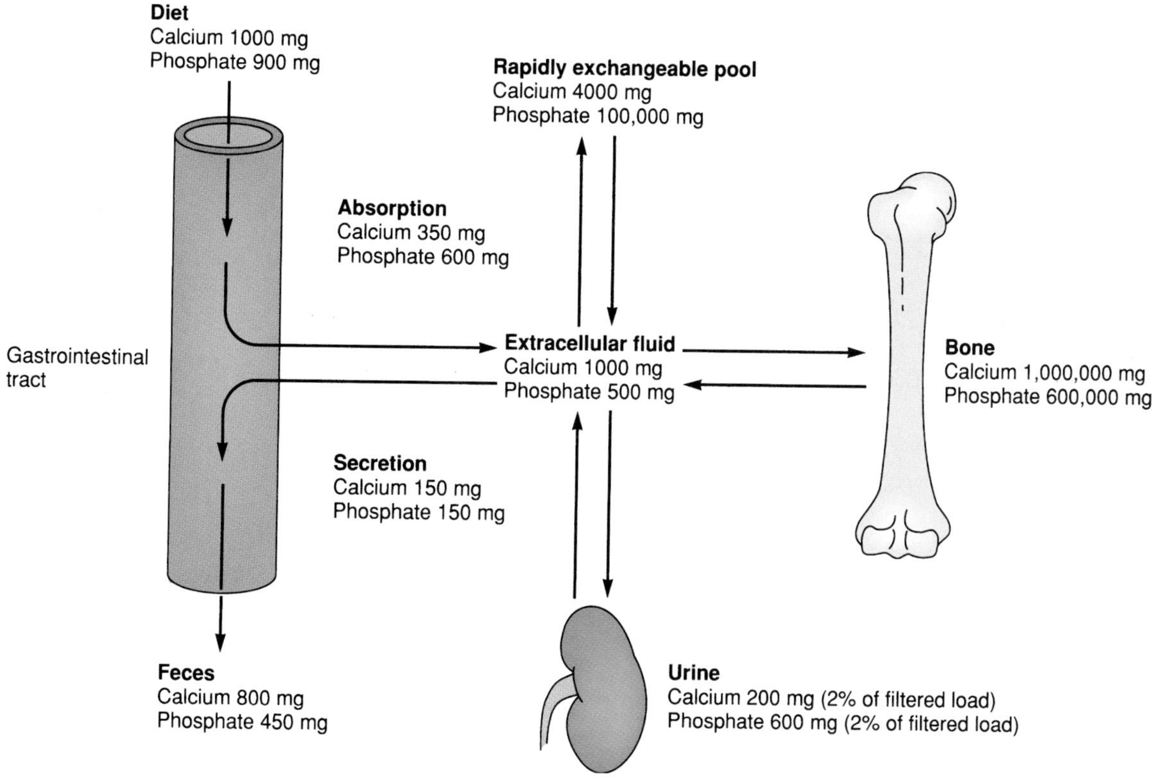

FIGURE 78.4 Average daily calcium and phosphate turnover in humans. (After Aurbach GD, Marx SJ, Spiegel AM, et al. Parathyroid hormone, calcitonin, and the calciferols. In: Wilson JD, Foster DW, eds. *Textbook of endocrinology,* 7th ed. Philadelphia: WB Saunders, 1985, p. 1144, with permission.)

and calcitonin. The actions of each of these hormones in the organs are summarized in Table 78.1.

Parathyroid Hormone

Parathyroid hormone (PTH) is the single most important hormonal regulator of calcium and phosphate metabolism in humans. It has direct effects on the skeleton and kidney and indirect effects on the intestine, mediated through vitamin D.

TABLE 78.1

HORMONAL REGULATION OF CALCIUM AND PHOSPHATE METABOLISM

Location	Parathyroid hormone	Vitamin D	Calcitonin
Gastrointestinal tract	No direct effect	Stimulates calcium and phosphate absorption	No direct effect
Skeleton	Stimulates calcium and phosphate resorption	Stimulates calcium and phosphate resorption	Inhibits calcium and phosphate resorption
Kidneys	Stimulates calcium resorption	No direct effect	Inhibits calcium and phosphate resorption

In target tissues, PTH binds first to membrane receptors, activating adenyl cyclase to generate cyclic adenosine monophosphate (cAMP), which regulates other intracellular enzymes.

In bone, the effects of PTH are complex, stimulating both resorption and the formation of new bone. However, sustained elevations of PTH stimulate osteoclasts and inhibit osteoblasts. Osteocytes, in the matrix of cortical bone, may also act to reabsorb matrix in response to PTH, a process referred to as *osteocytic osteolysis*. Calcium and phosphate mobilization in response to PTH occurs in two phases. Initially, mineral is mobilized from areas of rapid equilibrium. This phase is followed by a more sustained release mediated by newly synthesized lysosomal and hydrolytic enzymes. In the kidney, PTH increases the reabsorption of extracellular fluid calcium at any given concentration, although excess secretion, because of hypercalcemia, increases the net daily amount of urinary calcium excretion. Reabsorption in the proximal tubule and loop of Henle is linked with sodium transport such that factors that alter sodium transport concomitantly alter calcium reabsorption. In contrast, reabsorption in the distal nephron is independent of sodium and directly influenced by PTH. PTH also increases phosphate excretion. This action is accompanied by enhanced bicarbonate secretion. PTH probably has only indirect effects on the gastrointestinal tract, by stimulating the hydroxylation of 25-hydroxyvitamin D to 1,25-dihydroxyvitamin D in the kidney.

PTH is synthesized initially as a precursor, preproPTH, which is sequentially cleaved in the parathyroid gland to proPTH and then to PTH (Fig. 78.5). Secretion of this 84-amino acid molecule is controlled by a negative feedback loop with extracellular fluid calcium. Most PTH is secreted in this form and then cleaved in the liver into N- and C-terminal fragments. The N-terminus contains most of the biologic activity and is rapidly degraded by the liver, whereas the inactive C-terminus is slowly metabolized by the kidney.

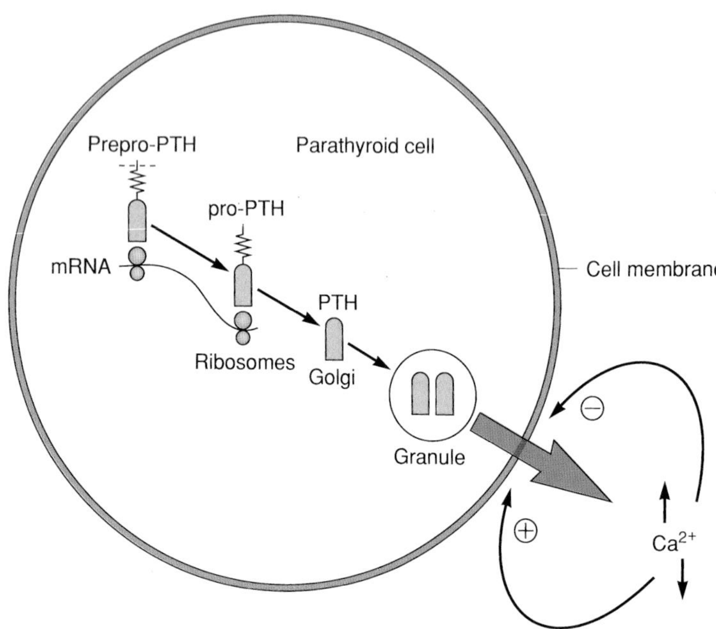

FIGURE 78.5 The parathyroid gland produces a precursor of parathyroid hormone (PTH), prepro-PTH, that is sequentially cleaved to pro-PTH and PTH. PTH secretion is controlled by the extracellular fluid volume. (After Klee GG, Kao PC, Heath H. Hypercalcemia. *Endocrinol Metab Clin North Am.* 1988;17:573.)

Vitamin D

Vitamin D acts at two major sites. It increases intestinal absorption of calcium and phosphate. In addition, in the skeleton, it promotes mineralization and enhances PTH-mediated mobilization of calcium and phosphate. It probably has no direct effect on the kidney.

Vitamin D_3, or cholecalciferol, is produced normally by the action of sunlight on 7-dehydrocholesterol in the skin (Fig. 78.6). It is then hydroxylated in the liver (25 position) and kidney

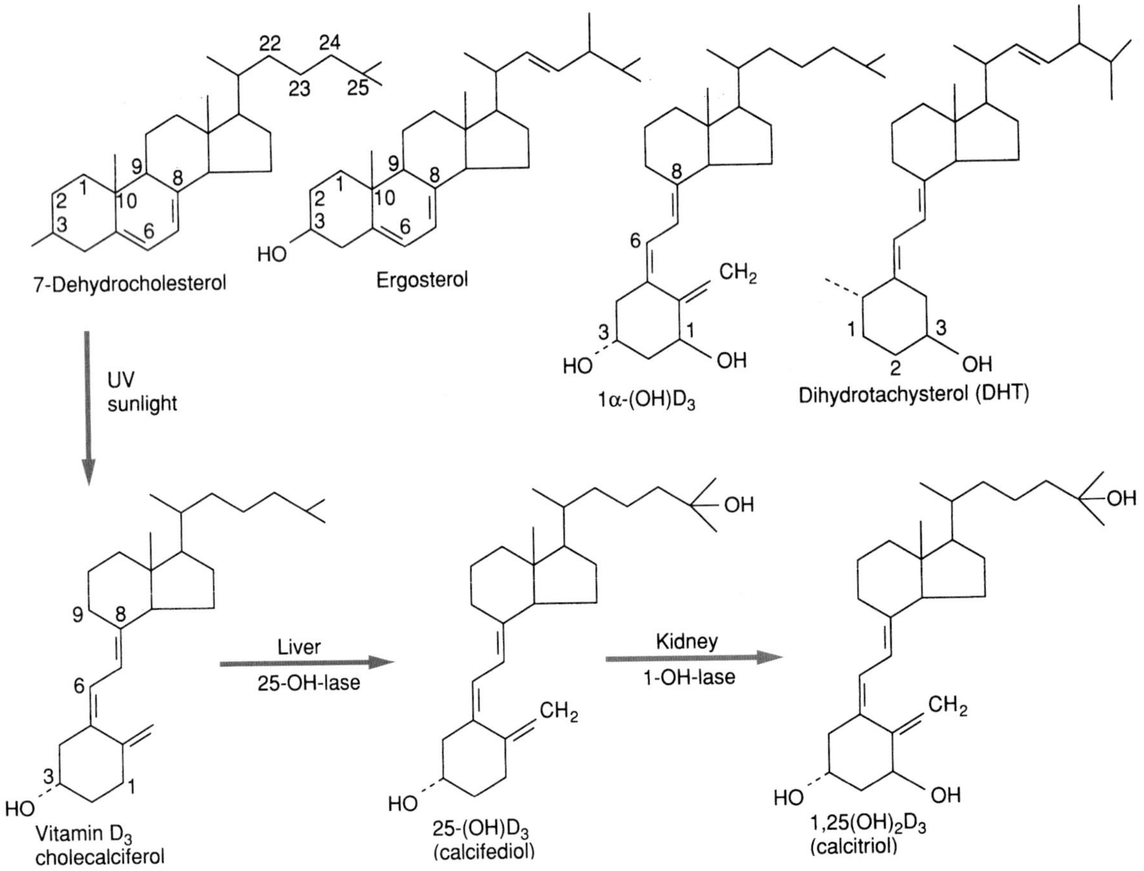

7-Dehydrocholesterol

Ergosterol

1α-$(OH)D_3$

Dihydrotachysterol (DHT)

UV sunlight

Vitamin D_3 cholecalciferol

Liver 25-OH-lase

25-$(OH)D_3$ (calcifediol)

Kidney 1-OH-lase

$1,25(OH)_2D_3$ (calcitriol)

FIGURE 78.6 Schematic illustration of the synthesis of vitamin D_3. Ergosterol, 1-g-hydroxyvitamin D_3, and dihydrotachysterol are synthetic preparations of vitamin D. (After Klee GG, Kao PC, Heath H. Hypercalcemia. *Endocrinol Metab Clin North Am* 1988;17:573.)

(1 position) to form the active 1,25-dihydroxyvitamin D_3 (calcitriol). Vitamin D_2 is normally present in yeast and fungi but not in humans. It is the major pharmacologic source of vitamin D. Pharmaceutical preparations include vitamin D_2 (ergocalciferol), 25-hydroxycholecalciferol (calcifediol), and 1,25-dihydroxycholecalciferol (calcitriol). 1-Hydroxycholecalciferol and dihydrotachysterol are synthetic preparations that require only 25-hydroxylation for activity and so are useful for supplementation in patients with renal failure, who lack the 1-hydroxylase.

Calcitonin

Calcitonin is a 32-amino acid protein produced by the parafollicular C (calcitonin) cells of the thyroid. The C cells are embryologically derived from the neural crest and, in lower animals, are found in the ultimobranchial bodies, which are glandular structures derived from the lowest branchial pouch. In humans, these structures are incorporated into the superior and lateral aspects of the thyroid lobes.

Total thyroidectomy, with removal of all the C cells, is well tolerated. It appears that calcitonin is not essential for the normal control of calcium metabolism in adult humans. It does inhibit bone resorption and can produce hypocalcemia in experimental animals. It also increases urinary calcium and phosphate excretion. These effects are mediated primarily through cAMP. Several secretagogues for calcitonin have been identified, including catecholamines, gastrin, and cholecystokinin, but the most potent appear to be calcium and pentagastrin. Calcitonin can be useful pharmacologically, to reduce serum calcium levels.

Mineral Homeostasis

Under normal conditions, serum calcium and phosphate levels vary minimally during the course of the day. Regulation occurs primarily through PTH but also through a series of feedback loops involving vitamin D and calcitonin (Fig. 78.7). A fall in serum ionized calcium increases PTH secretion and stimulates the production of 1,25-dihydroxyvitamin D_3. Conversely, increases in serum calcium inhibit PTH secretion and the formation of active calciferol.

Pathophysiology

Diseases of the parathyroid glands present almost exclusively as disorders of calcium metabolism. Hypercalcemia is the most common manifestation, and in the patient who presents with an elevated serum calcium level, the differential diagnosis can be complex. A thorough understanding of both hypercalcemia and hypocalcemia is essential for the successful treatment of patients undergoing parathyroid surgery. Primary disorders of plasma phosphate are not usually related to surgical disease and are not discussed in detail here.

HYPERCALCEMIA

Hypercalcemia is a relatively common clinical problem.[3] In the general population and in hospital outpatients, the incidence is between 0.1% and 0.5%. Most patients in this group have primary hyperparathyroidism. In contrast, hypercalcemia is identified in almost 5% of hospitalized patients, and nearly two thirds of them have a malignancy.

Clinical Manifestations

The symptoms of hypercalcemia are varied and nonspecific (Table 78.2). Severity is a function of both the magnitude and rapidity of onset of the hypercalcemia. Many of the manifestations are subtle and are evident only in retrospect, after the patient has been successfully treated for the cause of the elevated calcium. Specific symptoms and diagnostic tests are addressed in more detail in the section on hyperparathyroidism.

Differential Diagnosis

Although the diagnosis of primary hyperparathyroidism can, after appropriate investigation, be established with confidence in most patients, all causes of hypercalcemia must be considered and excluded. The multiple causes of hypercalcemia are listed in Table 78.3.

Etiology

Hyperparathyroidism

The diagnosis of hyperparathyroidism is discussed in detail later. Patients typically have elevated plasma concentrations of calcium and PTH, increased urinary excretion of calcium, and a low plasma concentration of phosphate.

Malignancy

Generally, patients with hypercalcemia and malignancy (humoral hypercalcemia of malignancy) can be classified into two groups.[4]) Patients with solid tumors, such as lung carcinoma (25% of all cases of humoral hypercalcemia of malignancy); breast carcinoma (20%); squamous cell carcinoma of the head, neck, esophagus, or female genital tract (19%); or renal cell cancer (8%), account for three fourths of all cases. Humoral hypercalcemia of malignancy in this setting generally appears late in the disease, with nearly all patients having known, or readily evident, malignancy. These patients have elevated levels of serum calcium, low levels of serum phosphorus, and elevated levels of urinary cAMP, consistent with increased PTH activity but normal or low serum PTH levels.

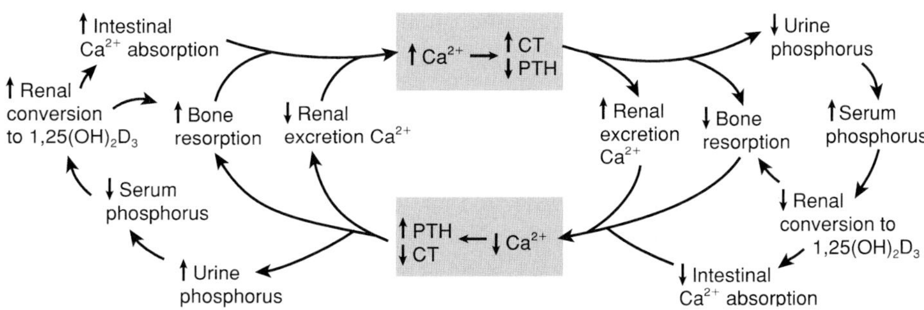

FIGURE 78.7 Feedback loops involved in the regulation of serum calcium and phosphorus. PTH, parathyroid hormone; CT, calcitonin.

TABLE 78.2 DIAGNOSIS

CLINICAL FEATURES OF HYPERCALCEMIA

Neurologic
- Lethargy
- Confusion
- Coma
- Headache
- Depression
- Paranoia
- Muscle weakness
- Hyporeflexia
- Incontinence
- Memory loss
- Hearing loss
- Ataxia

Gastrointestinal
- Constipation
- Anorexia
- Nausea and vomiting
- Polydipsia
- Weight loss
- Pancreatitis
- Peptic ulcer
- Abdominal pain

Cardiovascular
- Electrocardiogram changes (short QT interval, widened T-wave)
- Bradycardia
- Heart block
- Hypertension

Renal
- Polyuria
- Uremia
- Renal colic
- Nephrocalcinosis

Other
- Band keratopathy
- Conjunctivitis
- Change in vision
- Pruritus
- Thrombosis
- Myalgia

TABLE 78.3 ETIOLOGY

CAUSES OF HYPERCALCEMIA

- Hyperparathyroidism
- Malignancy
- Vitamin A or D intoxication
- Thiazide diuretics
- Hyperthyroidism
- Milk–alkali syndrome
- Sarcoidosis and other granulomatous diseases
- Familial hypocalciuric hypercalcemia
- Immobilization
- Paget disease
- Lithium therapy
- Addisonian crisis
- Idiopathic hypercalcemia of infancy

The hypercalcemia is now known to be caused by PTH-related protein secreted by the tumor, rather than by the bony metastases that many of these patients have because of the advanced nature of their cancers. In the second group, accounting for one fourth of cases, are patients with hematologic malignancies, such as multiple myeloma, certain lymphomas and leukemias, and a subset of the patients with breast cancer. These patients have elevated levels of serum calcium, but in contrast to most patients with solid tumors and humoral hypercalcemia of malignancy, they have elevated levels of serum phosphate and low levels of urinary cAMP. These patients always have lytic bony lesions and histologically demonstrate-increased osteoclast bone resorption adjacent to tumor cells. This osteoclast-activating activity is an effect of cytokines, mainly interleukin-1 beta and tumor necrosis factor-beta (lymphotoxin). These cytokines promote local net bone resorption and thus produce hypercalcemia and hyperphosphatemia.

Vitamin D and Vitamin A Intoxication

When administered in excess, vitamins A and D can produce hypercalcemia. Affected patients tend to have normal or elevated serum phosphate levels associated with a low PTH level. Metastatic calcification may occur.

Thiazide Diuretics

Thiazides may increase serum calcium levels to a mild degree, primarily through hemoconcentration and decreased renal excretion. Serum phosphate may also be depressed. It often takes several weeks for the hypercalcemia to resolve after the medication is discontinued.

Hyperthyroidism

Hyperthyroidism is associated with increased bone resorption. Often, the plasma PTH is low, and a history of other thyrotoxic symptoms can be elicited. The hypercalcemia usually resolves as the patient becomes euthyroid.

Milk–Alkali Syndrome

Typically, the milk–alkali syndrome occurs in patients with peptic ulcers who consume large quantities of milk and absorbable antacids. Usually, some degree of renal failure is present. PTH levels are low. This syndrome has become much less common with the increased use of nonabsorbable antacids and histamine 2-receptor antagonists.

Sarcoidosis and Other Granulomatous Diseases

These syndromes are associated with hypersensitivity to vitamin D. Apparently, the granulomas can convert the inactive vitamin D to its active form. Patients have elevated plasma globulins and low PTH levels. The administration of large doses of cortisone for 10 days usually reduces the hypercalcemia. Biopsy of lymph nodes or the liver may confirm the diagnosis.

Familial Hypocalciuric Hypercalcemia

This disease is an asymptomatic, autosomal dominant condition characterized by mild to moderate hypercalcemia, hypocalciuria, and normal or only slightly elevated PTH levels. It develops in people heterozygous for a mutation in the calcium-sensing receptor.[5] The mutation causes an increase in the set point for extracellular calcium concentration, so that the "normal" calcium level is higher in these people than in the normal population. No treatment is necessary, although people with this disease should receive genetic counseling. Neonatal severe hyperparathyroidism, which can be fatal, develops in children homozygous for mutations in this receptor. Treatment for neonates with this disease is controversial, but they appear to benefit from early surgical management.[6]

Immobilization

Immobilization produces hypercalcemia by increasing the ratio of bone resorption to bone formation. These patients can usually be distinguished by history, although on laboratory evaluation they have elevated serum levels of calcium and phosphate and a decreased serum concentration of PTH. Often, hypercalciuria is present, which may lead to the development of renal stones. Treatment is early mobilization and forced diuresis.

Other Causes

A variety of other diseases may produce hypercalcemia. For example, Paget disease (osteitis deformans) typically causes mild elevations in serum calcium. Paget disease can be diagnosed on the basis of the characteristic radiographic lesion. Adrenal insufficiency may be associated with hypercalcemia, although the symptoms are typically those of the primary abnormality. Lithium therapy appears to produce hypercalcemia by altering the parathyroid set point for inhibition by calcium, and, over long courses of therapy, may also be associated with hyperparathyroidism. Idiopathic hypercalcemia of infancy is a rare disorder that is probably the result of hypersensitivity to vitamin D. It occurs in infants with mental retardation and is satisfactorily treated with glucocorticoids. Other causes include aluminum-induced renal osteomalacia and a host of analytic errors related to improper specimen collection with prolonged tourniquet times, tube contamination, and instrument drift.

Medical Treatment

Although the choice of therapy is tailored to the cause of the hypercalcemia, several general measures can prove effective.[7]

For the patient with mild hypercalcemia, a trial of a decrease in dietary calcium is indicated. A reduction in intake of milk and other dairy products is suggested, along with discontinuation of thiazide diuretics and vitamin D preparations. Mobilization prevents bone demineralization.

Patients with more marked hypercalcemia or severe symptoms should be admitted to the hospital for treatment, with careful observation and monitoring. In the patient with severe hyperparathyroidism, although the definitive therapy is surgical, it is unwise to proceed with neck exploration until the calcium has been reduced to near-normal levels. The mainstay of therapy is intravenous hydration, preferably with normal saline solution in sufficient quantities to maintain the urine output above 100 mL per hour. These patients are often dehydrated before therapy, and fluid can be administered intravenously at a rate of 200 mL per hour. Caution must be exercised in older patients, whose cardiac reserve may be marginal. This therapy exploits the parallel handling of calcium and sodium by the kidneys. The diuretic furosemide also increases sodium and calcium excretion but should not be used until the patient is well hydrated.

The end points of therapy are a decrease in the serum calcium level and a reduction of symptoms. Diuresis with saline solution is usually effective when the hypercalcemia results from hyperparathyroidism or a benign cause. In contrast, the hypercalcemia of malignancy may produce severe symptoms associated with extremely high serum calcium levels that are difficult to control. In this setting, a variety of other measures may be considered (Table 78.4). Some of the agents used to treat hypercalcemia cause significant toxicity, and close patient monitoring is required during treatment. Calcitonin is a fairly weak hypocalcemic agent, but it acts rapidly and is associated with less toxicity than many of the other drugs. Salmon calcitonin is the most potent preparation. Glucocorticoids may be particularly efficacious in patients with sarcoidosis and other granulomatous diseases. Plicamycin has proved useful in patients with hypercalcemia of malignancy, but it causes a cumulative toxicity (thrombocytopenia, hepatotoxicity, and nephrotoxicity). Biphosphonates inhibit osteoclast activity directly. These agents are given intravenously and are particularly efficacious, although long-term use may be associated with significant osteomalacia. Prostaglandin synthetase inhibitors were initially considered useful, but their efficacy has proved to be limited. Intravenous phosphates and chelating agents have largely been abandoned because of their severe toxicity; however, oral phosphates may be beneficial in patients requiring prolonged therapy.

TABLE 78.4 TREATMENT

TREATMENT OF HYPERCALCEMIA

Therapy of Primary Disease
- Tumor resection (hypercalcemia of malignancy)
- Parathyroidectomy (primary hyperparathyroidism)

Expansion of extracellular volume
- Infusion of saline solution
- Enhancement of urinary calcium excretion
- Extracellular volume expansion
- Loop diuretics (furosemide and ethacrynic acid)

Inhibition of Bone Resorption
- Calcitonin
- Glucocorticoids
- Plicamycin (mithramycin)
- Bisphosphonates
- Gallium nitrate

Reduction of Intestinal Calcium Absorption
- Low-calcium diet
- Glucocorticoids

Other Treatments
- Dialysis
- Mobilization
- Oral phosphate
- Estrogens or progestogens (postmenopausal women with primary hyperparathyroidism)
- Chloroquine (sarcoidosis)

Modified from Attie MF. Treatment of hypercalcemia. *Endocrinol Metab Clin North Am.* 1989;18:802.

HYPOCALCEMIA

Hypocalcemia can occur as a consequence of various acquired and hereditary diseases.[8] Generally, these disorders produce a deficiency or defect in the action of either PTH or vitamin D. It is most commonly a significant clinical problem after neck operation for thyroid disease. Vitamin D deficiency is associated with compensatory PTH excess. The end result is rickets in children or osteomalacia in adults.

Clinical Features

The major signs and symptoms of hypocalcemia are a direct consequence of the reduction in plasma levels of ionized calcium, which increases neuromuscular excitability (Table 78.5). The earliest clinical manifestations are numbness and tingling in the circumoral area, fingers, and toes. Mental symptoms are also common. Patients become anxious, depressed, and occasionally confused. Tetany may develop, characterized by carpopedal

TABLE 78.5 DIAGNOSIS

CLINICAL FEATURES OF HYPOCALCEMIA

Neurologic
- Circumoral paresthesia
- Light-headedness
- Depression
- Anxiety
- Confusion
- Chvostek's sign
- Trousseau's sign
- Irritability
- Laryngeal spasm
- Seizures

Musculoskeletal
- Tetany
- Cramps
- Involuntary twitching
- Osteomalacia

Cardiovascular
- Electrocardiogram changes (prolonged QT interval, T-wave peaking)
- Arrhythmia
- Tachycardia, hypotension

Other Features
- Lenticular cataracts

spasm, tonic–clonic convulsions, and laryngeal stridor. The magnitude of symptoms at any given plasma concentration of ionized calcium varies from patient to patient. On physical examination, contraction of the facial muscles is elicited by tapping anterior to the ear, over the facial nerve (Chvostek's sign), although this sign may be present in 10% of normal patients. Trousseau's sign is elicited by occluding blood flow to the forearm for 3 minutes. The development of carpal spasm indicates hypocalcemia, although the test is unpleasant and clinically impractical.

Etiology

Some of the causes of hypocalcemia are listed in Table 78.6. The most common cause of hypocalcemia by far is excision of or damage to the parathyroid glands during thyroid surgery.

Postoperative Hypoparathyroidism

Postoperative hypoparathyroidism commonly develops after total thyroidectomy for malignancy. Most patients undergoing operation on the thyroid experience some alteration in serum calcium, although they often are asymptomatic; the low calcium probably represents contusion or temporary alteration of the blood supply to the parathyroid glands. The hypocalcemia is usually transient and is not treated unless significant symptoms develop. Occasionally, in hyperparathyroid patients who have parathyroidectomy and significant bone disease, a marked skeletal deposition of calcium and symptomatic hypocalcemia occurs, so-called *bone hunger*. The plasma calcium usually reaches its nadir at 48 to 72 hours after surgery and then slowly returns to normal within several days. These patients may require calcium and vitamin D therapy for weeks or months after parathyroidectomy.

TABLE 78.6 ETIOLOGY

CAUSES OF HYPOCALCEMIA

- Hypoparathyroidism
- Vitamin D deficiency
- Pseudohypoparathyroidism
- Hypomagnesemia
- Malabsorption
- Pancreatitis
- Hypoalbuminemia
- Chelation of calcium
- Osteoblastic metastases
- Toxic shock syndrome
- Hyperphosphatemia

Idiopathic Hypoparathyroidism

A less common form of hypoparathyroidism is idiopathic lack of function. It occurs both sporadically and in families. In some cases, it develops as part of a polyglandular disorder and is thought to have an autoimmune basis. DiGeorge syndrome is a congenital disorder involving the branchial pouches that produces agenesis of the thymus and parathyroid glands. Hypoparathyroidism may also develop in newborns as a result of prenatal suppression of the fetal parathyroid glands as a consequence of maternal hypercalcemia. It is also common in otherwise normal but premature infants.

Vitamin D Deficiency

Vitamin D deficiency may occur as a result of dietary deficiency or lack of exposure to the sun. Likewise, renal disease produces a decrease in the 1-hydroxylase activity necessary for the formation of active vitamin D_3. The result is a decrease in calcium absorption and an increased secretion of PTH by the stimulated parathyroid glands. Osteomalacia, abnormal fractures, and the deformities of rickets may result.

Pseudohypoparathyroidism

Pseudohypoparathyroidism is a familial disease characterized by a rotund appearance, shortening of the extremities, and sometimes mental deficiency. The defect is not in PTH secretion; in fact, most patients have elevated plasma levels of PTH with evidence of increased bone resorption. Rather, the kidney is unresponsive to the hormone, and as a consequence, hypocalcemia and hyperphosphatemia develop. The deficit appears to be in the renal adenyl cyclase system.

Hypomagnesemia

This unusual deficit may result from chronic alcoholism, malabsorption, parenteral nutrition, or increased renal clearance during therapy with aminoglycosides. The deficit appears to block the physical response to PTH in addition to its release from the parathyroid gland.

Other Causes

In short-gut syndrome, after extensive small-bowel resection or bypass, vitamin D and calcium may be absorbed in insufficient quantities. In pancreatitis, the massive soft-tissue destruction and saponification that occur with hemorrhagic disease may sequester significant amounts of calcium in the retroperitoneum. Some undefined systemic factor also appears to contribute to hypocalcemia in these patients. Hypoalbuminemia causes a reduction in the total plasma calcium level, although the level of ionized calcium remains within the normal range and patients are asymptomatic. Circulatory substances, such as the citrate used to anticoagulate banked blood and radiographic contrast media, may bind to calcium. In patients with osteoblastic metastases, particularly associated with prostate carcinoma, hypocalcemia has been attributed to increased

TABLE 78.7 TREATMENT

TREATMENT OF HYPOCALCEMIA

Symptom or goal	Treatment
Symptomatic hypocalcemia	Oral calcium carbonate or intravenous calcium gluconate, and possibly vitamin D supplements to increase the efficiency of absorption of oral supplements
Symptomatic tetany	Intravenous calcium gluconate
Correction of hypomagnesemia	Intravenous magnesium chloride
Vitamin D supplementation	Ergocalciferol, calcifediol (liver disease), calcitriol (renal disease)
Long-term therapy	Calcium carbonate; low-phosphate, low-oxalate diet; parathyroid grafting (immunosuppressed or cryopreserved autograft)

calcium flux into the lesions. Toxic shock syndrome is sometimes associated with hypocalcemia, but the mechanism has not been defined. Acute hyperphosphatemia, as a consequence of exogenous administration of phosphate or during the cytolytic chemotherapy of highly responsive tumors (e.g., Burkitt lymphoma and acute lymphoblastic leukemia), may produce symptomatic hypocalcemia associated with soft-tissue calcification.

Treatment

The treatment of hypocalcemia is summarized in Table 78.7. For acute symptomatic hypocalcemia, calcium should be administered intravenously. Calcium gluconate is less irritating to the veins than calcium chloride, and the calcium release is slower, without a risk for overcorrection. Usually, 20 to 30 mL of 10% solution is infused over a 15- to 20-minute period, and then 50 to 100 mL is administered over the next 12 hours in adults. A practical guide after an initial bolus dose includes 60 mL of 10% calcium gluconate in a 500 mL bag of dextrose 5% in water, infused at 1 mL/kg/h, and adjusted every 4 hours based on the serum level of calcium and patient symptoms. Bicarbonate precipitates any calcium infused through the same intravenous line. Serum magnesium should always be measured, and hypomagnesemia should be corrected if present. In patients with convulsions from advanced tetany, diphenylhydantoin therapy is useful, but symptoms should never be allowed to progress to this point.

Long-term therapy is gauged on the basis of symptoms. In the postoperative patient, the continued stimulus of mild hypocalcemia to any remaining parathyroid tissue may prove useful. Concomitant therapy with calcium and vitamin D is effective in a timely fashion. A starting dose of 2 g of oral calcium carbonate per day in divided doses is usually well tolerated. Vitamin D can be administered as calcitriol, a synthetic vitamin D analogue. Most adults respond to a dose of 0.5 to 2.0 mg per day; reduced doses may be necessary for patients with renal dysfunction.

HYPERPARATHYROIDISM

Definitions

Parathyroid neoplasms are rarely identified by physical enlargement but rather are sought because of the peripheral effects of excess hormone. Primary hyperparathyroidism develops spontaneously, without apparent cause but possibly in response to exogenous stimuli. When the normal control of serum calcium is disturbed and the autonomous production of PTH is increased, the state is referred to as *primary hyperparathyroidism*. This category includes both benign single- and multiple-gland enlargements and the much rarer parathyroid carcinoma. In some cases, the disease is familial. In contrast, *secondary hyperparathyroidism* occurs when a defect in mineral homeostasis leads to a compensatory increase in parathyroid function. This occurs most commonly in response to renal disease but may also develop as a consequence of the hypocalcemia associated with some diseases of the gastrointestinal tract, bones, or other endocrine organs. Occasionally, with prolonged secondary stimulation, the hyperfunctioning glands are no longer physiologically responsive to an increase in ionized calcium. This uncommon (affecting about 2% of patients after renal transplantation), relatively autonomous state referred to as *tertiary hyperparathyroidism*, develops most commonly after renal transplantation when the defect in calcium homeostasis is corrected.

Incidence

The advent in the 1970s of the widespread assessment of serum calcium as part of automated multichannel analysis has considerably altered our understanding of hyperparathyroidism. Before that time, primary hyperparathyroidism was thought to be a relatively rare condition. Most patients presented with symptoms of disease, usually renal stones or bony manifestations. Today, most patients are asymptomatic or have only vague symptoms or signs that can be related to hyperparathyroidism.[9,10] Occasionally, patients recognize that they had symptoms only after their well being improves following parathyroidectomy. Incidence varies with both age and gender (Table 78.8), but hyperparathyroidism is believed to develop in about 50 to 100 people per 100,000 in the general population, with approximately 50,000 new cases occurring annually in the United States.[9] Marked variations have been noted worldwide; the reasons for these differences remain unclear.

Etiology

The cause of primary hyperparathyroidism is not known. Although the sequence of progression from secondary to tertiary disease in response to chronic stimulation has a logical appeal, it is difficult to draw parallels with primary disease. Most patients with primary hyperparathyroidism have disease of a single rather than of multiple glands, which is not what

TABLE 78.8

AGE-SPECIFIC AND GENDER-SPECIFIC INCIDENCE OF PRIMARY HYPERPARATHYROIDISM

	New cases per 100,000	
Age (y)	Men	Women
<39	5	8
40–50	26	104
>60	92	189
Total	18	56

After Heath H III, Hodgson SF, Kennedy MA. Primary hyperthyroidism: incidence, morbidity, and potential economic impact in a community. *N Engl J Med.* 1980;302:189.

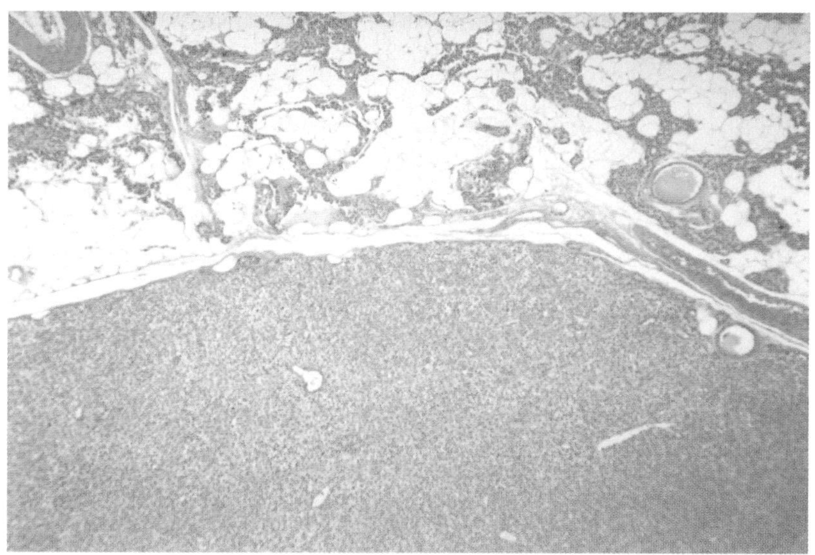

FIGURE 78.8 Parathyroid adenoma. The tumor consists of sheets of neoplastic chief cells and is separated from normal parenchyma by a thin capsule. (From Rubin E, Farber JL. *Pathology*, 3rd ed. Philadelphia: Lippincott Williams & Wilkins, 1999.)

might be predicted if an external stimulus were part of the pathophysiology. Hyperparathyroidism is most common in postmenopausal women, the population group with the highest incidence of osteoporosis and the most significant alterations in calcium and phosphate metabolism. Loss of renal function with aging is associated with elevations in PTH and decreases in phosphate clearance. It has been suggested but not demonstrated that a renal calcium leak, if sufficient, might result in a chronic calcium deficit stimulating the parathyroid glands.

Genetic studies of parathyroid adenomas have described an oncogene (*PRAD1*) that may be one step in the path to neoplasia in these tumors. Ongoing research indicates that overexpression of the normal *PRAD1* gene, also known as *cyclin D1*, allows progression of the cell cycle from the G1 phase to the S phase, thus promoting cellular growth and division. *PRAD1* is overexpressed in only a subset of parathyroid adenomas; further research may reveal other genetic alterations that contribute to the neoplastic growth.[10,11]

Hyperparathyroidism occurs in several familial forms. It is a major component of the multiple endocrine neoplasia (MEN) syndromes types I and IIA. The parathyroid disease of MEN-1 syndrome is multiple parathyroid adenomas that appear with increasing frequency over the patient's lifetime.[12] In other families, hyperparathyroidism is inherited in an autosomal dominant fashion without other manifestations of MEN-I or MEN-II; some have osseous abnormalities (tumor–jaw syndrome) and some apparently have isolated disease.

Pathology

Single-gland versus Multiple-gland Disease

Microscopically, the cell most commonly involved in primary hyperparathyroidism is the chief cell.[13] Less frequently, the oxyphil cell is the predominant cell type. Diseased glands typically have an increase in the proportion of stromal cells and a reduction in the proportion of stromal fat. Single diseased glands, or adenomas, have been classically described with a predominance of chief cells centering in a single focus, with a compressed rim of surrounding normal tissue (Fig. 78.8). In contrast, parathyroid hyperplasia has been characterized as a diffuse proliferation of clear cells in multiple glands, with little remaining normal tissue (Fig. 78.9). These criteria have

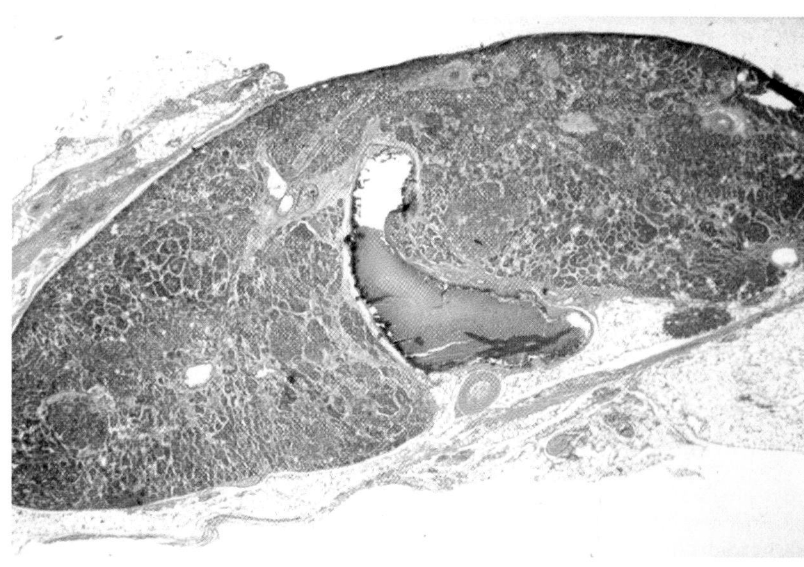

FIGURE 78.9 Primary parathyroid hyperplasia. The normal adipose tissue of the gland has been replaced by sheets and trabeculae of hyperplastic chief cells. (From Rubin E, Farber JL. *Pathology*, 3rd ed. Philadelphia: Lippincott Williams & Wilkins, 1999.)

TABLE 78.9

GLAND ENLARGEMENT IN 66 CONSECUTIVE PATIENTS WITH PRIMARY HYPERPARATHYROIDISM

Pathology	Patient, *n*	Percentage
Adenoma	50	76%
Double adenoma	4	6%
Hyperplasia	12	18%

From Lowney JK, Weber B, Johnson S, et al. Minimal incision parathyroidectomy: cure, cosmesis, and cost. *World J Surg*. 2000;24:1442–1445.

proved totally unreliable. Although pathologic studies can usually distinguish parathyroid glands from other tissue, they may not prove useful beyond this capacity.. Intraoperative decisions frequently depend on recognizing disease of one or more parathyroid glands, and in this regard, the histologic description of adenoma or hyperplasia is generally unreliable in primary hyperparathyroidism.

Patients with multiple-gland disease may have one gland that appears to be an adenoma and another that appears diffusely involved or even histologically normal with gross enlargement. Other methods of identifying normal glands, including staining of intracellular fat, measurement of glandular density, and flow cytometric analysis of cellular DNA content, have all been used with some reported success, although none provides unequivocal differentiation between normal and abnormal glands.

The most reliable index of abnormality is the determination of glandular enlargement by visual inspection. The incidence of single- and multiple-gland enlargement as judged by visual inspection in 66 consecutive patients with hyperparathyroidism is shown in Table 78.9. The visual assessment and judgment of the experienced surgeon have proved to be an effective basis for intraoperative decisions. This approach requires that all four parathyroid glands be evaluated at the time of operation. However, the recent ability to rapidly measure PTH during operation has provided a method to assess gland function rather than size. This experience indicates that there may be more enlarged glands than there are hyperfunctioning glands.[14]

Carcinoma

Parathyroid carcinoma is a rare entity, and the histologic diagnosis can be exceedingly difficult. The surgeon may suspect the diagnosis when dense invasion and scarring are encountered, although this may also be secondary to some other inflammatory disease in the neck. Pathologic criteria include marked mitotic activity, dense fibrous stroma, and evidence of local invasion into the capsule or surrounding vessels. Malignant-appearing tumors, however, may pursue an apparently benign clinical course; the converse is less frequently true. An aneuploid pattern by flow cytometric analysis of tumor DNA content may help to distinguish carcinoma from atypical adenoma in borderline cases.[15] The only reliable criteria of malignancy are metastases, most commonly to the lymph nodes, lung, or liver, and true local invasion.

Systemic Effects

The use of automated technology for determining serum calcium has changed not only the estimated incidence of hyperparathyroidism but also the usual mode of presentation.[16] Before screening, three fourths of patients presented with renal disease, particularly nephrolithiasis; one third to one half had skeletal manifestations, and rare patients had both. Most recent series suggest that at least half of the patients in whom hyperparathyroidism is diagnosed do not have renal or osseous disease and many are minimally symptomatic or asymptomatic. Manifestations of the disease are protean but generally nonspecific, and they may be difficult to elicit in the history. A significant proportion of patients present without a readily quantifiable index of disease severity. This finding has created some controversy about the need for surgery in the asymptomatic patient and particularly for the elderly or high-risk patient.[17,18]

The earliest complaints are often the vague symptoms of hypercalcemia. These vary with the magnitude of plasma calcium elevation and can include muscle weakness, anorexia, nausea, constipation, polyuria, and polydipsia. These nonspecific symptoms may or may not cause the patient to seek medical attention.[19] Some symptomatic patients have evidence of chronic disease involving the kidney or skeleton. Usually, only one of these systems is significantly involved in any individual patient. The treatment of hyperparathyroidism is designed to eliminate or halt the progression of the complications of the disease. Symptomatic patients can be divided into two groups. Members of the first group have renal manifestations, a slower onset of symptoms, and generally lower serum calcium concentrations. Patients in the second group have a more rapid onset of symptoms, higher serum calcium levels, and significant bone disease. No recognizable histologic or physiologic characteristics distinguish patients with renal disease from those with bone disease.

Renal Manifestations

Renal complications develop because the hypercalcemia leads to an increase in urinary calcium excretion and because PTH increases the excretion of phosphate and produces urinary alkalosis. Both these events predispose to stone formation. Urinary stones may be treated surgically or with lithotripsy, and subsequent definitive treatment of the hyperparathyroidism reduces the rate of re-formation. Of patients who present for the first time with renal colic, 5% to 10% are found to have primary hyperparathyroidism. Nephrocalcinosis (Fig. 78.10) is

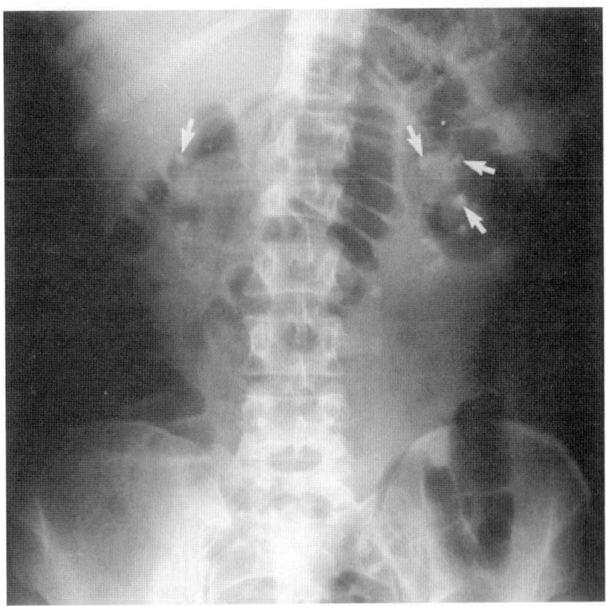

FIGURE 78.10 Abdominal film demonstrating nephrocalcinosis, or diffuse calcification of the renal parenchyma (*arrows*).

calcification of the renal parenchyma and occurs in 5% to 10% of patients with hyperparathyroidism. It causes more significant renal damage than nephrolithiasis does. In general, the more severe the renal damage, the less likely it is that nephrocalcinosis will regress after parathyroidectomy.

The incidence of hypertension in hyperparathyroidism increases with the degree of renal impairment. Hypertension may be a significant cause of the morbidity associated with hyperparathyroidism, but although a decrease in blood pressure has been demonstrated in some patients after parathyroidectomy, the correlation between the two conditions is not clear.

Skeletal Manifestations

Parathyroid bone disease in its most classic and severe form, osteitis fibrosa cystica, is seldom encountered; however, 5% to 15% of patients with parathyroid bone disease present with significant symptoms of skeletal disease. Most commonly, these symptoms include bone pain and pathologic fractures.

Bone changes are often demonstrable on detailed plain radiographs of the hands (Fig. 78.11). Characteristically, subperiosteal resorption is evident on the radial aspect of the middle phalanx of the second or third finger. Because of tufting of the distal phalanges, clubbing may be evident on physical examination. Other findings that typically involve the skull and long bones include bone cysts, "brown" tumors (i.e., localized proliferations of osteoclasts), and diffuse demineralization or granularity. More subtle bone loss can be detected by iliac crest bone biopsy or dual energy x-ray absorptiometry scan. The risk of bone fracture increases with increasing severity of bone loss.

Gastrointestinal Manifestations

Hypercalcemia is clearly associated with nonspecific gastrointestinal complaints, including nausea, vomiting, constipation, and anorexia, but attempts to demonstrate a definite relation between hyperparathyroidism and either peptic ulcer disease or pancreatitis remain unconvincing. Hypercalcemia stimulates gastric acid secretion experimentally and clinically and has been associated with pancreatitis. Therefore, a theoretic rationale for the complex of hyperparathyroidism and gastrointestinal symptoms does exist.

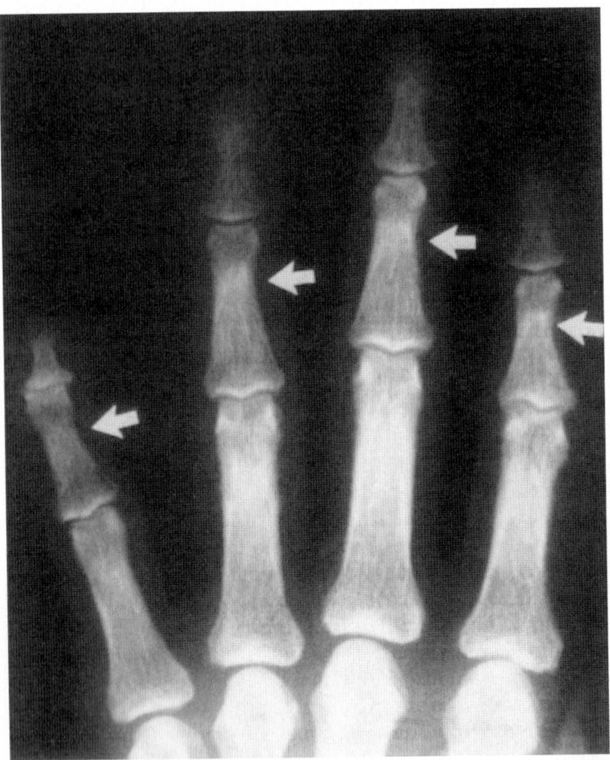

FIGURE 78.11 Magnification radiograph of the fingers in hyperparathyroidism. Subperiosteal cortical resorption (*arrows*) typically is most visible on the radial aspect of the middle phalanges.

Neuromuscular Manifestations

Neurologic and muscular complaints are those of hypercalcemia in general. Fatigability and proximal muscle weakness are among the most debilitating manifestations. Atrophy of type II muscle fibers, consistent with a neuropathic and not a myopathic cause, has been demonstrated. Sensory complaints include dysesthesia, a reduced vibratory sense, and stocking–glove sensory deficits.

Psychological Manifestations

The emotional disturbances of hyperparathyroidism are often subtle and difficult to quantify. As with other forms of hypercalcemia, they range from depression or anxiety to psychosis and coma. Patients undergoing parathyroidectomy frequently experience a sense of well-being and relief from fatigue and dullness postoperatively, even if they may have had no noticeable complaints preoperatively.

Other Manifestations

A variety of signs and symptoms of soft-tissue calcification have been described. Nonspecific arthralgia, particularly involving the proximal interphalangeal joints of the hands, is characteristic. The incidence of chondrocalcinosis is increased. Pruritus, vascular and cardiac calcification, and band keratopathy of the cornea have all been noted. Several reports have suggested an increased incidence of malignancy, but they remain unsubstantiated.

Physical Findings

Except in patients with the classic deformities of advanced bone disease, the physical examination is seldom helpful. Diseased parathyroid glands are infrequently palpable, except in patients with parathyroid carcinoma. A mass in the anterior neck in a patient with primary hyperparathyroidism is most commonly a thyroid nodule.

Laboratory Findings

Tests for calcium, PTH, phosphate, bicarbonate, and magnesium, in addition to other laboratory tests, are useful to establish the diagnosis of hyperparathyroidism.

Calcium. Hypercalcemia is the single most important diagnostic finding; however, particularly in early or mild cases, serial analysis may show fluctuations in and out of the normal range. Coexistent hypoalbuminemia and acidosis may produce an apparently normal total serum calcium, even though the ionized fraction is actually elevated. Serum concentrations of ionized calcium may be helpful in the patient with intermittent or mild hypercalcemia.

Parathyroid Hormone. In the United States, PTH measurement has become an important method for establishing the diagnosis of hyperparathyroidism. Because of the heterogeneity of the various circulating forms of PTH, conflicting and confusing results were often obtained during the initial clinical experience with radioimmunoassays. The methodology continues to be refined, and most current assays are sufficiently sensitive, specific, and reliable and are in wide clinical use. Intact hormone assays and whole molecule assays, as opposed

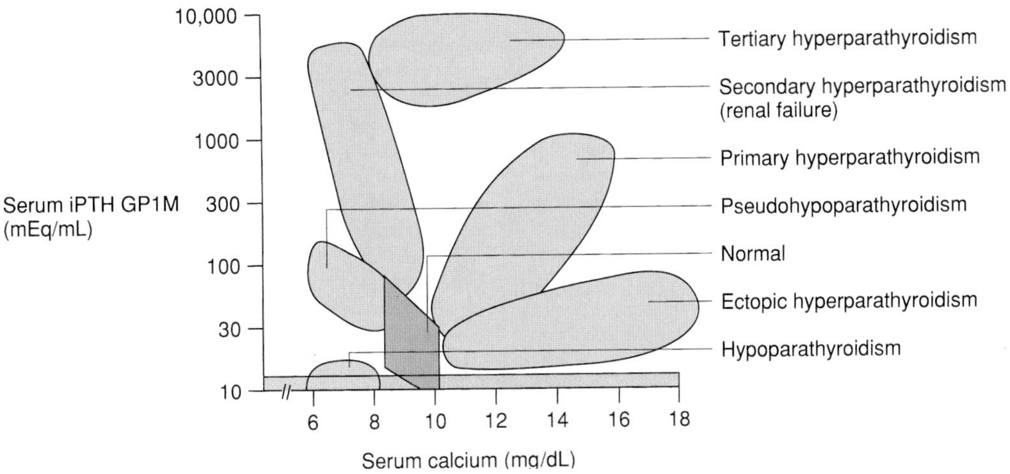

FIGURE 78.12 Relation between serum immunoreactive parathyroid hormone and serum calcium in patients with hypoparathyroidism, pseudohypoparathyroidism, ectopic hyperparathyroidism, and primary, secondary, and tertiary hyperparathyroidism. GP1M, guinea pig antiserum 1M. (After Clark OH, Way LW. Thyroid and parathyroid. In: Way LW, ed. *Current surgical diagnosis and treatment*, 8th ed. Norwalk, CT: Appleton & Lange, 1989, p. 249.)

to amino terminus or carboxyl terminus assays, are the most dependable. The demonstration of an elevated plasma PTH concentration alone does not establish the diagnosis of hyperparathyroidism. With a simultaneous elevated serum calcium level, this finding is virtually diagnostic (Fig. 78.12).

Phosphate. PTH increases renal phosphate excretion and, in about half of patients, produces hypophosphatemia. In the presence of renal disease, however, the serum phosphate levels may be normal or significantly elevated.

Bicarbonate. PTH also increases bicarbonate excretion, so that a hyperchloremic metabolic acidosis may develop. It has been suggested that the finding of an elevated serum chloride-to-phosphate ratio may be helpful in the differential diagnosis of hypercalcemia. A ratio greater than 30 is considered highly suggestive of hyperparathyroidism.

Magnesium. Hypomagnesemia develops in 5% to 10% of patients with hyperparathyroidism. After parathyroidectomy, if both hypocalcemia and hypomagnesemia are present, it may be difficult to correct the calcium until the serum magnesium has been corrected.

Other Diagnostic Tests. A variety of special diagnostic tests for hyperparathyroidism are available. None is more specific than the measurement of serum concentrations of calcium and PTH, although they may be useful in equivocal cases. For example, the 24-hour urinary calcium excretion is usually elevated in patients with hyperparathyroidism, although the finding is not specific for this disease. This test is helpful in identifying patients with familial hypercalcemic hypocalciuria, in whom the rate of urinary calcium excretion is low. Measurements of tubular reabsorption of phosphate below 30% suggest primary hyperparathyroidism. Urinary cAMP is generated specifically as a consequence of PTH activation of renal tubular adenyl cyclase. Increased urinary concentrations are identified in most patients with primary hyperparathyroidism. These measurements are rarely necessary because of the reliability of the intact PTH measurement.

Localization with Imaging Techniques

In order to try to simplify the operative approach to hyperparathyroidism, attempts have been made to localize enlarged glands preoperatively. In the hands of an experienced surgeon, the cure rate for hyperparathyroidism at the initial operation without preoperative localization exceeds 95% with the conventional full neck exploration. However, recent technologic developments have led surgeons to pursue alternatives to the full neck exploration. These innovations are increasingly accurate preoperative localization with ^{99m}technetium sestamibi scintigraphy or high-resolution ultrasound and intraoperative intact PTH measurement that allows termination of the operation without visualization of all four parathyroid glands. Surgeons have used these technologies in various combinations to limit the extent of the neck exploration. All the current alternative strategies, however, depend on a preoperative parathyroid localization study to direct the exploration.

The study most frequently used for imaging previously unoperated patients is ^{99m}technetium sestamibi scintigraphy (Fig. 78.13). Sestamibi scanning can identify the site of abnormal tissue in 75% to 80% of patients but has limitations in patients with small adenomas or multiple-gland disease. Sestamibi was originally developed for cardiac imaging. It also images parathyroid tissue on delayed scans and has been used recently for noninvasive parathyroid imaging. The use of a single nuclide with a short half-life and a high-energy profile has advantages in lateral, oblique, and three-dimensional

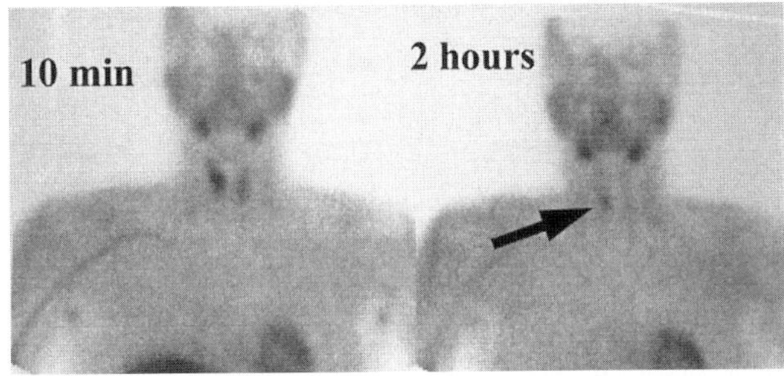

FIGURE 78.13 ^{99m}Technetium sestamibi scan of a patient with a parathyroid adenoma. The radionuclide is present in both thyroid and parathyroid tissue on the 10-minute film; however, by 2 hours, the radionuclide has washed out of the thyroid and remains only in the right-sided parathyroid gland. This scan shows a 794-mg right upper parathyroid adenoma (*arrow*).

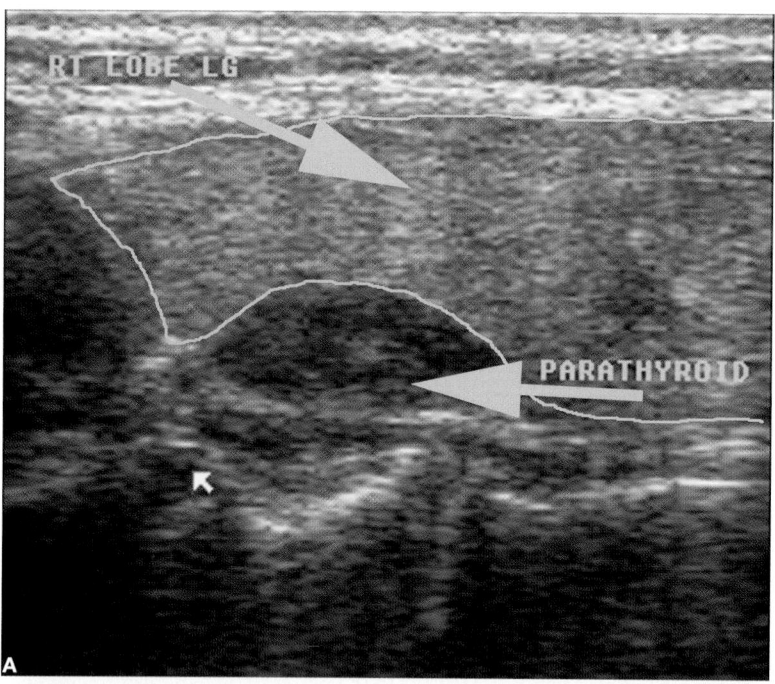

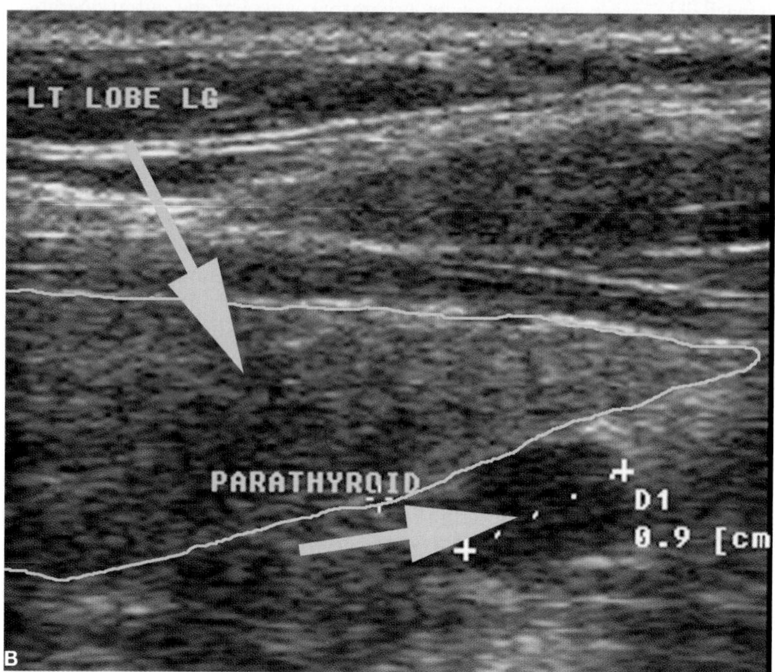

FIGURE 78.14 Ultrasound views of parathyroid adenomas. (*A*) Saggital image of the upper pole of the right lobe of the thyroid gland, demonstrating a hypoechoic parathyroid adenoma posterior to the thyroid parenchyma. (*B*) Saggital image of the lower pole of the lower pole of the left lobe of the thyroid gland with an adjacent hypoechoic parathyroid adenoma measuring 9 mm in greatest dimension.

imaging that technetium-thallium scanning, which was formerly used, does not provide.

High-resolution ultrasound examination of the neck has been used increasingly for localization of abnormal parathyroid tissue, particularly when it is available for use by the clinician. The current machines scan at high frequencies (10 to 13 MHz) that allow demonstration of small abnormalities in the neck (Fig. 78.14). The examination is best done by a clinician in real time, as that allows the most complete assessment of the neck, rather than scans performed by a technician for later review of still pictures by the physician. The sensitivity of cervical ultrasound for abnormal parathyroid glands is about the same as for sestamibi scanning. Ultrasonography is an operator-dependent technique. It is rapid and relatively inexpensive and can direct fine-needle aspiration for cytologic confirmation and immunoassay for PTH.

In patients with persistent or recurrent hyperparathyroidism, preoperative imaging is important to guide the exploration. High-resolution real-time ultrasonography, computed tomography (CT), magnetic resonance imaging (MRI), and sestamibi scanning all appear to have comparable sensitivities of 50% to 60%.[20–22] The results of these examinations may be less successful at centers without significant experience in their use.

Computed tomography is more expensive but less operator-dependent than ultrasonography. It clearly is superior in identifying deeper structures and for examining the retrosternal mediastinum. MRI is considerably more expensive than CT and has not been shown to be superior. Most surgeons prefer to have results of two or more imaging tests that confirm an abnormality before exploration in the reoperative setting.

Treatment

Indications for Surgery

Generally, the only practical therapeutic option is surgery. Nephrolithiasis, bone disease, and neuromuscular symptoms all respond well to surgical intervention. In contrast, surgery in patients with renal failure, hypertension, and psychiatric symptoms is not so uniformly successful, although it benefits some patients and is usually indicated in all except those at highest risk. The question of how to manage the large group of patients with apparently asymptomatic disease requires particularly careful consideration.

Management of Asymptomatic Hyperparathyroidism

A large proportion of patients with the diagnosis of hyperparathyroidism are minimally symptomatic or asymptomatic. The appropriate treatment for these patients remains controversial. Although little evidence indicates that irreversible complications, such as renal failure, eventually develop in patients with asymptomatic mild disease, the natural history of the disease remains incompletely defined. Many of the manifestations of this disease may go unrecognized until they are corrected surgically. Still unanswered is the question of how much asymptomatic disease may contribute to generalized osteopenia in this predominantly postmenopausal female population.

One study followed a group of 142 asymptomatic patients without operation.[23] At the end of the 10-year study, more than 20% of the patients had required surgery for an increase in serum calcium to above 11 mg/dL or for specific complications attributable to the disease. Another 20% were lost to or declined follow-up. The remaining patients either died of unrelated causes or had persistent asymptomatic disease. The authors concluded that because of the large percentage (about 40%) of patients who either required operation or were lost to follow-up, they could not reliably recommend conservative management.

A more recent report detailed the 10-year natural history of 121 patients with asymptomatic hyperparathyroidism.[10] Operation was recommended for those in whom symptoms or findings developed, according to the guidelines of the National Institutes of Health Consensus Conference (see later). During the monitoring period, indications for operation developed in 27% of the patients, and biochemical normalization and increased bone mass were observed in those who underwent surgery. However, although the patients who did not undergo operative correction continued to have biochemical abnormalities, renal stones or fractures did not develop in any of them. These data confirm the impression of most clinicians that mild hyperparathyroidism rarely takes a precipitously worsening clinical course; thus the risks and discomforts of management must remain appropriate to the disease.

In October 1990, a National Institutes of Health Consensus Development Conference reviewed the available evidence regarding the management of asymptomatic primary hyperparathyroidism.[24] After interval developments, a panel of experts reconvened in 2002, and revisited this issue.[17] The panel agreed that operation is the indicated treatment for all patients with symptoms; however, they recognized a subgroup of patients who have no symptoms attributable to hyperparathyroidism, and their conclusions included several indications for surgical intervention in these asymptomatic patients (Table 78.10).

The panel mandated close (every 6 months) follow-up for those patients not treated by operation. In addition, they recommended surgery for cases in which medical surveillance is neither desirable nor suitable, such as when a patient requests surgery, consistent follow-up is unlikely, coexistent illness complicates management, or a patient is younger than age 50 years.

This remains an area of considerable controversy, and complete resolution of the question requires a randomized, controlled trial. The complication rate of operation by an experienced surgeon is very low. Within a short period, the financial cost of medical follow-up exceeds that of treatment by operation. Based on these considerations, most patients should undergo operation, and those who do not must be closely followed.

TABLE 78.10 INDICATIONS/CONTRAINDICATIONS

NATIONAL INSTITUTES OF HEALTH CONSENSUS DEVELOPMENT CONFERENCE'S INDICATIONS FOR SURGICAL INTERVENTION IN PATIENTS WITH ASYMPTOMATIC PRIMARY HYPERPARATHYROIDISM

- Markedly elevated serum calcium (>1.0 mg/dL above normal)
- History of an episode of life-threatening hypercalcemia
- Reduced creatinine clearance
- Presence of one or more kidney stones detected by abdominal radiography
- Markedly elevated 24-hour urinary calcium excretion
- Substantially reduced bone mass as determined by direct measurement (dual energy X-ray absorptiometry T-score <−2.5)

ENDOCRINE

Principles of Surgical Correction

Although neck exploration for hyperparathyroidism may be straightforward, it sometimes becomes an arduous procedure requiring considerable patience because of the variability in both the location and the number of diseased glands. Persistent hyperparathyroidism and the necessity for reexploration can usually be avoided by a meticulous initial procedure. Reoperation is predictably more difficult than the initial operation, and the risks for damage to the recurrent laryngeal nerves and hypoparathyroidism are greater during reoperation.

It is essential that the surgeon be confident of the preoperative diagnosis and prospectively discuss the procedure with the patient. The potential complications of damage to either the recurrent laryngeal nerve or the superior laryngeal nerve and the development of hypocalcemia require discussion. Likewise, the possibility of an unsuccessful initial operation must be explained, and the patient should recognize that reexploration, including median sternotomy, may be required. Although alternatives to full neck exploration are often now applied, no patient should be explored by a surgeon who is unfamiliar with the principles and techniques of the conventional full neck exploration.

For a full neck exploration, the patient is placed under general anesthesia with a roll beneath the shoulders and the neck extended. The neck is opened through a transverse incision overlying the thyroid isthmus, and the platysma is similarly divided. Superior and inferior flaps are developed. The strap muscles are separated in the midline and retracted laterally; division is unnecessary. One lobe of the thyroid is chosen and rotated medially. Important landmarks include the tracheoesophageal groove, the recurrent laryngeal nerve, the inferior and superior thyroid arteries, and the middle thyroid vein (Fig. 78.15). In most patients, the nerve lies in the tracheoesophageal groove or

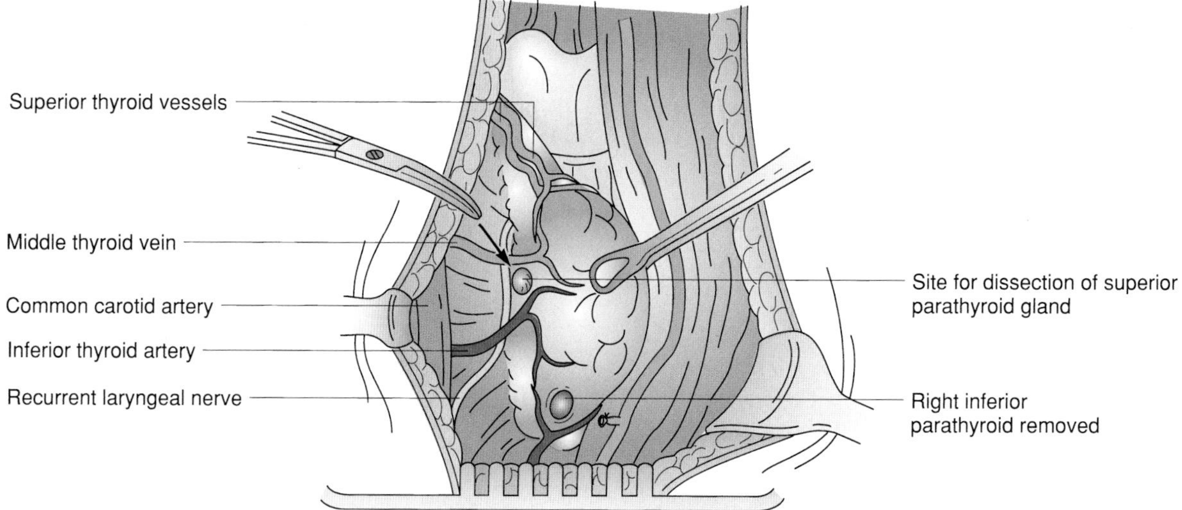

FIGURE 78.15 Lateral view of the right side of the neck after rotation of the thyroid lobe. The important anatomic landmarks are emphasized.

just laterally. Occasionally, it may be situated more anteriorly. Uncommonly, it may originate directly from the vagus without passing around the right subclavian artery. Both these variations make the recurrent nerve more susceptible to injury. The external branch of the superior laryngeal nerve, which innervates the cricothyroid muscle, usually lies medial to the superior thyroid vessels and should be carefully preserved.

For a full neck exploration, all four glands should be identified at the initial exploration because of the possibility of multiple-gland disease. Supernumerary glands may be present and should be sought at the initial procedure. Although frozen section has not been helpful in differentiating diseased from normal glands, it is generally reliable for confirming the presence or absence of parathyroid tissue. Small, thin biopsy specimens are sharply incised from the gland, with extreme care taken to avoid damaging its delicate blood supply. Most surgeons use frozen section selectively to confirm suspected abnormal parathyroid tissue or to document difficult or confusing situations.[25]

The upper glands are usually located far dorsally on the surface of the thyroid lobe at the level of the upper two thirds of the gland. The lower glands are less constant and may be located anywhere from well above the thyroid to the anterior mediastinum. The lower glands are most typically in the region where the thyrothymic ligament attaches to the lower pole of the thyroid lobe. If the inferior glands cannot be localized, the thymic pedicle should be carefully examined and mobilized. Because of their common embryologic origin, the inferior gland is frequently associated with the thymic remnant. Parathyroid glands within the mediastinum sometimes can be removed by mobilizing the thymus through the cervical incision. If this technique is unsuccessful in identifying the parathyroid gland, the thyroid lobe on the side of the missing gland is mobilized and palpated. Intraoperative ultrasonographic examination may identify an intrathyroidal parathyroid gland. As a last resort, excision of the thyroid lobe may be indicated.

If after meticulous exploration of all these areas three or four parathyroid glands have been identified, none of which is enlarged, most surgeons would favor terminating the operation.

Limited Surgical Exploration

With the availability of accurate preoperative localization methods, it has become routinely possible to identify abnormal parathyroid glands prior to operation for most patients. This allows the surgeon to know where to start the exploration. Then, intraoperative PTH measurement can be used to confirm removal of all hyperfunctioning parathyroid tissue, that is, when to stop the operation. This strategy of directed, limited neck exploration is applicable to about 75% of initial parathyroid explorations, and has about the same success rate as full neck exploration.[26–30] The preoperative localization can be done by either ^{99m}technetium sestamibi nuclear medicine scan or by high-resolution ultrasound. The intraoperative PTH measurement is first assessed at the outset of the procedure, and/or immediately preceding parathyroid gland excision (the pre-excision baseline). Blood samples are obtained at time intervals after parathyroid gland resection. A decrease of the PTH level by 50% from the higher of the incision or pre-excision baseline predicts long-term normocalcemia.[28] Other investigators use more sensitive criteria for the detection of multigland disease, including reduction of the PTH level into the normal range and kinetic assessments of the rate of PTH decrease.[31] This increase in sensitivity comes with the cost of decreased specificity, however. Blood samples can be obtained either centrally or peripherally.[32–34]

The limited nature of this operative approach also makes it easier to perform this operation under regional or local anesthetic in an ambulatory setting. However, because of the possibility of multiple gland disease or inaccurate preoperative localization, all surgeons undertaking this approach should also be skilled in the full neck exploration for hyperparathyroidism.[33,35,36]

Extent of Resection

The operative procedure performed has been based on the number of enlarged glands identified for full neck explorations, however, with the use of intraoperative PTH monitoring, it has become clear that not all enlarged parathyroid glands are hyperfunctioning.[14,37] In contrast, nearly all hyperfunctioning glands are enlarged and hypercellular. The full neck exploration experience has demonstrated that removing all enlarged glands is a highly successful approach to curing hyperparathyroidism, and in the absence of PTH monitoring, this remains an accepted approach. Typically, single-gland disease has been treated by simple excision, whereas any combination of two- or three-gland enlargement is treated by resecting the diseased tissue and leaving the normal glands in place. The question of whether two- or three-gland enlargement implies the presence of disease in all glands (hyperplasia) has not been resolved. If one gland is large and the remaining three are normal in size, resection of the single parathyroid cures virtually all patients. Of 76 patients with two- or three-gland disease treated by excising the large glands and leaving the normal glands, only eight (10.5%) had recurrent hypercalcemia, which tended to be mild (follow-up of 12 to 140 months postoperatively). This approach seems satisfactory in most patients.[38]

Treating patients with four-gland disease has been more difficult. In many of these patients, the disease occurs as a component of one of the familial syndromes, particularly MEN-I. Patients with four-gland parathyroid hyperplasia can be treated by subtotal parathyroidectomy (removing three and a half glands) or by total parathyroidectomy with autotransplantation of some parathyroid tissue into the nondominant forearm. Both operations depend on meticulous identification of all parathyroid tissue for adequate results. The putative advantage of the subtotal parathyroidectomy is that it leaves the remaining parathyroid tissue with its native blood supply. Total parathyroidectomy with autograft has the advantage of removing all the abnormal parathyroid tissue from the neck and placing it in a site where reoperation for recurrent hyperparathyroidism is simpler.

The reported incidence of recurrent hypercalcemia after subtotal parathyroidectomy for nonfamilial parathyroid hyperplasia is 0 to 16%; the incidence of permanent hypoparathyroidism is 4% to 5%. Total parathyroidectomy with autograft is associated with a similar risk for permanent hypoparathyroidism in the sporadic setting (5%) and a higher reported risk for recurrent hypercalcemia (20%). Reoperation for recurrent hypercalcemia is greatly simplified by the approach of total parathyroidectomy with autotransplantation. Thus, given the current data, sporadic parathyroid hyperplasia can be acceptably treated by either operation.[38–40]In patients with MEN-I, the disease is not the same as sporadic hyperplasia. Rather, defects in the MEN-1 gene cause multiple parathyroid adenomas that arise independently over the life of the patient.[41] The operative results reflect this independent capability of all parathyroid tissue in these patients to become neoplastic. The hypercalcemia recurrence rate is 26% to 36% with long-term follow-up after subtotal parathyroidectomy, and similar after total parathyroidectomy with autograft. However, the incidence of permanent hypoparathyroidism after autograft in MEN-1 is also significant (reported as high as 46%). While both approaches are currently accepted, most experienced centers now advocate subtotal parathyroidectomy as the initial operation in MEN-1 hyperparathyroidism, and anticipate that recurrent disease is likely, manageable, and less problematic than permanent hypocalcemia.[42–46]

Technique of Parathyroid Autotransplantation

The parathyroid gland is sliced into 15 to 20 pieces and autografted into a forearm muscle bed. The sites are marked with silk sutures. This location permits easy subsequent access under local anesthesia if recurrent hypercalcemia develops. Function of the autograft is documented by (a) normocalcemia, with the autograft as the only source of PTH, (b) by measuring higher concentrations of hormone in the antecubital vein draining the graft bed than in the corresponding vein in the opposite arm, or (c) "transient parathyroidectomy," by placing a venous occlusive tourniquet on the arm above the graft, and measuring changes over several minutes in the PTH levels drawn from the contralateral arm.[47] Lack of function is unusual outside of the MEN-1 patients; hypoparathyroidism develops in about 5% of patients. Glands should also be viably frozen in dimethyl sulfoxide and serum. If in the postoperative period it becomes clear that the patient is aparathyroid, the cryopreserved tissue can be reimplanted under local anesthesia.

Special Situations

Persistent or Recurrent Hyperparathyroidism

Persistent hyperparathyroidism occurs in fewer than 5% of patients after exploration by an experienced surgeon. Most commonly, it is the result of a single diseased gland remaining in the neck or the mediastinum. Recurrent disease develops after an interval of normocalcemia and may be the result of regrowth of diseased tissue, implantation from a tumor broken at the initial procedure, or even recurrent parathyroid carcinoma.

In the evaluation of these patients, it is essential to document that the initial diagnosis was correct. Familial hypocalciuric hypercalcemia should be excluded by measuring urinary calcium excretion.

Reviewing the original operative notes and pathology reports may provide clues to the position of missed glands. The locations of parathyroid tumors not found at the initial operation but identified on subsequent exploration in one large series are shown in Fig. 78.16.

It is generally agreed that localization studies do have a place in the management of recurrent disease. Noninvasive methods are used first, and if these are unsuccessful in identifying the diseased gland, selective angiography and venous sampling for PTH are used. The utility of the techniques vary across institutions, dependent on local experience, expertise and preference. Selective angiography localizes 50% to 80% of parathyroid glands that cannot be detected by any other modality. Venous sampling may also be helpful in some patients, although interpretation can be complicated by the collateralization that occurs postoperatively. Because it provides no direct image but indicates the side of the neck where the hyperfunctioning tissue is located, it may help to direct the exploration to one or the other side of the neck. Both these invasive radiographic techniques require considerable expertise. Transient cortical blindness, transverse myelitis, and cerebrovascular accidents have all been reported as complications of arteriography. Angiographic ablation of mediastinal parathyroid tissue with large doses of ionic contrast has been successful in selected patients. This technique may be used in some patients with mediastinal parathyroid adenomas who

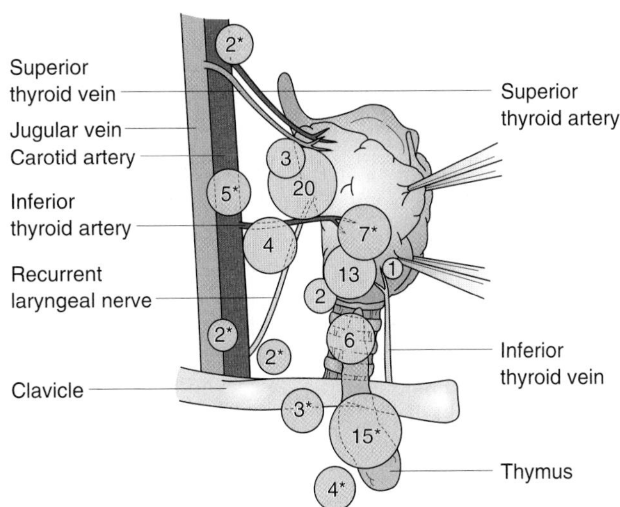

FIGURE 78.16 Location of parathyroid tumors missed on initial exploration but identified on subsequent operation. (After Jaskowiak N, Norton JA, Alexander HR, et al. A prospective trial evaluating a standard approach to reoperation for missed parathyroid adenoma. *Ann Surg* 1996;224:308–320.)

are at increased surgical risk and who have other functional parathyroid tissue remaining.[48]

Surgical reexploration can be a difficult procedure. The neck should almost always be reexplored first. If the thymic remnant has not already been removed, it should be excised at this time. Two adjunctive techniques, intraoperative ultrasonography to locate glands and intraoperative measurement of PTH to document the adequacy of resection, may be useful in patients undergoing operation for persistent disease.[49]

If the gland is not identified in the neck by means of the maneuvers described, the mediastinum is examined; most surgeons do this only if there is imaging evidence of disease in the mediastinum, rather than blind explorations. Median sternotomy and exploration are necessary in only 1% to 2% of patients with hyperparathyroidism. Successful transcervical mediastinal exploration is sometimes possible with use of the Cooper thymectomy retractor, a substernal retractor that permits more extensive mediastinal exploration and thymectomy through a cervical incision.[50] Any remaining thymic tissue is first isolated and examined. Inferior parathyroid glands most commonly migrate into the anterior mediastinum. If the results of this exploration are negative, the area posterior and lateral to the trachea is then explored. The location of superior parathyroid glands may be as far posterior as the esophagus and as far superior as the pharynx.

Surgical reexploration is successful in experienced hands in 60% to 80% of cases. The incidence of complications is increased. Unilateral recurrent nerve injury occurs in 5% to 10% of patients postoperatively, and permanent hypoparathyroidism in 10% to 20% of patients. Cryopreservation of excised tissue is an important component of the management of these patients because it allows later autotransplantation if the patient becomes hypoparathyroid postoperatively. The risks of these complications must be clearly outweighed by the clinical improvement in patients with advanced disease. Reoperation in asymptomatic patients with mild disease is controversial.

Hypercalcemic Crisis

Occasionally, patients with hyperparathyroidism become acutely hypercalcemic with severe symptoms. The pathogenesis appears to involve a vicious cycle of uncontrolled PTH secretion followed by hypercalcemia and secondary polyuria, dehydration, and reduced renal function, which exacerbate the hypercalcemia. Serum calcium concentrations may reach the range of 16 to 20 mg/dL, and the syndrome is manifested by rapidly developing muscle weakness, nausea and vomiting, lethargy, fatigue, and even coma. If the diagnosis of hyperparathyroidism is in question, ultrasonography or CT may help to identify the enlarged gland.

Definitive treatment involves resecting the diseased parathyroid tissue, which is almost always curative. Generally, however, it is safer to lower the serum calcium level before operation.

Hyperparathyroidism in Pregnancy

Hyperparathyroidism in pregnancy is a rare disorder that not only causes hypercalcemia in the mother but also is associated with increased morbidity and mortality rates in the fetus. Even the newborn is at risk for the development of tetany. The risk for fetal complications is higher if the hyperparathyroidism is left untreated. The mother should undergo operation in the second trimester.[51–54]

Neonatal Hyperparathyroidism

Neonatal hyperparathyroidism occurs in infants who are homozygous for a mutation of the calcium-sensing receptor and is characterized by hypotonia, poor feeding, constipation, and respiratory distress.[6] Each parent of these children is affected by familial hypocalciuric hypercalcemia. The 1-year survival rate in children with symptoms is less than 50%, and patients without symptoms appear to have significant bone disease. Total parathyroidectomy with autotransplantation is the treatment of choice.[55]

Secondary Hyperparathyroidism

Secondary hyperparathyroidism develops as a consequence of chronic renal failure. Phosphate retention and hyperphosphatemia reduce the serum calcium levels. This effect is aggravated by the reduction in 1-hydroxylase activity in the kidney, necessary for the activation of vitamin D_3. The secondary increase in PTH levels to compensate for the hypocalcemic effects is exacerbated by aluminum accumulation in bone. Aluminum, present both in the dialysate water and in phosphate-binding medications, contributes to the osteomalacia (renal osteodystrophy) that develops in all these patients after several years of dialysis. Therapy includes controlling the hyperphosphatemia with dietary restriction and phosphate-binding gels, calcium supplementation orally and in the dialysate bath, correction of acidosis, administration of vitamin D sterol, and reduction in aluminum intake in both the dialysate and the diet. Therapy should be initiated carefully because metastatic soft-tissue calcification may occur. Indications for surgical therapy include persistent, symptomatic hypercalcemia that cannot be controlled medically, particularly in prospective renal transplant patients; bony pain and abnormal fractures; ectopic calcification; and intractable pruritus. Subtotal parathyroidectomy and total parathyroidectomy with heterotopic autotransplantation both appear to be acceptable options, although reexploration for recurrent disease is less complicated after total parathyroidectomy with autotransplantation. Parathyroidectomy can actually enhance aluminum deposition, so any excess should be corrected preoperatively through chelation.

Parathyroid Carcinoma

Parathyroid carcinoma is a rare condition, accounting for less than 1% of all cases of hyperparathyroidism. Histologic criteria remain controversial, and the diagnosis is securely made only on the basis of local invasion or distant metastases. In comparison with patients with benign disease, these patients tend to be somewhat younger and more symptomatic. In contrast to the marked female predominance in benign disease, the male-to-female ratio in carcinoma is equal. Serum calcium, PTH, and alkaline phosphatase levels are relatively more elevated, and patients often have an elevated level of human chorionic gonadotropin. Patients may have manifestations of both renal and bone disease. The affected gland is palpable in almost half of patients.

Initial treatment should include radical resection of the involved gland, ipsilateral thyroid lobe, and regional lymph nodes. Neither chemotherapy nor radiation therapy has shown any benefit. If the disease recurs, resection should be attempted because without treatment these patients usually succumb to uncontrolled hypercalcemia. The long-term prognosis is poor, and the opportunity for survival depends on complete initial resection.[56]

MULTIPLE ENDOCRINE NEOPLASIA

Although these familial disorders are typically characterized by a predisposition to the development of tumors of multiple endocrine organs, the parathyroid is characteristically involved in two of them. The disorders are all inherited in an autosomal dominant fashion, and the tumors tend to be multicentric. The tumors may be benign or malignant and may occur metachronously or synchronously. MEN-I is characterized by the concurrence of parathyroid hyperplasia, pancreatic islet cell tumors, and pituitary adenomas. MEN-IIA consists of medullary thyroid carcinoma (MTC), pheochromocytoma, and parathyroid hyperplasia. MEN-2B includes MTC, pheochromocytoma, mucosal neuromas, and a distinctive marfanoid habitus. Together these syndromes encompass much of the spectrum of endocrine neoplasia.

Pathogenesis

A unifying hypothesis for the MEN syndromes was offered by Pearse[57] based on both embryologic and cytochemical studies. He suggested that these tumors arise in cells that embryologically derive from the neural crest and are characterized by amine precursor uptake and decarboxylase activity. According to this theory, some defect in the development of the neural crest might explain the development of multicentric tumors in multiple organs. Although the theory could account for the development of MTC, pheochromocytomas, pituitary tumors, and the widespread nervous system hypertrophy of MEN-IIB, the endocrine cells of the parathyroid and pancreas do not appear to be of neural crest origin. Another unifying hypothesis, developed subsequently, whereby a tumor in one organ secretes endocrine products that secondarily stimulate neoplasia in other glands, has not been accepted. Although some evidence has suggested the presence of a mitogenic factor in the serum of patients with MEN-I, direct attempts to define the pathophysiology have not proved rewarding. As a result, investigators in this area have taken a different approach, attempting to map the diseased gene through modern molecular genetic techniques.

The genetic abnormality in MEN-I has been identified and described in detail.[58,59] As a tumor-suppressor gene, the first mutation is inherited and becomes unmasked only when a second mutation, in some cases a deletion, develops in susceptible tissues. The resulting complete loss of the tumor suppressor allows neoplasia to develop. The occurrence of multiple second mutations explains the characteristic multicentric involvement of these diseases. Direct genetic testing is now available for some families with known mutations.

Mutations of the *RET* protooncogene are the cause of MEN-IIA.[60,61] Genetic testing is now available to identify affected family members and provide the opportunity for early treatment of MTC in affected persons.

Clinical Features and Management of Multiple Endocrine Neoplasia Type I

Characteristically, MEN-I develops in the third and fourth decades, without any gender predilection.[62] The gene is transmitted with nearly complete penetrance, and autopsy studies suggest that all three organs are affected in more than 90% of patients. The phenotype varies, however; more than 90% of patients have hyperparathyroidism, but evidence of islet cell neoplasms (30% to 80%) and pituitary tumors (15% to 50%) is less common. The cause of death in carriers of the MEN-I mutation is related to MEN-I in about 45% of patients and often caused by malignant islet cell or carcinoid tumors.[63]

Parathyroid Disease

Hypercalcemia secondary to hyperparathyroidism is usually the first biochemical abnormality detected in MEN-I and represents the best screening study for members of affected kindreds until direct genetic screening is available. Many of these patients are asymptomatic and have relatively mild hypercalcemia. When symptoms do develop, they typically involve the urinary tract rather than the skeleton.

Typically, the patients have four-gland disease, which may be particularly difficult to manage. The disease is characterized by metachronous development of multiple parathyroid adenomas.[41] There is no curative operation; the two accepted approaches (subtotal parathyroidectomy and total parathyroidectomy with autograft) each have faults (see earlier). Over time, the subtotal parathyroidectomy approach is becoming the preferred choice by most surgeons.

Pancreatic Tumors

In patients with pancreatic tumors, multicentric and diffuse hyperplasia of the pancreatic islets may occur in areas distant from any grossly evident tumor. The management of these tumors is controversial because although some patients have aggressive, malignant tumors, many patients have a fairly benign course. No reliable criteria are available to detect malignant tumors. Tumor size is often cited as a useful marker of prognosis, but substantial overlap has been noted between the sizes of primary benign and malignant tumors (Fig. 78.17).[64] Because of the difficulty in identifying the more aggressive subset, some authors have chosen a liberal policy of early operation to try to prevent metastasis and death.[65,66] The detection of these tumors can also be difficult; testing with meal stimulation can be used if an intervention plan supports the diagnosis at this early phase.[67] Some evidence indicates that measuring serum concentrations of pancreatic polypeptide may provide a general screening measure for a variety of islet cell tumors.[68] Pancreatic tumors are typically multicentric and frequently malignant. Somatostatin receptor scintigraphy can be a useful imaging technique to demonstrate the extent of tumor[69] (Fig. 78.18).

Gastrinoma is the most common functional tumor in MEN-I; typically, a severe ulcer diathesis (Zollinger-Ellison syndrome) develops that is associated with secretory diarrhea. Serum gastrin levels are usually markedly elevated (>100 pg/mL); when levels are equivocal (250 to 1,000 pg/mL), provocative testing with secretin (2 m/kg) may be useful. An absolute serum gastrin

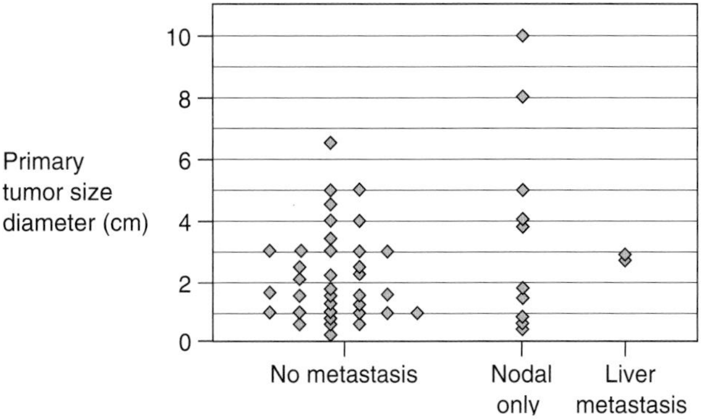

FIGURE 78.17 Scatter plot of largest primary tumor size versus metastatic status in 43 patients with pancreatic islet cell tumors associated with multiple endocrine neoplasia type I. Each point represents a single patient. Tumor size is not correlated with the presence of liver or lymph node metastases. (From Lowney JK, Frisella MM, Lairmore TC, et al. Islet cell tumor metastasis in multiple endocrine neoplasia type I: correlation with primary tumor size. *Surgery* 1998; 124:1043–1049.)

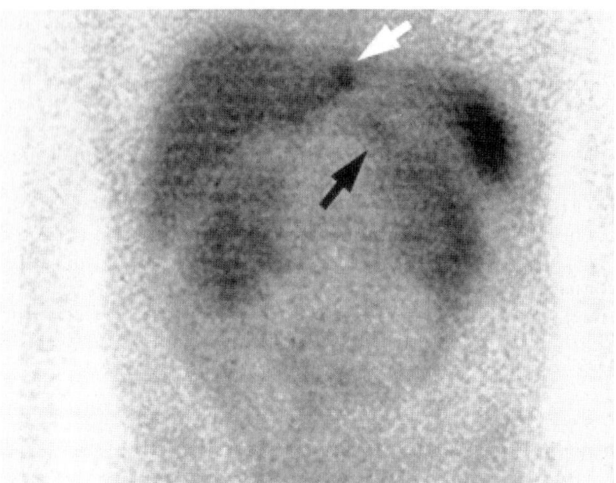

FIGURE 78.18 Somatostatin receptor scintigraphy in a patient with multiple endocrine neoplasia type I. This scintiscan detected an otherwise unrecognized metastasis to the left lateral segment of the liver (*white arrow*), which was resected along with the small primary tumor (*black arrow*).

increase of 200 pg/mL is diagnostic. The primary tumors are often in the submucosa of the duodenal wall.

Biochemical cure of these gastrinomas is almost never possible, as it is in sporadic gastrinomas, although exploration can reduce the need for antisecretory medications and may reduce the risk for liver metastasis. Histamine 2-receptor antagonists or proton pump inhibitors are effective in controlling acid secretion, although very high doses may be necessary; the malignant disease is often indolent. Total gastrectomy is no longer ever necessary to eliminate acid secretion.[70,71]

Insulinoma is the next most common pancreatic neoplasm. These tumors are usually small and multicentric. Patients present with a history of sweating, dizziness, confusion, and syncope, consistent with neuroglycopenia; these symptoms are relieved by consuming carbohydrates. The diagnosis is verified by documenting fasting hypoglycemia associated with inappropriately elevated plasma insulin levels. Preoperative tumor localization is usually achieved by a combination of CT and arteriography. Calcium is injected into various pancreatic arteries and plasma insulin levels in the hepatic vein plasma are measured to detect a gradient after the injection of specific pancreatic arteries.

Because the available medical therapy for insulinoma is limited, patients are treated operatively. Lesions in the tail of the gland can be enucleated if they are small; however, distal pancreatectomy carries little morbidity. Tumors of the head can usually be enucleated, so that pancreaticoduodenectomy can be avoided. In patients with malignant disease, metastases may respond to streptozocin, diazoxide, verapamil, or octreotide may successfully reduce insulin secretion and control symptoms. A diet of complex carbohydrates can also help stabilize serum glucose levels in the hyperinsulinemic patient.[70,71] Other islet cell lesions occur only rarely in association with MEN-I.

Pituitary Adenomas

Prolactin-secreting tumors occur most commonly in this setting, although Cushing disease or acromegaly develops in an occasional patient. Symptoms may result from compression of the optic chiasm, which produces bitemporal hemianopsia, or from prolactin excess, which produces amenorrhea and galactorrhea in female patients and hypogonadism in male patients.

Bromocriptine inhibits prolactin secretion and shrinks many prolactinomas. Refractory tumors and those producing other hormones can be managed by pituitary ablation or radiation.

Other Tumors

MEN-I is associated much less frequently with adrenocortical tumors and benign thyroid adenomas. Lipomas and carcinoid tumors may also occur.

Clinical Features and Management of Multiple Endocrine Neoplasia Type II

Like MEN-I, the MEN-II syndromes are inherited in an autosomal dominant fashion with complete penetrance but variable phenotype. Bilateral MTC occurs in every affected patient. More frequently than the other syndromes, MEN-IIB may arise as a new mutation that can be transmitted to subsequent generations.

Medullary Thyroid Carcinoma

Medullary thyroid carcinoma accounts for about 10% of all thyroid malignancies, and 20% of cases occur in the familial setting of MEN-IIA, MEN-IIB, or familial non-MEN MTC. It is usually the first tumor that develops in these patients and typically appears in the second or third decade. Tumors are virtually always bilateral and develop in multiple areas of the middle and upper portions of the thyroid lobe (Fig. 78.19). Occasionally, in young people, a diffuse proliferation of parafollicular C cells, termed *C-cell hyperplasia*, is present without frankly invasive carcinoma.[72] This finding is highly suggestive of one of the familial MTC syndromes.

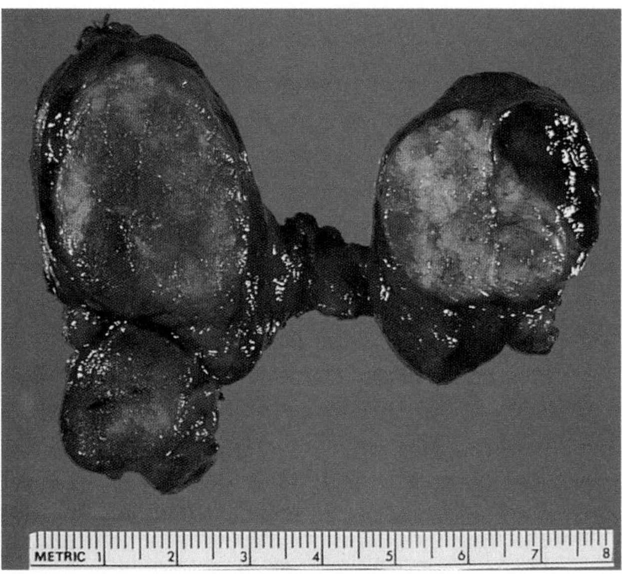

FIGURE 78.19 Medullary thyroid carcinoma. Coronal section of a total thyroid resection shows bilateral involvement by a firm, pale tumor. (From Rubin E, Farber JL. *Pathology*, 3rd ed. Philadelphia: Lippincott Williams & Wilkins, 1999.)

Patients typically present with a neck mass and may have hoarseness, dysphagia, or palpable cervical adenopathy. MTC may produce a variety of hormones, including calcitonin, adrenocorticotropic hormone, prostaglandin, and serotonin. The hypercalcitoninemia is often asymptomatic, although severe diarrhea can develop.

By detecting minimal elevations of plasma calcitonin, it is possible to diagnose MTC at a clinically occult stage.[73] Basal plasma calcitonin levels in normal subjects are in the range of 30 to 100 pg/mL. An increase to levels of 150 to 200 pg/mL occurs, however, after the administration of the potent secretagogues calcium and pentagastrin. The plasma calcitonin levels of patients with MTC show striking increases (>1,000 pg/mL) after provocative testing, so that they can be identified readily. Patients with occult disease may have only minimally elevated basal calcitonin levels that increase in response to secretagogues. The combined infusion of calcium and pentagastrin was the most effective screening test for familial MTC before genetic testing became available. By means of provocative testing in kindred members at risk for disease, MTC was diagnosed at a preclinical stage, and a greater percentage of these patients were cured by surgical therapy. With genetic testing now available, prophylactic thyroidectomy to prevent the development of MTC is possible for all affected people.

Postoperatively, the presence of residual MTC can be readily detected by provocative testing. Recent reports have suggested that meticulous reoperation in patients with recurrent or persistently elevated plasma calcitonin levels postoperatively, including mediastinal dissection on occasion, can normalize elevated plasma calcitonin levels and apparently cure many of them.[74] For the patient with unresectable metastases, few therapeutic options are available. Neither radiation nor chemotherapy is of significant benefit.

The clinical course of patients with the MEN-II syndromes is determined primarily by the status of their MTC. In the setting of MEN-IIA, the tumors are often indolent and survival prolonged, even in the presence of metastatic disease. By contrast, the tumors in patients with MEN-IIB occur at an earlier age and are generally more aggressive neoplasms. Patients may succumb to the disease at a young age. As a consequence of this aggressiveness, the size of kindreds with the disease is typically small, and usually only a few generations are affected.

Pheochromocytoma

Pheochromocytomas are usually detected during the initial screening or follow-up of patients in whom MTC has already been diagnosed. They typically appear in the second or third decade of life, and about 80% are bilateral. Usually, pheochromocytomas are benign but multicentric, and they almost always arise in the adrenal medulla. In patients with MEN-IIA or MEN-IIB, hyperplasia of the adrenal medulla may develop first, grossly characterized by thickening of the medullary tissue in both adrenal glands.

Pheochromocytomas may be asymptomatic, but most commonly, patients have pounding frontal headaches, episodic diaphoresis, palpitations, or anxiety. Hypertension also occurs and is often episodic.

The diagnosis is made by measuring the plasma concentration of metanephrines.[75–78] Patients with MEN-IIA or MEN-IIB and MTC should be evaluated for pheochromocytoma before they undergo thyroidectomy. If a patient is found to have both lesions, adrenalectomy should be performed first, followed by neck exploration in 1 to 2 weeks. If urinary excretion rates are equivocal, CT of the abdomen can identify lesions 1 cm or larger, and sometimes hyperplasia is recognized. Scintigraphy with ^{131}I-metaiodobenzylguanidine is used because this agent, which is similar to norepinephrine, is taken up and stored in neurotransmitter vesicles. Normal glands are not demonstrated, whereas about 90% of pheochromocytomas can be imaged. MRI is also sensitive for pheochromocytomas and has the advantage of allowing the differentiation of pheochromocytoma from benign adenoma based on T_2-weighted imaging characteristics.

Preoperatively, α-adrenergic blockade is induced with phenoxybenzamine. β-Adrenergic blockade with propranolol may be necessary if tachyarrhythmia subsequently develops, but it should not be initiated until after α-adrenergic blockade because of the risk for unopposed vasoconstriction (termed *unopposed-α effect*). Intraoperative hypertension is controlled with a vasodilator, such as sodium nitroprusside or phentolamine. The abdomen is explored through a bilateral subcostal incision or, more typically, with a laparoscope.[79] Bilateral pheochromocytomas are treated by bilateral adrenalectomy. In patients with MEN-IIA or MEN-IIB and a unilateral pheochromocytoma, only the diseased adrenal gland is removed. In about 30% of patients treated in this manner, a tumor eventually develops in the opposite gland. In the remaining patients, this approach avoids the need for glucocorticoid and mineralocorticoid replacement and the risk for addisonian crisis.[80] After unilateral adrenalectomy, patients are carefully screened at 6-month or 1-year intervals with plasma metanephrine measurements.

Parathyroid Disease

Hyperparathyroidism develops in about one third of patients with MEN-IIA, although it is usually asymptomatic. Occasionally, nephrolithiasis develops. Bone disease is unusual. Frequently, enlarged parathyroid glands are found at operation for MTC, although the patient is still normocalcemic. Multiglandular chief cell hyperplasia is the predominant histologic finding in MEN-IIA. Significant parathyroid disease rarely develops in MEN-IIB.[81]

Total parathyroidectomy and heterotopic autotransplantation are performed in hypercalcemic patients with MEN-IIA. In normocalcemic patients with MEN-IIA undergoing thyroidectomy for MTC, a total parathyroidectomy and heterotopic autotransplantation are performed in one session to ensure that the complete thyroidectomy does not compromise the parathyroid blood supply and to avoid reoperation in the neck for subsequent hyperparathyroidism. Evidence suggests that these patients are more easily treated, with a lower incidence of recurrent hyperparathyroidism, than patients with MEN-I.

Nonendocrine Manifestations of Multiple Endocrine Neoplasia Type IIB

In addition to MTC and pheochromocytoma, marked abnormalities of the nervous and musculoskeletal systems develop in patients with MEN-IIB. The classic phenotype is characterized by thick lips and a thin, marfanoid habitus (Fig. 78.20 A, B). The incidence of associated skeletal abnormalities is high; these include kyphosis, pectus excavatum, pes planus or cavus, and congenital dislocation of the hip. Diffuse autonomic nervous hypertrophy is another feature. Mucosal neuromas appear on the tongue (Fig. 78.20 C), eyelids, lips, and pharynx. Slit-lamp examination may reveal hypertrophied corneal nerves. Ganglioneuromatosis develops in the submucosal and myenteric plexuses of the gastrointestinal tract. Constipation is common, and radiographic findings may suggest megacolon or Hirschsprung disease.

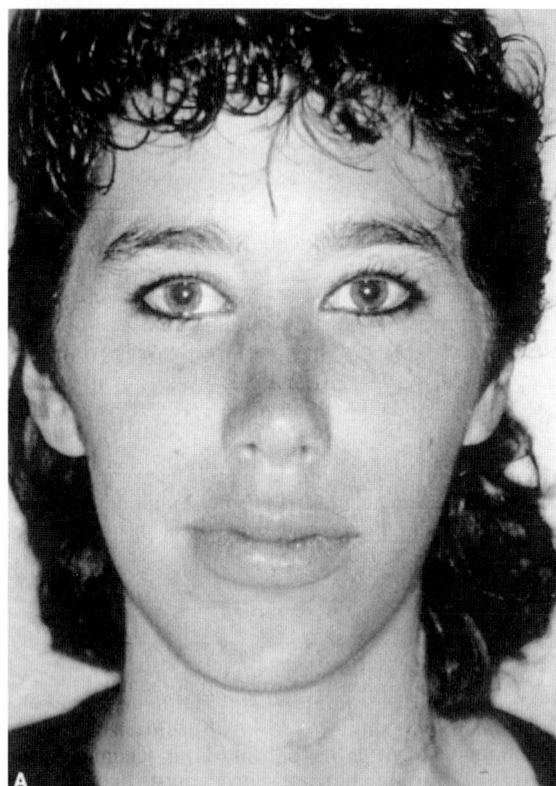

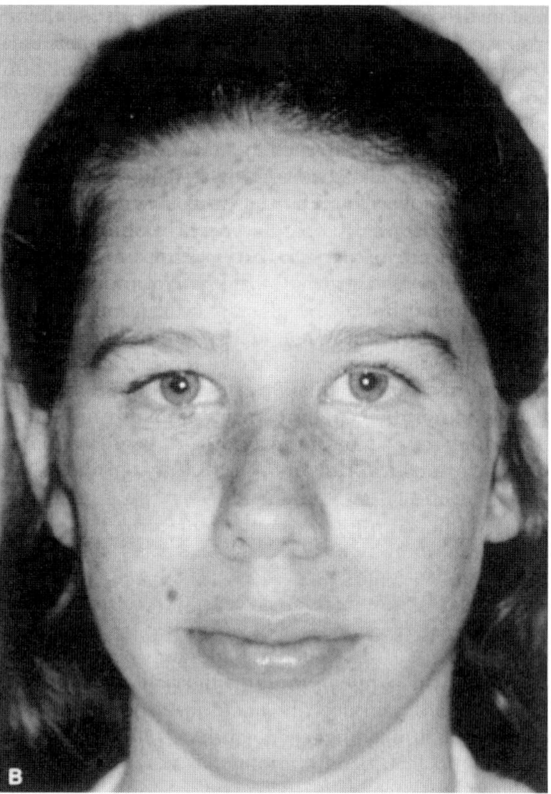

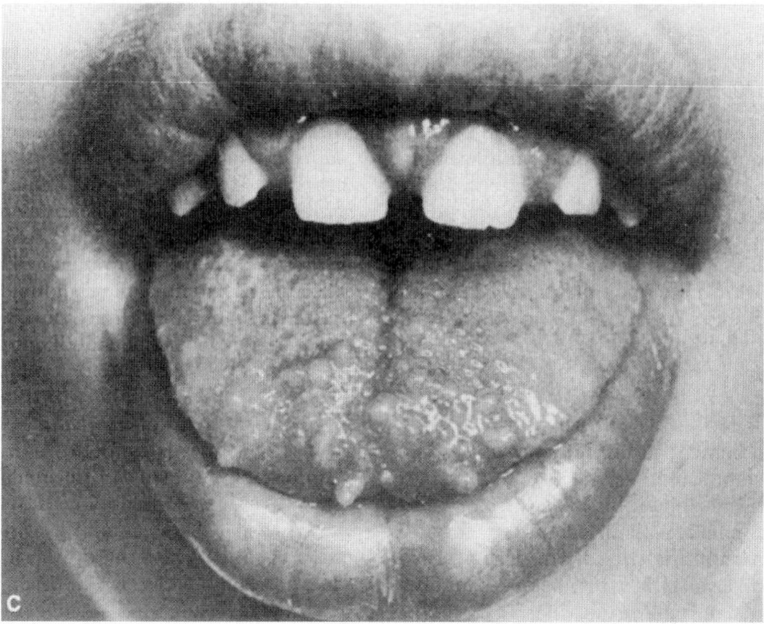

FIGURE 78.20 (*A* and *B*) Characteristic appearance of patients with multiple endocrine neoplasia type IIB, including thick lips. (*C*) Multiple mucosal neuromas on the tongue of a patient with MEN-IIB. (From Norton JA, Froome LC, Farrell FE, et al. Multiple endocrine neoplasia type 2b: the most aggressive form of medullary thyroid carcinoma. *Surg Clin North Am* 1979;59:109.)

KEY POINTS

- The normal parathyroid glands are flat, ovoid, and red-brown to yellow. Their dimensions are 5 to 7 mm × 3 to 4 mm × 0.5 to 2 mm, and they weigh between 30 and 50 mg each.
- Parathyroid hormone is the single most important hormonal regulator of calcium and phosphate metabolism in humans with direct effects on the skeleton and kidney and indirect effects on the intestine, mediated through vitamin D.
- The demonstration of an elevated plasma parathyroid hormone concentration alone does not establish the diagnosis of hyperparathyroidism; with a simultaneous elevated serum calcium level, this finding is virtually diagnostic.
- A large proportion of patients with the diagnosis of hyperparathyroidism are minimally or asymptomatic and

the appropriate treatment for these patients remains controversial.

- **It is routinely possible to identify abnormal parathyroid glands prior to operation for most patients allowing the surgeon to know where to start the exploration; intraoperative parathyroid hormone measurement can be used to confirm removal of all hyperfunctioning parathyroid tissue, that is, when to stop the operation.**

References

1. Akerstrom, G, Malmaeus J, Bergstrom R. Surgical anatomy of human parathyroid glands. *Surgery* 1984;95:14–21.
2. Mallette LE. Regulation of blood calcium in humans. *Endocrinol Metabol Clin N Am.* 1989;18:601–610.
3. Nussbaum SR. Pathophysiology and management of severe hypercalcemia. *Endocrinol Metabol Clin N Amer.* 1993;22:343–362.
4. Strewler GJ, Nissenson RA. Hypercalcemia in malignancy. West J Med. 1990;153:635–640.
5. Pollak M R, Brown EM, Chou Y-HW, et al. Mutations in the human Ca-sensing receptor gene cause familial hypocalciuric hypercalcemia and neonatal severe hyperparathyroidism. *Cell* 1993;75:1297–1303.
6. Pollak MR, ChouY-HW, Marx SJ, et al. Familial hypocalciuric hypercalcemia and neonatal severe hyperparathyroidism: effects of mutant gene dosage on phenotype. *J Clin Invest.* 1994;93:1108–1112.
7. Bilezikian JP. Management of acute hypercalcemia. *N Engl J Med.* 1992; 326:1196–1203.
8. Tohme, M. F. and Bilezikian, J. P. Hypocalcemic emergencies. *Endocrinol Metabol Clin N Amer.* 1993;22:363–375.
9. Heath H, Hodgson SF, Kennedy MA. Primary hyperparathyroidism: incidence, morbidity and potential economic impact in a community. *N Engl J Med.* 1980;302:189–193.
10. Arnold A. Molecular mechanisms of parathyroid neoplasia. *Endocrinol Metabol Clin N Am.* 1994;23:93–107.
11. Palanisamy N, Imanishi Y, Rao PH, et al. Novel chromosomal abnormalities identified by comparative genomic hybridization in parathyroid adenomas. *J Clin EndocrinolMetab.* 1998;83:1766–1770,.
12. Doherty GM, Lairmore TC, DeBenedetti MK. Multiple endocrine neoplasia type 1 parathyroid adenoma development over time. *World J Surg.* 2004;28(11):1139–1142.
13. Roth SI. Recent advances in parathyroid gland pathology. *Am J Med.* 1994;50:612–622.
14. Gauger PG. Agarwal G, England BG, et al. Intraoperative parathyroid hormone monitoring fails to detect double parathyroid adenomas: a 2-institution experience. *Surgery* 2001;130:1005–1010,.
15. Levin KE, Chew KL, Ljung BM, et al. Deoxyribonucleic acid cytometry helps identify parathyroid carcinomas. *J Clin Endocrinol Metab.* 1994; 67:779–784.
16. Heath H. Clinical spectrum of primary hyperparathyroidism: evolution with changes in medical practice and technology. *J Bone Miner Res.* 1991;6(suppl 2):S63–S70.
17. Bilezikian JP, PottsJT Jr, Fuleihan Gel H, et al. Summary statement from a workshop on asymptomatic primary hyperparathyroidism: a perspective for the 21st century. *J Clin Endocrinol Metab.* 2002;87:5353–5361.
18. Silverberg SJ, Shane E, JacobsTP, et al. A 10-year prospective study of primary hyperparathyroidism with or without parathyroid surgery. *N Engl J Med.* 1999;341:1249–1255.
19. Wells SA Jr, Leight GS, RossAJ 3rd. Primary hyperparathyroidism. *Curr Prob Surg.* 1980;17:398–463.
20. Miller DL, Doppman JL, Krudy AG, et al. Localization of parathyroid adenomas in patients who have undergone surgery. Part II. Invasive procedures. *Radiology* 1987;162:138–141.
21. Miller DL, Doppman JL, ShawkerTH, et al.. Localization of parathyroid adenomas in patients who have undergone surgery. Part I. Noninvasive imaging methods. *Radiology* 1987;162:133–137.
22. Weber CJ, Vansant J, Alazraki N, et al. Value of technetium 99m sestamibi iodine 123 imaging in reoperative parathyroid surgery. *Surgery* 1993;114:1011–1018.
23. Scholz DA, Purnell DC. Asymptomatic primary hyperparathyroidism: 10 year prospective study. *Mayo Clin Proc.* 1981;56: 473–478..
24. Potts JT Jr, Ackerman IP, BarkerCF, et al. Diagnosis and management of asymptomatic primary hyperparathyroidism: consensus development conference statement. *Ann Intern Med.* 1991;114:593–597.
25. Oertli D, Richter M, Kraenzlin M, et al. Parathyroidectomy in primary hyperparathyroidism: preoperative localization and routine biopsy of unaltered glands are not necessary. *Surgery* 1995;117:392–396.
26. Chen H, Sokoll LJ, Udelsman R. Outpatient minimally invasive parathyroidectomy: A combination of sestamibi-SPECT localization, cervical block anesthesia, and intraoperative parathyroid hormone assay. *Surgery* 1999;126:1016–1022.
27. Carty S, Worsey M, Virji M, et al. Concise parathyroidectomy: The impact of preoperative SPECT ^{99m}Tc sestamibi scanning and intraoperative quick parathormone assay. *Surgery* 1997;122:1107–1116.
28. Carneiro D M, SolorzanoCC, Nader MC, et al. 3rd Comparison of intraoperative iPTH assay (QPTH) criteria in guiding parathyroidectomy: which criterion is the most accurate? *Surgery* 2003;134: 973–979; discussion 979–981.
29. Carneiro DM, Irvin GL 3rd. Late parathyroid function after successful parathyroidectomy guided by intraoperative hormone assay (QPTH) compared with the standard bilateral neck exploration. *Surgery* 2000; 128: 925–929; discussion 935–936, .
30. Sfaniakis GN, Irvin GL III, Foss J, et al. Efficient parathyroidectomy guided by SPECT-MIBI and hormonal measurements. *J Nucl Med.* 1996; 37:798–804.
31. Gauger PG, Mullan MH, Thompson NW, et al. An alternative analysis of intraoperative parathyroid hormone data may improve the ability to detect multiglandular disease. *Arch Surg.* 2004;139: 164–169.
32. Carty SE, Worsey J, Virji MA, et al Concise parathyroidectomy: the impact of preoperative SPECT ^{99m}Tc sestamibi scanning and intraoperative quick parathormone assay. *Surgery* 1997;122:1107–1114; discussion 1114–1116.
33. Woodrum DT, Saunders BD, England BG, et al. The influence of sample site on intraoperative PTH monitoring during parathyroidectomy. *Surgery* 2004;136:1169–1175.
34. Boggs JE, Irvin GL 3rd, Molinari AS, et al. Intraoperative parathyroid hormone monitoring as an adjunct to parathyroidectomy. *Surgery* 1996; 120: 954–958.
35. Irvin GL 3rd, Sfakianakis G, Yeung L, et al. Ambulatory parathyroidectomy for primary hyperparathyroidism. *Arch Surg.* 1996;131:1074–1078.
36. Lowney JK, WeberB, Johnson S, et al. Minimal incision parathyroidectomy: cure, cosmesis, and cost. *World J Surg.* 2000;24:1442–1445.
37. Clerici T, Brandle M, Lange J, et al. Impact of intraoperative parathyroid hormone monitoring on the prediction of multiglandular parathyroid disease. *World J Surg.*2004;28:187–192.
38. Wells SA, Leight GS, Hensley M, et al. Hyperparathyroidism associated with the enlargement of two or three parathyroid glands. *Ann Surg.* 1985; 202:533–538.
39. Goretzki PE, Dotzenrath C, Roeher HD. Management of primary hyperparathyroidism caused by multiple gland disease. *World J Surg.* 1991; 15:693–697.
40. Wells SA Jr, Farndon JR, Dale JK, et al. Long-term evaluation of patients with primary parathyroid hyperplasia managed by total parathyroidectomy and heterotopic autotransplantation. *Ann Surg.* 1980;192: 451–458.
41. Doherty GM, Lairmore TC, DeBenedetti MK. Multiple endocrine neoplasia type 1 parathyroid adenoma development over time. *World J Surg.* 2004;28:1139–1142.
42. Marx SJ, Simonds WF, Agarwal SK, et al. Hyperparathyroidism in hereditary syndromes: special expressions and special managements. *J Bone Min Res* 2002;17(suppl 2):N37–43.
43. Elaraj DM, Skarulis MC, Libutti SK, et al. Results of initial operation for hyperparathyroidism in patients with multiple endocrine neoplasia type 1. *Surgery* 2003;134:858–864; discussion 864–855, .
44. Arnalsteen LC, Alesina PF, Quiereux JL, et al. Long-term results of less than total parathyroidectomy for hyperparathyroidism in multiple endocrine neoplasia type 1. *Surgery* 2002;132:1119–1124; discussion 1124–1125.
45. Hubbard J G, Sebag F, Maweja S, et al. Primary hyperparathyroidism in MEN 1—how radical should surgery be? *Langenbecks Archives of Surgery* 2002;386: 553–557.
46. Goudet P, Cougard P, Verges B, et al. Hyperparathyroidism in multiple endocrine neoplasia type I: surgical trends and results of a 256-patient series from Groupe D'etude des Neoplasies Endocriniennes Multiples Study Group. *World J Surg.* 2001;25:886–890.
47. Casanova D, Sarfati E, De Francisco A, et al. Secondary hyperparathyroidism: diagnosis of site of recurrence. *World J Surg.* 11991;5:546–549; discussion 549–550.
48. Doherty GM, Doppman JL, Miller DL, et al. Results of a multidisciplinary strategy for management of mediastinal parathyroid adenoma as a cause of persistent primary hyperparathyroidism. *Ann Surg.* 1992;215: 101–106.
49. Irvin GL III, Molinari AS, Figueroa C, et al. Improved success rate in reoperative parathyroidectomy with intraoperative PTH assay. Ann Surg. 1999;229:874–878; discussion 878–879.
50. Wells SA Jr, Cooper JD. Closed mediastinal exploration in patients with persistent hyperparathyroidism. *Ann Surg* 1991;214:555–561.
51. Amaya Garcia M, Acosta Feria M, Soto Moreno A, et al. Primary hyperparathyroidism in pregnancy. Gynecol Endocrinol. 2004;19: 111–114.
52. Ip P. Neonatal convulsion revealing maternal hyperparathyroidism: an unusual case of late neonatal hypoparathyroidism. Arch Gynecol Obstetr. 2003;268:227–229.
53. Schnatz PF, Curry SL. Primary hyperparathyroidism in pregnancy: evidence-based management. Obstet Gynecol Surv. 2002;57:365–376.
54. Haenel LC IV, Mayfield RK. Primary hyperparathyroidism in a twin pregnancy and review of fetal/maternal calcium homeostasis. *Am J Med Sci.* 2000;319:191–194..

55. Key LL, Thorne M, Pitzer B, et al. Management of neonatal hyperparathyroidism with parathyroidectomy and autotransplantation. *J Ped.* 1990;116:923–926.
56. Wang C, Gaz RD. Natural history of parathyroid carcinoma. Diagnosis, treatment, and results. *Am J Surg.* 1985;149:522–527.
57. Pearse AGE. Common cytochemical and ultrastructural characteristics of cells producing polypeptide hormone (the APUD series) and their relevance to the thyroid and ultimobranchial C-cells and calcitonin. *Proc R Soc Lond (Biol).* 1968;170:71–80.
58. Chandrasekharappa SC, Guru SC, Manickam P, et al. Positional cloning of the gene for multiple endocrine neoplasia-type 1. *Science* 1997;276: 404–407.
59. Mutch MG, Dilley WG, Sanjurjo F, et al. Germline mutations in the multiple endocrine neoplasia type 1 gene: evidence for frequent splicing defects. *Hum Mutat.* 1999;13:175–185.
60. Mulligan LM, Kwok JBJ, Healey CS, et al. Germ-line mutation of the RET proto-oncogene in multiple endocrine neoplasia type 2A. *Nature* 1993;363:458–460.
61. Donis-Keller H, Dou S, Chi D, et al. Mutations in the RET proto-oncogene are associated with MEN 2A and FMTC. *Hum Mol Genet* 1993;2: 851–856.
62. Doherty GM. Multiple endocrine neoplasia type 1. J Surg Oncol. 2005;89:143–150.
63. Doherty GM, Olson JA, Frisella MM, et al. Lethality of multiple endocrine neoplasia type I. *World J Surg.* 1998;22:581–586; discussion 586–587.
64. Lowney JK, Frisella MM, Lairmore TC, et al. Islet cell tumor metastasis in multiple endocrine neoplasia type I: Correlation with primary tumor size. *Surgery* 1998;124:1043–1049.
65. Skogseid B, Oberg K, Eriksson B, et al. Surgery for asymptomatic pancreatic lesion in multiple endocrine neoplasia type 1. *World J Surg.* 1996; 20:872–877.
66. Skogseid B, Grama D, Rastad J, et al. Operative tumour yields obviates preoperative pancreatic tumor localization in multiple endocrine neoplasia type 1. *J Intern Med.* 1995;238:281–288.
67. Skogseid B, Oberg K. Experience with multiple endocrine neoplasia type 1 screening. *J Intern Med.* 1995;238:255–261.
68. Mutch MG, Frisella MM, DeBenedetti MK, et al. Pancreatic polypeptide is a useful plasma marker for radiographically evident pancreatic islet cell tumors in patients with multiple endocrine neoplasia type 1. *Surgery* 1997;122:1012–1019; discussion 1019–1020.
69. Yim JH, Siegel BA, DeBenedetti MK, et al. Prospective study of the utility of somatostatin-receptor scintigraphy in the evaluation of patients with multiple endocrine neoplasia type 1. *Surgery* 1998;124: 1037–1042.
70. Doherty GM. Multiple endocrine neoplasia type 1: duodenopancreatic tumors. *Surg Oncol.* 2003;12:135–143.
71. Hausman MS Jr, Thompson NW, Gauger PG, et al. The surgical management of MEN-1 pancreatoduodenal neuroendocrine disease. *Surgery* 2004;136:1205–1211.
72. Wells SA Jr, Chi DD, Toshima K, et al. Predictive DNA testing and prophylactive thyroidectomy in patients at risk for multiple endocrine neoplasia type 2A. *Ann Surg.* 1994;220:237–247.
73. Cance WG, Wells SA Jr. Multiple endocrine neoplasia. Type IIa. *Curr Probl Surg.* 1985;22:1–56.
74. Moley JF, Wells SA Jr, Dilley WG, et al. Reoperation for recurrent or persistent medullary thyroid cancer. *Surgery* 1993;114:1090–1096.
75. Sawka AM, Jaeschke R, Singh RJ, et al. A comparison of biochemical tests for pheochromocytoma: measurement of fractionated plasma metanephrines compared with the combination of 24-hour urinary metanephrines and catecholamines.[comment]. *J Clin Endocrinol Metab.* 2003;88: 553–558.
76. Eisenhofer G. Editorial: biochemical diagnosis of pheochromocytoma—is it time to switch to plasma-free metanephrines? *J Clin Endocrinol Metab.* 2003;88:550–552.
77. Eisenhofer G, Lenders JW, Linehan WM, et al. Plasma normetanephrine and metanephrine for detecting pheochromocytoma in von Hippel-Lindau disease and multiple endocrine neoplasia type 2. *N Engl J Med.* 1999; 340:1872–1879.
78. Eisenhofer G, Keiser H, Friberg P, et al. Plasma metanephrines are markers of pheochromocytoma produced by catechol-O-methyltransferase within tumors. *J Clin Endocrinol Metabol.* 1998;83:2175–2185.
79. Brunt LM, Lairmore TC, Doherty GM, et al. Adrenalectomy for familial pheochromocytoma in the laparoscopic era. *Ann Surg.* 2002;235:713–720.
80. Lairmore TC, Ball DW, Baylin SB, et al. Management of pheochromocytomas in patients with multiple endocrine neoplasia type 2 syndromes.

CHAPTER 79 ■ ADRENAL GLANDS

JOHN A. OLSON, JR.

ANATOMY

The adrenal glands are bilateral, retroperitoneal, endocrine organs located adjacent to the superior pole of each kidney. These glands appear grossly as flat, triangular structures each weighing approximately 4 g. Each adrenal gland is composed of two distinct endocrine organs, the cortex and medulla. The outer adrenal cortex is bright yellow and nodular, whereas the adrenal medulla is red-brown in color and is sandwiched between the thin layers of the cortex. The adrenals are embedded in retroperitoneal perinephric fat but can be identified as distinct structures by their golden brown, nodular appearance. The right adrenal gland abuts the inferior vena cava medially and lies in close proximity to the diaphragmatic crus posteriorly and the liver anteriorly. The left adrenal gland resides between the kidney and aorta, immediately deep to the tail of the pancreas and spleen.

Embryologically, fetal and definitive adrenal cortices arise from coelomic mesoderm near the urogenital ridge during the fourth to sixth weeks of gestation. Postnatally, the fetal cortex involutes, leaving only the definitive cortex to differentiate into the three adult zonae, the glomerulosa, fasciculata, and reticularis. The adrenal medulla develops from the neural crest during the fifth gestational week and migrates along paraaortic and paravertebral routes to join the developing cortex. Ectopic adrenal cortex and medulla may be found anywhere along their respective paths of embryologic migration. Most neural crest tissue regresses, however, extra-adrenal neural crest derivatives may be found along the retroperitoneum and at the aortic bifurcation (organ of Zuckerkandl).

The adrenal cortex is composed of three distinct zones. The outer zona glomerulosa, located just beneath the fibrous gland capsule, is the site of mineralocorticoid production. The middle zona fasciculata, composed of linear arrays of large, foamy cells with lipid inclusions, is the predominant site of glucocorticoid and adrenal sex steroid biosynthesis. The inner zona reticularis is the primary location of synthesis of adrenal androgens. Both the zona fasciculata and zona reticularis respond to stimulation by adrenocorticotropic hormone (ACTH). The adrenal medulla is smaller than the cortex. Cells of the adrenal medulla appear as homogeneous sheets, with large, irregular, atypical-looking nuclei. The cytoplasm of these cells has numerous secretory granules containing

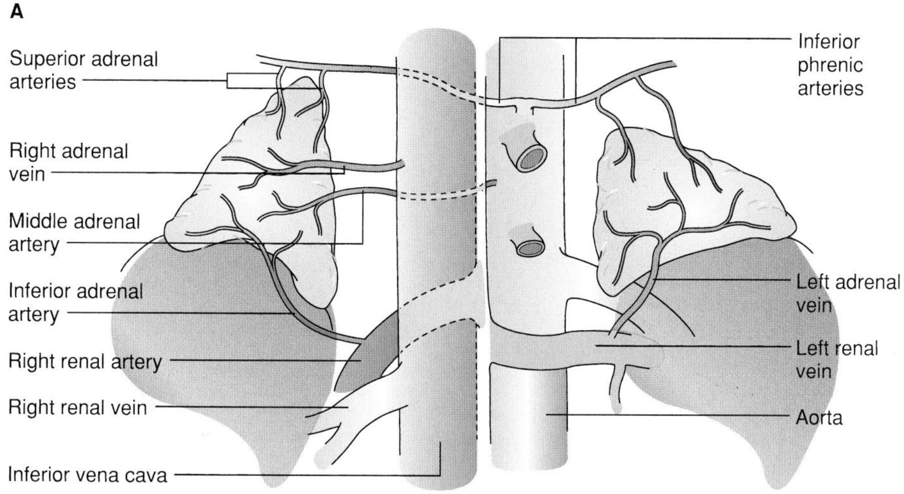

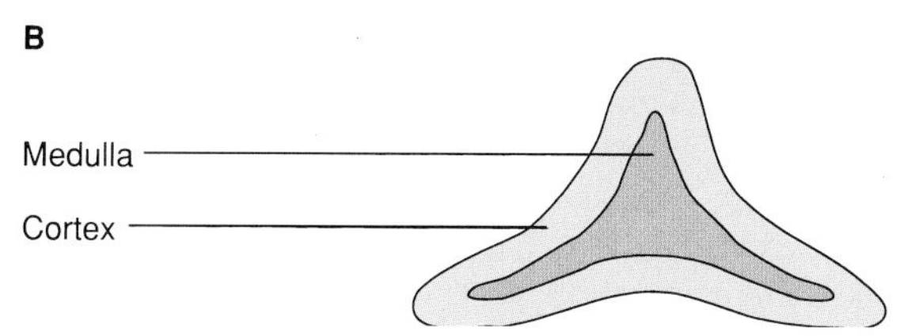

FIGURE 79.1 (*A*) Arterial (dark shaded) and venous (light shaded) anatomy of the adrenal glands. (*B*) Schematic showing outer adrenal cortex (light shaded) and inner adrenal medulla (dark shaded).

catecholamines, neuron-specific enolase, and chromogranin. Catecholamines in these granules precipitate chromium salts, which is the basis for the term *chromaffin cells*.

The adrenal glands have an extensive vascular supply derived from branches of the inferior phrenic artery superiorly, the aorta medially and the renal artery inferiorly. Venous return from the right adrenal gland empties directly into the inferior vena cava through a wide but short central vein. Venous drainage from the left adrenal gland empties into a smaller vein that shares a common trunk with the left phrenic vein. Together they join the left renal vein (Fig. 79.1).

BIOCHEMISTRY AND PHYSIOLOGY

Adrenal Cortex

Adrenocortical steroid hormones, glucocorticoids, mineralocorticoids, and androgenic steroids are all synthetic derivatives of cholesterol that are either extracted from plasma or synthesized intracellularly (Fig. 79.2). In mitochondria of cells in the adrenal cortex, cholesterol is converted by desmolase (CYP11A1) to delta-5-pregnenolone, the common parent compound for all adrenal cortex steroids. Pregnenolone is then shunted to the three biosynthetic pathways, each compartmentalized within the adrenal according to synthetic capabilities within each zone. In the zonae fasciculata and reticularis, pregnenolone is either converted to progesterone by 3-beta-hydroxysteroid dehydrogenase or is oxidized at position 17 by 17-alpha hydroxylase (CYP17) to form 17-hydroxypregnenolone. In the zona fasciculata, progesterone is hydroxylated by CYP17 at position 17 to form 17-hydroxyprogesterone. Subsequently, 17-hydroxyprogesterone is sequentially hydroxylated at the 21 position by 21-beta hydroxylase (CYP21A2) and at position 11 by 11-beta hydroxylase (CYP11B1) to form cortisol. In the zona reticularis, the androgenic steroids dehydroepiandrostenedione (DHEA) and androstenedione are made from 17-hydroxypregnenolone and 17-hydroxyprogesterone, respectively. Collectively, the glucocorticoid and androgenic steroids are known as *17-hydroxy corticosteroids and 17-hydroxy ketosteroids*. In the zona glomerulosa, progesterone is not hydroxylated at the 17 position owing to the lack of enzyme at this location. Instead aldosterone is made from progesterone by a sequential series of hydroxylation steps at position 21 by CYP21A2, position 11 by CYP11B1, and position 18 by aldosterone synthase (CYP11B2 and P450c11as). The zona glomerulosa is well suited to aldosterone biosynthesis because of the relative lack of 17-hydroxylase and the exclusive expression of aldosterone synthase, required for the conversion of corticosterone to aldosterone.

Cortisol

Cortisol is the predominant glucocorticoid in humans. Production and release of cortisol is tightly regulated by a complex feedback relationship between the hypothalamus, corticotrophs of the anterior pituitary, and cells of the adrenal cortex zonae fasciculata and reticularis. This endocrine system is called the *hypothalamic-pituitary-adrenal (HPA) axis*. Communication within the HPA axis is mediated by synthesis and secretion of corticotrophin-releasing hormone (CRH) by the hypothalamus and ACTH production by corticotrophs of the anterior pituitary (Fig. 79.3). ACTH is a cleavage product of a precursor polipeptide, proopiomelanocortin (POMC) that is built of 241 amino acid residues within corticotroph cells of the anterior and intermedate lobes of the pituitary. Several derivatives of POMC are important biologically active substances, including ACTH. Under stimlation of hypothalamic CRH stimulus, POMC can be cleaved into ACTH and β-lipotropic hormone in the anterior lobe. ACTH acts directly on the adrenal to regulate cortisol production by cells within the zonae fasciculata and reticularis. Feedback loops involving

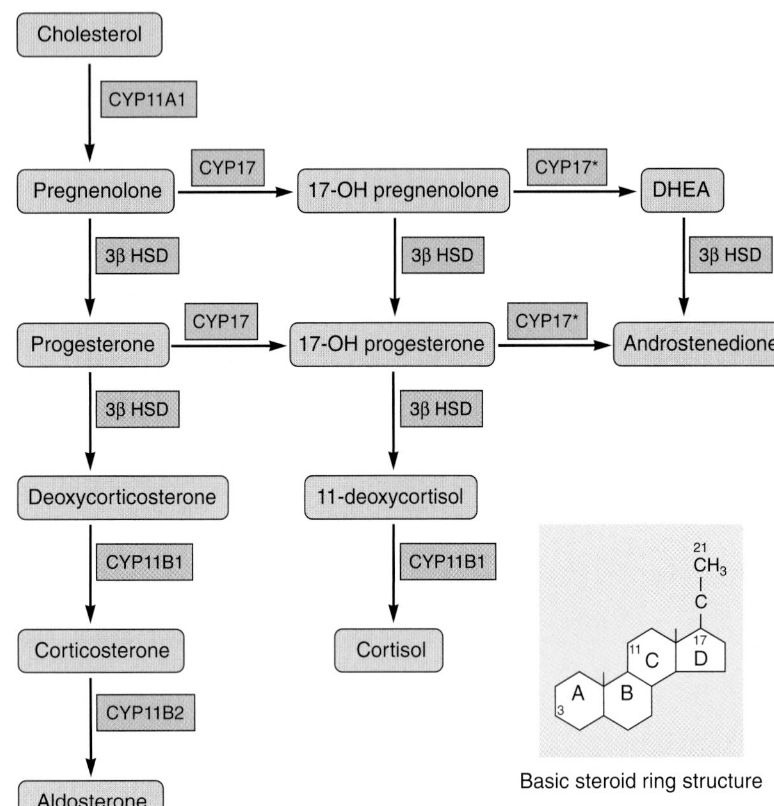

FIGURE 79.2 Steroid biosynthetic pathways in the adrenal cortex. Steroids and precursors are shown in square boxes. Enzymes are shown in stippled boxes. Enzyme gene symbol designations are: CYP11A1, desmolase; CYP17, 17α hydroxylase ($\pm$17,20 lyase*); 3β HSD, 3β Hydroxysteroid dehydrogenase; CYP21A2, 21 hydroxylase; CYP11B1, 11β hydroxylase; CYP11B2, Aldosterone synthase. *Inset*: Basic steroid ring structure. The four basic carbon rings are designated A, B, C, and D. Individual carbons at sites of steroidegenic enzyme activity are designated numerically.

cortisol, hypothalamic CRH, and pituitary ACTH keep the concentration of cortisol in plasma within a narrow range of 10 to 15 μg/dL. Typical daily production of cortisol in humans ranges between 10 to 30 mg and can increase to as high as 300 mg per day under conditions of maximal stress.

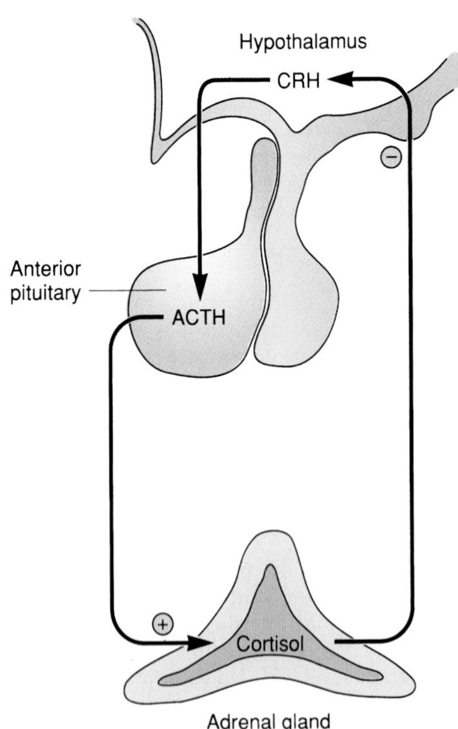

FIGURE 79.3 Schematic of hypothalamic-pituitary-adrenal axis for cortisol. Regulatory feedback relationships are designated with arrows.

In circulation, cortisol is protein bound to transcortin and albumin with a small percentage of free cortisol available to target tissues. The half-life of cortisol in circulation is 90 minutes. Cortisol is metabolized in the liver to the inactive metabolites dihydrocortisol and tetrahydrocortisol, which become conjugated to glucuronidate and excreted in the urine. These urinary metabolites, collectively known as *17-hydroxycorticosteroids*, as well as free cortisol, can be measured in the urine.

Cortisol binds to specific intracellular cytoplasmic receptors, causing translocation of activated receptor-ligand complexes to the nucleus. Biologic effects result from transcriptional activation of genes and may be grouped into intermediary metabolism, immunomodulation, and regulation of intravascular volume (Table 79.1). Important effects of cortisol on intermediary metabolism center on raising blood glucose directly and indirectly by providing substrate for gluconeogenesis by the liver. These effects include (a) stimulation of glucagon and inhibition of insulin-stimulated glucose uptake by cells; (b) decrease in peripheral protein synthesis and increase in proteolysis, thus delivering gluconeogenic amino acids to the liver; and (c) stimulation of peripheral lipolysis. In effect, cortisol acts anabolically in vital organs to preserve glucose supply and catabolically in peripheral tissues to mobilize gluconeogenic substrates. Cortisol also possesses profound antiinflammatory and immunosuppressive activities. Impairment of cellular immunity is due to inhibition of interleukin production, impairment of monocyte and neutrophil chemotaxis despite raised leukocyte counts, and reduction of T-cell activation. Humoral immunity is inhibited by inhibition of T-cell stimulation of B cells and by direct inhibition of B-cell proliferation and activation. These immunomodulatory effects may also underlie the impairment of normal wound healing seen in states of cortisol excess. Cortisol also regulates intravascular volume through renal retention of sodium and maintains blood pressure through inotropic and chronotropic effects on the heart as well as by increasing peripheral vascular resistance. In bone, glucocorticoids promote osteopenia by inhibition of bone formation by osteoblasts.

TABLE 79.1

SYSTEMIC EFFECTS OF CORTISOL

Function	Normal amounts	Excessive amounts
Metabolic		
Protein	Proteolysis	Muscle wasting
Glucose	Gluconeogenesis	Hyperglycemia
Fat	Low-use peripheral lipolysis	Limb thinness
	Central lipogenesis	Truncal obesity
Gastrointestinal	Mucosal cells	Ulceration
	Prostaglandin	Pancreatitis(?)
Cardiovascular	Chronotropic, inotropic	Hypertension
	Vascular resistance	
Renal	Sodium resorption	Hypertension
Bone	Osteoblastic development	Osteoporosis
Inflammatory and immune	Circulating cells	Infection
	Soluble mediators	
	Antigen processing	
Wound healing	Fibroblasts	Striae
	Epithelial cell	Dehiscence

Aldosterone

Aldosterone is the principle mineralocorticoid in humans. Aldosterone secretion by the cells of the adrenal zona glomerulosa is regulated by the renin-angiotensin system and by plasma potassium (Fig. 79.4). Aldosterone is also regulated to a lesser degree by ACTH and plasma sodium concentration. Juxtaglomerular myoepithelial cells lining afferent arterioles of the kidney sense renal blood flow and pressure, and they secrete renin in response to decreased perfusion. Renin enzymatically activates angiotensinogen to the inactive decapeptide precursor,

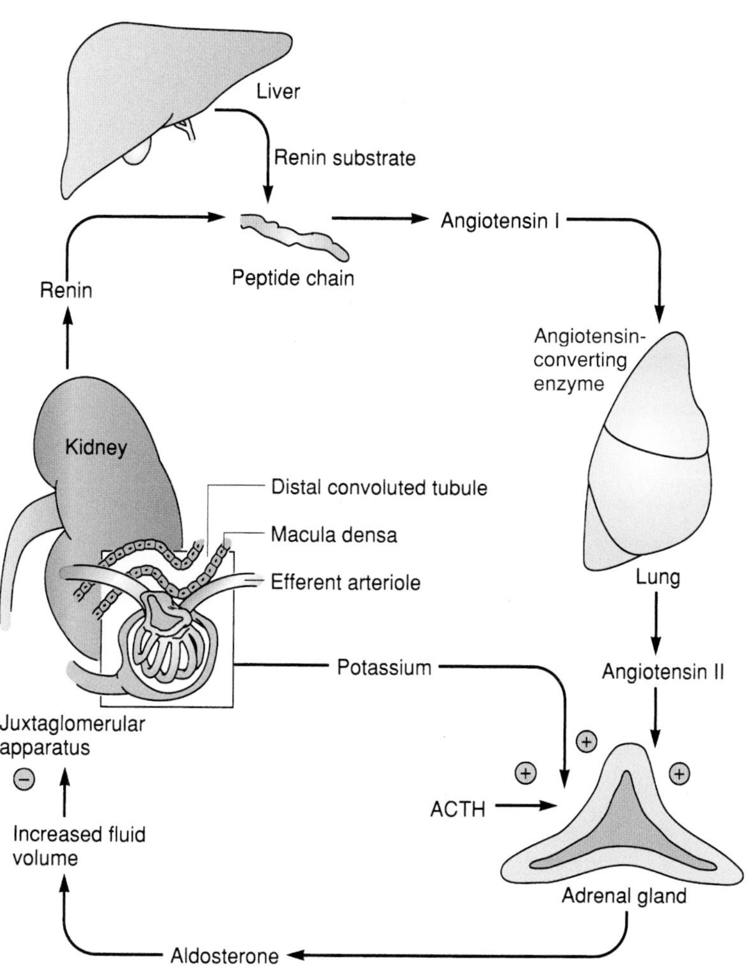

FIGURE 79.4 Regulatory relationships of renin, the angiotensins, and their sites of production and enzymatic conversion.

angiotensin I. Angiotensin I is converted to angiotensin II by angiotensin converting enzyme in the lung. Angiotensin II has three major effects: (a) arteriolar vasoconstriction; (b) renal sodium retention; and (c) increased aldosterone biosynthesis, each of which results in sodium retention and potassium excretion by the kidney. These effects work together to maintain arterial blood pressure as well as blood volume. Physiologic conditions that stimulate the renin-angiotensin cascade and aldosterone release include dehydration, upright posture and hemorrhage. Inhibitory factors include volume repletion. Postural changes in renin-angiotensin and aldosterone are mediated by the sympathetic nervous system.

Under normal circumstances, aldosterone secretion is controlled by total body sodium and potassium levels. Excess sodium intake suppresses renin activity and leading to decreased aldosterone levels and increased renal excretion of sodium. Conversely, sodium depletion stimulates the renin-angiotensin system and aldosterone production, which promotes sodium retention by the kidney. Increased potassium intake directly decreases renin release and aldosterone production; decreasing potassium intake increases renin release. Humans with normal sodium intake typically produce 100 to 150 mg of aldosterone per day.

In circulation, aldosterone is bound to albumin and transcortin with a small percentage of free aldosterone available to target tissues. The half-life of aldosterone in plasma is 15 minutes. Aldosterone is metabolized rapidly in the liver and conjugated to glucuronidate, which is excreted in the urine. In liver failure, metabolism of aldosterone is impaired leading to elevated levels and fluid retention.

Aldosterone is the major regulator of extracellular fluid volume and potassium homeostasis (Table 79.2). Aldosterone binds to high affinity aldosterone receptors in target tissues, including cells of the distal convoluted tubule in the kidney (the major site of action), the salivary glands, and colonic mucosa (minor sites). Stimulation of these cells results in retention of sodium and excretion of potassium. Retention of sodium in the kidney leads to passive reabsorption of water and an increase in extracellular fluid volume. To balance aldosterone-mediated retention of positively charged sodium ions the kidney epithelium releases intracellular potassium into the distal convoluted tubule for excretion in the urine. Hydrogen ion is also released causing acidification of the urine.

Adrenal Androgens

Adrenal C-19 androgenic steroids, include DHEA and delta-4 androstenedione, are synthesized in cells of the zona reticularis. These steroids promote secondary sexual characteristics in men and virilization in women. DHEA is the major adrenal androgen, while androstenedione is relatively minor. Both are relatively weak androgens and exert their effects on target tissue after local tissue conversion to testosterone. Unlike gonadal androgens, adrenal androgens are regulated by ACTH, not gonadotropins, and can therefore be inhibited by glucocorticoid administration.

TABLE 79.2

EFFECTS OF ALDOSTERONE SECRETION

Tubular action	Normal amounts	Excessive amounts
Increased resorption of sodium	Protects against low-volume states	Hypertension Positive sodium balance Hyporeninemia
Decreased resorption of potassium	Protects against hyperkalemia	Hypokalemia Metabolic alkalosis Hyperglycemia Nocturia, polyuria Muscle weakness

Adrenal Medulla

Catecholamines of the adrenal medulla include epinephrine, norepinephrine, and dopamine. These vasoactive hormones are synthetic derivatives of the amino acid tyrosine (Fig. 79.5). The biosynthetic pathway that converts tyrosine to active catecholamines involves four sequential enzymatic reactions: (a) tyrosine is converted to L-dihydroxyphenylalanine (dopa) by tyrosine hydroxylase; (b) dopa is converted to dopamine by aromatic-L-amino acid decarboxylase; (c) dopamine is converted to norepinephrine by dopamine beta hydroxylase; and (d) norepinephrine is converted to epinephrine by phenylethanolamine-N-methyltransferase (PNMT). Epinephrine is the major (80%) catecholamine stored in the adrenal medulla, followed by norepinephrine (20%) and dopamine (<1%). Tissue expression of the enzyme PNMT is limited to cells of either the adrenal medulla or organ of Zuckerkandl, located near the aortic bifurcation, thus most extraadrenal pheochromocytomas produce norepinephrine, rather than epinephrine.

A complex regulatory network governs synthesis and secretion of catecholamines. Factors that increase catecholamine release include splanchnic nerve stimulation, stress, and glucocorticoids. The metabolic milieu within the adrenal medulla also greatly influences catecholamine synthesis by regulating enzymatic activity: glucocorticoids, phospholipids, cyclic adenosine monophosphate, adenosine triphosphate, protein kinase, and magnesium increase activity of PNMT and decrease catecholamine negative feedback. Catecholamines are stored

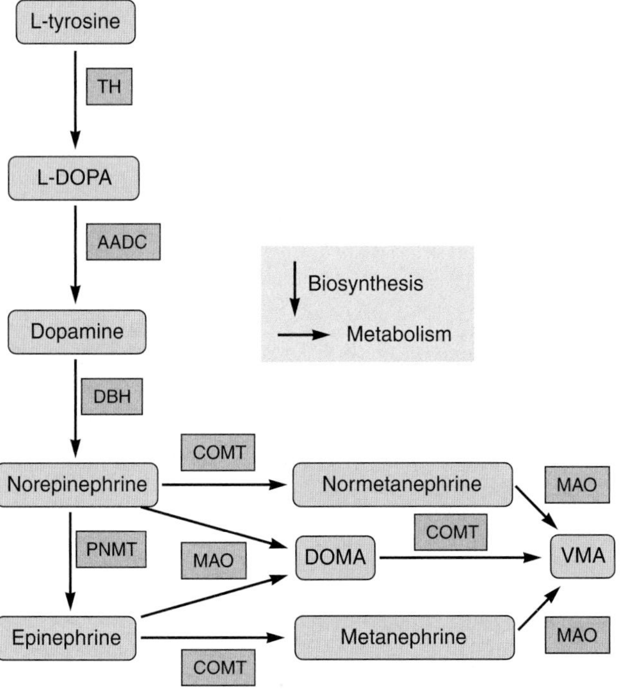

FIGURE 79.5 Catecholamine biosynthetic and metabolism pathways. Precursors, catecholamines, and metabolites are shown in square boxes. Enzymes are shown in stippled boxes. Enzyme gene symbol designations are: TH, tyrosine hydroxylase; AADC, aromatic-L-amino acid decarboxylase; DBH, dopamine β hydroxylase; PNMT, phenylethanolamine-N-methyltransferase; COMT, catechol-O-methyl- transferase; MAO, monoamine oxidase. VMA, 3-methoxy-4-hydroxy-mandelic acid.

TABLE 79.3

CATECHOLAMINE EFFECTS

Receptor class	Normal amounts	Excessive amounts
β_1	Chronotropic, inotropic Sweat glands Decreased glucose use	Tachycardia Sweating Hyperglycemia
β_2	Smooth muscle relaxation	Hypotension
α_1	Smooth muscle contraction Gluconeogenesis Glycogenolysis Suppressed insulin effects	Hypertension Hyperglycemia
α_2	Smooth muscle contraction[a]	Pallor

[a]Platelet aggregation.

and secreted from granules within cells of the medulla in association with the matrix protein chromogranin. Chromogranin A is measurable in the blood and their measurement may support the biochemical testing for pheochromocytoma, as well as other functional neuroendocrine tumors.

Catecholamines act on target tissues through membrane-bound receptors. Pharmacologic distinction of adrenergic receptors is made based on their relative responsiveness to natural and artificial bioamines. Alpha-adrenergic receptors show highest affinity for norepinephrine, less for epinephrine, and least for isoproterenol. Beta-adrenergic receptors are most responsive to isoproterenol and least to norepinephrine. In addition, specific antagonists recognize each receptor class: alpha-receptors are antagonized by phentolamine and phenoxybenzamine, and beta-receptors are blocked by propranolol and related compounds. Beta-adrenergic receptor subtypes include beta-1, which is present in cardiac muscle, adipose tissue, and small intestine, and beta-2 receptors, which are found in vascular, tracheal, and uterine smooth muscle, skeletal muscle, and liver. Alpha-adrenergic receptors are similarly subdivided: alpha-1 receptors mediate vasoconstriction whereas alpha-2 receptors modulate presynaptic norepinephrine release and platelet aggregation. (Table 79.3)

Metabolism of catecholamines occurs through three mechanisms: by specific uptake by sympathetic neurons, by nonspecific uptake and degradation by peripheral tissues, and by excretion in the urine. Catecholamines are metabolized in liver and kidney by two enzymes, monoamine oxidase and catechol-O-methyltransferase (Fig. 79.5). In these tissues, monoamine oxidase and catechol-O-methyltransferase convert epinephrine or norepinephrine to normetanephrine, and metanephrine, 3,4-dihydroxy-mandelic acid, and 3-methoxy-4-hydroxy-mandelic acid. These inactive metabolites are excreted by the kidney and are measurable in the urine either as free compounds or as conjugates of glucuronide or sulfate.

DISEASES OF THE ADRENAL CORTEX

Hypercortisolism

The term *hypercortisolism* refers to the physiologic state of glucocorticoid excess. This disorder is rare, with an estimated incidence of 10 per million population. The most common cause of hypercortisolism is the administration of exogenous steroids as immunosuppressive therapy for inflammatory disorders or after organ transplantation. Endogenous hypercortisolism, or Cushing syndrome, in all cases is caused by increased adrenal production of cortisol, which may be ACTH dependent (ACTH elevated) or independent (ACTH suppressed). Some patients with major depression or chronic alcoholism have abnormally high cortisol secretion and may appear to have clinical and biochemical features of Cushing syndrome. Pseudo-Cushing syndrome responds to treatment of the underlying disorder.

Cushing syndrome is ACTH dependent in 80% to 90% of cases. Such ACTH-dependent hypercortisolism is most often (80% to 90% of cases) caused by an ACTH-secreting pituitary adenoma (termed *Cushing disease*). Ectopic ACTH-producing nonendocrine tumors (mostly non-small cell lung cancer and bronchial carcinoids) represent 10% to 20% of cases of ACTH-dependent Cushing syndrome. All causes of ACTH-dependent Cushing syndrome involve bilateral adrenal hyperplasia in response to ACTH stimulation.

Of patients with endogenous Cushing syndrome, 10% to 25% have ACTH-independent disease caused by a primary adrenal cause. A solitary adrenal adenoma is present in 80% to 90% of these patients and is often associated with atrophy of both adjacent and contralateral adrenocortical tissue. Nodular cortical hyperplasia of both glands causes the remaining cases of primary adrenal Cushing syndrome. Although nodular hyperplasia represents a diffuse process, one or more distinct nodules may simulate adenomas. Rarely tumors secrete CRH ectopically, leading to ACTH-independent (though ACTH is elevated) Cushing syndrome with secondary adrenal hypertrophy.

Signs and Symptoms

Clinical features of cortisol excess are listed in Table 79.1. Truncal obesity (*orange on toothpicks*), accumulation of fat around the head and neck (*moon facies* and *buffalo hump*), and muscle wasting are present in most patients. Patients often have purple striae and purpura on the abdomen and extremities. Hirsutism may be present in women. High blood pressure is common and is usually moderate, although malignant hypertension has been observed. Muscle weakness and bone pain, particularly backache, are also common. Weakness is caused part to proximal muscle wasting but also to hypokalemia. Osteoporosis is common and pathologic fractures are observed in advanced cases. Neurologic symptoms, including headache, emotional lability, depression, and even psychosis may be observed. Glucose intolerance is common but can often be managed by alterations in diet alone. The serum potassium level may be low secondary to the weak mineralocorticoid properties of cortisol.

Autonomous glucocorticoid production without specific signs and symptoms of Cushing syndrome is termed subclinical Cushing syndrome. This condition is being diagnosed with increased frequency because of the detection of adrenal incidentalomas by routine CT. A substantial percentage of incidentalomas are hormonally active, with 5% to 20% of the tumors producing glucocorticoids. The estimated prevalence of subclinical hypercortisolism is 79 cases per 100,000 persons, substantially higher than classic Cushing syndrome. Depending on the amounts of glucocorticoids secreted by the tumor, the clinical spectrum ranges from slightly attenuated diurnal cortisol rhythm to atrophy of the contralateral adrenal gland. Patients with subclinical Cushing syndrome lack the classical stigmata of hypercortisolism but have a high prevalence of obesity, hypertension, and type 2 diabetes.

Diagnosis

The investigation of suspected Cushing syndrome should answer two questions: (a) Does the patient have hypercortisolism? (b) If the answer is yes, then what is the cause? It is worthwhile to emphasize that the diagnosis of Cushing syndrome is biochemical. Radiologic investigations should not be undertaken until Cushing syndrome has been confirmed and its likely etiology characterized biochemically.

Hypercortisolism insensitive to suppression by administration of exogenous glucocorticoid is the *sine qua non* of Cushing syndrome. The low-dose dexamethasone suppression test is the best test in patients with suspected Cushing syndrome. For this test, 1 mg of dexamethasone is administered orally at 11 PM and plasma cortisol is obtained at 8 AM the following day. Normal individuals suppress cortisol to below 5 μg/dL. Patients with Cushing syndrome fail to suppress below 5 μg/dL. False-positive test results occur in 10% to 15% of cases with the overnight test and occur especially in patients with obesity or alcoholism or in those taking estrogens or phenytoin. Measurement of free cortisol (not metabolites) in three consecutive 24-hour collections of urine is also a good screening test for Cushing syndrome. Collections should include concurrent creatinine measurement to evaluate the completeness of the collection. A 24-hour urinary free cortisol level greater than 100 μg is diagnostic of Cushing syndrome. This test may be less sensitive than the low-dose dexamethasone suppression test in mild hypercortisolism. Plasma cortisol levels can normally vary considerably during a 24-hour period, so a single random plasma cortisol level is not helpful in establishing a diagnosis of Cushing syndrome.

Once the presence hypercortisolism is established, the next task is to determine ACTH-dependent (pituitary or ectopic source) from ACTH-independent (primary adrenal) causes. Measurement of basal ACTH by immunoradiometric assay is the best test to make this distinction. Plasma ACTH levels are normally between 10 and 100 pg. Suppression of the absolute level of ACTH below 5 pg per mL is nearly diagnostic of adrenocortical neoplasms, which secrete high levels of cortisol and inhibit ACTH release by the pituitary. Patients with pituitary neoplasms and secondary bilateral adrenocortical hyperplasia have ACTH levels that may range from the upper limits of normal (15 pg. per mL) to 500 pg per mL. The highest plasma levels of ACTH (more than 1000 pg per mL) are in patients with ACTH-producing nonendocrine tumors such as non-small cell lung cancer.

Although 80% to 90% of patients with ACTH-dependent Cushing syndrome have Cushing disease, a high dose dexamethasone suppression test may be required to exclude ectopic ACTH syndrome. Hypercortisolism caused by to ACTH-secreting pituitary adenomas is suppressed at least partially by high dexamethasone, whereas hypercortisolism caused by adrenal tumors and ectopic ACTH-producing tumors is not suppressed. For this test 2 mg dexamethasone is administered orally every 6 hours for 2 days, and a 24-hour urine collection for free cortisol is taken during the second day. About 90% of patients with pituitary source Cushing disease have a 50% reduction in urine free cortisol. The specificity of the test can be improved to 100% for diagnosing pituitary disease if more than 90% suppression in urinary free cortisol is used.

Biochemical testing of suspected Cushing syndrome is followed by radiologic studies. Pituitary adenomas are best imaged with gadolinium-enhanced MRI of the sella turcica, which has a sensitivity approaching 100%, although small pituitary microadenomas may be missed. Patients with ACTH-independent Cushing syndrome require thin-section CT or MRI of the adrenal, which identifies adrenal abnormalities with more than 95% sensitivity. CT or MRI of the chest may identify a source of ectopic ACTH and should be undertaken in patients with elevated ACTH and hypercortisolism that cannot be suppressed by high-dose dexamethasone.

Despite the accuracy of biochemical testing and radiographic localization, a pituitary versus ectopic source of ACTH sometimes cannot be determined. Bilateral inferior petrosal sinus sampling is the best test to settle this issue. Simultaneous bilateral petrosal sinus and peripheral blood samples are obtained before and after peripheral intravenous injection of 1 μg per kg CRH. An inferior petrosal sinus to peripheral plasma ACTH ratio of 2.0 at basal stimulated or of 3.0 after CRH administration is 100% sensitive and specific for pituitary adenoma. Comparison of right and left inferior petrosal sinus ratios may also lateralize the adenoma.

The laboratory approach to the diagnosis of Cushing syndrome is summarized in Algorithm 79.1. A careful history and physical examination form the basis for suspecting this condition. A low-dose dexamethasone suppression test and/or

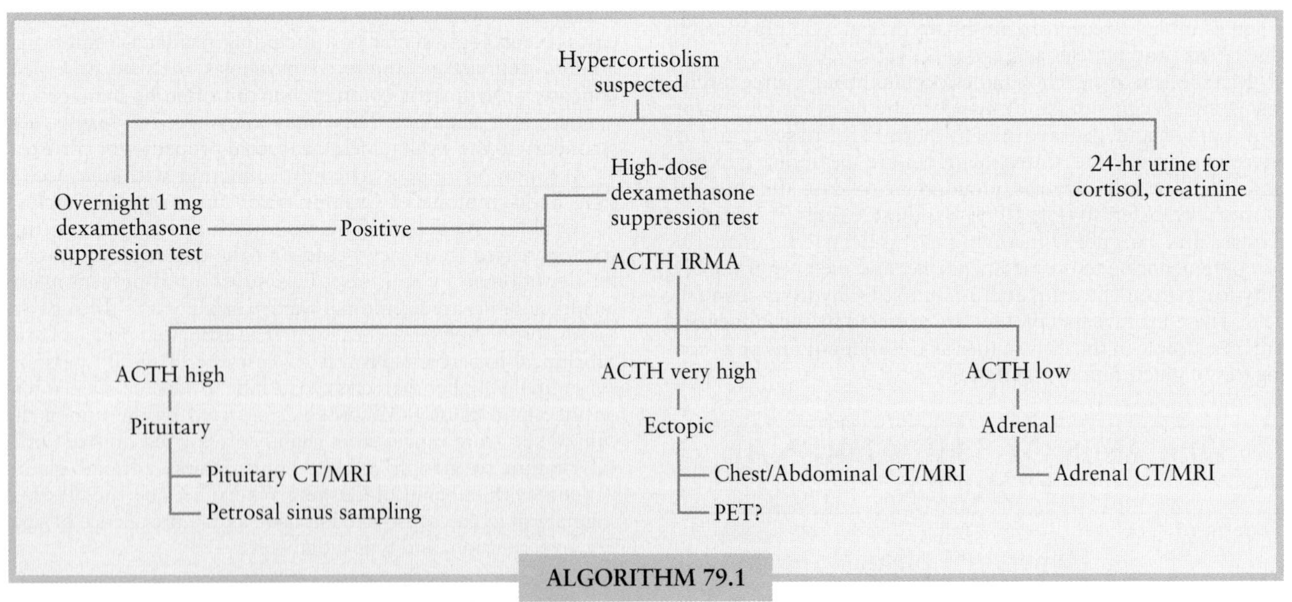

ALGORITHM 79.1 Diagnosis of hypercortisolism. ACTH, adrenocorticotropic hormone; IRMA, immunoradiometric assay; CT, computed tomography; MRI, magnetic resonance imaging; PET, positron emission tomography.

urinary free cortisol measurement provide initial evidence for the diagnosis. Plasma ACTH determination and the high-dose dexamethasone suppression test are then used to identify the underlying cause of excess cortisol production by the adrenal cortex. Imaging studies support the cause of Cushing syndrome suggested by biochemical testing and localize the site for subsequent treatment.

Treatment

ACTH-dependent Cushing syndrome is best treated by removing the source of ACTH excess. In the case of Cushing disease, transsphenoidal resection of the pituitary microadenoma is successful in 80% or more of cases. If a microadenoma is not found, then hemihypophysectomy may be performed with the understanding that fertility may be impaired. Pituitary irradiation is a good treatment option when fertility is desired, when a tumor is not found or is unresectable, or cure is not achieved by transsphenoidal resection of a tumor. Debulking of unresectable primary lesions or recurrences with or without bilateral adrenalectomy may provide palliation in some patients. Treatment of ectopic ACTH syndrome involves removal of the primary lesion. Medical adrenalectomy with metyrapone, aminoglutethimide, and mitotane has been used to suppress production of corticosteroid in inoperable cases for both pituitary and ectopic sources of ACTH. Bilateral adrenalectomy is a good option for patients intolerant of mitotane.

ACTH-independent Cushing syndrome is best treated by removal of the adrenal tumor and affected gland. Small lesions, less than 6 cm. in diameter, may be resected laparoscopically. Lesions larger than 6 cm or those suspected of being carcinoma require an anterior open approach. Resection of cortisol-producing benign adrenal adenomas is curative and prognosis is good following resection. Cortisol-producing adrenocortical carcinomas recur frequently following adrenalectomy, heralded by the reemergence of hypercortisolism. Micronodular pigmented hyperplasia and macronodular adrenal hyperplasia may involve both adrenal glands. These conditions are cured only by bilateral adrenalectomy. Medical adrenalectomy with mitotane or agents interfering with cortisol production is not currently recommended.

Whether patients with subclinical Cushing syndrome should undergo adrenalectomy is unclear. Adrenalectomy for subclinical Cushing is reasonable in young patients (<50 years), in patients with suppressed plasma ACTH, and in patients with a recent history of weight gain, substantial obesity, arterial hypertension, diabetes mellitus, and osteopenia. Truly asymptomatic patients with normal plasma ACTH concentrations and the elderly or unfit may be observed. Demonstration of the benefits of surgery versus conservative treatment in patients with subclinical Cushing syndrome will require a randomized prospective trial.

All patients who undergo adrenalectomy for Cushing syndrome require perioperative and postoperative glucocorticoid replacement, since the contralateral gland is suppressed. Replacement therapy with hydrocortisone, 12 mg/m^2 per day, may be required as long as 2 years postoperatively. Adequacy of replacement is monitored clinically. The duration of replacement therapy is guided by normalization of the ACTH stimulation test.

Hyperaldosteronism

Hyperaldosteronism is a syndrome of hypertension and hypokalemia caused by autonomous adrenal secretion of the mineralocorticoid aldosterone. Hyperaldosteronism may be primary, as a result of an adrenal neoplasm with suppressed plasma renin, or may be secondary, as a result of elevated plasma renin. Primary hyperaldosteronism is twice as common in women as in men, and it usually occurs between the ages of 30 and 50 years. Screening of hypertensive patients with plasma aldosterone and plasma renin activity (PRA) has suggested that primary hyperaldosteronism may be the underlying cause of up to 15% of cases of essential hypertension.

An aldosterone-producing adrenal adenoma (Conn syndrome) is the source of primary hyperaldosteronism in 60% to 70% of cases. Idiopathic bilateral adrenal hyperplasia causes the remaining cases of primary hyperaldosteronism. Adrenocortical carcinoma is a rare cause of primary hyperaldosteronism. Autosomal dominant glucocorticoid-suppressible hyperaldosteronism is a rare cause of hyperaldosteronism resulting from the fusion of the ACTH-responsive 11-beta hydroxylase gene promoter to the aldosterone synthase gene in cells of the adrenal cortex.

Secondary hyperaldosteronism is a physiologic response of the renin-angiotensin system to decrease renal perfusion renal artery stenosis, cirrhosis, congestive heart failure, and normal pregnancy. The adrenal cortex functions normally and secretes aldosterone in response to the elevated plasma renin and angiotensin caused by these conditions. Secondary hyperaldosteronism responds to treatment of the underlying cause.

Signs and Symptoms

Clinical manifestations of primary hyperaldosteronism are attributable to hypersecretion of aldosterone by the adrenal gland (Table 79.2). Aldosterone-mediated retention of sodium and excretion of potassium and hydrogen ion by the kidney causes moderate diastolic hypertension. Edema is absent. Hypokalemia occurs spontaneously in 80% to 90% of patients with primary hyperaldosteronism but may be normal. Hypokalemia is easily provocable in the remaining patients. Potassium depletion frequently causes symptoms of muscle weakness and fatigue, polyuria and polydipsia, as well as impaired insulin secretion and fasting hyperglycemia. Primary hyperaldosteronism should be suspected in hypertensive patients with spontaneous hypokalemia (serum concentration <3.5 mEq/L), moderate hypokalemia (serum potassium concentration <3.0) during diuretic therapy despite concomitant use of oral potassium or potassium-sparing diuretics, or refractory hypertension without explanation.

Diagnosis

The clinical hallmarks of primary hyperaldosteronism are (a) diastolic hypertension without edema; (b) suppression of plasma renin in the face of volume depletion; and (c) hypersecretion of aldosterone that fails to suppress with intravascular volume expansion. Diagnostic evaluation must establish primary hyperaldosteronism, discern surgically correctable adrenal adenoma from medically treatable idiopathic hyperplasia, and localize an adrenal tumor (Algorithm 79.2).

Demonstration of an elevated plasma aldosterone concentration (PAC) in the setting of suppressed PRA is the best test to establish primary hyperaldosteronism. The ratio in normal subjects and patients with essential hypertension is 4 to 10 compared with more than 30 in most patients with primary hyperaldosteronism. A PAC of greater than 20 ng/dL and a PAC/PRA ratio of greater than 30 are diagnostic for aldosteronoma with almost 90% sensitivity. A serum potassium value less than 3.5 mEq/L and urinary potassium excretion greater than 30 mEq per day also support a diagnosis of primary hyperaldosteronism. Hypokalemia and inappropriate kaliuresis are often but not always present as well. Before biochemical evaluation, patients need to be potassium repleted and have an adequate sodium intake. Medications including ACE inhibitors and spironolactone should be withheld for at least 4 weeks before study.

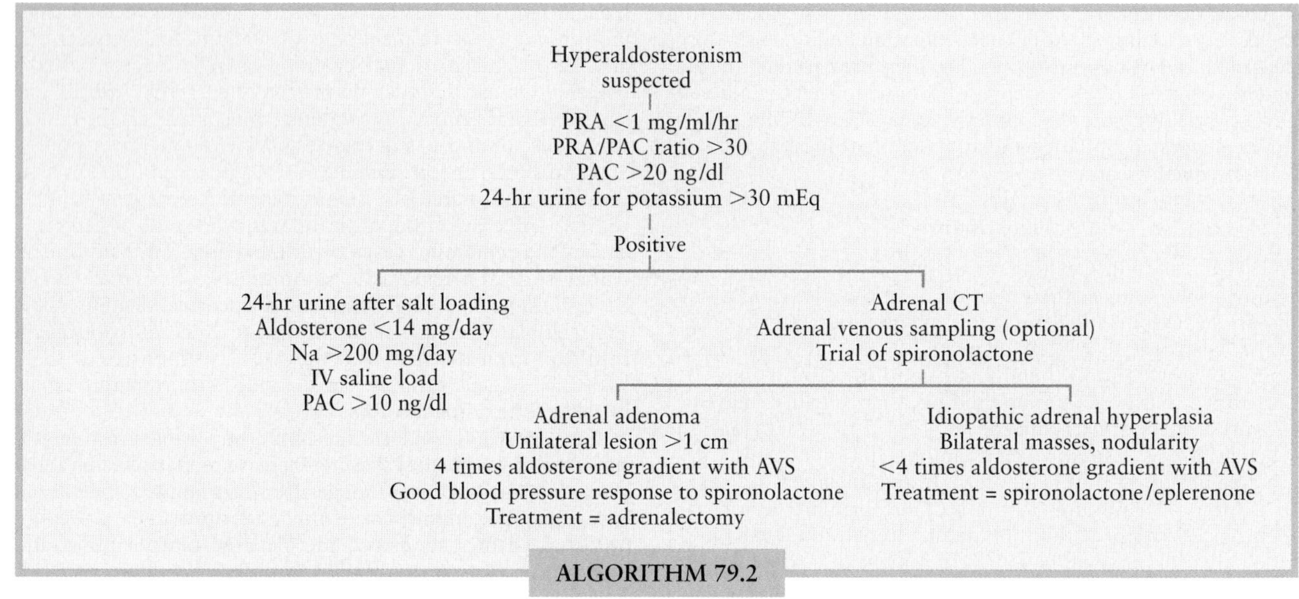

ALGORITHM 79.2 Diagnosis and management of hyperaldosteronism. PRA, plasma renin activity; PAC, plasma aldosterone concentration; CT, computed tomography; AVS, bilateral adrenal venous sampling.

An elevated PAC/PRA ratio alone does not establish the diagnosis of primary hyperaldosteronism, which must be confirmed by demonstrating inappropriate aldosterone secretion with salt loading. This involves a 24-hour urine collection for sodium and aldosterone after 3 days of a high-sodium diet. The 24-hour urinary excretion of aldosterone should be less than 14 μg. per 24 hours after a high-salt diet. An intravenous saline infusion test or captopril challenge test is also a reliable method to confirm primary hyperaldosteronism. These tests are not usually required.

After the diagnosis of primary hyperaldosteronism is made, distinction must be made between an aldosteronoma and idiopathic adrenal hyperplasia. The first test measures aldosterone in blood collected at 8 AM from a patient who has been supine overnight. Laboratory studies are repeated 4 hours later after the patient has been upright. Aldosterone secretion in patients with an aldosteronoma is unaffected by postural changes (<20 ng/dL), whereas, in patients with idiopathic adrenal hyperplasia, plasma aldosterone levels are elevated 33% (>20 ng/dL) or more by postural changes.

High-resolution adrenal computed tomography (CT) is the best test for localization of an adrenal tumor (Fig. 79.6). CT will detect an aldosterone-producing adenoma in 90% of cases overall. The presence of a unilateral adenoma greater than 1 cm on CT and supportive biochemical evidence of an aldosteronoma are generally all that is needed to make the diagnosis in most patients over 40 years of age. The contralateral adrenal gland must be examined in patients presumed to have an aldosterone-producing adenoma to ensure that bilateral hyperplasia is not present. Magnetic resonance imaging (MRI) is less effective and more costly but may be useful during pregnancy or in situations in which intravenous contrast medium injection is undesirable. The test of 6-[beta](131I)-iodo-methyl-19-norcholesterol (NP-59) scintigraphy identifies functional tumors and discriminates aldosteronoma from adrenal hyperplasia with an overall accuracy of approximately 75%, but requires a tumor of sufficient size (>1 cm) for imaging to be dependable.

Adrenal vein sampling to lateralize the source of aldosterone production is useful in patients with hyperaldosteronism when there is no adrenal abnormality on CT or MRI or when both adrenal glands are abnormal but asymmetric. Further, patients older than 40 years, in whom the possibility of a nonfunctioning adenoma is statistically higher, may benefit from routine sampling. Percutaneous transfemoral cannulation of both adrenal veins is performed and intravenous ACTH (50 μ/hr) is administered. Simultaneous adrenal vein blood samples for aldosterone and cortisol are taken before and after ACTH injection, and their ratios are determined. The PAC is markedly higher (at least fourfold) on the side of an adenoma, whereas there is little or no left–right gradient

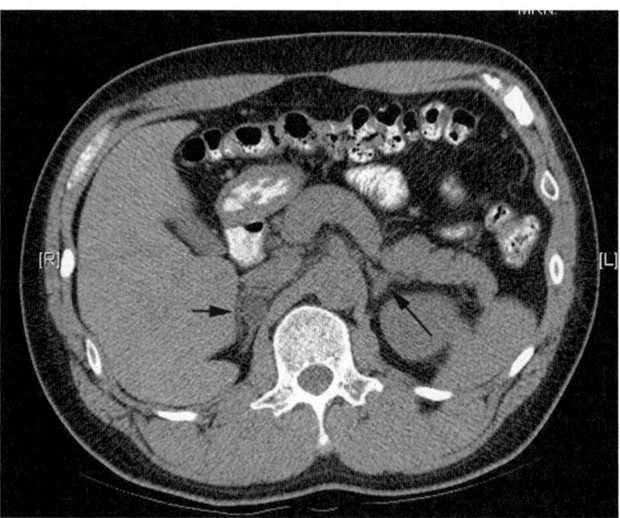

FIGURE 79.6 Computed tomography scan of right adrenal aldosteronoma. *Short arrow* shows aldosteronoma. *Long arrow* shows normal contralateral adrenal gland.

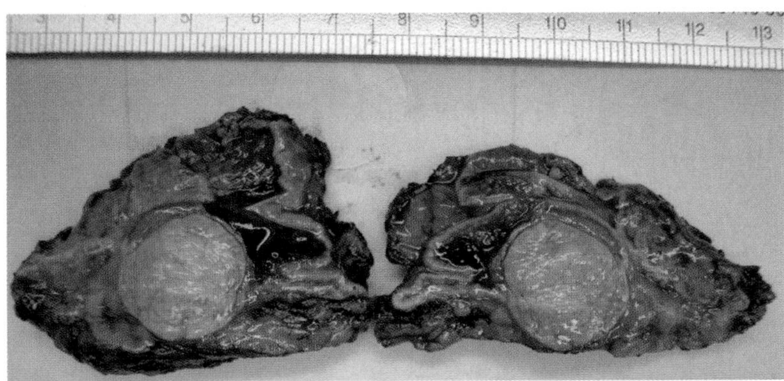

FIGURE 79.7 Aldosteronoma within right adrenal gland shown in Figure 79.8.

present in cases of bilateral adrenal hyperplasia. A 10-fold gradient of cortisol in adrenal veins to a peripheral sample ensures adequacy adrenal vein cannulation. This study is greater than 90% accurate and has been shown to alter management in 30% to 50% of patients, even in those with an apparent unilateral adenoma. This test is technically difficult and may be unsuccessful in 25% of patients. Emerging data suggest that adrenal vein sampling may be superior to CT in differentiating the source of aldosterone production in patients with hyperaldosteronism.

Treatment

Surgical removal of an aldosterone-secreting adenoma (Fig. 79.7) results in durable improvement of hypertension and hypokalemia in 70% to 90% of patients. Laparoscopic adrenalectomy is the preferred approach to remove these tumors. Morbidity and mortality following these procedures are almost negligible. Preoperative spironolactone or eplerenone and potassium are given to replenish potassium stores and correct alkalosis before anesthesia. Preoperatively, a significant fall in blood pressure with aldosterone receptor antagonists predicts a successful outcome after adrenalectomy. Response to adrenalectomy is also influenced by the duration and severity of hypertension and by the presence of histologic changes in the kidney. Age greater than 50 years, male sex, and the presence of multiple nodules within the adrenal is also associated with a poor response to surgery.

Management of idiopathic adrenal hyperplasia is medical because fewer than 20% to 30% of patients with this disease are cured by adrenalectomy. Idiopathic adrenal hyperplasia is treated with spironolactone or with newer aldosterone antagonist eplerenone. Other potassium sparing diuretics may be used including triamterene and amiloride. Treatment of glucocorticoid-suppressible hyperaldosteronism includes dexamethasone 0.5 to 1.0 mg daily. Glucocorticoids are used in small doses to avoid Cushing syndrome.

Congenital Adrenal Hyperplasia

The congenital adrenal hyperplasias are autosomal recessive conditions resulting from inherited defects of one or several of the enzymes necessary for cortisol biosynthesis (Fig. 79.8). Cortisol deficiency leads to ACTH overproduction and secondary hyperplasia of the adrenal cortex with shunting of cortisol precursors into adrenal androgen pathways. Peripheral tissues convert the excess adrenal androgens to testosterone, which causes virilization of the patient.

Most cases (>90%) of congenital adrenal hyperplasia are secondary to deficiency of 21-hydroxylase (CYP21A2) resulting from mutation of the gene on the short arm of chromosome 6. Two forms of this deficiency are recognized; partial or complete. The complete form is characterized by androgen excess at birth, with virilization, hypovolemia, hyponatremia, hyperkalemia, and hyperpigmentation. The partial form is characterized by virilization only and may present in adolescence or adulthood.

Of the remaining causes of congenital adrenal hyperplasia, 11-beta-hydroxylase deficiency (CYP11B1) is the second-most common cause, followed by 3-beta-hydroxydehydrogenase and 17-hydroxylase (CYP17) deficiency. Congenital lipoid adrenal hyperplasia is the most severe form of congenital adrenal hyperplasia and is often fatal (Table 79.4).

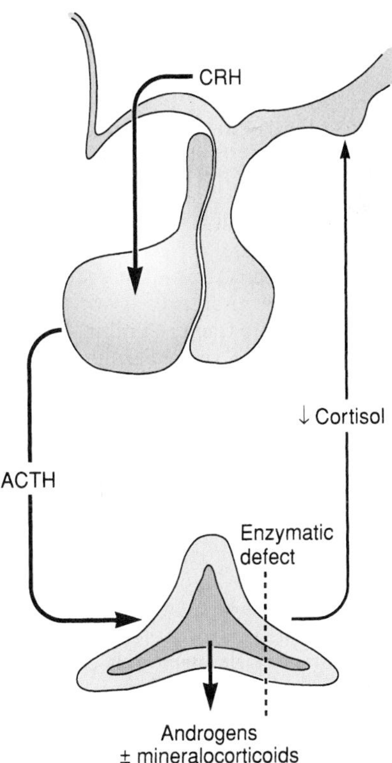

FIGURE 79.8 Schematic representation of the mechanism underlying congenital adrenal hyperplasias. Enzymatic defects in the adrenal gland prevent normal production of cortisol with resulting loss of negative feedback to the hypothalamus and pituitary. Chronic adrenocorticotropic hormone stimulation of the adrenal gland shunts steroid precursors through androgenic and mineralocorticoid pathways, leading to the overproduction of androgens and mineralocorticoids. The most common deficiencies are CYP21A2 (21-hydroxylase), CYP11B1 (11β-hydroxylase), and 3-β-HSD (3-β-hydroxysteroid dehydrogenase).

TABLE 79.4

CONGENITAL ADRENAL HYPERPLASIAS

Disease	21-Hydroxylase deficiency	11β-Hydroxylase deficiency	Aldosterone synthase deficiency	17α-Hydroxylase deficiency	3β-Hydroxysteroid dehydrogenase deficiency	Lipoid hyperplasia
Defective gene	*CYP21*	*CYP11B1*	*CYP11B2*	*CYP17*	*HSD3B2*	*STAR*
Ambiguous genitalia	Females	Females	No	Males	Males	Males
Addisonian crisis	Present	Rare	Salt wasting only	Absent	Present	Present
Incidence (general population)	1:10–18,000	1:100,000	Rare	Rare	Rare	Rare
Hormones						
Glucocorticoids	Reduced	Reduced	Normal	Corticosterone normal	Reduced	Reduced
Mineralocorticoids	Reduced	Elevated	Reduced	Elevated	Reduced	Reduced
Androgens	Elevated	Elevated	Normal	Reduced	Reduced (males) Elevated (females)	Reduced
Estrogens	Reduced (females)	Reduced in females	Normal	Reduced	Reduced	Reduced
Physiology						
Blood pressure	Reduced	Elevated	Reduced	Elevated	Reduced	Reduced
Na balance	Reduced	Elevated	Reduced	Elevated	Reduced	Reduced
K balance	Elevated	Reduced	Elevated	Reduced	Elevated	Elevated
Acidosis	Present	Absent	Present	Absent	Present	Present
Elevated metabolites	17-OHP	DOC, 11-deoxycortisol	Corticosterone ± 18-hydroxy-corticosterone	DOC corticosterone	DHEA, 17Δ^5 preg	None

OHP, hydroxyprogesterone; DOC, deoxycorticosterone; DHEA, dehydroepiandrostenedione.
(Modified from White PC, Speiser PW. Congenital adrenal hyperplasia due to 21-hydroxylase deficiency. *Endocr Rev.* 2000;21:245–291.)

Signs and Symptoms

Prenatal adrenal virilization in females produces ambiguous external genitalia (female pseudohermaphrodism). The ovaries, fallopian tubes, and uterus develop normally and patients are fertile. Postnatal congenital adrenal hyperplasia causes virilization of females and precocious puberty of males. Females develop hirsutism, polycystic ovaries, and irregular menses. Male patients exhibit secondary sexual characteristics by age 2 or 3 years. Fertility is often impaired. Both sexes experience rapid somatic growth and short stature. Virilization, salt wasting, and hyperpigmentation are variably present with the non-21-hydroxylase forms of congenital adrenal hyperplasias.

Diagnosis

Elevated plasma 17-hydroxyprogesterone is the most characteristic abnormality found in 21-hydroxylase deficiency. Both plasma cortisol and 24-hour free urinary cortisol excretion are variably reduced. Diagnosis of other forms of the disease involves demonstration of elevated levels of enzyme substrate: corticosterone and 11-deoxycortisol for 11-beta hydroxylase; dehydroepiandrosterone and 17 delta-5 hydroxypregnenolone for 3-beta hydroxydehydrogenase; and deoxycorticosterone and corticosterone for 17 beta-hydroxylase deficiency (Table 79.4).

Treatment

The treatment of 21-hydroxylase deficiency is glucocorticoid and mineralocorticoid replacement. Clinical management is often complicated by inadequately treated hyperandrogenism or iatrogenic hypercortisolism, or both. New treatment approaches under investigation include combination therapy to block androgen action and inhibit estrogen production, and bilateral adrenalectomy in the most severely affected patients. Female patients with ambiguous genitalia may require surgical correction as infants. Treatment of congenital adrenal hyperplasias caused by other enzyme deficiencies includes steroid and electrolyte replacement and surgical correction of the external genitalia in affected female infants.

Virilizing and Feminizing Adrenal Tumors

Excess production of adrenal androgens by an adrenal adenoma or carcinoma can produce virilizing features either alone or more commonly in addition to Cushing syndrome. Development of an adrenal virilizing tumor in women causes hirsutism and masculinization. Males with these tumors may present late with signs and symptoms of tumor enlargement or distant metastases develop. Virilizing tumors secrete androgen precursor, dehydroepiandrosterone, which can be measured either directly in plasma or in urine as a 17-ketosteroid. Feminizing adrenal neoplasms are extremely rare. Abdominal CT is subsequently used to localize the lesion. Resection of tumor and involved adrenal gland is the primary treatment for patients with adrenal virilizing tumors. Tumor recurrence is heralded by return of virilization or by detection of increased 17-ketosteroids in the urine. Tumor debulking or inhibition of steroidogenesis with aminoglutethimide or mitotane may be useful in controlling signs and symptoms in patients with metastatic disease.

Adrenocortical Carcinoma

Adrenocortical carcinoma is a rare malignancy with an estimated incidence of 0.5 to 2 cases per million per year.

Presentation peaks in the first and fifth decades of life. The prevalence is higher in females than in males (1.4 to 2:1). The cause of adrenocortical carcinoma is unknown, although somatic mutations in P53 and inheritance of this tumor in patients with germline mutations in P53 (Li Fraumeni syndrome) implicate this tumor suppressor gene in its pathogenesis.[1]

Signs and Symptoms

Adrenocortical carcinoma is a very aggressive malignancy, and most patients (up to 75%) present with locoregionally advanced or distant disease. Syndromes of adrenal hormone overproduction are frequent (up to 60%) and may include hypercortisolism, hyperaldosteronism, or virilization. Patients with rapidly progressive Cushing syndrome or mixed presentations with signs of both Cushing syndrome and virilization should be suspected of having adrenocortical carcinoma. Nonfunctioning adrenocortical carcinomas present most commonly as abdominal pain or mass with vague symptoms of nausea, weight loss, and fatigue.

Diagnosis

Patients with suspected adrenocortical carcinoma should have biochemical testing to identify hormone overproduction followed by staging investigations including cross-sectional imaging and bone scans. Contrast-enhanced CT of the abdomen and chest is important to preoperatively diagnose local tumor invasion and metastatic lesions as well as to confirm a functioning contralateral kidney (Fig. 79.9). In the absence of distant metastases or local invasion, preoperative distinction between large adenomas and carcinomas can be difficult, although large (>6 cm) adrenal masses that extend to nearby structures on CT scanning should be approached as carcinomas. Biopsy of adrenal lesions suspected of being adrenocortical carcinoma is unnecessary and should be avoided. The risk of seeding and the inability of histologic examination to distinguish between adenoma and carcinoma underlie this approach. Biopsy of extraadrenal lesions may be performed to confirm metastatic disease.

A definitive diagnosis of adrenocortical carcinoma requires pathologic demonstration of tumor invasion to adjacent organs or spread to lymph nodes or distant sites. Practically, any adrenal neoplasm larger than 6 cm or weighing more than 100 g should be considered malignant. Histologic features of tumor necrosis, hemorrhage, and local invasion are gross pathologic evidence of carcinoma, while cells with large, hyperchromatic nuclei and more than 20 mitoses per high-power field suggest malignancy.

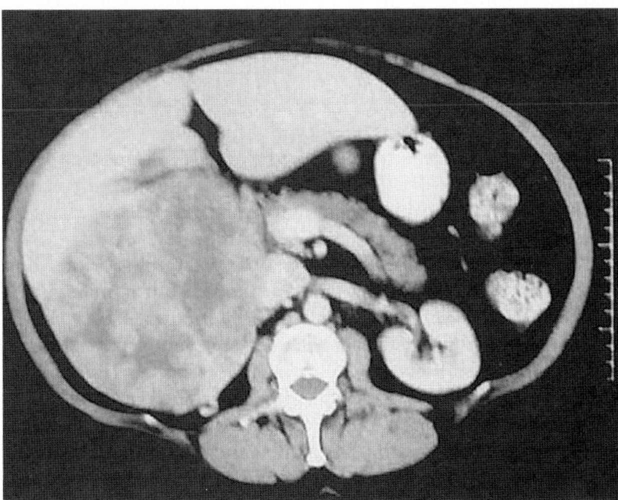

FIGURE 79.9 Computed tomography scan of right adrenocortical carcinoma showing invasion of liver and inferior vena cava. Note that a contralateral kidney is present and functioning.

TABLE 79.5 STAGING

AMERICAN JOINT COMMITTEE ON CANCER STAGING OF ADRENOCORTICAL CARCINOMA, WITH 5-YEAR SURVIVAL RATES

Stage	Criteria
Tumor	
T1	Tumor <5 cm, no invasion
T2	Tumor >5 cm, no invasion
T3	Tumor with invasion to fat
T4	Tumor with organ invasion
Lymph nodes	
N0	No lymph node metastasis
N1	Lymph node metastasis present
Metastasis	
M0	No distant metastasis
M1	Distant metastasis present

Stage group	TNM	5-year survival rate
I	T1 (<5 cm) N0M0	30%–45%
II	T2 (>5 cm) N0M0	12%–57%
III	T1-2, N1, M0 T3N0M0	5%–18%
IV	Any T, any N, M1 T3–4N1M0	0

Treatment

Surgical resection is the mainstay of treatment for all stages of adrenocortical carcinoma. Complete resection of locally confined tumor is the only chance for cure from adrenocortical carcinoma. However, distant or local spread is evident in 65% of cases at presentation and a minority of patients is resectable with curative intent. Recurrence rates after surgery range from 38 to 85%, depending on stage at presentation (Table 79.5).

Many patients with adrenocortical carcinoma present with metastatic disease, involving the lung, lymph nodes, liver, or bone. Resection or surgical debulking of locally advanced or metastatic lesions may provide symptomatic relief for select patients, especially those with low-grade, slow-growing, hormonally productive cancers. Symptomatic recurrent or metastatic disease is best treated by resection when feasible.

Chemotherapy for adrenocortical carcinoma usually includes mitotane, although no controlled studies have established its efficacy in this disease. Partial responses to mitotane occur in less than a third of patients, and survival is unchanged. Adjuvant chemotherapy with mitotane after complete resection for adrenocortical carcinoma is unproven and toxic so that many oncologists reserve its use for recurrent, unresectable or metastatic disease. Cisplatin in combination with mitotane or doxorubicin and 5-fluoruracil have been applied in metastatic disease with partial responses noted.

The prognosis of adrenocortical carcinoma is poor. Median survival following diagnosis for all patients is approximately 18 months. Overall survival following resection for all stages of adrenocortical cancer is 15% to 47% at 5 years. Stage-specific 5-year survival is 30% to 45% for stage I, 12% to 57% for stage II, 5% to 18% for stage III, and 0 for stage IV disease.

DISEASES OF THE ADRENAL MEDULLA

Pheochromocytoma

Pheochromocytomas are functional adrenal tumors that arise from neuroectodermal cells of the adrenal medulla or in certain extraadrenal sites. These tumors are uncommon, occurring in 0.005% to 0.1% of persons, but occur with increased frequency in hypertensive populations (0.2% incidence) and in heritable endocrine tumor syndromes. The peak incidence of pheochromocytoma occurs during the fourth and fifth decades of life, and men and women are affected about equally. The *rule of tens* is a useful way to characterize pheochromocytoma: tumors are bilateral in 10% of cases, extraadrenal in 10%, familial in 10%, multicentric in 10%, and malignant in 10% and occur in children in 10% of cases.

Approximately 10% of pheochromocytomas are extraadrenal, although most (98%) are still located within the abdomen. Extraadrenal pheochromocytomas can occur at any site in the abdomen where chromaffin tissue is located and have been found in the paravertebral ganglia, the organ of Zuckerkandl, and the urinary bladder. Clues to the presence of extraadrenal pheochromocytoma are predominance of norepinephrine because extraadrenal sites lack the enzyme necessary to convert norepinephrine to epinephrine.

Familial pheochromocytoma is a component of two autosomal dominant syndromes: von Hippel-Lindau syndrome and multiple endocrine neoplasia (MEN)-2. Patients with von Hippel-Lindau syndrome have pheochromocytoma (usually bilateral), retinal angiomas, cerebellar hemangioblastoma, epididymal cystadenoma, renal and pancreatic cysts, and renal cell carcinoma. Patients with MEN 2A develop pheochromocytoma (usually bilateral), medullary carcinoma of the thyroid (MTC), and primary parathyroid hyperplasia. Patients with MEN 2B develop pheochromocytoma (usually bilateral), MTC, mucosal neuromas, intestinal ganglioneuromatosis, and have a characteristic marfanoid body habitus. Pheochromocytoma also occurs in neurofibromatosis type 1 and familial paraganglioma. The frequency of pheochromocytoma in these disorders is 10% to 20% in von Hippel-Lindau syndrome, 50% in MEN-2, and 0.1 to 5.7% with neurofibromatosis type 1.

In some families, patients with pheochromocytomas have no other clinical abnormalities, suggesting the existence of a separate disease limited to the formation of adrenal medullary tumors. In a study of three generations of an affected kindred, a novel mutation was found in the von Hippel-Lindau gene even though there were no other clinical manifestations of this disorder. Patients with bilateral pheochromocytoma, young patients with pheochromocytoma, and patients with paraganglioma should be screened for MEN2 and von Hippel-Lindau syndrome.

The etiology and pathogenesis of pheochromocytoma is unknown. A genetic component seems certain because pheochromocytoma occurs not only as a part of familial syndromes but also as an isolated disorder because of mutation in the RET gene or the MEN2 gene. Familial pheochromocytoma as well as sporadic pheochromocytoma occurs also with mutations in the succinate dehydrogenase complex, subunit B, iron sulfur protein (SDHB). Either germline or somatic mutations in the SDHD gene is another cause of pheochromocytoma.[2]

Signs and Symptoms

Symptoms of pheochromocytoma are attributable to the effects of excessive circulating catecholamines on target tissues (Table 79.3). The classic triad of symptoms in patients with a pheochromocytoma is episodic headache, sweating, and tachycardia. Hypertension is common with pheochromocytoma and is sustained in roughly half of patients, is paroxysmal in one third, and is absent in one fifth. Orthostatic hypotension results from diminished plasma volume and blunted autonomic reflexes. Other symptoms include palpitations, anxiety, and tremulousness. Cardiovascular sequelae include myocardial infarction, cardiac dysrhythmias, and stroke. Gastrointestinal motility is also impaired. Asymptomatic patients with functioning tumors are rare, and nonfunctioning tumors are distinctly uncommon. Sudden death has been reported in patients with pheochromocytoma who have undergone surgical procedures or childbirth.

Diagnosis

Elevation of catecholamines and their metabolites in either urine or blood is essential for the diagnosis of pheochromocytoma. Determination of plasma-fractionated metanephrines is probably the best test for diagnosis of pheochromocytoma. Alternatively, measurement catecholamines and their metabolites in a single 24-hour urine collection may be performed to make or exclude this diagnosis. Measurement of plasma catecholamines is not as useful in distinguishing patients with pheochromocytoma from those with essential hypertension. Measurement of plasma chromogranin A is nonspecific and a poor diagnostic but potentially helpful confirmatory test.

Many medications alter or interfere with measurement or either plasma or urine catecholamines. Such medications should be discontinued to ensure accurate testing. These drugs include acetaminophen, labetolol, clonidine withdrawal, tricyclic antidepressants, antipsychotics and ethanol. To control blood pressure, other antihypertensives such as calcium channel blockers may be substituted.

In normotensive or mildly hypertensive patients with elevated plasma catecholamine levels (1,000 to −2,000 pg/mL), a clonidine suppression test may be used to distinguish from pheochromocytoma. An oral 0.3-mg dose of clonidine suppresses centrally mediated release of catecholamines to less than 500 pg/mL within 2 to 3 hours but does not affect release of catecholamines by a pheochromocytoma.

Biochemical confirmation of the diagnosis should be followed by radiologic evaluation to locate the tumor. Pheochromocytomas are best imaged with CT or MRI. Contrast-enhanced CT readily detects tumors 1 cm and larger and has sensitivity of 87% to 100% for pheochromocytoma (Fig. 79.10A). MRI is similarly sensitive, and a T2-weighted image brightness three times greater than liver is highly specific for pheochromocytoma (Fig. 79.10B, C). MRI is useful in suspected malignant pheochromocytoma to evaluate for inferior vena cava thrombus or liver invasion.

Functional nuclear imaging with iodine-131-metaiodobenzylguanidine (131-I MIBG) is a useful adjunct to cross sectional imaging for pheochromocytoma (Fig. 79.10D). MIBG resembles norepinephrine and is taken up by adrenergic tissues including pheochromocytoma. An MIBG scan can detect tumors not detected by CT or MRI or multiple tumors when CT or MRI is positive. Multiinstitutional experience with this technique has demonstrated an overall sensitivity of 77% to 87% and a specificity of 96% to 100%. This test is usually not necessary for sporadic pheochromocytoma unless urinary or plasma catecholamines and metabolites are marginally elevated, or if malignant or extraadrenal pheochromocytoma is suspected. 131-I MIBG scanning is also useful to screen patients with metastatic pheochromocytoma for high dose 131I MIBG therapy. 111-In-pentetreotide scintigraphy may also identify pheochromocytoma and can be used therapeutically as with 131-I MIBG.

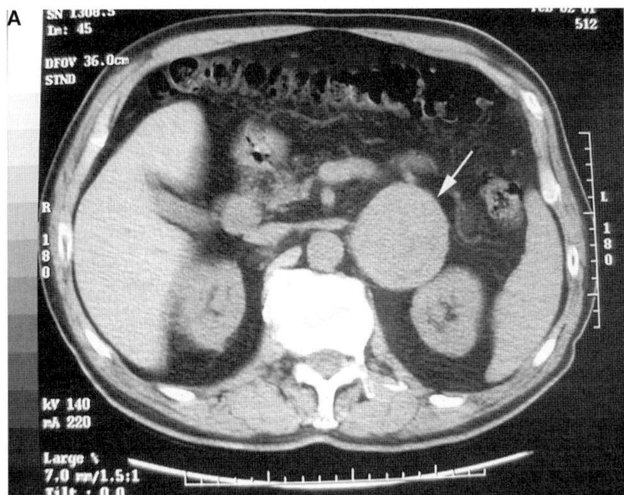

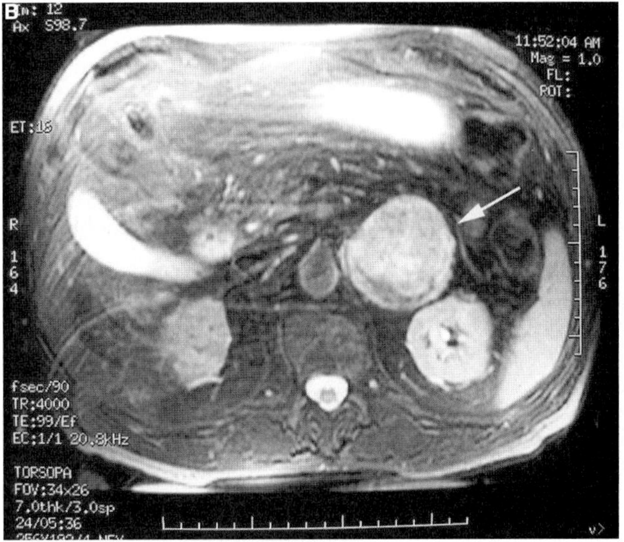

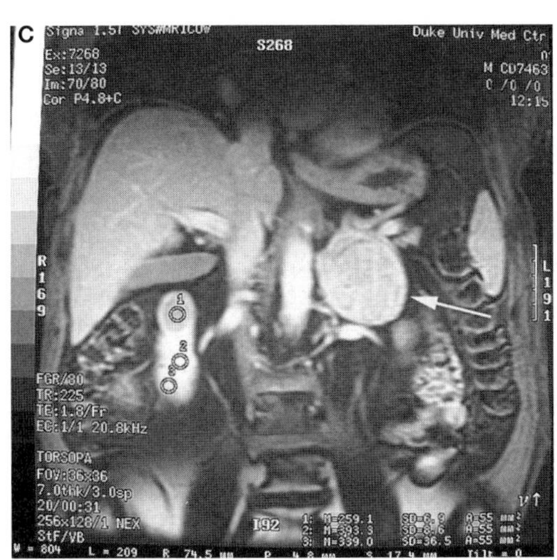

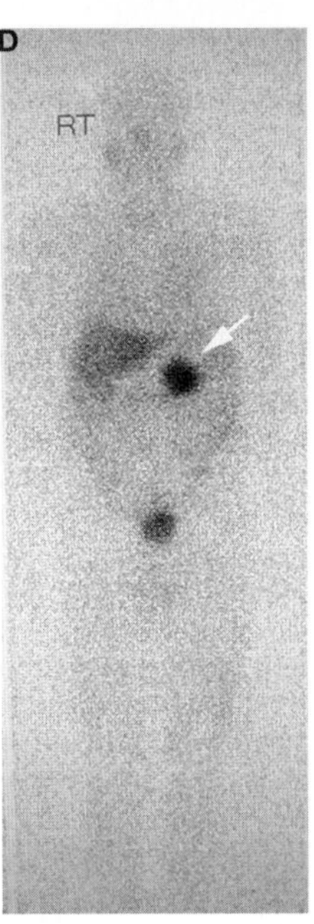

FIGURE 79.10 Imaging of pheochromocytoma (*arrows*). (*A*) Computed tomography scan shows well-circumscribed left adrenal mass. (*B*) T2-weighted magnetic resonance imaging shows the mass to be heterogeneously bright consistent with pheochromocytoma. (*C*) and (*D*) Coronal contrast enhanced MRI and near-simultaneous ^{131}I-metaiodobenzylguanine (^{131}I-MIBG) scanning show location of the pheochromocytoma and relationship to surrounding structures.

Treatment

Surgical resection is the only cure for pheochromocytoma. When the diagnosis of pheochromocytoma has been established and localization studies are completed, preoperative preparation of the patient centers on blood pressure control. Usually 1 to 3 weeks before operation alpha-adrenergic blockade is performed first with phenoxybenzamine, starting at 10 mg twice a day and increasing by 10 to 20 mg per day until blood pressure normalizes. Side effects of alpha blockade include postural hypotension, reflex tachycardia, nasal congestion, and an inability to ejaculate. Preoperative alpha blockade also reverses the relative hypovolemia that is usually present in patients with pheochromocytoma and also prevents severe blood pressure swings during intraoperative manipulation of the tumor. Metyrapone added preoperatively to phenoxybenzamine can achieve a greater degree of sympathetic blockade.

Beta-adrenergic blockade with propranolol added after alpha blockade can manage patients who develop tachycardia or who have inducible cardiac arrhythmias or ischemia. Propranolol may enhance pressor response to endogenous norepinephrine and thus should not be given until adequate alpha blockade has been established. Propranolol can also produce profound bradycardia, myocardial depression, and congestive heart failure. Newer drug regimens to manage hypertension in pheochromocytoma include selective alpha-1-adrenergic antagonists (terazosin and doxazosin) and calcium channel blockers (nifedipine and nicardipine).

Patients with pheochromocytoma can be expected to have blood pressure volatility and high intravascular volume requirements during and immediately after surgery. Elderly patients or those with history of heart disease may require pulmonary catheter insertion and arterial line placement for careful monitoring of blood pressure and arterial pH. Anesthetic agents may trigger the release of catecholamines from pheochromocytomas. The anesthetic plane is now considered more important than the choice of agent, and both enflurane and isoflurane have been used successfully. Magnesium administration during surgery is an effective way to control blood pressure in patients with pheochromocytoma. Intraoperative hypertension is best treated with a sodium nitroprusside drip, and cardiac arrhythmias are best managed with short-acting beta-blockers (esmolol) or lidocaine.

Formerly, an anterior approach through either a midline or bilateral subcostal incisions was used exclusively to resect pheochromocytomas. Today, CT, MRI, and nuclear scans permit preoperative localization of tumor in 95% or more of cases, so that the surgical approach may be more directed using a laparoscopic approach. Regardless of approach, important common principles include minimal handling of the tumor, early isolation and ligation of the adrenal vein, and avoidance of capsular rupture. Recurrence following resection of benign pheochromocytoma is infrequent, and its presence indicated malignancy.

Recurrent, malignant pheochromocytoma can include locally advance disease or metastasis to bone, liver, lymph nodes, lungs, and the central nervous system. Treatment of malignant pheochromocytoma involves resection of metastases when feasible and medical control of hypertension. Radiation therapy may be helpful to ameliorate pain from bony metastases. Ablative therapy with 131-I MIBG may also produce partial responses and palliation of hormonal symptoms. Radiofrequency ablation of hepatic and bone metastases can be effective in selected patients. Combination chemotherapy with cyclophosphamide, vincristine, and dacarbazine can also be effective. Overall 5-year survival for patients with malignant pheochromocytoma ranges from 36% to 60%.

Metastasis to the Adrenal Glands

The adrenal glands are frequent sites for metastases from many cancers. Carcinoma of the lung and breast account for most adrenal metastases; however, virtually any cancer including melanoma, lymphoma, and kidney and ovarian carcinoma can spread to the adrenals. Autopsy series of patients with carcinoma show that the adrenal glands are involved in more than 25% of cases. Among cancer patients, 50% to 75% of newly discovered adrenal masses represent metastases. Usually, either a primary site is obvious, or widespread disease is apparent. Biopsy of adrenal masses in patients with a history of carcinoma may be performed after pheochromocytoma is excluded. Resection of isolated adrenal metastases in select patients with long disease free intervals from lung cancer, renal cell carcinoma and melanoma can be considered, although subsequent extraadrenal disease usually develops. Median survival after complete resection of isolated adrenal metastases from a variety of tumors ranges from 13 to 60 months with actuarial 2- and 5-year survival of 40% to 50% and 20%, respectively.

Incidental Adrenal Mass

Clinically inapparent adrenal masses (also called *adrenal incidentalomas*) have become commonplace over the past 20 years with the increased use of abdominal imaging such as CT and MRI. The estimated prevalence of incidental adrenal neoplasms varies by population studied and method of detection. Unsuspected adrenal masses are detected by CT in between 0.6% and 1.9% of healthy patients, a figure that is somewhat lower than the estimated prevalence of up to 8.7% based on unselected autopsy data. Patients with a prior history of malignancy have a prevalence of adrenal masses of up to 4.4%. Adrenal masses increase in frequency with advancing age, ranging from 3% in midlife to 10% in the elderly. The combination of an aging population and increased application of abdominal imaging promises to create a significant public health challenge.

Over the past 10 years, increased awareness of morbidity associated with subclinical hormone overproduction as well the increased availability of minimally invasive, laparoscopic adrenalectomy has resulted in a lower threshold for treatment of adrenal masses. The goal of evaluation is to distinguish and remove those adrenal masses that are functioning or likely to be malignant versus those that are neither and may be observed.

Expectations of the yield for the workup of adrenal masses may be informed by epidemiologic reports and reports of pathologic findings in resected incidentalomas. Epidemiologic data indicate that up to 6.5% of incidentalomas are pheochromocytoma, 7% produce aldosterone, 0.035% produce cortisol, and 0.06% is carcinoma. A recent review of 44 reports describing over 3,000 such cases reported that 41% were cortical adenomas, 19% were metastases from other primary cancers, 10% were adrenocortical carcinomas, and 8% were pheochromocytomas, with the remainder including myelolipomas and cysts.

Diagnosis

The evaluation of incidental adrenal masses, previously considered controversial, can now be standardized. Two simple questions must be answered: Is it functional? Is it malignant? The diagnostic approach should proceed to answer these questions sequentially (Table 79.6). Current opinion is that all asymptomatic patients with adrenal masses should be screened for pheochromocytoma, hypercortisolism, and hyperaldosteronism (Algorithm 79.3).

All patients require a complete history and physical examination, biochemical evaluation of pertinent hormones, and select imaging studies. Attention must be paid to episodes of hypertension, tachycardia, and anxiety that suggest pheochromocytoma. Physical findings such as muscle wasting, purple striae, hirsutism, and gynecomastia may suggest either Cushing syndrome or a virilizing tumor. Secondary metastases from underlying malignancy must be considered and evaluated with appropriate history, physical examination, and select tests including mammograms in women and chest radiography in all patients, especially smokers.

Biochemical testing should routinely exclude pheochromocytoma, hypercortisolism, and hyperaldosteronism. Pheochromocytoma is evaluated either by 24-hour urine collection for catecholamines, metanephrines, and 3-methoxy-4-hydroxymandelic acid, or by plasma fractionated metanephrines. Subclinical or clinically apparent Cushing syndrome is best evaluated with the overnight 1 mg dexamethasone suppression test. Hyperaldosteronism is best assessed by concurrent measurement of serum or plasma aldosterone and PRA.

Imaging studies usually include cross-sectional imaging with either CT or MRI. CT is the best test for identifying and characterizing most adrenal masses. Using a fast scanner and 1-m scanning intervals, both adrenal glands can be identified in 97% to 99% of patients and lesions as small as 5 mm can be readily identified. Currently, attenuation values expressed in Hounsfield units (HU) have better performance than size or other criteria to differentiate adenomas from adrenal malignancy and nonadenomas such as pheochromocytoma. Adenomas are usually lipid rich and have attenuation values less than 18 HU on unenhanced CT, a threshold with high sensitivity and specificity (85% to 95% and 93% to 100%, respectively). Generally,

TABLE 79.6 DIAGNOSIS

SUMMARY OF TESTS FOR EVALUATION OF INCIDENTAL ADRENAL MASS

Question	Best test	Alternative test	Diagnosis
Is it functioning?	Plasma fractionated metanephrines	24-hr urine for catecholamines, metanephrines, VMA	Pheochromocytoma
	1 mg dexamethasone suppression test	24-hour urine for cortisol	Hypercortisolism
	Serum potassium Plasma renin/plasma aldosterone ratio	24-hour urine for potassium	Hyperaldosteronism
Is it malignant?	Computed tomography	Magnetic resonance imaging	Cortical adenoma Adrenocortical Carcinoma Pheochromocytoma Myelolipoma Cyst
	Fine Needle Aspiration		Metastasis

further workup is unnecessary when an adrenal lesion has an attenuation of less than 10 HU suggesting lipid-rich adrenal adenoma. A notable exception is lipid poor adenoma, which has higher HU density. In these cases, rapid washout of intravenous contrast suggests an adenoma. Using a 10- to 15-minute delayed enhanced CT, a washout value of 50% to 60% of the initial enhancement is used to distinguish adenoma from nonadenoma.

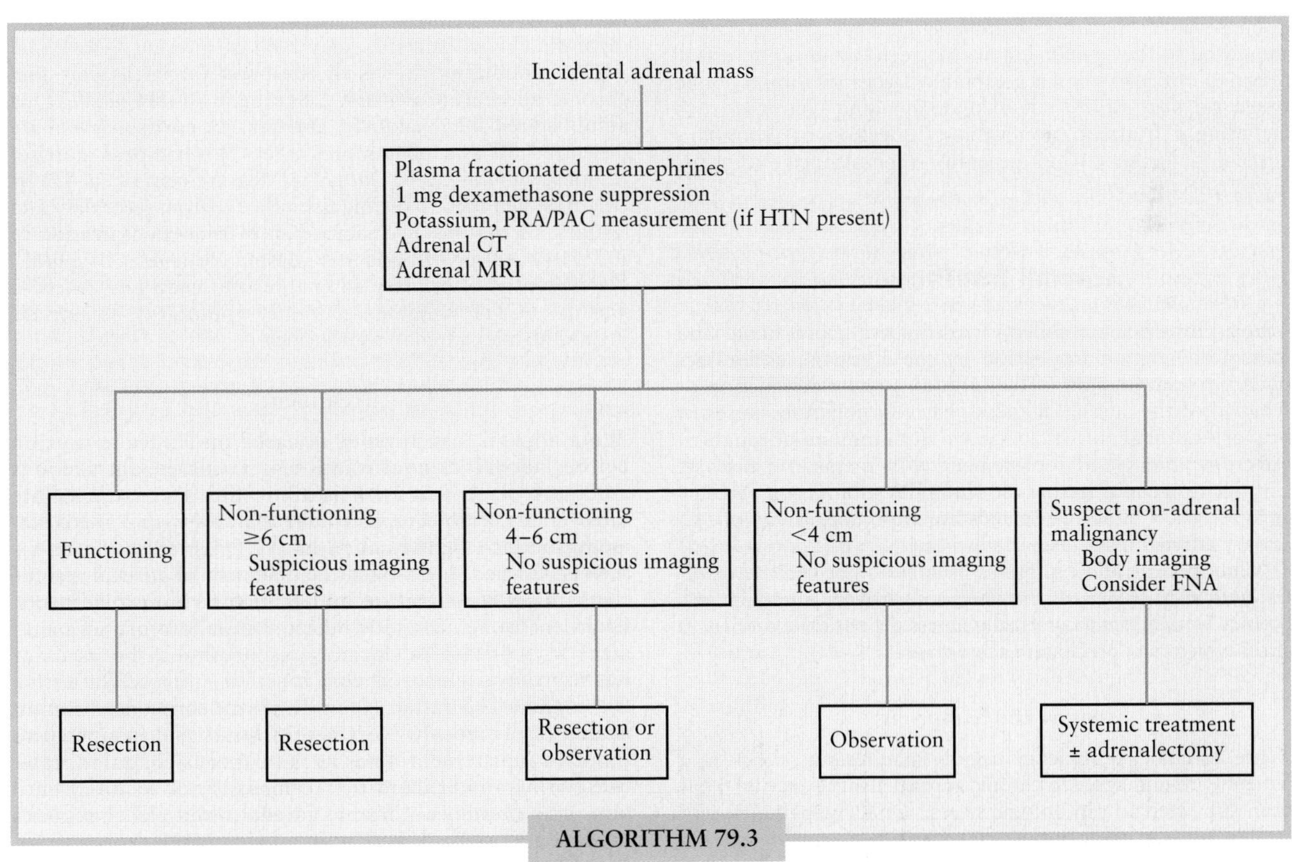

ALGORITHM 79.3 Diagnosis and management of the incidental adrenal mass. PRA, plasma renin activity; PAC, plasma aldosterone concentration; HTN, hypertension; CT, computed tomography; MRI, magnetic resonance imaging; FNA, fine needle aspiration.

MRI can differentiate adenomas, metastases and pheochromocytomas, although the best MRI technique for evaluating adrenal masses is complex and controversial. Adenomas usually show a loss in signal intensity on chemical shift MRI because of high lipid content. Malignant masses tend to be bright on T2-weighted images because of higher fluid content. Secondary metastases to the adrenal are hypointense to liver on T1-weighted images and are brighter than liver on T2-weighted images. Metastases also typically show strong contrast enhancement. Pheochromocytomas most often have low lipid content and high water content, giving low T1 signal intensities and very bright T2 signal intensities. Comparison of the adrenal mass to liver and spleen intensities on various sequences adds to specificity and sensitivity of the test.

Masses that appear cystic may be aspirated under CT guidance. Fine-needle aspiration biopsy may be of value in patients with known extraadrenal malignancy; however, it is not indicated in the evaluation of primary adrenal neoplasms and is contraindicated if pheochromocytoma is suspected.

Treatment

Resection is indicated for all functioning adrenal incidentalomas and those suspected of harboring primary adrenal cancer. Size cutoff for resecting adrenal incidentalomas has drifted to include smaller and smaller lesions. The prevalence of primary adrenal carcinoma in adrenal incidentalomas is related to mass size. The risk of primary adrenal carcinoma is less than 2% in lesions under 4 cm while the incidence rises to 25% for lesions larger than 6 cm. Lesions larger than 6 cm and smaller lesions with suspicious criteria on imaging should be resected. Lesions smaller than 4 cm with benign imaging characteristics should be followed. For lesions between 4 and 6 cm, either resection or observation is acceptable. Decisions should not be based on size alone, but also on imaging characteristics including CT attenuation values. Resection of secondary adrenal malignancy is not generally recommended except for highly select patients.

Adrenal Insufficiency

Adrenal insufficiency reflects inadequate glucocorticoid and mineralocorticoid production by the adrenals, either secondary to suppression of the HPA axis or by destruction or removal of the adrenal glands. The most common causes of primary adrenal insufficiency are autoimmune adrenalitis, infection, and gland replacement with metastatic disease. Chronic exogenous steroid use with HPA suppression and surgical resection of adrenal glands are important causes of secondary adrenal insufficiency.

Clinical signs and symptoms usually do not become manifest until at least 90% of the gland is destroyed. Adrenal insufficiency usually occurs gradually unless the patient experiences stress which may precipitate acute crisis.

Signs and Symptoms

Acute adrenal insufficiency usually manifests as shock in a patient with undiagnosed chronic adrenal insufficiency who has been subjected to physiologic stress. Similarly, patients with established adrenal insufficiency caused by exogenous steroid use may experience crisis if they do not increase glucocorticoid replacement during times of stress or illness. Symptoms of adrenal insufficiency reflect glucocorticoid and mineralocorticoid deficiencies. Signs and symptoms of acute insufficiency include fever, nausea, vomiting, refractory hypotension, and lethargy (Table 79.7). Acute adrenal insufficiency is a medical emergency and should be suspected in stressed patients with a history of either adrenal insufficiency or exogenous steroid use. Chronic adrenal insufficiency presents more subtly, with fatigue, weight loss, anorexia, nausea and vomiting, abdominal pain, and diarrhea.

TABLE 79.7 DIAGNOSIS

SYMPTOMS AND SIGNS OF ACUTE ADRENAL INSUFFICIENCY

Symptoms
Lethargy
Confusion or disorientation
Nausea and vomiting
Abdominal pain
Signs
Hypotension
Hyponatremia, hyperkalemia, azotemia,
Hypoglycemia
Fever
Anemia

Diagnosis

Laboratory findings of adrenal insufficiency include hyponatremia, hyperkalemia, azotemia, and fasting or reactive hypoglycemia. Hypercalcemia may also be present. The rapid ACTH stimulation test is the best test for both acute and chronic adrenal insufficiency. Synthetic ACTH (250 μg) is administered intravenously, and plasma cortisol levels are measured 30 and 60 minutes later. Normal peak cortisol response should exceed 20μg/dL. Measurement of ACTH by IRMA is then used to distinguish primary from secondary and tertiary adrenal insufficiency. High plasma concentration of ACTH (>200 pg/dL) and low plasma cortisol (<10 mg/dL) are diagnostic of primary adrenal insufficiency. Low levels of plasma ACTH indicate secondary (pituitary) or tertiary (hypothalamic) adrenal insufficiency.

Treatment

Acute adrenal insufficiency is based on clinical suspicion before laboratory confirmation is available. Intravenous volume replacement with isotonic fluids and immediate intravenous steroid replacement therapy with 4 mg dexamethasone is essential. A rapid ACTH stimulation test is then performed to establish the diagnosis of adrenal insufficiency after resuscitation and corticosteroid replacement. Hydrocortisone acetate is detected in laboratory measurement for cortisol so dexamethasone should be used for replacement of glucocorticoid function until ACTH testing is complete. Thereafter, 100 mg of hydrocortisone is administered intravenously every 6 to 8 hours and is tapered to standard replacement doses as the patient's condition stabilizes. Mineralocorticoid replacement is not required until oral intake resumes. Chronic adrenal insufficiency requires both corticosteroid and mineralocorticoid replacement. Usual daily dosing is 12 mg/m^2 of hydrocortisone and 0.05 to 0.10 mg fludrocortisone.

Patients who have known adrenal insufficiency or who have received supraphysiologic doses of corticosteroid for at least 1 week in the year preceding surgery should receive perioperative stress-dose corticosteroids. Administration of 100 mg hydrocortisone the morning of major surgery followed by 100 mg of hydrocortisone every 8 hours during the perioperative 24 hours is usually more than sufficient. Steroids can be rapidly tapered to replacement levels as the patient's condition permits.

Adrenalectomy. Surgical approaches to the adrenal glands include the laparoscopic approach, the anterior transabdominal approach, and less commonly, the combined thoracoabdominal approach or posterior retroperitoneal approach. Either adrenal gland can be removed using any of these approaches. The choice of approach depends on the suspected pathology, the size of the adrenal lesion, and the expertise of the surgeon. Small benign appearing tumors that are localized with confidence by imaging studies are resected using a laparoscopic or posterior approach. Posterior retroperitoneal adrenalectomy, once the most common method of adrenalectomy is less commonly used since most lesions amenable to this approach can be removed laparoscopically. Large adrenal masses and those that may harbor malignancy should be resected using an anterior approach to adequately explore the entire abdomen and gain sufficient exposure for safe resection. Very large adrenocortical carcinomas may require a thoracoabdominal approach for *en bloc* resection with involved adjacent structures.

Laparoscopic adrenalectomy. Laparoscopic adrenalectomy is now the preferred approach to most small, benign adrenal lesions including functioning and nonfunctioning adenomas and pheochromocytomas. Enthusiasm for the laparoscopic approach is based on the expectation of decreased postoperative pain, faster rehabilitation, and fewer complications. Numerous studies have shown the efficacy and safety of this procedure for tumors up to 6 cm. Larger lesions can be approached by experienced surgeons in select circumstances. Importantly, expertise in open adrenalectomy is absolutely necessary for the laparoscopic surgeon to convert to an open procedure and promptly rectify any intraoperative laparoscopic complications.

Laparoscopic adrenalectomy begins with induction of general anesthesia, placement of a urinary catheter and orogastric tube, and positioning of the patient in the lateral decubitus position with the affected side up. Exposure is facilitated by extension of the operating table at the patient's waist. A total of three or four intraperitoneal ports (one camera, one retractor particular for the right side, and two working ports) are placed at least 5 cm apart in a transverse line from the lateral edge of the rectus sheath to the midaxillary line between the costal margin and iliac crest (Fig. 79.11A). Four-quadrant exploration of the peritoneal cavity is first performed with the videoscope through the medialmost port, and the videoscope is then transferred to the middle port. A retractor is placed through the medialmost port to retract the viscera medially. Operating instruments are alternately placed within the abdomen through the lateral ports.

Laparoscopic adrenalectomy proceeds similar to the open anterior approach. Right adrenalectomy begins with mobilization of the liver to open the retroperitoneum and allow retraction of the right lobe of anteriorly and medially using the most medial port. The adrenal gland is then identified posterolateral to the inferior vena cava and superior to the kidney. Dissection usually begins by developing the plane between right adrenal and inferior vena cava using careful blunt dissection, with small vessels sequentially coagulated using electrosurgical or harmonic energy. The right adrenal vein is identified, carefully dissected and then doubly clipped and divided (Fig. 79.12A). Dissection then continues circumferentially around the gland with additional small vessels coagulated or clipped. The adrenal gland subsequently is placed in a bag and removed through an expanded port.

Left adrenalectomy is performed with mirror-image patient and port site orientation as right adrenalectomy. After port placement, dissection begins with mobilization of the splenic flexure of the colon and spleen from the left retroperitoneum. Subsequent medial retraction of the spleen, tail of the pancreas, and stomach is accomplished with the fan or similar retractor if necessary. Often after full mobilization, no retractor is necessary, and thus only 3 ports are needed. The left adrenal gland is identified in perinephric fat at the superior renal pole. Intraoperative laparoscopic ultrasound can be useful for this on the left side, particularly in Cushing syndrome with the associated increased truncal fat. Once identified, left adrenal gland dissection proceeds circumferentially around the gland, with identification, ligation and division of the left adrenal vein at the inferiormost aspect of the dissection (Fig. 79.12B). Care is needed to identify and avoid the inferior phrenic vein, which courses along the medial aspect of the left adrenal gland. Following circumferential dissection, the gland is removed.

Anterior approach. Anterior, open adrenalectomy begins with positioning the patient in reverse Trendelenburg position with elevation of the right flank. An ipsilateral or bilateral subcostal incision allows access to either adrenal and facilitates exploration of the abdomen (Fig. 79.11B). The abdomen is opened and explored for evidence of metastatic disease, including biopsy or excision of suspicious lesions. Resection of the right adrenal gland proceeds with full mobilization and anteromedial retraction of the right hepatic lobe (Fig. 79.13A). It is important to fully expose the retrohepatic inferior vena cava. In order to uncover the inferior vena cava, the right kidney and the right adrenal gland, the hepatic flexure and transverse colon and are retracted inferiorly, usually without need for extensive mobilization. A Kocher maneuver of the duodenum is seldom necessary as the adrenal gland is superior to this area. The retroperitoneal space is entered behind the liver to expose the adrenal gland. Dissection of the gland proceeds from its inferomedial aspect, where small feeding arteries are individually clipped and divided. The vena cava is carefully dissected along its lateral border, which allows identification of the right adrenal vein where it drains directly into the inferior vena cava from the anterior aspect of the adrenal gland. The adrenal vein is ligated and divided close to the vena cava. If necessary because of hemodynamic changes during an operation for a pheochromocytoma, the adrenal vein is identified and ligated early to avoid catecholamine surges and blood pressure fluctuations during manipulation of the gland. Once the adrenal vein is ligated, arterial feeding vessels are clipped and divided sequentially, beginning at the superolateral aspect of the gland and continuing medially.

Resection of the left adrenal gland requires mobilization of the spleen, tail of pancreas and left colon. The left colon is freed from its peritoneal attachments and is reflected inferiorly. The spleen is then delivered from the left upper quadrant medially, and the splenocolic ligament is divided. The spleen, stomach, and pancreatic tail are retracted medially *en bloc* to expose the left kidney and adrenal (Fig. 79.13B). The left adrenal vein is ligated and divided at its junction with the left renal vein. The gland is dissected and the arterial vessels are ligated and divided sequentially, beginning at the superolateral aspect of the gland and continuing medially.

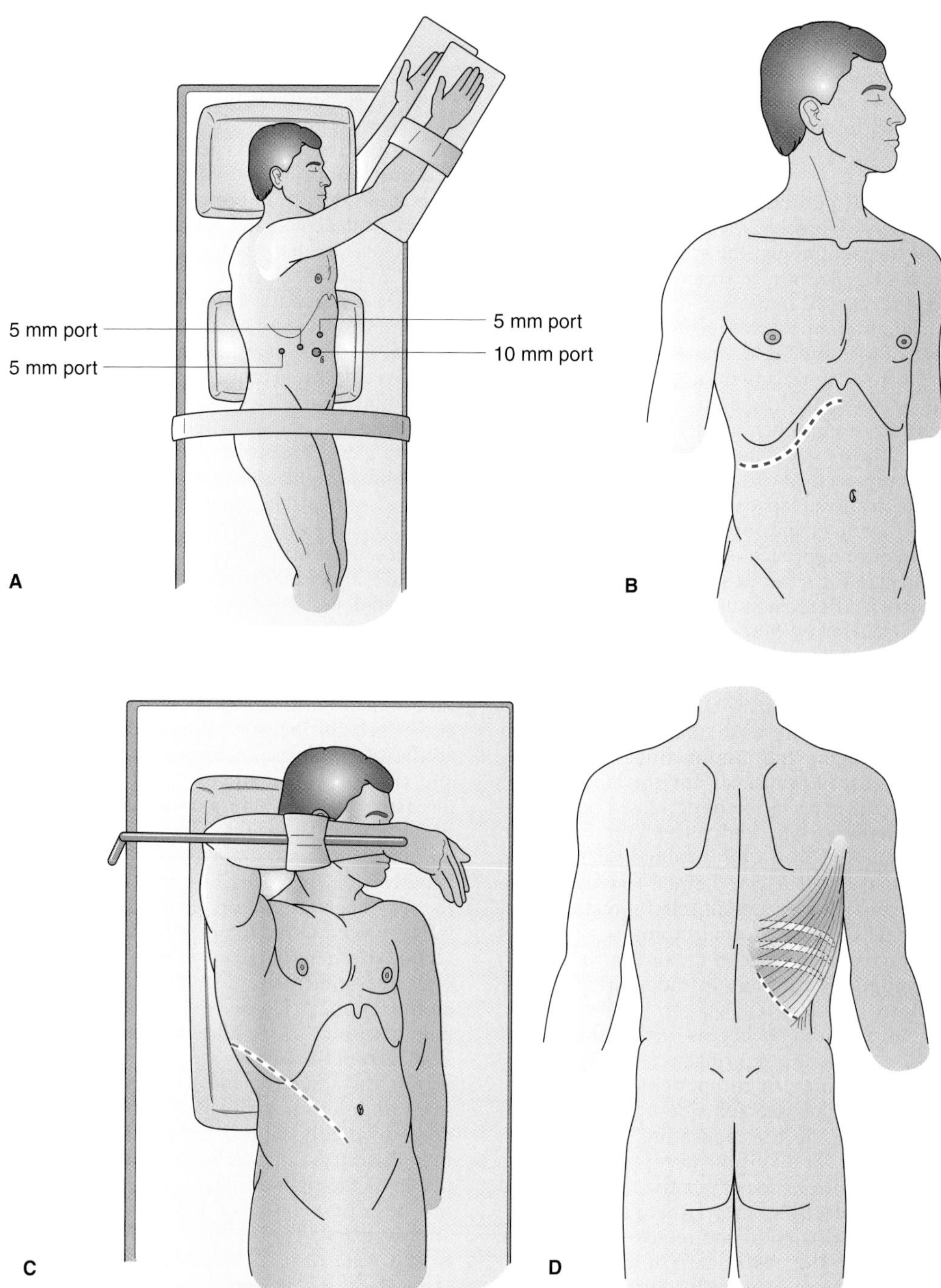

FIGURE 79.11 Incisions for right adrenalectomy. Shown are typical incisions for (*A*) laparoscopic approach, (*B*) open, anterior approach, (*C*) posterior, open approach, and (*D*) thoracoabdominal approach. Incisions for left adrenalectomy are positioned opposite.

Thoracoabdominal approach. The thoracoabdominal approach is used for large adrenal lesions with invasion of surrounding structures including the liver and diaphragm on the right side, and the spleen, pancreatic tail, stomach, and diaphragm on the left. The patient is positioned with the ipsilateral flank raised and arm extended cephalad. Incision is made in the tenth or eleventh intercostal space beginning at the posterior axillary line and is extended toward the midline of the abdomen (Fig. 79.11C). Retractors are placed and subsequent adrenalectomy is performed as for the anterior approach.

Posterior approach. With the advent of laparoscopic adrenalectomy, the posterior approach is infrequently used. When laparoscopic adrenalectomy is not an option, typically because of extensive prior transperitoneal operations, the posterior approach is better tolerated and allows faster postoperative

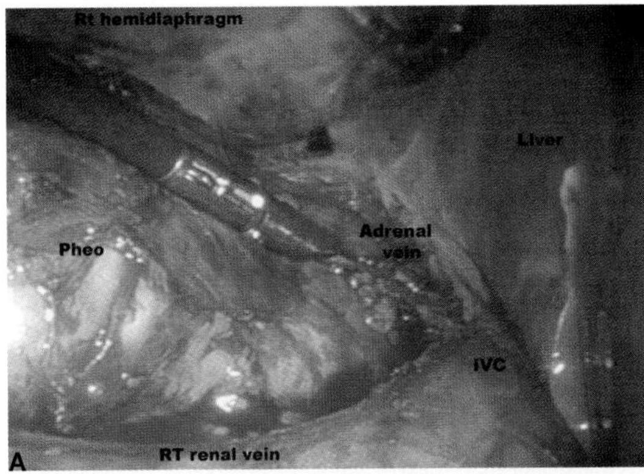

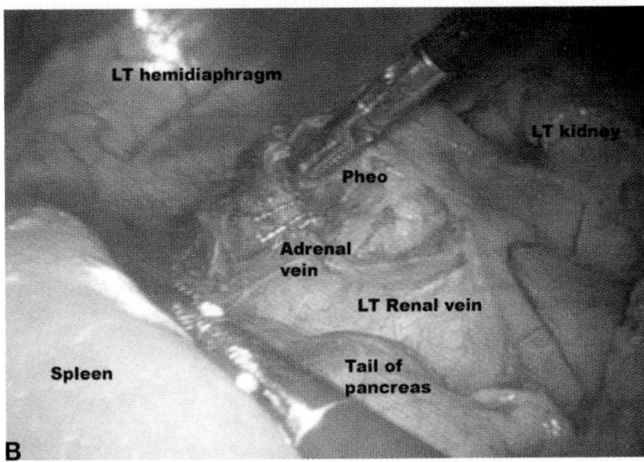

FIGURE 79.12 Laparoscopic adrenalectomy. Shown are intraoperative views of exposed right (*A*) and left (*B*) adrenal pheochromocytomas (pheo) in a patient with multiple endocrine neoplasia (MEN)-2A. Note clips on each adrenal vein. IVC, inferior vena cava.

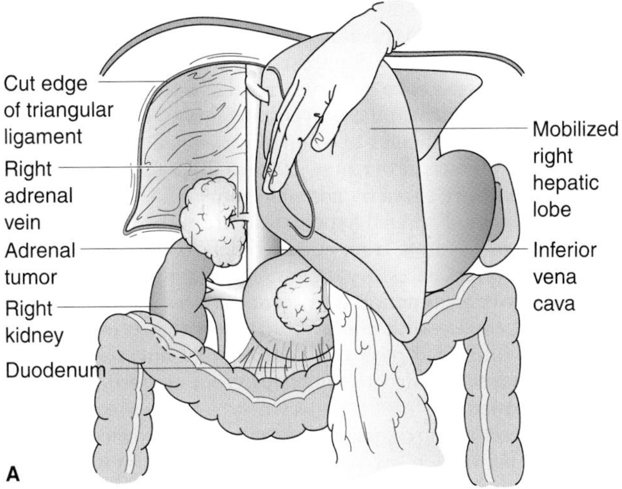

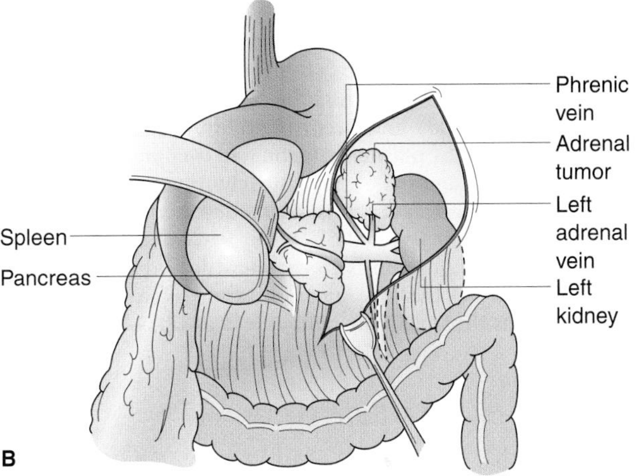

FIGURE 79.13 Anterior approach to right (*A*) and left (*B*) adrenalectomy. Note position of phrenic vein in relationship to the left adrenal vein and tumor.

recovery compared with the anterior approach. A posterior approach becomes increasingly more difficult as tumor size increases and is not recommended for excision of large pheochromocytomas, adrenal tumors greater than 6 cm, or adrenal carcinoma.

The patient is placed prone on the operating table and flexed at the waist, which allows the abdominal contents to fall away from the retroperitoneum. The incision is made from the midline at the tenth rib and is extended inferolaterally to the superior border of the posterior iliac crest (Fig. 79.11D). Dissection proceeds through the subcutaneous fat and latissimus dorsi muscle to the lumbodorsal fascia. This fascia is incised longitudinally, and the underlying sacrospinalis muscle. The sacrospinalis muscle is retracted medially, and the twelfth rib and vascular bundle are resected as far medially as possible. The twelfth intercostal nerve is preserved and gently retracted superiorly. The retroperitoneum is entered and the diaphragm is bluntly elevated from Gerota's fascia, the pleura are separated from the diaphragm, and the diaphragm is then divided. Gerota's fascia is incised, and the kidney is retracted inferiorly to expose the adrenal gland. The arterial blood supply is controlled first by clipping and ligating numerous arterial vessels, which course posteriorly. The adrenal vein, located deep to the arteries, is ligated as it is encountered. On the right, the adrenal vein exits from the anterior aspect of the gland and courses to the inferior vena cava. Once the adrenal vein is divided the gland is then freed circumferentially from its lateral to medial aspect. The inferior border of the gland is dissected last to maintain attachment to the kidney and allow inferior retraction of the gland. Finally, repair of the diaphragm and any incidental pleural defects, reapproximation of the lumbodorsal fascia, and closure of the skin.

KEY POINTS

- **Adrenocortical steroid hormones, glucocorticoids, mineralocorticoids, and androgenic steroids are all synthetic derivatives of cholesterol that is either extracted from plasma or synthesized intracellularly.**
- **Catecholamines of the adrenal medulla include epinephrine, norepinephrine, and dopamine, the vasoactive synthetic derivatives of the amino acid tyrosine.**
- **Cushing syndrome is adrenocorticotropic hormone dependent in 80% to 90% of cases, most often because of an ACTH-secreting pituitary adenoma, though ectopic ACTH-producing nonendocrine tumors (mostly non-small cell lung cancer and bronchial carcinoids) represent 10% to 20% of cases of ACTH-dependent Cushing syndrome; the remainder have a primary adrenal cause of hypercortisolism.**
- **An aldosterone-producing adrenal adenoma (Conn syndrome) is the source of primary hyperaldosteronism in 60% to 70% of cases while idiopathic bilateral adrenal hyperplasia causes most of the remaining cases of primary**

hyperaldosteronism; adrenocortical carcinoma is a rare cause of primary hyperaldosteronism.

- Surgical removal by laparoscopic adrenalectomy of an aldosterone-secreting adenoma results in durable improvement of hypertension and hypokalemia in 70% to 90% of patients; management of idiopathic adrenal hyperplasia is medical, because fewer than 20% to 30% of patients with this disease are cured by adrenalectomy.
- The congenital adrenal hyperplasias are autosomal recessive conditions resulting from inherited defects of one or several of the enzymes necessary for cortisol biosynthesis leading to ACTH overproduction and secondary hyperplasia of the adrenal cortex with shunting of cortisol precursors into adrenal androgen pathways; peripheral conversion of the excess adrenal androgens to testosterone causes virilization of the patient.
- Adrenocortical carcinoma has an estimated incidence of 0.5 to 2 cases per million per year, is very aggressive (most patients present with locoregionally advanced or distant disease), and hormone overproduction syndromes are frequent including hypercortisolism, hyperaldosteronism, or virilization.
- The *rule of tens* is a useful way to characterize pheochromocytoma: tumors are bilateral in 10% of cases, extraadrenal in 10%, familial in 10%, multicentric in 10%, and malignant in 10% and occur in children in 10% of cases; determination of plasma-fractionated metanephrines is the best test for diagnosis of pheochromocytoma.
- Unsuspected adrenal masses are detected by computed tomography in between 0.6% and 1.9% of healthy patients; the goal of evaluation is to distinguish and remove those adrenal masses that are functioning or likely to be malignant versus those that are neither and can be observed.

References

1. OMIM Online Mendelian Inheritance in Man [database online] #202300. Baltimore, MD: Johns Hopkins; 2005. Available at: http://www.ncbi.nlm.nih.gov/entrez/dispomim.cgi?id5202300. Access June 9, 2005.
2. OMIM Online Mendelian Inheritance in Man [database online] #171300. Baltimore, MD: Johns Hopkins; 2005. Available at: http://www.ncbi.nlm.nih.gov/ entrez/dispomim.cgi?id5171300). Access June 9, 2005.

Suggested Readings

Bravo EL, Tagle R. Pheochromocytoma: state-of-the-art and future prospects. *Endocr Rev*. 2003;24:539–553.

Brunt LM, Lairmore TC, Doherty GM, et al. Adrenalectomy for familial pheochromocytoma in the laparoscopic era. *Ann Surg*. 2002;235: 713–720.

Findling JW, Raff H. Diagnosis and differential diagnosis of Cushing syndrome. *Endocrinol Metab Clin North Am*. 2001;30:729–747.

Harrison LE, Gaudin PB, Brennan MF. Pathologic features of prognostic significance for adrenocortical carcinoma after curative resection. *Arch Surg*. 1999;134:181–185.

Kalady MF, McKinlay R, Olson JA Jr, et al. Laparoscopic adrenalectomy for pheochromocytoma. A comparison to aldosteronoma and incidentaloma. *Surg Endosc*. 2004;18:621–625.

Lenders JW, Pacak K, Walther MM, et al. Biochemical diagnosis of pheochromocytoma: which test is best? *JAMA* 200220;287:1427–1434.

Magill SB, Raff H, Shaker JL, et al. Comparison of adrenal vein sampling and computed tomography in the differentiation of primary aldosteronism. *J Clin Endocrinol Metab*. 2001;86:1066–1071.

Mansmann G, Lau J, Balk E, et al. The clinically inapparent adrenal mass: update in diagnosis and management. *Endocr Rev*. 2004;25: 309–340.

Mulatero P, Stowasser M, Loh KC, et al Increased diagnosis of primary aldosteronism, including surgically correctable forms, in centers from five continents. *J Clin Endocrinol Metab*. 2004;89:1045–1050.

Ng L, Libertino JM. Adrenocortical carcinoma: diagnosis, evaluation and treatment. *J Urol*. 2003;169:5–11.

NIH state-of-the-science statement on management of the clinically inapparent adrenal mass ("incidentaloma"). *NIH Consens State Sci Statements* 2002;19:1–25.

Orth DN. Adrenal insufficiency. *Curr Ther Endocrinol Metab*. 1994;5: 124–130.

Pacak K, Linehan WM, Eisenhofer G, et al. Recent advances in genetics, diagnosis, localization, and treatment of pheochromocytoma. *Ann Intern Med*. 2001;134:315–329.

Reincke M. Subclinical Cushing syndrome. *Endocrinol Metab Clin North Am*. 2000;29:43–56.

Shen WT, Sturgeon C, Duh QY. From incidentaloma to adrenocortical carcinoma: the surgical management of adrenal tumors. *J Surg Oncol*. 2005;89: 186–192.

Speiser PW, White PC. Congenital adrenal hyperplasia. *N Engl J Med*. 2003;349:776–788.

Stojadinovic A, Ghossein RA, Hoos A, et al. Adrenocortical carcinoma: clinical, morphologic, and molecular characterization. *J Clin Oncol*. 2002;20: 941–950.

Werbel SS, Ober KP. Acute adrenal insufficiency. *Endocrinol Metab Clin North Am*. 1993;22:303–328.

White PC, Speiser PW. Congenital adrenal hyperplasia due to 21-hydroxylase deficiency. *Endocr Rev*. 2000;21:245–291.

Young WF Jr. Minireview: primary aldosteronism—changing concepts in diagnosis and treatment. *Endocrinology* 2003;144:2208–2213.

CHAPTER 80 ■ PITUITARY GLAND

WILLIAM F. CHANDLER, RICARDO V. LLOYD, AND ARIEL L. BARKAN

The pituitary gland, or hypophysis, is a remarkably complex way station in the connection between the brain and a wide range of organs throughout the body. The hypothalamus of the brain is the principal integrating organ for regulating the internal environment of the body, and the pituitary is its major link with the organs outside the nervous system. The pituitary has been called the "master gland"; even with advances in modern neuroendocrinology, it remains worthy of that description.

EMBRYOLOGY, ANATOMY, AND PHYSIOLOGY

By the fourth week of gestation, an evagination develops in the roof of the stomodeal depression that is lined by ectodermal cells of the cavity destined to become the pharynx (Fig. 80.1). This structure is known as *Rathke's pouch*. At the same time, a depression develops in the floor of the diencephalon; this is

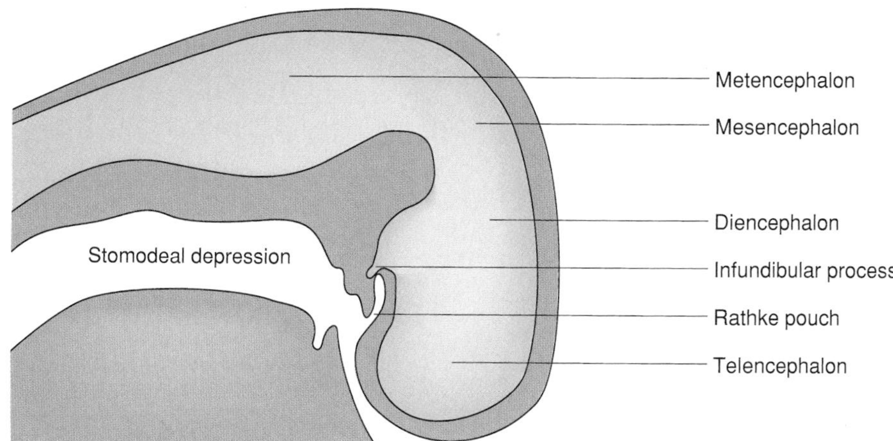

FIGURE 80.1 Diagram of a 4-week-old embryo illustrating how Rathke's pouch meets the infundibular process to form the anterior and posterior lobes, respectively, of the pituitary gland.

called the *infundibular process*. It too is lined with ectodermal cells. These are cells of the future diencephalic portion of the brain and, therefore, are more similar to the cells of central nervous system tissue. During a period of weeks, the two structures grow to meet each other—the infundibular process forming the neurohypophysis (pars neuralis) and Rathke's pouch forming the adenohypophysis (pars distalis). In lower animals, an intermediary lobe (pars intermedia) also forms, but in humans this is present only as a minor cleft. As the adenohypophysis enlarges, its upper portion (pars tuberalis) partially surrounds the stalk connecting the pituitary to the brain. Eventually, the connection between the adenohypophysis and the oral cavity disappears, but occasionally ectopic remnants of nonfunctioning pituitary cells, known as *pharyngeal pituitary tissue*, are left along its path.

In an adult, the dimensions of the hypophysis are 6 × 9 × 12 mm, and it weighs about 0.6 g. It enlarges during pregnancy and weighs up to 1 g in multiparous women. The adenohypophysis constitutes 80% of the gland and contains the pars distalis, pars tuberalis, and the remnant of the pars intermedia. The pars distalis is the major functional portion of the adenohypophysis, and in this chapter, it is considered synonymous with the adenohypophysis, or anterior pituitary. The neurohypophysis, or posterior pituitary, is small and is virtually as an extension of the hypothalamus of the brain.

The combined neurohypophysis and adenohypophysis are connected to the base of the brain by a common stalk (Fig. 80.2A). The stalk blends into the median eminence of the hypothalamus and serves to transport both hormone-rich portal blood to the adenohypophysis and nerve fibers to the neurohypophysis. The optic chiasm lies directly above the pituitary, just anterior to the stalk; thus, it is vulnerable to compression by a pituitary tumor. The supraoptic and paraventricular nuclei of the hypothalamus are depicted in Figure 80.2A because they are the principal locations of cell bodies with axons directed toward the neurohypophysis.

The median eminence is where hormonal contributions from axons originating in various nuclei of the hypothalamus enter blood destined for the adenohypophysis (Fig. 80.2B). Blood reaches this region primarily through the superior hypophyseal artery and flows into gomitoli, which are small capillary plexuses within the median eminence through which hormones enter the blood. The blood then travels through the portal system to the adenohypophysis, where the hormones modulate the activity of secretory cells. These cells, in turn, secrete hormones into the general circulation to stimulate end organs. This system comprises the hormones listed in Table 80.1. Each of these hormonal combinations constitutes a feedback system in which the brain (hypothalamus) senses the level of end-organ hormone output and, in turn, positively or negatively adjusts the secretion of the various hypothalamic hormones into the portal system.

The neurohypophysis differs significantly from the adenohypophysis in that it does not receive controlling hormones by means of the portal system but rather by direct transport through nerve fibers. The principal input into the neurohypophysis is via the supraoptic–hypophyseal tract, which arises from cells within the supraoptic and paraventricular nuclei. The tuberohypophyseal tract, which originates from the central and posterior portions of the hypothalamus, also contributes input to the neurohypophysis. These tracts carry both antidiuretic hormone (ADH; vasopressin) and oxytocin. ADH is secreted into the general circulation and causes the kidneys to absorb free water. Elevated levels of ADH (syndrome of inappropriate ADH secretion) cause water retention and hyponatremia, and inadequate levels of ADH (diabetes insipidus) cause dehydrtion and hypernatremia. Interestingly, surgical loss of the neurohypophysis does not usually result in diabetes insipidus because the stalk itself can still secrete ADH into the circulation. The feedback mechanism to the brain for release of ADH is mainly serum osmolarity, with hyperosmolar conditions causing the release of ADH and retention of water. Blood volume also affects the release of ADH; thus, hemorrhage causes water retention. Oxytocin functions only during pregnancy and causes both uterine contractions and milk letdown within the breasts.

The gross surgical anatomy of the pituitary is also critical to the surgeon because the pituitary is closely surrounded by a number of important structures. Figure 80.3A illustrates the coronal cross-section of the anatomy of the pituitary as seen from the front. The pituitary sits within the bony confines of the sella turcica ("Turkish saddle") and is bordered laterally by the cavernous sinuses (venous), inferiorly and anteriorly by the sphenoid sinus (air), posteriorly by the dorsum sellae, and superiorly by the membranous diaphragma sellae. The cavernous sinuses each contain the siphon region of the internal carotid artery and portions of cranial nerves III, IV, V, and VI, all within a venous plexus. The optic chiasm lies immediately above the diaphragma sellae. Directly below the anterior and inferior portions of the sella is the aerated sphenoid sinus. This is sufficiently large in 97% of patients to allow a transnasal, transsphenoidal surgical approach to the pituitary (Fig. 80.3B).

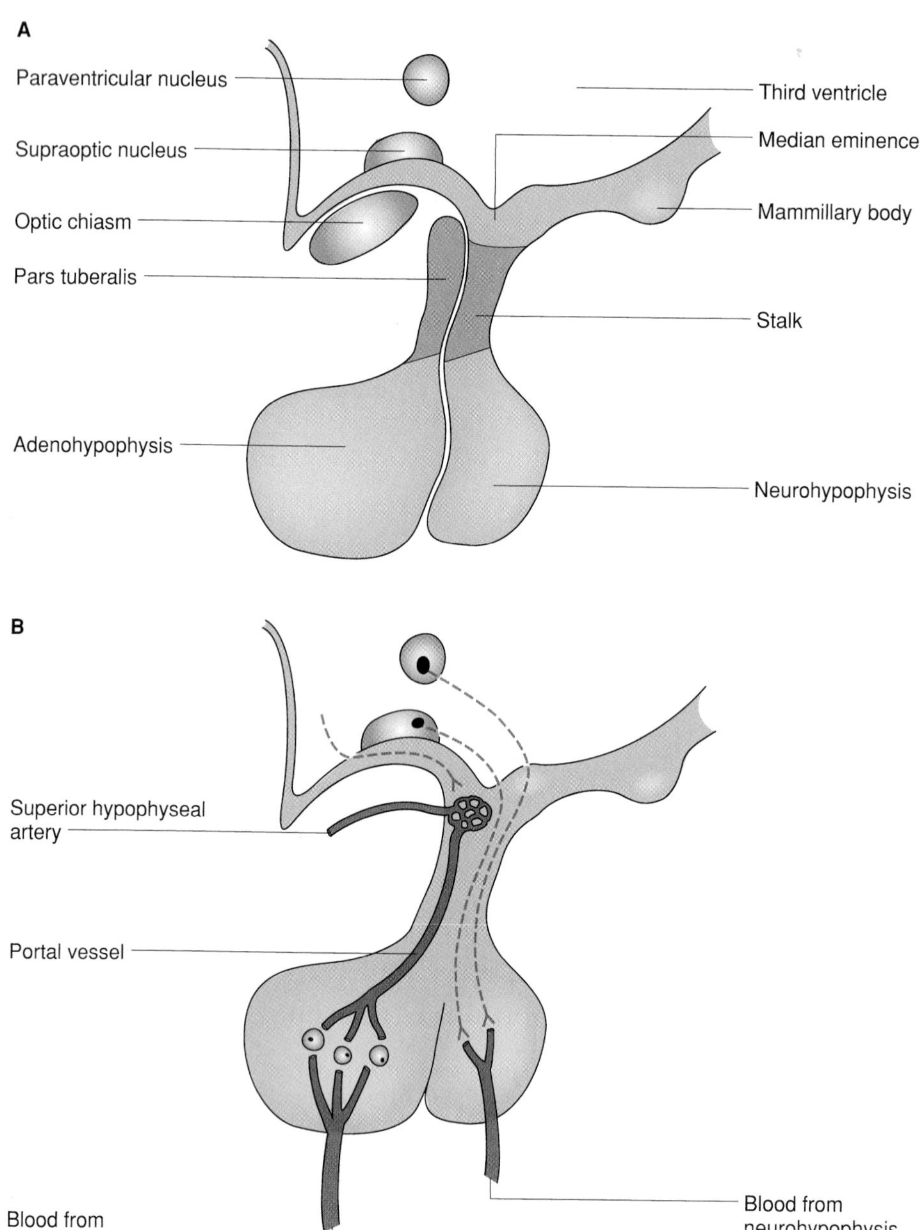

FIGURE 80.2 (*A*) Schematic diagram of the pituitary and floor of the third ventricle as seen in a midline sagittal view. Anterior is to the left. (*B*) Physiology of hormone release. The adenohypophysis receives releasing hormones through a portal venous system, and the neurohypophysis receives hormones directly from hypothalamic nuclei by means of neurons.

TABLE 80.1 DIAGNOSIS

HORMONES INVOLVED IN END-ORGAN STIMULATION

Hormone	Function
Thyrotropin-releasing hormone (TRH)	Stimulates the secretion of thyroid-stimulating hormone (TSH)
Corticotropin-releasing hormone (CRH)	Stimulates the release of adrenocorticotropic hormone (ACTH)
Growth hormone–releasing hormone (GHRH)	Stimulates the secretion of growth hormone (GH)
Gonadotropin-releasing hormone (GnRH)	Stimulates the secretion of luteinizing hormone (LH) and follicle-stimulating hormone (FSH)
Prolactin-inhibitory factor (dopamine)	Inhibits secretion of prolactin
Somatostatin	Inhibit the secretion of GH and, in part, TSH

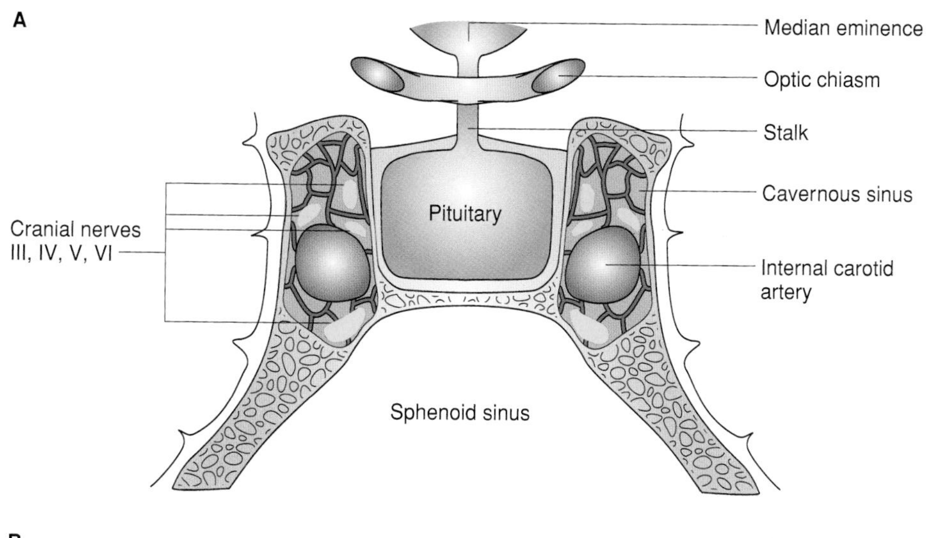

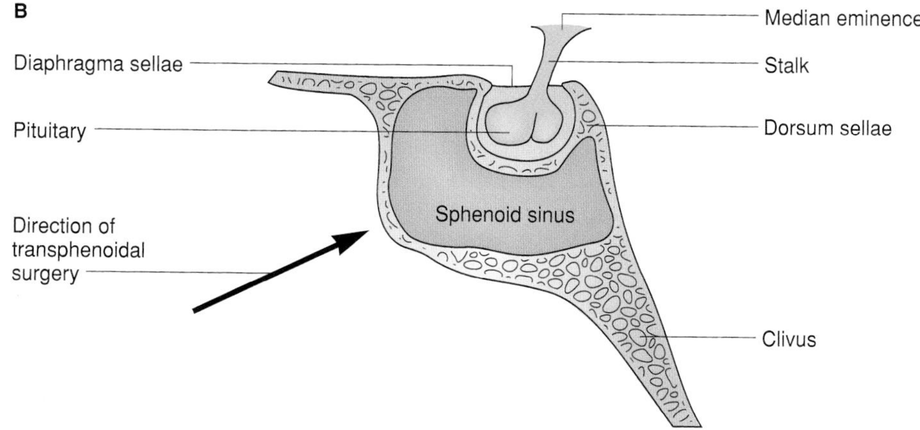

FIGURE 80.3 (*A*) Midpituitary coronal view of parasellar region. The sphenoid sinus is below and the cavernous sinuses are lateral. (*B*) Midsagittal view of pituitary and surrounding bony structures. Note the approach for transsphenoidal surgery. Anterior is to the left.

METHODS OF CELL ANALYSIS

Pituitary adenomas have been classified historically as acidophilic, basophilic, and chromophobic. Adenomas may show a variable staining pattern with conventional hematoxylin and eosin dyes, so it is difficult to classify adenomas based on these stains. For example, prolactinomas and sparsely granulated growth hormone adenomas may be acidophilic or chromophobic after hematoxylin and eosin staining (Table 80.2). Immunohistochemistry, ultrastructural studies, and *in situ* hybridization analyses for specific hormones are the most reliable methods of classifying pituitary adenomas today.

Other conventional stains that help in the analysis of pituitary adenomas include the reticulin stain, which helps to distinguish between pituitary hyperplasia and adenomas. The normal reticulin pattern is retained in hyperplasia and is similar to that seen in normal pituitary tissue, but it becomes disrupted in neoplasia. The periodic acid–Schiff reaction stains carbohydrates in ACTH-producing adenomas and in TSH- and follicle-stimulating hormone/luteinizing hormone (FSH/LH)-producing tumors.

The ultrastructural analysis of pituitary adenomas provides a great deal of information about size and type of secretory granules, cellular synthetic activity, and unique features of specific adenoma subtypes. For example, misplaced exocytosis is seen in prolactin-producing tumors, type I microfilaments are present in ACTH-producing tumors, and abundant mitochondria are characteristic of oncocytic null cell adenomas. The unique honeycomb pattern of the Golgi complex is a distinct morphologic feature of FSH/LH-producing adenomas in women.[1] Because of the pleomorphism and variations in size that are typical of secretory granules, the classification of adenomas is more reliably based on immunohistochemical findings at the light microscopic and ultrastructural levels than on the ultrastructural morphologic appearance of secretory granules.

The immunohistochemical staining of pituitary adenomas with specific antibodies is a reliable method for classifying adenomas according to the hormones that are being produced (Fig. 80.4). Highly purified polyclonal and monoclonal antibodies against prolactin, growth hormone (GH), ACTH, FSH-β,

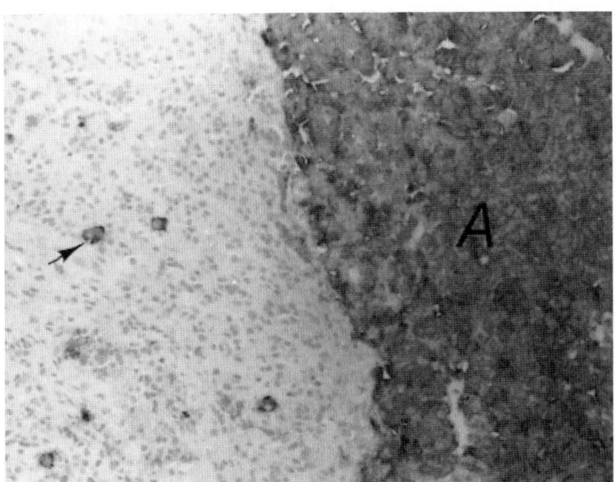

FIGURE 80.4 Immunohistochemical staining of an adrenocorticotropic hormone (*ACTH*)–producing adenoma (*A*) from a patient with Cushing disease. The normal pituitary tissue on the left contains a few ACTH-positive cells (*arrow*). Magnification ×250.

TABLE 80.2

FUNCTIONAL PITUITARY ADENOMAS: PATHOLOGIC FINDINGS

Adenoma type	Incidence (%)	Staining[a]	Immunoreactivity	Ultrastructure
PRL-secreting				
Sparsely granulated	28	C	PRL	Few SG 150–500 nm Misplaced exocytosis
Densely granulated	1	A	PRL	SG 400–1,200 nm
GH-secreting				
Sparsely granulated	5	C-A	GH	SG 300–600 nm Fibrous bodies
Densely granulated	5	A	GH	SG 100–250 nm
Mixed GH cell-PRL cell	5	A-C	GH, PRL	Variable pattern
Mixed GH cell-PRL cell	1	A	GH, PRL	SG 150–450 nm and 350–1,000 nm
ACTH-secreting	10	B	ACTH	SG 250–700 nm Prominent type I microfilaments
Gonadotrope cell	7–10	C-B	FSH, LH	SG 50–150 nm Distinct female pattern of honeycomb, golgi region
Thyrotrope cell	1	C-B	TSH	SG 50–250 nm

[a]Conventional H&E staining: A, acidophil; B, basophil; C, chromophobe;
ACTH, adrenocorticotropic hormone; FSH, follicle-stimulating hormone; GH, growth hormone; LH, luteinizing hormone; PRL, prolactin; SG, secretory granules; TSH, thyroid-stimulating hormone.

LH-β, and TSH-β are available for immunohistochemical staining. Many studies with these antibodies have revealed that some pituitary tumors are composed of several cell types that produce various hormones.[1] Ultrastructural immunohistochemistry provides a further degree of refinement in the classification and study of adenomas, because the exact site of hormone storage in secretary granules and the subcellular sites of production and processing in the rough endoplasmic reticulum and Golgi regions can be visualized with this technique.

Some adenomas may not store specific hormones, so immunohistochemical staining may be weak or absent. Messenger ribonucleic acid (mRNA) is usually present in the cytoplasm of adenomas. The localization of mRNA for specific protein hormones is becoming more widely used in the study and classification of pituitary adenomas. *In situ* hybridization studies have shown that many GH-producing adenomas in patients with acromegaly also express prolactin mRNA.[2] *In situ* and Northern hybridization studies have contributed to the understanding of adenoma subtypes. Null cell adenomas, which constitute up to 15% of pituitary neoplasms, commonly express the mRNA for gonadotropic hormones.

IMAGING OF THE PITUITARY AND PARASELLAR REGION

Modern, computerized imaging technology now provides remarkably detailed multiplanar images of the pituitary and parasellar structures. Magnetic resonance imaging (MRI) has evolved as the first choice for diagnostic imaging and is often the only test needed to make a therapeutic decision. With the intravenous infusion of a paramagnetic substance (e.g., gadolinium), MRI demonstrates intrasellar tumors as small as 5 mm and shows the growth pattern of larger tumors. It reveals the extent of suprasellar and sphenoid sinus extension, in addition to lateral extension into the cavernous sinuses (Fig. 80.5). Cysts and hemorrhage can be differentiated, as can blood flowing within an aneurysm.

Computed tomography (CT) also has a place in pituitary imaging and, if MRI is unavailable, may well suffice as the only mode of imaging. CT shows calcification better than MRI and, thus, is often helpful in imaging a craniopharyngioma. CT, even with intravenous contrast, cannot differentiate an aneurysm, so that MRI or angiography must be performed if this is suspected.

Plain skull radiographs are not needed if the diagnosis has been reached by CT or MRI, but they remain an important way to identify incidental lesions. A pituitary macroadenoma (>10 mm) causes enlargement of the sella turcica, which can easily be observed on a plain lateral skull radiograph. If this finding is noted on a radiograph performed for any reason (e.g., trauma), a more detailed study (e.g., MRI or CT) should be obtained.

Angiography is performed only if an aneurysm is suspected or if a lesion is so large that occlusion or compression of the internal carotid artery is in question.

CLINICAL AND ENDOCRINE EVALUATION

General Clinical Signs and Symptoms

Patients with pituitary lesions may present with symptoms and signs related to a mass effect on the pituitary and its surrounding structures, hypersecretion of hormones by the lesion itself, or a combination of both. Tumors or other mass lesions are generally larger than 1 cm before they produce symptoms related to compression. As a lesion enlarges, it may cause a loss of pituitary function, usually manifested by a decrease in hormone secretion from the adenohypophysis. This may result in a loss of TSH and subsequent hypothyroidism. A decrease in ACTH results in low serum cortisol levels, and a decrease in LH and FSH causes amenorrhea. A decline in GH is noted only in children with a loss of normal

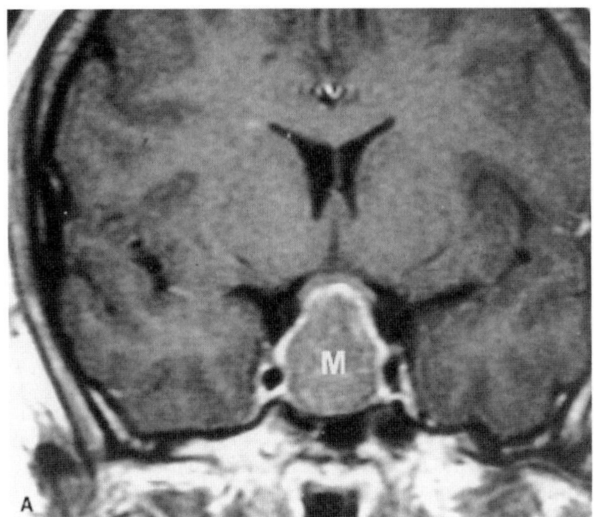

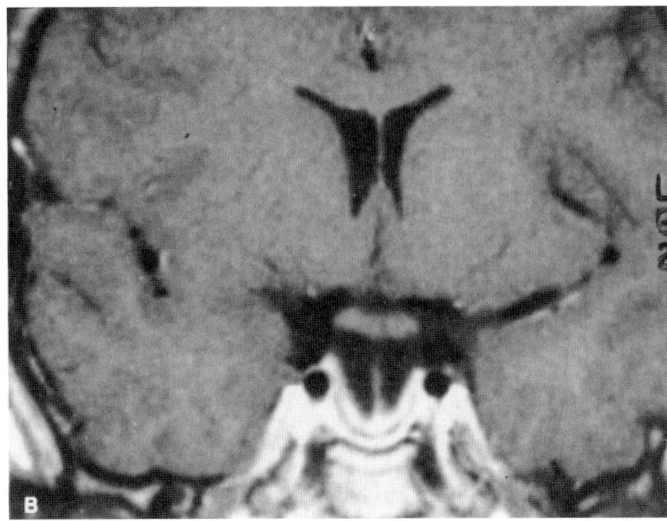

FIGURE 80.5 (*A*) Midpituitary coronal magnetic resonance imaging (MRI) shows a pituitary macroadenoma (*M*). (*B*) Postoperative MRI demonstrates gross total resection of tumor with cerebrospinal fluid in the sella.

growth progress. The one exception to this pattern is that generalized pituitary compression may cause a rise in prolactin levels because the activity of prolactin-inhibitory factor (dopamine) from the hypothalamus may be compromised by the compression. Generalized compression from within the sella rarely results in a loss of ADH from the neurohypophysis and subsequent diabetes insipidus. Lesions that originate in the region of the pituitary stalk, however, often present with early signs of diabetes insipidus. Symptoms related to a loss of pituitary function are usually insidious in onset, exception for those of sudden hemorrhage within the sella, or so-called pituitary apoplexy. Such hemorrhages are usually associated with a pituitary adenoma.

When mass lesions in the region of the pituitary enlarge, they may compress or invade nearby structures and cause symptoms unrelated to endocrine function. As tumors or other lesions grow laterally from the sella, they encounter the various contents of the cavernous sinuses. These include the third, fourth, first two divisions of the fifth, and sixth cranial nerves, in addition to the internal carotid artery. Compression of cranial nerves III, IV, or VI causes diplopia, and compression of cranial nerve V causes ipsilateral facial numbness. Invasion or constriction of the carotid may cause occlusion of this vessel, which in rare cases results in cerebral infarction. Upward growth of a tumor, which is relatively unrestricted, is much more common and often results in compression of the optic chiasm and loss of vision, typically a bitemporal hemianopsia. Extensive upward intracranial growth may compress the hypothalamus or the third ventricle and cause hydrocephalus. Rarely, intracranial extension results in cortical irritation and associated seizures. Downward growth of tumors into the sphenoid sinus is common but causes no clinical symptoms or signs.

The syndromes associated with hypersecretion of pituitary hormones include Cushing disease (ACTH), acromegaly (GH), hyperprolactinemia (prolactin), and Nelson syndrome (ACTH after adrenalectomy). Rare cases of TSH-secreting adenomas have been documented. Traditionally, pituitary adenomas have been divided into nonfunctioning and functioning tumors, but it has become clear through immunohistochemical studies that many nonfunctioning tumors are in fact endocrinologically active. Although secreted hormones may not cause clinical symptoms or signs, they may serve as a marker for the presence of a tumor before and after treatment.

General Endocrine Evaluation

The extent of the endocrine evaluation of a patient with a pituitary lesion depends on the urgency of the situation (e.g., impaired vision) and whether a hypersecretory state is suspected. If time permits, a careful evaluation of the endocrine status is warranted, including testing of pituitary reserve. Although this is most critical after treatment, it is ideal to obtain a complete pretreatment evaluation for comparison. A pituitary endocrine evaluation should include baseline values for prolactin, GH, insulinlike growth factor (IGF)-1, LH, FSH, testosterone, morning cortisol, ACTH, electrolytes, and glucose. Thyroid function tests, including TSH and free T4, should be performed. Because baseline values may not reflect the ability of the pituitary to respond to stress, it is sometimes indicated to test the reserve capacity of the pituitary. The most efficient way to do this is to administer insulin to induce hypoglycemia. Provided the patient has no contraindication to transient hypoglycemia (i.e., ischemic heart disease, cerebrovascular disease, or seizure disorder), insulin is given in a dose of 0.10 to 0.15 IU/kg, such that the serum glucose falls below 40 mg/dL. In the patient with normal pituitary function, transient hypoglycemia causes a rise in cortisol to above 20 μg/dL and a rise in GH to above 10 μg/L. In patients with compromised ACTH or GH production, a response is not noted.

If urgent surgical decompression is indicated, the previously mentioned baseline values are obtained, and the patient is prepared for surgery with sufficient hydrocortisone to cover the possibility of inadequate cortisol response to stress. Careful postoperative evaluation is then carried out to determine if long-term replacement therapy is needed. If the patient receives postoperative radiation therapy, the status of the pituitary should be checked periodically during the following years because pituitary function may slowly decline after radiation exposure.

If diabetes insipidus is suspected, urine osmolality and serum sodium should be assessed, and fluid intake and output should be carefully evaluated.

Cushing Disease

Although the diagnosis of hypercortisolism (Cushing syndrome) is often determined after physical examination by an astute physician, sometimes the physical manifestations are not obvious. Often, the precise cause of hypercortisolism is difficult to ascertain, even with detailed endocrine testing and imaging. The findings of Cushing syndrome often include central obesity, hypertension, hirsutism, fatigue, easy bruising, striae, moonlike facies, dorsal fat pad, and often depression or other mental changes. Less common abnormalities include headache, osteoporosis, diabetes mellitus, galactorrhea, and amenorrhea. Often, a patient presents without the classic cushingoid appearance and complains only of severe fatigue or depression.

The cause of hypercortisolism is an ACTH-secreting pituitary adenoma (Cushing disease) in up to 80% of cases; the remainder are caused by an adrenocortical tumor or an endocrine tumor that secretes ACTH or corticotropin-releasing hormone. Pituitary-dependent hypercortisolism is much more common in women (80%), and an ectopic cause is more common in men (80%). Thus, if an adult man presents with a rapid onset of Cushing syndrome, particularly with weight loss, hypertension, edema, or hypokalemia, an ectopic neoplasm must be strongly considered. Increased cortisol levels may be seen in patients with primary depression, alcoholism, obesity, or drugs such as estrogens and phenytoin.

Because imaging studies are nondiagnostic in up to 60% of patients with pituitary disorders, the diagnosis is often based completely on the results of endocrine testing.[3] Multiple measurements of cortisol and ACTH to evaluate the diurnal pattern are important but often misleading. They are mainly of value when clearly elevated. Urinary free cortisol excretion over 24 hours is an extremely important measurement, but it may also be elevated in cases of depression or alcoholism. Undetectable plasma or urinary cortisol in a patient with clinically florid Cushing syndrome is unequivical evidence of exogenous steroid therapy ("iatrogenic Cushing syndrome"). When the result of the overnight dexamethasone screening test (1 mg at 10:00 PM) is an 8:00 AM serum cortisol level below 1.8 μg/dL, hypercortisolism is rarely present. The differential diagnosis starts with measurements of plasma cortisol and ACTH: undetectable ACTH in a patient with clinical Cushing syndrome and elevated cortisol establishes the diagnosis of a cortisol-producing adrenal tumor. Plasma ACTH above 200 pg/mL and certainly above 500 pg/mL strongly suggests an ectopic source of ACTH. Most patients with Cushing disease have ACTH within the normal or slightly elevated range. The overlap with the cases of ectopic ACTH secretion, however, is significant and that poses the greatest diagnostic difficulty. Generally, the cortisol level of patients with a pituitary cause of hypercortisolism is not suppressed with the low-dose dexamethasone test (0.5 mg given every 6 hours for 2 days), but is with the higher dose (2 mg every given 6 hours for 2 days). The cortisol level of patients with adrenal or ectopic disorders classically is not suppressed with either dose. Exceptions are seen with both these tests (Algorithm 80.1).

When metyrapone is given, a rise in serum 11-deoxycortisol (or urinary 17-hydroxycortisteroids) is seen in normal patients or those with Cushing disease, but not in those with adrenal tumors of ectopic ACTH secretion. A positive response, however, does not absolutely rule out an adrenal or ectopic source of hypercortisolism. The most specific differential diagnostic test to distinguish an ectopic ACTH source from Cushing disease is the measurement of ACTH levels in both inferior petrosal sinuses by transfemoral catheterization, along with simultaneous measurement of peripheral blood levels. This provides convincing evidence for the existence of an ACTH-secreting pituitary tumor.[4] Inferior petrosal sinus sampling should be carried out in every case of suspected Cushing disease when MRI results are not *definitive* for a tumor. If the results of standard endocrine testing are conclusive for hypercortisolism and indicate a pituitary source and if MRI clearly shows a tumor, then invasive petrosal sinus sampling is not necessary before surgery.

Nelson's Syndrome

In 1958, Nelson and colleagues identified a syndrome of progressive hyperpigmentation, visual field loss, and amenorrhea associated with elevated ACTH levels related to a functional pituitary adenoma in a patient who had undergone bilateral adrenalectomy for hypercortisolism.[5] This syndrome today generally represents a missed diagnosis of Cushing disease that has been treated with adrenalectomy. Often these tumors are aggressive or occasionally malignant.

Acromegaly

Like Cushing syndrome, acromegaly can be diagnosed clinically when patients present with advanced stages of the disease. The enlargement of the facial features and extremities may be subtle, and the presenting symptoms may be nonspecific headaches, fatigue, arthralgias, decreased libido, or amenorrhea. Patients often have hypertension, diabetes mellitus, and an early onset of atherosclerotic cardiovascular disease. It is critical that this disease be diagnosed and treated because the associated mortality rate is 50% above normal per decade beyond the age of 40 years. With rare exceptions, the cause of acromegaly is a GH-secreting pituitary adenoma. Like other functioning adenomas, the tumors may be either small or large and invasive. Patients with larger tumors may present with visual loss. Rarely, elevated GH levels are secondary to the production of GH-releasing hormone by an ectopic tumor.

The endocrine diagnosis now rests largely on serum levels of IGF-1, also known as *somatomedin C*. Even though 90% of patients with acromegaly have GH levels higher than 10 ng/mL, and although GH in a resting, nonstressed patient is normally below 5 ng/mL, both normal patients and patients with acromgaly may have levels below 5 ng/mL. IGF-1, which mediates the effect of GH on peripheral tissues, should be measured in *all* circumstances in which acromegaly is suspected (Algorithm 80.2).

Hyperprolactinemia

Because 60% to 70% of prolactin-secreting pituitary adenomas are microadenomas, most patients present with endocrine symptoms rather than local mass effects. Hyperprolactinemia in women usually causes amenorrhea and often galactorrhea; thus, young women have a reason to seek medical evaluation while the tumor is still at an early stage. Because men do not have these early warning signs, they almost invariably present with macroadenomas associated with loss of libido, infertility, or loss of vision. The finding of amenorrhea or galactorrhea together with an elevated prolactin level does not always indicate the presence of a pituitary tumor. Table 80.3 lists other possible causes of hyperprolactinemia. Most important among these are renal failure, hypothyroidism, and the use of various drugs. Compression of the pituitary stalk by any type of mass lesion results in an increased secretion of prolactin. If the prolactin level is above 150 ng/mL, a pituitary tumor is almost invariably the cause, but microadenomas are often associated with prolactin levels below 100 ng/mL. The size of pituitary adenomas has been shown to correlate with the degree of prolactin elevation; levels may reach thousands of nanograms per milliliter. No reliable provocative tests are available to differentiate prolactinomas from other causes of hyperprolactinemia, so the diagnosis relies on ruling out other causes and imaging the adenoma (Algorithm 80.3).

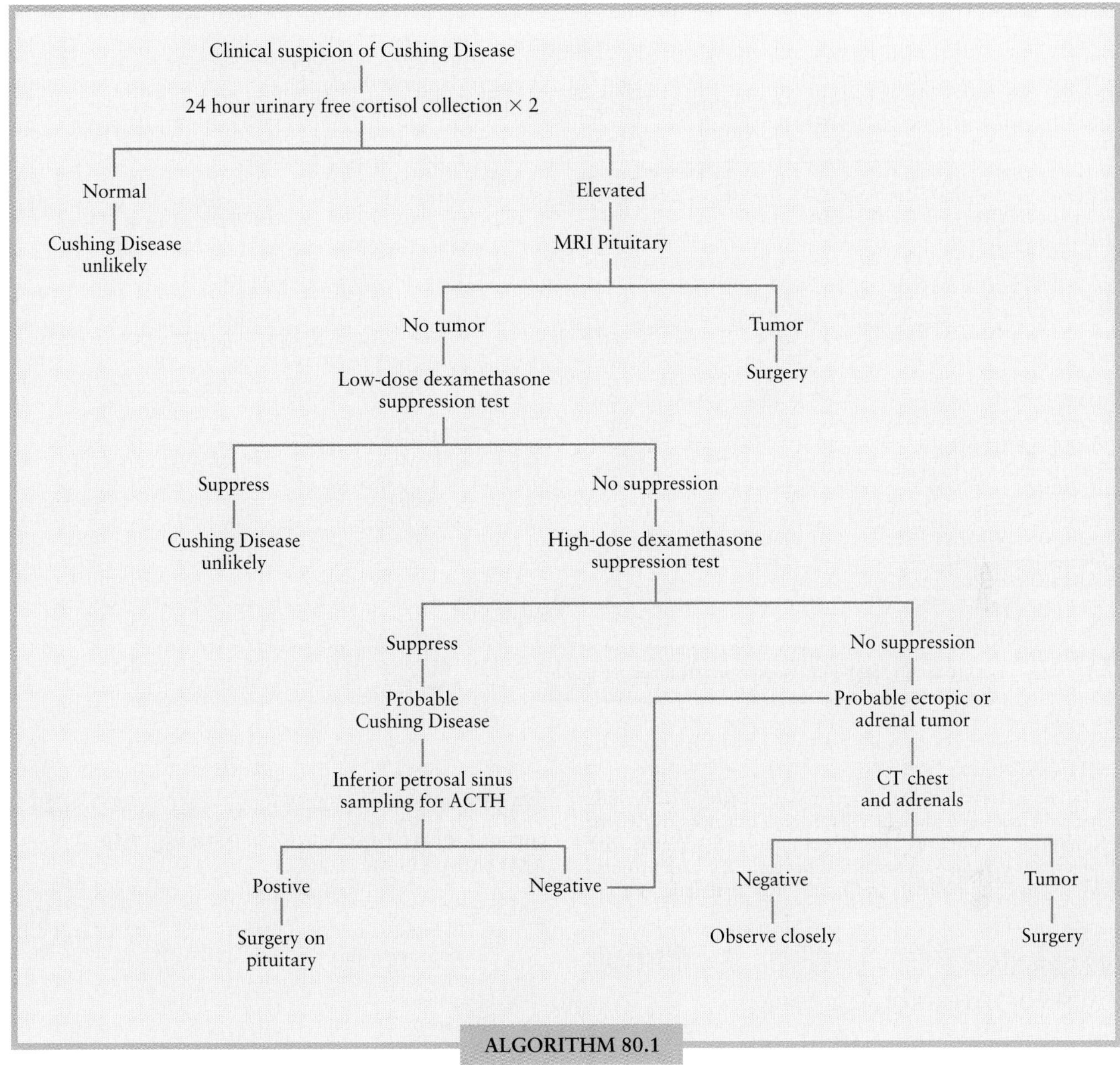

ALGORITHM 80.1 Workup and treatment of Cushing disease.

DIFFERENTIAL DIAGNOSIS

Table 80.4 lists the possible lesions that may occur within the sella or in the parasellar region. Pituitary adenomas head the list, because they are the most common lesion in this region and constitute 8% to 10% of all intracranial tumors. Occasionally, they are cystic and confused with other lesions. Craniopharyngiomas are the next most common tumor, and although more often suprasellar in location, they may be exclusively intrasellar. They are more common in children, but up to one third occur in adults. They are usually cystic and are calcified in 70% of children and 40% of adults. Meningiomas are also more commonly suprasellar and enhance strongly on CT and MRI. Germinomas, or so-called ectopic pinealomas, generally involve the pituitary stalk and often causes diabetes insipidus. If a patient presents with diabetes insipidus, the lesion is likely something other than a pituitary adenoma. Metastatic malignancies, commonly from lung and breast primary tumors, may be found in the pituitary, with 70% residing in the posterior pituitary. Optic nerve gliomas and hypothalamic gliomas may occasionally be confused with pituitary adenomas, as can the rare granular cell tumor (choristoma). Dermoids and epidermoids may occur within the sella, and fifth nerve neuromas may compress the sella.

Rathke's cysts are benign congenital remnants that develop within the sella and can cause a loss of pituitary function by local compression. These can be confused on imaging studies with cystic adenomas or craniopharyngiomas, and biopsy and surgical decompression are required.

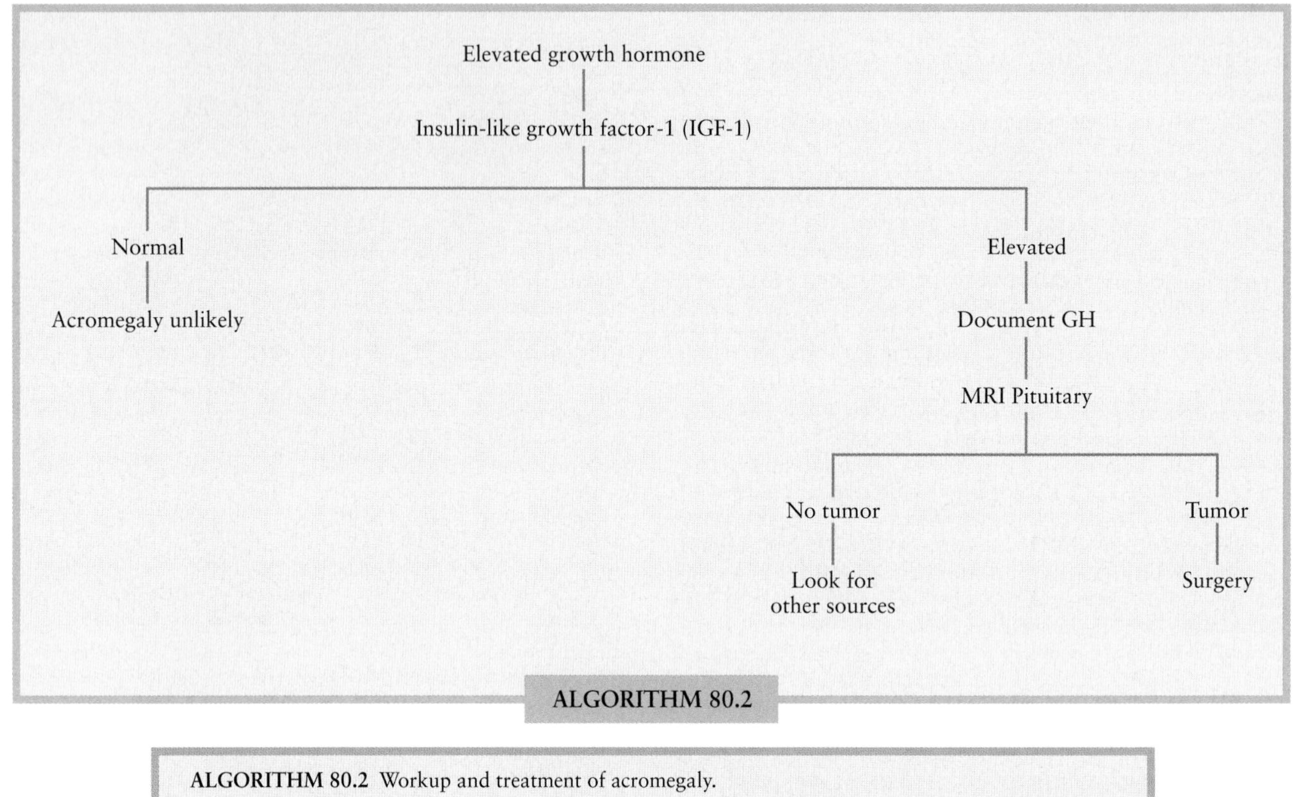

ALGORITHM 80.2 Workup and treatment of acromegaly.

Inflammatory and granulomatous processes can include bacterial abscesses within the sella. Sarcoidosis may involve the pituitary or its stalk, as can the granulomas associated with Langerhans cell histiocytosis (histiocytosis X). Hamartomas may involve the pituitary stalk and hypothalamus and are

TABLE 80.3 ETIOLOGY

CAUSES OF HYPERPROLACTINEMIA

Pituitary disease
Prolactinoma
Growth hormone-secreting adenoma
Pituitary stalk section (any concomittent structural lesion)
Empty sella syndrome
Hypothalamic disease
Tumors
Sarcoidosis
Radiation
Primary hypothyroidism (severe)
Chronic renal failure
Hepatic disease
Drugs
Phenothiazines
Metoclopramide
Tricyclic antidepressants
Estrogen
Opiates
Reserpine
Verapamil
Others
Pregnancy
Stress

TABLE 80.4 DIAGNOSIS

DIFFERENTIAL DIAGNOSIS OF INTRASELLAR AND PARASELLAR LESIONS

Tumors
Pituitary adenoma
Craniopharyngioma
Meningioma
Lymphoma
Germinoma
Chordoma
Granular cell tumor (choristoma)
Neuroma (arising from cranial nerve V)
Metastatic
Optic nerve glioma
Epidermoid
Dermoid
Infundibuloma
Hypothalamic glioma
Cysts
Rathke's cleft cyst
Pituitary cyst
Inflammatory and granulomatous lesions
Bacterial abscess
Sarcoidosis
Eosinophilic granuloma (histiocytosis X)
Tuberculosis
Mycoses
Granulomatous hypophysitis
Aneurysm
Hamartoma
Empty sella syndrome
Pituitary apoplexy

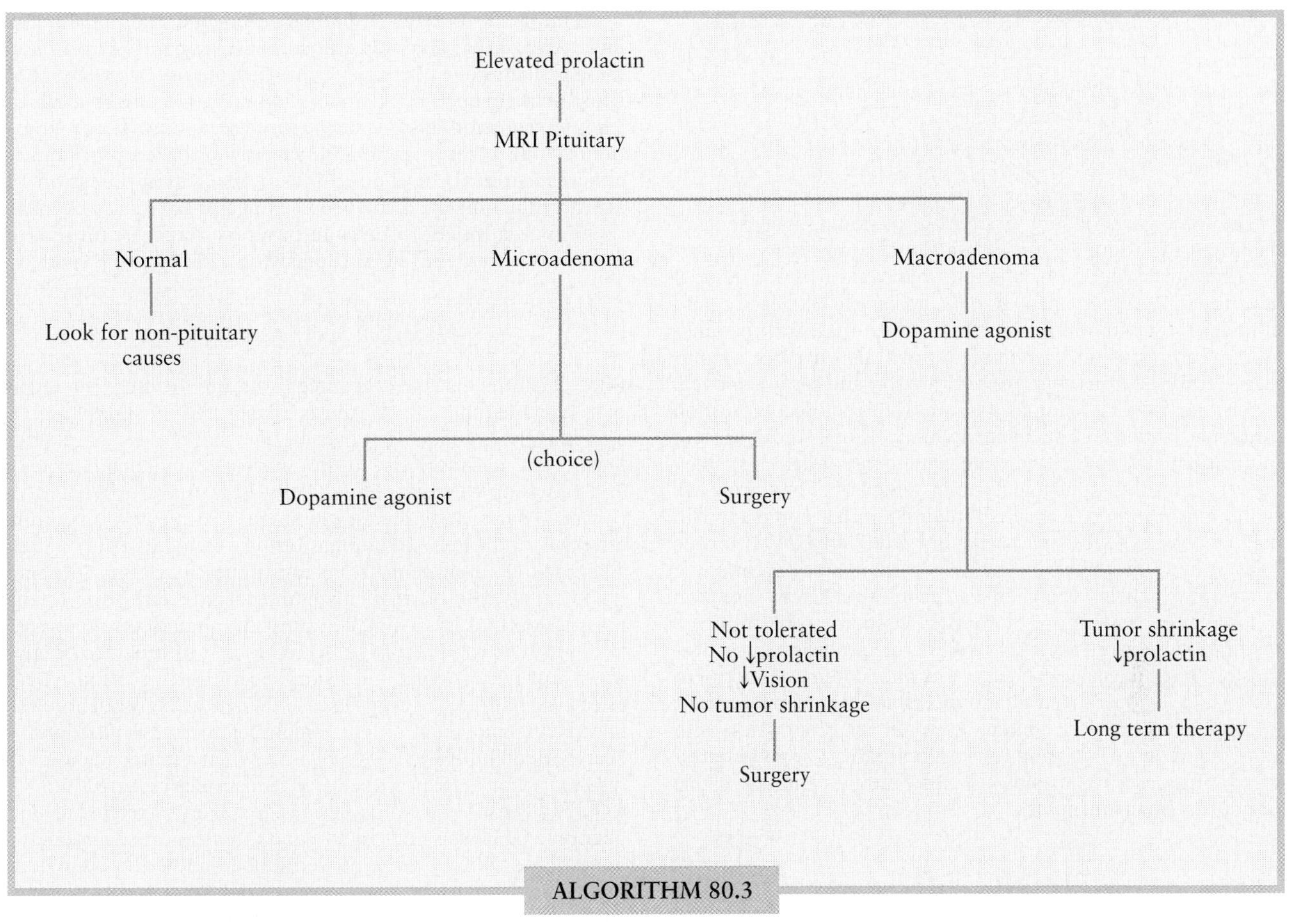

ALGORITHM 80.3 Diagnostic tests and treatment for hyperprolactinemia.

impossible to differentiate from invasive gliomas on imaging studies.

Aneurysms, usually from the internal carotid arteries but occasionally from the basilar artery, may appear within the sella and must be ruled out preoperatively with MRI or angiography.

The empty-sella syndrome is generally an anatomic variation that rarely causes symptoms. If a patient with headaches or head trauma undergoes skull radiography or CT, an enlarged sella may be found. With high-resolution CT or MRI, usually the elongated stalk is seen to reach the sellar floor, so that a cystic lesion can be ruled out. A contrast cisternogram may be used to visualize cerebrospinal fluid within the sella if necessary.

Pituitary apoplexy occurs symptomatically only rarely but may cause a profound and emergent situation. Infarction and hemorrhage, usually in a pituitary adenoma, cause a sudden intrasellar expansion with severe headache and a rapid loss of pituitary function, resulting in hypotension. A sudden loss of vision and other cranial nerve palsies may also develop. Treatment in severe cases involves the administration of steroids and surgical decompression of the sella.

TREATMENT AND RESULTS

The treatment of primary pituitary adenomas is generally surgical, although there are certain exceptions. Even with modern imaging techniques, the unequivocal diagnosis of an adenoma is not reached until tissue is obtained. As in Table 80.4, the list of possible parasellar lesions is extensive. Along with surgical removal or decompression of pituitary adenomas, additional treatment in the form of radiation or medical therapy is often indicated. In addition to treatment directed at the primary lesion, it is critical to assess pituitary function thoroughly before and after treatment to decide whether hormone replacement is indicated.

More than 95% of pituitary adenomas can be approached by the transsphenoidal route, usually through a transnasal approach to the sphenoid sinus using the operating microscope. Once the sphenoid sinus is entered, the anterior wall of the sella is carefully drilled away, and the dura surrounding the pituitary is identified. The dura is opened, and if a macroadenoma is present, the tumor is usually seen directly beneath the dura. If a microadenoma is present, the surgeon must carefully dissect around and often through the pituitary to identify the small tumor. In selected cases, it is helpful to use a frameless stereotactic system to define the anatomy of the sella and to localize a small tumor. This requires a special preoperative CT or MRI scan that can be entered into one of several commercially available frameless stereotactic systems. This three-dimensional precise localizing system adds to the safety of the transpphenoidal approach and reduces the chance of injury to surrounding structures, such as the carotid arteries or the cavernous sinuses.

Contraindications to the transsphenoidal approach, and therefore indications for a craniotomy, include massive suprasellar extension, extensive lateral intracranial extension, and the rare dumbbell-shaped tumor with a tight construction at the level of the diaphragma sellae. If a craniotomy is necessary, a right subfrontal approach to the optic nerve and chiasm is required; the tumor is removed in a piecemeal fashion with use of the operating microscope and microinstruments.

NONFUNCTIONING ADENOMAS

Because patients with nonfunctioning adenomas usually present with the effects of a mass lesion, these tumors are rarely microadenomas. Although their location can be either exclusively intrasellar or extensively suprasellar, almost all these tumors are currently approached via the transsphenoidal route.

The three goals of surgery for nonfunctioning macroadenomas are establishment of a diagnosis, decompression of surrounding structures, and gross total removal of tumor tissue if possible. The first goal is usually accomplished easily, and although most tumors turn out to be adenomas, surprise findings are not unusual. Decompression is also usually accomplished readily because most tumors are soft and easily removed. Fewer than 5% of adenomas are so fibrous that decompression is difficult. Evidence of adequate decompression is the consistent finding that 75% to 80% of patients with visual field loss show recovery after transsphenoidal tumor removal.[6] The third goal, total tumor resection, is much more difficult to accomplish with macroadenomas. Most macroadenomas (88% to 94%) invade at least the dura mater, and many grossly invade surrounding structures. Such invasion makes complete surgical resection impossible and, therefore, these patients need to be followed indefinitely with high-quality imaging to monitor tumor progression or recurrence. Whereas it was once common practice to administer postoperative radiation to all macroadenomas, most neurosurgeons are now content to watch for progression with high-resolution imaging and reserve local radiation for progression or recurrence.[7] Currently, no medical treatment is available for nonfunctional adenomas.

CUSHING DISEASE

Once it has been established that the cause of a patient's hypercortisolism is a pituitary lesion, the treatment of choice is transsphenoidal exploration of the pituitary. Only 40% of such patients have positive results on imaging studies and, therefore, careful and systematic exploration of the sellar contents by an experienced pituitary surgeon is required in many cases.[3] Microadenomas secreting ACTH may be very small and are often located deep within the gland itself. If a tumor is not evident when the dura is opened and all surfaces of the pituitary are examined, then incisions must be made into the gland and an internal exploration carried out. These microadenomas are usually located in one of the lateral aspects of the pituitary gland, and the initial choice of which side to explore can be guided by the results of preoperative petrosal sinus sampling for ACTH levels, as described earlier. If no tumor is identified, then a decision must be made regarding whether to resect all or a portion of the gland. If the endocrine evidence is convincing for a pituitary origin and the patient has no desire to have children, then total hypophysectomy is warranted. If petrosal sinus sampling clearly indicates laterality of the ACTH secretion, then an appropriate hemiresection of the gland is carried out. Macroadenomas are treated with maximal tumor resection, but endocrine remission is, of course, more difficult to accomplish in these situations. Obviously, patients with adrenal or ectopic lesions are treated by resection of tumors in these locations. Microadenomas are the source of ACTH secretion in about 75% of patients.[3,8,9] The postoperative remission rate in these patients is 88% to 96%, and the long-term recurrence rate appears to be no more than 5%. Therefore, selective microsurgical tumor resection in patients with microadenomas is clearly the current treatment of choice. Postoperative plasma cortisol concentrations below 1 μg/dL are a very good predictor of surgical cure, and the likelihood of recurrence is very low. If cortisol levels are not undetectable or in the normal range, a long-term cure is unlikely and the chance of recurrence goes up.

Some 10% to 20% of patients who undergo exploration have macroadenomas, and postoperative remission rates in these patients have been reported to be from 33% to 61%.[3,8–11] Most of them require postoperative radiation therapy, which leads to remission in some of the surgical failures. Those whose tumors fail to remit after both surgery and radiation require either a surgical adrenalectomy or medical suppression of adrenal function. In a small percentage of patients who have undergone adrenalectomy, the pituitary tumors continue to grow and secrete ACTH (Nelson syndrome).

ACROMEGALY

Like Cushing disease, acromegaly is a condition that ultimately threatens life. For this reason, it must be treated aggressively, even at the expense of normal pituitary function. During the past two decades, a variety of medical, surgical, and radiation therapies have evolved that have proved effective in lowering GH levels. No single treatment is uniformly effective, and often a combination of treatments is necessary. The goals of treatment are to lower the circulating GH and IGF-1 levels to a normal range and to reduce the size of the mass lesion that is causing compression-related symptoms.

Only 20% to 34% of GH-secreting tumors are microadenomas, however, so that microsurgical tumor resection is less effective than in Cushing disease. When a microadenoma is selectively removed transsphenoidally, endocrine remission may be expected in 80% to 88% of cases. When a macroadenoma is resected, immediate postoperative remission is reported in 30% to 68% of cases.[12] Remission rates are inversely related to preoperative GH levels and the size and invasiveness of tumors.

Radiation therapy has proved moderately effective in conjunction with partial surgical resection. Proton beam heavy-particle therapy was reported in 510 patients, 428 of whom had been observed for 1 to 20 years.[13] Analysis of these patients revealed a progressive fall in GH levels beginning immediately after treatment and continuing for up to 20 years. After 2 years, 47.5% of patients had GH levels below 10 ng/mL; at 4, 10, and 20 years, the rates were 65%, 87.5%, and 97.5%, respectively. A GH level below 5 ng/mL is achieved in 75% of patients at 10 years and 92.5% of patients at 20 years. Conventional radiation therapy provides comparable results (10-year posttreatment levels below 10 ng/mL in 81% and below 5 ng/mL in 69%). A recent review of our own patients, however, showed that after an average follow-up of 6.8 years, normalization of IGF-1 levels was attained in only 2 of 36 patients who received radiation (45 to 50 Gy) after surgical failure.[14] The remaining 34 patients had persistently elevated IGF-1 levels (219 ± 26% of upper normal limit) despite plasma GH levels averaging 4.6 ± 1.1 μg/L. A report by Landolt et al. suggests that stereotactic radiosurgery may be more effective than fractionated radiotherapy for persistant acromegaly after failed surgical treatment, but there is currently no conclusive evidence that focused radiosurgery is more effective than fractionated radiotherapy.[15]

Bromocriptine, a dopamine receptor agonist, lowered GH levels in 71% of 126 patients.[16] GH levels below 10 ng/mL, however, were achieved in only 14% of patients in this study. Bromocriptine does not appear to be an effective primary treatment for acromegaly, but may help to control GH and IGF-1 levels as an adjuvant therapy.

Somatostatin analogues have been demonstrated to reduce GH and IGF-1 levels significantly in most patients, and may provide tumor shrinkage, but GH levels rise again immediately after cessation of the drug. A newly approved GH-receptor blocker, pegvisomant, has proved useful in lowering IGF-1 levels in patients whose disease cannot be controlled by surgery or somatostatin analogues. Because this drug works peripherally, there is risk that the pituitary tumor may grow and enlarge during this treatment.

Given the variety of treatment modalities, a rational therapeutic approach is to resect tumors surgically when possible and to provide medical and radiation therapy to those patients in whom a remission cannot be achieved. The recurrence rate of GH-secreting tumors appears to be only 4% after successful surgery and less than 1% after radiation.[15]

PROLACTINOMAS

Prolactin-secreting adenomas are the most common functioning pituitary tumors but remain somewhat controversial with regard to treatment. The controversy exists because, unlike ACTH- or GH-secreting adenomas, prolactinomas can be treated medically with dopamine agonists, with excellent results. The treatment options include medical therapy, usually with a dopamine agonist; transsphenoidal surgical resection; radiation therapy; or, in some cases, no treatment. Because treatment considerations depend on tumor size, the treatments are discussed on that basis.

Macroadenomas

The goal in treating a patient with a large, prolactin-secreting adenoma is to decompress the optic pathways if they are involved and to reduce the prolactin levels to normal concentrations. Surgery is effective in improving vision in 80% of cases, but vision has also been reported to improve in patients treated with dopamine agonists. The success of surgery in reducing prolactin levels to normal has generally been disappointing. The uniform finding of various investigators has been that the likelihood of normalizing prolactin levels is greatly reduced if the initial concentration is above 200 ng/mL or if the macroadenoma is larger than 10 mm.

The administration of dopamine agonists to patients with macroadenomas reduces prolactin levels significantly in almost all instances, and reductions to normal ranges have been reported in more than 46%.[17] In 90% of patients, the size of the tumor is decreased to some degree and, in many, the reduction is dramatic. With rare exceptions, however, the tumor returns to its original size once bromocriptine is stopped. It is recognized that up to 25% of patients with macroadenomas experience an increase in tumor size during pregnancy, whereas this is true in fewer than 1% of patients with microadenomas.[17]

In most instances today patients with macroprolactinomas are treated initially with a dopamine agonist and surgery is reserved for the rare situation in which the patient is not responsive to this medication. Occassionally, patients with prolactinomas present with significant hemorrhage within the tumor and require surgical debulking of the hemorrhage and surrounding tumor.

Microadenomas

Primary medical treatment with a dopamine agonst is safe and effective and is currently the treatment of choice for most patients with a prolactin secreting microadenoma. As in macroadenomas, long-term continued therapy is indicated because prolactin levels rapidly rise with cessation of dopamine agonists in most patients. Pregnancy is of less risk to the patient with a microadenoma because tumor expansion and visual loss are rare.

The surgical treatment of prolactin-secreting microadenomas results in postoperative remission in a much higher percentage of patients. Two large series reported remission in 77%[18] and 72%[19] of patients. In the latter report, 88% were in remission, with prolactin levels below 100 ng/mL, and only 50% in those who had prolactin levels above 100 ng/mL. The incidence of new postoperative hypogonadism was only 1%. The recurrence rate in patients initially in remission after microsurgical tumor removal, however, has been disappointing compared with the rates after removal of other functioning tumors. Recurrences have uniformly been found to be higher in patients with postoperative prolactin levels in the upper end of the normal range. Recurrence rates of 17% to 50% during 5 years have been reported. Radiation therapy does not play a role in the treatment of microadenomas unless they recur in an aggressive manner.

ENDOCRINE

KEY POINTS

- **The hypothalamus of the brain is the principal integrating organ for regulating the internal environment of the body, and the pituitary is its major link with the organs outside the nervous system.**
- **The adenohypophysis constitutes 80% of the gland and contains the pars distalis, pars tuberalis, and the remnant of the pars intermedia.**
- **The neurohypophysis, or posterior pituitary, is small and is virtually an extension of the hypothalamus of the brain.**
- **MRI has evolved as the first choice for diagnostic imaging of the pituitary and is often the only test needed for a therapeutic decision to be made.**
- **The findings of Cushing syndrome often include central obesity, hypertension, hirsutism, fatigue, easy bruising, striae, moonlike facies, dorsal fat pad, and often depression or other mental changes. The cause of hypercortisolism is an ACTH-secreting pituitary adenoma (Cushing disease) in up to 80% of cases; the remainder are caused by an adrenocortical tumor or an endocrine tumor that secretes ACTH or corticotropin-releasing hormone.**
- **The goals of treatment of adenomas secreting growth hormone are to lower the circulating GH and IGF-1 levels to a normal range and to reduce the size of the mass lesion that is causing compression-related symptoms.**
- **The three goals of surgery for nonfunctioning macroadenomas are establishment of a diagnosis, decompression of surrounding structures, and gross total removal of tumor tissue, if possible.**

References

1. Kovacs K, Horvath E. Tumors of the pituitary gland. In: Hartmann WH, ed. *Atlas of tumor pathology*, series 2, fascicle 21. Washington, DC: Armed Forces Institute of Pathology, 1986:192.
2. Lloyd RV, Cano M, Chandler WF, et al. Human growth hormone- and prolactin-secreting pituitary adenomas analyzed by in situ hybridization. *Am J Pathol.* 1989;134:605.
3. **Chandler WF, Schteingart DE, Lloyd RV, et al. Surgical treatment of Cushing's disease. *J Neurosurg.* 1987;66:204.**
4. Oldfield EH, Chrousos GP, Schulte HM, et al. Preoperative lateralization of ACTH-secreting pituitary microadenomas by bilateral and simultaneous inferior petrosal venous sinus sampling. *N Engl J Med.* 1985;312: 100–103.
5. Nelson DH, Meakin JW, Dealy JB, et al. ACTH-producing tumor of the pituitary gland. *N Engl J Med.* 1958;259:161.
6. Ebersold MJ, Quast LM, Laws ER, et al. Long-term results in transsphenoidal removal of nonfunctioning pituitary adenomas. *J Neurosurg.* 1986;64:713.
7. Park P, Chandler WF, Barkan AL, et al. The role of radiation therapy after surgical resection of nonfunctional pituitary macroadenomas. *Neurosurgery* 2004;55:100–107.
8. Boggan JE, Tyrrell JB, Wilson CB. Transsphenoidal microsurgical management of Cushing's disease. *J Neurosurg* 1983;59:195.
9. Hardy J. Cushing's disease: 50 years later. *Can J Neurol Sci* 1982;9:375.
10. Kuwayama A, Kageyama N. Current management of Cushing's disease: Ppart II. *Contemp Neurosurg* 1985;7:1.
11. Salassa RM, Laws ER, Carpenter PC, et al. Cushing's disease: 50 years later. *Trans Am Clin Climatol Assoc.* 1982;94:122.

12. Tindall GT, Tindall SC. Transsphenoidal surgery for acromegaly: long-term results in 50 patients. In: Black PM, Zervas NT, Ridgeway EC, et al., eds. *Secretory tumors of the pituitary gland.* New York: Raven Press, 1984, p. 175.
13. Kliman B, Kjellberg RN, Swisher B, et al. Proton beam therapy of acromegaly: a 20-year experience. In: Black PM, Zervas NT, Ridgeway EC, et al., eds. *Secretory tumors of the pituitary gland.* New York: Raven Press, 1984, p. 191.
14. Barkan AL, Halasz I, Dornfeld KJ, et al. Pituitary irradiation is ineffective in normalizing plasma insulin-like growth factor I in patients with acromegaly. *J Clin Endocrinol Metab.* 1997;82:3187–3191.
15. Landolt AM, Haller D, Lomas N, et al. Stereotactic radiosurgery for recurrent surgically treated acromegaly: comparison with fractionated radiotherapy. *J Neurosurg.* 1998;88:1002–1008.
16. Besser GM, Wass JAH. The medical management of acromegaly. In: Black PM, Zervas NT, Ridgeway EC, et al., eds. *Secretory tumors of the pituitary gland.* New York: Raven Press, 1984, p. 155.
17. Thorner MO, Evans WS, Vance ML. Medical management of prolactinomas: I. In: Black PM, Servas NT, Ridgeway EC, et al., eds. *Secretory tumors of the pituitary gland.* New York: Raven Press, 1984, p. 53.
18. Hardy J. Transsphenoidal microsurgery of prolactinomas. In: Black PM, Zervas NT, Ridgeway EC, et al., eds. *Secretory tumors of the pituitary gland.* New York: Raven Press, 1984, p. 73.
19. Randall RV, Laws ER, Abboud CF, et al. Transsphenoidal microsurgical treatment of prolactin-producing pituitary adenomas. *Mayo Clin Proc.* 1983;58:108.

SECTION L
LUNG NEOPLASMS

CHAPTER 81 ■ LUNG NEOPLASMS

ANDREW C. CHANG, JOCEYNE MARTIN, AND VALERIE W. RUSCH

Although population estimates of both the incidence and mortality of lung cancer have begun to decline, lung cancer remains the leading cause of cancer-related death in the United States, with 172,570 new cases and 163,510 deaths projected for 2005. Lung cancer was second only to cardiovascular disease in causes of mortality reported for 2002.[1] As of 2001, the most recent year for which data are available, the majority (53%) of patients presented with distant disease, with merely 16% presenting with localized disease only.[2] The best predictor of survival for patients with lung cancer is still tumor stage. However, even among patients who have undergone complete curative resection for early stage disease, as determined using pathologic tumor-node-metastasis (TNM) criteria, a substantial number will have recurrence of their cancer.[3]

Surgical resection remains the mainstay in the treatment of lung cancer, yet only approximately 20% of all patients diagnosed with lung cancer are considered resectable (stages I to IIIA). Until recently, adjuvant chemotherapy did not appear to provide any benefit over surgery alone for early lung cancer. However, several groups in the past year have demonstrated that adjuvant chemotherapy with platinum-based chemotherapy may confer significant advantage in overall survival even in completely resected early-stage non–small cell lung cancer.[4–6] As understanding of the molecular changes that occur in lung cancer evolves, new strategies that allow for early detection and classification of lung cancer will provide valuable information for the treatment of patients.

HISTORY

Ferdinand Sauerbruch, whose interests included the physiology of pneumothorax and who is considered one of the pioneers of thoracic surgery, reported the first successful lobectomy for lung carcinoma in 1920. At that time, it was believed that only total pneumonectomy would provide a cure for lung cancer. Although this was neither the first pulmonary resection nor pneumonectomy, Dr. Evarts A. Graham performed the first successful single-stage pneumonectomy for a left upper lobe bronchogenic carcinoma,[7] establishing the modern era of thoracic surgery for lung cancer. Ultimately, Dr. Graham succumbed to lung cancer in 1957 and was outlived by his patient, Dr. James L. Gilmore, who had continued to smoke.[8]

EPIDEMIOLOGY

Recently, population studies have demonstrated a continued decline in lung cancer incidence among men (83.5 cases per 100,000) and stabilization of disease incidence among women (49.2 per 100,000) as of 2001. African American men continue to have the greatest incidence of lung cancer, in excess of nearly 50% (124.5 per 100,000) of the cases reported for all men.[2] The decline in overall incidence may be due in part to public health efforts to promote smoking cessation. In a follow-up to the Seven Countries Study of smoking-related mortality, follow-up analysis of the initial cohorts studied from Europe, the United States, and Japan confirmed that cigarette smoking increased the risk for death due to lung cancer at a hazard ratio of 4.2 per pack cigarettes smoked. Furthermore, the death rates due to lung cancer decreased to that of never-smokers among former smokers after 10 years of smoking cessation.[9] Exposure to environmental "second-hand" cigarette smoke also may contribute to increased risk of lung cancer.[10] Within the European prospective investigation into cancer and nutrition (EPIC), a recent nested case-control study of a cohort of 123,479 EPIC enrollees demonstrated that former smokers and subjects with environmental smoke exposure were at greater risk for developing lung cancer over a median follow-up period of 7 years.[11]

PATHOLOGIC CLASSIFICATION

Uniform classification of lung cancer is important both to provide consistent treatment for patients and to allow standardization in reports of epidemiologic, clinical, and basic scientific studies. Currently, the classification is largely histologic, based on light microscopy findings determined from specimens obtained by surgical resection or needle biopsy, permitting wide application among surgical pathology laboratories where more advanced techniques might not be readily available. Nevertheless, immunohistochemical and electron microscopy analyses are important, particularly in the diagnosis of neuroendocrine tumors, or distinguishing between primary bronchogenic adenocarcinoma and metastatic lesions. The most recent revision of the World Health Organization (WHO) classification (Table 81.1), entitled the "WHO/International Association for the Study of Lung Cancer (IASLC) Histological Classification of Lung and Pleural Tumours," was published in 1999.[12] Guidelines for defining preinvasive lesions, such as squamous dysplasia and carcinoma *in situ,* are provided. Recognition and definition of the heterogeneity among adenocarcinomas is reflected in the subclassification of this group, including more restrictive definitions for bronchioloalveolar carcinoma. Definitions for the spectrum of neuroendocrine tumors, ranging from typical and atypical carcinoid to small cell lung cancer (SCLC) and large cell neuroendocrine carcinomas, are provided.

TUMOR BIOLOGY

Genetic alterations in several regulatory pathways including apoptosis, cell cycle, and mitogenic signaling have been identified in tumors of patients with NSCLC. Chromosomal loss of heterozygosity (LOH) or allelic gain appears to occur more frequently among patients with adenocarcinoma and history of tobacco exposure than among patients without any smoking history. Mutations among the *Ras* oncogenes, particularly *K-ras*, are characterized by the accumulation of DNA adducts within these genes, predominantly among patients with a history of tobacco use.[13] This has been attributed to the exposure to tobacco carcinogens such as benzo[a] pyrene (BaP); its activated form, benzo[a] pyrene diol epoxide (BPDE); and N-nitrosamines. These genes encode GTP-binding proteins, which participate in cellular signal transduction; such mutations result in constant *Ras* activation. Another family of oncogenes, *Myc*, encoding several transcription factors, is activated by gene amplification, primarily in SCLC.[13]

The tumor suppressor gene, *p53*, is the most frequently mutated gene in human cancer. Among patients with a history of tobacco use, mutations within *p53* were identified in more than 50% of patients with NSCLC, particularly SCC and

TABLE 81.1 CLASSIFICATION

HISTOLOGIC CLASSIFICATION OF LUNG TUMORS

WHO[a]	WPL-LCSC[b]
1. Squamous cell carcinoma	01 Carcinoma *in situ*
Variants: 1.1 Papillary	
1.2 Clear cell	10 Squamous cell carcinoma
1.3 Small cell	11 Well-differentiated
1.4 Basaloid	12 Moderately differentiated
	13 Poorly differentiated
2. Small cell carcinoma	20 Small cell
Variant: 2.1 Combined small cell carcinoma	21 Lymphocyte-like or oat cell
	22 Intermediate
3. Adenocarcinoma	30 Adenocarcinoma
3.1 Acinar adenocarcinoma	31 Well differentiated
3.2 Papillary adenocarcinoma	32 Moderately differentiated
3.3 Bronchioloalveolar carcinoma	33 Poorly differentiated
3.4 Solid carcinoma with mucin	34 Bronchiolar or alveolar
3.5 Adenocarcinoma with mixed subtypes	
4. Large cell carcinoma	40 Large cell undifferentiated
Variants: 4.1 Large cell neuroendocrine carcinoma	41 Giant cell
4.2 Others	
5. Adenosquamous carcinoma	50 Poorly differentiated carcinoma
6. Carcinoma with pleomorphic, sarcomatoid, or sarcomatous elements	60 Bimulticomponent or multidifferentiated
7. Carcinoid	70 Carcinoid
7.1 Typical	
7.2 Atypical	
8. Carcinoma of salivary gland type	80 Bronchial gland tumors
8.1 Mucoepidermoid carcinoma	81 Adenoid cystic
8.2 Adenoid cystic carcinoma	82 Mucoepidermoid
8.3 Others	83 Mixed tumors
9. Unclassified	

[a]World Health Organization. Adapted from: Histological typical of lung tumours. *Tumori* 1981; 67:253.
[b]Working Party for the Study of Lung Cancer. Modified by Lung Cancer Study Group, National Cancer Institute.

non-BAC adenocarcinoma.[14,15] Among patients with stage I tumors, those with mutations, particularly truncating, structural, or those that abolished DNA contact, demonstrated significantly worse actuarial survival in comparison with patients who had wild-type *p53*, whereas those patients with missense mutations did not demonstrate significantly different survival from those with wild-type *p53*. In patients with more advanced stage tumors, mutations in *p53* did not identify patients at risk for worse outcomes, suggesting that the effects of *p53* mutation in later stage tumors may be diluted by the accumulation of mutations at loci important in later stages in the progression of tumorigenesis.[14] Interestingly, investigators have also identified p53 protein expression, determined by immunohistochemical analysis, as a predictor of poor outcome in patients with stage I NSCLC.[16] Furthermore, *p53* expression is also associated with tumors that are more likely to demonstrate distant metastases.[17] Although mutational analyses were not reported in these immunohistochemical studies, these findings may be particularly concordant, because it is possible that mutations of *p53* may result in greater steady-state levels of p53 protein, allowing for increased detection by immunohistochemistry.[18]

Epigenetic mechanisms of gene regulation also appear to participate in tumorigenesis of lung cancer. In particular gene promoter inactivation by hypermethylation may be an important mechanism in the inactivation of tumor suppressor genes such as *p16*^{INK4a}(*p16*), an inhibitory regulator in the cyclin D-retinoblastoma cell cycle pathway. In patients with premalignant lesions such as squamous dysplasia and carcinoma *in situ*, both allelic loss and hypermethylation of *p16* have been identified, with associated decrease in p16 protein expression,[19] suggesting that loss of *p16* may be an important early event in NSCLC tumorigenesis.[20]

More recently, investigators have attempted to identify, genomewide, the molecular events occurring in lung cancer and to relate these changes to tumor classification, patient prognosis, or even response to therapy. Microarray analyses, comprising a multitude of methodological approaches, have the potential to provide the investigator with an abundance of data describing changes in gene or protein expression.[21,22] Several groups have demonstrated that large-scale gene expression studies can identify patterns of expression distinguishing squamous cell carcinoma, adenocarcinoma, and small cell lung cancer.[23,24] Furthermore, within groups of patients with bronchogenic adenocarcinoma, tumor heterogeneity can be identified, distinguishing not only tumor grade and differentiation but also patient outcomes.[24,25] These studies, although largely retrospective, demonstrate the potential for gene and protein expression "profiles" to be used as diagnostic and prognostic tools in the treatment of lung cancer. However, before these techniques can be broadly applied, even in prospective clinical trials, issues of reproducibility between institutions and across analytic platforms must be addressed.[26] Defining those genes that appear to be causally involved in lung cancer tumorigenesis from those genes that may be secondary, participating in subsequent events, is critical for our understanding of this disease and the identification of the best targets for therapeutic intervention.

Historically, clinical trials demonstrated that only 10% to 19% of patients with chemotherapy-refractory advanced NSCLC responded to treatment with the tyrosine kinase inhibitor, gefitinib. Furthermore, the addition of gefitinib to standard chemotherapy yielded no demonstrable benefit.[27] As proof of concept for targeted molecular therapy, two groups recently demonstrated that tumors obtained from patients who exhibited rapid and dramatic tumor response to gefitinib were more likely to have mutations in the epidermal growth factor receptor (*EGFR*).[27,28] In contrast, gefitinib-insensitive tumors did not contain similar mutations. Supporting this finding, retrospective analyses of patients with NSCLC indicated that patients with adenocarcinoma of bronchioloalveolar subtype and "never-smokers," defined as patients with less than 100 cigarette lifetime smoking history, were more likely to respond to treatment with gefitinib,[29] and mutational analysis of these gefitinib-sensitive tumors contained similar somatic mutations.[30] Whether these findings can be confirmed prospectively remains unknown. However, these data represent an exciting potential application of gene expression profiling for use in patient prognosis and in the clinical management of lung cancer to prevent either overtreatment or undertreatment of patients.

NON–SMALL CELL LUNG CANCER

The diagnosis of lung cancer should be directed by the presumed stage of disease at patient presentation. Accurate and reproducible TNM staging of lung cancer allows clinicians to provide consistent treatment of lung cancer and provides the basis for uniform reporting of clinical research across institutions and study groups. In 1997, revisions in the International System for Staging Lung Cancer were adopted by the American Joint Committee on Cancer (AJCC) and the Union Internationale Contre le Cancer (UICC), based on 5,319 cases of lung cancer.[3]

The aims of the initial evaluation of a patient with NSCLC are to determine whether distant metastatic disease is present and to assess the extent of intrathoracic disease. A multidisciplinary approach, involving input from pulmonary medicine, chest radiology, oncology, and thoracic surgery, should be undertaken in the selection of the most suitable testing for any individual patient (Algorithm 81.1). A thorough history and physical examination, combined with a plain chest radiograph and baseline laboratory data (complete blood cell count and measurement of serum sodium, calcium, alkaline phosphatase, and lactate dehydrogenase levels), may suggest the presence of metastatic disease. Common metastatic sites include the brain, supraclavicular nodes, contralateral lung, bones, liver, and adrenal glands. Abnormal findings are then investigated further with computed tomographic (CT) and, more recently,[18] F-2-fluoro-2-deoxy-D-glucose-positron emission tomography (FDG-PET) body scans. If necessary, needle aspiration biopsy or open biopsy can be performed to determine the extent of disease.

If the initial clinical evaluation does not suggest the presence of distant disease, the extent of further evaluation by various scans is controversial. Some physicians always perform a complete metastatic workup with CT of the chest and abdomen, CT or MRI of the brain, and FDG-PET scan. CT of the chest and upper abdomen has become standard, as much to evaluate the extent of the primary tumor and the status of the mediastinal lymph nodes as to detect metastases in the ipsilateral or contralateral lung, liver, or adrenals. Additional scans in asymptomatic patients may detect the 5% to 10% of metastases that are occult, but these scans are not clearly cost effective in patients with clinical stage I or II tumors.

Patients presenting with suspected NSCLC and a pleural effusion should undergo thoracentesis, followed by thoracoscopy if the initial cytology is nondiagnostic. Patients presenting with metastatic (stage IV) disease involving a solitary distant site should obtain tissue confirmation at the site of metastasis, if technically feasible. However, if noninvasive testing demonstrates multiple metastases (e.g., multiple liver, brain, or bone lesions), then diagnosis of the primary lesion might provide the most efficient means of diagnosis, followed by the initiation of palliative chemotherapy.[31] In patients who are suitable candidates for operation, who have a suspicious

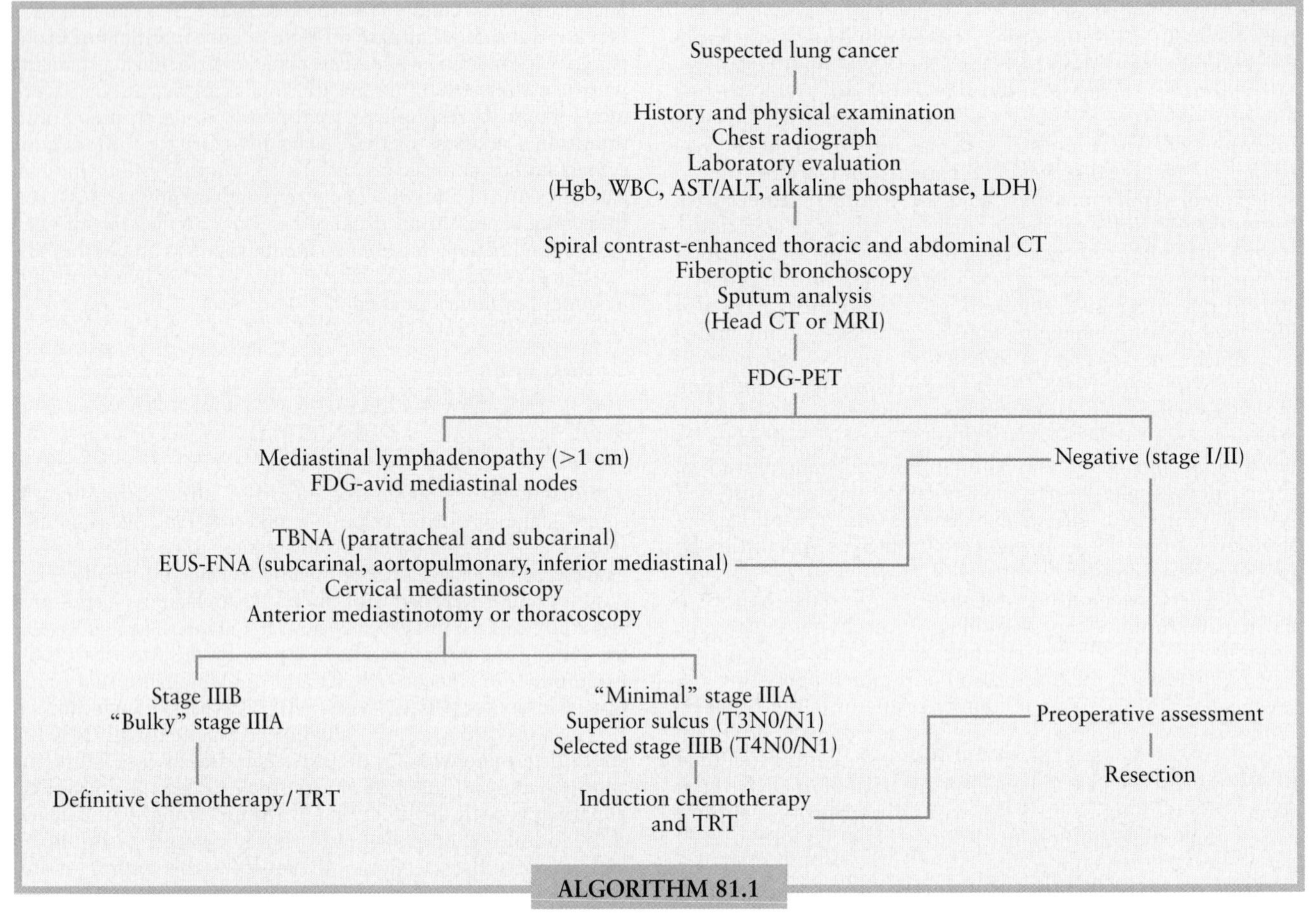

ALGORITHM 81.1 Decision making in patients who present with a solitary pulmonary nodule.

solitary pulmonary nodule that is of indeterminate origin despite appropriate evaluation, excisional biopsy and subsequent lobectomy of resectable lung cancer should be pursued.[32]

Recent multiinstitutional studies have indicated a benefit for a combined-modality approach in the treatment of stage IIIA NSCLC, consisting of neoadjuvant chemotherapy and radiation followed by surgical resection (North American Intergroup0139/ RTOG9309). Therefore tissue confirmation of mediastinal nodal involvement has implications not only for the staging but also for the management of patients who are otherwise candidates for surgical resection of locoregionally advanced NSCLC (Tables 81.2 and 81.3).[33]

Chest CT provides only anatomic clues for tumor involvement of mediastinal lymph nodes (enlargement greater than 10 mm), as demonstrated in a recent metaanalysis of more than 3,400 evaluable patients, with a pooled sensitivity of 57% and specificity of only 82%. This metaanalysis also demonstrated that FDG-PET scanning appears to provide increased sensitivity of 84% and specificity of 89% in over 1,100 patients studied for the detection of mediastinal malignancy.[34] Several single-institution prospective studies have also indicated the superior diagnostic accuracy of FDG-PET imaging.[35–37] A recent multiinstitutional trial involving 271 patients confirmed these findings. Although the overall sensitivity and specificity of FDG-PET staging was 61% and 84%, respectively, there was a significant improvement with FDG-PET over chest CT in the detection of both hilar (N1) lymph node (42% vs. 13%, $p = 0.0177$) and mediastinal (N2 and N3) tumor involvement (58% vs. 32%, $p = 0.004$).[38] However, although advanced detection modalities such as FDG-PET scanning may increase the suspicion of malignancy, its negative predictive value for mediastinal lymph node involvement does not appear to be sufficient, with a false–negative rate reported as high as 13%.[38] Integrated CT-PET imaging, in which concurrently performed chest CT provides anatomic correlation for positive PET findings, appears to provide more precise staging, particularly regarding tumor and nodal status,[39] and may also be used to guide further invasive testing in the accurate staging of lung cancer.

Ultimately tissue confirmation of noninvasive findings must be obtained, particularly in the setting of large, prospective trials being undertaken to determine the efficacy of neoadjuvant and adjuvant therapy.[40] Noninvasive techniques for clinical staging, particularly chest CT, have a reported false-negative rate of approximately 10% to 15%. FDG-PET scan also has a reported false-positive rate of as high as 50%.[35] Clinical staging of NSCLC, particularly of mediastinal lymph node involvement, can be accomplished by needle aspiration techniques from several approaches: transbronchial (TBNA), transthoracic, or transesophageal. Transesophageal endoscopic ultrasound with fine-needle aspiration appears to be particularly useful for sampling of posterior mediastinal nodes in the subcarinal, periesophageal, or aortopulmonary window station, particularly in patients with mediastinal

TABLE 81.2 CLASSIFICATION

TNM CLASSIFICATION FOR STAGING SYSTEM OF NON–SMALL CELL LUNG CANCER

Stage	TNM status
IA	T1 NO MO
IB	T2 NO MO
IIA	T1 N1 MO
IIB	T2 N1 MO
	T3 NO MO
IIIA	T3 N1 MO
	T1–3 N2 MO
IIIB	T4 Any N MO
	Any T N3 MO
IV	Any T any N M1

TNM definitions

T	TX	Positive malignant cell, but primary tumor not visualized by imaging or bronchoscopy
	T0	No evidence of primary tumor
	Tis	Carcinoma *in situ*
	T1	Tumor ≤3 cm, surrounded by lung or visceral pleura, without bronchoscopic evidence of invasion more proximal than the labor bronchus[a]
	T2	Tumor with any of the following features of size or extent: >3 cm in greatest dimension Involves main bronchus, ≥2 cm distal to the carina Invades the visceral pleura Associated with atelectasis or obstructive pneumonitis that extends to the hilar region but does not involve the entire lung
	T3	Tumor of any size that directly invades any of the following: chest wall (including superior sulcus tumors), diaphragm, mediastinal pleura, parietal pericardium; or tumor in the main bronchus <2 cm distal to the carina, but without involvement of the carina; or associated atelectasis or obstructive pneumonitis of the entire lung
	T4	Tumor of any size that invades any of the following: mediastinum, heart, great vessels, trachea, esophagus, vertebral body, carina; or tumor with a malignant pleural or pericardial effusion, or with satellite tumor nodule(s) within the ipsilateral primary tumor lobe of the lung[b]
N	NX	Regional lymph nodes cannot be assessed
	NO	No regional lymph node metastasis
	N1	Metastasis to ipsilateral peribronchial and/or ipsilateral hilar lymph nodes, and involvement in intrapulmonary nodes by direct extension of the primary tumor
	N2	Metastasis to ipsilateral mediastinal and/or subcarinal lymph node(s)
	N3	Metastasis to contralateral mediastinal, contralateral hilar, ipsilateral or contralateral scalene, or supraclavicular lymph node(s)
M	MX	Presence of distant metastasis cannot be assessed
	MO	No distant metastasis
	M1	Distant metastasis present [including metastatic tumor nodule(s) the ipsilateral non-primary tumor lobe(s) of the lung]

[a]The uncommon superficial tumor of any size with its invasive component limited to the bronchial wall that may extend proximal to the main bronchus is classified as T1.

[b]Most pleural effusions associated with lung cancer are caused by tumor. There are, however, some few patients in whom the pleural fluid (more than one specimen) is negative for tumor on cytopathologic examination and in whom the fluid is nonbloody and is not an exudate. In cases in which these elements and clinical judgment dictate that the effusion is not related to the tumor, the patient should be staged T1, T2, or T3, with effusion excluded as a staging element. Pericardial effusion is classified according to the same rules.

lymphadenopathy in regions that are not approachable by standard mediastinoscopic techniques. Diagnostic yield is improved with practitioner experience, sampling needle size, and on-site cytology examination to determine adequacy of the obtained samples.

Cervical mediastinoscopy remains the gold standard for tissue diagnosis of mediastinal lymphadenopathy with procedural sensitivity greater than 90% and specificity of 100%.[41] A recent retrospective review of a single institution's experience with routine mediastinoscopy, including 1,745 patients with known or suspected lung cancer, demonstrated overall sensitivity of 85%, with most false-negative results due to lymph node involvement in regions inaccessible to standard mediastinoscopic technique, morbidity of 0.6%, and perioperative mortality of 0.05%. Furthermore, of the patients found to have N2 or N3 disease at mediastinoscopy, only 6.6% (28/422) subsequently underwent surgical resection, including several patients treated on neoadjuvant protocol.[42] For patients with clinically suspicious aortopulmonary lymph node involvement (stations 5 and 6), an area that is generally not accessible by standard mediastinoscopy, anterior mediastinotomy, extended cervical mediastinoscopy, or more recently thoracoscopy can be performed.

One recent goal in the diagnosis of lung cancer has been the early detection of tumors arising in asymptomatic high-prevalence populations, that is, older patients with a history of tobacco use. Whether such efforts actually alter the natural history of disease remains controversial.[43,44] Although newer modalities of noninvasive imaging, such as FDG-PET imaging, have improved the accuracy of staging for lung cancer,[38] these techniques still rely on factors such as tumor cell volume, tumor density, and metabolic activity. Current staging procedures do not detect all lymph node or distant hematogenous metastases.

Risk Assessment

Having established that surgical resection is feasible, a significant number of patients with lung cancer cannot undergo operation due to associated comorbidity that increases operative mortality and postoperative morbidity. Age alone should not preclude patients with resectable disease from operation. However, in a population with a high prevalence of prior or continuing tobacco use, and therefore a predisposition to atherosclerotic cardiovascular disease, preoperative cardiovascular risk assessment and subsequent perioperative evaluation with noninvasive testing or coronary angiography, if indicated, is mandatory.[45]

Preoperative spirometry, particularly the forced expiratory volume in 1 sec (FEV_1), as an assessment of patients' suitability for pulmonary resection, is essential. Measurement of the diffusing capacity of the lung for carbon monoxide (DLCO) provides complementary data to standard spirometry, particularly for patients with evidence of interstitial lung disease or exertional dyspnea. Generally, if a patient demonstrates FEV_1 of greater than 2L (>60% predicted) or DLCO greater than 50% predicted, further evaluation of pulmonary capacity prior to resection, including pneumonectomy, is not necessary.[46] However, patients with limited pulmonary reserve, including those with FEV_1 less than 1.2L (40% predicted) or DLCO 35% to 40% predicted, are at high risk for significant morbidity or mortality following anatomic resection and should undergo further evaluation.[47]

Preoperative room-air arterial blood gas testing can identify patients at greater risk for perioperative complications or death. In particular, patients with arterial oxygen concentration less than 60 mm Hg, $PaCO_2$ greater than 45 mm Hg, or oxygen saturation less than 90% may be at greater risk for pulmonary resection. Quantitative perfusion scanning allows the assessment of predicted postoperative (ppo) lung function in patients with marginal pulmonary function and can be calculated as follows: ppo FEV_1(% predicted) = preoperative FEV_1(% predicted) × (1 − fraction of total number of anatomic segments to be resected). Patients with ppoFEV_1 less than 0.8 L, or 35% to 40% predicted, are likely at substantially increased risk for perioperative death or complication.[48,49]

If available, further testing with formal cardiopulmonary exercise testing (CPET) to calculate maximal oxygen consumption (VO_2 max) may allow further risk stratification in such marginal patients, although limited data support this approach. In small series, patients with VO_2 max less than 10 to 15 mL/kg per minute were at very high risk for postoperative complication, whereas those with VO_2 max greater than 20 mL/kg per minute underwent operation without complication or death.[49]

Informal exercise testing, particularly stair-climbing, may also aid the clinician in determining a patient's suitability for resection. Patients who are able to climb five flights of stairs will likely tolerate pneumonectomy, whereas those who cannot climb a single flight will likely not tolerate pulmonary resection. Furthermore, oxygen desaturation greater than 4% during exercise testing may also be an indicator for increased risk of perioperative complication. Careful preoperative physiologic assessment allows the clinician to identify patients at increased risk for perioperative complication or death and allow such patients to make an informed decision regarding operation.[50] Measures to minimize postoperative complications, including aggressive efforts to encourage smoking cessation, preoperative and postoperative chest physiotherapy including the use of incentive spirometry, early extubation and mobilization, and the use of postoperative thoracic epidural analgesia, although important for all patients undergoing pulmonary resection, may be of particular importance in patients with marginal pulmonary function who elect to undergo operation.

Treatment

Pulmonary resection, with definitive tumor staging, remains the mainstay of treatment for stages I and II NSCLC. The extent of resection, lobectomy, bilobectomy, or pneumonectomy, is determined by the location and size of the primary tumor and also by whether adjacent bronchopulmonary nodes are involved. At operation, tumor extent can be determined with examination of the parietal pleura, pericardium, and mediastinal structures. Complete resection must achieve microscopically negative bronchial and vascular margins.

If a tumor extends directly into the chest wall, diaphragm, or pericardium, an *en bloc* resection of the adjacent involved structure should be performed with the pulmonary resection. Reconstruction is performed as necessary (Fig. 81.1). On the other hand, if extensive endobronchial involvement is present but there is no involvement of the surrounding vascular or lymphatic structures, the tumor can sometimes be removed completely by lobectomy with segmental resection of the bronchus and/or pulmonary artery (bronchovascular sleeve resection), thus preserving lung function.

For peripherally located clinical stage I tumors, particularly among patients with limited pulmonary reserve, or those at high risk otherwise, segmental or nonanatomic "wedge" resection can be performed, although such patients are at greater risk for locoregional recurrence, as high as 25% to 50% in several reported series.[51–54] With centrally located tumors, patients should undergo sleeve lobectomy rather than pneumonectomy if complete resection can be achieved. Several institutional retrospective studies[55–59] have demonstrated that operative mortality is reduced among patients undergoing sleeve lobectomy (0% to 5.2%) when compared with those patients undergoing pneumonectomy (1.7% to 8.9%). Moreover, overall 5-year survival is improved among patients undergoing sleeve resection, particularly among those with N0 or N1 nodal status.

Although noninvasive techniques for preoperative assessment of mediastinal nodes have improved, for example with the advent of combined CT-PET, clinical staging is still inaccurate. Therefore, nodal status should be confirmed by intraoperative mediastinal lymph node sampling or mediastinal lymph node dissection. Accurate pathologic staging not only provides prognostic information but also clarifies the decision whether to proceed with adjuvant chemotherapy. Systematic sampling should include, for right-sided resections, at least one subcarinal, right paratracheal, and tracheobronchial angle lymph node each, and for left-sided resections, at least one subcarinal and paraaortic or aortopulmonary lymph node each, using standard nomenclature and numbering as depicted in Table 81.3. Several groups advocate complete mediastinal lymph node dissection, with *en bloc* removal of the nodal packets from the same levels as in systematic sampling.[60] Although nodal dissection may be as accurate as systematic sampling with similar morbidity, whether mediastinal lymph

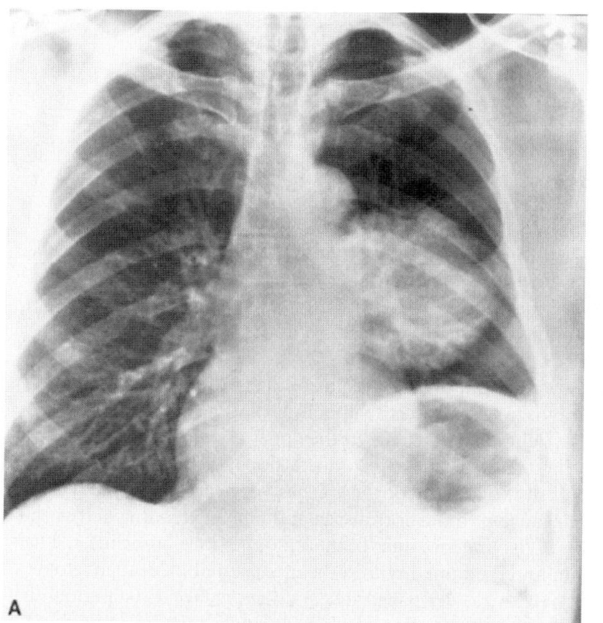

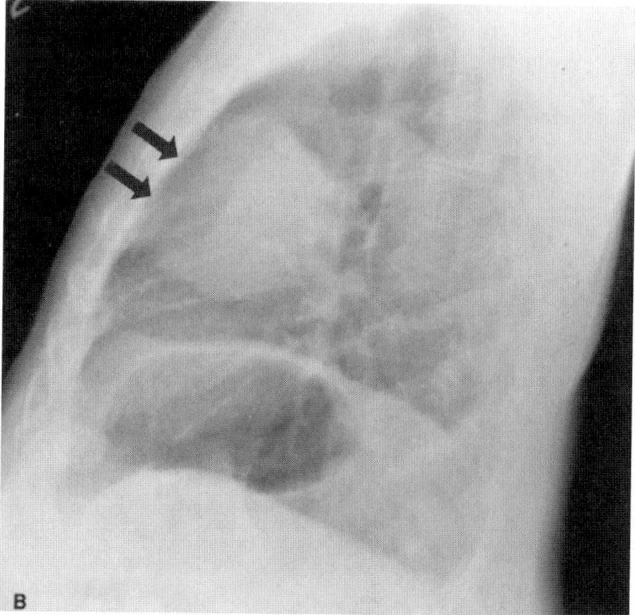

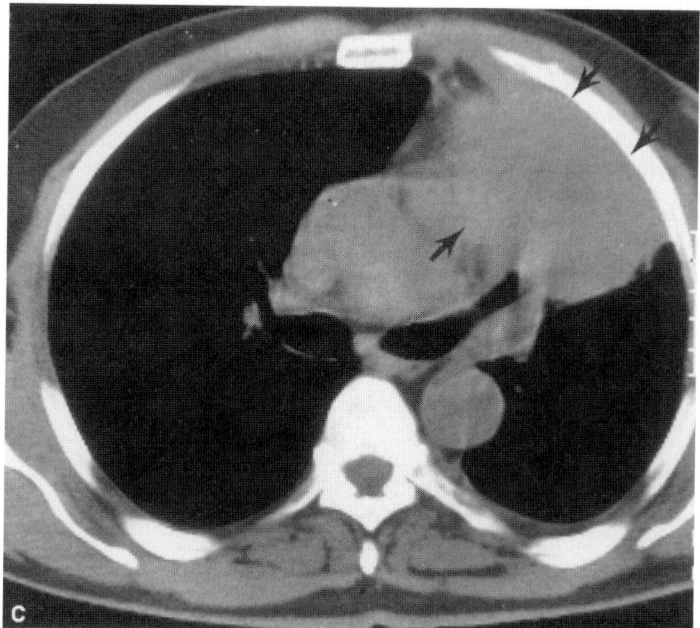

FIGURE 81.1 (*A*) Posteroanterior chest radiograph shows an elevated left hemidiaphragm, suggestive of phrenic nerve involvement by the mass. (*B*) Lateral chest radiograph shows extension of the mass to the anterior chest wall (*arrows*). (C) Computed tomography suggests both pericardial and chest wall involvement (*arrows*). At thoracotomy, the chest wall, phrenic nerve, and pericardium were found to be involved. All were resected *en bloc* with the tumor.

node dissection rather than sampling confers a survival advantage among patients undergoing major pulmonary resection remains controversial and is one of the questions addressed in a recently completed multicenter clinical trial, Z0030, conducted by the American College of Surgeons Oncology Group (ACOSOG).

Survival

The long-term survival after surgical resection for NSCLC is linked to the pathologic stage of disease. The overall 5-year survival rates are shown in Table 81.4 and range from 60% to 70% for stage I tumors, from 40% to 50% for stage II tumors, and from 15% to 30% for stage IIIA tumors. Nodal involvement has the strongest adverse influence on survival. Large peripheral tumors that extend directly into the chest wall without nodal involvement (T3N0) are associated with a 5-year survival rate of 40% after complete resection, whereas involvement of hilar or mediastinal nodes is associated with only a 20% survival rate. The status of the primary tumor has a lesser but still important effect on survival. Within stage I, for instance, T1N0 tumors are associated with a 5-year survival rate of 70%, substantially better than the 5-year survival rate of 60% associated with T2N0 tumors.

Some series suggest that histology also affects survival. In stage I or II NSCLC, the North American LCSG consistently observed a better disease-free and overall survival for squamous cell cancer than for nonsquamous tumors.[61] The influence of histology has not been reported in all series and is not seen in stage III and stage IV tumors. However, T and N status and histology provide only a crude estimate of outcome. Within a given TNM category and histology, it is still impossible to discern which individual patients will

TABLE 81.3

THE MOUNTAIN–DRESLER LYMPH NODE MAP

Nodal station	Anatomic landmarks
N2 nodes: All N2 nodes lie within the mediastinal pleural envelope	
1. Highest mediastinal nodes	Nodes lying above a horizontal line at the upper rim of the brachiocephalic (left innominate) vein where it ascends to the left, crossing in front of the trachea at its midline.
2. Upper paratracheal nodes	Nodes lying above a horizontal line drawn tangential to the upper margin of the aortic arch and below the inferior boundary of No. 1 nodes.
3. Prevascular and retrotracheal nodes	Prevascular and retrotracheal nodes may be designated 3A and 3P; midline nodes are considered to be ipsilateral.
4. Lower paratracheal nodes	The lower paratracheal nodes on the right lie to the right of the midline of the trachea between a horizontal line drawn tangential to the upper margin of the aortic arch and a line extending across the right main bronchus at the upper margin of the upper lobe bronchus, and contained within the mediastinal pleural envelope; the lower paratracheal nodes on the left lie to the left of the midline of the trachea between a horizontal line drawn tangential to the upper margin to the aortic arch and a line extending across the left main bronchus at the level of the upper margin of the left upper lobe bronchus, medial to the ligamentum arteriosum and contained within the mediastinal pleural envelope. Researchers may want to designate the lower paratracheal nodes as No. 4s (superior) and No. 4i (inferior) subsets for study purposes; the No. 4s nodes may be defined by a horizontal line extending across the trachea and drawn tangential to the cephalic border of the azygos vein; the No. 4i nodes may be defined by the lower boundary of No. 4s and the lower boundary of No. 4 as described above.
5. Subaortic (aortopulmonary window)	Subaortic nodes are lateral to the ligamentum arteriosum or the aorta or left pulmonary artery and proximal to the first branch of the left pulmonary artery and lie within the mediastinal pleural envelope.
6. Para-aortic nodes (ascending aorta or phrenic)	Nodes lying anterior and lateral to the ascending aorta and the aortic arch or the innominate artery, beneath a line tangential to the upper margin of the aortic arch.
7. Subcarinal nodes	Nodes lying caudal to the carina of the trachea but not associated with the lower lobe bronchi or arteries within the lung.
8. Paraesophageal nodes (blow carina)	Nodes lying adjacent to the wall of the esophagus and to the right or left of the midline, excluding subcarinal nodes.
9. Pulmonary ligament nodes	Nodes lying within the pulmonary ligament, including those in the posterior wall and lower part of the inferior pulmonary vein.
N1 nodes: All N1 nodes lie distal to the mediastinal pleural reflection and within the visceral pleura	
10. Hilar nodes	The proximal lobar nodes, distal to the mediastinal pleural reflection and the nodes adjacent to the bronchus intermedius on the right; radiographically, the hilar shadow may be created by enlargement of both hilar and interlobar nodes.
11. Interlobar nodes	Nodes lying between the lobar bronchi.
12. Lobar nodes	Nodes adjacent to the distal bronchi.
13. Segmental nodes	Nodes adjacent to the segmental bronchi.
14. Subsegmental nodes	Nodes around the subsegmental bronchi.

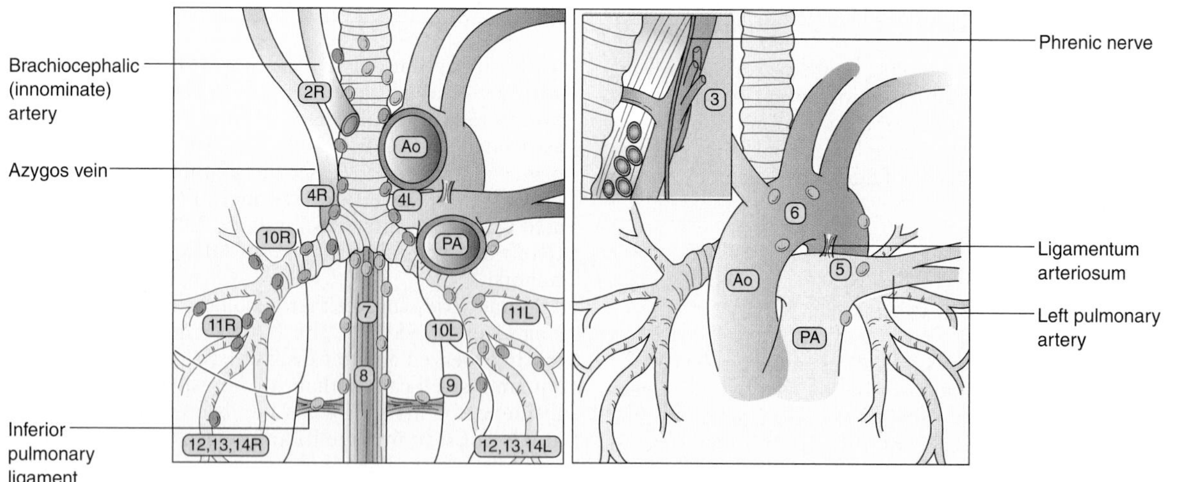

In this newer map, a stricter definition of the anatomic boundaries for each lymph node region facilitates correlation between findings at operation and findings on chest computed tomography (After Mountain CF, Dresler CM. Regional Lymph node classification for lung cancer staging. *Chest* 1997;111:1718).

TABLE 81.4 RESULTS

NEW STAGE DATA BASE: CUMULATIVE PERCENTAGE SURVIVING 5 YEARS BY CLINICAL AND SURGICAL TNM SUBSETS

	Clinical		Surgical	
TNM subset	No. patients	Patients surviving (%)	No. patients	Patients surviving (%)
T1 NO MO	687	61	511	67
T2 NO MO	1,189	38	549	57
T1 N1 MO	29	34	76	55
T2 NI MO	250	24	288	39
T3 NO MO	107	22	87	38
T3 N1 MO	40	9	55	25
T1–3N2 MO	471	13	344	23
T4 NO–2 MO	458	7	—	—
Any N3 MO	572	3	—	—
Any M1	1,427	1	—	—
TOTAL	5,230		1,910	

Adapted from Mountain CF. Revisions in the international system for staging lung cancer. *Chest* 1997; 111:1710.

experience relapse. A better understanding of lung cancer biology is needed to define which patients are truly at risk for recurrence.

Patterns of Recurrence

The predominant sites of relapse for all stages of NSCLC after surgical resection are distant metastases. Approximately 30% of recurrences are locoregional with tumors of both squamous and nonsquamous histology.[53] For all stages of disease, the brain is the single most common site of relapse, and brain metastases occur more frequently with nonsquamous tumors. Other common metastatic sites include bone, ipsilateral or contralateral lung, liver, and the adrenal glands.[53,62]

At least 60% of recurrences develop in the first 2 years after operation, and virtually all recurrences related to the original primary tumor occur within 5 years after surgery. Even the small proportion of patients with stage II or III disease who survive 5 years are likely to survive 10 years or more postoperatively. Most stage I patients, particularly those with T1N0 tumors, do experience long-term survival. The North American LCSG followed 907 patients with TlN0 tumors for a minimum of 5 years after operation.[62] Recurrences of the original primary tumor were rare after 5 years, and after that time, the occurrence of new pulmonary cancers becomes the dominant problem. The risk for development of a second lung cancer in patients who survive resection of a NSCLC is approximately 2% to 3% per patient per year.[63] Patients also face a consistent risk for the development of new, nonpulmonary primary cancers during the first 5 years after operation and thereafter. New, nonpulmonary malignancies develop in a wide variety of sites, but breast, colon, and prostate cancers are the most common.[53]

These facts underscore the importance of long-term follow-up after resection of early-stage NSCLC. Traditionally, most thoracic oncologists see lung cancer patients every 3 to 4 months during the first 2 years after operation, then every 6 months until 5 years after operation, and annually thereafter. There is no single way to detect recurrence, so follow-up includes a combination of history, physical examination, serial chest radiographs, and spiral chest CT. The cost effectiveness of this approach is unproved,[64] but clearly the primary physician following a patient should be aware of the risk for second primary tumors.

Adjuvant Therapy

The risk for recurrent disease, even after resection of early-stage NSCLC, has led to efforts to improve overall survival rates through the use of adjuvant therapy, even though no specific method is available to identify which patients will relapse. Various types of adjuvant therapy have been tested, including immunotherapy, radiation, chemotherapy, and combined chemotherapy and radiation.

In the early 1970s, a single-institution, nonrandomized study suggested that immunotherapy with intrapleural bacillus Calmette-Guérin (BCG) might improve survival after resection of stage I lung cancer. Subsequently, two early prospective, randomized large trials, from the North American LCSG[65] and the Ludwig Cancer Study Group[66] failed to demonstrate any survival advantage for patients treated with nonspecific adjuvant intrapleural immunotherapy. However, several studies of systemic immunotherapy have been performed. Ratto et al.[67] randomized 113 patients to receive either chemotherapy and radiation or adoptive immunotherapy with tumor-infiltrating lymphocytes and interleukin-2 after resection of stage II or III NSCLC. Immunotherapy led to an improved 3-year survival, particularly among patients with stage IIIB NSCLC. These results are not definitive because no true control arm was included in this trial, the number of patients accrued was small, and the patient population was heterogeneous.

Radiation has been extensively evaluated as adjuvant therapy. Retrospective series suggesting that postoperative radiation therapy (PORT) potentially improves overall survival[68–70] led to randomized trials comparing adjuvant radiation with no further treatment after pulmonary resection. These studies randomized relatively small numbers of patients with tumors of various stages and histologic types, using a wide range of doses and techniques.[71–75] None showed a significant difference in overall survival. Distant metastases remain the most common form of recurrent disease and are not affected by PORT to the mediastinum. However, several of these trials[71,72,74,75] showed that radiation significantly decreases the risk for locoregional recurrence in tumors of all histologic types (Table 81.5). A meta-analysis of several randomized controlled studies of PORT suggested an adverse effect on survival, particularly among patients treated with PORT with early-stage (I or II) lung cancer.[76] Therefore, postoperative radiation may be appropriate adjuvant treatment for patients who are at high risk for locoregional recurrence, either because of bulky nodal disease or close margins.

Because distant metastases are the predominant mode of relapse after resection of early-stage NSCLC, multiple randomized trials (Table 81.6) have been performed to determine whether postoperative adjuvant chemotherapy improves survival. Initial trials used chemotherapeutic agents, including nitrogen mustards, cyclophosphamide (Cytoxan), methotrexate, and nitrosourea, now known to have no activity in NSCLC.[77–80] Since the 1970s, all chemotherapy regimens have been cisplatin based. A meta-analysis of 9,387 patients entered into 52 randomized clinical trials showed a 5% survival benefit at 5 years for adjuvant cisplatin-based chemotherapy in comparison with surgery alone. Trials comparing adjuvant radiation with radiation plus chemotherapy showed an absolute survival benefit of 4% at 2 years in favor of combined-modality treatment.[81] Several of these trials have shown that approximately half of all patients actually receive the full dose of chemotherapy planned.[82,83] Intensive chemotherapy is probably better tolerated preoperatively, not when patients are recovering from a major operation.

TABLE 81.5 RESULTS

SUMMARY OF REPRESENTATIVE RANDOMIZED TRIALS COMPARING RADIATION WITH NO FURTHER TREATMENT AFTER SURGICAL RESECTION OF EARLY STAGE NON–SMALL CELL LUNG CANCER

Study	No. patients	NSCLC stage[a]	Radiation dose (Gy)	Overall survival difference
Van Houtte et al., 1980[67]	224	I, II	60	NS
LCSG. 1986[66]	210	II, IIIA	50	NS
Lafitte et al., 1996 [65]	132	IB	45–60	NS
MRC, 1996[64]	308	II, IIIA	40 (15 fractions)	NS
Smolle-Juettner et al., 1996[63]	155	I–IIIA	50–56	NS
Mayer et al., 1997[62]	155	IA–IIIA	50–56	NS

[a]The stages are listed according to the 1997 international system for staging lung cancer.
LCSG, Lung Cancer Study Group; MRC, medical Research Council; NS, not statistically significant; NSCLC, non–small cell lung cancer.

Recent trials of adjuvant chemotherapy in patients with completely resected NSCLC appear to indicate a therapeutic benefit. Initial studies from the West Japan Study Group indicated that postoperative treatment with uracil-tegafur (UFT), a well-tolerated oral analogue of fluorouracil, confers a survival advantage.[84] However, a recent randomized phase III trial from this same group failed to demonstrate a survival advantage among patients with resected stage I adenocarcinoma or squamous cell carcinoma. However, subset analysis of patients with pT1N0M0 tumors suggested a significant improvement in overall survival.[85] Although fluorouracil is not usually considered an active drug against NSCLC, prolonged low-dose administration used in this trial appears to have a significant antitumor effect.

The multicenter, multinational International Adjuvant Lung Cancer Trial evaluated the effect of cisplatin-based adjuvant chemotherapy on survival after complete resection of non–small cell lung cancer. A total of 1,867 patients with resected stage I, II, or III NSCLC were randomized to receive cisplatin-based chemotherapy, cisplatin-based chemotherapy and radiation, radiation alone, or no adjuvant treatment. Individual institutions administered additional chemotherapeutic agents at their discretion ("open-choice design"), with nearly half of the treated patients receiving cisplatin (100 mg/m^2) and etoposide for three or four cycles. The total dose delivered of cisplatin was greater than 240 mg/m^2 for 73.8% of treated patients. Additional agents used were vinorelbine, vinblastine, or vindesine. Cisplatin dosing varied from 80 to 120 mg/m^2/cycle, for a total expected dose of 300 to 400 mg/m^2. Statistically significant benefits were observed for both overall (absolute difference 4.1%) and disease-free (absolute difference 5.1%) survival at 5 years, for patients treated with cisplatin-based chemotherapy, with or without adjuvant radiation.[4] In subgroup analysis, the benefits of cisplatin-based adjuvant chemotherapy appeared to confer the greatest benefit on patients with stage III NSCLC. Planned radiotherapy did not appear to provide any added benefit.

Two recent studies, reported in abstract only, support the use of adjuvant chemotherapy in early-stage lung cancer. The Cancer and Leukemia Group B (CALGB) 9633 trial reported 344 patients, undergoing pulmonary resection for T2N0M0 (stage IB) NSCLC, randomized either to adjuvant therapy with paclitaxel and carboplatin or to observation.

TABLE 81.6 RESULTS

SUMMARY OF REPRESENTATIVE RANDOMIZED TRIALS TESTING THE BENEFIT OF ADJUVANT CHEMOTHERAPY AFTER SURGICAL RESECTION OF EARLY-STAGE NON–SMALL CELL LUNG CANCER

Study	No. patients	NSCLC stages[a]	Chemotherapy agents	Overall survival difference
Hughes and Wiggins, 1962[77]	1,002	Not stated	HN2 vs. no Rx	NS
Slack, 1970[78]	1,192	Not stated	HN2 vs. no Rx	NS
Shields et al., 1977[79]	417	Not stated	Cytoxan vs. Cytoxan + MTX	NS
Shields et al., 1982[80]	865	Not stated	CCNU + hydroxyurea vs. no Rx	NS
Feld et al., 1993[82]	269	I–IIA	CAP vs. no Rx	NS
Pisters et al., 1994[95]	72	IIIA	VP + RT vs. RT	NS
Dautzenberg et al., 1995[179]	267	I–IIIA	COPAC, RT vs. RT	NS
Wada et al., 1996[84]	323	I–IIIA	VP, UFT vs. UFT vs. no Rx	$p = 0.053$
Keller et al., 2000[83]	488	II, IIIA	EP + RT vs. RT	NS
Scagliatti et al., 2003[180]	1,209	I–IIIA	MVP vs. no Rx	NS
IALT, 2004[4]	1,867	I–IIIA	CDDP-based ± RT vs. RT vs. no Rx	Overall, $p < 0.03$; DFS, $p < 0.003$
Strauss et al., 2004[5]	344	IB	Carboplatin, paclitaxel vs. no Rx	Overall, $p = 0.028$; DFS, $p = 0.035$
Winton et al., 2004[6]	482	IB–II	CDDP, Vnb vs. no Rx	Overall, $p = 0.011$; DFS, $p = 0.0003$
Nakagawa et al., 2005[85]	332	I	UFT vs. no Rx	Overall, NS; T1N0, $p = 0.036$

[a]The stages are listed according to the 1997 international system for staging lung cancer.[3]
CAP: cyclophosphamide. doxorubicin. cisplatin; CCNU, J-12-chlorethyl)-3-cyclohexyl-J nitrosourea; CDDP, cisplatin; COPAC: cyclophosphamide, doxorubicin, cisplatin, vincristine, lomustine; Cytoxan, cyclophosphamide; DFS, disease-free survival; EP: etoposide, cisplatin; HN2, nitrogen mustard; IALT, International Adjuvant Lung Cancer Trial; M, mitomycin C; MTX, methotrexate; NS, not significant; no Rx, no adjuvant treatment; RT, radiation therapy; UFT, tegafur plus uracil; Vnb, vinorelbine; VP: vindesine, cisplatin.

Overall survival (4-year) improved from 59% to 71% with adjuvant chemotherapy. There was also significant reduction in both cancer-specific mortality and mortality from all causes.[5] In the second trial, recently reported by the National Cancer Institute of Canada-Clinical Trials Group (JBR.10), prolonged overall and disease-free survival for patients with resected stage IB or II (excluding T3N0M0) NSCLC treated adjuvantly with vinorelbine and cisplatin.[6] These survival differences were demonstrated despite poor patient compliance, with only 50% of patients completing their prescribed regimen of adjuvant therapy.[86]

Treatment of Stage III Disease

Stage III NSCLC indicates locoregionally advanced disease that encompasses several anatomic subsets that vary considerably in the likelihood that resection will provide durable oncologic benefit. Stage IIIB is generally considered unresectable. There is no role for resection for patients with T4 (stage IIIB) disease due to malignant pleural or pericardial effusion or infiltration of the heart or vertebra or for those with contralateral or supraclavicular nodal metastases (N3). However, several small series from specialized centers have demonstrated that surgery can be considered for selected patients with invasion of mediastinal structures, such as the superior vena cava, left atrium, carina, or aorta, with consideration for induction chemoradiation to "downstage" such tumors.[87,88] These series indicate that complete resection is essential to obtain survival benefit from this approach.

Stage IIIA includes patients with extrapulmonary disease involving the ipsilateral hemithorax (i.e., T3N1 and T1-3N2). The management of patients with stage IIIA disease as a result of mediastinal nodal involvement (N2) continues to evolve and is discussed in the following sections.

Role of Surgical Resection

The most controversial and complex part of the treatment of stage IIIA NSCLC is the management of patients with N2 disease. Reported 5-year survival rates after resection for N2 disease are usually 20% to 30% but range from 0% to 40%. This variation reflects the extent of mediastinal nodal involvement, the T status of the primary tumor, and the ability to perform a complete resection. With respect to mediastinal nodal involvement, adverse prognostic factors include the presence of extracapsular nodal disease, multiple levels of involved lymph nodes, and superior mediastinal nodal metastases.[89,90]

Historically, several series presented an inappropriately optimistic view of the benefit of surgical resection for N2 disease, because they focused on highly selected patients. The experience reported by Martini and Flehinger[91] from Memorial Sloan-Kettering Cancer Center places surgical resection for N2 disease in perspective because it examines the outcome of treatment of all patients with N2 disease and not just a small subset. From 1974 to 1981, a total of 1,598 patients with NSCLC, of whom 706 had mediastinal nodal metastases, were seen by the thoracic service. Only 151 patients, or 21% of all patients with N2 disease, had technically complete resections of the primary tumor and all accessible mediastinal lymph nodes. The overall survival of these 151 patients was 29% at 5 years. Moreover, 33 of 151 patients had "clinical" N2 disease (mediastinal nodal involvement extensive enough to be visible on chest radiography or bronchoscopy) with only an 8% survival rate at 3 years. Thus, only 16.7% of all patients potentially benefited in the long term from surgical resection. Overall survival was also influenced by the T status of the primary tumor; patients with T2 or T3 tumors fared significantly worse than those with Tl tumors. Based on these and other data, most surgeons consider for resection only those patients who have a Tl or T2 primary tumor and single-level intranodal N2 disease.

Two small randomized clinical trials further challenge the concept of surgical resection as the primary treatment for any patient with N2 disease. Rosell et al.[92] randomized 60 patients with stage IIIA NSCLC (16 of whom did not have N2 disease) to undergo surgical resection or to receive three cycles of cisplatin-based chemotherapy followed by surgical resection. The median survival of the patients who received preoperative chemotherapy was significantly longer (26 months vs. 8 months) than the survival of patients who underwent only surgical resection. A study of similar design from the M. D. Anderson Cancer Center corroborated these results.[93] Both trials were stopped early because of highly significant differences between the two study arms. These two studies suggest that it is appropriate to consider all patients with N2 disease diagnosed at mediastinoscopy for induction chemotherapy. Unfortunately, because pretreatment mediastinoscopy was not mandated in either trial, some patients who did not have N2 disease were included. The results of these trials are not universally accepted because of the small numbers of patients enrolled, the lack of systematic pretreatment staging, and the unusually poor survival of the patients in the control arms.

Rationale for Neoadjuvant Therapy

Although some patients with "minimal" N2 disease survive for long periods of time after surgical resection, most have more extensive nodal involvement and do not benefit from surgery as their primary treatment. Until the 1980s, the standard treatment for such patients was radiation. The reported survival rates after radiation are harder to interpret than those after surgical resection because most series include a mixture of stages IIIA and IIIB patients and do not define the precise extent of nodal involvement. Sequential trials by the Radiation Therapy Oncology Group (RTOG) showed that high-dose, continuous radiation yields the best chance of local control.[94] Many attempts have been made to intensify radiation dose without increasing radiation side effects, either by altering radiation fractionation schemes or by using three-dimensional conformal treatment planning. On the whole, these efforts have led to minimal improvements in both local control and survival because most patients relapse in distant sites, just as they do after surgical resection. For this reason, postoperative chemotherapy has been used as adjuvant therapy to surgery and radiation therapy in patients with N2 disease, although no benefit in survival has been shown.[95] The poor long-term survival and the risk for distant metastatic disease prompted an investigation of neoadjuvant multimodality therapy for stage III NSCLC.

Early Trials of Neoadjuvant Therapy

The concept of preoperative therapy followed by surgical resection (*neoadjuvant therapy*) dates back to 1955, when Bromley and Szur[96] used radiation (at an average dose of 47 Gy) to treat 66 patients before surgical resection. At operation, no viable tumor was found in 29 of 62 (47%) patients, but 10 patients died of complications in the first month, and only two patients survived to 5 years after operation. At the time, the natural history of NSCLC was not well understood, the methods of staging before resection were not very accurate, and the risk for distant metastases was not fully recognized. Effective chemotherapy did not exist, and it was hoped that an approach that increased resectability might lead to better long-term survival. Thus, early neoadjuvant trials focused on the use of preoperative radiation.

Several subsequent studies further explored this approach.[97] All these trials were flawed by a lack of pretreatment staging, by the use of widely varying amounts of radiation, and by excessively long intervals between irradiation and surgical resection. Nonetheless, it became apparent that aggressive local treatment did not improve long-term survival, even though radiation could sterilize tumor in a significant number of patients. The development of distant metastases in 50% to 80% of patients during or shortly after treatment underscored the need for systemic therapy in stage III NSCLC.

Recent Trials of Neoadjuvant Therapy

Because of a better understanding of the natural history of early-stage lung cancer and the revision of the international staging system in 1986, recent trials have defined more uniform patient populations, so that it has been easier to interpret trial results. Although many different treatment regimens have been used in neoadjuvant trials, they can be grouped into three major categories: (a) chemoradiation without surgical resection, (b) chemotherapy followed by surgical resection, and (c) chemoradiation followed by surgical resection.

Trials of Chemoradiation without Surgical Resection. These trials cannot be equated with trials of neoadjuvant therapy that include surgical resection because patients entered into nonsurgical trials are staged clinically without the benefit of mediastinoscopy. Therefore, nonsurgical trials include a mix of patients with stages IIIA and IIIB cancers, and they may even include some patients with earlier stage disease who are thought erroneously to have stage III disease because of benign mediastinal adenopathy diagnosed only by CT.

With the acceptance of chemotherapy and radiation as standard treatment, attention has focused recently on the optimal means to deliver both modalities. A study suggests that concurrent treatment is superior to sequential chemoradiotherapy. Furuse et al.[98] randomized 314 patients with stage III NSCLC to MVP (cisplatin, 80 mg/m^2 on day 1; mitomycin, 8 mg/m^2 on days 1 and 29; and vindesine on days 1, 8, 29, and 36) with concurrent split-course radiation or to MVP followed by standard radiation. Patients who received concurrent treatment had a significantly better response and survival.

The results of several phase III randomized trials comparing radiation alone with either sequential or concurrent chemotherapy and radiation are shown in (Table 81.7). These trials confirm the feasibility of combined-modality treatment and overall have shown that patients receiving chemoradiation have a better survival than those receiving either standard fractionated or hyperfractionated radiation alone. In most studies, the addition of chemotherapy improved median survival from between 9 and 10 months to 14 months and 5-year survival from 5% to between 15% and 20%. The somewhat variable results among these trials are related to several factors, including differences in total radiation dose and method of administration (split vs. continuous course); differences in chemotherapy dose, especially with respect to cisplatin; and differences in patient selection based on staging criteria.

Trials of Neoadjuvant Therapy with Surgical Resection

These trials have used two different treatment strategies: induction chemotherapy alone or concurrent chemoradiation before surgical resection. The rationale for chemotherapy alone as induction treatment is that it potentially allows the use of a more intense dose and also the use of some drugs, such as mitomycin, that cannot be administered in conjunction with radiation. Proponents of this approach also believe that chemotherapy is as effective as induction treatment as combined chemoradiation is and that separating the two modalities allows irradiation to be used postoperatively, when a higher total dose can be given. Proponents of concurrent preoperative chemoradiation believe that this approach provides adequate systemic treatment of micrometastatic disease and more effective control of bulky primary and mediastinal tumors.

Neoadjuvant Trials of Chemotherapy Alone Before Surgical Resection. One of the best-known early trials to demonstrate the feasibility of combining induction chemotherapy with subsequent pulmonary resection in patients with stage III NSCLC was developed by Martini et al.[99] In 1984, they initiated a trial of high-dose, cisplatin-based (120 mg/m^2) chemotherapy followed by surgical resection for patients with clinical N2 disease. Vindesine or vinblastine and subsequently mitomycin were added to form the so-called MVP regimen. Postoperative radiation was given to patients who had persistent mediastinal nodal tumor at thoracotomy, and all patients received two additional cycles of chemotherapy postoperatively. In 136 patients treated from 1984 to 1991, the major response rate to induction chemotherapy was 77% (105/136), and the complete resection rate was 65% (89/136). A complete pathologic response was noted in 19 patients (21%) at the time of resection. The overall survival at 5 years was 17% and the median survival was 19 months, a distinct improvement over the historical survival for this group of patients. Seven treatment-related deaths (5%) occurred in this study, five of which were postoperative.

A phase II trial, reported by the CALGB in 1995, of induction chemotherapy enrolled 74 patients, treated with two cycles of cisplatin (100 mg/m^2 on days 1 and 29) and vinblastine (5 mg/m^2 per week) without mitomycin followed by surgical resection for patients with mediastinoscopy-proved stage IIIA N2 disease.[100] In addition, two cycles of chemotherapy and 81-4 Gy of radiation were given postoperatively. Sixty-three patients (85%) had either an objective response or stable disease after induction therapy and underwent thoracotomy, with operative mortality rate of 3.2%. Twenty-three patients (37% of thoracotomies, 31% of all patients) had a complete resection, with 3-year survival of 46%. The overall 3-year survival was 23%. The lower resectability rate in this trial than in the study potentially reflects both the multiinstitutional nature of this trial and the use of a less intensive chemotherapy regimen (primarily because of the omission of mitomycin). However, the overall long-term survival appears similar for the two trials.

Two small randomized trials, initially reported in 1994[92,93] and subsequently updated,[101,102] compared surgical resection alone with cisplatin-based induction chemotherapy followed by surgery. Both studies demonstrated a significant overall survival benefit with the use of neoadjuvant chemotherapy. In the trial reported by Rosell et al.,[92] 60 patients with stage III NSCLC were randomized to surgery alone or to three cycles of neoadjuvant chemotherapy (mitomycin, ifosfamide, cisplatin) followed by surgical resection. The overall survival was significantly longer with the combined-modality therapy than with surgery alone, with median survival of 26 months versus 10 months, and 3-year survival of 20% versus 5%. No survivors were reported at 5 years following operation alone.[101] Roth et al.[93] conducted a similar study in which 60 patients with pathologically determined N2 disease or unequivocal T3 disease were randomized to surgery alone or to three cycles of induction chemotherapy with cyclophosphamide, etoposide, and cisplatin followed by surgery and additional postoperative chemotherapy. Although the rates of complete resection were similar in each study arm (31% for surgery, 39% for combined modality), the median and 3-year overall survival rates were significantly better in the combined-modality arm (21 vs. 14 months and 43% vs. 19%, respectively).[102] Several weaknesses in study design, including the small number of patients, the lack of uniform pretreatment staging, and the unusually poor survival of patients in the surgery-only arm, have raised doubts about the validity of the results of both of

TABLE 81.7 RESULTS

RESULTS OF PHASE III TRIALS COMPARING RADIOTHERAPY ALONE WITH CHEMORADIOTHERAPY FOR STAGE III NON–SMALL CELL LUNG CANCER

Study	No. patients	CT	RT(Gy)	Group	Median survival (mo)	Survival at 2 yr (%)	P
Trials Showing No Advantage							
Trovo et al., 1990[181]	111	CAMP	45 (seq)	CT-RT	11.7	17[a]	ND
				RT	10.0	19[a]	
Morton et al., 1991[182]	114	MACC	60 (seq)	CT-RT	10.6	21	>.2
				RT	10.4	16	
Le Chevalier et al., 1991[183]	353	VCPC	65 (seq)	CT-RT	12.0	21	.08
				RT	10.0	14	
Blanke et al., 1995[184]	214	CDDP	60–65 (con)	CT-RT	10.0	18	.35
				RT	10.7	13	
Trials in Favor of Combined Therapy							
Schaake-Konig et al., 1992[185]	331	CDDP	55 (con)	CT daily–RT	—	26	.01
				CT wkly–RT	—	19	ND
				RT	—	13	
Jeremic et al., 1995[186]	169	Carbo +VP-16	64.8 (con)	CT (wkly)-HXFRT	18.0	23[b]	.003
				CT (other wk)-HXFRT	13.0	16	ND
				HXFRT	8.0	6.6	
Dillman et al., 1996[187]	155	CDDP +Vbl	60 (seq)	CT-RT	13.7	26	.01
				RT	9.6	13	
Sause et al., 2000[188]	458	CDDP +Vbl	60 (seq)	CT-RT	13.2	32	.04
				HFXRT (69.6 Gy)	12.0	24	ND
				RT	11.4	21	

[a]From survival curve.
[b]Survival at 3 years.
CAMP: cyclophosphamide, doxorubicin, methotrexate, procarbazine; MACC: methotrexate, doxorubicin, cyclophosphamide, lomustine; VCPC: vindesine, cyclophosphamide, cisplatin, lomustine; CDDP. cisplatin; VP-16, etoposide; Vbl, vinblastine; ND, no difference; CT, chemotherapy; RT, radiotherapy; HFXRT, hyperfractionated radiation therapy; seq, sequential; con, concurrent.

these trials. Unfortunately, it is unlikely that larger trials of similar design will be performed in the future to corroborate these results.

Trials of Induction Chemoradiation Followed by Surgical Resection. The second approach to combined-modality therapy and surgical resection for stage III NSCLC has been to combine chemotherapy and radiation preoperatively (Table 81.8). This strategy aims to control micrometastatic disease while utilizing the synergism of concurrent radiation and chemotherapy to reduce tumor bulk in the primary site and mediastinum. In one of the first trials of this type, performed by the North American LCSG, 39 patients with stage III NSCLC received three cycles of chemotherapy with cyclophosphamide, doxorubicin, and cisplatin (CAP) and 1,500 cGy of radiation in 300-cGy fractions given concurrently with cycles 2 and 3 of the chemotherapy. The overall response rate to induction therapy was 51% (20/39), and 33% (13/39) of patients had a complete resection at thoracotomy. However, the overall 2-year survival was only 8%, with a median survival of 11 months. No treatment-related deaths occurred.[103]

The LCSG subsequently performed another phase II induction trial of cisplatin, 5-fluorouracil, and partially concurrent low-dose radiation (3,000 cGy in 15 fractions) in 85 patients with stage IIIA N2 or stage IIIB NSCLC.[104] Although the cisplatin dose in this trial was higher than in the previous study (75 instead of 60 mg/m^2 per dose, respectively), the overall response rate and complete resection rates were similar (56% and 34%, respectively). The median survival was 13 months. Four of 54 patients (7%) died postoperatively.

Faber et al.[105] performed two sequential phase II neoadjuvant trials of 5-fluorouracil and low-dose cisplatin (60 mg/m^2) plus 4,000 cGy of split-course radiation administered concurrently with the four cycles of induction chemotherapy. The second group of 74 patients also received etoposide in addition to the cisplatin and 5-fluorouracil. Of the 130 patients entered into these trials, 85 were candidates for surgery after induction therapy, and 62 (73%) underwent thoracotomy. The complete resection rate was 68% (58/85), and the overall survival rate was 40% at 3 years, with a median survival of 22 months. Induction therapy was associated with significant toxicity, but only one treatment-related death occurred. Operative mortality rate was 5% (3/62). The excellent results of these trials may reflect the inclusion of some patients who did not have N2 disease but were considered at that time to have stage III NSCLC by virtue of T3 (chest wall) N0 tumor status.

A neoadjuvant trial of similar design was performed by the CALGB in which high-dose cisplatin (100 mg/m^2), vinblastine, and 5-fluorouracil were given with 3,000 cGy of continuous

LUNG

TABLE 81.8 RESULTS

RESULTS OF REPRESENTATIVE NEOADJUVANT TRIALS FOR STAGE III NON-SMALL CELL LUNG CANCER: INDUCTION CHEMORADIOTHERAPY FOLLOWED BY SURGICAL RESECTION

				Survival	
Study	No. patients	Chemotherapy	Radiotherapy (Gy)	Median (mo)	2y (%)
Rush-Presbyterian, Faber et al., 1989[105]	IIIA: 85 (including 19 N0)	CDDP (60 mg/m^2) + 5-FU – VP-16 × 4	40(S), 20 fractions	21.7	40 (3 y)
LCSG, Weiden et al., 1991[104]	IIIA, IIIB: 85	CDDP (75 mg/m^2) + 5-FU × 2	30(C), 5 fractions	13	22[a]
CALGB, Strauss et al., 1992[106]	IIIA: 41 (including 8 N0-1)	CDDP (100 mg/m^2) + Vbl +5-FU × 2	30(C), 15 fractions	15.5	30[a]
SWOG, Albain et al., 1995[107]	IIIA, IIIB:126	CDDP (50 mg/m^2 days 1 and 8) + VP-16×2	45(C), 30 fractions	13(IIIA) 17 (IIIB)	37(IIIA) 39 (IIIB)
M.D. Anderson, Taylor et al., 2004[112]	IIIA: 107 (including 21 N1)	CDDP-based or carboplatin/paclitaxel	none	31	33 (5 y)
		CDDP + Vbl CDDP + VP-16	daily, 60–63(C) 69.6 (H)	27	30 (5 y)
North American Intergroup, Albain et al., 2003[113]	IIIA:				
	201, resection	CDDP (50 mg/m^2) + VP-16 × 4; 2 cycles consolidation	45(C)	22.0 (OS), 13.4 (PFS)	3y: 37 (OS), 27 (PFS)
	191, no surgery		61(C)	22.3 (OS), 11.8 (PFS)	3y: 34 (OS), 19 (PFS)

[a]From survival curve.

CALGB, Cancer and Leukemia Group B; LCSG, Lung Cancer Study Group; RTOG, Radiation Therapy Oncology Group; SWOG, Southwest Oncology Group; 5-FU, 5-fluorouracil; CDDP, cisplatin; Vbl, vinblastine; VP-16, etoposide; (C), continuous course; (H), Hyperfractionated; (S), split course.

radiation in 15 fractions to patients with stage IIIA disease.[106] The overall response rate was 51% (21/41), and the complete resection rate was 61% (25/41). The median survival was 15.5 months. Significant toxicity occurred, and treatment-related mortality was high at 15% (6/41).

The largest reported phase II neoadjuvant trial of concurrent chemotherapy and radiation was a multiinstitutional study performed by the Southwest Oncology Group.[107] Both stage IIIA and stage IIIB patients were entered, although, notably, pathologic documentation of the initial tumor stage, usually by mediastinoscopy, was required. The induction regimen included two cycles of cisplatin (50 mg/m^2 on days 1 and 8) and etoposide with 4,500 cGy of concurrent radiation in 25 fractions. All patients underwent thoracotomy unless their disease progressed. The objective response rate to induction therapy in the 126 eligible patients was 59%. The resectability rates were 85% for the IIIA N2 group and 80% for the IIIB group. Nearly two thirds of the patients had no viable tumor or only minimal residual foci of tumor in their surgical specimens. The 3-year survival rate was 27% for the IIIA group and 24% for the IIIB group, with median survival of 13 and 17 months, respectively. The best predictor of survival after surgery was the absence of tumor in the mediastinal nodes at surgery (3-year survival of 44%). The majority of recurrences were distant, and the brain was the single most common site. The operative mortality rate was 6%, and the overall treatment-related mortality was 10%. An important finding of SWOG 8805 was that survival was the same for patients with stage IIIB NSCLC by virtue of T4 tumor status and patients with stage IIIA N2 disease. However, patients with N3 disease had a poor overall survival. Importantly, the long-term follow-up of this study shows that the survival rates at 3 years are sustained at 6 years.[108]

Important differences between the Southwest Oncology Group trial and earlier neoadjuvant trials were the careful documentation of pretreatment stage, the use of a higher dose of continuous radiation (4,500 cGy rather than 3,000 cGy of continuous or 4,000 cGy of split-course radiation), and the fully concurrent manner in which the chemotherapy and radiation were administered. Early attempts to intensify this therapeutic approach by increasing or accelerating the radiation were associated with unacceptable toxicity. Two small single-institution trials illustrate this problem. Yashar et al.[109] treated 36 patients who had stage IIIA N2 disease with two cycles of cisplatin (25 mg/m^2 per day for 4 days) and etoposide and 55 Gy of concurrent radiation. All patients underwent exploratory thoracotomy, and 31 (86%) underwent resection, 27 with pneumonectomy. Although the overall 3-year survival rate was 34%, two operative deaths (5.6%) occurred, six patients required prolonged intubation because of postoperative adult respiratory distress syndrome (ARDS), and a bronchial stump leak developed in three patients.

In the second study, Fowler et al.[110] treated 13 patients who had stage IIIA N2 disease with two cycles of cisplatin (20 mg/m^2 per day for 4 days), 5-fluorouracil, and etoposide and 60 Gy of concurrent radiation in 30 fractions. Six patients then underwent lobectomy, and seven patients underwent pneumonectomy. The complication rate was unacceptably high; ARDS developed in one of the lobectomy patients and in five of the pneumonectomy patients and was fatal in two patients. Bronchial stump leaks developed in three pneumonectomy patients, of whom one died. The trial was closed prematurely after 13 patients had been accrued because of the excessive morbidity and mortality. An additional 27 patients who received the same induction therapy but did not undergo thoracotomy tolerated the treatment without major problems.

Two additional trials have tested concurrent induction chemoradiation in stage III NSCLC. Milstein et al.[111] conducted a phase II trial in which 36 patients (10 with T3N0 or T3Nl disease and 11 with IIIB disease) received two cycles of cisplatin (25 mg/m^2) and etoposide plus concurrent radiation to 50 Gy during 28 sessions. Twenty-four patients (21 with IIIA and three with IIIB disease) underwent thoracotomy, with complete resection in 20 (86%). Three of the 21 IIIA patients had complete tumor sterilization. The overall survival at 2 years was 39% (57% for resectable patients and 15% for unresectable patients), and the median survival was 15 months. One death from sepsis occurred during the induction treatment, and two postoperative deaths resulted from ARDS and bronchopleural fistula. This attempt to intensify induction chemoradiation by increasing the dose of radiation was not successful.

One recent study addresses the question of whether radiation augments the benefit of induction chemotherapy before surgical resection.[112] This retrospective review identified 107 patients who underwent resection for stage IIIA disease. Patients had been treated with induction chemotherapy (55 patients) with cisplatin-based (100 mg/m^2) or carboplatin/paclitaxel (Taxol), concurrent chemoradiation (15 patients) with cisplatin (75 mg/m^2) and vinblastine plus daily radiation to 60 to 63 Gy, or concurrent chemoradiation (37 patients) with cisplatin (50 mg/m^2) and etoposide plus hyperfractionated radiation to 69.6 Gy. Postoperatively, 35 patients treated with induction chemotherapy received adjuvant radiation therapy.

A recently completed intergroup clinical trial in North America sought to determine whether neoadjuvant therapy including surgical resection is superior to nonsurgical treatment with chemotherapy and higher-dose radiation in patients with stage IIIA NSCLC. In the Intergroup 0139/RTOG 9309 trial,[113] patients with proved pN2, stage IIIA NSCLC were randomized to receive neoadjuvant chemotherapy with concurrent thoracic radiation therapy (TRT) followed by operation or continuation with definitive TRT. Of 429 patients accrued over 92 months, 392 patients were considered eligible and were treated with cisplatin (50 mg/m^2) on days 1 and 8; and etoposide (50 mg/m^2) on days 1 to 5, every 3 weeks for 2 cycles, as well as 45 Gy TRT. Patients randomized to resection (n = 201) underwent operation 4 to 6 weeks later. Patients randomized to definitive radiation (n = 191) continued without break off cord to a total of 61 Gy. Following operation or completion of TRT, consolidation with two cycles of cisplatin and etoposide was given. Of note, less than two thirds of patients undergoing operation received consolidation treatment, compared with over 75% of patients receiving chemoradiation only. There was no mortality in either group during induction chemoradiation. Surgical mortality was 7%, with 12 of 14 deaths occurring in patients undergoing pneumonectomy.

Progression-free survival (PFS) was improved from a median of 11.8 months to 13.4 months, and 3-year PFS from 19% to 27% with the addition of surgery. There appeared to be improved local control with the addition of surgery, with local failure occurring in only 5% of surgically treated patients compared with 16% in the nonsurgical group, although this was not statistically significant. However, no statistically significant differences were seen in overall survival, with 3-year survival of 34% and 37% for the chemoradiation alone and chemoradiation and surgery groups, respectively. Survival for patients undergoing complete resection in this study has not yet been published. This study indicates that carefully selected patients with N2-positive stage IIIA NSCLC can be treated with multimodality therapy including surgical resection. Parenchymal-preserving bronchoplastic techniques may be considered for patients who require pneumonectomy, because the preliminary data indicate that those patients are at greater risk for early mortality. However, whether such techniques should be undertaken in the setting of recent RT has not been established.

Stimulated by the promising results of the Southwest Oncology Group 8805 trial for patients with T4 disease, Grunenwald et al.[88] performed a phase II trial of similar design for stage IIIB T4 NSCLC. The induction regimen consisted of cisplatin (100 mg/m^2), 5-fluorouracil, and vinblastine with 45 Gy of concurrent hyperfractionated (twice daily) radiation. Of 25 patients enrolled, 16 were subsequently eligible for surgery, and 12 had complete surgical resection. No induction treatment–related or operative deaths occurred. This study confirms that complete resection after induction therapy is feasible in a significant number of stage IIIB T4 tumors, a subset of stage IIIB tumors previously considered inoperable under any circumstances.

Current Status of Neoadjuvant Therapy and Surgical Resection

Taken as a whole, neoadjuvant therapy trials have demonstrated the feasibility of induction chemotherapy and surgical resection for the treatment of stage III NSCLC. Most studies show improved rates of resectability and survival in comparison with the historical experience for surgical resection or radiation alone. However, the optimal treatment approach to these locally advanced tumors has not yet been fully defined, especially because neoadjuvant trials vary with respect to eligibility criteria, inclusion of both stage IIIA and stage IIIB tumors, accuracy of pretreatment staging, and type of induction regimens. Moreover the response, resectability, and survival rates are not uniformly reported. In some cases, instead of reporting results as a percentage of the total number of patients entered into the study, the authors report resectability rates as a percentage of the patients with a radiographic response, and only the survival rates of patients who underwent resection are emphasized.

The potential toxicity of neoadjuvant regimens should not be overlooked. Induction regimens in which high-dose cisplatin ($\geq$100 mg/m^2) or radiation doses of 4,000 to 4,500 cGy are used have been well tolerated, but radiation doses of 5,500 cGy or higher have been associated with an excessive risk for postoperative ARDS and bronchial stump leak. Good response rates have been achieved with newer chemotherapeutic agents, such as paclitaxel, docetaxel, gemcitabine, and carboplatin, and they are better tolerated by patients. Determining the contribution of these agents in combined-modality therapy will require further trials, especially as the major form of relapse continues to be distant metastatic disease.

Future Directions

In addition to new chemotherapeutic agents, new radiation techniques, such as hyperfractionated or accelerated schedules, also merit further exploration in neoadjuvant trials with concurrent chemotherapy. Adelstein et al.[114] conducted a study in which 45 patients with stage IIIA or IIIB NSCLC received induction cisplatin, paclitaxel, and 30 Gy of accelerated hyperfractionated radiation therapy (1.5-Gy fraction twice daily). Surgery was then performed approximately 4 weeks after induction. The overall response rate was 54%. Forty patients (89%) proceeded to surgery, and 32 patients (71 %) underwent complete resection. Five complete pathologic remissions were seen. Fourteen patients overall were downstaged. Patients received a consolidation dose of chemotherapy and additional radiation to a total of 60 to 63 Gy. The 2-year relapse-free survival rate was 47%, and the 2-year survival rate was 65%. No apparent therapy-related deaths occurred, but the toxicity was high, with 89% of patients experiencing significant mucositis and 20% experiencing esophagitis of grade 3 or worse. Another new radiation technique is three-dimensional conformal therapy; higher radiation dosing (>70 Gy) of the tumor is possible while surrounding normal lung is spared, so that the possibility of local control is improved.[115,116]

The management of stage III NSCLC is complex and still evolving. Many trials indicate that resectability and survival rates are probably improved with the use of combined-modality therapy than with radiation or surgical resection alone. Regimens incorporating high-dose cisplatin with or without moderate-dose radiation have achieved the best results with acceptable levels of toxicity. Careful patient management leads to complete resection, and the operative risk is comparable with that of standard pulmonary resection. Very importantly, combined-modality treatment requires close collaboration among medical oncologists, radiation oncologists, surgeons, pulmonologists, and anesthesiologists. In the future, three key areas warrant further investigation: (a) the optimal combination and sequencing of newer, less toxic chemotherapeutic agents and a variety of new radiation techniques require further study; (b) clinical trials will need to determine whether concurrent chemoradiation is superior to chemotherapy alone as preoperative induction therapy; and (c) ongoing and future investigations of the molecular biologic features of tumors that dictate response to individual chemotherapeutic agents will allow a more individualized selection of induction treatment regimens and may in turn lead to improved long-term outcome.

Superior Sulcus Tumors

Tumors of the superior sulcus, described in detail by H. K. Pancoast in 1932,[117] represent an uncommon (3%) and challenging subset of NSCLC (Fig. 81.2). Tumors frequently involve the brachial plexus, subclavian vessels, or spine and typically fall into two categories: T3N0-1 (stage IIB or IIIA) or T4N0-1 (stage IIIB).[118] Until the 1950s these tumors were thought to be almost universally fatal, with no benefit provided by surgical resection. In 1961, Shaw and Paulson[119] demonstrated that preoperative thoracic radiation followed by surgical resection was potentially curative. For the subsequent 30 to 35 years, reports demonstrated 5-year survival of approximately of 25% to 30%. In a single-institutional experience, spanning 24 years, during which 225 patients underwent thoracotomy, 5-year survival for patients undergoing resection for stages IIB, IIIA, and IIIB superior sulcus tumors was 46%, 0%, and 13%, respectively.[120] In this retrospective study, the mode of preoperative therapy with radiation and/or chemotherapy, or adjuvant therapy did not appear to affect survival, which was influenced only by completeness of resection and tumor (T) and nodal (N) status in a multivariate analysis. As in other retrospective series, locoregional recurrence was the most common form of relapse, occurring in 40% of patients.[121]

Spurred by reports of the apparent success of neoadjuvant chemotherapy and thoracic radiation in achieving improved local control and survival for patients with locoregionally advanced NSCLC, the Southwestern Oncology Group coordinated a phase II trial, the first prospective, multicenter trial (SWOG 9416/Intergroup 0160) for superior sulcus tumors.[122] Of 111 patients eligible, including 31 patients with T4 disease, 102 completed induction chemoradiation and 95 were eligible for operation. Patients with mediastinal lymph node metastases (N2) were excluded from this trial. Of the 88 patients who underwent thoracotomy, over 90% had a complete resection, with 65% of patients demonstrating complete pathologic response (R0) or minimal residual disease (R1). Overall treatment mortality was 4.5%, including an operative mortality of 2.4%. Of note, intracranial and other distant metastases were more common (22% each) than locally recurrent disease only (11%). Overall 2- and 5-year survival was 55% and 41%, respectively, for all patients enrolled, and 70% and 53%, respectively, for patients with complete response.

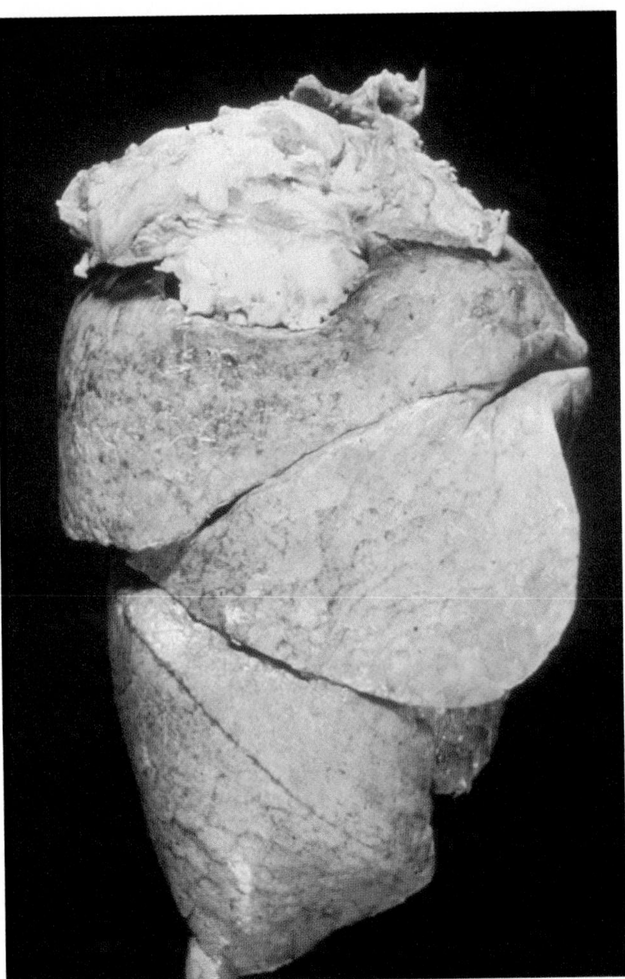

FIGURE 81.2 Gross figure of a squamous cell carcinoma showing a superior sulcus tumor (Pancoast tumor) arising from apex of the right lung. (From Cagle PT. *Color atlas and text of pulmonary pathology. Philadelphia*: Lippincott Williams & Wilkins, 2005.)

NEUROENDOCRINE TUMORS

Neuroendocrine tumors of the lung, which comprise a varied group of lesions, range from tumors with low-grade malignant potential (typical carcinoid) to SCLC, which is among the most rapidly growing and aggressive of human tumors. Between those two extremes, atypical carcinoid and large cell neuroendocrine carcinoma have been defined.[123]

Typical and Atypical Carcinoid Tumors

Carcinoid tumors, which are neoplasms with a low-grade malignant potential, account for about 2% of lung tumors in the United States. They arise from neuroendocrine stem cells of the bronchial epithelium and are classified as either typical or atypical. Histologically, typical carcinoids consist of uniform polygonal cells with round nuclei and fine granular chromatin (Fig. 81.3). Mitotic figures are rare. Atypical carcinoids

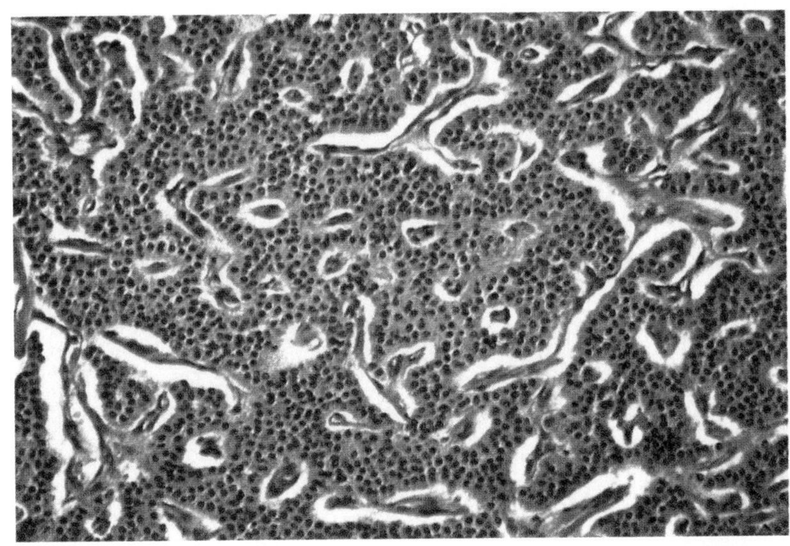

FIGURE 81.3 Typical carcinoid tumor of the lung. A microscopic view shows ribbons of tumor cells embedded in a vascular stroma. (From Rubin E, Farber JL. *Pathology,* 3rd ed. Philadelphia: Lippincott Williams & Wilkins, 1999.)

show increased mitotic activity, nuclear pleomorphism and areas of disorganization of the architecture and tumor necrosis[124] (Fig. 81.4).

Carcinoid tumors occur equally in both sexes and at a median age of 55 years. Half of patients present with pulmonary symptoms, including hemoptysis, dyspnea, and recurrent or persistent pneumonitis because 40% of lesions are centrally located in the main or lobar bronchi (Figs. 81.5 and 81.6). The lesions may be diagnosed by bronchoscopy, appearing as pink or purple friable endobronchial masses covered by intact epithelium. In the other half of patients, carcinoid tumors are diagnosed when radiologic abnormalities are detected on a chest radiograph as part of a routine examination.[125]

Lymph node metastases occur in approximately 10% to 15% of patients at diagnosis but are more frequent in atypical carcinoids. The carcinoid syndrome is associated with bronchial carcinoids in only 2% of cases, usually in patients with metastatic disease, particularly of the liver. The most common sites of metastases are lung, bone, liver, adrenal glands, and brain.[125]

The standard treatment of bronchial carcinoid is complete surgical resection, despite the presence of nodal involvement, with mediastinal lymph node sampling or dissection.[126] Lobectomy is required in about 50% of patients. Lesser resection (segmentectomy, sleeve resection) is adequate for complete resection in about 20% of patients. Endoscopic resection is invariably associated with local recurrence and should be used only as a palliative maneuver in patients whose general medical condition precludes thoracotomy and pulmonary resection.[125]

The long-term survival rate after surgical resection exceeds 90% in patients with typical carcinoids, even when hilar or mediastinal nodal metastases are present. In contrast, patients with atypical carcinoids have a 5-year survival rate of 60% after complete resection. The outcome is more closely linked to histology than to tumor size and location or nodal involvement. Recurrence is more frequent with tumors larger than 3 cm and in patients who present with lymph node metastases.[125]

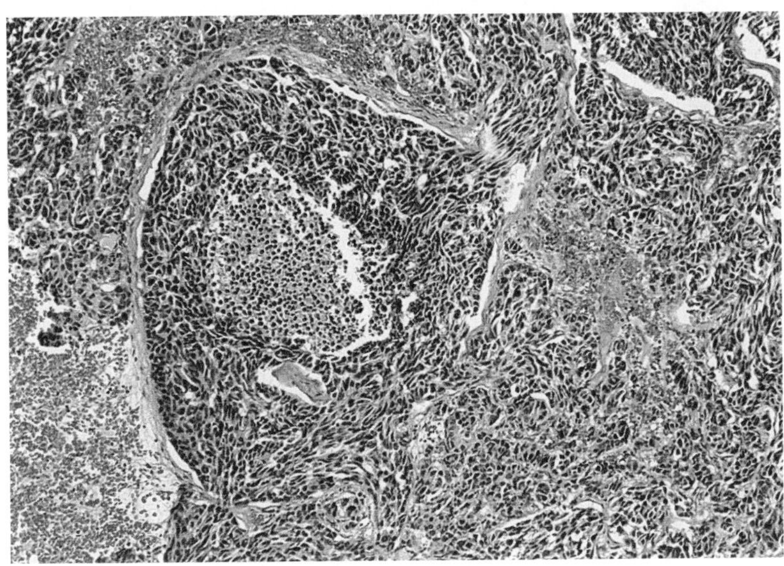

FIGURE 81.4 Atypical carcinoid tumor of the lung. A cellular tumor shows central necrosis and a disorganized architecture. (From Rubin E, Farber JL. *Pathology,* 3rd ed. Philadelphia: Lippincott Williams & Wilkins, 1999.)

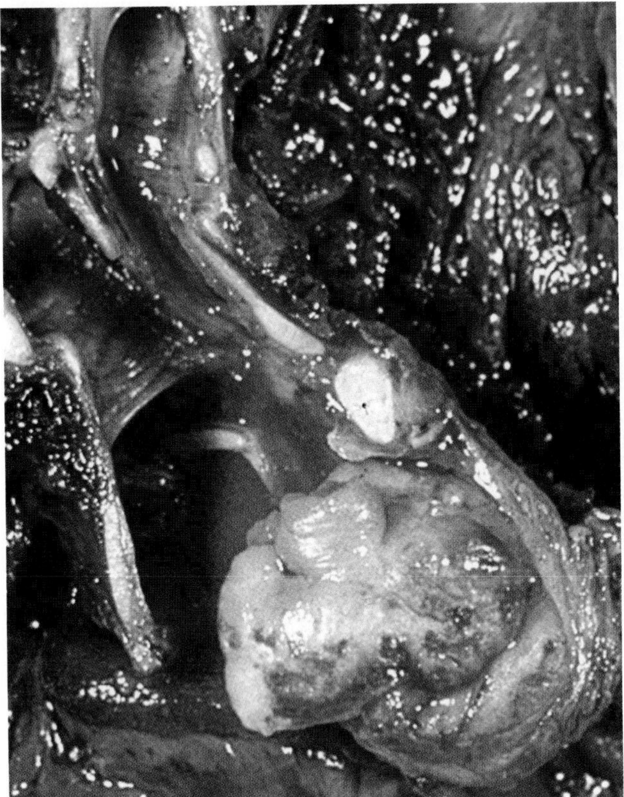

FIGURE 81.5 Gross figure of carcinoid tumor protruding into bronchial lumen. (From Cagle PT. *Color atlas and text of pulmonary pathology.* Philadelphia: Lippincott Williams & Wilkins, 2005.)

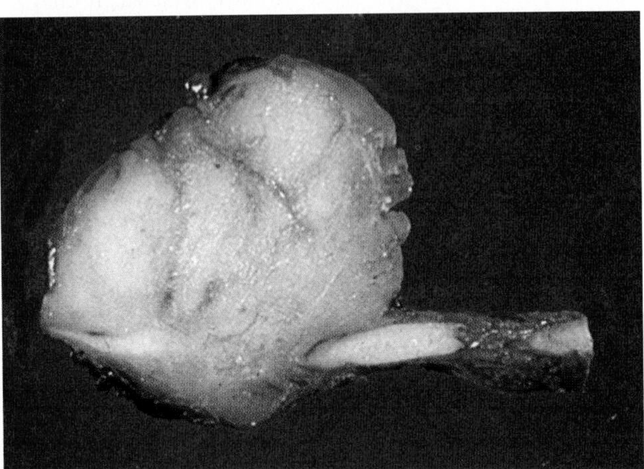

FIGURE 81.6 Gross figure of resected carcinoid tumor cut in cross section to show invasion through bronchial cartilage. (From Cagle PT. *Color atlas and text of pulmonary pathology.* Philadelphia: Lippincott Williams & Wilkins, 2005.)

Large Cell Neuroendocrine Carcinomas

Large cell neuroendocrine carcinoma is characterized by the microscopic features of neuroendocrine tumors, but the tumor cells are large, have a high mitotic rate, and frequently show necrosis[123,124] (Fig. 81.7). According to Travis et al.,[127,128] large cell neuroendocrine carcinomas are related to smoking,

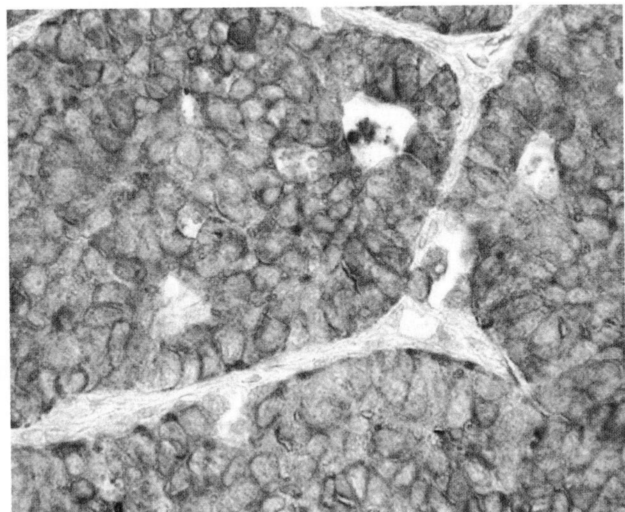

FIGURE 81.7 Large cell neuroendocrine carcinoma of lung shows positive immunostaining with synaptophysin antibody. (From Cagle PT. *Color atlas and text of pulmonary pathology.* Philadelphia: Lippincott Williams & Wilkins, 2005.)

as is SCLC, and are also high-grade tumors, with 5- and 10-year survival rates of 27% and 9%, respectively, despite complete resection. Few data are available concerning adjuvant therapy. For the time being, the management of large cell neuroendocrine carcinoma is identical to that of NSCLC.[129]

Small Cell Lung Cancer

Small cell carcinoma of the lung has the most aggressive clinical course of any type of pulmonary tumor and is often widely disseminated by the time of diagnosis. In contrast to non-small cell tumors, these lesions are notably responsive to chemotherapy and are rarely within the domain of the surgeon. The staging system for SCLC was developed by the Veterans Administration Lung Cancer Staging Group and divides patients into those with limited disease and those with extensive disease. This distinction was first based on what could be encompassed by a tolerable radiation portal. After clarification by the International Association for the Study of Lung Cancer, limited disease includes patients with tumors confined to one hemithorax and regional lymph nodes (hilar, ipsilateral, and contralateral mediastinal nodes and ipsilateral and contralateral supraclavicular nodes) and patients with ipsilateral pleural effusion, regardless of whether the cytology is positive or negative. On the other hand, both pericardial and bilateral pulmonary involvement are considered extensive disease.[130]

Common sites of distant metastases are bone, liver, bone marrow, and the central nervous system, and therefore the metastatic evaluation includes a bone scan and CT of the chest, abdomen, and brain. Some oncologists also perform bone marrow biopsies, but because the marrow is the sole site of extensive disease in fewer than 5% of patients, biopsies are usually judged unnecessary. After the staging process, approximately 30% to 40% of patients are found to have limited disease.

For patients with limited disease, response rates of 85% to 90% and complete response rates of 50% to 60% can be expected with the combination of etoposide and cisplatin and radiation therapy.[131] The median survival is 18 to 24 months, and the 2-year survival rates are 40% to 50% (5% more than before the use of radiation therapy).[132,133] In extensive SCLC treated with chemotherapy, response rates reach 75% to 85%, although complete response is seen in only 15% to 25% of patients. The median survival is between 7 and 11 months, with a 2-year survival near zero. The prognosis in SCLC depends primarily on the anatomic extent of disease, but after a review of prognostic variables in its 2,580-patient SCLC data base, the Southwest Oncology Group determined that the two-stage system should be extended into a four-stage system, with serum lactate dehydrogenase level, age, and pleural effusion used as additional staging criteria.[134]

The small numbers of patients with SCLC seen by surgeons represent fewer than 10% of all patients with SCLC. They have peripheral tumors with no nodal involvement or only hilar nodal involvement, which would be classified as T1–2 N0–1 tumors in the NSCLC staging system. In the past, such tumors were often diagnosed at exploratory thoracotomy for an asymptomatic coin lesion, but with the increasing use of diagnostic percutaneous needle aspiration, more patients with early-stage SCLC are now identified preoperatively. Such patients should be evaluated in conjunction with a medical oncologist, and surgical resection should be considered after distant disease has been excluded by a complete metastatic evaluation. For such cases, it has been suggested that the TNM classification be used in future trials and studies.[135]

Retrospective series have demonstrated a 5-year survival rate of 30% to 50% after resection of T1N0 or T2N0 SCLC.[135–137] Because of the propensity for small cell cancers to disseminate, adjuvant chemotherapy has traditionally been given to patients after surgical resection, even though, by virtue of the small numbers of patients available, no prospective, randomized trials have demonstrated whether this is of benefit.[137] Relapse in the primary site, which is a problem for most patients with limited-stage SCLC, is distinctly uncommon after complete resection of these early tumors.[138] Radiation therapy to the chest has been suggested after surgically complete resection, but because insufficient information is available in the literature and local relapse is uncommon, it cannot be considered a standard treatment.[136,137]

Because the role of surgical resection in patients with mediastinal nodal involvement (N2 disease) is questionable, mediastinoscopy should be considered mandatory to exclude mediastinal nodal disease.[139] This should ideally be performed separately from thoracotomy because it can be difficult for the pathologist to diagnose small cell cancer on a frozen section. The intraoperative management of SCLC is not significantly different from that of NSCLC, and an incomplete resection does not benefit the patient.

The addition of surgical resection after a response to induction chemotherapy has been proposed by some surgeons to cure a small number of patients with limited SCLC without mediastinal involvement.[140] To date, the LCSG has performed the only prospective, randomized trial evaluating the role of surgery in limited SCLC.[141] All patients enrolled in that study received chemotherapy, and those in whom at least a partial response was achieved were randomized to undergo or not undergo surgery. Because the survival rate was the same in both groups, this trial did not support the addition of pulmonary resection to the multimodality treatment of SCLC. Finally, the occurrence of a second primary lung carcinoma after treatment for SCLC is reported in the few patients with prolonged survival. It should not be assumed that the new tumor is of small cell histology, and these patients should be evaluated for the possibility of surgical resection.[142] The average risk for the development of a second lung cancer in patients who survive SCLC is approximately 6% per patient per year.[63]

BRONCHIAL GLAND CARCINOMAS

Bronchial gland carcinomas are rare primary tumors of the lung. They constitute about 1% of all lung neoplasms and 2% of the tumors for which surgical resection is performed. These tumors are also called primary salivary gland–type tumors of the lung because the tracheal and bronchial airway submucosa and the salivary glands contain serous and mucous glands that are histologically similar.[143] Often, they are called bronchial adenomas, but this term is misleading because they are malignant. Care must be taken to separate these primary tumors from metastases of primitive salivary gland tumors.[144] This group of carcinomas includes adenoid cystic carcinoma, mucoepidermoid carcinoma and the even rarer mixed tumor (pleomorphic adenoma). The only truly benign tumors are mucous gland adenomas.

The symptomatology of these tumors is determined essentially by their location and size.[144] Peripheral tumors, which are less frequent, are asymptomatic, generally presenting as a nodule on routine chest radiography. Proximally located tumors present with symptoms of bronchial irritation and obstruction, including cough, shortness of breath, hemoptysis, recurrent infection, wheezing, and stridor. Some patients have constitutional symptoms, such as weight loss and pain. On chest radiography, the nodule may again be seen, with pneumonia or atelectasis. Because of the slow growth of these tumors, signs and symptoms may develop over a period of years. Incompletely obstructing tumors frequently masquerade as asthma for prolonged periods of time. Smoking does not seem to be a risk factor for these tumors.

Peripheral tumors are diagnosed by percutaneous needle aspiration biopsy or at the time of thoracotomy. Tumors in major airways are diagnosed by bronchoscopy. Other studies, such as CT, are rarely required to make the diagnosis but may be of value in planning therapy. Because most of these tumors do not metastasize, complete excision, with preservation of as much pulmonary tissue as possible, is the goal. Whenever possible, sleeve resection of main bronchi is performed to preserve pulmonary tissue.

Adenoid Cystic Carcinoma

Adenoid cystic carcinomas are slowly growing malignant tumors that arise from the submucosal glands of the trachea and main bronchi (Fig. 81.8). They have also been called cylindromas, adenoid cystic basal cell carcinomas, adenomyoepitheliomas, and pseudoadenomatous basal cell carcinomas. Adenoid cystic carcinomas behave much like the major and minor salivary gland tumors of the same name, to which they are microscopically identical. An important aspect of their clinical behavior is that they tend to spread in the submucosal plane along the perineural lymphatics, well beyond the obvious endoluminal component of the tumor (Fig. 81.9). In a small biopsy specimen, it can be difficult to distinguish adenoid cystic carcinoma from a conventional adenocarcinoma. Immunohistochemical stains may help the pathologist differentiate the two by showing the presence of the myoepithelial cell immunophenotype in adenoid cystic carcinoma.[144]

Whenever possible, total excision by tracheal resection or tracheobronchial resection is the treatment of choice.[145] This is not always possible because of the extensive submucosal spread of tumor. In such cases, palliative resection may be necessary. Postoperative radiation is indicated because these tumors are radiation sensitive.

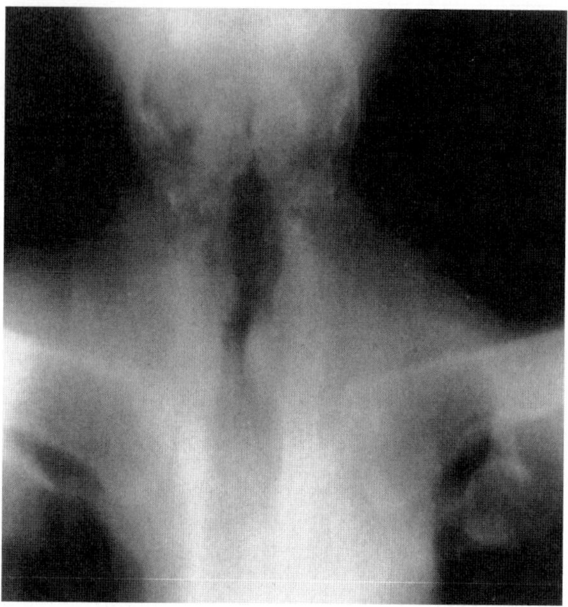

FIGURE 81.8 Tracheogram demonstrating airway obstruction by an adenoid cystic carcinoma of the upper trachea.

When no surgical resection is feasible because of the extent of the lesion, a palliative treatment option is endoscopic laser removal, followed by radiation (brachytherapy, external beam irradiation, or both). When complete surgical resection is possible, the prognosis is excellent. However, because of the slow-growing nature of the tumor and its responsiveness to radiation, prolonged survival is possible even with incomplete resection or palliative measures. Patients frequently live 10 years or more with persistent disease, including pulmonary metastases. In such cases, repeated efforts at palliation are indicated.

Mucoepidermoid Carcinoma

Mucoepidermoid carcinomas may be of low- or high-grade malignancy and have the same microscopic appearance as mucoepidermoid tumors of salivary gland origin. These tumors also arise in the glandular submucosa, presenting as submucosal lesions. The distinction between low-grade and high-grade tumor is based on mitotic activity, cellular necrosis, and nuclear pleomorphism.[143]

The principles of treatment of mucoepidermoid tumors are similar to those of carcinoid tumors. The more malignant variety must be treated as bronchogenic carcinoma. Some authors even think that adenosquamous carcinoma is the same entity as mucoepidermoid carcinoma but arising in the periphery of the lung.[143] The outlook for these tumors depends on the grade of malignancy and the stage of the disease. High-grade tumors have the same prognosis as bronchogenic carcinoma. Complete surgical resection is the mainstay of treatment. Mucoepidermoid tumors are too rare to permit an evaluation of combined modality therapy for more aggressive, high-grade tumors.[143]

Mucous Gland Adenoma

Mucous gland adenomas are rare submucosal tumors that arise from mucous glands. They are also known as *bronchial cysts* and *papillary cystadenomas*. Because of their totally benign behavior, they can usually be treated by endoscopic excision. Thoracotomy and surgical resection are indicated only if the distal lung has been destroyed by chronic infection or if endoscopic removal is technically contraindicated or incomplete.

OTHER MALIGNANT TUMORS OF THE LUNG

The lung comprises epithelial, mesodermal, and endodermal cells, and malignant tumors may arise from any of these cells. This group represents less than 1% of all primary lung cancers

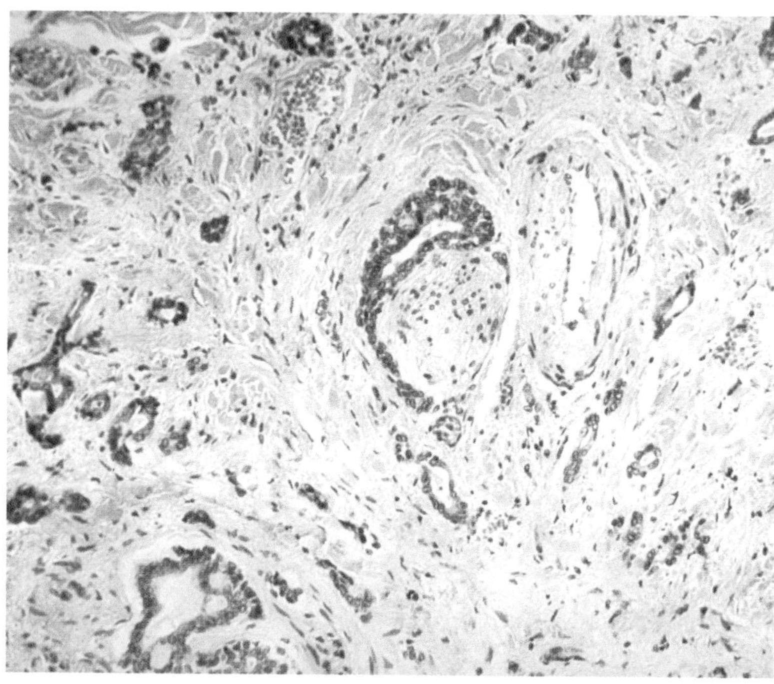

FIGURE 81.9 Adenoid cystic carcinoma. A photomicrograph shows perineural infiltration by the tumor. (From Rubin E, Farber JL. *Pathology*, 3rd ed. Philadelphia: Lippincott Williams & Wilkins, 1999.)

and is usually subdivided into lymphoid tumors, soft-tissue sarcomas, mixed epithelial/mesenchymal tumors, and ectopic tissue tumors.[146,147] Primary pulmonary lymphomas usually are excised for confirmatory diagnosis. Sarcomas arising from soft tissue or large vessels are treated in a similar fashion to sarcomas occurring elsewhere. Treatment of the other rare tumors, including pulmonary blastomas, primary melanomas of the bronchus, and malignant teratomas, primarily involves complete surgical resection. Radiation and chemotherapy do not have well-defined roles in the treatment of any of these tumors but are occasionally used in particular situations.

SURGICAL RESECTION OF PULMONARY METASTASES

Historical Background

The first report of the resection of a pulmonary metastasis performed as a separate procedure is attributed to Divis in 1926. In North America, the most quoted case of lobectomy for a metastatic carcinoma was that performed by Barney and Churchill in 1939.[148] Their patient underwent nephrectomy for an adenocarcinoma and was known to have a pulmonary mass. After the renal resection, the pulmonary tumor did not respond to radiation treatment and increased in size. Following exploration and resection of the pulmonary lesion, the patient survived disease-free for more than 20 years.

From 1940 to the mid-1960s, pulmonary metastasectomy was performed infrequently and only in highly selected patients. A total of 169 pulmonary metastasis resections were performed on 165 patients at the Mayo Clinic from 1941 to 1959.[149] This large number of operations may reflect the high volume of cases seen at the Mayo Clinic rather than the common use of surgical resection at that time. The first principles of pulmonary resection for metastatic disease were offered: complete removal of the primary disease, no evidence of recurrence or metastatic disease other than the lung lesion, and the patient in good general condition. Multiple lesions were not considered a contraindication to resection (Fig. 81.10), but it was thought that bilateral disease indicated a poor prognosis and should not be resected. Surgeons were already convinced that the resection should be as conservative of lung function as possible.

Since then, experience from several institutions suggests that more liberal indications for pulmonary metastasectomy are appropriate.[150] A striking example was the treatment of metastatic osteogenic sarcoma at Memorial Sloan-Kettering Cancer Center. From 1940 to 1965, only five such patients were treated surgically. During the same period, only 24 of 145 patients (17%) survived 5 years after resection of their primary tumors, and 118 of these patients (81%) died of pulmonary metastases. This experience prompted a more aggressive approach to the management of pulmonary metastases. Starting in 1965, a consecutive series of 22 patients with osteogenic sarcoma underwent pulmonary metastasectomy. Patients were considered for operation even if they had bilateral metastases or required multiple thoracotomies to remove all gross tumor. A total of 59 thoracotomies were performed in these 22 patients, with an overall 5-year survival rate of 32%. The dramatic improvement in survival in comparison with the historical experience strongly supported the aggressive use of pulmonary metastasectomy in these patients.[151]

During the past 30 years, surgical resection has become a widely accepted treatment for certain pulmonary metastases; however, some of the criteria for patient selection remain controversial. In addition, advances in chemotherapy have changed the indications for surgical resection. With some

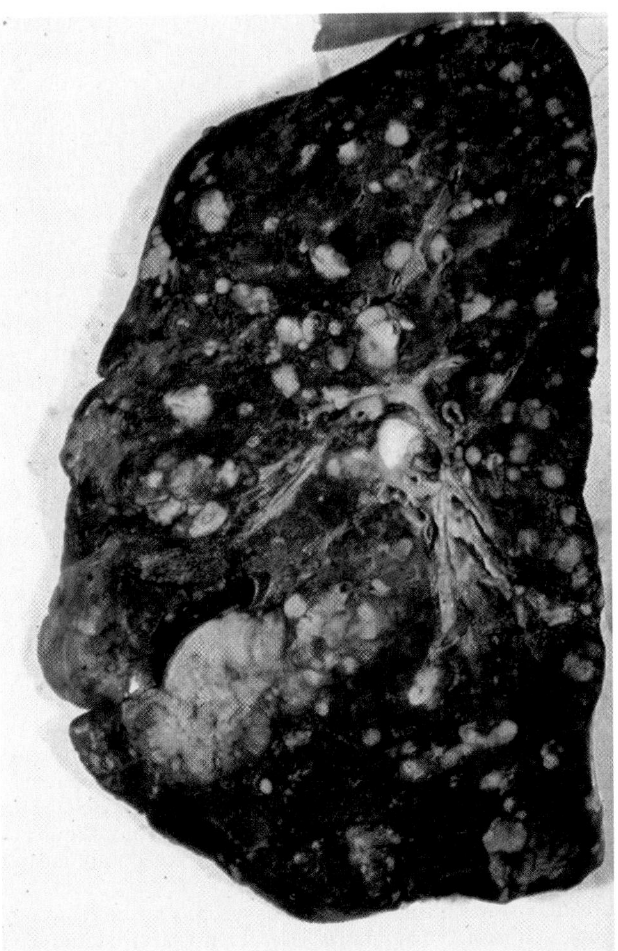

FIGURE 81.10 Metastatic carcinoma of the lung. A section through the lung shows numerous nodules of metastatic carcinoma, corresponding to "cannon ball" metastases seen radiologically. (From Rubin E, Farber JL. *Pathology*, 3rd ed. Philadelphia: Lippincott Williams & Wilkins, 1999.)

cancers, pulmonary metastasectomy is performed to prolong life expectancy, whereas with others, it serves mainly to restage disease or to provide adjuvant treatment after initial chemotherapy. The role of pulmonary metastasectomy will undoubtedly continue to evolve as improvements in systemic treatment are made.

Clinical Presentation and Diagnosis

Metastases are asymptomatic 85% of the time and are usually detected on a routine chest radiograph. Patients who undergo resection of a primary tumor with a known tendency to metastasize to the lung should have a chest radiograph as part of their routine follow-up care. On a chest radiograph, metastases usually present as well-circumscribed, spherical, solid masses with well-defined borders (Fig. 81.11). Cavitation is occasionally seen in large lesions with central necrosis, mostly squamous cell cancers. The distribution of lung metastases is predominantly subpleural or in the outer third of lung fields.[152]

Metastases to the lung usually arise in the pulmonary parenchyma. Endobronchial metastases are uncommon but occur most typically with renal cell, colon, and breast cancers. Even with endobronchial metastases, half of patients are

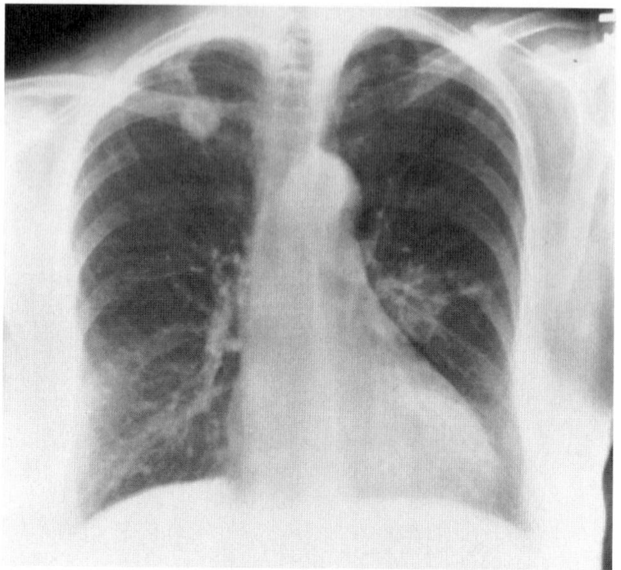

FIGURE 81.11 Chest radiograph of a patient with bilateral pulmonary metastases from endometrial cancer. The mass in the right upper lobe is well circumscribed and has the radiographic appearance typical of a metastasis.

asymptomatic.[153] More often, endobronchial disease represents an extension of contiguous parenchymal disease. The extent of endobronchial tumor can affect the approach to surgical resection. For these reasons, bronchoscopy should be performed before thoracotomy, especially if centrally located metastases are present.

Hilar or mediastinal nodal involvement sometimes accompanies pulmonary metastases. Several retrospective series have indicated that metastatic nodal involvement is a poor prognostic indicator, independent of disease-free interval or number of nodules.[154,155] However, the determinants of nodal involvement and the prognostic and therapeutic implications remain poorly understood. Lymphangitic spread can occur with or without concomitant pulmonary nodules. This happens most frequently in breast cancer and produces a characteristic radiographic appearance of diffusely increased interstitial markings and a clinical presentation of severe dyspnea that is out of proportion to the radiographic findings.

When pulmonary metastases are thought to be present on a chest radiograph, CT should be performed to determine their number, location, size, and potential resectability. Plain chest radiographs detect only lesions at least 9 mm in size. New lesions of this size seen on a chest radiograph in a patient already treated for a malignancy have a 90% chance of being malignant.[156] Even though CT can identify lesions as small as 3 mm, it often underestimates the number of pulmonary metastases (Fig. 81.12). When radiologic and surgical findings are correlated, only 75% of malignant nodules are detected by CT. Fifteen percent of CT studies overestimate the number of lung metastases for an accurate radiologic assessment of 61%.[157,158] FDG-PET scan appears to have a role as well in the preoperative evaluation of resectable pulmonary metastases, enhancing the detection of extrathoracic or mediastinal involvement that might preclude complete resection.[159]

Patients who present with multiple pulmonary nodules in the setting of a previously treated malignancy rarely pose a diagnostic dilemma. Patients who present with solitary pulmonary nodules are more problematic. Generally, a solitary lesion is more likely to be a metastasis if the primary tumor was a sarcoma or a melanoma. If the primary tumor originated in the head, neck, or breast, it is more likely to be a new primary lung cancer.[160] It has an equal chance of being a metastasis or a new primary if the initial tumor was of gastrointestinal or genitourinary origin. Percutaneous fine-needle aspiration biopsy usually yields a tissue diagnosis, but the necessity of a biopsy in the case of a solitary lesion is questionable. If the patient fits the criteria for resection, a biopsy of the lesion is best performed as an excisional biopsy. Because the findings on needle biopsy do not alter the recommendations for excision of a solitary lesion, this procedure should be undertaken only if the patient is not an operative candidate, if an alternative method of treatment is indicated, or if the patient requests that the diagnosis be established before consenting to operation.

Criteria for Surgical Resection

The disease-free interval, number of metastatic nodules, and tumor doubling time have been used as criteria for the surgical resection of pulmonary metastases. Each of these remains controversial with respect to its effect on long-term outcome.[161] The disease-free interval is defined as the time from resection of the primary tumor to the diagnosis of metastases. The length of the disease-free interval is thought to be of prognostic significance and varies greatly among published reports from 7 months to 5 years.[162]

The number of metastatic nodules resected has also been considered predictive of survival. In sarcomas, some have reported that the presence of four nodules is a significant breakpoint in survival; however, the significance of the number of nodules varies among reported series. Most consider the completeness of resection the best predictor of survival.[163] Obviously, when a shower of numerous, tiny (1- to 2-mm) lesions is encountered, complete resection is not possible.

Tumor doubling time is a measure of the aggressiveness of tumor growth. The prognostic importance of tumor doubling time, however, is questioned because various doubling times, from 20 to 136 days, have been found to be significant in different studies.[162] Many do not consider this a criterion for surgical resection. The disease-free interval, number of metastatic nodules, and tumor doubling time in fact reflect the intrinsic tumor biology.

In 1991, the International Registry of Lung Metastases was established. With regard to prognostic variables, 5,206 cases of pulmonary metastases were analyzed retrospectively.[157] Multivariate analysis showed a better prognosis for patients with germ cell tumors, a disease-free interval of 36 months or more, a single metastasis, and complete resection. A simple system of classification into prognostic groups was designed (Table 81.9).

Several guidelines must be met before a patient is considered for resection of pulmonary metastases: control of the primary tumor, absence of extrathoracic metastases, a general medical condition that permits thoracotomy, pulmonary function that allows complete resection of all metastases, and a lack of more effective systemic treatment. Resection should be undertaken only if complete resection is considered technically feasible.[164]

If the metastatic lesion is found at the same time as a recurrence of the primary site, the recurrent primary tumor should be treated before the metastatic disease is treated to prevent further seeding of the metastatic site. When the primary tumor and the metastasis are diagnosed simultaneously, lung resection may precede operation for the primary disease if it is doubtful whether the pulmonary disease can be completely resected and immediate subsequent resection of the primary tumor is planned.

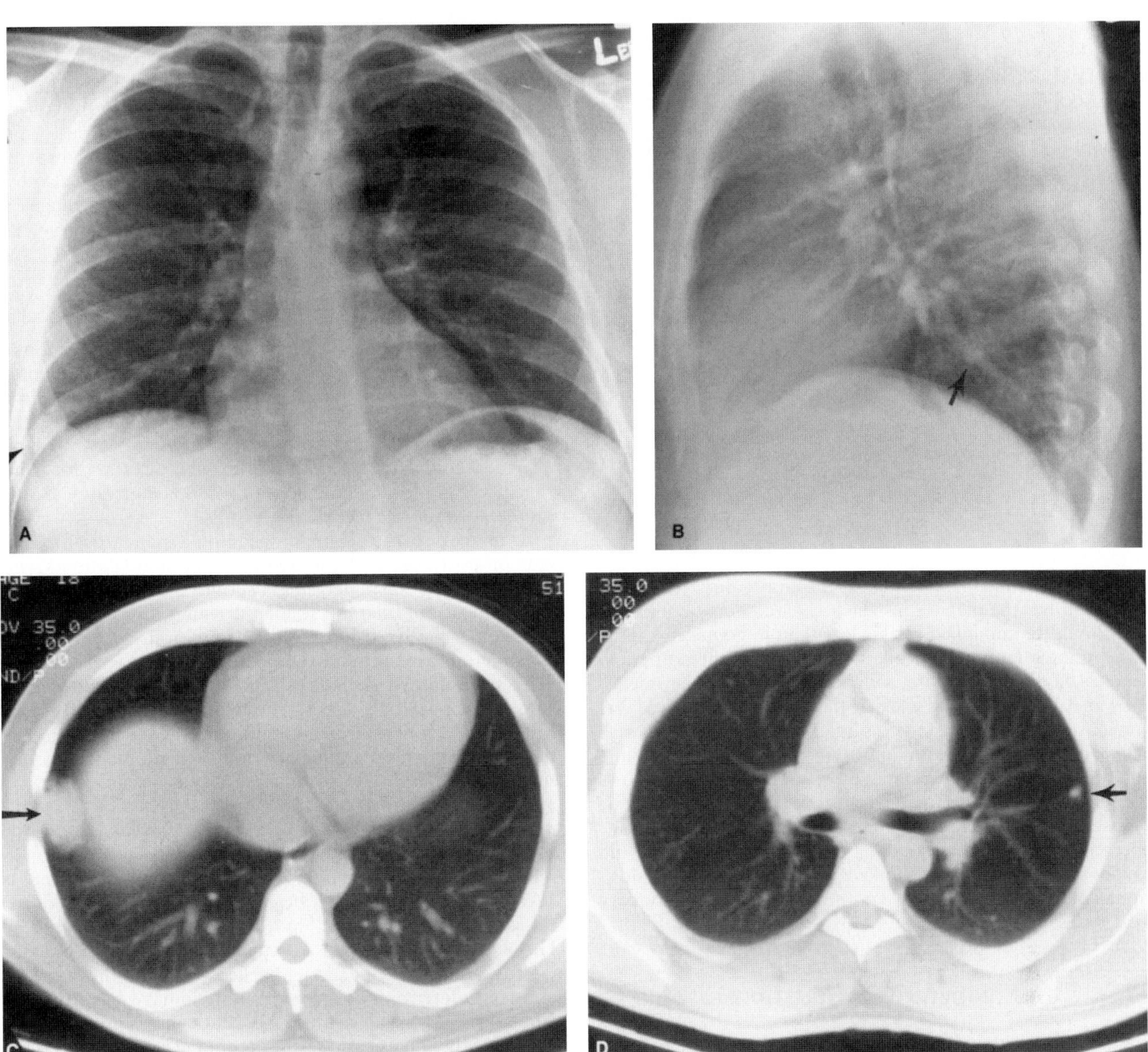

FIGURE 81.12 Imaging studies from a patient with metastatic embryonal rhabdomyosarcoma. Chest radiographs show a mass in the right lower lobe (*arrow*, A) that is best seen on the lateral view (*arrow*, B). Computed tomography (CT) confirmed the presence of this mass (*arrow*, C) and showed an additional nodule in the left upper lobe (*arrow*, D). At surgical exploration, however, multiple bilateral pulmonary metastases were found that measured less than 5 mm and therefore could not be seen on CT.

When a patient meets the criteria for resection of one or more pulmonary metastases, the natural history of the tumor and whether effective systemic therapy is available must be considered. Experience in breast cancer, testicular cancer, and osteogenic sarcoma illustrate this point.[165] In contrast to metastatic sarcoma, which is usually confined to the lungs, metastatic breast cancer to the lungs signals the development of widely disseminated disease. Although effective systemic therapy is available, patients with a solitary metastatic lesion, long disease-free interval following treatment for the primary breast cancer, and good performance status appear to have longer median and 5-year survival following pulmonary resection.[166,167]

The most striking example is the germ cell cancer. The advent of effective chemotherapy radically altered the management of pulmonary metastases of germ cell cancer and rendered an incurable disease curable. Chemotherapy is now the primary form of treatment. Surgical resection is reserved for patients who have a complete serologic response (normal levels of β-human chorionic gonadotropin and (α-fetoprotein) with residual pulmonary lesions, evidence of persistent intrathoracic disease with elevated markers despite a full course of chemotherapy, or lesions that do not respond or progress with chemotherapy.[168] Approximately one third of the resected pulmonary lesions contain viable tumor, one third contain fibrosis or necrosis, and one third are teratomas. Residual tumors are found mostly in patients with positive serology, and the prognosis is usually not as good as when no residual disease is present. A teratoma is removed to prevent it from degenerating to a more malignant form of germ cell tumor and to avoid the potential complications of local tumor growth. Thus, surgical resection plays a strictly adjuvant role in the treatment of malignant germ cell tumors.

The development of more effective chemotherapy regimens for sarcomas, especially osteogenic sarcomas, has also altered the management of pulmonary metastases in this disease.

TABLE 81.9 RESULTS

SURVIVAL BY PROGNOSTIC GROUP: THE INTERNATIONAL REGISTRY OF LUNG METASTASES

Groups	Median survival (mo)
I. Resectable, no risk factor (DFI ≥36 mo and single metastasis)	61
II. Resectable, 1 risk factor (DFI <36 mo or multiple metastases)	34
III. Resectable, 2 risk factors (DF) >36 mo and multiple metastases)	24
IV. Unresectable	14

DFI, disease-free interval.
From Pastorino U, Buyse M, Friendel G, et al. Long-term results of lung metastasectomy: prognostic analyses based on 5,206 cases. *J. Thorac Cardiovasc Surg* 1997; 11:34–49.

Surgical resection is part of a multimodality treatment approach, but the manner in which chemotherapy and resection should be combined is less clear than in germ cell cancer. The timing of an operation in relation to chemotherapy depends on the number, size, and location of pulmonary metastases at diagnosis and on whether the patient has received any previous chemotherapy. Often, surgical resection is performed between cycles of chemotherapy, with the aim of controlling both gross and micrometastatic disease. This approach allows the sensitivity of the patient's tumor to chemotherapy to be assessed, and the advisability of continuing the regimen postoperatively can be determined. The thoracic surgeon should collaborate with the medical oncologist in planning a multidisciplinary treatment program for the patient with pulmonary metastases of sarcoma.

Preoperative Evaluation

The preoperative evaluation of the patient undergoing resection of pulmonary metastases is similar to that of the patient undergoing removal of a primary lung cancer. Tests including pulmonary function, measurement of arterial blood gases, and, if necessary, ventilation-perfusion lung scanning are performed to be sure that the patient has sufficient reserve to tolerate complete resection of the metastases. The pulmonary function of patients who received chemotherapy may be substantially reduced. This is particularly true of patients treated with bleomycin and mitomycin, which can markedly diminish the diffusion capacity and, occasionally and unpredictably, cause an adult respiratory distress—type syndrome postoperatively. Maintaining patients on 35% or less inspired oxygen intraoperatively is thought to help prevent this complication. Like patients with primary lung cancers, these patients should stop smoking. Patients who smoke actively up to the time of operation are at risk for postoperative atelectasis or pneumonia.

It is also important to assess the patient's general medical condition and cardiovascular status. Older patients may have underlying coronary artery disease that requires preoperative treatment and additional perioperative monitoring. The cardiac function of patients who previously received chemotherapy, especially doxorubicin, may be impaired. A preoperative radionuclide scan or echocardiogram should be performed to determine the left ventricular ejection fraction and assess whether intraoperative hemodynamic monitoring is necessary. Other drugs, such as cisplatin, can impair renal or neurologic function and may influence perioperative management.

If a patient has recently undergone chemotherapy, the timing of surgery should be planned after consultation with the medical oncologist, so that the operation is not performed when the patient is neutropenic or thrombocytopenic. Resumption of chemotherapy postoperatively should also be a joint decision between the surgeon and medical oncologist so that it does not compromise wound healing.

Surgical Technique

Two principles guide the approach to resecting pulmonary metastatic lesions: complete resection of disease and maximal sparing of functioning lung tissue. Wedge resections should be performed whenever possible. A lobectomy or even a pneumonectomy may be performed when wedge resection will not provide a complete resection. This may be necessary for recurrences (completion pneumonectomy), centrally located tumors, or multiple metastases.[169,170]

Unilateral disease is approached by a standard anterolateral or posterolateral thoracotomy incision. Patients with bilateral pulmonary metastases should have a simultaneous resection of the bilateral lesions if technically feasible. This can be accomplished by a median sternotomy or a clamshell incision (bilateral anterior thoracotomy with or without transverse sternotomy). A clamshell incision provides better exposure to the posterior aspects of the lungs, particularly the left lower lobe, which is difficult to access by a median sternotomy.[171] Bilateral pulmonary nodules may require sequential posterolateral thoracotomies if they are centrally located and good exposure of the hilar vessels is needed.

The role of video-assisted thoracic surgery (VATS) in the management of patients with isolated suspected pulmonary metastasis is clear when performed for diagnostic purposes. VATS wedge resection can be carried out with a high degree of success and minimal morbidity or inconvenience.[172] However, the inability to palpate the entire lung adequately with the thoracoscope alone markedly impairs the surgeon's ability to determine whether all lesions have been resected when surgery is performed for metastatic disease. The value of VATS for the therapeutic resection of lung metastases is therefore questioned.[173]

Results

Surgical resection remains the mainstay of treatment for pulmonary metastases from many solid tumors that cannot be treated effectively with chemotherapy. These include colon cancers, renal cell cancers, melanomas, head and neck tumors, and endometrial cancers. The histologic subtypes of the pulmonary metastases in the International Registry of Lung Metastases are listed in Table 81.10.[157]

Globally, the actuarial survival after complete metastasectomy is 36% at 5 years and 26% at 10 years (median survival 35 months).[157] An experience in the resection of pulmonary metastases from renal cell carcinoma, head and neck tumors, colorectal cancers, testicular germ cell tumors, and soft-tissue sarcoma is summarized in (Table 81.11). These results again demonstrate that complete resection of metastatic disease is associated with prolonged survival in carefully selected patients. Furthermore, patients who are persistently free of disease at the primary tumor location but who have recurrent resectable metastatic disease of the lung also benefit from repeated surgery.[174] Mortality rates of pulmonary metastasectomy do not differ from those of thoracic surgery performed for lung cancers, varying between 0.6% and 2%.[150,168,175]

TABLE 81.10

HISTOLOGIC SUBTYPES FROM THE INTERNATIONAL REGISTRY OF LUNG METASTASES

Histologic groups	No. patients (%)	Subtypes
Carcinoma	2,260 (47)	Breast Lung Bowel Kidney Uterus Head and neck
Sarcoma	2,173 (45)	Osteosarcoma Other bone sarcomas Histiocytoma Leiomyosarcoma Synovial sarcoma Other soft tissue sarcoma
Other types	328 (8)	Wilms' tumor Teratoma Embryonal carcinoma Other germ cell tumor Melanoma

From Pastorino U, Buyse M, Friedel G, et al. Long-term results of lung metastasectomy: prognostic analyses based on 5,206 cases. *J Thorac Cardiovasc Surg* 1997; 113:37–49.

TABLE 81.11 RESULTS

RESULTS OF PULMONARY RESECTIONS FOR METASTASES AT MEMORIAL SLOAN-KETTERING CANCER CENTER

	No. patients	Survival (5 yr, %)
Renal cell carcinoma (1980–1993)189		
Solitary metastasis	50	54
Head and neck cancer (1966–1995)175		
Squamous cell	41	34
Glandular tumors	36	64
Overall	83	50
Colorectal cancer (1965–1988)190		
Overall	144	44
Soft-tissue sarcoma (1982–1997)191a		
Complete resection	161	46
Incomplete resection	52	23
No resection	473	17
Unknown	33	
Overall	719	25
Testicular germ cell tumors (1967–1995)(168)		
1967–1974	22	41
1975–1984	69	65
1984–1995	66	82
Overall	157	68

[a]Survival at 3 years

The surgical removal of pulmonary metastases is widely accepted, but its role has changed as more effective chemotherapy has become available for some cancers. It is important that the surgeon understand the indications for operation, the potential side effects of initial chemotherapy, and the ways in which surgical resection should be integrated into the overall treatment plan for these patients.

BENIGN TUMORS OF THE LUNG

Benign tumors of the lung are rare neoplasms. Few series are found in the literature, but in a 10-year surgical review (1958 to 1968) from the Mayo Clinic, 130 patients were found to have benign tumors.[176] Like malignant tumors, benign tumors arising from epithelial, mesodermal, or endodermal cell lines can develop in the lung. They may present as endobronchial lesions but more commonly as peripheral nodules.[177] Endobronchial tumors present with signs and symptoms related to airway obstruction or bleeding. Tumors arising in peripheral airways or within pulmonary parenchyma usually present as undiagnosed asymptomatic solitary pulmonary nodules. Types of benign lung tumors are listed in Table 81.12.

Hamartoma

The most frequent benign tumors are hamartomas, which represent 75% of benign lesions. They show a predilection for men.[178] A hamartoma consists of an abnormal arrangement of normal cells. In the lung, the most frequent component is cartilage. A hamartoma usually presents as a solitary pulmonary nodule with an extremely slow growth pattern. Classically, the radiographic appearance is that of a well-circumscribed nodule

TABLE 81.12 CLASSIFICATION

BENIGN TUMORS OF THE LUNG

EPITHELIAL
Polyps
Papilloma
Mucous gland adenoma

MESENCHYMAL
Vessel
- Sclerosing hemangioma
- Lymphangioma

Nerve
- Granular cell tumor
- Neurilemoma
- Neurofibroma

Muscle
- Leiomyoma

Miscellaneous
- Hamartoma
- Teratoma
- Clear cell (sugar) tumor

Others
- Lipoma
- Chondroma
- Fibroma

INFLAMMATORY PSEUDOTUMORS
Plasma cell granuloma
Pulmonary hyalinizing granuloma

that may contain popcorn calcification. If previous chest radiographs are available, these tumors are found to have been present for many years. Their growth pattern is variable but generally slow. These lesions can be diagnosed by CT if appropriate calcification is demonstrated. Needle aspiration is frequently diagnostic of a cartilaginous benign lesion.

Controversy exists regarding whether these lesions should be excised for pathologic diagnosis. Certainly, they do not require excision unless they are proximally located and cause symptoms related to endobronchial obstruction or unless carcinoma cannot be ruled out. If transthoracic needle aspiration biopsy confirms the presence of a hamartoma, many surgeons elect to follow patients with annual chest radiography rather than surgical excision. Occasionally, significant growth during follow-up necessitates excision.

Other Benign Tumors

Other benign tumors may present as endobronchial lesions (commonly fibromas, lipomas, chondromas, and granular cell myoblastomas). These tumors may be removed endoscopically, but frequently they also require surgical excision when the diagnosis is in doubt or when endoscopic excision has been incomplete. Peripheral tumors often are removed for diagnosis.

KEY POINTS

- **Lung cancer remains the leading cause of cancer-related death in the United States.**
- **Surgical resection remains the mainstay in the treatment of lung cancer, yet only about 20% of all patients diagnosed with lung cancer are considered resectable (stages I to IIIA).**
- **Taken as a whole, neoadjuvant therapy trials have demonstrated the feasibility of induction chemotherapy and surgical resection for the treatment of stage III NSCLC. Most studies show improved rates of resectability and survival in comparison with the historical experience for surgical resection or radiation alone.**
- **In addition to new chemotherapeutic agents, new radiation techniques, such as hyperfractionated or accelerated schedules, also merit further exploration in neoadjuvant trials with concurrent chemotherapy.**
- **Common sites of distant metastases are bone, liver, bone marrow, and the central nervous system; therefore, the metastatic evaluation includes a bone scan and CT of the chest, abdomen, and brain.**
- **Patients with multiple pulmonary nodules in the setting of a previously treated malignancy rarely pose a diagnostic dilemma. Patients who present with solitary pulmonary nodules are more problematic. Generally, a solitary lesion is more likely to be a metastasis if the primary tumor was a sarcoma or a melanoma. If the primary tumor originated in the head, neck, or breast, it is more likely to be a new primary lung cancer.**

References

1. Jemal A, Murray T, Ward E, et al. Cancer Statistics, 2005. *CA Cancer J Clin.* 2005;55:10–30.
2. Jemal A, Clegg LX, Ward E, et al. Annual report to the nation on the status of cancer, 1975–2001, with a special feature regarding survival. *Cancer* 2004;101:3–27.
3. Mountain C. Revisions in the International System for Staging Lung Cancer. *Chest* 1997;111:1710–1717.
4. **The International Adjuvant Lung Cancer Trial Collaborative Group. Cisplatin-based adjuvant chemotherapy in patients with completely resected non-small-cell lung cancer. *N Engl J Med.* 2004;350:351–360.**
5. Strauss GM, Herndon J, Maddaus MA, et al. Randomized Clinical Trial of adjuvant chemotherapy with paclitaxel and carboplatin following resection in Stage IB Non-Small Cell Lung Cancer (NSCLC): Report of Cancer and Leukemia Group B (CALGB) Protocol 9633 (abstract). *J Clin Oncol.* 2004;22:621-c-.
6. Winton TL, Livingston R, Johnson D, et al. Vinorelbine plus Cisplatin vs. Observation in Resected Non–Small-Cell Lung Cancer. *N Engl J Med.* 2005;352:2589–2597.
7. Graham EA, Singer JJ. Successful removal of an entire lung for carcinoma of the bronchus. *JAMA* 1933;101:1371–1374.
8. Warren WH. Historical facets of thoracic surgery emphasizing lung cancer. In Gruhn JG, Rosen ST, eds. *Lung cancer: the evolution of concepts.* New York: Field and Wood Medical Publishers, Inc.; 1989:73–106.
9. **Jacobs DR Jr, Adachi H, Mulder I, et al. Cigarette smoking and mortality risk: twenty-five-year follow-up of the Seven Countries Study. *Arch Intern Med.* 1999;159:733–740.**
10. Vineis P, Alavanja M, Buffler P, et al. Tobacco and cancer: recent epidemiological evidence. *J Natl Cancer Inst.* 2004;96:99–106.
11. Vineis P, Airoldi L, Veglia P, et al. Environmental tobacco smoke and risk of respiratory cancer and chronic obstructive pulmonary disease in former smokers and never smokers in the EPIC prospective study. *BMJ* 2005;330:277.
12. Brambilla E, Travis WD, Colby TV, et al. The new World Health Organization classification of lung tumours. *Eur Respir J.* 2001;18: 1059–1068.
13. Sanchez-Cespedes M. Dissecting the genetic alterations involved in lung carcinogenesis. *Lung Cancer* 2003;40:111–121.
14. Ahrendt SA, Hu Y, Buta M, et al. p53 mutations and survival in stage I non-small-cell lung cancer: results of a prospective study. *J Natl Cancer Inst.* 2003;95:961–970.
15. Ahrendt SA, Chow JT, Yang SC, et al. Alcohol consumption and cigarette smoking increase the frequency of p53 mutations in non-small cell lung cancer. *Cancer Res.* 2000;60:3155–3159.
16. D'Amico TA, Aloia TA, Moore M-BH, et al. Molecular biologic substaging of stage I lung cancer according to gender and histology. *Ann Thorac Surg.* 2000;69:882–886.
17. **D'Amico TA, Aloia TA, Moore M-BH, et al. Predicting the sites of metastases from lung cancer using molecular biologic markers. *Ann Thorac Surg.* 2001;72:1144–1148.**
18. Carbone DP, Mitsudomi T, Chiba H, et al. p53 Immunostaining positivity is associated with reduced survival and is imperfectly correlated with gene mutations in resected non-small cell lung cancer: A preliminary report of LCSG 871. *Chest* 1994;106:377S–381S.
19. Belinsky SA, Nikula KJ, Palmisano WA, et al. Aberrant methylation of p16INK4a is an early event in lung cancer and a potential biomarker for early diagnosis. *PNAS* 1998;95:11891–11896.
20. Esteller M, Corn PG, Baylin SB, et al. A gene hypermethylation profile of human cancer. *Cancer Res.* 2001;61:3225–3229.
21. Meyerson M, Franklin W, Kelley M. Molecular classification and molecular genetics of human lung cancers. *Semin Oncol.* 2004;31:4–19.
22. Chang AC, Beer DG, eds. *Lung cancer genetic profiling.* Philadelphia: Lippincott Williams and Wilkins, 2004.
23. Garber ME, Troyanskaya OG, Schluens K, et al. Diversity of gene expression in adenocarcinoma of the lung. *PNAS* 2001;98:13784–13789.
24. Bhattacharjee A, Richards WG, Staunton J, et al. Classification of human lung carcinomas by mRNA expression profiling reveals distinct adenocarcinoma subclasses. *PNAS* 2001;98:13790–13795.
25. **Beer DG, Kardia SL, Huang CC, et al. Gene-expression profiles predict survival of patients with lung adenocarcinoma. *Nat Med.* 2002;8: 816–824.**
26. Parmigiani G, Garrett-Mayer ES, et al. A cross-study comparison of gene expression studies for the molecular classification of lung cancer. *Clin Cancer Res.* 2004;10:2922–2927.
27. Lynch TJ, Bell DW, Sordella R, et al. Activating mutations in the epidermal growth factor receptor underlying responsiveness of non-small-cell lung cancer to gefitinib. *N Engl J Med.* 2004;350:2129–2139.
28. Paez JG, Janne PA, Lee JC, et al. EGFR mutations in lung cancer: correlation with clinical response to gefitinib therapy. *Science* 2004;304: 1497–1500.
29. Miller VA, Kris MG, Shah N, et al. Bronchioloalveolar pathologic subtype and smoking history predict sensitivity to gefitinib in advanced non-small-cell lung cancer. *J Clin Oncol.* 2004;22:1103–1109.
30. Pao W, Miller V, Zakowski M, et al. EGF receptor gene mutations are common in lung cancers from "never smokers" and are associated with sensitivity of tumors to gefitinib and erlotinib. *PNAS* 2004;101:13306–13311.
31. Postmus PE, Rocmans P, Asamura H, et al. Consensus report IASLC workshop Bruges, September 2002: pretreatment minimal staging for non-small cell lung cancer. *Lung Cancer* 2003;42:3–6.
32. Rivera MP, Detterbeck F, Mehta AC. Diagnosis of lung cancer: the guidelines. *Chest* 2003;123:129S–136S.
33. Mountain C, Dresler C. Regional lymph node classification for lung cancer staging. *Chest* 1997;111:1718–1723.
34. Toloza EM, Harpole L, McCrory DC. Noninvasive staging of non-small cell lung cancer: a review of the current evidence. *Chest* 2003;123:137S–146S.
35. Gonzalez-Stawinski GV, Lemaire A, Merchant F, et al. A comparative analysis of positron emission tomography and mediastinoscopy in staging non-small cell lung cancer. *J Thorac Cardiovasc Surg.* 2003;126:1900–1904.

36. Kernstine KH, McLaughlin KA, Menda Y, et al. Can FDG-PET reduce the need for mediastinoscopy in potentially resectable nonsmall cell lung cancer? *Ann Thorac Surg.* 2002;73:394–402.
37. Vesselle H, Pugsley JM, Vallieres E, et al. The impact of fluorodeoxyglucose F 18 positron-emission tomography on the surgical staging of non-small cell lung cancer. *J Thorac Cardiovasc Surg.* 2002;124:511–519.
38. Reed CE, Harpole DH, Posther KE, et al. Results of the American College of Surgeons Oncology Group Z0050 trial: the utility of positron emission tomography in staging potentially operable non-small cell lung cancer. *J Thorac Cardiovasc Surg.* 2003;126:1943–1951.
39. Cerfolio RJ, Ojha B, Bryant AS, et al. The accuracy of integrated PET-CT compared with dedicated PET alone for the staging of patients with non-small cell lung cancer. *Ann Thorac Surg.* 2004;78:1017–1023.
40. Krasna MJ, Reed CE, Nugent WC, et al. Lung cancer staging and treatment in multidisciplinary trials: cancer and leukemia group B cooperative group approach. *Ann Thorac Surg.* 1999;68:201–207.
41. Toloza EM, Harpole L, Detterbeck F, et al. Invasive staging of non-small cell lung cancer: a review of the current evidence. *Chest* 2003;123:157S–166S.
42. **Hammoud ZT, Anderson RC, Meyers BF, et al. The current role of mediastinoscopy in the evaluation of thoracic disease. *J Thorac Cardiovasc Surg.* 1999;118:894–899.**
43. Swensen SJ, Jett JR, Sloan JA, et al. Screening for lung cancer with low-dose spiral computed tomography. *Am J Respir Crit Care Med.* 2002;165:508–513.
44. Henschke CI, McCauley DI, Yankelevitz DF, et al. Early Lung Cancer Action Project: overall design and findings from baseline screening. *Lancet* 1999;354:99–105.
45. Eagle KA, Berger PB, Calkins H, et al. ACC/AHA guideline update for perioperative cardiovascular evaluation for noncardiac surgery—executive summary. A report of the American College of Cardiology/American Heart Association Task Force on Practice Guidelines (Committee to Update the 1996 Guidelines on Perioperative Cardiovascular Evaluation for Noncardiac Surgery). *Circulation* 2002;105:1257–1267.
46. Datta D, Lahiri B. Preoperative evaluation of patients undergoing lung resection surgery. *Chest* 2003;123:2096–2103.
47. Pate P, Tenholder MF, Griffin JP, et al. Preoperative assessment of the high-risk patient for lung resection. *Ann Thorac Surg.* 1996;61:1494–1500.
48. Cerfolio RJ, Allen MS, Trastek VF, et al. Lung resection in patients with compromised pulmonary function. *Ann Thorac Surg.* 1996;62:348–351.
49. Burke JR, Duarte IG, Thourani VH, et al. Preoperative risk assessment for marginal patients requiring pulmonary resection. *Ann Thorac Surg.* 2003;76:1767–1773.
50. Beckles MA, Spiro SG, Colice GL, et al. The physiologic evaluation of patients with lung cancer being considered for resectional surgery. *Chest* 2003;123:105S–114S.
51. Ginsberg RJ, Rubinstein LV. Randomized trial of lobectomy versus limited resection for T1 N0 non-small cell lung cancer. *Ann Thorac Surg.* 1995;60:615–622.
52. Landreneau R, Sugarbaker D, Mack M, et al. Wedge resection versus lobectomy for stage I (T1 N0 M0) non-small-cell lung cancer. *J Thorac Cardiovasc Surg.* 1997;113:691–700.
53. Martini N, Bains MS, Burt ME, et al. Incidence of local recurrence and second primary tumors in resected stage I lung cancer. *J Thorac Cardiovasc Surg.* 1995;109:120–129.
54. Yano T, Yokoyama H, Yoshino I, et al. Results of a limited resection for compromised or poor-risk patients with clinical stage I non-small cell carcinoma of the lung. *J Am Coll Surg.* 1995;181:33–37.
55. Deslauriers J, Gregoire J, Jacques LF, et al. Sleeve lobectomy versus pneumonectomy for lung cancer: a comparative analysis of survival and sites or recurrences. *Ann Thorac Surg.* 2004;77:1152–1156.
56. Gaissert H, Mathisen D, Moncure A, et al. Survival and function after sleeve lobectomy for lung cancer. *J Thorac Cardiovasc Surg.* 1996;111:948–953.
57. Okada M, Yamagishi H, Satake S, et al. Survival related to lymph node involvement in lung cancer after sleeve lobectomy compared with pneumonectomy. *J Thorac Cardiovasc Surg.* 2000;119:814–819.
58. Suen H-C, Meyers BF, Guthrie T, et al. Favorable results after sleeve lobectomy or bronchoplasty for bronchial malignancies. *Ann Thorac Surg.* 1999;67:1557–1562.
59. Yoshino I, Yokoyama H, Yano T, et al. Comparison of the surgical results of lobectomy with bronchoplasty and pneumonectomy for lung cancer. *J Surg Oncol.* 1997;64:32–35.
60. Keller SM, Adak S, Wagner H, et al. Mediastinal lymph node dissection improves survival in patients with stages II and IIIa non-small cell lung cancer. Eastern Cooperative Oncology Group. *Ann Thorac Surg.* 2000;70: 358–365; discussion 365–356.
61. Feld R, Rubinstein LV, Weisenberger TH. Sites of recurrence in resected stage I non-small-cell lung cancer: a guide for future studies. *J Clin Oncol.* 1984;2:1352–1358.
62. Thomas P, Rubinstein L. Cancer recurrence after resection: T1 N0 non-small cell lung cancer. Lung Cancer Study Group. *Ann Thorac Surg.* 1990;49:242–246.
63. Johnson BE. Second lung cancers in patients after treatment for an initial lung cancer. *J Natl Cancer Inst.* 1998;90:1335–1345.
64. Virgo KS, Naunheim KS, McKirgan LW, et al. Cost of patient follow-up after potentially curative lung cancer treatment. *J Thorac Cardiovasc Surg.* 1996;112:356–363.
65. Gail MH. A placebo-controlled randomized double-blind study of adjuvant intrapleural BCG in patients with resected T1N0, T1N1, or T2N0 squamous cell carcinoma, adenocarcinoma, or large cell carcinoma of the lung. LCSG Protocol 771. *Chest* 1994;106:287S–292S.
66. Ludwig Lung Cancer Study Group. Adverse effect of intrapleural *Corynebacterium parvum* as adjuvant therapy in resected stage I and II non-small cell carcinoma of the lung. *J Thorac Cardiovasc Surg.* 1985;89:842–847.
67. Ratto GB, Zino P, Mirabelli S, et al. A randomized trial of adoptive immunotherapy with tumor-infiltrating lymphocytes and interleukin-2 versus standard therapy in the postoperative treatment of resected nonsmall cell lung carcinoma. *Cancer* 1996;78:244–251.
68. Green N, Kurohara SS, George FW III, et al. Postresection irradiation for primary lung cancer: The impact of surgical adjuvant thoracic radiation therapy for patients with nonsmall cell lung carcinoma with ipsilateral mediastinal lymph node involvement. *Radiology* 1975;116:405–407.
69. Kirsh M, Rotman H, Argenta L, et al. Carcinoma of the lung: results of treatment over ten years. *Ann Thorac Surg.* 1976;21:371–377.
70. Sawyer TE, Bonner JA, Gould PM, et al. The impact of surgical adjuvant thoracic radiation therapy for patients with nonsmall cell lung carcinoma with ipsilateral mediastinal lymph node involvement. *Cancer* 1997;80: 1399–1408.
71. Mayer R, Smolle-Juettner FM, Szolar D, et al. Postoperative radiotherapy in radically resected non-small cell lung cancer. *Chest* 1997;112:954–959.
72. Stephens RJ, Girling DJ, Bleehen NM, et al. The role of post-operative radiotherapy in non-small-cell lung cancer: a multicentre randomised trial in patients with pathologically staged T1-2, N1-2, M0 disease. Medical Research Council Lung Cancer Working Party. *Br J Cancer* 1996;74:632–639.
73. Lafitte JJ, Ribet ME, Prevost BM, et al. Postresection irradiation for T2 N0 M0 non-small cell carcinoma: a prospective, randomized study. *Ann Thorac Surg.* 1996;62:830–834.
74. **The Lung Cancer Study Group. Effects of postoperative mediastinal radiation on completely resected stage II and stage III epidermoid cancer of the lung. *N Engl J Med.* 1986;315:1377–1381.**
75. Van Houtte P, Rocmans P, Smets P, et al. Postoperative radiation therapy in lung caner: a controlled trial after resection of curative design. *Int J Rad Oncol Biol Phys.* 1980;6:983-986.
76. **PORT Meta-analysis Trialists Group. Postoperative radiotherapy in non-small-cell lung cancer: systematic review and meta-analysis of individual patient data from nine randomised controlled trials. *Lancet* 1998;352: 257–263.**
77. Hughes FA, Higgins G. Veterans Administration Surgical Adjuvant Lung Cancer Chemotherapy Study: present status. *J Thorac Cardiovasc Surg.* 1962;44:295–304.
78. Slack NH. Bronchogenic carcinoma: nitrogen mustard as a surgical adjuvant and factors influencing survival. University surgical adjuvant lung project. *Cancer* 1970;25:987–1002.
79. Shields TW, Humphrey EW, Eastridge CE, et al. Adjuvant cancer chemotherapy after resection of carcinoma of the lung. *Cancer* 1977;40: 2057–2062.
80. Shields TW, Higgins GA Jr, Humphrey EW, et al. Prolonged intermittent adjuvant chemotherapy with CCNU and hydroxyurea after resection of carcinoma of the lung. *Cancer* 1982;50:1713–1721.
81. Non-small Cell Lung Cancer Collaborative Group. Chemotherapy in non-small cell lung cancer: a meta-analysis using updated data on individual patients from 52 randomised clinical trials. *BMJ* 1995;311: 899–909.
82. Feld R, Rubinstein L, Thomas PA. Adjuvant chemotherapy with cyclophosphamide, doxorubicin, and cisplatin in patients with completely resected stage I non-small-cell lung cancer. The Lung Cancer Study Group. *J Natl Cancer Inst.* 1993;85:299–306.
83. **Keller SM, Adak S, Wagner H, et al. A randomized trial of postoperative adjuvant therapy in patients with completely resected stage II or IIIA non-small-cell lung cancer. *N Engl J Med.* 2000;343:1217–1222.**
84. Wada H, Hitomi S, Teramatsu T. Adjuvant chemotherapy after complete resection in non-small-cell lung cancer. West Japan Study Group for Lung Cancer Surgery. *J Clin Oncol.* 1996;14:1048–1054.
85. Nakagawa M, Tanaka F, Tsubota N, et al. A randomized phase III trial of adjuvant chemotherapy with UFT for completely resected pathological stage I non-small-cell lung cancer: the West Japan Study Group for Lung Cancer Surgery (WJSG)—the 4th study. *Ann Oncol.* 2005;16:75–80.
86. Alam N, Shepherd FA, Winton T, et al. Compliance with post-operative adjuvant chemotherapy in non-small cell lung cancer: An analysis of National Cancer Institute of Canada and intergroup trial JBR.10 and a review of the literature. *Lung Cancer* 2005;47:385–394.
87. Rendina EA, Venuta F, De Giacomo T, et al. Induction chemotherapy for T4 centrally located non-small cell lung cancer. *J Thorac Cardiovasc Surg.* 1999;117:225–233.
88. Grunenwald DH, Andre F, Le Pechoux C, et al. Benefit of surgery after chemoradiotherapy in stage IIIB (T4 and/or N3) non-small cell lung cancer. *J Thorac Cardiovasc Surg.* 2001;122:796–802.
89. Okada M, Tsubota N, Yoshimura M, et al. Prognosis of completely resected pN2 non-small cell lung carcinomas: What is the significant node that affects survival? *J Thorac Cardiovasc Surg.* 1999;118:270–275.
90. Sagawa M, Sakurada A, Fujimura S, et al. Five-year survivors with resected pN2 nonsmall cell lung carcinoma. *Cancer* 1999;85:864–868.
91. Martini N, Flehinger BJ. The role of surgery in N2 lung cancer. *Surg Clin North Am.* 1987;67:1037–1049.

92. **Rosell R, Gomez-Codina J, Camps C, et al. A randomized trial comparing preoperative chemotherapy plus surgery with surgery alone in patients with non-small-cell lung cancer. *N Engl J Med.* 1994;330: 153–158.**
93. Roth J, Fossella F, Komaki R, et al. A randomized trial comparing perioperative chemotherapy and surgery with surgery alone in resectable stage IIIA non-small-cell lung cancer. *J Natl Cancer Inst.* 1994;86:673–680.
94. Perez CA, Pajak TF, Rubin P, et al. Long-term observations of the patterns of failure in patients with unresectable non-oat cell carcinoma of the lung treated with definitive radiotherapy. Report by the Radiation Therapy Oncology Group. *Cancer* 1987;59:1874–1881.
95. Pisters KM, Kris MG, Gralla RJ, et al. Randomized trial comparing postoperative chemotherapy with vindesine and cisplatin plus thoracic irradiation with irradiation alone in stage III (N2) non-small cell lung cancer. *J Surg Oncol.* 1994;56:236–241.
96. Bromley LL, Szur L. Combined radiotherapy and resection for carcinoma of the bronchus; experiences with 66 patients. *Lancet* 1955;269:937–941.
97. Payne DG. Is preoperative or postoperative radiation therapy indicated in non-small cell cancer of the lung? *Lung Cancer* 1994;10:S205–212.
98. Furuse K, Fukuoka M, Kawahara M, et al. Phase III study of concurrent versus sequential thoracic radiotherapy in combination with mitomycin, vindesine, and cisplatin in unresectable stage III non-small-cell lung cancer. *J Clin Oncol.* 1999;17:2692–2699.
99. Martini N, Kris M, Flehinger B, et al. Preoperative chemotherapy for stage IIIa (N2) lung cancer: the Sloan- Kettering experience with 136 patients. *Ann Thorac Surg.* 1993;55:1365–1373.
100. Sugarbaker DJ, Herndon J, Kohman LJ, et al. Results of cancer and leukemia group B protocol 8935:A multi-institutional phase II trimodality trial for stage IIIa (N2) non-small-cell lung cancer. *J Thorac Cardiovasc Surg.* 1995;109:473–485.
101. Rosell R, Gomez-Codina J, Camps C, et al. Preresectional chemotherapy in stage IIIA non-small-cell lung cancer: a 7-year assessment of a randomized controlled trial. *Lung Cancer* 1999;26:7–14.
102. Roth JA, Atkinson EN, Fossella F, et al. Long-term follow-up of patients enrolled in a randomized trial comparing perioperative chemotherapy and surgery with surgery alone in resectable stage IIIA non-small-cell lung cancer. *Lung Cancer* 1998;21:1–6.
103. Eagan RT, Ruud C, Lee RE, et al. Pilot study of induction therapy with cyclophosphamide, doxorubicin, and cisplatin (CAP) and chest irradiation prior to thoracotomy in initially inoperable stage III M0 non-small cell lung cancer. *Cancer Treat Rep.* 1987;71:895–900.
104. Weiden P, Piantadosi S. Preoperative chemotherapy (cisplatin and fluorouracil) and radiation therapy in stage III non-small-cell lung cancer: a phase II study of the Lung Cancer Study Group. *J Natl Cancer Inst.* 1991;83:266–273.
105. Faber L, Kittle C, Warren W, et al. Preoperative chemotherapy and irradiation for stage III non-small cell lung cancer. *Ann Thorac Surg.* 1989;47:669–675.
106. Strauss G, Herndon J, Sherman D, et al. Neoadjuvant chemotherapy and radiotherapy followed by surgery in stage IIIA non-small-cell carcinoma of the lung: report of a Cancer and Leukemia Group B phase II study. *J Clin Oncol.* 1992;10:1237–1244.
107. Albain KS, Rusch VW, Crowley JJ, et al. Concurrent cisplatin/etoposide plus chest radiotherapy followed by surgery for stages IIIA (N2) and IIIB non-small-cell lung cancer: mature results of Southwest Oncology Group phase II study 8805. *J Clin Oncol.* 1995;13:1880–1892.
108. Albain K, Rusch V, Crowley J, et al. Long-term survival after concurrent cisplatin/etoposide (PE) plus chest radiotherapy (RT) followed by surgery in bulky, stages IIIA(N2) and IIIB non-small cell lung cancer (NSCLC): 6-year outcomes from Southwest Oncology Group Study 8805. *Proc of the Am Soc Clin Oncol.* 1999;18:467a.
109. Yashar J, Weitberg A, Glicksman A, et al. Preoperative chemotherapy and radiation therapy for stage IIIa carcinoma of the lung. *Ann Thorac Surg.* 1992;53:445–448.
110. Fowler W, Langer C, Curran W Jr, et al. Postoperative complications after combined neoadjuvant treatment of lung cancer. *Ann Thorac Surg.* 1993;55:986–989.
111. Milstein D, Kuten A, Saute M, et al. Preoperative concurrent chemoradiotherapy for unresectable stage III nonsmall cell lung cancer. *Int J Rad Oncol Biol Phys.* 1996;34:1125–1132.
112. Taylor NA, Liao ZX, Cox JD, et al. Equivalent outcome of patients with clinical stage IIIA non-small-cell lung cancer treated with concurrent chemoradiation compared with induction chemotherapy followed by surgical resection. *Int J Rad Oncol Biol Phys.* 2004;58:204–212.
113. Albain KS, Scott CB, Rusch VR, et al. PL-4 phase III study of concurrent chemotherapy and full course radiotherapy (CT/RT) versus CT/RT induction followed by surgical resection for stage IIIA (pN2) non-small cell lung cancer (NSCLC): First outcome analysis of North American Intergroup trial 0139 (RTOG 93-09). *Lung Cancer* 2003;41:S4.
114. Adelstein DJ, Rice TW, Rybicki LA, et al. Accelerated hyperfractionated radiation, concurrent paclitaxel/cisplatin chemotherapy and surgery for stage III non-small cell lung cancer. *Lung Cancer* 2002;36:167–174.
115. Weil MD, Roach I, Mack, Pickett B, et al. 3D conformal radiotherapy in the sagittal plane for centrally located thoracic tumors. *Med Dosim.* 1995;20:11–14.
116. Hayman JA, Martel MK, Ten Haken RK, et al. Dose escalation in non-small-cell lung cancer using three-dimensional conformal radiation therapy: update of a phase I trial. *J Clin Oncol.* 2001;19:127–136.
117. **Pancoast H. Superior pulmonary sulcus tumor: tumor characterized by pain, Horner's syndrome, destruction of bone and atrophy of hand muscles. *JAMA* 1932;99:1391–1396.**
118. Vallieres E, Kraut M, Thomas C. Pancoast (superior sulcus) neoplasms. *Curr Prob Canc.* 2003;27:81–104.
119. Shaw R, Paulson D, Kee JJ. Treatment of the superior sulcus tumor by irradiation followed by resection. *Ann Surg.* 1961;154:29–40.
120. Rusch V, Parekh K, Leon L, et al. Factors determining outcome after surgical resection of T3 and T4 lung cancers of the superior sulcus. *J Thorac Cardiovasc Surg.* 2000;119:1147–1153.
121. Detterbeck FC. Pancoast (superior sulcus) tumors. *Ann Thorac Surg.* 1997;63:1810–1818.
122. Rusch V, Giroux D, Kraut M, et al. Induction chemoradiation and surgical resection for non-small cell lung carcinomas of the superior sulcus: Initial results of Southwest Oncology Group Trial 9416 (Intergroup Trial 0160). *J Thorac Cardiovasc Surg.* 2001;121:472–483.
123. Travis WD, Linnoila RI, Tsokos MG, et al. Neuroendocrine tumors of the lung with proposed criteria for large-cell neuroendocrine carcinoma. An ultrastructural, immunohistochemical, and flow cytometric study of 35 cases. *Am J Surg Pathol.* 1991;15:529–553.
124. Vuitch F, Sekido Y, Fong K, et al. Neuroendocrine tumors of the lung. Pathology and molecular biology. *Chest Surg Clin N Am.* 1997;7:21–47.
125. McCaughan B, Martini N, Bains M. Bronchial carcinoids. Review of 124 cases. *J Thorac Cardiovasc Surg.* 1985;89:8–17.
126. Martini N, Zaman MB, Bains MS, et al. Treatment and prognosis in bronchial carcinoids involving regional lymph nodes. *J Thorac Cardiovasc Surg.* 1994;107:1–7.
127. Jiang S-X, Kameya T, Shoji M, et al. Large cell neuroendocrine carcinoma of the lung: a histologic and immunohistochemical study of 22 cases. *Am J Surg Pathol.* 1998;22:526–537.
128. Travis WD, Rush W, Flieder DB, et al. Survival analysis of 200 pulmonary neuroendocrine tumors with clarification of criteria for atypical carcinoid and its separation from typical carcinoid. *Am J Surg Pathol.* 1998;22:934–944.
129. Zacharias J, Nicholson AG, Ladas GP, et al. Large cell neuroendocrine carcinoma and large cell carcinomas with neuroendocrine morphology of the lung: prognosis after complete resection and systematic nodal dissection. *Ann Thorac Surg.* 2003;75:348–352.
130. Stahel RA, Ginsberg R, Havemann K, et al. Staging and prognostic factors in small cell lung cancer: a consensus report. *Lung Cancer* 1989;5: 119–126.
131. **Shepherd FA. The role of chemotherapy in the treatment of small cell lung cancer. *Chest Surg Clin N Am.* 1997;7:113–133.**
132. **Pignon JP, Arriagada R, Ihde DC, et al. A meta-analysis of thoracic radiotherapy for small-cell lung cancer. *N Engl J Med.* 1992;327:1618–1624.**
133. Warde P, Payne D. Does thoracic irradiation improve survival and local control in limited- stage small-cell carcinoma of the lung? A meta-analysis. *J Clin Oncol.* 1992;10:890–895.
134. Albain K, Crowley J, LeBlanc M, et al. Determinants of improved outcome in small-cell lung cancer: an analysis of the 2,580-patient Southwest Oncology Group data base. *J Clin Oncol.* 1990;8:1563–1574.
135. Inoue M, Miyoshi S, Yasumitsu T, et al. Surgical results for small cell lung cancer based on the new TNM staging system. *Ann Thorac Surg.* 2000;70: 1615–1619.
136. Kreisman H, Wolkove N, Quoix E. Small cell lung cancer presenting as a solitary pulmonary nodule. *Chest* 1992;101:225–231.
137. Brock MV, Hooker CM, Syphard JE, et al. Surgical resection of limited disease small cell lung cancer in the new era of platinum chemotherapy: its time has come. *J Thorac Cardiovasc Surg.* 2005;129:64–72.
138. Shepherd F, Evans W, Feld R, et al. Adjuvant chemotherapy following surgical resection for small-cell carcinoma of the lung. *J Clin Oncol.* 1988;6:832–838.
139. Shah S, Thompson J, Goldstraw P. Results of operation without adjuvant therapy in the treatment of small cell lung cancer. *Ann Thorac Surg.* 1992;54:498–501.
140. Shepherd F, Ginsberg R, Patterson G, et al. Is there ever a role for salvage operations in limited small-cell lung cancer? *J Thorac Cardiovasc Surg.* 1991;101:196–200.
141. Lad T, Piantadosi S, Thomas P, et al. A prospective randomized trial to determine the benefit of surgical resection of residual disease following response of small cell lung cancer to combination chemotherapy. *Chest* 1994;106:320S–323S.
142. Inoue H, Iwasaki M, Ogawa J, et al. Surgical resection of a second primary lung carcinoma in a survivor of small cell carcinoma. *Ann Thorac Surg.* 1993;56:1160–1161.
143. Heitmiller R, Mathisen D, Ferry J, et al. Mucoepidermoid lung tumors. *Ann Thorac Surg.* 1989;47:394–399.
144. Moran CA. Primary salivary gland-type tumors of the lung. *Semin Diagn Pathol.* 1995;12:106–122.
145. Chin H, DeMeester T, Chin R, et al. Endobronchial adenoid cystic carcinoma. *Chest* 1991;100:1464–1465.
146. Miller DL, Allen MS. Rare pulmonary neoplasms. *Mayo Clin Proc.* 1993;68:492–498.
147. Berho M, Moran CA, Suster S. Malignant mixed epithelial/mesenchymal neoplasms of the lung. *Semin Diagn Pathol.* 1995;12:123–139.
148. Barney JD, Churchill ED. Adenocarcinoma of the kidney with metastases to the lung cured by nephrectomy and lobectomy. *J Urol.* 1939;42: 269–276.

149. Clagett OT, Woolner LB. Surgical treatment of solitary metastatic pulmonary lesion. *Med Clin North Am.* 1964;48:939–943.
150. Mountain C, McMurtrey M, Hermes K. Surgery for pulmonary metastasis: a 20-year experience. *Ann Thorac Surg.* 1984;38:323–330.
151. Martini N, Huvos A, Mike V, et al. Multiple pulmonary resections in the treatment of osteogenic sarcoma. *Ann Thorac Surg.* 1971;12:271–280.
152. Crow J, Slavin G, Kreel L. Pulmonary metastasis: a pathologic and radiologic study. *Cancer* 1981;47:2595–2602.
153. Heitmiller R, Marasco W, Hruban R, et al. Endobronchial metastasis. *J Thorac Cardiovasc Surg.* 1993;106:537–542.
154. Loehe F, Kobinger S, Hatz RA, et al. Value of systematic mediastinal lymph node dissection during pulmonary metastasectomy. *Ann Thorac Surg.* 2001;72:225–229.
155. Ercan S, Nichols FC III, Trastek VF, et al. Prognostic significance of lymph node metastasis found during pulmonary metastasectomy for extrapulmonary carcinoma. *Ann Thorac Surg.* 2004;77:1786–1791.
156. Johnson H Jr, Fantone J, Flye MW. Histological evaluation of the nodules resected in the treatment of pulmonary metastatic disease. *J Surg Oncol.* 1982;21:1–4.
157. Pastorino U, Buyse M, Friedel G, et al. Long-term results of lung metastasectomy: prognostic analyses based on 5206 cases. *J Thorac Cardiovasc Surg.* 1997;113:37–49.
158. McCormack P, Ginsberg K, Bains M, et al. Accuracy of lung imaging in metastases with implications for the role of thoracoscopy. *Ann Thorac Surg.* 1993;56:863–865.
159. Pastorino U, Veronesi G, Landoni C, et al. Fluorodeoxyglucose positron emission tomography improves preoperative staging of resectable lung metastasis. *J Thorac Cardiovasc Surg.* 2003;126:1906–1910.
160. Deleyiannis F, Thomas D. Risk of lung cancer among patients with head and neck cancer. *Otolaryngol Head Neck Surg.* 1997;116:630–636.
161. Robert JH, Ambrogi V, Mermillod B, et al. Factors influencing long-term survival after lung metastasectomy. *Ann Thorac Surg.* 1997;63: 777–784.
162. Rusch V. Pulmonary metastasectomy. Current indications. *Chest* 1995;107: 322S–331S.
163. Girard P, Baldeyrou P, Le Chevalier T, et al. Surgery for pulmonary metastases. Who are the 10-year survivors? *Cancer* 1994;74:2791–2797.
164. McCormack P. Surgical resection of pulmonary metastases. *Semin Surg Oncol.* 1990;6:297–302.
165. La Quaglia MP. Osteosarcoma. Specific tumor management and results. *Chest Surg Clin N Am.* 1998;8:77–95.
166. Singletary SE, Walsh G, Vauthey J-N, et al. A role for curative surgery in the treatment of selected patients with metastatic breast cancer. *Oncologist* 2003;8:241–251.
167. Friedel G, Pastorino U, Ginsberg RJ, et al. Results of lung metastasectomy from breast cancer: prognostic criteria on the basis of 467 cases of the international registry of lung metastases. *Eur J Cardiothorac Surg.* 2002;22: 335–344.
168. Liu D, Abolhoda A, Burt ME, et al. Pulmonary metastasectomy for testicular germ cell tumors: A 28-year experience. *Ann Thorac Surg.* 1998;66:1709–1714.
169. Putnam J Jr, Suell D, Natarajan G, et al. Extended resection of pulmonary metastases: is the risk justified? *Ann Thorac Surg.* 1993;55: 1440–1446.
170. Koong HN, Pastorino U, Ginsberg RJ. Is there a role for pneumonectomy in pulmonary metastases? *Ann Thorac Surg.* 1999;68:2039–2043.
171. Bains M, Ginsberg R, Jones W II, et al. The clamshell incision: an improved approach to bilateral pulmonary and mediastinal tumor. *Ann Thorac Surg.* 1994;58:30–32.
172. Liu H, Lin P, Hsieh M, et al. Application of thoracoscopy for lung metastases. *Chest* 1995;107:266–268.
173. McCormack PM, Bains MS, Begg CB, et al. Role of video-assisted thoracic surgery in the treatment of pulmonary metastases: results of a prospective trial. *Ann Thorac Surg.* 1996;62:213–216.
174. Kandioler D, Kromer E, Tuchler H, et al. Long-term results after repeated surgical removal of pulmonary metastases. *Ann Thorac Surg.* 1998;65:909–912.
175. Liu D, Labow DM, Dang N, et al. Pulmonary metastasectomy for head and neck cancers. *Ann Surg Oncol.* 1999;6:572–578.
176. Arrigoni M, Woolner L, Bernatz P, et al. Benign tumors of the lung. A ten-year surgical experience. *J Thorac Cardiovasc Surg.* 1970;60:589–599.
177. Oldham HN Jr. Benign tumors of the lung and bronchus. *Surg Clin North Am.* 1980;60:825–834.
178. Hansen C, Holtveg H, Francis D, et al. Pulmonary hamartoma. *J Thorac Cardiovasc Surg.* 1992;104:674–678.
179. Dautzenberg B, Chastang C, Arriagada R, et al. Adjuvant radiotherapy versus combined sequential chemotherapy followed by radiotherapy in the treatment of resected nonsmall cell lung carcinoma: A randomized trial of 267 patients. GETCB (Groupe d'Etude et de Traitement des Cancers Bronchiques). *Cancer* 1995;76:779–786.
180. Scagliotti GV, Fossati R, Torri V, et al. Randomized study of adjuvant chemotherapy for completely resected stage I, II, or IIIa non-small-cell lung cancer. *J Natl Cancer Inst.* 2003;95:1453–1461.
181. Trovo MG, Minatel E, Veronesi A, et al. Combined radiotherapy and chemotherapy versus radiotherapy alone in locally advanced epidermoid bronchogenic carcinoma. A randomized study. *Cancer* 1990;65:400–404.
182. Morton RF, Jett JR, McGinnis WL, et al. Thoracic radiation therapy alone compared with combined chemoradiotherapy for locally unresectable non-small cell lung cancer. A randomized, phase III trial. *Ann Int Med.* 1991;115:681–686.
183. Le Chevalier T, Arriagada R, Quoix E, et al. Radiotherapy alone versus combined chemotherapy and radiotherapy in nonresectable non-small-cell lung cancer: first analysis of a randomized trial in 353 patients. *J Natl Cancer Inst.* 1991;83:417–423.
184. Blanke C, Ansari R, Mantravadi R, et al. Phase III trial of thoracic irradiation with or without cisplatin for locally advanced unresectable non-small-cell lung cancer: a Hoosier Oncology Group protocol. *J Clin Oncol.* 1995;13:1425–1429.
185. Schaake-Koning C, van den Bogaert W, Dalesio O, et al. Effects of concomitant cisplatin and radiotherapy on inoperable non-small-cell lung cancer. *N Engl J Med.* 1992;326:524–530.
186. Jeremic B, Shibamoto Y, Acimovic L, et al. Randomized trial of hyperfractionated radiation therapy with or without concurrent chemotherapy for stage III non-small-cell lung cancer. *J Clin Oncol.* 1995;13:452–458.
187. Dillman R, Herndon J, Seagren S, et al. Improved survival in stage III non-small-cell lung cancer: seven-year follow-up of cancer and leukemia group B (CALGB) 8433 trial. *J Natl Cancer Inst.* 1996;88:1210–1215.
188. Sause W, Kolesar P, Taylor S IV, et al. Final results of phase III trial in regionally advanced unresectable non-small cell lung cancer: Radiation Therapy Oncology Group, Eastern Cooperative Oncology Group, and Southwest Oncology Group. *Chest* 2000;117:358–364.
189. Kavolius J, Mastorakos D, Pavlovich C, et al. Resection of metastatic renal cell carcinoma. *J Clin Oncol.* 1998;16:2261–2266.
190. McCormack PM, Burt ME, Bains MS, et al. Lung resection for colorectal metastases. 10-year results. *Arch Surg.* 1992;127:1403–1406.
191. Billingsley KG, Burt ME, Jara E, et al. Pulmonary metastases from soft tissue sarcoma: analysis of patterns of diseases and postmetastasis survival. *Ann Surg.* 1999;229:602–610.

CHAPTER 82 ■ CHEST WALL, PLEURA, MEDIASTINUM, AND NONNEOPLASTIC LUNG DISEASE

MICHAEL T. JAKLITSCH, LAMBROS ZELLOS, AND DAVID J. SUGARBAKER

ANATOMY OF THE CHEST WALL

The bony thorax consists of the 12 thoracic vertebrae, 12 pairs of ribs, the sternum, and the clavicles. The three articulating joints of the ribs create a noncollapsible, dynamic structure that provides respiration, protection of internal organs, and support for the upper extremities.

The first six ribs are considered true ribs because they articulate directly with the sternum, whereas the next four ribs are considered false because they articulate with the cartilage above them. Additionally, ribs 11 and 12 are considered floating ribs in that they articulate with only the vertebrae (Fig. 82.1).[1] Each rib has a head, a neck, and a shaft. The head has two facets. The upper one is used for articulation with the upper vertebrae, whereas the lower one is used to articulate with its vertebrae creating the costovertebral joint. The costotransverse joint is formed by the facet tubercle of the neck and the transverse process of its vertebra (Fig. 82.2). The shaft contains the costal groove at its inferior aspect, where the intercostal vein, artery, and nerve run. Procedures such as thoracentesis and chest tube placement should avoid the inferior aspect of the rib.

Three different muscles span the intercostal space (Fig. 82.3). From innermost to outermost they are the transverse thoracic, the internal intercostal, and the external intercostal muscles. The intercostal neurovascular bundle lies beneath the internal intercostal muscle, and the internal mammary (or internal thoracic) artery lies between the internal intercostal and the transverse thoracic muscle.

The sternum is flat and has three parts: the manubrium, body, and xiphoid bone. The sternum has a total length of 15 to 20 cm (Fig. 82.1B). The manubrium articulates with the clavicles and first costal cartilage at its superior lateral aspect. The manubrium articulates with the body of the sternum at its inferior aspect forming the angle of Louis. On a plain chest radiograph the angle of Louis corresponds to the junction of the second rib anteriorly and the fourth thoracic vertebra posteriorly.

The anterior and posterior intercostal arteries supply the intercostal space (see Fig. 82.3). The first two posterior intercostal arteries arise from the subclavian artery and the remain-

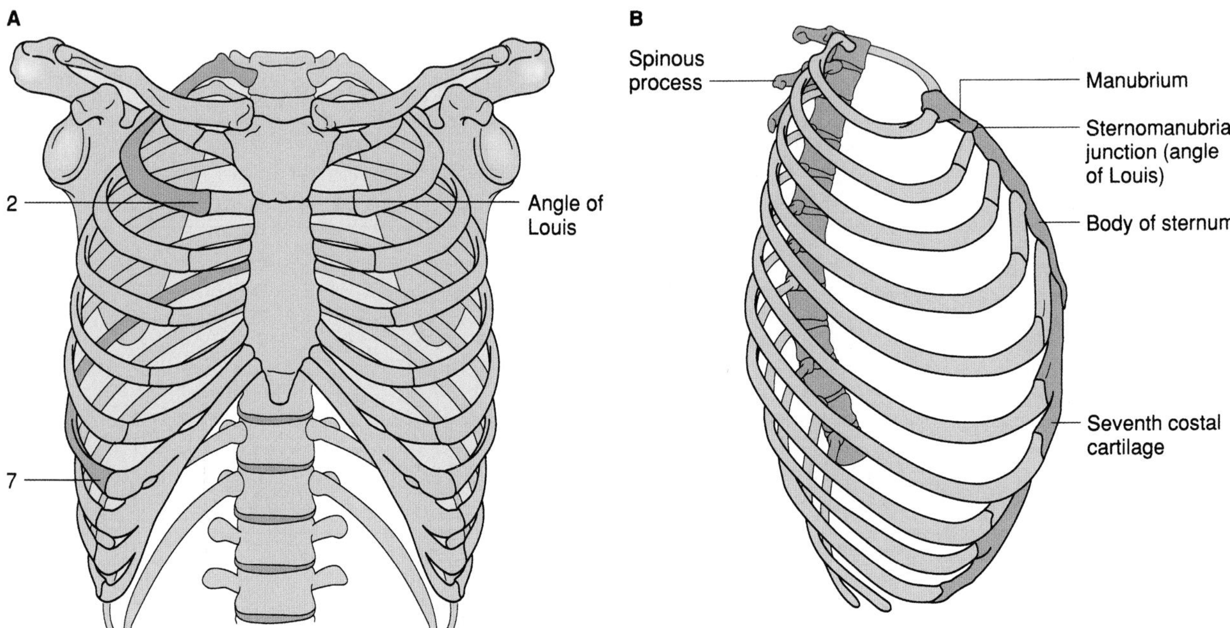

FIGURE 82.1 Skeletal support of the thorax. Anterior (*A*) and lateral (*B*) views. Note the anterior cartilaginous component of the upper 10 ribs, the fused costal cartilages of ribs 7 through 10, the location of the sternomanubrial junction (angle of Louis) at the level of the second rib, and the oblique course of the ribs laterally from posterior to anterior.

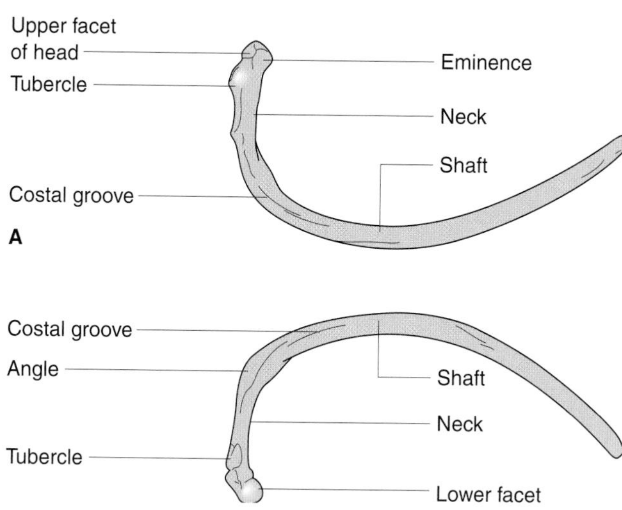

FIGURE 82.2 Anatomy of the rib as viewed from above (*A*) and below (*B*).

ing arteries arise from the thoracic aorta. The anterior intercostal arteries are branches of the internal mammary arteries and form an anastomosis with the posterior intercostal arteries.

The intercostal veins follow the course of the arteries along the inferior aspect of each rib and drain into the azygous and hemiazygous veins. The lymphatic drainage of the anterior part of the rib drains into the internal mammary nodes, and the lymphatic system of the posterior part of the rib drains into the vertebral nodes and the thoracic duct.

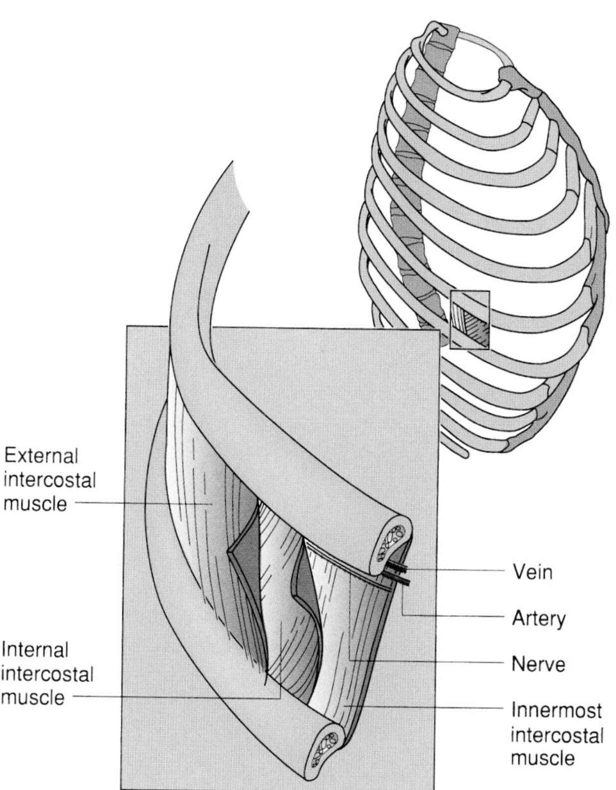

FIGURE 82.3 Anatomy of the intercostal space. The major intercostal muscles are the external and internal. The neurovascular bundle courses in the costal groove along the inferior aspect of the rib.

The muscles covering the bony thorax are divided into primary and secondary muscles of respiration. The diaphragm and the intercostal muscles constitute the primary respiratory muscles, and the secondary muscles are the latissimus, serratus, pectorals, trapezius, scalenes, and deltoid. The deltoid, pectoralis, and latissimus muscles help fixate the upper extremities and facilitate inspiration. In normal breathing, the diaphragm does approximately 75% of the total work of breathing and the intercostal muscles do the remaining 25% of the work. During periods of respiratory distress, the secondary muscles are used as well. Inspiration is an active process and expiration is passive, facilitated by the elastic recoil of the lungs. Active expiration is accomplished with contraction of the abdominal muscles (Figs. 82.4 and 82.5).

CONGENITAL CHEST WALL DEFORMITIES

A wide variety of chest wall abnormalities have been reported, most commonly involving the sternum. Most patients are asymptomatic. However, the most severe defects do cause cardiopulmonary compromise and are associated with other congenital malformations.

Depression Deformities/Pectus Excavatum

Depression deformity/pectus excavatum is the most common chest wall deformity; it consists of sternal depression because of abnormalities of the lower costal cartilages and occurs in 1 out of 700 children (Fig. 82.6).[2] There is a 3.4:1 male to female ratio, and 37% of cases occur in families with history of chest wall defects.[4] The sternum is posteriorly displaced and often rotated. There are varying degrees of depression arising from differential growth of the lower costal cartilage. The deepest depression is usually seen near the xiphoid and it can be mild or, in its worst form, the sternum can be in contact with the vertebral column. In addition, up to 20% of patients may have other musculoskeletal abnormalities, such as scoliosis and Marfan syndrome, whereas 2% to 3% of patients also have congenital heart disease.[2,4,5]

Many patients with pectus excavatum report decreased exercise tolerance, fatigability, dyspnea on exertion, and sternal pain. In addition, palpitations and multiple respiratory tract infections are reported. However, most patients present to their physicians with the complaint of cosmetic deformity rather than symptomatology.[6]

Cardiovascular and pulmonary work-up includes echocardiography, pulmonary function testing, exercise studies, and quantitative ventilation-perfusion scans.[7] Decreased cardiac index, increased oxygen uptake at rest, and decreased stroke volume have been described. These hemodynamic changes are more pronounced when testing patients in the sitting instead of supine position. Various methods have been developed to objectively grade the severity of the defect based on measurements derived from lateral chest radiographs.[8] One of these methods developed by Shamberger uses the ratio of two measured distances of the sternum from the vertebrae. These measurements along with the angle of the sternum are used to develop a score. Usually these two distances are measured from the angle of Louis to the T3 vertebrae and from the xiphoid to the T9 vertebrae.

Operative correction should be undertaken to improve cosmesis, self-image, respiratory or cardiovascular compromise, and exercise tolerance. Repair should be ideally undertaken before adolescence.[9] However, less than 15% of

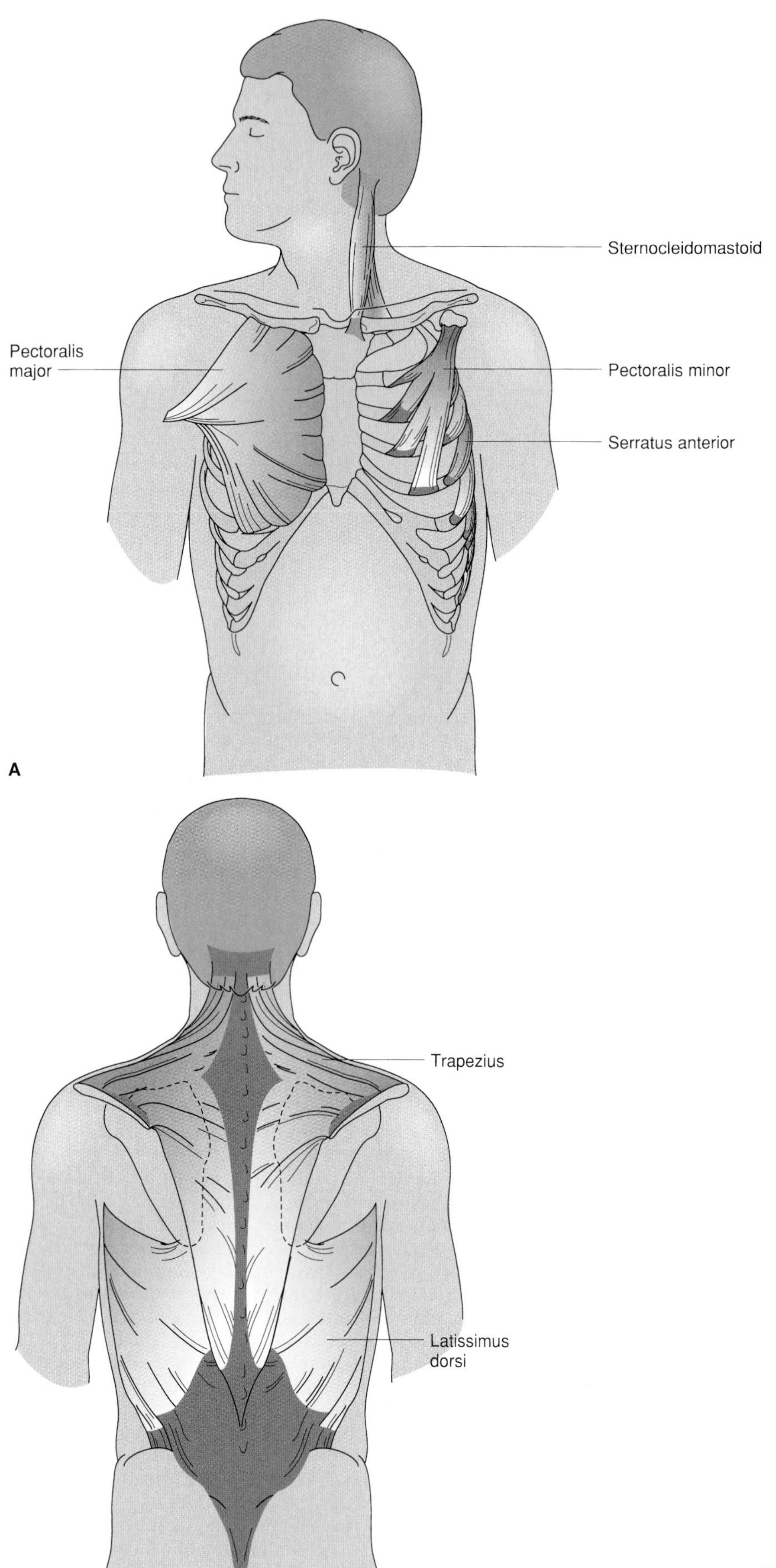

FIGURE 82.4 Thoracic musculature. Anterior (*A*) and posterior (*B*) views.

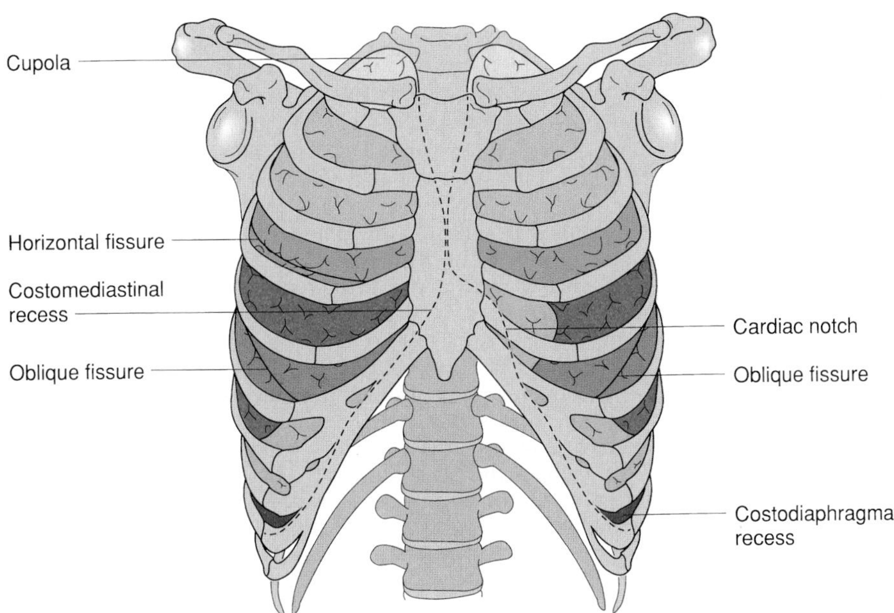

FIGURE 82.5 Topographic relations of the pleura to the chest wall. Laterally, the pleura extends to the level of the 11th to 12th ribs. The anterior reflection of the mediastinal and costal pleurae forms the costomediastinal recess, whereas the reflections of the costal and diaphragmatic pleurae form the costodiaphragmatic recess.

patients with pectus excavatum deformities undergo surgical repair. In a study by Fonkalsrud et al.[2] of 375 pectus excavatum repairs, only 47% had repair by age 11 years and 10% were age 20 years or older at the time of repair.

Since the Ochsner and DeBakey[10] series in 1939, various techniques have been developed to repair the pectus. Operative approaches can be classified into procedures that use no special support mechanism for sternal reconstruction and methods that use some type of support. Support can be either internal (vascularized and nonvascularized bone struts, metal struts, and Marlex) or external.[11] The most popular approach currently involves transverse inframammary incision or a midline incision, exposure of the sternum and cartilages, subperichondrial resection of the cartilages, sternal osteotomy, and anterior displacement of the sternum with or without strut support. Another technique involves 180-degree

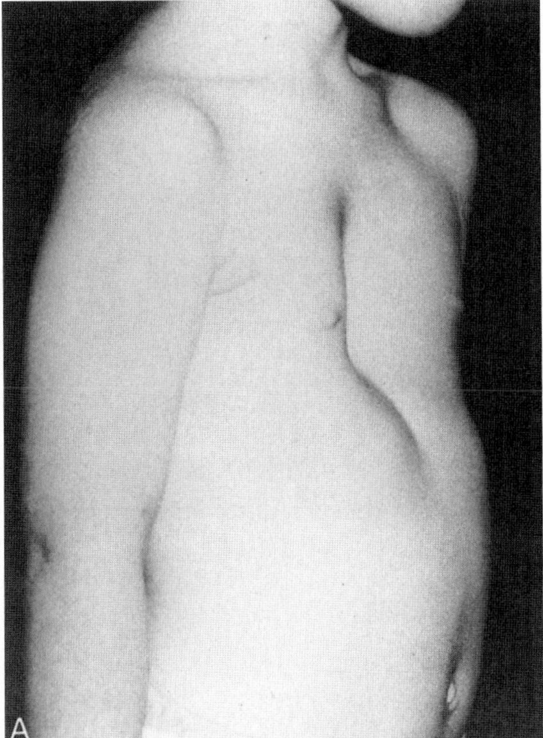

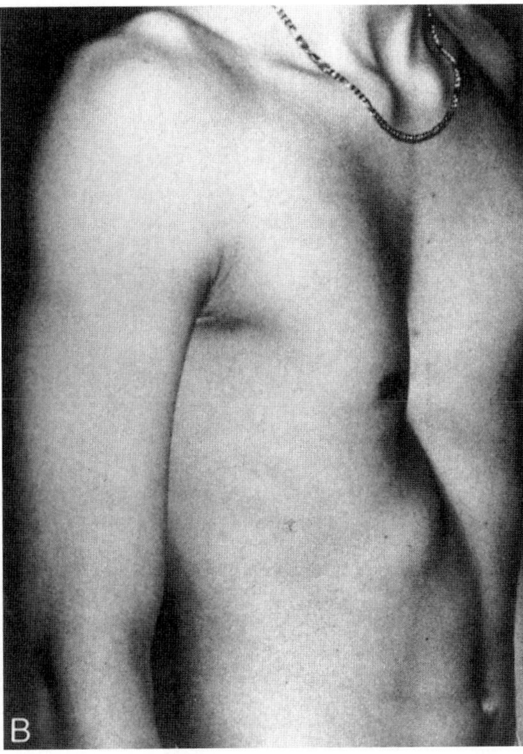

FIGURE 82.6 Photograph of (*A*) a 4.5-year-old girl with a symmetric pectus excavatum deformity and (*B*) a 16-year-old boy with pectus excavatum. Note that the depression extends to the sternal notch. (Adapted with permission from Shamberger RC. Chest wall deformities. In: Shields TW, ed. *General Thoracic Surgery.* 4th ed. Baltimore: Williams & Wilkins, 1994:529–557.)

rotation of the sternum and cartilages while preserving the internal mammary arteries.[12] One final technique popularized because of its simplicity involves placement of a subcutaneous silicone implant to correct the cosmetic defect, but without correction of the sternal displacement and hence none of the hemodynamic benefits.[13] Excellent results have been reported with each technique. The main postoperative complications are wound infection and a 1% incidence of pneumothorax. More than 90% of patients report excellent cosmetic results and improvement in cardiopulmonary function. The largest series reported recurrences of less than 10%.[7,14,15] Nuss et al.[16]) have reported on 42 patients (age 15 months to 15 years) who underwent correction of their deformity by a minimally invasive technique. At a mean follow-up of 4.6 years, results are encouraging, and this technique has become preferred at a number of major centers.

Long-term follow-up is required, especially with regard to recurrences during the rapid growth phase of puberty that can dramatically alter the appearance of the chest wall. Fonkalsrud and Bustorff-Silva[17]reported on their experience with pectus repair in 23 adults age 20 years and older who presented with poor exercise tolerance. Although the procedure was more difficult than when performed in younger patients, results were similar, with improved exercise tolerance and no recurrence.

Protrusion Deformities/Pectus Carinatum

Pectus carinatum (pigeon breast) is an anterior protrusion defect of the sternum and costal cartilages (Fig. 82.7).[3] Like pectus excavatum, this condition affects more males than females (3.6:1), but is less common than pectus excavatum by a ratio of 1:5.[18] This defect may not be apparent until the first decade of life. Similar to pectus excavatum, a familial predisposition is noted in 26% of cases and is associated with musculoskeletal defects, such as scoliosis (15%) and congenital heart disease.[18]

Protrusion deformities can be classified into three types. The most frequent type is the chondrogladiolar prominence variant (keel chest), which is an anterior displacement of the body of the sternum and symmetrical concavity of the costal cartilages. The sternum is elongated and the sternoxiphoidal junction is prominent. The second type is the lateral pectus carinatum, which occurs as a unilateral protrusion of the costal cartilages and is usually accompanied by sternal rotation about its long axis to the opposite side. The third and least common type is termed the *pouter pigeon breast* or chondromanubrial prominence and presents as a protrusion of the manubrium and depression of the sternal body.

Symptoms of pectus carinatum become more common as the patient ages and chest wall rigidity increases. These symptoms include exertional dyspnea or cardiac arrhythmia. Evaluation of cardiopulmonary function includes pulmonary function tests, echocardiography, and exercise testing.

An operative technique similar to the one for excavatum repair is used. The sternum and cartilage are exposed followed by subperichondrial resection of the cartilages. Sternal osteotomies may not be necessary except to correct sternal angulation (Fig. 82.8).[18] Postoperative complications are uncommon and include wound infection, wound dehiscence, and pneumothorax. Most patients achieve excellent results with few recurrences.

Poland Syndrome

Poland syndrome described in 1841 is a constellation of abnormalities that include hypoplasia of the breast and subcutaneous tissues, absence of the pectoralis major muscles, absence or hypoplasia of the pectoralis minor, and absence of costal cartilages. In addition, syndactyly, brachydactyly, or absence of phalanges has been described. The clinical manifestation of this defect can be quite variable. This rare defect is present in 1:30,000 births. Unlike pectus deformities, it does not appear to have a familial predisposition, but it also has variable degrees of severity.[19] Most commonly this defect is repaired using a latissimus dorsi myocutaneous flap with the addition of a breast implant in women. (Fig. 82.9).[3,20–25]

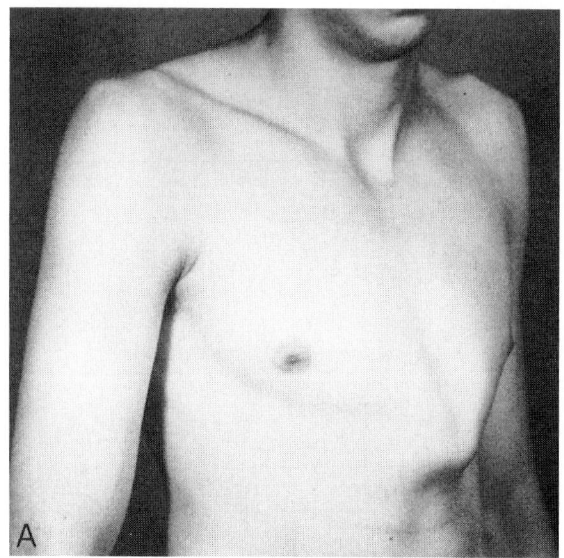

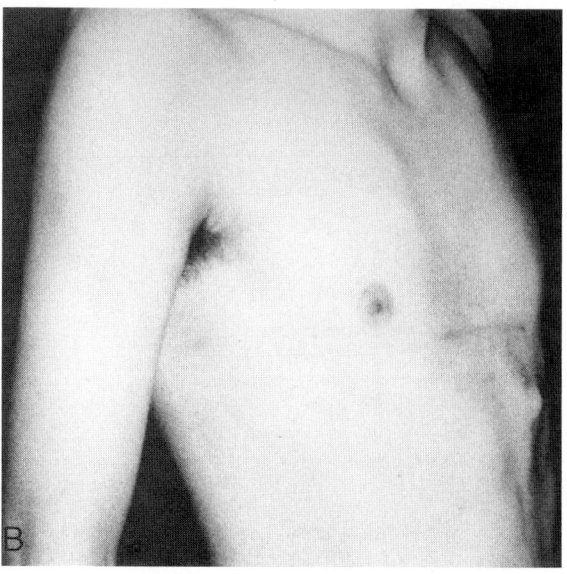

FIGURE 82.7 Photograph of (*A*) symmetric chondrogladiolar pectus carinatum in a 19-year-old man. Postoperative photograph (*B*) shows correction of the protruding sternum and costal cartilages. (Adapted with permission from Shamberger RC. Chest wall deformities. In: Shields TW, ed. *General Thoracic Surgery*. 4th ed. Baltimore: Williams & Wilkins, 1994:529–557.)

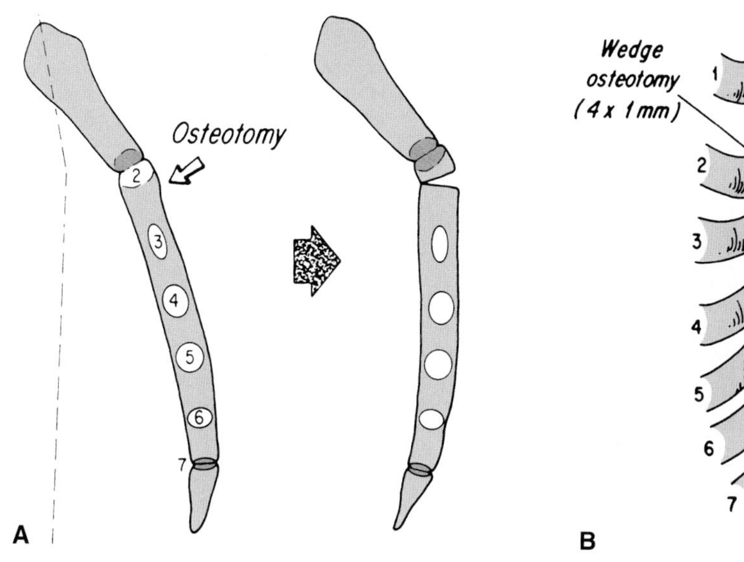

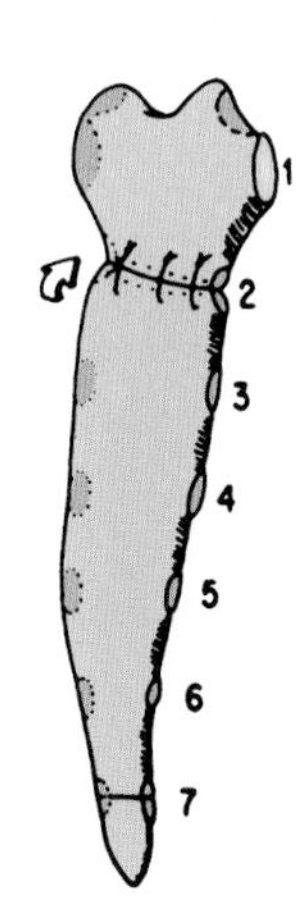

FIGURE 82.8 (*A*) A single or double osteotomy after resection of the costal cartilages allows posterior displacement of the sternum to an orthotopic position. (*B*) The mixed pectus deformity is corrected by full and symmetric resection of the third to seventh costal cartilages followed by transverse offset—0 to 10 degrees—wedge-shaped sternal osteotomy. Closure of this defect permits both anterior displacement and rotation of the sternum.

Sternal Clefts

A superior sternal cleft has a V- or U-shape appearance that can extend to the fourth costal cartilage. This defect can be repaired by direct apposition of the two sternal bands after oblique chondrotomies. If the defect is broad enough, hypotension may occur during apposition and prosthetic material would have to be used to diminish the constriction of mediastinal structures (Fig. 82.10).[26]

Complete sternal clefts involve the entire sternum, but also are associated with a crescentic anterior diaphragmatic defect and diastasis recti, which results in free communication between the peritoneal and pericardial cavities. Repair is accomplished with approximation of the pericardium and recti muscles, and prosthetic material is used to cover the sternal gap.

Distal sternal clefts are the most extensive defects and are associated with Cantrell's pentalogy, which includes distal cleft in the sternum, omphalocele, diaphragmatic cleft, pericardial defect and congenital heart defect (ventricular septal defect, tetralogy of Fallot). Primary sternal closure can be accomplished.[27–29]

CHEST WALL TUMORS

Chest wall tumors are rare. Most arise in the ribs (85%) with the remainder arising from the scapula, sternum, and clavicle.[30] These neoplasms can be classified as benign or malignant tumors of bone and soft tissue (Table 82.1)[31] and as primary versus metastatic malignant tumors. Metastatic tumors to the ribs are the most common malignant chest wall tumors, and primary bone tumors account for approximately 7% to 8% of all chest wall tumors.

Most chest wall tumors start as asymptomatic nodules that slowly enlarge and eventually cause pain. Pain signifies periosteal invasion and is more common with malignant tumors.[32] Appropriate evaluation of these patients includes thorough history and physical examination, computed tomography (CT) scan, and bone scan to rule out multiple lesions. Sagittal images from either magnetic resonance imaging (MRI) or three-dimensional CT scan are very helpful.

Pathologic diagnosis is confirmed by an excisional rather than incisional biopsy so that low-grade malignancies are not misdiagnosed. If malignancy is confirmed, wide resection is needed. The effect of resection margins on recurrences was analyzed in the Mayo Clinic series. Twice as many recurrences were noted with a 2-cm resection margin than with a 4-cm margin.[33–35]

Benign Bone Lesions

Fibrous Dysplasia

Fibrous dysplasia is a slow-growing lesion of the rib shaft that accounts for more than 30% of benign chest wall tumors. Most common during the third and fourth decade of life with no sex predisposition, fibrous dysplasia has a characteristic "soap bubble" or "ground glass" appearance on chest radiograph (Fig. 82.11). Fibrous dysplasia may cause pain as it enlarges, and pathologic fractures can develop. Fibrous dysplasia can also occur as part of Albright syndrome, in which the lesions are multiple and are associated with precocious puberty and skin pigmentation. Excision is indicated for symptom relief and to confirm the diagnosis.

Chondroma

Chondromas tend to occur during the second or third decade of life. They are also asymptomatic slow-growing tumors, but they tend to occur at the costochondral junction anteriorly. They have equal frequency in men and women and account for 15% to 20% of benign lesions of the chest wall. They can be divided into two types. The enchondroma arises in the medulla, and periosteal chondroma arises in the periosteum.

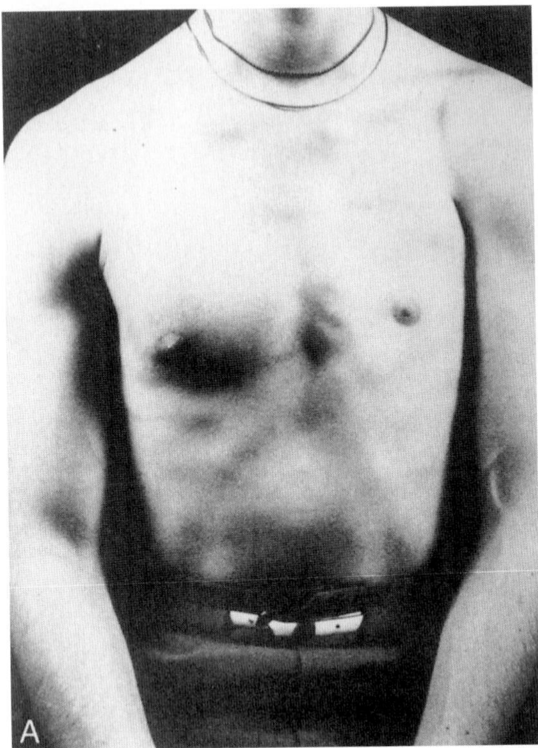

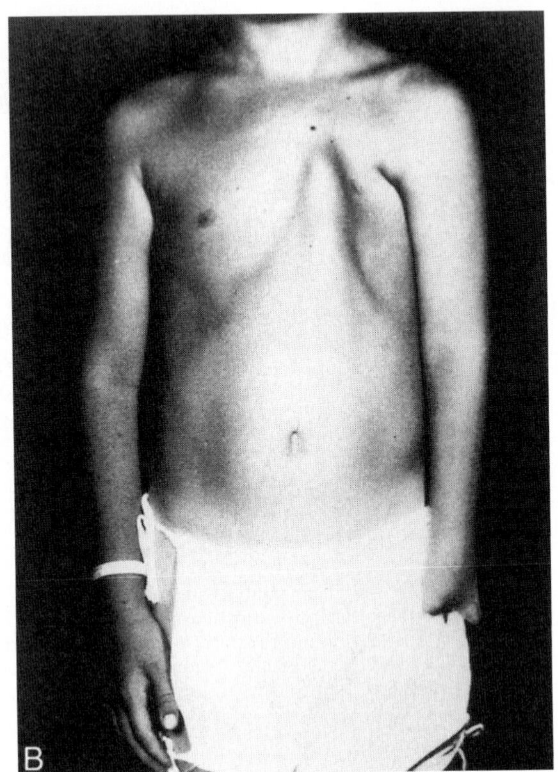

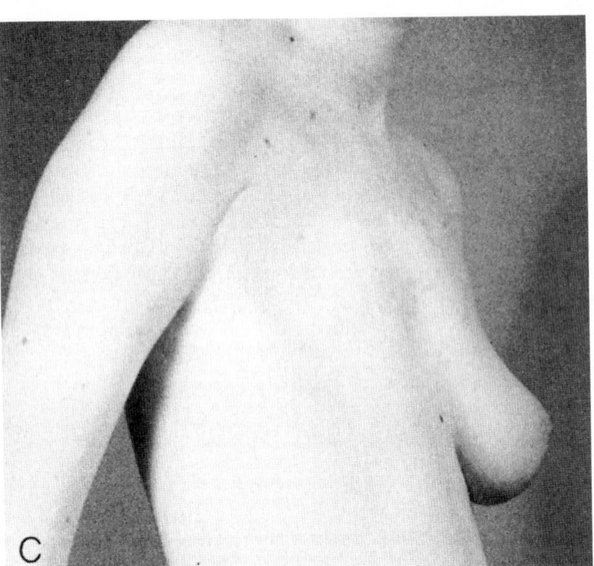

FIGURE 82.9 (*A*) muscular 15-year-old boy with loss of the left axillary fold, orthotopic sternum, and normal cartilages. He compensates adequately for loss of the pectoralis major and minor muscles. Surgery is not indicated in males with these findings. (*B*) An 8-year-old boy with Poland's syndrome. The pectoralis major and minor muscles and the serratus to the level of the fifth rib are absent. The boy has sternal obliquity and the third to fifth ribs are short, ending in points. The corresponding cartilages are absent. The endothoracic fascia lies beneath a thin layer of subcutaneous tissue. Note the hypoplastic nipple and ectromelia of the ipsilateral hand. (C) A 14-year-old girl with Poland's syndrome. Note the high position of the right nipple, amastia, sternal rotation, and depressed right anterior chest. The second to fourth ribs and cartilages were missing, reconstructed with rib grafts. Breast augmentation will be required at full growth. (From Shamberger RC. Chest wall deformities. In: Shields TW, ed. *General Thoracic Surgery*. 4th ed. Baltimore: Williams & Wilkins, 1994:529–557.)

Chondromas appear as lytic lesions with sclerotic margins on chest radiograph and are difficult to distinguish from chondrosarcomas either radiographically or histologically. Excisional biopsy is always recommended.[36]

Osteochondroma

An osteochondroma presents as a painless mass in young men (male to female ratio of 3:1). The mass originates from the cortex of the rib and has a characteristic appearance on a chest radiograph of a pedunculated bony mass capped with viable cartilage (Fig. 82.12).Familial osteochondromatosis is a variant that presents with multiple lesions. Resection is indicated for symptomatic and enlarging lesions. Recurrences are rare.

Eosinophilic Granuloma

Eosinophilic granuloma is a benign condition that primarily affects men. Multiple lesions of skull and rib are common. On plain radiographs they appear as expansile bone lesions. A solitary lesion can be excised, and radiotherapy is best for patients with multiple lesions.

Osteoid Osteomas

Osteoid osteomas are rare tumors that also affect men more frequently. They arise in the bony cortex of the rib or vertebral bodies and tend to be symptomatic especially at night. A small, radiolucent nidus encircled by a sclerotic margin is frequently seen on chest radiography. Rib resection provides relief of symptoms.

A

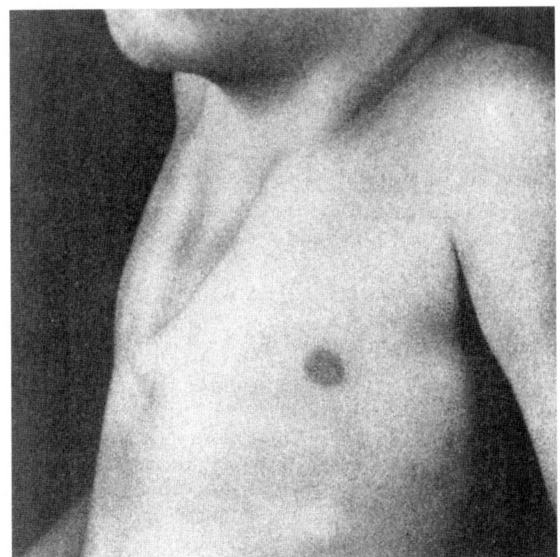

B

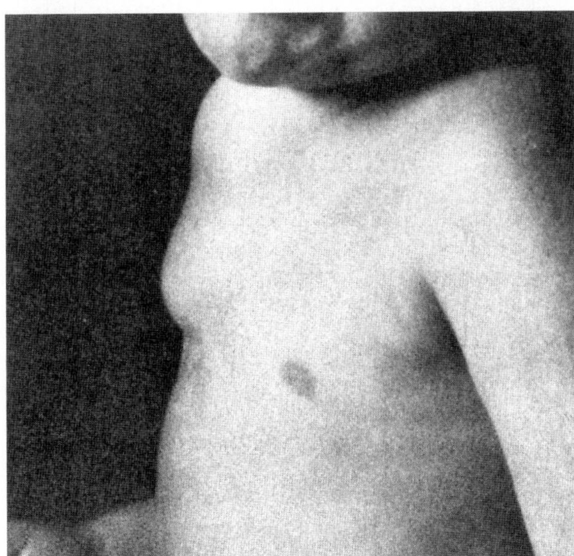

FIGURE 82.10 Cleft sternum at rest (*A*) and during forced expiration (*B*). Superior clefts of the sternum are variously V- or U-shaped. The appearance of the child as he cries explains the term *ectopia cordis*, although the heart is actually not misplaced. In the newborn, defects of this kind can be corrected by direct apposition of the sternal halves. In this child, closure of the defect was made possible by sliding chondrotomies on either side. (From Sabiston DC Jr. The surgical management of congenital bifid sternum with a partial ectopia cordis. *J Thorac Surg*. 1958;35:118.)

Malignant Bone Lesions

Chondrosarcoma

Chondrosarcoma is the most common of the chest wall malignant tumors, accounting for 20% of such tumors. Usually seen after the fourth decade of life, these lesions can arise after local trauma to the chest or secondary to malignant degeneration of benign chondromas or osteochondromas. They tend to present as an anterior chest mass and usually involve the anterior costochondral junctions of the sternum.[36,37] On chest radiography, they tend to have a similar appearance to benign chondromas. Resection with wide margins provides the best chance of local control, and 4 cm is recommended. Five-year survival rates of 70% have been reported after complete excision.[36,37]

TABLE 82.1 CLASSIFICATION

PRIMARY CHEST WALL TUMOR

MALIGNANT
Myeloma
- Malignant fibrous histiocytoma
- Chondrosarcoma
- Rhabdomyosarcoma
- Ewing's sarcoma
- Liposarcoma
- Neurofibrosarcoma
- Osteogenic sarcoma
- Hemangiosarcoma

Leiomyosarcoma
- Lymphoma

BENIGN
Osteochondroma
Chondroma
Desmoid
Fibrous dysplasia
Lipoma
Fibroma
Neurilemoma

From Pairolero P. Chest wall tumors. In: Shields TW, Locicero J, Ponn R, eds. *General thoracic surgery*, 5th ed. Philadelphia: Lippincott Williams & Wilkins, 2000, pp. 589–598.

Osteogenic Sarcoma

Although it is more common in the extremities, osteogenic sarcomas do occur in the ribs and account for 10% to 15% of malignant tumors. Chest radiographs reveal the characteristic

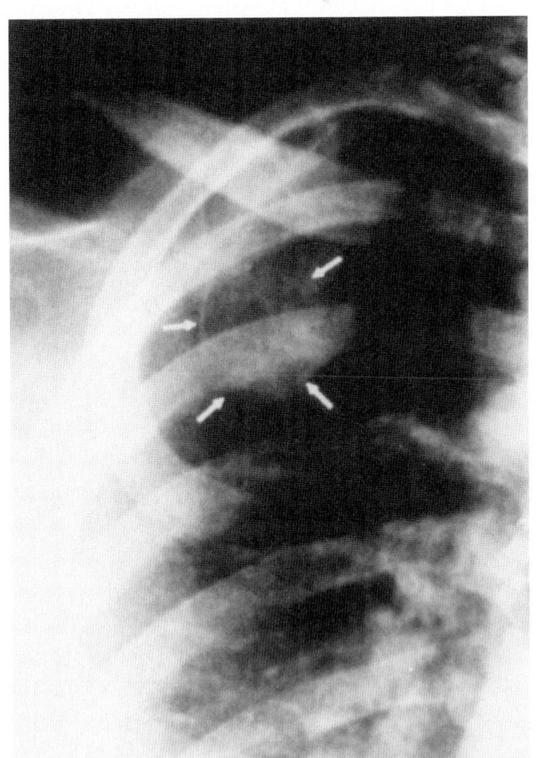

FIGURE 82.11 Fibrous dysplasia of the rib. Note the characteristic expansion and thinning of the cortex (*arrows*) and the central ground-glass appearance.

LUNG

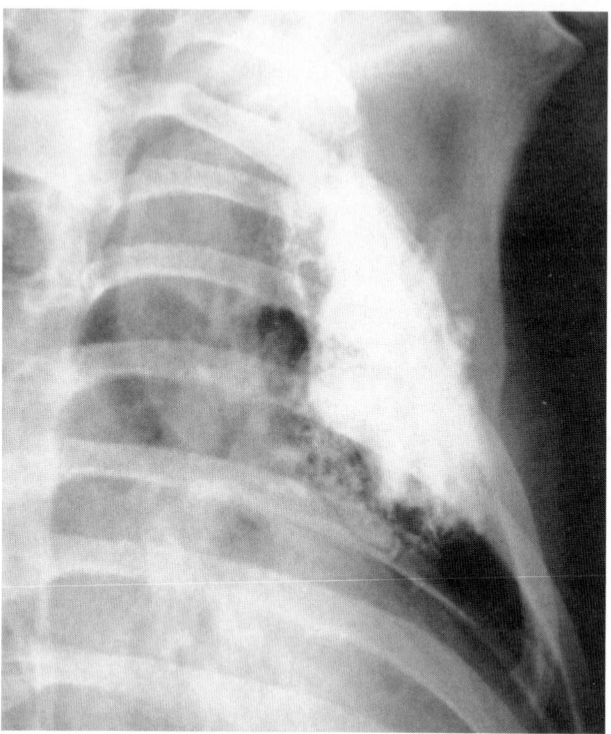

FIGURE 82.12 Osteochondroma of left second rib. The stippled calcification within the tumor and the intact cortex of the rib are characteristic.

"sunburst" pattern. Unlike chondrosarcomas, they tend to enlarge rapidly, and metastases are often present at initial evaluation. Chest and abdominal CT scan and bone scan are indicated for assessment of metastatic disease. Five-year survival following complete excision only can be as low as 20%, whereas survival after surgery and adjuvant chemotherapy rises to 60%.[38]

Ewing's Sarcoma

Ewing's sarcoma is the third most common malignant chest wall tumor (5% to 10%). It occurs more frequently in children and young men and has 2:1 male to female ratio. Patients complain of intermittent pain, and often there is an inflammatory response with fever and leukocytosis. Chest radiographs show the characteristic "onion peel" appearance. Similar to osteogenic sarcoma, metastases are common at initial presentation, displaying a preference for the lung and central nervous system. Five-year survival has improved to 50% using multimodality therapy (surgery followed by chemotherapy and radiotherapy).[39–42]

Solitary Plasmacytoma

Solitary plasmacytoma is a rare tumor arising from plasma cells. Many believe that this tumor is a harbinger of multiple myeloma, and often patients diagnosed with solitary plasmacytoma eventually develop systemic disease. Age at presentation is usually older than 50 years, and there is a male predisposition. Symptoms of pain with no palpable mass are common. Patients usually have an abnormal serum protein electrophoresis, Bence-Jones protein in the urine and bone marrow aspiration demonstrate cellular atypia. Biopsy will confirm the diagnosis (Fig. 82.13). A small solitary plasmacytoma should be completely resected. Whether to undertake extensive reconstructive procedures for this disease is controversial because differentiation from multiple myeloma can be quite difficult. Radiotherapy is the primary mode of therapy with a reported 5-year survival of 30%, although favorable results with radical excision have also been reported.[43,44]

Soft Tissue Tumors

Sarcomas are the most common malignant soft tissue chest wall tumors. Surgical excision is the preferred mode of therapy. Biopsy establishes the diagnosis, and, similar to sarcomas at other sites, mitotic rate, cellular pleomorphism, and nuclear to cytoplasmic ratio are used to classify them as low or high grade. Resection with wide margins and reconstruction is indicated. Adjuvant chemoradiation protocols are routinely used.

Metastatic Tumors

Hematologic dissemination is the most common cause of metastatic disease to the chest wall. Often radiation therapy is used for palliation. Surgical resection of an isolated rib metastasis, however, can provide excellent palliation in a shorter period of time and frequently with less morbidity.

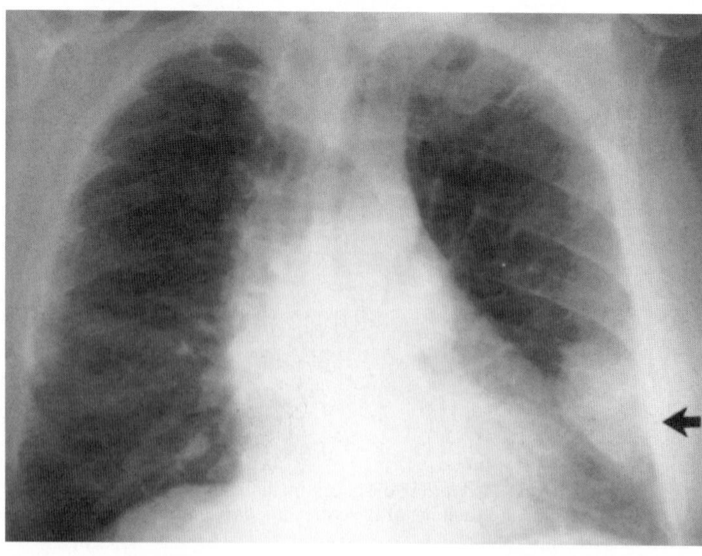

FIGURE 82.13 Plasmacytoma of the left seventh rib, showing characteristic cortical destruction and relatively large soft tissue component projecting into the chest.

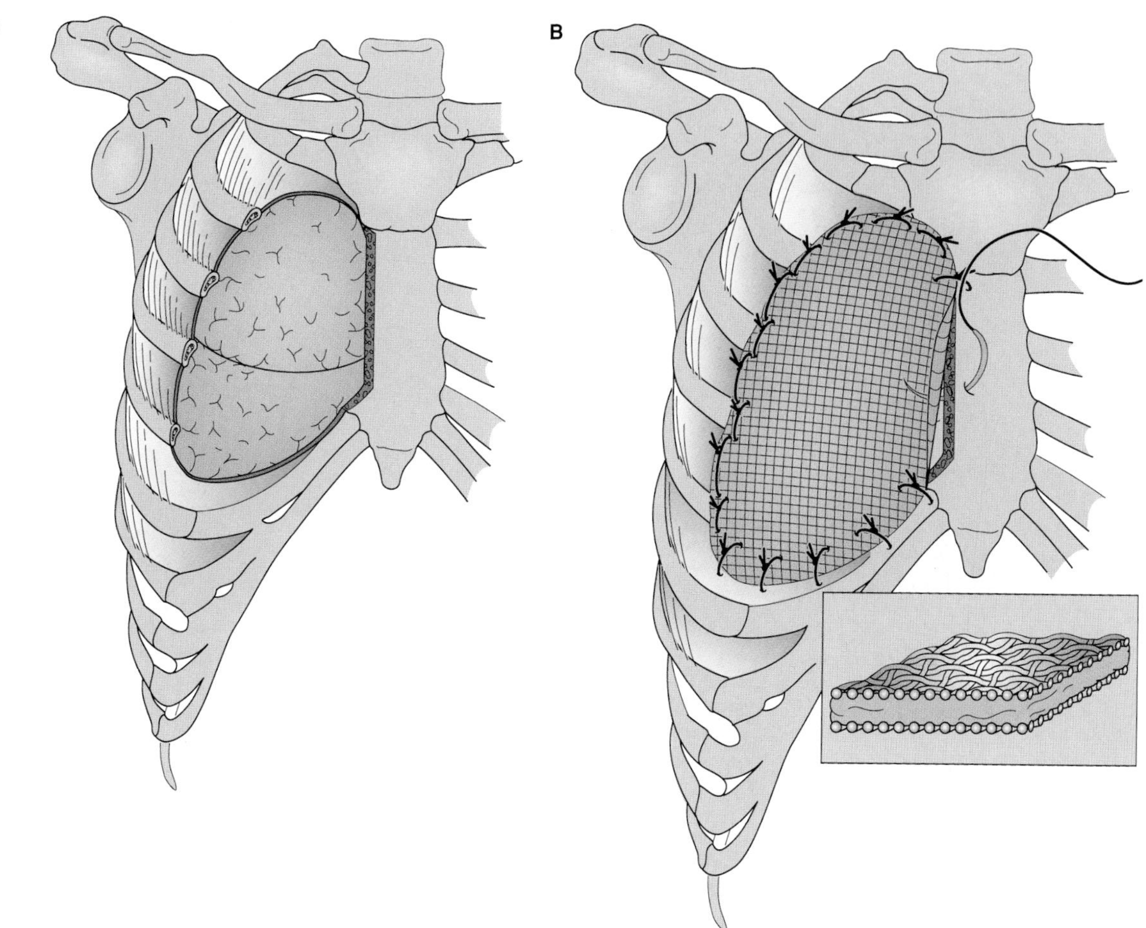

FIGURE 82.14 Marlex methylmethacrylate sandwich technique for chest wall reconstruction. (*A*) Upper anterior chest wall defect resulting from resection of ribs two to five and a portion of sternum. (*B*) Marlex methylmethacrylate prosthesis being sutured in place. Heavy, nonabsorable sutures either encircling the ribs or passed through the sternum are used to anchor the prosthesis in place. *Insert*: Detail of prosthesis showing sandwich of hardened methylmethacrylate between two sheets of Marlex.

Direct extension of breast and lung cancer to the chest wall is relatively common. In breast cancer, locoregional recurrence involving the chest wall can occur in more than 10% of stage II lesions following mastectomy.[45,46] Recurrences are treated with resection and adjuvant chemoradiotherapy.

CHEST WALL RECONSTRUCTION

The principal goals of chest wall reconstruction are protection of the intrathoracic organs, support of respiration by preventing paradoxical movement, and an acceptable cosmetic result without compromising the cancer operation. Reconstruction of the chest wall involves two parts: the bony thorax and the soft tissues.

The bony thorax is reconstructed on the basis of size and location of the defect. If the defect is small (less than 5 cm), then reconstruction may not be needed. If the defect is located posteriorly and deep to the scapula, then defects up to 10 cm in diameter may not need to be reconstructed. On the other hand, mesh closure of moderate sized (more than 5 cm) bony defects is straightforward, provides good cosmesis, and prevents scapular entrapment. A variety of prosthetic materials are available for reconstruction of the rib cage, such as Prolene mesh, Gore-Tex (W. L. Gore, Flagstaff, AZ), and methylmethacrylate-impregnated mesh (Fig. 82.14). These materials can be anchored to the surrounding chest wall to provide stability and the necessary rigidity for protection and respiration. Drainage of the subcutaneous tissues and chest cavity depends on the type of mesh used and its permeability to fluid. Iliac crest free bone grafts can provide excellent reconstructions of sternal body defects.

A variety of myocutaneous flaps have been developed. The latissimus dorsi flap, is the largest muscle of the thorax and hence can cover the largest defects (Fig. 82.15) . This flap can cover defects around a semicircle with the radius based on the origin of the thoracodorsal neurovascular supply. The pectoralis major flap, based on the thoracoacromial neurovascular supply, is the second largest muscle and has become the flap of choice for sternal defects (Fig. 82.16). Extra reach for both of these flaps can be achieved by dividing the tendonous insertion of the muscle while preserving the vascular pedicle. The rectus abdominis muscle is based on the internal mammary vessels and is mainly used for defects of the lower anterior chest wall and sternum (Fig. 82.17). The external oblique and serratus anterior muscles can also be used, but offer less coverage than the other flaps. Other options include the omentum and free flaps such as tensor fascia lata, but free flaps are more complicated and the omentum does not provide adequate coverage of large defects.[47–51]

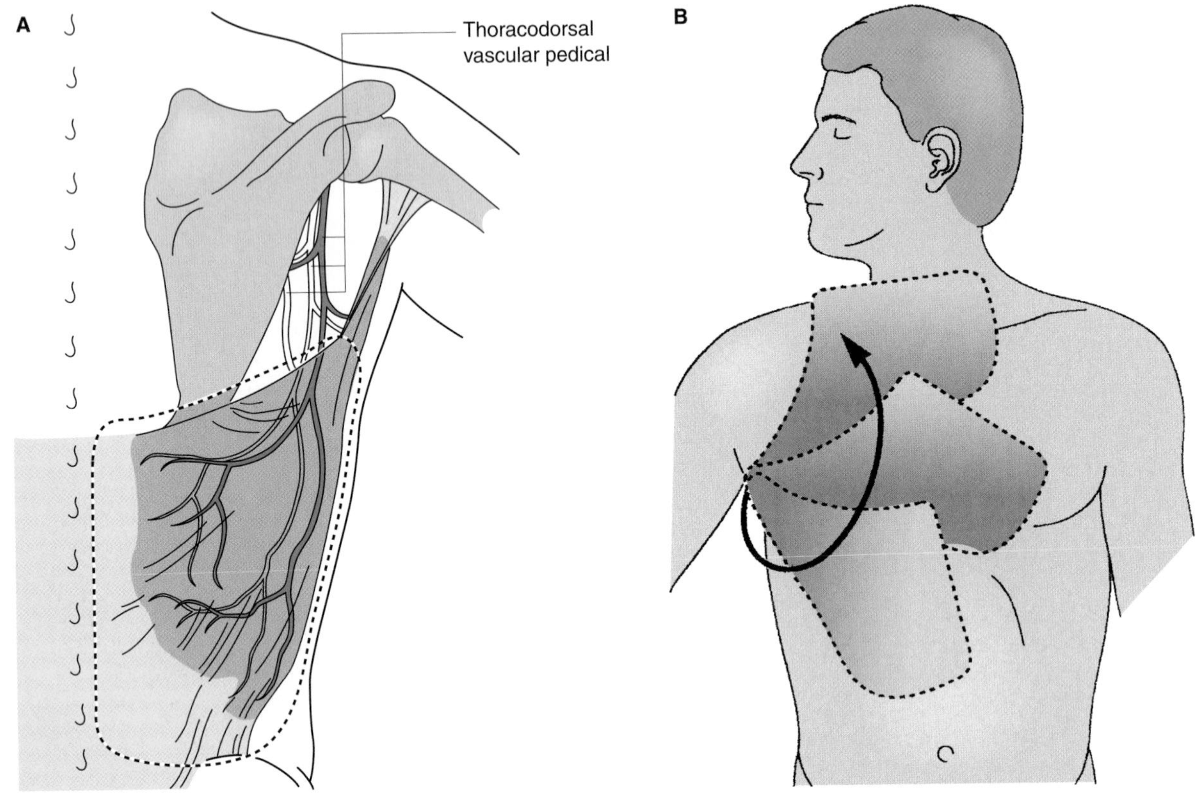

FIGURE 82.15 Latissimus dorsi muscle rotation flap for chest wall reconstruction. (*A*) Posterior view showing detachment of the origins of the muscle. The dominant blood supply, the thoracodorsal artery, is preserved. (*B*) Anterior view showing the extent to which the mobilized muscle reaches.

Thoracic Outlet Syndrome

Thoracic outlet syndrome (Fig. 82.18).[52] refers to compression of neurovascular structures at the thoracic outlet. The neurovascular structures involved are the subclavian artery and vein and the sympathetic and peripheral nerve components of the brachial plexus. The axillary vein courses posterior to the costocoracoid ligament and pectoralis minor tendon, eventually becoming the subclavian vein; it travels between the anterior scalene muscle and clavicle. The subclavian artery exits the chest behind the sternoclavicular joints, and, along with the trunks of the brachial plexus, it passes between the anterior and middle scalene muscles. Distal to the pectoralis tendon, the brachial cords form the motor and sensory nerves of the upper extremity.

The neurovascular structures can be compressed at three anatomic sites: the interscalene triangle, the costoclavicular space, and the subcoracoid area. In addition, numerous other factors such as cervical rib, scalene muscles, fibrous bands, spinal transverse processes, and trauma can cause compression (Table 82.2)[52–56]

The syndrome usually affects women. Neurologic complaints are more commonly seen than vascular ones, although a combination of both can be present. Pain and paresthesias are the most common symptoms followed by motor weakness and possibly atrophy of thenar and hypothenar muscles secondary to ulnar nerve compression. Compression of the median nerve results in index and middle finger paresthesias. Symptoms of vascular compromise include upper extremity claudication, coolness, and fatigue. Thrombosis and distal embolization are occasionally reported with the vascular compression syndrome. Repetitive arm motion can result in subclavian vein thrombosis, also known as Paget-Schroetter syndrome.[57]

For diagnostic purposes, four clinical maneuvers are used to reproduce the symptoms of the patient with thoracic outlet syndrome: the Adson or scalene test (Fig. 82.19), the costoclavicular or military test (Fig. 82.20), the hyperabduction test (Fig. 82.21), and the Roos test.[58] The Roos test involves abduction of the arm 90 degrees with external rotation of the shoulder while quickly opening and closing the fist for 3 minutes. All of these maneuvers, however, lack satisfactory sensitivity and specificity.

Plain radiographs are useful in detecting bony abnormalities. MRI can rule out cervical disease as the cause of the symptoms, whereas Doppler studies with provocative testing and an angiogram may be needed to assess vascular involvement. Nerve conduction velocities are useful to determine the site of compression.[59] A brachial plexus MRI with images obtained at rest and with arm abduction has been the most reliable diagnostic test in our hands.

Management

The majority of patients with thoracic outlet syndrome improve with physiotherapy such as posture training and stretching exercises.[60,61] Indications for surgery include persistent symptoms and continuing neurovascular problems, such as delayed conduction velocities. In addition, persistent vascular lesions like stenosis of the subclavian artery or aneurysms are indications for surgery. The procedure of choice is the transaxillary resection of the first rib and cervical rib when present. This procedure has good cosmetic results with excellent relief for neurologic symptoms. Recurrence of

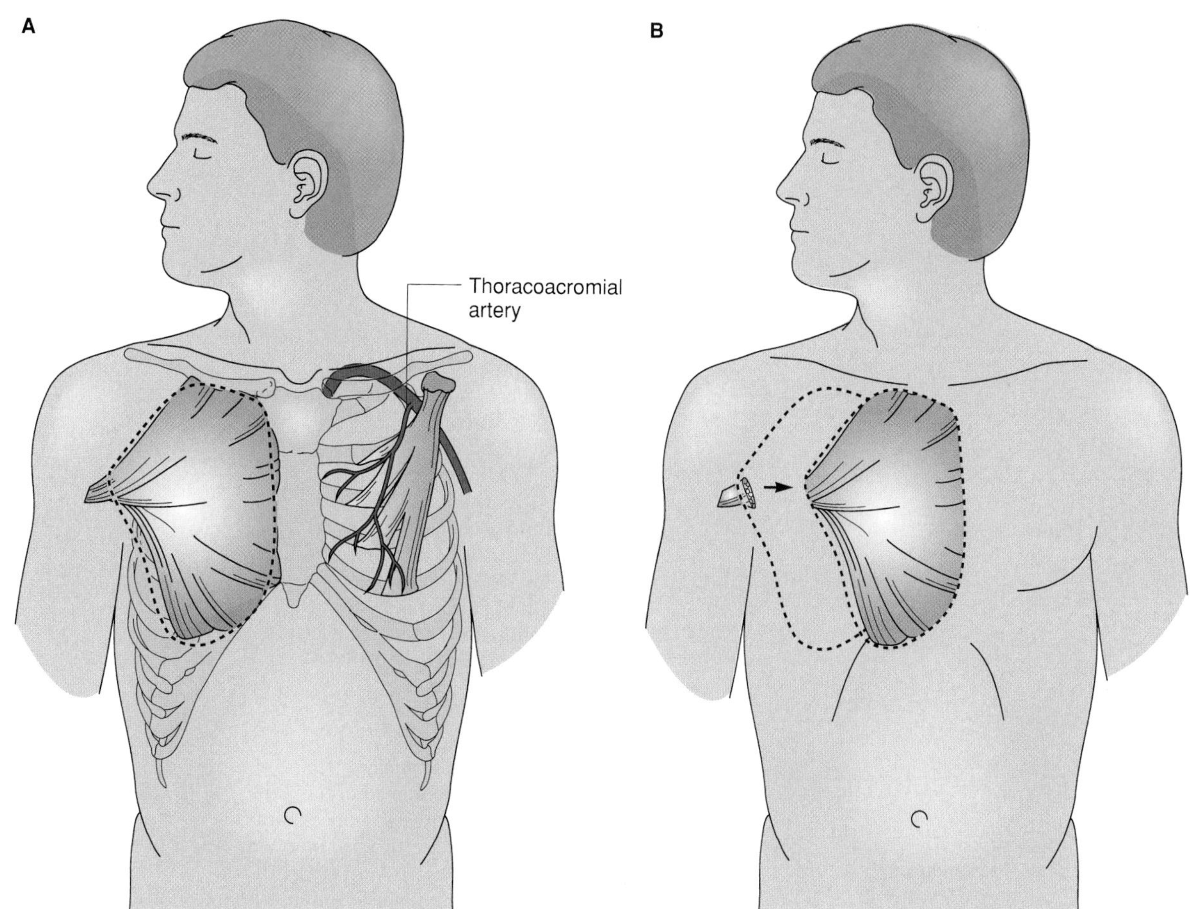

FIGURE 82.16 Pectoralis major muscle rotation flap. (*A*) Mobilization of the flap by detaching the clavicular, sternal, and chest wall origins as well as the insertion of the muscle on the greater tubercle of the humerus. The dominant blood supply, the thoracoacromial artery, which arises from the axillary artery medial to the proximal border of the pectoralis minor muscle is shown on the left side, where the pectoralis major muscle has been removed. (*B*) Medial transposition of the muscle flap, preserving the thoracoacromial neurovascular bundle.

symptoms has been reported in 2% to 30% of patients usually secondary to excessive scar formation or inadequate resection of the rib. Every effort should be made to resect the rib fully from the transverse process of the T1 vertebrae to the costomanubrial junction. Better results are reported in patients whose occupations do not require physical labor.[55,62–64] Complications include neurovascular injury, infection, incomplete resection of the cervical or first rib, and resection of the second rib instead of the first. Aneurysms of the subclavian artery can be addressed with saphenous or prosthetic graft bypass. Subclavian vein thrombosis should be treated with thrombolytic agents followed by first rib resection. Vein patch angioplasty via an anterior approach or balloon catheter dilation of the vein may be needed.

PLEURA

Anatomy

The pleural space is a potential space between the visceral pleura that envelops the lung and the parietal pleura that lines the chest wall. A small amount of fluid secreted by the mesothelial cells of the pleura normally lubricates the two surfaces. The visceral pleura is intimately adherent to the lung. The parietal pleura can be stripped from the ribs and mediastinum, but not from the central tendon of the diaphragm or the pericardium. The intercostal nerves innervate the visceral pleura including the diaphragmatic portion. They are rich in sensory innervations. The visceral pleura receives sympathetic and parasympathetic components, but it has no sensory component. The lymphatic drainage of the visceral pleura is directed toward the mediastinal lymph nodes, and the parietal pleura lymphatics drain into the regional nodes. Thus, the cervical pleura can drain into the axillary nodes, the costal pleura can drain into the intercostal and sternal nodes, the diaphragmatic pleura drains into the phrenic nodes, and the mediastinal pleura drains into the mediastinal nodes.

Pleural Effusions

A pleural effusion is an abnormal accumulation of fluid in the pleural space secondary to pleural or systemic disease. Normally only a small amount of fluid is present in the pleural space, although a liter of fluid is secreted daily by the parietal pleura and absorbed by the visceral pleura. Pleural effusions

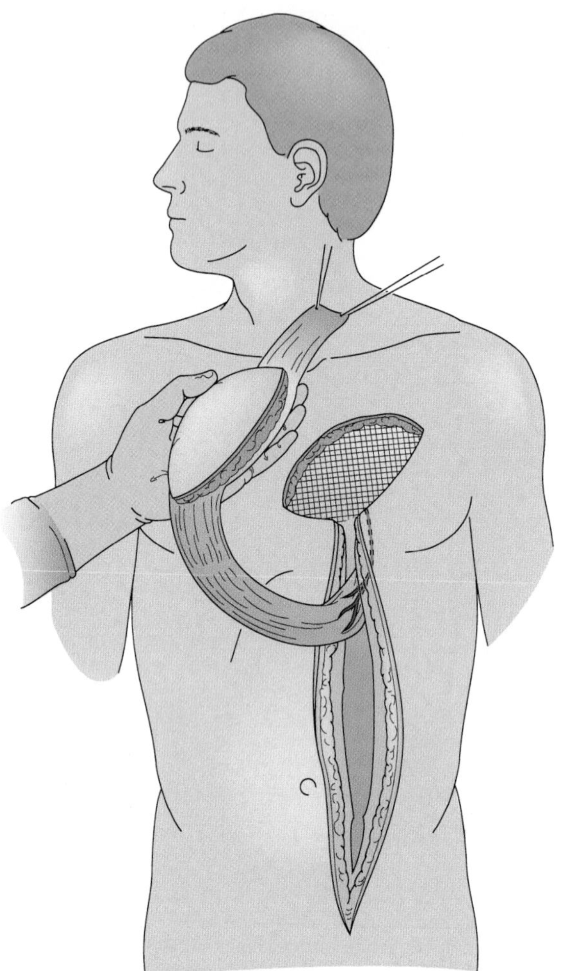

FIGURE 82.17 Rectus abdominis muscle rotation flap. Shown is the mobilization of the rectus abdominis muscle, which is based on the superior epigastric artery (the continuation of the internal thoracic artery), and rotation of the muscle and overlying skin to fill an anterior chest wall defect.

TABLE 82.2 ETIOLOGY

ETIOLOGIC FACTORS OF NEUROVASCULAR COMPRESSION SYNDROMES

ANATOMIC
Potential sites of neurovascular compression
Interscalene triangle
Costoclavicular space
Subcoracoid area
CONGENITAL
Cervical rib and its fascial remnants
Rudimentary first thoracic rib
Scalene muscles
Anterior
Middle
Minimus
Adventitious fibrous bands
Bifid clavicle
Exostosis of first thoracic rib
Enlarged transverse process of C7
Omohyoid muscle
Anomalous course of transverse cervical artery
Brachial plexus postfixed
Flat clavicle
TRAUMATIC
Fracture of clavicle
Dislocation of head of humerus
Crushing injury to upper thorax
Sudden, unaccustomed muscular efforts involving shoulder girdle muscles
Cervical spondylosis and injuries to cervical spine
ATHEROSCLEROSIS

From Urschel HC Jr, Razzuk MA. Thoracic outlet syndrome. In: Sabiston DC Jr, Spencer FC, eds. *Surgery of the chest*. Philadelphia: WB Saunders, 1990, pp. 536–553.

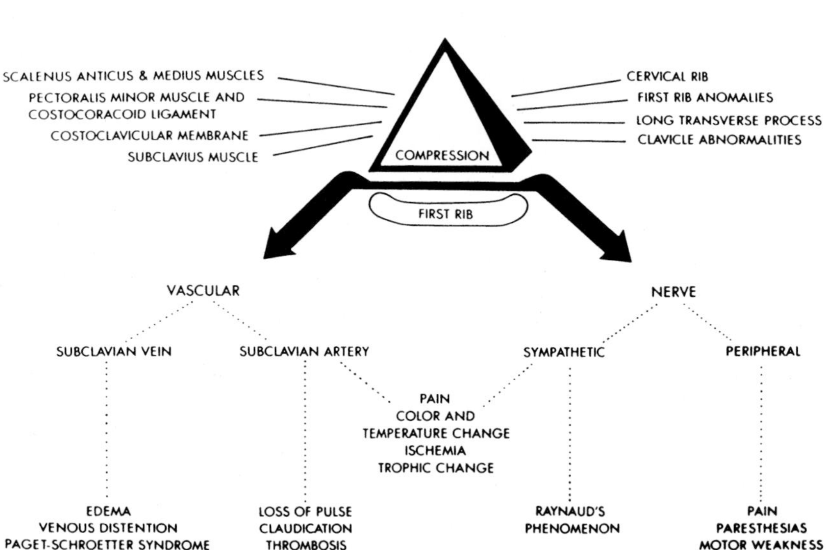

FIGURE 82.18 Schematic diagram showing the relation of muscle, ligament, and bone abnormalities in the thoracic outlet that may compress neurovascular structures against the first rib. (From Urschel HC Jr, Razzuk MA. Thoracic outlet syndrome. In: Sabiston DC Jr, Spencer FC, eds. *Surgery of the chest*. Philadelphia: WB Saunders, 1990, pp. 536–553.)

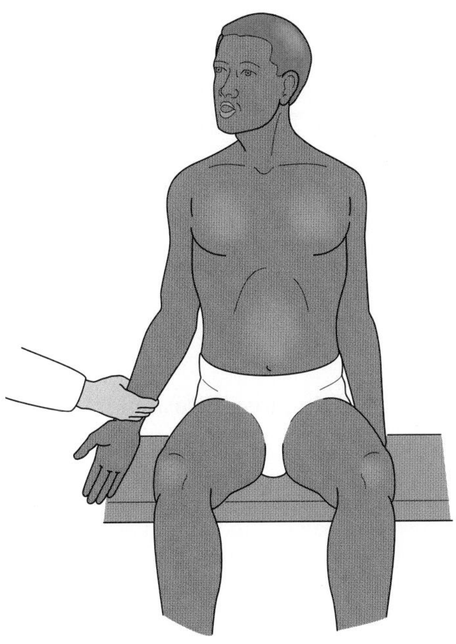

FIGURE 82.19 Adson's maneuver. Relation of scalene triangle to the neurovascular bundle.

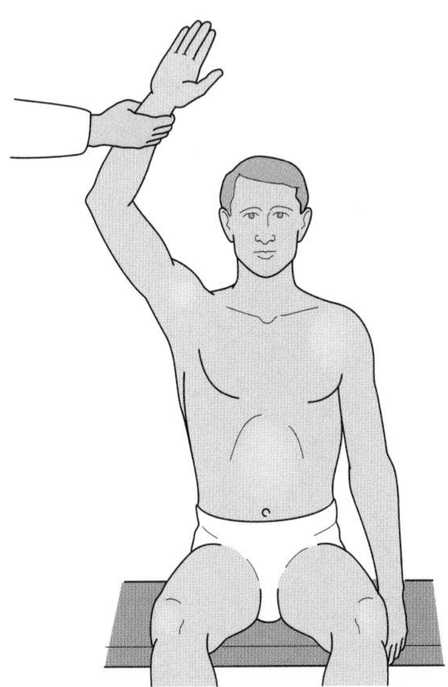

FIGURE 82.21 Hyperabduction maneuver. Relation of neurovascular bundle to pectoralis minor tendon, coracoid process, and humeral head (pulley effect).

may result from either increased hydrostatic pressure in adjacent capillary beds, increased negative intrapleural pressure, increased capillary permeability, decreased plasma oncotic pressure, or interrupted lymphatic drainage.

Pleural effusions can be asymptomatic or can present with pleuritic chest pain, dyspnea, and fever if secondary to an inflammatory process or with constant pain if secondary to malignancy. The first sign of a pleural effusion on an upright chest radiograph is blunting of the costophrenic angle; this requires more than 250 cc of fluid accumulation. Lateral decubitus films can demonstrate these effusions in patients who cannot sit upright. Chest CT scan often provides a better estimate of the volume of an effusion than chest radiograph.

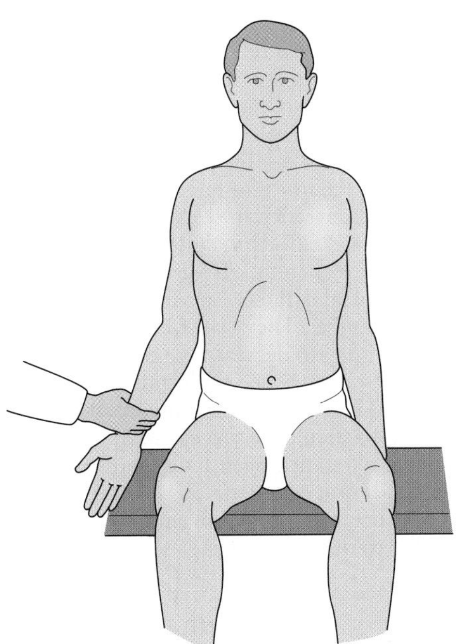

FIGURE 82.20 Costoclavicular maneuver (military position). Relation of costoclavicular space to neurovascular bundle.

Pleural effusions are either benign or malignant in origin and can be divided for diagnostic purposes into transudative or exudative categories. The distinction between transudates and exudates (Table 82.3)[65] is based on serum and pleural fluid ratios for lactate dehydrogenase (LDH) and protein (Table 82.4). Transudative effusions form because of changes in the dynamics of pleural fluid absorption or secretion. Exudative effusions, in contrast, result from changes in lymphatic vessel or pleural integrity and therefore are rich in protein. Effusions should also be tested routinely for the presence of bacteria and malignant cells. Measurement of pH, glucose, lipids, and amylase should also be done to help differentiate among the etiologies in Table 82.4.

Transudative Effusions

Transudative effusions tend to be benign. They usually do not become loculated and are free flowing. Common causes include systemic diseases such as congestive heart failure, cirrhosis, nephrotic syndrome, and hypoalbuminemia. Systemic conditions tend to result in bilateral effusions. Local processes that can cause transudative effusions include lobar collapse and pulmonary embolism. If these effusions remain untreated and become longstanding, they may develop exudative features. If an effusion is determined to be transudative, it can be treated usually by thoracentesis because of benign and treatable causes. Control of the systemic process that led to the effusion is of paramount importance to prevent fluid reaccumulation. If control of the systemic processes is suboptimal, which is often the case, then recurrent pleural effusions can be a problem. Repeat thoracentesis can be used, but the patient may need multiple treatments to control symptoms. Potential complications such as pneumothorax can be minimized with the use of ultrasound guidance at the time of drainage. However, loculations can eventually form with repeated thoracentesis from the pleural inflammatory response, and become infected secondarily. Alternatively, pleurodesis can be

TABLE 82.3 DIAGNOSIS

DIFFERENTIAL DIAGNOSIS OF PLEURAL EFFUSIONS

TRANSUDATIVE PLEURAL EFFUSIONS
Congestive heart failure
Pericardial disease
Cirrhosis
Nephrotic syndrome
Peritoneal dialysis
Superior vena cava obstruction
Myxedema
Pulmonary emboli
Sarcoidosis
Urinothorax

EXUDATIVE PLEURAL EFFUSIONS
Neoplastic diseases
- Metastatic disease
- Mesothelioma

Infectious diseases
- Bacterial infections
- Tuberculosis
- Fungal infections
- Viral infections
- Parasitic infections
- Pulmonary embolization

Gastrointestinal disease
- Esophageal perforation
- Pancreatic disease
- Intraabdominal abscess
- Diaphragmatic hernia
- Postabdominal surgery
- Endoscopic variceal sclerotherapy

Collagen vascular diseases
- Rheumatoid pleuritis
- Systemic lupus erythematosus
- Drug-induced lupus erythematosus
- Immunoblastic lymphadenopathy
- Sjögren syndrome
- Wegener granulomatosis
- Churg-Strauss syndrome

Postcardiac injury syndrome
Asbestos exposure
Sarcoidosis
Uremia
Meigs' syndrome
Yellow nail syndrome
Drug-induced pleural disease
- Nitrofurantoin
- Dantrolene
- Methysergide
- Bromocriptine
- Procarbazine
- Amiodarone

Trapped lung
Radiotherapy
Electric burns
Urinary tract obstruction
Iatrogenic injury
Ovarian hyperstimulation syndrome
Chylothorax
Hemothorax

carried out via chest tube insertion or thoracoscopically by instilling doxycycline or talc into the pleural space. The resulting inflammation tends to obliterate the potential pleural space, preventing reaccumulation of fluid.

TABLE 82.4

CRITERIA FOR EXUDATIVE EFFUSIONS BASED ON RATIO OF PLEURAL FLUID PROTEIN AND LDH CONCENTRATIONS TO SERUM CONCENTRATION

Protein/serum protein >0.5
LDH/serum LDH >0.6
Pleural LDH 1.67 times normal serum LDH

LDH, lactate dehydrogenase.

Exudative Effusions

The most common cause of an exudative effusion is malignancy. Causes other than neoplastic disease include pulmonary infections that can result in empyemas, collagen vascular diseases, Dressler syndrome, subdiaphragmatic intraperitoneal infections, and pulmonary infarction. The tumors most commonly involved with malignant pleural effusions are lung and breast cancer, lymphoma, ovarian, renal, and colon cancer.

Malignant Pleural Effusions

Most of these effusions are secondary to metastatic deposits on the pleura. These effusions can be free of malignant cells. Small asymptomatic effusions do not require treatment once the diagnosis has been established and usually decrease if the underlying malignancy responds to chemotherapy. Symptomatic malignant effusions need intervention. This intervention is best accomplished by addressing both the effusion and the neoplastic disease responsible for the effusion. Initially diagnostic and therapeutic thoracentesis should be used. Chemotherapy or irradiation can be used to treat the systemic malignancy. Radiotherapy is effective against many tumors causing lymphatic obstruction such as lymphoma. Radiation can take several weeks to relieve lymphatic obstruction, however, and hence will not provide immediate symptomatic relief.

Effusions that reaccumulate despite initial drainage and systemic therapy can be treated either by chest tube or thoracoscopic pleurodesis. Thoracoscopic pleurodesis has several advantages over that achieved with chest tube insertion. These include better distribution of the pleurodesing agent because of the ability to break up any loculations and to directly visualize the distribution. Also, biopsy of lesions can be performed if needed. Particularly in the breast cancer patient with negative fluid cytology, biopsy of the pleura under direct vision can provide tissue for receptor and biomarker analysis. Talc pleurodesis prevents recurrence in 93% of malignant effusions. Other management methods include pleuroperitoneal shunts in patients with recurrent effusions despite pleurodesis. Pleural and peritoneal catheters are inserted and connected to a valved pump chamber. The patient has to pump the chamber several times each day to decrease the effusion. More recently, there is a growing experience with indwelling catheters that allow the fluid to be removed and discarded on a daily basis. This strategy is particularly successful at controlling symptoms in patients with entrapped lung, and thus pleurodesis is not possible. Complications of these interventions include pneumothorax, hemothorax, empyema, loculations, and lung entrapment due to inexpansile lung.

Empyema

Although empyema is not as common as it was during the preantibiotic era, it is still a disease that often requires surgical intervention. Empyema is an infection of the pleural space, most commonly secondary to a pneumonic infectious process. It can also occur because of mediastinal infections as in esophageal perforation, hematogenous spread due to sepsis from an infectious process at another site, or secondary to surgery or trauma. Common organisms isolated include a variety of anaerobic organisms, as well as pneumococcus and other streptococcal organisms. Gram-negative organisms and fungi are also commonly isolated especially in trauma and immunosuppressed patients. Tuberculosis is seen more commonly in recent years as a consequence of the emergence of resistant strains and survival of a variety of patients who are immunocompromised. Cultures from patients who have been on antibiotics may remain negative.

Empyemas are diagnosed with aspiration of pus from the pleural cavity, although not all empyemas will have this characteristic appearance. The aspirated fluid may be only cloudy. Diagnosis can be assisted by measuring the effusion pH, protein content, cell counts, LDH, glucose, and amylase, and with a Gram stain of the fluid. The most sensitive test is fluid pH, with a pH less than 7.0 pathognomonic of empyema.

Empyemas are classified into three phases: the exudative or acute phase, the fibrinopurulent or transitional phase, and the organizing or chronic phase. During the acute phase, the effusion has a low viscosity and cell count. The fibrinopurulent or transitional phase is characterized by increased viscosity and cellularity along with fibrin deposition on the pleural surfaces. The lung becomes less expandable, and loculations begin to form. During the organizing or chronic phase, there is ingrowth of capillaries and fibroblasts. At this stage the pleural fluid is viscous and composed mainly of sediment. There is pleural thickening, and the lung becomes entrapped. The chronic phase can be seen as early as 1 week after onset of symptoms. Symptoms start during the acute or transitional phase, and the patient complains of fever, cough, sputum production, chest pain, and sweats. Chest radiographs will demonstrate the pleural effusion, but CT scan will show the pleural effusion and the loculations. The extent of pleural thickening can be demonstrated on CT scan. Systemic therapy with antibiotics and drainage of the effusion is essential in all phases. Surgical intervention for drainage of the effusion varies according to the phase of the empyema.

Untreated empyema can decompress through the chest wall (*empyema necessitans*) and can involve the mediastinum, the pericardium, and the vertebrae, and result in CNS infections or in lung entrapment by the thick pleura.

Multiple open drainage procedures have been described. These include rib resection at the most dependent part of the effusion and thoracotomy with decortication depending on the patient's state of health and disease history. Although these operations were designed in the preantibiotic era, they remain useful for severely ill patients that may not tolerate thoracotomy.

Thoracentesis is the treatment of choice for acute-phase empyemas. The low-viscosity fluid of acute empyema can be drained in its entirety and the diagnosis verified.

If the fluid is too viscous for the thoracentesis needles, then chest tube drainage may still successfully treat the empyema and produce pleural apposition. Chest tube drainage and antibiotics can be effective for acute- and transitional-phase empyemas. Furthermore, chest tube drainage can be assisted by the delivery of tissue plasminogen activator (tPA) through the tube. A 10 mg vial can be broken into 2 doses of 5 mg each, diluted in 60 cc to 100 cc of saline. The drug is allowed to dwell in the chest cavity for 20 to 40 minutes. If successful, there will be an increase in chest tube output and improvement in the chest radiograph within 2 doses given 12 hours apart. However, if significant loculations have already formed, chest tube drainage with tPA will also be ineffective, and operative drainage either by open or via video-assisted thoracic surgery (VATS) is indicated.[66–67]

VATS has been shown to be effective for drainage of loculated effusions and for pleural débridement. Organized chronic empyemas, however, with extensive pleural thickening may be inadequately débrided with VATS, and open thoracotomy with decortication may be required for full lung expansion.

Wounds resulting from open pleural drainage can be packed open and managed like any other open wound. Management can be combined with chest tube drainage if visceral and parietal pleura are not adherent. A mobilized skin flap (Eloesser flap) or Clagett window can be used to keep the cavity open. Both techniques involve the removal of a short segment of rib. The Clagett window technique then sews the pleura to the skin to marsupialize the wound and prevent premature closure. The Eloesser flap raises a myocutaneous flap that is then rotated over the rib above the defect and sewn to the pleura. If the cavity is cleared of infection and systemic disease has been eradicated, then extrathoracic muscle flap closure can be used to obliterate the cavity.[68–70]

Chylothorax

Chylothorax is a fatty effusion that accumulates in the pleural space secondary to some compromise of the thoracic duct or its collaterals. This accumulation can occur secondary to congenital causes, trauma (iatrogenic and otherwise) to branches of the thoracic duct, malignancies, infections, and thrombosis of the venous system.

Chylous fluid has high concentrations of fatty acids, cholesterol, and phospholipids, which gives chylous fluid its milky white color. The predominant cellular constituent is lymphocytes. Volume and content of fat within the chylous fluid varies with the composition of meals consumed. When the patient has not eaten for a few hours, chylous fluid will be clear.

The thoracic duct has a variable anatomic course. The most common anatomic relationship is found in approximately 50% of patients. The thoracic duct originates at the cisterna chyli between T10 and L3 and enters the chest through the aortic hiatus to the right of the aorta (Fig. 82.22).[71] It courses anterior to the vertebral bodies between the aorta and the azygos vein and posterior to the esophagus. At the level of the fifth thoracic vertebra the thoracic duct turns to the left as it passes posterior to the aortic arch. In the neck, it drains into the left jugulosubclavian junction. Two or more ducts can be present at any part of its course. Also, lymphatic collateral branches from the intercostal neurovascular bundles enter the duct from beneath each rib. The two most common causes of chylothorax are trauma and malignancy. Blunt trauma can result in chylothorax secondary to hyperextension of the spine and rupture of the thoracic duct, usually just above the diaphragm. Penetrating injury is usually associated with injuries of the aorta or esophagus. Iatrogenic trauma can occur during surgeries of the esophagus, aorta, subclavian vessels and base of the left neck. Importantly, injury below the fifth thoracic vertebra most commonly results in right-sided chylothorax, while injury above this level results in left-sided chylothorax.

Malignant etiologies are responsible for more than half of nontraumatic spontaneous chylous effusions in adults. Thoracic and abdominal malignancies can invade the thoracic duct with rupture of the duct due to erosion or obstruction. The resulting effusions can be unilateral or bilateral. Lymphoma is the most common malignancy that causes spontaneous chylothorax. Of the benign lesions, lymphangiomas, cystic hygromas and pulmonary lymphangiomatosis have most commonly been associated with chylous effusions.

Symptoms of chylothorax mimic those of other pleural effusions and include shortness of breath, chest pain, fatigue, and symptoms of the disease that caused the effusion such as

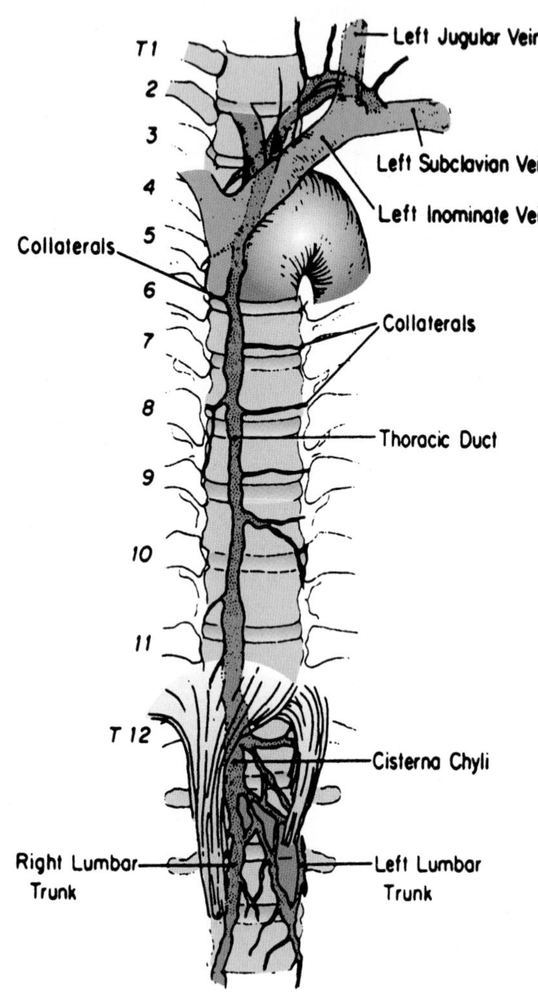

FIGURE 82.22 Schematic drawing of the most usual pattern and course of the thoracic duct. The single duct that enters the chest through the aortic hiatus between T12 and T10 is a relatively consistent finding and the usual site for surgical ligation.

an infectious or neoplastic disease. In addition, nutritional deficiencies can occur due to loss of fat, protein, and vitamins. Replacing the volume drained is essential to avoid volume depletion as well as to avoid nutritional deficiencies. Symptoms of pericardial tamponade can occur with chylous leaks into the pericardium.

Chylothorax is suspected when aspiration reveals a milky type effusion. The cell count reveals a predominance of lymphocytes, and this is quite helpful diagnostically. Effusions with a triglyceride level greater that 110 mg/dL have a 99% chance of being chylous, whereas those with a level less than 50 mg/dL have only a 5% chance of being chylous. Administering cream to the patient and observing the change in the character of the drainage can confirm the diagnosis in certain patients.

The initial management of chylous effusions consists of lung reexpansion via chest tube drainage and nutritional support with volume replacement of the daily losses. A fat-free enteral diet with medium-chain triglycerides that are absorbed directly by the venous system can be used to decrease the output of the effusion, but frequently requires several days to weeks to take effect. Intravenous alimentation can also result in an even further decrease in the daily output of the effusion. Radiation is particularly useful for chylous effusions secondary to lymphomas. Subcutaneous injections of somatostatin in addition to the parenteral nutrition have been used with success to treat chylous effusions in patients who did not respond to initial parenteral nutrition. Nonoperative management was previously recommended for up to 2 weeks in the pre–minimally invasive era. Newer techniques provide better alternatives to this strategy. Percutaneous embolization of the thoracic duct has been attempted and has been successful in selected patients with demonstrable thoracic duct leak.

Surgical approaches can be used for chronic chylous effusions unresponsive to other interventions such as cavernous lymphangiomas. These include pleuroperitoneal shunts, VATS or open thoracotomy with repair, fibrin glue application, or ligation of the thoracic duct. Operation on the same side as the effusion is usually preferred. Postoperative effusions following esophagectomy are best approached from the right side, with ligation of the duct above the diaphragm. Administration of cream preoperatively can help to identify the site of injury during surgery.

Pleuroperitoneal shunts have been advocated to avoid the nutritional and immunologic sequelae of a chylous leak as well as to reduce hospital length of stay. The advent of VATS, however, has popularized earlier operative treatment for patients who do not appear to respond immediately to conservative treatment. VATS thoracic duct clipping, pleurodesis, and fibrin glue application have all been described and may result in resolution of the effusion and hospital discharge within 10 days.[72–75]

Pneumothorax

Pneumothorax is the presence of air in the pleural space, which causes deflation of the lung (Fig. 82.23). Pneumothoraces are either spontaneous or acquired. Spontaneous pneumothoraces can be further subdivided into primary or secondary. A primary spontaneous pneumothorax refers to pneumothoraces occurring in patients without known underlying pulmonary disease, and secondary pneumothorax occurs in patients with a known predisposing process.[75] Acquired pneumothoraces can occur as a complication of numerous procedures, such as central venous access, thoracentesis, mechanical ventilation, surgery, or diagnostic lung biopsy.

Lung parenchyma injury with free egress of air into the pleural space results in loss of the negative intrapleural space that is needed for lung inflation. The lung begins to collapse with compromise of ventilation. Arterial hypoxemia can occur with 50% collapse of the lung due to the continuing perfusion of poorly ventilated lung. The extent of hypoxemia seen varies according to the underlying condition of the lung. Increasing positive intrapleural pressure is transmitted to mediastinal structures, and pressures as low as 15 to 20 cm H_2O can compromise venous return to the heart with decreasing cardiac output. These physiologic sequelae are collectively called *tension pneumothorax*. Failure to immediately address a tension pneumothorax can result in death.

Patients with pneumothorax most commonly complain of chest pain, usually pleuritic. This can occur even with small pneumothoraces and typically is felt most severely in the ipsilateral shoulder. Dyspnea is not usually seen in smaller pneumothoraces. Other symptoms, such as orthopnea and cough with occasional hemoptysis, are also seen with pneumothorax.

The physical examination is usually normal with small pneumothoraces. With larger pneumothoraces, decreased breath sounds are evident along with decreased chest wall motion and hyperexpansion of the chest. Percussion reveals

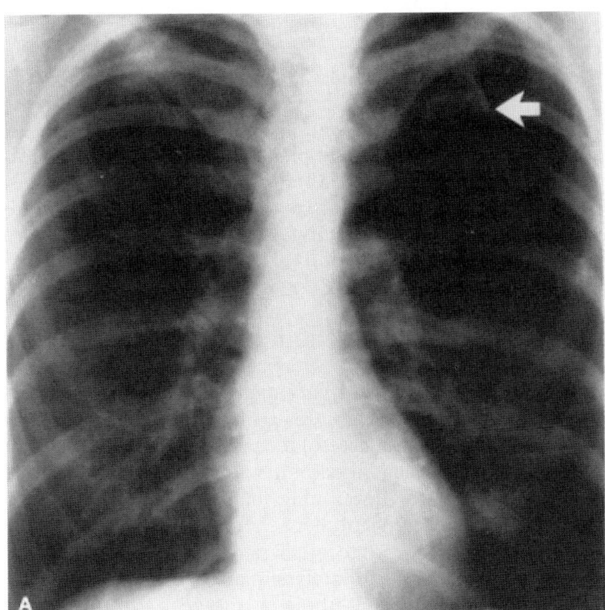

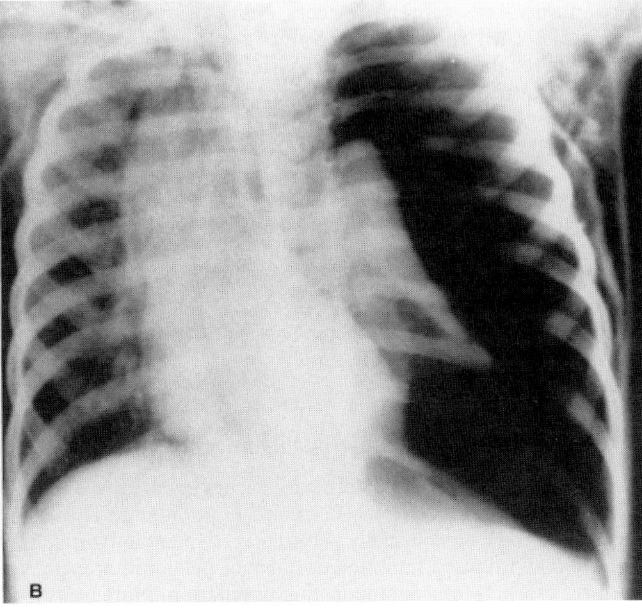

FIGURE 82.23 (*A*) A 40% left-sided spontaneous pneumothorax (*arrow*). (*B*) Progression of simple pneumothorax to a tension pneumothorax, showing the characteristic radiographic findings—virtual collapse of the entire involved lung, shift of the mediastinum to the contralateral side, and compression of the contralateral lung. Subcutaneous air dissecting along the left chest wall is also evident.

hyperresonance. Cyanosis can be seen especially in patients with underlying lung disease. Subcutaneous emphysema can be present in patients with traumatic pneumothoraces.

Posteroanterior chest radiographs can demonstrate the pneumothorax as a hyperlucent area with an absence of pulmonary markings. Depending on radiographic presentation, the pneumothoraces can be classified according to size into small (less than 20%), moderate (20% to 40%), and large (more than 40%). Displacement of the mediastinum and diaphragm signal the presence of tension pneumothorax. The posteroanterior radiograph may miss a large anterior pneumothorax. It can be readily seen, however, on lateral films. In addition, if a pneumothorax is suspected but not evident on posteroanterior and lateral films, an end expiratory film may facilitate the diagnosis. Patients with chronic obstructive pulmonary disease (COPD) may have apical bullae misdiagnosed as a pneumothorax due to a similar appearance on chest radiograph and resultant chest tube insertion into the bullae. Chest CT can be used to differentiate between these conditions.

Chest tube insertion to the apex of the hemithorax has been traditionally used for decompression of a pneumothorax and lung expansion. The usual approach is at the fourth, fifth, or sixth intercostal space in the midaxillary line. Digital palpation should be used to confirm entry into the chest cavity and to break up any adhesions. If the patient is ventilated, a short opening of the vent circuit may allow the lung to fall away from the chest wall and facilitate apical placement of the tube. Potential complications include intercostal vessel injury, lung parenchymal injury, intraabdominal placement of the chest tube with visceral injury, infection, and reexpansion pulmonary edema after rapid reexpansion of the lung.

Pigtail catheter (thoracic vent aspiration) of pneumothoraces is becoming more popular.[76] Similar principles to that of chest tube drainage apply except that the size of the catheter is much smaller. These are usually placed using the Seldinger technique and a guide wire. Special one-way Heimlich valves are also available so patients can be treated as outpatients after initial decompression.

Primary Spontaneous Pneumothorax

Primary spontaneous pneumothorax (Fig. 82.23) is a disease of young adults with more than 85% of cases seen in patients younger than age 40 years. The typical patient is tall, thin, and perhaps a smoker, with a family history of pneumothoraces. The cause of the pneumothorax is rupture of a subpleural apical bleb and commonly follows coughing or straining. In 10% of cases bilateral pneumothoraces can occur; in 5% of cases, rupture of a lower lobe bleb is responsible. Patients present with acute onset of chest pain that can subside within 24 hours despite persistence of the pneumothorax. Typical signs and symptoms of pneumothorax are present and include tachycardia, and decreased breath sounds if the pneumothorax is large enough. Chest radiographs confirm the diagnosis and chest CT can detect the blebs.

Treatment of primary spontaneous pneumothorax depends on its size and whether it is a first-time event. Healthy patients with small, first-time pneumothoraces have numerous options. They can be observed if minimally symptomatic, or they can have the pneumothorax decompressed by aspiration or chest tube insertion. If the CT scan shows a bleb, they can even choose thoracoscopic bullectomy. If observation is chosen, a repeat chest film within 4 hours is needed to document lack of progression. Reabsorption of air occurs at a rate of 1% to 2% per day. Persistent air leak occurs in fewer than 20% of patients.

With moderate-size pneumothoraces, aspiration or chest tube insertion is recommended to ensure full reexpansion, whereas patients with a large-size pneumothorax should be decompressed with a chest tube. A review of 11 studies over 30 years comprising 1,242 patients treated for primary spontaneous pneumothorax with needle aspiration or chest tube insertion demonstrated a 30% recurrence rate.[77] Patients who had a persistent leak or recurrence following initial aspiration had a 72% chance of recurrence.

Indications for surgery are persistent air leak, bilateral pneumothoraces, tension pneumothorax, recurrence, occupations involving acute environmental pressure changes (such as pilots and divers), and remote accessibility of medical care. The procedure of choice is VATS with stapling of the bleb responsible for the pneumothorax. With improved equipment and further decrease in the morbidity of VATS, surgical intervention may be offered to patients with a single occurrence, but blebs on CT scan. Mechanical pleurodesis by pleural shredding or thoracoscopic pleurectomy should be performed at the same time so that recurrences will be reduced. Complications include prolonged air leak or recurrence from missed blebs, incomplete lung expansion, bleeding, and Horner syndrome. Recurrence after VATS has been reported to be as low as 4%. If symptoms do occur, a chest CT scan should be used to check for recurrent blebs of the superior segment of the lower lobe and the posterior surface of the apical segment of the upper lobe.[78–79]

Secondary Spontaneous Pneumothorax

Secondary spontaneous pneumothorax occurs in patients who have underlying localized or generalized lung disease. These patients tend to be older, usually between ages 45 and 65 years, and have compromised lung function. Small pneumothoraces, therefore, can be symptomatic in this population. Numerous causes of secondary pneumothoraces exist. COPD is the most common; other common etiologies include cystic fibrosis and interstitial lung disease and infections.[71] Malignant disease, such as bronchogenic carcinoma can also present with a pneumothorax. Metastatic disease, such as sarcomas and especially osteogenic sarcomas in children, are known to predispose to this event as well. Catamenial pneumothorax occurs in women between the ages of 30 and 40 years, usually within the first 3 days after onset of menses, and most commonly involves the right side. Pulmonary or pleural endometriosis is thought to be one of the etiologies of this type of pneumothorax.

A disease process, such as pneumonia, causes a progressive destruction of alveolar walls and decrease of the elastic recoil of the lung with resulting slow collapse. Obstructive disease can result in hyperexpansion of distal air spaces with air dissecting into the interstitial tissues, the hilum, and mediastinum, causing pneumomediastinum and pneumothorax.

Patients may present with sudden onset of dyspnea, cough, and chest pain. However, it may be difficult to distinguish these symptoms from an exacerbation of the underlying pulmonary disease. The size of the pneumothorax that results in significant symptoms depends on the severity of the underlying disease process and pulmonary function reserve that each patient may have. As with primary pneumothorax, tension pneumothorax can also occur in these patients with the aforementioned clinical signs and symptoms.

Chest radiographs are the first diagnostic test obtained. Both posteroanterior and lateral views should be obtained. Occasionally in patients with apical bullae, the diagnosis may be quite difficult to make and chest CT scan will be needed. Unlike patients with a primary pneumothorax, these patients are usually quite symptomatic and hypoxic. Observation is rarely a viable option. Patients can be treated with aspiration or chest tube insertion. Due to loss of elastic recoil, initial lung reexpansion may not be complete and may require more time to achieve than primary pneumothorax. Approximately two thirds of secondary pneumothoraces resolve within 1 week of chest tube drainage. Patients who have persistent air leaks or recurrent pneumothorax, patients with pneumonectomy and pneumothorax, and patients with continued pulmonary functional compromise despite chest tube drainage should undergo surgery if a surgically correctable lesion is present.

Resections of bullae, pleurodesis, and parietal pleurectomy are the main goals of operative intervention. These goals can be achieved with open thoracotomy or VATS. VATS is preferable due to less postoperative compromise in these patients. Double-lumen intubation can be done in most of these patients. Resection of the bullae decreases the chance of a future pneumothorax, whereas pleurodesis decreases the chance that a recurrence will be of a significant size should one occur. Pleurodesis can be done via pleural abrasion, talc, or parietal pleurectomy. Although pleurodesis is not a contraindication to future lung transplantation, aggressive approaches such as parietal pleurectomy are best avoided. Patients who are not able to tolerate single-lung ventilation for VATS may undergo open thoracotomy or axillary thoracotomy.[79]

Mesothelioma

Mesothelioma is a rare and very aggressive, primary malignant pleural tumor. It originates from the mesothelial cells that line the parietal and visceral pleura. Approximately 3,000 new cases occur in the United States annually. The most significant risk factor for developing mesothelioma is exposure to asbestos. Other environmental risk factors have been reported such as exposure to other naturally occurring fibers, radiation exposure, and possibly simian virus 40.[80] Asbestos fibers are divided into amphibole (five types) and serpentine fibers. The amphibole fibers are most clearly associated with mesothelioma. Serpentine fibers are associated with lung cancer. While smoking and asbestos exposure have a synergistic effect in the development of lung cancer, there is no association of smoking with the development of mesothelioma. Before its ban in the United States in 1986, the industries that used asbestos included shipbuilding, construction, brake pad manufacturers, and others. Because these materials are still in use in making floor tiles, paint, piping, and car parts,[81] workers in the shipping, construction, and car repair industries are still at risk for exposure, as are people living or working in buildings constructed before 1987. Worldwide exposure continues to be a serious concern.

The latency period between exposure and disease is quite long; the peak incidence for mesothelioma is during the sixth decade of life. Most cases are due to occupational exposure, and therefore mesothelioma is most common in men. Young patients have been seen with the disease including children of men who worked in occupations at risk.

Mesotheliomas can be classified based on the histologic type.[82] The types seen are the epithelial, sarcomatous, or mixed. Epithelial histology is present in half of patients. Mesothelioma can present as a localized or diffuse tumor, with diffuse tumors more common. Mesothelioma can be confused with metastatic adenocarcinoma. Immunohistochemistry and electron microscopy lead to a definitive diagnosis (Figs. 82.24 and 82.25[83]).

Mesotheliomas usually cause nonspecific symptoms in the early stages. These include chest pain and shortness of breath, usually due to the presence of a pleural effusion. A pleural effusion is present in the vast majority of patients at some point during their clinical course. Weight loss, fever, cough, hemoptysis, and anorexia are other signs and symptoms. Paraneoplastic syndromes such as hypoglycemia, hypercalcemia, and a syndrome of inappropriate antidiuretic hormone (SIADH) have been occasionally reported. Radiographically, a pleural effusion is the most common sign of these tumors. If the disease is advanced, pleural thickening can be visible on chest radiograph. Chest CT scan or MRI are more sensitive in assessing pleural thickening and detecting pleural-based masses. Transdiaphragmatic involvement, neurovascular involvement, and mediastinal invasion are best assessed with MRI. Echocardiography can also assist in assessing pericardial involvement. Recently, positron-emission tomography scanning has been evaluated for assessment of metastatic disease and has been shown to be more sensitive than either CT or MRI.

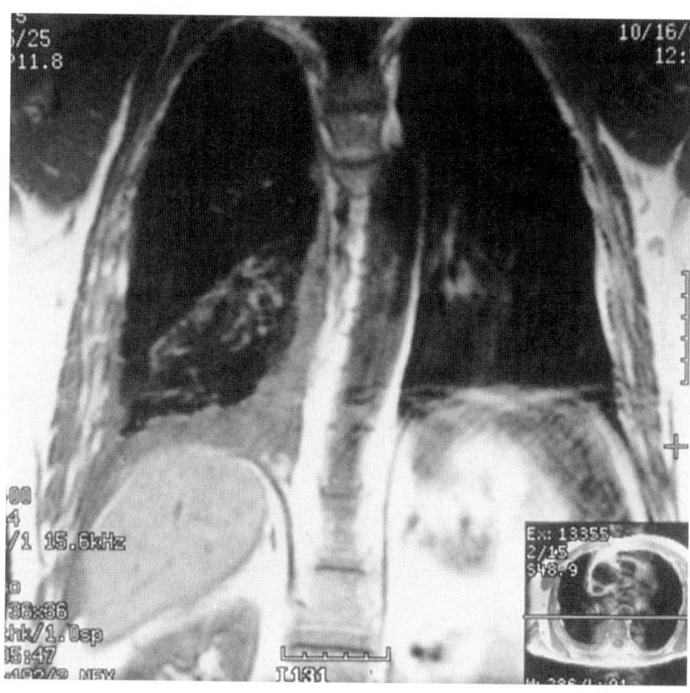

FIGURE 82.24 Magnetic resonance imaging of the patient in Figure 82.25 shows a large amount of tumor within the pleural space and into the diaphragmatic sulcus with no evidence of extension outside the hemithorax. (From Flores RM, Sugarbaker DJ. Malignant mesothelioma of the pleural space. *Ann Thorac Surg*. 2000;70:306.)

Pleural fluid can be obtained for cytologic and cytogenetic analysis and yields a diagnosis of mesothelioma in half of the cases. Percutaneous pleural biopsy provides enough tissue for diagnosis in about one third of patients. The tissue sample obtained is usually not enough to perform immunohistochemistry, or necessary electron microscopy studies.

For biopsy, thoracoscopy has a diagnostic yield of more than 80%, does not commit the patient to a major procedure, and provides enough tissue for all the studies needed. In cases in which the pleural space has been obliterated, thoracoscopy is not feasible and the procedure can be converted to an open biopsy. Half the patients are diagnosed within 8 weeks of onset of their symptoms if cytology is positive; however, if the cytology is negative, diagnosis is delayed, averaging 12 weeks from onset of symptoms.

Once diagnosis is confirmed, staging of the patient and treatment options present challenges. Several staging systems have been published, but are without universal acceptance. The commonly used staging systems include the Butchart (Table 82.5),[84] Brigham and Women's Hospital (Table 82.6),[85,86] and the new International TNM staging system (Table 82.7)[87] proposed by the International Mesothelioma Interest Group.

Treatment ranges from supportive care to multimodality therapy including aggressive surgery, chemotherapy, and radiotherapy. Survival with supportive care ranges from 4 to

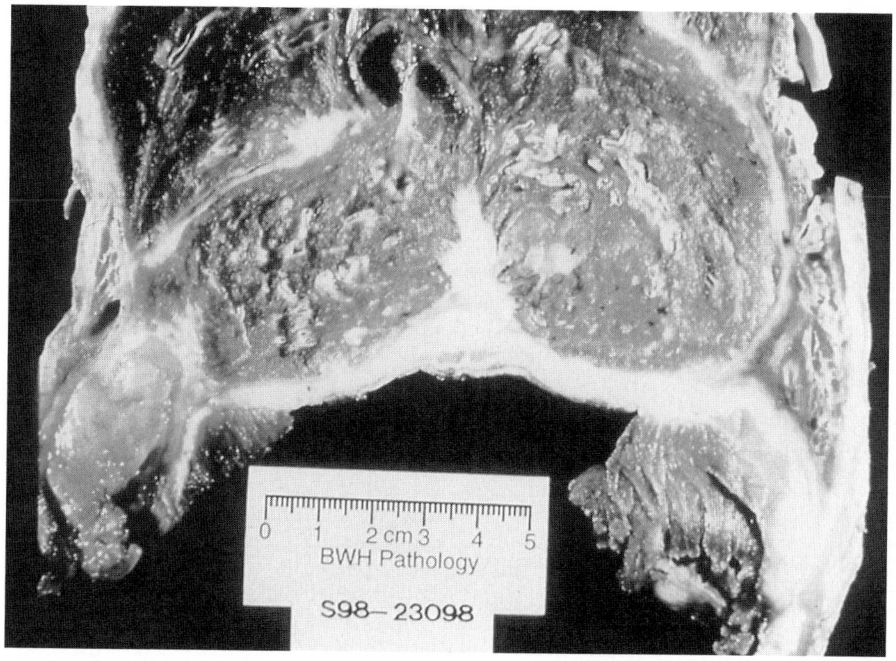

FIGURE 82.25 The gross pathologic specimen of the patient in Figure 82.24 following extrapleural pneumonectomy demonstrates an intact pleural envelope, inferiorly diaphragmatic muscle fibers remain intact, and tumor present within the pleural space with lung parenchymal invasion. The patient went on to receive chemotherapy and radiation. (From Flores RM, Sugarbaker DJ. Malignant mesothelioma of the pleural space. *Ann Thorac Surg*. 2000;70:306.)

TABLE 82.5 STAGING

THE BUTCHART STAGING SYSTEM

Stage	Definition
I	Within the capsule of the parietal pleura: ipsilateral pleura, lung, pericardium, diaphragm
II	Invading chest wall or mediastinum: esophagus, heart, opposite pleura Positive lymph nodes within the chest
III	Through diaphragm to peritoneum; opposite pleura Positive lymph nodes outside the chest
IV	Distant blood-borne metastases

Modified from Butchart EG, Ashcroft T, Barnsley WC, et al. Pleuropneumonectomy in the management of diffuse malignant mesothelioma of the pleura: experience with 29 patients. *Thorax* 1976;31:15–24.

12 months. Single-modality therapy has been ineffective whether it is radiation, chemotherapy, or surgery. Multimodality therapy including aggressive surgery has shown survival benefit in particular patients with some long-term survivors. The surgical procedures used in the management of mesothelioma include pleurodesis, pleurectomy with decortication, and extrapleural pneumonectomy (EPP). Surgery should be accompanied by chemotherapy and radiation in a multimodality setting. Cytoreductive surgery, such as pleurectomy and decortication, can provide palliation of the dyspnea secondary to lung encasement and chest wall pain. Pleurectomy with decortication followed by chemoradiation can result in a median survival as high as 21 months.[88,89] In the authors' experience, EPP is the procedure of choice whenever feasible because it is the most effective cytoreductive surgery, and with experienced surgeons EPP has a mortality rate close to 4%. EPP includes the en bloc removal of the affected lung, diaphragm, pericardium, and parietal pleura. Approximately one quarter of patients are candidates for EPP. Peritoneal invasion should be ruled out before undertaking EPP. When followed by chemoradiation, long-term survival is reported; however, EPP by itself does not offer a survival advantage.

TABLE 82.6 STAGING

THE REVISED BRIGHAM AND WOMEN'S HOSPITAL STAGING SYSTEM

Stage	Definition
I	Disease completely resected within the capsule of the parietal pleura without adenopathy: ipsilateral pleura, lung, pericardium, diaphragm, or chest wall disease limited to previous biopsy sites
II	All of stage I with positive resection margins and/or intrapleural adenopathy
III	Local extension of disease into chest wall or mediastinum; heart, or through diaphragm, peritoneum; or with extrapleural lymph node involvement
IV	Distant metastatic disease

Note: Butchart stage II and III (95) patients are combined into stage III. Stage I represents respectable patients with negative nodes. Stage II patients are respectable but have positive nodal status.

Numerous independent predictors of survival have been demonstrated in patients treated with EPP in the multimodality setting. They include age younger than 55 years, good performance status, epithelial histology, early stage disease, negative resection margins, and absence of lymph node involvement.[86] Results in 183 patients treated over 17 years were reviewed. These patients underwent EPP with postoperative chemotherapy (carboplatin/paclitaxel) and radiation (55 Gy). This series reported a 5-year survival of 46% with a median survival of 51 months for the subset of patients who had epithelial-type tumors with negative resection margins and absence of nodal involvement.[86]

For the patients who are not candidates for multimodality therapy with EPP, treatment options are being investigated; they include intracavitary chemotherapy, photodynamic therapy, and gene therapy.[90–92]

MEDIASTINUM

Anatomy

The mediastinum is bound by the thoracic inlet, the mediastinal pleura laterally, the diaphragm inferiorly, the sternum anteriorly, and the vertebrae posteriorly. The mediastinum is arbitrarily divided into anterosuperior, middle, and posterior (Fig. 82.26). The anterosuperior mediastinum is anterior to the pericardium and its reflection over the great vessels. The middle mediastinum is bound by the anterior and posterior edges of the pericardium. The posterior mediastinum is posterior to the pericardium.

The anterosuperior mediastinum contains the thymus, the ascending aorta, and the great vessels. Occasionally, ectopic parathyroid masses can be found here, arising because of the common embryologic origin with the thymus. The thyroid can also extend into this region when it enlarges. The middle mediastinum contains the heart, the pericardium, the tracheal bifurcation, the bronchi and their nodes, and the aortic arch. The posterior mediastinum contains the esophagus, the thoracic duct, the azygous vein, the descending aorta, and the sympathetic, parasympathetic, and intercostal nerves (Table 82.8) (Fig. 82.27[93]).

Mediastinal Masses

Epidemiology and Incidence

Numerous types of tumors can occur in the mediastinum. Tumor type varies by location and by patient age. When combining pediatric and adult populations, neurogenic tumors are the most common, followed by thymomas, cysts, and lymphomas. In the pediatric population, posterior mediastinal neurogenic tumors are more common, whereas in adults anterior mediastinal tumors predominate. In addition, the neurogenic tumors in children tend to be malignant (neuroblastomas), whereas the neurogenic tumors in adults tend to be benign.[94–96] In children, the most common mediastinal tumor is neuroblastoma followed by lymphoma and germ cell tumor. Other benign lesions can occur such as cysts of pericardial, aerodigestive, or thymic origin (Table 82.9).[97,98]

Anterior mediastinal lesions are more common in adults, with thymomas most common, followed by lymphomas and germ cell tumors. Series comparing patients from two different periods have shown that the incidence of malignancy in anterior mediastinal masses has more than doubled in recent years without any clear etiology.[99–104]

TABLE 82.7 STAGING

THE NEW INTERNATIONAL STAGING SYSTEM (IMIG)

T—TUMOR		
T1	1a	Tumor limited to the ipsilateral parietal pleura, including mediastinal and diaphragmatic pleura; no involvement of the visceral pleura
	1b	Tumor involving the ipsilateral parietal pleura, including mediastinal and diaphragmatic pleura; scattered foci of tumor also involving the visceral pleura
T2		Tumor involving each of the ipsilateral pleural surfaces (parietal, mediastinal, diaphragmatic, and visceral pleura) with at least one of the following features: Involvement of diaphragmatic muscle Confluent visceral pleural tumor (including the fissures) or extension of tumor from visceral pleura into the underlying pulmonary parenchyma
T3		Locally advanced but potentially respectable tumor; tumor involving all of the ipsilateral pleural surfaces (parietal, mediastinal, diaphragmatic, and visceral pleura) with at least one of the following features: Involvement of the endothoracic fascia Extension into the mediastinal fat Solitary, completely respectable focus of tumor extending into the soft tissues of the chest wall Nontransmural involvement of the pericardium
T4		Locally advanced technically unresectable tumor; tumor involving all of the ipsilateral pleural surfaces (parietal, mediastinal, diaphragmatic, and visceral) with at least one of the following features: Diffuse extension or multifocal masses of tumor in the chest wall, with or without associated rib destruction Direct transdiaphragmatic extension of tumor to the peritoneum Direct extension of tumor to the contralateral pleura Direct extension of tumor to one or more mediastinal organs Direct extension of tumor into the spine Tumor extending through to the internal surface of the pericardium with or without a pericardial effusion; or tumor involving the myocardium
N—LYMPH NODES		
NX		Regional lymph nodes cannot be assessed
N0		No regional lymph node metastases
N1		Metastases in the ipsilateral bronchopulmonary or hilar lymph nodes
N2		Metastases in the subcarinal or ipsilateral mediastinal lymph nodes, including the ipsilateral internal mammary nodes
N3		Metastases in the contralateral mediastinal, contralateral internal mammary, ipsilateral, or contralateral supraclavicular lymph nodes
M—METASTASES		
MX		Presence of distant metastases cannot be assessed
M0		No distant metastasis
M1		Distant metastasis present

Stage	Description
I	
Ia	T1aN0M0
Ib	T1bN0M0
II	T2N0M0
III	Any T3M0
	Any N1M0
	Any N2M0
IV	Any T4
	Any N3
	Any M1

Adopted with permission from RUSCH VW, the International Mesothelioma Interest Group. A proposed new international TNM staging system for malignant pleural mesothelioma. Chest 1995;108:1122–1128.

Symptoms and Signs

Symptoms at the time of diagnosis vary depending on the location and size of the mediastinal lesions. More than half of the lesions are symptomatic. Symptomatic lesions have a higher probability of malignancy. Patients' complaints include chest pain, dyspnea and cough, dysphagia, hoarseness, Horner syndrome, superior vena cava (SVC) syndrome, palpitations, malaise, weakness and weight loss, back pain, and signs of

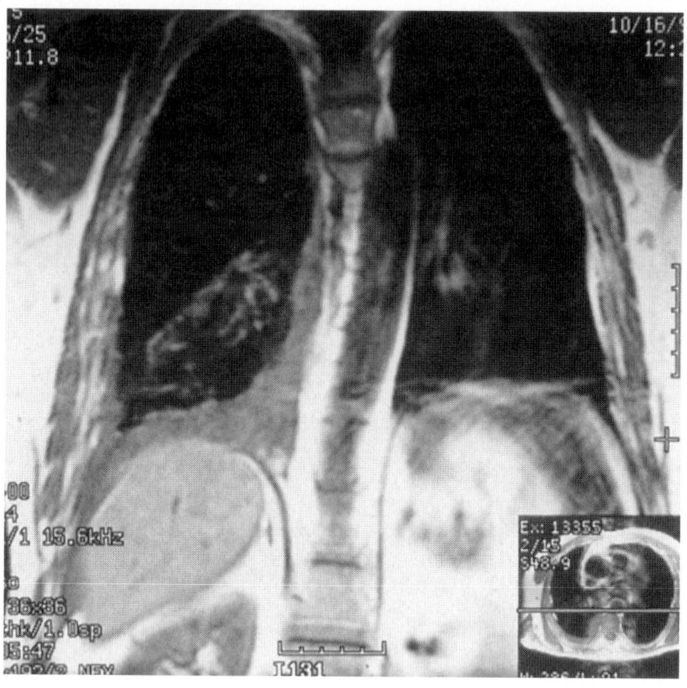

FIGURE 82.26 Compartments of the mediastinum. The superior and inferior mediastinum are separated by a line drawn from the sternomanubrial junction anteriorly on a lateral chest radiograph to the lower edge of the fourth vertebral body posteriorly. The inferior mediastinum is divided into anterior, middle, and posterior compartments by the pericardium.

spinal cord compression. Some mediastinal tumors have endocrine activity that may cause symptoms of hyperthyroidism, hyperparathyroidism, hypoglycemia, or paroxysmal malignant hypertension suggestive of pheochromocytoma.[95,98,103]

Diagnostic Approach

Most mediastinal masses can be seen on plain chest radiographs.[105] Chest CT scan will show the relationship of the mass to adjacent structures and better define its size and whether it is solid or cystic. MRI can provide additional information regarding neurovascular involvement and has largely replaced angiography in contemporary practice. In addition, MRI is used to assess intraspinal involvement of neurogenic tumors and has replaced CT myelograms.[106,107]

Human chorionic gonadotropin and α-fetoprotein are useful diagnostic and monitoring serologic markers when a germ cell tumor is suspected. Seminomas do not produce these markers. If an esophageal duplication cyst is suspected, then a barium esophagogram will rule out a communication with the esophagus.

Radionucleotide scanning is useful for the diagnosis of endocrine tumors. Technetium or iodine scanning may help in the evaluation of potential thyroid and hyperparathyroid masses. Gallium scans are useful in tumors, such as lymphomas and nonseminomatous germ cell tumors with an affinity for the isotopes. When mediastinal pheochromocytomas are sus-pected scanning with ^{131}I-metaiodobenzylguanidine (^{131}I-MIBG) is very useful in locating these extraadrenal paraganglionic tumors.[108]

Needle biopsy of the lesion in question can be performed under CT or ultrasound guidance or with transbronchial biopsy for middle mediastinal tumors.[109–111] Mediastinoscopy can be used in situations where a large tissue sample is needed for diagnosis as in the case of suspected lymphoma. Thoracoscopy is useful for lesions inaccessible by mediastinoscopy.[112,113]

TABLE 82.8

LOCATION OF PRIMARY MEDIASTINAL MASSES IN ADULTS AND CHILDREN

ANTEROSUPERIOR MEDIASTINUM
Thymoma
Lymphoma
Germ cell tumor
Lymphangioma
Hemangioma
Lipoma
Carcinoma
Thyroid adenoma
Parathyroid adenoma
MIDDLE MEDIASTINUM
Pericardial cyst
Bronchogenic cyst
Lymphoma
POSTERIOR MEDIASTINUM
Neurogenic tumor
Enteric cyst

Anterior Mediastinal Masses

Thymoma. Thymoma is the most common adult tumor of the anterosuperior mediastinum. Thymoma can occur at any age, but is rare in children and most common between the ages of 40 and 60 years. Thymoma originates from thymic epithelial cells. Patients may complain of chest pain or dyspnea due to the mass effect of the tumor. Thymomas are associated with systemic syndromes, such as myasthenia gravis, Cushing syndrome, hyper- and hypogammaglobulinemia, systemic lupus erythromatosus, rheumatoid arthritis, megaesophagus, red blood cell aplasia, or granulomatous myocarditis.[114] Differentiation of thymoma from lymphoma can be difficult.

Various classification systems have been proposed. Thymomas can be classified based on lymphocyte infiltration or resemblance to thymic medullary or cortical cells, whereas the Masaoka staging system[115–117] uses gross and microscopic invasion of capsule and adjacent structures to stage the thymomas (Table 82.10).

Treatment. Complete surgical resection via median sternotomy is the treatment of choice for thymomas that do not have widespread dissemination (Fig. 82.28). Other approaches, such as transcervical resection, have been described. However,

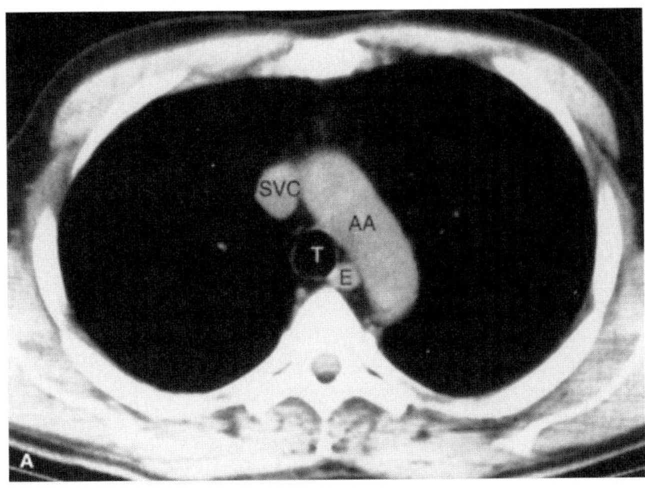

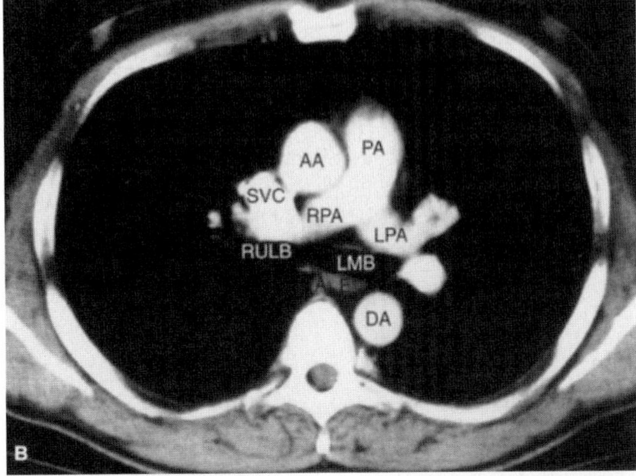

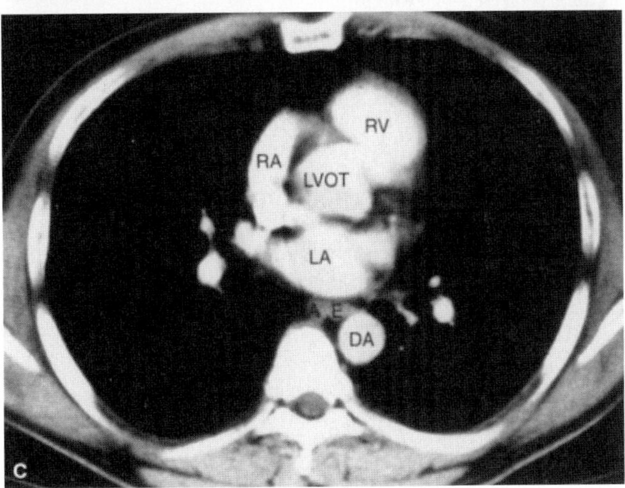

FIGURE 82.27 Normal mediastinal anatomy as shown with computed tomography scans. (*A*) Scan at level of the aortic arch and midtrachea. T, trachea; E, esophagus; AA, aortic arch; SVC, superior vena cava. (*B*) Scan at level of carina. RULB, right upper lobe bronchus; LMB, left mainstem bronchus; AA, ascending aorta; DA, descending aorta; A, azygos vein; E, esophagus; SVC, superior vena cava; PA, main pulmonary artery; LPA and RPA, left and right pulmonary arteries. (*C*) Scan at the level of the left atrium. LA, left atrium; RA, right atrium; LVOT, left ventricular outflow tract; RV, right ventricle; A, azygos vein; E, esophagus; DA, descending aorta.

complete excision of invasive thymomas is best achieved via sternotomy. Local recurrence can occur secondary to tumor seeding or drop metastases.[118] Radiotherapy for invasive thymomas improves local control. Chemotherapy is used for disseminated thymomas.[119–121]

The most common sites of recurrence are the lung, pleura, and mediastinum. For recurrent tumors, reexcision should be considered in addition to both chemotherapy and radiotherapy. Survival correlates with stage. The 10-year survival rate for patients with stage I disease is approximately 85%; for stage II, 60% to 84%; for stage III, 21% to 77%; and 26% to 47% for stage IV-A patients.[122–124] Involvement of great vessels has a negative impact on survival.

TABLE 82.9

MEDIASTINAL TUMORS IN CHILDREN

Type of tumor	Incidence reported in series (%)
Neurogenic	35
Lymphoma	25
Germ cell	11
Primary malignancy	2
Cysts	25

From Davis RD Jr, Oldham HN Jr, Sabiston DC Jr. The mediastinum. In: Sabiston DC Jr, Spencer FC, eds. *Surgery of the chest*, 5th ed. Philadelphia: WB Saunders, 1990, p. 507.

Myasthenia Gravis. Myasthenia gravis is the most common syndrome associated with thymoma. It has a prevalence of 0.5 to 14.2 per 100,000 population. It occurs more frequently in women, with a female to male ratio of 2:1.[125–127]

Fatigue and muscular weakness are the predominant symptoms. Facial muscles are most commonly involved. The patients can have ptosis, ophthalmoplegia, dysarthria, and dysphagia. Most patients with myasthenia gravis have thymic lymphoid hyperplasia; however 10% have thymoma. The incidence of myasthenia gravis in patients with thymoma increases with age and can be as high as 80% in patients older than 60 years.[128]

Diagnosis of myasthenia gravis is usually confirmed with the short-acting anticholinesterase edrophonium (Tensilon) test. Any intravenous dose of Tensilon results in improvement of muscle strength in patients with myasthenia gravis.

Treatment. The treatment of myasthenia gravis involves the administration of cholinesterase inhibitors, steroids, plasma-

TABLE 82.10

MASAOKA STAGING SYSTEM FOR THYMOMA

Stage	Definition
I	Macroscopically, completely encapsulated; microscopically, no capsular invasion
IIA	Macroscopic invasion in surrounding fatty tissues or mediastinal pleura
IIB	Microscopic invasion into the capsule
III	Macroscopic invasion into a neighboring organ, such as pericardium, great vessels, or lung
IVA	Pleural or pericardial dissemination
IVB	Hematogenous or lymphogenous metastases

Adapted from Masaoka A, Monden Y, Nakahara K, et al. Follow-up study of thymomas with special references to their clinical stages. *Cancer* 1981;48:2485, with permission.

pheresis, and surgery. Cholinesterase inhibitors increase the amount of acetylcholine available at the neuromuscular junction and improve the symptoms, but they do not affect the natural history of the disease. Steroids induce remission in the majority of patients; other immunosuppressants, such as azathioprine and cyclosporine, can induce remission where steroids have failed. Plasmapheresis is very useful for the control of acute severe symptoms and for preoperative preparation. The benefits of plasmapheresis can last from weeks to months.[129]

Thymectomy is associated with excellent clinical results and minimal morbidity, with up to 80% complete response. The chance of remission is best in young female patients who have a hyperplastic thymus and short duration of disease. Preoperative plasmapheresis facilitates perioperative management. Median sternotomy, transcervical and thoracoscopic approaches have been used for resection.[130–133]

Lymphomas. Lymphoma can present with disease in the chest 10% of the time. It is the second most common tumor of the anterosuperior and middle mediastinum in adults and the most common one in children. It rarely occurs in the posterior mediastinum. Hodgkin lymphoma of the nodular sclerosing type is most common.[98,134] Symptoms include chest pain, dyspnea, cough, and systemic symptoms, such as night sweats, fever, or weight loss. A large tissue sample may be needed to differentiate lymphoma from thymoma. Preoperative chest CT scan assists in the planning of the approach used for biopsy.

Treatment. Mediastinal lymphomas are treated primarily with radiation and chemotherapy. Resection of mediastinal lymphomas is not necessary because chemoradiation can achieve excellent results.[135]

Germ Cell Tumors. Primary germ cell tumors are the third most common anterosuperior mediastinal mass. Multiple types of germ cell tumors exist, including teratomas, teratocarcinoma, seminomas, embryonal cell carcinoma, choriocarcinoma, and endodermal sinus carcinoma. They arise from primordial germ cells that have migrated from the urogenital ridge. These tumors are not considered to be metastatic; however, scrotal evaluation with physical examination and sonogram is warranted to exclude a primary gonadal lesion.[136,137]

Although benign germ cell tumors occur with equal frequency in males and females, 90% of malignant tumors occur in young males. The most common mediastinal germ cell tumor is the benign teratoma. Seminoma is the most common malignant tumor, making up 50% of malignant tumors, followed by teratocarcinoma.[138]

Mediastinal teratoma. Most teratomas are benign tumors; approximately 10% are malignant. Dermoid cysts are the most common type of benign teratomas. They can contain hair, sweat glands, and sebaceous material.[139] Surgery is the treatment of choice, with excellent long-term results. These lesions do not tend to recur if completely resected.

Seminoma. CT scan of the chest, abdomen, and pelvis is required to evaluate the entire retroperitoneum and mediastinum. Serum **human chorionic gonadotropin** levels are elevated only in a minority of patients. Seminoma is a

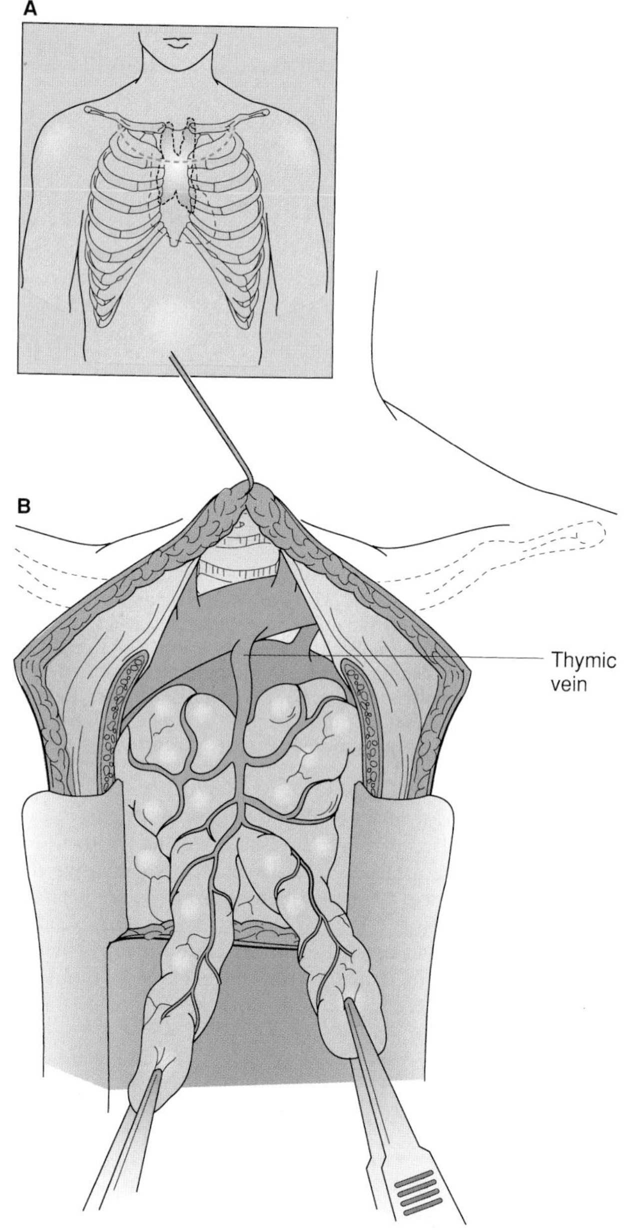

FIGURE 82.28 Technique of thymectomy. (*A*) Skin incision for partial sternotomy used to resect either a normal-sized thymus gland or one containing a small tumor. The incision placed over the sternomanubrial junction avoids a cervical scar and is more cosmetically appealing. After raising a skin and subcutaneous flap, the upper sternum is divided. (*B*) After the cervical extensions of the thymus glad are mobilized downward, the thymic vein is identified, ligated, and divided where it joins the innominate vein.

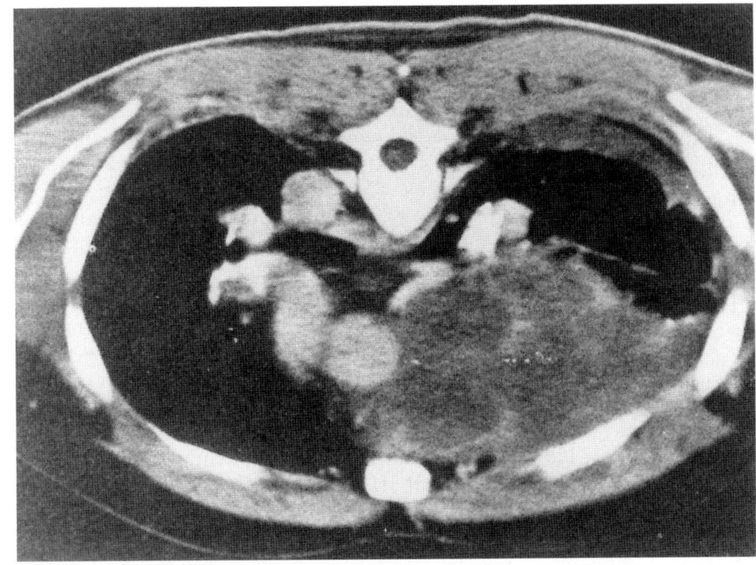

FIGURE 82.29 Computed tomography scan of a malignant nonseminomatous germ cell tumor of the anterior mediastinum reveals the inhomogeneous anterior mediastinal mass in contrast to the homogeneous density of a seminoma. Pleural effusion is also demonstrated in the right hemithorax. (From Shields TW. Primary lesions of the mediastinum and their investigation and treatment. In: Shields TW, ed. *General thoracic surgery*. Baltimore: Williams & Wilkins, 1994, pp. 1724–1769.)

radiosensitive tumor and radiation is the primary treatment modality. In patients who have significant thoracic tumor burden or extrathoracic disease, the addition of chemotherapy improves remission rates. Surgery is reserved for patients with persistent masses after chemotherapy to determine the need for further treatment if viable tumor is still present.[140,141]

Mediastinal nonseminomatous germ cell tumors. Nonseminomatous germ cell tumors of the mediastinum include malignant teratoma, embryonal cell carcinoma, choriocarcinoma, and endodermal tumors (Fig. 82.29).[142] These tumors produce α-fetoprotein and human chorionic gonadotropin, which are elevated in 90% of cases. They are useful markers for monitoring the adequacy of treatment and for surveillance. These tumors are difficult to treat. They are more aggressive than seminomas and they are not radiosensitive. Chemotherapy is the primary treatment modality. Relapses and development of secondary hematologic malignancies are not uncommon.[143,144]

Middle Mediastinal Masses

Mediastinal Cysts. Mediastinal cysts are the most common tumors of the middle mediastinum; they make up 20% of all mediastinal masses. The three most common in decreasing order are bronchogenic, pericardial, and enteric.

Bronchogenic cysts. Bronchogenic cysts are the most common type of mediastinal cysts. They can be found either within the lung parenchyma or in the mediastinum near the carina and the major bronchi (Fig. 82.30).[142] They can produce symptoms secondary to extrinsic compression of the airways or inflammation if they become infected. They can cause stridor, chest pain, cough, and dyspnea. They are more likely to be symptomatic in children.[145–147] CT scan confirms the diagnosis.

Symptomatic lesions should be excised. There are series supporting resection of asymptomatic lesions because many cysts eventually become symptomatic and resection of symptomatic lesions is associated with increased complications.[147–150] In addition, malignancy has been reported to arise from congenital cystic malformations from lung, including bronchogenic cysts. Occasionally bronchogenic cysts can be very adherent to major bronchi or vessels, and complete resection may not be possible. Partial resection is associated with recurrence. Ethanol sclerosis has been reported as treatment for mediastinal cysts.[151,152]

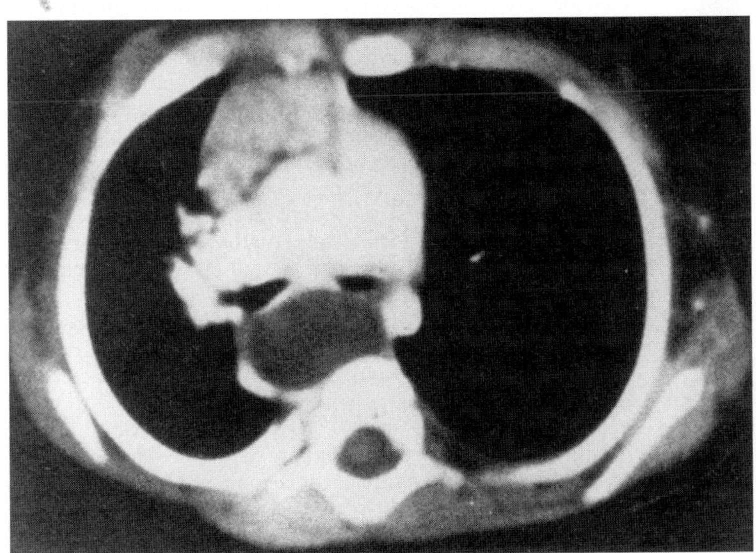

FIGURE 82.30 Computed tomography scan reveals a bronchogenic cyst located in the subcranial area with compression of the left mainstem bronchus with hyperinflation of the left lung and a mediastinal shift to the right. (From Shields TW. Primary lesions of the mediastinum and their investigation and treatment. In: Shields TW, ed. *General thoracic surgery*. Baltimore: Williams & Wilkins, 1994, pp. 1764–1769.)

Pericardial cysts. Most common at the right pericardiophrenic angle, these cysts may communicate with the pericardium. They are usually filled with clear fluid, hence the name "sweet water cyst." They are easily identified on CT scan because of their water-line consistency.[106,153] Resection is usually not required owing to lack of symptoms and absence of malignant potential. Larger cysts, however, can cause symptoms like chronic cough or costal margin pain. In such cases, resection is easily accomplished with thoracoscopic techniques.

Enteric cysts. Enteric cysts (or *duplication cysts* or *neuroenteric cysts*) can be associated with vertebral anomalies. These cysts usually have an inner lining of gastrointestinal epithelium. Esophageal lining is most common, although acid secreting gastric and intestinal epithelia are found as well (Fig. 82.31). These cysts usually become symptomatic in childhood. A duplication of the alimentary tract may coexist. Most often they are found in the right chest and occasionally they occur multiply. The most common symptom is dysphagia secondary to a mass effect on the esophagus. Those cysts with acid-secreting gastric mucosa can bleed and acutely enlarge.[154]

CT scan and endoscopic ultrasound have been used successfully for diagnosis. Technetium scans show uptake in the gastric mucosa. Surgical resection can be done by thoracoscopy if there is a defect in the esophageal muscle or mucosal defects requiring repair. Neuroenteric cysts can communicate with the dural space and can be associated with a variety of vertebral anomalies. Preoperative evaluation of the spinal column and dural anatomy via MRI is needed for an appropriately staged neurosurgical and thoracic approach if communication exists.[155,156]

Other Cysts. Thymic and other nonspecific cysts can occur in the mediastinum. Thymic cysts are benign, but can be confused with cystic degeneration of thymomas or teratomas. Excision for definitive diagnostic purposes should be performed.[157] Chyle-containing cysts, pancreatic pseudocysts, or cysts not otherwise specified can also occur.

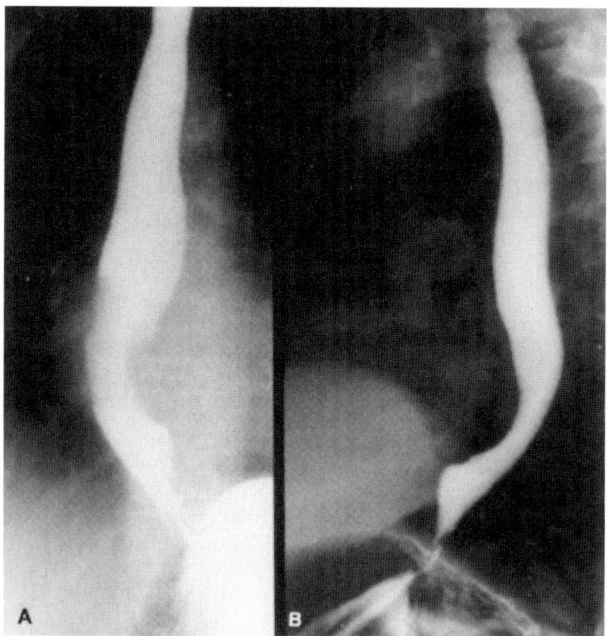

FIGURE 82.31 Barium esophagogram, posteroanterior (*A*) and lateral (*B*) views, showing an intramural esophageal duplication cyst.

Posterior Mediastinal Masses

Neurogenic Tumors. Neurogenic tumors are the most common neoplasms of the mediastinum, constituting 20% to 35% of all tumors. In adults, these tumors tend to be benign, whereas in the pediatric population they tend to be malignant. These tumors have multiple origins and include the nerve sheaths (neurilemomas, neurofibromas, and neurofibrosarcomas), the sympathetic ganglia (ganglioneuromas, ganglioneuroblastomas, and neuroblastomas), and the paraganglia cells (pheochromocytomas and chemodectomas).

Diagnosis. These tumors can present as asymptomatic masses incidentally found on diagnostic studies, or they can be symptomatic either because of mass effect and impingement on vital structures or due to systemic effects of hormonal activity. Mass effects can cause chest pain, back pain, dysphagia, cough, dyspnea, Horner syndrome, and Pancoast syndrome. Symptoms secondary to hormonal activity include hypertension, flushing, diarrhea, palpitations, headaches, sweating, and abdominal distention. Vasoactive substances secreted include catecholamines, vasoactive intestinal peptide, and insulin-like factors. Catecholamine-secreting tumors include paragangliomas, pheochromocytomas, neuroblastomas, and ganglioneuromas. Vasoactive intestinal peptide-secreting tumors include neurofibromas, neurofibrosarcomas, and ganglioneuromas. Insulin-like factor is secreted by neurofibrosarcomas.[158]

Dumbbell Tumors. Dumbbell tumors extend into the spinal column; they compose 10% of neurogenic tumors. Of all cases of dumbbell tumors, 60% are symptomatic with back pain or radicular pain. Spinal MRIs will define the tumor and its relationship to adjacent structures, especially spinal cord. Neurovascular involvement is best assessed with MRI. Catecholamine metabolic products can be measured in the urine.[159,160]

Nerve Sheath Tumors. Neurilemomas or Schwannomas are the most common neurogenic tumors followed by the neurofibromas. Schwannomas are well-encapsulated tumors; neurofibromas are not. They are both slow-growing benign lesions. They tend to occur between the third and fifth decades of life and can be associated with von Recklinghausen disease. Symptoms are usually caused by pressure on the affected nerves. Both types of tumor can undergo malignant degeneration into neurofibrosarcomas, also known as malignant nerve sheath tumors. Neurofibrosarcomas are fast-growing tumors that can invade adjacent structures. Hypoglycemic episodes have been described secondary to insulin-like substances produced by these tumors.[161]

Sympathetic Ganglia Tumors. This group of tumors is the second most common type of neurogenic mediastinal mass. These are most common in children and include benign and malignant lesions. Ganglioneuromas are benign, typically well-encapsulated elongated tumors. Ganglioneuroblastomas can occur as diffuse or composite subtypes. Although the diffuse type generally behaves as a benign tumor, it can metastasize in 5% of cases; the composite type has almost a 75% incidence of metastasis.

Neuroblastomas generally occur in children and usually in a child younger than age 4 years. They can secrete a variety of hormonally active substances and produce a characteristic neurologic opsoclonus-polymyoclonus syndrome with cerebellar and truncal ataxia.[162,163] Twenty percent of all neuroblastomas present within the thorax; the median age of the child at presentation with neuroblastoma is 11 months.[158]

Paraganglionic Tumors. Paragangliomas are vascular and hormonally active tumors. They are the least common type of neurogenic tumors. Patients who have functional tumors present with headaches, hypertension, and palpitations. Although the tumor is most commonly found in the paravertebral area, it can also be found in the middle mediastinum. Of all cases, 10% of paragangliomas are multiple and are associated with the multiple endocrine neoplasm syndrome.[164] Chemodactomas are less likely to be functional. Malignancy is determined by the clinical course of the patient. Diagnosis of hormonally active lesions is confirmed with measurement of urine catecholamine metabolites. These lesions appear on CT scan as vascular tumors that enhance with intravenous contrast. The MIBG scan can detect most of these lesions when CT scan fails.

Treatment. Surgery is the treatment of choice for neurogenic mediastinal lesions. Preoperative management includes functional assessment of these lesions in patients with suggestive symptoms and evaluation for intraspinal extension. Catecholamine-secreting tumors should be managed preoperatively in a manner similar to adrenal pheochromocytomas. If a lesion is determined to have an intraspinal component, it should be unroofed with a neurosurgeon followed by resection of the thoracic component by the thoracic team as a single stage procedure. Thoracoscopic resections have also been performed.[165–167] Complete surgical excision is essential. Although patient prognosis is excellent for benign tumors, prognosis depends on staging for the neuroblastomas, with chemotherapy included in the treatment regimen for advanced stage tumors.

Mediastinal Infections

Mediastinitis is one of the most serious infections that a surgeon may have to manage. The most common etiologies include esophageal perforations or postoperative esophageal anastomotic leaks, infections after median sternotomy for cardiac procedures, and extensions into the mediastinum of oropharyngeal, vertebral, pulmonary, or chest wall infections.

Postoperative wound infections after cardiac procedures occur in 2% of cases; they can range from a superficial cellulitis to severe sepsis with deep sternal and mediastinal involvement. Predisposing factors include diabetes, bilateral internal mammary artery harvesting, prolonged cardiopulmonary bypass and operative time, cardiogenic shock, and chest compressions during cardiopulmonary resuscitation.

Mediastinitis can present with fever, leukocytosis, sternal pain, chest pain, or neck pain depending on the initial site of the infection. Sternal instability may occur in patients with a median sternotomy. Patients with esophageal-related infections secondary to cervical anastomotic leaks or trauma present with neck pain, wound drainage, or subcutaneous emphysema. Perforations from foreign bodies or diagnostic esophagoscopy tend to occur at the level of the cricopharyngeal muscle, whereas therapeutic dilation of strictures or achalasia occur just above the site of intervention. Mediastinal esophageal perforations can cause chest pain, fever, and pleural effusion. On physical examination, varying degrees of superficial neck and sternal cellulitis can be present. Subcutaneous emphysema from esophageal perforation or descending mediastinal gas from oropharyngeal infections can be present. Differentiation between superficial wound infections and deep mediastinal infections is facilitated with the use of CT scan. Confirmation of esophageal perforation is recommended with either a water-soluble contrast esophagogram, barium esophagogram, or esophagoscopy.

Treatment

Treatment of these infections varies from local wound care to extensive débridement and flap reconstruction. In superficial sternal infections or localized neck infections secondary to esophageal leaks, local wound care with incision and adequate drainage will suffice as long as all fluid collections are drained. In more extensive cases with deep mediastinal involvement, extensive débridement of the mediastinal fascia is necessary. All necrotic cartilage, sternal bone, and ribs have to be removed. Irrigation with antibiotics is helpful. The wound can be closed with the use of closed irrigation systems if débridement was adequate, or it can be left open for continuous irrigation and débridement. Pectoralis, rectus, or omental flaps can be used for obliteration of dead space, once control of the ongoing infection has been obtained.

Mediastinal granulomatous infections are chronic infections with multiple causes, including all of the endemic mycoses, sarcoid, syphilis, tuberculosis, and fungus. In recent years, histoplasmosis has replaced tuberculosis as the most common cause of mediastinal granulomatous infection in the United States. A sequela of mediastinal histoplasmosis is the development of mediastinal fibrosis. One third of patients with chronic granulomatous disease progress to mediastinal fibrosis. In addition, airway compression and esophageal fistulas have been reported. Mediastinal fibrosis is the most common benign cause of SVC syndrome. The use of antifungal agents does not result in regression of this fibrosis. The predominant finding at surgery is extensive and dense fibrotic reaction involving the mediastinal structures. Surgery has been performed to relieve airway compromise, repair esophageal fistulas, and reconstruct the SVC.

Superior Vena Cava (SVC) Syndrome

The SVC syndrome refers to compression, invasion, or occlusion of the SVC lumen. The causes vary and include benign, malignant, and iatrogenic etiologies. Although benign disease was the main cause of this syndrome historically, malignant disease has become the most common etiology today representing about 90% of the cases.[168] Iatrogenic causes of SVC syndrome commonly occur secondary to indwelling intravenous pacemakers and intravenous catheters.[169]

Symptoms and Signs

Patients present with cough, and dyspnea on exertion; on physical examination there is facial and upper extremity edema with venous distention of the head, face, and chest wall. Symptoms may be minimal if the occlusion occurred gradually.

Malignant Etiology

Bronchogenic carcinoma is the most common malignant cause of SVC syndrome (75%), with 67% being non–small-cell and 33% small-cell histology. Lymphomas are the second most common malignant cause, followed by metastatic disease causing compression of two sides of the vena cava by mediastinal nodes.[170]

Benign Etiology

Multiple infectious diseases have been reported to cause the SVC syndrome, with *Histoplasmosis* the most common. Other causes of granulomatous reaction include blastomycosis, tuberculosis, nocardia infection, syphilis, actinomycosis, sarcoid tumors, and radiation therapy.[171,172] The latter does not require compression of two sides by nodes since mediastinal fibrosis is the underlying mechanism.

Diagnosis

The diagnosis of SVC syndrome begins with the physical examination and can be confirmed with contrast-enhanced CT or MRI; these have replaced other more invasive imaging methods. Histologic diagnosis guides therapy. Although this can be obtained with ultrasound-guided biopsies,[173] mediastinoscopy is generally more helpful in obtaining adequate tissue sample from nodes adjacent to large blood vessels.

Treatment

The average survival for untreated SVC syndrome is 7 months, but it is dependent on the etiology. Treatment consists of radiotherapy, chemotherapy, surgery, or thrombolysis specific to the etiology. Head elevation, diuretics, and O_2 are initial supportive measures. Radiotherapy is the most common treatment used, with excellent results in up to 90% of patients.[174]

Chemotherapy is used for malignancies known to respond, such as small-cell carcinomas or lymphomas.[175] Intravascular balloon dilatation and stenting is a highly effective intervention if other interventions cannot palliate symptoms in a timely manner. Other methods such as venous interposition grafting, replacement, bypass, thrombectomy, and thrombolysis have been used in patients who develop life-threatening symptoms.[176,177] Replacement or bypass of the vena cava has been more successful with autologous than prosthetic material.[178–181]

Thrombectomy and thrombolytic therapy have been used for catheter-induced syndromes, with the best results in patients who receive long-term anticoagulation and have the foreign body removed.

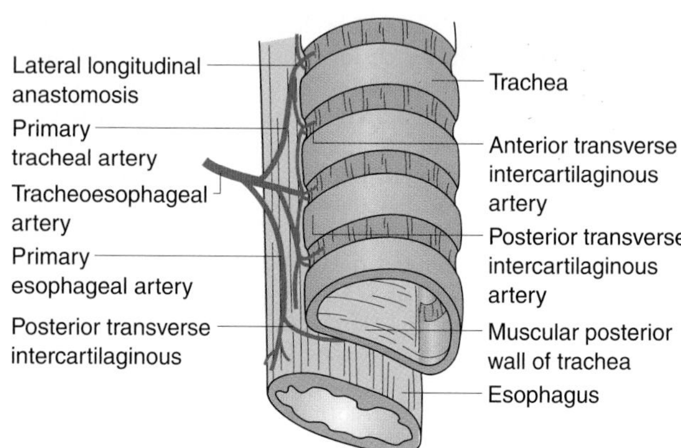

FIGURE 82.32 Semischematic view of the tracheal microscopical blood supply. Transverse intercartilaginous arteries derived from the lateral longitudinal anastomosis penetrate the soft tissues between each cartilage to supply a rich vascular network beneath the endotracheal mucosa. (After Salassa JR, Pearson BW, Payne WS, et al. Gross and microscopical blood supply of the trachea. *Ann Thorac Surg*. 1977;24:100–107.)

TRACHEA

Anatomy

The adult trachea extends from the anterior border of the cricoid cartilage to the carinal spur, with an average length of 11 cm. It has between 18 and 22 cartilaginous rings or two rings per centimeter. The rings are C-shaped with the cartilaginous portion making up the anterior and lateral walls and the membranous portion making up the posterior wall. The blood supply of the trachea has multiple sources that interconnect along the lateral walls of the trachea. The cervical trachea receives its blood supply from the inferior thyroid artery branches and tracheoesophageal branches of the subclavian artery. The thoracic trachea has a more variable blood supply, and numerous arteries may contribute branches from sources such as the innominate, internal thoracic, subclavian, and intercostal arteries (Fig. 82.32)[182] In general, the tracheobronchial angles are supplied by branches of the bronchial arteries.

Tracheal Tumors

Tumors involving the trachea may be either intrinsic or extrinsic. Extrinsic tumors are the same lesions that cause SVC syndrome. Malignant intrinsic tumors are more common than benign intrinsic tracheal tumors. The benign tumors are divided into papillomas, chondromas, fibromas, hemangiomas. The most common type of benign tumor is the papilloma, followed by chondroma, hamartoma, and fibroma. The small remaining miscellaneous group includes granular cell tumors, fibrous histiocytomas, glomus tumors, lipomas, leiomyomas, neurofibromas, and hamartomas.

Symptoms depend on the location of the tumor (distal versus proximal) and include voice changes, cough, hemoptysis, and airway obstruction with stridor or shortness of breath. Some patients have no symptoms at all.

Benign Intrinsic Tracheal Tumors

Papillomas. Papillomas are associated with the human papilloma viruses 6 and 11. They occur mainly in the larynx and have an irregular gross appearance. They can undergo malignant degeneration, especially in adults. Resection is indicated for lesions causing symptoms at any age and in adults to avoid malignancy. A variety of methods have been used, with laser resection increasing in popularity.

Chondromas. Chondromas originate from cartilage and tend to occur mainly in adults. They also have a tendency to recur, although not as commonly as papillomas. Surgical resection is the treatment of choice.

Hamartomas. Hamartomas also contain cartilage and in addition have epithelial and lymph tissue. It is a benign overgrowth of normal tissue components of the trachea. Resection is the treatment of choice because they cannot be differentiated from carcinoma without histology. These lesions rarely recur, and resections margins can be small.

Fibromas. Fibromas and fibrous histiocytomas tend to occur proximally, but unlike papillomas they have a smooth appearance. Resection can be accomplished bronchoscopically for fibromas, but fibrous histiocytomas have a tendency for recurrence, necessitating complete surgical resection.

Hemangiomas. Hemangiomas can occur at any age, but they represent the most common type of tracheal lesion in the pediatric population. They also have a female predilection. They tend to occur proximally, and, like other hemangiomas at other sites, they can enlarge and cause threatening airway obstruction. Unlike other benign tracheal lesions, they do often regress spontaneously, and observation is the initial treatment. Biopsy is to be avoided because hemorrhage is a common sequela. Surgery is reserved for persistent lesions.[183] If the hemangioma is too extensive, tracheostomy and stenting may be necessary for palliation of the threatened airway.

Malignant Intrinsic Tracheal Tumors

Malignant tumors of the trachea are more common that benign tumors, but still represent only 1% to 2% of all lung carcinomas. Primary tumors typically are squamous cell, adenoid cystic, and carcinoid lesions. Multiple other types of primary tumors have been described, but these three types are the most common. Common secondary malignant tumors include laryngeal, thyroid, lung, and esophageal cancers.

Primary malignant tumors have similar clinical presentations to the benign lesions. Cough, hemoptysis, and airway obstruction are commonly seen. Biopsy establishes the diagnosis.[184] Complete surgical resection, if possible, is the treatment of choice for these primary tumors. Adjuvant chemoradiation is offered, although its role has not been established in randomized series due to the low number of accrued cases.

Squamous Cell Carcinoma. Squamous cell carcinoma of the trachea presents typically as a single lesion fairly well localized superficially infiltrating lesion. Metastases to local nodes are seen in almost one third of the patients at presentation. Squamous cell carcinoma of the trachea occurs more commonly in males, with a male to female ratio of 3:1.

Adenoid Cystic Carcinoma. Adenoid cystic carcinomas are slow-growing tumors that can also involve a significant part of the trachea. They have a tendency to grow submucosally and involve more of the trachea than is clinically evident. Metastases to regional nodes occur. This tumor has a tendency to displace rather than invade adjacent structures even when large. It occurs with equal frequency in males and females.

Carcinoids. Carcinoids tend to occur as focal lesions in the tracheobronchial angles. Systemic symptoms of carcinoid such as flushing and diarrhea occur in 10% of cases. For completely resected lesions, 5-year survival rates of up to 90% have been reported.

Secondary Malignant Tumors. Laryngeal, thyroid, lung, and esophageal cancer can involve the trachea by direct extension. Tracheoesophageal fistulas are more common with esophageal cancer, and mediastinal nodal recurrence of lung cancer. These fistulas usually involve the left main bronchus. Tracheal involvement usually indicates unresectable disease, with the notable exception of limited tracheal involvement and negative mediastinal lymph nodes. Palliation for thyroid and laryngeal carcinomas with tracheal extension can occasionally be achieved with resection.

Surgical Airways

Surgical airways can be established either via tracheostomy (percutaneous or open) or cricothyroidotomy. The indications for a surgical airway are: airway obstruction at or above the larynx, inability to control airway secretions with other methods, and need for chronic ventilatory support for respiratory failure for relief of upper airway obstruction.

Tracheostomy

Controversy exists regarding the timing of tracheostomy for chronic ventilatory support. Laryngeal complications of orotracheal intubation have been described as early as 2 to 5 days after intubation, hence early tracheostomy should be considered.

Multiple techniques of tracheostomy have been described. These have been performed via horizontal or vertical skin incisions, or cruciate, vertical, horizontal, or flap-creating tracheal incisions. No technique has proven superior. The important technical aspects of this procedure are placement of the tracheal incision over the second, third, or fourth tracheal rings but not lower; avoidance of a large tracheal incision; and limiting dilation of the incision to no more than the actual tube size. The larger the tracheal incision the greater the chance for tracheal stenosis. A low tracheal incision places the tracheotomy tube close to the innominate artery and increases the potential for tracheoinnominate fistula formation. Percutaneous tracheostomy has gained popularity in recent years. Reviews of the experience with this procedure show a tracheal stenosis rate of 1.6% to 6%.[185,186]

Cricothyroidotomy

The main indication for cricothyroidotomy is the establishment of a surgical airway in an emergency situation. It is faster and easier to perform than tracheostomy because less dissection is needed. A tube as large as 8 mm can be inserted through an incision in the cricothyroid membrane. With this procedure, there is greater chance for an injury to the vocal cords and for subglottic stenosis, which is a difficult problem to correct. Cricothyroidotomies should be converted to a tracheostomy within 48 hours when possible. This procedure should also be avoided in children younger than 12 years.

Complications of Surgical Airways

Common complications of surgical airways are infection, hemorrhage, tracheal stenosis, and, rarely, tracheoesophageal fistulas. Tracheostomies are typically colonized with both gram-positive and gram-negative organisms, such as *Staphylococcus*, *Streptococcus*, and *Pseudomonas*. These organisms can cause cellulitis, mediastinitis, tracheobronchitis, and pneumonitis. Meticulous skin care and stoma care is essential.

Early postoperative bleeding usually occurs from the divided thyroid isthmus. This bleeding can be controlled with epinephrine-soaked sponges or topical anticoagulants. If unsuccessful, the patient should be returned to the operating room intubated through the larynx, and then the tracheal device removed for hemostasis. Late bleeding is usually secondary to granulation or tracheal erosions. The most serious bleeding occurs from erosion of the cuff or the tip of the tube into the innominate artery. It is a particular risk with low-placed tracheostomies or a high artery. Immediate control of the bleeding is essential to prevent exsanguination. Repair of this fistula involves reconstruction of the artery without prosthetic materials and tracheal repair with or without resection (Fig. 82.33).

Tracheoesophageal fistula can occur (Fig. 82.34) with either orotracheal or tracheostomy tubes. Either the cuff or the tube tip can erode posterior into the esophagus. The unsupported weight of the ventilator tubing may contribute to this, as does a concomitant nasogastric tube in the esophagus. Signs include impaired ventilation and reflux of gastric contents into the tracheobronchial tree. The fistula should be initially controlled with a larger volume low-pressure cuff or by advancing the tube further. Any esophageal tube should be removed and a gastrostomy performed with definite correction when the patient no longer requires endotracheal intubation. Tracheal stenosis occurs even with modern low-pressure cuffs if they are overinflated. The longer the period of endotracheal intubation, the higher the chance of such an injury. Large tracheal incisions for tracheostomy and hypotension have been implicated in the pathogenesis of this lesion.

Patients with tracheal stenosis can be asymptomatic early on, presenting years later with wheezing, dyspnea, or stridor, and be misdiagnosed with adult-onset asthma. In addition, segments of the trachea between the stoma and the cuff level can become malacic and collapse with respiratory effort. Treatment of tracheal stenosis involves initial dilation of the stenosis or tracheostomy below a high stenosis to relieve airway obstruction and elective resection of the lesion with adequate mobilization to ensure a tension-free end-to-end anastomosis.[187]

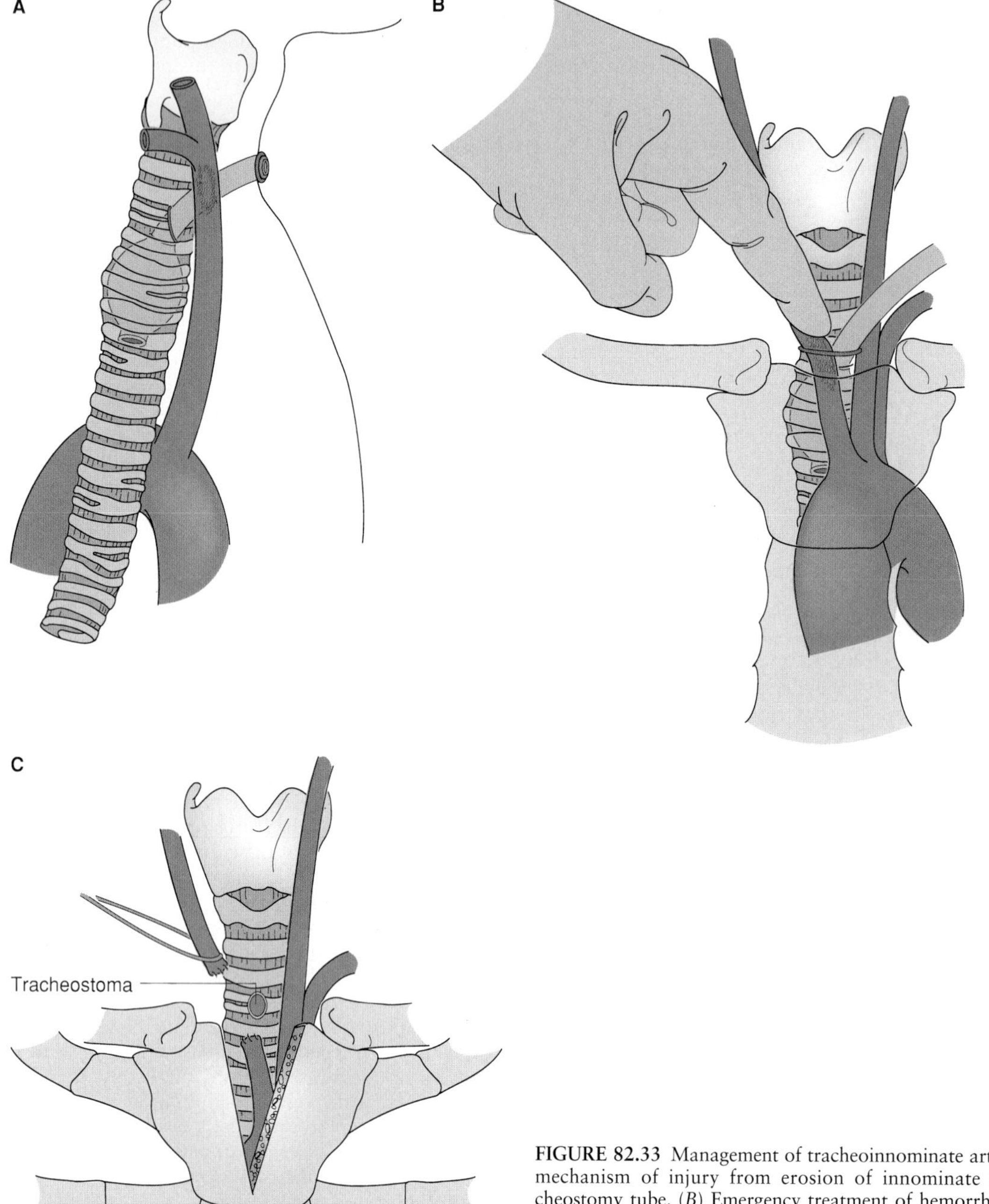

FIGURE 82.33 Management of tracheoinnominate artery fistula. (*A*) Common mechanism of injury from erosion of innominate artery by adjacent tracheostomy tube. (*B*) Emergency treatment of hemorrhage involves insertion of an endotracheal tube into the tracheostomy stoma, inflation of the cuff and downward and outward pressure on the fistula by the finger inserted through the tracheostomy incision to further tamponade the bleeding. (C) Through a partial upper sternal split, the segment of involved innominate artery is resected, and the oversewn ends covered with adjacent mediastinal fat or muscle. Tracheal resection is usually not necessary. A new tracheostomy tube may have to be inserted higher in the trachea or, if possible, the tracheostomy tube removed and the stoma covered with a sternohyoid muscle flap.

LUNG INFECTIONS

Abscess

Since the advent of effective antibiotics beginning with the penicillins in the 1940s, many fewer pneumonic processes progress to abscess formation. Mortality rates of 30% with residual chronic symptoms in 30% of patients prior to the introduction of the antibiotics have been greatly reduced. However, with the increasing incidence of solid organ transplantation requiring immunosuppression, bone marrow transplantation, cancer treatment, HIV infection, and other immune deficiencies, there is an increasing incidence of abscesses with a different pathogenesis and microbiologic flora.

Pathogenesis

Lung abscesses occur as a result of aspiration of infected material from the oropharynx, usually in patients with altered mental status or suppressed cough reflexes. There is often poor oral hygiene and gingival disease. Liquefaction necrosis occurs from the proliferation of anaerobic bacteria, forming a necrotic

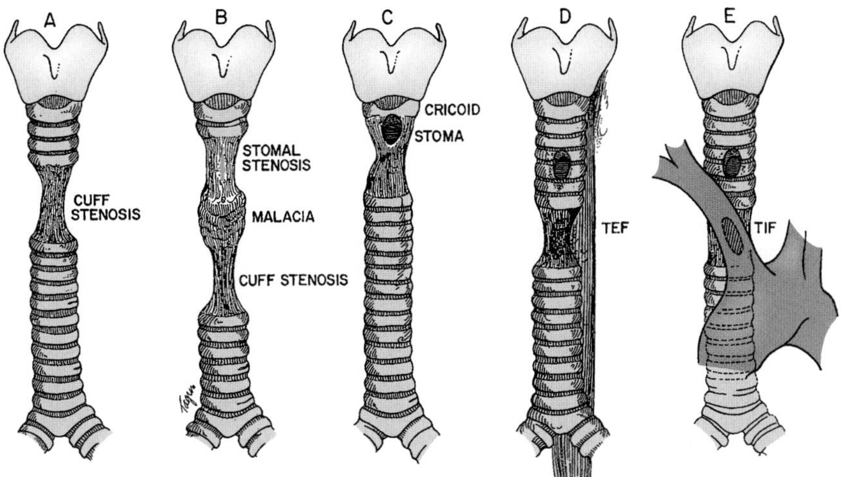

FIGURE 82.34 Diagrams of principal postintubation tracheal lesions. (*A*) Cuff stenosis from the cuff of an endotracheal tube. (*B*) Cuff stenosis from the cuff of a tracheostomy tube, usually lower in the trachea than that from an endotracheal tube. Stomal stenosis also occurs at the site of the tracheostomy itself. Malacia may occur either at the level of the cuff or in the segment between the stoma and the cuff stenosis. (*C*) Cuff stenosis at the site of a high tracheostomy stoma, which has eroded into the lower margin of the cricoid cartilage. In older patients, this may erode back further into the subglottic larynx, producing a laryngotracheal stenosis. A stoma placed in the cricothyroid membrane will, by definition, produce an intralaryngeal stenosis. (*D*) Tracheoesophageal fistula (TEF) produced by pressure of the cuff against the "party wall," often abetted by an indwelling firm nasogastric tube. (*E*) One type of tracheoinnominate fistula (TIF) as the result of a high pressure cuff erosion. The more common type, but also rare, is that seen with a low-placed tracheostomy stoma, which rests against the innominate artery itself. (From Grillo HC. Surgical treatment of postintubation tracheal injuries. *J Thorac Cardiovasc Surg*. 1979;78:860–875.)

cavity (Fig. 82.35). Even though abscesses can occur in any part of the lung, there is a predilection for the posterior segment of the right upper lobe and the superior segment of the right lower lobe since these are the most dependent segments while the patient is supine. Lung abscesses in immunocompromised patients are often hospital acquired; they tend to be multiple rather than single. *Staphylococcus* species, *Escherichia coli, Pseudomonas* species, and fungal organisms are all potential pathogens. If there is adequate communication between the bronchus and the

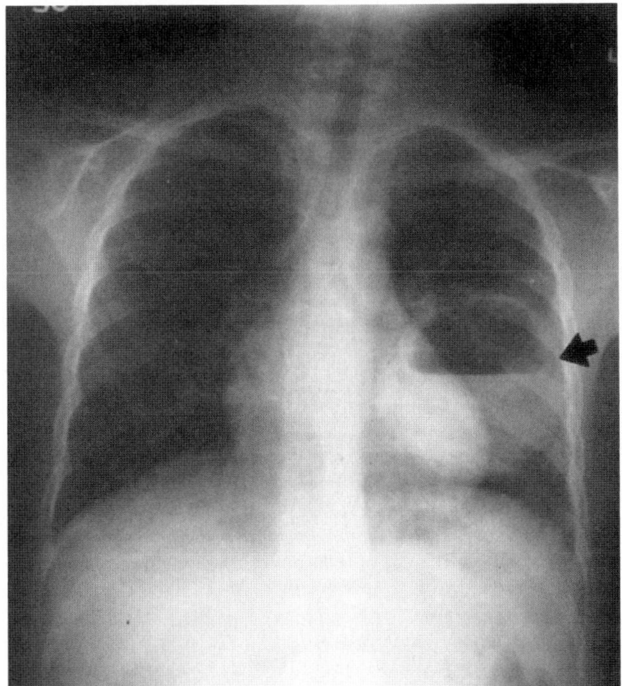

FIGURE 82.35 Chest radiograph showing a large abscess of the left lung with an air-fluid level (*arrow*).

abscess, the lesion can resolve with postural drainage, chest physiotherapy, and antibiotics. Inadequate communication results in incomplete drainage and chronic cavity formation.

Presentation

Typical symptoms are fever, cough, chest pain, occasional hemoptysis, and purulent sputum production. As the cavity erodes into adjacent bronchial segments, it may partially decompress with temporary improvement of symptoms. As the new communication becomes occluded, the symptoms recur. Chest radiographs show consolidation early on with the characteristic air-fluid level in the upright chest radiograph as the disease progresses and establishes communication with a bronchus.

Treatment

Antibiotic therapy with efficacy against anaerobic organisms, postural drainage, and chest physiotherapy are the initial therapies. In immunocompromised patients, broader coverage is needed. Bronchoscopy for cultures, drainage, and to rule out foreign bodies or neoplasm should be performed. Most abscesses less than 3 cm diameter will resolve with these interventions. Operative treatment is reserved for patients who do not respond to antibiotics or in the setting of sepsis, a large residual abscess cavity, empyema, or bronchopleural fistula. Percutaneous aspiration of the cavity can be used for patients who are not candidates for an extensive pulmonary resection. The resultant bronchopleural fistula will heal if adequate drainage of the cavity is established. Mortality rates have decreased significantly compared to the preantibiotic era and are now less than 5%. Abscesses caused by opportunistic organisms have a higher mortality rate, reflecting the immunocompromised state of the patient.

Bronchiectasis

Bronchiectasis (stasis in the bronchus) is an abnormal dilation of the distal bronchi that can be either congenital or acquired.[188]

Of all cases, 75% are acquired and occur as sequelae from chronic bacterial or viral infection. These infections result in obstruction of the distal airways from retained secretions and mucous plugs that lead to dilation and recurrent acute infection. Cystic fibrosis is a common cause of acquired bronchiectasis. There are three types of bronchiectasis based on the gross appearance of the bronchi: varicose, cylindrical, and saccular, with varicose the most common. Most patients present with chronic foul sputum production, fever, and hemoptysis. CT scan and bronchoscopy are used for diagnosis, to rule out extrinsic lesions, and to obtain sputum specimens to guide antibiotic therapy.

Treatment

The treatment for bronchiectasis is mainly nonoperative and consists of antibiotics, chest physiotherapy, and postural drainage. Patients with multisegment disease tend to have more chronic disease and tend to respond less to either medical or surgical treatment. Surgery is reserved for those patients who do not respond after a prolonged course of antibiotics and nonoperative management. It is essential to localize the area to be resected preoperatively. Extensive resections such as pneumonectomy are rarely required in the modern era of antibiotics, but bilateral staged resections are occasionally needed. Double-lumen intubation is useful to avoid intraoperative spillage to the unaffected side.[189] Bronchiectasis was a common mode of death in this country during the preantibiotic era. Today, the disease is rarely seen.

KEY POINTS

- **Pectus excavatum is most common chest wall deformity; it consists of sternal depression because of abnormalities of the lower costal cartilages and occurs in one out of 700 children.**
- **Chest wall tumors are rare. Most arise in the ribs (85%) with the remainder arising from the scapula, sternum, and clavicle.**
- **Chondrosarcoma is the most common of the chest wall malignant tumors, accounting for 20% of such tumors.**
- **Thoracic outlet syndrome refers to compression of neurovascular structures at the thoracic outlet. The neurovascular structures involved are the subclavian artery and vein, and the sympathetic and peripheral nerve components of the brachial plexus.**
- **Pleural effusions are either benign or malignant in origin and can be divided for diagnostic purposes into transudative or exudative categories.**
- **Pneumothorax is the presence of air in the pleural space, which causes deflation of the lung. Pneumothoraces are either spontaneous or acquired. Spontaneous pneumothoraces can be further subdivided into primary or secondary.**
- **Thymoma is the most common adult tumor of the anterosuperior mediastinum.**
- **Mediastinitis is one of the most serious infections that a surgeon may have to manage.**
- **The main indication for cricothyroidotomy is the establishment of a surgical airway in an emergency situation.**

References

1. Iannettoni MD, Orringer MB. Chest wall, pleura, mediastinum, and nonneoplastic lung disease. In: Greenfield LJ, Mulholland MW, Oldham KT, et al., eds. *Surgery: Scientific Principles and Practice,* 2nd ed. Philadelphia: Lippincott–Raven, 1997:1440–1482.
2. Fonkalsrud EW, Dunn JCY, Atkinson JB. Repair of pectus excavatum deformities: 30 years of experience with 375 patients. *Ann Surg.* 2000;231: 443–448.
3. Shamberger RC. Chest wall deformities. In: Shields TW, ed. *General thoracic surgery,* 4th ed. Baltimore: Williams & Wilkins, 1994:529–557.
4. Shamberger RC, Welch KJ. Surgical repair of pectus excavatum. *J Pediatr Surg.* 1988;23:615–622.
5. hamberger RC, Welch KJ, Castaneda AR, et al. Anterior chest wall deformities and congenital heart disease. *J Thorac Cardiovasc Surg.* 1988;96: 427–432.
6. Peterson RJ, Young WC Jr, Godwin JD, et al. Noninvasive assessment of exercise cardiac function before and after pectus excavatum repair. *J Thorac Cardiovasc Surg.* 1985;90:251–260.
7. Ellis DG. Chest wall deformities. *Pediatr Rev.* 1989;11:147–151.
8. Shamberger RC. Congenital chest wall deformities. *Curr Probl Surg.* 1996;33:469–542.
9. Shamberger RC, Welch KJ. Chest wall deformities. In: Ashcraft KW, Holder TM, eds. *Pediatric Surgery,* 2nd ed. Philadelphia: WB Saunders, 1993:146.
10. Ochsner A, DeBakey M. Chone-chondrosternon: report of a case and review of the literature. *J Thorac Surg.* 1939;8:469.
11. Robicsek F, Fokin A. Surgical correction of pectus excavatum and carinatum. *J Cardiovasc Surg.* 1999;40:725–731.
12. Taguchi, TK, Mochizuki T, Nakagaki M, et al. A new plastic operation for pectus excavatum: sternal turnover surgical procedure with preserved internal mammary arteries. *Chest.* 1975;67:606–608.
13. Sirensen JL. Subcutaneous silicone implants in pectus excavatum. *Scand J Plast Reconstr Surg.* 1987;22:173–176.
14. Baue AE. Chest wall, pleura, lungs, and diaphragm. In: Davis JH, Drucker WR, Gann DS, et al., eds. *Clinical Surgery*. St. Louis: Mosby, 1987:1190.
15. Kowalewski J, Brocki M, Zolynski K. Long-term observation in 68 patients operated on for pectus excavatum: surgical repair of funnel chest. *Ann Thorac Surg.* 1999;67:821–824.
16. Nuss D, Kelly RE, Croitoru DP, et al. A 10-year review of minimally invasive technique for the correction of pectus excavatum. *J Pediatr Surg.* 1998;33:545–552.
17. Fonkalsrud EW, Bustorff-Silva J. Repair of pectus excavatum and carinatum in adults. *Am J Surg.* 1999;177:121–124.
18. Shamberger RC, Welch KJ. Surgical correction of pectus carinatum. *J Pediatr Surg.* 1987;22:48–53.
19. **Beiser GD, Epstein SE, Stampfer M, et al. Impairment of cardiac function in patients with pectus excavatum, with improvement after operative correction. *N Engl J Med.* 1972;287:267–272.**
20. Seyfer AE, Icochea R, Graeber GM. Poland's anomaly: natural history and long-term results of chest wall reconstruction in 33 patients. *Ann Surg.* 1988;208:776–782.
21. Shamberger RC, Welch KJ, Upton J Jr. Surgical treatment of thoracic deformity in Poland's syndrome. *J Pediatr Surg.* 1989;24:760–766.
22. Hurwitz DJ, Stofman G, Curtin H. Three-dimensional imaging of Poland's syndrome. *Plast Reconstr Surg.* 1994;94:719–723.
23. Gatti JE. Poland's deformity reconstructions with a customized, extrasoft silicone prosthesis. *Ann Plast Surg.* 1997;39:122–130.
24. **Urschel HC Jr. Poland's syndrome. *Chest Surg Clin North Am.* 2000; 10:393–403.**
25. Marks MW, Iacobucci J. Reconstruction of congenital chest wall deformities using solid silicone onlay prostheses. *Chest Surg Clin North Am.* 2000;10:341–355.
26. Sabiston DC Jr. The surgical management of congenital bifid sternum with a partial ectopia cordis. *J Thorac Surg.* 1958;35:118.
27. Cantrell JR, Haller JA, Ravitch MM. A syndrome of congenital defects involving the abdominal wall, sternum, diaphragm, pericardium, and heart. *Surg Gynecol Obstet.* 1958;107:602–614.
28. Knox L, Tuggle D, Knott-Craig CJ. Repair of congenital sternal clefts in adolescence and infancy. *J Pediatr Surg.* 1994;29:1513–1516.
29. Daum R, Zachariou Z. Total and superior sternal clefts in newborns: a simple technique for surgical correction. *J Pediatr Surg.* 1999;34: 408–411.
30. Anderson BO, Burt ME. Chest wall neoplasms and their management. *Ann Thorac Surg.* 1994;58:1774–1781.
31. Pairolero PC. Chest wall tumors. In: Shields TW, ed. *General Thoracic Surgery,* 4th ed. Baltimore: Williams & Wilkins, 1994:579–589.
32. Graeber GM, Jones DR, Pairolero PC. Primary neoplasms. In: Pearson FG, Deslauriers J, Ginsberg RJ, et al., eds. *Thoracic surgery*. New York: Churchill Livingston, 1995:1237.
33. King RM, Pairolero PC, Trastek VF, et al. Primary chest wall tumors: factors affecting survival. *Ann Thorac Surg.* 1986;41:597–601.
34. Liptay MJ, Fry WA. Malignant bone tumors of the chest wall. *Semin Thorac Cardiovasc Surg.* 1999;11:278–284.
35. Dang NC, Siegel SE, Phillips JD. Malignant chest wall tumors in children and young adults. *J Pediatr Surg.* 1999;34:1773–1778.
36. Burt M, Fulton M, Wessner-Dunlap S, et al. Primary bony and cartilaginous sarcomas of the chest wall: results of therapy. *Ann Thorac Surg.* 1992;54:226–232.
37. Somers J, Faber LP. Chondroma and chondrosarcoma. *Semin Thorac Cardiovasc Surg.* 1999;11:270–277.
38. Douglas YI, Meuzelaar KJ, Van Der Lei B, et al. Osteosarcoma of the sternum. *Eur J Surg Oncol.* 1997;23:90–91.

39. Miser JS, Kinsela TJ, Triche TJ, et al. Preliminary results of treatment of Ewing's sarcoma of bone in children and young adults: six months of intensive combined modality therapy without maintenance. *J Clin Oncol.* 1988;6:484–490.
40. Schuck A, Hofmann J, Rube C, et al. Radiotherapy in Ewing's sarcoma and PNET of the chest wall: results of the trials CESS 81, CESS 86, and EICESS 92. *Int J Radiat Oncol Biol Phys.* 1981;42:1001–1006.
41. Saenz NC, Hass DJ, Meyers P, et al. Pediatric chest wall: Ewing's sarcoma. *J Pediatr Surg.* 2000;35:550–555.
42. Shamberger RC, LaQuaglia MP, Krailo MD, et al. Ewing sarcoma of the rib: results of an intergroup study with analysis of outcome by timing of resection. *J Thorac Cardiovasc Surg.* 2000;119:1154–1161.
43. Faber LP, Somers J, Templeton AC. Chest wall tumors. *Curr Probl Surg.* 1995;32:661–747.
44. Sabanathan S, Shah R, Mearns AJ. Surgical treatment of primary malignant chest wall tumours. *Eur J Cardiothorac Surg.* 1997;11:1011–1016.
45. Pairolero PC, Arnold PG. Chest wall reconstruction. *Ann Thorac Surg.* 1981;32:325–326.
46. McCormack PM, Bains MS, Burt ME, et al. Local recurrent mammary carcinoma failing multimodality therapy. *Arch Surg.* 1989;124:158–161.
47. Mathes SJ. Chest wall reconstruction. *Clin Plast Surg.* 1995; 22: 187.
48. Deschamps C, Tirnaksiz BM, Darbandi R, et al. Early and long-term results of prosthetic chest wall reconstruction. *J Thorac Cardiovasc Surg.* 1999;117:588–591.
49. Pairolero PC. Extended resections for lung cancer: how far is too far? *Eur J Cardiothorac Surg.* 1999;16 (suppl 1):S48–S50.
50. Seyfer AE. Breast cancer invasion into the chest wall with resection and reconstruction. *Semin Thorac Cardiovasc Surg.* 1999;11:285–292.
51. Lardinois D, Muller M, Furrer M, et al. Functional assessment of chest wall integrity after methylmethacrylate reconstruction. *Ann Thorac Surg.* 2000;69:919–923.
52. Urschel HC Jr, Razzuk MA. Thoracic outlet syndrome. In: Sabiston DC Jr, Spencer FC, eds. *Surgery of the Chest.* Philadelphia: WB Saunders, 1990:536–553.
53. Harding A, Silver D. Thoracic outlet syndrome. In: Sabiston DC Jr, ed. *Textbook of Surgery: the Biological Basis of Modern Surgical Practice.* 14th ed. Philadelphia: WB Saunders, 1991:1757.
54. Urschel HC. Thoracic outlet syndromes. In: Baue AE, Geha AS, Hammond GL, et al., eds. *Glenn's Thoracic and Cardiovascular Surgery.* 6th ed. Stamford, CT: Appleton & Lange, 1996:567.
55. Urschel HC, Razzuk M. Upper plexus thoracic outlet syndrome: optimal therapy. *Ann Thorac Surg.* 1997;63:935–939.
56. Abe M, Ichinohe K, Nishida J. Diagnosis, treatment, and complications of thoracic outlet syndrome. *J Orthop Sci.* 1999;4:66–69.
57. Mackinnon SE, Patterson GA, Novak CB. Thoracic outlet syndrome: a current overview. *Semin Thorac Cardiovasc Surg.* 1996a;8:176–182.
58. Netter FH. Clinical symposia. CIBA-GEIGY Corporation, 1971.
59. Ryan GM. Thoracic outlet syndrome. *J Shoulder Elbow Surg.* 1998; 7:440.
60. Pang D, Wessel HB. Thoracic outlet syndrome. *Neurosurgery.* 1988;22: 105–121.
61. Novak CB. Conservative management of thoracic outlet syndrome. *Semin Thorac Cardiovasc Surg.* 1996;8:201–207.
62. Mackinnon SE, Patterson AG. Supraclavicular first rib resection. *Semin Thorac Cardiovasc Surg.* 1996;8:208.
63. Goff CD, Parent FN, Sato DT, et al. A comparison of surgery for neurogenic thoracic outlet syndrome between laborers and nonlaborers. *Am J Surg.* 1998;176:215–218.
64. **Urschel HC Jr, Razzuk MA. Neurovascular compression in the thoracic outlet: changing management over 50 years. *Ann Surg.* 1998;228: 609–617.**
65. Light RW. The physiology of pleural fluid production and benign pleural effusion. In: Shields TW, ed. *General Thoracic Surgery,* 4th ed. Malvern, PA: Williams & Wilkins, 1994:676.
66. Jerjes-Sanchez C, Ramirez-Rivera A, Elijalde JJ, et al. Intrapleural fibrinolysis with streptokinase as an adjunctive treatment in hemothorax and empyema: a multicenter trial. *Chest.* 1996;109:1514–1519.
67. **Chin NK, Lim TK. Controlled trial of intrapleural streptokinase in the treatment of pleural empyema and complicated parapneumonic effusions. *Chest.* 1997;111:275–279.**
68. Wait MA, Sharma S, Hohn J, et al. A randomized trial of empyema therapy. *Chest.* 1997;111:1548–1551.
69. Davies CW, Kearny SE, Gleeson FV, et al. Predictors of outcome and long-term survival in patients with pleural infection. *Am J Respir Crit Care Med.* 1999;160:1682–1687.
70. Huang HC, Chang HY, Chen CW, et al. Predicting factors for outcome of tube thoracostomy in complicated parapneumonic effusion for empyema. *Chest.* 1999;115:751–756.
71. DeMeester TR, Lafontaine E. The pleura. In: Sabiston DC Jr, Spencer FC, eds. *Surgery of the chest,* 5th ed. Philadelphia: WB Saunders, 1990: 444–497.
72. Rimensberger PC, Muller-Schenker B, Kalangos A, et al. Treatment of a persistent postoperative chylothorax with somatostatin. *Ann Thorac Surg.* 1998;66:253–254.
73. Cope C, Salem R, Kaiser LR. Management of chylothorax by percutaneous catheterization and embolization of the thoracic duct: prospective trial. *J Vasc Intervent Radiol.* 1999;10:1248–1254.
74. Kelly RF, Shumway SJ. Conservative management of postoperative chylothorax using somatostatin. *Ann Thorac Surg.* 2000;69:1944–1945.
75. **Sassoon CS. The etiology and treatment of spontaneous pneumothorax. *Curr Opin Pulm Med.* 1995;1:331–338.**
76. Martin T, Fontana G, Olak J, et al. Use of pleural catheter for the management of simple pneumothorax. *Chest.* 1996;110:1169–1172.
77. Schramel FMNH, Postmus PE, Vanderschueren RGJRA. Current aspects of spontaneous pneumothorax. *Eur Respir J.* 1997;10:1372–1379.
78. Cardillo G, Facciolo F, Giunti R, et al. Videothoracoscopic treatment of primary spontaneous pneumothorax: a 6-year experience. *Ann Thorac Surg.* 2000;69:357–362.
79. **Hatz RA, Kaps MF, Meimarakis G, et al. Long-term results after video-assisted thoracoscopic surgery for first-time and recurrent spontaneous pneumothorax. *Ann Thorac Surg.* 2000;70:253–257.**
80. Rusch VW. Diffuse malignant mesothelioma. In: Shields TW, LoCicero J III, Ponn RB, eds. *General thoracic surgery,* 5th ed. Philadelphia: Lippincott Williams & Wilkins, 2000, pp. 767–782.
81. Nicholson WJ, Perket G, Selikoff IJ. Occupational exposure to asbestos: population at risk and projected mortality 1980–2030. *Am J Ind Med.* 1982;3:259–311.
82. Hammar SP, Bolen JW. Pleural neoplasms. In: Dail DH, Hammar SP, eds. *Pulmonary Pathology.* New York: Springer, 1988:979.
83. Flores RM, Sugarbaker DJ. Malignant mesothelioma of the pleural space. *Ann Thorac Surg.* 2000;70:306.
84. Butchart EG, Ashcroft T, Barnsley WC, et al. Pleuropneumonectomy in the management of diffuse malignant mesothelioma of the pleura: experience with 29 patients. *Thorax.* 1976;31:15–24.
85. Sugarbaker DJ, Strauss GM, Lynch TJ, et al. Node status has prognostic significance in the multimodality therapy of diffuse, malignant mesothelioma. *J Clin Oncol.* 1993;11:1172–1178.
86. **Sugarbaker DJ, Flores RM, Jaklitsch MT, et al. Resection margins, extrapleural nodal status, and cell type determine postoperative long-term survival in trimodality therapy of malignant pleural mesothelioma: results in 183 patients. *Thorac Cardiovasc Surg.* 1999;117:54–65.**
87. Rusch VW, The International Mesothelioma Interest Group. A proposed new international TNM staging system for malignant pleural mesothelioma. *Chest.* 1995;108:1122–1128.
88. Wanebo JH, Martini N, Melamed MR, et al. Pleural mesothelioma. *Cancer.* 1976;38:2481–2488.
89. Rusch VW. Pleurectomy/decortication in the setting of multimodality treatment for diffuse malignant pleural mesothelioma. *Semin Thorac Cardiovasc Surg.* 1997;9:367–372.
90. Kaiser LR. New therapies in the treatment of malignant pleural mesothelioma. *Semin Thorac Cardiovasc Surg.* 1997;9:383–390.
91. Rusch VW, Venkatraman ES. Important prognostic factors in patients with malignant pleural mesothelioma managed surgically. *Ann Thorac Surg.* 1999;68:1799–1804.
92. Jablons D. Positron emission tomography with F18-fluorodeoxyglucose in the staging and preoperative evaluation of malignant pleural mesothelioma. *J Thorac Cardiovasc Surg.* 2000;120:128–133.
93. Esposito C, Romeo C. Surgical anatomy of the mediastinum. *Semin Pediatr Surg.* 1999;8:50–53.
94. Heimburger IL, Battersby JS, Vellios F. Primary neoplasms of the mediastinum: a fifteen-year experience. *Arch Surg.* 1963;978–984.
95. Azanow KS, Pearl RH, Zurcher R, et al. Primary mediastinal masses: a comparison of adult and pediatric populations. *J Thorac Cardiovasc Surg.* 1993;106:67–72.
96. Billmire DF. Germ cell, mesenchymal, and thymic tumors of the mediastinum. *Semin Pediatr Surg.* 1999;8:85–91.
97. **Haller JA, Mazur DO, Morgan WM. Diagnosis and management of mediastinal masses in children. *J Thorac Cardiovasc Surg.* 1969; 58:385.**
98. Davis RD, Oldham HN, Sabiston DC. Primary cysts and neoplasms of the mediastinum: recent changes in clinical presentation, methods or diagnosis, management and results. *Ann Thorac Surg.* 1987;44:229–237.
99. Rubush JL, Gardner IC, Boyd WK, et al. Mediastinal tumors: review of 186 cases. *J Thorac Cardiovasc Surg* 1973;65:216–222.
100. **Lousta R, Koikkalainen K, Jyrala A, et al. Mediastinal tumors: a follow-up of 208 patients. *Scand J Thorac Cardiovasc Surg.* 1978;12: 253–259.**
101. Ovum E, Birkeland S. Mediastinal tumors and cysts: a review of 191 cases. *Scand J Thorac Cardiovasc Surg.* 1983;86:727.
102. Mullen B, Richardson JD. Primary anterior mediastinal tumors in children and adults. *Ann Thorac Surg.* 1986;42:338–345.
103. Cohen AJ, Thompson L, Edwards FH, et al. Primary cysts and tumors of the mediastinum. *Ann Thorac Surg.* 1991;41:378–386.
104. **Whooley BP, Urschel JD, Antkowiak JG, et al. Primary tumors of the mediastinum. *J Surg Oncol.* 1999;70:95–99.**
105. Harris GJ, Harmon PK, Trinkel JK, et al. Standard biplane roentgenography is highly sensitive in documenting mediastinal masses. *Ann Thorac Surg.* 1987;44:238–241.

106. Pugatch RD, Faling LJ, Robbins AH, et al. CT diagnosis of benign mediastinal abnormalities. *AJR* 1980;134:685.
107. VonSchulthess GK, McMurdok, Tscholakoff D, et al. Mediastinal masses: MR imaging. *Radiology.* 1986;158:259–289.
108. Shapiro B, Sisson J, Kalff V, et al. The location of a middle mediastinal pheochromocytoma. *J Thorac Cardiovasc Surg.* 1984;87:814–820.
109. Helio A. Tumors in the mediastinum: US-guided histologic core core-needle biopsy. *Radiology* 1993;189:143.
110. D'Agostino HB, Sanchez RB, Laoide RM, et al. Anterior mediastinal lesions: transsternal biopsy with CT guidance work in progress. *Radiology.* 1993;189:703.
111. Bressler EL, Kirkham JA. Mediastinal masses: alternative approaches to CT-guided needle biopsy. *Radiology.* 1994;191:391–396.
112. Mack M, Landreneau R. Thoracoscopy for the diseases of the mediastinum including thymectomy for myasthenia gravis. *Semin Laparosc Surg.* 1996;3:245–252.
113. Roviaro G, Varoli F, Nucca O, et al. Videothoracoscopic approach to primary mediastinal pathology. *Chest.* 2000;117:1179–1183.
114. Morgenthaler TI, Brown LR, Colby TV, et al. Thymoma. *Mayo Clin Proc.* 1993;68:1110–1123.
115. Masaoka A, Monden Y, Nakahara K, et al. Follow-up study of thymomas with special references to their clinical stages. *Cancer.* 1981;48:2485.
116. Kirchen T, Muller-Hermelink HK. New approaches to the diagnosis of thymic epithelial tumors. *Prog Surg Pathol.* 1989;70:167–189.
117. Weide LG, Ulbright TM, Loehrer PJ, et al. Thymic carcinoma: a distinct clinical entity responsive to chemotherapy. *Cancer.* 1993;71: 1219–1223.
118. Nakahara K, Ohno K, Hashimoto J, et al. Thymoma: results with complete resection and adjuvant postoperative irradiation in 141 consecutive patients. *J Thorac Cardiovasc Surg.* 1988;95:1041–1047.
119. Urgesi A, Monetti V, Ross G, et al. Role of radiation therapy in locally advanced thymoma. *Radiother Oncol.* 1990;19:273–280.
120. Loeher PJ Sr, Perez CA, Roth LM, et al. Chemotherapy for advanced thymoma: preliminary results of an intergroup study. *Ann Intern Med.* 1990;113:520–524.
121. Thomas CR, Wright CD, Loehrer PJ. Thymoma: state of the art. *J Clin Oncol.* 1999;17:2280–2289.
122. Gripp S, Hilgers K, Wurm R, et al. Thymoma: prognostic factors and treatment outcomes. *Cancer.* 1998;83:1495–1503.
123. Okumura M, Miyoshi S, Takeuchi Y, et al. Results of surgical treatment of thymomas with special reference to the involved organs. *J Thorac Cardiovasc Surg.* 1999;117:605–613.
124. Wilkins KB, Sheikh E, Green R, et al. Clinical and pathologic predictors of survival in patients with thymoma. *Ann Surg.* 1999;230:562–572.
125. Treves TA, Rocca WA, Menoeghin F. Epidemiology of myasthenia gravis. In: Anderson DW, Schoenberg DG, eds. *Neuroepidemiology: a tribute to Bruce Schoenberg.* Boston: CRC Press,1991:297.
126. Phillips LH, Torner JC. Has the natural history of myasthenia gravis changed over the past 40 years? An analysis of the epidemiological literature. *Neurology.* 1993;43:A386.
127. Phillips LH. The epidemiology of myasthenia gravis. *Neurol Clin North Am.* 1994;12:263–271.
128. Hopkins LC. Clinical features of myasthenia gravis. *Neurol Clin North Am.* 1994;12:243–261.
129. Saunders DB, Scoppetta C. The treatment of patients with myasthenia gravis. *Neurol Clin North Am.* 1994;12:343–368.
130. Crucitti F, Doglietto GB, Bellanone R, et al. Effects of surgical treatment in thymoma with myasthenia gravis: our experience in 103 patients. *J Surg Oncol.* 1992;50:43–46.
131. Nussbaum MS, Rosenthal GJ, Saunders KJ, et al. Management of myasthenia gravis by extended thymectomy with anterior mediastinal dissection. *Surgery.* 1992;112:681–688.
132. Sugarbaker DJ. Thoracoscopy in the management of anterior mediastinal masses. *Ann Thorac Surg.* 1993;56:653–656.
133. Defilippi VJ, Richman DP, Ferguson MK. Transcervical thymectomy for myasthenia gravis. *Ann Thorac Surg.* 1994;57:194–197.
134. Yellin A. Lymphoproliferative diseases. *Chest Surg Clin North Am.* 1992;2:107–120.
135. Glick RD, La Quaglia MP. Lymphomas of the anterior mediastinum. *Semin Pediatr Surg.* 1999;8:69–77.
136. Kuhn MW, Weissbach L. Localization, incidence, diagnosis, and treatment of extratesticular germ cell tumors. *Urol Int.* 1985;40:166–172.
137. Chaganti RSK, Rodriguez E, Mathew S. Origin of adult male mediastinal germ cell tumors. *Lancet.* 1994;343:1130–1132.
138. Dulmet EM, Macchiavini P, Suc B, et al. Germ cell tumors of the mediastinum: a 30 year experience. *Cancer* 1993;72:1895–1901.
139. Mandelbaum I. Germ cell tumors of the mediastinum. *Chest Surg Clin North Am.* 1992;2:203–211.
140. Jain KK, Bols GJ, Bains MS, et al. The treatment of extragonadal seminoma. *J Clin Oncol.* 1984;2:820–827.
141. Motzer R, Bosl G, Heelan R, et al. Residual mass: an indication for further therapy in patients with advanced seminoma following systemic chemotherapy. *J Clin Oncol.* 1987;5:1065–1070.
142. Shields TW. Primary lesions of the mediastinum and their investigation and treatment. In: Shields TW, ed. *General Thoracic Surgery.* Baltimore: Williams & Wilkins, 1994:1724–1769.
143. Kantoff O. Surgical and medical management of germ cell tumors of the chest. *Chest.* 1993;103:331S–335S.
144. Nichols CR, Roth BJ, Heerema N, et al. Hematologic neoplasia associated with primary germ cell tumors. *N Engl J Med.* 1990;322:1425–1429.
145. Patel SR, Meeker DP, Biscotti CV, et al. Preservation and management of bronchogenic cysts in the adult. *Chest.* 1994;106:79–85.
146. Coran AG, Drongowski R. Congenital cystic disease of the tracheobronchial tree in infants and children: experience with 44 consecutive cases. *Arch Surg.* 1994;129:521–527.
147. Bolton JW, Shahian DM. Asymptomatic bronchogenic cysts: what is the best management? *Ann Thorac Surg.* 1992;53:1134–1137.
148. Hazelrigg SR, Landreneau RJ, Mack MJ, et al. Thoracoscopic resection of mediastinal cysts. *Ann Thorac Surg.* 1993;56:569–660.
149. Suen HC, Mathisen DJ, Grillo HC, et al. Surgical management and radiological characteristics of bronchogenic cysts. *Ann Thorac Surg.* 1993;55: 476–481.
150. Martinoid E, Pons F, Azorin J, et al. Thoracoscopic excision of mediastinal bronchogenic cysts: results in 20 cases. *Ann Thorac Surg.* 2000;69:1525–1528.
151. Bennheim J, Griffel B, Versano S, et al. Mediastinal leiomyosarcoma in the wall of a bronchogenic cyst. *Arch Pathol Lab Med.* 1980;104:221.
152. Malde HM, Kedar RP, Chadda DJ. Ethanol sclerosis of a mediastinal cyst. *Can Assoc Radiol J.* 1993;44:310–312.
153. Feigin DS, Fenoglis JJ, McAllister HA, et al. Pericardial cysts: a radiologic– pathologic correlation and review. *Diagn Radiol.* 1977;125:15.
154. Whitaker JA, Deffenbaugh LD, Cooke AR. Esophageal duplication cyst. *Am J Gastroenterol.* 1980;73:329.
155. D'Almeida AC, Steward DH Jr. Neuroenteric cysts: case report and literature review. *Neurosurgery.* 1981;8:596–599.
156. Allen MS, Payne WS. Cystic foregut malformation in the mediastinum. *Chest Surg Clin North Am.* 1992;2:89–106.
157. Rastegar H, Arger P, Harlan AH. Evaluation and therapy of mediastinal thymic cysts. *Ann Surg.* 1980;46:236.
158. Adams GA, Schochat SJ, Smith EI, et al. Thoracic neuroblastoma: a pediatric Oncology Group study. *J Pediatr Surg.* 1993;28:372–378.
159. Ricci C, Rendina EA, Venuto F, et al. Diagnostic imaging and surgical treatment of dumbbell tumors of the mediastinum. *Ann Thorac Surg.* 1990;50:586–589.
160. Moon WK, Jung-Gi I, Hau MC. Malignant schwannomas of the thorax: CT findings. *J Comp Assist Tomogr.* 1993;17:274–276.
161. Wain JC. Neurogenic tumors of the mediastinum. *Chest Surg Clin North Am.* 1992;2:121–136.
162. Zajtchuk R, Bowen TD, Seyfer AD, et al. Intrathoracic ganglioneuroblastoma. *J Thorac Cardiovasc Surg.* 1980;80:605–612.
163. Joshi VV, Cantor AB, Altshuler G, et al. Age-linked prognostic categorization based on a new histologic grading system of neuroblastomas: a clinicopathologic study of 211 cases from the Pediatric Oncology Group. *Cancer.* 1992;8:2197–2211.
164. Olson JL, Salyer WR. Mediastinal paragangliomas (aortic body tumors): a report of four cases and a review of the literature. *Cancer.* 1978;41:2405–2412.
165. Akwari OE, Payne NS, Onofrio BM, et al. Dumbbell neurogenic tumors of the mediastinum. *Mayo Clin Proc.* 1978;53:353–358.
166. Grillo HC, Ojemann RG, Scannell JG, et al. Combined approach to "dumbbell" intrathoracic and intraspinal neurogenic tumors. *Ann Thorac Surg.* 1983;36:402.
167. Landreneau RJ, Dowling RD, Ferson PF. Thoracoscopic resection of a posterior mediastinal neurogenic tumor. *Chest.* 1992;102:1288–1290.
168. Parish JM, Marschke RF, Dines DE, et al. Etiologic considerations in superior vena cava syndrome. *Mayo Clin Proc.* 1981;56:407–413.
169. Mazzetti H, Dussant A, Tentori C. Superior vena cava occlusion and/or syndrome related to pacemaker leads. *Am Heart J.* 1993;125:831.
170. Nieto AF, Doty DB. Superior vena cava obstruction: clinical syndrome, etiology, and treatment. *Curr Probl Cancer.* 1986;10:441–484.
171. Mahajan V, Strimlan V, VanOrdstran HC, et al. Benign superior vena cava syndrome. *Chest.* 1975;68:32.
172. Lagerstrom CF, Mitchell HG, Graham BS, et al. Chronic fibrosing mediastinitis and superior vena caval obstruction from blastomycosis. *Ann Thorac Surg.* 1992;54:764–765.
173. Ko J, Yang P, Yuan A, et al. Superior vena cava syndrome: rapid histologic diagnosis by ultrasound guided transthoracic needle aspiration biopsy. *Am J Respir Crit Care Med* 1994;149:783–787.
174. Abner A. Approach to the patient who presents with superior vena cava obstruction. *Chest* 1993;103:394S–394S.
175. Perez-Soler R, McLaughlin P, Velasquez WS, et al. Clinical features and results of management of superior vena cava syndrome secondary to lymphoma. *J Clin Oncol* 1984;2:260–266.
176. Ferguson TB, Burford TH. Mediastinal granuloma: a 15 year experience. *Ann Thorac Surg.* 1965;1:125.

177. Dodds GA, Harrison JK, O'Laughlin MO, et al. Relief of superior vena cava syndrome due to fibrosing mediastinitis using the Palmaz stent. *Chest* 1994;106:315.
178. Doty DB, Doty JR, Jones KW. Bypass of superior vena cava: 15 years experience with spiral vein graft for obstruction of superior vena cava caused by benign disease. *J Thorac Cardiovasc Surg.* 1990;99:889–896.
179. Moore WM Jr, Hollier LH, Pickett TK. Superior vena cava and central venous reconstruction. *Surgery* 1991;110:35–41.
180. Roberts JR, Bueno R, Sugarbaker DJ. Multimodality treatment of malignant superior vena cava syndrome. *Chest.* 1999;116:835–837.
181. Yim CD, Sane SS, Bjarnason H. Superior vena cava stenting. *Radiol Clin North Am.* 2000;38:409–424.
182. Salassa JR, Pearson BW, Payne WS, et al. Gross and microscopical blood supply of the trachea. *Ann Thorac Surg.* 1977;24:100–107.
183. Mathisen DJ. Tracheal tumors. *Chest Surg Clin North Am.* 1996;6:875–898.
184. Grillo HC, Mathisen DJ. Primary tracheal tumors: treatment and results. *Ann Thorac Surg.* 1990;49:69–77.
185. Kearney PA, Griffen MM, Ochoa JB, et al. A single-center 8-year experience with percutaneous dilational tracheostomy. *Ann Surg.* 2000;231:701–709.
186. Norwood S, Vallina VL, Short K, et al. Incidence of tracheal stenosis and other late complications after percutaneous tracheostomy. *Ann Surg.* 2000;232:233–241.
187. Mathisen DJ. Surgery of the trachea. *Curr Probl Surg.* 1998;35:455–542.
188. Bolman RM III, Wolfe WG. Bronchiectasis and bronchopulmonary sequestration. *Surg Clin North Am.* 1980;60:867–881.
189. Johnson PC, Sarosi GA. The endemic mycoses: surgical considerations. *Semin Thorac Cardiovasc Surg.* 1995;7:95–103.

SECTION M
ARTERIAL SYSTEM: BASIC CONSIDERATIONS IN VASCULAR DISEASE

CHAPTER 83 ■ CONGENITAL HEART DISEASE

ERIC J. DEVANEY, RICHARD G. OHYE, JENNIFER C. HIRSCH, AND EDWARD L. BOVE

HISTORY

Cardiac surgery as a specialty is notable for the developments and rapid technical advances that have been made during the past few decades. Much of the original interest was focused on attempts to treat congenital heart defects associated with cyanosis and early mortality. The first successful treatment of a congenital lesion was the closure of a patent ductus arteriosus (PDA) by Gross and Hubbard in 1938.[1] The description of the subclavian artery-to-pulmonary artery (PA) shunt by Blalock and Taussig in 1945[2] opened the way to the palliation of many complex cyanotic lesions—most notably, tetralogy of Fallot (TOF). The 1950s represented the decade of greatest advances, which laid the foundation for the field of cardiac surgery. Lewis and Taufic in 1952[3] performed the first open closure of an atrial septal defect (ASD) by using surface hypothermia and inflow occlusion. In 1953, Gibbon[4] performed the first repair of an ASD with the use of a pump oxygenator that became the model for modern cardiopulmonary bypass. Next, Warden et al.[5] used controlled cross-circulation with an adult as the oxygenator during intracardiac repairs. Building on the work of Gibbon, Kirklin et al.[6] then published the first series of eight intracardiac operations performed at the Mayo Clinic with the use of cardiopulmonary bypass. With these landmark efforts, focused on congenital heart disease, the field of cardiac surgery was established.

ATRIAL SEPTAL DEFECT

Cardiac septation occurs between the third and sixth weeks of fetal development. The septum primum, which arises from the roof of the common atrium and descends inferiorly, initially divides the common atrium. The ostium primum is the opening below the inferior edge of septum primum, which is obliterated as the septum primum fuses with the endocardial cushions. The ostium secundum forms in the mid-portion of the septum primum prior to closure of the ostium primum. The septum secundum also arises from the roof of the atrium and descends along the right side of the septum primum and covers the ostium secundum. This creates a flap valve whereby blood from the inferior vena cava may preferentially stream beneath the edge of septum secundum and through the ostium secundum into the left atrium. After birth, the increase in left atrial pressure usually closes this pathway.

An ASD is a hole in the atrial septum (Fig. 83.1).ASDs are the third most common congenital heart defect, occurring in 1 out of 1,000 live births and representing 10% of congenital heart defects.[7] The most common ASD is the secundum defect, which occurs when the ostium secundum is too large for complete coverage by the septum secundum. Ostium secundum defects account for about 80% of ASDs. An ostium primum ASD, representing 10% of ASDs, occurs as a result of failure of fusion of the septum primum with the endocardial cushions. The ostium primum defect is discussed later in the section on atrioventricular septal defects (AVSDs). A third type of ASD is the sinus venosus defect, seen in about 10% of cases. Sinus venosus ASDs are caused by abnormal fusion of the venous pathways with the atrium and are characterized by defects high in the atrial septum near the orifice of the superior vena cava or, less commonly, low in the atrial septum near the inferior vena cava. Sinus venosus defects are frequently associated with partial anomalous pulmonary venous connection, usually with the right upper pulmonary vein draining into the superior vena cava near the cavoatrial junction. The rarest type of ASD is the unroofed coronary sinus septal defect. This occurs when there is loss of the common wall

A

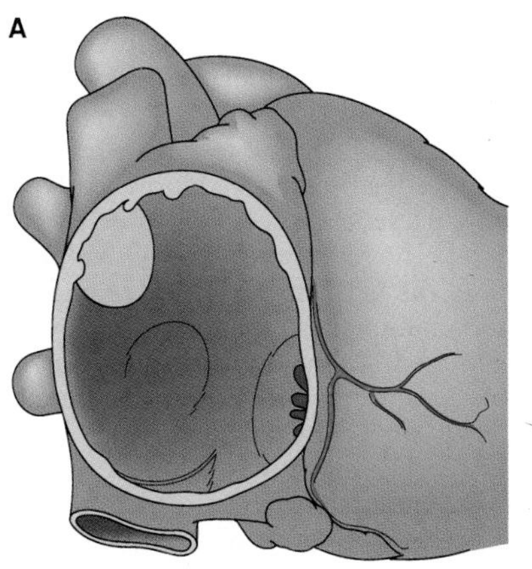

B

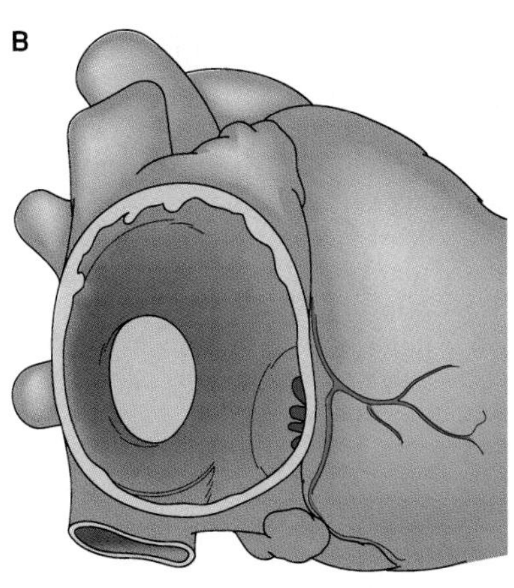

C

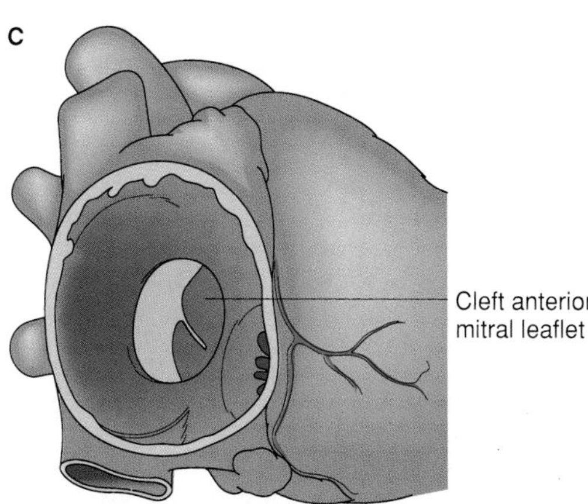

FIGURE 83.1 The anatomy of atrial septal defects. In the sinus venosus type (*A*), the right upper and middle pulmonary veins frequently drain to the superior vena cava or right atrium. (*B*) Secundum defects generally occur as isolated lesions. (*C*) Primum defects are part of a more complex lesion and are best considered as incomplete atrioventricular septal defects.

between the coronary sinus and the left atrium adjacent to the atrial septum. This unroofing of the coronary sinus leads to a communication between the right and left atria at the site of the coronary sinus.

Failure of postnatal fusion of the septum secundum to the septum primum results in a persistent slit-like communication known as a patent foramen ovale (PFO). PFOs are extremely common in the general population, and autopsy studies have demonstrated a prevalence of 27%.[8] PFOs are generally considered separate from other ASDs due to the absence of significant shunting, but they remain important clinically due to the occurrence of paradoxical embolization. A paradoxical embolus is a blood clot arising from a systemic vein that would normally pass to the lungs but, in the presence of a septal defect, may instead cross into the systemic circulation.

ASDs lead to increased pulmonary blood flow (PBF) secondary to left-to-right shunting. Shunting at the atrial level is determined by the size of the defect and by the relative ventricular compliance (i.e., blood preferentially fills the more compliant ventricle). At birth, both chambers are equally compliant, but as pulmonary vascular resistance (PVR) falls, the right ventricle remodels and becomes more compliant. Shunting across the atrial septum causes a volume load on the right heart. A volume load is created by additional venous return to a chamber during diastole.

The volume overload from an ASD is usually well tolerated, and patients are frequently asymptomatic. Symptoms tend to develop when the ratio of pulmonary to systemic blood flow (Q_p/Q_s) exceeds two. The most common symptoms are fatigue, shortness of breath, exercise intolerance, and recurrent respiratory infections. Older patients with untreated ASDs tend to develop atrial dysrhythmias, and adults may develop congestive heart failure (CHF) and right ventricular dysfunction. Pulmonary vascular obstructive disease may develop rarely as a late complication of untreated ASD. Paradoxical embolization is also an important potential complication of ASD.

The classic physical findings in patients with ASDs include fixed splitting of the second heart sound and a systolic ejection murmur at the left upper sternal border due to relative pulmonary stenosis (PS) (increased flow across a normal pulmonary valve). A diastolic flow murmur across the tricuspid valve is occasionally audible. A prominent right ventricular lift and increased intensity of the pulmonary component of the second heart sound may occur with pulmonary hypertension. Chest radiography shows cardiomegaly, with enlargement of the right atrium, right ventricle, and PA. Electrocardiography frequently demonstrates right axis deviation and an incomplete right bundle branch block. When right bundle branch block occurs with a leftward or superior axis, the diagnosis of AVSD should be considered. Echocardiography confirms the diagnosis of ASD and defines the anatomy. Cardiac catheterization is important in selected cases to assess PVR in older patients, but it is used more frequently with therapeutic intent for device closure of ASDs.

Due to the long-term complications associated with ASD, repair is recommended for all patients with symptomatic defects and in asymptomatic patients in whom the Q_p/Q_s is greater than 1.5. Repair is usually performed in children prior to school age. Closure of ASDs may be performed surgically or using a device deployed in the cardiac catheterization laboratory.

Surgical repair is usually recommended for large secundum defects and for most other types of ASDs. The heart is usually exposed by median sternotomy. Other surgical approaches have been proposed, including minimally invasive techniques, but there are technical drawbacks associated with each of the alternative approaches. In most cases, a limited midline incision with a partial lower sternal split provides adequate exposure and a cosmetically acceptable scar. The heart is carefully inspected for anomalies of systemic and pulmonary venous return.

Cardiopulmonary bypass is required with cooling to between 32°C and 35°C. The superior and inferior vena cava are separately cannulated for venous drainage, and the arterial cannula is placed in the ascending aorta. Following aortic clamping and arrest of the heart with cardioplegia, the atrial septum is exposed through a right atriotomy. Small secundum defects or PFOs may sometimes be closed primarily by suturing the edge of septum primum to the edge of septum secundum. More commonly, larger defects are closed using a patch (polytetrafluorethylene or autologous pericardium) and a running polypropylene suture. When anomalous pulmonary venous drainage is present, a baffle is created to redirect the flow across the ASD. In all cases, care is taken to de-air the left atrium to avoid the complication of air embolization. Surgical closure of an ASD can be accomplished with a mortality approaching zero and minimal morbidity.[9] Common postoperative complications include atrial fibrillation and post-pericardiotomy syndrome.

The first transcatheter device closure of an ASD was performed in 1976.[10] A number of devices are currently available for percutaneous closure of secundum ASDs,[11] and success rates for device deployment range from 80% to 95%.[12,13] Device closure has the advantages of fewer complications and a shorter hospitalization. Device closure of small to moderate secundum ASDs and PFOs has now become the standard of care at most large centers.

The long-term survival for patients undergoing ASD repair in childhood is normal.[14,15] The major long-term complication following surgical closure of ASD is the development of supraventricular arrhythmias, although the risk is lowered when the ASD is closed in childhood.[15,16] The persistence of this risk despite relief of right-sided volume overload is thought to be related to incomplete atrial remodeling or due to the presence of the atriotomy scar. Longer follow-up will be required to determine whether device closure alters the risk of atrial dysrhythmias.

Occasionally, adults will present with a newly diagnosed ASD. Many studies have confirmed that ASD closure in adults over the age of 40 increases survival and limits the development of heart failure.[17,18] When the Q_p/Q_s is less than 1.5 and the ratio of pulmonary to systemic vascular resistance (R_p/R_s) is greater than 0.7, significant pulmonary vascular obstructive disease is usually present. A PVR in excess of 10 to 12 Woods units·m^2 represents a contraindication to ASD closure.

VENTRICULAR SEPTAL DEFECT

Ventricular septation is a complex process that requires accurate development and alignment of a number of structures including the muscular interventricular septum, the atrioventricular (AV) septum (arising from the endocardial cushions), and the infundibular septum (which divides the outflow tracts of the right and left ventricles). The membranous septum is a fibrous portion of the ventricular septum that is adjacent to the central fibrous body (where the mitral, tricuspid, and aortic valve annuli make contact).

Ventricular septal defects (VSDs) are the most common congenital heart anomalies (with the exception of bicuspid aortic valve, which occurs in about 1.3% of the population). VSDs are present in about 4 of 1,000 live births and represent about 40% of congenital heart defects.[7] VSDs are classified based on their location in the ventricular septum (Fig. 83.2). The most common defects are perimembranous (80%), which are located in the area of the membranous septum. Inlet defects (5%) are located beneath the septal leaflet of the tricuspid valve and are sometimes called AV canal-type defects. Defects located high in the ventricular septum are outlet defects (10%). Outlet VSDs are typically adjacent to both the pulmonary and aortic valves. Outlet defects are also known by several other names, including supracristal, infundibular, or doubly committed subarterial. Outlet defects are more common in the Asian population. Trabecular (or muscular) VSDs (5%) are completely bordered by muscle. Trabecular VSDs are frequently multiple and may be associated with perimembranous or outlet defects. The size of VSDs varies. By definition, a VSD is nonrestrictive when its size (or the cumulative size of multiple defects) is greater than or equal to the size of the aortic annulus.

A VSD causes increased PBF due to left-to-right shunting primarily during systole. This creates a volume load on the left heart (the left atrium and ventricle receive the increased venous return during diastole). The right ventricle is not volume loaded (blood is ejected from the left ventricle (LV) through the VSD and directly into the pulmonary circulation); however, it does experience a pressure load. The volume of shunt flow is determined by the size of the defect and by the ratio of pulmonary to systemic vascular resistance. After birth the PVR is still high and shunting across a VSD is sometimes minimal. Over the first several weeks of life, shunting tends to increase as the PVR normally falls. Therefore, a patient with a large VSD may be asymptomatic at birth but eventually develop severe CHF.

The natural history for patients with isolated VSDs is highly variable. Most VSDs are restrictive and tend to close spontaneously during the first year of life. Large VSDs are nonrestrictive, resulting in right ventricular and pulmonary pressures that are systemic or nearly systemic, and high PBF with Q_p/Q_s ratios greater than 2.5 to 3. Moderate VSDs are restrictive, with pulmonary pressures that are one-half systemic (or less) and Q_p/Q_s ratios of 1.5 to 2.5. Small VSDs are highly restrictive; right ventricular pressures remain normal, and the Q_p/Q_s is less than 1.5. Patients with large VSDs tend to develop symptoms of CHF by 2 months of age. Untreated, excessive PBF leads to pulmonary vascular obstructive disease by the second year of life. The histologic changes associated with pulmonary vascular obstructive disease have been classified by Heath and Edwards based on severity.[19] Grade 1 consists of medial hypertrophy; grade 2 reflects intimal proliferation; grade 3 is characterized by intimal fibrosis and vascular occlusion; grades 4 through 6 describe progressive vessel dilatation, angiomatoid malformation, and necrotizing arteritis. Grades 1 and 2 are considered reversible, whereas the latter stages are irreversible. Patients with smaller VSDs may remain asymptomatic. In patients with outlet VSDs, prolapse of the aortic valve may occur, producing aortic insufficiency.[20]

Signs of heart failure in infants with large VSDs include tachypnea, hepatomegaly, poor feeding, and failure to thrive. On physical examination, there is a holosystolic murmur at the left sternal border. Usually, the murmur is louder with smaller defects. The precordium is active. The pulmonary component of the second heart sound is accentuated in the presence of pulmonary hypertension. Chest radiography shows increased pulmonary vascular markings and cardiomegaly. Electrocardiography is significant for right ventricular hypertrophy.

Patients with small VSDs have little shunting and are usually asymptomatic, having only a pansystolic murmur. Patients with moderate VSDs manifest symptoms and signs that are proportional to the degree of shunting.

In patients who have developed significant pulmonary vascular obstructive disease, the volume of left-to-right shunting is decreased, and the murmur may disappear. Eisenmenger's physiology results when the shunt flow reverses to right-to-left, creating cyanosis.

The diagnosis of VSD is confirmed by echocardiography, which accurately defines the anatomy and excludes the presence of associated defects. Cardiac catheterization is used selectively in older children and adults in whom elevated PVR is suspected. PVR is calculated by the following formula:

$$PVR = (PA_{mean} - LA)/Q_p$$

where PA_{mean} is the mean pulmonary artery pressure and LA is the left atrial pressure. The units of resistance by this formulation

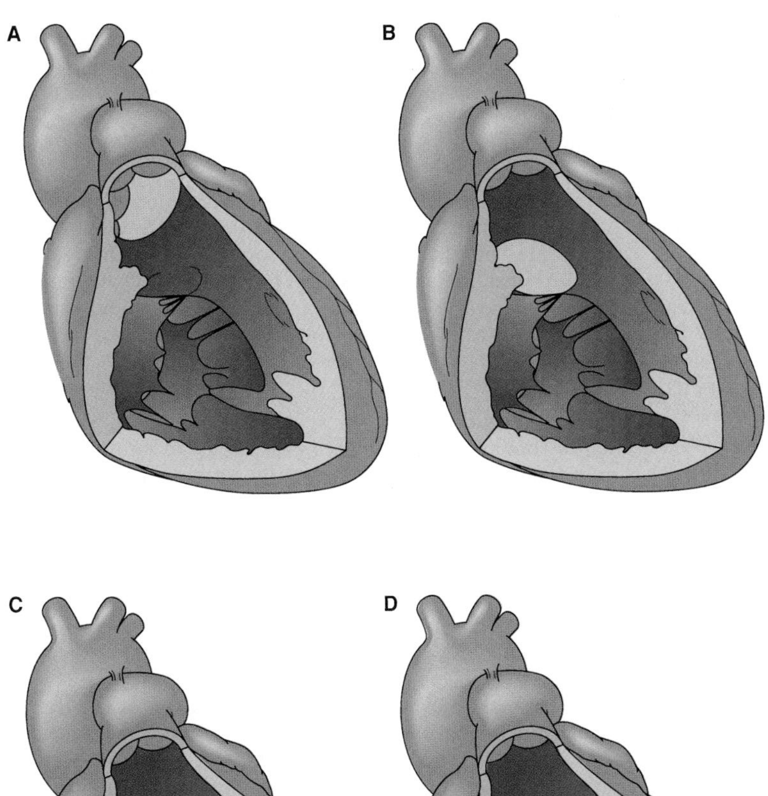

FIGURE 83.2 The anatomy of ventricular septal defects (VSDs) as seen through the right ventricle. (*A*) Outlet, or subarterial, VSDs are generally bordered superiorly by the pulmonary valve annulus. (*B*) Perimembranous VSDs are most common, extending from the membranous septum into the infundibular septum. (C) Inlet defects are located predominantly beneath the septal leaflet of the tricuspid valve. (*D*) Muscular VSDs are situated away from the valves, toward the cardiac apex.

(using pressures in millimeters of mercury and pulmonary flow in liters per minute) are Woods units (which can be expressed in dynes·sec/cm^5 by multiplying by 80). In the pediatric population, vascular resistance is frequently calculated using the cardiac output indexed to the body surface area (in square meters) with the resulting indexed resistance units of Woods units·m^2. PVR may be fixed or reactive, and, at the time of cardiac catheterization, response to various pulmonary vasodilators may be assessed.

The management of a patient with a VSD depends on the size of the defect, the type of the defect, the shunt volume, and the PVR. In general, patients with large defects who have intractable CHF or failure to thrive should undergo early surgical repair. If the congestive symptoms can be moderated by medical therapy, then surgery may be deferred until 6 months of age. Patients with moderate VSDs may be safely followed. If closure has not occurred by school age, then surgical closure is indicated. Small VSDs with Q_p/Q_s of less than 1.5 do not require closure. There is a small long-term risk of endocarditis for these patients, but this can be minimized with the appropriate use of prophylactic antibiotics.[21] Patients with outlet VSDs have a significant risk of developing aortic insufficiency due to leaflet prolapse, and, therefore, all of these patients should undergo surgical closure.[22] Older children and adults must undergo catheterization to assess the pulmonary circulation. When there is a fixed PVR greater than 8 to 10 Woods units·m^2, then surgery is contraindicated.

Surgical closure is performed through a median sternotomy. Cardiopulmonary bypass is utilized with bicaval cannulation, and the patient is typically cooled to between 28°C and 32°C. After aortic cross-clamping, cold cardioplegia is delivered through the aortic root to arrest the heart. Exposure of the ventricular septum is most often achieved by making a right atriotomy and retracting the leaflets of the tricuspid valve. This provides access to perimembranous, inlet, and most trabecular VSDs. Outlet VSDs are frequently best exposed via a pulmonary arteriotomy because the defect lies just beneath the valve. Trabecular VSDs located near the ventricular apex can be very difficult to expose, and an apical ventriculotomy may be necessary. Once the defect is exposed, it is closed using a polytetrafluoroethylene patch and a running polypropylene suture, although other centers may prefer other patch material or interrupted suture technique. It is important to understand the anatomy of the conduction tissue when closing VSDs. The AV node is an atrial structure that lies at the apex of an anatomic triangle (known as the triangle of Koch) formed by the coronary sinus, the tendon of Todaro (a prominent band leading from the inferior vena cava and inserting in the atrial septum), and the septal attachment of the tricuspid valve. The node then gives rise to the bundle of His, which penetrates the AV junction beneath the membranous septum. The bundle of His then bifurcates into right and left bundle branches, which pass along either side of the muscular ventricular septum. In the presence of a perimembranous VSD, the bundle of His passes along the posterior and inferior rim of the defect, generally on the left ventricular side. In this critical area, sutures must be placed superficially on the right ventricular side a few millimeters from the edge of the defect. The bundle of His also tends to run along the posterior and inferior margin of inlet VSDs. The conduction tissue is usually remote from outlet and trabecular VSDs.

PA banding is a palliative maneuver that is used to protect the pulmonary circulation from excessive blood flow. PA banding is currently performed only in patients who are felt to be poor candidates for VSD closure, either due to associated illness or due to anatomic complexity, such as multiple trabecular VSDs ("Swiss cheese" septum). Banding is performed without the need for cardiopulmonary bypass. A band is placed around the main PA and tightened to achieve a distal PA pressure of about one-half systemic. The band is secured to the adventitia of the PA to prevent its migration. Distal migration may result in narrowing and poor growth of one or both branch pulmonary arteries, whereas proximal migration can cause deformity of the pulmonary valve. Later, when the patient is a candidate for VSD closure, the band must be removed. Repair of the main PA at the band site is also usually necessary and can typically be accomplished by scar resection and primary closure or patch repair.

Recently, transcatheter devices have been developed to allow closure of some VSDs in the cardiac catheterization laboratory.[23]

Surgical closure of a VSD is associated with a mortality of about 1%.[24] Potential complications include injury to the conduction tissue and injury to the tricuspid or aortic valves. Transient heart block may result from tissue swelling or injury from retraction, but permanent heart block occurs in only about 1% to 2% of cases. When heart block develops after surgery, patients are usually observed for a period of 7 to 10 days prior to permanent pacemaker implantation. Closure of perimembranous and inlet VSDs may result in distortion of the tricuspid valve, which may cause significant regurgitation. Aortic valve injury may occur as a result of inaccurate suturing, especially in perimembranous and outlet defects. A residual VSD is seen in about 5% of cases, and reoperation is indicated when significant shunting persists ($Q_p/Q_s > 1.5$). The Q_p/Q_s ratio can be calculated by measuring oxygen saturations and using the following formula derived from the Fick equation:

$$Q_p/Q_s = (\text{Ao} - \text{SVC})/(\text{PV} - \text{PA})$$

where Ao is the aortic (or systemic) saturation, SVC is the saturation in the superior vena cava, PV the saturation in the pulmonary veins (which is usually estimated to be 95% to 100%), and PA the saturation in the pulmonary arteries. Intraoperative echocardiography is used routinely to identify residual defects, which can then be repaired before the patient leaves the operating room.

AORTIC STENOSIS

Aortic stenosis (AS) refers to a form of left ventricular outflow tract obstruction that may occur at a valvar (70%), subvalvar (25%), or supravalvar (5%) level (Fig. 83.3). AS occurs in about 4% of patients with congenital heart disease.[7] The severity of AS may be graded as mild (peak pressure gradient less than 50 mm Hg), moderate (50 to 75 mm Hg), or severe (greater than 75 mm Hg).

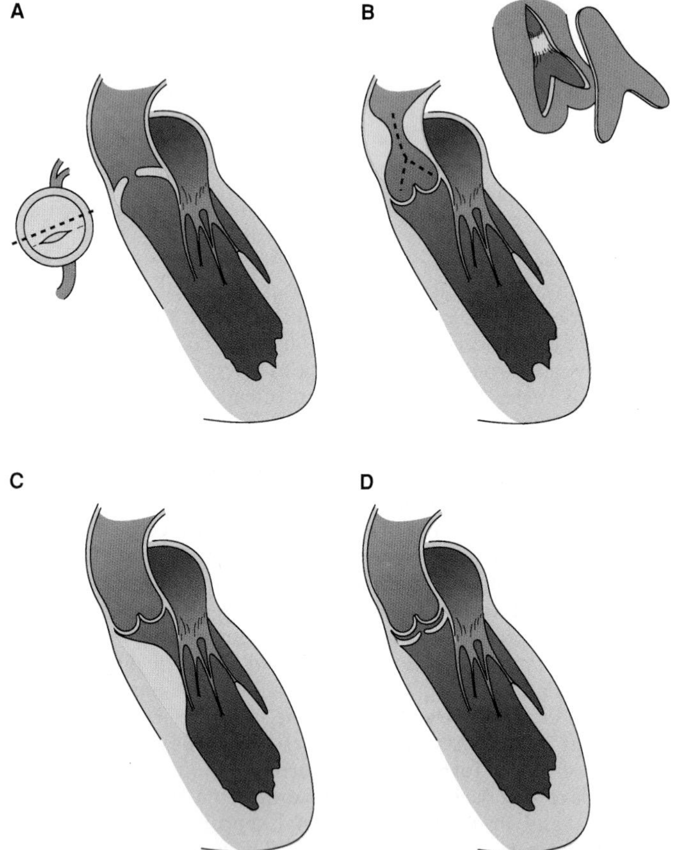

FIGURE 83.3 Anatomy of the types of congenital aortic stenosis. (*A*) Valvar aortic stenosis. (*B*) Supravalvar aortic stenosis and its repair (*inset*). (C) Diffuse (tunnel) subvalvar aortic stenosis. (*D*) Discrete subvalvar aortic stenosis.

Valvar AS occurs secondary to maldevelopment of the aortic valve. Most commonly, a bicuspid valve is present, although tricuspid and unicuspid valves are also represented. In valvar AS, the leaflets are thickened and frequently dysmorphic, and there is a variable degree of leaflet fusion along the commissures. The aortic annulus may be hypoplastic. In 20% of cases, valvar AS is associated with other cardiac defects, most commonly coarctation of the aorta, PDA, VSD, or mitral stenosis. Males with valvar AS outnumber females by a ratio of 4:1. There is a wide spectrum of clinical presentation of valvar AS, but patients tend to present in one of two groups: younger patients (neonates and infants) with severe AS develop symptoms of rapidly progressive CHF, whereas older patients, with less severe obstruction at birth, have a more indolent course.

Severe AS is usually well tolerated during fetal development. Although left ventricular output and antegrade flow across the aortic valve are decreased, the right ventricle compensates with increased output, and systemic perfusion is maintained by flow across the ductus. After birth, there is increased venous return to the left heart, and this exacerbates the pressure load created by the stenotic aortic valve, leading to left ventricular dysfunction. As the ductus closes during postnatal life, systemic malperfusion may develop with resulting hypotension, acidosis, and oliguria. Coronary perfusion is also impaired due to the combination of systemic hypotension and elevated left ventricular end-diastolic pressures. Patients with critical AS typically exhibit severe left ventricular dysfunction. These patients usually show signs of distress soon after birth. On examination, there is impaired distal perfusion with poor capillary refill and diminished, thready pulses. A systolic ejection murmur may be absent if the cardiac output is severely diminished. Differential cyanosis may be observed due to perfusion of the lower body with desaturated blood shunting through the ductus. The ECG shows left ventricular hypertrophy, and the chest radiograph displays cardiomegaly and pulmonary congestion. Echocardiography establishes the diagnosis.

The neonate or infant with critical AS represents a true emergency. Endotracheal intubation and inotropic support is routine. Ductal patency is maintained with prostaglandins, and acidosis is corrected. All patients with critical AS require some form of urgent intervention. The approach is determined by the valve morphology and by the presence of associated defects. In its most extreme form, critical AS may be associated with underdeveloped left-sided cardiac chambers and therefore may represent a form of hypoplastic left heart syndrome. In these cases, single ventricle palliation must be undertaken. For patients with adequate left-sided chambers, relief of AS may be achieved by one of the following three approaches: percutaneous balloon valvuloplasty, surgical valvotomy, or aortic valve replacement. Balloon valvuloplasty is generally considered the procedure of choice when the aortic valve annulus is adequate and there are no associated cardiac defects. Alternatively, surgical valvotomy may be accomplished by closed or open techniques. The closed approach is performed using cardiopulmonary bypass but without aortic cross-clamping. Dilators of increasing size are passed through a ventriculotomy in the left ventricular apex and advanced across the aortic valve. Some centers prefer open surgical valvotomy, which allows a precise valvotomy under direct vision, although aortic cross-clamping with cardioplegia is necessary. In all cases, the goal of therapy is to relieve stenosis without creating excessive aortic insufficiency. Dramatic clinical improvement is expected following balloon or surgical valve valvotomy, and early survivals of greater than 80% have been reported.[25,26] The incidence of aortic insufficiency is slightly higher following balloon valvotomy. In most cases, however, stenosis will recur and repeat valvotomy or aortic valve replacement will eventually be required. Aortic valve replacement is problematic in the neonate due to small patient size. In these cases, many consider the best valve replacement to be a pulmonary autograft (Ross procedure)[27] with enlargement of the aortic annulus (Konno aortoventriculoplasty).[28] The Ross-Konno procedure has been used successfully for neonates with critical AS in whom the aortic annulus is hypoplastic and for selected patients in whom valvuloplasty was unsuccessful. Survival following the Ross-Konno procedure in infants has been shown to be excellent.[29] Growth of the pulmonary autograft has been documented, thereby making it an ideal valve replacement for children. Unfortunately, as part of the Ross procedure, the pulmonary valve must be replaced using a cryopreserved homograft that does not grow, and homograft replacement must be anticipated at intervals as the patient grows.

In contrast to infants with critical AS, older children with valvar AS usually present with less severe stenosis (mild or moderate), and most are asymptomatic. Symptoms of angina, syncope, and CHF are not commonly reported. Congenital valvar AS is a progressive lesion, however, and survival is dependent on the severity of stenosis and its rate of its progression. Sudden cardiac death is the most common cause of mortality. Endocarditis occurs in less than 1% of patients. The diagnosis of valvar AS in older children can frequently be made on physical exam. There is a classic systolic crescendo-decrescendo murmur at the upper sternal border, which radiates to the neck. An ejection click is often present. A visible apical impulse is suggestive of significant left ventricular hypertrophy. In severe cases, the pulse may be weak and delayed (pulsus tardus et parvus). The ECG shows left ventricular hypertrophy. The chest radiograph is usually normal. Echocardiography accurately defines the level of stenosis and its severity. Using Doppler techniques, the pressure gradient across the stenotic valve may be estimated using a simplified form of Bernoulli's equation $P = 4V^2$, where P is the pressure gradient and V is the peak flow velocity. Cardiac catheterization is generally reserved for therapeutic intervention.

All patients with severe valvar AS should undergo intervention, as should all symptomatic patients with moderate stenosis. Asymptomatic patients with mild or moderate stenosis are generally observed. As described previously for critical AS, the techniques used to relieve AS in older patients include percutaneous balloon valvuloplasty, surgical valvulotomy, and valve replacement. Balloon valvuloplasty is usually performed as the primary intervention, and is associated with a success rate of nearly 90% and a mortality of less than 1%.[30] Open surgical valvotomy is an alternative approach with similar results.[31] For valves that are severely dysplastic, develop restenosis after intervention, or become insufficient as a result of prior intervention, valve replacement may be necessary. For older children, there are more options for valve replacement. The choices include mechanical prostheses, bioprosthetic valves, and tissue substitutes, such as porcine xenografts, cryopreserved human allografts, and pulmonary autografts (Ross procedure). The mechanical valves are the most durable but require chronic anticoagulation. The bioprosthetic and tissue valves do not require long-term anticoagulation but tend to deteriorate over time (with the exception of the pulmonary autograft). The pulmonary autograft has the potential advantage of growth but the homograft used to replace the pulmonary valve will require replacement. Selection of the appropriate replacement valve is a complex decision that requires input from all involved parties.

Subvalvar AS occurs below the level of the aortic valve and may be discrete (80%) or diffuse (20%). Discrete (or membranous) subaortic stenosis is rarely seen in infants and tends to progress over time. This lesion consists of a crescentic or circumferential fibrous or fibromuscular membrane that protrudes into the left ventricular outflow tract. The pathogenesis of discrete subaortic stenosis is unknown, but it is thought to be an acquired lesion which develops secondary to a congenital abnormality of the left ventricular outflow tract in which abnormal flow patterns lead to endocardial injury with resultant fibrosis. Although the aortic valve leaflets are usually normal in discrete subaortic stenosis, the turbulent flow created by the obstruction can cause leaflet thickening and progressive aortic insufficiency. Diffuse subaortic stenosis is a more severe form of stenosis that creates a long, tunnel-like obstruction. Diffuse subaortic stenosis should be distinguished from hypertrophic cardiomyopathy. Both forms of subaortic stenosis are associated with a high risk of endocarditis. The clinical findings in subvalvar AS are similar to those for valvar stenosis.

Intervention for discrete subvalvar stenosis is usually undertaken when the gradient exceeds 30 to 50 mm Hg or when aortic insufficiency is present. In these patients, resection of the membrane is readily performed by a transaortic approach. To reduce the incidence of restenosis, many centers advocate concurrent performance of a septal myomectomy to alter the geometry of the left ventricular outflow tract. Operative mortality approaches zero. The recurrence rate of discrete stenosis following membrane resection and myomectomy has been reported to be as low as 4%.[32]

The indications for operative intervention in diffuse subaortic stenosis are similar to those for valvar stenosis. When diffuse subaortic stenosis is associated with hypoplasia of the aortic annulus, repair is best achieved with a Konno aortoventriculoplasty, whereby an incision is carried across the aortic annulus and subjacent ventricular septum, the opening patched, and an aortic valve implanted. Patients with an adequate aortic annulus may undergo a septoplasty (modified Konno), in which the septal incision is confined to the immediate subvalvar area, and a patch is used to widen the left ventricular outflow tract without replacing the aortic valve. Despite the technical complexity of repair of diffuse subaortic stenosis, excellent results have been reported with high survival and freedom from reoperation.[33]

Supravalvar AS is characterized by thickening of the wall of the ascending aorta. The lesion may be localized (80%) to the region of the sinotubular ridge (at the level of the valve commissures), creating an hourglass deformity, or it may be more diffuse (20%), extending into the aortic arch and its branches. In both varieties, the aortic valve leaflets may be abnormal. The free edges of the aortic valve leaflets may adhere to the aortic wall in the region of intraluminal thickening, and this may lead to reduced coronary blood flow during diastole. Aortic wall thickening may also extend into the coronary ostia and further impair coronary blood flow. Associated cardiac lesions are common, particularly branch PA stenoses. A genetic basis for supravalvar AS has been established.[34] About 50% of cases of supravalvar AS are associated with Williams' syndrome, in which a partial deletion of chromosome 7 (including the elastin gene) leads to the triad of supravalvar stenosis, mental retardation, and a characteristic "elfin" facies. Isolated mutations in the elastin gene have also been shown to produce familial supravalvar AS with an autosomal dominant pattern of transmission. There is a significant incidence of endocarditis in patients with supravalvar AS. Sudden death is frequently reported and is probably related to coronary obstruction.

The signs and symptoms of supravalvar AS are similar to those in other forms of left ventricular outflow tract obstruction. The diagnosis is made by echocardiography, but cardiac catheterization [and more recently magnetic resonance imaging (MRI)] is essential to define the aortic, coronary, and pulmonary arterial anatomy prior to surgical intervention.

Operative intervention is indicated for patients with supravalvar AS in whom the gradient exceeds 50 mm Hg. A number of operations have been proposed for the treatment of localized supravalvar stenosis. The classical repair involves a longitudinal incision across the obstruction in the ascending aorta, which is extended into the noncoronary sinus. The thickened, hypertrophic ridge is resected by endarterectomy and the aortotomy is augmented with an elliptical patch. A variation of this repair involves creation of an inverted-Y aortotomy with one limb of the Y extended into the noncoronary sinus and the other into the right coronary sinus. A Y-shaped patch is then used to augment the aortotomy. Finally, the Brom repair is performed by transection of the ascending aorta beyond the supravalvar ridge. Separate incisions are then made through the supravalvar ridge into each sinus of Valsalva. Triangular patches are placed to augment each of these incisions, thereby relieving the supravalvar obstruction. Reconnection of the aortic root to the ascending aorta completes the repair. The repair of the diffuse type of supravalvar stenosis is performed under circulatory arrest with extensive patching of the ascending aorta, transverse arch, and involved arch arteries. Branch pulmonary stenoses are best managed using transcatheter techniques.

The results of surgery for localized supravalvar AS are generally good with low operative mortality and excellent long-term survival.[35–37] The diffuse form is more difficult to treat, and recurrence is more likely. Overall results are much worse when severe bilateral PA stenoses are present.

TETRALOGY OF FALLOT

TOF is the most common cyanotic congenital heart defect. It occurs in 0.6 per 1,000 live births and has a prevalence of about 5% among all patients with congenital heart disease.[7] The pathologic anatomy is frequently described as having four components: VSD, overriding aorta, PS, and right ventricular hypertrophy (Fig. 83.4). Embryologically, the anatomy of TOF is thought to result from a single defect: anterior malalignment of the infundibular septum.[38] The infundibular septum normally separates the primitive outflow tracts and fuses with the ventricular septum. Anterior malalignment of the infundibular septum creates a VSD due to failure of fusion with the ventricular septum and also displaces the aorta over the VSD and right ventricle. Infundibular malalignment also

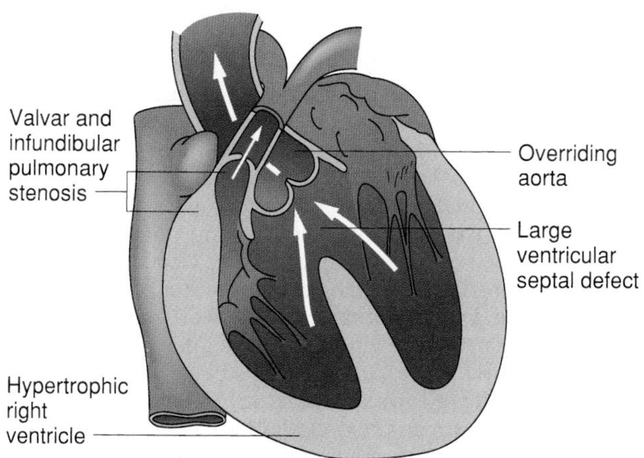

FIGURE 83.4 The four anatomic features of tetralogy of Fallot. The primary morphologic abnormality, anterior and superior displacement of the infundibular septum, results in a malalignment ventricular septal defect, overriding of the aortic valve, and obstruction of the right ventricular outflow. Right ventricular hypertrophy is a secondary occurrence.

crowds the right ventricular outflow tract, causing PS and, secondarily, right ventricular hypertrophy. Prominent muscle bands also extend from the septal insertion of the infundibular septum to the right ventricular free wall and contribute to the obstruction of the right ventricular outflow tract. The pulmonary valve is usually stenotic and is bicuspid in 58% of cases.[39] Pulmonary atresia occurs in about 7% of cases of TOF. The branch pulmonary arteries in TOF may exhibit mild diffuse hypoplasia or discrete stenosis (most frequently of the left PA at the site of ductal insertion). Coronary artery anomalies are frequently present. The origin of the left anterior descending from the right coronary artery, which occurs in 5% of cases, is clinically important because the vessel crosses the right ventricular infundibulum and is vulnerable to injury at the time of surgery. A right aortic arch is present in 25% of patients with TOF. Associated defects include ASD, complete AVSD, PDA, or multiple VSDs.

Patients with TOF develop cyanosis due to right-to-left shunting across the VSD. The degree of cyanosis depends on the severity of obstruction of the right ventricular outflow tract. Frequently, cyanosis is mild at birth and may remain undetected for weeks or months. Neonates with severe infundibular obstruction or pulmonary atresia will develop symptoms shortly after birth and will require a prostaglandin infusion to maintain ductal patency to ensure adequate PBF. In other patients, the right ventricular outflow tract obstruction is minor, and the predominant physiology is that of a large VSD with left-to-right shunting and CHF.

The occurrence of intermittent cyanotic spells is a well-known feature of tetralogy. The etiology of spelling is still controversial but is clearly related to a transient imbalance between pulmonary and systemic blood flow. A spell may be triggered by hypovolemia or peripheral vasodilation (e.g., after a bath or vigorous physical exertion). Spells may occur in neonates but are most frequently reported in infants between the ages of 3 and 18 months. Most spells resolve spontaneously within a few minutes, but some spells may be fatal. Older children have been observed to spontaneously squat to terminate spells. The squatting position is thought to increase systemic vascular resistance, which thereby favors PBF.

Cyanosis is the most frequent physical finding in tetralogy. Auscultation reveals a normal first heart sound and a single second heart sound. A systolic ejection murmur is present at the left upper sternal border. Older children may develop clubbing of the fingers and toes. Chest radiography typically demonstrates a boot-shaped heart due to elevation of the cardiac apex from right ventricular hypertrophy. Pulmonary vascular markings are usually reduced. A right aortic arch may be present. An ECG shows right ventricular hypertrophy. Echocardiography is definitive, and catheterization is not necessary in most cases.

The medical management of TOF is directed toward the treatment and prevention of cyanotic spells. The immediate treatment of the spelling patient includes administration of oxygen, narcotics for sedation, and correction of acidosis. Transfusion is indicated for anemic infants. Alpha-agonists are useful for increasing systemic vascular resistance (which favors PBF). Some centers have used beta-blockers as a form of long-term therapy to suppress the incidence of spells.

All patients with TOF should undergo surgical repair. Asymptomatic patients should be repaired electively between 4 and 6 months of age. Early repair is indicated for neonates with severe cyanosis and for infants who have had a documented spell or worsening cyanosis.

Classically, the repair of TOF was accomplished in two stages. During the first stage, PBF was augmented by creating a connection (or shunt) between a systemic artery and the PA. At the second stage, the shunt was taken down, and a complete repair was performed. The first shunt procedure was the Blalock-Taussig shunt, in which the subclavian artery was mobilized and divided distally, and an end-to-side anastomosis was created between the inferiorly deflected subclavian and the ipsilateral PA. Other shunt operations were subsequently developed and involved connections between the ascending aorta and right PA (Waterston shunt) or between the descending aorta and left PA (Potts shunt). The modified Blalock-Taussig shunt is the most common type of shunt used today and consists of an interposition graft (polytetrafluoroethylene) between the innominate or subclavian artery and the ipsilateral PA. Creation of a shunt may be accomplished with or without the use of cardiopulmonary bypass.

Currently, one-stage repair of TOF is preferred by most centers. Initial palliation with a shunt is still indicated for some patients who present a high risk for complete repair, such as those with multiple congenital anomalies, severe concurrent illness, or an anomalous coronary artery crossing a hypoplastic infundibulum.

Complete repair of TOF is performed using a median sternotomy and cardiopulmonary bypass with bicaval venous cannulation. By a transatrial approach, the right ventricular outflow tract can be examined through the tricuspid valve. Muscle bundles obstructing the right ventricular outflow tract are divided or resected. The VSD is closed with a patch. Pulmonary valvotomy is performed, when indicated, via a vertical incision in the main PA. When the pulmonary valve annulus or infundibulum is severely hypoplastic, a transannular outflow tract patch may be necessary to relieve the obstruction. When an anomalous coronary artery crosses the infundibulum, a transannular incision may be contraindicated. In these cases, and in patients with pulmonary atresia, placement of a conduit (cryopreserved homograft or bioprosthetic heterograft) between the right ventricle (via a separate ventriculotomy) and main PA will be necessary. Patients who undergo construction of a transannular patch develop pulmonary insufficiency as a consequence. This is surprisingly well tolerated in most infants, as long as the tricuspid valve is competent. As these patients grow older, some will develop right ventricular failure due to chronic pulmonary insufficiency, and pulmonary valve implantation may be necessary.[40,41]

The early mortality following repair of TOF is between 1% and 5%.[39,42] The results are worse for patients with TOF and pulmonary atresia. Long-term complications include recurrent obstruction of the right ventricular outflow tract and development of right ventricular dysfunction due to chronic pulmonary insufficiency. Actuarial survival at 20 years is 86% with excellent functional status.[43]

TRANSPOSITION OF THE GREAT ARTERIES

Transposition of the great arteries (TGA) is a congenital cardiac anomaly in which the aorta arises from the right ventricle and the PA originates from the LV (ventriculoarterial discordance; Fig. 83.5). The looping refers to the right or left looping of the primitive heart tube during fetal development, which determines whether the atria and ventricles are concordant (right atrium attaches to right ventricle and left atrium attaches to LV) or discordant. l-TGA is associated with AV discordance (right atrium attaches to LV and left atrium attaches to right ventricle), and is also termed congenitally corrected TGA. l-TGA is a rare variant of TGA and is beyond the scope of this chapter, which will focus on d-TGA. The defect can be subdivided into d-TGA with intact ventricular septum (IVS) (55% to 60%) and d-TGA with VSD (40% to 45%), one third of which are hemodynamically insignificant. Pulmonic stenosis (PS), causing significant left ventricular outflow tract

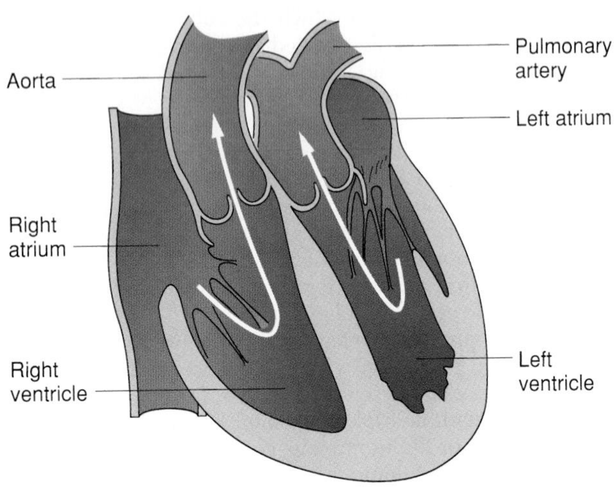

FIGURE 83.5 Anatomy of the most common type of transposition of the great arteries. The location of the ascending aorta is usually anterior to and to the right of the pulmonary artery.

obstruction, occurs rarely with an IVS and in approximately 10% of d-TGA/VSD.[44]

d-TGA is a relatively common cardiac anomaly and is the most common form of congenital heart disease presenting as cyanosis in the first week of life. The malformation accounts for approximately 10% of all congenital cardiovascular malformations in infants.[45] The degree of cyanosis depends on the amount of mixing between the pulmonary and systemic circulations. In TGA, oxygenated pulmonary venous blood is returned to the lungs and desaturated systemic blood is returned to the body. Because the two circulations exist in parallel, some mixing between them must occur to allow oxygenated blood to reach the systemic circulation and the desaturated blood to reach the lungs. Mixing may occur at a number of levels, most commonly at the atrial level through an ASD or a PFO. Generally, two levels of mixing are necessary to maintain adequate systemic oxygen delivery with a VSD or PDA serving as an additional site for cardiac mixing. In TGA, there can be no fixed shunt in one direction without an equal amount of blood passing in the other direction; otherwise, one circulation would eventually empty into the other. Therefore, the amount of desaturated blood reaching the lungs (effective PBF) must equal the amount of saturated blood reaching the aorta (effective systemic blood flow). Clinical characteristics are dependent on the degree of mixing and the amount of PBF. These factors relate to the specific anatomic subtype of d-TGA. Neonates with d-TGA with IVS (or small VSD) have mixing limited to the atrial level and PDA. The ASD may be restrictive and the PDA generally will close over the first days to week of life. As the degree of mixing decreases, the patient becomes increasingly cyanotic and will eventually suffer cardiovascular collapse. Fortunately, the majority of these neonates will manifest cyanosis early in life, which is recognized by nurse or physician within the first hour in 56% and in the first day in 92%.[46] In d-TGA with a large VSD, there is additional opportunity for mixing and increased PBF. The neonate with d-TGA/VSD may only manifest mild cyanosis, which may be initially overlooked. However, generally within 2 to 6 weeks signs and symptoms of CHF will emerge. Tachypnea and tachycardia become prominent, whereas cyanosis may remain mild. Auscultatory findings are consistent with CHF with increased PBF, including a pansystolic murmur, third heart sound, mid-diastolic rumble, gallop, and narrowly split second heart sound with increased pulmonary component. Neonates with d-TGA and significant PS present with severe cyanosis at birth. Lesser degrees of PS will result in varying levels of cyanosis. In cases of TGA, the ECG is normal at birth, demonstrating the typical pattern of right ventricular dominance. Although the classic chest radiographic appearance of an egg-shaped heart with a narrow superior mediastinum may be seen, this finding is often obscured by an enlarged thymic shadow. The abnormal ventriculoarterial connection is clearly seen on echocardiography, which demonstrates that the posterior great vessel arising from the LV is a PA that bifurcates soon after its origin. The anterior great vessel is the aorta and arises from the right ventricle. Associated lesions, including VSD, left ventricular outflow tract obstruction, and coarctation, may also be diagnosed. Although used less frequently, cardiac catheterization may be helpful to confirm the basic anatomy, discern associated lesions, define the coronary anatomy, and improve cardiac mixing by means of balloon atrial septostomy.

The infant with TGA and severe cyanosis requires prompt diagnosis and treatment to improve mixing and increase the arterial oxygen saturation. The first intervention to improve mixing in a cyanotic newborn suspected of having TGA is to ensure ductal patency by beginning an infusion of prostaglandin E1 (PGE1). In the presence of a restrictive ASD, a balloon atrial septostomy, a technique developed by William Rashkind[47] in 1966, is performed. The procedure involves inserting a balloon-tipped catheter across the foramen ovale into the left atrium. Inflation and forcible withdrawal of the catheter tears the septum primum and enlarges the ASD. Mixing generally increases immediately, with a substantial increase in arterial oxygen saturation.

Without intervention, d-TGA is universally fatal. Untreated, 30% of neonates will die in the first week of life, 50% by the first month, 70% within 6 months, and 90% by 1 year.[48] The definitive surgical treatment of patients with TGA has changed dramatically in the past decade with the advent of the arterial switch operation. Before this procedure, repair of TGA was generally delayed until patients were at least 6 months of age. Historically, palliative procedures were often necessary to improve the systemic saturation or protect the pulmonary vascular bed before definitive repair. If balloon atrial septostomy failed to enlarge the ASD adequately, a Blalock-Hanlon septectomy was performed. Rarely used today, this operation is a method of surgically enlarging the ASD without cardiopulmonary bypass. In patients with large VSDs, significant CHF and pulmonary hypertension are present early in life. Historically, the main PA was banded to reduce distal PA pressure and prevent the development of pulmonary vascular occlusive disease. Changes of pulmonary vascular disease may develop in about 25% of patients with hemodynamically large VSDs by 3 months of age; therefore, early reduction of PA pressure was essential. In those cases of transposition with severe left ventricular outflow tract obstruction, total pulmonary flow is reduced and systemic-to-PA shunting was undertaken until definitive repair could be accomplished.

Historically, definitive repair was achieved by redirecting venous inflow at the atrial level. First successfully performed by Senning[49] in 1959, the operation was simplified by Mustard[50] in 1964 (Fig. 83.6). In both techniques, the atrial septum is repositioned such that superior and inferior vena caval blood is rerouted to the mitral valve and then to the LV and PA. Pulmonary venous blood is redirected to the tricuspid valve and right ventricle. The right ventricle then ejects the oxygenated blood to the systemic circulation. The Mustard operation uses a large patch of pericardium or prosthetic material to create the intraatrial baffle. In the Senning procedure, the patient's atrial tissue is used, and little or no foreign material is necessary. Although physiologic repair at the

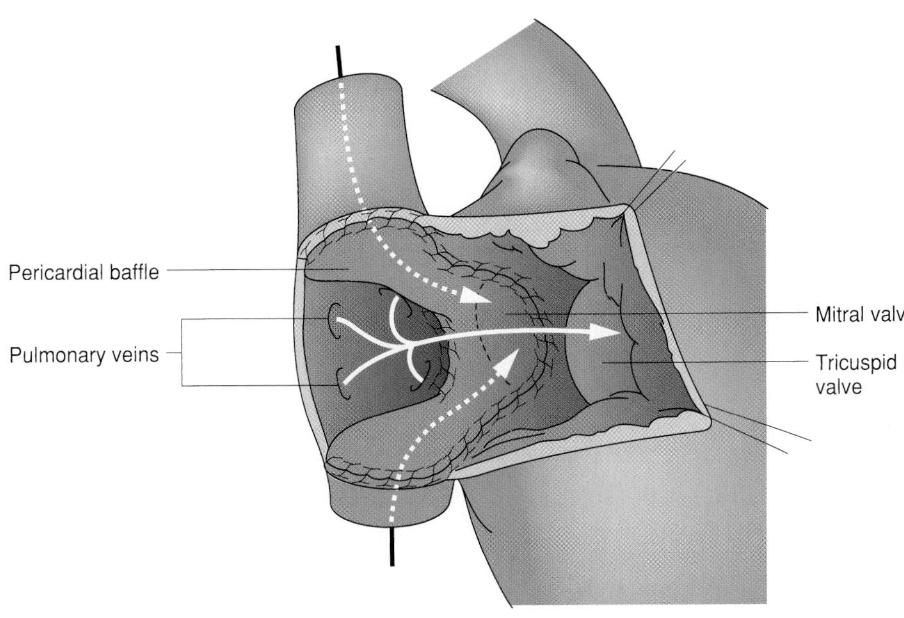

FIGURE 83.6 The Mustard operation for transposition of the great arteries. In this procedure, the atrial septum is excised and replaced with a pericardial baffle, so that pulmonary venous blood is redirected over the baffle to the tricuspid valve. Superior and inferior vena caval blood then drains to the mitral valve.

atrial level is associated with a low operative mortality rate (<5%), even in infants, a number of late problems have occurred. Obstruction to vena caval inflow, particularly at the junction of the superior vena cava and the right atrium, still occurs in about 5% of patients and may be more common when the procedure is performed in an infant. Additionally, pulmonary venous obstruction may develop and is often difficult to repair. Perhaps because of the complex atrial suture lines, atrial dysrhythmias are common and occur in more than half of patients observed on a long-term basis. In addition, pacemakers may be necessary for troubling bradyarrhythmias in as many as 10% of these patients.

The most serious long-term complication of repair by either the Senning or Mustard technique has been right ventricular dysfunction. Right ventricular failure with an enlarged, poorly contractile chamber and secondary tricuspid regurgitation has been found in a significant number of these patients in long-term follow-up studies. The true incidence of significant right ventricular failure in these cases remains difficult to define and is clearly influenced by an earlier era of operation with different methods of myocardial protection and surgical technique. The fact that many of these infants underwent definitive repair after many months of significant cyanosis may also have influenced right ventricular function.

The long-term complications of atrial repair prompted a reexamination of direct arterial repair for transposing the great arteries. The "arterial switch" operation, first successfully performed by Jatene in 1975, has become the optimal surgical procedure for infants with this condition.[51] Current techniques have reduced the operative mortality to levels comparable with those of atrial repair. Additionally, because the operation is performed early in life, this approach has virtually eliminated the interim morbidity and mortality associated with postponement of surgery until at least 6 months of age. The operative technique involves transection of both great vessels and direct reanastomosis to reestablish ventriculoarterial concordance (Fig. 83.7). Additionally, the coronary arteries are removed from the anterior aorta and relocated to the posterior great vessel (neoaorta). The extensive experience gained with this procedure has confirmed that any variant of coronary artery anatomy can be successfully repaired, although certain unusual forms clearly impose a higher risk. Because many patients with TGA have an IVS, left ventricular pressure falls early in life as PVR decreases. In this situation, it is essential that the arterial repair be performed within the first 2 to 3 weeks of life, while the LV is still able to meet systemic workloads. In patients presenting later, the LV can be retrained with a preliminary PA banding and aorticopulmonary shunt followed by the definitive arterial repair. Although patients with large VSDs do not require early repair because of their decreased left ventricular pressure, experience has indicated that, even in this subgroup, the operation is best performed within the first month of life, before secondary complications such as pulmonary hypertension, CHF, or infection develop.

Patients with fixed left ventricular outflow tract obstruction are not candidates for the arterial repair because correction would result in systemic ventricular outflow tract obstruction. Most of these patients also have large VSDs. Palliation early in life with systemic-to-PA shunting is an option, with definitive repair postponed until somatic growth results in cyanosis as the shunt is outgrown. At that time, the Rastelli procedure is performed, in which left ventricular blood is redirected through the VSD and to the anterior aorta by placement of an intraventricular patch (Fig. 83.8). The PA is ligated, and right ventricle-to-distal PA continuity is reestablished with a valve-bearing conduit. An increasing number of experienced centers currently recommend early complete repair in the neonatal period using a Rastelli procedure. Early repair eliminates the interim morbidity and mortality associated with a systemic-to-PA shunt and chronic cyanosis.

Current hospital survival for the ASO ranges from approximately 90% to 95%.[44,52–54] D-TGA/IVS generally has a lower mortality than d-TGA/VSD or d-TGA/VSD/PS. Hospital mortality for d-TGA/IVS ranges from 3.5–7.6%, compared to 9.4–13.1% for d-TGA/VSD.[52,53] Long-term survival at 5 to 10 years and 15 years range from 87.9a5 to 93% and 86% to 88%, respectively.[52–54] The most common cause for reintervention is supravalvar pulmonic stenosis, occurring in 3.9% to 16%.[52,54]

DOUBLE-OUTLET RIGHT VENTRICLE

Double-outlet ventricle includes a variety of malformations in which, by 50% or more, both great arteries arise from one ventricle. Although double-outlet LVs occur, a far more common anomaly is the double-outlet right ventricle (DORV). A VSD is usually present in DORV, in addition to other defects, including

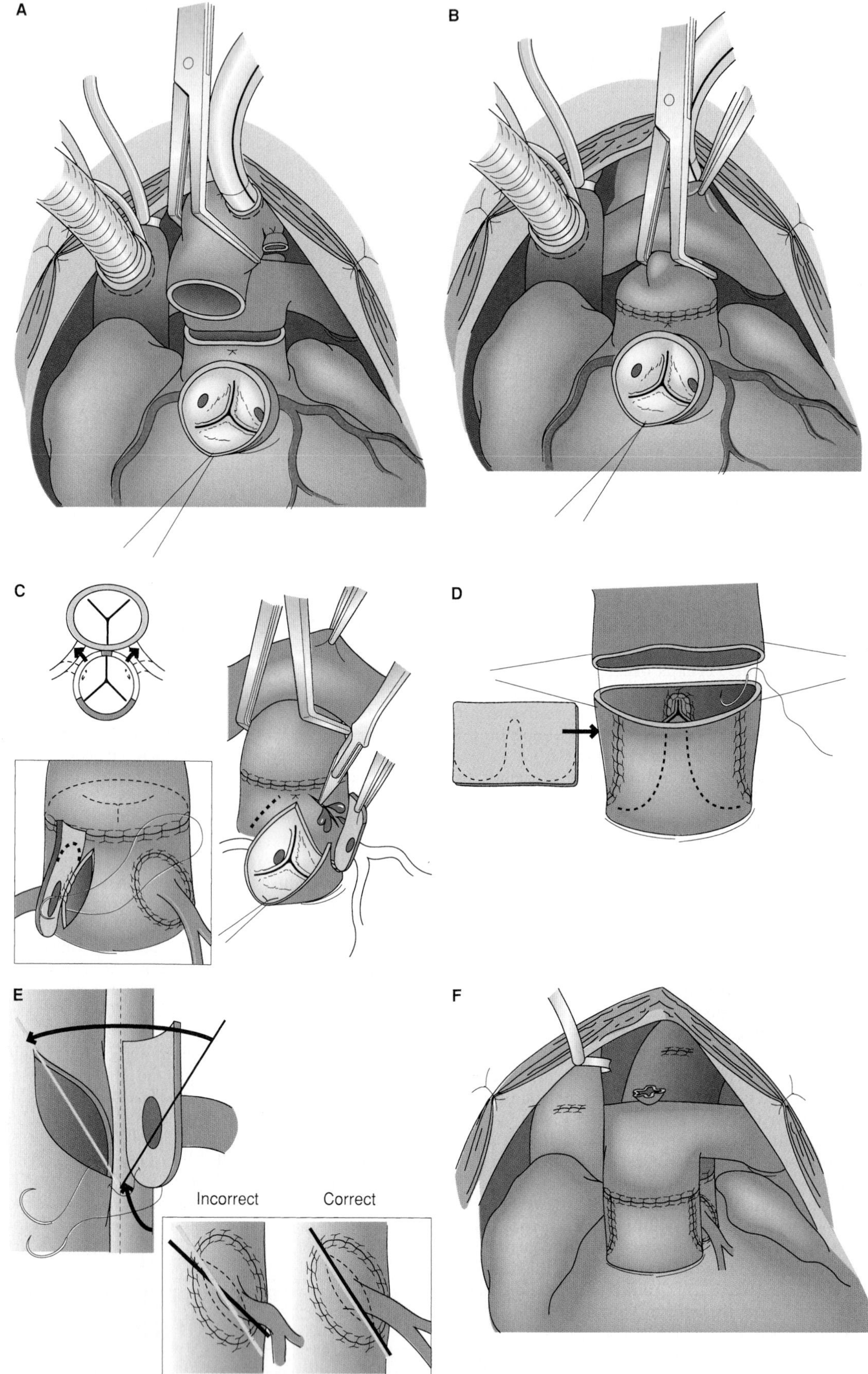

FIGURE 83.7 Arterial switch procedure for transposition of the great arteries. (*A*) Division of aorta and pulmonary artery. (*B*) LeCompte maneuver; posterior translocation of the aorta. (*C*) Mobilization of the coronary arteries. (*D*) Placement of pantaloon-shaped pericardial patch. (*E*) Proper alignment of the coronary arteries on the neoaorta. (*F*) Completed repair.

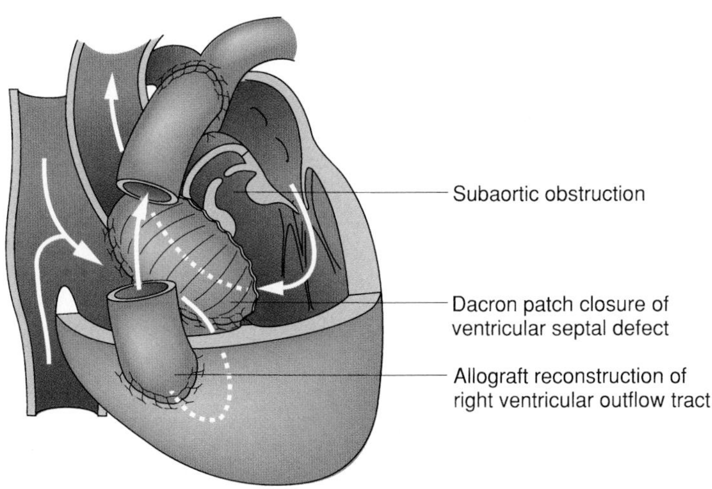

FIGURE 83.8 The Rastelli procedure for transposition of the great arteries with ventricular septal defect and pulmonary stenosis. A prosthetic patch placed within the right ventricle directs left ventricular blood through the defect to the aorta. The main pulmonary artery is ligated, and right ventricular blood then passes through a conduit to the distal pulmonary arteries.

discordant ventriculoarterial connections, valvar or subvalvar stenosis of the PA and aortic outflow, and single ventricle.

The physiologic consequences of DORV vary depending on the associated defects. The three most critical factors determining the net effects on the circulation are the size of the VSD, the presence or absence of PS, and the presence and degree of left-sided obstruction. As a result, DORV may clinically resemble an isolated VSD, TOF, or TGA.

The size and location of the VSD are important considerations in planning operative management. The VSD may be primarily directed toward the aorta, toward the PA, equally toward both arteries (doubly committed), or remote from both great vessels (noncommitted). The location of the VSD affects the direction of flow of oxygenated blood and thus affects the degree of cyanosis. VSDs in DORV seldom close spontaneously. This is fortunate, as closure would result in severe hemodynamic decompensation or death.

If the VSD is large, nonrestrictive and committed to the aorta, it can be closed with a tunnel-like patch that directs left ventricular flow into the aorta. A restrictive VSD must be enlarged to avoid creating subaortic stenosis. For patients with DORV and PS, repair requires right ventricular outflow tract reconstruction with a patch or a valved allograft conduit, in addition to patch closure of the VSD.

DORV with transposition-type physiology (malposed great vessels with the VSD committed to the PA) may be treated by a variety of methods, depending on the specific anatomic details. The preferred approach would be to perform an arterial switch operation, thus making the VSD committed to the aorta, and baffling the left ventricular outflow from the VSD to this neoaorta. Another preferred approach, which depends on a favorable orientation of the two great vessels and VSD, would be an intraventricular tunnel from the VSD to the aorta. A third approach utilizes the Damus-Kaye-Stanzel operation (DKS). During the DKS, the proximal PA is anastomosed end-to-side into the aorta. The VSD is baffled to both semilunar valves, which both connect to the aorta. An extracardiac conduit is then placed to reconstruct right ventricle-to-PA continuity. This approach may also be useful when the VSD is doubly or noncommitted, so that making a direct connection to either single great vessel is problematic.

The current results for correction of DORV with subaortic VSD are excellent, with a 15-year survival, including hospital mortality, of 96%.[55,56] Mortality for the more complex repairs tends to be slightly higher. Hospital mortality for an arterial switch operation with VSD closure for DORV range from 3.7% to 14.3%.[57,58]

TRUNCUS ARTERIOSUS

Truncus arteriosus is a rare anomaly that accounts for 0.4% to 4% of all cases of congenital heart disease.[59–61] A single arterial vessel arises from the heart, overriding the ventricular septum, and gives rise to the systemic, coronary, and pulmonary circulations. Two classification schemes have been proposed—one by Collett and Edwards[62] in 1949 and the other by Van Praagh and Van Praagh[63] in 1965 (Fig. 83.9). The Collett and Edwards classification focused on the origin of the pulmonary arteries from the common arterial trunk (Table 83.1).The system offered by Van Praagh and Van Praagh, a somewhat more surgically oriented scheme, is based on the presence or absence of a VSD, the degree of formation of the aorticopulmonary septum, and the status of the aortic arch (Table 83.2).

Persistent truncus arteriosus is the result of failed development of the aorticopulmonary septum and subpulmonary infundibulum (conal septum). Normal septation leads to the development of both pulmonary and systemic outflow tracts, division of the semilunar valves, and formation of the aorta and pulmonary arteries. Failure of septation results in a VSD (absence of the infundibular septum), a single semilunar valve, and a single arterial trunk. Most cases are associated with a VSD reminiscent of the VSD associated with TOF. However, in this anomaly, the superior margin of the defect is formed by the truncal valve. The truncal valve leaflets are generally dysmorphic, and their motion may be restricted. Leaflet number is highly variable, with about 65% tricuspid, 22% quadricuspid, 9% bicuspid, and rarely unicuspid or pentacuspid.[64] As a result of these abnormally developed valve leaflets, a moderate or greater degree of truncal insufficiency is present in 20% to 26% of patients.[65,66] Mild stenosis is common, significant stenosis is present in only 4% to 7%.[65,66] Significant obstruction is predicted by gradients of more than 30 mm Hg in the presence of normal cardiac output.[67] The PAs are usually of normal size and most often arise from the left posterolateral aspect of the truncal artery, often in close proximity to the truncal valve and ostium of the left coronary artery.

Other cardiac anomalies are common, with a PFO usually present. A true ASD is found in 9% to 20%, a persistent left superior vena cava in 4% to 9%, and mild tricuspid valve stenosis in 6%.[68,69] An interrupted aortic arch, most commonly type B, is present in association with truncus arteriosus (Van Praagh type A4/B4) in approximately 10% to 20%.[70,71] The arch is rightward, generally with mirror image branching, in 21% to 36%.[68,71] Aberrant origins of the brachiocephalic vessels are

VASCULAR

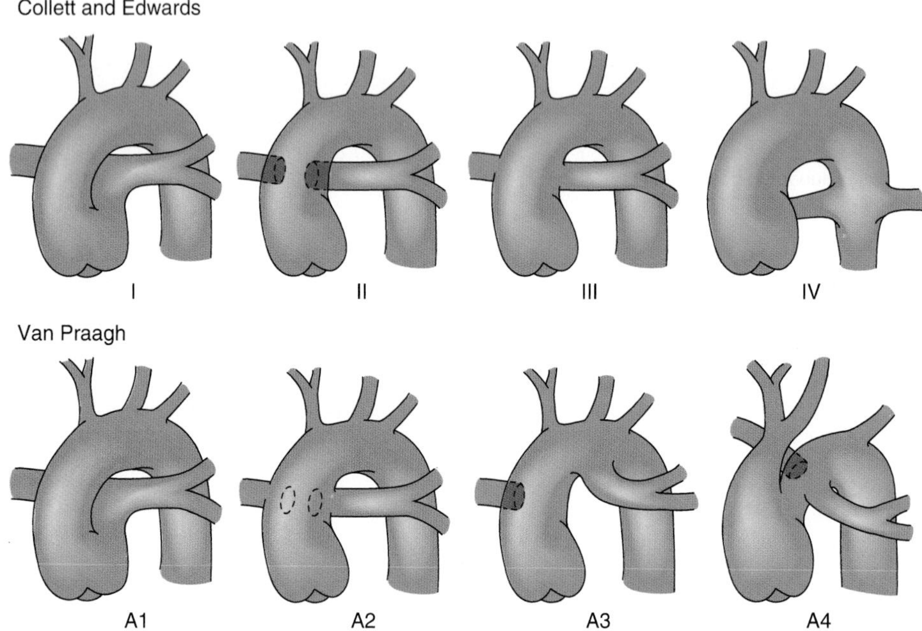

FIGURE 83.9 Truncus arteriosus: classification schemes as described by Collett and Edwards[62] and by Van Praagh and Van Praagh.[63] (From Hernanz-Schulman M, Fellows KE. Persistent truncus arteriosus: pathologic, diagnostic, and therapeutic considerations. *Semin Roentgenol.* 1985;20:121, with permission.)

reported, most commonly an aberrant right subclavian artery in 4% to 10%.[68,72] Coronary ostial abnormalities are of particular surgical significance and occur in 37% to 49% of cases.[73] The left coronary artery is frequently noted to have a high origin, not uncommonly near the takeoff of the pulmonary arteries. Rarely, the left coronary can originate from the main pulmonary trunk or a branch PA.[72] Extracardiac anomalies are reported in approximately 28% of patients with truncus arteriosus.[65] Described abnormalities include skeletal, genitourinary, and gastrointestinal deformities. As mentioned earlier, monoallelic microdeletion of chromosome 22q11 is common, with DiGeorge syndrome diagnosed in at least 11%.[65]

The anatomy of truncus arteriosus results in the obligatory mixing of systemic and pulmonary venous blood at the level of the VSD and truncal valve, which produces arterial saturations of 85% to 90%. The systemic arterial saturation depends on the volume of PBF, which in turn is determined by the PVR. As the PVR begins to fall, excessive pulmonary circulation ensues and leads to pulmonary congestion and signs and symptoms of CHF. This nonrestrictive left-to-right shunt may cause early development of irreversible pulmonary vascular obstructive disease.

The presence of truncal valve abnormalities poses further hemodynamic burdens. Truncal valve regurgitation leads to ventricular dilatation and low diastolic coronary perfusion pressures that can result in myocardial ischemia. Truncal valve stenosis promotes ventricular hypertrophy, increases the myocardial oxygen demand, and limits coronary and systemic perfusion, especially with the large volume of runoff into the pulmonary vascular bed.

Neonates with truncus arteriosus present with signs of CHF and collapsing peripheral pulses. Chest radiography shows marked cardiomegaly; pulmonary plethora, often with minimal thymus shadow; and a right aortic arch. The ECG most often depicts biventricular hypertrophy. Echocardiography is the diagnostic procedure of choice and can demonstrate the truncal vessel, the structure and function of the truncal valve, associated lesions such as interrupted aortic arch, and often the pulmonary arterial anatomy. Cardiac catheterization is

TABLE 83.1 CLASSIFICATION

COLLETT AND EDWARDS CLASSIFICATION OF TRUNCUS ARTERIOSUS

Type	Description
I	Common arterial trunk gives rise to a main pulmonary artery and the aorta
II	Right and left pulmonary arteries arise directly and in close proximity from the posterior wall of the truncus
III	Right and left pulmonary arteries arise from more widely separated orifices on the posterior truncal wall
IV	Branch pulmonary arteries are absent. Pulmonary blood flow is derived from aorticopulmonary collaterals

TABLE 83.2 CLASSIFICATION

VAN PRAAGH AND VAN PRAAGH CLASSIFICATION OF TRUNCUS ARTERIOSUS

Type	Description
A	With a VSD
B	Without a VSD
1	The aorticopulmonary septum is partially developed (partially separate main pulmonary artery)
2	The aorticopulmonary septum is absent (no main pulmonary artery segment); both branch pulmonary arteries arise from the common trunk
3	Either branch pulmonary artery is absent
4	Hypoplasia, coarctation, atresia, or absence of the aortic isthmus is associated with a large PDA

PDA, patent ductus arteriosus; VSD, ventricular septal defect.

not performed unless the anatomy is unclear, further information is needed about the status of the truncal valve, or the status of the pulmonary vasculature is unclear (i.e., infants older than 3 months at diagnosis).

The natural history of patients born with truncus arteriosus is early demise. Approximately 40% of infants are dead within 1 month, 70% by 3 months and 90% by 1 year.[74] Early death is caused by CHF. Survivors may do well for a period of time until the development of pulmonary vascular obstructive disease and Eisenmenger's syndrome. The ultimate treatment of truncus arteriosus is surgical correction in the neonatal period. Medical treatment is palliative and directed toward controlling CHF with fluid restriction, diuretics, digitalis, and afterload reduction. Complete repair entails separating the pulmonary arteries from the truncus, repairing the resulting defect in the aorta, closing the VSD, and restoring the continuity of the right ventricular outflow tract with an extracardiac conduit. Severe truncal valve regurgitation requires truncal valve replacement, which is best done with a cryopreserved allograft. An associated interrupted aortic arch is repaired by constructing a primary end-to-end anastomosis of the distal ascending aorta with proximal augmentation if necessary.

The results of truncus arteriosus repair have improved greatly during the last two decades. Before the importance of early operation to avoid irreversible PVR was appreciated, patients underwent repair at most institutions at an average age of 2 to 5 years with high mortality rates. Ebert showed that repair in the first 6 months of life is not only possible, but preferable, reporting a mortality rate of 9%.[75] Current hospital mortality for the neonatal repair of truncus arteriosus ranges between 4.3% to 17%, with the majority of deaths occurring in complex truncus arteriosus or in truncus arteriosus with associated severe truncal valve regurgitation.[65–67,76,77] Risk factors for poor outcome identified in various studies include significant truncal regurgitation, need for truncal valve replacement, birth weight less than 2.5 kg, presence of interrupted aortic arch or coronary artery anomalies, pulmonary reconstruction with a technique other than valved heterograft or allograft, and age greater than 100 days.[65–67,76–79] Other recent studies have demonstrated that interrupted aortic arch has been neutralized as a risk factor.[67,77]

CORONARY ARTERY ANOMALIES

Coronary artery anomalies occur in between 0.3% and 1.3% of the population.[80,81] They can be classified as minor, secondary, or major based on their clinical significance.[82] Minor defects have no functional significance and are usually detected as incidental findings at cardiac catheterization. Secondary defects have no intrinsic significance but alter surgical management when they are present. An example of a secondary defect is an anomalous origin of the left anterior descending artery from the right coronary artery that crosses the hypoplastic infundibulum in a patient with TOF. The presence of this vessel may prevent the safe performance of a transannular incision and thereby mandate the use of a conduit. Major defects are the most important form of coronary anomaly, because they exert an intrinsically adverse effect on the myocardium. Major anomalies can be subdivided based on anatomy: coronary arteriovenous fistula, anomalous pulmonary origin of a coronary artery, anomalous aortic origin of a coronary artery, myocardial bridging, or coronary artery aneurysm.

Coronary arteriovenous fistula is the most common major coronary anomaly. An abnormal connection exists between a coronary artery (usually the right) and another vascular structure (usually one of the right heart chambers). Most fistulas are isolated and solitary. The fistula leads to left-to-right shunting, which can produce CHF. Other symptoms include angina, endocarditis, myocardial infarction, arrhythmia, and sudden death. The diagnosis is suggested by echocardiography and confirmed by catheterization. All symptomatic fistulas should be occluded, either surgically or by transcatheter techniques. In some cases, coronary bypass grafting may be necessary when distal flow is compromised by fistula occlusion. Treatment of asymptomatic fistulas is controversial, but occlusion should probably be undertaken when significant left-to-right shunting is present.

The second most common major coronary anomaly is origin of a coronary artery from the PA. The most common manifestation is the anomalous left coronary artery arising from the pulmonary artery (ALCAPA). The right coronary (or both coronaries) may also arise anomalously from the PA, but only in very rare cases. ALCAPA is usually well tolerated during fetal development, but after birth, the pulmonary systolic pressure usually drops (following ductal closure and decline in PVR) and the anomalous coronary is perfused with desaturated blood at low pressure. Collateral vessels develop between the normal right coronary artery and the abnormal left coronary, but the benefit is negated due to the development of coronary steal, whereby the collateral blood shunts left-to-right by retrograde flow in the anomalous coronary into the low-pressure PA. Most patients will present between 6 weeks and 3 months of life. Typical symptoms include irritability, difficulty in feeding, and other signs of CHF. Untreated, ALCAPA is nearly always fatal. Rarely, patients will survive to adulthood and present with symptoms of angina or sudden death. On examination, patients with ALCAPA frequently have a holosystolic murmur of ischemic mitral regurgitation. The pulmonary component of the second heart sound may be pronounced due to pulmonary hypertension. Chest radiography is significant for cardiomegaly and pulmonary edema. Electrocardiographic evidence of ischemia and infarction is usually present. Echocardiography is usually diagnostic and is useful for assessing the severity of left ventricular dysfunction and ischemic mitral regurgitation, which are commonly present. Catheterization is occasionally necessary to clarify the anatomy, but this technique is used less frequently due to the risk of inducing life-threatening arrhythmias.

Surgical repair is indicated for all patients with ALCAPA. Historically, the initial surgical approach involved ligation of the proximal left coronary artery. This served to eliminate coronary steal and allow perfusion of the left coronary system by collaterals from the right. Despite the ease of simple ligation, most centers have abandoned this approach in favor of establishment of a two-coronary system, which offers better long-term freedom from ischemia. In older patients, this may be achieved by proximal ligation of the left coronary artery in conjunction with coronary artery bypass, ideally with a left internal mammary graft. Coronary bypass is technically difficult in neonates, and a number of alternative operations have been devised to create a direct connection between the aorta and the anomalous coronary artery. Most commonly, this can be achieved by removing the origin of the left coronary artery (along with a button of adjacent PA) and reimplanting the vessel directly into the side of the aorta. Another approach involves creation of a side-to-side connection between the aorta and PA with placement of an intrapulmonary baffle to direct flow from this connection to the anomalous left coronary ostium. Survival following surgical repair of ALCAPA has improved over the years.[83] Recent reports have suggested an operative mortality of 6% or less.[84,85] Ventricular function tends to normalize after surgery.[86] In most patients, mitral valve function also improves,[84,86] but for patients with severe mitral regurgitation, concurrent mitral valve repair is usually indicated.

Anomalous aortic origins of the coronary arteries are usually minor defects, but a potentially dangerous abnormality exists when the left main coronary artery arises from the right coronary sinus and passes between the PA and aorta. This defect has been associated with cardiac symptoms and sudden death, as has the origin of the right coronary artery from the left coronary sinus (usually when the right coronary is dominant).[87,88] The etiology of ischemia in both defects is thought to be related to the acute angle of origin and slit-like orifice of the anomalous vessel and the extrinsic compression created by the apposing walls of the aorta and PA. These defects usually present in older patients. Symptomatic patients are treated surgically by coronary artery bypass.

Myocardial bridging occurs when a segment of an epicardial coronary artery (usually the left anterior descending) takes an intramyocardial course over a short segment. Although this is a common incidental finding at cardiac catheterization, this defect has been associated in some cases with myocardial ischemia. Treatment involves dividing the muscle bridge to free the coronary, coronary bypass beyond the bridge, or transcatheter stenting.

Coronary aneurysms occur rarely, usually in conjunction with an inflammatory condition such as Kawasaki syndrome, polyarteritis nodosa, Takayasu arteritis, or syphilis. Coronary aneurysms may thrombose or lead to distal coronary stenosis or embolization. Rupture occurs uncommonly. Treatment ranges from antiplatelet therapy to coronary bypass grafting.

PATENT DUCTUS ARTERIOSUS

The ductus arteriosus is a normal fetal vascular structure that allows blood from the right ventricle to bypass the high-resistance pulmonary vascular bed and pass directly to the systemic circulation. The ductus communicates between the main PA (or proximal left PA) and the proximal descending thoracic aorta. Histologically, the media of the ductus contains a predominance of smooth muscle cells, whereas the media of the aorta and PA contain well-developed elastic fibers. Vasocontrol of the ductus is mediated by two important mechanisms: oxygen tension and prostaglandin levels. During fetal development, low oxygen tension and high levels of circulating prostaglandin maintain ductal patency. During the final trimester, the ductus becomes less sensitive to prostaglandins and more sensitive to the effects of oxygen tension. Following birth, the rise in oxygen tension and a fall in prostaglandins (which were previously supplied principally by the placenta) lead to ductal closure, which is usually complete by 12 to 24 hours. After closure, the ductus becomes a fibrous cord known as the ligamentum arteriosum. Failure of closure of the ductus leads to the condition called PDA. PDA occurs in about 1 out of 1,200 live births and accounts for 7% of congenital heart defects.[7] The incidence is much higher in premature infants (greater than 20%).[89] This elevated incidence is thought to be related to immaturity of the ductal wall resulting in impaired sensitivity to oxygen tension.

PDA may occur as an isolated defect, or it may occur in association with a number of other anomalies. Patency of the ductus arteriosus is desirable in a number of defects in which there is either inadequate PBF (such as pulmonary atresia) or inadequate systemic blood flow (as in severe coarctation of the aorta). The discovery that extrinsic delivery of prostaglandins can maintain ductal patency has played a critical role in improving the survival of these patients.[90]

The physiologic manifestation of PDA is shunting of blood across the ductus. The shunt volume is determined by the size of the ductus and by the ratio of pulmonary to systemic vascular resistance. At birth, the PVR drops dramatically and continues to decline over the first several weeks of life. As a result, shunting across a PDA is from left-to-right. Excessive PBF can lead to CHF. In extreme cases, hypotension and systemic malperfusion may result. Patients with a large PDA who survive infancy tend to develop pulmonary vascular obstructive disease. Eisenmenger's physiology results when the PVR exceeds the systemic vascular resistance, producing a reversal of shunting across the ductus to right-to-left. This leads to cyanosis and, eventually, right ventricular failure. Small PDAs may persist to adulthood without producing any symptoms or physiologic derangement. Endocarditis and endarteritis have been reported as long-term complications of PDA.[91]

In patients with PDA, symptoms are proportional to the shunt volume and the presence of associated defects. Left-to-right shunting produces volume overload of the left heart. Infants with CHF demonstrate symptoms of tachypnea, tachycardia, and poor feeding. Older children may present with recurrent respiratory infections, fatigue, and failure to thrive. Physical findings include a widened pulse pressure and a continuous "machinery" murmur heard best along the left upper sternal border. Chest radiography shows increased pulmonary vascular markings and left heart enlargement. Left ventricular hypertrophy and left atrial enlargement may be evident on the ECG. Echocardiography is the diagnostic method of choice. Diagnostic cardiac catheterization is performed only in older patients with suspected pulmonary hypertension to evaluate for pulmonary vascular obstructive disease. More frequently, catheterization is utilized for transcatheter occlusion of the ductus in selected cases.

PDA closure is performed for all symptomatic patients. Closure is also recommended for asymptomatic patients due to the risk of heart failure, pulmonary hypertension, and endocarditis. Closure of the ductus may be accomplished by one of three approaches: pharmacologic, surgical, and endovascular. Indomethacin, which is a prostaglandin inhibitor, stimulates PDA closure in premature infants.[92] It is rarely effective in full-term infants. The dosing regimen is 0.1 to 0.2 mg/kg intravenously at 12- or 24-hour intervals for a total of three doses. This is effective in about 80% of premature babies.[93] Due to its side effects, indomethacin is contraindicated in patients with sepsis, renal insufficiency, intracranial hemorrhage, or bleeding disorders. Failure of indomethacin after two complete courses results in referral for surgical closure.

The surgical approach to PDA is through a left posterolateral thoracotomy via the third or fourth intercostal space. The pleura is incised over the proximal descending thoracic aorta. This allows medial retraction of the vagus nerve. The recurrent laryngeal nerve curves behind the ductus and should be protected throughout the procedure. Dissection is then performed to demonstrate the pertinent anatomy. In many cases, the ductus is the largest vascular structure present, and it must not be confused with the aorta. Ductal tissue is extremely friable, so direct manipulation is minimized. In premature infants, the ductus is controlled with a single surgical clip; this procedure is commonly performed in the neonatal intensive care unit, thereby avoiding problems associated with patient transfer.[94,95] In older patients, occlusion of the ductus is achieved with simple silk ligature, or, preferably, by division between ligatures to minimize recurrence.

Recently, thoracoscopic techniques have been developed to perform PDA ligation.[96] This approach has the potential benefits of decreased pain and quicker recovery. Disadvantages include a substantial learning curve and increased operating time.

A number of endovascular devices have been developed for the purpose of transcatheter occlusion of the PDA.[97–99] This approach is very successful in older infants, children, and adults with small and moderate-sized PDAs and has become the treatment of choice at many centers. Surgical therapy is reserved for PDAs having a large diameter or very short length.

Rarely, an adult will present with a significant PDA. These patients must be carefully evaluated for the presence of pulmonary vascular obstructive disease prior to ductal closure. If the patient is not a candidate for device closure, surgical closure can be problematic. Calcification of the ductal wall is common in adults, and this makes ligation hazardous. In some cases, cardiopulmonary bypass may be required with closure of the ductus from within the PA.[100,101]

Closure of the ductus by surgical or transcatheter techniques is achieved with a mortality that approaches zero.[94] Potential complications include pneumothorax, recurrent laryngeal nerve injury, and chylothorax (from injury to the thoracic duct). Long-term survival should be normal following PDA ligation in most patients. Survival in premature infants depends primarily on the extent of prematurity with its attendant complications.

ATRIOVENTRICULAR SEPTAL DEFECT

Defects in the embryologic development of the endocardial cushions may result in a variety of morphologic abnormalities in the AV valves and the atrial and ventricular septa. These anomalies range from the ostium primum ASD to the complete AVSD (or AV canal defect), with a spectrum of intermediate forms. PDA and TOF are occasionally seen in association with these defects. A high percentage of patients with abnormalities of the AV structures have Down syndrome.

Complete AVSD is an anomaly characterized by a common AV orifice, rather than separate mitral and tricuspid orifices, and a deficiency of endocardial cushion tissue, which results in an ASD and an inlet type of VSD. Complete AVSDs were subclassified by Rastelli et al.[102] into three types according to the morphology of the anterior leaflet of the common AV valve (Table 83.3). Incomplete AVSDs are variants in which there is partial fusion of the AV valves, resulting in separate right and left AV valve orifices. The ostium primum ASD is a type of incomplete AVSD in which VSD component is absent.

When both left and right AV valves equally share the common AV valve orifice, the AVSD is termed balanced. Occasionally, the orifice may favor the right AV valve (right dominance) or the left AV valve (left dominance). In marked right dominance, the left AV valve and LV are hypoplastic, and frequently coexist with other left-sided abnormalities including AS, hypoplasia of the aorta, and coarctation. Conversely, marked left dominance results in a deficient right AV valve with associated hypoplasia of the right ventricle, pulmonary stenosis or atresia, and TOF. Patients with severe imbalance require staged single ventricle reconstruction.

The conduction tissue is displaced in an ASVD and is at risk during the surgical repair. The AV node is located posteriorly and inferiorly of its normal position toward the coronary sinus in what has been termed the nodal triangle. This triangle is bounded by the coronary sinus, the posterior attachment of the inferior bridging leaflet, and the rim of the ASD. The bundle of His courses anteriorly and superiorly to run along the leftward aspect of the crest of the VSD, giving off the left bundle branch and continuing as the right bundle branch.

A number of other cardiac anomalies are associated with AVSDs including a PDA (10%) and TOF (10%).[69] Important abnormalities of the left AV valve include single papillary muscle (parachute mitral valve) (2% to 6%) and double orifice mitral valve (8% to 14%).[103] A persistent left superior vena cava with or without an unroofed coronary sinus is encountered in 3% of patients with an AVSD. DORV (2%) significantly complicates or may even preclude complete surgical correction.[69] Left ventricular outflow tract obstruction from subaortic stenosis or redundant AV valve tissue occurs in 4% to 7%.[104,105]

Patients with an incomplete AVSD generally present in a similar fashion as a patient with a large secundum ASD. Patients with a complete AVSD with both atrial and ventricular level shunting generally present early in infancy with signs and symptoms of CHF. In addition, moderate or severe left AV valve regurgitation occurs in approximately 10% of patients with an AVSD worsening the clinical picture. On physical examination, the precordium is hyperactive, often with a prominent thrill. Auscultatory findings include a systolic murmur along the left sternal border, a high-pitched murmur at the apex from left AV valve regurgitation, and a mid-diastolic flow murmur across the common AV valve. In the presence of elevated PVR, there may be a split first heart sound. Significant cardiomegaly and pulmonary overcirculation are found on the chest radiograph. ECG reveals biventricular hypertrophy, atrial enlargement, prolonged PR interval, leftward axis, and counterclockwise frontal plane loop. Doppler/echocardiography is diagnostic, defining the atrial and ventricular level shunting, valvular anatomy, and any associated anomalies. Cardiac catheterization should be performed for patients older than the age of 1 year, for patients with signs or symptoms of increased PVR, or in some cases to further evaluate other associated major cardiac anomalies. If the PVR is high, it is important to remeasure it while the child is breathing 100% oxygen with and without nitric oxide. If the pulmonary resistance falls, it implies that much of the elevated resistance is dynamic and can be managed in the perioperative period by ventilatory manipulation, supplemental oxygen, and nitric oxide. More recently, sildenafil has been shown to decrease elevation in PVR in children with CHF.[106] Markedly elevated pulmonary resistance (greater than 10 Woods units × m^2) that does not respond to oxygen administration is generally considered a contraindication to repair.

Operative treatment is almost always necessary as soon as symptoms are observed to prevent further clinical deterioration. Even in the absence of symptoms, operation is best performed before 6 months of age. PA banding, which permits delaying the repair until the child is larger, is no longer used today except in select complex or single ventricle cases, extremely low birth weight or prematurity, and very poor clinical condition. This approach exposes the child to the risks of two operations, and the overall mortality exceeds that of primary repair in infancy.

Correcting AVSDs requires patch closure of both septal defects, with any necessary valve reconstruction. Separate atrial and ventricular patches or a single patch for both chambers can be used.[107] During closure of the ventricular defect, the surgeon must carefully avoid injury to the conduction system, which passes along the posterior and inferior rim of the ventricular septum.

The short- and long-term success of the operation is highly dependent on the status of the PVR and the surgeon's ability to maintain competence of the mitral valve. In developed countries, it is fortunately relatively uncommon for patients to present late in the course of an AVSD with refractory PVR elevations.

TABLE 83.3 CLASSIFICATION

RASTELLI CLASSIFICATION OF ATRIOSEPTAL VENTRICULAR DEFECTS

Type	Description
A	The anterior bridging leaflet is divided and attached to the septum by multiple chordae
B	The anterior bridging leaflet is attached to a papillary muscle in the right ventricle
C	The anterior bridging leaflet is free-floating, with no attachments except to the valve annulus

Although earlier reports recommend that the cleft in the left AV valve should not be closed and the valve treated as a trileaflet structure, most authors now believe that closure of the cleft is an important mechanism in preventing postoperative left AV valve regurgitation. Significant AV valve regurgitation at the conclusion of surgery, severe dyplasia of the left AV valve, and failure to close the cleft of the left AV valve have been identified as important risk factors for reoperation.[108] Significant postoperative left AV valve regurgitation is also a risk factor for operative and long-term mortality.[104,108] The cleft should not be completely closed in the presence of a single papillary muscle to avoid causing left AV valve stenosis. In the case of a double orifice valve, the bridging tissue should not be divided to create a single opening in the valve.

Operative mortality is related largely to associated cardiac anomalies and left AV valve regurgitation. Mortality for repair of uncomplicated incomplete AVSDs ranges from 0% to 0.6%, and the addition of left AV valve regurgitation increases mortality to 4% to 6%.[104,109] For complete AVSDs the mortality without left AV valve regurgitation is approximately 5%, compared with 13% when significant degrees of regurgitation are present.[104]

The majority of reoperations after repair of AVSD are due to left AV valve regurgitation. Significant postoperative AV valve regurgitation occurs in 10% to 15% of patients, necessitating reoperation for valve repair or replacement in 7% to 12%.[108,110,111]

COARCTATION OF THE AORTA

Coarctation of the aorta is a narrowing of the proximal descending thoracic aorta distal to the origin of the left subclavian artery, near the insertion of the ductus arteriosus (or ligamentum arteriosum). The severity of luminal narrowing and the length of the aorta affected are variable. Coarctation is thought to occur as a result of ectopic tissue from the ductus arteriosus, which migrates into the wall of the adjacent aorta. After birth, as the ductus closes, the ectopic tissue in the aorta also constricts. Frequently, a posterior shelf of tissue is present at the point of most severe obstruction. The aortic obstruction caused by coarctation creates a pressure load on the LV.

The incidence of coarctation is about 0.5 per 1,000 live births, and its prevalence is 5% of congenital heart defects.[7] Coarctation is commonly associated with other heart defects including bicuspid aortic valve (in more than 50% of cases), PDA, and VSD. Other left-sided obstructive lesions may also be present, such as aortic arch hypoplasia, AS, mitral stenosis, and left ventricular hypoplasia. Coarctation is also recognized to occur in association with Turner's syndrome.

Patients with severe coarctation present in the newborn period. Aortic obstruction is so significant that perfusion of the lower body is dependent on flow from the ductus arteriosus. Spontaneous ductal closure typically worsens the aortic obstruction and may lead to malperfusion of tissues distal to the coarctation. The pressure load on the LV may precipitate CHF. Patients may develop shock with severe acidosis, oliguria, and diminished distal pulses. Infants with severe coarctation will generally not survive without intervention.

Older children with coarctation are usually asymptomatic. The diagnosis is commonly made on the basis of hypertension in the upper extremities with decreased pulses in the lower extremities. Noninvasive blood pressure measurements in all four extremities help to quantify the severity of aortic obstruction. These older patients tend to develop extensive collateral arteries that bypass the obstruction. Life expectancy for these patients is limited due to the development heart failure later in life. Other long-term complications of coarctation include endocarditis (frequently involving a bicuspid aortic valve), endarteritis (in the post-stenotic area of the aorta at the site of the jet of turbulent flow), aortic dissection, aortic aneurysm, and intracranial hemorrhage (from Berry aneurysms, which occur more commonly in patients with coarctation).[112]

The diagnosis of coarctation can usually be made clinically. The infant with significant coarctation is frequently asymptomatic at birth, but following closure of the ductus develops signs of heart failure such as irritability, tachypnea, and poor feeding. Lower extremity pulses are absent, and upper extremity pulses may be weak. Chest radiography shows cardiomegaly and pulmonary venous congestion. There is a left ventricular strain pattern on the ECG. Echocardiography is usually diagnostic, demonstrating narrowing of the aorta at the coarctation site with a loss of pulsatility in the descending aorta.

In older children and adults with coarctation, there is usually a pressure gradient between the arms and legs, which can be demonstrated by measuring cuff pressures in all four extremities. On chest radiography, rib notching may be evident, secondary to erosion of the inferior rib borders from the development of large intercostals collateral vessels. Echocardiography usually confirms the diagnosis. Anatomic details may also be clarified with computed tomography and magnetic resonance imaging. Cardiac catheterization is usually not necessary.

Generally, all patients with coarctation should undergo surgical repair. For neonates, the acute medical management includes initiation of PGE1 for the purpose of reopening the ductus; this maneuver partially relieves the aortic obstruction and augments perfusion of the lower body due to improved antegrade flow across the arch as well as right-to-left flow across the ductus. Prostaglandins are usually effective for reopening the ductus when initiated within 7 to 10 days of life but are less successful thereafter.

Surgical repair of coarctation is usually performed through a left posterolateral thoracotomy via the third or fourth intercostal space. The descending thoracic aorta, ductus (or ligamentum), transverse aortic arch, and brachiocephalic vessels are mobilized. Care is taken to preserve the vagus nerve and its recurrent laryngeal branch. The preferred surgical approach to coarctation in infants and children is a resection with end-to-end anastomosis.[113] In older children and adults, it may not be possible to perform a resection with primary repair without creating excessive tension on the anastomosis, which may lead to hemorrhage or scarring with recurrent coarctation. An alternative strategy is necessary in these cases. Patch aortoplasty may be performed in children in whom further growth is anticipated.[114,115] The subclavian flap repair augments the narrowed aorta using native arterial tissue. Blood flow to the left arm is maintained by collateral vessels, although long-term studies have demonstrated a slight discrepancy in limb length in some patients. Prosthetic patch material may also be used. By avoiding circumferential prosthetic material, growth potential of the native aorta is preserved. The disadvantage of patch repair is a high risk of aneurysm formation. In adults, in whom growth is no longer an issue, resection of the coarctation may be performed with subsequent placement of a prosthetic interposition graft (either Dacron or polytetrafluoroethylene).

One of the principal concerns during coarctation repair is interruption of distal aortic blood flow, especially to the spinal cord. The anterior spinal artery is fed by major radicular branches from intercostal arteries. In patients without well-formed collaterals, ischemia of the spinal cord may be precipitated by aortic cross-clamping, and paraplegia may result. Protective measures include induction of mild hypothermia, maintenance of a high proximal aortic pressure, and minimization of cross-clamp time. In older patients, distal aortic perfusion may be maintained by the technique of left heart bypass, in which oxygenated blood is taken from the left atrium and delivered to the femoral artery or distal aorta using a centrifugal pump.[116] Overall, the incidence of paraplegia following coarctation repair is less than 1%.[117]

Following repair, patients may develop severe hypertension. This can be managed using intravenous beta-blockers (e.g., esmolol) or vasodilators (e.g., sodium nitroprusside). Uncontrolled hypertension can lead to the complication of mesenteric arteritis. Hypertension usually resolves within days to weeks after repair, although older children and adults may require lifelong antihypertensive therapy. Repair of coarctation during infancy is thought to minimize the risk of late hypertension.[118]

Transcatheter therapy has been proposed for the primary therapy of coarctation, but this approach is controversial due to the incidence of recurrent coarctation, need for multiple interventions, injury to the femoral vasculature (for access), and aneurysm formation.[119–121] On the other hand, balloon angioplasty is widely accepted for the treatment of recurrent coarctation following surgery, in which the success rate is on the order of 90%.[122–124]

The early mortality following repair of coarctation in neonates is 2% to 10%, whereas the risk in older children and adults is about 1%.[113,125] The incidence of recurrent coarctation following resection and end-to-end repair is about 4% to 8%.[113,126] The long-term survival following repair of coarctation is determined by the presence of associated defects and the persistence of hypertension.

UNIVENTRICULAR HEART

In the univentricular heart, only one ventricular chamber is connected to the atria. To be classified as a ventricle, a chamber must receive at least half of an inlet valve. In the most common form of univentricular heart, both the mitral and tricuspid valves connect to a morphologic LV (double-inlet LV), which ejects blood through a hypoplastic outlet chamber and then, due to malposition of the great arteries, to the aorta. The outlet chamber is not considered to be a ventricle, regardless of its size, because it does not receive an inlet valve. Similarly, the intracardiac communication is not termed a VSD, but a bulboventricular foramen. Univentricular hearts are frequently associated with malpositions of the great vessels and varying degrees of obstruction to the PBF. In double-inlet LV, the aorta is usually anterior and to the left of the PA.

The presentation of infants with univentricular heart is variable, depending on the amount of PBF.[127] When the pulmonary flow is excessive, cyanosis may be mild, and the dominant feature is CHF. Associated PS decreases the PBF, and the degree of cyanosis is increased. Associated lesions may further complicate the picture, such as coarctation, subaortic stenosis, or a restrictive ASD. Patients with moderate PS may achieve a well-balanced circulation with acceptable systemic oxygenation and normal PA pressure. These patients may be symptom-free well into adolescence. Most patients, however, require intervention early in life to reduce excessive PBF or to increase it in the presence of significant PS. Pulmonary vascular obstructive disease develops early when PBF is excessive. With the possible exception of patients in whom the pulmonary and systemic blood flow is well balanced, the prognosis for patients with unoperated univentricular hearts is poor. More than half die early of CHF or dysrhythmias.

In the presence of excessive PBF and pulmonary hypertension, operation should be performed early in life to control PBF and prevent the development of pulmonary vascular occlusive disease. Options include PA banding or division of the main PA in conjunction with a controlled aorticopulmonary shunt. PA banding is a less complicated procedure; however, it is often difficult to adjust the pulmonary flow accurately, and too proximal or too distal a band can lead to distortion of the pulmonary valve or branch pulmonary arteries, which further complicates later operations. Simple division of the PA with placement of a modified Blalock-Taussig shunt can be undertaken in the presence of an adequate bulboventricular foramen providing unobstructed flow to the aorta. This option avoids the problems associated with a PA band, and more accurately controls the PBF. Another similar technique is division of the main PA, side-to-side anastomosis of the proximal PA with the native aorta, and placement of a modified Blalock-Taussig shunt (modified Damus-Kaye-Stanzel procedure). It is not uncommon for the bulboventricular foramen to decrease in size over time. Maintaining continuity from both the outlet chamber and the LV eliminates the possibility of subaortic obstruction, which can occur when the systemic blood flow depends entirely on egress through a bulboventricular foramen. In infants who are well balanced and can be safely managed medically until the age of 4 to 6 months, a hemi-Fontan or bidirectional Glenn, in which the superior vena caval flow is directed into the pulmonary arteries, can be used to increase the effective PBF. This procedure maximizes pulmonary flow without causing a volume overload to the single ventricle. It is most commonly used as part of an interim stage to a complete atriopulmonary connection or Fontan procedure.

The ultimate goal of surgical correction in patients with a univentricular heart is the total diversion of all vena caval blood directly into the pulmonary arteries. The Fontan procedure was first successfully performed in a patient with tricuspid atresia but has since evolved as an excellent way to establish physiologic repair for patients with more complex forms of univentricular heart.[128] The superior vena caval blood returns directly via an end-to-side anastomosis with the PA (bidirectional Glenn) or through a right atrial-PA connection (hemi-Fontan). The inferior vena caval flow is directed to the PA with an intraatrial baffle (lateral tunnel technique, Fig. 83.10) or an extracardiac conduit. All oxygenated pulmonary venous flow empties into the ventricular chamber through the AV valves to be ejected to the systemic circulation, while superior and inferior vena caval blood flows directly to the lungs to acquire oxygen prior to returning to the heart. For the Fontan procedure to be performed with a low operative mortality and an acceptable functional result, certain criteria must be met. Normal PA pressure (<20 mm Hg) and PVR (<2 Woods units·m^2) are the most important prerequisites. Additionally, it is essential that ventricular function and AV valve function be normal. Many of the criteria originally proposed, including normal cardiac rhythm, right atrial hypertrophy, normal systemic venous return, and age older than 4 years, are of little or no importance. Although the Fontan procedure cannot be considered a truly corrective operation, it offers benefits that cannot be equaled by those of any of the other palliative procedures. The major advantages include restoration of normal systemic oxygen saturation and reduction of ventricular volume overload.

Ventricular septation procedures have also been successfully performed in patients with univentricular hearts. The subset of patients with a double-inlet LV, anterior and leftward aorta, nonrestrictive outlet foramen, and mild or no PS are best suited for septation. This anatomy allows placement of a relatively direct and straight prosthetic patch in the ventricle that separates the pulmonary and systemic circulations. The septation procedure has been associated with a relatively high morbidity, primarily related to complete heart block, so that its overall effectiveness is reduced. Few centers have continued to apply this procedure in carefully selected patients.

The current results for the Fontan are excellent with hospital mortality ranging from 2% to 9%.[129–131] The condition of survivors is generally good and most attain a functional status of New York Heart Association class I or II. The long-term results have been reported with a 93% 5-year survival and a 91% 10-year survival.[131] Although long-term results are

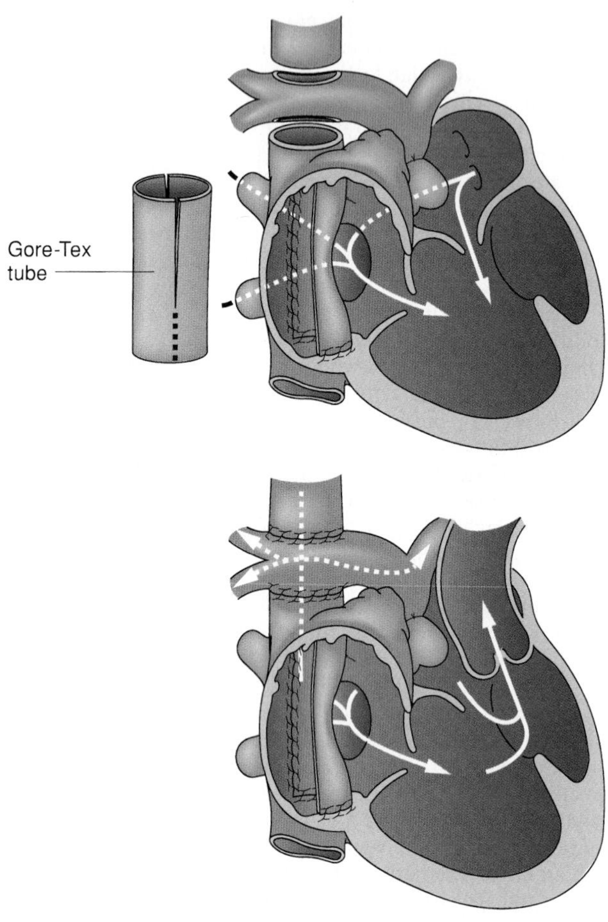

FIGURE 83.10 Total cavopulmonary connection for univentricular heart. The internal orifices of the superior and inferior venae cavae are connected in the right atrium with a patch cut from a Gore-Tex tube. The superior vena cava is divided just above its junction with the right atrium, and both ends are anastomosed to the right pulmonary artery. The main pulmonary artery is ligated.

encouraging, late complications may be seen. Continued surveillance for arrhythmias, CHF, protein-losing enteropathy, and hepatic dysfunction remains important.

HYPOPLASTIC LEFT-HEART SYNDROME

Hypoplastic left-heart syndrome (HLHS) refers to a constellation of congenital cardiac anomalies characterized by marked hypoplasia or absence of the LV and severe hypoplasia of the ascending aorta. The systemic circulation is dependent on the right ventricle via a PDA and there is obligatory mixing of pulmonary and systemic venous blood in the right atrium. There is associated aortic valve stenosis or atresia, and mitral valve stenosis or atresia. The descending aorta is essentially a continuation of the ductus arteriosus, and the ascending aorta and aortic arch are a diminutive branch from this vessel. Initial management includes a prostaglandin infusion to maintain ductal patency and correction of metabolic acidosis. The patient may require intubation and ventilator adjustment to reduce supplemental oxygen and maintain a PCO_2 of about 40 mm Hg to avoid excessive pulmonary flow.

Alternative approaches to the treatment of this problem include cardiac transplantation and staged reconstructive surgery. Transplantation for HLHS is generally performed with the same techniques that are standard for transplantation in older children and adults. However, it is necessary to have a generous amount of donor aortic arch that can be used to augment the tiny recipient arch. Results of transplantation in neonates have been excellent in centers with extensive experience in this area, and a 2-year survival as high as 70% has been reported.[132] In the context of improving results for staged reconstruction, risks of immunosuppression, and limited donor availability, competing risk analysis favors staged repair, and most centers pursue this option as primary therapy for HLHS.[133] Transplantation is generally reserved for very high-risk patients, such as those with depressed right ventricular function of severe tricuspid regurgitation.

The first successful palliation of HLHS was reported by Norwood on a series of infants operated on between 1979 and 1981.[134] This procedure has been technically refined over the years, but three essential components remain: atrial septectomy, anastomosis of the proximal PA to the aorta with homograft augmentation of the aortic arch, and aortopulmonary shunt (Fig. 83.11). As described previously for the univentricular heart, subsequent reconstructive management of HLHS includes an interim hemi-Fontan procedure or bidirectional Glenn anastomosis at 4 to 6 months of age, followed by a Fontan procedure at about 18 to 24 months.

Universally fatal only two decades ago, tremendous strides have been made in improving the outcomes for patients with HLHS. Of the three stages, the highest risk stage of the repair remains the Norwood operation. During the 1990s, the hospital survival for the Norwood procedure across the United States was approximately 40%.[135] Currently, select centers have reported hospital survivals of 90% or greater.[136–139] Reported survivals for the hemi-Fontan and Fontan procedures have also been excellent at 98% for both operations.[130,140]

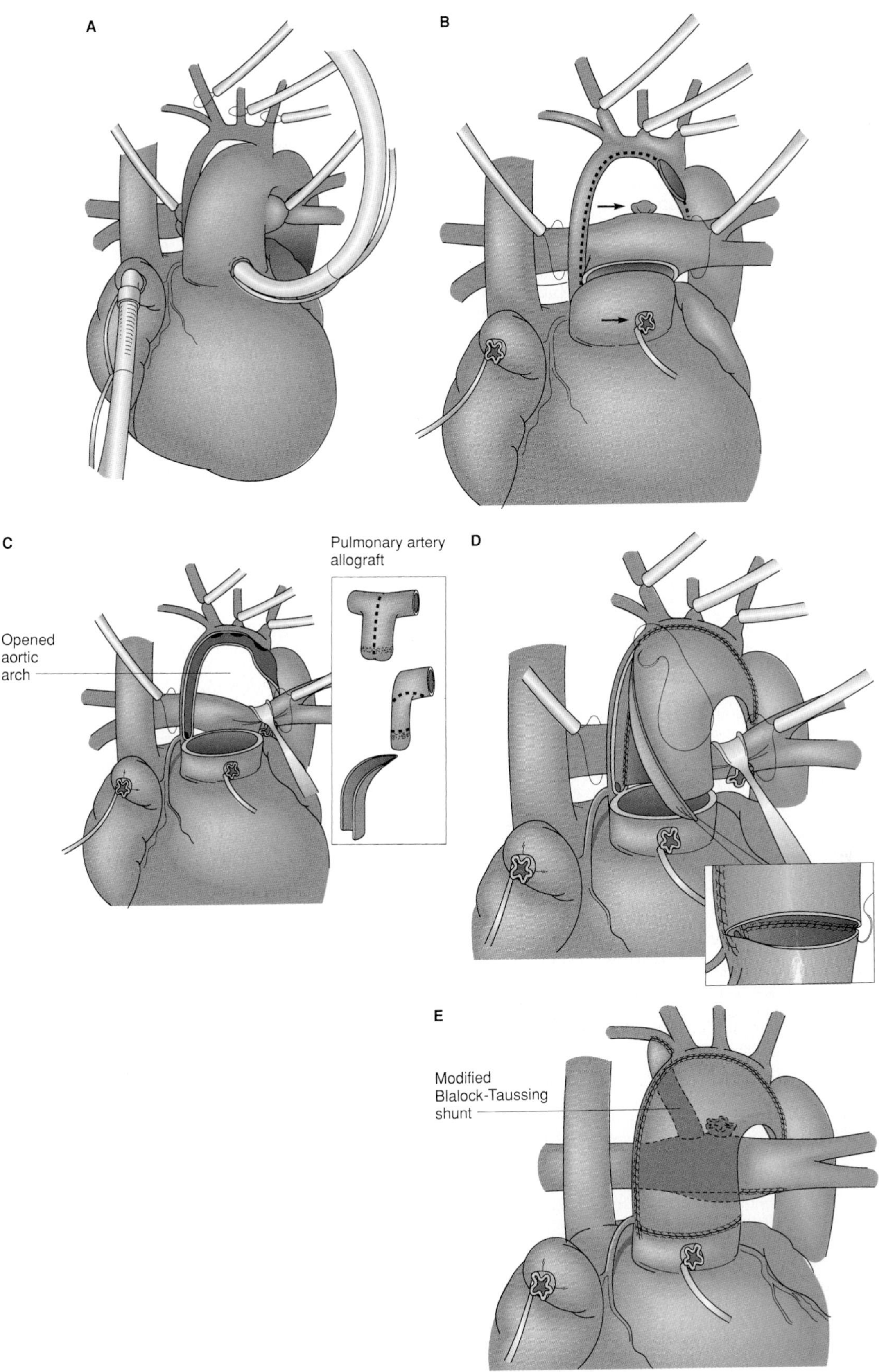

FIGURE 83.11 Steps in the Norwood procedure for hypoplastic left-heart syndrome. (*A*) Cannulation for bypass. (*B*) Division of pulmonary artery and ductus arteriosus. (*C*) Aortic arch opened from the origin to beyond the ductus. (*D*) Pulmonary allograft used to enlarge arch and connect to ventricle. (*E*) Completed repair.

KEY POINTS

- Much of the original interest was focused on attempts to treat congenital heart defects associated with cyanosis and early mortality. The first successful treatment of a congenital lesion was the closure of a patent ductus arteriosus by Gross and Hubbard in 1938.
- An atrial septal defect (ASD) is a hole in the atrial septum. ASDs are the third most common congenital heart defect, occurring in 1 out of 1,000 live births and representing 10% of congenital heart defects.
- Ventricular septal defects (VSDs) are the most common congenital heart anomalies (with the exception of bicuspid aortic valve, which occurs in about 1.3% of the population).
- Tetralogy of Fallot (TOF) is the most common cyanotic congenital heart defect. It occurs in 0.6 per 1,000 live births and has a prevalence of about 5% among all patients with congenital heart disease. The pathologic anatomy is frequently described as having four components: ventricular septal defect, overriding aorta, pulmonary stenosis, and right ventricular hypertrophy.
- Coronary arteriovenous fistula is the most common major coronary anomaly.

References

1. **Gross R, Hubbard J. Surgical ligation of a patent ductus arteriosus. *JAMA* 1939;112:729.**
2. **Blalock A, Taussig H. The surgical treatment of malformations of the heart in which there is pulmonary stenosis or atresia. *JAMA* 1945;128:189.**
3. Lewis F, Taufic M. Closure of atrial septal defects with the aid of hypothermia: experimental accomplishments and the report of one successful case. *Surgery* 1953;33:53.
4. **Gibbon J. Application of a mechanical heart-lung apparatus to cardiac surgery. *Minn Med.* 1954;37:171.**
5. Warden E, Cohen M, Read C. Controlled cross-circulation for open intracardiac surgery: physiologic studies and results of creation and closure of ventricular septal defects. *J Thorac Surg.* 1954;28:331.
6. Kirklin J, DuShane J, Patrick R. Intracardiac surgery with the aid of a mechanical pump-oxygenator system (Gibbon type): report of eight cases. *Proc Staff Meet Mayo Clin.* 1955;30:201.
7. Hoffman JI, Kaplan S. The incidence of congenital heart disease. *J Am Coll Cardiol.* 2002;39:1890.
8. Hagen PT, Scholz DG, Edwards WD. Incidence and size of patent foramen ovale during the first 10 decades of life: an autopsy study of 965 normal hearts. *Mayo Clin Proc.* 1984;59:17.
9. Hopkins RA, Bert AA, Buchholz B, et al. Surgical patch closure of atrial septal defects. *Ann Thorac Surg.* 2004;77:2144; author reply 2149.
10. King TD, Thompson SL, Steiner C, Mills NL. Secundum atrial septal defect. Nonoperative closure during cardiac catheterization. *JAMA* 1976;235:2506.
11. O'Laughlin MP. Catheter closure of secundum atrial septal defects. *Tex Heart Inst J.* 1997;24:287.
12. Cowley CG, Lloyd TR, Bove EL, et al. Comparison of results of closure of secundum atrial septal defect by surgery versus Amplatzer septal occluder. *Am J Cardiol.* 2001;88:589.
13. Du ZD, Koenig P, Cao QL, et al. Comparison of transcatheter closure of secundum atrial septal defect using the Amplatzer septal occluder associated with deficient versus sufficient rims. *Am J Cardiol.* 2002; 90:865.
14. Murphy JG, Gersh BJ, McGoon MD, et al. Long-term outcome after surgical repair of isolated atrial septal defect. Follow-up at 27 to 32 years. *N Engl J Med.* 1990;323:1645.
15. Roos-Hesselink JW, Meijboom FJ, Spitaels SE, et al. Excellent survival and low incidence of arrhythmias, stroke and heart failure long-term after surgical ASD closure at young age. A prospective follow-up study of 21–33 years. *Eur Heart J.* 2003;24:190.
16. Gatzoulis MA, Freeman MA, Siu SC, et al. Atrial arrhythmia after surgical closure of atrial septal defects in adults. *N Engl J Med.* 1999;340:839.
17. Attie F, Rosas M, Granados N, et al. Surgical treatment for secundum atrial septal defects in patients >40 years old. A randomized clinical trial. *J Am Coll Cardiol.* 2001;38:2035.
18. Konstantinides S, Geibel A, Olschewski M, et al. A comparison of surgical and medical therapy for atrial septal defect in adults. *N Engl J Med.* 1995;333:469.
19. Heath D, Edwards JE. The pathology of hypertensive pulmonary vascular disease; a description of six grades of structural changes in the pulmonary arteries with special reference to congenital cardiac septal defects. *Circulation* 1958;18:533.
20. Momma K, Toyama K, Takao A, et al. Natural history of subarterial infundibular ventricular septal defect. *Am Heart J.* 1984;108:1312.
21. Dajani AS, Taubert KA, Wilson W, et al. Prevention of bacterial endocarditis. Recommendations by the American Heart Association. *Circulation* 1997;96:358.
22. Backer CL, Idriss FS, Zales VR, et al. Surgical management of the conal (supracristal) ventricular septal defect. *J Thorac Cardiovasc Surg.* 1991;102:288; discussion 295.
23. Hijazi ZM. Device closure of ventricular septal defects. *Catheter Cardiovasc Intervent.* 2003;60:107.
24. Mavroudis C, Backer CL, Jacobs JP. Ventricular septal defect. In: Mavroudis C, Backer CL, eds. *Pediatric cardiac surgery.* Philadelphia: Mosby; 2003.
25. McCrindle BW, Blackstone EH, Williams WG, et al. Are outcomes of surgical versus transcatheter balloon valvotomy equivalent in neonatal critical aortic stenosis? *Circulation* 2001;104:I152.
26. Cowley CG, Dietrich M, Mosca RS, et al. Balloon valvuloplasty versus transventricular dilation for neonatal critical aortic stenosis. *Am J Cardiol.* 2001;87:1125, A1110.
27. **Ross DN. Replacement of aortic and mitral valves with a pulmonary autograft. *Lancet* 1967;2:956.**
28. **Konno S, Imai Y, Iida Y, et al. A new method for prosthetic valve replacement in congenital aortic stenosis associated with hypoplasia of the aortic valve ring. *J Thorac Cardiovasc Surg.* 1975;70:909.**
29. Ohye RG, Gomez CA, Ohye BJ, et al. The Ross/Konno procedure in neonates and infants: intermediate-term survival and autograft function. *Ann Thorac Surg.* 2001;72:823.
30. Moore P, Egito E, Mowrey H, et al. Midterm results of balloon dilation of congenital aortic stenosis: predictors of success. *J Am Coll Cardiol.* 1996;27:1257.
31. Chartrand CC, Saro-Servando E, Vobecky JS. Long-term results of surgical valvuloplasty for congenital valvar aortic stenosis in children. *Ann Thorac Surg.* 1999;68:1356; discussion 1359.
32. Rayburn ST, Netherland DE, Heath BJ. Discrete membranous subaortic stenosis: improved results after resection and myectomy. *Ann Thorac Surg.* 1997;64:105.
33. Jahangiri M, Nicholson IA, del Nido PJ, et al. Surgical management of complex and tunnel-like subaortic stenosis. *Eur J Cardiothorac Surg.* 2000;17:637.
34. Chowdhury T, Reardon W. Elastin mutation and cardiac disease. *Pediatr Cardiol.* 1999;20:103.
35. McElhinney DB, Petrossian E, Tworetzky W, et al. Issues and outcomes in the management of supravalvar aortic stenosis. *Ann Thorac Surg.* 2000;69:562.
36. Stamm C, Kreutzer C, Zurakowski D, et al. Forty-one years of surgical experience with congenital supravalvular aortic stenosis. *J Thorac Cardiovasc Surg.* 1999;118:874.
37. Brown JW, Ruzmetov M, Vijay P, Turrentine MW. Surgical repair of congenital supravalvular aortic stenosis in children. *Eur J Cardiothorac Surg.* 2002;21:50.
38. Van Praagh R, Van Praagh S, Nebesar RA, et al. Tetralogy of Fallot: underdevelopment of the pulmonary infundibulum and its sequelae. *Am J Cardiol.* 1970;26:25.
39. Hirsch JC, Bove EL. Tetralogy of Fallot. In: Mavroudis C, Backer CL, eds. *Pediatric cardiac surgery.* Philadelphia: Mosby; 2003:xx.
40. de Ruijter FT, Weenink I, Hitchcock FJ, et al. Right ventricular dysfunction and pulmonary valve replacement after correction of tetralogy of Fallot. *Ann Thorac Surg.* 2002;73:1794; discussion 1800.
41. Discigil B, Dearani JA, Puga FJ, et al. Late pulmonary valve replacement after repair of tetralogy of Fallot. *J Thorac Cardiovasc Surg.* 2001; 121:344.
42. Karl TR, Sano S, Pornviliwan S, Mee RB. Tetralogy of Fallot: favorable outcome of nonneonatal transatrial, transpulmonary repair. *Ann Thorac Surg.* 1992;54:903.
43. Bacha EA, Scheule AM, Zurakowski D, et al. Long-term results after early primary repair of tetralogy of Fallot. *J Thorac Cardiovasc Surg.* 2001;122:154.
44. Kirklin J. Complete transposition of the great arteries. In: Kirklin J, ed. *Cardiac surgery.* New York: Churchill Livingston; 1993:1383–1467.
45. Fyler D. Report of the New England Regional Infant Cardiac Program. *Pediatrics* 1980;65:375.
46. Levin DL, Paul MH, Muster AJ, et al. d-Transposition of the great vessels in the neonate. A clinical diagnosis. *Arch Intern Med.* 1977;137:1421.
47. Rashkind WJ. Historical aspects of surgery for congenital heart disease. *J Thorac Cardiovasc Surg.* 1982;84:619.
48. **Liebman J. Natural history of transposition of the great arteries: anatomy and birth and death characteristics. *Circulation* 1969;40:237.**
49. Senning A. Surgical correction of transposition of the great vessels. *Surgery* 1959;45:966.
50. **Mustard W. Successful two stage correction of transposition of the great vessels. *Surgery* 1964;55:469.**
51. Jatene AD, Fontes VF, Paulista PP, et al. Successful anatomic correction of transposition of the great vessels. A preliminary report. *Arq Bras Cardiol.* 1975;28:461.

52. Haas F, Wottke M, Poppert H, Meisner H. Long-term survival and functional follow-up in patients after the arterial switch operation. *Ann Thorac Surg*. 1999;68:1692.
53. Brown JW, Park HJ, Turrentine MW. Arterial switch operation: factors impacting survival in the current era. *Ann Thorac Surg*. 2001;71:1978.
54. Losay J, Touchot A, Serraf A, et al. Late outcome after arterial switch operation for transposition of the great arteries. *Circulation* 2001; 104:I121.
55. Belli E, Serraf A, Lacour-Gayet F, et al. Biventricular repair for double-outlet right ventricle. Results and long-term follow-up. *Circulation* 1998; 98:II360; discussion II365.
56. Kirklin JW, Pacifico AD, Blackstone EH, et al. Current risks and protocols for operations for double-outlet right ventricle. Derivation from an 18 year experience. *J Thorac Cardiovasc Surg*. 1986;92:913.
57. Walters HI, Pacifico A. Double outlet ventricles. In: Mavroudis C, Backer CL, eds. *Pediatric cardiac surgery*. Philadelphia: Mosby; 2003:408–441.
58. Musumeci F, Shumway S, Lincoln C, Anderson RH. Surgical treatment for double-outlet right ventricle at the Brompton Hospital, 1973 to 1986. *J Thorac Cardiovasc Surg*. 1988;96:278.
59. Rowe R, Freedom R, Mehrizi A. *The neonate with congenital heart disease*. Philadelphia: WB Saunders; 1981.
60. Calder L, Van Praagh R, Van Praagh S, et al. Truncus arteriosus communis. Clinical, angiocardiographic, and pathologic findings in 100 patients. *Am Heart J*. 1976;92:23.
61. Tandon R, Hauck AJ, Nadas AS. Persistent truncus arteriosus. A clinical, hemodynamic, and autopsy study of nineteen cases. *Circulation* 1963;28:1050.
62. Collett R, Edwards J. Persistent truncus arteriosus: a classification according to anatomic type. *Surg Clin North Am*. 1949;29:1245.
63. Van Praagh R, Van Praagh S. The anatomy of common aorticopulmonary trunk (truncus arteriosus communis) and its embryologic implications: a study of 57 necropsy cases. *Am J Cardiol*. 1965;16:406.
64. Fuglestad SJ, Puga FJ, Danielson GK, Edwards WD. Surgical pathology of the truncal valve: a study of 12 cases. *Am J Cardiovasc Pathol*. 1988;2:39.
65. Urban AE, Sinzobahamvya N, Brecher AM, et al. Truncus arteriosus: ten-year experience with homograft repair in neonates and infants. *Ann Thorac Surg*. 1998;66:S183.
66. Lacour-Gayet F, Serraf A, Komiya T, et al. Truncus arteriosus repair: influence of techniques of right ventricular outflow tract reconstruction. *J Thorac Cardiovasc Surg*. 1996;111:849.
67. Bove EL, Lupinetti FM, Pridjian AK, et al. Results of a policy of primary repair of truncus arteriosus in the neonate. *J Thorac Cardiovasc Surg*. 1993;105:1057; discussion 1065.
68. Marcelletti C, McGoon DC, Danielson GK, et al. Early and late results of surgical repair of truncus arteriosus. *Circulation* 1977;55:636.
69. Bharati S, Kirklin JW, McAllister HA Jr, Lev M. The surgical anatomy of common atrioventricular orifice associated with tetralogy of Fallot, double outlet right ventricle and complete regular transposition. *Circulation* 1980;61:1142.
70. Nath PH, Zollikofer C, Castaneda-Zuniga W, et al. Persistent truncus arteriosis associated with interruption of the aortic arch. *Br J Radiol*. 1980;53:853.
71. Butto F, Lucas RV Jr, Edwards JE. Persistent truncus arteriosus: pathologic anatomy in 54 cases. *Pediatr Cardiol*. 1986;7:95.
72. Bharati S, McAllister HA Jr, Rosenquist GC, et al. The surgical anatomy of truncus arteriosus communis. *J Thorac Cardiovasc Surg*. 1974;67:501.
73. Shrivastava S, Edwards JE. Coronary arterial origin in persistent truncus arteriosus. *Circulation* 1977;55:551.
74. Kirklin J, Barrat-Boyes B. *Cardiac surgery*. New York: John Wiley & Sons; 1993:1179.
75. Ebert PA, Turley K, Stanger P, et al. Surgical treatment of truncus arteriosus in the first 6 months of life. *Ann Surg*. 1984;200:451.
76. Brown JW, Ruzmetov M, Okada Y, et al. Truncus arteriosus repair: outcomes, risk factors, reoperation and management. *Eur J Cardiothorac Surg*. 2001;20:221.
77. Thompson LD, McElhinney DB, Reddy M, et al. Neonatal repair of truncus arteriosus: continuing improvement in outcomes. *Ann Thorac Surg*. 2001;72:391.
78. Hanley FL, Heinemann MK, Jonas RA, et al. Repair of truncus arteriosus in the neonate. *J Thorac Cardiovasc Surg*. 1993;105:1047.
79. Rajasinghe HA, McElhinney DB, Reddy VM, et al. Long-term follow-up of truncus arteriosus repaired in infancy: a twenty-year experience. *J Thorac Cardiovasc Surg*. 1997;113:869; discussion 878.
80. Alexander RW, Griffith GC. Anomalies of the coronary arteries and their clinical significance. *Circulation* 1956;14:800.
81. Yamanaka O, Hobbs RE. Coronary artery anomalies in 126,595 patients undergoing coronary arteriography. *Cathet Cardiovasc Diagn*. 1990;21:28.
82. Dodge-Khatami A, Mavroudis C, Backer CL. Congenital Heart Surgery Nomenclature and Database Project: anomalies of the coronary arteries. *Ann Thorac Surg*. 2000;69:S270.
83. Dodge-Khatami A, Mavroudis C, Backer CL. Anomalous origin of the left coronary artery from the pulmonary artery: collective review of surgical therapy. *Ann Thorac Surg*. 2002;74:946.
84. Huddleston CB, Balzer DT, Mendeloff EN. Repair of anomalous left main coronary artery arising from the pulmonary artery in infants: long-term impact on the mitral valve. *Ann Thorac Surg*. 2001;71:1985; discussion 1988.
85. Ando M, Mee RB, Duncan BW, Drummond-Webb JJ, et al. Creation of a dual-coronary system for anomalous origin of the left coronary artery from the pulmonary artery utilizing the trapdoor flap method. *Eur J Cardiothorac Surg*. 2002;22:576.
86. Schwartz ML, Jonas RA, Colan SD. Anomalous origin of left coronary artery from pulmonary artery: recovery of left ventricular function after dual coronary repair. *J Am Coll Cardiol*. 1997;30:547.
87. Basso C, Maron BJ, Corrado D, Thiene G. Clinical profile of congenital coronary artery anomalies with origin from the wrong aortic sinus leading to sudden death in young competitive athletes. *J Am Coll Cardiol*. 2000;35:1493.
88. Frommelt PC, Frommelt MA. Congenital coronary artery anomalies. *Pediatr Clin North Am*. 2004;51:1273.
89. Siassi B, Blanco C, Cabal LA, Coran AG. Incidence and clinical features of patent ductus arteriosus in low-birthweight infants: a prospective analysis of 150 consecutively born infants. *Pediatrics* 1976;57:347.
90. Elliott RB, Starling MB, Neutze JM. Medical manipulation of the ductus arteriosus. *Lancet* 1975;1:140.
91. Campbell M. Natural history of persistent ductus arteriosus. *Br Heart J*. 1968;30:4.
92. Heymann MA, Rudolph AM, Silverman NH. Closure of the ductus arteriosus in premature infants by inhibition of prostaglandin synthesis. *N Engl J Med*. 1976;295:530.
93. Gersony WM, Peckham GJ, Ellison RC, et al. Effects of indomethacin in premature infants with patent ductus arteriosus: results of a national collaborative study. *J Pediatr*. 1983;102:895.
94. Coster DD, Gorton ME, Grooters RK, et al. Surgical closure of the patent ductus arteriosus in the neonatal intensive care unit. *Ann Thorac Surg*. 1989;48:386.
95. Taylor RL, Grover FL, Harman PK, et al. Operative closure of patent ductus arteriosus in premature infants in the neonatal intensive care unit. *Am J Surg*. 1986;152:704.
96. Burke RP, Jacobs JP, Cheng W, et al. Video-assisted thoracoscopic surgery for patent ductus arteriosus in low birth weight neonates and infants. *Pediatrics* 1999;104:227.
97. Cowley CG, Lloyd TR. Interventional cardiac catheterization advances in nonsurgical approaches to congenital heart disease. *Curr Opin Pediatr*. 1999;11:425.
98. Goyal VS, Fulwani MC, Ramakantan R, et al. Follow-up after coil closure of patent ductus arteriosus. *Am J Cardiol*. 1999;83:463, A410.
99. Patel HT, Cao QL, Rhodes J, Hijazi ZM. Long-term outcome of transcatheter coil closure of small to large patent ductus arteriosus. *Catheter Cardiovasc Intervent*. 1999;47:457.
100. Omari BO, Shapiro S, Ginzton L, et al. Closure of short, wide patent ductus arteriosus with cardiopulmonary bypass and balloon occlusion. *Ann Thorac Surg*. 1998;66:277.
101. Goncalves-Estella A, Perez-Villoria J, Gonzalez-Reoyo F, et al. Closure of a complicated ductus arteriosus through the transpulmonary route using hypothermia. Surgical considerations in one case. *J Thorac Cardiovasc Surg*. 1975;69:698.
102. Rastelli G, Kirklin JW, Titus JL. Anatomic observations on complete form of persistent common atrioventricular canal with special reference to atrioventricular valves. *Mayo Clin Proc*. 1966;41:296.
103. Draulans-Noe HA, Wenink AC, Quaegebeur J. Single papillary muscle ("parachute valve") and double-orifice left ventricle in atrioventricular septal defect convergence of chordal attachment: surgical anatomy and results of surgery. *Pediatr Cardiol*. 1990;11:29.
104. Studer M, Blackstone EH, Kirklin JW, et al. Determinants of early and late results of repair of atrioventricular septal (canal) defects. *J Thorac Cardiovasc Surg*. 1982;84:523.
105. Piccoli GP, Ho SY, Wilkinson JL, et al. Left-sided obstructive lesions in atrioventricular septal defects: an anatomic study. *J Thorac Cardiovasc Surg*. 1982;83:453.
106. Schulze-Neick I, Hartenstein P, Li J, et al. Intravenous sildenafil is a potent pulmonary vasodilator in children with congenital heart disease. *Circulation* 2003;108[Suppl 1]:II167.
107. Weintraub RG, Brawn WJ, Venables AW, Mee RB. Two-patch repair of complete atrioventricular septal defect in the first year of life. Results and sequential assessment of atrioventricular valve function. *J Thorac Cardiovasc Surg*. 1990;99:320.
108. Puga FJ. Reoperation after repair of atrioventricular canal defects. *Semin Thorac Cardiovasc Surg Pediatr Card Surg Annu*. 1998;1:123.
109. Stewart S, Alexson C, Manning J. Partial atrioventricular canal defect: the early and late results of operation. *Ann Thorac Surg*. 1987;43:527.
110. Minich LL, Tani LY, Pagotto LT, et al. Size of ventricular structures influences surgical outcome in Down syndrome infants with atrioventricular septal defect. *Am J Cardiol*. 1998;81:1062.
111. Hanley FL, Fenton KN, Jonas RA, et al. Surgical repair of complete atrioventricular canal defects in infancy. Twenty-year trends. *J Thorac Cardiovasc Surg*. 1993;106:387; discussion 394.
112. Reifenstein GH, Levine SA, Gross RE. Coarctation of the aorta. A review of 104 autopsied cases of the "adult type," 2 years of age or older. *Am Heart J*. 1947;33:146.
113. Backer CL, Mavroudis C, Zias EA, et al. Repair of coarctation with resection and extended end-to-end anastomosis. *Ann Thorac Surg*. 1998; 66:1365; discussion 1370.

114. Backer CL, Paape K, Zales VR, et al. Coarctation of the aorta. Repair with polytetrafluoroethylene patch aortoplasty. *Circulation* 1995;92:II132.
115. **del Nido PJ, Williams WG, Wilson GJ, et al. Synthetic patch angioplasty for repair of coarctation of the aorta: experience with aneurysm formation. *Circulation* 1986;74:I32.**
116. Wong CH, Watson B, Smith J, et al. The use of left heart bypass in adult and recurrent coarctation repair. *Eur J Cardiothorac Surg.* 2001;20:1199.
117. Brewer LA 3rd, Fosburg RG, Mulder GA, Verska JJ. Spinal cord complications following surgery for coarctation of the aorta. A study of 66 cases. *J Thorac Cardiovasc Surg.* 1972;64:368.
118. Seirafi PA, Warner KG, Geggel RL, et al. Repair of coarctation of the aorta during infancy minimizes the risk of late hypertension. *Ann Thorac Surg.* 1998;66:1378.
119. Tynan M, Finley JP, Fontes V, et al. Balloon angioplasty for the treatment of native coarctation: results of Valvuloplasty and Angioplasty of Congenital Anomalies Registry. *Am J Cardiol.* 1990;65:790.
120. Ovaert C, McCrindle BW, Nykanen D, et al. Balloon angioplasty of native coarctation: clinical outcomes and predictors of success. *J Am Coll Cardiol.* 2000;35:988.
121. Cooper RS, Ritter SB, Rothe WB, Chen CK, et al. Angioplasty for coarctation of the aorta: long-term results. *Circulation* 1987;75:600.
122. Hellenbrand WE, Allen HD, Golinko RJ, et al. Balloon angioplasty for aortic recoarctation: results of Valvuloplasty and Angioplasty of Congenital Anomalies Registry. *Am J Cardiol.* 1990;65:793.
123. Hijazi ZM, Fahey JT, Kleinman CS, Hellenbrand WE. Balloon angioplasty for recurrent coarctation of aorta. Immediate and long-term results. *Circulation* 1991;84:1150.
124. Yetman AT, Nykanen D, McCrindle BW, et al. Balloon angioplasty of recurrent coarctation: a 12-year review. *J Am Coll Cardiol.* 1997;30:811.
125. van Heurn LW, Wong CM, Spiegelhalter DJ, et al. Surgical treatment of aortic coarctation in infants younger than three months: 1985 to 1990. Success of extended end-to-end arch aortoplasty. *J Thorac Cardiovasc Surg.* 1994;107:74; discussion 85.
126. Presbitero P, Demarie D, Villani M, et al. Long term results (15–30 years) of surgical repair of aortic coarctation. *Br Heart J.* 1987;57:462.
127. Hawkins JA, Thorne JK, Boucek MM, et al. Early and late results in pulmonary atresia and intact ventricular septum. *J Thorac Cardiovasc Surg.* 1990;100:492.
128. **Fontan F, Fernandez G, Costa F, et al. The size of the pulmonary arteries and the results of the Fontan operation. *J Thorac Cardiovasc Surg.* 1989;98:711; discussion 719.**
129. Cetta F, Feldt RH, O'Leary PW, et al. Improved early morbidity and mortality after Fontan operation: the Mayo Clinic experience, 1987 to 1992. *J Am Coll Cardiol.* 1996;28:480.
130. Bove EL. Current status of staged reconstruction for hypoplastic left heart syndrome. *Pediatr Cardiol.* 1998;19:308.
131. Stamm C, Friehs I, Mayer JE Jr, et al. Long-term results of the lateral tunnel Fontan operation. *J Thorac Cardiovasc Surg.* 2001;121:28.
132. Bailey LL, Gundry SR, Razzouk AJ, et al. Bless the babies: one hundred fifteen late survivors of heart transplantation during the first year of life. The Loma Linda University Pediatric Heart Transplant Group. *J Thorac Cardiovasc Surg.* 1993;105:805; discussion 814.
133. Jenkins PC, Flanagan MF, Sargent JD, et al. A comparison of treatment strategies for hypoplastic left heart syndrome using decision analysis. *J Am Coll Cardiol.* 2001;38:1181.
134. **Norwood WI, Lang P, Casteneda AR, Campbell DN. Experience with operations for hypoplastic left heart syndrome. *J Thorac Cardiovasc Surg.* 1981;82:511.**
135. Gutgesell HP, Gibson J. Management of hypoplastic left heart syndrome in the 1990s. *Am J Cardiol.* 2002;89:842.
136. Azakie A, Martinez D, Sapru A, et al. Impact of right ventricle to pulmonary artery conduit on outcome of the modified Norwood procedure. *Ann Thorac Surg.* 2004;77:1727.
137. Mair R, Tulzer G, Sames E, et al. Right ventricular to pulmonary artery conduit instead of modified Blalock-Taussig shunt improves postoperative hemodynamics in newborns after the Norwood operation. *J Thorac Cardiovasc Surg.* 2003;126:1378.
138. Pizarro C, Malec E, Maher KO, et al. Right ventricle to pulmonary artery conduit improves outcome after stage I Norwood for hypoplastic left heart syndrome. *Circulation* 2003;108[Suppl 1]:II155.
139. Sano S, Ishino K, Kawada M, et al. Right ventricle-pulmonary artery shunt in first-stage palliation of hypoplastic left heart syndrome. *J Thorac Cardiovasc Surg.* 2003;126:504; discussion 509.
140. Douglas WI, Goldberg CS, Mosca RS, et al. Hemi-Fontan procedure for hypoplastic left heart syndrome: outcome and suitability for Fontan. *Ann Thorac Surg.* 1999;68:1361.

CHAPTER 84 ■ VALVULAR HEART DISEASE AND CARDIAC TUMORS

MARTINUS T. SPOOR AND STEVEN F. BOLLING

In 1953, with the introduction of the pump oxygenator by Gibbons, the first of many valvular operations was performed, but results, especially for valvular insufficiency, were often suboptimal. In 1963, the Starr-Edwards ball-valve prosthesis was introduced, and this marked the new era of valve surgery. Since then many modifications and different forms of prosthetic heart valves have been developed, and today more than 100,000 operations for valve repair or replacement are performed in the United States each year. Over the past 15 years, marked improvements in the clinical outcome of patients with valvular heart disease have been achieved. It is impossible to attribute this success to any one specific factor, but improvements in noninvasive monitoring of ventricular function, improvements in prosthetic valves, advances in reconstructive techniques, and the development of guidelines for timing of surgical intervention are all contributing factors in the improved prognosis from valvular heart disease.

All valvular heart disease places a hemodynamic burden on one or both ventricles, which may initially be tolerated as the cardiovascular system compensates for the overload. Eventually, however, hemodynamic overload leads to right or left ventricular dysfunction and congestive heart failure and ultimately may result in death.

VALVULAR ANATOMY

Proper valve function is one of the most critical elements that determine efficient cardiac function. The aortic valve mechanism may be described as passive, whereas the mitral valve has an active component consisting of papillary muscle contraction, which facilitates leaflet alignment. The aortic valve shares important anatomic relations to the mitral valve, the interventricular septum and the conduction system (Fig. 84.1).

The aortic valve comprises three leaflets. The leaflets are semilunar; the attachments of the leaflets to the aorta are in one plane and are crescent shaped. Although a normal aortic valve is described as having three equally sized leaflets; 50% of the population will have one leaflet that is slightly larger than the others.[1] There is no true aortic valve annulus; however, the

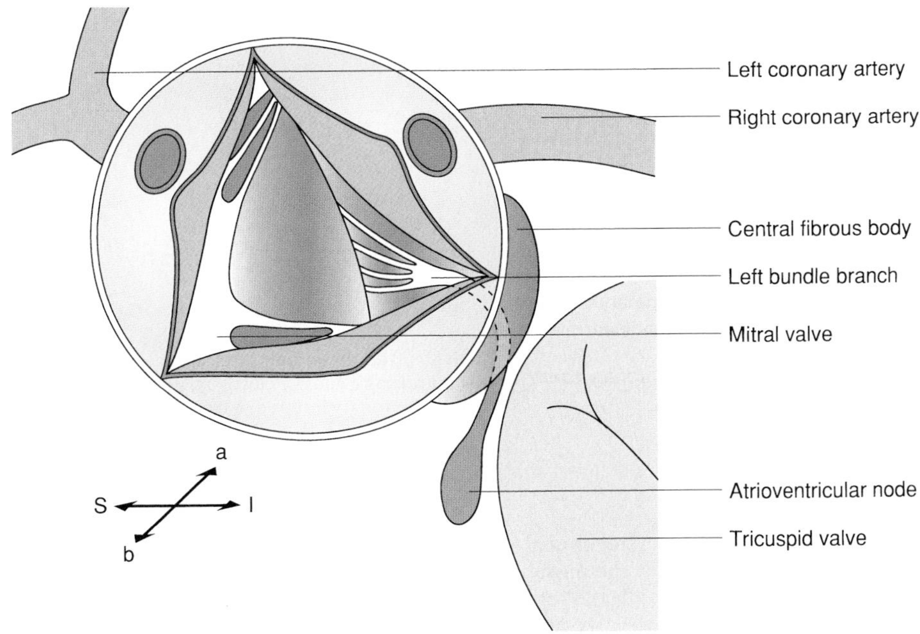

FIGURE 84.1 Schematic diagram of the anatomic relations of the aortic valve. The mitral valve is shown posterolaterally and the septum medially. (After Wilcox BR, Anderson RN. *Surgical anatomy of the heart.* New York: Raven Press, 1985.)

surgical annulus of the aortic valve is situated at the junction between the ventricular chamber and the aorta. Its location is defined by the semilunar attachments to the aortic valve leaflets.[2] The sinuses of Valsalva are defined as the areas between the aorta and the valve leaflet edge when the valve is open. The wall of the aorta in the sinuses is thinner than the distal aorta and the aortic tissue balloons out at the sinuses.[3]

The fibrous skeleton of the heart forms the posterior wall of the left ventricular outflow tract. The right fibrous trigone is continuous with the membranous portion of the septum. It forms the central fibrous body that is located at the junction between the noncoronary and right coronary leaflets, through which the atrial ventricular conduction tissue passes to the crest of the ventricular septum[2] (Fig. 84.2).

The mechanical properties of the aortic valve must allow the valve to open with minimal transvalvar gradient and to close completely with minimal flow reversal. Under normal circumstances the leaflets offer little or no obstruction to flow because the specific gravity of the leaflets is equal to that of blood.[4] The mechanism responsible for the opening and closing of the valve is passive, responding to the pressure fluctuations of the cardiac cycle and pressure differences between the left ventricle (LV) and aorta.

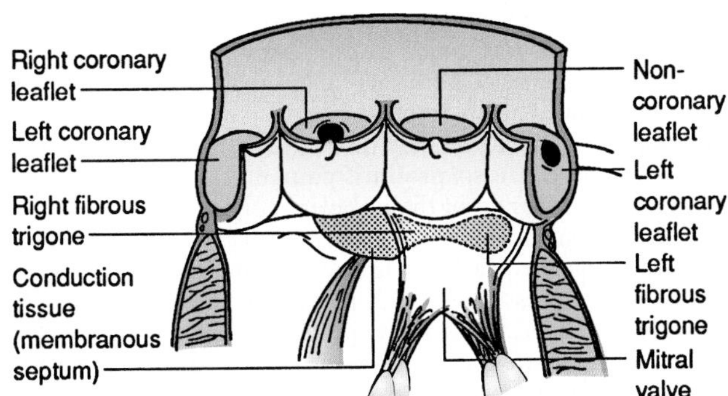

FIGURE 84.2 Schematic diagram of the relationship of the aortic valve leaflets to the structures underlying the commissures.

In contrast to the aortic valve, the mitral valve anatomy is more complex. Mitral valve competence depends on the coordinated function of its components: the leaflets, annulus, papillary muscles, chordae tendineae, and the entire LV.

The mitral valve is the "inlet" to the LV. The mitral valve consists of two leaflets, the anterior (aortic) and posterior (mural) leaflets. The two leaflets are separated at the annulus by the posteromedial and anterolateral commissures. The anterior leaflet is semicircular and spans the distance between the two commissures. It is attached to the anterolateral wall of the LV in direct continuity with the fibrous skeleton of the heart and with the left leaflet and part of the noncoronary aortic valve leaflet.[5,6] The posterior leaflet is rectangular in shape and is divided into three portions by clefts in the leaflet (Fig. 84.3).[7]

The mitral annulus represents the junction of the fibrous and muscular tissue that joins the left atrium and ventricle. The average human mitral annular cross-sectional area is 5 to 11 cm.[2,8] The annulus has two major collagenous structures: the right fibrous trigone (located at the intersection of the membranous septum, mitral and tricuspid valves, and aortic root) and the left fibrous trigone (located at the posterior junction of the mitral valve and left coronary leaflet of the aortic valve). During systole the annulus assumes an elliptical shape and is able to contract and decrease in diameter, whereas in diastole it assumes a more circular shape.[8] Annular flexibility allows for increased leaflet coaptation during systole and increased annular orifice area during diastole. The anterior aspect of the annulus, which is in continuity with the fibrous skeleton of the heart, has limited flexibility, whereas the posterior aspect of the annulus, which is not attached to any rigid surrounding structures, has more flexibility. In mitral regurgitation (MR), dilation typically occurs along the more flexible posterior aspect of the annulus.

The anterolateral and posteromedial papillary muscles arise directly from the apical and midportion of the ventricular wall and give rise to chordae tendineae that go to both leaflets.[7] The anterolateral papillary muscle receives a dual blood supply from the left anterior descending artery and from either a diagonal or marginal branch of the circumflex artery. In contrast, the posteromedial papillary muscle has a

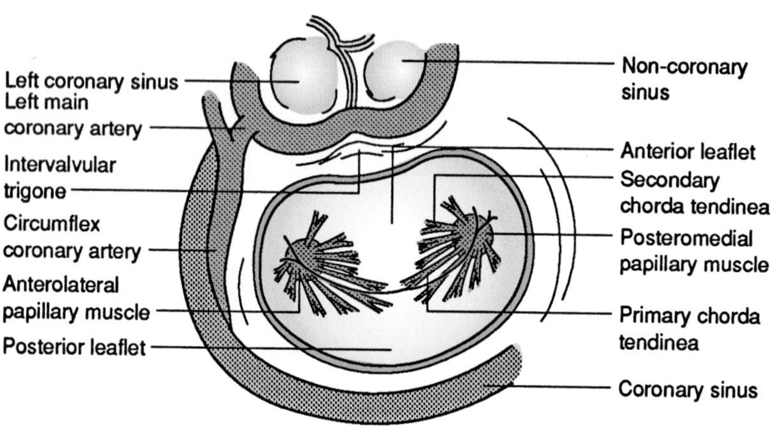

FIGURE 84.3 Important surgical anatomic features of the mitral valve and the closely related aortic valve, circumflex coronary artery, and coronary sinus.

singular blood supply, either from the right coronary or the circumflex artery, and is therefore more susceptible to ischemia and infarction.[9,10] The posterior aspect of the LV wall and the papillary muscles together play a very important role in valvular competence and leaflet coaptation. The dynamics of both papillary muscles closely mimic the dynamics of the LV, and during LV contraction the leaflets are pulled downward and together. The LV wall geometry and mechanics play a more significant role in valve competence than the papillary muscles alone. Dilatation of the LV may alter the alignment and tension on the papillary muscles and therefore may contribute to valvular incompetence.

The chordae tendineae are made up of fibrous connective tissue and attach the leaflets to either the papillary muscles or the LV wall directly. The chordae are divided into three groups. The primary chordae attach directly to the free edge of the leaflet and ensure that the leaflets coapt without prolapse or flail. The secondary chordae are more prominent on the anterior leaflet, attach to the leaflet along the line of coaptation, and are important in maintenance of ventricular function. Tertiary chordae are present only on the posterior leaflet and attach directly to the ventricular wall or to the trabeculae carnae. In addition, there are commissural chordae, which arise directly from either of the papillary muscles and attach to both leaflets.[11]

Maintenance of the chordal, annular, and subvalvar continuity and mitral geometric relationships is important in the preservation of overall ventricular function and may be even more important in patients with compromised function. Secondary MR is observed in patients with either idiopathic or ischemic cardiomyopathy and can be caused by many factors. In patients with nonischemic dilated cardiomyopathy, in the absence of intrinsic mitral valve disease MR is the result of a progressive dilation of the annular-ventricular apparatus with altered ventricular geometry and subsequent loss of leaflet coaptation.[12] In patients with ischemic cardiomyopathy, the mechanisms that contribute to MR are more complex. They may include a combination of both dilation of the annular-ventricular apparatus and LV wall/papillary muscle dysfunction, again with the net result being failure of leaflet coaptation secondary to altered left ventricular geometry.[12] It is important to remember that secondary MR related to primary LV cardiomyopathy is a ventricular-based disease that requires specialized valvular surgical techniques. A large leaflet area is required for coaptation because the mitral leaflet area is two time times greater than the area of the mitral orifice. As more leaflet tissue is used for coverage of the enlarging orifice, a critical reduction in tissue available for coaptation is reached, such that leaflet coaptation becomes ineffective, and a central regurgitant jet of functional or secondary insufficiency develops.[12] Therefore, the most significant determinant of mitral valve coaptation, leaflet orifice area, and MR are the dimensions of the mitral valve annulus. The LV dimension is less important in functional MR, because chordal and papillary muscle length is not significantly altered in individuals with idiopathic cardiomyopathy with or without MR.

DIAGNOSIS

The initial assessment of patients with valvular heart disease depends on a careful history and physical examination, which will reveal information regarding the type of valvular disease. It also provides an estimate of the severity, duration, and prognosis of the dysfunction. This is then supplemented by data obtained from the chest radiograph, 12-lead electrocardiogram, echocardiogram, and the cardiac catheterization. Many now advocate surgical intervention without catheterization, providing the patient does not have any risk factors for coronary artery disease, as the reliability of noninvasive procedures improves.

Physical Examination

Cardiac examination includes inspection, observation, palpation, and auscultation, with provocative maneuvers as appropriate. Examination of the peripheral arterial pulses, inspection of the jugular venous pattern, and a thorough search for systemic findings such as edema, ascites, or jaundice must be conducted.

The classic midsystolic murmur of aortic stenosis (AS) is produced by the turbulent, high-velocity flow across the narrowed aortic valve. This murmur is heard best at the base of the heart and usually radiates to both carotid arteries. A sustained, forceful, nondisplaced apical impulse may be palpable, produced by prolonged ventricular ejection through the stenotic valve. High-grade lesions can also produce palpable vibrations (thrills) owing to transmission of the turbulent aortic flow.

Aortic insufficiency (AI) characteristically produces a hyperdynamic circulation with marked increases in systemic arterial pulse pressure. A high-pitched, decrescendo diastolic murmur that is best heard in expiration at the left sternal border is characteristic for AI. Acute AI may produce only a short diastolic murmur because rapid equalization of aortic and ventricular diastolic pressures limits the amount of regurgitant flow. Additionally, peripheral signs of low cardiac output, such as cold, vasoconstricted extremities, can be produced.

MR, like AI, produces a hyperdynamic circulation. Unlike AI, the peripheral findings of MR are otherwise unremarkable. The cardiac auscultatory findings of MR include a widely split S_2 resulting from early aortic valve closure. The holosystolic murmur of MR is a constant, blowing murmur heard best at the apex and usually radiating to the axilla. A diastolic murmur caused by diastolic reflow across the mitral valve can also be present. The mid to late systolic click murmur of mitral valve prolapse is more variable than the murmur of MR.

Mitral stenosis (MS) produces few peripheral signs on physical examination but many cardiac findings. Abrupt tensing of the fibrotic mitral valve produces the opening snap. Both the opening snap and the first heart sound are decreased as the valve becomes increasingly calcified and immobile. Presystolic accentuation is caused by the increased flow associated with atrial contraction and is therefore usually lost with the onset of atrial fibrillation. Rales are associated with the onset of pulmonary congestion.

Tricuspid regurgitation (TR) can be associated with a pulsatile liver, ascites, edema, right ventricular heave, and jugular venous distention. The pansystolic murmur of TR is localized more to the left lower sternal border.

Electrocardiogram

The 12-lead electrocardiogram is useful in assessing rhythm disturbances and specific chamber enlargement that can be associated with valvular disease. More often, the data obtained are nonspecific indicators of overall cardiac function. Increased QRS voltage associated with LV hypertrophy is a common finding associated with valvular heart disease. Atrial ectopic activity and atrial fibrillation are also common findings.

Imaging Techniques

Chest Radiograph

The routine posteroanterior and lateral chest radiographs provide relatively nonspecific information about cardiac chamber enlargement and pulmonary congestion that may be useful in assessing the physiologic impact of valvular heart disease. The ready availability and low expense of the chest radiograph make it a useful means of observing the patient with valvular heart disease, despite the introduction of more precise means of cardiac imaging such as echocardiography.

Echocardiography

The practice of echocardiography rests on the principle that air, blood, and tissue reflect sound waves with different efficiency based on different impedances. The echo transducer transmits sound waves and receives reflected signals from the targeted structure. These reflected signals are then used to construct an image of the structure being scanned.

Cardiac echocardiography has revolutionized the diagnosis of valvular heart disease. M-mode and two-dimensional (2D) echocardiography allow real-time assessment of chamber size, wall thickness, and valve appearance and motion. Doppler echo with color Doppler overlay on the 2D image provides bedside physiologic data regarding blood flow across stenotic or regurgitant valves. Transesophageal echocardiography allows for even more accurate evaluation of valvular morphology.

Doppler echocardiography uses basic Doppler principles to measure the velocity of red blood cells in a targeted area. The two most commonly used formats are continuous-wave Doppler and gated, or pulsed, Doppler. Continuous-wave Doppler samples all sound waves returned along the course of the transducer beam. Instantaneous mean velocity and direction of blood flow are determined from the frequency shift of the returning signal. Pulsed Doppler samples blood velocity at a specific point along the beam course, known as the sample volume. A disadvantage of continuous-wave Doppler is that it lacks the ability to indicate where along the Doppler path the blood velocity is being reported. The chief disadvantage of pulsed Doppler is a phenomenon known as aliasing, which makes it difficult to accurately measure high-speed blood velocities. Continuous-wave Doppler is therefore most useful for measuring high-speed blood flow, such as that found in aortic stenosis; pulsed Doppler is used to assess flow at a specific point. Modification of the Bernoulli principle, which relates velocity change to pressure drop across points of fixed resistance, allows quantification of pressure gradients across a stenotic valve orifice. Accurate correlation with subsequent catheterization data has been demonstrated. The assessment of regurgitant flow is less accurate. Qualitative determination of the severity of regurgitant flow can be made with pulsed Doppler by measuring how far the high-flow jet extends from the incompetent valve. Doppler techniques are especially applicable for the assessment of tricuspid regurgitation because of the technical limitations of other studies.

Cardiac Catheterization

Cardiac catheterization may be used to obtain a wide range of intracardiac and great vessel pressures and hemodynamic parameters (Table 84.1). Access to the left side of the heart can be obtained by way of percutaneous introduction of catheters through either the femoral or brachial arteries. Right-sided access can be made via the femoral or jugular veins. About 5% of severely stenotic aortic valves cannot be crossed with this retrograde approach. In these instances, a catheter can be passed from the venous circulation across the atrial septum to the left side of the heart. This technique is also useful in the presence of severe MR, when pulmonary capillary wedge pressure does not adequately estimate left ventricular end-diastolic pressure (LVEDP), and in the presence of a tilting-disc aortic valve prosthesis.

TABLE 84.1

NORMAL CARDIAC HEMODYNAMIC PRESSURES AND VALUES

	Systolic	End diastolic	Mean
Pressure (mm Hg)			
Right atrium			0–8
Right ventricle	15–30	0–8	
Pulmonary artery	15–0	3–12	9–16
Pulmonary artery wedge/left atrium			
Left ventricle	100–140	3–12	
Aorta	100–140	60–90	70–105
Cardiac output index (L/min/m^2)		2.6–4.2	
Resistance (dynes s/cm^2)			
Pulmonary		20–130	
Systemic		700–1600	

Modified from Grossman W. Barry WH. Cardiac catheterization. In: Braunwald E, ed. *Heart disease: a textbook of cardiovascular medicine.* Philadelphia: WB Saunders, 1988, 287.

Regurgitant lesions are graded qualitatively on a 1+ to 4+ scale based on contrast injections made upstream from the lesion in question; for example, an aortic root injection is used to assess aortic insufficiency (AI). Regurgitation of scale 1 + corresponds to a regurgitant fraction of about 20%, 2 + about 20% to 40%, 3 + between 40% and 60%, and 4 + greater than 60%. Fractions exceeding 30% to 40% (2+ or greater) are considered hemodynamically significant. The most troublesome lesion in this regard is TR, because no direct access to the right ventricle is technically feasible except across the valve itself. Artifactual TR can be caused by the catheter crossing the valve or by ventricular ectopic activity induced by right ventricular injections.

Radionuclide Angiography

Radionuclide angiography yields visual and numeric data regarding cardiac function and valvular disease. Combined with ^{99m}technetium, it is useful in measuring forward flow in patients with regurgitation. Serial determination of ventricular function with radionuclide cineangiography is now a mainstay in the long-term follow-up of many valvular heart disease patients.

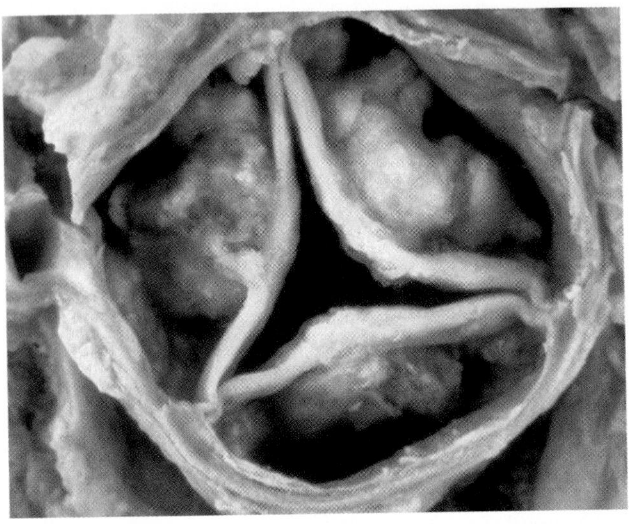

FIGURE 84.4 Calcific aortic stenosis. Large deposits of calcium salts are evident in the cusps and the free margins of the thickened aortic valve, as viewed from above. (From Rubin E, Farber JL. *Pathology*, 3rd ed. Philadelphia: Lippincott Williams & Wilkins, 1999.)

AORTIC STENOSIS

In the adult population of the United States the most common cause of aortic stenosis (AS) is thickening (degeneration) and deposition of calcium within the aortic leaflets (Table 84.2).[13,14] The overall impact of a lifetime of leaflet stress with each cardiac contraction causes shearing forces that may produce small deposits of calcium within the leaflets (Fig. 84.4). This normal aging process can be accelerated by rheumatic heart disease. Aortic stenosis occurs more frequently in the presence of a congenitally bicuspid aortic valve, and in these instances leaflet calcification can occur as early as age 20 to 30 years and may become symptomatic between the ages of 30 and 60 years. When the disease is acquired in a previously normal tricuspid valve, stenosis typically occurs in the sixth to eighth decades of life. Despite the etiology of the AS, the pathophysiologic consequences are the same.

AS may be defined as a point of resistance between the left ventricular cavity and the aorta that prevents proper ejection of blood. The normal aortic valve orifice is approximately 3.0 to 4.0 cm^2. For any significant changes in the circulation to occur, the valve area must be reduced to one fourth its normal size. The aortic valve becomes a point of fixed resistance in the left ventricular outflow tract at the smaller orifice area. Hemodynamic data have been used to grade the degrees of AS as mild (>1.5 cm^2), moderate (1.0 to 1.5 cm^2), or severe (≤1.0 cm^2).[15] When AS is severe and cardiac output is normal, the mean transvalvar gradient generally exceeds 50 mm Hg and this is a rough cut-off for operative intervention. Some patients with severe AS may remain asymptomatic, whereas others with only moderate AS may develop symptoms. Therapeutic decisions, particularly those related to surgical intervention, are based largely on the presence or absence of symptoms, and not on the absolute valve area or transvalvar gradient.[15] A decrease in the effective orifice area yields a progressive obstruction of flow from the LV. Disturbance of the normal flow pattern through the outflow tract can contribute to further deterioration of valvular mechanical efficiency. In addition, ventricular adaptations to the increased resistance occur and can lead to ventricular hypertrophy or dysfunction.

Because of the increased resistance created by the stenotic valve, the pressure is greater in the LV than in the aorta and can cause structural changes over time within the ventricle. Left ventricular hypertrophy is the principal pathophysiologic consequence of AS, and this results in the development of a stiff LV because of the increase in wall thickness. This is the normal adaptive response to the increased work demand imposed by the valvar stenosis. Over time, the hypertrophy affects both systolic and diastolic function and can be detrimental.[16,17] Left ventricular systolic pressures increase with the increasing level of stenosis, and an adequate cardiac output and normal systemic pressures are maintained until late in the course of AS. Left ventricular systolic pressures as high as 300 mm Hg can develop, and hypertrophic hearts can weigh as much as 500 to 700 g. These alterations eventually lead to a decrease in ventricular compliance, increased left ventricular end-diastolic pressure, and pulmonary congestion. Diastolic

TABLE 84.2 ETIOLOGY

CAUSES OF LEFT VENTRICULAR OUTFLOW TRACT OBSTRUCTION

Valvular (Aortic Stenosis)
- Acquired
  - Rheumatic disease
  - Degenerative (fibrocalcific) disease
    - Tricuspid valve
    - Congenital bicuspid valve
  - Infective endocarditis
  - Other
- Congenital
  - Tricuspid valve with commissural fusion
  - Unicuspid unicommissural valve
  - Hypoplastic annulus

Supravalvular
- Membranous
- Hourglass
- Hypoplastic

Subvalvular
- Hypertrophic cardiomyopathy
- Discrete (membranous) subaortic stenosis
- Tunnel subaortic stenosis

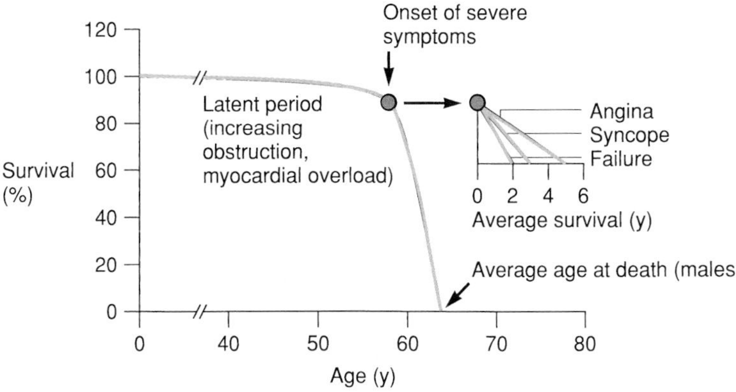

FIGURE 84.5 Natural history of aortic stenosis without surgical intervention.

dysfunction is one of the major causes of congestive heart failure and can occur in 15% to 40% of cases. In AS, diastolic dysfunction may precede systolic dysfunction. The ventricular function in these patients ultimately is characterized by an afterload mismatch between the ventricle and the systemic circulation, which contributes to the development of congestive heart failure. Relief of the obstructive process may reverse these adverse ventricular adaptations.[18]

The pressure difference that occurs across the aortic valve can be used to determine the degree of valvular stenosis. Echocardiography with Doppler examination of the aortic valve provides an accurate assessment of the transvalvar gradient and the area of the aortic valve. The product of the cross-sectional area and bloodstream velocity is flow, and as the bloodstream reaches a point of narrowing the velocity must increase for flow to remain constant. The increase in velocity can then be detected by the Doppler technique and be translated into a pressure gradient. The measured velocity can also be used in the continuity equation (based on the Bernoulli equation) to estimate aortic valve area. Echocardiographic assessment is also useful in determining the extent of left ventricular hypertrophy (LV mass) and in estimating left ventricular ejection fraction (EF). The severity of AS can be measured accurately with noninvasive studies; because many of the patients with AS are elderly and are at risk for coronary disease, however, cardiac catheterization with coronary angiography is usually performed prior to valve replacement. From catheterization data, two techniques are used to assess the severity of AS; one measures pressure on both sides of the aortic valve and the second uses a pullback catheter to measure left ventricular pressure and a pressure measurement above the aortic valve. The transvalvar pressure gradient can then be used in the Gorlin calculation of the aortic valve area. As the transvalvar gradient increases, the correlation with degree of stenosis also increases.[18]

Ejection fraction is the most commonly used index to measure left ventricular systolic function. The EF is affected by both preload and afterload and therefore may not accurately measure intrinsic ventricular contractility. Careful assessment of EF is needed to determine the severity of AS. Poor EF due to afterload mismatch must be differentiated from poor EF caused by intrinsic or end-stage myocardial disease.

The natural history of AS in the adult consists of a prolonged latent period during which the morbidity and mortality rates are low. The rate of progression of the stenotic lesion has been estimated in a number of studies, and the average rate of change is approximately 0.10 cm^2 per year. The systolic pressure gradient across the valve may increase by as much as 10 to 15 mm Hg per year.[15] Progression of AS is thought to be more rapid in patients with degenerative calcific disease than in those with congenital or rheumatic disease. During this time hypertrophy normalizes left ventricular wall stress, and ultimately symptoms will develop as the stenosis progresses. The classic symptoms of AS are angina, syncope, and congestive heart failure, and most patients with moderate to severe AS are symptomatic. Average survival after onset of angina is 4 to 5 years, after syncope 2 to 3 years, and after congestive heart failure 1 to 2 years[18,19] (Fig. 84.5). Symptomatic patients with significant uncorrected AS have 1-year and 2-year mortality rates of 25% and 50%, respectively.[20] The majority of patients with AS succumb to heart failure. The risk of sudden death due to a ventricular arrhythmia in a truly asymptomatic patient with severe AS is not well defined but appears to be approximately 1% to 2%. Aortic valve replacement for AS is clearly indicated in the symptomatic patient; however, it is not strictly indicated in the asymptomatic patient with severe AS to prevent sudden death.[15]

Angina occurs in approximately 35% to 50% of patients with AS, in the absence of coronary artery disease, and the risk of an acute MI is increased in this population. In patients with hypertrophic hearts, there is an increased myocardial oxygen demand because of the increase in muscle mass and high afterload, which ultimately lowers the threshold for ischemia. In addition, coronary perfusion occurs predominantly during diastole, and the increase in intramyocardial pressure and LVEDP both present resistance to flow and therefore reduce coronary flow reserve, therefore limiting myocardial oxygen supply.[21,22,23]

Syncope, which can occur in up to 25% of patients with symptomatic AS, is related to limitations in cardiac output and a decrease in cerebral perfusion. Syncope is usually associated with exertion and its etiology remains controversial. According to one theory, exercise induces a decrease in total peripheral resistance that goes uncompensated because the stenotic valve restricts cardiac output.[23,24] Additional studies have indicated that the initial event in a syncopal episode results from a drop in blood pressure thought to arise secondary to an arrhythmia.[18]

Symptoms of heart failure in AS may stem from circulatory or myocardial failure (systolic or diastolic dysfunction). Circulatory failure caused by decreased cardiac output can produce systemic acidosis from anaerobic metabolism. The lactic acidosis causes hyperventilation that produces symptoms of dyspnea and fatigue. Patients with AS have a fixed cardiac output, and when systemic vasodilation occurs there is a decrease in arterial pressure. Tachycardia is poorly tolerated in patients with AS because prolonged ejection times are required to maintain adequate flow through the stenotic valve. Eventually an adequate pressure gradient across the stenotic valve can no longer be maintained and left ventricular failure ensues. Death occurs in 10% to 20% of patients secondary to heart failure.

No proven medical therapy exists for AS. The only effective relief of this mechanical obstruction to blood flow is aortic valve replacement. There has been some recent interest in the role of statins for the secondary prevention of AS progression.

Although we have means to accurately determine the severity of AS, it is not the severity of the lesion that determines the optimal timing for surgical intervention; rather, it is based on the presence of symptoms in combination with the severely stenotic valve that determines the timing of intervention. Asymptomatic patients with AS should undergo a baseline 2D echocardiogram with Doppler to confirm the presence of the aortic pathology, assess the transvalvar gradient, measure the area of the aortic valve, determine left ventricular size and function as well as degree of hypertrophy, and evaluate for the presence of any additional valvular disease. In some instances the patient may need to undergo cardiac catheterization and coronary angiography if a discrepancy exists between the clinical and echocardiographic findings or if the patient is symptomatic and at risk for coronary artery disease.[15]

Exercise testing in patients with AS has been discouraged because of safety concerns and should not be used in patients who are symptomatic. The frequency of follow-up for the asymptomatic patient is determined by the severity of the stenotic lesion. Most patients with mild AS undergo annual evaluation, and if symptoms develop a prompt evaluation should be performed. Serial echocardiograms are helpful to assess changes in left ventricular hypertrophy and function or changes in valve area. Patients with severe AS should undergo at least annual evaluation. In patients with moderate AS, a serial study every 2 years is adequate, whereas in patients with mild AS serial studies can be performed every 5 years.[15]

About 75% of patients with symptomatic AS will die within 3 years after the onset of symptoms unless aortic valve replacement is performed.[25] Typically a gradient of more than 50 mm Hg or a valve area of less than 1.0 cm^2 indicates critical stenosis that is capable of causing symptoms and death. These are not absolute values; some patients with larger valve areas or smaller gradients may have symptoms that are related to the presence of the AS and should therefore undergo valve replacement. Aortic valve replacement in symptomatic patients with severe AS is indicated, and increased survival has been demonstrated in this population. Many of these patients have a depressed EF due to excess afterload, and in these patients ventricular function improves following valve replacement. Asymptomatic patients with severe AS and left ventricular dysfunction should also undergo aortic valve replacement. The relief of the obstruction will reduce the left ventricular afterload and may eventually lead to restoration of contractile function. In asymptomatic patients with mild or moderate AS the natural course may be benign, and these patients should be followed serially with noninvasive studies to assess for any progression of the stenosis or evidence of left ventricular dysfunction. A controversial group of patients with AS are those with a low EF and a low transvalvar gradient. Studies in this population have shown a high operative mortality and persistence of symptoms even after valve replacement.[26,27] The criteria for deciding which patients in this group should have aortic valve replacement are evolving. Some studies indicate that patients in this group may have favorable outcomes if both cardiac output and the gradient are increased with either inotropic stimulation or the administration of nitroprusside. Those patients who demonstrate an increase in cardiac output without an increase in transvalvar gradient, possibly indicating loss of ventricular contractile reserve, may not benefit from valve replacement.[28,29] In addition, patients with severe AS who are undergoing coronary revascularization should undergo simultaneous aortic valve replacement.

Balloon aortic valvotomy for acquired AS is now thought to be useful only for palliation of the disease. The rate of complications, including death, stroke, aortic rupture, aortic insufficiency (AI), and vascular injury, exceeds 10%. In addition, the mortality rate following this procedure is similar to that of the untreated population with AS.[30] This procedure may be useful, however, in alleviating symptoms in patients who are clearly not operative candidates because of other precluding medical conditions. Balloon valvotomy has also been used successfully as a bridge to valve replacement in very sick patients.

AORTIC INSUFFICIENCY

Aortic insufficiency (AI) results from failure of proper leaflet coaptation resulting from either an intrinsic leaflet abnormality or a distortion of the aortic root. Common causes of leaflet abnormalities that result in AI include infective endocarditis and rheumatic fever. Aortic root causes of AI include annuloaortic ectasia, Marfan syndrome, aortic dissection, collagen vascular disease, and syphilis (Table 84.3). The causes of AI can be grouped according to the structural components of the valve. Both calcific aortic valve disease and rheumatic disease may prevent an inflexible valve from closing properly or the leaflets may become destroyed in endocarditis. Enlargement of the aortic root with dilation of the commissures may cause the effective valve orifice to be greater than the surface area of the leaflets.[31] Rheumatoid diseases, degenerative diseases, collagen-vascular diseases, and loss of commissural support from an acute aortic dissection may all produce an incompetent valve and result in similar hemodynamic consequences.[32]

The inability of the valve leaflets to coapt fully provides an effective opening between the aorta and the LV during diastole that allows blood that has been ejected to flow retrograde into the left ventricular chamber. The effective stroke volume is then less than the volume ejected with each heartbeat. This state produces both a volume and pressure overload state in

TABLE 84.3 ETIOLOGY

CAUSES OF AORTIC INSUFFICIENCY

	Pathology		
Cause	Leaflet	Aortic root	Loss of commissural support
Common			
Rheumatic disease	+	−	−
Congenital disease	+	−	±
Endocarditis	+	−	±
Less Common			
Syphilis	±	+	−
Connective tissue disease (e.g., Marfan syndrome)	+	+	−
Aortic dissection	−	+	+
Uncommon			
Trauma	+	+	+
Hypertension	±	±	±
Inflammatory disease (ankylosing spondylitis, Reiters syndrome)	+	+	−

Modified from Greenberg BH. Acquired aortic valve disease. In: Greenberg BH, Murphy E, eds. *Valvular heart disease*. Littleton, MA: PSG Publishing, 1987:157.

the LV, which results in eccentric hypertrophy of the LV (left ventricular wall thickness increases in proportion to the increase in ventricular diameter) such that the radius between wall thickness and chamber radius remains normal. The volume overload is caused by regurgitant flow, and the pressure overload results from the increased volume of blood ejected.

With the increased diastolic loading of the LV and left ventricular chamber enlargement, the LV follows the law of Laplace, which states that the left ventricular wall tension will increase proportionately with the increase in left ventricular radius. The increase in wall tension produces a compensatory increase in left ventricular wall thickness to volume ratio and therefore allows a normal amount of noncontractile systolic work to be performed. The amount of subendocardial ischemia and angina in patients with AI is therefore less than that in AS.

Aortic insufficiency can yield the greatest increase in ventricular mass produced by any of the valvular lesions. The left ventricular chamber enlargement and hypertrophy allow for increased cardiac output and stroke volumes in severe AI. Total cardiac outputs (not effective cardiac output) can be as high as 20 to 30 L/min in well-compensated chronic AI. A significant part of the volume returned will return to the heart as regurgitant flow, and ejection fraction may remain normal. The diastolic retrograde blood flow into the LV can cause dramatic decreases in systemic blood pressure, and myocardial failure then progresses even before onset of severe symptoms. Limitations in the cardiac output produce symptoms of fatigue and weakness when the end-stages of the disease are reached. Cardiac failure ensues when any of the additional regurgitant volume cannot be ejected and left ventricular end-diastolic pressure rises and forward flow decreases.

Acute AI is seen in traumatic aortic injury, acute aortic dissection, and endocarditis. In acute AI the LV does not have the opportunity to adapt to the increased volume load and therefore cannot accommodate the large volume of reversed blood flow. The regurgitant volume results in a rapid rise in LVEDP and left atrial pressure, which is then transmitted back to the pulmonary circulation and produces fulminant pulmonary congestion. Overall, the hemodynamic effects of acute AI produce a low cardiac output state or cardiovascular collapse, characterized by an elevated end-diastolic ventricular pressure, tachycardia, peripheral vasoconstriction, and systemic hypotension.[21,33]

Echocardiography is indispensable in confirming the presence of both acute and chronic AI, delineating the severity of regurgitation, determining the cause of AI, estimating the degree of pulmonary hypertension, and determining whether there is equilibration of aortic and left ventricular diastolic pressures. Death from pulmonary edema, ventricular arrhythmias, electromechanical dissociation, and circulatory collapse is common in acute, severe AI. Early surgical intervention with aortic valve repair or replacement is advocated. Peripheral vasodilators (nitroprusside, dobutamine, and dopamine) can be used to augment forward flow and reduce LVEDP. They may be useful in the preoperative management of these patients.[15] Intraaortic balloon counterpulsation is contraindicated in this setting because of the further exacerbation of AI.

Patients with chronic AI gradually accommodate to the reversal of flow through the aortic orifice. Consequently, large end-diastolic volumes are present. Despite these increases, these patients are able to maintain an adequate EF. Patients with chronic AI may remain well compensated and asymptomatic until late in their clinical course, despite the excessive volume load on the LV. Eventually deterioration in left ventricular systolic function develops. EF and cardiac output decline and end-systolic volumes increase. The mechanism for the onset of the left ventricular dysfunction is controversial and may be associated with inadequate hypertrophy with afterload mismatch or primary myocardial dysfunction. Once the symptoms of dyspnea, orthopnea, angina, presyncope, or syncope develop the average survival is only 3 to 5 years.[15,21]

Many patients with AI have angina, but angina occurs less frequently than in patients with AS. The oxygen demand in hearts with AI is very high because of large stroke volumes and slightly increased ejection pressures. Therefore, AI increases myocardial oxygen consumption, but the endocardium becomes ischemic with increased demand and decreased oxygen delivery owing to the decreased diastolic perfusion pressure.[34] In the presence of stenotic coronary arteries this effect may be even more pronounced. The use of vasodilating agents (sodium nitroprusside, hydralazine, nifedipine) has been proposed as a means to improve forward stroke volume and decrease regurgitant volume in patients with chronic severe AI. Theoretically, these afterload-reducing agents facilitate a reduction in left ventricular end-diastolic volume and wall stress, which results in preservation of left ventricular function and decreased left ventricular mass. From a practical standpoint, these agents prolong the compensated phase in asymptomatic patients who have volume overload with normal systolic function.[35]

In the evaluation of a patient with chronic AI, the echocardiogram plays an important role. Measurements of end-systolic and end-diastolic volumes, wall thickness, EF, and shortening fraction can be obtained. This information is useful in evaluating for irreversible changes in the LV. The echocardiogram is also a useful noninvasive means of following AI over time. Cardiac catheterization is used to determine the severity of insufficiency, as well as for any concomitant coronary artery disease. A calculation of the regurgitant volume can be made as well as a direct measure of left ventricular end-diastolic pressure.[15,18]

In contrast to acute AI, compensated chronic AI can be well tolerated.[36] Several studies have attempted to identify the optimal timing of aortic valve surgery for chronic AI, and from these studies a number of prognostic indicators have been identified. Asymptomatic or minimally symptomatic patients with AI should be identified early and should be followed yearly with echocardiography to assess for a deterioration in left ventricular function (EF $<40\%$), increases in the end-systolic dimension to greater than 55 mm, or decreases in fractional shortening to less than 30%, with the understanding that waiting for symptomatic decompensation may compromise postoperative outcome. Proposed operative criteria for AI suggest ventricular decompensation, increased end-systolic left ventricular diameter greater than 55 mm, fractional shortening less than 30%, ejection fraction less than 50%, and increase left ventricular end-diastolic volume[35] (Fig. 84.6). Sudden death occurred with an average mortality of less than 0.2% per year.[15,37,38] The rate of progression to symptoms or LV systolic dysfunction, or both, averaged 4.3% per year.[15] An exercise tolerance test can ensure that patients are not masking symptoms by limiting their own activity.

Patients with depressed LV function tend to develop symptoms within 2 to 3 years, with the average rate of onset of symptoms being greater than 25% per year. Patients who are symptomatic with New York Heart Association (NYHA) class 3 or 4 heart failure, angina, or syncope with normal systolic function should undergo aortic valve replacement. Patients in NYHA functional class 2, 3, or 4 with mild to moderate LV dysfunction should also undergo aortic valve replacement. Patients with NYHA class 4 failure symptoms represent a significant higher operative risk population because of the lower likelihood of recovery of systolic function following valve replacement; however, valve replacement is still a better alternative than medical management alone.[15,35] Nonoperative management of patients with severe AI and abnormal left ventricular function is associated with a 50% mortality rate at

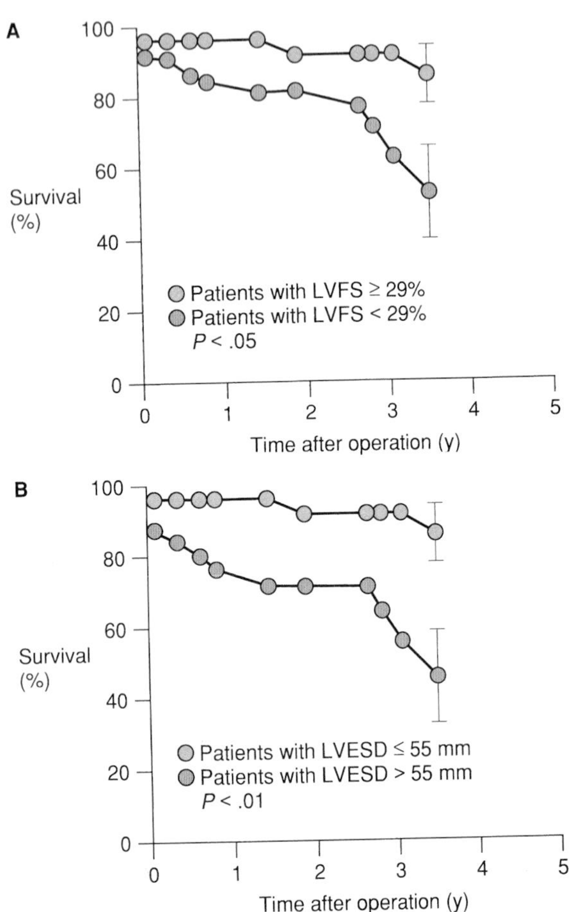

FIGURE 84.6 Survival after operation for aortic regurgitation as a function of left ventricular fractional shortening (*LVFS*; *A*) and left ventricular end-systolic diameter (*LVESD*; *B*). Both early and late survival are improved with improved LV function. (After Bonow RO, Rosing DR, Kent KM, et al. Timing of operation for chronic aortic regurgitation. Am J Cardiol. 1982;50:325.)

TABLE 84.4 — TREATMENT

MANAGEMENT OF AORTIC INSUFFICIENCY

Severity of aortic regurgitation	Symptoms	Left ventricular function	Management
Mild-moderate	No	Normal	No medical therapy
Severe	No	Normal	Vasodilator therapy
Severe	No	Depressed	Aortic valve replacement
Severe	Yes	Normal	Aortic valve replacement
Severe	Yes	Depressed	Aortic valve replacement
Severe	Severe	Severely depressed	Medical therapy followed by aortic valve replacement

TABLE 84.5 — ETIOLOGY

CAUSES OF MITRAL STENOSIS

Valvular
Rheumatic disease
Nonrheumatic disease
  Infective endocarditis
  Congenital mitral stenosis
  Single papillary muscle (parachute valve)
  Mitral annular calcification

Supravalvular
Myxoma
Left atrial thrombus
Other

1 year.[39] Ideally, valve replacement should take place well before irreversible damage to the LV occurs (Table 84.4).[15,35]

MITRAL STENOSIS

Mitral stenosis (MS) is almost exclusively the direct sequela of rheumatic heart disease and tends to affect women more frequently than men. In developed countries there has been a steady decline in the incidence of rheumatic fever, resulting in a reduced incidence of MS (Table 84.5). Nonrheumatic causes of MS include severe mitral annular and leaflet calcification, endocarditis, and congenital lesions.[40,41] Both rheumatic fever and MS remain common in third-world and developing countries. Mitral stenosis is a continuous and progressive lifelong disease, usually consisting of a slow, stable course with progressive acceleration later in life (Fig. 84.7). There is typically a long latent period between the development of rheumatic fever and the onset of symptoms. In the asymptomatic patient, survival at 10 years is 80%, with 60% of patients having no progression of symptoms. Once significant limiting symptoms occur, there is a dismal 10-year survival rate of 0 to 15%. Mortality in these patients results from heart failure (60% to 70%), systemic embolism (20% to 30%), pulmonary emboli (10%), or infection (1% to 5%).[15]

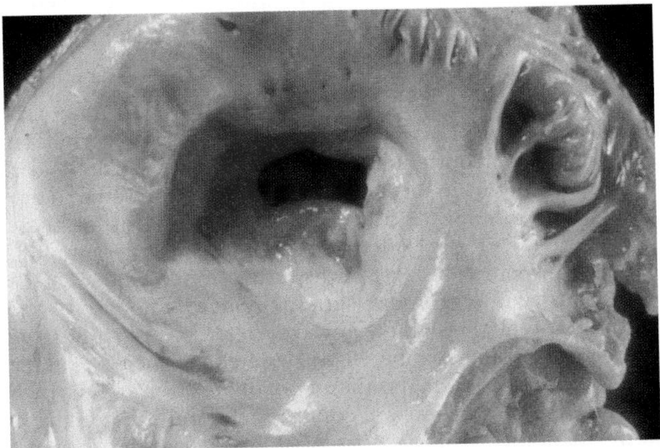

FIGURE 84.7 A view of the mitral valve from the left atrium shows rigid, thickened, and fused leaflets with a narrow orifice, creating the characteristic "fish mouth" appearance of rheumatic mitral stenosis. (From Rubin E, Farber JL. *Pathology*, 3rd ed. Philadelphia: Lippincott Williams & Wilkins, 1999.)

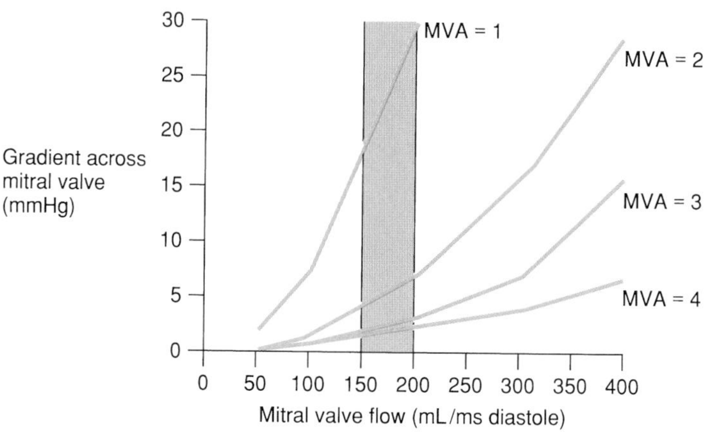

FIGURE 84.8 Mitral valve gradient as a function of mitral flow. Blue area represents normal transvalvular flow. Gradient increases exponentially with decreases in mitral valve area.

The normal adult mitral valve area is 4 to 5 cm^2. Reduction of this orifice area to less than 2.5 cm^2 represents mild MS. This is the point at which a transvalvar gradient first develops (Fig. 84.8). At an orifice area of 1 cm^2, the MS is considered critical and the transvalvar gradient required to maintain a normal resting cardiac output is 20 mm Hg. This pressure gradient is then transmitted back through the pulmonary venous network and leads to signs and symptoms of pulmonary congestion. The transvalvar gradient can be exacerbated by any increase in cardiac output and transmitral flow. Thus exercise, stress, infection, pregnancy, or atrial fibrillation with a rapid ventricular response often precipitates the first symptoms of dyspnea in patients with mild MS. Normal atrial contraction, as seen in sinus rhythm, augments diastolic filling of the ventricle by up to 30% in patients with MS. Loss of atrial augmentation of LV filling, as seen in atrial fibrillation, which develops in 30% to 40% of patients with MS,[15] results in at least a 20% decrease in cardiac output. The concomitant increase in heart rate associated with atrial fibrillation leads to further impaired filling of the left ventricle, decreased cardiac output, and increased left atrial pressure, which may result in development of acute pulmonary edema.[42,23] Aggressive rate control with digoxin, β blocking agents or calcium channel blockers is therefore warranted. An increased incidence of atrial fibrillation is correlated with increased age and left atrial dilation. The dilation of the atrium is associated with fibrosis and disorganization of the atrial fibers leading to disparate atrial conduction times. Mural thrombi and thromboembolism are serious sequelae of MS and are directly related to the presence of atrial fibrillation. The emboli can enter the cerebral circulation, coronary arteries, or renal, splanchnic, or peripheral circulation and multiple emboli can occur in up to 25% of the cases.[15,42,44] Anticoagulant therapy, therefore, is required because of the high risk of embolism in patients with chronic atrial fibrillation and mitral stenosis.

MS is the most sparing of the left-sided valvar lesions in terms of ventricular function. The pathophysiologic signs and symptoms of MS are related to the pressure buildup and stasis upstream from the point of valvar obstruction. In long-standing MS, pulmonary artery pressures can exceed systemic pressures. At pressures greater than 70 mm Hg, impedance to right heart outflow frequently results in right-sided failure, with right ventricular dilation, TR, and pulmonic insufficiency. Further decreases in left heart preload result, and a low cardiac output syndrome can develop.

Patients with MS typically have symptoms of left-sided heart failure, dyspnea on exertion, orthopnea, and paroxysmal nocturnal dyspnea. Less frequently they have hemoptysis, hoarseness, and symptoms of right-sided failure.[42] Frequently, the patient remains asymptomatic until atrial fibrillation develops or pregnancy occurs, and then dyspnea and orthopnea become more pronounced. The symptoms of MS arise from the increase in left atrial pressure and reduced cardiac output resulting from a mechanical obstruction of filling of the LV. Although the symptoms are of left-sided ventricular failure, contractility of the LV is usually normal.[45] In some instances there may be a reflexive increase in systemic vascular resistance and a decrease in EF. Right ventricular function becomes impaired, because it has to overcome the pulmonary congestion and increased resistance of the stenotic mitral valve. Right ventricular function is compromised due to two mechanisms: first by the afterload imposed on it by high left atrial pressure and second by the development of secondary pulmonary vasoconstriction.

Echocardiography is the diagnostic tool of choice for assessing the severity of MS. Use of the echocardiogram can help assess leaflet mobility and thickness, calcification, subvalvar fusion, and appearance of the commissures. In addition, the hemodynamic severity of the obstruction can be assessed with Doppler evaluation, and the valve area can be calculated.[46] The mean transmitral gradient can be measured from the continuous-wave Doppler signal across the mitral valve, and it can be used to estimate the pulmonary artery systolic pressure.

For the asymptomatic patient, in sinus rhythm, with mild MS (valve area >1.5 cm^2 and gradient <5 mm Hg) prophylaxis against endocarditis is the only medical therapy indicated. These patients will remain stable for a number of years. Yearly reevaluation and follow-up is recommended, but a yearly echocardiogram is not warranted unless a change in symptoms occurs.[15,21]

If the symptoms are mild or there is evidence that pulmonary hypertension is beginning to develop, mechanical relief of MS is indicated because further delay may worsen the prognosis.[47] Percutaneous balloon valvotomy provides good relief with prolonged benefits, unlike valvotomy in AS. Balloon valvotomy should not be used in the presence of heavy annular calcification, severe subvalvar distortion, atrial fibrillation or clot, and mild to moderate MR. In this instance open commissurotomy, valve reconstruction, or mitral valve replacement improves survival and reduces symptoms.[48,49] Some controversy still remains in the management of patients with MS who remain asymptomatic except for the presence of atrial fibrillation. Some advocate the combination of an appropriate operative intervention on the mitral valve in combination with the Cox maze procedure to ensure the maintenance of sinus rhythm postoperatively.[50,51]

MITRAL REGURGITATION

The most common causes of mitral regurgitation (MR) are infective endocarditis, myxomatous degeneration of the mitral valve (Barlow's syndrome, mitral valve prolapse), collagen vascular disease, spontaneous rupture of the chordae tendineae, rheumatic fever, ischemic disease, or secondary to cardiomyopathy (Table 84.6).

The primary pathophysiologic feature of MR is systolic unloading of the LV into the left atrium. With the onset of systole, left ventricular pressure rises and exceeds left atrial pressure long before it reaches aortic root pressure, and therefore more than half of the left ventricular volume can be ejected through the incompetent mitral valve before the aortic valve has opened. Mitral regurgitation itself leads to a cycle of continuing volume overload of the already dilated ventricle, progression of annular dilation, increased LV wall tension, increasing degrees of MR, and worsening congestive heart failure (CHF). Patients with MR refractory to medical therapy have a poor long-term survival. In a study of 28 patients with MR, cardiomyopathy, and an ejection fraction of less than 25%, the 1-year survival without transplantation was 46%.[52]

The pathophysiology of acute severe MR from chordal rupture, endocarditis, blunt chest trauma, or myocardial infarction is different from that of chronic MR. In acute MR, the acute presence of the volume overload causes an increase in end-diastolic volume and an increase in left ventricular preload. Afterload is reduced because of the presence of the new pathway for the ejection of blood into the left atrium, and therefore end-systolic volume is reduced. There is an acute increase in the EF; however, because the stroke volume is regurgitated back into the left atrium, the forward flow stroke volume and cardiac output are ultimately reduced. In addition, the left atrium is normal with a low compliance, and the acute increase in left atrial pressure can lead to pulmonary edema. In the acute setting, the hemodynamic overload often is not tolerated and mitral valve repair or replacement must be performed on an urgent basis. This is not the case in chronic and secondary MR, where the compensatory changes occur slowly and lead to gradual changes.

In MR, the regurgitant volume ejected into the left atrium is dependent on mitral orifice size, ventricular to atrial pressure gradient, and heart rate.[53] In compensated chronic MR, the regurgitant flow into the left atrium increases left atrial pressure, which leads to atrial enlargement and an increase in compliance. Left atrial pressures rise during systole and decline in diastole. At end diastole, left atrial pressure remains mildly elevated, representing a flow gradient. In this setting, with only mild elevations in left atrial pressures, increases in pulmonary vascular resistance usually do not occur. The impedance to LV emptying (afterload) is reduced and allows the ventricle to adapt to the regurgitant volume by increasing total cardiac output to maintain an adequate forward output. The increases in LV preload, wall tension, diastolic volume, and stroke volume represent ventricular adaptations to severe MR. In compensated MR the patient may remain asymptomatic even with exercise, and this phase may last for years.

The prolonged burden of the volume overload will eventually result in left ventricular dysfunction and the transition to decompensated MR. As the LV begins to fail and end-systolic volumes increase, contractile dysfunction impairs ejection and end-systolic volume increases. The increase in preload eventually leads to LV dilation and a change in the shape of the ventricle from an ellipse to a sphere. The dilated ventricle leads to further increases in the regurgitant fraction, a decrease in forward stroke volume, and subsequent pulmonary congestion. The favorable loading conditions of MR tend to maintain the EF in the low-normal range despite the presence of significant left ventricular dysfunction. Correction of MR should be timed to occur before advanced left ventricular decompensation.

TABLE 84.6 ETIOLOGY

CAUSES OF MITRAL REGURGITATION

Disorders of the Mitral Value Leaflets
Loss of contracture of valvular tissue
- Rheumatic fever
- Endocarditis
- Systemic lupus erythematosus

Congenital
- Cleft leaflet (isolated)
- Endocardial cushion defect

Connective tissue disorders
Other

Disorders of the Mitral Annulus
Calcification
Dilatation
Destruction

Disorders of the Chordae Tendineae
Rupture of the chordae tendineae
- Endocarditis
- Myocardial infarction
- Connective tissue disorder
- Other

Thickening of fusion of the chordae tendineae
Elongation of the chordae tendineae

Disorders of the Paillary Muscles
Dysfunction of rupture of papillary muscle
- Ischemia or infarction
- Endocarditis
- Inflammatory disorder

Malalignment
- Left ventricular dilatation
- Hypertrophic cardiomyopathy
- Infiltrative cardiomyopathy

Other

Modified from Silverman ME, Hurst JW. The mitral complex: clues to its afflictions. *Cardiovasc Clin North Am.* 1973;5:35.

With elimination of the regurgitant volume, the ventricle no longer has to expend an excessive amount of work on flow that is going in the reverse direction. In cases of severe myocardial dysfunction, the positive effects of the elimination of the regurgitant flow may be even more pronounced. In secondary MR, ventricular mass also increases and the degree of LV hypertrophy correlates with the amount of chamber dilation. The ratio of LV mass to LV end-diastolic volume remains normal. In the setting of decreased afterload, the EF may remain in the normal range, even in the presence of significantly impaired intrinsic LV contractility.[54] Many of the commonly used indices of cardiac pump performance are dependent on both preload and afterload and therefore are not as reliable in the setting of MR. LV end-systolic volume is a better parameter because it reflects changes in systolic ventricular function, is independent of preload, and varies directly with afterload.[55]

Various interventions can alter the size of the regurgitant orifice area. An increase in preload or afterload or a decrease in contractility will result in dilation of the LV and an increase in regurgitant orifice area. In a study of patients with severe CHF who were managed medically (with diuretics, nitrates, and afterload-reduction agents), the observed decrease in filling pressure and systemic vascular resistance led to a reduction in the MR associated with their failure. This was attributed to reduction in the regurgitant orifice area related to the decrease in LV volume and annular distension.[56] This complex relationship between mitral annular area and leaflet coaptation may explain why in myopathy performing a "valvular" repair with an undersized annuloplasty ring can help with a ventricular "muscular" problem. This, in fact, this represents a ventricular solution for a ventricular problem (Fig. 84.9).

Secondary MR also impacts on coronary flow characteristics. Coronary flow reserve is limited in patients with MR because of an increase in baseline coronary flow and flow velocity that was related to LV volume overload, hypertrophy, and preload (LV wall stress). The restriction in coronary flow reserve improved following valve reconstruction because of a reduction in the baseline coronary flow and flow velocity once the LV preload, work, and mass were reduced.[7] Based on this study, in patients with secondary MR, a restriction in the coronary flow reserve would seem probable, and an improvement in flow reserve and velocity would be expected following mitral valve repair. Ultimately mitral valve repair in this setting would lead to improvement in LV geometry.

In the setting of chronic CHF, cardiac reserve is depressed and a number of compensatory mechanisms are activated and may account for many symptoms of failure and contribute to its further progression. Some of these mechanisms are responsible for the vasoconstriction seen in heart failure and include stimulation and activation of the neuroendocrine and sympathetic nervous systems. Increases in circulating norepinephrine levels are documented in CHF. Additionally, studies have shown that proinflammatory cytokines (tumor necrosis factor (TNF)-α, IL-1, IL-2 and IL-6) may be responsible for the myocardial depression in heart failure. TNF-α has been shown to be produced by the heart under stress, has negative inotropic effects, and may play a role in the development of LV dysfunction, dilated cardiomyopathy, hypotension, and pulmonary edema, all of which can be seen in advanced CHF.[57,58]

Chronic MR is compensated by the development of eccentric cardiac hypertrophy, and cardiac enlargement becomes apparent on physical examination. Echocardiography will provide an estimation of both left atrial and ventricular volume, estimation of EF, and assessment of the severity of the regurgitation and may delineate the anatomic cause of the patient's clinical condition.

Transesophageal echocardiography is the study of choice used to delineate the anatomic cause of the MR and can help direct successful repair of the valve in addition to assessing the severity of the MR. In MR, left ventricular performance can best be gauged by assessing the diameter to which the LV can contract at end-systole. Echocardiography can measure end-systolic dimension, which is less dependent on preload than

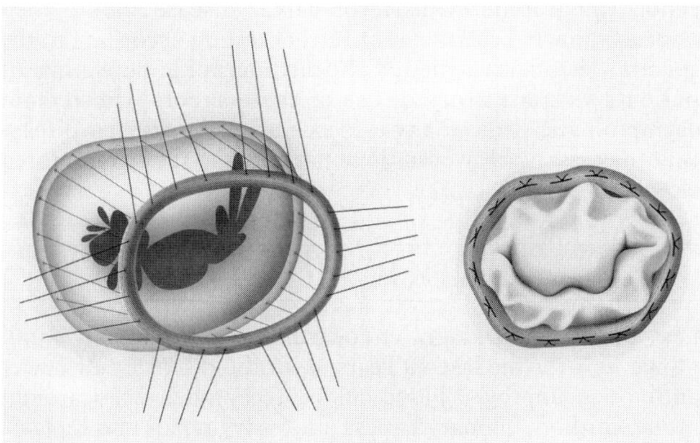

FIGURE 84.9 Mitral valve annuloplasty ring, used to overcorrect and undersize the mitral valve annulus.

EF is and can be used as a measure of left ventricular contractile function.[59] When the end-systolic dimension exceeds 45 mm, the prognosis worsens.[60] Therefore, patients should be referred for consideration of surgical intervention when mild symptoms develop or if the EF is depressed (less than 60%) or the end-systolic dimension exceeds 45 mm, even in the absence of symptoms. In patients with compromised right ventricular function, indicative of pulmonary hypertension, there is an even worse prognosis.[61]

Cardiac catheterization is necessary when a discrepancy exists between clinical and noninvasive findings. It is also performed when surgery is being planned, to assess the extent and severity of coronary artery disease before surgical intervention. Ventriculography does provide an additional method to assess left ventricular dilation and function and to gauge severity of MR. In addition, right heart catheterization should be performed if there is concern regarding pulmonary hypertension.

In asymptomatic patients with mild MR and no evidence of left ventricular enlargement or dysfunction or of pulmonary hypertension, yearly reassessment should be performed. Performance of echocardiography at that time will be based on any evidence of clinical progression of the regurgitation.[15]

Management of asymptomatic patients with moderate to severe MR is somewhat controversial. Historically, this group of patients would be followed with annual echocardiography to assess for any changes in left ventricular function, and only with the onset of left ventricular dysfunction would surgical intervention be considered. Today, with the improved techniques of mitral valve reconstruction, earlier surgical intervention, before the onset of left ventricular dysfunction, should be advocated.[15]

Patients with acute severe MR are almost always symptomatic at presentation. The initial goal in management of these patients is to decrease the amount of MR and, in turn, increase forward flow and decrease pulmonary congestion. Ventricular preload reduction with diuretics and nitrates will help with pulmonary congestion. Preload and afterload reduction with vasodilators will reduce MR by decreasing the gradient across the mitral valve. Inotropic agents can also be used to decrease the regurgitant orifice size by improving myocardial contractility. In addition, an intraaortic balloon pump can be effective as a temporizing measure before surgical intervention. No studies, however, have demonstrated that afterload reduction agents safely reduce or delay the need for surgery or improve outcomes. In patients with MR who develop symptoms with preserved left ventricular function, surgical intervention is the most appropriate therapy. In patients who develop atrial fibrillation, heart rate should be aggressively controlled with digoxin, calcium channel blocking agents or β-blocking agents, and there is an increased risk, although less than with MS, of embolism.[15]

Patients who are asymptomatic or symptomatic with evidence of left ventricular dysfunction (EF <60% or ESD >45 mm) should also undergo operative intervention. The EF, ideally, should not be allowed to fall into the low-normal range in patients with chronic MR before referral for mitral valve surgery. Even in the face of advanced left ventricular dysfunction, surgical intervention should still be performed, because symptoms are likely to improve and further deterioration of left ventricular function can be prevented.[15]

Two different operative interventions exist for MR: mitral valve repair and mitral valve replacement. It has been demonstrated in a number of studies that the preservation of the annulus-papillary muscle continuity is of paramount importance to preservation of left ventricular function.[62] Mitral valve repair has a better late outcome and lower operative mortality than mitral valve replacement, and therefore repair should be performed preferentially when feasible.[63,64,65] Even when the valve is replaced, an attempt to preserve all the chordal structures and connections should be made. Historically, with mitral valve replacement the operative mortality was high because of the destruction of the mitral valve apparatus. Preservation of the chordal and subvalvar apparatus enhances postoperative survival and helps with preservation of left ventricular function.

With improved and newly modified surgical techniques, postoperative survival after a well-timed mitral valve reconstruction approaches that of the general population. This procedure preserves the patient's native valve without a prosthesis and avoids the need for anticoagulation or the risk of valve failure late after surgery. Preservation of the mitral valve apparatus leads to better postoperative left ventricular function and survival. Mitral valve repair is technically more challenging and requires special expertise to be performed, and may on occasion fail in the long term. In general, rheumatic disease of the mitral valve and severe annular calcification are associated with less likelihood of repair.

Between 1992 and 2004 at the University of Michigan, 289 patients with an EF of 30% or less and operated on by a single surgeon received an undersized complete mitral annuloplasty ring as their MVR procedure. Of these, 170 patients had a flexible complete ring. In follow-up, 16 "flexible" patients (9.4%) required a repeat procedure for significant recurrent geometric MR and CHF (10 replacements, 3 re-repairs, 3 transplants). The average time to reoperation was 2.4 years. In contrast, 119 patients with an EF of 30% or less received an MVR using an undersized nonflexible complete ring. Only 1 "nonflexible" patient required a repeat MVR and two patients required a transplant (2.5%). The time to reoperation was 4.0 years. A significant difference in reoperation rates, for recurrent MR, occurred between the two groups ($p = 0.012$). There were no differences between groups, in terms of age, ring size used, preoperative EF, LV size, MR grade, or NYHA class.

MITRAL VALVE PROLAPSE

Mitral valve prolapse (MVP) is the most common form of valvular heart disease and occurs in 2% to 6% of the population. It often appears as a clinical entity without significant MR; however, it has become the most common cause of MR in the United States, as a result of the decline in rheumatic heart disease.[53,66] The cause of mitral valve prolapse is likely congenital with defective fibroelastic connective tissue in the leaflets, chordae, and annulus.[67] Only 5% to 10% of patients with MVP develop MR.[68] Moderate to severe MR may eventually result in LV dysfunction and development of CHF. Pulmonary hypertension may develop with the onset of right ventricular failure.

The most useful noninvasive test for defining MVP is 2D Doppler echocardiography. Leaflet redundancy is often associated with an enlarged mitral annulus and elongated chordae tendineae. Patients with MVP who remain asymptomatic should be clinically evaluated every 3 to 5 years. Serial echocardiography is not necessary and should be performed only if cardiac symptoms develop. These patients should have antibiotic prophylaxis for the prevention of infective endocarditis during procedures associated with bacteremia. Surgical intervention for MVP is reserved for patients who progress to MR or those who develop a flail leaflet secondary to a ruptured chordae. The majority of these valves are amenable to surgical repair.[15]

TRICUSPID VALVE DYSFUNCTION

Tricuspid valve dysfunction can occur with anatomically normal or abnormal valves. The most common cause of tricuspid valve regurgitation is right ventricular enlargement with secondary dilation of the tricuspid annulus. Right ventricular systolic hypertension occurs in MS, pulmonic valve stenosis, and pulmonary hypertension. Right ventricular diastolic hypertension occurs in dilated cardiomyopathy and right ventricular failure of any etiology.

Echocardiography is used to assess valve structure and motion, measuring annular size and identifying other abnormalities that might influence tricuspid valve function. Doppler imaging is able to assess the severity of TR, right ventricular systolic pressure, and the tricuspid valve diastolic gradient. In patients with severe MS and TR, relief of the MS alone will facilitate a decrease in the pulmonary artery pressure and may result in a significant decrease in the degree of TR. Patients with severe TR from any cause have poor long-term outcomes because of right ventricular dysfunction or systemic venous congestion. Annuloplasty is typically the approach to patients with severe TR. Tricuspid valve and chordal reconstruction has been performed in cases of TR caused by endocarditis and trauma. When the leaflets themselves are destroyed or grossly abnormal, valve replacement with a low-profile bioprosthetic valve is recommended.[69] There is a very high rate of thromboembolic complications with the use of mechanical valve prosthesis in the tricuspid position.[15]

VALVE DISEASE ASSOCIATED WITH ANORECTIC DRUGS

In 1997, the association between valvular heart disease and the combination of fenfluramine and phentermine was reported in 24 patients. Abnormal valve morphology and associated regurgitation were identified in both right- and left-sided heart valves. All 24 patients were symptomatic and had newly diagnosed heart murmurs; however, the frequency of valvular pathology in asymptomatic patients receiving the drug combination could not be determined.[70] The U.S. Food and Drug Administration has reported in echocardiographic prevalence surveys a 32% incidence of significant AI or MR in patients who received the combination of fenfluramine and phentermine for 6 to 24 months. In light of these data, these drugs have been withdrawn from the market.

From recent studies, it appears that the prevalence of significant valvar regurgitation is related to duration of exposure to the drugs, and patients who were exposed only for a brief period have a much lower risk of developing valvar regurgitation. The Committee on Management of Patients with Valvular Heart Disease recommends that all patients with a history of use of these agents should undergo a thorough cardiovascular physical examination. Echocardiography is reserved for patients with symptoms, heart murmurs, or other physical evidence of cardiac involvement. Patients with clinical and echocardiographic evidence of valvar disease should then undergo directed treatment or further testing according to the specific lesion identified. Echocardiographic screening of patients with a history of use of these agents who remain asymptomatic without any evidence of cardiovascular disease is not necessary. However, these patients should be monitored closely.[15]

ENDOCARDITIS

Less than 50 years ago, endocarditis was uniformly fatal. However, over the last 40 years, with the discovery of newer antibiotics, improved blood culture techniques, echocardiography, cardiopulmonary bypass, and valve repair and replacement procedures, the mortality is now between 10% and 15%. The patients' ability to survive results from technological advancements and a better understanding of the disease process by the treating physicians. The overall incidence of infective endocarditis is estimated to range from 1 to 6 per 100,000 per year.[71]

Both diseased native heart valves and prosthetic heart valves are at increased risk for the development of endocarditis; in addition, infection of normal valves can occur. Preexisting heart disease has been discovered in a significant percentage of patients with endocarditis. In one study of patients with endocarditis, 24% had rheumatic heart disease, 23% had congenital abnormalities, and 32% had normal heart valves.[72] A history of previous endocarditis has also been demonstrated to be a risk factor and was identified in 11% to 15% of patients.[73] Endocarditis affects left-sided heart valves more frequently than right-sided valves. Right-sided endocarditis is often associated with intravenous drug use, and tricuspid valve involvement was identified in 46% to 92% of patients with endocarditis associated with a history of drug abuse.[74,75] Hypertrophic cardiomyopathy and mitral valve prolapse are also associated with an increased risk of development of endocarditis.

Endocarditis of diseased heart valves can be precipitated by anything that can cause a transient bacteremia. Commonly reported portals of entry include dental infection and procedures, surgery, endoscopy, intravenous catheters, intravenous drug abuse, and infections of the skin, lungs, bowel, and urinary tract. Endocarditis of previously diseased valves tends to run an indolent, subacute course, whereas involvement of normal valves usually presents as a fulminant process. *S. aureus* and alpha-hemolytic streptococcal infections, with *Streptococcus viridans,* are the most commonly cultured organisms.[73,75,76] Alpha-hemolytic streptococcal infections are most often associated with dental procedures. Infection with *S. aureus* is associated with a shorter time interval to diagnosis, a higher morbidity, and a more virulent course. *Enterococcus* has been reported in 5% to 17% of the cases and gram-negative rod infections are rare comprising 1% to 9% of cases.[75]

Prosthetic valve endocarditis, which encompasses 15% to 30% of all cases of endocarditis, is reported to occur in 1% to 2% of all valve implants. Prosthetic valve endocarditis is associated with an overall higher mortality rate than native valve endocarditis.[75,77] Prosthetic valve endocarditis that occurs in the early postoperative period (within the first 2 months) is frequently due to staphylococcal epidermidis, either from a break in technique during the procedure or from skin contamination. Late-onset prosthetic valve endocarditis follows the profile of native valve endocarditis and is related to bacteremic seeding of the valve. Fungal infections tend to occur in patients with prosthetic valves who are immunocompromised and intravenous drug users. Culture-negative endocarditis can occur and is related to prior antibiotic treatment before blood cultures were obtained as well as in fungal infections and noninfective endocarditis, as seen in patients with systemic lupus erythematosus. The recommended antibiotic regimen in these cases is a full 6-week course of vancomycin and gentamicin.[15]

The aortic (Fig. 84.10) and mitral valves are affected with almost equal frequency, and simultaneous involvement of both valves occurs in 5% to 15% of cases.[77,78] Abscess formation is the most commonly reported perivalvar complication, occurring in 20% of cases, and is most often caused by *S. aureus.* Perivalvar involvement is most frequently reported with aortic valve infection. Other complications of endocarditis include systemic emboli, leaflet tears, chordal rupture, aortic mycotic infections, conduction defects, sinus of Valsalva aneurysms, intrapericardial rupture with pyogenic pericarditis, and valve thrombosis. Fungal vegetations, because of their bulky size, can produce valvular stenosis.

Aortic valve disease remains the most common predisposing cause of aortic valve endocarditis. The proportion of rheumatic lesions has decreased from about 40% to 10% and has been primarily replaced by sclerotic lesions. Up to 20% of cases occur in patients with a bicuspid aortic valve.[79] The aortic valve is the most common site for prosthetic valve endocarditis. In prosthetic valve endocarditis, *Staphylococcus epidermidis, S. aureus,* and gram-negative rods are most frequently responsible for the early form of infection, whereas streptococcal, staphylococcal, and gram-negative rod infections are seen more frequently in t late infections. In mitral valve endocarditis, the infection is primarily localized to the leaflet. Predisposing mitral valvular pathology includes annular calcification, chordal rupture, chordal shortening, and mitral stenosis. Extension beyond the valve into the annular tissue is common.[80]

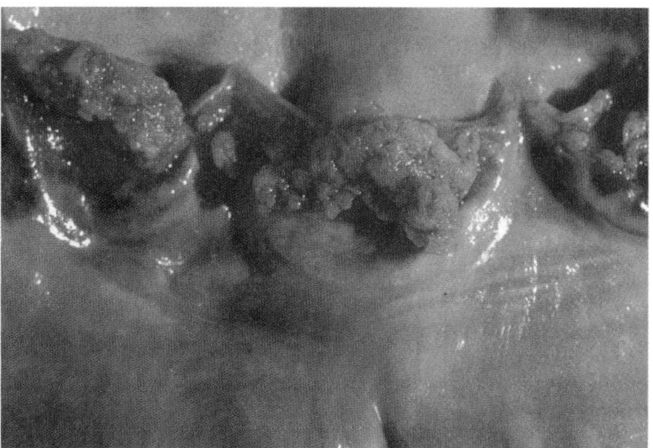

FIGURE 84.10 Bacterial endocarditis. The aortic valve of an intravenous drug abuser displays adherent vegetations. (From Rubin E, Farber JL. *Pathology,* 3rd ed. Philadelphia: Lippincott Williams & Wilkins, 1999.)

The clinical diagnosis of infective endocarditis requires a multifaceted approach. Physical examination, microbiological results, laboratory testing, and invasive and noninvasive imaging procedures all combine to aid in the diagnosis of infective endocarditis. The most common presenting symptoms for endocarditis are fever, fatigue, malaise, and dyspnea. Pyrexia, newly noted heart murmur, and microscopic hematuria are the most common clinical signs. Of all patients, 30% present with septic emboli, which produce a variety of symptoms. Left-sided emboli can involve the spleen, kidneys, cerebral vasculature, and coronary system, resulting in ischemia. Septic emboli from tricuspid valve endocarditis can produce a picture of patchy infiltrates on chest radiograph. Blood cultures are the mainstay of diagnosis and are accurate in over 90% of cases. False-negative results occur in the presence of previous antibiotic treatment, intramyocardial abscesses, and fungal infections.

Echocardiography is useful in the diagnosis of endocarditis, as well as in the detection and characterization of the hemodynamic and pathologic consequences of infection. The consequences include the presence of vegetations on the valve leaflets, valvular regurgitation, ventricular dysfunction, the presence of abscesses, aneurysm formation, leaflet perforation or destruction, fistula formation, shunts, and ruptured chordae. Echocardiographic information also plays a useful role in monitoring therapy and in defining the need for, as well as assessing the results of, surgical intervention. Transesophageal echocardiography is more accurate than transthoracic echocardiography in the detection of valvular vegetations.[81] Two different sets of clinical criteria for diagnosis of endocarditis have been established: the Von Reyn criteria (1981) and more recently the Duke criteria (1994), which take into account echocardiographic criteria for diagnosis.[82]

The mainstay of therapy for endocarditis is medical management with the appropriate antibiotic therapy. The antibiotics need to reach bactericidal levels for a period of 4 to 6 weeks. Factors associated with increased mortality and increased risk of medical failure include older patient age, infection with *S. aureus,* the presence of emboli, and the degree of heart failure at presentation.[77] Medical therapy is effective in sterilizing 35% to 65% of prosthetic valve endocarditis cases. Continued medical therapy in the face of cardiac decompensation carries a mortality rate as high as 90%. The primary cause of death in endocarditis is from congestive heart failure and AI.

Indications for surgical intervention in endocarditis include the presence of new-onset unmanageable congestive heart failure or cardiogenic shock due to surgically treatable valvular heart disease with or without the established diagnosis of endocarditis. Surgical intervention should not be delayed in the presence of acute infective endocarditis when CHF ensues. Surgical intervention is not indicated when complications (severe embolic cerebral damage) or other comorbid conditions make the prospect of recovery remote. Additional indications for surgical intervention in the hemodynamically stable patient with endocarditis include the failure of antimicrobial therapy as demonstrated by persistently positive blood cultures. Other indications for operative intervention include valvular insufficiency, perivalvar abscess formation, and pericarditis. Fungal and gram-negative rod infections are associated with a very high failure rate of medical therapy, and therefore surgical intervention is often advocated earlier.[15]

Aortic valve endocarditis has the highest rate of associated complications, and surgical intervention is most often advocated in these cases. Treatment consists of excision of the infected valve, débridement of perivalvar abscess, and valve replacement, preferably with an aortic tissue allograft. In the surgical treatment of mitral valve endocarditis, mitral valve repair, rather than replacement, has demonstrated good functional results with a low risk of recurrent disease. Valvular repair techniques include anterior and posterior leaflet resection, leaflet patching, and direct suture. Pagani et al.[83] demonstrated that reconstructive techniques including débridement of infected tissue, leafletoplasty, and implantation of a prosthetic annuloplasty ring could be performed in the setting with low operative mortality and morbidity. Tricuspid valve endocarditis has been treated with valve excision alone; however, most patients should undergo valve repair and reconstruction, because long-term survivors of tricuspid valvectomy eventually require a tricuspid valve replacement.[69]

Valve replacement in hemodynamically stable patients results in a favorable outcome in 80% to 95% of cases. A reinfection rate of 1% to 13% can be expected. David et al.[84] reported on[62] patients undergoing operative intervention for active endocarditis, with a 0% operative mortality rate for native valve endocarditis and a 12.5% mortality rate for prosthetic valve endocarditis.

PROSTHETIC HEART VALVES

The development of prosthetic heart valves has changed the care of patients with valvular heart disease. Significant progress has been made in the design and manufacturing of materials for both the mechanical and biologic tissue valves, with the ultimate goal being the production of the ideal valve prosthesis. The characteristics of the ideal valve include adequate flow characteristics or hemodynamics, durability, biocompatibility, resistance to thrombosis, ease of insertion, and silence. A number of valve substitutes are available today for clinical use, and each type of prosthesis possesses its own inherent advantages and disadvantages. The prosthetic valves available are of two primary categories: mechanical and tissue (biologic) valves. The mechanical prostheses include the caged-ball, tilting-disc, and bileaflet valves. Tissue valves include porcine (stented and stentless) and pericardial valves. In addition, allografts (tissue homografts) are available for use in both the aortic and mitral positions, and autografts (pulmonic valve) are available for use in the aortic position.

Mechanical Valve Substitutes

Despite the increasing age of patients undergoing valve replacement in the United States today and the trend toward implantation of bioprostheses in older patients, mechanical valves still predominate over bioprostheses in the United States. The first successful mechanical prosthesis clinically implanted was the Starr-Edwards Silastic ball prosthesis (Fig. 84.11), which was the gold standard for over 20 years. The performance of this valve is well documented.[85] The Starr-Edwards valve is easy to implant, but it requires a generous amount of room for insertion because of the large size of the cage and therefore is not used in patients with a small left ventricle or narrow aorta.[86] The hemodynamics of the valve are adequate; with the larger sizes, however, the transvalvar gradient with this valve is consistently higher than those of equal diameter of the bileaflet and tilting-disc varieties.[87] The thromboembolic rates with the Starr-Edwards valve have also been reported to be slightly higher than those of the bileaflet and titling-disc valves used today. Long-term experience with this valve for up to 20 years demonstrates excellent durability statistics; however, because of its higher transvalvar gradient and increased risk of thromboembolism, this valve is rarely used today.

In 1969 the Bjork-Shiley monostrut mechanical prosthesis was introduced (Fig. 84.12). This is a monoleaflet valve with a free-floating central tilting disc that is retained by a pair of struts. Hemodynamics with this valve are superior to those of the cage-ball valves,[88] especially in the smaller sizes; however, the incidence of thromboembolic complications is similar to that of the Starr-Edwards valve.[89] Valve thrombosis has occurred in a small percentage of patients, particularly with valves in the mitral position. In 1976, in an attempt to improve on the design of the valve, the original flat disc was made slightly convexoconcave. This new valve had improved hemodynamics and had virtually eliminated the incidence of thrombosis; however, a number of patients experienced the catastrophic complication of strut fracture and disc escape. This occurred more frequently with the larger-size valves and was more common with the 70-degree convexoconcave valve. This led to the recall of all convexoconcave valves from the market in 1986.[90]

The St. Jude bileaflet valve was fist implanted clinically in 1977 (Fig. 84.13). This valve has two semicircular carbon discs that open to 85 degrees with a pivot mechanism. Therefore, the need for struts is eliminated. This valve has excellent hemodynamics, because the central leaflet opening provides for a large effective orifice area. The pressure gradients across these valves are among the least associated with any of the mechanical prostheses.[91] Thromboembolic rates (2% per patient-year) are similar to those with other mechanical valves. The St. Jude valve is less prone to the development of valve thrombosis than are other titling-disc valves, and in some instances only one leaflet may be involved in the thrombotic process, which allows time for reoperation before the development of cardiovascular collapse.[92] Durability with this valve is excellent with a limited number of failures occurring at 10-year follow-up.[93] Recently, St. Jude introduced a modification of this valve, which incorporated a Silzone coating into the sewing ring of the valve. Silzone, a silver-based material, was used to decrease the incidence of endocarditis and infection. Unfortunately, preliminary results from a large prospective multicenter clinical trial demonstrate that these valves have

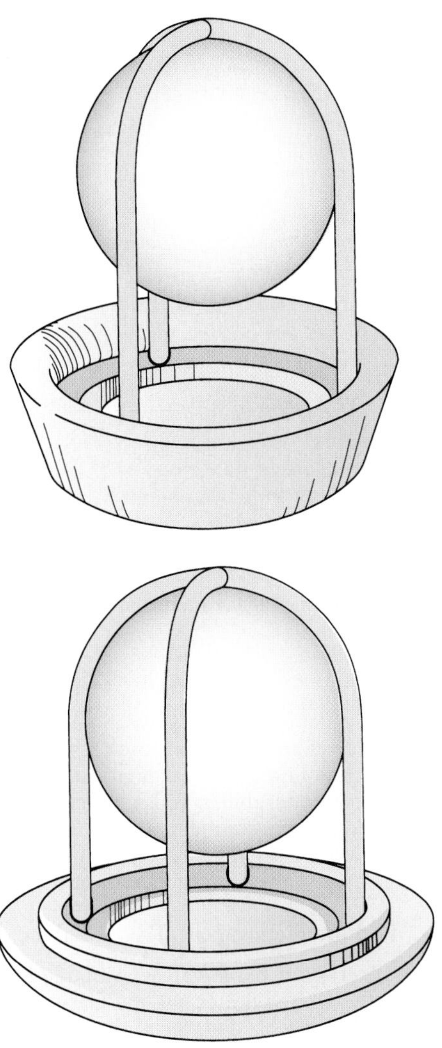

FIGURE 84.11 Starr-Edwards aortic caged-ball valve.

a higher incidence of perivalvar leak, and this has led to the voluntary removal of this valve product from the market.[94]

The CarboMedics prosthetic valve (Fig. 84.14) was first implanted in the United States in 1993. This is a bileaflet valve with two carbon-coated discs that open to 78 degrees. This valve is similar to the St. Jude valve, but it possesses a different design of the hinges and mechanism of valve closure. The incidence of thrombosis and the transvalvar gradients with this valve are slightly higher than for the St. Jude valve. The incidence of thromboembolic complications is similar to that of the St. Jude valve, and no structural problems have been reported.[95]

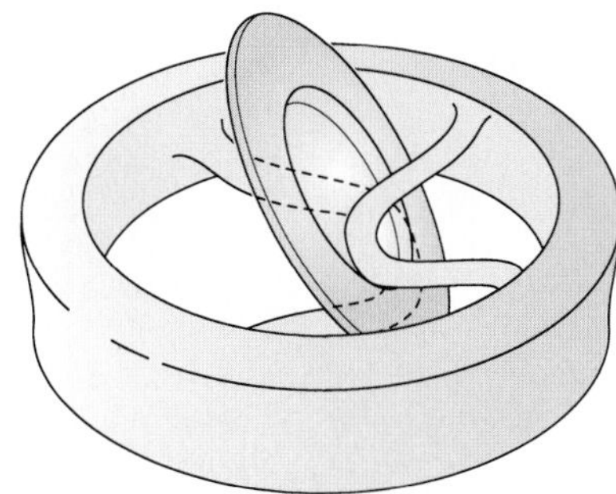

FIGURE 84.12 Bjork-Shiley tilting-disc valve.

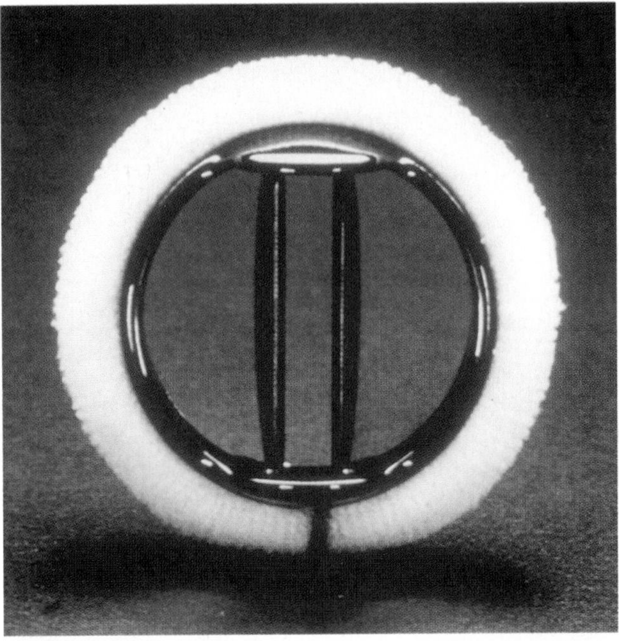

FIGURE 84.13 St. Jude bileaflet valve.

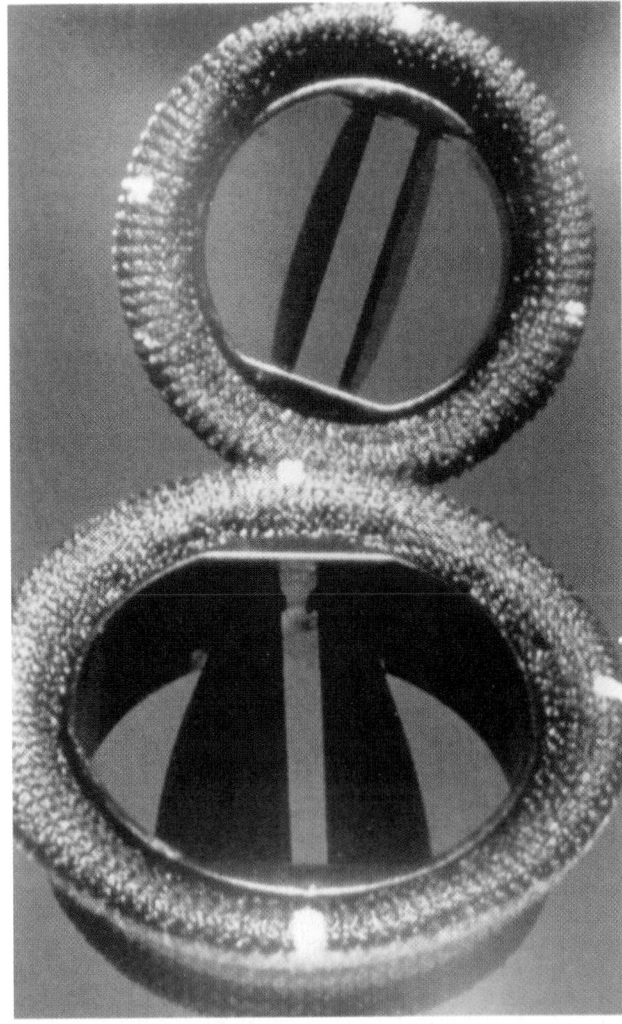

FIGURE 84.14 CarboMedics mechanical prosthesis.

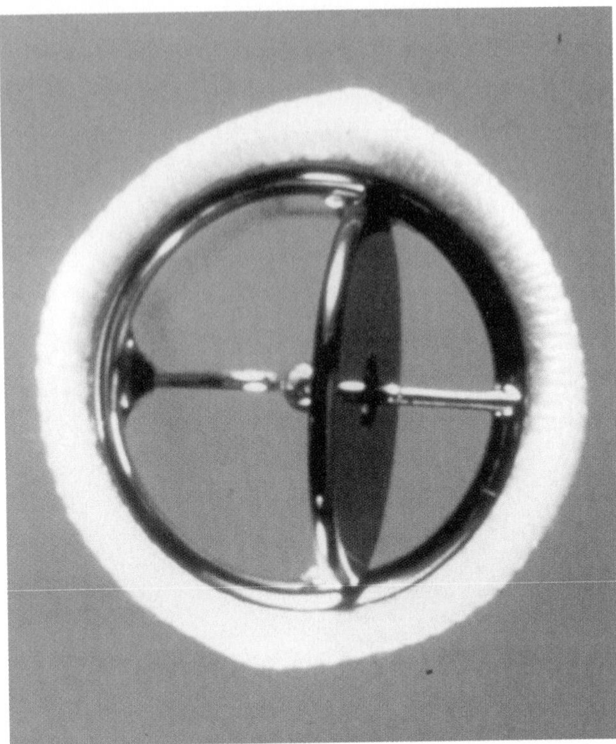

FIGURE 84.15 Medtronic-Hall mechanical prosthesis.

The Medtronic-Hall valve (Fig. 84.15) was first implanted clinically in 1977. This was a newly designed type of tilting-disc valve that uses a guiding rod through an opening in the center of the disc. The disc opens to a large angle, and therefore this valve possesses excellent flow characteristics, having hemodynamics similar to those of the St. Jude valve. Thromboembolic complication rates are similar to those of other titling-disc prostheses. There is a small incidence of thrombotic occlusion with is valve. The durability of the valve is excellent, with no structural failures reported to date.[96]

All the mechanical valves share the advantage of long-term durability; an increased risk of thromboembolism; and a risk of bleeding secondary to the need for anticoagulation.[97] Rates of thrombotic complications are low (<1%) when the patient is adequately anticoagulated. The incidence of thromboembolism in adequately anticoagulated patients with a valve in the aortic position is 0.5% to 3% per patient-year and in the mitral position is 0.5% to 5%. Anticoagulation-related bleeding remains one of the most common causes of valve-related morbidity (1% to 3% per patient-year) and mortality (0.1% to 0.5% per patient-year).[98]

Tissue Valves

A variety of different tissue valve types have been developed over the past 30 years, and most of these valves have been proved unacceptable because of the rapidity with which they degenerate and become incompetent. In 1969, Carpentier introduced the use of glutaraldehyde for tissue valve preservation.[99] Glutaraldehyde enhances the formation of collagen covalent cross-linkage bonds, increases tissue strength, renders the tissue nonviable, and reduces the tissue antigenicity. One of the newer changes in the manufacture of tissue valves is based on the finding that fixation at pressures greater than 4 mm Hg causes severe alterations in the collagen fiber geometry that lead to earlier degeneration of the valve. Some of the manufacturers of tissue valves are now using low-pressure or zero-pressure fixation techniques, and preliminary long-term viability studies indicate better durability. Today, different fixation techniques, newer mounting techniques, and the addition of agents to retard calcification mark the differences among the commercially available tissue valves for implantation.

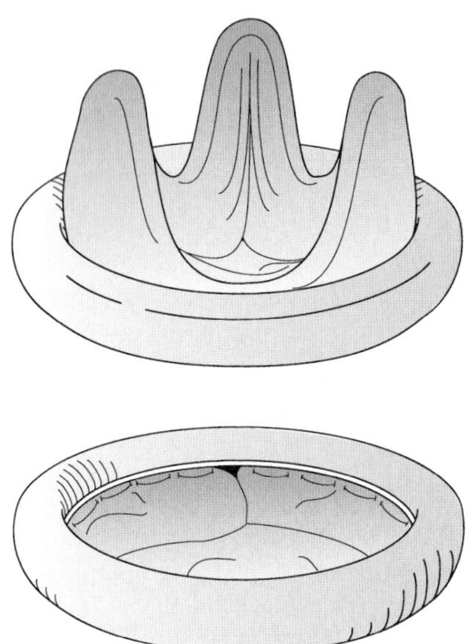

FIGURE 84.16 Carpentier-Edwards porcine bioprosthetic valve.

Porcine Heterograft Tissue Valves

The porcine heterograft tissue valves available for implantation today in the United States are the Carpentier-Edwards (Fig. 84.16) and Hancock (Fig. 84.17) valves. Both of these valves are fixed with glutaraldehyde, but they differ in strut design and construction. Porcine aortic valves are limited in their effective orifice area owing to the presence of a shelf of myocardial tissue at the base of the right coronary cusp that is inherent in all porcine valves. The Carpentier-Edwards valve in its construction attempted to overcome this additional shelf of muscle tissue by creation of an asymmetric stent. Overall,

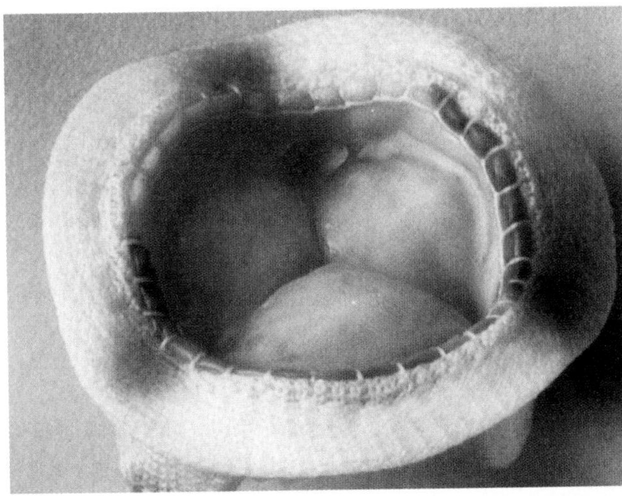

FIGURE 84.17 Hancock II porcine bioprosthesis.

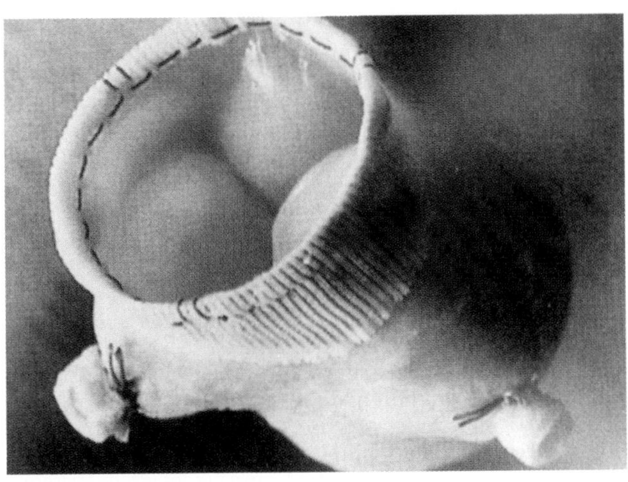

FIGURE 84.18 Medtronic Freestyle valve.

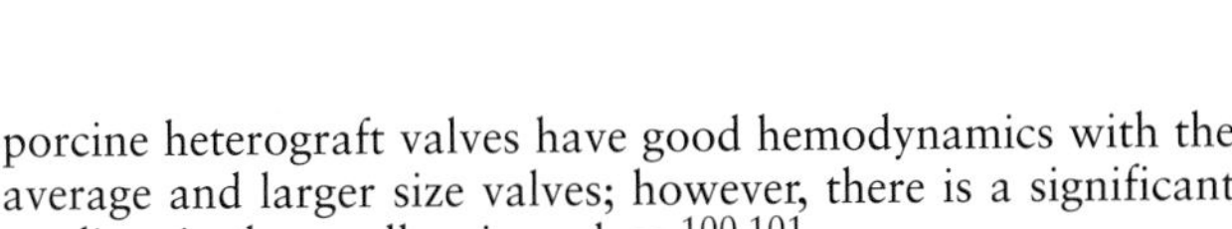

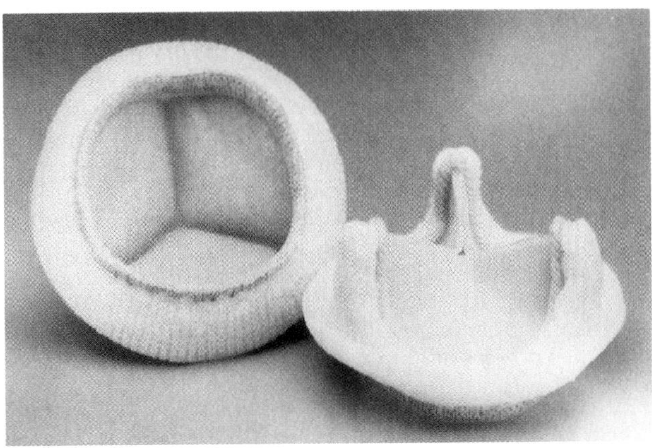

FIGURE 84.20 Carpentier-Edwards Perimont pericardial bioprosthesis.

porcine heterograft valves have good hemodynamics with the average and larger size valves; however, there is a significant gradient in the smaller size valves.[100,101]

A significant advantage of these tissue valves is the lack of need for anticoagulation. They have a very low thromboembolic complication rate; however, the risk does exist. There is an increased risk of thromboembolic complications in patients with atrial fibrillation, an enlarged left atrium, history of previous emboli, presence of a left atrial clot, or significantly reduced left ventricular function. These patients should be considered for anticoagulation therapy.[101]

The main problem with the porcine heterograft tissue valve is tissue degeneration, and the risk of valve failure increases over time. At 10 years, there is a 70% failure rate for these valves, and this rate is accelerated in younger patients.[102,103] Some of these durability issues may be improved with the new low-pressure fixation techniques now being used. With fixation of the valve leaflets at pressures greater than 4 mm Hg, alterations in the collagen were noted and may lead to early degradation of the valves.

Stentless Heterograft Valves

Stentless heterograft porcine valves are currently available for use in the aortic position (Figs. 84.18 and 84.19). One advantage of these valves is excellent hemodynamics owing to a larger effective orifice area than for stented tissue valves. There is demonstrated ability for postoperative long-term ventricular remodeling, little early calcification with good early durability results, and no need for anticoagulation. These stentless valves provide the same opportunities as allograft valves for implantation using the subcoronary technique or for complete root replacement (Medtronic Freestyle, Baxter PRIMA valve). The distinct disadvantages of these newer valves are that there is a steep learning curve for the surgeon in terms of implantation and slightly longer cross-clamp times are required for the implantation in comparison to those for the stented valves.[104]

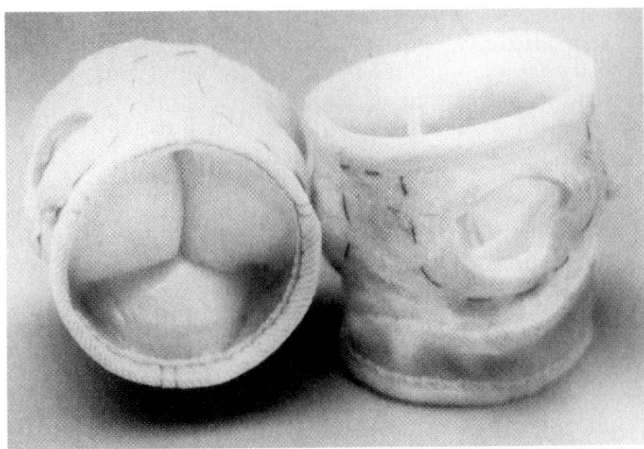

FIGURE 84.19 Baxter Prima valve.

Pericardial Bioprostheses

The original pericardial tissue valves were made of glutaraldehyde-preserved bovine pericardium, fashioned in a three-cusp valve mounted on a cloth-covered frame. These valves offer a larger effective orifice and therefore have excellent hemodynamics, especially in the smaller size valves. This feature makes these valves very attractive for use in patients with a small aortic root. In 1991 the Carpentier-Edwards pericardial bioprostheses was introduced (Fig. 84.20) commercially. This valve is fixed in glutaraldehyde at 0 pressure. This valve has better hemodynamics than the porcine heterograft valves, and long-term durability studies are still being conducted.[80]

Aortic Allografts

Aortic allografts have been used for aortic valve replacement since the 1960s. These valves are harvested and then cryopreserved with antibiotic solutions. Allografts have very low thromboembolic complication rates and are associated with a very low incidence of endocarditis, with freedom from degeneration at 10 years being 95%. Indications for allograft use include patients with contraindications for anticoagulation and a life expectancy greater than 10 years, and native or prosthetic valve endocarditis or abnormal aortic root morphology. The disadvantages of this valve are its limited availability, increased cost, and increased technical complexity of insertion.[105]

Pulmonary Valve Autograft (Ross Procedure)

In 1967, Ross introduced pulmonary autograft for aortic root reconstruction and aortic valve replacement. This procedure involves careful harvesting and transfer of the pulmonary valve and proximal pulmonary artery to the aortic position. The pulmonary valve autograft can be implanted as a free valve or as an entire root. A pulmonary allograft is then used for reconstruction of the continuity of the right ventricle and pulmonary artery. Its use today is primarily in infants and children where growth of the pulmonary autograft has been documented.[106] It is also used in selected young adults with contraindications for anticoagulation. Ross reported 339 cases, with 85% freedom from valve replacement at 20 years.[107] Performance of this procedure requires significant technical expertise.

All of the tissue valves have the advantage of a low risk of thromboembolism and usually do not require anticoagulation. They all have limited durability; at 6 to 7 years valve failure—free rates in adults are 90% to 95%; by 10 years they are approximately 70% to 80%.[101,108] Embolic rates with tissue valves range from 0.2% to 3.8% per year for aortic valves and 0.3% to 5.1% for mitral valves.[109] Failure rates increase with younger patient age.

Selection of Valve Prosthesis

Selection of the appropriate valve prosthesis is dependent on both the surgical procedure and patient factors (i.e., age, any risk for anticoagulation, and presence of infection). Once the decision is made to perform valve replacement, it is important to evaluate the valve annulus carefully and to choose the correct valve size for the patient. The overall objective with sizing of the valve is typically to use the largest valve size and design for the patient, because prosthetic valve orifices are effectively smaller than the native counterparts. The cavity size of the chamber in which the valve will be situated is also very important. In a narrow aortic root, a low-profile valve is preferred. In the mitral position, the size of the left ventricular chamber in systole should be considered because it must accommodate the prosthesis.

Among patient factors, age is a critical factor in selection of the most appropriate prosthesis for insertion. Mechanical valves, with their increased durability over tissue valves, are preferred in the younger patient. The current trend is toward the use of bioprosthetic valve in patients over age 70 years and mechanical valves in younger patients.[110] Anticoagulation is advisable for all mechanical valves in all positions, and therefore any contraindication to anticoagulation must be considered when selecting a valve prosthesis.[88,109] Psychosocial factors are also important in consideration of valve choice: patient compliance with anticoagulation or the desire of a young woman to bear children should be considered. Although many factors need to be considered in valve prosthesis selection, some general guidelines can be stated. Bioprosthetic valves are recommended for patients older than 65 to 70 years or when life expectancy is less than 10 years. Mechanical prosthetic valves are recommended for younger patients, those without contraindications to anticoagulation, and those with smaller aortic annuli.

ANTICOAGULATION

Anticoagulation in patients with native valve disease or in patients with prosthetic valves is indicated when the risk of thromboembolism associated with these conditions exceeds the morbidity of hemorrhagic complications caused by the anticoagulant therapy. A second caveat of anticoagulant therapy is that lower rates of thromboembolism must be demonstrated with treatment.

Indications

Data from several large studies stratify the relative risk of thromboembolism for specific valvular disease. Rheumatic heart disease carries the highest risk of thromboembolism. Patients with mitral rheumatic disease have a 20% risk of developing clinically significant emboli, and a 10% to 15% mortality rate without treatment.[44] Patients with mitral valve disease and atrial fibrillation have a four to seven times risk of thromboembolism when compared with similar patients in normal sinus rhythm. More specifically, patients in atrial fibrillation with MS have about a 50% greater risk of thromboembolism than patients with MR, or 31.5% versus 22%, respectively (Table 84.7).[111] Whereas thromboemboli occur in only 8% of patients with MS or MR who are in sinus rhythm, patients who develop a single embolic event do have a 30% to 65% chance of having recurrent episodes; more than half of these occur within 6 months. Patients with large atria (diameter larger than 55 mm) are at increased risk for developing atrial fibrillation and therefore should be considered for prophylactic anticoagulation. In addition, advanced age and decreased cardiac index are also risk factors for thromboembolism. Anticoagulant therapy is therefore recommended for patients with atrial fibrillation and associated systemic emboli, mitral valve disease, and cardiomyopathy.[112]

Valvular lesions other than mitral valve disease carry a relatively low risk of embolism. Calcific emboli do not appear to be prevented by warfarin therapy. Anticoagulation is therefore not indicated for mitral valve prolapse, mitral annular calcification, or aortic valve disease without other risk factors. Emboli associated with endocarditis are usually not thrombotic in nature, and anticoagulation is not indicated for endocarditis unless other indications exist (e.g., prosthetic valve endocarditis).

Reliable data from randomized trials of anticoagulant therapy in patients with prosthetic heart valves are sporadic, but some specific recommendations are available (Table 84.8). Initial experiences with the Starr-Edwards ball valve showed an average embolic risk of 6% per year, ranging up to a 30% risk over the course of one study in which anticoagulants were not used. Anticoagulant therapy reduces this risk by threefold to sixfold. The new generation of low-profile tilting-disc valves, although thought to have lower thrombosis potential, still demonstrates thromboembolic rates without anticoagulation of up to 3% per year. Bioprosthetic tissue valves have a low potential for thromboembolism, on the order of 2% per year. Half of all tissue valve thromboembolic episodes occur in the first 12 weeks after surgery. Lifelong anticoagulation is therefore recommended for all patients with mechanical valves, and an initial period of anticoagulation is recommended by some authors for patients with bioprosthetic valves to cover the early period of neointimal deposition. Antiplatelet therapy with either aspirin or dipyridamole (Persantine) may be an effective alternative treatment to lower thromboembolic risk, but the data are not well supported. These agents may be useful as an adjunct to warfarin in cases in which single-drug therapy is ineffective in preventing embolic complications.

Summarizing all prosthetic valve data, Edmunds [113] concluded that the cumulative risk of thromboembolism for mechanical valves with anticoagulation and prosthetic valves without anticoagulation was about equal at 2% per year. Anticoagulated patients with mechanical valves assume the added risk of bleeding complications, but 10% of patients with tissue valves in the aortic position, and up to 40% to 60% of patients with bioprosthetic mitral valves, eventually require warfarin anticoagulation, thus partially negating the benefit of the tissue prosthesis.

Complications

Data derived from patients with prosthetic valves who are on warfarin therapy suggest a uniform risk of major bleeding

TABLE 84.7

ASSOCIATION OF THROMBOEMBOLISM WITH ATRIAL FIBRILLATION AND AGE IN PATIENTS WITH MITRAL VALVE DISEASE[a]

Age (y)	Sinus rhythm	Atrial fibrillation	Total
Mitral Stenosis			
≤35	4.5	27.5	9.0
>35	11.3	32.3	23.9
Total	7.9	31.5	19.0
Mitral Regurgitation			
≤35	3.7	15.8	8.6
>35	16.7	25.0	23.2
Total	7.6	22.2	16.7

[a]Incidence of thromboembolism in percentage of total patients studied.
Modified from Coulshed N, Epstein EJ, McKindrich CS, et al. Systemic embolisation in mitral valve disease. *Br Heart* J. 1970;32:26.

TABLE 84.8 TREATMENT

ANTICOAGULANT RECOMMENDATIONS

Indication	Recommended prothrombin time elevation with warfarin administration
Prosthetic Heart Valves	
Mechanical	1.5–2
Bioprosthetic	1.3–1.5 (3 mo postoperatively)
Native Valve Disease	
Rheumatic mitral valve	
Previous embolism	1.5–2 (1.3–1.5 after 1 y)
Atrial fibrillation	1.3–1.5
Dilated left atrium (>55 mm in diameter)	1.3–1.5
Aortic valve disease	No treatment[a]
Mitral valve prolapse	No treatment[a]
Mitral annular calcification	No treatment[a]
Infective endocarditis	No treatment[a]
Atrial Fibrillation	
Previous embolism	1.5–2 (1.3–1.5 after 1 y)
Mitral valve disease	1.3–1.5
Cardiomyopathy	
Dilated	1.3–1.5
Hypertrophic	1.3–1.5
Thyrotoxicosis	1.3–1.5[b]
Lone atrial fibrillation	No treatment[a]
Cardioversion	1.3–1.5b

[a]Unless other indications exist.
[b]Maintain therapy for 2 to 4 weeks after conversion to sinus rhythm.

episodes of 1% to 2% per year, with a mortality rate of 0.17% per year for patients on anticoagulant therapy. Bleeding complications most commonly involve the central nervous, genitourinary, or gastrointestinal system, including the retroperitoneum. Fatal bleeds usually involve the central nervous system. Trauma is frequently an inciting cause. Previous recommendations that prothrombin time be maintained at 2 to 2.5 times control appear to be excessive, and fewer bleeding complications can be expected at the newly recommended levels of 1.3 to 1.5 times control for most patients.[49,51,112,114]

Patients who have suffered an embolic cerebrovascular accident thought to be cardiac in origin should undergo urgent computed tomography of the brain. Anticoagulant therapy should be instituted immediately if the scan is negative. If a large or hemorrhagic infarct is observed, therapy should be postponed for 1 week.

Few studies address the management of patients requiring interruption of anticoagulation because of bleeding complications or because major surgery is planned. The authors believe that anticoagulation should be reversed by withholding warfarin several days before operation and allowing prothrombin time to decrease to about 14 to 15 seconds. Therapy should be resumed 1 to 2 days postoperatively in low-risk patients. High-risk patients should be switched to heparin preoperatively once the prothrombin time reaches subtherapeutic levels. The heparin can be discontinued immediately before operation and resumed as soon as 12 hours postoperatively if operative bleeding is not an issue. Rapid reversal of anticoagulation should be made with fresh frozen plasma transfusions, if necessary. Vitamin K administration makes subsequent warfarin therapy more difficult and should be avoided. The benefits of aspirin use through the perioperative period remain unconfirmed.

Contraindications

Anticoagulant therapy is specifically contraindicated in any patient with a predisposition for bleeding complications, from either systemic disease (e.g., active ulcer disease) or coagulopathy; in those likely to incur trauma through occupation or pastime; in those likely to be poorly compliant; and in those with a desire for future pregnancy.

Anticoagulation in the pregnant patient is a significant problem. Warfarin is a small molecule that readily crosses the placental barrier. The immature fetal liver is susceptible to the effects of warfarin, and a protracted hypocoagulable state develops. Fetal clotting factors can take 2 to 3 weeks to return to normal after cessation of warfarin therapy. Warfarin is also a known fetal teratogen, especially with use during the first trimester. A fetal loss rate over 30% and a rate of premature labor over 50% have been reported with warfarin use during pregnancy.[115] Use of warfarin late in pregnancy can produce fetal neurologic complications as a result of intracranial hemorrhage, and the trauma of delivery is a significant problem in this regard. Heparin is not transferred across the placental barrier but can produce fetal loss through placental hemorrhage. Conversely, the pregnant woman is in a hypercoagulable state, with elevated levels of clotting factors and decreased fibrinolytic activity. Cessation of anticoagulation during pregnancy can lead to an incidence of cerebral events as high as 25%. Antiplatelet agents are not as toxic to the fetus as warfarin but do not confer adequate protection to the mother.

The best solution to this problem is the use of a bioprosthesis in patients wishing to become pregnant, with use of antiplatelet agents during pregnancy. If an unforeseen pregnancy develops in a patient with a mechanical valve, a regimen including subcutaneous low-molecular-weight heparin is now advocated.

CARDIAC TUMORS

The most common cardiac tumors are secondary tumors, usually originating from the lung in men and from the breast in women. Primary cardiac tumors are rare in all age groups, with the incidence being variably quoted as 1.7 to 10 per 100,000. They are mainly benign (65% to 80%), but early detection is essential because successful resection is possible only if cardiac function is preserved. Small cardiac tumors, apart from myxomas, usually lie intramurally and cause dysrhythmias by interfering with the conduction tissue. Bradyarrhythmias and tachyarrhythmias may occur. Larger tumors project into the cardiac cavities and cause obstruction of the valves, the cavities, and the ventricular outflow tracts. Presentation is thus often nonspecific, and a high index of suspicion must be maintained; unexplained murmurs, congestive cardiac failure, and dysrhythmias may be the first signs.

Electrocardiography is usually normal or nonspecifically abnormal. Chest radiography is also usually normal, though chamber enlargement and tumor calcification may be seen. Echocardiography is the best screening investigation, allowing assessment of the size, shape, location, attachment, and mobility of the tumor, as well as displacement of the coronary arteries by the tumor mass. However, echocardiography may miss large tumors in various chambers, possibly due to the relative homogeneous state of certain tumors and to the lack of normal tissue interfaces because of the large tumor size. Thus the gold standard still remains cardiac catheterization.

Treatment is by surgical resection. When complete excision cannot be achieved, relief of the obstruction alone can give good long-term results. Enucleation or conservative resection of ventricular tumors should be undertaken. Atrial tumors can be radically excised and the defect in the atrial wall repaired with pericardium.

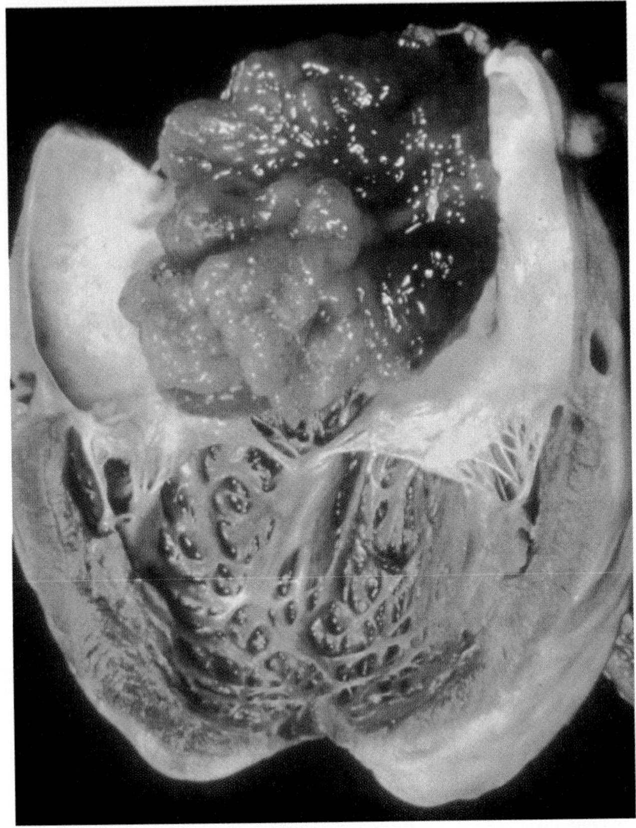

FIGURE 84.21 Cardiac myxoma. The left atrium contains a large, polypoid tumor, which protrudes into the mitral valve orifice. (From Rubin E, Farber JL. *Pathology*, 3rd ed. Philadelphia: Lippincott Williams & Wilkins, 1999.)

Myxoma

This is the most common tumor of the heart, comprising 50% of benign tumors. It is more common in women and rare before adulthood, though it has been described in a newborn. They are usually solitary, although biatrial myxomas with a common attachment at the fossa ovalis have been described, as have complex and familial forms.[116] These last syndromes are associated with earlier development of tumors at atypical and multiple locations. Recurrences are also more common. In the complex myxoma syndrome, cutaneous lentigos, myxomas at various sites, and endocrine tumors accompany the cardiac tumor.

Cardiac myxomas usually originate in the left atrium (75%; Fig. 84.21); 20% are seen in the right atrium and 4% in the ventricles. Other sites have been reported (both atrioventricular valves, inferior vena cava, and both ventriculoarterial valves), but the stalk usually originates from the inferior rim of the fossa ovalis. Pathologically they are soft, semitranslucent tumors; histologically they contain large amounts of amorphous matrix with syncytial groups of elongated cells, closely related to thin-walled capillaries. In the past, there was some question over the origin of these tumors, with some claiming that they are areas of organized thrombus rather than true neoplasms and hence better called Lambi's excrescences. This theory does not now appear appropriate.

Myxomas may present with cardiac failure resulting from valve obstruction or regurgitation and impingement into the cardiac chambers. This may be further manifested as pulmonary hypertension. They may also present with embolization, either systemic or pulmonary, because of thrombotic embolization or fragmentation of the tumor.[116] Constitutional symptoms (e.g., fever, malaise, weight loss) are also common, probably owing to an autoimmune phenomenon. Physical examination is often unrewarding, though the murmur of mitral stenosis is a classic finding. Diagnosis is best achieved by echocardiography; catheterization is best avoided because of the risk of tumor fragmentation. When the diagnosis has been made, surgery should be undertaken urgently in view of the risk of embolization. Since the first report of successful resection in 1954, the surgical mortality rate has fallen to 5%. Care must be taken in handling the tumor to ensure that no fragments are left behind, and all four cardiac chambers must be examined because multiple tumors may occur. Excision should be wide around the base of the stalk, because local recurrence is possible and the tumor may become locally invasive. If this precaution is taken, single tumors rarely recur, although this is more common in the complex syndrome, which is associated with an overall recurrence rate of 6.3%. The 20-year survival is 91%, but occasionally the tumor may metastasize to brain and bone.

Hamartomas

Of hamartomas, 85% occur in infants and children, usually in the free wall of the left ventricle or the interventricular septum. They comprise 5% of primary cardiac tumors and are usually single, round, firm, well-encapsulated masses, with a false capsule that allows enucleation. They are entirely benign and show no malignant transformation. On cutting, the surface bulges convexly and the fibrous tissue intermingled with muscle has a whorled appearance. Occasionally they calcify. They often interfere with the conduction system so that sudden death is common, occurring in 30% of patients.

Rhabdomyomas

This tumor is primarily a tumor of childhood. Fifty percent of patients die within the first month of life, and 80% die by 1 year. In 50% of patients, it is associated with tuberous sclerosis. Rhabdomyomas are often multiple in the interventricular septum and adjacent free wall; diffuse myocardial disease leads to heart failure and death. The tumors are usually well-circumscribed, nonencapsulated, whitish nodules, and they may grow to a large size, projecting into the ventricular cavities.[117] The individual cells are large and vacuolated, with delicate radiating strands of cytoplasm. They are filled with glycogen. Whether they are true neoplasms or simply overgrowths of the Purkinje cells, and thus hamartomas, remains uncertain, but spontaneous regression has been described. They are certainly congenital, because intrauterine diagnosis has been confirmed at neonatal operation.

Lipoma

This very uncommon tumor usually occurs in adults. Most often it is located subendocardially and appears as a yellow mass projecting into the cardiac chamber.[118] Rarely, it is intramural and unencapsulated. It is slow growing and may calcify following fat necrosis. Microscopically it comprises fatty tissue with interlacing muscle fibers.

In children the most common benign cardiac tumors are rhabdomyoma, fibroma, hemangioma, and teratoma. In adults, the most common benign cardiac tumors are myxoma, fibroma, hemangioma, granular cell tumor, lipoma, paraganglioma, hamartoma, histiocytoma, and hemangioendothelioma. The most common malignant tumors in children are rhabdomyosarcoma, fibrous histiocytoma, angiosarcoma, fibrosarcoma, and myxoid sarcoma. In adults, the most common malignant cardiac tumors are angiosarcoma, fibrous histiocytoma, leiomyosarcoma, osteosarcoma, fibrosarcoma, myxoid sarcoma, rhabdomyosarcoma, and liposarcoma.[119]

In children, hemangiomas and benign teratomas occur infrequently. Primary malignant tumors are extremely rare; when they do occur, they are usually hemangiosarcomas and small cell sarcomas.[120] Early death is usually to the result of rapid growth and dissemination.

The more common metastatic cardiac tumors originate from bronchogenic carcinoma of the breast, lymphoma, leukemia, esophagus, uterus, melanoma, stomach, sarcomas, germ cell tumors, and, in further decreasing frequency, tumors of the oral pharynx, colorectal, kidney, thyroid, larynx, urinary system, hepatobiliary system, prostate, pancreas, and ovary.[121]

KEY POINTS

- **Proper valve function is one of the most critical elements that determine efficient cardiac function.**
- **Initial assessment of patients with valvular heart disease depends on a careful history and physical examination, which will reveal information regarding the type of valvular disease. It also provides an estimate of the severity, duration, and prognosis of the dysfunction.**
- **The severity of AS can be measured accurately with noninvasive studies. However, because many of the patients with AS are elderly and are at risk for coronary disease, cardiac catheterization with coronary angiography is usually performed prior to valve replacement.**
- **There is no proven medical therapy for AS. The only effective relief of this mechanical obstruction to blood flow is aortic valve replacement.**
- **Aortic insufficiency can yield the greatest increase in ventricular mass produced by any of the valvular lesions.**
- **Acute AI is seen in traumatic aortic injury, acute aortic dissection, and endocarditis.**
- **Mitral stenosis (MS) is almost exclusively the direct sequelae of rheumatic heart disease and tends to affect women more frequently.**
- **The primary pathophysiologic feature of MR is systolic unloading of the LV into the left atrium.**
- **Transesophageal echocardiography is the study of choice used to delineate the anatomic cause of the MR and can help direct successful repair of the valve in addition to assessing the severity of the MR.**
- **Less than 50 years ago, endocarditis was uniformly fatal. However, over the last 40 years, with the discovery of newer antibiotics, improved blood culture techniques, echocardiography, cardiopulmonary bypass, and valve repair and replacement procedures, the mortality rate is now between 10% and 15%.**
- **The most common cardiac tumors are secondary tumors, usually originating from the lung in men and from the breast in women.**

References

1. Silver MA, Roberts WC. Detailed anatomy of the normally functioning aortic valve in hearts of normal and increased weight. *Am J Cardiol.* 1985;55:454.
2. Anderson RH, Devine WA, Ho SY, et al. The myth of the aortic annulus: the anatomy of the subaortic outflow tract. *Ann Thorac Surg.* 1991; 52:640.
3. Thubrikar MJ, Nolan SP, Aouad J, et al. Stress sharing between the sinus and leaflets of canine aortic valve. *Ann Thorac Surg.* 1986;42:434.
4. Zimmerman J. The functional and surgical anatomy of the aortic valve. *Isr J Med Sci.* 1969;5:862.
5. Davila JC, Plamer ET. The mitral valve: anatomy and pathology for the surgeon. *Arch Surg.* 1962;84:174.
6. Walmsley R. Anatomy of human mitral valve in adult cadaver and comparative anatomy of the valve. *Br Heart J.* 1978;40:351.
7. Ranganathan N, Lam JH, Wigle ED, et al. Morphology of the human mitral valve. II. The valve leaflets. *Circulation* 1970;41:459.
8. Pollick C, Pitman M, Filly K, et al. Mitral and aortic valve orifice area in normal subjects and in patients with congestive cardiomyopathy: determination by two dimensional echocardiography. *Am J Cardiol.* 1982; 49:1191.
9. Fenster MS, Feldman MD. Mitral regurgitation: an overview. *Curr Probl Cardiol.* 1995;20:193.
10. Voci P, Bilotta F, Caretta Q, et al. Papillary muscle perfusion pattern: a hypothesis for ischemic papillary muscle dysfunction. *Circulation* 1995;91:1714.
11. Lam JH, Ranganathan N, Wigle ED, et al. Morphology of the human mitral valve. I. Chordae tendineae: a new classification. *Circulation* 1970;41:449.
12. Boltwood CM, Tei C, Wong M, et al. Quantitative echocardiography of the mitral complex in dilated cardiomyopathy: the mechanism of functional mitral regurgitation. *Circulation* 1983;68:498.
13. Passik CS, Ackermann DM, Pluth JR, et al. Temporal changes in the causes of aortic stenosis: a surgical pathologic study of 646 cases. *Mayo Clin Proc.* 1987;62:119.
14. Waller B, Howard J, Fess S. Pathology of aortic valve stenosis and pure aortic regurgitation: a clinical morphologic assessment. *Clin Cardiol.* 1994; 17:85.
15. **Bonow RO, Carabello B, de Leon AC, et al. ACC/AHA guidelines for the management of patients with valvular heart disease. Executive summary. *J Heart Valve Dis.* 1998;7:672.**
16. Hess OM, Ritter M, Schneider J, et al. Diastolic stiffness and myocardial structure in aortic valve disease before and after valve replacement. *Circulation* 1984;69:855.

17. Huber D, Grimm J, Koch R, et al. Determinants of ejection performance in aortic stenosis. *Circulation* 1981;64:126.
18. Maier GW, Wechsler AS. Pathophysiology of aortic valve disease. In: Edmunds LH, ed. *Cardiac surgery in the adult.* New York: McGraw-Hill, 1997, p. 835.
19. Lester SJ, Heilbron B, Gin K, et al. The natural history and rate of progression of aortic stenosis. *Chest* 1998;113:1109.
20. Chizner MA, Pearle DL, de Leon AC Jr. The natural history of aortic stenosis in adults. *Am Heart J.* 1980;99:419.
21. **Marcus ML, Doty DB, Hiratzka LF, et al. Decreased coronary reserve: a mechanism for angina pectoris in patients with aortic stenosis and normal coronary arteries. *N Engl J Med.* 1982;307:1362.**
22. **Carabello BA, Crawford FA. Medical progress: valvular heart disease. *N Engl J Med.* 1997;337:32.**
23. Otto CM. Aortic stenosis: clinical evaluation and optimal timing of surgery. *Cardiol Clin.* 1998;16:353.
24. Richards AM, Nicholls MG, Ikram H, et al. Syncope in aortic valvular stenosis. *Lancet* 1984;2:1113.
25. O'Keefe JH Jr, Vlietstra RE, Bailey KR, et al. Natural history of candidates for balloon aortic valvuloplasty. *Mayo Clin Proc.* 1987;62:986.
26. Carabello BA, Green LH, Grossman W, et al. Hemodynamic determinants of prognosis of aortic valve replacement in critical aortic stenosis and advanced congestive heart failure. *Circulation* 1980;62:42.
27. Brogan WC III, Grayburn PA, Lange RA, et al. Prognosis after valve replacement in patients with severe aortic stenosis and low transvalvular pressure gradient. *J Am Coll Cardiol.* 1993;21:1657.
28. Cannon JD Jr, Zile MR, Crawford FA Jr, et al. Aortic valve resistance as an adjunct to the Gorlin formula in assessing the severity of aortic stenosis in symptomatic patients. *J Am Coll Cardiol.* 1992;20:1517.
29. deFilippi CR, Willett DL, Brickner ME, et al. Usefulness of dobutamine echocardiography in distinguishing severe from nonsevere valvular aortic stenosis in patients with depressed left ventricular function and low transvalvular gradients. *Am J Cardiol.* 1995;75:191.
30. Otto CM, Mickel MC, Kennedy JW, et al. Three-year outcome after balloon aortic valvuloplasty: insights into prognosis of valvular aortic stenosis. *Circulation* 1994;89:642.
31. Bellhouse BJ, Bellhouse F, Abbott JA, et al. Mechanism of valvular incompetence in aortic sinus dilatation. *Cardiovasc Res.* 1973;7:490.
32. Carter JB, Sethi S, Lee GB, et al. Prolapse of semilunar cusps as causes of aortic insufficiency . *Circulation* 1971;43:922.
33. Mann T, McLaurin L, Grossman W, et al. Assessing the hemodynamic severity of acute aortic regurgitation due to infective endocarditis. *N Engl J Med.* 1975;293:108.
34. Vinten-Johansen J, Weiss HR. Regional O_2 consumption in canine left ventricular myocardium in experimental acute aortic valvular insufficiency. *Cardiovasc Res.* 1981;15:305.
35. Bonow RO. Chronic aortic regurgitation. Role of medical therapy and optimal timing for surgery. *Cardiol Clin* 1998;16:449.
36. Goldschlager N, Pfeifer J, Cohn K, et al. The natural history of aortic regurgitation: a clinical and hemodynamic study. *Am J Med.* 1973;54:577.
37. Henry WL, Bonow RO, Rosing DR, et al. Observations on the optimum time for operative intervention for aortic regurgitation. *Circulation* 1980;61:484.
38. Bonow RO, Lakatos E, Maron BJ, et al. Serial long-term assessment of the natural history of asymptomatic patients with chronic aortic regurgitation and normal left ventricular systolic function. *Circulation* 1991;84:1625.
39. Aronow WS, Ahn C, Kronzon I, et al. Prognosis of patients with heart failure and unoperated severe aortic valvular regurgitation and relation to ejection fraction. *Am J Cardiol.* 1994;74:286.
40. Waller BF, Howard J, Fess S. Pathology of mitral valve stenosis and pure mitral regurgitation, part I. *Clin Cardiol.* 1994;17:330.
41. Waller BF, Howard J, Fess S. Pathology of mitral valve stenosis and pure mitral regurgitation, part II. *Clin Cardiol.* 1994;17:395.
42. Wood P. An appreciation of mitral stenosis. *Br Med J.* 1954;1:1051.
43. Thompson ME, Shaver JA, Leon DF. Effect of tachycardia on atrial transport in mitral stenosis. *Am Heart J.* 1977;94:297.
44. Neilson GH, Galea EG, Hossack KF. Thromboembolic complications of mitral valve disease. *Aust NZ J Med.* 1978;8:372.
45. Gash AK, Carabello BA, Kent RL, et al. Left ventricular performance in patients with coexistent mitral stenosis and aortic insufficiency. *J Am Coll Cardiol.* 1984;3:703.
46. Martin RP, Rakowski H, Kleiman JH, et al. Reliability and reproducibility of two dimensional echocardiograph measurement of the stenotic mitral valve orifice area. *Am J Cardiol.* 1979;43:560.
47. Carabello BA. Timing of surgery for mitral and aortic stenosis. *Cardiol Clin.* 1991;9:229.
48. Reyes VP, Raju BS, Wynne J, et al. Percutaneous balloon valvuloplasty compared with open surgical commissurotomy for mitral stenosis. *N Engl J Med.* 1994;331:961.
49. Wilkins GT, Weyman AE, Abascal VM, et al. Percutaneous balloon dilation of the mitral valve: an analysis of echocardiographic variables related to outcome and the mechanism of dilatation. *Br Heart J.* 1988;60:299.
50. Kobayashi J, Kosakai Y, Isobe F, et al. Rationale of the Cox maze procedure for atrial fibrillation during redo mitral valve operations. *J Thorac Cardiovasc Surg.* 1996;112:1216.
51. Kawaguchi AT, Kosakai Y, Sasako Y, et al. Risks and benefits of combined maze procedure for atrial fibrillation associated with organic heart disease. *J Am Coll Cardiol.* 1996;28:985.
52. Stevenson LW, Fowler MB, Schroeder JS, et al. Poor survival of patients with idiopathic cardiomyopathy considered too well for transplantation. *Am J Med.* 1987;83:871.
53. Fenster MS, Feldman MD. Mitral regurgitation: an overview. *Curr Probl Cardiol.* 1995;20:193.
54. Starling MR, Kirsh MM, Montgomery DG, et al. Impaired left ventricular contractile function in patients with long-term mitral regurgitation and normal ejection fraction. *J Am Coll Cardiol.* 1993;22:239.
55. Carabello BA, Willimans H, Gash AK, et al. Hemodynamic predictors of outcome in patients undergoing valve replacement. *Circulation* 1986; 74:1309.
56. Rosario LB, Stevenson LW, Solomon SD, et al. The mechanism of decrease in dynamic mitral regurgitation during heart failure treatment: importance of reduction in regurgitant orifice size. *J Am Coll Cardiol.* 1998;32:1819.
57. Torre-Amione G, Kapadia S, Benedict C, et al. Proinflammatory cytokine levels in patients with depressed left ventricular ejection fraction: a report from the Studies of Left Ventricular Dysfunction (SOLVD). *J Am Coll Cardiol.* 1996;27:1201.
58. Herrera-Garza EH, Stetson SJ, Cubillos-Garzon A, et al. Tumor necrosis factor-(: A mediator of disease progression in the failing human heart. *Chest* 1999;115:1170.
59. Carabello BA. Clinical assessment of systolic dysfunction. *ACC Curr J Rev.* 1994;3:25.
60. Zile MR, Gaasch WH, Carroll JD, et al. Chronic mitral regurgitation: predictive value of preoperative echocardiographic indexes of left ventricular function and wall stress. *J Am Coll Cardiol.* 1984;3:235.
61. Hochreiter C, Niles N, Devereux RB, et al. Mitral regurgitation: relationship of noninvasive descriptors of right and left ventricular performance to clinical and hemodynamic findings and to prognosis in medically and surgically treated patients. *Circulation* 1986;73:900.
62. **David TE, Uden DE, Strauss HD. The importance of the mitral apparatus in left ventricular function after correction of mitral regurgitation. *Circulation* 1983;68:II-76.**
63. Gallino A, Jenni R, Hurni R, et al. Early results after mitral valvuloplasty for pure mitral regurgitation. *Eur Heart J.* 1987;8:902.
64. Rankin JS, Feneley MP, Hickey MS, et al. A clinical comparison of mitral valve repair versus replacement in ischemic mitral regurgitation. *J Thorac Cadiovasc Surg.* 1988; 95:165.
65. Akins CW, Hilgenberg AD, Buckley MJ, et al. Mitral valve reconstruction versus replacement for degenerative or ischemic mitral regurgitation. *Ann Thorac Surg.* 1994;58:668.
66. Olson LJ, Subramanian R, Ackermann DM, et al. Surgical pathology of the mitral valve: a study of 712 cases spanning 21 years. *Mayo Clin Proc.* 1987;62:22.
67. Roberts WC, McIntosh CL, Wallace RB. Mechanisms of severe mitral regurgitation in mitral valve prolapse determined from analysis of operatively excised valves. *Am Heart J.* 1987;113:1316.
68. Barlow JB, Pocock WA. Mitral valve prolapse, the specific billowing mitral leaflet syndrome, or an insignificant non-ejection systolic click. *Am Heart J.* 1979;97:277.
69. Sons H, Dausch W, Kuh JH. Tricuspid valve repair in right-sided endocarditis. *J Heart Valve Dis.* 1997;6:636.
70. Connolly HM, Crary JL, McGoon MD, et al. Valvular heart disease associated with fenfluramine-phentermine. *N Engl J Med.* 1997;337:581.
71. Hogevik H, Olaison L, Anderson R, et al. Epidemiologic aspects of infective endocarditis in an urban population: a 5-year prospective study. *Medicine* 1995;74:324.
72. Bayliss R, Clarke C, Oakley CM, et al. Incidence, mortality, and prevention of infective endocarditis. *J R Coll Physicians London* 1986;20:15.
73. **Edmunds LH Jr, Clark RE, Cohn LH, et al. Guidelines for reporting morbidity and mortality after cardiac valvular operations. *Ann Thorac Surg.* 1996;62:932.**
74. Skehan JD, Murray M, Mills PG. Infective endocarditis: incidence and mortality in the North East Thames Region. *Br Heart J.* 1988;59:62.
75. Steusse DC, Vlessis AA. Epidemiology of native valve endocarditis. In: Vlessis AA, Bolling SF, eds. *Endocarditis: a multidisciplinary approach.* Armonk, NY: Futura, 1999, p. 77.
76. Vlessis AA, Khaki A, Grunkemeier GL, et al. Risk, diagnosis and management of prosthetic valve endocarditis: a review. *J Heart Valve Dis.* 1997; 6:443.
77. Vlessis AA, Hovaguimian H, Jaggers J, et al. Infective endocarditis: Ten-year review of medical and surgical therapy. *Ann Thorac Surg.* 1996;61:1217.
78. Hogevik H, Olaison L, Andersson R, et al. Epidemiologic aspects of infective endocarditis in an urban population: a 5-year prospective study. *Medicine* 1995;74:324.
79. **Aklog L, Gobezie R, Adams DH. Aortic valve endocarditis. In: Vlessis AA, Bolling SF, eds. *Endocarditis: a multidisciplinary approach.* Armonk, NY: Futura, 1999, p. 235.**
80. **Schwartz CF, Bolling SF. Mitral valve endocarditis. In: Vlessis AA, Bolling SF, eds. *Endocarditis: a multidisciplinary approach.* Armonk, NY: Futura, 1999, p. 263.**

81. Bach DS. Echocardiographic diagnosis and findings in infective endocarditis. In: Vlessis AA, Bolling SF, eds. *Endocarditis: a multidisciplinary approach*. Armonk, NY: Futura, 1999, p. 135.
82. Armstrong WS, Shea M. Clinical diagnosis of infective endocarditis. In: Vlessis AA, Bolling SF, eds. *Endocarditis: a multidisciplinary approach*. Armonk, NY: Futura, 1999, p. 107.
83. Pagani FD, Monaghan HL, Deeb GM, et al. Mitral valve reconstruction for active and healed endocarditis. *Circulation* 1996;94:II133.
84. David TE, Bos J, Christakis GT, et al. Heart valve operations in patients with active infective endocarditis. *Ann Thorac Surg.* 1990;49:701.
85. Cobanoglu A, Jamieson WR, Miller DC, et al. A tri-institutional comparison of tissue and mechanical valves using a patient-oriented definition of "treatment failure." *Ann Thorac Surg.* 1987;43:245.
86. Pelletier L, Carrier M, Leclerc Y, et al. The Carpentier-Edwards pericardial bioprosthesis: clinical experience with 600 patients. *Ann Thorac Surg.* 1995;60:S297.
87. Miller DC, Oyer PE, Mitchell RS, et al. Performance characteristics of the Starr-Edwards Model 1260 aortic valve prosthesis beyond ten years. *J Thorac Cardiovasc Surg.* 1984;88:193.
88. Bjork VO, Henze A. Ten years' experience with the Bjork-Shiley tilting disc valve. *J Thorac Cardiovasc Surg.* 1979;78:331.
89. Borkon AM, Soule L, Baughman KL, et al. Ten-year analysis of the Bjork-Shiley standard aortic valve. *Ann Thorac Surg.* 1987;43:39.
90. Hiratzka LF, Kouchoukos NT, Grunkemeier GL, et al. Outlet strut fracture of the Bjork-Shiley 60 degrees convexo-concave valve: current information and recommendations for patient care. *J Am Coll Cardiol.* 1988;11:1130.
91. Czer LS, Matloff J, Chaux A, et al. A 6 year experience with the St. Jude Medical valve: Hemodynamic performance, surgical results, biocompatibility and follow-up. *J Am Coll Cardiol.* 1985;6:904.
92. Czer LS, Chaux A, Matloff JM, et al. Ten-year experience with the St. Jude Medical valve for primary valve replacement. *J Thorac Cardiovasc Surg.* 1990;100:44.
93. Crawford FA Jr, Kratz JM, Sade RM, et al. Aortic and mitral valve replacement with the St. Jude Medical prosthesis. *Ann Surg.* 1984;199:753.
94. Company Press Release: St. Jude Medical Inc. St. Jude Medical recalling heart valve products with Silzone coating. January 24, 2000.
95. Copeland JG III. An International experience with the CarboMedics prosthetic heart valve. *J Heart Dis.* 1995;4:56.
96. Beaudet RL, Poirier NL, Doyle D, et al. The Medtronic-Hall cardiac valve: 7-1/2 years' clinical experience. *Ann Thorac Surg.* 1986;42:644.
97. Akins CW. Results with mechanical cardiac valvular prostheses. *Ann Thorac Surg.* 1995;60:1836.
98. Hammermeister KE, Henderson WG, Burchfiel CM, et al. Comparison of outcome after valve replacement with a bioprosthesis versus a mechanical prosthesis: initial 5 year results of a randomized trial. *J Am Coll Cardiol.* 1987;10:719.
99. **Carpentier A, Lemaigre G, Robert L, et al. Biological factors affecting long-term results of valvular heterografts. *J Thorac Cardiovasc Surg.* 1969; 58:467.**
100. Chaitman BR, Bonan R, Lepage G, et al. Hemodynamic evaluation of the Carpentier-Edwards porcine xenograft. *Circulation* 1979;60:1170.
101. Wernly JA, Crawford MH. Choosing a prosthetic heart valve. *Cardiol Clin.* 1998;16:491.
102. Edwards TJ, Livesey SA, Simpson IA, et al. Biological valves beyond fifteen years: the Wessex experience. *Ann Thorac Surg.* 1995;60:S211.
103. Bernal JM, Rabasa JM, Lopez R, et al. Durability of the Carpentier-Edwards porcine bioprosthesis: role of age and valve position. *Ann Thorac Surg.* 1995;60:S248.
104. Doty JR, Flores JH, Millar RC, et al. Aortic valve replacement with Medtronic freestyle bioprosthesis: operative technique and results. *J Card Surg.* 1998; 13:208.
105. O'Brien MF, Stafford EG, Gardner MA, et al. Allograft aortic valve replacement: long-term follow-up. *Ann Thorac Surg.* 1995;60:S65.
106. **Elkins RC, Knott-Craig CJ, Ward KE, et al. Pulmonary autograft in children: realized growth potential. *Ann Thorac Surg.* 1994;57:1387.**
107. **Ross D. The versatile homograft and autograft valve. *Ann Thorac Surg.* 1989;48:S69.**
108. Hammond GL, Geha AS, Kopf GS, et al. Biological versus mechanical valves: analysis of 1,116 valves inserted in 1,012 adult patients with a 4,818 patient-year and a 5,327 valve-year follow-up. *J Thorac Cardiovasc Surg.* 1987;93:182.
109. Gohlke-Barwolf C, Acar J, Oakley C, et al. Guidelines for prevention of thromboembolic events in valvular heart disease. *Eur Heart J.* 1995; 16:1320.
110. Burr LH, Jamieson WR, Munro AI, et al. Porcine bioprosthesis in the elderly: clinical performance by age groups and valve positions. *Ann Thorac Surg.* 1995;60:264.
111. Coulshed N, Epstein EJ, McKendrick CS, et al. Systemic embolism in mitral valve disease. *Br Heart J.* 1970;32:26.
112. Levine HJ, Pauker SG, Eckman MK. Antithrombotic therapy in valvular heart disease. *Chest* 1995;108:360S.
113. Edmunds LH Jr. Thromboembolic complications of current cardiac valvular prostheses. *Ann Thorac Surg.* 1982;34:96.
114. Stein PD, Kantrowitz A. Antithrombotic therapy in mechanical and biological prosthetic heart valves and saphenous vein bypass grafts. *Chest* 1989;95:107S.
115. Sareli P, England MJ, Berk MR, et al. Maternal and fetal sequelae of anticoagulation during pregnancy in patients with mechanical heart valve prostheses. *Am J Cardiol.* 1989;63:1462.
116. **Reynen K. Cardiac myxomas. *N Engl J Med.* 1995;333:1610–1617.**
117. Butany J, Nair V, Ahluwalia MS, et al. Papillary fibroelastoma of the interatrial septum. *J Card Surg.* 2004;19:349–353.
118. Gaerte SC, Meyer CA, Winer-Muram HT, et al. Fat-containing lesions of the chest. *Radiographics* 2002;22:S61–78.
119. Donsbeck AV, Ranchere D, Coindre JM, et al. Primary cardiac sarcomas: an immunohistochemical and grading study with long-term follow-up of 24 cases. *Histopathology* 1999:34:295–304.
120. Roberts WC. Cardiac neoplasms. In: Topol EJ, ed. *Textbook of cardiovascular medicine*. Philadelphia: Lippincott-Raven, 1998, pp. 971–974.
121. Schvartzman PR, White RD. Imaging of cardiac and paracardiac masses. *J Thorac Imaging* 2000;15:265–73
122. Shapiro LM. Cardiac tumours: diagnosis and management. *Heart* 2001;85:218–222

CHAPTER 85 ■ ISCHEMIC HEART DISEASE

MARTIN LEBOUTILLIER III AND VERDI J. DISESA

CORONARY CIRCULATION

Coronary Anatomy

The right and left coronary arteries originate from the aorta just above the aortic valve cusps (Fig. 85.1). The orifices of the two arteries within the sinuses of Valsalva designate the right and left coronary cusps. The third aortic valve cusp is referred to as the *noncoronary cusp*.

The left main coronary artery travels posterolaterally to the left behind the pulmonary artery and divides (usually within 10 mm) into two main branches, the left anterior descending (LAD) coronary artery and the left circumflex coronary artery.

The LAD coronary artery emerges from behind the pulmonary artery to course anteriorly within the interventricular groove down to the cardiac apex, sometimes wrapping around it onto the posterior interventricular groove. The initial branches of the LAD coronary artery are usually the first diagonal, which takes off at an acute angle and runs over the anterolateral surface of the left ventricle, and the first septal perforator, which emerges at a right angle from the LAD artery and penetrates the interventricular septum. The continuation of the LAD artery may give off several more diagonal and septal branches. By means of this arborization, the LAD

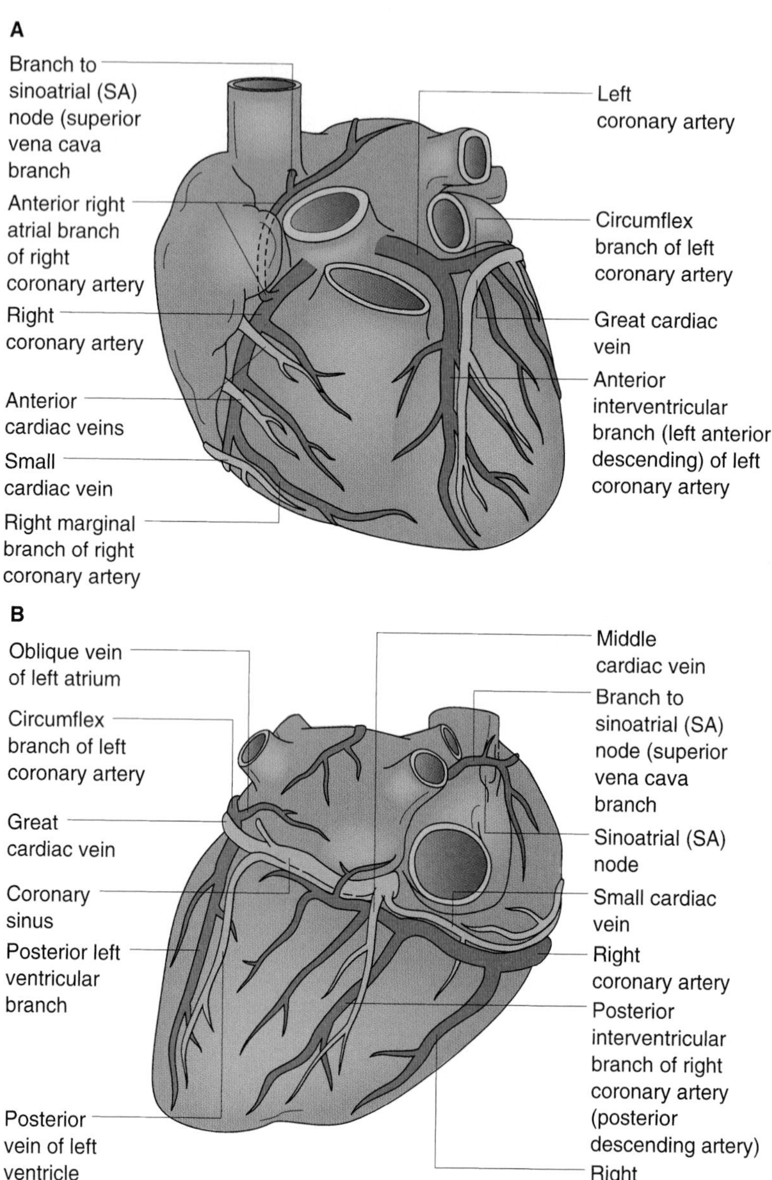

FIGURE 85.1 Anatomy of the coronary arteries and cardiac veins. (*A*) Anterior view. The origin of the left main coronary artery is left lateral and somewhat posterior with respect to the aorta; it courses behind the pulmonary artery and then divides into the left anterior descending and circumflex coronary arteries. The origin of the right coronary artery is almost directly anterior, and it runs in the atrioventricular groove. (*B*) Posterior view. The great, middle, and small cardiac veins all come together at the level of the coronary sinus, which lies in the left inferior atrioventricular groove and empties into the right atrium.

artery nourishes the anterior, anterolateral, septal, and apical walls of the left ventricle.

The circumflex coronary artery descends posteriorly from the left main coronary and runs within the posterior atrioventricular groove. In about 80% to 85% of persons, it terminates with branches to the posterolateral wall of the left ventricle. In the remainder, it extends to the crux of the heart and gives off the posterior descending artery (PDA), which runs in the posterior interventricular groove. The usual branches of the circumflex are referred to as *obtuse marginal branches* because they cover myocardium where, as seen in the left anterior oblique projection, the lateral wall and posterior wall of the heart form an angle of more than 90 degrees.

The right coronary artery descends in the right atrioventricular groove to the crux, where in 80% to 85% of cases it gives off the PDA, occasionally continuing and terminating as posterior left ventricular branches. The right ventricular free wall is fed by acute marginal branches from the right coronary artery, which feed the heart where (as seen in the left anterior oblique projection) it forms an angle of less than 90 degrees as it turns onto the diaphragm.

Whichever artery is responsible for supplying the PDA (i.e., the right coronary or left circumflex artery) determines whether the coronary circulation is *right dominant* or *left dominant*. The PDA gives off the atrioventricular nodal artery, and occlusion of this artery can result in heart block.

Cardiac Veins

The following three venous systems drain the coronary circulation:

1. The coronary sinus, located in the posterior atrioventricular groove, receives blood from the great, middle, and small cardiac veins and from the posterior veins of the left ventricle. It empties into the right atrium. The great cardiac vein ascends along the LAD artery in the interventricular groove and then turns posteriorly to follow the circumflex coronary artery to empty into the coronary sinus. The middle

cardiac vein returns from the apex along the posterior interventricular groove, and the small cardiac vein follows the right coronary artery. Both these veins empty at the level of the crux into the coronary sinus.

2. The thebesian veins are tiny venous orifices that drain the myocardium, emptying directly into any of the four chambers of the heart.
3. The anterior cardiac veins drain the right ventricular coronary system, traversing the right ventricular free wall and crossing the atrioventricular groove to empty directly into the right atrium or a correlating vein at its base.

Coronary Blood Flow

Perfusion of any organ provides oxygen and nutrients to support function. Every minute, the heart uses about 8 to 10 mL of oxygen per 100 g of myocardium. Given the fact that myocardial blood flow is 70 to 90 mL/min per 100 g and oxygen delivery is about 14 to 18 mL/min, myocardial oxygen extraction is high, and the oxygen content in the coronary sinus is only 4 to 6 mL/100 mL of blood. This corresponds to an oxygen pressure of about 20 mm Hg and a hemoglobin saturation of about 30%. Therefore, even at rest, the heart extracts oxygen maximally, and increased oxygen demand cannot be met by increased oxygen extraction. Rather, the coronary circulation has the ability to increase blood flow dramatically and must meet increased oxygen needs by increasing delivery.[1]

Physical Regulation

Under the usual circumstances, perfusion pressure determines blood flow. Because most myocardial blood flow occurs in diastole, as diastolic pressure increases, so does myocardial perfusion. Excessive elevation in diastolic pressure secondarily causes coronary vasoconstriction, which prevents unnecessary blood flow. Conversely, at low diastolic pressures, the coronary arteries dilate to decrease vascular resistance and increase flow. Coronary flow may decrease as a result of coronary spasm, intramural clot, or coronary atherosclerosis. In general, clinically significant obstruction that limits flow occurs only with more than a two-thirds reduction in luminal diameter.

During systole, increased cavitary pressure compresses intramyocardial vessels and virtually eliminates forward flow. As mentioned, myocardial perfusion, particularly of the left ventricle, occurs during diastole, so that myocardial blood flow depends on coronary arterial patency, diastolic pressure, and length of diastole. That is why tachycardia, for example, can lead to ischemia, not only by increasing oxygen demand but also by limiting perfusion time.

Metabolic Regulation

The autoregulatory ability of the coronary circulation produces an increase in blood supply proportional to any increment in myocardial oxygen requirements. The most important metabolic regulator of this phenomenon is adenosine, a potent vasodilator. Adenosine is a breakdown product of adenosine triphosphate, a crucial high-energy phosphate metabolic intermediate.[2] Increased myocardial oxygen demands increase adenosine triphosphate metabolism and directly cause an increase in adenosine concentration. This results in coronary vasodilation and increased oxygen delivery.

In general, prostaglandins produce decreases in coronary vascular resistance, but only thromboxane A_2 is thought to play a major role as a coronary vasoconstrictor. Thromboxane A_2 is released by platelets, particularly in the setting of angina and myocardial infarction (MI).[3]

Stimulation of the cardiac sympathetic nerves directly constricts the coronary arteries. This effect is usually overwhelmed by the autoregulatory vasodilator response to increased myocardial oxygen demand caused by sympathetic stimulation. Although acetylcholine, which is released by parasympathetic or vagal stimulation, produces coronary vasodilation directly, it lowers the heart rate and decreases contractility, so that oxygen requirements are diminished and vasoconstriction results.

CORONARY ATHEROSCLEROSIS

The Lesion

Although atherosclerotic plaques are not uniform within a person or throughout a population, certain common characteristics can be identified. In all cases, atherosclerosis represents a combination of smooth muscle cell proliferation, formation by the smooth muscle cells of tissue matrix consisting of collagen, elastin, and proteoglycans, and the accumulation of intracellular and extracellular lipid. The lesions characteristically occur within the intima, the innermost wall of the artery, and progress from benign "fatty-streak" lesions to complicated plaques.

As early as childhood, fatty-streak lesions consisting of lipid-laden macrophages and smooth muscle cells may line the arterial intima (Fig. 85.2). This process may occur in the aorta during the first decade of life, but coronary arterial lesions generally do not appear until the second or third decade of life. Fatty streaks are nonobstructive and frequently progress no further. In populations at risk, however, a whitish fibrous plaque may then develop. These lesions protrude into the arterial lumen and may obstruct. The subintimal proliferation of smooth muscle cells is the factor most responsible for such protrusion. The fibrous surface of the lesion is the result of the buildup of connective tissue matrix and intracellular and extracellular lipid.

The advanced, complicated lesion develops from an aging fibrous plaque. The necrotic core of the plaque may enlarge and become calcified. Hemorrhage into the plaque can disrupt the smooth, fibrous surface, with resulting ulcerations that are thrombogenic. The organization of clot on the plaque surface increases the degree of protrusion into the arterial lumen and further decreases flow.

Risk Factors

Although the characteristics, locations, and severity of lesions in each person can vary, a number of established risk factors appear to predispose to atherosclerosis.[4] These include advanced age, genetic predisposition, male sex, hypertension, diabetes mellitus, hyperlipidemia, and cigarette smoking. The presence of one risk factor increases the likelihood that the disease will develop at an earlier age, and the presence of more than one risk factor accelerates the process even further.

The association of aging with the development of atherosclerotic coronary disease is complex; many of the other risk factors, such as hypertension, hyperglycemia, and hyperlipidemia, are also associated with aging. Genetic factors play a major role, with direct effects on vascular endothelial biology and arterial wall structure. Indirectly, genetic factors predispose patients to risk factors with a genetic basis, such as hypertension, hyperlipidemia, and diabetes. It was once accepted dogma that male sex was a well-documented major risk for the development of coronary disease. Recently, it has become increasingly apparent that coronary artery disease is an equally important health problem in women. Historically, however, ischemic heart disease has been underdiagnosed and less aggressively treated in women. Consequently, women often face higher risks of death and disability from MI than do men.

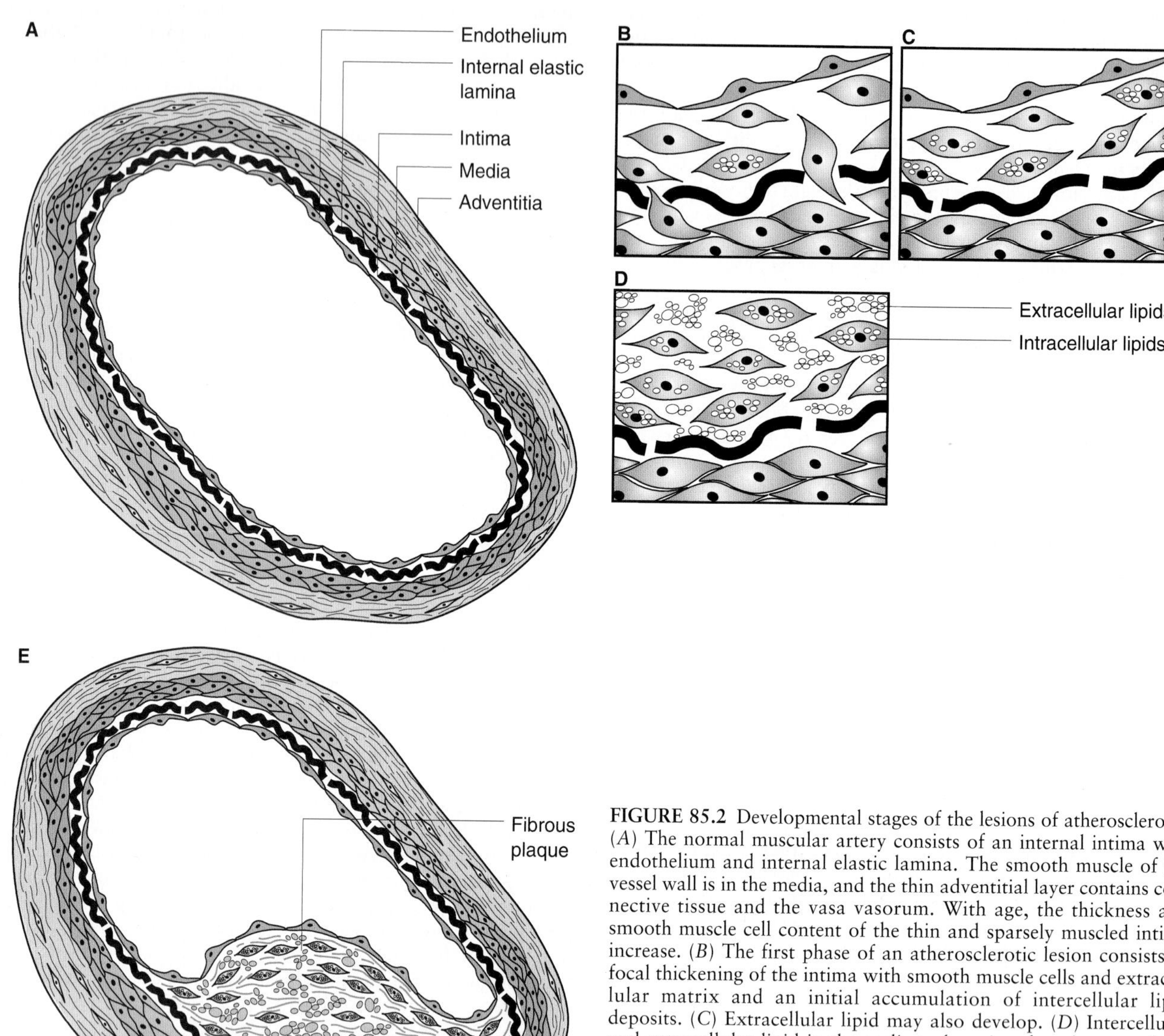

FIGURE 85.2 Developmental stages of the lesions of atherosclerosis. (*A*) The normal muscular artery consists of an internal intima with endothelium and internal elastic lamina. The smooth muscle of the vessel wall is in the media, and the thin adventitial layer contains connective tissue and the vasa vasorum. With age, the thickness and smooth muscle cell content of the thin and sparsely muscled intima increase. (*B*) The first phase of an atherosclerotic lesion consists of focal thickening of the intima with smooth muscle cells and extracellular matrix and an initial accumulation of intercellular lipid deposits. (*C*) Extracellular lipid may also develop. (*D*) Intercellular and extracellular lipid in the earliest phase is referred to as a fatty streak. (*E*) A fibrous plaque results as fibroblasts that cover the proliferating smooth muscle cells laden with lipids and cell debris continue to accumulate. The lesion becomes more complex as continuing cell degeneration leads to an ingress of blood constituents and calcification. (After Glomset JA, Ross R. Atherosclerosis and the arterial smooth-muscle cells. *Science* 1973;180:1332, with permission.)

Hypertension

Although the mechanism is uncertain, high blood pressure exerts a profound influence on the development of ischemic heart disease. It has been suggested that an increase in shear stress at particular vessel locations may alter the vascular endothelium such that it is predisposed to fatty deposition and the development of plaque. The risk for coronary artery disease increases with increasing blood pressure; in middle-aged men with blood pressures higher than 160/95 mm Hg, the incidence of coronary disease is five times greater than in normotensive men. Control of hypertension decreases this risk, with the greatest benefit seen in patients whose diastolic blood pressure exceeds 105 mm Hg before treatment.

Diabetes Mellitus

A clear association is seen between diabetes mellitus and atherosclerosis. In both insulin-dependent and non–insulin-dependent diabetic patients, the risk for coronary artery disease is at least doubled, and the risk is even higher in patients with juvenile-onset diabetes and in diabetic women. Unfortunately, although hyperglycemia and atherosclerosis are strongly linked, rigorous control of elevated blood glucose concentrations by insulin does not appear to affect coronary mortality.

Hyperlipidemia

Both hypercholesterolemia and hypertriglyceridemia are important risk factors for coronary artery disease. The Lipid Research Clinics Trial[5] demonstrated a direct association between plasma lipoprotein levels, cholesterol levels, and morbidity and mortality from coronary artery disease. Furthermore, the risk in treated patients was decreased in direct proportion to the degree of cholesterol lowering. Hypertriglyceridemia appears to affect the incidence of coronary artery disease specifically in patients with familial combined hyperlipidemia, and accentuates the risk in diabetics and smokers.

High-density lipoproteins (HDL) contain about 20% of total plasma cholesterol. The HDL level is inversely proportional to the risk for the development of coronary artery disease. HDL levels are about 25% higher in women than in men, are raised by exercise and estrogens, and are decreased by androgens and cigarette smoking. High HDL levels offer some protection against the development of coronary artery disease.

Cigarette Smoking

Cigarette smoking is one of the most important risk factors for coronary artery disease. Smoking clearly accelerates the disease process, and smoking cessation clearly decreases the risk. In men who smoke one pack of cigarettes per day, the death rate from coronary artery disease is 70% higher and the incidence of the disease is three to five times greater than in nonsmokers. Cigarette smoking appears to potentiate other risk factors, such as hypertension and diabetes mellitus.

Prevention

Angina pectoris and MI are late manifestations of coronary artery disease. Because atherosclerosis, as evidenced by fatty streaks and early complicated lesions, has been found in men as early as the second decade of life, primary prevention of this disease must begin early. The importance of understanding the risk factors for coronary disease and eliminating or modifying those that can be controlled cannot be overemphasized.

Clinical Presentation

The clinical manifestations of ischemic heart disease result from an imbalance between coronary arterial blood flow and the capacity of the blood to transport oxygen (supply), and myocardial oxygen demands. Atherosclerotic disease directly compromises coronary blood flow. When significant coronary obstructive disease is present, any of the three interrelated ischemic clinical syndromes can result—angina pectoris, MI, and ischemic cardiomyopathy.

The clinical presentation of coronary artery disease can take many forms. As many as 25% of patients who have positive results on exercise testing because of coronary occlusive disease have no clinical symptoms of typical angina pectoris. Similarly, some acute MIs are silent; patients may have electrocardiographic (ECG) or other evidence of past myocardial injury but no prior history of a clinical syndrome consistent with MI. In some patients, sudden death is the first and only manifestation of ischemic heart disease.

In another subset of patients without typical symptoms, progressive heart failure develops. Evaluation may show a diffuse loss of ventricular function associated with significant coronary obstruction. This entity is often referred to as *ischemic cardiomyopathy.* Patients who have had multiple symptomatic MIs and progress to severe heart failure resulting from the loss of ventricular muscle can be said to have ischemic cardiomyopathy.

Symptoms of Coronary Artery Disease

Symptomatic angina pectoris is the classic presentation of coronary artery disease. The typical description of angina is pressure or heaviness felt in the middle of the chest, sometimes radiating to the left shoulder and down the left arm. Patients typically clench their fists in the middle of the chest as they describe this discomfort. Other, less typical syndromes may signal the presence of significant coronary obstruction and myocardial ischemia. Patients may complain of abdominal pain, nausea, or belching or feel only vague anxiety or feelings of doom. These kind of symptoms may be more typical of those experienced by women with coronary artery disease. Other symptoms include back pain or pain in one or both shoulders, jaw pain, or hand heaviness or numbness. Stable angina pectoris is brought on by reproducible increases in myocardial demand for oxygen. Patients report that certain levels of activity, emotional stress, or excitement can trigger angina, which is subsequently relieved by rest or relaxation.

The clinical presentations of patients with angina pectoris, therefore, vary considerably. The diagnosis of myocardial ischemia is suggested by the presence of angina pectoris but requires documentation of ECG changes of ischemia during chest pain or during exercise testing (Fig. 85.3). The differential diagnosis of angina includes esophagitis secondary to gastrointestinal reflux, peptic ulcer disease, biliary colic, visceral arterial ischemia, pericarditis, pleurisy, thoracic aortic dissection, and many musculoskeletal disorders. Furthermore, so-called angina equivalents develop in some patients with the onset of myocardial ischemia. These include shortness of breath caused by sudden reductions in ventricular contractility and compliance. Other patients have episodes of silent or

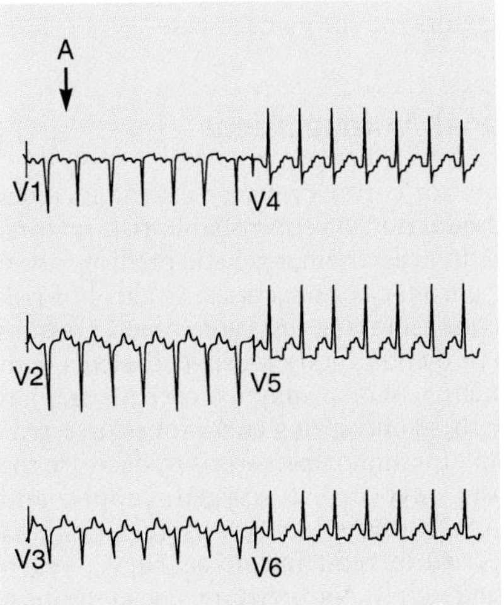

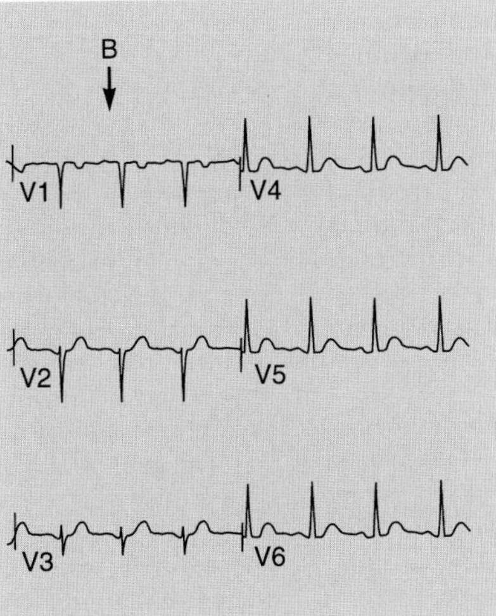

FIGURE 85.3 Electrocardiogram from a 60-year-old man during an exercise test showing the standard precordial leads, V_1 through V_6. (*A*) During exercise, depression of the ST segment and ischemia are seen in leads V_4 through V_6. (*B*) These resolve after exercise is stopped. (After Wagner GS. Ischemia due to increased myocardial demand. In: *Marriott's practical electrocardiography,* 9th ed. Baltimore: Williams & Wilkins, 1994, with permission.)

asymptomatic myocardial ischemia, documented only by continuous ECG monitoring.

In unstable angina, today frequently classified as one of the acute coronary syndromes (ACSs), these symptoms may occur at rest or when the patient is sleeping, and myocardial ischemia typically develops without demonstrable changes in myocardial oxygen demand. In these cases, the *supply* of blood to the myocardium may be so marginal that spontaneous coronary reactivity alone may lead to symptoms. The term *unstable angina* also is applied to patients with new-onset angina pectoris or a marked increase in the frequency or severity of episodes of angina pectoris after a stable period.

A less typical form of angina is Prinzmetal's or variant angina. This type of angina occurs at rest or during sleep. It is thought to result from coronary arterial spasm. Such spasm may be mediated by the autonomic nervous system or by local vasoconstrictive agents. It may also result from smooth muscle irritation or contraction caused by adjacent plaques. Spasm is almost always associated with underlying fixed atherosclerotic disease. Patients may have ST-segment elevation, rather than the more typical ST-segment depression that occurs during episodes of classic angina.

Physicians often grade angina according to the Canadian Heart Association scheme. Class I patients do not have symptoms. Class II patients have angina on significant exertion. Class III patients have angina on mild exertion, and class IV patients have symptoms at rest. A similar classification from the New York Heart Association is used to describe the severity of heart failure. Patients in New York Heart Association class I have no symptoms of heart failure. Class II patients have symptoms on significant exertion. Class III patients have symptoms on mild exertion, such as during normal daily activities, and class IV patients have symptoms at rest.

Physical Examination Findings

Usually, no signs of coronary artery disease are detected during the physical examination, but evidence of associated conditions may be found. Peripheral vascular disease may be manifested by a loss of pulses or the presence of bruits in the carotid arteries, abdomen, or femoral arteries. Other signs, such as ocular xanthomas or hypertensive retinal changes, may provide corroborative evidence in patients at risk for coronary disease.

Diagnostic Studies

Laboratory studies may be useful for detecting cardiac risk factors, such as diabetes mellitus, hyperlipidemia, or hyperthyroidism. In addition, several markers have been identified as helpful in identifying patients at risk for the development of coronary artery disease. These include serum homocysteine and C-reactive protein (CRP) levels. Hyperhomocysteinemia has been found to be an independent risk factor for cardiovascular disease. Elevated levels of CRP, a nonspecific marker of systemic inflammation, may also identify patients with increased risk of developing ischemic heart disease. Anemia in the presence of subcritical or borderline coronary obstruction may precipitate angina; myocardial ischemia results from the reduced oxygen-carrying capacity of blood.

The ECG pattern is frequently normal but may reveal evidence of old MI. Typically, these changes include Q waves or loss of R-wave progression in the precordial leads. Chronic ST-segment and T-wave changes may be suggestive of underlying coronary disease but are not specific.

Stress testing may be useful for detecting the presence of coronary disease or assessing the functional significance of coronary lesions. In the standard test, a patient undergoes graded exercises on a treadmill with ECG monitoring. If signs or symptoms of angina pectoris develop in association with typical ischemic ECG changes, the test result is considered positive. The most diagnostic ECG changes are downward sloping ST-segment depressions. The accuracy of the test is reduced when the patient has underlying ECG abnormalities. Specificity may be improved if the test is combined with the administration of thallium. Thallium is a radioactive isotope that is distributed intracellularly, like potassium. When thallium is injected during exercise, if coronary ischemia develops, the involved area of myocardium fails to take up thallium and a defect is apparent on a myocardial scan. As the patient recovers from exercise and the ischemia is relieved, the previous defect fills in. In patients who cannot exercise, thallium imaging can be performed after the administration of dipyridamole. Dipyridamole, a coronary vasodilator, may reveal areas of relative underperfusion, and a thallium defect appears on scanning, as with exercise testing. When exercise or the administration of dipyridamole is considered unsafe, a rest–redistribution thallium myocardial scan may reveal evidence of borderline regional myocardial perfusion. In this test, scanning is performed early after injection with thallium and again several hours later. A defect noted on the early scan that fills in later is considered a sign of significant coronary obstruction. A defect that never fills in on thallium scanning is a sign of irreversibly scarred, nonviable myocardium.

Coronary arteriography, which is an invasive diagnostic procedure, is the only way to make a definitive diagnosis of significant coronary obstruction. Coronary arteriography is indicated for patients with atypical presentations and borderline or normal stress test results in whom a definitive diagnosis of coronary artery disease is needed. When classic anginal symptoms and ECG changes make the diagnosis of coronary disease fairly certain, patients should undergo coronary angiography if they are refractory to medical therapy or are candidates for revascularization. Regardless of symptoms, patients suspected of having severe coronary artery disease, such as stenosis of the left main coronary artery or severe proximal three-vessel coronary disease, should undergo coronary arteriography to document their condition because of the survival benefits that accrue with revascularization. Diagnostic coronary arteriography is also indicated when cardiac surgery is being planned for patients with other cardiac disease, such as valvular heart disease, in whom concomitant coronary disease is suspected. Examples include patients with aortic stenosis who have angina as part of the presentation. Patients with valvular heart disease who do not have angina but nonetheless have risk factors for coronary disease should also undergo angiography before surgery. These include men older than 45 to 50 years with one or more risk factors for coronary disease.

Medical Management

The medical management of coronary artery disease includes the identification and reduction of controllable risk factors. Obviously, patients can do little about a genetic predisposition for the development of coronary obstructions. Control of risk factors by weight reduction, smoking cessation, blood pressure control, and limitation of dietary fats is sensible. Patients with hyperthyroidism or anemia, which may exacerbate anginal symptoms, should have these underlying conditions corrected.

The goal of all therapy for angina pectoris is to decrease the imbalance between the myocardial oxygen supply and demand. Most of the medications that are useful in angina pectoris are more effective in reducing myocardial oxygen demand than in increasing supply. *Nitroglycerin,* one of the most commonly used agents, primarily dilates venous capacitance vessels, but, at higher doses, it may also cause systemic arterial dilation. Although nitrate compounds do not appear to increase coronary blood flow in the normal heart, these drugs may dilate the coronary arterioles to some extent, so that coronary collateral blood flow improves in patients with extensive atherosclerotic obstructive disease. The primary benefit of nitrates, however, appears to be that they reduce myocardial oxygen demand by reducing ventricular work. This is the consequence of a reduction in systemic vascular resistance and dilation of venous capacitance vessels, which lowers ventricular filling pressures, ventricular wall stress or tension, and contractile work.

Beta adrenergic blockers also reduce myocardial oxygen demand by decreasing both cardiac contractility and heart rate. These agents may also reduce blood pressure and systemic vascular resistance, and so further reduce the work of the heart. *Calcium channel blockers,* such as nicardipine and diltiazem, have more complex cardiac and vascular effects; these include a reduction in ventricular contractility, variable degrees of vasodilation, and possibly a direct protection of myocytes when these cells become hypoxic. Calcium channel blockers may be particularly effective in patients with a component of coronary vasospastic disease. *Angiotensin-converting enzyme (ACE) inhibitors* decrease systemic vascular resistance or impedance to left ventricular outflow by blocking the conversion of angiotensin I to angiotensin II (a potent vasoconstrictor), which decreases both the workload of the heart and myocardial oxygen demand. *Statins* help to control cholesterol levels, especially of low-density lipoprotein (LDL) cholesterol, elevated levels of which are important risk factors for atherosclerosis.

All patients with known coronary artery disease should be taking aspirin. The antiplatelet therapy of aspirin has been found to reduce the risk of subsequent vascular events when administered after a heart attack or other ischemic event and continued on a long-term basis.

ACUTE MYOCARDIAL INFARCTION

Acute MI is the direct result of an interruption in the blood supply to the myocardium. It is not the result of increased myocardial oxygen demand but rather of loss of oxygen supply. It usually occurs after a coronary artery thrombosis at the site of a stenosis of caused by a vulnerable plaque. The stenosis itself may not be severe until the plaque ruptures and clot totally occludes the vessel. Although the acute event associated with MI is thrombosis, studies in which cardiac catheterization was used have shown that about 20% to 30% of culprit coronary arteries are patent again within a few days of infarction. This is more common in nontransmural than in transmural MIs.[6]

One major determinant of the prognosis after acute MI is the amount of ventricular myocardium that undergoes necrosis. For patients with post-MI ejection fractions of more than 50%, the 3-year survival is nearly 90%, but when the ejection fraction falls below 37%, the 3-year survival rate is only 50% (Fig. 85.4). The loss of 25% of the ventricular myocardium leads to symptomatic cardiac dysfunction, whereas the acute loss of more than 40% is frequently associated with cardiogenic shock and death. Efforts to treat patients who are experiencing MI are therefore focused on decreasing myocardial loss by improving flow to the area at risk as quickly as possible. Interestingly, collateral vessels, when present, may supply enough blood to limit markedly the amount of myocardium lost. Thus, although well-developed collaterals may not prevent demand-induced angina, they may significantly diminish the loss of myocardium after an acute coronary occlusion.

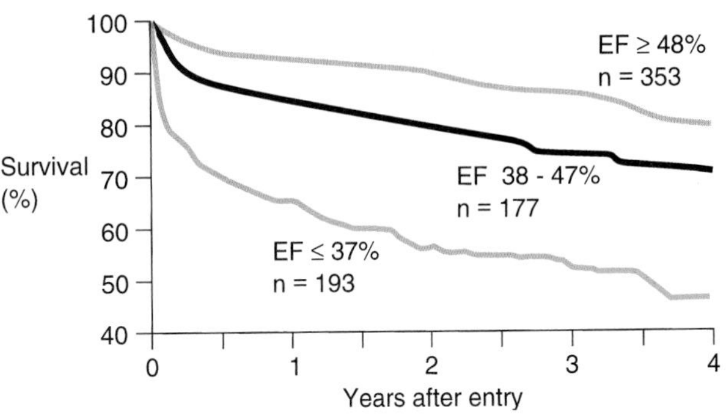

FIGURE 85.4 Survival of patients in the Multicenter Investigation on Limitation of Infarct Size. The probability of survival is reduced in patients with a poor ejection fraction at the time of admission for a myocardial infarction. (After Braunwald E. *Circulation* 1987;76 [suppl II]:406, with permission.)

Presentation

Pain is the most common presenting complaint in patients with MI. It is deep, visceral, and frequently described as heavy or crushing. However, pain is by no means universally present, and 20% to 25% of patients (most often diabetic or elderly patients) do not have symptoms. The combination of substernal chest pain lasting for more than 20 to 30 minutes and diaphoresis is strongly suggestive of MI. Interestingly, anterior MIs (usually involving the LAD coronary artery) result in sympathetic hyperactivity, with tachycardia and hypertension, whereas inferior MIs (involving the right coronary artery) frequently result in parasympathetic activity, with bradycardia and hypotension.

Diagnosis

The classic ECG picture of an acute MI is the development of elevated ST segments (early), and Q waves (late), in leads reflecting the affected area (Fig. 85.5). Clinicians frequently characterize MIs by the associated ECG changes. Transmural infarctions usually cause Q waves, whereas subendocardial or nontransmural infarctions are characterized by transient ST-segment changes and evolving T-wave inversion but not the development of Q waves. MIs are frequently referred to by these ECG changes and are called either *Q-wave* (transmural) or *non–Q-wave* (nontransmural or subendocardial) *infarctions.*

At the time of MI, enzymes are released by necrotizing myocytes in large enough quantities to be detected in the serum. As a result, enzyme elevations have become the sine qua non of the diagnosis of MI: specifically, serum levels of creatine kinase and troponin. Creatine kinase, a cardiac enzyme involved in high-energy phosphate metabolism, is increased after myocardial cell death and rises substantially within 8 to 24 hours, returning to normal within 1 to 2 days. Creatine kinase has several tissue-specific isoenzymes; the isoenzyme found specifically in cardiac tissue is denoted as CK-MB. Because creatine kinase is found in brain (CK-BB) and muscle (CK-MM) and can rise significantly after stroke, surgery, cardiac catheterization, or simply an intramuscular injection, it is crucial to measure the specific isoenzyme CK-MB when ruling out MI. Characteristic elevations of CK-MB occur in 95% of patients with clinically proven MI. Cardiac troponin (cTnI or cTnT), a cardiac marker with greater specificity, rises rapidly following myocardial injury. Troponin levels peak at 12 to 24 hours and may remain elevated for over 1 week. Because of their high

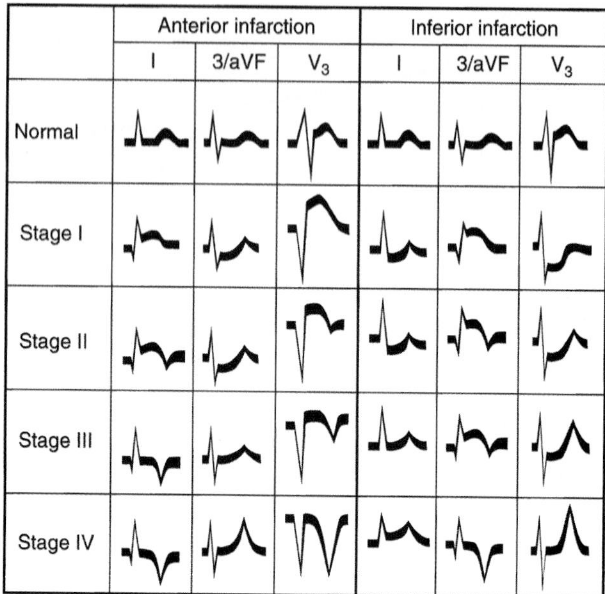

FIGURE 85.5 The pattern of evolution of the electrocardiogram in acute myocardial infarction. In the first stage, acute ST elevations are present in the leads reflecting the affected area of myocardium. Reciprocal ST depressions are seen in leads away from the site of the infarct. In stage 2, T-wave inversion begins, which deepens in stage 3. ST-segment elevations are no longer present. A Q wave may develop early, but Q waves are present by stage 4, and persistent T-wave inversions, which may be deep, are seen. (After Marriott HJL. Myocardial infarction. In: *Practical electrocardiography,* 7th ed. Baltimore: Williams & Wilkins, 1983, p. 379, with permission.)

specificity and early elevation they are a tremendous adjunct to CK-MB in early detection of myocardial injury or ACS.

Medical Management

During the early phase of MI, it may not be clear whether the patient has ACS, a potentially reversible process, or whether the symptoms indicate a process leading to irreversible myocardial injury. The ECG may be unrevealing, and cardiac isoenzymes may be unavailable. In this situation, oxygen should be administered, heart rhythm should be monitored, and lidocaine should be given to prevent ventricular fibrillation if warning arrhythmias occur. *Early evolving MI* is the term used to describe the condition of patients within 4 to 6 hours after the onset of continued chest pain. This state is important to recognize because ischemic myocardium may still be salvaged before irreversible necrosis develops.

The goal of initial treatment should be to control pain, most frequently with intravenous morphine. Reducing anxiety and pain may have a significant therapeutic effect by decreasing myocardial oxygen demand and limiting infarct size. Intravenous nitroglycerin, begun at a low dose of 0.2 mg/kg per minute to prevent the side effects of hypotension and headache, may diminish infarct size, prevent sudden death, and reduce the likelihood of congestive heart failure (CHF).[7] The use of beta-blockers is not uniformly agreed on, although they too have been shown to limit infarct size and decrease early mortality.[8] Hypotension and bradyarrhythmias occur more frequently with beta-blockers than with intravenous nitroglycerin. Giving them to patients with acute MI who have increased sympathetic tone, however, is probably a safe and beneficial practice. Unlike beta-blockers, calcium channel blockers are of little benefit in the setting of acute MI.[9]

Thrombolytic agents convert plasminogen to plasmin, a powerful thrombolysin. It was hypothesized that administration of thrombolytic agents would lead to the dissolution of coronary thrombi and reverse the process that leads to MI. In the late 1970s, a European trial of one thrombolytic agent, streptokinase, revealed a significant benefit when the drug was given within 12 hours of acute MI.[10] Thrombolytic trials in the 1980s involving thousands of patients established the benefit of this approach, showing that thrombolysis reopens acutely occluded coronary arteries in most cases, restoring flow and reducing mortality.[11]

Three intravenous thrombolytic agents have been approved by the Food and Drug Administration: streptokinase, recombinant tissue-type plasminogen activator (rTPA), and anisoylated plasminogen streptokinase activator complex (APSAC). The most widely used is streptokinase, which has been effective in several large trials[12] and is inexpensive. APSAC was developed to enable treating physicians to administer intravenous therapy as a bolus within a few minutes, with the effect maintained for a few hours, rather than as a continuous intravenous infusion, which is necessary with streptokinase and rTPA. However, results are not significantly better than with the other two drugs; furthermore, APSAC is expensive, and its prolonged half-life and thrombolytic effect can be a significant drawback rather than a benefit. Recombinant DNA techniques are used to produce rTPA, which is significantly more expensive than streptokinase. Although it generates less of a systemic fibrinolytic effect than either streptokinase or APSAC, its patency rates are higher.[13]

Systemic intravenous thrombolytic therapy unquestionably decreases morbidity and mortality after MI. The earlier the treatment, the greater the impact, with the greatest benefit accruing in patients treated within 1 to 2 hours after the onset of symptoms.[14] Furthermore, morbidity is decreased secondary to a reduction in arrhythmias and failure of ventricular power. Heparin and antiplatelet drugs such as aspirin provide an added benefit when combined with thrombolytic therapy, particularly in the case of rTPA, which has a short half-life and little antithrombin effect because it does not generate excessive amounts of fibrin degradation products.

Hemorrhage is a major problem with all lytic agents, commonly developing at a site of vascular access. Stroke occurs in fewer than 1% of patients but may be catastrophic because of its hemorrhagic nature. Bleeding and stroke occur most frequently in elderly, female, hypertensive, and small patients. This strategy is becoming less common as the already wide availability of emergency percutaneous transluminal coronary angioplasty (PTCA) continues to grow.

More commonly patients with myocardium in jeopardy are placed on glycoprotein IIb/IIIa inhibitors, which affect ADP-mediated platelet adhesion, and are typically required for catheter-based interventional procedures. There are three groups of IIb/IIIa inhibitors: reversible, nonreversible, and monoclonal antibodies. The half-life of the reversible inhibitors, eptifibatide (Integrillin) and tirofiban (Aggrastat), is approximately 8 hours. In this setting, these shorter-acting agents are preferable given the possibility of the need for emergency surgical revascularization. Ticlidopine (Ticlid) and clopidogrel (Plavix) bind irreversibly to platelets and last for the lifetime of the platelets. For this reason, surgical intervention may have to be delayed for 3 to 5 days due to the potential for bleeding complications related to platelet inhibition. Abciximab (ReoPro) is a Fab antibody fragment that binds to the IIb/IIIa receptor inhibiting platelet adhesion with a half-life of 30 minutes.

Bivalirudin (Angiomax) is a direct and reversible thrombin inhibitor also used in the acute setting of MI. It is primarily used in the setting of PTCA, but it has been used for systemic anticoagulation for surgical intervention in patients with heparin allergies. Coagulation returns to near baseline an hour following discontinuation of the infusion. This drug is currently being examined as a superior alternative to standard heparin protocols for PTCA.

Indications for Mechanical Intervention

The use of thrombolytic therapy with early recanalization of the culprit vessel responsible for the MI has had a tremendous impact on the treatment and prognosis of patients experiencing acute MI. The issue then becomes whether anything more need be done acutely; despite reperfusion, significant residual stenoses remain. The Thrombolysis in Myocardial Infarction phase II trial compared elective catheterization and PTCA within the first 2 days of lytic therapy for MI versus cardiac catheterization and PTCA only if ischemia developed later in the hospital course.[15] The more invasive approach failed to provide a benefit with respect to early or late mortality and, in fact, increased risk significantly. Based on the results of this and other trials, cardiac catheterization and PTCA should be withheld in most patients who have no symptoms after thrombolytic therapy for an acute MI. A more invasive approach is justified in patients who exhibit residual ischemia during their hospital stay, either during convalescence or at a predischarge exercise stress test. PTCA may be appropriate, but if cardiac catheterization shows coronary artery disease in multiple vessels or anatomy more suitable for bypass than for PTCA, surgery should be carried out. The early and long-term results in patients operated on within 30 days of acute MI are excellent.[16]

In centers where emergency intervention is available, patients who present to the emergency room with a diagnosis of early evolving MI can be brought immediately to the catheterization laboratory for intervention in the culprit vessel. American College of Cardiology (ACC) target guidelines currently call for a maximum of 90 minutes for "door to reperfusion time." Abciximab or other antiplatelet agent is usually started in the emergency room and continued through catheterization. In most cases, the occluded vessel can be reopened and an intracoronary stent deployed rapidly, thus allowing for maximal preservation of threatened myocardium.

Postinfarction Angina

Chest pain recurs in 10% to 15% of patients after acute MI, a frequency that increases dramatically if thrombolytic therapy is used. In that situation, the incidence of angina after MI may be as high as 30% to 35%. Postinfarction angina is an indication that myocardial cells are ischemic, and it often occurs when a patient is at rest. This generally indicates that residual myocardial tissue at risk for infarct extension, a complication that can and should be avoided. After MI, the mortality rate may increase by 15% to as much as 40% if infarct extension occurs.[17] In fact, infarct extension may be the most powerful predictor of mortality after MI; the average 1-year mortality increases from about 18% to 65% if infarct extension occurs. Thus, postinfarction angina is an indication for cardiac catheterization, with mechanical intervention, such as PTCA or coronary bypass surgery, if indicated. This is particularly relevant because the mortality rate associated with coronary bypass surgery after MI is extremely low, less than 4% in most advanced centers.[16]

Cardiogenic Shock

The development of cardiogenic shock after MI is uncommon. In the multicenter investigation for the limitation of infarct size, cardiogenic shock developed in only 60 of 845 patients with acute MI.[18] That group had a 65% mortality rate, whereas in the group in which shock did not develop, the mortality rate was only 4%. Infarct extension occurred in 23% of the shock group, and in 7% of the group without shock. More importantly, in 50% of affected patients, shock developed more than 24 hours after admission. Evaluation of these patients revealed that age above 65 years, ejection fraction below 35% on admission, a large MI as indicated by the magnitude of the CK-MB leak, a history of diabetes mellitus, and a history of previous MI are all risk factors for the development of shock. When three of these risk factors were present, the in-hospital mortality rate was 18%; when all five risk factors were present, the in-hospital mortality rate was 55%.[18]

Animal studies have shown that even in the face of prolonged regional myocardial ischemia, intervention with emergency revascularization may decrease the amount of damage sustained by the myocardium. These studies have focused on ways to decrease energy expenditure during early reperfusion and ways to tailor the initial reperfusate so as to decrease cellular swelling, provide intermediary cellular metabolic substrates, and decrease oxidant injury. In this way, myocardial damage resulting from an ischemic insult can be drastically reduced.[19] A prospective study has evaluated the effect on mortality of emergency coronary bypass surgery in patients in cardiogenic shock after MI.[20] Emergency coronary bypass was performed on 80 consecutive patients in cardiogenic shock who were being maintained on vasopressors and intraaortic balloon pumps (IABPs) after MI. When surgery was performed within 18 hours of the onset of shock, the mortality rate was 7%; when surgery was performed after 18 hours, the mortality rate was 31%. This represents a definite improvement over the results of medical therapy (65% mortality) for this severe complication of MI. In centers capable of performing surgery of this kind, it may be the ideal approach to patients in shock after MI. These results, which have not been duplicated by other institutions, must be viewed as preliminary.

Ventricular Septal Defect

Ventricular septal defects (rupture) occur in about 2% of patients after MI and are becoming increasingly rare as interventional techniques continue to improve. In general, this complication develops at a time when the myocardium is at its weakest, about 7 to 10 days after MI. It is more common in anterior than in posterior MIs, and with medical treatment alone the associated mortality rate is more than 90%. At greatest risk for the development of this complication are elderly hypertensive women with transmural infarction. Clinically, hypotension develops with CHF. Emergency cardiac catheterization reveals an oxygen step-up in the right ventricle, indicating a left-to-right shunt. Echocardiography can clearly document the lesion and is the early diagnostic tool of choice. Medical therapy involves decreasing the afterload as much as possible; an IABP is invariably used, in addition to vasodilator therapy if possible. The preload is optimized, and surgery should be performed immediately. Previous approaches involved the stabilization of patients for a prolonged period in the hope that the infarcted area of myocardium would become firmer and hold sutures better. During the 3 weeks that were generally allowed for this process, however, irreversible failure of multiple organ systems frequently developed as a result of shock and sepsis.

When these patients present with signs and symptoms of rapid onset of CHF and early cardiogenic shock several days after acute MI, physical examination reveals a loud holosystolic murmur. An echocardiogram should be obtained immediately to establish the diagnosis. Once the diagnosis of septal rupture is made, an IABP should be inserted promptly. Intubation may be required. During this time, hemodynamic and metabolic resuscitation should be undertaken. The patient is then brought directly to the operating room and the lesion is repaired. Early operation before end-organ complications occur carries a much better survival rate than medical therapy alone. In most studies, hospital mortality ranges from 26% to 50%. Surgical opinion clearly favors early intervention for this complication.[21]

Acute Mitral Regurgitation

Papillary muscle rupture with acute mitral regurgitation also occurs infrequently, in fewer than 2% of patients. Like ventricular septal defect, it develops between the third and fifth days, when infarcted myocardium is at its weakest. Posteroinferior MIs lead to this complication more frequently than anterior infarctions, almost certainly because the circumflex artery and PDA provide the most crucial blood supply to the papillary muscles. Clinically, this complication can present with signs and symptoms similar to those of a ventricular septal defect. A new murmur and symptoms of CHF with hypotension develop. The pulmonary capillary wedge pressure tracing, however, shows prominent V waves, and no right ventricular oxygen step-up occurs. Immediate medical therapy involves decreasing the afterload with an IABP. Surgery, although it poses an added risk, leads to a better survival than continued medical therapy and decreases the mortality from more than 90% to less than 50%. Evidence has shown that, if total mitral valve excision can be avoided and all or part of the subvalvular mitral apparatus saved, the mortality rate can be decreased even further, from 20% with mitral valve replacement to 5% if the mitral valve apparatus is preserved with either repair or replacement. Long-term survival is also improved. In one series, the 4-year survival rate was 89% in the group of patients in whom the mitral apparatus was conserved; it was 59% in the group of patients who underwent mitral valve replacement with total excision of the native valve.[22]

Free Wall Rupture

Ventricular free wall rupture after MI occurs also at a time when the myocardium is at its weakest, between the third and sixth days after infarction. The incidence is not well known, but the medical mortality rate is exceedingly high (>90%). The benefits of surgical intervention are undocumented. A variety of case reports cite the dramatic rescue of some patients, but circumstances must be ideal. The free wall rupture must be small and contained, so that time is available for diagnosis and operative intervention. Most commonly, free wall rupture leads to death. In some cases, it is contained and may go unrecognized until a pseudoaneurysm develops, which is diagnosed at a later date.

MECHANICAL INTERVENTIONS

Catheter-based Coronary Revascularization

PTCA is a cardiac catheterization technique designed to reduce the degree of myocardial obstruction and improve regional coronary blood flow. In 1977 Gruentzig and Hoff designed a balloon dilation catheter for use in the coronary arteries and initiated this important treatment option for patients with ischemic heart disease. PTCA is performed in a standard cardiac catheterization laboratory. The technique is similar to coronary angiography. Under fluoroscopic guidance, a catheter is directed into the coronary artery to be treated. A guide wire is then placed across the obstructing lesion. A balloon catheter is passed over the guide wire and the balloon positioned in the midportion of the obstructing lesion. Under fluoroscopic control, the balloon is inflated to a pressure of 4 to 10 atmospheres for 20 to 60 seconds to reduce the degree of coronary obstruction. Balloon inflation may be repeated several times. It is unclear whether the beneficial effect of this treatment is compression or fracture of the plaque or fracture of the more pliable part of the coronary vessel circumference. After the balloon catheter is withdrawn, coronary angiography is undertaken immediately to assess the degree of dilation and to look for dilation-related complications, such as arterial dissection or acute thrombosis. Since the first successful coronary angioplasty was reported in 1977, the number of PTCA procedures has increased dramatically, to more than 400,000 cases per year in the United States.

In addition to transluminal angioplasty, several other techniques have been developed that can be applied in percutaneous catheter-based systems. These include the placement of intracoronary stents, which are wire mesh cylinders similar in design to the stents placed in other locations, including stenotic major vessels. The systems have been miniaturized so that they can be deployed in the coronary system. The results of initial, nonrandomized studies are encouraging in regard to rates of acute thrombosis and stent failure. Stents appear to be more effective for treating coronary dissections and abrupt vessel closures in the catheterization laboratory. On a long-term basis, the rates of restenosis appear to be lower with stents than with balloon angioplasty. The long-term results of bare or heparin-coated stents are disappointing with patients requiring multiple interventions for restenosis. Drug eluding stents are the latest answer to the problem of in-stent restenosis. These stents are coated with a time-released drug (paclitaxel or sirolimus available in the United States), which prevents cell proliferation and has been shown to decrease the rate of in-stent restenosis at up to 1 year.[23] Thus far, no data exist to support the long-term benefits of these newer devices. Atherectomy devices are useful in severely calcified coronary lesions in which inflation of a balloon is not effective. These are similar to high-speed rotating drill bits and literally drill a hole through obstructed and calcified coronary lesions over a guide wire. Multiple lasers have been developed for use in coronary revascularization. The results have been extremely varied to date, and, as of yet, no laser has been accepted as a standard of care.

Indications

The indications for PTCA are the same as those for coronary artery bypass surgery, the main alternative revascularization technique. Patients with intractable symptoms and those with proximal coronary stenoses that place a large amount of myocardium at risk are potential candidates for angioplasty. The ideal lesion for angioplasty is a symmetric focal stenosis in an epicardial vessel. Long, asymmetric stenoses or those adjacent to bends in the artery or branch points are less likely to be treated successfully. In general, PTCA is contraindicated if significant disease is present in the left main coronary artery, the target coronary artery is less then 2 mm in luminal diameter, multiple significant obstructive lesions are present in the same artery, or the obstructive lesions are complex, such as those involving or straddling arterial bifurcations.

Complications

The primary risk of angioplasty is dissection of the coronary vessel with acute closure. This occurs in about 3% of cases and usually requires emergency coronary bypass surgery.[24] MI may result but can be aborted by immediate surgical revascularization. Other risks are similar to those of coronary angiography and include cerebral vascular accident and local arterial trauma. Improvements in balloon catheter design and fabrication have enhanced the success rate of PTCA and made it possible to achieve more extensive dilation in patients with multiple-vessel or complex coronary artery disease.

Results

Successful primary dilation of favorable coronary arterial obstructive lesions is accomplished in more than 90% of PTCA/stent procedures, with an immediate complication rate of about 3%. The most significant long-term problem with PTCA/stent is the high incidence of restenosis. Restenosis is probably the result of postdilation proliferation of intimal and smooth muscle cells in response to the angioplasty. In-stent restenosis rates of between 20% and 40% within the first 6 months after stenting have been reported in patients with initially successful dilation for simple lesions.[25] Restenosis rates as high as 60% have been reported for patients with complex lesions that required multiple dilations. Although restenting of recurrent stenotic lesions may be carried out successfully, many of these patients ultimately require bypass grafting. As noted, early data from trials with drug eluting stents show improved results at 6 months and 1 year, but long-term data are not yet available.[23]

In the 1990s, several large, randomized trials were completed that compared balloon angioplasty with coronary artery bypass surgery in the treatment of multiple-vessel coronary artery disease.[25–33] As in most large, randomized clinical studies, large numbers of patients were screened, and a relative minority fulfilled the criteria for enrollment. In other words, the final patient cohort was highly selected. Nonetheless, the overall results of half a dozen of these studies in several thousand patients indicate that short- and intermediate-term results for angioplasty and surgery are similar. Mortality rates were the same for the two procedures, although patients treated with angioplasty tended to be discharged from the hospital sooner. Patients who underwent angioplasty also had a higher rates of repeated intervention and crossover to surgical intervention. In several subgroup analyses, patients with diabetes appeared to be treated best with coronary bypass grafting.[30–32] Although initial reports of the use of stents, lasers, and atherectomy devices are encouraging, the results of large, randomized trials are still pending. Furthermore, even in single-vessel disease, including proximal high-grade LAD artery disease, it appears that intervention of some kind, whether revascularization by catheter-based techniques or by coronary artery bypass surgery, improves long-term outcomes.[33]

Coronary Artery Bypass Surgery

Coronary artery bypass grafting (CABG) is among the most commonly applied major surgical operations in the United States, with more than 250,000 procedures performed yearly. The goals of CABG are identical to the goals of medical treatment and PTCA—to treat ischemic heart disease by relieving the imbalance of myocardial oxygen supply and demand. The indications for CABG versus medical treatment or PTCA in an individual patient may be controversial. Choosing the optimal therapy for a given patient necessitates weighing variables, such as the pattern of coronary artery obstruction, ventricular function, severity of symptoms, initial response to medical therapy, and presence of noncardiac disease. Patients require individual evaluation to determine the potential short- and long-term benefits of surgical revascularization versus medical treatment or less invasive angioplasty.[26]

Indications

Patients are said to have *single-*, *double-*, or *triple-vessel* disease if significant atherosclerotic narrowing is present in one, two, or all three of the major arteries (i.e., LAD, circumflex, and right coronary arteries). In general, data from clinical trials and retrospective studies suggest that as the number of diseased major coronary arterial segments increases, the survival benefit of surgical therapy over medical therapy alone becomes greater (Table 85.1). This observation in general terms has been borne out by the three major prospective, randomized coronary bypass studies—the Coronary Artery Surgery Study (CASS),[35] the Veterans Administration Cooperative Study,[51] and a European report[52] (see later). In patients with stable angina, the presence of severe, proximal, triple-vessel disease, especially in those with impaired left ventricular function, generally is an indication for surgical revascularization.

TABLE 85.1 INDICATIONS/CONTRAINDICATIONS

INDICATIONS FOR CORONARY BYPASS SURGERY

ANATOMY
- Left main coronary artery disease
- Triple-vessel disease involving the proximal left anterior descending coronary artery with normal or diminished ejection fraction
- Double-vessel disease involving the proximal left anterior descending coronary artery with normal or diminished ejection fraction

SYMPTOMS
- Unstable (crescendo) angina
- Postmyocardial infarction angina
- Acute coronary occlusion after percutaneous transluminal coronary angioplasty
- Symptoms unsuccessfully controlled with medical therapy
- Controlled symptoms, but with unacceptable lifestyle

Another well-accepted indication for CABG is the presence of significant stenosis of the left main coronary artery.[53] Both the Veterans Administration Cooperative Study[51] and the CASS[35] provide overwhelming evidence for improved survival with surgical treatment in patients with left main artery disease. Most cardiologists and cardiac surgeons also believe a surgical benefit exists for patients with normal or depressed left ventricular function and two-vessel disease associated with a high-grade proximal obstruction of the LAD artery.[52]

Above all, the most common indication for CABG continues to be the relief of disabling angina refractory to medical therapy. Bypass surgery reduces or eliminates angina in more than 90% of patients, and those patients with the most severe anginal syndromes derive the greatest benefit. The randomized studies[35,51,52] have provided strong evidence that CABG is more effective than medical treatment in relieving angina and improving the capacity for physical work and overall quality of life. Finally, the survival of patients with silent ischemia (i.e., patients without symptoms who have significant atherosclerotic disease and myocardial ischemia demonstrated by ECG changes, exercise stress testing, and coronary angiography) is improved after CABG.

Patients with unstable angina are a heterogeneous group. In general, the occurrence of unstable (or crescendo) angina suggests that the patient is at risk for MI and death. These patients require aggressive medical therapy, including nitrates, adrenergic blockers, and calcium antagonists, in addition to heparin anticoagulation to forestall coronary arterial thrombosis. If the patient continues to experience unstable or rest angina despite maximal medical treatment, urgent coronary angiography is indicated in preparation for revascularization.[32] Collective outcome data from several series of patients with unstable angina who underwent surgical revascularization demonstrated increased rates of perioperative MI, postoperative low cardiac output, and death in comparison with patients who underwent CABG for chronic stable angina. Nonetheless, patients with unstable angina had *late* outcomes after CABG similar to those of patients with chronic stable angina; relief of angina was excellent, the late MI rate was low, and, most importantly, long-term survival was similar.

Although the role of CABG in the setting of acute MI is not unequivocal, the development of recurrent angina early after infarction has become an accepted indication for operative intervention. These patients are at risk for infarct extension or for a second infarction. Even mild postinfarction angina mandates an aggressive response, with coronary angiography and consideration of revascularization (see earlier).

As mentioned, emergency CABG is necessary in the approximately 3% of patients in whom coronary occlusive complications develop during PTCA.[24] Most of these occlusions result from coronary dissections proximal or distal to the site of dilation. Emergency CABG is indicated as soon as it is apparent that an acute coronary occlusion has developed, an event heralded by the onset of chest pain, ECG changes, and often hemodynamic instability. It is usually possible to verify the presence and nature of the acute coronary occlusion by immediate repeated coronary angiography, which allows the diagnosis to be confirmed.

In most cases of an evolving MI, the ischemic injury is somewhat attenuated and hemodynamic stability is better if intraaortic balloon counterpulsation is established promptly in the catheterization laboratory before the patient is transported to the operating room. If severe hemodynamic instability develops despite balloon pump support, portable cardiopulmonary bypass perfusion with femoral arterial and venous cannulation may provide sufficient stabilization so that the patient can be transported to the operating room. In general, these patients should be placed on cardiopulmonary bypass as quickly as possible to initiate cardioplegic arrest and myocardial cooling and prevent further extension of the infarction.

Standard Surgical Technique

In coronary artery surgery, the diseased coronary artery is bypassed by creating an alternative conduit to deliver blood beyond the coronary stenosis. Grafts are constructed by making an end-to-side anastomosis to the coronary artery distal to the obstruction. The proximal end of a vein graft is usually sutured end-to-side to the ascending aorta. When the aorta is diseased, the origin of the innominate artery is sometimes used. The vein most commonly used as a graft is the greater saphenous vein, although the lesser saphenous vein is sometimes employed. Today, the greater saphenous vein increasingly is harvested using an endoscopic approach, allowing removal of long segments of vein via a small incision near the knee. This technique has been shown to reduce significantly the incidence of postoperative leg wound infections, markedly reduce postoperative pain, and improve wound healing.[36] The patency rates of endoscopically harvested conduit appear to be similar to that of the open technique. The cephalic vein from the arm is practically never used because its long-term patency is extremely poor. Cryopreserved saphenous vein is the rarely used conduit of last resort because of the high rate of closure.

The use of arterial grafts has increased. The most commonly used arterial graft is the left internal mammary artery (IMA). It is used most often as a pedicle graft, with its origin at the subclavian artery retained. The distal end is anastomosed end-to-side to the coronary artery. The artery most commonly grafted with the left IMA is the LAD coronary artery. When multiple arterial grafts are desired, the right IMA can be used either as a pedicle graft or as a free graft, with the proximal anastomosis made on the ascending aorta or on the left IMA. More limited use has been made of the gastroepiploic artery and the inferior epigastric artery. Use of the radial artery has been increasing recently. This conduit may be brought off the mid point on the left IMA, or the aorta, and grafted to vessels on the lateral wall. Performance of radial artery grafts appears to be better when the target vessel stenosis is at least 70%. Vasodilators like calcium channel blockers or nitrates are necessary to prevent radial artery spasm and early graft closure. Endoscopically harvested radial arteries appear to have equivalent patency rates with those harvested via the open method.[37] The main benefit of these arterial grafts is improved long-term patency. The actuarial probability of vein graft patency at 10 years is 50%. In contrast, the probability that the left IMA will be patent at 10 years is 90% to 95%. Also, evidence suggests that early mortality is reduced when at least one mammary artery graft is used,

To construct accurate anastomoses, a quiet, bloodless field is created in most cases with the use of cardiopulmonary bypass and cardioplegia for the purpose of arresting the heart (Fig. 85.6). With the patient on bypass and the heart empty, the distal ascending aorta is cross-clamped, and potassium cardioplegia solution is injected into the aortic root to cause nearly instantaneous cardiac arrest. Cardioplegic solution at a temperature of 4°C to 10°C induces rapid myocardial cooling along with cardiac arrest in diastole. In addition, many surgeons apply cold saline solution directly to the surface of the heart, either intermittently or continuously, to maintain the myocardial temperature between 10°C and 15°C during aortic cross-clamping. The most important components of cardioplegia are cold and potassium (usually 15 to 20 mEq/L), which causes depolarization of the myocardial membrane and arrest of the heart in diastole. Myocardial temperatures of 10°C to 15°C decrease the metabolic rate of the heart by 80%, and arrest lowers the metabolic rate to as little as 5% of that of the normothermic, working heart.

A number of cardioplegia solutions are available, although the ones most commonly used are based on a dilute blood solution with potassium and often other additives. Some techniques employ initial warm induction of arrest followed by cold cardioplegia. A warm dose of cardioplegia before removal of the cross-clamp has been advocated. This may be particularly useful in patients with significant preoperative ischemic insults. Warm cardioplegia reperfusion supplies oxygen and substrates while maintaining diastolic arrest with the attendant decreases in metabolic demand. Some surgeons prefer to perform the entire operation with the patient and the heart kept warm while cardioplegia is administered continuously.[54] The administration of cardioplegia is more commonly antegrade, with injection of the solution into the aortic root proximal to the cross-clamp. It has been shown that the retrograde administration of cardioplegia through a cannula placed in the coronary sinus can enhance myocardial protection because significant coronary arterial stenosis may prevent the homogenous delivery of cardioplegia, a problem avoided by the retrograde approach.[56–58] There is a risk, however, that protection of the right ventricle may be jeopardized with retrograde cardioplegia alone. The combination of antegrade and retrograde cardioplegia may thus be optimal in some cases. The retrograde cardioplegia technique is often applied in patients who have previously undergone CABG, in an effort to avoid the complication of atheromatous embolization in diseased bypass grafts.[58] Retrograde cardioplegia is also helpful in the presence of significant aortic insufficiency.

CABG is performed with the aid of optical 2.5 to 3.5 × magnification. Monofilament sutures are used by most surgeons, and specific techniques vary from a single continuous running anastomosis to multiple interrupted sutures. In addition to individual vein or mammary artery graft anastomoses to specific arterial branches, two or more distal anastomoses can be constructed from a single vein or mammary artery. These sequential grafts are especially favored when anastomoses are planned at multiple distal sites or when suitable conduit material is in short supply.

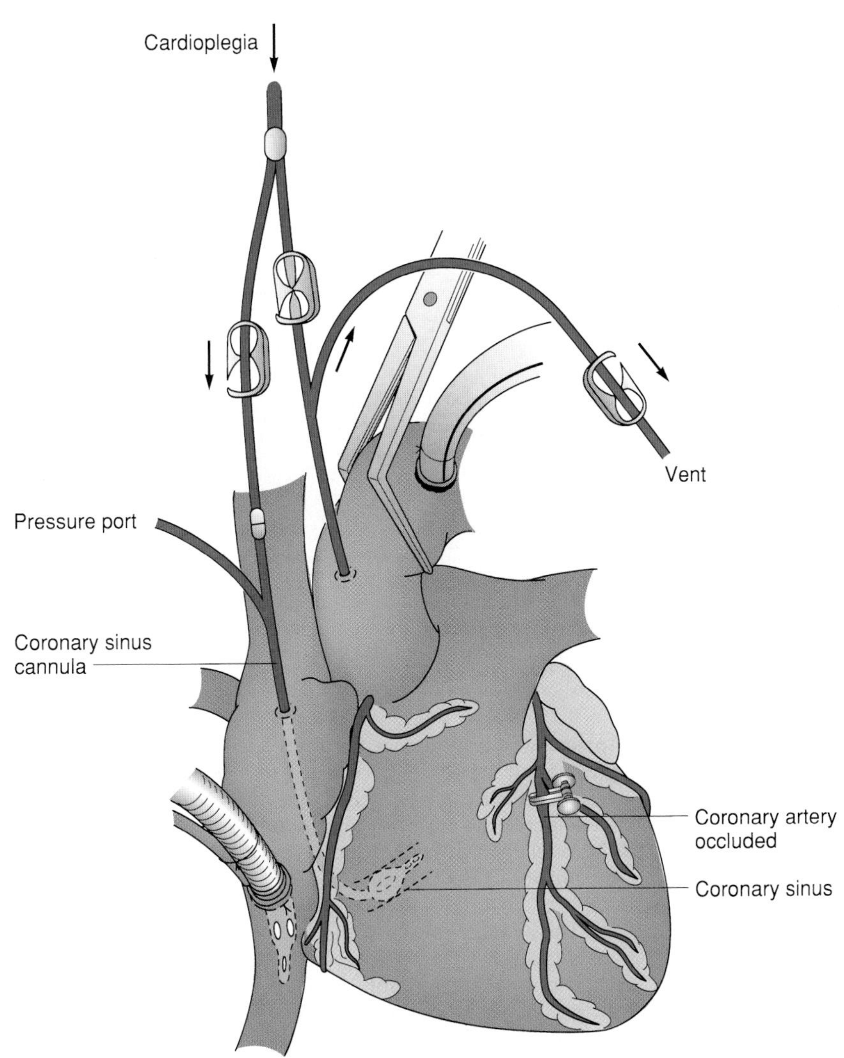

FIGURE 85.6 Cardiac instrumentation for retrograde administration of cardioplegic solution through the coronary sinus. A catheter with an occlusive balloon tip has been placed within the coronary sinus through the right atrium. The cardioplegic solution can be administered through the coronary sinus or the aortic root (antegrade). A pressure-measuring side port on the coronary sinus catheter can be used to prevent excessive distention of the coronary venous system. (After Partington MT, et al. Studies of retrograde cardioplegia I. *J Thorac Cardiovasc Surg.* 1989;97:613, with permission.)

When the distal anastomoses are completed, the aortic clamp is released. After reperfusion is initiated, ventricular fibrillation may develop, but cardioversion is usually accomplished with a single, biphasic electric shock. If a partially occluding clamp is placed on the ascending aorta, the proximal aorta—saphenous vein graft anastomoses can be constructed as myocardial perfusion is maintained through the native circulation and the newly constructed mammary anastomoses (Fig. 85.7). In some cases, especially in reoperation, the proximal anastomoses are made during ischemic time with the cross-clamp still in place, so that the partially occluding clamp, which can be difficult to place and can cause atherosclerotic embolism in the presence of old grafts, is not needed.

When CABG is performed, if diffuse atherosclerotic changes are present or if the site chosen for a distal anastomosis is heavily diseased, the surgeon may need to perform an endarterectomy to allow for a more reliable graft-to-artery anastomosis. The data regarding the safety and efficacy of coronary endarterectomy are conflicting; endarterectomy sites are more prone to early thrombosis and reocclusion. Endarterectomy of the distal right coronary artery, the most common site for endarterectomy, appears to be safe and well tolerated, in part because the right coronary artery is often already nearly totally occluded. Data comparing the long-term comparative value of endarterectomy of the LAD coronary artery versus grafting alone are not available. Endarterectomy should not be performed unless distal disease is so severe that it is necessary

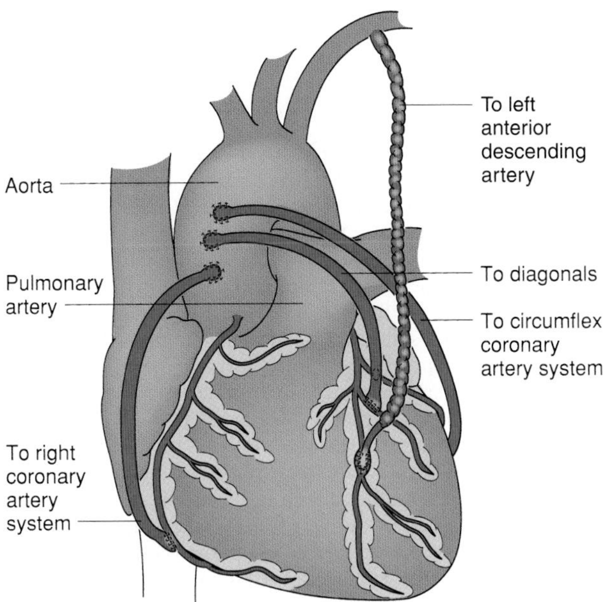

FIGURE 85.7 Most patients require multiple-vessel grafting and typically have a combination of vein grafts and a mammary artery graft. The most common site for use of the left internal mammary artery is the left anterior descending artery.

for distal flow. Because patients with diffuse distal disease are already likely to have a poor outcome, it has proved difficult to demonstrate a beneficial effect of coronary endarterectomy.

New and Future Techniques

In standard CABG, described previously, a heart—lung machine and cardioplegia are used to achieve cardiac arrest and maintain a motionless, bloodless, operative field. Recently, the trend has been to perform CABG on the beating heart.[38–49] It is ironic that the first coronary bypass procedures were performed on the beating heart. Now, however, with the development of epicardial stabilization devices and advances in technology, surgery performed on the beating heart is becoming commonplace. Kolessov,[43] a Russian investigator, reported coronary bypass surgery on a beating heart in 1967, but since then, surgery on the beating heart has rarely been reported until recently. Off-pump coronary artery bypass surgery (OPCAB), as the name implies, is CABG performed on the beating heart. Minimal-access cardiac surgery is the use of an incision smaller than full median sternotomy for the purpose of cardiac surgery. Minimally invasive direct coronary artery bypass (MID CAB) has gained favor recently.[44] Another term is *left anterior small thoracotomy* (LAST) for CABG.[45,46] Clearly, the semantics and nomenclature can rapidly become confusing. To keep it simple, we refer to two separate entities. In the first, off-pump CABG, the heart–lung machine and the associated systemic inflammatory response are avoided. In the second, minimally invasive or port access cardiac surgery, various incisions are used that are smaller than a standard sternotomy incision.

Off-pump heart surgery has been a recent trend. The standard technique of cardiopulmonary bypass is associated with a rate of stroke of 3% to 7%, and a temporary neurocognitive decline occurs in 65% of patients.[32] Furthermore, the comorbid conditions, age, and noncardiac risk factors of patients undergoing coronary bypass grafting have been increasing in recent years. Finally, technologic advances have created devices that can be used to stabilize the epicardial surface of the heart and have advanced the wide applicability of off-pump surgery.

Cardiopulmonary bypass results in a systemic inflammatory response involving the activation of the complement system, inflammatory cytokines, monocytes, neutrophils, and platelets and the inhibition of the coagulation system.[47–49] This total-body inflammatory response associated with cardiopulmonary bypass results in temporary organ dysfunction and tissue edema. Usually, these changes are inconsequential. However, if a patient is elderly or has a comorbid condition, such as severe emphysema, the cardiopulmonary bypass machine may mean the difference between a poor and a good outcome. Off-pump coronary bypass grafting is now considered appropriate for any patient with suitable anatomic features (coronary arteries of sufficient size and quality in approachable locations). Patients with preserved ventricular function and anterolateral diseased vessels requiring bypass are the best candidates. Patients who require intracardiac procedures, such as valve replacement, are not candidates.

The technique of off-pump coronary bypass involves stabilization of the epicardial surface with one of several devices. The devices fall into two categories—those that push and those that pull. A reusable suction stabilization system (Estech, Danville CA) is used at our institution, where approximately 40% of operations are performed off-pump (Fig. 85.8). This is a suction system that latches onto the epicardial surface and stabilizes it without impinging on ventricular filling; therefore, hemodynamic parameters are more easily maintained. Only half the dose of heparin used in conventional coronary bypass grafting is used with this system. Small clamps or silastic tapes are used to occlude the coronary arteries while grafts are sewn in place. With the pericardium retracted and the apex of the heart tipped vertically or rotated to the right, all coronary arterial systems can be reached with this technique.

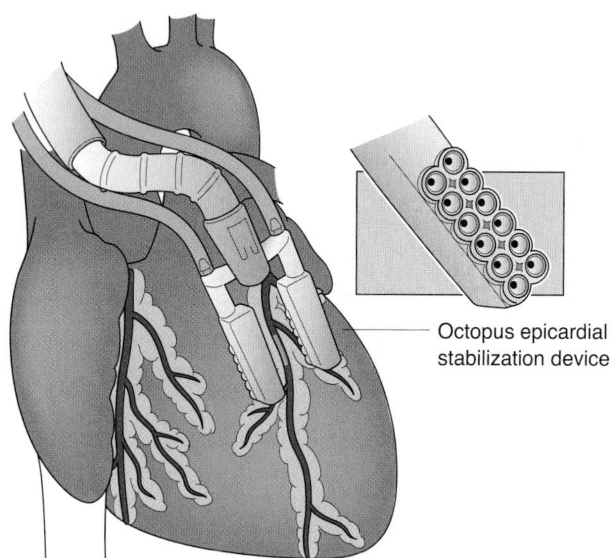

FIGURE 85.8 The Octopus epicardial stabilization device supplies suction to the surface of the heart and allows the surgeon to create a precise anastomosis on the beating heart.

The outcomes for off-pump coronary bypass grafting have been excellent. Mortality rates are comparable with those of conventional CABG. The need for transfusion is reduced. Length of hospital stay may be reduced. Cost is reduced as well. The neurocognitive decline seen after on-pump coronary bypass grafting appears to occur less often. This issue, however, is under investigation. To date, results have been excellent, but longer follow-up is needed.[50]

Minimally invasive or portaccess cardiac surgery has also been a recent trend.[32] We are convinced that the size of the incision and whether the operation is performed on- or off-pump are two different issues, although they are often discussed together. Minimally invasive incisions include partial sternotomies, small thoracotomies, and combined partial sternotomies and thoracotomies. Initial small series and reports indicate that these incisions can be used for both coronary bypass grafting and valve surgery. They appear to reduce patient discomfort and length of hospital stay. The overall risk of the procedure, however, remains the same. Minimally invasive surgery has gained attention in the lay press and on the Internet. However, it is not generally accepted as standard practice.

Transmyocardial revascularization (TMR) with CABG or alone is a surgical procedure that uses a CO_2 laser to create 1-mm channels in the left ventricle of the heart. TMR is useful in the subset of patients with large areas of ischemic myocardium that are not supplied by a vessel suitable for PTCA or bypass grafting.. The creation of these small transmyocardial channels appears to promote local neoangiogenesis by an unknown mechanism. This has been found to provide superior angina relief compared to CABG alone in patients with diffuse coronary artery disease.[51] One study has shown superior myocardial perfusion in areas of the heart which have undergone TMR.[52]

The use of videoscope- and robot-assisted heart surgery is under investigation.[54–56] Advances in computer and robotic technologies have been used to improve image quality and reduce tremors and cardiac motion, so that it has become possible to create coronary artery anastomoses on the beating heart endoscopically. Such procedures have been demonstrated in the laboratory within a satisfactory time frame. The control console used by the surgeon can be placed at a site remote from the operative field. This technique, which is also investigational, combines the best of both worlds in that minimally invasive surgery and off-pump techniques are applied together.

In summary, several new technologies and techniques for the treatment of coronary artery disease are on the horizon. Initial results, especially for off-pump surgery, appear promising. Off-pump surgery provides several advantages over the standard and well-tested technique of coronary artery bypass by avoiding use of a cardiopulmonary bypass machine. However, randomized trials demonstrating improved outcomes have not been completed to date. As always, time and careful analysis of patient outcomes will help us to choose appropriate therapies

TABLE 85.2 ETIOLOGY

CAUSES OF LOW CARDIAC OUTPUT

Inadequate preload
Excessive afterload
Poor ventricular contractility
Perioperative ischemia
Poor myocardial preservation
Arrhythmia
Severe acidosis
Tension pneumothorax
Tamponade

Postoperative Management

Postoperative cardiac surgical management is based on hemodynamic monitoring in an intensive care unit setting. Arterial blood pressure, central venous pressure, pulmonary capillary wedge pressure, cardiac output, and urine output all provide valuable information regarding the adequacy of arterial circulation, tissue perfusion, and organ function, and these parameters should be followed closely. In addition, arterial blood gases, complete blood cell counts, electrolytes, and the ECG should be evaluated at regular intervals. A chest radiograph should be performed when the patient arrives in the intensive care unit to check for the position of the endotracheal tube, nasogastric tube, chest tubes, and Swan-Ganz catheter. Also, pleural effusion, pneumothorax, and mediastinal widening should be ruled out, and a follow-up chest film should be obtained 8 to 12 hours later. Mediastinal and chest tube drainage should be recorded hourly. Shed blood can be autotransfused to minimize the use of banked blood products. Patients should be weighed daily to assist in fluid management. In all patients, a capillary leak syndrome develops after cardiopulmonary bypass that results in fluid accumulation, and a marked increase in total body sodium with a weight gain of 5 to 10 kg is typical. After extubation, which is normally between 4 and 12 hours postoperatively, pulmonary toilet should be vigorous. Most patients who have undergone CABG can be transferred to a step-down unit on the day after surgery, where they are monitored for arrhythmias. Diuresis is begun gradually so that the weight returns to the preoperative level, and a regular diet is started. Early ambulation is desirable.

Common causes of reduced cardiac output in the early postoperative period are hypovolemia and an increase in systemic vascular resistance as a consequence of persistent hypothermia or increased circulating catecholamines. Arrhythmias, bradycardia (secondary to resolving hypothermia), heart block (thought to be secondary to a transient but persistent effect of cardioplegia), or a supraventricular tachyarrhythmia (primarily atrial fibrillation), can also contribute to a low cardiac output. Management is more often directed at correcting such alterations than at increasing ventricular contractility. Patients are vigorously rewarmed, given adequate crystalloid or colloid solution to optimize cardiac filling pressures, and are often treated with a vasodilator, such as sodium nitroprusside or nicardipine, to maintain the mean blood pressure between 65 to 75 mm Hg in an effort to reduce systemic vascular resistance. Arrhythmias should be treated and bradycardia managed with atrial or atrioventricular pacing.

Low Cardiac Output. The causes of low cardiac output are listed in Table 85.2. If the calculated cardiac index is less than 2 L/min per square meter despite optimization of the heart rhythm, preload (cardiac filling pressures), and afterload (systemic vascular resistance), an inotropic agent may be indicated to enhance contractility. Poor ventricular contractility immediately after operation may be secondary to stunning from intraoperative ischemia or to preoperative ventricular dysfunction. Other correctable factors, such as poor oxygenation or persistent acidosis, may be responsible. If a low cardiac output continues after acidosis and inadequate oxygenation have been corrected, an inotropic drug is used. Appropriate first selections are milrinone, epinephrine, and occasionally dobutamine.

If a postoperative patient remains in cardiogenic shock despite significant inotropic support, placement of an IABP may be necessary. The balloon is inserted percutaneously into the femoral artery and positioned in the thoracic descending aorta. Balloon inflation and deflation are timed according to the ECG signals, with the balloon inflated during diastole and deflated during systole. IABP increases coronary artery perfusion because balloon inflation raises the intraaortic pressure during diastole, and active balloon deflation at the commencement of systole maximally decreases the afterload.

Rarely, if hemodynamic instability and shock continue despite these aggressive measures, a left ventricular assist device should be considered. The cause of a persistently low cardiac output state should be pursued aggressively before this step is taken because persistent cardiac dysfunction may be a consequence of inadequate coronary revascularization, early graft occlusion, or an unrecognized intracardiac or valvular mechanical defect. Support with a left ventricular assist device is extremely labor-intensive and costly and should be considered only if myocardial failure is thought to be reversible or if the patient is a candidate for transplantation.

Bleeding. Platelet function and blood clotting factors can be altered after cardiopulmonary bypass and may not normalize for up to 36 hours postoperatively. The average postoperative blood loss is 400 to 800 mL, and much of this shed blood can be reinfused. Continued bleeding at a rate faster than 200 mL/ho for 4 hours or more postoperatively is considered excessive, and in these cases, specific abnormalities in coagulation should be corrected aggressively. It is simple and safe to give additional protamine to reverse residual heparin activity. Transfusion of platelets, fresh frozen plasma, or cryoprecipitate should be considered if the results of coagulation studies indicate that they are needed. Reexploration is required if bleeding continues after correction of coagulopathy.

Tamponade. Cardiac tamponade is a potentially lethal cause of low cardiac output early after operation. Clinical features include a decreasing output in the presence of a narrowed pulse pressure, rising cardiac filling pressures, pulsus paradoxus, a widened mediastinal silhouette on chest film, and decreased urine output. These classic signs may be absent or equivocal. Sudden cessation of chest tube drainage in cases of excessive bleeding should alert the physician to the possibility of tamponade. Transesophageal echocardiography can establish this diagnosis immediately and can assess ventricular function in addition to preload, an extremely useful parameter in treating the patient in shock.

Late cardiac tamponade can develop up to several weeks after operation and can be caused by hemopericardium or a transudative pericardial effusion. Presenting symptoms, which may be obvious but frequently are subtle, include lethargy, malaise, mild respiratory distress, nonspecific chest discomfort, fluid retention, and hepatomegaly. The diagnosis is made by echocardiography, and the tamponade nearly always can be managed successfully with either percutaneous or operative drainage.

Infection. The major wound complications after coronary artery surgery are sternal infection, dehiscence, and mediastinitis, problems that occur in 0.5% to 2% of patients. The wound infection rate is somewhat higher in patients who undergo bilateral mammary artery grafting, especially if they are elderly or diabetic. *Staphylococcus* species are the responsible organisms in most cases, and in an increasing number of these patients, the bacteria are methicillin-resistant. Risk factors associated with postoperative wound infections are diabetes, a preoperative hospital stay of longer than 2 days, chronic obstructive pulmonary disease with prolonged ventilator support, the use of bilateral IMA grafts, and low cardiac output.

Sternal dehiscence and mediastinitis may occur even in the absence of an apparent superficial wound infection or drainage. Helpful clinical features of these initially occult infections are fever, elevated white blood cell count, and sternal tenderness or instability. Once the diagnosis is made, however, immediate mediastinal reexploration and aggressive débridement of infected bone and cartilage are necessary because mediastinitis with sepsis can cause rapid deterioration. Primary reclosure of the wound is sometimes possible, but it is often necessary to use pectoral or rectus muscle flaps for wound closure, not only to bring in a good blood supply but also to fill the void left by the débrided sternum.

Stroke. Cerebral vascular accident, or stroke, can be a devastating complication after bypass surgery. Stroke is usually caused by atherosclerotic emboli that frequently originate in the aorta and are loosened by cannulation, cross-clamping, or the construction of proximal anastomoses. Underlying cerebral vascular disease in conjunction with alterations in cerebral blood flow patterns resulting from cardiopulmonary bypass may also play a role. Strokes occur in 1% to 2% of low-risk patients after bypass surgery but in up to 10% of the elderly. The need to evaluate the extracranial cerebral circulation before bypass surgery is controversial. No data suggest that the investigation of asymptomatic carotid bruits and subsequent endarterectomy, if significant stenosis is found, reduce the incidence of stroke after bypass operation. In general, only symptomatic or severe carotid stenoses should be addressed before bypass surgery. The issue of the timing of endarterectomy and CABG (i.e., whether they should be performed sequentially or as a combined procedure) is also controversial. If the carotid disease is asymptomatic, factors affecting the timing of coronary surgery usually take precedence.

Postpericardiotomy Syndrome. Postpericardiotomy syndrome is a delayed pericardial inflammatory reaction characterized by fever, anterior chest pain, and a pericardial friction rub. It occurs in up to 30% of cardiac surgery patients postoperatively. The syndrome is associated with the development of pericardial effusions, which rarely lead to cardiac tamponade. In addition, postpericardiotomy syndrome can result in mediastinal fibrosis and premature graft closure. Treatment with nonsteroidal antiinflammatory agents for 2 weeks or more usually eliminates the symptoms of postpericardiotomy syndrome, but corticosteroids may be required in patients with recurring episodes.

TABLE 85.3

PREDICTION OF THE RISK FOR OPERATIVE MORTALITY[a]

	Low	Medium	High
Age (y)	60	75	75
Gender	Male	Female	Female
Diabetes	No	Yes	Yes
Unstable angina	Yes	No	Yes
Ejection fraction	65%	35%	25%
Three-vessel disease	Yes	Yes	Yes
Operative incidence	First	First	Redo
Predicted mortality rate	0.8%	3.4%	12%

[a]Based on the Society of Thoracic Surgery National Cardiac Database Risk Stratification Algorithm.

Risk Factors for Operative Mortality

The assessment and analysis of risk factors for operative mortality after coronary bypass surgery are important components of the preoperative evaluation of patients with coronary disease (Table 85.3). Furthermore, as an increasing number of interested parties scrutinize the results of bypass surgery, preoperative risk stratification is crucial. Among the many factors that affect outcome after CABG are the patient's state of general health and the potential for complete revascularization. Incomplete revascularization secondary to either severe distal coronary artery disease or inadequate conduits for bypass grafting is associated with a higher operative mortality rate and an uncertain long-term outcome. Likewise, patients with concurrent medical problems, such as cerebrovascular, pulmonary, or renal insufficiency, are much more likely to sustain additional complications during CABG and have a higher operative risk.[65]

Poor ventricular function is among the most important factors increasing the mortality risk of bypass surgery. Operative risk also is increased when the patient requires additional operative intervention, such as valve repair or replacement. Furthermore, when ventricular function is not improved by bypass grafting or when mitral valve replacement or ventricular reconstruction is required because of complications of previous infarction, the long-term outlook is noticeably worsened.[65,69]

Several reports have documented increased morbidity and mortality in elderly patients undergoing CABG. In the CASS, the operative mortality rate in patients 70 years of age or older was nearly 8%, compared with an overall estimated mortality rate of about 3% in lower risk, younger patients. An important observation made in elderly patients is that their increased mortality is the result of postoperative complications, such as stroke, respiratory failure, renal failure, or sepsis and rather than cardiac failure. Although age is an incremental risk factor for early death after coronary bypass surgery, it is not a contraindication to surgery.[65,66]

The influence of the patient's sex on surgical outcome is less clear, despite several reports suggesting a higher operative risk for women. In many of these studies, the women undergoing CABG were older, with a higher incidence of unstable angina, preoperative CHF, hypertension, and diabetes. Some reports have attributed the increased risk of bypass surgery in women to their smaller physical stature, with a correspondingly smaller coronary arterial bed and the technical limitations this poses. However, the higher risk for women is more likely a consequence of increased risk factors, such as advanced age and severity of the anginal syndrome.[67]

Other factors that increase operative risk include renal insufficiency, diabetes mellitus, peripheral vascular disease, cerebral vascular disease, respiratory insufficiency, and obesity. Most of these conditions are also associated with premature or accelerated atherosclerosis and a high incidence of generalized cardiovascular disease secondary to hypertension, hyperlipidemia, and abnormal carbohydrate metabolism. The operative morbidity in patients with end-stage renal disease is increased, often as a result of bleeding and infection. Mortality is also increased. Patients with a functioning kidney transplant have a better outcome than patients requiring long-term hemodialysis.

Reoperative CABG has become increasingly more frequent during the past several years and accounts for an increasing proportion of all CABG procedures carried out in the United States. Reoperative surgery is associated with a slightly higher operative mortality than primary bypass procedures. This is a consequence of the technical difficulty of the procedure, which results from pericardial adhesions and scar formation, and of the fact that patients who undergo reoperation are older and have more advanced coronary disease, and revascularization is more likely to be incomplete.[68]

Long-term Outcomes

Controlled clinical trials have shown that surgical revascularization provides significant relief of anginal symptoms.[34,61,70,71] Most series show initial elimination of angina in about 90% of patients, with about 70% of patients remaining free of cardiac events for 1 to 3 years. In one report, 67% of surviving patients were free of angina 20 years after surgery.[69] Reoperation improved survival in patients with recurrent symptoms.[68]

Several studies suggest that CABG may enhance ventricular function, both in the immediate postoperative period and late after surgery. Nonetheless, controversy continues regarding the long-term functional effects of bypass surgery, especially on systolic function, with some reports suggesting a deterioration in ventricular performance. In a few controlled clinical trials, functional improvement was documented both at rest and during exercise 8 months postoperatively. In addition, improvement in the left ventricular ejection fraction was demonstrated in one study and could be attributed to improved contractility in myocardial regions that had been ischemic during exercise before surgery.[72] Clinical improvement after coronary bypass surgery, including cessation of angina, stabilization of ventricular function, and, most importantly, enhanced survival, depends on short- and long-term graft patency. In a follow-up study that included postoperative coronary angiography, 82% of patients with at least one graft patent on the 1-year coronary angiogram were alive 12 years after surgery, compared with only 42% of the patients who had no patent grafts 1 year after operation. Vein graft occlusion within the first few months of surgery is almost certainly caused by poor blood flow, poor coronary arterial runoff, injury to the graft during preparation, competitive flow from the native circulation, or faulty surgical technique. Vein graft stenosis or graft failure within the first few years is associated with neointimal hyperplasia, a process that is demonstrable angiographically in up to 75% of vein grafts after 1 year. The overall occlusion rates for saphenous vein grafts are 5% to 20% during the first postoperative year, and 2% to 4% annually for the next 4 years; they reach 22% to 30% at 5 years and 50% at 10 years.

Use of the IMA graft has become increasingly favored because it greatly improves late patency. Patency rates for IMA grafts are 95% at 1 year, 94% at 8 years, and 85% or better at 10 years. This improved IMA graft patency has been reported for both pedicle and free IMA grafts. Excellent late IMA graft patency clearly correlates with increased patient survival, reduced symptom recurrence, and fewer reoperations. In a study from the Cleveland Clinic, where IMA grafts have been used extensively, 10-year survival rates in patients with saphenous vein grafts for single-, double-, and triple-vessel disease were 88%, 79.5%, and 71%, respectively, compared with 93.4%, 90%, and 82.6% in a comparable group of patients who had IMA grafts to the LAD artery.[32,69] Radial arteries may also have higher long term patency rates than vein grafts.

About 90% of patients survive 5 years after a primary CABG, 80% survive 10 years and about 58% survive 15 years. Use of the IMA graft improves long-term survival to 89% at 10 years. For all patients in the three major clinical trials, long-term surgical survival was 58% at 11 years in the Veterans Administration Study,[57] 71% at 12 years in the European study,[58] and 87% at 8 years in the CASS.[35] At 5 years, 10% of the surgically treated patients in the CASS had died. One fourth of these deaths were sudden coronary, 47% were not sudden but of cardiac cause, and 28% were noncardiac deaths. In the European trial, the 5-year surgical survival rate in patients with stable angina and good left ventricular function was 92%; this decreased to 71% at 12 years. Medical therapy in a matched group of patients resulted in 83% survival at 5 years and 67% at 12 years. The difference between medical and surgical therapy at 12 years is still significant, but of less magnitude, possibly because of the fact that the patients received only saphenous vein grafts. Better long-term survival should result from mammary grafting, which is now universally performed.

About one in seven patients who had vein grafts required reoperation after 15 years, twice the reoperation rate of patients who received at least one mammary artery bypass. As mentioned earlier, patients who undergo reoperation have at least double the operative risk of primary elective CABG patients because the operation is technically more difficult, the patients' average age is higher, and atherosclerotic disease is more advanced. In addition, long-term results after reoperation are poorer because of these factors and because revascularization may not be as complete. Symptom relief is usually of shorter duration.

Principles Derived from Cooperative Studies

Although the clearest indication for a mechanical intervention such as PTCA or CABG is unstable angina on maximal medical therapy, improvement in long-term survival in certain anatomic patterns of coronary disease provides another indication for bypass surgery. The three prospective, randomized trials comparing coronary bypass with medical therapy were carried out in the 1970s. Both surgical and medical management of coronary artery disease have improved dramatically since that time. For example, the use of IMA grafts was negligible during the time period of these studies, as was the use of PTCA and platelet-inhibiting drugs. Nonetheless, important principles derived by these studies still shape the clinical approach to coronary artery disease.

Veterans Administration Cooperative Study. The Veterans Administration Cooperative Study[28] randomly assigned 686 male patients (average age 50 years) to initial medical versus surgical therapy. All patients had medically stable angina, single-vessel disease or worse, and an ejection fraction of more than 30%. Despite a much higher operative mortality rate than was acceptable, even at that time, the study revealed a tremendous benefit derived from surgery for patients with left main artery disease.[57] In these patients, the 3-year survival rate was 93% in the surgery group and 68% in the medical group. Furthermore, patients with a history of hypertension, previous MI, abnormal resting ECG, and increasingly severe symptoms (high clinical risk), in addition to patients with three-vessel disease and decreased left ventricular function (high anatomic risk), fared significantly better with surgery.

European Coronary Surgery Study. The European Coronary Surgery Study[58] examined only men younger than 65 years who had mild to moderate angina, normal left ventricular function, and at least two-vessel disease. At 8 years of follow-up, surgery improved survival in the population as a whole (89% vs. 80%), in patients with three-vessel disease (92% vs. 77%), and in patients with two-vessel disease involving the proximal LAD artery (90% vs. 79%). Immediate surgery provided no benefit in single-vessel disease, even if it involved the proximal LAD artery (but the IMA was not used).

Coronary Artery Surgery Study. The CASS was a prospective, randomized study[35] carried out between 1975 and 1979 in the United States in men and women younger than 65 years who had symptoms no more severe than mild angina. At 10 years of follow-up, the group as a whole had derived no benefit from surgery. In patients with an ejection fraction between 30% and 50%, however, surgery conferred an increased survival (79% vs. 61%). Furthermore, in the observational studies that were part of this project, surgery provided a survival advantage in all patients with three-vessel disease, but patients who had the more severe anatomic disease with the worst ventricular function benefitted the most. Although it appears that surgery provides the greatest benefit to those with left ventricular dysfunction, CHF is a major determinant of *poor* surgical outcome. When heart failure, not angina, is the predominant symptom, surgery yields a poor result. Pulmonary rales, use of diuretics and digitalis, and an enlarged heart are predictors of increased operative risk.[65] Nonetheless, in patients with significant angina, although left ventricular dysfunction increases the surgical risk and decreases long-term survival, bypass surgery bestows the greatest benefit in terms of improved long-term survival.

Coronary Bypass Surgery for Heart Failure

Patients with severely impaired ventricular function may be referred for bypass surgery when severe associated coronary obstructions are detected. Often, it is difficult to decide whether the patient who is at severely increased risk because of ventricular dysfunction is a candidate for bypass surgery, or whether transplantation should be pursued. In patients with ischemic but viable myocardium, ventricular function may improve after bypass surgery once adequate blood flow is restored. The term *hibernating myocardium* has been used to describe ventricular dysfunction secondary to inadequate coronary flow even in the absence of ECG changes or anginal symptoms.[72] The term *ischemic cardiomyopathy* implies irreversible myocardial dysfunction associated with extensive myocyte necrosis and infarction. Surgical revascularization improves the contractile function of hibernating muscle, whereas little functional benefit is derived from revascularization in ischemic cardiomyopathy if the myocardium is extensively scarred or infarcted.

In deciding whether to recommend transplantation or bypass surgery to a patient at high risk because of severely depressed left ventricular function, it is therefore important to determine the viability of the myocardium. Anginal symptoms suggestive of reversible ischemia are often a useful indicator of viable myocardium that would benefit from revascularization. Patients whose only symptom is heart failure should be approached with caution. Myocardial viability may be assessed better with positron emission tomography, but this is not widely available. Some cardiologists and surgeons find it useful to perform thallium scanning, either during exercise, with dipyridamole, or at rest, to assess myocardial viability. Muscle that takes up thallium (early or late) is presumed to be viable. Radionuclide scanning provides data with which to estimate the potential for improved ventricular function after revascularization in patients with coronary obstructive disease and significant left ventricular dysfunction because it can identify poorly functioning but viable ischemic areas. A thallium defect during exercise or even at rest that subsequently fills on the delayed images is evidence that viable myocardium is present despite poor function. In a patient with these findings, especially if angina is present, bypass surgery rather than transplantation is generally indicated if operable coronary disease is present. The postoperative outcome in these patients is acceptable, and left ventricular function is usually improved. These results can be enhanced by new ventricular reconstructive procedures which can be combined with CABG surgery and provide a means to deal with irreversibly damaged areas of the heart. One increasingly applicable technique is surgical anterior ventricular restoration (SAVR). In this operation, infarcted anterior-apical left ventricular myocardium is resected. The resulting defect is closed with a patch in such a way as to restore a more normal elliptical shape and better function to the ventricle.[73] In patients with CHF and no evidence of reversible ischemia, bypass surgery entails a high risk and provides little benefit, and transplantation should be considered.

KEY POINTS

- **Although the characteristics, locations, and severity of lesions in each person can vary, a number of established risk factors appear to predispose to atherosclerosis. These include advanced age, genetic predisposition, male sex, hypertension, diabetes mellitus, hyperlipidemia, and cigarette smoking.**
- **Cigarette smoking is one of the most important risk factors for coronary artery disease.**
- **Symptomatic angina pectoris is the classic presentation of coronary artery disease.**
- **Angina pectoris and MI are late manifestations of coronary artery disease.**
- **No signs of coronary artery disease are detected during the physical examination.**
- **Medical management of coronary artery disease includes the identification and reduction of controllable risk factors.**
- **Systemic intravenous thrombolytic therapy unquestionably decreases morbidity and mortality after MI.**
- **In coronary artery surgery, the diseased coronary artery is bypassed by creating an alternative conduit to deliver blood beyond the coronary stenosis.**
- **Although the clearest indication for a mechanical intervention such as PTCA or CABG is unstable angina on maximal medical therapy, improvement in long-term survival in certain anatomic patterns of coronary disease provides another indication for bypass surgery.**

References

1. Messer JV, Wagman RJ, Levine HJ, et al. Patterns of myocardial oxygen extraction during rest and exercise. *J Clin Invest.* 1962;41:725.
2. Berne RM. The role of adenosine in the regulation of coronary blood flow. *Circ Res.* 1980;47:807.
3. Robertson RM, Robertson D, Roberts LJ, et al. Thromboxane A_2 in vasotonic angina pectoris. *N Engl J Med.* 1981;304:998.
4. McGill H. Risk factors for atherosclerosis. *Adv Exp Med Biol.* 1977;104:273.

5. The Lipid Research Clinics Program. The Lipid Research Clinics Coronary Primary Prevention Trial results. II. The relationship of reduction in incidence of coronary heart disease to cholesterol lowering. *JAMA* 1984; 251:365.
6. DeWood MA, Spores J, Notske R, et al. Prevalence of total coronary occlusion during the early hours of transmural myocardial infarction. *N Engl J Med.* 198;303:897.
7. **Flaherty JT, Becker LC, Bulkley BH, et al. A randomized prospective trial of intravenous nitroglycerin in patients with acute myocardial infarction. *Circulation* 1976;54:766.**
8. **Herlitz J, Elmfeldt D, Hjalmarson A, et al. Effect of metoprolol on indirect signs of the size and severity of acute myocardial infarction. *Am J Cardiol.* 1983;51:1282.**
9. Yusuf S, Held P, Fuberg C. Update of effects of calcium antagonists in myocardial infarction or angina in light of the second Danish verapamil infarction trial (DAVIT-II) and other recent studies. *Am J Cardiol.* 1991; 67:1295.
10. **European Cooperative Study Group for Streptokinase Treatment in Acute Myocardial Infarction. Streptokinase in acute myocardial infarction. *N Engl J Med.* 1979;301:797.**
11. Fry ETA, Sobel BE. Coronary thrombosis. In: Zipes DP, Rowlands DJ, eds. *Progress in cardiology,* vol 2. Philadelphia: Lea & Febiger; 1990:199.
12. Yusuf S, Collins R, Peto R, et al. Intravenous and intracoronary fibrinolytic therapy in acute myocardial infarction: overview of results on mortality, reinfarction and side effects from 33 randomized control trials. *Eur Heart J.* 1985;6:556.
13. White HD, Rivers JT, Maslowski AH, et al. Effect of intravenous streptokinase as compared with that of tissue plasminogen activator on left ventricular function after first myocardial infarction. *N Engl J Med.* 1989; 320:817.
14. Tiefenbrunn AJ, Sobel BE. The impact of coronary thrombolysis on myocardial infarction. *Fibrinolysis* 1989;3:1.
15. **TIMI Study Group. Comparison of invasive and conservative strategies after treatment with intravenous tissue plasminogen activator in acute myocardial infarction: results of the Thrombolysis in Myocardial Infarction (TIMI) phase II trial. *N Engl J Med.* 1989;320:618.**
16. **Naunheim KS, Kessler KA, Kanter KR, et al. Coronary artery bypass for recent infarction: predictors of mortality. *Circulation* 1988;78[Suppl I]:1.**
17. Maisel AS, Ahnve S, Gilpin E, et al. Prognosis after extension of myocardial infarct: the role of W wave on non-Q wave infarction. *Circulation* 1985; 71:211.
18. Hands ME, Rutherford JD, Muller JE, et al. The in-hospital development of cardiogenic shock after myocardial infarction: incidence, predictors of occurrence, outcome, and prognosis factors. *J Am Coll Cardiol.* 1989; 14:40.
19. Allen BS, Okamoto F, Buckberg GD, et al. Studies of controlled reperfusion after ischemia. XIII. Reperfusion conditions: critical importance of total ventricular decompression during regional reperfusion. *J Thorac Cardiovasc Surg.* 1986;92:605.
20. Allen BS, Rosenkranz E, Buckberg GD, et al. Studies on prolonged acute regional ischemia. IV. Myocardial infarction with left ventricular failure. *J Thorac Cardiovasc Surg.* 1989;98:691.
21. Agnihotri AK, Madsen JC, Daggett WM. Surgical treatment of complications of acute myocardial infarction: postinfarction ventricular septal defect and free wall rupture. In: Cohn LH, Edmunds LH, eds. *Cardiac surgery in the adult,* 4th ed. New York: McGraw-Hill; 2003:681.
22. David TE, Ho WL. The effect of preservation of chordae tendineae on mitral valve replacement for postinfarction mitral regurgitation. *Circulation* 1986;74[Suppl I]:116.
23. **Holmes DR, Leon MB, Moses JW, et al. Analysis of 1-year clinical outcomes in the SIRIUS trial: a randomized trial of a sirolimus-eluting stent versus a standard stent in patients at high risk for coronary restenosis. *Circulation* 2004;109:634.**
24. **Green MA, Gray LA Jr, Slater AD, et al. Emergency aortocoronary bypass after failed angioplasty. Ann Thorac Surg. 1991;51:194.**
25. King SB III, Talley JD. Coronary arteriography and percutaneous transluminal coronary angioplasty: changing patterns of use and results. *Circulation* 1989;79[Suppl I]:19.
26. Pocock SJ, Henderson RA, Rickards AF, et al. Meta-analysis of randomised trials comparing coronary angioplasty with bypass surgery. *Lancet* 1995; 346:1184.
27. **King SB III, Lembo NJ, Weintraub WS, et al. A randomized trial comparing coronary angioplasty with coronary bypass surgery. *N Engl J Med.* 1994;331:1044.**
28. Hamm CW, Reimers J, Ischinger T, et al. A randomized study of coronary angioplasty compared with bypass surgery in patients with symptomatic multivessel coronary disease. *N Engl J Med.* 1994;331:1037.
29. Alderman EL, Andrews K, Bost J, et al. The Bypass Angioplasty Revascularization Investigation (BARI) Investigations: comparison of coronary bypass surgery with angioplasty in patients with multivessel disease. *N Engl J Med.* 1996;335:217.
30. Barsness GW, Peterson ED, Obman EM, et al. Relationship between diabetes mellitus and long-term survival after coronary bypass and angioplasty. *Circulation* 1997;97:2551.
31. Weintraub WS, Stein B, Kosinski A, et al. Outcome of coronary bypass surgery versus coronary angioplasty in diabetic patients with multivessel coronary artery disease. *J Am Coll Cardiol.* 1998;31:10.
32. **Eagle KA, Guyton RA, Davidoff R, et al. ACC/AHA guidelines for coronary artery bypass graft surgery: executive summary and recommendations—a report of the American College of Cardiology/American Heart Association task force on practice guidelines (committee to revise the 1991 guidelines for coronary artery bypass graft surgery). *Circulation* 1999; 100:1464.**
33. Jones RH, Kesler D, Phillips HR III, et al. Long-term survival benefits of coronary artery bypass grafting and percutaneous transluminal angioplasty in patients with coronary artery disease. *J Thorac Cardiovasc Surg.* 1996;111:1013.
34. Nwasokwa ON, Koss JR, Friedman GH, et al. Bypass surgery for chronic stable angina: predictors of survival benefit and strategy for patient selection. *Ann Intern Med.* 1991;114:1035.
35. Myers WO, Marshfield WI, Gersh BJ, et al. Medical versus early surgical therapy in patients with triple-vessel disease and mild angina pectoris: a CASS registry study of survival. *Ann Thorac Surg.* 1987;44:471.
36. Carpino PA, Khabbaz KR, Bojar RM, et al. Clinical benefits of endoscopic vein harvesting in patients with risk factors for saphenectomy wound infections undergoing coronary artery bypass grafting. *J Thorac Cardiovasc Surg.* 2000;119:69.
37. Connolly MW, Torrillo LD, Stauder MJ, et al. Endoscopic radial artery harvesting: results of first 300 patients. *Ann Thorac Surg.* 2002; 74:502.
38. Benetti FJ, Naselli G, Wood M, et al. Direct myocardial revascularization without extracorporeal circulation: experience in 700 patients. *Chest* 1991;100:312.
39. Benetti FJ, Ballester C, Sani G, et al. Video-assisted coronary bypass surgery. *J Cardiovasc Surg.* 1995;10:620.
40. Westaby S. Coronary surgery without cardiopulmonary bypass. *Br Heart J.* 1995;73:203.
41. Grundeman PF, Borst C, van Herwaarden JA, et al. Hemodynamic changes during displacement of the beating heart by the Utrecht Octopus method. *Ann Thorac Surg.* 1997;63:S88.
42. Wan S, LeClerc JL, Vincent JL. Inflammatory response to cardiovascular bypass: mechanisms involved and possible therapeutic strategies. *Chest* 1997;112:676.
43. Kolessov VI. Mammary artery—coronary artery anastomosis as method of treatment for angina pectoris. *J Thorac Cardiovasc Surg.* 1967;54: 535.
44. Subramanian VA. Less invasive arterial CABG on a beating heart. *Ann Thorac Surg.* 1997;63:S68.
45. Calafiore AM, Di Giammarco G, Teodori G, et al. Left anterior descending coronary artery grafting via left anterior small thoracotomy without cardiopulmonary bypass. *Ann Thorac Surg.* 1996;61:1658.
46. Lloyd CT, Calafiore AM, Wilde P, et al. Integrated left anterior small thoracotomy and angioplasty for coronary artery revascularization. *Ann Thorac Surg.* 1999;68:908.
47. Wan S, Izzat MB, Lee TW, et al. Avoiding cardiopulmonary bypass in multivessel CABG reduces cytokine response and myocardial injury. *Ann Thorac Surg.* 1999;68:52.
48. Struber M, Cremer JT, Gohrbandt B, et al. Human cytokine responses to coronary artery bypass grafting with and without cardiopulmonary bypass. *Ann Thorac Surg.* 1999;68:1330.
49. Downing SW, Edmunds LH. Release of vasoactive substances during cardiopulmonary bypass. *Ann Thorac Surg.* 1992;54:1236.
50. Connolly MW. Current results of off-pump coronary artery bypass surgery. *Sem Thorac Cardiovasc Surg.* 2003;15:45.
51. Allen KB, Dowling RD, Schuch DR, et al. Adjunctive transmyocardial revascularization: five-year follow-up of a prospective, randomized trial. *Ann Thorac Surg.* 2004;78:458.
52. Frazier OH, March RJ, Horvath KA. Transmyocardial revascularization with a carbon dioxide laser in patients with end-stage coronary artery disease. *N Engl J Med.* 1999;341:1021.
53. Stevens JH, Burdon TA, Peters WS, et al. Port access coronary artery bypass grafting: a proposed surgical method. *J Thorac Cardiovasc Surg.* 1996; 111:567.
54. Stephenson ER Jr, Ducko ST, Sankholkar S, et al. Computer-assisted endoscopic coronary artery bypass anastomoses: a chronic animal study. *Ann Thorac Surg.* 1999;68:838.
55. Shennib H, Bastawisy A, Mack MJ, et al. Computer-assisted telemanipulation: an enabling technology for endoscopic coronary artery bypass. *Ann Thorac Surg.* 1998;66:1060.
56. Stephenson ER Jr, Sankholkar S, Ducko CT, et al. Robotically assisted microsurgery for endoscopic coronary artery bypass grafting. *Ann Thorac Surg.* 1998;66:1064.
57. Detre KM, Takaro T, Hultgren H, et al., and the study participants. Long-term mortality and morbidity results of the Veterans Administration randomized trial of coronary artery bypass surgery. *Circulation* 1985;72 [Suppl V]:84.
58. Varnauskas E, and the European Coronary Surgery Study Group. Twelve-year follow-up of survival in the randomized European Coronary Surgery Study. *N Engl J Med.* 1988;319:332.

59. Takaro T, Pifarre R, Fish R. Left main coronary artery disease. *Prog Cardiovasc Dis.* 1985;28:229.
60. Akins CW. Controversies in myocardial revascularization: coronary artery surgery for single-vessel disease. *Semin Thorac Cardiovasc Surg.* 1994; 6:109.
61. Hammermeister KE, Morrison DA. Coronary bypass surgery for stable angina and unstable angina pectoris. *Cardiol Clin.* 1991;9:133.
62. Gundry SR, Wang N, Bann D, et al. Retrograde continuous warm blood cardioplegia: maintenance of myocardial homeostasis in humans. *Ann Thorac Surg.* 1993;55:358.
63. Noyez L, van Son JA, van der Werf T, et al. Retrograde versus antegrade delivery of cardioplegic solution in myocardial revascularization: a clinical trial in patients with three-vessel coronary disease who underwent myocardial revascularization with extensive use of the internal mammary artery. *J Thorac Cardiovasc Surg.* 1993;105:854.
64. Rosengart TK, Krieger K, Lang SJ, et al. Reoperative coronary artery bypass surgery: improved preservation of myocardial function with retrograde cardioplegia. *Circulation* 1993;88[Suppl II]:330.
65. Grover FL, Johnson RR, Marshall G, et al. Factors predictive of operative mortality among coronary artery bypass subsets. *Ann Thorac Surg.* 1993; 56:1296.
66. Smith JM, Rath R, Feldman DJ, et al. Coronary artery bypass grafting in the elderly: changing trends and results. *J Cardiovasc Surg.* 1992;33:468.
67. Barbir M, Lazem F, Ilsley C, et al. Coronary artery surgery in women compared with men: analysis of coronary risk factors and in-hospital mortality in a single centre. *Br Heart J.* 1994:71:408.
68. Lytle BW, Loop FD, Taylor PC, et al. The effect of coronary reoperation on the survival of patients with stenoses in saphenous vein bypass grafts to coronary arteries. *J Thorac Cardiovasc Surg.* 1993;105:605.
69. Lawrie GM, Morris GC Jr, Earle N. Long-term results of coronary bypass surgery: analysis of 1,698 patients followed 15 to 20 years. *Ann Surg.* 1991;213:355.
70. Myers WO, Schaff HV, Gersh BJ, et al. Improved survival of surgically treated patients with triple vessel coronary disease and severe angina pectoris. *J Thorac Cardiovasc Surg.* 1989;98:487.
71. Nwasokwa ON, Koss JR, Friedman GH, et al. Bypass surgery for chronic stable angina: predictors of survival benefit and strategy for patient selection. *Ann Intern Med.* 1991;114:1035.
72. Braunwald E, Rutherford JD. Reversible ischemic left ventricular dysfunction: evidence for the hibernating myocardium. *J Am Coll Cardiol.* 1986; 8:1467.
73. Mickleborough LL. Left ventricular reconstruction for ischemic cardiomyopathy. *Sem Thorac Cardiovasc Surg.* 2002;14:144.

CHAPTER 86 ■ MECHANICAL CIRCULATORY SUPPORT

FRANCIS D. PAGANI AND KEITH D. AARONSON

The spectrum of mechanical circulatory support has changed dramatically since Cooley first implanted an orthotopic cardiac prosthesis as a bridge to heart transplant[1] and DeVries first implanted a total artificial heart as a permanent replacement for the failing native heart.[2] Since then, numerous technologic advances and rigorous scientific investigations have dramatically improved the availability, durability, and safety of mechanical cardiac support devices.

Mechanical circulatory support is indicated in situations in which the heart can no longer pump blood and meet oxygen requirements commensurate with the needs of the body. "A variety of devices, ranging from the widely available intraaortic balloon pump (IABP) to the sophisticated total artificial heart, are used to treat patients with failing hearts. The appropriate support system is always that device that can provide the best potential results in the simplest possible manner."[3]

INDICATIONS AND DEVICE SELECTION

The spectrum of mechanical circulatory support is complex due to the multiple, intended indications for use and the availability of numerous types of mechanical support devices. Currently, there are three accepted, intended indications for mechanical circulatory support. The first indication applies to patients who have sustained a reversible myocardial injury and there exists reasonable expectation that myocardial function will recover over a short period of circulatory support (generally less than 2 weeks) and require short-term temporary mechanical circulatory support as a "bridge to myocardial recovery." Examples of reversible forms of myocardial injury include an acute myocardial infarction, acute viral myocarditis, or postcardiotomy cardiogenic shock with failure to wean from cardiopulmonary bypass following open heart cardiac procedures. Under these circumstances there are several types of devices that can be utilized to provide temporary mechanical circulatory support and include an IABP, extracorporeal ventricular assist device (VAD) (either pulsatile or nonpulsatile, that provides either univentricular or biventricular circulatory support), and extracorporeal membrane oxygenation [ECMO or preferably referred to as extracorporeal life support (ECLS)]. The second indication applies to patients in whom myocardial function is unlikely to recover and are considered possible future candidates for heart transplantation (longstanding ischemic, valvular, or idiopathic cardiomyopathy with refractory end-stage heart failure, severe acute myocardial infarction, or myocarditis). Longer-term circulatory support devices that are implantable and permit greater patient mobility, rehabilitation, and discharge to home are more appropriate under a "bridge to transplant" indication. The third indication applies to patients with chronic refractory end-stage heart failure due to irreversible forms of nonischemic or ischemic cardiomyopathy and who are not eligible for heart transplantation and require permanent circulatory support as "destination therapy." Implantable circulatory support devices with long-term reliability and approved by the U.S. Food and Drug Administration (FDA) for this indication are appropriate devices in this clinical situation.[4,5] The survival and quality of life benefit of mechanical circulatory support for destination therapy for the treatment of end-stage refractory heart failure has been demonstrated in the prospective, randomized trial REMATCH (Randomized Evaluation of Mechanical Assistance in the Treatment of Congestive Heart Failure).[4,5]

In the near future, an additional group of patients may require consideration for mechanical circulatory support. These patients include those in whom long-term circulatory support (weeks to months) will be required for ventricular remodeling and recovery from various types of cardiomyopathies. Anecdotal observations from the cumulative experience with long-term circulatory support for bridge to transplant indication and recent small clinical studies have demonstrated that long-term circulatory support (weeks to months), associated with sustained mechanical unloading of the left ventricle, can improve myocardial function in those patients thought to have irreversible, dilated, end-stage cardiomyopathies.[6–9] Several studies have demonstrated that long-term mechanical circulatory support can restore ventricular geometry;[10–12] improve myocyte function, orientation, and size;[13–17] reduce myocyte apoptosis;[18] reduce myocardial cytokine gene and protein expression;[19,20] reverse abnormal neurohormonal patterns associated with advanced heart failure;[21,22] and improve myocardial mitochondrial function.[23] These observations have led clinicians to consider mechanical circulatory support alone or in conjunction with other future possible therapies (gene therapy, myocyte or stem cell implantation), as a potential modality to reverse end-stage cardiomyopathy. Whether these observations hold under future rigorous experimental scrutiny remains unknown at this time.

Thus, the intended use and clinical indication for mechanical circulatory support has significant influences on the appropriate device selection and the justification for use. The decision to initiate mechanical circulatory support therefore must include an analysis of the intended use, clinical setting, type of mechanical circulatory devices available, and patient variables.

Importantly, there are no absolute hemodynamic criteria to meet to initiate mechanical circulatory support for any indication. For patients presenting with an acute cardiovascular event, evidence of cardiogenic shock manifest by a cardiac index less than 1.8 to 2.2 L/min/m^2, systolic blood pressure less than 90 mm Hg, pulmonary capillary wedge pressure or left atrial pressure greater than 15 to 20 mm Hg, right atrial pressure greater than 18 to 20 mm Hg, and evidence of poor tissue perfusion, reflected by oliguria, rising creatinine and liver transaminases, mental status changes, and cool extremities, despite the use of optimal pharmacologic therapy, are general guidelines to initiate mechanical circulatory support. Patient history and overall clinical setting also needs to be considered in the decision to initiate mechanical circulatory support. When patients reach this degree of hemodynamic compromise, the risk of death is substantial and is in excess of 50% at 30 days.[24,25] This high mortality occurs despite the availability of optimal pharmacologic therapy, invasive circulatory monitoring, thrombolysis, and IABP support. Thus, in appropriate clinical settings and when utilized in an optimal time setting, mechanical circulatory support can be lifesaving.

More subtle indications to initiate mechanical circulatory support may be present, particularly in the group of patients suffering from chronic refractory end-stage heart failure secondary to an ischemic or nonischemic cardiomyopathy. These indications include progressive organ dysfunction or persistent significant symptoms despite optimal medical management with or without inotrope therapy. The deterioration in end-organ function or progressive decline in functional performance may occur even though hemodynamic parameters may not have significantly changed (chronic adaptation to low cardiac output). In addition, patients who do not tolerate optimal medical management for heart failure and experience renal insufficiency or hypotension in the setting of optimal dosages of angiotensin-converting enzyme (ACE) inhibitors or beta-blockers may need consideration for VAD therapy. Patients who do not tolerate inotrope therapy as a result of refractory ventricular arrhythmias or have life-threatening coronary anatomy and unstable angina not amenable to revascularization and are at risk of immanent death (hours, days, or weeks) may be considered for mechanical circulatory support without necessarily meeting hemodynamic criteria. For patients being considered for "destination therapy," specific criteria to meet have been defined by the REMATCH trial and by the Centers for Medicare and Medicaid Services (CMS).[5] These criteria include symptoms of congestive heart failure consistent with New York Heart Association class IV symptoms for the past 60 days, VO_2 of less than 12 mL/kg/min, left ventricular ejection fraction of less than 25%, and on optimal medical therapy.[5]

PATIENT SELECTION AND TIMING OF INTERVENTION

Patient selection is perhaps the single most crucial factor in determining outcome of patients who receive mechanical circulatory support. Patients should be excluded for consideration for mechanical circulatory support if they have significant contraindications to mechanical circulatory support or if they have significant contraindications to heart transplantation in situations in which they are unlikely to wean from circulatory support once it has been initiated and the intended use is as a bridge to recovery or heart transplantation. Contraindications to initiating mechanical circulatory support include irreversible renal, hepatic, or respiratory failure, sepsis, or a significant cognitive deficit. Severe obstructive or restrictive pulmonary disease is also a contraindication to mechanical circulatory support. Perioperative hypoxia as a result of significant underlying lung disease can contribute to pulmonary vasoconstriction with right-sided circulatory failure. Often, patients with severe pulmonary disease have an elevated pulmonary vascular resistance that is fixed (not responsive to pulmonary artery vasodilators). Fixed pulmonary vascular resistance represents a contraindication to heart transplantation. Moderate elevations in pulmonary vascular resistance can be encountered in patients with cardiogenic shock and does not preclude successful use of mechanical circulatory support if reversibility (lowering) of the pulmonary vascular resistance is documented during therapy with inotropes or pulmonary vasodilators. Acute renal failure requiring dialysis is a relative contraindication to initiating mechanical circulatory support. In the setting of cardiogenic shock with acute renal failure, establishing normal hemodynamics with mechanical circulatory support may resolve the renal failure in a relatively short period. Thus, the degree and duration of cardiogenic shock along with the patient's baseline renal function must be considered in estimating the probability of recovery of renal function. This is important in considering whether the patient will be a transplant candidate or not, in the event that native heart function does not recover while the patient is mechanically supported. Similarly, improvement in hepatic congestion and recovery of synthetic functions of the liver can occur with institution of mechanical circulatory support. The presence of portal hypertension or liver cirrhosis is an absolute contraindication to initiating mechanical circulatory support. Development of risk stratification models have supported the observation that patients with increasing degrees of significant multiorgan failure do poorly following intervention with mechanical circulatory support.[26–30]

In addition to the degree of organ dysfunction, age is an important risk factor for survival for patients on mechanical circulatory support. Age can represent an absolute contraindication to initiate mechanical support if the patient is unlikely to wean and is too old to qualify for heart transplantation. Data from the American Society for Artificial Internal Organs–International Society for Heart & Lung Transplantation (ASAIO-ISHLT) registry have demonstrated that patients older than 70 years have a decreased survival on mechanical circulatory support.[30] However, the probability of weaning from mechanical circulatory support is not affected by age.[30]

Timing the initiation of mechanical circulatory support is also crucial to patient outcome. In the setting of postcardiotomy shock, data from the Abiomed BVS 5000 registry demonstrate that delay in initiating mechanical circulatory support for greater than 6 hours after the initial weaning from cardiopulmonary bypass is associated with a significant decrease in survival, 44% versus 14%.[31,32] Delay in instituting mechanical circulatory support also increases the need for biventricular support as opposed to just univentricular support, because patients requiring biventricular support have a decreased survival.[30–34] As the severity of illness and organ dysfunction increases, patients are more likely to require biventricular support.[34,35] An episode of cardiac arrest prior to the initiation of mechanical circulatory support significantly reduces survival, 47% versus 7%.[31,32] In a 6-year experience from the Heinemann University Hospital, Samuels et al.[36] reported on 45 patients supported with the Abiomed BVS 5000. Overall, 22 (49%) patients weaned from support and 14 (31%) survived to hospital discharge. For patients that received optimal timing of insertion by establishing a weaning algorithm, outcomes were improved with 60% of patients weaning from device support and 43% surviving to hospital discharge.[36]

Selection of the appropriate mechanical circulatory device is also critical to a successful outcome and is dependent on a number of factors (Tables 86.1 to 86.4). These factors include the cause of the circulatory failure, the duration of support, whether biventricular or univentricular support is required, whether combined cardiac and pulmonary failure is present, the size of the patient, the intended use for the device, and the current FDA restrictions and regulations for a particular device. Consideration of all these factors help to define the endpoint of therapy, which may include bridge to recovery, bridge to heart transplant, and destination therapy.

TABLE 86.1 INDICATIONS/CONTRAINDICATIONS

CONSIDERATIONS IN INSTITUTING MECHANICAL CIRCULATORY SUPPORT

What is the likelihood of reversibility of the myocardial injury?
What is the probable duration of support needed?
What is the urgency of the need for support (minutes, hours, days)? (e.g., cardiac arrest vs. advanced chronic heart failure)
To what degree is myocardial performance impaired?
What degree of circulatory support and device invasiveness is needed? (e.g., IABP vs. LVAD)
Is univentricular or biventricular support needed?
(Right heart failure indicated by right atrial pressure greater than 20 mm Hg, severe tricuspid regurgitation, presence of hepatic failure, coagulopathy, renal dysfunction)
Is cardiac or combined cardiopulmonary support needed?
What is the patient's size?
What device will offer the patient the greatest degree of mobility and potential for rehabilitation during circulatory support?
What are the current FDA-approved indications for this device?

FDA, U.S. Food and Drug Administration; IABP, intraaortic balloon pump; LVAD, left ventricular assist device.

TABLE 86.2

CURRENT BODY SURFACE AREA LIMITATIONS FOR MECHANICAL CIRCULATORY SUPPORT DEVICES

Device	BSA limitation (m^2)
HeartMate XVE LVAD	1.5
Thoratec pVAD	0.8–1.0
Abiomed BVS 5000	0.8–1.0
AbioCor TRH[a]	1.7
CardioWest TAH	1.7
Novacor LVAS	1.5
DeBakey LVAD[a]	1.2
HeartMate II[a]	1.2–1.4

BSA, body surface area.
[a]Investigational device.

OTHER IMPORTANT MEDICAL CONSIDERATIONS IN INSTITUTING MECHANICAL CIRCULATORY SUPPORT

Valvular Heart Disease

Abnormalities of the cardiac valves have important adverse consequences in patients being considered for mechanical circulatory support and may require repair or replacement to initiate successful mechanical circulatory support or achieve weaning from support. Mild to moderate aortic stenosis in the absence of insufficiency is not a contraindication to placement of a VAD. Severe aortic stenosis should be corrected prior to placement of a VAD, preferably with a bioprosthetic or homograft valve, to facilitate future weaning or optimize native heart function in the event of device failure. The presence of even mild to moderate aortic insufficiency can have a significant impact on the effectiveness of VADs. In the cases in which left ventricular assistance is initiated with left atrial to aortic cannulation, aortic insufficiency will result in left ventricular distention in the presence of significant left ventricular dysfunction. Left ventricular distention adversely affects subendocardial blood flow and can ultimately prevent weaning from circulatory support. In cases in which left ventricular assistance is initiated with devices that require left ventricular apical to aortic cannulation, reductions in left ventricular pressure elicited by mechanical assistance increase the pressure gradient across the aortic valve and increases the degree of aortic insufficiency. Thus, blood pumped into the aortic root by the device will flow backward across the incompetent aortic valve (aortic insufficiency), thereby decreasing net forward flow and compromising end-organ perfusion. Even mild to moderate aortic insufficiency may become severe with initiation of mechanical support from a left VAD (LVAD), because the elevated left ventricular end-diastolic pressure will be significantly reduced by the emptying of the left ventricular cavity by the device and the aortic root pressure will be elevated above baseline because of device flow. The significance of the regurgitant volume of blood can

TABLE 86.3

ANTICOAGULATION REQUIREMENTS FOR MECHANICAL CIRCULATORY SUPPORT DEVICES

Device	Anticoagulation protocol
Centrifugal (BioMedicus, St. Jude, Sarns)	Heparin/antiplatelet therapy
ECMO (extracorporeal life support)	Heparin
Abiomed BVS 5000	Heparin/antiplatelet therapy
CardioWest TAH	Heparin/antiplatelet therapy followed by warfarin (Coumadin)/antiplatelet therapy for long-term support
Thoratec pVAD	Heparin/antiplatelet therapy followed by warfarin/antiplatelet therapy for long-term support
Novacor LVAS	Heparin/antiplatelet therapy followed by warfarin/antiplatelet therapy for long-term support
HeartMate XVE LVAD	Antiplatelet therapy

easily be determined by measuring cardiac output with a thermodilution catheter and comparing it to device flow. In cases in which device flow exceeds the cardiac output, measured by thermodilution technique, of greater than 1.5 to 2 L/min, the volume of regurgitation is considered significant. In addition, the presence of significant aortic insufficiency can be confirmed by echocardiography. Patients with a mechanical valve prosthesis in the aortic valve position should have the mechanical valve replaced with a bioprosthetic valve prior to institution of left ventricular assistance. During complete unloading of the left ventricle by a VAD, the aortic valve may not open and is prone to thrombus formation.

TABLE 86.4 TREATMENT

CLASSIFICATION AND INDICATIONS OF MECHANICAL CIRCULATORY SUPPORT DEVICES

Pump type	Intended duration of support	FDA status	Indications or potential uses
Intraaortic balloon pump	Short-term	Approved	1. Short-term bridge to recovery
EXTRACORPOREAL NONPULSATILE			
ECMO	Short-term	Approved[1]	1. Short-term bridge to recovery (centrifugal pumps are FDA-approved for short-term support of less than 6 hours. Longer periods of support are considered "off-label" use.)
Centrifugal pumps	Short-term	Approved[1]	
TandemHeart	Short-term	Approved[1]	
EXTRACORPOREAL PULSATILE			
Thoratec pVAD	Short or long-term	Approved[1,2]	1. Short-term bridge to recovery
Abiomed BVS 5000	Short-term	Approved[1]	2. Bridge to transplant
IMPLANTABLE PULSATILE			
HeartMate IP1000 LVAD	Long-term	Approved[1]	1. Bridge to transplant
HeartMate XVE LVAS	Long-term	Approved[1,2]	2. Destination therapy
Novacor LVAS	Long-term	Approved[1]	
LionHeart LVAS	Long-term	Investigative[2]	
IMPLANTABLE NONPULSATILE			
HeartMate II	Long-term	Investigative[1,2]	1. Bridge to transplantation
HeartMate III	Long-term	Investigative[1,2]	2. Destination therapy
DeBakey LVAD	Long-term	Investigative[1,2]	
Jarvik 2000	Long-term	Investigative[1,2]	
TOTAL ARTIFICIAL HEART			
CardioWest	Long-term	Approved[1]	1. Bridge to transplantation
AbioCor	Long-term	Investigative[2]	2. Destination therapy

[1,2] See Indications in last column of table.

Patients with significant preexisting mitral stenosis at the time of initiation of device support may require correction of the valvular problem before implantation of the device depending on device selection and site of cannulation. In the setting of significant mitral stenosis, left ventricular filling is impaired. VADs that utilize apical ventriculotomy for cannula placement for ventricular drainage may experience limitations in device filling due to the mitral stenosis. This problem can be circumvented by either choosing a device that can utilize left atrial drainage or by correcting the underlying valvular pathology (mitral valve repair or replacement with a bioprosthetic valve). Mitral regurgitation does not have an impact on the filling of a VADs. In situations in which weaning from mechanical circulatory support may be feasible, correction of the mitral pathology, either stenosis or regurgitation, is necessary to optimize ventricular function.

Adequate right heart function is extremely important to maintain LVAD flow in the early postoperative period in patients on univentricular support. Severe tricuspid regurgitation can significantly impair the forward flow of blood on the right side particularly in situations of high pulmonary vascular resistance. Further, severe tricuspid regurgitation contributes to elevated central venous pressure, hepatic congestion, and renal dysfunction. Severe tricuspid regurgitation may be present preoperatively in the setting of volume overload and biventricular failure or may develop following institution of LVAD support as a consequence of right ventricular dilation from leftward shift of the interventricular septum.[37–39] If severe tricuspid regurgitation is present during the initiation of LVAD support, tricuspid valve repair should be performed to improve right ventricular performance.

Coronary Artery Disease

Patients that have significant obstructive coronary artery disease or patients with postcardiotomy shock following failed coronary bypass operations may continue to experience angina during mechanical circulatory support. Generally, coronary artery disease does not have adverse hemodynamic consequences during the period of device support. However, the presence of obstructive coronary disease with ongoing ischemia may limit the degree of myocardial recovery and significantly impact the ability to wean from device support.

Perioperative ischemia of the right ventricle may be of hemodynamic significance during institution of LVAD support. Right ventricular ischemia causing myocardial stunning or infarction that occurs during or soon after implantation of a LVAD can elicit right-sided circulatory failure, resulting in decreased flow to the LVAD. In patients who have had coronary bypass surgery and are candidates for mechanical circulatory support, patent bypass grafts, particularly to the right coronary artery or left anterior descending coronary artery, should be preserved to reduce the risk of perioperative right-sided circulatory failure and arrhythmias. In selected situations it may be important to perform a coronary artery bypass to the right coronary artery or left anterior descending coronary artery systems to optimize right heart function in the perioperative period if significant obstructive coronary lesions amenable to bypass are present in the distribution of the these arteries.

Arrhythmias

Atrial and ventricular arrhythmias are common in patients with cardiogenic shock and underlying ischemic heart disease or idiopathic cardiomyopathies. These arrhythmias generally persist in the immediate postoperative period and subsequently resolve with time as the hemodynamic condition of the patient improves and inotropic therapy is weaned. Some patients will have persistent arrhythmias due to their underlying pathology (e.g., giant cell myocarditis). Severe ventricular arrhythmias have traditionally been thought to be a contraindication to univentricular support. However, recent experience has revealed that the hemodynamic consequences in patients in whom these arrhythmias develop in the late postoperative period are generally not life threatening.[40–42] In the absence of pulmonary hypertension and elevated pulmonary vascular resistance in the postoperative period, patients maintain adequate LVAD flows during ventricular fibrillation. This situation is analogous to a Fontan (systemic vein to pulmonary artery) circulation. In the early perioperative period, some patients with refractory ventricular arrhythmias may require biventricular support until the pulmonary vasculature resistance drops and a Fontan circulation is tolerated. The addition of right ventricular support for hemodynamic compromise due to refractory ventricular arrhythmia is unusual. In situations in which weaning from mechanical support is feasible or planned, elimination of the ventricular arrhythmias with antiarrhythmic therapy is essential.

Atrial fibrillation and flutter hinders right ventricular filling but is reasonably well-tolerated in recipients of VADs. Early electrical or pharmacologic cardioversion is indicated to avoid thrombus formation and improve exercise tolerance. Anticoagulation is indicated in patients with persistent atrial or ventricular arrhythmias to prevent thrombus formation (even for those devices for which anticoagulation is otherwise unnecessary).

Intracardiac Shunts

Potential intracardiac shunts such as a patent foramen ovale or atrial septal defect should be closed at the time of initiation of LVAD support to prevent right-to-left shunting. These anomalies should be identified prior to surgery using transesophageal echocardiogram.[43] During the initiation of left ventricular assistance, left atrial pressure is reduced compared to right atrial pressure. This gradient causes shunting of deoxygenated blood from the right atrium into the left resulting in significant systemic hypoxemia. In cases in which a patent foramen ovale or atrial septal defect has been missed, treatment includes administering pulmonary vasodilators and inotropic agents to decrease the shunt by improving right heart function and lowering right atrial pressure. If significant hypoxia persists, reoperation to close the anomaly is required.

MANAGEMENT AND COMPLICATIONS OF MECHANICAL CIRCULATORY SUPPORT

Bleeding, right-sided circulatory failure, air embolism, and progressive multisystem organ failure are the most frequent complications that occur in the early postoperative period following initiation of mechanical circulatory support. Complications most common in the late postoperative period include infection, thromboembolism, and device failure.

Bleeding

Bleeding is a frequent, early complication in patients supported by mechanical assist devices and generally requires reoperation in the early postoperative period. Risk factors for bleeding include preoperative hepatic congestion and failure, poor preoperative nutritional status, prolonged cardiopulmonary bypass times, extensive surgical dissection, reoperative surgery, multiple cannulation sites, decreased platelet function, and induction of fibrinolysis as a result of contact with biomaterial surfaces during cardiopulmonary bypass and mechanical circulatory support devices. In the early experience of mechanical circulatory support, about 50% of patients required reoperation for bleeding. The risk of major hemorrhage has decreased substantially with the use of the serine protease inhibitor, aprotinin and supplemental administration of vitamin K prior to operation.[44,45] Meticulous surgical technique is also an important factor to reduce hemorrhagic complications.

Right-Sided Circulatory Failure

Right-sided circulatory failure occurs in approximately 10% to 20% of patients supported by left ventricular assistance. The etiology of right-sided circulatory failure is multifactorial and includes primary pathologies within the pulmonary vascular bed and/or right ventricle. Frequently, the occurrence of right-sided circulatory failure is a consequence of both. Factors contributing to right-sided circulatory failure include impaired right ventricular function as a result of intraoperative air embolism, myocardial stunning as a result of poor intraoperative myocardial protection, ischemia and infarction from coronary artery disease, arrhythmias, volume loading, and alteration of right ventricular septal geometry induced by left ventricular unloading. Several studies have demonstrated that factors, such as elevated central venous pressure, transpulmonary gradient greater than 16 mm Hg, acute decrease in pulmonary artery pressures equal to or greater than 10 mm Hg at the onset of LVAD support, degree of preoperative pulmonary edema, and increased need for perioperative transfusions, all increase the need for right ventricular mechanical support following LVAD implantation.[26,27,35,46,47] Multiple perioperative transfusions elicit the expression and release of numerous inflammatory cytokines, including interleukin-1 beta, interleukin-6, and tumor necrosis factor-alpha (TNF-α).[48] TNFα can induce pulmonary hypertension and its effect may be mediated by platelet activating factor, a potent vasoconstrictor of the pulmonary circulation.[49] Acute unloading of the left ventricle by mechanical assist may cause the septum to shift leftward, increasing right ventricular volume loading and reducing its function.[37–39] The negative consequences of this phenomenon may be offset by the reduction in pulmonary artery pressures and right ventricular afterload caused by device-mediated left ventricular decompression.[37–39] Hemodynamic stability can be attained with isolated left ventricular support in about 90% of patients without the need for right ventricular assistance, even in those patients with substantial right ventricular dysfunction, if there is effective replacement of left-sided heart function and aggressive treatment of pulmonary hypertension. More recently, improved perioperative management of elevated pulmonary vascular resistance including the use of inhaled nitric oxide, a specific, potent pulmonary vasodilator, in combination with milrinone, isoproterenol, or dobutamine have significantly reduced the need for placement of a right VAD (RVAD).[50–52] In patients with marked elevation of central venous pressure, multiorgan failure, and severe right ventricular dysfunction with low pulmonary artery pressures, early biventricular support may be indicated.[53]

Thromboembolism and Anticoagulation Management

The occurrence of thromboembolic events following mechanical circulatory support is variable and depends on a number of factors including the type of device, duration of support, location and number of cannulation sites, and the presence of prosthetic valves within the heart. Overall, approximately 10% of patients receiving mechanical circulatory support with implantable devices will experience a thromboembolic event.[5] This rate is probably higher, in the range of 20%, for patients on short-term extracorporeal devices. Improvement in the rate of thromboembolic events has come from more aggressive antiplatelet therapy in conjunction with warfarin, improved device design, and more frequent use of left ventricular apical as compared to left atrial cannulation. In patients supported for short durations only, anticoagulation is usually achieved with heparin and antiplatelet therapy. Longer term support usually requires transition to warfarin and antiplatelet therapy for most, but not all devices.

The single, most significant technologic advance in preventing thromboembolic events in patients on long-term left ventricular assistance has been attributed to the use of textured blood contacting surfaces within the devices. This technology has been applied in the HeartMate (Thoratec Inc., Pleasanton, CA) series of implantable LVADs.[54,55] The interior surfaces of this LVAD have been textured using sintered titanium microspheres on the rigid metallic surfaces and integrally textured polyurethane on the movable diaphragm (Fig. 86.1).

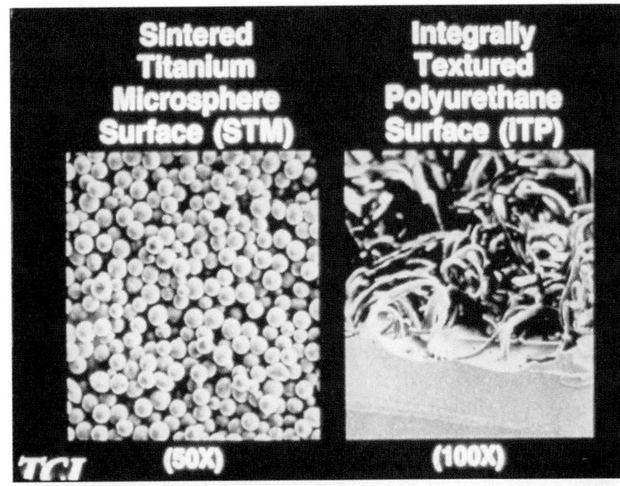

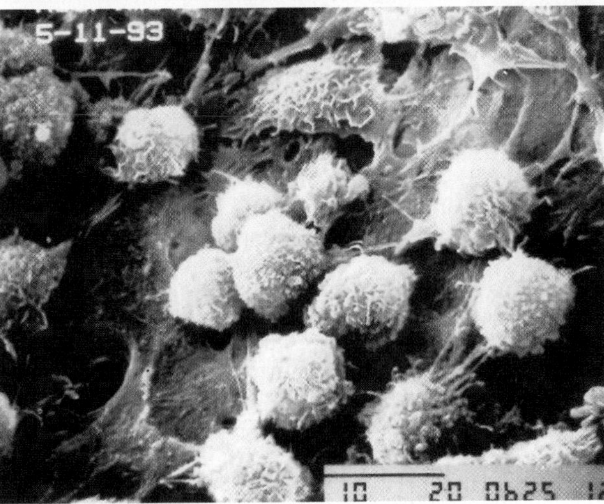

FIGURE 86.1 Sintered titanium microsphere surface and integrally textured polyurethane surface incorporated in the HeartMate LVAS (Photograph courtesy of Thoratec, Inc., Pleasanton, CA.)

This design feature permits a uniform autologous tissue lining to establish on all the blood-contacting surfaces of the pump, minimizing thrombus formation and bacterial colonization. The tightly adherent fibrin-cellular matrix, once mature, contains macrophages, mesenchymal cells, endothelial cells, and other blood components. This densely adherent neointima eliminates direct contact between the device and blood elements, substantially reducing the risk of embolization. Most thromboembolic events occur either perioperatively due to air emboli or occur remotely from the time of device implantation in association with device infection, particularly device fungal infection. Patients supported with the HeartMate LVAD require antiplatelet therapy with aspirin alone but do not require systemic anticoagulation with heparin or warfarin as with other forms of mechanical circulatory support (Table 86.3).

Infection

Infections can be device-related [e.g., device endocarditis, driveline or cannula site infection, pocket infection (infection external to an implanted device)] or non–device-related (e.g., pneumonia, urinary tract infection). The incidence of early nosocomial non–device- or device-related infections in patients undergoing mechanical circulatory support is approximately 30% to 40% in many series and is related to the acuity of illness in this population of patients.[56–65] Patients with persistent or recurrent sepsis and those patients with device-related infections tend to have a higher mortality than patients without these complications.[60] In patients on long term (greater than 2 weeks) mechanical circulatory support, infection remains the single, most significant obstacle to successful outcome. Infection was the most common cause of mortality during LVAD support seen in the REMATCH trial, with infection contributing to 41% of deaths.[5] Within 3 months after implantation, the probability of infection with the device was 28%. Most of these late infections began in the percutaneous tube (driveline) tract and pocket of the device. However, clinical experience has revealed that LVAD infection rates can be minimized with attention to infection control guidelines, optimal implantation techniques, and meticulous wound care.[66,67]

Risk factors for development of infection that are present before device insertion include preoperative infection at remote sites (not in the area of implantation), malnutrition, prolonged hospitalization, immobilization, broad-spectrum antibiotic therapy, immunosuppressive medications (e.g., steroids), mechanical ventilation, and the presence of nontunneled central venous catheters (especially for more than 5 to 7 days). In LVAD recipients, predisposing factors for local wound necrosis, apart from age, diabetes, and chronic debilitation, usually are tension on the wound edges, recurrent trauma to the driveline exit site, and localized hematoma of the device pocket followed by bacterial colonization and subsequent infection. The percutaneous tube of the device can be a portal of entry for bacterial and fungal pathogens. Intracorporeal device infections can occur within the pumps themselves and on their outer surfaces, which are generally caused by biofilm-forming bacteria and fungi (e.g., *Staphylococcus* spp.). Device-related infections can sometimes be successfully treated with antibiotic suppression and device exchange or removal. Infections involving the preperitoneal pocket (subfascial space created for device placement) surrounding implantable LVAD require more aggressive treatment, including open drainage, débridement, and rerouting of the driveline through a fresh exit site. However, patients that are device-dependent and awaiting transplantation, generally cannot tolerate device removal as a therapeutic option to eradicate the infection. Antibiotic suppression and transplantation remain the only chance for cure of device-related infections in some instances. Fortunately, these infections do not generally preclude heart transplantation, and transplant outcomes and survival are generally not significantly affected in this situation.[59,68]

Recent data have also demonstrated that patients maintained on long-term mechanical circulatory support have significant derangements in their immune system secondary to patient–device interactions. These data suggest that LVAD implantation is accompanied by progressive defects in cellular immunity that seem to be the result of an aberrant state of T-cell activation involving the CD95 (FAS) pathway and activation-induced cell death of CD4 T-cells.[69,72] These defects predispose recipients of LVADs to fungal infections and other systemic infections as a result of defects in their cellular immunity.[69–72]

Sensitization to HLA Antigens

Recent evidence demonstrates that recipients of long-term mechanical circulatory support develop prominent B-cell activation as evidenced by heightened production of anti–human leukocyte antigen (HLA) and antiphospholipid antibodies. The incidence of antibody development to HLA class I or II antibodies may be as high as 80 percent.[72,73] This enhanced B-cell reactivity is thought to be secondary to activation-induced cell death of CD4 T-cell as noted previously.[69,72–74]

The presence of preformed lymphocytotoxic antibodies reactive against donor lymphocytes in recipient serum detected in a routine cross-match is considered a significant obstacle to successful solid organ transplantation. The presence of preformed lymphocytotoxic antibodies is associated with a high incidence of humoral allograft rejection, early graft failure, and poorer patient survival.[74,75] These antibodies are primarily directed against donor major histocompatability complex (MHC) class I HLA antigens constitutively expressed by the allograft endothelium, because nonactivated endothelium does not express MHC class II HLA antigens. Consequently, the risk for early graft failure (i.e., within the first 24 to 48 hours) is significantly higher in the presence of a positive cross-match. In addition, the real risk for early graft failure after a positive cross-match appears to reside in the IgG fraction of donor-specific antibodies. An IgM-positive cross-match can result from the presence of antilymphocytic autoantibodies, which do not specifically react with donor HLA allotypes, and their presence generally does not lead to early graft failure.

Device Malfunction

As with any mechanical device, malfunction is an anticipated occurrence. The types and severity of device malfunctions vary with each of the devices. Many devices have built-in back-up systems that, in the event of catastrophic device failure, provide support to the patient. In addition, most patients supported by a LVAD have enough residual left ventricular function to help sustain them until corrective measures can be taken. Device malfunctions in total artificial hearts are more problematic, because there is no native heart to provide hemodynamic support in the event of a total device failure. Stringent quality control measures in fabrication and testing and very low mechanical failure rates are therefore even more essential with total artificial hearts.

CONSIDERATIONS IN WEANING PATIENTS FROM MECHANICAL CIRCULATORY SUPPORT

A number of factors must be considered when weaning patients from mechanical circulatory support. First and foremost is the consideration of any pathologic abnormalities of the heart, such as valvular disease or severe coronary disease, that have not been addressed and corrected. If the underlying pathology that has caused the patient to require mechanical circulatory support is not corrected, then the chances of weaning from mechanical circulatory support will be negligible. Cardiac tamponade must also be excluded. Bleeding is a major early complication of mechanical circulatory support and reoperation for cardiac tamponade and bleeding is frequent. Transesophageal echocardiogram may not reliably identify cardiac tamponade in the early postoperative period. Thus, a high index of suspicion and low threshold for reoperation is critical to rule out tamponade. Volume status, preload and afterload, cardiac rhythm, and degree of inotropic support should be optimized for weaning. Noncardiac causes can contribute to failure to wean from mechanical circulatory support. Pulmonary edema, elevated pulmonary vascular resistance, acute respiratory distress syndrome (ARDS), and pneumonia may hinder right ventricular function.

Once a patient's status has been optimized, weaning from mechanical circulatory support with the use of transesophageal echocardiogram is ideal. As device flows are reduced, transesophageal echocardiogram provides information on ventricular filling and performance and valve function. If patients can maintain satisfactory hemodynamics with reduction of pump flow, they can be considered for weaning. In the setting of biventricular support, it is important that device flows on the right side be reduced prior to turning down left-sided device flows to prevent pulmonary edema in the event of inadequate left-sided ventricular function. As device flows are reduced, native heart function will be begin to support the circulation and monitoring of the systemic arterial waveform will demonstrate native heart contractions in synchronization with the electrocardiogram.

If hemodynamics are unsatisfactory during the weaning trial, the patient will require continued support and subsequent weaning trials. In cases in which weaning from mechanical circulatory support is not possible, patients should be evaluated for heart transplantation and bridged to a mechanical device with long-term support capabilities when feasible.

MECHANICAL CIRCULATORY SUPPORT DEVICES

Intraaortic Balloon Pump

The IABP was first introduced in 1962 by Moulopolous and colleagues.[76] The first clinical use of the IABP was reported by Kantrowitz et al.[77] in 1968, who described the use of the pump in three patients suffering from postinfarction cardiogenic shock refractory to medical therapy. Since that time, the IABP has become one of the simplest, most affordable, and most utilized circulatory assist devices available to support patients in cardiogenic shock (Fig. 86.2). The IABP can be inserted percutaneously and may augment cardiac output by as much as 10% to 25% depending on a number of factors that include balloon size, patient size, degree of aortic compliance, cardiac rhythm, blood pressure, and IABP settings and timing. Patients with ischemic cardiomyopathy have the greatest increase in

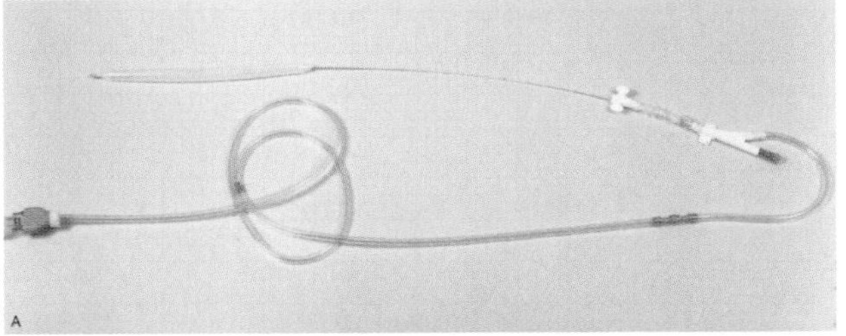

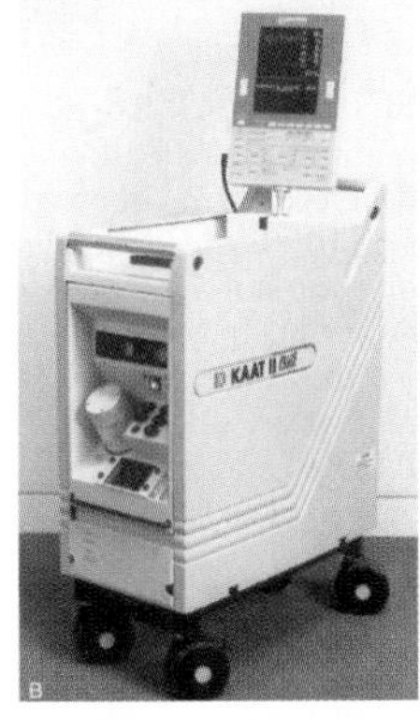

FIGURE 86.2 Intraaortic balloon pump. (*A*) Catheter-mounted balloon is typically positioned within the thoracic aorta through a percutaneous insertion in the groin. (*B*) Console for the intraaortic balloon pump.

cardiac output, with improved cardiac contractility resulting from enhanced coronary perfusion. The IABP has become a standard in coronary care and cardiac surgery centers in the treatment of left ventricular dysfunction and cardiogenic shock that is refractory to medical management.

The concept for the IABP was first developed from the realization that the area under the arterial pressure trace (time-tension index) was an indirect estimation of the heart's oxygen consumption and that by decreasing the area during systole by reducing afterload would effectively support the failing heart. Harken et al.[78] described a device that lowered the time-tension index by withdrawing blood from the arterial tree just before ventricular systole, returning it to the circulation in diastole. In 1962, Moulopolous et al.[76] described a catheter-based balloon that produced hemodynamic effects similar to the Harken pump, but without an extracorporeal pump. Moulopolous passed a balloon into the aorta that inflated during ventricular diastole, thereby augmenting diastolic blood pressure. Deflation just before ejection effectively decreased the afterload of the heart afterload and thus the work of the heart during systole.

The major hemodynamic effects of the IABP are a decrease in left ventricular afterload and an increase in coronary artery perfusion pressure. Cardiac output improves from enhanced myocardial contractility as a result of increased coronary blood flow and reduced afterload and preload. The IABP is positioned with the tip of the balloon lying just distal to the left subclavian artery. The balloon should fill the aorta so that during the inflation cycle it nearly occludes the vessel. In adults, balloon volumes of 30 to 40 mL are optimal. Inflation should be timed to coincide with closure of the aortic valve, which, is obtained by identifying the dicrotic notch of aortic blood pressure trace (Fig. 86.3). Deflation should occur as late as possible to maintain the duration of the augmented diastolic blood pressure but before the aortic valve opens and the ventricle ejects. Deflation is timed to occur with the onset of the electrocardiographic R wave. A regular heart rate with an easily identified R wave or a good arterial pulse tracing with a discrete

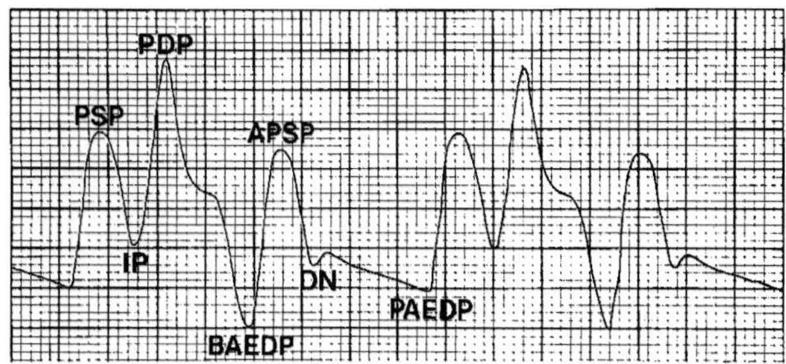

FIGURE 86.3 Aortic pressure tracing during intraaortic balloon pump support. Balloon counterpulsation is occurring after every other heartbeat (1:2 counterpulsation). With correct timing, balloon inflation (IP) begins immediately after aortic valve closure, signaled by the dicrotic notch (DN). Compared with unassisted ejection, the pump augments diastolic blood flow by increasing peak aortic pressure during diastole (PDP). Balloon deflation before systole decreases ventricular afterload, with lower aortic end-diastolic pressure (BAEDP vs. PAEDP) and lower peak systolic pressure (APSP vs. PSP). (Courtesy of St. Jude Medical, Inc., Cardiac Assist Division, Minneapolis, MN.)

aortic dicrotic notch optimizes performance of the IABP. Current balloon pumps trigger off the electrocardiographic R wave or from the arterial pressure tracing. During tachycardia, the IABP is usually timed to inflate every other beat. In unstable patients, obtaining a regular rhythm or regular paced rhythm optimizes proper timing of the IABP.

The IABP can be inserted into the common femoral artery either by the percutaneous technique, using a modified Seldinger technique, or by surgical cut-down. A cut-down is generally performed during cardiopulmonary bypass when the arterial pulse is absent due to nonpulsatile flow. During insertion, a guide wire is introduced into the femoral artery then followed by dilating catheters and the balloon. After passage of the flexible guide wire, the soft tissue tract and vessel are progressively dilated until an appropriately sized sheath can be inserted. Sheathless IABP catheters are available. Next, the furled catheter (standard size 9.5-Fr, 40-mL balloon) is passed proximally until its tip rests in the thoracic aorta just distal to the left subclavian. In situations in which the common femoral or iliac arteries cannot be used because of occlusive disease and an inability to advance the guide wire, the axillary artery, exposed below the middle third of the clavicle may be used as an alternative entry site. Alternatively, in situations of postcardiotomy failure to wean, the ascending aorta may be utilized as an insertion site. Fluoroscopy or transesophageal echocardiography should be utilized to ensure proper positioning of the guide wire. The balloon should be positioned so that, during inflation, it does not occlude the left subclavian artery. Heparin is recommended if the IABP remains in place for more than 24 hours. Weaning of the IABP entails observing the clinical response to reducing the ratio assisted heart beats to total beats from 1:1 to 1:3 or 1:4. At the time of removal of the IABP, every effort should be made to flush out any thrombus as the balloon catheter is removed. Hemostasis should be obtained by application of direct pressure to the entry site for at least 30 to 45 minutes. Removal of the IABP placed through a cut-down on the femoral artery may require repair of that artery and concomitant embolectomy if there have been signs of ischemia of the lower extremity.

Complications from use of the IABP include leg ischemia, balloon rupture, thrombosis within the balloon, sepsis, infection at the insertion site, bleeding, false aneurysm formation, lymph fistula, femoral neuropathy, vessel perforation with hemorrhage, and aortic dissection from catheter passage below the intima. Depending on the extent of peripheral vascular disease, balloon position can occlude major branches of the aorta and elicit ischemia of the tissues supplied by these vessels. Examples of this scenario include intestinal "angina" from occlusion of the mesenteric vessels and upper extremity symptoms when the balloon impinges on the left subclavian artery. Female gender, peripheral vascular disease, diabetes, smoking, advanced age, obesity, and cardiogenic shock are risk factors for the development of leg ischemia. Balloon rupture is usually indicated by the appearance of blood within the balloon catheter. Leg ischemia, balloon rupture, and sepsis are an indication for removal of the IABP. If the patient is balloon dependent, a replacement balloon can be inserted in a new site. The IABP has several disadvantages. In the best of circumstances, cardiac output is augmented by 25% as compared to LVADs that can augment cardiac output by three to five times baseline flows. The IABP offers no significant support to the right heart. Mobilization and ambulation of the patient is limited while the IABP is being utilized.

Extracorporeal, Continuous Flow Circulatory Support Devices

Extracorporeal Life Support

ECLS, traditionally referred to as ECMO, is a temporary form of mechanical circulatory support that provides circulatory assistance, as well as oxygenation and carbon dioxide removal from blood.[79–81] The ECLS circuit is similar in concept to cardiopulmonary bypass routinely used in the operating room for cardiac procedures. However, with ECLS, safe application for extended periods of time (days) has required certain modifications, particularly the inclusion of membrane oxygenators. The first successful use of prolonged ECLS was reported by Hill in 1972.[82] Subsequently, ECLS has been used in an increasing number of indications including neonatal, pediatric, and adult respiratory support; neonatal, pediatric, and adult postcardiotomy support; and as a bridge to LVAD or heart and lung transplantation.

ECLS supports the circulation by unloading the right ventricle and draining blood from the venous circulation, oxygenating it, then returning it to the arterial circulation. ECLS does not unload the left ventricle, although left ventricular preload is reduced by decreasing pulmonary venous return. In patients with severe left ventricular dysfunction, the use of an IABP helps reduce left ventricular afterload during systole and improves myocardial contractility. The use of the IABP and inotropic therapy can maintain sufficient cardiac contractility to prevent stasis within the ventricle where clot formation is possible.[83] If left ventricular function is so severely reduced that there is no ejection, an atrial septostomy can be performed to vent pulmonary venous return. Alternatively, a left-sided vent can be connected to the venous line to relieve ventricular distention. It is important during ECLS support to maintain some degree of pulmonary blood flow to prevent thrombosis. Additionally, it is important to continue ventilation of the lungs to maintain the oxygen saturation of the blood ejected from the left ventricle above 90%. Poorly oxygenated blood ejected from the left ventricle will perfuse the coronary arteries and add hypoxic damage to the already injured heart. Venovenous ECLS, unlike venoarterial ECLS, maintains flow through the heart. Venoarterial ECLS is used primarily for cardiac or cardiorespiratory support, whereas venovenous ECLS is used for pulmonary support.

Current ECLS circuits typically comprise a centrifugal pump with either a hollow fiber or membrane oxygenator, oxygen blender, pump console, heat exchanger, and pump cart. A roller pump is used by some centers. Cannulation for ECLS is extremely variable and depends on the clinical situation and whether venoarterial or venovenous circuit is desired.

In emergent situations in which institution of mechanical circulatory support is needed within minutes (acute cardiac and/or respiratory arrest), percutaneous cannulation of the femoral vein and artery can be performed. In less urgent situations, cut-down on the internal jugular and carotid artery or femoral vessels can be performed. In cases of postcardiotomy failure in the operating room, venous access can be obtained by insertion of cannula in the right atrium and arterial outflow obtained by cannulation of the ascending aorta.

ECLS is usually continued for several days to weeks and during this time, patients are vigorously diuresed or undergo continuous venovenous hemofiltration (CVVH) to remove excess third-space fluid. Right atrial and left atrial pressures and pump flows are monitored, and mixed venous saturations are maintained above 75%, which is an accurate reflection of the adequacy of systemic flows. A sudden decrease in venous drainage is usually manifested by chugging of the venous lines with wide respiratory fluctuations and flow; causes include hypovolemia, cannula kinking or malposition, pneumothorax, and pericardial tamponade. Centrifugal pumps are afterload sensitive, and kinking of the inflow cannula will result in decreased flow.

Although the results of ECLS are very encouraging, the use of ECLS is associated with significant side effects, including bleeding, stroke, infection, hematologic abnormalities, and initiation of a whole-body inflammatory response that occurs in response to circulatory bypass. Complement activation through the alternative pathway is a well-documented response to hemodialysis and cardiopulmonary bypass. Circulating C3a and C5a lead to neutrophil adherence, aggregation, and activation; activated neutrophils in turn release free radicals, proteases, and arachidonic acid metabolites that, among other things, damage the integrity of cellular membranes. Additionally, the complexity of ECMO requires continuous intensive care unit monitoring by skilled personnel.

Numerous large clinical series have reported successful use of ECLS for cardiac and/or respiratory support in adult, pediatric, and neonatal patients. In the largest series reported to date, Bartlett et al.[84] at the University of Michigan reported on the outcome of 1,000 patients supported with ECLS from 1980 through 1998. For patients with cardiac failure, 33% of adult patients (31 cases) and 48% of pediatric patients (105 cases) survived to hospital discharge. Survival in adult patients was improved by utilizing ECLS as a bridge to longer-term implantable devices in patients who did not demonstrate early recovery of myocardial function.[85,86] Conversely, the availability of long-term implantable devices has extended the use of ECLS in situations in which recovery of myocardial function is unlikely.[85–87] Smedira et al.[88] reported on the clinical experience of 202 adult patients receiving ECLS for cardiac failure at the Cleveland Clinic. Survival at 24 hours, 30 days, and 1 year was 90%, 38%, and 29%, respectively. For patients alive at 30 days, survival at 5 years was 63%. Complications occurring during ECLS support were significant. Infectious complications occurred in 49% of patients. Forty percent of patients required dialysis, neurologic complications occurred in 33%, and limb complications occurred in 25%. Risk factors for death included older age, thoracic aortic operations, reoperations, decompensated heart failure, and nonuse of an IABP. The authors recommended concomitant IABP support for all patients requiring ECLS support to improve myocardial recovery and improve organ function with pulsatile flow. Magovern and Simpson[89] reported on the outcome of 92 adult patients following institution of ECLS support. Twenty of 55 (36%) patients survived to hospital discharge following ECLS support for postcardiotomy failure to wean. Twenty-three of 27 (85%) patients survived ECLS support following percutaneous interventions in the catheterization laboratory, and 2 of 4 (50%) survived ECLS for primary cardiac allograft failure. No patient (of 6) survived ECLS support for cardiac resuscitation.

Centrifugal Pumps

Centrifugal pumps are extracorporeal systems that provide short-term mechanical circulatory support (Fig. 86.4).[90,91] The systems are easy to operate, widely available, disposable, and relatively inexpensive compared to most other forms of mechanical circulatory assist. These systems are most commonly used in cardiopulmonary bypass to support open heart operations. Worldwide, numerous centrifugal pumps are available or are in development for clinical use. However, in the United States, until recently only three centrifugal pumps have been commercially available. All are disposable and are relatively simple to operate. The Sarns centrifugal pump (Terumo Inc., Ann Arbor, MI) uses a spinning impeller system to impart a rotary motion to incoming perfusate. The St. Jude Medical Lifestream centrifugal pump (St. Jude Medical, Inc. Cardiac Assist Division, Chelmsford, MA) employs a curved vane design and angled egress blood flow path that purports to minimize turbulence, decrease hemolysis, and reduce periods of flow stasis. The BioMedicus Bio-pump (Medtonic BioMedicus, Inc., Eden Prairie, MN) centrifugal pump head consists of valveless rotator cones that impart a circular motion to incoming blood by viscous drag and constrained vortex principles generating pressure and flow. The Carmeda BioMedicus Bio-pump (Medtronic Inc., Minneapolis, MN) has heparin covalently bonded to the blood exposed surfaces. These three disposable pump heads can be magnetically coupled to an electric motor, which is controlled by a computerized console. Control of flow is accomplished by adjusting the revolutions per minute of the spinning pump head. Short-term (generally limited to hours to days) ventricular or pulmonary support can be provided with centrifugal pumps. It can be used for femoral-femoral bypass, conventional cardiopulmonary bypass, left and/or right ventricular assistance, and extracorporeal membrane oxygenation (ECLS).

The most common use of the centrifugal pump, other than for conventional cardiopulmonary bypass operations for open heart procedures, is for patients who have had postcardiotomy failure and cardiogenic shock.[90–92] Postcardiotomy cardiac failure occurs in 2% to 6% of patients who have cardiac procedures.[90] However, with the advent of newer technologies, the use of these circuits for postcardiotomy cardiac failure has significantly declined. Results of a voluntary registry reporting the use of the centrifugal pump as right, left, or biventricular assist devices have shown that approximately 25% of patients were weaned from the device and eventually discharged.[92] The centrifugal pump can be used to provide left, right, or biventricular assistance. Cannulation for left ventricular assistance is most commonly performed through the right superior pulmonary vein into the left atrium with return into the ascending aorta. Right ventricular assistance is provided by cannulation of the right atrium and pulmonary artery. The pulmonary artery catheter is either placed through the right ventricle and threaded through the pulmonary valve or inserted directly into the pulmonary artery. Cannulas are secured in place with two purse string pledgeted sutures and tourniquets.

Tandem Heart pVAD

The Tandem Heart pVAD (Cardiac Assist Technologies, Inc, Pittsburgh, PA) is a percutaneous left atrial-to-femoral artery VAD (Fig. 86.5). The pump is a low speed, continuous flow, centrifugal pump that has a very low potential for hemolysis and thromboembolism. It is a dual-chamber pump composed of an upper housing and a lower housing assembly. The upper housing provides a conduit for inflow and outflow of blood. The lower housing assembly provides communication with the controller; the means for rotating the impeller of the VAD; and an anticoagulation infusion line integral to the pump to

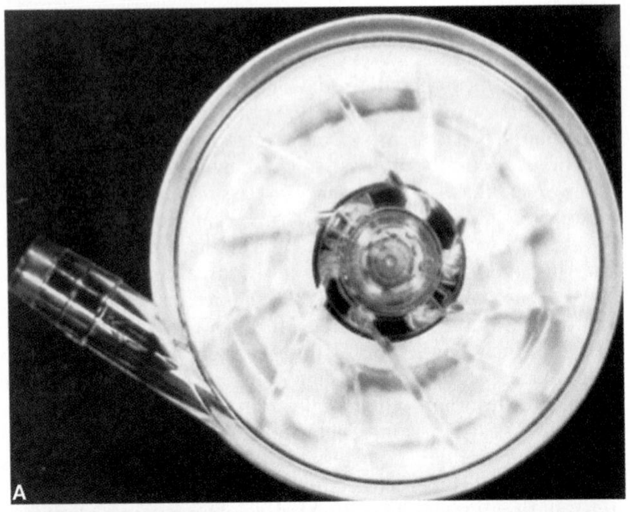

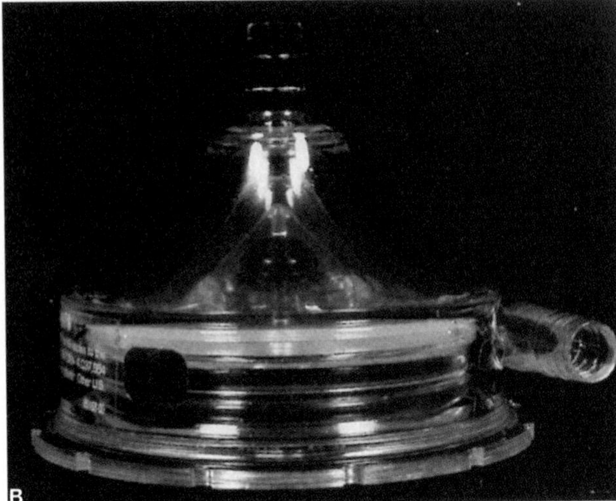

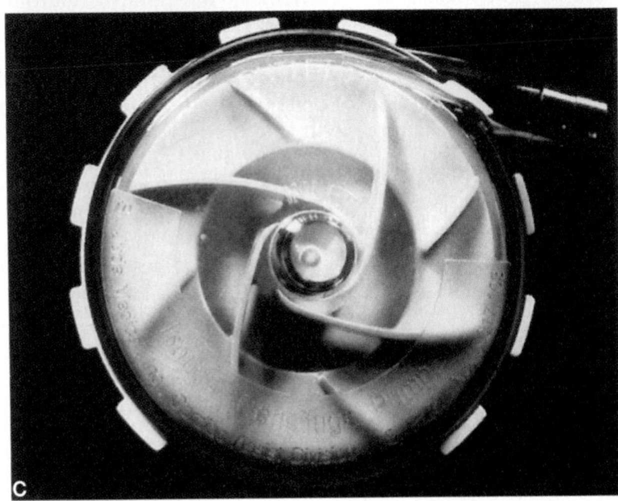

FIGURE 86.4 (*A*) Sarns centrifugal pump head. (*B*) BioMedicus Biopump centrifugal pump head. (*C*) St. Jude Medical Lifestream centrifugal pump head.

provide a hydrodynamic bearing, cooling of the bearing, and local anticoagulation. The controller is a microprocessor-based electromechanical drive and infusion system that is designed to operate on alternating current (AC) current or on internal batteries.

Implantation of the device is performed percutaneously through the right femoral vein (Fig. 86.6). A standard Brockenbrough catheter is inserted into the superior vena cava and the interatrial septum is punctured in the fossa ovalis using a Ross needle. The Brockenbrough catheter is then exchanged for a stiff guide wire with a distal soft wire loop identical to the device used for mitral valvuloplasty by the Inoue method. The transseptal puncture site is then dilated to 21 Fr with a two-stage dilator followed by insertion of a venous inflow cannula, which is sutured to the skin of the thigh. An arterial perfusion catheter of 14 Fr to 19 Fr is inserted percutaneously into the right femoral artery or two arterial perfusion catheters of 12 Fr into both femoral arteries.

Thiele et al.[93] reported on the use of the Tandem Heart pVAD in 18 patients presenting in cardiogenic shock. Mean duration of support was 4 ± 3 days. Following percutaneous placement of the device, mean cardiac index improved from 1.7 ± 0.3 L/min/m^2 to 2.4 ± 0.6 L/min/m^2. Mean device flow during support was 3.2 ± 0.6 L/min. Pulmonary wedge pressure decreased from 31 ± 8 mm Hg to 23 ± 6 mm Hg. Survival at 30 days was 56%. The Tandem Heart pVAD has been recently FDA-approved for temporary circulatory support for cardiogenic shock in patients refractory to optimal medical therapy and IABP.

Extracorporeal Pulsatile Flow Circulatory Support Devices

Thoratec Ventricular Assist System

The Thoratec pVAD (Thoratec Laboratories Inc., Pleasonton, CA) is a paracorporeal, pneumatically powered, pulsatile system configured for univentricular or biventricular support that consists of a seamless polyurethane blood sac contained within a rigid polycarbonate housing (Fig. 86.7).[94–97] An external drive console sends pressurized air to the pump, which compresses the blood sac and causes blood to be ejected. Bjork-Shiley concavoconvex tilting-disk valves within the inflow and outflow conduits ensure unidirectional blood flow. The device has a stroke volume of approximately 65 mL and a maximum output of 7 L/min. For left ventricular support, the pump inflow cannula can be placed in the left ventricular apex or the left atrium, and the pump outflow conduit is anastomosed to the ascending aorta. For right ventricular support, a large-bore cannula is placed in the right atrium, and the outflow conduit is sewn to the main pul-

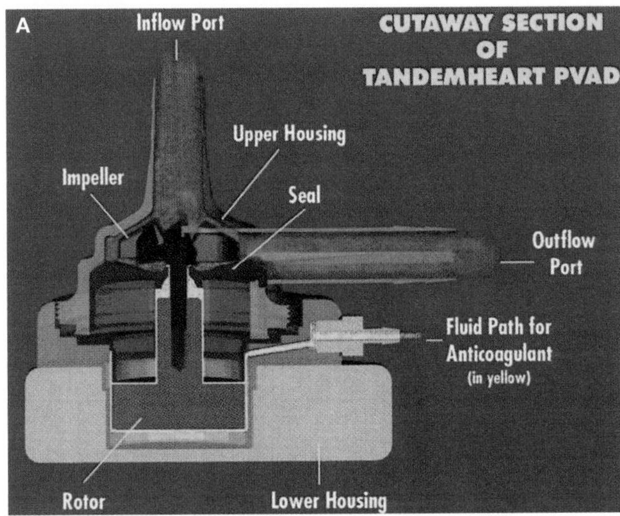

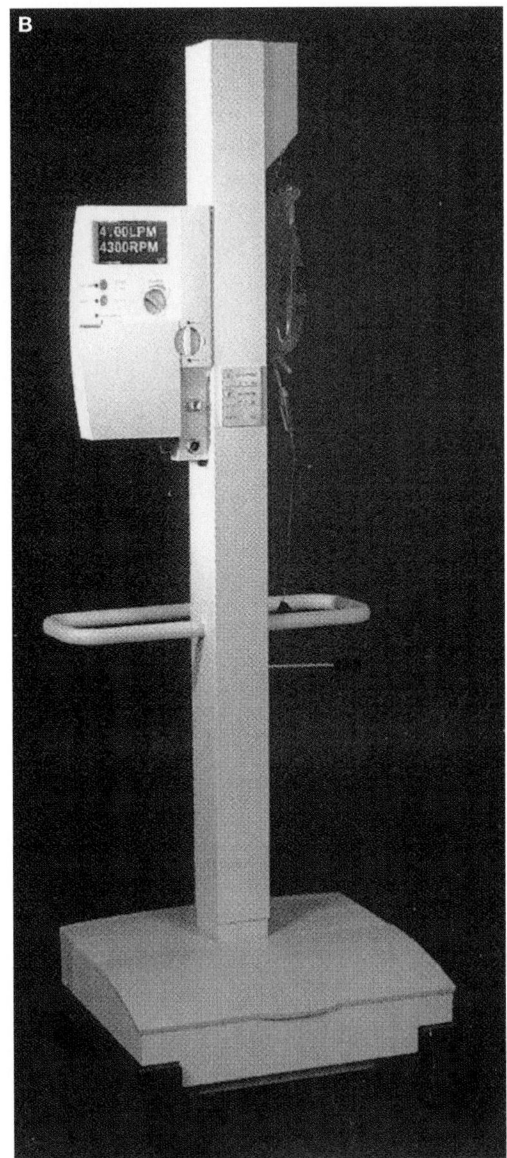

FIGURE 86.5 (*A*) Internal view of the Tandem Heart pVAD centrifugal pump demonstrating upper and lower housing and internal impeller. (*B*) Electrical control console for the Tandem Heart pVAD centrifugal pump. (Photographs courtesy of Cardiac Assist, Inc., Pittsburgh, PA.)

monary artery. When biventricular support is needed, right pump flow is adjusted so that it is less than left pump flow to prevent excessive pulmonary congestion. After the cannulas have been externalized subcostally, the inflow and outflow cannulas are connected to the pump(s), which reside externally on the anterior surface of the abdomen. During the support period, anticoagulation with dextran, heparin, warfarin, and dipyridamole is required. Patients may be ambulatory, but their mobility is limited by the size of the drive console and the paracorporeal position of the pump(s). The Thoratec pVAD can be operated in fixed-rate, volume, or synchronous mode. Volume mode is preferred because it maximizes support of the cardiac output. In the synchronous mode, the pump empties when triggered by the R-wave obtained from the patient's electrocardiogram. In this mode, weaning may be achieved by adjusting the device rate to a heart rate ratio in the range of 1:1 to 1:3. Synchronous mode is intended for weaning patients from support. Although the console can function automatically to achieve maximum pump flows, the operator must adjust the systolic driving pressure and diastolic vacuum pressure. The FDA has approved the Thoratec pVAD for use as a bridge to recovery and bridge to transplantation. New system designs to the paracorporeal Thoratec VAD currently include a small, portable drive console that enhances patient mobility and permits discharge from the hospital.[96]

Abiomed BVS 5000

The Abiomed BVS 5000 (Abiomed Inc., Danvers, MA) support system is an automated ventricular support device intended to provide complete temporary left and or right heart support (Fig. 86.8).[31,32,98] The Abiomed BVS 5000 is FDA-approved for short-term mechanical circulatory support as a bridge to recovery in cases of cardiogenic shock due to postcardiotomy failure to wean, acute myocarditis, and myocardial infarction.

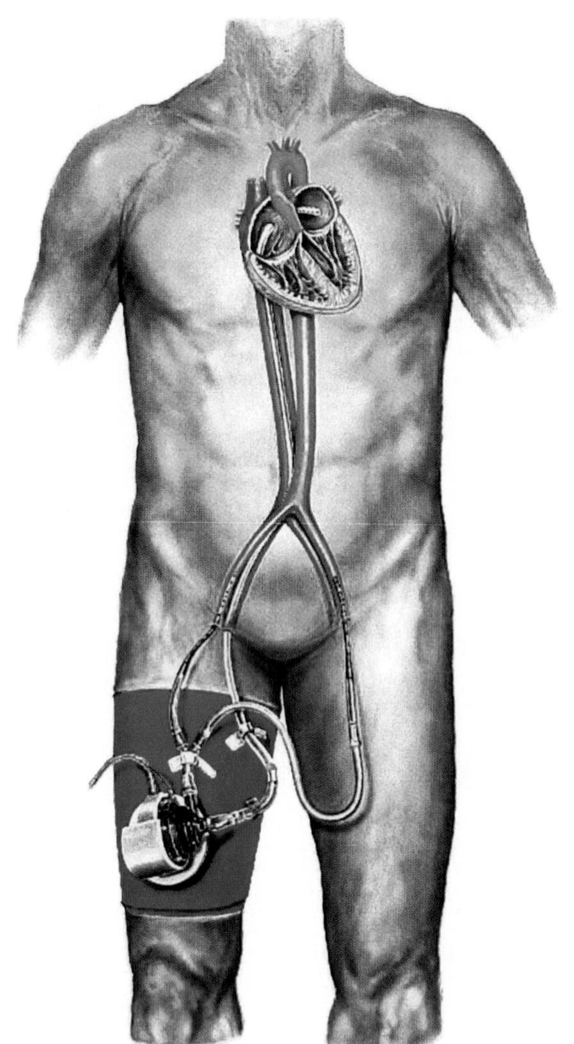
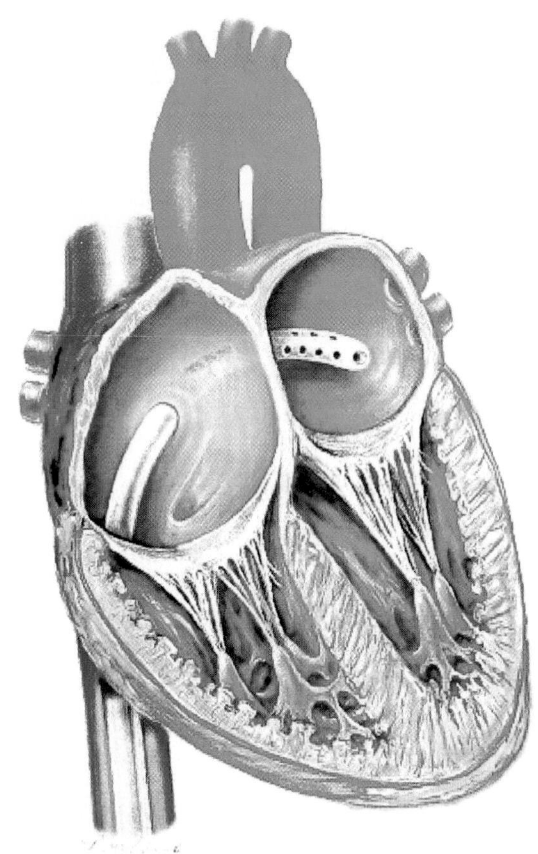

FIGURE 86.6 Schematic representation of the cannulation of the femoral artery and femoral vein with transseptal placement of the inflow catheter within the left atrium from the femoral vein. The Tandem Heart pVAD is secured to the patient's right thigh. (Photograph courtesy of Cardiac Assist, Inc., Pittsburgh, PA.)

Positioned externally, this pulsatile system simulates normal physiologic mechanical cardiac function. A microprocessor-based drive console is used to supply power to a disposable, pneumatically driven two-chambered blood pump that supports one side of the heart. Left atrial blood inflow is returned to the ascending aorta and right atrial inflow is returned to the pulmonary artery. Transthoracic cannulas are used to connect the external system with the patient. Each blood pump consists of two Angioflex polyurethane atrioventricular-like chambers (Fig. 86.9). Tri-leaflet polyurethane valves are strategically positioned to separate (a) atrial and ventricular bladders and (b) ventricular bladders and outflow cannulas. One or two disposable blood pumps are operated by a single BVS console, which automatically adjusts beat rate and systolic/diastolic ratio based on compressed air flow into and out of the external system. The pump is placed at the bedside and blood drains from the patient's left or right atrium by gravity, without the use of vacuum pressure, into the top of the pump and returns to the patient's aorta or pulmonary artery from the bottom of the pump. Filling of the blood pump chambers can be regulated by adjusting the height of the blood pump relative to the patient's heart. The blood pump is a dual-chamber device that incorporates an atrial (filling) chamber and a ventricular (pumping) chamber. Unidirectional flow is ensured by two trileaflet polyurethane valves fabricated from Angioflex, a biomaterial. The durations of pump systole and diastole are calculated automatically by the microprocessor to optimize pump filling and maintain a stroke volume of 83 mL. The console drives and adjusts left and right sides independently of each other. System controls are essentially limited to "on" and "off."

In addition to the traditional blood pumps and console, new blood pump designs and console, designated the AB5000,

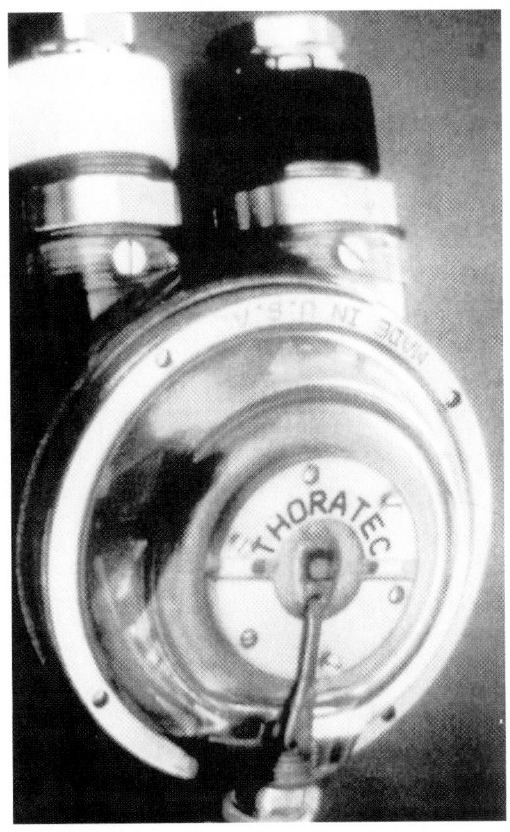

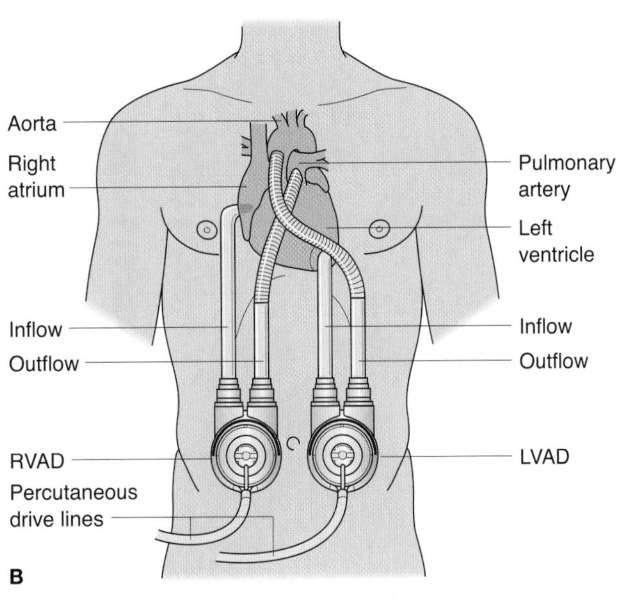

FIGURE 86.7 (*A*) Thoratec pVAD. (*B*) The Thoratec Ventricular Assist System in the biventricular support configuration. RVAD, right ventricular assist device (right atrium to pulmonary artery); LVAD, left ventricular assist device (left ventricular apex to aorta).

have recently been introduced and approved by the FDA for short-term circulatory support (Fig. 86.10).

Implantable Pulsatile Flow Circulatory Support Devices

HeartMate XVE LVAS

The HeartMate LVAD (Thoratec Laboratories Inc., Pleasonton, CA) is an implantable, pulsatile LVAD designed for long term circulatory support and is approved by the FDA as a bridge to heart transplantation and destination therapy (Fig. 86.11).[99–103] The unique feature of this device is that its blood-contacting surfaces of the pump are textured with sintered titanium spheres on the rigid surface and integrally textured polyurethane on the movable surfaces to encourage the deposition of circulating cells (see section on thromboembolism) (Fig. 86.12). In addition to the unique surface design, the pusher plate of the pump moves the diaphragm in a way that creates a wandering vortex in the blood chamber. This feature prevents stagnation of blood in any part of the chamber. Presently, there are two versions of the HeartMate in clinical use: an older pneumatic version (IP- 1000 LVAS) and a more recent vented electric version (XVE-LVAS). The HeartMate blood pump consists of a flexible polyurethane diaphragm within a ridged outer titanium alloy housing. The inflow and outflow conduits of the HeartMate device each contain a 25-mm porcine valve within a titanium cage to ensure unidirectional blood flow. The outflow conduit is extended by a 20-mm woven Dacron graft. With the XVE-LVAS, diaphragm movement and blood ejection depend on an electric motor positioned below the diaphragm (Fig. 86.13). The electric rotary motor within the titanium housing drives a cam up and down (translational movement) causing diaphragm movement. An external vent equalizes the air pressure and permits emergency pneumatic actuation in the event of electrical failure. The external system controller and batteries in the XVE-LVAS are small and lightweight, allowing the patient nearly unlimited mobility. The drive line is covered with a polyester velour that promotes tissue bonding and anchoring to the skin and reduces the risk of infection. The XVE-LVAS is powered by two rechargeable batteries that provide 4 to 6 hours of charge and are usually worn in a shoulder holster, vest, or belt. The wearable electrical devices currently available have external backup mechanisms to continue support without the need for reoperation in case of failure of the device. If the device should fail, the native heart is able to provide systemic support until the device can be examined. Because the electronic control unit is outside the body, it can easily be repaired should failure of the software, chip, or electronics occur (Fig. 86.14). Finally, if the motor device fails, the single-pusher-plate device can be pneumatically activated with a handheld portable pump or with the 75-lb pneumatic console that operates the IP-1000 model.

The HeartMate is implanted through an extended median sternotomy incision with the aid of cardiopulmonary bypass. The pump is positioned below the left hemidiaphragm, either within the peritoneal cavity or in a preperitoneal pocket. The inflow tube crosses the diaphragm and is inserted in the apex of the left ventricle. The outflow graft exits from the pocket, crosses the diaphragm, and is anastomosed to the ascending

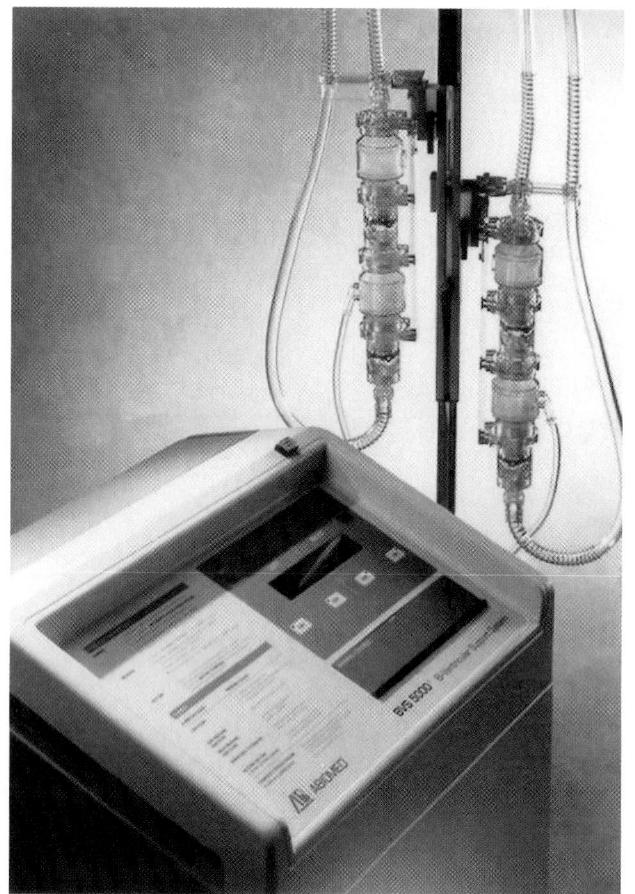

A

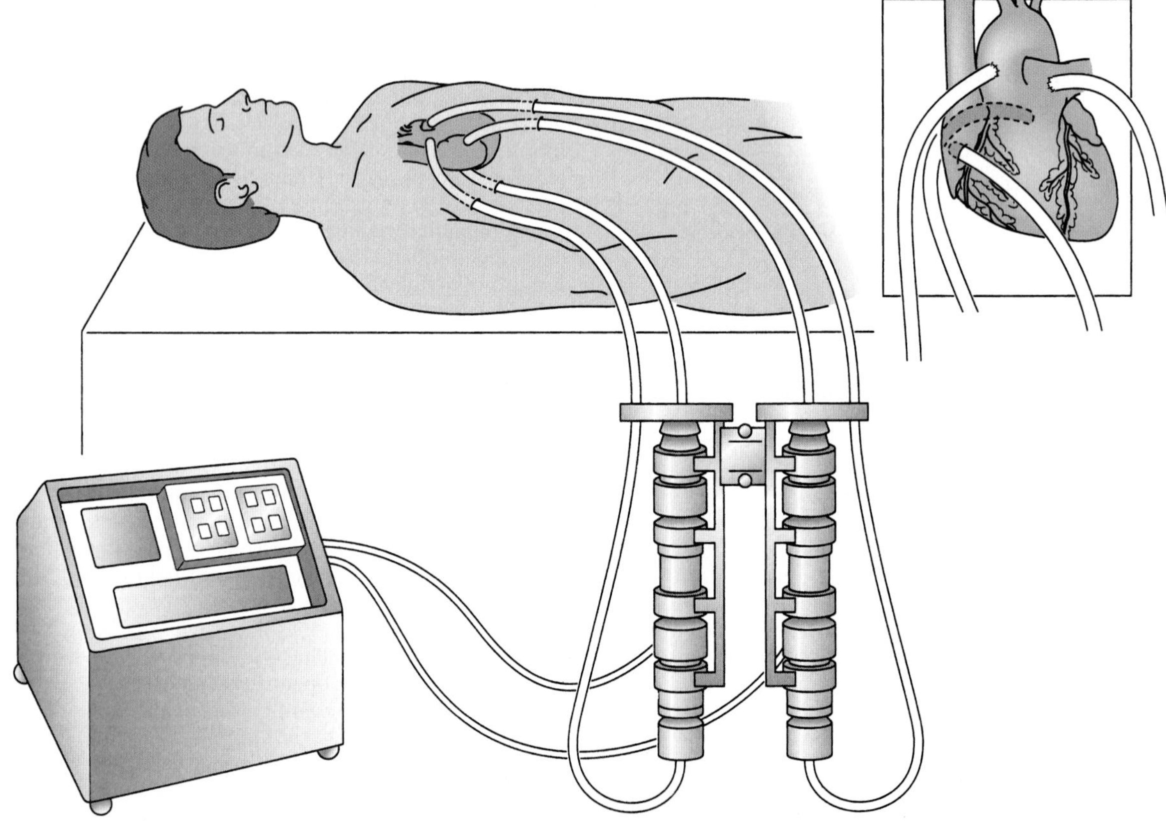

B

FIGURE 86.8 (*A*) Abiomed BVS 5000 biventricular assist device. Shown are the drive console (*left*) with blood pumps (*right*). (*B*) Schematic representation of the Abiomed BVS 5000 with biventricular support configuration (see inset).

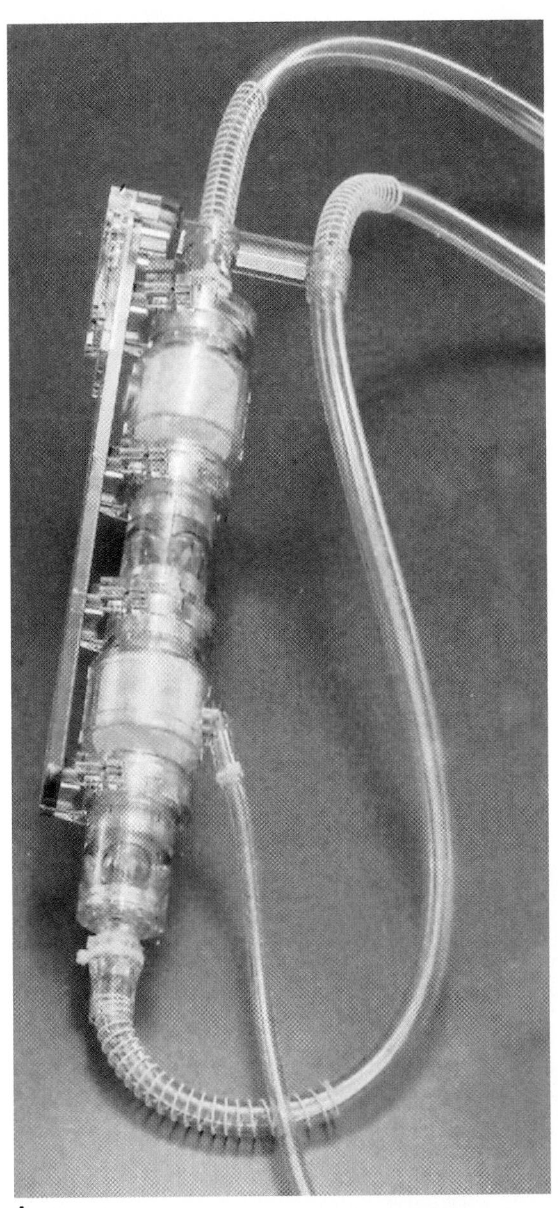

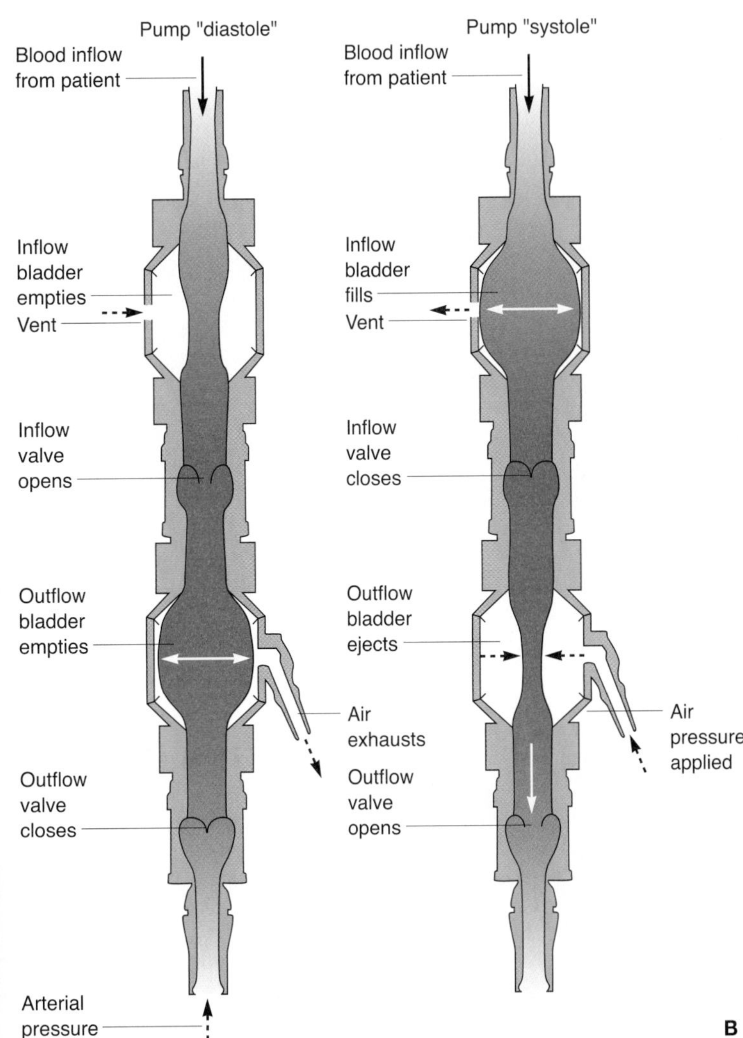

FIGURE 86.9 (*A*) Abiomed blood pump. (*B*) Mechanism of Abiomed blood pump action.

aorta. The driveline is externalized through the right or left abdominal wall and connected to the external power and control unit. The maximum pump flow is 11.6 L/min for the IP-1000 LVAS and 9.6 L/min for the XVE-LVAS. The HeartMate device can be operated either in a fixed-rate mode or, more often, in an automatic mode that more closely resembles normal physiologic conditions. In the automatic mode, the device ejects when the pump is 90% full or when it senses a decreased rate of filling. As the patient's activity increases, the pump fills faster and the rate (or stroke volume) automatically increases, resulting in an increase in pump output. With a decrease in activity, pump filling and output decrease. Because the aortic valve rarely opens when the heart is fully supported by a LVAD, pump output is synonymous with cardiac output. During normal operation, the pump completely unloads the left ventricle and supports cardiac output at physiologic levels. Because of the portability and ease of operation of the HeartMate XVE-LVAS, patients can be discharged to await heart transplantation outside the hospital.

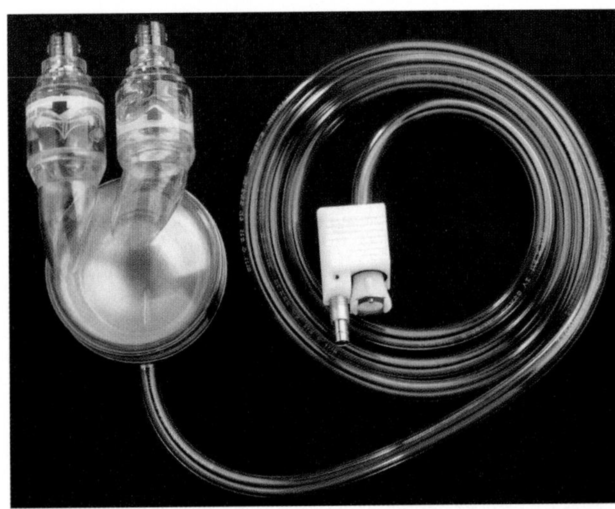

FIGURE 86.10 New Abiomed blood pump design.

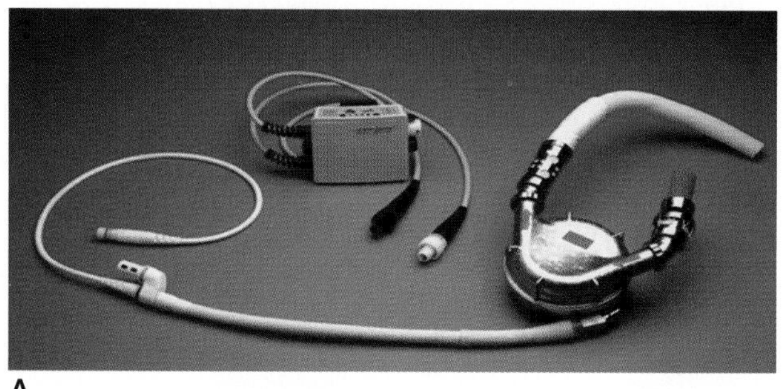

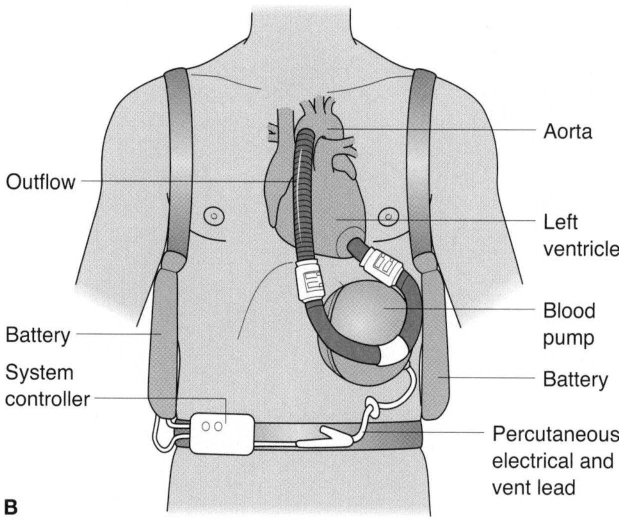

FIGURE 86.11 (*A*) The HeartMate XVE LVAS. (*B*) Schematic representation of preperitoneal pump placement for left ventricular assist and percutaneous driveline, external controller, and power source (batteries).

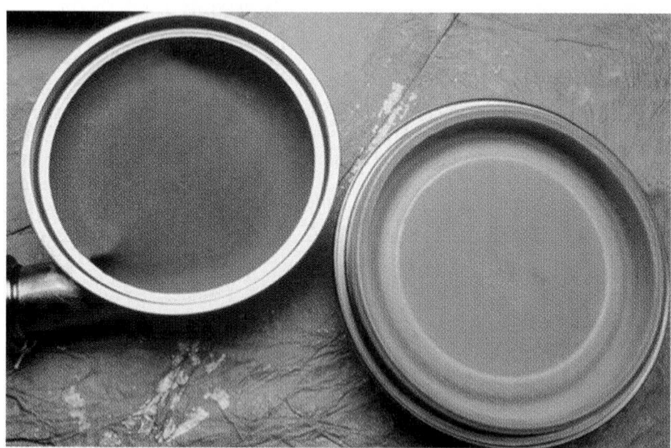

FIGURE 86.12 The HeartMate XVE LVAS demonstrating the textured surfaces of the metal housing (*left*) and diaphragm surfaces (*right*).

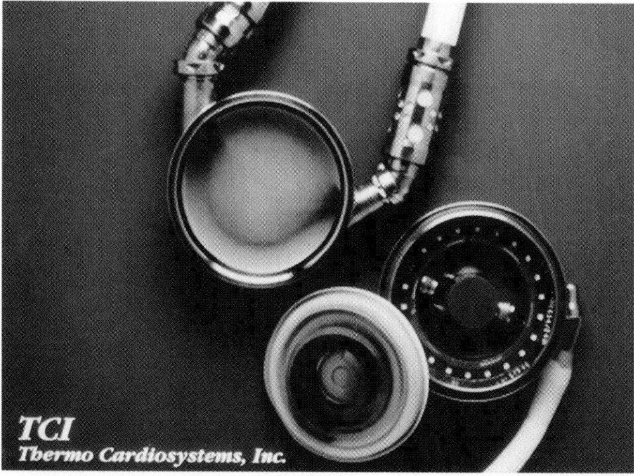

FIGURE 86.13 The HeartMate XVE LVAS demonstrating the internal rotary motor (*right*) that drives the movable diaphragm (*middle*).

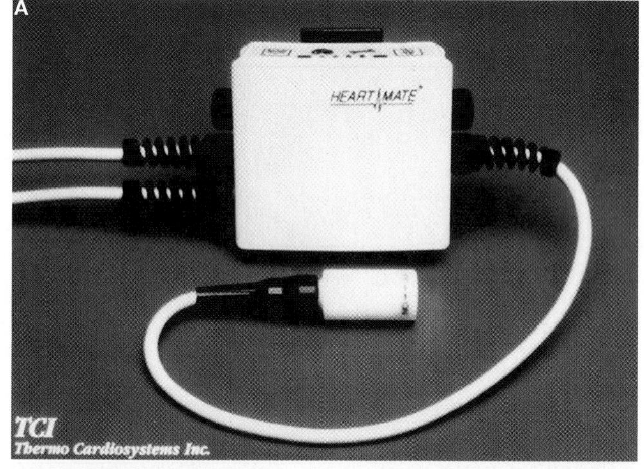

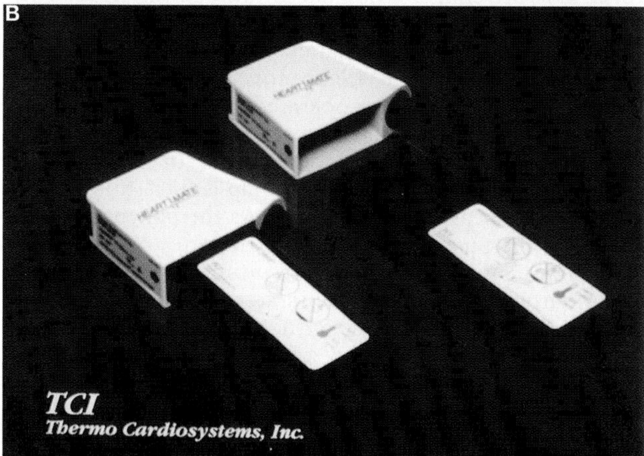

FIGURE 86.14 (*A*) The computer controller for the HeartMate XVE LVAS. (*B*) Power source (batteries).

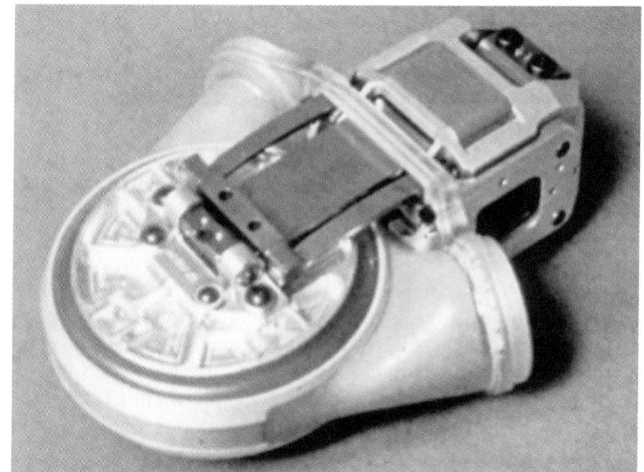

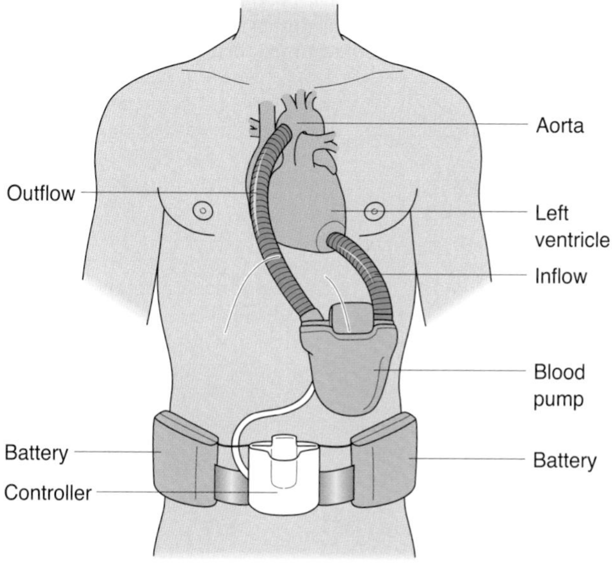

FIGURE 86.15 (*A*) The Novacor LVAD. (*B*) Schematic representation of preperitoneal placement of the Novacor LVAD for left ventricular assist and external computer and power source (batteries).

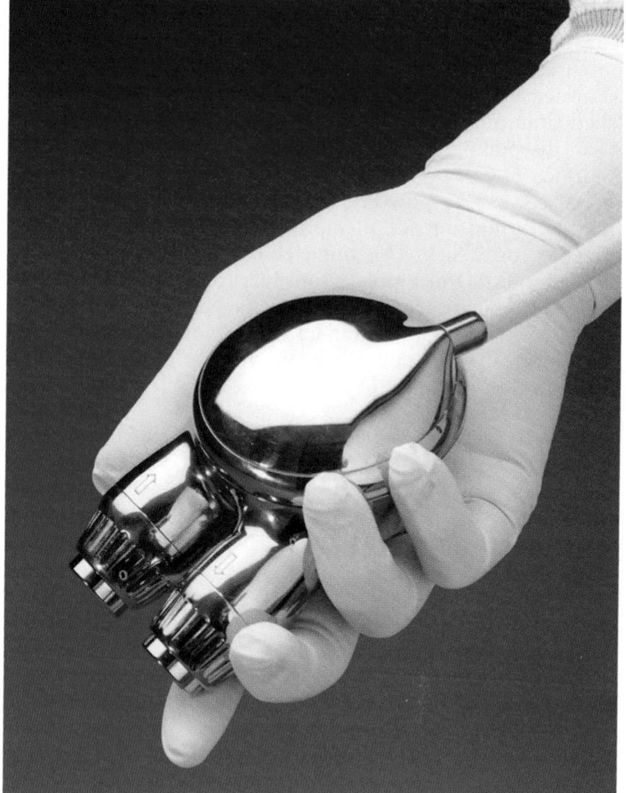

FIGURE 86.16 The Thoratec IVAD.

Novacor LVAS

The Novacor LVAD (WorldHeart, Inc., Ottawa, Ontario) is a portable, implantable LVAD designed for long-term circulatory support (Fig. 86.15).[104–106] It differs significantly from the HeartMate in its mode of pump actuation and use of a smooth blood-contacting surfaces. During pump systole, two opposing pusher plates compress a seamless polyurethane blood sac, causing ejection of blood. Unidirectional flow is ensured by use of 21-mm bioprosthetic valved conduits at the inlet and outlet orifices. The device produces a maximum stroke volume of 70 mL and is monitored by an external drive console. An internal solenoid converts the electric energy from the console to mechanic energy, compressing the pusher plates and pressurizing the pump sac for blood ejection. A percutaneous lead contains the necessary electrical wires and a vent to transfer air. In 1993, the Novacor LVAS was converted from a console-operated system into a wearable system to enhance patient mobility. The wearable system eliminates the need for a bulky console by incorporating a compact controller and rechargeable power packs that are worn on the patient's belt. The wearable system is designed for out-of-hospital use and can be monitored with a bedside monitor. The Novacor is implanted through an extended median sternotomy incision. The pump is positioned in the abdominal wall just anterior to the posterior rectus sheath between the left iliac crest and the costal margin. Cardiopulmonary bypass support is necessary during placement of the left ventricular apical inflow conduit and anastomosis of the outflow graft to the ascending aorta. A percutaneous drive line is brought out through the right lateral abdominal wall and is connected to the cable from the controller. The external controller provides power and allows control and monitoring of the pump. The system can be operated in either a fixed-rate, synchronous, or fill-to-empty mode. The synchronized mode maximizes cardiac unloading. In this mode, an electrocardiographic signal causes pump diastole to correspond with cardiac systole, allowing the heart to fill the pump with little effort. Alternatively, pump output may be maximized by means of the fill to empty mode in which the pumping rate is adjusted automatically depending on the filling rate of the pump. Finally, the system may also be operated in a fixed rate mode in which the operator sets a constant pumping rate. During device use, anticoagulation with heparin and later with warfarin and antiplatelet therapy is necessary to prevent thromboembolism. During long-term support, ambulatory patients can be discharged and live outside the hospital while awaiting a suitable donor heart. The Novacor LVAS is approved by the FDA for use in bridge to heart transplant indication.

Thoratec IVAD

A small, simple, and versatile implantable ventricular assist device (IVAD) based on the paracorporeal Thoratec pVAD has recently been developed and approved for circulatory assist as a bridge to heart transplantation or recovery (Fig. 86.16).[107] The IVAD has the same blood flow path and Thoralon polyurethane blood pumping sac as the paracorporeal Thoratec VAD, but the housing is a smooth contoured, polished titanium alloy. The IVAD has a new sensor to detect when the pump is full and empty and is controlled with the Thoratec TLC-II portable VAD driver, which is a small, briefcase-sized, battery-powered, pneumatic control unit. A small flexible (9-mm outside diameter) percutaneous pneumatic driveline for each VAD is tunneled out of the body from the LVAD or RVAD in a pre- or intraperitoneal position. Small size and simplicity are the major advantages of the new device. The IVAD weight (339 g) and implanted volume (252 mL) are approximately one half that of the current implantable pulsatile electromechanical LVAD systems.

LionHeart LVD2000 LVAS

The Arrow LionHeart LVD2000 LVAS (Fig. 86.17) is a completely implantable device that has been under development at the Pennsylvania State University for more than 15 years with the collaborative research efforts of Arrow International (Reading, PA) and is the first system to undergo clinical testing as a device exclusively designed as means of destination support.[108] The LionHeart device was designed to operate without percutaneous wires or vents, requiring the patient only to carry a rechargeable, extracorporeal battery pack. A roller-screw mechanism moves the pump's titanium pusher plate back and forth permitting ejection and passive filling of a 70-mL blood sac. The seamless blood sacs are solution cast from segmented polyurethane. Tilting Delrin disk valves ensure unidirectional blood flow. An intrathoracic compliance chamber and implanted controller/backup battery are included. The intrathoracic compliance chamber eliminates the need for percutaneous venting and allows for the displacement of the actuating air during device diastole and consists of a flexible chamber. The flexible chamber is in contact with the lung tissue, which is in turn in contact with atmospheric pressures thus eliminating the need for a percutaneous vent. The transcutaneous energy transmission system (TETS) (see Fig. 86.17) is used to power the pump's brushless direct current

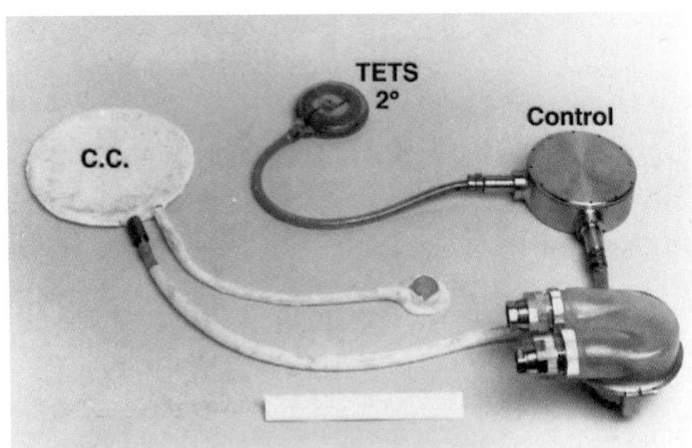

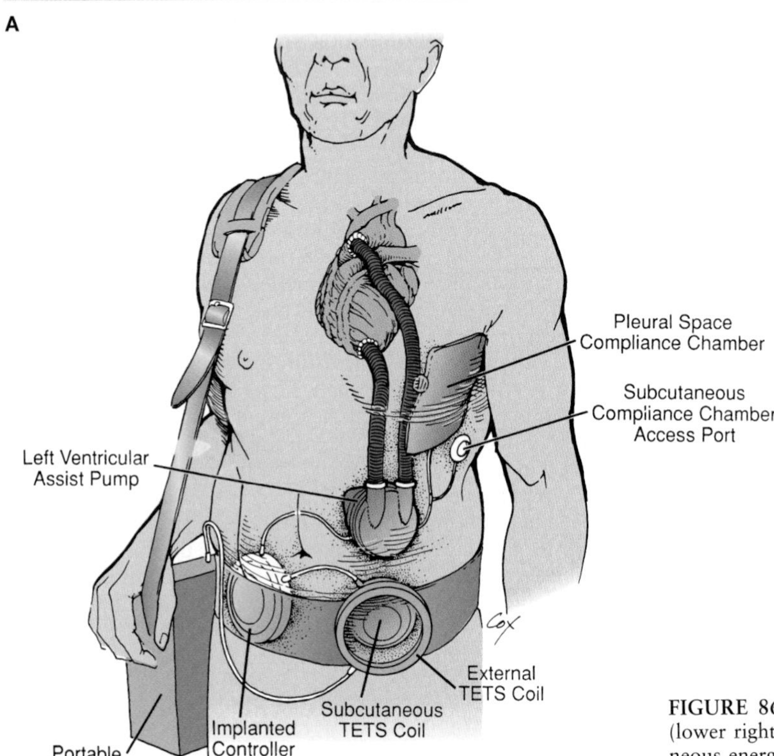

FIGURE 86.17 (*A*) The Lion Heart LVAD, demonstrating pump (lower right-hand corner), internal controller ("control"), transcutaneous energy transmission system (TETS), and internal compliance chamber (CC). (*B*) Schematic representation of placement of the Lion Heart LVAD and internal components for left ventricular assist.

(DC) motor as well as to modify the internal controller's algorithm if desired. The TETS transfers power from an external source across intact skin and tissue to the device using electromagnetic induction. This is accomplished using a pair of wire coils, one implanted subcutaneously and one located directly over the implanted coil on the skin surface. By selecting an appropriate operating frequency and coil geometry, a coupling coefficient suitable for power transfer across intact skin and tissue can be obtained. System telemetry occurs by means of an implanted radio frequency transmitter. The pump is placed in the preperitoneal position, and cannulas pass into the mediastinum through the diaphragm. The system is currently undergoing human investigation.

Implantable Continuous Flow Circulatory Assist Devices (Rotary Pumps with Axial Flow Design)

Implantable, continuous flow, rotary pumps with axial flow design are currently under going experimental animal investigation or early human trials and offer several advantages over pulsatile flow pumps. These advantages include smaller size, fewer moving parts, enhanced simplicity and durability, absence of valves to direct blood flow, smaller blood contacting surfaces, and reduced energy requirements. The ability to design smaller pumps using axial flow technology is a result of the elimination of a large blood chamber necessary with pulsatile systems. An additional important feature of these pumps is the lack of need for a compliance chamber. This feature alleviates the problem of internal compensation that is associated with conventional pulsatile pumps that, to date, has significantly hindered total internalization.

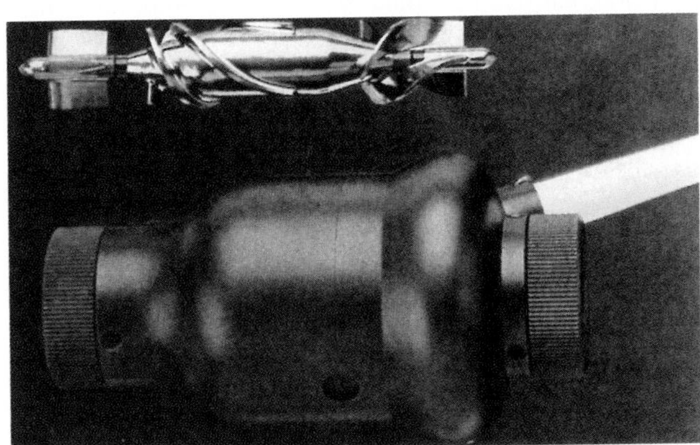

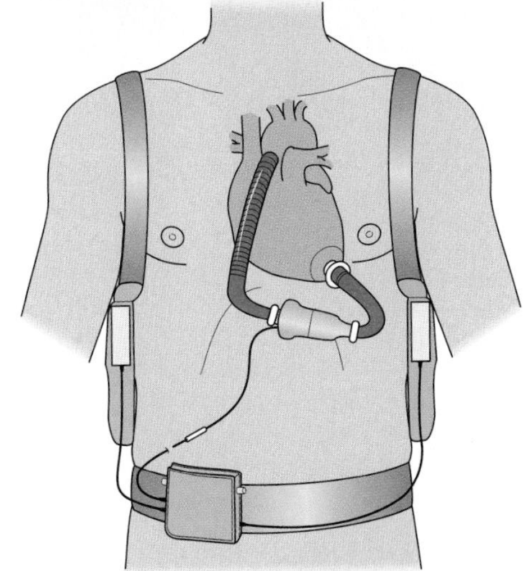

FIGURE 86.18 (*A*) The Lion Heart LVAD, demonstrating pump (*bottom*) and internal pump rotor (*top*). (*B*) Schematic representation of the HeartMate II LVAD in the preperitoneal position with associated external controller and power source (batteries).

HeartMate II

The HeartMate II is a small integrated pump-motor assembly that connects into the circulatory system through an apical cannula whose inlet orifice draws blood flow from the left ventricular apex, and an outflow cannula that is anastomosed to the ascending aorta (Fig. 86.18).[109–111] The pump is placed below the left costal margin under the left rectus abdominal muscle. The inflow cannula exits the left ventricular apex and crosses the diaphragm in the costophrenic angle, entering the subrectus pocket under the left rib margin to attach to the pump. The outflow cannula is tunneled back under the sternum to the ascending aorta. The pump consists of a 12-mm diameter straight duct and uses 14-mm diameter grafts for both the inlet and outlet cannulas. On entering the pump, blood passes through inlet stator vanes. After exiting the stator vanes, the blood flow is energized by the pump rotor that imparts tangential velocity and kinetic energy. Blood flow leaving the rotor then passes through a set of exit stator vanes that turn and diffuse the stream velocity, recovering kinetic energy in the process. The net action results in generation of a net pressure rise across the pump. Torque required to drive the pump rotor is developed by an integral electric motor. The pump's 12-mm diameter duct is actually a thin-walled tube that passes through the bore of the motor's coil windings. The motor's rotor is a permanent magnet located in the hub of the pump's rotor. The location of the pump rotor in the tube places the motor magnet in the proper position with respect to the coils, which is at the centerline of the winding's axis, and centered longitudinally with respect to the coil's length. Excitation current sequentially commutated to the coils creates a spinning magnetic field, thereby imparting torque and angular velocity to the motor magnet. The pump rotor spins on two bearings located at either end. Both bearings react against radial and axial thrust forces. Each bearing's stationary element is located in the hub of the respective inlet and outlet stators; the bearings themselves are similar to standard ball-cup jewel bearings. The outer boundary of the bearing's adjacent static and moving surfaces are washed directly by the main blood flow. Under normal operation, inlet pressure to the axial flow pump will be cyclic and vary with the systolic-diastolic phases of the left ventricle. Pressures developed within the left ventricle during systole depend on cardiac contractility and the overall flow demand of the patient. In the clinical situation of compromised cardiac contractility, with the pump operating at some nominal speed, systolic contractions of the heart will generate a pressure rise at the pump inlet, followed during diastole, by inlet pressures falling to its lowest level. This leads to a changing differential pressure across the pump, which in turn causes a corresponding fluctuation of flow delivered to the aorta. Thus, under most circumstances, the rotary pump will generate some pulsatility. Totally nonpulsatile flow would occur if the heart is in fibrillation, a state that cannot be tolerated chronically, or if the pump is operated at too high a speed or negative inflow pressure causing left ventricular collapse. The HeartMate II is currently in human testing.

Jarvik 2000

The Jarvik 2000 Heart (Jarvik Heart, Inc., New York, NY) is a compact axial flow impeller pump (Fig. 86.19).[112–116] The

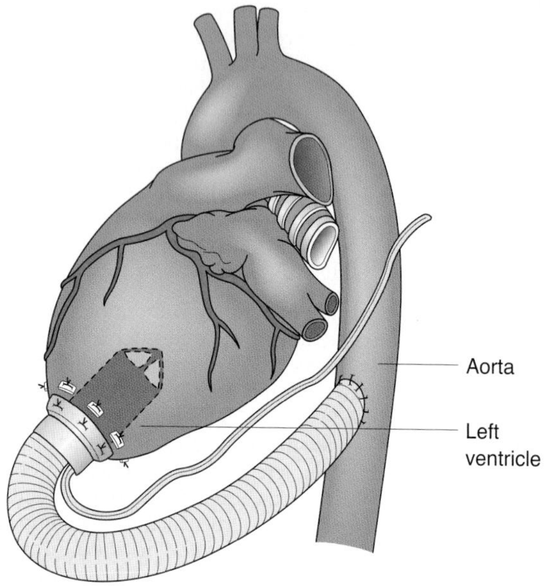

FIGURE 86.19 Schematic representation of placement of the Jarvik 2000 LVAD within the left ventricle.

outflow orifice of the pump is attached to a Dacron graft for anastomosis to the descending thoracic aorta. The Jarvik 2000 pump is inserted through a sewing cuff sewn into the apex of the left ventricle. The current adult version of the Jarvik 2000 measures 2.5 cm in diameter by 5.5 cm in length, with a weight of 85 g and a displacement volume of 25 mL. The pediatric iteration of the device measures 1.4 cm in diameter by 5 cm in length, with a weight of 18 g and displacement volume of 5 mL. The pump rotor contains the permanent magnet of a brushless direct current motor and mounts the impeller blades. A titanium shell accommodates the rotor and suspends it at each end by tiny, blood-immersed ceramic bearings. The adult pump functions at speeds of 8,000 to 12,000 rpm, achieving blood flow up to 8 L/min. The pediatric version of the Jarvik 2000 achieves pump flows of up to 3 L/min. Noise and hemolysis are minimal with each device. Percutaneous power is delivered from external batteries via a controller unit. Internal electrical wires are brought via the left pleural cavity to the apex of the chest and then subcutaneously across the neck to the base of the skull, where a percutaneous titanium pedestal transmits fine electrical wires through the skin of the scalp. The Jarvik 2000 LVAD is currently in human trials.

DeBakey LVAD

The DeBakey LVAD is an axial flow pump that measures approximately 86 mm long and 25 mm wide (about the size of an AA battery) (Fig. 86.20).[117–121] It weighs 95 g and has a displacement of 15 cm^3. Within the flow tube, the components consist of an inducer-impeller (the only moving part), a fixed flow straightener that acts as the front-bearing support for the inducer-impeller, and a fixed rear diffuser, that provides the rear bearing of the inducer-impeller. The diffuser retards the highly tangential blood flow velocity by redirecting it axially, an action that results in fluid pressure build. Rare earth magnets, which are embedded in the blades of the impeller, act as the rotor of the brushless motor, causing it to spin in a magnetic field. The pump is designed to produce flows of 5 L/min against 100 mm Hg pressure with a rotor speed of 10,000 rpm with less than 10 W of power. Extensive computational fluid

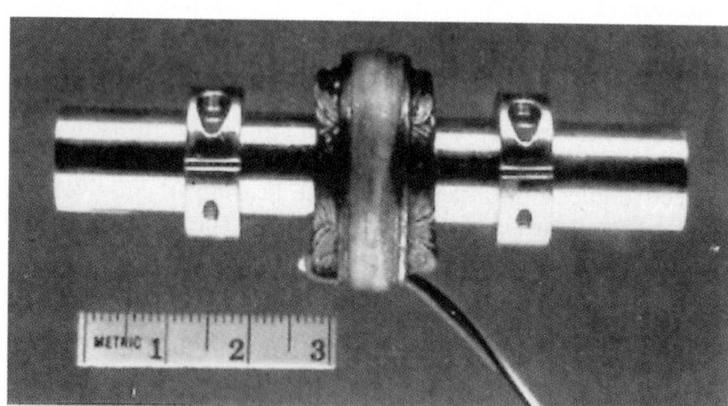

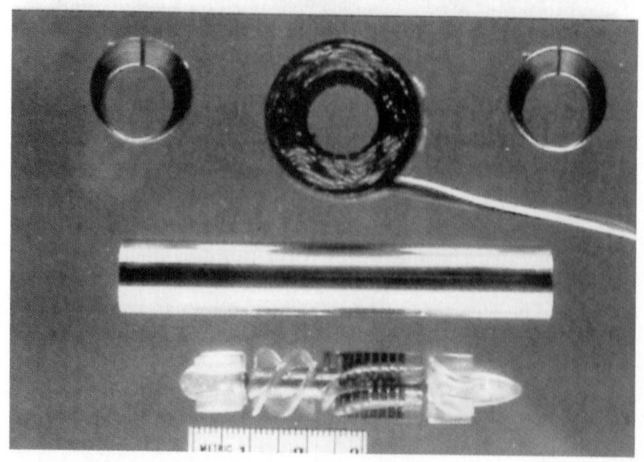

A

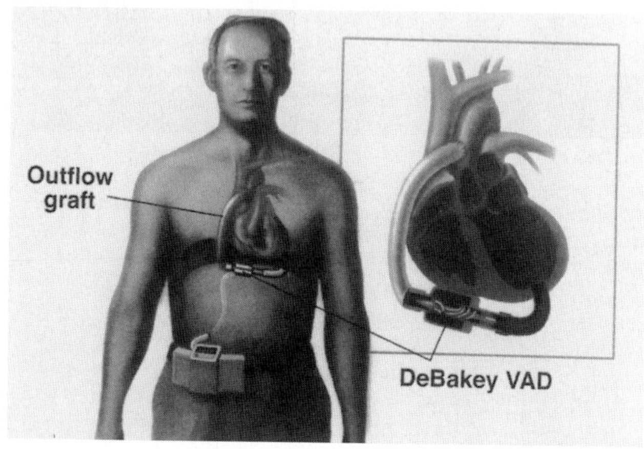

B

FIGURE 86.20 (*A*) The DeBakey LVAD demonstrating pump (*top*) with internal components including pump rotor (*bottom*). (*B*) Schematic representation of placement of the DeBakey LVAD with external controller and power source (batteries).

dynamics analyses were performed jointly with NASA-Ames Research Center to optimize the hydraulic performance and minimize hemolysis of the pump. The DeBakey LVAD is currently under investigation in human trials.

Implantable Continuous Flow Circulatory Assist Devices (Rotary Pumps with Centrifugal Flow Design)

Rotary pumps of centrifugal flow design represent the third generation of VADs. These devices are somewhat larger than rotary pumps with axial flow design and provide nonpulsatile flow at rotational speeds that are much slower, about 2,000 to 4,000 rpm compared to 8,000 to 15,000 rpm for pumps with axial flow design. The same general advantages and disadvantages of design features that apply to rotary pumps with axial flow design apply to centrifugal flow design. The major feature of the third generation of rotary pumps with centrifugal flow design is that the impeller is rotated and levitated in a magnetic field eliminating the need for bearings with subsequent problems associated with bearing wear (Fig. 86.21). Thus, these devices have a great potential for very long durability. Currently, there are three devices in animal and human testing, the HeartMate III (Thoratec, Inc., Pleasanton, CA) (see Fig. 86.21), DuraHeart (Terumo, Inc., Ann Arbor, MI), and HeartQuest (MedQuest, Inc., Salt Lake City, UT).

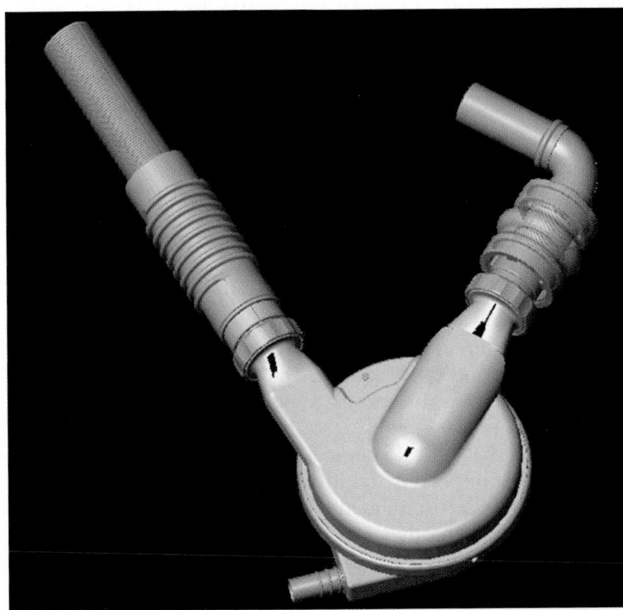

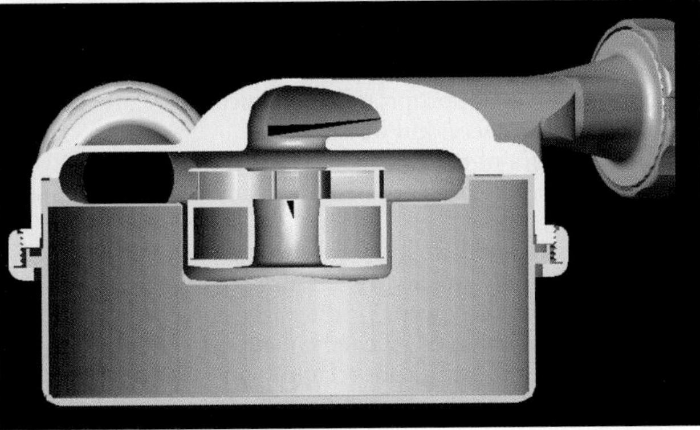

FIGURE 86.21 The HeartMate III LVAD.

Total Artificial Hearts

CardioWest C-70 Total Artificial Heart

The CardioWest C-70 total artificial heart (SynCardia Systems, Inc., Tucson, AZ), formerly called the Jarvik or Symbion total

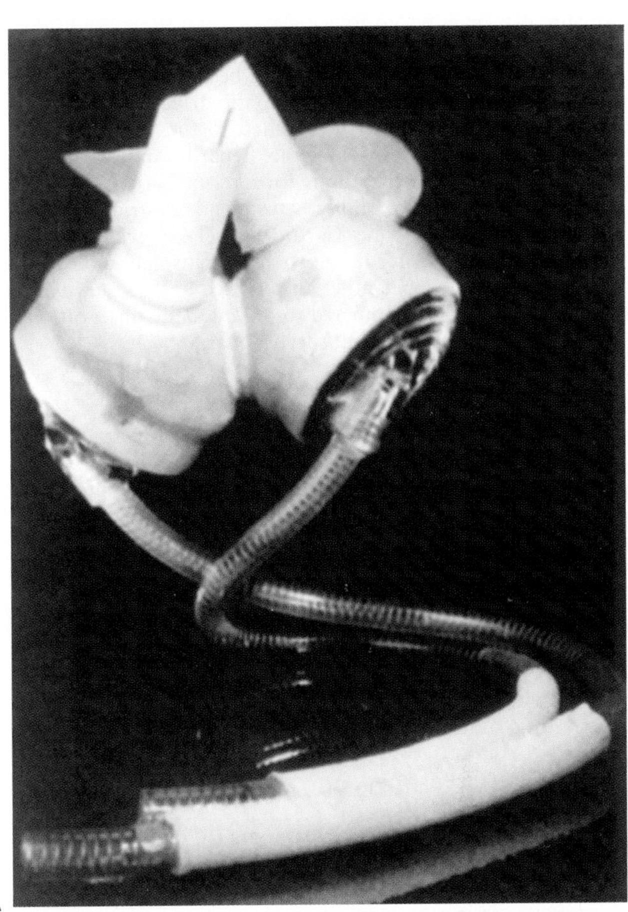

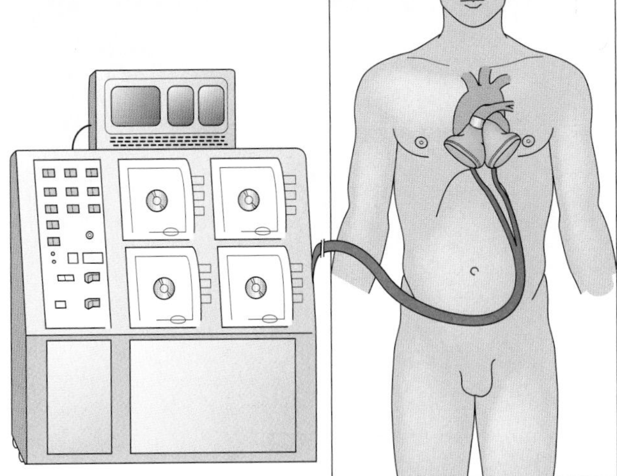

FIGURE 86.22 (*A*) The CardioWest total artificial heart. (*B*) Schematic representation of orthotopic placement of the CardioWest total artifical heart with percutaneous drive line connected to the pneumatic drive console.

artificial heart, is a pulsatile biventricular cardiac replacement system (Fig. 86.22).[122–125] The rigid polyurethane pump contains a smooth, flexible polyurethane diaphragm that separates the blood and air chambers. Two Medtronic-Hall mechanical valves located at the inflow and outflow orifices ensure unidirectional blood flow. Compressed air from the external drive console moves the diaphragm upward, pressurizing the blood chamber and causing ejection of blood. The pump has a maximum stroke volume of 70 mL and a maximum flow rate of 15 L/min, although the average flow rate is less than 8 L/min. Pump rate, duration of systole, and driving pressure can be adjusted to achieve optimal flow conditions. The total artificial heart is surgically implanted in the mediastinal space after the ventricles have been excised, while the atrial cuffs are retained. The pneumatic drivelines are externalized percutaneously and attached to the drive console. Anticoagulation with dipyridamole, heparin, and warfarin is necessary to prevent thrombus formation. Patients may be ambulatory, but their mobility is frequently restricted by the large drive console. The CardioWest TAH was recently approved by the FDA for bridge to heart transplant indication. In a recent study, Copeland et al. reported a 79% survival to heart transplantation compared to 46% for the observational arm. One-year posttransplant survival was 86%.

Abiomed Total Replacement Heart

The AbioCor (Fig. 86.23) total artificial heart system (Abiomed, Inc., Danvers, MA) is an orthotopically positioned blood pump that alternately ejects blood into the pulmonary and systemic vasculature.[126] The system uses brushless DC motors that are powered by TETS. Implanted nickel-cadmium batteries can also drive the system in case the external coils detach. The Abiomed total artificial heart shifts hydraulic fluid to pump blood in a one to one fashion. A unidirectional centrifugal pump combined with a rotating valve transmits hydraulic fluid against one of the pump's diaphragm while withdrawing fluid from the contralateral side. In this fashion, alternating filling and emptying of the pumps with blood occurs.

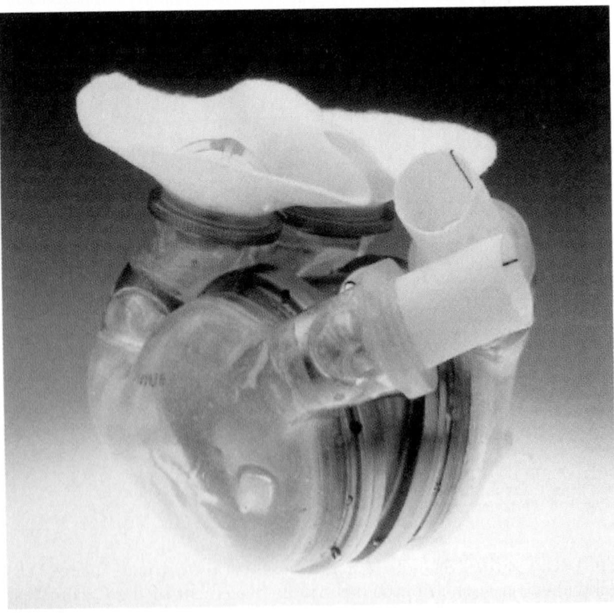

FIGURE 86.23 The AbioCor Total Replacement Heart.

The Abiomed total replacement heart is cast from a solution of proprietary polyetherurethane and then externally reinforced to provide rigidity. The system incorporates 24-mL polyetherurethane trileaflet valves in both the inlet and outlet orifices. The control schemes of this system demonstrate so called Starling behavior so that increases in venous return elicit a commensurate increase in left pump output until a maximum output is reached. The Abiomed total artificial heart modulates motor speed as the principal way to control cardiac output. Optimal pumping rate is made a function of right atrial pressure, inferred from transducer-measured pressure readings within the right hydraulic chamber. Compensation for right and left flow imbalances depends on a flexible, 20-mL hydraulic chamber positioned against the left atrium. This compliance chamber, in continuity with the right pump's hydraulic chamber, exerts negative feedback on right pump filling. As left atrial pressure rises, hydraulic fluid shifts into the right hydraulic chamber limiting the passive diastolic filling of the right pump's blood chamber. Less blood is then delivered to the left side until left atrial pressure decreases.

FUTURE DIRECTIONS

Recent rapid technologic advancements and successful clinical applications of mechanical circulatory support have made the future of this field optimistic but uncertain. It is now very likely that long-term mechanical circulatory support will become a viable alternative to heart transplantation and medical therapy for patients with advanced congestive heart failure in the immediate future. Due to technologic advancements, it will be difficult to predict what devices will ultimately prove to be most efficacious. It is likely that a variety of devices will become available for use depending on clinical circumstances and patient characteristics.

KEY POINTS

- **Mechanical circulatory support is indicated in situations in which the heart can no longer pump blood and meet oxygen requirements commensurate with the needs of the body.**
- **The spectrum of mechanical circulatory support is complex due to the multiple, intended indications for use and the availability of numerous types of mechanical support devices.**
- **The intended use and clinical indication for mechanical circulatory support has significant influences on the appropriate device selection and the justification for use. There are no absolute hemodynamic criteria for initiating mechanical circulatory support for any indication.**
- **Patient selection is perhaps the single most crucial factor in determining outcome of patients who receive mechanical circulatory support.**
- **Age is an important risk factor for survival for patients on mechanical circulatory support.**
- **Selection of the appropriate mechanical circulatory device is critical to a successful outcome.**
- **Abnormalities of the cardiac valves have important adverse consequences in patients being considered for mechanical circulatory support.**
- **Bleeding, right-sided circulatory failure, air embolism, and progressive multisystem organ failure are the most frequent complications that occur in the early postoperative period following initiation of mechanical circulatory support.**
- **The single most significant technologic advance in preventing thromboembolic events in patients on long-term left ventricular assistance has been attributed to the use of textured blood-contacting surfaces within the devices.**

References

1. **Cooley DA, Liotta D, Hallman GL, et al. Orthotopic cardiac prosthesis for two-staged cardiac replacement. *Am J Cardiol.* 1969;24:723.**
2. **DeVries WC, Anterson JL, Joyce LD, et al. Clinical use of the total artificial heart. *N Engl J Med.* 1984;310:273.**
3. Sapirstein JS, Pierce WS. Mechanical circulatory support. In: Lazar J, Greenfield MW, Mulholland KT, et al., eds. *Surgery: scientific principles and practice*, 2nd ed. Philadelphia: Lippincott-Raven Publishers; 1997: 1550–1565.
4. **Rose EA, Moskowitz AJ, Packer M, et al., for the REMATCH Trial. Rationale, design, and end points. *Ann Thorac Surg.* 1999;67:723.**
5. **Rose EC, Gelijns AC, Moskowitz AJ, et al., for the REMATCH Study Group. Long-term use of a left ventricular assist device for end-stage heart failure. *N Engl J Med.* 2001;345:1435.**
6. Frazier OH, Myers TJ. Left ventricular assist system as a bridge to myocardial recovery. *Ann Thoracic Surg.* 1999;68:734.
7. Dipla K, Mattiello JA, Jeevanandam V, et al. Myocyte recovery after mechanical circulatory support in humans with end-stage heart failure. *Circulation* 1998;97:2316.
8. Mueller J, Wallukat G, Weng Y-G, et al. Weaning from mechanical cardiac support in patients with idiopathic dilated cardiomyopathy. *Circulation* 1997;96:542.
9. Westaby S, Jin XY, Katsumata T, et al. Mechanical support in dilated cardiomyopathy: signs of early left ventricular recovery. *Ann Thorac Surg.* 1997;64:1303.
10. **Levin HR, Oz MC, Chen JM, et al. Reversal of chronic ventricular dilation in patients with end-stage cardiomyopathy by prolonged mechanical unloading. *Circulation* 1995;91:2717.**
11. Nakatani T, Sasako Y, Kobayashi J, et al. Recovery of cardiac function by long-term left ventricular support in patients with end-stage cardiomyopathy. *ASAIO J.* 1998;44:M516.
12. Hetzer R, Muller J, Weng Y, et al. Cardiac recovery in dilated cardiomyopathy by unloading with a left ventricular assist device. *Ann Thorac Surg.* 1999;68:742.
13. Scheinin SA, Capek P, Radovencevic B, et al. The effect of prolonged left ventricular support on myocardial histopathology in patients with end-stage cardiomyopathy. *ASAIO J.* 1992;38:M271.
14. Jacquet L, Zerbe T, Stein KL, et al. Evolution of human cardiac myocyte dimension during prolonged mechanical support. *J Thoracic Cardiovasc Surg.* 1991;101:256.
15. McCarthy PM, Nakatani S, Vargo R, et al. Structural and left ventricular histologic changes after implantable LVAD insertion. *Ann Thoracic Surg.* 1995;59:609.
16. Nakatani S, McCarthy PM, Kottke-Marchant K, et al. Left ventricular echocardiographic and histologic changes: impact of chronic unloading by an implantable ventricular assist device. *J Am Coll Cardiol.* 1996;27:894.
17. Zafeiridis A, Jeevanandam V, Houser SR, et al. Regression of cellular hypertrophy after left ventricular assist device support. *Circulation* 1998;98:656.
18. Milting H, Bartling B, Schumann H, et al. Altered levels of mRNA of apoptosis-mediating genes after mid-term mechanical ventricular support in dilative cardiomyopathy-first results of the Halle Assist Induced Recovery Study (HAIR). *Thorac Cardiovasc Surg.* 1999;47:48.
19. Altemose GT, Gritsus V, Jeevanandam V, et al. Altered myocardial phenotype after mechanical support inhuman beings with advanced cardiomyopathy. *J Heart Lung Transplantation* 1997;16:765.
20. Torre-Amione G, Stetson SJ, Youker KA, et al. Decreased expression of tumor necrosis factor-alpha in failing human myocardium after mechanical circulatory support: a potential mechanism for cardiac recovery. *Circulation* 1999;100:1189.
21. James KB, McCarthy PM, Thomas JD, et al. Effect of the implantable left ventricular assist device on neuroendocrine activation in heart failure. *Circulation* 1995;92[Suppl II]:II-191.
22. Delgado R III, Radovancevic B, Massin EK, et al. Neurohormonal changes after implantation of a left ventricular assist system. *ASAIO J.* 1998;44:299.
23. Lee SH, Doliba N, Osbakken M, et al. Improvement of myocardial mitochondrial function after hemodynamic support with left ventricular assist devices in patients with heart failure. *J Thorac Cardiovasc Surg.* 1998;116:344.
24. Hochman JS, Sleeper LA, Webb JG, et al. Early revascularization in acute myocardial infarction complicated by cardiogenic shock. *N Engl J Med.* 1999;341:625.
25. Norman JC, Cooley DA, Igo SR, et al. Prognostic indices for survival during postcardiotomy intra-aortic balloon pumping. *J Thorac Cardiovasc Surg.* 1977;74:709.
26. Oz MC, Goldstein DJ, Pepino P, et al. Screening scale predicts patients successfully receiving long-term implantable left ventricular assist devices. *Circulation* 1995;92[Suppl II]:II-169.
27. Rao V, Oz MC, Flanney MA, et al. Revised screening scale to predict survival after insertion of a left ventricular assist device. *J Thorac Cardiovasc Surg.* 2003;125:855.
28. Deng MC, Loebe M, El-Banayosy A, et al. Mechanical circulatory support for advanced heart failure: effect of patient selection on outcome. *Circulation* 2001;103:231.
29. Pennington DG, McBride LR, Peigh PS, et al. Eight year's experience with bridging to cardiac transplantation. *J Thorac Cardiovasc Surg.* 1994;107:472.
30. Pae WE. Ventricular assist devices and total artificial hearts: a ASAIO-ISHLT Registry experience. *Ann Thorac Surg.* 1993;55:295.
31. Guyton RA, Schonberger J, Everts P, et al. Postcardiotomy shock: clinical evaluation of the BVS 5000 biventricular support system. *Ann Thorac Surg.* 1993;56:346–356.
32. Jett GK. Postcardiotomy support with ventricular assist devices: selection of recipients. *Semin Thorac Cardiovasc Surg.* 1994;6:136.
33. Pennington DG, Merjavy JP, Swartz MT, et al. The importance of biventricular failure in patients with postoperative cardiogenic shock. *Ann Thorac Surg.* 1985;39:16.
34. Farrar DJ, Hill JD, Pennington DG, et al. Preoperative and postoperative comparison of patients with univentricular and biventricular support with the Thoratec ventricular assist device as a bridge to cardiac transplantation. *J Thorac Cardiovasc Surg.* 1997;113:202.
35. Kormos RL, Gasior TA, Kawai A, et al. Transplant candidate's clinical status rather than right ventricular function defines the need for univentricular versus biventricular support. *J Thorac Cardiovasc Surg.* 1996;111:773.
36. Samuels LE, Holmes EC, Thomas MP, et al. Management of acute cardiac failure with mechanical assist: experience with the Abiomed BVS 5000. *Ann Thorac Surg.* 2001;71:S67.
37. Santamore WP, Gray LA. Left ventricular contributions to right ventricular systolic function during LVAD support. *Ann Thorac Surg.* 1996;61:350.
38. Pavie A, Leger P. Physiology of univentricular versus biventricular support. *Ann Thorac Surg.* 1996;61:347.
39. Mandarino WA, Winowich S, Gorcsan J, et al. Right ventricular performance and left ventricular assist device filling. *Ann Thorac Surg.* 1997;63:1044.
40. Aria H, Swartz MT, Pennington DG, et al. Importance of ventricular arrhythmias in bridge patients with ventricular assist devices. *ASAIO Trans.* 1991;37:M427.
41. Oz MC, Rose EA, Slater JP, et al. Malignant ventricular arrhythmias are well tolerated in patients receiving long-term left ventricular devices. *J Am Coll Cardiol.* 1994;24:1688.
42. Salzberg SP, Lachat ML, Zünd G, et al. Left ventricular assist device (LVAD) enables survival during 7 h of sustained ventricular fibrillation. *Eur J Cardiothorac Surg.* 2004;26:444.
43. Shapiro GC, Leibowitz DW, Oz MC, et al. Diagnosis of patent foramen ovale with transesophageal echocardiography in a patient supported with a left ventricular assist device. *J Heart Lung Transplantation* 1995;14:594.
44. Goldstein DJ, Seldomridge JA, Chen JM, et al. Use of aprotinin in LVAD recipients reduces blood loss, blood use, and perioperative mortality. *Ann Thorac Surg.* 1995;59:1063.
45. Kaplon RJ, Gillinov AM, Smedira NG, et al. Vitamin K reduces bleeding in left ventricular assist device recipients. *J Heart Lung Transplantation* 1999;18:346.
46. Nakatani S, Thomas JD, Savage RM, et al. Prediction of right ventricular dysfunction after left ventricular assist device implantation. *Circulation* 1996;94[9 Suppl]:II-216.
47. Fukamachi K, McCarthy PM, Smedira NG, et al. Preoperative risk factors for right ventricular failure after implantable left ventricular assist device insertion. *Ann Thorac Surg.* 1999:68:2181.
48. Shenkar R, Coulson WF, Abraham E. Hemorrhage and resuscitation induce alterations in cytokine expression and the development of acute lung injury. *Am J Respir Cell Mol Biol.* 1994;10:290.
49. Horvath CJ, Ferro TJ, Jesmok G, et al. Recombinant tumor necrosis factor increases pulmonary vascular permeability independent of neutrophils. *Proc Natl Acad Sci USA.* 1988;85:9219.
50. **Argenziano M, Choudhri AF, Moazami N, et al. Randomized, double-blind trial of inhaled nitric oxide in LVAD recipients with pulmonary hypertension. *Ann Thorac Surg.* 1998;65:340.**
51. Salamonsen RF, Kaye D, Esmore DS. Inhalation of nitric oxide provides selective pulmonary vasodilation, aiding mechanical cardiac assist with the Thoratec left ventricular assist device. *Anaesth Intensive Care* 1994;22:209.
52. Hare JM, Shernan SK, Body SC, et al. Influence of inhaled nitric oxide on systemic flow and ventricular filling pressure in patients receiving mechanical circulatory assistance. *Circulation* 1997;95:2250.
53. **Ochiai Y, McCarthy PM, Smedira NG, et al. Predictors of severe right ventricular failure after implantable left ventricular assist device insertion: analysis of 245 patients. *Circulation* 2002;106:198.**
54. Rose EA, Levin HR, Oz MC, et al. Artificial circulatory support with textured interior surfaces: A counterintuitive approach to minimizing thromboembolism. *Circulation* 1994;90[Suppl II]:II-87.
55. Rafii S, Oz MC, Seldomridge JA, et al. Characterization of hematopoietic cells arising on the textured surface of left ventricular assist devices. *Ann Thorac Surg.* 1995;60:1627.
56. Holman WL, Fix RJ, Foley BA, et al. Management of wound and left ventricular assist device pocket infection. *Ann Thorac Surg.* 1999;1080.
57. McKellar SH, Allred BD, Marks JD, et al. Treatment of infected left ventricular assist device using antibiotic-impregnated beads. *Ann Thorac Surg.* 1999;67:554.

58. Arabia FA, Copeland JG, Smith RG, et al. Infections with the CardioWest total artificial heart. *ASAIO J.* 1998;44:M336.
59. Argenziano M, Catanese KA, Moazami N, et al. The influence of infection on survival and successful transplantation in patients with left ventricular assist devices. *J Heart Lung Transplantation* 1997;16:822.
60. Hermann M, Weyand M, Greshake B, et al. Left ventricular assist device infection is associated with increased mortality but is not a contraindication to transplantation. *Circulation* 1997;95:814.
61. Fischer SA, Trenholme GM, Costanzo MR, et al. Infectious complications in left ventricular assist device recipients. *Clin Infect Dis.* 1997;24:18.
62. Springer WE, Wasler A, Radovancevic B, et al. Retrospective analysis of infection in patients undergoing support with left ventricular assist systems. *ASAIO J.* 1996;42:M763.
63. McCarthy PM, Schmitt SK, Vargo RL, et al. Implantable LVAD infections: Implications for permanent use of the device. *Ann Thorac Surg.* 1996; 61:359.
64. Holman EL, Murrah CP, Ferguson ER, et al. Infections during extended circulatory support: University of Alabama at Birmingham experience 1989 to 1994. *Ann Thorac Surg.* 1996;61:366.
65. Gordon SM, Schmitt SK, Jacobs M, et al. Nosocomial bloodstream infections in patients with implantable left ventricular assist devices. *Ann Thorac Surg.* 2001:72;725.
66. Holman WL, Park SJ, Long JW, et al, for the REMATCH Investigators. Infection in permanent circulatory support: experience from the REMATCH trial. *J Heart Lung Transplantation* 2004;23:1359.
67. Dembitsky WP, Tector AJ, Park S, et al. Left ventricular assist device performance with long-term circulatory support: lessons from the REMATCH trial. *Ann Thorac Surg.* 2004;78:2123.
68. Poston RS, Husain S, Sorce D, et al. LVAD bloodstream infections: therapeutic rationale for transplantation after LVAD infection. *J Heart and Lung Transplantation* 2003;22:914.
69. Ankersmit HJ, Tugulea S, Spanier T, et al. Activation-induced T-cell death and immune dysfunction after implantation of left ventricular assist device. *Lancet* 1999;354:550.
70. Deng MC, Erren M, Tjan TD, et al. Left ventricular assist system support is associated with persistent inflammation and temporary immunosuppression. *Thorac Cardiovasc Surg.* 1999;47[Suppl 2]:326.
71. Goldstein DJ, el-Amir NG, Ashton RC, et al. Fungal infections in left ventricular assist device recipients. Incidence, prophylaxis, and treatment. *ASAIO J.* 1995;41:873.
72. Itescu S, John R. Interactions between the recipient immune system and the left ventricular assist device surface: immunological and clinical implications. *Ann Thorac Surg.* 2003;75:S58.
73. Nader M, Itescu S, Williams MR, et al. Platelet transfusions are associated with the development of anti-major histocompatibility complex class I antibodies in patients with ventricular assist support. *J Heart Lung Transplantation* 1998;17:876.
74. Itescu S, Tung TC, Burke EM, et al. Preformed IgG antibodies against major histocompatibility complex class II antigens are major risk factors for high-grade cellular rejection in recipients of heart transplantation. *Circulation* 1998;98:786.
75. Kobashigawa JA, Sabad A, Drinkwater D, et al. Pretransplant panel reactive-antibody screens. Are they truly a marker for poor outcome after cardiac transplantation? *Circulation* 1996;94:II-294.
76. Moulopoulos SD, Topaz S, Kolff WJ. Diastolic balloon pumping (with carbon dioxide) in the aorta: a mechanical assistance to the failing circulation. *Am Heart J.* 1962;63:669.
77. **Kantrowitz A, Tjonneland S, Freed PS, et al. Initial clinical experience with intraaortic balloon pumping in cardiogenic shock. *JAMA* 1968; 203:135.**
78. **Claus RH, Birtwell WC, Albertal G, et al. Assisted circulation, the arterial counterpulsator. *J Thorac Cardiovasc Surg.* 1961;41:447.**
79. Muehrcke DD, McCarthy PM, Stewart RW, et al. Extracorporeal membrane oxygenation for postcardiotomy cardiogenic shock. *Ann Thorac Surg.* 1996;61:684.
80. Smedira NG, Wudel JH, Hlozek CC, et al. Venovenous extracorporeal life support for patients after cardiotomy. *ASAIO J.* 1997;43:M444.
81. McGovern GJ, Magovern JA, Benckart DH, et al. Extracorporeal membrane oxygenation-preliminary results in patients with postcardiotomy cardiogenic shock. *Ann Thorac Surg.* 1994;57:1462.
82. Hill JD, O'Brien TG, Murray JJ, et al. Extracorporeal oxygenation for acute post-traumatic respiratory failure. *N Engl J Med.* 1972;286:629.
83. Bavaria JE, Furukawa S, Kreiner G. Effect of circulatory assist devices on stunned myocardium. *Ann Thorac Surg.* 1990;49:123.
84. **Bartlett RH, Roloff DW, Custer JR, et al. Extracorporeal life support: the University of Michigan experience. *JAMA* 2000;283:904.**
85. **Pagani FD, Lynch W, Swaniker F, et al. Extracorporeal life support to left ventricular assist device bridge to heart transplant: a strategy to optimize survival and resource utilization. *Circulation* 1999;100:II206.**
86. Pagani FD, Aaronson KD, Dyke DB, et al. Assessment of an extracorporeal life support to LVAD bridge to heart transplant strategy. *Ann Thorac Surg.* 2000;70:1977.
87. Bowen FW, Carboni AF, O'Hara ML, et. al. Application of "double bridge mechanical" resuscitation for profound cardiogenic shock leading to cardiac transplantation. *Ann Thorac Surg.* 2001;72:86.
88. Smedira NG, Moazomi N, Golding CM, et. al. Clinical experience with 202 adults receiving extracorporeal membrane oxygenation for cardiac failure: survival at five years. *J Thorac Cardiovasc Surg.* 2001;122:92.
89. Magovern GJ, Simpson KA. Extracorporeal membrane oxygenation for adult cardiac support: the Allegheny experience. *Ann Thorac Surg.* 1999;68:655.
90. Noon GP, Lafuente JA, Irwin S. Acute and temporary ventricular support with BioMedicus centrifugal pump. *Ann Thorac Surg.* 1999;68:650.
91. Curtis JJ, Walls JT, Wagner-Mann CC, et al. Centrifugal pumps: description of devices and surgical techniques. *Ann Thorac Surg.* 1999;68:666.
92. Mehta SM, Aufiero TX, Pae WE, et al. Results of mechanical ventricular assistance for the treatment of postcardiotomy cardiogenic shock. *ASAIO J.* 1996;42:211.
93. Thiele H, Lauer B, Hambrecht R, et al. Reversal of cardiogenic shock by percutaneous left atrial-to-femoral arterial bypass assistance. *Circulation* 2001;104:2917.
94. McBride LR, Naunheim KS, Fiore AC, et al. Clinical experience with 111 Thoratec ventricular assist devices. *Ann Thoracic Surg.* 1999;67:1233.
95. El-Banayosy A, Korfer R, Arusoglu L, et al. Bridging to cardiac transplantation with the Thoratec ventricular assist device. *Thorac Cardiovasc Surg.* 1999;47[Suppl 2]:307.
96. Farrar DJ, Buck KE, Coulter JH, et al. Portable pneumatic biventricular driver for the Thoratec ventricular assist device. *ASAIO J.* 1997;43:M631.
97. El-Banayosy A, Arusoglu L, Kizner L, et al. Predictors of survival in patients bridged to transplantation with the Thoratec VAD device: a single-center retrospective study on more than 100 patients. *J Heart Lung Transplantation* 2000;19:964.
98. Gray LA, Champsaur GG. The BVS 5000 biventricular assist device. The worldwide registry experience. *ASAIO J.* 1994;40:M460.
99. Frazier OH, Myers TJ, Radovancevic B. The HeartMate left ventricular assist systems—overview and 12 year experience. *Texas Heart Institute J.* 1998;25:265.
100. McCarthy PM, Smedira NO, Vargo RL, et al. One hundred patients with the HeartMate left ventricular assist device: evolving concepts and technology. *J Thorac Cardiovasc Surg.* 1998;115:904.
101. Frazier OH, Rose EA, Oz MC, et al. Multicenter clinical evaluation of the HeartMate vented electric left ventricular assist system in patients awaiting heart transplantation. *J Thorac Cardiovasc Surg.* 2001;122:1186.
102. Morgan JA, John R, Rao V, et al. Bridging to transplant with the HeartMate left ventricular assist device: the Columbia Presbyterian 12-year experience. *J Thorac Cardiovasc Surg.* 2004;127:1309.
103. Long JW. Advanced mechanical circulatory support with the HeartMate left ventricular assist device in the year 2000. *Ann Thorac Surg.* 2001;71:176.
104. Robbins RC, Oyer PE. Bridge to transplant with the Novacor left ventricular assist system. *Ann Thorac Surg.* 1999;68:695.
105. El-Banayosy A, Deng M, Loisance DY, et al. The European experience of Novacor left ventricular assist (LVAS) therapy as a bridge to transplant: a retrospective multi-centre study. Eur *J Cardiothorac Surg.* 1999;15:835.
106. Murali S. Mechanical circulatory support with the Novacor LVAS: worldwide clinical results. *Thorac Cardiovasc Surg.* 1999;47[Suppl 2]:321.
107. Reichenbach SH, Farrar DJ, Hill JD. A versatile intracorporeal ventricular assist device based on the Thoratec VAD system. *Ann Thorac Surg.* 2001;71:S171.
108. Mehta SM, Pae WE, Rosenberg G, et al. The LionHeart LVD-2000: a completely implanted left ventricular assist device for chronic circulatory support. *Ann Thorac Surg.* 2001;71:S156.
109. Thomas DC, Butler KC, Taylor LP, et al. Progress on development of the Nimbus-University of Pittsburgh axial flow left ventricular assist system. *ASAIO J.* 1998;44:M521.
110. Butler KC, Dow JJ, Litwak P, et al. Development of the Nimbus/University of Pittsburgh Innovative Ventricular Assist System. *Ann Thorac Surg.* 1999;68:790.
111. Griffith BP, Kormos RL, Borovetz HS, et al. HeartMate II left ventricular assist system: from concept to first clinical use. *Ann Thorac Surg.* 2001;71:116.
112. Westaby S, Katsumata T, Evans R, et al. The Jarvik 2000 Oxford System: increasing the scope of mechanical circulatory support. *J Thorac Cardiovasc Surg.* 1997;114:467.
113. Westaby S, Katsumata T, Houel R, et al. Jarvik 2000 Heart: potential for bridge to myocyte recovery. *Circulation* 1998;98:1568.
114. Frazier OH, Myers TJ, Gregoric ID, et al. Initial clinical experience with the Jarvik 2000 implantable axial-flow left ventricular assist system. *Circulation* 2002;105:2855.
115. Westaby S, Frazier OH, Beyersdorf F, et al. The Jarvik 2000 Heart. Clinical validation of the intraventricular position. *Eur J Cardiothorac Surg.* 2002;22:228.
116. Frazier OH, Myers TJ, Westaby S, Gregoric ID. Clinical experience with an implantable, intracardiac, continuous flow circulatory support device: physiologic implications and their relationship to patient selection. *Ann Thorac Surg.* 2004;77:133.
117. Salzberg S, Lachat M, Zünd G, et al. Left ventricular assist device as bridge to heart transplantation—lessons learned with the MicroMed DeBakey axial blood flow pump. *Eur J Cardiothorac Surg.* 2003;24:113.
118. DeBakey ME. Development of a ventricular assist device. *Artificial Organs* 1997;21:1149.
119. DeBakey ME. A miniature implantable axial flow ventricular assist device. *Ann Thorac Surg.* 1999;68:637.

120. Fossum TW, Morley D, Benkowski R, et al. Chronic survival of calves implanted with the DeBakey ventricular assist device. *Artificial Organs* 1999;23:802.
121. Wieselthaler GM, Schima H, Hiesmayr M, et al. First clinical experience with the DeBakey VAD continuous-axial-flow pump for bridge to transplantation. *Circulation* 2000;101:356.
122. Arabia FA, Copeland JG, Pavie A, et al. Implantation technique for the CardioWest total artificial heart. *Ann Thorac Surg.* 1999;68:698.
123. Copeland JG, Smith RG, Arabia FA, et al. Cardiac replacement with a total artificial heart as a bridge to transplantation. *N Engl J Med.* 2004;351:859.
124. Copeland JG, Smith RG, Arabia FA, et al. Total artificial heart bridge to transplantation: a 9-year experience with 62 patients. *J Heart Lung Transplantation* 2004;23:823.
125. Copeland JG, Arabia FA, Tsau PH, et al. Total artificial hearts: bridge to transplantation. *Cardiol Clin.* 2003;21:101.
126. Dowling RD, Gray LA, Etoch SW, et al. The AbioCor implantable replacement heart. *Ann Thorac Surg.* 2003;75:93.

CHAPTER 87 ■ PERICARDIUM

SCOTT M. BRADLEY

EMBRYOLOGY AND ANATOMY

The pericardium forms during the fifth week of gestation, when the two pleuropericardial membranes fuse with each other and the root of the lungs to divide the primitive thoracic cavity into the pericardial cavity and the pleural spaces.[1] The pleuropericardial membranes contain the cardinal veins and phrenic nerves and, in the adult, form the fibrous pericardium. After development, the serous pericardium, consisting of a single layer of mesothelial cells, lines the fibrous pericardium. Together, the serous and fibrous pericardiums comprise the parietal pericardium. The visceral pericardium, or epicardium, covers the heart and intrapericardial great vessels. The phrenic nerves lie in the parietal pericardium. Hence, diaphragm paralysis can complicate operations on the pericardium. The pericardium superiorly merges with the adventitia of the great vessels and inferiorly is attached to the central tendon of the diaphragm. The oblique sinus is a blind cul-de-sac located behind the left atrium, and the transverse sinus is a tubular space between the aorta and main pulmonary artery anteriorly and the right and left atria posteriorly (Fig. 87.1). The vascular supply of the pericardium is from the internal thoracic arteries via the pericardiophrenic branches and from the descending aorta. Venous drainage is to the internal thoracic veins and azygos system. Lymphatic drainage is to the local bronchial and tracheal nodes and to the thoracic duct. Innervation is by the sympathetic trunks and the phrenic and vagus nerves. The pericardium normally contains 15 to 50 mL of serous fluid. This fluid is an ultrafiltrate of plasma with a protein content lower than plasma.[2]

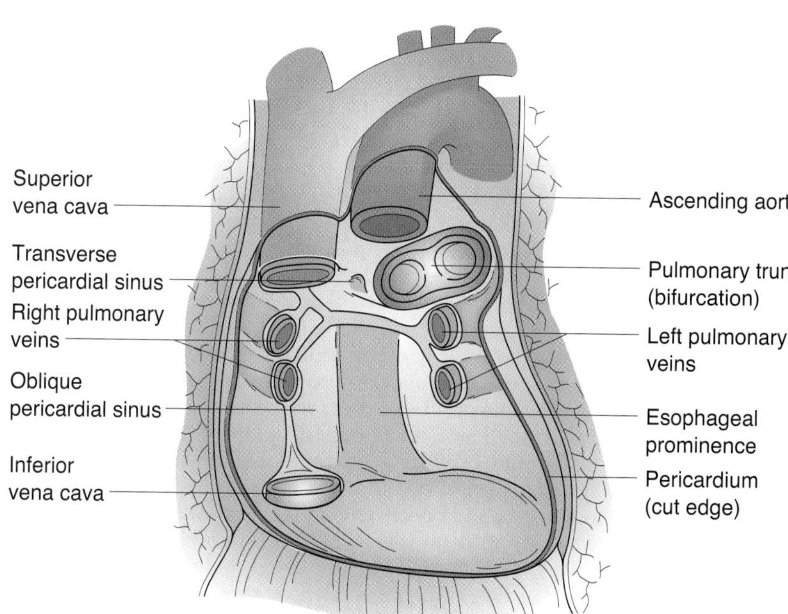

FIGURE 87.1 Diagrammatic illustration of the pericardial attachments to the great vessels and pulmonary veins after removing the heart. The transverse sinus is a free space behind the aorta and main pulmonary artery. The oblique sinus lies behind the left atrium.

VASCULAR

NORMAL PHYSIOLOGY

Not all of the functions of the pericardium are well understood, and people can do well with congenital absence or after surgical removal of the pericardium. Structural functions appear to include mechanically protecting and anchoring the heart, preventing acute cardiac distention, and serving as a barrier to infection.[2] The pericardium contributes to diastolic coupling of the ventricles. Diastolic coupling links pressure rises in the right ventricle to the left ventricle, coordinating movement of the two ventricles along their respective Starling curves. The pericardium also functions as an absorptive surface, transmitting fluid to both the thoracic duct system and the pleural spaces. Regulatory functions include mechanoreceptors, which govern blood pressure and heart rate. Pericardial fluid exhibits fibrinolytic activity, which opposes the clotting of intrapericardial blood.

Pericardial disease produces characteristic changes in hemodynamics and systemic venous pulsations. Normal intrapericardial pressure is essentially the same as pleural pressure, and at end-expiration is about 2 mm Hg below atmospheric pressure. During inspiration, pericardial pressure decreases slightly. The normal hemodynamic effect of inspiration is to increase right-sided venous return, right ventricular preload, right ventricular stroke volume, pulmonary arterial flow, and pulmonary vascular bed capacity. Inspiration decreases pleural pressure and pericardial pressure. Pooling of blood in the lungs causes a decrease in pulmonary capillary wedge pressure, left-sided venous return, left ventricular stroke volume, systemic arterial pressure, and aortic flow. The decrease in arterial pressure seen during normal inspiration is less than 10 mm Hg. Increased right ventricular filling during inspiration also causes a leftward shift of the interventricular septum, further decreasing left ventricular volume and stroke volume.

Normal jugular venous pulsations show three positive pulse waves, the a, c, and v waves, and two negative waves, the x and y descents (Fig. 87.2). The a wave results from normal atrial contraction. Its peak corresponds to S_4. The c wave is due to the bulging of the atrioventricular valve into the atrium during isovolumic ventricular systole. It begins at S_1. The x descent (systolic collapse) is due to the downward displacement of the base of the heart during ventricular systole and atrial relaxation. Its lowest point is in midsystole. The v wave is due to passive atrial filling from the vena cavae and occurs just after S_2. The y descent (diastolic collapse) follows the opening of the atrioventricular valve and during passive ventricular filling. The effects of respiration are that during inspiration, with decreasing intrathoracic pressure, the x descent is lower than the y. During expiration, with more positive intrathoracic pressure and lower systemic venous return, the y descent is equal to or lower than the x.

DIAGNOSTIC STUDIES

The electrocardiogram is usually nonspecific but can contribute to the diagnosis of pericardial disease. QRS voltage may be decreased in the presence of a large pericardial effusion. Electrocardiographic changes in pericarditis typically go through four stages, which are believed to be due to generalized superficial myocarditis (Table 87.1). Progression through the first three stages takes several days, whereas the fourth stage occurs weeks or months later.[3]

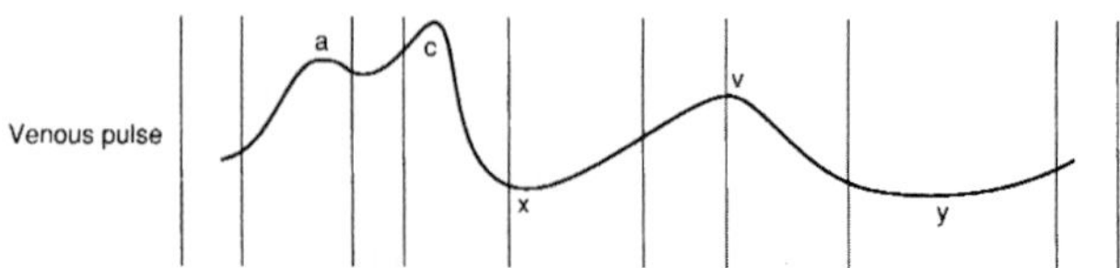

FIGURE 87.2 The jugular venous pulse contour.

TABLE 87.1 DIAGNOSIS

STAGES OF ELECTROCARDIOGRAPHIC CHANGES IN PERICARDITIS

1. Diffuse ST-segment elevation in all leads except aVR and V_1, without reciprocal depression
2. Normalization of ST segments with flattening of T waves
3. T-wave inversion
4. Normalization of T waves

The chest radiograph may show pericardial calcifications in chronic constrictive pericarditis, especially if caused by tuberculosis. The cardiac silhouette may be enlarged or irregular in the presence of effusion, cyst, or tumor. In the presence of a large pericardial effusion, the cardiac silhouette takes on the shape of a water bottle. Pneumopericardium may also be seen on chest radiograph.

The echocardiogram is the most useful noninvasive modality in pericardial disease. Echocardiography (either transthoracic or transesophageal) can demonstrate structural changes in the pericardium including effusion, thickening, and masses, as well as accompanying cardiac pathology. It is extremely sensitive for pericardial fluid, being able to detect as little as 15 mL. Echocardiography can also demonstrate the functional changes caused by pericardial disease and can help to differentiate tamponade, constriction, and restriction. Echocardiography is very helpful in guiding pericardiocentesis.

Computed tomography (CT) and magnetic resonance imaging (MRI) are occasionally useful to define pericardial masses and thickening.[4] CT provides better definition of calcification and is more expedient in an unstable patient. MRI can provide better definition of masses and does not require intravenous contrast.

Cardiac catheterization provides the hemodynamic pressure tracings, which can distinguish tamponade, constriction, and restriction. Catheterization also provides an opportunity for endomyocardial biopsy to diagnose myocardial disease, including restrictive cardiomyopathy.

CARDIAC (PERICARDIAL) TAMPONADE

Cardiac tamponade can be defined as hemodynamically significant cardiac compression due to accumulating pericardial contents (effusion, blood, pus, gas, or tumor) that evoke and defeat compensatory mechanisms.[3] Cardiac compression by the contents of the pericardial space prevents adequate filling of the heart, decreases stroke volume and cardiac output, and increases systemic and pulmonary venous pressures. The occurrence of tamponade is dependent on both the volume and rate of accumulation of pericardial contents. Rapid accumulation of a small amount of pericardial fluid (100 to 200 mL in an adult) may produce acute tamponade, whereas slow accumulation of liters of fluid can occur in a chronic effusion before tamponade occurs. Cardiac tamponade results when pericardial pressure rises to 20 to 30 mm Hg. Cardiac filling pressures, namely right and left atrial, pulmonary artery diastolic and wedge, and right and left ventricular end-diastolic pressures become equal to each other and to the pericardial pressure. Right atrial pressure in tamponade is usually 15 to 35 mm Hg.

However, with accompanying hypovolemia, such as occurs during postoperative bleeding or traumatic tamponade, central venous pressures may be lower.

Cardiac tamponade can be caused by neoplastic disease; any of the causes of pericarditis (see later); or intrapericardial bleeding due to anticoagulants, procedures, surgery, or trauma. Trauma may be either penetrating or blunt. Tamponade may result from myocardial rupture during myocardial infarction or aortic rupture due to aneurysmal disease or dissection. Clinical findings in tamponade include dyspnea and tachycardia. The three classic signs of acute tamponade (Beck's acute cardiac compression triad) are (a) falling arterial pressure, (b) rising venous pressure, and (c) a small, quiet heart.[5] In actuality, the systemic blood pressure may be low, normal, or even elevated in patients with chronic hypertension. Blood pressure is more likely to be normal when pericardial fluid has accumulated gradually and low with acute tamponade. The neck veins are typically distended and peripheral cyanosis, particularly in the face, reflects venous congestion. However, venous distention may be minimal or absent with accompanying hypovolemia. The heart sounds may also be normal rather than faint.

Tamponade produces characteristic changes in jugular venous pulsations: the x descent (systolic collapse) remains, whereas the y descent (diastolic collapse) disappears.[6] With tamponade, there is typically a fall in systolic blood pressure of more than 10 mm Hg during inspiration, or "pulsus paradoxus." Pulsus paradoxus may be absent if there is accompanying left ventricular dysfunction, in the presence of an atrial septal defect, during regional (postoperative) tamponade, and if the patient is receiving positive-pressure ventilation. Causes of pulsus paradoxus other than tamponade include chronic obstructive pulmonary disease, asthma, pulmonary embolism, right ventricular heart failure or infarction, obesity, and tense ascites.

Echocardiography can be very useful in the diagnosis of cardiac tamponade. It may reveal the presence of pericardial fluid. More specific echocardiographic signs of tamponade include right atrial compression, right ventricular diastolic collapse, and abnormal inspiratory decreases in left ventricular dimensions, mitral valve excursion, and mitral valve inflow. Localized atrial compression (usually postoperative) may cause tamponade without these characteristic echocardiographic features.

Cardiac tamponade is only definitively diagnosed when removal of pericardial fluid improves the clinical picture. Removal of as little as a few milliliters of fluid may result in significant improvement in cardiac output. When tamponade produces falling systemic blood pressure, emergency pericardiocentesis is indicated. Needle pericardiocentesis with hemodynamic monitoring and echocardiographic guidance is optimal. Placement of a drainage catheter into the pericardial space over a guidewire (Seldinger technique) can provide ongoing fluid drainage and allow monitoring of the rate of fluid accumulation. Surgical drainage, including placement of a pericardiostomy tube via a subxiphoid approach, creation of a pericardial window, or pericardial resection, are alternatives when pericardiocentesis fails or tamponade recurs.

Postoperative Cardiac Tamponade

Tamponade after cardiac surgery can occur in the absence of many, or all, of the classic signs of tamponade. Accompanying hypovolemia may limit the absolute rise in filling pressures, and positive pressure ventilation may mask pulsus paradoxus. Tamponade should always be included in the differential diagnosis of low cardiac output after any closed or open-heart operation. It should be particularly suspected in the presence of rising filling pressures and falling systemic blood pressure, urine output, and cardiac output poorly responsive to volume, inotropes, vasopressors, and diuretics. Mediastinal chest tube drainage that abruptly increases, or ceases, is highly suggestive. Chest radiography may show an enlarged cardiac silhouette or more subtle findings, such as shifting of epicardial markers (e.g., temporary pacemaking wires) away from the edge of the pericardium. However, postoperative tamponade may result from the accumulation of relatively small amounts of intrapericardial blood, and the chest radiograph is most often unhelpful. Echocardiography is less sensitive for intrapericardial blood than for serous fluid. More specific echocardiographic signs of tamponade may be absent if clotted intrapericardial blood causes localized atrial compression. Reexploration of the chest is the only definitive method of diagnosing acute postoperative tamponade and is indicated in any patient with low cardiac output of unclear origin. Late postoperative tamponade typically occurs in patients on anticoagulants and may present insidiously.

PERICARDIAL CONSTRICTION

Pericardial constriction occurs when the heart is constrained by a thickened, fibrotic pericardium. The pericardial space may either be obliterated or contain effusion (effusive-constrictive pericarditis). Constrictive pericarditis typically progresses over months to years. The clinical picture may include dyspnea, orthopnea, cough, fatigue, pleural effusions, abdominal swelling and discomfort, hepatomegaly, ascites, peripheral edema, fatigue, and pulsus paradoxus. Kussmaul's sign is an increase in jugular venous distention with inspiration. Rapid diastolic ventricular filling may produce a loud third heart sound (a "pericardial knock"). Electrocardiographic changes of low voltage and nonspecific T-wave changes may be seen. Up to 25% of patients will have atrial fibrillation or flutter. Fibrotic obstruction of the right ventricular outflow tract may produce an electrocardiographic (ECG) pattern of right ventricular hypertrophy. Chest radiograph shows a normal heart size and clear lung fields. Pericardial calcification is essentially pathognomonic but is present in only about 40% of cases. Echocardiography shows small ventricles with good systolic function. Ventricular expansion shows an abrupt halt during diastole. The inferior vena cava is dilated. Doppler interrogation may show an abnormal inspiratory increase in tricuspid flow and decrease in mitral flow. Patients with effusive-constrictive pericarditis are more likely to have cardiomegaly on chest radiograph and pericardial fluid on echocardiogram. Beck's chronic cardiac compression triad is: high venous pressure, ascites, and a small, quiet heart.[5]

Unlike cardiac tamponade, pericardial constriction produces no restriction of early diastolic filling but a sudden restriction in late diastole.[6] Rapid ventricular filling during early diastole quickly reaches the limit of ventricular distensibility. Late diastolic restriction produces an early diastolic dip, followed by a rapid increase and plateau (square root sign) in the right ventricular pressure tracing (Fig. 87.3). Jugular venous pulsations show prominent x and y descents, with a y descent (diastolic collapse) that is deeper and more rapid than normal. Right atrial pressure, pulmonary artery diastolic and wedge pressures, and both right and left ventricular end-diastolic pressures are elevated (15 to 30 mm Hg) and within 5 mm Hg of each other. In effusive-constrictive pericarditis, right atrial and ventricular pressure tracings more closely resemble those seen in tamponade: There is a deep x descent and small y descent in the right atrium and no early diastolic dip in the right ventricle. Once the pericardial fluid is removed, the pressure tracings revert to those of constrictive pericarditis, with prominent x and y descents in the atrium and a prominent early diastolic dip in the ventricle.

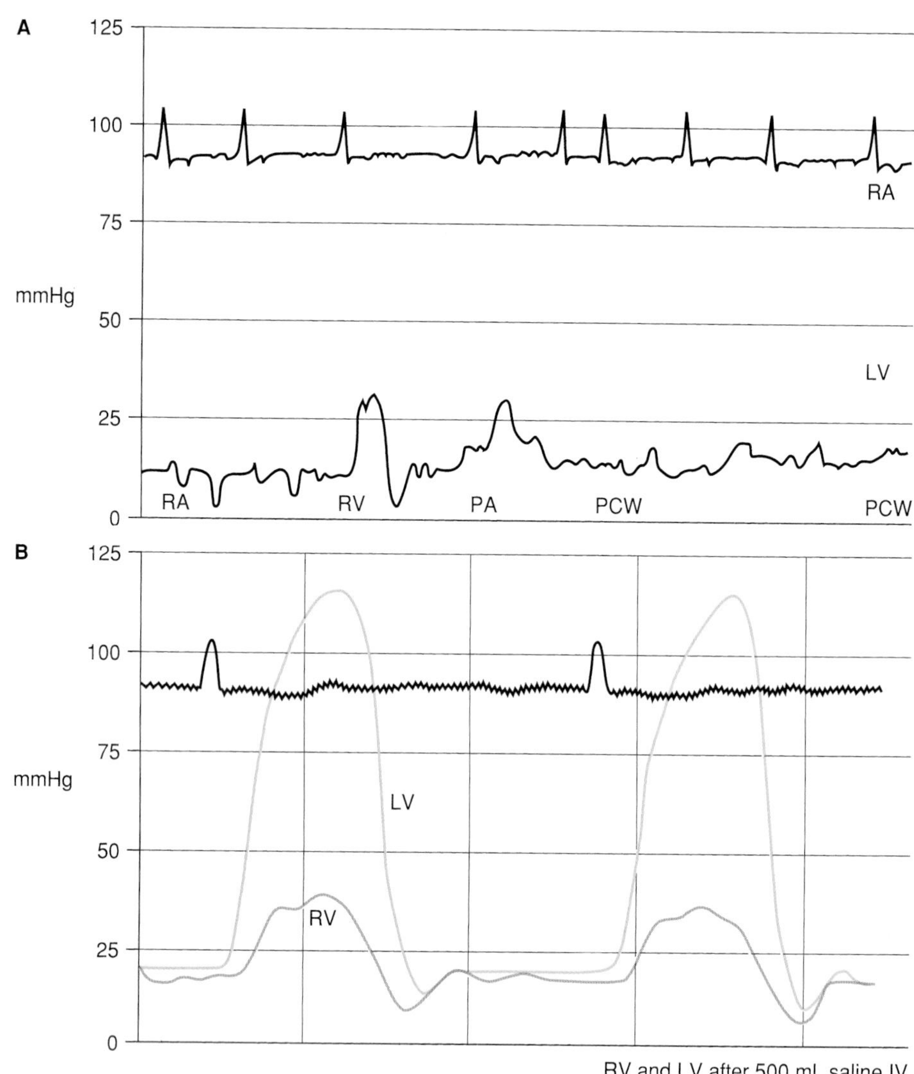

FIGURE 87.3 Pressure recordings from a patient with constrictive pericarditis. (*A*) The right atrial (RA) tracing shows elevated mean pressure and a prominent y descent. The right ventricular pressure (RV) shows the dip and plateau pattern (square root sign). There is equalization of the RA, RV diastolic, pulmonary artery (PA) diastolic, pulmonary capillary wedge (PCW), and left ventricular (LV) diastolic pressures. (*B*) RV and LV diastolic pressures increase and equalize after the administration of 500 mL of saline. (After Brockington GM, Zebede J, Pandian NG. Constrictive pericarditis. *Cardiol Clin.* 1990;8:649.)

The diagnosis of constrictive pericarditis is made by the typical clinical and hemodynamic findings in the presence of pericardial thickening (at least 4 mm by CT or MRI). Differentiation between pericardial constriction and restrictive cardiomyopathy may be difficult. Patients with restrictive cardiomyopathy do not have pericardial thickening. They are also more likely to show impairment of systolic ventricular function, mitral and tricuspid regurgitation, left-sided pressures that are higher than right-sided pressures, slower early and mid-diastolic filling, and left and right ventricular pressures that move in the same direction, rather than opposite directions, with inspiration.[7] Patients with pericardial constriction are more likely to have equalization of right and left ventricular end-diastolic pressure, a right ventricular systolic pressure ≤50 mm Hg, and a right ventricular end-diastolic pressure that is greater than one third of right ventricular systolic pressure.[8]

Constriction may be a late sequela of any type of acute pericarditis. Other causes include mediastinal irradiation, cardiac surgery, amyloidosis, scleroderma, hemochromatosis, neoplastic disease, sarcoidosis, and trauma. Patients with constriction and accompanying ascites and peripheral edema may also be confused with patients who have primary liver disease (such as Budd-Chiari syndrome or cirrhosis), or other causes of right-sided heart failure. In some cases, pericardial and/or myocardial biopsy may be necessary to make the appropriate diagnosis. The definitive treatment of constrictive pericarditis is pericardiectomy (see later).

CONGENITAL ABNORMALITIES

Congenital deficiency of the pericardium may be complete but is more often partial and occurs on the left side. Such deficiency is more common in males. Partial absence is usually asymptomatic. However, with partial defects on the right, herniation of the right atrium, right ventricle, and right lung have been reported. CT and MRI can demonstrate pericardial defects. Symptomatic herniation can be treated by completion pericardiectomy or patch closure of the pericardial defect with bovine pericardium or PTFE (Gore-Tex). Congenital total absence is also usually asymptomatic and an incidental finding at operation or autopsy.

Pericardial cysts range from 1 to 15 cm in size. Most occur at the right cardiophrenic angle, are asymptomatic, and noticed on chest radiographs done for other reasons. However, pericardial cysts may (rarely) cause mediastinal compression with respiratory or hemodynamic collapse in neonates. Diagnosis can be confirmed by CT scan, which shows a cyst adjacent to the pericardium containing homogeneous fluid of water density. The differential diagnosis of a pericardial cyst includes foramen of Morgagni hernia, bronchogenic cyst, lipoma, and other homogeneous neoplasms of the mediastinum. Surgical removal should be undertaken if the cyst increases in size or is symptomatic or if the diagnosis is in doubt.

NEOPLASTIC PERICARDIAL DISEASE

Primary neoplasms of the pericardium are rare. Malignant tumors include sarcomas, teratomas, and mesotheliomas; benign tumors include fibromas, lipomas, hemangiomas, lymphangiomas, leiomyomas, and neurofibromas. Primary malignancies of the mediastinum, lung, or esophagus may directly extend to the pericardium. Metastatic neoplasm is the most common source of neoplastic pericardial disease and remains the most common cause of pericardial effusion. Of patients dying of cancer, 5% to 10% have cardiac involvement (85% of these are pericardial). Metastatic lung cancer, breast cancer, lymphoma, leukemia, and melanoma are the most common. Many cases present as cardiac tamponade. Diagnosis is by echocardiogram, CT or MRI, and identification of tumor cells in aspirated pericardial fluid. Cytologic analysis of pericardial fluid may be negative in 20% to 50% of cases, and pericardial biopsy may then be helpful in establishing a diagnosis. Treatment can include radiotherapy, direct instillation of antineoplastic agents into the pericardium, and tube drainage for relief of effusion and tamponade. Sclerosing agents, such as doxycycline, can also give good control of malignant pericardial effusions.

PERICARDITIS

Pericarditis includes any inflammatory or infectious process affecting the pericardium. It has a wide range of causes and may be either acute or chronic in course. The clinical picture of acute pericarditis may mimic, and must be differentiated from, myocardial ischemia and infarction. The predominant symptom of acute pericarditis is chest pain. Like angina pectoris, the pain is precordial or retrosternal and may radiate to the left shoulder and arm. Unlike angina, chest pain due to pericarditis is typically pleuritic in nature and can last for a period of days. The pain is worsened by deep breathing, lying down, or turning and improved by sitting up or leaning forward. Fever, which is usually low-grade, may be seen, along with nonspecific symptoms such as anorexia. Dyspnea and syncope may occur. Physical examination may reveal a diphasic (systolic and diastolic) pericardial friction rub, which is scratchy or creaky in nature. The electrocardiogram may show the characteristic four-stage progression discussed previously. In contrast, the electrocardiographic changes seen with myocardial ischemia are less generalized, ST-segment elevation is accompanied by reciprocal ST depression, and pathologic Q waves develop. In patients with pericarditis, echocardiography can show pericardial fluid and diagnose cardiac tamponade. The symptoms of chronic pericarditis usually reflect either cardiac tamponade due to pericardial effusion or pericardial constriction.

Idiopathic and Viral Pericarditis

Other than neoplastic disease, idiopathic or nonspecific pericarditis is the most common cause of pericardial effusion. Symptoms are due to acute pericardial inflammation or pericardial effusion. Chest pain, fever, and nonspecific malaise are common. Cardiac tamponade occurs rarely. The erythrocyte sedimentation rate is typically elevated. A viral source can only be definitively identified in a minority (15% to 20%) of cases. The most common viral pathogens are Coxsackievirus, echovirus, adenovirus, and influenza. Treatment is with nonsteroidal antiinflammatory drugs or aspirin. Corticosteroids may be used as second-line therapy. Pericardiocentesis, surgical drainage, or pericardiectomy may be necessary for cases unresponsive to medical therapy or for constriction.

Uremic Pericarditis

Pericarditis may occur in up to 50% of patients with untreated renal disease and 20% of patients undergoing hemodialysis. It is less common in those undergoing peritoneal dialysis. The exact pathogenesis remains unclear, and occurrence is not directly related to the levels of blood urea nitrogen and creatinine. Chest pain is less common than in idiopathic pericarditis, so that delay in diagnosis is common. Treatment is with increased dialysis, nonsteroidal antiinflammatory drugs and, if necessary, corticosteroids. Pericardiocentesis or surgical drainage may be necessary for effusions that are hemodynamically significant or unresponsive to medical therapy. The pericardial fluid is usually bloody. Pericardiectomy is reserved for continued reaccumulation of fluid or late constriction.

Purulent Pericarditis

Bacteria may enter the pericardium by direct injury, by extension from contiguous pneumonia or peritonitis, or by hematogenous or lymphatic spread during sepsis. Clinical findings are chest pain, fever, and elevation of the white blood cell count. Inciting organisms in adults are commonly *Staphylococcus* and gram-negative bacteria. In children, *Staphylococcus* and *Haemophilus influenzae* are typical. Less commonly, fungal or nocardial infection may involve the pericardium by lymphatic spread or direct extension. Treatment is by pericardiocentesis (both diagnostic and therapeutic) and antibiotics. Surgical drainage with a pericardial tube or even pericardiectomy may be necessary for thick, purulent drainage (often seen with *H. influenzae*) or recalcitrant cases.

Parasitic pericarditis is rare. Amoebic infection may occur by intrapericardial rupture of a liver abscess and can result in tamponade. Echinococcal pericarditis is caused by rupture of a myocardial cyst into the pericardium. The clinical results range from localized pericardial inflammation to rapid cyst multiplication with cardiac compromise.

Tuberculous Pericarditis

Pericarditis may be seen in 1% to 2% of cases of tuberculosis. In countries where pulmonary tuberculosis has declined, tuberculous pericarditis is also uncommon. However, pericarditis due to atypical organisms (*Mycobacterium avium* or *Mycobacterium intracellulare*) may be seen in immunocompromised patients. In nonindustrialized countries, tuberculous pericarditis remains common. Organisms usually reach the pericardium by hematogenous spread, although lymphatic spread and direct extension from neighboring lymph nodes or the lung are also possible. Four stages of tuberculous pericarditis are recognized: fibrinous pericarditis, effusive pericarditis (nonconstrictive), fibrous (nonconstrictive), and fibrous (constrictive, calcific). Diagnosis is by staining or culture of pericardial fluid or tissue (pericardial biopsy). Treatment is by multidrug antituberculous chemotherapy, and pericardiocentesis. Corticosteroids are generally of no benefit.[9,10] Open pericardial drainage should be avoided. The development of pericardial constriction is avoided by early diagnosis, closed drainage, and chemotherapy. If late constriction does develop, pericardiectomy may be necessary.

Acquired Immunodeficiency Syndrome

Up to 20% of AIDS patients may have pericardial effusions. Pericarditis may be associated with tuberculosis and other mycobacterial infections, lymphoma, and Kaposi's sarcoma. The inflammation may also be nonspecific.

Dressler and Postpericardiotomy Syndrome

Pericarditis occurs during the evolution of acute myocardial infarction in 3% to 5% of patients (Dressler syndrome).[11] A similar syndrome occurs in 10% to 40% of patients undergoing cardiac surgery and may also be seen after blunt or penetrating cardiac trauma and permanent pacemaker placement. Symptoms are chest pain, fever, and malaise. A pericardial friction rub is generally present. Laboratory studies show lymphocytosis and elevation of the erythrocyte sedimentation rate. Pericardial effusion and tamponade may develop. The syndrome typically develops 10 days to 2 months after cardiac surgery. The pathogenesis of Dressler and postpericardiotomy syndrome is thought to involve an inflammatory reaction to intrapericardial blood, viral activation, or antimyocardial autoantibodies. Treatment is with nonsteroidal antiinflammatory drugs, aspirin, and occasionally steroids. Pericardiocentesis or pericardiectomy may be required for symptomatic effusion, recurrent effusions, or late pericardial constriction.

Vasculitis, Connective Tissue Disease, and Drugs

Pericarditis may be seen in patients with acute rheumatic fever, rheumatoid arthritis, systemic lupus erythematosus, scleroderma, Wegener granulomatosis, polyarteritis nodosa, dermatomyositis, ankylosing spondylitis, Reiter syndrome, Behçet disease, and familial Mediterranean fever. Large pericardial effusions may be seen in acute rheumatic fever and rheumatoid arthritis. Treatment is by management of the underlying disease and appropriate approaches to effusion or tamponade. A variety of drugs has been implicated in pericarditis; these include procainamide, hydralazine, dantrolene, methysergide, and cromolyn sodium.

PERICARDIOCENTESIS

Pericardiocentesis may be used for both diagnostic and therapeutic purposes. Diagnostic pericardiocentesis is indicated for a newly discovered pericardial effusion if the clinical picture suggests an infectious or neoplastic etiology. In this setting, the results of pericardiocentesis guide subsequent therapy. Diagnostic pericardiocentesis may also be useful in the setting of a persistent or unresolved effusion. Therapeutic pericardiocentesis is indicated in the clinical setting of acute cardiac tamponade.

Pericardiocentesis is optimally performed in the cardiac catheterization laboratory so that the hemodynamic response can be monitored. Echocardiography is very useful for directing pericardiocentesis, as well as for monitoring successful evacuation of pericardial contents. Using local anesthesia and sterile technique, a long needle (16- to 22-gauge, depending on the patient's size and the anticipated viscosity of the pericardial fluid) attached to a syringe is introduced into the pericardial space. The most common approach is subxiphoid, starting just to the left of the xiphoid process and aiming posteriorly at a 45-degree angle for the patient's left shoulder or midscapular area (Fig. 87.4). If echocardiography shows the preponderance of effusion to be anterior, rather than inferior, a parasternal approach may be used instead. The needle is introduced 1 to 2 cm to the left of the sternum, in the fourth or fifth intercostal space, and directed posteriorly at 90 degrees to the body. With either approach, the needle is slowly advanced until fluid is aspirated. An ECG lead may be attached to the needle to monitor for an "injury current" (negative deflection of the QRS complex), indicating contact with the epicardium. However, with echocardiographic guidance, this is now rarely used. If the pericardiocentesis is diagnostic, aspirated fluid is sent for bacteriologic, chemical, hematologic, and cytologic analyses, and the needle is removed. If ongoing drainage of pericardial fluid is desired, a guidewire may be passed through the needle and a soft, multiholed drainage catheter introduced using Seldinger technique.

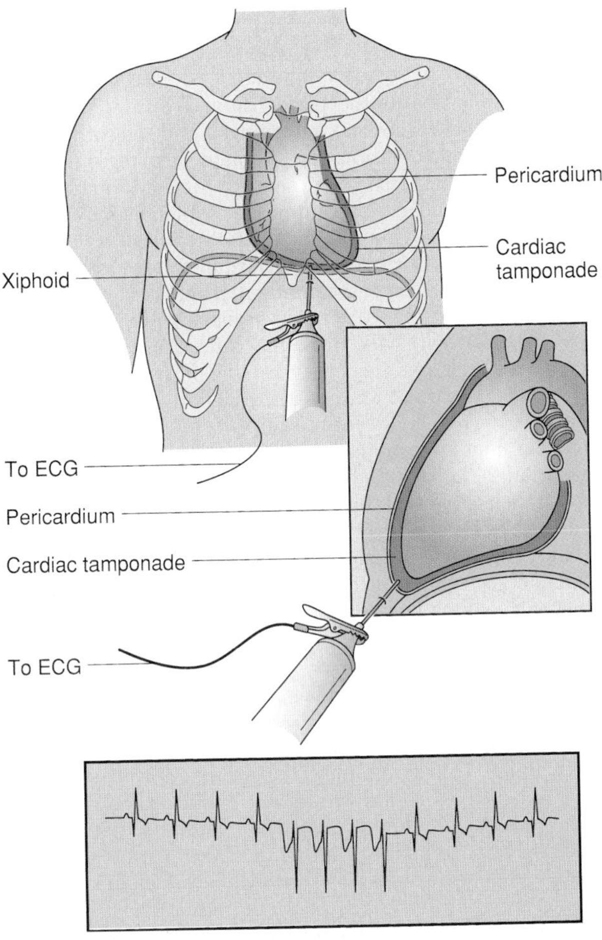

FIGURE 87.4 Pericardiocentesis. The needle is inserted to the left of the xiphoid and directed toward the left shoulder or midscapular area, posteriorly at a 45-degree angle. An electrocardiographic lead may be attached to the needle, and the negative deflection of the QRS complex represents contact with the epicardium.

Potential complications of pericardiocentesis include puncture or laceration of the heart or coronary arteries, the lung or the upper abdominal organs. Arrhythmias are also possible, although usually self-limited on withdrawal of the needle. Echocardiography is quite effective in showing the location of the pericardial fluid and whether the needle is the pericardial space, reducing the likelihood of complications. Pericardiocentesis as well as drainage via a small tube may be ineffective for highly viscous pericardial effusions, such as seen in purulent pericarditis or bloody (postoperative) effusions. Open surgical drainage may be required in such cases.

Analysis of pericardial fluid obtained through pericardiocentesis can be diagnostic of a variety of pericardial disorders. Neoplastic pericardial disease is diagnosed by cytologic studies. Gram stain and cultures reveal the source of purulent pericarditis. Tuberculous pericarditis is diagnosed by the presence of acid-fast bacilli in the pericardium. Uremic pericarditis is characterized by bloody pericardial fluid. Rheumatic pericarditis is marked by fluid high in protein and leukocytes and low in glucose. Pericardial fluid seen in myxedema, tuberculosis, and rheumatoid arthritis may contain cholesterol crystals. Pericardial fluid due to systemic lupus erythematosus shows a high protein content, a normal to low glucose, a low complement level, and lupus cells may be seen. Viral or nonspecific pericarditis is diagnosed by excluding other causes.

PERICARDIAL BIOPSY AND SURGICAL DRAINAGE

Pericardial biopsy may be required to establish a diagnosis if pericardiocentesis is unsuccessful or unrevealing. This is particularly common in cases of neoplastic pericardial disease and tuberculous pericarditis. Biopsy may be via a subxiphoid approach under local or general anesthesia, or an anterior thoracotomy under general anesthesia. A small incision is made, the pericardium is grasped with a clamp, and a small piece is excised for pathologic examination (Fig. 87.5). Any fluid present is sent for analysis, and, if indicated, a tube may be placed in the pericardium for ongoing drainage. If the approach is via anterior thoracotomy, the pericardium is left open to drain into the left pleural space, and a pleural chest tube placed.

Open surgical drainage may be necessary for viscous pericardial effusions, as in purulent pericarditis or bloody effusions, or for recurrent or recalcitrant effusions. A subxiphoid approach allows placement of a pericardiostomy tube as well as excision of a piece of pericardium for analysis. This approach avoids contamination of the pleural spaces, which may be desirable in cases of purulent pericarditis. Chronic effusions, particularly if malignant, may be better dealt with via an anterior thoracotomy or median sternotomy, with excision of a large segment of pericardium, leaving the effusion to drain into the left pleural space. Such partial pericardial resection is also termed a pericardial "window."

General anesthesia in the presence of pericardial compression may be poorly tolerated. The induction of anesthesia removes many of the patient's compensatory mechanisms and can produce a precipitous fall in blood pressure. Preinduction pericardiocentesis and/or volume loading may prevent this response. Patients undergoing anesthesia for drainage of hemodynamically compromising pericardial fluid should be prepped and draped, with the surgeon gowned and gloved, prior to induction of anesthesia.

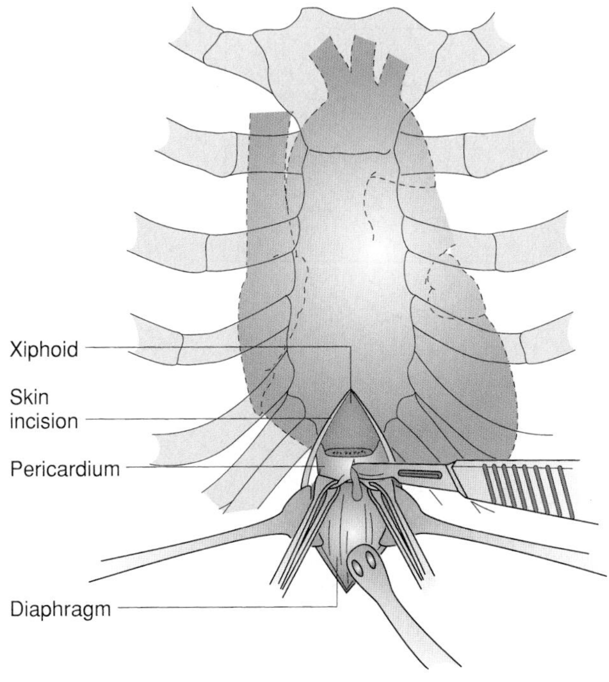

FIGURE 87.5 Open pericardial biopsy or drainage. The xiphoid is exposed through a midline incision and either retracted or removed. Limited exposure to the pericardium is achieved.

PERICARDIECTOMY

Surgical removal of the pericardium is most commonly performed for constrictive pericarditis. It may also be used for chronic malignant effusions or recalcitrant pericardial effusion due to other causes and unresponsive to less aggressive measures. The approach is via median sternotomy or left anterior thoracotomy (Figs. 87.6 and 87.7). Resection aided by thoracoscopy has also been reported with good results.[12] Cardiopulmonary bypass may be used for safety if the pericardial dissection is particularly difficult or for hemodynamic

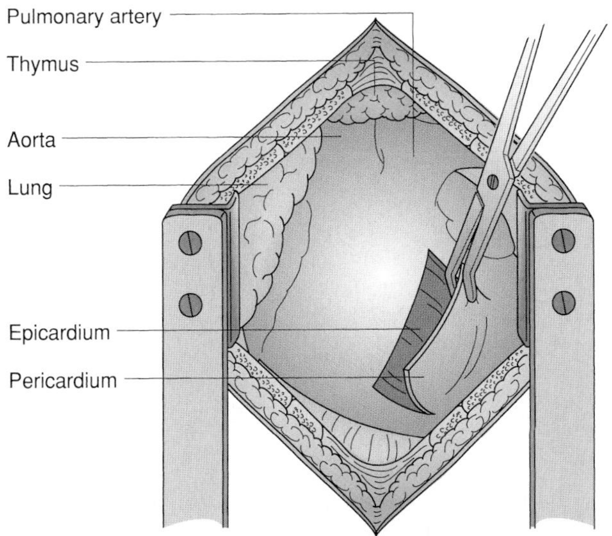

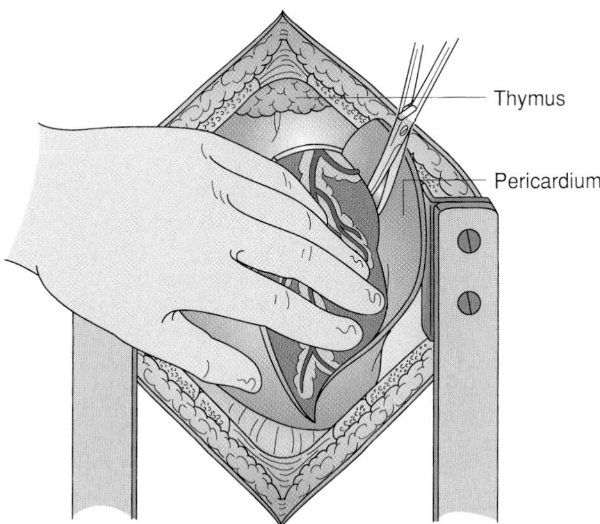

FIGURE 87.6 Pericardiectomy via a median sternotomy. (*A*) The pericardium is incised and a dissection plane established between the fibrous pericardium and the epicardium. (*B*) The heart is retracted to the right so that complete pericardiectomy from one phrenic nerve to the other can be achieved.

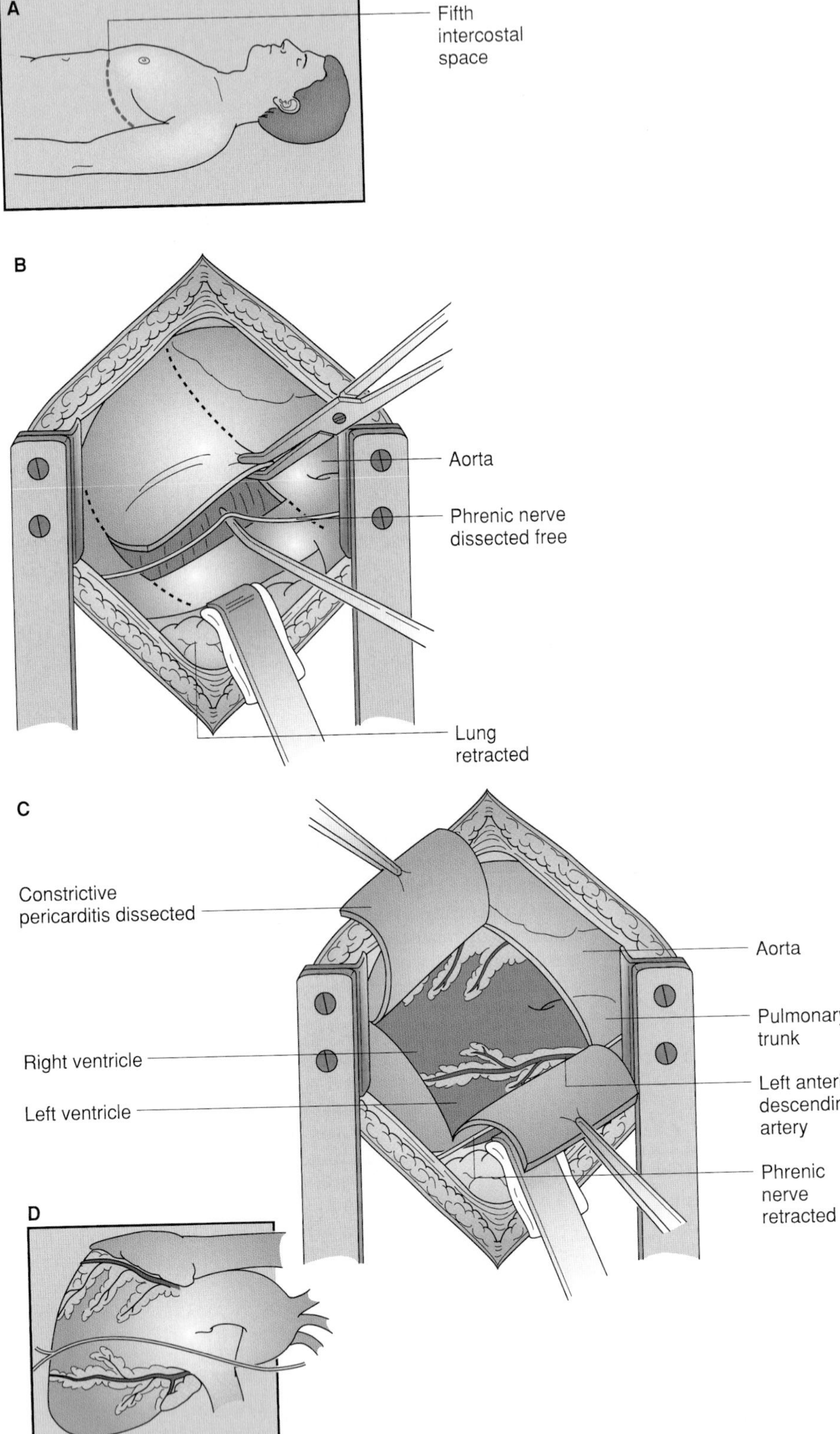

FIGURE 87.7 Pericardiectomy via an anterolateral left thoracotomy in the fifth interspace. The appropriate dissection plane is established and the phrenic nerve mobilized (usually on a 2- to 3-cm pedicle of pericardium) to allow removal of the posterolateral pericardium overlying the left ventricle. (After Kirklin JW, Barratt-Boyes BG. *Cardiac surgery.* New York: John Wiley & Sons; 1986, p. 1438.)

support if extensive cardiac manipulation is required. However, its use is associated with an increased risk of bleeding, and it should only be used if necessary. The anterior thoracotomy approach is traditional, and allows resection of the pericardium over the left ventricle with minimal cardiac manipulation. However, use of cardiopulmonary bypass generally requires femoral cannulation, with its attendant risks. Due to its familiarity, the median sternotomy approach is more commonly used today.[13] It allows relatively easy institution of cardiopulmonary bypass via the chest. However, the sternal approach does require more extensive cardiac manipulation to reach the pericardium overlying the left ventricle. The recommended technical approach is to resect the pericardium overlying the left ventricle before the right to avoid the right ventricle pumping unimpeded in the presence of a still constricted left ventricle, which can result in pulmonary edema. In practice, especially when working via a sternotomy, this sequence of resection may not be feasible. Regardless of approach, pericardium should be removed from phrenic nerve to phrenic nerve anteriorly, as well as posterior to the left phrenic nerve.

Operative mortality for pericardiectomy is closely related to the patient's preoperative status.[14] In the Mayo Clinic's extensive experience, mortality was 1% for patients in preoperative NYHA class I or II, 10% for class III, and 46% for class IV.[15] The majority (70%) of operative mortality was due to low cardiac output. Operative survivors fared well, with 5- and 15-year survivals of 84% and 71%, respectively; 99% of late survivors were in NYHA class I or II. Constriction secondary to radiation treatment may also have a worse outlook, perhaps due to accompanying radiation-induced myocardial injury.

INTRAOPERATIVE CLOSURE OF THE PERICARDIUM

Closure of an otherwise normal pericardium at the end of an open heart operation may have the advantage of removing the heart from the sternum and of facilitating sternal reentry in the event of reoperation via median sternotomy.[16] However, it may also have the disadvantage of depressing cardiac function in the early postoperative period. In one study of 10 patients after cardiac valve replacement, pericardial closure (with the sternum still open) produced significant decreases in mean stroke volume (72 to 51 mL) and cardiac output (5.1 to 3.7 L/min).[17] In the same 10 patients, cardiac function was measured before and after reopening the pericardium (by removing a sliding pericardial suture) with the chest closed. Reopening the pericardium resulted in increases in mean stroke volume (53 to 67 mL) and cardiac output (4.1 to 5.3 L/min). Thus, closure of the pericardium after an open heart operation should be avoided in patients whose cardiac function is already compromised.

KEY POINTS

- **Not all of the functions of the pericardium are well understood, and people can do well with congenital absence or after surgical removal of the pericardium.**
- **The electrocardiogram is usually nonspecific but can contribute to the diagnosis of pericardial disease.**
- **The echocardiogram is the most useful noninvasive modality in pericardial disease.**
- **Cardiac tamponade can be defined as hemodynamically significant cardiac compression due to accumulating pericardial contents that evoke and defeat compensatory mechanisms.**
- **Cardiac tamponade is only definitively diagnosed when removal of pericardial fluid improves the clinical picture.**
- **Primary neoplasms of the pericardium are rare.**
- **Echocardiography is very useful for directing pericardiocentesis, as well as monitoring successful evacuation of pericardial contents.**

References

1. Sadler TW. *Langman's medical embryology,* 7th ed. Baltimore: Williams & Wilkins; 1995, p. xx.
2. **Spodick DH. Macrophysiology, microphysiology, and anatomy of the pericardium: a synopsis. *Am Heart J.* 1992;124:1046.**
3. Spodick DH. The normal and diseased pericardium: current concepts of pericardial physiology, diagnosis and treatment. *J Am Coll Cardiol.* 1983;1:240.
4. Moncada R, Kotler MN, Churchill RJ, et al. Multimodality approach to pericardial imaging. *Cardiovasc Clin.* 1986;17:409.
5. Beck CS. Two cardiac compression triads. *JAMA* 1935;104:714.
6. Shabetai R, Fowler NO, Gunteroth WG. The hemodynamics of cardiac tamponade and constrictive pericarditis. *Am J Cardiol.* 1970;26:480.
7. Hatle LK, Appleton CP, Popp RL. Differentiation of constrictive pericarditis and restrictive cardiomyopathy by Doppler echocardiography. *Circulation* 1989;79:357.
8. **Vaitkus PT, Kussmaqul WG. Constrictive pericarditis versus restrictive cardiomyopathy: a reappraisal ans update of diagnostic criteria. *Am Heart J.* 1991;122:1431.**
9. Quale JM, Lipschik GY, Henrich AE. Management of tuberculous pericarditis. *Ann Thorac Surg.* 1987;43:653.
10. Sagrista-Sauleda J, Permanyer-Miralda G, Soler-Soler J. Tuberculous pericarditis: ten year experience with a prospective protocol for diagnosis and treatment. *J Am Coll Cardiol.* 1988;11:724.
11. **Dressler W. A post-myocardial infarction syndrome: preliminary report of a complication resembling idiopathic recurrent, benign pericarditis. *JAMA* 1956;160:1379.**
12. Hazelrigg SR, Mack MJ, Landreneau RJ, et al. Thoracoscopic pericardiectomy for effusive pericardial disease. *Ann Thorac Surg.* 1993;56:792.
13. **DeValeria PA, Baumgartner WA, Casale AS, et al. Current indications, risks, and outcome after pericardiectomy. *Ann Thorac Surg.* 1991; 52:219.**
14. **Seifert FC, Miller DC, Oesterle SN, et al. Surgical treatment of constrictive pericarditis: analysis of outcome and diagnostic error. *Circulation* 1985; 72[suppl. II]:II-264.**
15. McCaughan BC, Schaff HV, Piehler JM, et al. Early and late results of pericardiectomy for constrictive pericarditis. *J Thorac Cardiovasc Surg.* 1985; 89:340.
16. Rao V, Komeda M, Weisel RD, et al. Should the pericardium be closed routinely after heart operations? *Ann Thorac Surg.* 1999;67:484.
17. Hunter S, Smith GH, Angelini GD. Adverse hemodynamic effects of pericardial closure soon after open heart operation. *Ann Thorac Surg.* 1992; 53:425.

CHAPTER 88 ■ ATHEROSCLEROSIS AND THE PATHOGENESIS OF OCCLUSIVE DISEASE

ANTON N. SIDAWY, NITEN SINGH, SUBODH ARORA, AND ALEXANDER W. CLOWES

Atherosclerosis is a disease of the intima of large arteries that causes luminal narrowing, thrombosis, and occlusion associated with ischemia of the end organ. Throughout much of its course, the disease is not detectable. Thrombosis, including vascular occlusion and embolization, produces the clinical events of importance, such as myocardial infarction, stroke, and ischemic gangrene of the extremities. The widespread prevalence of lesions in arteries of asymptomatic people, the chronicity of the process, the suddenness of the terminal vascular events, and the lack of a single etiologic factor make it impossible to give a simple explanation for atherogenesis and atherosclerosis progression. In fact, atherosclerosis might be a form of nonspecific adaptation on the part of large blood vessels to a variety of harmful stimuli and that the clinical consequences, or what we might call the true disease process, appear when the compensatory mechanisms are overwhelmed.

NORMAL STRUCTURE OF BLOOD VESSELS

Normal arteries and veins, both large and small, are formed from endothelium, smooth muscle, and extracellular matrix synthesized by these vascular wall cells. The vascular wall is invariably organized into layers (Fig. 88.1). The intima, defined as the part of the wall between the blood and the internal elastic lamina, is composed of a monolayer of endothelium at the luminal surface and may overlie one or more layers of smooth muscle. The media, lying beneath the intima, constitutes the bulk of the vessel and contains smooth muscle cells arranged in layers and dispersed in a matrix made of elastin, collagen, and proteoglycan. The adventitia lies outside the external elastic lamina and forms the outer coat. It is composed of loose connective tissue, fibroblasts, capillaries, neural fibers, and occasional leukocytes. In very large arteries with greater than 28 elastic layers, a microvasculature (vasa vasorum) penetrates the media from the adventitial side and provides an alternative nutrient supply to the flux from the luminal surface.[1] In thickened, atherosclerotic vessels the vasa vasora are extensive and penetrate into the diseased intima.[2,3]

In the fetus, the vessel wall is derived from mesoderm. A brief review of this process is of interest because many aspects of wound healing and atherogenesis in adult vessels represent a recapitulation of the fetal program of vasculogenesis and angiogenesis. The earliest vascular primordia in the embryo are isolated "hemangioblasts" that display endothelial and hematopoietic immunologic markers.[4,5] The hemangioblasts cluster and form cords and, later, tubes that become the major vascular conduits. Some of the clusters become blood islands, the precursors for hematopoietic tissues. These structures sprout, grow, and remodel to form the primitive vascular system.[6]

Endothelial cells probably play a central role in the organization and building of vascular structures. They are derived from the hemangioblasts, organize at sites of later vessel development, and are followed by local mesenchymal cells that form the outer layers of the emerging blood vessels. These mesenchymal cells are the precursors of smooth muscle cells and fibroblasts. Once associated with the vessel wall, many of these cells begin to express smooth muscle specific alpha actin. This pattern of endothelial invasion followed by smooth muscle recruitment is reactivated in later life during angiogenesis in the presence of tumors and in wounds undergoing repair.

The adult form of blood vessels appears to be established by birth. In large vessels, the number of elastic and smooth muscle layers remains constant although wall mass increases due to smooth muscle proliferation and matrix synthesis.[7,8] The vascular architecture is probably genetically determined because alterations in animal size by hormonal manipulations (e.g., excess growth hormone) are associated with increased wall mass but no change in the number of cell layers.[9] It is likely that the primitive endothelial cell regulates wall architecture because it is involved in the recruitment of the corresponding primitive smooth muscle cell. These activities of the endothelial cell in the embryo presage its role in determining vascular diameter and mass in normal and diseased adult arteries.

These observations on the embryologic origin of vascular wall cells and the development of blood vessels provide many insights into vascular wall organization and function in the adult and provoke numerous questions for which at present there are few answers. What determines the initial organization of the hemangioblasts (the primitive endothelium)? Are they tracking some kind of predetermined scaffolding? What are the signals that regulate proliferation of these cells? How do they go about recruiting the primitive smooth muscle cells? How do the endothelial cells then regulate smooth muscle number and function? Does the molecular language of endothelial-smooth muscle cell discourse extend to other types of cell interactions (e.g., between leukocytes or platelets and vascular wall cells)? In the last decade, the answers to these questions and a rudimentary understanding of how vascular cells interact in normal and disease states have begun to be realized. In the next section, recent evidence that vascular wall function as well as structure depend absolutely on cell—cell interactions is reviewed.

This chapter is based in part on Clowes AW. Theories of atherosclerosis. In: White RA, ed. *Atherosclerosis and arteriosclerosis: human pathology and experimental animal methods and models.* Boca Raton, FL: CRC Press, 1989, p. 3.

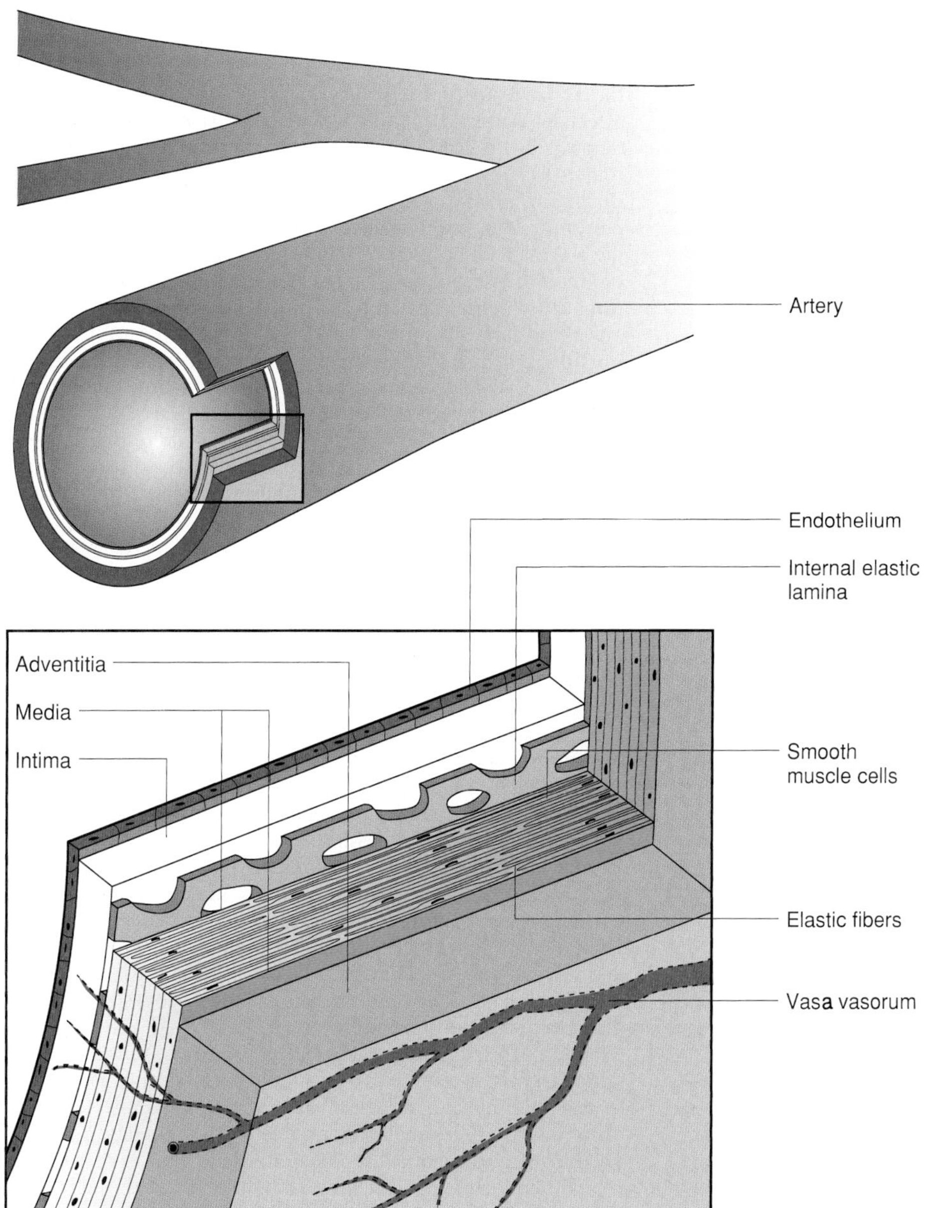

FIGURE 88.1 The artery wall is made of multiple layers (intima, media, and adventitia) that vary in composition depending on the artery.

REGULATION OF LUMENAL AREA

This description of the usual arterial wall anatomy gives no clue to how a vessel adjusts its mass and dimensions in response to external stimuli (hypertension, increased blood flow, vascular injury) or to how it maintains a nonthrombogenic state at the luminal surface. For this, the array of possible physiologic functions of the wall and its cellular components under normal and abnormal conditions must be considered.

Blood vessels, both large and small, become larger during growth and development and as a compensatory mechanism to increased blood flow or more appropriately increased blood velocity (Fig. 88.2). A particularly striking example of this is found in an artery proximal to an arteriovenous fistula; if the fistula is not treated, the artery can become frankly aneurysmal.[10] Similarly, a vessel undergoing stenosis experiences an increase in blood velocity at the point of luminal narrowing. When the stenosis is attributable to intimal thickening or to an atherosclerotic plaque, the vessel dilates at the site of the lesion. For example, a diseased coronary vessel dilates and can maintain the correct luminal dimensions despite changes in wall structure as long as the intimal lesion does not occupy more than 40% of the area inside the internal elastic lamina (Fig. 88.3).[11] At this point, pathologic narrowing begins to take place. Why vessels should dilate in each of these instances when the velocity of flow increases has not been determined. One possibility is that the cells in the wall, particularly the endothelium, are somehow capable of sensing changes in blood velocity and shear and can translate this biomechanical information into biochemical signals that then regulate the contractile state of the artery.[12–15] The effect of shear stress on the regulation of arterial vasomotility is described in more detail later in this section. Endothelial cell secretory products play a critical role in smooth muscle cell function.[16] They secrete vasodilating (prostaglandin I_2 and E_2, adenosine, and nitric oxide) and vasoconstricting substances (endothelin).

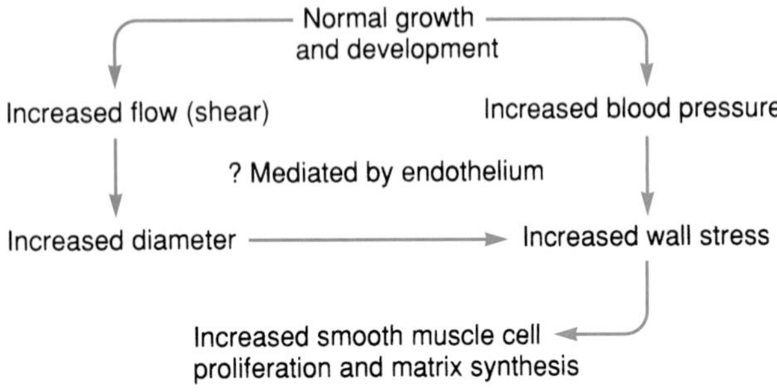

FIGURE 88.2 Changes in blood flow and pressure can have profound effects on arterial wall structure. In part, the response to hemodynamic changes might be mediated by the endothelium (After Clowes AW. Theories of atherosclerosis. In: White RA, ed. *Atherosclerosis and arteriosclerosis: human pathology and experimental animal methods and models*. Boca Raton, FL: CRC Press; 1989, p. 3, with permission.)

Where endothelium is damaged or absent, adherent platelets release the vasoconstrictor thromboxane A_2.

Nitric oxide, previously called endothelium-dependent relaxing factor, is an important regulator in normal and diseased vessels.[17] It is a short-acting substance that is derived from the metabolic breakdown of arginine.[18–20] A number of factors stimulate endothelial cells to secrete nitric oxide, including thrombin, acetylcholine, bradykinin, serotonin, and products of platelet release. Hence, when the endothelium is present and functional, neighboring thrombotic events are likely to cause vasodilation, whereas when the endothelium is absent or dysfunctional these same factors cause vasoconstriction. Moreover, when the endothelium is missing the vessel does not respond normally to changes in blood flow, either in the short-term or the long term.[21] Changes in blood flow affect wall mass.[22–24] In this regard, it is interesting to note that various factors that affect smooth muscle contraction or relaxation also modulate growth (nitric oxide, endothelin, thrombin, and prostaglandins).[25–29] These observations may be the first preliminary evidence that transient signals affecting the diameter of vessels might have, in the long term, more permanent effects on wall structure. Certain pathologic conditions in which either endothelium is missing or is abnormal are associated with acute and chronic vasospasm; it is quite possible that the acute problems of atypical angina (coronary vasospasm) and cerebrovasospasm after cerebral hemorrhage are manifestations of abnormal endothelial function and decreased nitric oxide.[30] There is a relationship among shear stress exerted on the arterial lumen, the production of nitric oxide, and the development of atherosclerosis. Normal shear stress in arteries (usually higher than 15 dyne/cm^2) is protective, whereas low shear stress (less than 4 dyne/cm^2) induces the formation of atherosclerotic lesions.[31] In addition, Malek et al.[32] have found that increasing shear stress led to an increase in the expression of endothelial nitric oxide synthase (eNOS) mRNA, leading to an increase in nitric oxide production resulting in vasodilatation. Areas of low shear stress in the arterial tree, such as the carotid bifurcation, are foci for the formation of atherosclerotic lesions.[31]

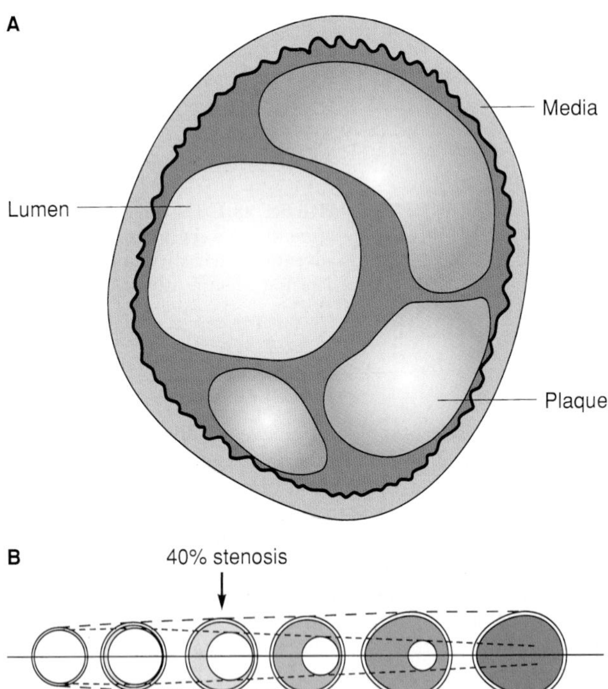

FIGURE 88.3 (*A*) Coronary arteries dilate as atherosclerotic plaques form and maintain normal luminal dimensions Luminal narrowing begins only after the plaque occupies more than 40% of the cross-sectional area within the internal elastic lamina and bulges outward at sites of medial atrophy. (*B*) The course of lesion formation and luminal narrowing. (After Glagov S, Weisenberg E, Zarins CK, et al. Compensatory enlargement of human atherosclerotic coronary arteries. *N Engl J Med*. 1987;316:1371, with permission.)

Endothelial dysfunction underlies and is the earliest change in the development and progression of atherosclerosis. This role of endothelial dysfunction has been emphasized recently. It probably begins in childhood and extends through clinical events later in life. Most studies have shown that impaired endothelial function exists very early in the development of atherosclerosis, before the appearance of visible lesions. In children of parents with genetic defects of lipid transport or in children living with smokers, there is clear evidence of endothelial dysfunction. As these children grow, the endothelial dysfunction becomes more pronounced, and it continues to exist after atherosclerosis is established.[33] It is present in numerous conditions associated with an increased risk for cardiovascular disease including hypertension, hypercholesterolemia, cigarette smoking, diabetes mellitus, and estrogen deficiency in postmenopausal women.[34]

The endothelium is a very active organ. Endothelial cells have the ability to transduce signals from the flow of blood and from chemicals and then to convert these signals into actions in the underlying vessel wall. The surface of endothelial cells has a wide variety of receptors, including those for shear stress, oxidized low-density lipoproteins (LDL), and inflammatory mediators, to name a few. Through these receptors, endothelial cells orchestrate actions that affect not only the endothelium but also the entire vascular wall. In diseased state, such actions include adverse changes in vascular tone, proliferation of smooth muscle cells resulting in hypertrophy, and recruitment and adhesion of mononuclear cells, which are early steps in the development and progression of atherosclerosis. One of the most important defenses that the endothelium possesses for maintaining vascular health is nitric oxide, which has been shown to inhibit the expression of receptors that mediate substances implicated in the formation of atherosclerosis, such as oxidized LDL, inflammatory mediators, and angiotensin II.[35] The chief role of nitric oxide in reversing pathologic changes appears to be its ability to counteract oxidative stress, a common pathogenic pathway for most major risk factors for atherosclerosis. Reduced eNOS may be the result of reactive oxygen species (ROS) that form peroxynitrite, which leads to oxidation of LDL. In addition peroxynitrite leads to degradation of tetrahydrobiopterin (BH_4), an essential cofactor of eNOS.[36,37] The classical atherosclerotic risk factors, such as hypertension, smoking, and hyperlipidemia, all act at the endothelial level by increasing oxidative stress, which inactivates nitric oxide and upsets the balance between endogenous vasodilators and vasoconstrictors, growth promoters and growth inhibitors, antiinflammatory and proinflammatory mediators, and other factors important to endothelial function and vascular health.[38]

The normal endothelium functions in an inhibitory mode, maintaining relaxed vascular tone and inhibiting smooth muscle cell growth, platelet and leukocyte adhesion and aggregation, and thrombosis. In hypertensive, hypercholesterolemic, and diabetic patients, endothelial dysfunction has been associated with decreased production or decreased activity of nitric oxide.[39] In studies of apolipoprotein E knockout mice, eNOS was ablated and accelerated atherosclerosis was noted.[40] Endothelial dysfunction is associated with most of the known risk factors for atherosclerosis and cardiovascular disease and may constitute a contributing cause for such disease. This concept has important clinical implications, especially in terms of preventive strategies.

Angiotensin-converting enzyme (ACE) acts both to produce angiotensin II, a potent vasoconstrictor, from angiotensin I and to degrade bradykinin. Angiotensin II is highly atherogenic, stimulating the synthesis of various growth and chemotactic factors and promoting superoxide anion generation, which degrades nitric oxide. In contrast, bradykinin is a vasodilator that exerts its effect via nitric oxide. Within the endothelium, excess angiotensin II is not only a vasoconstrictor but also a promoter of smooth muscle cell proliferation and a potent stimulator of inflammatory mediators and growth factors, such as tumor necrosis factor-alpha (TNF-α), interleukin (IL)-1, IL-6, IL-8, insulinlike growth factor 1 (IGF-β), platelet-derived growth factor (PDGF), transforming growth factor-β (TGF-β), and basic fibroblast growth factor (bFGF).[41] All these processes can be inhibited or reversed by ACE inhibition therapy because it decreases the level of angiotensin II and inhibits the degradation of bradykinin. ACE inhibitors prevent not only the adverse effects of hypertension but also the effects of oxidative stress from other mechanisms. Clinical trials have shown that 6 months of ACE inhibition therapy, using quinapril, is associated with a significant improvement in endothelial function in normotensive patients with coronary artery disease.[42] ACE inhibition at the tissue level appears to be critical to prevent oxidative stress within the endothelium. This is the reason why tissue-avid ACE inhibitors, like quinapril, may have advantages over other drugs in their class. Restoring endothelial function through ACE inhibitors has become an attractive therapeutic target.

REGULATION OF MEDIAL AND INTIMAL THICKENING

Earlier it was observed that, for embryonic vessels to form, primitive endothelial cells must migrate and become aligned and then recruit smooth muscle precursors from the surrounding mesenchyme. Because endothelial cells grow as a monolayer, they can proliferate only when the vascular structure is enlarging in circumference, during vascular elongation (angiogenesis), or when injured endothelium is being replaced. Massive denudation and endothelial loss is not a normal event and probably occurs only during pathologic degeneration of the intima or during surgical instrumentation of the vessel. In any event, endothelial proliferation does not contribute significantly to an increase in wall mass. Smooth muscle cell proliferation does.

Under several circumstances, vessels of adult animals respond by becoming thicker. In hypertensive animals and humans, arteries exhibit medial thickening, whereas after endothelial denudation or in the presence of hypercholesterolemia, they develop a thick intima.[43,44] Exactly how these responses are regulated is not clear although it is certain that in each instance proliferation of smooth muscle cells and accumulation of extracellular matrix are important components. In addition, in hypercholesterolemic subjects, the accumulation of lipid and lipid-filled macrophages contributes to the intimal lesion.[45]

Vessel wall mass is largely determined by the accumulation of smooth muscle cells and matrix synthesized by smooth muscle cells. Hence, how smooth muscle number is regulated needs to be considered.[46] Under normal circumstances, smooth muscle cells proliferate in the vessels of young animals and enter a quiescent state at maturity. For example, smooth muscle cells in adult rat carotid artery do not increase in number and turn over at a rate of 0.06 % per day.[47] In animal models of disease, these cells can readily be stimulated to enter the growth cycle by induction of hypertension or direct vascular injury. Observations made in these models provide us with insights into possible mechanisms for initiation and progression of vascular disease in humans.

Although hypertension has its greatest impact on the small "resistance vessels," in fact large arteries are equally affected. In response to increased pressure the wall thickens.[43,48] Morphometric studies have shown that this increase is largely a medial process and involves all components of the vessel wall, including the mass of smooth muscle cells and matrix. In some forms of hypertension, there is an increase in smooth muscle number, whereas in others there is an increase in the DNA content per cell. Tetraploid and octaploid cells have been detected. In venous grafts transposed from a relatively hypotensive venous environment into the normotensive arterial circulation, there is an increase in wall thickness and a corresponding increase in smooth muscle number.[46] In each instance the change in pressure affects the mass of cells and associated matrix.

How a change in pressure might induce smooth muscle cells to proliferate, to change their ploidy or to synthesize matrix is not known. In some circumstances (e.g., severe hypertension, vein grafting), there is a detectable but small amount of endothelial loss.[49] However, this is not a usual feature in more moderate or chronic forms of hypertension. Glagov and associates have suggested that increased tension and stretch have a direct effect on matrix protein synthesis, but not on cell proliferation.[50] Alternatively, increased wall tension might affect the endothelium, and the endothelium might in turn secrete factors regulating smooth muscle mass.

Of the models of smooth muscle growth *in vivo*, perhaps the best studied is the balloon injury model first developed by Baumgartner.[47,51,52] In this model, smooth muscle proliferation is stimulated by the passage of an inflated balloon catheter along an artery. The artery is at once stretched and denuded of its endothelium. Immediately thereafter, platelets begin to adhere to the wall wherever endothelium is missing; they then spread and degranulate. In most situations, endothelial denudation and platelet adherence are followed 1 to 2 days later by the onset of medial smooth muscle proliferation. In the ballooned rat carotid (Fig. 88.4), this can be a most dramatic response with a three-log increase in the thymidine labeling index (a measure of proliferation). This early proliferation in the media does not lead to an increase in wall thickness; the wall thickens only after smooth muscle cells migrate from the media and proliferate in the intima. In normal animals, this process continues for a period of time and subsides spontaneously whether or not endothelium reappears at the luminal surface. The intimal mass is further increased by the accumulation of extracellular matrix synthesized by the smooth muscle cells.[53]

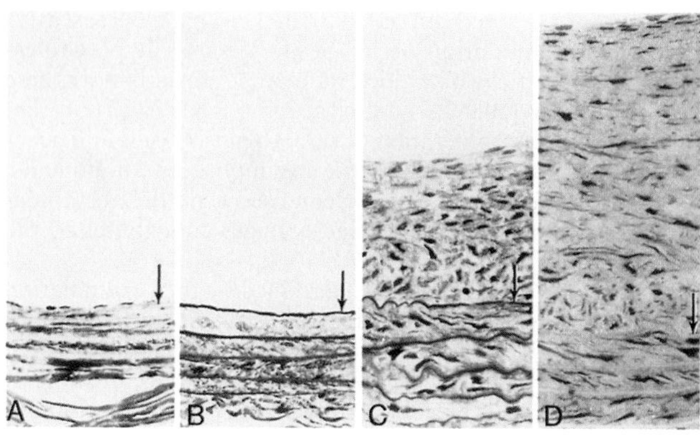

FIGURE 88.4 Elastic arteries injured by the passage of a balloon embolectomy catheter develop substantial intimal thickenings. In this series of histologic cross-sections of rat carotid artery before (*A*) and after ballooning (*B–D*), the endothelium is stripped away and the inner layer of medial smooth muscle cells is damaged (*B*). (C) By 2 weeks, the intima is thickened by the migration and proliferation of smooth muscle cells derived from the media. The mass of cells does not change significantly after this time; nevertheless, the intima is thicker at 3 months (*D*) because of matrix synthesis and accumulation. (From Clowes AW, Reidy MA, Clowes MM. Kinetics of cellular proliferation after arterial injury. I. Smooth muscle growth in the absence of endothelium. *Lab Invest.* 1983:49:327, with permission.)

A link between smooth muscle proliferation and earlier platelet granule release has been proposed. Among the proteins released are several growth factors including PDGF, TGF-β, and an epidermal growth factor-like protein.[54] Where these granule proteins go after being released from the platelets is not known. One hypothesis suggests that these factors accumulate in the artery wall and stimulate subsequent smooth muscle growth.[44] This hypothesis (the reaction to injury hypothesis) was first proposed many decades ago as a general mechanism for atherogenesis and has been refined in view of recent information. Although attractive in theory, it is based on rather slim evidence mainly derived from experiments in thrombocytopenic animals.[54] Injured arteries in these animals show very little intimal thickening.

The hypothesis that the decrease in intimal thickening in injured arteries of thrombocytopenic animals is attributable to decreased proliferation of smooth muscle cells has proven to be incorrect.[55] In the ballooned rat carotid model, even though intimal thickening is diminished in thrombocytopenic animals, smooth muscle proliferation and early cell cycle gene expression are the same as in controls. The interpretation of these findings is that platelet products play a role in the movement of smooth muscle cells from one vascular compartment to the next (media to intima) but do not affect the initiation of proliferation. Whether platelet factors can influence the growth of intimal smooth muscle has yet to be determined.

Although little is known of what starts or stops the intimal thickening process, there are several observations that are interesting and are perhaps important when we consider the current theories of atherosclerosis. The first is that the surface of the injured artery accumulates a single layer of platelets. Fibrin and microthrombi are seen only at the luminal surface when the artery is reinjured after an intimal thickening has formed or in small craters in association with adherent macrophages in hypercholesterolemic animals.[56–59] Active, fulminant thrombosis is not a usual feature of injured vessels; when it occurs, it must represent a major aberration of vessel function. Second, in models demonstrating early reendothelialization or partial deendothelialization without medial injury, intimal thickening does not develop, although one or two rounds of medial smooth muscle proliferation can occur.[60] This result suggests that endothelium might play a role in suppressing smooth muscle growth and migration from the media to the intima. It is known that smooth muscle growth inhibitors can be extracted from the vessel wall, that endothelium can synthesize a heparin-like molecule which inhibits SMC growth *in vitro,* and that heparin itself can suppress both proliferation and migration of SMC *in vitro* and *in vivo*.[61] Taken together, these findings suggest that the endothelium can inhibit smooth muscle proliferation and that the quiescent state of smooth muscle cells in the normal arteries of adult animals might be an actively maintained one rather than one attributable to the lack of growth factors (Fig. 88.5).

REGULATION OF SMOOTH MUSCLE GROWTH

Platelets have long been considered the major source of mitogen for proliferating smooth muscle. However, smooth muscle cells are able to proliferate in injured and hypertensive arteries when platelets are absent. If platelet factors are not important, what, then, is the stimulus for smooth muscle growth? Three alternatives present themselves: (a) growth factors from vascular wall cells or resident leukocytes; (b) exogenous, neuroendocrine factors; or (c) loss of local inhibitors of smooth muscle proliferation. All three mechanisms might be important. Let us consider the first alternative. It is of some interest that when a rat carotid is denuded of endothelium with a balloon catheter, a substantial fraction of the medial smooth muscle cells proliferate (around 20% to 30%), but when denudation is accomplished with a fine nylon wire there is very little proliferation (around 2% to 4%).[62] These procedures differ only in regard to the degree to which the media is damaged. Ballooning destroys 20% of the medial smooth muscle, as well as the endothelium, whereas passage of the nylon wire destroys only the endothelium. The observations become more interesting if we note that cultured cells, when damaged, release growth promoting activity.[63,64] The predominant growth promoting activity is due to fibroblast growth factors (FGFs).[65,66] These factors have been found in a wide variety of tissues and cell types and are synthesized by endothelium and smooth muscle cells. They are distinguished from other polypeptide mitogens by their ability to bind strongly to heparin. Furthermore, both acidic and basic FGF are potent smooth muscle mitogens *in vitro*. Finally, FGF can bind to heparin-like molecules so that released FGF might readily be "stored" in the heparan sulfate proteoglycan-containing matrix at sites of cell death.[67] The experiments of Lindner and Reidy provide strong evidence to support the conclusion that basic FGF is the important growth factor for the first wave of proliferation in balloon injured rat carotid artery.[68,69] This mechanism of tissue repair is probably quite relevant for the development of the fibrous cap in advanced atherosclerotic lesions. At these sites, toxic oxidized lipids accumulate, and there is clear evidence of injury and necrosis.[45] The release of cellular FGF could provide the stimulus for smooth muscle proliferation in the overlying fibrous cap.

Because cell death is not necessarily a prominent feature of growing tissues, there must be other means for controlling smooth muscle proliferation. Smooth muscle cells not only respond to factors from dead cells, platelets (PDGF, TGF-β, EGF-like molecules), and plasma (thrombin, lipoproteins, IGF-1) but also synthesize and respond to their own secreted factors.[46] Both endothelial and smooth muscle cells, as well as macrophages, are potential sources of mitogen. In addition to the FGFs, these cell types synthesize and secrete PDGF, IL-1, TGF-β, and IGF-1.

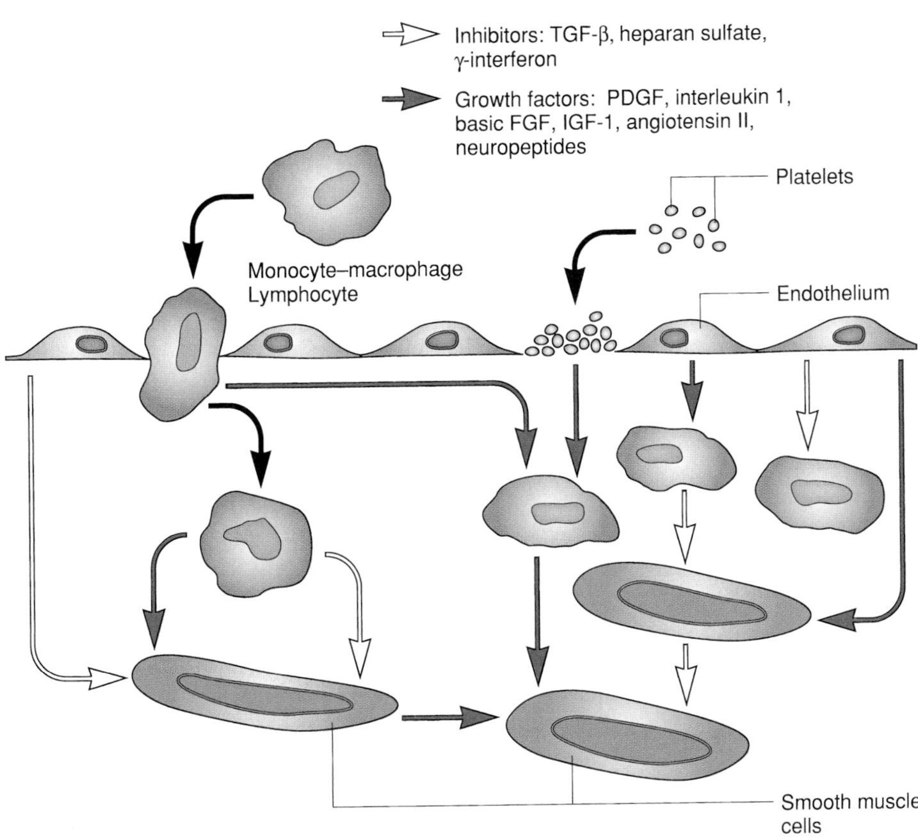

FIGURE 88.5 Diagram depicts the complexity of the interactions between vascular wall cells (endothelium and smooth muscle), platelets, and blood-borne leukocytes (monocyte/macrophage and lymphocyte). Each cell is capable of synthesizing and releasing several smooth muscle growth factors and inhibitors.

PDGF in particular has been studied in detail.[70] The original studies on PDGF stemmed from the observation that serum prepared from whole blood contains substantially more growth promoting activity than serum prepared from plasma. These findings led to the discovery of PDGF, a basic dimeric protein with a molecular weight of approximately 30,000. It is transported in the blood in the alpha granule of the platelet and is released along with other alpha granule proteins. PDGF is by itself extremely potent and is active as a smooth muscle mitogen in trace amounts (nanogram per milliliter). It also exhibits a range of other activities on smooth muscle and other types of cells (stimulates smooth muscle migration, contraction, and matrix synthesis) although it is not a mitogen for endothelium. When placed in a wound chamber *in vivo*, it induces a granulation tissue response.[71]

An important development in the field of growth factor research in the last decade was the demonstration that the structure of the gene for PDGF is nearly identical to that of the oncogene v-sis, a gene associated with cellular transformation by the simian sarcoma virus.[72,73] This discovery, coupled with the finding that a variety of cells including normal cells synthesize and secrete active PDGF, raises the possibility that normal wound healing and malignant, unscheduled growth of tumor cells might have striking similarities with subtle differences in gene regulation. It also led to a search for growth factors in vascular wall cells. We now have solid evidence that endothelium, smooth muscle cells, and leukocytes, including macrophages, can express the PDGF gene (c-sis or PDGF B chain) *in vitro* and *in vivo*.[70] PDGF research is complicated by the observation that PDGF is not a single molecule but is either a heterodimer or homodimer of two isoforms, PDGF A and PDGF B. The cellular receptors are also dimers of two isoforms, alpha and beta, such that PDGF B binds to both alpha and beta, but PDGF A binds only to the alpha form of the receptor. The implications of this complexity of growth factor and receptor expression have yet to be understood. At present, we know that human platelets transport mainly PDGF AB, whereas cultured SMC from human plaques, baboon graft intima, and injury-induced rat intimal thickening express mainly PDGF A chain mRNA. This observation is probably not an artifact of cell culture because the primary lesions from which the cells are derived contain relatively large amounts of A chain mRNA. Macrophages in atherosclerotic lesions express PDGF B protein. What role PDGF plays in wall function remains to be determined. It is not clear how the expression of the protein is regulated nor is it clear whether regulation also occurs at the level of receptor expression. These findings suggest the intriguing possibility that the vascular wall cells, as well as the platelets, are a source of growth factors in the artery wall, and through the endogenous production of growth factors thus might be able to regulate their own growth (autocrine control) or their neighbor's growth (paracrine control). Alternatively, PDGF might control some other function than proliferation. At least after injury and in atherosclerotic mouse arteries, PDGF may act as a chemoattractant and regulate the movement of SMC from the media into the intima or from the wall into the overlying thrombus.[74,75] In smooth muscle cell migration, PDGF uses a different signaling pathway than that used for proliferation.[76]

Another alternative for regulation, in addition to factors from the blood and the cells themselves, is neuroendocrine control of smooth muscle growth.[77,78] Several neurotransmitters affect smooth muscle hypertrophy and proliferation (serotonin, neurokinin A, substance K, substance P). Furthermore, sympathectomy or inhibitors of sympathetic nerve function inhibit the increase in DNA in the media of developing arteries and arteries subjected to hypertension.[79,80] In injury models, prazosin (an alpha-1 antagonist) and cilazapril (an ACE inhibitor) both inhibit intimal thickening.[81,82] These recent observations provide some support for the possibility that neuroendocrine factors also influence intimal smooth muscle proliferation.

Although smooth muscle mass may be determined in large measure by the presence or absence of growth factors, that is, positive effectors of growth, smooth muscle mass might also be influenced by endogenous inhibitors. Growth might be viewed as release from quiescence. Earlier, it was pointed out that endothelial regeneration in injured arteries is associated with cessation of underlying intimal smooth muscle growth. On the other hand, in healing vascular grafts, intimal smooth muscle cells proliferate only underneath the newly formed endothelial surface.[83] These observations are in parallel with studies of endothelial and smooth muscle cells in culture demonstrating that vascular wall cells can synthesize and secrete both inhibitors and promoters of smooth muscle growth.[13] The growth promoting factors have already been described. Both cell types synthesize heparan sulfate, which, when released from the larger proteoglycan, can inhibit the growth of cultured smooth muscle cells.[84,85] Both cell types synthesize and secrete a TGF-β precursor,[86] and TGF-β can be found in the arterial wall after injury.[87] The precursor molecule can then be activated. In general, TGF-β acts as an inhibitor, although at times it can promote smooth muscle growth. Antibody to TGF-β administered to rats suppresses injury-induced intimal thickening.[88] There are other growth inhibitors *in vivo* that might be released by leukocytes present in the vascular wall. Although this mechanism is not important for the regulation of mass in normal artery, it is probably very important in diseased vessels. In atherosclerotic plaques there are large numbers of macrophages and lymphocytes. Hansson et al.[89] have shown that resident T cells secrete gamma interferon and induce the expression of class II major histocompatibility antigens. Gamma interferon also inhibits smooth muscle growth in culture, and in the injured rat carotid, there is a significant population of I_a-positive, growth-inhibited intimal smooth muscle cells.[90] Although smooth muscle cells make up the bulk of the intimal thickening, 1% or less of the intimal cells are T cells. Because I_a expression is absolutely dependent on the presence of gamma interferon, these observations strongly support the view that gamma interferon is an endogenous regulator of intimal smooth muscle growth. A recent study of the effects of gamma interferon refutes this conclusion and suggests that it may at times promotes smooth muscle cell growth.[91] Finally, growth of vascular wall cells might be regulated not only by secreted soluble factors but also by direct cell—cell contact. This inhibitory mechanism is very important for endothelium and perhaps less so for smooth muscle cells.

These growth factors exert their effects via specific receptors located in the cell membrane. The majority of growth factors receptors belong to a family of peptide receptors called receptor tyrosine kinases (RTKs). A growth factor's function can be endocrine, paracrine, or autocrine in nature. A growth factor's function is said to be endocrine when it is released in the circulation and exerts its function after attaching to receptors located on cells in a distant organ. A growth factor acts in a paracrine manner when it effects cells located in the vicinity of the cell that secreted it. A growth factor can also causes its effect on the same cell that secretes it in an autocrine manner. In each of these situations, the growth factor interacts with its own specific receptors located on distant cells, adjacent cells, or on the same cells that secreted it. The paracrine and autocrine functions are important in case of arterial injury. When endothelial cells and smooth muscle cells are injured, they secrete growth factors, such as PDGF, that bind to receptors on the same or adjacent cells causing smooth muscle cell proliferation and migration to form intimal hyperplasia.[44]

Once the growth factor binds to the extracellular domain of its receptor, the kinase function becomes activated and phosphorylates specific cytoplasmic substrates to activate pathways required for the function of the growth factor. Various growth factor receptors use different specific substrates for their actions and the same growth factor may use a different substrate depending on the ultimate action required whether it is cell division, motion, or differentiation. Therefore, the most important events in signal transduction take place in the cytoplasm of the cell.[92] Triggered by growth factor attachment, the intracellular domains interact on a molecular level. Then intracellular protein molecules belonging to various protein families bind to specific sites along the intracellular cytoplasmic domain of the phosphorylated receptor. These proteins carry specific recognition sites that allow a certain family of proteins to bind to a specific area of the intracellular domain. By doing so, various cellular signaling pathways are activated. Each pathway controls a specific function of the growth factor. The recognition sites found on the cellular proteins are called src homology-2 (SH-2) or src homology-3 (SH-3) domains. In addition, the SH-2 and SH-3 phosphorylated sites of the protein serve to bind them to other cellular proteins that belong to the signaling cascade. Proteins that are involved in these pathways include guanosine triphosphatase activating protein (GAP), phospholipase-C (PLC), and phosphatidylinositol-3 kinase (Pl-3K) binding protein. These cascades of phosphorylation and specific protein binding eventually lead to a specific function of the growth factor; the function may be one of differentiation, proliferation, cell shape changes, or motility.[93]

The signaling pathways or cascades rely on the proteins' phosphorylation for the signal to be transmitted to the nucleus and cause gene activation. One of these pathways is called Ras pathway. Once the growth factor attaches to its receptor, the receptor phosphorylates itself. Ras, a protein that attaches to the cytoplasmic aspect of the cellular membrane, undergoes phosphorylation and activates Raf-1 protein, which indirectly phosphorylates mitogen-activated protein kinase (MAPK). MAPK phosphorylates transcription factors inside the nucleus (e.g., Myc, jun) that stimulate gene activity.[93] Jak-STAT pathway is another important signaling pathway that was recently described.[94,95] Signal transducers and activators of transcription (STATs) are families of protein that have been found to phosphorylate by Jaks, kinase enzymes activated in response to growth factor interaction with its receptor. The two pathways, Ras and Jak-STAT, may intersect on the way to the nucleus to cause gene activation. It is believed that MAPK from the Ras pathway enhances STAT activity by causing additional phosphorylation.[96]

Direct cell-to-cell communication and the presence of gap junctions have been demonstrated in monolayers of endothelium[97] and in mixed cell population between endothelium and smooth muscle cells.[98] The significance of these direct links has not been defined, although a recent study has demonstrated that cultured pericytes or smooth muscle cells can inhibit endothelial growth when the cells are in contact with one another. *In vivo* capillary endothelial cells appear to grow when pericytes are absent and to stop growing when the pericytes reappear. Endothelial cells can also regulate the growth of one another. Plasma membrane preparations from confluent large vessel endothelium actively inhibit growing endothelial cells.[99] The intercellular links might help to regulate endothelial proliferation and endothelial-mediated vascular relaxation in collateral vessels by propagating signals from one cell to the next upstream from a large vessel occlusion. Direct cell—cell communication would also provide a mechanism for a local response in a vessel without the need for the release and wide dissemination of potent vasoactive or growth regulatory substances.

In summary, the size of a vessel wall is dependent on the mass of cells and matrix. Because smooth muscle cells and associated matrix proteins make up the bulk of the tissue, an understanding of the regulation of smooth muscle growth during development and in diseased states is extremely important. Smooth muscle number and distribution are affected by growth factors from the blood (particularly from platelets and leukocytes), growth factors and inhibitors from the vascular wall cells themselves, and neuroendocrine factors particularly from sympathetic innervation of the vessel wall. Smooth muscle quiescence in normal adult artery might be maintained by heparin-like inhibitors synthesized by vascular wall cells or the absence of growth factor. Growth initiation might be due to a shift in the balance of these negative and positive stimuli (see Fig. 88.5). For example, any condition causing injury of vascular wall cells or inducing the influx of macrophages would be expected to set up a favorable environment for smooth muscle growth. Hypercholesterolemia, a significant risk factor for atherosclerosis, is associated with macrophage migration and the accumulation of toxic oxidized LDL in susceptible large arteries. Release of endogenous FGF from dying foam cells as well as release of other growth factors (possibly PDGF) from stimulated endothelium, smooth muscle, and macrophages would increase the local concentration of growth promoting activity. Smooth muscle cells would be expected to respond by proliferating and migrating into the intima; if collections of these cells were already present in the intima as a consequence of fetal development, they might be even more responsive. These factors might also regulate the traffic of other leukocytes (macrophages, T cells) in and out of the wall, and these activated cells would in turn amplify or retard the initial smooth muscle response by the production of growth factors or inhibitors. The extent and complexity of these interactions between the cells of the wall and the blood have yet to be unraveled.

REGULATION OF THE ANTICOAGULATED STATE

Blood does not clot in normal arteries even when flow is stopped for prolonged periods. On the other hand, endothelial injury or loss provokes a dramatic thrombotic response. These observations define the importance of the endothelial layer in the maintenance of the anticoagulated state.[100,101] Studies performed primarily on cultured cells have demonstrated that endothelial cells possess an array of anticoagulant and antithrombotic functions, and it is certain that many of these are of importance *in vivo*. Endothelial cells also have several procoagulant functions, and the balance between procoagulant and anticoagulant functions is regulated by signals from the blood, as well as from neighboring cells.

On the anticoagulant side of the balance, the endothelium synthesizes a membrane-associated heparan sulfate that, like heparin, increases the affinity of antithrombin III for thrombin.[102] Because this interaction requires the binding of heparan sulfate to the antithrombin III, the complex must be active at the level of the endothelial surface. Heparan-antithrombin III then rapidly inactivates circulating thrombin and other activated serine proteases in the clotting cascade including VII, IX, and X. Thus, endothelial derived heparan sulfate can act to impede two aspects of the injury response: the activation of the clotting cascade and the stimulation of smooth muscle proliferation, which we referred to earlier. In addition, endothelial cells can inhibit clotting by means of the protein C pathway.[103] Endothelium synthesizes and secretes a protein called thrombomodulin, which in turn is bound to a surface receptor. The receptor-thrombomodulin complex binds thrombin and in so doing inactivates the proteolytic activity for fibrinogen. The thrombomodulin-thrombin complex activates protein C, and the activated protein C binds to protein S on the endothelial surface. The protein C-protein S complex then can inactivate factor Va, thereby inhibiting the clotting cascade. That this pathway is important is amply demonstrated in homozygous protein C deficient patients who develop spontaneous thrombosis. Finally, endothelial cells can inhibit platelet adhesion and aggregation through the synthesis of prostaglandin I_2 (PGI_2) and can degrade formed fibrin by activating plasminogen to plasmin.

On the procoagulant side, endothelial cells synthesize and secrete tissue factor, platelet activating factor, a plasminogen activator inhibitor, and von Willebrand factor, and they express a number of receptors for factors of the clotting cascade.[100] When the cells are exposed to a variety of inflammatory mediators derived from the blood or from resident macrophages (e.g., endotoxin, IL-1, TNF), endothelial cells respond by changing the balance of anticoagulant-procoagulant activities to favor coagulation. As well, the cells synthesize and express IL-1, which potentially could affect the underlying smooth muscle cells.[104] At present, these conclusions are largely based on *in vitro* experiments; although they have relevance mainly for the microvasculature, they also may prove to be important for large vessels in view of the recent evidence that not only macrophages but also different populations of lymphocytes are present in the atherosclerotic plaque. Furthermore, the ability of the vascular wall cells to maintain the anticoagulant state at the luminal surface must have a direct bearing on the thrombotic complications associated with end-stage atherosclerosis.

LESIONS OF ATHEROSCLEROSIS

Atherosclerosis is a disease of the intima characterized by the accumulation of smooth muscle cells and lipid.[104,105] The earliest lesion appears to be a local accumulation of lipid in the vessel wall located either in the extracellular matrix or inside "foam cells" (lipid-filled smooth muscle cells or macrophages). The relationship between the so-called fatty streak (Fig. 88.6) made up of foam cells and the pathologic process of atherosclerosis, the fibrous plaque and the complicated lesion, has been the subject of some debate.[106] Fatty streaks are found even in young children. Although atherosclerosis has a predilection for certain countries, the extent of fatty streaks of the aorta and coronary arteries in young people is about the same in countries that have low mortality rates from heart attack as in countries with high rates. The lipid streaks have been found to be just as common in females as in males, although atherosclerosis is more prevalent in males. Finally, even though the lipid streaks are distributed throughout the aorta, end-stage disease is mostly confined to the abdominal segment. Hence, if the fatty streak is the precursor of the more advanced lesion then there must either be a selection process or the whole concept must be wrong. The issue remains unresolved.

An alternative precursor for the atherosclerotic plaque is the intimal cell mass.[107,108] These focal accumulations of smooth muscle cells are frequently found in the vessels of children in locations that later develop fibrous plaques. In fat-fed swine, the intimal cell masses enlarge and become atherosclerotic.[109] Although the concept of the intimal cell masses as the initial lesion is attractive, there are several problems with it. First, this initial lesion is present in people throughout the world regardless of eventual risk for atherosclerosis. Second, as a general rule there is a gradual thickening of the intima throughout the arterial tree as part of the aging process; this has little to do with atherosclerosis. Finally, it has been difficult to find animal models of atherosclerotic change in intimal masses, whereas the formation of fibrofatty lesions from fatty streaks has been rather easily modeled by cholesterol feeding in a number of species. For these reasons, support for the intimal cell mass as the initial lesion has not achieved wide acceptance.

Whatever the initial lesion might be in atherosclerosis, it is widely agreed that the lesions characteristic of late atherosclerosis are the fibrous and the complicated plaques. The fibrous plaque is characterized by a thick fibrous luminal cap containing smooth muscle cells and leukocytes overlying a central core of necrotic debris and lipid (the "atheroma"). Animal studies have suggested that there might be either denudation or nondenuding injury of the endothelium at the surface.[58] The functional state of the endothelial and smooth muscle cells and leukocytes in these lesions is not known. Macrophages, by becoming foamy, clearly play a role in the metabolism of lipid, and activated macrophages also secrete a range of factors that modulate the metabolic and growth state of the vascular wall cells. Macrophages also proliferate locally in the lesions.[110,111] In addition, other leukocytes particularly T lymphocytes, are present; because some adjacent smooth muscle cells express the class II antigen HLA-DR, they must be exposed to gamma interferon presumably derived from the neighboring T cells.[112] In addition to inducing the expression of HLA-DR, gamma interferon inhibits smooth muscle proliferation. Hence, in the advanced atherosclerotic lesion these leukocytes might play a critical role in regulating smooth muscle proliferation and accumulation.[113,114]

The complicated lesion of atherosclerosis is a fibrous plaque with the additional features of ulceration, luminal thrombosis, calcification, and wall hemorrhage (see Fig. 88.6).

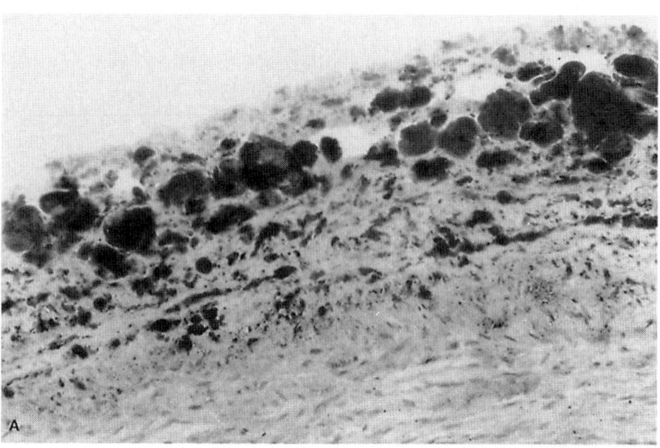

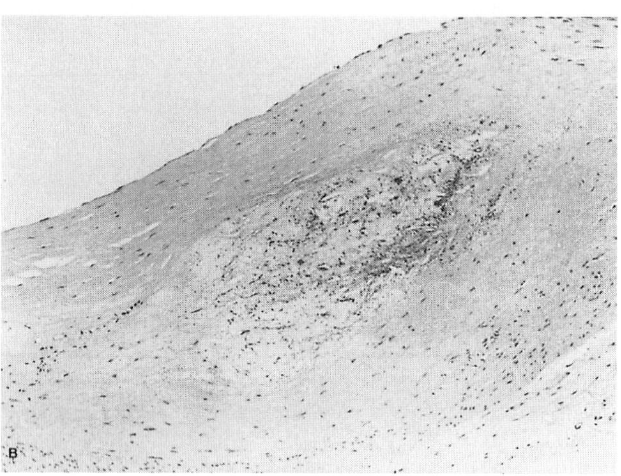

FIGURE 88.6 Histologic cross-sections of a fatty streak containing foam cells stained dark with oil Red O (*A*) and atherosclerotic plaque with fibrous cap (*B*). (Courtesy of David Gordon, M.D., Department of Pathology, University of Washington School of Medicine, Seattle, WA.)

It is the source of the thromboembolic activities associated with symptomatic disease. Why a fibrous lesion evolves into a complicated plaque is not understood. This process might be accelerated by such risk factors as hypertension, whereas atherogenesis might be affected more by hypercholesterolemia and cigarette smoking. More importantly, the advent of the inflammatory cells and the release of potent mediators of inflammation must play a role in the development of the complicated lesion. Earlier it was pointed out that growth factors for smooth muscle not only were liberated from platelets but were also synthesized and secreted by macrophages and the vascular wall cells themselves. In addition, potent cytokines, such as IL-1, TNF, and gamma interferon alter the growth state and metabolism of the vascular wall cells. In particular, the balance of anticoagulation-coagulation at the surface of the endothelium might be shifted away from anticoagulation and toward coagulation. In the plaque, large amounts of tissue factor and plasminogen activator-1 (PAI-1) are present.[115–117] These changes, in addition to frank endothelial desquamation in response to injurious agents, including oxidized LDL, homocystinemia, and tobacco products, could promote thrombosis in the vessel, an event that is decidedly unusual. Small accretions of thrombus with subsequent fibrotic remodeling together with hemorrhage from new blood vessels in the ischemic central region of the plaque could account for the relatively rapid increase in plaque size and luminal narrowing that has been observed in some arterial beds.

THEORIES OF ATHEROSCLEROSIS

Some of the information on vascular wall structure and function might be relevant to general theories of atherosclerosis. From the foregoing, it should be evident that an artery is not just an inert nonthrombogenic conduit for blood; rather, it is an organ whose structure and function are very carefully modulated by interactions between vascular wall cells themselves and between vascular wall cells and the blood. Bearing this in mind, we can reexamine the prevailing theories of atherosclerosis.

Over the last century, a number of theories have been advanced to explain how atherosclerosis evolves. In reality, these theories attempt to account for one or more aspects of the disease and are therefore not mutually exclusive. Much of the controversy over these theories has to do with individual opinion concerning which of the aspects of atherosclerosis is most important.

Lipid Insudation Hypothesis

Perhaps the oldest hypothesis termed the "lipid insudation" hypothesis states that the lipid in the atherosclerotic lesion is derived from lipoproteins in the blood;[45,118] it thereby links the risk factor hypercholesterolemia directly to the development of the plaque foam cell, the atheroma, and eventually the complicated lesion. There is good evidence now that the lipid in the plaque comes from the blood; there is also substantial evidence correlating the severity of hypercholesterolemia (particularly elevated LDL cholesterol) with the severity of atherosclerosis both in human and in animal models. When animals are made hyperlipidemic, the initial change is a migration of macrophages through the endothelium into the subintima and media. These cells then engorge the lipids carried into the wall by lipoproteins to form foam cells. These foam cells presumably secrete chemoattractants, growth factors, and cytokines, which trigger off complex events that lead to the formation of an atherosclerotic plaque.[119] The most important study to demonstrate that blood cholesterol level is a risk factor for coronary artery disease and hence atherosclerosis is the

Framingham study. A large group of healthy men and women were studied and it was found that the risk for developing clinically evident coronary artery disease was related to cholesterol levels.[120] Although a high level of LDL cholesterol is an important risk factor for atherosclerosis, epidemiologic studies have shown that levels of apolipoprotein B, the primary protein constituent of LDL, very low density lipoprotein (VLDL), and chylomicrons, correlate more accurately with the risk of atherosclerosis. Particles resembling VLDL and intermediate LDL have been identified within the atherosclerotic plaque.[121] High-density lipoproteins (HDLs) oppose the deposition of cholesterol by transporting cholesterol to the liver. Thus, low levels of HDL correlate with an increased risk of atherosclerosis and high levels of HDL are protective. The lipid insudation theory states that the lipid in the atherosclerotic lesion is derived from the lipoproteins in the blood.[45,122] The earliest lesions induced by elevated plasma cholesterol levels are the fatty streaks, which have an impressive accumulation of lipids in them. For a considerable period of time it was thought that the lipid containing foam cells were derived from smooth muscle cells, but there is considerable evidence now that most of these cells originate from circulating monocytes/macrophages and only a fraction represent cholesterol laden smooth muscle cells. Although not all fatty streaks become fibrous plaques, results from the Pathological Determinants of Atherosclerosis in Youth program have shown that atherosclerosis commences as a fatty streak, which progresses to the complicated lesion, namely the fibrous plaque.[123]

It is still unclear as to how the monocytes penetrate the endothelium to reach the subendothelial space. The endothelial injury hypothesis postulates that there is endothelial denudation that allows this penetration, but a number of experimental studies have failed to show any damage to the endothelium over the fatty streaks. Once in the subendothelial space of the intima, the monocytes take up lipoprotein cholesterol to become foam cells. Denudation of endothelial cells probably occurs later in the development of the lesion, exposing the underlying foam cells. Brown et al.,[124] however, showed that even the highest concentration of LDL could not induce the accumulation of cholesterol in monocytes/ macrophages or in smooth muscle cells, the precursors of arterial foam cells. Thus, it is not the circulating LDL that causes lipid accumulation in the monocytes/macrophages, but it is oxidized LDL that is taken up avidly by the macrophages. Oxidized LDL is more atherogenic than native LDL and in animal models antioxidant compounds can slow the rate of atherosclerotic lesion progression by 50% or more.[125] In addition, two antioxidant enzymes are associated with HDL, paraoxonase and platelet activating factor acetylhydrolase. These factors are believed to degrade deleterious oxidized phospholipids associated with LDL.[126] There is a good deal of epidemiologic evidence correlating high intake of antioxidant vitamins with decreased risk of coronary artery disease in humans.[127] However, the results of randomized clinical trials have not demonstrated a decrease in progression of atherosclerosis. These trials have failed to demonstrate a consistent significant effect of single or multivitamin regimens on the incidence of death from coronary vascular disease.[128,129]

Regarding the role of genetic background in the development and progression of atherosclerosis, Dansky et al.[130] have demonstrated that expression of the human apo A-I transgene on the apo E-deficient background increases HDL cholesterol and greatly diminishes fatty streak lesion formation. They also demonstrated that increases in apo A-I and HDL cholesterol inhibit foam cell formation in apo E-deficient/human apo A-I transgenic mice at a stage following lipid deposition, endothelial activation, and monocyte adherence, without increases in HDL-associated paraoxonase.

The role of "statins" in delaying the progression of the atherosclerotic lesion has been investigated. Several studies, such as the Coronary Primary Prevention trial and the Helsinki Heart Study have shown a relation between reduction in the lipoprotein profile and a reduction in the cardiac events. In the first study, a 20% reduction in LDL cholesterol yielded a more than 30% reduction in coronary events, and in the second study, gemfibrozil reduced LDL cholesterol by 8% and triglycerides by more than 35%, while causing a 15% increase in HDL and reduced coronary events by 34%.[131,132]

The discovery of the statin (e.g., Simvastatin, Lovastatin) group of drugs was a major advance in the pharmacologic management of hypercholesterolemia. The statins are analogues of HMG CoA reductase; therefore they block its action and inhibit the synthesis of cholesterol. Statins are highly effective agents for the primary and secondary prevention of coronary artery disease. Although lowering of cholesterol, especially LDL cholesterol, appears to be the most important mechanism for the beneficial effects of statins, other effects including improvement in endothelial function may also play an important role. The inhibition of cholesterol synthesis increases hepatic expression of the LDL receptor, leading to increased clearance of circulating LDL. Several studies have shown that lipid lowering statin therapy leads to a reduction in cardiovascular events and mortality from cardiac events.[133] These studies also showed a reduction in the incidence of stroke, which has a relatively weak association with cholesterol levels. In the preliminary results of the Heart Protection Study there is evidence that long-term statin use reduces the incidence in cardiovascular events in patients with coronary artery disease, carotid artery disease, peripheral vascular disease, or diabetes regardless of baseline LDL cholesterol level. [134,135] Simvastatin and lovastatin have been shown to reduce vascular injury from experimental stroke in a rodent model, independent of lipid changes.[136] Decreasing inflammation by lowering LDL cholesterol, and thus oxidized LDL cholesterol, is one theory on the mechanism of action of statins. Studies using C-reactive protein (CRP) as a marker of inflammation have shown a decrease in CRP along with a decrease in LDL in patients on statin therapy. However, other studies have not shown the same correlation and this has fostered a lipid independent theory. Further studies are being conducted to elucidate the mechanism of the statins effect.[137]

The Encrustation Hypothesis

Like the lipid insudation hypothesis, the encrustation hypothesis focuses on one aspect of the disease.[138] This hypothesis proposes that plaque initiation and progression is the consequence of repeated cycles of thrombosis and remodeling. However, autopsy studies of vessels of children and experiments with cholesterol-fed animals have shown that thrombosis is not the initial event in atherogenesis; in fact, thrombosis appears to be a feature of advanced disease. Hence, this hypothesis is applicable only to the problem of plaque progression. Furthermore, it does not explain how lipid and smooth muscle cells accumulate in the lesion.

The Reaction to Injury Hypothesis

This hypothesis attempts to explain how smooth muscle growth is regulated in atherogenesis.[44] As originally proposed, it stated that the initial event is some form of injury to the endothelium. In regions denuded of endothelium platelets adhere and release growth factors; these growth factors accumulate in the wall and stimulate medial smooth muscle proliferation and migration into the intima. As discussed previously, this theory is based on the observation that platelets carry potent smooth muscle mitogens in their granules and that the injury-induced arterial lesion closely resembles the fibrous cap found in the atherosclerotic plaque. A modified version of this theory suggests that injuries to the endothelium, which do not produce denudation, might also cause smooth muscle growth by stimulating damaged endothelium to synthesize and release growth factors. Alternatively, monocytes might be attracted to the zone of injury; the monocyte/macrophage might then be activated and start to elaborate growth promoting activity. The reaction to injury hypothesis suggests a possible mechanism for the accumulation of connective tissue cells and matrix; it fails to provide an explanation for the lipid accumulation or the monoclonal nature of the advanced atherosclerotic plaque.

The Monoclonal Hypothesis

This hypothesis focuses attention on smooth muscle accumulation in the lesion.[139] It states that the cells of any particular plaque are likely to arise as a clone from a single progenitor smooth muscle cell. This hypothesis is based on the observation that individual plaques of human females heterozygote for the X-linked marker glucose-6-phosphate dehydrogenase (G-6-PD) frequently exhibit one, but not both, of the G-6-PD isotypes. At a certain moment in time, single cells might be stimulated to enter the growth cycle and undergo several rounds of division leading to the formation of a monoclonal lesion. The mechanism of cell activation leading to such lesions is not evident as yet; the only other known monoclonal cell masses in humans are neoplasias (e.g., leiomyomas). This would tend to suggest carcinogens or possibly viruses as possible etiologic agents and thereby might explain the link between cigarette smoking and atherosclerosis. An alternative to carcinogenesis as an explanation for monoclonality is the possibility of activation of a susceptible population of stem cells.[140,141] Smooth muscle cells might have limited replicative capacity, and there might be only a small population of stem cells in the wall capable of responding to growth factors. Whatever the mechanism of activation might be, any theory attempting to provide a mechanism for the accumulation of smooth muscle cells in atherosclerotic plaques must take into account this observation of monoclonality.

The Intimal Cell Mass Hypothesis

This hypothesis was mentioned earlier and states that the accumulations of intimal smooth muscle cells are one of the two possible initial lesions in atherosclerosis.[107,108] These small accumulations of smooth muscle cells are found in children at sites where atherosclerosis later develops. How they happen to get there is unclear, nor is it evident what makes them susceptible to atherogenic stimuli. It could be that these cells are primordial rests and really are a form of stem cell capable of responding to external mitogenic stimuli. Because the intimal cell masses are found in the vessels of children throughout the world regardless of the prevalence of atherosclerosis, it is likely that the atherosclerotic change is largely determined by extrinsic risk factors such as hypercholesterolemia.

The Infection Hypothesis

Although the role of infection in the development of atherosclerosis has been debated for many years, only recently this role has been emphasized due to a panel convened by the National Heart, Lung, and Blood Institute (NHLBI).[142] The expert panel examined the evidence linking infections to the development of the atherosclerotic process, in particular the role of cytomegalovirus (CMV) and *Chlamydia pneumoniae*. The panel reported on the seroepidemiologic evidence and the reports localizing those infectious agents to the human plaque. In addition, they examined animal studies aiming to show cause and effect among CMV, *C. pneumoniae*, and the development of atherosclerotic lesions in animal models.

CMV belongs to the herpesvirus family, which also includes the Epstein-Barr virus. Approximately 15% of adolescents, 50% of adults by age 35, and 70% of patients older than 75 years have evidence of past infection with this virus.[143] Melnick et al.[144] found significantly higher titers of CMV antibodies in patients undergoing coronary artery bypass surgery (70%) compared to matched controls (43%). Cardiac transplant recipients with CMV exposure, as evidenced by increased serum CMV IgG antibodies, are more likely to develop post-transplantation atherosclerosis than patients without exposure to CMV.[145] CMV infection has been associated with restenosis following coronary angioplasty.[146] In addition, CMV has also been implicated in the development of carotid atherosclerosis. CMV antigens have been isolated from carotid plaque, and increased levels of CMV antibody titers are associated with carotid intimal-medial thickening.[147] Although it has been difficult to culture viral particles from atherosclerotic lesions, this by itself does not constitute a strong evidence against the role of CMV infection in atherosclerosis because it is possible that the virus trigger the infection without persisting in the tissue.[143,144,148] Because of the ubiquitous nature of CMV, it is difficult to ascertain whether it is a pathogen in atherosclerosis.[149]

Three species of *Chlamydia, Chlamydia trachomatis, Chlamydia psittaci,* and *C. pneumoniae,* which are gram-negative bacteria, are known to cause human disease. *C. pneumoniae* cause upper respiratory infections and 10% of all cases of pneumonia. The prevalence of antibodies to *C. pneumoniae* is around 50% in adults.[149] *C. pneumoniae* organisms have been isolated from atherosclerotic plaque from both carotid and coronary arteries.[150,151] In a rabbit model, infection with *C. pneumoniae* has been shown to accelerate the formation of the atherosclerotic lesion. In addition, treatment with azithromycin prevented the formation of the lesion.[152] To gain insight into the mechanism by which *C. pneumoniae* infection affect the process of atherogenesis, Libby's group studied atherosclerotic plaques for the presence of chlamydial heat shock protein 60 (HSP60).[153,154] Studying plaques from human carotid atherosclerotic arteries, these investigators found that chlamydial and human HSP60 colocalize within macrophages located in the atherosclerotic lesions. They have also shown that both chlamydial and human HSP60 induced the production of TNF-α and matrix metalloproteinase (MMP) by macrophages. They concluded that, by inducing the production of such factors by macrophages, chlamydial HSP 60 may represent the mechanism by which infection with *C. pneumoniae* promotes atherosclerosis.[153] In addition, the same investigators have shown that chlamydial and human HSP60 activate human endothelial cells, smooth muscle cells, and macrophages to secrete factors [e.g., E-selectin, intercellular adhesion molecule-1 (ICAM-1), and vascular cell adhesion molecule-1 (VCAM-1)] important to the pathophysiology of atherosclerosis.[154]

In addition to CMV and *Chlamydia, Helicobacter pylori* and herpes simplex virus are also being investigated as possible agents in atherosclerosis.[155] More work needs to be done to definitively establish the relationship between these and other agents and atherosclerosis. Establishing the role of infectious agents in the development of atherosclerosis is very important because it suggests that antiinfectious agents, such as known antibiotics, may play a role in preventing or slowing the atherosclerotic process.

Inflammatory and Immune Hypothesis

Mediators of inflammation, such as cytokines and growth factors, have been found in the atherosclerotic plaques. These mediators are involved in the synthesis and degradation of collagen by vascular smooth muscle cells. Such mediators include TGF-α and gamma interferon.[156] IL-2 receptors are markers suggesting the activation of T lymphocytes, and gamma interferon is produced and secreted by activated T lymphocytes.[157]

The involvement of macrophages and T lymphocytes in atherogenesis also suggests both an immune as well as an inflammatory response. The lymphocytes found in atherosclerotic lesions are polyclonal, indicating that these cells do not develop in response to a single antigen. Several different subclasses of T lymphocytes have been identified in atherosclerotic plaque, including both CD4 (helper-inducer cells) and CD8 (cytotoxic T cells).[158] In addition, accelerated coronary artery atherosclerosis is a unique variant of atherosclerosis that develops and progresses rapidly in transplanted hearts, suggesting an immunologic etiology. The lesions seen in transplanted hearts involve the entire coronary tree, and these lesions contain all the cellular elements characteristic of atherosclerosis; in addition, they have increased numbers of T lymphocytes and macrophages compared to the typical atherosclerotic lesion.[159] Mouse transplant models, using heterotopic heart transplants and arterial interposition grafts, produced arterial lesions that resembled transplant arteriosclerosis.[160,161]

Activation of the complement system is an important step in the immune process causing immune complexes to deposit in the arterial wall or precipitating the binding of specific antibodies to antigens found in vascular tissues. Cholesterol particles are potent activators of the complement system.[162] This activation of the complement system results in the production of proinflammatory molecules and the terminal membrane attack complex (MAC), which has been known to stimulate the production of cytokines, such as TNFβ and IL-8, and growth factors, such as basic FGF and PDGF by vascular smooth muscle (VSMC) and endothelial cells.[162] MAC has been identified in atherosclerotic lesions, particularly fibrous plaque.[163]

Most complications related to atherosclerotic lesions may be due to plaque disruption or rupture. Plaque disruption exposes the circulating blood to its lipid core with subsequent formation of thrombus (Fig. 88.7), leading to acute arterial occlusion.[164,165] Plaque stability is very important in preventing plaque rupture. This stability is provided by the integrity of the extracellular matrix within the plaque. Plaque instability is related to the degree of inflammation because inflammatory cells produce cytokines that decrease the production of collagen or increase its degradation.[166] Therefore, the balance between the production of MMPs, which degrade collagen, and that of tissue inhibitors of metalloproteinases (TIMPs) regulates plaque stability.[167] The expression of both MMPs and TIMPs can be demonstrated in atheromas. TIMPs have been found in macrophages present within plaques.[167] Inflammatory cytokines such as IL-1 and TNF can induce the expression of MMPs by macrophages.[168] In addition, gamma interferon produced by T lymphocytes decreases collagen production again leading to weakening of plaque extracellular matrix and rupture.[169] The foam cells express tissue factor on their surface and activate factor VII, which leads to thrombin formation and platelet aggregation with subsequent conversion of fibrinogen to fibrin leading to thrombosis.[170] Interestingly, lipid lowering strategies led to a decrease in plaque content of macrophages and a decrease in expression of MMP-1 increasing collagen production and retention, which improve plaque stability.[168,171]

Inflammation appears to be a common factor in all theories of atherosclerosis and more research is being performed in this area and isolating inflammatory mediators that may be involved.[172] Each of these hypothesis attempts to explain one or more aspects of atherogenesis. It is reasonable to conclude that each might be applicable at a different time during the development of the lesion (Fig. 88.8).

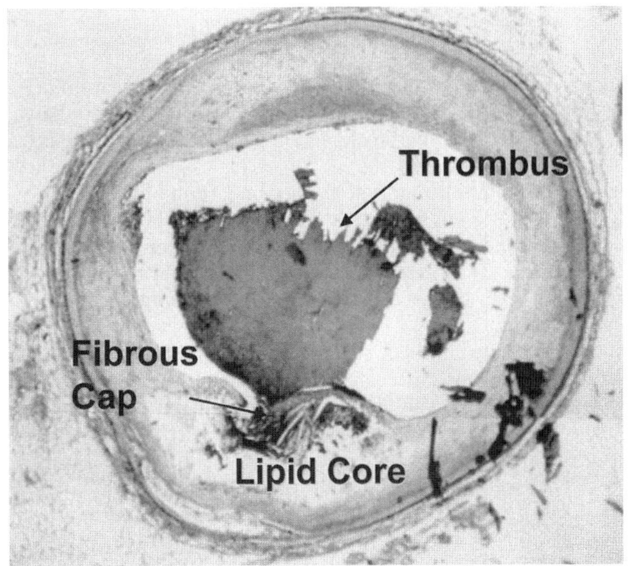

FIGURE 88.7 Plaque cap rupture exposing the lipid core of the atheroma and leading to thrombus formation. (Courtesy of Dr. Maria de Lourdes Higuchi, Department of Pathology, University of São Paulo, Brazil.)

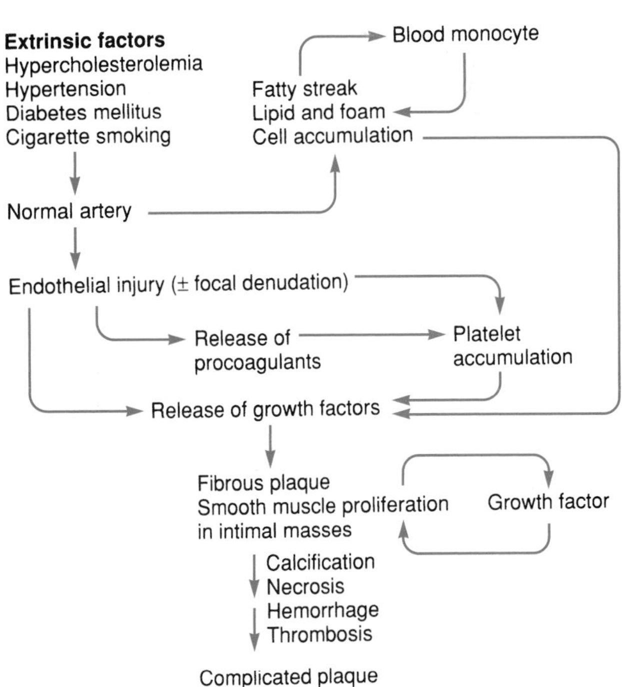

FIGURE 88.8 Atherogenesis and progression of atherosclerosis is probably the consequence of multiple factors acting on the arterial wall. (After Clowes AW. Theories of atherosclerosis. In: White RA, ed. *Atherosclerosis and arteriosclerosis: human pathology and experimental animal methods and models.* Boca Raton, FL: CRC Press; 1989, p. 3, with permission.)

KEY POINTS

- Susceptibility to atherosclerosis might be determined by both intrinsic (numbers of intimal masses) and extrinsic factors (hypercholesterolemia, hypertension, diabetes, cigarette smoking).
- The initial event might be the accumulation of lipid by insudation in regions of increased susceptibility. This would lead to the production of macrophage chemotactic factors and the influx of monocytes from the blood that together with the smooth muscle cells would sequester lipid and become foam cells.
- LDL oxidized in the wall as well as other extrinsic injurious agents could produce some degree of endothelial injury and perhaps later even limited denudation. Growth factors might then be released from the endothelium, activated macrophages and other leukocytes, and the smooth muscle cells as well as from adherent platelets
- Growth factors could them stimulate proliferation and migration of susceptible smooth muscle cells to form isolated smooth muscle clones and fibrous lesions.
- Further production of matrix by the smooth muscle would permit continued accumulation of lipid.
- Like a growing tumor, these lesions would enlarge, develop ischemic cores, and thereby induce an angiogenic response.
- The thickened plaque with its necrotic lipid core (the atheroma) might not withstand the rigors of continued arterial pulsation and might develop hemorrhage within the lesion on account of the shearing forces on the new capillaries.
- Breakdown of the surface and a change in the coagulation function of the endothelium would render the plaque more thrombogenic. Such changes would lead to the terminal thrombotic event, the hallmark of all ischemic complications in atherosclerotic patients.

References

1. Wolinsky H, Glagov S. Nature of species differences in the medial distribution of aortic vasa vasorum in mammals. *Circ Res.* 1967;20:409.
2. Heistad DD, Armstrong ML. Blood flow through vasa vasorum of coronary arteries in atherosclerotic monkeys. *Arteriosclerosis* 1986;6:326.
3. Barger AC, Beeuwkes R III, Lainey LL, et al. Hypothesis: vasa vasorum and neovascularization of human coronary arteries. *N Engl J Med.* 1984;310:175.
4. Coffin JD, Poole TJ. Embryonic vascular development: Immunohistochemical identification of the origin and subsequent morphogenesis of the major vessel primordia in quail embryos. *Development* 1988;102:735.
5. Pardanaud L, Altmann C, Kitos P, et al. Vasculogenesis in the early quail blastodisc as studied with a monoclonal antibody recognizing endothelial cells. *Development* 1987;100:339.
6. Le Douarin NM. Cell migrations in embryos. *Cell* 1984;38:353.
7. Wolinsky H, Glagov S. A lamellar unit of aortic medial structure and function in mammals. *Circ Res.* 1967;20:99.
8. Wolinsky H, Glagov S. Structural basis for the static mechanical properties of the aortic media. *Circ Res.* 1964;14:400.
9. Dilley RJ, Schwartz SM. Vascular remodeling in the growth hormone transgenic mouse. *Circ Res.* 1989;65:1233.
10. Zarins CK, Zatina MA, Giddens DP, et al. Shear stress regulation of artery lumen diameter in experimental atherogenesis. *J Vasc Surg.* 1987;5:413.
11. **Glagov S, Weisenberg E, Zarins CK, et al. Compensatory enlargement of human atherosclerotic coronary arteries. *N Engl J Med.* 1987;316:1371.**
12. Frangos JA, Eskin SG, McIntire LV, Ives CL. Flow effect on prostacyclin production by cultured human endothelial cells. *Science* 1985;227:1477.
13. **Gibbons GH, Dzau VJ. The emerging concept of vascular remodeling. *N Engl J Med.* 1994;330:1431.**
14. Davies PF, Tripathi SC. Mechanical stress mechanisms and the cell. An endothelial paradigm. *Circ Res.* 1993;72:239.
15. Resnick N, Collins T, Atkinson W, et al. Platelet-derived growth factor B chain promoter contains a cis-acting fluid shear-stress-responsive element. *Proc Natl Acad Sci U S A.* 1993;90:4591.
16. **Vanhoutte PM. The endothelium: modulator of vascular smooth-muscle tone. *N Engl J Med.* 1988;319:512.**
17. Furchgott RF. Role of endothelium in responses of vascular smooth muscle. *Circ Res.* 1983;53:557.
18. Ignarro LJ, Buga GM, Wood KS, et al. Endothelium-derived relaxing factor produced and released from artery and vein is nitric oxide. *Proc Natl Acad Sci U S A.* 1987;84:9265.
19. **Palmer RMJ, Ferrige AG, Moncada S. Nitric oxide release accounts for the biological activity of endothelium-derived relaxing factor. *Nature* 1987;327:524.**
20. Ignarro LJ. Biological actions and properties of endothelium-derived nitric oxide formed and released from artery and vein. *Circ Res.* 1989;65:1.
21. Langille BL, O'Donnell F. Reductions in arterial diameter produced by chronic decreases in blood flow are endothelium-dependent. *Science* 1986;231:405.
22. Kohler TR, Jawien A. Flow affects development of intimal hyperplasia after arterial injury in rats. *Arterioscler Thromb.* 1992;12:963.
23. Kohler TR, Kirkman TR, Kraiss LW, et al. Increased blood flow inhibits neointimal hyperplasia in endothelialized vascular grafts. *Circ Res.* 1991;69:1557.
24. Geary RL, Kohler TR, Vergel S, et al. Time course of flow-induced smooth muscle cell proliferation and intimal thickening in endothelialized baboon vascular grafts. *Circ Res.* 1994;74:14–23.
25. Shultz PJ, Knauss TC, Mené P, et al. Mitogenic signals for thrombin in mesangial cells: Regulation of phospholipase C and PDGF genes. *Am J Physiol.* 1989;257:F366.
26. Bobik A, Grooms A, Millar JA, et al. Growth factor activity of endothelin on vascular smooth muscle. *Am J Physiol Cell Physiol.* 1990;258:C408.
27. Libby P, Warner SJC, Friedman GB. Interleukin 1: a mitogen for human vascular smooth muscle cells that induces the release of growth-inhibitory prostanoids. *J Clin Invest.* 1988;81:487.
28. Nakaki T, Nakayama M, Yamamoto S, Kato R. Endothelin-mediated stimulation of DNA synthesis in vascular smooth muscle cells. *Biochem Biophys Res Commun.* 1989;158:880.
29. Garg UC, Hassid A. Nitric oxide-generating vasodilators and 8-bromo-cyclic guanosine monophosphate inhibit mitogenesis and proliferation of cultured rat vascular smooth muscle cells. *J Clin Invest.* 1989;83:1774.
30. Freiman PC, Mitchell GG, Heistad DD, et al. Atherosclerosis impairs endothelium-dependent vascular relaxation to acetylcholine and thrombin in primates. *Circ Res.* 1986;58:783.
31. Malek AM, Alper SL, Izumo S. Hemodynamic shear stress and its role in atherosclerosis. *JAMA* 1999;282:2035.
32. Malek AM, Izumo S, Alper SL. Modulation by pathophysiological stimuli of the shear stress-induced up-regulation of endothelial nitric oxide synthase expression in endothelial cells. *Neurosurgery* 1999;45:334.
33. Stary HC, Chandler AB, Dinsmore RE, et al. A definition of advanced types of atherosclerotic lesions and a histological classification of atherosclerosis—a report from the Committee on Vascular Lesions of the Council on Arteriosclerosis, American Heart Association. *Circulation* 1995;92:1355.
34. Celermajer DS, Sorensen KE, Gooch VM, et al. Non-invasive detection of endothelial dysfunction in children and adults at risk of atherosclerosis. *Lancet* 1992;340:1111.
35. Zeiher AM, Fisslthaler B, Schray-Utz B, et al. Nitric oxide modulates the expression of monocyte chemoattractant protein 1 in cultured human endothelial cells. *Circ Res.* 1995;76:980.
36. Griendling KK, Fitgerald, GA. Oxidative stress and cardiovascular injury. Part I: Basic mechanism and in vivo monitoring of ROS. *Circulation* 2003;108:1912.
37. Milstien S, Katusic Z. Oxidation of tetrahydrobiopterin by peroxynitrite: Implication for vascular endothelial function. *Biochem Biophys Res Commun.* 1999;263:681.
38. Griendling KK, Alexander RW. Oxidative stress and cardiovascular disease [editorial; comment]. *Circulation* 1997;96:3264.
39. Vane JR, Anggard EE, Botting RM. Regulatory functions of the vascular endothelium. *N Engl J Med.* 1990;323:27.
40. Knowles JW, Reddick RL, Jennette JC, et al. Enhanced atherosclerosis and kidney dysfunction in eNOS (-/-)ApoE (-/-) mice are ameliorated by enalapril treatment. *J Clin Invest.* 2000;105:451.
41. Weiss D, Sorescu D, Taylor WR. Angiotensin II and Atherosclerosis. *Am J Cardiol.* 2001;72:453–461.
42. Mancini GB, Henry GC, Macaya C, et al. Angiotensin-converting enzyme inhibition with quinapril improves endothelial vasomotor dysfunction in patients with coronary artery disease. The TREND (Trial on Reversing ENdothelial Dysfunction) Study [see comments] [published erratum appears in *Circulation* 1996;94:1490]. *Circulation* 1996;94:258.
43. Wolinsky H. Long-term effects of hypertension on the rat aortic wall and their relation to concurrent aging changes: morphological and chemical studies. *Circ Res.* 1972;30:301.
44. **Ross R. Pathogenesis of atherosclerosis—an update. *N Engl J Med.* 1986;314:488.**
45. Steinberg D, Parthasarathy S, Carew TE, et al. Modifications of low-density lipoprotein that increase its atherogenicity. *N Engl J Med.* 1989;320:915.
46. Schwartz SM, Campbell GR, Campbell JH. Replication of smooth muscle cells in vascular disease. *Circ Res.* 1986;58:427.
47. **Clowes AW, Reidy MA, Clowes MM. Kinetics of cellular proliferation after arterial injury. I. Smooth muscle growth in the absence of endothelium. *Lab Invest.* 1983;49:327.**

48. Owens GK. Control of hypertrophic versus hyperplastic growth of vascular smooth muscle cells. *Am J Physiol.* 1989;257:H1755.
49. Zwolak RM, Adams MC, Clowes AW. Kinetics of vein graft hyperplasia: association with tangential stress. *J Vasc Surg.* 1987;5:126.
50. Leung DY, Glagov S, Mathews MB. Cyclic stretching stimulates synthesis of matrix components by arterial smooth muscle cells in vitro. *Science* 1976;191:475.
51. Baumgartner HR, Studer A. Consequences of vessel catheterization in normal and hypercholesterolemic rabbits. *Pathol Microbiol.* 1966;29:393.
52. Kumagai H, Suzuki H, Matsukawa S, et al. Captopril therapy following percutaneous transluminal angioplasty for bilateral renal artery stenosis. *Arch Intern Med.* 1989;149:1973.
53. Bowen-Pope DF, Ross R, Seifert RA. Locally acting growth factors for vascular smooth muscle cells: endogenous synthesis and release from platelets. *Circulation* 1985;72:735.
54. Friedman RJ, Stemerman MB, Wenz B, et al. The effect of thrombocytopenia on experimental atherosclerotic lesion formation in rabbits. Smooth muscle cell proliferation and re-endothelialization. *J Clin Invest.* 1977;60:1191.
55. Fingerle J, Johnson R, Clowes AW, et al. Role of platelets in smooth muscle cell proliferation and migration after vascular injury in rat carotid artery. *Proc Natl Acad Sci U S A.* 1989;86:8412.
56. Groves HM, Kinlough-Rathbone RL, Richardson M, et al. Thrombin generation and fibrin formation following injury to rabbit neointima. Studies of vessel wall reactivity and platelet survival. *Lab Invest.* 1982;46:605.
57. Hatton MWC, Moar SL, Richardson M. Deendothelialization in vivo initiates a thrombogenic reaction at the rabbit aorta surface. Correlation of uptake of fibrinogen and antithrombin III with thrombin generation by the exposed subendothelium. *Am J Pathol.* 1989;135:499.
58. Faggiotto A, Ross R. Studies of hypercholesterolemia in the nonhuman primate. II. Fatty streak conversion to fibrous plaque. *Arteriosclerosis* 1984;4:341.
59. Faggiotto A, Ross R, Harker L. Studies of hypercholesterolemia in nonhuman primate. I. Changes that lead to fatty streak formation. *Arteriosclerosis* 1984;4:323.
60. Reidy MA. A reassessment of endothelial injury and arterial lesion formation. *Lab Invest.* 1985;53:513.
61. Clowes AW, Clowes MM. Regulation of smooth muscle proliferation by heparin in vitro and in vivo. *Int Angiol.* 1987;6:45.
62. Clowes AW, Clowes MM, Fingerle J, Reidy MA. Regulation of smooth muscle cell growth in injured artery. *J Cardiovasc Pharmacol.* 1989; 14[Suppl 6]:S12.
63. Gajdusek CM, Schwartz SM. Comparison of intracellular and extracellular mitogen activity. *J Cell Physiol.* 1984;121:316.
64. Gajdusek CM, Carbon S. Injury-induced release of basic fibroblast growth factor from bovine aortic endothelium. *J Cell Physiol.* 1989;139:570.
65. Burgess WH, Maciag T. The heparin binding (fibroblast) growth factor family of proteins. *Annu Rev Biochem.* 1989;58:575.
66. Gospodarowicz D, Neufeld G, Schwiegerer L. Fibroblast growth factor: structural and biological properties. *J Cell Physiol.* 1987;[suppl 5]:15.
67. Vlodavsky I, Folkman J, Sullivan R, et al. Endothelial cell-derived basic fibroblast growth factor: synthesis and deposition into subendothelial extracellular matrix. *Proc Natl Acad Sci U S A.* 1987;84:2292.
68. Lindner V, Lappi DA, Baird A, et al. Role of basic fibroblast growth factor in vascular lesion formation. *Circ Res.* 1991;68:106–113.
69. Lindner V, Reidy MA. Proliferation of smooth muscle cells after vascular injury is inhibited by an antibody against basic fibroblast growth factor. *Proc Natl Acad Sci U S A.* 1991;88:3739.
70. Raines EW, Bowen-Pope DF, Ross R. Platelet-derived growth factor. In: Sporn MB, Roberts AB, eds. *Handbook of experimental pharmacology: peptide growth factors and their receptors.* Heidelberg, Germany: Springer-Verlag; 1989, p. xx.
71. Sprugel KH, McPherson JM, Clowes AW, et al. Effects of growth factors in vivo. I. Cell ingrowth into porous subcutaneous chambers. *Am J Pathol.* 1987;129:601–613.
72. Doolittle RF, Hunkapillar MW, Hood LE, et al. Simian sarcoma virus oncogene, v-sis, is derived form the gene (or genes) encoding a platelet-derived growth factor. *Science* 1983;221:275.
73. Waterfield MD, Scrace GT, Whittle N, et al. Platelet-derived growth factor is structurally related to the putative transforming protein p28-sis of simian sarcoma virus. *Nature* 1983;304:35.
74. Ferns GAA, Raines EW, Sprugel KH, et al. Inhibition of neointimal smooth muscle accumulation after angioplasty by an antibody to PDGF. *Science* 1991;253:1129.
75. Jawien A, Bowen-Pope DF, Lindner V, et al. Platelet-derived growth factor promotes smooth muscle migration and intimal thickening in a rat model of balloon angioplasty. *J Clin Invest.* 1992;89:507.
76. Bornfeldt KE, Raines EW, Graves LM, et al. Platelet-derived growth factor. Distinct signal transduction pathways associated with migration versus proliferation. *Ann N Y Acad Sci.* 1995;766:416.
77. Blaes N, Boissel JP. Growth-stimulating effect of catecholamines on rat aortic smooth muscle cells in culture. *J Cell Physiol.* 1983;116:167.
78. Dalsgaard CJ, Hultgardh-Nilsson A, Haegerstrand A, et al. Neuropeptides as growth factors. Possible roles in human disease. *Regul Pept.* 1989;25:1.
79. Bevan RD. Trophic effects of peripheral adrenergic nerves on vascular structure. *Hypertension* 1984;6:III-19.
80. Bevan RD, Tsuru H. Functional and structural changes in the rabbit ear artery after sympathetic denervation. *Circ Res.* 1981;49:478.
81. Powell JS, Clozel JP, Muller RKM, et al. Inhibitors of angiotensin-converting enzyme prevent myointimal proliferation after vascular injury. *Science* 1989;245:186.
82. Jackson CL, Bush RC, Bowyer DE. Inhibitory effect of calcium antagonists on balloon catheter-induced arterial smooth muscle cell proliferation and lesion size. *Atherosclerosis* 1988;69:115.
83. Clowes AW, Reidy MA. Mechanisms of graft failure. The role of cellular proliferation. *Ann N Y Acad Sci.* 1987;516:673.
84. Fritze LMS, Reilly CF, Rosenberg RD. An antiproliferative heparan sulfate species produced by postconfluent smooth muscle cells. *J Cell Biol.* 1985;100:1041.
85. Castellot JJ Jr, Addonizio ML, Rosenberg R, et al. Cultured endothelial cells produce a heparin-like inhibitor of smooth muscle cell growth. *J Cell Biol.* 1981;90:372.
86. Antonelli-Orlidge A, Saunders KB, Smith SR, et al. An activated form of transforming growth factor b is produced by cocultures of endothelial cells and pericytes. *Proc Natl Acad Sci U S A* 1989;86:4544.
87. Majesky MW, Lindner V, Twardzik DR, et al. Production of transforming growth factor β_1 during repair of arterial injury. *J Clin Invest.* 1991; 88:904.
88. Wolf YG, Rasmussen LM, Ruoslahti E. Antibodies against transforming growth factor-β_1 suppress intimal hyperplasia in a rat model. *J Clin Invest.* 1994;93:1172.
89. Hansson GK, Jonasson L, Seifert PS, et al. Immune mechanisms in atherosclerosis. *Arteriosclerosis* 1989;9:567.
90. Hansson GK, Jonasson L, Holm J, et al. Gamma interferon regulates vascular smooth muscle proliferation and Ia expression in vitro and in vivo. *Circ Res.* 1988;63:712.
91. Tellides G, Tereb DA, Kirkiles-Smith NC, et al. Interferon-gamma elicits arteriosclerosis in the absence of leukocytes. *Nature* 2000;403:207.
92. Aaronson SA. Growth factors and cancer. *Science* 1991;254:1146.
93. Brugge JS. New intracellular targets for therapeutic drug design. *Science* 1993;260:918–919.
94. Schindler C, Shuai K, Prezioso VR, Darnell JE. Interferon-dependent tyrosine phosphorylation of a latent cytoplasmic transcription factor. *Science* 1992;257:809.
95. Zhong Z, Wen Z, Darnell JE. Stat3: a stat family member activated by tyrosine phosphorylation in response to epidermal growth factor and interleukin. *Science* 1994;264:95.
96. Baringa M. Two major signaling pathways meet at MAP-kinase. *Science* 1995;269:1673.
97. Larson DM, Haudenschild CC, Beyer EC. Gap junction messenger RNA expression by vascular wall cells. *Circ Res.* 1990;66:1074.
98. Orlidge A, D'Amore PA. Inhibition of capillary endothelial cell growth by pericytes and smooth muscle cells. *J Cell Biol.* 1987;105:1455.
99. Heimark RL, Schwartz SM. The role of membrane-membrane interactions in the regulation of endothelial cell growth. *J Cell Biol.* 1985; 100:1934.
100. Hawiger JJ. Hemostasis, bleeding, and thromboembolic complications of trauma and infection. In Clowes GHA Jr, ed. *Trauma, sepsis and shock. The physiological basis of therapy.* New York: Marcel Dekker; 1988, pp. 123–159.
101. Rodgers GM. Hemostatic properties of normal and perturbed vascular cells. *FASEB J.* 1990;2:116.
102. Marcum J, McKenney J, Rosenberg R. The acceleration of thrombin-antithrombin III complex formation in rat hind quarters via heparin-like molecules bound to endothelium. *J Clin Invest.* 1984;74:341.
103. Esmon CT. The roles of protein c and thrombomodulin in the regulation of blood coagulation. *J Biol Chem.* 1989;264:4743.
104. Cotran RS, Kumar V, Robbins SL. *Robbins pathologic basis of disease.* Philadelphia: WB Saunders; 1989:553–595.
105. Benditt EP, Gown AM. Atheroma: the artery wall and the environment. *Int Rev Exp Pathol.* 1980;21:55.
106. McGill HC Jr. Persistent problems in the pathogenesis of atherosclerosis. *Arteriosclerosis* 1984;4:443.
107. Velican C, Velican D. Intimal thickening in developing coronary arteries and its relevance to atherosclerotic involvement. *Atherosclerosis* 1976; 23:345.
108. Velican C, Velican D. The precursors of coronary atherosclerotic plaques in subjects up to 40 years old. *Atherosclerosis* 1980;37:33.
109. Thomas WA, Kim DN. Atherosclerosis as a hyperplastic and/or neoplastic process. *Lab Invest.* 1983;48:245.
110. Gordon D, Reidy MA, Benditt EP, Schwartz SM. Cell proliferation in human coronary arteries. *Proc Natl Acad Sci U S A.* 1990;87:4600.
111. O'Brien ER, Alpers CE, Stewart DK, et al. Proliferation in primary and restenotic coronary atherectomy tissue: Implications for antiproliferative therapy. *Circ Res.* 1993;73:223.
112. Jonasson L, Holm J, Skalli O, et al. Expression of class II transplantation antigens on vascular smooth muscle cells in human atherosclerosis. *J Clin Invest.* 1985;76:125.
113. Stemme S, Rymo L, Hansson GK. Polyclonal origin of T lymphocytes in human atherosclerotic plaques. *Lab Invest.* 1991;65:654.
114. Sharrett AR, Patsch W, Sorlie PD, et al. Associations of lipoprotein cholesterols, apolipoproteins A-I and B, and triglycerides with carotid

atherosclerosis and coronary heart disease: the atherosclerosis risk in communities (ARIC) study. *Arterioscler Thromb.* 1994;14:1098.
115. Wilcox JN, Smith KM, Schwartz SM, Gordon D. Localization of tissue factor in the normal vessel wall and in the atherosclerotic plaque. *Proc Natl Acad Sci U S A.* 1989;86:2839.
116. Schneiderman J, Sawdey MS, Keeton MR, et al. Increased type 1 plasminogen activator inhibitor gene expression in atherosclerotic human arteries. *Proc Natl Acad Sci U S A.* 1992;89:6998.
117. Lupu F, Bergonzelli GE, Heim DA, et al. Localization and production of plasminogen activator inhibitor-1 in human healthy and atherosclerotic arteries. *Arterioscler Thromb.* 1993;13:1090.
118. Page JH. Atherosclerosis. An introduction. *Circulation* 1954;10:1.
119. Masuda J, Ross R. Atherogenesis during low level hypercholesterolemia in the nonhuman primate. I. Fatty streak formation. *Arteriosclerosis* 1990;10:164.
120. Castelli WP. Epidemiology of coronary heart disease: the Framingham study. *Am J Med.* 1984;76:4.
121. Rapp JH, Harris HW, Hamilton RL, et al. Particle size distribution of lipoproteins from human atherosclerotic plaque: a preliminary report. *J Vasc Surg.* 1989;9:81.
122. Breslow JL. Insights into lipoprotein metabolism from studies in transgenic mice. *Annu Rev Physiol.* 1994;56:797.
123. Strong JP, Malcom GT, Oalmann MC, Wissler RW. The PDAY Study: natural history, risk factors, and pathobiology. Pathobiological Determinants of Atherosclerosis in Youth. *Ann N Y Acad Sci.* 1997; 811:226; discussion 235–237.
124. Brown MS, Basu SK, Falck JR, et al. The scavenger cell pathway for lipoprotein degradation: specificity of the binding site that mediates the uptake of negatively-charged LDL by macrophages. *J Supramol Struct.* 1980;13:67.
125. Steinberg D. A critical look at the evidence for the oxidation of LDL in atherogenesis. *Atherosclerosis* 1997;131[suppl]:S5.
126. Libby P. Managing the risk of atherosclerosis: the role of high-density lipoprotein. *Am J Cardiol.* 2001;88:3N.
127. Rimm EB, Stampfer MJ. The role of antioxidants in preventive cardiology. *Curr Opin Cardiol.* 1997;12:188.
128. Steinberg D, Witzum JL. Is the oxidative modification hypothesis relevant to human atherosclerosis? Do antioxidant trials conducted to date refute the hypothesis? *Circulation* 2002;105:2107.
129. Salonen RM, Nyyssonen K, Kaikonen J, et al. Six year effect of combined vitamin C and E supplementation on atherosclerosis progression. The Antioxidant Supplementation in Atherosclerosis Prevention (ASAP) Study. *Circulation* 2003;107:947.
130. Dansky HM, Charlton SA, Barlow CB, et al. Apo A-I inhibits foam cell formation in Apo E-deficient mice after monocyte adherence to endothelium. *J Clin Invest.* 1999;104:31.
131. Lipid Research Clinics Program [Letter]. *JAMA* 1984;252:2545.
132. Frick MH, Elo O, Haapa K, et al. Helsinki Heart Study: primary-prevention trial with gemfibrozil in middle-aged men with dyslipidemia. Safety of treatment, changes in risk factors, and incidence of coronary heart disease. *N Engl J Med.* 1987;317:1237.
133. Randomised trial of cholesterol lowering in 4444 patients with coronary heart disease: the Scandinavian Simvastatin Survival Study (4S). *Lancet* 1994;344:1383.
134. Collins R, Peto R, Armitage J. The MRC/BHF Heart Protection Study preliminary results. *Int J Clin Pract.* 2002;56:53.
135. Fonarow GC, Watson KE. Effective strategies for long-term statin use. *Am J Cardiol.* 2003;92:27i.
136. Endres M, Laufs U, Huang Z, et al. Stroke protection by 3-hydroxy-3-methylglutaryl (HMG)-CoA reductase inhibitors mediated by endothelial nitric oxide synthase. *Proc Natl Acad Sci U S A.* 1998;95:8880.
137. Kinlay S, Selwyn AP. Effects of statins on inflammation in patients with acute and chronic coronary syndromes. *Am J Cardiol.* 2003;91:9B.
138. Duguid JB. Thrombosis as a factor in the pathogenesis of aortic atherosclerosis. *J Pathol Bacteriol.* 1948;60:57.
139. Benezra M, Vlodavsky I, Ishai-Michaeli R, et al. Thrombin-induced release of active basic fibroblast growth factor-heparan sulfate complexes from subendothelial extracellular matrix. *Blood* 1993;81:3324.
140. Schwartz SM, Reidy MA, Clowes AW. Kinetics of atherosclerosis, a stem cell model. *Ann N Y Acad Sci.* 1985;454:292.
141. Murray CE, Gipaya CT, Bartosek T, et al. Monoclonality of smooth muscle cells in human atherosclerosis. *Am J Pathol.* 1997;151:697.
142. Libby P, Egan D, Skarlatos S. Roles of infectious agents in atherosclerosis and restenosis: an assessment of the evidence and need for future research. *Circulation* 1997;96:4095.
143. Melnick JL, Adam E, DeBakey ME, et al. Possible role of cytomegalovirus atherogenesis. *JAMA* 1990;263:2204.
144. Melnick JL, Adam E, DeBakey ME. Cytomegalovirus and atherosclerosis. *Eur Heart J.* 1993;14[suppl K]:30.
145. Grattan MT, Moreno-Cabral CE, Starnes VA, et al. Cytomegalovirus infection is associated with cardiac allograft rejection and atherosclerosis. *JAMA* 1989;261:3561.
146. Epstein SE, Speir E, Zhou YF, et al. The role of infection in restenosis and atherosclerosis: focus on cytomegalovirus. *Lancet* 1996;348[suppl 1]:s13.
147. Nieto FJ, Adam E, Sorlie P, et al. Cohort study of cytomegalovirus infection as a risk factor for carotid intimal-medial thickening, a measure of subclinical atherosclerosis [see comments]. *Circulation* 1996; 94:922.
148. Galloway DA, McDougall JK. The oncogenic potential of herpes simplex viruses: evidence for a 'hit- and-run' mechanism. *Nature* 1983;302:21.
149. Kuvin JT, Kimmelstiel CD. Infectious causes of atherosclerosis. *Am Heart J.* 1999;137:216.
150. Grayston JT, Kuo CC, Coulson AS, et al. Chlamydia pneumoniae (TWAR) in atherosclerosis of the carotid artery [see comments]. *Circulation* 1995;92:3397.
151. Kuo CC, Shor A, Campbell LA, et al. Demonstration of Chlamydia pneumoniae in atherosclerotic lesions of coronary arteries. *J Infect Dis.* 1993;167:841.
152. Muhlestein JB, Anderson JL, Hammond EH, et al. Infection with Chlamydia pneumoniae accelerates the development of atherosclerosis and treatment with azithromycin prevents it in a rabbit model. *Circulation* 1998;97:633.
153. Kol A, Bourcier T, Lichtman AH, et al. Chlamydial and human heat shock protein 60s activate human vascular endothelium, smooth muscle cells, and macrophages. *J Clin Invest.* 1999;103:571.
154. Kol A, Sukhova GK, Lichtman AH, et al. Chlamydial heat shock protein 60 localizes in human atheroma and regulates macrophage tumor necrosis factor-alpha and matrix metalloproteinase expression. *Circulation* 1998;98:300.
155. Danesh J, Collins R, Peto R. Chronic infections and coronary heart disease: is there a link? *Lancet* 1997;350:430.
156. Amento EP, Ehsani N, Palmer H, et al. Cytokines and growth factors positively and negatively regulate interstitial collagen gene expression in human vascular smooth muscle cells. *Arterioscler Thromb.* 1991; 11:1223.
157. Hansson GK, Holm J, Jonasson L. Detection of activated T lymphocytes in the human atherosclerotic plaque. *Am J Pathol.* 1989;135:169.
158. Libby P, Hansson GK. Involvement of the immune system in human atherogenesis: Current knowledge and unanswered questions. *Lab Invest.* 1991;64:5.
159. Salomon RN, Hughes CC, Schoen FJ, et al. Human coronary transplantation-associated arteriosclerosis. Evidence for a chronic immune reaction to activated graft endothelial cells. *Am J Pathol.* 1991;138:791.
160. Russell PS, Chase CM, Winn HJ, Colvin RB. Coronary atherosclerosis in transplanted mouse hearts. I. Time course and immunogenetic and immunopathological considerations. *Am J Pathol.* 1994;144:260.
161. Shi C, Russell ME, Bianchi C, et al. Murine model of accelerated transplant arteriosclerosis. *Circ Res.* 1994;75:199.
162. Torzewski J, Bowyer DE, Waltenberger J, Fitzsimmons C. Processes in atherogenesis: complement activation. *Atherosclerosis* 1997;132:131.
163. Rus HG, Niculescu F, Constantinescu E, et al. Immunoelectron-microscopic localization of the terminal C5b-9 complement complex in human atherosclerotic fibrous plaque. *Atherosclerosis* 1986;61:35.
164. Richardson PD, Davies MJ, Born GV. Influence of plaque configuration and stress distribution on fissuring of coronary atherosclerotic plaques. *Lancet* 1989;2:941.
165. Cheng GC, Loree HM, Kamm RD, et al. Distribution of circumferential stress in ruptured and stable atherosclerotic lesions: a structural analysis with histopathological correlation. *Circulation* 1993;87:1179.
166. Kinlay S, Selwyn AP, Libby P, et al. Inflammation, the endothelium, and the acute coronary syndromes. *J Cardiovasc Pharmacol.* 1998;32[suppl 3]:S62.
167. Fabunmi RP, Sukhova GK, Sugiyama S, et al. Expression of tissue inhibitor of metalloproteinases-3 in human atheroma and regulation in lesion-associated cells: a potential protective mechanism in plaque stability. *Circ Res.* 1998;83:270.
168. Libby P, Aikawa M. New insights into plaque stabilisation by lipid lowering. *Drugs* 1998;56[suppl 1]:9.
169. Libby P, Schoenbeck U, Mach F, et al. Current concepts in cardiovascular pathology: the role of LDL cholesterol in plaque rupture and stabilization. *Am J Med.* 1998;104:14S.
170. Dandona P, Aljada A. A rational approach to pathogenesis and treatment of type 2 diabetes mellitus, insulin resistance, inflammation, and atherosclerosis. *Am J Cardiol.* 2001;90:27G.
171. Aikawa M, Rabkin E, Okada Y, et al. Lipid lowering by diet reduces matrix metalloproteinase activity and increases collagen content of rabbit atheroma: a potential mechanism of lesion stabilization. *Circulation* 1998; 97:2433.
172. Libby P. Vascular Biology of atherosclerosis overview and state of the art. *Am J Cardiol.* 2003;91:3A.

CHAPTER 89 ■ VASCULAR DIAGNOSTICS

SERGIO X. SALLES-CUNHA AND THOMAS W. WAKEFIELD

The essentials of vascular diagnostics cover a range of common pathologies, testing objectives, and technologies available. The pathologies considered in detail are cerebrovascular with special emphasis given to extracranial carotid stenosis, peripheral arterial, aortic and aortic branches, and peripheral venous. Obstructive and aneurysmal diseases are the primary focus of the arterial sections. The section on the aorta and its branches focuses on abdominal aortic aneurysms (AAAs), mesenteric ischemia, and renal artery stenosis. Peripheral venous diseases are distinctly subdivided into detection of acute thrombosis, chronic obstruction, and chronic valvular insufficiency.

The objectives of testing are addressed according to the pathology and may dictate the technology employed. The examinations may be performed for screening, definitive diagnosis, preoperative mapping, intraoperative imaging, patient monitoring, and treatment follow-up.

The primary technologies employed are physiologic testing, ultrasonography (US), x-ray angiography, computed tomography (CT) and/or computed tomography angiography (CTA), and magnetic resonance angiography (MRA) and/or magnetic resonance imaging (MRI). These technologies are selected according to test objectives and pathology being addressed.

EXTRACRANIAL CAROTID STENOSIS

Obstructive and embolic diseases located at the carotid artery bifurcation in the neck are treated to avoid stroke. Multicenter, randomized trials have demonstrated the advantages of carotid endarterectomy for both symptomatic and asymptomatic patients.[1,2] The effectiveness and indications of carotid stenting are being investigated.[3] Screening of patients at risk is warranted, and, consequently, duplex US has become the most commonly used technology.[4] Examinations with blind, continuous-wave Doppler without US imaging and oculoplethysmography are not recommended. Screening should identify not only patients with severe carotid stenosis who are candidates for surgery but also subjects with mild or moderate stenosis who are candidates for medical treatment. Significant differences exist between simple protocols used for screening and exams required for definitive diagnosis and preoperative mapping. Although duplex US may be sufficient as a preoperative examination, some centers perform a second, confirmatory evaluation prior to treatment. For this purpose, MRA and four-vessel arch cerebral angiography have been used. MRA often complements MRI, and CTA may complement CT in the evaluation of the symptomatic patient. US imaging has also been employed intraoperatively and is the preferred method for monitoring patients with mild or moderate carotid stenosis and for treatment follow-up. Details of distinct protocols for each objective are described.

Screening

Screening is performed with US scanners of varying technologic sophistication. The common, external, and internal carotid arteries are scanned with gray scale and/or color flow imaging (Fig. 89.1). Peak-systolic velocity (PSV) measured at the site of stenosis is the most common parameter evaluated during a screening test. A PSV greater than 125 cm/sec suggests a hemodynamic significant stenosis greater than 50% diameter reduction (Fig. 89.2). Variability in velocity measurements, however, is around 20%. Therefore, a velocity criterion of 100 cm/sec increases sensitivity and is particularly useful in an elderly population with decreased cardiac hemodynamics. Direct imaging may take precedence over indirect velocity determinations. A transverse section at the site of maximum stenosis provides information not obtained by other imaging means (Fig. 89.3). In contrast, velocities may be affected by anatomic configuration, whereas angiography may not portray the minimal lumen dimension. MRA imaging may be affected by protocol and velocity profiles as well.

In summary, a percent stenosis measured in transverse section greater than 50% and/or a PSV greater than 100 cm/sec at the site of a carotid stenosis, is a positive screening warranting further evaluation. Patients with mild plaquing of less than 50% are candidates for medical treatment. The test should be deemed "inconclusive" if a high-quality image and/or velocity measurement cannot be obtained due to instrument deficiencies, acoustic shadowing caused by calcification, extremely high bifurcation in the neck, vessel tortuosity, fat, short neck, or even lack of patient cooperation during the US.

Definitive Diagnosis

A definitive diagnostic examination is commonly performed with high-quality US and focuses on symptomatic patients, asymptomatic patients at risk, or subjects with a positive screening test. Carotid arteriography, MRA, and perhaps CTA are more expensive alternatives for definitive diagnosis and are often used if US is inconclusive or if the vascular laboratory fails to provide the minimum quality required for Intersocietal Commission for Accreditation of Vascular Laboratories (ICAVL) accreditation. These techniques provide a more general view of the aortic arch and intracranial arteries than images commonly obtained with US. MRA and perhaps CTA can be incorporated effectively in the evaluation of symptomatic patients requiring MRI or CT of the brain.[5]

The US scan covers the cervical carotid arteries from the proximal common to the distal internal carotid artery. Color-flow/gray scale scans are performed to create both transverse and longitudinal US images. To comply with ICAVL norms, blood velocities must be measured at the proximal and distal common carotid artery, the proximal and distal internal carotid artery, and the proximal external carotid artery. A single velocity waveform from each vertebral artery is required. If a stenosis is imaged, velocities must be obtained before, at, and immediately past the site of maximum narrowing.

Velocity criteria for a positive test vary according to the degree of stenosis selected to represent a severe stenosis (e.g., 60%, or 70%) and the instrument being used. ICAVL recommends that velocity criteria be validated in each laboratory.

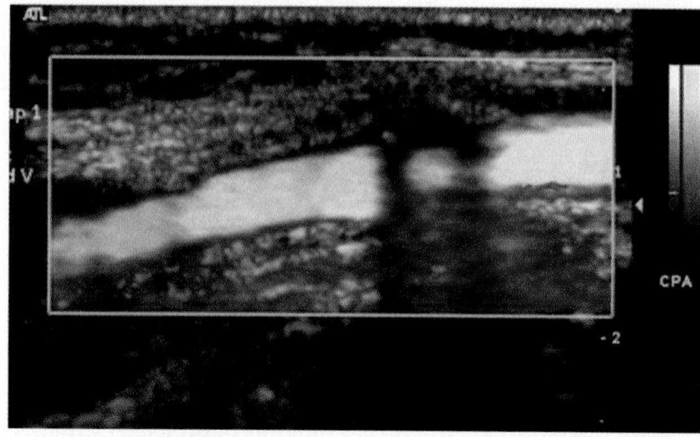

A

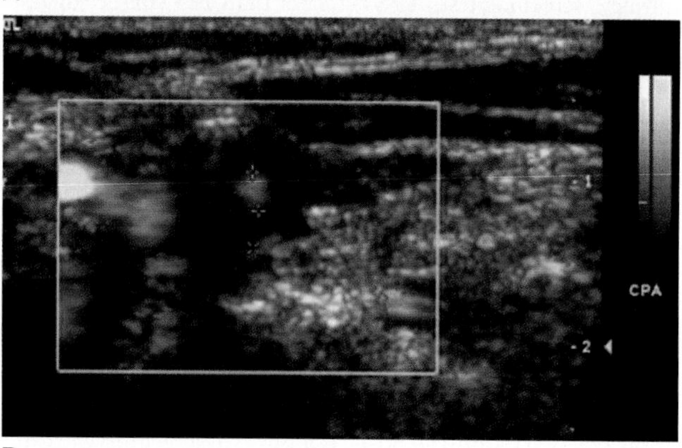

B

FIGURE 89.1 Longitudinal (*A*) and transverse (*B*) images of common and internal (*A*) carotid arteries obtained with power Doppler, a variant of color flow ultrasonography. The attenuation in the ultrasound signal in the longitudinal image is commonly ascribed to wall calcification. High sensitivity of power Doppler permits detection of lumen inside calcified plaques. A lumen of 2.4 mm in a bulb of 7.5 mm resulted in a 68% measurement of local stenosis. This stenosis represents a borderline 60% stenosis by the NASCET/ACAS method. With a circular lumen in transverse imaging, only a single arteriographic projection may be needed to confirm the stenosis.

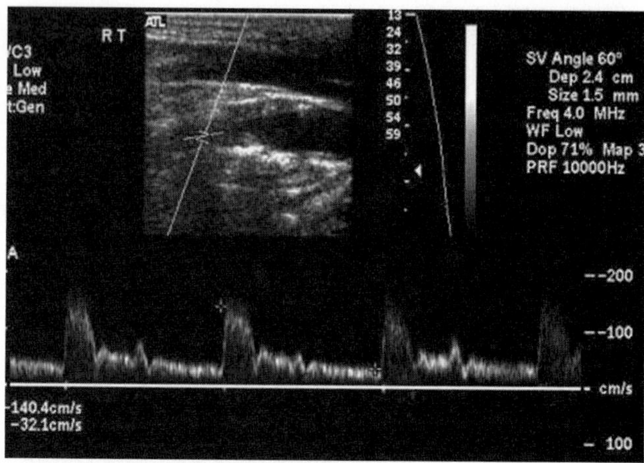

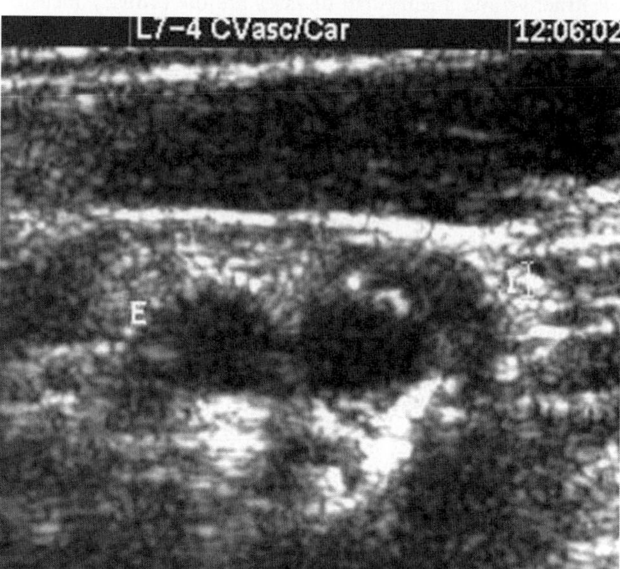

FIGURE 89.2 Peak-systolic velocity equal to 140 cm/sec in the internal carotid artery suggests a hemodynamic significant stenosis greater than 50% diameter reduction. Percent stenosis measurements from the transverse image of an internal carotid artery (the vessel to the right of the reader) were 52% in the vertical and 35% in the horizontal direction. Depending on the direction of the projection, the arteriogram could provide a reading greater or lesser than 50%. An ultrasound reading of 50% to 79% based on the velocity measurement could be misleading. Measurement variability of 20% for velocities and 10% for arteriographic or ultrasonographic imaging should be taken into consideration during the interpretation.

Referring physicians should be aware of the vascular laboratory practices to validate velocity criteria. A definitive diagnosis focuses on measurement of velocity determinations along with percent stenosis based on US imaging.

To calculate percent stenosis, the residual lumen can be compared to the normal lumen distal to the carotid bulb or to the original diameter at the site of stenosis. Comparison to the normal, distal lumen has been the technique adopted by the NASCET and ACAS trials.[1,2] Although the method employed in these trials is effective for surgical decision making, it results in underestimation of mild or moderate stenoses, the most common findings during carotid US evaluation. In these cases, comparison with the local original diameter gives a better parameter for stenosis follow-up.[6] Furthermore, 80% and 70% local stenoses correlate well with a 70% NASCET and a 60% ACAS stenosis, respectively.[6] Based on arteriographic and US resolution (close to 0.2 mm), other technical limitations and physiologic variability, it is recommended that carotid stenosis be interpreted as a 10% interval (a 65% measurement indicates a 60% to 70% stenosis range). Simple velocity parameters suggested for discrimination of severe stenosis include (a) PSVs in excess of 250 cm/second,[7] (b) end-diastolic velocities above 100 cm/second,[8] and (c) ratio of PSV measured at the internal carotid plaque and PSV at the common carotid artery greater than 4.[9]

Plaque characterization is a debatable topic that needs further investigation.[10–12] Evaluation of plaque heterogeneity, intraplaque hemorrhage, and plaque surface irregularity may eventually predict symptoms or CT or MRI brain defects better than percent diameter reduction. Based on US plaque echogenicity, the ICARUS project has described accurate prediction of plaque embolization during carotid stenting.[10] Plaque characterization, however, is subjective and dependent on instrument settings. Until computer programs to analyze plaque echogenicity in two dimensions and three dimensions become readily available, plaque characterization should be interpreted cautiously and used as secondary information.

MRA can be acquired rapidly, without contrast agents or with nonnephrotoxic or nonallergic contrast materials.[5] Multiple projections (Fig. 89.4) and three-dimensional (3D)

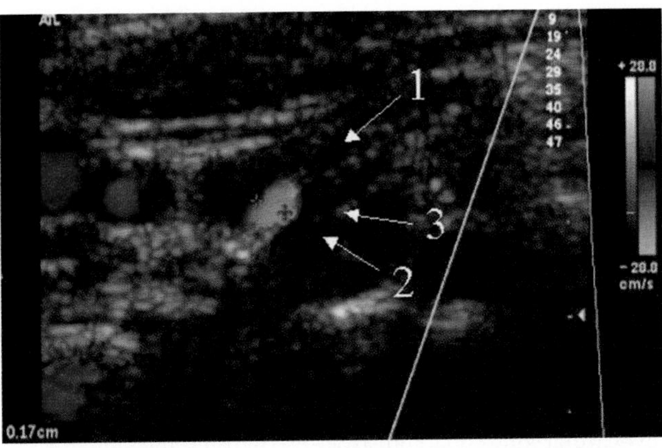

FIGURE 89.3 Transverse images of the internal (vessel to the right of the reader) and external carotid arteries and jugular vein (*left*) obtained with a transducer placed in the lateral aspect of the neck. An horizontal line would represent a anteroposterior arteriographic projection. Residual lumen in the projection of arrow 1 is 1.7 mm and of arrow 2 is 3.4 mm. The internal and external carotid arteries would be superimposed in an arteriogram taken in the direction of arrow 3. A transverse section demonstrates why arteriography in different projections result in different degrees of stenosis and could redirect arteriographic projections to avoid superimposition of the carotid arteries.

processing are possible. MRA, however, is limited by patient motion, several artifacts, and implants, such as pacemakers. MRA findings are also dependent on method selection, interpretation, and presentation. The noncontrast methods most commonly used in clinical practice are two-dimensional (2D) or 3D time-of-flight (TOF). Gadolinium or contrast-enhanced 3D MRA may be less susceptible to artifacts and may image larger volumes in a single acquisition, but the timing following intravenous infusion must be properly controlled. Limiting the field of view (FOV) may improve resolution of carotid bifurcation images. The common practice of presenting several MRA projections showing small images, sometimes only 3 mm in diameter, adversely affects the accuracy of carotid stenosis measurements. Flow voids caused by high velocities or changes in direction of flow often affect interpretation, increasing interobserver disagreement. Due to lack of sensitivity to slow velocity or low volumetric flow, internal carotid occlusion by MRA needs to be confirmed by another technique.

CTA provides multiple projections, transverse images, and information on plaque characteristics.[5,12] Disadvantages include the need for contrast, ionizing radiation, and limitations imposed by bone. Although temporal and contrast resolutions are improved, dependency on preprocessing and postprocessing may alter actual resolution of anatomic measurements, may create artifacts interpreted as disease, or may mask disease.

Contrast arteriography provides detailed imaging of the aortic arch, carotid bifurcation, and intracranial vessels. Nephrotoxicity, allergic reactions, a small but possible risk of stroke, vessel superposition, and subestimation of stenosis in certain projections are disadvantages that can be overcome by noninvasive techniques. The use x-ray currently necessary for the performance of carotid stent placement.

In summary, definitive diagnosis of extracranial carotid stenosis can be performed with US in most patients and includes estimates of percent diameter reduction based on transverse and longitudinal US images along with velocity measurements. Heterogeneous plaques with irregular surfaces and intraplaque anomalies may be considered as potential source of emboli, particularly if no other source of symptoms

VASCULAR

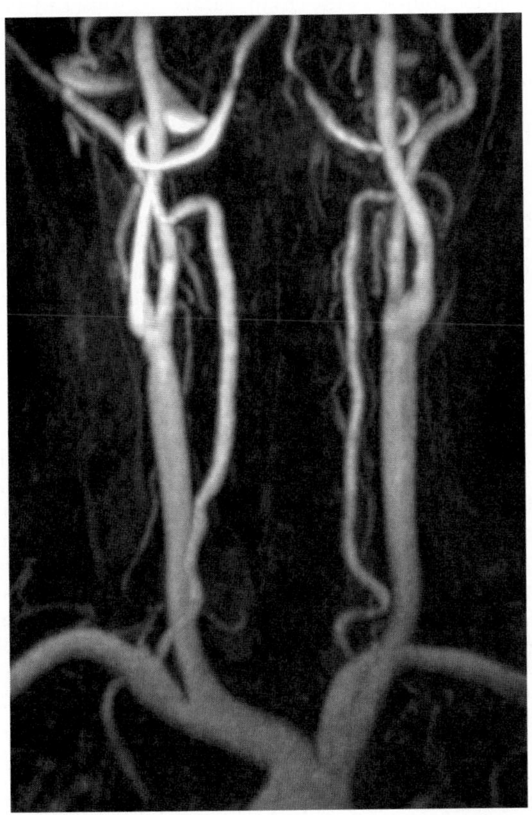

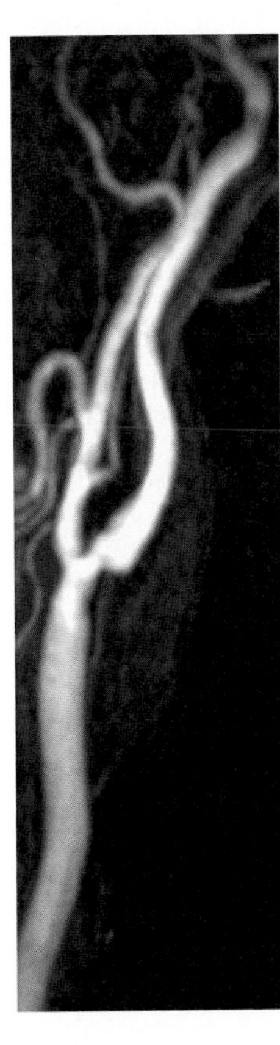

FIGURE 89.4 Magnetic resonance angiography (MRA) of the extracranial cerebral arteries. (*A*) Three-dimensional reconstruction of the entire MRA data set. (*B*) Subvolume reconstruction that demonstrates a 30% to 40% stenosis at the common carotid bifurcation that extends distally into the proximal internal carotid artery. (Courtesy of Frank J Londy, R.T.(R), University of Michigan Medical Center.)

is identifiable. The most common use of MRA and CTA is to validate US findings. Internal carotid total occlusion should be confirmed by a second examination. MRA and CTA may also be complementary in the evaluation of the symptomatic patient. Use of x-ray catheter arteriography is being limited to indeterminate cases.

Preoperative Mapping

Cost-effectiveness supports the primary use of US in asymptomatic patients. In principle, carotid endarterectomy of a severe stenosis can be performed based on US alone. Increased reliability and screening for or definitive diagnosis of other pathologies may dictate additional cerebral and aortic arch imaging.

High-quality US must be employed to be effective as a preoperative mapping modality. In addition to the information described in the "definitive diagnosis" section, US can provide exact locations of the carotid bifurcation, the proximal beginning of the carotid plaque, and the distal ending of the plaque. The latter is associated with demonstration of a patent, nondiseased, distal, nonkinked, cervical internal carotid artery.[13] All measurements can be referred to the ear lobe, and/or plaque location can be marked over the neck skin. Plaque location may be depicted so well on the surface of the skin that the surgical incision may be optimized and minimized accordingly.

Intraoperative Imaging

Completion arteriography documents patency of a treated carotid artery, potential thrombosis, and technical defects that require prompt correction. This technique, however, is not free of complications and may be insensitive to defects that do not affect the flow lumen. Vascular surgeons trained in ultrasonography may opt for completion studies performed with intraoperative US probes rather than arteriography.[14] US provides additional information on the arterial wall, flaps, dissection, and other abnormalities in addition to the flow lumen itself. One of the difficulties of intraoperative US is to determine what findings must be repaired.

Carotid stenting is commonly performed under fluoroscopy. US may be used to determine appropriate stent deployment and the fate of the treated atheroma. Reports of carotid stenting performed under US guidance will appear in the near future.

High-end equipment or portable/lap top devices have been employed in surgery. Technically, the US probe is placed inside a sleeve full of gel. The surgeon then holds the US probe against the vessel of interest over a saline pool. Liquid-gel continuity must exist from the probe to the vessel to avoid disruption of the US signal. A second person is needed to operate the US scanner or the keyboard may be isolated for the surgeon to manipulate the commands.

Patient Monitoring

A US examination is usually recommended within 6 months for patients with moderate carotid stenosis who are not yet candidates for surgical treatment. Patients with mild stenosis are commonly followed on a yearly basis.

Treatment Follow-Up

US is a cost effective method to follow patients after carotid endarterectomy or stenting. Follow-up examinations are recommended at 6 weeks, 6 months, 1 year, and yearly thereafter. As a newer technique, carotid stenting should be followed at shorter intervals. After carotid stent placement, carotid velocity measurements may be altered in comparison to nonstented carotid arteries. Usual velocity criteria for stenosis determination need to be confirmed by imaging findings. One practical reason to follow patients after carotid intervention is to monitor for the development of carotid plaque on the side contralateral to a carotid endarterectomy.

PERIPHERAL ARTERIAL DISEASE

Peripheral arterial disease (PAD) is underrecognized and undertreated, despite its significant prevalence in the elderly and its association with high mortality and morbidity from myocardial infarction and stroke.[15] Diabetes and smoking are strongly linked to PAD. Screening can be expeditiously performed with physiologic testing. Definitive diagnosis is achieved by expert clinical examination, physiologic quantification documenting progression of disease or effects of treatment, and extent of disease corroborated by duplex US imaging.[16] Although US preoperative mapping has been accomplished in trained vascular laboratories,[17] the standard imaging for treatment decisions is arteriography. MRA and CTA have been used recently for detailed imaging of the arteries of the lower extremity.[18–20] Experts claim that US, MRA, and CTA can be as sensitive or better than arteriography to detect crural and pedal arteries. Such results, however, are operator and method (e.g., MRA sequence) dependent. Examination details according to testing objectives are described later.

Screening

The measurement of ankle pressures is a common screening procedure for PAD (Fig. 89.5A). With the patient supine, a pneumatic cuff is wrapped around the ankle and is inflated to suprasystolic pressures. Systolic pressure is measured with the Doppler technique as the disappearance or onset of flow is detected at the posterior tibial or dorsal pedal (anterior tibial) artery while the cuff is inflated or deflated. Systolic ankle pressure is then compared with the highest systolic brachial pressure. The ankle-brachial index (ABI) is the ratio of ankle to brachial pressure. A normal ABI is greater than 1.0. Taking into consideration physiologic and measurement variances, an ABI less than 0.9 is considered abnormal. An ABI less than 0.5 is associated with moderate or severe ischemia and vascular consultation for possible revascularization is recommended.

The ABI is a rapid and effective screening method, but it may fail in the renal dialysis or the diabetic patient, particularly one that has been treated with insulin for many years. These patients may have rigid, calcific arteries that are not totally compressible by cuff inflation. A second screening alternative is to evaluate the Doppler waveforms directly. A normal Doppler waveform is triphasic with a major flow wave moving in the direction of the foot, followed by a smaller reverse wave toward the heart, and then by another small forward wave toward the periphery (see Fig. 89.5B upper tracings). In the presence of a severe proximal obstruction, the flow waveform becomes monophasic, having only one rounded wave with low amplitude and abnormally prolonged systolic duration (see Fig. 89.5B lower tracings). Toe pressures may be measured using small cuffs and a photoplethysmograph to detect flowing blood. Details, such as toe temperature and rate of inflation/deflation, influence toe pressure measurement. Measuring pressure with the toe at approximately 28°C and on cuff inflation is recommended. A normal toe-brachial systolic pressure ratio, or toe-brachial index (TBI), is 0.7 to 0.8. Significant ischemia is suspected for TBI less than 0.4.

A

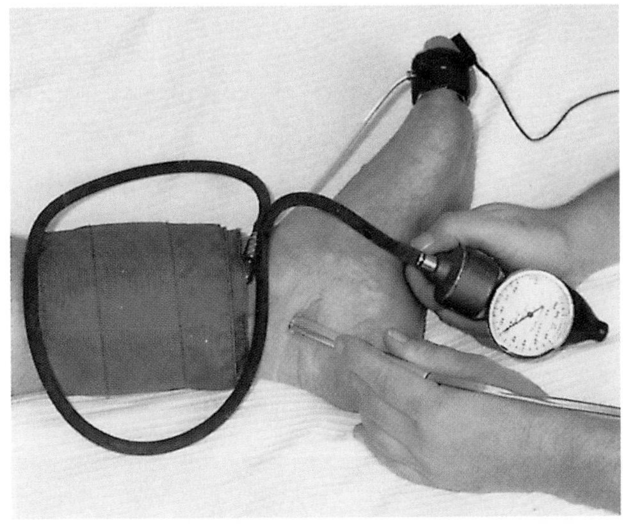

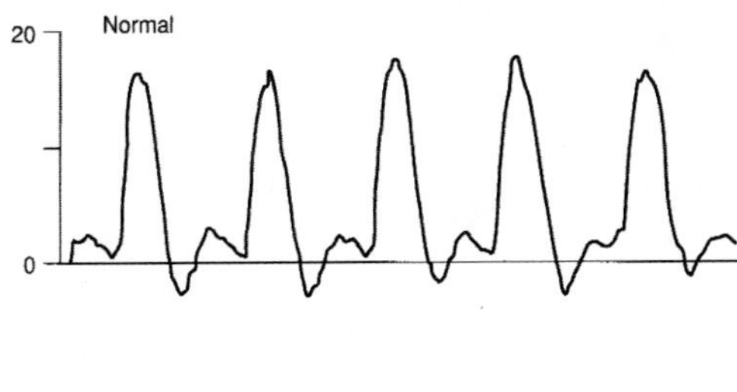

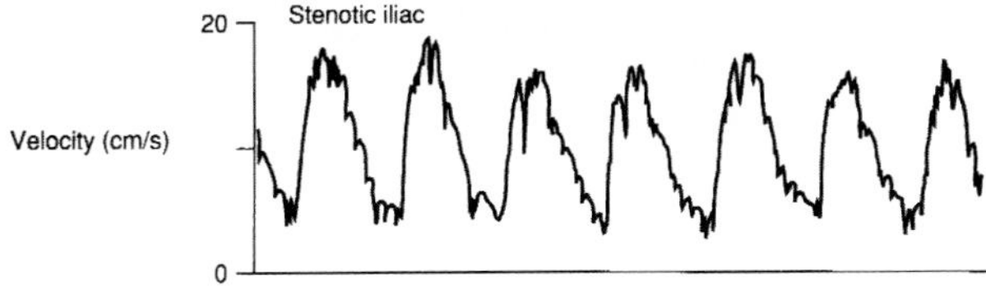

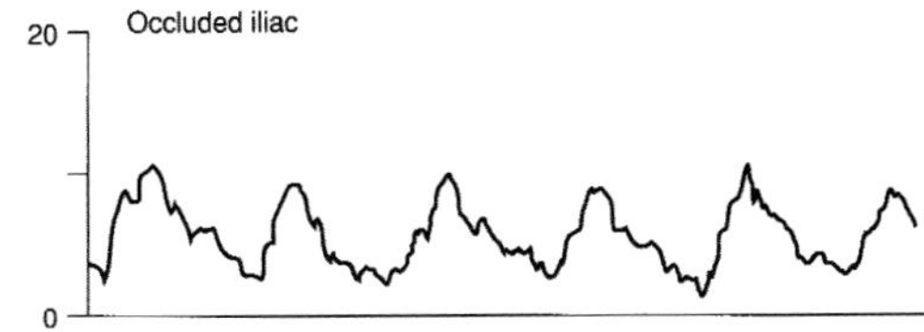

B

FIGURE 89.5 Screening for peripheral arterial disease (PAD). (*A*) Ankle pressure measurement. A continuous-wave Doppler ultrasound probe, aimed at the posterior tibial artery, detects arterial flow signals. A pneumatic cuff wrapped around the ankle or toe is used to measure ankle or toe pressures. Foot is rotated to place toe at heart level. Toe pulses are detected with a photoplethysmograph. (*B*) Analogue recordings of Doppler signals obtained from the common femoral artery of a normal subject, a patient with an iliac artery stenosis, and a patient with occlusion of the iliac artery.

Definitive Diagnosis

Several physiologic tests have been used for definitive diagnosis of PAD: segmental pressures, Doppler waveforms, and pulse volume recording (PVR). To measure segmental pressures, cuffs are placed around the ankle, upper calf, and thigh. Decreased pressure in relation to the proximal cuff or to the contralateral pressure at the same level is an indicator of PAD proximal to measuring site. A 20 to 30 mm Hg difference in cuff pressures is significant. At least two papers describing work performed in modern laboratories deemed segmental pressures unnecessary.[21,22] It has been demonstrated that thigh and upper calf pressures may give redundant information once segmental Doppler waveforms and ankle pressures were obtained.[22]

Doppler waveforms are obtained at the common femoral, mid superficial femoral, popliteal, posterior tibial, and anterior tibial (or dorsal pedal) arteries. Triphasic waveforms suggest absence of PAD but cannot exclude stenosis that may become hemodynamic significant in conditions of increased flow. Specifically, common femoral triphasic waveforms have masked hemodynamic significant iliac stenosis. Monophasic waveforms indicate PAD proximal to the site of measurement. Localized increase in Doppler velocities indicates the presence of a moderate or severe stenosis (Fig. 89.6). Lack of Doppler velocity signal indicates either total occlusion, poor sensitivity of the instrument, or misplacement of the sample volume away from the intended artery.

PVR obtains waveforms at the thigh, upper calf, ankle, and foot levels. Toe tracings may also be recorded. A pneumatic cuff wrapped around the limb is inflated to 60 mmHg. A pressure transducer connected to the cuff records the pulse volume waveforms (Fig. 89.7). Disappearance of the dicrotic notch suggests mild PAD, decreased amplitude with prolonged duration of the systolic pulse correlates with moderate obstruction, and a flat PVR tracing represents severe disease proximal to the recording cuff. In contrast to ankle pressures, PVR waveforms may not be affected by arterial calcification because PVR tracings represent pulsations in the entire calf segment, including perfusion beyond the major arteries. Issues, such as inconsistent calibration between instrument manufacturers and poor sensitivity once arterial pressure drops below cuff pressure, have yet to be addressed. With modern instrumentation, PVRs are less dependent than Doppler on the experience of the technologist.

Presently, it is recommended to obtain Doppler waveforms with a duplex US scanner. Origin of the Doppler signal is clearly determined and training toward arterial mapping can be accomplished with this approach. In summary, segmental flow and pressure dynamics have been used to diagnose aortoiliac, femoropopliteal, and infrapopliteal PAD. A well-trained person can predict the sites of major obstruction in 80% to 85% of the cases.[22]

Preoperative Mapping

Color-flow, duplex US has been employed to map the lower extremity arterial tree prior to infrainguinal reconstruction.[16,17] The examination, however, must be performed by someone trained in vascular US and knowledgeable of the vascular surgeon who referred the patient to the arterial mapping. Poor mapping of the iliac and proximal infrapopliteal arterial segments in large patients can be a significant deficiency of US mapping. Expert arterial mapping compares favorably to arteriography in the femoropopliteal segments and may have higher sensitivity to detect patent distal tibial arteries in the presence of proximal occlusions. Bypasses have been performed successfully in patients deemed candidates for leg amputation based on arteriography. US contrast agents may also be useful in these situations. These substances, injected intravenously, improve US echo reflection thus increasing sensitivity to detection of small, patent arteries or arteries with slow or poor flow distal to major occlusions.

A complete examination includes the aorta, iliacs, femorals, popliteals, and infrapopliteal arteries all the way to the arteries in the foot. A complete examination may last longer than

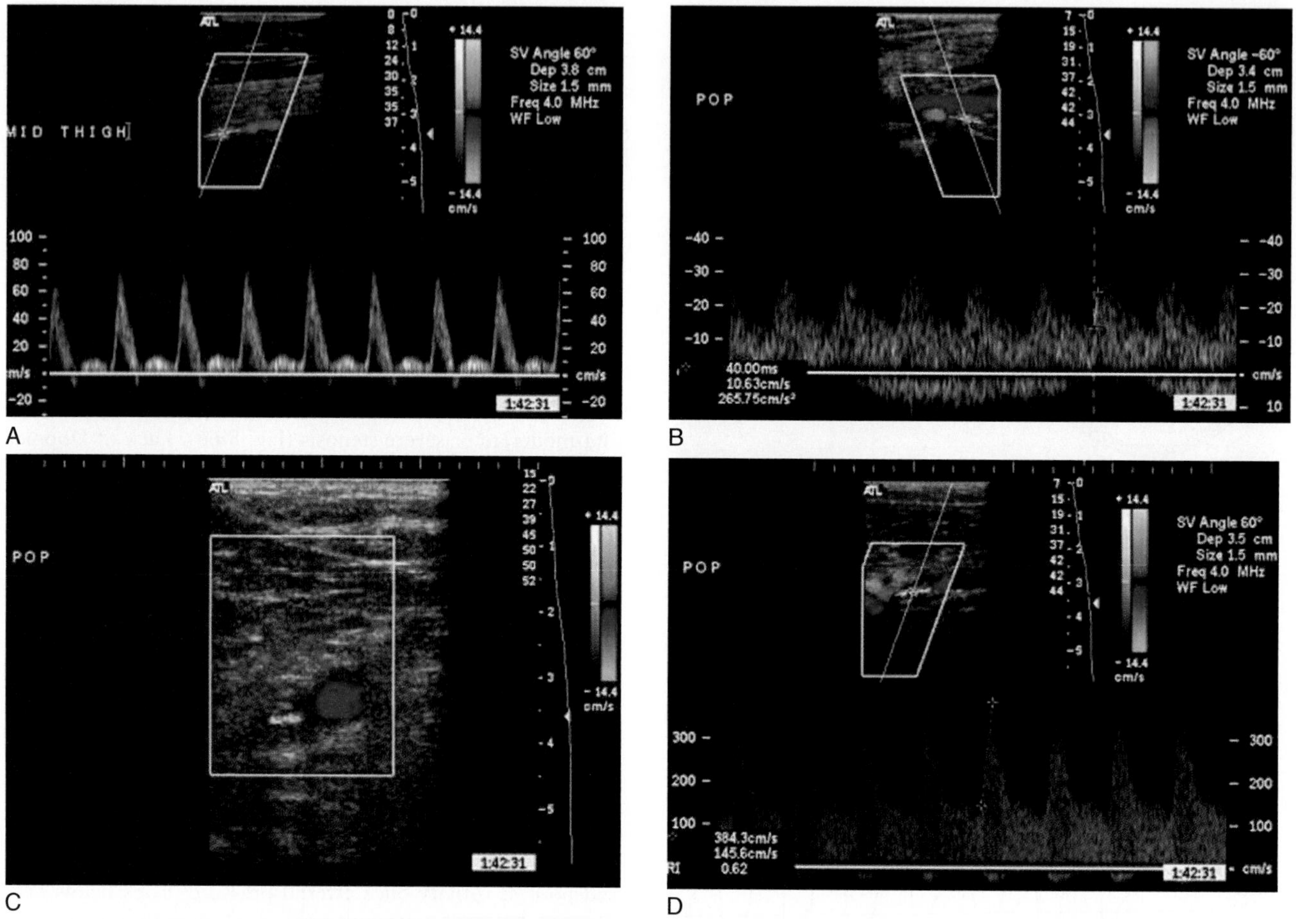

FIGURE 89.6 (*A*) Triphasic, normal duplex Doppler flow velocity waveform at mid superficial femoral artery; peak-systolic velocity (PSV): 80 cm/s. (*B*) Monophasic, abnormal waveform at distal popliteal artery; PSV = 40 cm/s, end-diastolic velocity (EDV) = 11 cm/s. (*C*) Transverse image showing severe stenosis of popliteal artery and normal popliteal vein. (*D*) Elevated velocities at the popliteal artery stenosis; PSV = 384 cm/s and EDV = 146 cm/s.

1 hour. A scan from the proximal iliac artery may be stopped once a significant stenosis or occlusion is found, most likely in the superficial femoral artery. Mapping of the popliteal artery should always be attempted. Such mapping may be sufficient to direct endovascular or surgical treatment of the femoropopliteal segment, particularly in the claudicant. If the patient is a candidate for an infrapopliteal reconstruction, then US mapping restarts at the foot level. US scanning is performed toward the popliteal artery via patent tibial and peroneal arteries until significant obstructions are detected. Severe stenosis often causes a doubling or tripling in velocities through the narrowed lumen. This finding, however, may be attenuated if the stenosis is distal

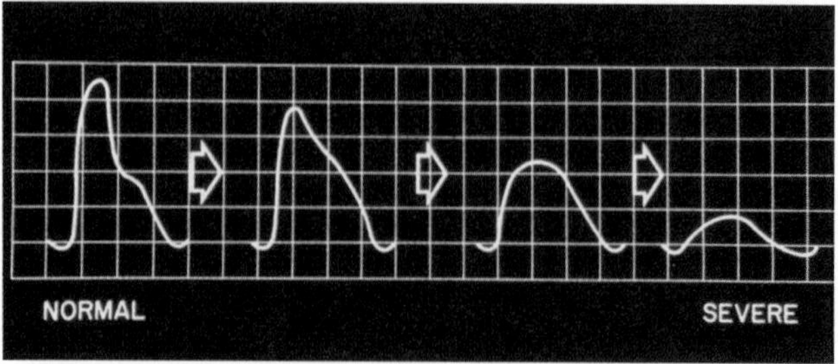

FIGURE 89.7 Arterial pulse volume recorded with a pneumatic cuff wrapped around a limb segment. Alterations in waveforms correspond to severity of disease.

to an occlusion or to another significant stenosis. An experienced sonographer then interprets color flow and B-mode gray scale imaging to grade the stenosis.

A particular advantage of US mapping is the detailed localization of an anastomotic site (Fig. 89.8). The patient can go to the operating room with a skin mark, no longer than 2 inches, where a native artery is patent and has soft walls. Dissection and exposure are efficiently performed based on the knowledge of arterial depth, appropriate run-off, and other periarterial anatomic information.

US mapping has been compared to arteriography with operative decision-making based on US mapping.[23] Patients have been scheduled for surgery based on US and intraoperative arteriography has been performed to confirm US findings or to alter the operative plan. Bypasses have been performed based on preoperative US mapping, and completion arteriography has documented the effectiveness of the operation or determined the need for repair. Finally, intraoperative US has also been used as a substitute to completion arteriography.

In addition, vein mapping in search of a conduit is a complementary part of arterial US mapping.[24,25] The great and/or small saphenous veins and the cephalic and the basilic veins can be mapped. Patency, lack of thrombosis, absence of vein wall thickness, diameter measurements, and length of available vein are determined during vein mapping for arterial revascularization. An arm vein of 2 mm in diameter usually dilates to become a 4-mm graft, whereas saphenous vein dilatation with arterial pressure is not as accentuated.

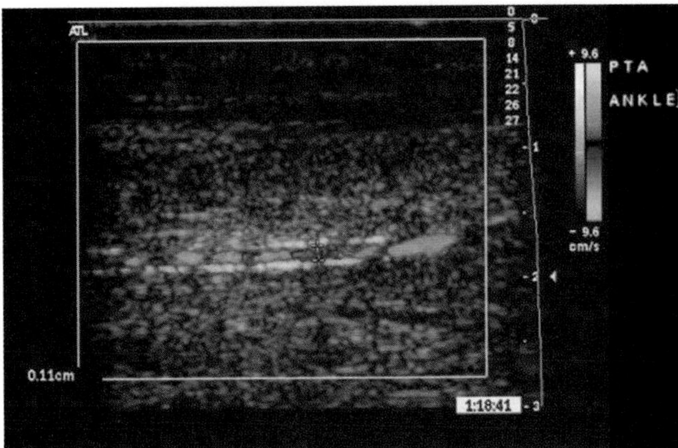

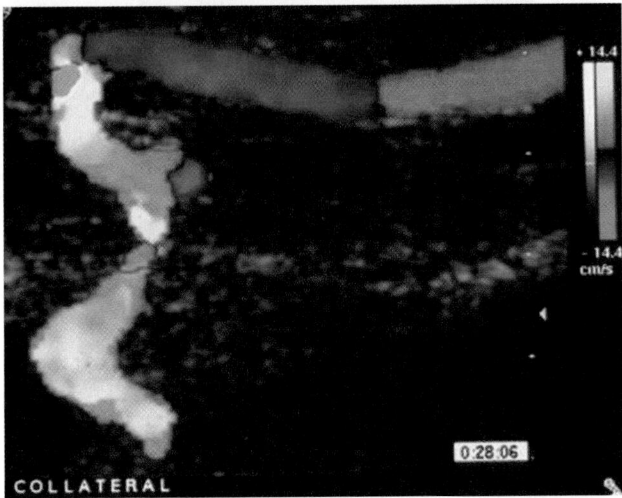

FIGURE 89.8 Selection of the distal anastomosis based on ultrasonography (US) mapping. (*A*) Thickened anterior tibial arterial wall, not the first choice for a distal anastomosis. (*B*) A thin-walled distal segment of a posterior tibial artery distal to a collateral reentry can be appropriately selected with US imaging as the site for a distal anastomosis.

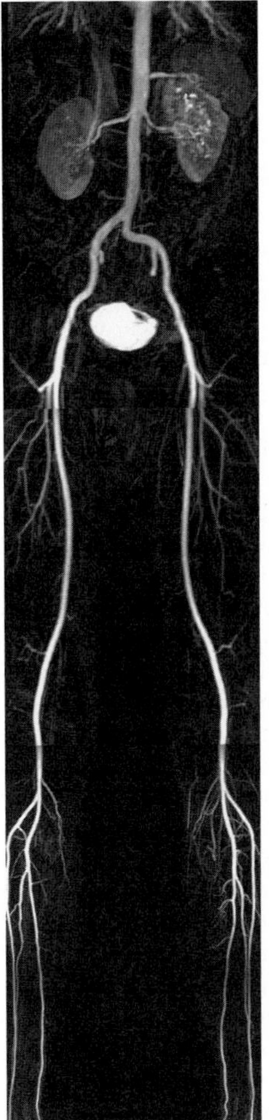

FIGURE 89.9 Magnetic resonance angiography (MRA) of the aorta and lower extremity arterial circulation. Composite image obtained from images taken at three "stations" or image volumes: from suprarenal aorta to below the bifurcation of the common femoral artery, from the proximal superficial femoral to the proximal popliteal artery, and from the proximal popliteal artery to the ankle level. This examination was performed with two contrast injections. The distal station was initially imaged with the first contrast injection and the proximal and middle stations were then imaged with the second contrast injection. This explains the contrast material apparent in the bladder. (Courtesy of Frank J Londy, R.T.(R), University of Michigan Medical Center.)

US arterial mapping, at present, is limited to a few dedicated centers, as arteriography remains the most common imaging technique prior to leg revascularization. Despite potential for nephrotoxic, allergic, and arterial puncture complications, particularly in the renal and diabetic patient, arteriography provides a detailed, long FOV that can be easily and promptly interpreted. Often, multiple injections are needed to image the aortoiliac, femoropopliteal, and crural-pedal arteries adequately. MRA and CTA have become noninvasive alternatives.[18–20]

In contrast to US, MRA is a noninvasive technique that depicts a long FOV, demonstrating the entire vasculature of the leg in one longitudinal image (Fig. 89.9). MRA quality is dependent on the method and sequence selected.[26] 2D TOF is still used in many centers. TOF imaging time may take longer than 1 hour to perform and suppression of venous flow artifacts requires special pulse sequencing and software. Modern 3D, contrast-enhanced MRA has certain advantages over 2D TOF. Imaging the three segments, aortoiliac, thigh, and calf, can be tricky. The bolus of MRA contrast needs to be chased down the leg. One method uses slow injection of contrast, while images are obtained in three stages. Another method uses three separate injections and requires image subtraction software to eliminate MR signals from previous injections. Combination of these techniques with 2D TOF may be needed for improved imaging of distal calf and foot arteries. MRA has become sensitive enough to image distal arteries not visualized by arteriography; the reverse, however, may also occur. Proper detection, quantification, and interpretation of stenosis and signals caused by arteriovenous fistulas and extremely high or low flows need further investigation. Restricting MRA to small FOVs may improve imaging details. Several other methods are currently under investigation.

Modern CTA can collect data from the abdominal aorta to the foot arteries in less than 1 minute.[20] Computer hardware, multiple x-ray detectors, mathematical algorithms, x-ray generators, and tube and table movement have contributed to this accomplishment. The problem, however, lies in the interpretation of hundreds of images produced. Automatic 3D imaging may help, but several decisions require manual, individual human interpretation. A multitude of 3D rendering software exists, and there is no consensus about which one to use in specific applications. Differences of volume versus surface rendering exemplify this difficulty. Calcification, contrast, and bone may not be distinguishable and expert interpretation is variable. Venous contamination at the calf and foot can occur, particularly in patients with inflammation. Administration of large doses of iodinated contrast material is a risk for many elderly patients with PAD.

In summary, arteriography continues to be the most used preoperative imaging modality. Centers with expertise in US mapping, MRA, and CTA have demonstrated advantages of these techniques. Distal arteries can be detected with one of these techniques while undetectable by others. The decision to amputate a leg should not be based on a single imaging modality that may fail to demonstrate viable distal arteries.

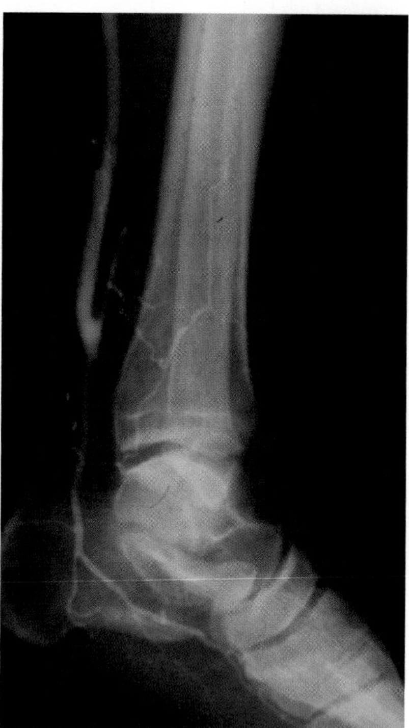

FIGURE 89.10 Completion arteriography of a femorotibial bypass graft. (Courtesy of George Andros, MD.)

Intraoperative Imaging

Completion arteriography remains the standard to evaluate bypass grafts. The arteriographic image is limited to the distal portion of the graft, the distal anastomosis, and the run-off arteries (Fig. 89.10). Endovascular procedures to treat femoral, popliteal, and infrapopliteal arteries are performed under fluoroscopy. Duplex US has been employed intraoperatively with advantages for detection of defects at the anastomoses, arterial wall, and vein valve sinuses (Fig. 89.11).[27] Endovascular treatment of the superficial femoral artery under US visualization is also possible (Fig. 89.12).

Technical details of US intraoperative imaging have been described in the section about carotid intraoperative mapping. The diseased arteries and veins that may be used as an arterial conduit can be scanned to confirm preoperative findings. The bypass graft or other revascularization may be scanned at any time during the procedure. *In situ* bypass graft verification may be performed to be certain that valve leaflets have been disrupted and are not obstructing blood flow. Ligation of all tributaries must be confirmed. Distal outflow may be evaluated at the completion of the distal anastomosis.

An alternative means to evaluate the procedure is intraoperative, intraarterial pressure measurements. This technique is most effective after the distal revascularization has been performed and flow is increased through the iliac arteries. This increased flow exacerbates the significance of an iliac stenosis. If arterial pressure proximal to the reconstruction is decreased by more than 10 to 20 mm Hg in relation to brachial pressure, then a significant iliac stenosis is present and treatment by balloon dilatation and/or stenting is considered.

Another application of pressure measurements is when an arteriovenous fistula is constructed at or near the distal anastomosis to improve flow through a prosthetic graft. Pressure is measured at the distal end of the graft. If this pressure is less than 100 mm Hg, then banding of the venous side of the fistula is performed to minimize steal and to guarantee an acceptable driving pressure toward the ischemic periphery.

Patient Monitoring

Medically or surgically treated patients can be followed with standard, noninvasive diagnostic examination. Ankle pressures should remain stable after medical treatment and should improve after surgical treatment, remaining stable thereafter. Likewise, plethysmographic pulses and Doppler velocity waveforms should improve immediately after surgical treatment. A strong factor to monitor patients surgically treated is to monitor the contralateral extremity. Direct monitoring of the treatment performed is usually done with duplex US as described later.

Treatment Follow-Up

Duplex US surveillance with correction of progressive lesions is recommended after lower extremity bypass, angioplasty, and stenting.[28] Bypass grafts of the lower extremity are commonly followed postoperatively at 3, 6, 9, 12, 18, and 24 months and yearly thereafter. Evaluation of other vascular reconstructions in general and endovascular treatment in particular should adhere to a similar schedule. Complete scanning of proximal arteries, bypass graft, and distal arteries may be performed initially or only when a sensitive physiologic parameter deteriorates. Clinical signs and symptoms, ankle pressures, and PVR may not be sensitive enough to detect graft or other arterial defects early. Decreased blood velocity or blood flow rate have been used to detect arterial obstruction at an early stage. For *in situ* bypasses to the popliteal or tibial arteries, a systolic velocity below 45 cm/sec indicates graft and/or arterial obstruction. In general, a decrease of 20% to 30% in blood velocity or flow rate through the graft is an indicator for complete mapping of the graft and inflow and outflow arteries. At the area of maximal stenosis, the velocity will increase some twofold to threefold above the velocity either just proximal or just distal to the stenosis. One pitfall that must be avoided is to concentrate on

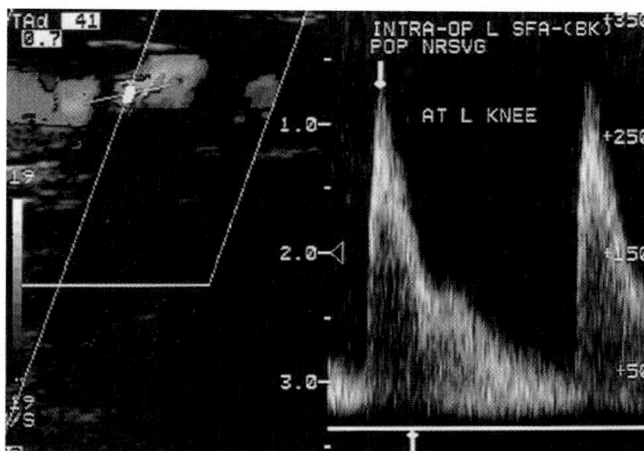

FIGURE 89.11 Vein valve defect of a femoropopliteal bypass detected by ultrasonography (US). Note the wall imaging and the increased velocity (275 cm/s) at the abnormal site. (From Johnson BL, Bandyk DF, Back MR, et al. Intraoperative duplex monitoring of infrainguinal vein bypass procedures. *J Vasc Surg*. 2000;31:678, with permission.)

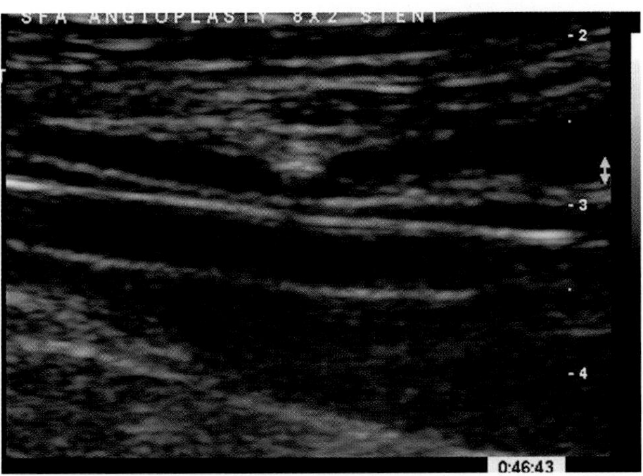

FIGURE 89.12 Superficial femoral artery balloon dilatation and stenting under ultrasonography (US) guidance. The image shows a balloon catheter within the stent. At the level of the depth scale, on the reader's right side of the image, the proximal wall of the stent is at 3 cm deep, the catheter is at approximately 3.2 cm and the distal wall of the stent is at 3.5 cm. (Courtesy of Enrico Ascher, MD, and Natalie Marks, MD.)

one defect and stop searching for a second or multiple problems. On occasion, multiple obstructions may occur throughout the arterial network.

A low-flow condition through a bypass graft may not necessarily be due to an obstruction of a native artery or of the lower extremity bypass graft. Low flow may be indicative of heart failure and may be a marker of increased mortality risk in the elderly.

PERIPHERAL ANERUYSMS

This section covers iliac and popliteal intrinsic aneurysms and false aneurysm following arterial puncture or trauma. Similar basic principles may be applied to other arterial aneurysms of the upper and lower extremities.

Screening

Iliac, popliteal, and false aneurysms are usually screened by physical examination and palpation. Serendipitous detection of an iliac or popliteal aneurysm warrants evaluation of the contralateral iliac or popliteal artery and the aorta. Conversely, the incidence of femoral and popliteal aneurysms in patients with aortic aneurysms may be greater than noted previously, justifying US screening.[29]

Definitive Diagnosis

Unless the patient is obese, US alone is sufficient to diagnose the presence and to estimate the size of peripheral aneurysms. In particular, US can detect small, partially thrombosed popliteal aneurysms that are difficult to be identified with flow imaging techniques such as angiography and MRA.[30] These aneurysms are often masked by the concomitant presence of arterial occlusive disease, atherosclerotic obstruction, and segmental thrombosis of infrapopliteal arteries. Screening and subsequent definitive diagnosis for peripheral arterial occlusive disease, embolic or atherosclerotic, is recommended. US can detect false aneurysms, particularly of the common femoral and proximal superficial femoral arteries, is simple and can combine definitive diagnosis and preoperative mapping in one examination.

Preoperative Mapping

Preoperative imaging follows procedures similar to those described for PAD. Preoperative mapping, particularly US, is facilitated if the patient does not have PAD. Technical conditions and leg positioning during arteriography may hinder visualization of arteries distal to a popliteal aneurysm, forcing an unwanted repetition of the examination. This drawback may be avoided with MRA, whereas US allows for repeat examination with the leg in different positions.

The type of treatment of iatrogenic false aneurysms is dependent on aneurysm size, location, number of lobes, and neck length and diameter. Small false aneurysms with long necks may be observed until they thrombose spontaneously. Thrombin injection has replaced US probe compression.[31] If thrombin injection is considered, neck diameter and length must be carefully determined. Although no dimensions have been determined precisely, neck diameter greater than 3 or 4 mm and neck length shorter than 5 mm may increase the risk of thrombin leak to the native artery. Surgical contraindications versus complications of a large thrombosed mass influence the decision on how to treat large false aneurysms.

Intraoperative Imaging

Intraoperative evaluation is similar to that described for PAD, unless a false aneurysm is being treated with thrombin injection. In this case, US is performed under sterile conditions of the groin. US is used to delineate the aneurysm, to guide the needle, to monitor thrombin injection and to determine treatment effectiveness. Thrombin injection is monitored with either color flow or B-mode, gray scale imaging. Although a bolus injection is often used, slow injection with creation of small "blobs" of thrombus at the tip of the needle, appropriate placement of such thrombi, and additional slow injections may minimize drug delivery. Adjunct compression with the US probe may facilitate the process of thrombosis, while minimizing the quantity of thrombin administered. Most importantly, US guides the injection and documents that the native arteries did not receive thrombin, remain patent, do not thrombose, and do not have a floating thrombus. Complications of this procedure can be devastating if thrombin is injected in the artery feeding the false aneurysm.

Patient Monitoring

If the patient has associated arterial obstructive disease, patient monitoring should follow the protocols mentioned in the previous PAD section. If the disease is primarily aneurysmal, the patient should be followed for development of aneurysms in other peripheral arteries and the aorta. Untreated small aneurysms are commonly followed every 6 to 12 months. The follow-up routine is not as rigid as that recommended for PAD, is age dependent, and can be associated with medical examination for other cardiovascular reasons.

Treatment Follow-Up

Bypass grafts should be followed as prescribed for PAD patients. Because the natural history of endovascular treatment is still undefined, and the endovascular grafting technology is rapidly changing, follow-up intervals shorter than those prescribed for bypass grafts are recommended. Patency of native arteries and thrombosis of false aneurysms treated with thrombin injections should be confirmed with a postoperative US surveillance 1 to 2 days after the procedure.

AORTIC ANEURYSMS

This section focuses on abdominal aortic aneurysms (AAA) with particular emphasis on screening and follow-up of endovascular treatment.

Screening

Screening for AAA in smokers, hypertensive men 60 years of age and older, and relatives of subjects with known aneurysms is recommended. Screening patients of both genders with PAD may also uncover popliteal and/or AAA. US is an effective screening tool unless the patient is too large or has too much gas in the abdomen. The examination should be performed in the morning, after 10 hours of fasting, without smoking, and preferentially after antigas treatment if appropriate. Although surgical or endovascular treatment is reserved for aneurysms greater than 5.5 cm in diameter, screening protocols also detect smaller aneurysms. Aortas with diameters greater than 3 cm or with an enlargement of 50% or more are considered aneurysmal. Patients with small aneurysms are candidates for medical treatment and US follow-up.

US screening usually provides an estimation of maximum diameter measured in an undefined anatomic position, not necessarily in the anteroposterior or lateral directions. It is commonly believed that US dimensions may underestimate AAA diameter when compared to CT. With the proliferation of screening programs performed outside the hospital, a definitive diagnosis test in a qualified laboratory is recommended to confirm and expand on the screening findings.

Definitive Diagnosis

Rarely an additional imaging modality besides US is necessary to accomplish the definitive diagnosis of an AAA. Usually US also determines if the AAA is infrarenal and if associated iliac artery aneurysms are present. Evaluation for PAD is also recommended.

Preoperative Mapping

US may be adequate if open AAA repair is being considered. Clear documentation of the renal arteries in relation to the neck of the aneurysm is required. The US examination must report on the quality of such finding. Arteriography and perhaps MRA provide additional information not readily available with US.[32]

Although endovascular treatment of AAA has been performed based on traditional arteriography, modern tendency is to employ 3D reconstructions from contrast CT films.[33] CT has advantages over MRI in the detection of calcification in the aortic neck, an important descriptor of the endograft sealing zone. Interinstitution variability is apparently lower for CT than for MR examinations. Gadolinium-enhanced CT can be performed to avoid nephrotoxic contrast. CT scan slices, however, need to be small. A 2-mm slice is currently recommended, for example, for precise delineation of renal artery origin. 3D modeling (Fig. 89.13) emphasizes several deficiencies of standard 2D imaging.

Neck diameter is a crucial measurement for endograft selection and proper sealing. Horizontal slices depict the "cross-section" area of an angulated aorta as elliptical when in reality the section transverse to the longitudinal direction of the vessel is circular. Excessive neck angulation is a contraindication for endografting. Neck angulation can be quantitated precisely after selection of greatest angle by rotation of the 3D model. The length of the prosthesis must adapt to the aortoiliac length, usually underestimated by arteriography and standard CT. Length measurement can be performed at the center of the vessel accounting for curvatures in all directions using 3D modeling. Simulations for selection of the appropriate endoprosthesis can be performed using the computer model. This 3D model, however, is not created by automatic reconstruction of aneurysms alone. Expert identification of vessels and other anatomic structures, performed manually in the computer, may be needed.

Intraoperative Imaging

Standard arteriographic and fluoroscopic imaging is performed during endovascular repair of AAAs. US may facilitate puncture of the common femoral artery in situations of difficult anatomy, weak arterial pulses, and small arteries. Minimum requirements for fluoroscopy, particularly for endovascular repair, include a portable C-arm with a 12-inch image intensifier capable of digital subtraction angiography (DSA), road-mapping, and measurements.[34] DSA eliminates bones and other static structures, emphasizing the arteries. Road-mapping registers live fluoroscopic images simultaneously with a semitransparent image of a previous DSA sequence or run. Positioning and deployment of an endograft is then performed in relation to the anatomy of the aorta and renal arteries. Calibrated catheters facilitate measurements.

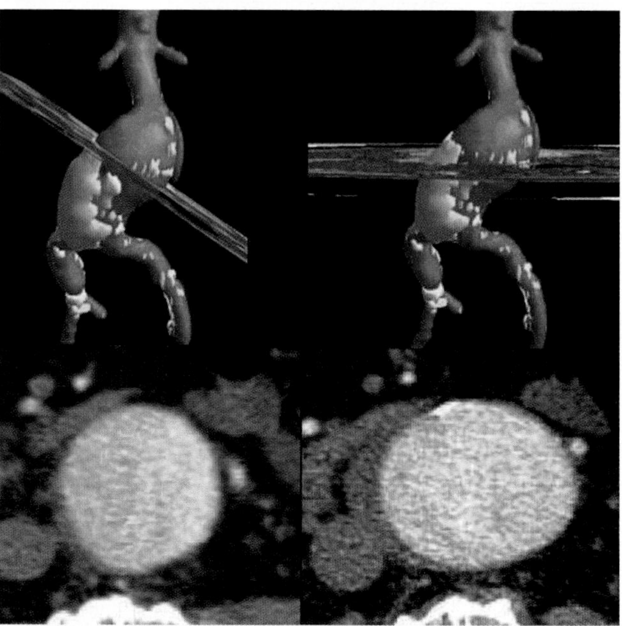

FIGURE 89.13 Evaluation of abdominal aortic aneurysm (AAA) for endovascular graft repair based on three-dimensional (3D) model configurations reconstructed from computed tomography (CT) slices. The model has different color codes for blood, thrombus, calcium, and virtual endograft. CT planar images can be reconstructed in any direction. Diameter may be measured in circular rather than elliptical images of the aorta. Neck length and angulation can be calculated. Necessary length of an endograft can be estimated. (Courtesy of HG Beebe, MD.)

Parallax errors caused by the conic shape of x-ray beams or by the surgeon's position in relation to the monitor must be avoided for precise measurements and device deployment. Completion arteriography is recommended, preferably in more than one projection. Delayed images are taken to demonstrate lack of late endoleaks into the aneurysm sac.

Intravascular ultrasound (IVUS) imaging may add information not available with arteriography.[35] Most commonly, the IVUS catheter has a rotating ultrasound element in its tip and produces a cross-sectional image from inside out, demonstrating the lumen and arterial wall. Before placement of an endograft, IVUS imaging of the pathway from femoral to aorta may reveal arterial wall thrombus, calcification, or a stenosis with a smaller lumen than expected. IVUS is also employed to view the thoracic aorta and to detect dissections.[35] Diameter measurements can be confirmed with IVUS. After placement, IVUS may show correct or incomplete juxtaposition between an endograft or a stent and the arterial wall. IVUS can rule out or detect dissections, flaps, and pseudoaneurysms in the arteries proximal and distal to the endovascular device.

Pressure measurement at the distal iliac arteries may also be performed to investigate obstructions caused, for example, by kinks, external compression, dissections, or intimal flaps.

Patient Monitoring

Patients with small aneurysms are monitored regularly at 6- to 12-month intervals. Patients who had their AAA treated with an open procedure are rarely monitored for this purpose alone. However, a small percentage of these patients may develop suprarenal or thoracic aneurysms or even iliac aneurysms. Most likely, these patients will be followed according to other cardiovascular diseases.

Treatment Follow-Up

Aortofemoral or aortoiliac bypass grafts may occlude or develop false aneurysms, most likely at a distal anastomotic site. Thrombosis is usually limited to one of the limbs of the graft. The incidence of such complications is low, detection is usually by clinical examination, and routine vascular laboratory follow-up with ABI is recommended.

Follow-up of endografts, however, is frequent and often depends on investigational protocols. The most common follow-up is done with CT and the most complete examination includes 3D modeling. Endoleaks, endograft migration, and aneurysm size are commonly monitored. Recording pressure in the aneurysmal sac is being investigated as a means of predicting posttreatment rupture or endograft migration. Migration can be detected with standard x-ray that clearly depicts the stent component of the endograft. 3D volume measurement has demonstrated that aortic diameter is an insensitive indicator of size changes.[36] Therefore, aneurysm size should be monitored based on volumetric determinations. Endoleak detection by CT requires contrast injection and delayed detection. Occasionally, only 3D modeling can determine the actual pathway of the perceived endoleak. The various types of endoleaks are type I, arterial—aneurysm sac at the proximal and/or distal ends of the endograft; type II, peripheral lumbar/mesenteric arteries–aneurysm sac; type III, endograft defect—aneurysm sac, caused by an endograft hole or limb disconnection; and type IV, seepage through the graft material.

High-quality US, particularly with US contrast agents, is a cost-effective and sensitive means of detecting endoleaks.[37] Flow waveforms detected by duplex US are also unique in differentiating endoleaks. Some endoleaks behave like false aneurysms with flow in and out of a pocket inside the aneurysm (Fig. 89.14A), whereas others behave like a channel of flow between a source and a drainage point (see Fig. 89.14B). Still other endoleaks have a direct flow into the aneurysm (see Fig. 89.14C). Whereas the first two types of endoleaks described may regress or cause aneurysm expansion, the third type probably results in rapid expansion of the aneurysm with increased risk of rupture. Slow seepage of blood into the aneurysm sac is possible and may be undetectable by any available technique. For example, an aneurysm can grow as much as 1 cm in diameter in 1 year, at a rate of less than 0.03 mm per day! This expansion can be perceived only by measurements of aneurysm size. Continued pressure in the aneurysm sac when this occurs is called endotension.

AORTA AND BRANCHES

This section covers aortoiliac occlusive disease, mesenteric ischemia, and renal artery stenosis. All abdominal US examinations require fasting, no smoking, and antigas therapy for at least 10 hours prior to the test.

Screening

Aortoiliac occlusive disease is included in the screening of patients with PAD. Additionally, an abnormal, monophasic Doppler waveform at the common femoral artery is indicative of aortoiliac obstruction. A normal, triphasic waveform, however, does not rule out stenosis. No reliable protocol has been devised for screening of mesenteric and renal arteries. US methods described in the definitive diagnosis section may be interpreted as screening tests prior to arteriography.

Definitive Diagnosis

Aortoiliac Arteries

Obstruction of the aorta and iliac arteries can be detected with US if the patient is not obese. The patient needs to be prepared as described for the AAA US protocol. Occlusions are detected by color flow image and stenoses are graded as moderate or severe by a twofold to threefold increase in velocity at the site of narrowing. This procedure is often associated with infrainguinal arterial mapping.

Arteriography remains the standard imaging modality. US findings may aid clinical decision making prior to arteriography in the aortoiliac or infrainguinal segments.[38] Single-projection arteriography can miss the narrowest lumen dimension of an iliac artery if the residual lumen is not circular. MRA can be reformatted in multiple projections to avoid this drawback. 3D CTA modeling also allows for appropriate reconstruction of the aortoiliac system.

Pressure measurements performed via the common femoral artery, particularly under conditions of increased flow, are reliable determinants of the effects of iliac stenoses. Pressure measurements performed after a distal infrainguinal bypass or after injection of a vasodilatory substance, such as papaverine, is sensitive in exposing an iliac stenosis.

Mesenteric Arteries

Stenosis or occlusion of the celiac artery (CA), superior mesenteric artery (SMA), and inferior mesenteric arteries can be detected with US.[39,40] PSV greater than 275 or 200 cm/s predicts an SMA or CA stenosis of at least 70%, respectively. Retrograde flow in the hepatic artery is indicative of CA

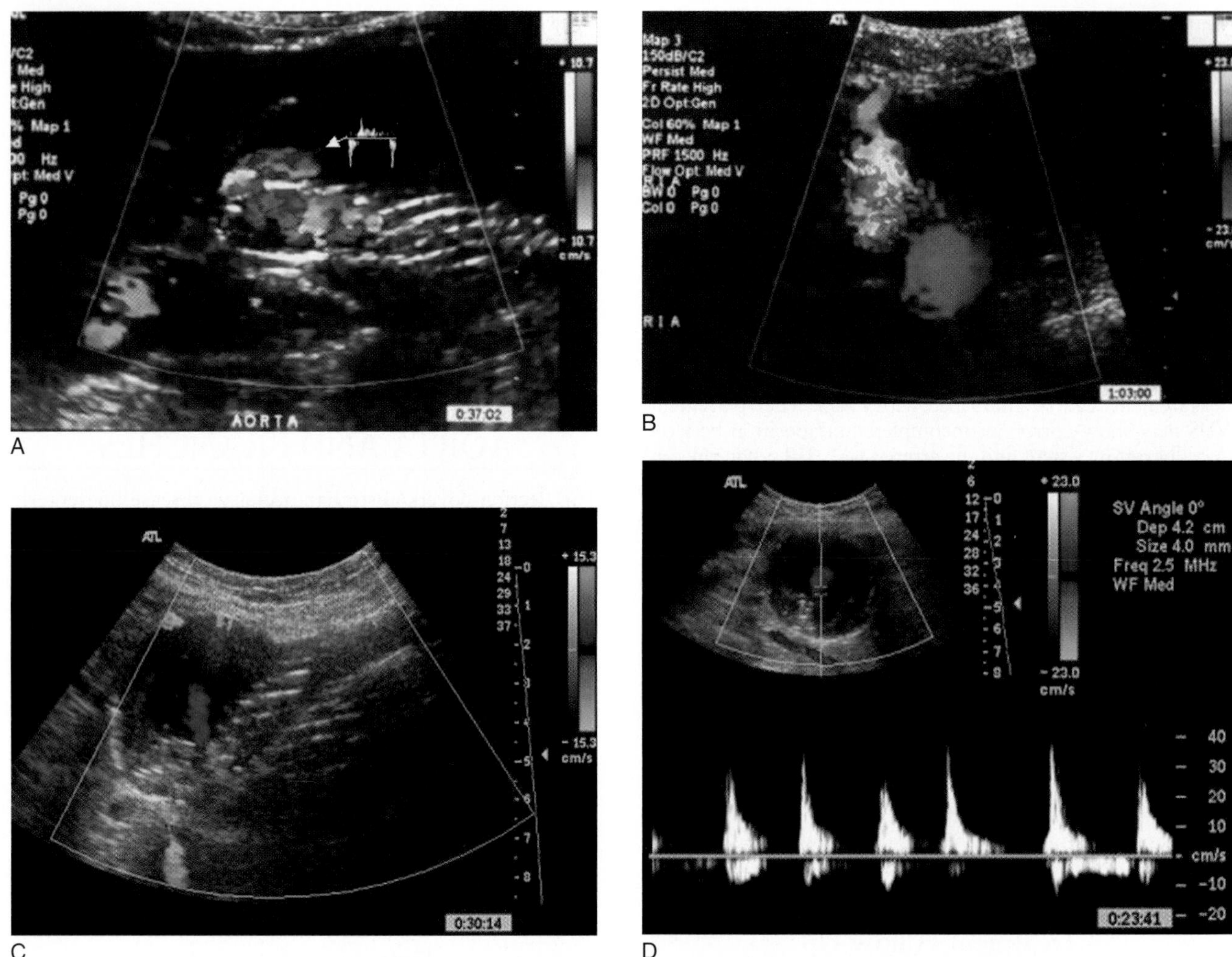

FIGURE 89.14 Examples of endoleak detected by ultrasonography. (*A*) A type I endoleak with flow in and out of the aneurysmal sac, behaving like an pseudoaneurysm within the aneurysm is shown to the reader's left. (*B*) Another type I endoleak caused a flow channel through the aneurysm, from the graft to a small perianeurysm, artery is shown on the right. (*C* and *D*) A type III endoleak with direct flow into the aneurysmal sac.

severe stenosis or occlusion. A differential diagnosis, including median arcuate ligament syndrome, may be evaluated with US. Median arcuate ligament syndrome of the CA is not caused by a typical atherosclerotic obstruction but by external compression of the CA by anatomic positioning or a hypertrophic ligament. In this condition, US does not show a plaque but may show high velocities or low velocities when the measurement is performed on the patient standing or exhaling.

The standard mesenteric artery examination is arteriography. The multitude of branches, potential collateralization, and changes in direction of flow associated with extended mesenteric occlusions create a burden for adequate MRA and CTA.[32] These techniques, however, may be adequate for definitive diagnosis of stenosis located in the CA and SMA.

Renal Arteries

US evaluates flow waveforms in the renal arteries and in the kidneys and estimates kidney length. A renal artery to aorta peak-systolic velocity ratio (RAR) greater than 3.5 is indicative of a renal artery stenosis of at least 60%. Duration of the systolic onset longer than 100 mseconds also suggests renal artery stenosis. Kidneys less than 8 to 9 cm or a size difference of 2 cm between the right and the left kidney suggest poor kidney perfusion by the renal arteries. Fibromuscular dysplasia and renal artery aneurysms can also be detected with US. However, complete visualization of the renal arteries is not always possible, and the duration of the US is quite variable depending of the quality of US imaging obtainable and positional/probe compression maneuvers to obtain adequate visibility of the renal structures. Often, accessory renal arteries are not detected.

Resistance to flow in the kidneys can also be evaluated with the calculation of renal resistive indices (RIs). Normal renal flow waveforms have diastolic flow velocities that are at least 30% of PSVs. The RI is calculated as the quotient of the difference between systolic and diastolic velocity and the systolic velocity. An RI greater than 0.8 indicates kidney damage enough to undermine any potential benefit of a renal artery revascularization.

In addition to US imaging of the renal arteries, kidney perfusion, renal length, and parenchymal thickness, MRA/MRI can detect other causes of hypertension, including adrenal and juxtaglomerular cell tumors.[41] Renal accessory arteries may be missed with MRA. Arteriography is the standard procedure to evaluate the renal arteries.

Normal arteries and normal kidneys of a potential kidney transplant donor can be performed by all of the imaging modalities described previously. Venous evaluation needs to be added to the arterial examination. The anatomic position and the arterial and venous anastomoses, most commonly to iliac vessels, facilitate US examination of the transplanted kidney.

Intraoperative Imaging

Arteriography is the standard procedures associated with the performance of endovascular treatment and at the completion of surgical procedures. Intraoperative US has contributed to optimization of technical success and improved outcome related to visceral revascularization.[42] Minor and major defects, such as kinks, residual stenosis, residual flaps, thrombus, and bidirectional flow have been detected. Occlusions, intimal defects, extrinsic tissue bands, and graft anastomotic stenosis have been detected with color-flow duplex US and corrected during open renal revascularization.[43] Imaging and increased velocities are criteria employed in the analysis of these procedures with intraoperative US techniques similar to those described in the extracranial carotid section.

Patient Monitoring

Most of these patients are followed clinically for various, diverse medical conditions. Patients with aortoiliac occlusive disease may be directed to an exercise-rehabilitation program. Their potential risk for cardiac, carotid, and infrainguinal atherosclerotic disease directs requests for appropriate noninvasive evaluation.

Treatment Follow-Up

Revascularization procedures have been followed without an approved consensus. Vascular laboratory examinations have been requested based on individual signs and symptoms. Routine monitoring of stented renal arteries is recommended (Fig. 89.15). The transplanted kidney has been monitored for technical defects, stenosis or thrombosis of the feeding artery, or draining vein. Kidney acceptance/rejection has been monitored based on kidney perfusion detected with color flow, power Doppler or US contrast agents. Doppler waveforms from the various regions of the kidney have been used to identify a variety of conditions.

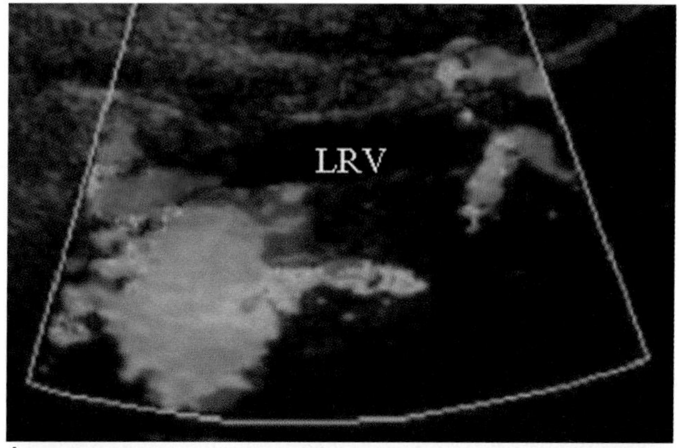

A

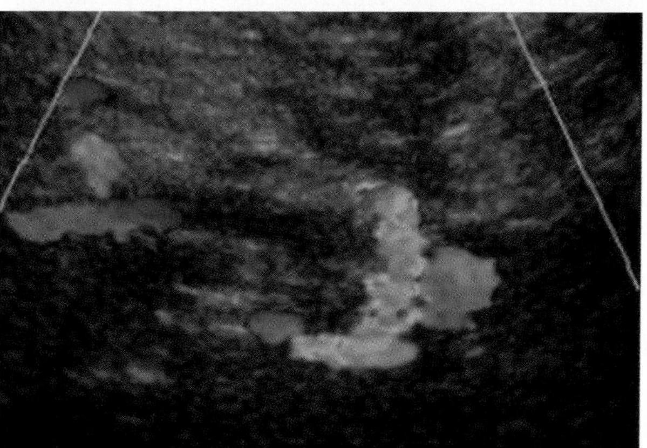

B

C

FIGURE 89.15 Monitoring left renal artery stenting. (*A*) Transverse image of the aorta, proximal left renal artery and left renal vein (LRV). (*B*) The stent is visualized entering the aorta; the stent was 5 mm in diameter and 2 cm long. (*C*) The ultrasound plane cuts the stent obliquely; the echoes apparently inside the stent are actually created by the stent surface. Velocity waveforms were within normal limits.

PERIPHERAL VENOUS DISEASE

Although vascular laboratory accreditation can be obtained based on femoropopliteal US for deep venous thrombosis (DVT), this section emphasizes the growing importance of detecting deep and superficial venous insufficiency and of differentiating between acute venous thrombosis from chronic venous thrombosis or chronic venous obstruction.

DEEP VENOUS THROMBOSIS

DVT of the major peripheral veins requires definitive diagnosis and immediate treatment. However, questions about unilateral versus bilateral examination, need for detection of calf venous thrombosis, follow-up of thrombolytic therapy, and detection of nonvenous findings that cause signs and symptoms are issues that warrant discussion.

Screening

A vascular laboratory may be accredited based on US examination limited to unilateral femoropopliteal imaging and evaluation of the contralateral common femoral vein. Although this protocol may be considered a definitive diagnosis in large vein DVTs, it can also be characterized as a screening procedure that fails to provide a complete diagnosis. Effective screening may be limited to probe compression in search of incompressible venous segments. Screening may be extended with Doppler waveforms obtained at the common femoral, midfemoral, and popliteal veins. Normal venous flow is phasic with respiration. Continuous flow suggests proximal obstruction. Such an obstruction may be caused by nonocclusive thrombus or by external compression. Absent flow is consistent with thrombosis and should match findings of venous incompressibility.

Definitive Diagnosis

In addition to evaluation of the femoropopliteal segment, a complete examination is extended to the iliac veins as proximal as feasible, inferior vena cava, and infrapopliteal veins, including the muscular veins.[44] Infrapopliteal veins must be carefully evaluated in patients who have had orthopedic surgery. Venous compressibility by US probe and venous flow phasicity with respiration as detected by duplex demonstrate patency of the venous system. Partial or totally incompressible vein segments, partially filled veins as detected by color flow Doppler, and continuous or absent flow signals are consistent with venous thrombosis.

Differentiation between acute (recent) thrombosis and chronic obstruction is determined based on the factors outlined in Table 89.1 (Fig. 89.16). Evaluation of thrombus elasticity by US may improve quantification of thrombus aging.[45]

If the patient presents with localized calf pain, examination of this region may identify thrombus in a muscular or infrapopliteal vein or a hypoechoic or hyperechoic mass, such as a hematoma or seroma. Discomfort behind or around the knee may be caused by a Baker's cyst. Other pathologies, such as popliteal arterial aneurysms, false aneurysms, or enlarged lymph nodes, may be detected by US. A common finding is reflux or valvular incompetence of either the saphenous or femoropopliteal veins. All these abnormal findings should be routinely searched for and reported during a venous examination. Simply stating that the extremity does not have DVT results in additional testing and delayed diagnosis. Therefore, the physician requesting an US test for DVT should also inquire about other potential causes of the patient's signs and symptoms.

Evaluation of the upper extremity and jugular veins follows the basic principles of lower extremity protocols with a few significant differences. The axillary and subclavian veins are not compressible with an US probe. Diagnosis is based on imaging and characteristics of flow waveforms. The innominate veins must be evaluated with special sector transducers having lower frequencies for deeper penetration of the US signal. In-dwelling venous catheters have become a major risk factor for DVT in the upper extremity. Thrombus may be detected around the catheter or a catheter-like image caused by the thrombus may be detected after catheter removal.

US has become so dominant in the evaluation of peripheral veins that venography or any other method are rarely performed. Drawbacks of venography, besides cost and risk, include nonvisualization of vein segments and poorly interpretable images in the blood–contrast interface region.[46] About half of the infrapopliteal venous segments not demonstrated by venography can be patent by US. Due to lack of pertinent anatomic references, thrombus in deep calf veins may be interpreted as superficial thrombosis and vice versa. Nonoccluding common femoral vein thrombus may be masked by poor contrast filling and blood flow artifact.

CT venography, in addition to being more expensive than US, is specific but not sensitive to detect DVT of the lower extremities.[47] In contrast, magnetic resonance venography (MRV) is commonly requested to document central thrombus extent in patients with US diagnosis of femoral and/or iliac thrombosis.[48] Venous thrombosis is associated with inflammation, which can be detected by gadolinium-enhanced MRV. Comparison of signal intensity around the vein and in the core of the vein may provide additional information

TABLE 89.1 DIAGNOSIS

DIFFERENCES BETWEEN ACUTE (RECENT) THROMBOSIS AND CHRONIC OBSTRUCTION

Acute thrombosis	Chronic obstruction
Veins are dilated in relation to proximal segments or to the contralateral venous segment	Veins are shrunken and have a decreased diameter
Nonechoic or hypoechoic	May be as hyperechoic as the surrounding tissue
Elastic and may be floating in the middle of the vein	Inelastic and is adhered to the venous wall, often creating a characteristic wall thickness
Proximal end may be bullet shaped or may conform to the venous flow coming from a tributary	Less well defined proximal ending
Collaterals and venous recanalization not common	Collaterals and venous recanalization often observed

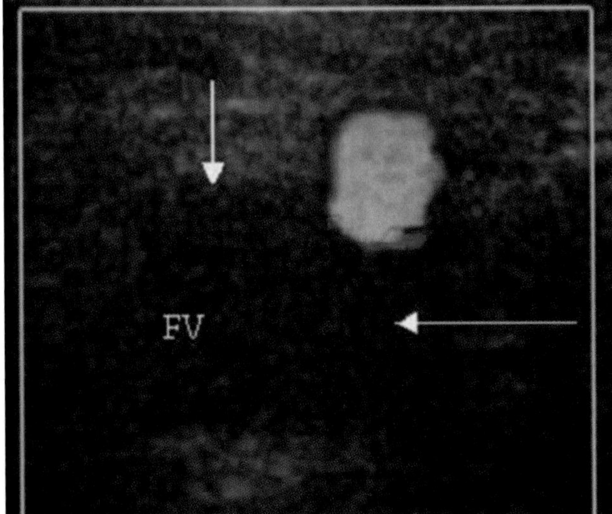

A

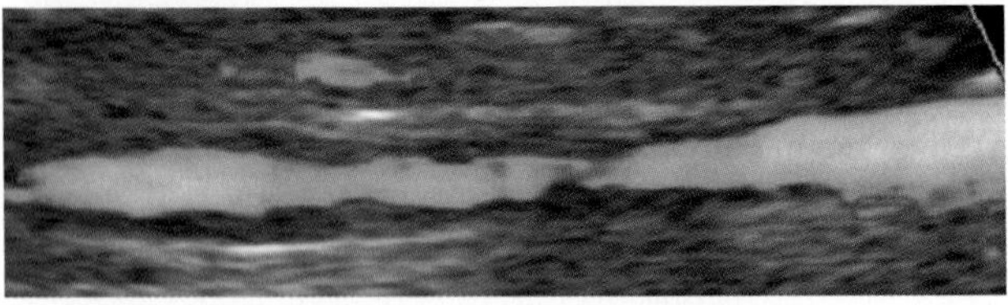

B

FIGURE 89.16 Differentiation between acute and chronic deep venous thrombosis (DVT). (*A*) An enlarged femoral vein is barely imaged underneath the femoral artery at mid to upper thigh; thrombus is hypoechoic, the vein is incompressible and no venous flow was detected. (*B*) A power Doppler image of a femoral vein with old thrombus and reflux; note the thickening of the venous wall.

about thrombus age. Detection of compression syndrome by the iliac arteries may require transcutaneous or intravascular US and MRV.[49]

MRV is a preferred technique to study the abdominal veins. MRV can elucidate thrombus in the abdominal veins versus tumors (Fig. 89.17).

Peritreatment Imaging

Although feasible and perhaps indicated as cost-effective, US imaging has not been exploited appropriately as a monitoring imaging modality during venous thrombolysis. Endovascular treatment of iliocaval compression syndrome has been monitored with intravascular US and venography (Fig. 89.18).[49]

A growing application of transcutaneous and intravascular US is in the bedside insertion of inferior vena cava filters (Fig. 89.19).[50] US permits localization of the renal arteries and veins, visualization of the guide wire, and catheter and device deployment and is not limited by body habitus or bowel gas. Double or single puncture techniques have been employed. With either technique, the objective is to identify the delivery position below the renal veins. With the single puncture technique, the delivery sheath is placed under IVUS guidance, the IVUS catheter is removed, the delivery catheter is inserted into the sheath, and the filter is deployed.

Patient Follow-Up

Patients at risk of developing DVT or pulmonary embolism have been tested numerous times during their hospitalization. Usually three negative tests in a period of 7 days indicate that the patient is a low risk for DVT. However, one complete negative examination has been found adequate to withhold anticoagulation. If the patient's conditions change during hospitalization, US should be repeated. Monitoring thrombus propagation after treatment has helped in decision making related to placement of a filter in the inferior or superior vena cava.

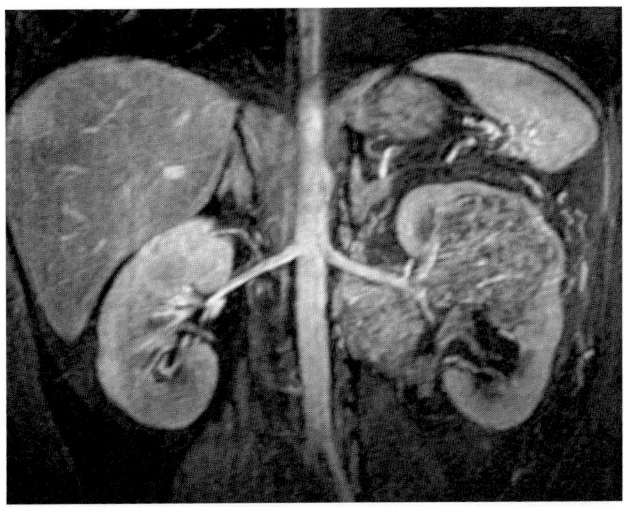

A

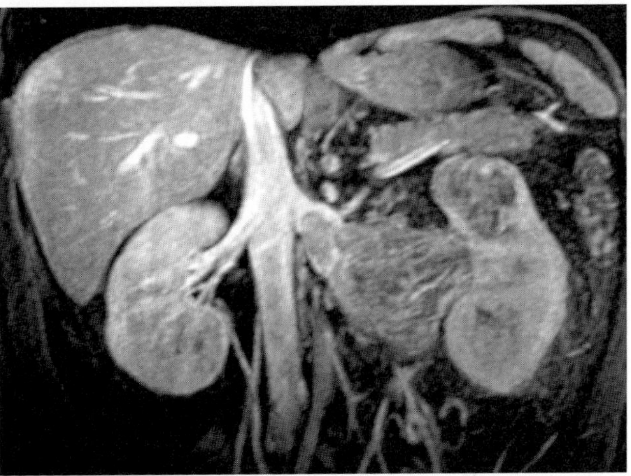

B

FIGURE 89.17 Magnetic resonance angiography (MRA): tumor invading the left renal vein. Arterial phase demonstrates presence of a tumor (*A*) while the venous phase image (*B*) further defines the tumor location to be in the left renal vein and also delineates the venous dilation secondary to tumor growth. (Courtesy of Frank J Londy, R.T.(R), University of Michigan Medical Center.)

CHRONIC VENOUS INSUFFICIENCY

The advent of endovascular treatment of the saphenous veins with laser or radiofrequency ablation has perked the interest of many medical specialists. Telangiectasias (spider veins), reticular veins, varicose veins, and perforating veins can be treated with a variety of techniques. Banding, ligation, stripping, endovascular or percutaneous foam or liquid sclerotherapy, and endovascular ablation or obliteration have been used to treat the saphenous vein. Perforating veins have been treated with subfascial endoscopic perforator surgery (SEPS), sclerotherapy, ligation, or disruption. The ease of application of many of these therapies may lead to unnecessary treatment if proper diagnostic and preoperative mapping protocols are not followed rigorously. Proper classification of patients and detailed US mapping are recommended. The *c*linical-*e*tiological-*a*natomic-*p*athophysiology (CEAP) classification is recommended to record clinical, etiologic, anatomic, and pathophysiologic aspects of chronic venous insufficiency (CVI) of the lower extremities (Table 89.2).[51]

Screening

US screening for chronic venous obstruction includes evaluation of the common femoral, midfemoral, popliteal, above-knee great saphenous, below-knee great saphenous, and small saphenous veins. Patency, obstruction, and reflux should be recorded. Standard recommendation is to perform the US examination with the patient standing. If the disease is advanced, however, the examination is performed in the supine position after lowering the foot-side of the bed about 10 to 20 degrees. This reverse Trendelenburg position improves venous filling with blood and facilitates visualization of otherwise collapsed veins. Patency is documented with color flow. Obstruction is demonstrated with B-mode, gray scale imaging. Partial obstruction is shown by a combination of color flow and B-mode findings. Reverse flow is observed following compression proximal to the site of observation or following release of distal compression, while the patient is standing. Reverse flow is considered reflux if longer than 1 second in the deep veins and longer than 0.5 second in the superficial veins.[52]

Definitive Diagnosis

Definitive diagnosis requires expansion of US imaging to properly document extension of venous obstruction. Detection of

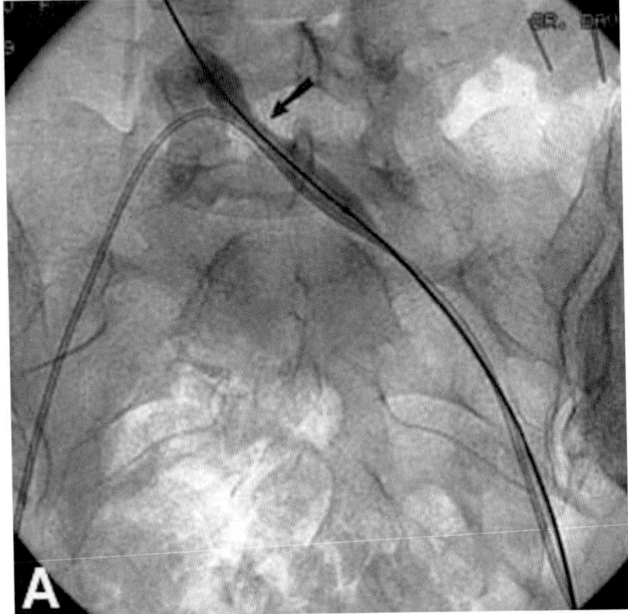

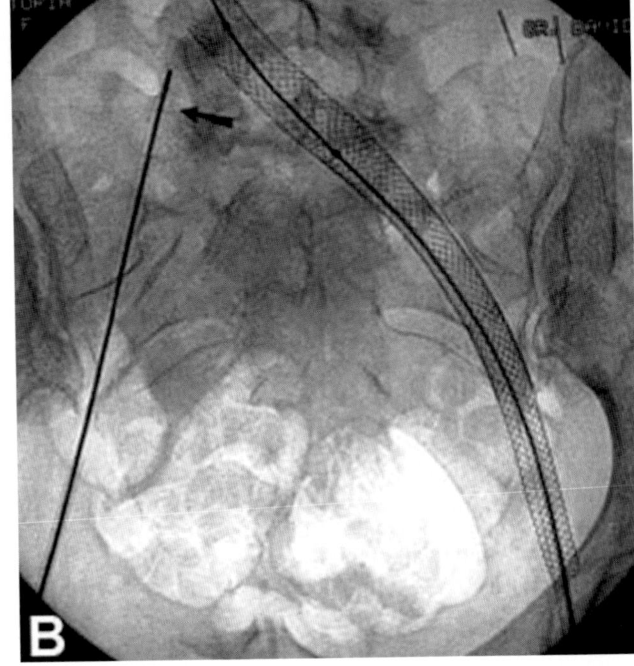

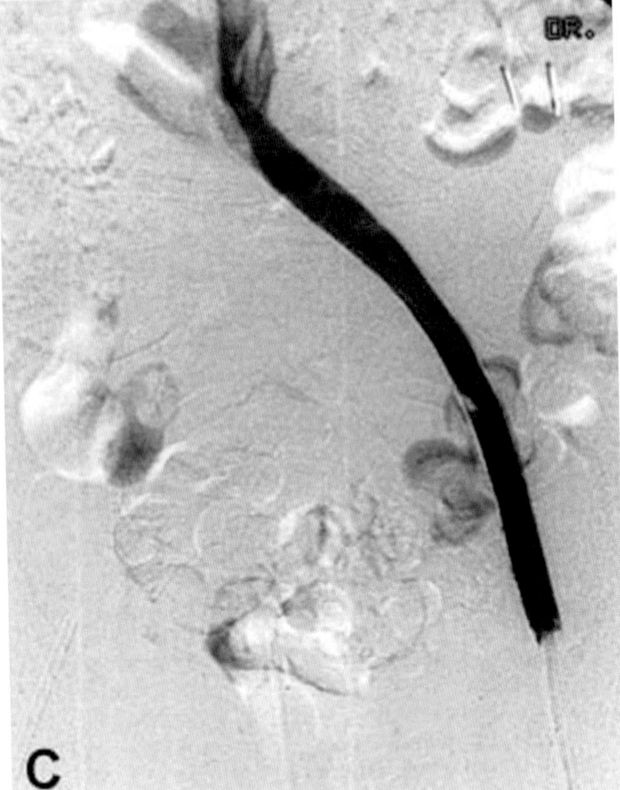

FIGURE 89.18 (*A*) Balloon angioplasty of left common iliac vein stenosis (*arrows*) with 10 × 4-mm balloon catheter (patient 2). (*B*) Postdeployment radiograph of 14/40 mm, 10/68 mm, and 10/38 mm Wall stents in left common and external iliac veins with reduction of gradient from 4 to 0 mm Hg. Note intravenous ultrasound (IVUS) catheter in right common iliac vein (*arrow*), which was used to monitor placement of the caval end of common iliac vein stent. (*C*) Postdeployment venogram demonstrating widely patent left common and external iliac veins with no residual stenosis. (From Hurst DR, Forauer AR, Bloom JR, et al. Diagnosis and endovascular treatment of iliocaval compression syndrome. *J Vasc Surg*. 2001;34:106, with permission.)

reflux is expanded to include the evaluation of the saphenofemoral and saphenopopliteal junctions. Observation of reflux in superficial veins in the anterior, lateral, and posterior aspects of the calf and thigh complement the evaluation of the saphenous veins. Evaluation of nonsaphenous veins approaching the gluteal and pelvic regions may lead to the suspicion of pelvic congestion syndrome.

Perforating veins are evaluated in the medial, anterior, lateral, and posterior aspects of the calf and thigh.[53] Most commonly, perforating veins are detected in the medial aspect. Perforating and communicating veins may belong to a complex network of superficial vessels. Following all abnormal, visible, superficial veins is tedious, time consuming, and unnecessary. Documentation of nonvisible, nonpalpable varicose veins in the groin, thigh, and even the calf is recommended.

Photo-plethysmography (PPG) is another noninvasive technique that can aid in characterizing venous insufficiency. Local changes in skin blood flow are detected by a probe placed on the leg with a light-sensitivity diode. Red blood cells within the dermis absorb maximum light when the pressure is

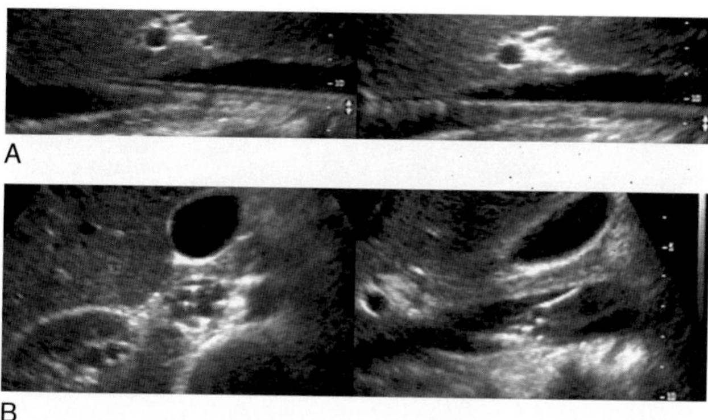

FIGURE 89.19 Inferior vena cava filter deployment under ultrasound guidance. (*A*) Catheter and device inside vein. (*B*) The filter already deployed in transverse (*left*) and longitudinal (*right*) sections. (Courtesy of Andrew Seiwert, MD, and Linda Jones, RVT.)

high and the veins are full, and it is this fact that drives this test. PPG has high sensitivity but only intermediate specificity for diagnosing CVI. If positive, further characterization is necessary and an aggressive intervention is anticipated, such as surgical intervention. If negative, it is strongly predictive of the absence of venous reflux. The level of venous reflux is determined using tourniquets on specific areas of the leg.

Air-plethysmography (APG) is a more discriminating study.[54,55] It has the ability to measure venous reflux, calf muscle pump function, and the presence or absence of outflow obstruction. This test has both high sensitivity and specificity. The concept of APG is that the leg is surrounded by a polyurethane sleeve, which contains expandable air-filled chambers that are connected to a pressure transducer. This allows volume measurements to be made with accuracy based on pressure transduction calibrations. Volume changes are measured once the patient changes from a supine to a standing position.

Measurements made with APG include indices of reflux, specifically venous volume (VV) and venous filling index (VFI), with and without superficial occlusion. VFI is a measurement of volume change per unit time. Increasing VFI is highly associated with the prevalence of skin changes and ulceration. Calf muscle pump function can be assessed with ejection volume and ejection fraction. To obtain the ejection fraction, the patient is asked to perform a toe raise. The ejection fraction, like the VFI, is an important predictor of which patients will develop skin ulceration. Residual volume is measured after 10 toe raises. The residual volume fraction is most correlated with ambulatory venous pressure. Finally, venous outflow is assessed measuring the outflow fraction with the patient supine. Venous flow is obstructed with cuff inflation at the thigh level. The outflow fraction per unit time, measured after cuff deflation, indicates degree of resistance to venous outflow. The benefit of APG in clinical practice is that it provides an understanding of the different components contributing to the overall severity of venous insufficiency including reflux, calf muscle pump function, and obstruction. It is an objective evaluation of nonoperative therapies, or pre- and postoperative hemodynamic assessments. For example, it was demonstrated, using APG assessment, that various compression stockings are more effective in controlling reflux compared with calf muscle function in patients with less severe CVI. Patients with more severe CVI benefited more from improved calf muscle pump function than reflux control.[56]

TABLE 89.2 CLASSIFICATION

CEAP CLASSIFICATION OF CHRONIC VENOUS INSUFFICENCY

Grade	Description
CLINICAL PRESENTATION	
C1	Telangiectasias and reticular veins
C2	Varicose veins
C3	Edema
C4a	Skin pigmentation or eczema
C4b	Lipodermatosclerosis or atrophic blanch
C5	Healed or
C6	Nonhealed ulcers
ETIOLOGY	
Ec	Congenital
Ep	Primary or unknown
Es	Secondary to thrombosis, trauma, or other known cause
ANATOMY	
Ad	Deep
As	Superficial
Ap	Perforating veins
PATHOPHYSIOLOGY	
Po	Obstruction[a]
Pr	Reflux

[a]Obstructive disease should be clearly separated from primary valvular insufficiency.

Preoperative Mapping

Detailed documentation of sources and drainage of saphenous vein reflux affects the type of treatment performed. Multiple types of great saphenous vein reflux have been described (Table 89.3 and Fig. 89.20). A similar classification has been described for the small saphenous vein. In addition, the vein of Giacomini, the extension of the small saphenous vein into the thigh, must be evaluated in conjunction with the small saphenous vein.

Patterns of reflux are associated with changes in vein diameter.[57] Veins with diffuse or proximal reflux have larger diameters than veins with segmental or distal reflux. Reflux is probable in saphenofemoral junction (SFJ) greater than 8 mm in diameter, thigh segments of the great saphenous greater than 6 mm and calf veins, saphenous or perforating, greater than 4 mm.

Almost half of the women with telangiectasias have reflux in the saphenous vein. Segmental reflux is the most common pattern of reflux in women and men with telangiectasias or simple varicose veins. The SFJ is rarely refluxing. As the disease progresses causing edema and skin changes, involvement of a refluxing SFJ becomes more common. In patients with lipodermatosclerosis one should expect abnormal, refluxing perforating veins.

Intraoperative Imaging

US imaging is an integral part of laser or radiofrequency ablation protocols. The vein being treated is cannulated, the catheter is positioned (e.g., near the SFJ), and the results of the ablation are checked under US visualization (Fig. 89.21). Sclerotherapy of varicose or perforating veins, foam therapy

VASCULAR

TABLE 89.3 CLASSIFICATION

CLASSIFICATION OF GREAT SAPHENOUS VEIN REFLUX

Type	Description
Perijunction	From the saphenofemoral junction of a vein other than the great saphenous or from a tributary of the saphenofemoral junction to the great saphenous or other veins in the vicinity of the junction
Proximal	From the saphenofemoral junction to a tributary or perforating vein in the thigh or even upper calf
Distal	From a tributary or perforating vein down to the ankle level
Segmental	From a tributary or perforating vein proximally to another tributary or perforating vein distally
Multiple segmental	Including or not including the saphenofemoral junction
Diffuse	From the saphenofemoral junction to the ankle level

of saphenous veins, and perforating vein ligation or disruption can also be performed under US guidance.

Patient Follow-Up

Regardless of the treatment performed, recurrence has been documented. The unknown is what type, when, where, and how bad clinically is the recurrence. The channels of stripped or ablated saphenous veins have reopened, at least partially. Neovascularization or vessel networks composed of small arteries and veins have been described.[58] New telangiectasias have surfaced. Reverse flow can be detected in recanalized or untreated segments with constituting pathologic reflux. Thrombus has been detected in the immediate or late postoperative period. Arterialized, pulsatile flow with high diastolic component has been detected inside or alongside partially thrombosed veins. Thrombus has expanded to the common femoral vein after ablation without ligation. Overall, however, highly successful treatment has resulted in the disappearance of the vein with most symptomatic patients being pleased following ablation therapy. Follow-up is still too short to properly evaluate the long-term effects of new endovascular treatments.

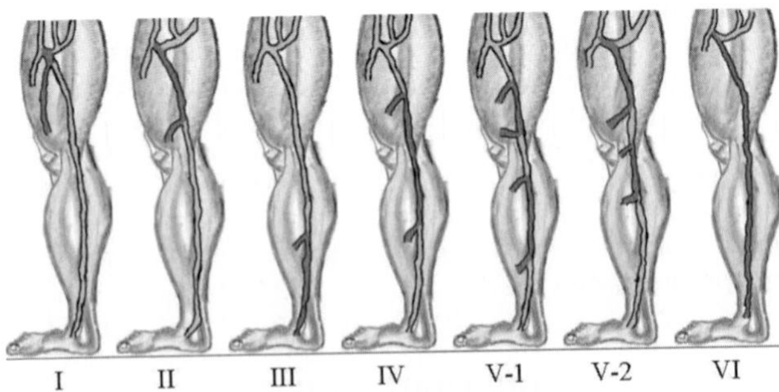

FIGURE 89.20 Types of great saphenous vein (GSV) reflux. Left to right: I: Perijunction, not involving the GSV; II: Proximal; III: Distal; IV: Segmental; V-1: Multisegmental, not involving the saphenofemoral junction (SFJ); V-2: Multisegmental with the SJF as the main source; and VI: Diffuse from the SFJ to the ankle level. (Drawings courtesy of Monique Salles-Cunha.)

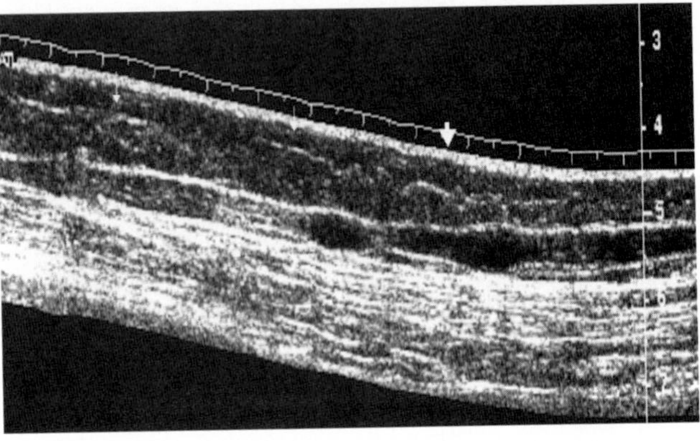

FIGURE 89.21 Ultrasound expanded field of view demonstrating atretic segments (*thin arrows*) and thrombosed sinus (*thick arrow*) after radiofrequency ablation of a refluxing great saphenous vein in the thigh. (From Salles-Cunha SX, Rajasinghe H, Dosick SM, et al. Fate of great saphenous vein after radio-frequency ablation: detailed ultrasound imaging. *Vasc Endovasc Surg.* 2004;38:339–344, with permission.)

Importantly, although CVI may often be ameliorated with a single treatment, it may require multiple treatment sessions.

KEY POINTS

- **Vascular imaging can be performed with a variety of technologies.**
- **US as a screening method is capable of providing definitive diagnosis for most vascular pathologies of peripheral vessels.**
- **Although preoperative mapping of the extracranial carotid and peripheral arteries has been successfully performed in select centers, arteriography remains the standard.**
- **MRA and CTA are emerging noninvasive technologies with a broad range of applications.**
- **US may replace or complement completion arteriography in the operating room.**
- **US has been employed successfully during endovascular procedures, particularly for the treatment of saphenous vein reflux.**
- **US has achieved dominance in all testing objectives regarding peripheral veins but remains inadequate for complete evaluation of the abdominal vasculature.**
- **MRV has definite advantages for evaluation of abdominal veins.**
- **US remains cost-effective in the follow-up of the vascular patient.**
- **Three-dimensional CTA models have emerged as the most informative method of preoperative mapping and follow-up of the patient with abdominal aortic aneurysms.**

References

1. Beneficial effect of carotid endarterectomy in symptomatic patients with high-grade carotid stenosis. North American Symptomatic Carotid Endarterectomy Trial Collaborators. *N Engl J Med.* 1991;325:445.
2. Endarterectomy for asymptomatic carotid artery stenosis. Executive Committee for the Asymptomatic Carotid Atherosclerosis Study. *JAMA* 1995;273:1421.
3. Hobson RW II. Rationale and status of randomized controlled clinical trials in carotid artery stenting. *Semin Vasc Surg.* 2003;16:311.
4. Lavenson GS Jr, Pantera RL, Garza RM, et al. Development and implementation of a rapid, accurate, and cost-effective protocol for national stroke prevention screening. *Am J Surg.* 2004;188:638.
5. Ahmed M, Masaryk TJ. Imaging of acute stroke: state of the art. *Semin Vasc Surg.* 2004;17:181.

6. Beebe HG, Salles-Cunha SX, Scissons RP, et al. Carotid arterial ultrasound scan imaging: a direct approach to stenosis measurement. *J Vasc Surg.* 1999; 29:838.
7. Fillinger MF, Baker RJ Jr, Zwolak RM, et al. Carotid duplex criteria for a 60% or greater angiographic stenosis: variation according to equipment. *J Vasc Surg.* 1996;24:856.
8. Faught WE, Mattos MA, van Bemmelen PS, et al. Color-flow duplex scanning of carotid arteries: new velocity criteria based on receiver operator characteristic analysis for threshold stenoses used in the symptomatic and asymptomatic carotid trials. *J Vasc Surg.* 1994;19:818.
9. Moneta GL, Edwards JM, Chitwood RW, et al. Correlation of North American Symptomatic Carotid Endarterectomy Trial (NASCET) angiographic definition of 70% to 99% internal carotid artery stenosis with duplex scanning. *J Vasc Surg.* 1993;17:152.
10. Biasi GM, Froio A, Diethrich EB, et al. Carotid plaque echolucency increases the risk of stroke in carotid stenting: the Imaging in Carotid Angioplasty and Risk of Stroke (ICAROS) study. *Circulation* 2004;110:756.
11. Kramer CM. Magnetic resonance imaging to identify the high-risk plaque. *Am J Cardiol.* 2002;90(10C):15L.
12. Cinat M, Lane CT, Pham H, et al. Helical CT angiography in the preoperative evaluation of carotid artery stenosis. *J Vasc Surg.* 1998;28:290.
13. Wain RA, Lyon RT, Veith FJ, et al. Accuracy of duplex ultrasound in evaluating carotid artery anatomy before endarterectomy. *J Vasc Surg.* 1998; 27:235.
14. Valenti D, Gaggiano A, Berardi G, et al. Intra-operative assessment of technical defects after carotid endarterectomy: a comparison between angiography and colour duplex scan. *Cardiovasc Surg.* 2003;11:26.
15. Criqui MH. Peripheral arterial disease—epidemiological aspects. *Vasc Med.* 2001;6[3 suppl]:3.
16. Salles-Cunha SX, Andros G. Preoperative duplex scanning prior to infrainguinal revascularization. *Surg Clin North Am.* 1990;70:41.
17. Ascher E, Hingorani A, Markevich N, et al. Role of duplex arteriography as the sole preoperative imaging modality prior to lower extremity revascularization surgery in diabetic and renal patients. *Ann Vasc Surg.* 2004;18:433.
18. Eiberg JP, Lundorf E, Thomsen C, et al. Peripheral vascular surgery and magnetic resonance arteriography: a review. *Eur J Vasc Endovasc Surg.* 2001;22:396.
19. Schoenberg SO, Londy FJ, Licato P, et al. Multiphase-multistep gadolinium-enhanced MR angiography of the abdominal aorta and runoff vessels. *Invest Radiol.* 2001;36:283.
20. Pierce G. Basics of computed tomography angiography of the lower extremity vessels. *Semin Vasc Surg.* 2004;17:102.
21. Moneta GL, Yeager RA, Lee RW, Porter JM. Noninvasive localization of arterial occlusive disease: a comparison of segmental Doppler pressure and arterial duplex mapping. *J Vasc Surg.* 1993;17:578.
22. Gale SS, Scissons RP, Salles-Cunha SX, et al. Lower extremity arterial evaluation: are segmental arterial blood pressures worthwhile? *J Vasc Surg.* 1998;27:831.
23. Ascher E, Salles-Cunha SX, Hingorani A, Markevich N. Duplex ultrasound arterial mapping before infrainguinal revascularization. In: Mansour A, Labropoulos N, eds. *Vascular diagnosis.* Philadelphia: Elsevier-Saunders, 2004, p. 237.
24. Kupinski AM, Evans SM, Khan AM, et al. Ultrasonic characterization of the saphenous vein. *Cardiovasc Surg.* 1993;1:513.
25. Salles-Cunha SX, Andros G, Harris RW, et al. Preoperative, noninvasive assessment of arm veins to be used as bypass grafts in the lower extremities. *J Vasc Surg.* 1986;3:813.
26. Sands MJ, Levitin A. Basics of magnetic resonance imaging. *Semin Vasc Surg.* 2004;17:66.
27. Johnson BL, Bandyk DF, Back MR, et al. Intraoperative duplex monitoring of infrainguinal vein bypass procedures. *J Vasc Surg.* 2000;31:678.
28. Roth SM, Bandyk DF. Duplex imaging of lower extremity bypasses, angioplasties, and stents. *Semin Vasc Surg.* 1999;12:275.
29. Diwan A, Sarkar R, Stanley JC, et al. Incidence of femoral and popliteal artery aneurysms in patients with abdominal aortic aneurysms. *J Vasc Surg.* 2000;31:863.
30. Ascher E, Markevich N, Schutzer RW, et al. Small popliteal artery aneurysms: are they clinically significant? *J Vasc Surg.* 2003;37:755.
31. Gale SS, Scissons RP, Jones L, Salles-Cunha SX. Femoral pseudoaneurysm "thrombinjection." *Am J Surg.* 2001;181:379.
32. Prince MR, Narasimham DL, Stanley JC, et al. Gadolinium-enhanced magnetic resonance angiography of the abdominal aortic aneurysms. *J Vasc Surg.* 1995;21:656.
33. Beebe HG, Kritpracha B. Computed tomography scanning for endograft planning: evolving toward three-dimensional, single source imaging. *Semin Vasc Surg.* 2004;17:126.
34. Fillinger MF, Weaver JB. Imaging equipment and techniques for optimal intraoperative imaging during endovascular interventions. *Semin Vasc Surg.* 1999;12:315.
35. Lee JT, White RA. Basics of intravascular ultrasound: an essential tool for the endovascular surgeon. *Semin Vasc Surg.* 2004;17:110.
36. Kritpracha B, Beebe HG, Comerota AJ. Aortic diameter is an insensitive measurement of early aneurysm expansion after endografting. *J Endovasc Ther.* 2004;11:184.
37. Bendick PJ, Zelenock GB, Bove PG, et al. Duplex ultrasound imaging with an ultrasound contrast agent: the economic alternative to CT angiography for aortic stent graft surveillance. *Vasc Endovascular Surg.* 2003;37:165.
38. Schneider PA, Ogawa DY. Is routine preoperative aortoiliac arteriography necessary in the treatment of lower extremity ischemia? *J Vasc Surg.* 1998;28:38.
39. Zwolak RM. Can duplex ultrasound replace arteriography in screening for mesenteric ischemia? *Semin Vasc Surg.* 1999;12:252.
40. Moneta GL. Screening for mesenteric vascular insufficiency and follow-up of mesenteric artery bypass procedures. *Semin Vasc Surg.* 2001;14:186.
41. Prince MR, Schoenberg SO, Ward JS, et al. Hemodynamically significant atherosclerotic renal artery stenosis: MR angiographic features. *Radiology* 1997;205:128.
42. Oderich GS, Panneton JM, Macedo TA, et al. Intraoperative duplex ultrasound of visceral revascularizations: optimizing technical success and outcome. *J Vasc Surg.* 2003;38:684.
43. Dougherty MJ, Hallett JW Jr, Naessens JM, et al. Optimizing technical success of renal revascularization: the impact of intraoperative color-flow duplex ultrasonography. *J Vasc Surg.* 1993;17:849.
44. Salles-Cunha SX, Beebe HG. Direct noninvasive tests (duplex scan) for evaluation of acute venous disease. In: Gloviczki P, Yao JST, eds. *Handbook of venous disorders,* 2nd ed. Guidelines of the American Venous Forum. London: Arnold; 2001:110.
45. Emelianov SY, Chen X, O'Donnel M, et al. Triplex ultrasound: elasticity imaging to age deep venous thrombosis. *Ultrasound Med Biol.* 2002;28:757.
46. Muller C, Muller R, Andros G, Salles-Cunha SX. Pitfalls in the comparison of phlebographic and ultrasonic-based diagnosis in the evaluation of the lower extremity. *J Vasc Technol.* 1992;16:136.
47. Peterson DA, Kazerooni EA, Wakefield TW, et al. Computed tomographic venography is specific but not sensitive for diagnosis of acute lower-extremity deep venous thrombosis in patients with suspected pulmonary embolism. *J Vasc Surg.* 2001;34:798.
48. Froelich JB, Prince MR, Greenfield LJ, et al. "Bull's-eye" sign on gadolinium-enhanced magnetic resonance venography determines thrombus presence and age: a preliminary study. *J Vasc Surg.* 1997;26:809.
49. Hurst DR, Forauer AR, Bloom JR, et al. Diagnosis and endovascular treatment of iliocaval compression syndrome. *J Vasc Surg.* 2001;34:106.
50. Garrett JV, Passman MA, Guzman RJ, et al. Expanding options for bedside placement of inferior vena cava filters with intravascular ultrasound when trans-abdominal ultrasound imaging inadequate. *Ann Vasc Surg.* 2004;18:329.
51. Eklof B, Rutherford RB, Bergan JJ, et al, for the American Venous Forum International Ad Hoc Committee for Revision of the CEAP Classification. Revision of the CEAP classification for chronic venous disorders: consensus statement. *J Vasc Surg.* 2004;40:1248.
52. Labropoulos N, Tiongson J, Pryor L, et al. Definition of venous reflux in lower-extremity veins. *J Vasc Surg.* 2003;38:793.
53. Sandri JL, Barros FS, Pontes S, et al. Diameter-reflux relationship in perforating veins of patients with varicose veins. *J Vasc Surg.* 1999;30:867.
54. Christopoulos D, Nicolaides AN, Szendro G. Venous reflux: quantification and correlation with the clinical severity of chronic venous disease. *Br J Surg.* 1988;75:352.
55. Bays RA. Healy DA. Atnip RG, et al. Validation of air plethysmography, photoplethysmography, and duplex ultrasonography in the evaluation of severe venous stasis. *J Vasc Surg.* 1994;20:721.
56. Zaijkowski PJ, Proctor MC, Wakefield TW, et al. Compression stockings and venous function. *Arch Surg.* 2002;137:1064.
57. Engelhorn C, Engelhorn A, Salles-Cunha S, et al. Relationship between reflux and greater saphenous vein diameter. *J Vasc Technol.* 1997;21:167.
58. Salles-Cunha SX, Comerota AJ, Tzilinis A, et al. Ultrasound findings after radiofrequency ablation of the great saphenous vein: descriptive analysis. *J Vasc Surg.* 2004;40:1166.

CHAPTER 90 ■ ENDOVASCULAR TREATMENT OF DISEASE

MATTHEW J. EAGLETON AND SUNITA D. SRIVASTAVA

The treatment of vascular disease has progressed significantly over the past several years with the evolution and application of endovascular procedures. In particular, the endovascular treatments of aortic aneurysmal disease and carotid artery stenosis have received intense scrutiny. Intravascular treatment of disease, however, is not a new concept. In the 1960s, radiologist Charles Dotter pioneered the concept of endovascular therapy.[1] He conceived the idea of using dilators of varying diameters to serially expand stenotic atherosclerotic lesions in the iliac arteries. Since then, the technology has continued to evolve. The development of guide wire-directed catheter technology has allowed physicians to percutaneously access nearly any blood vessel in the body. This combined with the development of the angioplasty balloon revolutionized percutaneous interventions and allowed for the treatment of stenotic lesions through a percutaneous arterial puncture. This procedure has been further enhanced by the development of metallic stents to assist in maintaining long-term patency of percutaneous angioplasty. With advancing technology, more endovascular procedures are being applied to the treatment of peripheral vascular disease. The goal of this chapter is to outline many of the applications of endovascular therapies for the treatment peripheral vascular disease including technical aspects, complications, and outcomes.

BASIC CONCEPTS

The basic concept of most endovascular procedures is to obtain percutaneous access of a blood vessel and then to gain access across the lesion (either a stenosis or aneurysm) with a guide wire. This allows for endovascular treatment of the problem. Most arterial and venous access is obtained through a percutaneous puncture over the femoral vessels. From this location, most other branches of the arterial tree can be reached. Access from the femoral vessels, however, is not always possible or ideal, and in those instances percutaneous access is generally obtained through a brachial vessel puncture. Once blood vessel access is obtained, a guide wire is inserted through the needle and into the artery or vein. Generally, the needle is then removed and a sheath is placed into the vessel over the wire. A sheath is a specialized piece of equipment, with a valve on one end, which allows continuous access to the blood vessel. This allows for continued introduction and removal of a variety of pieces of equipment while protecting the vessel wall from repeated trauma. Sheaths are available in a variety of sizes and a variety of shapes, and the exact sheath used depends on the procedure being performed and the blood vessel being accessed (Fig. 90.1).

The next tool to consider once a secured entry into the blood vessel is obtained is the guide wire, which allows remote access across the lesion. Guide wires are constructed in a variety of sizes; the three most commonly used sizes are 0.035-, 0.018-, and 0.014-inch diameter. The length of the guide wire is also important and generally varies from 145 to 300 cm. The guide wire length needs to be long enough to cover the cumulative distance required both inside and outside the patient. This will vary based on lesion location, the type of procedure performed, and the type of other pieces of technology being used. There are several factors that are important in guide wire construction and include the stiffness of the wire, the coating on the wire, and the tip shape (see Fig. 90.1). Some of these factors affect the steerability and trackability of the wire. Steerability refers to the ability to direct the intravascular tip of the wire by manipulating the extravascular portion, and trackability refers to the ability of the wire to allow a catheter to follow its course. The tip of the wire may be straight, angled, or J-tipped, and the tip may be stiff or floppy, making it less traumatic. Many wires have a tightly wound inner steel core that confers differing magnitudes of stiffness to the body of the guide wire. A surrounding wrap of lighter, more flexible wire helps prevent fracture and fragmentation while the guide wire is in use. Most guide wires have a hydrophilic coating of either polytetrafluoroethylene or silicone, which decreases the coefficient of friction during catheter exchange or while traversing a stenosis.

Catheters are another vital piece of equipment important in performing endovascular procedures. They are used to perform diagnostic procedures, maintain access across a lesion while a more suitable wire is exchanged, and support devices such as balloons and stents that are delivered to the lesion attached to the catheter. Catheters are constructed from a variety of materials including polyurethane, polyethylene, polypropylene, and nylon. Catheters are also available in a variety of diameters [measured in French (F)] and lengths. Catheters constructed from polyethylene have a low coefficient of friction and are pliable with good shape memory. They are useful for selective catheterization. Polyurethane catheters are softer, more pliable, and follow guide wires more easily but have a higher coefficient of friction. Nylon catheters are stiffer but tolerate higher flow rates. The construction of the catheter affects several important properties that include trackability (the ability of the catheter to follow the direction of the wire), pushability (the ability of force applied on one end of the catheter to induce movement on the other end), crossability (the facility with which a catheter will follow the wire across a lesion), and steerability. The shape of the catheter's head is variable and dictates the catheter's function (see Fig. 90.1). Functionally catheters are classified as selective or non-selective. Nonselective catheters, also known as flush catheters, often have multiple side holes that allow large amount of contrast to exit in a short period of time. These catheters' head shapes are usually either straight or curved. Selective catheters have only one end hole but are available in a variety of shapes, including straight, angled, reverse curved, and double-curved. The choice of catheter used depends on the type of procedure being performed.

An important tool in endovascular procedures is the angioplasty balloon. This is a balloon mounted on the end of a

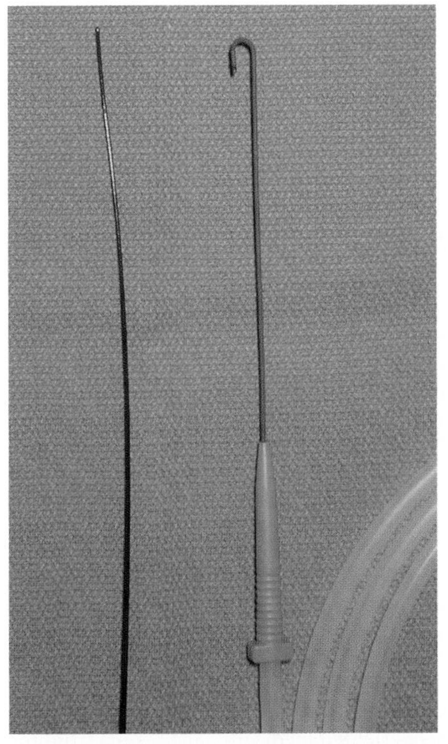

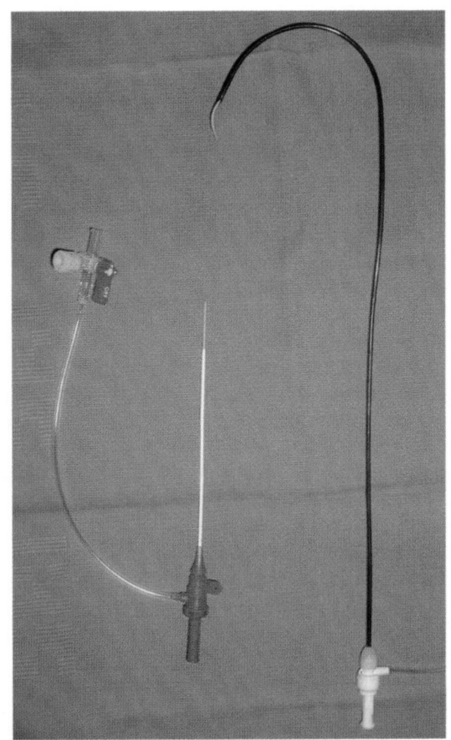

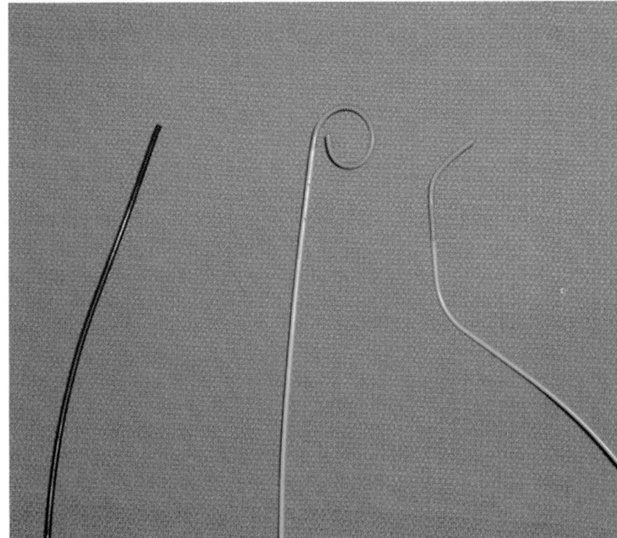

FIGURE 90.1 (*A*) An example of two different endovascular wires. The one on the left has a straight tip, and it is coated with a hydrophilic substance, which increases its maneuverability in stenotic lesions. The wire on the right has a J-tip on the end, which allows it to be less traumatic to the arterial wall. (*B*) An example of two different types of sheaths. The smaller sheath on the left is representative of the standard access sheath used for many endovascular procedures, whereas the larger one on the right demonstrates a more specialized sheath of a larger size with a preshaped curve. (C) An example of angiographic catheters. The catheter on the left represents a straight catheter that is hydrophilic coated. It is an end-hole catheter that is used for selective catheterization of vessels. The catheter in the middle is a nonselective catheter that has a "pigtail" shape. It has multiple side holes and is most generally used for nonselective angiography. The catheter on the right is also a selective catheter that has a preformed shape that allows the interventionalist the ability to access vessels in unique anatomic locations.

catheter that has the ability to be inflated and deflated through a port on the extravascular portion of the catheter (Fig. 90.2). The function of the angioplasty balloon is to provide a dilating force on the endoluminal surface of a blood vessel. As with all catheters, angioplasty balloon catheters are constructed with a number of variables, most specific to the balloon itself. Balloons vary in sizes that range from 1.5 to 40 mm, and they are selected with the intent to slightly overdilate the vessel being treated. The length of the balloon is also variable and can range from one to several centimeters in length. Typically there are radiopaque markers on either end of the balloon that allow for accurate placement at the site of the lesion. The rounded area of the balloon that extends beyond the markers is termed the "shoulder" of the balloon. The length of the shoulders of the balloon varies from balloon type to balloon type. In addition, balloons are constructed of a variety of types of material, which alters the way in which the balloons respond to inflation. Most balloons are constructed of polyethylene, polyethylene terephthalate, or other low-compliance polymers. These allow for a low or noncompliant balloon, which allows the balloon at high inflation pressures to exert more radial force without increasing the balloon diameter. Other balloons, particularly those used in aortic endografting, are more compliant and will continue to change diameter with increase pressure, thus reducing the radial force applied.

As discussed in more detail later, balloon angioplasty is often supplemented with the placement of an intravascular stent. The evolution of stents has occurred along two fundamental design philosophies: balloon-expandable stents and self-expanding stents (see Fig. 90.2). Stents are composed of a variety of metals including steel, nitinol, tantalum, platinum, and various metal alloys. The construction is also variable and includes laser-cut, woven, knitted, coiled, or welded. The construction of the stent helps to determine its properties. The ideal stent properties are high radial force, minimal induction of neointimal hyperplasia, longitudinal flexibility, high radiopacity, radial elasticity, ability to conform to the vessel, low profile with high expansion ratio, no foreshortening, durable, and affordable.[2] Balloon-expandable stents are best exemplified by the prototypical Palmaz stent. The basic mechanism is a metal tube (stent) placed around a balloon. The balloon is expanded thus dilating the metal tube, which then maintains the nominal diameter of the balloon. Most are made of stainless steel alloy providing greater radial and hoop strength with minimal foreshortening, which allows for exact placement. These same properties, however, allow little flexibility and render the stents susceptible to irreversible deformation when subjected to external compressive forces. The prototype of the self-expanding stents is the Wallstent. These stents function on the principle of elasticity, as the stents self-expand to their nominal diameter when released from a constrained state within the delivery catheter. A stent of a larger nominal diameter than the target vessel is chosen so that it exerts a continuous outward expansile force. The final diameter is the equilibrium that is reached between the elastic recoil of the vessel and the expansile force of the stent. Some general properties of self-expanding stents are that they are flexible, track better than balloon-expandable stents, and have crush resistance. Unfortunately, these stents foreshorten during placement and thus can only be accurately positioned at one end. With improving technology and the development of better alloys (e.g., nitinol, a nickel and titanium alloy), many of the adverse properties of both balloon- and self-expanding stents are overcome and they approach closer the properties of the ideal stent. As discussed in more detail later, the specific choice of stent to use in a given situation depends on the procedure being performed.

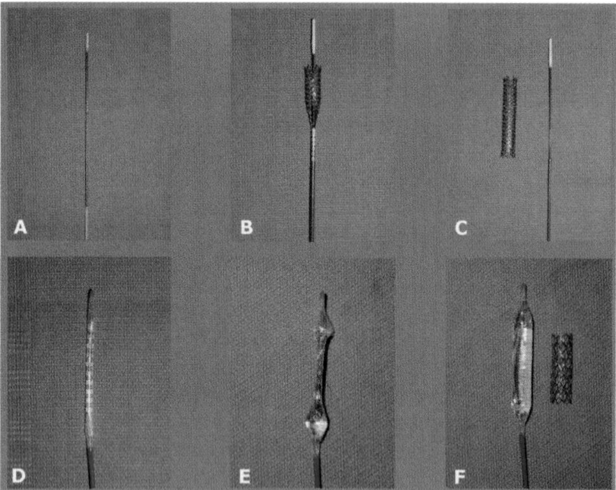

FIGURE 90.2 (*A, B, C*) These pictures depict a self-expanding stent at various stages of deployment. (*A*) The stent ensheathed on the catheter prior to deployment. (*B*) The stent partially deployed. Note the expansion of the stent in the unsheathed portion. (*C*) The self-expanding stent fully deployed. (*D, E, F*) These pictures depict a balloon-expandable stent at various stages of deployment. (*D*) The balloon-expandable stent mounted on a catheter prior to deployment and (*E*) at the start of expansion. (*F*) A fully expanded balloon-expandable stent adjacent to the inflated balloon used to deploy it.

CAROTID ARTERY INTERVENTIONS

Stroke occur in nearly 700,000 patients annually in the United States resulting in an estimated 164,000 deaths and contributing $54 billion in health-care costs.[3] Nearly one third of strokes are attributable to carotid artery stenosis, and nearly 200,000 carotid endarterectomies (CEAs) are performed each year in the United States to help prevent this debilitating problem.[4] The value of CEA to reduce the risk of stroke has been proven in a number of randomized, prospective clinical trials. CEA has been documented to reduce the incidence of both stroke and combined stroke and death in symptomatic patients with a stenosis greater than 70%.[5] In the North American Symptomatic Carotid Endarterectomy Trial, life-table estimates of the cumulative risk of any ipsilateral stroke at 2 years were 26% in patients treated with aspirin alone versus 9% in those patients treated with CEA. For major or fatal ipsilateral stroke the estimates were 13.1% and 2.5% for medical versus surgical treatment, respectively. For patients with asymptomatic disease, although the results are not as dramatic, there is a significant decrease in stroke risk with CEA versus medical therapy. The Asymptomatic Carotid Atherosclerosis Study randomized 4,657 patients with greater than 60% stenosis to receive either CEA or medical therapy.[4] The aggregate risk over 5 years for ipsilateral stroke and any perioperative stroke or death was 5.1% for surgical patients and 11.0% for patients treated medically. The results from the Asymptomatic Carotid Surgery Trial were very similar.[6] CEA has also proven durable, with reoperation for recurrent stenosis reported from as low as 1% to as high as 9%.

Endovascular treatment of carotid artery stenosis is less invasive and thus may be associated with a lower morbidity and mortality compared with CEA. The underlying indications for treatment of carotid artery stenosis do not change with the application of percutaneous techniques. However, carotid artery stenting must at least demonstrate clinical equipoise with CEA to become an accepted alternative. In the United States, most applications of carotid artery stenting currently are reserved for patients that are characterized as "high risk" for conventional CEA or in patients that are enrolled in ongoing clinical trials.

Percutaneous treatment of carotid artery stenosis was first described in 1980 by Kerber et al.[7] at which time they described the application of percutaneous transluminal balloon angioplasty (PTA) of an atherosclerotic lesion. Since that time the procedure has evolved tremendously and now includes the application of either a balloon-expandable or self-expanding stent. Currently, patients are premedicated with aspirin and either ticlopidine or clopidogrel at least 1 day prior to the procedure. Heparin anticoagulation is standard once arterial access has been obtained. The majority of the procedure does not differ significantly from the performance of PTA and stent placement at other sites. Percutaneous arterial access is obtained through a common femoral artery puncture. Brachial artery access is possible, although more difficult, if femoral access is prohibitive. Selective catheterization of the common carotid artery is performed utilizing one a variety of preformed catheters that best fit the anatomic variability. The common carotid artery is cannulated with a 6-F or 7-F introducer sheath or guide catheter. An inability to access the common carotid artery with these devices due to vessel tortuosity or anatomic variation is the principle cause of procedure failure. During advancement of the sheath, distal guide wire access is maintained in the external carotid artery. Guide wire access across the lesion in the internal carotid artery is then obtained. Occasionally, the lesion requires predilation with a smaller angioplasty balloon to facilitate placement of the stent. Little outcome variability has been described when comparing the placement of a balloon-expandable versus self-expanding stent, although most often self-expanding stents are placed due to the balloon-expandable stents vulnerability to compression.[8] If necessary, the stent is extended from the internal carotid artery into the common carotid artery effectively "jailing" the external carotid artery ostia.

One of the most catastrophic complications of carotid artery stenting is stroke, which is most often due to atheroemboli or thromboemboli dislodged at the time of the procedure. Unfortunately, unlike in peripheral interventions when a surgical therapy can often be used to correct an interventional complication, it is rare that an operation can correct distal cerebral embolization. To decrease the incidence of these complications, several cerebral protection devices have been developed and are utilized at the time of stent placement. Several series evaluating the efficacy of cerebral protection devices have shown up to an 80% reduction in the rate of acute neurologic events related to embolic complications compared with unprotected procedures.[9–12] There are a number of different types of cerebral protection devices, including distal occlusive balloons, distal filter systems, and proximal protection systems. The distal protection devices must cross the lesion prior to stent placement and before they are opened, thus some embolization may occur as they cross the lesion. Distal occlusive balloons consist of a 0.014-inch guide wire with the balloon on the distal portion. The balloon is inflated in the extracranial internal carotid artery distal to the lesion occluding blood flow (Fig. 90.3). After placement of the stent, stagnant blood and debris is suctioned from the region before blood flow is resumed by deflating the balloon. Distal filter systems are placed in a similar location but allow for continuous blood flow through the filter while it traps emboli. Proximal protection systems provide protection by occluding flow in the common carotid artery and external carotid artery. The collateral flow through the circle of Willis then provides a "back-pressure" that prevents distal embolization during the procedure. After stent placement, the blood in the internal carotid artery is then evacuated to prevent embolization of debris when antegrade flow is reestablished.

Carotid artery stent placement complications can be divided into three stages.[13] Stage I complications occur primarily during access of the common carotid artery. Stage II complications occur during positioning of the distal protection device in a straight cervical segment of the internal carotid artery. Stage III complications occur during predilation, stent deployment, and postdilation of the stent. When a neurologic event does occur, one should have an understanding of the cerebral circulation to proceed with neurologic rescue procedures.[14] In patients with a transient ischemic attack (TIA) or minor stroke and a normal angiogram, medical management should ensue. In patients with minor or major strokes and evidence of occlusion of an intracranial vessel, catheter-directed thrombolysis should be initiated and glycoprotein platelet receptor antagonists administered.[13]

As was stated earlier, in order for carotid artery stenting to gain full acceptance, it must provide clinical outcomes that rival CEA. Most of our knowledge about carotid stent outcomes is derived from single institution case series and registries. The first large series reported was by Yadav et al.[15] and included 126 carotid stenting procedures performed in 107 patients that were at high risk for CEA due to medical comorbidities. The 30-day incidence of ipsilateral major stroke and death was only 1.6%. At 6 months, however, there was a 4.9% incidence of asymptomatic restenosis. Lal et al.[15a] reported their results from 122 carotid stent procedures performed in 118 patients. Similarly, there was a low 30-day stroke and death rate of 3.3%. This analysis applied Kaplan-Meier curves and predicted cumulative in-stent restenosis, defined as a recurrent

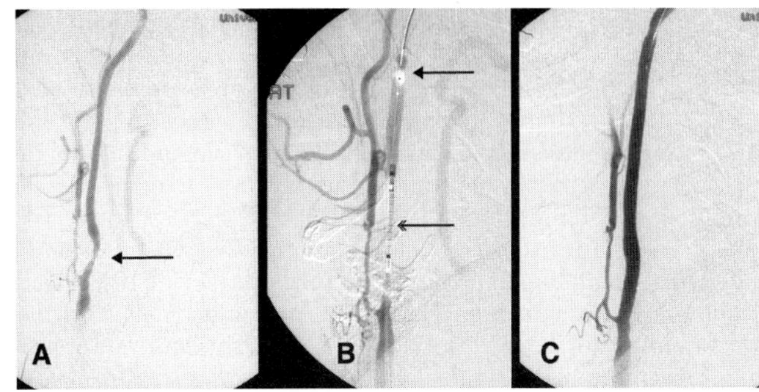

FIGURE 90.3 Angiograms from a patient undergoing a carotid artery stent. (*A*) There is an 85% recurrent stenosis within the internal carotid artery (*arrow*). The patient had undergone a carotid endarterectomy 1 year prior. (*B*) After wire access was obtained across the lesion, a balloon occlusion protection device was placed prior to angioplasty and stenting. This current angiogram shows placement of a self-expanding stent at the site of the internal carotid narrowing (*top arrow*). The balloon occlusion device can be seen in the distal internal carotid artery (*bottom arrow*). Note the absence of contrast beyond the protection device. After stent deployment and prior to balloon deflation, the contents of the common carotid artery and proximal internal carotid artery will be aspirated and discarded. (C) After stent deployment, there is resolution of the internal carotid artery narrowing.

stenosis greater than 80%, in 6.4% of the patients at 5 years. None was associated with onset of symptoms.

The largest collection of patients undergoing carotid artery stenting comes from a review of the Global Carotid Artery Stent Registry.[16] This report, from 53 participating centers in Europe, South and North America, and Asia, is based on a survey questioning the performance and complications of carotid artery stenting. The registry began in 1997 and since then has accrued 12,392 procedures in 11,243 patients. The technical success rate was 98.9%, with technical success defined as less than 30% residual stenosis. Thirty-day complication rates were 3.07% for TIA, 2.14% for minor strokes, 1.2% for major strokes, and 0.64% for deaths. Thirty-day combined stroke and procedure-related death rate was 3.98%. In support of the use of cerebral protection devices, 4,221 patients underwent carotid artery stenting with cerebral protection resulting in a stroke and procedure related death rate of 2.23% compared with 6,753 patients who underwent a procedure without cerebral protection and had a rate of 5.29%. This difference was consistent even when patients were stratified into those that were treated for symptomatic disease and those that were asymptomatic. Restenosis rates of 5.6% were reported at 48 months, although because of the registry format Kaplan-Meier curves were not possible. A 48-month neurologic event rate was reported at 4.5%. Multiple other registries, including ARCHER (Acculink for Revascularization of the Carotids in High Risk Patients), CABERNET (Carotid Artery Revascularization using the Boston Scientific EPI Filter Wire EX/EZ and the EndoTex Nex Stent), BEACH (Boston Scientific EPI-A Carotid Stenting Trial for High Risk Surgical Patients), SHELTER (Stenting of High Risk Patients Extracranial Lesions with Emboli Removal), and MAVERIC (Evaluation of the Medtronic AVE Self-Expanding Carotid Stent with Distal Protection in the Treatment of Carotid Stenosis), are based on high-risk entry criteria.

To better evaluate the outcomes of carotid artery stenting, in particular compared with CEA, several randomized trials have been organized and are currently underway. The first large trial of carotid angioplasty was the Carotid and Vertebral Artery Transluminal Angioplasty Study (CAVATAS).[17] This study enrolled a total of 504 patients; however, only 55 of the 251 patients treated percutaneously underwent stent placement and in no patient was cerebral protection used. The most recent randomized trial to present results was the Stenting and Angioplasty with Protection in Patients at High Risk for Endarterectomy (SAPPHIRE).[18] The goal of this trial was to compare the safety and effectiveness of carotid artery stenting with embolic protection to CEA in high-risk patients. Patients were eligible if they had a greater than 50% stenosis and were symptomatic or had a greater than 80% stenosis and were asymptomatic. High-risk was defined as patients with at least one of the following criteria: contralateral carotid artery occlusion, radiation therapy to the neck, previous CEA with recurrent stenosis, contralateral laryngeal nerve injury, difficult surgical access, heart failure, open heart surgery within the previous 6 weeks, myocardial infarction within preceding 4 weeks, unstable angina, severe pulmonary disease, tandem lesions, or age greater than 80 years. The primary outcome evaluated were rates of death, stroke or myocardial infarction at 30 days. At 30 days, the CEA group (n = 151) had a composite endpoint rate of 12.6%, whereas the carotid stent group (n = 156) (performed with cerebral protection) had a rate of 5.8% (P = .047). When stratified into groups that were symptomatic and asymptomatic, the trends followed that of the whole group but did not reach statistical significance. The main goal of the trial was to show that carotid artery stenting was not inferior to CEA in these high-risk patients, and this goal was met.

Randomized trials comparing the outcomes in patients considered to be of conventional risk, either symptomatic or asymptomatic, are underway. The Carotid Revascularization Endarterectomy versus Stent Trial (CREST) is a prospective randomized trial of symptomatic patients with carotid stenosis of greater than 50% by angiography or greater than 80% by duplex ultrasound (US). As of March 2004, 840 patients had been enrolled and 186 patients randomized at 55 centers. The Stent-Protected Percutaneous Angioplasty of the Carotid versus Endarterectomy (SPACE) is a European study comparing carotid artery stenting with CEA in symptomatic patients. As of December 2003, 581 had been enrolled. Both trials are ongoing and no definitive outcomes are yet available.

MESENTERIC ARTERY INTERVENTIONS

Chronic and acute mesenteric ischemia are well described conditions resulting from occlusive disease of the splanchnic vessels. The prevalence of mesenteric occlusive disease among the elderly has been reported at 17.5%.[19] Symptomatic disease is usually a result of occlusion or stenosis of two of the three mesenteric vessels. A delay in diagnosis and treatment of this clinical syndrome can result in bowel infarction and death. Surgical therapy with revascularization and bowel resection has been the traditional mode of treatment. Endoluminal treatment is emerging as a quicker and less morbid alternative to surgery.

Percutaneous therapy for mesenteric occlusive disease was first described in 1980 by Furer and Ulflacker in two separate reports.[20,21] Furer reported the first balloon angioplasty of an superior mesenteric lesion with success. The early experience with percutaneous treatment favored balloon angioplasty, and several small series reported excellent initial results.[22–24] They were limited, however, by early restenosis ranging from 17% to 25% with mean follow-up of 25 to 39 months. Failures were attributed to extrinsic compression, elastic recoil, and refractory disease. This led to the application of primary stenting particularly in the setting of ostial disease.

Early series evaluating the efficacy of mesenteric stenting were limited by the small numbers of patients and short follow-up.[25–27] Later series have emerged with larger numbers of patients and interventions. The Cleveland Clinic experience reported by Kasirajian et al.[27a] compared outcomes in 28 patients treated with endovascular therapy to 85 patients treated with open surgical therapy. Both groups were matched in comorbid risk factors, number of occlusive vessels involved, and duration of symptoms. They differed, however, in the age of onset and presentation. The median age for the endovascular group was 72, whereas in the open surgery group it was 65. Although both groups had similar postprocedure complication rates and 3-year restenosis rates, the percutaneous group had a higher incidence of recurrent symptoms. This may have been related to the number of lesions treated in the percutaneous group, which was one compared to the surgical group who had more than one vessel revascularized. Rose et al.[28] found similar results in 1995 in their retrospective review of surgical and percutaneous revascularization modes in patients. The mortality and complication rates were similar and the open surgical group underwent multivessel revascularization in the Kasirajian review.[27a] Long-term pain relief was 67% at 9 months in the endovascular group and 82.7% at 34.5 months in the surgical group. The authors suggested that the differences in symptomatic relief stemmed from the number of vessels revascularized. A series by Sharafuddin et al. retrospectively evaluated 25 patients in whom 28 procedures were performed with 96% technical success and found no difference in clinical outcome or patency rates in patients who were treated for simple stenotic lesions, occlusions, or complex lesions. The patency rates and complication rates were similar to other recent studies.[29,30]

With the advent of lower profile sheaths, wires, and stents, percutaneous interventions have become more feasible and often the first-line treatment in the setting of mesenteric occlusive disease (Fig 90.4). As with renal disease, the lesions are often ostial and respond best to stent placement. In the setting of multiocclusive lesions, solitary treatment of the superior mesenteric lesion will often suffice.

RENAL ARTERY INTERVENTIONS

Renovascular hypertension is the most common cause of secondary hypertension, and obstructive renal lesions account for 5% of such cases.[31,32] Without treatment, such lesions can result in progressive renal dysfunction with ischemic nephropathy, congestive heart failure, and renal atrophy.[33] Renal revascularization options include both surgical and percutaneous

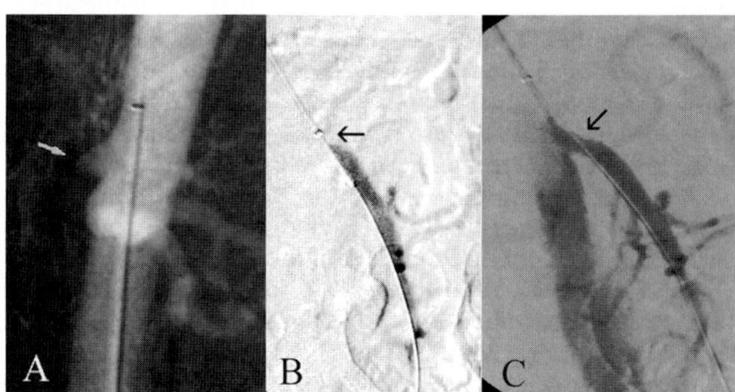

FIGURE 90.4 (*A*) Lateral aortogram demonstrating occlusion of the superior mesenteric artery (*SMA, arrow*) in a patient with post-prandial abdominal pain and weight loss. (*B*) The occlusion was crossed with a guide-wire (*arrow*) and subsequently balloon angioplastied and stented. (C) Completion angiography reveals resolution of the occlusion with antegrade flow in the SMA. The patient's symptoms resolved.

interventions. Although both therapies offer similar technical results, the morbidity and mortality of surgical revascularization ranges from 17% to 31% and 2% to 7%, respectively.[34–37] Transcatheter therapy offers similar patency, with fewer complications and shorter hospital stay.

Percutaneous transluminal angioplasty is the treatment of choice for nonorificial atherosclerotic lesions and fibromuscular dysplasia. The first percutaneous transluminal angioplasty of the renal artery was reported by Gruntzig et al. in 1978.[38] Technical success for percutaneous transluminal angioplasty in this setting has been reported at 90% in several series.[39–41] The incidence of restenosis in the setting of angioplasty, however, is high. Reports from Martin and Weibull in separate series have reported a 30% incidence of restenosis.[34,39] Elastic recoil and extensive atherosclerotic aortic and orificial plaque limit the application of balloon angioplasty in patients with ostial disease and account for the high recurrence rate afterwards.

Selective placement of stents in the renal arteries (Fig. 90.5) evolved following the first report by Palmaz et al.[42] in animal models. Although first used in the setting of elastic recoil or dissection after balloon angioplasty, the use of stenting has become a primary modality for renal artery stenosis, particularly in the setting of ostial disease.[43,44] Several studies have evaluated the efficacy of stenting for ostial disease. The ERASME study prospectively assessed the safety and results of Palmaz stent of the renal artery in 10 centers with 106 patients. The investigators demonstrated technical success in 95% of arteries and 16.9% restenosis rate at 8 months of which 10 out of 15 lesions were successfully redilated.[45] Rees et al.[46] reported similar success in the United States with a multicenter trial evaluating the Palmaz stent in ostial renal stenosis. Single center reports have also verified the high technical success rate of primary stenting with restenosis rates of 15% to 20%.[47,48]

Despite the high procedural success rate and lower restenosis rate than balloon angioplasty, the effects of renal artery stenting on hypertension and renal function have varying results. Improvement in hypertension control after renal artery stenting have been demonstrated in several series and vary from 49% to 80%, whereas azotemic benefit is more variable with most centers reporting stabilization of renal function rather than improvement.[44,47,49–51] A multicenter registry report by Dorros et al.[50] evaluated the 4-year follow-up in 1,058 patients and found significant improvement in blood pressure control, decrease in number of antihypertensive medications from 2.4 to 1.9 and stabilization of serum creatinine levels.

Results from surgical revascularization and renal interventions are comparable. Higher complication rates are reported with concurrent repair of aneurysmal disease or other visceral stenosis.[47,52] Cambria et al.[53] reviewed 285 renal revascularizations and reported an operative mortality of 5.6% and an 8.1% mortality in procedures that involved an aortic anastomosis. Hallett et al.[36] documented an operative mortality of 7.1% in a series of 652 renal operations. In contrast, complications related to renal interventions are most commonly groin hematoma and puncture site trauma although atheroembolic phenomena and contrast nephropathy also occur.[45,54] Lower profile systems, embolic protection devices, meticulous technique, increased experience, and nonnephrotoxic radiographic agents have been used to reduce the incidence of emboli and renal failure.[55–57]

Renal artery interventions have been shown to have excellent technical results and patency comparable to open surgical revascularization. The modest recurrent stenosis rate can be treated adequately with repeat intervention and balloon angioplasty. However, its long-term effect on preservation of renal function remains to be proven. Long-term outcomes with both surgery and percutaneous therapy are better in patients with normal renal function and success with either intervention is limited in the setting of parenchymal loss and elevated serum creatinines.[58–60]

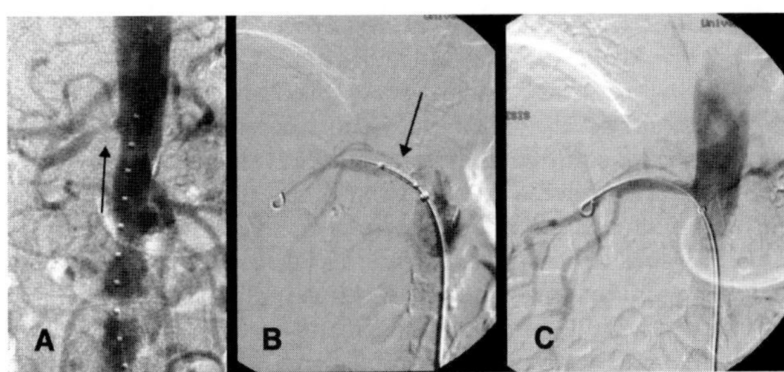

FIGURE 90.5 Angiograms from a patient undergoing angioplasty and stenting of a right renal artery stenosis. (*A*) Flush aortogram that reveals a high-grade right renal artery stenosis (*arrow*). (*B*) Wire access is obtained across the lesion, and a sheath is advanced up to the origin of the renal artery. A balloon-expandable stent (arrow, prior to deployment) is placed at the level of the stenosis (*arrow*). (*C*) After deployment of the stent, there is no residual stenosis.

AORTIC INTERVENTIONS

Endografting for Aortic Aneurysms

Abdominal aortic aneurysm (AAA) repair has had favorable results, but a less invasive procedure with fewer physiologic stresses has evolved over time. Parodi et al.[61] reported the first clinical use of endovascular AAA repair. Since that time, the application of aortic endografting for the treatment of AAA has significantly progressed and continues to do so. The current indications for endovascular repair of AAA remain the same as for conventional operative repair. It provides many potential benefits over conventional repair, however. It requires small groin incisions instead of a large abdominal one, which may decrease the incidence of postoperative pulmonary complications. There is decreased retroperitoneal dissection and thus a lower risk of perioperative bleeding. There is no or minimal aortic occlusion, which reduces the intraoperative hemodynamic stresses compared with open aneurysm repair.[62] These benefits may broaden the scope of aneurysm repair to patients who previously were deemed untreatable due to comorbidities.

Endograft Construction

The design of an aortic endograft can greatly affect the ability to place the device in a patient. One design component that is important for effective endograft placement is the delivery system. This is the equipment that houses the endograft in a compact fashion allowing it to be delivered to the proper anatomic location. Most endografts are placed through the common femoral artery and iliac artery system. The size of the delivery system must be smaller than lumen through which it must pass. Inadequate vessel diameter or the presence of extensive calcifications can inhibit endograft placement. The majority of available endografts easily traverse an iliofemoral segment of 7 to 8 mm in diameter. Another feature of the endograft delivery system is its flexibility, which allows it to traverse a tortuous iliac artery. Some tortuosity can be corrected or "straightened" with the use of a stiff guide wire; however, this is not always possible or desirable. Delivery systems composed of long, flexible, tapered tips pass more easily than those with short, stiff, blunt tips.[63]

Two general classifications of endograft construction exist: unibody and modular. A unibody device is a single piece graft. This single piece includes the main body and both limbs. This composition decreases the risk of endoleaks as there are fewer sites of component apposition. However, a larger delivery system is often required, and there is less flexibility in obtaining the correct length of the graft. The modular system includes endografts that are comprised of two to three pieces. Generally there is a main body that may have one attached limb and one or two docking limbs. These types of devices can be introduced through smaller delivery systems and offer a greater degree of flexibility with regard to placement. With multiple sites of graft-graft apposition, however, there is increased risk of endoleak.

Graft composition further varies by the material that is used to construct the graft, and the metal "skeleton" that is used to support it. Graft material ranges from thin-walled polytetrafluorethylene to polyester. The graft material is supported by a metal framework (stent) that is composed of stainless steel, elgiloy, or nitinol. The graft support can be placed inside the graft material, an endoskeleton, or outside the graft material, an exoskeleton. Grafts can be fully supported, having stent material throughout, or only partially supported, with portions of the graft having only material and no metallic support. The graft skeleton provides several key elements to endograft construction. The metal skeleton provides some degree of radial force that helps to provide a seal to prevent blood flow around the graft and a point of fixation. Some devices have hooks or barbs in the proximal aspect of the skeleton that help to anchor the graft onto the aortic wall and prevent migration. Other grafts have a bare stent that extends above the level of the fabric that helps to anchor the graft in the pararenal and suprarenal portion of the aorta, at a point where less disease may be present. The other function of the metal skeleton is to provide columnar strength to the graft, which helps to prevent migration. The skeleton may play an important role in prevention of graft kinking as it crosses tortuous anatomy, but the lack of a skeleton may be important in allowing a graft to adapt more readily to morphologic changes that occur after aneurysmal exclusion, without dislodgment of attachment sites.

Anatomic Requirements for Graft Placement

There are several anatomic requirements for the successful placement of an aortic endograft. Exact requirements vary with specific device design, but the key aspects remain the same. These include an appropriate aortic neck, a distal sealing zone, and a suitable path for the endograft to be placed through. The aortic neck is defined as the area of the aorta cephalad to the aneurysm, below the level of the renal arteries, in which the aortic endograft will be placed. This area is important for two reasons: (a) it is the site of proximal fixation that will prevent the device from migrating distally and (b) a circumferential seal must be obtained in this region to prevent blood leakage around the graft and into the aneurysm sac. In general, a 15-mm length of aortic neck is required below the level of the most caudal renal artery and above the level of the aneurysm to meet these needs. Several devices employ the use of a suprarenal, uncovered stent to provide additional protection against graft migration. Other aortic neck characteristics are important in determining whether a patient is an ideal endograft candidate. These include neck angulation, the shape of the neck, and the quality of the neck. Acute angulation of the neck can greatly affect the ability to obtain a proximal seal. Aortic neck angulation greater than 60 degrees compared with the centerline is often considered prohibitive for endovascular aneurysm repair. The shape of the aortic neck will also affect the ability to obtain a seal and fixation. A conical shaped neck, defined as an increase in diameter over the course of 15 mm by more than 10%, is felt to be a contraindication to routine aortic endografting. In addition, the presence of circumferential thrombus or severe aortic wall calcification can negatively affect the ability to obtain a seal and fixation.

The iliofemoral arterial system is important for endograft placement because it provides the route for graft placement, as well as the site for obtaining a distal seal. Many of the features important in an aortic neck for obtaining a seal and fixation are also important in the iliac arteries. The presence of thrombus, calcification, and tortuosity can significantly hinder the iliac limb seal. Most available endograft systems require at least a 15-mm segment of iliac artery to be of adequate caliber and free of significant disease to obtain a distal seal.

Endograft Placement

The most important aspects of aortic endograft placement take place prior to graft placement in determining whether a patient is indeed a suitable candidate for endograft placement, choosing an appropriate endograft device, and properly determining the size graft to be placed. These determinations are best made based on thin-cut helical computed tomography scans and in some cases with the addition of diagnostic angiography. The majority of endografts are placed through the femoral arteries that have been operatively exposed. The aorta is cannulated with a guide wire and catheter. Small boluses of contrast agent are delivered to identify the renal arteries to avoid covering them. Due to the often angulated nature of an aneurysmal aorta, it can be necessary to focus the image intensifier at an oblique cranial-caudal view to obtain the best view of the renal arteries. The device is generally placed over a stiff guide wire and positioned to allow the most extensive coverage within the aortic neck without intruding on the ostia of the renal arteries. Every device has its own unique deployment instructions and discussion of them is beyond the scope of this chapter. Depending on the construction of the endograft, following deployment of the main body (which may include an attached ipsilateral limb), the ipsilateral limb and contralateral limbs are placed.

Postoperative surveillance is extremely important in patients undergoing endovascular AAA repair. Complications may be asymptomatic at first and not present clinically for several years.[64–66] Protocols for graft surveillance vary from institution to institution, but most entail four-view abdominal plain film radiographic evaluation and intravenous contrast, thin-cut computed tomography (CT) scanning. Major imaging generally occurs at 1 month, 6 months, 12 months, and then yearly thereafter. From these images, assessment can be made to evaluate for migration, changes in aneurysm size, and the presence of endoleaks. An alternative method used to track aneurysms following endograft repair is via calculation of aneurysm volume. Aneurysm volume is determined from three-dimensional reconstructions of spiral CT scans. Aneurysm morphology can change after endograft exclusion, and thus a measurement of the volume may be a more accurate assessment of changes in aneurysm size.[67,68] Duplex US would provide a less invasive and less costly means of following aortic aneurysms following endovascular exclusion, but it does not yet provide the sensitivity and specificity obtained by CT scans.[69] The addition of US contrast agents may improve its efficacy; however, its use currently is not routine.[70]

Complications Associated with Aortic Endograft Placement

A number of problems can arise during the placement of an aortic endograft, and there are several that can arise in the follow-up period. The following paragraphs outline some of the more common problems encountered.

Iliac Artery Disease. As the primary route of insertion for most endografts is via the iliofemoral arterial system, the presence of atherosclerotic disease, aneurysmal disease, and tortuosity in the iliac arteries can greatly affect the ease with which these grafts are placed. In cases of iliac artery lumen narrowing secondary to atherosclerotic disease and severe vessel tortuosity, advancement of the device despite the presence of resistance can result in vessel rupture. Iliac rupture occurs in 1% to 2% of cases of endograft placement.[71,72] Occasionally, iliac artery narrowing can be dealt with by predilation of an occlusive lesion with balloon angioplasty. Preprocedural iliac stent placement, however, can be prohibitive to endograft placement and is discouraged. An alternative is to use an iliac conduit. An iliac conduit involves suturing a prosthetic graft to the iliac artery (and occasionally the aorta), even if it is aneurysmal. The device is placed through the conduit and into the aorta. The ipsilateral limb is then "landed" in the conduit and the end of the conduit is anastomosed to the common femoral artery. The distal end of the common iliac artery can be oversewn at a level to allow continued perfusion of the hypogastric artery in a retrograde fashion. Alternatively, the hypogastric artery can be anastomosed to the iliac conduit.

Iliac artery ectasia and aneurysmal disease can cause a problem obtaining a distal seal. Enlarged common iliac arteries are present in up to 30% of patients presenting for endovascular aneurysm repair.[73–75] Some endografts allow for the placement of larger iliac limbs, or flared limbs, that can obtain seals in ecstatic iliac arteries. In those that do not, however, the distal seal may need to be obtained in the external iliac artery. This generally requires sacrifice of the hypogastric artery by coil embolization prior to the procedure. The presence of a hypogastric artery aneurysm requires the same approach. Rarely is bilateral hypogastric artery exclusion required, but, when it is, it is performed in a staged fashion. Hypogastric embolization is associated with side effects in up to 50% of patients. Buttock claudication is the predominant complaint, occurring in 12% to 50% of patients, but it generally resolves within several months.[73–75] Patients requiring embolization of the more distal branches of the hypogastric artery are at an increased risk for developing symptoms, although bilateral hypogastric embolization has not been.[75,76] Coil embolization of the hypogastric artery is not necessary in the presence of a common iliac artery aneurysm provided that there is a 5-mm neck of iliac artery proximal to the hypogastric origin as well as a 15-mm neck in the external iliac artery.[77] This anatomic arrangement allows for an adequate seal and can be successful in up to two thirds of patients requiring coverage of the hypogastric artery.

Endoleaks. An endoleak is the persistence of blood flow outside of the endograft within the aneurysm sac. Endoleaks are classified according to their etiology, and currently five different types have been described.[78–80] Type I endoleaks arise from inadequate sealing at either proximal aortic (allowing antegrade flow) or distal iliac (allowing retrograde flow) attachment sites. Type II endoleaks arise from patent branch vessels off of the aortic sac that allow for retrograde flow into the aneurysm. Such branches include patent lumbar arteries and a patent inferior mesenteric artery (Fig. 90.6). Type III endoleaks develop from defects in the fabric of the graft or at the junction zone between modular components. Type IV endoleaks develop secondary to diffuse "leaking" of blood between the interstices of the fabric or where the graft is sutured to a stent. Type V endoleaks are applied to the scenario in which the aneurysm sac remains pressurized resulting in subsequent aneurysmal enlargement despite no demonstrable evidence of blood flow into the aneurysm sac. The pressure applied to the aneurysm sac causing it to continue to expand, in this situation, has been termed endotension.[81] Controversy with regard to this concept exists. Some argue that this merely represents a type I, II, III, or IV endoleak in which the defect is large enough to allow blood flow into the aneurysm sac, but it either occurs intermittently or is too small to be visualized by conventional means.[63]

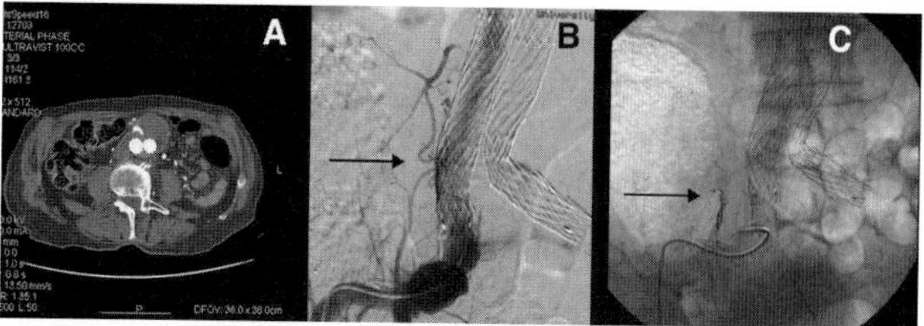

FIGURE 90.6 These are radiologic images from a patient who underwent an endograft repair of an abdominal aortic aneurysm (AAA). The patient had a known type II endoleak but subsequently developed an increase in the size of the aneurysm. (*A*) Computed tomography scan revealing a type II endoleak. (*B*) Angiogram revealing the branch off the hypogastric artery that was contributing to the endoleak (*arrow*). (*C*) Subsequent coil embolization of this vessel (*arrow*) led to resolution of the endoleak.

Types I and III endoleaks are associated with an increased risk of aneurysm expansion and possible rupture, and thus they should be treated.[82,83] Treatment of these lesions can be accomplished with the placement of an extension cuff over the site of the leak. Alternatively, if it is a type I leak, placement of a large balloon-expandable stent at the level of the leak may increase the radial force at that level and seal the leak. Failure to resolve a type I or III endoleak in an endovascular fashion should result in the conversion to an open procedure with standard repair of the aneurysm and removal of the endovascular device. Type II endoleaks are rarely associated with aneurysm rupture.[84] At least 10% to 15% of patients will be identified with a type II endoleak during follow-up.[85–88] Type II endoleaks are generally observed unless they are associated with an increase in aneurysm size or are associated with aortic pulsatility on physical exam. Arteriography is the next step in the evaluation of a patient with a type II endoleak associated with these findings. Superselective arterial canalization can be performed with embolization of feeding vessels. An alternative approach is via direct aneurysm sac puncture, during which sac pressures can be measured as well as the injection of contrast to identify the feeding vessels precisely.[89] Sac pressure measurements may be an indicator of the presence of an endoleak, even if it is not detected by routine imaging. The use of implantable intrasac pressure transducers to monitor patients following endovascular repair is currently under investigation.[90]

Limb Thrombosis. Thrombosis of an iliac limb of an aortic endograft occurs in up to 11% of patients.[91–94] There are a number of factors that have been suggested to place patients at increased risk for developing graft limb thrombosis. The lack of stent support within an iliac limb has been shown to increase the risk of thrombosis by nearly eightfold compared with intrinsically supported limbs.[93] Intuitively, the presence of atherosclerotic disease and luminal narrowing within the iliac artery increases the risk of limb thrombosis.[92] Oversizing of the iliac limb causes the graft material to have a significant amount of infolding, thus narrowing the intraluminal diameter and placing the limb at increased risk for thrombosis.[94] Extension of the limb into the external iliac artery can contribute to the risk of limb thrombosis due to the change in vessel diameter, as well as due to kinking caused by the acute angulation the artery takes as it exits the pelvis.[92] Most patients present with limb thrombosis within the first 6 months following endograft repair. Management of patients with acute limb thrombosis is dictated by the presenting symptoms. As many as one third of patients remain asymptomatic and require no intervention.[92] Most patients, however, are symptomatic and are managed with a femoral-femoral artery bypass. Few patients are successfully treated with thrombolysis or graft thrombectomy followed by endovascular repair of the underlying problem.

Migration. Stent graft migration complicates abdominal aortic endograting in 9% to 45% of cases.[88,95–97] Migration is a known risk factor for the delayed development of a type I endoleak and subsequent delayed aneurysm rupture or late conversion.[97] Blood flow is the main displacing force that causes graft migration. This force is counteracted by the frictional forces of the graft against the aortic wall, particularly at the aneurysm neck. These frictional forces can be affected by the length of the neck or the presence of thrombus and calcifications. Albertini et al.[96] evaluated their patients that developed migration or a delayed type I endoleak. Neck angulation and neck diameter were the two factors associated with their development. Morphologic changes in the aortic aneurysm and aneurysm neck have been suggested to contribute to graft migration. Aneurysm neck dilation occurs mostly in the first 2 years after graft placement and has been shown to be independently associated with device migration.[97,98] This finding, however, has not been supported by all series.[99]

Outcomes

Endograft repair of AAA has a low mortality rate (less than 3%) and subsequent rates of aneurysm rupture are reduced to 1% per year.[83,88,100,101] The need for a secondary intervention, however, is not insignificant.[102] In the Eurostar registry, reporting on 1,023 patients with follow-up of 12 months or longer, 186 (18%) of patients required a secondary intervention. The majority of these (76%) were accomplished through a transfemoral approach, and the rest required an intraabdominal or extraanatomic procedure. The rates of freedom from intervention at 1, 3, and 4 years were 89%, 67%, and 62%, respectively. Mortality was higher in those patients requiring a secondary procedure and was more frequently associated with those requiring an intraabdominal intervention. Similar results have been reported from single institution series. Montefiore Medical Center reported secondary procedure rates of 10%, whereas the Cleveland Clinic Foundation had a secondary intervention rate of 15%.[100,103] Univariate analysis revealed that secondary procedures were more common in patients with large major and minor sac axes, in patients who received a large aortic stent because of a proximal endoleak present at the initial repair, and in patients who received treatment later in the course of the review. This latter finding is thought to be secondary to the increased complexity of cases.

There have been several studies comparing the results of aortic endograft repair of AAA with conventional surgery. None of these studies have been prospective, randomized trials but have compared the outcomes of endografting with historic controls or a concomitant surgical arm. In addition, the long-term durability of aortic endograft repair of AAA is not known and only currently are data being collected. It does appear, however, that endovascular repair is associated with a shorter initial hospital stay compared with open surgery. This difference, however, is negated if the total number of hospital days, including subsequent ones for secondary procedures, is taken into consideration.[104] Schermerhorn et al.[105] evaluated quality-adjusted life expectancy after endovascular AAA repair compared with open surgical repair using a Markov decision-analysis model. Endovascular data was derived from the EUROSTAR registry, whereas the open aneurysm repair data came from the 1995 Medicare claims for elective repair of nonruptured AAA. A case-base analysis of 70-year-old men revealed the life expectancy after endovascular AAA repair was 7.09 quality-adjusted life years compared with open AAA repair of 7.03 quality-adjusted life years. This represents a difference of approximately 3 weeks. Sensitivity analysis, however, revealed that for individuals younger than 64 years, open surgical repair results in a significantly greater quality-adjusted life expectancy. As newer grafts are designed and long-term outcomes evaluated, we will have a better understanding about the future role of aortic endografting.

Aortoiliac Angioplasty and Stenting

Endovascular treatment of aortoiliac occlusive disease has become increasingly prominent over the past several years and has assumed a dominant role in the treatment of this disease. Factors including decreased morbidity compared with conventional surgery, shorter hospital stays, and equivalent patency rates have contributed to this change.

The specific indications for treatment of aortoiliac occlusive disease are independent of the approach to treatment, either endovascular or conventional surgery. This is covered in more detail in Chapter 95, but an intervention is generally indicated if disabling claudication or limb-threatening ischemia is present. Clinically, pain starts in the thighs and buttocks and is often present in combination with lower extremity discomfort. Erectile dysfunction may be present in men. Weakened femoral pulses and decreased segmental blood pressures are indications of proximal disease. Indications for PTA, as opposed to PTA with primary stenting, are changing. Historically, PTA was the first approach and the application of a stent was reserved for suboptimal results of primary PTA, defined as a persistent reduction of the lumen diameter of 30% or more. A resting mean blood pressure gradient of 5 mm of Hg or greater or a systolic blood pressure gradient exceeding 10 mm Hg are also considered significant. Provocative testing performed by the intra-arterial injection of vasodilatory agent (25 mg papaverine or 100 to 200 μg of nitroglycerine) may unmask a lesion and reveal a significant blood pressure gradient. Other indications for stent placement include eccentric stenosing plaque, arterial dissection, and when recanalization of an occluded segment is performed. With the ease with which stent placement can be performed, a more liberal approach to stenting is occurring.

Balloon dilation of iliac arteries is a relatively simple procedure. A retrograde transfemoral approach is the most widely used approach, although crossover procedures from the contralateral side can be performed. Following the use of angiography to identify the site of the lesion, a guide wire is advanced across the lesion. Once this is performed, the dilation balloon, sized to match or slightly exceed the normal vessel diameter, is inflated. The inflation device allows for the measurement of pressure within the PTA balloon, and often dilations to a pressure of 6 to 8 atmospheres of pressure are performed. Balloon dilation causes a fracture in the arterial plaque creating a local dissection, stretching the media and adventitia. Completion arteriography with or without pressure measurements is generally performed. The exact mechanism of stent deployment varies depending on the type of stent placed (balloon-expandable or self-expanding) and the manufacturer. Stents are advanced across a lesion in a "protected" fashion. This entails the advancement of a sheath across the lesion, the advancement of the stent within the sheath to the level of the lesion, and then the retraction of the sheath. This protects the stent from being dislodged as it crosses a tight stenosis. If primary stent placement is considered, predeployment balloon angioplasty may be necessary to allow for advancement of the sheath and the stent.

Percutaneous treatment of chronic iliac artery occlusions is technically feasible. This is approached in a similar fashion as in a stenotic, nonocclusive lesion. Access to the artery is obtained in either a retrograde or antegrade fashion. The rate-limiting step in this scenario is obtaining wire access across the lesion. This is often accomplished with a combination of a catheter and a hydrophilic wire. Long areas of occlusion, as well as densely calcified lesions, can hinder the technical feasibility. Once wire access across the lesion is obtained, the stenosis can undergo balloon angioplasty to obtain a flow channel. This is best supported with the use of a stent after predilation.

Aortic bifurcation lesions present a unique situation as balloon angioplasty or stent placement in the origin of a common iliac artery may cause occlusion of the contralateral artery orifice. To overcome this problem, a technique termed "kissing balloon" or "kissing stent" placement is used (Fig. 90.7). This is the simultaneous placement of PTA balloons or stents that traverse the ostia of both common iliac arteries. If stents are used, it is mandatory that the proximal ends of both stents are parallel so that the flow into one stent is not hindered by the other. In most cases, the use of noncompressable, balloon-expandable stents are most beneficial in this procedure. Below the level of the aortic bifurcation, however, self-expanding stents are perfectly acceptable.

Iliac artery stent placement is technically successful in up to 97% of patients.[106] Technical complications occur in less than 6% of interventions and include subintimal dilation, dissection, arterial rupture, inability to cross the lesion with a wire, and distal embolization. Belli et al.[107] reported in their series that only 2.8% of patients developed complications requiring surgery, and only 0.9% required reconstructive bypass. Clinically significant distal embolization occurs in up to 1% of patients undergoing iliac artery PTA and stent placement. Silent peripheral embolization has been detected by Doppler US in 90% of patients immediately following iliac artery PTA, but this decreases with time.[108] Symptomatic embolization can be treated by a variety of endovascular methods including suction thrombectomy and thrombolytic therapy. If these methods are unsuccessful, surgical thromboembolectomy is necessary.

Iliac artery dissection during PTA is reported in less than 1% of patients.[109] Half of the patients develop significant lumen compromise. Dissections are treated with prolonged balloon inflation to "tack down" the flap, or with placement of an intraarterial stent. If endovascular therapy is unsuccessful, operative treatment includes iliac endarterectomy, iliofemoral artery bypass, femoral-femoral artery bypass, and aortobifemoral artery bypass grafting. Arterial dissection has been reported in 10% of patients undergoing iliac artery stent placement.[110] Nearly two thirds of the dissections caused a flow-limiting lesion that required the placement of an additional stent. Vessel injury is related to balloon oversizing and the degree of arterial calcification. Iliac artery rupture during balloon dilation and stent placement has been reported in up to 0.9% of cases.[111,112] Vessel disruption can present with uncontained hemorrhage, contained hemorrhage, or pseudoaneurysm formation. The key to initial management is to maintain guide wire access across the site of disruption. Control of the hemorrhage can be obtained with the insertion of an angioplasty balloon to tamponade the site of injury. If prolonged balloon tamponade does not achieve hemostasis, the placement of a covered stent is warranted. Uncontrolled hemorrhage demands operative intervention, but balloon occlusion proximal to the site of injury can afford time to prepare for surgery. Risk factors for rupture are similar to those for dissection and include the presence of a high-grade stenosis with heavy calcifications. Other risk factors include the use of oversized balloons and manual inflation without manometric control.

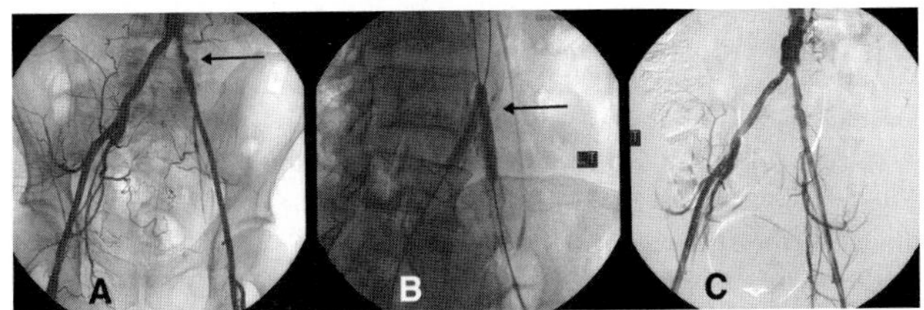

FIGURE 90.7 Angiograms from a patient who presented with disabling claudication of his left lower extremity. (*A*) Aortogram revealed an area of stenosis in the proximal common iliac artery on the left (*arrow*). A pressure gradient was measured across this lesion and was found to be 30 mm Hg. (*B*) The patient underwent placement of a balloon-expandable left iliac artery stent. To preserve the lumen of the right common iliac artery, a "kissing" balloon technique was performed in which a balloon was expanded in the right common iliac artery as the balloon-expandable stent was placed in the left common iliac artery (*arrow*). (C) Angiographic resolution of the stenosis. There was also resolution of the pressure gradient.

Results of iliac artery balloon angioplasty have been well documented. Johnston et al.[112a] prospectively analyzed the results of 984 patients that underwent PTA, 684 of whom had aortoiliac angioplasty. Outcomes were assessed by Kaplan-Meier analysis. Twelve percent of the patients were treated for iliac artery occlusions, and the rest had nonocclusive stenoses. Initial success, defined as a combination of clinical factors and ankle-brachial index, was achieved in 88.6% of patients. This dropped to 48.2% at 60 months. Predictors of success included the indication for operation (with better results in patients treated for claudication vs. limb-threatening ischemia), site of angioplasty (common iliac artery lesions favoring external iliac artery lesions), and lesion severity (stenoses favoring occlusions). Becker et al.[113] report a meta-analysis involving 2,679 procedures. Five-year patency rates for this group were 72%. More recently, Tegtmeyer et al.[106] reported a single institution experience in 200 patients with a technical success rate of PTA alone of 88% and a 5-year patency of 85%.

Outcomes from treatment of iliac artery stenosis with PTA and stent placement have also been evaluated with long-term clinical data. The outcome from the use of the self-expanding Wallstent in 140 patients was evaluated by Martin et al.[114] Primary patency was 81% at 1 year and 71% at 2 years, and secondary patency was 91% and 86%, respectively. Similar results were obtained by Vorwerk et al.[115] They followed 118 patients with primary patency rates of 95% at 1 year, 88% at 2 years, and 82% at 4 years, and secondary patency rates were 96%, 93%, and 91%, respectively. Palmaz et al.[111] evaluated the outcomes of the use of the balloon-expandable Palmaz stent in 486 patients enrolled in a multicenter trial. Technical success occurred in 99% of patients with clinical follow-up patency of 90% at 1 year and 84% after 2 years. A meta-analysis evaluating outcomes of iliac artery PTA and stent placement in 1,300 patients, with a variety of types of stents, was performed by Bosch and Hunink.[116] Four-year primary patency rates were 77% for stenotic lesions treated with iliac stenting and 61% for occlusive lesions in patients with claudication, and 67% and 53%, respectively, in patients with limb-threatening ischemia. The risk of long-term failure was reduced by 39% after stent placement compared with PTA alone. Iliac artery stent patency rates are significantly lower in women and in patients with renal insufficiency and critical limb ischemia.[117]

LOWER EXTREMITY ARTERIAL INTERVENTIONS

Lower extremity atherosclerotic disease affects a substantial portion of the population. For a more in-depth discussion on the pathophysiology and clinical presentation of the disease please refer to Chapter 96. Patients presenting with disabling claudication and have failed nonoperative therapy, or those patients presenting with limb threatening ischemia, are considered for more invasive intervention. Treatment has traditionally been bypass grafting for femoral artery, popliteal artery, and tibial artery disease. With the development of improved angioplasty and stent technology, more and more endovascular procedures are being applied to infrainguinal arterial disease.

Femoropopliteal Angioplasty and Stenting

The approach to femoropopliteal artery interventions can proceed via one of three routes. The antegrade approach via an antegrade puncture of the ipsilateral common femoral artery is perhaps one of the most utilized approaches. Alternatively, a retrograde approach through the contralateral common femoral artery can be used, with the catheters and wires traversing the aortic bifurcation. This approach, however, is often reserved for the treatment of short occlusions at or near the origin of the superficial femoral artery. Otherwise, the distance from the point of access becomes too long, and there is increased difficulty manipulating the catheters and wires. A less frequently used approach is via puncture of the ipsilateral popliteal artery. This approach is often used in patients that have had a failed attempt at an antegrade approach or in those that have severe stenotic or occlusive changes in the proximal part of the superficial femoral artery. Once arterial access is obtained, principles of wire access, balloon dilation, and stent placement (when necessary) are similar to those described for aortoiliac artery PTA and stent placement.

There have been mixed results reported for outcomes of patients treated with percutaneous balloon angioplasty of femoropopliteal artery stenosis. Initial technical success occurs in 88% to 93% of patients.[118–122] Primary patency rates for femoropopliteal interventions have been reported as 43% to 58% at 1 year, 41% to 46% at 2 years, 38% to 41% at 3 years, and 26% to 38% at 5 years.[118–123] Several factors have been shown to affect outcome of femoropopliteal angioplasty. The length of the lesion has a negative effect on long-term patency. Lofberg et al.[122] evaluated outcomes of 92 patients who underwent 121 PTA procedures. They reported a primary patency at 5 years of only 12% in those with occlusions longer than 5 cm and 32% in those with occlusions shorter than 5 cm. Similar results were found by Matsi et al.,[118] but they had some success with PTA of lesions up to 10 cm in length. Others have shown that treatment of patients with stenoses faired better than those with occlusions, and those with claudication faired better than those with limb threatening ischemia.[120,124] The quality of outflow also affects outcome.[123] Due to the poor outcomes of femoropopliteal PTA, some argue that it should not be recommended as a first-line treatment in patients with infrainguinal occlusive disease but reserved for those who would not tolerate surgery or have no surgical options. Others, however, argue that it does not preclude surgery and may be a viable first option, reserving surgery for those that eventually fail PTA. Given the poor outcomes of PTA, few studies have attempted to evaluate whether the placement of a stent, either primarily or after failed PTA, would improve outcomes of endovascular procedures in the femoropopliteal arteries. Outcomes from many of these studies have not been shown to significantly improve patency rates. Primary patency rates for femoropopliteal artery stenting have been reported as 54% to 86% at 1 year and 29.9% to 48% at 3 years.[125–128] Secondary patency rates at 3 years increases to 68.3%.[128] Complications during PTA and stenting of the femoropopliteal arteries include arterial disruption, thrombosis, distal embolization, and arterial dissection. Complications occur more frequently in this branch of the arterial tree as compared with the aortoiliac system, and half of these complications require operative intervention.

Another technique to revascularize the lower extremity in a percutaneous fashion is the use of percutaneous intentional extraluminal (or subintimal) angioplasty and recanalization. This method overcomes some of the problems associated with conventional PTA in that the subintimal plane that is developed has a smooth neolumen, which may be less prone to thrombosis. The technique was originally described in 1990 by Bolia et al.[129] This procedure is accomplished by using a wire to enter the subintimal space of a native artery proximal to an area of hemodynamic significant stenosis or occlusion. The wire is advanced in this plane past an area of severe disease and then reenters the true lumen. The channel is then enlarged by balloon angioplasty. In the femoropopliteal region it has been specifically applied to long lesions, greater than 10 cm in length. Initial technical success rate of the procedure has varied from 82% to 90%.[130–133] Initial failure of the procedure is primarily due to inability to gain reaccess to the true lumen. Primary patency rates have been reported to be 27% to 62% at 1 year. Long-term patency rates are not known, and the application of this technique is controversial. It generally carries a low morbidity and may represent a mode of revascularization in patients with limb-threatening ischemia who do not have a surgical option.

Many failures of PTA and stenting are due to the development of neointimal hyperplasia leading to recurrent in-stent stenosis. In an attempt to address this problem, stents covered with graft material have been placed. Saxon et al.[134] reported the largest experience as part of a U.S. multicenter prospective randomized trial of PTA versus PTA and expanded polytetrafluoroethylene (ePTFE)-covered stents. The total number of patients treated was only 28, with 13 patients receiving PTA alone and 15 patients randomized to PTA and covered stent placement. At 2-year follow-up, primary patency in the covered stent group was 87%, whereas in the PTA alone group it was only 25% ($P = .002$). Further investigation is certainly warranted into the application of this technology. In addition, drug-eluting stents are being investigated for the treatment of femoropopliteal disease. One such study evaluated the use of sirolimus-eluting stents.[135] Sirolimus acts as an antiinflammatory and cytostatic antiproliferative agent that diminishes smooth muscle cell proliferation, which may prevent the development of neointimal hyperplasia. Duda et al.[135] reported on the outcome of 36 patients recruited for the participation in a randomized, double-blind, prospective trial evaluating drug-eluting stents versus uncoated stents in the treatment of femoropopliteal occlusive disease. The in-stent mean lumen diameter was significantly larger in the sirolimus-eluting stent group compared with the uncoated stent at 6 months. Long-term patency rates are not yet known, and further investigation with this stent, as well as others, is underway.

Crural Artery Angioplasty and Stenting

Treatment of critical limb ischemia resulting from tibial vessel occlusion remains a challenge. In most situations, patients are elderly or have multiple comorbidities, which place them at high risk for surgery. Early application of angioplasty and stenting techniques to tibial vessel lesions was limited. With increased experience; however, the lack of emergent surgery to "rescue" tibial interventions has led to wider application. The technical aspects of the procedure do not differ too significantly from angioplasty in other arterial locations. Guide wire access is obtained across the lesion. Typically, a smaller guide wire is required such as one that is of 0.018 or 0.014 inches in diameter. Angioplasty is performed primarily, with stents rarely being placed as the risk of thrombosis is too great. Immediate technical success occurs in 87% to 92% of patients.[136,137] Complications related to tibial PTA that subsequently require emergent surgical intervention only occur in 0.7% of patients.

The two largest series reported on the outcomes of tibial PTA were reported by Faglia et al.[136] in 2002 and by Dorros et al.[137] in 2001. Faglia reported on the outcomes of 191 tibial PTA procedures performed in patients with critical limb ischemia (rest pain or tissue loss). Clinical recurrence occurred in 7.3% of patients at a mean time to recurrence of 4.6 months. The majority of these recurrences were successfully treated with repeat angioplasty. Major amputation was required in only 5.2% of patients. Dorros reported on the outcome of 270 PTA procedures in patients with critical limb ischemia. Over a 5-year follow-up, only 8% required a subsequent surgical revascularization and only 9% required a major amputation. Survival, however, was only 56% at 5 years. In some centers, tibial PTA for isolated tibial lesions is being considered as the primary intervention prior to tibial artery bypass, particularly in patients with multiple comorbidities. As more experience is gained with this procedures, a better understanding of its outcomes and its potential applications will be attained.

VENOUS INTERVENTIONS

The pathophysiology of chronic disease is complex and generally results from a combination of contributing factors, such as reflux, as well as outflow obstruction. The application of angioplasty and stenting to the venous circulation is gaining increased popularity. In particular, it is being applied to the treatment of iliac venous outflow obstruction. The etiology of outflow obstruction may be secondary to previous iliac vein thrombosis or due to a primary cause of obstruction, such as May-Thurner syndrome. A more thorough discussion of venous disease is presented in Chapter 105. The technique of venous angioplasty and stenting is similar to that applied to the arterial system. Guide wire access is obtained across the area of stenosis and PTA performed to eliminate the obstruction. Placement of a stent is often necessary, and intravascular US can play an instrumental role in accurate placement (Fig. 90.8).[138]

Raju et al.[139] reviewed the results of balloon dilation and stent placement for the relief of iliac vein stenosis in 304 patients with symptomatic iliac vein stenosis. Of these patients, 57% had symptoms that were also associated with symptoms attributable to reflux disease. Approximately half of the patients had stenoses due to nonthrombotic causes (i.e., May-Thurner syndrome), whereas the other half were postthrombotic in nature. Forty-four limbs required a reintervention because of restenosis of the treated segment. Primary and secondary patency rates at 24 months were 71% and 97%, respectively. Patients with venous ulceration had healing in 62% of patients by 2 years, and after stent placement limbs that were free from swelling increased from 12% to 47%, and limbs that were free from pain increased from 17% to 71%. Treatment of patients with occluded iliac veins is technically feasible. In general, however, these procedures require the stenting of longer segments (mean length 22 cm) and multiple in-line stents (mean stents = 3).[140]

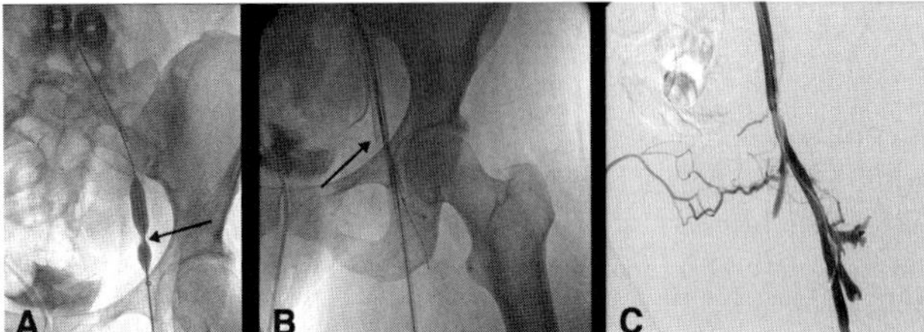

FIGURE 90.8 Venograms from a patient who presented with left common iliac vein thrombosis. After thrombolysis, areas of residual stenosis were placed in the left common iliac and external iliac veins. (*A*) Balloon angioplasty of a stricture noted in the left external iliac vein. Note the "waist" depicting the stenosis that is being treated during the balloon angioplasty (*arrow*). (*B*) Self-expanding stents were placed in the left common iliac and external iliac veins. Depicted is the deployment of the most distal self-expanding stent (*arrow*). (*C*) Completion venogram shows resolution of the stenosis and excellent flow within the venous system.

THROMBOLYSIS

Thrombolytic therapy is generally used to treat acute arterial or venous occlusions. There are a variety of agents that have been used for thrombolytic therapy, including streptokinase compounds, urokinase compounds (UK), tissue plasminogen activator and its recombinant forms (rt-PA). These agents are all plasminogen activators, which do not directly degrade fibrinogen but rather are trypsinlike serine proteases that have high specific activity directed at the cleavage of a single peptide bond in the plasminogen zymogen, converting it to plasmin. Plasmin is the molecule that then cleaves fibrin polymer resulting in the dissolution of thrombus. In the majority of cases of peripheral vascular disease in which thrombolytic agents are used, it is delivered in a catheter-directed fashion. Access to the blood vessel is obtained either on the contralateral side or in an "upstream" location. Best results are obtained if the area of thrombosis can be crossed with an infusion wire or catheter and the thrombolytic agent delivered directly into the thrombus burden. Specialized catheters and wires, with multiple small side holes, have been developed to allow for this. Other techniques of thrombolysis include the delivery of low-dose continuous infusion, the delivery of high-dose graded infusion, or pulse spray infusion in which periodic forceful injection of the drug into the clot are performed. Progress is assessed angiographically on a regular basis until thrombolysis is complete or no further progress is attained. In cases of acute limb ischemia, thrombolysis can generally be applied safely only to patients with category I and IIa limb ischemia, as it takes several hours to attain lysis. Patients with more severe ischemia may not tolerate the delay in recanalization and thus may require more urgent surgical intervention.

There have been two major randomized trials evaluating the use of thrombolytic therapy for lower extremity ischemia: Surgery versus Thrombolysis for Ischemia of the Lower Extremity (STILE) and Thrombolysis or Peripheral Artery Surgery (TOPAS).[141,142] In the STILE trial thrombolytic therapy was successful at restoring patency in 81% of bypass grafts and 69% of native arteries. One of the successes of thrombolytic therapy was that it reduced the extent of the planned surgical procedure in 55.8% of the patients. At 6-month follow-up, only 5.7% of patients undergoing thrombolysis required an amputation, whereas 17.9% of those randomized directly to surgery required one. In the TOPAS trial, complete lysis was obtained in 67.9% of patients. Of those treated with thrombolysis, approximately one third had underlying lesions treated percutaneously and avoided a conventional operation.

Treatment was most effective in patients whose thrombosis was less than 14 days in duration.

The main risks associated with the use of thrombolytic therapy are due to the increased risk of bleeding. In the STILE and TOPAS trials, complications occurred at an incidence of 22% to 41% of patients and included hemorrhage, distal embolization, and catheter-related problems. Life-threatening hemorrhage occurred in 6.2% of patients undergoing thrombolytic therapy in the STILE trial and in 12.5% of patients treated with thrombolytics in the TOPAS trial. The TOPAS trial did reveal that when aspirin and therapeutic heparin were withheld during thrombolytic therapy the rate of intracranial hemorrhage was decreased from 5% to 0.5%. In addition, aggressive control of hypertension is also beneficial at decreasing the risk of intracranial hemorrhage.[143] An analysis of data collected in a prospective, single-institution registry at the Cleveland Clinic Foundation revealed an overall complication rate of 55.9% in patients undergoing thrombolytic therapy for both arterial and venous disease. Complications rates were also analyzed according to the type of thrombolytic agent used (either UK or rt-PA). In patients receiving thrombolytic therapy for arterial disease the complications reported were the development of a hematoma or pseudoaneurysm (30.6% UK vs. 57.7% rt-PA), any bleeding requiring a transfusion (11.9% UK vs. 18.7% rt-PA), and intracranial bleeding (0.8% UK vs. 1.6% rt-PA). Mortality rates were 2.9% for UK and 1.6% for rt-PA. For patients treated with venous thrombolysis, the complications reported were hematoma formation (18.4% UK vs. 28.6% rt-PA) and any bleeding requiring a transfusion (14.3% UK vs. 42.9% rt-PA). There were no cases of intracranial bleeding in patients undergoing venous thrombolysis.

To minimize the risks of thrombolytic therapy, several criteria have been universally accepted as contraindications to its use. Absolute contraindications include stroke or TIA within the past 2 months, gastrointestinal bleeding within the past 10 days, and neurosurgery or intracranial trauma within the past 3 months. Relatively major contraindications include cardiopulmonary resuscitation within the past 10 days, major nonvascular surgery or trauma within the past 10 days, uncontrolled hypertension, intracranial tumor, and recent eye surgery. From a technical standpoint, the use of micropuncture needles and small catheters may decrease the risk of bleeding complications. Monitoring of laboratory values, such as fibrinogen levels, have been of no value in predicting which patients are at increased risk of bleeding.[144] In the presence of hemorrhage, heparin and thrombolytic agent should be discontinued. If necessary, thrombolytic agents can be reversed with cryoprecipitate, fresh frozen plasma, tranexamic acid, aminocaproic acid, or aprotinin. These interventions are rarely necessary as most thrombolytic agents have short half-lives, in the range of minutes.

SUMMARY

Endovascular therapy is an exciting field that offers an alternate modality of treatment to patients with a variety of peripheral vascular disorders. In most cases, the indications for the procedure are the same whether an open or endovascular option are being considered. The field of endovascular therapy continues to grow at a rapid pace and will continue to do so with the development of improving technologies. These improvements may, in the future, allow many procedures to attain clinical equipoise with open surgical procedures and in such instances may replace them. In cases in which this is not the true, the endovascular interventions may remain the procedure of choice in high-risk patients.

KEY POINTS

- **The treatment of vascular disease has progressed significantly over the past several years with the evolution and application of endovascular procedures.**
- **Endovascular treatment of carotid artery stenosis is less invasive and thus may be associated with a lower morbidity and mortality compared with CEA.**
- **In order for carotid artery stenting to gain full acceptance, it must provide clinical outcomes that rival CEA.**
- **With the advent of lower profile sheaths, wires, and stents, percutaneous interventions have become more feasible and often the first-line treatment in the setting of mesenteric occlusive disease.**
- **Percutaneous transluminal angioplasty is the treatment of choice for nonorificial atherosclerotic lesions and fibromuscular dysplasia.**
- **Results from surgical revascularization and renal interventions are comparable.**
- **The most important aspects of aortic endograft placement take place prior to graft placement in determining whether a patient is indeed a suitable candidate for endograft placement, choosing an appropriate endograft device, and properly determining the size graft to be placed.**
- **Postoperative surveillance is extremely important in patients undergoing endovascular AAA repair.**
- **Endovascular treatment of aortoiliac occlusive disease has become increasingly prominent over the past several years and has assumed a dominant role in the treatment of this disease.**
- **There have been mixed results reported for outcomes of patients treated with percutaneous balloon angioplasty of femoropopliteal artery stenosis.**

References

1. **Dotter C, Judkins M. Transluminal treatment of arteriosclerotic obstruction: description of a new technique and preliminary report of its application. *Circulation* 1969;30:645.**
2. Leung D, Spinosa D, Hagspiel K, et al. Selection of stents for treating iliac arterial occlusive disease. *J Vasc Interv Radiol.* 2003;14:137.
3. American Heart Association. Heart disease and stroke statistics—2004 update. *Am Heart Assoc.* 2003;x:1.
4. Executive Committee for the Asymptomatic Carotid Atherosclerosis Study. Endarterectomy for asymptomatic carotid artery stenosis. *JAMA* 1995;273:1421.
5. North American Symptomatic Carotid Endarterectomy Trial Collaborators. Beneficial effect of carotid endarterectomy in symptomatic patients with high-grade carotid stenosis. *N Engl J Med.* 1991;325:445.
6. MRC Asymptomatic Carotid Surgery Trial (ACST) Collaborative Group. Prevention of disabling and fatal strokes by successful carotid endarterectomy in patients without recent neurological symptoms: randomised controlled trial. *Lancet* 2004;363:1491.
7. Kerber C, Hornwell L, Lowden O. Catheter dilation of proximal carotid stenosis during distal bifurcation endarterectomy. *Am J Neuroradiol.* 1980;1:348.
8. Wholey M, Wholey M, Tan W, et al. A comparison of balloon-mounted and self-expanding stents in the carotid arteries: immediate and long-term results of more than 500 patients. *J Endovasc Ther.* 2003;10:171.
9. Castriota F, Cremonesi A, Manetti R, et al. Impact of cerebral protection devices on early outcome of carotid stenting. *J Endovasc Ther.* 2002; 9:786.
10. Wilentz J, Chati Z, Krafft V, et al. Retinal embolization during carotid angioplasty and stenting: mechanisms and role of cerebral protection systems. *Catheter Cardiovasc Interv.* 2002;56:320.
11. Macdonald S, McKevitt F, Venables G, et al. Neurological outcomes after carotid stenting protected with the Neuroshield filter compared to unprotected stenting. *J Endovasc Ther.* 2002;9:777.
12. Martin J, Pache J, Treggiari-Venzi M, et al. Role of the distal balloon protection technique in the prevention of cerebral embolic events during carotid stent placement. *Stroke* 2001;32:479.
13. Wholey M, Jarmolowski C, Wholey M, et al. Carotid artery stent placement—ready for prime time? *J Vasc Interv Radiol.* 2003;14:1.
14. Wholey M, Wholey M, Tan W, et al. Management of the neurologic complications of carotid artery stenting. *J Endovasc Ther.* 2001;8:341-353.

15. **Yadav J, Roubin G, Iyer S, et al. Elective stenting of the extracranial carotid arteries. *Circulation* 2004;95:376.**
15a. Lal BK, Hobson RW, Goldstein J, et al. In-stent recurrent stenosis after carotid artery stenting: life table analysis and clinical relevance. *J Vasc Surg*. 2003;38:1162.
16. **Wholey M, Al-Mubarek N, Wholey M. Updated review of the global carotid artery stent registry. *Catheter Cardiovasc Interv.* 2003;60:259.**
17. **CAVATAS Investigators. Endovascular versus surgical treatment in patients with carotid stenosis in the Carotid and Vertebral Artery Transluminal Angioplasty Study (CAVATAS): a randomized trial. *Lancet* 2001;357:1729.**
18. **Yadav J, Wholey M, Kuntz R, et al. Protected carotid-artery stenting versus endarterectomy in high-risk patients. *N Engl J Med.* 2004;351:1493.**
19. Hansen K, Wilson D, Craven T, et al. Mesenteric arterial disease in the elderly. *J Vasc Surg*. 2004;40:45.
20. Furer J, Gruntzig A, Kugelmeier J, et al. Treatment of abdominal angina with percutaneous dilation for an arteria mesentterica superior stenosis. Preliminary communication. *Cardiovasc Intervent Radiol*. 1980;3:43.
21. Uflacker R, Goldany M, Constant S. Resolution of mesenteric angina with percutaneous transluminal angioplasty of a superior mesenteric artery stenosis using a balloon catheter. *Gastrointest Radiol*. 1980;5:367.
22. Allen R, Martin G, Rees C, et al. Mesenteric angioplasty in the treatment of chronic mesenteric intestinal ischemia. *J Vasc Surg*. 1996;24:415.
23. Hallisey M, Deschaine J, Illescas F, et al. Angioplasty for the treatment of visceral ischemia. *J Vasc Intervent Radiol*. 1995;6:785.
24. Matsumoto A, Tegtmeyer C, Fitzcharles E. Percutaneous transluminal angioplasty of visceral artery stenoses: results and long term clinical follow-up. *J Vasc Intervent Radiol*. 1995;6:165.
25. Sheeran S, Murphy T, Khwaja A, et al. Stent placement for treatment of mesenteric artery stenoses or occlusions. *J Vasc Intervent Radiol*. 1999;10:861.
26. Nyman U, Ivancev K, Lindh M, et al. Endovascular treatment of chronic mesenteric ischemia: Report of five cases. *Cardiovasc Intervent Radiol*. 1998;21:305.
27. Kandarpa K, Becker G, Huniak M, et al. Transcatheter interventions for the treatment of peripheral atherosclerotic lesions: Part I. *J Vasc Intervent Radiol*. 2001;12:695.
28. Rose S, Quigley T, Raker E. Revascularization for chronic mesenteric ischemia: comparison of operative arterial bypass grafting and percutaneous transluminal angioplasty. *J Vasc Intervent Radiol*. 1995;6:339.
28a. Kasirajian K, O'Hara PJ, Gray BH, et al. Chronic mesenteric ischemia: open surgery versus percutaneous angioplasty and stenting. *J Vasc Surg*. 2001;33:63.
29. Steinmetz E, Tatou E, Favier-Biavoux C, et al. Endovascular treatment as first choice in chronic intestinal ischemia. *Ann Vasc Surg*. 2002;16:693.
30. Matsumoto A, Angle J, Spinosa D, et al. Percutaneous transluminal angioplasty and stenting in the treatment of chronic mesenteric ischemia: results and longterm follow. *J Am Coll Surg*. 2002;194:S22.
31. Dean R, Tribble R, Hansen K, et al. Evolution of renal artery insufficiency in ischemic nephropathy. *Ann Surg*. 1991;213:446.
32. Sos T, Trost D. Renal vascular disease as a cause of hypertension. *Curr Opin Nephrol Hyperten*. 1995;4:76.
33. Dean R, Tribble R, Hansen K, et al. Prevalence of ischemic nephropathy in the atherosclerotic population. *Am J Kidney Dis*. 1994;24:615.
34. Weibull H, Bergqvist D, Bergentz S, et al. Percutaneous transluminal renal angioplasty versus surgical reconstruction of atherosclerotic renal artery stenosis: a prospective randomized study. *J Vasc Surg*. 1993;18:841.
35. Hansen K, Starr S, Sands E, et al. Contemporary surgical management of renovascular disease. *J Vasc Surg*. 1992;16:319.
36. Hallett JJ, Fowl R, O'Brien P. Renovascular operations in patients with chronic renal insufficiency: do the benefits justify the risks? *J Vasc Surg*. 1987;5:633.
37. Novick A, Ziegelbaum M, Vidt D, et al. Trends in surgical revascularization for renal artery disease: ten years' experience. *JAMA* 1987;257:498.
38. **Gruntzig A, Kuhlmann U, Vetter W. Treatment of renovascular hypertension with percutaneous transluminal dilatation of a renal artery stenosis. *Lancet* 1978;1:801.**
39. Martin L, Cork R, Kaufman S. Long term results of angioplasty in 110 patients with renal artery stenosis. *J Vasc Intervent Radiol*. 1992; 3:619.
40. Losinno F, Zuccala A, Busato F, et al. Renal artery angioplasty for renovascular hypertension and preservation of renal function: long tern angiographic and clinical follow-up. *AJR Am J Roentgenol*. 1994;162:853.
41. Klow N, Palusen D, Vatne K, et al. Percutaneous renal artery angioplasty using the coaxial technique: ten years of experience from 591 procedures in 419 patients. *Acta Radiol*. 1998;39:594.
42. Palmaz J, Kopp D, Hayashi H. Normal and stenotic renal arteries: experience with balloon expandable intraluminal stenting. *Radiology* 1987; 164:705.
43. **Blum U, Krimme B, Flugel P, et al. Treatment of ostial renal artery stenoses with vascular endoprostheses after unsuccessful balloon angioplasty. *N Engl J Med.* 1997;336:459.**
44. White C, Ramee S, Collins T, et al. Renal artery stent placement: utility in lesions difficult to treat with balloon angioplasty. *J Am Coll Cardiol*. 1997;30:1445.
45. Bakker J, Goffette P, Henry M, et al. The Erasme study: a multicenter study on the safety and technical results of the Palmaz stent used for the treatment of atherosclerotic ostial renal artery stenosis. *Cardiovasc Intervent Radiol*. 1999;22:468.
46. Rees C, Palmaz J, Becker G, et al. Palmaz stent in the atherosclerotic stenoses involving the ostia of the renal arteries: preliminary report of a multi-center study. *Radiology* 1991;181:721.
47. Bush R, Najibi S, MacDonald M, et al. Endovascular revascularization of renal artery stenosis: technical and clinical results. *J Vasc Surg*. 2001;33:1041.
48. Ivanovic V, McKusick M, Johnson C, et al. Renal artery stent placement: complications at a single center tertiary care center. *J Vasc Intervent Radiol*. 2003;14:225.
49. Yutan E, Glickerman D, Caps M, et al. Percutaneous transluminal revascularization for renal artery stenosis: Veterans Affair Puget Sound health care system experience. *J Vasc Surg*. 2001;34:685.
50. Dorros G, Jaff M, Mathiak L, et al. Multicenter Palmaz stent renal artery stenosis revascularization registry report: four year follow up of 1058 successful patients. *Catheter Cardiovasc Intervent*. 2002;55:182.
51. Henry M, Amor M, Henry I. Stents in the treatment of renal artery stenosis: long term follow up. *J Endovasc Ther*. 1999;6:42.
52. Xue F, Bettmann M, Langdon D, et al. Outcome and cost comparison of percutaneous transluminal renal angioplasty, renal arterial stent placement and renal artery bypass grafting. *Radiology* 1999;212:378.
53. Cambria R, Brewster D, L'Italien G, et al. The durability of different reconstructive techniques for atherosclerotic renal artery disease. *J Vasc Surg*. 1994;20:76.
54. Beek F, Kaate R, Beutler J, et al. Complications during renal artery stent placement for atherosclerotic ostial stenosis. *Cardiovasc Intervent Radiol*. 1997;20:184.
55. Spinosa D, Matsumoto A, Angle J, et al. Safety of CO_2 and gadodiamide enhanced angiography for the evaluation and percutaneous treatment of renal artery stenosis in patients with chronic renal insufficiency. *AJR Am J Roentgenol*. 2001;176:1305.
56. Feldman R, Wargovich T, Bitti J. No touch technique for reducing aortic wall trauma during renal artery stenting. *Catheter Cardiovasc Intervent*. 1999;46:245.
57. Henry M, Henry I, Klonaris C, et al. Renal angioplasty and stenting under protection: the way of the future? *Catheter Cardiovasc Intervent*. 2003;60:299.
58. Cambria R, Brewster D, L'Italien G, et al. Renal artery reconstruction for the preservation of renal function. *J Vasc Surg*. 1996;24:371.
59. Sivamurthy N, Surowiec S, Culakova E, et al. Divergent outcomes after percutaneous therapy for symptomatic renal artery stenoses. *J Vasc Surg*. 2004;39:365.
60. Steinbach F, Novick A, Campbell S, et al. Long term survival after surgical revascularization for atherosclerotic renal artery disease. *J Urol*. 1997; 158:36–41.
61. **Parodi J, Palmaz J, Barone H. Transfemoral intraluminal graft implantation for abdominal aortic aneurysms. *Ann Vasc Surg*. 1991;5:491.**
62. Baxendale B, Baker D, Hutchinson A, et al. Haemodynamic and metabolic response to endovascular repair of infra-renal aortic aneurysms. *Br J Anaesth*. 1996;77:581.
63. Ouriel K, Greenberg R, Clair D. Endovascular treatment of aortic aneurysms. *Curr Prob Surg*. 2002;39:242.
64. White R, Donayre C, Walot I, et al. Abdominal aortic aneurysm rupture following endoluminal graft deployment: report of a predictable event. *J Endovasc Ther*. 2000;7:257.
65. **Harris P, Vallavhaneni S, Desgranges P, et al. Incidence and risk factors of late rupture, conversion, and death after endovascular repair of infrarenal aortic aneurysms: the EUROSTAR experience. *J Vasc Surg*. 2000;32:739.**
66. Whitaker S. Imaging of abdominal aortic aneurysm before and after endoluminal stent-graft repair. *Eur J Radiol*. 2001;39:3.
67. Harris P, Brennan J, Martin J, et al. Longitudinal aneurysm shrinkage following endovascular aortic aneurysm repair: a source of intermediate and late complications. *J Endovasc Surg*. 1999;6:11.
68. Wolf Y, Tillich M, Lee W, et al. Changes in aneurysm volume after endovascular repair of abdominal aortic aneurysm. *J Vasc Surg*. 2002; 36:305.
69. Golzarian J, Murgo S, Dussaussois L, et al. Evaluation of abdominal aortic aneurysm after endoluminal treatment: comparison of color Doppler sonography with biphasic helical CT. *AJR Am J Roentgenol*. 2002; 178:623.
70. Bendick P, Bove P, Long G, et al. Efficacy of ultrasound scan contrast agents in the noninvasive follow-up of aortic stent grafts. *J Vasc Surg*. 2003;37:381.
71. **Zarins C, White R, Schwarten D, et al. AneuRx stent graft versus open surgical repair of abdominal aortic aneurysm: multicenter prospective clinical trial. *J Vasc Surg*. 1999;29:292.**
72. **May J, White G, Waugh R, et al. Improved survival after endoluminal repair with second-generation prostheses compared with open repair in the treatment of abdominal aortic aneurysms: a 5-year concurrent comparison using life table method. *J Vasc Surg*. 2001;33:S21.**
73. Lee W, O'Dorisio J, Wolf Y, et al. Outcome after unilateral hypogastric artery occlusion during endovascular aneurysm repair. *J Vasc Surg*. 2001;33:921.
74. Schoder M, Zaunbauer L, Holzenbein T, et al. Internal iliac artery embolization before endovascular repair of abdominal aortic aneurysms: frequency, efficacy, and clinical results. *Am J Radiol*. 2001;177:599.

75. Mehta M, Veith F, Ohki T, et al. Unilateral and bilateral hypogastric artery interruption during aortoiliac aneurysm repair in 154 patients: a relatively innocuous procedure. *J Vasc Surg.* 2001;33:S27.
76. Kritpracha B, Pigott J, Price C, et al. Distal internal iliac artery embolization: a procedure to avoid. *J Vasc Surg.* 2003;37:943.
77. Wyers M, Shermerhorn M, Fillinger M, et al. Internal iliac artery occlusion without coil embolization during endovascular abdominal aortic aneurysm repair. *J Vasc Surg.* 2002;36:1138.
78. White G, Yu W, May J. Endoleak: a proposed new terminology to describe incomplete aneurysm exclusion by an endoluminal graft. *J Endovasc Surg.* 1996;3:124.
79. White G, May J, Waugh R, et al. Type I and type II endoleaks: a more useful classification for reporting results of endoluminal AAA repair. *J Endovasc Surg.* 1998;5:189.
80. White G, May J, Waugh R, et al. Type III and type IV endoleaks: toward a complete definition of blood flow in the sac after endoluminal AAA repair. *J Endovasc Surg.* 1998;5:305.
81. Gilling-Smith G, Brennan J, Harris P, et al. Endotension after endovascular aneurysm repair: definition, classification, and strategies for surveillance and interventions. *J Endovasc Surg.* 1999;6:305.
82. Zarins C, White R, Hodgson K, et al. Endoleak as a predictor of outcome after endovascular aneurysm repair. *J Vasc Surg.* 2000;32:90.
83. Holzenbein T, Kretschmer G, Thurnher S, et al. Midterm durability of abdominal aortic aneurysm endograft repair: a word of caution. *J Vasc Surg.* 2001;33:S46.
84. Buth J, Harris P, van Marrewijk C, et al. The significance and management of different types of endoleaks. *Semin Vasc Surg.* 2003;16:95.
85. Chuter T, Faruqi R, Sawhney R, et al. Endoleak after endovascular repair of abdominal aortic aneurysms. *J Vasc Surg.* 2001;34:98.
86. Buth J, Laheji R. Early complications and endoleaks after endovascular abdominal aortic aneurysm repair: report of a multicenter study. *J Vasc Surg.* 2000;31:134.
87. Dattilo J, Brewster D, Fan C-M, et al. Clinical failures of endovascular abdominal aortic aneurysm repair: incidence, causes, and management. *J Vasc Surg.* 2002;35:1137.
88. Zarins C. The US AneuRx clinical trial: 6-year clinical update 2002. *J Vasc Surg.* 2003;37:904.
89. Baum R, Cope C, Fairman R, et al. Translumbar embolization of type 2 endoleaks after endovascular repair of abdominal aortic aneurysms. *J Vasc Interv Radiol.* 2001;12:111.
90. Ellozy S, Carroccio A, Lookistein R, et al. First experience in human beings with a permanently implantable intrasac pressure transducer for monitoring endovascular repair of abdominal aortic aneurysms. *J Vasc Surg.* 2004;40:405.
91. Fairman R, Baum R, Carpenter J, et al. Limb intervention in patients undergoing treatment with an unsupported bifurcated aortic endograft system: a review of the phase II EVT trial. *J Vasc Surg.* 2002;36:118.
92. Carroccio A, Faries P, Morrissey N, et al. Predicting iliac limb occlusion after bifurcated aortic stent grafting: anatomic and device-related causes. *J Vasc Surg.* 2002;36:679.
93. Baum R, Shetty S, Carpenter J, et al. Limb kinking in supported and unsupported abdominal aortic stent-grafts. *J Vasc Interv Radiol.* 2000;11:1165.
94. Amesur N, Zajko A, Orons P, et al. Endovascular treatment of iliac limb stenosis or occlusion in 31 patients treated with the Ancure endograft. *J Vasc Interv Radiol.* 2000;11:421.
95. Resch T, Ivancev K, Brunkwall J, et al. Distal migration of stent-grafts after endovascular repair of abdominal aortic aneurysms. *J Vasc Interv Radiol.* 1997;10:257.
96. Albertini N, Kalliafas S, Travis S, et al. Anatomical risk factors for proximal perigraft endoleak and graft migration following endovascular repair of abdominal aortic aneurysms. *Eur J Endovasc Surg.* 2000;19:308.
97. Cao P, Verzini F, Zannetti S, et al. Device migration after endoluminal abdominal aortic aneurysm repair: analysis of 113 cases with a minimum follow-up period of 2 years. *J Vasc Surg.* 2002;35:229.
98. Badran M, Gould D, Raza I, et al. Aneurysm neck diameter after endovascular repair of abdominal aortic aneurysms. *J Vasc Interv Radiol.* 2002;13:887.
99. Lee J, Lee J, A [illegible] et al. Stent-graft migration following endovascular repair of aneurysms with large proximal necks: anatomical risk factors and long-term sequelae. *J Endovasc Ther.* 2002;9:652.
100. Sampram E, Karafa M, Mascha E, et al. Nature, frequency, and predictors of secondary procedures after endovascular repair of abdominal aortic aneurysm. *J Vasc Surg.* 2003;37:930.
101. Becker G, Kovacs M, Mathison M, et al. Risk stratification and outcomes of transluminal endografting for abdominal aortic aneurysm: 7-year experience and long-term follow-up. *J Vasc Intervent Radiol.* 2003;12:1033.
102. **Laheji R, Buth J, Harris P, et al. Need for secondary interventions after endovascular repair of abdominal aortic aneurysms. Intermediate-term follow-up results of a European collaborative registry (EUROSTAR).** ***Br J Surg.*** **2000;87:1666.**
103. Ohki T, Veith F, Shaw P, et al. Increasing incidence of midterm and long-term complications after endovascular graft repair of abdominal aortic aneurysms: a note of caution based on a 9-year experience. *Ann Surg.* 2001;234:323.
104. Carpenter J, Baum R, Barker C, et al. Durability of benefits of endovascular versus conventional abdominal aortic aneurysm repair. *J Vasc Surg.* 2002;35:222.
105. **Schermerhorn M, Finlayson S, Fillinger M, et al. Life expectancy after endovascular versus open abdominal aortic aneurysm repair: results of a decision analysis model on the basis of data from EUROSTAR.** ***J Vasc Surg.*** **2002;36:1112.**
106. Tegtmeyer C, Hartwell G, Selby J, et al. Results and complications of angioplasty in aortoiliac disease. *Circulation* 1991;83:I53.
107. Belli A, Cumberland D, Knox A, et al. The complication rate of percutaneous peripheral balloon angioplasty. *Clin Radiol.* 1990;41:380.
108. Al-Hamali S, Baskerville P, Fraser S, et al. Detection of distal emboli in patients with peripheral arterial stenosis before and after iliac angioplasty: a prospective study. *J Vasc Surg.* 1999;29:345.
109. Gardiner G Jr, Meyerovitz M, Stokes K, et al. Complications of transluminal angioplasty. *Radiology* 1986;159:201.
110. Ballard J, Sparks S, Taylor F, et al. Complications of iliac artery stent deployment. *J Vasc Surg.* 1996;24:545.
111. Palmaz J, Laborde J, Rivera F, et al. Stenting of iliac arteries with the Palmaz stent: experience from a multicenter trial. *Cardiovasc Intervent Radiol.* 1992;15:291.
112. Allaire E, Melliere D, Poussier B, et al. Iliac artery rupture during balloon dilation: what treatment? *Ann Vasc Surg.* 2003;17:306.
112a. Johnston KW, Roe M, Hogg-Johnston SA, et al. 5-Year results of a prospective study of percutaneous transluminal angioplasty. *Ann Surg.* 1987;206:403.
113. Becker G, Katzen B, Dake M. Non-coronary angioplasty. *Radiology* 1989;170:921.
114. **Martin E, Katzen B, Benenati J, et al. Multicenter trial of the Wallstent in the iliac and femoral arteries.** ***J Vasc Intervent Radiol.*** **1995;6:843.**
115. Vorwerk D, Gunther R, Schurmann K, et al. Aortic and iliac stenoses: follow-up results of stent placement after insufficient balloon angioplasty in 118 cases. *Radiology* 1996;198:45.
116. Bosch J, Hunink M. Meta-analysis of the results of percutaneous transluminal angioplasty and stent placement for aortoiliac occlusive disease. *Radiology* 1997;204:87.
117. Timaran C, Stevens S, Freeman M, et al. Predictors for adverse outcome after iliac angioplasty and stenting for limb-threatening ischemia. *J Vasc Surg.* 2002;36:507.
118. Matsi P, Manninen H, Soder H, et al. Percutaneous transluminal angioplasty in femoral artery occlusions: primary and long-term results in 107 claudicant patients using femoral and popliteal catheterization techniques. *Clin Radiol.* 1995;50:237.
119. Stanley B, Teague B, Raptis S, et al. Efficacy of balloon angioplasty of the superficial femoral artery and popliteal artery in the relief of leg ischemia. *J Vasc Surg.* 1996;23:679.
120. Matsi P, Manninen H, Vanninen R, et al. Femoropopliteal angioplasty in patients with claudication: primary and secondary patency in 140 limbs with 1–3 year follow up. *Radiology* 1994;191:727.
121. Golledge J, Ferguson K, Ellis M, et al. Outcome of femoropopliteal angioplasty. *Ann Surg.* 1999;229:146.
122. Lofberg A, Karacagil S, Ljungman C, et al. Percutaneous transluminal angioplasty of the femoropopliteal arteries in limbs with chronic lower limb ischemia. *J Vasc Surg.* 2001;34:114.
123. Johnston K. Femoral and popliteal arteries: reanalysis of results of balloon angioplasty. *Radiology* 1992;183:767.
124. **Hunink M, Donaldson M, Meyerovitz M, et al. Risks and benefits of femoropopliteal percutaneous balloon angioplasty.** ***J Vasc Surg.*** **1993; 17:183.**
125. Jahnke T, Voshage G, Muller-Hulsbeck S, et al. Endovascular placement of self-expanding nitinol coil stents for the treatment of femoropopliteal obstructive disease. *J Vasc Intervent Radiol.* 2002;13:257.
126. Cheng S, Ting A, Wong J. Endovascular stenting of superficial femoral artery stenosis and occlusions: results and risk factor analysis. *Cardiovasc Surg.* 2001;9:133.
127. Strecker E, Boos I, Gottmann D. Femoropopliteal artery stent placement: evaluation of long-term success. *Radiology* 1997;205:375.
128. Gordon I, Conroy R, Arefi M, et al. Three-year outcome of endovascular treatment of superficial femoral artery occlusion. *Arch Surg.* 2001; 136:221.
129. Bolia A, Miles K, Brennan J, et al. Percutaneous transluminal angioplasty of occlusions of the femoral and popliteal arteries by subintimal dissection. *Cardiovasc Intervent Radiol.* 1990;13:357.
130. Harthun N, Cage D, Spinosa D. Subintimal recanalization is safe and effective in treating chronic critical limb ischemia in selected patients. *Am Surg.* 2004;70:479-483.
131. Desgranges P, Boufi M, Lapeyre M, et al. Subintimal angioplasty: feasible and durable. *Eur J Vasc Endovasc Surg.* 2004;28:138.
132. Laxdal E, Jenssenn G, Pedersen G, et al. Subintimal angioplasty as a treatment of femoropopliteal artery occlusion. *Eur J Vasc Endovasc Surg.* 2003;25:578.
133. Tisi P, Mirnezami A, Baker S, et al. Role of subintimal angioplasty in the treatment of chronic lower limb ischemia. *Eur J Endovasc Surg.* 2002;24:417.
134. Saxon R, Coffman J, Gooding J, et al. Long-term results of ePTFE stent-graft versus angioplasty in the femoropopliteal artery: single center experience from a prospective, randomized trial. *J Vasc Intervent Radiol.* 2003;14:303.

135. Duda S, Bosiers M, Pusich B, et al. Endovascular treatment of peripheral artery disease with expanded PTFE-covered nitinol stents: interim analysis from a prospective controlled study. *Cardiovasc Intervent Radiol.* 2002;25:413.
136. Dorros G, Jaff M, Dorros A, et al. Tibioperoneal (outflow lesion) angioplasty can be used as primary treatment in 235 patients with critical limb ischemia: five year follow up. *Circulation* 2001;104:2057.
137. Faglia E, Mantero M, Caminiti M, et al. Extensive use of peripheral angioplasty, particularly infrapopliteal, in the treatment of ischaemic diabetic foot ulcers: clinical results of a multicentric study of 221 consecutive diabetic subjects. *J Intern Med.* 2002;252:225.
138. Hurst D, Forauer A, Bloom J, et al. Diagnosis and endovascular treatment of iliocaval compression syndrome. *J Vasc Surg.* 2001;34:106.
139. Raju S, Owen S, Neglen P. The clinical impact of iliac venous stents in the management of chronic venous insufficiency. *J Vasc Surg.* 2002;35:8.
140. Raju S, McAllister S, Neglen P. Recanalization of totally occluded iliac and adjacent venous segments. *J Vasc Surg.* 2002;36:903.
141. The STILE Investigators. Results of a prospective randomized trial evaluating surgery versus thrombolysis for ischemia of the lower extremity. *Ann Surg.* 1994;220:251.
142. Ouriel K, Veith F, Sasahara A, et al. A comparison of recombinant urokinase with vascular surgery as initial treatment for acute arterial occlusion of the legs. *N Engl J Med.* 1998;338:1105.
143. McNamara T, Goodwin S, Kandarpa K. Complications of thrombolysis. *Semin Intervent Radiol.* 1994;11:134.
144. Ouriel K, Gray B, Clair D, et al. Complications associated with the use of urokinase and recombinant tissue plasminogen activator for catheter-directed peripheral arterial and venous thrombolysis. *J Vasc Intervent Radiol.* 2000;11:295.

CHAPTER 91 ■ VASCULAR INFECTIONS

G. PATRICK CLAGETT

Vascular infections are among the most challenging and difficult problems encountered by vascular surgeons. Patients are often elderly, frail, desperately ill with multiple medical comorbid conditions, and unable to tolerate the extensive, complex operations usually required to treat the problem. Medical treatment based on specific antibiotic therapy is rarely successful when used alone, and complete resection and excision of all infected vascular structures are usually necessary to eradicate infection. Immediate restoration of blood flow to critical vascular beds by alternate anatomic routes or with replacement vascular conduits that minimize the risk for recurrent infection present additional challenges that tax the skill and ingenuity of vascular surgeons. Despite a great deal of progress in the treatment of vascular infections, morbidity and mortality remain among the highest of all vascular conditions.[1–3]

VASCULAR PROSTHETIC INFECTIONS

Pathogenesis

Vascular prostheses are foreign bodies that can be primarily infected by contamination at the time of placement or secondarily infected after implantation by hematogenous, lymphatic, or contiguous spread of microorganisms. The overall incidence of clinically overt prosthetic infection varies according to anatomic site. Aortic prostheses confined to the abdominal or thoracic cavity rarely become infected; the incidence ranges from 0.5% to 2%.[2] The incidence is higher, from 2% to 6%, in proximal or distal anastomotic sites at the femoral level (e.g., aortofemoral or femoral-popliteal bypasses).[4]

Several features of the femoral area predispose to infectious complications. The groin is a relatively dirty area that is difficult to clean, and incisions placed in the groin are prone to infection and healing problems. Vertical groin incisions cut obliquely across the inguinal crease, tend to gape, and in obese patients lie buried in moist folds of skin. Furthermore, superficial inguinal lymph nodes are usually transected during exposure of the common femoral artery and, if not ligated, will bathe a vascular prosthesis in lymph fluid that may contain bacteria. Potential sources of prosthetic contamination in this circumstance include open, infected ischemic ulcers of a lower extremity, gangrenous toes, and wounds in any other area drained by the inguinal lymphatics, such as the perineum and perianal area. Another factor implicating the groin wound in the etiology of vascular prosthetic infections is transient local ischemia during placement of an aortic cross-clamp, which may render the wound more susceptible to infection.

Most authorities agree that the majority of vascular prosthetic infections are initiated at the time of operation.[2,3,5] Although direct proof of this tenet is difficult to obtain, the prevalence of *Staphylococcus epidermidis* among offending organisms suggests that skin contamination with the patient's own flora is an important mechanism.[6,7] Mucosal colonization of nasal, oropharyngeal, and gastrointestinal sites are also potential sources of *S. epidermidis* and other coagulase-negative staphylococci bacteremia and contamination.[8]

The presence of *Staphylococcus aureus* and other nosocomially acquired bacteria is also common and points to environmental sources of contamination. Other intraoperative sources of contamination include intestinal flora when the gastrointestinal tract is entered or when operations, such as cholecystectomy, are performed concomitantly. Laminated thrombus lining the wall of aneurysms has been implicated as a source of contamination and, when cultured, yields bacteria in about 10% of specimens. *S. epidermidis* is the most common isolate.[9,10]

Postoperative sources of vascular prosthetic infection include wound complications, urinary tract infections, and invasive line sepsis. Early and late hematogenous seeding of prostheses can occur during transient bacteremia associated with remote, noncontiguous infections or dental procedures.

Although bacteria are most often cultured from infected arterial prostheses, other, less common microorganisms, such as fungi, *Mycoplasma*, and *Mycobacterium* have been encountered. *S. epidermidis* is the most common pathogen reported in modern series and outnumbers *S. aureus* infections two to one. Gram-negative and polymicrobial infections are increasingly encountered but remain less prevalent than gram-positive infections. In many cases, negative cultures are reported despite convincing local evidence of infection, including a nonincorporated prosthesis surrounded by grossly purulent fluid.[11] These cases are most likely due to *S. epidermidis* or other low-virulence organisms that are exposed to perioperative antibiotics at the time of sampling and require fastidious microbiologic techniques for growth. Sonication of infected prosthetic material, growth in tryptic soy broth, and prolonged incubation for several days have been reported to increase the yield of cultures positive for *S. epidermidis*.[12]

The presence of a foreign body, such as an implanted device, increases the risk for infection. Early investigations documented that it takes only 10^2 *S. aureus* organisms to cause an abscess at the site of a subcutaneous silk suture but 10^6 organisms to cause an infection in normal skin with no foreign body present. The explanations of why foreign materials are prone to infection involve physicochemical properties of the material, impairment of host defenses, and special properties of bacteria that facilitate their growth in the presence of a biomaterial.[13]

The biologic reaction to an implanted vascular prosthesis comprises an acute inflammatory response in the early stages and progresses to formation of a fibrous capsule or tissue growth into porous materials. Neutrophils rapidly become associated with any implanted biomaterial *in vivo*, become prematurely activated by contact with the material, and rapidly lose the capacity to become activated in response to subsequent stimuli, such as the presence of bacteria. Neutrophils in contact with biomaterials rapidly lose their ability to produce superoxide and other reactive oxygen species and become relatively impotent in their microbicidal activity.[14,15] In a sense, the biomaterial becomes a massive "decoy" that averts and diverts the ability of neutrophils to respond normally to bacteria in the microenvironment. In addition, neutrophil products released in these circumstances may promote dysfunction of new neutrophils entering the microenvironment.[16]

Vascular prosthetic biomaterials may vary in their susceptibility to infection by different microorganisms. Highly textured or rough-surfaced biomaterials, such as textiles manufactured from Dacron (woven or knitted), are more prone to bacterial adherence than smooth-surfaced biomaterials, such as expanded polytetrafluoroethylene (ePTFE) or polyurethane.[17] *In vivo*, adherence of platelets, plasma proteins, and other blood constituents and varying conditions of shear may dramatically alter the responses of different biomaterials to microorganisms, and all biomaterials remain susceptible to infection.[18,19]

The principal organism responsible for infections of all implanted medical devices, including vascular prostheses, is *S. epidermidis*. It is one species of coagulase-negative staphylococci that is a major cause of nosocomial infections and of nosocomial bacteremias in particular.[20] The organism is a ubiquitous skin commensural of relatively slow growth and low virulence. It causes chronic infections with local manifestations but little or no systemic toxicity. Pivotal in the pathogenesis of *S. epidermidis* infection is the production of multilayered biofilms composed of exopolysaccharides, usually referred to as "slime."

The elaboration of biofilms takes place following the adherence of *S. epidermidis* to biomaterials and usually occurs when organisms adhere to one another in microcolonies.[21] Both adherence of organisms to polymer surfaces and to each other (cell-cell adhesion) is mediated by capsular polysaccharide adhesins.[21,22] Mutant bacteria that do not produce adhesins lack cell-cell adhesion and do not produce biofilms.[23] Once elaborated, biofilms form a protective shield that allows continued bacterial growth in relatively hostile environments. Bacterial nutrients and metabolic wastes freely traverse the polysaccharide biofilm but antibiotics do not. Biofilms also alter inflammatory changes, impair host defenses, and promote tenacious adherence of microbial colonies to the biomaterial.[24] *S. epidermidis* infections tend to be persistent and refractory to antibiotics, and the implant must be removed to clear the infection.

Once established, bacterial infection spreads throughout a vascular prosthesis and eventually involves anastomotic sites. The eventual destruction of vascular tissue leads to the formation of an anastomotic false aneurysm. The first manifestation of a vascular prosthetic infection is often an anastomotic false aneurysm or its most frequent complication, prosthetic limb thrombosis in the case of an aortobifemoral bypass. When the false aneurysm involves the aortic anastomosis, rupture into the duodenum may occur and produce an aortoduodenal fistula with catastrophic hemorrhage.

Although all microorganisms producing vascular prosthetic infections are associated with false aneurysms, they vary in their propensity to destroy vascular tissue. Gram-negative organisms, such as *Pseudomonas aeruginosa, Proteus species*, and *Escherichia coli* are particularly notorious for their ability to digest vascular tissue.[25] These organisms elaborate elastase and alkaline protease, which break down elastin, collagen, fibronectin, and fibrin. *S. epidermidis* and other coagulase-negative staphylococci also secrete proteolytic proteins that can degrade vascular tissue. The mechanisms underlying protease elaboration and activation is highly regulated and complex.[26] In addition to causing vascular disruption and the formation of false aneurysms, many bacteria produce substances that are highly thrombogenic and may induce thrombosis that is the first manifestation of a vascular prosthetic infection.

Clinical Presentation

The clinical presentations of vascular prosthetic infections can be protean and subtle, so that the diagnosis is difficult. The tempo and severity of the clinical manifestations often depend on the microorganism. A patient whose infection is caused by a virulent organism, such as *S. aureus, P. aeruginosa,* or *E. coli* presents with systemic signs of sepsis. As an example, a patient with a vascular prosthesis who has persistent fever, chills, and an elevated white blood cell count with a left shift should be suspected of having a vascular prosthetic infection. Virulent microorganisms also tend to cause earlier manifestations of infection, with the interval between implantation of the prosthesis and diagnosis of infection often being months. Very early prosthetic infections, diagnosed within weeks of implantation, are most often associated with wound infections that involve the vascular prostheses by contiguous spread.

In contrast, patients with infection caused by a low-virulence organism, such as *S. epidermidis*, present later, often years after placement.[7] Systemic signs and symptoms are usually mild or absent. These patients most often present with local manifestations, such as a chronic groin sinus that discharges small amounts of pus, a chronic wound infection exposing the prosthesis, femoral anastomotic false aneurysm, or aortofemoral bypass limb thrombosis. They may have low-grade fever and mild constitutional symptoms, but overt systemic signs of sepsis are absent. The white blood cell count is usually normal or only mildly elevated, but the erythrocyte sedimentation rate is often abnormal. A patient presenting with a femoral anastomotic false aneurysm or limb thrombosis who has an elevated erythrocyte sedimentation rate should be suspected of having a vascular prosthetic infection.

Patients presenting with massive gastrointestinal hemorrhage from aortoduodenal or aortoenteric fistula frequently have had lesser episodes of bleeding hours to days before the major episode. These are often referred to as "herald" or "sentinel" episodes of bleeding and offer a window of opportunity for diagnosis and management that may avert exsanguinating hemorrhage. Any patient with an intraabdominal vascular prosthesis who has an episode of upper or lower gastrointestinal bleeding should be suspected of having an underlying aortoenteric fistula, and an expeditious workup is important.

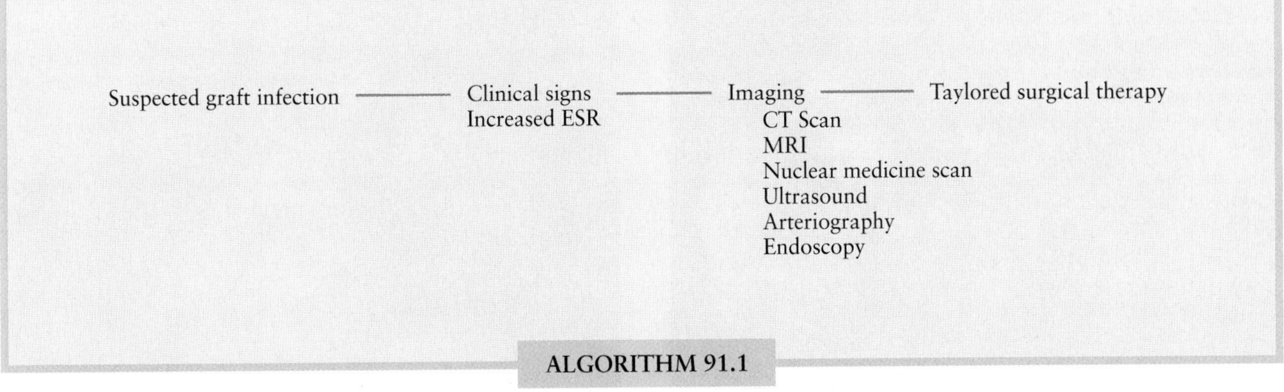

ALGORITHM 91.1 Diagnosis and treatment of prosthetic infection.

Chronic gastrointestinal bleeding can also occur in patients with an aortoenteric fistula but is more often associated with an enteric erosion. This condition, often referred to as "graft-enteric erosion," differs from aortoenteric fistula in that the body or limb of the vascular prosthesis erodes into bowel and the aortic suture line is not involved. This produces chronic bleeding from the eroded bowel mucosa, analogous to bleeding from an ulcer, and patients may present with chronic anemia. The diagnosis should be suspected in a patient with an intraabdominal vascular prosthesis who has anemia, stool positive for occult blood on guaiac testing, and fever.

Another manifestation of aortofemoral and aortoiliac prosthetic infections is hydroureteronephrosis. This can develop if the ureter becomes obstructed as a result of periprosthetic inflammation and may be bilateral or unilateral, depending on the extent of infection. It is unusual for hydroureteronephrosis to be the initial manifestation of vascular prosthetic infection because the urologic condition is usually asymptomatic. This complication most often is noted during the workup of a patient with an infected vascular prosthesis who presents with other symptoms, such as a groin sinus or gastrointestinal bleeding.

Diagnosis

Because the manifestations of vascular prosthetic infections are so varied and subtle and because the consequences of a missed diagnosis may be lethal, imaging tests are important (Algorithm 91.1).[27] The types of imaging and other diagnostic tests used are based on the clinical presentation. Computed tomography (CT) scanning has long been the mainstay of diagnostic imaging for suspected vascular prosthetic infection. CT findings suggestive of infection include ectopic gas, periprosthetic fluid, loss of tissue planes, periprosthetic inflammatory changes, thickening of adjacent bowel, hydroureteronephrosis, and anastomotic false aneurysm (Fig. 91.1).[28] These findings are most specific and useful for late infections. During the immediate period following implantation, periprosthetic fluid, air, and inflammatory changes may be present for 2 to 3 months. After 3 months, postoperative hematoma and gas should resolve and tissue planes return to normal.[29]

Magnetic resonance imaging (MRI) has provided an alternative to CT scanning for cross-sectional imaging. In addition to demonstrating the same features seen on CT (periprosthetic air, fluid and structural abnormalities), MRI is particularly helpful in assessing periprosthetic inflammatory changes. These are seen as high-intensity signals on T2-weighted images in the tissues surrounding the prosthesis and accurately portray tissue edema (Fig. 91.2).[30] Such images can be particularly helpful in assessing the extent of infection, which may determine the operative approach. For example, in a patient with an infection localized to a single, distal limb of an aortobifemoral bypass, removal of the entire prosthesis may not be required for adequate treatment of the infection.

Radionuclide scanning has also been used in the diagnosis of vascular prosthetic infections. Scintigraphy with the use of autologous white blood cells labeled with indium oxine In^{111} is the most common technique currently used, although the use of white cells labeled with ^{67}gallium, technetium, and other isotopes have been reported.[31,32] In addition, scintigraphy based on labeled human immunoglobulin G has been used and may be more sensitive than scintigraphy with white blood cells.[33] A problem with all scintigraphic methods in diagnosing vascular prosthetic infections is a lack of specificity caused by uptake in other organs or tissues that may be contiguous. In addition, faint or no uptake in the presence of limited or low-virulence infection can result in false-negative results. Scintigraphy is most helpful when occult prosthetic infection is suspected. An example would be a patient with a vascular prosthesis presenting with a fever of unknown origin or a complex of other nonspecific symptoms in whom white blood cell scintigraphy "lights up" the prosthesis.

Ultrasonography can be useful and is noninvasive and inexpensive. The finding of an echo-lucent rim or "halo" sign surrounding a vascular prosthesis is highly suggestive of a vascular prosthetic infection (Fig. 91.3). In addition, duplex ultrasonography may uncover other findings such as anastomotic

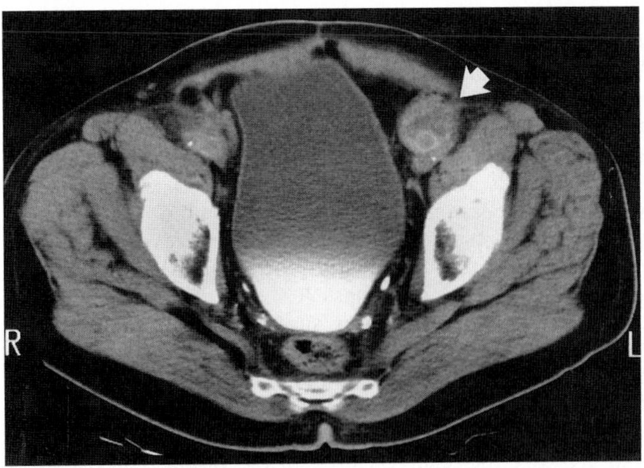

FIGURE 91.1 Computed tomography (CT) scan of lower pelvis demonstrating fluid and an enhancing ring around the left limb of an aortobifemoral bypass (*arrow*).

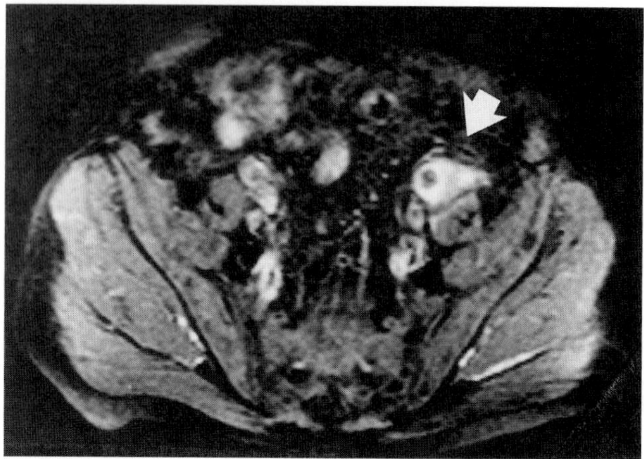

FIGURE 91.2 Magnetic resonance imaging (MRI) of the lower pelvis of the patient in Figure 91.1. The arrow points to high intensity signals on T2-weighted images characteristic of inflammation and tissue edema.

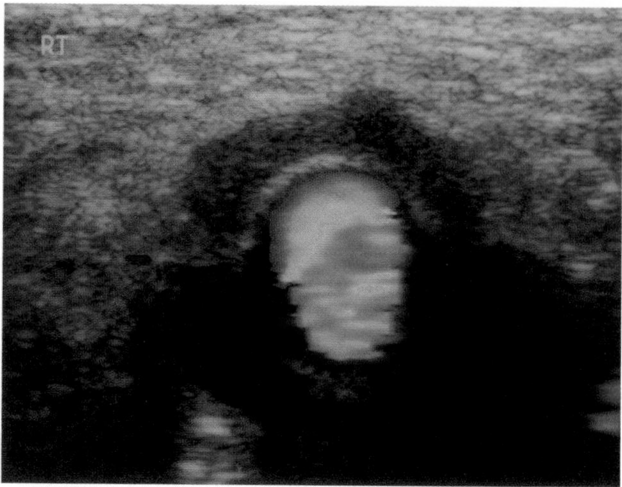

FIGURE 91.3 Duplex, color-flow scan demonstrating echo lucent rim or "halo" sign surrounding the limb of an aortofemoral bypass graft.

false aneurysms that are frequently associated with vascular prosthetic infections.

Arteriography is of limited usefulness in the diagnosis of vascular prosthetic infection, but it may, on occasion, demonstrate an aortic false aneurysm or even active leakage of contrast into the bowel lumen, which is pathognomonic for aortoenteric fistula. Arteriography is helpful in planning reconstruction after removal of the prosthesis and is most useful in late infection, when the vascular anatomy may have been altered by progressive occlusive disease.

In patients presenting with gastrointestinal bleeding and suspected aortoenteric fistula, complete upper gastrointestinal endoscopy with visualization of the third and fourth portions of the duodenum, the most common site of fistula, is necessary. Even if this study is incomplete, with inability to visualize the distal duodenum or the finding of gastrointestinal lesions (e.g., chronic peptic ulcer) that are not actively bleeding, an aortoenteric fistula may still be present. Continued, unexplained bleeding mandates operative exploration to rule out aortoenteric fistula. At the time of operation, the duodenum, proximal jejunum, and any other bowel in contact with a vascular prosthesis must be dissected free to make or exclude this diagnosis.

Treatment

The primary goals of treatment are to save life and limb, and this is best accomplished by eradicating infection and maintaining adequate circulation to portions of the body perfused by the infected prosthesis. Secondary goals include minimizing morbidity, restoring normal function, and maintaining long-term function without the need for repeated intervention and risk of amputation.

These goals are best achieved by excision of all infected prosthetic material and vascular tissues combined with appropriate arterial reconstruction. The currently favored methods of arterial reconstruction for aortic prosthetic infection include extraanatomic bypass[34–50] and *in situ* replacement with the use of autogenous superficial femoral popliteal veins,[48,51–58] arterial allografts,[59–71] and vascular prostheses that are often treated or soaked in antibiotic solutions.[48,72–76] Pooled outcome data from contemporary series reported since 1985 are presented in Table 91.1. Direct comparisons of these data to judge the relative success of the various approaches is difficult because of the heterogeneity of patients with different degrees of illness and different comorbid conditions in the reported series. All of these approaches are valid and useful depending on patient-specific characteristics and circumstances. It is a mistake to think that a single surgical approach is applicable to all patients with this condition. These complicated and multifaceted patients with varying degrees of illness require individualized attention. The pros and cons of each approach are also outlined in Table 91.1.

Extraanatomic bypass, usually involving an axillofemoral bypass, is an excellent choice for infected aortoiliac recon-

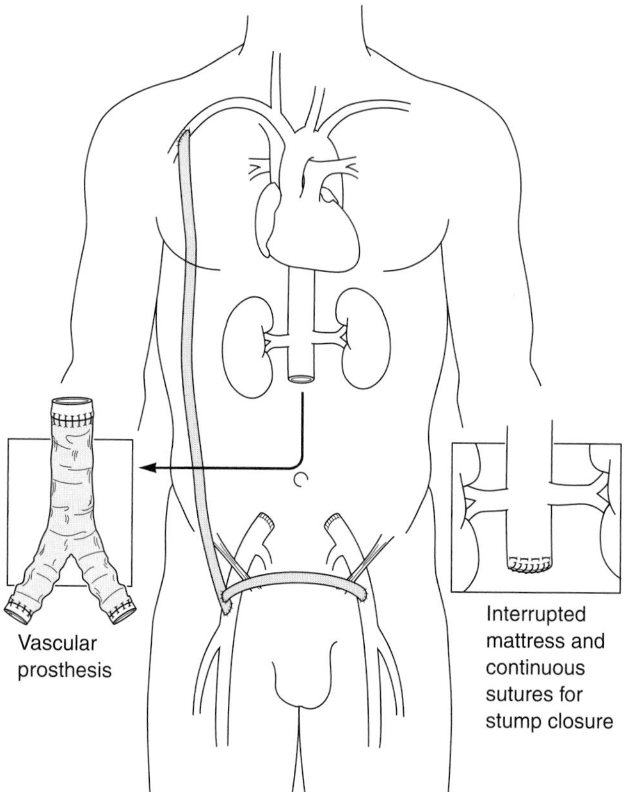

FIGURE 91.4 Standard treatment for an infected aortic vascular prosthesis. An axillobifemoral bypass is performed first. This is followed a few days later by removal of the infected aortic prosthesis and careful oversewing of the aortic stump as illustrated. This operation has its greatest usefulness in patients with infected aortoiliac prostheses and who have femoral areas free of infection and good runoff.

TABLE 91.1

TREATMENT OF AORTIC PROSTHETIC INFECTIONS[a]

	References	No. patients	Mortality (range) %	Major amputation (range) %	Reinfection/ anastomotic or vascular disruption %	Five-year primary patency %	Five-year assisted/ secondary patency %	Advantages	Disadvantages
Extra-anatomic bypass	34–50	590	21.2 (5.0–40.6)	10.7 (0–15.6)	16.0	30–73	65–90	Procedure can be staged. Less physiologic stress.	Poor patency, high long-term amputation rate. Thrombectomy, revision often required. Potential for reinfection of bypass and aortic stump blowout.
In situ superficial femoral-popliteal vein replacement	48, 51–58	147	11.0 (6.7–20.0)	5.4 (4.9–6.7)	0.6	84	98–100	Autogenous reconstruction, resists infection. Excellent patency, low long-term amputation rate.	Complex procedure. Long ischemia time. Fasciotomy may be required in up to 20%.
In situ allograft replacement	59–71	684	22.0 (8.3–36.4)	2.0 (0–3.0)	9.7	?	?	Expeditious procedure. No aortic stump.	Reinfection. Allograft deterioration and disruption. Unavailability of allografts.
In situ prosthetic replacement	48, 72–76	126	13.0 (8.0–21.7)	0	10.3	?	?	Expeditious procedure. No aortic stump.	Reinfection rate high and unpredictable. Indefinite antibiotic therapy.

[a]Pooled data from major series reported since 1985.

structions in which femoral sites are free of sepsis and arterial run-off is good (Fig. 91.4). It is also possibly less of a physiologic insult than other procedures, particularly when the operations can be staged so that extraanatomic bypass precedes removal of the infected aortic prosthesis by a period of days.[35] This approach has the advantage of preserving lower extremity blood flow during removal of the aortic prosthesis, so that ischemic time is minimized.

Unfortunately, the durability of an extraanatomic bypass is limited in patients with multilevel occlusive disease and poor runoff. Most patients with infected aortic prostheses have an aortobifemoral bypass, and extraanatomic bypass in such patients usually requires bilateral axillofemoral procedures with distal anastomoses to diseased and, often, small profunda femoral or popliteal arteries. These are disadvantaged reconstructions with poor long-term patency despite the administration of antithrombotic agents (Table 91.1). They are prone to sudden thrombotic occlusion without warning, and amputation rates are high, even after thrombectomy and multiple revisions. In one large series, one third of patients required major amputation during long-term follow-up.[36] In addition, reinfection of the extraanatomic bypass prostheses occurs in 10% to 20% of patients, and this condition is often lethal. A final problem with extraanatomic bypass is continuing infection at the site of aortic closure, or aortic "stump." Although an infrequent occurrence (<10% of cases), aortic stump blowout is almost always fatal.

Dissatisfaction with the long-term patency of extraanatomic bypass led to the development of *in situ* autogenous venous reconstruction.[48,51–58] Early experiences were with greater saphenous veins, but the use of superficial femoropopliteal veins rapidly evolved because of their large caliber and superior patency (Figs. 91.5 and 91.6).[51] This reconstruction is most applicable in patients with extensive occlusive disease and poor runoff, a circumstance in which the patency of an autogenous venous reconstruction would theoretically be better than the patency of a prosthetic bypass. The situation is analogous to the use of vein grafts for femoropopliteal and distal bypasses because of their superior patency in comparison with prosthetic conduits. This advantage has been realized, with excellent 5-year cumulative rates of 85% to 90% for primary patency and 100% for secondary/assisted patency in superficial femoropopliteal vein aortofemoral reconstructions.[53,58] Long-term amputation rates have been reported to be correspondingly low.

The principal disadvantage of using superficial femoropopliteal veins for aortofemoral reconstruction is that the procedure is technically demanding and long. The lower extremity ischemic time is longer than with other approaches but can be minimized by carefully sequencing the procedure to shorten aortic cross-clamp time. To minimize open body cavity exposure and lower extremity ischemia, the operation is carried out in the following order: (a) dissect superficial femoropopliteal veins and leave *in situ* until needed, (b) isolate and

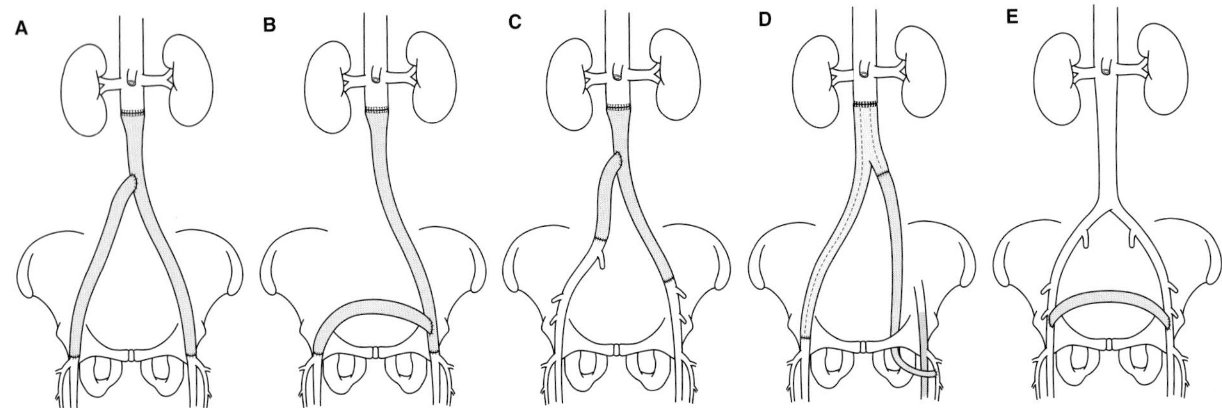

FIGURE 91.5 Multiple reconstructions using the superficial femoropopliteal vein after removal of an infected vascular prosthesis. (*A*) Standard *in situ* aortobifemoral replacement. (*B*) Left *in situ* aortofemoral bypass with left-to-right femoral crossover bypass. (*C*) *In situ* aortoiliac reconstruction. (*D*) Unilateral transobturator aorta profunda bypass. (*E*) Femoral crossover bypass.

control femoral vessels, (c) enter abdomen and obtain aortic control, (d) remove infected prosthesis, and (e) perform reconstruction with superficial femoropopliteal veins.[77]

Acute venous hypertension can result in the need for leg fasciotomy in up to 20% of limbs following harvest of the superficial femoral-popliteal vein.[78] Special risk factors that predict the need for fasciotomy include preexisting, advanced limb ischemia (preoperative ankle-brachial index <0.40) and concomitant ipsilateral harvest of the greater saphenous vein. Acute muscle swelling from venous hypertension coupled with ischemia-reperfusion injury are major pathogenetic factors.[78]

Long-term lower extremity venous morbidity is also a potential drawback to harvesting the superficial femoropopliteal veins. However, venous morbidity has been surprisingly infrequent and mild.[53,58] The benign course following removal of the superficial femoropopliteal veins is a consequence of several compensating mechanisms.[79] First, the junction of the profunda femoral and common femoral veins is carefully preserved after disconnection of the proximal superficial femoral vein to allow unimpeded drainage via the profunda system. Second, several anatomic collateral connections are found between the remaining distal popliteal vein and the profunda system, and many of these collaterals enlarge to accommodate the increase in volume flow following removal of the superficial femoropopliteal vein. Finally, the valves in the tibial veins and collateral circuits remain functional, so that distal venous reflux does not occur.

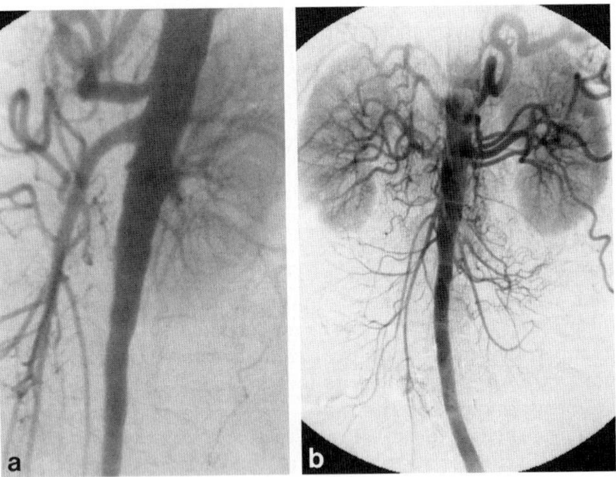

FIGURE 91.6 Lateral (*A*) and anteroposterior (*B*) arteriogram of a superficial femoropopliteal vein *in situ* replacement after removal of an infected aortobifemoral bypass. The left-to-right femoral crossover bypass with superficial femoropopliteal vein is not shown. The figure illustrates the excellent size match between the large-caliber superficial femoropopliteal vein and the infrarenal aorta.

A final concern is that placing superficial femoropopliteal veins in an infected field may lead to reinfection and disruption. Experience with this approach has documented that these vein grafts resist gram-positive, gram-negative, and fungal infections, and disruption of anastomoses has been rare. Long-term aneurysmal degeneration has also been studied for up to 10 years after placement of these vein grafts, and has not occurred.[53]

In situ allograft replacement has been reported with varying degrees of success.[59–71] Acute and delayed aortic allograft disruption has been reported and is a distinct limitation of using allografts in infected fields[61,80] (Table 91.1). In addition, long-term deterioration leading to thrombosis and aneurysmal degeneration has been reported. Ready availability of allograft material is another limitation of this approach in situations in which emergency or urgent operations are often required.

Replacement of the infected aortic prosthesis with a new prosthesis has also been reported.[48,72–76] Most often, the new prosthesis is soaked in an antibiotic solution, usually rifampin (60 mg/mL for 15 minutes), before implantation.[74,75] This approach is most often successful in patients with limited infections of low virulence following aggressive débridement of all infected vascular and surrounding tissues to create a clean field. Despite these precautions, the potential for reinfection is a serious drawback,[44] and patients treated in this manner require close and vigilant follow-up with frequent imaging studies such as CT or MRI. They also are usually treated with lifelong oral antibiotics.

In situ prosthetic and allograft reconstructions may be most useful in very ill and unstable patients and in those with actively bleeding aortoenteric fistulae. Expeditious *in situ* replacement in these circumstances can be lifesaving and may be used as a "bridge" procedure, with definitive reconstruction (extraanatomic or superficial femoropopliteal vein) carried out at a later date when the patient has been rendered fit for such a reconstruction.

Conservative approaches that do not involve removal of the infected prostheses have also been reported.[81–86] These are based on aggressive drainage and debridement of infected tissues; intensive, culture-specific antibiotic therapy; meticulous wound care to achieve coverage of exposed prosthetic material; and coverage of exposed prosthetic material with muscle flaps. Conservative approaches are most appropriately used when infection is extracavitary and limited in extent, systemic signs of sepsis are absent, the virulence of the infecting organisms is low, and anastomotic sites are uninvolved.[84] Elderly and frail patients with multiple medical comorbidities who would most likely not survive conventional operations for aortic graft infection should be considered selectively for less invasive procedures.[85] Like those who have undergone *in situ* prosthetic replacement, these patients require close follow-up and indefinite oral antibiotic treatment.

If an infection involves only one limb of a bifurcated aortic prosthesis, the limb is usually resected.[12,87–90] Revascularization is often carried out via obturator bypass or another prosthetic reconstruction performed in a clean field. Autogenous superficial femoropopliteal or greater saphenous veins have also been used for this purpose.[89] It is important that the extent of infection be assessed with imaging studies in addition to direct visual inspection. In the case of a unilateral femoral infection of an aortofemoral bypass, the general approach is to begin the operation by inspecting the intraabdominal portion of the prosthesis. If the infection grossly involves the main body of the bifurcated prosthesis, complete removal is necessary. If the suspected limb is well incorporated and free of gross infection, division of the limb, closure of the tunnel, and obturator or other extraanatomic bypass are performed. The final portion of this operation is removal of the infected limb from below, with care taken to prevent cross-contamination of other, freshly placed incisions that have been closed.

Infection of Femoropopliteal/Distal Prosthetic Bypasses

In general, the management principles for infected infrainguinal prosthetic bypasses are similar to those for infected aortic prostheses. Excision of all infected prosthetic material and creation of a new bypass through clean tissue planes are optimal.[91] Venous autografts are preferable to vascular prostheses because of the low risk of reinfection. Unfortunately, many of these patients have limited sources of adequate vein for a new vein graft bypass. Additionally, because of the limited anatomic area, cross-contamination and infection of a new prosthetic conduit are probable. The overall mortality of patients undergoing operations for infected prosthetic infrainguinal bypasses approaches 20% and may be higher in patients undergoing limb salvage procedures.[91,92] These considerations have led some experts to recommend excision of the infected prosthesis and amputation in circumstances in which the limb remains in jeopardy after removal of the infected prosthesis. The rate of major amputation is approximately 40%.[91,92] If assessment with Doppler ultrasonography indicates that the limb remains viable (audible arterial signals present at the ankle level), removal of the infected prosthesis with vein patch closure of anastomotic sites is preferred. If only a limited portion of the prosthesis is involved, nonresectional, conservative measures have been successfully used.[81,93] Results with this approach are best when virulence of the infection is low, sepsis is absent, and anastomoses are free of infection.

Prevention of Vascular Prosthetic Infections

The benefit of short-term antibiotic prophylaxis in preventing wound infections after vascular surgery has been demonstrated in randomized trials.[94–96] Most often, a first generation cephalosporin is administered intravenously shortly before operation, during operation if blood loss is extensive or the operation is prolonged, and 2 hours after operation. Evidence suggests that a more prolonged course, for up to 4 to 5 days after operation or until all invasive lines have been removed, may provide additional protection.[97] When patients have infected ischemic lesions of a lower extremity, culture-specific antibiotics should be administered perioperatively. Also, the use of more specific prophylactic antibiotic therapy should be considered in hospitals where certain organisms are prevalent, especially when exposure is increased by prolonged preoperative hospitalization.

Attention to intraoperative factors is also important in preventing vascular prosthetic infections. Patients undergoing repeated and emergency operations are especially prone to wound infections and present additional risks. Meticulous attention to hemostasis and avoidance of wound hematomas and seromas that can become secondarily infected are important surgical tenets that are often difficult to achieve in patients given anticoagulants during the operation and who are also taking antithrombotic agents, such as aspirin or clopidogrel. If possible, these agents should be discontinued 1 week before the operation. Ligation and control of the femoral lymphatics are also probably important technical features in preventing vascular prosthetic infections. Electrocautery of lymphatic tissue leads to coagulation necrosis of lymphatic vessels but does not prevent extravasation of lymph fluid.

Patients undergoing aortic operations are prone to intraoperative hypothermia, and this condition has been shown to impair neutrophil function and increase the incidence of postoperative wound infection.[98] Maintenance of normal body temperature should be the goal during major vascular operations. Additional procedures on the gastrointestinal or biliary tract that may result in intraoperative contamination of a vascular prosthesis should be avoided unless the additional procedure is deemed necessary to avoid life-threatening postoperative complications. Hematogenous seeding of a vascular prosthesis is a continuing risk for as long as the prosthesis is in place. Dental work, procedures on the gastrointestinal and genitourinary tracts, and angiographic procedures should be carried out with the patient protected by prophylactic antibiotics.

INFECTED (MYCOTIC) ANEURYSMS

Pathogenesis

In the late 19th century, Osler first used the term *mycotic* to describe the peripheral, infected aneurysms occurring in patients with bacterial endocarditis.[99] The beaded gross appearance of the multiple aneurysms in these patients resembled a fungus growth, hence the term *mycotic*. However, he delineated the pathogenesis to be destruction of the arterial wall subsequent to embolization of bacteria-laden material from the heart. In the era before antibiotics, the presence of such lesions indicated a malignant form of endocarditis because death was inevitable.

Mycotic aneurysms, as described by Osler, are now rare, and a more comprehensive term is *infected aneurysm* or *microbial arteritis*.[100] Infected aneurysms encompass preexisting aneurysms that are secondarily infected by hematogenous or contiguous spread and infections of the arterial wall that subsequently cause aneurysmal degeneration.[101] When the arterial wall is completely disrupted and a contained rupture is present, the aneurysm may be termed an infected false- or pseudoaneurysm. Currently, less than 10% of infected aneurysms are caused by bacterial endocarditis.[102]

It is difficult to infect the normal arterial wall during bacteremia, but such a mechanism has been postulated in severely immunocompromised patients. Special risk factors for microbial arteritis include long-term steroid use, chemotherapy for malignancy, severe alcoholism, chronic renal failure, and extensive radiation therapy.[103,104] Such infections may be initiated by hematogenous spread of bacteria through the vasa vasorum. Much more common is infection of abnormal arterial walls with irregular luminal surfaces, to which microorganisms attach during bacteremia.[100] Arterial wall defects and irregularities associated with infected aneurysms include atherosclerotic plaque, degenerative arterial aneurysms, and congenital abnormalities such as aortic coarctation and patent ductus arteriosus. Host compromise, malnutrition, and advanced age are also seen in many of these patients.

Contiguous spread of infection is common in infected aortic aneurysms and is seen in such conditions as spinal osteomyelitis, pancreatitis, and retroperitoneal abscess associated with diverticulitis and other gastrointestinal and severe urinary infections.[100] Trauma is becoming an increasingly common mechanism by which infected aneurysms develop; bacteria are introduced at the time of intraarterial drug injection with contaminated needles (drug abuse)[105] or the placement of arterial catheters for diagnostic and therapeutic interventions or for monitoring.[106] Almost all infected arterial aneurysms associated with trauma are false aneurysms in which arterial wall continuity is lost.

In reports of infection of preexisting aortic aneurysms, gram-positive organisms predominate over gram-negative organisms and are present in about 60% of cases.[100,107] Of these, *Staphylococcus* species are the most prevalent with *S. aureus* being the most commonly encountered overall. Streptococci are also etiologic agents, with *Streptococcus viridans* being the most common subtype. In iatrogenic arterial infections associated with indwelling arterial catheters, methicillin-resistant *S. aureus* and other nosocomial organisms are being seen with increasing frequency.

Salmonella is the most prevalent organism associated with infection of a nonaneurysmal aorta.[100,104,107,108] The diseased, plaque-ridden aorta has a unique susceptibility to *Salmonella* infections. *Salmonella choleraesuis* and *Salmonella enteritidis*, especially the subtype *Salmonella typhimurium,* account for more than half of reported cases of *Salmonella* aortitis.[100]

Gram-negative arterial infections are much more virulent than gram-positive infections, and arteries infected with gram-negative organisms are much more prone to rupture. Gram-negative organisms, such as *P. aeruginosa*, can elaborate alkaline proteinase and a variety of elastases that cause vascular wall neurosis.[25] In addition, many bacteria, both gram-positive and gram-negative, produce collagenases.[109–111] Bacteria can also up-regulate collagenases and metalloproteinases in inflammatory cells associated with aneurysms.[111] Recent interest has centered on neutrophil elastase in the pathogenesis of aneurysms.[112] According to this view, bacteria may play an indirect role, acting principally through the recruitment of acute inflammatory cells, which subsequently release neutrophil elastase.

Once the arterial wall is infected, rapid, focal and progressive deterioration occurs. This process results in the characteristic saccular or multiloculated appearance of these aneurysms and often leads to locally contained rupture and the formation of a false aneurysm. In aortas without a preexisting aneurysm, infected aneurysms tend to occur in the posterior wall of the suprarenal or supraceliac aorta[100,103,104] (Fig. 91.7). When a preexisting aortic aneurysm becomes secondarily infected, the infrarenal location is the most common site.[107,113,114]

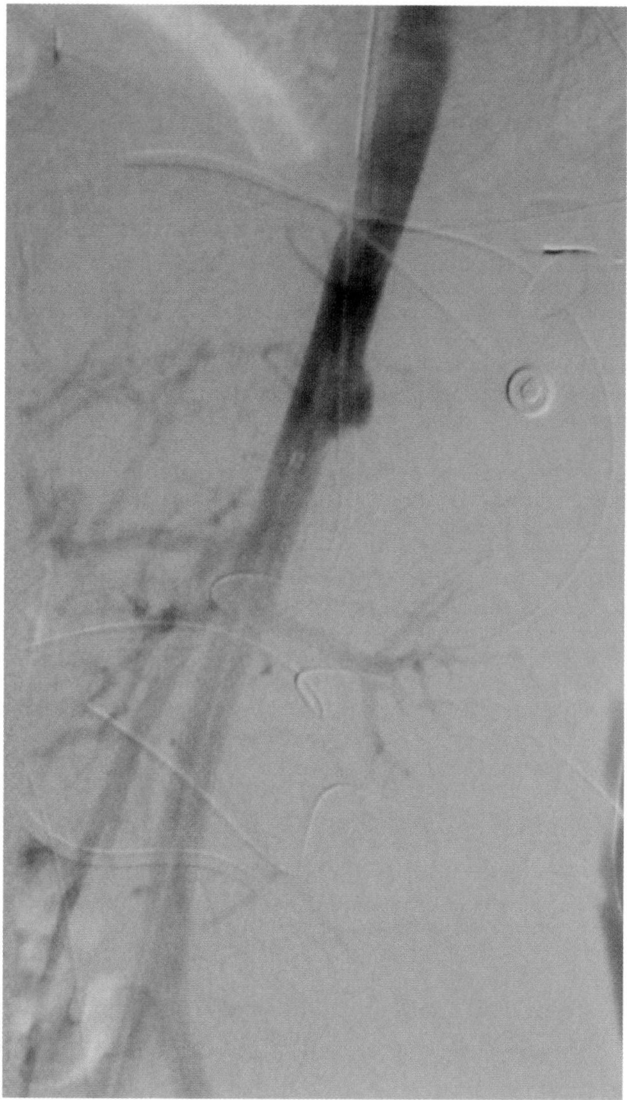

FIGURE 91.7 Infected aneurysm involving the posterior wall of the supraceliac aorta.

Clinical Presentation

The clinical presentation of an infected aneurysm depends on the virulence of the organism, the anatomic location, and the duration of infection. *Salmonella* aortic infections may appear after a febrile gastrointestinal illness. The presence of a tender abdominal aortic aneurysm in such a patient in association with continued fever and positive blood cultures strongly suggests this diagnosis. Infection of a preexisting aortic aneurysm may present as fever of unknown origin, malaise, or back and flank pain. Such patients are frequently debilitated, malnourished, and immunocompromised as the result of chronic illness, and the presence of an aortic aneurysm and positive blood cultures in this setting should arouse suspicion of an infected aneurysm. Chronic osteomyelitis or other retroperitoneal infectious processes contiguous to the aorta may also be present.

Infected aortic aneurysms are prone to rupture, even when small.[107,108] They may have been unsuspected before rupturing, and the diagnosis of infection may not be obvious at the time of emergency operation.[113] The diagnosis should be entertained in a patient presenting with a ruptured aortic aneurysm who has a fever and an elevated white blood cell count, especially when the aneurysm is small (<5 cm in diameter). At operation, additional clues include the presence of chronically inflamed retroperitoneal tissues with indistinct dissection planes and a focal aneurysm with relatively normal aorta above and below the site. Gram stains of smears from involved tissues and thrombus may be diagnostic, and cultures should be obtained even if the results of Gram stains are negative.

In contrast to aortic and other central aneurysms, peripheral infected aneurysms are usually readily apparent and the diagnosis obvious. A painful, cellulitic, warm pulsatile mass over a major artery in a febrile patient is a common clinical presentation.[105] An elevated white blood cell count and positive blood cultures are usual. The patient may have a history of drug abuse, and inadvertent or deliberate arterial injection with a contaminated needle should be suspected.[105] The common femoral artery is the most common site, and a prior history of arterial catheterization or the presence of an indwelling angiographic catheter or sheath for endovascular procedures is being increasingly seen.[106] Many of these procedures require repeated angiography and manipulation during prolonged periods, and femoral arterial sheaths or catheters are left in place for access. This increases the opportunity for arterial infection, and the risk is proportional to catheter residence time. Femoral puncture closure devices may also be sources of infection.[106]

Diagnosis

Infected aortic aneurysms can be difficult to diagnose. Leukocytosis is sensitive, but not specific, for an infected aneurysm. Blood cultures are important but may be negative in as many as 50% of patients with an infected aortic aneurysm.[100] Positive blood cultures in the presence of an abdominal aortic aneurysm should be considered evidence of an infected aneurysm until they are proven otherwise.

Radiologic studies are useful in confirming the diagnosis; CT and aortography are the most important tests.[108] MRI may also be helpful. CT and MRI will demonstrate the aneurysm and may show perivascular retroperitoneal inflammation and edema. A contained rupture may be present and suggests the diagnosis. The presence of periaortic air along with inflammatory changes is diagnostic (Fig. 91.8). Arteriography may aid in the diagnosis but is most useful in planning arterial reconstruction. A saccular aneurysm in an otherwise normal-appearing vessel or a multilobulated aneurysm strongly suggests the presence of aortic infection (Fig. 91.9).[100]

Treatment

Although culture-specific antibiotic therapy is important in the treatment of an infected aneurysm, surgical therapy is almost always necessary and lifesaving. Antibiotic therapy is started preoperatively and continued for at least 6 weeks after operation.[103] Surgical treatment must be expeditious because of the risk for aneurysm rupture and death. In stable patients who are dramatically improving on antibiotic therapy, withholding surgical treatment for a period to minimize, and possibly eliminate, local infection may be appropriate. However, there are reports of rupture during prolonged antibiotic therapy and the timing of operative intervention is a matter of careful judgment.[100]

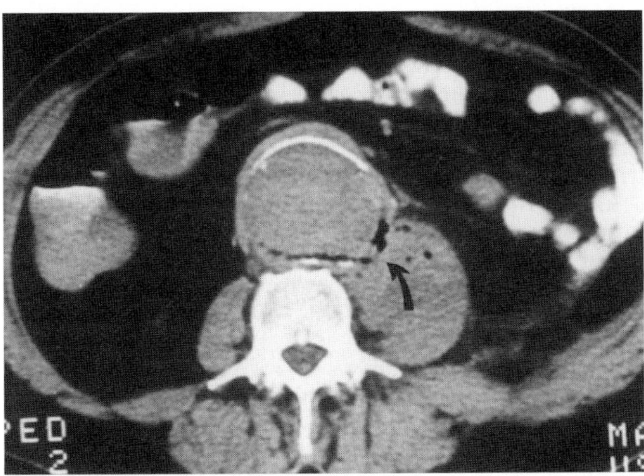

FIGURE 91.8 Computed tomography scan of infected aortic aneurysm with gas (*arrow*) present within the aorta and adjacent soft tissue.

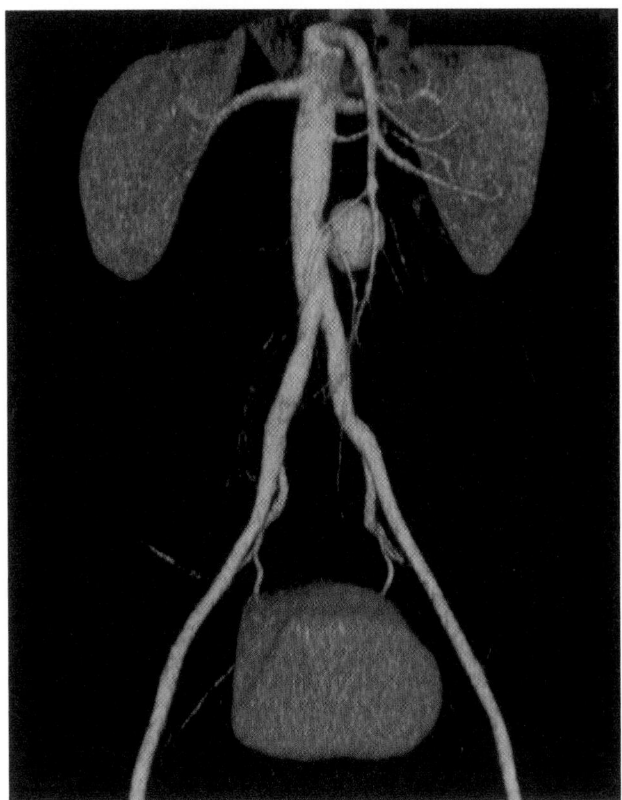

FIGURE 91.9 Computed tomography (CT) angiogram demonstrating focal, saccular infrarenal aortic aneurysm infected with *Staphylococcus aureus* in an HIV-positive patient.

The principles of treatment for an infected aneurysm are similar to those of surgical therapy of an infected arterial prostheses: eradication of infection by resection of the infected aneurysm and surrounding tissues and creation of a new bypass to restore circulation. Most authorities favor creating a new bypass through clean tissues. For infected aortoiliac aneurysms, axillofemoral bypass is most commonly performed.[102,104,108,113–115] For infected femoral aneurysms, an obturator bypass from the common iliac to the distal superficial femoral artery with a vascular prosthesis or vein graft routed through the obturator foramen successfully avoids the infected groin and restores distal circulation (Fig. 91.10).[105,106]

Prosthetic reconstruction *in situ* has been successfully used for infected aortic aneurysms when gross purulence is absent and contamination is minimal.[103,107,114,116–119] It is especially appropriate in patients with an aortic aneurysm that ruptures into the overlying duodenum, a condition usually referred to as *primary aortoduodenal fistula.* Contamination is minimal in this condition, and long-term results with prosthetic reconstruction *in situ* are good.[107,116–120] Patients treated in this manner require close follow-up because of the risk for recurrent infection, and most should be treated with lifelong oral antibiotics. Prosthetic reconstruction *in situ* is usually necessary for unstable patients with ruptured, infected aortic aneurysms.[107] Extraanatomic bypass is not feasible in this circumstance because of the prolonged lower extremity

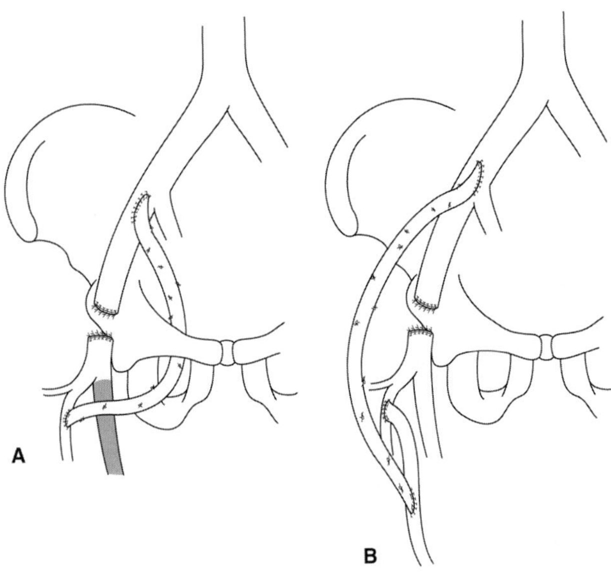

FIGURE 91.10 Extraanatomic bypass options using superficial femoral popliteal vein grafts for restoring lower extremity circulation for treatment of infected femoral aneurysms.

ischemia time, especially when hypotension has been present. Overall mortality for patients with an infected aortic aneurysms is approximately 25% and is higher when rupture is present.[100]

A promising new approach involves harvesting superficial femoral popliteal veins to reconstruct the aortoiliac system after resection of an infected aneurysm and debridement of retroperitoneal tissues.[53] These vein grafts have also been used to replace infected common femoral arterial aneurysms associated with drug abuse[105,106] (see Fig. 91.10). The large vein grafts appear to be resistant to infection by most organisms, and disruption when they are placed in infected fields has not been reported. Because of the additional operative time for harvesting veins, reconstruction *in situ* with superficial femoral popliteal veins should be used in relatively stable patients.

SEPTIC THROMBOPHLEBITIS

Septic thrombophlebitis most commonly involves upper extremity and neck veins after the insertion of intravenous catheters and needles or intravenous drug abuse. However, venous thrombi can become secondarily infected during bacteremia or contiguity with areas of infection. Examples of contiguous infection include pelvic septic thrombophlebitis developing after obstetric infections,[121] internal jugular thrombophlebitis associated with severe pharyngitis and peritonsillar abscesses,[122] and visceral thrombophlebitis stemming from appendicitis. *S. aureus* is the most common organism cultured from patients with peripheral septic thrombophlebitis, and gram-negative and polymicrobial infections are common when a contiguous infection is the cause. Regardless of the source, infected thrombus propagates throughout the lumen of the involved vein, and septicemia with high spiking fevers and chills quickly develops. An intense perivascular inflammatory response accompanies the spread of intraluminal infection and is clinically manifested by marked edema, pain, tenderness, and erythema overlying the involved vein. *S. aureus* and other virulent organisms infecting clot can rapidly form an intravascular abscess. In this circumstance, the lumen of the vein becomes a "closed space," and excision or surgical drainage is necessary to treat the infection. Propagation of the infected clot can also give rise to septic pulmonary embolism resulting in pneumonia, metastatic pulmonary abscess, and septic pleural effusion.

The clinical diagnosis is readily apparent when peripheral veins in the extremities are involved. In addition to pain, swelling, and redness along the course of the vein, pus may be expressed at the site of catheter or needle insertion. When deep or central veins are involved, the diagnosis is more difficult. These patients may present with clinical signs of severe sepsis and occasionally with complications of septic pulmonary embolization. CT or MRI can be particularly helpful and may demonstrate enlarged, dilated veins with intravenous thrombus and perivascular inflammatory changes. These imaging modalities are most useful for septic thrombophlebitis involving ileofemoral, caval, axillary-subclavian, and pelvic veins.

The treatment of septic thrombophlebitis depends on its anatomic location. Along with antibiotic therapy, excision of a superficial vein in an extremity is curative.[123–125] One must take care to remove the entire length of involved vein to eradicate infection. When deep veins of an extremity or central veins of the chest or pelvis are involved, vein excision is difficult and associated with large losses of blood and severe morbidity. The mainstays of therapy for septic deep or central vein thrombophlebitis are intensive antibiotic therapy and heparin anticoagulation to halt the thrombotic process and prevent embolization.[126] Therapy may have to be continued for 2 to 3 weeks and is successful in most cases. If it is not successful and sepsis continues despite medical therapy, surgical intervention is indicated. Venous thrombectomy and vein excision have been reported to be successful in cases refractory to medical therapy.[121] When thrombectomy of the iliocaval system is undertaken, placement of a stainless steel caval filtration device (Greenfield filter) for protection against pulmonary embolism may be advisable.[127] Sepsis does not preclude placement of these devices. In advanced cases in which abscess forms within large veins that cannot be subjected to thrombectomy because of organization of thrombus and vein scarring, abscess drainage and débridement are indicated.

KEY POINTS

- **Vascular infections are among most challenging and difficult problems encountered by surgeons.**
- **Overall incidence of clinically overt prosthetic infection varies according to anatomic site.**
- **Majority of vascular prosthetic infections are initiated at the time of operation.**
- **The principal organism responsible for infections of all implanted medical devices, including vascular prostheses, is *S. epidermidis*.**
- **The clinical presentations of vascular prosthetic infections can be protean and subtle, so that the diagnosis is difficult.**
- **Imaging tests are important because the consequences of a missed diagnosis may be lethal.**
- **The primary goals of treatment are to save life and limb, and this is best accomplished by eradicating infection by excision of all infected prosthetic material and vascular tissues combined with appropriate arterial reconstruction.**

References

1. Balas P. An overview of aortofemoral graft infection. *Eur J Vasc Endovasc Surg.* 1997;14[Suppl A]:3.
2. Kearney RA, Eisen HJ, Wolf JE. Nonvalvular infections of the cardiovascular system. *Ann Intern Med.* 1994;121:219.
3. O'Brien T, Collin J. Prosthetic vascular graft infection. *Br J Surg.* 1992;79:1262.
4. **Lorentzen JE, Nielsen OM, Arendrup H, et al. Vascular graft infection: an analysis of sixty-two graft infections in 2411 consecutively implanted synthetic vascular grafts. *Surgery* 1985;98:81.**

5. Seabrook GR. Pathobiology of graft infections. *Semin Vasc Surg.* 1990;3:81.
6. Bandyk DF, Berni GA, Thiele BL, Towne JB. Aortofemoral graft infection due to Staphylococcus epidermidis. *Arch Surg.* 1984;119:102.
7. Jones L, Braithwaite BD, Davies B, et al. Mechanism of late prosthetic vascular graft infection. *Cardiovasc Surg.* 1997;5:486.
8. Costa SF, Miceli MH, Anaissie EJ. Mucosa or skin as source of coagulase-negative staphylococcal bacteraemia? *Lancet Infect Dis.* 2004;4:278.
9. Schwartz JA, Powell TW, Burnham SJ, Johnson Jr G. Culture of abdominal aortic aneurysm contents. *Arch Surg.* 1987;122:777.
10. Ernst CB, Campbell HC, Daugherty ME, et al. Incidence and significance of intra-operative bacterial cultures during abdominal aortic aneurysmectomy. *Ann Surg.* 1977;185:626.
11. Padberg FT Jr, Smith SM, Eng RHK. Accuracy of disincorporation for identification of vascular graft infection. *Arch Surg.* 1995;130:183.
12. **Bandyk DF, Bergamini TM, Kinney EV, et al. In situ replacement of vascular prostheses infected by bacterial biofilms. *J Vasc Surg.* 1991;13:575.**
13. Merritt K, Hitchins VM, Neale AR. Tissue colonization from implantable biomaterials with low numbers of bacteria. *J Biomed Mater Res.* 1999;44:261.
14. Kaplan SS, Basford RE, Jeong MH, Simmons RL. Mechanisms of biomaterial-induced superoxide release by neutrophils. *J Biomed Mater Res.* 1994;28:377–386.
15. Kaplan SS, Basford RE, Jeong MH, Simmons RL. Biomaterial-neutrophil interactions: dysregulation of oxidative functions of fresh neutrophils induced by prior neutrophil-biomaterial interaction. *B Biomed Mater Res.* 1996;30:67.
16. Kaplan SS, Heine RP, Simmons RL. Defensins impair phagocytic killing by neutrophils in biomaterial-related infection. *Infect Immun.* 1999;67:1640.
17. Brunstedt MR, Sapatnekar S, Rubin KR, et al. Anderson JM. Bacterial/blood/material interactions. I. Injected and preseeded slime-forming Staphylococcus epidermidis in flowing blood with biomaterials. *J Biomed Mater Res.* 1995;29:455.
18. Wang I, Anderson JM, Jacobs MR, Marchant RE. Adhesion of Staphylococcus epidermidis to biomedical polymers: contributions of surface thermodynamics and hemodynamic shear conditions. *J Biomed Mater Res.* 1995;29:485.
19. Shive MS, Hasan SM, Anderson JM. Shear stress effects on bacterial adhesion, leukocyte adhesion, and leukocyte oxidative capacity on a polyetherurethane. *J Biomed Mater Res.* 1999;46:511.
20. von Eiff C, Peters G, Heilmann C. Pathogenesis of infections due to coagulase-negative staphylococci. *Lancet Infect Dis.* 2002;2:677.
21. Veenstra GC, Cremers FFM, van Dijk H, Fleer A. Ultrastructural organization and regulation of a biomaterial adhesion of Staphylococcus epidermidis. *J Bacteriol.* 1996;178:537.
22. Mack D, Riedewald J, Rohde H, et al. Essential functional role of the polysaccharide intercellular adhesion of Staphylococcus epidermidis in hemagglutination. *Infect Immun.* 1999;67:1004.
23. Rupp ME, Ulphani JS, Fey PD, et al. Characterization of the importance of polysaccharide intercellular adhesin/hemagglutinin of Staphylococcus epidermidis in the pathogenesis of biomaterial-based infection in a mouse foreign body infection model. *Infect Immun.* 1999;67:2627.
24. Henke PK, Bergamini TM, Watson AL, et al. Bacterial products primarily mediate fibroblast inhibition in biomaterial infection. *J Surg Res.* 1998;74:17.
25. **Geary KJ, Tomkiewicz ZM, Harrison HN, et al. Differential effects of a gram-negative and a gram-positive infection on autogenous and prosthetic grafts. *J Vasc Surg.* 1990;11:339.**
26. Rzychon M, Sabat A, Kosowska K, et al. Staphostatins: an expanding new group of proteinase inhibitors with a unique specificity for the regulation of staphopains, Staphylococcus spp. cysteine proteinases. *Mol Microbiol.* 2003;49:1051.
27. Modrall JG, Clagett GP. The role of imaging techniques in evaluating possible graft infections. *Semin Vasc Surg.* 1999;12:339.
28. Low RN, Wall SD, Jeffrey RB, et al. Aortoenteric fistula and perigraft infection: evaluation with CT. *Radiology* 1990;175:157.
29. Qvafordt PG, Reilly LM, Mark AS, et al. Computerized tomographic assessment of graft incorporation after reconstruction. *Am J Surg.* 1985;150:227.
30. Auffermann W, Olofsson PA, Rabahie GN, et al. Incorporation versus infection of retroperitoneal aortic grafts: MR imaging features. *Radiology* 1989;172:359.
31. Brunner MC, Mitchell RS, Baldwin JC, et al. Prosthetic graft infection: limitations of indium white blood cell scanning. *J Vasc Surg.* 1986;3:42.
32. Fiorani P, Speziale F, Rizzo L, et al. Detection of aortic graft infection with leukocytes labeled with technetium 99m-hexametazime. *J Vasc Surg.* 1993;17:87.
33. LaMuraglia GM, Fischman AJ, Strauss HW, et al. Utility of the indium 111-labeled human immunoglobulin G scan for the detection of focal vascular graft infection. *J Vasc Surg.* 1989;10:20.
34. **O'Hara PJ, Hertzer NR, Beven EG, Krajewski LP. Surgical management of infected abdominal aortic grafts: review of a 25-year experience. *J Vasc Surg.* 1986;2:725.**
35. **Reilly LM, Stoney RJ, Goldstone J, Ehrenfeld WK. Improved management of aortic graft infection: the influence of operation sequence and staging. *J Vasc Surg.*** 1987;5:421.
36. Quinones-Baldrich WJ, Hernandez JJ, Moore WS. Long-term results following surgical management of aortic graft infection. *Arch Surg.* 1991; 126:507.
37. Ricotta JJ, Faggioli GL, Stella A, et al. Total excision and extra-anatomic bypass for aortic graft infection. *Am J Surg.* 1991;162:145.
38. Leather RP, Darling III RC, Chang BB, Shah DM. Retroperitoneal in-line aortic bypass for treatment of infected infrarenal aortic grafts. *Surg Gynecol Obstet.* 1992;175:491.
39. Olah A, Vogt M, Laske A, et al. Axillo-femoral bypass and simultaneous removal of the aorto-femoral vascular infection site: is the procedure safe? *Eur J Vasc Surg.* 1992;6:252.
40. Bacourt F, Koskas F, and the French University Association for Research in Surgery. Axillobifemoral bypass and aortic exclusion for vascular septic lesions: a multicenter retrospective study of 98 cases. *Ann Vasc Surg.* 1992;6:119.
41. Lehnert T, Gruber HP, Maeder N, Allenberg JR. Management of primary aortic graft infection by extra-anatomic bypass reconstruction. *Eur J Vasc Surg.* 1993;7:301.
42. Sharp WJ, Hoballah JJ, Mohan CR, et al. The management of the infected aortic prosthesis: a current decade of experience. *J Vasc Surg.* 1994;19:844.
43. Kuestner LM, Reilly LM, Jicha DL, et al. Secondary aortoenteric fistula: contemporary outcome with use of extraanatomic bypass and infected graft excision. *J Vasc Surg.* 1995;21:184.
44. Hannon RJ, Wolfe JHN, Mansfield AO. Aortic prosthetic infection: 50 patients treated by radical or local surgery. *Br J Surg.* 1996;83:654.
45. Schmitt DD, Seabrook GR, Bandyk DF, Towne JB. Graft excision and extra-anatomic revascularization: the treatment of choice for the septic aortic prosthesis. *J Cardiovasc Surg.* 1990;31:327.
46. Bunt TJ. Vascular graft infections: a personal experience. *Cardiovasc Surg.* 1993;1:489.
47. Yeager RA, Taylor LM, Moneta GL, et al. Improved results with conventional management of infrarenal aortic infection. *J Vasc Surg.* 1999;30:76.
48. **Bandyk DF, Novotney ML, Back MR, et al. Expanded application of in situ replacement for prosthetic graft infection. *J Vasc Surg.* 2001;34:411.**
49. **Seeger JM, Pretus HA, Welborn MB, et al. Long-term outcome after treatment of aortic graft infection with staged extraanatomic bypass grafting and aortic graft removal. *J Vasc Surg.* 2000;32:451.**
50. Dorigo W, Pulli R, Azas L, et al. Early and long-term results of conventional surgical treatment of secondary aorto-enteric fistula. *Eur J Vasc Endovasc Surg.* 2003;26:512.
51. **Clagett GP, Bowers BL, Lopez-Viego MA, et al. Creation of a neo-aortoiliac system from lower extremity deep and superficial veins. *Ann Surg.* 1993;218:239.**
52. Nevelsteen A, Lacroix H, Suy R. Autogenous reconstruction with the lower extremity deep veins: an alternative treatment of prosthetic infection after reconstructive surgery for aortoiliac disease. *J Vasc Surg.* 1995;22:129.
53. **Clagett GP, Valentine RJ, Hagino RT. Autogenous aortoiliac/femoral reconstruction from superficial femoral-popliteal veins: feasibility and durability. *J Vasc Surg.* 1997;25:255.**
54. Franke S, Voit R. The superficial femoral vein as arterial substitute in infections of the aortoiliac region. *Ann Vasc Surg.* 1997;11:406.
55. Brown Jr, PM, Kim VB, Lalikos JF, et al. Autologous superficial femoral vein for aortic reconstruction in infected fields. *Ann Vasc Surg.* 1999;13:32.
56. Cardozo MA, Frankini AD, Bonamigo TP. Use of superficial femoral vein in the treatment of infected aortoiliofemoral prosthetic grafts. *Cardiovasc Surg.* 2002;10:304.
57. Gibbons CP, Ferguson CJ, Fligelstone LJ, Edwards K. Experience with femoro-popliteal vein as a conduit for vascular reconstruction in infected fields. *Eur J Vasc Endovasc Surg.* 2003;25:424.
58. Daenens K, Fourneau I, Nevelsteen A. Ten-year experience in autogenous reconstruction with the femoral vein in the treatment of aortofemoral prosthetic infection. *Eur J Vasc Endovasc Surg.* 2003;25:240.
59. Kieffer E, Bahnini A, Koskas F, et al. In situ allograft replacement of infected infrarenal aortic prosthetic grafts: results in forty-three patients. *J Vasc Surg.* 1993;17:349.
60. Vogt PR, Pfammatter T, Schlumph R, et al. In situ repair of aortobronchial, aortoesophageal, and aortoenteric fistulae with cryopreserved aortic homografts. *J Vasc Surg.* 1997;26:11.
61. Ruotolo C, Plissonnier D, Bahnini A, et al. In situ arterial allografts: a new treatment for aortic prosthetic infection. *Eur J Vasc Endovasc Surg.* 1997;14[suppl A]:102.
62. Nevelsteen A, Feryn T, Lacroix H, et al. Experience with cryopreserved arterial allografts in the treatment of prosthetic graft infections. *Cardiovasc Surg.* 1998;4:378.
63. Chiesa R, Astore S, Piccolo G, et al. Fresh and cryopreserved arterial homografts in the treatment of prosthetic graft infections: experience of the Italian Collaborative Vascular Homograft Group. *Ann Vasc Surg.* 1998;12:457.
64. Leseche G, Castier Y, Petit MD, et al. Long-term results of cryopreserved arterial allograft reconstruction in infected prosthetic grafts and mycotic aneurysms of the abdominal aorta. *J Vasc Surg.* 2001;34:616.
65. Verhelst R, Lacroix V, Vraux H, et al. Use of cryopreserved arterial homografts for management of infected prosthetic grafts: a multicentric study. *Ann Vasc Surg.* 200;14:602.

66. Vogt PR, Brunner-LaRocca HP, Lachat M, et al. Technical details with the use of cryopreserved arterial allograft for aortic infection: influence on early and midterm mortality. *J Vasc Surg.* 2002;35:80.
67. **Noel AA, Gloviczki P, Cherry Jr KJ, et al., and Members of the United States Cryopreserved Aortic Allograft Registry. Abdominal aortic reconstruct in infected fields: early results of the United States Cryopreserved Aortic Allograft Registry. *J Vasc Surg.* 2002;35:847.**
68. Gabrial M, Pukacki F, Dzieciuchowicz L, et al. Cryopreserved arterial allografts in the treatment of prosthetic graft infections. *Eur J Vasc Endovasc Surg.* 2004;27:590.
69. Teebken OE, Pichlmaier MA, Brand S, Haverich A. Cryopreserved arterial allografts for in situ reconstruction of infected arterial vessels. *Eur J Vasc Endovasc Surg.* 2004;27:597.
70. Lavigne JP, Postal A, Kolh P, Limet R. Prosthetic vascular infection complicated or not by aortoenteric fistula: comparison of treatment with and without cryopreserved allograft (homograft). *Eur J Vasc Endovasc Surg.* 2003;25:416.
71. Kieffer E, Gomes D, Chiche L, et al. Allograft replacement for intrarenal aortic graft infection: early and late results in 179 patients. *J Vasc Surg.* 2004;39:1009.
72. Walker WE, Cooley DA, Duncan JM, et al. The management of aortoduodenal fistula by in situ replacement of the infected abdominal aortic graft. *Ann Surg.* 1987;205:727.
73. Speziale F, Rizzo L, Sbarigia E, et al. Bacterial and clinical criteria relating to the outcome of patients undergoing in situ replacement of infected abdominal aortic grafts. *Eur J Vasc Endovasc Surg.* 1997;13:127.
74. Hayes PD, Nasim A, London NJM, et al. In situ replacement of infected aortic grafts with rifampicin-bonded prostheses: the Leicester experience (1992 to 1998). *J Vasc Surg.* 1999;30:92.
75. Young RM, Cherry KJ Jr, Davis PM, et al. The results of in situ prosthetic replacement for infected aortic grafts. *Am J Surg.* 1999;178:136.
76. Batt M, Magne JL, Alric P, et al. In situ revascularization with silver-coated polyester grafts to treat aortic infection: early and midterm results. *J Vasc Surg.* 2003;38:983.
77. Clagett GP. Aortic graft infections. In: Towne JB, ed. *Complications in vascular surgery*, 2nd ed. New York: Marcel Dekker, 2003, p. 317.
78. Modrall JG, Sadjadi J, Ali AT, et al. Deep vein harvest: predicting the need of fasciotomy. *J Vasc Surg.* 2004;39:387.
79. Wells JK, Hagino RT, Bargmann KM, et al. Venous morbidity after superficial femoral-popliteal vein harvest. *J Vasc Surg.* 1999;29:282.
80. Koskas F, Plissonnier D, Bahnini A, et al. In situ arterial allografting for aortoiliac graft infection: a 6-year experience. *Cardiovasc Surg.* 1996;4:495.
81. Calligaro KD, Veith FJ, Schwartz ML, et al. Selective preservation of infected prosthetic arterial grafts. Analysis of a 20-year experience with 120 extracavitary-infected grafts. *Ann Surg.* 1994;220:461.
82. Morris GE, Friend PJ, Vassallo DJ, et al. Antibiotic irrigation and conservative surgery for major aortic graft infection. *J Vasc Surg.* 1994; 20:88.
83. Belair M, Soulez G, Oliva VL, et al. Aortic graft infection: the value of percutaneous drainage. *Am J Radiol.* 1998;171:119.
84. Calligaro KD, Veith FJ. Graft-preserving methods for managing aortofemoral prosthetic graft infection. *Eur J Vasc Endovasc Surg.* 1997;14[suppl A]:38.
85. Calligaro KD, Veith FJ, Yuan JG, et al. Intra-abdominal aortic graft infection: complete or partial graft preservation in patients at very high risk. *J Vasc Surg.* 2003;38:1199.
86. Tambyraja AL, Chalmers RT. Conservative management of MRSA periaortic graft abscess. *Ann Vasc Surg.* 2003;17:676.
87. Becquemin JP, Qvarfordt P, Kron J, et al. Aortic graft infection: is there a place for partial graft removal? *Eur J Vasc Endovasc Surg.* 1997;14[suppl A]:53.
88. Miller JH. Partial replacement of an infected arterial graft by a new prosthetic polytetrafluoroethylene segment: a new therapeutic option. *J Vasc Surg.* 1993;17:546.
89. Towne JB, Seabrook GR, Bandyk D, et al. In situ replacement of arterial prosthesis infected by bacterial biofilms: long-term follow-up. *J Vasc Surg.* 1994;19:226.
90. Sladen JG, Chen JC, Reid JDS. An aggressive local approach to vascular graft infection. *Am J Surg.* 1998;176:222.
91. **Mertens RA, O'Hara PJ, Hertzer NR, et al. Surgical management of infrainguinal arterial prosthetic graft infections: review of a thirty-five year experience. *J Vasc Surg.* 1995;21:782.**
92. Kikta MJ, Goodson SF, Bishara RA, et al. Mortality and limb loss with infected infrainguinal bypass grafts. *J Vasc Surg.* 1987;5:566.
93. Cherry KJ, Roland CF, Pairolero PC, et al. Infected femorodistal bypass: is graft removal mandatory? *J Vasc Surg.* 1992;15:295.
94. Kaiser AB, Clayson KR, Mulherin JL, et al. Antibiotic prophylaxis in vascular surgery. *Ann Surg.* 1978;188:283.
95. Pitt HA, Postier RG, MacGowan WAL, et al. Prophylactic antibiotics in vascular surgery: topical, systemic, or both? *Ann Surg.* 1980;192:356.
96. Hasselgren P, Ivarsson L, Risberg B, Seeman T. Effects of prophylactic antibiotics in vascular surgery: a prospective, randomized, double-blind study. *Ann Surg.* 1984;200:86.
97. Hall JC, Christiansen KJ, Goodman M, et al. Duration of antimicrobial prophylaxis in vascular surgery. *Am J Surg.* 1998;175:87.
98. Kurz A, Sessler DL, Lenhardt R, Study of Wound Infection and Temperature Group. Perioperative normothermia to reduce the incidence of surgical-wound infection and shorten hospitalization. *N Engl J Med.* 1996;334:1209.
99. Osler W. The Gulstonian lectures on malignant endocarditis. *Br Med J.* 1885;1:467.
100. Reddy DJ, Ernst CB. Infected aortic aneurysms: recognition and management. *Semin Vasc Surg.* 1988;1:174.
101. Patel S, Johnston KW. Classification and management of mycotic aneurysms. *Surg Gynecol Obstet.* 1977;144:691.
102. Dean RH, Waterhouse G, Meacham PW, et al. Mycotic embolism and embolomycotic aneurysms. *Ann Surg.* 1986;204:300.
103. Chan FY, Crawford ES, Coselli JS, et al. In situ prosthetic graft replacement for mycotic aneurysm of the aorta. *Ann Thorac Surg.* 1989;47:193.
104. Oz MC, Brener BJ, Buda JA, et al. A ten-year experience with bacterial aortitis. *J Vasc Surg.* 1989;10:439.
105. Benjamin ME, Cohn EJ, Purtill WA, et al. Arterial reconstruction with deep leg veins for the treatment of mycotic aneurysms. *J Vasc Surg.* 1999;30:1004.
106. Bell C, Ali A, Brawley JG, D'Addio VJ, et al. Arterial reconstruction of infected femoral artery pseudoaneurysms using superficial femoral-popliteal vein. *J Am Coll Surg.* 2005;200:831.
107. Fichelle JM, Tabet G, Cormier P, et al. Infected infrarenal aortic aneurysms: when is in situ reconstruction safe? *J Vasc Surg.* 1993;17:635.
108. Gomes MN, Choyke PL, Wallace RB. Infected aortic aneurysms. A changing entity. *Ann Surg.* 1992;215:435.
109. McGregor JA, Lawellin D, Franco-Buff A, et al. Protease production by microorganisms associated with reproductive tract infection. *Am J Obstet Gynecol.* 1986;154:109.
110. Tilson MD, Newman KM. Proteolytic mechanisms in the pathogenesis of aortic aneurysms. In: Yao JST, Pearce WH, eds. *Aneurysms: new findings and treatments.* Norwalk, CT: Appleton & Lange, 1994, p. 3.
111. Pierce RA, Sandefur S, Doyle GA, Welgus HG. Monocytic cell type-specific transcriptional induction of collagenase. *J Clin Invest.* 1996; 97:1890.
112. Buckmaster MJ, Curci JA, Murray PR, et al. Source of elastin-degrading enzymes in mycotic aortic aneurysms: bacteria or host inflammatory response? *Cardiovasc Surg.* 1999;7:16.
113. Reddy DJ, Shepard AD, Evans JR, et al. Management of infected aortoiliac aneurysms. *Arch Surg.* 1991;126:873.
114. Sessa C, Farah I, Voirin L, et al. Infected aneurysms of the infrarenal abdominal aorta: diagnostic criteria and therapeutic strategy. *Ann Vasc Surg.* 1997;11:453.
115. Moneta GL, Taylor LM Jr, Yeager RA, et al. Surgical treatment of infected aortic aneurysm. *Am J Surg.* 1998;175:396.
116. Robinson JA, Johansen K. Aortic sepsis: is there a role for in situ graft reconstruction? *J Vasc Surg.* 1991;13:677.
117. Kyriakides C, Kan Y, Kerle M. et al. 11-year experience with anatomical and extraanatomical repair of mycotic aortic aneurysms. *Eur J Vasc Endovasc Surg.* 2004;27:585.
118. Oderich GS, Panneton JM, Bower TC, et al. Infected aortic aneurysms: aggressive presentation, complicated early outcome, but durable results. *J Vasc Surg.* 2001;34:900.
119. Hsu RB, Chen RJ, Wang SS, Chu SH. Infected aortic aneurysms: clinical outcome and risk factor analysis. *J Vasc Surg.* 2004;40:30.
120. Daugherty M, Shearer GG, Ernst CB. Primary aortoduodenal fistula: extraanatomic vascular reconstruction not required for successful management. *Surgery* 1979;86:399.
121. Kniemeyer HW, Grabitz K, Buhl R, et al. Surgical treatment of septic deep venous thrombosis. *Surgery* 1995;118:49.
122. Bach MC, Roediger JH, Rinder HM. Septic anaerobic jugular phlebitis with pulmonary embolism: problems in management. *Rev Infect Dis.* 1988;10:424.
123. Leonard JD, Printen KJ. Thrombophlebitis in the elderly. *Am Surg.* 1980;46:441.
124. Munster AM. Septic thrombophlebitis: a surgical disorder. *JAMA* 1974;230:1010.
125. Pruitt BA Jr, McManus WF, Kim SH, Trat RC. Diagnosis and treatment of cannula-related intravenous sepsis in burn patients. *Ann Surg.* 1980;191:546.
126. Ang AK, Brown OW. Septic deep vein thrombosis. *J Vasc Surg.* 1986;4:563.
127. Hoffman MJ, Greenfield LJ. Central venous septic thrombosis managed by superior vena cava Greenfield filter and venous thrombectomy: a case report. *J Vasc Surg.* 1986;4:606.

CHAPTER 92 ■ CEREBROVASCULAR OCCLUSIVE DISEASE

JOHN S. LANE AND LOUIS M. MESSINA

Cerebrovascular disease encompasses a variety of clinical disorders of the extracranial cerebral arteries that can cause transient cerebral ischemia or stroke. Most causes of stroke used to be considered untreatable. Significant advances in the surgical treatment of extracranial cerebrovascular disease, however, have contributed greatly to reducing the mortality associated with stroke.

The first carotid endarterectomy took place in 1954. By 1984, carotid endarterectomy had become the most frequently performed vascular surgical procedure and the third most frequently performed operation in the United States. Nonetheless, much controversy surrounded the operation, owing to the publication of a number of clinical reports showing a wide variability in mortality and morbidity rates after carotid endarterectomy. Prospective, randomized studies that compared the efficacy of carotid endarterectomy plus optimal medical treatment versus optimal medical treatment alone have established unambiguously the efficacy of carotid endarterectomy in the management of cerebrovascular disease. Recently, endovascular therapy has attracted attention and enthusiasm as a potentially equivalent alternative treatment for cerebrovascular disease in select patients. This chapter reviews the epidemiology, anatomy, pathophysiology, diagnosis, and treatment of cerebrovascular disease of the extracranial arteries.

EPIDEMIOLOGY

Stroke remains the third most common cause of death in the United States, and atherosclerotic occlusive disease of the extracranial portion of the carotid artery is the most common cause of stroke. Stroke is a devastating illness in every respect. Each year, 500,000 people suffer strokes, and of these, 200,000 die as a consequence of stroke (Fig. 92.1). Of the remaining patients who survive a stroke, two thirds are disabled, and one third require prolonged hospitalization because of residual disability (Table 92.1). Neurologic deficits resulting in paralysis, blindness, and aphasia compromise the stroke victim's ability to perform many normal daily functions and live a satisfying existence. The cumulative public health cost for the disabilities caused by strokes is enormous, exceeding $16 trillion a year.[1]

ANATOMY

Although the brain constitutes only 2% of the total body weight, it takes up 17% of the cardiac output and 20% of the available oxygen supply.[2] A clinical implication of the high oxygen requirements of neural tissue is that the tissue can become necrotic within minutes of a loss of arterial circulation.

In adults, the ascending aorta rises from the left ventricle and courses anteriorly in the mediastinum. The branches of

TABLE 92.1 RESULTS

RESIDUAL DISABILITY IN 119 STROKE SURVIVORS: FRAMINGTON STUDY

Disability level	Occurrence (%)
Institutionalized	16
Dependent in self-care activities	31
Dependent for mobility	20
Dependent for vocational activity	71
Decreased socialization	62

(Adapted from Gresham GE, Fitzpatrick TE, Wolf PA, et al. Residual disability in stroke survivors: the Framingham study. *N Engl J Med* 1975;293:954, with permission.)

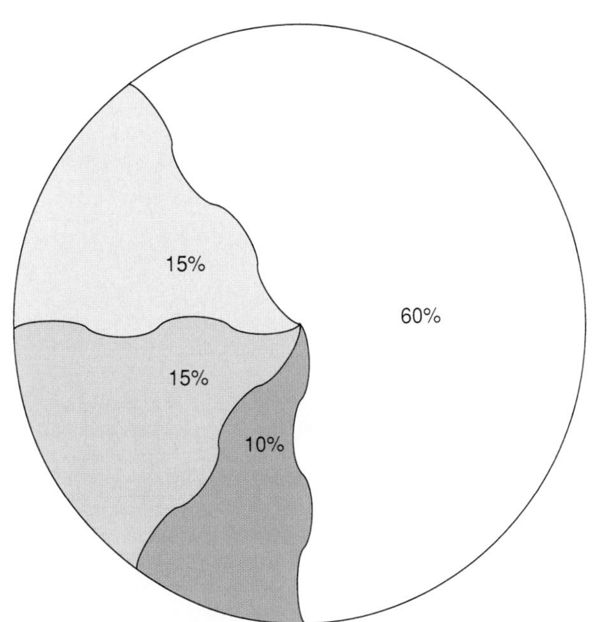

FIGURE 92.1 The precise distribution of the causes of stroke varies among reports, but the most common causes are thromboembolic events originating in the extracranial arteries, heart, and intraparenchymal or subarachnoid hemorrhage.

VASCULAR

aortic arch are the brachiocephalic (innominate) artery, the left common carotid artery, and the left subclavian artery. These arteries supply blood to the head and neck, both upper extremities, and the proximal trunk. The aortic arch crosses the upper mediastinum obliquely from a right anterior to a left posterior position. The brachiocephalic artery is the first and most anterior branch of the aortic arch. Beneath the head of the right clavicle, the brachiocephalic artery bifurcates to form the right subclavian artery and the right common carotid artery. It is because of this anterior position that the brachiocephalic artery is accessible for reconstruction through a median sternotomy. The left common carotid artery arises within 1 cm of the brachiocephalic artery and courses posteriorly into the left side of the base of the neck. In 10% of the normal population, the left common carotid artery arises directly from the brachiocephalic artery. Finally, the left subclavian artery arises from a posterior location at the distal end of the aortic arch. Because of its distal and posterior location, it is not easily reached through a median sternotomy and is best approached through a high left anterior or anterolateral thoracotomy.

The brain is supplied by paired internal carotid arteries anteriorly and the vertebral arteries posteriorly (Fig. 92.2). Under normal conditions, the paired internal carotid arteries supply about 80% to 90% of the total cerebral blood flow, and the paired vertebral arteries supply 10% to 20% of the total cerebral flow. The common carotid artery bifurcates at the level of the angle of the mandible into the internal and external carotid arteries. The branches of the external carotid artery include the ascending pharyngeal artery, the superior thyroid, lingual, occipital, and posterior auricular arteries. Its terminal branches are the internal maxillary and superficial temporal arteries.

The internal carotid artery can be divided into four segments: cervical, intrapetrosal, intracavernous, and supraclinoid. The cervical, extracranial portion of the internal carotid artery usually has no branches. The intracavernous and supraclinoid portions are referred to clinically as the carotid siphon. The first major branch of the internal carotid artery is the ophthalmic artery. The supraclinoid portion of the internal carotid artery gives rise to the major branches of the internal carotid artery, including the ophthalmic, posterior communicating, and anterior choroidal arteries. Eventually, the internal carotid artery bifurcates into its terminal branches, the anterior cerebral and middle cerebral arteries. The anterior communicating artery joins the comparable vessel from the contralateral hemisphere, whereas the posterior communicating artery provides anterior-posterior communication between the carotid system and the ipsilateral posterior cerebral branches of the basilar artery. Together, these branches form the circle of Willis (Fig. 92.3). Variations in the anatomy of the circle of Willis occur in 50% to 80% of the normal population. About 15% of the population have no anastomoses between the anterior and the posterior cerebral circulations, and as many as 35% lack the anastomotic channels between the anterior and posterior circulations or between the right and left hemispheric circulations. A deficiency of this collateral pathway has important clinical consequences when one of the four major cerebral arteries becomes occluded.

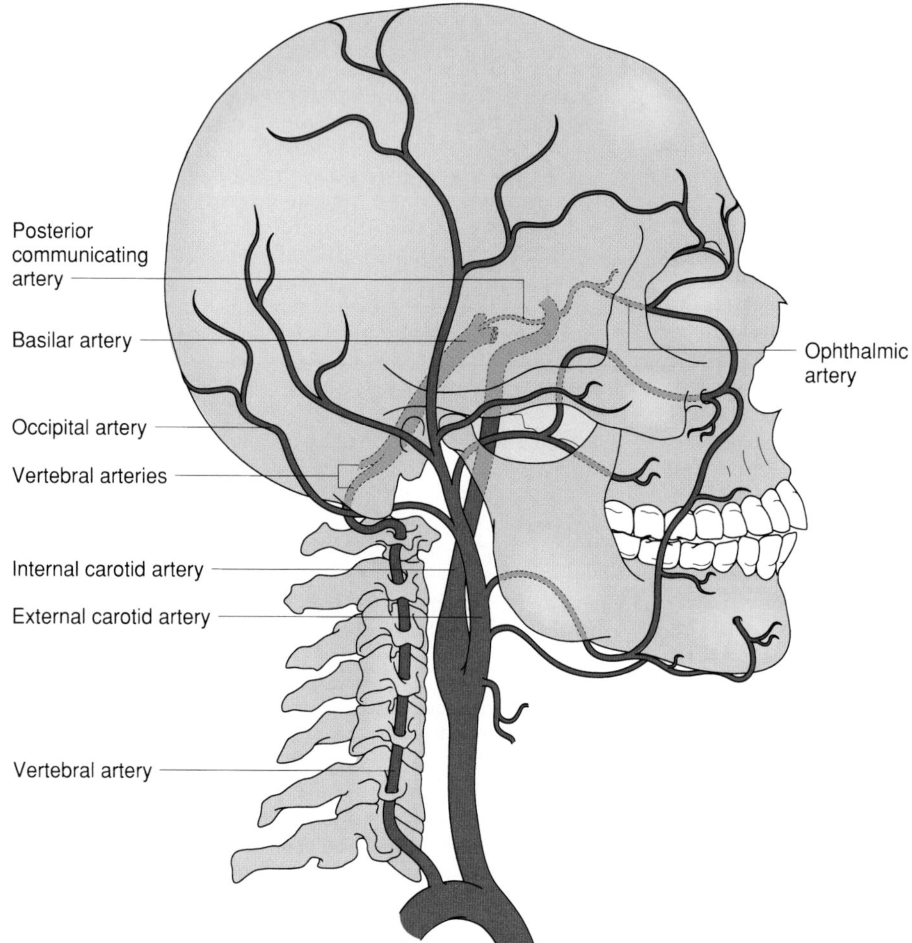

FIGURE 92.2 The paired carotid and vertebral arteries supply blood to the brain. Extensive extracranial collaterals between the external carotid and vertebral systems allow for antegrade perfusion when a proximal occlusion develops in either vessel. Likewise, periorbital collaterals allow for retrograde flow through the ophthalmic artery to the internal carotid artery in the presence of a cervical internal carotid artery occlusion. Extensive side-to-side collaterals are found between the right and left external carotid arteries and right and left vertebral arteries.

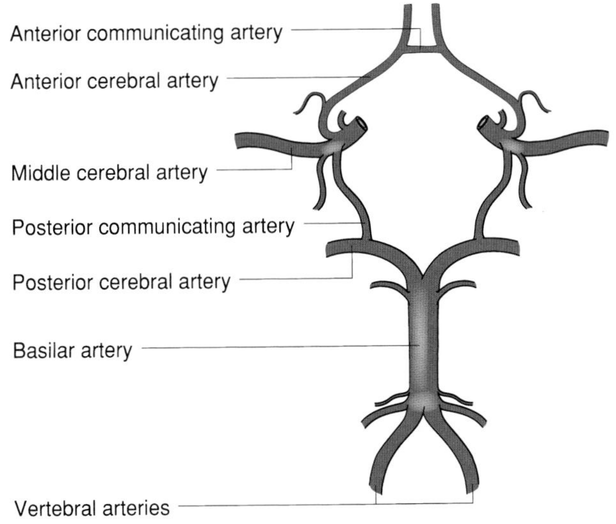

FIGURE 92.3 The circle of Willis is a highly efficient intracranial collateral network; however, multiple important variations occur, and an incomplete circle producing an isolated hemisphere is not uncommon.

The vertebral arteries arise from the first portion of the subclavian artery and enter the transverse cervical process at the level of the sixth cervical vertebra and ascend in the transverse foramen. Eventually the vertebral arteries pierce the posterior allantoid-occipital membrane and course into the posterior fascia through the foramen magnum. They then travel along the lateral border of the medulla and unite to form the basilar artery. The extracranial portion of the vertebral artery has segmental spinal and muscular branches. The basilar artery terminates as the right and left posterior cerebral arteries, which give rise to the posterior communicating arteries of the circle of Willis.

A number of clinically important collateral pathways exist between cerebral arteries. These collaterals become significant sources of arterial flow to the brain when arterial occlusive disease develops in one of the four major arteries supplying blood to the brain. Branches of the external carotid artery (facial, internal maxillary, and superficial temporal arteries) can anastomose with the infraorbital and supraorbital arteries. These anastomotic networks become important sources of blood flow into the intracranial portions of the internal carotid artery when a hemodynamic stenosis develops in the extracranial circulation. Communications between the branches of the external carotid artery and the ophthalmic artery are the most important of the collateral networks. Similarly, the vertebral artery gives off numerous muscular branches in the neck. If the proximal vertebral artery becomes occluded, collateral branches from the external carotid artery can anastomose to the distal vertebral artery by way of these branches. If the common carotid artery becomes occluded, blood can flow from the vertebral artery through the external carotid artery branches into the internal carotid artery, so that antegrade blood flow in the internal carotid artery is maintained. Finally, branches of the left and right external carotid arteries can anastomose freely across the face.

PATHOPHYSIOLOGY

Although stroke has many causes (Table 92.2), most are the result of a few distinct pathologic processes. Whereas atherosclerosis remains the most common cause of stroke in adults, other nonatherosclerotic causes of stroke exist. These less common pathologic processes include aneurysms of the internal carotid artery, carotid coils (loops or gentle curves in the internal carotid artery), and carotid kinks (acute bends in the internal carotid artery cause the carotid artery to fold up on itself).

Fibromuscular dysplasia is a vessel wall abnormality that occurs typically in women 30 to 50 years of age and involves the cervical internal carotid artery distal to the carotid bifurcation.[3,4] Fibromuscular dysplasia is pathologically subdivided into four categories: intimal fibroplasias, medial fibroplasias, medial hyperplasia, and perimedial dysplasia. In its most common form, the internal carotid artery becomes alternatingly thickened and thinned and acquires a beaded appearance on angiography. Stroke can be the result of emboli or a low-flow state. Fibromuscular disease can affect a number of arteries systematically and is also associated with congenital intracranial (Berry) aneurysms.

An inflammatory disorder that occurs more commonly in women is Takayasu's arteritis. This inflammatory arteritis can affect any branch of the aorta or pulmonary arteries. When this entity causes symptoms and signs of cerebrovascular insufficiency, it usually affects the three branches of the aortic arch. Temporal arteritis, a condition typically seen in the elderly, most commonly affects muscular arteries, such as the superficial temporal artery, and is characterized clinically by headache, monocular visual symptoms, low-grade fever, and tenderness of the superficial femoral artery. If left untreated, it can result in permanent blindness.

Both spontaneous arterial dissections and aneurysms can affect the intracranial portion of the carotid artery, although these are rare.[5] Spontaneous dissection of the internal carotid artery usually originates just distal to the carotid bifurcation and reenters at the most distal aspect of the extracranial portion of the internal carotid artery. Spontaneous dissection can occur as a result of fibromuscular dysplasia. False aneurysms of the carotid artery are also uncommon and most often are caused by a traction injury to the internal carotid artery at the base of the skull associated with forceful flexion and extension of the neck. Spontaneous dissections and aneurysms of the internal carotid artery are most frequently complicated by thromboembolic events causing transient ischemia or stroke.

Atherosclerosis is the pathologic process most often responsible for symptoms of cerebrovascular insufficiency. The cause of atherosclerosis in the cerebral arterial circulation remains incompletely understood.[6] Clinically, atherosclerosis tends to be a segmental disease. It usually develops at areas of local turbulence (e.g., vessel bifurcations) and causes focal vessel wall injury. The origins of the great vessels at the aortic arch or their proximal cervical bifurcations are involved frequently. Typically, the common carotid artery is spared. The carotid bifurcation is the most common location of atherosclerotic lesions in the cerebral circulation. This tendency is most likely the consequence of a variety of hemodynamic changes.[7] Atherosclerotic plaques tend to occur along the outer wall of the carotid bifurcation, and often involve only the most proximal portion of the external carotid artery. At the outer wall of the carotid bifurcation, disruption of normal laminar blood flow results in flow separation, turbulence, flow stasis, prolonged particle residence time, and increased shear stress (alternating areas of high and low shear stress). Grossly, the atherosclerotic plaque is thickest at the carotid bifurcation and extends 2 cm into the distal internal carotid artery. The plaque occupies the media and intima, sparing the outer media and adventitia. Usually, the plaque tapers from the media into the normal intima. Such tapering often permits a smooth surface after endarterectomy. Finally, atherosclerotic stenosis can develop at the origins of the anterior and middle cerebral arteries, but these lesions are significantly less common than those found in the cervical portion of the internal carotid artery.

Atherosclerotic plaque at the carotid bifurcation initially appears as a fatty streak. Uncomplicated, mature atheroscle-

TABLE 92.2 ETIOLOGY

CAUSES OF CEREBRAL ISCHEMIA AND INFARCTION

ISCHEMIC

Atherothromboembolic
High-grade stenoses and occlusions
Emboli
Plaque
Platelet-fibrin debris
Intraplaque hemorrhage

Cardioembolic
Arrhythmias (atrial fibrillation, other arrhythmias)
Myocardial infarction with mural thrombus
Mitral valve prolapse, calcified annulus
Rheumatic heart disease (valvular, nonvalvular)
Prosthetic heart valves
Other (myopathy, atrial myxoma, subacute bacterial endocarditis, paradoxic emboli)

Systemic
Cardiac arrest and resuscitation
Profound shock
Cardiopulmonary bypass

Venous thromboses
Dural venous sinuses
Bilateral jugular vein occlusions

Miscellaneous causes
Lacunar infarcts
Lipohyalinosis
Fibrinoid necrosis
Charcot-Bouchard aneurysms
Migraine and vasospasm
Diabetes
Moyamoya
Kawasaki syndrome
Amyloid degeneration
Fibromuscular disease
Giant cell arteritis
Spontaneous dissections
Trauma (extracranial cerebral vessels)
  Blunt
  Penetrating
Hypercoagulable states
Binswanger's encephalopathy
Substance abuse

HEMORRHAGIC

Intraparenchymal hemorrhage
Hypertensive encephalopathy
Amyloid angiopathy
Arteriovenous malformation
Trauma

Subarachnoid hemorrhage
Berry aneurysms
Arteriovenous malformations
Trauma

Extracranial
Atherosclerosis
  Great vessels
  Carotid artery
Fibromuscular dysplasia
Trauma

TABLE 92.2 (Continued) ETIOLOGY

CAUSES OF CEREBRAL ISCHEMIA AND INFARCTION

Aortic aneurysms
  Dissecting
  Atherosclerotic
  Traumatic
Takayasu's panarteritis
Temporal arteritis
Carotid dissections
  Spontaneous
  Trauma
Carotid aneurysms

(Modified from Zelenock GB. The brain. In: *Clinical ischemic syndromes: mechanisms and consequences of tissue injury.* St Louis: Mosby, 1990, p. 350.)

rotic plaques are characterized by a heterogenous core, covered by a fibrous cap. Disruption of the fibrous cap is often the precipitating event that causes embolization or thrombosis. The disruption of a fibrous cap can be secondary to a number of processes, including progressive growth of the atherosclerotic lesion, an increase in blood flow velocity and shear stress, hemorrhage into the plaque, or rupture of the vasa vasorum. Loss of a fibrous cap results in a loss of endothelial cell coverage, so that the underlying necrotic core of the plaque is exposed to the circulating blood. These changes promote platelet deposition and thrombus formation on the ulcerated surface. The disruption of a mature, complex plaque can then result in stroke following the embolization of atheromatous debris or platelet-fibrin aggregates (Fig. 92.4). Alternatively, thrombosis of the artery can result in embolization or distal ischemia (Fig. 92.5). Recently, elevated serum levels of matrix metalloproteinase-9, a zinc-dependent endopeptidase involved in tissue remodeling, was associated with plaque instability and increased risk of embolization.[8,9]

Carotid duplex scanning can reveal some of these pathologic changes. A mature plaque is calcified and highly echogenic. A complicated plaque with intraplaque hemorrhage is usually anechoic, in which case it is called soft plaque. Some prospective studies have shown a correlation between the presence of soft plaque and transient ischemia and stroke, whereas the presence of hard, calcified plaque is characterized by a lack of associated symptoms.[10,11]

Clinical risk factors for the development of carotid artery atherosclerotic lesions are the same as those for coronary artery disease and include increased age, hypertension, diabetes mellitus, hyperlipidemia, hypercoagulable states, positive family history, and tobacco use. A strong correlation between carotid plaque and elevated plasma homocysteine levels has been identified.[12]

Stroke secondary to cerebrovascular disease can occur by either of two distinct mechanisms: ischemia associated with a low-flow state or embolism. Cerebral ischemia in a low-flow state is the consequence of the development of hemodynamically significant stenoses involving multiple cerebral arteries or stenosis in an artery supplying a vascular territory with a poor collateral network. Although the earliest reports linking stroke and extracranial carotid occlusive disease were published in the 19th century, it was not until the 1950s that Fisher et al.[13] and Millikan[14] established the correlation between extracranial carotid artery occlusive disease and stroke. These investigators showed that most strokes associated with carotid artery occlusive disease are caused by cholesterol or platelet-fibrin emboli that dislodge from atherosclerotic plaques within the extracranial carotid artery and subsequently occlude distal branches of the internal carotid artery. Their hypothesis differed substantially

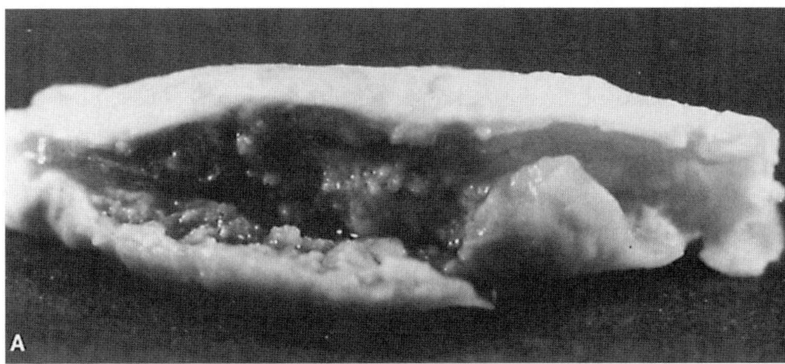

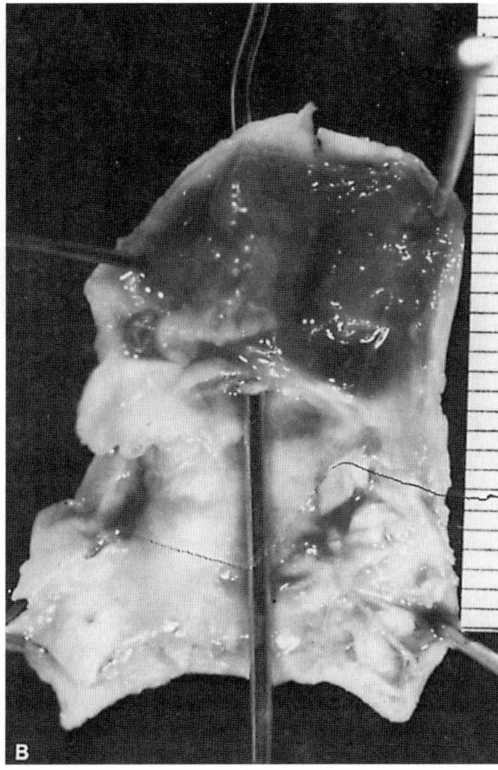

FIGURE 92.4 Endarterectomy specimens. (*A*) The thickened atherosclerotic plaque is almost totally occluded by intraluminal thrombus. This patient had symptoms of repeated embolism. (*B*) Hemorrhage is seen within the plaque, not in the lumen. If this hemorrhagic plaque excavates into the lumen, an ulceration will form.

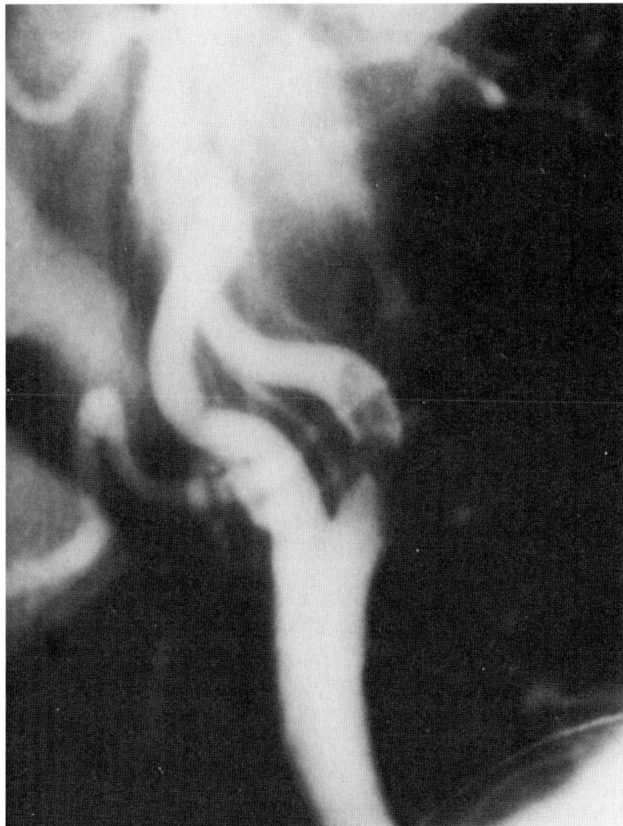

FIGURE 92.5 An isolated atherosclerotic lesion at the origin of the internal carotid artery. Free-floating intraluminal thrombus can be seen distal to the atherosclerotic plaque in this patient with crescendo transient ischemic attacks.

from the conventional dogma that most strokes were caused by cerebral ischemia secondary to reduced cerebral perfusion. This hypothesis was established by the identification of Hollenhorst plaques, which are platelet-fibrin aggregates or cholesterol crystals obstructing branches of the retinal artery.[15]

CLINICAL PRESENTATION

Transient ischemic attack (TIA) and hemispheric stroke are the most common clinical presentations of extracranial cerebrovascular occlusive disease. A TIA is the sudden onset of a focal neurologic deficit that resolves completely within 24 hours of onset. It can be manifested as a transient hemispheric event or as transient mononuclear blindness. A transient hemispheric attack presents clinically as a contralateral combined (motor and sensory) deficit or as a purely motor or purely sensory deficit. The specific clinical presentation depends on the anatomic location of the area of cerebral ischemia. Transient mononuclear blindness, also known as amaurosis fugax, is a transient loss of vision secondary to mechanical obstruction of a branch of the retinal artery (e.g., a cholesterol crystal resulting in a Hollenhorst plaque).[15] In most patients undergoing ophthalmologic examination immediately after an episode of amaurosis fugax, however, the retinal circulation is found to be normal. When ischemia occurs transiently in the distal distribution of the posterior circulation of the brain, it causes transient vertebrobasilar insufficiency. This can present as binocular visual loss, drop attacks (in which the patient does not lose consciousness but collapses to the floor), dysarthria, vertigo, dysphasia, incoordination, or other signs of cerebellar insufficiency. When atheromatous emboli are the cause of TIAs, symptoms generally last less than 15 minutes. Interestingly, serial computed tomography (CT) in patients with TIAs has shown that as many as 25% have had strokes in the area corresponding to the distribution of their symptoms.[16] Finally, vasospasm or migraine headaches can also present as transient ischemia.

A stroke is an acute neurologic deficit that lasts more than 24 hours. Like TIAs, most strokes are the result of embolic occlusion of a branch of the middle cerebral artery by atheromatous debris or a platelet-fibrin aggregate. Alternatively, a minority of strokes occur because of a low-flow state after internal carotid artery occlusion. These infarcts occur in "watershed" areas of the brain, located at the border between the anterior and posterior cerebral circulation. These typically are situated between the superior parietal and posterior temporooccipital lobes of the ipsilateral hemisphere. These strokes are characterized clinically by a contralateral sensorimotor deficit that is more pronounced in the proximal than in the distal limb, a prominent visual field defect, aphasia, and features of partial inattention.[17]

The anatomic distribution of ischemic strokes can be distinguished by the presentation of clinical deficits. Stroke in the distribution of the anterior cerebral artery is characterized by weakness or paralysis in the contralateral limbs, with sparing of the face, numbness and tingling in the contralateral limbs, dyspraxia, and abnormalities of higher cerebral function. Strokes in the distribution of the middle cerebral artery are characterized by sensorimotor deficits in the contralateral limbs and homonymous hemianopsia. If the dominant hemisphere is involved, aphasia may be present. Strokes in the distribution of the anterior choroidal artery are characterized by contralateral hemiplegia, hypesthesia, and homonymous hemianopsia.

Anterior circulation strokes should be distinguished from lacunar strokes and vertebrobasilar strokes. Lacunar strokes are usually characterized by pure motor or sensory dysfunction in the contralateral limb in patients with hypertension. The term *lacunar*, derived from the Latin word for "hole" or "cavity," refers to the appearance of infarcted tissue within the substance of the brain on gross examination. The pathophysiologic basis of lacunar strokes is usually disease of small (200 μm) arterioles. Vertebrobasilar strokes present with ipsilateral cranial nerve deficits, contralateral sensorimotor deficits, and signs of cerebellar insufficiency, including ataxia, vertigo, nystagmus, diplopia, and drop attacks. Symptoms of global cerebral ischemia can be difficult to distinguish from those of vertebrobasilar dysfunction.

DIAGNOSIS

Despite the development of various sophisticated diagnostic technologies, the clinical diagnosis of patients with symptomatic cerebrovascular occlusive disease remains centered on the careful performance of a neurologic examination. Of paramount importance is to differentiate between focal and nonfocal neurologic deficits. The history and physical examination should localize the area of cerebral ischemia responsible for the neurologic deficit. A complete physical examination should be performed to determine the presence of vascular occlusive disease in either the coronary or peripheral circulation. Review of systems should focus on risk factors for cardiovascular disease and predisposing factors for stroke, such as hypertension and cardiac arrhythmias.

A wide variety of noninvasive and invasive diagnostic studies can be performed to determine the causes and effects of stroke. In color-flow duplex scanning, real-time B-mode ultrasonography and color-enhanced pulsed Doppler flow measurements are used to determine the extent of carotid stenosis with high sensitivity and specificity.[18,19] Real-time B-mode imaging permits the localization of disease and determination of the presence or absence of calcification within plaque. Determination of the extent of stenosis is based largely on velocity criteria. Because stenosis increasingly obliterates the lumen of a vessel, the velocity of the blood flow must increase in the area of stenosis so that the total volume of flow remains constant within the vessel. Thus, velocity correlates with the extent of stenosis (Fig. 92.6). Typically, the internal carotid artery velocity profile is one of low resistance characterized by significant blood flow during diastole (Fig. 92.7). In contrast, the external carotid artery reflects a signal typical of a high-resistance muscular artery, in which little blood flow occurs during diastole.

Performing and interpreting a carotid duplex scan requires considerable skill and experience. Duplex scanning is most accurate in assessing carotid artery stenoses in which the luminal diameter is reduced by more than 50%. Color-flow duplex scanning has been refined sufficiently such that some clinicians now proceed to carotid endarterectomy without preoperative angiography. As mentioned earlier, the presence of calcium within the carotid wall, indicated by increased echogenicity, may be of prognostic significance. Furthermore, plaque heterogeneity may predict the presence of neurologic symptoms more accurately than the degree of carotid stenosis.[20] A shortcoming of duplex scanning is its inability to image anatomically inaccessible areas, such as the great vessel origins, distal internal carotid artery, or intracranial vasculature.

Transcranial Doppler

In transcranial Doppler studies, a low-frequency directional Doppler probe is focused through the thin temporal bone on the anterior, middle, and posterior cerebral arteries. Transcranial Doppler is of particular clinical value in patients with vasospasm after subarachnoid hemorrhage. In patients with cerebrovascular disease, transcranial Doppler complements duplex scanning by identifying significant intraarterial stenoses and revealing patterns of collateral flow. Transcranial color-flow duplex imaging is also available.

Angiography

Angiography has traditionally been considered the gold standard for the diagnosis of cerebrovascular disease. Angiography allows a complete and detailed visualization of both the intracranial and extracranial arterial circulations. Nonetheless, angiography remains painful for the patient and poses serious inherent risks. These include dye allergy, renal toxicity (particularly in patients with diabetes mellitus), and neurologic complications, such as stroke (1% to 4% of patients). Digital subtraction angiography has reduced the need for selective carotid artery catheterization and therefore has reduced the risk of neurologic complications.

Computed Tomography and Magnetic Resonance Imaging

Computed tomography of the brain is a valuable test for patients with TIAs or stroke. Contrast-enhanced scans assess density changes and the presence of edema, which can determine the location and extent of a stroke. CT of the brain distinguishes accurately between cerebral hemorrhage and infarction. Hemorrhage is associated with areas of increased density on CT, whereas infarction is associated with areas of decreased density that do not appear until at least 8 hours after the stroke has occurred. CT angiography can give nearly the same anatomic detail as contrast arteriography with added information regarding plaque morphology. It requires a significant contrast load, however, and its routine use to identify cerebrovascular disease has not been validated.

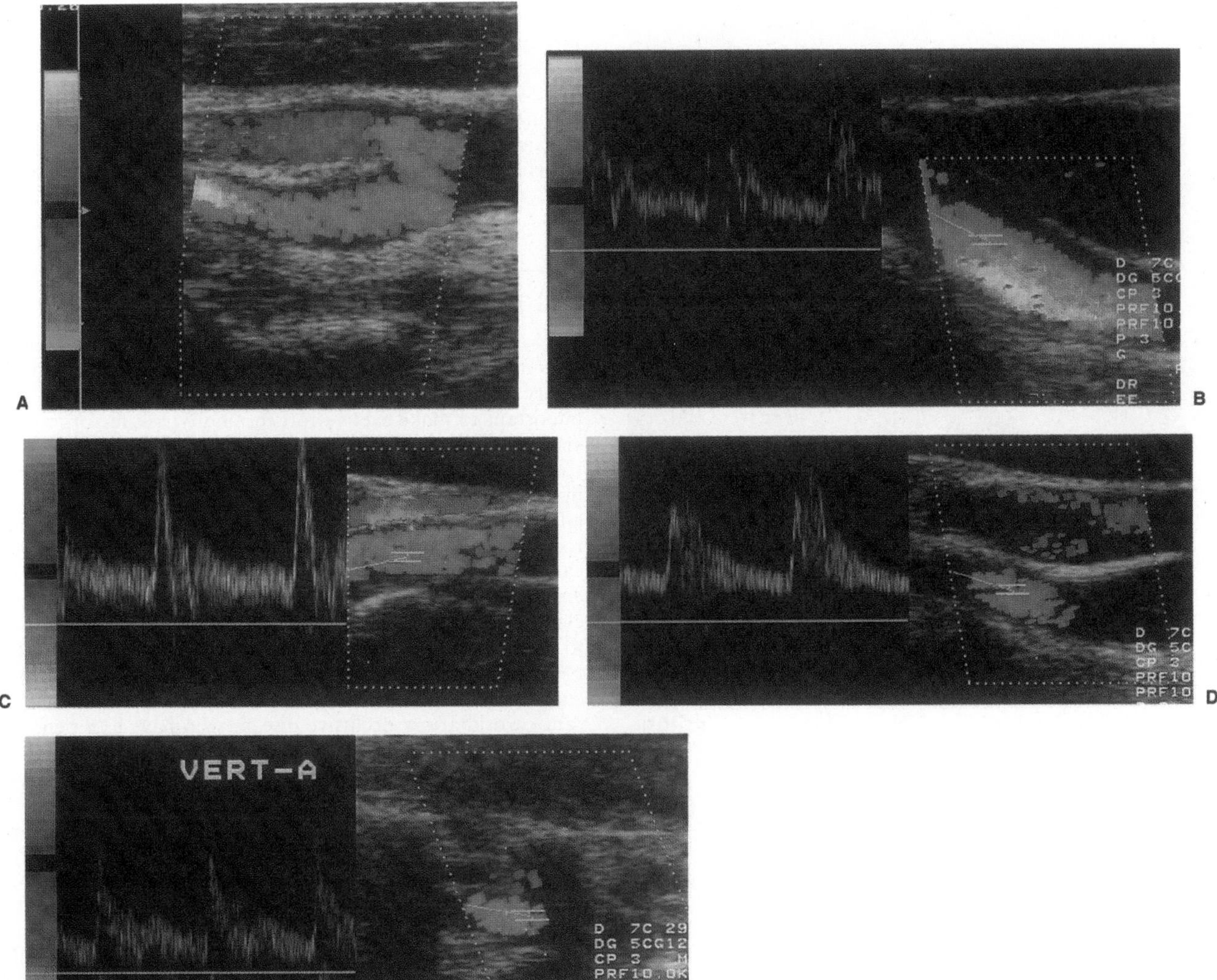

FIGURE 92.6 (*A*) Color-flow duplex scan showing a normal carotid artery bifurcation, the external carotid artery, and the internal carotid artery. (*B* to *D*) Duplex B-mode and analogue waveform of the common carotid artery (*B*), external carotid artery (*C*), and internal carotid artery (*D*). Note typical high-resistance waveform of the external carotid artery, which has reversal of flow in early diastole and minimal diastolic flow. In contrast, the internal carotid artery has a classic low-resistance waveform characterized by continuous flow throughout diastole. (*E*) Color-flow duplex image and analogue waveform of the vertebral artery.

Magnetic resonance imaging (MRI) and MR angiography (MRA) are highly sensitive techniques for the evaluation of patients with symptomatic cerebrovascular disease. MRI is more sensitive than CT in detecting an acute stroke. MRI can detect a stroke immediately after the infarction has occurred, whereas CT cannot. Cerebral hemorrhage, however, is less well identified by MRI than by CT. MRA permits evaluation of both the extracranial and intracranial cerebral circulations. Although techniques in MRA are rapidly evolving, the current precision of MRA in determining the extent of carotid stenosis is inferior to conventional angiography. MRA can be used as an adjunct to duplex ultrasound to delineate the anatomy of the great vessels and intracranial vessels, complementing confounding duplex ultrasound results and increasing the diagnostic accuracy of carotid stenoses. In combination with duplex ultrasound, MRI or MRA may obviate the need for the risks of contrast arteriography.[21,22] As technology improves, its precision may approach contrast arteriography.

NATURAL HISTORY OF CAROTID ARTERY OCCLUSIVE DISEASE

Symptomatic Disease

Many studies have attempted to define the natural history and clinical consequences of TIA and stroke. Despite limitations of these studies, it is clear that the risk for stroke is substantial after a carotid territory TIA or stroke. In community-based studies, the risk for stroke in the first 3 years after a TIA varied from 12% to 17%.[23,24] In hospital-based studies, the risk for stroke following a TIA varied from 10% to 30% in the first year, with a 6% risk for stroke in the subsequent 5 years. The cumulative risk for stroke at 5 years after a TIA was 30% to 50%. Moreover, these patients were at high risk for death from coronary artery disease. One third of the patients died within 5 years after TIA, usually of coronary occlusive

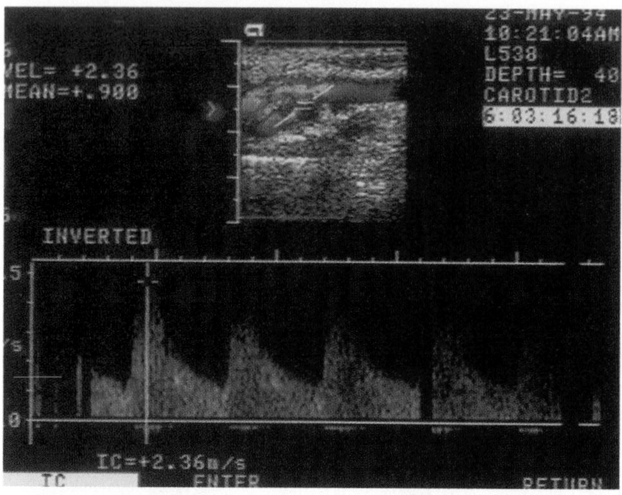

FIGURE 92.7 Color-flow duplex scan and analogue waveform of a high-grade internal carotid artery stenosis. Note acoustic shadowing in the region of the stenosis caused by calcification of the artery wall. Doppler scan taken at midstream of the jet of flow through the stenosis shows marked elevation of the peak systolic velocity (236 cm/s).

disease. The natural history of ischemic stroke is ominous. The initial stroke carries a 20% to 30% hospital mortality rate. The risk for recurrent stroke is high, ranging from 5% to 40%, and 30% of these are fatal.[25,26]

Asymptomatic Disease

Only 10% of patients who experience a stroke from any cause have had an antecedent TIA. Asymptomatic carotid bruits have been reported to occur in about 5% of the population older than 50 years.[27] Carotid bruits, however, are not diagnostic of a significant carotid artery stenosis. Bruits can represent a radiation of cardiac murmurs or denote the presence of mild carotid artery disease associated with calcification of the arterial wall. In fact, the poor correlation between the presence of a bruit and stenosis is illustrated by the fact that only 23% of patients identified to have bruits on physical examination have a significant (>50%) carotid stenosis.[28] With the wide availability of noninvasive carotid duplex studies, a carotid bruit is of little significance in predicting a neurologic event. A carotid bruit, however, remains a significant predictor of symptomatic, life-threatening coronary artery disease.

Carotid duplex ultrasonography has been used to determine the prevalence of asymptomatic carotid stenoses. The overall prevalence of internal carotid artery stenosis is 30% in patients older than 50 years. The prevalence of stenoses greater than 50% is only 3.7%, however, and greater than 80% is only 0.9%

Studies of the natural history of patients with asymptomatic carotid artery stenosis do not provide a clear and definitive estimate of their risk for stroke. The risk for stroke, however, appears to be proportional to the degree of carotid stenosis. Patients at highest risk are those in whose luminal diameter is reduced by more than 80%. Furthermore, the degree of stenosis is progressive in 85% of patients receiving serial duplex examinations. For patients found to have a stenosis of 75% to 80%, the risk for stroke varied from 18% and 46%.[29,29]

The risk of stroke is also elevated in patients undergoing major surgical procedures, such as coronary artery bypass grafting or peripheral vascular surgery.[30] Perioperative stroke after coronary artery bypass grafting is not increased with unilateral asymptomatic high-grade stenosis.[31–34] It is recommended, however, that prophylactic repair be considered when bilateral, asymptomatic high-grade stenosis is present. Controversy exists over the timing of carotid endarterectomy (CEA) and coronary artery bypass grafting. Meta-analysis suggests simultaneous and staged approaches carry a similar risk of stroke. Patient morbidity varies on which procedure is done first.

MANAGEMENT

Medical Treatment

The majority of asymptomatic and symptomatic carotid artery occlusive disease is caused by atherosclerosis. It is important to make every effort to modify risk factors to prevent progression of atherosclerotic disease. This includes control of hypertension, cessation of smoking, management of lipid disorders and diabetes, attainment of ideal body weight, and regular exercise. No drug therapy has been shown to reduce the risk for stroke in patients with asymptomatic carotid artery occlusive disease. A number of studies have examined the role of antiplatelet drugs (aspirin, ticlopidine, clopidogrel, and dipyridamole) and anticoagulation therapy to reduce the risk for stroke in patients after TIA or stroke.[1] No study has provided definitive evidence that systemic anticoagulation reduces the risk for stroke in patients with significant carotid artery occlusive disease who have experienced a TIA and stroke. The efficacy of aspirin in preventing stroke is also controversial. Aspirin, by reducing platelet adhesion and aggregation, has been shown to reduce morbidity and mortality from symptomatic coronary artery occlusive disease. When the endpoints of stroke and death are combined, a number of studies have shown a benefit in patients treated with aspirin. A recent meta-analysis of antiplatelet therapy in patients with a history of TIA or stroke demonstrated a 22% risk reduction in recurrent TIA or stroke, myocardial infarction, or vascular death (17.8%) compared with untreated controls (22.4%).[35] Ticlopidine and clopidogrel have also been studied in randomized prospective clinical trials. Ticlopidine has a marginal benefit compared with aspirin in preventing recurrent TIA or stroke, myocardial infarction, or vascular death, but is associated with significant side effects. Clopidogrel has a relative risk reduction of recurrent stroke, myocardial infarction, or death of 7.3% compared with aspirin in patients with a history of TIA or stroke, with a safety profile similar to aspirin.[36] The combination of clopidogrel and aspirin shows no benefit to clopidogrel alone and is associated with increased bleeding. A number of serious methodologic criticisms of these studies have been made. Because these studies use a composite endpoint (TIA, stroke, myocardial infarction, or death), it is unclear whether antiplatelet therapy reduces recurrent TIA or stroke alone. Considering most patients with extracranial cerebrovascular disease have concomitant cardiac and peripheral vascular disease, however, antiplatelet therapy should be recommended.

Surgical Treatment

Indications for carotid surgery include TIA, stroke (with minimal residual neurologic deficit), and high-grade asymptomatic carotid artery stenosis. Less common indications include global cerebral ischemia, caused by hemodynamically significant stenosis of three of the four major cerebral arteries. Such patients should undergo an extensive evaluation to detect other possible causes of their global symptoms, such as cardiac arrhythmia and middle ear abnormalities.

Technique of Carotid Endarterectomy

During carotid endarterectomy general endotracheal anesthesia, regional cervical block, or local anesthesia can be used. Proponents of general anesthesia emphasize a greater ability to control intraoperative blood pressure and improved surgical exposure in a motionless patient. In addition, general anesthesia reduces the cerebral metabolic rate and may increase the threshold for ischemia. Proponents of regional or local anesthesia emphasize accurate cerebral perfusion assessment in an awake patient, thereby reducing the need for intraoperative shunting. In addition, perioperative myocardial infarction risk may be reduced.

Surgical exposure of the carotid artery can be achieved through an incision along the medial border of the sternocleidomastoid muscle or by an oblique transverse incision through a skin crease. During dissection of the carotid bifurcation, manipulation should be minimized to prevent embolization of atherosclerotic plaque. After the administration of systemic heparin, the carotid artery is clamped, and a lateral arteriotomy is made from the common carotid artery to the distal extent of the plaque in the internal carotid artery (Fig. 92.8). The feasibility of carotid endarterectomy depends on the localization of the atherosclerotic plaque, which usually occupies the intima and inner medial, with sparing of the outer media and adventitia. In addition, atherosclerotic plaque is segmental in nature and tapers from within the deep media into the intima of the diseased artery distally. The cleavage plane for the endarterectomy is chosen at the thickest portion of the plaque, usually in the carotid bulb. This plane is then extended proximally, and the proximal plaque is circumferentially transected. As the endarterectomy is extended toward the internal carotid artery, it is important to identify the transition zone of the plaque from within the deep media to the intima. This usually allows the plaque to be feathered distally, with a naturally molded arterial wall left in the distal internal carotid artery. The operation is completed by performing an eversion endarterectomy of the portion of the plaque that extends into the proximal external carotid artery. The plaque in the external carotid artery usually ends at the first bifurcation point. After completion of the endarterectomy, any loose medial muscle fragments are removed. If a residual shelf is noticed at the distal endpoint, attempts should be made to continue the endarterectomy until a smooth transition is achieved. As a last resort, inverted tacking sutures are placed to prevent a flap from being raised during restoration of blood flow.

The use of routine patch angioplasty is supported by the Asymptomatic Carotid Atherosclerosis Study (ACAS), in which restenosis rates were reduced from 21% to 7% with the use of a patch.[37] Other benefits of patch angioplasty include a reduced risk of perioperative thrombosis, early and late stroke, and late restenosis. The type of patch has not been shown to alter outcome.

After completion of the endarterectomy, an objective technique should be used to determine the adequacy of the surgical repair. Techniques include continuous-wave Doppler with B-mode ultrasonography and intraoperative arteriography.

An alternative surgical technique is eversion carotid endarterectomy. This procedure involves dividing the internal carotid artery at the bifurcation. The adventitia and media of the internal carotid is then everted cranially with removal of the atheromatous plaque. A standard endarterectomy is performed in the common carotid artery. The internal carotid is then reapproximated with the carotid bifurcation with continuous suture. Advantages of this procedure include shorter clamp time and avoidance of a patch. Using this technique, recurrent stenoses usually occur at the proximal suture line.[38] However, some studies report lower restenosis rates.[39] The use of intraoperative shunts can be cumbersome with this approach.

Depending on the surgeon's preference, a variety of methods can be used to monitor the adequacy of cerebral perfusion during the period of internal carotid artery occlusion. These include neurologic assessment of the awake patient under local or regional cervical block, assessment of the internal carotid artery back pressure in the anesthetized patient, or continuous bilateral electroencephalographic monitoring. Cerebral protection during carotid cross-clamping involves optimal maintenance of systemic hemodynamics. Shunt placement during the period of carotid clamping is essential in some patients. Some surgeons use shunts in all patients, whereas others do so selectively. In large series, results do not vary between practitioners who never use a shunt, those who always do, and those who do so selectively.

Postoperatively, the patient should be monitored carefully for the first 12 to 24 hours after endarterectomy to evaluate hemodynamic stability and monitor neurologic status. Most patients tolerate this procedure well and can be discharged 24 to 72 hours postoperatively.

COMPLICATIONS OF CAROTID ENDARTERECTOMY

Neurologic Complications

Stroke can occur during or after carotid endarterectomy secondary to a variety of mechanisms, including inadequacy of collateral blood flow to the brain during temporary internal carotid artery occlusion, embolization during dissection of the carotid artery, or embolism or thrombosis of the reconstruction during the early postoperative period. Thrombosis after carotid endarterectomy usually is a result of sudden intimal dissection secondary to a loose flap or an inadequate distal endarterectomy endpoint. Embolization after carotid endarterectomy is usually secondary to the formation of platelet aggregates on the surface of the endarterectomized vessel. If neurologic deficit occurs within 24 hours of surgery, immediate reexploration is warranted to exclude a technical problem. Finally, stroke can be caused by intracerebral hemorrhage, which appears to be more common in patients with multiple-vessel involvement. It tends to occur on the second or third postoperative day and should be excluded by CT scan. Recent analysis of North American Symptomatic Carotid Endarterectomy Trial (NASCET) data found that the risk of perioperative stroke or death after endarterectomy for symptomatic stenosis was increased in patients with contralateral carotid occlusion, a left-sided procedure, hemispheric TIA, ipsilateral ischemic lesion on CT scan, and an ulcerated plaque.[40]

Postoperative cranial nerve dysfunction can develop in up to 39% of patients undergoing carotid endarterectomy.[41] Only 60% of these injuries produce clinical symptoms, such as hoarseness, difficulty in swallowing, or a change in speech patterns. Common cranial nerve injuries are to the recurrent laryngeal nerve, causing hoarseness; the hypoglossal nerve, causing the tongue to deviate toward the side of the injury; and the superior laryngeal nerve, causing the voice to become fatigued easily. The marginal mandibular nerve is less commonly injured but can result in facial drooping and loss of the ipsilateral nasolabial fold. The greater auricular nerve, spinal accessory nerve, and glossopharyngeal nerve are also vulnerable to injury.

Most cranial nerve injuries resolve completely within 6 months after the operation. All patients who undergo carotid endarterectomy should have a careful cranial nerve examination before and after the operation. Bilateral recurrent laryngeal nerve injuries can cause vocal cord palsy and loss of a patent airway. A patient

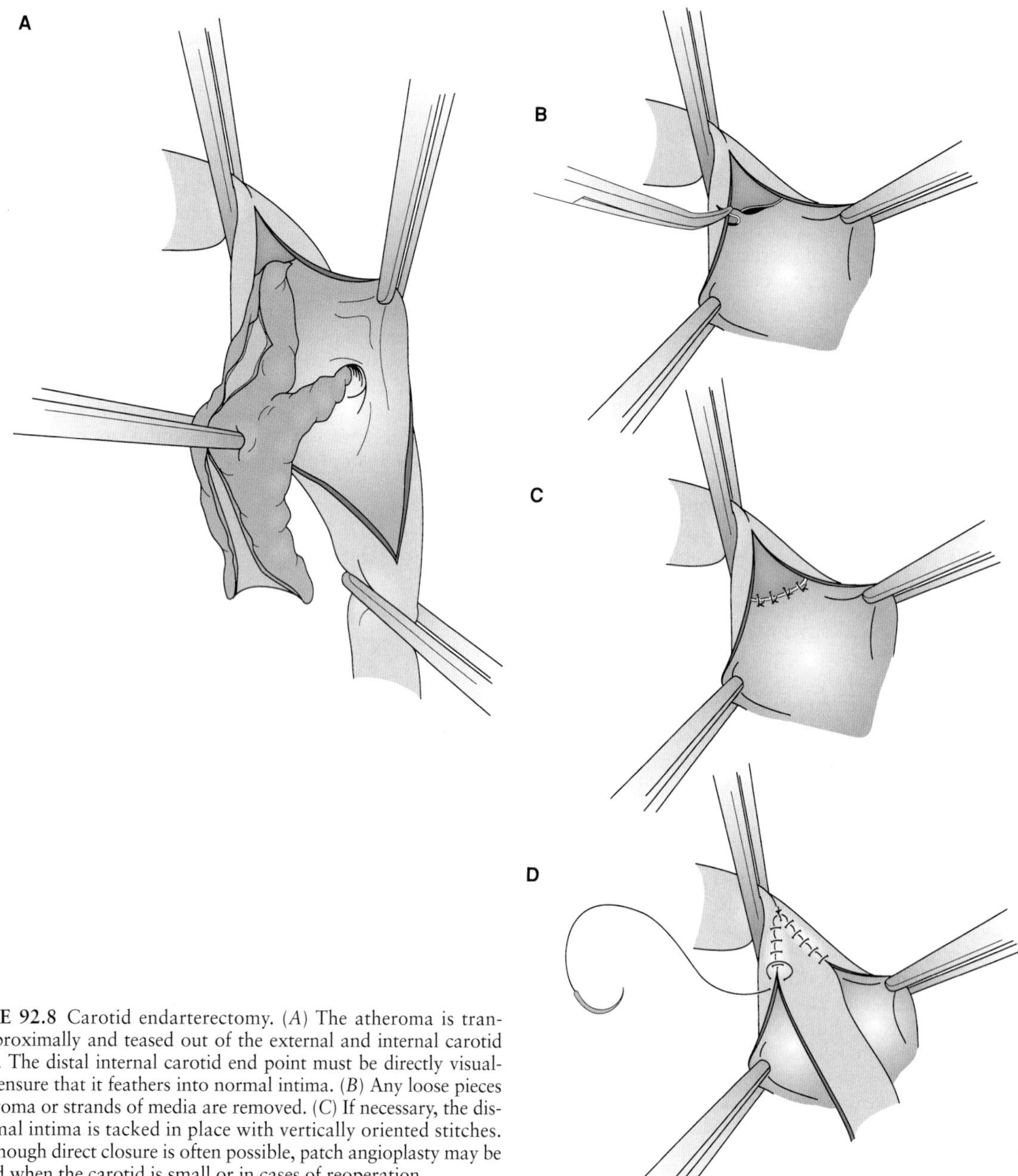

FIGURE 92.8 Carotid endarterectomy. (*A*) The atheroma is transected proximally and teased out of the external and internal carotid arteries. The distal internal carotid end point must be directly visualized to ensure that it feathers into normal intima. (*B*) Any loose pieces of atheroma or strands of media are removed. (*C*) If necessary, the distal normal intima is tacked in place with vertically oriented stitches. (*D*) Although direct closure is often possible, patch angioplasty may be required when the carotid is small or in cases of reoperation.

who sustains a bilateral recurrent laryngeal nerve injury may require an emergency tracheostomy. In patients undergoing second-stage contralateral carotid endarterectomies, it is common to perform preoperative indirect laryngoscopy to assess the vocal cord ipsilateral to the previous operation.

Non-neurologic Complications

Significant hemorrhage occurs after carotid endarterectomy in about 1% to 5% of patients. A somewhat higher rate of postoperative hemorrhage is noted in patients who receive aspirin perioperatively.

Patients may also experience episodes of hypertension and hypotension.[42] Hypotension and bradycardia occur secondary to increased baroreceptor reflex activity during dissection of the carotid artery or stimulation of the sinus nerve after removal of a rigid atheromatous plaque. This can be treated by local injection of 1% lidocaine into the tissue adjacent to the carotid sinus, thereby blocking the sinus nerve. Hypertension may develop if the carotid sinus nerve is interrupted, either by transection or by changing in arterial wall compliance. Episodes of severe hypertension or hypotension are associated with an increased risk for neurologic events.[44]

Myocardial infarction remains the most common cause of morbidity and mortality after carotid endarterectomy. Death from myocardial infarction accounts for 20% to 100% of all deaths after carotid endarterectomy.[43] The 10-year cumulative survival rate after carotid endarterectomy in patients with coronary artery disease who undergo coronary artery bypass grafting before carotid endarterectomy is 55%, but is only 32% in patients whose coronary disease remains uncorrected.[44]

Recurrent carotid stenosis is a relatively common complication after carotid endarterectomy (Fig. 92.9). Residual or recurrent carotid artery stenosis can be detected in up to 30% of patients undergoing careful postoperative surveillance with

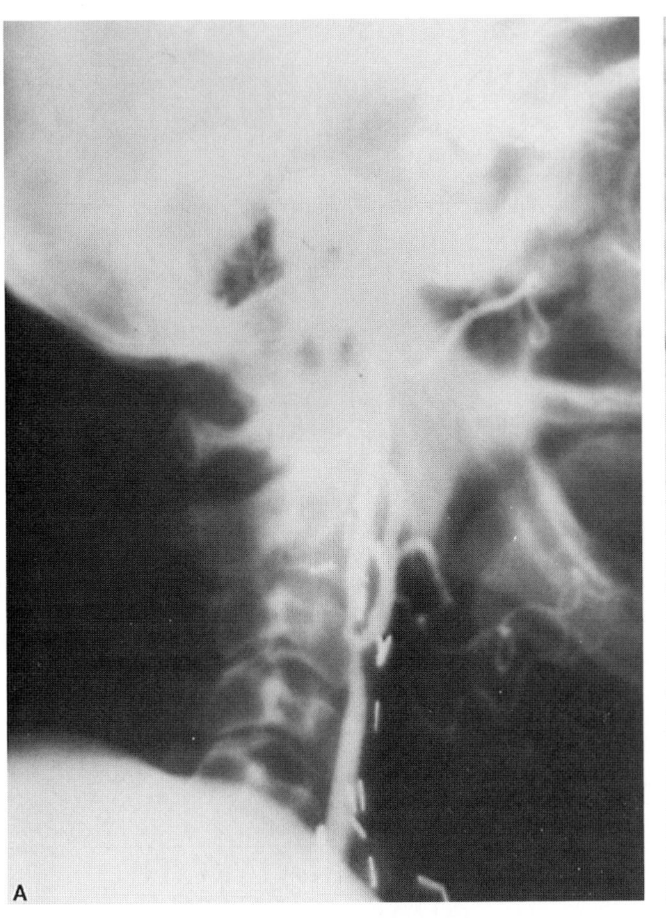

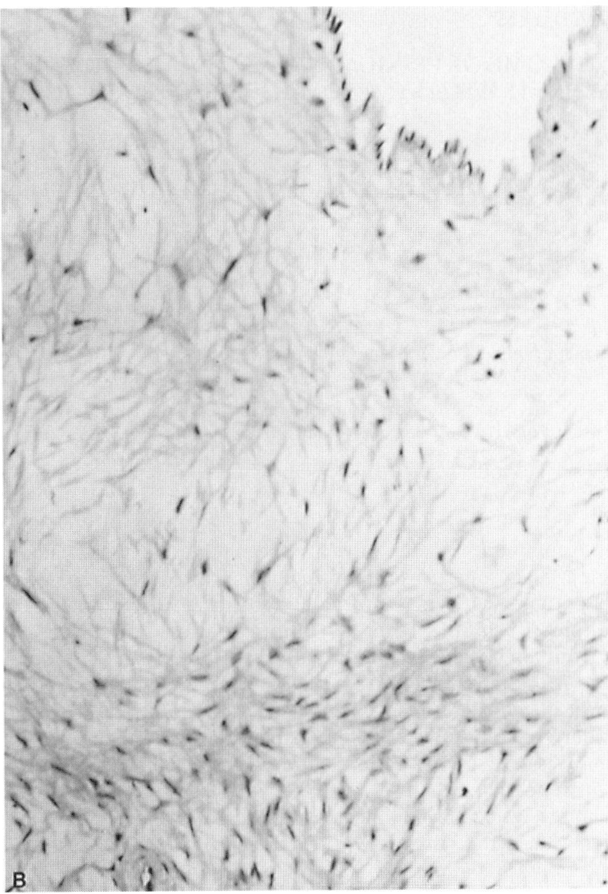

FIGURE 92.9 (*A*) Angiogram showing recurrent carotid stenosis. (*B*) Histology demonstrates a fibrous hyperplastic lesion, which was excised at reoperation.

carotid duplex scanning. Less than 3% of patients, however, experience symptomatic recurrence. Two forms of recurrent disease have been identified.[45] Carotid stenosis that recurs within 6 months of the initial endarterectomy usually is secondary to intimal hyperplasia, which is characterized by the proliferation of vascular smooth muscle and an increase in matrix deposition. When stenosis recurs 2 years or more after endarterectomy, recurrent atherosclerosis is usually found at the time of reoperation. The risk for recurrent carotid stenosis has been documented to be higher in women and in patients with hypercholesterolemia.

EFFICACY OF CAROTID ENDARTERECTOMY IN THE PREVENTION OF STROKE

The efficacy of carotid endarterectomy in preventing stroke has been the subject of considerable controversy. The controversy arose in part from wide variations (1% to 24.4%) in the reported rates of stroke after carotid endarterectomy.[46] In response to this controversy, a number of prospective, randomized studies examining the efficacy of carotid endarterectomy were undertaken. Three studies have established unambiguously the efficacy of carotid endarterectomy in preventing stroke in symptomatic patients with carotid stenosis[47–49] (Table 92.3).

The NASCET evaluated patients with recent hemispheric, retinal TIA, or nondisabling stroke. Subjects were randomized to the best available medical management or to an experimental group that received the best medical management plus carotid endarterectomy.[49] The patients were stratified according to degree of stenosis, 30% to 69% and 70% to 99%. Although the study was to include a 5-year follow-up, it was stopped prematurely, because of superior results in patients with 70% to 99% stenosis receiving endarterectomy. This conclusion was based on an interim analysis of 328 patients undergoing carotid endarterectomy and 331 receiving best medical therapy alone. At 18 months, the incidence of stroke in the surgical patients was 9%, and it was 26% in the patients receiving medical therapy alone. This represented an absolute risk reduction of 17% and a relative risk reduction of 65%. An even greater risk reduction was seen in the group of patients who experienced major or fatal ipsilateral stroke; an 81% relative risk reduction was observed in the patients who underwent carotid endarterectomy. Moreover, the benefit of surgery was seen within 3 months of operation. The implication of this finding is that many of the strokes occurred soon after randomization. Thus, when a patient is identified as having a symptomatic high-grade carotid artery stenosis, evaluation for surgery should begin immediately. The NASCET findings were supported by the results of the European Carotid Surgery Trial, and the Veterans Administration Cooperative Study 309. The nearly identical results found in these studies further substantiated the efficacy of carotid endarterectomy in symptomatic patients.[50,51]

TABLE 92.3 RESULTS

OUTCOME OF CLINICAL TRIALS OF CAROTID ENDARTERECTOMY IN PATIENTS WITH SYMPTOMATIC HIGH-GRADE CAROTID ARTERY STENOSIS

		Ipsilateral stroke rate (%)		Risk reduction (%)	
Study	Mean follow-up	Surgical	Nonsurgical	Absolute	Relative
NASCET	2y	9[a]	26[b]	17	65
ECST	3y	12.3[a]	21.9[b]	9.6	56
VACSP 2309		7[a]	19.4[b]	11.7	63

[a]Significantly different from nonsurgery, $P<.05$.
[b]Included episodes of crescendo transient ischemic attack in addition to stroke as major endpoint of study.

NASCET, North American Symptomatic Carotid Endarterectomy Trial; ECST, European Carotid Surgery Trial; VACSP, VA Cooperative Study.

A number of studies have also been undertaken to evaluate the efficacy of carotid endarterectomy in preventing stroke in patients with asymptomatic carotid artery stenosis[50–52] (Table 92.4). The Veterans Administration Asymptomatic Carotid Stenosis Trial was a multicenter prospective, randomized trial in which 440 patients who had asymptomatic carotid stenosis of 50% or more were randomized to carotid endarterectomy plus aspirin or aspirin alone.[53] At the time of analysis, 8% of the patients undergoing carotid endarterectomy experienced a TIA or stroke, whereas 20.6% of patients who received aspirin alone experienced a neurologic complication. When the patients who experienced TIA were excluded and only the patients who experienced ipsilateral stroke were examined, no significant difference between the two groups was identified. However, there was considerable crossover from the medical to the surgical arm in patients experiencing TIAs. This was the first prospective, randomized study showing that carotid endarterectomy plus aspirin is more effective than aspirin alone in reducing the frequency of TIA or stroke in patients with asymptomatic carotid stenosis.

The Asymptomatic Carotid Artery Stenosis Trial (ACAS), a prospective randomized trial sponsored by the National Institutes of Health, examined outcomes in asymptomatic carotid disease using stroke as the primary endpoint.[54] Patients with asymptomatic stenosis of 60% or more were randomized to either carotid endarterectomy and aspirin or aspirin alone. This study was also interrupted because of a significant benefit identified in patients undergoing carotid endarterectomy compared with medical therapy. At the time the study was interrupted, a relative reduction in the stroke rate of 50% had been observed in patients undergoing carotid endarterectomy. The benefit was much greater in men than in women. These prospective, randomized studies established the role of carotid endarterectomy in preventing stroke in patients with both symptomatic and asymptomatic high-grade carotid artery stenosis.

TABLE 92.4 RESULTS

OUTCOME OF CLINICAL TRIALS OF CAROTID ENDARTERECTOMY IN PATIENTS WITH ASYMPTOMATIC CAROTID STENOSIS

	Rate of ipsilateral neurological events (%)		Risk reduction (%)	
Study	Surgical	Nonsurgical	Absolute	Relative
VACSP[a]	8[c]	20.6	12.6	38
ACAS[b]	4.8[c]	10.6	5.8	55

[a]Transient ischemic attacks and stroke were endpoints.
[b]Stroke was the only end point.
[c]$P<.05$ compared with nonsurgical group

VACSP, Veterans Administration Cooperative Studies Program (carotid stenosis ≥50%); ACAS, Asymptomatic Carotid Artery Study (carotid stenosis ≥60%).

EXTERNAL CAROTID ENDARTERECTOMY

External carotid endarterectomy with division of the internal carotid artery is recommended for patients with ipsilateral internal carotid artery occlusion presenting with ipsilateral retinal or hemispheric TIA or stroke. In these cases, a large cul-de-sac in the proximal internal carotid artery may serve as a source of emboli that travel through an "internalized" external carotid artery (Fig. 92.10).

DIRECT AORTIC ARCH RECONSTRUCTION

Atherosclerotic lesions at the origin of the great vessels can result in TIA or stroke. Most commonly involved are the brachiocephalic and left common carotid arteries. When such lesions are identified, they can be repaired by direct reconstruction through a median sternotomy. For patients with lesions of the brachiocephalic artery, the options of endarterectomy or aortobrachiocephalic bypass grafting with a synthetic graft are available. Often, it is necessary to undertake revascularization of both the brachiocephalic and left common carotid arteries. Despite the complexity of these operations, they are in general attended by low complication rates and a neurologic morbidity rate of 2% or less.

VERTEBRAL ARTERY RECONSTRUCTION

Atherosclerosis at the origin of the vertebral arteries can become symptomatic, causing TIA or stroke in the posterior cerebral circulation. When appropriate indications exist, a

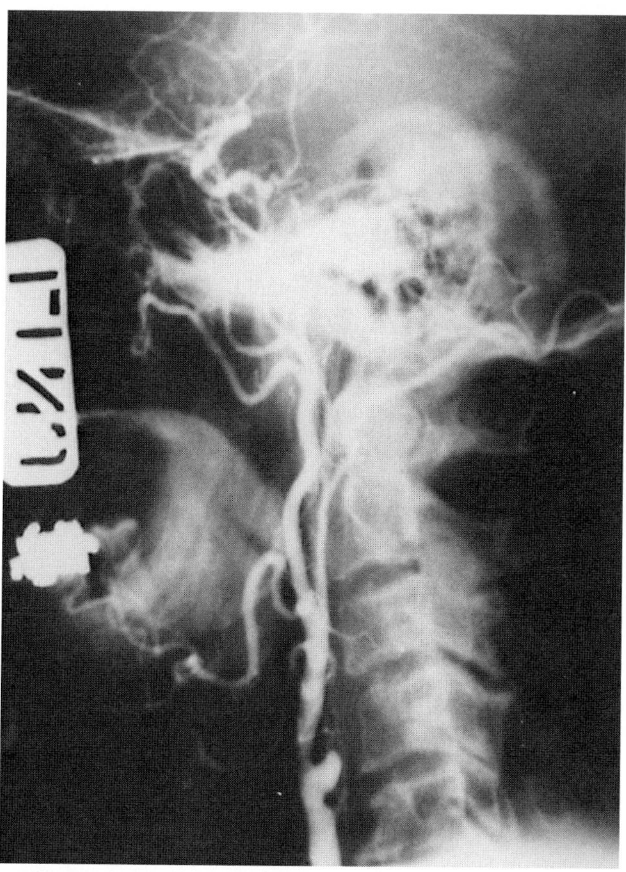

FIGURE 92.10 A totally occluded internal carotid artery with a residual stump can be a source of emboli. Note the periorbital collateral circulation.

variety of techniques are available for reconstruction of the vertebral arteries. Vertebral artery endarterectomy can be undertaken through an arteriotomy in the subclavian artery. Alternatively, the vertebral artery can be ligated at its origin and transposed to a normal ipsilateral common carotid artery. Less commonly, distal vertebral artery reconstructions are accomplished with a carotid-vertebral bypass using saphenous vein.

EXTRA-ANATOMIC BYPASS

Patients with atherosclerotic stenosis at the origin of the aortic arch vessels can present with neurologic symptoms and symptoms related to ischemia of the upper extremities. For patients who are not candidates for direct aortic arch reconstruction, a variety of alternative, extra-anatomic bypasses can be undertaken. These include subclavian-carotid, carotid-subclavian, axillary-axillary, carotid-carotid, and femoral-axillary bypass. Choice of conduit for these reconstructions includes Dacron, polytetrafluoroethylene (PTFE), and saphenous vein. Most of these extraanatomic reconstructions have good long-term patency rates.

ENDOVASCULAR THERAPY

Carotid artery angioplasty and stenting is a minimally invasive, technically feasible approach to treat extracranial cerebrovascular disease. Proponents of this procedure emphasize decreased morbidity compared with endarterectomy because of the avoidance of surgical complications. The possibility of embolism from angioplasty of a friable and complex atherosclerotic lesion, however, is concerning. Cerebral embolic protection devices are now routinely used, in the form of a filter or balloon catheter placed distal to the lesion before angioplasty.

Although the potential benefits of this less-invasive approach are obvious, questions remain regarding the efficacy of these procedures in preventing later strokes. At present, data from four prospective, randomized clinical trials comparing carotid artery angioplasty and stenting with endarterectomy are available (Table 92.5). Three of the trials were conducted in adequate risk patients and one in high-risk patients for carotid endarterectomy.

The Carotid and Vertebral Artery Transluminal Angioplasty Study (CAVATAS) compared surgery with angioplasty for symptomatic carotid and vertebral disease.[53] A total of 504

TABLE 92.5 RESULTS

OUTCOME OF CLINICAL TRIALS COMPARING CAROTID ARTERY ANGIOPLASTY AND STENTING TO CAROTID ENDARTERECTOMY

	30-day rate of death or stroke (%)		All stroke or death rate (%)	
Study	CAS	CEA	CAS	CEA
CAVATAS	10	10	14.3[a]	14.2[a]
Wallstent[b]	12.1[c]	4.5	12.1[c,e]	3.6[e]
SAPPHIRE	4.8[d]	9.8[d]	5.5[e] (12.2)[c,f]	8.4[e] (20.1)[f]

CAS, carotid artery stenting; CEA, carotid endarterectomy.

[a]Death and disabling stroke only at 3 years.
[b]Symptomatic patients only.
[c]$P < .05$ compared to CEA.
[d]Includes myocardial infarction as end point.
[e]At 1 year.
[f]Primary end point death stroke or myocardial infarction at 30 days plus ipsilateral stroke or death from neurologic causes within 31 days to 1 year.

CAVATAS: Carotid and Vertebral Artery Transluminal Angioplasty Study.

SAPPHIRE: Stenting and Angioplasty with Protection in Patients at High Risk for Endarterectomy trial.

symptomatic patients considered suitable candidates for carotid endarterectomy were randomized and followed for 3 years. Of these patients, 90% had symptoms within 6 months of randomization. Of patients in the angioplasty group, 25% had stents placed. The 30-day stroke and death rates and 3-year disabling stroke and death rates were comparable in each group (Table 92.5). The authors concluded endovascular therapy was similar to carotid endarterectomy in the prevention of stroke at 3 years. The major criticism of this study was the high complication rates seen in the endarterectomy group, which exceeded the 30-day stroke and death rate reported in the NASCET or ECST studies. Furthermore, this study primarily involved angioplasty alone and no embolic protection device was used.

A second randomized study compared angioplasty and stenting with endarterectomy in symptomatic patients at suitable risk for surgery.[54] This study was halted prematurely because of higher than expected complication rates seen in the carotid stenting group. Five of the seven patients in the carotid stenting group had a stroke within 30 days. Limitations of this study include the small sample size and inadequate credentialing of the operators.

A third randomized study, the Wallstent study,[55] sought to establish the equivalency of carotid artery stenting with endarterectomy in symptomatic carotid artery stenosis. The primary endpoint of the study was ipsilateral stroke, procedure-related death, or vascular death within 1 year. Here, 219 patients were randomized (107 stent and 112 endarterectomy). Stroke or death was four times greater in the carotid stenting group (see Table 92.5). Major stroke was observed in 3.7% in the stenting group and 0.9% in the endarterectomy group. Based on these results, the study was halted. The authors concluded carotid artery stenting was not equivalent to carotid endarterectomy. This study, however, has been criticized for flaws in its methodology.

A fourth randomized study, Stenting and Angioplasty with Protection in Patients at High Risk for Endarterectomy trial (SAPPHIRE), was the first to employ cerebral embolic protection devices.[56] Here, 310 high-risk patients were randomized and followed for 1 year. Asymptomatic patients with stenoses greater than 80% (68%) and symptomatic patients with stenoses greater than 50% (32%) were included in the trial. Patients with recurrent stenosis from prior endarterectomy were also included (30%). The composite endpoint was death, stroke, or myocardial infarction within 30 days and death or ipsilateral stroke at 1 year. Outcomes were similar between groups at 1 year (Table 92.5). However, 30-day stroke, death, or myocardial infarction rates were 39% lower in the stenting group. The investigators concluded stenting was not inferior to surgery in this high-risk population. Asymptomatic patients, however, had equally unsatisfactory results with carotid stenting or endarterectomy in this study. The 1-year stroke rates for asymptomatic patients approached the 5-year stroke rates in the medical arm of ACAS, suggesting medical therapy may be appropriate for asymptomatic high-risk patients. In addition, the difference seen in the treatment groups may be secondary to the inclusion of myocardial infarction (most non-Q wave) as part of the primary endpoint. Myocardial infarction was not included as a primary endpoint in many of the carotid endarterectomy trials. Nonetheless, the U.S. Food and Drug Administration approved carotid artery stenting with embolic protection for SAPPHIRE-eligible patients, based on the results of this study.

Carotid artery stenting is a rapidly evolving procedure whose results are approaching those of carotid endarterectomy. The periprocedural rates of stroke, myocardial infarction, and death continue to decline. The long-term efficacy and durability of carotid artery stenting is unknown, however, whereas carotid endarterectomy has an established record of durability. Further randomized trials are in progress to address suitability for average risk patients. At present, carotid artery stenting should be limited to high-risk patients (Table 92.6). The application of carotid artery stenting to patients at suitable risk to undergo endarterectomy should be limited to ongoing randomized clinical trials.

TABLE 92.6 INDICATIONS/CONTRAINDICATIONS

HIGH-RISK PATIENTS TO BE CONSIDERED FOR CAROTID ARTERY STENTING

MEDICAL COMORBIDITY
Age >80
Coronary artery disease
Acute myocardial infarction in prior 4 weeks
CABG within prior 6 months
Congestive heart failure (class III/IV)
Ejection fraction <30%
Dialysis dependent renal failure
Severe chronic obstructive pulmonary disease
FEV_1 <1.0L
LOCAL FACTORS
Carotid restenosis after carotid endarterectomy
Anatomically high lesion (above second cervical vertebrae)
Contralateral internal carotid artery occlusion
Contralateral laryngeal nerve palsy
Radiation induced internal carotid artery stenosis
Prior neck dissection
Permanent tracheal stoma
Cervical scarring

CABG, coronary artery bypass graft.

KEY POINTS

- **Significant advances in the surgical treatment of extracranial cerebrovascular disease have contributed greatly to reducing the mortality associated with stroke.**
- **Stroke remains the third most common cause of death in the United States, and atherosclerotic occlusive disease of the extracranial portion of the carotid artery is the most common cause of stroke.**
- **Atherosclerosis is the pathologic process most often responsible for symptoms of cerebrovascular insufficiency.**
- **Clinical risk factors for the development of carotid artery atherosclerotic lesions are the same as those for coronary artery disease: increased age, hypertension, diabetes mellitus, hyperlipidemia, hypercoagulable states, positive family history, and tobacco use.**
- **The most common clinical presentations of extracranial cerebrovascular occlusive disease are transient ischemic attack (TIA) and hemispheric stroke.**
- **The majority of asymptomatic and symptomatic carotid artery occlusive disease is caused by atherosclerosis. It is therefore important to modify risk factors to prevent progression of atherosclerotic disease.**
- **Prospective, randomized studies have established the role of carotid endarterectomy in preventing stroke in patients with both symptomatic and asymptomatic high-grade carotid artery stenosis.**
- **Carotid artery stenting is a rapidly evolving procedure whose results are approaching those of carotid endarterectomy.**
- **At present, carotid artery stenting should be limited to high-risk patients. The application of carotid artery stenting to patients at suitable risk to undergo endarterectomy should be limited to ongoing randomized clinical trials.**

Acknowledgment

We thank Nayan Sivamurthy, Fellow of the UCSF Division of Vascular Surgery, for assistance with preparing this chapter.

References

1. Marshall RS, Mohr JP. Current management of ischaemic stroke. *J Neurol Neurosurg Psychiatry* 1993;56:6.
2. Carpenter MB. *Core text of neuroanatomy*. Baltimore: Williams & Wilkins, 1974.
3. Stanley JC, Gerwertz BL, Bove EL. Arterial fibrodysplasia, histopathological character, and current etiologic concepts. *Arch Surg.* 1975;11:561.
4. Effeney DJ, Ehrenfeld WK, Stoney RJ. Why operate on carotid fibromuscular dysplasia? *Arch Surg.* 1980;115:1261.
5. Ehrenfeld WK, Wylie EJ. Spontaneous dissection of the internal carotid artery. *Arch Surg.* 1976;111:1294.
6. Ross R. The pathogenesis of atherosclerosis: a perspective for the 1990s. *Nature* 1993;362:801.
7. Zarins CK, Ernst CB, Stanley JC. *Current therapy in vascular surgery*. Philadelphia: BC Dekker, 1991.
8. Loftus IM, Naylor AR, Bell PR, et al. Plasma MMP-9—a marker of carotid plaque instability. *Eur J Vasc Endovasc Surg.* 2001;21:17–21.
9. Alvarez B, Ruiz C, Chacon P, et al. Serum values of metalloproteinase-2 and metalloproteinase-9 as related to unstable plaque and inflammatory cells in patients with greater than 70% carotid artery stenosis. *J Vasc Surg.* 2004;40:469–475.
10. **Tegos TJ, Stavropoulos P, Sabetai MM, et al. Determinants of carotid plaque instability: echoicity versus heterogeneity. *Eur J Vasc Endovasc Surg.* 2001;22:22–30.**
11. Mathiesen EB, Bonaa KH, Joakimsen O. Echolucent plaques are associated with high risk of ischemic cerebrovascular events in carotid stenosis. The Tromso Study. *Circulation* 2001;103:2171–2175.
12. Selhub J, Jaques PF, Bostom AG. Association between plasma homocysteine concentrations and extracranial carotid artery stenosis. *N Engl J Med.* 1995;332:286.
13. **Fisher CM, Pritchard JE, Mathews WH. Arteriosclerosis of the carotid arteries. *Circulation* 1952;6:457.**
14. Millikan CH. The pathogenesis of transient focal cerebral ischemia. *Circulation* 1965;32:438.
15. Hollenhorst RW. Significance of bright plaques in the retinal arteries. *JAMA* 1961;178:23.
16. Norris JW, Zhu CA. Silent stroke and carotid stenosis. *Stroke* 1992;23:483.
17. Mohr JP, Barnett HJM, Barnett HJM, et al. *Stroke: pathophysiology, diagnosis, and management*. New York: Churchill Livingstone, 1986.
18. **Moneta GL, Edwards JM, Chitwood RW. Correlation of North American Symptomatic Carotid Endarterectomy Trial (NASCET) angiographic definition of 70% to 99% internal carotid artery stenosis with duplex scanning. *J Vasc Surg.* 1993;17:152.**
19. Londrey GL, Spadone DP. Does color flow imaging improve the accuracy of duplex carotid evaluation? *J Vasc Surg.* 1991;13:659.
20. AbuRahma AF, Wulu JT, Crotty B. Carotid plaque ultrasound heterogeneity and severity of stenosis. *Stroke* 2002;33:1772–1775.
21. Back MR, Rogers GA, Wilson JS, et al. Magnetic resonance angiography minimizes need for arteriography after inadequate carotid duplex ultrasound scanning. *J Vasc Surg.* 2003;38:422–430
22. Nederkoorn PJ, van der Graaf Y, Hunink MG. Duplex ultrasound and magnetic resonance angiography compared with digital subtraction angiography in carotid artery stenosis: a systematic review. *Stroke* 2003;34:1324–1332.
23. Friedman GD, Wilson WS, Mosier JM. Transient ischemic attacks in a community. *JAMA* 1969;210:1428.
24. Whisnant JP, Matsumoto N, Elveback LR. Transient cerebral ischemic attacks in a community. *Mayo Clin Proc.* 1973;48:194.
25. Matsumoto N, Whisnant JP, Kurland LT. Natural history of stroke in Rochester, Minnesota, 1955 through 1969: an extension of a previous study, 1945 through 1954. *Stroke* 1973;4:20.
26. Bardin JA, Bernstein EF, Humbert PB. Is carotid endarterectomy beneficial in prevention of recurrent stroke? *Arch Surg.* 1982;117:1401.
27. Mohr JP. Asymptomatic carotid artery disease. *Stroke* 1982;13:431.
28. Chambers BR, Norris JW. Outcome in patients with asymptomatic neck bruits. *N Engl J Med.* 1986;315:860.
29. Roederer GO, Langlois YE, Jager KA. The natural history of carotid arterial disease in asymptomatic patients with cervical bruits. *Stroke* 1984;15:605.
30. Barnes RW, Marzalek PB. Asymptomatic carotid disease in the cardiovascular surgical patient: is prophylactic endarterectomy necessary? *Stroke* 1981;12:497.
31. Brener BJ, Brief DK, Alpert J. The risk of stroke in patients with asymptomatic carotid stenosis undergoing cardiac surgery: a follow-up study. *J Vasc Surg.* 1987;5:269.
32. Breslau PJ, Fell G, Ivey TD. Carotid arterial disease in patients undergoing coronary artery bypass operations. *J Thorac Cardiovasc Surg.* 1981; 82: 765.
33. Ivey TD, Strandness DJ, Williams DB. Management of patients with carotid bruit undergoing cardiopulmonary bypass. *J Thorac Cardiovasc Surg.* 1984;87:183.
34. McCann RL. Surgical management of carotid artery atherosclerotic disease. *South Med J.* 1993;86:2. S23.
35. Antithrombotic Trialists' Collaboration. Collaborative meta-analysis of randomised trials of antiplatelet therapy for prevention of death, myocardial infarction and stroke in high risk patients. *BMJ* 2002;324:71–86.
36. **CAPRIE Steering Committee. A randomised, blinded, trial of clopidogrel versus aspirin in patients at risk of ischaemic events (CAPRIE). *Lancet* 1996;348:1329–1339.**
37. Moore WS, Kempczinski RF, Nelson JJ. Recurrent carotid stenosis: results of the Asymptomatic Carotid Atherosclerosis Study. *Stroke* 1998;29:2018.
38. Green RM, Greenberg R, Illig K, et al. Eversion endarterectomy of the carotid artery: technical considerations and recurrent stenoses. *J Vasc Surg.* 2000;32:1052–1061.
39. Cao P, Giordano G, De Rango P, et al. Eversion versus conventional carotid endarterectomy: late results of a prospective multicenter randomized trial. *J Vasc Surg.* 2000;31:19–30.
40. Ferguson GG, Eliasziw M, Barr HW, et al. The North American Symptomatic Carotid Endarterectomy Trial: surgical results in 1415 patients. *Stroke* 1999;30:1751–1758.
41. Hertzer NR, Rutherford RM. *Vascular surgery*. Philadelphia: WB Saunders, 1984.
42. Bove EL, Fry WJ, Gross WS. Hypotension and hypertension as consequences of baroreceptor dysfunction following carotid endarterectomy. *Surgery* 1979;85:633.
43. O'Donnell TF, Callow AD, Willett C. The impact of coronary artery disease on carotid endarterectomy. *Ann Surg.* 1983;198:705.
44. Hertzer NR, Arison R. Cumulative stroke and survival ten years after carotid endarterectomy. *J Vasc Surg.* 1985;2:661.
45. Stoney RJ, String ST. Recurrent carotid stenosis. *Surgery* 1976;80:705.
46. Easton JP, Sherman DG. Stroke and mortality rate in carotid endarterectomy: 228 consecutive operations. *Stroke* 1977;8:565.
47. Beneficial effect of carotid endarterectomy in symptomatic patients with high-graft carotid stenosis. *N Engl J Med.* 1991;325:445.
48. MRC European Carotid Surgery Trial: interim results for symptomatic patients with severe (70%–99%) or with mild (0%–29%) carotid stenosis. *Lancet* 1991;337:1235.
49. Mayberg MR, Wilson SE, Yatsu F. Carotid endarterectomy and prevention of cerebral ischemia in symptomatic carotid stenosis. *JAMA* 1991;266: 3289.
50. Carotid surgery vs. medical therapy in asymptomatic carotid stenosis. *N Engl J Med.* 1993;328:221.
51. Hobson RW, Weiss DG, Fields WS. Efficacy of carotid endarterectomy for asymptomatic carotid stenosis. *N Engl J Med.* 1993;328:221.
52. Endarterectomy for asymptomatic carotid artery stenosis. *JAMA* 1995; 273:1421.
53. Brown MM, Rogers J, Bland JM, and the CAVATAS Investigators. Endovascular versus surgical treatment in patients with carotid stenosis in the carotid and vertebral artery transluminal angioplasty study (CAVATAS): a randomized trial. *Lancet* 2001;357:1729–1737.
54. Naylor AR, Bolia A, Abbott RJ, et al. Randomized study of carotid angioplasty and stenting versus carotid endarterectomy: a stopped trial. *J Vasc Surg.* 1998;28:326–334.
55. Alberts MJ. Results of a multicenter prospective randomized trial of carotid artery stenting vs. carotid endarterectomy. *Stroke* 2001;32:325.
56. **Yadav JS, Wholey MH, Kuntz RE, et al. Protected carotid-artery stenting versus endarterectomy in high-risk patients. *N Engl J Med.* 2004;351: 1493–1501.**

CHAPTER 93 ■ UPPER EXTREMITY OCCLUSIVE DISEASE

JAMES S. T. YAO

A wide spectrum of arterial occlusive diseases in an upper extremity can cause ischemic symptoms. An accurate diagnosis requires a thorough history, careful physical examination, and the liberal use of ancillary tests. Appropriate surgical treatment depends on the location of the occlusive lesion and the nature of the underlying occlusive process. In general, proximal lesions involving the subclavian, axillary, and brachial arteries are more amenable to reconstructive surgery.

HISTORY TAKING

Taking an appropriate history is the most important initial step in the workup of a patient with upper extremity ischemia. In addition to a careful delineation of the patient's symptoms, an appropriate inquiry should include occupational, pharmacologic, and athletic risks and a pertinent medical history. Table 93.1 lists conditions and activities that can be related to the development of upper extremity ischemic symptoms.

SYMPTOMS

The presenting symptoms of upper extremity occlusive disease include evidence of arterial emboli, Raynaud's phenomenon, pain, and exercise-related forearm fatigue. Embolic symptoms include gangrene of the tips of the fingers, petechiae of the skin, splinter hemorrhages of the nail bed, and livedo reticularis. The term "*Raynaud's phenomenon*" refers to episodic digital color changes provoked by stimuli, such as cold or emotion. The digits first exhibit pallor, then cyanosis, and followed by reactive hyperemia. The pathophysiology of the color changes from white to blue to red is thought to be digital ischemia (resulting from vasospasm), followed by desaturation of hemoglobin (which produces cyanosis), and then by a reactive hyperemia. Raynaud's phenomenon should not be confused with Raynaud's disease. The former is a secondary process, whereas the latter is a primary disease without a known cause. The diagnosis of primary Raynaud's disease is made only after all the etiologic factors listed in Table 93.1 have been excluded and after symptoms persist for at least 2 years in the absence of other conditions that might be causal. Raynaud's phenomenon secondary to an underlying cause can be unilateral or bilateral. In patients with unilateral Raynaud's phenomenon, organic arterial occlusive disease should be suspected. In contrast, bilateral symptoms are often the consequence of a systemic disease that causes vasospasm. The precise classification of primary and secondary Raynaud's phenomenon is often difficult, and the terminology is imprecise. Many physicians prefer to use the term "Raynaud's syndrome" to characterize all patients with episodic vasospastic disease of the hands. Raynaud's phenomenon should also be distinguished from acrocyanosis, a disorder characterized by painless, persistent, diffuse cyanosis of the fingers and hands.

CLINICAL EXAMINATION

The physical examination should include an examination of the thoracic outlet and the entire upper extremity. Palpation of the supraclavicular region may help to detect the presence of a subclavian aneurysm or a cervical rib. Auscultation of the subclavian artery with the stethoscope placed just below the midclavicular region and listening for a bruit with the patient's arm placed in a neutral position (or abduction) and external rotation (or hyperabduction) help to establish the diagnosis of thoracic outlet compression to the artery. Palpation of pulses begins with the subclavian artery in the supraclavicular fossa and continues with the axillary artery under the armpit, the brachial artery at the upper arm and elbow, and the radial and ulnar arteries at the wrist level. A decreased or absent pulse in any site other than the supraclavicular fossa indicates major artery occlusion. Conversely, a readily palpable pulse in the supraclavicular fossa can represent a subclavian artery aneurysm.

Examination of the hand is not complete unless an Allen test is performed. The examiner stands beside or facing the subject. The radial and ulnar arteries of one wrist are compressed by the examiner's fingers. The subject is asked to open and close the hand rapidly for 1 minute to empty blood out of the hand and then to extend the fingers quickly. The radial or the ulnar artery is released, and the hand is observed for capillary refilling and return of color. The test result is judged normal if refilling of the hand is complete within a short period (<6 seconds). Any portion of the hand that does not blush is an indication of incomplete continuity of the arch. Hyperextension of the fingers must be avoided because it produces a false-positive result. In addition to the Allen test, examination of the hand must include palpation of the palm for a pulsatile mass or excess scar tissue.

NONINVASIVE TESTING

Several noninvasive tests, including plethysmography, transcutaneous Doppler examination, and duplex scan, are available for the objective evaluation of patients with upper extremity ischemia.[1] Of these, Doppler examination is the most straightforward and consists of audible signal interpretation, waveform recording with spectral analysis, and systolic pressure measurements. Bilateral examinations should be performed for comparative purposes. Because many of the diseases affecting the hand are symmetric, the asymptomatic hand often will have significant disease.[2] This is especially true in patients with systemic disease causing hand ischemia.

Because both the axillary and brachial arteries are superficial vessels, they are amenable to Doppler examination (Algorithm 93.1). Any change from normal signals (triphasic) to abnormal signals (monophasic) indicates the presence of an occlusive lesion. Distal to the elbow, arterial signals are more difficult to obtain. At the wrist, both the radial and ulnar

TABLE 93.1 ETIOLOGY

CONDITIONS AND RISKS FOR UPPER EXTREMITY ISCHEMIA

OCCUPATIONAL INJURY
Vibration syndrome
Pneumatic tools
Chain saws
Grinders
Electrical burns
Hypothenar hammer syndrome
Mechanical work or auto repair
Lathe operation
Carpentry
Electrical work
Occupational acroosteolysis—polyvinylchloride exposure
ATHLETIC ACTIVITIES
Thoracic outlet compression
Baseball pitching
Kayaking
Weight lifting
Rowing
Butterfly swimming
Golfing
Hand ischemia
Baseball catching
Frisbee
Karate
Handball
PHARMACOLOGIC HISTORY
Ergot poisoning
Beta blockers
Drug abuse, cocaine use
Cytotoxic drugs
Dopamine overdose
MEDICAL CONDITIONS
Atherosclerosis
Arteritis
Collagen disease
Scleroderma
Rheumatic arteritis
Systemic lupus erythematosus
Dermatomyositis
Allergic necrotizing arteritis
Takayasu's disease
Giant cell arteritis
Blood dyscrasias
Cold agglutinins
Cryoglobulins
Polycythemia vera
Behçet's syndrome
Antiphospholipid syndrome
Thoracic outlet syndrome
Congenital arterial wall defects
Pseudoxanthoma elasticum
Ehlers-Danlos syndrome
Fibromuscular dysplasia
Iatrogenic injury
Arterial blood gas and pressure monitoring
Cardiac catheterization
Arteriography
Frostbite
Renal transplantation and related problems
Azotemic arteriopathy
Hemodialysis shunts
Radiation
Breast carcinoma
Hodgkin's disease
Aneurysms of the upper extremity

arteries become superficially situated once again. Palpation of the ulnar artery can be difficult, and Doppler examination is helpful in determining the patency of this artery. In the hand, Doppler examination of the palmar arches is performed best at the midthenar and hypothenar regions. The common digital vessels should be examined at the base of the fingers where they divide into the proper digital arteries, which lie along the shaft of the proximal phalanx of each finger. Waveform recording is useful in both analysis and record keeping.

For segmental upper extremity pressures, a pneumatic cuff is placed at the upper arm, as in routine blood pressure recording. The brachial artery blood pressure reflects the pressure in all proximal arteries, and the value should be within 10 to 20 mm Hg of that in the opposite extremity. A greater difference signifies innominate, subclavian, axillary, or brachial stenosis. If brachial artery occlusion is suspected, a pressure cuff is applied to the forearm and the pressure recorded in a similar manner, with the radial artery used for signal detection. A pressure drop of 20 to 30 mm Hg signifies an obstruction distal to the brachial artery. For finger pressure measurement, a 2.5-cm cuff is placed at the base of the finger, and the return of Doppler signals after cuff deflation is monitored at the fingertip. An arterial occlusion distal to the palmar arch is defined by a pressure gradient between the fingers of more than 15 mm Hg or a wrist-to-digit difference of 30 mm Hg.

The Doppler technique is of particular value in determining palmar arch patency in a patient who is unconscious or uncooperative in performing an Allen test. Before arterial line placement, this simple test may help to avoid hand ischemia. In the modified Allen test, the Doppler probe is placed over the radial artery while the ulnar artery is compressed. If the signal disappears, the arch depends on the ulnar artery for supply. If the signal remains strong, the arch is complete. A similar maneuver is repeated over the ulnar artery while the radial artery is compressed.

The plethysmograph is used to record finger pulse contours for analysis and to differentiate between a normal state and obstructive or vasospastic disease.[1] The duplex scan is helpful in establishing the diagnosis of aneurysm.

LABORATORY TESTING

In severe bilateral hand ischemia, a systemic cause of the arterial lesions should be sought. Laboratory tests include serologic, immunologic, and hematologic studies to help establish the diagnosis (Table 93.2). The erythrocyte sedimentation rate remains a useful screening test to aid in the diagnosis of various forms of arteritis. A positive antinuclear antibody test result suggests connective tissue disease or other arteritides. When the antinuclear antibody titer is abnormal, immunofluorescent pattern analysis of antibodies can help to establish the diagnosis of various connective tissue disorders. The speckled pattern antibody is more specific for systemic lupus erythematosus. A nucleolar pattern suggests scleroderma. A positive anticardiolipin antibody is diagnostic for antiphospholipid syndrome, which is characterized by thromboembolic events in young adults.[3]

RADIOLOGIC TESTING

A combination of laboratory and radiologic testing may be needed to establish the proper diagnosis of systemic disease. The radiologic examination includes soft-tissue radiography of the hand, chest roentgenography, esophageal barium swallow and motility test, and arteriography. The soft-tissue radiograph of the hand may reveal calcinosis, which is diagnostic for the CREST (calcinosis cutis, Raynaud's phenomenon,

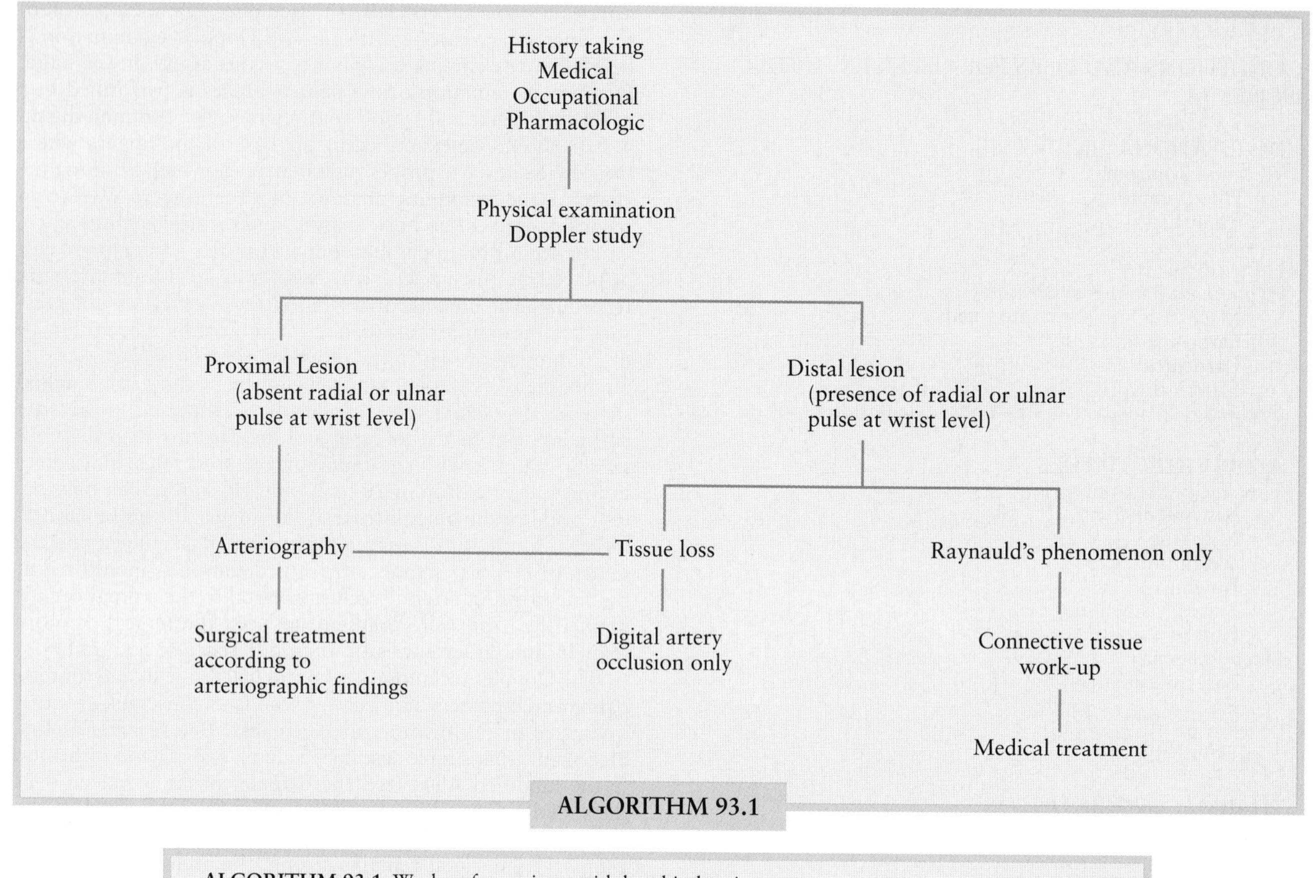

ALGORITHM 93.1 Workup for patients with hand ischemia.

esophageal motility disorder, sclerodactyly, and telangiectasia) syndrome, or diffuse calcified arteries in diabetic or azotemic arteriopathy (Fig. 93.1). The chest film is essential to detect bony anomalies of the thoracic outlet, such as cervical ribs (Fig. 93.2), anomalous first ribs, and healed fractures of the first rib or clavicle. Pulmonary fibrosis on the chest film is another indication of systemic sclerosis.

Arteriography is useful in defining the vascular anatomy of the hand and calculating the degree of peripheral ischemia. In the investigation of upper extremity ischemia, arteriography must include all arteries from the aortic arch to the hand. The anatomic variability of the upper extremity arteries, especially the palmar arches (superficial and deep), is well known,[4] and incomplete palmar arches play a significant role in ischemic disease and contribute to digital ischemia. In general, the deep palmar arch is formed primarily by the terminal part of the radial artery, and the superficial arch by the ulnar artery. According to the manner in which the contributing arteries join, arches are categorized as complete or incomplete. In a study of 500 hand arteriograms, the deep palmar arch appeared complete in 95.2% of cases.[5] Because the ulnar artery predominates in supplying blood to the hand, the completeness of the superficial palmar arch is the determining factor in hand ischemia. In contrast to the deep arch, the superficial palmar arch exhibits many variations (Fig. 93.3). Six types of complete arch are known; however, a complete superficial palmar arch was seen in only 42.4% of cases.[5]

TABLE 93.2 DIAGNOSIS

LABORATORY STUDIES PERFORMED IN PATIENTS WITH SUSPECTED UPPER EXTREMITY ARTERIAL DISEASE

Erythrocyte sedimentation rate
Rheumatoid factor
Antinuclear antibody
Immunoglobulin electrophoresis
Cryoglobulins
Cold agglutinins
VDRL test
Complement (C3, C4)
Anticardiolipin antibody
Blood cell counts

DIAGNOSIS

The diagnosis of large-artery upper extremity occlusion is usually not difficult, and a careful pulse examination often helps to establish it. In distal arterial lesions causing hand or finger ischemia, the use of noninvasive testing to detect digital artery occlusion helps to distinguish Raynaud's phenomenon from Raynaud's disease. The diagnosis of primary Raynaud's disease should not be made until secondary causes of Raynaud's phenomenon have been eliminated. Furthermore, because the onset of Raynaud's phenomenon may precede other manifestations of underlying systemic disease by many years, the diagnosis of Raynaud's disease is usually not made until 2 years

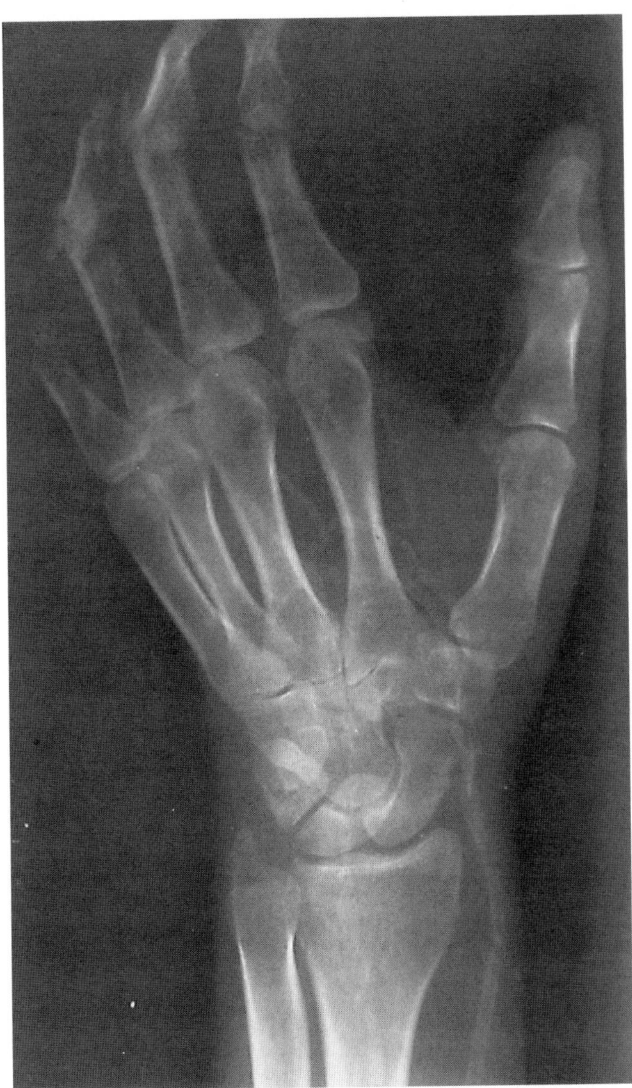

FIGURE 93.1 Typical appearance of azotemic arteriopathy (calciphylaxis) in a diabetic patient with a renal transplant. All the digital arteries are distinctly seen on plain film. The radial artery has a "pipe stem" appearance. An arteriogram shows multiple digital artery occlusions. (From Yao JST. Arterial surgery of the upper extremity. In: Haimovici H, Callow AD, DePalma RG, et al., eds. *Vascular Surgery: Principles and Techniques*, 3rd ed. Norwalk, CT: Appleton & Lange, 1989:863, with permission.)

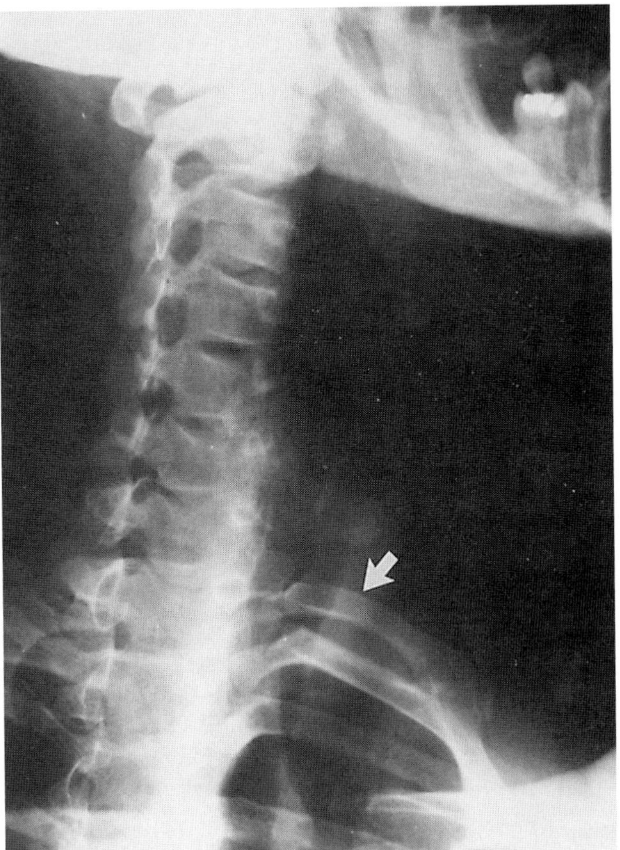

FIGURE 93.2 Cervical rib (*arrow*) in a patient with subclavian aneurysm caused by thoracic outlet compression.

have elapsed with no appearance of systemic disease. If this strict criterion is followed, most patients will be found to have Raynaud's phenomenon (secondary) rather than Raynaud's disease (primary).

PROXIMAL ARTERIAL LESIONS

Atherosclerosis is the most common cause of upper extremity occlusive lesions. The most common site of involvement is the first part of the subclavian artery. The innominate artery is also a common site of disease. Lesions include total occlusion with or without associated steal phenomena, high-grade stenoses, and ulcerating plaques causing distal embolism.

Forms of arteritis producing upper extremity ischemic symptoms include such diverse processes as Takayasu's arteritis, giant cell arteritis, temporal arteritis, and polymyalgia rheumatica. Takayasu's arteritis is a nonspecific inflammatory process of unknown cause that segmentally affects the aorta and its main branches. The disease process can involve the carotid, subclavian, axillary, and pulmonary arteries and is noted most often in young women from 10 to 30 years of age.[6]

The most frequently recognized clinical features of giant cell arteritis (cranial, temporal, and granulomatous arteritis) are related to involvement of the cranial arteries. In temporal arteritis and polymyalgia rheumatica, the subclavian or axillary arteries are common sites of involvement.[7] In addition to upper extremity ischemic symptoms, patients with arteritis often present with fever, malaise, headache, and joint pain. The erythrocyte sedimentation rate is often elevated. The results of some serologic tests can also be positive, but none of the tests are sufficiently sensitive or specific for findings to be considered diagnostic.

Arteriographic examination in patients with upper extremity occlusive symptoms is often diagnostic. The involvement of multiple arteries and a well-developed network of collaterals are characteristic of Takayasu's disease; the pulmonary artery is affected in more than 45% of patients. Characteristic arteriographic findings in giant cell arteritis include long segments of smooth arterial stenosis, alternating with areas of normal or increased caliber, smoothly tapered occlusions, and the absence of irregular plaques and ulcerations (Fig. 93.4).

Thoracic outlet syndrome is by far the most common condition producing upper extremity vascular complications in young adults. Possible sites of compression include the costoclavicular space, formed by the first thoracic rib and clavicle; the interscalene triangle; the angle between the insertion of the pectoralis minor tendon and the coracoid process in the axilla; and the head of the humerus in extreme external rotation. Thoracic outlet compression may be caused by bony anomalies,

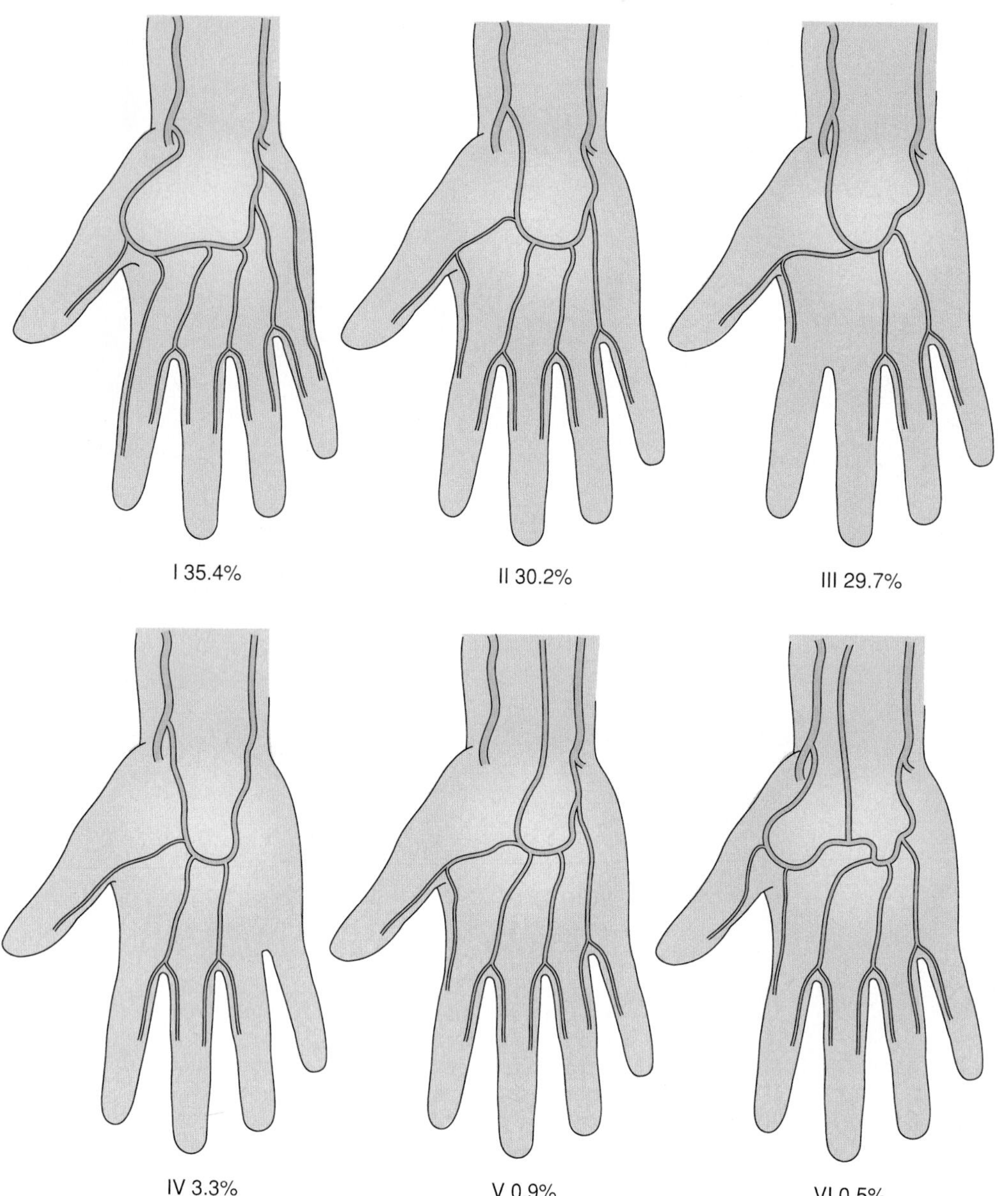

FIGURE 93.3 Different types of complete superficial palmar arch found on 500 hand arteriograms. (From Janevski BK. *Angiography of the Upper Extremity*. Amsterdam: Martinus Nijhoff, 1982, with permission.)

such as a cervical rib or an abnormal first thoracic rib, or it may be secondary to hypertrophy of the anterior scalene muscle. Although a cervical rib is found in 0.5% to 1% of the population, fewer than 10% of such persons have symptoms of neurovascular compression (Fig. 93.5). Arterial complications include aneurysm formation, poststenotic dilation, thrombosis, and distal embolism. The latter can cause digital gangrene or severe hand ischemia. Aneurysm formation is not confined to the subclavian or axillary arteries. It is now recognized that aneurysm formation in both the anterior and, more commonly, the posterior circumflex arteries caused by repetitive athletic activities is responsible for severe hand ischemia resulting from distal embolization.[8] Tethering of the axillary artery between the chest and the loop of circumflex arteries, around the humeral neck, can produce a traction injury resulting in intimal damage with subsequent thrombosis or aneurysm formation. Distal embolization occurs because of retrograde clot extrusion from the side branch aneurysm with persistent excessive activity of the upper extremity. Such injury has been observed in baseball pitchers and volleyball players.[9–11] The circumflex artery is not the only one affected; aneurysm formation in the suprascapular and subscapular arteries has also been reported.[11] Additionally, direct trauma from the head of the humerus can cause compression to the axillary artery with similar sequelae.[9,12] Neurologic symptoms and upper extremity venous thrombotic complications are more common presentations of thoracic outlet syndrome than are arterial complications, but the latter are more threatening to limb and function and are always an urgent indication for arteriography.

DISTAL ARTERIAL LESIONS

Several collagen vascular disorders produce ischemia of the distal upper extremity, including scleroderma, rheumatoid arthritis, systemic lupus erythematosus, polyarteritis nodosa, and dermatomyositis. All cause systemic symptoms and present with upper extremity symptoms ranging from Raynaud's phenomenon to gangrene of the digits. Extensive involvement of the palmar arches or digital arteries is common (Fig. 93.6).

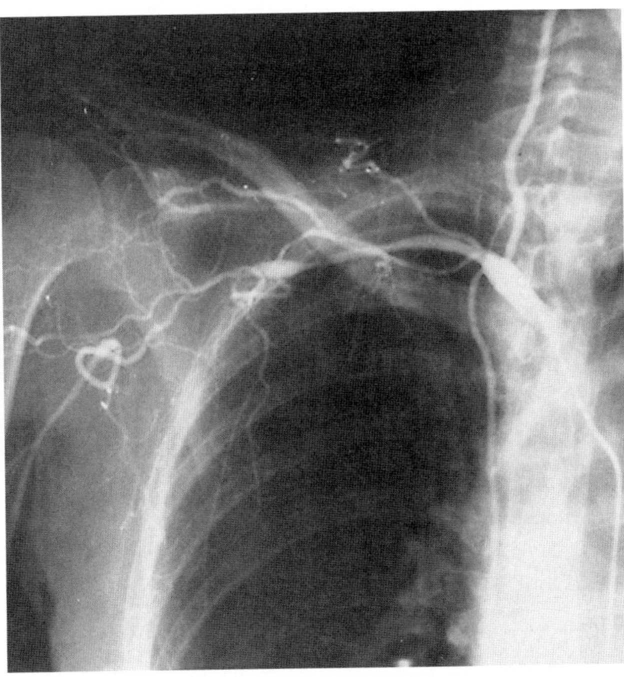

FIGURE 93.4 Characteristic long, segmental narrowing of the subclavian artery in a patient with giant cell arteritis. (From Yao JST. Arterial surgery of the upper extremity. In: Haimovici H, Callow AD, DePalma RG, et al., eds. *Vascular Surgery: Principles and Techniques,* 3rd ed. Norwalk, CT: Appleton & Lange, 1989, p. 858, with permission.)

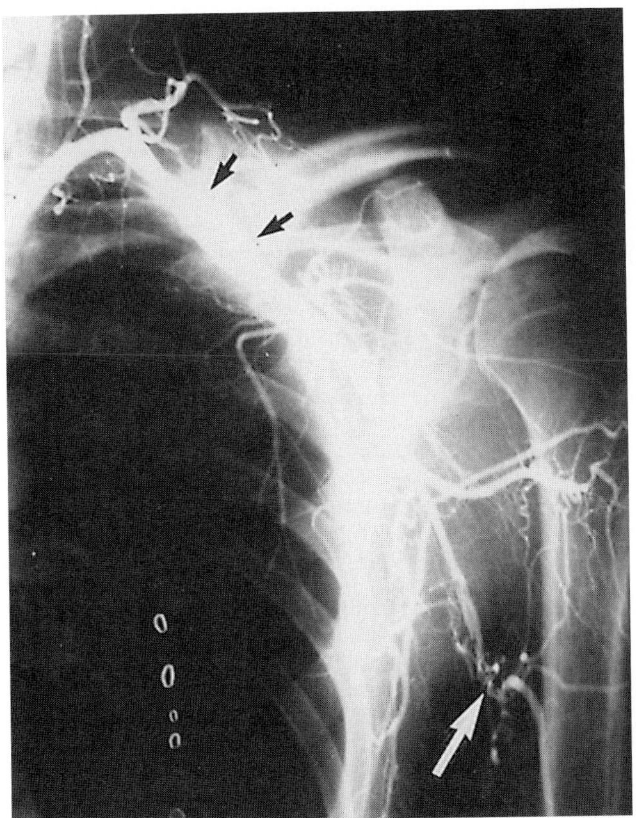

FIGURE 93.5 Arteriogram in a patient with subclavian aneurysm (*black arrows*) caused by a cervical rib. Multiple distal arterial occlusions have developed as a result of embolism (*white arrow*).

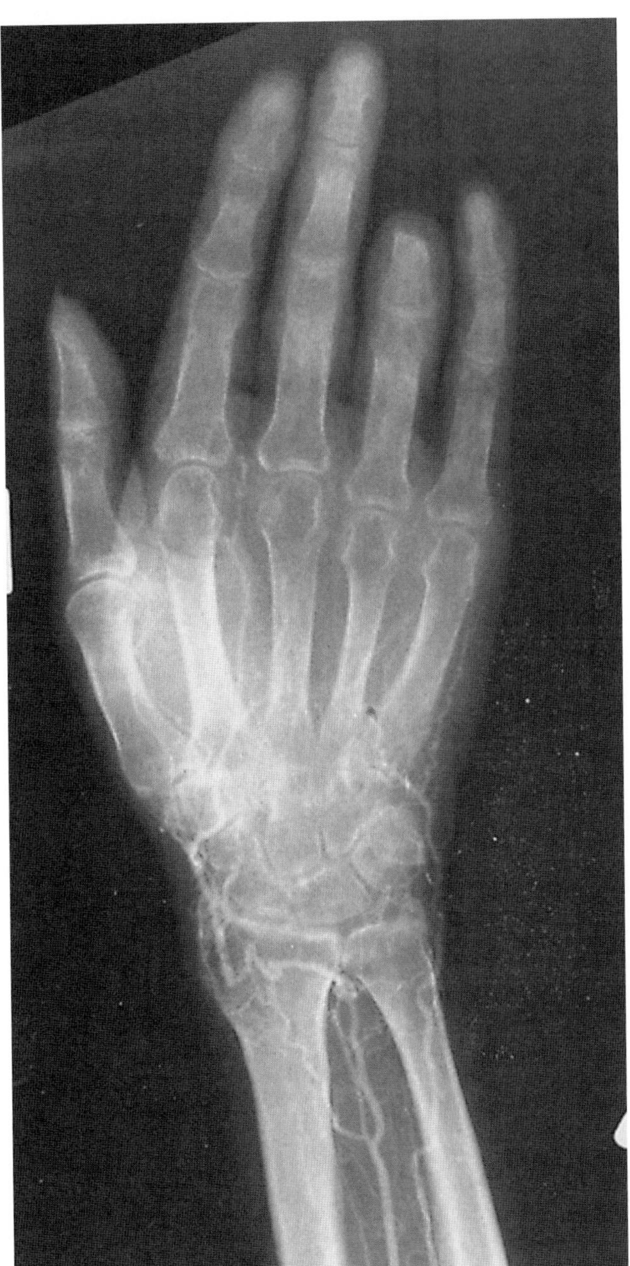

FIGURE 93.6 Arteriogram of a patient with scleroderma and digital gangrene. Extensive small-artery occlusion involves the palmar arch and digital arteries.

Buerger's disease (thromboangiitis obliterans) was first described in 1879, but its existence as a distinct entity is still questionable. It was initially described in male patients of Mediterranean origin who presented with digital gangrene but no occlusion of the larger arteries; however, contemporary practice recognizes that men and women of many ethnic backgrounds can be affected. A persistent characteristic of the disease is a strong association with heavy smoking of a particularly addictive nature. The diagnosis of Buerger's disease is based on histologic evidence of the involvement of both arteries and veins. Venous involvement can be manifested clinically as migrating phlebitis. Characteristic arteriographic findings are occlusion of the small arteries of the digits and the presence of abundant collaterals. The typical corkscrew appearance of the collaterals and lack of the large-vessel plaques characteristic of atherosclerosis are strongly suggestive of Buerger's disease. Like the symptomatic hand, the asymptomatic hand may demonstrate digital artery occlusions.

Polycythemia vera, cryoglobulinemia, and the presence of cold agglutinins are the most common forms of blood dyscrasia associated with occlusion of the arteries of the hand. Occlusion of the small arteries is generally thought to be caused by local thrombosis or embolism. Specific immunologic and blood tests help to establish the diagnosis.

Catheter injuries to the radial and brachial arteries have become more common because of the increasing use of diagnostic and therapeutic procedures involving catheterization. These are especially troublesome when an incomplete palmar arch is not recognized before placement of a catheter in the radial artery. Gangrene or severe ischemia can result from the injury.

Vibration syndrome, characterized by blanching and numbness of the hands after the use of pneumatic drills, is a well-recognized clinical entity causing hand ischemia. The so-called vibratory white finger is a form of occupational trauma. Repetitive trauma to the digital arteries that initially causes spasm, but ultimately causes thrombosis and permanent occlusion, is believed to be the primary factor responsible for ischemic symptoms.

Hypothenar hammer syndrome is another form of occupational trauma, commonly seen in mechanics and carpenters. The mechanism of injury is the repetitive use of the palm of the hand in activities that involve pounding, pushing, or twisting. The anatomic location of the ulnar artery at the area of hypothenar eminence makes it vulnerable to stress. When this area is repeatedly traumatized, ulnar artery occlusion or aneurysm formation can result (Fig. 93.7). Digital artery occlusion is a consequence of embolism from the injured artery.

Calciphylactic arteriopathy (heavily calcified arteries) in patients with diabetes or chronic renal failure can lead to gangrene or severe ischemia of the hand. Azotemic arteriopathy (calciphylaxis) is characterized by calcification of the media of the digital arteries, which produces a "pipe stem" pattern on plain film.5

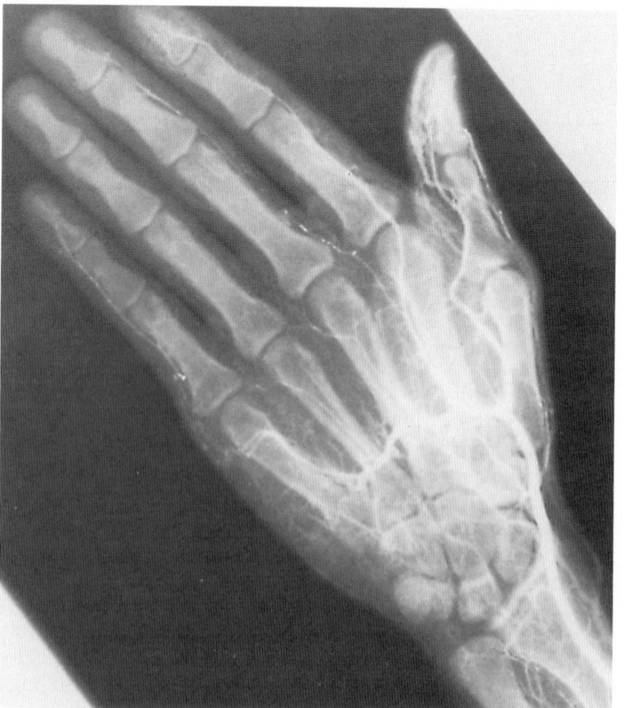

FIGURE 93.7 Occlusion of the ulnar artery over the hamate bone in a patient with hypothenar hammer syndrome.

TREATMENT

The treatment of upper extremity ischemic vascular disorders is directed toward the underlying cause. Stenosis or embologenic lesions of proximal large vessels usually require surgical therapy. The type of reconstructive procedure depends on the nature and location of the lesion. Arterial complications of thoracic outlet obstruction often require a bypass procedure after resection of the subclavian aneurysm and removal of the cervical rib.[13] A bypass graft with autogenous vein (saphenous or cephalic) often relieves occlusion of the brachial artery and its major branches.[14] A short segmental occlusion of either the radial or ulnar artery is best treated by thrombectomy or endarterectomy with a vein patch. An aneurysm in the hand can be resected and continuity restored by end-to-end anastomosis or an interposed vein graft.

The results of bypass grafting in the upper extremity are similar to those of lower extremity revascularization—that is, proximal grafts fare better than distal grafts. In a recent report, the overall 5-year patency was 52.2% in 43 patients.[15] The patency rate for anastomosis proximal to the brachial artery bifurcation was better than that for more distal placement (61.9% vs. 34.8%). Major amputation is not often required, even after graft occlusion, as it is in lower extremity surgery.

Steroid therapy may be needed if arteritis is causing systemic symptoms. Iatrogenic drug-induced ischemia must be treated by cessation of the drug. Dramatic improvement can occur in patients with ergot poisoning.

Distal lesions with occlusion at or distal to the palmar arch are unlikely to be amenable to direct surgical treatment. In these patients, conservative treatment with the use of a calcium blocker (e.g., nifedipine) may reduce the severity and frequency of attacks. A host of medications have been recommended.[16] None, however, has proved consistently effective.

In all patients with upper extremity ischemia of any cause, smoking cessation is an important step. Many of the constituents of tobacco smoke cause adverse vascular effects, particularly vasoconstriction, and this effect seems especially prominent in the upper extremity. Likewise, general protective measures, such as avoiding exposure to cold temperatures and mechanical trauma, have beneficial effects when scrupulously applied.

KEY POINTS

- **Presenting symptoms of upper extremity occlusive disease include evidence of arterial emboli, Raynaud's phenomenon, pain, and exercise-related forearm fatigue.**
- **Physical examination should include the thoracic outlet and the entire upper extremity.**
- **Several noninvasive tests, including plethysmography, transcutaneous Doppler examination, and duplex scan, are available for the objective evaluation of patients with upper extremity ischemia.**
- **In severe bilateral hand ischemia, a systemic cause of the arterial lesions should be sought.**
- **Atherosclerosis is the most common cause of upper extremity occlusive lesions.**
- **Thoracic outlet syndrome is by far the most common condition producing upper extremity vascular complications in young adults.**

References

1. Sumner DS. Noninvasive assessment of upper extremity ischemia. In: Bergan JJ, Yao JST, eds. *Evaluation and treatment of upper and lower extremity circulatory disorders*. Orlando, FL: Grune & Stratton, 1984, pp. 75–95.
2. Erlandson EE, Forrest ME, Shields JJ, et al. Discriminant arteriographic criteria in the management of forearm and hand ischemia. *Surgery* 1981;90:1025–1036.
3. Levine JS, Branch DW, Rauch J. The antiphospholipid syndrome. *N Engl J Med*. 2002;346:752–763.
4. **Coleman SS, Ansun BJ. Arterial patterns in the hand based upon a study of 650 specimens. *Surg Gynecol Obstet*. 1961;113:409–424.**
5. Janevski BK. *Angiography of the Upper Extremity*. Amsterdam: Martinus Nijhoff, 1982.
6. Mishima Y. Leriche Memorial Lecture at 24th World Congress: Takayasu's arteritis in Asia. *Cardiovasc Surg*. 2001;9:3–10.
7. **Weyand CM, Goronzy JJ. Medium- and large-vessel vasculitis. *N Engl J Med*. 2003;349:160–169.**
8. **McCarthy WJ, Yao JST, Schafer MF, et al. Upper extremity arterial injury in athletes. *J Vasc Surg*. 1989;9:317–327.**
9. Rohrer MJ, Cardullo PA, Pappas AM, et al. Axillary artery compression and thrombosis in throwing athletes. *J Vasc Surg*. 1990;11:761–768.
10. Reekers JA, den Hartog BMG, Kuyper CF, et al. Traumatic aneurysm of the posterior circumflex humeral artery: A volleyball player's disease? *J Vasc Interv Radiol*. 1993;4:405–408.
11. Kee ST, Dake MD, Wolfe-Johnson B, et al. Ischemia of the throwing hand in major league baseball pitchers: embolic occlusion from aneurysms of axillary artery branches. *J Vasc Interv Radiol*. 1995;6:979–982.
12. **Durham JR, Yao JST, Pearce WH, et al. Arterial injuries in the thoracic outlet syndrome. *J Vasc Surg*. 1995;21:57–70.**
13. **Yao JST, Flinn WR, McCarthy WJ, et al. Upper extremity revascularization. In: Bergan JJ, Yao JST, eds. *Techniques in arterial surgery*. Philadelphia: WB Saunders, 1990. pp. 328–338.**
14. **McCarthy WJ, Flinn WR, Yao JST, et al. Result of bypass grafting for upper limb ischemia. *J Vasc Surg*. 1986;3:741–746.**
15. Mesh CL, Yao JST. Upper extremity bypass: five-year follow-up. In: Yao JST, Pearce WH, eds. *Long-term results in vascular surgery*. Norwalk, CT: Appleton & Lange, 1993, pp. 353–365.
16. Bowling JCR, Dowd PM. Raynaud's disease. *Lancet* 2003;361:2078–2080.

CHAPTER 94 ■ SPLANCHNIC VASCULAR OCCLUSIVE AND ANEURYSMAL DISEASE

GERALD B. ZELENOCK AND JAMES C. STANLEY

Occlusive and aneurysmal diseases of the splanchnic vessels are relatively uncommon problems in clinical practice. However, it is important that physicians recognize the clinical presentations of these diseases and be knowledgeable regarding contemporary diagnostic studies and newer treatment options. For example, a past classic diagnostic study of choice, aortography with selective visceral arteriography, is being replaced with fast (32-slice) and ultrafast (64-slice) computed tomographic angiography (CTA) or high-quality magnetic resonance angiography. In addition, endovascular techniques are displacing conventional open surgical treatment modalities for patients with these diseases.

The complex functions of the splanchnic viscera are subserved by a circulation uniquely adapted for absorbing and distributing nutrients. Persistence or regression of parts of the primitive visceral circulation result in important variations in the splanchnic arteries and their collateral circulation. Thus, a common celiacomesenteric trunk, replaced hepatic branches from the celiac artery to the superior mesenteric artery (SMA), or a persistent ventral anastomosis producing an arch of Bühler are anatomic variations that are relevant in assessing both occlusive and aneurysmal diseases of the splanchnic circulation.

The vascular anatomy of the splanchnic viscera follows well-described patterns[1] (Figs. 94.1 to 94.4); however, the right hepatic artery has a replaced origin from the SMA in approximately 15% to 20% of the population and the left hepatic artery is derived from the left gastric artery in about 25% of the population. In the event of occlusion or stenosis of either the celiac artery or SMA, the gastroduodenal artery becomes an important collateral vessel.

The SMA originates from the anterior surface of the aorta 1 or 2 cm below the celiac trunk. Extensive large-vessel anastomotic arcades occur among the 10 to 20 jejunal and ileal SMA branches. In addition, a well-defined anastomosis exists between the middle and left colic branches of the SMA and inferior mesenteric artery in the region of the splenic flexure. The inferior mesenteric artery arises 5 to 6 cm below the SMA, typically supplying the left half of the transverse colon and the entire descending colon through the left colic artery. The inferior mesenteric artery gives off a variable number of sigmoid branches and terminates as the paired superior hemorrhoidal arteries. The marginal artery of Drummond and the arch of Riolan are discrete branch vessels capable of significant enlargement, as important collateral vessels, in the face of occlusion or stenosis of the proximal splanchnic arteries.

The venous anatomy of the gastrointestinal tract tends to parallel the arterial blood supply and drains into the portal venous system perfusing the liver. The anastomosis of the splenic vein with the superior mesenteric vein forms the portal vein. Hepatic venous blood is drained by right, middle, and left hepatic veins, which enter the vena cava. Portal-systemic anastomoses are common and are of considerable importance in the presence of portal hypertension.

Intestinal blood flow in humans has been estimated to be between 500 and 1,200 mL/min, or about 10% to 20% of the cardiac output. Duplex arterial scanning, combining Doppler blood flow velocity determinations with B-mode ultrasonography, allows precise measurement of cross-sectional areas and enables calculation of volumetric flows (Fig. 94.5). Baseline intestinal blood flow and the response to standard meals have been established, with significant increases in SMA blood flow 20 to 30 minutes after the ingestion of food that persist for up to 90 minutes. Changes in celiac artery blood flow occur with all meal types; however, these changes are not significant.

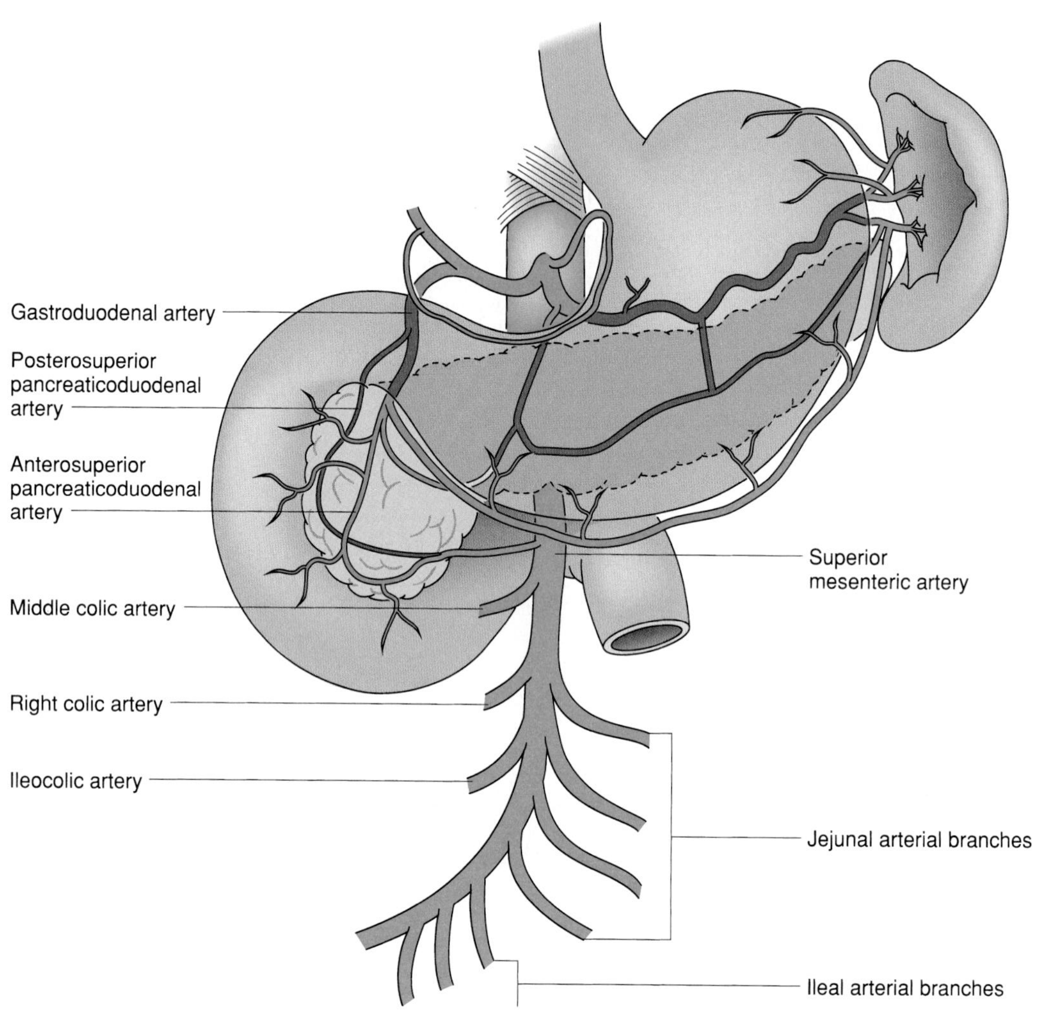

FIGURE 94.1 The celiac artery distributes blood to the stomach, duodenum, pancreas, liver, and spleen; in addition, the gastroduodenal artery and pancreaticoduodenal arcades provide important collateral flow between the celiac and superior mesenteric arteries. The superior mesenteric artery is retropancreatic but crosses anteriorly to the fourth portion of the duodenum. It supplies blood to the duodenum and head of the pancreas, jejunum, ileum, ascending colon, and right half of the transverse colon (see Fig. 94.2). Large anastomotic arcades course between the jejunal and ileal branches.

The intestinal mucosa represents 50% of the mass of the intestine, but receives 75% of the resting blood flow. The muscular and serosal layers of the intestine receive the remaining 25%. Control of blood flow in the splanchnic circulation is affected by the sympathetic nervous system and also by metabolic, myogenic, and extrinsic factors. Stimulation of sympathetic nerves increases vascular tone and decreases splanchnic blood flow, where as parasympathetic nerve stimulation appears to have little direct effect on blood flow. Numerous intrinsic hormones, such as secretin, gastrin, cholecystokinin, glucagon, and vasoactive intestinal peptide, in addition to substances such as histamine, serotonin, bradykinin, and the prostaglandins, all have physiologic roles in regulating intestinal blood flow. Other substances such as epinephrine, norepinephrine, and angiotensin, as well as many commonly used pharmaceuticals, also have important effects on the splanchnic circulation (Table 94.1).

The potential for bacterial translocation and toxin absorption add to the complexity of ischemia and reperfusion within the gut. These adverse effects exacerbate local injury and have important systemic effects, including myocardial depression and increased capillary permeability with edema formation and organ dysfunction.[2–6] Loss of mucosal barrier function is clearly present in acute splanchnic ischemia, with three predisposing factors: (a) physical disruption of the mucosa, (b) a change in the normal intestinal microflora (usually resulting from treatment with broad-spectrum antibiotics), and (c) impairment of host immune defenses. The repair of mucosal damage and enhancement of host defenses appear to be facilitated by early enteral feeding, and by specific nutrients, such as glutamine.

The splanchnic ischemic syndromes are most conveniently categorized as acute or chronic. However, the designation of chronic ischemia is perhaps a misnomer because even in this setting, the underlying pathophysiology is characterized by repetitive, near critical ischemic events. Acute splanchnic syndromes include mesenteric arterial embolism, mesenteric arterial thrombosis, nonocclusive mesenteric ischemia, iatrogenic ischemia, and venous thrombosis. Splanchnic ischemia severe enough to cause intestinal infarction is three times as lethal as myocardial infarction and five times as lethal as a stroke. Chronic splanchnic ischemic syndromes include arteriosclerotic mesenteric occlusive disease and the median arcuate ligament syndrome.

ACUTE SPLANCHNIC ISCHEMIA

Mesenteric Arterial Embolism

Approximately half of acute mesenteric ischemia cases are caused by an embolus, typically from a cardiac source. Atrial fibrillation and myocardial infarction with mural thrombus formation are the most common embolic sources; however, any arrhythmia or anatomic cardiac defect may result in a mesenteric embolus. Embolism of an intracardiac tumor, such

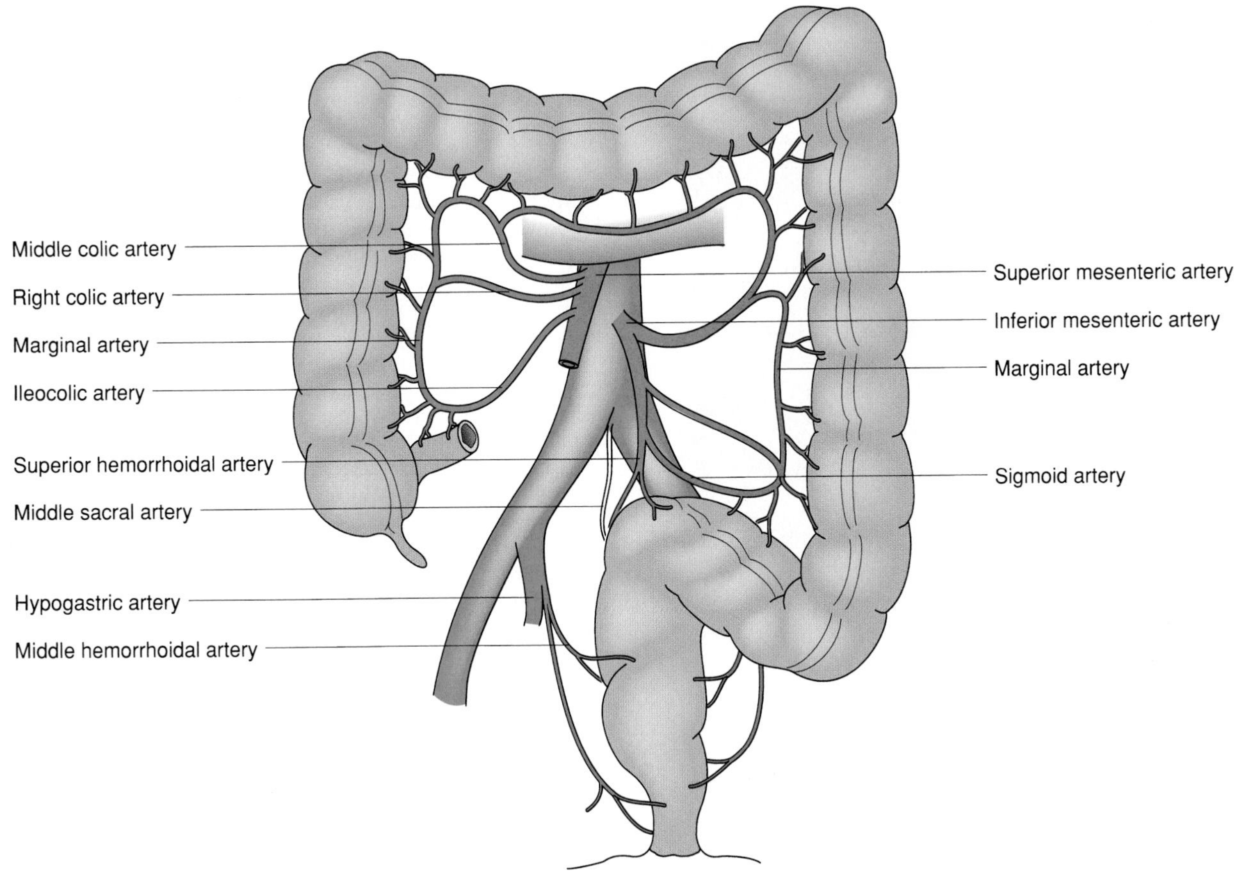

FIGURE 94.2 The inferior mesenteric artery (IMA) supplies blood to the left half of the transverse colon and the entire descending colon, including the sigmoid colon and rectum (via sigmoid and superior hemorrhoidal branches). The left branch of the middle colic artery, from the superior mesenteric artery, and the ascending portion of the left colic artery, from IMA, form a collateral network in the region of the splenic flexure. The IMA serves as an important source of collateral blood supply when the proximal two visceral vessels are occluded.

as an atrial myxoma or a paradoxic embolus, is a rare causes of mesenteric ischemia.

Acute mesenteric embolism usually results in sudden and severe epigastric or midabdominal pain, followed promptly by evacuation of the gut, with emeses or explosive diarrhea. The patient can often precisely pinpoint the onset of pain, and fully 25% of patients have had previous embolic events. The underlying cardiac disorder, as a source of the embolus, may be evident with an irregularly irregular rhythm indicating atrial fibrillation, the classic murmur of mitral stenosis, or an enlarged heart. The abdominal examination may be normal initially, with signs of an acute abdomen evolving later. Slight to moderate abdominal distension is common. Bowel sounds are highly variable, and not useful as a diagnostic finding. The classic presentation of acute mesenteric ischemia is severe abdominal pain that is out of proportion to minimal or absent physical findings. Peritoneal signs or blood in the stool are late and ominous signs, implying intestinal infarction.

No laboratory tests are pathognomonic of acute mesenteric ischemia. Standard hematologic and biochemical studies are unrewarding early in the clinical course.[7] Later, hemoconcentration, acidosis, leukocytosis, and elevated serum phosphorus or transaminases may be evident, yet none of these abnormalities need be present, even with a major mesenteric embolus. The diagnosis usually depends on clinical suspicion followed by characteristic anatomic findings demonstrated by angiography, computed tomography (CT) scan, or occasionally by ultrasound. Embolic lodging in the SMA is often just past the inferior pancreaticoduodenal and middle colic arteries, thus isolating the small bowel from its major collateral circulation (Fig. 94.6).

In the case of a suspected diagnosis, the patient should be anticoagulated with heparin, volume-resuscitated, and taken to the operating room for an emergent embolectomy. Prophylactic antibiotics and full hemodynamic monitoring are mandatory. The SMA is exposed beneath the transverse mesocolon, proximal and distal control are obtained, and a Fogarty catheter embolectomy through either a transverse or longitudinal arteriotomy is performed. Patch closure of the SMA is used if the artery is small or a longitudinal incision has been made. Intestinal viability is assessed after restoration of blood flow.

Acute Mesenteric Thrombosis

A less common cause of acute splanchnic ischemia follows thrombosis of an underlying diseased SMA. The presentation is that of an acute intestinal catastrophe less abrupt than seen with an SMA embolus, with eventual development of severe midabdominal pain. These symptoms may occur *de novo* or be superimposed on a background of chronic intestinal angina. A history of motility disturbances causing nausea, diarrhea, or constipation are common but of no diagnostic value.

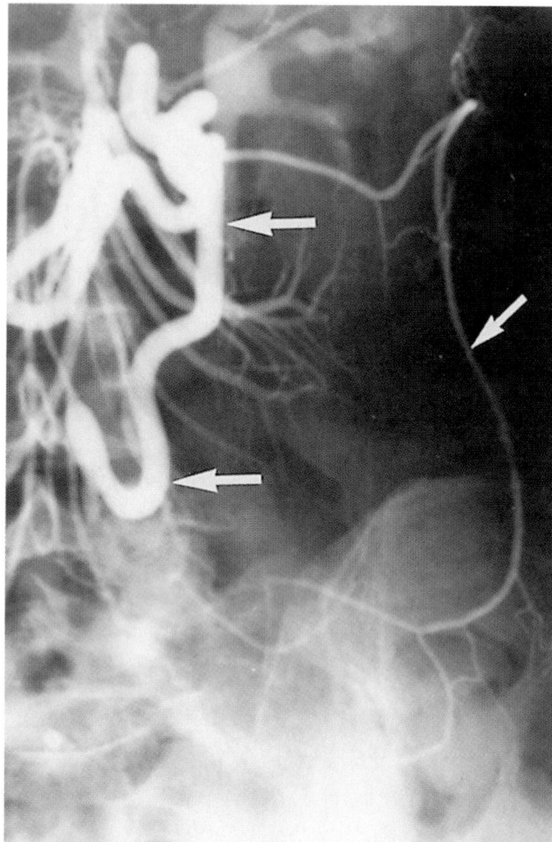

FIGURE 94.3 Selective inferior mesenteric artery angiography demonstrates the marginal artery of Drummond and the larger, more functionally important arc of Riolan, or central anastomotic artery. (From Zelenock GB. Splanchnic arteriosclerotic disease and intestinal angina. *Arch Surg.* 1980;115:497–501.)

Urgent angiography with lateral aortography in addition to standard anteroposterior views, is appropriate to establish a diagnosis of mesenteric thrombosis (Fig. 94.7). The occlusive process is usually more extensive than apparent on angiography. Ultrafast CTA is being used more frequently to recognize mesenteric ischemia and holds considerable promise, yet its sensitivity and specificity remain to be defined.

Reperfusion of the splanchnic circulation is the major priority in these acutely ill patients. Recent weight loss with its attendant nutritional, would-healing, and immunologic compromise, makes any operative procedure hazardous. Reperfusion may be accomplished by infusion of thrombolytic agents, and an angioplasty with stent placement. Used selectively, however, these endovascular interventions have potential benefit, even if an open revascularization were required at a later time. Nevertheless, this approach is not appropriate when peritoneal signs suggest frankly necrotic bowel requiring resection.

Operations for an acute SMA thrombosis must be individualized. Contemporary opinion favors multiple-vessel revascularization and the use of short antegrade conduits whenever possible. Nevertheless, in the acute setting, a variety of alternative surgical techniques, including single-vessel revascularization and the use of retrograde bypasses, have resulted in survival and are appropriate in certain circumstances. In the presence of frankly necrotic bowel requiring resection, autogenous conduits are preferred for these revascularization.

Low-Flow Nonocclusive Mesenteric Ischemia

Nonocclusive mesenteric ischemia remains a problem in contemporary practice.[8,9] Vasoconstriction of the mesenteric blood vessels is common, occurring in response to diminished cardiac output, shock, hypovolemia, dehydration, or the use of vasoactive medications (Table 94.2). This form of intestinal ischemia occurs most often in critically ill patients who are hemodynamically unstable secondary to shock or congestive heart failure. Gastrointestinal mucosal sloughing and bleeding may be present. A diagnosis in these instances may be established with angiography (Fig. 94.8). The focus of intervention is on pharmacologic support of the circulation with relief of splanchnic vasoconstriction. Treatments include optimizing hemodynamic and volume status, correcting contributing medical conditions, and when possible eliminating adverse pharmacologic agents. Selective intraarterial infusion of vasodilators is appropriate,[10] including intraarterial papaverine (30 to 60 mg/h) and intravenous glucagon (2 to 4 mg/h), which selectively increases splanchnic blood flow, have been advocated in treating this form of intestinal ischemia.[11]

Iatrogenic Acute Splanchnic Ischemia

An increasingly common cause of acute ischemia is complications of certain catheter-related procedures and operations. Diagnostic or therapeutic angiography may cause iatrogenic splanchnic ischemia as a consequence of an arterial dissection or embolization,

Aortic aneurysm resection is the prototypic surgical procedure associated with iatrogenic intestinal ischemia.[12] Its potential for compromising colonic and small bowel circulation is underappreciated. Intestinal ischemia is more common with ruptured aneurysms, when occlusive and aneurysmal disease coexist, and when important collateral vessels are compromised by the aortic procedure itself (Fig. 94.9). After an aortic aneurysm repair, colonic ischemia is clinically apparent in 1% to 2% of cases and has been detected endoscopically in 6% to 8% of cases. These patients often present with diarrhea, and the stool is usually grossly bloody or guaiac-positive. When such occurs, immediate colonoscopy is indicated. If the ischemia is confined to the mucosa and submucosa and subsequently heals, a stricture may form (Fig. 94.10). If the ischemia is more profound and transmural infarction occurs, resection is required, and the mortality rate approaches 60%.

Other Types of Acute Splanchnic Ischemia

Ischemia of the intestines may also accompany aortic dissections, traumatic injuries, or the inflammatory arteritides. The clinical presentation and diagnosis depends on the underlying cause, with superimposed symptoms of abdominal distension, an acute abdomen, or gastrointestinal bleeding.[13,14] Treatment must be highly individualized. In the setting of acute aortic dissection, branch revascularization or fenestration is essential. Traumatic injuries also require urgent surgical intervention. Inflammatory arteritides require treatment of the underlying medical condition, with operation reserved only for resection of clearly nonviable bowel. Intraoperative recognition of intestinal viability, the appropriate limits to resection, and consideration of a "second-look" procedure are critical.[15–17] Clinical parameters of color, spontaneous peristalsis, and

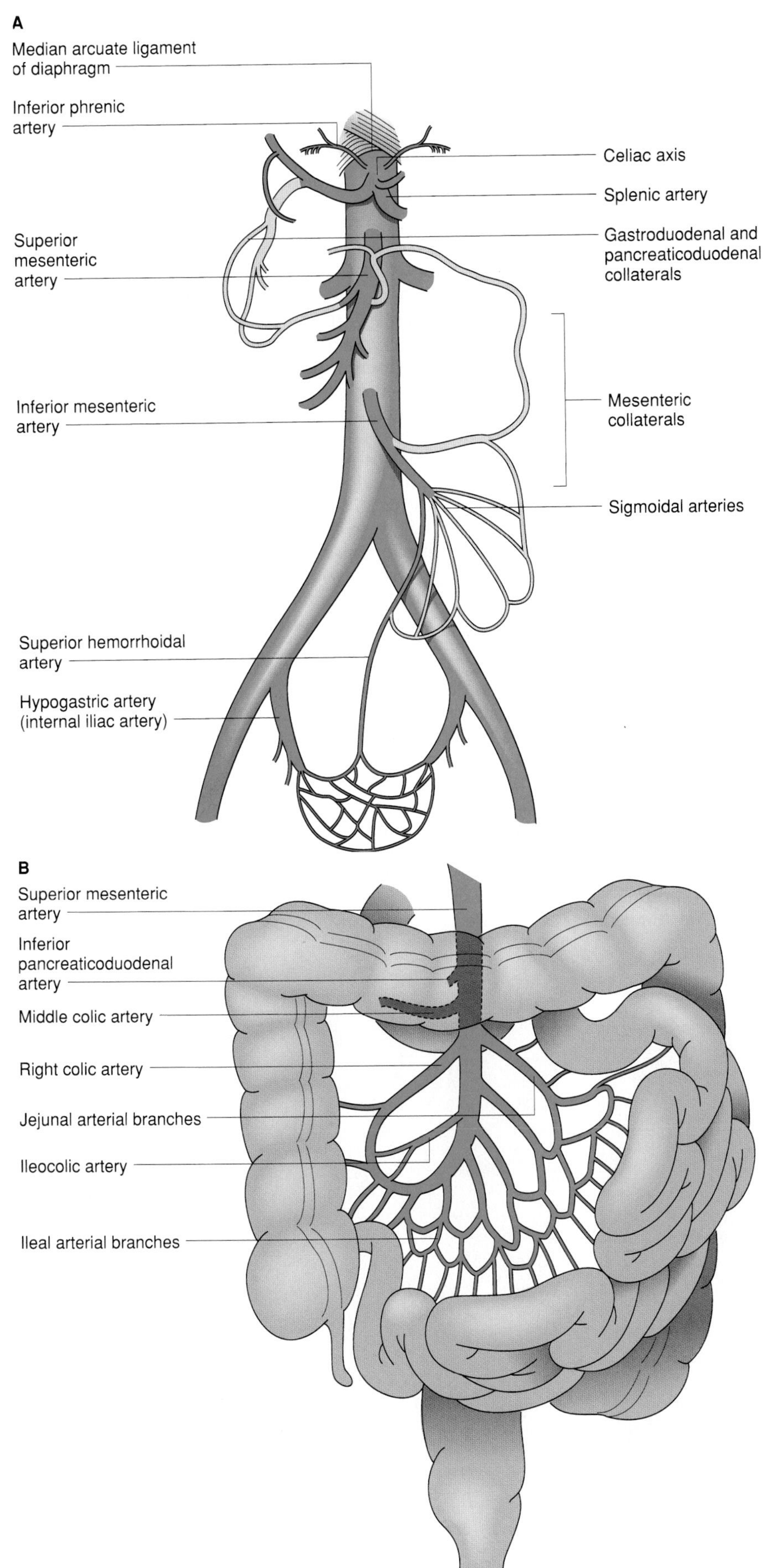

FIGURE 94.4 (*A*) The collateral circulation to the intestine occurs at several levels. Well- recognized visceral-visceral and visceral-parietal collateral branches and anastomoses are important. The unnamed intestinal arcades (*B*) and the intramural anastomoses.

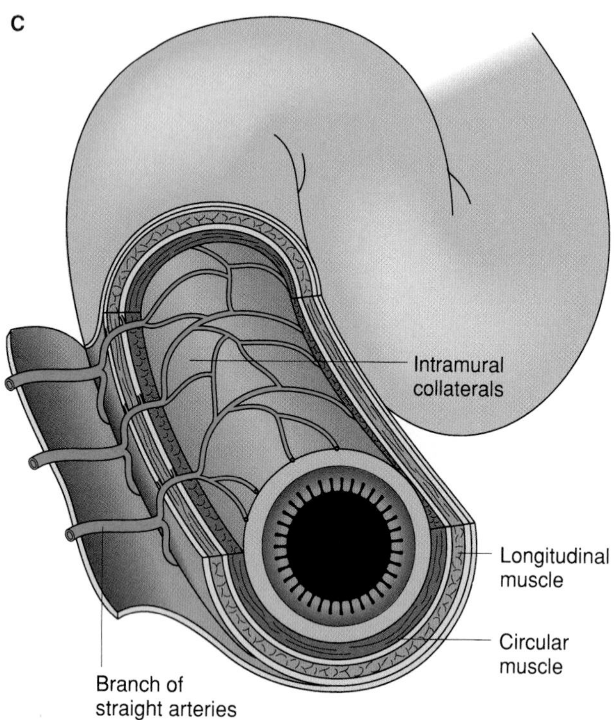

FIGURE 94.4 (*Continued*) (C) are effective short-segment collaterals.

palpable pulses are not sensitive or specific enough to provide a basis for precise and confident clinical decisions. The most common adjunctive technique to determine the extent of necessary bowel resection is Doppler ultrasonography. Fluorescein dye or Wood's lamp analyses are also frequently used to assess bowel viability.

If large segments of ischemic small bowel are resected, the potential exists for the development of short-gut syndrome, in which insufficient intestine remains for adequate nutrient absorption. Contemporary clinical practice is to not resect marginally viable intestine and resect only unequivocally necrotic tissue at the initial operation. A planned "second-look" surgical procedure 24 to 48 hours later, is undertaken to evaluate the status of the remaining intestine.

Mesenteric Venous Thrombosis

Thrombosis of mesenteric veins is most often subacute in its presentation. A vague prodrome of crampy abdominal pain, abdominal distention, nausea, and malaise may occur for a few days to several weeks before the disease is recognized. However, in the presence of widespread and major venous occlusions, the presentation can be acute and catastrophic. Mesenteric venous thrombosis may be secondary to an associated condition, including: an intraabdominal inflammatory process, peritonitis, portal hypertension, a hypercoagulable state, and the use of oral contraceptives. Plain films often reveal bowel wall edema. The venous phase of a selective mesenteric arteriogram may reveal the thrombus, and CT studies often demonstrate thrombus within the portal and superior mesenteric veins. In many instances, the diagnosis is made intraoperatively, with the presence of bloody ascites, dusky-appearing intestine that is thick and rubbery. The small mesenteric veins are often cordlike and exude clot when cut. Surgical therapy consists of resection of nonviable intestine, occasional large-vessel venous thrombectomy, and administration of anticoagulants. Correction of any predisposing hypercoagulable state is mandatory, such as deficiency of antithrombin III and proteins C and S, as well as the presence of factor V Leiden, anticardiolipin antibodies (the lupus anticoagulant). In cases of primary mesenteric venous thrombosis, postoperative anticoagulant therapy is continued indefinitely, because if untreated venous thrombosis recurs in 30% to 40% of patients. Anticoagulation reduces the incidence of recurrence to 3% to 5%. In cases secondary to a treatable cause, such as peritonitis, relatively short-term anticoagulation is recommended, similar to that used when treating venous thrombosis.

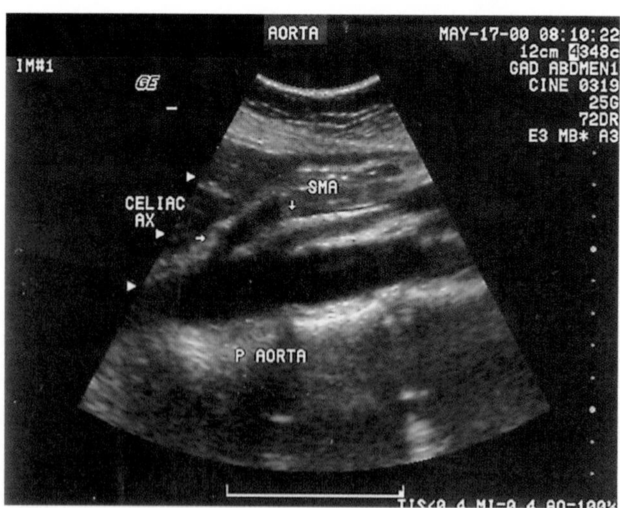

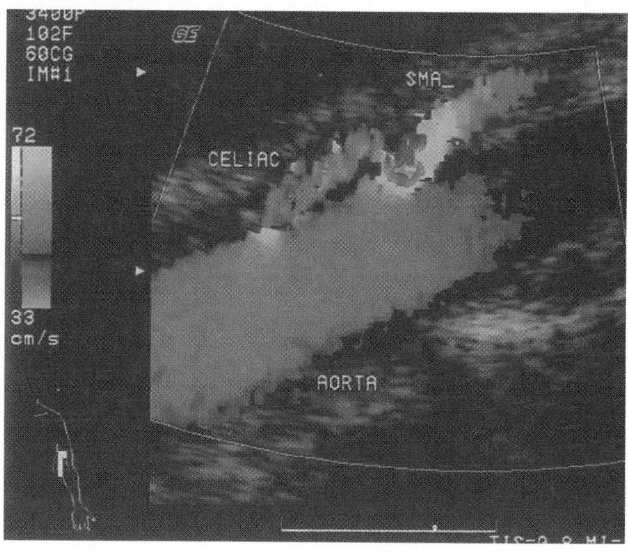

FIGURE 94.5 (*A*) Duplex scan of the aorta and celiac and superior mesenteric arteries. Vessel diameter, flow velocity, calculated volumetric blood flow, spectral analysis, and the response to physiologic stimuli allow a precise assessment of the visceral circulation. (*B*) Color-flow Doppler scanning allows rapid identification of flow disturbances. (Courtesy of Dr. Phillip Bendick, William Beaumont Hospital, Royal Oak, MI.)

TABLE 94.1

DUPLEX MEASUREMENT OF INTESTINAL BLOOD FLOW

Vessel	Average diameter (range)	Characteristics on duplex scan	Calculated fasting volume flow (mL/min)	Calculated volume flow change from fasting by type of meal[a] (%)					
				Mixed	Cholesterol	Fat	Protein	Mannitol	Water
Celiac artery	0.66 cm (0.4–0.8 cm)	Continuous forward flow; no reverse flow: end-diastolic velocity about one-third peak systolic velocity No significant changes with meals	1,083 ± 75	18 ± 4	1±4	10 ± 8	21 ± 6	37± 19	14± 5
Superior mesenteric artery	0.59 cm (0.44–0.68 cm)	Early diastolic flow reversal; forward diastolic flow; end-diastolic velocity about zero After eating, loss of reverse flow and increased peak systolic and end-diastolic velocities noted	538 ± 37	164± 30	118 ± 23	117± 25	78 ± 15	48± 11	24± 8

[a]Calculated volume flow changes that occurred after meals were not significantly increased in the celiac artery but were significantly increased with all meals except water in the superior mesenteric artery.

From Moneta GL, Taylor DC, Heiton WS, et al. Duplex ultrasound measurement of postprandial intestinal blood flow: effect of meal composition. *Gastroenterology* 1988;95:1294.

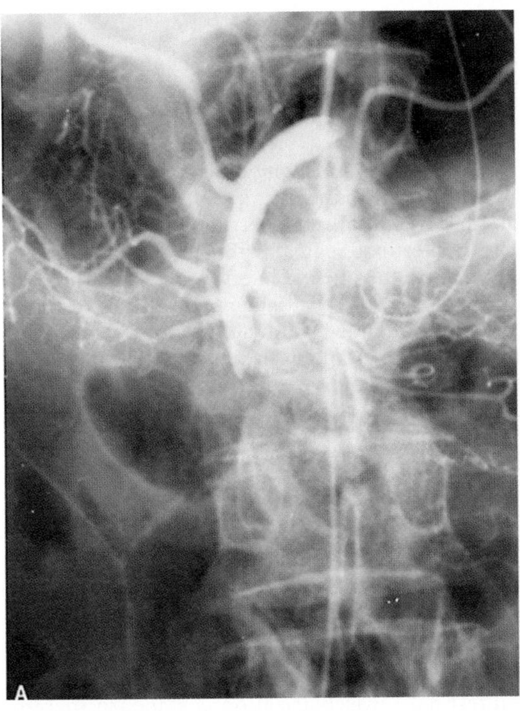

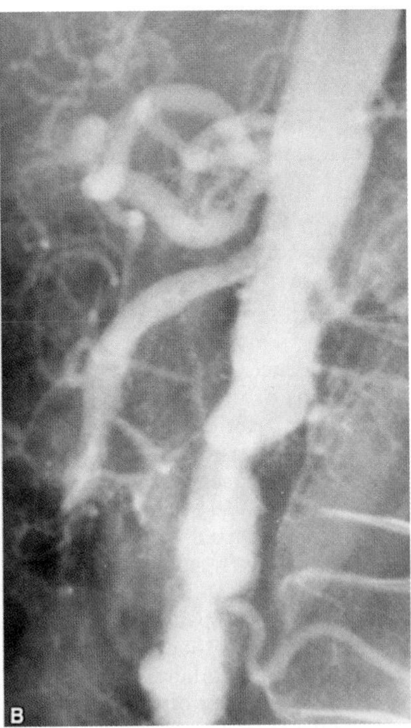

FIGURE 94.6 (*A*) Anteroposterior view of a typical superior mesenteric artery (SMA) embolus lodged distal to the origin of the middle colic artery and first jejunal branches of the SMA. The pattern of injury typically spares the first few inches of the jejunum and the colon distal to the min-transverse portion. (*B*) Lateral aortogram demonstrates embolus with sparing of proximal SMA. This pattern is distinct from SMA thrombosis.

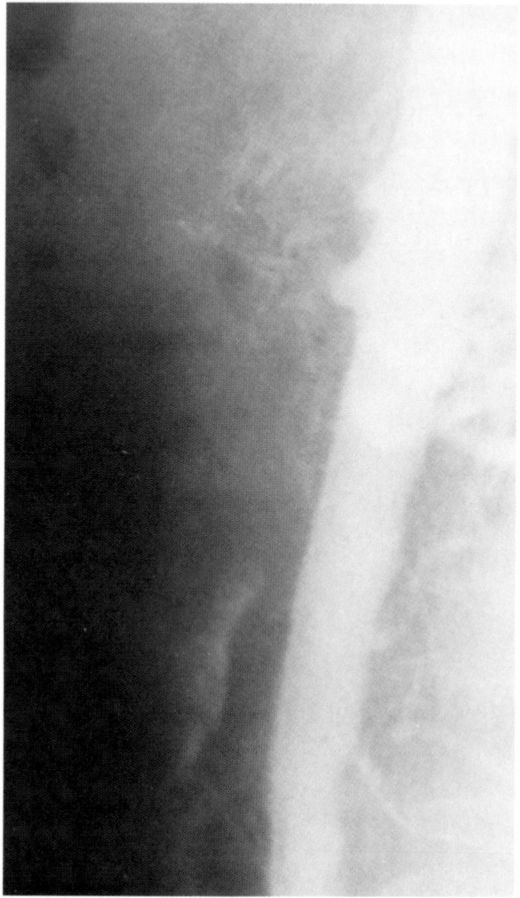

FIGURE 94.7 Lateral aortogram demonstrating acute celiac and superior mesenteric artery thrombosis, which results in widespread necrosis of the abdominal viscera.

TABLE 94.2

EFFECTS OF VARIOUS SUBSTANCES ON MESENTERIC CIRCULATION AND MOTOR ACTIVITY

Substance	Intestinal blood flow	Intestinal O_2 uptake	Intestinal motility
Acetylcholine	Increase	Increase	Increase
Adenosine	Increase	Variable	—
Angiotensin II	Decrease	—	Increase
Bradykinin	Variable	—	Increase
Ca^{2+}, high levels	Decrease	—	Increase
Ca^{2+} antagonists	Increase	—	Decrease
Dopamine	Variable	Decrease	—
Epinephrine	Variable	Variable	—
Gastrin	Increase	Increase	Increase
Glucagon	Increase	Increase	Decrease
Histamine	Increase	Increase	Increase
Isoproterenol	Increase	Variable	—
K^+ high levels	Decrease	—	Increase
Mg^{2+}	Increase	—	—
Nitroprusside	Increase	—	—
Norepinephrine	Decrease	Decrease	—
Papaverine	Increase	No change	—
PGE_1	Increase	Increase	—
PGF_{2a}	Decrease	Variable	Increase
PGI_2	Increase	—	—
Secretin	Variable	No change	—
Serotonin	Variable	Variable	Variable
Somatostatin	Decrease	—	Decrease
Vasopressin	Decrease	Decrease	Variable
Vasoactive intestinal polypeptide	Increase	Increase	—

PG, prostaglandin.
From Wakefield TW, Stanley JC. The intestine. In: Zelenock GB, D'Alecy LG, Schlafer M, et al., eds. *Clinical ischemic syndromes: mechanisms and consequences of tissue injury*, St. Louis: Mosby, 1990.

CHRONIC SPLANCHNIC ISCHEMIA

Chronic Arteriosclerotic Splanchnic Ischemia

Intestinal angina is most often a consequence of aortic spillover arteriosclerosis affecting the origins of the celiac, superior mesenteric, and inferior mesenteric arteries. The responsible anatomic lesions invariably involve at least two of these three arteries (Fig. 94.11). The occlusive process may also be widespread throughout the mesenteric arcades, especially in diabetics. The patient is either typically affected with generalized clinical overt arteriosclerosis or a relatively young woman with an extensive cigarette-smoking habit.

These patients develop "food fear" and modify their pattern of eating so that they only consume small quantities of food at any one time. Intestinal angina may manifest as periumbilical discomfort, developing 15 to 30 minutes after eating and often lasting 1 to 4 hours. Patients with chronic splanchnic ischemia almost always have a profound weight loss, which raises the specter of an intraabdominal malignancy. Many times, gastrointestinal contrast studies, endoscopy, various scans, and nonproductive exploratory laparotomies have been undertaken before a diagnosis of intestinal ischemia is considered.

The progression from minor symptoms to intestinal infarction is unpredictable. Frequently, patients with intestinal infarction are discovered, in retrospect, to have had preexisting symptoms of intestinal angina. Although delayed recognition is commonplace, therapeutic interventions must proceed expeditiously, in that if intestinal angina progresses to transmural infarction it is attended by an 80% mortality rate.

Duplex scanning, MRA and CT scans support the diagnosis of this form of intestinal vascular disease. Aortography, including both anteroposterior and lateral views, however, has most commonly been used to assess this disease (Fig. 94.12). In some clinical series, 85% of the celiac, superior mesenteric, and inferior mesenteric arteries were totally occluded or severely stenosed.[18] Although often diseased, the inferior mesenteric artery frequently serves as the major remaining source of blood flow to the gut, with an occluded celiac artery and SMA. At the very least, duplex scanning of the aorta and visceral vessels should be undertaken in suspected cases. MRA, CTA, or conventional angiography can then be pursued when appropriate.[19–21]

Elective intestinal revascularization is standard therapy in the treatment of arteriosclerotic chronic mesenteric ischemia.[13,22–31] Multiple-vessel revascularization with short, antegrade conduits of either autogenous saphenous vein or prosthetic material are favored (Fig. 94.13). A variety of other bypass techniques have also resulted in long-term relief of

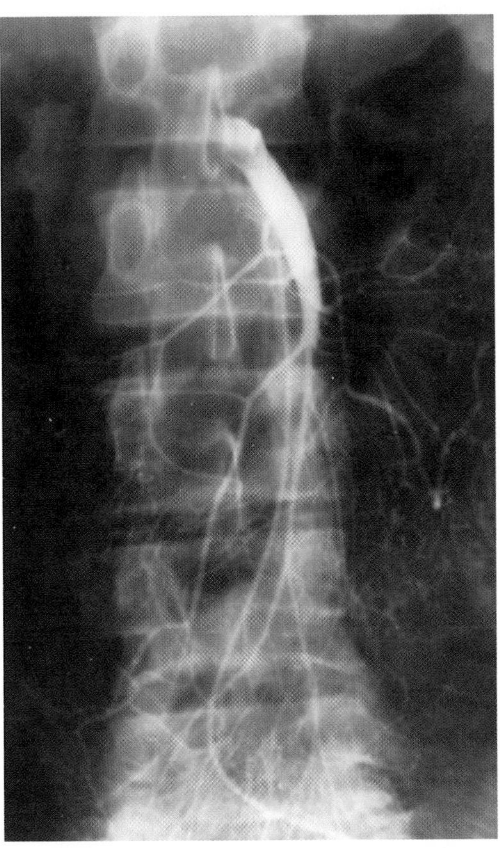

FIGURE 94.8 Low-flow nonocclusive ischemia causes profound vasoconstriction within the mesenteric arcades, which may be sufficient to cause mucosal necrosis or transmural infarction if not relieved.

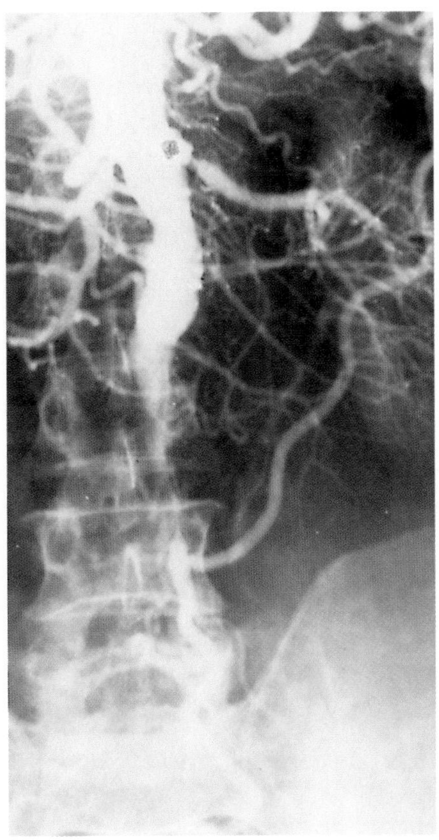

FIGURE 94.9 The multiple causes of iatrogenic visceral ischemia include medications, diagnostic and therapeutic angiographic procedures, and surgical procedures. A common surgical cause is aortic aneurysm resection. Coexistent aneurysmal and occlusive disease, seen in this aortogram, identify a patient at high risk.

symptoms (Fig. 94.14). Endarterectomy through a "trapdoor" aortotomy with a thoracoabdominal exposure (Figs. 94.15 and 94.16), is particularly effective when multiple proximal intestinal arterial stenoses or occlusions, as well as concomitant renal artery lesions, are present. Percutaneous angioplastic procedures with endoluminal stenting are often used, but long-term follow-up and collected series of patients treated in this fashion are still lacking.[32,33]

Median Arcuate Ligament Syndrome

Symptomatic entrapment of the celiac artery by the median arcuate ligament is controversial. Symptoms include postprandial periumbilical abdominal pain, but this symptom may or may not represent intestinal ischemia. Arteriography in these patients reveals a significant compression of the celiac artery by the median arcuate ligament of the diaphragm (Fig. 94.17). Lysis of the overlying median arcuate ligament and surrounding neural tissue affords relief of symptoms in approximately half of these patients, with celiac axis revascularization required, either surgical or endovascular, in an occasional case.

SPLANCHNIC ARTERY ANEURYSMAL DISEASE

Splanchnic artery aneurysms are uncommon, but the more frequent use of CT, magnetic resonance imaging (MRI), and ultrasonography has resulted in an increase in their clinical recognition. These aneurysms are clearly important considering that nearly 22% present as surgical emergencies, including 8.5% that result in the patient's death. The splanchnic vessels involved with these macroaneurysms, in decreasing order of frequency, are the splenic, hepatic, superior mesenteric, celiac, gastric– gastroepiploic, jejunal–ileal–colic, pancreaticoduodenal–pancreatic, and gastroduodenal arteries (Table 94.3). The general clinical manifestations, and management of these aneurysms, including the more widespread use of endovascular interventions have been addressed in a number of recent reviews.[34–43] However, the specifics of each of these splanchnic artery aneurysms deserve individual consideration.

Splenic Artery Aneurysm

Splenic artery aneurysms account for 60% of all splanchnic artery aneurysms. The occurrence of these lesions in the general population is probably similar to the 0.78% incidence in nearly 3600 consecutive patients undergoing abdominal arteriographic studies for reasons other than suspected aneurysmal disease.[44] Women are four times more likely than men to develop splenic artery aneurysms.

The predilection for these aneurysms to affect the splenic artery reflects a peculiar group of associated disorders having an effect on the vasculature. Three distinct factors may contribute to the development of splenic artery aneurysms, including two that account for their unusual female predilection. The first factor is medial fibrodysplasia, which usually occurs in women and is most often manifested by renal artery stenosis and secondary hypertension. Approximately 2% of patients with renal artery fibrodysplasia have splenic artery

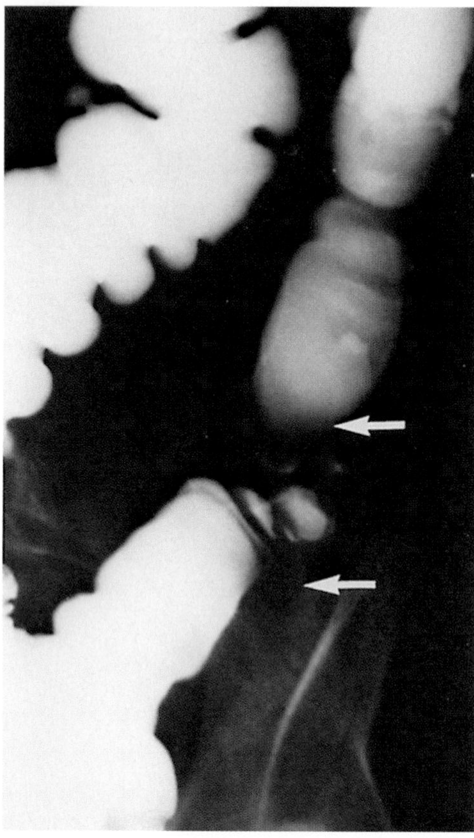

FIGURE 94.10 Stricture formation resulting from sigmoid colon ischemia after repair of a ruptured aortic aneurysm. A loss of haustrations is seen through the descending colon and the fixed narrowing in the midportion of the sigmoid colon (*arrows*).

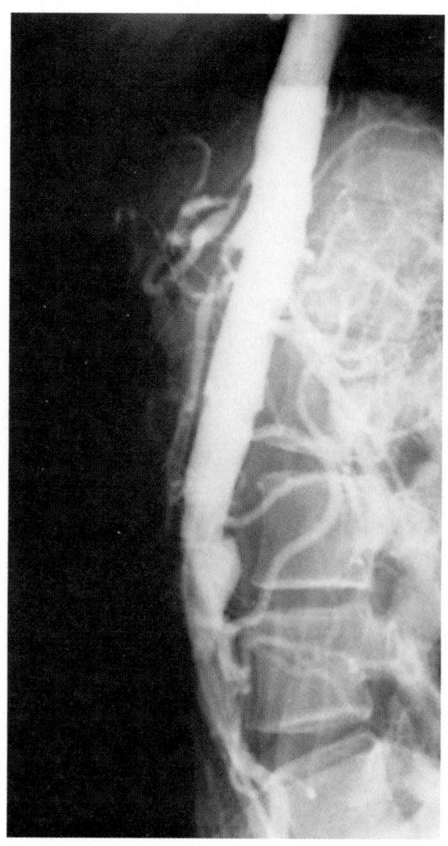

FIGURE 94.11 High-grade stenosis of the celiac and superior mesenteric arteries are apparent in this lateral aortogram. (From Zelenock GB. Splanchnic arteriosclerotic disease and intestinal angina. *Arch Surg*. 1980;115:497–501.)

aneurysms, and all of these patients have been women.[44] Systemic hypertension may contribute to aneurysm expansion in these patients. The second factor relates to the vascular consequences of pregnancy, with its known increase in splenic blood flow and reproductive hormone–related changes in elastic tissue. This factor becomes a particular problem with repeated pregnancies. Approximately 40% of women harboring these lesions have completed six or more pregnancies.[44,45] The third factor is evident in the nearly 10% of patients with portal hypertension and splenomegaly who develop splenic artery aneurysms.[44,46,47] In these cases, the vessel wall integrity may be compromised by increased splenic blood flow[118,49] and excessive estrogen activity occurring as a consequence of the underlying cirrhosis. Although splenic artery aneurysms have been described with regularity among patients after orthotopic liver transplantation,[50–53] it is speculative as to whether these represent preexisting aneurysms associated with portal hypertension or have arisen as a consequence of the transplant and attendant drug therapy, such as steroids.[50] Aneurysms in the latter patients are more likely to affect women, and appear directly related to the severity of the pre-existing portal hypertension.[52] Rare splenic artery aneurysms appear associated with developmental anomalies of the foregut arterial circulation.[54,55]

Certain splenic artery aneurysms exhibit extensive arteriosclerosis (Fig. 94.18). The fact that calcific arteriosclerotic changes appear limited to the aneurysm and not the intervening artery suggests that this is more likely a secondary event, rather than a primary etiologic process (Fig. 94.19). Arterial disruptions caused by periarterial inflammatory disease, such as chronic pancreatitis, or penetrating trauma are less common causes of these aneurysms. Microaneurysms of smaller intraparenchymal splenic arteries are usually caused by a systemic vasculitis, such as polyarteritis nodosa, and appear to be of less clinical importance as a vascular disease than extraparenchymal aneurysms attributed to other causes.

Most aneurysms involving the distal splenic artery are saccular and occur at branchings. At such sites, discontinuities exist in the internal elastic lamina of normal vessels, and any subsequent degenerative events involving elastic tissue, as might occur with arterial fibrodysplasia or pregnancy, are likely to produce aneurysmal changes (Fig. 94.20). Such aneurysms are multiple 20% of the time, in contrast to those in patients undergoing liver transplantation for cirrhosis-related portal hypertension where multiple aneurysms occur in 90% of patients. Proximal aneurysms of the main splenic artery are usually solitary and are frequently associated with arterial erosions by pancreatitis-related pseudocysts (Fig. 94.21).

Vascular calcifications on plain abdominal radiographs may be the first clinical evidence of a splenic artery aneurysm. The most characteristic of these findings are signet-ring calcifications (Fig. 94.22). However, contemporary diagnoses of splenic artery aneurysms usually follow their arteriographic demonstration during studies for nonvascular diseases. Color-flow Doppler ultrasonography, CT, and MRI, often establish the presence of these lesions and are often useful in identifying

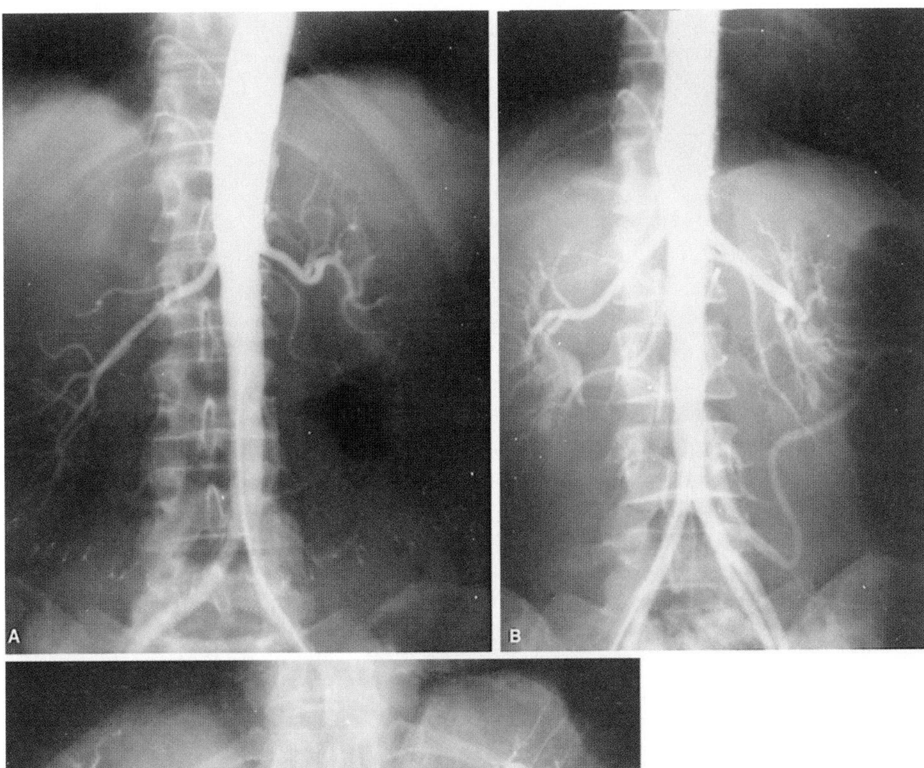

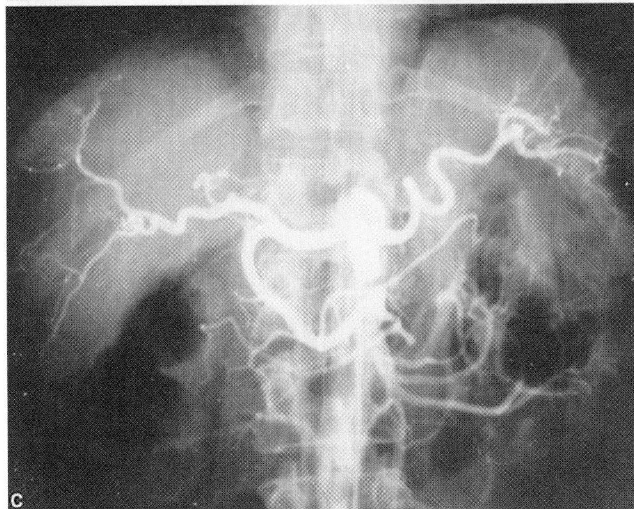

FIGURE 94.12 Chronic visceral ischemia produces visceral angina when multiple occlusions of major splanchnic blood vessels are present. Lack of apparent intestinal blood flow (*A*) and an unusually prominent inferior mesenteric artery (*B*) are angiographic sighs of chronic visceral ischemia. Selective celiac injection (*C*) also fills the superior mesenteric artery distribution secondary to occlusions of the proximal superior and inferior mesenteric arteries.

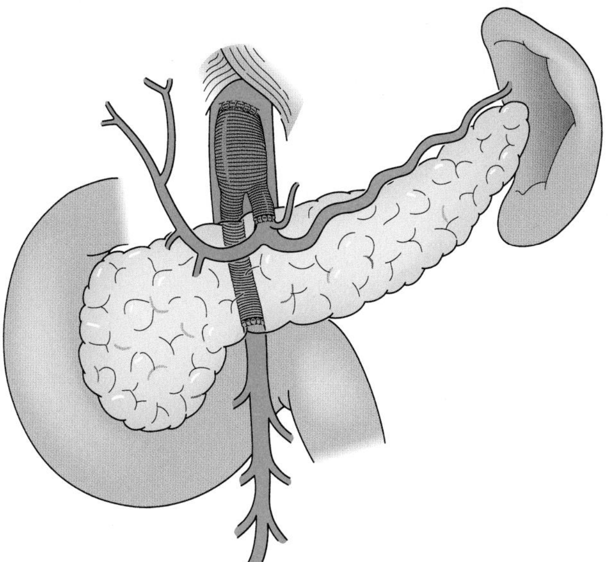

FIGURE 94.13 Bypass grafts to the visceral vessels may originate from the supraceliac aorta. Short antegrade conduits and multiple-vessel revascularization are favored.

bleeding aneurysms.[56,57] These studies are also useful in following asymptomatic splenic artery aneurysms.

Left upper quadrant or epigastric pain may occur in patients with an intact splenic artery aneurysm. In a recent review, nearly half the patients with these aneurysms complained of abdominal pain.[41] However, the literature tends to include more spectacular cases and most bland aneurysms are likely to be asymptomatic.

In cases of splenic artery aneurysm rupture, bleeding is usually initially contained within the lesser sac, with later hemorrhage into the peritoneal cavity and causes vascular collapse. This represents the so-called double-rupture attributed to splenic artery aneurysms. Pancreatitis-related aneurysms are not usually associated with intraperitoneal bleeding. They are more commonly a source of intestinal hemorrhage after rupture into the stomach or pancreatic ductal system.[58–62] Arteriovenous fistula formation after splenic artery aneurysm rupture into an adjacent splenic vein is rare.[63] Gastrointestinal hemorrhage from esophageal varices due to left-sided portal hypertension may accompany these fistulas.

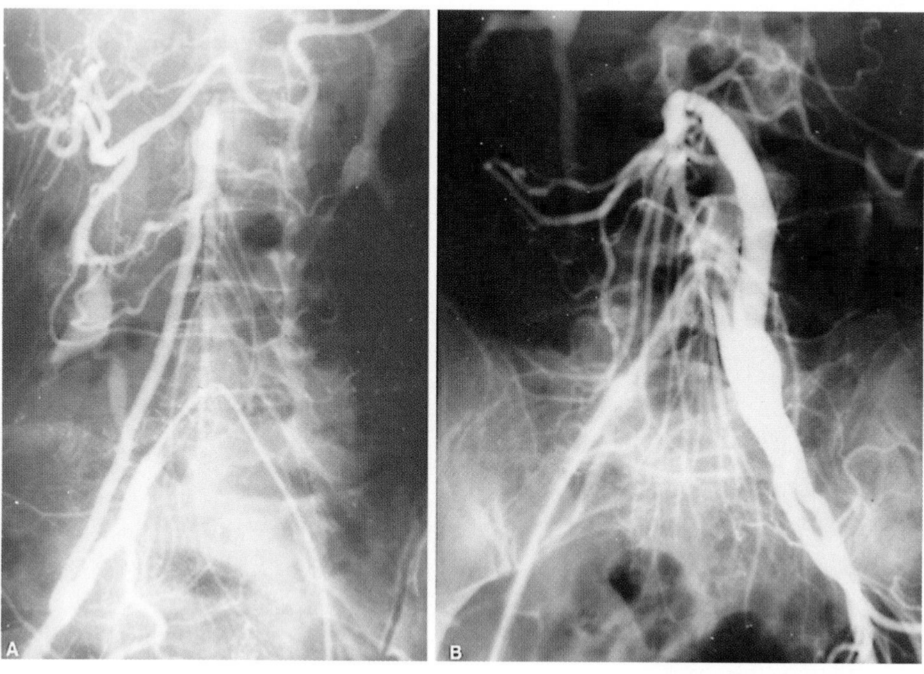

FIGURE 94.14 Retrograde conduits are an alternative bypass, and even single-vessel revascularization may provide effective long-term relief of symptoms in selected circumstances. (*A*) Retrograde right external iliac artery to superior mesenteric artery (SMA) vein graft. Filling is excellent throughout the distribution of the SMA and in the branches of the celiac artery as a result of collateral flow through the gastroduodenal artery. (*B*) A left common iliac artery-SMA bypass.

The risk of splenic artery aneurysm rupture depends on a number of confounding and poorly defined factors. In general, rupture of bland aneurysms occurs in less than 2% of cases.[44] Contrary to prior tenets, rupture appears just as likely when the aneurysm is calcified, occurs in a normotensive patient, or occurs in the very elderly patient. Bland aneurysms associated with liver transplants rupture twice as often as in other patients,[50,51] and such is a fatal complication in over half of transplant patients.[64]

Nearly 95% of aneurysms recognized during pregnancy have ruptured.[44,65–68] The maternal mortality rate approaches 75%, and the fetal mortality rate exceeds 95% in these cases.[69] Pregnancy-related rupture occurs most often during the third

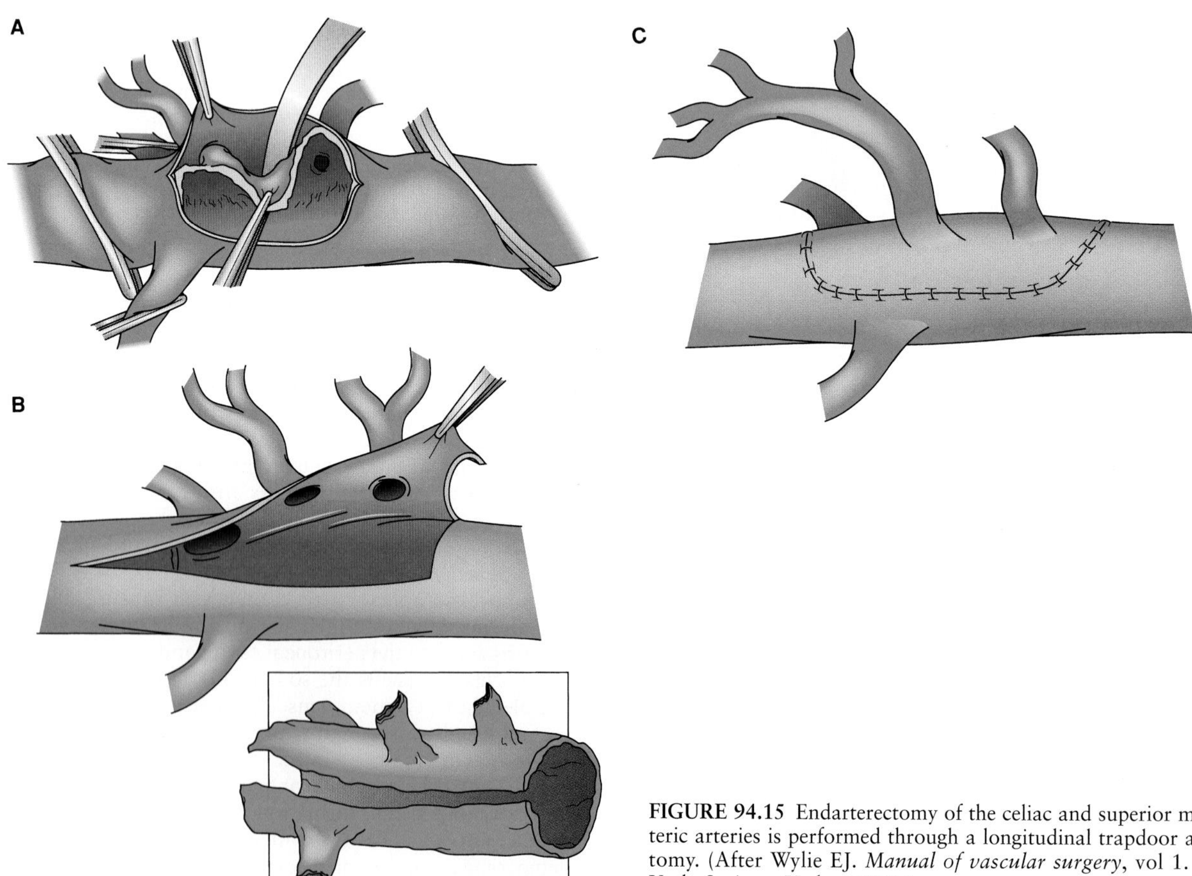

FIGURE 94.15 Endarterectomy of the celiac and superior mesenteric arteries is performed through a longitudinal trapdoor aortotomy. (After Wylie EJ. *Manual of vascular surgery*, vol 1. New York: Springer-Verlag, 1980.)

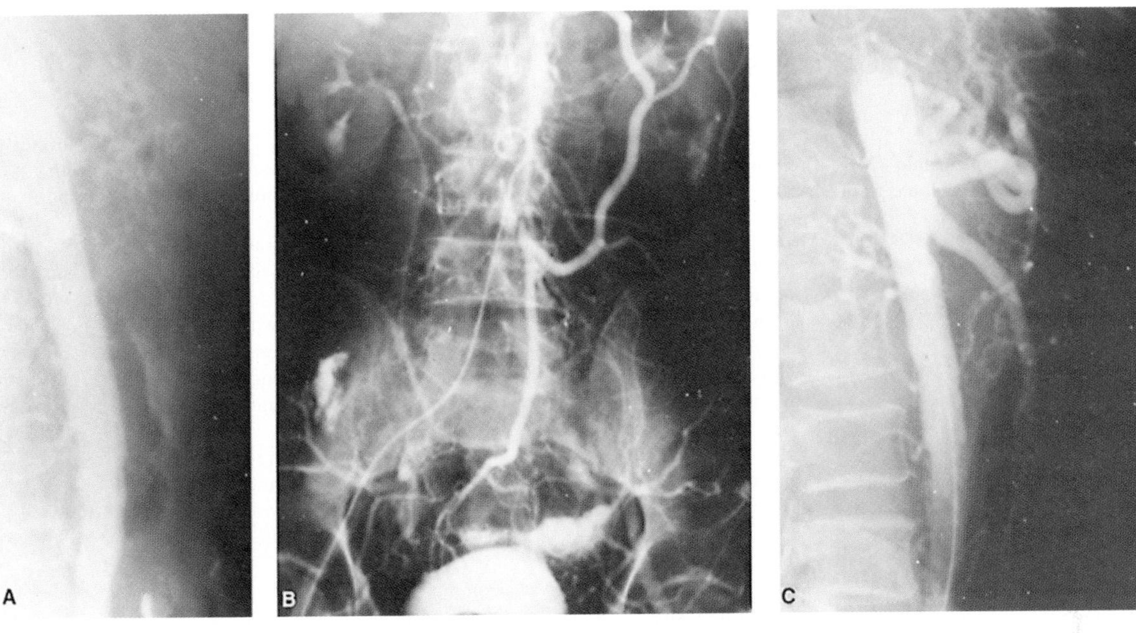

FIGURE 94.16 (*A*) Preoperative lateral aortogram demonstrates total occlusion of the celiac and superior mesenteric arteries. (*B*) Anteroposterior view with selective injection demonstrates large inferior-to-superior mesenteric artery collateral flow. (C) Postoperative angiography demonstrates widely patent celiac and superior mesenteric arteries after transaortic endarterectomy.

trimester (69%) and is less common during the first two trimesters (12%), during labor (13%), or postpartum (6%).[67] Given the fact that most women develop these aneurysms with repeated pregnancies, it is reasonable to assume that most aneurysms in pregnant women go unrecognized and do not

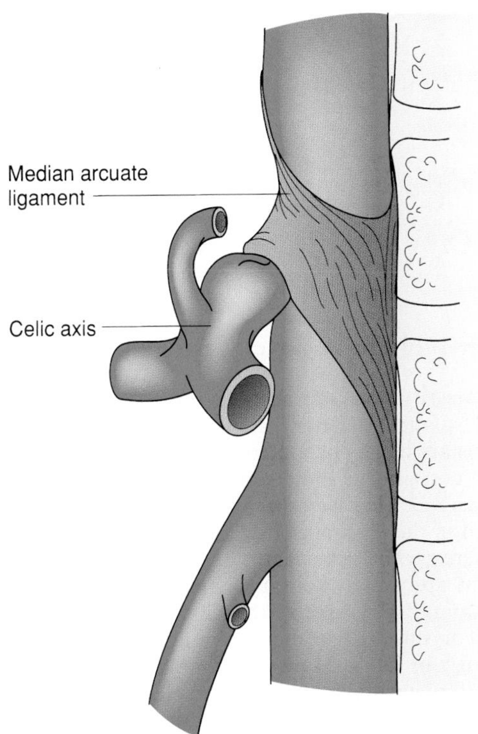

FIGURE 94.17 The median arcuate ligament syndrome is controversial. The anatomic fibrous tissue within the crura of the diaphragm is extraordinarily strong and may significantly narrow the celiac axis.

rupture. Nevertheless, splenic artery aneurysms in pregnant patients must be considered a threat to the life of the mother and fetus.

The reported mortality rate accompanying an open operation for rupture of a bland splenic artery aneurysm unassociated with pregnancy is 25%.[45] Thus, it would seem ill advised to undertake elective operative intervention for an asymptomatic splenic artery aneurysm if the surgical mortality rate exceeds 0.5%. This latter figure represents the product of the predicted 2% rupture rate of bland aneurysms, and the known 25% risk of operative death when treating a patient following aneurysmal rupture. If intervention becomes necessary in higher risk patients, then percutaneous transcatheter embolization of the aneurysm may represent a more appropriate therapy.

Splenectomy has been the most common form of open surgical therapy for splenic artery aneurysms in the past. However, because of the immunologic importance of the spleen even in the aged, simple ligature obliteration or excision of these aneurysms appears preferable to splenectomy.[70] Laparoscopic ligation of these aneurysms in certain instances may prove quite feasible.[71–73] Treatment of splenic artery aneurysms embedded in pancreatic tissue, especially those associated with pancreatitis may require distal pancreatectomy.[74] In some of these cases, especially false aneurysms caused by pseudocyst erosion into the artery, treatment may entail incising the aneurysmal sac and ligating entering and exiting vessels from within. Pancreatic resection or cyst drainage in these latter cases must be individualized and depends on the extent and chronicity of the associated pancreatic inflammatory disease.

Percutaneous transcatheter embolization of splenic artery aneurysms often is preferred over an open operative intervention.[75–78] However, careful follow-up of endovascular-treated patients is mandatory. Splenic infarction and late rupture is a concern, as is transient obliteration of the aneurysm, or coil migration and erosion into the adjacent viscera.[79,80] Stent graft exclusion of an aneurysm with maintenance of splenic artery flow has been used in select cases.[81–83]

TABLE 94.3

SPLANCHNIC ARTERY MACROANEURYSMS

Aneurysm location	Frequency within splanchnic circulation	M:F ratio	Contributing factors	Frequency of reported rupture (%)	Site of rupture	Mortality with rupture
Splenic artery	60%	1:4	Medial degeneration; arterial fibrodysplasia; multiple pregnancies; portal hypertension; chronic pancreatitis with arterial erosion by pseudocysts	2% (bland aneurysms)	Intraperitoneal within lesser sac; intragastric with pancreatitis-related inflammatory aneurysms	25% bland and unassociated with pregnancy; during pregnancy 70% maternal, 75% fetal
Hepatic artery	20%	2:1	Medial degeneration; blunt and penetrating liver trauma; infection related to intravenous substance abuse	20%	Intraperitoneal and biliary tract with equal frequency	35%
Superior mesenteric artery	5.5%	1:1	Infection related to bacterial endocarditis, often associated with nonhemolytic streptococci and more recently with intravenous substance abuse; medial degeneration	Uncommon (thrombosis more common)	Intraperitoneal and retroperitoneal	50%
Celiac artery	4%	1:1	Medial degeneration	13%	Intraperitoneal	50%
Gastric and gastroepiploic arteries	4%	3:1	Periarterial inflammation; medial degeneration	90%	Intraperitoneal (30%), intestinal tract (70%)	70%
Jejunal, ileal, and colic arteries	3%	1:1	Medial degeneration; connective tissue diseases	30%		
Pancreaticoduodenal, pancreatic, and gastroduodenal arteries	2%	4:1	Pancreatitis-related arterial necrosis and arterial erosion by pseudocysts (60% of gastroduodenal, 30% of pancreaticoduodenal artery aneurysms); medial degeneration	75% inflammatory, 50% noninflammatory	Intestinal tract (85%); intraperitoneal (15%)	50%

M:F, male to female.

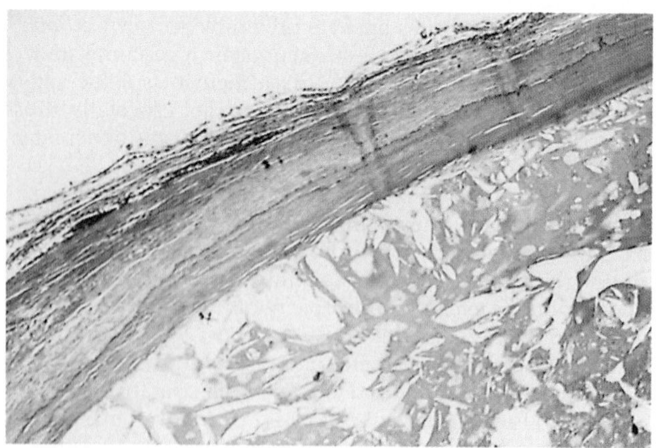

FIGURE 94.18 Splenic artery aneurysm exhibiting marked fibrosis cholesterol clefts and with calcific arteriosclerosis (hematoxylin-eosin, decalcified, X32).

Hepatic Artery Aneurysm

Hepatic artery aneurysms account for 20% of all previously reported splanchnic artery aneurysms (Fig. 94.23). These aneurysms are being encountered more frequently in contemporary times, and in some series outnumber splenic artery aneurysms.[41,84] Men have been twice as likely to be affected as women in the past, although gender differences are not as apparent in recent experiences.[41,85] Hepatic artery macroaneurysms are usually solitary. Large aneurysms tend to be saccular, and aneurysms less than 2 cm are usually fusiform. These aneurysms are extrahepatic in nearly 80% of cases and intrahepatic in 20%. More than one third of patients with hepatic artery aneurysms have other splanchnic aneurysms.[86]

Most noninfectious and nontraumatic hepatic artery aneurysms are usually recognized after the sixth decade of life. The cause of many hepatic artery aneurysms is poorly defined. Two facts regarding the cause of these aneurysms are notewor-

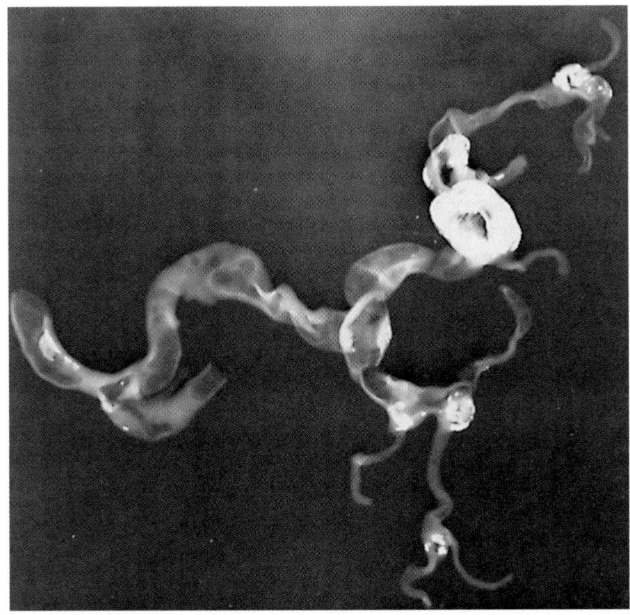

FIGURE 94.19 Splenic artery aneurysm. Marked calcific arteriosclerosis limited to splenic artery aneurysms occurring at vessel bifurcations (specimen roentgenogram) is seen. Intervening arterial segments are unaffected by advanced arteriosclerotic changes. (Stanley JC, Thompson NW, Fry WJ. Splanchnic artery aneurysms. *Arch Surg.* 1970;101:689–697, with permission.)

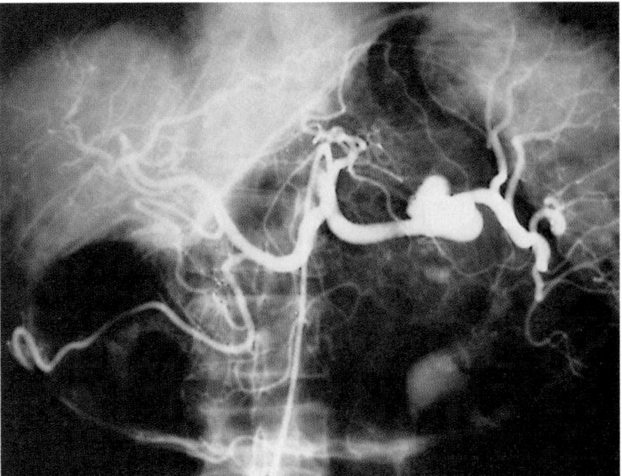

FIGURE 94.21 Splenic artery aneurysm. Arteriogram documents a pancreatitis-related aneurysm affecting the mid-splenic artery. (Stanley JC, Frey CF, Miller TA, et al. Major arterial hemorrhage: a complication of pancreatic pseudocysts and chronic pancreatitis. *Arch Surg.* 1976; 111:435–440, with permission.)

thy. First, arteriosclerosis most likely represents a secondary event rather than a primary cause of these aneurysms. Most of these lesions probably occur as a result of medial degeneration. Second, with increasing societal violence and intravenous substance abuse, the number of reported traumatic and infection-related aneurysms has markedly increased[41] (Fig. 94.24). Another common cause of intrahepatic pseudoaneurysms is arterial injury accompanying invasive percutaneous diagnostic and therapeutic procedures involving penetration of the liver.[87,88] Nearly 17% of these aneurysms encountered more recently have occurred in orthotopic liver transplant patients.[41] Systemic arteriopathies, such as periarteritis nodosa, have been incriminated as a cause of occasional macroaneurysms, but are more often associated with intraparenchymal microaneurysms.[89]

Hepatic artery aneurysms may be suspected because of displacement of or indentations on intestinal structures noted on barium contrast studies. Most contemporary diagnoses of these aneurysms result from their incidental recognition during arteriography, CT, or ultrasonography for nonvascular disease. Few hepatic artery aneurysms are symptomatic. When they become symptomatic, most present with right upper quadrant or epigastric pain. Rapid expansion of these aneurysms may cause severe discomfort similar to that of acute pancreatitis. Large aneurysms have been reported to cause obstructive jaundice, although most hepatic artery aneurysms are too small to compress the major bile ducts. These lesions rarely present as pulsatile abdominal masses.

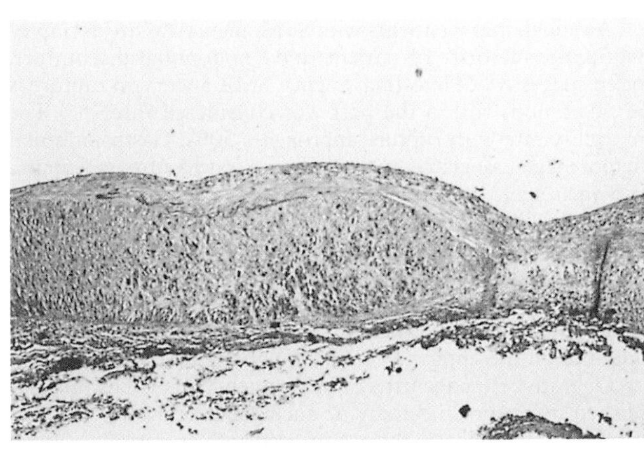

FIGURE 94.20 Splenic artery aneurysm exhibiting fragmentation of internal elastic lamina and medial dysplasia in a patient having renal arterial fibrodysplasia (Masson stain, X32).

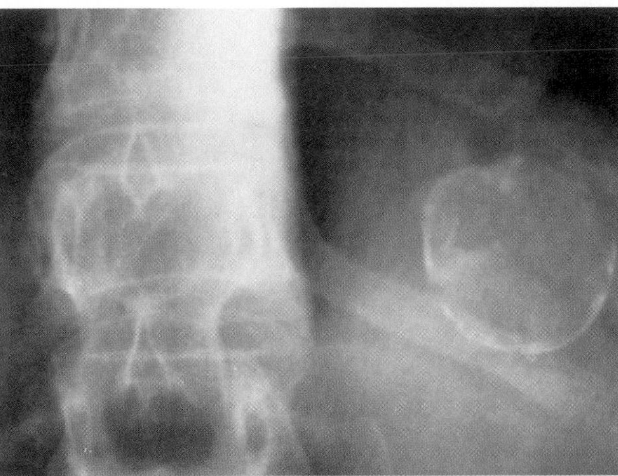

FIGURE 94.22 Splenic artery aneurysm. Curvilinear signet ring–like calcification in the left upper quadrant characteristic of a splenic artery aneurysm. (Stanley JC, Thompson NW, Fry WJ. Splanchnic artery aneurysms. *Arch Surg.* 1970;101:689–697, with permission.)

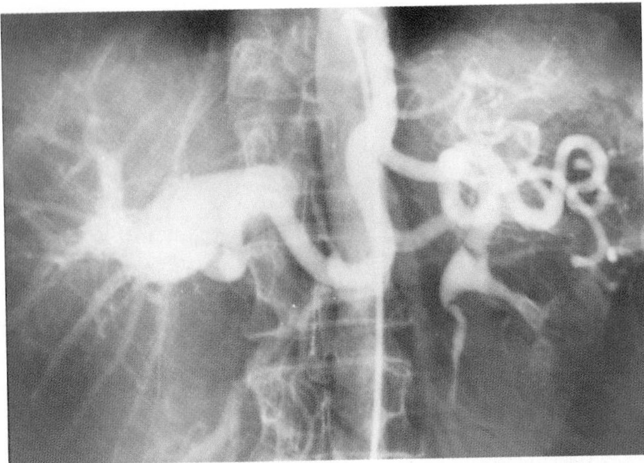

FIGURE 94.23 Hepatic artery aneurysm. Selective celiac arteriogram demonstrates a large saccular aneurysm at the bifurcation of the proper hepatic artery. (Zelenock GB, Stanley JC. Splanchnic artery aneurysms. In: Rutherford RB, ed. *Vascular surgery*. Philadelphia, WB Saunders, 2000;1369, with permission.)

The reported incidence of hepatic artery aneurysm rupture approaches 20%, but the contemporary rate may be less. It is certainly less than the often-quoted rupture rate of 44% in cases reported a few decades ago.[45] Aneurysm rupture is associated with a 35% mortality rate, although in recent times the mortality appears less.[41] Bleeding from a ruptured hepatic artery aneurysm occurs with equal frequency into the biliary tract and peritoneal cavity. Hemobilia accompanies the former, being manifest by biliary colic, hematemesis, and jaundice.[90] Chronic, relatively asymptomatic hemorrhage is an uncommon sequela of aneurysm rupture into the biliary tract. Intraperitoneal bleeding is usually caused by rupture of inflammatory-related false aneurysms.

Common hepatic artery aneurysms are often be treated by aneurysmectomy or aneurysm exclusion, without arterial reconstruction. The extensive hepatic arterial collateral circulation and parallel portal venous circulation often ensure adequate blood flow to the liver with interruption of the proximal common hepatic artery. Liver necrosis is more likely to follow ligation of arteries in the more distal hepatic circulation. Nevertheless, even in the latter vessels, complex arterial reconstructions should be avoided and simple ligation undertaken if temporary intraoperative occlusion of the involved artery does not result in obvious hepatic ischemia. If liver blood flow appears inadequate with such a maneuver, then hepatic artery reconstruction should be undertaken using either prosthetic or autologous vein grafts. In the case of rapidly bleeding ruptured intraparenchymal aneurysms, hepatic territory resection may be necessary therapy.

Percutaneous transcatheter obliteration of hepatic artery aneurysms with balloons, coils, or thrombogenic particulate matter is often a preferred alternative to open surgical intervention.[41,75,88,91,92] One must realize that transcatheter embolization may be transiently successful, and repeated embolization or surgical therapy may subsequently be required to adequately treat these patients.[77,91] Transcatheter thrombin injection[93] and endograft exclusion of select aneurysms may prove useful in carefully chosen patients.[94,95]

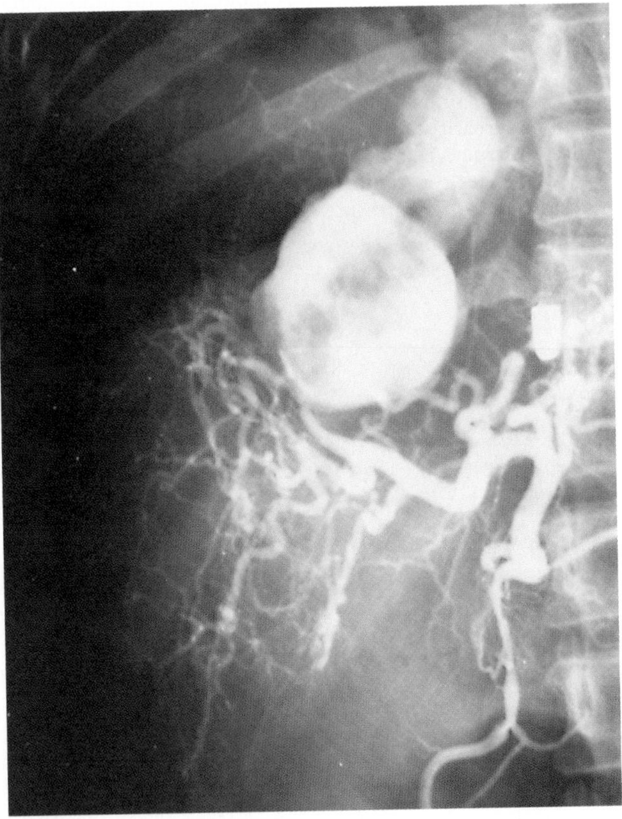

FIGURE 94.24 Traumatic hepatic artery aneurysm. Blunt abdominal injury and gunshot wounds cause most traumatic lesions. (Whitehouse WM Jr, Graham LM, Stanley JC. Aneurysms of the celiac, hepatic, and splenic arteries. In: Bergan JJ, Yao JST, eds. *Aneurysms: diagnosis and treatment*. New York, Grune & Stratton, 1981:405, with permission.)

Superior Mesenteric Artery Aneurysm

Aneurysms of the proximal SMA account for 5.5% of all splanchnic artery aneurysms. These lesions affect men twice as often as women. Infection from a cardiac source has been a common cause of these aneurysms in the past,[45,96] but are less common in recent times.[97] Nonhemolytic streptococci, as well as many common pathogens accompanying parenteral substance abuse, cause bacterial endocarditis and are the underlying source of infection in most cases. Many of these aneurysms are associated with intramural dissections (Fig. 94.25).[98] SMA aneurysms may also be caused by medial degeneration, periarterial inflammation, and trauma. Arteriosclerosis, as in the case of other splanchnic aneurysms, is usually a secondary process. SMA aneurysms are often recognized during arteriographic studies for nonvascular disease.[42,97]

Although many patients with SMA aneurysms are asymptomatic, the majority of patients have abdominal discomfort, often suggestive of intestinal angina. SMA aneurysm rupture is not common, and in the past was considered rare.[97,98] The mortality rate with rupture approaches 50%. Gastrointestinal hemorrhage associated with these aneurysms often accompanies their acute occlusion with bleeding into areas of intestinal infarction. Location of most aneurysms near the origins of the inferior pancreaticoduodenal and middle colic arteries isolates the distal mesenteric circulation when dissections or occlusions occur. In these circumstances, intestinal ischemia develops because the usual collateral network from the adjacent celiac and inferior mesenteric arterial circulations is obstructed.

Operative management of SMA aneurysms is best accomplished by aneurysmectomy or aneurysm exclusion, followed by intestinal revascularization if needed with an aortomesenteric graft. Because of potential infection when bowel ischemia is present, autologous vein or artery is favored over prosthetic conduits for these reconstructions. SMA aneurysm ligation without arterial reconstruction may be successful in patients who have

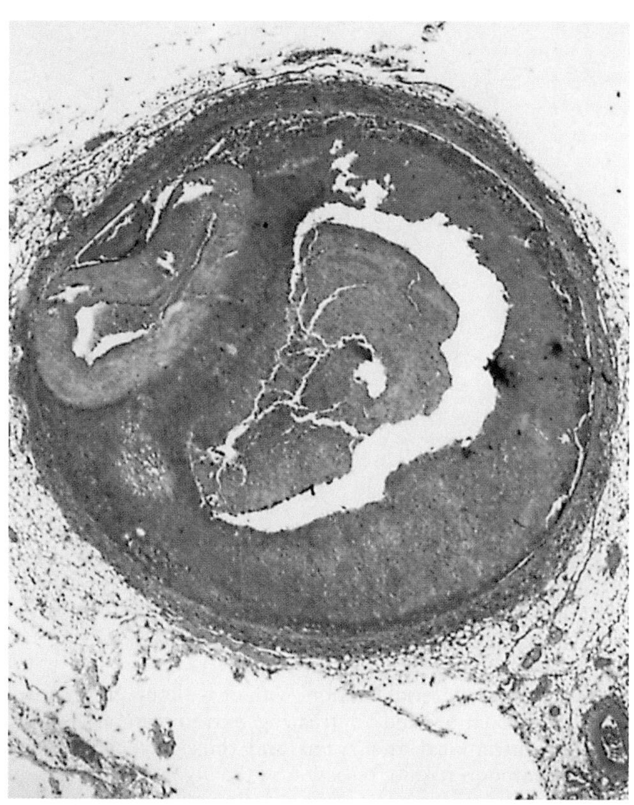

FIGURE 94.25 Superior mesenteric artery aneurysm. Microscopic cross-section of a dissecting aneurysm affecting the proximal superior mesenteric artery (hematoxylin-eosin, X20).

developed an adequate collateral circulation to their midgut. In fact, ligation and aneurysmorrhaphy have been the most commonly reported means of managing these aneurysms.[100–103] Temporary intraoperative occlusion of the SMA with Doppler documentation of adequate intestinal blood flow should be undertaken before proceeding with SMA ligation.

Endovascular stent graft placement for select SMA aneurysms has appeal,[104,105] although infection and thrombosis may compromise this type treatment. Obliteration of these aneurysms by coils or direct thrombin injection may be preferred in high-risk patients having discrete aneurysm necks and adequate collateral circulation to the distal SMA.[97,106]

Celiac Artery Aneurysm

Celiac artery aneurysms account for 4% of all splanchnic artery aneurysms. Men and women appear equally affected. Those aneurysms encountered before 1950 were usually infectious in etiology, but in contemporary times have been associated with medial degeneration.[107,108] Arteriosclerosis is a common histologic finding that is considered a secondary event rather than an etiologic process. Other splanchnic artery aneurysms affect nearly 40% of these patients. Celiac artery aneurysms are usually saccular, and most are located in the distal vessel (Fig. 94.26).

Most celiac artery aneurysms are asymptomatic or appear to be associated with vague abdominal discomfort.[41,45] These aneurysms are usually recognized during ultrasonography, angiography, or other imaging studies for nonvascular diseases. In more recent times, rupture has affected 13% of these aneurysms and carried a mortality rate of 50%.[107] In contrast, rupture rates published before 1950 were often higher than 80%. Rupture usually causes exsanguinating intraperitoneal hemorrhage. Although rare, gastrointestinal bleeding may follow rupture of the aneurysm into the stomach or pancreatic ductal system.

Aneurysmectomy with celiac artery reconstruction is the preferred treatment for these lesions, although aneurysm exclusion with ligation of its branches has been performed successfully in select patients.[107–110] When simple ligature is undertaken, the adequacy of the liver's collateral circulation must be documented. If liver ischemia is apparent after temporary intraoperative celiac artery occlusion, then hepatic revascularization becomes mandatory. An aortoceliac or aortohepatic artery bypass in these circumstances is best performed with either an autologous vein or prosthetic graft. Surgical therapy of celiac artery aneurysmal disease has been successful in more than 90% of cases.

Endovascular obliteration of a celiac artery aneurysm is not often considered because of the need to occlude the hepatic, splenic and left gastric arteries, and perhaps the inferior phrenic arteries, in order to isolate the aneurysms. Nevertheless, in select cases catheter-based therapy may be successful.[111]

Gastric and Gastroepiploic Artery Aneurysms

Gastric and gastroepiploic artery aneurysms account for 4% of all splanchnic artery aneurysms (Fig. 94.27). Gastric artery aneurysms occur 10 times more often than gastroepiploic artery aneurysms. Men are three times more likely than women to develop these aneurysms. Most of these perigastric lesions have been encountered in patients more than 50 years of age. These aneurysms usually are solitary, occurring as a result of periarterial inflammation or medial degeneration. In many cases, there is an antecedent history of peptic ulcer disease. Arteriosclerosis, when present, is considered a secondary event, not a cause of these lesions.

Most reported gastric or gastroepiploic artery aneurysms have been symptomatic when initially recognized, frequently presenting as emergencies.[112–114] Rupture has accompanied more than 90% of reported cases, with gastrointestinal bleeding occurring slightly more than twice as often as intraperitoneal hemorrhage. Rupture carries a 70% mortality rate.[45]

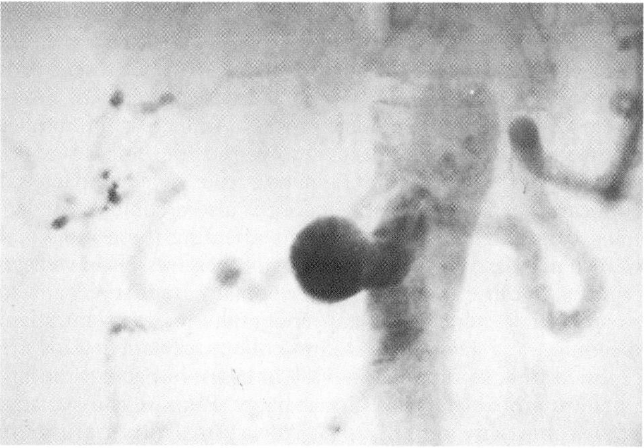

FIGURE 94.26 Celiac artery aneurysm. Aortogram reveals saccular aneurysm that exhibited medial degenerative changes and secondary arteriosclerosis. (Stanley JC, Whitehouse WM Jr. Aneurysms of the splanchnic and renal arteries. In: Bergan JJ, Yao JST, eds. *Surgery of the aorta and its body branches*. Orlando, Grune & Stratton, 1979:497, with permission.)

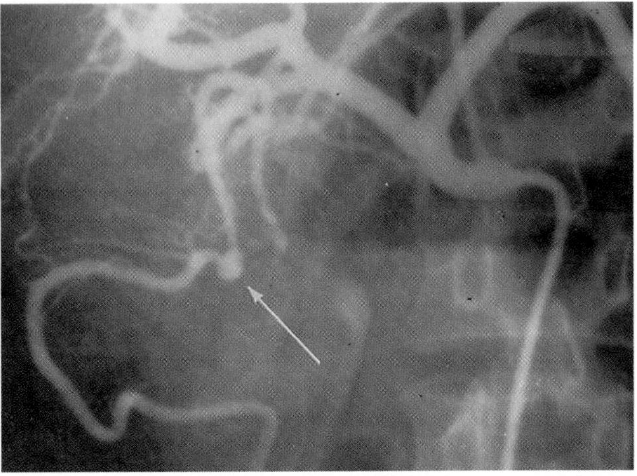

FIGURE 94.27 Gastroepiploic artery aneurysm. Selective celiac arteriogram revealing small aneurysm responsible for massive gastrointestinal hemorrhage. (Stanley JC, Thompson NW, Fry WJ. Splanchnic artery aneurysms. *Arch Surg*. 1970;101:689–697, with permission.)

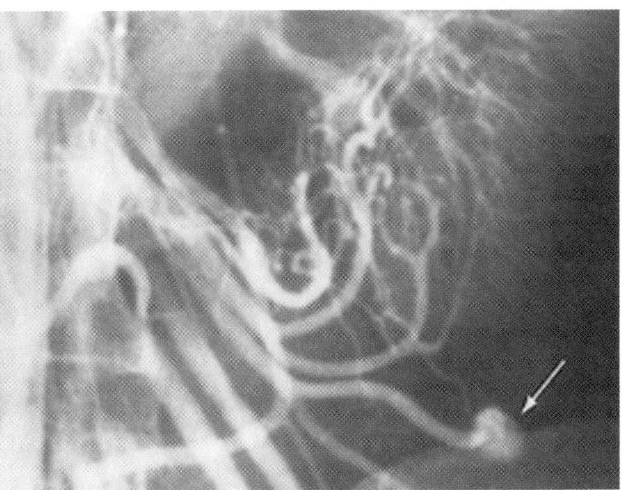

FIGURE 94.28 Ileal artery aneurysm. Mesenteric arteriogram documenting saccular aneurysm of distal ileal artery (Zelenock GB, Stanley JC: Splanchnic artery aneurysms. In: Rutherford RB, ed. *Vascular surgery*. Philadelphia, WB Saunders, 2000;1369, with permission.)

These figures may overestimate the seriousness of these aneurysms, with reported cases often spectacular and unrepresentative of the usual case.

Surgical treatment is recommended for all gastric and gastroepiploic artery aneurysms.[7] Vascular reconstructive surgery is not required in these cases. Intramural gastric aneurysms may be excised with a small segment of involved stomach, whereas extramural aneurysms can be treated by arterial ligation alone, with or without aneurysm excision. Certain lesions may be treated by a laparoscopic approach.[115] Intraoperative identification of these small aneurysms is often tedious if preoperative localization has not been established by arteriographic studies. Endovascular occlusion of life-threatening bleeding from a ruptured aneurysm may be appropriate as a prelude to definitive open surgical aneurysmectomy in select cases.

Jejunal, Ileal, and Colic Artery Aneurysms

Aneurysms of the jejunal, ileal, and colic arteries account for 3% of all splanchnic artery aneurysms (Fig. 94.28). They usually occur in patients more than 60 years of age. Men and women are affected equally. Multiple aneurysms have been encountered in 10% of cases. Acquired medial defects cause most of these lesions. Although arteriosclerosis is present with 20% of these aneurysms, it is considered to represent a secondary event, not an etiologic process. An increasing number of mycotic aneurysms affect these vessels, developing as the sequela of infected emboli originating from subacute bacterial endocarditis.[116] Periarteritis nodosa is also a common underlying cause of multiple aneurysms affecting these intestinal branch arteries.[117] Most aneurysms of these vessels have been reported to cause abdominal pain, yet many are first recognized as incidental findings during arteriography for gastrointestinal bleeding.[45,118] Jejunal, ileal, and colic artery aneurysms are reported to have ruptured in 30% of cases, but actual rupture rates are probably a third of that figure. Rupture is associated with a mortality rate of 20%. Aneurysmal rupture usually occurs into the gastrointestinal tract. Rupture into the mesentery or peritoneal cavity is uncommon.

Operation for intestinal branch aneurysms is recommended in all instances, except for bland aneurysms associated with connective-tissue diseases. Expeditious surgical therapy requires careful preoperative localization with arteriographic studies. Arterial ligation, with or without aneurysmectomy, is recommended in treating extraintestinal lesions, whereas intramural aneurysms and those associated with bowel infarction require resection of the involved intestine. In select patients transcatheter embolization may be undertaken, although intestinal necrosis with perforation or late stricture formation is a recognized complication of such therapy.[119]

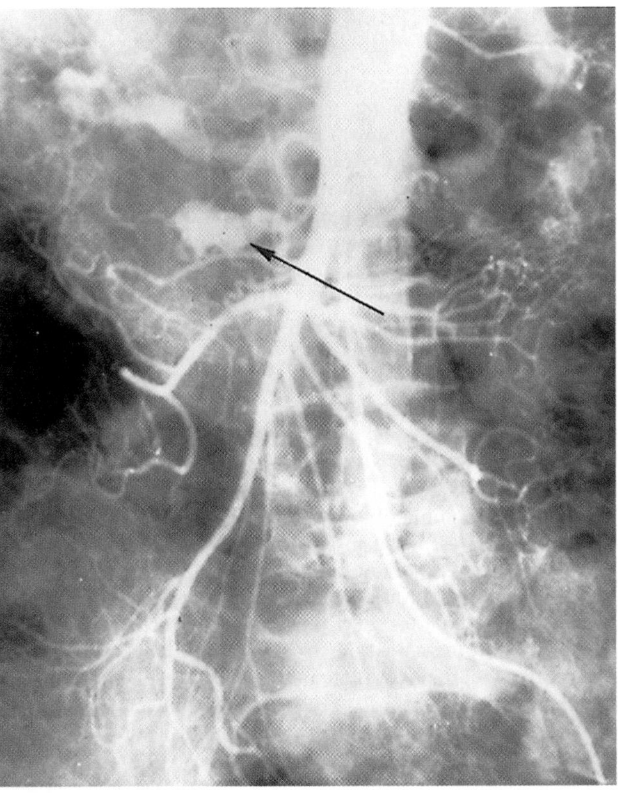

FIGURE 94.29 Inferior pancreaticoduodenal artery aneurysm. Selective superior mesenteric arteriogram revealing false aneurysm secondary to pseudocyst erosion of artery. (Stanley JC, Frey CF, Miller TA, et al. Major arterial hemorrhage: a complication of pancreatic pseudocysts and chronic pancreatitis. *Arch Surg*. 1976;111:435–440, with permission.)

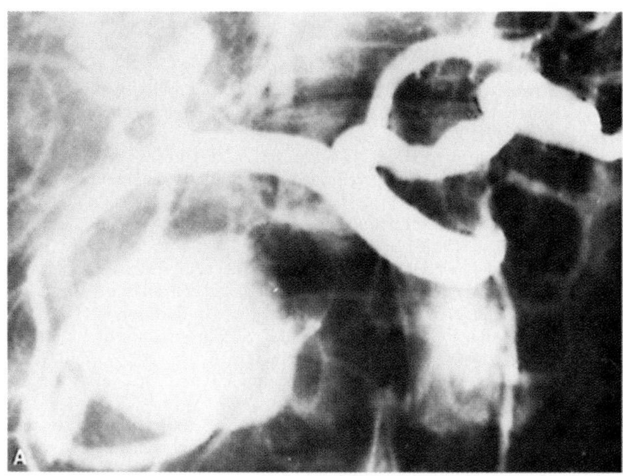

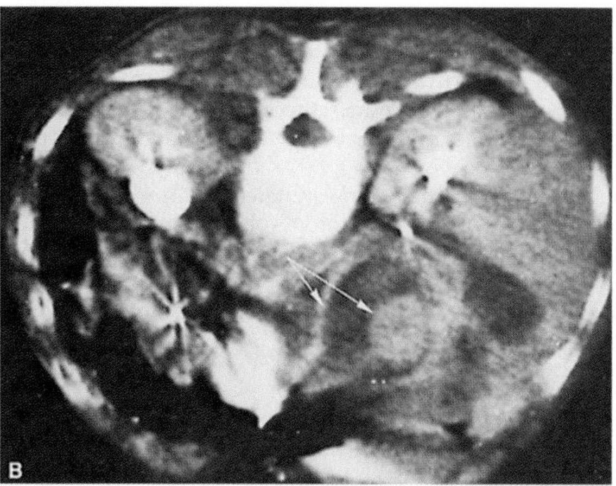

FIGURE 94.30 Gastroduodenal artery aneurysm. (*A*) Selective celiac arteriogram. (*B*) Computed tomography scan of a pancreatic pseudocyst (*short arrow*) containing the aneurysm (*long arrow*). (Eckhauser FE, Stanley JC, Zelenock GB, et al. Gastroduodenal and pancreaticoduodenal artery aneurysms: a complication of pancreatitis causing spontaneous gastrointestinal hemorrhage. *Surgery* 1980;88:335–344, with permission.)

Inferior mesenteric artery aneurysms represent a unique subset of these mesenteric aneurysms.[120,121] They are quite rare and their etiology so varied that the clinical importance of them has not been clearly established.

Pancreaticoduodenal, Pancreatic, and Gastroduodenal Artery Aneurysms

Pancreatic and pancreaticoduodenal artery aneurysms (Fig. 94.29) account for 2% of all splanchnic artery aneurysms, and gastroduodenal artery aneurysms (Fig. 94.30) represent an additional 1.5% of these aneurysms. Men are four times more likely than women to develop these lesions. Most patients with these aneurysms are older than age 50 years. Most of these lesions are associated with pancreatitis-related vascular necrosis or vessel erosion by an adjacent pancreatic pseudocyst. Medial degeneration and trauma are less common causes of these aneurysms. Arteriosclerosis is invariably a secondary, not a causative, process. Many recently reported aneurysms have been associated with celiac artery stenoses or occlusions, and likely represent the effect of inordinately high volume blood flow on branchings of the collateral circulation,[89,91] where pre-existing discontinuities of elastin are known to exist in normal arteries. A similar scenario contributing to aneurysm formation may exist in instances of an SMA occlusion or severe stenosis.[124]

Pancreatitis-related aneurysms are often difficult to diagnose and treat. Most are associated with epigastric pain and discomfort, which may be caused by the underlying pancreatic inflammatory disease that accompanies about 60% of gastroduodenal and 30% of pancreaticoduodenal artery aneurysms. Arteriography usually establishes the presence of these aneurysms, but CT scanning and MRI are of increasing importance in their recognition. These latter noninvasive studies are especially important in detecting rupture or associated pancreatic pathology.

Gastroduodenal and pancreaticoduodenal aneurysm rupture has affected more than 50% of the reported cases, occurring in 75% of inflammatory and 50% of noninflammatory lesions. Hemorrhage usually occurs into the stomach, the biliary tract, or pancreatic ductal system. Bleeding of pancreatitis-related aneurysms into the peritoneal cavity is less likely, affecting approximately 15% of cases. The overall mortality rate with rupture, including pancreatitis-related aneurysms, approaches 25% despite operative intervention, but is nearly double that figure in the case of true pancreaticoduodenal artery aneurysms.

Surgical intervention is appropriate in all but the poorest risk patients with gastroduodenal, pancreaticoduodenal, or pancreatic arterial aneurysms.[45,125–129] Pancreatitis-related false aneurysms are usually treated by arterial ligation from within the aneurysmal sac, rather than extraaneurysmal arterial ligation. Extensive dissection of the pancreas affected by dense inflammatory adhesions in such circumstances is hazardous. In situations in which a pancreatic pseudocyst or abscess has eroded the artery, a drainage procedure should be undertaken. Distal pancreatectomy, or even pancreaticoduodenectomy, may be the safest mode of treatment in select cases.

Transcatheter embolization and electrocoagulation have an important role in treating very high-risk patients.[130–134] Thrombin injection may serve as another means of occluding small aneurysms.[135,136] Nevertheless, rebleeding and late aneurysmal rupture with these therapies can occur and restrict their universal use.[125,136] In select patients, however, endovascular occlusion of the bleeding aneurysm may be an appropriate life-saving measure, followed by a later definitive open resection.

KEY POINTS

- **Occlusive and aneurysm diseases of the splanchnic vessels are relatively uncommon problems in clinical practice.**
- **Approximately 50% of acute mesenteric ischemia cases are caused by an embolus, typically from a cardiac source. Atrial fibrillation and a myocardial infarction with mural thrombus formation are the most common embolic sources.**
- **Acute mesenteric embolism usually results in sudden and severe epigastric or midabdominal pain, followed promptly by evacuation of the gut, with emeses or explosive diarrhea.**
- **Complications of certain catheter-related procedures and operations are an increasingly common cause of acute ischemia.**

- **Intestinal angina is most often a consequence of aortic spillover arteriosclerosis affecting the origins of the celiac, superior mesenteric, and inferior mesenteric arteries.**
- **In patients with chronic mesenteric ischemia, the progression from minor symptoms to intestinal infarction is unpredictable.**
- **Splanchnic artery aneurysms are uncommon, but the more frequent use of computed tomography, magnetic resonance imaging, and ultrasonography has resulted in an increase in their clinical recognition.**
- **Splenic artery aneurysms are the most common splanchnic artery aneurysm accounting for 60% of all splanchnic artery aneurysms.**

References

1. Reuter SR, Redman HC. *Gastrointestinal Angiography*. 2nd ed. Philadelphia: WB Saunders; 1971.
2. Deitch EA. The role of intestinal barrier failure and bacterial translocation in the development of systemic infection and multiple organ failure. *Arch Surg*. 1990;125:403–404.
3. Harward T, Brooks D, Flynn T, et al. Multiple organ dysfunction after mesenteric artery revascularization. *J Vasc Surg*. 1993;18:459–469.
4. Jamieson W, DeRose G, Harris K, et al. Myocardial and circulatory performance during the ischemic phase of superior mesenteric artery occlusion. *Can J Surg*. 1993;36:435–439.
5. Pargger H, Staender S, Studer W, et al. Occlusive mesenteric ischemia and its effects on jejunal intramucosal pH, mesenteric oxygen consumption, and oxygen tensions from surfaces of the jejunum in anesthetized pigs. *Intensive Care Med*. 1997;23:91–99.
6. Park PO, Haglund U, Bulkley GB, et al. The sequence of development of intestinal tissue injury after strangulation ischemia and reperfusion. *Surgery* 1990;107:574–580.
7. Thompson JS, Bragg LE, West WW. Serum enzyme levels during intestinal ischemia. *Ann Surg*. 1990;211:369–373.
8. Landreneau RJ, Fry WJ. The right colon as a target organ of nonocclusive mesenteric ischemia. *Arch Surg*. 1990;125:591–594.
9. Levy PJ, Krausz MM, Manny J. Acute mesenteric ischemia: improved results-a retrospective analysis of ninety-two patients. *Surgery* 1990;107: 372–380.
10. Mesh CL, Gewertz BL. The effect of hemodilution on blood flow regulation in normal and post-ischemic intestine. *J Surg Res*. 1990;48: 183–189.
11. Oshima A, Kitajima M, Sakai N, et al. Does glucagon improve the viability of ischemic intestine? *J Surg Res*. 1990;49:524–533.
12. **Zelenock GB, Strodel WE, Knol JA, et al. A prospective study of clinically and endoscopically documented colonic ischemia in 100 patients undergoing aortic reconstructive surgery with aggressive colonic and direct pelvic revascularization, compared with historic controls. *Surgery* 1989; 106:771–780.**
13. Rutherford R, Taylor L, eds. Mesenteric ischemia. *Semin Vasc Surg*. 1990;3:141.
14. Taylor LM Jr. Mesenteric ischemia. *Semin Vasc Surg*. 1990;3:141.
15. Ballard J, Stone W, Hallett J, et al. A critical analysis of adjuvant techniques used to assess bowel viability in acute mesenteric ischemia. *Am Surg*. 1993;59:309–311.
16. Brolin RE, Semmlow JL, Sehonanda A, et al. Comparison of five methods of assessment of intestinal viability. *Surg Gynecol Obstet*. 1989;168:6–12.
17. Levy PJ, Krausz MM, Manny J. The role of second-look procedures in improving survival time for patients with mesenteric venous thrombosis. *Surg Gynecol Obstet*. 1990;170:287–291.
18. **Zelenock GB, Graham LM, Whitehouse WM Jr, et al. Splanchnic arteriosclerotic disease and intestinal angina. *Arch Surg*. 1980;115: 497–501.**
19. Burkart D, Johnson C, Reading C, et al. MR measurement of mesenteric venous flow: prospective evaluation in healthy volunteers and patients with suspected chronic mesenteric ischemia. *Radiology* 1995;194:801–806.
20. Moneta G, Lee R, Yeager R, et al. Mesenteric duplex scanning: a blinded prospective study. *J Vasc Surg*. 1993;17:79–86.
21. Moneta GL, Taylor DC, Helton WS, et al. Duplex ultrasound measurement of postprandial intestinal blood flow: effect of meal composition. *Gastroenterology* 1988;95:1294–1301.
22. Beebe H, MacFarlane S, Raker E. Supraceliac aortomesenteric bypass for intestinal ischemia. *J Vasc Surg*. 1987;5:749–754.
23. Bjorck M, Acosta S, Lindberg F, et al. Revascularization of the superior mesenteric artery after acute thromboembolic occlusion. *Br J Surg*. 2002;89:923–927.
24. Foley MI, Moneta GL, Abou-Zamzam AM Jr, et al. Revascularization of the superior mesenteric artery alone for treatment of intestinal ischemia. *J Vasc Surg*. 2000;32:37–47.
25. Gentile A, Moneta G, Taylor L, et al. Isolated bypass to the superior mesenteric artery for intestinal ischemia. *Arch Surg*. 1994;129:926–932.
26. Geroulakos G, Tober JC, Anderson L, et al. Antegrade visceral revascularization via a thoracoabdominal approach for chronic mesenteric ischaemia. *Eur J Vasc Endovasc Surg*. 1999;17:56–59.
27. Jimenez JG, Huber TS, Ozaki CK, et al. Durability of antegrade synthetic aortomesenteric bypass for chronic mesenteric ischemia. *J Vasc Surg*. 2002;35:1078–1084.
28. **Kasirajan K, O'Hara PJ, Gray BH, et al. Chronic mesenteric ischemia: open surgery versus percutaneous angioplasty and stenting. *J Vasc Surg*. 2001;33:63–71.**
29. Kazmers A. Operative management of chronic mesenteric ischemia. *Ann Vasc Surg*. 1998;12:299–308.
30. Stoney RJ, Schneider PA. Technical aspects of visceral arterial revascularization. In: Bergan JJ, Yao JST, eds. *Techniques in arterial surgery*. Philadelphia: WB Saunders, 1990.
31. Stoney RJ, Reilly LM, Ehrenfeld WK. Chronic mesenteric ischemia and surgery for chronic visceral ischemia. In: Wilson SE, Veith FJ, Jobson RW, et al., eds. Vascular surgery: principles and practice. New York: McGraw-Hill, 1987.
32. Matsumoto AH, Angle JF, Spinosa DJ, et al. Percutaneous transluminal angioplasty and stenting in the treatment of chronic mesenteric ischemia: results and long-term followup. *J Am Coll Surg*. 2002;194:S22–S31.
33. McShane M, Proctor A, Spencer P, et al. Mesenteric angioplasty for chronic intestinal ischemia. *Eur J Vasc Surg*. 1992;6:333–336.
34. Carmeci C, McClenathan J. Visceral artery aneurysms seen in a community hospital. *Am J Surg*. 2000;179:486–489.
35. **Carr SC, Pearce WH, Vogelzang RL, et al: Current management of visceral artery aneurysms. *Surgery* 1996; 120:627–634.**
36. Gabelmann A, Gorich J, Merkle EM. Endovascular treatment of visceral artery aneurysms. *J Endovasc Ther*. 2002;9:38–47.
37. Jorgensen BA. Visceral artery aneurysms: a review. *Dan Med Bull*. 1985;32: 237–242.
38. Panayiotopoulos YP, Assadourian R, Taylor PR. Aneurysms of the visceral and renal arteries. *Ann Roy Coll Engl*. 1996;412–419.
39. Pilleul F, Dugougeat F. Transcatheter embolization of splanchnic aneurysms/pseudoaneurysms: Early imaging allows detection of incomplete procedure. *J Comput Assist Tomogr*. 2002;26:107–112.
40. Rokke O, Sondenaa K, Amundsen SR, et al. Successful management of eleven splanchnic artery aneurysms. *Eur J Surg*. 1997;163:411–417.
41. **Shanley CJ, Shah NL, Messina LM: Common splanchnic artery aneurysms: splanic, hepatic and celiac. *Ann Vasc Surg*. 1996;10:315–322.**
42. **Shanley CJ, Shah NL, Messina LM. Uncommon splanchnic artery aneurysms: Pancreaticoduodenal, gastroduodenal, superior mesenteric, inferior mesenteric and celiac. *Ann Vasc Surg*. 1996;10:506–515.**
43. Wagner WH, Allins AD, Treiman RL, et al. Ruptured visceral artery aneurysms. *Ann Vasc Surg*. 1997;11:342–347.
44. Stanley JC, Fry WJ. Pathogenesis and clinical significance of splenic artery aneurysms. *Surgery* 1974;76:898–909.
45. **Stanley JC, Thompson NW, Fry WJ. Splanchnic artery aneurysms. *Arch Surg*. 1970;101:689–697.**
46. Lee PC, Rhee RY, Gordon RY, et al. Management of splenic artery aneurysms: the significance of portal and essential hypertension. *J Am Coll Surg*. 1999;189:483–490.
47. Puttini M, Aseni P, Brambilla G, et al. Splenic artery aneurysms in portal hypertension. *J Cardiovasc Surg*. 1982;23:490–493.
48. Nishida O, Moriyasu F, Nakamura T, et al. Hemodynamics of splenic artery aneurysm. *Gastroenterology* 1986;90:1042–1046.
49. Ohta M. Hashizume M, Ueno K, et al. Hemodynamic study of splenic artery aneurysm in portal hypertension. *Hepatogastroenterology* 1994;41:181–184.
50. Ayalon A, Wiesner RH, Perkins JD, et al. Splenic artery aneurysms in liver transplant patients. *Transplantation* 1988;45:386–389.
51. Bronsther O, Merhav H, Van Thiel D, Starzl TE. Splenic artery aneurysms occurring in liver transplant recipients. *Transplantation* 1991;52:723–724.
52. Kobori L, van der Kolk MJ, de Jong KP, et al. Splenic artery aneurysms in liver transplant patients. Liver Transplant Group. *J Hepatol*. 1997;27: 890–893.
53. Robertson AJ, Rela M, Karani J, Heaton ND. Splenic artery aneurysm and orthotopic liver transplantation. *Transplant Internat*. 1999;12:68–70.
54. Ailawadi G, Cowles RA, Stanley JC, et al. Common celiacomesenteric trunk: Aneurysmal and occlusive disease. *J Vasc Surg*. 2004;40:1040–1043.
55. Settembrini PG, Jausseran JM, Roveri S, et al. Aneurysms of anomalous splenomesenteric trunk: clinical features and surgical management in two cases. *J Vasc Surg*. 1996;24:687–692.
56. Ishida H, Konno K, Hamashima Y, et al. Splenic artery aneurysm: value of color Doppler and the limitation of gray-scale ultrasonography. *Abdom Imag*. 1998;23:627–632.
57. Martin KW, Morian JP Jr, Lee JK, et al. Demonstration of a splenic pseudoaneurysm by MR imaging. *J Comput Assist Tomogr*. 1985;9: 190–192.
58. De Vries JE, Schattenkerk ME, Malt RA. Complications of splenic artery aneurysm other than intraperitoneal rupture. *Surgery* 1982;91:200–204.
59. Harper PC, Gamelli RL, Kaye MD. Recurrent hemorrhage into the pancreatic duct from a splenic aneurysm. *Gastroenterology* 1984;87:417–420.
60. Stabile BE, Wilson SE, Debas HT. Reduced mortality from bleeding pseudocysts and pseudoaneurysms caused by pancreatitis. *Arch Surg*. 1983;118:45–51.

61. Stanley JC, Frey CF, Miller TA, et al. Major arterial hemorrhage: a complication of pancreatic pseudocysts and chronic pancreatitis. *Arch Surg.* 1976;111:435–440.
62. Wagner WH, Cossman DV, Treiman RL, et al. Hemosuccus pancreaticus from intraductal rupture of a primary splenic artery aneurysm. *J Vasc Surg.* 1994;19:158–164.
63. Brothers TE, Stanley JC, Zelenock GB: Splenic arteriovenous fistula: Review of the literature with four new case reports. *Int Surg.* 1995;80:189–194.
64. Gaglio PJ, Regenstein F, Slakey D, et al. Alpha-1 antitrypsin deficiency and splenic artery aneurysm rupture. An association? *Am J Gastroenterol.* 2000;95:1531–1534.
65. Angelakis EJ, Bair WE, Barone JE, et al. Splenic artery aneurysm rupture during pregnancy. *Obstet Gynecol.* 1993;48:145–148.
66. Lowry SM, O'Dea TP, Gallagher DI, et al. Splenic artery aneurysm rupture: the seventh instance of maternal and fetal survival. *Obstet Gynecol.* 1986; 67:291–292.
67. Macfarlane JR, Thorbjarnarson B. Rupture of splenic artery aneurysm during pregnancy. *Am J Obstet Gynecol.* 1966;95:1025–1037.
68. O'Grady JP, Day EJ, Toole AL, et al. Splenic artery aneurysm rupture in pregnancy. A review and case report. *Obstet Gynecol.* 1977;50:627–630.
69. Caillouette JC, Merchant EB. Ruptured splenic artery aneurysm in pregnancy. Twelfth reported case with maternal and fetal survival. *Am J Obstet Gynecol.* 1993;168:1810–1813.
70. Taylor JL, Woodward DA. Splenic conservation and the management of splenic artery aneurysm. *Ann R Coll Surg Engl.* 1987;69:179–180.
71. Arca MJ, Gagner M, Heniford BT, et al. Splenic artery aneurysms: methods of laparoscopic repair. *J Vasc Surg.* 1999;30:184–188.
72. Hashizume M, Ohta M, Ueno K, et al. Laparoscopic ligation of splenic artery aneurysm. *Surgery* 1993;113:352–354.
73. Hashizume M, Ohta M, Ueno K, et al. Laparoscopic ligation of splenic artery aneurysm. *Surgery* 1993;113:352–354.
74. de Perrot M, Buhler L, Schneider PA, et al. Do aneurysms and pseudoaneurysms of the splenic artery require different surgical strategy? *Hepatogastroenterology* 1999;46:2028–2032.
75. Baker KS, Tisnado J, Cho SR, et al. Splanchnic artery aneurysms and pseudoaneurysms: transcatheter embolization. *Radiology* 1987;163: 135–139.
76. McDermott VG, Shlansky-Goldberg R, Cope C. Endovascular management of splenic artery aneurysms and pseudoaneurysms. *Cardiovasc Intervent Radiol.* 1994; 17:179–184.
77. Salam TA, Lumsden AB, Martin LG, et al. Nonoperative management of visceral aneurysms and pseudoaneurysms. *Am J Surg.* 1992;164:215–219.
78. Waltman AC, Luers PR, Athanasoulis CA, et al. Massive arterial hemorrhage in patients with pancreatitis: complementary roles of surgery and transcatheter occlusive techniques. *Arch Surg.* 1986;121:439–443.
79. Takahashi T, Shimada K, Kobayashi N, et al: Migration of steel-wire coils into the stomach after transcatheter arterial embolization for a bleeding splenic artery pseudoaneurysm: Report of a case. *Surg Today.* 2001;31: 458–462.
80. Wholey MH, Chamorro HA, Rao G, et al. Splenic infarction and spontaneous rupture of the spleen after therapeutic embolization. *Cardiovasc Radiol.* 1978;1:249–253.
81. Arepally A, Dagli M, Hofmann LV, et al. Treatment of splenic artery aneurysm with use of stent-graft. *J Vasc Interv Radiol.* 2002;13:631–633.
82. Brountzos EN, Vagenas K, Apostolopoulou SC, et al. Pancreatitis-associated splenic artery pseudoaneurysm: Endovascular treatment with self-expandable stent-grafts. *Cardiovasc Intervent Radiol.* 2003;26:88–91.
83. Yoon H-K, Lindh M, Uher P, et al. Stent-graft repair of a splenic artery aneurysm. *Cardiovascular Intervent Radiol.* 2001;24: 200–203.
84. *Guida PM, Moore SW.* Aneurysm of the hepatic artery: report of five cases with a brief review of the previously reported cases. Surgery 1966;60:299–310.
85. Lumsden AB, Mattar SG, Allen RC, et al. Hepatic artery aneurysms: The management of 22 patients. *J Surg Res.* 1996; 60:345–350.
86. **Abbas MA, Fowl RJ, Stone WM, et al. Hepatic artery aneurysm. Factors that predict complications. *J Vasc Surg.* 2003;38:41–45.**
87. Czerniak A, Thompson JN, Hemingway AP, et al. Hemobilia: a disease in evolution. *Arch Surg.* 1988;23:718–721.
88. Okazaki M, Higashihara H, Ono H, et al. Percutaneous embolization of ruptured splanchnic artery pseudoaneurysms. *Acta Radiol.*1991;32:349–354.
89. Parangi S, Oz MC, Blume RS, et al. Hepatobiliary complications of polyarteritis nodosa. *Arch Surg.* 1991;126:909–912.
90. Stauffer JT, Weinman MD, Bynum TE. Hemobilia in a patient with multiple hepatic artery aneurysms: a case report and review of the literature. *Am J Gastroenterol.* 1989;84:59–62.
91. Kadir S, Athanasoulis CA, Ring EJ, et al. Transcatheter embolization of intrahepatic arterial aneurysms. *Radiology* 1980;134:335–339.
92. Thibodeaux LC, Deshmukh RM, Hearn AT, et al. Management options for hepatic artery aneurysms. *Ann Vasc Surg.* 1995;9:285–288.
93. Patel JV, Weston MJ, Kessel DO, et al. Hepatic artery pseudoaneurysm after liver transplantation: treatment with percutaneous thrombin injection. *Transplantation* 2003;75:1755–1757.
94. Bürger T, Halloul Z, Meyer F, et al. Emergency stent-graft repair of a ruptured hepatic artery secondary to local postoperative peritonitis. *J Endovasc Ther.* 2000;7:324–327.
95. **Larson RA, Solomon J, Carpenter JP: Stent graft repair of visceral artery aneurysms. *J Vasc Surg.* 2002;36:1260–1263.**
96. Friedman SG, Pogo GJ, Moccio CG. Mycotic aneurysm of the superior mesenteric artery. *J Vasc Surg.* 1987;6:87–90.
97. Stone WM, Abbas M, Cherry KJ, et al. Superior mesenteric artery aneurysms: Is presence an indication for intervention? *J Vasc Surg.* 2002; 36:234–237.
98. Cormier F, Ferry J, Artru B, et al. Dissecting aneurysms of the main trunk of the superior mesenteric artery. *J Vasc Surg.* 1992;15:424–430.
99. Blumenberg RM, David D, Slovak J. Abdominal apoplexy due to rupture of a superior mesenteric artery aneurysm: clip aneurysmorrhaphy with survival. *Arch Surg.* 1974;108:223–226.
100. Olcott C, Ehrenfeld WK. Endoaneurysmorrhaphy for visceral artery aneurysms. *Am J Surg.* 1977;133:636–639.
101. DeBakey ME, Cooley DA. Successful resection of mycotic aneurysm of superior mesenteric artery: case report and review of the literature. *Am J Surg.* 1953;19:202.
102. Geelkerken RH, van Bockel JH, de Roos WK, et al. Surgical treatment of intestinal artery aneurysms. *Eur J Vasc Surg.* 1990;4:563–567.
103. Kopatsis A, D'Anna JA, Sithian N, et al. Superior mesenteric artery aneurysm: 45 years later. *Am Surg.* 1998;64:263–266.
104. Appel N, Duncan JR, Schuerer DJE. Percutaneous stent-graft treatment of superior mesenteric and internal iliac artery pseudoaneurysms. *J Vasc Interv Radiol.* 2003;14:917–922.
105. Cowan S, Kahn MB, Bonn J, et al. Superior mesenteric artery pseudoaneurysm successfully treated with polytetrafluoroethylene covered stent. *J Vasc Surg.* 2002;35:805–807.
106. Hama Y, Iwasaki Y, Kaji T, et al. Coil compaction after embolization of the superior mesenteric artery pseudoaneurysm. *Eur Radiol.* 2002; 12(suppl 3):S189–191.
107. **Graham LM, Stanley JC, Whitehouse WM Jr, et al. Celiac artery aneurysms: historical (1745–1949) versus contemporary (1950–1984) differences in etiology and clinical importance. *J Vasc Surg.* 1985;2: 757–764.**
108. Stone WM, Abbas MA, Gloviczki P, et al. Celiac arterial aneurysms. *Arch Surg.* 2002;137:670–674.
109. Hertzer NR, Mullally PH. Celiac artery aneurysmectomy with hepatic artery ligation. *Arch Surg.* 1972;104:337–339.
110. Parfitt J, Chalmers RT, Wolfe JH. Visceral aneurysms in Ehlers-Danlos syndrome: Case report and review of the literature. *J Vasc Surg.* 2000;31:1248–1251.
111. Schoder M, Cejna M, Langle F, et al. Glue embolization of a ruptured celiac trunk pseudoaneurysm via the gastroduodenal artery. *Eur Radiol.* 2000;10:1335–1337.
112. Funahashi S, Yukizane T, Yano K, et al. An aneurysm of the right gastroepiploic artery. *J Cardiovasc Surg.* 1997;38:385–388.
113. Jacobs PP, Croiset van Ughelen FA, Bruyninckx CA, Hoefsloot F. Haemoperitoneum caused by a dissection aneurysm of the gastroepiploic artery. *Eur J Vasc Surg.* 1994;8:236–237.
114. Witte JT, Hasson JE, Harms BA, et al. Fatal gastric dissection and rupture occurring as a paraesophageal mass: a case report and literature review. *Surgery* 1990;107:590–594.
115. Uchikoshi F, Sakamoto T, Imabunn S, et al. Aneurysm of the right gastroepiploic artery: a case report of laporoscopic resection. *Cardiovasc Surg.* 1993;1:550–551.
116. Trevisani MF, Ricci MA, Michaels RM, et al. Multiple mesenteric aneurysms complicating subacute bacterial endocarditis. *Arch Surg.* 1987; 122:823–824.
117. Sellke FW, Williams GB, Donovan DL, et al. Management of intra-abdominal aneurysms associated with periarteritis nodosa. *J Vasc Surg.* 1986;4:294–298.
118. Sarcina A, Bellosta R, Magnaldi S, et al. Aneurysm of the middle colic artery—case report and literature review. *Eur J Vasc Endovasc Surg.* 2000;20:198–200.
119. Naito A, Toyota N, Ito K. Embolization of a ruptured middle colic artery aneurysm. *Cardiovasc Intervent Radiol.* 1995;18:56–58.
120. Graham LM, Hay MR, Cho KJ, et al. Inferior mesenteric artery aneurysms. *Surgery* 1985;97:158–163.
121. Raso AM, Rispoli P, Maggio D, et al. Post stenotic aneurysm of the interior mesenteric artery: case report and discussion. *J Cardiovasc Surg.* 1996;37:359–362.
122. **Coll DP, Ierardi R, Kerstein MD, et al. Aneurysms of the pancreaticoduodenal arteries: A change in management. *Ann Vasc Surg.* 1998;12: 286–291.**
123. Suzuki K, Kashimura H, Sato M, et al. Pancreaticoduodenal artery aneurysms associated with celiac axis stenosis due to compression by median arcuate ligament and celiac plexus. *J Gastroenterol.* 1998;33: 434–438.
124. Gouny P, Fukui S, Aymard A, et al. Aneurysm of the gastroduodenal artery associated with stenosis of the superior mesenteric artery. *Ann Vasc Surg.* 1994;8:281–284.
125. de Perrot M, Berney T, Deleaval J. Management of true aneurysms of the pancreaticoduodenal arteries. *Ann Surg.* 1999;229:416–420.
126. **Eckhauser FE, Stanley JC, Zelenock GB, et al. Gastroduodenal and pancreaticoduodenal artery aneurysms: a complication of pancreatitis causing spontaneous gastrointestinal hemorrhage. *Surgery* 1980;88:335–344.**

127. Chiou AC, Josephs LG, Menzoian JO. Inferior pancreaticoduodenal artery aneurysm: report of a case and review of the literature. *J Vasc Surg*. 1993; 17:784–789.
128. Gadacz TR, Trunkey D, Kieffer RF. Visceral vessel erosion associated with pancreatitis: case reports and a review of the literature. *Arch Surg*. 1978; 113:1438–1440.
129. Iyomasa S, Matsuzaki Y, Hiei K, et al. Pancreaticoduodenal artery aneurysm: a case report and review of the literature. *J Vasc Surg*. 1995; 22:161–166.
130. Carr JA, Cho JS, Shepard AD, et al. Visceral psuedoaneurysms due to pancreatic pseudocysts: Rare but lethal complications of pancreatitis. *J Vasc Surg*. 2000;32:722–730.
131. Mandel SR, Jaques PF, Mauro MA, et al. Nonoperative management of peripancreatic arterial aneurysms: a 10-year experience. *Ann Surg*. 1987;205:126–128.
132. Nyman U, Svendsen P, Jivegard L, et al. Multiple pancreaticoduodenal aneurysms: treatment with superior mesenteric artery stent-graft placement and distal embolization. *J Vasc Interv Radiol*. 11:1201–1205.
133. Thakker RV, Gajjar B, Wilkins RA, et al. Embolization of gastroduodenal artery aneurysm caused by chronic pancreatitis. *Gut* 1983;24: 1094–1098.
134. Vujic I, Anderson MC, Meredith HC, et al. Successful embolization of the dorsal pancreatic artery to control massive upper gastrointestinal hemorrhage. *Ann Surg*. 1980;46:184–186.
135. Manazer JR, Monzon JR, Dietz PA, et al. Treatment of pancreatic pseudoaneurysm with percutaneous transabdominal thrombin injection. *J Vasc Surg*. 2003;38:600–602.
136. McIntyre TP, Simone ST, Stahlfeld KR. Intraoperative thrombin occlusion of a visceral artery aneurysm. *J Vasc Surg*. 2002;36:393–395.

CHAPTER 95 ■ AORTOILIAC DISEASE

DANIEL J. REDDY AND ALEXANDER D. SHEPARD

Atherosclerotic occlusive disease of the aorta and iliac arteries is one of the most common problems encountered by vascular surgeons. Alone or in combination with more common femoropopliteal or tibial occlusive disease, it is the most frequent cause of chronic lower extremity arterial insufficiency. Because a greater number of muscle groups are affected by aortoiliac atherosclerosis than by infrainguinal disease, the resulting symptoms may be particularly disabling. The treatment of symptomatic aortoiliac disease also represents one of the major success stories of modern vascular surgery. Since the first reconstructive procedures on the abdominal aorta were performed nearly five decades ago, treatment has undergone significant progress. Advances in noninvasive vascular diagnosis, arteriography, preoperative assessment,anesthesia, and critical care in addition to those in surgical technique have contributed to improved outcomes. Reconstructive procedures for aortoiliac disease have become routine, with low perioperative morbidity and mortality and excellent early and long-term outcomes. The excellent durability of such reconstructions is undoubtedly in large part related to the large caliber and high flow rates of the vessels involved.

Depending on the pattern of the occlusive process and patient risk, a variety of revascularization techniques are currently available. Selection of a patient-specific treatment strategy from an increasing array of alternatives, although challenging, frequently will alleviate symptoms, avoid an amputation, and prevent or reverse organ dysfunction.

ANATOMY

The arteries supplying blood to the lower extremities are frequently divided into abdominal, or "inflow," arteries (the aorta and iliac arteries) and infrainguinal, or "outflow," arteries (the femoropopliteal and tibial arteries). The aorta enters the abdomen from the chest through the aortic hiatus, located between the 12th thoracic and first lumbar vertebrae, and ends at the level of the fourth lumbar vertebra, where it bifurcates into the right and left common iliac arteries. This terminal bifurcation roughly corresponds to the level of the umbilicus. Each common iliac artery curves posteriorly into the sacral hollow and divides into an internal and an external iliac branch. The external iliac then curves anteriorly and continues along the psoas muscle under the inguinal ligament to become the common femoral artery, which in turn bifurcates into the superficial and deep (profunda) femoral arteries. The internal iliac (hypogastric) artery follows the curve of the pelvic side wall and branches repeatedly to supply the pelvic viscera and gluteal musculature (Fig. 95.1).

The branches of the abdominal aorta can be divided in three groups:

1. Three unpaired arteries to the gut arise from its anterior wall; the celiac trunk supplies the foregut, the superior mesenteric artery supplies the midgut, and the inferior mesenteric perfuses the hindgut.
2. Arteries to the three paired genitourinary glands arise close together from the lateral wall of the aorta—the adrenal, renal, and gonadal branches.
3. Branches to the "roof" and walls of the abdominal cavity include the phrenic, lumbar, and median sacral arteries. These branches assume varying degrees of importance in the formation of collateral perfusion channels around occlusive lesions in the aorta and iliac arteries.

Because the abdominal aorta and its iliac branches are retroperitoneal structures coursing through the deepest portions of the abdominal cavity, a sophisticated operative technique is required to expose them. The proximal (suprarenal) abdominal aorta is rendered particularly inaccessible by the overlying stomach, pancreas, and colon. Occlusive lesions of this portion of the aorta are relatively uncommon, however, in comparison with those of the distal (infrarenal) aorta. The crossing left renal vein serves as a useful surgical landmark defining the usual boundary between these two segments of the abdominal aorta. Although transabdominal exposure of the infrarenal aorta is fairly routine, it requires reflection of the transverse colon superiorly and of the small bowel and its mesentery and distal duodenum to the right. The iliac bifurcations can also be difficult to expose because of their location deep in

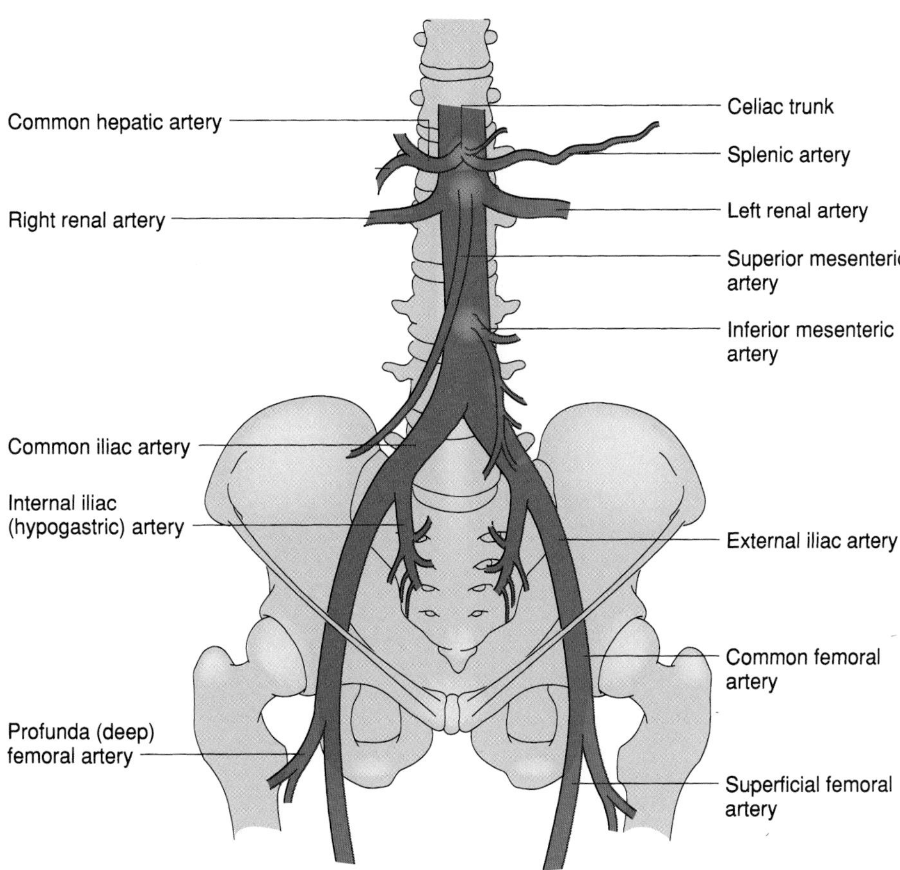

FIGURE 95.1 Anatomy of the abdominal aorta and iliac arteries.

the pelvis; in addition, the bifurcation of the left iliac artery lies directly behind the sigmoid colon.

PATHOPHYSIOLOGY

Although atherosclerosis is a generalized disease, the earliest and most severe lesions tend to occur at arterial bifurcations and in areas of relative fixation, where the disruption of normal laminar flow is greatest. The aortic bifurcation is in fact the location where the earliest atherosclerotic changes are first noted in most young adults. In persons predisposed to the development of more advanced disease, plaque gradually extends proximally into the infrarenal aorta and distally into the common iliac arteries, usually along the posterior wall first. With progressive worsening of the occlusive process, hemodynamic alterations lead to the enlargement of a network of auxiliary or collateral channels around the involved segments. Important collateral arterial pathways around the aortic bifurcation and common iliac segments are the intercostal and lumbar arteries to circumflex iliac and iliolumbar arteries, the superior to inferior epigastric arteries, and the superior and inferior mesenteric arteries to rectal and internal pudendal arteries. Collateral pathways around occlusive lesions of the external iliac arteries include the hypogastric-to-circumflex femoral channels (Figs. 95.2 and 95.3).

With slowly developing occlusive lesions, this collateral network is usually sufficient to provide enough blood flow to meet the resting metabolic needs of the lower extremities. These channels, however, do not have the capacity to increase blood flow to the levels necessary to meet the exercise demands of the leg musculature. *Claudication* (from the Latin verb *claudicare*, "to limp") is the term used to denote the characteristic exercise-induced, cramping pain in the muscles of the lower extremity that results. With acute arterial occlusions and multiple-level disease (occlusive disease in both the aortoiliac and infrainguinal segments), collateral pathways may be inadequate to meet even the basal metabolic needs of nonexercising tissue. The outcome is critical limb ischemia associated with pain at rest, tissue loss (gangrene, nonhealing ulceration), and threatened limb viability.

PRESENTATION

The risk factors for aortoiliac occlusive disease are those for atherosclerosis in general—smoking, hypertension, lipid abnormalities, diabetes mellitus, male sex, older age, and genetic predisposition. Smoking appears to be a particularly important risk factor for the development of lower extremity atherosclerotic occlusive disease.[1] Patients with symptoms of aortoiliac occlusive disease usually present in their 50s and 60s, whereas patients with symptoms of infrainguinal disease are generally in their 70s.[2] Patients with critical limb ischemia secondary to multiple-level disease are also generally in this older age group.

Claudication is the most common presenting symptom of patients with significant aortoiliac disease. Induced by ambulation and quickly relieved by rest, claudication is usually described as a cramping pain, tiredness, or easy fatigability of the involved muscle groups. Although patients with aortoiliac disease classically present with claudication of the thighs, hips, and buttocks, a significant minority may complain of only calf claudication. Erectile dysfunction in men secondary to reduced hypogastric perfusion is another common complaint.

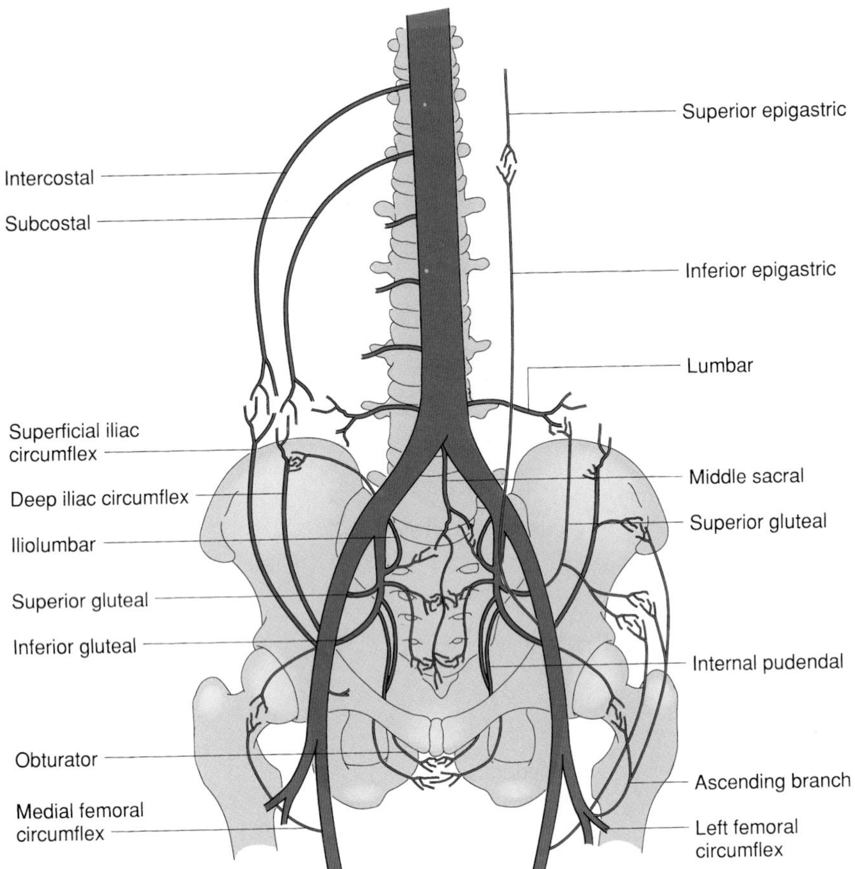

FIGURE 95.2 Major pathways of parietal–visceral collateral circulation in aortoiliac occlusive disease.

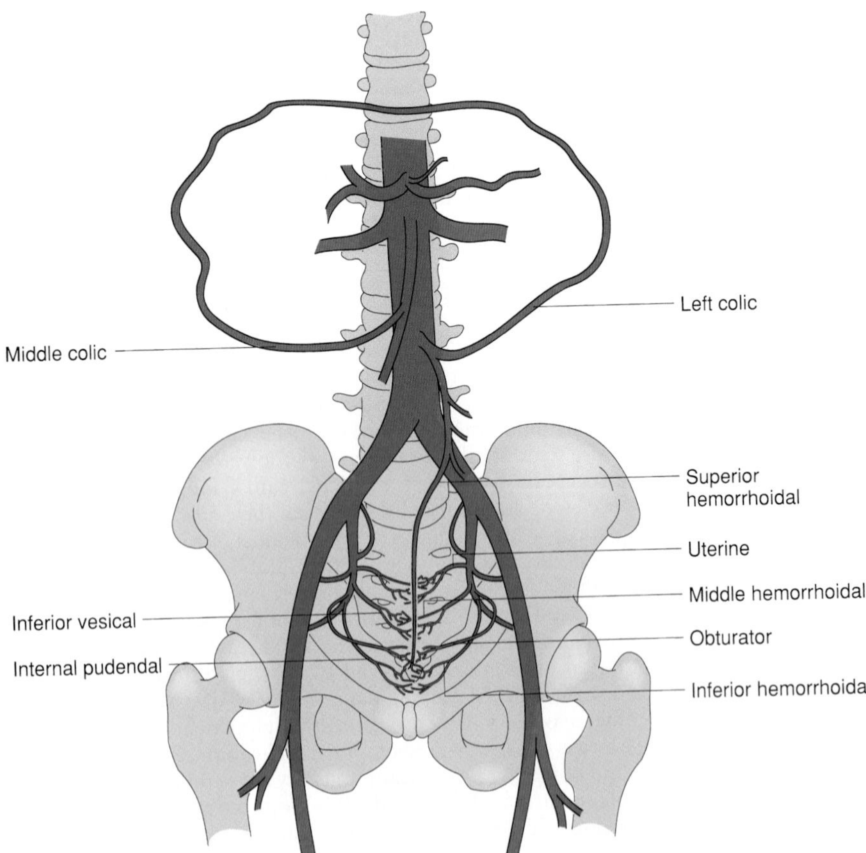

FIGURE 95.3 Major visceral collateral network available to compensate for occlusive aortoiliac disease.

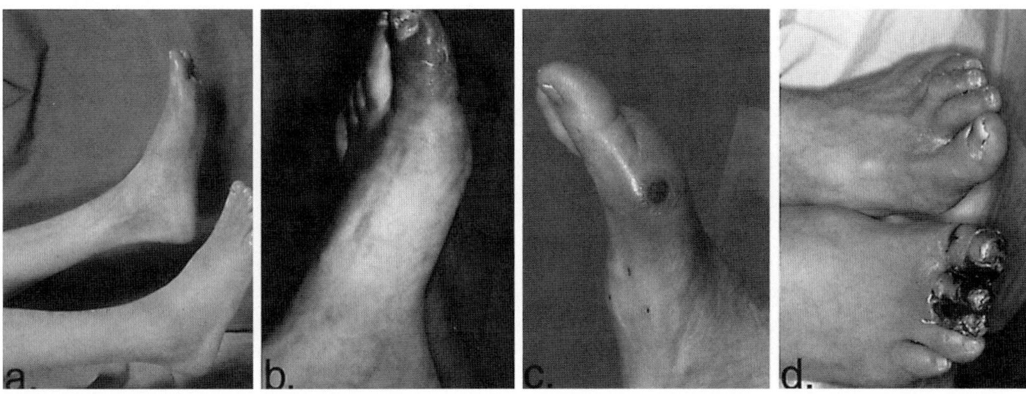

FIGURE 95.4 Clinical manifestations of critical limb ischemia. (*A*) Patient with ischemic rest pain. Note the absence of hair on the atrophic shiny skin of the feet and the rubor at dependency. (*B*) First-toe ischemia and dermal discoloration of blue-toe syndrome. (*C*) Ischemic ulceration. (*D*) Digital gangrene.

The combination of bilateral lower extremity claudication, atrophy of the leg muscles, impotence, and diminished or absent femoral pulses is known as "Leriche's syndrome," after the French physician who first described these classic manifestations of aortoiliac disease.[3] Critical limb ischemia associated with rest pain or tissue loss may be a manifestation of aortoiliac occlusive disease but almost always occurs in combination with more distal femoropopliteal disease (Fig. 95.4). In the absence of infrainguinal disease, aortoiliac collaterals are almost always able to maintain adequate resting tissue perfusion. An exception to this rule is atheroembolic disease, or "blue toe" syndrome. Degenerative plaque(s) in the aortoiliac (or any proximal arterial) segment can ulcerate or rupture to release platelet microthrombi and atheromatous debris into the arterial lumen. Downstream embolization into the microcirculation of the lower extremities can produce digital ischemia and gangrene and dermal discoloration in a characteristic reticular pattern (livedo reticularis) (Fig. 95.4). Such patients usually have palpable pedal pulses.

Physical examination typically reveals diminished or absent femoral pulses. Severely diseased, calcified femoral arteries may be palpable as firm, tubular masses. Normal femoral and distal pulses may be palpable, however, even in the presence of hemodynamically significant aortoiliac stenoses. Such pulses rapidly disappear following ambulation as the increased flow demands of the exercising leg muscles lead to lowered peripheral vascular resistance. Bruits heard over the lower abdomen or groins suggest the presence of turbulent flow resulting from occlusive plaque. Patients with long-standing aortoiliac atherosclerosis may have disuse atrophy of the lower extremity musculature. Other common signs of lower extremity arterial occlusive disease include trophic changes, such as hair loss on the legs or toes and thin, shiny skin on the feet, in addition to rubor on limb dependency coupled with pallor on elevation. Such chronic advanced changes in addition to gangrene and nonhealing ulceration(s) are unusual in the absence of multiple-level disease.

Different patterns of aortoiliac disease have been identified on preoperative arteriographic studies (Fig. 95.5).[4] Disease confined to the distal infrarenal aorta and common iliac arteries, classified as type I, accounts for only 10% of patients with inflow disease. Patients with type I disease are younger and more frequently female than patients with other forms of aortoiliac disease, and they usually present with complaints of disabling claudication in the buttocks, hips, and thighs.[5] Such localized disease may be amenable to endarterectomy or percutaneous transluminal angioplasty. More extensive disease is the rule; atherosclerotic plaque extends distally into the external iliac artery and not infrequently to the common femoral bifurcation in more than 80% of patients. In somewhat less than half this group, no significant occlusive disease is present in the femoropopliteal and tibial segments (type II disease) (Fig. 95.6). Such patients experience worse claudication than persons with more localized, type I disease. In the remaining patients, occlusive disease in the aortoiliac segment is combined with femoropopliteal or tibial disease (type III disease) (Fig. 95.7). As outlined previously, patients with such multiple-level disease are usually older than those in the other two groups and more frequently present with symptoms of critical limb ischemia.

In all three groups, the atherosclerotic process progresses unpredictably, but the end result in a small percentage of patients (approximately 5% to 6% in our experience) is occlusion of the terminal infrarenal aorta with propagation of clot proximally to the levels of the renal arteries (Fig. 95.8 and 95.9). In the absence of significant renal artery stenoses, propagation proximally to the renal arteries is an unusual event. One other pattern worthy of mention is aortoiliac hypoplasia, an uncommon variant usually encountered in young to middle-aged women who smoke cigarettes. The infrarenal aorta and iliac arteries are unusually small in caliber and hence prone to significant narrowing, even with modest disease. Operative treatment in such patients can be particularly challenging.

EVALUATION

In the overwhelming majority of cases, a diagnosis of significant aortoiliac occlusive disease can be made on the basis of the history and physical examination alone. A clinical diagnosis can and should be supplemented by noninvasive vascular testing. Such testing provides valuable information to the treating clinician by confirming the presence of disease and objectively documenting the degree of ischemia and the arterial segment(s) involved. A baseline is established according to which the patient can be followed and interventions planned. Treatment results can be assessed by repeated testing. Such information is particularly useful in a patient with an equivocal history or pulse examination. Arteriography can then be reserved for those patients considered suitable candidates for operative or endovascular (catheter-based) intervention.

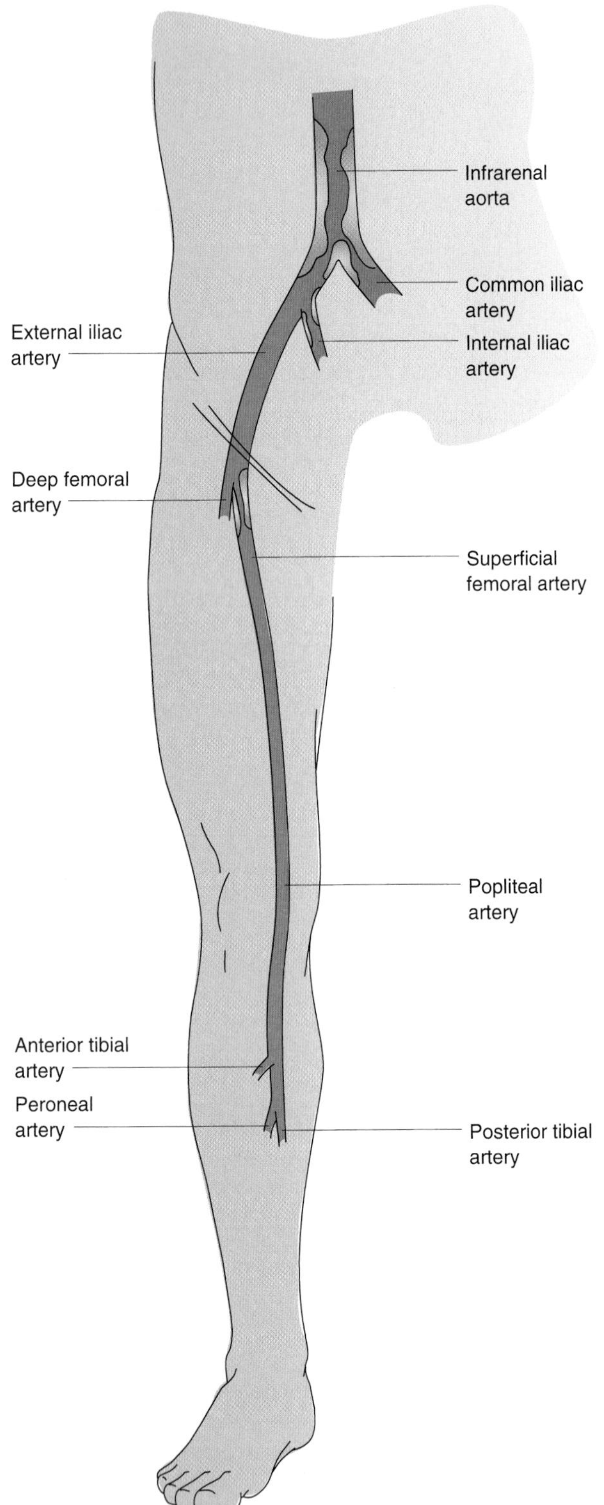

FIGURE 95.5 Common sites of arteriosclerotic lesions in aortoiliofemoral occlusive disease. Although often a generalized process, partially segmental distribution of major disease, most prominent at arterial bifurcations, usually allows surgical revascularization.

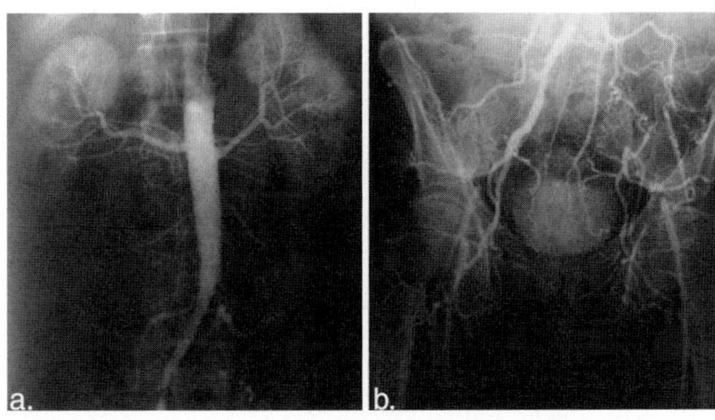

FIGURE 95.6 Abdominal aortograms demonstrating type II disease. Left common and external iliac occlusion can be seen, with reconstitution of the ipsilateral internal iliac and common femoral arteries through visceral and lumbar collaterals. The right external iliac artery is also occluded, and the right common femoral artery is reconstituted through right hypogastric-to-circumflex femoral channels.

Segmental Pressure Measurements

Measurement of the systolic arterial pressures at different levels of the lower extremity with a hand-held, pencil-sized, continuous-wave Doppler flow probe is the simplest and most useful noninvasive method to assess arterial occlusive disease. The ratio of the ankle systolic pressure to the brachial systolic pressure is the ankle–brachial index (ABI), or pressure ratio, and is a good indicator of the degree of ischemia present. With the Doppler probe used as an ultrasonic stethoscope, the systolic pressures in the dorsalis pedis and posterior tibial artery are measured at the ankle, and each of these values is then the numerator of a simple fraction in which the higher of the two brachial pressures is the denominator. Normal ABIs are generally equal to or slightly greater than 1. Patients with claudication usually have ABIs ranging from 0.5 to 0.9, whereas patients with rest pain and tissue loss have ABIs of less than 0.5.

Determination of limb systolic pressures at different locations (with the "four-cuff" technique, pressures are measured at the upper thigh, lower thigh, calf, and ankle) provides information about which arterial segment(s) are involved with occlusive disease (Figs. 95.10 and 95.11). A pressure drop of more than

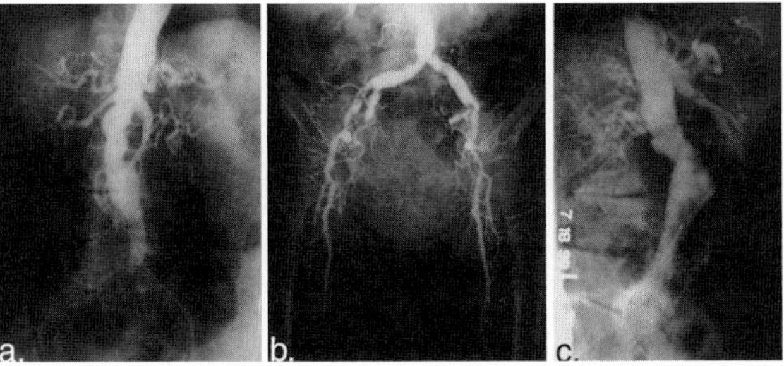

FIGURE 95.7 Abdominal aortograms demonstrating type III disease. (*A*) Extensive atherosclerotic disease has produced both ulcerated plaques and aneurysmal degeneration in the aorta and common iliac arteries bilaterally. (*B*) Preocclusive stenoses in the proximal right external and internal iliac arteries and in the left internal iliac artery. (*C*) The superficial femoral arteries are occluded bilaterally.

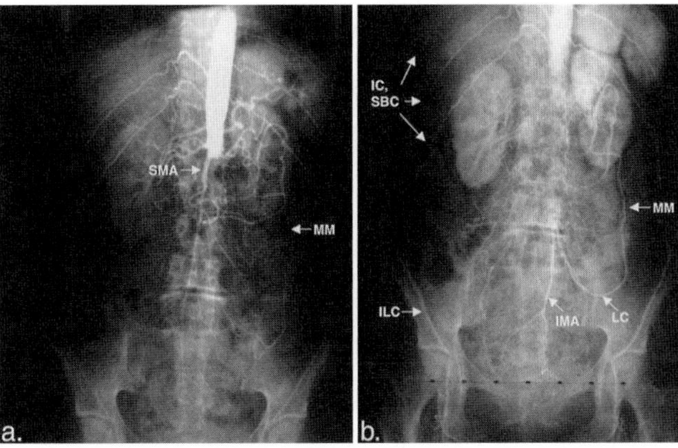

FIGURE 95.8 Abdominal aortograms demonstrating juxtarenal aortic occlusion and an extensive collateral network reconstituting the femoral arterial segments. SMA, superior mesenteric artery; MM, meandering mesenteric, IC, intercostal; SBC, subcostal; ILC, iliac circumflex; IMA, inferior mesenteric artery; LC, left colic.

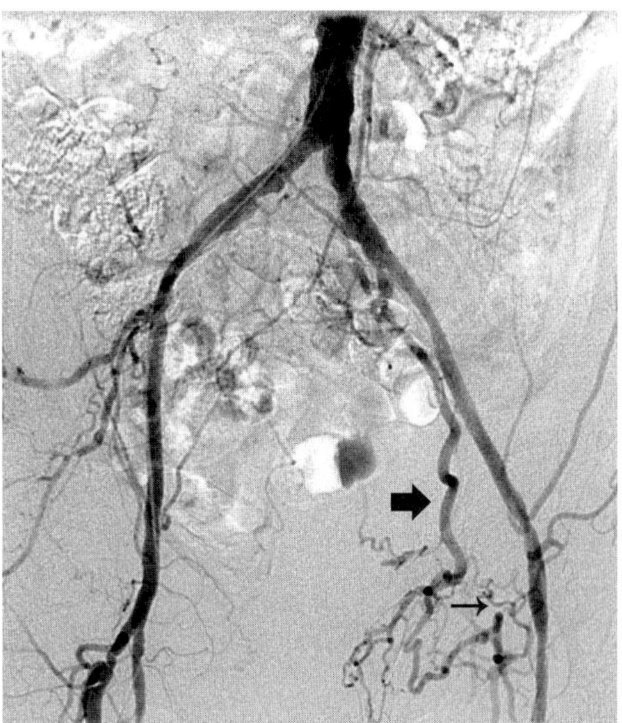

FIGURE 95.9 Pelvic aortogram showing a large collateral from the left hypogastric artery to left profunda artery.

20 mm Hg between consecutive levels is indicative of significant disease within the intervening arterial segment. A reduced upper thigh pressure signifies occlusive disease in the aortoiliac or common femoral segments.

In patients with extensive calcification in the walls of the tibial arteries (as is frequently seen in diabetes mellitus or end-stage renal disease), the ankle pressures may not be interpretable because the vessels are too "stiff" to be compressed by the externally applied cuff. In this situation, the pressure in the digital arteries of the great toe can be measured because these small vessels are generally spared calcification. A toe pressure of less than 30 mm Hg indicates severe ischemia. Inspection of the Doppler-derived arterial waveforms can provide additional information when tibial vessels are incompressible.

Patients with claudication occasionally have normal or nearly normal ABI. As described previously, in such cases the arterial stenosis is not severe enough to cause a pressure drop while the limb is at rest but does produce a hemodynamic effect under conditions of higher rates of flow, as during exercise. Higher rates of flow through a moderately stenotic segment increase the energy lost at the site, so that a significant distal pressure drop results. Exercise stress testing can be used to evaluate patients suspected of having such disease. ABIs are measured before and after a treadmill exercise protocol; a drop of 15% or more in the ABI following exercise is indicative of hemodynamically significant occlusive disease.

Duplex Scanning

Duplex scanning of the aorta and iliac arteries has been advocated by some as a more precise noninvasive diagnostic tool.[6] Some authorities have even suggested that duplex scanning can be used to plan therapeutic interventions without the need for arteriography. Imaging of the abdominal arteries, however, is difficult because of their deep retroperitoneal and pelvic locations. Many patients are not candidates for such studies because of body habitus and overlying bowel gas; even in experienced hands, this procedure is time-consuming. These problems have limited the widespread use of this modality.

DIFFERENTIAL DIAGNOSIS

The diagnosis of aortoiliac disease is usually straightforward, but occasional diagnostic confusion may arise when other causes of lower extremity pain are present. Irritation of lumbosacral nerve roots by spinal stenosis or intervertebral disk herniation may cause buttock and leg pain that is associated with activity. Such symptoms (neurogenic claudication), however, usually cannot be reproduced at the same level of activity and frequently occur when the patient is standing, so that the patient must sit or lie down to obtain relief. In addition, the pain is usually in a classic sciatic distribution. Degenerative arthritis of the hip joints may produce similar buttock, hip, and referred thigh pain. The physical examination typically reveals pain directly over the hip joint that is exacerbated by movement of the joint. Peripheral neuropathy, particularly that associated with diabetes mellitus, may masquerade as ischemic rest pain. In all these situations, segmental limb pressure measurements, with or without stress testing, can be helpful in determining the contribution of arterial occlusive disease to the patient's symptoms.

TREATMENT

The aims of therapy in aortoiliac occlusive disease are to relieve symptoms and, in cases of critical limb ischemia, prevent limb loss (Algorithm 95.1). Medical therapy should be instituted in all patients with symptomatic disease, but is insufficient as sole therapy in patients with limb-threatening ischemia.

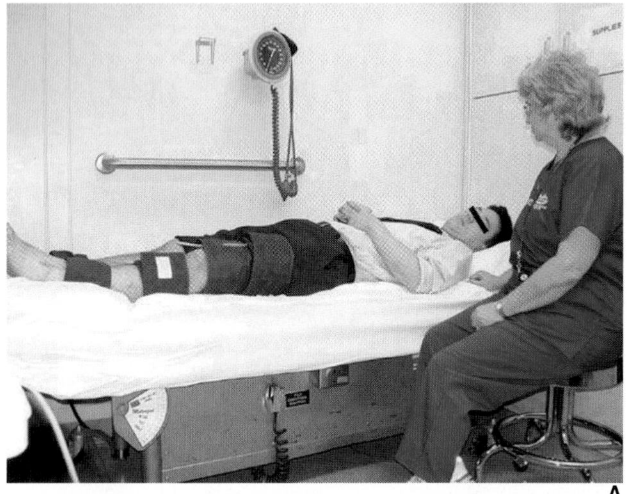

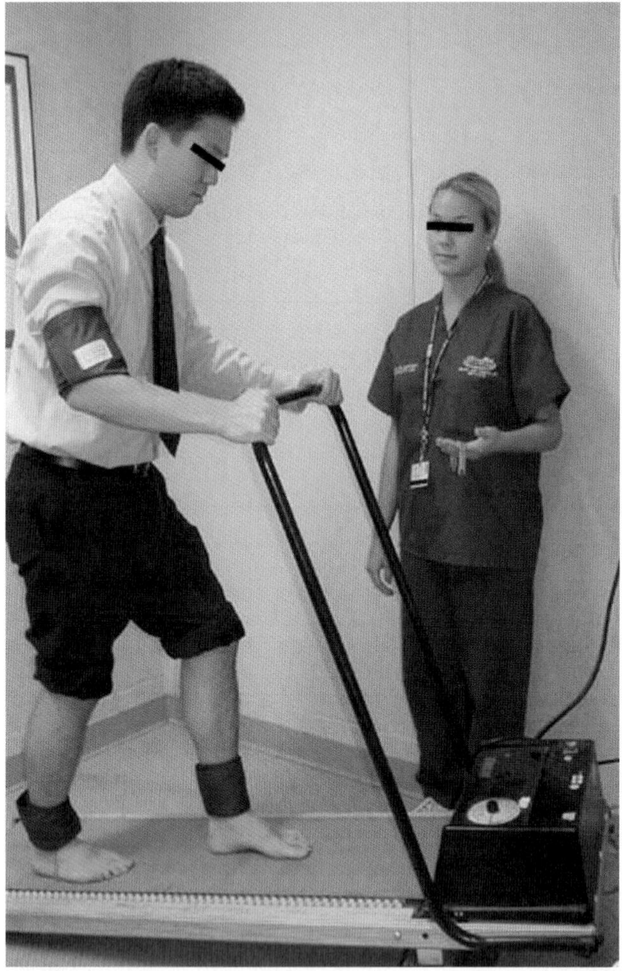

FIGURE 95.10 Noninvasive testing to evaluate lower extremity ischemia. (*A*) Segmental pressure measurements with cuffs placed at the upper thigh, lower thigh, calf, and ankle. (*B*) Stress testing with treadmill ergometry.

Medical Therapy

Risk factor modification, including smoking cessation and the follow-up and treatment of diabetes mellitus, systemic arterial hypertension, and hyperlipidemia should be an important component of primary care for all these patients.[7] Although control of these factors will not reverse the atherosclerotic process, it may limit the progression of disease. Furthermore, some data indicate that smoking cessation lessens the severity of symptoms in many patients. Also, a daily exercise program of regular walking may improve collateral development and increase the anaerobic tolerance of ischemic skeletal muscle. Finally, pharmacotherapy with medications such as pentoxifylline and cilostazol can be a valuable adjunct in selected patients.[8,9] Although the mechanisms of action of these agents are unclear, both have effected a modest but significant reduction in claudication symptoms in controlled trials. Some form of platelet inhibition, usually with aspirin, should also be considered for all patients. Although no specific data have demonstrated that antiplatelet therapy is helpful in the treatment of lower extremity arterial occlusive disease, abundant evidence has shown it to be beneficial in the treatment of atherosclerotic occlusive disease in other vascular territories (e.g., coronary and cerebral vessels).

Revascularization

Indications

Revascularization is clearly indicated in patients with critical limb ischemia; without intervention, the vast majority progress to limb loss in a fairly short period of time. Patients with significant or repetitive atheroembolism from an aortoiliac source represent another group who clearly benefit from operative therapy. Removal or bypass of the culprit lesion(s) eliminates the risk for further macroembolism and microembolism. The treatment for patients with claudication secondary to aortoiliac occlusive disease remains somewhat controversial and must be individualized. Patients with mild to moderate symptoms can be treated medically with satisfactory results. Patients with severe, disabling, lifestyle-limiting symptoms of claudication can benefit from revascularization therapy. The current safety and long-term durability of direct aortic reconstruction make this approach acceptable even for older, higher-risk patients with significant symptoms. For patients who cannot tolerate such procedures, a variety of other methods of revascularization are available that have had good long-term success rates.

Arteriography

Once a decision has been made to proceed with revascularization therapy, contrast arteriography, either cut film or digital subtraction, is used for a detailed anatomic evaluation of the arterial circulation of the lower extremities. Such information is necessary to choose the most appropriate method of revascularization (operative or endovascular) and plan the procedure. Biplane abdominal aortography with demonstration of the arterial tree below the inguinal ligament ("runoff") is required. This procedure is most commonly performed from the femoral artery with the best pulse by means of a retrograde Seldinger technique. When neither femoral artery is available, a transaxillary or translumbar approach provides good access. Anteroposterior views of the aortoiliofemoral segments demonstrate the extent of the occlusive process and the pattern of collateral formation. Oblique views of the iliac and femoral arteries are frequently necessary to document posterior wall plaque and stenoses t the origins of the deep femoral arteries. Lateral aortography provides information about the origins of the visceral arteries, whereas anteroposterior views demonstrate the renal arteries. Views of the runoff to at least the midcalf level are required to assess the degree of

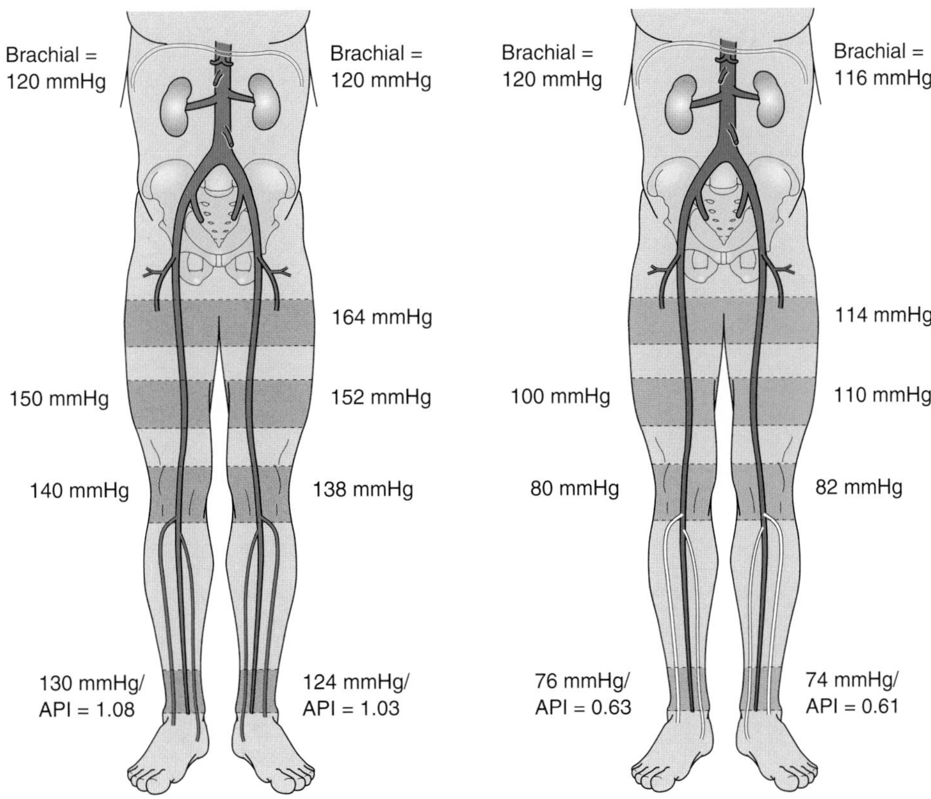

FIGURE 95.11 Segmental pressure measurements typical of normal results (*A*) and aortoiliac occlusive disease (*B*).

associated occlusive disease; in cases of critical limb ischemia, visualization of the pedal circulation is usually necessary.

Occasionally, the hemodynamic effect of a stenosis or series of stenoses along an iliac arterial segment may be difficult to determine, even with oblique views. When the significance of a stenosis remains in question, pressures proximal and distal to the lesion(s) can be measured. A drop of more than 5 to 10 mm Hg across the stenosis is indicative of a hemodynamically significant lesion. For borderline cases, distal pressure measurements can be obtained before and after interarterial injection of a vasodilator, such as tolazoline (Priscoline), to simulate the hyperemic hemodynamics of exercise. A pressure drop of 20 mm Hg or more during hyperdynamic flow is considered to indicate hemodynamic significance.

The information supplied by arteriography is crucial to the success of a revascularization procedure. In addition to providing a detailed "road map" of the exact arterial segments involved and the pathology present, arteriography identifies associated anatomic variations (e.g., accessory renal arteries) and aortic wall characteristics (e.g., extensive calcification, ulcerated plaque), which may alter the operative approach and the conduct of the procedure. For example, an operating surgeon who knows that the aortic wall just below the renal arteries is heavily diseased with ulcerated plaque may decide to control the aorta at a more proximal level rather than risk dislodging atheromatous debris with standard infrarenal aortic clamping. Similarly, documented occlusive lesions in the visceral or renal arteries (e.g., a patent inferior mesenteric artery with a large "meandering mesenteric artery") may best be addressed at the time of aortic reconstruction or require particular attention to avoid complications.

The major risks of arteriography, allergic reactions and contrast-induced renal dysfunction, have been greatly reduced during the last several years by the introduction of newer nonionic contrast agents and recognition of the importance of adequate hydration before the procedure. Nevertheless, interest has been increasing in the use of magnetic resonance imaging (MRI) to avoid these and other complications of angiography. Current MR angiography (MRA) technology, although promising, does not provide sufficient detail or accuracy to supplant traditional angiography in the evaluation of aortoiliac occlusive disease.[10] We currently utilize MRA in patients with moderately severe renal dysfunction (serum creatinine $\geq$3.0 mg/dL), for whom the burden of radioactive contrast in a complete aortogram with runoff study is considered too risky. Any questions remaining after MRA can be answered by a more focused arteriographic study with a smaller load of radioactive contrast.

Choice of Revascularization Technique

A variety of procedures, both endovascular and surgical, are available for revascularization of the patient with aortoiliac occlusive disease. Selection depends on a number of factors, including the pattern of the occlusive process, patient risk, and surgeon experience. Commonly used techniques include (a) catheter-based balloon dilation, with or without luminal

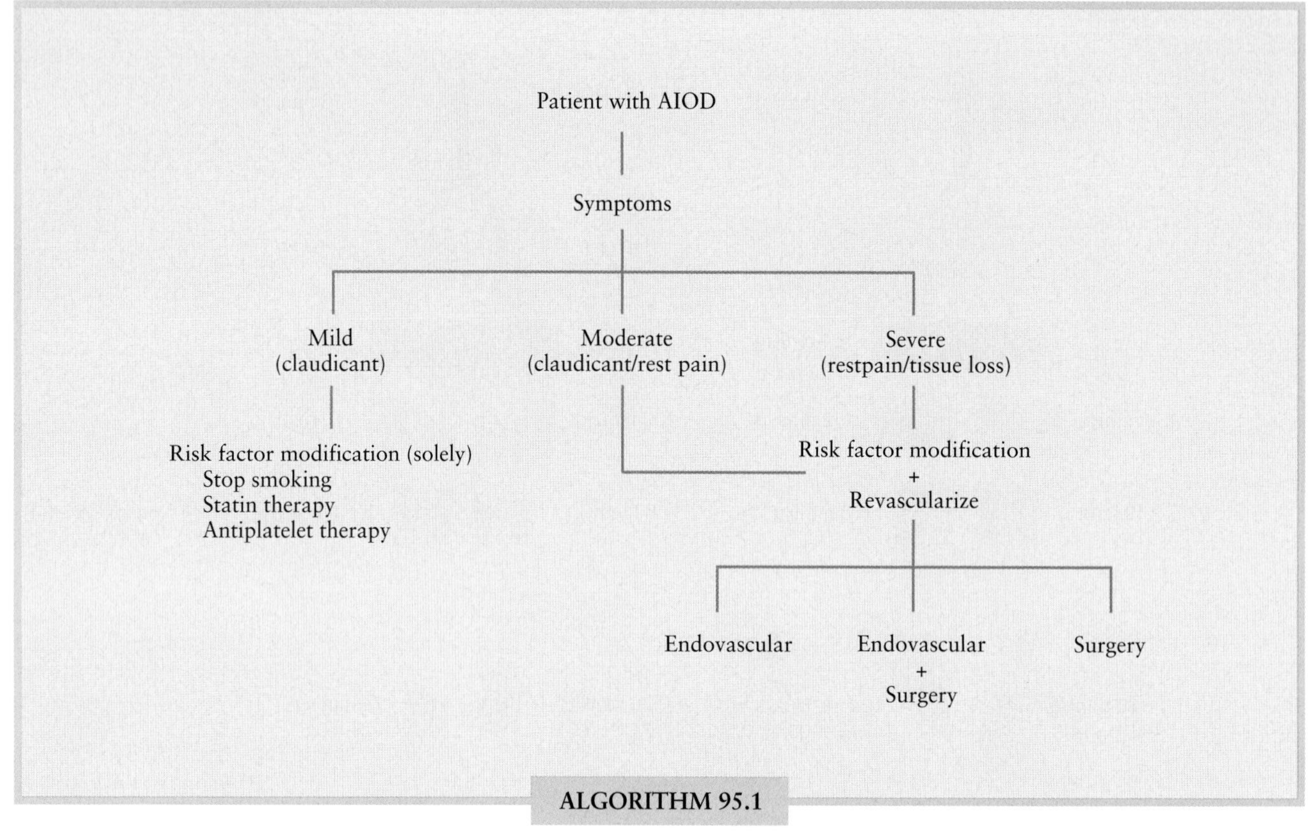

ALGORITHM 95.1 Management of aortoiliac disease.

stenting, (b) aortoiliac endarterectomy, (c) arterial reconstruction with an anatomically placed bypass prosthesis (aortofemoral or iliofemoral), and (d) arterial reconstruction with a remote or extraanatomically placed bypass prosthesis (axillofemoral or bifemoral, femorofemoral, thoracofemoral). Catheter-based techniques are best suited for focal lesions of the common iliac arteries. Endarterectomy is limited to good-risk patients with focal occlusive disease at the aortic bifurcation and common iliac arteries. Prosthetic aortobifemoral bypass is the procedure of choice for most patients with advanced, extensive aortoiliac involvement and is considered the gold standard technique for aortoiliac revascularization. Axillofemoral or bifemoral bypass is reserved for the small subpopulation of patients in whom standard direct aortic reconstruction is considered too risky, either for medical reasons (usually severe pulmonary or cardiac disease) or technical reasons (aortic reoperations, multiple prior abdominal procedures with dense adhesions, prior abdominal irradiation, prosthetic graft infections). The descending thoracic aorta can be considered as an alternative arterial source for the construction of a thoracofemoral bypass in good-risk patients with a "hostile" abdomen.[11] Femorofemoral or iliofemoral bypass can be used in poor-risk patients with diffuse unilateral iliac disease or bilateral iliac involvement when the stenosis in one of the iliac arteries can be appropriately treated by balloon angioplasty, with or without intraluminal stenting.

Preoperative Evaluation

The evaluation of patients for whom aortoiliac reconstruction is being considered should include a careful assessment of overall operative risk. Age *per se* is not a contraindication to a standard direct aortic reconstruction, if it is needed. A "lesser" procedure of more limited durability, however, may provide a similarly excellent outcome in a patient with reduced life expectancy. Patients with significant aortoiliac disease may have atherosclerotic occlusive disease in other vascular territories (e.g., coronary, cerebral) that affects their operative risk. The detection and treatment of significant coronary artery disease is particularly important because myocardial infarction is the leading cause of both perioperative and late mortality.[12] More than 50% of patients with aortoiliac occlusive disease have clinical or electrocardiographic evidence of coronary disease.[13] Selected patients may require cardiac catheterization and even occasional coronary angioplasty or bypass grafting before undergoing aortic reconstruction. Pulmonary and renal function should also be routinely assessed because of the higher mortality associated with postoperative dysfunction of these organ systems.

Endovascular Treatment

Since the very first transarterial dilation procedures, percutaneous transluminal angioplasty (PTA) has become the most commonly performed and, in some cases, the preferred therapy for iliac artery occlusive disease. Like operative reconstruction, PTA when properly selected in this anatomic segment is likely to be successful owing to the large caliber of the vessels and high rates of flow in the aortoiliac segment. Acceptance of endovascular treatment by surgeons and patients for aortoiliac disease continues to advance at a rapid pace. Many factors must be taken into consideration before selecting aortoiliac angioplasty or stent placement for the treatment of aortoiliac occlusive disease. The continuum from claudication to limb-threatened ischemia, and patient comorbities are primary consideration. Usually patients with mild to moderate aortoiliac disease are easily amenable to angioplasty or stent. The best results are obtained with short, focal, nonocclusive lesions in the common iliac arteries.[14] Patients with severe atherosclerotic lesions, long (>10 cm) and complex aortoiliac stenosis or occlusions would benefit from revascularization, although many anecdotes illustrate short-term success with endovascular approaches. Complications (thrombosis, dissection, perforation, and distal embolism) in experienced hands are uncommon and can frequently be remedied with intraluminal stenting or thrombolytic therapy. Stents have made it possible to apply angioplasty in a larger number of lesions (e.g., longer occlusions) and may improve long-term patency rates by reducing rates of restenosis.[15] This technique is particularly useful in high-risk patients, those with critical ischemia secondary to multiple-level disease, and patients in whom iliac PTA can be combined with an infrainguinal bypass for limb salvage. Even in good-risk patients with focal iliac disease, however, PTA may be the preferred initial approach, with surgical intervention reserved for the more difficult circumstances following endovascular failures. If the presence of an appropriate lesion is suspected, PTA may be considered at the same time that the diagnostic arteriogram is performed. Open surgery involves an "up-front" risk in the initial stages, with anesthesia and longer hospital stays. The endovascular model involves the continued surveillance and initial lower "up-front" risk. These patients will require follow-up angiography and repeat interventions as the disease continues to progress and ultimately more investment in time and resources. Complications are usually local. Long-term results depend on the initial extent of aortoiliac disease, but usually will not be as good as open surgery. Results from angioplasty of iliac arteries range from 70% to 90% over a 3-year span. This continues to decrease to as low as 50% patency at 5 years. Iliac artery occlusion with resultant endovascular recanilization shows patency of 70% at 1 year to 60% at 3 years. Open surgery involving a aortobifemoral bypass has been a durable operation for decades. Patency is usually greater than 85% at 5 years.

A combined open operation with endovascular surgery appears to have promising results and demonstrate that ideal patient care outcomes remain in the hands of the vascular surgeon (Fig. 95.12). Preliminary results show that infrainguinal bypass with concomitant aortoiliac angioplasty or stenting, or both, have a slightly higher patency of the distal bypass.[16] With the continued advancement of stents, smaller delivery devices, fluoroscopy equipment, and operator skills, endovascular intervention will continue to be a major component of care of the patient with aortoiliac occlusive disease.

Endarterectomy

Endarterectomy was more commonly performed in the era before prosthetic graft conduits were developed. Currently, direct arterial repair is reserved for the management of focal atheroocclusive disease (type I) limited to the distal aorta and common iliac arteries (Figs. 95.13 and 95.14). When performed for this specific indication, aortoiliac endarterectomy can produce excellent long-term results, similar to those of aortofemoral grafting. Endarterectomy is less well suited for disease extending in the external iliac arteries and is to be avoided when aneurysmal degeneration complicates the primary atheroocclusive aortoiliac process.

The aorta and common iliac arteries are exposed and vascular control is secured. During dissection, care is taken to preserve the autonomic nerves overlying the aortic bifurcation so that normal sexual function is not disturbed. The patient is then heparinized and atraumatic occlusion clamps or tapes are applied. Arteriotomies are made over the aorta and the common iliac arteries to expose the diseased lumen. The atherosclerotic plaque, along with the overlying intima and inner portion of the involved media, is removed. Good "breakoff" points for the removed plaques are needed to prevent postoperative thrombosis that results from the formation of an occluding flap of retained atheroma. The arteriotomies are closed by direct suture or with patch angioplasty, depending on vessel caliber.

Aortofemoral Prosthesis

Aortofemoral bypass is the most durable and reliable of all treatment options, for which reason it is the reference standard for the reconstruction of advanced aortoiliac occlusive disease (Figs. 95.15 and 95.16). The operative sequence starts with exposure of the abdominal aortic segment between the renal and inferior mesenteric arteries by means of appropriate retroperitoneal dissection and cephalad mobilization of the fourth portion of the duodenum and the left renal vein. Care is taken during dissection to avoid injury to the lumbar veins. Moreover, gentle handling of the dissected segment may lessen the risk for atheroembolism during the operation. The common, superficial, and deep femoral arteries are secured through separate groin incisions. Retroperitoneal tunnels are then developed between the exposed infrarenal aorta and the groins by means of blunt dissection. Care is taken to avoid injury to the bowel, particularly the rectosigmoid on the left. The tunnels are directed posterior to the ureter to avoid postoperative obstructive uropathy from graft limb compression of the ureter. A prosthesis of the appropriate size (polytetrafluoroethylene or Dacron) is selected, and the patient is heparinized. With an occluding clamp below the renal arteries and another just above the inferior mesenteric artery, the proximal anastomosis is performed as either an end-to-end or end-to-side graft to the aorta. The end-to-side technique has been found to be just as good, depending on the pattern of occlusive lesions and opportunity to perfuse the internal iliac arteries. The proximal anastomosis is placed as close to the renal arteries as practical to prevent future compromise of the bypass resulting from progression of atherosclerosis in the remaining infrarenal cuff. The limbs of the prosthesis are then

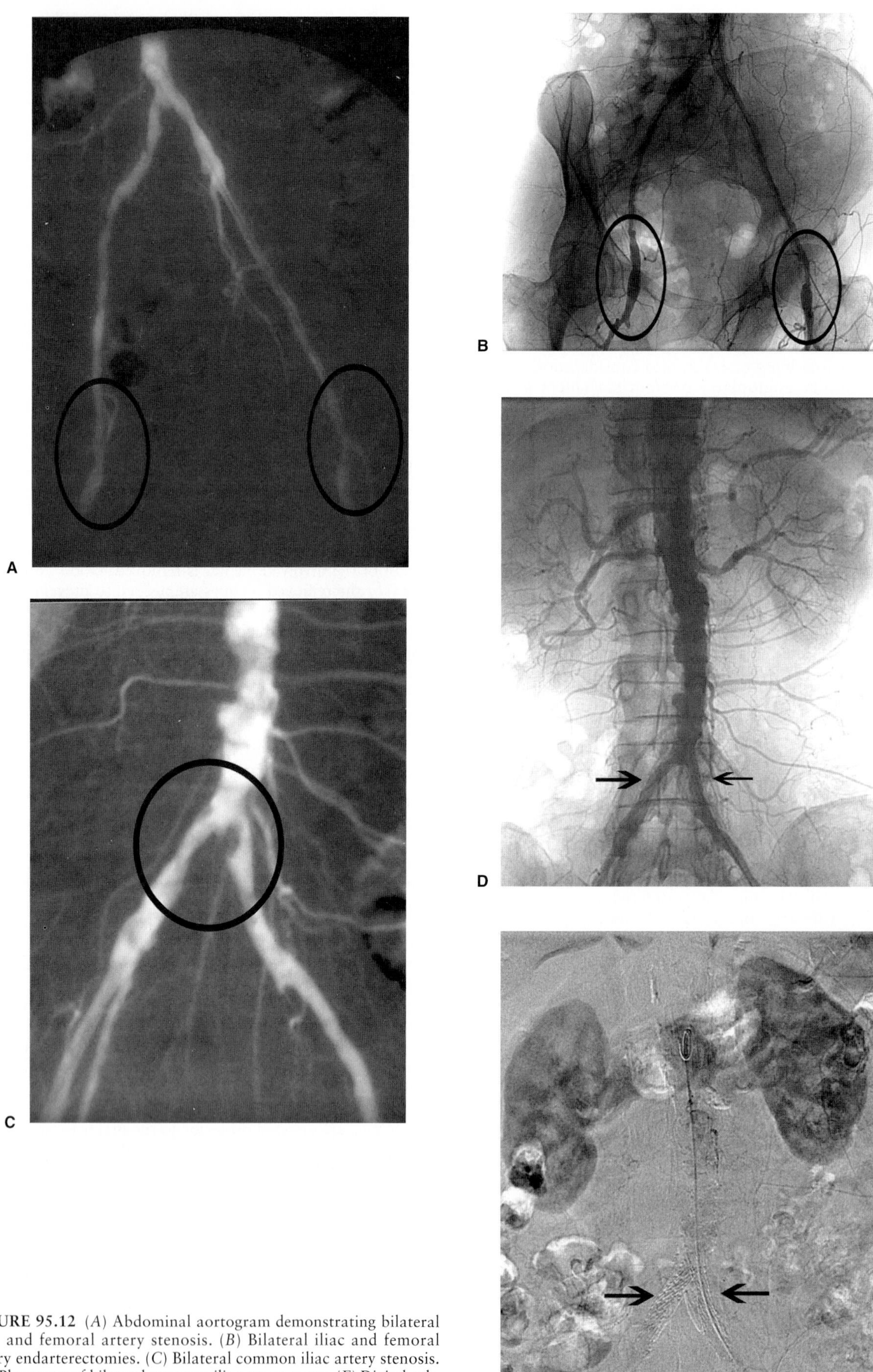

FIGURE 95.12 (*A*) Abdominal aortogram demonstrating bilateral iliac and femoral artery stenosis. (*B*) Bilateral iliac and femoral artery endarterectomies. (C) Bilateral common iliac artery stenosis. (*D*) Placement of bilateral common iliac artery stents. (*E*) Digital subtraction view of bilateral common iliac artery stents.

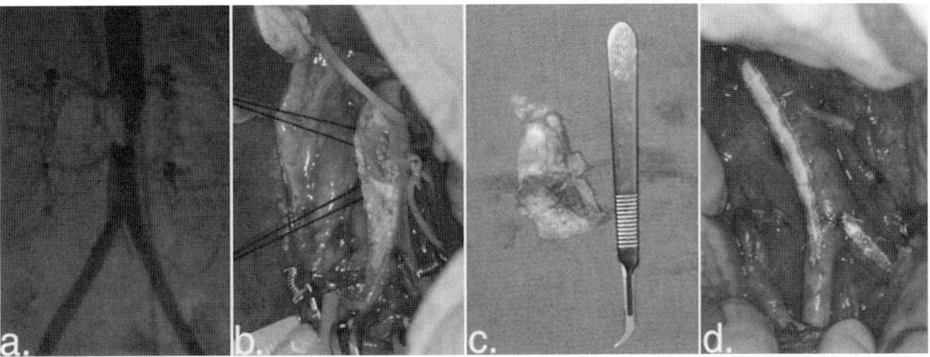

FIGURE 95.14 (*A*) Preoperative angiogram demonstrates severe stenosis of the infrarenal aorta with mild stenosis bilaterally at the origin of the common iliac arteries (type I disease). (*B*) Long arteriotomy over the infrarenal aorta and proximal right common iliac artery reveals advanced ulcerated luminal disease. A second, separate arteriotomy over the left common iliac artery was also created to approach plaque in that vessel. (*C*) Aortic component of the atherosclerotic plaque. (*D*) The two arteriotomies are closed, and polytetrafluoroethylene patches are used for angioplasty.

delivered through the retroperitoneal tunnels into the groins. The distal anastomoses are performed to the common femoral arteries and may be carried into the deep femoral arteries as needed. The technique for distal femoral anastomosis is chosen to ensure adequate graft outflow, particularly if superficial femoral artery disease is present. In the patient with tissue loss secondary to type III or multiple-level aortoiliac disease associated with occluded superficial femoral arteries and compromised deep collaterals, concomitant distal reconstruction should rarely be required (Fig. 95.17).

Aortofemoral bypass has excellent 5- and 10-year graft patency rates of approximately 85% and 75%, respectively. Perioperative morbidity and mortality are reported to be below 10% and 5%, respectively, in many centers.[12,17]

Axillofemoral Prosthesis

Axillofemoral extraanatomic reconstruction has been used for revascularization in poor-risk patients and in those with a hostile abdomen and has been reported to be an acceptable alternative to aortofemoral prosthesis. The axillary artery supplying the arm with the higher systolic blood pressure is usually chosen as the inflow vessel. The operative sequence starts with exposure of the most proximal part of the axillary artery through an infraclavicular incision and splitting of the pectoralis major muscle between its sternal and clavicular heads. The common, superficial, and deep femoral arteries are then dissected through groin incisions. The axillary or long limb of an externally supported polytetrafluoroethylene graft is then advanced behind the pectoralis major muscle and through a subcutaneous tunnel in the anterior axillary line connecting the axillary artery and the ipsilateral groin. Next, a cross-femoral- to-femoral limb of the graft is delivered through a subcutaneous suprapubic tunnel connecting the two groins. An anastomosis between the proximal axillary artery and the prosthesis is constructed in an end-graft to side-of-artery fashion. The graft is positioned parallel to the axillary artery and behind the pectoral muscles for the first 10 cm, before it enters the subcutaneous channel along the anterior axillary line. Following this plan seems to minimize traction on the anasto-

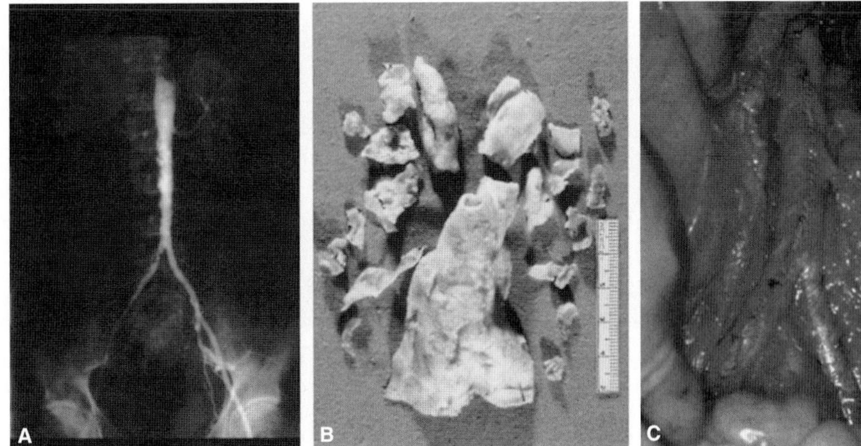

FIGURE 95.13 (*A*) Preoperative angiogram revealing diffuse infrarenal aorta atherosclerosis with severe right common iliac stenosis and right internal iliac occlusion (type I disease). (*B*) Atherosclerotic plaque is removed. (*C*) Long arteriotomy over the entire length of the infrarenal aorta and right common iliac artery is closed after the endarterectomy is complete.

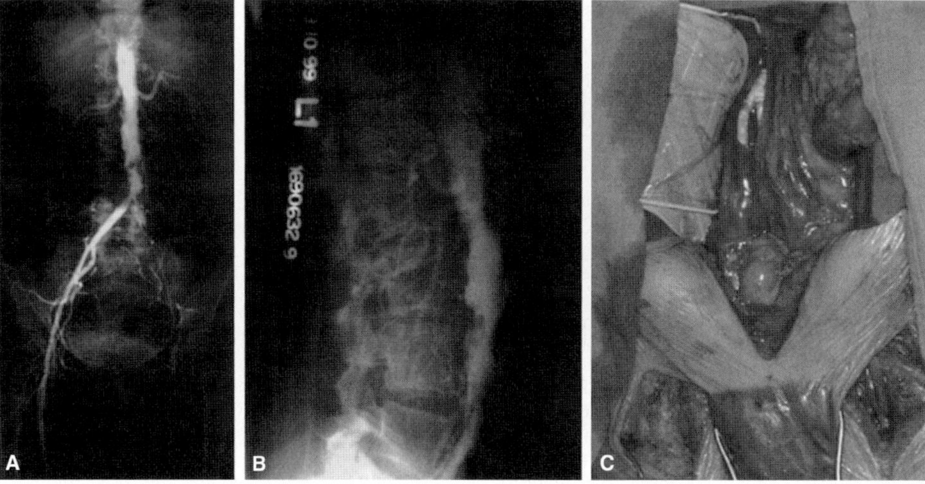

FIGURE 95.15 (*A* and *B*) Preoperative biplane aortograms demonstrates advanced preocclusive disease of the infrarenal aorta and its bifurcation with occlusion of the left common and external iliac arteries (type II disease). (*C*) The patient was treated with placement of an aortobifemoral prosthesis. The short shaft and limbs of the prosthesis are in a retroperitoneal location and are partially covered with a layer of posterior parietal peritoneum. The two groin incisions are kept open to display the anastomoses of the two limbs to the common femoral arteries.

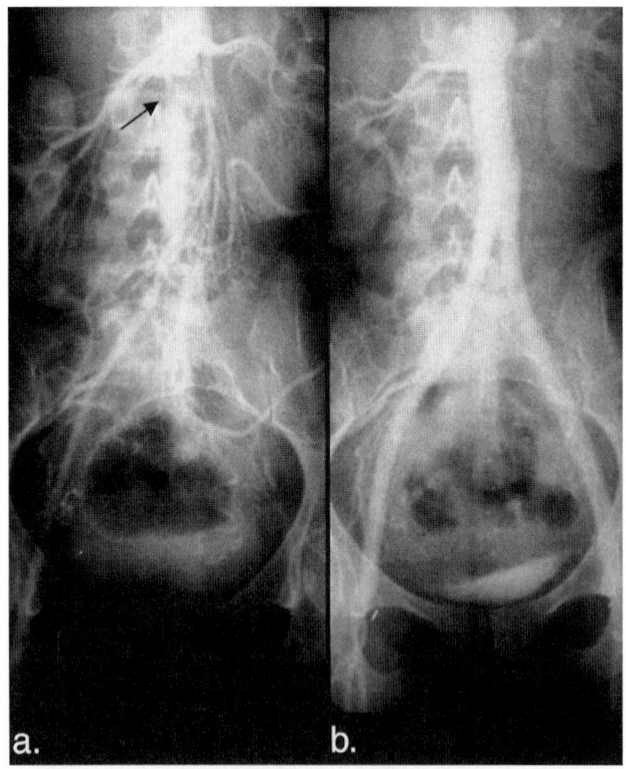

FIGURE 95.16 (*A*) Preoperative aortogram demonstrates advanced preocclusive disease of the infrarenal aorta and its bifurcation with occlusion of the left common and external iliac arteries (type II disease). (*B*) Aortogram after placement of an aortobifemoral prosthesis.

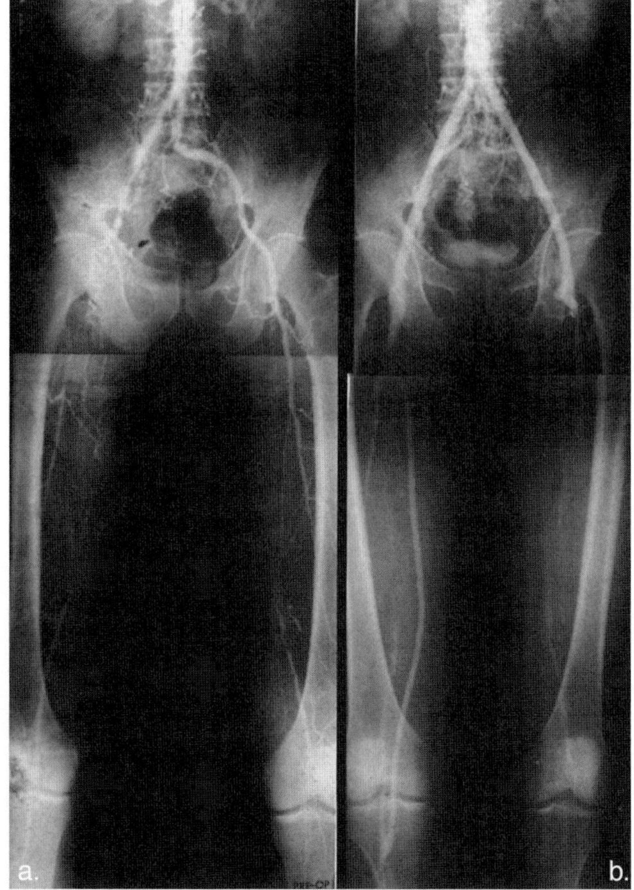

FIGURE 95.17 This diabetic patient presented with gangrene of the right first and second toes. (*A*) The preoperative angiogram revealed aortic bifurcation disease, right external iliac and superficial femoral arterial occlusion, and reconstitution of a heavily diseased right deep femoral artery. On the left, occlusion of the superficial femoral artery is seen, with a patent left deep femoral artery supplying the left leg (multiple-level type III disease). (*B*) The patient underwent an aortobifemoral bypass with a concomitant right femoral-to-below knee popliteal bypass to bring pulsatile flow to the diseased forefoot.

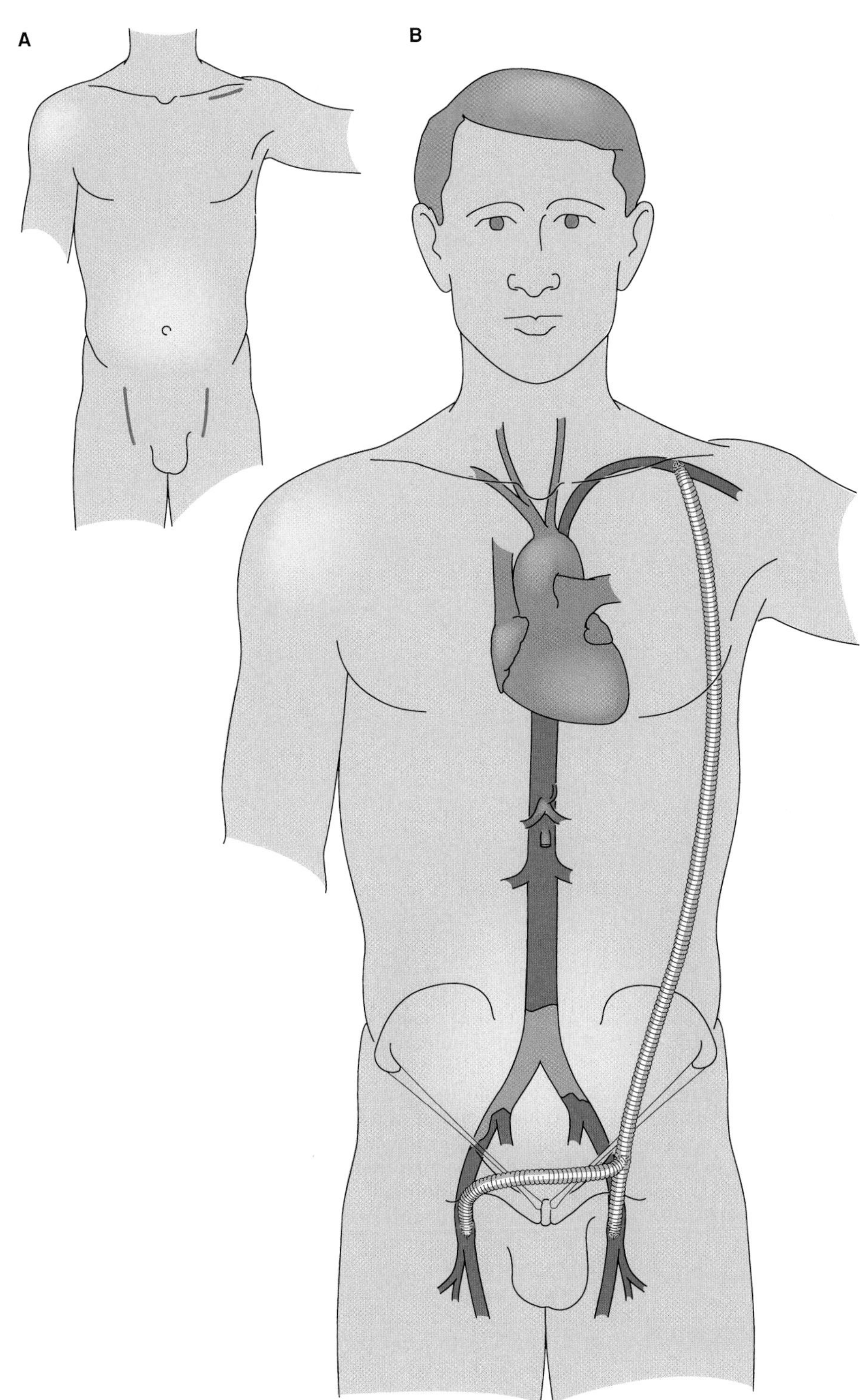

FIGURE 95.18 A unilateral axillary to upsilateral femoral artery bypass graft is supplemented with a crossfemoral-to-femoral artery bypass graft limb. This extraanatomic graft is frequently implanted on the right (although the artist's depiction shows the left) to allow unimpeded access to the thoracoabdominal aorta when necessary.

mosis during arm movement and reduces the incidence of anastomotic disruption. The distal anastomoses are performed to the common femoral arteries and may be carried over or onto the deep femoral arteries to ensure adequate graft outflow (Fig. 95.18).

The reported 5-year patency of the axillofemoral graft varies widely (30% to 80%) but is generally accepted to be lower than the patency of an aortofemoral prosthesis. The axillobifemoral bypass should therefore be reserved for patients with bilateral advanced aortoiliac disease who are either poor surgical risks or have a hostile abdomen.[18]

Other Prosthetic Reconstructions

For high-risk patients with diffuse advanced disease limited to one iliac artery, unilateral femorofemoral or iliofemoral bypass may be used to revascularize the ischemic extremity. If

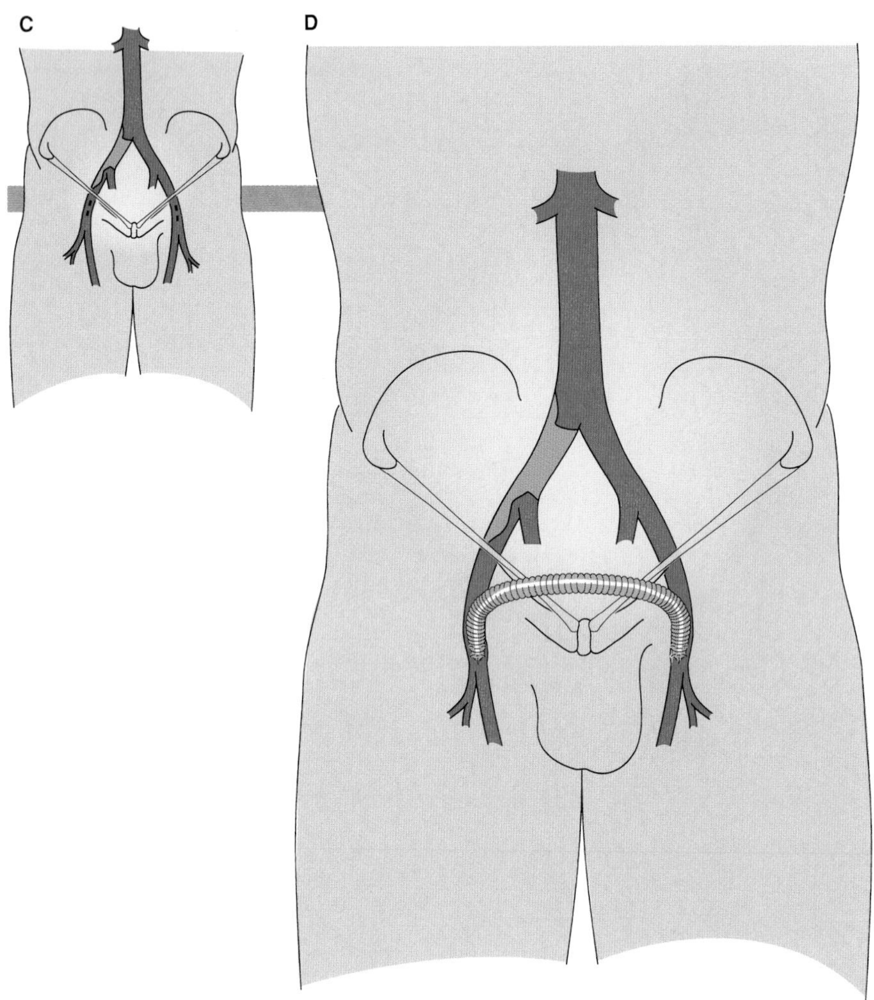

FIGURE 95.19 The crossfemoral-to-femoral artery bypass graft is well tolerated and can be performed with the patient under regional anesthesia.

the contralateral iliac artery is normal or bears a lesion that is well treated by angioplasty or stenting, crossfemoral-to-femoral artery bypass is worthy of consideration. Iliofemoral bypass has a modest graft patency advantage over femorofemoral bypass (70% vs. 60%, respectively), but the main advantage is avoidance of a second groin incision and its associated complications. Femorofemoral bypasses are reserved for patients with occluded or heavily diseased common iliac arteries, in whom iliofemoral bypass is not advisable (Fig. 95.19).

KEY POINTS

- **Atherosclerotic occlusive disease of the aorta and iliac arteries is one of the most common problems encountered by surgeons.**
- **The aortic bifurcation is the location where the earliest atherosclerotic changes are first noted in most young adults.**
- **Risk factors for aortoiliac occlusive disease are those for atherosclerosis in general: smoking, hypertension, lipid abnormalities, diabetes mellitus, male sex, older age, and genetic predisposition.**
- **Smoking appears to be a particularly important risk factor for the development of lower extremity atherosclerotic occlusive disease.**
- **Claudication is the most common presenting symptom of patients with significant aortoiliac disease.**
- **Physical examination typically reveals diminished or absent femoral pulses in patients with aortoiliac occlusive disease.**
- **In the majority of cases, a diagnosis of significant aortoiliac occlusive disease can be made on the basis of the history and physical examination alone.**
- **Since the very first transarterial dilation procedures, percutaneous transluminal angioplasty (PTA) has become the one most commonly performed and, in some cases, the preferred therapy for iliac artery occlusive disease.**
- **Aortofemoral bypass is the most durable and reliable of all treatment options, for which reason it is the reference standard for the reconstruction of advanced aortoiliac occlusive disease.**
- **A combined open operation with endovascular surgery appears to have promising results in the treatment of aortoiliac occlusive disease.**

References

1. Kannel WB, Shurtleff D. The Framingham study: cigarettes and the development of intermittent claudication. *Geriatrics* 1973;28:61–68.
2. Hughson WG, Mann JI, Garrod A. Intermittent claudication: prevalence and risk factors. *Br Med J.* 1978;1:1379–1381.
3. Leriche R, Morel A. The syndrome of thrombotic obliteration of the aortic bifurcation. *Ann Surg.* 1948;127:193–206.
4. **DeBakey ME, Lawrie GM, Glaeser DH. Patterns of atherosclerosis and their surgical significance. *Ann Surg.* 1985;201:115–131.**

5. **Brewster DC, Darling RC. Optimal methods of aortoiliac reconstruction. *Surgery* 1978;84:739.**
6. Kohler TR, Nance DR, Cramer MM, et al. Duplex scanning for diagnosis of aortoiliac and femoropopliteal disease: a prospective study. *Circulation* 1987;76:1074–1080.
7. Girolami GB, Bernardi E, Prins MH, et al. Treatment of intermittent claudication with physical training, smoking cessation, pentoxifylline, or nafronyl: a meta-analysis. *Arch Intern Med.* 1999;159:337–345.
8. Porter JM, Cutler BS, Lee BY, et al. Pentoxifylline efficacy in the treatment of intermittent claudication: multicenter controlled double-blind trial with objective assessment of chronic occlusive arterial disease patients. *Am Heart J.* 1982;104:66–71.
9. Money SR, Herd JA, Isaacsohn JL, et al. Effects of cilostazol on walking distances in patients with intermittent claudication caused by peripheral vascular disease. *J Vasc Surg.* 1998;27:267–275.
10. Haney TF, Debatin JF, Leung DA, et al. Evaluation of the aortoiliac and renal arteries: comparison of breath-hold, contrast-enhanced, three-dimensional MR angiography with conventional angiography. *Radiology* 1997;204: 357–362.
11. Passman MA, Farber MA, Criado E, et al. Descending thoracic aortoiliofemoral artery bypass grafting: a role for primary revascularization for aortoiliac occlusive disease? *J Vasc Surg.* 1999;29:249–258.
12. **Szilagyi DE, Elliott JP Jr, Smith RF, et al. A thirty-year survey of the reconstructive surgical treatment of aortoiliac occlusive disease. *J Vasc Surg.* 1986;3:421–436.**
13. Hertzer NR, Young JR, Kramer JR, et al. Routine coronary angiography prior to elective aortic reconstruction: results of selective myocardial revascularization in patients with peripheral vascular disease. *Arch Surg.* 1979;114:1336–1344.
14. Johnston KW, Rae M, Hogg-Johnston SA, et al. Five-year results of a prospective study of percutaneous transluminal angioplasty. *Ann Surg.* 1987;206:403–413.
15. **Henry M, Amor M, Ethevenot G, et al. Palmaz stent placement in iliac and femoropopliteal arteries: primary and secondary patency in 310 patients with 2- to 4-year follow-up. *Radiology* 1995;197:167.**
16. **Schneider P. Iliac angioplasty and stenting in association with infrainguinal bypass: timing and techniques. *Semin Vasc Surg.* 2003;16:291–299.**
17. Brewster DC. Current controversies in the management of aortoiliac occlusive disease. *J Vasc Surg.* 1997;25:365–379.
18. Passman MA, Taylor LM, Moneta GL, et al. Comparison of axillofemoral and aortofemoral bypass for aortoiliac occlusive disease. *J Vasc Surg.* 1996;23:263–269; discussion 269–271.
19. **Dotter C, Judkins M. Transluminal treatment of arteriosclerotic obstruction: description of a new technic and a preliminary report of its application. *Circulation* 1964;30:654–670.**

CHAPTER 96 ■ FEMOROPOPLITEAL AND TIBIAL OCCLUSIVE DISEASE

MATTHEW T. MENARD AND MICHAEL BELKIN

Arterial occlusive disease is highly prevalent in Western society and constitutes the leading overall cause of death in the United States. With the aging of the American population, the prevalence of lower extremity occlusive disease has steadily increased in recent decades. Not surprisingly, therefore, the clinical manifestations and complications of atherosclerosis are the most common therapeutic challenge encountered and treated by vascular surgeons.

The tendency for atherosclerotic lesions to develop at specific anatomic sites and follow recognizable patterns of progression was first appreciated in the late 1700s by the British anatomist and surgeon John Hunter. Considered one of the forefathers of vascular surgery, his dissections of atherosclerotic aortic bifurcations are preserved at the Hunterian museum in London and presage the disease process that Leriche would give his name to 150 years later.[1] The modern era of surgical reconstruction for complex atherosclerotic occlusive disease began in earnest in 1947, when the Portuguese surgeon J. Cid dos Santos successfully endarterectomized a heavily diseased common femoral artery.[2] Four years later, building on the pioneering work of Alexis Carrel,[3] Kunlin[4] would report the first long-segment vein bypass in the lower extremity. It would be another 10 years before the initial efforts to extend vein grafting to the tibial level were described by McCaughan.[5] Tremendous advances in both the understanding of atherosclerosis biology and the ability to treat arterial occlusive disease percutaneously have had a dramatic impact on the treatment algorithms for arterial insufficiency in recent years.

Although a diverse range of technical skill is required of the contemporary vascular surgeon, it is worth noting that infrainguinal arterial bypass surgery remains the signature operation distinguishing vascular surgeons from other specialists involved in the treatment of peripheral vascular disease. This distinction stems primarily from the fact that the outcome of infrainguinal reconstruction is highly dependent on the judgment and technical skill of the surgeon, with the end result being either successful limb salvage or major limb amputation. This chapter reviews the surgical management of femoropopliteal and tibial arterial occlusive disease and details standard and advanced techniques underlying successful infrainguinal operative revascularization.

INFRAINGUINAL ARTERIAL OCCLUSIVE DISEASE

Chronic obliterative atherosclerosis of the infrainguinal vessels is the most prevalent manifestation of arterial occlusive disease encountered by the vascular surgeon. Claudication, the reproducible ischemic muscle pain resulting from inadequate oxygen delivery during exercise, is the cardinal presenting symptom and affects 5% of people older than age 55 years. Another 10% of those in this age group have asymptomatic peripheral atherosclerotic disease, whereas 1% have critical leg ischemia in the form of rest pain or gangrene.[6] Natural history studies indicate patients with claudication have increased rates of cardiovascular mortality, but an overall low risk of associated limb loss.[7,8] Most patients with claudication demonstrate a stable pattern of disease throughout their lifetime or have improvement in their symptoms as a result of risk factor modification, whereas 20% to 30%

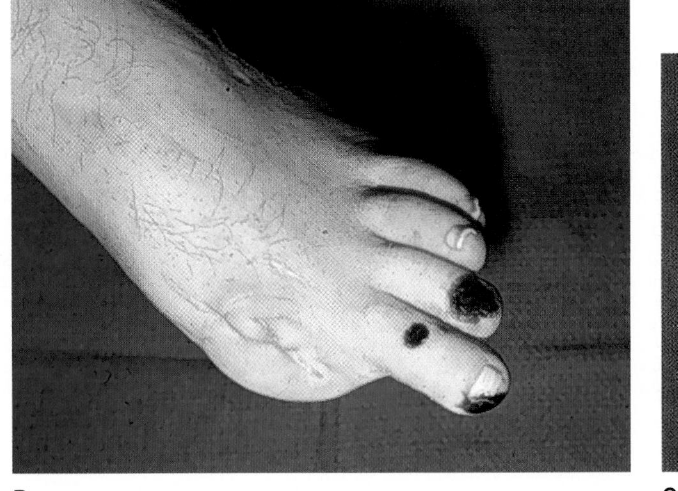

A B C

FIGURE 96.1 Examples of digital ischemic ulcerations resulting from progressive arterial insufficiency.

undergo operation within 5 years as a result of disease progression. The annual rates of mortality and limb loss in patients with claudication are approximately 5% and 1%, respectively.[9]

The most common lesion seen below the inguinal ligament is that of a short-segment total occlusion of the superficial femoral artery. Although isolated disease of this nature typically presents as calf muscle claudication, it is not uncommon for patients with hemodynamically significant single-level lesions, even those with long-segment arterial occlusions, in the superficial femoral artery or more distal arterial beds to be only minimally symptomatic or even asymptomatic. Although this finding can sometimes be the result of exercise limitations imposed by concomitant coronary arterial disease or other physiologic impairments such as lung disease or arthritis, it is more often a result of compensatory collateral flow. For example, collateral perfusion from the profunda femoral artery around a heavily diseased or occluded superficial femoral artery frequently reconstitutes the distal superficial femoral artery or popliteal artery with enough well perfused arterial blood to ensure sufficient resting tissue perfusion. Similarly, the rich network of geniculate collaterals can compensate for a diseased popliteal arterial segment to a sufficient degree to prevent rest pain or overt tissue loss.

In contrast, patients with more extensive single vessel involvement of the femoral, popliteal, or tibial arteries sometimes manifest rest pain or ischemic tissue loss. Similarly, those patients with multilevel disease involving the femoropopliteal system in combination with occlusive disease of the aortoiliac vessels or the infrageniculate runoff, can present with a range of symptoms from mild claudication to more severe levels of critical ischemia or gangrene.[10] Rest pain occurs when blood flow is inadequate to meet metabolic requirements. In the lower extremity, ischemic rest pain is localized to the forefoot and should be easily distinguishable from benign muscle cramps in the calf commonly seen in older patients. Patients with rest pain are often awakened by severe discomfort in the forefoot and hang the affected extremity over the edge of the bed for temporary symptomatic relief. Trophic changes, such as muscle wasting, thinning of skin, thickening of nails and hair loss are frequently also seen in the distal affected limb. Rest pain is an ominous symptom and usually requires revascularization given the tendency for progression to tissue loss.

Ischemia ulcerations usually begin as small, dry ulcers of the toes or heel area, and progress to frankly gangrenous changes of the forefoot or heel with greater degrees of arterial insufficiency (Fig. 96.1). Patients with diabetes or renal failure are more susceptible to the development of ischemic pedal ulcers. Such progressive disease, affecting multiple levels of the peripheral vasculature tree, is also more frequently encountered in the elderly. Approximately one third of patients operated on for symptomatic aortoiliac occlusive disease have orificial profunda femoris occlusive disease and more than 40% have superficial femoral artery occlusions.

Several identifiable patterns of infrainguinal occlusive disease are well recognized. Patients with an extensive history of cigarette smoking typically have lesions limited to the superficial femoral artery and corresponding symptoms of calf claudication (Fig. 96.2). Diabetes, in contrast, most often targets the tibial vessels, and patients may present with frank tissue necrosis in the presence of a palpable popliteal pulse and no prior history of claudication. Alternatively, the so-called "blue toe syndrome" is a situation in which atherosclerotic debris breaks free from a more proximal source, for example, an aortoiliac or femoropopliteal plaque or a thrombus lined aneurysm, and embolizes to the distal vessels.[11,12] Wire manipulation during coronary or peripheral angiographic procedures and cross-clamping across a calcific aortic plaque during cardiac surgery are common sources of such emboli. The terminal target of the microembolic particles, whether cholesterol crystals, calcified plaque, thrombus or platelet aggregates, is typically the small vessels of the toes and heel.

A particularly virulent form of atherosclerotic arterial disease is often found in young female smokers.[13,14] Radiographic imaging in this subset of patients typically reveals atretic, narrowed vasculature with diffusely calcific atherosclerotic changes. Such patients invariably have an extensive smoking history, with or without other typical risk factors for atherosclerosis. Given the diminutive size of the inflow and outflow vessels, the durability of endovascular intervention is generally inferior in these patients, particularly in the face of continued cigarette use.

Typically half of patients proceeding to surgery for arterial occlusive disease have significant coronary artery disease, even more have hypertension, and almost 80% are current or prior cigarette smokers.[15,16] The low mortality and morbidity associated with operative intervention in recent years is in large part a result of advances in the management of concomitant coronary disease. Specifically, the importance and benefit of better preoperative identification of patients in need of initial coronary revascularization, awareness of the benefit of waiting an interval period following coronary stenting prior to proceeding with major noncoronary vascular surgery, improved perioperative pharmacologic management of

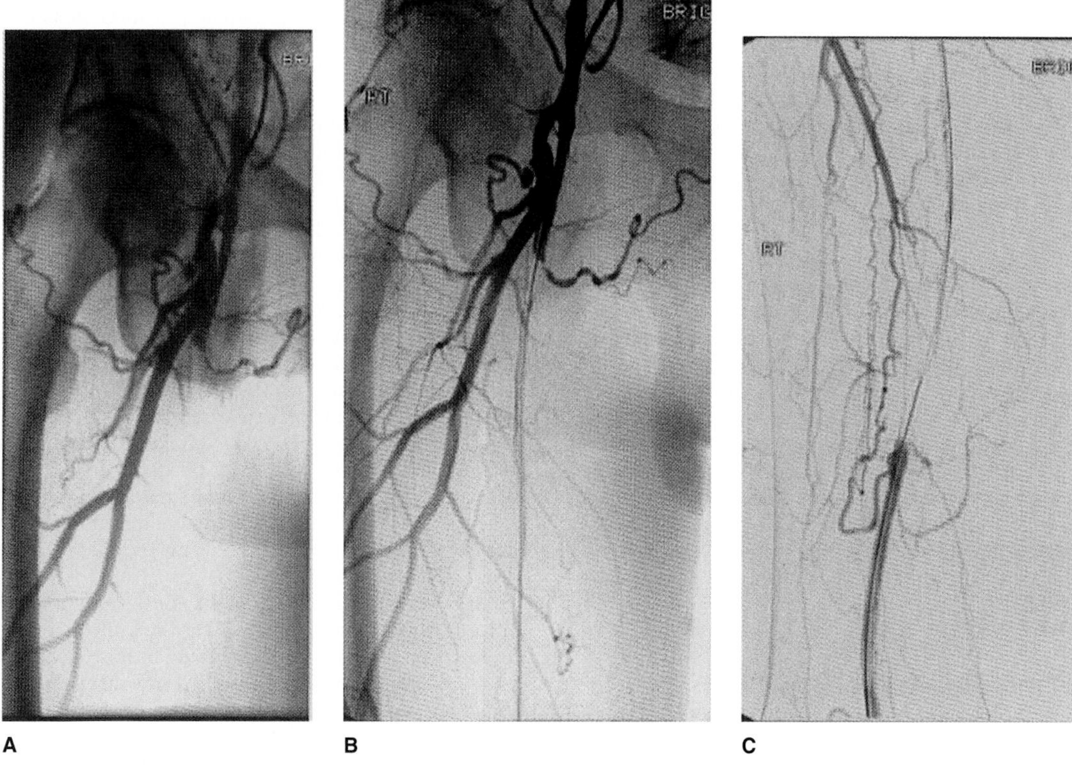

FIGURE 96.2 Long-segment total occlusion of superficial femoral artery in a patient with a long history of cigarette smoking and severe claudication.

patients with impaired myocardium and more focused efforts to tailor operative and postoperative fluid administration to the individual patient's myocardial reserve are all well recognized.[17,18] General advances in postoperative management, including pulmonary care, infection control, and blood product utilization, have further contributed to the progress seen.

Diagnosis

The diagnosis of infrainguinal occlusive disease is generally based on patient symptomatology, physical examination, and noninvasive tests, such as segmental pressure measurements and pulse volume recordings. Following the diagnosis of lower extremity disease and the decision to pursue intervention, further imaging is warranted. In this regard, duplex ultrasonography, magnetic resonance angiography (MRA) and computed tomographic angiography (CTA) are increasingly being utilized as first line modalities in planning the optimal revascularization approach, and have supplanted contrast angiography as the initial imaging study of choice.

Although growing literature supports the use of duplex scanning as a stand-alone preoperative mapping modality,[19] this use requires a highly dedicated vascular laboratory and to date has not gained wide acceptance. CTA is increasingly being utilized as a preoperative road mapping technique in institutions able to provide high-quality three-dimensional reconstructions. MRA is also particularly useful as a noninvasive screening test to determine the suitability for percutaneous therapy, as advances have solved many of the technical limitations of earlier studies (Fig. 96.3). Should a lesion amenable to percutaneous therapy be identified, angiography is then pursued. Alternatively, in some instances of femoropopliteal level reconstruction, operative planning may be

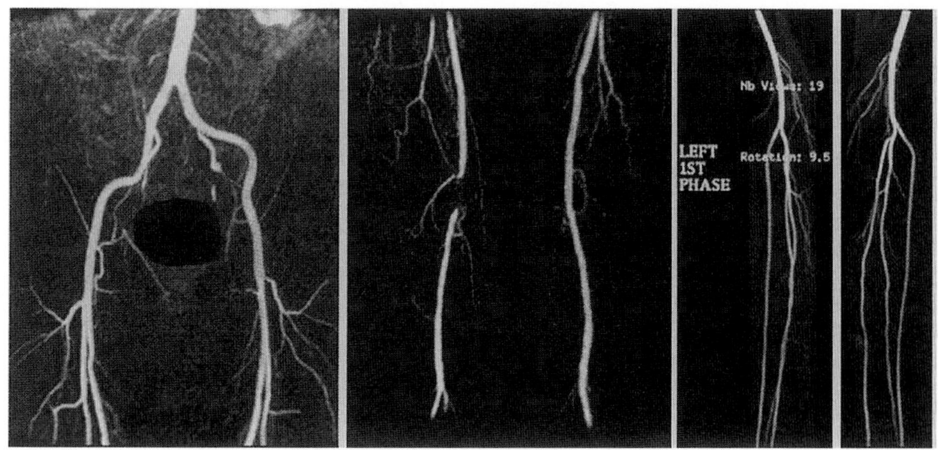

FIGURE 96.3 Magnetic resonance angiogram identifying short-segment occlusion of right superficial femoral artery, a lesion amenable to attempt at percutaneous therapy.

based solely on MRA scanning if high-quality time of flight and gadolinium enhanced images are obtained.[20–22] In many case, however, surgeons are reluctant to proceed to surgery without the confirmation afforded by standard contrast angiography. This reluctance is particularly true if the distal target is at the tibial or pedal level, where CTA and MRA technology remains more limited.

When digital subtraction angiography is undertaken for preoperative planning, a retrograde femoral approach is typically utilized from the contralateral limb. In patients in whom noninvasive imaging indicates a widely patent common femoral and proximal superficial femoral artery and body habitus is not prohibitive, an antegrade approach can serve as useful alternative. In ambiguous lesions, pull-back pressure measurements, both before and after the administration of a systemic vasodilator, such as papaverine or nitroglycerine, or the application of a tourniquet to induce reactive hyperemia, can be useful in documenting the hemodynamic significance of a particular stenotic zone.[23] The utilization of gadolinium[24] or carbon dioxide[25] as contrast agents in patients with compromised renal function, although perhaps less effective in the periphery than in the aortoiliac vasculature, can minimize or eliminate the nephrotoxic effects associated with standard iodinated contrast medium.

Indications for Treatment

Risk factor modification remains a cornerstone of the management of lower extremity occlusive disease. Smoking cessation, blood pressure control, and aggressive efforts at cholesterol lowering should be addressed with every patient with atherosclerotic disease. Lipid-lowering therapy involves both dietary modification and more recently, increasing utilization of hydroxymethylglutaryl-coenzyme A reductase inhibitor. Strong evidence exists supporting the benefit of a structured walking program[26] in increasing the walking distance of patients with claudication. The benefit of walking outside of a structured regimen with close follow up is more debatable.[27] Medical management with pentoxifylline or, more recently, cilostazol, has benefit in a subset of patients and remains a reasonable first-line approach to improve claudication symptoms.[28] Finally, antiplatelet therapy, either aspirin or clopidogrel, is a critically important element of the treatment of established occlusive disease,[29] given its documented ability to prevent thrombosis and embolization and possibly even to arrest the progression of atherosclerosis.

Infrainguinal reconstruction for the treatment of peripheral vascular occlusive disease has been increasingly successful for both long-term palliation of intermittent claudication and for the salvage of limbs threatened by critical ischemia. Although there are certainly cases in which primary amputation represents the safest and most advisable solution in the face of irreversible ischemia, particularly for cases in which extensive infection or tissue necrosis is present, an attempt at reconstruction is almost always indicated when a limb is threatened by severe ischemia. Improvements in perioperative management and surgical technique have allowed progressively more distal reconstructions to be successfully completed in an older, sicker, and challenging patient population.[17] In general, high rates of relief for claudication and up to an 80% to 90% limb salvage rate may be anticipated for patients with critical ischemia at institutions devoted to peripheral bypass surgery.[30,31] The two major indications for intervention of infrainguinal arterial occlusive disease are claudication and limb-threatening critical ischemia. Less common indications for infrainguinal arterial reconstruction include trauma-related vessel disruption, popliteal artery entrapment syndrome. and femoropopliteal arterial aneurysm with thromboembolism. Claudication is a relative indication for intervention given the natural history of the disease, and it remains a subjective assessment on the part of both patient and surgeon as to the relative degree of disability a particular level of claudication pain represents. For example, two-block claudication in a younger patient whose livelihood depends on walking tolerance constitutes a more significant disability than the same degree of claudication in an older, retired individual able to attend to his or her daily affairs without significant consequence.

Thus, proximal above-knee reconstruction in a patient with disabling claudication and a patent popliteal artery with intact runoff may be justified in view of its minimal operative mortality, excellent long-term palliation, and absence of added risk of limb loss beyond that expected from the natural history of the disease process. In contrast, patients with claudication with diffuse superficial femoropopliteal and tibioperoneal disease are usually not suitable candidates for revascularization because long-distance reconstruction does not necessarily provide symptomatic relief and graft failure may result in distal arterial thrombosis and a jeopardized limb. Because most patients with claudication remain stable for years, it is important to allow sufficient time for collaterals to develop; some patients may improve to such an extent that intervention proves unnecessary.[6]

In contrast, critical ischemia is associated with inevitable amputation for most patients unless surgical correction is undertaken. As is true with claudication, ischemic rest pain must be carefully distinguished from other sources of pain in the elderly population, most commonly arthralgia and neuropathy. Although tissue necrosis and gangrene are usually self-evident when caused by critical ischemia, similar lesions associated with venous stasis, severe anemia, decubitus ulcers and diabetic neuropathy must be excluded.

Role of Percutaneous Transluminal Angioplasty

Of relevance in any discussion of infrainguinal occlusive disease is the notable shift in the indications for percutaneous intervention witnessed in recent years. As the associated risks of balloon angioplasty and stenting have fallen and the relative success rates have risen, the threshold for offering endovascular treatment to patients with claudication has significantly decreased. Patients once considered appropriate only for risk factor modification, exercise therapy, and medical treatment are now increasingly being offered percutaneous revascularization as a secondary or even primary treatment option. Similarly, occlusive disease of the tibial vessels, once thought to be the exclusive domain of operative bypass, is increasingly being treated percutaneously.

The impact of these trends on the natural history of occlusive disease, and to what extent the expanding reach of percutaneous therapy will affect subsequent operative management in a given patient, remains to be seen. Certainly, as the enthusiasm for less-invasive options has spread to include the infrapopliteal level, the relative roles of surgical and percutaneous intervention are actively being redefined. Whether these changes will significantly affect the number of patients proceeding to open surgery remains to be seen. As the escalating use of renal and aortoiliac angioplasty and stenting has led to a considerable drop in open surgical reconstructions in these vascular beds, the rising popularity and success of femoral and tibial wire-based interventions may similarly reduce the volume, or ultimately just delay the timing of, subsequent infrainguinal reconstructive surgery.

A marked increase in the number and versatility of available balloons and stents has helped to fuel the increasing application of percutaneous technology. Newer generation atherectomy devices, cold balloon angioplasty and flexible stents designed to withstand the unique torsional forces of the leg or with drug-eluting capability may significantly improve the patency and durability rates currently seen.[32,33] Until the efficacy of infrainguinal percutaneous intervention is better defined, however, surgical revascularization remains the gold standard for any patient with critical limb ischemia. For patients with favorable anatomy and significant operative risk, and for the treatment of claudication in general, percutaneous therapy has assumed a more primary role.

Percutaneous transluminal angioplasty is generally performed under local anesthesia with minimal intravenous sedation and as either a day surgical procedure or involving an overnight admission. Associated morbidity and mortality has significantly declined in recent years. Importantly, overall complication rates are low, and technical failure rarely changes the available surgical options. Contrast-induced acute renal failure remains the most common complication. With the development of hypoosmolar and isoosmolor contrast agents; the overall incidence has fallen to less than 6%,[34] although higher rates are found in patients with preexisting renal failure and diabetes.[35,36]

Access site complications, predominately pseudoaneurysms and arteriovenous malformations (AVF), occur in 1% of patients.[37] Most of them can be managed conservatively, with close observation, serial hematocrit checks, and fluid and blood product replacement. Surgery is reserved for those patients with ongoing bleeding effecting hemodynamic instability or distal ischemia, or pseudoaneurysms or AVFs that fail to resolve on serial ultrasound imaging with several weeks of careful observation. Stable pseudoaneurysms in patients without coagulopathy can also be managed with ultrasound-guided compression therapy; more recently, ultrasound-guided thrombin injection into the sac has been used with good success.[38] Infection related to the placement of newer percutaneous closure devices, such as the Perclose (Abbott Laboratories, Abbott Park, IL) and the AngioSeal (St. Jude Medical, St. Paul, MN), which are quickly becoming the preferred means of puncture site control, typically present several weeks to months after the percutaneous procedure. Rarely, maldeployment of these devices can lead to embolic or thrombotic sequelae causing compromise of distal flow.[39]

When medical therapy or percutaneous treatment has proven inadequate or is technically inadvisable, open surgical revascularization remains the gold standard for those patients with disabling claudication, ischemic rest pain and ischemic ulceration or gangrene. Successful infrainguinal bypass grafting requires adequate arterial inflow. While aortobifemoral, femorofemoral and axillofemoral bypass grafting remain routinely performed inflow procedures, aortoiliac angioplasty and stenting is increasingly becoming the preliminary procedure performed to attain sufficient inflow prior to construction of a more distal bypass graft. At times, the necessity of improving the inflow to support an infrainguinal graft is determined intraoperatively, either by direct visual assessment of the arterial flow at the desired donor site or by comparison of a transduced pressure tracing from the donor site with that of a systemic pressure tracing, typically obtained from a radial arterial line. Of equal importance to the outcome of any infrainguinal graft is target vessel selection. In general, the target vessel should be the least diseased artery that is the dominant supply to the foot. If tissue necrosis is present, restoration of pulsatile flow to the foot is often required to obtain full and sustained wound healing.

Operative Management

Infrainguinal surgical bypass can be performed under general anesthesia, or in the appropriate patient, regional spinal or epidural anesthesia. In cases involving multiple sites of dissection, such as those necessitating more tedious arm vein or lesser saphenous vein harvesting, the procedures are particularly amenable to a two-team approach, with the time saved having direct benefit in minimizing the total anesthetic load and physiologic insult. The patient is sterilely prepped and draped from the midabdomen down to the foot. Typically, the site proposed for the distal anastomosis is explored first in order to ascertain whether the preoperative imaging was accurate in predicting the suitability of the target vessel. On occasion, the operation is begun with an on-table angiogram to clarify the anatomy if preoperative imaging was deferred or ambiguous.

The above-knee popliteal vessel is easily exposed through a medial thigh incision, with subsequent posterolateral retraction of the sartorious muscle. The popliteal artery with its accompanying vein and nerve is found just posterior to the femur. The vessel is palpated to determine the presence of atherosclerotic plaque, which will guide the extent of dissection and the optimal bypass target site. The below-knee popliteal artery is also exposed through a medial incision in the proximal calf (Fig. 96.4). If the saphenous vein is to be harvested, the incision is made directly over the vein to minimize the creation of devascularized skin flaps. With the exposed vein carefully protected, the incision is carried through the deep muscular fascia and the medial head of the gastrocnemius is reflected posterolaterally to expose the below-knee popliteal fossa. The distal popliteal artery is then dissected free from the adjacent tibial nerve posteriorly and popliteal vein medially. If the distal target is the tibioperoneal trunk, the dissection is continued along the anteromedial surface of the distal popliteal artery after dividing the origin of the soleus muscle from the tibia (Fig. 96.5). In instances in which the below-knee popliteal artery has previously been exposed or where sepsis is involved, a lateral approach with excision of a segment of proximal fibula is a useful alternative approach to the below-knee popliteal artery.

Although exposure of the proximal posterior tibial and peroneal vessels can be gained by extending the tibioperoneal trunk dissection distally, more distal exposure of these vessels is best gained through targeted medial incisions. The posterior tibial artery is found beneath the divided musculotendinous origin of the soleus muscle, and the peroneal artery is deeper and more lateral. The posterior tibial artery at the level of the ankle is a relatively easier target given the proximity of the vessel to

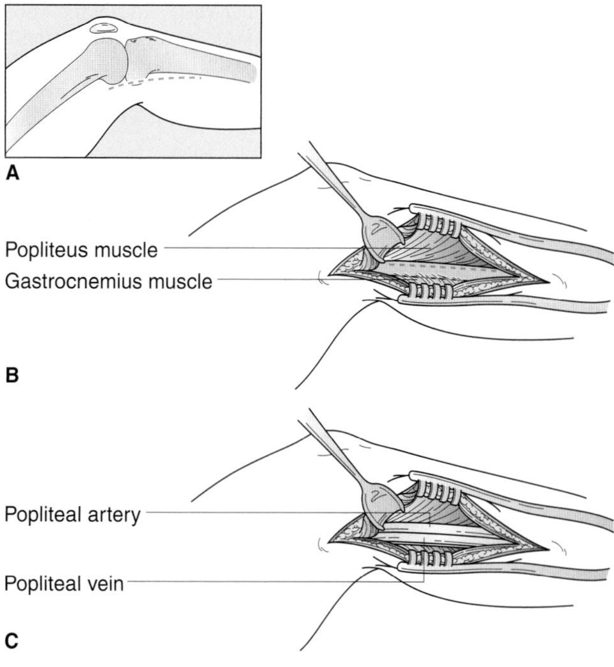

FIGURE 96.4 Exposure of the popliteal artery below the knee. The medial incision is made directly overlying the course of the greater saphenous vein.

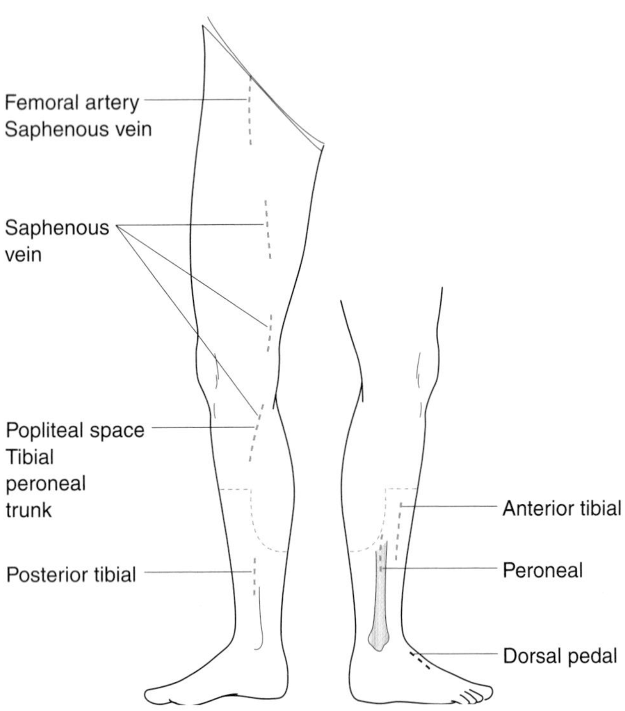

FIGURE 96.5 Placement of incisions for femoropopliteal and femorotibial bypass and for greater saphenous vein harvest. These should avoid the incision lines for a below-knee amputation.

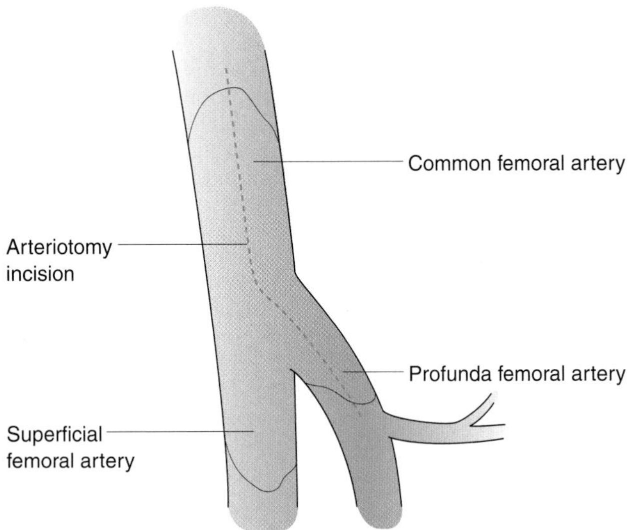

FIGURE 96.6 In the setting of orificial profunda femoral artery disease, extending the common femoral arteriotomy into the origin of the profunda and performing a profundaplasty will maximize profunda flow in the event of graft thrombosis.

the skin surface. The initial incision is made just posterior to the medial malleolus, and the artery exposed by division of the overlying retinaculum. Further distal dissection allows access to the bifurcation and medial and lateral plantar branches.[40] The more distal peroneal artery may be approached laterally via an incision placed over the distal fibula. Excision of a short segment of fibula will expose the underlying artery.

The anterior tibial artery is typically approached from the anterolateral aspect of the calf (Fig. 96.5) and is found deep within the anterior compartment with the adjacent deep peroneal nerve and anterior tibial veins. It is best identified by developing the intermuscular plane between the tibialis anterior muscle belly medially and the extensor digitorum longus laterally. The dorsalis pedis artery is easily exposed through an axial incision on the dorsum of the foot just lateral to the extensor hallucis longus tendon (see Fig. 96.5). The artery lies just deep to the extensor retinaculum.

Following exposure of the distal anastomotic target vessel, the site of the proximal anastomosis is dissected. For patients with superficial femoral artery disease, this dissection is most commonly at the level of the common femoral artery. This vessel is exposed through a longitudinal or oblique incision centered directly over the femoral pulse. Lymphatic tissue overlying the femoral vessels is best ligated and divided to prevent the postoperative development of lymph fistulas or lymphoceles. The severity of any concomitant common femoral and profunda femoral disease and the level of reconstruction planned dictate the extent of exposure of the femoral vessels. In most instances, the dissection extends from the inguinal ligament to the common femoral artery bifurcation, where the origins of the superficial and profunda femoral arteries are individually isolated.

If a profundaplasty is required, the dissection is extended distally along a sufficient length of the profunda femoral artery to attain an endpoint suitable for clamping and sewing (Fig. 96.6). Similarly, the inguinal ligament can be partially divided to facilitate access to the distal external iliac artery in cases in which a more extensive proximal endarterectomy is necessary. In these circumstances, it is customary to close the endarterectomized bed with a vein, bovine pericardial or Dacron patch, onto which the proximal anastomosis can subsequently be attached.[41] In patients with a hostile groin crease from prior surgery or radiation therapy or in obese, diabetic patients with an intertriginous rash at the inguinal crease, meticulous skin preparation, close attention to draping, careful surgical technique, and judicious use of a short course of intravenous antibiotic therapy help minimize the chances of a postoperative wound or graft infection.

If all or part of the superficial femoral artery is spared of significant atherosclerotic involvement, the proximal anastomosis can be moved distally as dictated by the particular anatomic pattern of disease, and a so-called "distal origin graft" can be fashioned[42] (Fig. 96.7). This situation is particularly applicable to the diabetic population, in whom infrapopliteal disease is the rule and sparing of the superficial femoral and popliteal arteries is not uncommon. It is also utilized in situations in which conduit is sparse, and a moderately diseased proximal vessel is accepted as an inflow source for a more distal origin bypass graft in the interests of performing a fully autologous vein graft rather than utilizing prosthetic material. An increasingly popular approach when only limited conduit is available is to combine, either concurrently in the operating room or as a staged preoperative procedure, catheter based treatment of the superficial femoral or popliteal artery inflow with more distal bypass.[42]

Autogenous Vein Bypass

In general, infrainguinal bypass surgery is best performed with autogenous vein conduit, preferably the ipsilateral greater saphenous vein if available.[43] This preference is particularly true for grafts extending below the knee, where prosthetic conduits of Dacron or polytetrafluoroethylene (r)have significantly poorer patency rates. The first report of a femoropopliteal bypass graft using autogenous greater saphenous vein in a reversed orientation was by Kunlin in 1951.[4] Given the orientation of the vein valves, the vein is reversed such that the distal end of the vein is sewn to the proximal inflow artery and the larger proximal end of the vein is sewn to the distal outflow artery. The vein is harvested through a long incision overlying the course of the vein or by more tedious but less invasive sequential skip incisions with intervening cutaneous skin bridges (see Fig. 96.5). All side branches are ligated and after harvest, the vein is cannulated and gently dilated with a solution containing heparin and papaverine to assess its suitability.

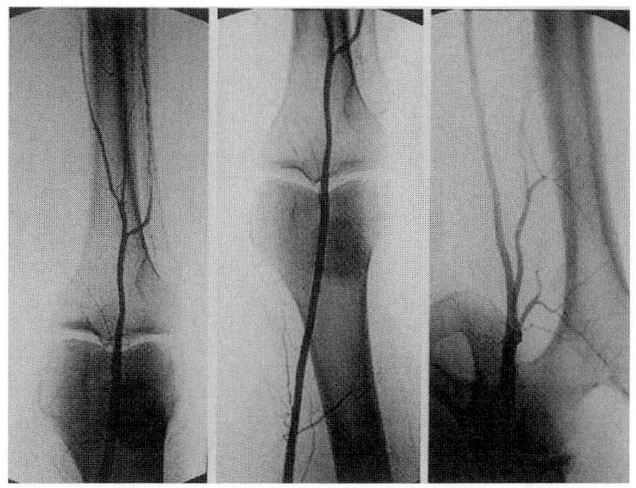

A

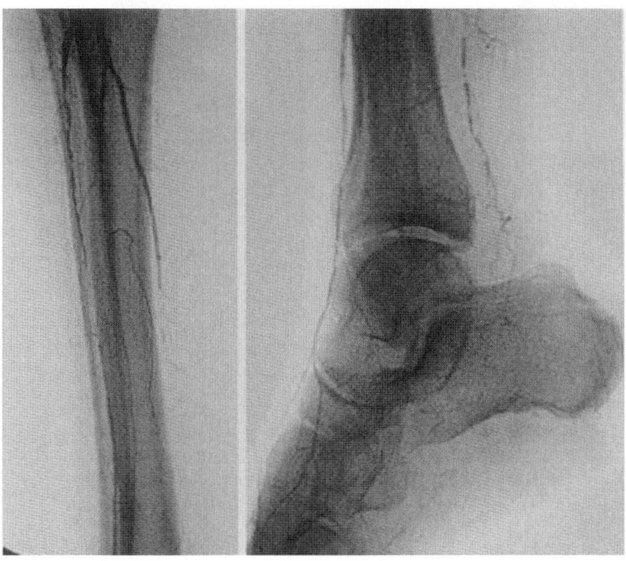

B

FIGURE 96.7 Arteriogram indicating preservation of the superficial femoral artery and popliteal arteries with mid-calf occlusions of all three infrageniculate vessels. This anatomic pattern of disease is amenable to "distal origin" vein grafting from the below-knee popliteal or proximal posterior tibial artery to the dorsalis pedis artery.

Veins with chronic fibrosis or that fail to dilate to a diameter of 3 mm or greater will likely have poor long-term function.

An alternative and less invasive approach to saphenous vein harvest involves the use of endoscopic technology. In the case of harvesting of the greater saphenous vein, small skin incisions are made over the saphenofemoral junction and the distal vein, and guided by a videoscope inserted distally and advanced proximally, the side branches of the vein are serially identified and either cauterized or clip-ligated. The vein is then divided distally and proximally and removed, leaving the overlying skin undisturbed. Advocates of this method cite a significant reduction in wound complication rates and reduced rates of hospital stay.[44] Although it has not been widely adopted by vascular surgeons, the technique does have particular theoretical appeal in cases, for example, when contralateral saphenous vein is to be utilized or the healing potential of the donor leg is compromised.

For prosthetic grafts, a tunnel is usually fashioned through the subsartorial plane between the groin incision and the above-knee popliteal space in the interests of protecting the graft from subsequent infection. For vein conduits, it remains the surgeon's preference as to whether the graft is tunneled deeply or in a superficial location in the subcutaneous space. The more superficial configuration greatly facilitates ongoing clinical examination and ultrasonographic surveillance as well as later surgical revision, but carries a risk of graft exposure should there be wound healing problems. Occlusion from trauma to grafts placed superficially has been of theoretic, but not practical concern.

The order of anastomoses is surgeon dependent, with strong feelings expressed for and against both. Prior to occluding the target vessel, the patient is systemically anticoagulated with 5,000 to 10,000 units of heparin. Additional heparin is given throughout the procedure to maintain the activated clotting time near the target range of 250 to 300 seconds. After allowing sufficient time for the heparin to circulate, atraumatic vascular clamps are placed proximally and distally and the artery is incised. The vein is then spatulated and a beveled anastomosis carried out. Typically a no. 5-0 monofilament suture of polypropylene is used for the femoral anastomosis, a no. 6-0 used at the popliteal level and a very fine no. 7-0 suture used at the tibial or pedal level. If the target tibial vessel is deep within the calf and visibility is challenging, a technique of "parachuting" the heel of the distal anastomosis is often employed. After completing the first anastomosis, the graft is carefully tunneled under antegrade pressure. Some surgeons prefer to mark the distended graft to ensure against mechanical twisting or kinking of the graft during the tunneling process. One of the benefits of performing the proximal anastomosis first is that adequacy of flow through the graft can be assessed, both before and after tunneling, with brief release of the clamp.

Occasionally, such extensive calcification of the target vessel is encountered that the risk of a significant injury from clamping, even with the minimally traumatic clamps in use today, is prohibitively high. In such cases, proximal inflow and distal artery backbleeding can be controlled by occlusion balloons placed intralumenally. For distal anastomoses at the knee or more distal level, another alternative technique is the use of a proximally placed sterile pneumatic tourniquet. This technique is particularly advantageous when sewing to diminutive distal tibial or pedal targets, where the impact of a crush injury or plaque dislodgment on graft function could be considerable. Removing the need for clamps by the using the tourniquet has two further advantages. First, it improves the operative visibility. Second, and more importantly, given that less longitudinal and circumferential dissection is needed, the degree of vessel spasm and venous bleeding that frequently accompanies vessel exposure at this level is kept to a minimum.

Flow through the graft and the outflow arteries is assessed following completion of the bypass with a continuous-wave Doppler. Ideally, a contrast angiogram is also performed after directly cannulating the proximal graft (Fig. 96.8); this allows for immediate repair of any technical defects that are identified, such as intraluminal thrombus, twisting or kinking of the graft or retained valve cusps.[45] Intraoperative completion duplex ultrasonography is an additional sensitive screen for hemodynamically significant abnormalities within the graft,[46,47] and its use further serves to prevent early graft loss caused by correctable technical problems.

Current reports of the 5-year results of reversed saphenous vein graft using modern techniques have been excellent, with primary and secondary patency rates of up to 75% and 80% respectively and limb salvage rates as high as 90%[48–50] (Table 96.1).

In Situ Grafting

There has been ongoing enthusiasm in some circles for *in situ* vein bypass grafting, whereby except for its proximal and distal extent, the greater saphenous vein is left undisturbed in its native bed. This technique was first described in 1962,[51] but was later popularized by Leather and Karmody in the late

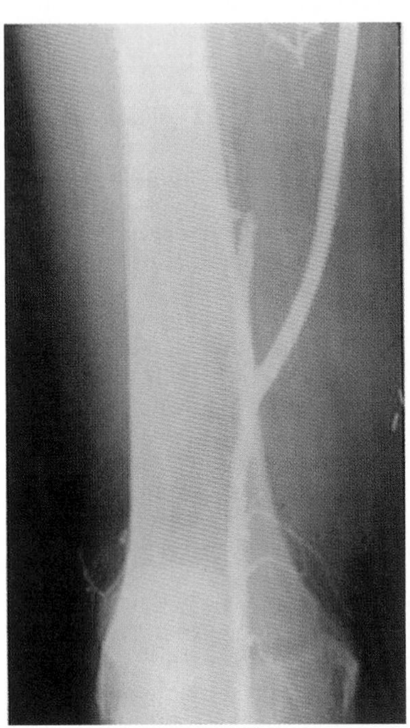

A

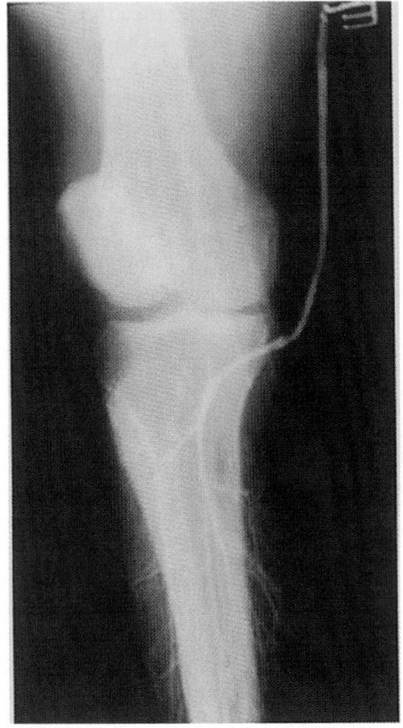

B

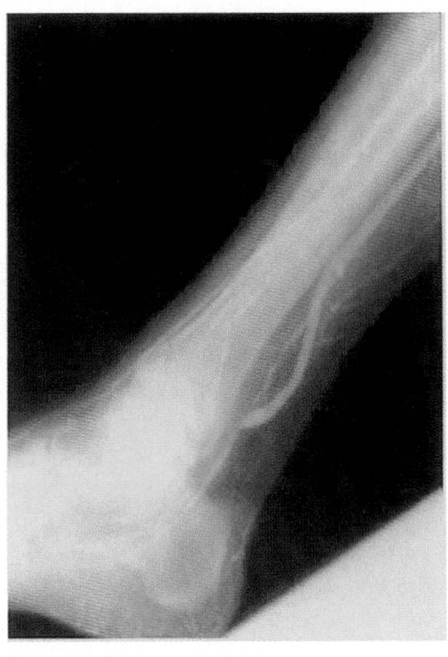

C

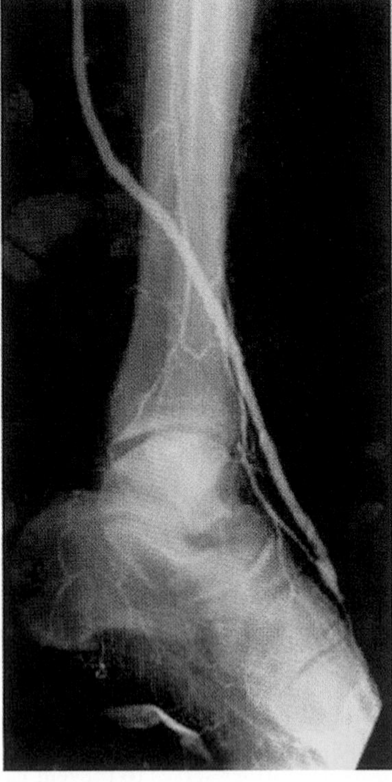

D

FIGURE 96.8 Intraoperative completion arteriograms of distal anastomoses to the above-knee popliteal (*A*), below-knee popliteal (*B*), distal posterior tibial (*C*), and dorsalis pedis (*D*) arteries.

1970s.[52] Recent reports of *in situ* saphenous vein grafting have indicated 5-year graft patency rates of up to 80% and limb salvage rates of 84% to 95%[30,31,49,53–55] (Table 96.1).

The *in situ* approach minimizes trauma to the vein during excision and handling and in theory enhances preservation of the vasovasorum and endothelium. It further lowers the considerable risk of wound healing complications seen with traditional vein harvesting, increases vein utilization, and facilitates the creation of more technically precise anastomoses because the proximal and distal vein diameters are more closely matched to those of the inflow and outflow target vessels (Fig. 96.9). The extent of the proximal vein mobilization is dictated by the location of the saphenofemoral junction relative to the proposed site of the proximal anastomosis. It may at times be necessary to perform an endarterectomy of the superficial femoral artery if the length of proximal vein is insufficient. Lysis of the valve cusps is obligatory given the nonreversed configuration, and is facilitated by newer, less traumatic valvulotomes that function safely through the blinded segments of undissected graft. Critics of this technique argue that the advantages listed above have not translated into improved graft function or patency. They further argue that the time required and dissection involved in finding and ligating substantial side branches that can develop into physiologically important arteriovenous fistulae that "steal" distal flow obviates the stated benefits of this approach. Newer techniques using angioscopy and endoluminal coiling[56] of larger side branches may help to minimize these concerns.

Angioscopic assisted valve lysis has been employed for over a decade, but has not gained widespread favor. Although there is a significant learning curve with this technology and operative times, at least initially, are significantly prolonged, advocates cite fewer wound complications, shorter hospital stays, and decreased recuperative periods as potential benefits. Proponents of routine angioscopy for direct visualization of valve lysis stress its particular utility in demonstrating such unsuspected endoluminal venous pathology as phlebitic strictures, webs and fibrotic valve cusps.[57] This adjunct may be particularly useful in cases in which arm vein is used because endoluminal pathology is more frequently encountered and is presumably responsible in part for suboptimal results.[58]

Nonreversed Saphenous Vein Grafts

Recognizing the many practical advantages inherent to the *in situ* technique, some surgeons have modified the approach to infrainguinal bypass grafting with venous conduit to incorporate several of the same principles.[30] In particular, if the harvested

TABLE 96.1 RESULTS

FIVE-YEAR PATENCY AND LIMB SALVAGE RESULTS OF INFRAINGUINAL BYPASS GRAFTING

Study	Patients, *n*	Conduit	Primary patency	Secondary patency	Limb salvage
Conte, 2001[50]	1642	Autogenous vein	63	73	85
Belkin, 1996[30]	568	*In situ* vein	72	82	90
	189	Nonreversed vein	65	65	82
Shah, 1995[31]	2058	*In situ* vein	72	81	95
Taylor, 1990[48]	564	Reversed vein	75	81	90
Veith, 1986[43]	338	PTFE to popliteal	38		70
	254	PTFE to tibial	12[a]		61[a]

[a] 4-year data.
PTFE, polytetrafluoroethylene.

vein is tapered to any significant extent, it is used in a nonreversed fashion. By optimizing the size matching between the artery and vein at both the proximal and distal anastomosis sites as discussed previously, one can often accept for use smaller veins than would be suitable for reversed vein grafting. The non-reversed configuration also allows preservation of the saphenous vein hood, which both extends the available conduit length and is especially beneficial when the femoral artery is thick-walled and diseased.

The vein is harvested and dilated in a similar fashion to reversed vein grafts and the cusps of the proximal valve of the

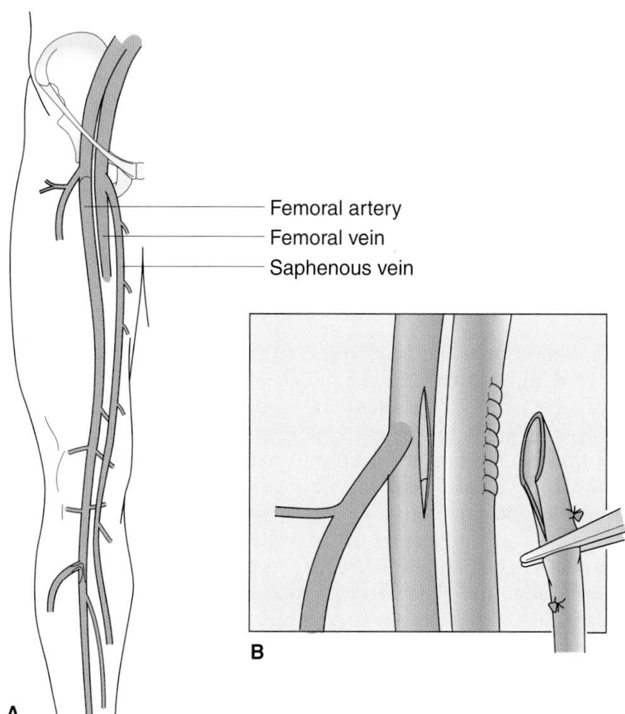

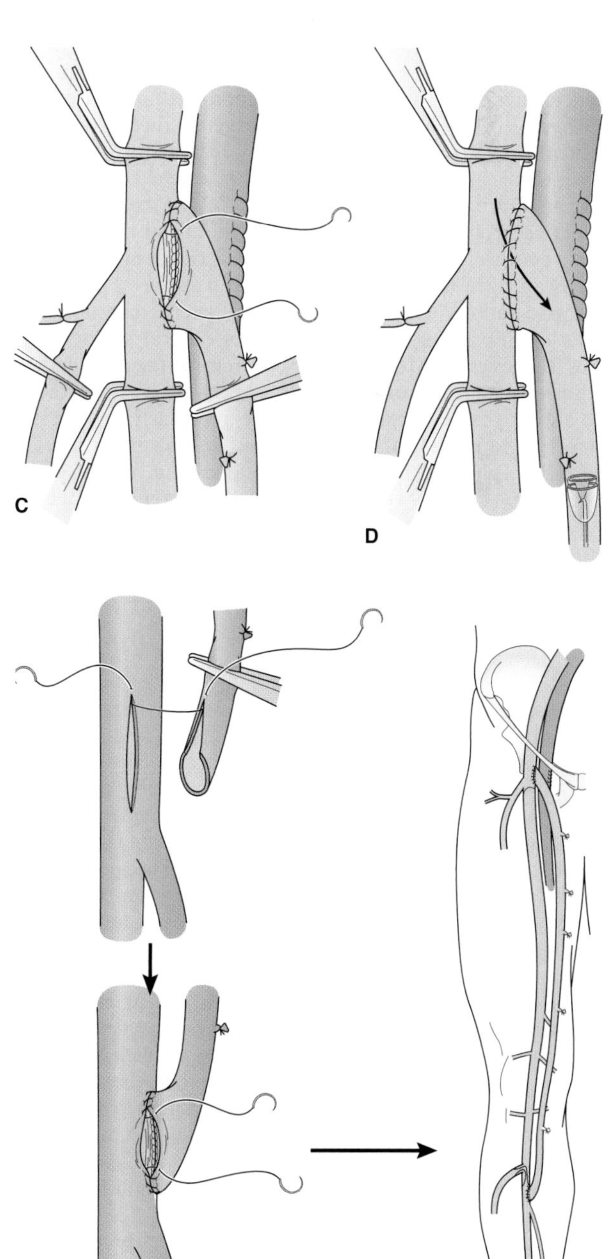

FIGURE 96.9 (*A*) In the *in situ* method of infrainguinal reconstruction, the saphenous vein is left undisturbed in its native bed except for at the proximal and distal anastomotic sites, in this case the common femoral artery and the tibioperoneal trunk, respectively. (*B*) The saphenofemoral junction is transected in the groin, the venotomy in the femoral vein is oversewn and the proximal end of the saphenous vein spatulated in prepared for anastomosis. (C) After the first venous valve is excised under direct vision, the graft is anastomosed end-to-side to the femoral artery. Flow is then restored through the vein graft and the valvulotome passed from the distal end to lyse the residual valves (*D*) before the distal anastomosis is performed (*E*).

VASCULAR

greater saphenous vein are excised under direct vision with fine Potts scissors. There are currently two main types of valvulotomes available. The modified Mills valvulotome is a short, metal, hockey stick-shaped cutter that can be introduced through the distal end of the vein or through the side branches. After the proximal anastomosis is performed, and with the perfused conduit on gentle stretch, the valves are carefully lysed in a sequential fashion by pulling the valvulotome inferiorly. An alternative, recently designed self-centering valvulotome allows lysis of all valves in a single pass and is thought by some to be less traumatic. Once acceptable pulsatile flow is ensured, the distal anastomosis is performed in the standard fashion.

It is important to note that similar patency rates have consistently been demonstrated regardless of which technique is applied,[54,55] and so surgeon preference and comfort level is an acceptable reason for choosing one method over another.

Prosthetic Bypass

It is recommended that infrainguinal bypass surgery be performed with saphenous vein or an autologous substitute whenever feasible given the clearly demonstrated enhanced patency rates.[30,59] Some institutions more frequently rely on prosthetic grafts. When the distal target is the above-knee popliteal artery and the tibial outflow is relatively well preserved, this is an acceptable approach, as patency rates in this situation approach those of vein grafts.[60] A variety of surgical adjunctive procedures, from patching the distal anastomotic target vessel to the creation of a distal arteriovenous fistula or various autogenous vein cuffs interposed between the distal prosthetic and the target artery, have all been attempted as a means of improving the patency rates of grafts extending below the knee.[61] More recently, flared grafts designed to minimize turbulence and shear stress between the prosthetic and native vessel have gained some popularity. Polyester (Dacron) and polytetraflouroethylene (Teflon) grafts are the two main types of prosthetic available and, as in other anatomic positions, available data shows generally equal results with either choice. The entire procedure is carried out through two small proximal and distal incisions between which the graft is tunneled anatomically. The selection of a 6- or 8-mm graft is dictated by the size of the native vessels.

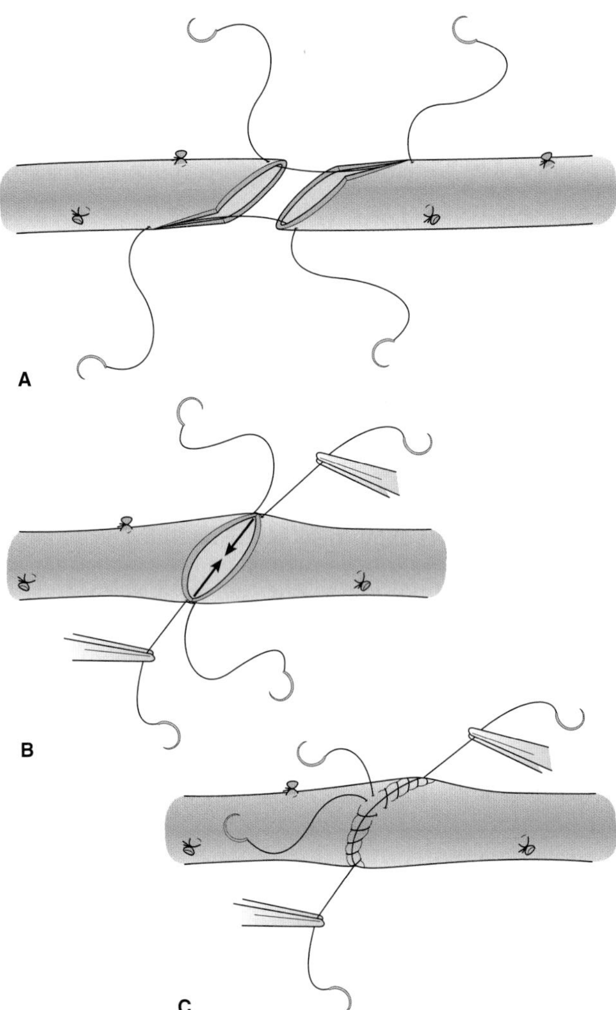

FIGURE 96.10 Creation of a composite graft from two or more segments of arm vein or lesser saphenous vein is sometimes necessary to obtain the desired length of fully autogenous conduit for infrainguinal bypass. A widely spatulated venovenostomy is optimal.

Reoperative Bypass Surgery

As the patient population treated by vascular surgeons has increased in age, and more and more challenging cases are accepted for primary treatment, there has been a corresponding increase in the incidence of reoperative bypass surgery performed for infrainguinal arterial occlusive disease. Such reoperative procedures are particularly challenging, both because of the scarring present at the inflow and outflow target sites and because there is typically a lack of ipsilateral greater saphenous vein. Whenever possible, the first problem is addressed by choosing anastomotic sites just above or below the previous touchdown points, thereby avoiding dissection through often densely scarred tissue planes. When ipsilateral greater saphenous vein is absent because of prior infrainguinal or coronary artery bypass surgery or prior saphenous vein stripping, there are a number of alternative conduit sites available. Investigators examining the consequence of using the contralateral greater saphenous vein in these situations found it to be the optimal conduit; despite the presumably high incidence of contralateral lower extremity as well as coronary occlusive disease in this population, the short- and long-term impact was found to be minimal.[62]

In the absence of any greater saphenous vein, preoperative venous duplex ultrasonography is employed to evaluate the cephalic and basilic veins of the arms and the lesser saphenous veins of the legs in an effort to determine the best conduit available. Often the veins distal to the antecubital crease are scarred and of small caliber, but their more proximal counterparts are often of excellent size and quality. The use of arm veins in general can be extremely technically challenging and for that reason has not been universally adopted. The dissection of the basilic vein can be particularly tedious as it has multiple side branches and lies adjacent to several important nerves. As arm veins are often relatively short, a venovenostomy is often required to create composite grafts long enough to complete the arterial reconstruction (Fig. 96.10). This is performed with generous spatulation of each vein hood to create a widely patent vein-to-vein anastomosis. Given their thin-walled nature, arm vein grafts are also quite prone to twisting and kinking, and special care must to taken during the tunneling process to avoid these problems. The more proximal arm veins can be relatively large, and it is often advantageous to use one or more of the segments in a nonreversed fashion to better match the graft to the inflow vessel size.

Not surprisingly, the results of reoperative infrainguinal bypass surgery do not match those of primary reconstruction. With autogenous vein, 5-year patency rates of 60% and limb salvage rates of 70% to 80% have been reported.[16,62] Coumadin is often used postoperatively in patients with compromised outflow or in who the conduit was of marginal quality and has been associated with improved long-term patency.[63]

Postreconstruction Management

Many patients undergoing surgical reconstruction for arterial insufficiency require one or more adjunctive operative procedures of their foot. Small, uninfected ulcerations of the toe or foot often can be safely managed conservatively. However, larger, gangrenous lesions of the toe, forefoot, or heel usually require débridement of all necrotic tissue at the completion of the revascularization procedure. If the ischemia is particularly severe or infection is present, a toe or transmetatarsal amputation may be necessary in order to achieve a margin of healthy tissue. This is particularly important in patients with diabetes or end-stage renal disease, in whom persistent infection or necrosis can result in limb loss despite the presence of a well-revascularized extremity. The wounds are usually left open and treated with saline wet-to-dry dressings or newer, vacuum sponge dressings. Serial débridements on the ward or in the operating room are often necessary for the larger wounds, which can then be surgically closed after an interval healing period or allowed to slowly close via secondary intention over time.

Unless otherwise contraindicated, all patients are maintained indefinitely on an antiplatelet regimen with either aspirin or clopidogrel following surgical bypass. As stated previously, in cases in which a graft is at increased risk of failure, such as in the setting of reoperation or in cases in which compromised outflow or a marginal conduit was accepted, the antiplatelet agent may be supplemented with heparin and then warfarin.[63] Patients with distal calf or pedal incisions should be placed on bed-rest with leg elevation in the early postoperative period to minimize leg swelling and wound healing complications. Thereafter, aggressive rehabilitation maximizes the chances of and shortens the time to a return to full function after extensive reconstructive surgery. Ongoing risk factor modification in the form of smoking cessation, lipid reduction, exercise, blood pressure management, and diabetic blood sugar control is of further paramount importance in minimizing the risk of disease progression or recurrence.[64]

Graft Failure and Surveillance

Postoperative graft failures are typically classified according to the time interval from surgery as early, intermediate, or late. Graft thrombosis occurring within 30 days, so-called "early graft failures," are generally thought to be a result of technical or judgment errors by the surgeon. Included in this list would be such technical errors as twists, kinks, incompletely lysed valves or anastomotic defects, as well as judgment errors in using a poor quality vein or targeting an outflow vessel with inadequate runoff to support the graft. Intermediate graft failures include those between 30 days and 2 years and are generally attributed to the proliferation of intimal hyperplasia at the anastomoses or prior valve sites within the graft (Fig. 96.11). Randomized trials are currently underway to determine the impact of molecular modulation of vein grafts on the development of intimal hyperplasia, and hold some progress in reducing or minimizing this significant cause of vein graft failure.[65] Late graft failures occurring beyond 2 years are typically a result of the progression of atherosclerotic occlusive disease within the inflow or outflow arteries.

Given the known incidence of graft failure and the potentially dire consequence in terms of limb salvage or preservation of limb function in a patient with limited options for secondary or tertiary bypass, the ability to maintain graft patency through early identification and prompt correction of graft stenoses is of paramount importance.[66] Serial postoperative surveillance scanning with a duplex ultrasound has proven an excellent means of accurately identifying hemodynamically significant stenoses within the vein graft that threaten the graft patency.[67] Velocity criteria have been developed for high-grade lesions that may warrant either more intensive surveillance or prophylactic intervention. Absolute velocities less than 40 cm/sec or greater than 300 cm/sec or a three-fold increase in velocity in one segment compared with that of an adjacent segment are all indicative of impending graft failure. Confirmation by angiography and expeditious treatment by percutaneous cutting balloon angioplasty, surgical patch angioplasty or interposition grafting of such significant lesions minimizes the risk of graft thrombosis and ensures optimal long term graft patency.

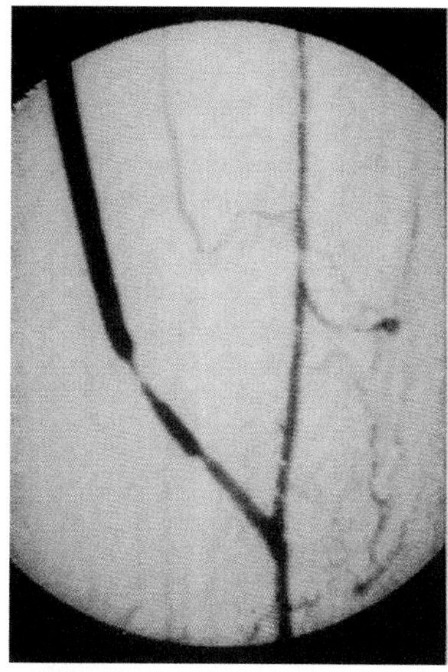

FIGURE 96.11 Arteriogram demonstrating severe stenosis of distal graft from intimal hyperplasia, likely at prior valve site.

Complications

The most commonly seen major complications of infrainguinal bypass surgery are cardiac in nature, and include myocardial infarction, congestive heart failure and arrhythmias. In a recent review spanning 20 years and involving more than 1600 procedures, the perioperative myocardial infarction rate was 3%, and the rate of cerebrovascular accident was 1%.[50] Patients with diabetes mellitus or preoperative renal insufficiency are at particular risk for developing postoperative renal failure (defined as an elevation of serum creatinine >3 mg/dL, doubling of the serum creatinine or the need for hemodialysis), which is seen in up to 2% of patients overall. Patients undergoing lower extremity revascularization are also prone to wound complications, given the length of incisions and the prolonged operating times often required. Wound infection, including cellulitis, abscess formation, wound dehiscence and skin flap necrosis, are most commonly seen and can best be avoided by gentle handling of the tissue and the use of skin bridges and careful avoidance of skin flaps during vein harvesting. Postoperative hematomas, usually caused by slow capillary or venous oozing, or seromas are seen in 5% of patients, and less commonly encountered hemorrhage, typically a result of either a slipped vein branch ligature or anastomotic disruption, is seen in less than 1% of cases.

KEY POINTS

- Infrainguinal arterial bypass surgery remains the signature operation distinguishing vascular surgeons from other specialists involved in the treatment of peripheral vascular disease.
- Chronic obliterative atherosclerosis of the infrainguinal vessels is the most prevalent manifestation of arterial occlusive disease encountered by the vascular surgeon.
- The most common lesion seen below the inguinal ligament is that of a short segment total occlusion of the superficial femoral artery.
- A particularly virulent form of atherosclerotic arterial disease is often found in young female smokers.
- Typically half of patients proceeding to surgery for arterial occlusive disease have significant coronary artery disease, even more have hypertension, and almost 80% are current or prior cigarette smokers.
- The diagnosis of infrainguinal occlusive disease is generally made based on patient symptomatology, physical examination, and noninvasive tests, such as segmental pressure measurements and pulse volume recordings.
- The impact of these trends on the natural history of occlusive disease and the extent to which the expanding reach of percutaneous therapy will affect subsequent operative management in a given patient remains to be seen.
- When medical therapy or percutaneous treatment has proven inadequate or is technically inadvisable, open surgical revascularization remains the gold standard for those patients with disabling claudication, ischemic rest pain, and ischemic ulceration or gangrene.
- Infrainguinal bypass surgery is best performed with autogenous vein conduit, preferably the ipsilateral greater saphenous vein if available.
- Many of the patients undergoing surgical reconstruction for arterial insufficiency will require one or more adjunctive operative procedures of their foot.

References

1. Gray EA. *Portrait of a surgeon. A biography of John Hunter*. London: Robert Hale; 1952.
2. dos Santos JC: Sur la desobstion des thromboses arterielles anciennes. *Mem Acad Chir*. 1947;73:409.
3. **Carrel A. The surgery of blood vessels, etc. *John Hopkins Hosp Bull*. 1907;190:18.**
4. Kunlin J. Le traitement de l'ischemie arteritique par la greffe veineuse longue. *Rev Chir* 1951;70:206.
5. McCaughan JJ Jr. Surgical exposure of the distal popliteal artery. *Surgery* 1958;44:536.
6. Halperin JL. Evaluation of patients with peripheral vascular disease. *Thromb Res*. 2002;106:303.
7. Imparato AM, Kim GE, Davidson T, et al. Intermittent claudication: Its natural course. *Surgery* 1975;78:795.
8. McAllister FF. The fate of patients with intermittent claudication managed conservatively. *Am J Surg*. 1976;132:593.
9. **Walsh DB, Gilbertson JJ, Zwolak RM, et al. The natural history of superficial femoral artery stenoses. *J Vasc Surg*. 1991;14:299.**
10. **Brewster DC, Perler BA, Robison JG, et al. Aortofemoral graft for multilevel occlusive disease: predictors of success and need for distal bypass. *Arch Surg*. 1982;117:1593.**
11. Wingo JP, Nix ML, Greenfield LJ, et al. The blue toe syndrome: hemodynamic and therapeutic correlates of outcome. *J Vasc Surg*. 1986;3:475.
12. Karmody AM, Powers SR, Monaco VJ, et al. "Blue toe" syndrome. *Arch Surg*. 1976;111:1263.
13. Cronenwett JL, Davis JT, Gooch JB, et al. Aortoiliac occlusive disease in women. *Surgery* 1980;88:775.
14. Caes F, Cham B, Van den Brande P, et al. Small artery syndrome in women. *Surg Gynecol Obstet*. 1985;161:165.
15. **Hertzer NR, Beven EG, Young JR, et al. Coronary artery disease in peripheral vascular patients: A classification of 1000 coronary angiograms and results of surgical management. *Ann Surg*. 1984;199:223.**
16. Belkin M, Conte MS, Donaldson MC, et al. Preferred strategies for secondary infrainguinal bypass: lessons learned from 300 consecutive reoperations. *J Vasc Surg*. 1995;21:282.
17. Whittemore AD, Clowes AW, Hechtman HB, et al. Aortic aneurysm repair: Reduced operative mortality associated with maintenance of optimal cardiac performance. *Ann Surg*. 1980 192:414–21.
18. Kaluza GL, Joseph J, Lee JR, et al. Catastrophic outcomes of noncardiac surgery soon after coronary stenting. *J Am Coll Cardiol*. 2000;35:1288.
19. Grassbaugh JA, Nelson PR, Rzucidlo EM, et al. Blinded comparison of preoperative duplex ultrasound scanning and contrast arteriography for planning revascularization at the level of the tibia. *J Vasc Surg*. 2003;37:1186.
20. Carpenter JP, Owen RS, Holland GA, et al. Magnetic resonance angiography of the aorta, iliac and femoral arteries. *Surgery* 1994116:17.
21. **Baum RA, Rutter CM, Sunshine JH, et al. Multicenter trial to evaluate vascular magnetic resonance angiography of the lower extremity. *JAMA* 1995;274:875.**
22. Koelemay MJ, Lijmer JG, Stoker J, et al. Magnetic resonance angiography for the evaluation of lower extremity arterial disease: A meta-analysis. *JAMA*. 2001285:1338.
23. Udoff EJ, Barth KH, Harrington DP, et al. Hemodynamic significance of iliac artery stenosis: pressure measurements during angiography. *Radiology* 1979;132:289.
24. Spinosa DJ, Kaufmann JA, Hartwell GD. Gadolinium chelates in angiography and interventional radiology: a useful alternative to iodinated contrast media for angiography. *Radiology* 2002;223:319.
25. Back MR, Caridi JG, Hawkins IF, et al. Angiography with carbon dioxide (CO_2). *Surg Clin North Am*. 1998;78:575.
26. Nehler MR, Hiatt WR. Exercise therapy for claudication. *Ann Vasc Surg*. 1999;13:109.
27. Regensteiner JG, Meyer TJ, Krupski WC. Hospital versus home-based exercise rehabilitation for patients with peripheral arterial occlusive disease. *Angiology* 1997;48:291.
28. Dawson DL, Cutler BS, Hiatt WR, et al. A comparison of Cilostazol and Pentoxifylline for treating intermittent claudication. *Am J Med*. 2000;109:523.
29. Antiplatelet Trialists' Collaboration. Collaborative overview of randomised trials of antiplatelet therapy—II. Maintenance of vascular graft or arterial patency by antiplatelet therapy. *BMJ*. 1994;308:159–168.
30. **Belkin M, Knox J, Donaldson MC, et al. Infrainguinal arterial reconstruction with nonreversed greater saphenous vein. *J Vasc Surg*. 1996;24:957.**
31. **Shah DM, Darling RC, Chang BB, et al. Long-term results of in situ saphenous vein bypass: analysis of 2058 cases. *Ann Surg*. 1995;222:438.**
32. Faries PF, Morrissey NJ, Teodorescu V, et al. Recent advances in peripheral angioplasty and stenting. *Angiology* 2002;53:617.
33. Duda SH, Poerner TC, Wiesinger B, et al. Drug-eluting stents: Potential applications for peripheral arterial occlusive disease. *J Vasc Interv Radiol*. 2003;14:291.
34. Berkseth RO, Kjellstrand CM. Radiologic contrast-induced nephropathy. *Med Clin North Am*. 1984;68:351.
35. Kandzari DE, Rebeiz AG, Wang A, et al. Contrast nephropathy: an evidence-based approach to prevention. 2003;3:395.
36. MacNeill BD, Harding SA, Bazari H, et al. Prophylaxis of contrast-induced nephropathy in patients undergoing coronary angiography. *Catheter Cardiovasc Interv*. 2003;60:458.
37. Knight CG, Healy DA, Thomas RL. Femoral artery pseudoaneurysms: risk factors, prevalence, and treatment options. *Ann Vasc Surg*. 2003;17: 503.
38. Lonn L, Olmarker A, Geterud K, et al. Prospective randomized study comparing ultrasound-guided thrombin injection to compression in the treatment of femoral pseudoaneurysms. *J Endovasc Ther*. 2004;11:570.
39. Quinn SF, Kim J. Percutaneous femoral closure following stent-graft placement: Use of the Perclose Device. *Cardiovasc Intervent Radiol*. 2004;27:231.
40. Ascher E, Veith FJ, Gupta SK. Bypasses to plantar arteries and other tibial branches: An extended approach to limb salvage. *J Vasc Surg*. 1988;8:434.
41. Malone JM, Goldstone J, Moore WS. Autogenous profundaplasty: The key to long-term patency in secondary repair of aortofemoral graft occlusion. *Ann Surg*. 1978;188:817.
42. Reed AB, Conte MS, Belkin M, et al. Usefulness of autogenous bypass grafts originating distal to the groin. *J Vasc Surg*. 2002;35:48.
43. Veith FJ, Gupta SK, Ascer E, et al. Six-year prospective multicenter randomized comparison of autologous saphenous vein and expanded polytetraflouroethylene graft in infrainguinal arterial reconstruction. *J Vasc Surg*. 1986;3:104.
44. Rosenthal D. Endoscopic in situ bypass. *Surg Clin N Am*. 1995;75:703.
45. Baxter BT, Rizzo RJ, Flinn WR, et al. A comparative study of intraoperative angioscopy and completion arteriography following femorodistal bypass. *Arch Surg*. 1990;125:997.
46. Gilbertson JJ, Walsh DB, Zwolak RM, et al. A blinded comparison of angiography, angioscopy, and duplex scanning in the intraoperative evaluation of in situ saphenous vein bypass grafts. *J Vasc Surg*. 1992;15:121.
47. Bandyk D, Johnson B, Gupta A, et al. Nature and management of duplex abnormalities encountered during infrainguinal vein bypass grafting. *J Vasc Surg*. 1996;24:430.
48. Taylor LM, Edwards JM, Porter JM. Present status of reversed vein bypass grafting: Five-year results of a modern series. *J Vasc Surg*. 1990;11:193.
49. Fogle MA, Whittemore AD, Couch NP, et al. A comparison of in situ and reversed saphenous vein grafts for infrainguinal reconstruction. *J Vasc Surg*. 1987;5:46.

50. **Conte MS, Belkin M, Upchurch GR, et al. Impact of increasing comorbidity on infrainguinal reconstruction: A 20-year perspective. *Ann Surg.* 2001;233:445.**
51. Hall KV. The great saphenous vein used "in situ" as an arterial shunt after extirpation of vein valves. A preliminary report. *Surgery* 1962;51: 492.
52. Leather RP, Powers SR, Karmody AM. A reappraisal of the in situ saphenous vein arterial bypass: Its use in limb salvage. *Surgery* 1979;86:453.
53. Donaldson MC, Mannick JA, Whittemore AD. Femoral-distal bypass with in situ greater saphenous vein: Long term results using Mills valvulotome. *Ann Surg.* 1991;213:457.
54. Moody AP, Edwards PR, Harris PL. In situ versus reversed femoropopliteal vein grafts: Long-term follow-up of a prospective, randomized trial. *Br J Surg.* 1992;79:750.
55. Wengerter KR, Veith FJ, Gupta SK, et al. Prospective randomized multicenter comparison of in situ and reversed vein infrapopliteal bypasses. *J Vasc Surg.* 1991;13:189.
56. Rosenthal D, Dickson C, Rodriquez FJ, et al. Infrainguinal endovascular in situ saphenous vein bypass: Ongoing results. *J Vasc Surg.* 1994;20: 389.
57. Panetta TF, Marin ML, Veith FJ, et al. Unsuspected pre-existing saphenous vein pathology: An unrecognized cause of vein bypass failure. *J Vasc Surg.* 1992;15:102.
58. Marcaccio EJ, Miller A, Tannenbaum GA, et al. Angioscopically directed interventions improve arm vein bypass grafts. *J Vasc Surg.* 1993;17:994.
59. Whittemore AD, Kent KC, Donaldson MC, et al. What is the proper role of polytetrafluoroethylene grafts in infrainguinal reconstruction? *J Vasc Surg.* 1989;10:299.
60. Quinones-Baldrich WJ, Prego AA, Ucelay-Gomez R, et al. Long-term results of infrainguinal revascularization with polytetrafluoroethylene: A ten-year experience. *J Vasc Surg.* 1992;16:209.
61. Miller JH, Foreman RK, Ferguson L, et al. Interposition vein cuff for anastomosis of prosthesis to small artery. *Aust NZ J Surg.* 1984;54:283.
62. Chew DK, Owens CD, Belkin M, et al. Bypass in the absence of ipsilateral greater saphenous vein: safe superiority of the contralateral greater saphenous vein. *J Vasc Surg.* 2002;35:1085.
63. Sarac TP, Huber TS, Back MR, et al. Warfarin improves the outcome of infrainguinal vein bypass grafting at high risk for failure. *J Vasc Surg.* 1998;28:446.
64. Creager MA. Medical management of peripheral arterial disease. *Cardiol Rev.* 2001;9:238.
65. **Mann MJ, Whittemore AD, Donaldson MC, et al. Ex-vivo gene therapy of human vascular bypass grafts with E2F: the PREVENT single-centre, randomized, controlled trial. *Lancet* 1999;354:1493.**
66. Veith FJ, Weiser RK, Gupta SK, et al. Diagnosis and management of failing lower extremity arterial reconstructions prior to graft occlusion. *J Cardiovasc Surg.* 1984;25:381.
67. Bandyk DF, Schmitt DD, Seabrook GR, et al. Monitoring functional patency of in situ saphenous vein bypasses: The impact of a surveillance protocol and elective revision. *J Vasc Surg.* 1989;9:286.

CHAPTER 97 ■ LOWER EXTREMITY AMPUTATION

JOSEPH GIGLIA AND MARCUS D. JARBOE

Surgeons are often involved in treating patients requiring lower extremity amputation. In fact, more than 115,000 lower extremity amputations are performed in the United States alone each year (Table 97.1). Clinical judgment is critical to a successful outcome. Factors to consider are primary amputation, revascularization, repeat revascularization, level of amputation, and timing of amputation. The surgeon must remember that the goal is to maintain maximal function of the patient not necessarily maximal length of the limb. Consequently, experience of the surgeon has been shown to be key to a successful outcome.[1]

TABLE 97.1

TOTAL AMPUTATIONS EACH YEAR IN THE UNITED STATES

Type of amputation	No.	Percentage
Phalangeal	36,800	32
Foot	11,500	10
Below-knee	33,350	29
Above-knee	33,350	29
Total	115,000	100

From Frang RD, Tayor LM, Porter JM. Amputations. In: Porter JM, Taylor LM, eds. Basic Data Underlying Clinical Decision Making in Vascular Surgery. St. Louis: Quality Medical, 1994:153.

INDICATIONS

Most lower extremity amputations are performed for complications of diabetes or arterial insufficiency (Table 97.2). Chronic infection and trauma account for less than 10% of the total number of amputations. Other indications include neuroma, frostbite, malignancy, chronic pain, arterial embolization, venous insufficiency, and cryoglobulinemia.[2]

TABLE 97.2 INDICATIONS/CONTRAINDICATIONS

INDICATIONS FOR LOWER EXTREMITY AMPUTATION

Indication	Percentage
Complications of diabetes mellitus	60–80
Nondiabetic infection with ischemia	15–25
Ischemia without infection	5–10
Chronic osteomyelitis	3–5
Trauma	2–5
Miscellaneous (neuroma, frostbite, tumor, pain nonhealing wound)	5–10

From Malone JM. Lower extremity amputation. In: Moore WS, ed. *Vascular surgery: a comprehensive review.* Philadelphia: WB Saunders 1993:810.

Elective lower extremity amputation in diabetic and vascular patients is indicated for gangrene (dry gangrene), gangrene with infection (wet gangrene), unremitting and unreconstructable rest pain, and nonhealing ulcers. The goal of the operation is to remove all nonviable tissue, relieve ischemic rest pain, ensure primary wound healing, and facilitate rehabilitation. A surgeon capable of performing the procedure should perform elective amputation only following an evaluation for revascularization and a potential limb salvage procedure. Veith and colleagues[3] reported that 96% of patients who underwent lower extremity arteriography for limb-threatening infrainguinal arteriosclerosis were candidates for arterial reconstruction. Not all patients are candidates for arteriography, including those with organic brain syndrome, nonfunctional limbs, fixed joint contractures, insensate feet, and those with extensive gangrene.

Spinal cord stimulation (SCS) may offer a chance for limb salvage for patients with chronic ischemia in whom reconstruction is not an option. Based on Melzack and Wall's theory for treatment of chronic pain,[4] the mechanism of pain relief and increased blood flow in end-stage peripheral vascular disease is unclear. Despite this, there is peripheral vasodilatation on the microvascular level which leads to pain relief,[5] increased claudication distance,[6] ulcer healing,[7] and possible limb salvage.[5,8,9] The 1-year foot salvage rate is 60% to 70% on average, according to a review of the literature.[10] SCS is only appropriate when surgery for revascularization is no longer possible. Furthermore, SCS only dilates microvasculature and does nothing for the underlying, progressive peripheral vascular disease that is causing the ischemia. SCS, therefore, is only a temporizing measure, but can potentially give an extended functional period with a procedure that is well tolerated and relatively simple to perform.[10]

Emergent amputation is indicated in the face of uncontrolled or ascending infection. In the case of uncontrolled sepsis, it can even be a life-saving maneuver. A diabetic patient with a foot abscess is a surgical emergency. Frequently, incision and drainage with or without a toe or a combined toe and metatarsal resection is sufficient to control the acute problem. If the process has extended proximal to the foot, an open amputation of the leg is indicated. An above-knee amputation (AKA) is indicated in patients with infection involving the entire leg, a fixed knee contracture, or those with a nonfunctional limb.

Primary amputation is occasionally indicated in cases of treatment for lower extremity trauma. Both penetrating and blunt injuries of the lower extremities are frequently associated with vascular, nerve, bone, and extensive soft tissue injuries. A decision for treatment with primary amputation is extremely difficult and requires extensive clinical judgment and multidisciplinary input. Contributing factors include the severity of the injury, the overall clinical status, and the ultimate rehabilitation potential of the patient.

Several treatment guidelines have been developed for lower extremity trauma. Lange[11] recommended primary amputation for open tibial fractures with associated vascular injuries if the posterior tibial nerve was disrupted in an adult or if the duration of warm ischemia was greater than 6 hours in a crush injury. In addition, he suggested that primary amputation was relatively indicated in patients with polytrauma, severe ipsilateral foot injuries, and in those with an expected protracted postoperative course. These suggestions are supported in work by Bosse et al.[12] demonstrating, in the case of high energy lower extremity trauma, amputation and reconstruction have equal functional outcomes at 2 years. Additional guidelines have been provided by Johansen and colleagues[13] who devised a Mangled Extremity Severity Score to predict the need for amputation based on the extent of skeletal or soft tissue damage, limb ischemia, shock, and age.

EVALUATION FOR REVASCULARIZATION

Modern vascular surgery techniques allow successful limb salvage in situations not previously possible. All patients who present for possible lower extremity amputation should be considered for revascularization. The evaluation may require only a thorough history and physical examination if there is an obvious contraindication to revascularization (e.g., nonfunctional limb, severe organic brain syndrome). Conversely, contrast angiography with selected lower extremity injections may be necessary to fully define the patient's anatomy and suitability for reconstruction. Even in cases where high-quality contrast angiography cannot visualize an adequate target vessel, successful limb salvage has been obtained with a pedal bypass if duplex examination or magnetic resonance angiography (MRA) identifies a preserved dorsalis pedis.

Upper extremity[14] and cryopreserved cadaver vein[15] have increased the options for conduit in limb salvage situations. Prosthetic grafts with vein cuffs[16,17] provide other alternatives when appropriate autogenous conduit is not available. An operation for limb salvage should never be denied *only* for lack of conduit.

Revascularization is often performed in conjunction with a limited amputation, either simultaneously or as a staged procedure. This allows management of the acute problem of sepsis and the underlying chronic ischemia. In extreme cases, a limited amputation can be combined with revascularization and a tissue transfer (free or rotational flap) to achieve limb salvage.[18,19]

CHOICE OF AMPUTATION LEVEL

General

The choice of amputation level depends on the indication for the procedure, the condition of the patient, and the rehabilitation potential of the patient. The most common amputation levels are illustrated in Fig. 97.1. Because most amputations are performed for complications of diabetes or arterial insufficiency, the selected level must remove all nonviable, painful tissue, allow primary healing, and maximize rehabilitation potential. Selection of the amputation level for malignant disease is dependent on the biologic characteristics of the neoplasm and will not be discussed further.

The general medical condition and the rehabilitation potential of the patient are important factors in deciding to proceed with amputation and in selecting the appropriate level. If a patient is ambulatory and independent preoperatively, the level with the greatest likelihood of maintaining function should be selected. If the patient is not ambulatory or has significant co-morbid conditions, the primary wound-healing rate should be the determining factor.

Specific Situations

Aggressive attempts to salvage a distal amputation level are not indicated for patients who are unlikely to ambulate with a prosthesis.[20] For example, patients with fixed joint contractures greater than 15 degrees at the knee or 10 degrees at the hip are unlikely to ambulate with a prosthesis. Below-knee amputations are relatively contraindicated in patients with paraplegia because flexion contractures at the knee can lead to stump ulceration.

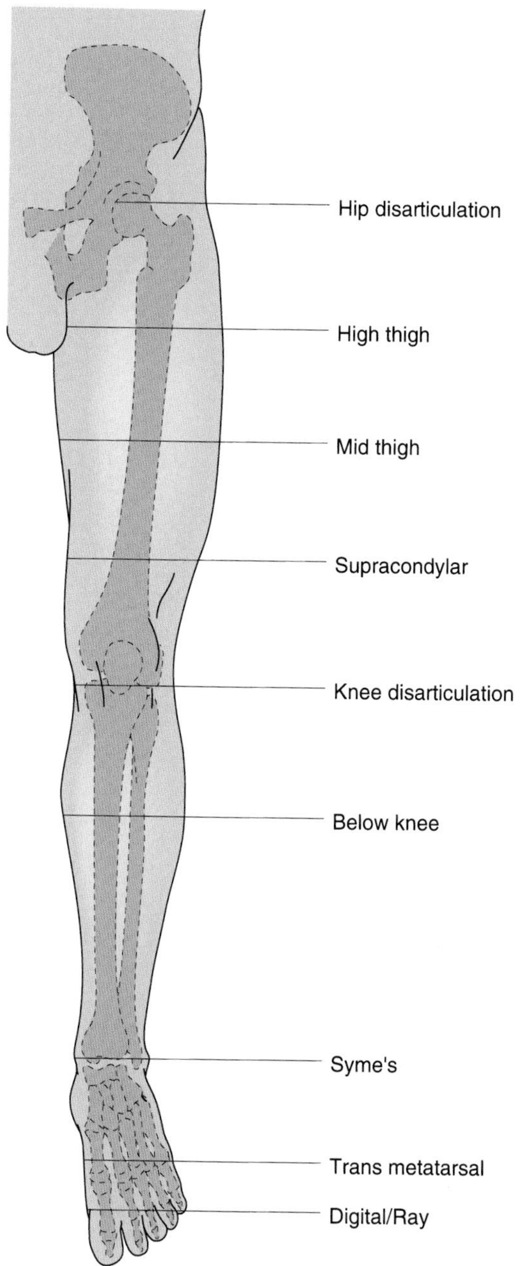

FIGURE 97.1 Common amputation levels for the lower extremity.

Energy Requirement

The energy required to ambulate following a lower extremity amputation increases with ascending level of amputation. The more proximal the amputation, the less likely a patient will be able to ambulate postoperatively. Table 97.3 illustrates the increased energy cost of the common lower extremity amputations. In clinical practice, the most significant increase is between a below-knee amputation (BKA) and an AKA. Ambulation on an above-knee prosthesis requires the use of muscle groups poorly suited for that purpose. These increased energy costs are minor issues for young trauma or cancer patients; however, they represent a considerable obstacle for the older diabetic or vascular patient.

TABLE 97.3

REHABILITATION ENERGY COST OF AMPUTATION AT VARIOUS LEVELS

Amputation level	Energy cost
Digital or ray	Minimal (except first ray)
Transmetatarsal	Minimal during normal walking
Below-knee	30%–60% increase in energy required for ambulation
Above-knee	60%–100% increase in energy required for ambulation
Hip disarticulation	100%–110% increase in energy required for ambulation

Clinical Assessment

The primary preoperative consideration for wound healing is the status of the skin and muscle blood flow. Operative technique, the patient's nutritional status, and the presence of infection also affect wound healing. Clinical judgment by an experienced surgeon accurately predicts healing of a BKA in approximately 80% of cases.[21] A palpable pulse at the level immediately proximal to the proposed amputation essentially ensures healing;[22] however, the converse is not true. Noninvasive arterial testing is the most common adjunctive test used to predict healing of a specific amputation level. Its usefulness is limited when medial sclerosis prevents vessel compression, a condition common in diabetic patients. Because the digital vessels are often spared from this process, digital pressure readings may be helpful in this setting.

A variety of nuclear medicine techniques[23,24] has been used to assess skin perfusion at the proposed amputation level; however, reproducibility among centers is lacking. Fluorescein skin blood flow measurements did not correlate with amputation healing in a blinded study.[25] Transcutaneous oxygen measurement has been shown to predict primary healing; however, the technique is not widely used as it is not widely available.[26,27] Laser Doppler velocimetry,[28] photoplethysmography,[29] theromography,[30] and pulse volume recordings[31] have all been applied with mixed results. Tables 97.4 to 97.7 summarize the

TABLE 97.4 RESULTS

PREOPERATIVE LEVEL SELECTION: TOE AMPUTATION

Selection criteria	Successful healing, primary and secondary per total
Empiric	86/115 (75%)
Presence of pedal pulses	357/365 (98%)
Doppler toe pressure >30 mm[a]	47/60 (78%)
Doppler ankle pressure >35 mm[a]	44/46 (96%)
Photoplethysmographic digit or [a]TMA pressure >20 mm	20/20 (100%)
^{133}Xe skin blood flow >2.6 mL/100 g of tissue/min	5/6 (83%)

[a]Systolic pressure (mm Hg).
TMA, transmetatarsal.
From Durham JR. Lower extremity amputation levels: indications, methods of determining appropriate level, technique, prognosis. In: Rutherford RB, ed. *Vascular surgery*, 3rd ed. Philadelphia: WB Saunders, 1989:1693.

TABLE 97.5 RESULTS

PREOPERATIVE LEVEL SELECTION: FOOT AND FOREFOOT AMPUTATION

Selection criteria	Successful healing, primary and secondary per total
Empiric	11/24 (46%)
	36/50 (72%)
Doppler ankle systolic pressure	
<40 mm Hg	5/9 (56%)
>40 mm Hg	20/60 (33%)
40–60 mm Hg	4/5 (80%)
>50 mm Hg	14/21 (66%)
>60 mm Hg	68/91 (75%)
>70 mm Hg	70/93 (75%)
Doppler toe systolic pressure	4/5 (80%)
>30 mm Hg	
Doppler ankle-brachial pressure index	
>0.45 (nondiabetic)	
>0.50 (diabetic)	58/60 (97%)
Photoplethysmographic toe systolic pressure	
>55 mm Hg	14/14 (100%)
>45 and <55 mm Hg	2/8 (25%)
<45 mm Hg	0/8 (0%)
Fiberoptic fluorometry (dye fluorescence index >44)	18/20 (90%)
Laser Doppler velocimetry	2/6 (33%)
^{125}I-iodopyrine skin blood flow	
>8 mL/100 g of tissue/min	18/18 (100%)
^{133}Xe skin blood flow	23/25 (92%)
>2.6 mL/100 g of tissue/min	
Transcutaneous Po_2	
>10 mm (or a >10-mm increase on Fio_2 = 1.0)	6/8 (75%)
>28 mm Hg	3/3 (100%)
Transcutaneous Pco_2	
<40 mm Hg	3/3 (100%)

From Durham JR. Lower extremity amputation levels: indications, methods of determining appropriate level, technique, prognosis. In: Rutherford RB, ed. Vascular Surgery, 3rd ed. Philadelphia: WB Saunders, 1989:1695.

TABLE 97.6 RESULTS

PREOPERATIVE LEVEL SELECTION: BELOW-KNEE AMPUTATION

Selection criteria	Successful healing, primary and secondary per total
Empiric	794/974 (82%)
Doppler ankle systolic pressure	
>30 mm Hg	66/70 (94%)
Doppler calf systolic pressure	
>50 mm Hg	36/36 (100%)
>68 mm Hg	96/97 (99%)
Doppler thigh systolic pressure	
>100 mm Hg	31/31 (100%)
>80 mm Hg	104/113 (92%)
Fluorescein dye	24/30 (80%)
Fiberoptic fluorometry (dye fluorescence index >44)	12/12 (100%)
Laser Doppler velocimetry	8/8 (100%)
Skin perfusion pressure	
^{99m}Tc-pertechnetate	24/26 (92%)
^{131}I- or ^{125}I-antipyrine >30 mm	60/62 (97%)
Photoelectric skin perfusion pressure >20 mm	60/71 (85%)
^{133}Xe skin blood flow	
Epicutaneous >0.9 mL/100 g of tissue/min	14/15 (93%)
Intradermal >2.4 mL/100 g of tissue/min	83/89 (93%)
Intradermal >1 mL/100 g of tissue/min	11/12 (92%)
Transcutaneous Po_2 = 0	0/3 (0%)
>10 mm Hg (or >10-min increase on Fio_2 = 1.0)	76/80 (95%)
>10 and <40 mm Hg	5/7 (71%)
>20 mm Hg	25/26 (96%)
>35 mm Hg	51/51 (100%)
Transcutaneous Po_2 index >0.59	17/17 (100%)
Transcutaneous Pco_2 <40 mm Hg	7/8(88%)

From Durham JR. Lower extremity amputation levels: indications, methods of determining appropriate level, technique, prognosis. In: Rutherford RB, ed. Vascular Surgery, 3rd ed. Philadelphia: WB Saunders, 1989:1700.

results of various preoperative tests to predict wound healing for toe, foot and forefoot, below-knee, and above-knee amputations, respectively.

OPERATIVE TECHNIQUE

General Considerations

Diabetic patients who present septic require adequate fluid resuscitation broad-spectrum antibiotics (including anaerobic coverage), and an emergent operation. Whereas maintenance of limb length and function is admirable, control of sepsis and wide débridement of all nonviable tissue is essential and potentially lifesaving. All patients require atraumatic tissue handling. Avoid forceps on the skin edge. Excessive skin flaps and dead space are also not desired. Amputations done in the face of active infection are kept open and treated with dressing changes. Consider delayed primary closure in cases where perfusion is intact.

Postoperatively, the limb is elevated to minimize tissue edema and promote healing. Ambulation is delayed until healing is assured. This sedentary patient population requires effective prophylaxis against deep venous thrombosis.

Digital and Ray Amputations

Digital amputations are indicated for gangrene or osteomyelitis localized distal to the middle phalanx. The technique is illustrated in Fig. 97.2A. A circumferential skin incision is made over the

TABLE 97.7 RESULTS

PREOPERATIVE LEVEL SELECTION: ABOVE-KNEE AMPUTATION

Selection criteria	Successful healing, primary and secondary per total
Empiric	390/430 (91%)
Fiberoptic fluorometry (dye fluorescence index >44)	6/7 (86%)
Laser Doppler velocimetry	6/6 (100%)
Photoelectric skin perfusion pressure >21 mm	19/19 (100%)
Skin perfusion pressure (^{131}I- or ^{125}I-antipyrine)	44/48 (92%)
^{133}Xe skin blood flow intradermal >2.6 mL/100 g of tissue/min	20/20 (100%)
Transcutaneous PO_2	
>10 mm (or 10-mm increase on FIO_2 = 1.0)	15/23 (65%)
>20 mm	12/12 (100%)
>23 mm	2/2 (100%)
>35 mm	21/24 (100%)
Transcutaneous PCO_2 <38 min	5/5 (100%)

From Durham JR. Lower extremity amputation levels: indications, methods of determining appropriate level, technique, prognosis. In: Rutherford RB, ed. Vascular-Surgery, 3rd ed. Philadelphia: WB Saunders, 1989:1707.

distal end of the proximal phalanx, and carried down to bone. Nerves and tendons are transected under tension and allowed to retract. The proximal phalanx is divided with bone shears and the transected end is smoothed with a rongeur. The wound is closed in layers and, postoperatively, the patient is kept at bed rest for several days.

A ray amputation is indicated when the disease process extends to the digital crease. The technique is similar to a digital amputation and is illustrated in Fig. 97.2B. A circumferential incision is made at the base of the involved toe and extended proximally on the dorsum of the foot over the metatarsal. The incision is extended to bone. The periosteum is cleared circumferentially and the bone is transected at a level that will allow tension-free closure of the wound. In the case of the first or fifth toe, the incision is extended on the medial or lateral aspect of the foot, respectively.

In selected cases of neuropathic ulcers, the metatarsal head can be resected leaving the toe intact. A dorsal longitudinal incision is made over the metatarsal bone and a counterincision is made at the region of the ulcer on the plantar aspect of the foot. The distal portion of the metatarsal and the metatarsal head are then resected. The wound is packed in a through-and-through fashion until significant healing has occurred.

Transmetatarsal Amputation

Transmetatarsal amputation (TMA) is a useful procedure that maintains a patient's ability to ambulate without the aid of a prosthesis. It is indicated when the gangrenous or infectious process involves multiple digits or the forefoot. It is contraindicated when the underlying process extends to the proposed skin incision or the plantar aspect of the foot is affected. In the latter situation, an open amputation through the metatarsal bones can be performed. The wound is allowed to close secondarily or covered with a skin graft. Skin grafts in this position, however, are susceptible to breakdown secondary to the pressure related to ambulation.

The technique is demonstrated in Fig. 97.3. A skin incision is made on the dorsum of the foot immediately proximal to the metatarsal heads and extended medially and laterally to a point midway between the plantar and dorsal surfaces. The plantar incision is made along the digital crease and extended diagonally medially and laterally to connect to the dorsal incision. The dorsal incision is deepened to the periosteum, which is cleared with a small periosteal elevator. The metatarsal bones are transected 0.5 cm proximal to the dorsal skin incision. The plantar flap is fashioned by continuing the dissection just superficial to the metatarsal heads. Care is taken to maintain plantar flap thickness. The nerves and tendons are transected sharply under tension and allowed to retract. The plantar flap is rotated anteriorly and assessed for length. Excess tissue is excised sharply and the deep tissue is approximated with absorbable suture. The skin is closed without tension using monofilament suture.

Ambulation is delayed for 1 month to allow adherence of the plantar flap. Either a soft dressing or a short leg cast can be used for a postoperative dressing.

Syme Amputation

The Syme amputation is an uncommon foot amputation that preserves limb length and the epiphyseal growth plates, and allows ambulation without a prosthesis. It is indicated in cases of extensive foot trauma. It is relatively contraindicated for patients with neurotrophic sensory changes and in vascular patients.

The procedure can be performed in one or two stages, as illustrated in Fig. 97.4. When a Syme amputation is performed in two stages the stump is less bulky and thus easier to fit with a prosthesis and visually more appealing.

The initial steps for both procedures are identical, except that the skin incision for the two-stage procedure is located 1.5 cm more distally. The skin incision for the one-stage procedure extends from the medial to the lateral malleolus in the horizontal and vertical planes. The dorsal incision is extended to the bone, and the tendons are transected under tension. The anterior tibial artery is identified, divided, and suture ligated. The dissection is carried into the tibiotalar joint space as the foot is forcibly plantar flexed. The ligaments are transected and the talus is dislocated. The plantar aspect of the incision is deepened to the calcaneus, and the calcaneus is sharply dissected from the plantar fascia. The plantar fascia is densely adherent and care must be taken to prevent damage to the heel pad, especially at the level of the Achilles tendon. The posterior tibial artery must be preserved, because it perfuses the heel pad. The foot is then removed. The two procedures differ from this point forward.

In the one-stage procedure, the medial and lateral malleoli are transected flush with the tibiotalar joint space, and the heel pad is rotated over the ends of the tibia and fibula. The deep fascial layers are approximated with absorbable suture and the skin is closed with monofilament suture. In the two-stage procedure, the heel pad is similarly positioned and the wound is closed without further bone transection. In 6 weeks, elliptical incisions are made over the medial and lateral malleoli and the distal ends of the tibia and fibula are transected flush with the ankle joint. In addition, the distal flares of the tibia and fibula are transected, creating the rectangular stump of the two-stage procedure. The wound is closed in a similar fashion. For both procedures, weight bearing is delayed for at

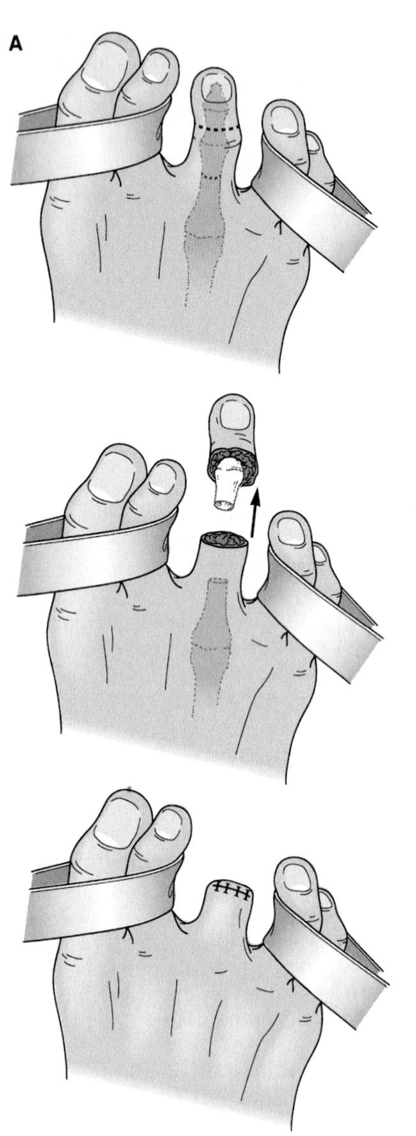

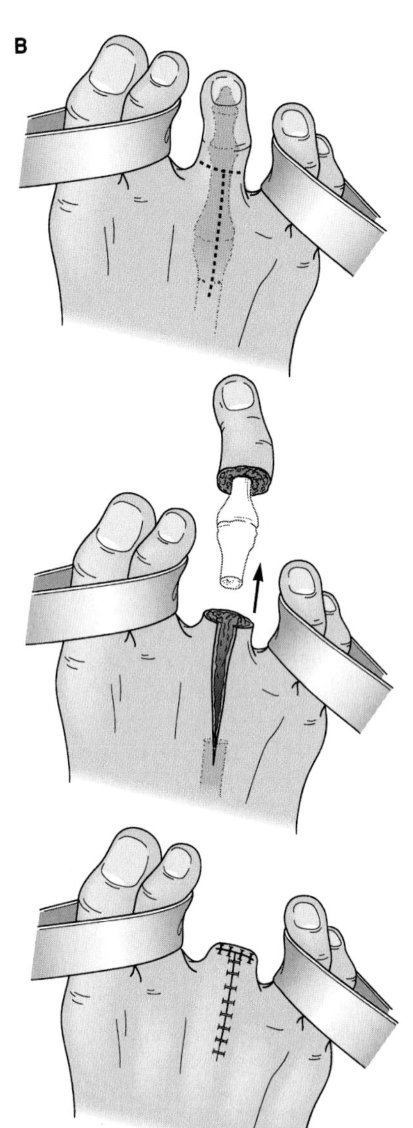

FIGURE 97.2 (*A*) Digital amputation. A circumferential skin incision is made proximal to the gangrenous process. The proximal phalanx is transected and the soft tissue approximated. (*B*) Metatarsal head resection (ray amputation). A racquet-shaped skin incision is made with the circular component extending circumferentially around the digit and the longitudinal component extending proximal to the metatarsal head. The metatarsal is transected proximal to the head and the soft tissue approximated.

least 4 weeks to allow heel pad fixation. A soft dressing or a short leg cast can be used.

Below-Knee Amputation

The complications of diabetes and arterial insufficiency constitute most of the indications for below-knee amputations. Table 97.8 outlines the criteria used to decide between a BKA and an above knee amputation in this setting.

The most common technique, using a long posterior flap, is illustrated in Fig. 97.5. When gangrene, wounds, or incisions preclude the use of a posterior flap, equal anteroposterior or sagittal flaps can be used; however, the posterior flap is associated with the highest incidence of primary healing and is thus preferred whenever possible. This higher rate of healing presumably reflects the fact that the posteriorly located gastrocnemius and soleus muscles are supplied by the sural arteries that originate proximal to the knee.

The proposed skin incision is drawn on the leg with a marker. The tibia should be transected 10 cm distal to the tibial tuberosity and the anterior aspect of the skin incision should be 1 cm distal to the site selected for the tibial transection. The anterior incision is extended medially and laterally. The length of the anterior incision should equal two thirds of the circumference of the leg at the proposed level of the tibial transection. The incision is then extended longitudinally along the medial and lateral aspects of the leg. The length of the longitudinal incisions should equal one third of circumference of the leg at the level of the tibial transection. Distally, the medial and lateral incisions are connected posteriorly. Curving the distal corners of the posterior flap prevents the accumulation of redundant tissue at the medial and lateral aspects of the completed amputation. The skin incisions should be down to the fascia to allow separation of the skin edges. This step decreases the chance of inadvertent injury to the posterior flap later in the procedure; however, the greater and lesser saphenous veins may be transected and need to be ligated.

The anterior aspect of the incision is deepened through the periosteum of the tibia. The muscles of the anterior compartment are divided at the level of the skin incision and the anterior tibial neurovascular bundle is identified and suture ligated. The proximal tibia is circumferentially cleared of periosteum, and transected 1 cm proximal to the skin incision. The anterior aspect of the tibia is cut on a 45-degree angle. The fibula is cleared and transected 1 cm proximal to the transected tibia.

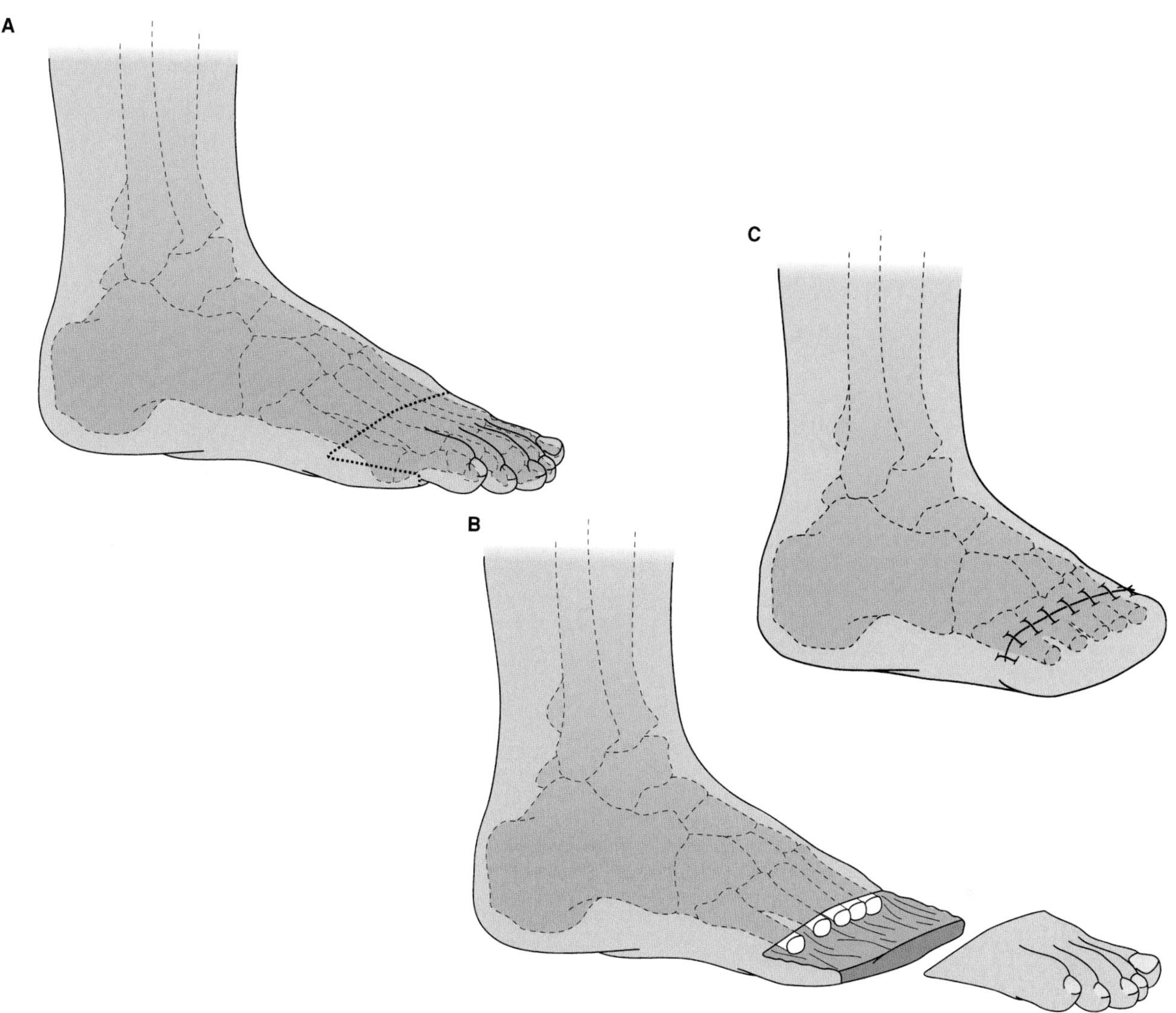

FIGURE 97.3 (*A*) The skin incision for the transmetatarsal amputation is made on the dorsum of the foot immediately proximal to the metatarsal heads and on the plantar surface within the digital crease. (*B*) The metatarsal heads are transected proximal to the skin incision and separated from the plantar soft-tissue flap along a plane adjacent to the bone. (*C*) The plantar soft-tissue flap is rotated anteriorly and approximated.

The bones are divided with either a power-driven reciprocating saw, or a manual saw. Regardless, care must be taken to avoid trauma to the anterior skin flap.

The posterior tibial and peroneal neurovascular bundles are identified and suture ligated. The tibia is retracted anteriorly and the posterior musculature is divided along the plane of the longitudinal skin incisions using an amputation knife. Extreme caution must be taken to avoid injury to the skin edges of the posterior flap during this step. Often a scalpel is needed to complete the division of the gastrocnemius tendon distally. The specimen is removed and manual compression achieves temporary hemostasis while the remaining vascular structures are identified and ligated. The nerve is retracted distally, ligated, transected, and allowed to retract. The posterior flap is rotated anteriorly to assess thickness and length. Frequently, the musculature needs to be debulked to allow a tension-free closure. Rough edges of the bones are filed smooth and the wound is irrigated. Bone wax is not used. The end of the tibia is covered and stabilized using absorbable 2-0 sutures placed medially, laterally, and anteriorly. The fascia is closed using absorbable suture, and the skin is closed with monofilament suture or staples.

The length of the BKA may be shortened if required by the infectious or gangrenous process. Although not ideal, a short BKA is functionally superior to an AKA. In the extreme case, the tibia can be transected at the level of the tibial tuberosity and the stump can still be fit with a prosthesis. If a BKA is necessary at this level, the biceps tendon and collateral ligament should sutured to the tibia, the common peroneal nerve should be transected above the knee, and the fibula should be removed.

In the face of extensive foot infection, an open (guillotine) amputation should be performed as the first part of a staged procedure. A circumferential incision is made in the distal leg just proximal to the malleoli. The fascia is divided, and the tibia and fibula are dissected free. The bones are divided at the level of the skin incision. All major neurovascular bundles are suture ligated and the remaining soft tissue is divided to complete the amputation. Several sutures are placed through the skin and underlying fascia to prevent retraction. The wound is left open and dressed. A definitive BKA is delayed until the infectious process has resolved, which typically occur within a week.

Rarely, a patient may require an emergent amputation, yet have overwhelming medical problems that preclude any operative intervention. As a temporizing maneuver, a tourniquet is

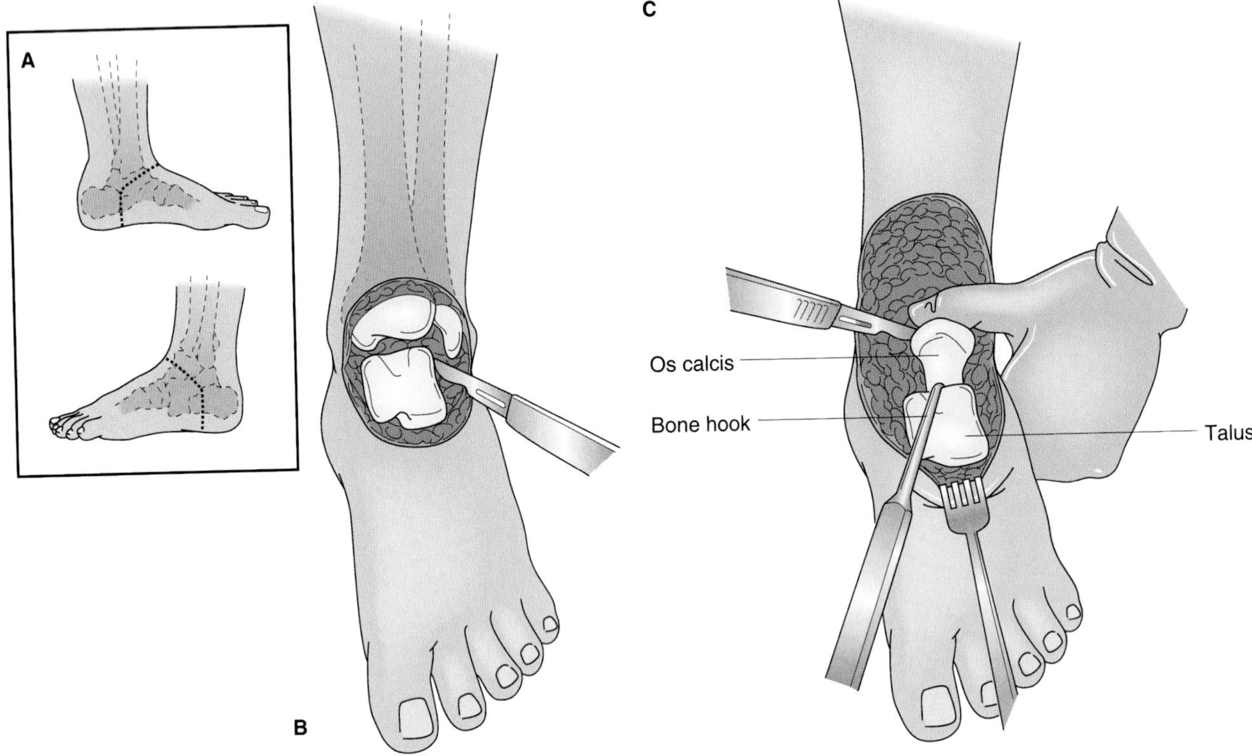

FIGURE 97.4 (*A*) The skin incision for the one-stage Syme amputation connects the medial and lateral malleoli in both the horizontal and vertical planes. The skin incision for the two-stage procedure is located approximately 1.5 cm further distally. (*B*) The incision is extended into the tibial—talar joint space, and the foot is placed in forced plantar flexion. (*C*) The calcaneus is sharply dissected from the adherent plantar fascia along a plane adjacent to the bone.

placed proximal to the infectious or gangrenous process and the extremity is packed in dry ice. This prevents the systemic release of muscle degradation products and allows the required procedure to be delayed while the patient's condition can be stabilized.

Above-Knee Amputation

An AKA is indicated for patients requiring an amputation with a fixed-knee contracture or a nonfunctional limb. Typically, a transverse fish mouth incision is made in the lower thigh. Take care to carry the initial skin incision to the subcutaneous tissue. This step will decrease the likelihood of inadvertent injury to the posterior skin flap during transection of the posterior muscle groups. The dissection is carried down to the femur that is cleared using a periosteal elevator to a level 2 to 3 cm proximal to the skin incision. The superficial femoral artery is dissected free and suture ligated. The bone is transected with a reciprocating or manual saw, and the posterior muscle flap is divided with an amputation knife. Manual compression with a laparotomy pad on the newly divided stump will easily control hemorrhage while vessels are identified and ligated or electrocoagulated. Alternative incisions can be made to accommodate surgical wounds. Most AKA wounds will heal even when the femoral pulse is nonpalpable. More proximal thigh amputations are performed when arterial perfusion is in question.

Hip Disarticulation

Lower extremity amputation at the level of the hip is an uncommon operation.

The indications include malignancy, trauma, and infection and, rarely, because of complications of arterial insufficiency. Hip disarticulation performed for an ischemic AKA is often associated with complications in the absence of revascularization.[32] The technique is well described.

Other Lower Extremity Amputations

Two additional mid-foot amputations have been well described. Although these are not often indicated in the vascular patient with atherosclerosis, they may have a role in selected cases.[33] A Lisfranc amputation is performed at the tarsometatarsal joint level and may be an option if there is inadequate soft tissue coverage for a transmetatarsal amputation.[34] A Chopart amputation is performed at the level of the calcaneocuboid–talonavicular bones. A modified Chopart amputation includes a percutaneous heel cord lengthening.[35] Knee disarticulation is a useful amputation for patients with immature growth plates. It is superior to an AKA and allows end weight bearing, improved proprioception, and improved prosthetic control. The required prosthesis is bulky and less cosmetically appealing than that used for a BKA. The technique is well described.[36] Rotationplasty is an uncommon procedure performed primarily for

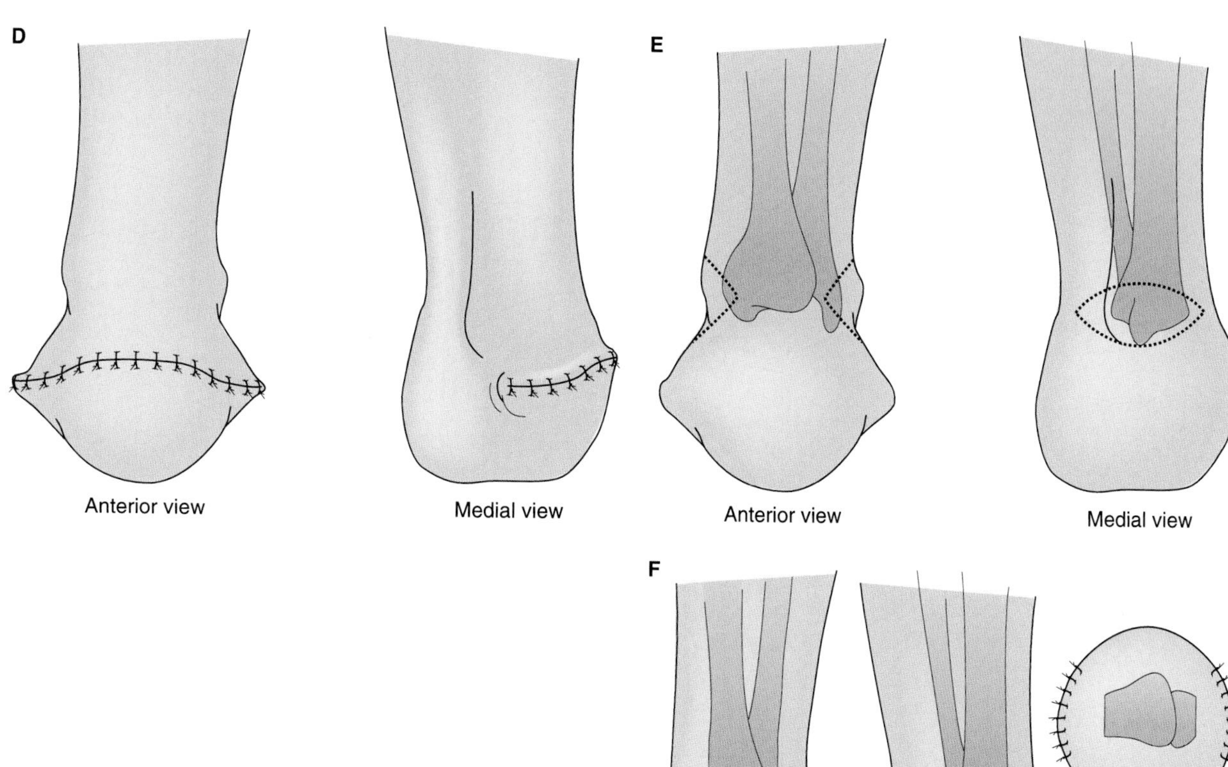

FIGURE 97.4 (*Continued*) (*D*) The heel pad is rotated anteriorly and approximated after the calcaneal dissection in the two-stage procedure and after the additional transection of the medial and lateral malleoli in the one-stage procedure. (*E*) Elliptic incisions are made over the medial and lateral malleoli during a second operation for the staged procedure. The medial and lateral malleoli are transected flush with the ankle joint, and the distal flares of the tibia and fibula are removed. (*F*) The two-stage procedure results in a less bulbous, more cosmetically acceptable residual limb.

treatment of osteogenic sarcoma of the thigh.[37] It involves nerve-sparing resection of the femur and knee, 180-degree rotation of the leg, and reattachment of the leg. This results in a functional, sensate foot that can easily be fit with a prosthesis.

Wound Dressings

An important consideration after amputation is the type of wound dressings applied to the stump. Two important factors in the success of an amputation are time to rehabilitation and complete wound healing, both of which are influenced by postoperative wound care.[38] With transtibial amputations, there are a number of options, such as soft gauze dressings with elastic wrap, rigid plaster dressings without immediate prosthesis, rigid plaster with immediate postoperative prosthesis, and prefabricated pneumatic postoperative prosthesis. Several studies have compared two of more of these options. End points are not standardized, however, and most studies are not randomized and prospective, making comparisons and meta-analysis difficult.[38]

TABLE 97.8 RESULTS

AMPUTATION MORTALITY

Category	Percentage	Number
Below-knee	2	25/1,200
Above-knee	9	54/609
Diabetic vs. nondiabetic	No difference	
After amputation revision	5.5	12/218

From Frang RD, Tayor LM, Porter JM. Amputations. In: Porter JM, Taylor LM, eds. Basic Data Underlying Clinical Decision Making in Vascular Surgery. St. Louis: Quality Medical, 1994:154.

Benefits and drawbacks are found for each postoperative option.[38] Gauze dressings with elastic wrap are simple and low cost and provide good accessibility to evaluate wound healing. On the other hand, they may lead to higher rates of joint contraction, increased time to ambulation, and risk pressure ischemia from poorly placed elastic wrap. Despite these drawbacks, no convincing data show that soft gauze dressings are inferior to other options.[38,39]

Rigid plaster helps with joint contracture and helps protect the wound from trauma. With addition of a temporary prosthesis, the rigid plaster also promotes early ambulation. The plaster, however, does not provide easy access to evaluate and care for the wound and if not fitted properly will result in sheer stress and thereby break down the wound. Consequently, a level of skill in plaster placement is required of the surgical team to make appropriate and often frequent plaster changes.[38]

Finally, a prefabricated pneumatic postoperative prosthesis allows early ambulation and weight bearing, easy wound

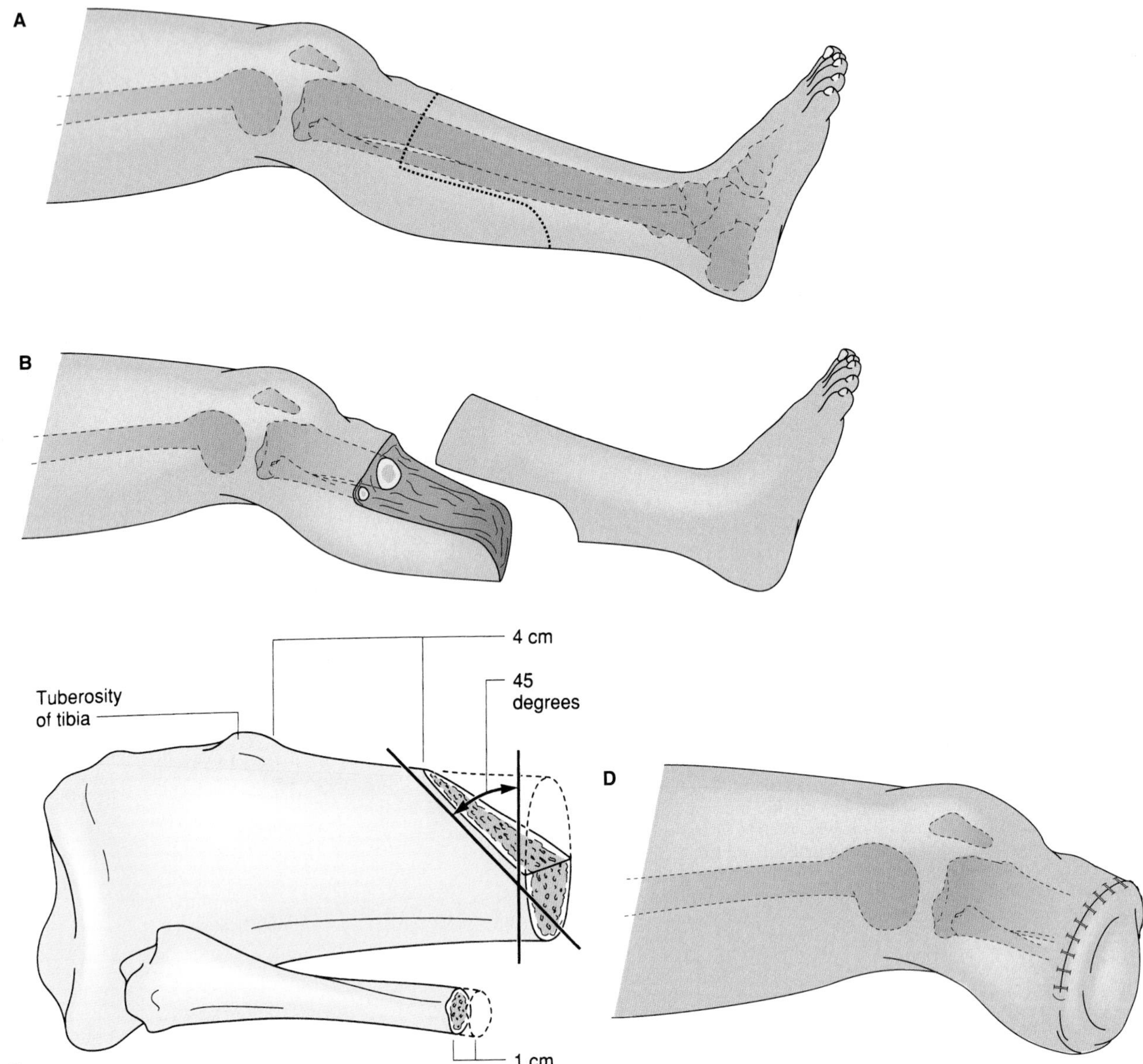

FIGURE 97.5 (*A*) The skin incision for a below-knee amputation based on a posterior flap is made 11 cm distal to the tibial tuberosity and extended medially and laterally to the midpoint of the calf. The length of the posterior flap is about 2 cm longer than the diameter of the calf at the point of the proximal incision. (*B*) The tibia is transected 1 cm proximal to the skin incision. The fibula is transected an additional 1 cm proximal to the level of the tibial transection, and the posterior calf muscles are incised along the plane of the skin incision. (*C*) The anterior aspect of the tibia is beveled at an angle of about 45 degrees, and the bone edges are filed. (*D*) The posterior flap is rotated anteriorly and approximated.

access for examination, prevention of joint contracture, and wound protection. The prosthesis, however, is bulky and upfront is more expensive that the simple gauze. Prospective studies have demonstrated statistically fewer postoperative complications with the pneumatic prosthesis and statistically fewer limbs requiring higher revisions.[40]

Complications

Mortality

Operative mortality depends on the indication and the level. Mortality rates for major lower extremity amputations in vascular and diabetic patients have been reported to be between 0 and 35%.[41] Combined mortality rates from multiple series are shown in Table 97.8.[42] Cardiovascular causes account for two thirds of these deaths, with myocardial infarction responsible for one third.[42] These review data are further supported by recent studies by Sandnes et al.[43] and Aulivola et al.[44]

Long-term survival following amputation in the vascular population is shown in Table 97.9. The 5-year survival rate is only 37% compared with 85% for age-matched controls.[45]

Deep Venous Thrombosis and Pulmonary Embolism

The incidence of deep venous thrombosis following lower extremity amputation ranges from 4% to 38%.[46–48] Prophylactic measures including subcutaneous heparin, early mobilization, and pneumatic compression devices are mandatory.

TABLE 97.9

SURVIVAL AFTER AMPUTATION FOR ISCHEMIA

Time (y)	Survival rate (%)
1	75
2	60
3	50
4	45
5	37

From Frang RD, Taylor LM, Porter JM. Amputations. In: Porter JM, Taylor LM, eds. *Basic data underlying clinical decision making in vascular surgery.* St. Louis: Quality Medical, 1994:115, with permission.

Stump Complications

Stump complications include nonhealing, infection, hematoma, contractures, ulceration, phantom pain, and trauma. Although most amputations heal primarily, a small percentage do not. Amputation at a more proximal level usually is successful. Postoperative infections complicate 12% to 28% of all amputations with the percentage higher in cases performed for infection.[49] Local wound care with drainage, débridement and dressing changes, and systemic antibiotics should be instituted. Wound hematomas are best treated with prevention. Meticulous homeostasis and avoidance of subcutaneous cavities decrease their incidence. Closed-suction drains are inadequate to drain blood and have been reported to increase the incidence of wound infection. Hematomas should be treated in the operating room with evacuation, irrigation, and closure of the wound.

Joint contractures complicate 1% to 3% of all amputations.[41,45] These contractures can occur rapidly postoperatively and are best treated by prevention. Rehabilitation specialists and physical therapists should evaluate patients preoperatively. Active and passive range of motion should be initiated immediately postoperatively. Adequate pain medication, ideally with patient-controlled or epidural anesthesia,[50,51] is crucial. Pillows and bed positions that result in hip or knee flexion are to be strictly avoided.

Ulcers tend to develop over bony prominences. Poorly fitting prostheses or shoes are the most common causes. Diabetic patients with peripheral neuropathy are especially susceptible to the development of ulcers following toe and limited foot amputations. They can also form on the anterior aspect of AKAs secondary to the disproportional contraction of the hip flexors relative to the hip extensors. Local wound care and bedrest usually lead to healing if the ulcer is superficial. Deep skin ulcers with involvement of the soft tissue and the underlying bone are more complicated. They often suggest borderline perfusion of the stump and require formal revision to a higher level to treat definitively.

Another option in complicated wound closure is negative-pressure wound dressing, which has been used for a wide range of difficult to heal lesions. Studies indicate that this dressing technique decreases wound volume, whereas traditional moist gauze dressings do not.[52] The dressings result in granulation tissue and healing in otherwise difficult tissue beds, such as diabetic foot ulcers[53] and decubitus pressure ulcers.[54] Although one study in swine demonstrated no difference between negative pressure dressing and wet-to-dry dressing,[55] other studies have shown increased vascularity and granulation tissue.[56] In addition to helping contract the size of the wound, negative-pressure dressings also decrease the number and frequency of dressing changes drastically when compared with wet-to-dry dressings.

Neuromas are regenerative nerve tissue that forms in response to transection. They can lead to pain if trapped in the fibrous scar or if irritated by a prosthesis. Proximal nerve division under tension during the original operation decreases the incidence of this complication. Symptomatic neuromas should be treated with proximal resection of the nerve because local excision of the neuroma is rarely adequate.

Some element of phantom extremity pain occurs in nearly all amputations,[57] although these complaints are not always directed to the treating surgeon. It is necessary to describe these common symptoms to the patient and specifically inquire about their presence. The pain is disabling in 5% to 30%[58] of patients surveyed. Currently, pain is felt to be a component of a central pain syndrome and unrelated to either a neuroma or the perception of an intact extremity. Although there is no universally effective treatment, Malone[41] has reported a low incidence with an aggressive rehabilitation program, including immediate prosthetic fitting. Recently, electroconvulsive therapy has been suggested as an effective treatment for refractory cases of phantom pain.[59]

Trauma to a limb following an amputation can convert a healed amputation to a nonhealing wound requiring more a proximal amputation. Perioperatively patients with a BKA have to be observed closely to prevent attempted ambulation. Diabetic patients with retinopathy should not walk barefoot following toe and foot amputations secondary to the risk that minor trauma may lead to a major wound healing problem.

Additional Amputation

The incidence of future amputation in vascular patients is significant. Little et al.[60] reported that a more proximal amputation was required in 75% of all vascular patients within 3.5 years after toe amputation. The incidence of contralateral limb loss in vascular and diabetic patients has been reported to be between 15% to 33% 5 years after a major lower extremity amputation.[61] These dismal figures reflect the systemic nature of the underlying diseases and emphasize the importance of appropriate foot care, patient education, close follow-up, and early intervention.[62] A concerted multidisciplinary approach can dramatically decrease the incidence of initial and subsequent lower extremity amputation.[63]

Special Situations

In selected cases, hyperbaric oxygen (HBO) therapy can provide benefit in treating nonhealing amputations sites. Patients require thorough evaluation of their cardiopulmonary status before initiating such treatment. In addition, the treating vascular surgeon has to determine that revascularization is completed or is not indicated. Patients may benefit from treatment if there is a substantial increase in transcutaneous oxygen pressure ($TcPO^2$) near the wound with administration of 100% oxygen. Daily treatments are typically continued for 30 days. Platelet-derived growth factor (becaplermin, Regranex) is approved for use in the United States and has been effective in the management of diabetic foot ulcers and following open foot amputations or débridements. The wound must be clear of all necrotic tissue before initiating therapy.

REHABILITATION AND PROSTHETIC MANAGEMENT

General Considerations

Rehabilitation must be individualized. For some patients, successful rehabilitation means ambulation on a prosthesis and resumption of an independent lifestyle. For others, success may mean being able to pivot on the contralateral limb to be

TABLE 97.10

AMBULATION AFTER LOWER EXTREMITY AMPUTATION FOR DIABETES OR OCCLUSIVE DISEASE

Amputation level	Postoperative ambulation (%)
Digit or ray	100
Transmetatarsal	100
Syme amputation	90–100
Below-knee	75
Above-knee	39
Hip disarticulation	<100

From Frang RD, Taylor LM, Porter JM. Amputations. In: Porter JM, Taylor LM, eds. *Basic data underlying clinical decision making in vascular surgery.* St. Louis: Quality Medical, 1994:155, with permission.

able to assist with transfer. Ambulating with a prosthesis depends on the physiologic status of the patient. Table 97.3 illustrates the dramatic increase in energy requirement with increasing level of the amputation. As expected, the chance of ambulating on a prosthesis decreases with ascending amputation level. The percentages of diabetic and vascular patients who can ambulate with amputations at various levels are shown in Table 97.10. In addition, the likelihood of ambulating postoperatively is inversely related to the patient's age and the length of the rehabilitation process.[64]

Specific Considerations

Digital and Ray Amputations

All patient who were ambulatory preoperatively should be able to achieve their preoperative functional status following a digital or ray amputation. The first digit and metatarsal head are important for weight bearing and for power. A shoe orthosis should effectively compensate for these functions when the patient has some training.

The most important component of postoperative rehabilitation for patients following a digital or ray amputation is education. The rate of repeat amputation (other toe, more proximal level, contralateral limb) is extremely high. Several studies have indicated that the rate of repeat amputation is diminished with a coordinated education program.[65,66]

Transmetatarsal Amputation

A transmetatarsal amputation does not increase the energy requirement of ambulation, therefore, postoperative ambulation is expected following successful healing. The absence of the toes and metatarsal heads results in the loss of some forward thrust during the push-off phase of ambulation. This deficit can be overcome with either a steel-shank or a rigid, roller-soled shoe. The void in the distal shoe is filled with an insert.

Syme Amputation

The prognosis for return to bipedal ambulation following a Syme amputation is excellent. The required energy expenditure is only 10% more than baseline.[67] A significant advantage of this amputation is the ability to ambulate on the stump with only a cup slipper. Even though this activity is permitted on only a limited basis in the home, it is much more convenient for the patient, especially when arising at night. For routine activity the patient uses a prosthesis composed of a nonmotion foot attached to a leg shaft. The shaft has a cutout on the medial aspect to allow passage of the flared distal end of the stump. The configuration of the distal end of the stump results in a bulbous ankle, which is less aesthetically pleasing than the typical below-knee prosthesis.

Below-Knee Amputation

The rehabilitation potential following a BKA is very good. Even when the indication for amputation is arterial insufficiency, approximately 75% of patients are able to ambulate with a prosthesis.[42] Multiple design options are available, however, the patellar tendon and the medial and lateral tibial flares are the weight-bearing surfaces for most prostheses. A variety of foot designs are possible to permit extension, flexion, rotation, and energy storage.

Above-Knee Amputation

Ambulation on an above-knee prosthesis is achieved by less than 40% of patients with arterial insufficiency.[42] In this patient population, the rate of ambulation on bilateral above-knee prostheses is less than 10%.[68] Most above-knee prostheses use the ischial tuberosity as the primary weight-bearing surface and are secured either by a belt or a suction socket. For younger patients, a suction socket works well. Patients with groin scars from previous revascularization attempts may benefit from a belt mechanism. The knee design depends on the patient's general condition and thigh strength. A knee that engages during the stance phase of gait is more stable and is frequently used in older patients.

KEY POINTS

- **More than 115,000 lower extremity amputations are performed in the United States alone each year.**
- **The vast majority of lower extremity amputations are performed for complications of diabetes or arterial insufficiency.**
- **Emergent amputation is indicated in the face of uncontrolled or ascending infection.**
- **Primary amputation is occasionally indicated in cases of treatment for lower extremity trauma.**
- **The energy required to ambulate following a lower extremity amputation increases with ascending level of amputation.**
- **Revascularization is often performed in conjunction with a limited amputation, either simultaneously or as a staged procedure.**
- **The choice of amputation level depends on the indication for the procedure, the condition of the patient, and the rehabilitation potential of the patient.**

References

1. Falstie-Jensen N, Christensen K. A model for prediction of failure in amputation of the lower limb. *Dan Med Bull.* 1990;37:283.
2. Sanmugarajah J, Hussain S, Schwartz J, et al. Monoclonal cryoglobulinemia with extensive gangrene of all four extremities—a case report. *Angiology* 2000;51(May):431–434.
3. Veith F, Gupta S, Samson R. Progress in limb salvage by reconstructive arterial surgery combined with new or improved adjunctive procedures. *Ann Surg.* 1981;194:386.
4. Melzack R, Wall P. Pain mechanisms: a new theory. *Science* 1965;150:971–979.
5. Augustinsson LE, Carlsson CA, Holm J, et al. Epidural electrical stimulation is severe limb ischemia. Pain relief, increased blood flow, and a possible limb-saving effect. *Ann Surg.* 1985;202:104–110.
6. Tallis RC, Illis LS, Sedgwick EM, et al. Spinal cord stimulation in peripheral vascular disease. *J Neurol Neurosurg Psychiatry* 1983;46:478–484.
7. Meglio M, Cioni B, Dal Lago A, et al. Pain control and improvement of peripheral blood flow following epidural spinal cord stimulation: case report. *J Neurosurg.* 1981;54:821–823.
8. Horsch S, Claeys L. Epidural spinal in the treatment of severe peripheral arterial occlusive disease. *Ann Vasc Surg.* 1994;5:468–474.

9. Ubbink DT, Spincemaille GH, Prins MH, et al. Microcirculatory investigations to determine the effect of spinal cord stimulation for critical leg ischemia: the Dutch multicenter randomized controlled trial. *J Vasc Surg.* 1999;30:236–244.
10. Huber SJ, Vaglienti RM, Huber JS. Spinal cord stimulation in severe, inoperable peripheral vascular disease. *Neuromodulation* 2000;3:131–143.
11. Lange R. Limb reconstruction versus amputation decision making in massive lower extremity trauma. *Clin Orthop.* 1989;(Jun):92–109.
12. **Bosse MJ, et al. An analysis of outcomes of reconstruction or amputation of leg-threatening injuries. *N Engl J Med.* 2002;347:1924–1931.**
13. **Johansen K, Daines M, Howey T, et al. Objective criteria accurately predict amputation following lower extremity trauma. *J Trauma* 1990;30(May): 568–572; discussion 572–573.**
14. Harwood T, Coe E, Flynn T, et al. The use of arm vein conduits during infrageniculate arterial bypass. *J Vasc Surg.* 1992;16:420–423.
15. Leseche G, Penna C, Bouttier S, et al. Femorodistal bypass using cryopreserved venous allografts for limb salvage. *Ann Vasc Surg.* 1997;11(3): 230–236.
16. Raptis S, Miller J. Influence of vein cuff on polytetrafluoroethylene grafts for primary femoropopliteal bypass. *Br J Surg.* 1995;82:478–491.
17. Stonebridge P, Prescott R, Ruckley C. Randomized trial comparing infrainguinal polytetrafluoroethylene bypass grafting with and without vein interposition cuff at the distal anastomosis. The Joint Vascular Research Group. *J Vasc Surg.* 1997;26(Oct):543–550.
18. Lepantalo M, Tukiainen E. Combined vascular reconstruction and microvascular muscle flap transfer for salvage of ischaemic legs with major tissue loss and wound complications. *Eur J Vasc Endovasc Surg.* 1996;12: 65–69.
19. Briggs S, Banis JJ, Kaebnick H, et al. Distal revascularization and microvascular free tissue transfer: an alternative to amputation in ischemic lesions of the lower extremity. *J Vasc Surg.* 1985;2(Nov):806–811.
20. Biancari F, Kantonen I, Alback A, et al. Limits of infrapopliteal bypass surgery for critical leg ischemia: when not to reconstruct. *World J Surg.* 2000;24(Jun):727–733.
21. **Keagy B, Schwartz J, Kotb M, et al. Lower extremity amputation: the control series. *J Vasc Surg.* 1986;4(Oct):321–326.**
22. **Dwars B, Van Den Broek T, Ravwerda J, et al. Criteria for reliable selection of the lowest level of amputation in peripheral vascular disease. *J Vasc Surg.* 1992;15:536.**
23. Avci S, Musdal Y. Skin blood flow level and stump healing in ischemic amputations. *Orthopedics* 2000;23(Jan):33–36.
24. Moore W. Determination of amputation level: measurement of skin blood flow with xenon-133 clearance. *Arch Surg.* 1973;107:798.
25. Burnham S, Wagner W, Keagy B, et al. Objective measurement of limb perfusion by dermal fluorometry: a criterion for healing of below knee amputation. *Arch Surg.* 1990;125:513.
26. **Malone J, Anderson G, Halka S, et al. Prospective comparison of noninvasive techniques for amputation level selection. *Am J Surg.* 1987;154:179.**
27. Misuri A, Lucertini G, Nanni A, et al. Predictive value of transcutaneous oximetry for selection of the amputation level. *J Cardiovasc Surg.* 2000;41(Feb):83–87.
28. Holloway G, Watkins B. Laser Doppler measurement of cutaneous blood flow. *J Invest Dermatol.* 1977;69:300.
29. Schwartz J, Schuler J, O'Connor R, et al. Predictive value of distal perfusion pressure in the healing of amputation of the digits and forefoot. *Surg Gynecol Obstet.* 1982;154:865.
30. Golbranson F, Yu E, Gelberman R. The use of skin temperature determinations in lower extremity amputation level selection. *Foot Ankle Int.* 1982;3(Nov-Dec):170–172.
31. Gibbons G, Wheelock F, Hoar C, et al. Predicting success of forefoot amputations in diabetics by noninvasive testing. *Arch Surg.* 1979;114:1034.
32. Endean ED, Schwarcz TH, Barker DE, et al. Hip disarticulation: factors affecting outcome. *J Vasc Surg.* 1991;(Sep)14(3): 398–404.
33. Chang B, Bock D, Jacobs R, et al. Increased limb salvage by the use of unconventional foot amputations. *J Vasc Surg.* 1994;19:341–349.
34. Roach J, Deutsch A, McFarlane D. Resurrection of the amputations of Lisfranc and Chopart for diabetic gangrene. *Arch Surg.* 1987;122:931–934.
35. Leiberman J, Jacobs R, Goldstock L, et al. Chopart amputation with percutaneous heel cord lengthening. *Clin Orthop.* 1993;292:245–249.
36. Burgess E. Disarticulation of the knee: a modified technique. *Arch Surg.* 1977. 112:1250.
37. Merkel K, Gebhardt M, Springfield D. Rotationplasty as a reconstructive operation after tumor resection. *Clin Orthop.* 1991;270:231–236.
38. Smith DG, McFarland LV, Sangeorzan BJ, et al. Postoperative dressing and management strategies for transtibial amputations: a critical review. *J Rehabil Res Dev.* 2003;40(3):213–224.
39. Kane TJ, Pollack EW. The rigid versus soft postoperative dressing controversy: a controlled study in vascular below-knee amputees. *Am J Surg.* 1980;46:244–247.
40. Schon LC, Short KW, Soupiou O, et al. Benefits of early prosthetic management of transtibial amputees: a prospective clinical study of a prefabricated prosthesis. *Foot Ankle Int.* 2002;23:509–514.
41. Malone J. Lower extremity amputation. In: Moore W, ed. *Vascular surgery: a comprehensive review.* Philadelphia: WB Saunders, 1993, p. 809.
42. Frang R, Taylor L, Porter J. Amputations. In: Porter J, Taylor L, eds. *Basic data underlying clinical decision making in vascular surgery.* St. Louis: Quality Medical Publishing, 1994, p. 153.
43. Sandnes DK, Sobel M, Flum DR. Survival after lower extremity amputation. *J Am Coll Surg.* 2004;199:394–402.
44. Aulivola B, et al. Major lower extremity amputation. *Arch Surg.* 2004;139: 395–399.
45. Roon A, Moore W. Below-knee amputations: a modern approach. *Am J Surg.* 1977;134:153.
46. Williams J, Britt L, Eades T, et al. Pulmonary embolism after amputation of the lower extremity. *Surg Gynecol Obstet.* 1975;140(Feb):246–248.
46. Yeager R, Moneta G, Edwards J, et al. Deep vein thrombosis associated with lower extremity amputation. *J Vasc Surg.* 1995;22(Nov):612–615.
48. Burke B, Kumar R, Vickers V, et al. Deep vein thrombosis after lower limb amputation. *Am J Phys Med Rehab.* 2000;79(Mar-Apr):145–149.
49. Fisher DJ, Clagett G, Fry R, et al. One-stage versus two-stage amputation for wet gangrene of the lower extremity: a randomized study. *J Vasc Surg.* 1988;8(Oct):428–433.
50. Enneking F, Morey T. Continuous postoperative infusion of a regional anesthetic after an amputation of the lower extremity. A randomized clinical trial [letter; comment]. *J Bone Joint Surg.* 1997;79(Nov):1752–1753.
51. Pinzur M, Garla P, Pluth T, et al. Continuous postoperative infusion of a regional anesthetic after an amputation of the lower extremity. A randomized clinical trial [see comments]. *J Bone Joint Surg.* 1996;78(Oct):1501–1505.
52. Eginton MT, Brown KR, Seabrook GR, et al. A prospective randomized evaluation of negative-pressure wound dressings for diabetic foot wounds. *Ann Vasc Surg.* 2003;17(6):645–649.
53. Armstrong DG, Lavery LA, Abu-Rumman P, et al. Outcomes of subatmospheric pressure dressing therapy on wounds of the diabetic foot. *Ostomy Wound Management* 2002;48(4):64–68.
54. Ford CN, Reinhard ER, Yeh D, et al. Interim analysis of a prospective, randomized trial of vacuum-assisted closure versus the healthpoint system in the management of pressure ulcers. *Ann Plast Surg.* 2002;(Jul) 49(1): 55–61.
55. Miller Q, Bird E, Bird K, et al. Effect of subatmospheric pressure on the acute healing wound. *Curr Surg.* 2004;(Mar-Apr)61(2):205–208.
56. Morykwas MJ, Argenta LC, Shelton-Brown EI, et al. Vacuum-assisted closure: a new method for wound control and treatment: animal studies and basic foundation. *Ann Plast Surg.* 1997;(Jun) 38(6):553–562.
57. Iacono R, Linford J, Sandyk R. Pain management after lower extremity amputation. *Neurosurgery* 1987;20(Mar):496–500.
58. Sherman R, Sherman C, Parker L. Chronic phantom and stump pain among American veterans: results of a survey. *Pain* 1984;18:83.
59. Rasmussen K, Rummans T. Electroconvulsive therapy for phantom limb pain. *Pain* 2000;85(Mar):297–299.
60. Little J, Stephen M, Zylstra P. Amputation of the toes for vascular disease: fate of the affected leg. *Lancet* 1976;2:1318.
61. Whitehouse F, Jurgensen C, Block M. The later life of the diabetic amputee: another look at the fate of the second leg. *Diabetes* 1968;17:520.
62. Powell T, Burnham S, Johnson, GJ. Second leg ischemia. Lower extremity bypass versus amputation in patients with contralateral lower extremity amputation. *Am J Surg.* 1984;50(Nov):577–580.
63. Van Gils C, Wheeler L, Mellstrom M, et al. Amputation prevention by vascular surgery and podiatry collaboration in high-risk diabetic and nondiabetic patients. The Operation Desert Foot experience. *Diabetes Care* 1999;22(May):678–683.
64. Harris W. Lower-extremity amputation in elderly patients. *Can J Surg.* 1987;30(Sep):315.
65. Bild D, Selby J, Sinnock P, et al. Lower-extremity amputation in people with diabetes. Epidemiology and prevention. *Diabetes Care* 1989;12(Jan):24–31.
66. Del Aguila M, Reiber G, Koepsell T. How does provider and patient awareness of high-risk status for lower-extremity amputation influence foot-care practice? *Diabetes Care* 1994;17(Sep):1050–1054.
67. Waters R, Perry J, Antonelli D, et al. Energy cost of walking amputees: the influence of level of amputation. *J Bone Joint Surg.* 1976;58A:42.
68. Malone J. Above the knee amputation and hip disarticulation. In: Ernst C, Stanley C, eds. *Current therapy in vascular surgery.* Philadelphia: BC Decker, 1991, p. 699.

CHAPTER 98 ■ PATHOGENESIS OF ANEURYSMS

B. TIMOTHY BAXTER AND JASON MACTAGGART

An aneurysm is a permanent, localized dilation encompassing all three layers of a blood vessel wall. The Committee for Reporting Standards of the major North American vascular societies more precisely defines an aneurysm as a 50% increase in the diameter of a vessel in comparison with its expected normal diameter.[1] Aneurysms are usually classified based on their etiology and anatomic location. The most common etiology of an aneurysm is vessel wall degeneration. Other less common causes include: infection, poststenotic dilation, trauma, arteritis, and various connective tissue defects (e.g., the high incidence of thoracic aneurysms in Marfan syndrome). Despite the occurrence of aneurysms throughout the arterial tree, the predominant extracranial location for aneurysms is the infrarenal aorta. Intracranial aneurysms, although common, appear to be etiologically distinct from extracranial aneurysms. This chapter focuses on the pathogenesis of the degenerative, infrarenal, abdominal aortic aneurysm (AAA).

CLINICAL RISK FACTORS

Large-scale studies have shown that patients with AAA possess many of the same risk factors as those who develop atherosclerosis. Increasing age, male gender, and smoking are the three chief risk factors for AAA recently identified within the aneurysm detection and management cohort (ADAM).[2] Of all the risk factors implicated in this cohort, the strongest modifiable risk factor appeared to be smoking. Although not all studies of AAA concur, other clinical features associated with aneurysms include hypertension, the presence of coronary artery disease, hyperlipidemia, and chronic obstructive pulmonary disease.[3–9]

AAA and Atherosclerosis

Until recently, degenerative AAAs were usually referred to as *atherosclerotic* because of the strong clinical and histopathologic associations between the two disease processes. AAA and atherosclerosis share many of the same clinical risk factors, and atherosclerotic plaque is almost always present in resected aneurysm wall.[10] Some arteries are also known to undergo compensatory remodeling in response to atherosclerotic luminal narrowing.[11] Furthermore, in human autopsy studies, increasing amounts of atherosclerotic plaque in the infrarenal aorta were associated with localized aortic dilation and thinning of the aortic media.[12,13]

Animal experiments lend support to the hypothesis that AAA may be caused by atherosclerosis. In monkeys, Zarins et al.[14] demonstrated that withdrawal of an atherogenic diet resulted in aortic atherosclerotic plaque regression and an associated development of AAAs. In another model primarily used to study atherosclerosis, transgenic mice with apolipoprotein E deficiency are found to spontaneously develop aortic aneurysms.[15] This characteristic can be augmented by giving prolonged subcutaneous infusions of angiotensin II.[16]

Although atherosclerosis may appear to be directly linked with AAA, other evidence suggests that AAA may be its own distinct pathologic process. In 1980, Tilson and Stansel[17] pointed out four important clinical differences seen in groups of AAA and aortic occlusive disease patients. They observed that AAA patients (a) exhibit a higher ratio of men to women; (b) are 10 years older on the average; (c) rarely manifest symptoms of lower extremity vascular insufficiency; and (d) rarely experience problems with late graft patency compared with the aortic occlusive disease patients. In addition to these observations, multiple studies have also failed to show a consistent, positive association linking AAA with diabetes mellitus, one of the principle modifiable risk factors for atherosclerosis.[2–4] In fact, the aforementioned aneurysm detection and management cohort trial found a negative relationship between AAA and diabetes mellitus.

Examination of pathologic specimens reveal histologic differences as well. Whereas AAA is found to be a transmural process, atherosclerosis is mainly confined to the intima, with some erosion into the media in advanced disease. Some researchers have proposed that atherosclerosis may even be an incidental finding in AAA, citing specimens obtained from poststenotic and syphilitic aneurysms that can show atherosclerotic changes as well.[18]

In summary, it appears that the development of AAA is not simply the end result of the atherosclerotic process. Most likely, other factors of equal or greater importance are influencing aneurysm formation. Although the potential role of atherosclerosis in initiating a local inflammatory process that could lead to AAA in susceptible individuals should not be dismissed, other avenues of research aimed at sorting out this susceptibility may prove to be more fruitful in understanding the pathogenesis of AAA.

CLINICAL AND BASIC SCIENCE RESEARCH IN AAA PATHOGENESIS

AAA as a Distinct Pathologic Entity

Recognizing AAA as a distinct pathologic entity with significant morbidity, mortality, and health care costs, the National Heart, Lung, and Blood Institute has sponsored efforts to further understand its pathogenesis. These efforts are focused on four areas: (a) molecular genetics; (b) inflammation and immune responses; (c) proteolytic degradation of the aortic wall connective tissue; and (d) biomechanical wall stress.[19] The remainder of this chapter highlights past and current research in each of these four areas.

Problems in Aneurysm Research

Before a discussion of AAA research can be fully understood and appreciated, there are two important problems that must be considered. The first is that almost all of the human AAA tissue available for study is sampled late in the course of the disease. The early changes in the human aorta during AAA pathogenesis are essentially unknown and can only be approximated through the use of animal models. The second problem is the lack of a single, well-accepted animal model that reproduces the entire spectrum of pathology found in human AAA. Currently, there are a variety of animal models, each of which develops an aneurysm through a different inciting mechanism. Although many of the models and even late stage human AAA disease seem to ultimately converge to similar end-stage processes, the events leading to the end-stage disease may in fact be very different. Consequently, all AAA research should be evaluated within the context of these two problems and the limitations of this research should be recognized.

MOLECULAR GENETICS

The study of the genetics of AAA serves two purposes. The first is that by locating and characterizing genes suspected in AAA pathogenesis, investigators may uncover additional pathways for more detailed study. These pathways may also provide potential new targets for pharmacologic intervention. The second, and perhaps most important purpose, is to develop a means for genetic testing to help identify patients at risk for developing AAA early in the course of the disease.

Although clinicians treating large numbers of patients with AAA were undoubtedly aware of clusters of aneurysms within families, Clifton[20] was the first to describe three affected siblings in 1977. Data supporting this observation did not appear until 7 years later, when Tilson and Seashore[21] described 50 families with more than one affected member. In 1986, Johansen and Koepsell[22] reported the incidence of AAA at 19% among first-degree relatives of matched controls. A more recent study examining first-degree relatives using ultrasonography corroborated these findings, with 18% of affected siblings older than age 60 years harboring AAAs.[23]

Although these studies demonstrated a familial tendency to develop AAA, they did not use genetic models to determine the specific inheritance pattern of AAA. Two of the more conclusive studies to date have used segregation analyses of large pedigrees and both have concluded that the genetic transmission of AAA is best explained by a single gene rather than by multiple factors. However, these studies do not agree on whether the gene inheritance is recessive[24] or dominant.[25] In contrast, Kuivaniemi et al.[26] published their pedigree analysis of 233 families with at least two affected members in 2003. They concluded that AAA is a multifactorial disorder without a single inheritance mode.

In addition to traditional pedigree analysis, new techniques in molecular biology and computer technology have become available to help investigators study the genetic aspects of AAA formation. Two studies using cDNA microarrays analyzed the gene expression profiles of human AAA tissue compared to normal and atherosclerotic aortas. AAA tissue demonstrated a pattern showing chronic inflammation, smooth muscle cell depletion, atherosclerosis, and extracellular matrix degradation that was significantly different from the normal aortas.[27,28] Another study using whole genome scanning and linkage analysis of 36 AAA families found possible susceptibility loci on chromosomes 4 and 19, recommending further study of nearby candidate genes.[29]

In searching for a gene that might explain AAA, considerable work has focused on the genes regulating matrix protein metabolism, inflammation, and immune function. With the exception of rare cases of collagen mutations,[30] no known mutations in matrix proteins can account for the majority of AAAs.[19] Research has implicated a multitude of polymorphisms in protease, cytokine, and other immunoregulatory genes thought to be associated with AAA (Table 98.1). However, most of these studies are small and lack the statistical power to provide definitive information, so the contribution of each factor to AAA pathogenesis remains to be clarified.

INFLAMMATION AND IMMUNE RESPONSES

Importance of Inflammation

Histologic examination of human AAA tissue demonstrates an inflammatory cell infiltrate consisting of T-cells, B-cells, dendritic cells, plasma cells, and macrophages.[31–33] These cells are typically located throughout the intima, media, and adventitia, and in extreme cases produce what is termed *inflammatory AAA*. In contrast to the panmural inflammation of AAA, the microscopic appearance of an atherosclerotic aorta shows an infiltrate of T-cells and macrophages located within the intima and media.[33] In comparing larger versus smaller AAAs, Freestone et al.[34] found that as aneurysm size increased, so did the intensity of the inflammatory cell infiltrate.

Animal models of AAA confirm the importance of inflammation in the aorta during aneurysm formation. In the elastase infusion model, transient infusion of the infrarenal rat aorta with porcine pancreatic elastase immediately renders the aorta slightly larger than it's preperfusion diameter through the mechanical disruption of the elastic lamellae. The aorta then remains stable in size for nearly 3 days. When examined after 3 days, however, a 300% increase in size is seen with a concurrent inflammatory cell infiltrate.[35] This model has been adapted to mice, with the inflammation and secondary enlargement occurring closer to 2 weeks following elastase infusion.[36] A second commonly used mouse model employing the periaortic application of calcium chloride also shows an intense inflammatory cell infiltrate preceding aortic enlargement.[37] Further evidence that invading inflammatory cells play a key role in AAA progression comes again from the elastase infusion model. In these experiments, rats treated with either cyclosporine or methylprednisolone failed to develop aortic inflammation and subsequently did not develop AAAs in comparison to placebo treated control rats.[38]

VASCULAR

Recruitment of the Inflammatory Cell Infiltrate

The stimulus for the recruitment of the inflammatory cells into the aorta is currently unknown and is an area of ongoing research. The elastin degradation product hypothesis suggests that as the elastin in the aortic wall breaks down, specific epitopes are exposed generating an immune response with subsequent inflammatory cell invasion. Supporting experimental evidence comes from Hance et al.,[39] who studied soluble elastin degradation fragments from human AAA tissue. They found that these peptides are able to attract mononuclear phagocytes in vitro through a specific interaction with a 67-kd elastin binding protein receptor on the phagocytes. Elastin degradation products have also been found to induce angiogenesis in the adventitia of rat aortas.[40] What remains to be explained is the inciting event leading to elastin breakdown and whether these peptides initiate or help amplify the immune response in AAAs.

Studies of human AAA tissue reveal characteristics consistent with an autoimmune process, namely large amounts of immunoglobin G[41] and the presence of plasma cells.[31] Additionally, a proposed autoantigen has been identified and characterized by Gregory et al.[42] It is a 40kd protein similar to an extracellular matrix component that specifically binds to antibodies isolated from human AAA. However, two more

TABLE 98.1

POLYMORPHISMS ASSOCIATED WITH ABDOMINAL AORTIC ANEURYSM

Reference	Polymorphism	Patients with AAA	Patients without AAA
Schillinger[114]	Heme oxygenase-1 promotor gene	Homozygous or heterozygous for less than 25 GT repeats, 41%	Homozygous or heterozygous for less than 25 GT repeats, 59%
Pola[115]	Angiotensin converting enzyme gene	Normotension: DD genotype frequency, 70%; II genotype frequency, 5% Hypertension: DD genotype frequency, 32%; II genotype frequency, 21%	Normotensive controls DD genotype frequency, 25% II genotype frequency, 32%
Gerdes[116]	Apolipoprotein E gene	E3E3 genotype: expansion rate, 2.1 mm/y E3E4 genotype: expansion rate, 1.3 mm/y E2E3 genotype: expansion rate, 3.1 mm/y E2E4 genotype: expansion rate, 4.2 mm/y	
Rossaak[117]	Plasminogen activator inhibitor-1 gene promoter	Familial AAA 4G4G genotype frequency, 20% 5G5G genotype frequency, 26% Nonfamilial AAA 4G4G genotype frequency, 38% 5G5G genotype frequency, 14%	Healthy control subjects 4G4G genotype frequency, 35% 5G5G genotype frequency, 13%
Wang[118]	TIMP-1 and TIMP-2 genes	Female TIMP-1 nt 434 C allele frequency, 62% T allele frequency, 38% Male TIMP-2 nt 573 G allele frequency, 91% A allele frequency, 9%	Female TIMP-1 nt 434 C allele frequency, 27% T allele frequency, 73% Male TIMP-2 nt 573 G allele frequency, 79% A allele frequency, 21%
Kotani[119]	Endothelial nitric oxide synthase gene	Patients with AAA requiring operation 5 repeat intron 4 allele frequency, 79% 4 repeat intron 4 allele frequency, 21% Patients with AAA under observation 5 repeat intron 4 allele frequency, 96% 4 repeat intron 4 allele frequency, 4%	Healthy control subjects 5 repeat intron 4 allele frequency, 90% 4 repeat intron 4 allele frequency, 10%
Rasmussen[120]	HLA-DR B1 gene	Patients with inflammatory AAAs HLA DR B1*15 allele frequency, 47% HLA DR B1*0404 allele frequency, 14%	Healthy control subjects HLA DR B1[a] allele frequency, 27% HLA DR B0404 allele frequency, 3%
Jones[121]	MMP-9 gene	MMP-9 nt 1562 CC genotype frequency 62% CT genotype frequency 35% TT genotype frequency 2.9%	MMP-9 nt 1562 CC genotype frequency 72% CT genotype frequency 28% TT genotype frequency 0.5%
Brown[122]	IL-10 gene	IL-10 nt 1082 G allele frequency 41% A allele frequency 59%	IL-10 nt 1082 G allele frequency 53% A allele frequency 47%
Strauss[123]	MTHFR gene	MTHFR nt 677 C allele frequency 63% T allele frequency 37%	MTHFR nt 677 C allele frequency 79% T allele frequency 21%

Adapted from Ailawadi G, Eliason JL, Upchurch GR Jr. Current concepts in the pathogenesis of abdominal aortic aneurysm. *J Vasc Surg*. 2003;38:584–588

[a]AAA, abdominal aortic aneurysm; GT, genotype; TIMP, tissue inhibitors of metalloproteinases; HLA, human leukocyte antigen; IL, interleukin; MTHFR,

recent studies have cast doubt on this autoimmune hypothesis, characterizing the immune response in AAA tissue as relatively nonspecific.[43,44]

Infection with *Chlamydia pneumoniae* has been suggested as a possible contributor in the formation of AAA. In one early study, investigators found that chlamydial antigens were present in a majority of human AAA tissue samples compared with healthy control aortas.[45] Subsequent studies have confirmed that chlamydia, or chlamydial antigens, are frequently present in AAA tissue.[46,47] In another study by Tambiah and Powell[48] using a rabbit model of AAA, topical treatment of the aorta with chlamydial antigens enhanced aneurysm formation through a process that could be attenuated by treatment with azithromycin. In this instance, the mere presence of the chlamydial antigens was sufficient to enhance aneurysm development without active infection, leading the investigators to suggest that azithromycin most likely worked through an antiinflammatory mechanism. All together however, considering the high prevalence of chlamydial infection in the general population,[49] strong evidence of specificity for AAA is currently lacking.

Another possible recruitment mechanism involves the action of chemokines, a related family of low molecular weight cytokines that control leukocyte trafficking. Compared with controls, human AAA tissue contains greater amounts of the chemokines interleukin-8 (IL-8) and monocyte chemoattractant protein-1.[50] In mice, work using the elastase infusion model has demonstrated an increased production of the chemokine monocyte chemoattractant protein-1 and chemokines regulated on activation, normal T-expressed and secreted) in aneurysmal tissue. Notably, the expression of these chemokines by the aortic smooth muscle cells preceded the influx of inflammatory cells during the experimental AAA development.[51]

Cytokines and AAA

Once inflammatory cells are present in the aorta, they can produce a multitude of effects. One of the most critical functions is that of coordination and direction of the ongoing immune response. This effect is achieved through the action of cytokines, which can be produced both by invading inflammatory cells and also by resident mesenchymal cells. The cytokine profile of human AAA tissue has been extensively examined. Studies of homogenized AAA tissue, as well as AAA tissue culture explants, have found overexpression of proinflammatory cytokines, such as tumor necrosis factor-alpha, IL-6 and IL-1β.[52,53] The Th1 cytokine interferon gamma (IFN-γ) has also been implicated in human AAA,[52] and elevated circulating levels of IFN-γ appear to correlate with more rapid aneurysm expansion.[54] Furthermore, a recent study using the calcium chloride AAA model in mice demonstrated that transgenic mice deficient in IFN-γ were unable to produce aneurysms. The ability to generate aneurysms was regained with the transplantation of splenocytes capable of producing IFN-γ.[55]

These findings contrast with recent work implicating the Th2 cytokine response. Schonbeck et al.[56] examined the cytokine profile of human AAA tissue and found no evidence for Th1 or IFN-γ pathway activation, but rather an abundance of IL-4, IL-5, and IL-10, all Th2 cytokines.[56] Extending these observations into an animal model, researchers transplanted wild type mouse aortas into mice deficient in IFN-γ receptors. Despite the absence of IFN-γ receptors in all cells save for the transplanted aorta, these chimeric mice were able to form large aneurysms. Upon treatment with anti-IL-4 antibody however, these transplanted mice were unable to form aneurysms, a finding confirmed in IL-4 knockout mice.[57] These findings suggest that invading inflammatory cells depend on Th2 signaling pathways for aneurysm development.

Smooth Muscle Cell Depletion

The presence of inflammatory cells and the cytokine environments they produce are thought to be responsible for another unique feature found in AAA—decreased medial smooth muscle cell density. Histologic examination of AAA specimens reveal a paucity of medial smooth muscle cells compared with normal and atherosclerotic aortas.[58,59] In addition, many of the smooth muscle cells present show features consistent with apoptosis.[58] The significance of these findings is clear, as smooth muscle cells are primarily responsible for the deposition and maintenance of the aorta's normal extracellular matrix. This concept was recently illustrated using an aortic xenograft rat model, where seeding of the graft with vascular smooth muscle cells resulted in protection of the graft from inflammation, proteolysis, and aneurysm formation.[60]

Role of Prostaglandins

Several studies have examined the role of prostaglandin E2 (PGE_2) in aneurysm formation. In these studies, researchers have found an increased expression of cyclooxygenase-2 (Cox-2) localizing primarily to infiltrating macrophages. Cox-2 is thought to be responsible for the increased PGE_2 levels found in both human aneurysm tissue and conditioned media from aortic tissue culture.[61,62] PGE_2 may be important in aneurysm pathogenesis by virtue of its ability to alter matrix metalloproteinase (MMP) activity, cytokine expression, and smooth muscle cell viability. Indomethacin, a nonspecific cyclooxygenase inhibitor, decreases PGE_2 in aortic tissue culture and also has been shown to decrease the size of experimental aneurysms in the rat elastase infusion model.[63]

Oxidative Stress

Inflammatory cells can also be a significant source of reactive oxygen species. These toxic substances, which may also be produced by mesenchymal cells and endothelial cells, are capable of inducing apoptosis of smooth muscle cells and activating proteases.[64,65] Miller et al.[66] have shown that reactive oxygen species and evidence of oxidative damage are increased in human AAA tissue. In rats, using the elastase infusion model, investigators have shown that genes associated with oxidative stress, such as those coding inducible nitric oxide synthase and heme oxygenase, are upregulated during aneurysm development.[67] In addition, using the same rat model, inhibition of inducible nitric oxide synthase, one of many enzymes capable of producing nitric oxide, attenuated aneurysm development.[68] Researchers studying mice using the elastase infusion model have confirmed that elevated inducible nitric oxide synthase expression and nitric oxide mediated tissue damage are seen during aneurysm formation. However, this same study also found that mice lacking the gene for inducible nitric oxide synthase were able to form aneurysms in a similar manner to controls, casting doubt on the importance of this enzyme in AAA pathogenesis.[69]

Protease Production

Finally, and possibly most importantly, invading inflammatory cells are capable of producing proteases, or inducing surrounding mesenchymal cells to produce proteases, that have the ability to destroy the extracellular matrix structures necessary for maintaining aortic wall integrity. This concept has been extensively studied and is another one of the main categories of AAA pathogenesis research.

PROTEOLYTIC DEGRADATION OF AORTIC WALL CONNECTIVE TISSUE

The two principle functions of the aorta, blood transport and transmission of pulsatile energy, demand both tensile strength and elasticity in its structure. These properties are provided mainly by collagen and elastin, two connective tissue proteins synthesized and maintained primarily by resident mesenchymal cells in the aortic wall. Because the normal structure and function of the aorta are so dependent upon these two proteins, the study of elastin, collagen, and their metabolism has provided valuable insight into the pathogenesis of AAA.

Collagen

Collagen is present both in the aortic media and the adventitia, and is chiefly responsible for imparting tensile strength to the aorta.[70] The predominant forms of collagen in the aorta are types I and III.[71] When comparing human AAA tissue with normal control aorta and aortas with occlusive disease, it is clear that the expression of both type I and type III collagens are increased in aneurysmal tissue.[72, 73] Moreover, the mass of collagen has been shown to increase progressively with increasing aneurysm size.[74] This increased expression, which appears to be regulated by a soluble tissue factor,[74] localizes to adventitial fibroblasts, medial smooth muscle cells adjacent to inflammatory infiltrates, and to transformed myofibroblasts within atherosclerotic plaque.[75] Further evidence of increased collagen metabolism in AAA was demonstrated by finding elevated plasma levels of the aminoterminal propeptides of type III procollagen, a marker of type III collagen turnover, in AAA patients compared to controls.[76] Mutations in type III collagen have been identified and linked to AAA,[30] however, these mutations are rarely the cause of degenerative AAA.[19]

Elastin

Elastin, which comprises approximately 50% of the dry weight of the normal aorta,[77] is the other major aortic connective tissue protein and is responsible for the aorta's viscous and elastic properties.[78] It is synthesized and secreted as a soluble monomer, tropoelastin, which is organized and cross-linked into insoluble fibers on a preformed scaffold of microfibrillar proteins forming the medial lamellae.[79] The unique structure of elastin fibers confers resistance to proteolytic degradation and the half-life of elastin in human tissues is measured in decades.[80] Most elastin is thought to be produced by the early postnatal period, although elastin production does continue at very low levels into adulthood.[73] Recently, Krettek et al.[81] identified macrophages within human AAA tissue as a source of additional tropoelastin synthesis. This elastogenesis appeared ineffective however, as markers of mature, organized elastin were greatly diminished.

In examining histologic sections of human AAA tissue, one of the most striking features is the fragmentation of the medial lamellae and the decreased concentration of elastin.[82,83] Paradoxically, biochemical studies looking at the absolute mass of elastin in aneurysmal aortas compared with normal aortas have shown larger amounts of elastin in the diseased tissue.[84,85] This finding is most likely explained by poor uptake of stain by the newly synthesized and unorganized elastin and also by the redistribution of the elastin over a larger aortic diameter. Nevertheless, despite an overall increase in elastin content, the increase does not keep pace with aortic expansion and its concentration is markedly decreased relative to that of collagen.[82,85] This effect results in increased stiffness in the aneurysmal aortic wall.

Proteolytic Enzymes

Because disruption of collagen and elastin is necessary for and well documented in AAA pathogenesis, investigators have focused intensely on studying the enzymes capable of degrading them. In the early 1980s, researchers began studying the proteolytic activity within human AAA tissue.[86–88] Since then, numerous studies have demonstrated the importance of the enzymatic degradation of the aortic wall in the development of AAA (Table 98.2). Although there are many enzymes capable of degrading these proteins in vivo, particular emphasis has been placed on the study of MPs.

Matrix Metalloproteinases

MMPs are a family of structurally related enzymes that are capable of digesting the various components of the extracellular matrix. They are produced by most of the cell types native to the aorta, such as endothelial cells, smooth muscle cells and adventitial fibroblasts, and are also produced by invading inflammatory cells, such as macrophages. The normal physiologic function of these enzymes is thought to be primarily extracellular matrix remodeling, although participation in other functions, such as cell motility and cell signaling are also known.[89] Most MMPs are secreted from cells in a proenzyme form and require some form of processing to become fully activated. Other MMPs are anchored to cell surfaces to help concentrate their activities close to the cell. Regulation of MMP synthesis and activity occurs through a number of mechanisms. MMP synthesis is primarily regulated at the level of transcription. Activity level may be regulated by the processing of the proenzyme form to its active form. Endogenous inhibitors (tissue inhibitors of metalloproteinases) and interaction with specific extracellular matrix components can also affect activity.[90] Dysregulation of MMP activity has been linked not only with vascular disease, but also malignancy, rheumatoid arthritis and a host of other pathologic conditions.

Matrix Metalloproteinase-9. MMP-9, also known as *gelatinase B*, is one of the most extensively studied MMPs within AAA research. MMP-9 has the capacity to degrade both elastin and partially hydrolyzed collagen. Using zymography and immunohistochemistry, studies of human AAA tissue have demonstrated increased amounts of MMP-9 compared with control tissue.[91] Furthermore, this MMP-9 localizes to areas surrounding infiltrating macrophages in the aortic wall. Using the elastase infusion model in mice, Pyo et al.[36] showed that mice lacking the gene for MMP-9 were resistant to AAA formation. In addition, they were able to show that the key source of MMP-9 was in fact the infiltrating macrophage, as infusion of bone marrow cells from mice with the MMP-9 gene into the MMP-9 knockout mice permitted aneurysm formation.

Matrix Metalloproteinase-2. MMP-2, also known as gelatinase A, is another MMP found to be important in AAA pathogenesis. MMP-2 has the capacity to degrade elastin, but unlike MMP-9, MMP-2 can degrade intact fibrillar collagen.[92] MMP-2 also differs from MMP-9 in that processing of MMP-2 to its activated form requires the presence of other membrane-bound MMPs.[89] Like MMP-9, MMP-2 levels and activity have been found to be greater in human AAA tissue compared with controls;[93,94] however, whereas MMP-9 is typically not present in disease free aortas,[91] MMP-2 is constitutively produced by resident mesenchymal cells even in histologically normal aortas.[93] Confirmation of the importance of MMP-2 to AAA development has come from the calcium chloride mouse model of AAA. In this study, Longo et al.[37] were able to show that the targeted deletion of the MMP-2 gene inhibited AAA formation and that the key source of MMP-2 production was not invading inflammatory cells but resident mesenchymal cells. The stimulus for the increased production and activation of MMP-2 in aneurysmal aortas remains unknown.

Other Matrix Metalloproteinases. MMP-12, also referred to as *macrophage elastase*, is also elevated in human AAA tissue compared with controls. Importantly, immunohistochemical analysis has localized the enzyme to areas of elastin destruction.[95] In contrast to MMP-9 and MMP-2, however, MMP-12 has not been shown to be absolutely required for aneurysm generation in knockout mice.[36] Levels of other MMPs are altered in AAA as well, but current studies have not documented a definitive role for these enzymes in AAA development.

Other Proteases

In addition to MMPs, other proteases and their endogenous inhibitors have been suggested as potential contributors to AAA pathogenesis. Cystatin C, an endogenous inhibitor of cysteine proteases, appears to be reduced in human AAA

TABLE 98.2

ENZYMES ALTERED IN ABDOMINAL AORTIC ANEURYSM

Reference	Enzyme	Primary substrate	Alteration in AAA	Cells of origin
MATRIX METALLOPROTEINASES				
Irizarry[125]	MMP-1	Collagen I, III	Increased protein localized to adventitia	Epithelial, inflammatory, mesenchymal cells
Davis[94]	MMP-2 (gelatinase A)	Collagen I, IV, elastin	Increased mRNA and protein localized to mesenchymal cells	SMCs, fibroblasts
Carrell[126]	MMP-3	Collagen	Increased mRNA	Macrophages
Thompson[91]	MMP-9 (gelatinase B)	Collagen, elastin	Increased protein localized to aortic macrophages	Macrophages, SMCs
Curci[95]	MMP-12	Elastin	Increased mRNA and protein localized to aortic macrophages	Macrophages
Mao[127]	MMP-13	Collagen I, II, III, IV	Increased mRNA and protein localized to mesenchymal cells	SMCs
Nollendorfs[128]	MT-MMP-1 (MMP-14)	Activates pro-MMP-2	Increased mRNA and protein localized to macrophages and SMCs	Macrophages, SMCs
Tamarina[129] et al., 1997	TIMP-1	Inhibitor of MMPs	Increased mRNA levels	SMCs
Tamarina[129]	TIMP-2	Inhibitor of MMP-2	Increased mRNA levels	SMCs
Carrell[126]	TIMP-3	Inhibitor of MMPs	Increased mRNA levels	Macrophages
CYSTEINE PROTEASES				
Shi[96]	Cathepsin S	Elastin	Increased protein	Macrophages, SMCs
Shi[96]	Cathepsin K	Elastin	Increased protein	Macrophages, SMCs
Gacko[130]	Cathepsin D	Not elastin or collagen	Increased activity in AAA tissue	Inflammatory cells?
Gacko[130]	Cathepsin L	Not elastin or collagen	Increased activity in AAA tissue	Inflammatory cells?
Shi[96]	Cystatin C	Inhibitor of cysteine proteases	Decreased protein	SMCs, fibroblasts
SERINE PROTEASES				
Jean-Claude[131]	Plasmin	Activates MMPs	Increased protein	Macrophages
Reilly[132]	Tissue-plasminogen activator	Activates MMPs, plasminogen	Increased protein	Macrophages
Schneiderman[133]	Urokinase-plasminogen activator	Activates MMPs, plasminogen	Increased mRNA	Macrophages

Adapted from Ailawadi G, Eliason, JL, Upchurch GR Jr. Current concepts in the pathogenesis of abdominal aortic aneurysm. *J Vasc Surg.* 2003;38:584–588.
AAA, abdominal aortic aneurysm; SMC, smooth muscle cell; MMP, matrix metalloproteinase; TIMP, tissue inhibitors of metalloproteinases.

tissue.[96] Serine proteases, particularly neutrophil elastase, have been hypothesized to play a role in AAA formation because of their potent elastase activities. However, there is currently no supporting experimental evidence. Other serine proteases, such as those from the plasminogen activator family, have been shown to play a role in AAA formation, although the main pathogenic mechanism involving these enzymes appears to be activation of MMPs.[97]

Potential Medical Therapy with Matrix Metalloproteinases

In addition to adding to the basic knowledge of AAA pathogenesis, the study of MMPs has also lead to the realization that inhibition of their activity may prevent or slow aneurysm growth. Tetracycline and its derivatives are potent inhibitors of MMPs *in vitro*[98] and in animal studies have inhibited aneurysm expansion.[99,100] Small trials in human AAA patients have been performed;[101,102] however, definitive evidence for their efficacy awaits large-scale randomized trials. Thus, medical therapy for the treatment of AAA, especially smaller aneurysms, may very well be an alternative to surgical therapy in the future.

BIOMECHANICAL WALL STRESS

Unique Conditions in the Infrarenal Aorta

The infrarenal aorta is subjected to unique hemodynamic flow patterns and also possesses specific structural characteristics that are thought to predispose it towards aneurysm formation. Reflected pressure waves from the aortic bifurcation and the presence of large renal and splanchnic artery takeoffs result in disturbed flow patterns.[103] The elastin to collagen ratio decreases distally, translating into increased stiffness in this section of the aorta.[104] In addition, the absence of vasa vasorum in the normal abdominal aortic media[105] and the presence of a thick intraluminal thrombus are thought to impair oxygen and nutrient delivery to the aneurysmal aorta.[106] All of these observations are plausible reasons for the development and progression of disease in the infrarenal aorta.

Aortic Wall Stress

Stress on the aortic wall is one of the key factors involved in the rupture of AAAs. The law of Laplace is often used to explain the propensity for larger aneurysms to rupture because it predicts wall tension to be directly proportional to the product of the radius of a tubular, thin-walled structure (AAA diameter) and its intraluminal pressure (patient blood pressure). This explanation may be an oversimplification, however, because AAAs are often asymmetrical, thick-walled, and become more spherical in shape as their size increases.[107] Because of these factors, researchers are developing improved methods to help determine patterns of stress on the aneurysmal aortic wall as well as the effect of stress on the pathogenesis of AAA.

Raghavan et al.[108] have recently used a method termed *finite element analysis* to noninvasively determine AAA wall stress distribution and AAA rupture risk. Application of this method comparing calculated stress values obtained from patients near the time of AAA rupture, with patients who have size-matched electively repaired AAA showed significantly elevated stress values in the ruptured AAA group.[109] Although still investigational, these methods could have an important impact on determining the indications for operative repair of AAAs in the future.

Hemodynamics

In addition to influencing rupture, hemodynamic factors may also play an important role in aneurysm initiation and growth. Using the elastase infusion model in rats, research has established that increases in flow through the injured aorta decrease macrophage infiltration into the aortic media[110] and increase macrophage antioxidative gene expression.[111] AAAs in these high flow groups also demonstrated a significant reduction in diameter compared with the low and normal flow groups. Expression of MMPs[112] and reactive oxygen species[113] are also influenced by hemodynamic factors in experimental aneurysm formation.

CONCLUSION

Significant progress has been made over the past 20 years in delineating the pathogenesis of AAA. Both clinicians and basic scientists will continue to play important roles in studying this disease process. It is hoped that by enhancing our knowledge of the underlying pathology of AAA, new and improved methods of diagnosis and treatment will follow.

KEY POINTS

- The principle risk factors for abdominal aortic aneurysm (AAA) are smoking, increasing age, male gender, and family history of AAA.
- Population studies reveal a strong genetic predisposition to AAA formation, the mechanism of which is currently unknown.
- AAAs are the result of aortic wall degeneration and defective aortic wall remodeling.
- Chronic inflammation, macrophages in particular, play a key role in the degenerative process.
- Digestion of elastin and collagen by proteolytic enzymes, such as the matrix metalloproteinases, is crucial to aneurysm formation.
- Structural and hemodynamic factors unique to the infrarenal abdominal aorta most likely play a role in aneurysm pathogenesis.

References

1. Johnston KW, Rutherford RB, Tilson MD, et al. Suggested standards for reporting on arterial aneurysms. Subcommittee on Reporting Standards for Arterial Aneurysms, Ad Hoc Committee on Reporting Standards, Society for Vascular Surgery and North American Chapter, International Society for Cardiovascular Surgery. *J Vasc Surg.* 1991;13:452–458.
2. **Lederle FA, Johnson GR, Wilson SE, et al. The aneurysm detection and management study screening program: validation cohort and final results. Aneurysm Detection and Management Veterans Affairs Cooperative Study Investigators. *Arch Intern Med.* 2000;160:1425–1430.**
3. Pleumeekers HJ, Hoes AW, van der Does E, et al. Aneurysms of the abdominal aorta in older adults. The Rotterdam Study. *Am J Epidemiol.* 1995;142:1291–1299.
4. Goldberg RJ, Burchfiel CM, Benfante R, et al. Lifestyle and biologic factors associated with atherosclerotic disease in middle-aged men. 20-year findings from the Honolulu Heart Program. *Arch Intern Med.* 1995;155: 686–694.
5. Alcorn HG, Wolfson SK, Jr, Sutton-Tyrrell K, et al. Risk factors for abdominal aortic aneurysms in older adults enrolled in The Cardiovascular Health Study. *Arterioscler Thromb Vasc Biol.* 1996;16:963–970.
6. Rodin MB, Daviglus ML, Wong GC, et al. Middle age cardiovascular risk factors and abdominal aortic aneurysm in older age. *Hypertension.* 2003;42:61–68.
7. Vardulaki KA, Walker .M, Day NE, et al. Quantifying the risks of hypertension, age, sex and smoking in patients with abdominal aortic aneurysm. *Br J Surg.* 2000;87:195–200.
8. Bengtsson H, Bergqvist D, Ekberg O, et al. A population based screening of abdominal aortic aneurysms (AAA). *Eur J Vasc Surg.* 1991;5:53–57.
9. Smith FC, Grimshaw GM, Paterson IS, et al. Ultrasonographic screening for abdominal aortic aneurysm in an urban community. *Br J Surg.* 1993;80:1406–1409.
10. Zarins CK, Glagov S. Artery wall pathology in atherosclerosis. In: Rutherford RB, ed. *Vascular Surgery.* 5th ed. Philadelphia: WB Saunders; 2000:313–330.
11. Zarins CK, Weisenberg E, Kolettis G, et al. Differential enlargement of artery segments in response to enlarging atherosclerotic plaques. *J Vasc Surg.* 1988;7:386–394.
12. Xu C, Zarins CK, Glagov S. Aneurysmal and occlusive atherosclerosis of the human abdominal aorta. *J Vasc Surg.* 2001;33:91–96.
13. Zarins CK, Xu C, Glagov S. Atherosclerotic enlargement of the human abdominal aorta. *Atherosclerosis.* 2001;155:157–164.
14. Zarins CK, Xu C, Glagov S. Aneurysmal enlargement of the aorta during regression of experimental atherosclerosis. *J Vasc Surg.* 1992;15: 90–98101.
15. Tangirala RK, Rubin EM, Palinski W. Quantitation of atherosclerosis in murine models: correlation between lesions in the aortic origin and in the entire aorta, and differences in the extent of lesions between sexes in LDL receptor-deficient and apolipoprotein E-deficient mice. *J Lipid Res.* 1995;36:2320–2328.
16. Daugherty A, Manning MW, Cassis LA. Angiotensin II promotes atherosclerotic lesions and aneurysms in apolipoprotein E-deficient mice. *J Clin Invest.* 2000;105:1605–1612.
17. Tilson MD, Stansel HC. Differences in results for aneurysm vs occlusive disease after bifurcation grafts: results of 100 elective grafts. *Arch Surg.* 1980;115:1173–1175.
18. **Tilson MD. Aortic aneurysms and atherosclerosis. *Circulation.* 1992;85: 378–379.**
19. Tromp G, Wu Y, Prockop DJ, et al. Sequencing of cDNA from 50 unrelated patients reveals that mutations in the triple-helical domain of type III procollagen are an infrequent cause of aortic aneurysms. *J Clin Invest.* 1993;91:2539–2545.
20. Clifton MA. Familial abdominal aortic aneurysms. *Br J Surg.* 1977;64: 765–766.
21. Tilson MD, Seashore MR. Fifty families with abdominal aortic aneurysms in two or more first-order relatives. *Am J Surg.* 1984;147:551–553.
22. Johansen K, Koepsel T. Familial tendency for abdominal aortic aneurysms. *JAMA.* 1986;256:1934–1936.
23. Baird PA, Sadovnick AD, Yee IM, et al. Sibling risks of abdominal aortic aneurysm. *Lancet.* 1995;346:601–604.
24. Majumder PP, St Jean PL, Ferrell RE, et al. On the inheritance of abdominal aortic aneurysm. *Am J Hum Genet.* 1991;48:164–170.
25. Verloes A, Sakalihasan N, Koulischer L, et al. Aneurysms of the abdominal aorta: familial and genetic aspects in three hundred thirteen pedigrees. *J Vasc Surg.* 1995;21:646–655.
26. **Kuivaniemi H, Shibamura H, Arthur C, et al. Familial abdominal aortic aneurysms: collection of 233 multiplex families. *J Vasc Surg.* 2003;37: 340–345.**
27. Armstrong PJ, Johanning JM, Calton WC Jr, et al. Differential gene expression in human abdominal aorta: aneurysmal versus occlusive disease. *J Vasc Surg.* 2002;35:346–355.
28. Tung WS, Lee JK, Thompson RW. Simultaneous analysis of 1176 gene products in normal human aorta and abdominal aortic aneurysms using a membrane-based complementary DNA expression array. *J Vasc Surg.* 2001;34:143–150.

29. Shibamura H, Olson JM, van Vlijmen-Van Keulen C, et al. Genome scan for familial abdominal aortic aneurysm using sex and family history as covariates suggests genetic heterogeneity and identifies linkage to chromosome 19q13. *Circulation.* 2004;109:2103–2108.
30. Kontusaari S, Tromp G, Kuivaniemi H, et al. A mutation in the gene for type III procollagen (COL3A1) in a family with aortic aneurysms. *J Clin Invest.* 1990;86:1465–1473.
31. Beckman EN. Plasma cell infiltrates in atherosclerotic abdominal aortic aneurysms. *Am J Clin Pathol.* 1986;85:21–24.
32. Bobryshev YV, Lord RS, Parsson H. Immunophenotypic analysis of the aortic aneurysm wall suggests that vascular dendritic cells are involved in immune responses. *Cardiovasc Surg.* 1998;6:240–249.
33. Koch AE, Haines GK, Rizzo RJ, et al. Human abdominal aortic aneurysms. Immunophenotypic analysis suggesting an immune-mediated response. *Am J Pathol.* 1990;137:1199–1213.
34. **Freestone T, Turner RJ, Coady A, et al. 1995. Inflammation and matrix metalloproteinases in the enlarging abdominal aortic aneurysm. *Arterioscler Thromb Vasc Biol.* 1995;15:1145–1151.**
35. Anidjar S, Dobrin PB, Eichorst M, et al. Correlation of inflammatory infiltrate with the enlargement of experimental aortic aneurysms. *J Vasc Surg.* 1992;16:139–147.
36. **Pyo R, Lee JK, Shipley JM, et al. Targeted gene disruption of matrix metalloproteinase-9 (gelatinase B) suppresses development of experimental abdominal aortic aneurysms. *J Clin Invest.* 2000;105:1641–1649.**
37. **Longo GM, Xiong W, Greiner TC, et al. Matrix metalloproteinases 2 and 9 work in concert to produce aortic aneurysms. *J Clin Invest.* 2002; 110:625–632.**
38. Dobrin PB, Baumgartner N, Anidjar S, et al. Inflammatory aspects of experimental aneurysms. Effect of methylprednisolone and cyclosporine. *Ann N Y Acad Sci.* 1996;800:74–88.
39. Hance KA, Tataria M, Ziporin SJ, et al. Monocyte chemotactic activity in human abdominal aortic aneurysms: role of elastin degradation peptides and the 67-kD cell surface elastin receptor. *J Vasc Surg.* 2002;35: 254–261.
40. Nackman GB, Karkowski FJ, Halpern VJ, et al. Elastin degradation products induce adventitial angiogenesis in the Anidjar/Dobrin rat aneurysm model. *Surgery.* 1997;122:39–44.
41. Brophy CM, Reilly JM, Smith GJ, et al. The role of inflammation in nonspecific abdominal aortic aneurysm disease. *Ann Vasc Surg.* 1991;5: 229–233.
42. Gregory AK, Yin NX, Capella J, et al. Features of autoimmunity in the abdominal aortic aneurysm. *Arch Surg.* 1996;131:85–88.
43. Yen HC, Lee FY, Chau LY. Analysis of the T cell receptor V beta repertoire in human aortic aneurysms. *Atherosclerosis.* 1997;135:29–36.
44. Walton LJ, Powell JT, Parums DV. Unrestricted usage of immunoglobulin heavy chain genes in B cells infiltrating the wall of atherosclerotic abdominal aortic aneurysms. *Atherosclerosis.* 1997;135:65–71.
45. Juvonen J, Juvonen T, Laurila A, et al. Demonstration of Chlamydia pneumoniae in the walls of abdominal aortic aneurysms. *J Vasc Surg.* 1997;25:499–505.
46. Halme S, Juvonen T, Laurila A, et al. Chlamydia pneumoniae reactive T lymphocytes in the walls of abdominal aortic aneurysms. *Eur J Clin Invest.* 1999;29:546–552.
47. Meijer A, van Der Vliet JA, Roholl PJ, et al. Chlamydia pneumoniae in abdominal aortic aneurysms: abundance of membrane components in the absence of heat shock protein 60 and DNA. *Arterioscler Thromb Vasc Biol.* 1999;19:2680–2686.
48. **Tambiah J, Powell JT. Chlamydia pneumoniae antigens facilitate experimental aortic dilatation: prevention with azithromycin. *J Vasc Surg.* 2002;36:1011–1017.**
49. Kalayoglu MV, Libby P, Byrne GI. Chlamydia pneumoniae as an emerging risk factor in cardiovascular disease. *JAMA.* 2002;288:2724–2731.
50. Koch AE, Kunkel SL, Pearce WH, et al. Enhanced production of the chemotactic cytokines interleukin-8 and monocyte chemoattractant protein-1 in human abdominal aortic aneurysms. *Am J Pathol.* 1993;142: 1423–1431.
51. Colonnello JS, Hance KA, Shames ML, et al. Transient exposure to elastase induces mouse aortic wall smooth muscle cell production of MCP-1 and RANTES during development of experimental aortic aneurysm. *J Vasc Surg.* 2003;38:138–146.
52. Szekanecz Z, Shah MR, Pearce WH, et al. Human atherosclerotic abdominal aortic aneurysms produce interleukin (IL)-6 and interferon-gamma but not IL-2 and IL-4: the possible role for IL-6 and interferon-gamma in vascular inflammation. *Agents Actions.* 1994;42:159–162.
53. Newman KM, Jean-Claude J, Li H, et al. Cytokines that activate proteolysis are increased in abdominal aortic aneurysms. *Circulation.* 1994; 90:II224–227.
54. Juvonen J, Surcel HM, Satta J, et al. Elevated circulating levels of inflammatory cytokines in patients with abdominal aortic aneurysm. *Arterioscler Thromb Vasc Biol.* 1997;17:2843–2847.
55. Xiong W, Zhao Y, Prall A, et al. Key roles of CD4+ T cells and IFN-gamma in the development of abdominal aortic aneurysms in a murine model. *J Immunol.* 2004;172:2607–2612.
56. Schonbeck U, Sukhova GK, Gerdes N, et al. T(H)2 predominant immune responses prevail in human abdominal aortic aneurysm. *Am J Pathol.* 2002;161:499–506.
57. Shimizu K, Shichiri M, Libby P, et al. Th2-predominant inflammation and blockade of IFN-gamma signaling induce aneurysms in allografted aortas. *J Clin Invest.* 2004;114:300–308.
58. Henderson EL, Geng YJ, Sukhova GK, et al. Death of smooth muscle cells and expression of mediators of apoptosis by T lymphocytes in human abdominal aortic aneurysms. *Circulation.* 1999;99:96–104.
59. Lopez-Candales A, Holmes DR, Liao S, et al. Decreased vascular smooth muscle cell density in medial degeneration of human abdominal aortic aneurysms. *Am J Pathol.* 1997;150:993–1007.
60. Allaire E, Muscatelli-Groux B, Mandet C, et al. Paracrine effect of vascular smooth muscle cells in the prevention of aortic aneurysm formation. *J Vasc Surg.* 2002;36:1018–1026.
61. Holmes DR, Wester W, Thompson RW, et al. Prostaglandin E2 synthesis and cyclooxygenase expression in abdominal aortic aneurysms. *J Vasc Surg.* 1997;25:810–815.
62. Walton LJ, Franklin IJ, Bayston T, et al. Inhibition of prostaglandin E2 synthesis in abdominal aortic aneurysms: implications for smooth muscle cell viability, inflammatory processes, and the expansion of abdominal aortic aneurysms. *Circulation.* 1999;100:48–54.
63. Miralles M, Wester W, Sicard GA, et al. Indomethacin inhibits expansion of experimental aortic aneurysms via inhibition of the cox2 isoform of cyclooxygenase. *J Vasc Surg.* 1999;29:884–883.
64. Li PF, Dietz R, von Harsdorf R. Reactive oxygen species induce apoptosis of vascular smooth muscle cell. *FEBS Lett.* 1997;404:249–252.
65. Rajagopalan S, Meng XP, Ramasamy S, et al. Reactive oxygen species produced by macrophage-derived foam cells regulate the activity of vascular matrix metalloproteinases in vitro. Implications for atherosclerotic plaque stability. *J Clin Invest.* 1996;98:2572–2579.
66. Miller FJ, Jr, Sharp WJ, Fang X, et al. Oxidative stress in human abdominal aortic aneurysms: a potential mediator of aneurysmal remodeling. *Arterioscler Thromb Vasc Biol.* 2002;22:560–565.
67. Yajima N, Masuda M, Miyazaki M, et al. Oxidative stress is involved in the development of experimental abdominal aortic aneurysm: a study of the transcription profile with complementary DNA microarray. *J Vasc Surg.* 2002;36:379–385.
68. Johanning JM, Franklin DP, Han DC, et al. Inhibition of inducible nitric oxide synthase limits nitric oxide production and experimental aneurysm expansion. *J Vasc Surg.* 2001;33:579–586.
69. Lee JK, Borhani M, Ennis TL, et al. Experimental abdominal aortic aneurysms in mice lacking expression of inducible nitric oxide synthase. *Arterioscler Thromb Vasc Biol.* 2001;21:1393–1401.
70. Dobrin PB, Baker WH, Gley WC. Elastolytic and collagenolytic studies of arteries. Implications for the mechanical properties of aneurysms. *Arch Surg.* 1984;119:405–409.
71. Barnes MJ. Collagens in atherosclerosis. *Coll Relat Res.* 1985;5:65–97.
72. McGee GS, Baxter BT, Shively VP, et al. Aneurysm or occlusive disease–factors determining the clinical course of atherosclerosis of the infrarenal aorta. *Surgery.* 1991;110:370–376.
73. Mesh CL, Baxter BT, Pearce WH, et al. Collagen and elastin gene expression in aortic aneurysms. *Surgery.* 1992;112:256–262.
74. Minion DJ, Wang Y, Lynch TG, et al. Soluble factors modulate changes in collagen gene expression in abdominal aortic aneurysms. *Surgery.* 1993;114:252–257.
75. Hunter GC, Smyth SH, Aguirre ML, et al. Incidence and histologic characteristics of blebs in patients with abdominal aortic aneurysms. *J Vasc Surg.* 1996;24:93–101.
76. Satta J, Juvonen T, Haukipuro K, et al. Increased turnover of collagen in abdominal aortic aneurysms, demonstrated by measuring the concentration of the aminoterminal propeptide of type III procollagen in peripheral and aortal blood samples. *J Vasc Surg.* 1995;22:155–160.
77. Parks WC, Pierce RA, Lee KA, et al. Elastin. *Adv Mol Cell Biol.* 1993;6:133–182.
78. Boucek R. *Contributions of elastin and collagen organization to passive mechanical properties of arterial tissue.* Boca Raton, FL: CRC Press. 1988.
79. Mecham R, Broekelmann T, Davis E, et al. Elastic fibre assembly: macromolecular interactions. *Ciba Foundn Symp.* 1995;192:172—184.
80. Shapiro SD, Endicott SK, Province MA, et al. Marked longevity of human lung parenchymal elastic fibers deduced from prevalence of D-aspartate and nuclear weapons-related radiocarbon. *J Clin Invest.* 1991;87:1828–1834.
81. Krettek A, Sukhova GK, Libby P. Elastogenesis in human arterial disease: a role for macrophages in disordered elastin synthesis. *Arterioscler Thromb Vasc Biol.* 2003;23:582–587.
82. Rizzo RJ, McCarthy WJ, Dixit SN, et al. Collagen types and matrix protein content in human abdominal aortic aneurysms. *J Vasc Surg.* 1989;10:365–373.
83. Baxter BT, McGee GS, Shively VP, et al. Elastin content, cross-links, and mRNA in normal and aneurysmal human aorta. *J Vasc Surg.* 1992; 16:192–200.
84. Sumner DS, Hokanson DE, Strandness DE Jr. Stress-strain characteristics and collagen-elastin content of abdominal aortic aneurysms. *Surg Gynecol Obstet.* 1970;130:459–466.
85. Minion DJ, Davis VA, Nejezchleb PA, et al. Elastin is increased in abdominal aortic aneurysms. *J Surg Res.* 1994;57:443–446.
86. Busuttil RW, Abou-Zamzam AM, Machleder HI. Collagenase activity of the human aorta. A comparison of patients with and without abdominal aortic aneurysms. *Arch Surg.* 1980;115:1373–1378.

87. Busuttil RW, Rinderbriecht H, Flesher A, et al. Elastase activity: the role of elastase in aortic aneurysm formation. *J Surg Res.* 1982;32:214–217.
88. Cannon DJ, Read RC. Blood elastolytic activity in patients with aortic aneurysm. *Ann Thorac Surg.* 1982;34:10–15.
89. Visse R, Nagase H. Matrix metalloproteinases and tissue inhibitors of metalloproteinases: structure, function, and biochemistry. *Circ Res.* 2003;92:827–839.
90. Nagase H, Woessner JF Jr. Matrix metalloproteinases. *J Biol Chem.* 1999; 274:21491–21494.
91. Thompson RW, Holmes DR, Mertens RA, et al. Production and localization of 92-kilodalton gelatinase in abdominal aortic aneurysms. An elastolytic metalloproteinase expressed by aneurysm-infiltrating macrophages. *J Clin Invest.* 1995;96:318–326.
92. Aimes RT, Quigley JP. Matrix metalloproteinase-2 is an interstitial collagenase. Inhibitor-free enzyme catalyzes the cleavage of collagen fibrils and soluble native type I collagen generating the specific 3/4- and 1/4-length fragments. *J Biol Chem.* 1995;270:5872–5876.
93. McMillan WD, Patterson BK, Keen RR, et al. In situ localization and quantification of seventy-two-kilodalton type IV collagenase in aneurysmal, occlusive, and normal aorta. *J Vasc Surg.* 1995;22:295–305.
94. Davis V, Persidskaia R, Baca-Regen L, Itoh Y, et al. Matrix metalloproteinase-2 production and its binding to the matrix are increased in abdominal aortic aneurysms. *Arterioscler Thromb Vasc Biol.* 1998;18:1625–1633.
95. Curci JA, Liao S, Huffman MD, et al. Expression and localization of macrophage elastase (matrix metalloproteinase-12) in abdominal aortic aneurysms. *J Clin Invest.* 1998;102:1900–1910.
96. Shi GP, Sukhova GK, Grubb A, et al. Cystatin C deficiency in human atherosclerosis and aortic aneurysms. *J Clin Invest.* 1999;104:1191–1197.
97. Carmeliet P, Moons L, Lijnen R, et al. Urokinase-generated plasmin activates matrix metalloproteinases during aneurysm formation. *Nat Genet.* 1997;17:439–444.
98. Liu J, Xiong W, Baca-Regen L, et al. Mechanism of inhibition of matrix metalloproteinase-2 expression by doxycycline in human aortic smooth muscle cells. *J Vasc Surg.* 2003;38:1376–1383.
99. Prall AK, Longo GM, Mayhan WG, et al. Doxycycline in patients with abdominal aortic aneurysms and in mice: comparison of serum levels and effect on aneurysm growth in mice. *J Vasc Surg.* 2002;35:923–929.
100. Petrinec D, Liao S, Holmes DR, et al. Doxycycline inhibition of aneurysmal degeneration in an elastase-induced rat model of abdominal aortic aneurysm: preservation of aortic elastin associated with suppressed production of 92 kD gelatinase. *J Vasc Surg.* 1996;23:336–346.
101. Mosorin M, Juvonen J, Biancari F, et al. Use of doxycycline to decrease the growth rate of abdominal aortic aneurysms: a randomized, double-blind, placebo-controlled pilot study. *J Vasc Surg.* 2001;34:606–610.
102. **Baxter BT, Pearce WH, Waltke EA, et al. Prolonged administration of doxycycline in patients with small asymptomatic abdominal aortic aneurysms: report of a prospective (Phase II) multicenter study. *J Vasc Surg.* 2002;36:1–12.**
103. Moore JE, Jr, Ku DN, Zarins CK, et al. Pulsatile flow visualization in the abdominal aorta under differing physiologic conditions: implications for increased susceptibility to atherosclerosis. *J Biomech Eng.* 1992;114: 391–397.
104. Peterson L, Jensen RE, Parnell J. Mechanical properties of arteries in vivo. *Circ Res.* 1960;8:622–633.
105. Wolinsky H, Glagov S. Comparison of abdominal and thoracic aortic medial structure in mammals. Deviation of man from the usual pattern. *Circ Res.* 1969;25:677–686.
106. Vorp DA, Lee PC, Wang DH, et al. Association of intraluminal thrombus in abdominal aortic aneurysm with local hypoxia and wall weakening. *J Vasc Surg.* 2001;34:291–299.
107. **Vorp DA, Raghavan ML, Webster MW. Mechanical wall stress in abdominal aortic aneurysm: influence of diameter and asymmetry. *J Vasc Surg.* 1998;27:632–639.**
108. Raghavan ML, Vorp DA, Federle MP, et al. Wall stress distribution on three-dimensionally reconstructed models of human abdominal aortic aneurysm. *J Vasc Surg.* 2000;31:760–769.
109. Fillinger MF, Raghavan ML, Marra SP, et al. In vivo analysis of mechanical wall stress and abdominal aortic aneurysm rupture risk. *J Vasc Surg.* 2002;36:589–597.
110. Sho E, Sho M, Hoshina K, et al. Hemodynamic forces regulate mural macrophage infiltration in experimental aortic aneurysms. *Exp Mol Pathol.* 2004;76:108–116.
111. Nakahashi TK, Hoshina K, Tsao PS, et al. Flow loading induces macrophage antioxidative gene expression in experimental aneurysms. *Arterioscler Thromb Vasc Biol.* 2002;22:2017–2022.
112. Grote K, Flach I, Luchtefeld M, et al. Mechanical stretch enhances mRNA expression and proenzyme release of matrix metalloproteinase-2 (MMP-2) via NAD(P)H oxidase-derived reactive oxygen species. *Circ Res.* 2003;92: e80–86.
113. Howard AB, Alexander RW, Nerem RM, et al. Cyclic strain induces an oxidative stress in endothelial cells. *Am J Physiol.* 1997;272:C421–427.
114. Schillinger M, Exner M, Mlekusch W, et al. Heme oxygenase-1 gene promoter polymorphism is associated with abdominal aortic aneurysm. *Thromb Res.* 2002;106:131–136.
115. Pola R, Gaetani E, Santoliquido A, et al. Abdominal aortic aneurysm in normotensive patients: association with angiotensin-converting enzyme gene polymorphism. *Eur J Vasc Endovasc Surg.* 2001;21:445–449.
116. Gerdes LU, Lindholt JS, Vammen S, et al. Apolipoprotein E genotype is associated with differential expansion rates of small abdominal aortic aneurysms. *Br J Surg.* 2000;87:760–765.
117. Rossaak JI, Van Rij AM, Jones GT, et al. Association of the 4G/5G polymorphism in the promoter region of plasminogen activator inhibitor-1 with abdominal aortic aneurysms. *J Vasc Surg.* 2000;31: 1026–1032.
118. Wang X, Tromp G, Cole CW, et al. Analysis of coding sequences for tissue inhibitor of metalloproteinases 1 (TIMP1) and 2 (TIMP2) in patients with aneurysms. *Matrix Biol.* 1999;18:121–124.
119. Kotani K, Shimomura T, Murakami F, et al. Allele frequency of human endothelial nitric oxide synthase gene polymorphism in abdominal aortic aneurysm. *Intern Med.* 2000;39:537–539.
120. Rasmussen TE, Hallett JW Jr, Schulte S, et al. Genetic similarity in inflammatory and degenerative abdominal aortic aneurysms: a study of human leukocyte antigen class II disease risk genes. *J Vasc Surg.* 2001;34: 84–89.
121. Jones GT, Phillips VL, Harris EL, et al. Functional matrix metalloproteinase-9 polymorphism (C-1562T) associated with abdominal aortic aneurysm. *J Vasc Surg.* 2003;38:1363–1367.
122. Bown MJ, Burton PR, Horsburgh T, et al. The role of cytokine gene polymorphisms in the pathogenesis of abdominal aortic aneurysms: a case-control study. *J Vasc Surg.* 2003;37:999–1005.
123. Strauss E, Waliszewski K, Gabriel M, et al. Increased risk of the abdominal aortic aneurysm in carriers of the MTHFR 677T allele. *J Appl Genet.* 2003;44:85–93.
124. Ailawadi G, Eliason JL, Upchurch GR Jr. Current concepts in the pathogenesis of abdominal aortic aneurysm. *J Vasc Surg.* 2003;38:584–588.
125. Irizarry E, Newman KM, Gandhi RH, et al. Demonstration of interstitial collagenase in abdominal aortic aneurysm disease. *J Surg Res.* 1993;54:571–574.
126. Carrell TW, Burnand KG, Wells GM, et al. Stromelysin-1 (matrix metalloproteinase-3) and tissue inhibitor of metalloproteinase-3 are overexpressed in the wall of abdominal aortic aneurysms. *Circulation.* 2002;105: 477–482.
127. Mao D, Lee JK, VanVickle SJ, et al. Expression of collagenase-3 (MMP-13) in human abdominal aortic aneurysms and vascular smooth muscle cells in culture. *Biochem Biophys Res Commun.* 1999;261:904–910.
128. Nollendorfs A, Greiner TC, Nagase H, et al. The expression and localization of membrane type-1 matrix metalloproteinase in human abdominal aortic aneurysms. *J Vasc Surg.* 2001;34:316–322.
129. Tamarina NA, McMillan WD, Shively VP, et al. Expression of matrix metalloproteinases and their inhibitors in aneurysms and normal aorta. *Surgery.* 1997;122:264–262.
130. Gacko M, Glowinski S. Cathepsin D and cathepsin L activities in aortic aneurysm wall and parietal thrombus. *Clin Chem Lab Med.* 1998;36: 449–452.
131. Jean-Claude J, Newman KM, Li H, et al. Possible key role for plasmin in the pathogenesis of abdominal aortic aneurysms. *Surgery.* 1994;116: 472–478.
132. Reilly JM, Sicard GA, Lucore C. Abnormal expression of plasminogen activators in aortic aneurysmal and occlusive disease. *J Vasc Surg.* 1994;19: 865–872.
133. Schneiderman J, Bordin GM, Engelberg I, et al. Expression of fibrinolytic genes in atherosclerotic abdominal aortic aneurysm wall. A possible mechanism for aneurysm expansion. *J Clin Invest.* 1995;96: 639–645.

CHAPTER 99 ■ CAROTID AND UPPER EXTREMITY ANEURYSMS

JOHN W. HALLETT, JR. AND TODD E. RASMUSSEN

Aneurysms of the innominate, extracranial carotid, subclavian, and axillary arteries are rare in comparison with other types of peripheral aneurysms, accounting for less than 5% of all aneurysms.[1] Nonetheless, their recognition and management present several unique challenges for the surgeon. Their causes are diverse. These aneurysms generally present as a thromboembolic event; rarely do they rupture. Exposure and repair of these aneurysms can be problematic, testing the judgment and skill of the most experienced surgeon.

ANATOMIC CONSIDERATIONS

During embryologic development, the aortic arch and brachiocephalic arteries evolve from paired dorsal aortae, which lie on either side of the trachea proximally and fuse in the thorax. The normal sequence of aortic arch branches is present in 80% of the population (Fig. 99.1). In approximately 10% of patients, the brachiocephalic trunk and left common carotid artery have a common origin from the aortic arch. An origin of the left vertebral artery from the aortic arch between the left common carotid artery and the left subclavian artery occurs in about 6% of patients. A less common aberration, found in one of every 200 autopsies, is an anomalous origin of the right subclavian artery (see Fig. 99.1).[2] As the aberrant right subclavian artery courses toward the right upper extremity, its position is retroesophageal in 80% of patients, between the trachea and the esophagus in 15%, and anterior to the trachea in 5%,[3,4] In addition to arterial abnormalities, extraneous cervical and malformed first ribs are associated with subclavian aneurysms related to thoracic outlet syndrome.[5,6]

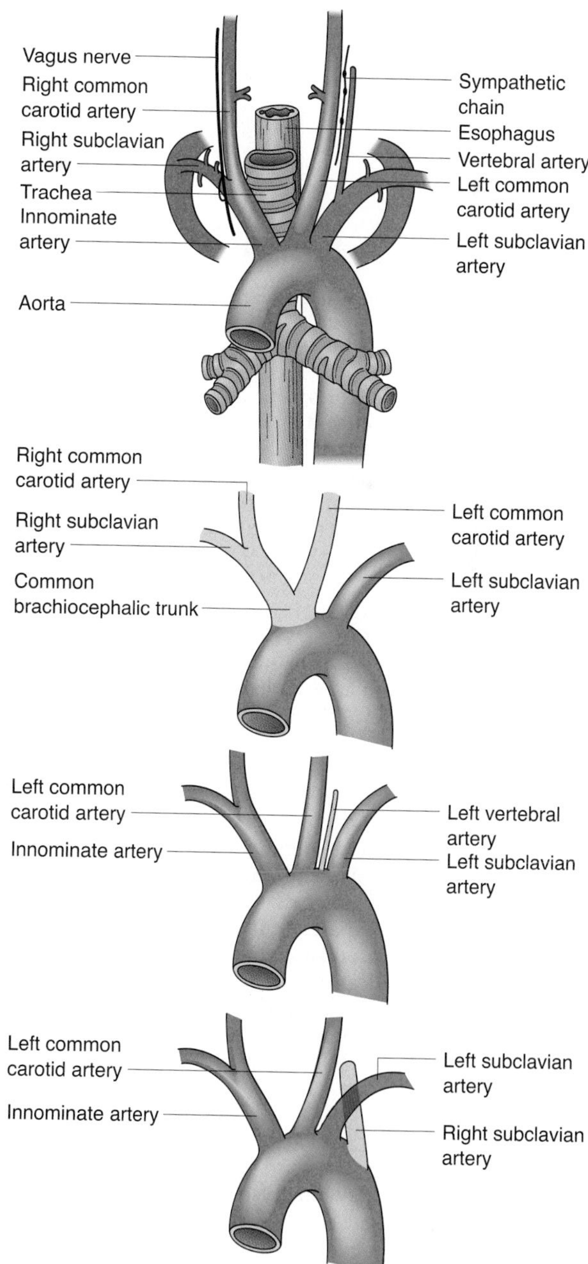

FIGURE 99.1 (Top) Normal anatomy of the aortic arch, present in 80% of patients. (Bottom) The three most common anatomic variations. 1. Common origin of left common carotid artery and brachiocephalic trunk. 2. Anomalous origin of the left vertebral artery. 3. Anomalous origin of right subclavian artery.

PREVALENCE OF BRACHIOCEPHALIC ANEURYSMS

Various clinical studies have emphasized the rarity of brachiocephalic aneurysms, which account for approximately 2% of all peripheral aneurysms and for less than 1% of all surgically treated peripheral aneurysms. In a 40-year review from the Mayo Clinic, the most common type of brachiocephalic aneurysm was subclavian (56%), followed by extracranial carotid (34%) and innominate aneurysms (10%) (Fig. 99.2).[7] More specifically, approximately 250 carotid endarterectomies for occlusive disease are performed for every one carotid artery aneurysm repair.[8,9]

ETIOLOGY

Atherosclerosis, which is highly prevalent in aortic, iliac, and femoropopliteal aneurysms, is not as common in aneurysms of the brachiocephalic arteries. In many ways, the pathogenesis is specific to the brachiocephalic artery. Both true and false

VASCULAR

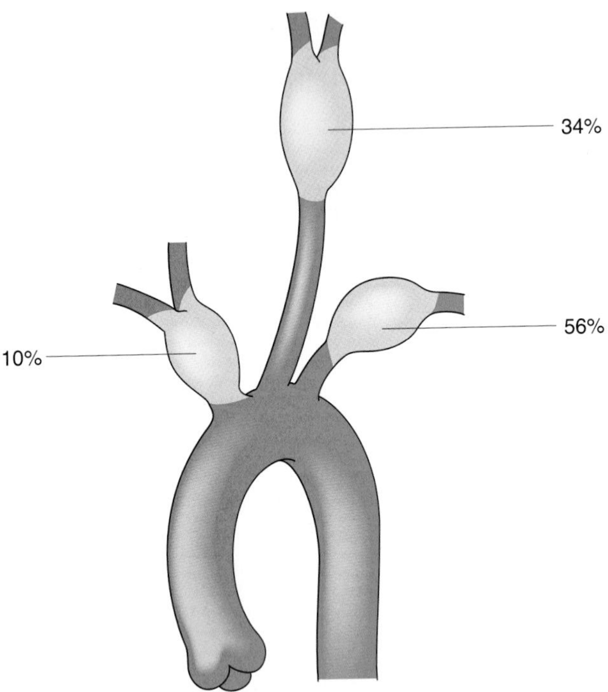

FIGURE 99.2 Relative frequencies of brachiocephalic aneurysms.

aneurysms play etiologic roles, and their relative prevalence depends on the local practice. For example, busy trauma centers more frequently report false aneurysms from blunt and penetrating trauma. Tertiary medical centers have larger series of brachiocephalic aneurysms related to atherosclerosis, thoracic outlet syndrome, and degenerative arterial dysplasias.[1,10]

Innominate Artery

Isolated innominate artery aneurysms are extraordinarily rare. Most are associated with atherosclerosis, hypertension, and a history of smoking. A few others are mycotic.[7]

Carotid Artery

Only one third of carotid artery aneurysms appear to be related to atherosclerosis, and they usually occur at the carotid bifurcation. The other two thirds usually involve the internal carotid artery and are evenly distributed among cases of fibromuscular dysplasia, spontaneous dissection, congenital abnormalities, and trauma.[9,11,12] Postendarterectomy pseudoaneurysm is another type of carotid aneurysm that has become more prevalent with the increased use of carotid artery patching.[13]

Subclavian Artery

Proximal subclavian artery aneurysms are usually atherosclerotic. They account for fewer than half of all subclavian artery aneurysms. A more prevalent cause of subclavian artery aneurysm is thoracic outlet compression and chronic injury of the artery caused by an abnormal cervical or first rib.[5,6,14] Although less common, an aberrant artery, most commonly found on the right, is another cause of subclavian aneurysm. Like other congenitally persistent arteries, an aberrant subclavian artery is prone to aneurysmal degeneration.[3,4,15]

Axillary Artery

Extensive reviews of aneurysms in the axillary–subclavian region reveal that the vast majority of cases involve the subclavian artery (88%), whereas solitary axillary artery aneurysms are much less common (12%).[16,17] In elderly patients, atherosclerosis is the cause of solitary axillary artery aneurysms. In younger patients, some type of trauma, such as the use of a crutch, precedes most cases of axillary artery aneurysm.[16,17]

CLINICAL FEATURES

Several general clinical features distinguish brachiocephalic aneurysms from other peripheral arterial aneurysms.[1] First, brachiocephalic aneurysms are detected over a much wider age range. Although the mean age of patients is about 50 years, the range extends from the second to the ninth decade of life. Like lower extremity aneurysms, atherosclerotic brachiocephalic aneurysms usually occur in the sixth or seventh decade of life. In contrast, subclavian artery aneurysms related to thoracic outlet compression and internal carotid artery aneurysms caused by fibromuscular disease occur in patients in the third or fourth decade of life.

Second, the sex distribution is variable and depends on aneurysm location. Proximal innominate, subclavian, and common carotid aneurysms are at least twice as common in men. Distal subclavian artery aneurysms related to thoracic outlet syndrome and internal carotid aneurysms caused by fibromuscular disease are observed predominantly in women.[1,6]

Third, brachiocephalic aneurysms are much more likely to be symptomatic at presentation than are peripheral femoral or popliteal aneurysms. In fact, two thirds of patients with brachiocephalic aneurysms are symptomatic at recognition.[7]

Finally, brachiocephalic atherosclerotic aneurysms are commonly associated with other aneurysms.[7–9] In one fourth to one half of patients, an additional aneurysm is present or develops later.[10,16] In addition to these general clinical features, aneurysms in each anatomic brachiocephalic region have some unique clinical features.

Innominate Artery Aneurysm

Innominate artery aneurysms are symptomatic in more than one half of patients and are associated with three basic clinical presentations: local compressive symptoms of regional nervous or venous structures, transient ischemic attacks or strokes resulting from thromboembolism, or upper extremity ischemia. Because these lesions usually lie behind the sternum, they may not be palpable.[10] However, a large pulsatile and expansive supraclavicular mass should arouse suspicion of an innominate artery aneurysm.

Subclavian Artery Aneurysm

Subclavian artery aneurysms are related most commonly to thoracic outlet compression. Many patients have an abnormal cervical rib.[6] Frequently, they present with digital embolization. Recognition of the offending arterial aneurysm or ulcerative plaque is often delayed because it is hidden behind the clavicle. Other manifestations of subclavian artery aneurysms include supraclavicular or shoulder pain, shoulder and arm paresthesias, and upper extremity claudication following aneurysm thrombosis.[14,16,18] Subclavian artery aneurysms rarely rupture.

Aberrant Subclavian Artery Aneurysm

Aberrant subclavian artery aneurysms occur more often in men and may present over a wide age range. Various clinical presentations include esophageal or tracheal compression; obstruction of the venous outflow of the head, neck, and upper extremities; thromboembolism; and rupture. The most common symptom is dysphagia, which has been termed *dysphagia lusoria*.[1,4,15] In general, one third of patients present with dysphagia and another third with dyspnea and respiratory problems; the remainder are asymptomatic.[4] These aneurysms are more likely to rupture than most other brachiocephalic aneurysms, and rupture is the clinical outcome in approximately 10% to 15% of such patients.[15]

Carotid Artery Aneurysm

Approximately 70% of carotid artery aneurysms involve the internal carotid artery, and the remaining 30% affect the carotid bifurcation. Their main risk is thromboembolic.[12] The risk for transient ischemic attack or stroke depends on associated stenosis and thrombus formation in the aneurysm.[11] Other symptoms associated with carotid artery aneurysms include cranial nerve dysfunction, neck or ear pain, and headache.[7,19]

Axillary Artery Aneurysm

Isolated axillary artery aneurysms generally present with thromboembolic complications. Acute thrombosis often precipitates a vascular emergency.[16] Distal thrombus propagation or thromboembolism may cause severe hand ischemia.

DIAGNOSIS AND EVALUATION

The sternum and clavicles prevent palpation of most innominate or proximal subclavian artery aneurysms. Even carotid artery aneurysms may lie deep in the neck and not be palpable until they are large. Cervical common carotid aneurysms must be differentiated from enlarged lymph nodes, head or neck malignancies, and carotid body tumors.[1,13] In elderly, hypertensive women, the proximal right common carotid artery may be tortuous and easily mistaken for an aneurysm.

Initial diagnostic tests depend on the clinical presentation of the patient. Computed tomography of the chest, supraclavicular fossa, and neck is usually definitive. Duplex ultrasonography can detect carotid artery aneurysms and most subclavian or axillary aneurysms. Gadolinium-enhanced magnetic resonance imaging or multislice, helical computed tomographic angiography can provide adequate initial anatomic information for most patients. Standard catheter arteriography with views of the aortic arch, great vessels, and intracranial circulation is essential when an endovascular repair is undertaken (Fig. 99.3).[1,19,20]

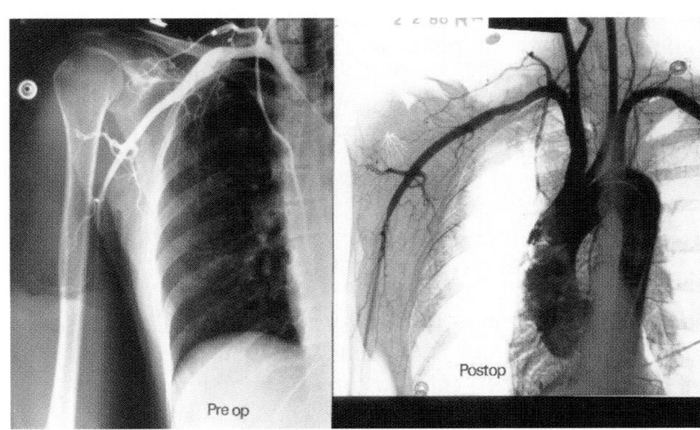

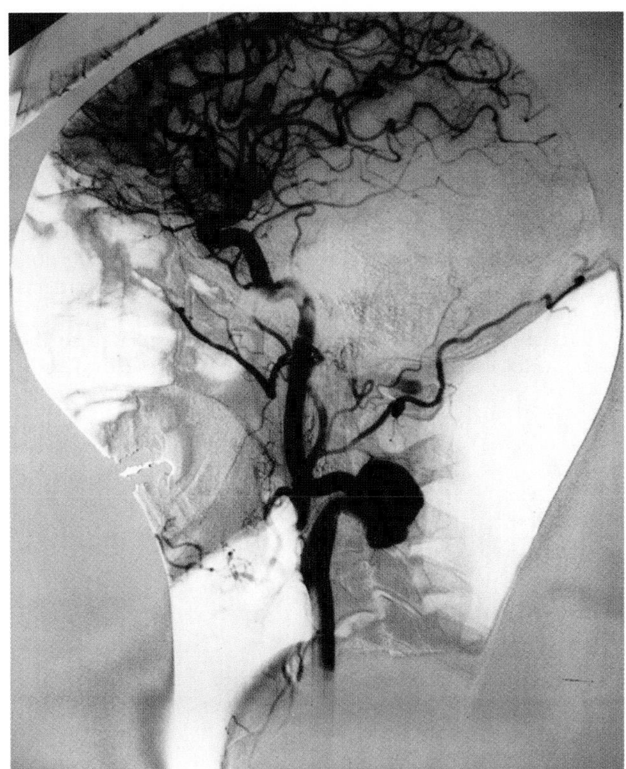

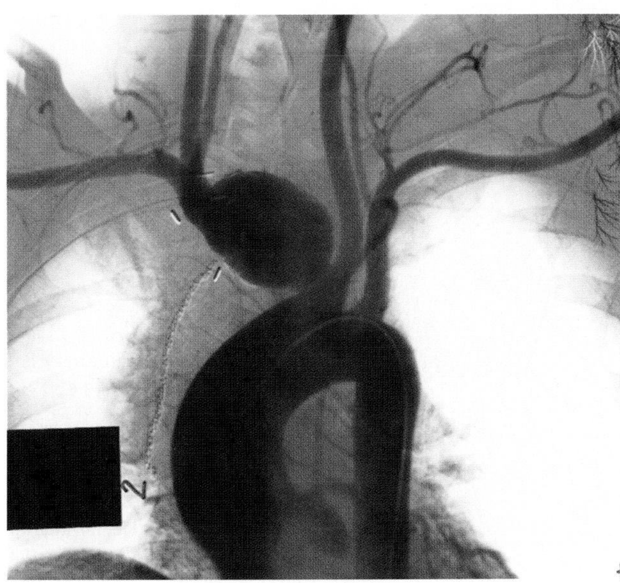

FIGURE 99.3 (*A*) Arteriography of subclavian artery aneurysm preoperatively and postoperatively. (*B*) Arteriography of carotid artery aneurysm. (*C*) Arteriography of innominate artery aneurysm.

SURGICAL AND ENDOVASCULAR TREATMENT

Surgical resection with arterial reconstruction is indicated for most patients with brachiocephalic aneurysms. Although endovascular stent grafts have been placed percutaneously to treat isolated cases of brachiocephalic aneurysms, their safety and durability remain controversial.[21–23] Asymptomatic brachiocephalic aneurysms in patients with poor health or adverse anatomic situations are usually observed. Each type of aneurysm presents its own unique therapeutic challenge.

Innominate Artery Aneurysm

Isolated innominate artery aneurysms are approached through a median sternotomy, with extension of the incision into the neck or right supraclavicular region as needed (Fig. 99.4A). They are generally replaced with an 8- to 10-mm single-limb prosthetic distal aorta–innominate artery graft (Fig. 99.5A). The need to shunt rarely arises during these reconstructions, but intraoperative electroencephalography or measurement of common carotid stump pressures is a useful adjunct to determine the adequacy of collateral cerebral blood flow. If the innominate artery aneurysm is infected, direct in-line reconstruction with autogenous material, such as arterial homografts, internal iliac or superficial femoral arteries, or superficial femoral veins, can be performed.

Subclavian Artery Aneurysm

Proximal intrathoracic atherosclerotic subclavian artery aneurysms are approached through a median sternotomy, with extension of the incision into the right supraclavicular area for right-sided aneurysms (see Fig. 99.4A).[24] Isolated left intrathoracic subclavian artery aneurysms are best approached through a left posterolateral thoracotomy. A synthetic graft is generally necessary for reconstruction.[24] In selected patients, a covered stent graft may suffice.

Patients with subclavian artery aneurysms related to thoracic outlet compression require aneurysm resection, graft replacement, and concomitant resection of the abnormal cervical or anomalous first rib (Fig. 99.5B). This reconstruction can generally be accomplished through two incisions, one supraclavicular and one infraclavicular (Fig. 99.4A). Occasionally, transaxillary incision is necessary for adequate removal of an offending first rib. An alternative is a single incision with resection of the clavicle. This approach provides excellent exposure but may leave the patient with some cosmetic deformity and occasional shoulder discomfort. The subclavian artery can be replaced with saphenous vein, hypogastric artery, or a synthetic graft, depending on the size of the artery (see Fig. 99.5B).

Axillary artery aneurysms are generally exposed through a subpectoral and medial upper arm incision (see Fig. 99.4B). An interposition vein graft is generally appropriate.

Aberrant Subclavian Aneurysm

The surgical approach to aberrant subclavian artery aneurysms depends on the pathology of both the aberrant artery and the adjacent aorta. Although a variety of surgical approaches have been described, a single operation performed in two stages is most common.[4] Initially, a supraclavicular approach is used to reimplant the normal distal subclavian artery into the ipsilateral right common carotid artery. A posterolateral thoracotomy is then performed to obliterate the origin of the aberrant artery and repair the aorta (Fig. 99.5C). The proximal aberrant subclavian artery may be associated with a large, conical duct of Kommerell, which makes aortic control more difficult. In such patients, aortic cross-clamping is generally necessary for safe repair. Although simple cross-clamping with thoracic aortic repair may be possible in 50% of such patients, the remaining patients may require cardiopulmonary bypass or hypothermic circulatory arrest.[4] Recently, an endovascular approach has been described.[29]

Carotid Artery Aneurysm

Repair of a common carotid artery aneurysm is accomplished by aneurysm resection or endoaneurysmorrhaphy combined with either primary end-to-end anastomosis or an interposition prosthetic or autogenous graft (Fig. 99.5D). A standard cervical neck

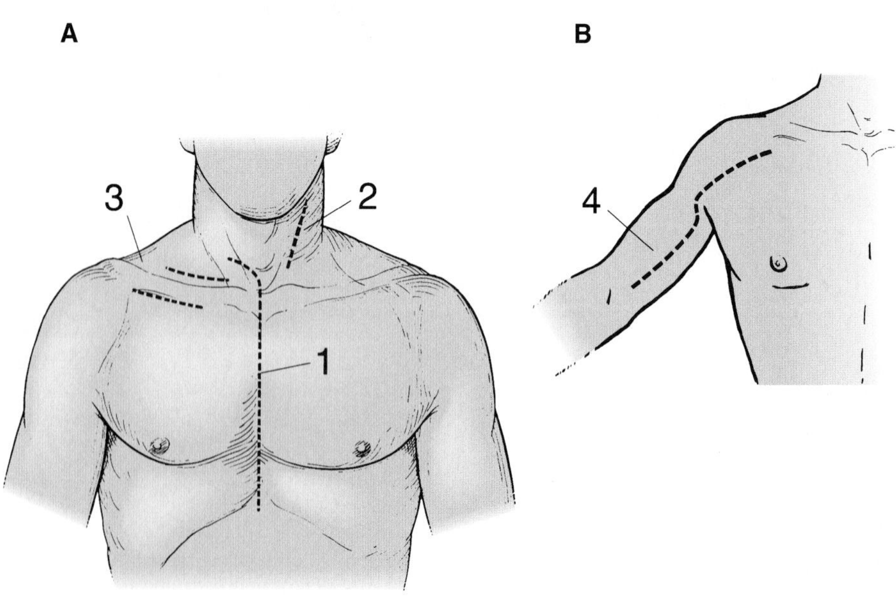

FIGURE 99.4 (*A*) Approach No. 1: Median sternotomy with extension into cervical or right supraclavicular incision as approach to innominate artery aneurysm. Approach No. 2: Cervical incision as approach to carotid artery aneurysm. Approach No. 3: Supraclavicular incision to proximal portion of right subclavian artery and infraclavicular incision to middle and distal portions of subclavian artery. (*B*) Approach No. 4: Surgical incision to approach distal subclavian or axillary artery aneurysm. Patient's arm is away from side. Note that the medial extent can become the infraclavicular incision in approach No. 3 if more proximal exposure is necessary.

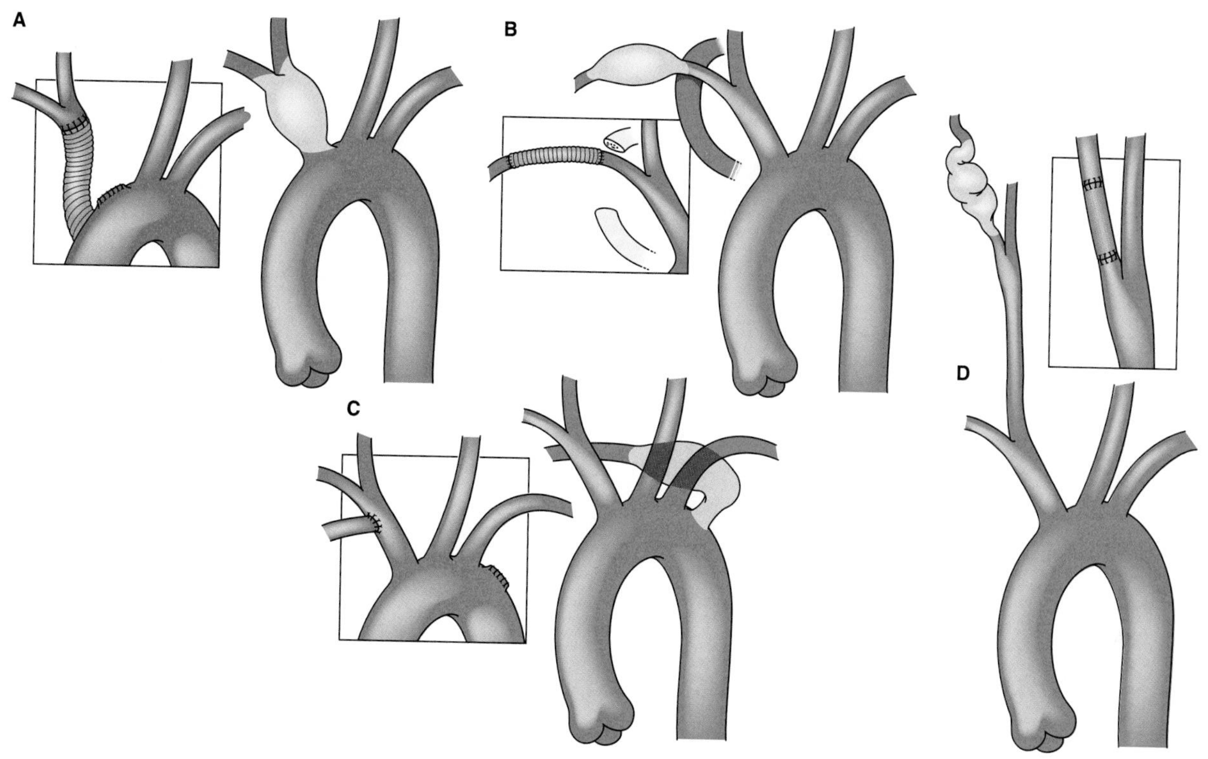

FIGURE 99.5 (*A*) Schematic representation of aneurysm resection and graft replacement for an innominate artery aneurysm. (*B*) Schematic representation of subclavian artery aneurysm resection, graft replacement, and rib resection for subclavian artery aneurysm related to thoracic outlet obstruction. (*C*) Schematic representation of an aberrant right subclavian artery aneurysm. Repair involves two steps: reimplantation of normal distal subclavian artery into right common carotid artery through supraclavicular approach, followed by left posterolateral thoracotomy to obliterate origin of the aberrant subclavian artery and repair the aorta. (*D*) Schematic representation of extracranial right carotid artery aneurysm with subsequent resection and interposition grafting.

incision along the anterior border of the sternocleidomastoid muscle is suitable for aneurysms at the bifurcation or proximal internal carotid artery (Fig. 99.4A). Exposure of high cervical internal carotid aneurysms is more difficult and may be facilitated by adjuncts, such as nasotracheal intubation with or without subluxation of the jaw, mobilization of the parotid gland, and division of the posterior belly of the digastric muscle, styloid mandibular ligament, and styloid process.[25] Distal carotid control in high cervical aneurysms may require an aneurysm clip, the bulb tip of a shunt, or an indwelling small-balloon occlusion catheter. In reported cases, the distal internal carotid artery has been ligated, and an extracranial–intracranial bypass has been performed to the middle cerebral artery or its M2 segment.[25]

Outcome of Open Surgical Therapy

Elective repair of brachiocephalic aneurysms is associated with a mortality of 0% to 8%.[6,7,12] Most deaths occur in patients undergoing simultaneous cardiovascular procedures, such as coronary revascularization or aortic arch reconstruction.[1] The risk of stroke depends on the aneurysm type. Perioperative neurologic deficits are more common in patients with atherosclerotic carotid artery aneurysms than in those with aneurysms that are not atherosclerotic (10% to15% versus 5%). Most surgical series report a neurologic complication rate higher than routine carotid endarterectomy. For high carotid artery aneurysms, cranial nerve injury is problematic and affects as many as 15% of patients.[12,13] Glossopharyngeal nerve injury is considered the most morbid complication, as a permanent gastrostomy is occasionally required.

Late Survival

All factors considered, late survival for patients with brachiocephalic arterial aneurysms is favorable. In a large series from the Mayo Clinic, 5- and 10-year survival rates were 81% and 61%, respectively (Fig. 99.6A).[7] Aneurysm location affects late survival. Patients who undergo repair of carotid artery aneurysms have a 10-year survival of 80%, which is no different from that of age- and sex-matched controls (Fig. 99.6B). However, patients with atherosclerotic subclavian artery aneurysms have a significantly shorter survival than matched controls.[7] This difference is generally related to associated cardiovascular morbidity.

Endovascular Therapy

Recently, endovascular approaches have been reported for brachiocephalic aneurysms. These have included a combination of embolization and stent grafts. Endovascular therapy has generally been reserved for patients who are not good surgical candidates (e.g., irradiated fields, multiple previous operations, or areas anatomically difficult to approach surgically). Although successful in some cases, embolization and early stent thrombosis have been problematic.[21–29] Increasing experience with endovascular approaches to vascular disease in general is likely to expand the use of endovascular therapy for brachiocephalic aneurysms.

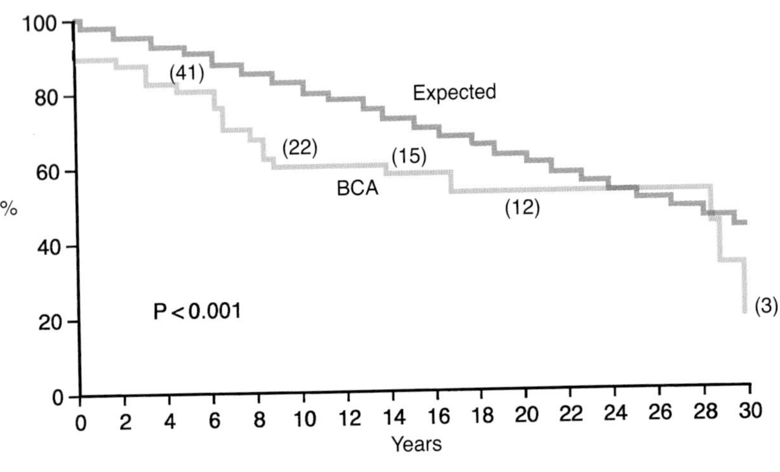

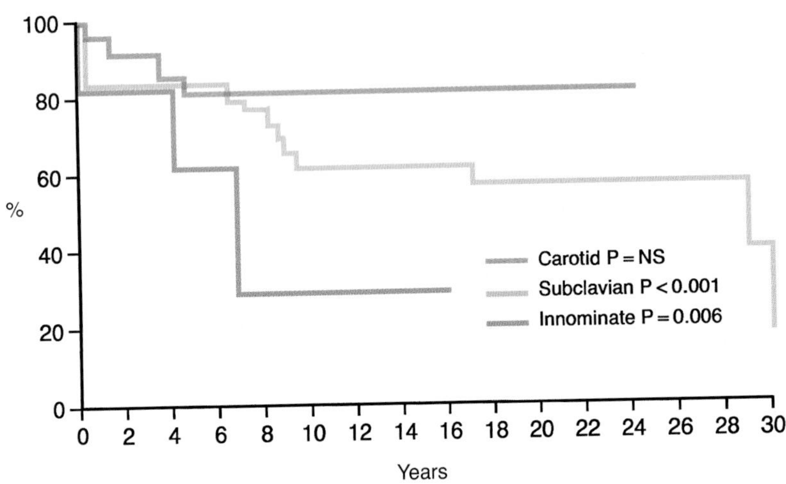

FIGURE 99.6 (*A*) Survival of patients with brachiocephalic aneurysms in comparison with expected survival adjusted for age, sex, and year of operation. (*B*) Survival for each group of brachiocephalic aneurysms. (From Bower TC, Pairolero PC, Hallett JW Jr, et al. Brachiocephalic aneurysm: the case for early recognition and repair. *Ann Vasc Surg.* 1991;5: 125–132.)

KEY POINTS

- **Upper extremity aneurysms are rare in comparison with other types of peripheral aneurysms.**
- **The etiology of brachiocephalic artery aneurysms is diverse.**
- **Surgical resection with arterial reconstruction is indicated for most patients with brachiocephalic aneurysms.**
- **Late survival for patients with brachiocephalic arterial aneurysms is favorable.**
- **Increasing experience with endovascular approaches to vascular disease in general is likely to expand the use of endovascular therapy for brachiocephalic aneurysms.**

References

1. Bower TC. Aneurysms of the great vessels and their branches. *Semin Vasc Surg.* 1996;9:134–146.
2. **Bosniak MA. An analysis of some anatomic—roentgenologic aspects of the brachiocephalic vessels. *Am J Roentgenol.* 1964;91:1222–1231.**
3. Stone WM, Brewster DC, Moncure AC, et al. Aberrant right subclavian artery: varied presentations and management options. *J Vasc Surg.* 1990;11:812–817.
4. Kieffer E, Bahnini A, Koskas F. Aberrant subclavian artery: surgical treatment in thirty-three adult patients. *J Vasc Surg.* 1994;19:100–111.
5. Hood DB, Kuehne J, Yellin AE, et al. Vascular complications of thoracic outlet syndrome. *Am Surg.* 1997;63:913–917.
6. Nehler MR, Taylor LM Jr, Moneta GL, et al. Upper extremity ischemia from subclavian artery aneurysm caused by bony abnormalities of the thoracic outlet. *Arch Surg.* 1997;132: 527–532.
7. Bower TC, Pairolero PC, Hallett JW Jr, et al. Brachiocephalic aneurysm: the case for early recognition and repair. *Ann Vasc Surg.* 1991;5: 125–132.
8. Painter TA, Hertzer NR, Beven EG, et al. Extracranial carotid aneurysms: report of six cases and review of the literature. *J Vasc Surg.* 1985;2: 312–318.
9. Zwolak RM, Whitehouse WM Jr, Knake JE, et al. Atherosclerotic extracranial carotid artery aneurysms. *J Vasc Surg.* 1984;1:415–422.
10. Brewster DC, Moncure AC, Darling RC, et al. Innominate artery lesions: problems encountered and lessons learned. *J Vasc Surg.* 1985;2:99–112.
11. Schievink WI, Piepgras DG, McGaffrey TV, et al. Surgical treatment of extracranial internal carotid artery dissecting aneurysms. *Neurosurgery* 1994;35:809–816.
12. Moreau P, Albat B, Thevenet A. Surgical treatment of extracranial internal carotid artery aneurysms. *Ann Vasc Surg.* 1994; 8:409–416.
13. **Faggioli GL, Freyrie A, Stella A, et al. Extracranial internal carotid artery aneurysms: results of a surgical series with long-term follow-up. *J Vasc Surg.* 1996;23:578–595.**
14. Cormier JM, Amrane M, Ward A, et al. Arterial complications of the thoracic outlet syndrome: fifty-five operative cases. *J Vasc Surg.* 1989;9: 778–787.
15. Kiernan PD, Dearani J, Byrne WD, et al. Aneurysm of an aberrant right subclavian artery: case report and review of the literature. *Mayo Clin Proc.* 1993;68:468–474.
16. Pairolero PC, Walls JT, Payne WS, et al. Subclavian–axillary artery aneurysms. *Surgery* 1981;90:757–763.
17. Abbott WM, Darling RC. Axillary artery aneurysms secondary to crutch trauma. *Am J Surg.* 1973;125:515–520.
18. Dougherty MJ, Calligaro KD, Savarese RP, et al. Atherosclerotic aneurysm of the intrathoracic subclavian artery: a case report and review of the literature. *J Vasc Surg.* 1995;21:521–529.
19. Coffin O, Maiza D, Galateau-Salle F, et al. Results of surgical management of internal carotid artery aneurysm by the cervical approach. *Ann Vasc Surg.* 1997;11:482–490.
20. Laitt RD, Thompson JF, Goddard P, et al. Subclavian artery aneurysm: the role of magnetic resonance imaging. *Cardiovasc Surg.* 1994;2:612–614.
21. **May J, White G, Waugh R, et al. Transluminal placement of a prosthetic graft—stent device for treatment of subclavian artery aneurysm. *J Vasc Surg.* 1993;18:1056–1059.**
22. Beregi JP, Prat A, Willoteaux S, et al. Covered stents in the treatment of peripheral arterial aneurysms: procedural results and midterm follow-up. *Cardiovasc Intervent Radiol.* 1999;22:13–19.

23. Parodi JC, Schonholz C, Ferreira LM, et al. Endovascular stent—graft treatment of traumatic arterial lesions. *Ann Vasc Surg.* 1999;13:121–129.
24. **Coselli JS, Crawford ES. Surgical treatment of aneurysms of the intrathoracic segment of the subclavian artery. *Chest* 1987;91:704–708.**
25. Sundt TM Jr, Pearson BW, Piepgras DG, et al. Surgical management of aneurysms of the distal extracranial internal carotid artery. *J Neurosurg.* 1986;64:169–182.
26. Puech-Leao P, Orra HA. Endovascular repair of an innominate artery aneurysm. *J Endovasc Ther.* 2002;8:429–432.
27. Mukherjee D, Roffi M, Yadov. Endovascular treatment of carotid artery aneurysms with stent grafts. *J Invasive Cardiol.* 2002;14:269–272.
28. Terramani TT, Workman MJ, Loberman Z et al. Adjunctive endovascular techniques in the management of postoperative carotid artery pseudoaneurysms. *Vasc Endovascular Surg.* 2003;37:207–212.
29. Corral JS, Zuniga CG, Sanchez JB et al. Treatment of aberrant right subclavian artery aneurysm with endovascular occlusion and adjunctive surgical bypass. *J Vasc Interv Radiol.* 2003;14:789–792.

CHAPTER 100 ■ THORACIC AORTIC ANEURYSMS

SUSAN D. MOFFATT-BRUCE AND R. SCOTT MITCHELL

Aneurysmal disease of the thoracic aortic is a disease entity that is often associated with high morbidity and mortality. By definition an aortic aneurysm is an abnormal fusiform or saccular dilation of the aorta. It can affect the ascending, arch, descending or entire thoracoabdominal component of the aorta. The patient population ranges from younger patients with extensive connective tissue disease to the frail elderly. Treatment decisions concerning operative intervention in terms of both timing and extent of resection are difficult and often involve multidisciplinary management.

The modern surgical treatment of aortic disease began in the 1950s when successful segmental resection and graft replacement of a thoracic aneurysm was reported by Swam et al.,[1] Lam and Aram.,[2] and De Bakey and Cooley.[3] In 1956, De Bakey and Cooley[3] reported the first successful resection of an ascending aortic aneurysm using cardiopulmonary bypass.[4] With enhanced diagnostic modalities, improved surgical techniques and better perioperative management, surgical results have continued to improve. Furthermore, an improved understanding of the pathophysiology and natural history of thoracic aortic disease has facilitated treatment decisions.

PREVALENCE, DIAGNOSTIC EVALUATION, AND NATURAL HISTORY

The true prevalence of thoracic aortic aneurysms is likely underreported. However, in a very extensive Swedish study with a population autopsy rate of 83%, the incidence of thoracic aortic aneurysms was reported as 489 per 100,000 men and 437 per 100,000 women with a median age of 77.7 years for men and 85.3 years for women.[5] Approximately 50% of all thoracic aortic aneurysms are located in the descending aorta; these aneurysms most commonly arise at the level of the left subclavian artery and are often associated with atherosclerosis.[6] Aneurysms associated with Marfan syndrome typically present in the ascending aorta. During the first half of the 20th century, thoracic aneurysms were far more common than abdominal aortic aneurysms because of the predominance of infectious aneurysm in the thoracic aorta. By 1964 however, the ratio had declined to less than 1 to 1, primarily as a result of the decline in the incidence of syphilitic aortitis.[7]

Although the vast majority of thoracic aneurysms are asymptomatic, enlarging thoracic aneurysms can present with hoarseness caused by stretching of the left recurrent laryngeal nerve, stridor from tracheal compression, dysphagia from esophageal impingement, dyspnea or hemoptysis from compression of the lung or edema from compression of the superior vena cava. Patients with aneurysms of the ascending aorta may also present with signs and symptoms of aortic insufficiency. Acute presentation may be caused by atypical chest pain either from expansion of the aneurysm or dissection of the aortic wall. Thoracic aortic aneurysms are often detected only after workup for another complaint, often involving a plain chest radiograph that reveals mediastinal enlargement. The mean age at time of diagnosis ranges between 59 and 69 years, with men predominating over women with a ratio of between 2:1 and 4:1.

Diagnostic modalities for thoracic aortic aneurysm include chest radiograph, catheter-based angiography, computed tomography (CT), magnetic resonance imaging (MRI), and transesophageal echocardiography (TEE).[8] Catheter-based angiography is invasive, utilizes nephrotoxic contrast agents, and effectively images only the flow lumen. However, little information pertaining to the aortic wall or surrounding structures is acquired. To a limited extent, exposure to contrast media can be minimized by the use of CO_2 and gadolinium.

CT although requiring radiation exposure and nephrotoxic contrast material, is widely available. Using angiographic enhancement, CT provides detailed information about the size, location, and extent of aortic disease as well as involvement of the mediastinal structures and pericardial and pleural spaces. This is the most common means of evaluating the thoracic aorta both at presentation and for follow-up (Figure 100.1).

MRI offers many of the advantages of CT but does not require ionizing radiation or nephrotoxic contrast media. However, MRI suites are not always available, frequently require lengthy image acquisition times, and have physically restrictive access.

TEE offers excellent visualization of the ascending and descending thoracic aorta as well as cardiac structures, pericardium, and pleural spaces. Tracheal shadowing, however, limits visualization of the proximal and distal aortic arch. In addition, the technical expertise to perform TEE is not always readily available.

Once a thoracic aortic aneurysm has been diagnosed, the management strategy is dictated by aneurysm size and rate

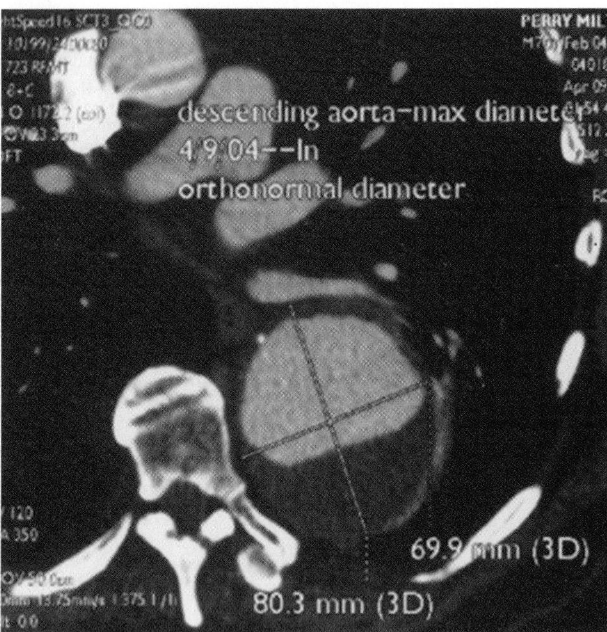

FIGURE 100.1 Computed tomography with angiographic enhancement of descending thoracic aortic aneurysm.

of growth. Enlarging aortic aneurysms are at risk of both dissection and rupture. Aortic dissection involves an intimal tear that initiates a high-pressure entry point into the subadventitial layer, which then propagates and can lead to aortic rupture or branch vessel compromise. Rupture rates correlate with size and in the early 1970s aortic rupture accounted for up to 77% of deaths in patients with aneurysms associated with dissection.[9] More recently, the Olmstead County, Minnesota, registry reported that the actual incidence of thoracic aneurysms had increased threefold but that the natural history was less perilous with a rupture rate of 16% at 3 years for 6-cm aneurysms compared to 31% for 7-cm aneurysms.[10] Juvonen et al.[11] from Mount Sinai in New York have identified clinical variables associated with rupture with the most important being increasing age, presence of chronic obstructive pulmonary disease (COPD), maximal thoracic and abdominal diameter, and the presence of pain. Utilizing a multivariable equation, the risk of rupture at 1 year can be calculated for any patient.

$$\text{Ln}\lambda = -21.055 + 0.0093\,(\text{age}) \text{ and } 0.841\,(\text{pain}) + 1.282\,(\text{COPD}) + 0.643\,(\text{descending diameter}) + 0.405\,(\text{abdominal diameter})$$

Probability of rupture within 1 year $= e^{-\lambda(365)}$

Diameters are entered in centimeters and pain and COPD are 0 if absent and 1 if present.

The Yale Aortic Diseases Group has reported rupture or dissection of ascending or arch aneurysms at a median size of 6 cm as compared to 7.2 cm for descending and thoracoabdominal aneurysms. Overall long-term survival of patients with thoracic aneurysms at 1 and 5 years was 85% and 64%, respectively. Patients with descending thoracic aneurysms had lower long-term survival than did patients with ascending aneurysms.[6] Furthermore, they have found that the mean rate of rupture or dissection is 2% per year for small aneurysms, 3% for aneurysms 5.0 to 5.9 cm, and 6.9% for aneurysms of 6.0 cm or greater in diameter. Even more striking, when using proportional hazards regression, the odds ratio for rupture is more than 25 times higher in patients with aneurysms of 6.0 cm or greater compared to aneurysms in the 4.0 to 4.9 cm size range.[12,13]

In three of the largest aortic aneurysm studies, of those patients who did not undergo operation at the time of diagnosis, rupture of the aneurysm was the most common cause of death, with rates ranging from 42% to 70%.[7,9,14] In all three series, the rate of rupture for aneurysms complicated by dissection substantially exceeded the rate for nondissecting aneurysm.[15] The 5-year survival rate ranged from 13% to 39%. It has been found that thoracic aneurysms enlarge at a more rapid rate than abdominal aneurysms and that aneurysms of the arch grow the fastest.[7,15]

TYPES AND PATHOGENESIS

Atherosclerotic Aneurysms

There has been a long-standing belief that aortic aneurysms may represent a late degenerative stage of atherosclerotic disease.[6] This concept, however, has been seriously challenged in recent years and aortic aneurysms are now being viewed in terms of genetic and molecular mechanisms. Atherosclerotic disease is so prevalent in the general population that it is now often thought to be associated with, rather than causative of, aneurysmal disease. Aneurysms associated with atherosclerosis of the aorta most commonly involve the descending or thoracoabdominal segments. Abnormal proteolysis, the presence of elastolytic serum enzymes and deficiencies of collagen and elastin have been implicated as factors contributing to the development of these aneurysms.[7] Atherosclerotic lesions of the thoracic aorta may ulcerate and penetrate the internal elastic lamina of the aortic wall, which can result in hemorrhage within the layers of the media and the formation of intramural hematoma. Saccular and fusiform aneurysms may develop, and dissection, rupture and embolization can also occur. Once aneurysmal dilatation of the aorta has begun, it tends to progress. Whether this is due to a gradual but constant increase in size or episodic incremental increases is unknown. Associated COPD and hypertension increase the rate of aneurysm growth.

Degenerative Aneurysms

Aneurysms classified as degenerative are those thought to be secondary to inborn errors of metabolism, resulting in defective production of collagen, the fibrous ground substance that is the main constituent of skin, tendons, ligaments, and blood vessels. Two major disease entities included are Marfan syndrome and Ehlers-Danlos syndrome. In Marfan syndrome, there are specific abnormalities of fibrillin-1, the main component of extracellular microfibrils. The defective gene FBN1 is responsible for fibrillin-1 and is located on the long arm of chromosome 15. The molecular defects in the fibrillin-1 gene are responsible for the impaired structural integrity of the skeletal, ocular and cardiovascular systems. Cardinal features of the disorder include tall stature, ectopia lentis, mitral valve prolapse, aortic root dilatation and aortic dissection. About three quarters of patients have an affected parent and new mutations account for the remainder of cases. Cardiovascular involvement is the most serious problem associated with the Marfan syndrome. The prevalence of aortic dilatation in Marfan syndrome is 70% to 80% and most commonly involves the aortic root and sinuses of Valsalva. It presents at an early age and tends to be more common in men than women (Figure 100.2).

Not all degenerative aneurysms can be associated with a known disease entity. Those that fail the criteria for Marfan syndrome or other distinguishable disease entities have also been studied. Histologic examination of these aneurysms reveals fragmentation and degeneration of elastic fibers in the

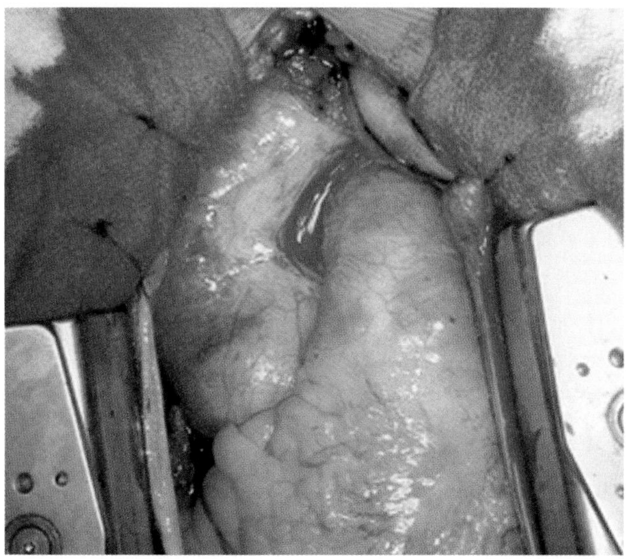

FIGURE 100.2 Ascending aortic aneurysm in a patient with Marfan syndrome.

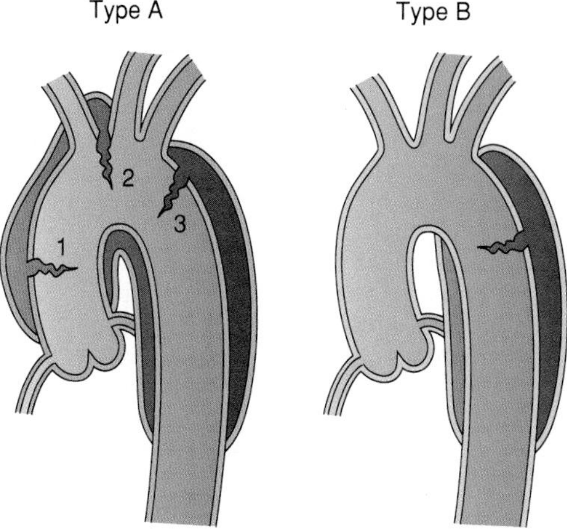

FIGURE 100.3 Stanford classification of aortic dissections based on the presence or absence of involvement of the ascending aorta. Numbers indicate the locations of the site of primary intimal tear. (After Miller DC, Stinson EB, Oyer PE, et al. Operative treatment of aortic dissection. *J Thorac Cardiovasc Surg*. 1979;78:365–382.)

arterial media.[6] The mechanisms for this degeneration are unknown. Others have suggested that loss of structural integrity of the adventitia, not the media, is required for aneurysm formation. These pathologic changes must be differentiated from the normal aging process, in which elastic fibers fragment, smooth muscle cells diminish, collagen becomes more prominent and ground substance increases, thus rendering the aorta less distensible and gradually more weakened.

Aneurysms Associated with Dissections

Aortic dissection results when blood separates the layers of the aortic media, usually through a tear in the intima. This tear occurs most commonly in the aorta at the non-coronary sinus, resulting in ascending aortic involvement, referred to as a *Stanford type A dissection*, or in the descending thoracic aorta originating at or after the subclavian artery, referred to as a *Stanford type B dissection* (Fig. 100.3).

Hypertension would appear to be the single most important risk factor for thoracic aortic dissection.[7] The majority of patients with Stanford type A dissections are treated as surgical emergencies since survival is less than 10% at 3 months without treatment. Stanford type B dissections are usually treated medically with anti-impulse therapy and long-term antihypertensive management. Operative intervention is required for complicated Stanford type B dissections, including rupture or impending rupture, malperfusion syndromes, intractable pain, or rapid expansion. Any dissected aorta can progress to become aneurysmal mandating very good follow up of all patients with aortic dissections.

Traumatic Aneurysms

Trauma is the most common cause of nondegenerative disease affecting the thoracic aorta. During sudden deceleration, the untethered aortic arch and descending aorta can flex anteriorly, stretching the aorta against the ligamentum, with a resultant partial or complete circumferential intimal disruption. According to autopsy series, 36% to 54% of disruptions occur at the aortic isthmus, 8% to 27% involve the ascending aorta, 8% to 18% occur in the arch, and 11% to 21% involve the distal descending aorta.[16,17] For the 10% to 20% of patients who survive this acute event, the rupture is partially contained by the aortic adventitia and pleura. Of those that survive traumatic injury to the aorta, aneurysmal formation around the site of injury can occur and often dilates faster because it is an unsuspected injury.

Mycotic Aneurysms

Mycotic aneurysms are rare and can be caused by bacterial, fungal, spirochetal, or viral agents. Before antibiotics, syphilis accounted for approximately 75% of aneurysms. Since the discovery of antibiotic treatment, however, syphilitic aneurysms have become rarities. Mycotic aneurysms occur at the sites of localized infections in the aortic or arterial walls, usually as the result of metastatic infection from septicemia, which is commonly caused by infective endocarditis. Infection of atherosclerotic plaques themselves can also result in mycotic aneurysms. Infection may also spread to blood vessel walls from contiguous sepsis, particularly infected lymph nodes or trauma. Preexisting aortic aneurysms may also become infected, usually from bloodstream seeding. Although any pathogen may infect aneurysms, *Salmonella* species show a special proclivity for vascular tissues. Treatment consists of long-term antibiotics before and after aneurysm resection.

OPERATIVE MANAGEMENT

The natural history of thoracic aneurysms has shown a propensity to increase in size until they rupture.[6,12] The approach to the timing of surgical intervention has been the subject of much debate.[12,18,19] The Yale Aortic Diseases Group has extensively studied growth rates of aneurysms and has reported that the annual growth rate varies from 0.08 cm/year for small (4.0 cm) aneurysms to 0.16 cm/year for large (8.0 cm) aneurysms. The annual growth rates for patients suffering from chronic dissections are significantly higher, ranging from 0.24 cm/year for small aneurysms to 0.48 cm/year from large aneurysms.[12]

Therefore it has been suggested that preemptive surgical therapy be applied at a size of 5.5 cm for ascending and arch aneurysms and 6.5 cm for descending aortic aneurysms.[12,18] These surgical threshold criteria should be modified for patients with Marfan syndrome or connective tissue disease in which preemptive surgery is appropriate at 5.0 cm for ascending and arch aneurysms and 6.0 cm for descending aneurysms.[19] Furthermore, any patients with symptoms or rapid growth as seen on sequential CT scans should have surgical intervention in a timely manner.

Once the necessity for operative intervention has been determined, a full cardiac evaluation must be completed. This evaluation often involves stress testing and angiographic evaluation of coronary arteries as indicated. The basic premise of operative repair for aneurysms, regardless of the situation, is replacement with an interposition graft with or without cardiopulmonary bypass. Cardiac anesthetic management is essential with central venous pressure and arterial monitoring as well as large-volume intravenous infusion lines. Intraoperative transesophageal echocardiography is often very helpful for monitoring cardiac performance throughout the operation.

Ascending Aortic Aneurysm

Operations to replace an ascending aortic aneurysm are approached via a median sternotomy. All pathologic segments of the aorta are evaluated and replaced if abnormal, including the aortic valve, sinuses of Valsalva, the tubular portion of the ascending aorta, and the aortic arch. Cardiopulmonary bypass is established through atrial cannulation and either femoral arterial cannulation or axillary artery cannulation. The heart is vented via the pulmonary artery or left atrium. Axillary artery cannulation allows for selective antegrade cerebral perfusion during the replacement of the aorta.[20] Technically, the axillary artery can be accessed by making a 4 cm incision 2 cm below the clavicle. Carrying the incision down through the deltoid muscle, the axillary vein and artery can be dissected and isolated. A 6-mm Dacron graft is anastomosed onto the artery after the administration of 5000 units of heparin and then connected to the aortic cannula (Fig. 100.4). Myocardial protection is achieved by infusion of antegrade blood cardioplegia into the coronary ostia and retrograde cardioplegia into the coronary sinus accompanied by a cooling jacket for topic hypothermia.

If the aneurysm is contained to the root and does not involve the arch and head vessels the heart can be arrested with the cross clamp proximal to the innominate artery. At this time, the aortic valve is also assessed and if insufficient will have to be replaced prior to replacement of the aorta (Fig. 100.5). If however, the dilation of the aorta extends up into the arch, clamping the aorta is not possible and an "open distal anastomosis" is required. Hypothermic circulatory arrest is used for visceral protection, and cerebral protection attained using antegrade cerebral perfusion via the right axillary cannula and a balloon catheter in the left carotid artery. The distal anastomosis, using a monofilament suture, is then performed in a timely manner with only selective antegrade perfusion. The cross clamp is then reapplied to the graft and full cardiopulmonary bypass can then resume. The proximal anastomosis is then completed encompassing all diseased portions of the ascending aorta and the aortic root.

Aortic Arch Aneurysms

Operations involving replacement of the thoracic aortic arch are approached from a median sternotomy using hypothermic circulatory arrest with selective antegrade cerebral perfusion. The use of selective antegrade cerebral perfusion during operations of the aortic arch has reduced the risk of embolism and associated morbidity.[21] Separate arterial cannulation of

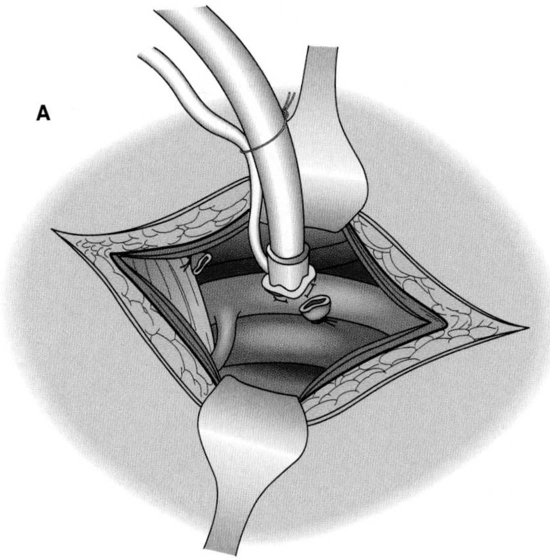

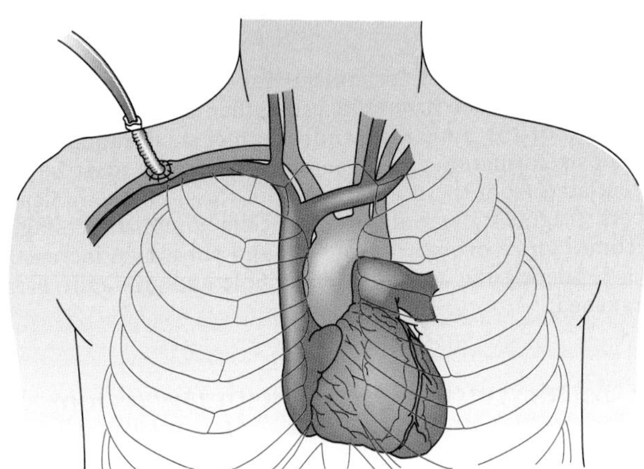

FIGURE 100.4 Cannulation of the right axillary artery with direct arterial cannulation (*A*) or with the use of a side graft (*B*). Once established, axillary artery cannulation can allow for antegrade cerebral perfusion throughout the aortic replacement procedure. (From Sabik JF, Nemeh H, Lytle BW, et al. Cannulation of the axillary artery with a side graft reduces morbidity. *Ann Thorac Surg.* 2004;77: 1315–1320.)

non-diseased arch vessels can be used as well to help ensure good cerebral perfusion. Replacement of the arch often involves reimplantation of arch vessels. This procedure can be accomplished as implanting an island of vessels or alternatively, using a trifurcated graft with individual vessel implantation excising diseased origins of the arch vessels (Fig. 100.6).[21,22] Reimplantation of individual arch vessels has been suggested to reduce the risk of embolization.[22]

Descending Aortic Aneurysms

Operative repair of the descending thoracic aneurysm is performed through a left posterolateral thoracotomy with a double lumen endotracheal tube in place for single lung ventilation. Prior to operation, most patients have lumbar drains placed in the operating room and have continuous cerebral spinal fluid (CSF) pressure monitoring during the case. CSF drains are placed to help reduce the incidence of paraparesis and paraplegia caused by spinal cord ischemia which can

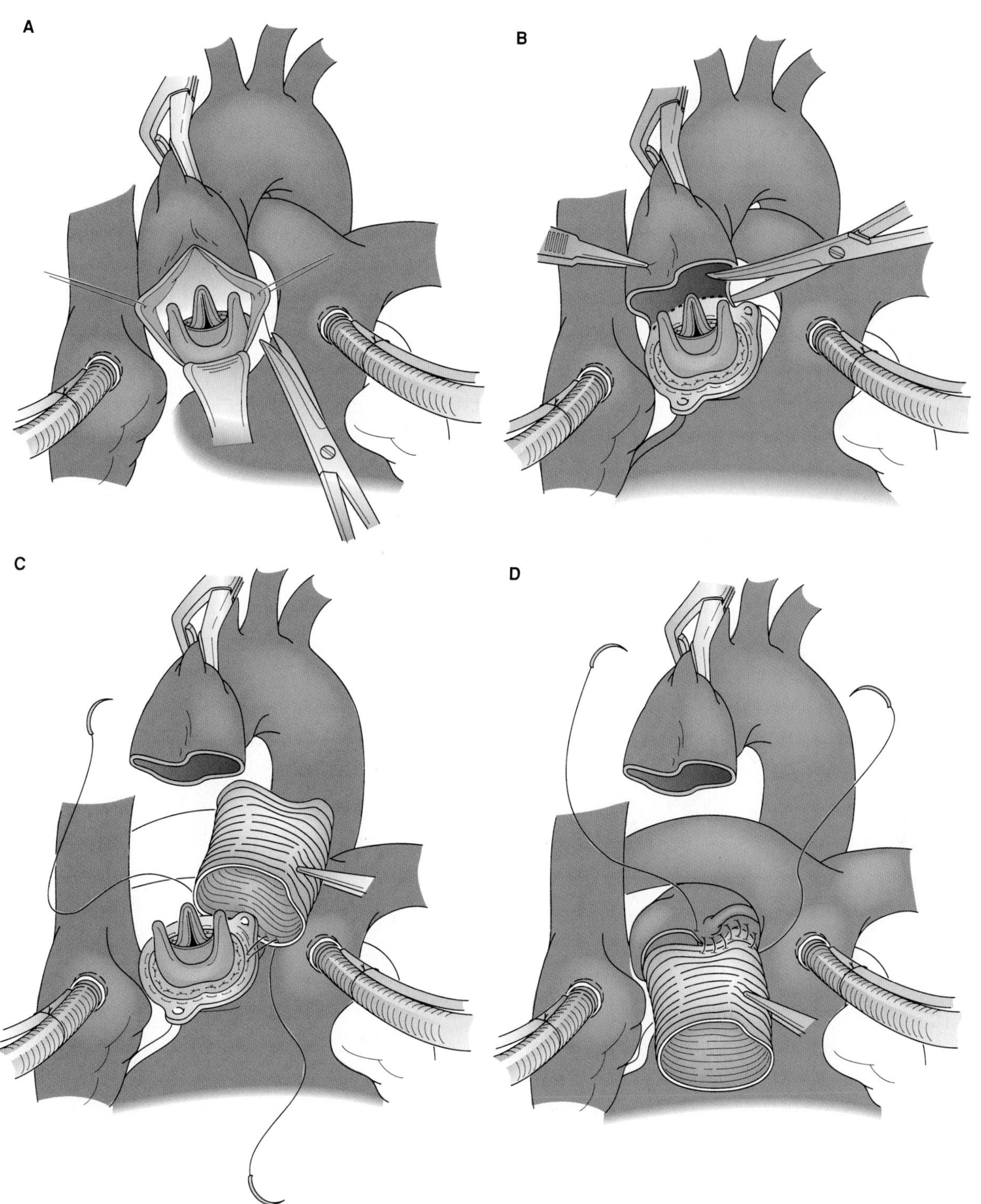

FIGURE 100.5 Operative repair of an ascending aortic aneurysm with distal clamping of the aorta. (*A*) Valve replacement, when indicated, is performed after cardioplegic arrest. (*B*) A full-thickness cuff of proximal aorta is developed and the aorta is transected just distal the coronary ostia. (*C*) The posterior suture line begins to the left of the left main coronary ostium and proceeds rightward, over the ostium. (*D*) Completion of the distal suture line is performed prior to release of the cross clamp. Careful measurement of the graft length ensures a tension-free distal anastomosis. (After Frist WH, Miller DC. Repair of ascending aortic aneurysms and dissections. *J Cardiac Surg*. 1986;1:33–52.)

accompany resection of aorta in the peridiaphragmatic area.[23] Pharmacologic agents are also used during the case, including barbiturates, naloxone, and steroids, to help reduce neurological injury. Two operative strategies may be employed. For patients in whom the transverse arch cannot be safely clamped, profound hypothermic circulatory arrest is used for both cardiac, and central and peripheral nervous system protection. If the arch can be safely clamped, as determined by inspection, palpation, TEE visualization, and epiaortic ultrasound, moderate hypothermia is employed with sequential aortic clamping, reimplantation of critical intercostals arteries, and the distal anastomosis constructed with peripheral

VASCULAR

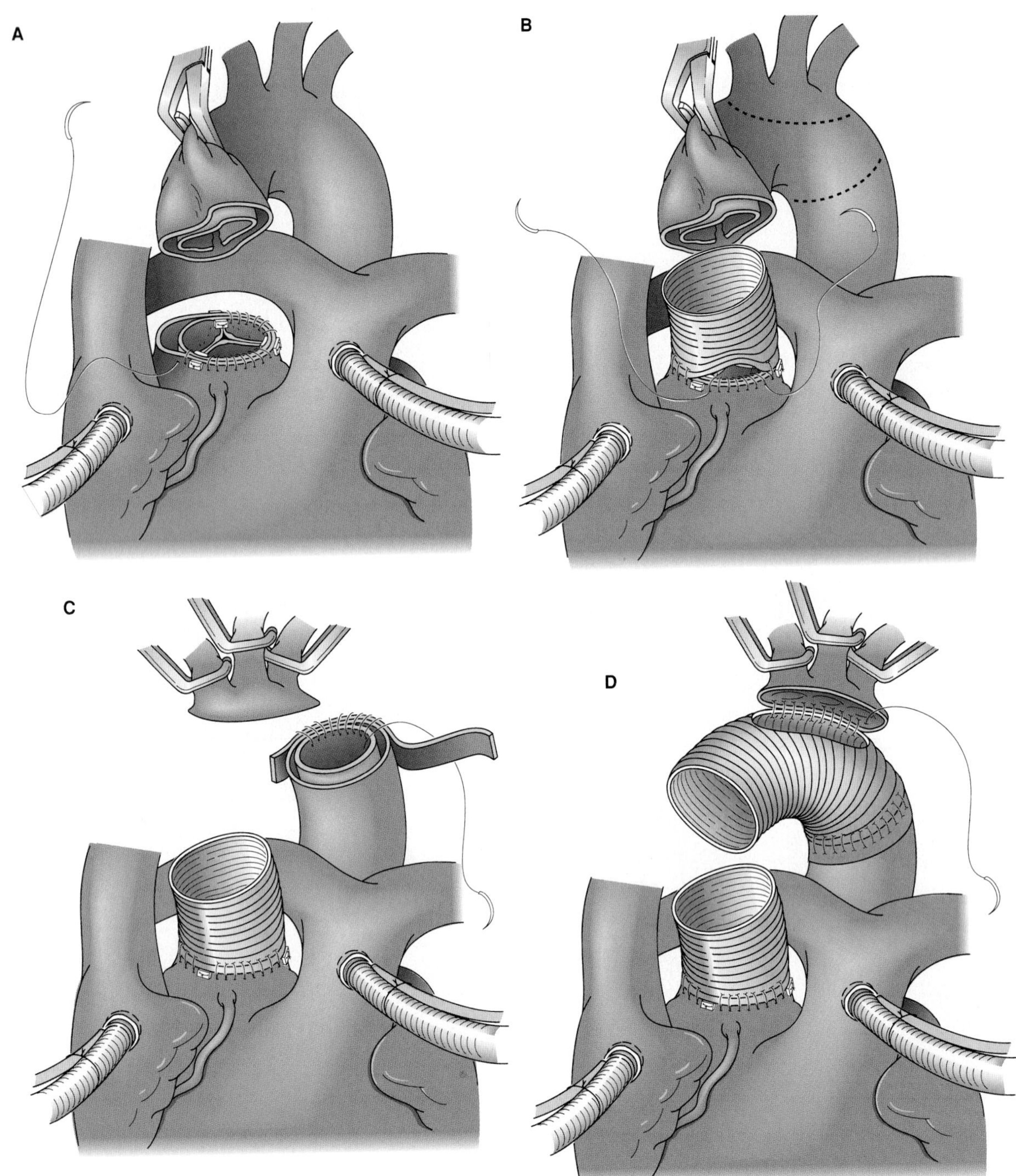

FIGURE 100.6 Repair of ascending and arch aneurysm with dissection. (*A*) The ascending aorta is repaired first with the cross-clamp in place. (*B*) While the ascending graft is placed proximally the patient is cooled. (C) During a period of hypothermic circulatory arrest (18°C), the distal aortic suture line is completed. (*D*) A button of aorta containing the cerebral vessels can be fashioned or alternatively, reanastomosed separately to a trifurcated graft. (*Continued*)

perfusion via the femoral artery (Fig. 100.7).[24,25,26] Other modalities used to help reduce paraparesis and paraplegia include monitoring of sensory evoked potentials and motor evoked potentials.[23] Epidurals for pain control are typically placed the night before the operation and are not used until the patient is extubated and moving all extremities.

The extent of the arch involvement helps to dictate the mode of perfusion used in these cases. If the arch is relatively spared and enough normal aorta can be identified distal to the left common carotid artery, a proximal clamp can be placed which allows for left heart bypass. In using left heart bypass, the left atrium and femoral artery are cannulated. A centrifugal pump, heparin-bonded shunts, and minimal heparinization can be used, which may be attractive in that the bleeding and inflammatory complications of fully heparinized cardiopulmonary bypass are avoided. However, full cardiopulmonary bypass with cannula-

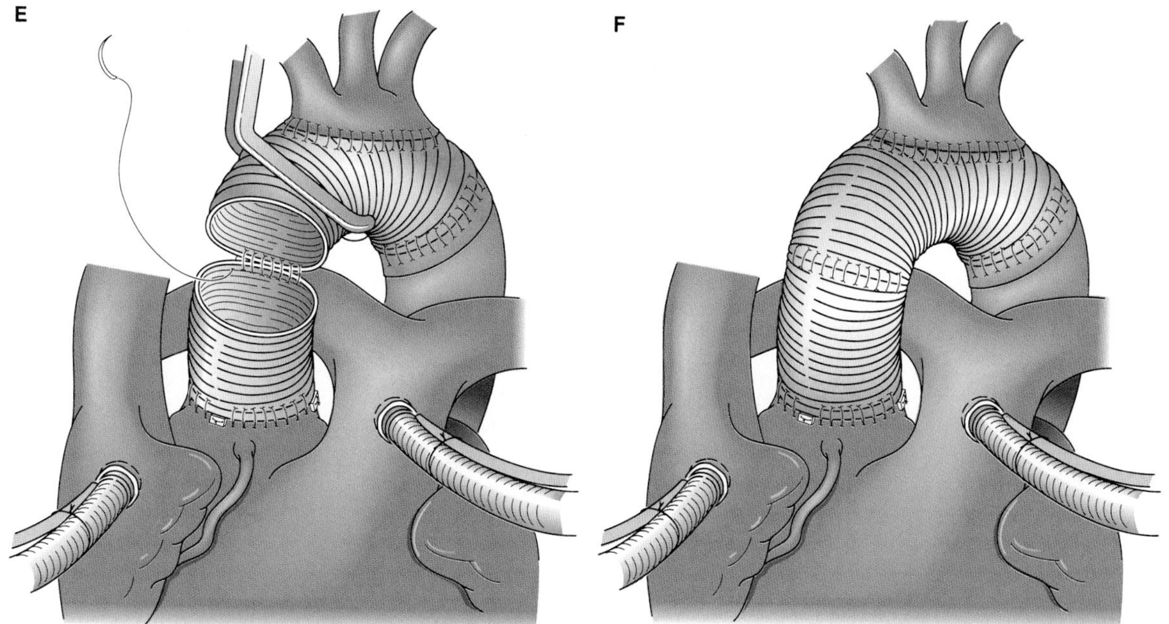

FIGURE 100.6 (*Continued*) (*E*) The cross-clamp is placed proximally, rewarming of the patient is instituted and the proximal and distal grafts are joined. (*F*) The repair as seen prior to decannulation. (After Griepp RB, Stinson EB, Hollingsworth JF, et al. Prosthetic replacement of the aortic arch. *J Thorac Cardiovasc Surg*. 1975;70:1051–1063.)

tion of the femoral artery and femoral vein and use of an oxygenator allows for good distal perfusion. Cooling of the patient is also possible so that if the arch is involved, profound circulatory arrest can be used to perform an open proximal anastomosis while continuing to perfuse distally. Debates concerning the appropriateness of partial versus full cardiopulmonary bypass continue, with all concerted efforts aimed at reducing the associated morbidity associated with these extensive aortic replacement surgeries.[27,28]

Once the extent of the aneurysm has been ascertained, the proximal and distal full-thickness cuffs are fashioned and an interposition graft is sutured in place with a monofilament suture. Lumbar artery pairs identified via thin slice computed tomographic aortography are also reimplanted into the interposition graft. This process can often take more than 30 minutes, which mandates cardiopulmonary bypass as opposed to the "clamp-and-sew" technique and its associated increased risk of paraplegia.[23] Once the affected portion of aorta has been successfully replaced, the patient can be appropriately warmed, and hemostasis assured. The deflated lung is reinflated and the patient is removed from cardiac support when hemodynamically permissible. The thoracic incision is closed by reapproximating the ribs and primary closure of the affected thoracic musculature.

Operative Outcomes

Despite of continued improvement in surgical technique and postoperative care, operative morbidity and mortality remains high for patients with thoracic aortic aneurysms. These patients, in addition to aneurysmal disease, often have associated comorbidities including renal dysfunction, chronic obstructive lung disease and ischemic heart disease. Preoperative assessment and management is paramount to facilitating good operative outcomes.

Multiple studies have demonstrated the adverse effect on survival of emergent versus elective operation. Hospital mortality rates for emergency thoracic aneurysm repair can be as high as 30%, whereas elective mortality rates approach zero.[29] In order to predict risk after elective repair of ascending and aortic arch aneurysms, the Mount Sinai group analyzed multiple variables.[30] They found that the presence of diabetes and manifestations of atherosclerosis emerge as extremely important risk factors for adverse outcome after ascending and arch surgery, displacing age.

Groups looking at descending thoracic aortic replacement outcomes have shown that patients who underwent atriofemoral or venofemoral bypass had favorable results compared with the "clamp-and-sew" techniques. Although renal failure was reduced by distal perfusion, rates of paraplegia and paraparesis remain dependent on the extent of repair and clamp time.[29,30] Nonetheless, use of combined adjuncts including CSF drainage reimplantation of intercostals arteries, and distal aortic perfusion have reduced the overall early neurologic deficits rate from 7% to a low of 0.9%.[30,31]

ENDOVASCULAR THERAPY

The main objective of surgical therapy for thoracic aortic aneurysms is to prevent aortic rupture. Surgical procedures on the thoracic aorta are fraught with significant mortality and morbidity, particularly surgery involving the descending thoracic aorta. In an effort to reduce associated complications, endovascular repair has been explored and developed over the past decade. Endovascular repair is attractive because stent-graft devices can be introduced from a peripheral site eliminating disabling laparotomies and thoracotomies, and aortic cross clamping with its associated physiologic perturbations. Parodi introduced the concept of balloon-expandable stents attached to the ends of vascular grafts for the repair of abdominal aortic aneurysms.[34] The initial endovascular approach at Stanford Medical Center was a combined effort between the division of interventional radiology and the department of cardiovascular surgery.[35,36] An Institutional Review Board approval was initially obtained for endovascular treatment of high risk patients with descending thoracic aneurysms who were deemed nonsurgical candidates.

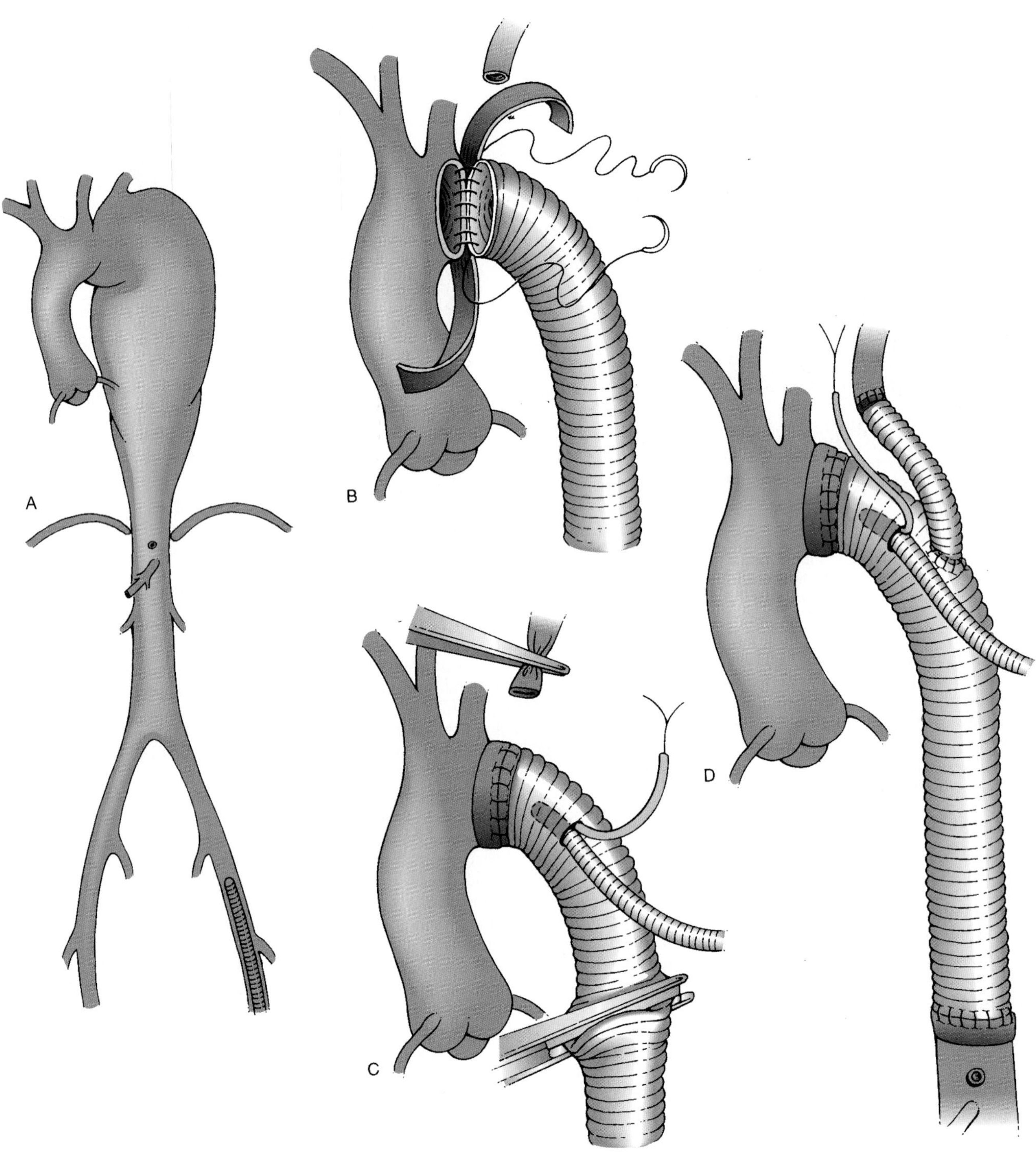

FIGURE 100.7 Distal arch and descending aortic aneurysm repair. (*A*) Femoral artery perfusion with hypothermic circulatory arrest. (*B*) Distal arch is replaced under hypothermic circulatory arrest. (C) The cross-clamp is reapplied and graft is recannulated to perfuse the head. (*D*) The subclavian artery can be reattached and the distal repair completed. (From Aneurysm of the aortic arch. In: Cohn LH, Edmunds LH, eds. *Cardiac surgery in the adult*, 2nd ed. New York: McGraw-Hill, 2003, p. 1163.)

Contrast-enhanced CT with three-dimensional reconstruction is the primary diagnostic tool for planning an endovascular intervention. Aneurysm size and extent can be evaluated as well as distance from critical side branches. Stent grafts are oversized by approximately 10% to 15% from the CT cross-sectional diameter in an effort to obtain sufficient radial force to achieve an endoseal and prevent stent graft migration. A minimum of 2 cm of normal aorta at the proximal and distal ends of the aneurysm must exist for adequate fixation. The anatomic features of descending thoracic aneurysms that make them ideal for endovascular repair is that they often arise distal to the subclavian artery and proximal to the celiac artery, allowing for adequate landing zones. Femoral or iliac arteries are normally required to be at least 8 mm in size to allow passage of a 24-Fr sheath. Because the endovascular devices are limited to 40 mm, the aorta must be 37 mm or less (Fig. 100.8).

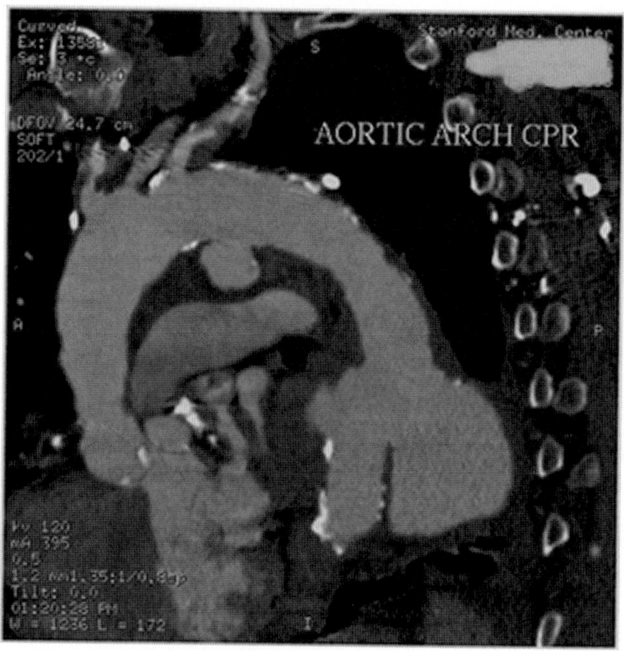

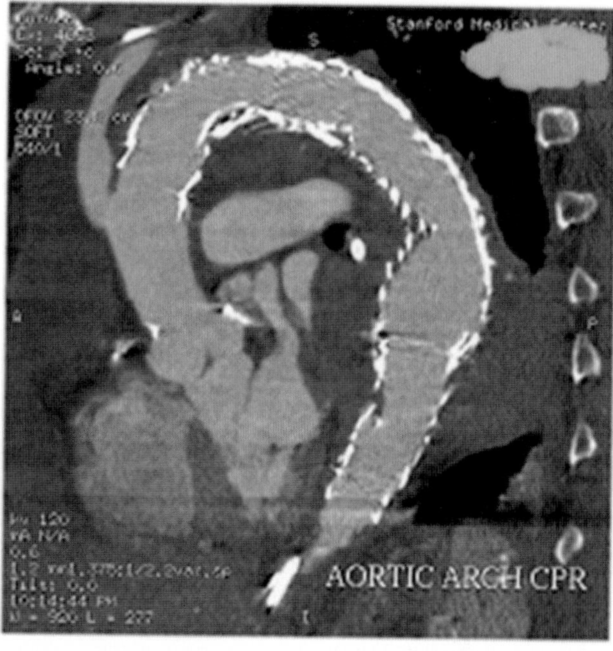

A B

FIGURE 100.8 (*A*) Thoracic angiogram of a thoracic aortic aneurysm suitable for stent graft repair. (*B*) Thoracic angiogram illustrating successful exclusion of the aneurysm sac with a endovascular stent graft.

In the first 103 Stanford patients, 60% of whom were absolute non-operative candidates, operative mortality was 10%. Embolic strokes occurred in seven patients, likely secondary to atheroemboli dislodged during guide wire or sheath manipulation within the aorta arch. Subsequent design modifications of the Gore (WL Gore & Associates Inc., Flagstaff, AZ) and Medtronic (Medtronic, Minneapolis, MN) devices have significantly increased catheter flexibility and improved stent graft delivery, eliminating the necessity for passing the introducer sheath into the aortic arch. Although spinal cord injury was considered a risk, because critical intercostals T8 to T12 would often be covered, paraplegia or paraparesis occurred in only three patients, and these patients had had previous or simultaneous abdominal aortic repairs.[35,36]

Since the first generation homemade stents, commercially produced second- and third-generation stent grafts have become more flexible, have a lower profile and increased conformability with greater ease of insertion and deployment. However, questions concerning device failure and migration and long-term results with respect to endoluminal exclusion remain unanswered. The most recent data from the Gore TAG multicenter trial show favorable implant characteristics, with decrease blood loss, intensive care unit stay, and total hospital stay compared to a nonrandomized cohort of open surgical patients.[37] Late follow-up to 2 years show a low rate of migration (3%), low appearance of late endoleaks (9%) with most managed with new endografts, and a 17% incidence of increase in size of the aneurysm sac. There has been one open conversion, and no late ruptures, prompting the conclusion that for anatomically suitable patients, stent graft repair produced similar long-term event-free survival, and was associated with less perioperative morbidity.

CONCLUSIONS

Aneurysmal disease of the thoracic aorta is a disease that affects both young and old. The morbidity and mortality associated with treatment of this disease is significant and therefore involves careful diagnosis, timely intervention and rigorous follow-up. Surgical intervention, when appropriate, requires careful planning and meticulous visceral protection in order to provide good outcomes. Endovascular techniques are being devised that may eventually provide appropriate treatment with less morbidity than that associated with open surgical treatment. The best outcomes for all patients who suffer from aneurysmal disease of the thoracic aorta are provided by a multidisciplinary approach with a firm understanding of the pathogenesis and natural history of this disease.

KEY POINTS

- **Aneurysmal disease of the thoracic aorta is a disease that affects both young and old.**
- **The morbidity and mortality associated with treatment of thoracic aortic aneurysms is significant and therefore involves careful diagnosis, timely intervention and rigorous follow-up.**
- **Surgical intervention, when appropriate, requires careful planning and meticulous visceral protection in order to provide good outcomes.**
- **Endovascular techniques are being devised that may eventually provide appropriate treatment with less morbidity than that associated with open surgical treatment.**
- **The best outcomes for all patients who suffer from aneurysmal disease of the thoracic aorta are provided by a multidisciplinary approach with a firm understanding of the pathogenesis and natural history of the disease.**

References

1. Swan H, Maaske C, Johnson M, et al. Arterial homografts, II: resection of thoracic aortic aneurysm using a stored human arterial transplant. *Arch Surg.* 1950;61:732–737.
2. Lam CR, Aram HH. Resection of a descending thoracic aorta for aneurysm: a report of the use of a homograft in a case and an experimental study. *Ann Surg.* 1951;134:743–752.

3. De Bakey ME, Cooley DA. Successful resection of aneurysm of thoracic aorta and replacement by graft. *JAMA* 1953;152:673–676.
4. Cooley DA, De Bakey ME. Resection of entire ascending aorta in fusiform aneurysm using cardiac bypass. *JAMA* 1956;162:1158–1159.
5. Svensjo S, Bengtsson H, Bergqvist D, et al. Thoracic and thoracoabdominal aortic aneurysm and dissection: an investigation based on autopsy. *Br J Surg*. 1996;83:68–71.
6. Coady MA, Rizzo JA, Goldstein LJ, et al. Natural history, pathogenesis, and etiology of thoracic aneurysms and dissections. *Cardiol Clin North Am*. 1999;17:615–635.
7. Kouchoukos NT, Dougenis D. Surgery of the thoracic aorta. *N Engl J Med*. 1997;336:1876–1888.
8. Nguyen BT. Computed tomography diagnosis of thoracic aortic aneurysm. *Semin Roentgenol*. 2001;36:309–324.
9. Pressler V, McNamara JJ. Thoracic aortic aneurysm: natural history and treatment. *J Thorac Cardiovasc Surg*. 1980;79:489–498.
10. Clouse WD, Hallett J, Schaff H, et al. Improved prognosis of thoracic aortic aneurysms: a population-based study. *JAMA* 1998;280:1926–1929.
11. Juvonen T, Ergin MA, Galla JD, et al. Prospective study of the natural history of thoracic aortic aneurysms. *Ann Thorac Surg*. 1997;63:1533–1545.
12. Coady MA, Rizzo JA, Elefteriades JA. Developing surgical intervention criteria for thoracic aortic aneurysms. *Cardiol Clin North Am*. 1999;17: 827–839.
13. Davies RR, Goldstein LJ, Coady MA, et al. Yearly rupture or dissection rates for thoracic aortic aneurysms: simple prediction based on size. *J Cardiovasc Surg*. 1997;113:476.
14. Perko MJ, Norgaard M, Herzog TM, et al. Unoperated aortic aneurysm: a survey of 170 patients. *Ann Thorac Surg*. 1995;59:1204–1209.
15. Griepp RB, Ergin A, Galla JD, et al. Natural history of descending thoracic and thoracoabdominal aneurysms. *Ann Thorac Surg*. 1999;67:1927–1930.
16. Williams JS, Graff JA, Uku JM, et al. Aortic injury in vehicular trauma. *Ann Thorac Surg*. 1994;57:726–730.
17. Razzouk AJ, Gundry SR, Wang N, et al. Repair of traumatic aortic rupture: a 25-year experience. *Arch Surg*. 2000;135:913–919.
18. Davies RR, Goldstein LJ, Coady MA, et al. Yearly rupture or dissection rates for thoracic aortic aneurysms: simple prediction based on size. *Ann Thorac Surg*. 2002;73:17. Coady MA, Rizzo JA, Hammond GL, et al. What is the appropriate size criterion for resection of thoracic aortic aneurysms? *J Thorac Cardiovasc Surg*. 1997;113:476–491.
19. Di Eusanio M, Schepens M, Morshuis W, et al. Brain protection using antegrade selective cerebral perfusion: a multicenter study. *Ann Thorac Surg*. 2003;76:1181–1189.
20. Strauch JT, Spielvogel D, Lauten A, et al. Technical advances in total aortic arch replacement. *Ann Thorac Surg*. 2004;77:581–590.
21. Spielvogel D, Mathur MN, Lansman SL, et al. Aortic arch reconstruction using a trifurcated graft. *Ann Thorac Surg*. 2003;75:1034–1036.
22. Gharagozloo F, Neville RF, Cox JL. Spinal cord protection during surgical procedures on the descending thoracic and thoracoabdominal aorta: a critical overview. *Semin Thorac Cardiovasc Surg*. 1998;10:73–86.
23. Rokkas CK, Kouchoukos NT. Profound hypothermia for spinal cord protection in operations on the descending thoracic and thoracoabdominal aorta. *Semin Thorac Cardiovasc Surg*. 1998;10:57–60.
24. Kouchoukos NT, Daily BB, Rokkas CK, et al. Hypothermic bypass and circulatory arrest for operations on the descending thoracic and thoracoabdominal aorta. *Ann Thorac Surg*. 1995;60:67–77.
25. Kouchoukos NT, Rokkas CK. Hypothermic Cardiopulmonary bypass for spinal cord protection: rationale and clinical results. *Ann Thorac Surg*. 1999;67:1940–1958.
26. Coselli JS, LeMaire SA, Conklin LD, et al. Left heart bypass during descending thoracic aortic aneurysm repair does not reduce the incidence of paraplegia. *Ann Thorac Surg*. 2004;77:1298–1303.
27. Coady MA, Mitchell RS. Femoro-femoral partial bypass in the treatment of thoracoabdominal aneurysms. *Semin Thorac Cardiovasc Surg*. 2003;15: 340–344.
28. Kawachi Y, Nakashima A, Kosuga T, et al. Comparative study of the natural history and operative outcome in patients 75 years and older with thoracic aortic aneurysm. *Circ J*. 2003;67:592–596.
29. Hagl C, Galla JD, Spielvogel D, et al. Diabetes and evidence of atherosclerosis are major risk factors for adverse outcome after elective thoracic aortic surgery. *J Thorac Cardiovasc Surg*. 2003;126:1005–1012.
30. Svensson LG, Crawford ES, Hees KR, et al. Variables predictive of outcome in 832 patients undergoing repairs of the descending thoracic aorta. *Chest* 1993;104:1248–1253.
31. Estrera AL, Rubenstein FS, Miller CC, et al. Descending thoracic aortic aneurysm: surgical approach and treatment using the adjuncts cerebrospinal fluid drainage and distal aortic perfusion. *Ann Thorac Surg*. 2001;72:481–486.
32. Safi HJ, Miller CC, Huynh TT, et al. Distal aortic perfusion and cerebrospinal fluid drainage for thoracoabdominal and descending thoracic aortic repair. *Ann Surg*. 2003;238:372–381.
33. Parodi JC, Palmaz JC, Barone HD. Transfemoral intraluminal graft implantation for abdominal aortic aneurysms. *Ann Vasc Surg*. 1991;5: 491–499.
34. Dake MD, Miller DC, Semba CP, et al. Transluminal placement of endovascular stent-grafts for the treatment of descending thoracic aortic aneurysm. *N Engl J Med*. 1994;331:1729–1734.
35. Mitchell RS, Miller DC, Dake MD, et al. Thoracic aortic aneurysm repair with an endovascular stent graft: the "first generation." *Ann Thoracic Surg*. 1999;67:1971–1980.
36. Makaroun MS, Dillavou ED, Kee ST, et al. Endovascular treatment of thoracic aortic aneurysms: Results of the phase II multicenter trial of the GORE TAG thoracic endoprosthesis. *J Vasc Surg*. 2005;41:1–9.

CHAPTER 101 ■ THORACOABDOMINAL AORTIC ANEURYSMS

HAZIM J. SAFI, TAM T. T. HUYNH, CHARLES C. MILLER III, ANTHONY L. ESTRERA, EYAL E. PORAT, AND ALI AZIZZADEH

Etheredge reported the first successful repair of a thoracoabdominal aortic aneurysm (TAAA) using a homograft tube, in 1955. A year later, DeBakey used a Dacron tube graft to replace the descending thoracic aorta and infrarenal abdominal aorta. Subsequently, Crawford introduced what became known as the *clamp-and-go technique,* encompassing three basic principles of aortic surgery: the inclusion technique, use of a Dacron tube graft conduit, and reimplantation of visceral and renal arteries. Initially, the operation to repair TAAA had to be performed with haste, to avoid extended periods of organ ischemia. TAAA surgery has since been transformed with the use of adjuncts that provide better organ protection and result in improved outcome; however, sudden fatal rupture of a TAAA remains a looming and unpredictable threat Although emergency repair of ruptured TAAA can save lives, the associated morbidity and mortality remain extremely high. Elective surgical repair of TAAA is the only effective treatment for eradicating the risk of aneurysm rupture and improving patient survival (Fig.101.1). This chapter provides a comprehensive approach to the diagnosis and management of TAAA as well as insight into the recent surgical results and advances in organ protection.

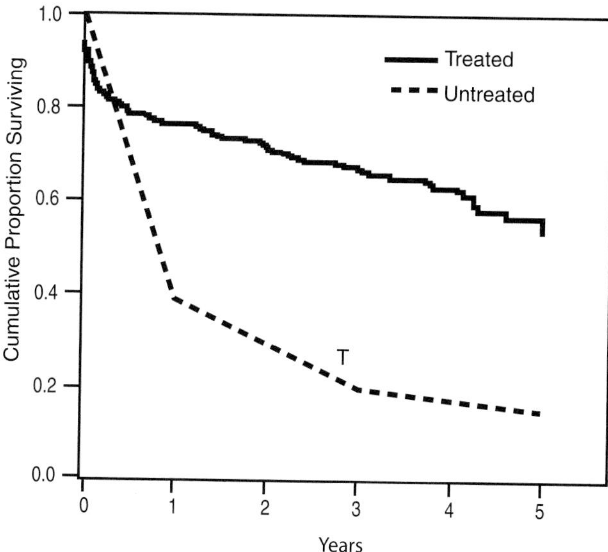

FIGURE 101.1 Thoracoabdominal aortic aneurysm: comparison of survival rates in untreated patients versus surgically treated patients.

EPIDEMIOLOGY

Abdominal aortic aneurysm remains the 13th leading cause of death in the United States. Improved imagining techniques, increasing mean age of the population, and overall heightened awareness, all contribute to an apparent increase in the prevalence of aortic aneurysms. However, the incidence of TAAA from population studies of the thoracic or abdominal aortic aneurysms can only be inferred. Infrarenal abdominal aortic aneurysms occur three to seven times more frequently than thoracic aortic aneurysms, but less than 1,000 TAAAs are repaired annually compared with approximately 50,000 infrarenal abdominal aortic aneurysms. The estimated prevalence of abdominal aortic aneurysms varies between 2.3% to 10.7% depending on the population studied and the size used to define an aneurysm.[1–3] The incidence of TAAAs is estimated to be 10.4 cases per 100,000 person-years.[4] The mean age of patients with a TAAA is between 59 and 69 years with a male-to-female predominance of between 2 and 4 to 1.[5]

Less than 40% of patients with untreated large TAAAs survive beyond 5 years, with most deaths caused by rupture.[5–8] TAAA studies have shown that rupture is more likely to occur when aneurysms exceed 5 cm in diameter and that the rate of rupture rises with increasing aneurysm size.[6, 9–12] The median size at which TAAAs rupture is around 7 cm.[13,14] Aneurysms equal to or greater than 8 cm have an 80% risk of rupture within 1 year of diagnosis.[15] The lifetime probability of rupture for any untreated aortic aneurysm is 75% to 80%, but the size at which the aneurysm will rupture and how long it will take to reach that point cannot be easily calculated. However, the average overall rate of growth for TAAAs is 0.10 to 0.42 cm per year with an exponential growth rate for aneurysms exceeding 5 cm in diameter.[9,14,16–18]

PATHOGENESIS

An aortic aneurysm is defined as a localized or diffuse dilatation that exceeds 50% of normal aortic diameter. Most TAAAs are degenerative, with an underlying pathology similar to the more frequently encountered infrarenal abdominal aortic aneurysm. Arteriosclerosis has long been implicated in the development of aortic aneurysm; however, arteriosclerosis primarily affects the intima and typically causes occlusive disease, whereas aneurysm disease usually involves the media and adventitia. Although the pathogenesis of arteriosclerotic occlusive disease and that of aneurysm disease have been shown to be distinct, the two conditions commonly occur together. Histologically, degenerative aortic aneurysms are characterized by thinning of the media with destruction of smooth muscle cells and elastin, infiltration of inflammatory cells, and neovascularization.[19–21] A chronic inflammatory infiltrate, comprised of macrophages as well as T and B lymphocytes, is consistently observed in the outer layer of aneurysm wall. The degree of vessel wall inflammation varies and the stimulus for cell migration remains unclear. These inflammatory cells, particularly macrophages, secrete proteases and elastases that can degrade the aortic wall; in turn, elastin degradation products may act as chemotactic agents for the influx of inflammatory cells.[19] The role of matrix metalloproteinases (MMPs), the most prominent type of elastases, in the development of aortic aneurysms has emerged from both clinical and experimental studies. Increased elastases MMP-2, MMP-9 and MMP-12 have been found in aortic aneurysmal aortic tissue.[19,22–24]

Familial clustering of aortic aneurysms is evident because up to 20% of patients with aneurysms have one or more first-degree relatives with the same affliction.[25–27] Marfan syndrome, characterized by skeletal, ocular, and cardiovascular abnormalities, is the most common inherited connective tissue disorder related to aortic aneurysm and dissection. Marfan syndrome occurs at a frequency of 1:5,000 worldwide. Aortic dilatation observed in Marfan patients has been linked to mutations in fibrillin-1. Other known genetic syndromes that predispose individuals to TAAA and dissection include Ehlers-Danlos syndrome, Turner syndrome, and polycystic kidney disease.[28–31] In addition, a familial syndrome in which multiple members have thoracic aortic aneurysm and dissection, with yet to be identified genetic abnormalities, has been reported in the literature.[32] In most of these families, the phenotype for TAAA and dissection is inherited in an autosomal dominant manner with marked variability in the age at onset of aortic disease and decreased penetrance.[32]

A small percentage of TAAAs are the result of infection (mycotic aneurysms) or trauma (pseudoaneurysms). An infected aneurysm frequently results from bacterial or septic emboli that seed an atherosclerotic aorta. Another mechanism is contiguous spread from empyema or adjacent infected lymph nodes. Although any organism can infect the aortic wall, *Salmonella, Haemophilus influenza, Staphylococcus, Mycobacterium tuberculosis* and *Treponema pallidum spirochetes* species are the most common.[33,34] Infected aortic aneurysms are usually saccular and thought to be at greater risk for rupture. Chronic traumatic pseudoaneurysm of the aorta related to previously unrecognized traumatic transection is also prone to rupture and surgical repair is warranted at the time of diagnosis.

Approximately 25% of TAAAs are associated with chronic aortic dissection. An estimated 20% to 40% of patients will develop aneurysms in the thoracoabdominal aorta within 2 to 5 years following acute aortic dissection.[35–37] Persistent patency of the false aortic lumen is reported to be a significant predictor of aneurysm formation.[38 39] However, the presence of chronic aortic dissection or patent false lumen has not been linked to a higher risk of aortic rupture.[40] Aneurysmal disease occurs in more than one part of the aorta in approximately 20% of cases. The so-called "mega" aorta is an "extensive" aortic aneurysm involving the ascending, transverse arch, and the entire thoracoabdominal aorta. Although associated factors include Marfan syndrome and chronic aortic dissection, the cause of extensive aortic aneurysm remains unknown.

CLINICAL MANIFESTATIONS

Aortic aneurysms can cause compressive symptoms although most do not until they reach a large size. The most frequent complaint is an ill-defined chronic back pain, although pain can also occur in the chest, flank or epigastrium. Acute changes in the characteristics and severity of pain can indicate sudden expansion or impending aortic rupture. Hoarseness, resulting from vocal cord paralysis caused by compression of the left recurrent laryngeal or vagus nerves, is frequently seen in patients with large aneurysms of the proximal descending thoracic aorta. Patients may also experience dyspnea related to compression of the tracheobronchial tree. A large aneurysm can exert pressure on the adjacent esophagus or duodenum, causing dysphagia or weight loss related to obstruction or early satiety. Direct erosion of the aneurysm into the adjacent tracheobronchial tree, esophagus, or both can cause exsanguination, presenting as massive hemoptysis or hematemesis, respectively. Less frequently, direct erosion can cause slow intermittent blood loss. Rarely, paraplegia or paraparesis can occur in patients with TAAA as a result of acute occlusion of the intercostal or spinal arteries. These findings are usually associated with acute aortic dissection, but can also result from thromboembolization. Although most aneurysms have a varying amount of mural thrombus, distal embolization causing acute mesenteric, renal or lower extremity ischemia is infrequent.

Rupture is thought to be the first clinical manifestation of a TAAA in as many as 10% to 20% of patients. The acute onset of severe chest, abdominal or back pain, associated with hypotension must raise the suspicion of a ruptured aneurysm. A pulsatile mass may be palpable in the abdomen, however, if the larger part of the TAAA is positioned deep within the thoracic cage, the aneurysm may not be apparent on physical examination. Although most ruptured aneurysms are fatal unless treated emergently, the ruptured arterial wall may temporarily seal for several hours or days before free rupture. In patients who are brought to the hospital alive, rupture is usually contained within the pleura or retroperitoneum. Free rupture is accompanied by severe hypotension and patients are more likely to die before reaching the hospital.

DIAGNOSTIC IMAGING

The diagnosis of TAAA can be confirmed by various imaging modalities. Currently, computed tomography angiography (CTA) is the imaging modality of choice in defining the extent of TAAA (Fig. 101.2) and for planning operative strategy. The diameter of the entire aorta, from the ascending segment to the bifurcation, can be accurately measured at various levels on axial images. The distinction between the false and true lumens in aortic dissection can be shown on CTA images. CTA can also detect thrombus or inflammatory changes in the aortic wall. Furthermore, the presence of free (or contained) fluid or blood can indicate free (or contained) rupture. Thin-slice CTA image acquisition can also identify patent intercostal arteries. Coronal reformatting or three-dimensional reconstruction of axial CT images provides additional views of TAAA (Fig. 101.3). Intravenous iodinated contrast can be omitted in patients with impaired renal function because it is not required for simple sizing of TAAA.

Magnetic resonance angiography (MRA) has become widely available and is frequently used as a screening test to detect diseases of the aorta and its branches. The principal advantage of MRA over CTA is that MRA does not require intravenous iodinated contrast and thus can be performed safely in patients with impaired renal function. Although MRA provides better contrast resolution, its spatial resolution is poorer than that of spiral CT. In addition, CT can better demonstrate aortic calcification and intramural thrombus compared with MRA. The time required to acquire images, claustrophobia, internal metallic hardware (e.g., pacemakers, orthopedic rods), and higher cost are other limiting factors of MRA.

Transesophageal echocardiography (TEE) can provide excellent imaging of the ascending and descending thoracic

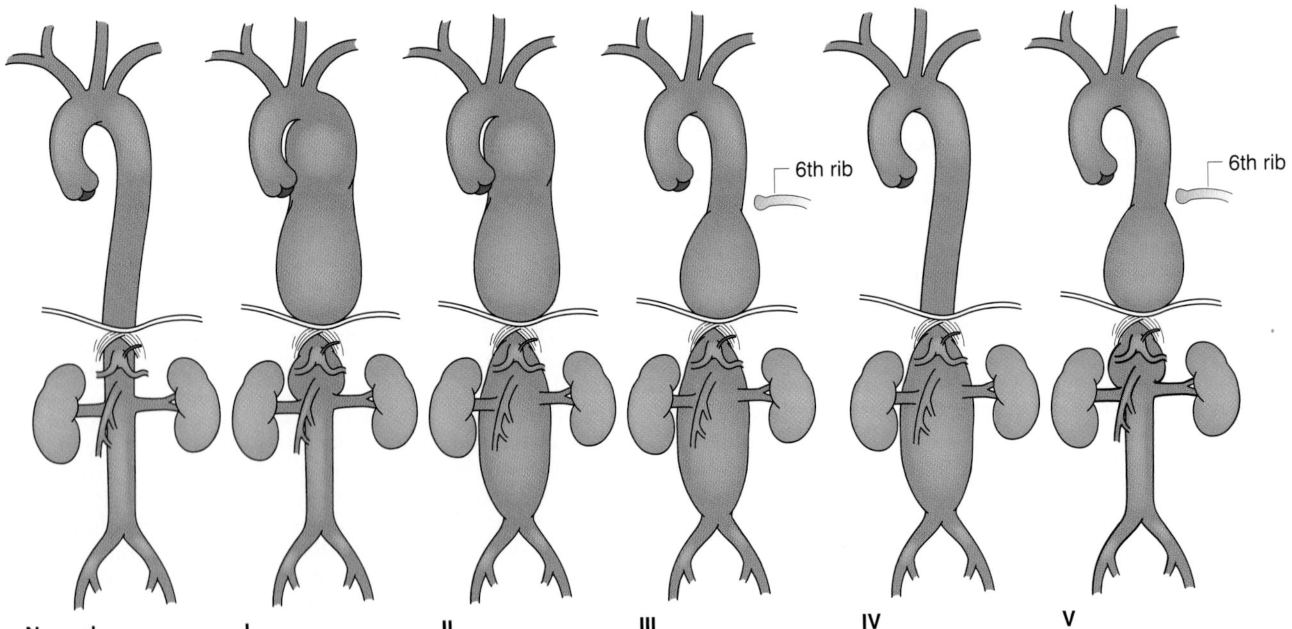

FIGURE 101.2 Thoracoabdominal aortic aneurysm classification. Extent I, distal to the left subclavian artery to above the renal arteries. Extent II, distal to the left subclavian artery to the below the renal arteries. Extent III, from the sixth intercostal space to below the renal arteries. Extent IV, the twelfth intercostal space to the iliac bifurcation (total abdominal aortic aneurysm). Extent V, below the sixth intercostal space to just above the renal arteries.

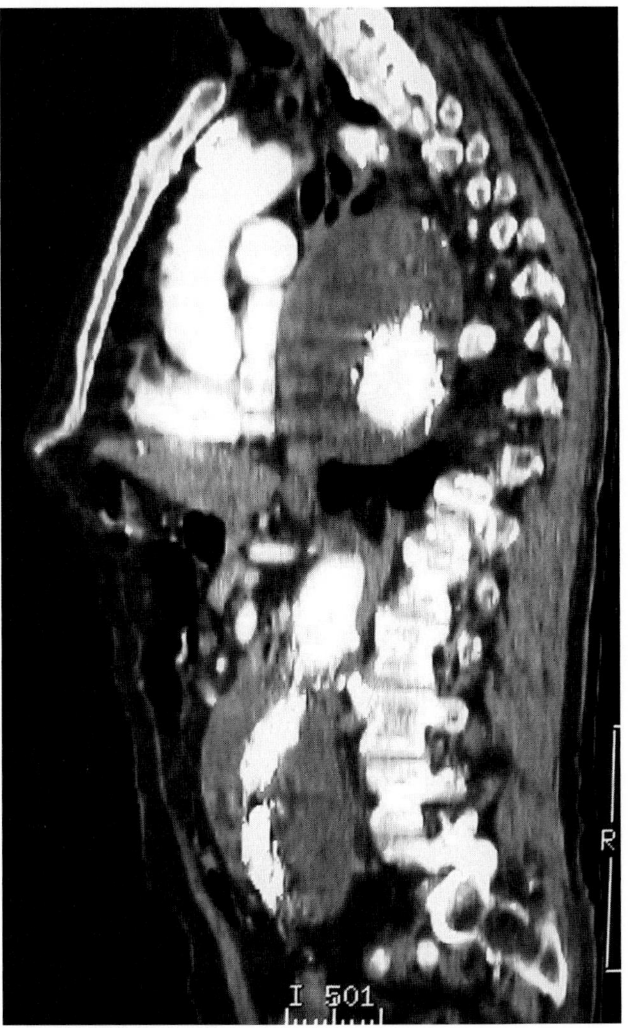

FIGURE 101.3 Sagittal computed tomography image of an extent II TAAA.

aorta. TEE can be performed at the bedside or in the operating room. TEE can be used in patients who are too unstable to be transported to the CT scanner. TEE can show aortic wall disease, differentiating arteriosclerotic plaque from intimal tear due to dissection. In the operating room, TEE can also be used to locate the optimal area for aortic cross-clamping and to assess cardiac function. However, TEE is an invasive modality and requires an experienced operator for optimal visualization and interpretation. Examination of the aorta by TEE is limited to the supra-diaphragmatic aorta because the ultrasound probe loses contact with the aorta as it crosses the gastroesophageal junction.

PREOPERATIVE EVALUATION

The initial consultation with the TAAA patient focuses on a thorough history and physical examination, primarily to detect comorbidities because there are generally few symptoms or physical signs related to the aneurysm itself. The extent of the TAAA is determined from imaging studies. Further evaluation of associated risk factors is performed, and consultation with a cardiologist, pulmonologist, or nephrologist is necessary to aid in the stratification of risks.

Ischemic heart disease is prevalent in this population and is the most common cause of death in patients with a TAAA. TEE provides an excellent estimate of cardiac function. Coronary artery revascularization, using either percutaneous intervention (balloon angioplasty or stent) or surgical bypass, may be indicated prior to TAAA surgery. For patients who must undergo coronary artery bypass prior to TAAA repair, the conduit of choice is the saphenous vein graft. The left internal mammary artery is avoided to obviate the possibility of cardiac ischemia should aortic cross-clamping proximal to the left subclavian artery be required during the TAAA repair. Moreover, the internal mammary artery may be an important collateral blood supply to the spinal cord and chest wall.

OPERATIVE TECHNIQUES

The patient is brought to the operating room and placed in the supine position on the operating table and prepared for surgery. The right radial artery is cannulated for continuous arterial pressure monitoring. General anesthesia is induced. Endotracheal intubation is established using a double lumen tube for selective one-lung ventilation during surgery. A sheath is inserted in the internal jugular vein, and a pulmonary balloon-tipped catheter is floated into the pulmonary artery for continuous monitoring of the central venous and pulmonary artery pressures. Large-bore central and peripheral venous lines are established for fluid and blood replacement therapy. Temperature probes are placed in the patient's nasopharynx, rectum, or bladder. Electrodes are attached to

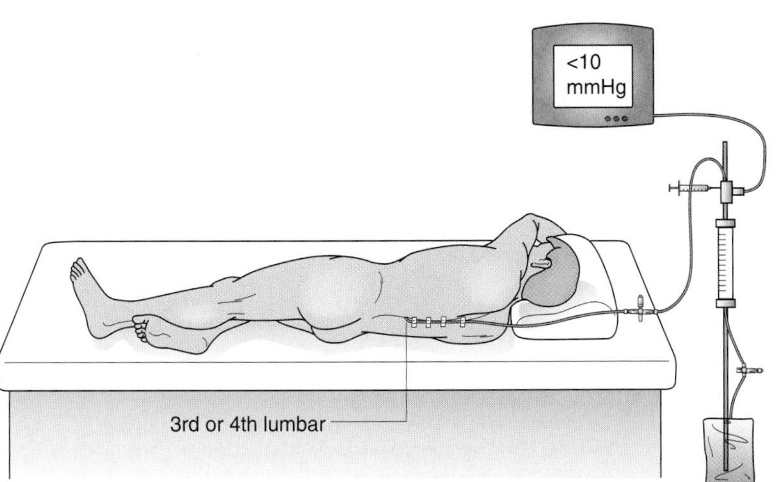

FIGURE 101.4 Placement of the lumbar catheter in the third or fourth lumbar space to provide cerebrospinal fluid drainage and pressure monitoring.

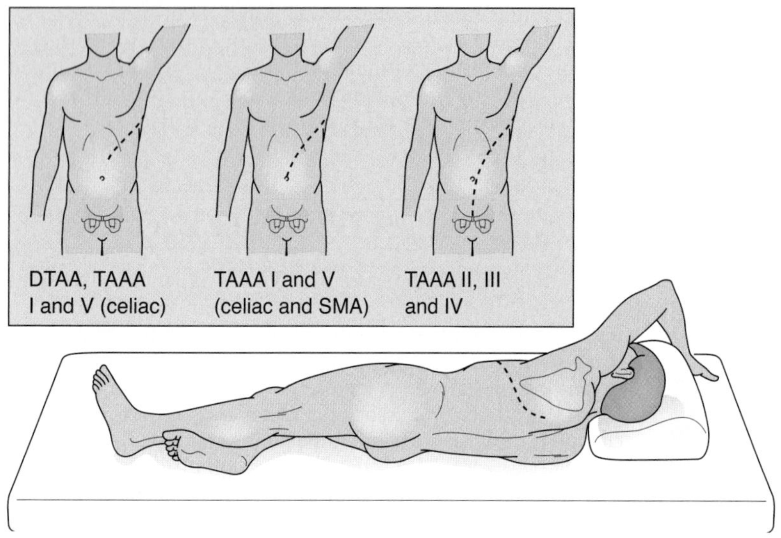

FIGURE 101.5 Tailoring of thoracoabdominal incisions for aneurysm extent. DTAA, descending thoracic aortic aneurysms; TAAA, thoracoabdominal aortic aneurysm; SMA, small mesenteric artery.

the scalp for electroencephalography and along the spinal cord for somatosensory evoked potential to assess the central nervous system and spinal cord function, respectively. The patient is then positioned on the right side with the hips and knees flexed to open the intervertebral spaces. A lumbar catheter is placed in the third or fourth lumbar space to provide cerebrospinal fluid (CSF) pressure monitoring and drainage (Fig. 101.4). The CSF pressure is kept at 10 mm Hg or less by gravity drainage of CSF fluid throughout the procedure. The patient is then repositioned in the right lateral decubitus position with the hips slightly turned to allow access to both groins. The operative field is scrubbed using standard aseptic solution and draped.

The incision is tailored to complement the extent of the aneurysm (Fig. 101.5). The full thoracoabdominal incision begins posteriorly between the tip of the scapula and the spinous process, curving along the sixth intercostal space to the costal cartilage, then obliquely to the umbilicus, and finally in the midline to above the symphysis pubis. The latissimus dorsi muscle is divided and the insertion of the serratus anterior muscle is mobilized. The left lung is deflated and the left thoracic cavity is entered. Resection of the sixth rib facilitates exposure and is routinely performed for all TAAA, except extent IV. Usually, a full thoracoabdominal exploration is necessary for extent II, III, and IV TAAA. A modified thoracoabdominal incision begins similar to the full thoracoabdominal incision, but ends at the costal cartilage or above the umbilicus. The modified thoracoabdominal incision provides excellent exposure for surgery involving the descending thoracic aorta, extent I, and extent V TAAA when the aneurysm ends above the superior mesenteric artery. The thoracoabdominal incision is extended to the level of the umbilicus, for extent I and V TAAAs that involve the superior mesenteric artery. A self-retaining retractor is placed firmly on the edges of the incision to maintain full thoracic and abdominal exposure during the procedure.

The dissection begins at the level of the hilum of the lung cephalad to the proximal descending thoracic aorta. The ligamentum arteriosum is identified and transected, taking care to avoid injury to the left recurrent laryngeal nerve. The extent of the distal abdominal aneurysm is assessed. The muscular portion of the diaphragm only is divided and the left phrenic nerve preserved (Fig. 101.6). A retroperitoneal plane is then developed, mobilizing the spleen, bowel loops, and left kidney to the right side of the abdominal aorta (medial visceral rotation). To prepare for distal aortic perfusion, the patient is anticoagulated using intravenous heparin (1 mg/kg body weight). The pericardium is opened posterior to the left phrenic nerve to allow direct visualization of the pulmonary veins and left atrium. The left atrium is cannulated through the left inferior pulmonary vein or atrial appendage. A centrifugal pump with an in-line heat exchanger is attached to the left atrial cannula and the arterial inflow is established through the left common

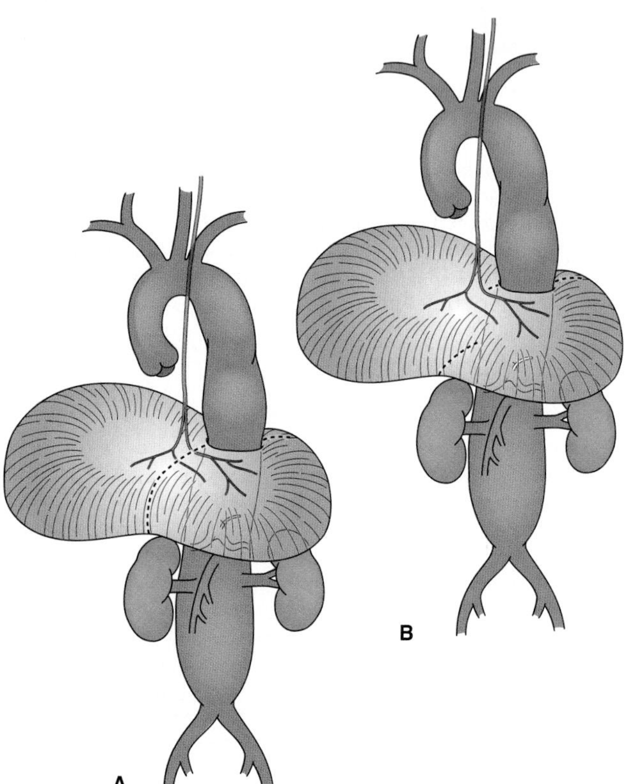

FIGURE 101.6 In previous surgical practice, the diaphragm was divided (*A*); currently only the muscular portion of the diaphragm is cut (*B*).

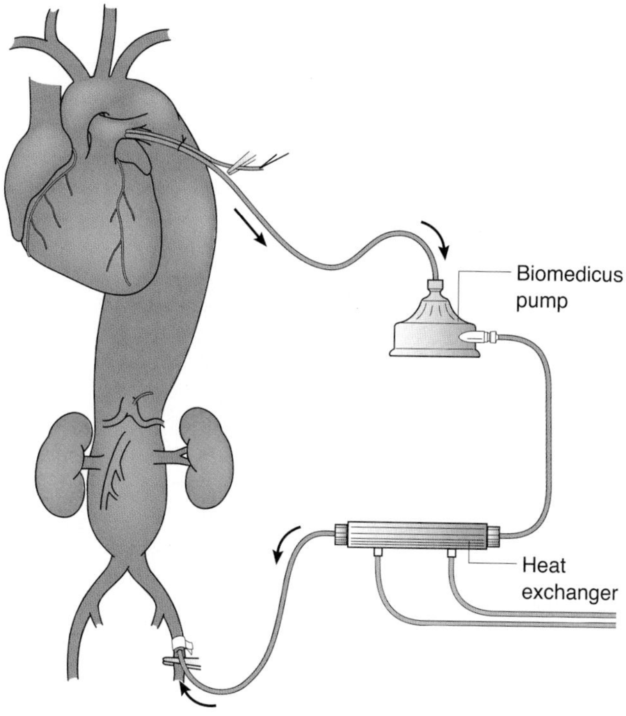

FIGURE 101.7 Distal aortic perfusion from the left inferior pulmonary vein to the left common femoral artery.

femoral artery, or the descending thoracic aorta, if the femoral artery is not accessible. Distal aortic perfusion is begun (Fig. 101.7).

Padded clamps are applied onto the proximal descending thoracic aorta just distal to the left subclavian artery and the mid-thoracic aorta. When the proximal extent of the aneurysm is too close to the left subclavian artery, the aorta between the left common and left subclavian arteries is clamped. The left subclavian artery is clamped separately. Because of the danger of graft-esophageal fistula, the inclusion technique for the proximal anastomosis is no longer used. Instead, the aorta is transected to separate it from the underlying esophagus (Fig. 101.8A). A woven Dacron graft impregnated with collagen or gelatin for replacement is preferred. The graft is sutured in an end-to-end fashion to the descending thoracic aorta, using a running 3-0 or 2-0 monofilament polypropylene suture. The anastomosis is checked for bleeding. Pledgeted polypropylene sutures for reinforcement are placed, if necessary. Sequential clamping is used for all TAAAs. After completion of the proximal anastomosis, the mid-descending aortic clamp is moved distally onto the abdominal aorta at the celiac axis to accommodate intercostal reattachment. Reattachment of patent, lower intercostal arteries (T8 to T12) is performed routinely, except in cases of occluded arteries, heavily calcified aorta, or acute aortic dissection. After completion of intercostal reattachment, the proximal clamp is released from the aorta and reapplied on the aortic graft beyond the intercostal patch, restoring pulsatile flow to the reattached intercostal arteries (Fig. 101.8B). The distal clamp is moved onto the infrarenal aorta, the abdominal aorta is opened, and the graft is passed through the aortic hiatus. The celiac, superior mesenteric, and renal arteries are identified and perfused using 9- or 12-Fr balloon-tipped catheters, depending on the size of the ostia (Fig 101.8C). The delivery of cold perfusate (4°C) to the viscera depends on the proximal aortic pressure, which is maintained between 300 and 600 mL/min. Renal temperature is directly monitored and kept at approximately 15°C. The visceral vessels are usually reattached using the inclusion technique. On completion of this anastomosis, the proximal clamp is moved beyond the visceral patch, restoring pulsatile flow to the viscera and kidneys (Fig. 101.8D). The final graft anastomosis is then completed at the aortic bifurcation. In most cases an island patch accommodates reattachment of the celiac, superior mesenteric, and both renal arteries. If the right or left renal artery is located at too great a distance from other arteries, its reattachment usually requires a separate interposition bypass graft. A visceral patch is no longer used for Marfan patients because of the high incidence of recurrent patch aneurysms in such cases. Instead, a woven Dacron graft is used with side-arm grafts of 10 mm and 12 mm for separate attachment of the celiac, superior mesenteric and the left and right renal arteries.

The patient is weaned from partial bypass once the core body or nasopharyngeal temperatures reaches 36°C to 37°C. Protamine is administered (1 mg/1 mg heparin), and the atrial and femoral cannulae are removed. Once hemostasis is achieved, two or sometimes three 36-Fr chest tubes are placed in the pleural cavity for drainage. The diaphragm is reapproximated using running 1-0 polypropylene suture. The left lung is reinflated. Closure of the incision is done in a standard fashion. The patient is placed in the supine position, and a single lumen endotracheal tube is exchanged for the double lumen tube. If the vocal cords are swollen, the double lumen tube is kept in place until the swelling resolves. The patient is then transferred to the intensive care unit (ICU). Figure 101.9 shows an extent II TAAA before and after surgery.

Elephant Trunk Technique for Extensive Aortic Aneurysms

Single stage repair of extensive aneurysms involving the ascending, arch, and thoracoabdominal aorta greatly increases operative risks. The patient undergoes a lengthy procedure that requires multiple incisions, a daunting array of protective surgical adjuncts, protracted clamp times, and considerable blood loss. Staged repair is a practical solution. Prior to the introduction of the elephant trunk technique by Borst in 1983, staged repair was fraught with complications, particularly excessive bleeding from the pulmonary artery and thoracic aorta in the second stage repair of the thoracic or thoracoabdominal aorta. The elephant trunk technique resolves this problem because it allows the surgeon to avoid surgical manipulation and cross-clamping the proximal native descending thoracic aorta in the second stage.

The first stage of the elephant trunk technique is performed, in a similar fashion to standard surgery of the ascending aorta and transverse arch, with the exception that an inverted distal graft is inserted (Fig. 101.10A). The folded edge of the inverted graft is sutured to the descending thoracic aorta just distal to the left subclavian artery. When the distal anastomosis is completed, the inner portion of the graft is retrieved. A side hole is made in the graft, and the aortic island containing the great vessels is reimplanted. The proximal anastomosis to the ascending aorta is completed, and the distal portion of the graft, or "elephant trunk," is left dangling in the proximal descending aorta. In the first stage, cardiopulmonary bypass, profound hypothermia, circulatory arrest, and retrograde cerebral perfusion provide protection to the brain and guard against stroke.

The second stage of the elephant trunk technique is much like standard TAAA repair, using the adjuncts distal aortic perfusion and CSF drainage. After initiation of the pump, the

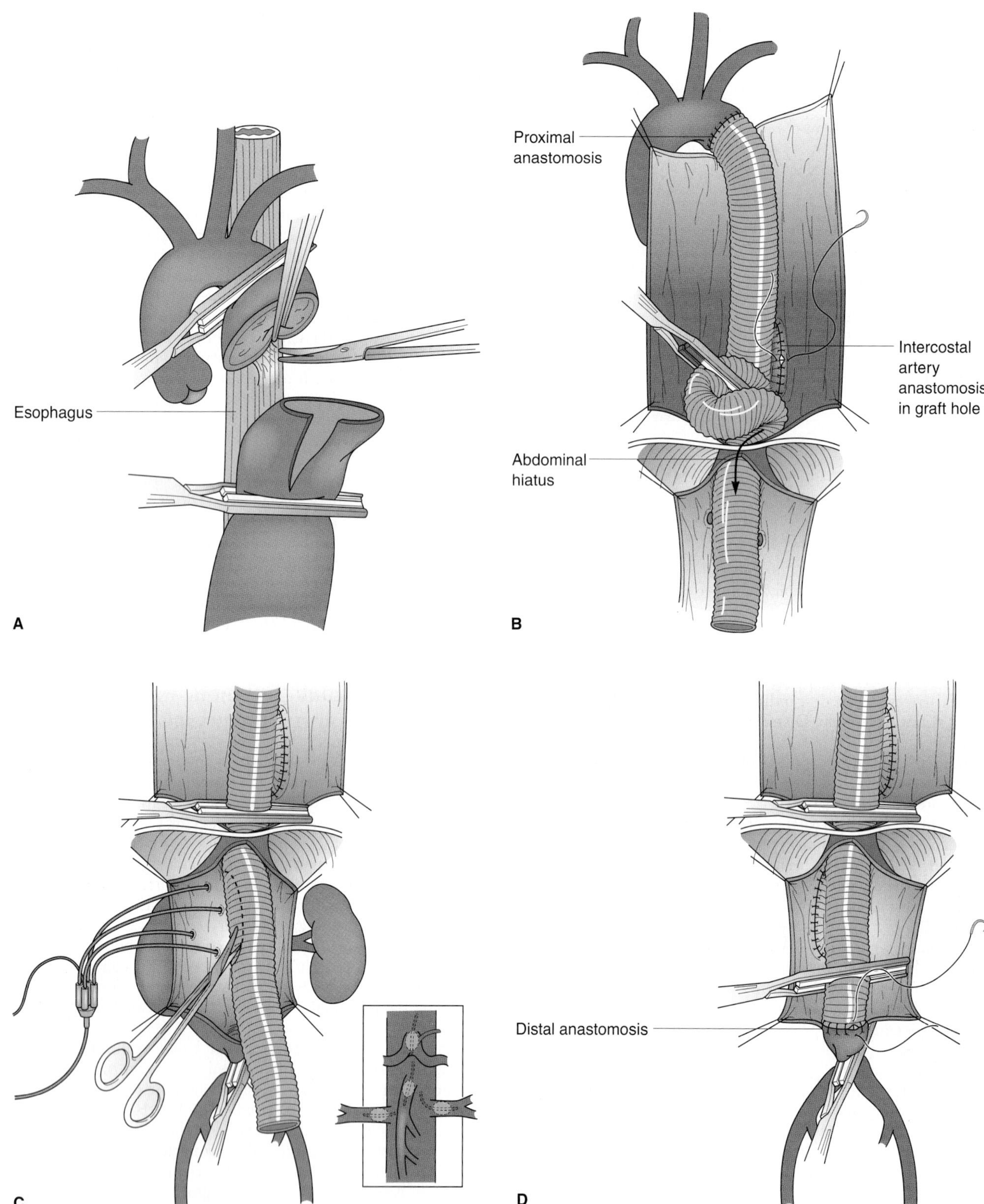

FIGURE 101.8 Sequential clamping and graft replacement. Padded clamps are placed on the proximal and mid-distal descending thoracic aorta. (*A*) The proximal part of the aneurysm is opened. The aortic neck is completely transected and separated from the esophagus. The proximal anastomosis is fashioned. Subsequently, the patent lower intercostal arteries are reattached via an elliptical hole in the graft. (*B*) The proximal clamp is then moved onto the graft to restore pulsatile flow to the intercostal arteries, and the graft is pulled through the hiatus into the abdomen. The distal clamp is reapplied onto the infrarenal aorta. The remaining of the aneurysm is opened. Balloon-tipped catheters are inserted into the celiac, superior mesenteric, and renal arteries to permit perfusion. (*C*) An elliptical hole is made in the graft for reimplantation of the visceral and renal arteries. (*D*) Pulsatile flow is then restored to the visceral and renal arteries, and the distal anastomosis is completed.

distal clamp is applied at the mid-descending thoracic aorta. The proximal third of the descending thoracic aorta is opened without a proximal clamp. The elephant trunk portion of the graft, inserted in the descending thoracic aorta during stage 1, is grasped quickly and clamped (Fig. 101.10B and C). The new graft is sutured to the "elephant trunk" to replace the remaining aneurysm.

POSTOPERATIVE MANAGEMENT

In the ICU, the patient's hemodynamic status is monitored very closely. The patient is awakened as quickly as possible to check neurologic status. However, most patients are kept on mechanical ventilation the first postoperative night. Blood loss is liberally replaced using banked blood products. The patient's mean arterial pressure is maintained between 90 and 100 mm Hg to ensure good organ perfusion, particularly to the spinal cord. CSF pressure is continuously monitored. Approximately 10 to 15 mL of CSF is drained hourly to keep CSF pressure at 10 mm Hg or less. Ideally, the patient is weaned off the ventilator on the first postoperative day. Oral diet is resumed when the patient is extubated and has bowel sounds. If the patient requires longer mechanical ventilation, then a nasoduodenal feeding tube is placed and enteral feeding begins on the second or third postoperative day, when bowel activity returns. Some patients may develop postoperative ileus and require total parenteral nutrition. After the patient recovers from anesthesia and is moving all extremities, potential delayed neurologic deficit is monitored. Warning signs for delayed neurologic deficit are unstable arterial blood pressure, hypoxemia, low hemoglobin (<10 g/dL), or increased CSF pressure (>15 mm Hg). CSF drainage is discontinued on the third postoperative day. The length of stay in the ICU is about 3 or 4 days, depending on the neurologic and pulmonary status of the patient. The patient is subsequently transferred to the telemetry floor. Physical therapy is initiated in the ICU and continued throughout the patient's hospital stay. The median length of stay for patients following TAAA is 15 days.[41] Annual CT scan follow-up is recommended to screen for the development of new aneurysm or graft-related pseudoaneurysm formation. The frequency of follow-up visits or CT scans varies based on TAAA etiology. For example, patients with remaining unoperated aortic dissection, connective tissue disorders (Marfan syndrome), a family history of aortic aneurysm, or concurrent aneurysms may need closer surveillance.

SURGICAL OUTCOMES

Mortality rates for patients undergoing TAAA and descending thoracic aortic aneurysm repair range between 4% and 21%.[10,42–44] The variable success rates are partly related to

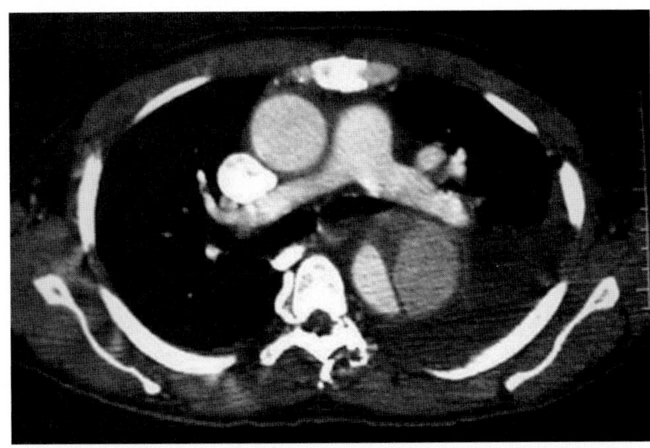
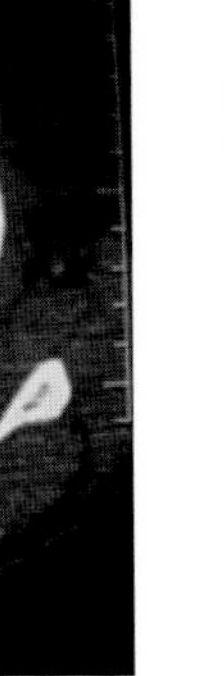
A

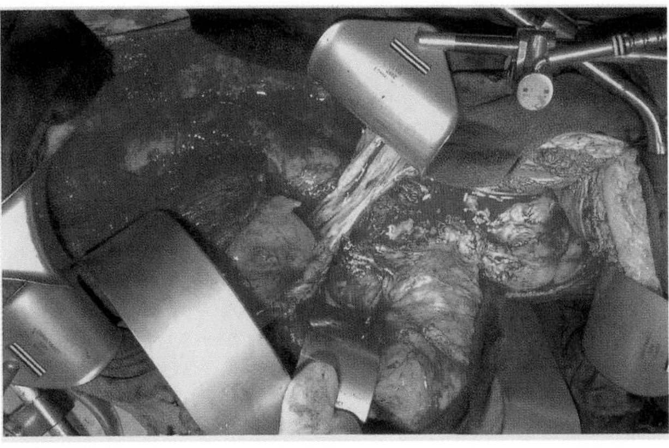
B

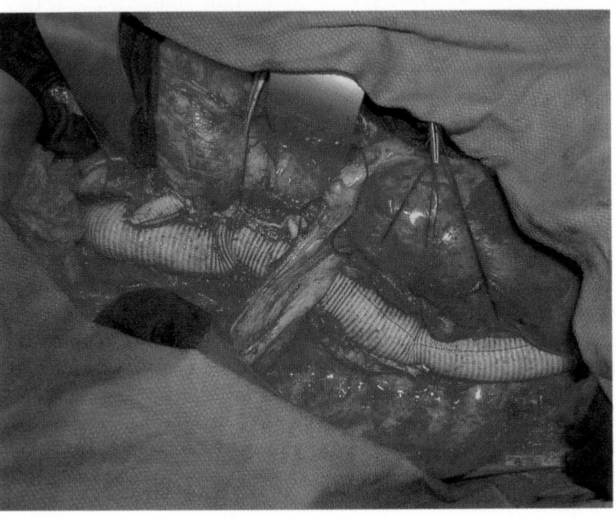
C

FIGURE 101.9 Example of TAAA extent II repair. (*A*) Preoperative computed tomography showing proximal part of the aneurysm with chronic dissection. Intraoperative photograph of the thoracoabdominal aortic aneurysm before (*B*) and after (*C*) graft replacement. The proximal anastomosis was just distal to the left subclavian artery; the patent lower intercostal arteries were reattached; the celiac, superior mesenteric and right renal arteries were reimplanted together; the left renal artery was reimplanted via an interposition bypass graft; and the distal anastomosis was to the aorta just above the bifurcation. The separate left renal artery graft was necessary because it was located far away from the remaining visceral arteries.

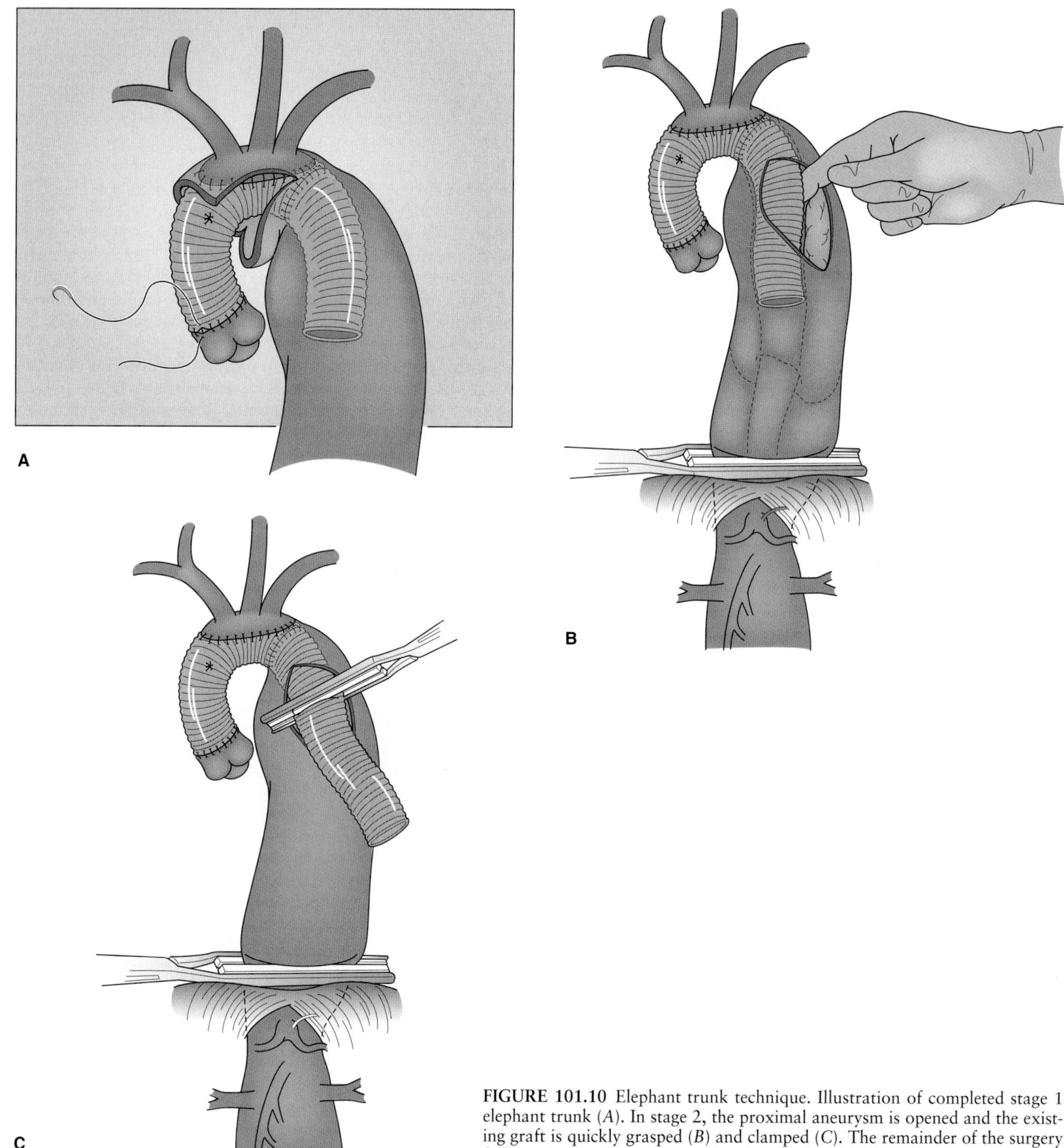

FIGURE 101.10 Elephant trunk technique. Illustration of completed stage 1 elephant trunk (*A*). In stage 2, the proximal aneurysm is opened and the existing graft is quickly grasped (*B*) and clamped (*C*). The remainder of the surgery follows the standard technique for thoracoabdominal aortic aneurysm.

the heterogeneity of the patient population and to the expertise of the treating team. In the cumulative experience of the authors of this chapter (from January 1991 to February 2003), 1,004 patients underwent TAAA and descending thoracic aortic aneurysm repair.[45] Of these patients, 63% were men with a median age of 65 years (range, 8 to 89 years). Approximately 7% of patients had emergency surgery for free or contained rupture of TAAA or descending thoracic aortic aneurysm. Currently, the 30-day mortality rate is approximately 14%. Using multivariable analysis, advanced age, renal failure, and paraplegia have been identified as important risk factors for mortality.[46] Patients age 79 years or older with at least one of three factors—emergency presentation, a history of diabetes, or congestive heart failure—have been identified as a particularly high-risk group with 30-day mortality as high as 50%.[41] Overall, 70% of patients recover from TAAA without significant postoperative complications.[47] The 5-year survival for patients after TAAA is between 60% and 70%. Recently, negative predictors for long-term survival were found to include advanced age, extent II TAAA, renal failure, emergency surgery, cerebrovascular disease and active tobacco smoking.[45]

Neurologic Outcome

Postoperative neurologic deficit remains the most devastating complication following TAAA repair. When the descending thoracic aorta is cross-clamped, the spinal cord is quickly rendered ischemic because of the immediate interruption of perfusion to the spinal cord and consequent increased CSF pressure. Therefore, in the "cross-clamp-and-go" era the single most important predictor of neurologic deficit was the length of clamp time. The rationale for the present method of protection is to increase the spinal cord perfusion pressure directly with distal aortic perfusion, and indirectly by reducing CSF pressure to 10 mm Hg or less. Animal and human studies have confirmed that CSF drainage reduces CSF pressure and can improve spinal cord perfusion during aortic cross clamping.[48–50] Since 1991, distal aortic perfusion and CSF drainage have been utilized as adjuncts for all patients undergoing elective repair of TAAA. Overall, in a total of 1004 patients, immediate postoperative neurologic deficit (paraplegia or paraparesis that occurs as the patient awakens from anesthesia) occurred in 2.4% of patients operated with adjuncts, and in 6.8% patients without adjuncts.[45] This combination of adjuncts has reduced the cumulative rate of neurologic deficits to 0.9% for descending thoracic aortic repair and to 3.3% for thoracoabdominal aortic repair.[45] Repair of the most extensive TAAAs, (extent II) has long been known to result in the highest incidence of neurologic deficits. In the cross-clamp and go era, this incidence was as high as 30% to 40%.[43] With the use of adjuncts, the rate of immediate neurologic deficits for extent II TAAA has been reduced to 6.6%.[45] (Fig. 101.11). In addition to the extent of the aneurysm, other perioperative risk factors for immediate neurologic deficits include age, emergency presentation, renal dysfunction, active smoking, and cerebrovascular disease. The use of intraoperative distal aortic perfusion and perioperative CSF drainage, in combination, prevents one neurologic deficit in twenty cases for all patients, and one in five for extent II TAAA.[45]

Also important in spinal cord protection is the reimplantation of intercostal arteries. During the era of cross-clamp and go reimplantation of intercostal arteries was found to be a risk factor for postoperative neurologic deficit.[51] This link was explained by the longer cross-clamp time required to reattach the intercostal arteries. The level at which the anterior radicular artery, known as the *artery of Adamkiewicz* or *arteria radicularis magna,* originates is known to be variable. Most commonly this artery branches from one of the lower intercostal arteries with or without additional collateral branches from nearby intercostal arteries. The anterior radicular artery is believed to be the major blood supply to the anterior spinal artery of the spinal cord. The relationship of neurologic deficit to ligation, reimplantation, and pre-existing occlusion of intercostal arteries in patients undergoing TAAA repair using adjuncts has been studied. It was found that ligation of patent lower intercostal arteries (T9 to T12) increased the risk of paraplegia.[52] Therefore, all patent lower intercostal arteries from T9 to T12 are reattached, either together as a patch to a side hole made in the Dacron graft, or when the intercostal arteries are too far apart, separately as buttons or using interposition bypass grafts. However, if the lower intercostal arteries are occluded, the patent upper intercostal arteries will be reimplanted, because these are thought to assume a more important role in the collateral system to the anterior spinal artery in this situation.

Adequate spinal cord perfusion pressure should be maintained with avoidance of hypotension during and after surgery. Intravenous nitroprusside, in particular, can precipitate systemic hypotension, and has been shown to cause a paradoxical increase of CSF pressure,[53] and therefore it is no longer used. A detailed account of the essential anesthetic care during TAAA repair is beyond the scope of this chapter. However, the importance of adequate maintenance of systemic arterial pressure with judicious blood transfusion cannot be overemphasized, as organ perfusion greatly depends on the systemic circulation. Clearly, the era of cross-clamp—and go is over, and the spinal cord must be provided with some form of protection.

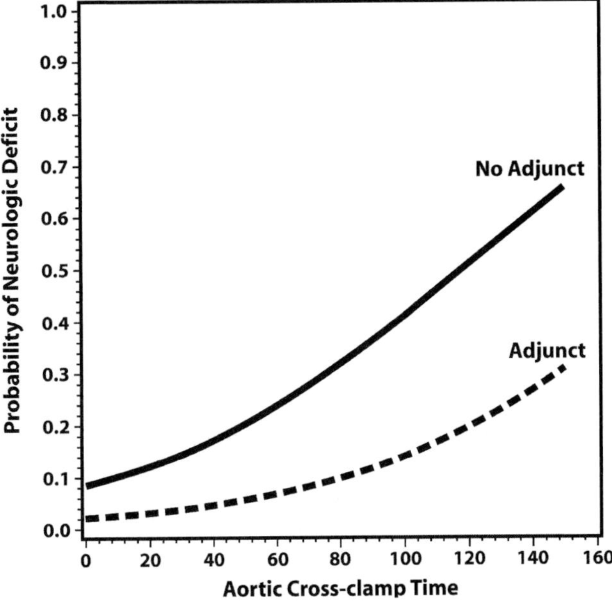

FIGURE 101.11 The probability of neurologic deficit increases with clamp time and is markedly higher in patients undergoing thoracoabdominal aortic aneurysm surgery without adjuncts.

Delayed Neurologic Deficits

Delayed neurologic deficit refers to the onset of paraplegia or paraparesis after a period of observed normal neurologic function. Delayed onset neurologic deficit after TAAA repair was first reported in 1988, at which time the condition was considered irreversible and beyond the surgeon's control.[54] Since then numerous reports have described improvements in patients' neurologic function by using CSF drainage for delayed onset neurologic deficits.[55–57] Delayed neurologic deficit has been observed as early as 2 hours and as late as 2 weeks following surgery (median, 3 days), in 2.7% of patients.[58] No single risk factor is responsible for delayed neurologic deficit. However, using multivariable analysis, acute dissection, extent II TAAA, and renal insufficiency were identified as significant preoperative predictors for delayed onset neurologic deficit.[58] In a subsequent case-control study, postoperative mean arterial pressure of less than 60 mm Hg and CSF drain complications were found to be predictors in the development of delayed onset neurologic deficit, independent of preoperative predictors[59] (Fig. 101.12).

As improved spinal cord protection during TAAA surgery has reduced the incidence of neurologic complications, delayed onset neurologic deficit has emerged as an important clinical entity. The exact mechanisms involved in the development of delayed neurologic deficit remain unknown. It is speculated that delayed neurologic deficit after TAAA repair may result from a 'second hit' phenomenon. Adjuncts can protect the spinal cord intraoperatively and reduce the incidence of immediate neurologic deficit, but the spinal cord remains

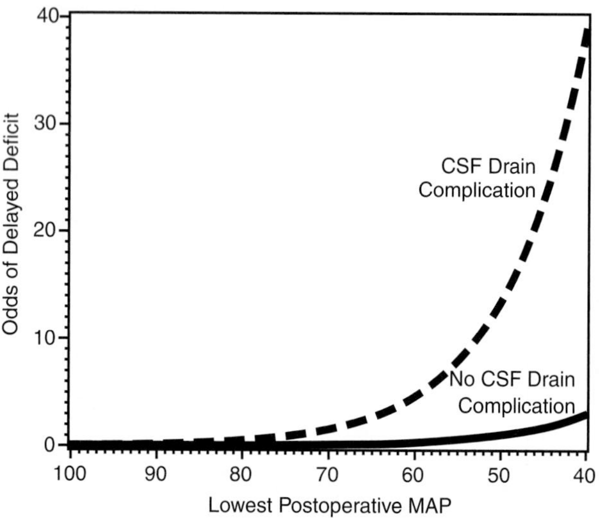

FIGURE 101.12 Odds of delayed neurologic deficit by lowest postoperative mean arterial blood pressure, with or without cerebrospinal fluid drain complication. Odds are referenced to one. For example, a patient with a mean arterial blood pressure of 40 mm Hg and a cerebrospinal fluid drain complication would have 40:1 odds of delayed neurologic deficit. CSF, cerebrospinal fluid.

vulnerable during the early postoperative period. Additional ischemic insults caused by hemodynamic instability, malfunction of the CSF drainage catheter, or both may constitute a "second hit," causing delayed neurologic deficit. Furthermore, in the rigid unyielding spinal column, any rise in CSF pressure could lead to an increase in compartment pressure, with consequent decreased spinal cord perfusion. Hence, CSF is drained freely when delayed neurologic deficit develops to relieve the compartment pressure.

To optimize postoperative spinal cord perfusion and oxygen delivery, mean arterial pressure is kept above 90 to 100 mm Hg, hemoglobin above 10 mg/dL, and cardiac index greater than 2.0 L/min. If delayed neurologic deficit occurs, measures to increase spinal cord perfusion are instituted immediately. The patient is placed flat in the supine position. The patency and function of the drain is ascertained at once. If the drain has been removed the CSF drainage catheter is reinserted immediately and CSF is drained freely until the CSF pressure drops below 10 mm Hg. The systemic arterial pressure is raised, blood transfusion is liberally infused, and oxygen saturation is increased, as indicated above. CSF drainage is continued for at least 72 hours for all patients with delayed onset neurologic deficit. Using this multifaceted approach to treating delayed onset neurologic deficit, an improvement in neurologic function is seen in 57% of patients.[60] When the CSF drain was still in place at the onset of delayed neurologic deficit 75% of patients recovered function; 43% recovered neurologic function if the CSF drain had to be reinserted at the time of the delayed neurologic deficit. Patients who developed delayed neurologic deficit but did not have CSF drainage failed to recover function.

Renal Failure

Acute postoperative renal failure is defined as an increase in serum creatinine of 1 mg/dL per day for 2 consecutive days or by the need for hemodialysis. The reported rate of acute renal failure from large series of patients undergoing TAAA repair falls within the range of 5% to 40% and is associated with mortality rates as high as 70%. Patients who develop acute renal failure more frequently sustain non-renal complications, such as respiratory failure, central nervous system dysfunction, sepsis, and gastrointestinal hemorrhage. For patients who develop postoperative renal failure early continuous venovenous hemodialysis or daily intermittent hemodialysis is initiated. In the experience of the authors of this chapter, approximately one third of patients who develop acute renal failure remain on hemodialysis, and predictably these patients have a prolonged length of hospital stay. Long-term survival for patients on hemodialysis is dismal. Preoperative chronic renal insufficiency and ruptured aneurysms are known predictors of acute postoperative renal failure. Although the authors of this chapter have theorized that patients with the most extensive extent II TAAA are at highest risk for the development of postoperative renal failure, extent of TAAA has not been shown to be a significant predictor.

The goals of perioperative renal protection are to maintain adequate renal oxygen delivery, reduce renal oxygen utilization, and reduce direct renal tubular injury. However, good strategies to protect renal function during surgical TAAA repair remain elusive. The benefit of cold temperatures for metabolic suppression in organ protection is well known. Local hypothermia has been shown to protect against renal ischemia and reperfusion injury in laboratory animals, and there is some evidence that patients with cold visceral perfusion have superior survival and recovery rates. However, this strategy has not decreased the incidence of acute renal failure. The incidence of postoperative renal failure remains troublesome and the pursuit of an optimal method of renal protection continues to be a top priority.

Cardiopulmonary Complications

The association between ischemic heart disease and decreased early and late survival following TAAA repair is well known. In Crawford's series of 1,509 patients undergoing TAAA surgery, a comparison of mortality rates for patients with and without coronary artery disease found a 31% incidence of coronary artery disease related to a 12% mortality rate and for patients without coronary artery disease an 8% mortality rate. The incidence of postoperative cardiac complications in this series was 12% and was also associated with increased early mortality (30% versus 5% without cardiac complications). Other cardiac complications include postoperative atrial arrhythmias, which occur in approximately 10% of patients. Treatment for atrial arrhythmias usually involves one or more pharmacologic agents (amiodarone, β-blockers, or calcium channel blockers). Occasionally, electrical cardioversion may be required in refractory cases or when there is associated hypotension.

The incidence of pulmonary complications after TAAA repair ranges from 20% to 50%. Respiratory failure is usually described as days of required postoperative mechanical ventilatory support. Predictors of prolonged postoperative respiratory failure include advanced age, aortic cross-clamp time (greater than 60 minutes), number of packed red blood cells transfused and tobacco use. Early tracheostomy is favored for patients who remain ventilator-dependent.

Elephant Trunk Technique

The authors of this chapter have performed the two-staged elephant trunk procedure in nearly 200 patients with extensive aortic aneurysms.[61] Mortality rates range from 5% to

9% after stage one, and 6% to 7% for stage two. During the interval between the two stages, (approximately 31 days to 6 weeks), mortality has averaged around 6.5%. When a 5-year follow-up of patients who failed to return for second-stage repair was performed, 32% had died. Although the exact cause of death was unable to be determined in many of these patients, it is likely that a significant percentage of deaths were a result of aneurysm rupture. Major complications for both stages have been relatively low, with stroke rates of 2% in the first stage and no neurologic deficits in the second. Determining the optimum length of recovery time between stages has been difficult. Because these patients are vulnerable to rupture, it is currently recommended that the second stage repair be performed after a 4- to 6-week period of recovery.

Impact of Aortic Dissection

Aortic dissection has long been considered a risk factor for neurologic deficit in patients undergoing repair of descending thoracic and TAAAs, particularly during the clamp-and-go era.[62–65] However, in a series of 729 patients operated on for descending thoracic and TAAAs, no differences were reported in neurologic outcome between patients with and those without chronic dissection; the rate of paraplegia was 3.6% with dissection versus 4.7% without dissection.[66] Several factors are likely responsible for the good neurologic outcome of patients with chronic dissection; they include better surgical techniques and anesthetic care, moderate hypothermia, and reimplantation of intercostal arteries. The key element in the improved spinal cord protection, however, has been the use of the adjuncts distal aortic perfusion and CSF drainage.

In acute aortic dissection, the risk of paraplegia following graft replacement of the descending thoracic or thoracoabdominal aorta remains substantial with a neurologic deficit rate of 32%.[67] An additional 16 patients with acute aortic dissection have been operated on with no neurologic complications. Nevertheless, acute dissection aneurysm patients are usually critically ill, undergoing surgery emergently with little time for preparation. The method of spinal cord protection employed during surgery for acute dissection is often not optimal. In particular, reimplantation of intercostal arteries is ill-advised because of the risk of catastrophic bleeding from the friable dissected tissues, and the use of the adjuncts distal aortic perfusion and CSF drainage may not be possible in the presence of hemodynamic instability.

Endoluminal Approach

Since the first successful reported thoracic endograft procedure in 1991,[68] endovascular management of thoracic aortic pathology has evolved at a rapid pace. Numerous centers have reported series of patients receiving thoracic endografts for a variety of conditions, including acute and chronic type B aortic dissections, traumatic thoracic transections, and descending thoracic and TAAAs.[69–71] A number of thoracic endograft devices are currently awaiting U.S. Food and Drug Administration approval. Although the short-term benefits of endovascular therapy are clear, with less morbidity and shorter length of hospital stay compared with conventional surgery, the reported mortality rates appear to replicate those from conventional surgery in large centers. The long-term effectiveness of endoluminal exclusion of aneurysms remains to be defined. Several cases of immediate and delayed paraplegia have been reported in the literature following thoracic endograft placement.[72,73] Patent intercostal arteries are a major source of type II endoleak, although the significance of which is undetermined. The development of fenestrated and branched endografts will allow reimplantation of patent intercostal, visceral and renal arteries. The next generation of endografts holds a promising future for endovascular treatment as an acceptable alternative to the open repair in selected patients with TAAA.

KEY POINTS

- **Remarkable progress has been made in the surgical treatment of thoracoabdominal aortic aneurysms.**
- **The decline in mortality and complication rates can be attributed to improvements in perioperative care and in surgical technique, particularly the adoption of adjunct distal aortic perfusion and cerebrospinal fluid drainage.**
- **Neurologic deficit is no longer a major threat to patients, because the use of adjuncts has lowered the incidence for all thoracoabdominal aortic aneurysms to 2.4%.**
- **Research needs to be continued that focuses on improving organ preservation, particularly for the most troublesome extent II thoracoabdominal aortic aneurysm.**

Acknowledgment

The authors of this chapter are grateful to Kirk Soodhalter, editor, and to Carl Clingman for his assistance with the illustrations.

References

1. Bickerstaff L, Hollier L, Peenen H, et al. Abdominal aortic aneurysms: The changing natural history. *J Vasc Surg.* 1984;1:6–12.
2. Wanhainen A, Bjorck M, Boman K, et al. Influence of diagnostic criteria on the prevalence of abdominal aortic aneurysm. *J Vasc Surg.* 2001;34:229–235.
3. Wilmink A, Quick C. Epidemiology and potential for prevention of abdominal aortic aneurysm. *Br J Surg.* 1998;85:155–162.
4. Clouse WD, Hallett JW Jr, Schaff HV, et al. Improved prognosis of thoracic aortic aneurysms: a population-based study. *JAMA* 1998;280:1926–1929.
5. Bickerstaff LK, Pairolero PC, Hollier LH, et al. Thoracic aortic aneurysms: a population-based study. *Surgery* 1982;92:1103–1108.
6. Perko MJ, Norgaard M, Herzog TM, et al. Unoperated aortic aneurysm: a survey of 170 patients. *Ann Thorac Surg.* 1995;59:1204–1209.
7. Pressler V, McNamara JJ. Thoracic aortic aneurysm: natural history and treatment. *J Thorac Cardiovasc Surg.* 1980;79:489–498.
8. **Crawford ES, DeNatale RW. Thoracoabdominal aortic aneurysm: observations regarding the natural course of the disease. *J Vasc Surg.* 1986;3:578–582.**
9. Cambria RA, Gloviczki P, Stanson AW, et al. Outcome and expansion rate of 57 thoracoabdominal aortic aneurysms managed nonoperatively. *Am J Surg.* 1995;170:213–217.
10. Elefteriades JA, Hartleroad J, Gusberg RJ, et al. Long-term experience with descending aortic dissection: the complication-specific approach. *Ann Thorac Surg.* 1992;53:11–20.
11. Lobato AC, Puech-Leao P. Predictive factors for rupture of thoracoabdominal aortic aneurysm. *J Vasc Surg.* 1998;27:446–453.
12. Juvonen T, Ergin MA, Galla JD, et al. Prospective study of the natural history of thoracic aortic aneurysms. *Ann Thorac Surg.* 1997;63:1533–1545.
13. **Coady MA, Rizzo JA, Hammond GL, et al. Surgical intervention criteria for thoracic aortic aneurysms: a study of growth rates and complications. *Ann Thorac Surg.* 1999;67:1922–1926.**
14. Davies RR, Goldstein LJ, Coady MA, et al. Yearly rupture or dissection rates for thoracic aortic aneurysms: simple prediction based on size. *Ann Thorac Surg.* 2002;73:17–27.
15. Dapunt OE, Galla JD, Sadeghi AM, et al. The natural history of thoracic aortic aneurysms. *J Thorac Cardiovasc Surg.* 1994;107:1323–1332.
16. Coady MA, Rizzo JA, Hammond GL, et al. What is the appropriate size criterion for resection of thoracic aortic aneurysms? *J Thorac Cardiovasc Surg.* 1997;113:476–491.
17. Masuda Y, Takanashi K, Takasu J, et al. Expansion rate of thoracic aortic aneurysms and influencing factors. *Chest* 1992;102:461–466.
18. Rizzo JA, Coady MA, Elefteriades JA. Procedures for estimating growth rates in thoracic aortic aneurysms. *J Clin Epidemiol.* 1998;51:747–754.
19. Ailawadi G, Eliason JL, Upchurch GR Jr. Current concepts in the pathogenesis of abdominal aortic aneurysm. *J Vasc Surg.* 2003;38:584–588.

20. Lopez-Candales A, Holmes DR, Liao S, et al. Decreased vascular smooth muscle cell density in medial degeneration of human abdominal aortic aneurysms. *Am J Pathol.* 1997;150:993–1007.
21. Pan JH, Lindholt JS, Sukhova GK, et al. Macrophage migration inhibitory factor is associated with aneurysmal expansion. *J Vasc Surg.* 2003;37:628–635.
22. Longo GM, Xiong W, Greiner TC, et al. Matrix metalloproteinases 2 and 9 work in concert to produce aortic aneurysms. *J Clin Invest.* 2002;110:625–632.
23. Annabi B, Shedid D, Ghosn P et al. Differential regulation of matrix metalloproteinase activities in abdominal aortic aneurysms. *J Vasc Surg.* 2002;35:539–546.
24. McMillan WD, Pearce WH. Increased plasma levels of metalloproteinase-9 are associated with abdominal aortic aneurysms. *J Vasc Surg.* 1999;29:122–127.
25. Biddinger A, Rocklin M, Coselli J, et al Familial thoracic aortic dilatations and dissections: a case control study. *J Vasc Surg.* 1997;25:506–511.
26. Coady MA, Davies RR, Roberts M, et al. Familial patterns of thoracic aortic aneurysms. *Arch Surg.* 1999;134:361–367.
27. Hasham SN, Willing MC, Guo DC, et al. Mapping a locus for familial thoracic aortic aneurysms and dissections (TAAD2) to 3p24-25. *Circulation* 2003;107:3184–190.
28. Hossack KF, Leddy CL, Johnson AM, et al. Echocardiographic findings in autosomal dominant polycystic kidney disease. *N Engl J Med.* 1988;319: 907–912.
29. Elsheikh M, Casadei B, Conway GS, et al. Hypertension is a major risk factor for aortic root dilatation in women with Turner's syndrome. *Clin Endocrinol (Oxf).* 2001;54:69–73.
30. Pepin M, Schwarze U, Superti-Furga A, et al. Clinical and genetic features of Ehlers-Danlos syndrome type IV, the vascular type. *N Engl J Med.* 2000;342:673–680.
31. Wenstrup RJ, Meyer RA, Lyle JS, et al. Prevalence of aortic root dilation in the Ehlers-Danlos syndrome. *Genet Med.* 2002;4:112–117.
32. Milewicz DM, Chen H, Park ES et al. Reduced penetrance and variable expressivity of familial thoracic aortic aneurysms/dissections. *Am J Cardiol.* 1998;82:474–479.
33. Jarrett F, Darling RC, Mundth ED, et al. Experience with infected aneurysms of the abdominal aorta. *Arch Surg.* 1975;110:1281–1286.
34. Bakker-de Wekker P, Alfieri O, et al. Surgical treatment of infected pseudoaneurysms after replacement of the ascending aorta. *J Thorac Cardiovasc Surg.* 1984;88:447–451.
35. Bachet JE, Termignon JL, Dreyfus G, et al. Aortic dissection. Prevalence, cause, and results of late reoperations. *J Thorac Cardiovasc Surg.* 1994; 108:199–205.
36. Bernard Y, Zimmermann H, Chocron S, et al. False lumen patency as a predictor of late outcome in aortic dissection. *Am J Cardiol.* 2001;87:1378–1382.
37. Elefteriades JA, Lovoulos CJ, Coady MA, et al. Management of descending aortic dissection. *Ann Thorac Surg.* 1999;67:2002–2005.
38. Bernard Y, Zimmermann H, Chocron S et al. False lumen patency as a predictor of late outcome in aortic dissection. *Am J Cardiol.* 2001;87:1378–1382.
39. **Marui A, Mochizuki T, Mitsui N, et al. Toward the best treatment for uncomplicated patients with type B acute aortic dissection: A consideration for sound surgical indication. *Circulation* 1999;100:275–280.**
40. Juvonen T, Ergin MA, Galla JD, et al. Risk factors for rupture of chronic type B dissections. *J Thorac Cardiovasc Surg.* 1999;117:776–786.
41. Huynh TTT, Miller CC III, Estrera AL, et al. Determinants of hospital length of stay after thoracoabdominal aortic aneurysm repair. *J Vasc Surg.* 2002;35:648–653.
42. Kouchoukos NT, Daily BB, Rokkas CK, et al. Hypothermic bypass and circulatory arrest for operations on the descending thoracic and thoracoabdominal aorta. *Ann Thorac Surg.* 1995;60:67–76.
43. **Svensson LG, Crawford ES, Hess KR, et al. Experience with 1509 patients undergoing thoracoabdominal aortic operations. *J Vasc Surg.* 1993;17:357–368.**
44. Cambria RP, Clouse WD, Davison JK, et al. Thoracoabdominal aneurysm repair: results with 337 operations performed over a 15-year interval. *Ann Surg.* 2002;236:471–479.
45. **Safi HJ, Miller CC III, Huynh TTT, et al. Distal aortic perfusion and cerebrospinal fluid drainage for thoracoabdominal and descending thoracic aortic repair: Ten years of organ protection. *Ann Surg.* 2003;238:372–381.**
46. Safi HJ, Campbell MP, Ferreira ML, et al. Spinal cord protection in descending thoracic and thoracoabdominal aortic aneurysm repair. *Semin Thorac Cardiovasc Surg.* 1998;10:41–44.
47. Miller CC III, Porat EE, Estrera AL, et al. Analysis of short-term multivariate competing risks data following thoracic and thoracoabdominal aortic repair. *Eur J Cardiothorac Surg.* 2003;23:1023–1027.
48. Jacobs MJ, de Mol BA, Elenbaas T, et al. Spinal cord blood supply in patients with thoracoabdominal aortic aneurysms. *J Vasc Surg.* 2002;35:30–37.
49. Hollier LH, Money SR, Naslund TC, et al. Risk of spinal cord dysfunction in patients undergoing thoracoabdominal aortic replacement. *Am J Surg.* 1992;164:210–213.
50. Coselli JS, Lemaire SA, Koksoy C, et al. Cerebrospinal fluid drainage reduces paraplegia after thoracoabdominal aortic aneurysm repair: results of a randomized clinical trial. *J Vasc Surg.* 2002;35:631–639.
51. Safi H, Miller CI, Carr C, et al. The importance of intercostal artery reattachment during thoracoabdominal aortic aneurysm repair. *J Vasc Surg.* 1998;27:58–68.
52. Safi H, Miller CI, Carr C, et al. The importance of intercostal artery reattachment during thoracoabdominal aortic aneurysm repair. *J Vasc Surg.* 1998;27:58–68.
53. Huynh TT, Miller CC III, Safi HJ. Delayed onset of neurologic deficit: significance and management. *Semin Vasc Surg.* 2000;13:340–344.
54. **Crawford ES, Mizrahi EM, Hess KR, et al. The impact of distal aortic perfusion and somatosensory evoked potential monitoring on prevention of paraplegia after aortic aneurysm operation [. *J Thorac Cardiovasc Surg.* 1988;95:357–67; published erratum in *J Thorac Cardiovasc Surg.* 1989 May;97:665]**
55. Widmann MD, DeLucia A, Sharp WJ, et al. Reversal of renal failure and paraplegia after thoracoabdominal aneurysm repair. *Ann Thorac Surg.* 1998;65:1153–1155.
56. Azizzadeh A, Huynh T, Miller CI, et al. Reversal of twice-delayed neurologic deficits with cerebrospinal fluid drainage after thoracoabdominal aneurysm repair: a case report and plea for a national database collection. *J Vasc Surg.* 2000;31:592–598.
57. Safi HJ, Miller CC III, Azizzadeh A, et al. Observations on delayed neurologic deficit after thoracoabdominal aortic aneurysm repair. *J Vasc Surg.* 1997;26:616–622.
58. Estrera AL, Miller CC III, Azizzadeh A, et al. Preoperative and operative predictors of delayed neurologic deficit following repair of thoracoabdominal aortic aneurysm. *J Thorac Cardiovasc Surg.* 2003;126:1288–1295.
59. Azizzadeh A, Huynh TT, Miller CC III, et al. Postoperative risk factors for delayed neurologic deficit after thoracic and thoracoabdominal aortic aneurysm repair: a case-control study. *J Vasc Surg.* 2003;37:750–754.
60. Estrera AL, Miller CC III, Azizzadeh A, et al. Predictors of delayed neurologic deficit following repair of thoracic and thoracoabdominal aortic aneurysm [abstract]. 2001.
61. **Safi HJ, Miller CC III, Estrera AL, et al. Staged repair of extensive aortic aneurysms: morbidity and mortality in the elephant trunk technique. *Circulation* 2001;104:2938–2942.**
62. Svensson LG, Crawford ES, Hess KR, et al. Variables predictive of outcome in 832 patients undergoing repairs of the descending thoracic aorta. *Chest* 1993;104:1248–1253.
63. Okita Y, Tagusari O, Minatoya K et al. Is distal anastomosis only to the true channel in chronic type B aortic dissection justified? *Ann Thorac Surg.* 1999;68:1586–1591.
64. Gilling-Smith GL, Worswick L, Knight PF, et al. Surgical repair of thoracoabdominal aortic aneurysm: 10 years' experience. *Br J Surg.* 1995; 82:624–629.
65. Dudra J, Shiiya N, Matsui Y, et al. Operative results of thoracoabdominal repair for chronic type B aortic dissection. *J Cardiovasc Surg (Torino).* 1997;38:147–151.
66. Safi HJ, Miller CC III, Estrera AL, et al. Chronic aortic dissection not a risk factor for neurologic deficit in thoracoabdominal aortic aneurysm repair. *Eur J Vasc Endovasc Surg.* 2002;23:244–250.
67. Safi HJ, Miller CC III, Reardon MJ, et al. Operation for acute and chronic aortic dissection: recent outcome with regard to neurologic deficit and early death. *Ann Thorac Surg.* 1998;66:402–411.
68. Volodos NL, Karpovich IP, Troyan VI, et al. Clinical experience of the use of self-fixing synthetic prostheses for remote endoprosthetics of the thoracic and the abdominal aorta and iliac arteries through the femoral artery and as intraoperative endoprosthesis for aorta reconstruction. *Vasa Suppl.* 1991;33:93–95.
69. Buffolo E, da Fonseca JH, de Souza JA, et al. Revolutionary treatment of aneurysms and dissections of descending aorta: the endovascular approach. *Ann Thorac Surg.* 2002;74:S1815–1817.
70. **Dake MD, Miller DC, Mitchell RS, et al. The "first generation" of endovascular stent-grafts for patients with aneurysms of the descending thoracic aorta. *J Thorac Cardiovasc Surg.* 1998;116:689–703.**
71. Greenberg R, Resch T, Nyman U, et al. Endovascular repair of descending thoracic aortic aneurysms: an early experience with intermediate-term follow-up. *J Vasc Surg.* 2000;31:147–156.
72. Kasirajan K, Dolmatch B, Ouriel K, Clair D. Delayed onset of ascending paralysis after thoracic aortic stent graft deployment. *J Vasc Surg.* 2000;31:196–199.
73. Gravereaux EC, Faries PL, Burks JA, et al. Risk of spinal cord ischemia after endograft repair of thoracic aortic aneurysms. *J Vasc Surg.* 2001; 34:997–1003.

CHAPTER 102 ■ ABDOMINAL AORTIC ANEURYSMS

THOMAS S. HUBER, W. ANTHONY LEE, C. KEITH OZAKI, AND JAMES M. SEEGER

Abdominal aortic aneurysms are a common problem in developed countries and represent a significant public health risk. Operative repair is the only accepted means to reduce the risk of rupture and the associated mortality. The treatment algorithm represents a balance between the estimated risk of operation and the future risk of rupture. The open operative technique has been refined during the past five decades since the first successful description by Dubost et al.[1] The past decade and a half has witnessed the rapid development of the endovascular approach that has revolutionized treatment. The commercial release of these devices has led to their widespread application, although their indications and long-term durability remain undefined.

DEFINITIONS AND CLASSIFICATIONS

An aneurysm is defined as a permanent, focal dilation of an artery that exceeds 1.5 times the normal, expected diameter.[2] The diameter of a normal abdominal aorta in an adult man is approximately 2 cm (range, 1.4 to 3.0 cm); therefore a 3-cm aorta would be considered aneurysmal.[3] The abdominal aorta is consistently larger in men than in women and increases slightly with age in both sexes.[4] Abdominal aortic aneurysms should be differentiated from other conditions in which the size of the aorta is increased, including ectasia and arteriomegaly. In *aortic ectasia*, the diameter is increased by less than 50% of the normal expected diameter. The term *arteriomegaly* refers to a diffuse (nonfocal) enlargement of several arterial segments with increases in diameter greater than 50% of the normal expected diameter. Arterial segments in patients with arteriomegaly may be considered aneurysmal if the diameter of a segment is increased by more than 50% of the diameter of an adjacent segment. The term *aneurysmosis* denotes the presence of multiple aneurysmal segments separated by either normal, occluded, or arteriomegalic segments.

Abdominal aortic aneurysms are classified primarily according to how far they extend cephalad (Fig. 102.1). More than 95% of all abdominal aortic aneurysms are classified as infrarenal.[5] These aneurysms start below the orifices of the renal arteries and usually have a 1.5- to 2-cm segment of normal infrarenal aorta. Approximately 10% to 20% of all abdominal aortic aneurysms are associated with aneurysms of the iliac arteries (common iliac, internal iliac, external iliac, in descending order of frequency).[6,7] The management of abdominal aortic aneurysms associated with common iliac artery aneurysms is similar to the management of abdominal aortic aneurysms alone, and these two patterns should be considered basically the same disease process. The only significant difference in the decision algorithm is the configuration of the graft for open repair (tube versus bifurcated) and the site of the distal anastomoses. Aneurysms classified as juxtarenal extend to the level of the renal arteries, and those classified as suprarenal extend proximally to the level of the superior mesenteric and/or celiac arteries. Aneurysms involving the thoracic and abdominal aorta are designated as thoracoabdominal aortic aneurysms and are classified (extent 1 through 4) according to how far they extend both cephalad and caudal. Aneurysms that extend above the renal arteries are significantly more complicated and associated with greater morbidity as might be predicted from the obligatory periods of renal and mesenteric ischemia associated with repair.

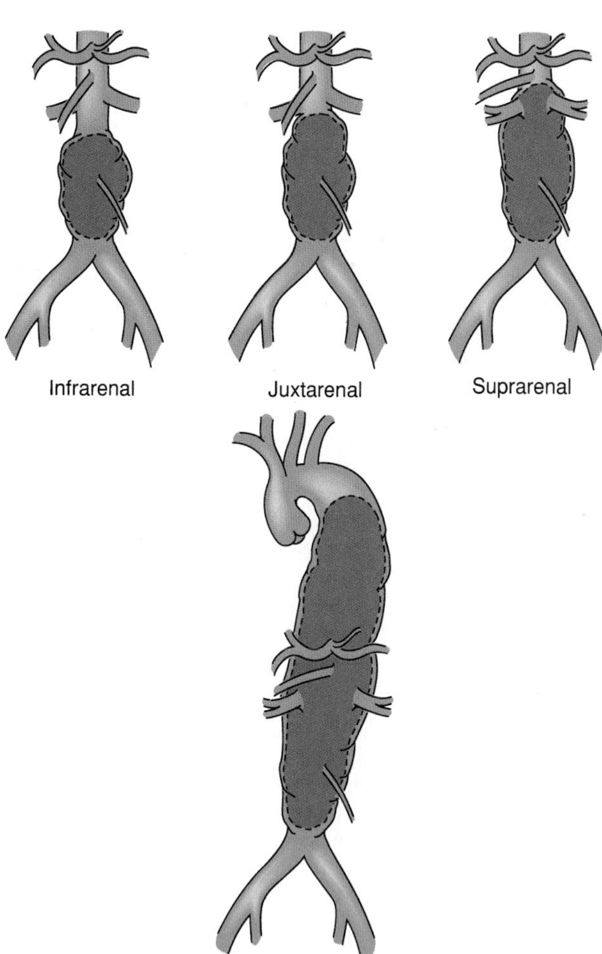

FIGURE 102.1 Classification of abdominal aortic aneurysms. More than 95% of all abdominal aortic aneurysms are infrarenal. Juxtarenal aneurysms extend cephalad to the level of the renal arteries, and suprarenal aneurysms to the level of the superior mesenteric and/or celiac arteries. Aneurysms involving the thoracic and abdominal portions of the aorta are designated as thoracoabdominal aortic aneurysms and are classified (extent 1 to 4) according to how far they extend cephalad and caudal.

MAGNITUDE OF THE PROBLEM

Abdominal aortic aneurysms and their sequelae are common problems in developed countries. The incidence of abdominal aortic aneurysms in the United States ranges from 1.5% in autopsy series to 3.2% among unselected adult patients screened with ultrasonography.[5] Predictably, the incidence increases among subsets of patients with defined risk factors for abdominal aortic aneurysms and approximates 50% among patients with either femoral or popliteal artery aneurysms.[5] It should be emphasized that these rates have been determined with the broad definition of an aneurysm provided previously (1.5 times the normal vessel diameter) and do not necessarily reflect aneurysms that are of sufficient size to merit repair. Furthermore, the incidence of abdominal aortic aneurysms appears to be increasing and this likely reflects an increase in the "true" incidence that cannot be simply attributed to an increase in detection, diagnosis or aging.[8] A total of 14,751 deaths were caused by abdominal aortic aneurysms and/or dissections during 2003 and this corresponded to death rate of 5.1/100,000 as reported by the Center for Disease Control and Prevention.[9] Notably, these numbers may be underestimates because a significant number of sudden deaths in elderly patients may be secondary to undiagnosed aortic aneurysms.

PATHOGENESIS AND RISK FACTORS

The pathogenesis of abdominal aortic aneurysms is unresolved although it remains an intense area of both experimental and clinical investigation. Multiple potential etiologic factors have been implicated including atherosclerosis,[10] hemodynamics,[11] collagen,[12] collagenase,[13] elastin,[14] elastase,[15] metalloproteinases,[16] protease inhibitors,[17] programmed cell death (apoptosis),[18] neutrophils,[19] and inflammatory mediators.[20] The etiology is likely multifactorial with interaction between both environmental and genetic factors. Unfortunately, investigation into the potential mechanisms has not resulted in any effective therapies. Elucidation of the pathogenesis has been complicated by the older age of patients at presentation and the absence of suitable animal models.

Multiple risk factors have been identified for the development of abdominal aortic aneurysms and include age, sex, smoking, hypertension, hyperlipidemia, peripheral vascular disease, myocardial infarction, and family history.[21,22] Identification of these risk factors is important to facilitate screening high-risk patient populations. Abdominal aortic aneurysms are a disease process of the elderly and are rare among persons younger than 50 years. Indeed, the mean age among patients undergoing repair across the United States was 72 ± 7 years (±SD) in a recent series making up a 20% national sample.[23] A meta-analysis of the population based screening studies for abdominal aortic aneurysms reported that male sex had the strongest association (odds ratio, 5.69).[21] The incidence of death resulting from abdominal aortic aneurysms for men 60 to 64 years of age is 11-fold higher than that for women of the same age, but it is only threefold higher for men between 85 and 90 years. Furthermore, men account for approximately 80% of all abdominal aortic aneurysm repairs performed nationally.[23] The Aneurysm Detection and Management Veterans Affairs Cooperative Study Group (ADAM) reported that smoking was the strongest risk factor associated with abdominal aortic aneurysms larger than 4 cm (odds ratio, 5.57) among the 73,451 veterans screened.[24] Similarly, Wilmink et al.[24,25] reported that abdominal aneurysms were 7.6 times more likely to develop in current smokers than in nonsmokers and that the duration of smoking rather than level of exposure appeared to correlate with their development. Johansen and Koepsell[26] reported the incidence of abdominal aortic aneurysms was 19.2% among first-degree relatives of patients with aneurysms, but only 2.4% among first-degree relatives of control patients with aortoiliac occlusive disease. Similarly, Darling et al.[27] prospectively analyzed patients undergoing repair of abdominal aortic aneurysms and reported that 15.1% had a first-degree relative with an abdominal aortic aneurysm, in contrast to 1.8% in the control group. Interestingly, the presence of a female family member with an aneurysm correlated with an increased risk for rupture.

The presence of an aneurysm in the aorta, iliac, femoral, or popliteal arteries dramatically increases the risk for development of a new or additional abdominal aortic aneurysm. In patients undergoing abdominal aortic or iliac artery aneurysm repair, the chance that an additional aneurysm will eventually develop in either the aorta or iliac vessels that merits intervention is approximately 5 to15%.[28,29] The second aneurysm may develop anywhere in the remaining native aorta, commonly within the residual infrarenal aortic cuff. Similarly, the incidence of aortoiliac aneurysms in patients with popliteal or femoral artery aneurysms is approximately 50%.[5] All patients found to have a peripheral artery aneurysm should undergo computed tomography (CT) of the entire aorta and iliac vessels to rule out a synchronous aneurysm in addition to being screened for other peripheral aneurysms. Interestingly, the reverse scenario is not true; patients with aortic or iliac artery aneurysms have a less than 5% chance of having a peripheral artery aneurysm, and evaluation beyond physical examination is likely not justified.[30]

The incidence of abdominal aortic aneurysm is increased among patients with an aortic dissection and among patients with heart transplants. Late or repeated operations are required in approximately 20% of patients by 10 years after an acute aortic dissection.[31] The aneurysms may develop in either the thoracic or abdominal aorta, although the former site is more commonly affected. The term *dissecting aneurysm* is frequently used although it is a misnomer; dissection and aneurysm are separate processes. Simply, a dissection is a tear within the aortic wall itself that extends for a variable length resulting in "true" and "false" lumen. The prevalence of abdominal aortic aneurysms and the rate of expansion are both increased among heart transplant patients.[32–34] The responsible mechanisms remain unclear, but the obligatory chronic immunosuppression may contribute. Interestingly, several transplant centers have initiated screening programs as part of their pretransplant evaluation.

It is notable that the risk factors for abdominal aortic aneurysm are similar to those associated with the development of atherosclerosis. Furthermore, atherosclerotic changes are found almost universally within the abdominal aorta at the time of repair. However, the processes of atherosclerosis and aneurysmal degeneration are likely separate and distinct. Simplistically, atherosclerosis is a process that leads to a narrowing of the vessel lumen, whereas aneurysmal degeneration leads to dilation. Aneurysms have historically been referred to as *atherosclerotic aneurysms* although this is likely a misnomer that has been appropriately replaced by the term *nonspecific aneurysms*.

PRINCIPLES OF MANAGEMENT

The treatment goals for patients with abdominal aortic aneurysms are to prolong life, relieve symptoms, and prevent rupture. Because surgical treatment is the only effective means to achieve these goals, the crucial question that must be answered is whether the patient should undergo operative repair. The decision algorithm is straightforward for patients with ruptured or symptomatic aneurysms, but more difficult for patients with asymptomatic, intact aneurysms. The decision to recommend operative intervention in the elective setting is contingent on the balance between the risk of operation and the risk of expectant or nonoperative management. Appropriate assessment of these risks requires an understanding of the size-associated risk for rupture, the growth rate, and the mortality associated with repair. However, it should be emphasized that repair of an asymptomatic, intact aneurysm is a prophylactic operation.

Understanding the natural history of untreated abdominal aortic aneurysm requires knowledge of the physics associated with the vessel wall. The tangential stress (t) of a fluid-filled cylindrical tube is determined by the following equation:

$$t = Pr/d$$

where P is the pressure exerted by the blood (dyne/cm^2), r is the internal radius (cm), and d is the thickness (cm) of the arterial wall.[35] The tangential stress of a cylinder 0.2-cm thick with an internal radius of 0.8 cm and a fluid pressure of 150 mm Hg is 8×10^5 dyne/cm^2 (Fig. 102.2). An increase in the internal radius (diameter) of the cylinder to 2.94 cm and a concomitant decrease in the wall thickness, as might occur with an aneurysm, would increase the tangential stress to 98×10^5 dyne/cm^2. Thus, a threefold increase in diameter would result in a 12-fold increase in the tangential stress. Aneurysms rupture when the tangential stress exceeds the tensile strength of the vessel wall. It should be emphasized that the tangential stress varies directly with the radius of the cylinder (vessel) but is independent of its length.

The diameter of an abdominal aortic aneurysm is the greatest predictor of rupture as would be predicted by the tangential stress of the vessel wall. The diameter of an aneurysm is determined by measuring its greatest diameter from outer wall to outer wall in any orientation (i.e., anterior to posterior, transverse) throughout the extent of the aneurysm. These measurements may be confounded by the tortuosity of the vessel so every attempt should be made to obtain a cross-sectional measurement perpendicular to its longitudinal axis. The collective

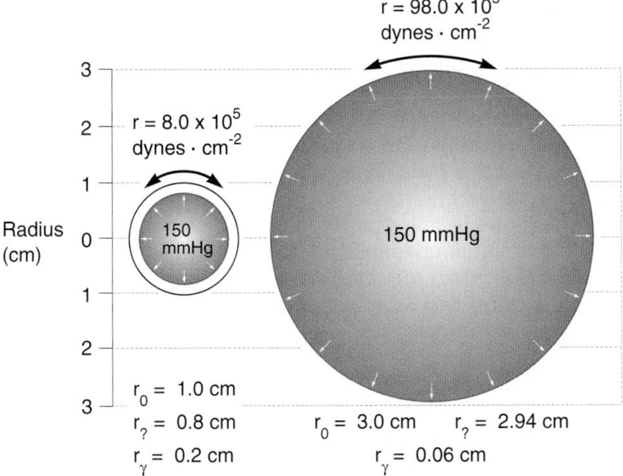

FIGURE 102.2 Cross-sectional view of a 2-cm-diameter cylinder that expands to a diameter of 6 cm while wall cross-sectional area remains constant. t, wall stress; d, wall thickness; r_i, inside radius; r_0, outside radius. Expansion of a 1-cm-diameter cylinder to a diameter of 3 cm with no change in wall cross-sectional area increases wall tensile stress 12-fold.

TABLE 102.1

ESTIMATED ANNUAL RUPTURE RISK OF ABDOMINAL AORTIC ANEURYSMS

Diameter (cm)	Rupture risk (%/yr)
<4	0
4–5	0.5–5
5–6	3–15
6–7	10–20
7–8	20–40
>8	30–50

(From Brewster DC, Cronenwett JL, Hallett JW Jr, et al. Guidelines for the treatment of abdominal aortic aneurysms. Report of a subcommittee of the Joint Council of the American Association for Vascular Surgery and Society for Vascular Surgery. *J Vasc Surg.* 2003;37:1106–17.)

annual rupture risks per aneurysm diameter are shown in Table 102.1.[36] Although there is some variability in the data, it is generally appreciated that the rupture risk for aneurysms less than 5 cm in diameter is small, but increases considerably for those greater than 6 cm. These data may be simplified by using the rule that the annual rupture risk is 5% or less for a 5-cm aneurysm, 10% for a 6-cm aneurysm, and 20% for a 7-cm aneurysm. These numbers correspond to an estimated 5-year rupture risk of 50% for 6-cm aneurysms and 100% for those that are 7 cm. Notably, both the ADAM[24] and UK Small Aneurysm Trial[37] that randomized patients with small aneurysms (4 to 5.5 cm) to open repair or surveillance reported that the rupture risk for surveillance was 1% or less per year.

A variety of other factors have also been reported to increase the aneurysm rupture risk, including female gender,[38] chronic obstructive pulmonary disease,[38,39] smoking,[38] hypertension,[38,39] family history,[40] and wall stress.[41] Notably, the UK Small Aneurysm Trial reported that the rupture risk was increased for female gender (hazard ratio, 3), current smoking (hazard ratio, 1.5), severe chronic obstructive pulmonary disease (hazard ratio, 0.6 per L forced expiratory volume in 1 second) and higher mean arterial pressure (hazard ratio, 1.2 per mm Hg). Fillinger et al.[42] have used finite element analysis to calculate the wall stress of abdominal aortic aneurysms and have reported that the wall stress of symptomatic/ruptured aneurysms exceeds those for elective aneurysms. The impact of the aneurysm growth rate on rupture risk remains unclear and has been difficult to separate from aneurysm diameter alone. However, an aneurysm expansion of 1 cm/year or more is generally considered worrisome and a potential risk factor for rupture.

The natural history of abdominal aortic aneurysms is to increase in size over time. An estimated 80% of all small aneurysms continue to grow.[2] The mean rate of growth has varied from 0.2 to 0.3 cm/year in population studies[43–46] to 0.4 cm/year in referral practices[47–49] with the latter figure (0.4 cm/year) generally quoted as a reasonable estimate. Several factors including female gender, current smoking, and larger original diameter have been associated with an increased rate of growth as might be predicted from their increased rupture rate.[43,46] It should be emphasized that these growth rates are mean values and that all aneurysms do not grow in a linear fashion as might be predicted. The growth curve may be somewhat erratic or "staccato" with no growth detected during consecutive 6-month intervals followed by a growth of 0.6 cm during the next one.[50] Furthermore, it should be emphasized that the past rate of growth does not predict future events; patients should not be lulled into a false sense of security if their aneurysm is relatively stable over time.

The mortality rate associated with repair of an abdominal aortic aneurysm primarily depends on the status of the aneurysm (intact/asymptomatic, intact/symptomatic, ruptured) and the method of repair (open vs. endovascular). A recent population study reported that the operative mortality rate for open repair of intact aneurysms in the United States was 4.2%.[23] Predictably, the operative mortality rate increased with age, ranging from 2.2% among persons age 50 to 59 years to 9.2% among those older than age 80 years. Interestingly, the operative mortality rate was significantly higher among women (6.1% versus 3.7%). The operative mortality rate for open repair in the randomized trials comparing operative repair with surveillance for small aneurysms (UK Small Aneurysm Trial, 5.8%; ADAM, 2.7%) and open repair with endovascular repair (Dutch Randomized Endovascular Aneurysm Management [DREAM] Trial, 4.6%; Endovascular Aneurysm Repair [EVAR] Trial 1, 4.6%)[51,52] were within the range of the nationwide series. Furthermore, a literature review examining the mortality rate of open abdominal aortic aneurysm repair encompassing 64 individual studies reported a collective rate of 5.5%.[53] A moderate degree of variability has been reported historically for the mortality rates of open, intact aneurysms repairs with values ranging from less than 4% among the best individual series to 10% among the state and community series.[5,54]

The operative mortality rate for endovascular repair of intact abdominal aortic aneurysms appears to be less than associated with open repair despite the equivocal results from the initial clinical trials.[55–59] Lee et al.[60] reported that the operative mortality rate was 3.8% for open repair and 1.3% for endovascular repair in 2001 across the United States. Notably, patients undergoing endovascular repair were both older and had more comorbidities. Similar findings were reported from the State of New York during the same year (open—4.9%, endovascular—1.5%).[61] Early results from the DREAM trial[52] and EVAR Trial[51] comparing open and endovascular repair have reported that the perioperative mortality rate is lower for endovascular repair (DREAM trial, 1.2% versus 4.6%; EVAR Trial, 1.7% versus 4.7%).

The operative mortality rate for open repair of intact/symptomatic aneurysms among patients undergoing emergent repair exceeds that for elective repair and has ranged from 9% to 19% in recent series.[5,62,63] Various explanations have been proposed for this increased mortality rate relative to that for intact/asymptomatic aneurysms, including failure to maximize preoperative medical conditions, increased incidence of inadvertent venous injuries, and less experienced operative teams, although the true explanation remains unclear. It is notable that the increased rate has been fairly consistent in the literature, in contrast to the mortality rate for intact/asymptomatic aneurysms, which has decreased gradually. Comparable data are not available for the emergent repair of intact/symptomatic aneurysms using the newer endovascular approach.

The actual mortality rate for ruptured abdominal aortic aneurysms is somewhat difficult to determine because a significant number of sudden deaths in elderly patients are likely secondary to ruptured aneurysms. It has been estimated that 50% of all patients with ruptured abdominal aortic aneurysms die before reaching the hospital, and that approximately 50% of those who actually undergo open repair do not survive.[5] Indeed, a recent meta-analysis spanning 50 years and 77 studies reported that the operative mortality rate of ruptured aneurysms was 48%.[64] These figures correspond to an overall mortality rate of approximately 80%, although this rate may be an underestimate. It is remarkable that the optimization of prehospital and emergency room care including a reduction in the mean transfer time from the emergency department to the operating room to 12 minutes has not resulted in a decrease of the mortality rate of ruptured aneurysms.[65] Furthermore, the operative mortality rate for ruptured aneurysms treated with the open approach has remained relatively stable during the past few decades.[64,66] Several recent reports have shown that it is feasible to treat select patients with ruptured aneurysms with the endovascular approach and that the associated operative mortality rate may be significantly less.[67–69] In one of the larger series, Castelli et al.[67] reported that the mortality rate for the endovascular approach was only 20%. Similarly, Lee et al.[68] reported that the initiation of an aggressive approach to treat all possible ruptured aneurysms with the endovascular approach resulted in a decrease in the associated operative mortality (37% versus 12%) and complication (84% versus 65%) although the differences did not achieve statistical significance.

CLINICAL PRESENTATION AND DIAGNOSIS

The overwhelming majority of abdominal aortic aneurysms are asymptomatic at the time they are discovered. Most aneurysms are detected not during physical examination but rather during abdominal and pelvic imaging studies, such as ultrasonography and CT, performed for other indications (e.g., chronic back pain, renal cysts). It is often difficult to feel an abdominal aortic aneurysm on physical examination, even when a concerted effort is made, because of its anatomic location in the posterior abdomen, and these difficulties are exacerbated by the frequent presence of truncal obesity. A recent literature review examining the accuracy of physical examination reported that the sensitivity ranged from 33% to 100%, the specificity ranged from 75% to 100% and the positive predictive value ranged from 14% to 100%.[70] Given these fairly broad ranges, the authors concluded that physical examination could not be relied upon to exclude an abdominal aortic aneurysm. Predictably, the accuracy of primary care physicians for detecting abdominal aortic aneurysms in patients with known aneurysms is only fair because of the limitations noted previously and the failure to actually evaluate the aorta during the routine physical examination. Intact abdominal aortic and iliac artery aneurysms may present with symptoms that lead to further investigation and the correct diagnosis. Enlargement of the aneurysm may cause vertebral erosion and chronic back pain. Additionally, thrombosis of an abdominal aortic aneurysm may cause acute ischemia in the lower torso, and aneurysms may be a source of arterial macroemboli or microemboli that cause acute ischemia of a lower extremity or digit, respectively.

Patients with intact/symptomatic or ruptured aneurysms present with abdominal or back pain related to the aneurysm itself. The etiology of the pain is unclear, but may be secondary to local nerve compression. The character of the pain is variable and ranges from dull to sharp. The pain is usually acute in onset and persistent. It may be superimposed on more chronic abdominal or back pain, but the presentation is usually not subtle, and the pain can be differentiated from more chronic complaints. Additionally, the pain may radiate from the abdomen to the back, flank, inguinal region, or genitalia. Approximately 10% of patients with ruptured abdominal aortic aneurysms present with signs and symptoms similar to those of ureteral colic or other acute urologic problems.[71] Indeed, the diagnosis of a ruptured aneurysm must be ruled out in a timely fashion in patients presenting with testicular pain who have normal results on both urinalysis and testicular examination.

The presentation of patients with a ruptured abdominal aortic aneurysm may range from hemodynamically stable to profound shock. The hemodynamic status depends on how effectively the tissues adjacent to the aorta tamponade the bleeding and the patient's physiologic status and ability to withstand acute hemorrhage. If the adjacent tissues effectively tamponade the bleeding, the patient may present in a hemodynamically stable state with essentially normal vital signs. However, it should be emphasized that this is usually a temporary situation, and health care providers should not be lulled into a false sense of security. A ruptured abdominal aortic aneurysm is a true medical emergency that requires immediate operative repair regardless of the patient's hemodynamic status. Furthermore, the vital signs may be misleading because patients can lose up to 15% of their blood volume (class 1 shock) without any appreciable change in their pulse rate or blood pressure. Patients with free intraperitoneal ruptures likely exsanguinate quickly and do not survive long enough to seek medical attention.

Patients with a ruptured abdominal aortic aneurysm may also present with either an aortoenteric or an aortocaval fistula although both are relatively rare. Patients with an aortoenteric fistula may present with massive intestinal bleeding. The aorta may rupture through any portion of the bowel although the duodenum and proximal small bowel are the most common sites. The overwhelming majority of aortoenteric fistulae result from the erosion of a prosthetic graft into the adjacent bowel (secondary aortoenteric fistula) rather than from an unrepaired aneurysm (primary aortoenteric fistula). However, the diagnosis of an aortoenteric fistula must be ruled out in all patients with gastrointestinal bleeding and either an abdominal aortic aneurysm or a previous aortic reconstruction. Patients with an aortocaval fistula present with high-output congestive heart failure, a continuous abdominal bruit, and edema of the lower extremities. The severity of the heart failure symptoms depends on the size of the fistula and the magnitude of the systemic shunt.

Several imaging studies are available to establish or confirm the diagnosis of an abdominal aortic aneurysm. Indeed, the introduction of endovascular techniques for aneurysm repair has resulted in an evolution of these modalities. The generic goals for imaging patients with an abdominal aortic aneurysm are to establish the diagnosis, determine the presence of rupture, determine the cephalad/caudal extent of the aneurysm, determine the feasibility of endovascular repair, appropriately size the aneurysm and access vessels for endovascular repair, screen for other visceral pathology, and screen for the presence of anatomic variants that would complicate operative repair, such as a left-sided vena cava or a horseshoe kidney. No imaging study is ideal for every application, and it is imperative to understand the strengths and weaknesses of the various tests.

Both plain radiographs of the abdomen and barium enemas have historically been used to diagnose abdominal aortic aneurysms. The aortic wall is frequently calcified and can occasionally be detected on these studies. The sensitivity of these studies is not very good, however, and they should not be used for this purpose because better imaging studies are available. They have no role in the evaluation of a patient with a potential ruptured abdominal aortic aneurysm and are actually detrimental because of the requisite imaging time and associated delay in diagnosis; however, these studies can be very useful for patients undergoing evaluation for abdominal pain or changes in their bowel habits. Furthermore, the status of the aorta should be determined during the routine review of these studies.

Abdominal ultrasound is a safe, simple, and inexpensive means of detecting abdominal aortic aneurysms (Fig. 102.3).

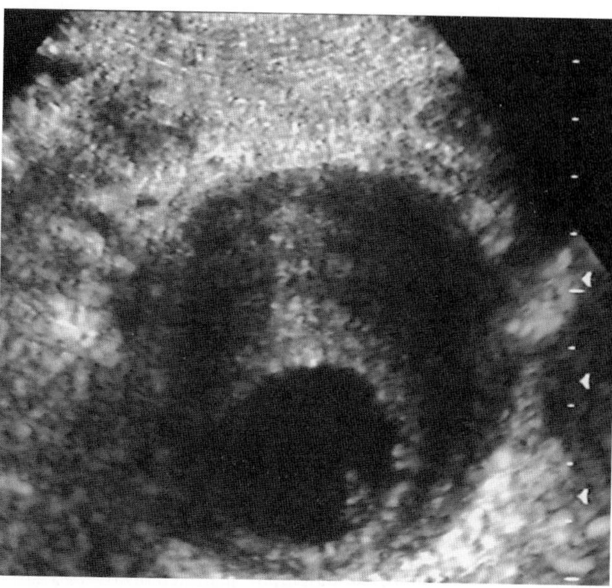

FIGURE 102.3 B-mode ultrasonogram showing a transverse view of an infrarenal abdominal aortic aneurysm. Note the vessel wall and the large quantity of intraluminal clot surrounding the smaller, blood-filled center (*dark circle*).

It is relatively inexpensive and does not require the use of ionizing radiation, intravenous contrast, or arterial cannulation. Furthermore, the ultrasound units are portable and almost universally available in the hospital setting. The sensitivity of ultrasound for detecting abdominal aortic aneurysms is good, and the technique is reproducible within 0.3 cm.[72] However, the technique is somewhat operator-dependent and potentially confounded by the presence of bowel gas. Ultrasound can accurately image the infrarenal aorta to its bifurcation but is less reliable for imaging the portions of the aorta proximal to the renal arteries and distal to the iliac vessels. Furthermore, it is not as reliable as CT for differentiating a ruptured from an intact aneurysm. It is an excellent tool for screening patients at high risk for an abdominal aortic aneurysm and for confirming the presence of an aneurysm suspected by physical examination or clinical presentation. Furthermore, ultrasound is a useful technique to follow patients with small aneurysms (<4 cm) for whom the exact measurement is not crucial. It should likely not be used to confirm the diagnosis of a ruptured aneurysm, nor should it be used as the sole imaging study before elective repair because it may not provide a complete image of the aorta and iliac arteries.

CT overcomes many of the limitations of ultrasound and is the current gold standard for imaging patients with abdominal aortic aneurysms (Fig. 102.4). The technique is more expensive than ultrasound, not as universally available, and potentially harmful because of the use of ionizing radiation and intravenous contrast. However, the allergic response to the contrast may be reduced by administering a steroid preparation, whereas the associated nephrotoxicity can be reduced by the use of acetylcysteine or sodium bicarbonate.[73,74] Needless, these potential risks can be avoided altogether by not using contrast. However, the quality of the noncontrast images is less than optimal and the diagnosis of a ruptured aneurysm potentially confounded. CT is very sensitive for detecting both intact and ruptured aneurysms, and the images are reproducible within 0.2 cm.[72] The quality of the CT images has continued to improve with each new generation of scanners, and the image acquisition times have decreased. Currently, it is possible

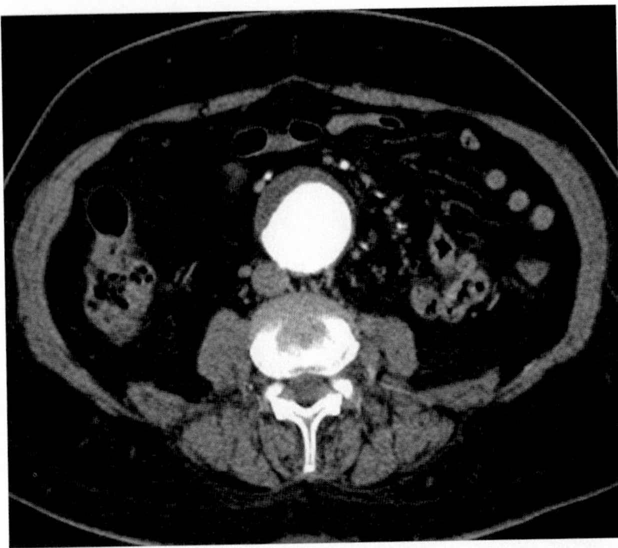

FIGURE 102.4 Computed tomography scan demonstrates a large abdominal aortic aneurysm. Note that the majority of the lumen is filled with contrast.

to image the aorta and iliac vessels from the ascending arch to the femoral vessels during a routine aneurysm scan with an image acquisition time of less than 45 seconds using 16- to 64-array multirow detectors. The quality of CT arteriograms likewise continues to improve and may soon replace the more traditional catheter-based diagnostic arteriogram. It is possible to reconstruct the axial CT images into three-dimensional (3D) images using special software and obtain images perpendicular to the centerline blood flow (Fig. 102.5). Indeed, these 3D CT images through the centerline path may improve the accuracy and consistency of sizing for endovascular repair and suffice as the only preoperative imaging study.[75] CT is excellent for determining the cephalad/caudal extent of an aneurysm and detecting involvement of the iliac vessels. It is also helpful for detecting other intraabdominal pathology or anatomic variants that may impact the operative approach. Specific concerns include the location of the left renal vein and other associated venous anomalies, the location and size of the kidneys, and the characteristics of the aneurysm wall. CT is currently the sole diagnostic test performed before open surgical repair in most cases and the imaging study of choice to confirm or refute the diagnosis of a ruptured abdominal aortic aneurysm. Additionally, CT is the serial imaging study of choice when aneurysms exceed 4 cm and approach the threshold for operative intervention.

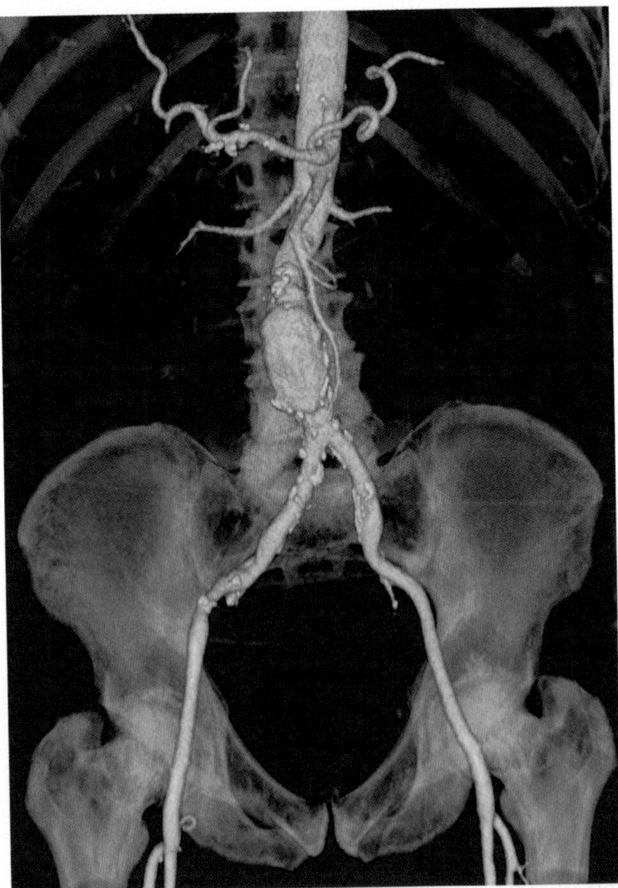

FIGURE 102.5 Three-dimensional computed tomography of the aorta and the iliac, femoral, and visceral arteries is shown. Note the infrarenal abdominal aortic aneurysm that extends to the aortic bifurcation.

Magnetic resonance imaging (MRI) is an alternative to CT. It has not been applied as extensively, but the image quality, sensitivity, and potential advantages relative to ultrasonography are almost comparable to those of CT. The technology is not as widely available as CT, and most surgeons are less familiar with interpreting the images. A generic contraindication to MRI is the presence of implanted ferromagnetic devices (e.g., pacemakers, joints), and the scanning of intubated, critically ill patients is cumbersome, if not prohibitive. One advantage of MRI relative to CT is the potential to differentiate "new" from "old" blood. This has proved beneficial in the rare patient with CT findings that are equivocal for a ruptured abdominal aortic aneurysm.

Catheter-based or invasive arteriography is frequently performed before abdominal aortic aneurysm repair although it should not be viewed as a diagnostic test. Admittedly, abdominal aortic aneurysms are frequently diagnosed during invasive aortography. However, arteriography simply visualizes the lumen of vessels (i.e., aorta, iliac and femoral arteries). Abdominal aortic aneurysms are frequently filled with laminated thrombus and have a fairly normal appearing vessel lumen. The "lumenogram" produced by the contrast reflects the patent lumen rather than the "true" lumen of the vessel and the actual size of the aneurysm. Preoperative arteriography may be beneficial before endovascular repair and help select the appropriate size device. Additionally, it may be helpful in a subset of patients undergoing open repair who have aortoiliac occlusive disease, poorly controlled hypertension/renal insufficiency, chronic mesenteric ischemia, and/or renal anomalies, including horseshoe kidneys. Invasive arteriography may also be helpful in patients with suprarenal or thoracoabdominal aortic aneurysms although this is only a relative indication. Invasive arteriography is not routinely used before open repair because the added information does not justify the expense and risk in most cases. The potential complications include arterial injury and embolization in addition to those associated with the administration of intravenous contrast and ionizing radiation as outlined previously. The role for invasive arteriography will likely further decrease with the evolution of the alternative, noninvasive arterial imaging studies such as CT arteriography.

The diagnostic approach and initial treatment for patients with a potential ruptured aneurysm merit further comment. Because of the high attendant mortality rate, a prompt diagnosis and emergent repair are required. In a study from the Cleveland Clinic Vascular Registry, the operative mortality rate associated with ruptured abdominal aortic aneurysms increased from 35% when the initial diagnosis was correct to a rate of 75% when the initial diagnosis was incorrect.[76]

Admittedly, the clinical presentation may be confusing, and delays in diagnosis are not uncommon. The classic triad of hypotension, abdominal pain, and a pulsatile abdominal mass was present in only 50% of patients with ruptured aneurysms in a single institutional series.[77]

Elderly patients who present to the emergency room in a hemodynamically *unstable* state with abdominal or back pain require emergent exploratory laparotomy in most cases. The potential causes of shock (i.e., hypovolemic, cardiogenic, septic, neurogenic) can usually be quickly differentiated by a brief history and physical examination. However, this clinical scenario is most suggestive of hypovolemic or hemorrhagic shock resulting from an intraabdominal catastrophe. The differential diagnosis is extensive and includes pancreatitis, mesenteric infarction, acute Addisonian crisis, and rupture of a visceral artery aneurysm in addition to rupture of an abdominal aortic aneurysm. A myocardial infarction can mimic a ruptured aneurysm in this patient population and potentially confounds the diagnosis, although it can usually be confirmed by the findings on electrocardiogram. Additional diagnostic imaging have not traditionally been considered necessary in this setting and, indeed, have been considered potentially harmful because of the obligatory delay in getting patients to the operating room. As a result of the dramatic reduction in CT acquisition times and the potential feasibility of endovascular repair, abdominal/pelvic CT scans are likely indicated in this scenario to confirm the diagnosis and plan the operative procedure provided they can be obtained expeditiously. This approach has the added advantage of potentially reducing the number of negative laparotomies in critically ill patients. A recent natural history study of patients with ruptured abdominal aortic aneurysms not offered operative repair reported that less than 15% of the patients died within 2 hours of hospital admission.[78] Based upon these findings, the authors concluded that most patients with ruptured aneurysms are sufficiently stable to undergo a CT scan and consideration for endovascular repair. Several findings on CT are suggestive of a ruptured abdominal aortic aneurysm including disruption of the calcium ring within the aortic wall, disruption of the aortic margins, retroperitoneal hematomas, mass lesions in the psoas region, displacement of the kidneys, abnormal soft tissues posterior to the aorta, effacement of the normal fat planes between the aorta and adjacent viscera, and abnormal retroperitoneal fluid collections (Fig. 102.6). It is should be noted that it is not necessary for patients to receive gastrointestinal contrast in this setting and that the obligatory delay for this preparation is likely detrimental.

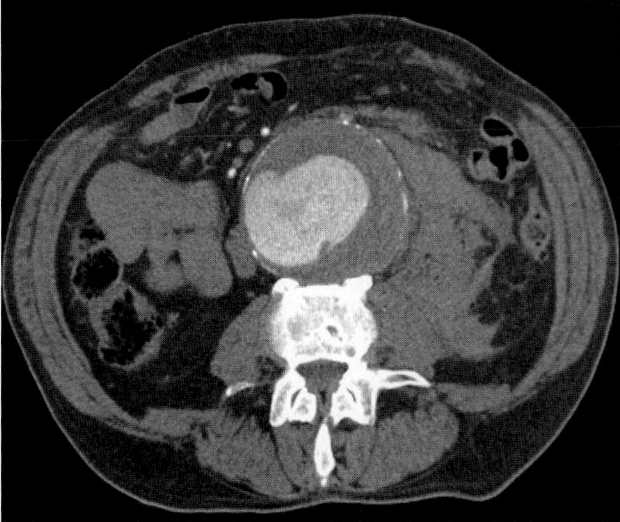

FIGURE 102.6 Contrast computed tomography demonstrates a ruptured abdominal aortic aneurysm. Note the large retroperitoneal hematoma and the loss of the normal fat plane anterior and lateral to the left psoas muscle.

Elderly patients who present to the emergency room hemodynamically *stable* with abdominal or back pain should be evaluated for a ruptured abdominal aortic aneurysm. Admittedly, the differential diagnosis for abdominal or back pain in this patient population is extensive, and the incidence of a ruptured abdominal aortic aneurysm is small. An expeditious history and physical examination can usually determine the cause of the pain. A pulsatile abdominal aortic mass, an unexplained low hematocrit, or hemodynamic instability before presentation are particularly worrisome and increase the level of suspicion. The diagnosis of an abdominal aortic aneurysm may be confirmed with a portable abdominal ultrasonogram in the emergency room. Indeed, the current trauma algorithms include abdominal ultrasonography as a diagnostic technique for blunt trauma, and many centers have ultrasound units assigned to the emergency room. If ultrasound confirms the diagnosis of an aneurysm, further evaluation with CT should be obtained to rule out rupture. Alternatively, CT may be obtained as the sole imaging study without ultrasound. Any findings consistent with a ruptured aneurysm on CT mandate direct transfer to the operating room and immediate repair. Aggressive fluid resuscitation should be avoided and mild hypotension (i.e., systolic pressure more than 80 mm Hg) tolerated in conscious patients because of the theoretical potential to cause the aneurysm to rupture into the peritoneal cavity and/or release the tamponade effect of the retroperitoneal tissue. If an intact aneurysm is found on CT without any suggestion of rupture, the next logical question is whether the aneurysm is the source of the pain. Symptomatic aneurysms are likely associated with an increased risk of rupture although the natural history remains poorly defined. Patients with symptomatic/intact aneurysms 5 cm in diameter or more should be admitted to a monitored setting and scheduled for urgent operative repair, usually the following day, provided no additional causes for the pain are identified. Additional sources of the abdominal pain should be sought in patients with aneurysms smaller than 4 cm in light of the small rupture risk. The appropriate treatment for patients with aneurysms 4 to 5 cm is less clear. These aneurysms have the potential to rupture although the risk is small. It is recommended that these patients be admitted and the source of their pain further investigated. However, urgent operative repair is recommended if no additional causes are identified.

The role of screening for abdominal aortic aneurysms in asymptomatic patients has been partially clarified. The United States Preventative Task Force has issued a position statement advocating a single screening ultrasound in males 65 to 75 years of age who have a smoking history.[79] These recommendations were based upon the results of a best-evidence systematic review that identified four population based randomized controlled trials demonstrating that screening resulted in a reduction of aneurysm related mortality in this subset of patients.[80] Notably, the Preventative Task Force stated that the literature did not substantiate screening for women even among those with a family history and stated that the harms of screening outweighed the risks. Screening for abdominal aortic aneurysms in this subset of elderly men has been shown to be both cost effective[81] and comparable to other screening programs in adult patients.[82] Despite the Preventative Task Force's recommendations, screening should likely be extended to other high risk patient populations including patients with a family history of a first degree relative with an abdominal aortic aneurysm, evidence of a peripheral artery aneurysm, and those undergoing evaluation for a heart transplantation. There is currently legislation pending in Congress sponsored by the Society of Vascular Surgery supporting a single screening ultrasound in adults. Interestingly, Kim et al.[83] predicted that the introduction of a national screening program would reduce the number of emergent aneurysm repairs while increasing the number of elective repairs. They estimated that this would translate into two additional elective repairs per month for a typical district, general hospital while saving 11 abdominal aortic aneurysm–related deaths per year

OPERATIVE INDICATIONS

All patients with symptomatic or ruptured abdominal aortic aneurysms should undergo operative repair unless they have an underlying medical condition, such as metastatic cancer, that precludes long-term survival or their quality of life is not sufficient to justify the intervention. The latter situation entails a difficult decision, but not offering operative repair should be considered in certain cases (e.g., a debilitated, demented patient in a nursing home) after the family has been consulted.

The operative decision-making process for intact/asymptomatic abdominal aortic aneurysms is a complex one that needs to be tailored to the individual patient. Indeed, there is no single parameter that merits repair. The operative indications are contingent upon the size of the aneurysm, life expectancy, comorbidities, preference, and anatomic configuration. It is important to remember that the repair of an intact/asymptomatic abdominal aortic aneurysm is a prophylactic operation that represents a balance between the operative risk and the future risk of rupture with the ultimate treatment goals to prolong life, relieve symptoms, and prevent rupture.

The diameter of the abdominal aortic aneurysm is the best predictor of rupture as stated previously and has been used as the most common indication for repair. There has been a change in the diameter-based operative criteria within the past few decades although this has been clarified more recently with level 1 evidence. It is interesting to note that the diameter threshold for good-risk patients has decreased from 6 cm to as low as 4 cm with latter recommendation from the guidelines of the governing national vascular surgical societies.[72] Both the UK Small Aneurysm Trial[37] and the ADAM trial[24] concluded that it was safe to follow patients with 4.0- to 5.5-cm aneurysms and that early operation did not confer any long-term survival benefit. As noted previously, the rupture risk for patients in the surveillance group was less than 1% per year. It is important to note that more than 60% of the patients in both studies ultimately underwent operative repair. A follow-up study from the UK Small Aneurysm Trial reported a survival benefit (7.2% lower estimated risk of death at 8 years) for the patients randomized to early surgery. However, only a small percentage (6%) of this difference was due to rupture of unrepaired aneurysms.[84] Notably, the risk of rupture was fourfold higher for women and the authors concluded that the diameter-threshold for repair might be too high for women. The proponents of using smaller diameter-based thresholds for repair (<5.5 cm) have justified their approach stating that even small aneurysms rupture, aneurysms continue to increase in diameter and will likely need to be repaired, the patients' medical conditions will likely deteriorate with age, and the operative mortality/morbidity rate for small aneurysms may be less. Although level 1 evidence does not support this lower threshold, it is important to note that the size discrepancy between a 5.2 cm and 5.5 cm aneurysm is very small and likely within the resolution of the imaging study.

TABLE 102.2

INDEPENDENT RISK FACTORS FOR OPERATIVE MORTALITY AFTER ELECTIVE ABDOMINAL AORTIC ANEURYSM REPAIR

Risk factor	Odds ratio	95% CI
Creatinine >1.8 mg/dL	3.3	1.5–7.5
Congestive heart failure	2.3	1.1–5.2
Electrocardiographic ischemia	2.2	1.0–5.1
Pulmonary dysfunction	1.9	1.0–3.8
Older age (per decade)	1.5	1.2–1.8
Female gender	1.5	0.7–3.0

(From Steyerberg et al. Kievit J, de Mol Van Otterloo JC, et al. Perioperative mortality of elective abdominal aortic aneurysm surgery. A clinical prediction rule based on literature and individual patient data. *Arch Intern Med.* 1995;155:1998–2004.)

The presence of medical comorbidities predictably impacts the perioperative mortality rate and threshold for aneurysm repair. Steyerberg et al.[85] identified several independent risk factors for operative mortality during open repair (Table 102.2) and these observations have been supported by multiple other reports. The dramatic impact of renal insufficiency was further emphasized by a national series that reported a ninefold increase in mortality among this subset of patients. Notably, the estimated glomerular filtration rate may be a better index of renal function than serum creatinine and, therefore, likely a better predictor of adverse outcome after aneurysm repair.[86] Life expectancy is inseparable from comorbidities, but it should be emphasized that the average life expectancy for a 60-year-old and 85-year-old man in the United States is 18 and 5 years respectively.[87]

Patient preference should be factored into the operative decision-making process. Although level 1 evidence suggests that it is likely safe to follow abdominal aortic aneurysms until they reach the 5.5-cm threshold, patients may not be willing to accept this small, finite risk and desire to have their aneurysm repaired a lower threshold. Indeed, patients often echo the justification for early repair proposed by surgeons.

Lastly, the anatomic configuration of the aneurysm and/or the associated structures should factor into the operative decision process. Any technical factors that complicate the repair likely increases the perioperative mortality/morbidity including the need for suprarenal clamp application due to the obligatory renal/visceral ischemia, venous anomalies (e.g. left-sided vena cava), renal anomalies (e.g., horseshoe kidney), and inflammatory aneurysms. Admittedly, many of these technical concerns are relevant only to the open approach and can be overcome or avoided by endovascular repair.

The introduction of the endovascular approach has further challenged the operative indications for intact and asymptomatic aneurysms. Indeed, the significant decrease in the perioperative mortality rate reported for the endovascular approach in both the DREAM trial[52] and EVAR Trial[51] appear to justify lowering the threshold. However, it is important to note that only perioperative outcomes have been reported from these trials and both initial reports concluded that changes in clinical practice should not be implemented until the longer-term results are available. Similarly, Finlayson et al.[54] used a decision analysis model to determine the optimal diameter for open and endovascular aneurysm repair and concluded that the endovascular approach lowers the operative threshold only for older patients in poor health.

The Joint Council of the American Association for Vascular Surgery and the Society for Vascular Surgery have released updated guidelines for the treatment of patients with abdominal aortic aneurysms that address the concerns highlighted previously.[36] They recommend that a diameter of 5.5 cm is an appropriate threshold for repair in the "average patient" with an intact infrarenal aneurysm, but emphasize the importance of individualizing each case. They state that rapid aneurysm expansion (>1 cm/year), symptoms related to the aneurysm, and female gender merit repair at a smaller diameter, whereas consideration should be given to earlier repair in young patients provided that the operative mortality rate is acceptable. Furthermore, they recommend that a larger diameter threshold is appropriate in higher risk patients and emphasize that there does not appear to be any justification to alter the operative threshold for the endovascular approach.

Patients who do not meet the threshold for operative repair should be followed closely in the outpatient clinic. It is important to educate the patients about their underlying disease process and emphasize the importance of long-term follow-up. Notably, Valentine et al.[88] reported that 32% of patients with small aneurysms managed by "watchful waiting" were noncompliant with their follow-up plan. Furthermore, it is important to counsel patients about the presence of symptoms associated with rupture and the importance of seeking urgent medical attention. Recent guidelines have suggested that patients with aneurysms less than 3 cm in diameter should be reimaged at 5 years, whereas aneurysms between 3.0 and 3.4 cm should be reimaged at 3 years and aneurysms between 3.5 and 3.9 cm should be reimaged at 1 year.[89] Aneurysms larger than 4.0 cm should likely be reimaged every 6 months. As noted previously, abdominal ultrasound is likely the most appropriate imaging study for aneurysms less than 4.0 cm with CT more appropriate above that threshold. It is important to note that up to 50% of the patients deemed a prohibitive operative risk and not offered elective repair will ultimately die from a ruptured aneurysm.[90–94] These patients who are not candidates for elective repair should not be offered emergent repair in the event that their aneurysm ruptures or becomes symptomatic.

CHOICE OF OPEN OR ENDOVASCULAR REPAIR

After the decision to recommend operative repair has been made, the technique for the repair must be determined. Admittedly, these decisions are somewhat interrelated because the decision to recommend operative repair in certain subsets of patients is often contingent on whether they are candidates for the endovascular approach. The past decade and a half has witnessed a rapid evolution of the endovascular technique, and, indeed, this evolution has helped define the surgical discipline. It has been clearly demonstrated that the technical success rates for endovascular graft deployment are excellent and the need for intraoperative conversion small. The perioperative events have been defined by level 1 evidence although the longer-term results remain undefined. Many of the technical limitations of the devices and approach have been identified and overcome. There are currently three commercially available devices (Excluder Bifurcated Endoprosthesis from W. L. Gore, Flagstaff, AZ; AneuRx AAA Stent Graft System from Medtronic Vascular, Santa Rosa, CA; and Zenith AAA Endovascular Graft from Cook Medical Incorporated, Bloomington, IN) and one device that has been removed (Ancure Endograft System from Guidant, Menlo Park, CA). Despite the limitations associated with the devices and their long-term outcome, the endovascular approach for treatment of abdominal aortic aneurysms has been widely used. Indeed, approximately one third of all intact abdominal aortic aneurysm repairs in the United States during 2001 were repaired using this newer technique.[60] The choice of open or endovascular repair is complicated and contingent upon several factors including feasibility, outcome, comorbidities, compliance, cost, and preference. It is imperative that these issues, including their respective advantages/disadvantages or strengths/weakness, be addressed with the patients during the decision process to insure proper informed consent.

The initial determinant of the approach is the anatomic configuration of the aorta, the aneurysm, and the access vessels. The endovascular devices are available in only a finite range of sizes and their application suitable only if specific anatomic conditions are satisfied. Notably, all three commercially available devices (Fig. 102.7) are similar and consist of a fabric graft (polyester or expanded polytetrafluoroethylene) and a metallic exoskeleton (stainless steel or nitinol) that facilitate proximal/distal fixation by radial force with or without hooks. They are modular devices consisting of either two components (main body and contralateral iliac limb) or three components (main body, contralateral iliac limb, ipsilateral iliac limb) with a variety of additional components that allow proximal or distal extensions at the aortic and iliac ends, respectively. The initial experience with aortoaortic or "tube graft" configurations were unsuccessful because of problems with the distal landing site at the aortic bifurcation and have been abandoned. Indeed, the current strategy is to seat the proximal component of the bifurcated system as close to the lowest renal artery as possible and the distal components as close to the iliac bifurcation as possible. Although there is some variability among the three commercially available devices in terms of their specific sizes and anatomic constraints, the general anatomic requirements are similar. The infrarenal abdominal aorta must have a suitable, nonaneurysmal landing zone for the endograft that measures 15 mm or more in length and more than 17 to 19 mm but less than 26 to 28 mm in diameter (ranges reflect differences between the commercial devices). Furthermore, the proximal neck angulation should be 45 degrees or less as measured by the intersection of the centerline of the infrarenal aorta at the landing zone site and the centerline of the aneurysm through the aortic bifurcation. The infrarenal neck should be relatively free of thrombus and calcification to facilitate a seal at the implantation site. It is notable that neck length requirements have increased from 1 cm or more to 1.5 cm or more since the original commercial release of the AneuRx and Ancure devices. Indeed, the longer the infrarenal neck length and, therefore, the longer the device seal zone the better. The iliac artery should have a suitable landing zone 20 mm or more with an associated diameter between 7 and 20 mm to facilitate both anchoring the graft in the iliac artery and passing the main device into the aorta. The distal landing zone for the iliac limbs is usually in the common iliac artery in an attempt to preserve the internal iliac artery although the anatomic constraints with regards to the size of the access vessels and introduction of the devices are relevant for both the common and external iliac vessels.

The percentage of patients that are anatomically suitable for an endograft remains unresolved and is likely contingent upon the nature of the individual surgeon/institution practice and the available devices. This percentage of suitable patients has been highly variable with report of 30% in nationwide series,[95] 55% in a regional series,[96] and 14% to 66% in institutional series.[97–99] Notably, the reasons cited for exclusion include a short infrarenal neck (54%), inadequate iliac vessels (47%), and a wide infrarenal neck (40%).[97]

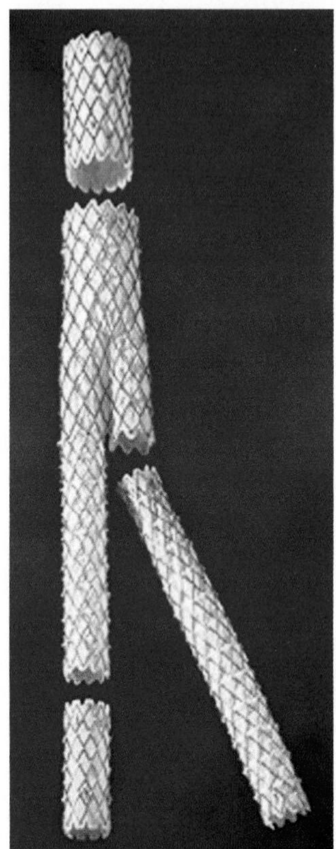

A

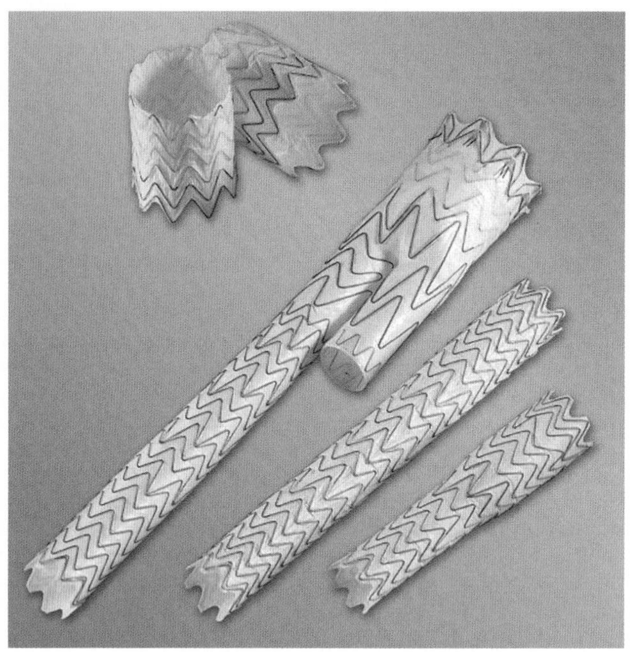

B

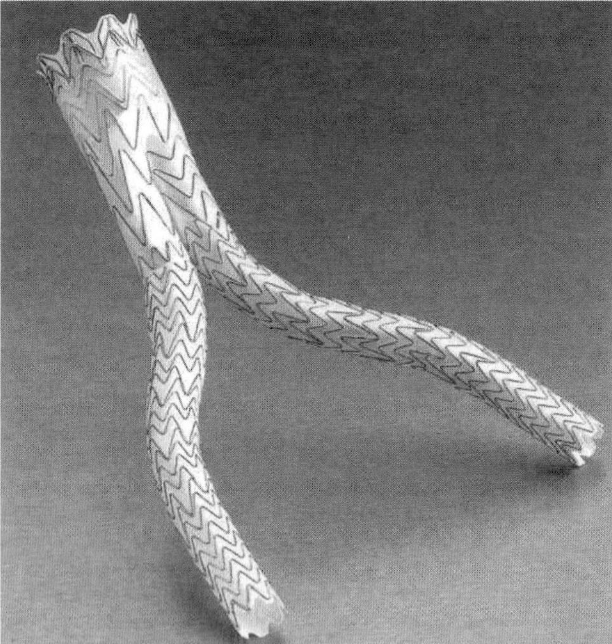

C

FIGURE 102.7 Commercially available endografts: AneuRx (*A*), Excluder (*B*), and Zenith (*C*). All three are similar and consist of a fabric graft (polyester or expanded polytetrafluoroethylene) and a metallic exoskeleton (stainless steel or nitinol) that facilitate proximal/distal fixation by radial force with or without hooks. They are modular devices consisting of either two (main body and contralateral iliac limb) or three (main body, contralateral iliac limb, ipsilateral iliac limb) components with a variety of additional ones that allow proximal or distal extensions at the aortic and iliac ends, respectively.

A variety of techniques have been described to overcome the anatomic limitations for endografting outlined previously thereby extending the feasibility of the approach. Indeed, some modification has been described to overcome almost every anatomic contraindication. Stenoses within the access vessels can be overcome by dilation (i.e., balloon angioplasty, Dotter dilational angioplasty) or by the use of a prosthetic conduit.[100] The prosthetic conduit is usually anastomosed to the bifurcation of the common iliac artery and then tunneled through the retroperitoneal space below the inguinal ligament. Alternatively, an aortouniiliac endograft can be configured and a femorofemoral bypass performed. Notably, the patency rates of the femorofemoral bypass graft in this setting have been reported to be excellent.[101,102] Aneurysmal degeneration of the common iliac artery can be overcome by a variety of techniques including simply using larger-diameter iliac graft limbs, using an aortic extension as a cuff ("bell bottom" technique), occluding/embolizing the internal iliac artery and seating the iliac limb in the external iliac artery or by bypassing the internal iliac artery (and seating the iliac

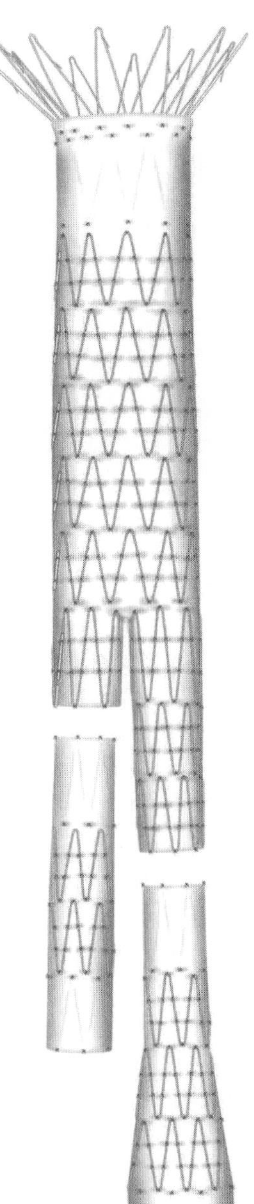

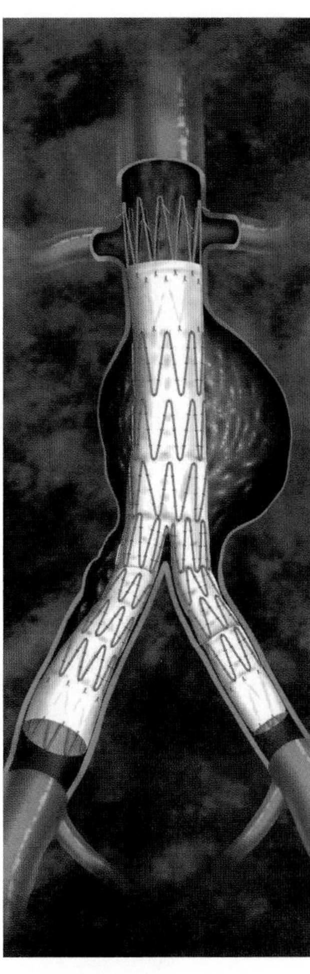

FIGURE 102.7 (*Continued*)

limb in the external iliac artery). Although relatively simple to perform, internal iliac artery embolization has been associated with a moderate incidence of complications including buttock/thigh claudication (30% to 40%), sexual dysfunction, neurologic deficit/paraplegia, pelvic ischemia, and gluteal compartment syndrome.[103,104] The claudication improves with time in most patients, but can be quite debilitating particularly in patients that do not have symptoms preoperatively. Many of the other complications, although somewhat rare, are not reversible and can be catastrophic. Because of these concerns, bilateral internal iliac artery occlusion/embolization should be avoided. Bypass of the internal iliac artery overcomes many of these limitations and has been associated with excellent results in terms of long-term graft patency although the procedure is somewhat challenging and adds significantly to the overall magnitude of the "less-invasive" procedure.[100] Unfortunately, extending the indications for endovascular repair beyond those recommend by the manufacturers has been associated with an increase in the incidence of adverse events including decreased survival and a higher need for reintervention.[105]

Consideration of the perioperative and long-term outcomes after endovascular aneurysm repair requires introduction of the concepts of endoleak and endotension. Simply, endoleak is the perfusion of the aneurysm sac outside the lumen of the endograft, whereas endotension is the persistent pressurization within the excluded aneurysm sac. Endoleaks have been classified as types 1 through 4 based on the mechanism of the leak (Fig. 102.8). Type 1 leaks originate at either the proximal or distal attachment sites. Type 2 leaks are from the collateral circulation originating in the lumbar or inferior mesenteric arteries. Type 3 leaks are caused by fabric tears or problems at the graft interfaces of the modular devices, whereas type 4 leaks are usually transient (<24 hours) trans graft extravasations and can result from the porosity of the graft and needle holes. It should be emphasized that the entire concept of an endoleak is predicated on the ability to detect contrast or blood flow outside the lumen of the endograft and is therefore contingent on the sensitivity and specificity of the various imaging techniques. The major concern about both endoleaks and endotension is that the pressure transmitted to the aneurysm wall will cause the aneurysm to rupture. The clinical significance of the various endoleak types is different. Both Type 1 and 3 endoleaks are considered major adverse outcomes associated with an increased risk of rupture that merit urgent/emergent treatment.[106] Type 2 endoleaks are generally considered less worrisome in terms of their rupture risk although they are associated with an increased risk for reintervention.[106] They can generally be followed with serial imaging studies, but merit evaluation/intervention if the aneurysm sac continues to enlarge. Type 4 endoleaks are self-limited and benign. The clinical significance of endotension is likewise unresolved. Indeed, the concept itself is somewhat ambiguous given the limitations of actually measuring the pressure within the aneurysm sac. It should be noted that freedom from endoleak does not necessarily mean freedom from endotension given the observation that aneurysms can continue to enlarge in the absence of an identifiable endoleak.[107]

The perioperative complication rates appear to be lower after endovascular repair. As noted previously, the randomized, controlled DREAM and EVAR trials and two population studies reported a significant decrease in the perioperative mortality rate.[51,52,60,61] The EVAR Trial also reported a trend towards a decrease in the combined operative mortality/severe complication rate (9.8% versus 4.7%, $p = 0.10$). Multiple clinical trials have reported that the overall major complication rates after both endovascular and open repair are approximately 15% although the magnitude of the complications is less for the endovascular approach and includes primarily vascular access complications (e.g., hematoma, femoral artery injury).[108] These clinical trials have likewise demonstrated that the total hospital length of stay, intensive care unit length of stay, operative blood loss, and time necessary to resume normal activities are all less for the endovascular approach.[108] Interestingly, the impact on sexual function remains unresolved. A survey of the DREAM trial participants demonstrated that sexual dysfunction was common after both endovascular and open repair, but returned to the baseline state at 3 months for both groups.[109] In contrast, Xenos et al.[110] reported significantly less orgasmic and erectile dysfunction after endovascular repair.

The long-term outcome after endovascular repair, including an overall mortality benefit, remains unknown and represents the major, current limitation of the technique. Indeed, the con-

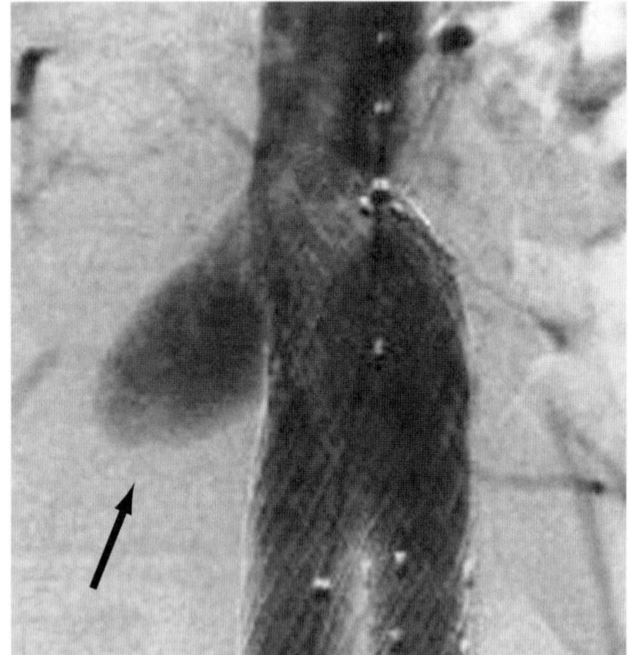

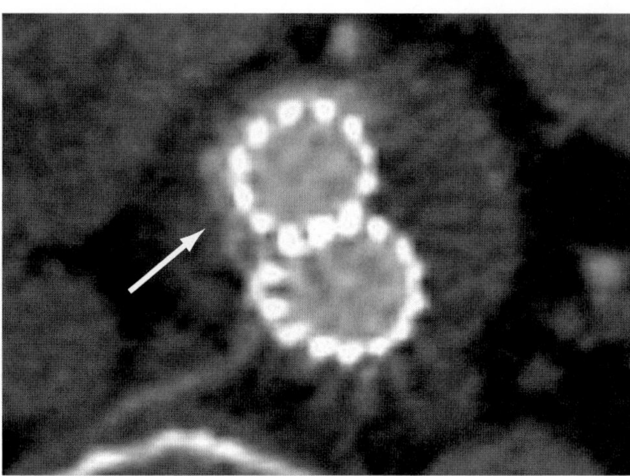

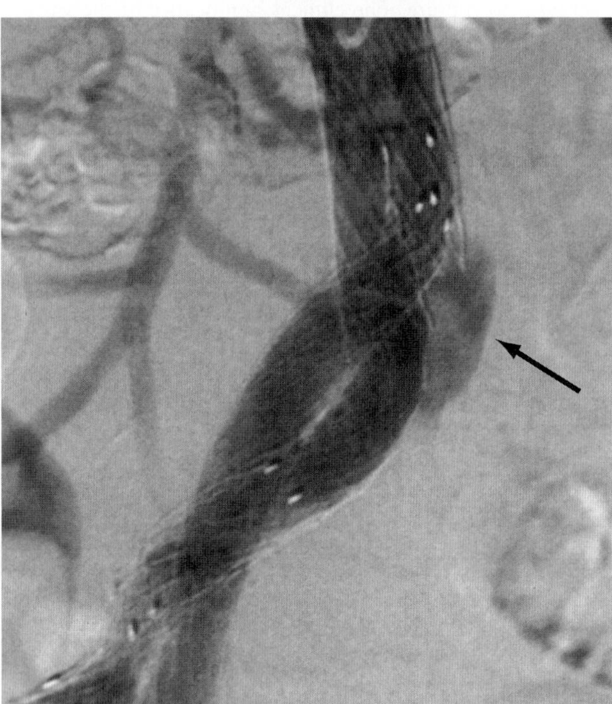

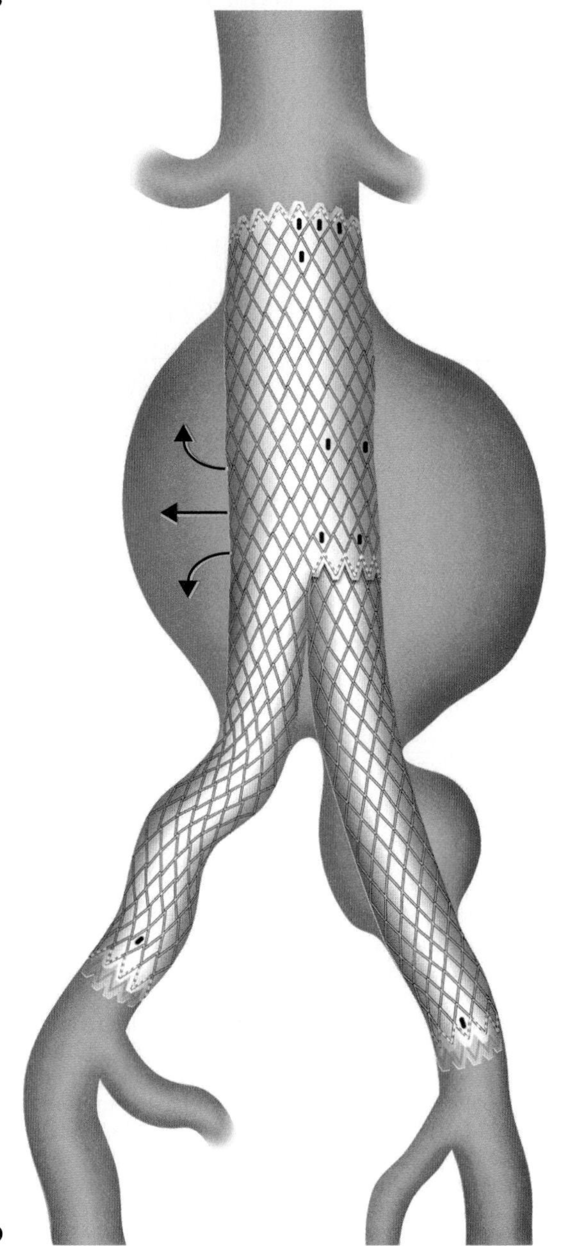

FIGURE 102.8 The various endoleaks are demonstrated. (*A*) Type 1 leaks originate at either the proximal or distal attachment sites. Note the large blush of contrast outside of the graft lumen at the proximal fixation site. (*B*) Type 2 leaks are from the collateral circulation originating in the lumbar or inferior mesenteric arteries. Note the contrast filled limbs of the graft and the rim of contrast outside the limbs of the graft, but within the lumen of the aorta. The other computed tomography images demonstrated that the leak originated from the inferior mesenteric artery. (*C*) Type 3 leaks are caused by fabric tears or problems at the graft interfaces of the modular devices. Note the contrast blush outside of the lumen of the graft at the modular interface. (*D*) Type 4 leaks are usually transient (<24 hours) transgraft extravasations and can result from the porosity of the graft and needle holes.

clusions from both the initial DREAM trial[111] and EVAR Trial[51] publications highlight this limitation. It is not surprising that this remains an outstanding issue since the technology has not been around long enough to withstand the proverbial "test of time." It is clear that the endovascular approach is not as secure a repair as the more traditional, open alternative. The endovascular repair is associated with ongoing rupture risk that likely approaches 1% per year.[108,112] The risk of rupture has been shown to be associated with poor patient selection, operator error, unrecognized/untreated endoleaks, large aneurysms, and device migration.[108,113] Interestingly, the mortality rate associated with rupture after endovascular repair may be less than for de novo ruptures.[114] Approximately 10% to 20% of patients develop an endoleak during the first year after endovascular repair and an additional 10% to 20% develop a new or late endoleak.[115–117] Admittedly, not all of these require remediation. The excluded aneurysms can continue to grow and thereby represent an ongoing rupture risk. This has been correlated with the presence of endoleak as noted previously but also with the specific device used for the repair and the baseline aneurysm size.[118,119] Additionally, some type of structural failure including fabric tears, hook fractures, and suture breakage has been reported for almost every device. Design modifications have been implemented to overcome many of these deficiencies although they represent an ongoing concern that may not be manifest for years after implantation. As a consequence of all these potential limitations, reintervention is necessary in about 15% of the patients/ year.[116] Most of these remedial procedures are catheter based with the risk of open conversion approximately 1% to 2% per year.[112] Unfortunately, the perioperative complication rate for open conversion likely exceeds that for open repair as might be predicted given its complexity. It is important to emphasize that open aneurysm repair is associated with a small incidence of graft-related complications and need for remedial procedures. Approximately 2% of patients undergoing open repair require reintervention within the first 5 years,[36] whereas graft-related complications and graft-related deaths have been reported in 15% and 2% of patients respectively at 15 years.[120]

The presence of significant comorbidities and advanced age favors the endovascular approach. Although the operative threshold in regards to the aneurysm diameter measurement is the same, the endovascular approach allows a subset of patients not considered suitable candidates for an open operation to have their aneurysms repaired. Indeed, endovascular aneurysm repair has been shown to be feasible in patients with hepatic insufficiency[121] and consistently safe in octogenarians.[122] Despite the potential nephrotoxicity associated with iodinated contrast, chronic renal insufficiency is not an absolute contraindication to endovascular repair. Strategies to reduce the associated risk can be employed including the administration acetylcysteine and sodium bicarbonate.[73,74] Alternatively, the procedure can be performed using intravascular ultrasound or the less nephrotoxic contrast agent gadolinium.[123]

The uncertainty about the long-term outcome after endovascular repair mandates indefinite postoperative surveillance. It is imperative that patients comply with the prescribed protocol and their ability/desire to fulfill these expectations should be factored into the specific choice of procedure. It is important to note that, although the incidence of complications declines with the number of negative postoperative CT scans, new endoleaks have been discovered as long as 7 years postprocedure. Similarly, it is imperative that all surgeons that offer endovascular aneurysm repair provide conscientious, long-term follow-up.

The cost comparisons between the open and endovascular approach have been somewhat inconclusive. The shorter hospital length of stay and lower incidence of major complications have predictably resulted in a reduction in some of the hospital costs. However, these have been offset by increases in other hospital-related costs with the cost of the device itself representing the single largest item. Notably, Sternbergh and Money[124] reported that the cost of the device accounted for 52% of the total cost of the endovascular repair and estimated that the costs of open and endovascular repair were $12,546 and $19,985 respectively in the AneuRx phase II clinical trial. Analysis of the hospital costs and reimbursement associated with endovascular repair among seven medical centers (three university hospitals and four community hospitals) demonstrated a net loss of $2,162.[124,125] However, other analyses have reported that the contribution to the hospital margin on a daily basis may be superior for endovascular repair given the associated shorter duration of stay that permits higher throughput, fuller overhead amortization, and better use of inpatient beds.[126] It is important to note that most of the analyses have focused on the hospital and device related costs, but have failed to include the associated professional fees and the costs associated with long-term follow-up that may be quite substantial. Indeed, it has been reported that the overall cost of endovascular repair may be twice that for the open approach.[108]

Despite the various advantages and disadvantages of the approaches outlined previously, patients seem to prefer the endovascular approach and this patient preference appears to be one of the driving forces for the widespread application of the technique. Indeed, it is uncommon for patients that are candidates for either approach to elect open repair. Notably, Williamson et al.[127] reported that 18% of all patients undergoing open repair would not undergo the procedure again. The potential to perform the endovascular repair completely percutaneously (i.e. no femoral artery exposure) will likely further increase the appeal of the approach.[128] However, a follow-up study from the DREAM trial reported that patients undergoing endovascular had a better quality of life initially after the procedure, but those undergoing open repair had a better quality at 6 months and beyond.[129]

The proverbial "bottom line" for the open versus endovascular debate remains unresolved. The Joint Council of the American Association for Vascular Surgery and the Society for Vascular Surgery have recommended that endovascular repair is most appropriate for patients at increased risk for open repair because of its uncertain long-term durability and need for surveillance.[36] The subset of patients at increased risk includes older, sicker patients and those with other mitigating anatomic concerns such as the proverbial "hostile abdomen." The recommendations further emphasize that extending the limits of the endovascular approach to patients that are poor anatomic candidates increases the incidence of adverse outcome. Notably, similar recommendations regarding the role of the endovascular approach were reached in a recent review article[108] and a decision analysis model using the EUROSTAR registry data.[130]

OPERATIVE REPAIR

Preoperative Evaluation

The preoperative evaluation of patients undergoing elective abdominal aortic aneurysm repair is similar to that of patients undergoing any major general or vascular surgical procedure. Patients undergoing endovascular repair should likely undergo the same preoperative work-up despite the perception that associated perioperative stresses are less. All patients should receive a complete history, and a physical examination, electrocardiogram, and a chest radiograph. Routine laboratory studies, including a complete blood cell count with platelets, measurement of serum creatinine and serum electrolyte levels, and coagulation studies, should be obtained. A specimen should be sent to the blood bank and the appropriate quantity of blood products cross-matched. This number can be determined from the historic operative transfusion requirements obtained from the blood bank but usually 2 to 4 units of packed red blood cells are sufficient. A thorough peripheral pulse examination should be included in the physical examination and validated with formal ankle–brachial indices. The anesthesiologist should see the patients preoperatively, and a bowel preparation with mechanical lavage should be performed the day before surgery. Additionally, patients should be started on a beta-blocker, an aspirin, and a statin (HMG CoA reductase inhibitors) agent if they are not already using them. The American College of Cardiology/American Heart Association Guideline Update on Perioperative Cardiovascular Evaluation for Noncardiac Surgery recommends that the beta-blockers be titrated to a target resting heart rate between 50 and 60 beats per minute based on the evidence that perioperative beta-blockade reduces perioperative ischemia and may reduce the incidence of myocardial infarction and death.[131] Although not part of the American College of Cardiology/American Heart Association Perioperative Guidelines, a recent study demonstrated that statins were associated with a decreased incidence of perioperative mortality and nonfatal myocardial infarction after aneurysm repair.[132] Indeed, all patients with atherosclerotic cardiovascular disease should likely be taking aspirin, beta-blockers, a lipid-lowering agent, and an angiotensin-converting enzyme inhibitor long-term as part of the American Heart Association/American College of Cardiology (AHA/ACC) Guidelines for Preventing Heart Attack and Death in Patients with Atherosclerotic Cardiovascular Disease.[133]

All active medical problems, including abnormalities identified during the preoperative evaluation, should be controlled as well as possible before elective aneurysm repair. However, extensive diagnostic testing is probably unnecessary. Routine pulmonary function tests and measurement of arterial blood gases are not indicated, although they may be beneficial in selected patients with advanced chronic obstructive pulmonary disease.[134] The presence of chronic obstructive pulmonary disease often complicates postoperative ventilator management, but it is unusual for a patient's pulmonary disease to be sufficiently severe to preclude operation.[135] Furthermore, the history and physical examination alone are sufficient to identify this small subset of patients. Similarly, timed urine collections for creatinine clearance and other assessments of renal function have not proved beneficial despite the dramatic impact of preoperative renal insufficiency on perioperative outcome although it may be beneficial to calculate the estimated glomerular filtration rate as noted previously.

The appropriate cardiac work-up before abdominal aortic aneurysm repair remains controversial and is somewhat institution-dependent. This controversy has been further complicated by the publication of the Coronary Artery Revascularization Prophylaxis (CARP). Trial that examined the role of coronary artery revascularization before major vascular surgery among patients with significant coronary artery disease.[136] Notably, the study reported that preoperative coronary artery revascularization did not reduce the incidence of either perioperative myocardial infarction or long-term mortality. It is important to emphasize that the overall objective of the preoperative cardiac workup is to optimize the cardiovascular system and thereby reduce both the perioperative and long-term risk of myocardial infarction and death. Admittedly, the prevalence of coronary artery disease among patients undergoing abdominal aortic aneurysm repair is quite high. Hertzer et al.,[137] in a landmark publication, reported that 25% of 1,000 patients undergoing evaluation for peripheral vascular surgery (cerebral vascular occlusive disease, lower extremity arterial occlusive disease, abdominal aortic aneurysm) had severe, surgically correctable lesions detected during cardiac catheterization; 6% had severe, uncorrectable disease, and only 8% had no evidence of disease. Interestingly, the incidence of surgically correctable disease was highest among patients undergoing evaluation for abdominal aortic aneurysm. The AHA/ACC Perioperative Guidelines include an extensive algorithm for cardiac assessment.[131] Briefly, patients with major clinical predictors of perioperative cardiovascular risk (unstable coronary syndromes, decompensated congestive heart failure, significant arrhythmias, and significant valvular disease) should be seen in consultation by a cardiologist and considered for catheterization with the subsequent care dictated by the findings. Patients with intermediate clinical predictors (mild angina, prior myocardial infarction, compensated congestive heart failure, diabetes) undergoing high-risk surgical procedures such as abdominal aortic aneurysm repair should undergo noninvasive cardiac testing and potentially cardiac catheterization/revascularization depending on the results. Patients with minor clinical predictors (advanced age, abnormal electrocardiogram, minor arrhythmias, history of stroke, poorly controlled hypertension) and moderate or excellent functional capacity (more than four metabolic equivalent levels) can undergo high-risk surgical procedures without further cardiac evaluation, but those with poor functional capacity should undergo noninvasive cardiac testing as outlined for patients with intermediate predictors. Unfortunately, the majority of patients undergoing evaluation for abdominal aortic aneurysm repair (high-risk surgical procedure) require noninvasive cardiac testing as part of the AHA/ACC algorithm. Notably, there is insufficient evidence to support a reduced cardiac workup for patients undergoing endovascular repair.[138] It is important to emphasize that although the cardiac risk of endovascular repair may be less, the subset of patients undergoing the procedure are often older and sicker than those undergoing open repair.

All patients should undergo some type of imaging modality as part of their preoperative evaluation to confirm the diagnosis and plan the operative procedure. Indeed, determining whether a patient is an endovascular candidate and appropriately sizing the device depend on the anatomic measurements obtained at the time of imaging. CT of the chest, abdomen, and pelvis is the optimal imaging study to visualize the aneurysm and is the only imaging study required in most cases. Abdominal ultrasonography is insufficient as the sole imaging study before aneurysm repair in light of its inability to accurately determine the cephalad extent of the aneurysm and the involvement of the iliac vessels. Preoperative arteriography may be helpful as an adjunct to standard CT among the subset of patients undergoing endovascular or standard surgical repair that have renal anomalies or occlusive disease in the renal, mesenteric, or aortoiliac vessels.

Open Repair of Intact Abdominal Aortic Aneurysms

Technique

A significant amount of preparation is required in the operating room before making the incision and this preparation needs to be coordinated among the surgical and anesthetic teams for both the open and endovascular approach. Although the decision about the choice of anesthesia is deferred to the anesthesiologists, inhalation agents and an endotracheal tube are used most frequently. Adjunctive epidural anesthesia may improve postoperative pain control[139] and may be beneficial in patients with severe pulmonary disease.[140] Adequate intravenous access should be established to facilitate resuscitation. Central venous access is usually obtained although not necessary. Electrocardiographic leads, an arterial catheter, and a Foley catheter should be placed for continuous monitoring of the electrocardiogram, arterial pressure, and urine output, respectively. Additionally, a nasogastric tube should be inserted. A Swan-Ganz pulmonary artery catheter or a transesophageal echocardiogram probe should be inserted in patients with significant cardiac disease. However, routine use of pulmonary artery catheters in patients undergoing aortic surgery is not recommended and may be associated with a higher rate of intraoperative complications.[141,142] Peripheral arterial pulses should be integrated with either palpation or continuous-wave Doppler ultrasound and marked to facilitate confirmation after restoration of lower extremity perfusion. Strategies to maintain core body temperature should be initiated.[141,143] Specifically, the room temperature should be increased, warming devices should be attached to all intravenous infusion lines, and either a recirculating alcohol blanket or forced-air blanket should be applied. Bush et al.[144] reported that hypothermia (<34.5°C) during abdominal aortic aneurysm repair was associated with multiple physiologic derangements and adverse outcomes. Use of an intraoperative autologous transfusion device should be considered. However, a recent meta-analysis of five randomized, controlled trials reported that there is insufficient evidence to recommend its use during vascular surgery including aortic surgery.[145] These devices should likely be used when a significant amount of blood loss is anticipated such as during suprarenal or thoracoabdominal aortic aneurysms. Furthermore, they can be helpful in patients who object to blood transfusions on religious principles. An extensive operative field from "nipples to toes" should be prepared with the use of topical antimicrobial agents. A first-generation cephalosporin or vancomycin should be administered prior to the incision.

Abdominal aortic aneurysms may be repaired through several different incisions/approaches including midline, retroperitoneal, or transverse (supraumbilical straight, infraumbilical straight, infraumbilical curvilinear, bilateral subcostal). The incisions/approaches must be viewed as complementary because not one is perfect for every clinical scenario. Indeed, surgeons should be familiar with the various approaches and select the optimal one for the clinical setting. The determinants of the incision include the cephalad/caudal extent of the aneurysm, body habitus, presence of prior abdominal incisions, presence of abdominal wall stomas, comorbidities, additional intraoperative pathology, inflammatory aneurysms, renal anomalies, requirements for concomitant procedures, urgency of aortic control, and surgeon preference. The midline approach is preferable for patients with ruptured abdominal aortic aneurysms because aortic control at the level of the diaphragm can be obtained rapidly. The bilateral subcostal approach provides the best exposure and is the incision of choice for obese patients, patients with extensive iliac artery aneurysms, patients requiring concomitant renal artery revascularization, and patients with juxtarenal aneurysms that require suprarenal aortic control. The retroperitoneal approach is optimal for patients with multiple previous abdominal incisions ("hostile abdomen"), abdominal wall stomas, suprarenal aneurysms, inflammatory aneurysms, and

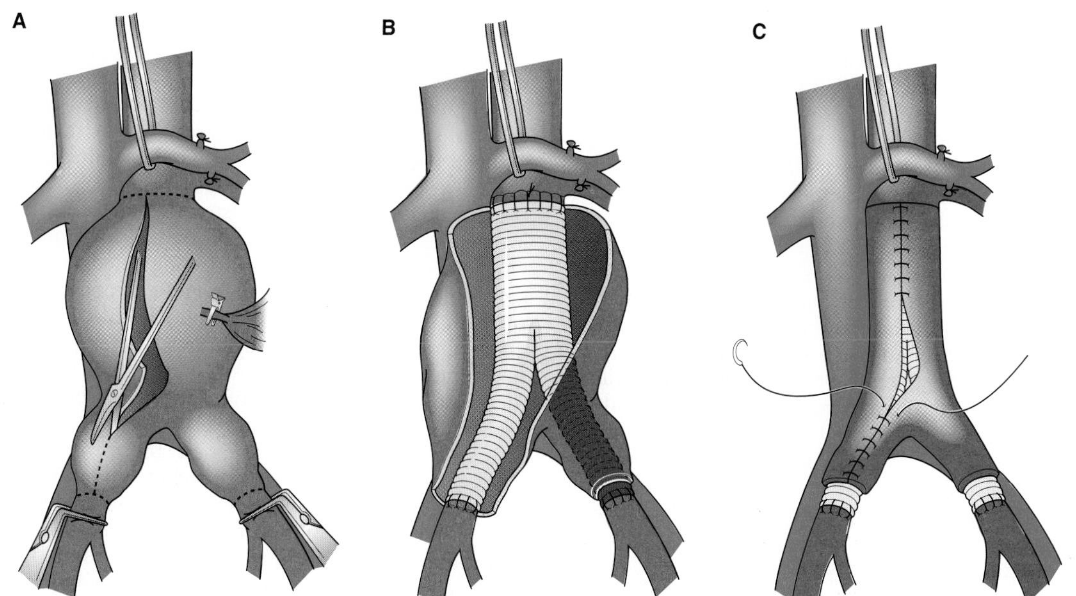

FIGURE 102.9 Steps involved in the standard repair of an infrarenal abdominal aortic aneurysm extending into the proximal common iliac arteries. (*A*) The proximal duodenum is mobilized and the retroperitoneum overlying the aorta incised. The infrarenal aorta immediately below the renal vein is dissected. The iliac bifurcations are exposed, and vascular clamps are applied to the infrarenal aorta and distal common iliac arteries after adequate heparinization. A longitudinal arteriotomy is extended from the infrarenal aorta onto the right common iliac artery. (*B*) Back bleeding from the lumbar arteries is controlled with figure-of-eight sutures. The proximal anastomosis is performed in an end-to-end configuration below the renal arteries. The distal anastomoses are performed at the common iliac bifurcation beyond the aneurysmal segments. The left limb of the graft is tunneled through the intact left common iliac aneurysm shell. (*C*) The residual aneurysm shell is closed over the prosthetic graft, and the retroperitoneum is reapproximated to prevent erosion of the graft into the overlying bowel.

horseshoe kidneys. However, the retroperitoneal approach is limited by the inability to assess the intraperitoneal structures adequately and the limited access to the right renal artery and right iliac vessels. It was previously argued that the retroperitoneal approach posed less of a physiologic insult than the transperitoneal approach and, therefore, was ideal for patients with advanced pulmonary or cardiac disease. However, this contention has not been supported by a prospective, randomized trial.[146] A detailed description of the retroperitoneal approach is beyond the context of this chapter but is available in most standard vascular surgical texts.

The sequence of steps used to repair an intact, infrarenal abdominal aortic aneurysm after a bilateral subcostal incision can be summarized (Fig. 102.9). The abdomen is explored after the peritoneal cavity is entered, and both the gallbladder and colon carefully examined. The lower abdominal wall flap is immobilized to either the drapes or the pubic towel with the use of penetrating towel clips. The small bowel is manually retracted laterally to the right, and the duodenum is mobilized by incising the ligament of Treitz. The inferior mesenteric vein may be suture-ligated at this juncture to facilitate exposure. The tissue adjacent to the inferior mesenteric vein should be palpated to rule out a large, meandering mesenteric artery. This artery is an important visceral collateral and should be preserved. The retroperitoneum over the aorta is incised with the electrocautery, and the left renal vein is exposed. Self-retaining Buckwalter retractors are then placed to facilitate further exposure. The small bowel is placed in a bowel bag, eviscerated, and retracted laterally to the right with the aid of malleable retractors for the Buckwalter. The transverse colon and superior abdominal wall flap are retracted cephalad while the lower abdominal wall is further retracted caudal. The aorta immediately inferior to the renal arteries is exposed and both renal arteries visualized. The infrarenal aorta at this location is dissected circumferentially to facilitate placement of a transverse aortic clamp. However, this step may be omitted if a vertical clamp is used. It is important to identify the course of the renal vein and any venous anomalies on the preoperative CT scan to prevent inadvertently injuring these structures at this stage of the procedure. In the presence of a retroaortic renal vein or circumaortic collar, the aortic neck should not be dissected circumferentially and vascular control should be obtained with a vertical clamp. The retroperitoneum over the aorta is then incised further caudally and the incision extended along the course of the right common iliac artery. The extent of the caudal dissection depends on the anatomic configuration of the aneurysm. If the aneurysm extends to the aortic bifurcation, it is sufficient to dissect only the common iliac arteries provided a suitable site for clamp application is identified. If the aneurysm extends to the distal common iliac arteries, both the internal and external iliac vessels should be dissected free. This may be facilitated on the left side by mobilizing the sigmoid colon along its peritoneal reflection and reflecting it medially. The inferior mesenteric artery is then dissected free and vascular control obtained with a vessel loop. Patients are administered 100 units of intravenous heparin per kilogram, and the activated clotting time is confirmed to be twice the baseline value. Supplemental doses of heparin are administered throughout the procedure as dictated by the activated clotting time. Interestingly, a recent randomized, controlled trial reported that heparin does not reduce thrombotic events or increase bleeding during aneurysm repair but is associated with a significant reduction in myocardial events.[147] Additionally, 0.5 mg of mannitol per kilogram is administered before clamp application.[148]

During the time required for adequate mixing of the heparin, the availability of the necessary equipment is reviewed and confirmed with the operating room personnel. The appropriately sized tube or bifurcated prosthetic graft is selected. The graft diameter is sized according to the infrarenal aortic neck by visual inspection or with calibrated sizers. The general "rule of thumb" is that the smaller graft should be selected when the aorta is between two graft sizes because the aorta always appears smaller after it is transected and redundant graft material at the proximal anastomosis is more difficult to correct than the opposite problem. A variety of vascular prostheses are available. Despite the contentions of the various manufacturers, there is no clear advantage for an individual graft and the choice should be determined by surgeon preference as dictated by ease of handling, cost, availability, and requirements for preclotting. The distal vascular clamps are applied to the external, internal, or common iliac vessels depending on the extent of the aneurysm and the character of the vessels. Occasionally, the iliac vessels are so calcified that they cannot be safely occluded with a clamp. Vascular control may be obtained intraluminally in this setting with the use of a balloon thromboembolectomy catheter after the aneurysm has been incised. The proximal aortic clamp is applied in sequence after the distal clamps. The clamp is applied immediately below the renal arteries to facilitate an anastomosis to the proximal infrarenal aorta. The length of the infrarenal aorta should be sufficient to permit a safe anastomosis. However, a long infrarenal cuff should be avoided because it may become aneurysmal over time. Either a vertical or horizontal aortic clamp may be used, although the latter is preferred because it simplifies the anastomosis. The aorta is then incised longitudinally, and the incision is extended down the right common iliac artery as necessary. Attempts should be made to preserve the autonomic nerves overlying the distal aorta and proximal left common iliac artery in potent men. This can usually be achieved by incising the left common iliac artery transversely beyond the aneurysmal portion and tunneling the limb of the graft through the residual shell. The intraluminal thrombus and debris are removed from within the aorta, and all back bleeding from the lumbar arteries is controlled with suture ligatures. The atheromatous debris within the aorta has been reported to be culture-positive in approximately 25% of cases, although this finding has not been associated with long-term graft infections.[149,150] The infrarenal aorta at the level of the planned proximal anastomosis may be completely transected, or the back wall may be left intact. Completely transecting the aorta makes the proximal anastomoses slightly easier although leaving the back wall intact reinforces the anastomosis and provides the equivalent of an autogenous pledget. The proximal anastomosis is performed in an end-end configuration with a running 3-0 cardiovascular suture. All leaks in the suture line are repaired with similar 4-0 sutures and felt pledgets as necessary. The distal anastomosis or anastomoses are performed to the aortic bifurcation, common iliac arteries, or iliac bifurcation as dictated by the anatomy of the aneurysm. A 3-0 cardiovascular suture is used for anastomoses at the aortic bifurcation, and a similar 4-0 suture is used for the common iliac arteries. All anastomoses are flushed before flow is restored to remove any intraluminal debris. Blood flow is restored to the pelvis and lower extremities in sequence. Attempts should be made to flush initially into the internal iliac circulation to prevent embolization to the lower extremities, which can be facilitated by manually compressing the common femoral arteries for tube graft configurations. The lower torso should be reperfused gradually (i.e., one vessel at a time and one extremity at a time) to prevent hypotension and other acute sequelae associated with the reperfusion of ischemic tissues. This process requires significant communication and coordination between the surgical and anesthetic teams. It is imperative that the patient is resuscitated prior to reperfusion and it is frequently necessary to delay this process to allow the anesthesiologists to achieve this objective. Reperfusion of the ischemic tissue causes the release of acid, potassium, and a variety of inflammatory mediators into the systemic circulation, all of which are potentially detrimental.

The inferior mesenteric artery should be reimplanted into either the body of the graft or the left limb if it is patent. Seeger et al.[151] reported that routine reimplantation of the inferior mesenteric artery resulted in decreased rates of colonic infarction and death after aortic reconstruction. The colon and lower extremities should be interrogated with the Doppler ultrasound after reperfusion, and heparin is reversed with intravenous protamine sulfate after confirmation of adequate signals. Protamine dose is estimated based on the effectiveness of protamine (1 mg of protamine per 100 units of heparin), the initial dose of heparin, the current activated clotting time, and the elapsed time from the administration of heparin. The protamine should be administered slowly to prevent any untoward hemodynamic events.[152] Notably, a recent randomized, controlled trial reported that protamine effectively reverses the heparin effect but provides no clinical benefit during peripheral vascular surgery, including aneurysm repair.[153] The shell of the aneurysm and the overlying retroperitoneum are both closed with absorbable suture after adequate hemostasis to provide a biologic tissue layer between the graft and the viscera. The retractors are then removed, the viscera are returned to their anatomic positions, the nasogastric tube is confirmed to be in the antrum, and the abdominal wall fascia is closed with standard technique. Interestingly, patients undergoing aortic reconstruction for aneurysmal disease have been reported to have a higher incidence of abdominal wall hernias than those undergoing reconstruction for occlusive disease.[154–156]

The configuration of the aortic reconstruction (aortoaortic, aortoiliac, aortofemoral) depends on the extent of aneurysmal involvement and the degree of occlusive disease. Aneurysmal involvement of the common iliac vessels should be considered an extension of the aortic process and treated appropriately. Specifically, common iliac arteries larger than 2.0 cm should be considered aneurysmal and replaced. The entire common iliac artery usually must be replaced, although it is possible to replace only the proximal segment if the aneurysmal involvement is isolated. Conversely, common iliac arteries smaller than 2.0 cm have a relatively benign natural history and do not need to be replaced because only a small percentage ultimately become aneurysmal and require treatment.[28,29] Despite the fact that a patient may be a candidate for an aortic tube graft, it is often easier to perform an aortobiiliac graft because the terminal aorta is often very calcified. Aortobifemoral bypass grafts should be reserved for the small subset of patients who truly have concomitant aneurysms and severe occlusive disease because the risks of wound complications and graft infections are significantly greater. Indeed, the risk for graft infections is less than 0.5% for aortobiiliac grafts but approximately 2% for aortobifemoral grafts.[28,29,157] It is imperative to remember the original indication for the procedure and choose the appropriate aortic reconstruction (aortobiiliac bypass for aortoiliac aneurysm, aortobifemoral bypass for aortoiliac occlusive disease). Admittedly, there is a role for aortobifemoral reconstructions in patients with aneurysmal disease, and it is futile to attempt an aortobiiliac reconstruction in patients with severe external iliac artery disease.

The postoperative care after open repair is fairly routine and predictable for the majority of patients. Patients are transferred directly from the operating room to the intensive care unit although selective use of the intensive care unit may be appropriate.[158] Most of the patients are extubated in the operating room or shortly after arrival in the intensive care unit. The intensive care unit length of stay is usually 1 to 2 days, and the median total length of stay is 8 days.[23] Patients are encouraged to get out of bed and begin ambulating in the early postoperative period (24 to 48 hours). Preoperative prophylactic antibiotics are continued for a total of 24 hours. Nasogastric decompression is continued until bowel function returns. Oral feedings are initiated after removal of the nasogastric tube and advanced quickly to solids. Patients are discharged when they are ambulatory, can tolerate a regular diet, have normal bowel function, and are sufficiently able to care for themselves. A small subset of people requires transfer to rehabilitation or extended care facility. Patients are usually seen in the clinic two weeks after discharge and then at 6 months. Additional clinic appointments may be necessary as dictated by any ongoing medical problems. Patients are not allowed to drive until their incisional pain has resolved and they have stopped taking pain medications. Furthermore, patients are discouraged from lifting objects heavier than 10 lbs for the first 6 months to reduce the incidence of an incisional hernia.

Complications and Outcome

Open repair of intact abdominal aortic aneurysms is associated with significant mortality and morbidity.[23,159,160] The attendant mortality rates have been discussed extensively in the preceding sections entitled Principles of Management and Choice of Open or Endovascular Repair. Briefly, the nationwide mortality rate is approximately 4%,[23] but it ranges from approximately 3% to 10% among the various surgeon, institution, state, and national series. The overall morbidity rate remains less clear, although the specific complications have been well defined. Huber et al.[23] reported that 33% of all patients undergoing repair of intact abdominal aortic aneurysms across the United States develop some type of complication as defined by the *International Classification of Diseases, Ninth Revision* (ICD-9), postoperative complication codes. Similarly, Hua et al.[161] reported from the National Surgical Quality Improvement Program—Private Sector that the overall incidence of morbidity after open repair was 35%.

Intraoperative complications can result from injury to the intraabdominal structures during dissection, although these technical complications are not necessarily specific to the aneurysm repair. The small bowel, colon, ureter, and major venous structures (inferior vena cava, iliac veins, left renal vein) are particularly susceptible. Iatrogenic bowel injury at the time of abdominal aortic aneurysm repair is particularly problematic because of the potential to infect the prosthetic graft. If the colon is injured before the aneurysm repair, the defect in the colon should be fixed and the aneurysm repair should be aborted. If the small bowel is injured before the aneurysm repair, the same course should likely be followed although this decision requires a modicum of clinical judgment. The infectious concerns must be balanced by the fact that the small bowel contents are sterile, patients usually receive a preoperative bowel preparation, a second procedure will be required to repair the aneurysm, and there is a small risk of aneurysm rupture during the intervening delay. Injury to the bowel during or after implantation of the aortic graft should be treated with repair of the defect, extensive irrigation, and prolonged antibiotics. Admittedly, these approaches are very conservative and it is noteworthy that multiple clinical series have attested to the safety of simultaneous aortic and gastrointestinal/urologic procedures.[162–165] The ureter is most susceptible to injury at the point where it crosses over the iliac bifurcation. Injury can be avoided by a heightened awareness of this anatomic location and dissection in the tissue plane immediately on top of the common iliac vessels. Inadvertent venous injury can be associated with significant bleeding, which can usually be controlled by direct pressure using sponge sticks and suture repair. The left renal vein may be transected if necessary. It should be transected near its juncture with the vena cava, and the gonadal, adrenal, and lumbar branches should be preserved to maintain venous outflow from the kidney. Although somewhat inelegant, division of the left renal vein does not appear to affect renal function after abdominal aortic aneurysm repair.[166] Transecting the iliac artery or infrarenal aorta may facilitate exposure of the iliac or retroaortic renal veins, respectively.

Excessive intraoperative bleeding may be encountered occasionally. Routine elective aneurysm repairs are usually associated with moderate intraoperative blood loss with a mean transfusion requirement of 1 to 2 units of packed red blood cells. Excessive bleeding may be caused by either the surgical trauma or coagulopathy. Reversal of the heparin with protamine may help correct the coagulopathic bleeding. Patients with significant bleeding and platelet counts less than 50,000/mL should receive a platelet transfusion, and it should be considered for coagulopathic bleeding and counts below 100,000/mL. Transfusions of fresh frozen plasma are indicated both for patients with either significant bleeding in conjunction with prolonged coagulation studies (>1.5 times control value) and for those with coagulopathic bleeding. Massive bleeding, defined as more than 100% of the blood volume, may induce a dilutional coagulopathy with prolongation of the coagulation studies. Additional blood products should be set up in the blood bank in the event of significant bleeding. This process may require an additional blood bank specimen. Intraoperative autologous transfusion devices should also be considered if not already in use.

Ischemia of the lower extremities has been reported to occur in approximately 3% of cases after open repair.[160] The causes are multiple and include distal embolization, thrombosis, clamp injury, and technical errors. The lumen of the aneurysm is frequently filled with both thrombus and atheroma that may serve as a source for both macroembolization and microembolization. The macroemboli usually lodge at a bifurcation of major vessels; the microemboli usually lodge in the digital vessels and, unfortunately, are not amenable to mechanical extraction. Thrombosis may result from inadequate heparinization, hypercoagulable conditions, or poor arterial runoff. The technical conduct of the operation outlined previously is designed to minimize the ischemic complications. The specific maneuvers include anticoagulation, selection of a suitable site for distal clamp application and anastomosis, intraluminal control of severely calcified vessels, flushing of the vessels before clamp removal, and sequential removal of the vascular clamps. Further intervention is mandatory if the lower extremities are found to be ischemic. Anastomotic defects should be corrected. Correction may simply require dissembling and redoing the anastomosis, but often requires relocating it further distal on the outflow artery. If no problems are identified at the distal anastomosis, the femoral vessels should be explored and thrombectomized. A transverse arteriotomy may be created in the common femoral artery if it is anticipated that only a thrombectomy will be required; a longitudinal incision should be created if a bypass (inflow or outflow) procedure is anticipated. The transverse arteriotomy can simply be closed with interrupted sutures without narrowing the lumen in the event that an additional bypass procedure is not necessary, whereas the longitudinal arteriotomy requires a patch closure. A bypass from the aortic graft to the femoral vessels is required if adequate inflow cannot be restored with thrombectomy alone. The popliteal artery below the knee should be explored and thrombectomized if the extremity is still ischemic after adequate inflow is restored. This may be facilitated by creating a longitudinal arteriotomy on the below knee popliteal artery to the tibioperoneal trunk to allow cannulation of all three crural vessels. A below knee popliteal or tibial artery bypass is required if adequate perfusion to the distal extremity is not restored after patch closure of the popliteal arteriotomy. Predictably, a complex lower extremity revascularization in addition to an aortic reconstruction is associated with a significant degree of morbidity and dramatically increases the mortality rate.[167] The decision to proceed with an infrainguinal bypass depends on the status of the extremity and requires clinical judgment. Aborting the procedure and allowing for a period of observation and rewarming is appropriate when popliteal Doppler signals are detected and the foot is cool yet not severely ischemic. Reoperation and definitive treatment may be necessary in the early postoperative period unless marked improvement is noted.

Many of the systemic complications that follow open aneurysm repair are not surprising, given the magnitude of the operation and the age/comorbidities of the patients. Cardiac complications (ischemia, infarction, arrhythmias, congestive heart failure) occur in up to 25%[159,160,168] and are the leading cause of death after open aneurysm repair in many series. Pulmonary complications (pneumonia, ventilatory dependence greater than 48 hours, acute respiratory distress syndrome) are also quite common and approximately 10% of the patients require prolonged ventilation.[159,160] Deterioration of renal function, defined by an increase in serum creatinine or blood urea nitrogen, occurs in approximately 5% of cases although acute renal failure requiring dialysis is rare (<1%).[160] The potential causes of renal insufficiency in the perioperative period are numerous and include contrast nephrotoxicity, hypovolemia, atheroembolization, and the inflammatory response from the lower torso ischemia/reperfusion injury. Postoperative bleeding requiring reexploration, intraabdominal abscess, and abdominal wound complications are all relatively infrequent complications and are associated with all major intraabdominal procedures.

Ischemic colitis has been reported to occur in approximately 2% to 13% of cases after open aneurysm repair.[169] The reported incidence depends on the diagnostic algorithm and modality (routine sigmoidoscopy versus selective sigmoidoscopy) and is dramatically increased after ruptured aneurysm repair. Indeed, the incidence of colonic ischemia after ruptured aneurysm repair in patients undergoing routine colonoscopy is approximately 25% to 40%.[169,170] The sigmoid colon is affected most frequently although all the sections of the colon may be involved. The ischemia may result from inadequate resuscitation, disruption of collaterals, and/or failure to revascularize a hemodynamically significant inferior mesenteric artery. Patients usually present with bloody diarrhea in the early postoperative period. However, the diagnosis should be considered in the absence of bloody diarrhea in patients with thrombocytopenia, multiple-organ dysfunction, increasing abdominal pain or peritonitis, and generalized failure to thrive. The diagnosis may be confirmed by endoscopy. Although sigmoidoscopy is used most frequently, a complete colonoscopy is likely optimal due to the potential involvement of the other colon segments. Treatment depends on the endoscopic findings and clinical setting. The endoscopic findings range from mucosal ischemia to transmural necrosis. Unfortunately, it is often difficult to differentiate diffuse mucosal ischemia from transmural necrosis. Patients with mucosal ischemia alone should be treated with bowel rest, broad-spectrum antibiotics, total parenteral nutrition, and serial endoscopic examinations. Many of these lesions resolve spontaneously without long-term sequelae although colonic strictures may develop in a subset of patients. Patients with transmural colonic necrosis should undergo laparotomy with resection of the involved segment, a proximal diverting colostomy, and a distal Hartmann pouch. After laparotomy, they should be maintained on broad-spectrum antibiotics and parenteral nutrition. The reported mortality rate in patients with transmural necrosis is approximately 85%.[169] Maintaining antegrade flow through the internal iliac vessels, routinely implanting the inferior mesenteric artery, and avoiding disruption of the colonic collateral circulation may largely prevent this adverse outcome.

Several other gastrointestinal complications are relatively common after standard infrarenal abdominal aortic aneurysm repair.[171] A postoperative ileus develops in essentially all patients. Bowel function usually returns within 3 to 5 days after repair, at which time the nasogastric tube is removed and oral feedings are initiated. An ileus may persist beyond this time period in a subset of patients although no additional specific therapy is usually required. Nasogastric decompression should be continued, narcotics minimized, electrolytes normalized, and ambulation encouraged. Either calculous or acalculous cholecystitis may develop after aneurysm repair. The mortality rates historically reported for postoperative cholecystitis were significant[172] and served as the catalyst for simultaneous cholecystectomy and aneurysm repair. Although this approach has been found to be safe and not associated with an increased risk for graft infections, it is usually reserved for patients with small stones or evidence of chronic cholecystitis. Pancreatitis may develop after abdominal aortic aneurysm repair although the incidence is surprisingly low in light of the obligatory manipulation of the pancreas during repair. The treatment of pancreatitis in this setting is conservative and includes bowel rest, parenteral nutrition, and serial imaging.

Sexual dysfunction is quite common after both open and endovascular aneurysm repair as noted previously. Erectile and/or orgasmic dysfunction have been reported to occur in 5% to 18% of men undergoing aortoiliac reconstruction.[173] The responsible mechanisms include interruption of the pelvic perfusion and injury to the autonomic nerves that overlie the distal aorta/proximal common iliac arteries. Injury to these autonomic nerves disrupts the internal sphincter mechanism of the bladder and results in retrograde ejaculation. Care should be exercised during aneurysm repair to maintain pelvic perfusion and avoid nerve injury to prevent these untoward complications. It is imperative that these potential complications be discussed with patients preoperatively.

Paraplegia after open infrarenal abdominal aortic aneurysm repair occurs with an incidence of 0.25%.[174] The potential mechanisms for this devastating complication include embolization, thrombosis of the spinal artery, and disruption of the spinal blood supply from a low-lying artery of Adamkiewicz or loss of prograde flow through the internal iliac arteries. Paraplegia after aneurysm repair is an irreversible injury. Maintaining adequate prograde pelvic perfusion may potentially minimize this complication.

The long-term outcome after open repair is generally favorable. Long-term survival is improved after aneurysm repair, although it falls short of that of age-matched controls with survival rates of approximately 90%, 65%, and 40% at 1, 5, and 10 years.[2,5,175] Cardiovascular causes account for the leading cause of death.[176] This underscores the importance of long-term medical follow-up and the AHA/ACC Guidelines for preventing myocardial infarction and death.[133,176] Prosthetic aortic grafts are associated with long-term complications with a reported incidence of approximately 10 to 15% at 15 years.[108,177,178] Notably, bifurcated grafts are associated with a higher incidence of complications (13%) than tube grafts (5%).[28] The long-term graft related complications include infection, aortoenteric fistula, thrombosis, and pseudoaneurysm formation. Additional aneurysms of a sufficient size to merit intervention develop in approximately 5% to 15% of patients in either the iliac vessels or the aorta above the prosthetic graft.[28,29] It is recommended that patients undergo CT of the complete aorta and iliac vessels 5 years postoperatively to screen for graft complications and additional aneurysms. Furthermore, patients with prosthetic aortic grafts should receive prophylactic antibiotics before undergoing invasive procedures, including colonoscopy and dental extractions.

Endovascular Repair of Intact Abdominal Aortic Aneurysms

Technique

The preoperative evaluation and preparation before endovascular abdominal aortic aneurysm repair is significantly more complicated than for the open approach. The various imaging studies must be analyzed before it can be determined whether the endovascular approach is even feasible. Appropriate measurements must be taken and the necessary devices/components selected. An operative plan must be generated including specific modifications of the standard approach to overcome the patient's anatomic limitations and thereby extend the feasibility of the technique. Indeed, "preoperative planning, preoperative planning, and preoperative planning" have facetiously been identified as the three most important components of a successful repair.

A variety of imaging techniques and combinations thereof have been employed to determine the feasibility of an aneurysm for endovascular repair and select the appropriate devices/components. These include conventional CT, arteriography with marker catheters, and 3D CT with centerline measurements. All of the methodologies are likely acceptable and offer some specific advantages/disadvantages.[179] It has been reported that 3D CT may improve the accuracy for the sizing and may be more helpful in complex cases.[179] It is important to emphasize that no imaging technique is perfect and, consequently, a certain degree of flexibility is necessary for the operative plan. Measurements obtained from the 3D CT tend to overestimate the actual renal–internal iliac artery length assumed by the graft when deployed in vivo. Similar sizing limitations are associated with the arteriogram/marker catheter technique and have been attributed to the course of the catheter, the presence of intraluminal thrombus, and the conformational changes in the aorta that result from the stiff guide wires and/or the device itself.

The various devices/components should be selected using the underlying principles that the main body of the device should sit as close to the orifices of the renal arteries as possible while the iliac limbs should extend to the orifices of the internal iliac arteries. Furthermore, the manufacturers' recommendations for sizing and device selection should be followed. Grafts seated well below the orifices of the renal arteries have been associated with proximal migration[180] while oversizing the graft diameter beyond that recommended has been associated with both graft migration and aneurysm reexpansion.[181] The endograft is sized according to the anatomic configuration of the aneurysm and adjacent arteries, and it must be performed in advance of the procedure to insure that the appropriate devices are available. The diameter and length of the infrarenal cuff, aneurysm, and iliac vessels must be measured precisely, in addition to the distance from the aortic bifurcation to the iliac landing site/common iliac bifurcation. The diameter of the proximal graft is chosen to oversize the aortic cuff and iliac arteries by approximately 10% to 20%. Additional devices should be ordered for each case including two iliac limbs and an aortic extension cuff to allow the necessary flexibility to deviate from the preoperative plan. Each endograft construction is essentially customized for an individual patient. Work sheets are available from the manufacturers to confirm the suitability of an aneurysm for endovascular repair and to aid in the selection of an appropriately sized device. Technical assistance is available from the various manufacturers to facilitate essentially every step of the process from initial assessment to component selection to deployment. Furthermore, physicians are required to complete a training course comprised of sizing exercises and monitored deployments.

The choice of the specific endovascular device is contingent upon the anatomic constraints of the aneurysm, device associated outcome, and surgeon preference. There are specific differences between the various grafts that lend themselves to different clinical scenarios. The specific considerations include neck diameter, neck length/angulation, renal–hypogastric artery distance, common iliac artery diameter, and access vessel diameter. For example, a graft with suprarenal fixation may be more suitable for a shorter neck while a lower profile system may be most appropriate for patients with smaller access (common femoral and external iliac arteries) vessels. Despite the initial concerns about compromising renal function, suprarenal fixation has consistently been shown to be safe.[182] Some decrease in renal function has been shown to occur after both open and endovascular repair,[183] but only 11% of patients have been reported to have a >20% decrease after endograft repair with suprarenal fixation.[184] Deployment of the various endografts is reasonably involved from a technical aspect, thus, it is not particularly surprising that most surgeons elect to concentrate their experience with one or two of the devices. The ease of deployment and the precision of the deployment with regard to the location of the renal artery orifices also likely contribute to the differences in surgeon preference.

The need for adjunctive procedures to facilitate the endovascular repair is usually determined by the preoperative imaging studies and should be factored into the overall plan. The major concerns include stenotic access vessels and the absence of a suitable common iliac artery landing zone because of aneurysmal enlargement. The remedial procedures for small access vessels or significant occlusive disease include serial dilation or a retroperitoneal iliac prosthetic conduit. Repeated attempts to pass the devices sheaths through a diseased native vessel should be discouraged and frequently result in vessel rupture at the common iliac bifurcation. Aneurysmal degeneration of the common iliac artery can be overcome by seating the iliac limb in the external iliac artery. This process necessitates either embolizing or bypassing the ipsilateral internal iliac artery. The internal iliac artery can be coil embolized, and the procedure can be performed in either staged (embolization first) or simultaneous approach. Alternatively, the iliac limb of the endograft can simply occlude the internal iliac artery flush provided the iliac bifurcation is sufficiently funneled.[185] Several reports have documented that accessory renal arteries may be covered at the time of the endograft with little clinical sequelae.

The intraoperative preparation for endovascular repair is similar to that for the open approach although there are several significant differences. The appropriate imaging equipment is mandatory. Ideally, this would entail a complete endovascular suite with a fixed fluoroscopic unit although a portable unit with the appropriate vascular software and an imaging table is sufficient. General endotracheal anesthesia is likely the standard although a variety of techniques have been employed including regional and local anesthesia. Indeed, the endovascular approach is well suited to these less invasive alternatives particularly considering the feasibility of a completely percutaneous approach. Intraoperative autologous transfusion devices and a nasogastric tube are unnecessary. It is currently quite rare to convert an endovascular repair at the time of the initial implantation despite the early experience that reported a rate of up to 5%.[55–57,59] However, it should be emphasized that endovascular aneurysm repair is a surgical procedure and should be performed in an operating room with strict adherence to aseptic technique.

Although the technique for implanting the various endografts is somewhat specific to the individual device, the basic steps for deploying a modular bifurcated device are illustrated in Figure 102.10. Briefly, the common femoral arteries are exposed bilaterally and an umbilical tape is wrapped circumferentially around the vessels at the level of the inguinal ligament to facilitate vascular control. A variety of femoral incisions are possible although a 2 to 3 cm transverse incision along the caudal border of the inguinal ligament is usually ideal and has been associated with a low incidence of postoperative wound complications. Approximately 2 cm of the common femoral artery is dissected free. It is not usually necessary to dissect its superficial and profunda femoral branches. While the dissection is being performed, the various device components are prepared on the back table by the surgical technologist. A purse string suture using a 5-0 cardiovascular suture can be placed on the anterior aspect of the common femoral artery and left untied until the completion of the procedure. The various catheters/sheaths may be introduced through the center of the purse string. This can facilitate rapid/simple closure of the artery at the completion of the procedure. The common femoral artery on the side chosen to introduce the main body of the device (ipsilateral groin) is punctured using an angiographic needle and a 0.035-inch standard working wire (e.g., Bentsen) is passed into the abdominal aorta using fluoroscopic guidance. A 5-Fr introducer sheath is advanced over the guide wire using a Seldinger technique and vessel entry is confirmed by manual contrast injection. The working wire is further advanced into the thoracic aorta and exchanged for a longer 0.035-inch stiffened guide wire (e.g., Meier) using a catheter. Attention is then directed to the contralateral groin and in a similar manner a stiff guide wire is advanced into the aorta and an appropriate size large-diameter introducer sheath is inserted over the guide wire into the body of the aneurysm at approximately the L3 vertebral space. An angiographic catheter is advanced to the L1 vertebral body through the contralateral sheath and the catheter connected to the power injector. The patient is then anticoagulated using a standard protocol (100 units/kg) and therapeutic anticoagulation (activated clotting time twice baseline) is maintained throughout the procedure. The main body delivery catheter is introduced over the stiff wire through the ipsilateral groin and the upper limit of the main body positioned between the L1 to L2 vertebral bodies. Devices that do not have an integral sheath as part of their delivery system require an 18- to 22-Fr sheath to be inserted prior to introduction of the actual delivery catheter. Radiopaque markers on the graft facilitate the positioning and orientation of the main body.

An aortogram is obtained and the location of the renal arteries identified. The fluoroscope should be adjusted to optimize visualization of the infrarenal neck. A 5- to 10-degree craniocaudal angulation is usually sufficient to account for the anterior angulation of the infrarenal neck caused by the natural lumbar lordosis of the spine and the posterior bulging of the aneurysm sac. The location of the renal arteries is marked on the imaging screen and the position of the main body finely adjusted. The main body is now deployed exposing the opening of the contralateral docking limb. Using a combination of a hydrophilic wire and a curved catheter, the contralateral docking limb is cannulated. This can be challenging at times and requires a modest degree of catheter skills. Various maneuvers including different fluoroscopic projections, different shaped

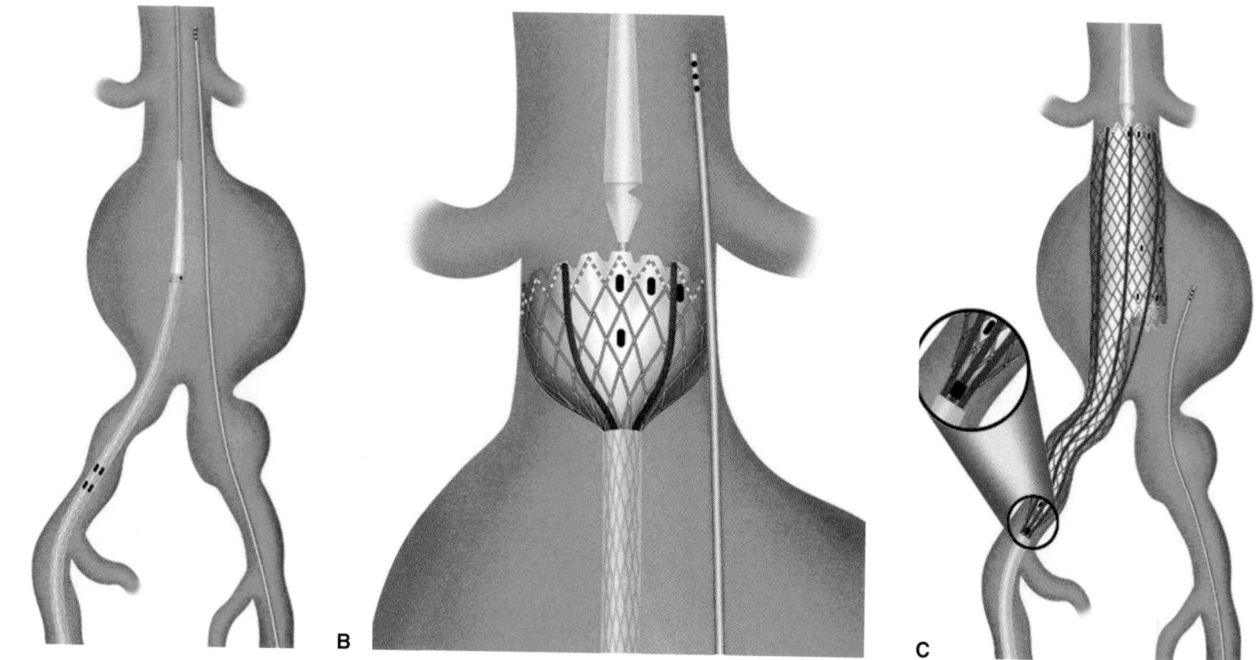

FIGURE 102.10 General steps involved in the endovascular repair of an abdominal aortic aneurysm. The common femoral arteries are exposed bilaterally and stiff wires are introduced into the thoracic aorta under fluoroscopic guidance. An appropriate size large-diameter introducer sheath is inserted over the stiff wire into the body of the aneurysm at approximately the L3 vertebral space on the side contralateral to the one chosen for the main device. (*A*) The main body delivery catheter is introduced over the stiff wire through the ipsilateral groin and the upper limit of the main body positioned between the L1 to L2 vertebral bodies. An aortogram is obtained and the location of the renal arteries identified. The location of the renal arteries is marked on the imaging screen and the position of the main body finely adjusted. (*B* and *C*) The main body is deployed exposing the opening of the contralateral docking limb. The contralateral docking limb is cannulated and a stiff wire advanced into the thoracic aorta. Deployment of the contralateral limb is started by obtaining a retrograde arteriogram through the contralateral sheath in the opposite oblique projection to identify the orifice of the internal iliac artery. (*Continued*)

catheters, and orientation of the contralateral docking limb prior to deployment of the main body device can facilitate this step. It is imperative to confirm that the intrastent passage of the cannulating guide wire. Confirmation can be rapidly performed by visualizing the guide wire in two orthogonal projections and confirming that the stents of the endograft can be seen on either side of the cannulating guide wire. Alternatively, an arteriogram can be performed using a catheter within the main body. The contralateral wire is advanced into the ascending thoracic aorta under fluoroscopic guidance and exchanged for a stiff wire using a catheter.

Deployment of the contralateral limb is started by obtaining a retrograde arteriogram through the contralateral sheath in the opposite oblique projection to identify the orifice of the internal iliac artery. The location of the orifice is marked on the imaging screen and a marker catheter is used to measure the distance from the contralateral docking limb to the origin to confirm that the choice of the contralateral limb is not too long. The contralateral limb is then introduced over the stiff wire, appropriately positioned relative to the docking limb and the orifice of the internal iliac artery, and the subsequently deployed.

After deployment of all the devices, a compliant aortic occlusion balloon is advanced over the ipsilateral stiff wire and inflated in the region of the infrarenal neck to mold the proximal attachment sites. The aortic balloon is then withdrawn and gently expanded at both distal (iliac) fixation sites. A completion arteriogram is then obtained using an angiographic catheter through one of the introducer sheaths (Fig. 102.11). The arteriogram should adequately evaluate the proximal/distal fixation sites and the orifices of the renal/internal iliac arteries. Additionally, it should include a delayed phase to help identify any late endoleaks. Problems identified on the completion study should be corrected if possible. The potential remedial procedures include balloon dilation or aortic/iliac extension cuffs.

All sheaths, catheters, and wires are removed after the completion arteriogram. The common femoral arteriotomy is closed using the purse string suture although additional hemostatic sutures are frequently necessary. The heparin is reversed with protamine (1 unit protamine/100 units heparin) after adequate signals are detected at the feet by Doppler ultrasound. The groin wounds are closed in layers with a continuous suture and the final skin later is closed with a subcuticular stitch.

The immediate postoperative course is fairly uneventful. Patients are transferred to the general care ward after recovery in the post anesthesia care unit. Patients are started on an appropriate diet the evening of the procedure and encouraged to get out of bed. Plain radiographs of the abdomen (four views, optimized for metal) are obtained on the first postoperative day, and patients are discharged thereafter. Patients are seen in the outpatient clinic at 1 month postoperatively with an abdominal/pelvic CT scan. It is important to note that mild

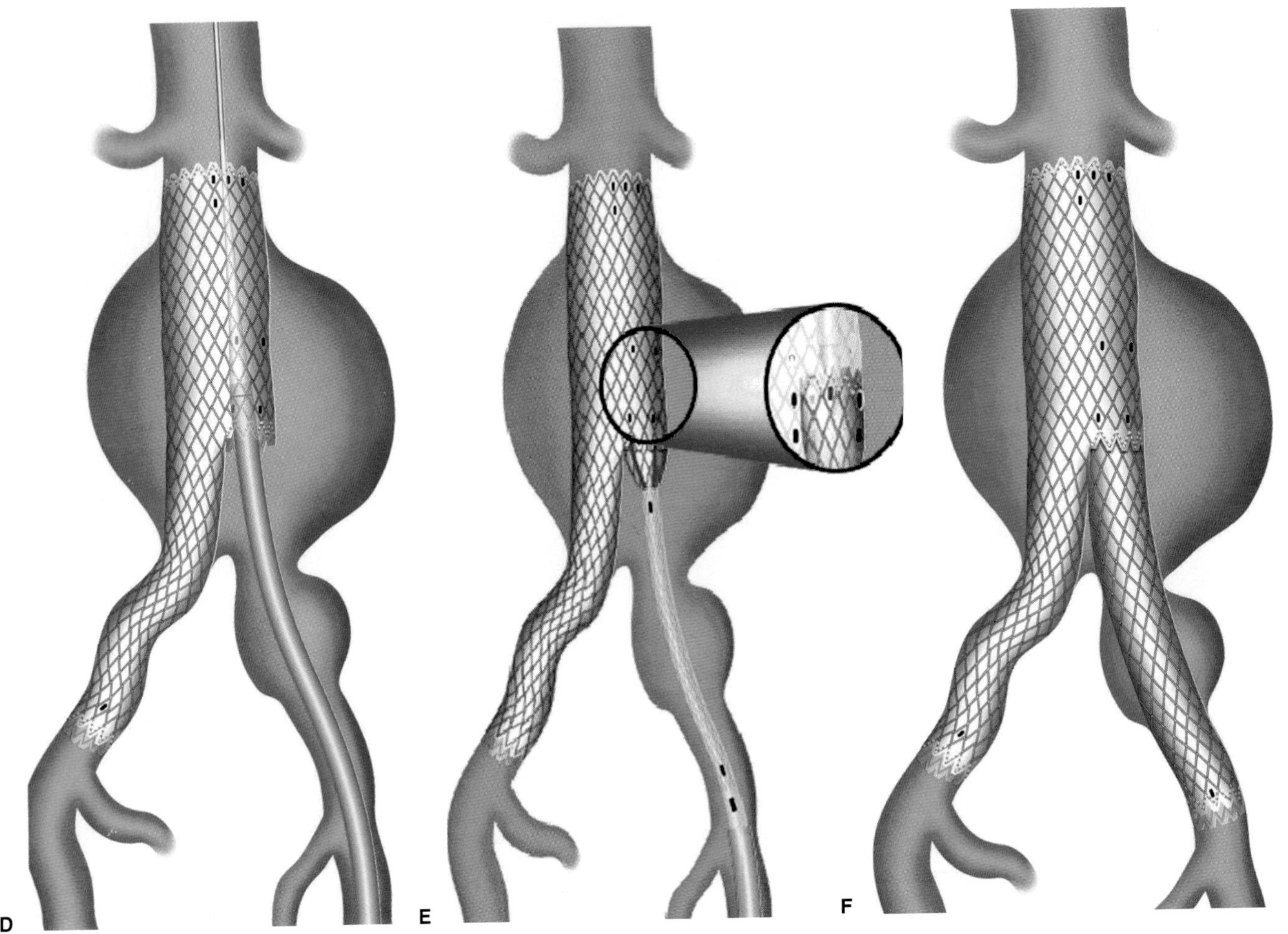

FIGURE 102.10 (*D, E,* and *F*) The location of the orifice is marked on the imaging screen and the contralateral limb is then introduced over the stiff wire, appropriately positioned, and deployed. A compliant aortic occlusion balloon is advanced over the ipsilateral stiff wire and inflated in the region of the infrarenal neck to mold the proximal and distal attachment sites.

fever and the finding of air around the graft on CT are common occurrences immediately after endograft repair and have not been associated with graft infection.[186]

It is imperative that patients are followed long-term given the uncertainty associated with the endovascular repair and the need for remedial procedures. As noted previously, new endoleaks have been identified as late as 7 years postoperatively.[187] A variety of protocols and imaging techniques have been described although an abdominal/pelvic CT scan and plain radiographs at 6 months postoperatively and then yearly thereafter seems reasonable. More frequent imaging may be indicated if the aneurysm continues to grow or there is evidence of an endoleak. The surveillance CT scans should include unenhanced images (i.e., no contrast) and biphasic contrast views with delayed images to help identify any late endoleaks.[188] Although not part of all surveillance protocols, plain radiographs are very helpful to identify structural changes/problems with the grafts (Fig. 102.12). Duplex ultrasound has been employed as a surveillance tool, but its accuracy is dependent on the local expertise of the technologist and vascular laboratory.[189–191]

Complications and Outcome

The overall mortality and complication rates after endovascular repair were reviewed in sections entitled Principles of Management and Choice of Open or Endovascular Repair. Briefly, the mortality rates in the recent randomized trials and national series is approximately 2%,[51,60,111] the rupture risk is approximately 1% per year,[108,112] and the incidence of remedial procedures approximately 10% per year.[116] The overall complication rate remains less defined, but a recent study from the National Surgical Quality Improvement—Private Sector reported an overall morbidity rate of 24%.[161] Many of the same complications that can occur after open repair can occur after endovascular repair. However, the relative incidence of the various complications is significantly different, and several complications inherent to the endovascular repair have been identified.

A variety of potential complications may arise during insertion of the delivery catheter or the large introducer sheath. Indeed, access problems secondary to iliac stenoses and/or tortuosity are the most common procedure related complication.

The maximum outer diameters of the three commercially available devices are 22 Fr for the AneuRx, 21 Fr for the Excluder, and 23 Fr for the larger Zenith sizes. These correspond to an outer diameter of approximately 7 mm (1 Fr corresponds to the circular cross-sectional diameter of $1/\pi$ mm, e.g., 24 Fr = 24/3.14 mm or 7.6 mm). A variety of techniques are available to correct or overcome the access vessel stenoses, and these should be factored into the preoperative plan. Excessive force during insertion of these large sheaths or delivery catheters can result in serious injury and perforation of the vessels. Predictably, this can lead to significant hemorrhage and hemodynamic changes. The diagnosis can be confirmed by arteriography and the bleeding controlled intraluminally with the device sheath or a balloon catheter. A variety of endovascular salvage techniques are possible in this setting including deployment of the main device or a covered stent over the disrupted artery. Indeed, nearly all major arterial disruptions, with possible exception of the proximal aorta, may be treated using endovascular techniques and should not necessarily lead to an emergent laparotomy. Safe conduct of an endovascular aneurysm repair is predicated by sufficient knowledge of the various salvage techniques, the necessary catheter and guide wire skills to execute them, and the availability of a necessary complement of ancillary equipment. However, prevention of the problem is the best treatment, and a low threshold for retroperitoneal iliac conduit should be maintained during preoperative planning. Dissection within the arterial wall of the iliac vessels or aorta may also result from misdirection or excessive force during cannulation of the vessels. It can usually be corrected by cannulating the "true" lumen and reestablishing its integrity by deployment of a peripheral (uncovered) stent.

Graft deployment can be associated with mechanical problems related to the delivery system or inappropriate positioning. A host of mechanical problems have been described, and the list will likely expand with widespread application of the devices and the introduction of newer systems. Many of the mechanical problems are device-specific and related to the actual sequence of events and manipulations required. Troubleshooting guidelines and specific recommendations are available from the manufacturers. Deployment of the endovascular graft below the proximal target site on the infrarenal aorta may be corrected by using an aortic extension or cuff. Attempting to reposition the graft further proximally after deployment has not been successful and is not recommended. Deployment of the endovascular graft across the orifices of the renal arteries can potentially be corrected by displacing the graft caudally. A guide wire can be passed over the flow divider and out the contralateral groin. The entire graft can then be retracted caudally by pulling on the wires. Alternatively, a large balloon can be inflated above the flow divider and retracted. Extreme care must be exercised during these maneuvers to prevent complete dislodgement of the proximal main body from the neck. Deployment of the graft across part of the renal orifice can be corrected by placing a stent within the lumen of the renal artery and, thereby, displacing part of the main body caudally. Deployment of the endograft across the lumen of one internal iliac artery is usually tolerated provided the contralateral vessel is patent and relatively free of occlusive disease. Indeed, it is relatively common to embolize a single internal iliac artery in patients with common iliac artery aneurysms to facilitate fixation of the graft limb in the external iliac artery. Occlusion of both internal iliac arteries or occlusion of one vessel in the presence of contralateral disease may render the pelvis ischemic. Occasionally one of the iliac limbs can be pushed cephalad using a sheath and its dilator. It should be emphasized that many of these remedial procedures are not manufacturer approved and should only be attempted by experienced endovascular surgeons. Because of the advanced age of many of these patients and their attendant comorbidities, open surgical conversion should be contemplated only as a last resort after exhausting appropriate endovascular options, once again emphasizing the need for advanced endovascular expertise during these procedures.

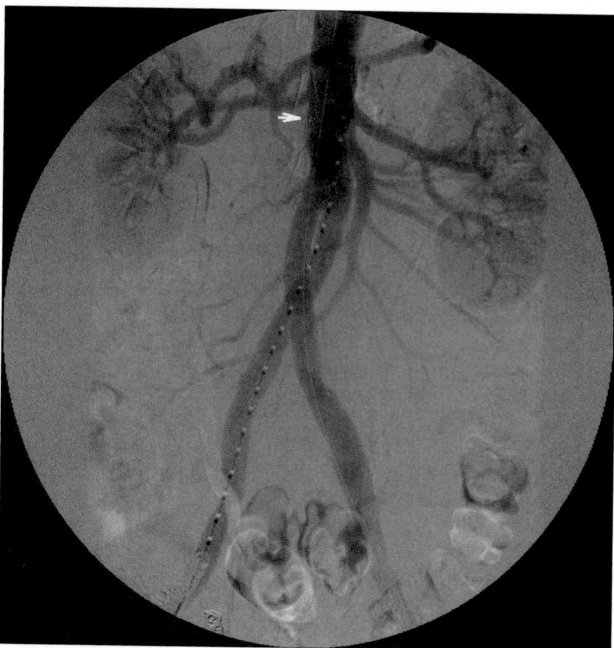

FIGURE 102.11 Completion arteriogram after an endovascular aneurysm repair is shown. The arrow marks the caudal extent of the stent graft. Note that the iliac limbs have been intentionally crossed to facilitate the cannulation of the contralateral gate.

It is relatively common to see an endoleak on the completion arteriogram. Treatment is contingent upon the specific type of leak and their associated natural history although the majority of these early endoleaks ultimately resolve.[192] The type 1 (attachment site) and type 3 (fabric tear or module interface) endoleaks are particularly concerning and every reasonable attempt to correct these defects should be made. The aneurysm sac is presumably still exposed to systemic pressure in the presence of a type 1 or type 3 endoleak, and, therefore, the rupture risk likely approaches that associated with the untreated aneurysm. Both the type 1 and 3 endoleaks can potentially be corrected by repeat balloon angioplasty at the proximal/distal attachment sites or at the modular interface. If these measures are not successful, additional extension devices can be deployed. With the exception of large proximal type 1 endoleaks completely resistant to standard maneuvers, it is reasonable to manage most perioperative endoleaks expectantly, especially since many seal spontaneously with reversal of anticoagulation within 6 months. Furthermore, it should be kept in mind that the inability to obtain a satisfactory exclusion of the aneurysm at the time of endograft implantation does not mandate a surgical conversion in the same setting. Consideration should be given to completing the procedure, allowing for a brief recovery, and discussing potential options in an elective, outpatient setting with the patient and their family. The potential options at this point include referral to another center of endovascular expertise, open surgical repair with removal of any or all implanted devices, or no further treatment if the patient is a poor surgical risk. Type

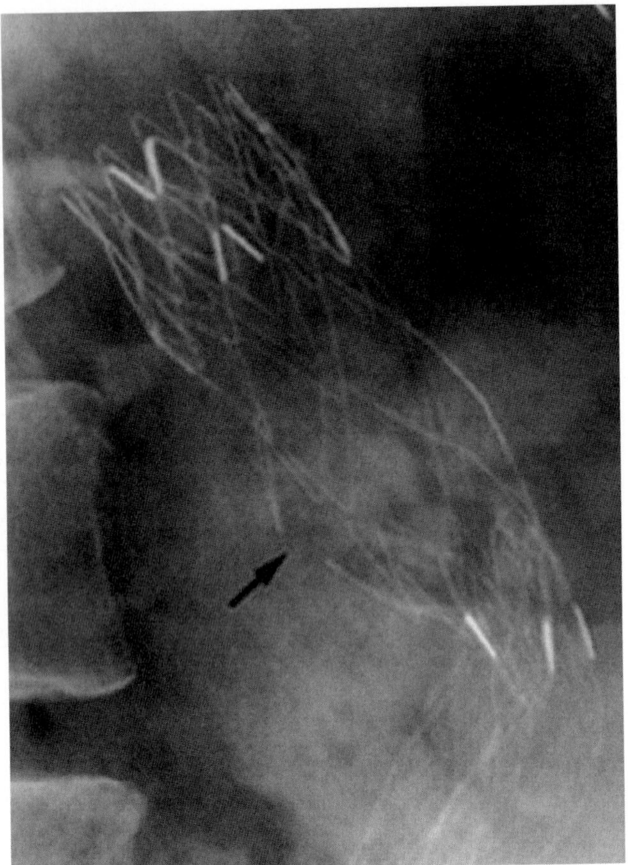

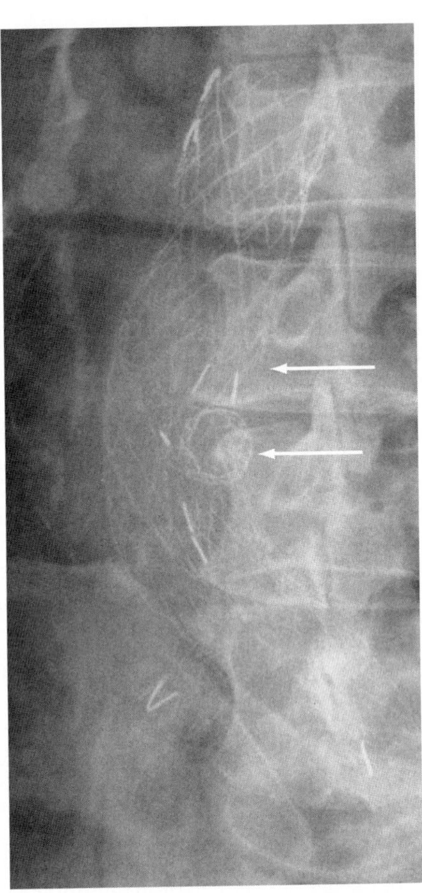

FIGURE 102.12 Plain radiographs of an endovascular graft demonstrating (*A*) strut fracture and (*B*) modular disruption. (From Magennis R, Joekes E, Martin J, et al. Complications following endovascular abdominal aortic aneurysm repair. *Br J Radiol.* 2002;75:700–707.)

2 endoleaks (retrograde branch vessel related) have a relatively benign natural history and do not merit aggressive intervention unless the aneurysm continues to increase in size over time. Type 4 (trans graft) endoleaks are self-limiting, and do not merit treatment at all. They are identified as a diffuse contrast "blush" at the time of the completion arteriography. They represent a diagnosis of exclusion and mandate that the more worrisome type 1 endoleak be ruled out.

The spectrum of immediate postoperative complications after endovascular aneurysm repair is comparable to that outlined for after open repair and will not be repeated. However, the incidence of major, systemic complications after endovascular aneurysm repair is quite small. It is noteworthy that the incidence of both paraplegia and bowel ischemia are comparable after endovascular and open repair although the mechanisms are different and likely due to atheroembolism.[193,194] Indeed, diffuse embolization to the small bowel has been reported after endovascular repair and is almost uniformly fatal.[193]

The long-term complications after endovascular repair include endoleak, structural failure, need for remedial procedures, need for open conversion and rupture. These ongoing risks further emphasize the importance of conscientious lifelong surveillance. All type 1 and 3 endoleaks identified during surveillance merit further evaluation and correction given their ongoing rupture risk. Device migration has been reported to lead to type 1 endoleaks and has been associated with neck length, site of deployment below the renal arteries, and surgeon/center experience.[180] The treatment of these late occurring type 1 and 3 leaks is identical to that for those occurring earlier and includes identification of the specific site and remediation with either balloon angioplasty or an additional endovascular devices, although the latter is most common. Type 2 endoleaks merit intervention and treatment if the aneurysm continues to increase in diameter. Identification of the type 2 endoleak can be challenging and may require selective catheterization of the superior mesenteric or internal iliac arteries.[195] A variety of approaches have been described to treat the type 2 endoleaks including coil embolization, laparoscopic ligation of the feeder vessels, and direct translumbar injection of the aneurysm sac with glue or other thrombotic agents.

Aneurysms that continue to increase in size after endovascular repair merit further intervention and may require open conversion due to their ongoing rupture risk. Continued aneurysm growth has been associated with the type of prosthesis and baseline size in addition to the presence of endoleak.[118] It should be emphasized that goal of aneurysm repair is to prevent rupture/death from rupture and that endoleak and even sac enlargement are surrogate markers of potential late failure of therapy. Indeed, even the clinical significance of an enlarging sac in the absence of a visible endoleak is controversial as long as a secure proximal and distal fixation of the endograft has been demonstrated. To confound the issue further, rupture of aneurysms without endoleak or change in sac diameter have also been reported, leading some to describe the phenomenon teleologically as endotension. An endoleak that is not detected on a properly performed contrast CT scan typically cannot be identified on arteriography. In contrast, if an endoleak that merits intervention is seen on surveillance imaging, proper diagnostic investigation should include all the fixation sites and the modular interfaces and selective injections of mesenteric and hypogastric arteries with sufficient contrast dose and proper acquisition techniques. It should be emphasized that open conversion and explant of the endovascular graft is technically more challenging than a de novo open repair and usually requires suprarenal or supraceliac aortic control. It is not always possible or necessary to remove the whole endovascular graft particularly when the device has suprarenal fixation. It is possible to transect the endovascular graft near the usual site of the infrarenal aortic anastomosis and incorporate the fabric/stents of the graft into the anastomosis. Temporary distal vascular control can be achieved by clamping the limbs of the endovascular graft. The limbs of a bifurcated surgical graft may be anastomosed directly to the endograft limbs if they are securely fixed to the iliac artery. Ideally, the limbs of the endograft should be removed and a standard aortobiiliac graft performed.

A variety of device-specific complications, including strut fracture, fabric tears, and buckling of the graft, have been identified, and the list will likely increase with the introduction of newer systems. These complications may present at any time throughout the postoperative period. An extensive discussion of all the potential device-related complications and their treatment is beyond the scope of this chapter. Disturbingly, regression of the aneurysm has been associated with significant conformational changes in the endografts and has resulted in limb thrombosis and disruption of the distal attachment sites.[196] These adverse outcomes in the presence of decrease in the aneurysm size have been termed the "paradox of success."

Repair of Ruptured Abdominal Aortic Aneurysms

Open Repair

The approach to the patient with a ruptured abdominal aortic aneurysm is similar to the elective approach, although several points merit further comment. It is important to realize that operative repair is the only acceptable treatment and the only effective means to prevent further hemorrhage. The diagnosis should be made in an expeditious fashion and the appropriate treatment initiated. Several series have documented successful endovascular aneurysm repair and this approach may represent the optimal treatment.[67–69] However, open repair remains the standard treatment across the country.

The patient should be taken emergently to the operating room once the diagnosis of a ruptured aneurysm has been made. Unnecessary delays to complete the preoperative evaluation should be avoided. Unfortunately, the diagnosis is not always made in a setting where an operating room is immediately available. Given this scenario, the patient should be transferred to a setting in which an operating room is available or the necessary resources should be mobilized. The decision to transfer or treat locally should be dictated by the ultimate time necessary to get the patient to the operating room and the institutional resources. The operating room and anesthesia personnel should be notified immediately upon diagnosis and instructed that the patient is en route. The necessary instrument trays should be opened, the room temperature in the operating room raised, adjunctive measures to maintain body temperature obtained, and the intraoperative autologous salvage device prepared. Indeed, hypothermia has been shown to be a strong, independent predictor of mortality after ruptured aneurysm repair.[197] The blood bank should be notified and instructed to send 6 units of blood to the operating room. The blood should be type O negative or type-specific if cross-matched units are not available. Furthermore, the blood bank should be instructed to expedite the cross-match of additional red blood cells, fresh frozen plasma, and platelets. The patient should be prepared and draped before intubation and the induction of anesthesia. Simultaneously, the surgeon and assistants should be prepared to make the incision at the time of induction. Patients with ruptured aneurysms frequently become hypotensive after the induction of anesthesia because of its vasodilator effect.

A midline incision should be made and supraceliac aortic control obtained. Control is facilitated by bluntly dissecting the gastrohepatic ligament, the crus of the diaphragm, and the connective tissue enveloping the aorta. The latter may be somewhat tenacious and require a moderate amount of force. Vascular control can be achieved manually by either occluding the aorta between the fingers and thumb or compressing it against the vertebral bodies. Definitive control should be obtained with an aortic clamp, which can be guided along the arm, hand, and digits. Care should be utilized during these maneuvers to prevent injury to the esophagus. Inexperienced surgeons may mistake the esophagus for the aorta in hypotensive patients. The presence of a nasogastric tube or pulse may aid in differentiating the aorta from the esophagus. Aortic control can also be achieved through a variety of other means: thoracotomy with occlusion of the descending thoracic aorta, intraluminal control of the infrarenal aorta with a Foley balloon, supraceliac control via a retroperitoneal approach, and intraluminal control with an aortic balloon catheter inserted through the femoral arteries. The aortic surgeon should be familiar with these various techniques because they can be helpful in certain clinical settings, but the midline approach with supraceliac control is recommended for most ruptured infrarenal aneurysms. After supraceliac aortic control has been obtained, the infrarenal aorta is dissected and vascular control is achieved below the level of the renal arteries. Often, the hematoma from the ruptured aneurysm facilitates the dissection by displacing the normal tissue planes. However, the normal tissues may be obscured, and care should be taken not to injure the venous structures, particularly the left renal vein. The supraceliac aortic clamp can be released after infrarenal control has been obtained, and flow can be restored to the visceral vessels. It is imperative that these various steps are coordinated with the anesthesia team, and it is recommended that the supraceliac clamp be left in position to facilitate reapplication if necessary. Distal vascular control can be achieved with either vascular clamps or intraluminal balloons, depending on the character of the iliac vessels.

Patients can be heparinized after proximal and distal vascular control has been obtained, provided that the patient is doing well and the case is proceeding expeditiously. However, the decision to anticoagulate the patient is contingent on a variety of factors, including the quantity of blood lost, presence of any coagulopathic bleeding, body temperature, and hemodynamic status. Anticoagulation potentially reduces thrombotic complications, but it exacerbates coagulopathic bleeding. Before completion of the distal anastomoses, thromboembolectomy catheters should be passed distally through the iliac vessels to remove any thrombus or debris. It is recommended that the inferior mesenteric artery be implanted if patent to reduce the risk of postoperative colonic ischemia.

The heparin effect can be reversed with protamine after confirmation of distal lower extremity arterial signals. The administration of fresh frozen plasma, platelets, or both should be considered at this point if any evidence of coagulopathic bleeding is noted.

The postoperative course after repair of a ruptured aneurysm is predictably more complicated and protracted than the course after elective repair.[198–202] Both the intensive care unit and total hospital length of stay are significantly increased. The mortality and complications rates are likewise significantly increased. As noted previously, the operative mortality rate for patients with ruptured abdominal aortic aneurysms who make it to the operating room is approximately 50%.[5] The spectrum of postoperative complications after repair of a ruptured aneurysm is essentially the same as after elective repair despite the increased overall incidence. The incidence of bowel ischemia may be as high as 40% and routine colonoscopy may be indicated.[170] Abdominal compartment syndrome[203] and adrenal insufficiency[204] have been reported after ruptured aneurysm repair and merit consideration in patients that are not doing well. Notably, adrenal insufficiency was identified in almost 70% of patients with unexplained postoperative hypotension after ruptured aneurysm repair.[204] Predictably, long-term survival is decreased relative to patients undergoing elective repair[200] although the overall quality of life is comparable.[205]

Endovascular Repair

The endovascular approach has the potential to impact the operative mortality rate for ruptured abdominal aortic aneurysms. Although the worldwide experience is very small, the initial findings are impressive particularly given the significant mortality/morbidity associated with the open repair that has remained relatively constant over the past few decades.[64] Despite the appeal of the endovascular approach, the application is likely not ready for widespread use and requires a defined protocol/approach consisting of an experienced endovascular surgeon, a committed team, an available operating room with the necessary imaging equipment, and a standing inventory of suitable devices. Furthermore, the patient must be an acceptable anatomic candidate for endovascular repair. Several recent studies have estimated that only approximately 20% to 40% of patients with ruptured aneurysms are anatomically suitable for endovascular repair although this number may increase to approximately 65% with larger diameter devices.[182,206,207] It should be emphasized that these percentages are somewhat device dependent and it is anticipated that they will increase with the introduction of newer ones.

The endovascular approach for the treatment of ruptured abdominal aortic aneurysms can be briefly summarized and has recently been described by Lee et al.[68] Patients with a presumed diagnosis of a ruptured abdominal aortic aneurysm that are hemodynamically stable as defined by a systolic blood pressure greater than 80 mm Hg and normal mentation should undergo a rapid CT to determine their suitability. Notably, aggressive fluid resuscitation should be avoided during this period to avoid the theoretical risk of releasing the retroperitoneal tamponade. The anatomic criteria for endovascular repair include an acceptable neck anatomy (length $\geq$10 mm, diameter $\leq$28 mm) and adequate access vessels ($\geq$7 mm diameter). The operative plan is generated and the appropriate devices selected based upon the CT findings and patients are taken directly to the operating room from the scanner. Oversizing of the aortic neck 20% or more and encroachment on the orifices of the renal arteries with adjunctive stenting are both tolerated in an attempt to limit the necessary inventory and increase the proximal fixation zone, respectively. Access to the common femoral arteries is obtained using a percutaneous approach with direct exposure and repair delayed until the completion of the procedure. The remaining conduct of the procedures is essentially the same as described in the elective setting. It is not usually necessary to occlude the aorta with an intraluminal balloon although one should be readily available in the event that the patients become hemodynamically unstable. It should be noted that the criteria for an acceptable result are less in the setting of a ruptured aneurysm and persistent attempts to achieve a perfect radiographic result should be avoided. The ultimate goal is to prevent further hemorrhage and to allow the patient to be resuscitated. Further interventions including conversion to open repair may be necessary at a later date, but these can usually be performed in an elective fashion.

ADDITIONAL CONSIDERATIONS

Isolated Iliac Artery Aneurysms

Isolated iliac artery aneurysms are rare and have been reported to occur with an incidence ranging from 0.03% in autopsy series[6] to 2.2% in single-institution series.[208] The common iliac artery is involved in approximately 70% of the cases, and the internal iliac artery in the remainder.[209] Aneurysmal involvement of the external iliac artery, either in combination with the common iliac artery or alone, is distinctly rare. These isolated iliac artery aneurysms should be differentiated from the common iliac artery aneurysms that occur concomitantly with abdominal aortic aneurysms. Simultaneous aneurysmal involvement of the aorta and common iliac arteries occurs in about 10% to 20% of all abdominal aortic aneurysms;[6,7] this pattern should be considered as one disease process and treated accordingly.

The natural history of isolated iliac artery aneurysms is poorly defined because of their low incidence. The clinical risk factors appear to be similar to those for abdominal aortic aneurysms with the highest incidence seen among elderly men. Unlike patients with abdominal aortic aneurysms, a significant proportion of patients with isolated iliac artery aneurysms present with symptoms.[209] These symptoms may result from either rupture or compression of adjacent structures including the bowel, ureters, iliac veins, and nerves. The clinical presentation of patients with a ruptured iliac artery aneurysm is similar to that of ruptured abdominal aortic aneurysms, and the diagnosis should be included in the differential for patients with genitourinary symptoms and normal findings on urinalysis and testicular examination. CT is optimal for confirming the diagnosis of an isolated iliac artery aneurysm. The utility of ultrasonography is limited by the posterior course of the iliac vessels and the overlying bowel. Large iliac artery aneurysms may occasionally be palpated during rectal or gynecologic examination, and ruptured iliac artery aneurysms may present with ecchymosis of the perineum.

The principles of treatment for asymptomatic, isolated iliac artery aneurysms are similar to those for abdominal aortic aneurysms, and operative repair is justified when the risk for rupture offsets the risk of repair. Unfortunately, the natural history of isolated iliac artery aneurysms and the appropriate threshold for repair remain unresolved. The reported growth rate for iliac artery aneurysms less than 3 cm is 0.11 cm/year while that for aneurysms 3 to 5 cm is 0.26 cm/year.[210] Although rupture has been reported for aneurysms smaller than 2 cm, it is rare for aneurysms smaller than 3 cm to rupture.[208] Operative repair is generally recommended for good risk patients with isolated iliac artery aneurysms 3.5 cm or more and surveillance recommended for smaller ones. The frequency of surveillance imaging studies should be dictated by the size of the aneurysm with yearly studies appropriate for aneurysms less than 3 cm with 6-month intervals appropriate for aneurysms between 3 to 3.5 cm.[208]

The treatment or repair of isolated iliac artery aneurysms depends on the specific vessel involved and the extent of the aneurysm. Theoretically, common iliac artery aneurysms can be repaired with an interposition graft or a covered stent provided that there is a sufficient proximal and/or distal neck to sew the anastomosis or seat the graft. However, this is rarely an option because the aneurysmal involvement of the vessel usually extends over its whole length. Therefore, repair necessitates replacing the whole common iliac artery with a bifurcated graft similar to the approach for patients with combined aortic and iliac artery aneurysms. Both open and endovascular approaches are available and the concerns about the individual choice (i.e., open versus endovascular) are likely similar to that outlined for abdominal aortic aneurysms. Additionally, the principles of treatment for both the open and endovascular approach of isolated iliac artery aneurysms are similar to abdominal aortic aneurysms. In the case of open repair, the proximal anastomosis should be performed immediately below the renal arteries to prevent subsequent aneurysmal degeneration of the infrarenal cuff while the distal anastomosis should be performed at the common iliac bifurcation on the involved side. The distal anastomosis on the uninvolved common iliac artery can be performed to a nonaneurysmal segment. For the endovascular repair, the graft should be seated immediately below the renal arteries and at the takeoff of the internal iliac artery on the side opposite the aneurysm. The iliac limb on the side of the aneurysm is seated in the external iliac artery and necessitates embolization or bypass of the ipsilateral internal iliac artery.

The treatment of internal iliac artery aneurysms is exclusion. This can be performed using either an endovascular or open approach, although the former is likely preferred because of its simplicity. Bypass of an internal iliac artery aneurysm is not usually possible because there is rarely a proximal or distal neck. Indeed, aneurysm involvement usually extends to the common iliac bifurcation and the distal aspect arborizes into multiple smaller vessels. The principles of the endovascular treatment include obliterating both the arterial inflow and the outflow of the aneurysm. The outflow is usually thrombosed using selective coil embolization although a variety of other agents have been described. Placing a covered stent across its orifice extending from the common to the external iliac vessels eliminates the inflow. The open approach requires vascular control of the distal common iliac and proximal external iliac arteries. The internal iliac artery is then opened by incising the aneurysm, and the branches are oversewn from within. The proximal internal iliac artery can be either oversewn at its takeoff, or the resultant defect at the common iliac bifurcation can be repaired with patch angioplasty. The appropriate treatment for patients with bilateral internal iliac arteries remains unclear. Exclusion of both vessels has the potential to cause severe pelvic ischemia that may not be remediable. A conservative approach is likely justified in this setting with a higher threshold for intervention appropriate before exclusion of the second vessel. Treatment options include excluding only the larger vessel, attempted revascularization, and staged exclusion after sufficient time has elapsed to facilitate potential collateral development. Regardless of the treatment option, it is important to assess the status of the pelvic circulation including the profunda femoral artery.

Inflammatory Abdominal Aortic Aneurysms

Approximately 5% of all abdominal aortic aneurysms are inflammatory.[211] They are characterized by a dense inflammatory response involving the anterior and lateral walls of the infrarenal aorta with sparing of its posterior aspect. The inflammatory response consists of a dense cellular infiltrate that has a white, glistening appearance on inspection. The inflammation results in an increase in wall thickness with the difference between the inner and outer diameters of the aorta ranging from 1 to 5 cm. The cause of the inflammatory process remains unresolved, but it may be an autoimmune phenomenon. Indeed, some type of autoimmune disorder has been reported in up to 20% of patients with inflammatory aneurysms.[212]

Patients with an inflammatory abdominal aortic aneurysm are predominantly men and frequently present with symptoms of back or abdominal pain. The triad of a pulsatile abdominal aortic mass, abdominal pain, and an elevated sedimentation rate has been described. Abdominal ultrasonography or CT may confirm the diagnosis. The anterior and lateral aspects of the aortic wall are thickened and hypoechoic on the sonogram. The CT findings are characteristic and include both thickening and contrast enhancement in the same distribution. An inexperienced observer may confuse the CT findings with those of a ruptured abdominal aortic aneurysm. Hydronephrosis with medial displacement of the ureters is frequently seen, and this contrasts with the usual lateral displacement seen with noninflammatory aneurysms. Indeed, this entity may share some pathogenetic pathways with retroperitoneal fibrosis.

The treatment of inflammatory abdominal aortic aneurysms is essentially the same as the treatment of the more common, noninflammatory variety. Nonoperative treatment with corticosteroids has been advocated in the past although this approach is likely ineffective and has largely been abandoned.[213] It has been suggested that the rupture risk of inflammatory abdominal aortic aneurysms is considerably less than the rupture risk of the noninflammatory variety because the wall thickness is increased. This is not true, however, and patients should not be lulled into a false sense of security. It should be noted that most aneurysms rupture through their posterior or posterolateral aspect, which is not involved in the inflammatory process. The open repair of an inflammatory abdominal aortic aneurysm is complicated by the fact that the adjacent structures, including the duodenum, colon, and ureters, may be involved in the process and densely adherent to the aortic wall. Indeed, a recent series reported an increased operative blood loss and procedure time for the open repair of inflammatory abdominal aortic aneurysms compared with the more common uninvolved type. These potential technical difficulties should likely be factored into the operative indications and size related threshold for the open approach.

The endovascular approach may be the optimal treatment for patients with inflammatory abdominal aortic aneurysms because of the concerns about the inflammatory process and adherent structures.[214–216] Surprisingly, the inflammatory process has been reported to regress after both open[217] and endovascular repair.[218] The technical difficulties associated with the open repair can be reduced by using a retroperitoneal approach. Inflammatory aneurysms can be repaired through a transperitoneal approach, and this scenario occasionally arises when the diagnosis is not made preoperatively. Regardless of the open approach, no attempt should be made to mobilize the adherent structures, specifically the duodenum, because of the potential for accidental injury. Proximal aortic control can be achieved either immediately above the renal arteries or above the visceral vessels. Alternatively, intraluminal aortic control can be achieved with a balloon catheter although this approach is less appealing. Distal control can usually be achieved at the common iliac arteries or at the level of their bifurcation. The duodenum and other adherent structures should be mobilized by incising the wall of the aneurysm and then reflecting them laterally. The proximal anastomosis can usually be performed to the infrarenal aorta after the aneurysm wall has been incised. The placement of preoperative ureteral catheters may facilitate identification of the ureters intraoperatively and can be helpful in patients with hydronephrosis. An increased incidence of anastomotic pseudoaneurysms has been demonstrated in patients with inflammatory aneurysms after open repair and likely justifies long-term surveillance.[219]

Juxtarenal and Suprarenal Abdominal Aortic Aneurysms

The management of aneurysms extending to the level of the renal arteries or further cephalad is more complicated as reflected by the increase in their associated morbidity and mortality rates.[220–222] The repair of these aneurysms is complicated by the obligatory period of renal and visceral ischemia associated with aortic occlusion during the proximal anastomosis. These increased morbidity and mortality rates should be factored into the decision algorithm and threshold for operative repair. Elective operative repair is usually recommended for patients with aneurysms 6 cm or larger in diameter in this setting although the 5.5 cm criterion may be appropriate for very good-risk patients and those with juxtarenal aneurysms who will require only a short period of suprarenal aortic occlusion.

Abdominal aortic aneurysms extending to the renal arteries or more cephalad may be repaired via either a retroperitoneal or a transperitoneal approach although the former is optimal. The retroperitoneal approach, with elevation of the left kidney, obviates the concerns about the left renal vein and simplifies exposure of the whole abdominal aorta. Furthermore, incising the diaphragm circumferentially and its crus may expose the descending thoracic aorta. Admittedly, the right renal artery is inaccessible from the retroperitoneal approach and exposure of the right common iliac artery and its bifurcation may be challenging. The proximal anastomosis may be fashioned as a large hood incorporating the orifices of the renal and visceral arteries. Separate revascularization of the left renal artery is occasionally necessary if the orifices of the renal arteries are splayed too far apart by the aneurysm. The transperitoneal repair of these proximal aneurysms requires exposure of the suprarenal aorta for clamp application. This procedure is facilitated by retracting the left renal vein inferiorly after ligating its adrenal, gonadal, and lumbar branches. As noted previously, the left renal vein may be ligated near its confluence with the cava without adverse sequelae. However, the named collaterals of the left renal vein (e.g., adrenal) should be preserved. The anterior surface of the aorta at the level of the visceral vessels is encased by dense neural tissue that can be incised. Incising the crus of the diaphragm that envelops the lateral aspect of the aorta further facilitates application of the aortic clamp. The configuration of the proximal anastomosis depends on the extent of the aneurysm and the vessels involved. Juxtarenal aneurysms can be repaired by obtaining suprarenal control and sewing the proximal anastomosis at the level of the renal orifices. The proximal anastomosis for suprarenal aneurysms can be performed by fashioning an anastomotic hood that incorporates most of the visceral vessels although this frequently requires separate revascularization of one renal artery.

Endovascular aneurysm repair has been reported to be feasible for juxtarenal and suprarenal abdominal aortic aneurysms.[223] There are no currently available commercial devices. However, the endovascular approach represents an active area of investigation that may represent the next frontier. Application of the technique is associated with a whole host of new engineering problems including designing a stent graft with properly positioned orifices for the visceral vessels through which additional covered stents can be deployed. Extraanatomic visceral revascularization (e.g., iliorenal bypass) combined with one of the commercially available grafts may offer an alternative endovascular approach to extend the limits of the technique without the added complexity of a branched vessel configuration.

Infected Abdominal Aortic Aneurysms

Infected abdominal aortic aneurysms comprise a small subset of all abdominal aortic aneurysms, accounting for less than 1% of all repairs.[224] The term *mycotic aneurysm* has traditionally been used to refer to infected aneurysms although it is a misnomer that has led to a significant amount of confusion. A newer classification system, proposed to clarify the situation, consists of four groups based on the underlying mechanism: (a) mycotic aneurysm, in which a septic embolus from the heart infects an artery; (b) microbial arteritis, in which bacteria infects an atherosclerotic but non-aneurysmal artery and cause aneurysmal degeneration; (c) existing aneurysms that become infected; and (d) traumatic pseudoaneurysm with concomitant bacterial inoculation.[225] Microbial arteritis resulting from hematogenous bacterial spread currently accounts for approximately 80% of all cases of infected aortic aneurysms.[226,227] *Salmonella* causes approximately 40% of all aneurysmal infections in contemporary series with the remainder caused by *Streptococcus, Staphylococcus, Bacteroides, Arizona hinshawii, Escherichia coli,* and *Pseudomonas aeruginosa*.[225]

The diagnosis of infected aortic aneurysm is often difficult and the clinical presentation insidious. Patients may present with fever, back/abdominal pain, or both. Physical examination is often remarkable for a palpable abdominal mass and the presence of peripheral emboli. Laboratory studies are notable for an elevated leukocyte count and positive blood cultures although the latter are present in only 50% of cases[227,228] and negative blood cultures do not exclude the diagnosis. CT is the most useful diagnostic study, and the features suggestive of an infected aneurysm include a periaortic mass, an aneurysm in an atypical location, periaortic fluid or gas, retroperitoneal inflammation, and frank rupture. The angiographic finding of a saccular or eccentric aneurysm in an atypical location is also suggestive of an infected aneurysm.

The treatment of an infected aneurysm requires control of hemorrhage in the presence of rupture, removal of all infected tissues, and restoration of perfusion to the viscera and lower torso. Patients should be started on broad-spectrum antibiotics when the diagnosis is first suspected although antibiotic therapy alone is not sufficient and the operative intervention should not be delayed in an attempt to sterilize the retroperitoneum. Patients with suspected rupture should undergo emergent exploration through either a transperitoneal or retroperitoneal approach. After vascular control has been obtained, the retroperitoneum should be explored, and intraoperative cultures with a stat Gram stain should be obtained. Several options for arterial reconstruction are available, including in situ replacement with a prosthetic graft, ligation of the infrarenal aorta with extra-anatomic bypass (axillofemoral configuration), or in situ replacement with staged extraanatomic bypass and subsequent removal of the in situ graft. The choice is contingent on the character of the aorta, degree of inflammation in the retroperitoneum, suspected organism, and hemodynamic status. In situ replacement of the infected aneurysm with a prosthetic graft is a reasonable option if retroperitoneal inflammation is minimal and the Gram stain is negative. Ligation of the infrarenal aorta with extra-anatomic bypass at the same session is the recommended approach in most settings although this is a major undertaking. The three-stage approach of in situ replacement followed by extra-anatomic bypass and graft explant is reserved for patients who cannot tolerate the simultaneous procedure because of underlying comorbidities or hemodynamic instability. The integrity of the aortic stump at the time of ligation and the potential for dehiscence or breakdown of the suture line are major concerns. The aorta should be débrided back to grossly uninvolved tissue and sutured in two layers with a running horizontal mattress and a simple continuous suture of nonabsorbable monofilament. A pedicle of omentum can be mobilized and approximated next to the aortic stump to help control the retroperitoneal inflammation and minimize the risk for stump dehiscence. When the diagnosis is suspected preoperatively and no evidence of rupture is found, the staged approach with extraanatomic bypass followed by graft removal is recommended. The procedures are usually performed 2 to 3 days apart to allow the patients a period of recovery. Patients should be anticoagulated between procedures to prevent thrombosis of the extraanatomic bypass resulting from competitive flow. Fortunately, the risk of graft thrombosis and graft infection during the intervening period is small. Endovascular repair of infected aortic aneurysm has been reported and should be considered an additional alternative.[229] Although the long-term safety of the endovascular approach remains unclear in this setting, it may serve as a temporizing approach that converts an urgent problem to an elective one. Mycotic aneurysms involving the suprarenal aorta pose a particularly challenging problem, but fortunately they are uncommon. In situ replacement with a prosthetic graft is frequently the only available option. Extraanatomic bypass (hepatorenal and splenorenal) of the renal arteries with ligation of the suprarenal aorta is an option but represents a significant undertaking and should be reserved for selected cases.

Patients with infected aneurysms, regardless of the arterial reconstruction, require long-term antibiotics and follow-up. Patients should receive intravenous antibiotics for 6 weeks, with the specific choice depending on the culture results. After completing the intravenous antibiotics, patients should be started on oral antibiotics although the duration of treatment remains unresolved. Patients should finish a course of at least 6 months of oral antibiotics; suppressive, lifelong therapy may be appropriate. Additionally, patients should undergo serial CT scans to assess the retroperitoneum and the status of the in situ graft when applicable. CT is usually performed 2 weeks postoperatively, then again 3 months and 6 months later. Patients with in situ revascularization should undergo imaging every 6 months indefinitely although this is not necessary for patients with extraanatomic revascularization in the absence of retroperitoneal inflammation. Predictably, the morbidity and mortality rates associated with infected abdominal aortic aneurysms are significant with a 40% mortality rate reported in a recent publication.[230]

Aortoenteric Fistulae

An aortoenteric fistula is a communication between the aorta and the bowel. The duodenum where it crosses anterior to the infrarenal aorta is involved most commonly, but the communication can develop between almost any portion of the small or large intestine. Primary aortic fistulae result when nonspecific abdominal aortic aneurysms erode into the bowel and are distinctly rare with a reported incidence of 0.04% to 0.07% in autopsy series.[231] Secondary aortic fistulae result from the erosion of a prosthetic aortic graft into the bowel; they are significantly more common, with a reported incidence of 0.1% to 2.0%.[232] Notably, they can occur after endovascular aneurysm repair.[233] The management of both primary and secondary aortic fistulae is the same.

The diagnosis of an aortoenteric fistula is often difficult and mandates a high index of suspicion. Patients usually present with gastrointestinal bleeding manifested as either hematemesis or melena. The initial episode of gastrointestinal bleeding is often self-limited and has been described as a "herald" bleed. The diagnosis of aortoenteric fistula should be foremost among the differential when a patient with a known aneurysm or prior aortic reconstruction presents with intestinal bleeding. Patients should undergo endoscopic evaluation of the upper and lower intestinal tract to determine the source of bleeding. It is imperative that the clinical suspicion of an aortoenteric fistula be communicated to the endoscopist to ensure that the third and fourth portions of the duodenum are adequately examined. The upper endoscopy occasionally requires the use of a pediatric colonoscope to facilitate examination of the fourth portion of the duodenum. The endoscopic findings of erosion, thrombus, active bleeding, or visible prosthetic graft in third or fourth portion of the duodenum are worrisome and/or diagnostic of an aortoenteric fistula and mandate emergent laparotomy. Mild duodenitis and gastritis are frequently seen at the time of endoscopy but do not exclude the diagnosis of an aortoenteric fistula. Notably, the findings of upper gastrointestinal endoscopy are normal in up to 30% of patients with a documented aortoenteric fistula.[234] Abdominal pelvic CT should be performed if the results of endoscopy are inconclusive. The findings on CT that suggest an aortoenteric fistula include inflammation within the retroperitoneum, an anastomotic pseudoaneurysm, close approximation of the bowel and the prosthetic aortic graft or aneurysm, and loss of the normal tissue planes between the third portion of the duodenum and the aorta or prosthetic graft. Occasionally, both endoscopy and CT are nondiagnostic despite the clinical suspicion of an aortoenteric fistula. Exploratory laparotomy is recommended in this setting for both diagnosis and treatment. Adherence of the bowel to the aorta at the time of the initial exploration suggests an aortoenteric fistula and mandates obtaining suitable proximal and distal control of the aorta, iliac vessels, or prosthetic graft before further dissection. The diagnosis cannot be excluded until the bowel is entirely separated from the retroperitoneum.

Treatment of an aortoenteric fistula requires repair of the defect in the gastrointestinal tract in addition to repair of the aneurysm or treatment of the infected prosthetic graft. Treatment of the gastrointestinal defect is usually straightforward and is based on standard surgical principles. After the fistula is disassembled, the edges of the bowel can be débrided and a primary closure performed with either a stapler or sutures. A limited bowel resection or diversion of the enteral tract may be necessary. The intraoperative and longer-term management of the aortic aneurysm or prosthetic graft is the same as that outlined previously for infected aortic aneurysms. Indeed, aortoenteric fistulae represent a variant of infected aortic aneurysms. In situ replacement of the prosthetic graft or infrarenal aorta, ligation of the infrarenal aorta with excision of the prosthetic graft and extraanatomic bypass, and in situ replacement with staged extraanatomic bypass and subsequent graft excision are all reasonable options. The clinical scenario usually dictates the choice. Ligation of the infrarenal aorta with excision of the graft and extraanatomic bypass is recommended in most cases. However, in situ repair is appropriate for patients who are older or sicker, who have minimal retroperitoneal inflammation or evidence of hemodynamic instability, or in whom ligation of the infrarenal aorta would compromise the renal arteries. Additionally, patients should be maintained on long-term antibiotics and undergo serial imaging studies, as outlined for infected aneurysms.

Venous Anomalies

Anomalies of the vena cava and renal veins are occasionally encountered at the time of aortic reconstruction. The common anomalies are related to the embryologic development of the iliac veins and vena cava. The four most clinically relevant anomalies include duplication of the inferior vena cava (0.2% to 3.0%), left-sided vena cava (0.2% to 0.5%), circumaortic left renal vein (1.5% to 8.7%), and retroaortic renal vein (1.2% to 2.4%).[235] Patients with a duplicated inferior vena cava have large veins that run parallel to the infrarenal aorta and join together either anterior or posterior to the aorta at the level of the renal vein. In the case of a left-sided inferior vena cava, a large vein runs parallel to the left side of the aorta, and a right-sided vena cava is absent. The left-sided vena cava crosses the aorta at the level of the renal vein to become the suprarenal inferior vena cava. The gonadal and adrenal veins on the right drain directly into the renal vein in a mirror image of the normal anatomy. The circumaortic renal vein is a collar of veins that surrounds the aorta at the level of the normal renal veins. In the case of a retroaortic left renal vein, a single vein runs posterior to the aorta at the usual location. Notably, both duplication of the inferior vena cava and left-sided vena cava can be associated with other venous anomalies, including a circumaortic or retroaortic renal vein.

The diagnosis of the various venous anomalies can usually be made preoperatively by CT. Identification of the vena cava and left renal vein should be part of the mental checklist used when the preoperative CT scans are reviewed. The various anomalies may not become evident immediately in the operating room if missed on the preoperative imaging studies. A very prominent left real vein at the usual location or slightly inferior is suggestive of a left-sided vena cava, whereas the absence of a left renal vein despite dissection along the anterior aspect of the aorta at the level of the superior mesenteric artery is suggestive of a retroaortic renal vein.

The open repair of an infrarenal abdominal aortic aneurysm in a patient with a venous anomaly is essentially the same as the standard approach, although additional care should be exercised to prevent inadvertent injury. Exposure of the infrarenal neck is more difficult in the presence of a duplicated or left-sided vena cava. However, sufficient exposure can usually be obtained by gentle dissection and mobilization of the venous structures. The presence of a duplicated or left-sided vena cava is a relative contraindication to the left retroperitoneal approach. A circumaortic renal collar or retroaortic renal vein presents a potential hazard when the proximal aortic clamp is applied. A vertical aortic clamp is recommended and obviates the dissection on the posterior aspect of the aorta. Transecting the aorta may facilitate exposure of a retroaortic renal vein when significant bleeding is encountered.

Renal Anomalies

Congenital variations in the renal anatomy may complicate the repair of an abdominal aortic aneurysm. Specifically, their presence may complicate the dissection during open repair because they are frequently associated with multiple renal arteries, aberrant venous return, and abnormally positioned ureters. The various congenital anomalies of the upper urinary system have been classified in an attempt to standardize the approach for vascular surgeons.[236] The anomalies have been broken down into abnormalities of position, including simple ectopia, and abnormalities of both form and fusion, including horseshoe kidney, crossed renal ectopia without fusion, and crossed renal ectopia with fusion. An ectopic kidney may be positioned anywhere from the pelvis to the thorax. Common forms of ectopic kidney include the pelvic kidney, located opposite the sacrum and below the aortic bifurcation; the lumbar kidney, located opposite the sacral promontory in the iliac fossa and anterior to the iliac vessels; the abdominal kidney, located above the iliac crest adjacent to the second lumbar vertebra; and the thoracic kidney, which can be located above the diaphragm in the posterior mediastinum. In a horseshoe kidney, two distinct renal masses are fused by either renal parenchyma or fibrous tissue; in the overwhelming majority, the lower poles are fused. In crossed renal ectopia, the kidney mass is located on the side opposite to its insertion in the bladder. Multiple configurations of crossed ectopia with and without fusion have been described.

The preoperative objective for the various renal anomalies is to image the renal mass adequately, delineate the course of the ureter, and establish the arterial and venous supply. The approach is simplified by the fact that most patients undergo abdominal/pelvic CT as part of the preoperative evaluation. The location and position of both the kidneys and ureters, like the position of the left renal vein, should be established as part of the review of every CT scan for patients with aneurysms. All patients with renal anomalies should likely undergo preoperative arteriography to confirm the location and number of renal arteries, and delayed images should be obtained at the time of arteriography to visualize the venous return and course of the ureters.

Patients with renal anomalies can safely undergo repair of an abdominal aortic aneurysm using either an open or endovascular approach.[237–239] However, the anomalies must be factored into the operative plan. The specific operative approach depends on the location of the renal mass, blood supply, course of the ureters, and presence of fusion. A left-sided retroperitoneal or transperitoneal approach with medial visceral rotation is the most helpful for open repair, particularly in patients with horseshoe kidney. A standard transperitoneal approach with transection of the fused parenchyma has been reported in patients with horseshoe kidney although this may be associated with significant bleeding and urine leak and, therefore, is discouraged. The frequently encountered multiple renal arteries can be handled most expeditiously by using a Carrel patch technique, in which a cuff of aorta including the renal artery orifices is reimplanted into the aortic graft after completion of the proximal anastomosis. Endovascular repair is possible in many cases with the feasibility dictated by the location of the renal arteries in addition to the other anatomic considerations. Use of the endovascular approach frequently requires covering some of the renal vessels and has been associated with loss of some renal parenchyma.[237]

Coexistent Renal or Visceral Artery Occlusive Disease

Coexistent renal or visceral artery occlusive disease is frequently found in patients undergoing abdominal aortic aneurysm repair. The true incidence is probably greater than appreciated because of the selective use of arteriography and reliance on CT. The optimal management of patients with coexistent lesions remains unresolved. The options include repair of the aneurysm alone, simultaneous repair of the aneurysm and revascularization of the renal or visceral vessels, and staged repair, with either aneurysm repair or revascularization performed first. Furthermore, the specific treatment options include both open and endovascular alternatives for the aneurysm repair and visceral/renal revascularization (i.e., angioplasty/stent). The rapid expansion of the endovascular technologies has afforded effective, safe approaches that have widely replaced open surgical revascularization for renal artery stenoses. The role of endovascular treatment for mesenteric artery occlusive disease remains less clear. It has been shown to be technically feasible although questions remain about its long-term durability. Regardless, the optimal approach represents a balance between the indications for the procedure and the associated added risk.

Renal/visceral revascularization is mandatory at the time of open aneurysm repair if the affected vessels are involved in the aneurysm, as in a suprarenal aneurysm or a horseshoe kidney. More commonly, a lower pole or accessory renal artery may come off the aneurysm. The decision to perform a concomitant revascularization with either reimplantation or a bypass graft in this setting depends on the size of the vessel and the quantity of kidney parenchyma it perfuses. Revascularization is recommended for larger vessels (>2 mm) that supply a significant portion of the renal mass. The presence of any accessory renal arteries should factor into the operative plan and the general feasibility for endovascular repair. Covering small, accessory renal arteries has been reported to be safe although it must be appreciated that this approach sacrifices some renal parenchyma.[240]

Combined aneurysm repair with renal/visceral artery revascularization may be justified if the traditional indications for renal or visceral artery revascularization are satisfied. The indications for renal revascularization include poorly controlled hypertension in a patient with a significant renal artery stenosis and rapidly progressive renal insufficiency in a patient with adequate renal mass and bilateral renal artery stenoses. The traditional indications for mesenteric revascularization include symptoms of chronic mesenteric ischemia and critical stenosis of either the superior mesenteric artery alone or two of the three visceral vessels. Endovascular renal revascularization can be safely performed simultaneous with endovascular aneurysm repair although it should likely be performed prior to open aneurysm repair. Simultaneous open aneurysm repair and renal artery bypass is associated with a significant increase in the operative mortality rate relative to the aneurysm repair alone.[241,242] Patients with chronic mesenteric ischemia and abdominal aortic aneurysms should have their visceral occlusive disease corrected prior to aneurysm repair. Repairing the aneurysm first potentially increases the risk of developing mesenteric infarction while the simultaneous open approach is likely prohibitive given the significant morbidity/mortality associated with open mesenteric revascularization alone.[243–245] The optimal means of visceral revascularization remains unresolved as noted previously although endovascular visceral artery revascularization prior to aneurysm repair is an attractive option.

The optimal treatment for patients with aneurysms and asymptomatic renal/visceral artery lesions remains even less clear. Natural history studies with the use of both arteriography[246] and duplex scanning[247] have suggested that significant renal artery stenoses are preocclusive lesions that may merit intervention. However, analysis of patients with asymptomatic renal artery stenosis who underwent aortic reconstruction found that the natural history of the renal artery lesions is fairly benign when untreated and is associated only with an increase in the antihypertensive requirements.[248] Little is known about the natural history of asymptomatic mesenteric occlusive lesions. However, a recent small report suggested that patients with asymptomatic severe mesenteric occlusive disease involving all three visceral vessels have a high incidence of bowel infarction.[249] Consideration should be given to mesenteric revascularization prior to aneurysm repair in patients with severe visceral artery occlusive disease because of the potential risk of mesenteric infarction at the time of aneurysm repair as noted previously.

Additional Concurrent Intraabdominal Disease

The finding of an abdominal aortic aneurysm and an additional intraabdominal process that may require operative repair is a relatively frequent event. A second surgical problem may be identified as part of the preoperative evaluation or discovered at the time of the exploratory laparotomy during open aneurysm repair. Alternatively, an abdominal aortic aneurysm may be identified during the surgical treatment of another problem. No algorithms have been defined for the management of such concurrent problems, and the overall approach requires a modicum of clinical judgment. Options include simultaneous repair or staged repair with repair of the abdominal aortic aneurysm as either the first or second procedure. The approach depends on the risk for aneurysm rupture, natural history of the second surgical problem, and potential for infection of the prosthetic graft during simultaneous repair. Notably, endovascular aneurysm repair has affected the approach to patients with these combined problems because of its reduced morbidity and mortality, which has allowed more rapid treatment.

The generic recommendation for patients with an abdominal aortic aneurysm and an additional intraabdominal surgical problem is that the most life-threatening or imminent problem be addressed first. The natural history of untreated abdominal aortic aneurysm has been defined reasonably well and has been outlined extensively earlier in this chapter. It has been reported that the risk for aneurysm rupture is increased after major intraabdominal surgery and is potentially related to an increase in collagenase activity.[250] However, this reported increased rupture risk is speculative and should not necessarily be factored into the decision algorithm. The management of concurrent colon cancer and abdominal aortic aneurysm is a frequent treatment dilemma that provides an excellent illustration of the approach to these problems. Indeed, the reported incidence of colon cancer and an abdominal aortic aneurysm occurring simultaneously ranges from 0.5% to 2.1%.[165] The treatment principles promulgated by Szilagyi et al.[251] include the following:

(a) aneurysm repair first in the presence of rupture; (b) colon resection first in the presence of hemorrhage, perforation, or obstruction; (c) aneurysm repair first in the presence of a large aneurysm and a small colon cancer; and (d) colon resection first in the presence of a large colon cancer and a small aneurysm.

Simultaneous abdominal aortic aneurysm repair and cholecystectomy is probably safe for patients with cholelithiasis or evidence of chronic cholecystitis. The safety of these simultaneous procedures has been documented in several series, and the concerns about an increased incidence of aortic graft infection have not been substantiated.[252] Advocates of the simultaneous approach justify the cholecystectomy by the potential requirement for a cholecystectomy in the future and the morbidity and mortality associated cholecystitis after aneurysm repair.[252] Although a consensus is not found in the literature, simultaneous abdominal aortic aneurysm repair and cholecystectomy are recommended only if evidence of chronic cholecystitis or multiple small stones is present. Regardless, the cholecystectomy and other simultaneous procedures should not be performed until after the aneurysm repair is completed and the retroperitoneum closed in an attempt to reduce the hypothetical risk for graft infection.

The safety and utility of other simultaneous procedures remain poorly defined although a wide range of procedures have been combined with open aneurysm repair.[162–165] The repair of ventral hernias is often mandatory to achieve a tension-free abdominal closure and should be viewed more as an extension of the aneurysm repair than as a simultaneous procedure. Inguinal hernias may be repaired at the time of aneurysm repair, but it is uncertain whether the small risk associated with a subsequent procedure at a later date offsets the obligatory additional time for the simultaneous repair. Appendectomy[253] and small-bowel excision for Meckel's diverticulum[252] have been reported to be safe when performed concomitantly with aneurysmectomy although the natural history of the associated underlying problems in the usual age group of patients undergoing abdominal aortic aneurysm repair is relatively benign.

KEY POINTS

- **An aneurysm is defined as a permanent, focal dilation of an artery that exceeds 1.5 times the normal, expected diameter.**
- **The treatment goals for patients with abdominal aortic aneurysms are to prolong life, relieve symptoms, and prevent rupture.**
- **The process of atherosclerosis and aneurysmal degeneration are likely separate and distinct.**
- **The actual mortality rate for ruptured abdominal aortic aneurysms is somewhat difficult to determine because a significant number of sudden deaths in elderly patients are likely secondary to ruptured aneurysms.**
- **The overwhelming majority of abdominal aortic aneurysms are asymptomatic at the time they are discovered.**
- **Perioperative complication rates appear to be lower after endovascular repair.**
- **The uncertainty about the long-term outcome after endovascular repair mandates indefinite postoperative surveillance.**
- **Open repair of intact abdominal aortic aneurysms is associated with significant mortality and morbidity.**
- **The long-term complications after endovascular repair include endoleak, structural failure, need for remedial procedures, need for open conversion and rupture.**
- **Isolated iliac artery aneurysms are rare and have been reported to occur with an incidence ranging from 0.03% in autopsy to 2.2% in single-institution series.**
- **The management of aneurysms extending to the level of the renal arteries or further cephalad is more complicated as reflected by the increase in the associated morbidity and mortality rates.**
- **The diagnosis of an aortoenteric fistula is often difficult and mandates a high index of suspicion.**
- **The generic recommendation for patients with an abdominal aortic aneurysm and an additional intraabdominal surgical problem is that the most life-threatening or imminent problem be addressed first.**

References

1. Dubost C, Allary M, Oeconomos N. Resection of an aneurysm of the abdominal aorta: reestablishment of the continuity by a preserved human arterial graft, with result after five months. *AMA Arch Surg.* 1952;64: 405–408.
2. Ernst CB. Abdominal aortic aneurysm. *N Engl J Med.* 1993;328:1167–1172.
3. Collin J, Araujo L, Walton J, et al. Oxford screening programme for abdominal aortic aneurysm in men aged 65 to 74 years. *Lancet* 1988;2: 613–615.
4. Ouriel K, Green RM, Donayre C, et al. An evaluation of new methods of expressing aortic aneurysm size: relationship to rupture. *J Vasc Surg.* 1992;15:12–18.
5. Taylor LM, Porter JM. Abdominal aortic aneurysms. In: Porter JM, Taylor LM, eds. *Basic data underlying clinical decision making in vascular surgery.* St. Louis: Quality Medical Publishing; 1994, pp. 98–100.
6. Brunkwall J, Hauksson H, Bengtsson H, et al. Solitary aneurysms of the iliac arterial system: an estimate of their frequency of occurrence. *J Vasc Surg.* 1989;10:381–384.
7. Lowry SF, Kraft RO. Isolated aneurysms of the iliac artery. *Arch Surg.* 1978;113:1289–1293.
8. Best VA, Price JF, Fowkes FG. Persistent increase in the incidence of abdominal aortic aneurysm in Scotland, 1981–2000. *Br J Surg.* 2003;90: 1510–1515.
9. Hoyert DL, Kung H, Smith BL. Deaths: preliminary data for 2003. *Natl Vital Stat Rep.* 2005 Feb 28;53:1–48.
10. Zarins CK, Glagov S. Aneurysms and obstructive plaques: differing local responses to atherosclerosis. In: Bergan JJ, Yao J, eds. *Aneurysms: diagnosis and treatment.* New York: Grune and Stratton; 1982, p. 61.
11. Sho E, Sho M, Hoshina K, et al. Hemodynamic forces regulate mural macrophage infiltration in experimental aortic aneurysms. *Exp Mol Pathol.* 2004;76:108–116.
12. Tilson MD, Elefteriades J, Brophy CM. Tensile strength and collagen in abdominal aortic aneurysm disease. In: Greenhalgh RM, Mannick JA, Powell JT, eds. *The cause and management of aneurysms.* Philadelphia: WB Saunders; 1990, p. 97.
13. Busuttil RW, Abou-Zamzam AM, Machleder HI. Collagenase activity of the human aorta. A comparison of patients with and without abdominal aortic aneurysms. *Arch Surg.* 1980;115:1373–1378.
14. Baxter BT, McGee GS, Shively VP, et al. Elastin content, cross-links, and mRNA in normal and aneurysmal human aorta. *J Vasc Surg.* 1992;16:192–200.
15. Lindholt JS, Jorgensen B, Klitgaard NA, et al. Systemic levels of cotinine and elastase, but not pulmonary function, are associated with the progression of small abdominal aortic aneurysms. *Eur J Vasc Endovasc Surg.* 2003;26:418–422.
16. Newman KM, Ogata Y, Malon AM, et al. Identification of matrix metalloproteinases 3 (stromelysin-1) and 9 (gelatinase B) in abdominal aortic aneurysm. *Arterioscler Thromb.* 1994;14:1315–1320.
17. Brophy CM, Marks WH, Reilly JM, et al. Decreased tissue inhibitor of metalloproteinases (TIMP) in abdominal aortic tissue: a preliminary report. *J Surg Res.* 1991;50:653.
18. Rowe VL, Stevens SL, Reddick TT, et al. Vascular smooth muscle cell apoptosis in aneurysmal, occlusive, and normal human aortas. *J Vasc Surg.* 2000;31:567–576.
19. Eliason JL, Hannawa KK, Ailawadi G, et al. Neutrophil depletion inhibits experimental abdominal aortic aneurysm formation. *Circulation,* 2005;112:232–240.
20. Newman KM, Jean-Claude J, Li H, et al. Cytokines that activate proteolysis are increased in abdominal aortic aneurysms. *Circulation* 1994;90:II224–II227.
21. Cornuz J, Sidoti PC, Tevaearai H, et al. Risk factors for asymptomatic abdominal aortic aneurysm: systematic review and meta-analysis of

population-based screening studies. *Eur J Public Health*. 2004;14: 343–349.

22. Lederle FA, Johnson GR, Wilson SE, et al. Prevalence and associations of abdominal aortic aneurysm detected through screening. Aneurysm Detection and Management (ADAM) Veterans Affairs Cooperative Study Group. *Ann Intern Med*. 1997;126:441–449.
23. Huber TS, Wang JG, Derrow AE, et al. Experience in the United States with intact abdominal aortic aneurysm repair. *J Vasc Surg*. 2001;33:304–310.
24. Lederle FA, Wilson SE, Johnson GR, et al. Immediate repair compared with surveillance of small abdominal aortic aneurysms. *N Engl J Med*. 2002;346:1437–1444.
25. Wilmink TB, Quick CR, Day NE. The association between cigarette smoking and abdominal aortic aneurysms. *J Vasc Surg*. 1999;30:1099–1105.
26. Johansen K, Koepsell T. Familial tendency for abdominal aortic aneurysms. *JAMA* 1986;256:1934–1936.
27. Darling RC III, Brewster DC, Darling RC, et al. Are familial aortic aneurysms different? *J Vasc Surg*. 1989;10:39–43.
28. Calcagno D, Hallett JW Jr, Ballard DJ, et al. Late iliac artery aneurysms and occlusive disease after aortic tube grafts for abdominal aortic aneurysm repair. A 35-year experience. *Ann Surg*. 1991;214:733–736.
29. Kalman PG, Rappaport DC, Merchant N, et al. The value of late computed tomographic scanning in identification of vascular abnormalities after abdominal aortic aneurysm repair. *J Vasc Surg*. 1999;29: 442–450.
30. Cutler BS. Arteriosclerotic femoral artery aneurysms. In: Ernst CB, Stanley JC, eds. *Current therapy in vascular surgery*. St. Louis: Mosby; 1995:315.
31. Haverich A, Miller DC, Scott WC, et al. Acute and chronic aortic dissections–determinants of long-term outcome for operative survivors. *Circulation* 1985;72:II22–II34.
32. Ammori BJ, Madan M, Bodenham AR. A review of the management of abdominal aortic aneurysms in patients following cardiac transplantation. *Eur J Vasc Endovasc Surg*. 1997;14:185–190.
33. Muluk SC, Steed DL, Makaroun MS, et al. Aortic aneurysm in heart transplant recipients. *J Vasc Surg*. 1995;22:689–694.
34. Vantrimpont PJ, van Dalen BM, van Riemsdijk-van Overbeeke IC, et al. Abdominal aortic aneurysms after heart transplantation. *J Heart Lung Transplant*. 2004;23:171–177.
35. Zierler RE, Strandness DE Jr. Hemodynamics for the vascular surgeon. In: Moore WS, ed. Vascular surgery: a comprehensive review. Philadelphia: WB Saunders; 2005, pp. 179–204.
36. Brewster DC, Cronenwett JL, Hallett JW Jr, et al. Guidelines for the treatment of abdominal aortic aneurysms. Report of a subcommittee of the Joint Council of the American Association for Vascular Surgery and Society for Vascular Surgery. *J Vasc Surg*. 2003;37:1106–1117.
37. Mortality results for randomised controlled trial of early elective surgery or ultrasonographic surveillance for small abdominal aortic aneurysms. The UK Small Aneurysm Trial Participants. *Lancet* 1998;352: 1649–1655.
38. Brown LC, Powell JT. Risk factors for aneurysm rupture in patients kept under ultrasound surveillance. UK Small Aneurysm Trial Participants. *Ann Surg*. 1999;230:289–296.
39. Cronenwett JL, Murphy TF, Zelenock GB, et al. Actuarial analysis of variables associated with rupture of small abdominal aortic aneurysms. *Surgery* 1985;98:472–483.
40. Verloes A, Sakalihasan N, Koulischer L, et al. Aneurysms of the abdominal aorta: familial and genetic aspects in three hundred thirteen pedigrees. *J Vasc Surg*. 1995;21:646–655.
41. Fillinger MF, Marra SP, Raghavan ML, et al. Prediction of rupture risk in abdominal aortic aneurysm during observation: wall stress versus diameter. *J Vasc Surg*. 2003;37:724–732.
42. Fillinger MF, Raghavan ML, Marra SP, et al. In vivo analysis of mechanical wall stress and abdominal aortic aneurysm rupture risk. *J Vasc Surg*. 2002;36:589–597.
43. Brady AR, Thompson SG, Fowkes FG, et al. Abdominal aortic aneurysm expansion: risk factors and time intervals for surveillance. *Circulation* 2004;110:16–21.
44. Collin J, Araujo L, Walton J. How fast do very small abdominal aortic aneurysms grow? *Eur J Vasc Surg*. 1989;3:15–17.
45. Nevitt MP, Ballard DJ, Hallett JW Jr. Prognosis of abdominal aortic aneurysms. A population-based study. *N Engl J Med*. 1989;321: 1009–1014.
46. Solberg S, Singh K, Wilsgaard T, et al. Increased growth rate of abdominal aortic aneurysms in women. The Tromso study. *Eur J Vasc Endovasc Surg*. 2005;29:145–149.
47. Bernstein EF, Chan EL. Abdominal aortic aneurysm in high-risk patients. Outcome of selective management based on size and expansion rate. *Ann Surg*. 1984;200:255–263.
48. Delin A, Ohlsen H, Swedenborg J. Growth rate of abdominal aortic aneurysms as measured by computed tomography. *Br J Surg*. 1985;72:530–532.
49. Guirguis EM, Barber GG. The natural history of abdominal aortic aneurysms. *Am J Surg*. 1991;162:481–483.
50. Kurvers H, Veith FJ, Lipsitz EC, et al. Discontinuous, staccato growth of abdominal aortic aneurysms. *J Am Coll Surg*. 2004;199:709–715.
51. Greenhalgh RM, Brown LC, Kwong GP, et al. Comparison of endovascular aneurysm repair with open repair in patients with abdominal aortic aneurysm (EVAR trial 1), 30-day operative mortality results: randomised controlled trial. *Lancet* 2004;364:843–848.
52. Prinssen M, Verhoeven EL, Buth J, et al. A randomized trial comparing conventional and endovascular repair of abdominal aortic aneurysms. *N Engl J Med*. 2004;351:1607–1618.
53. Hallin A, Bergqvist D, Holmberg L. Literature review of surgical management of abdominal aortic aneurysm. *Eur J Vasc Endovasc Surg*. 2001;22:197–204.
54. Finlayson SR, Birkmeyer JD, Fillinger MF, et al. Should endovascular repair lower the threshold for repair of abdominal aortic aneurysms? *J Vasc Surg*. 1999;29:973–985.
55. Becquemin JP, Lapie V, Favre JP, et al. Mid-term results of a second generation bifurcated endovascular graft for abdominal aortic aneurysm repair: the French Vanguard trial. *J Vasc Surg*. 1999;30:209–218.
56. Blum U, Voshage G, Lammer J, et al. Endoluminal stent-grafts for infrarenal abdominal aortic aneurysms. *N Engl J Med*. 1997; 336:13–20.
57. May J, White GH, Yu W, et al. Concurrent comparison of endoluminal versus open repair in the treatment of abdominal aortic aneurysms: analysis of 303 patients by life table method. *J Vasc Surg*. 1998;27:2 13–220.
58. Moore WS, Rutherford RB. Transfemoral endovascular repair of abdominal aortic aneurysm: results of the North American EVT phase 1 trial. EVT Investigators. *J Vasc Surg*. 1996;23:543–553.
59. Zarins CK, White RA, Schwarten D, et al. AneuRx stent graft versus open surgical repair of abdominal aortic aneurysms: multicenter prospective clinical trial. *J Vasc Surg*. 1999;29:292–305.
60. Lee WA, Carter JW, Upchurch G, et al. Perioperative outcomes after open and endovascular repair of intact abdominal aortic aneurysms in the United States during 2001. *J Vasc Surg*. 2004;39:491–496.
61. Anderson PL, Arons RR, Moskowitz AJ, et al. A statewide experience with endovascular abdominal aortic aneurysm repair: rapid diffusion with excellent early results. *J Vasc Surg*. 2004;39:10–19.
62. Haug ES, Romundstad P, Aadahl P, et al. Emergency non-ruptured abdominal aortic aneurysm. *Eur J Vasc Endovasc Surg*. 2004;28:612–618.
63. Soisalon-Soininen S, Salo JA, Perhoniemi V, et al. Emergency surgery of non-ruptured abdominal aortic aneurysm. *Ann Chir Gynaecol*. 1999;88: 38–43.
64. Bown MJ, Sutton AJ, Bell PR, et al. A meta-analysis of 50 years of ruptured abdominal aortic aneurysm repair. *Br J Surg*. 2002;89:714–730.
65. Johansen K, Kohler TR, Nicholls SC, et al. Ruptured abdominal aortic aneurysm: the Harborview experience. *J Vasc Surg*. 1991;13:240–245.
66. Katz DJ, Stanley JC, Zelenock GB. Operative mortality rates for intact and ruptured abdominal aortic aneurysms in Michigan: an eleven-year statewide experience. *J Vasc Surg*. 1994;19:804–815.
67. Castelli P, Caronno R, Piffaretti G, et al. Ruptured abdominal aortic aneurysm: endovascular treatment. *Abdom Imaging* 2005;30:263–269.
68. Lee WA, Hirneise CM, Tayyarah M, et al. Impact of endovascular repair on early outcomes of ruptured abdominal aortic aneurysms. *J Vasc Surg*. 2004;40:211–215.
69. Lombardi JV, Fairman RM, Golden MA, et al. The utility of commercially available endografts in the treatment of contained ruptured abdominal aortic aneurysm with hemodynamic stability. *J Vasc Surg*. 2004;40: 154–160.
70. Lynch RM. Accuracy of abdominal examination in the diagnosis of non-ruptured abdominal aortic aneurysm. *Accid Emerg Nurs*. 2004;12:99–107.
71. Moursi MM, Stanley JC. Surgical treatment of ruptured infrarenal aortic aneurysms. In: Ernst CB, Stanley JC, eds. *Current therapy in vascular surgery*. St. Louis: Mosby; 1995, pp. 224–226.
72. Hollier LH, Taylor LM, Ochsner J. Recommended indications for operative treatment of abdominal aortic aneurysms. Report of a subcommittee of the Joint Council of the Society for Vascular Surgery and the North American Chapter of the International Society for Cardiovascular Surgery. *J Vasc Surg*. 1992;15:1046–1056.
73. Liu R, Nair D, Ix J, et al. N-acetylcysteine for the prevention of contrast-induced nephropathy. A systematic review and meta-analysis. *J Gen Intern Med*. 2005;20:193–200.
74. Merten GJ, Burgess WP, Gray LV, et al. Prevention of contrast-induced nephropathy with sodium bicarbonate: a randomized controlled trial. *JAMA* 2004;291:2328–2334.
75. Sprouse LR, Meier GH III, Parent FN, et al. Is three-dimensional computed tomography reconstruction justified before endovascular aortic aneurysm repair? *J Vasc Surg*. 2004;40:443–447.
76. Hoffman M, Avellone JC, Plecha FR, et al. Operation for ruptured abdominal aortic aneurysms: a community-wide experience. *Surgery* 1982;91:597–602.
77. Wakefield TW, Whitehouse WM Jr, Wu SC, et al. Abdominal aortic aneurysm rupture: statistical analysis of factors affecting outcome of surgical treatment. *Surgery* 1982;91:586–596.
78. Lloyd GM, Brown MJ, Norwood MG, et al. Feasibility of preoperative computer tomography in patients with ruptured abdominal aortic

aneurysm: a time-to-death study in patients without operation. *J Vasc Surg*. 2004;39:788–791.
79. Screening for abdominal aortic aneurysm: recommendation statement. *Ann Intern Med*. 2005;142:198–202.
80. Fleming C, Whitlock EP, Beil TL, et al. Screening for abdominal aortic aneurysm: a best-evidence systematic review for the U.S. Preventive Services Task Force. *Ann Intern Med*. 2005;142:203–211.
81. Lindholt JS, Juul S, Fasting H, et al. Hospital costs and benefits of screening for abdominal aortic aneurysms. Results from a randomised population screening trial. *Eur J Vasc Endovasc Surg*. 2002;23:55–60.
82. Wilmink AB, Quick CR, Hubbard CS, et al. Effectiveness and cost of screening for abdominal aortic aneurysm: results of a population screening program. *J Vasc Surg*. 2003;38:72–77.
83. Kim LG, Scott RA, Thompson SG, et al. Implications of screening for abdominal aortic aneurysms on surgical workload. *Br J Surg*. 2005;92: 171–176.
84. Long-term outcomes of immediate repair compared with surveillance of small abdominal aortic aneurysms. *N Engl J Med*. 2002;346: 1445–1452.
85. Steyerberg EW, Kievit J, de Mol Van Otterloo JC, et al. Perioperative mortality of elective abdominal aortic aneurysm surgery. A clinical prediction rule based on literature and individual patient data. *Arch Intern Med*. 1995;155:1998–2004.
86. National Kidney Foundation. K/DOQI Clinical practice guidelines for chronic kidney disease: evaluation, classification, and stratification. *Am J Kidney Dis*. 2002;39:S76–S110.
87. Cronenwett JL. Factors influencing the long-term results of aortic aneurysm surgery. In: Yao J, Pearce WH, eds. Vascular surgery: long term results. East Norwalk: Appleton and Lange; 1993, pp. 171–179.
88. Valentine RJ, Decaprio JD, Castillo JM, et al. Watchful waiting in cases of small abdominal aortic aneurysms: Appropriate for all patients? *J Vasc Surg*. 2000;32:441–448.
89. McCarthy RJ, Shaw E, Whyman MR, et al. Recommendations for screening intervals for small aortic aneurysms. *Br J Surg*. 2003;90:821–826.
90. Conway KP, Byrne J, Townsend M, et al. Prognosis of patients turned down for conventional abdominal aortic aneurysm repair in the endovascular and sonographic era: Szilagyi revisited? *J Vasc Surg*. 2001;33: 752–757.
91. Englund R, Perera D, Hanel KC. Outcome for patients with abdominal aortic aneurysms that are treated non-surgically. *Aust NZ J Surg*. 1997;67:260–263.
92. Jones A, Cahill D, Gardham R. Outcome in patients with a large abdominal aortic aneurysm considered unfit for surgery. *Br J Surg*. 1998;85:1382–1384.
93. Tambyraja AL, Stuart WP, Sala TA, et al. Non-operative management of high-risk patients with abdominal aortic aneurysm. *Eur J Vasc Endovasc Surg*. 2003;26:401–404.
94. Walker EM, Hopkinson BR, Makin GS. Unoperated abdominal aortic aneurysm: presentation and natural history. *Ann R Coll Surg Engl*. 1983; 65:311–313.
95. Woodburn KR, Chant H, Davies JN, et al. Suitability for endovascular aneurysm repair in an unselected population. *Br J Surg*. 2001;88:77–81.
96. Arko FR, Filis KA, Seidel SA, et al. How many patients with infrarenal aneurysms are candidates for endovascular repair? The Northern California experience. *J Endovasc Ther*. 2004;11:33–40.
97. Carpenter JP, Baum RA, Barker CF, et al. Impact of exclusion criteria on patient selection for endovascular abdominal aortic aneurysm repair. *J Vasc Surg*. 2001;34:1050–1054.
98. Elkouri S, Martelli E, Gloviczki P, et al. Most patients with abdominal aortic aneurysm are not suitable for endovascular repair using currently approved bifurcated stent-grafts. *Vasc Endovascular Surg*. 2004;38:401–412.
99. Wolf YG, Fogarty TJ, Olcott C IV, et al. Endovascular repair of abdominal aortic aneurysms: eligibility rate and impact on the rate of open repair. *J Vasc Surg*. 2000;32:519–523.
100. Lee WA, Berceli SA, Huber TS, et al. Morbidity with retroperitoneal procedures during endovascular abdominal aortic aneurysm repair. *J Vasc Surg*. 2003;38:459–463.
101. Clouse WD, Brewster DC, Marone LK, et al. Durability of aortouniiliac endografting with femorofemoral crossover: 4-year experience in the Evt/Guidant trials. *J Vasc Surg*. 2003;37:1142–1149.
102. Hinchliffe RJ, Alric P, Wenham PW, Hopkinson BR. Durability of femorofemoral bypass grafting after aortouniiliac endovascular aneurysm repair. *J Vasc Surg*. 2003;38:498–503.
103. Lee WA, O'Dorisio J, Wolf YG, et al. Outcome after unilateral hypogastric artery occlusion during endovascular aneurysm repair. *J Vasc Surg*. 2001;33:921–926.
104. Lyden SP, Sternbach Y, Waldman DL, et al. Clinical implications of internal iliac artery embolization in endovascular repair of aortoiliac aneurysms. *Ann Vasc Surg*. 2001;15:539–543.
105. Greenberg RK, Clair D, Srivastava S, et al. Should patients with challenging anatomy be offered endovascular aneurysm repair? *J Vasc Surg*. 2003;38:990–996.
106. Buth J, Harris PL, van Marrewijk C, et al. The significance and management of different types of endoleaks. *Semin Vasc Surg*. 2003;16:95–102.
107. Gilling-Smith GL, Martin J, Sudhindran S, et al. Freedom from endoleak after endovascular aneurysm repair does not equal treatment success. *Eur J Vasc Endovasc Surg*. 2000;19:421–425.
108. Rutherford RB, Krupski WC. Current status of open versus endovascular stent-graft repair of abdominal aortic aneurysm. *J Vasc Surg*. 2004;39:1129–1139.
109. Prinssen M, Buskens E, Nolthenius RP, et al. Sexual dysfunction after conventional and endovascular AAA repair: results of the DREAM trial. *J Endovasc Ther*. 2004;11:613–620.
110. Xenos ES, Stevens SL, Freeman MB, et al. Erectile function after open or endovascular abdominal aortic aneurysm repair. *Ann Vasc Surg*. 2003;17:530–538.
111. Prinssen M, Verhoeven EL, Buth J, et al. A randomized trial comparing conventional and endovascular repair of abdominal aortic aneurysms. *N Engl J Med*. 2004;351:1607–1618.
112. Harris PL, Vallabhaneni SR, Desgranges P, et al. Incidence and risk factors of late rupture, conversion, and death after endovascular repair of infrarenal aortic aneurysms: the EUROSTAR experience. European Collaborators on Stent/graft techniques for aortic aneurysm repair. *J Vasc Surg*. 2000;32:739–749.
113. van Marrewijk CJ, Fransen G, Laheij RJ, et al. Is a type II endoleak after EVAR a harbinger of risk? Causes and outcome of open conversion and aneurysm rupture during follow-up. *Eur J Vasc Endovasc Surg*. 2004;27: 128–137.
114. May J, White GH, Stephen MS, et al. Rupture of abdominal aortic aneurysm: concurrent comparison of outcome of those occurring after endovascular repair versus those occurring without previous treatment in an 11-year single-center experience. *J Vasc Surg*. 2004; 40:860–866.
115. Lifeline Registry of Endovascular Aneurysm Repair: Registry data report. *J Vasc Surg*. 2002;35:616–620.
116. Laheij RJ, Buth J, Harris PL, et al. Need for secondary interventions after endovascular repair of abdominal aortic aneurysms. Intermediate-term follow-up results of a European collaborative registry (EUROSTAR). *Br J Surg*. 2000;87:1666–1673.
117. Schurink GW, Aarts NJ, van Bockel JH. Endoleak after stent-graft treatment of abdominal aortic aneurysm: a meta-analysis of clinical studies. *Br J Surg*. 1999;86:581–587.
118. Bertges DJ, Chow K, Wyers MC, et al. Abdominal aortic aneurysm size regression after endovascular repair is endograft dependent. *J Vasc Surg*. 2003;37:716–723.
119. Greenberg RK, Deaton D, Sullivan T, et al. Variable sac behavior after endovascular repair of abdominal aortic aneurysm: analysis of core laboratory data. *J Vasc Surg*. 2004;39:95–101.
120. Biancari F, Leo E, Ylonen K, et al. Value of the Glasgow Aneurysm Score in predicting the immediate and long-term outcome after elective open repair of infrarenal abdominal aortic aneurysm. *Br J Surg*. 2003;90: 838–844.
121. Hall J, Singh G, Hood D, et al. Management of an abdominal aortic aneurysm in a patient with end-stage liver disease. *Am J Transplant*. 2004;4:666–668.
122. Biebl M, Lau LL, Hakaim AG, et al. Midterm outcome of endovascular abdominal aortic aneurysm repair in octogenarians: a single institution's experience. *J Vasc Surg*. 2004;40:435–442.
123. Sam AD, Morasch MD, Collins J, et al. Safety of gadolinium contrast angiography in patients with chronic renal insufficiency. *J Vasc Surg*. 2003;38:313–318.
124. Sternbergh WC III, Money SR. Hospital cost of endovascular versus open repair of abdominal aortic aneurysms: a multicenter study. *J Vasc Surg*. 2000;31:237–244.
125. Bertges DJ, Zwolak RM, Deaton DH, et al. Current hospital costs and Medicare reimbursement for endovascular abdominal aortic aneurysm repair. *J Vasc Surg*. 2003;37:272–279.
126. Rosenberg BL, Comstock MC, Butz DA, et al. Endovascular abdominal aortic aneurysm repair is more profitable than open repair based on contribution margin per day. *Surgery* 2005;137:285–292.
127. Williamson WK, Nicoloff AD, Taylor LM Jr, et al. Functional outcome after open repair of abdominal aortic aneurysm. *J Vasc Surg*. 2001;33: 913–920.
128. Morasch MD, Kibbe MR, Evans ME, et al. Percutaneous repair of abdominal aortic aneurysm. *J Vasc Surg*. 2004;40:12–16.
129. Prinssen M, Buskens E, Blankensteijn JD. Quality of life endovascular and open AAA repair. Results of a randomised trial. *Eur J Vasc Endovasc Surg*. 2004;27:121–127.
130. Schermerhorn ML, Finlayson SR, Fillinger MF, et al. Life expectancy after endovascular versus open abdominal aortic aneurysm repair: results of a decision analysis model on the basis of data from EUROSTAR. *J Vasc Surg*. 2002;36:1112–1120.
131. Eagle KA, Berger PB, Calkins H, et al. ACC/AHA guideline update for perioperative cardiovascular evaluation for noncardiac surgery–executive summary a report of the American College of Cardiology/American Heart Association Task Force on Practice Guidelines (Committee to Update the 1996 Guidelines on Perioperative Cardiovascular Evaluation for Noncardiac Surgery). *Circulation* 2002;105:1257–1267.
132. Kertai MD, Boersma E, Westerhout CM, et al. A combination of statins and beta-blockers is independently associated with a reduction in the incidence of perioperative mortality and nonfatal myocardial infarction in

patients undergoing abdominal aortic aneurysm surgery. *Eur J Vasc Endovasc Surg*. 2004;28:343–352.

133. Smith SC Jr, Blair SN, Bonow RO, et al. AHA/ACC Guidelines for Preventing Heart Attack and Death in Patients With Atherosclerotic Cardiovascular Disease: 2001 update. A statement for healthcare professionals from the American Heart Association and the American College of Cardiology. *J Am Coll Cardiol*. 2001;38:1581–1583.
134. Jayr C, Matthay MA, Goldstone J, et al. Preoperative and intraoperative factors associated with prolonged mechanical ventilation. A study in patients following major abdominal vascular surgery. *Chest* 1993;103: 1231–1236.
135. Upchurch GR Jr, Proctor MC, Henke PK, et al. Predictors of severe morbidity and death after elective abdominal aortic aneurysmectomy in patients with chronic obstructive pulmonary disease. *J Vasc Surg*. 2003; 37:594–599.
136. McFalls EO, Ward HB, Moritz TE, et al. Coronary-artery revascularization before elective major vascular surgery. *N Engl J Med*. 2004;351:2795–2804.
137. Hertzer NR, Beven EG, Young JR, et al. Coronary artery disease in peripheral vascular patients. A classification of 1000 coronary angiograms and results of surgical management. *Ann Surg*. 1984;199:223–233.
138. Cuypers PW, Buth J. Does endovascular aortic aneurysm repair justify a reduced cardiology work-up? *J Cardiovasc Surg (Torino)*. 2003;44: 437–442.
139. Boylan JF, Katz J, Kavanagh BP, et al. Epidural bupivacaine-morphine analgesia versus patient-controlled analgesia following abdominal aortic surgery: analgesic, respiratory, and myocardial effects. *Anesthesiology* 1998; 89:585–593.
140. Major CP Jr, Greer MS, Russell WL, et al. Postoperative pulmonary complications and morbidity after abdominal aneurysmectomy: a comparison of postoperative epidural versus parenteral opioid analgesia. *Am Surg*. 1996;62:45–51.
141. Eagle KA, Berger PB, Calkins H, et al. ACC/AHA Guideline Update for Perioperative Cardiovascular Evaluation for Noncardiac Surgery–Executive Summary. A report of the American College of Cardiology/American Heart Association Task Force on Practice Guidelines (Committee to Update the 1996 Guidelines on Perioperative Cardiovascular Evaluation for Noncardiac Surgery). *Anesth Analg*. 2002;94:1052–1064.
142. Valentine RJ, Duke ML, Inman MH, et al. Effectiveness of pulmonary artery catheters in aortic surgery: a randomized trial. *J Vasc Surg*. 1998;27:203–211.
143. Elmore JR, Franklin DP, Youkey JR, et al. Normothermia is protective during infrarenal aortic surgery. *J Vasc Surg*. 1998;28:984–992.
144. Bush HL Jr, Hydo LJ, Fischer E, et al. Hypothermia during elective abdominal aortic aneurysm repair: the high price of avoidable morbidity. *J Vasc Surg*. 1995;21:392–400.
145. Alvarez GG, Fergusson DA, Neilipovitz DT, et al. Cell salvage does not minimize perioperative allogeneic blood transfusion in abdominal vascular surgery: a systematic review. *Can J Anaesth*. 2004;51:425–431.
146. Sicard GA, Reilly JM, Rubin BG, et al. Transabdominal versus retroperitoneal incision for abdominal aortic surgery: report of a prospective randomized trial. *J Vasc Surg*. 1995;21:174–3.
147. Thompson JF, Mullee MA, Bell PR, et al. Intraoperative heparinisation, blood loss and myocardial infarction during aortic aneurysm surgery: a Joint Vascular Research Group study. *Eur J Vasc Endovasc Surg*. 1996;12: 86–90.
148. Nicholson ML, Baker DM, Hopkinson BR, et al. Randomized controlled trial of the effect of mannitol on renal reperfusion injury during aortic aneurysm surgery. *Br J Surg*. 1996;83:1230–1233.
149. Marques DS, Lingaas PS, Geiran O, et al. Multiple bacteria in aortic aneurysms. *J Vasc Surg*. 2003;38:1384–1389.
150. van der Vliet JA, Kouwenberg PP, et al. Relevance of bacterial cultures of abdominal aortic aneurysm contents. *Surgery* 1996;119:129–132.
151. Seeger JM, Coe DA, Kaelin LD. Routine reimplantation of patent inferior mesenteric arteries limits colon infarction after aortic reconstruction. *J Vasc Surg*. 1992;15:635–641.
152. Wakefield TW, Hantler CB, Wrobleski SK, et al. Effects of differing rates of protamine reversal of heparin anticoagulation. *Surgery* 1996;119: 123–128.
153. Dorman BH, Elliott BM, Spinale FG, et al. Protamine use during peripheral vascular surgery: a prospective randomized trial. *J Vasc Surg*. 1995; 22:248–255.
154. Hall KA, Peters B, Smyth SH, et al. Abdominal wall hernias in patients with abdominal aortic aneurysmal versus aortoiliac occlusive disease. *Am J Surg*. 1995;170:572–575.
155. Liapis CD, Dimitroulis DA, Kakisis JD, et al. Incidence of incisional hernias in patients operated on for aneurysm or occlusive disease. *Am Surg*. 2004;70:550–552.
156. Raffetto JD, Cheung Y, Fisher JB, et al. Incision and abdominal wall hernias in patients with aneurysm or occlusive aortic disease. *J Vasc Surg*. 2003;37:1150–1154.
157. Yeager RA, Porter JM. Arterial and prosthetic graft infection. In: Porter JM, Taylor LM, eds. Basic data underlying clinical decision making in vascular surgery. St. Louis: Quality Medical Publishing; 2005, pp. 90–97.
158. Bastounis E, Filis K, Georgopoulos S, et al. Selective use of the intensive care unit after elective infrarenal abdominal aortic aneurysm repair. *Int Angiol*. 2003;22:308–316.
159. Akkersdijk GJ, Van der GY, Moll FL, et al. Complications of standard elective abdominal aortic aneurysm repair. *Eur J Vasc Endovasc Surg*. 1998;15:505–510.
160. Johnston KW. Multicenter prospective study of nonruptured abdominal aortic aneurysm. Part II. Variables predicting morbidity and mortality. *J Vasc Surg*. 1989;9:437–447.
161. Hua HT, Cambria RP, Chuang SK, et al. Early outcomes of endovascular versus open abdominal aortic aneurysm repair in the National Surgical Quality Improvement Program-Private Sector (NSQIP-PS). *J Vasc Surg*. 2005;41:382–389.
162. Georgopoulos S, Pikoulis E, Bacoyiannis C, et al. Combined abdominal aortic aneurysmectomy and other abdominal operations. *Scand J Surg*. 2004;93:61–63.
163. Grego F, Lepidi S, Bassi P, et al. Simultaneous surgical treatment of abdominal aortic aneurysm and carcinoma of the bladder. *J Vasc Surg*. 2003;37:607–614.
164. Illuminati G, Calio' FG, D'Urso A, et al. Simultaneous repair of abdominal aortic aneurysm and resection of unexpected, associated abdominal malignancies. *J Surg Oncol*. 2004;88:234–239.
165. Kiskinis D, Spanos C, Melas N, et al. Priority of resection in concomitant abdominal aortic aneurysm (AAA) and colorectal cancer (CRC): review of the literature and experience of our clinic. *Tech Coloproctol*. 2004;suppl 1:s19–s21.
166. Komori K, Furuyama T, Maehara Y. Renal artery clamping and left renal vein division during abdominal aortic aneurysm repair. *Eur J Vasc Endovasc Surg*. 2004;27:80–83.
167. Harward TR, Ingegno MD, Carlton L, et al. Limb-threatening ischemia due to multilevel arterial occlusive disease. Simultaneous or staged inflow/outflow revascularization. *Ann Surg*. 1995;221:498–503.
168. Blankensteijn JD, Lindenburg FP, Van der Graaf Y, et al. Influence of study design on reported mortality and morbidity rates after abdominal aortic aneurysm repair. *Br J Surg*. 1998;85:1624–1630.
169. Tollefson DF, Ernst CB. Colon ischemia following aortic reconstruction. In: Porter JM, Taylor LM, eds. *Basic data underlying clinical decision making in vascular surgery*. St. Louis: Quality Medical Publishing; 1994, pp. 111–115.
170. Champagne BJ, Darling RC III, Daneshmand M, et al. Outcome of aggressive surveillance colonoscopy in ruptured abdominal aortic aneurysm. *J Vasc Surg*. 2004;39:792–796.
171. Valentine RJ, Hagino RT, Jackson MR, et al. Gastrointestinal complications after aortic surgery. *J Vasc Surg*. 1998;28:404–411.
172. Ottinger LW. Acute cholecystitis as a postoperative complication. *Ann Surg*. 1976;184:162–165.
173. Yao J. Vasculogenic impotence. In: Ernst CB, Stanley JC, eds. *Current therapy in vascular surgery*. St. Louis: Mosby; 1995, pp. 397–400.
174. Szilagyi DE. A second look at the etiology of spinal cord damage in surgery of the abdominal aorta. *J Vasc Surg*. 1993;17:1111–1113.
175. Feinglass J, Cowper D, Dunlop D, et al. Late survival risk factors for abdominal aortic aneurysm repair: experience from fourteen Department of Veterans Affairs hospitals. *Surgery* 1995;118:16–24.
176. McFalls EO, Ward HB, Santilli S, et al. The influence of perioperative myocardial infarction on long-term prognosis following elective vascular surgery. *Chest* 1998;113:681–686.
177. Biancari F, Ylonen K, Anttila V, et al. Durability of open repair of infrarenal abdominal aortic aneurysm: a 15-year follow-up study. *J Vasc Surg*. 2002;35:87–93.
178. Hallett JW Jr, Marshall DM, Petterson TM, et al. Graft-related complications after abdominal aortic aneurysm repair: reassurance from a 36-year population-based experience. *J Vasc Surg*. 1997;25:277–284.
179. Parker MV, O'Donnell SD, Chang AS, et al. What imaging studies are necessary for abdominal aortic endograft sizing? A prospective blinded study using conventional computed tomography, aortography, and three-dimensional computed tomography. *J Vasc Surg*. 2005;41:199–205.
180. Zarins CK, Bloch DA, Crabtree T, et al. Stent graft migration after endovascular aneurysm repair: importance of proximal fixation. *J Vasc Surg*. 2003;38:1264–1272.
181. Sternbergh WC III, Money SR, Greenberg RK, et al. Influence of endograft oversizing on device migration, endoleak, aneurysm shrinkage, and aortic neck dilation: results from the Zenith Multicenter Trial. *J Vasc Surg*. 2004;39:20–26.
182. Ricotta JJ. What's new in vascular surgery. *J Am Coll Surg*. 2004;198: 600–625.
183. Mehta M, Cayne N, Veith FJ, et al. Relationship of proximal fixation to renal dysfunction in patients undergoing endovascular aneurysm repair. *J Cardiovasc Surg (Torino)*. 2004;45:367–374.
184. Grego F, Frigatti P, Antonello M, et al. Suprarenal fixation of endograft in abdominal aortic aneurysm treatment: focus on renal function. *Ann Surg*. 2004;240:169–178.
185. Wyers MC, Fillinger MF, Schermerhorn ML, et al. Endovascular repair of abdominal aortic aneurysm without preoperative arteriography. *J Vasc Surg*. 2003;38:730–738.

186. Velazquez OC, Carpenter JP, Baum RA, et al. Perigraft air, fever, and leukocytosis after endovascular repair of abdominal aortic aneurysms. *Am J Surg*. 1999;178:185–189.
187. Corriere MA, Feurer ID, Becker SY, et al. Endoleak following endovascular abdominal aortic aneurysm repair: implications for duration of screening. *Ann Surg*. 2004;239:800–805.
188. Rozenblit AM, Patlas M, Rosenbaum AT, et al. Detection of endoleaks after endovascular repair of abdominal aortic aneurysm: value of unenhanced and delayed helical CT acquisitions. *Radiology* 2003;227:426–433.
189. Elkouri S, Panneton JM, Andrews JC, et al. Computed tomography and ultrasound in follow-up of patients after endovascular repair of abdominal aortic aneurysm. *Ann Vasc Surg*. 2004;18:271–279.
190. Raman KG, Missig-Carroll N, Richardson T, et al. Color-flow duplex ultrasound scan versus computed tomographic scan in the surveillance of endovascular aneurysm repair. *J Vasc Surg*. 2003;38:645–651.
191. Wolf YG, Johnson BL, Hill BB, et al. Duplex ultrasound scanning versus computed tomographic angiography for postoperative evaluation of endovascular abdominal aortic aneurysm repair. *J Vasc Surg*. 2000;32: 1142–1148.
192. Matsumura JS, Moore WS. Clinical consequences of periprosthetic leak after endovascular repair of abdominal aortic aneurysm. Endovascular Technologies Investigators. *J Vasc Surg*. 1998;27:606–613.
193. Rockman CB, Riles TS, Landis R. Lower extremity paraparesis or paraplegia subsequent to endovascular management of abdominal aortic aneurysms. *J Vasc Surg*. 2001;33:178–180.
194. Zhang WW, Kulaylat MN, Anain PM, et al. Embolization as cause of bowel ischemia after endovascular abdominal aortic aneurysm repair. *J Vasc Surg*. 2004;40:867–872.
195. Kasirajan K, Matteson B, Marek JM, et al. Technique and results of transfemoral superselective coil embolization of type II lumbar endoleak. *J Vasc Surg*. 2003;38:61–66.
196. Harris P, Brennan J, Martin J, et al. Longitudinal aneurysm shrinkage following endovascular aortic aneurysm repair: a source of intermediate and late complications. *J Endovasc Surg*. 1999;6:11–16.
197. Janczyk RJ, Howells GA, Bair HA, et al. Hypothermia is an independent predictor of mortality in ruptured abdominal aortic aneurysms. *Vasc Endovascular Surg*. 2004;38:37–42.
198. Bradbury AW, Makhdoomi KR, Adam DJ, et al. Twelve-year experience of the management of ruptured abdominal aortic aneurysm. *Br J Surg*. 1997;84:1705–1707.
199. Halpern VJ, Kline RG, D'Angelo AJ, et al. Factors that affect the survival rate of patients with ruptured abdominal aortic aneurysms. J *Vasc Surg*. 1997;26:939–945.
200. Johnston KW. Ruptured abdominal aortic aneurysm: six-year follow-up results of a multicenter prospective study. Canadian Society for Vascular Surgery Aneurysm Study Group. *J Vasc Surg*. 1994;19:888–900.
201. Maziak DE, Lindsay TF, Marshall JC, et al. The impact of multiple organ dysfunction on mortality following ruptured abdominal aortic aneurysm repair. *Ann Vasc Surg*. 1998; 12:93–100.
202. van Dongen HP, Leusink JA, Moll FL, et al. Ruptured abdominal aortic aneurysms: factors influencing postoperative mortality and long-term survival. *Eur J Vasc Endovasc Surg*. 1998;15:62–66.
203. Papavassiliou V, Anderton M, Loftus IM, et al. The physiological effects of elevated intra-abdominal pressure following aneurysm repair. *Eur J Vasc Endovasc Surg*. 2003;26:293–298.
204. Parikshak M, Shepard AD, Reddy DJ, et al. Adrenal insufficiency in patients with ruptured abdominal aortic aneurysms. *J Vasc Surg*. 2004;39: 944–950.
205. Hennessy A, Barry MC, McGee H, et al. Quality of life following repair of ruptured and elective abdominal aortic aneurysms. *Eur J Surg*. 1998;164:673–677.
206. Reichart M, Geelkerken RH, Huisman AB, et al. Ruptured abdominal aortic aneurysm: endovascular repair is feasible in 40% of patients. *Eur J Vasc Endovasc Surg*. 2003;26:479–486.
207. Rose DF, Davidson IR, Hinchliffe RJ, et al. Anatomical suitability of ruptured abdominal aortic aneurysms for endovascular repair. *J Endovasc Ther*. 2003;10:453–457.
208. Richardson JW, Greenfield LJ. Natural history and management of iliac aneurysms. *J Vasc Surg*. 1988; 8:165–171.
209. Krupski WC, Bass A, Rosenberg GD, et al. The elusive isolated hypogastric artery aneurysm: novel presentations. *J Vasc Surg*. 1989;10: 557–562.
210. Santilli SM, Wernsing SE, Lee ES. Expansion rates and outcomes for iliac artery aneurysms. *J Vasc Surg*. 2000;31:114–121.
211. Money SR, Hollier LH. Surgical treatment of inflammatory abdominal aortic aneurysms. In: Ernst CB, Stanley JC, eds. *Current therapy in vascular surgery*. St. Louis: Mosby; 1995, pp. 229–231.
212. Haug ES, Skomsvoll JF, Jacobsen G, et al. Inflammatory aortic aneurysm is associated with increased incidence of autoimmune disease. *J Vasc Surg*. 2003;38:492–497.
213. Baskerville PA, Browse NL. Peri-aortic fibrosis: progression and regression. *J Cardiovasc Surg (Torino)*. 1987;28:30–31.
214. Chuter T, Ivancev K, Malina M, et al. Inflammatory aneurysm treated by means of transfemoral endovascular graft insertion. *J Vasc Interv Radiol*. 1997;8:39–41.
215. Nevelsteen A, Lacroix H, Stockx L, et al. Inflammatory abdominal aortic aneurysm and bilateral complete ureteral obstruction: treatment by endovascular graft and bilateral ureteric stenting. *Ann Vasc Surg*. 1999;13:222–224.
216. Ruppert V, Verrel F, Kellner W, et al. Endovascular repair of inflammatory abdominal aortic aneurysms: a valuable alternative? Case report and review of literature. *Ann Vasc Surg*. 2004; 18:357–360.
217. Bitsch M, Norgaard HH, Roder O, et al. Inflammatory aortic aneurysms: regression of fibrosis after aneurysm surgery. *Eur J Vasc Endovasc Surg*. 1997;13:371–374.
218. Ruppert V, Umscheid T, Rieger J, et al. Endovascular aneurysm repair: Treatment of choice for abdominal aortic aneurysm coincident with horseshoe kidney? Three case reports and review of literature. *J Vasc Surg*. 2004;40:367–370.
219. Bonati L, Rubini P, Japichino GG, et al. Long-term outcome after inflammatory abdominal aortic aneurysm repair: case-matched study. *World J Surg*. 2003;27:539–544.
220. Crawford ES, Beckett WC, Greer MS. Juxtarenal infrarenal abdominal aortic aneurysm. Special diagnostic and therapeutic considerations. *Ann Surg*. 1986;203:661–670.
221. Jean-Claude JM, Reilly LM, et al. Pararenal aortic aneurysms: the future of open aortic aneurysm repair. *J Vasc Surg*. 1999;29:902–912.
222. Martin GH, O'Hara PJ, Hertzer NR, et al. Surgical repair of aneurysms involving the suprarenal, visceral, and lower thoracic aortic segments: early results and late outcome. *J Vasc Surg*. 2000;31:851–862.
223. Greenberg RK, Haulon S, O'Neill S, et al. Primary endovascular repair of juxtarenal aneurysms with fenestrated endovascular grafting. *Eur J Vasc Endovasc Surg*. 2004;27:484–491.
224. Reddy DJ, Shepard AD, Evans JR, et al. Management of infected aortoiliac aneurysms. *Arch Surg*. 1991;126:873–878.
225. Ellenby MI, Ernst CB. Surgical treatment of infected abdominal aortic aneurysms. In: Ernst CB, Stanley JC, eds. *Current therapy in vascular surgery*. St. Louis: Mosby; 1995, pp. 232–235.
226. Brown SL, Busuttil RW, Baker JD, et al. Bacteriologic and surgical determinants of survival in patients with mycotic aneurysms. *J Vasc Surg*. 1984;1:541–547.
227. Oz MC, Brener BJ, Buda JA, et al. A ten-year experience with bacterial aortitis. *J Vasc Surg*. 1989;10:439–449.
228. Ewart JM, Burke ML, Bunt TJ. Spontaneous abdominal aortic infections. Essentials of diagnosis and management. *Am Surg*. 1983;49:37–50.
229. Koeppel TA, Gahlen J, Diehl S, et al. Mycotic aneurysm of the abdominal aorta with retroperitoneal abscess: successful endovascular repair. *J Vasc Surg*. 2004;40:164–166.
230. Fillmore AJ, Valentine RJ. Surgical mortality in patients with infected aortic aneurysms. *J Am Coll Surg*. 2003;196:435–441.
231. Taheri SA, Kulaylat MN, Grippi J, et al. Surgical treatment of primary aortoduodenal fistula. *Ann Vasc Surg*. 1991;5:265–270.
232. Pitrowski JJB. Management of vascular graft infection. In: Bernhard VM, Towne JB, eds. *Complications in vascular surgery*. St. Louis: Quality Medical Publishing; 1991, p. 235.
233. French JR, Simring DV, Merrett N, et al. Aorto-enteric fistula following endoluminal abdominal aortic aneurysm repair. *Aust NZ J Surg*. 2004;74:397–399.
234. Berman SS, Bernhard VM. Management of primary aortoenteric fistula. In: Ernst CB, Stanley JC, eds. *Current therapy in vascular surgery*. St. Louis: Mosby; 1995, pp. 262–264.
235. Giordano JM. Venous anomalies encountered during aortic reconstruction. In: Ernst CB, Stanley JC, eds. *Current therapy in vascular surgery*. St. Louis: Mosby; 1995, pp. 252–255.
236. Gaspar MR, Waters HJ, Averbook AW. Renal ectopia and renal fusion in patients requiring abdominal operations. In: Ernst CB, Stanley JC, eds. *Current therapy in vascular surgery*. St. Louis: Mosby; 1995, pp. 246–250.
237. Davidovic LB, Kostic DM, Jakovljevic NS, et al. Abdominal aortic surgery and horseshoe kidney. *Ann Vasc Surg*. 2004;18:725–728.
238. Jackson RW, Fay DM, Wyatt MG, et al. The renal impact of aortic stent-grafting in patients with a horseshoe kidney. *Cardiovasc Intervent Radiol*. 2004;27:632–636.
239. Kaplan DB, Kwon CC, Marin ML, et al. Endovascular repair of abdominal aortic aneurysms in patients with congenital renal vascular anomalies. *J Vasc Surg*. 1999;30:407–415.
240. Kim B, Donayre CE, Hansen CJ, et al. Endovascular abdominal aortic aneurysm repair using the AneuRx stent graft: impact of excluding accessory renal arteries. *Ann Vasc Surg*. 2004;18:32–37.
241. Benjamin ME, Hansen KJ, Craven TE, et al. Combined aortic and renal artery surgery. A contemporary experience. *Ann Surg*. 1996;223: 555–565.
242. Huber TS, Harward TR, Flynn TC, et al. Operative mortality rates after elective infrarenal aortic reconstructions. *J Vasc Surg*. 1995;22 :287–293.
243. Derrow AE, Seeger JM, Dame DA, et al. The outcome in the United States after thoracoabdominal aortic aneurysm repair, renal artery bypass, and mesenteric revascularization. *J Vasc Surg*. 2001;34:54–61.

244. Gentile AT, Moneta GL, Taylor LM Jr, et al. Isolated bypass to the superior mesenteric artery for intestinal ischemia. *Arch Surg.* 1994; 129:926–931.
245. Mateo RB, O'Hara PJ, Hertzer NR, et al. Elective surgical treatment of symptomatic chronic mesenteric occlusive disease: early results and late outcomes. *J Vasc Surg.* 1999;29:821–831.
246. Tollefson DF, Ernst CB. Natural history of atherosclerotic renal artery stenosis associated with aortic disease. *J Vasc Surg.* 1991;14:327–331.
247. Zierler RE, Bergelin RO, Isaacson JA, et al. Natural history of atherosclerotic renal artery stenosis: a prospective study with duplex ultrasonography. *J Vasc Surg.* 1994;19:250–257.
248. Williamson WK, Abou-Zamzam AM Jr, Moneta GL, et al. Prophylactic repair of renal artery stenosis is not justified in patients who require infrarenal aortic reconstruction. *J Vasc Surg.* 1998;28:14–20.
249. Thomas JH, Blake K, Pierce GE, et al. The clinical course of asymptomatic mesenteric arterial stenosis. *J Vasc Surg.* 1998;27:840–844.
250. Swanson RJ, Littooy FN, Hunt TK, et al. Laparotomy as a precipitating factor in the rupture of intra-abdominal aneurysms. *Arch Surg.* 1980;115:299–304.
251. Szilagyi DE, Elliott JP, Berguer R. Coincidental malignancy and abdominal aortic aneurysm. Problems of management. *Arch Surg.* 1967;95:402–412.
252. String ST. Management of concurrent intra-abdominal disease and abdominal aortic aneurysms. In: Ernst CB, Stanley JC, eds. *Current therapy in vascular surgery.* St. Louis: Mosby; 1995, pp. 235–237.
253. Oshner JL, Cooley DA, DeBakey ME. Associated intra-abdominal lesions encountered during resection of aortic aneurysms. *Dis Colon Rectum* 1960;3:485–490.

CHAPTER 103 ■ RENAL ARTERY OCCLUSIVE AND ANEURYSMAL DISEASE

JAMES C. STANLEY, GILBERT R. UPCHURCH, JR., AND PETER K. HENKE

Renal artery occlusive and aneurysmal disease has been recognized with increasing frequency with the advent of less invasive imaging modalities. The importance of elevated blood pressure as a contributor to cardiovascular arteriosclerosis is well recognized and renal artery stenoses may account for hypertension in many of these patients. In fact, this disease may be one of the most unrecognized and untreated vascular diseases in contemporary times. Renal artery aneurysms are relatively rare. Their clinical relevance is often questioned, although recent experience suggests that they too contribute to a hypertensive state in certain patients.

RENAL ARTERY OCCLUSIVE DISEASE

Renovascular hypertension secondary to renal artery occlusive disease is the most common form of surgically correctable hypertension. Systemic blood pressure elevations in these patients follow reductions in renal perfusion with activation of the renin–angiotensin system. Although this physiologic response tends to restore the renal artery perfusion pressures toward normal, it does so in a pathologic manner by producing hypertension in the systemic circulation.

Pathophysiology of Renovascular Hypertension

The physiologic basis of renovascular hypertension is relatively well defined. This form of hypertension was first recognized more than 60 years ago by Goldblatt et al.,[1] who produced sustained hypertension in dogs after gradual reductions in renal artery blood flow using an externally controlled vascular clamp. Subsequent studies have discounted the importance of renal ischemia per se as the cause of renovascular hypertension, with other hemodynamic signals appearing essential in increasing renin release, the most obvious being a decrease in mean renal artery perfusion pressure. A stenosis causing an 80% reduction in renal artery cross-sectional area (a so-called critical stenosis) induces a pressure gradient sufficient to cause increased renin release from the kidney. Renin and its effects on angiotensin and aldosterone account for the elevated blood pressure of renovascular hypertension (Fig. 103.1).

Renin is produced by the juxtaglomerular apparatus of the kidney. This anatomic area consists of a variety of cells, including *myoepitheloid cells* or *granular cells*, located on the wall of the afferent arterioles; the *macula densa,* which is composed of specialized tubular epithelial cells in the glomerular hilus at the transition of the loop of Henle to the distal convoluted tubule; and *lacis cells,* located in the region of the efferent glomerular arteriole and the macula densa. Lacis cells are intimately associated with the glomerulus and are anatomically similar to mesangial cells. The interrelations between the macula densa, glomerular arteriole vasomotion, and renal tubular function are important in understanding renin kinetics.

Regulation of renin production and its release from the kidney at the cellular and molecular level is complex. Renal baroreceptors, acting as stretch receptors, affect the release of renin from juxtaglomerular cells. Activation of these receptors appears to involve the calcium ion, with increasing evidence that renin release and intracellular levels of calcium are

VASCULAR

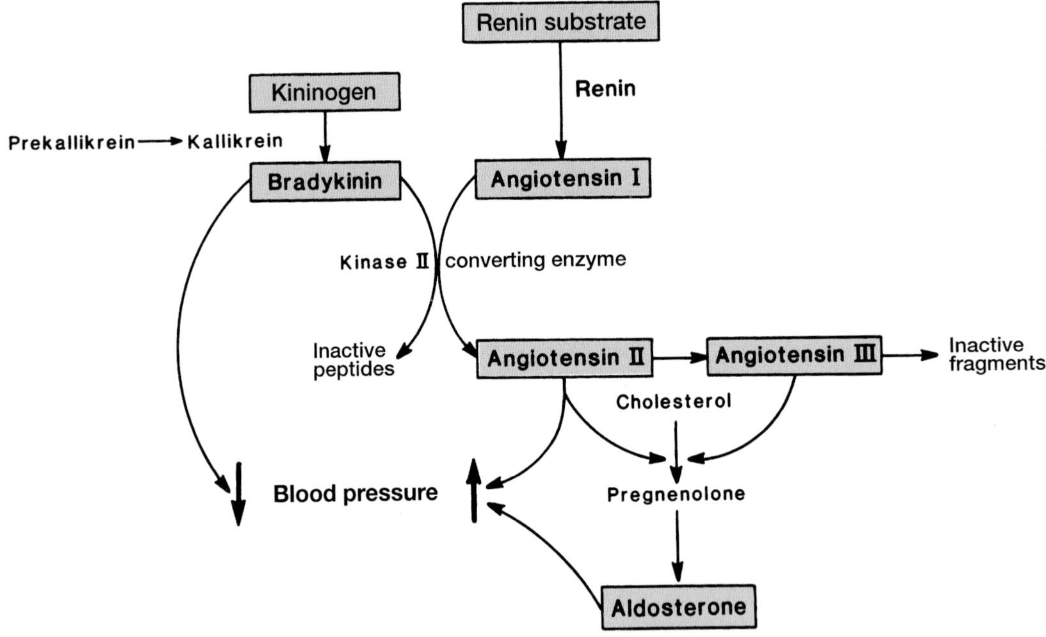

FIGURE 103.1 Renin–angiotensin system interrelation with aldosterone and bradykinin in regulation of blood pressure. (After Stanley JC, Graham LM, Whitehouse WM Jr. Renovascular hypertension. In: Miller TA, Rowland BJ, eds. *Physiologic basis of modern surgical care*. St Louis: CV Mosby, 1988, p. 734, with permission.)

inversely related. Alternatively, renin release can occur with changes in pressure at the afferent renal arteriole level, as well as with changes in renal interstitial volume and pressure.

Renin is a proteolytic enzyme, active at a neutral pH on its only known substrate, angiotensinogen. The renin gene is located on chromosome 1 (Figs. 103.2 and 103.3). This gene comprises nine exons and an additional miniexon, interrupted by eight introns. Transcription of the renin gene to renin mRNA is followed by its translation into a preprorenin molecule with a molecular weight of 45 kd. Subsequent cleavage and glycosylation of this molecule in the rough endoplasmic reticulum produces prorenin with a molecular weight of 47 kd. Prorenin is transferred into the Golgi complex, where it is secreted and processed to active renin. Renin is a single-chain polypeptide with a molecular weight of about 38 kd.[2] It is stored as granules within the juxtaglomerular cells and, in some instances, as granules within the arteriolar wall.

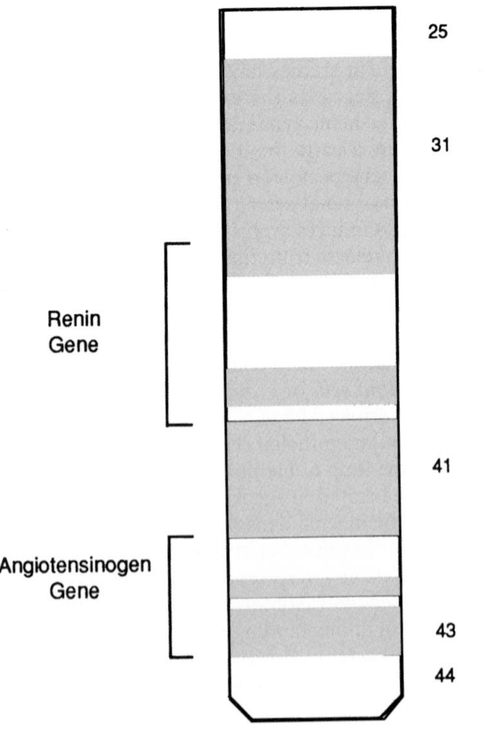

FIGURE 103.2 Chromosome 1 contains both the human renin and angiotensinogen genes.

Renin has a half-life of 20 to 30 minutes. Under usual circumstances of normal sodium balance, the sum of renin activity measured in both renal veins is about 48% greater than that in the infrarenal vena cava or peripheral arterial and venous circulations.[3] The renin levels in the peripheral circulation appear to be in a steady state because of this relatively constant 48% contribution of renin from the kidneys. The liver is the primary site for removal and clearance of renin.[4] Extrarenal renin or reninlike enzymes (isorenins) exist in the submaxillary salivary gland, uterus, placenta, and brain, but there is no evidence that these substances are functionally important in elevating blood pressure.

The biochemistry of the renin–angiotensin system has been well defined (Fig. 103. 4). The primary, if not sole, function of renin is the hydrolysis of renin substrate (a circulating peptide known as *angiotensinogen*) to form angiotensin I. Angiotensinogen is an α_2-globulin with a molecular weight of 60 kd. It is produced in the liver. The gene for angiotensinogen is located on chromosome 1 and is composed of five exons and four introns (Figs. 103.2 and 103.5). The nucleotides encoding for the angiotensin I peptide exist within the second exon. Expression of the angiotensinogen gene is subject to a variety of physiologic and pathophysiologic stimuli, including steroid hormones, angiotensin II, salt loading, and various drugs. Angiotensinogen itself has no vasoactive properties.

Angiotensin I, a decapeptide produced by the renin–renin substrate reaction, has little vasoactivity. It does exert an effect on the adrenal medulla, the sympathetic and central nervous

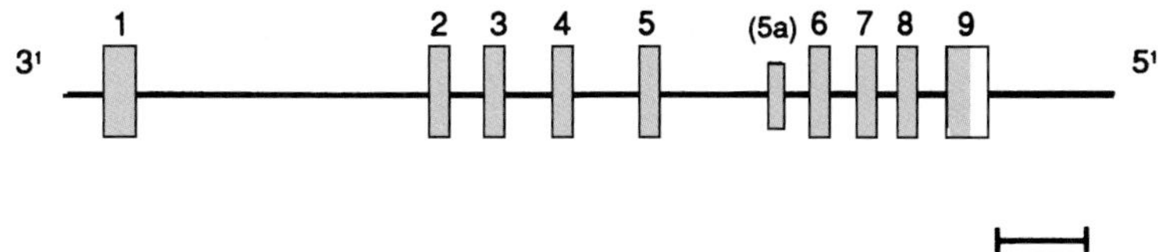

FIGURE 103.3 Human renin gene, consisting of nine exons and eight introns, with a 9–base pair miniexon (5a) of unknown function located between exons five and six. This gene is about 12.18 kb long. The coding sequence is contained in the second to eighth exons and in portions of the first and ninth exons.

systems, and the renal arterioles. Angiotensin II is formed when two C-terminal peptides are cleaved from angiotensin I by the carboxypeptidase, angiotensin-converting enzyme (ACE). Angiotensin II, an octapeptide, represents the vasoconstrictive element of renovascular hypertension. Although angiotensin II stimulates liver production of renin substrate, in normal subjects, it provides a continuous negative feedback on renal release of renin.[5] Angiotensin II has a half-life of about 4 minutes. Angiotensin III, a heptapeptide, is produced with the aminopeptidase cleavage of angiotensin II to I-desaspartyl-angiotensin II. Angiotensin III is known to inhibit angiotensin II, but its most relevant effect is to increase aldosterone synthesis. Nevertheless, angiotensin III has little biologic activity of physiologic importance.

Aldosterone is secreted from the zona glomerulosa of the adrenal cortex and represents the volume element of renovascular hypertension. The biosynthesis of this mineralocorticoid includes cleavage of a side chain of cholesterol to form pregnenolone. This step is facilitated by both angiotensin II and III. Aldosterone increases renal conservation of sodium and water, with a subsequent extracellular fluid volume expansion and an eventual increase in blood pressure.

ACE (dipeptidylcarboxypeptidase) is a zinc metallopeptidase responsible for producing angiotensin II from angiotensin I by removing C-terminal peptides from angiotensin I. The molecular weight of ACE is 150,000 to 180,000 kd. The ACE gene has been mapped to chromosome 17 in humans. ACE has its highest concentration in the endothelium of the pulmonary circulation. Conversion of angiotensin I to angiotensin II, at physiologic concentrations, occurs in a single passage through the lungs.[6] ACE has been found at lower levels in the blood and kidney as well as in other vascular beds. ACE is also important in the metabolism of the vasodepressor bradykinin. At least two enzymes appear to inactivate bradykinin. The first is kinase I, which acts by cleaving the carboxy-terminal arginine of bradykinin. The second, kinase II, acts by cleaving the carboxy-terminal dipeptide group, Phe-Arg. Kinase II and ACE appear to be similar in

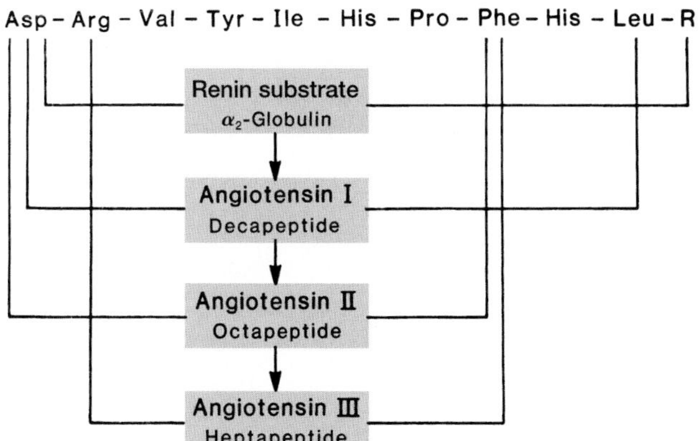

FIGURE 103.4 Biochemical composition of renin substrate and the angiotensins. (After Stanley JC, Graham LM: Renovascular hypertension. In: Miller TA, ed. *Physiologic basis of modern surgical care.* 2nd ed. St Louis: Quality Medical Publishing, 1998, p. 918, with permission.)

that they have nearly identical substrate specificities, cofactor requirements, and antigenic specificities.[7]

The most common means of determining plasma renin activity is the measurement of angiotensin I generation using a modified radioimmunoassay. Renin activity is expressed as the hourly amount of angiotensin I generated per volume of plasma assayed. The assay involves two phases: (a) an incubation of plasma to generate angiotensin I and (b) the actual radioimmunoassay of generated angiotensin I. Assay techniques vary among laboratories, often making interlaboratory comparisons difficult. Renin secretion is calculated as the renal arteriovenous difference in renin activity multiplied by renal plasma flow and is expressed as nanograms per milliliter per hour.

The actions of angiotensin on cardiac activity, vascular smooth muscle reactivity, and sodium and water metabolism contribute to increased arterial pressure (Fig. 103.6). The most important consequence of renal artery occlusive disease is the production of angiotensin II, which is one of the most potent pressor substances known. Angiotensin II acts directly on arteriolar smooth muscle of nearly all vascular beds; the splanchnic, renal, and cutaneous circulations are most sensitive to its effects. Despite an acceptance of the central importance of angiotensin in the generation of renovascular hypertension, the exact role of cellular or locally secreted renin and generated angiotensin in this clinical setting remains undetermined.

Hemodynamic responses to an activated renin–angiotensin system depend on the rate of alterations in renal blood flow as well as on whether one or both kidneys are affected. Acute reductions in renal blood flow result in rapid increases in plasma renin and blood pressure. In the case of unilateral renovascular disease with a normal opposite kidney, the hypertension is characterized by renin hypersecretion from the affected kidney and suppression of renin production in the contralateral kidney.[8,9] Sodium retention within the affected kidney is counterbalanced by continuous sodium excretion from the normal contralateral kidney, resulting in relative intravascular volume depletion. This vasoconstrictive form of hypertension is angiotensin II dependent and responds to ACE inhibitors.

Pathophysiologic alterations in the case of bilateral renovascular disease, or unilateral disease of a solitary kidney, relate to changes other than vasoconstriction. Angiotensin II causes sodium retention, diminutions in glomerular filtration, stimulation of aldosterone production, and stimulation of norepinephrine release from the adrenergic nervous system. In chronic bilateral or unilateral renovascular hypertension in patients with only one kidney, sodium retention accounts for late reductions in renin secretion, although it is possible that absolute renin activity is abnormally high with regard to the existing sodium balance. Blood pressure elevations do not appear as dependent on the renin–angiotensin system in sodium-replete chronic renovascular hypertension. In this setting, ACE inhibitors are more effective in reducing elevated blood pressures with sodium depletion.[10]

Pathology of Renal Artery Occlusive Disease

Different macrovascular occlusive diseases affect the renal arterial circulation.[11,12] The most common are arteriosclerosis and arterial fibrodysplasia. Developmental renal artery

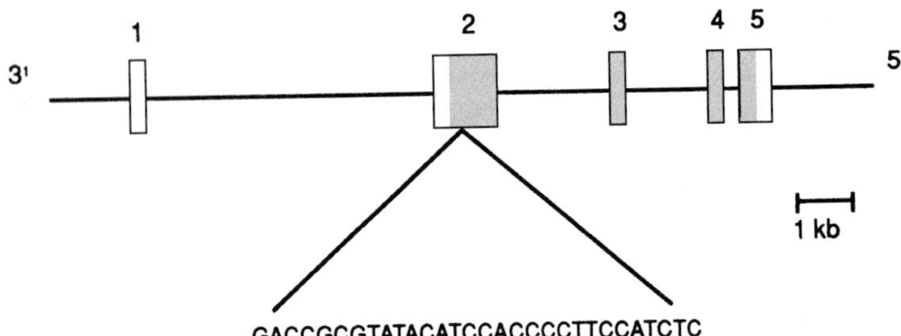

FIGURE 103.5 Human angiotensinogen gene, which consists of five exons and four introns. This gene is about 14.55 kb long. The coding sequence for angiotensinogen is contained in the second to fifth exon. The second exon contains the coding sequence for angiotensin I.

narrowings are a rare cause of renovascular hypertension. Although uncommon, renal artery emboli, spontaneous dissections, and traumatic occlusions are occasionally associated with acute renin-mediated hypertension.

Arteriosclerosis

Arteriosclerotic renal artery occlusive disease accounts for about 95% of reported cases of renovascular hypertension (Fig. 103.7). This type of renovascular hypertension may be even more common because most reported experiences are surgical series that exclude many older patients who are not operative candidates. Arteriosclerotic renovascular disease most commonly presents during the sixth decade of life. Men are affected twice as often as women. Although some degree of arteriosclerotic renal artery stenotic disease affects nearly half of the elderly population, it is not always associated with elevated blood pressures. Many of these patients exhibit occlusive disease of the coronary, cerebral, mesenteric, or extremity circulation.[13–15] This is particularly the case in black patients, who exhibit more severe extrarenal arteriosclerotic vascular disease.[16]

Arteriosclerotic renal artery occlusive disease characteristically affects the proximal third of the vessel in the form of eccentric or concentric stenoses. In nearly 80% of cases, these lesions occur as spillover of diffuse aortic atherosclerosis. Arteriosclerotic renal artery lesions are bilateral in three-quarters of patients. When unilateral, these lesions affect the right and left renal arteries with equal frequency, although the left renal artery often appears more severely diseased. Intimal and medial accumulations of cholesterol-laden foam cells and fibrous tissue are typical of these lesions. Necrosis, hemorrhage, calcification, and luminal thrombus are characteristic of complicated atherosclerotic plaques associated with more advanced disease.

Arterial Fibrodysplasia

Arterial fibrodysplasia is the second most common type of renal artery disease, accounting for about 5% of reported cases of renovascular hypertension.[11,12] Dysplastic renal artery stenoses represent a heterogenous group of lesions. They are classified by the specific pathologic process and vessel wall region most affected. Included among these lesions are intimal fibroplasia, medial fibroplasia, and perimedial dysplasia.[17] The last two entities appear to be a continuum of the same disease process. Each category has certain characteristic features deserving individual comment.

Intimal Fibroplasia. Intimal fibroplasia accounts for about 5% of all dysplastic renal artery stenoses (Fig. 102.8). These lesions occur in children and young adults more often than in the elderly, and they affect both genders equally. The cause of primary intimal fibroplasia is unknown but may be related to persistent embryonic myointimal cushions. Secondary intimal fibroplasia has been attributed to flow disturbances, blunt

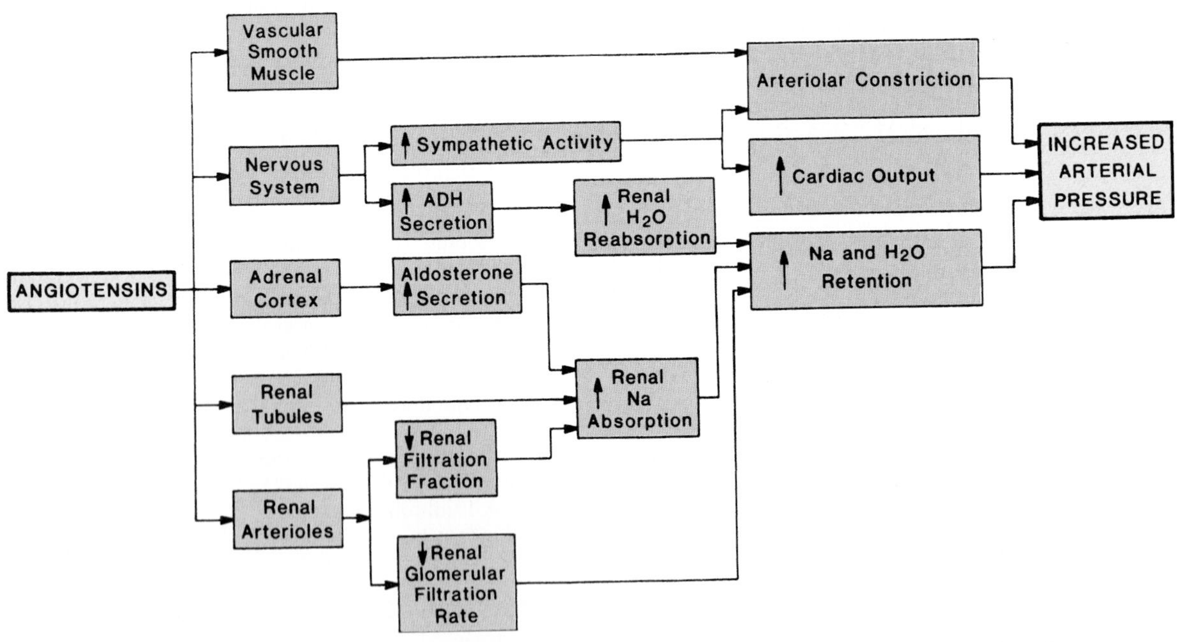

FIGURE 103.6 Effects of angiotensins contributing to increased arterial pressure. (After Stanley JC, Graham LM: Renovascular hypertension. In: Miller TA, ed. *Physiologic basis of modern surgical care.* 2nd ed. St Louis: Quality Medical Publishing, 1998, p. 918, with permission.)

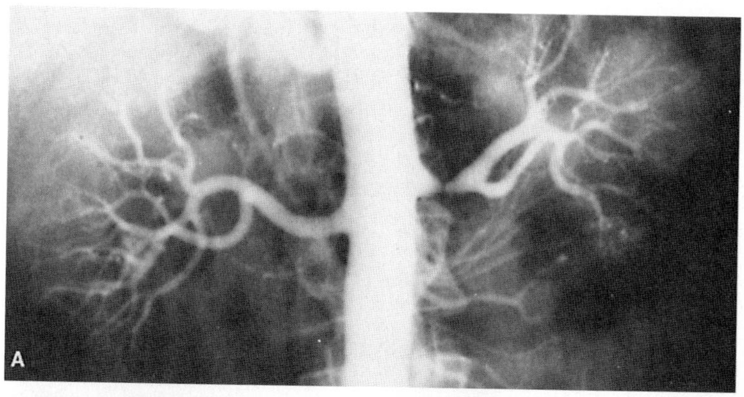

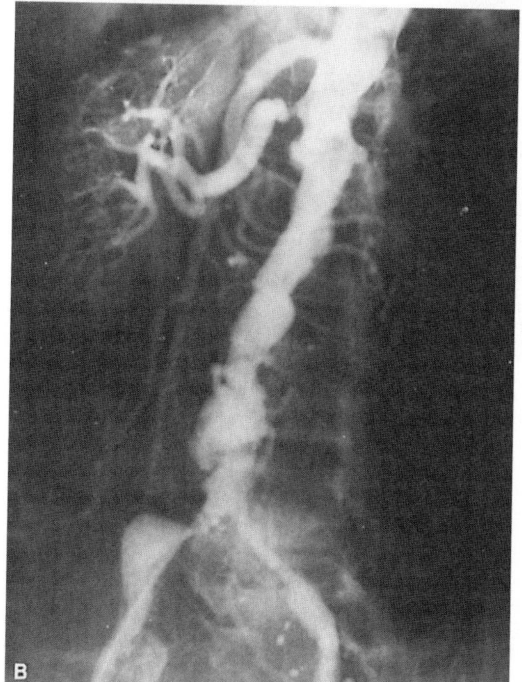

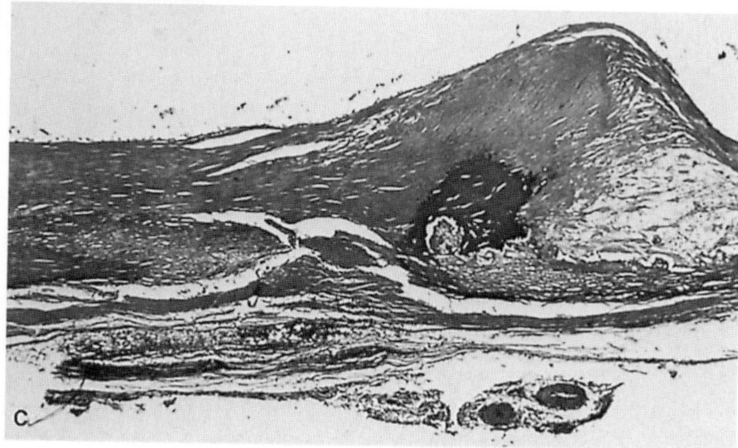

FIGURE 103.7 Renal artery arteriosclerosis. (*A*) Intrinsic focal lesion of proximal renal artery. (*B*) Severe aortic spill-over disease affecting renal artery orifice and entire abdominal aorta. (*C*) Complicated renal artery plaque exhibiting collections of cholesterol, extensive fibrosis, and calcification (hematoxin–eosin, X60). (*A* and *C* from Stanley JC. Morphologic, histopathologic and clinical characteristics of renovascular fibrodysplasia and arteriosclerosis. In: Bergan JJ, Yao JST, eds. *Surgery of the aorta and its body branches*. New York: Grune & Stratton; 1979, p. 355, with permission; *B* from Stanley JC, Graham LM, Whitehouse WM Jr. Renovascular hypertension. In: Miller TA, Rowland BJ, eds. *Physiologic basis of modern surgical care*. St Louis: CV Mosby; 1988, p. 734, with permission.)

abdominal trauma during childhood, and the sequela of an earlier arteritis, such as occurs with rubella. Progression of intimal fibroplasia may cause turbulent blood flow and an accelerated fibroproliferative response that rapidly compromises the arterial lumen.

Intimal fibroplasia usually presents as a smooth, focal stenosis of the distal main renal artery. In some patients, these lesions produce long, tubular stenoses, and in rare cases, they present as webs affecting segmental arteries. Proximal ostial lesions most often represent the secondary form of this disease, associated with abdominal aortic hypoplasia and coarctation. Subendothelial accumulations of irregularly arranged mesenchymal cells surrounded by loose fibrous connective tissue are typical of all intimal fibrodysplastic lesions. The internal elastic lamina is usually intact, but partial fragmentation may occur. Medial and adventitial structures are normal in primary intimal fibrodysplasia.

Medial Fibroplasias. Medial fibroplasia is the most commonly diagnosed dysplastic renal artery disease, accounting for 85% of these lesions (Fig. 103.9). Medial fibroplasia is invariably found in women, with cases in men being anecdotal. The clinical presentation of this disease is most common between 25 and 45 years of age. Medial fibroplasia appears to be a systemic arteriopathy, with the internal carotid and external iliac arteries representing the extrarenal vessels most often affected. The cause of medial fibroplasia remains poorly understood but appears to be associated with modification of smooth muscle to myofibroblasts caused by estrogenic stimuli during the reproductive years, unusual traction forces on affected vessels, and mural ischemia from impairment of vasa vasorum blood flow.[17] The physical forces contributing to medial fibroplasia may be attributed to ptotic kidneys with stretching of the renal arteries (Fig. 103.10). The fact that renal ptosis occurs more often in women than in men may

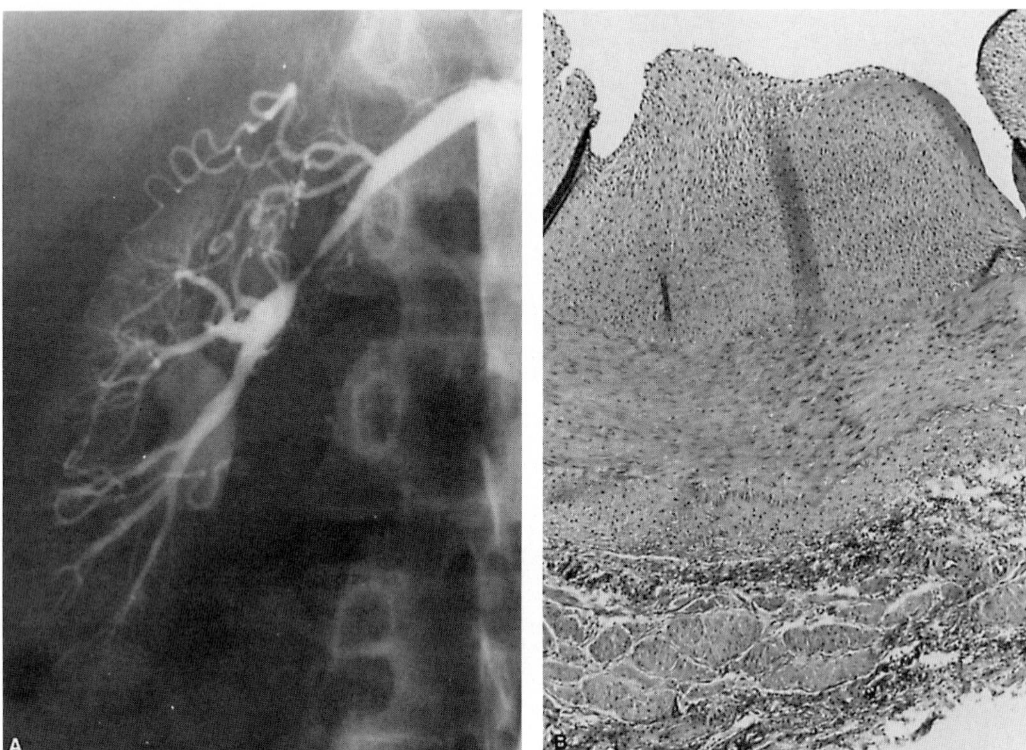

FIGURE 103.8 Intimal fibroplasia. (*A*) Focal stenosis of main renal artery mid-portion. (*B*) Subendothelial mesenchymal cells within a loose fibrous connective tissue matrix are noted above an intact internal elastic lamina, normal media, and normal adventitial tissues (hematoxin–eosin, X120). (*A* from Stanley JC, Fry WJ. Renovascular hypertension secondary to arterial fibrodysplasia in adults: criteria for operation and results of surgical therapy. *Arch Surg*. 1975;110:922–928, with permission; *B* from Stanley JC. Morphologic, histopathologic and clinical characteristics of renovascular fibrodysplasia and arteriosclerosis. In: Bergan JJ, Yao JST, eds. *Surgery of the aorta and its body branches*. New York: Grune & Stratton, 1979, p. 355, with permission.)

explain the almost unique involvement of the renal artery with medial fibroplasia in women.

Morphologic appearances of medial dysplasia range from solitary stenoses to multiple constrictions with intervening mural dilations affecting the middle and distal main renal artery. The latter are responsible for this lesion's classic string-of-beads appearance. Actual macrovascular aneurysms occurring at branchings affect a little more than 10% of patients with arterial fibrodysplasia. Stenotic disease of segmental branches occurs in about 25% of cases. Bilateral disease affects nearly 60% of patients and is usually most severe on the right. Unilateral lesions affect the left and right renal arteries in 10% and 30% of

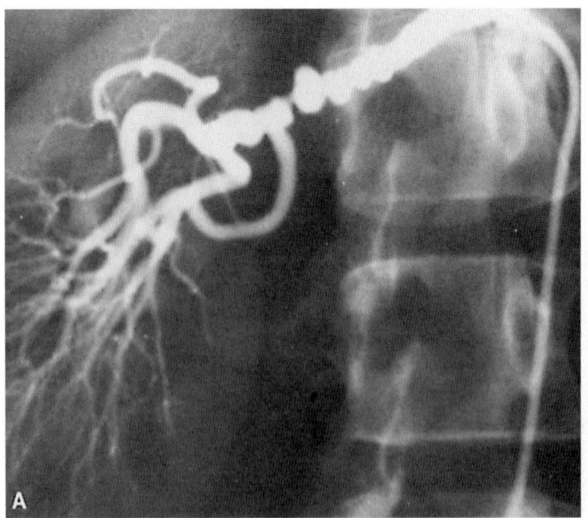

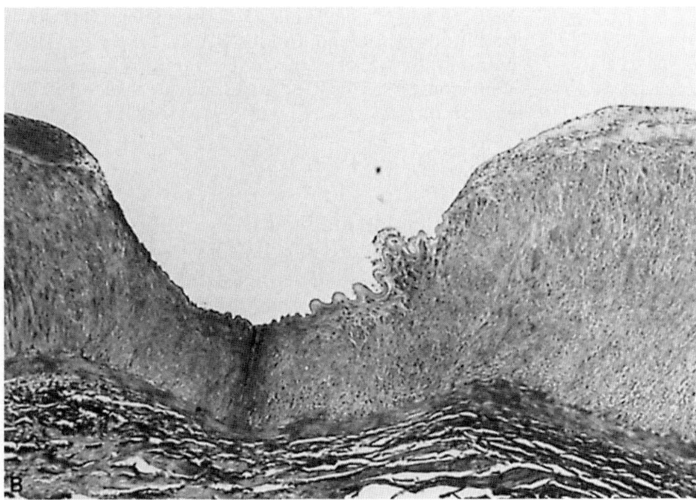

FIGURE 103.9 Medial fibroplasia. (*A*) Serial stenoses alternating with mural aneurysms, producing a string-of-beads appearance in the mid-portion and distal main renal artery. (*B*) Diffuse form of medial fibroplasia exhibiting regions of excess fibroproliferation with intervening area of medial thinning (Masson stain, X60, longitudinal section). (From Stanley JC. Morphologic, histopathologic and clinical characteristics of renovascular fibrodysplasia and arteriosclerosis. In: Bergan JJ, Yao JST, eds. Surgery of the aorta and its body branches. New York: Grune & Stratton; 1979, p. 355.)

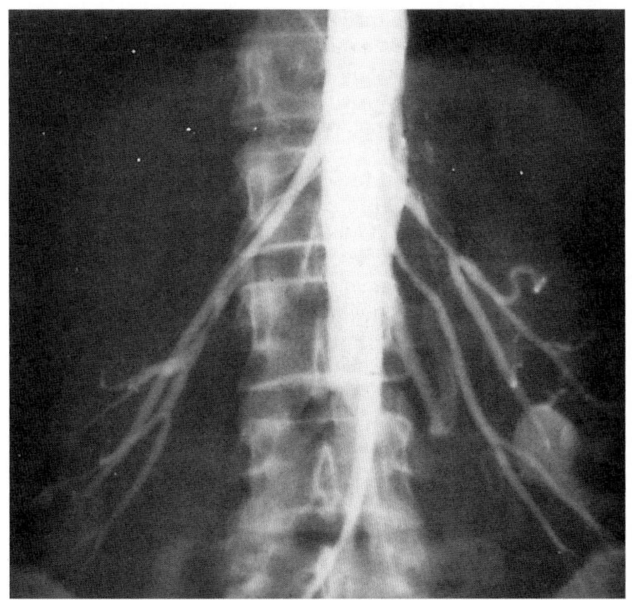

FIGURE 103.10 Medial fibrodysplasia manifested as irregular narrowings to ptotic kidneys affecting the mid-portion of the main renal arteries, which appear stretched during upright aortography. (From Stanley JC, Wakefield TW. Arterial fibrodysplasia. In: Rutherford RB, ed. *Vascular surgery*. 5th ed. Philadelphia, WB Saunders, 2000, p. 387, with permission.)

cases, respectively. Progression of disease occurs in about 20% of patients and is most evident among premenopausal women.

Gradations in medial fibroplasia exist, including diffuse and peripheral forms of the disease in the same vessel.[17] Diffuse medial fibroplasia is typified by severe disorganization of medial smooth muscle cells, which appear to be transformed to myofibroblasts.[18] These latter secretory cells generate accumulations of ground substances that encroach on the vessel lumen. These stenoses often alternate with areas of medial thinning and mural dilations. Peripheral medial fibroplasia is typified by a limitation of the fibroproliferative process to the outer portion of the media, causing stenoses less severe than those occurring with diffuse disease.

Perimedial Dysplasia. Perimedial dysplasia accounts for nearly 10% of dysplastic renal artery stenotic disease (Fig. 103.11). These lesions invariably occur in women, usually between the ages of 30 and 50 years. Perimedial dysplasia is bilateral in 20% of patients and appears to be more progressive than medial fibrodysplasia. Perimedial dysplasia is characterized by solitary or multiple constrictions, without intervening dilations. Most stenoses involve the distal main renal artery, without segmental branch involvement. Certain histologic features are common to both perimedial dysplasia and medial fibroplasia, and they may represent different manifestations of the same pathologic entity. Although unusual accumulations of elastic tissue in inner adventitial regions is the most prominent abnormality in perimedial dysplasia, increases in medial ground substances may also accompany this type of dysplastic disease.[17]

Developmental Renal Artery Disease

Developmental renal artery stenoses are a rare cause of renovascular hypertension[19,20] (Fig. 103.12). These lesions are encountered most often in children and young adults. About 40% of children with renovascular hypertension are thought to have developmental renal artery stenoses. Similarly, nearly 20% of adults with intimal fibroplastic renal artery disease have stenoses that can be attributed to developmental defects. Both genders are affected equally. These stenotic lesions represent

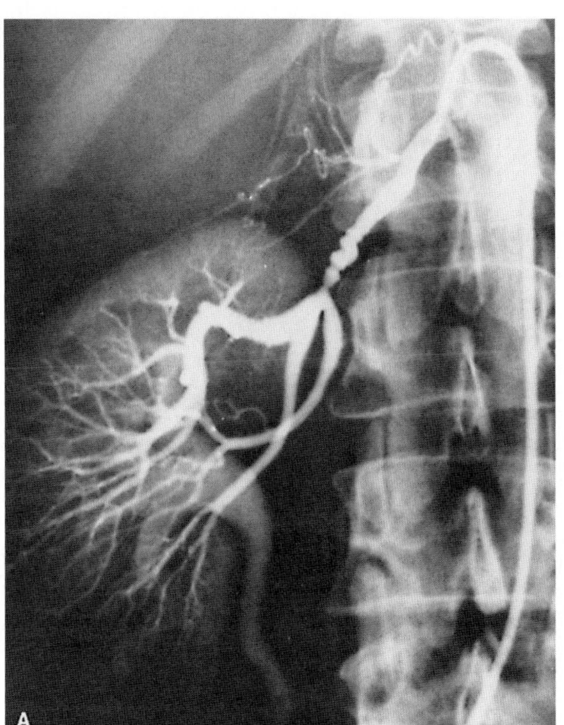

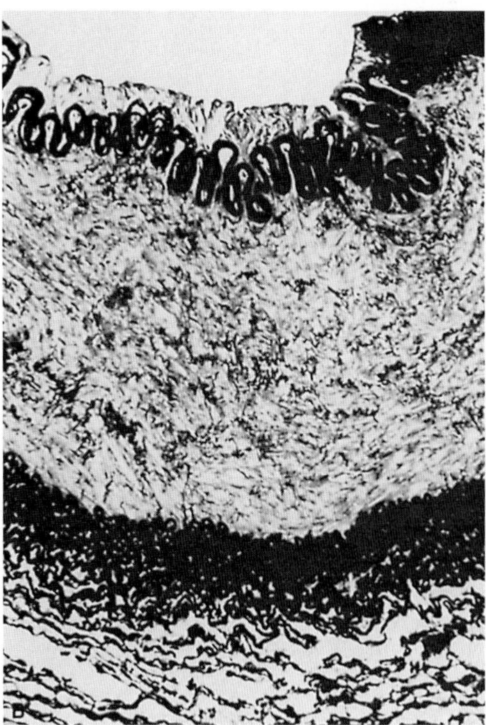

FIGURE 103.11 Perimedial dysplasia. (*A*) Multiple stenoses without mural aneurysms in the mid-portion of the renal artery are characteristic of these lesions. (*B*) These lesions are due to excessive accumulations of elastic tissue at medial–adventitial junction (Verhoeff stain, X120). (From Stanley JC. Morphologic, histopathologic and clinical characteristics of renovascular fibrodysplasia and arteriosclerosis. In: Bergan JJ, Yao JST, eds. *Surgery of the aorta and its body branches*. New York: Grune & Stratton, 1979, p. 355, with permission.)

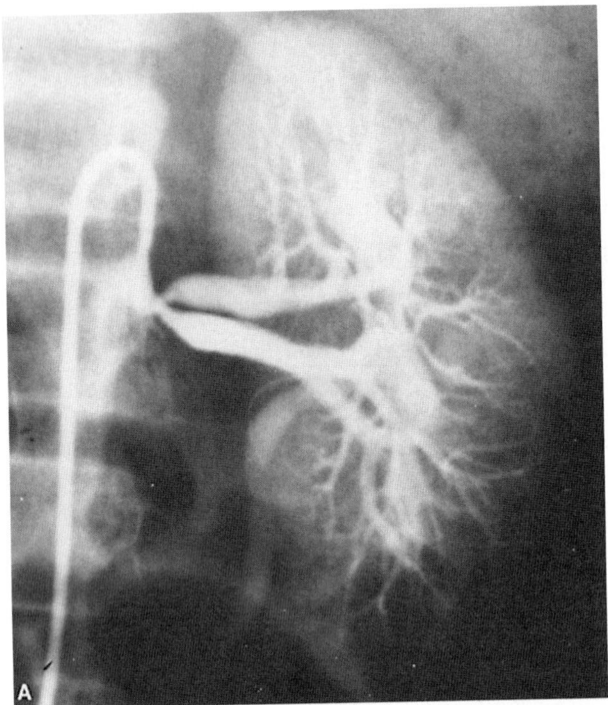

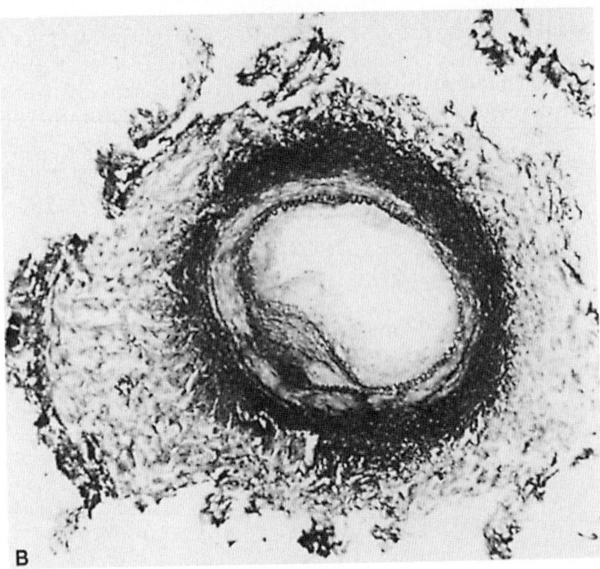

FIGURE 103.12 Developmental renal artery stenoses. (*A*) Proximal vessel stenosis in a patient with neurofibromatosis and infrarenal aortic hypoplasia. (*B*) Fragmentation and duplication of the internal elastic lamina and deficient medial tissues characterize these lesions. Intimal fibroplasia encroaches on the vessel lumen, which is less than 1 mm in diameter. Adventitial elastic tissues appear excessive (Movat stain, X100). (*A* from Stanley JC, Fry WJ. Pediatric renal artery occlusive disease and renovascular hypertension: etiology, diagnosis, and operative treatment. Developmental occlusive disease of the abdominal aorta and the splanchnic and renal arteries. *Arch Surg*. 1981;116:669–676, with permission; *B* from Stanley JC, Graham LM, Whitehouse WM Jr, et al. Developmental occlusive disease of the abdominal aorta and the splanchnic and renal arteries. *Am J Surg*. 1981; 142:190–196, with permission.)

true hypoplasia of the renal artery, exhibiting an external hourglass appearance. Developmental lesions usually occur at the aortic origin of the artery. Sparse medial tissue, intimal fibroplasia, fragmentation and duplication of the internal elastic lamina, and disproportionate excesses in adventitial elastic tissue are the most common histologic abnormalities in these diminutive vessels.[20,21]

Developmental renal artery narrowings may be attributed to certain embryonic events occurring as the two fetal dorsal aortas fuse and all but one of their lateral branches to the kidney regress. Abnormal transition of mesenchyme to medial smooth muscle at that time, or later impairment of its growth, can cause both aortic and renovascular anomalies. Vessels to the mesonephros within mesenchymal tissue around the two dorsal aortas are replaced during fetal growth by a more cephalic group of vessels to the metanephros. A solitary artery to each kidney evolves from these arteries in 75% of people because of an obligate hemodynamic advantage over adjacent channels. Flow changes in the region where single central renal arteries usually arise may afford coexisting polar arteries hemodynamic advantages that ensure their persistence. Supporting such a hypothesis concerning the cause of developmental lesions is the fact that multiple stenotic renal arteries exist in up to 70% of patients with central abdominal aortic coarctation or hypoplasia.

Clinical Features of Renovascular Hypertension

The frequency of renovascular hypertension among patients who have diastolic blood pressures higher than 100 mm Hg is about 2%. It is much more common in patients with more severe diastolic blood pressure elevations; as many as 5% of such patients are found to have a renovascular cause of their hypertension.

Findings suggestive of renovascular hypertension include systolic and diastolic upper abdominal bruits; initial diastolic blood pressures greater than 115 mm Hg; a sudden worsening of mild to moderate essential hypertension; development of hypertension during childhood; or rapid onset of high blood pressure after the age of 50 years. Hypertension resistant to drug therapy and malignant hypertension are also more likely to be associated with this form of secondary hypertension. Similarly, patients who exhibit deterioration in renal function while receiving multiple antihypertensive drugs, especially ACE inhibitors, may have underlying renal artery stenotic disease. The costs and errors incumbent to indiscriminate evaluations for this form of hypertension are prohibitive. A decision algorithm based on the presenting degree of hypertension and presence or absence of clinical and laboratory evidence of renovascular hypertension is necessary for contemporary practice (Algorithm 103.1).

Diagnosis of Renal Artery Stenosis and Secondary Hypertension

Most diagnostic and prognostic tests for renovascular hypertension assess either the anatomic stenosis or derangements of renal function attributed to the stenosis. The usefulness and limitations of these tests become relevant in the proper selection of patients for surgical intervention.

Conventional arteriography was central to the evaluation of patients in the past when renovascular hypertension was suspected. Oblique aortography and multiple-plane selective renal arteriography have improved the recognition of the morphologic character and extent of renal artery stenoses in this disease entity. Collateral vessels circumventing a renal artery stenosis are evidence of the lesion's hemodynamic importance. A pressure gradient of about 10 mm Hg is necessary for collateral vessel development, and the same degree of pressure change is associated with activation of the renin system. Thus, the functional importance of an otherwise benign-appearing stenosis is established when collateral vessels are evident (Fig. 103.13).

Intraarterial digital subtraction angiography is a common means of assessing the presence of renal artery stenotic disease.

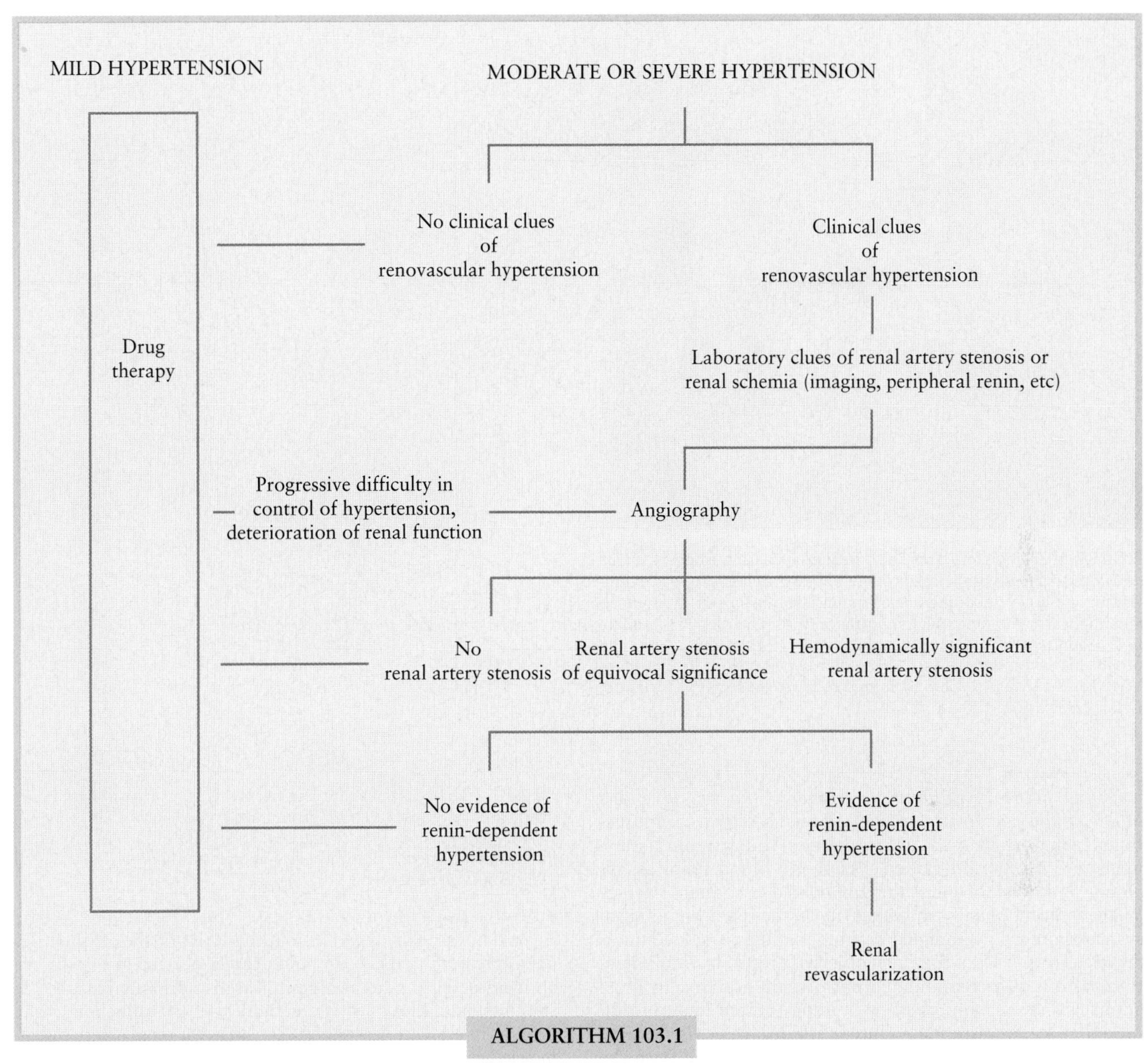

ALGORITHM 103.1 Management of renovascular hypertension. (After Stanley JC. Renal artery stenosis and hypertension. In: Brewster DC, ed. *Common problems in vascular surgery*. Chicago, Year Book, 1989, p. 187, with permission).

The latter allows use of smaller quantities of iodine contrast agents compared with conventional arteriography, and it lessens the potential of contrast-induced nephrotoxicity. This quality is of particular relevance in patients with compromised renal function. The use of carbon dioxide or gadolinium in the latter circumstances is also appealing, but may not always provide sufficient anatomic detail for clinical decision making in patients with segmental arterial disease.

Computed tomographic arteriography (CTA) is another frequently used means of assessing coexistent renal artery and aortic disease. It allows computer-generated visualization of the vessels from many different angles not possible with conventional biplanar studies. However, CTA carries the risk of contrast-induced nephrotoxicity.

Magnetic resonance angiography, especially with breath-hold techniques and gadolinium enhancement, provides high-resolution images of diseased renal arteries.[22,23] A normal study usually confirms absence of disease, but because of phase-dropout with vessel tortuosity, a study may appear abnormal in a patient having a relatively undiseased, nonstenotic artery. Nevertheless, its noninvasiveness and lack of nephrotoxicity make magnetic resonance angiography an attractive diagnostic test.

Deep abdominal renal artery ultrasonography may identify hemodynamically significant renal artery narrowings by defining the renal artery resistive index as directly imaging the renal arteries and characterizing flow velocity patterns through these vessels.[24,25] This study is a reasonable initial screening test. Existence of a stenosis appears established when peak systolic velocities are in the range of 180 to 200 cm/s and the ratio of these velocities to those in the aorta approaches 3.5. Unfortunately, ultrasonography does not discriminate among renal artery stenoses exceeding 60% cross-sectional narrowing. Failure to identify a main renal artery in the absence of any parenchymal flow signal suggests main renal artery occlusion. An occluded accessory or segmental renal artery, however, may not be recognized and, thus, contributes to this technology's false-negative assessments.

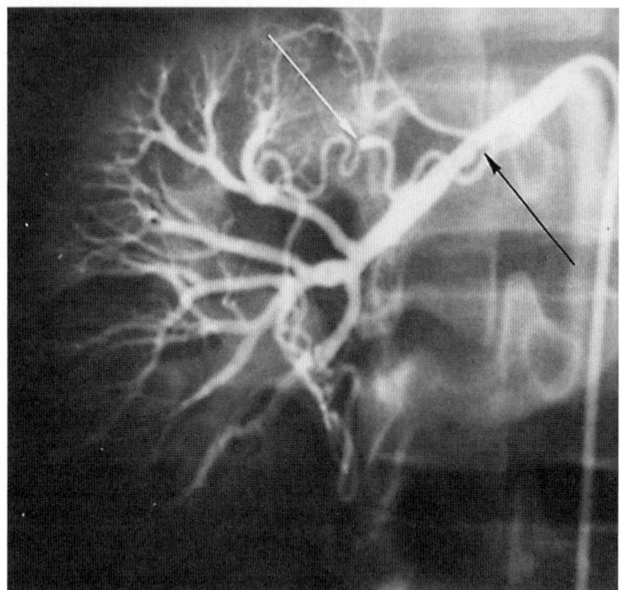

FIGURE 103.13 Arteriogram of a benign-appearing stenosis (*black arrow*) associated with a large collateral vessel (*white arrow*) circumventing the lesion, defining hemodynamic significance of the stenosis and implicating its functional importance. (From Stanley JC, Graham LM, Whitehouse WM Jr. Limitations and errors of diagnostic and prognostic investigations in renovascular hypertension. In: Bernhard VM, Towne JM, eds. *Complications in vascular surgery*. Orlando: Grune & Stratton, 1984, p. 213.)

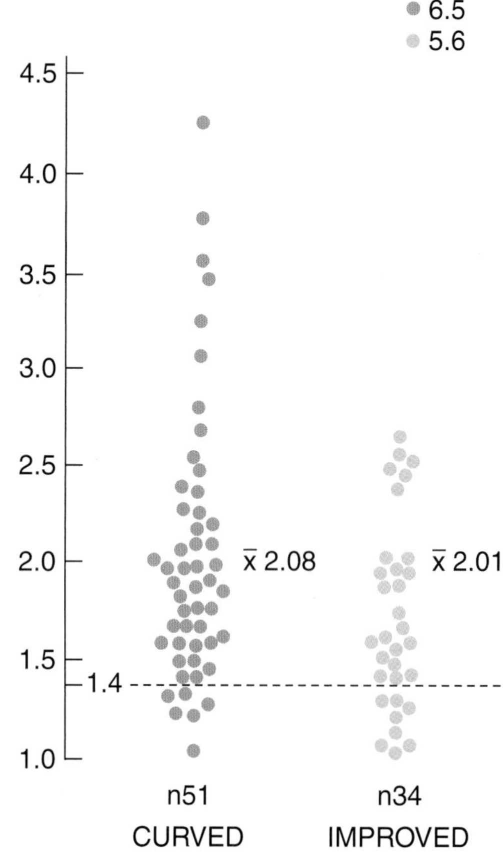

FIGURE 103.14 Renal vein renin ratios, reflecting their limited diagnostic and prognostic value. (From Stanley JC, Gewertz BL, Fry WJ. Renal:systemic renin indices and renal vein renin ratios as prognostic indicators in remedial renovascular hypertension. *J Surg Res*. 1976;20: 149–155, with permission.)

Renin activity comparing peripheral and renal venous blood, in the past, was a recognized means of detecting functionally important renal artery disease. Today, renin assessments are rarely undertaken. Peripheral blood renin assays alone are not useful unless they are related to sodium balance. When assessing renal vein renin activity, the renin–angiotensin system should be stimulated before sampling to reduce interpretive errors of data that may otherwise result from minimal fluctuations in nonstimulated basal renin activity. In most adults, this is accomplished by limiting sodium intake to 20 mEq/d and administering a diuretic for 3 days before testing. Blood samples for renin assays should be obtained with the patient tilted to an upright position. Renin-suppressing drugs, such as β-blockers, are discontinued before testing whenever possible. ACE inhibitors stimulate renin release, but the validity of doing this to increase the diagnostic accuracy in patients with renovascular hypertension is questionable. Renin activity is usually reported as either a ratio or an index.

The *renal vein renin ratio* (RVRR) is calculated by dividing the renin activity in venous blood from the affected kidney by that from the contralateral kidney. An RVRR of greater than 1.48 is indicative of functionally important renovascular stenotic disease.[8,9] Because this test compares one kidney to another, it may not be useful in patients with bilateral disease if both kidneys exhibit elevated, but equal degrees of abnormally high renin secretion. This is believed to be the case in the 15% of patients benefiting from operation in whom the RVRR is less than 1.48 (Fig. 103.14).The *renal:systemic renin index* (RSRI) is calculated by subtracting systemic renin activity from individual renal vein renin activity and dividing the remainder by systemic renin activity.[8] It is an expression of individual kidney renin release. In nonrenovascular essential hypertensive patients, renal vein renin activity from each kidney is usually 24% higher than systemic activity.[3,9] Thus, the total of both kidneys' activity is usually 48% higher than systemic activity and represents a steady state of renal renin release.

In renovascular hypertension, the RSRI of the affected kidney is greater than 0.24. In mild degrees of renal artery disease, an increase in ipsilateral renin release is normally balanced by suppression of the contralateral kidney renin production, with a drop in its RSRI to less than 0.24. Bilateral renal artery disease may cause this servomechanism to be lost, and the autonomous release of renin from both kidneys may cause the sum of the individual RSRIs to be considerably greater than 0.48. Renin production then exceeds the capacity of normal hepatic degradation, and a hyperreninemic form of hypertension evolves.

The usefulness of ischemic kidney renin hypersecretion (RSRI more than 0.48) and contralateral kidney renin suppression (RSRI less than 0.24, approaching 0) as a means of discriminating between expected cured and improved operative outcomes has been well established[26] (Fig. 103.15). The prognostic accuracy of RSRI appears limited in that a little less than 10% of patients who are cured do not exhibit contralateral renin suppression. Renin secretion from the nonoperated kidney must be suppressed if a cure is to be expected. Although the RSRI represents an important refinement in the use of renin data in managing renovascular hypertensive patients, these data must be applied cautiously to clinical decision making.

Hypertensive urography is not a good diagnostic test for renovascular hypertension because of its limited sensitivity.[27] Bilateral or segmental disease often interferes with the recognition of gross differences in contrast excretion between the two kidneys. Nevertheless, rapid-sequence urography may contribute to a diagnosis of renovascular hypertension in the following circumstances: (a) there is at least a 1-minute delay in contrast appearance within the collecting system of the affected

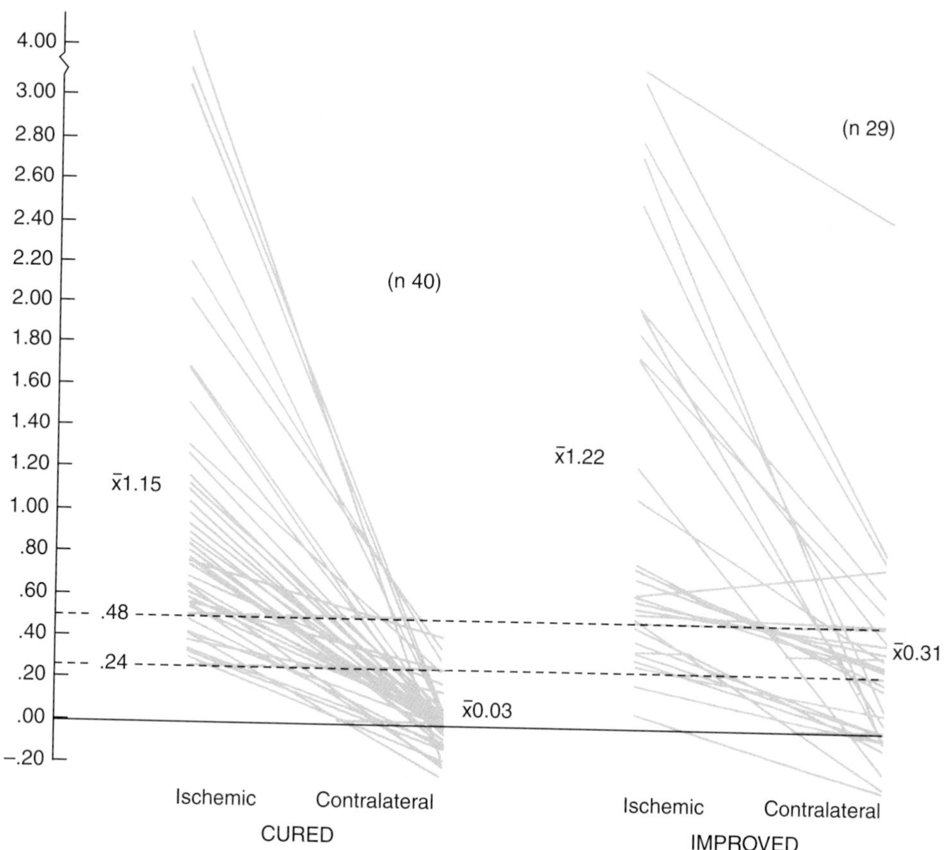

FIGURE 103.15 Renal–systemic renin indices, depicting their prognostic usefulness. (From Stanley JC, Fry WJ. Surgical treatment of renovascular hypertension. *Arch Surg.* 1977;1121291–1297, with permission.)

kidney compared with that of the contralateral kidney; (b) a discrepancy in renal length exists, with the right kidney being 2 cm shorter than the left or the left being 1.5 cm shorter than the right; and (c) there is hyperconcentration of contrast in the collecting system of the affected kidney evident on late radiographs. Ureteral or pelvic irregularities owing to the presence of large collateral vessels may accompany the aforementioned urographic findings. In a large series of patients with proven renovascular hypertension, urograms were abnormal in 27% of children, 48% of adults with arterial fibrodysplastic disease, and about 72% of adults with atherosclerotic lesions.[28] Thus, use of hypertensive urography as a diagnostic or prognostic test for renovascular hypertension appears unjustified.

Isotopic renography allows both renal imaging and analysis of the washout curve of a number of radioactive tracers. In the past, common compounds used for these studies have included ^{99m}technetium-diethylenetriamine pentaacetic acid, iodine 123-orthoidohippurate or iodine 131-orthoidohippurate, ^{99m}technetium mercaptoacetyltriglycine, ^{99m}technetium-dimercaptosuccinic acid, and ^{99m}glucoheptonate. These studies provide an assessment of renal blood flow as well as excretory function. Unfortunately, different states of hydration and intrarenal vascular resistance often contribute to flow abnormalities and false-positive studies in nonrenovascular hypertensives. The specificity and sensitivity of these studies are both about 75%. Administration of ACE inhibitors improves the sensitivity and specificity by blocking the compensatory change in glomerular filtration, causing it to fall in the affected kidney. The widespread use of this modified technology has not occurred, although some view ACE inhibitor-modified studies to be of greater value.[29] Renal perfusion/excretion ratios and more sophisticated computer analyses offer a potential means of increasing the predictive value of radionuclide screening for renovascular hypertension.

Treatment

Therapeutic results in the management of renovascular hypertension often relate to the proper execution of an appropriate intervention. Treatment options include drug therapy, percutaneous transluminal angioplasty (PTA) with or without stent placement, transcatheter renal ablation, arterial reconstructive surgery, and nephrectomy.

Drug Therapy

Antihypertensive drugs are often successful in the initial management of patients with renovascular hypertension. β-Blocking agents, such as propranolol and atenolol, are commonly used as first-line therapy. Refractory hypertension, especially that caused by bilateral disease or unilateral lesions with contralateral parenchymal disease, may respond to the addition of a thiazide diuretic, although with impaired renal function, the use of a loop diuretic, such as furosemide, is more effective. ACE inhibitors, such as captopril and enalapril, have proved to be the most effective drugs in treating renovascular hypertension. Unfortunately, ACE inhibitors may have a deleterious effect on renal function by preferentially dilating the glomerular efferent arterioles, critically decreasing intraglomerular blood pressure, and reducing glomerular filtration. Certainly, ACE inhibitors should be used cautiously when the entire renal parenchymal mass is at risk, as occurs in renovascular hypertensive patients who have bilateral disease or a solitary kidney. Use of angiotensin receptor blockers has not been well defined in this subgroup of hypertensive patients. Because stenotic disease of the renal artery often progresses with concomitant loss of renal mass and function, a definitive means of restoring normal renal blood flow may be more logical therapy than drug

RESULTS

TABLE 103.1

PERCUTANEOUS TRANSLUMINAL ANGIOPLASTY FOR FIBRODYSPLASTIC RENOVASCULAR HYPERTENSION

Institution failed	Patients	Follow-up mean (mo)	Postprocedural blood pressure response (%)		
			Cured	Improved	Failed
Mayo Clinic	105	43	22	41	37
University of Virginia	66	39	39	59	2
University Hospital, Zurich, Switzerland	28	15	50	39	11
University of Florida	23	6	52	22	26
University Hospitals, Leuven, Belgium	22	26	95	—	5
Hospital Broussais, Paris	20	19	68	16	15

treatment, once a diagnosis of renovascular hypertension has been established.

Percutaneous Transluminal Angioplasty

In 1978, Grüntzig et al.[30] were the first to report the use of PTA in the management renovascular hypertension. The minimally invasive nature of renal artery PTA offers certain advantages over operative intervention and this therapy is now widely in use.[31] Most renal artery stenoses can be traversed with a guide wire and subsequently dilated with or without a stent, with minimal morbidity and mortality. To justify PTA, the clinical significance of the renal artery stenosis should be documented prior to initiating endovascular therapy. In particular the patient should have adequate renal cortical reserve to recover renal function postintervention.

Arterial Fibrodysplasia. Patients with renal artery fibrodysplasia benefit the most and incur the fewest complications following renal PTA compared to those with other forms of renovascular disease. Medial dysplastic stenoses are most amenable to PTA, and this is often considered primary therapy for lesions limited to the main renal artery. Excellent early technical and clinical results usually follow renal artery PTA in these patients.[32–37] Similarly, these patients have experienced excellent long-term clinical results, with a primary patency rate of 87% after more than 3 years of follow-up (Table 103.1).[38]

Developmental Disease. In contrast, ostial lesions associated with developmental aortic anomalies in pediatric patients represent true hypoplastic vessels that are less likely to be successfully dilated.[39] In a like fashion, less common causes of renovascular hypertension in children, including arteritis, William syndrome, and neurofibromatosis, do not respond well to renal artery PTA.

Arteriosclerosis. The greatest experience with renal artery PTA is with arteriosclerotic disease.[40–48] The presence of aortic spillover arteriosclerosis versus isolated renal artery arteriosclerosis has an important impact on long-term clinical results. Historically, PTA alone, without stent placement, has resulted in a technical success rate of only 70% to 80%. Ostial spillover lesions, treated by PTA alone have technical success rate of only 30% to 50%. These latter stenoses often manifest excessive recoil and many exhibit acute dissections. As a result of high early post-PTA restenosis rates, stenting of atherosclerotic lesions is considered appropriate in many patients. Results following renal artery stenting for atherosclerotic disease vary depending on outcome definitions and the indication for intervention, yet many studies have good long-term technical results (Table 103.2). For example, Palmaz stents placed in 64 renal arteries in 59 patients, resulted in a 2-year secondary patency rate of 92%.[46] Others have documented 5-year primary and secondary patency rates of 84 and 92%, respectively.[41]

RESULTS

TABLE 103.2

PERCUTANEOUS TRANSLUMINAL ANGIOPLASTY WITH STENT PLACEMENT FOR ARTERIOSCLEROTIC RENOVASCULAR DISEASE

Institution	Patients	Postprocedural blood indication follow-up			Pressure response (%) mean (mo)		
		Hypertension	Renal insufficiency		Cured	Improved	Failed
Dorros-Feuer Foundation	76	76	48	6	6	46	48
University Hospital, Freiburg, Germany	68	68	29	27	16	62	22
Ochsner Clinic	66	66	Unknown	19	2	64	34
Polyclinique D'Essey	59	59	10	14	19	57	24
Hotel-Dieu de Montreal	33	33	17	13	6	61	33
University of Texas Health Center (multicenter study)	28	28	14	7	11	54	36

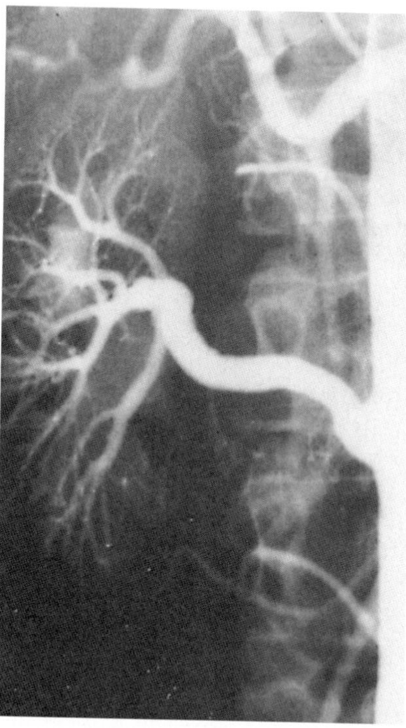

FIGURE 103.16 Autogenous saphenous vein aortorenal graft. (From Stanley JC, Graham LM. Renovascular hypertension. In: Miller DC, Roon AJ, eds. *Diagnosis and management of peripheral vascular disease*. Menlo Park, CA: Addison-Wesley, 1981, with permission.)

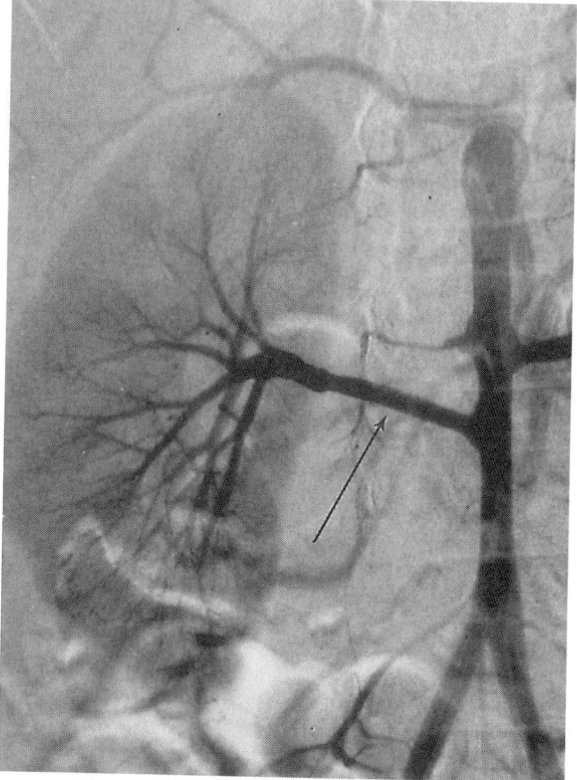

FIGURE 103.17 Autogenous iliac artery aortorenal graft in a child. (From Stanley JC, Zelenock GB, Messina LM, Wakefield TW. Pediatric renovascular hypertension: a thirty-year experience of operative treatment. *J Vasc Surg*. 1995;21:212–227, with permission.)

In treating hypertension, long-term benefits have been reported in 52% to 78% of patients (Table 103.2). PTA with stenting for progressive ischemic nephropathy is not as effective at reversing renal failure. In these cases, as with open surgical interventions, benefits appear related to the degree and duration of ischemic nephropathy prior to PTA, with those having a relative rapid onset of renal insufficiency and serum creatinine of less than 3 mg/dL demonstrating the best response.[49–53]

Complications accompanying renal artery PTA for either atherosclerotic or fibrodysplastic disease, are uncommon, with severe complications occurring in less than a few percent of cases. Intimal disruption occurs more often with proximal renal artery dilation, where the vessel elasticity is greater and medial disruption is less likely. Medial tears are more common with distal renal artery dilation where vessel elasticity is less. Surgery following failed renal artery PTA is much more hazardous than primary surgery alone,[54] being associated with a much higher incidence of emergent repair and nephrectomy. Blood pressure benefits after a failed renal artery PTA that necessitates secondary operation are significantly lower, being 57% after reoperation versus 89% for a primary operation.[54]

Arterial Reconstructive Surgery

Operative treatment of patients with renovascular occlusive disease has become relatively well defined.[11,12,26,28,55–60] It is important that the primary revascularization procedure be successful. This point is underscored by the fact that nephrectomy accompanies nearly half of the reoperations for failed initial reconstructions.[61] Operative details vary when treating the different subgroups of renal artery disease.

Aortorenal Bypass. Aortorenal bypass in adults with arteriosclerotic and fibrodysplastic occlusive disease is most often performed using autologous reversed saphenous vein (Fig. 103.16).[11,12] Dacron or expanded polytetrafluoroethylene conduits may also be used in reconstructing these vessels with similar results. Because vein grafts in children often become aneurysmal,[21,62] autologous hypogastric artery grafts and direct aortic reimplantations of the renal artery are favored in children[21] (Figs. 103.17 and 103.18).

Nonanatomic Bypass Procedures. Nonanatomic bypass procedures are important in treating certain patients with renovascular hypertension.[57,63–66] The hepatic artery or iliac arteries may be used as sites of origin for bypass grafts to the renal artery, especially when originating a graft from the aorta would entail unacceptable risks. Use of the splenic artery in situ for a left-sided splenorenal bypass is appropriate in adults, but only after ascertaining that this vessel and the celiac trunk are free of stenotic disease. Splenorenal bypasses are not recommended in children because of the potential existence of a celiac artery growth arrest that may not be evident at the time of reconstruction, but which may evolve later.

Ex Vivo Renal Artery Reconstruction. Ex vivo renal artery reconstruction is an alternative means of treating select cases of renovascular hypertension, especially those involving revascularization of multiple second- or third-order segmental branches.[60,67,68] Most renal artery reconstructions can be successfully performed in situ. Disadvantages of *ex vivo* reconstructions include the necessity to cool the kidney, longer operating times, and perhaps most important, the disruption of preexisting collateral channels.

Operative Arterial Dilation. Operative arterial dilation, alone or in conjunction with a bypass procedure, is useful in the treatment of fibrous intraparenchymal stenotic disease. In this setting, sequentially larger metal dilators are advanced through a transverse arteriotomy in the main renal artery after heparin anticoagulation. These dilators, increasing in size by 0.5-mm increments, must be advanced with care to avoid overdilating the vessel, lest intimal fracture occur.

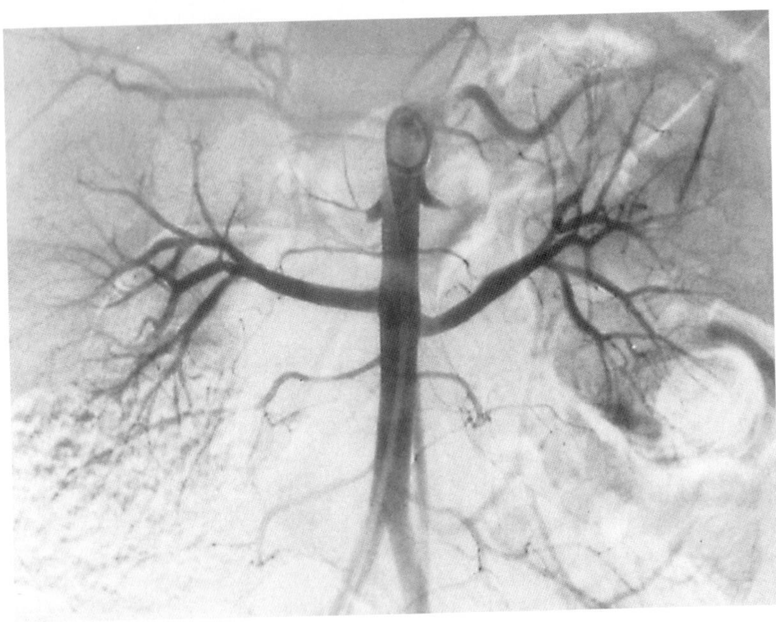

FIGURE 103.18 Aortic reimplantation of main renal arteries, beyond orificial stenoses in a child. (From Stanley JC, Zelenock GB, Messina LM, Wakefield TW. Pediatric renovascular hypertension: a thirty-year experience of operative treatment. *J Vasc Surg*. 1995;21: 212–227, with permission.)

Endarterectomy. Endarterectomy is often performed for proximal renal artery arteriosclerotic disease.[11,12,69–71] The two techniques most often used are: (a) transaortic renal endarterectomy through an axial aortotomy or the transected infrarenal aorta, and (b) direct renal artery endarterectomy. The extent of aortic and renal artery disease, as well as the need to perform coexistent aortic reconstructive surgery, dictates which of these procedures is most appropriate. In most cases, a linear aortotomy is begun just to the left of the superior mesenteric artery and extended in the midline to below the renal arteries. The diseased aortic intimal and medial tissues are elevated, and with gentle traction, the renal artery atheroma is extracted. This type of endarterectomy is particularly useful in treating bilateral disease (Fig. 103.19) or when the disease affects multiple renal arteries. Extensive plaque of the more distal renal artery, especially when involving bifurcations, may be better treated by a direct renal artery arteriotomy and endarterectomy with a patch-graft closure.

Results of Operative Therapy

Renal preservation and maintenance of renal function are important in assessing clinical experiences. Nephrectomy usually does not offer as much benefit as renal revascularization. Even when nephrectomy provides good results, it leaves the patient at considerable risk if contralateral disease occurs later. Cumulative primary and secondary nephrectomy rates in any given practice should not exceed 10%. Improved renal function after

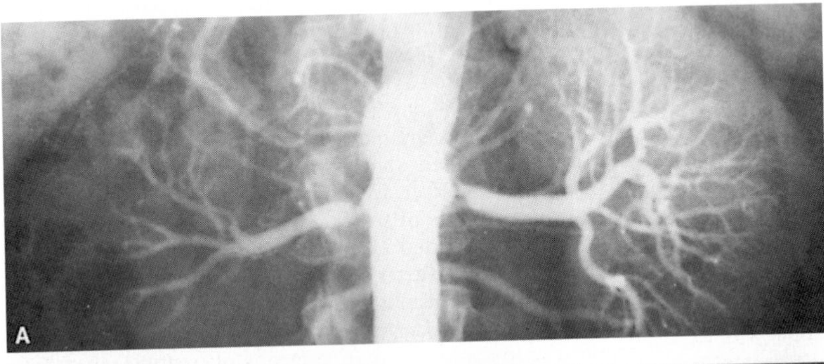

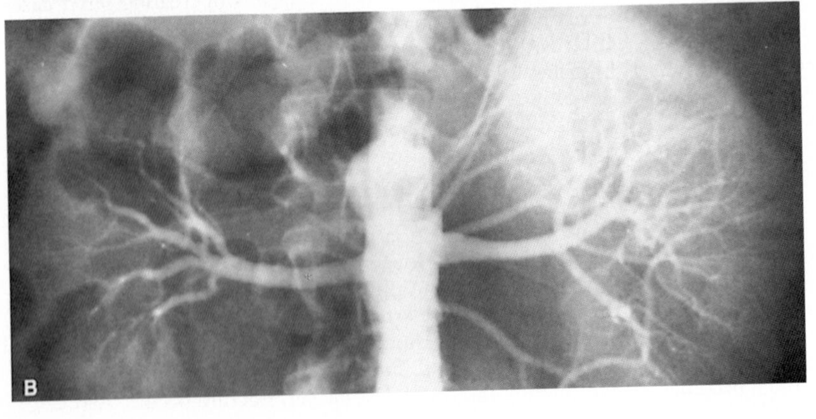

FIGURE 103.19 Transaortic bilateral renal artery endarterectomy. Preoperative (*A*) and postoperative (*B*) aortography. (From Stanley JC, Messina LM, Wakefield TW, et al. Renal artery reconstruction. In: Bergan JJ, Yao JST, eds. *Techniques in arterial surgery*. Philadelphia: WB Saunders; 1990, p. 247, with permission.)

TABLE 103.3

RESULTS

RESULTS OF SURGICAL TREATMENT OF RENOVASCULAR HYPERTENSION IN SPECIFIC PATIENT SUBGROUPS, UNIVERSITY OF MICHIGAN EXPERIENCE

Subgroup mortality	Patients	Postoperative status[a]			
		Cure rate (%)	Improvement rate (%)	Operative rate (%)	Failure rate (%)
Pediatric disease	34	85	12	3	0
Arterial fibrodysplasia	144	55	39	6	0
Arteriosclerosis					
Focal renal artery disease	64	33	58	9	0
Overt extrarenal disease	71	25	47	28	8.5

[a] Represents outcome of 415 operations (346 primary, 59 secondary), including initial nephrectomy in 17 patients.
Cure: Blood pressures were 150/90 mm Hg or less for a minimum of 6 months postoperatively, during which no antihypertensive medications were administered. *Improvement:* Normotensive while on drug therapy, or if diastolic blood pressures ranged between 90 and 100 mm Hg but were at least 15% lower than preoperative levels. *Failure*: Diastolic blood pressures greater than 90 mm Hg but less than 15% lower than preoperative levels or greater than 110 mm Hg. Lower pressure standards were used in evaluating children.
(From Stanley JC, Whitehouse WM Jr, Graham LM, et al. Operative therapy of renovascular hypertension. *Br J Surg.* 1982;63[Suppl]:S63, with permission.)

revascularization is well recognized and is most likely to occur among patients exhibiting arteriosclerotic disease with a relatively sudden onset of renal function impairment.

Surgical treatment of renovascular hypertension affords excellent outcomes.[11,12] Differences among most individual experiences reflect variations in the prevalence of different renovascular disease categories (Table 103.3). Renovascular hypertension in childhood is most likely to exhibit a salutary outcome after restoration of normal renal blood flow (Table 103.4). Arterial fibrodysplastic renovascular hypertension (Table 103.5) is more likely to benefit from operation than is arteriosclerotic renovascular hypertension (Table 103.6), which is probably a reflection of coexistent essential hypertension in older patients with arteriosclerotic disease. Arteriosclerotic renovascular hypertension occurs in two subgroups of patients: (a) those with focal renal artery disease whose only clinical manifestation of arteriosclerosis is secondary hypertension, and (b) those with clinically overt extrarenal arteriosclerosis affecting the coronary, carotid, aorta, or extremity vessels. The severity and duration of hypertension, age, and gender in these two subgroups are similar, yet the surgical outcome regarding amelioration of hypertension is worse in patients with overt extrarenal arteriosclerotic disease. Open revascularization of a kidney with an occluded renal artery offers recovery of renal function and improvement in blood pressure control in nearly half the patients.[73]

RENAL ARTERY ANEURYSMAL DISEASE

Aneurysms of the renal artery are unusual and poorly understood vascular lesions encountered with increasing frequency.[74–82] Complications of these aneurysms, often detected in the setting of other renal vascular disease, have been overestimated in reports that usually describe surgical series rather than population-based experiences. Other misperceptions regarding the importance of these aneurysms reflect unrecognized differences among their four principal categories: (a) true renal artery aneurysms, (b) dissecting renal artery aneurysms, (c) aneurysmal dilations occurring with medial fibrodysplastic disease, and (d) arteritis-related microaneurysms. The two renal artery macroaneurysms most relevant to clinical practice, true aneurysms and those associated with dissections, deserve individual discussion (Table 103.7).

True Renal Artery Aneurysms

The precise incidence of true renal artery aneurysms in the general population approaches 0.09%. This figure was derived in the mid-1970s from incidental demonstration of these

VASCULAR

TABLE 103.4

RESULTS

RENOVASCULAR HYPERTENSION IN CHILDREN

Institution	Patients	Operative outcome (%)			Surgical mortality rate (%)
		Cured	Improved	Failed	
University of Michigan	57	79	19	2	0
Cleveland Clinic	27	59	18.5	18.5	4
University of California, Los Angeles	26	84.5	7.5	4	4
Vanderbilt University	21	68	24	8	0
University of Pennsylvania	17	76.5	23.5	0	0
Argentinean Institute, Buenos Aires	15	53	13	27	7
University of California, San Francisco	14	86	7	0	7

(Modified from Stanley JC. The evolution of surgery for renovascular occlusive disease. *Cardiovasc Surg.* 1994;2:195–202, with permission.)

RESULTS

TABLE 103.5

FIBRODYSPLASTIC RENOVASCULAR HYPERTENSION IN ADULTS

Institution	Patients	Operative outcome (%) Cured	Improved	Failed	Surgical mortality rate (%)
University of Michigan	144	55	39	6	0
Baylor College of Medicine	113	43	24	33	0
Cleveland Clinic	92	58	31	11	Unstated
University of California, San Francisco	77	66	32	1.3	0
Mayo Clinic	63	66	24	10	Unstated
University Hospital Leiden, The Netherlands	53	53	34	13	2
Vanderbilt University	44	72	24	4	2.3
Columbia University	42	76	14	10	Unstated
Bowman Gray	40	33	57	10	0
University of Lund, Malmo, Sweden	40	66	24	10	0

(Modified from Stanley JC. The evolution of surgery for renovascular occlusive disease. *Cardiovasc Surg*. 1994;2:195–202, with permission.)

RESULTS

TABLE 103.6

ARTERIOSCLEROTIC RENOVASCULAR HYPERTENSION IN ADULTS

Institution	Patients	Operative outcome (%) Cured	Improved	Failed	Surgical mortality rate (%)
Wake Forrest University	500	12	73	15	4.6
University of Michigan	135	29	52	19	4.4
University of California, San Francisco	84	39	23	38	2.4
Cleveland Clinic	78	40	51	9	2
Columbia University	67	58	21	21	Unstated
University of Lund, Malmo, Sweden	66	49	24	27	0.9
Hospital Aiguelongue, Montpellier, France	65	45	40	15	1.1
Vanderbilt University	63	50	45	5	9

(Modified from Stanley JC. The evolution of surgery for renovascular occlusive disease. *Cardiovasc Surg*. 1994;2:195–202, with permission.)

TREATMENT

TABLE 103.7

TRUE AND DISSECTING RENAL ARTERY ANEURYSMS

Lesion	Males/females	Contributing factors	Rate of rupture	Mortality with rupture	Treatment
True aneurysm	1/1.2	Congenital defects, Arterial fibrodysplasia Hypertension	3%	10% (during pregnancy: 55% maternal, 55% fetal)	Aneurysmectomy with renal artery reconstruction, Aneurysmorrhaphy, Nephrectomy for ruptured aneurysms
Dissecting aneurysm	10/1	Blunt trauma, Arterial catheterization, Arterial fibrodysplasia, Arteriosclerosis	Uncommon	Undefined	Renal artery reconstruction

aneurysms in some 8500 patients subjected to arteriographic studies for non-renal disease at the University of Michigan.[81] Large reported series of these aneurysms are uncommon (Table 103.8). The group being studied bears greatly on the reported frequency of these lesions. For example, macroaneurysms have been identified in 0.7% of patients undergoing arteriographic studies directed at renal disease,[83] and in 2.5% of those being evaluated for hypertension.[81] The occurrence of these lesions in 9.2% of hypertensive adults with renal artery fibrodysplasia emphasizes the importance of patient selection in determining their incidence.[17] Women are affected with renal artery aneurysms 1.2 times more often than men. However, when aneurysms in patients with arterial fibrodysplasia are excluded, there appears to be no gender predilection.

TABLE 103.8 RESULTS

SELECTED EXPERIENCES WITH RENAL ARTERY ANEURYSMS

			Principal Surgical procedure				
	Patients (aneurysms)	Major symptoms	Excision and closure	Bypass	*Ex vivo* repair	Unplanned nephrectomy	Surgical mortality rate (%)
University of Michigan	168 (252)	26%	63	33	0	8	0
Heinrich-Heine University	94 (136)	Unknown	37	46	4	0	0
Wake Forrest University	62 (72)	11%	11	48	28	0	1.6
University of Toronto	56 (67)	51%	10	0	4	3	0
Vanderbilt University	39 (43)	15%	6	7	5	3	0
Mayo Clinic	32 (45)	34%	11	17	7	7	0

The predisposition of these aneurysms to affect the right renal artery may be a reflection of the greater incidence of right-sided medial fibrodysplastic disease in women.

Anatomy and Pathology

True renal artery aneurysms are usually located at renal artery bifurcations (Fig. 103.20). Most of these aneurysms are saccular. The average diameter of true aneurysms at the time of their clinical recognition is 1.5 cm. Extraparenchymal aneurysms are very common, accounting for more than 90% of these lesions, with more than 75% occurring at first- or second-order branchings of the main renal artery.

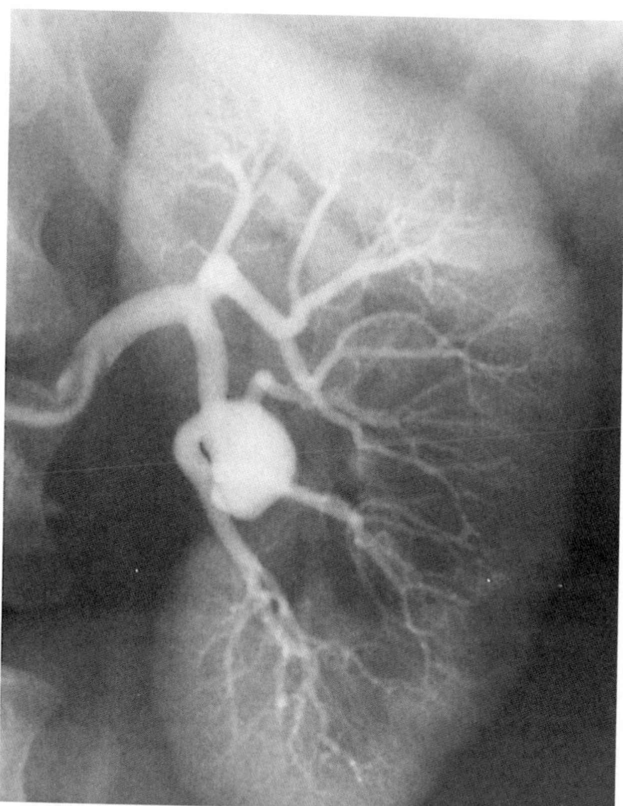

FIGURE 103.20 Renal artery aneurysm at a second-order branch. (Stanley JC, Whitehouse WM Jr. Renal artery macroaneurysms. In: Bergan JJ, Yao JST, eds. *Aneurysms*. New York: Grune & Stratton,1982, p. 417, with permission.)

Two distinct histologic categories of true renal artery aneurysms exist. The first type appears to be associated with a congenital elastic tissue defect or medial degenerative process (Fig. 103.21). Internal elastic lamina fragmentation, excessive accumulations of collagen and other ground substances, a paucity of medial elastic tissue, and a loss of recognizable medial smooth muscle characterize these lesions.

The second type of aneurysm exhibits arteriosclerosis (Fig. 103.22). Hemorrhage, calcium deposition, collections of cholesterol, necrotic debris, and a matrix of fibrous tissue typify these lesions. Such atheromatous changes often occur at irregular intervals in these aneurysms, with intervening areas composed of thin, collagenous acellular fibrous tissue. Severe arteriosclerosis of the adjacent nonaneurysmal renal artery is uncommon. When present in an aneurysm, arteriosclerosis is considered a secondary event rather than a primary etiologic event. The fact that arteriosclerotic changes affect some, but not all aneurysms in patients with multiple lesions suggests a nonarteriosclerotic cause of most renal artery aneurysms.

Both congenital and acquired factors appear to contribute to the formation of true renal artery aneurysms. Discontinuity of the internal elastic lamina is common at branchings of normal muscular arteries, and the fenestrations resulting from these discontinuities may contribute to the development of aneurysms considered congenital in origin. The reported increase in the frequency of aneurysms with age is a likely sequela of further loss of elastic tissue at these already weakened branchings.

The high incidence of renal artery aneurysms associated with medial fibrodysplasia is well recognized (Fig. 103.23). In the latter disease state, further fragmentation and disruption of elastic tissue with loss of smooth muscle at bifurcations leaves little more than a thin layer of fibrous connective tissue to contain blood flow. The greater incidence of aneurysms among patients with hypertension secondary to dysplastic renal artery stenoses, in comparison with those with arteriosclerotic stenoses, supports the tenet that arterial fibrodysplasia is a direct contributor to aneurysmal changes. Blood pressure elevations occur in 40% to 80% of patients with renal artery macroaneurysms and may contribute to aneurysm development. Increased mural tension in these cases, especially in the presence of preexisting internal elastic lamina deficiencies at bifurcations, may further compromise the structural integrity of the renal artery.

In the case of pediatric patients, most aneurysms occur in poststenotic locations. These latter aneurysms have an amorphous globular configuration with thinning of all vessel wall elements. The more typical saccular aneurysms occurring at bifurcations in older patients account for approximately a third of renal artery aneurysms in childhood.

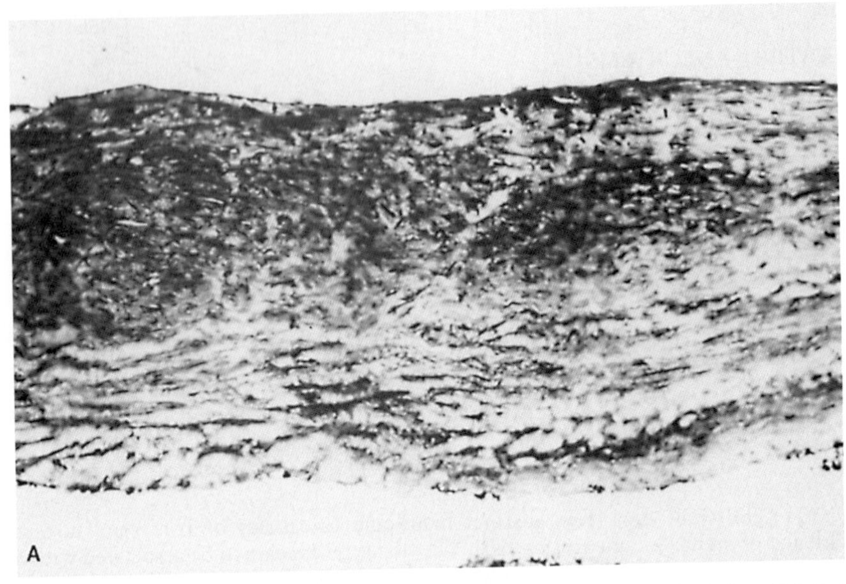

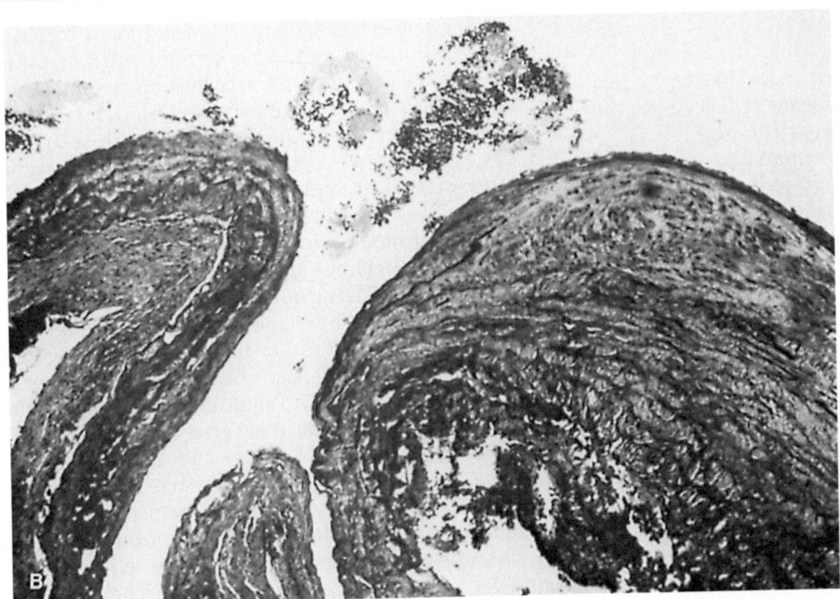

FIGURE 103.21 Renal artery aneurysm of undetermined etiology. (*A*) Excessive collagen and accumulation of ground substance with loss of smooth muscle characterize most such aneurysmal walls (Movat stain, X40). (*B*) Interruption of internal elastic lamina demonstrated at orifice of saccular renal artery aneurysm. Defects in elastic lamella have been related to the development of renal artery aneurysms (Movat stain, X60). (From Stanley JC, Rhodes EL, Gewertz BL, et al. Renal artery aneurysms: significance of macroaneurysms exclusive of dissections and fibrodysplastic mural dilations. *Arch Surg*. 1975;110:1327–1333, with permission.)

Clinical Manifestations

Most renal artery aneurysms appear to be asymptomatic and are discovered incidentally.[76–78,82] Aneurysmal expansion, compression of nearby structures, and renal infarction from dislodged thrombus may cause flank or abdominal pain. Hematuria and abdominal bruits have been attributed to some of these lesions, but in most instances, these findings result from nonaneurysmal disease. Although quite rare, covert rupture of renal artery aneurysms into an adjacent vein may be associated with hematuria and hypertension. Once suspected because of findings on radiographs, intravenous pyelography or computed tomography (CT), arteriography becomes the definitive diagnostic study. Gadolinium-enhanced magnetic resonance arteriography (MRA) and three-dimensional reconstructed CT scanning have a potential, but unproven, role in the anatomical delineation of these aneurysms.

The theory that renal artery aneurysms cause hypertension has been a subject of continual controversy.[76,77,79,80] Embolization of aneurysmal thrombus or thrombotic occlusion of an adjacent artery may result in renal ischemia and renovascular hypertension (Fig. 103.24), but this result is uncommon. Atheromatous plaque ulceration within large aneurysmal sacs may also predispose to embolic complications. If the kidney segment affected by embolization is totally infarcted, the patient may not become hypertensive. However, if the tissue simply becomes hypoperfused, then it may become the source of considerable renin production and the cause of severe secondary hypertension. Small aneurysms without calcific arteriosclerosis are less likely sources of such renal arterial occlusions.

Aneurysmal compression or kinking of a neighboring artery causing flow reductions has been proposed as a cause of renovascular hypertension but has been poorly documented in the literature. More often, coexisting renal artery occlusive disease in the vicinity of aneurysms may account for secondary hypertension in these patients. Because of this possibility, one should search for existence of occult stenoses in hypertensive patients with aneurysms. Assessments of renin activity with determination of renal:systemic renin indices among patients with hypertension and renal artery aneurysms may establish the presence of renovascular hypertension.

Rupture is the most serious complication attending renal artery aneurysms, though it occurs less commonly than does rupture of many splanchnic aneurysms. Exsanguinating hemorrhage from a ruptured renal artery aneurysm occurs

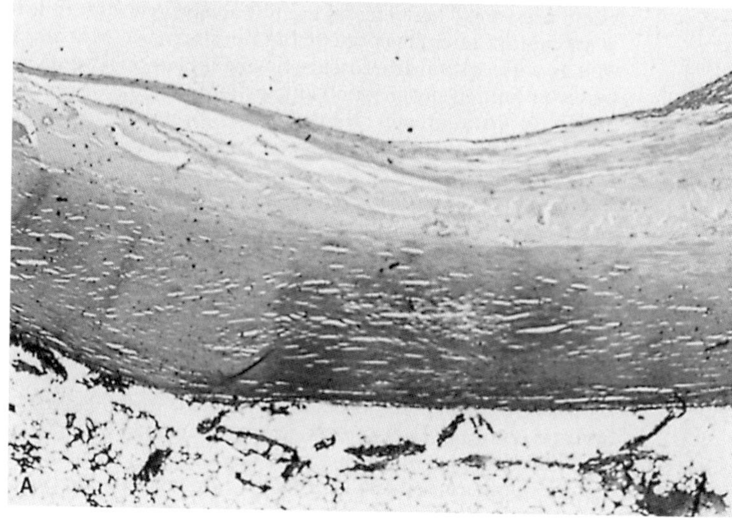

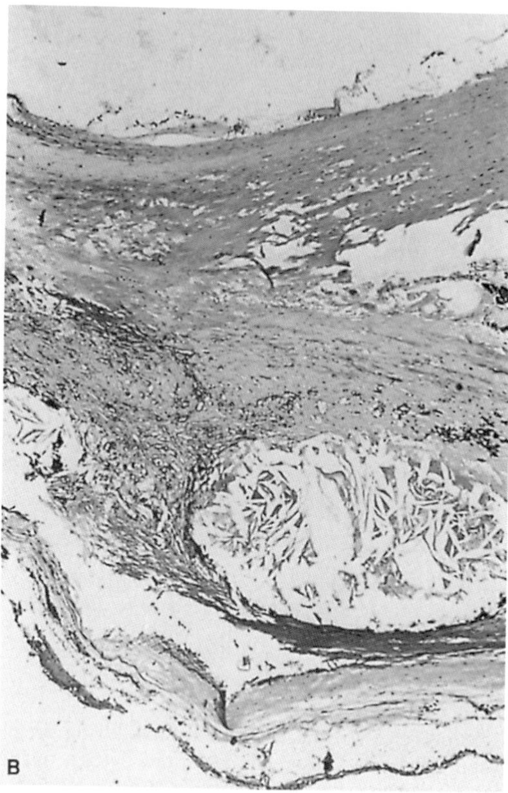

FIGURE 103.22 Arteriosclerotic renal artery aneurysm. (*A*) Fibrocollagenous aneurysm walls, with loss of all normal architecture, frequently alternated with areas exhibiting arteriosclerotic changes (hematoxylin-eosin, X40). (*B*) Calcium deposition and cholesterol clefts within the matrix of fibrous tissue are typical of many larger arteriosclerotic aneurysms (hematoxylin-eosin, X40). (From Stanley JC, Rhodes EL, Gewertz BL, et al. Renal artery aneurysms: Significance of macroaneurysms exclusive of dissections and fibrodysplastic mural dilations. *Arch Surg.* 1975; 110:1327–1333, with permission.)

rarely[76,84,85] The mortality rate with rupture is approximately 10%. Loss of a kidney is a near universal outcome of rupture. The relatively high reported rupture rate, approaching 3%, likely reflects the surgical nature of most published experiences. In fact, overt extraparenchymal rupture occurred in 2% of patients harboring these lesions, and covert rupture causing renal arteriovenous fistulas occurred in an additional 1.5% of one of the largest reported series from a surgical group.[76] Certainly, bland renal artery aneurysm rupture is likely to be considerably less than 3%.

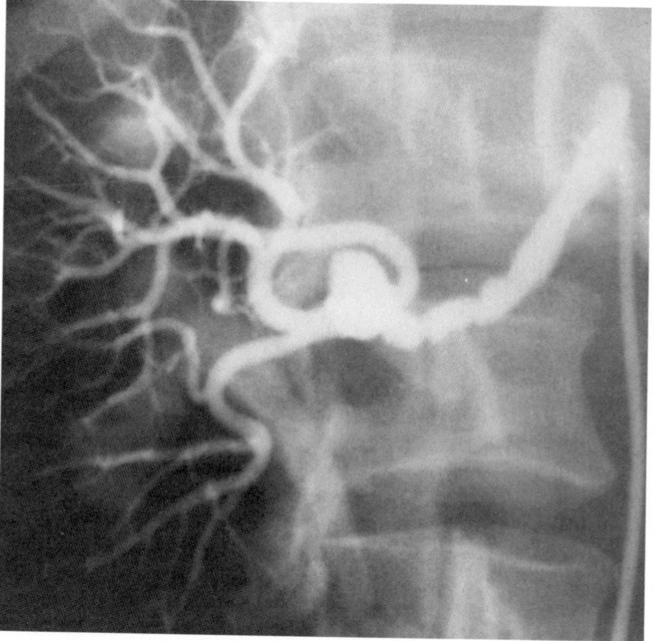

FIGURE 103.23 Saccular renal artery aneurysm occurring at the primary bifurcation of a main renal artery exhibiting medial fibroplasia. (From Stanley JC, Whitehouse WM Jr. Renal artery macroaneurysms. In: Bergan JJ, Yao JST, eds. *Aneurysms*. New York: Grune & Stratton;, 1982, p. 417, with permission.)

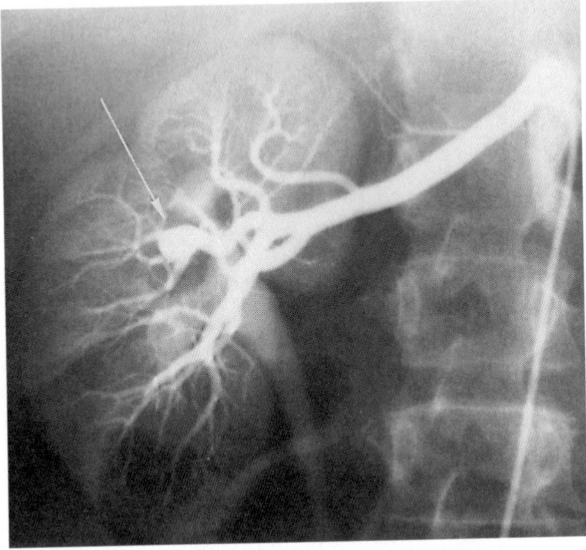

FIGURE 103.24 Small nonatherosclerotic intraparenchymal aneurysm associated with segmental thromboembolic renal ischemia and cortical infarct (*arrow*). (From Stanley JC, Whitehouse WM Jr. Renal artery macroaneurysms. In: Bergan JJ, Yao JST, eds. *Aneurysms*. New York: Grune & Stratton,1982, p. 417, with permission.)

Rupture of renal artery aneurysms during pregnancy is an exception to the generally accepted benign nature of most bland aneurysms.[86–88] Aneurysm rupture during pregnancy does not appear related to age, increased blood pressure, or number of pregnancies. Rupture of renal artery aneurysms is responsible for fetal death in nearly 85% of cases and is associated with a 55% maternal mortality rate.

An increased risk of renal artery aneurysm rupture has been attributed to large size, absence of calcification, and elevated blood pressure. These factors are not always relevant. In fact, overt rupture often has occurred in normotensive patients, as well as with calcific atherosclerotic aneurysms.[76,81] Similarly, size is of limited prognostic value as an indicator of rupture potential; with greater rupture rates occurring in larger aneurysms being inconsistently reported in the literature. Nevertheless, a larger size remains a logical reason to assign a greater risk of rupture.

Treatment

Indications for surgical intervention for true renal artery aneurysms are reasonably well defined. Operative intervention is indicated in the following situations: (a) aneurysms with functionally important renal artery stenoses; (b) aneurysms harboring thrombus, especially with evidence of distal embolization and cortical infarcts; (c) aneurysms in women who plan to have children; and (d) aneurysms with diameters greater than 1.5 cm in otherwise healthy patients. Size is a soft indication for surgical therapy, although the risk of rupture seems to correlate with size. Cautious surgical intervention by those experienced in renovascular surgery in properly selected patients with renal artery aneurysms appears justified because of the small, but unpredictable, incidence of rupture with its attendant loss of kidney and life.

The objective of surgical therapy is to eliminate the aneurysm without removing the kidney or compromising its function.[76,89,90] Most aneurysms are best approached with a transabdominal, extraperitoneal exposure of the renal vasculature following medial displacement of the overlying colon and foregut viscera. Large aneurysms of the main renal artery can usually be excised with simple primary closure of the artery, but excision of smaller aneurysms may require arterial closure with a vein patch (Fig. 103.25). More extensive renal artery reconstructions using autogenous saphenous vein or internal iliac artery as aortorenal grafts are favored for bifurcation aneurysms,

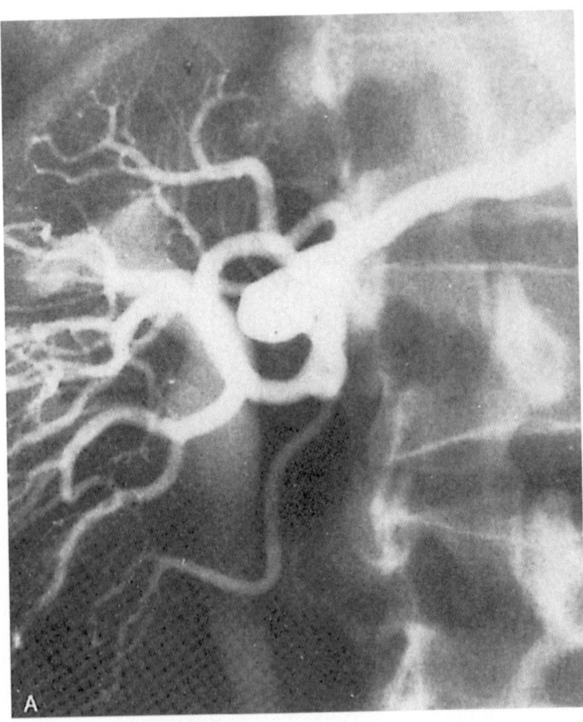

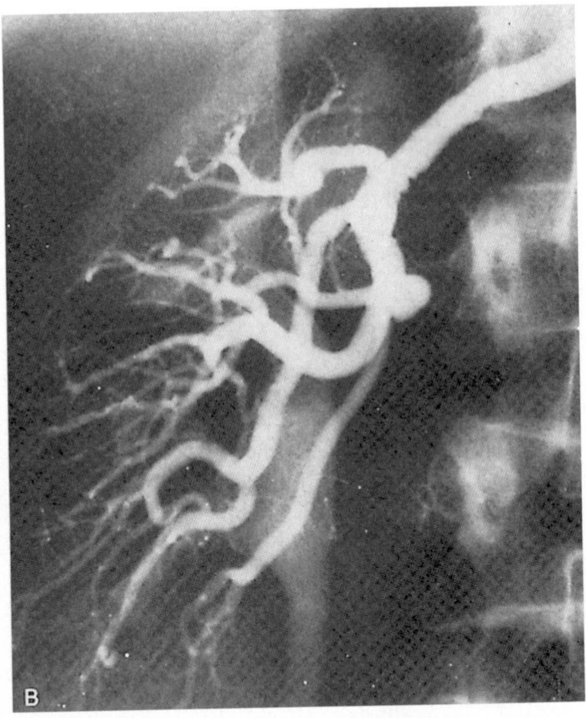

FIGURE 103.25 (*A*) Renal artery aneurysm located at bifurcation of main renal artery. (*B*) Surgical treatment included aneurysmectomy and vein patch graft closure of the artery. (From Stanley JC. Renal artery aneurysms and dissections. In: Veith FJ, ed. *Current critical problems in vascular surgery*, Vol 3. St. Louis: Quality Medical Publishing, 1991, p. 311, with permission.)

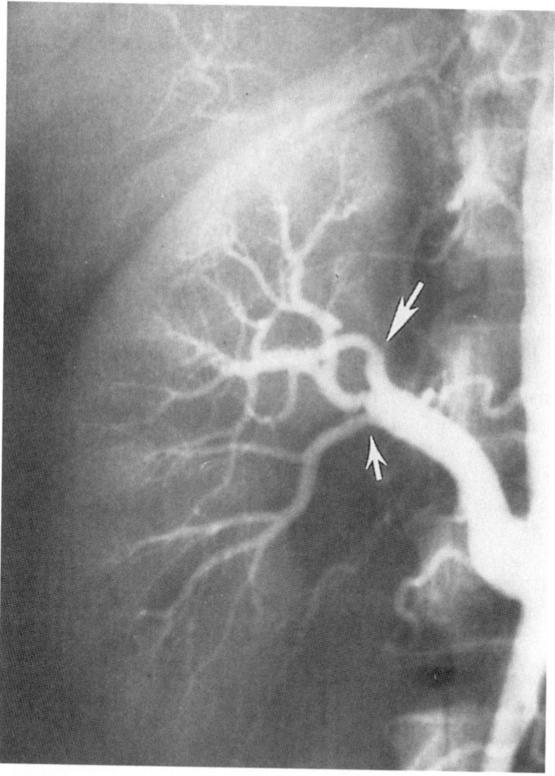

FIGURE 103.26 Aortorenal bypass with reversed autogenous saphenous vein, following excision of an aneurysm in a fibrodysplastic vessel, with end-to-end anastomosis to one first-order segmental branch (*large arrow*) and end-to-side implantation of the other first-order segmental branch (*small arrow*). (From Ernst CB, Stanley JC, Fry WJ. Multiple primary and segmental renal artery revascularization utilizing autogenous saphenous vein. *Surg Gynecol Obstet.* 1973;137:1023–1026, with permission.)

especially those associated with functionally important stenoses (Fig. 103.26).

Aneurysmectomy with reimplantation of the involved vessel or vessels into a normal adjacent or proximal renal artery is appropriate for treating many first-and second-order branch aneurysms (Fig. 103.27).[91,92] These procedures are usually undertaken in situ, although ex vivo reconstructions may be preferred in certain cases, especially with coexistent segmental renal artery stenotic disease. Last, renal artery aneurysms 2 to 3 mm in diameter may be plicated by way of a closed aneurysmorrhaphy using a fine running cardiovascular suture. These very small aneurysms are often encountered at operation as incidental lesions when treating larger aneurysms.

Nephrectomy is the usual therapy for managing ruptured aneurysms and extensive intraparenchymal aneurysms. Long-term outcome is actually quite good with this mode of therapy in carefully selected cases, with no patients treated in this manner at the University of Michigan requiring hemodialysis during a 20 year follow-up.[76] Nevertheless, arterial reconstruction should be considered in those instances in which the kidney does not appear to have been irreparably injured from ischemia caused by the rupture. In other cases, partial nephrectomy may be required when aneurysmal erosion has occurred into an adjacent vein causing a chronic arteriovenous fistula. Acute arteriovenous fistulas can occasionally be treated by conventional means with local excision and arterial reconstruction.

In general, renal artery aneurysms are not amenable to endovascular intervention. In part, this is because of their usual location at arterial bifurcations. In anecdotal cases, main renal artery aneurysms have been successfully excluded by stent graft placement, and peripheral branch aneurysms have been successfully embolized.[93–95] Embolization of intraparenchymal aneurysms is an appropriate alternative to partial nephrectomy in those patients with evidence of distal cortical infarction.

Renal artery aneurysms not treated by operation should be subjected to long-term surveillance. Duplex ultrasonography, CT, or MRA may prove useful in establishing an aneurysm's stability. Arteriography should be considered in patients who

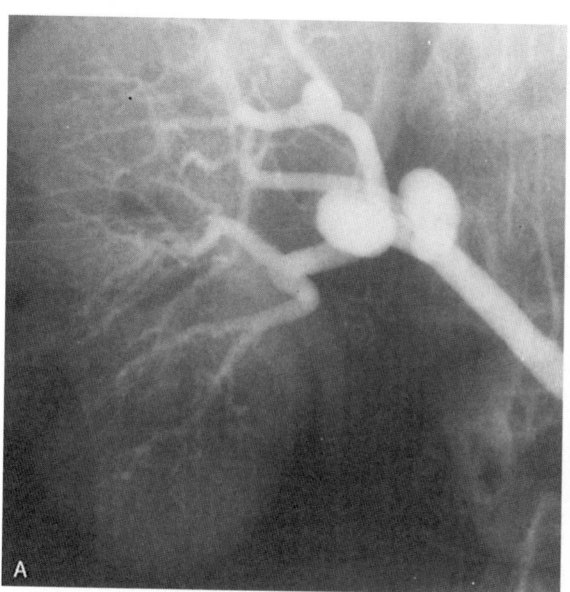

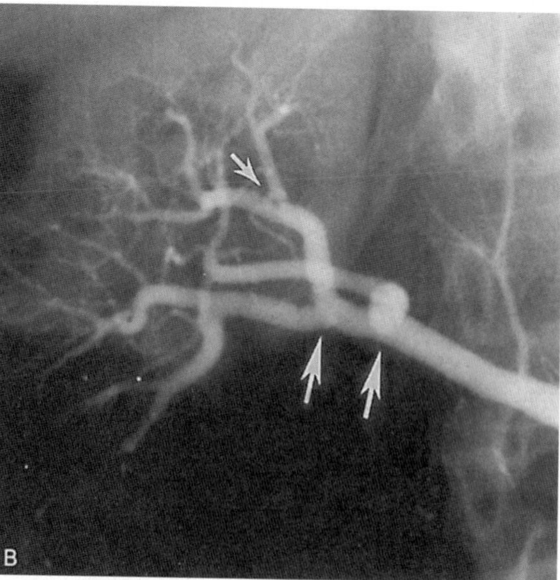

FIGURE 103.27 (*A*) Renal artery aneurysms involving multiple segmental artery branchings. (*B*) Surgical treatment included aneurysmectomy and end-to-side reimplantation (*large arrows*) of segmental vessels into the adjacent artery and closed aneurysmorrhaphy (*small arrow*). (From Stanley JC. Renal artery aneurysms and dissections. In: Veith FJ, ed. *Current critical problems in vascular surgery*, Vol 3. St. Louis, Quality Medical Publishing, 1991;311, with permission.)

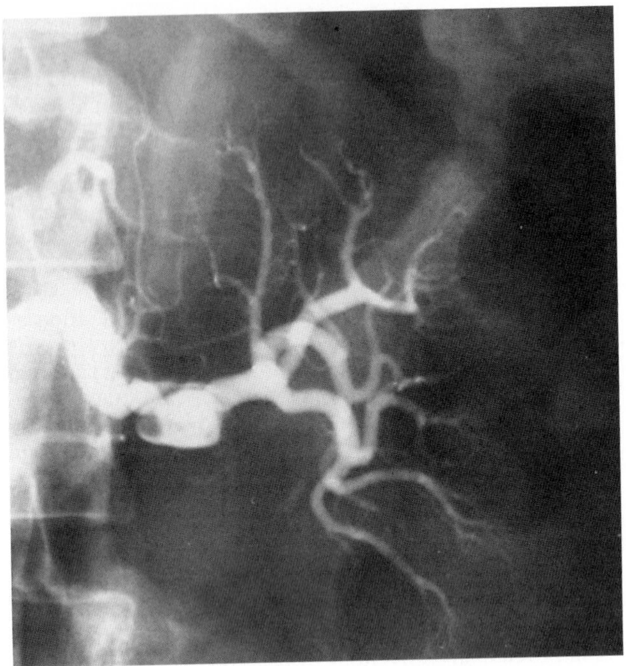

FIGURE 103.28 Saccular dissecting main renal artery aneurysm. (From Gewertz BL, Stanley JC, Fry WJ. Renal artery dissections. *Arch Surg*. 1977;112:409–414, with permission.)

develop symptoms suggestive of aneurysmal expansion, exhibit hematuria, or become hypertensive. Because of the relatively low incidence of complications attending most renal artery aneurysms, noninvasive studies performed on a regular basis are favored over repeated arteriographic studies, which may carry risks exceeding those of the aneurysmal disease.

Dissecting Renal Artery Aneurysms

Isolated renal artery dissections causing aneurysms are rare.[96–100] Dissections are usually classified into two categories—those due to blunt abdominal trauma or intraluminal catheter-induced injury and those occurring spontaneously (Fig. 103.28). Nearly one third of renal artery dissections are bilateral.

Anatomy of Pathology

Dissections of the renal artery affect men nearly 10 times as often as in women. In part, this reflects the greater likelihood of trauma-induced dissections that occur in men. Although an overall predilection for right renal artery involvement exists, trauma-related dissections more commonly affect the left renal artery. Blood viscosity, shear forces, and flow turbulence are common contributors to the propagation of all dissections, but inadequate structural integrity due to injury or disease may initiate a dissection. Other factors contributing to these aneurysms vary among the different categories of dissection.

Blunt abdominal trauma contributes to renal artery dissections by two specific mechanisms. The first is violent displacement of the kidney with deceleration causing marked stretching of the artery with fracture of the intima, which is the least-elastic vessel wall component. This event commonly results in subintimal dissections. The second mechanism relates to the unyielding posteriorly located vertebral bodies and direct arterial injury. In this setting traumatic compression of the renal arteries against the vertebra may cause deeper medial hemorrhage and false aneurysm formation because of vasa vasorum rupture or actual vessel wall disruption.

Iatrogenic, catheter-related, renal artery injury occurring during diagnostic arteriography is another recognized cause of these aneurysms. This complication is uncommon. Iatrogenic dissections usually occur within the inner media or subintimal tissues. Dissections accompanying therapeutic catheterizations, such as balloon angioplasty, are common, although only a few cause critical narrowings or occlusion of the renal artery. In these instances, stent placement often restores normal renal artery blood flow.

Primary or spontaneous dissections causing pseudoaneurysms, affect the renal arteries more than any other peripheral artery. Most are related to coexistent arteriosclerotic or dysplastic renovascular disease. A 0.5% incidence of dissections in patients with fibrodysplastic renal arteries has been reported.[97] Spontaneous dissections usually occur within the outer media adjacent to the external elastic lamina (Fig. 103.29). They occur less commonly within the inner or central media. In many instances, these dissections have been attributed to rupture of abnormal vasa vasorum. It is possible that the dissecting intramural hematoma in these circumstances increases medial ischemia and contributes to further aneurysm formation. Spontaneous renal artery dissections usually affect proximal vessels and terminate at branchings.

Clinical Manifestations

Flank and back pain, hematuria, ileus, and elevated blood pressure frequently accompany acute dissections regardless of the cause.[97,98] Chronic renal artery dissections, when clinically relevant, are usually associated with renovascular hypertension or impaired renal function. Certain dissections may be self-limited, asymptomatic, and of no functional importance.

An incorrect initial clinical diagnosis is common, occurring in more than half of patients having renal artery dissections. Intravenous pyelography has been advocated for evaluating patients suspected of serious renal hilar injuries including

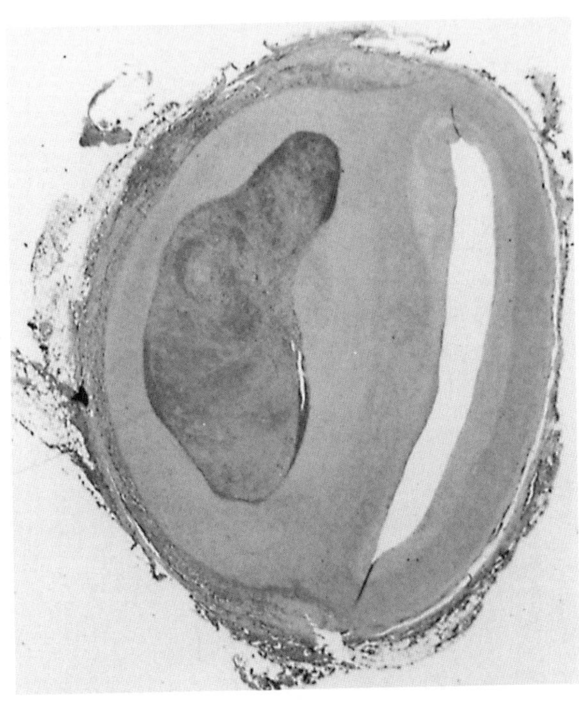

FIGURE 103.29 Dissection exhibiting deep mural hematoma and compression of adjacent lumen (hematoxylin-eosin, X60). (From Stanley JC. Pathologic basis of macrovascular renal artery disease. In: Stanley JC, Ernst CB, Fry WJ, eds. Renovascular *Hypertension*. WB Saunders, Philadelphia, 1984, p. 46, with permission.)

dissecting aneurysms. However, a false-negative excretory urogram occurs in approximately 10% of patients who have documented major renal artery injury. Furthermore, minor perirenal hematomas and cortical contusions frequently impair contrast excretion and may cause one third to one half these studies to be false-positive. Because of this fact and the need for prompt diagnosis to improve results of surgical therapy, intravenous urograms should be deferred in favor of earlier arteriographic examinations.

Arteriography is necessary to diagnose and define the extent of renal artery dissections. Dissection is radiographically diagnosed when the following are recognized: (a) luminal irregularities with aneurysmal dilatation or saccular dissections associated with segmental stenoses; (b) extension of the dissections to the first renal artery branching; (c) cuffing at branchings; and, (d) variable degrees of reversibility documented on serial arteriographic studies.

Trauma-related dissections warrant emergent primary arterial reconstructions once a hemodynamic narrowing or occlusion of the main renal artery or a major segmental branch is recognized. Delayed repair is necessary for less obvious trauma-related injuries if hypertension persists or renal function deteriorates. Spontaneous dissecting aneurysms, when acute, are technically easier to treat than traumatic lesions and should be subjected to surgical therapy soon after hemodynamically significant stenoses or occlusions are recognized. Operative intervention is also pursued for chronic spontaneous dissections associated with severe renovascular hypertension or deteriorating renal function. Again, endovascular stent placement is an appropriate alternative therapy for short proximal renal artery dissections with a defined distal endpoint.

Treatment

Kidney preservation is very important in patients with renal artery dissections, especially in blunt abdominal trauma patients, where renal artery injury of the contralateral kidney is often present. Nephrectomy under such circumstances should be avoided. Although many dissections are not amenable to operative repair, arterial reconstructions in the form of aortorenal bypass using autogenous saphenous vein or hypogastric artery, with ex vivo repairs in selected cases, provide reasonable kidney salvage rates.

KEY POINTS

- **Renal artery occlusive and aneurysmal disease has been recognized with increasing frequency with the advent of less invasive imaging modalities.**
- **Renovascular hypertension secondary to renal artery occlusive disease is the most common form of surgically correctable hypertension.**
- **The most important consequence of renal artery occlusive disease is the production of angiotensin II, which is one of the most potent pressor substances known.**
- **Arteriosclerotic renal artery occlusive disease accounts for about 95% of reported cases of renovascular hypertension.**
- **Arteriosclerotic renal artery occlusive disease characteristically affects the proximal third of the vessel in the form of eccentric or concentric stenoses.**
- **Medial fibroplasia is the most commonly diagnosed dysplastic renal artery disease, accounting for 85% of these lesions.**
- **Developmental renal artery stenoses are a rare cause of renovascular hypertension.**
- **Renovascular hypertension is much more common in patients with more severe diastolic blood pressure elevations; as many as 5% of such patients are found to have a renovascular cause of their hypertension.**
- **Therapeutic results in the management of renovascular hypertension often relate to the proper execution of an appropriate intervention.**
- **Surgical treatment of renovascular hypertension affords excellent outcomes.**
- **Aneurysms of the renal artery are unusual and poorly understood vascular lesions encountered with increasing frequency.**

References

1. Goldblatt H, Lynch J, Hanzal RF, et al. Studies on experimental hypertension. I. The production of persistent elevation of systolic blood pressure by means of renal ischemia. *J Exp Med.* 1934;59:347.
2. Pratt RE, Carleton JE, Richie JP, et al. Human renin biosynthesis and secretion in normal and ischemic kidneys. *Proc Natl Acad Sci USA.* 1987;84:7837–7840.
3. Sealey JE, Buhler FR, Laragh JH, et al. The physiology of renin secretion in essential hypertension: estimation of renin secretion rate and renal plasma flow from peripheral and renal vein renin levels. *Am J Med.* 1973; 55:391–401.
4. Schneider EG, Davis JO, Baumber JS, et al. The hepatic metabolism of renin and aldosterone: a review with new observations on the hepatic clearance of renin. *Circ Res.* 1970;26/27(suppl 1):175.
5. Samuels AI, Miller ED Jr, Fray JCS, et al. Renin-angiotensin antagonists and the regulation of blood pressure. *Fed Proc.* 1976;35:2512–2520.
6. Oparil S, Tregear GW, Koerner T, et al. Mechanism of pulmonary conversion of angiotensin I to II in the dog. Circ Res 1971;29:682–690.
7. Oshima G, Gecse A, Erdos EG. Angiotensin I–converting enzyme of the kidney cortex. *Biochim Biophys Acta.* 1974; 350:26–37.
8. Stanley JC, Gewertz BL, Fry WJ. Renal:systemic renin indices and renal vein renin ratios as prognostic indicators in remedial renovascular hypertension. *J Surg Res.* 1976;20:149–155.
9. Vaughan ED Jr, Buhler FR, Laragh JH, et al. Renovascular hypertension: renin measurements to indicate hypersecretion and contralateral suppression, estimate renal plasma flow, and score for surgical curability. *Am J Med.* 1973; 55:402–414.
10. Gavras H, Brunner HB, Vaughan ED Jr, et al. Angiotensin–sodium interaction in blood pressure maintenance of renal hypertensive and normotensive rats. *Science* 1973;180:1369–1371.
11. Stanley JC. The evolution of surgery for renovascular occlusive disease. *Cardiovasc Surg.* 1994;2:195–202..
12. **Stanley JC. David M. Hume memorial lecture. Surgical treatment of renovascular hypertension. *Am J Surg.* 1997;174:102–110.**
13. Louie J, Isaacson JA, Zierler RE, et al. Prevalence of carotid and lower extremity arterial disease in patients with renal artery stenosis. *Am J Hypertens.* 1994;7:436–439.
14. Valentine RJ, Clagett GP, Miller GL, et al. The coronary risk of unsuspected renal artery stenosis. *J Vasc Surg.* 1993;18:433–440.
15. Valentine RJ, Martin JD, Myers SI, et al. Asymptomatic celiac and superior mesenteric artery stenoses are more prevalent among patients with unsuspected renal artery stenoses. *J Vasc Surg.* 1991;14:195–199.
16. Novick AC, Zaki S, Goldfarb D, et al. Epidemiologic and clinical comparison of renal artery stenosis in black patients and white patients. *J Vasc Surg.* 1994;20:1–5.
17. Stanley JC, Gewertz BL, Bove EL, et al. Arterial fibrodysplasia: histopathologic character and current etiologic concepts. *Arch Surg.* 1975;110: 561–566.
18. Sottiurai V, Fry WJ, Stanley JC. Ultrastructure of smooth muscle, myofibroblasts and fibroblasts in human arterial dysplasia. *Arch Surg.* 1978; 113:1280–1288.
19. Graham LM, Zelenock GB, Erlandson EE, et al. Abdominal aortic coarctation and segmental hypoplasia. *Surgery* 1979; 86:519–529.
20. Stanley JC, Graham LM, Whitehouse WM Jr, et al. Developmental occlusive disease of the abdominal aorta and the splanchnic and renal arteries. *Am J Surg.* 1981;142:190–196.
21. **Stanley JC, Zelenock GB, Messina LM, et al. Pediatric renovascular hypertension: a thirty-year experience of operative treatment. *J Vasc Surg.* 1995;21:212–227.**
22. Hertz SM, Holland GA, Baum RA, et al. Evaluation of renal artery stenosis by magnetic resonance angiography. *Am J Surg.* 1994;168: 140–143.
23. Prince MR, Narasimham DL, Stanley JC, et al. Breath-hold 3D gadolinium MRA: new developments for imaging the abdominal aorta and its major branches. *Radiology* 1995;197:785–792.
24. Hansen KJ, Tribble RW, Reavis SW, et al. Renal duplex sonography: evaluation of clinical utility. *J Vasc Surg.* 1990; 12:227–236.
25. Kohler TR, Zierler RE, Martin RL, et al. Noninvasive diagnosis of renal artery stenosis by ultrasonic duplex scanning. *J Vasc Surg.* 1986;4:450–456.
26. Stanley JC, Fry WJ. Surgical treatment of renovascular hypertension. *Arch Surg.* 1977;112:1291–1297.

27. Thornbury JR, Stanley JC, Fryback DG. Hypertensive urogram: a nondiscriminatory test for renovascular hypertension. *AJR Am J Roentgenol.* 1982;138:43–49.
28. Stanley JC, Whitehouse WM Jr, Graham LM, et al. Operative therapy of renovascular hypertension. *Br J Surg.* 1982; 63(suppl):S63.
29. Meier GH, Sumpio B, Setaro JF, et al. Captopril renal scintigraphy: a new standard for predicting outcome after renal revascularization. *J Vasc Surg.* 1993;17:280–287.
30. Grüntzig A, Vetter W, Meier B, et al. Treatment of renovascular hypertension with percutaneous transluminal dilatation of a renal-artery stenosis. *Lancet* 1978;1:801–802.
31. Knipp BS, Dimick JB, Eliason JL, et al. Diffusion of new technology for the treatment of renovascular hypertension in the United States: surgical revascularization versus catheter-based therapy, 1988–2001. *J Vasc Surg.* 2004;40:717–723.
32. Bonelli FS, Mckusick MA, Textor SC, et al. Renal artery angioplasty: Technical results and clinical outcome in 320 patients. *Mayo Clin Proc.* 1995;70:1041–1052.
33. Cluzel P, Raynaud B, Beyssen B, et al. Stenoses of renal branch arteries in fibromuscular dysplasia: Results of percutaneous transluminal angioplasty. *Radiology* 1994;193:227–232.
34. Davidson R, Barri Y, Wilcox CS. Predictors of cure of hypertension in fibromuscular renovascular disease. *Am J Kidney Dis.* 1996; 28:334–338.
35. Luscher TF, Keller HM, Imhof HG, et al. Fibromuscular hyperplasia: Extension of the disease and therapeutic outcome. Results of the University Hospital Zurich Cooperative Study on Fibromuscular Hyperplasia. *Nephron* 1986;44(suppl 1):109–114.
36. Sos TA, Pickering TG, Sniderman K, et al. Percutaneous transluminal renal angioplasty in renovascular hypertension due to atheroma or fibromuscular dysplasia. *N Engl J Med.* 1983;309:274–279.
37. Tegtmeyer CJ, Kellum CD, Ayers C. Percutaneous transluminal angioplasty of the renal artery: results and long-term follow-up. *Radiology* 1984;153:77–84.
38. Tegtmeyer CJ, Selby JB, Hartwell GD, et al. Results and complications of angioplasty in fibromuscular disease. *Circulation* 1991;83(Suppl 2): 1155–1161.
39. Martin EC, Diamond NG, Casarella WJ. Percutaneous transluminal angioplasty in nonatherosclerotic disease. *Radiology* 1980;135:27–33.
40. **Ayerdi J, Hodgson KJ. Balloon angioplasty and stenting for renovascular occlusive disease. *Pers Vasc Surg Endovasc Ther.* 2004;16:25–42.**
41. Blum U, Krumme B, Flugel P, et al. Treatment of ostial renal artery stenoses with vascular endoprostheses after unsuccessful balloon angioplasty. *N Engl J Med.* 1997;336:459–465.
42. Boisclair C, Therasse E, Oliva VL, et al. Treatment of renal angioplasty failure by percutaneous renal artery stenting with Palmaz stents: midterm technical and clinical results. *AJR Am J Roentgenol.* 1997;168:245–251.
43. Dorros G, Jaff M, Jain A, et al. Follow-up of primary Palmaz-Schatz stent placement for atherosclerotic renal artery stenosis. *Am J Cardiol.* 1995;75:1051–1055.
44. Dorros G, Jaff M, Mathiak L, et al. Four-year follow-up of Palmaz-Schatz stent revascularization as treatment for renal artery stenosis *Circulation* 1998;98:642–647.
45. Harjai K, Khosla S, Shaw D, et al. Effect of gender on outcomes following renal artery stent placement for renovascular hypertension. *Cathet Cardiovasc Diagn.* 1997;42:381–386.
46. Henry M, Amor M, Henry I, et al. Stent placement in the renal artery: three-year experience with the Palmaz stent. *J Vasc Intervent Radiol.* 1996;7:343–350.
47. **Leertouwer TC, Gussenhoven EJ, Bosch JL, et al. Stent placement for renal arterial stenosis: Where do we stand? A meta-analysis. *Radiology* 2000;216:78–85.**
48. Rees CR, Palmaz JC, Becker GJ, et al. Palmaz stent in atherosclerotic stenoses involving the ostia of the renal arteries: Preliminary report of a multicenter study. *Radiology* 1991;181:507–514.
49. Dean RH, Lawson JD, Hollifield JW. Revascularization of the poorly functioning kidney. *Surgery* 1979;85:44–52.
50. Hansen KJ, Cherr GS, Craven TE, et al. Management of ischemic nephropathy: Dialysis-free survival after surgical repair. *J Vasc Surg.* 200032:472–48?
51. **Hansen KJ, Thomason RB, Craven TE, et al. Surgical management of dialysis-dependent ischemic nephropathy. *J Vasc Surg.* 1995;21:197–211.**
52. Jacobson HR. Ischemic renal disease: An overlooked clinical entity? *Kidney Int.* 198834:729–743.
53. Jamieson GG, Clarkson AR, Woodroffe AJ, Faris I. Reconstructive renal vascular surgery for chronic renal failure. *Br J Surg.* 1984;71:338–340.
54. Wong JM, Hansen KJ, Oskin TC, et al. Surgery after failed percutaneous renal artery angioplasty. *J Vasc Surg.* 1999;30:468–482.
55. Anderson CA, Hansen KJ, Benjamin ME, et al. Renal artery fibromuscular dysplasia: results of current surgical therapy. *J Vasc Surg.* 1995;22:207–217.
56. Cambria RP, Brewster DC, L'Italien G, et al. Simultaneous aortic and renal artery reconstruction: evolution of an eighteen-year experience. *J Vasc Surg.* 1994;21:916–925.
57. Cambria RP, Brewster DC, L'Italien GJ, et al. The durability of different reconstructive techniques for atherosclerotic renal artery disease. *J Vasc Surg.* 1994;20:76–87.
58. **Cherr GS, Hansen KJ, Craven TE, et al. Surgical management of atherosclerotic renovascular disease. *J Vasc Surg.* 200235:236–245.**
59. Hansen KJ, Starr SM, Sands RE, et al. Contemporary surgical management of renovascular disease. *J Vasc Surg.* 1992; 16:319–331.
60. Murray SP, Kent C, Salvatierra O, et al. Complex branch renovascular disease: management options and late results. *J Vasc Surg.* 1994;20: 338–346.
61. Stanley JC, Whitehouse WM Jr, Zelenock GB, et al. Reoperation for complications of renal artery reconstructive surgery undertaken for treatment of renovascular hypertension. *J Vasc Surg.* 1985;2:133–144.
62. Stanley JC, Ernst CB, Fry WJ. Fate of 100 aortorenal vein grafts: characteristics of late graft expansion, aneurysmal dilatation, and stenosis. *Surgery* 1973;74:931–944.
63. Chibaro EA, Libertino JA, Novick AC. Use of the hepatic circulation for renal revascularization. *Ann Surg.* 1984;199:406–411.
64. Khauli RB, Novick AC, Ziegelbaum M. Splenorenal bypass in the treatment of renal artery stenosis: experience with 69 cases. *J Vasc Surg.* 1985;2:547–551.
65. Novick AC, Stewart R, Hodge EE,. Use of the thoracic aorta for renal arterial reconstruction. *J Vasc Surg.* 1994;19:605–609.
66. Moncure AC, Brewster DC, Darling RC, et al. Use of the splenic and hepatic arteries for renal revascularization. *J Vasc Surg.* 1986;3: 196–203.
67. Brekke IB, Sodal G, Jakobsen A, et al. Fibromuscular renal artery disease treated by extracorporeal vascular reconstruction and renal autotransplantation: short- and long-term results. *Eur J Vasc Surg.* 1992; 6:471–476.
68. van Bockel JH, van den Akker PJ, Chang PC, et al. Extracorporeal renal artery reconstruction for renovascular hypertension. *J Vasc Surg.* 1991; 13:101–111.
69. Dougherty MJ, Hallett JW Jr, Naessens J, et al. Renal endarterectomy vs. bypass for combined aortic and renal reconstruction: is there a difference in clinical outcome? *Ann Vasc Surg.* 1995;9:87–94.
70. McNeil JW, String ST, Pfeiffer RB Jr. Concomitant renal endarterectomy and aortic reconstruction. *J Vasc Surg.* 1994;20:331–337.
71. Stoney RJ, Messina LM, Goldstone J, et al. Renal endarterectomy through the transected aorta: a new technique for combined aortorenal arteriosclerosis—a preliminary report. *J Vasc Surg.* 1989;9:224–233.
72. Oskin TC, Hansen KJ, Deitch JS, et al. Chronic renal artery occlusion: nephrectomy versus revascularization. *J Vasc Surg.* 1999;29:140–149.
73. Whitehouse WM Jr, Kazmers A, Zelenock GB, et al. Chronic total renal artery occlusions: effects of treatment on secondary hypertension and renal function. *Surgery* 1981;89:753–763.
74. Dzsinich C, Gloviczki P, McKusick MA, et al. Surgical management of renal artery aneurysm. *Cardiovasc Surg.* 1993;3:243–247.
75. English WP, Pearce JD, Craven TE, et al. Surgical management of renal artery aneurysms. J *Vasc Surg.* 2004;40:53–60.
76. **Henke PK, Cardneau JD, Welling TH III, et al. Renal artery aneurysms. A 35-year clinical experience with 252 aneurysms in 168 patients. *Ann Surg.* 2001;234:454–463.**
77. Henriksson C, Bjorkerud S, Nilson AE, et al. Natural history of renal artery aneurysm elucidated by repeated angiography and pathoanatomical studies. *Eur Urol.* 1985;11:244–248.
78. Henriksson C, Lukes P, Nilson AE, et al. Angiographically discovered, non-operated renal artery aneurysms. *Scand J Urol Nephrol.* 1984;18: 59–62.
79. Martin RS III, Meacham PW, Ditesheim JA, et al. Renal artery aneurysm: selective treatment for hypertension and prevention of rupture. *J Vasc Surg.* 1989;9:26–34.
80. Pfeiffer T, Reiher L, Grabitz K, et al. Reconstruction for renal artery aneurysm: operative techniques and long-term results. *J Vasc Surg.* 2003;37:293–300.
81. Stanley JC, Rhodes EL, Gewertz BL, et al. Renal artery aneurysms: significance of macroaneurysms exclusive of dissections and fibrodysplastic mural dilations. *Arch Surg.* 1975;110:1327–1333.
82. Tham G, Ekelund L, Herrlin K, et al. Renal artery aneurysms: natural history and prognosis. *Ann Surg.* 197:348–1983.
83. Edsman G. Angiography and suprarenal angiography. *Acta Radiol.* 1965;(Suppl 155):1–141.
84. Hidai H, Kinoshita Y, Murayama T, et al. Rupture of renal artery aneurysm. *Eur Urol.* 1985;11:249–253.
85. Schorn B, Valk V, Dalichau H, et al. Kidney salvage in a case of ruptured renal artery aneurysm: case report and literature review. *Cardiovasc Surg.* 1997;5:134–136.
86. Cohen JR, Shamash FS. Ruptured renal artery aneurysms during pregnancy. *J Vasc Surg.* 1987;6:51–59.
87. Love WK, Robinette MA, Vernon CP. Renal artery aneurysm rupture in pregnancy. *J Urol.* 1981;126:809–811.
88. Rijbroek A, Dijk AV, Roex AJM. Rupture of renal artery aneurysm during pregnancy. *Eur J Vasc Surg.* 1994;8:375–376.
89. Huppt T, Allenberg JR, Post K, et al. Renal artery aneurysms: surgical indications and results. *Eur J Vasc Surg.* 1992;6:477–486.
90. Mercier C, Piquet P, Piligian F, et al. Aneurysms of the renal artery and its branches. *Ann Vasc Surg.* 1986;1:321–327.
91. Bugge-Asperheim B, Sodal G, Flatmark A. Renal artery aneurysm: ex vivo repair and autotransplantation. *Scand J Urol Nephrol.* 1984;18: 63–66.

92. Dubernard JM, Martin X, Gelet A, et al. Aneurysms of the renal artery: surgical management with special reference to extracorporeal surgery and autotransplantation. *Eur Urol.* 1985;11:26–30.
93. Bui BT, Oliva VL, Leclerc G, et al. Renal artery aneurysm: Treatment with percutaneous placement of a stent-graft. *Radiology* 1995;195:181–182.
94. Centenera LV, Hirsch JA, Choi IS, et al. Wide-necked saccular renal artery aneurysm: Endovascular embolization with the Guglielmi detachable coil and temporary balloon occlusion of the aneurysm neck. *J Vasc Interv Radiol.* 1998;9:513–516.
95. Tateno T, Kubota Y, Sasagawa I, et al. Successful embolization of a renal artery aneurysm with preservation of renal blood flow. *Int Urol Nephrol.* 1996;28:283–287.
96. Edwards BS, Stanson AW, Holley KE, et al. Isolated renal artery dissection: presentation, evaluation, management and pathology. *Mayo Clin Proc.* 1982;57:564–571.
97. Gewertz BL, Stanley JC, Fry WJ. Renal artery dissections. *Arch Surg.* 1977;112:409–414.
98. Müller BT, Reiher L, Pfeiffer T, et al. Surgical treatment of renal artery dissection in 25 patients: Indications and results. *J Vasc Surg.* 2003;37:761–768.
99. Reilly LM, Cunningham CG, Maggisano R, et al. The role of arterial reconstruction in spontaneous renal artery dissection. *J Vasc Surg.* 1991;14:468–479.
100. Smith BM, Holcomb GW, Richie RE, et al. Renal artery dissection. *Ann Surg.* 1984;200:134–146.

CHAPTER 104 ■ LOWER EXTREMITY ANEURYSMS

LINDA M. GRAHAM

PERIPHERAL ANEURYSMS

Femoral and popliteal artery aneurysms, although far less common than abdominal aortic aneurysms, are the most frequently encountered peripheral aneurysms. Their significance comes from their potential for limb-threatening complications and their association with life-threatening abdominal aortic aneurysms.

Incidence

The exact incidence of femoral and popliteal aneurysms is difficult to define, but they are being recognized with increasing frequency. An aging population, increased arterial trauma, more common use of invasive therapies for vascular disease, and increased use of imaging modalities all contribute to the rise in number of peripheral aneurysms being diagnosed. In a screening study of men between the ages of 65 and 74 years, abdominal aortic aneurysms were identified in 4.9% of patients.[1] In patients with abdominal aortic aneurysms, 6.8 % had femoral artery aneurysms and 9.6% had popliteal artery aneurysms.[2] Screening of men between the ages of 65 and 80 years identified popliteal artery aneurysms in 1%.[3]

An increased number of false aneurysms are occurring coincident with the increased use of bypass surgery and catheter-based diagnostic and therapeutic procedures. The incidence of pseudoaneurysms is 0.3% after diagnostic procedures and 1.5% after therapeutic procedures,[4] although this may decrease with the use of suture closure devices after catheter-based interventions. False aneurysms can also arise from trauma during surgery, such as orthopaedic procedures. Femoral pseudoaneurysms develop after 0.08% of total hip arthroplasties, and popliteal aneurysms arise following 0.17% of total knee arthroplasties.[5]

Degenerative (often called atherosclerotic) femoral and popliteal artery aneurysms are encountered far more frequently in men than women. The male to female ratio in patients with femoral and popliteal aneurysms is about 30:1.[6,7] This predilection for men is markedly different from aortic aneurysms where male to female patient ratio is approximately 4:1.[2]

Pathogenesis

The cause of femoral and popliteal aneurysms has changed distinctly since they were first recognized centuries ago. Once primarily mycotic, syphilitic, or traumatic in origin, most true aneurysms have a degenerative cause (commonly called *atherosclerotic aneurysms*), whereas false aneurysms usually follow surgery or trauma. Tibial artery aneurysms are distinctly uncommon, but most often result from infection or trauma, either blunt or penetrating.

The cause of degenerative aneurysms of the femoral and popliteal vessels is not clear. One factor believed to contribute to aneurysm formation is turbulent flow beyond a relative stenosis resulting in poststenotic dilatation beyond the inguinal ligament at the groin or beyond the tendinous hiatus of the adductor magnus or the arcuate popliteal ligament and the heads of the gastrocnemius muscle at the popliteal level. Arterial wall fatigue resulting from vibration and turbulence proximal to a major branching or caused by stress during hip and knee flexion may also contribute to aneurysm formation.

The frequent occurrence of multiple peripheral aneurysms in the same patient suggests a systemic abnormality in the arterial wall, which promotes aneurysmal degeneration at locations where hemodynamic or mechanical factors put unusual stress on the arterial wall. The multiple factors that contribute to aneurysmal degeneration are reviewed in Chapter 103, and they are believed to contribute to degenerative femoral and popliteal aneurysms, as well as aortic aneurysm. The presence of an inflammatory infiltrate has been noted in the wall of femoral and popliteal aneurysms, similar to aortic aneurysms.[8] The exact role of this inflammatory process, with potential release of reactive oxygen species and matrix metalloproteinases, is unknown. Apoptosis of smooth muscle cells may also play a role in the formation of aneurysms by limiting the ability of the arterial wall to respond to the degenerative process.[9] These factors, however, do not explain the male predilection for femoral and popliteal aneurysm formation unless it is caused, in part, by a genetic abnormality that is carried on the X chromosome. There is no direct evidence of this abnormality in humans.

Clinical Manifestations

Femoral and popliteal aneurysms may be asymptomatic, being an incidental finding on routine physical examination. Both femoral and popliteal artery aneurysms, however, may be accompanied by symptoms of local fullness, pain caused by pressure on the adjacent nerve, limb edema, and venous distention or thrombophlebitis caused by compression of the adjacent vein. Patients may also present with lower extremity ischemia with intermittent claudication, rest pain, or gangrene secondary to complications of a femoral or popliteal aneurysm including thrombosis, distal embolization, or rupture. Because the natural history and complication rate in femoral and popliteal aneurysms differ, they are considered separately here.

FEMORAL ARTERY ANEURYSMS

Femoral artery aneurysms are the most common peripheral aneurysm if both true and false aneurysms are considered together. Their clinical importance rests in the fact that they are limb-threatening lesions and can jeopardize the viability of the leg if thrombosis, embolization, or rupture occurs. The vast majority of true aneurysms are degenerative lesions (commonly called *atherosclerotic aneurysms*), whereas false aneurysms include anastomotic, traumatic, and mycotic lesions. Rarely, femoral aneurysms develop secondary to connective tissue disorders. The femoral region is the most common site for both anastomotic aneurysms and mycotic aneurysms associated with trauma; so the presentation and surgical repair of these lesions are discussed.

Degenerative (Atherosclerotic) Aneurysms

Incidence

The exact incidence of degenerative (atherosclerotic) common femoral artery aneurysms in the general population remains undefined. They are found in 6.8% of all patients with abdominal aortic aneurysms, and 85% of patients with femoral artery aneurysms have abdominal aortic aneurysms.[2,6]

Pattern of Disease

Femoral aneurysms most frequently affect the common femoral artery. They may be classified as *type I*, those limited to the common femoral artery, or *type II*, those involving the orifice of the profunda femoris artery.[10] Type I and type II aneurysms occur with nearly equal frequency. This classification becomes important in reference to vascular reconstructive procedures, with type II aneurysms requiring more complex reconstructions to ensure continued patency of both the superficial and profunda femoris arteries. Isolated lesions of the profunda femoris artery are rare (2% of femoral artery aneurysms), and are prone to rupture because they are difficult to diagnose at the asymptomatic stage. Isolated superficial femoral artery aneurysms are also uncommon, but one third of patients present with rupture and one quarter with thrombosis.[11]

Femoral artery aneurysms can be limb-threatening lesions, and they are frequently associated with limb-threatening popliteal aneurysms and life-threatening abdominal aortic aneurysms. Multiple aneurysms are common in patients with femoral artery aneurysms. In a series of 100 patients with degenerative femoral artery aneurysms seen at a single institution, 72% of patients had bilateral femoral artery aneurysms.[6] In addition, aortoiliac aneurysms were detected in 85% of patients, thoracic aortic aneurysms in 6%, and popliteal aneurysms in 44%, of which 55% were bilateral.

Clinical Manifestations

The typical patient with a degenerative femoral artery aneurysm is a man in his sixties or seventies with the usual risk factors for atherosclerosis. Of these patients, 86% are cigarette smokers, 36% have hypertension, and 14% have diabetes mellitus.[6] Associated cardiovascular disease is common, with clinical manifestations of coronary artery disease and cerebrovascular disease present in 34% and 7%, respectively.

The clinical manifestations of femoral artery aneurysms cover the spectrum from asymptomatic to severe ischemia of the lower extremity. Although 40% of patients are asymptomatic at the time of diagnosis, the majority present with local symptoms or complaints of lower extremity ischemia.[6] Local pain or observation of a groin mass is the only complaint in 18% of patients. Lower extremity venous disease is present in 8%, being attributable to venous obstruction by the femoral artery aneurysm in 4%; but venous obstruction is rarely the sole sign of an aneurysm. Lower extremity ischemic symptoms of claudication, rest pain, or gangrene are present in 42% of patients and often lead to the diagnosis of the femoral artery aneurysm, but the ischemic symptoms are usually the result of associated arterial disease rather than the femoral aneurysm.

As with aneurysms in other locations, femoral artery aneurysms may be complicated by embolization, thrombosis, or rupture. Peripheral embolization may be identified incidentally on angiography or produce signs as mild as spotty discoloration of the toes and as severe as peripheral gangrene. Thrombosis usually produces significant ischemic symptoms but does not always acutely jeopardize limb viability. The reported rate at which complications occur spans a large range, with the higher numbers noted in series consisting primarily of patients from a surgical service. Although embolization is reported in about 10% of aneurysms, the femoral artery aneurysm is not necessarily the source of these emboli because many patients have a concomitant popliteal aneurysm.[6] In larger clinical series, 1% to 16% of patients with degenerative femoral artery aneurysms present with an acute thrombosis, whereas 1% to 16% have a chronically thrombosed lesion.[6,10] Rupture is reported in 1% to 14% of aneurysms.[6,10]

Natural History

The natural history of degenerative femoral artery aneurysms is poorly defined. Most publications have reviewed aneurysms that were treated surgically. A small asymptomatic femoral artery aneurysm does not appear to pose the same threat to the limb as does a popliteal artery aneurysm. In a series of 100 patients with atherosclerotic femoral artery aneurysms, serious limb-threatening complications were documented in only 2.9% of the 105 aneurysms followed nonoperatively.[6] This was, however, a preselected group in which many symptomatic or large aneurysms were excluded from follow-up because operative intervention was undertaken after the initial diagnosis.

Diagnosis

In most cases the diagnosis of femoral artery aneurysm is suspected by the finding of a pulsatile groin mass on routine physical examination or during evaluation for vascular disease. If the femoral artery aneurysm is small or thrombosed, detection on physical examination may be difficult. Although a radiograph of the region may occasionally demonstrate the calcified rim of the aneurysm, only ultrasonography, computed

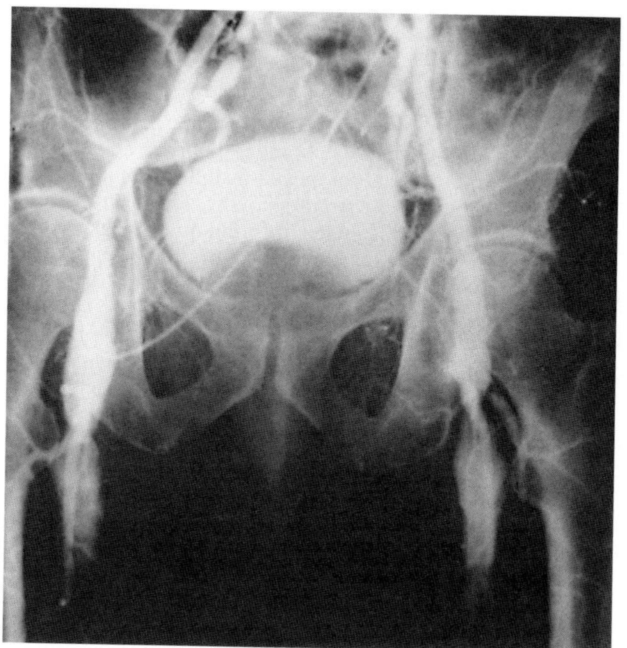

FIGURE 104.1 Arteriogram demonstrating bilateral femoral artery aneurysms that extend into the superficial femoral arteries. Unlike many patients with femoral artery aneurysms, this patient did not have an associated aortic aneurysm or popliteal aneurysms.

raphy (CT), or magnetic resonance imaging (MRI) can reliably establish the diagnosis of the femoral aneurysm. In addition, these modalities are useful in accurately defining the size of the lesion and evaluating associated aneurysmal disease in the distal aorta and popliteal regions. These findings are particularly important because life-threatening abdominal aortic aneurysms are missed on physical examination in 50% of patients with multiple aneurysms.[12] The diagnostic accuracy of arteriography is limited because it demonstrates only the residual lumen and an aneurysm filled with smooth mural thrombus may be missed, but the definition of the vascular anatomy of the lower extremity provided by angiography is helpful in planning the appropriate operative procedure (Fig. 104.1).

Treatment

Management of femoral artery aneurysms can be found in Algorithm 104.1. Operative treatment is indicated for aneurysms causing local symptoms and presenting with limb-threatening complications. Asymptomatic aneurysms greater than 2.5 cm in diameter should also be repaired unless the patient is a prohibitive risk for operative intervention. In patients with small, asymptomatic aneurysms, observation may be appropriate, particularly in the patient with multiple medical problems who would be high risk for surgery. When nonoperative management is selected, the size of the aneurysm should be documented by ultrasonography. The patient should be followed at regular intervals with ultrasound scans and careful examination for occult complications. Operative treatment should be undertaken without undue delay if the femoral aneurysm enlarges, produces symptoms, or is complicated by embolization, thrombosis, or rupture.

Surgical Strategy. The operative approach is individualized based on associated aneurysmal disease. In patients with multiple asymptomatic aneurysms, treatment is staged. The life-threatening aortic lesions are treated before limb-threatening popliteal lesions. Femoral artery aneurysms are addressed after popliteal lesions unless the femoral aneurysm is repaired in combination with treatment of the aortic or popliteal aneurysm. If an aortofemoral bypass is necessary, the femoral aneurysm should be treated at the same time, to avoid later

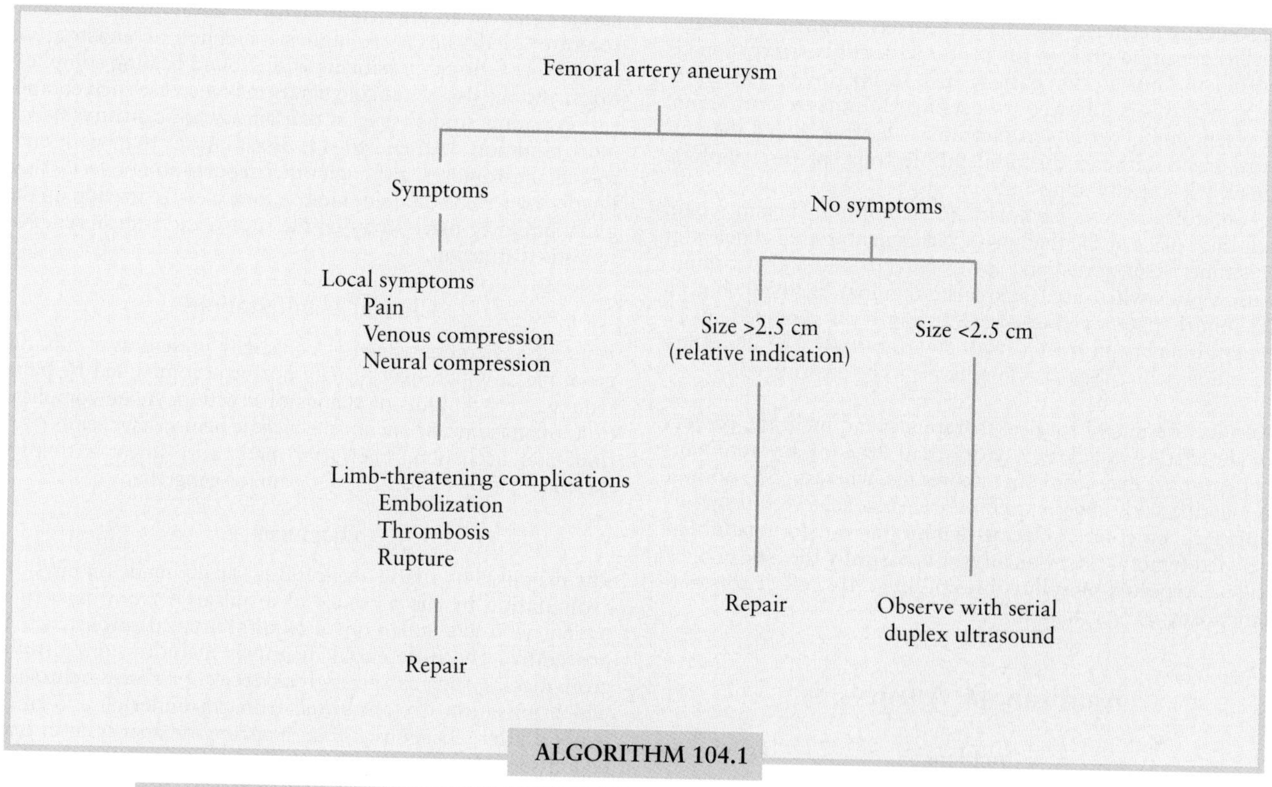

ALGORITHM 104.1 Management of femoral artery aneurysm.

anastomotic aneurysm formation. The graft limb can be anastomosed into an interposition graft that has replaced the femoral aneurysm. Similarly, if a stent graft is placed for treatment of an abdominal aortic aneurysm in a patient with femoral artery aneurysms, arterial access should be gained above the femoral aneurysm or the femoral aneurysm should be repaired subsequently with an interposition graft. The incidence of femoral artery aneurysm enlargement or pseudoaneurysm formation after using an aneurysmal femoral artery as the arterial access site, however, is not known. In patients with severe lower extremity ischemia, the femoral aneurysm is treated with an interposition graft, from which the proximal anastomosis of the required femoropopliteal or femorotibial bypass is based.

Technique. The operative procedure for treatment of an isolated femoral artery aneurysm is determined by aneurysmal involvement of the superficial and deep femoral arteries as well as by the existence of lower extremity occlusive disease. The femoral artery aneurysm is usually approached through a vertical groin incision. When addressing an unusually large aneurysm or a ruptured aneurysm, however, initial proximal control of the external iliac artery through a retroperitoneal approach is advisable. After proximal and distal arterial control is obtained, the aneurysm sac is opened and the atheromatous debris removed. Small aneurysms may be excised, but routine excision of large aneurysms in not recommended because these lesions can be adherent to the adjacent vein and nerve. For type I aneurysms, the preferred treatment is reconstruction with an interposition graft of Dacron or expanded polytetrafluoroethylene with the proximal anastomosis at the distal external iliac artery or proximal common femoral artery and the distal anastomosis at the femoral bifurcation.

For type II aneurysms with patent superficial and profunda femoris arteries, an interposition graft to the profunda femoris artery with reimplantation of the superficial femoral artery is one standard configuration. If the superficial femoral artery is chronically occluded and the patient has minimal symptoms, an interposition graft to the profunda femoris artery alone is sufficient; but if the patient has severe lower extremity ischemia, this is followed by a standard distal reconstruction. If recent emboli or *in situ* thrombosis have occluded the outflow tract, catheter thromboembolectomy or thrombolytic therapy is a useful adjuvant.

Stent grafts have been used for femoral aneurysm repair, but their place in the therapeutic armamentarium is unclear at this time. Stent grafts have lower patency and higher complication rates when used below the inguinal ligament, but an 18-month patency rate of 92% has been reported in 12 femoral aneurysm treated with stent grafts.[13] The durability of endovascular repairs also remains to be determined.

Results. Results of surgical therapy depend upon the patency of the distal vasculature. More than 80% of asymptomatic patients have excellent long-term results, whereas 68% of those presenting with lower extremity ischemia achieve satisfactory long-term outcomes.[6] Operative mortality rate for repair of an isolated femoral artery aneurysm is basically the risk of anesthesia. Reported mortality rates of up to 4% reflect concomitant aortic reconstruction.

Anastomotic Aneurysms

Incidence

Anastomotic aneurysms result from a disrupted suture line between a graft and the host artery. The incidence varies with the location of the anastomosis and the type of graft that is used. Anastomotic aneurysms at the femoral artery account for nearly 80% of these lesions, and 3% of all femoral anastomoses or 6% of femoral anastomoses after aortofemoral bypass develop this complication compared with 0.2% of aortic anastomoses.[14,15] Patient factors that are associated with increased likelihood of developing a femoral anastomotic aneurysm after aortofemoral bypass include chronic obstructive pulmonary disease, current smoking, and postoperative groin wound infection.[16] After infrainguinal bypass procedures, the incidence of anastomotic aneurysms is higher with prosthetic grafts then autogenous vein grafts with 6% of femoral anastomoses developing aneurysms when Dacron is used compared with 0.9% when a vein graft is placed.[14] Anastomotic aneurysms are a late complication of bypass procedures; the mean interval from primary procedure to recognition is more than 6 years.[17,18]

Pathogenesis

Several factors contributing to anastomotic aneurysm formation have been identified including weakness of the arterial wall, the type of graft material and suture utilized, the presence of infection, the method of construction of the anastomosis, and the stress on the suture line from hypertension, leg motion, or excess tension on the graft limb.[14,17,18] Progressive degeneration of the recipient artery accounts for most anastomotic aneurysms, and an increased incidence of anastomotic aneurysms has been noted following endarterectomy of the artery at the anastomosis. False aneurysms occur less frequently with saphenous vein grafts than synthetic vascular grafts, a reflection of more complete healing of autogenous tissue. With the use of monofilament synthetic suture, anastomotic aneurysms are rarely result from a loss of suture integrity, although occasionally a broken suture is a factor in pseudoaneurysm formation. Although most anastomotic aneurysms are not accompanied by overt graft infection, occult infections with coagulase-negative *Staphylococcus* species may be an important factor in development of anastomotic aneurysms.[18] A higher incidence of anastomotic aneurysms is noted in patients with wound healing complications, and the use of anticoagulants may increase such complications. Some studies suggest that anastomotic aneurysms are more common with end-to-side anastomoses than with end-to-end anastomoses, although other reports do not verify this. Finally, hypertension, joint motion, or excessive tension on the graft limb may place stress on the suture line and cause anastomotic disruption.

Clinical Manifestations

Femoral anastomotic aneurysms usually present as a pulsatile groin mass, which may or may not be accompanied by pain, redness, or symptoms of venous obstruction. Acute complications of anastomotic aneurysms include hemorrhage, embolization, and occlusion. The latter may cause lower extremity ischemia with claudication, rest pain, or gangrene.

Diagnosis

The diagnosis of a false aneurysm is usually made on physical examination by the presence of a pulsatile groin mass in a patient who has undergone a femoral arterial reconstructive procedure. The differential diagnosis includes nonpulsatile groin masses, such as hernia, lymphocele, or abscess, through which pulsation is transmitted from an underlying normal femoral artery. Diagnosis of an anastomotic aneurysm in one region should raise suspicion of other anastomotic aneurysms because multiple lesions are found in at least 30% of patients,[17] and their presence suggests infection. Evaluation of an anastomotic aneurysm includes ultrasonography or CT of all anastomoses of

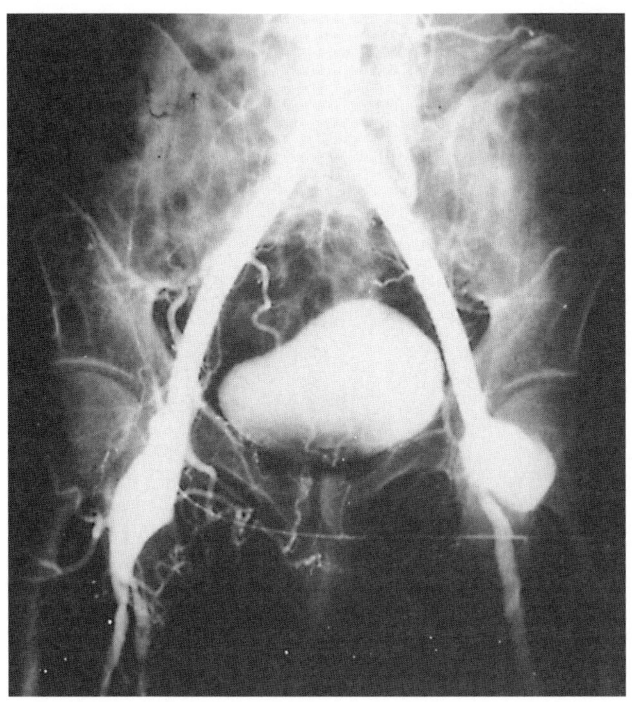

FIGURE 104.2 Arteriogram demonstrating bilateral femoral anastomotic aneurysms after an aortofemoral bypass and a left femoropopliteal bypass.

the graft. Angiography done prior to repair of the anastomotic aneurysm is helpful in defining the proximal and distal arterial anatomy (Fig. 104.2).

Treatment

Because of the progressive nature of anastomotic aneurysms, surgical treatment is undertaken for all lesions except small (<2 cm in diameter), stable, asymptomatic aneurysms in high-risk patients. Some anastomotic aneurysms, dependent upon anatomy, are amenable to endovascular treatment. Principles of surgical therapy are those of primary aneurysms: obtain proximal and distal control and replace the aneurysmal segment. Securing proximal control often requires dividing the inguinal ligament to isolate the graft limb. Distal control is most easily obtained using intraluminal balloon catheters. If intrinsic arterial disease requires extension of the graft distally on the profunda femoris or superficial femoral artery, these arteries can be identified by dissection through unscarred tissue distal to the previous exposure. After débridement of the degenerated artery, an interposition graft is placed between the prosthetic graft limb and the healthy native artery. Cultures of the graft and vessel wall are essential to exclude infection as an etiologic factor in the development of the anastomotic aneurysm. If infection is obvious at the time of surgery, the approach is the same as that of any infected graft with removal of infected prosthetic material and reestablishment of blood flow, if necessary, with a bypass through an uninfected tissue route, such as an obturator, lateral femoral, or axillofemoral bypass.

Results. Results of elective operations on uncomplicated anastomotic aneurysms are excellent with 2% operative mortality, 97.5% graft patency at 2 years, and 2% amputation within 2 years of surgery.[17] Recurrence is reported in less than 16% of cases.[14,15] Patients presenting with aneurysms complicated by hemorrhage, occlusion, or embolization have significantly increased operative morbidity and mortality.

Catheter-Induced Pseudoaneurysms

Incidence

The femoral artery is the preferred site of arterial access for both diagnostic angiography and interventional therapies including endovascular grafts. In recent years, diagnostic studies for coronary and peripheral artery occlusive disease have increased as have the subsequent endovascular interventions, which has resulted in an increased number of catheter-induced pseudoaneurysms. Because interventional techniques often require prolonged arterial cannulation, large-bore sheaths, and anticoagulation, they are accompanied by a higher rate of arterial complications than are diagnostic studies. Review of recent experience shows that pseudoaneurysms form after about 0.3% of diagnostic catheterizations and about 1.5% of catheter-based therapeutic procedures.[4] The use of percutaneous closure devices decreases the risk of developing a pseudoaneurysm at the arterial access site for an interventional procedure by a factor of 10 to an incidence of about 0.1%.[19,20] These pseudoaneurysms often require intervention.

Pathogenesis

Pseudoaneurysms from iatrogenic catheter trauma meet the classic definition for pseudoaneurysm in that they are collections of blood in continuity with the arterial system that are not enclosed by all three layers of the arterial wall. These lesions form because of failed hemostasis at the arterial wall defect created by catheter insertion. Normally, hemostasis, aided by direct focal application of pressure or hemostatic devices, seals the defect promptly, and the arterial wall repairs itself. When hemostasis is not successfully obtained, blood under arterial pressure leaks from the artery, dissects surrounding tissue planes, and forms what is perceived on physical examination to be a pulsatile mass. The gross findings at surgery are a blood-filled cavity surrounded by a capsule. The cavity is in direct continuity with the arterial lumen via a catheter-sized mural defect. Like all pseudoaneurysms, these lesions can cause symptoms by rupture or compression of surrounding structures.

Diagnosis

The diagnosis of catheter-induced pseudoaneurysm is suspected when a pulsatile groin mass is noted after arterial catheterization. The differential diagnosis includes hematoma, lymphadenopathy, and abscess. CT, MRI, or conventional and color-flow duplex scanning is used to establish the diagnosis, differentiate pseudoaneurysm from hematoma, and define the communication between the mass and the arterial lumen. Color-flow duplex scanning is relatively inexpensive and sensitive, and thus is the diagnostic test of choice. It provides accurate diagnosis, localization, and sizing of catheter-induced false aneurysms.

Natural History

Color-flow duplex scanning has been used to define the incidence and natural history of pseudoaneurysms after percutaneous transluminal coronary angioplasty.[21] Many pseudoaneurysms will thrombose spontaneously within 4 weeks, but thrombosis is less likely to occur in anticoagulated patients and in those with pseudoaneurysms more than 1.8 cm in diameter. About 30% of patients with pseudoaneurysms will require intervention.[22]

Treatment

Therapy of catheter-induced pseudoaneurysms is influenced by aneurysm size and symptoms, and whether the patient

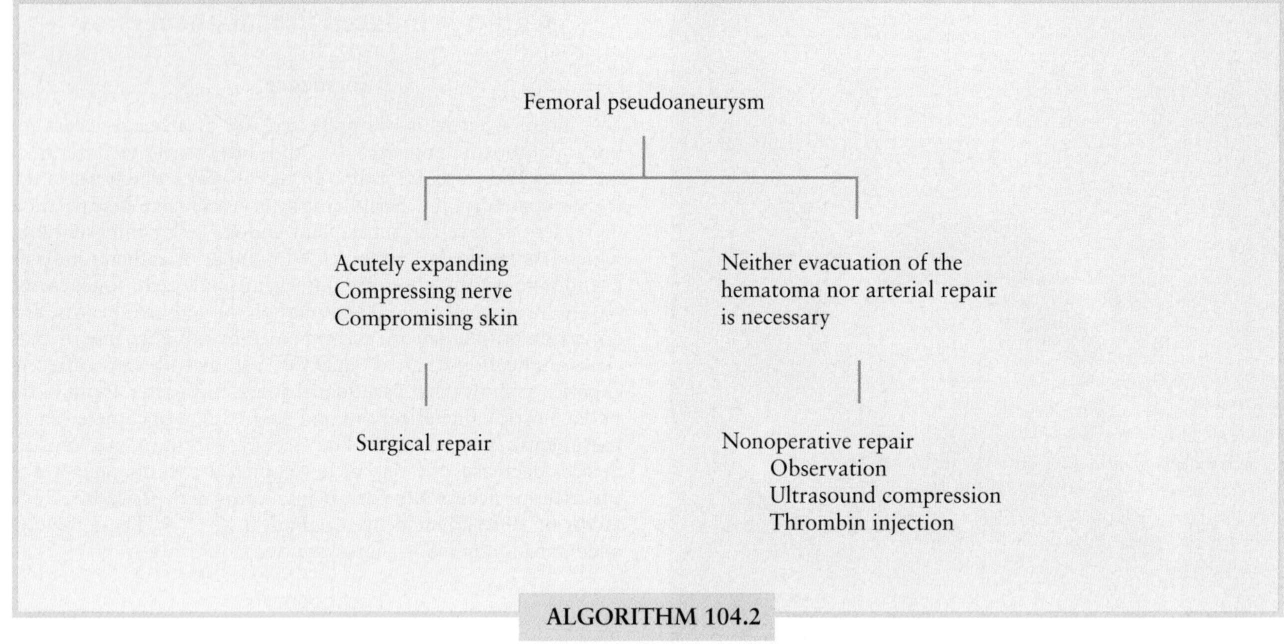

ALGORITHM 104.2 Management of femoral pseudoaneurysm.

requires continuous anticoagulation (Algorithm 104.2). Surgical therapy is mandatory for all catheter-induced pseudoaneurysms that are acutely expanding, compressing adjacent nerves, or compromising the overlying skin. Proximal and distal arterial control is obtained, and the arterial defect is repaired directly, rarely requiring placement of more than one to two sutures.

An excellent alternative to a surgical approach, when urgent evacuation of the hematoma and arterial repair is not required, is the use of ultrasound-directed compression therapy or thrombin injection into the false aneurysm. The pseudoaneurysm is identified with a color-flow scanner and then compressed with the scan head. Real-time observation of flow in the underlying artery allows compression of the pseudoaneurysm while maintaining flow in the native vessel to prevent arterial occlusion. Pseudoaneurysm thrombosis is documented by absence of flow signals on release of scan-head pressure in the case of compression therapy.

Another nonoperative treatment option of catheter-induced pseudoaneurysms is percutaneous ultrasound-guided injection of 0.5 to1.0 mL thrombin (1000 U/mL) into the pseudoaneurysm away from the neck of the aneurysm.[23–25] Thrombin injection avoids the discomfort of prolonged compression and is effective in anticoagulated patients. Continuous ultrasonographic imaging is used to monitor thrombosis of the pseudoaneurysm.

Results

The results of ultrasound-guided compression therapy for catheter-induced pseudoaneurysms is very good. Thrombosis of the pseudoaneurysm is obtained in 80% to 90% of cases. Initial success rate is similar in patients who are anticoagulated and in those who are not, but long-term success is better in patients not receiving anticoagulant therapy. In one of the largest series of pseudoaneurysms treated with ultrasound-guided compression, thrombosis was achieved in 86% of anticoagulated patients and in 98% of those not anticoagulated, with a 20% recurrence rate in less than 24 hours in anticoagulated patients.[26] Success using this therapeutic modality requires a knowledgeable ultrasonographer, meticulous post-compression follow-up, and early immobilization.

Thrombin injection to induce thrombosis of pseudoaneurysms is successful in 94% to 98% of patients with thrombosis occurring in less than 1 minute.[23–25] This technique can be complicated by arterial thrombosis, particularly if an excessive volume of thrombin is used, and may not be appropriate for pseudoaneurysms with large necks. Remote thromboembolic events are rare and probably are not a result of a systemic effect of the thrombin. Allergic reactions to bovine thrombin occasionally occur. Large pseudoaneurysm size (greater than 8 cm in diameter) and an associated arteriovenous fistula (AVF) are predictors of failure, and an AVF is a predictor of recurrence.[27] Initial success is lower for pseudoaneurysms that follow stent placement procedures, presumably because of the larger sheath placed in the artery and the larger resultant arterial defect.[28] These lesions may require surgical therapy.

Mycotic Aneurysms

The term *mycotic aneurysm* is currently used to refer to any infected aneurysm. Mycotic aneurysms today are often a complication of parental drug abuse, but can follow arterial trauma of any form, including invasive diagnostic and therapeutic procedures. In the past, septic emboli from bacterial endocarditis were a major cause of aneurysmal degeneration, but this is less common today. With the advent of antibiotics, aneurysms secondary to syphilis or tuberculosis are rare. With the change in cause, the location of mycotic aneurysms has shifted from central to peripheral arteries with the femoral artery being the most common site.[29,30] The importance of mycotic aneurysms comes from their propensity to rupture.

Pathogenesis

The pathogenesis of mycotic aneurysms can be divided into four major categories, although other less common causes also exist.[29] First, septic emboli from bacterial endocarditis may lodge in normal arteries, causing infection that weakens the arterial wall, resulting in aneurysm formation. These lesions are often multiple. Secondly, during an episode of bacteremia, microorganisms may lodge in a pre-existing atherosclerotic plaque or aneurysm and begin to multiply with the same result. A third cause of mycotic aneurysms is the contiguous spread of bacteria from a local abscess. The inflammatory process destroys the arterial wall, causing pseudoaneurysm formation. Finally, trauma to the artery with concomitant contamination may result in formation of an infected pseudoaneurysm. This mechanism of mycotic aneurysm formation is being seen more frequently, coincident with the increased use of catheter-based invasive diagnostic and therapeutic procedures. Bacteria may be introduced concomitantly with needle puncture or by migration during prolonged arterial catheterization. Mycotic aneurysms accompanying drug abuse may be secondary to direct contamination of the arterial wall, or they may result from destruction of the vessel wall by a local abscess.

The bacteriology of arterial infections depends upon the cause of the lesion. Aneurysms secondary to bacterial endocarditis grew *Pneumococcus*, *Streptococcus*, and *Enterococcus* species most frequently in the past; but recently staphylococci, *Salmonella*, *Escherichia coli*, and *Proteus* organisms also have been cultured.[30] *Staphylococcus aureus* is the most common pathogen in mycotic femoral artery aneurysms secondary to trauma and drug abuse, occurring in more than 65% of cases.[31] In this population, at least 50% of the *S. aureus* organisms are resistant to methicillin. Polymicrobial groin infections are also common in this group of patients.

Clinical Manifestations

The typical patient with a mycotic femoral aneurysm presents with a history of chills and fever, and a tender, enlarging, pulsatile groin mass. The patient may have a history of intravenous drug use, recent penetrating trauma, or bacterial endocarditis. Local signs of infection, including tenderness, erythema, and warmth are noted on physical examination. Lower extremity edema may occur secondary to venous obstruction. Petechial skin lesions, splinter hemorrhages, cutaneous abscesses, and septic arthritis may occur as a result of emboli originating from a mycotic aneurysm. A "sentinel bleed" may occur and signals impending rupture and life-threatening hemorrhage. Emergency surgery is indicated.

Diagnosis

The diagnosis of a mycotic aneurysm is usually straightforward, but distinguishing an abscess adjacent to the femoral artery from a femoral mycotic aneurysm may be difficult. In the patient with a pulsatile groin mass, laboratory findings including a leukocytosis, elevated erythrocyte sedimentation rate, and positive blood cultures are suggestive but not specific for a mycotic aneurysm. Multiple blood cultures or downstream arterial blood cultures may be necessary to yield positive results. Ultrasonography, CT, and MRI are helpful in establishing the diagnosis of an aneurysm (Fig. 104.3), but lack precision in distinguishing infected from bland aneurysms. Arteriography delineates the proximal and distal arterial anatomy to aid in planning the operative procedure. The diagnosis of a mycotic aneurysm is confirmed at operation by demonstration of organisms on Gram stain or by positive cultures of the aneurysm wall.

Treatment

Mycotic aneurysms represent a serious life- and limb-threatening disease because their natural history is one of expansion and rupture. Therefore, mycotic aneurysms should be addressed surgically. The goal of treatment is eradication of the infection by excision of the aneurysm and débridement of adjacent infected tissue as well as by long-term antibiotic therapy. Secondly, adequate distal circulation must be restored. Before operative intervention is performed, the patient is started on antibiotics that are modified based on sensitivity testing of intraoperative cultures. Stent grafts have been used in selected cases of mycotic aneurysms when other approaches were not feasible, but this is not advocated as a preferred treatment until larger series and longer follow-up is available.

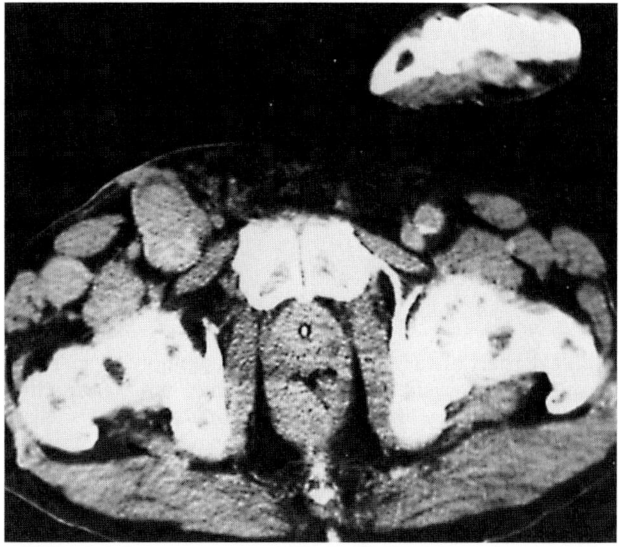

FIGURE 104.3 Computed tomography scan of an infected femoral anastomotic aneurysm that was diagnosed 5 years after aortofemoral graft placement.

The complexity of the operative procedure varies with the location and extent of the mycotic aneurysm. Although a direct approach to the femoral artery may be taken, a retroperitoneal exposure of the distal external iliac artery is sometimes preferred for large or proximal femoral lesions to avoid excessive hemorrhage. When an infected femoral artery aneurysm is confined to only one arterial segment (common, superficial, or deep femoral artery), the aneurysm is excised and the proximal and distal arteries are ligated. In these cases in which an isolated arterial segment is ligated, severe ischemia resulting in amputation is unusual. In more than 50% of cases, however, the mycotic aneurysm involves the femoral artery bifurcation, and treatment requires resection of the femoral bifurcation and débridement to healthy arterial wall. The distal external iliac or proximal common femoral artery, as well as the superficial and deep femoral arteries, are oversewn with nonabsorbable monofilament suture. This results in significant ischemia in most patients, but with the patient heparinized, symptoms gradually improve as collateral circulation increases. The majority of patients will not need revascularization for limb salvage,[32] but up to one third of patients will have limb-threatening ischemia.[31] In patients in whom sepsis can be adequately controlled at the initial procedure, aggressive débridement may be followed by immediate revascularization using autogenous saphenous vein graft as the conduit and covering the graft with a sartorius muscle flap.[31] Another option is to observe patients for 24 hours after arterial ligation and selectively revascularize only those patients in who limb-threatening ischemia persists. A saphenous vein graft is tunneled through uninfected tissue planes in a lateral femoral or obturator route. Use of prosthetic material is avoided because of the high incidence of early and late septic complications. Antibiotics are begun preoperatively and continued for 6 weeks postoperatively.

POPLITEAL ARTERY ANEURYSMS

Popliteal aneurysms are limb-threatening lesions, the vast majority of which are degenerative in etiology. Occasionally, anastomotic or traumatic popliteal aneurysms, and rarely mycotic aneurysms, are encountered in contemporary clinical practice. The remainder of this section addresses only popliteal aneurysms that are degenerative in etiology.

Incidence

Popliteal artery aneurysms are the most common degenerative peripheral aneurysm. They occur slightly more frequently than femoral artery lesions; however, popliteal aneurysms are relatively unusual compared to abdominal aortic aneurysms. Aortic aneurysms are diagnosed with about 10 times the frequency of popliteal aneurysms.[33,34]

Pattern of Disease

Like patients with femoral artery aneurysms, multiple aneurysms occur frequently in patients with popliteal aneurysms. About 60% to 70% of patients have bilateral popliteal aneurysms, and 55% have extrapopliteal aneurysms.[35,36] Abdominal aortic aneurysms are encountered in 40% to 50%, and are particularly common in patients with bilateral popliteal aneurysms, of whom about 70% have aortic aneurysms.[35–37] Femoral artery aneurysms occur in nearly 40% of patients.[36,37] The importance of this multiplicity of aneurysms is that they may be missed on physical examination. Therefore, their presence must be determined by other studies such as ultrasonography or CT so that potentially life-threatening abdominal aortic aneurysms and other limb-threatening lesions are identified and managed appropriately.

Clinical Manifestations

The typical patient with a popliteal aneurysm is a man in his sixties or seventies with the usual risk factors for atherosclerosis. These aneurysms occur almost exclusively in men. Of patients with popliteal aneurysms, 50% to 75% are smokers, 40% to 60% have hypertension, and about 15% have diabetes mellitus.[35–38] Other manifestations of cardiovascular disease are also common, with 10% of patients having manifestations of cerebrovascular disease and more than 40% having evidence of significant cardiac disease.[35]

The clinical manifestations of popliteal artery aneurysms range from an asymptomatic pulsatile mass to severe lower-extremity ischemia. About 40% of patients are asymptomatic at diagnosis.[7] More than 50% of patients present with symptoms of limb ischemia, usually claudication, but the ischemia may be more advanced and manifested as rest pain or gangrene. Local symptoms, including sensation of a mass, local pain, and leg swelling or phlebitis secondary to compression of the adjacent vein, account for the remainder of symptoms. A popliteal artery aneurysm may be complicated by thrombosis, embolization, or rupture. Thrombosis is reported in approximately 40% of patients,[36] and embolization occurs in about 25% of cases.[36] Some patients present with classic "blue toe syndrome," but more commonly, repeated episodes of embolization occlude the outflow vessels and result in thrombosis of the aneurysm. Thus, thrombosis may be the end result of embolization from a popliteal aneurysm. Rupture occurs in fewer than 5% of popliteal aneurysms;[35,36] and in these cases, the hemorrhage is usually confined to the popliteal space, thus permitting surgical intervention and arterial reconstruction.

Natural History

The natural history of popliteal aneurysms is not well defined because most series are composed primarily of aneurysms that have been treated surgically. In a review of 29 reports in the English literature published between 1980 and 1994, subgroups of patients were identified whose aneurysms had been observed.[7] A mean of 35% of patients with conservative follow-up developed ischemic complications, and 25% of these required amputation even with modern therapy. Thus, a significant percentage of popliteal aneurysms will develop a complication if left untreated, and although this is not synonymous with limb loss, the amputation rate is high.

Diagnosis

The diagnosis of popliteal aneurysm is usually first suspected on physical examination. Palpation of the popliteal space with the knee flexed reveals a pulsatile mass in approximately two thirds of patients. Small aneurysms may not be palpable on physical examination, and if thrombosis has occurred the mass may be nonpulsatile. Radiographs of the knee demonstrating a calcified arterial wall occasionally suggest the diagnosis of a popliteal artery aneurysm, but it must be confirmed by ultrasonography, CT, or MRI. These diagnostic modalities can establish diagnosis of popliteal artery aneurysms and exclude other entities that could be responsible for a nonpulsatile popliteal fossa mass (tumor or Baker's cyst). Ultrasonography, CT, or MRI is also useful in the detection of associated aneurysms, particularly abdominal aortic and femoral artery aneurysms. Angiography can be misleading in the diagnosis of aneurysms because intraluminal thrombus may obscure the true size of the vessel, but angiography is essential to define the distal vasculature before operative repair is undertaken (Fig. 104.4).

Treatment

Indications

Surgical treatment is indicated for all symptomatic and many asymptomatic aneurysms. Controversy exists regarding the optimal management of small asymptomatic popliteal aneurysms because the natural history is not well defined. The incidence of complications with popliteal artery aneurysms is high, and the occurrence of complications does not correlate with the size of the aneurysm because the most common complications are embolization and thrombosis, which are not size related. In fact, in some reports the average diameter of symptomatic aneurysms is smaller than asymptomatic lesions.[39] These considerations, and the significantly higher limb loss rate after complications development even when intervention is undertaken, has resulted in the recommendation for operative treatment when a popliteal aneurysm is diagnosed unless the patient is an inordinately high operative risk.

Conservative management is recommended by some physicians because the life expectancy of patients with popliteal aneurysms is lower than the normal age-matched population and combining thrombolytic therapy with bypass grafting has improved outcome in patients presenting with an acutely thrombosed popliteal aneurysm and a severely ischemic extremity. The use of a modeling system has suggested that improved results are seen with elective surgery compared to

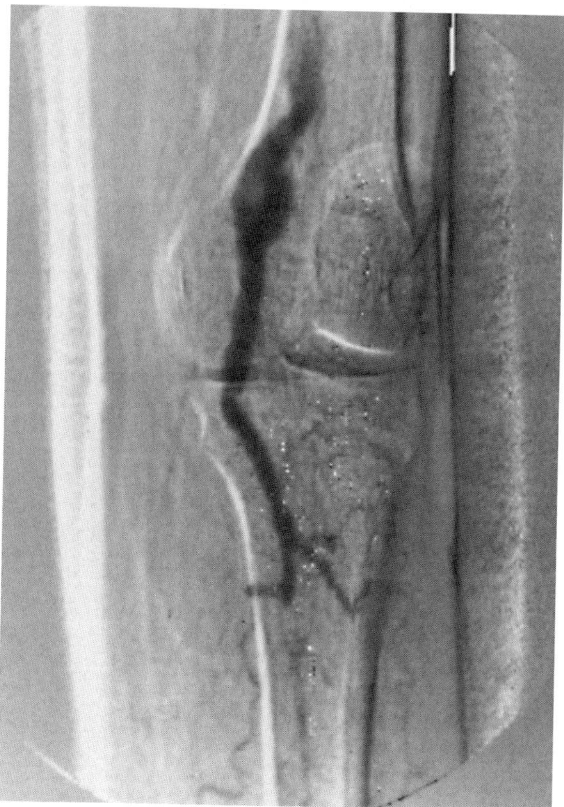

FIGURE 104.4 Arteriogram demonstrating a popliteal aneurysm associated with occlusion of the outflow tract presumably from repeated episodes of embolization. A bypass to the distal posterior tibial artery was successful.

conservative management at 1 to 2 years after presentation.[40] Thus, when the patient's life expectancy is severely compromised by another disease, conservative therapy is appropriate; but patients with a life expectancy of greater than 2 years benefit from operative treatment.

The goals of surgical treatment are to eliminate the potential for complications and to preserve or restore adequate blood flow to the limb. In patients with multiple aneurysms, the operative approach must be individualized. Generally, the life-threatening aortic aneurysm is treated first, followed by repair of the popliteal aneurysm. On the other hand, if a limb-threatening complication has occurred, treatment of the popliteal aneurysm usually takes precedence, followed by expeditious aortic aneurysm repair.

Surgical Technique

Most popliteal aneurysms are easily approached through standard medial thigh and calf incisions for exposure of the distal superficial femoral artery and the distal popliteal artery, respectively. Occasionally, the posterior approach is preferred for lesions confined to the popliteal fossa, especially when accompanied by symptoms due to compression of adjacent structures. Most aneurysms are left in situ, bypassed using a segment of saphenous vein, and ligated proximally and distally. The conduit of choice for bypass is autologous saphenous vein, which is harvested from the thigh, reversed, and tunneled along the course of popliteal artery. The proximal and distal anastomosis may be either end-to-end or end-to-side in configuration, with the aneurysm excluded from the circulation by proximal and distal ligatures. Ligation should be adjacent to the aneurysm to minimize the number of patent collaterals that are in continuity with the aneurysm.[41] Late expansion and rupture of a bypassed and ligated popliteal aneurysm can occur when patent geniculate arteries continue to perfuse and pressurize the aneurysm. When the distal popliteal and proximal tibial vessels are occluded with recent emboli, they can sometimes be cleared using a balloon catheter or intraoperative thrombolytic therapy. Frequently, bypass grafts must be carried to the distal tibial arteries. Extensive femoral and popliteal aneurysms may require a femoral-popliteal or femoral-tibial bypass using in situ saphenous vein, that originates from a prosthetic graft replacing a common femoral artery aneurysm. Popliteal aneurysms have been treated by an endovascular approach. Small series show a primary patency rate of about 50% at 14 to 18 months,[13,42] and a cumulative patency of 74%,[43] suggesting that this approach should be reserved for high risk patients who require intervention.

The patient who presents with an acutely ischemic extremity secondary to popliteal aneurysm thrombosis is a management challenge. Popliteal aneurysms often thrombose because of repeated episodes of emboli to the outflow vessels, which results in their occlusion. An expeditious arteriogram may identify a suitable outflow vessel for the bypass graft. If no target vessel is identified, intraarterial thrombolytic therapy should be initiated with the goal of lysing thrombus in the tibial arteries to identify a suitable outflow vessel for vascular reconstruction. Although the embolic process may be chronic, results with thrombolytic therapy followed by bypass of the aneurysm have been much better than surgical therapy alone for the patient with an acutely occluded aneurysm and severe leg ischemia.

Results

Excellent results are obtained in asymptomatic aneurysms with intact distal vasculature. Patients with thrombosed aneurysms or those in whom multiple episodes of embolization have occluded the tibial arteries have less optimal results. Operative mortality is in the 0% to 2% range, with asymptomatic patients fairing better than those presenting with acutely symptomatic lesions.[44,45] In patients undergoing revascularization before ischemic complications occur, 5- and 10-year graft patency rates are greater that 80% and limb salvage is 93% to 98%.[35,46] Graft patency rates in patients undergoing surgery after developing complications of their aneurysms are 60% and 48% at 5 and 10 years, respectively, and limb salvage rates are 60% to 80%.[35,46,47] Thrombolytic therapy, when successful, improves primary graft patency in patients presenting with acute limb ischemia.[48]

KEY POINTS

- **Femoral and popliteal aneurysms may be asymptomatic, being an incidental finding on routine physical examination, but they are potentially limb-threatening and are frequently associated with life-threatening abdominal aortic aneurysms.**
- **Femoral artery aneurysms are the most common peripheral aneurysm if both true and false aneurysms are considered together.**
- **Anastomotic aneurysms result from a disrupted suture line between a graft and the host artery.**
- **Catheter-induced pseudoaneurysms result from failed hemostasis.**
- **Popliteal aneurysms often develop limb-threatening complications if not treated, and results of surgical therapy are much better if treatment is undertaken prior to the development of complications.**
- **Thrombolytic therapy is a useful adjuvant in patients presenting with acute limb ischemia secondary to occlusion of a popliteal artery aneurysms and the outflow arteries.**

References

1. Ashton HA, Buxton MJ, Day NE, et al. The Multicentre Aneurysm Screening Study (MASS) into the effect of abdominal aortic aneurysm screening on mortality in men: a randomised controlled trial. *Lancet* 2002;360:1531–1539.
2. Diwan A, Sarkar R, Stanley JC, et al. Incidence of femoral and popliteal artery aneurysms in patients with abdominal aortic aneurysms. *J Vasc Surg.* 2000;31:863–869.
3. Trickett JP, Scott RA, Tilney HS. Screening and management of asymptomatic popliteal aneurysms. *J Med Screen.* 2002;9:92–93.
4. Lange P, Houe T, Helgstrand UJV. The efficacy of ultrasound-guided compression of iatrogenic femoral pseudo-aneurysms. *Eur J Vasc Endovasc Surg.* 2001;21:248–250.
5. Calligaro KD, Dougherty MJ, Ryan S, et al. Acute arterial complications associated with total hip and knee arthroplasty. *J Vasc Surg.* 2003;38: 1170–1177.
6. **Graham LM, Zelenock GB, Whitehouse WM Jr, et al. Clinical significance of arteriosclerotic femoral artery aneurysms. *Arch Surg.* 1980;115: 502–507.**
7. Dawson I, Sie RB, Van Bockel JH. Atherosclerotic popliteal aneurysm. *Br J Surg.* 1997;84:293–299.
8. Faggioli GL, Gargiulo M, Bertoni F, et al. Parietal inflammatory infiltrate in peripheral aneurysms of atherosclerotic origin. *J Cardiovasc Surg.* 1992;33: 331–336.
9. Thompson RW, Liao SX, Curci JA. Vascular smooth muscle cell apoptosis in abdominal aortic aneurysms. *Coronary Artery Dis.* 1997;8:623–631.
10. **Cutler BS, Darling RC. Surgical management of arteriosclerotic femoral aneurysms. *Surgery* 1973;74:764–773.**
11. Jarrett F, Makaroun MS, Rhee RY, et al. Superficial femoral artery aneurysms: an unusual entity? *J Vasc Surg.* 2002;36:571–574.
12. Dent TL, Lindenauer SM, Ernst CB, et al. Multiple arteriosclerotic artery aneurysms. *Arch Surg.* 1972;105:338–344.
13. Henry M, Amor M, Henry I, et al. Percutaneous endovascular treatment of peripheral aneurysms. *J Cardiovasc Surg.* 2000;41:871–883.
14. **Szilagyi DE, Smith RF, Elliott JP, et al. Anastomotic aneurysms after vascular reconstruction: problems of incidence, etiology, and treatment. *Surgery* 1975;78:800–816.**
15. **Szilagyi DE, Elliott JP Jr, Smith RF, et al. A thirty-year survey of the reconstructive surgical treatment of aortoiliac occlusive disease. *J Vasc Surg.* 1986;3:421–436.**
16. Ylönen K, Biancari F, Leo E, et al. Predictors of development of anastomotic femoral pseudoaneurysms after aortofemoral reconstruction for abdominal aortic aneurysm. *Am J Surg.* 2004;187:83–87.
17. Dennis JW, Littooy FN, Greisler HP, et al. Anastomotic pseudoaneurysms. A continuing late complication of vascular reconstructive procedures. *Arch Surg.* 1986;121:314–317.
18. Seabrook GR, Schmitt DD, Bandyk DF, et al. Anastomotic femoral pseudoaneurysm: An investigation of occult infection as an etiologic factor. *J Vasc Surg.* 1990;11:629–634.
19. Knight CG, Healy DA, Thomas RL. Femoral artery pseudoaneurysms: risk factors, prevalence, and treatment options. *Ann Vasc Surg.* 2003;17: 503–508.
20. La Perna L, Olin JW, Goines D, et al. Ultrasound-guided thrombin injection for the treatment of postcatheterization pseudoaneurysms. *Circulation* 2000;102:2391–2395.
21. Kresowik TF, Khoury MD, Miller BV, et al. A prospective study of the incidence and natural history of femoral vascular complications after percutaneous transluminal coronary angioplasty. *J Vasc Surg.* 1991;13:328–335.
22. Kent KC, McArdle CR, Kennedy B, et al. A prospective study of the clinical outcome of femoral pseudoaneurysms and arteriovenous fistulas induced by arterial puncture. *J Vasc Surg.* 1993;17:125–133.
23. Fram DB, Giri S, Jamil G, et al. Suture closure of the femoral arteriotomy following invasive cardiac procedures: a detailed analysis of efficacy, complications, and the impact of early ambulation in 1,200 consecutive, unselected cases. *Catheter Cardiovasc Interv.* 2001;53:163–173.
24. Mohler ER III, Mitchell ME, Carpenter JP, et al. Therapeutic thrombin injection of pseudoaneurysms: a multicenter experience. *Vasc Med.* 2001;6:241–244.
25. Maleux G, Hendrickx S, Vaninbroukx J, et al. Percutaneous injection of human thrombin to treat iatrogenic femoral pseudoaneurysms: short- and midterm ultrasound follow-up. *Eur Radiol.* 2003;13:209–212.
26. Cox GS, Young JR, Gray BR, et al. Ultrasound-guided compression repair of postcatheterization pseudoaneurysms: Results of treatment in one hundred cases. *J Vasc Surg.* 1994;19:683–686.
27. Kumins NH, Landau DS, Montalvo J, et al. Expanded indications for the treatment of postcatheterization femoral pseudoaneurysms with ultrasound-guided compression. *Am J Surg.* 1998;176:131–136.
28. Hertz SM, Brener BJ. Ultrasound-guided pseudoaneurysm compression: Efficacy after coronary stenting and angioplasty. *J Vasc Surg.* 1997;26: 913–916.
29. Anderson CB, Butcher HR Jr, Ballinger WF. Mycotic aneurysms. *Arch Surg.* 1974;109:712–717.
30. Brown SL, Busuttil RW, Baker JD, et al. Bacteriologic and surgical determinants of survival in patients with mycotic aneurysms. *J Vasc Surg.* 1984;1: 541–547.
31. Reddy DJ, Smith RF, Elliott JP, et al. Infected femoral artery false aneurysms in drug addicts: evolution of selective vascular reconstruction. *J Vasc Surg.* 1986;3:718–724.
32. Gan JP, Leiberman DP, Pollock JG. Outcome after ligation of infected false femoral aneurysms in intravenous drug abusers. *Eur J Vasc Endovasc Surg.* 2000;19:158–161.
33. **Szilagyi DE, Schwartz RL, Reddy DJ. Popliteal arterial aneurysms. Their natural history and management. *Arch Surg.* 1981;116:723–728.**
34. Ramesh S, Michaels JA, Galland RB. Popliteal aneurysm: morphology and management. *Br J Surg.* 1993;80:1531–1533.
35. Anton GE, Hertzer NR, Beven EG, et al. Surgical management of popliteal aneurysms: trends in presentation, treatment, and results from 1952 to 1984. *J Vasc Surg.* 1986;3:125–134.
36. Vermilion BD, Kimmins SA, Pace WG, et al. A review of one hundred forty-seven popliteal aneurysms with long-term follow-up. *Surgery* 1981;90: 1009–1014.
37. **Whitehouse WM Jr, Wakefield TW, Graham LM, et al. Limb-threatening potential of arteriosclerotic popliteal artery aneurysms. *Surgery* 1983;93: 694–699.**
38. Lowell RC, Gloviczki P, Hallett JW Jr, et al. Popliteal artery aneurysms: the risk of nonoperative management. *Ann Vasc Surg.* 1994;8:14–23.
39. Ascher E, Markevich N, Schutzer RW, et al. Small popliteal artery aneurysms: are they clinically significant? *J Vasc Surg.* 2003;37:755–760.
40. Michaels JA, Galland RB. Management of asymptomatic popliteal aneurysms: the use of a Markov decision tree to determine the criteria for a conservative approach. *Eur J Vasc Surg.* 1993;7:136–143.
41. Jones WT III, Hagino RT, Chiou AC, et al. Graft patency is not the only clinical predictor of success after exclusion and bypass of popliteal artery aneurysms. *J Vasc Surg.* 2003;37:392–398.
42. Gerasimidis T, Sfyroeras G, Papazoglou K, et al. Endovascular treatment of popliteal artery aneurysms. *Eur J Endovasc Surg.* 2003;26:506–511.
43. Tielliu IFJ, Verhoeven ELG, Prins TR, et al. Treatment of popliteal artery aneurysms with the Hemobahn stent-graft. *J Endovasc Ther.* 2003;10: 111–116.
44. Varga ZA, Locke-Edmunds JC, Baird RN, et al. A multicenter study of popliteal aneurysms. *J Vasc Surg.* 1994;20:171–177.
45. Reilly MK, Abbott WM, Darling RC. Aggressive surgical management of popliteal artery aneurysms. *Am J Surg.* 1983;145:498–502.
46. Roggo A, Brunner U, Ottinger LW, et al. The continuing challenge of aneurysms of the popliteal artery. *Surg Gynecol Obstet.* 1993;177: 565–572.
47. Dawson I, Van Bockel JH, Brand R, et al. Popliteal artery aneurysms: Long-term follow-up of aneurysmal disease and results of surgical treatment. *J Vasc Surg.* 1991;13:398–407.
48. Dorigo W, Pulli R, Turini F, et al. Acute leg ischaemia from thrombosed popliteal artery aneurysms: role of preoperative thrombolysis. *Eur J Vasc Endovasc Surg.* 2002;23:251–254.

SECTION N

VENOUS SYSTEM

CHAPTER 105 ■ VENOUS DISEASE

THOMAS W. WAKEFIELD AND MICHAEL C. DALSING

ACUTE VENOUS THROMBOEMBOLIC DISEASE

Incidence, Risk Factors, and Categories

Venous thromboembolism (VTE) including deep venous thrombosis (DVT) and pulmonary embolism (PE) is a national healthcare concern. DVT affects greater than 250,000 patients annually, whereas PE affects greater than 200,000 patients per year. The incidence has remained constant since 1980[1] and increases with age. The cost of treatment for both DVT and PE (termed VTE) is in the billions of dollars per year. Although Virchow's triad of stasis, vessel wall injury, and hypercoagulability has defined the events that predispose to DVT formation for the past 150 years, today the understanding of events that occur at the level of the vein wall including the influence of the inflammatory response on thrombogenesis is increasingly becoming recognized.

Acquired risk factors for VTE include increasing age, malignancy, immobilization, surgery and trauma, oral contraceptive use, hormone replacement therapy, pregnancy and the puerperium, neurologic disease, cardiac disease, obesity, and antiphospholipid antibodies.[2] Genetic risk factors include deficiencies of antithrombin, protein C and protein S, factor V Leiden, prothrombin 20210A, blood group non-O, dysfibrinogenemia, dysplasminogenemia, hyperhomocystinemia, reduced heparin cofactor II activity, elevated levels of clotting factors (e.g., factors XI, IX, VII, VIII, X, and II), and elevations in plasminogen activator inhibitor-1 (PAI-1).[3] When a patient presents with an idiopathic VTE, there is family history of VTE, there is recurrent thrombosis, or there is thrombosis in unusual locations, workup for a hypercoagulable state may be indicated (hypercoagulable testing, Table 105.1).[2,3] Hematologic diseases associated with VTE include heparin-induced thrombocytopenia and thrombosis syndrome (HITTS), disseminated intravascular coagulation (DIC), antiphospholipid antibody syndrome, thrombotic thrombocytopenic purpura (TTP), hemolytic uremic syndrome (HUS), and myeloproliferative disorders.

Most DVT affect the iliac, femoral, or popliteal lower limb veins. Presenting symptoms include unilateral leg pain and swelling, but some DVTs are silent, with the first manifestation a PE. A recent study of 5,451 patients with ultrasound confirmed DVT revealed the most common comorbidities to be hypertension, surgery within 3 months, immobility within 30 days, cancer, and obesity.[4]

Pathogenesis of Venous Thrombosis

After venous thrombosis, an acute to chronic inflammatory response occurs in the vein wall and thrombus leading to thrombus amplification, organization, and vein recanalization (but often at the expense of vein wall and vein valvular damage). Initially, there is an increase in neutrophils in the vein wall followed by monocytes/macrophages. Cytokines, chemokines, and

TABLE 105.1 ■ DIAGNOSIS

HYPERCOAGULABLE TESTING

Standard coagulation tests
APC resistance test
Factor V Leiden genetic analysis
Prothrombin 20210A genetic analysis
Homocysteine level
Protein C antigen/activity
Protein S antigen
Antithrombin antigen/activity
Antiphospholipid/anticardiolipin antibody
Platelet count/platelet aggregation testing
Factor VIII, XI, IX, VII, X, II levels
Functional plasminogen
Heparin antibodies (if indicated)
Mixing studies (if aPTT is elevated)

APC, activated protein C; aPTT, activated thromboplastin time.

inflammatory factors [e.g., tumor necrosis factor (TNF)] facilitate inflammation. The ultimate response of the vein wall depends on proinflammatory and antiinflammatory mediators. Selectins (P- and E-selectin) have been found to be intimately involved in this process. Selectins are the first up-regulated glycoproteins on activated platelets and endothelial cells. The P-selectin receptor is P-selectin glycoprotein ligand-1 (PSGL-1). This receptor, expressed on leukocytes, facilitates the initial rolling of inflammatory cells along stimulated vascular endothelium. Interactions between P-selectin and PSGL-1 mediate leukocyte-endothelial cell and leukocyte-platelet interactions. Even leukocyte-leukocyte interactions are facilitated by this mechanism. PSGL-1 has greatest affinity for P-selectin, and lesser affinity for E-selectin and another selectin (L-selectin). The role of P-selectin in venous thrombosis has been investigated and suggested by the study of a mouse with high circulating levels of P-selectin, the Delta CT mouse.[5] This mouse has a normal phenotype, but expresses circulating plasma P-selectin threefold to fourfold higher than wild-type mice. These mice are hypercoagulable based on clotting tests. A receptor antagonist against the P-selectin receptor (rPSGL-Ig) will reverse the hypercoagulability. Alternatively, wild-type mice administered soluble P-selectin become hypercoagulable. It has been hypothesized that microparticles (<1 micron fragments) are important for this effect. We have demonstrated in a mouse model of inferior vena cava (IVC) thrombosis that the Delta CT mouse has increased thrombosis, associated with elevated levels of microparticles.[6] It is believed that with initial thrombosis, selectin up-regulation leads to microparticle formation. These procoagulant microparticles are then recruited into the area of developing thrombosis, amplifying the process. Selectin inhibition, especially combined P-selectin and E-selectin gene deficiency, results in less microparticle formation and less thrombosis.

In a recent experimental study, the generation of procoagulant activity was shown to be dependent on P-selectin: PSGL-1 interactions related to microparticle formation.[7] These microparticles were labeled with a fluorescent tag and when injected intravenously were found to be recruited into a growing thrombus in the microcirculation of the mouse cremasteric muscle. They were not found in areas of the vessel free of thrombus. The procoagulant nature of these microparticles was demonstrated by their ability to normalize bleeding in factor VIII deficient mice.

There is also growing evidence that blood-borne tissue factor associated with leukocytes, or circulating in soluble form, is also involved with venous thrombogenesis. Leukocyte adhesion to platelets may trigger leukocyte activation causing recruitment of blood-borne tissue factor onto the surface of leukocytes associated with thrombus, or recruitment of tissue factor positive leukocytes onto the growing thrombus might provide the stimulus for coagulation propagation.[8] In a silicone shunt model of venous thrombosis, tissue factor has been found to be associated predominately with leukocytes within the thrombi. This may relate to the concept of encrypted tissue factor and the availability of tissue factor to be active in the process of thrombogenesis.

Venous thrombosis results in thromboembolization, luminal recanalization, or chronic occlusion with scarring. When rapid and complete thrombus resolution occurs, valvular function is better preserved and the sequela of chronic venous insufficiency (CVI) is lessened. If this does not occur, the thrombosed vein may recanalize, partially restoring the vessel lumen. However, the subsequent intraluminal scarring entraps the valvular mechanism resulting in valvular incompetence or leads to vein wall fibrosis, preventing the normal function of the valve mechanism. Finally, venous thrombosis more rarely results in complete fibrous luminal obliteration.

Inflammatory cells are important to the process of thrombus recanalization and organization. Although it may seem intuitive that a decrease in inflammation will decrease thrombogenesis, once clot forms, the presence of neutrophils is important for thrombus recanalization. In a study using an antibody to neutrophils, animals rendered neutropenic developed significantly larger thrombi.[9] Neutropenic cancer patients are not protected from DVT, and multiple neutropenic episodes were significantly associated with recurrent VTE in patients with malignant disease who required filter placement due to a failure of, or contraindication to, anticoagulation.[10] An inverse correlation between thrombus neutrophils and thrombus weight in mouse thrombi, especially prominent in the center of the thrombus, has been noted. The presence of monocytes and uPA has found to be important in later thrombus organization and recanalization. Injection of monocyte chemotactic protein-1 into thrombi in a rat DVT model resulted in enhanced thrombus resolution.[11] Thrombi have been found to contain increasing amounts of both tissue plasminogen activator (tPA) and urokinase-type plasminogen activator (uPA) activity as they resolve,[12] and this activity is expressed by invading monocytes.[13] In a recent study, mice gene deleted for uPA had impaired thrombus resolution with collagen deposition and cell infiltration restricted primarily to the margins of the thrombus, with few neovascular channels present. Mice gene deleted for tPA, however, were not similarly affected suggesting that uPA, not tPA, is responsible for this activity. Absence of uPA was also associated with delayed monocyte recruitment into the thrombus.[14] Taken together, the inflammatory cell data suggest that inflammation is important for thrombus organization and recanalization, with neutrophils setting the early stage for later monocyte activity.

Venous Thromboembolism Diagnosis

The diagnosis of DVT cannot be made on presenting symptoms and signs only. Up to 50% of patients with acute DVT present without symptoms. When symptoms are present, patients complain of a pain or ache in the calf or in the leg. The most common physical presentation is edema of the calf or ankle.[15] With extensive proximal DVT, massive edema, cyanosis, and dilated superficial collateral veins may be noted.

Objective tests must be used for DVT diagnosis. In the past, indirect tests such as impedance plethysmography (IPG) and fibrinogen scanning were used. Now, because of its high sensitivity, specificity, and reproducibility, duplex ultrasound imaging has become test of choice and has replaced contrast phlebography. Duplex ultrasound imaging includes both B-mode imaging and Doppler flow analysis. Venous segments are investigated for thrombus presence, venous dilation, and venous segment incompressibility with light probe pressure. Doppler flow findings suggestive of acute DVT are absence of spontaneous flow, loss of flow variation with respiration, and failure to increase flow with distal augmentation. Duplex imaging carries sensitivity and specificity rates greater than 95% for acute DVT.[16] Magnetic resonance imaging (MRI) may be helpful to diagnose pelvic vein and IVC thrombus, as may spiral CT imaging. However, even at the calf level, duplex imaging is an accurate test in symptomatic patients. Duplex ultrasound imaging is painless, requires no contrast, can be repeated, and is safely performed during pregnancy. The test is also able to detect other potential causes of symptoms. These facts support duplex imaging as the test of choice for DVT diagnosis. Importantly, a single complete and technically adequate negative compression duplex scan is accurate enough to withhold anticoagulation with minimal long-term adverse thromboembolic complications.[17] Combining clinical characteristics with a sensitive D-dimer assay may decrease the number of negative duplex scans.[18]

Other conditions may be confused with DVT. These include muscle strain, muscle contusion, and cellulitis. Iliac vein obstruction in the retroperitoneum by a tumor/mass may also result in unilateral massive leg swelling. A Baker's cyst may also produce unilateral leg pain and swelling, especially in the calf. Other causes of leg swelling, usually bilateral, include cardiac, renal, or hepatic causes.

Almost any pulmonary symptom can mimic PE. Changes on chest radiograph are infrequently present. By the time hemoptysis occurs, pulmonary infarction has occurred. In the past, tests used for PE included ventilation/perfusion scanning (V/Q) and pulmonary arteriography. The problem with V/Q scanning is that it is diagnostic in only approximately one third of cases, and pulmonary arteriography carries with it morbidity and even occasional mortality. Spiral (helical) CT scanning has thus been investigated and has shown promise. In many institutions, it has become the test of choice. A multicenter study evaluating its role in PE diagnosis is currently being conducted (PIOPED II). The results of this study should allow for an accurate determination of its utility as a diagnostic test for PE. Certain cardiac biomarkers of cardiac injury, including troponin and brain natriuretic peptide (BNP) have now been recognized to be useful for the diagnosis of acute PE.[19]

Treatment

The primary treatment of VTE is systemic anticoagulation (Algorithm 105.1). Effective anticoagulation reduces the risk of PE, the extension of VTE, and the recurrence of venous thrombosis. It is extremely important for anticoagulation to be instituted promptly, as it has been demonstrated that the recurrence rate for VTE is approximately fourfold to sixfold higher if anticoagulation is not therapeutic in the first 24 hours compared to it becoming therapeutic in the first 24 hours.[20] After adequate treatment of acute DVT, over an 8-year follow-up, recurrent DVT may still occur in up to one third of patients.[21]

Systemic intravenous unfractionated heparin (UFH) is usually used for 5 days during which time oral anticoagulation (with warfarin) is instituted. Because of the bleeding risks of UFH, which can occur in up to 10% of patients over the initial

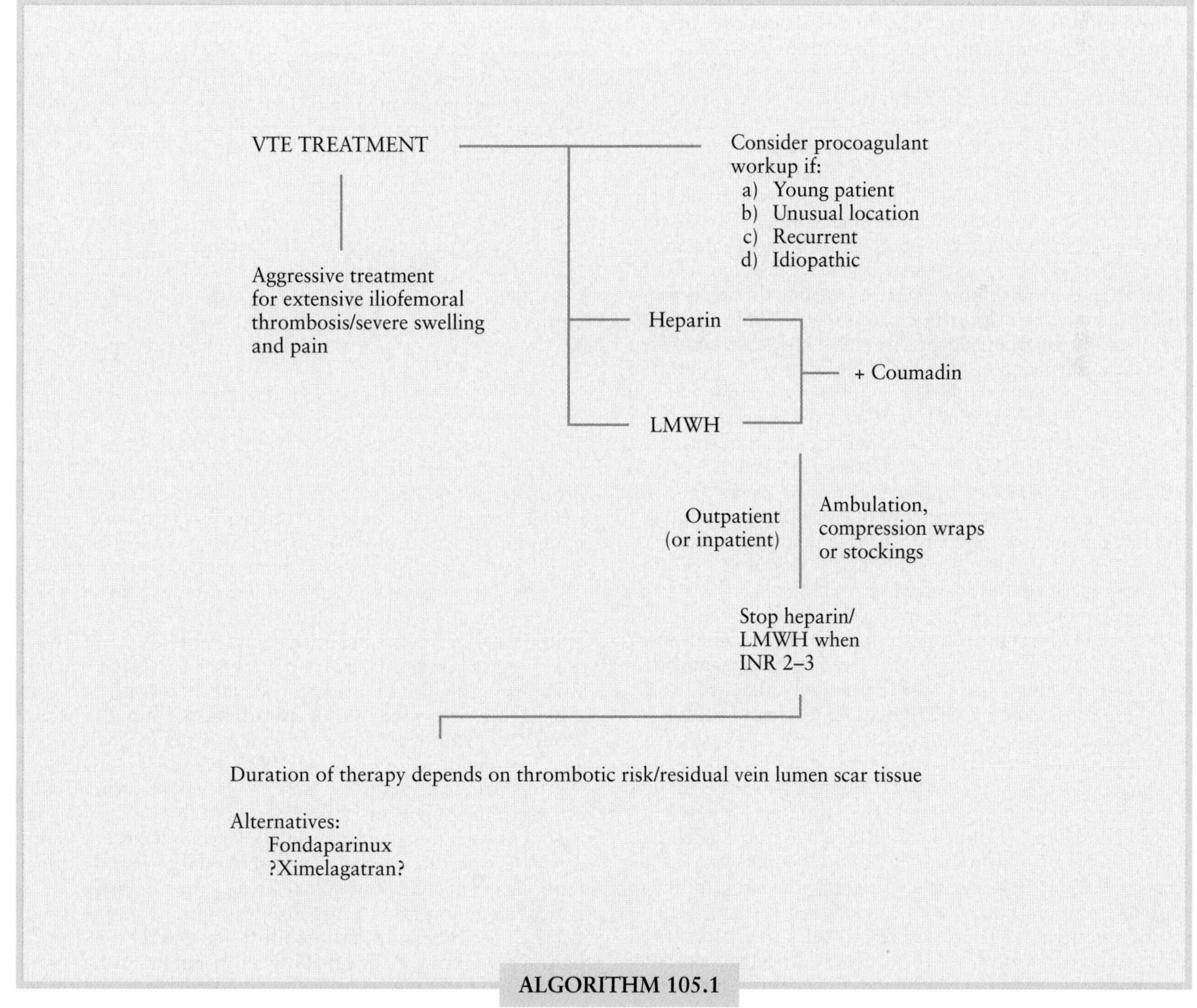

ALGORITHM 105.1 Treatment of venous thromboembolism.

5 days of treatment, along with need for close monitoring (due to variable anticoagulant response based on administered dose, related to nonspecific binding to cells and plasma proteins), low-molecular-weight heparin (LMWH) has been advanced. Multiple studies and meta-analyses have demonstrated that LMWHs are at least equivalent to standard UFH, if not slightly superior, regarding thrombus recurrence, with a lower risk for major hemorrhage and even an improvement in mortality.[22] LMWHs, derived from the lower molecular weight range of standard UFH, demonstrate greater anti–factor Xa activity and less direct anti–factor IIa (thrombin) inhibition. The advantages of LMWHs include less bleeding, less antiplatelet activity, a lower incidence of heparin-induced thrombocytopenia (HIT), less interference with protein C, a more predictable bioavailability, lower complement activation, a lower risk for osteoporosis, and importantly a more predictable dose-response (because of reduced binding to cells and plasma proteins). As LMWHs can be administered subcutaneously and are dosed weight-based, they may be given in the outpatient setting and do not require frequent monitoring except in certain circumstances, such as in renal insufficiency, morbid obesity, and perhaps pregnancy.[23]

Warfarin should be started only after anticoagulation is therapeutic with heparin/LMWH to prevent warfarin-induced skin necrosis. The goal for warfarin is an international normalized ratio (INR) between 2.0 to 3.0. The recommended duration of anticoagulation after a first episode of VTE is 3 to 6 months.[24] However, after a second episode of VTE, the usual recommendation is lifelong warfarin unless there are other mitigating factors to decrease this recommendation. Recurrent VTE is increased significantly with hypercoagulable states such as homozygous factor V Leiden and prothrombin 20210A mutation, protein C/S deficiency, antithrombin deficiency, antiphospholipid antibodies, and cancer.[3] One area of controversy involves heterozygous versus homozygous factor V Leiden and prothrombin gene variant. Heterozygous factor V Leiden and prothrombin 20210A patients do not demonstrate the same high risk of VTE recurrence. Thus, the length of oral anticoagulation may be shortened. However, combined heterozygous deficiency states are likely additive. Calf thrombi may be treated with 6 weeks to 3 months of warfarin, whereas idiopathic DVT requires at least 6 months of warfarin with longer intervals necessary. A recent multicenter trial suggested that for idiopathic DVT, low-dose warfarin (INR 1.5 to 2.0) was statistically superior to placebo over a 4-year follow-up (64% risk reduction for recurrent DVT after the completion of an initial 6 months of standard warfarin therapy).[25] However, a second study suggested that full-dose warfarin (INR 2.0 to 3.0) was superior to low-dose warfarin in these same types of patients without a difference in bleeding.[26] This suggest that idiopathic DVT requires long-term oral anticoagulation of some still to be defined duration. Recent studes suggest that residual scar tissue (thrombus burden) may also need to be taken into consideration when determining length of anticoagulation.[27]

The most common complications of heparin anticoagulation include bleeding and HIT. The bleeding risk has been suggested to be approximately 10% over the first 5 days. With warfarin dosed to a therapeutic INR of 2 to 3, the incidence of major bleeding is approximately 2% to 4% per year.[28] HIT occurs in 0.6% to 30% of patients receiving heparin. Although morbidity and mortality have been high, early diagnosis and appropriate treatment have decreased rates to 6% and 0%, respectively.[29] HIT is caused by a heparin-dependent antibody immunoglobulin G (IgG), which binds to platelets. This induces platelet aggregation, which begins 3 to 14 days after heparin administration.[30] Both bovine and porcine heparin, as well as LMWH, have been associated with HIT. However, the incidence with LMWH is much less. Both arterial and venous thromboses have been reported, and even small exposures to heparin have been known to cause the syndrome.[31] The diagnosis should be suspected in any patient who experiences a 50% drop in platelet count, when the platelet count decreases below 100,000/mm^3 during heparin therapy, or in any patient who experiences thrombosis (particularly in unusual sites) during heparin therapy.[2,32] The assay of choice is the enzyme-linked immunosorbent test, which detects the antiheparin antibody in the patient's plasma. The most important step, once the diagnosis is suspected, is cessation of heparin. Warfarin is contraindicated in this condition until adequate anticoagulation has occurred. The direct thrombin inhibitors lepirudin and argatroban are the treatment of choice, because these agents show no cross-reactivity to heparin antibodies.[33] LMWH has too high an incidence of cross-reactivity to be used in HIT without prior *in vitro* testing.

Special Issues in Deep Venous Thrombosis Treatment

The safety of LMWH compared to warfarin has led to a consideration of the long-term use of LMWH in replacement of oral vitamin K antagonists. Although there is absence of definitive evidence of superiority for LMWH, rates of vein segment recanalization have been reported to be higher in certain venous segments using LMWH versus traditional oral agents.[34] These segments were the common femoral, femoral, and popliteal veins. Additionally, the use of Fragmin has been found to be superior to warfarin in certain cancer patients when used for 6 months without differences in major bleeding.[35]

The use of once a day as compared to twice a day LMWH dosing has been assessed in a meta-analysis of greater than 1,500 patients.[36] There was no difference in the incidence of recurrent thromboembolism, thrombosis size, hemorrhagic events, and mortality. This suggests that the more convenient once-daily regimen is adequate for treatment in most but not all situations.

New Treatment

Two new therapeutic classes of agents have demonstrated the promise of greater efficacy with less bleeding risk for both VTE prophylaxis and treatment. These include direct thrombin inhibitors and specific factor Xa inhibitors. The direct thrombin inhibitor, ximelagatran/melagatran, (Exanta™, AstraZeneca), can be taken orally and may be an alternative to warfarin without the need for the same monitoring as warfarin. The oral ximelagatran is metabolized to the active melagatran. Its half-life is 4 to 5 hours in patients, and approximately 80% of its excretion is renal. There is no increase in bleeding potential with this agent. In a large prospective study comparing oral ximelagatran to placebo for 18 additional months after 6 months of standard anticoagulant treatment for DVT in 1,223 patients, the recurrent DVT/PE rate was reduced significantly from 12.6% to 2.8%.[37] Major and minor bleeding events were equivalent at 23.9% and 21.0%. Likewise, this agent has been found effective in DVT prophylaxis in orthopedic surgery patients. A concerning abnormality with the drug is an increase in liver function tests in approximately 6% of patients that appears to normalize over time.

The specific factor Xa inhibitor pentasaccharide [fondaparinux (Arixtra™; Sanofi-Synthelab)] potentiates approximately 300 times the neutralization of factor Xa by antithrombin, without inactivating thrombin. It has a half-life of 17 hours and has no nonspecific binding to plasma proteins. It is primarily exerted by the kidneys. Large prospective randomized studies for both DVT and PE treatment have also been conducted.[38,39] For DVT, with 2,205 patients (>30% outpatients), the recurrent DVT rate/major hemorrhage rate for pentasaccharide (3.9%/1.1%) was essentially equivalent compared to LMWH (4.1%/1.2%). For PE, with 2,213 patients (with >15% outpatients), recurrent PE/major hemorrhage rate for pentasaccharide (3.8%/1.3%) was equivalent to standard UF (5%/1.1%). Mortality rates were equal between pentasaccharide-treated patients and conventional-treated patients. In orthopedic surgical indications, this agent has also shown superiority to the best currently available DVT prophylaxis using LMWH. In fact, in hip fracture and knee reconstruction surgery, this agent has decreased the incidence of DVT by greater than 50% and in a meta-analysis of greater than 7,000 patients, the odds reduction for pentasaccharide as compared to enoxaparin was 55% with no difference in critical bleeding (although major bleeding was slightly greater).[40–42] It has also shown a significant decrease in DVT in prolonged prophylaxis in hip fracture patients after 7 days of in-hospital prophylaxis.[43] These two agents alone, and in addition to others, likely will revolutionize the prophylaxis and treatment of DVT. Other new alternative agents are in various stages of development, such as oral heparin, oral LMWH, defibrination agents, P-selectin inhibitors, factor VIIa inhibitors, tissue factor pathway inhibitors, PAI-1 inhibitors, and activated protein C (Table 105.2).

Thrombolytic and Surgical Procedures for Deep Venous Thrombosis/Pulmonary Embolism

Systemic thrombolytic therapy was initially investigated for use in acute DVT in the late 1970s and 1980s. A lack of benefit was primarily noted because of significantly increased risks of bleeding although two small studies suggested an improvement with systemic stretokinase.[44,45] Recombinant tPA has generally superseded urokinase and streptokinase in clinical use, although urokinase has been withdrawn from the market. Improved patient selection and the use of catheter-directed venous thrombolysis provide faster thrombus resolution, decreased bleeding risks, and decreased postthrombotic syndrome.[46,47] Early thrombolysis in massive iliofemoral DVT is indicated, especially if thrombus is less than 7 days old.[48–50] Venous patency after lysis over 2 years follow-up may be as high as 60% to 85%.[51]

The use of thrombolytic therapy for PE is also appealing. Thrombolysis has been shown to decrease right ventricular injury, right ventricular strain, and decrease pulmonary hypertension and perfusion deficits that persist after standard heparin anticoagulation for massive PE.[51,52] Catheter-directed thrombolysis may be safer than systemic administration for PE, although data for this approach are limited.[53]

Catheter-directed thrombolysis is well accepted for axillary and subclavian venous thrombosis, especially effort thrombosis in younger patients. More rapid thrombolysis decreases long-term swelling and dependence on venous collaterals for outflow.[54] Subclavian vein angioplasty/stenting for exertional axillary/subclavian venous thrombosis has been reported.[55] However, thoracic outlet decompression following thrombolysis is usually all that is needed, although angioplasty with or without stenting in this region may be necessary if there is venous damage resulting from the thoracic outlet compression. However, if stenting is used, it must not be performed until after the decompression has been accomplished. Patch venoplasty may be necessary if angioplasty is not successful. In cases of secondary axillary/subclavian or other upper extremity DVT, particularly due to indwelling catheters, anticoagulation and catheter removal is indicated. The duration of

TABLE 105.2 MANAGEMENT

ALTERNATIVE AGENTS FOR ANTICOAGULATION

Drugs	Mechanism of action
Oral heparins SNAC-UFH SNAD-LMWH	Heparin is bound noncovalently to carrier proteins enabling passage through GI mucosa
Defibrination agents	Serine protease that cleave fibrinopeptide A from fibrinogen, resulting in less stable fibrin clot
P-selectin inhibitors	Decrease amplification of thrombosis by reducing leukocyte/platelet interactions
Factor VIIa inhibitors	Compete with factor VIIa for TF binding
Tissue factor pathway inhibitors	Inhibit factor VIIa:TF complex
PAI-1 inhibitors	Inhibit the inhibitor to the fibrinolytic system, augmenting fibrinolysis
Activated protein C	Inactivate factor Va, VIIIa, as well as inhibitors of tPA
Direct thrombin inhibitors Recombinant hirudin and analogues Lepirudin (renal excretion) Argatroban (hepatic excretion) Bivalirudin (renal clearance/ proteolytic cleavage) Ximelagatran (renal excretion)	Bind to thrombin and inhibits its activity directly without need for cofactors (e.g., antithrombin III); ximelagatran (PO)/melagatran
Synthetic pentasaccharide	Inhibit factor Xa without inhibiting thrombin

GI, gastrointestinal; PAI-1, plasminogen activator inhibitor-1; PO, per os; SNAC, sodium N-(8-[2-hydroxybenzoyl]amino)coprylate-UFH, unfractionated heparin; SNAD, sodium N-(10[2-hydroxybenzoyl]amino)decanate -LMWH, low-molecular-weight heparin; TF, tissue factor; tPA, tissue plasminogen activator.

anticoagulation should be individualized, based on the patient's overall thrombotic risk.

Open catheter iliofemoral venous thrombectomy is not widely performed. This is due to the perceived morbidity of the procedure and the lack of well-confirmed benefit over anticoagulation. However, one randomized prospective study and other nonrandomized studies suggest improved long-term morbidity.[56,57] Although there are no data comparing the efficacy of catheter-directed thrombolysis versus open thrombectomy, experimentally thrombolysis leaves a less thrombogenic surface than open thrombectomy.[58] Postembolectomy rethrombosis may be decreased by employing a groin arteriovenous fistula and only performing this procedure for DVT less than 7 days old. The use of rotational thrombectomy extraction device may also be useful in this setting, either alone or additive to traditional therapies, although patient numbers are small.[59] Additional techniques include using catheters that break up, macerate, and suction out thrombus and combining mechanical and pharmacologic tehniques.[60]

Finally, strong data exist regarding ambulation and compression therapy associated with the treatment for DVT. The rate and severity of CVI after proximal DVT can be decreased in half by the use of compression stockings.[61,62] Walking with good compression does not increase the risk of PE, and it decreases significantly the incidence and severity of chronic venous disease (CVD).[63–65] The evidence today supports early ambulation and good compression in the treatment for DVT.

Superficial Thrombophlebitis

Superficial thrombophlebitis may appear spontaneously in patients with varicose veins, in pregnant or postpartum women, or in patients with rare conditions such as thromboangiitis obliterans and Behçet's disease. It may also occur related to intravenous lines and in areas of trauma. It has been estimated to exceed 125,000 cases per year.[66] The presence of superficial thrombophlebitis, especially if it occurs in a migratory pattern, suggests the presence of an abdominal cancer such as carcinoma of the pancreas (Trousseau's sign). In approximately 1% to 40% of cases, simultaneous DVT exists.[67–75] PE is rare unless extension into the deep venous system occurs, although in the literature the incidence has been reported between 0% to 17%.[68–70,72,75–78]

Patients usually present complaining of localized extremity pain and redness. They will demonstrate areas of induration, erythema, and tenderness corresponding to dilated and thrombosed superficial veins. Over time, a firm cord usually develops. Unless the deep veins become involved, patients do not demonstrate generalized swelling.[79] The presence of fever and shaking chills suggests septic/suppurative thrombophlebitis, usually from intravenous cannulation.

Superficial thrombophlebitis must be distinguished from a number of conditions including ascending lymphangitis, cellulitis, erythema nodosum, erythema induration, and panniculitis. Unlike these other disorders, superficial thrombophlebitis is well localized over a superficial vein.

Primary treatment of superficial thrombophlebitis is the administration of nonsteroidal antiinflammatory drugs, local heat, elevation, and support using either stockings or elastic wrap. Ambulation is encouraged. In most cases, symptoms will resolve or significantly improve within 7 to 10 days. Excision of the involved vein is recommended for recurrent phlebitis in the same vein segment, although the procedure is technically easier and the incisions tend to be smaller if the inflammation in the phlebitic vein is allowed to resolve its acute inflammation (usually waiting at least 6 months) before contemplating surgical excision. This obviously has to be modified if the indication for removal is septic/suppurative thrombophlebitis. If there is progressive proximal extension with involvement of the saphenofemoral junction (lower extremity) or cephalic-subclavian junction (upper extremity), ligation and resection of the vein at the junction should be performed. Alternatively, full-dose anticoagulation can be administered and the situation followed with monthly venous duplex scans. It is generally felt that medical management with anticoagulants versus surgical treatment is somewhat superior for minimizing complications and preventing subsequent DVT and PE development. On the other hand, surgical treatment with ligation at the saphenofemoral junction combined with stripping (with or without perforator interruption) appears to minimize superficial venous thrombus extension, which ultimately provides improved pain relief.[80]

Septic thrombophlebitis requires treatment with broad-spectrum intravenous antibiotics. If rapid resolution of the cellulitis occurs, no treatment beyond a short course of antibiotics and standard treatment for the superficial thrombophlebitis are required. However, if the patient becomes septic, excision of the infected vein is required. With positive blood cultures, an extended course of antibiotics specific for the identified organism is indicated additionally.

The majority of episodes of uncomplicated superficial thrombophlebitis respond to conservative management. However, the recurrence rate for superficial thrombophlebitis has been estimated between 15% to 20%.[70,71,77]

CHRONIC VENOUS DISEASE

Normal Venous Anatomy

The lower extremity venous system is composed of deep, perforating, and superficial veins (Fig. 105.1).[81] The common femoral, femoral, and deep (profunda) femoral veins, in addition to the popliteal and tibial veins, make up the deep system.

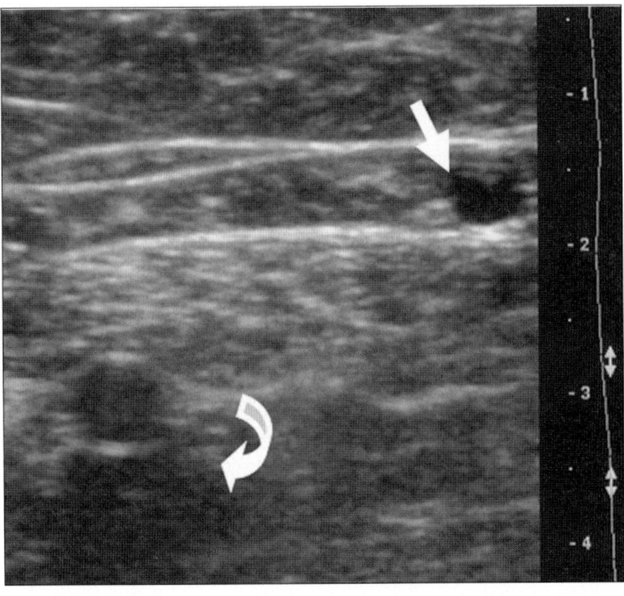

FIGURE 105.1 Duplex image demonstrating the superficial compartment, which contains the saphenous compartment with great saphenous vein (GSV) (straight arrow) lying within and the deep compartment with femoral vessels (curved arrow) lying within.

There is a concerted effort to replace the once named "superficial" femoral vein with simply "femoral vein" to alleviate the confusion the term "superficial" implies when treating conditions such as DVT. The deep veins lie beneath the investing fascia of the muscles of the leg and thigh (the deep compartment). The saphenous veins have similarly undergone a change in name to the great saphenous (GSV) and small saphenous vein (SSV) to standardize the abbreviations that are otherwise extremely confusing. It has also become clear that the GSV and SSV lie within the superficial compartment and also within a saphenous compartment. The saphenous nerve lies within the GSV compartment jeopardizing injury during surgery, but if the associated sensory loss occurs it appears to have little impact on the patient's quality of life.[82] The sural nerve lies in close proximity to the SSV within its compartment. The superficial veins outside the saphenous compartment are called accessory saphenous veins if they lie parallel to the GSV or SSV. The term *communicating vein* is now reserved for those veins that interconnect with other veins of the same system, and the term *perforating vein* is reserved for those that penetrate the muscular fascia to connect superficial to deep.[81] In the past, perforating veins with rather constant anatomic location have been named for their discoverer (e.g., Crockett's, Boyd's perforators), but more descriptive terms designating location are now preferred.[81]

The variability of the lower extremity venous system is well known, but only certain anatomic variations are of importance for current surgical practice. The popliteal and femoral veins have variable anatomy and are often duplicated much like the tibial veins. The deep femoral vein often connects directly or though tributaries to the popliteal vein. Although duplication of the GSV has been estimated to present in up to 50% of patients in some studies,[83] it is becoming evident that duplications of the true GSV lying within the saphenous compartment may be less common.[84] The saphenofemoral junction often has at least four branches in addition to the GSV but the arrangement and precise location of the branches is quite variable. The most cephalic branch is generally the superficial epigastric vein and is of some importance in new techniques for managing GSV reflux. The SSV is rarely duplicated (4%).[85] Although the SSV appears to pierce the deep fascia in the upper third of the calf, in reality the membranous layer forming the roof of the SSV compartment is thickened while the muscular fascia disappears, which positions the SSV between the gastrocnemius muscle bellies.[85] In only 62% of limbs does the SSV actually end in the popliteal fossa.[85] The anatomy of the perforating veins becomes extremely important when considering surgery aimed at preventing reflux in the lower leg. Certainly, removing the GSV may not prevent the impact of perforator reflux if one ignores the fact that the posterior tibial perforators connect the posterior accessory GSV with the posterior tibial veins rather than forming a direct connection with the GSV. Similarly, not recognizing the presence of paratibial perforators can result in an unsuccessful operation aimed at preventing calf perforator reflux.[86]

With the exception of foot veins, the valves promote blood flow from superficial to deep and from caudal to cephalad in direction. The valves are made of a fine connective tissue skeleton covered by endothelium and are generally bicuspid, delicate, and extremely strong. The tibial and peroneal veins contain about 7 to 19 valves each. The popliteal vein contains one or two valves and the femoral vein has generally three. About 70% of common femoral veins have a valve located within 1 cm of the inguinal ligament. Twenty-five percent of external iliac and 10% of the internal iliac veins have a valve.[87] The common iliac vein generally has no valves. Within like lengths of the superficial venous system when compared to the deep veins, fewer valves are found (approximately seven to nine in the GSV and SSV). Perforating veins and even larger venules have venous valves.[87]

Variable numbers of venous lakes (1 to 18 sinuses) are found in the soleus muscle. These sinuses are valveless, floppy channels linked to small-valved venous channels that prevent reflux to the superficial system. The sinuses empty into the posterior tibial vein in the proximal calf. Within the gastrocnemius muscle, there are interlacing valved venous networks that coalesce to form a pair of venous channels that empty into the popliteal vein. These intramuscular venous chambers store venous blood and are crucial to calf muscle pump function.

The veins of the abdomen and pelvis begin at the inguinal ligament as the external iliac joined medially by the internal iliac to form the common iliac vein. The internal iliac vein drains the pelvis via connections such as the obturator, gluteal, and internal pudendal veins and their interconnections. To the right of the fifth lumbar vertebrae and aorta, the common iliac veins join to form the IVC. Compression of the left iliac vein by the right common iliac artery can lead to a venous obstructive condition called the May-Thurner syndrome. The IVC typically ascends to the right of the aorta and vertebral column terminating in the right atrium. Its direct tributaries are the lumbar veins, the right gonadal vein, the renal veins, the right suprarenal vein, the right inferior phrenic vein, and the hepatic veins. Other named veins generally join one of these tributaries to empty into the IVC. Because of the embryonic evolutions that lead to the "normal" IVC and its branches, variations are common. Duplication of the IVC occurs in 0.2% to 0.3% of cases, transposition or a left-sided IVC can occur in 0.2% to 0.5% of cases, and a retroaortic left renal (1.2% to 2.4%) and circumaortic left renal vein (1.5% to 8.7%) have also been reported.[88] In the face of IVC occlusion, veins of the chest and abdominal wall, the azygos and hemiazygos systems, and vertebral plexuses may play a prominent role in venous decompression.

Normal Venous Physiology

Under conditions of low volume or external pressure, many veins lying within muscle are demonstrated by duplex scanning to collapse in an elliptical configuration with external pressure consistent with a thin vein wall and the lack of external support.[89] With muscular relaxation, veins within these compartments change from an elliptical to a circular configuration to accept venous blood being emptied from the superficial system and delivered to the lower extremity by arterial inflow. Compliance is very high, in fact, increasing the venous volume by over two and one half times results in only a 0 to 15 mm Hg increment rise in pressure.[90] This allows a significant amount of blood (500 mL plus in the standing position) to become sequestered in the lower limb without a significant buildup of intraluminal pressure. However, once a vein reaches its full circular shape, further increases in venous volume results in a proportional increase in intraluminal pressure. The capacitance of the venous system has been met and sustained venous hypertension results in decompensation noted as edema. Normally, modest exercise of the muscles will expel the blood volume and reset the capacitance of the venous system.

In contrast to intramuscular veins, duplex scanning demonstrates that large axial veins (e.g., femoral, popliteal) collapse in a circular manner. Supported/tethered on all sides by connective tissue, these veins are subject to equal external pressures along the vein wall and expand or collapse in a direct response to changes in volume.[91] Their compliance mimics that of an artery in that pressure changes are more reflective of volume changes. They are conduit rather than compliance vessels.

The calf muscle and possibly the thigh muscles act as a pump, the "peripheral heart," which can generate pressures of up to 300 mm Hg during exercise.[87] Muscle contraction propels the blood toward the heart and lungs via the cephalad conduit veins. The valves in the proximal superficial and deep veins open to allow blood to move forward. The perforating vein valves close to prevent venous blood reflux from deep to superficial veins thereby preventing high pressures generated in the deep system from affecting superficial structures (i.e., skin, soft tissues). In addition, blood moves centrally during exercise by compression of the superficial veins between the deep fascia and skin, but the pressure generated is only 100 to 150 mm Hg.[87] As the calf muscle relaxes, the flow/pressure gradient falls and proximal vein valve closure prevents reflux. Arterial blood then slowly fills the venous system; valves in the foot veins and perforating veins open to allow the deep veins to fill from the superficial system replenishing the calf muscle pump venous sinuses.

The vein valve functions in a four-phase cycle: opening, equilibrium, closing, and closed phase. During equilibrium, flow separation occurs at the valve edge, the flow splits into two streams with one of the streams directed into the valve sinus possibly aiding in a self-cleaning step (preventing stasis). When maximally open, the two cusps create about a 35% narrowing of the outflow lumen, which may aid in outflow.[92] Interestingly, the majority of the cycle has the valve in the open position. Valve closure normally occurs within 0.5[93] to 1.0[94] second in response to retrograde blood flow and the loss of a pressure/flow gradient. Closure time is somewhat dependent on the stimulus to closure and a flow velocity of at least 30 cm per second is required.[95]

An intravenous catheter placed into a foot vein can measure changes in venous pressure over time and with movement. These measurements reflect normal venous hemodynamics in the distal superficial venous system.[87] When laying flat, a person's normal lower extremity intravenous pressure is about 15 mm Hg, but with standing the pressure rises to reflect the hydrostatic pressure of a column of blood from the heart to the foot catheter most reflective of the patient's height (generally ±90 mm Hg). A hemodynamic study of venous function involves pressure measurements obtained during controlled exercise. The venous filling time (VFT) is the time required to arrive at a steady-state pressure after standing. Ten steps (one per second) causes a drop in pressure and the lowest pressure, called the ambulatory venous pressure (AVP), is generally less than 45 mm Hg. The venous refilling time (VRT) is the time required, following exercise, to reach the baseline erect pressure. It is normally greater than 20 seconds. This rather simplistic measurement reflects a complex interaction of the venous conduits, the property of the veins, and the action of the pump.[96] If one measures the venous pressure in deeper veins and in more central locations, the measurements would be considerably different, but such measurements are not commonly obtained in clinical practice.

Prevalence and Impact

CVD is a common, costly malady in Western countries. If one considers the entire spectrum of the disease, it affects more than 30 million Americans (more than half women).[97,98] Varicose veins are observed in 15% to 20% of the adult population.[99] Skin changes suggestive of venous disease are noted in 6 to 7 million U.S. citizens, and venous ulcers occur in up to 2% of those with CVI (approximately 500,000 patients).[97,100] Recent population studies confirm these earlier observations.[101] Furthermore, the annual cost to treat venous ulcers alone, as one aspect of CVD in the U.S. population, is estimated at greater than $1 billion.[102]

Pathophysiology and Etiology

Three pathophysiologic states exist: obstruction, valvular insufficiency, and calf muscle pump malfunction. These conditions reflect a failure of one or more of the components of the normal venous system and are not mutually exclusive.

Venous obstruction causes an increased resistance to blood exiting the lower extremity. It has been estimated to be the major hemodynamic problem in about 15% of lower extremity CVD,[103,104] but some question whether this may be an underestimation of its importance and prevalence.[105] The result is elevated intravenous pressure noted clinically as pain especially after exercise.[105] If the deep system is primarily involved, the increased pressure generated with each calf compression may impact the perforating veins resulting in valvular malfunction and lead to venous hypertension in the superficial system and its capillary network. Primary causes of venous obstruction are very uncommon, whereas secondary venous outflow obstruction is generally a sequela of DVT. Extrinsic causes include compression of the iliac and pelvic veins by tumor, fibrosis, or infection. Left common iliac vein compression by the right common iliac artery, as well as external iliac vein compression from the internal iliac artery on either side, have been described.[106,107] Contents of a femoral hernia can crush the femoral vein, as can soft tissue tumors of the thigh. Arterial aneurysms can impinge on the femoral vein. The popliteal vein can be obstructed by a popliteal aneurysm or Baker's cyst.[108] With the exception of venous thrombosis, intraluminal sources of outflow obstruction, are even less common. Aplasia of the vein or tumors of the vein wall have been described.[108,109] Intraluminal webs from repetitive trauma has been reported in 14% to 30% of symptomatic cases of the May-Thurner syndrome.[106]

Valvular insufficiency may occur in any part of the lower extremity venous systems. It accounts for 85% of symptomatic CVD cases with a 70% incidence of primarily superficial and 30% primarily deep venous insufficiency (DVI).[103,104] The resulting reflux allows the transmission of high venous pressures to the lower leg while standing that cannot be relieved by exercise. Primary valvular insufficiency may rarely be a consequence of congenital absence of valves.[110] More commonly, venous valve prolapse (elongated, floppy valves) or defects in the vein wall that cause the valve ring to dilate can result in malfunctioning valve cusps with retained valve architecture.[111,112] The muscle cell dilating effect of estrogens may explain the genesis of varicose veins noted in the first trimester. Prolonged exposure to high venous pressures can cause vein dilation as occurs from an arteriovenous fistula or occupations requiring prolonged periods of standing. Approximately 40% to 70% of deep vein valvular dysfunction occurs secondary to DVT, whereas the remainder appears to be of a primary etiology.[103,113] Inflammation and thrombosis associated with DVT tends to cause valve scarring, whether or not recanalization is complete, leaving a damaged valve architecture in contradistinction to primary valvular insufficiency. This classic differentiation between "primary" and "secondary" (or postthrombotic) pathology does not clearly exist when subjected to direct observation of the veins and valves at surgery. In fact, the two conditions can be present in the same patient as noted some 20 years ago.[114] In these cases, the vein wall is thickened/fibrotic at the valve station or there is thickening of the valve cusps and/or intima. Pathologic study of 11 such veins demonstrated clear postthrombotic changes in 6, but phlebosclerosis of a nonthrombotic origin in the remaining 5.[115] Clearly, preservation of a rather normal valve architecture can be explained if primary reflux and sustained high pressure on the wall is the cause of the changes noted. Another theory is that rapid resolution of acute thrombi, an event known to occur, may have allowed these valves to escape damage or the valve itself may not have been directly involved in the thrombotic process.[116] The fibrotic process involves only the vein wall and the valve cusps become floppy by virtue of a decrease in wall diameter resulting from a thickened, noncompliant vein wall.[115] The valve remains architecturally intact and can be repaired surgically, a situation once thought impossible in the postthrombosis patient.

Finally, there can be failure of calf muscle pump function. The pump becomes unable to generate the force needed to eject blood from the leg while standing, resulting in sustained venous hypertension. Patients with muscle disuse (e.g., paraplegia, traumatic injury, elderly or bedridden patients) may not have sufficient muscle for effective exercise. Pathologic conditions that result in muscle fibrosis (e.g., muscular dystrophy, multiple sclerosis) can destroy the calf muscle pump. Thrombus and scarring in the gastrocnemius and soleal veins can prevent blood from entering the pump resulting in a deficient ejection volume with contraction. With the exception of muscle rehabilitation, very little can be offered patients with some of these disorders.

Regardless of the etiology, the sequelae of venous hypertension/stasis are changes observed in the lower leg skin and subcutaneous tissues. Originally, ischemia from various causes was considered the etiology of the damage noted in the skin and soft tissue of the lower leg especially ulceration.[117] More recent observations suggest that far from being simply an ischemic event, the end-organ response to venous hypertension is highly dynamic. The final answer is likely to involve a complex interaction of multiple factors that favor either continued destruction or the ultimate healing of the ulcer. Leukocytes, the extracellular matrix, fibroblasts, and a host of other factors are recruited to heal the early endothelial injury and the more delayed soft tissue injury.[117] The soft tissue injury may result in a chronic ulcer that requires growth factors to force the process to healing.[118] Research in this area is active.

Clinical Signs and Symptoms

Venous disease presents in many ways. Spider veins, also known as *telangiectases*, appear as fine, blue-red branchings just underneath the skin surface that may or may not be accompanied by a larger, more deeply located, pathologic vein.

Hereditary varicose veins usually appear during the second decade of life. If a secondary etiology is involved (e.g., thrombosis, trauma), varicosities often present several years after the inciting event. These veins appear alone or in clusters as dilated, often bluish, serpentine, and palpable protrusions of branches of the GSV, SSV, or collateral veins lying beneath the skin within the subcutaneous tissues. Symptoms may be those associated with any type of CVD.

CVD can result in pain, edema, hyperpigmentation, stasis dermatitis or eczema, and/or venous ulcers. These changes often occur in the "gaiter" area just above the medial malleolus. Important perforating veins lay in this area. The observed hyperpigmentation is thought to result from extruded red blood cells that are degraded by macrophages leaving hemosiderin deposits.

Venous claudication is a pain syndrome experienced when walking and is associated with cyanosis, a sensation of increased swelling, and increased prominence of the superficial veins, which is relieved with rest in combination with elevation of the extremity.[105,119,120] It may be so severe in rare cases that amputation is requested.[107] The most severe form is observed when venous incompetence is associated with obstruction and when the obstructive process is in a more proximal locale.[121]

Critical to patient management and treatment evaluation is an accurate classification of the disease at any given time. Each patient should be stratified according to the *c*linical picture, the *e*tiology, the *a*natomic distribution, and the *p*athophysiology (CEAP) classification system.[122] This classification system helps the physician to define the venous disease being confronted so that a focused and appropriate management strategy can be made. An extension of the clinical portion of this classification system is available to quantify the extent of venous disease and therefore to evaluate the patient's treatment response.[123,124] If surgery is performed, the patient's clinical outcome score can be evaluated according to a grading scheme.[123] An improved method of determining a change in disease severity following intervention has been developed and awaits full clinical utilization.[124] Quality of life surveys are tools being developed specifically for patients with venous disease to help determine the impact of the disease on the patient's life and the effect therapy has on the patient's overall well-being.[125] Application of these surveys to the postsurgical outcome of patients has yet to be achieved, but when available will improve our ability to precisely determine the effect and true use of a given intervention.

Diagnostic Evaluation

The diagnosis of CVD begins with a thorough history and physical examination. The history is quite important to provide hints to familial coagulation disorders or events in the patient's history that may impact the care of the chronic disorder. Utilization of the CEAP clinical classification (Table 105.3) will provide a snapshot of the patient being examined, whereas use of the more detailed venous clinical severity score (Table 105.4) will allow some impression of how any therapy is performing on patient's behalf.

Venous duplex ultrasonography provides a B-mode image of the vein as well as spectral analysis of the blood flow within it. It is essential to clarify the etiology (E of CEAP; congenital, primary, or secondary), better define the anatomic location (A of CEAP; specific veins can be imaged with spectral analysis to determine reflux), and aid in determining the pathophysiology (P of CEAP; reflux, obstruction, or both) of the venous problem. Once considered unnecessary in the evaluation of patients with simple varicose veins, it has become common practice prior to intervention due to superficial and perforator venous system variability and the need for precise targeting of veins during endoluminal intervention.[83,126–128]

TABLE 105.3 CLASSIFICATION

CLINICAL CLASSIFICATION CHRONIC VENOUS DISEASE

Class	Description
0	No signs
1	Telangiectases/reticular veins
2	Varicose veins
3	Edema
4	Skin changes (hyperpigmentation, eczema, lipodermatosclerosis)
5	Class 4 and healed ulcers
6	Class 4 and active ulcers

TABLE 105.4 DIAGNOSIS

VENOUS CLINICAL SEVERTY SCORE

Attribute	Absent 0	Mild 1	Moderate 2	Severe 3
Pain	None	Occasional, not restricting activity or requiring analgesics	Daily, moderate activity limitation, occasional analgesics	Daily, severe limiting activities or requiring regular use of analgesics
Varicose veins*	None	Few, scattered: branch VVs	Multiple: GS varicose veins confined to calf or thigh	Extensive: thigh *and* calf or GS *and* LS distribution
Venous edema†	None	Evening ankle edema only	Afternoon edema, above ankle	Morning edema above ankle and requiring activity change, elevation
Skin pigmentation‡	None or focal, low intensity (tan)	Diffuse, but limited in area and old (brown)	Diffuse over most of gaiter distribution (lower 1/3) *or* recent pigmentation (purple)	Wider distribution (above lower 1/3) *and* recent pigmentation
Inflammation	None	Mild cellulitis, limited to marginal area around ulcer	Moderate cellulitis, involves most of gaiter area (lower 1/3)	Severe cellulitis (lower 1/3 and above) or significant venous eczema
Induration	None	Focal, circummalleolar (<5 cm)	Medial or lateral, less than lower third of leg	Entire lower third of leg or more
No. of active ulcers	0	1	2	>2
Active ulceration, duration	None	<3 mo	>3 mo, <1 y	Not healed >1 y
Active ulcer, size§	None	<2-cm diameter	2- to 6-cm diameter	>6-cm diameter
Compressive therapy‖	Not used or not compliant	Intermittent use of stockings	Wears elastic stockings most days	Full compliance: stockings + elevation

*"Varicose" veins must be >4-mm diameter to qualify so that differentiation is ensured between C1 and C2 venous pathology.
†Presumes venous origin by characteristics [e.g., brawny (not pitting or spongy) edema], with significant effect of standing/limb elevation and/or other clinical evidence of venous etiology (i.e., varicose veins, history of DVT). Edema must be regular finding (e.g., daily occurrence). Occasional or mild edema does not qualify.
‡Focal pigmentation over varicose veins does not qualify.
§Largest dimension/diameter of largest ulcer.
‖Sliding scale to adjust for background differences in use of compressive therapy.
GS, Greater saphenous; LS, lesser saphenous; VV, varicose vein.

From Rutherford RB, Padberg FT Jr, Comerota AJ, et al. Venous severity scoring: an adjunct to venous outcome assessment. *J Vasc Surg.* 2000;31:1307.

Venous duplex imaging clearly visualizes deep veins and valves as well.

Valvular insufficiency is defined as prolonged reflux time through a valve following a provocative test. A reflux time of more than 0.5 second is considered abnormal if a rapidly deflating distal cuff during the provocative test, whereas greater than 1.0 second is considered the cut-off following manual compression.[93,94] A recent study suggests that these values may be appropriate for the deep calf veins but that 1.0 second should be the cut-off for larger femoropopliteal veins even when using the rapidly deflating distal cuff method.[129] The latter has yet to be confirmed by other investigators. The examination is performed in the upright position in these reports. Many other provocative maneuvers to generate venous reflux exist (Valsalva, standardized Valsalva, etc.) in addition to performing the test in different positions (e.g., 15% Trendelenburg, sitting).[130] Each may be acceptable if standardized for an individual laboratory and supported by the literature. Venous obstruction is seen as thickened, scarred, and constricted veins with poor flow and diminished augmentation following distal and/or proximal compression. Respiratory variation is lost as a result of local disease or proximal occlusion. Similar imaging and spectral analysis can be performed to determine obstruction or insufficiency in the superficial and perforator veins. Reflux in the superficial system is considered abnormal with parameters similar to the deep calf veins and is determined by provocative compression.[130] Disease within the SSV should not be ignored because it can have a significant clinical impact as an isolated event.[131] Incompetent perforating veins are generally larger in diameter, thereby allowing a larger volume of blood flow during reflux, and are considered to demonstrate reflux with a reflux time greater than 0.5 second.[128] There is some thought that this cut-off should be decreased to 0.35 second, but currently the 0.5-second cutoff stands in most laboratories.[129] By imaging the entire lower leg venous system, the surgeon is provided a detailed roadmap of all veins with confirmation of obstruction or reflux if present within segments commonly separated by valves. Of course, isolated venous valvular insufficiency or obstruction may have little clinical impact on the patient, and therefore clinicians have attempted to quantify the pathology by adding up segmental disease, determining mean duration of reflux, determining peak reverse flow velocity, and so forth. [94,132] Although average scores correlate with disease severity, individual results have little predictive value and therefore these methods have not been widely adapted. The issue of common standards for the performance and interpretation of venous duplex studies still plagues efforts to define venous disease[130] but many find it the most versatile and reproducible imaging device currently available.[130,133] This is often the only diagnostic evaluation needed for superficial and even perforator disease requiring treatment as a first stage in patient management.

A difficult area of investigation from a noninvasive perspective is the pelvic, abdominal, and chest veins. CT and MRI can provide details of anatomy and the effect of surrounding structures in areas not visualized by duplex evaluation.[134–136] However, as with all vascular laboratory studies, clinical correlation is mandatory because anatomic presence does not necessarily translate into a clinical problem. For example, iliac vein compression is commonly seen in an asymptomatic population.[137] These studies are particularly useful in evaluating for pelvic congestion syndrome.[138]

Plethysmography assesses the overall hemodynamics of the lower extremity venous system. Air plethysmography (APG) can measure several venous hemodynamic parameters and is the most common study currently performed. A plastic cylinder filled with air is fitted over the calf and foot. Changes in leg volume with positional change or exercise are detected by pressure changes in the cylinder. The venous filling index is 90% of resting standing venous volume (VV) divided by the time it takes to reach 90% of VV as the patient shifts from the supine to standing position (mL/second). A venous filling index of 2 mL per second or less is indicative of competent venous system and higher values suggest venous insufficiency.[139,140] The use of tourniquets to separate superficial from deep or perforator disease has not been reliable,[141] but it can be useful in specific cases. After an erect baseline reading, patients exercise by dorsiflexion or heel raises to empty the calf veins. The ejection fraction is the amount of blood propelled cephalad with a single muscle contraction divided by VV. After a series of 10 ankle flexions, the volume remaining in the leg is referred to as the residual volume and when divided by the VV is called the residual volume fraction. An ejection fraction of greater than 60% and residual volume fraction of less than 35% suggests that the calf pump is working well.[142,143] The residual volume fraction is relatively equivalent to the AVP.[102,141] Significant outflow obstruction is determined by occluding venous outflow until a stable plateau is reached. The thigh cuff causing the venous occlusion is rapidly deflated, and the difference between maximal volume and that volume present 1 second later divided by the total calf volume is called the outflow fraction (OF). Normally, 38% or more of venous blood is expelled from the leg in one second.[140] Several other plethysmographic methods (e.g., impedance, photo) and even light reflex rheography have evaluated similar venous parameters. The ability of these techniques to completely eliminate the presence of significant venous occlusion in patients with CVD has come into question.[144] Although, these plethysmographic methods can differentiate patients with severe CVI (class 3 or greater) from those without disease,[130] stratification by symptom severity is not possible and therefore its use in the treatment of patients with minor symptoms, such as varicose veins or telangiectases, is questionable.[130] Because these studies do not provide an anatomic image of the venous system or evaluation of individual venous valve function, many physicians combine one of these studies as an estimate of global hemodynamics, in patients with advanced disease (clinical grade 3 or higher), with ultrasonography to complete the venous evaluation.

As in acute venous disease, venography has no significant role in the initial evaluation of patients with CVD. Ascending venography can suggest venous occlusion when duplex imaging clearly demonstrates an open system.[133] Even the presence of significant collaterals on transfemoral venography may underestimate the degree of venous occlusion documented by intravascular ultrasound.[105,145] The use of ascending venography is selectively used in specific cases to complement noninvasive studies when considering intervention in the deep venous system or in research protocols.

The technique of descending venography has been well described.[146] Descending venography is used to determine valve leaflet integrity, anatomic location, and demonstrate the extent of reflux.[146] Assessment of the competence of the profunda femoris venous system in addition to the femoral system is imperative. If it is a competent system, it may be a source for a valve transposition or may predict success with an isolated proximal femoral vein repair.[147–149] Certainly, descending venography is not infallible in determining the presence or absence of a normal valve.[115] Raju et al. report that descending venography misrepresented the presence of a valve in 11% of cases (a valve considered present was not at operation) and missed an intact valve in 25% of cases (a valve thought absent was actually present).[115] However, when combined with a careful venous duplex examination, it is currently the best method available to determine preoperatively if an *in situ* reconstruction will be possible.

Intravenous pressure measurements can aid in the diagnosis of venous disease but is invasive and generally used only when invasive surgery of the deep system is being considered. This study can help to determine of the overall magnitude of reflux.[102] AVP has been shown to correlate with the presence of venous ulceration, with each 10 torr increase above 30 torr corresponding to a 10% to 15% increase in the incidence of venous ulceration.[150] Direct lower limb intravenous pressure measurements obtained prior to and after thigh cuff compression and compared to arm intravenous pressure have been suggested as a method to determine the presence or absence of venous obstruction and to determine if obstruction is compensated or not.[115,151] The inventors of this intravenous measurement now question the reliability of this or any other hemodynamic studies to accurately rule out significant iliac obstruction and recommend intravenous ultrasonography to clarify the issue.[144] Although intravenous pressure measurements and venography were once the gold standard for evaluating venous disease, duplex scanning and plethysmographic techniques are the anatomic and functional tests of choice in current medical practice.[139]

Treatment Options and Results

Conservative Medical Therapy

The mainstay of CVD therapy has remained unchanged for decades (Algorithm 105.2). The goals are to manage clinical symptoms and to control venous hypertension. These therapeutic maneuvers can be inconvenient, uncomfortable, and difficult to perform for the elderly patient with dexterity problems, but compliance is mandatory for effective results. Wearing high-quality compressive stockings (graded 30 to 40 mm Hg at the ankle), elevating the legs when possible during the day, avoiding prolonged periods of standing or sitting, elevating the foot of the bed 4 to 6 inches while sleeping, and applying bandages to ulcerations when needed are all components of conservative therapy.[152,153] Compressive garments range from elastic bandage wraps and compressive stockings to firm relatively inelastic wraps that provide graduated compression from the distal ankle to the proximal portion of the leg. Historically, compression stockings use has been associated with poor patient compliance. However, the design of compression stocking has advanced significantly over recent years and are now available in various colors, styles, lengths, and degrees of compression. More recently, a structured exercise program has been shown to improve calf muscle pump function in patients with CVD and

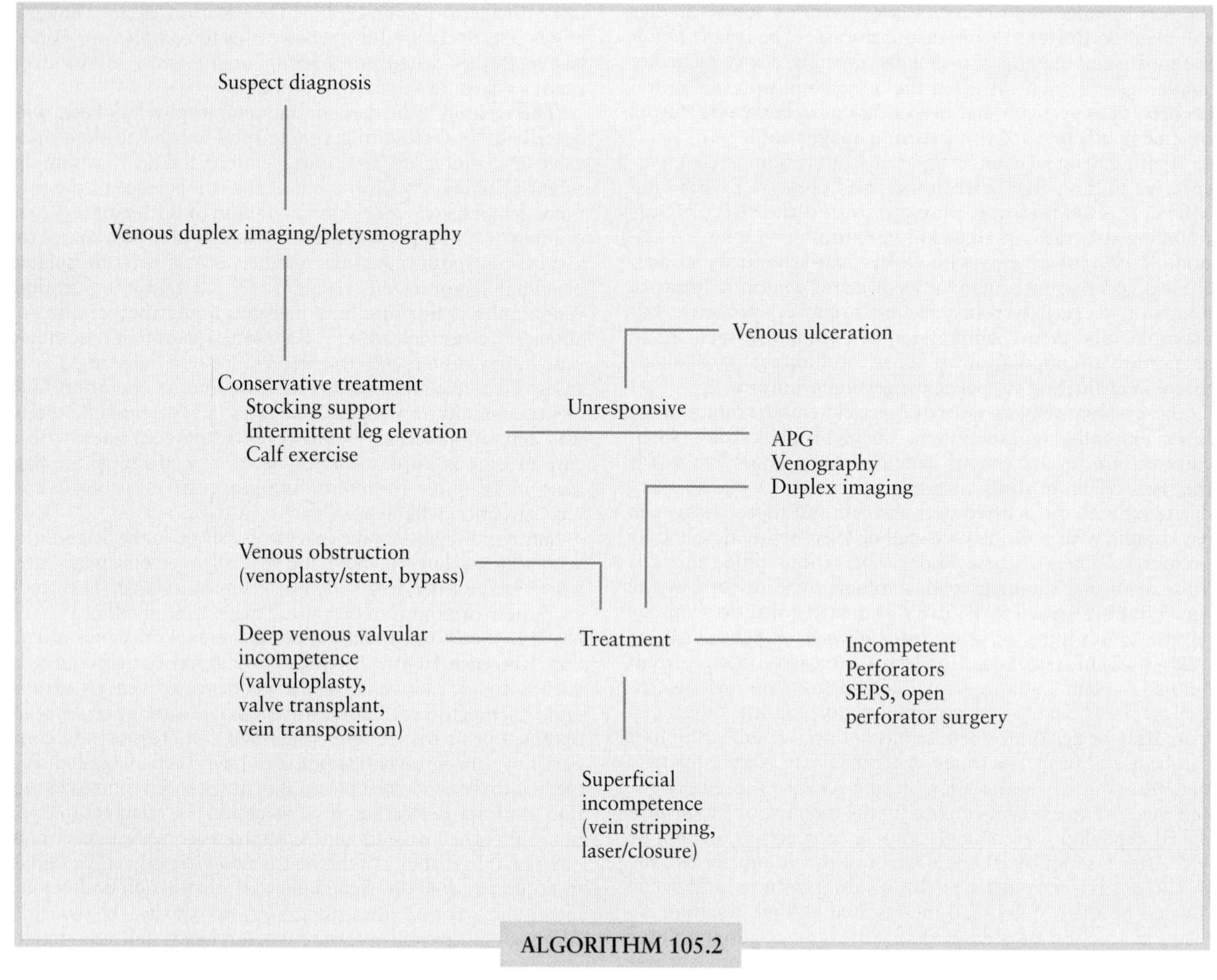

ALGORITHM 105.2 Treatment of chronic venous insufficiency.

should be considered in the overall conservative treatment of these patients.[154]

In Europe, various drugs (e.g., diosmin, rutosides) have been touted to improve the feeling of heaviness, fatigue, and even edema of CVD In one small randomized trial comparing rutosides to compression therapy, the latter was more effective in reducing leg edema and increasing venous refill times over the 4-month trial.[155]

Venous ulcer therapy has two goals: heal the ulcer and prevent recurrence. Elevation and compression to control edema are paramount. Pentoxifylline may provide a small incremental benefit, but appears to work best as an adjunct to compressive therapy.[156] Daflon has been shown in a European study to be of benefit in healing ulcers less than 10 cm in diameter.[157] However, it has not been approved by the U.S. Food and Drug Administration (FDA). The Unna paste boot is a dressing composed of gauze moistened with zinc oxide and calamine lotion containing glycerin and is a mainstay in the treatment of venous ulcers.[153] Newer wound care products provide a substitute to the Unna boot and aim to provide a warm, moist, and clean environment for ulcer healing. Multilayer dressings provide compression and absorbency to protect the ulcer bed from the wound fluid which can impede wound healing.[153] Most of these dressings have one absorbent layer and one to three elastic layers for compression. This group of dressings allow for weekly changes in most cases. Ulcers that have more copious amounts of drainage require more frequent dressing changes or the use of a hydrocolloid dressing. Such hydrocolloid and hydrogel dressings are able to absorb many times their weight in wound fluid. Therefore, these dressings can stay in place longer, while maintaining a drier environment for the ulcer and surrounding tissues. For resistant venous ulcers, skin grafting is an option. These ulcers can be extensive, and skin grafting allows for coverage of raw surfaces to speed the healing process. Once the ulcer has a clean base of granulation tissue, a split-thickness skin graft can be applied. There are reports on improved healing with skin grafting for chronic venous ulceration.[158] Skin grafting is generally considered only when ulcer healing has not occurred with diligent conservative management. A new allogenic cultured bilayer skin equivalent is being used for the treatment of venous stasis ulcers. Its advantages over autogenous skin include outpatient application and lack of donor site risks. One trial has demonstrated decreased time to ulcer closure and increased overall number of ulcers healed with its use.[159] It can also be used as a precursor to skin grafting.

Sclerotherapy

The failure of conservative measures triggers a surgical response. Sclerotherapy (needle injection of caustic solutions directly into superficial veins) has long been advocated for treating varicosities remaining after saphenous stripping, small isolated varicosities, and telangiectasias. Sclerotherapy alone appears an effective treatment for branch varicosities in patients without major saphenous reflux and appears effective when combined with GSV stripping to control branch varicosities.[160,161] Hamel-Desnos et al.[162] found GSV ultrasonography directed foam sclerotherapy to be 84% effective in eliminating reflux for 1 year. This is less than reported for other methods of GSV ablation and lacks long term follow-up but does demonstrate the technique's potential. The most common sclerosing agents are sodium tetradecyl sulfate and hypertonic saline with some use of polidocanol or a combination of 25% dextrose with 10% saline. All act to damage the vein endothelium inducing inflammation and scarring and resulting in lumen collapse.[163] The use of foam sclerotherapy, adding air to the sclerosing agent, appears to be the current technique of choice especially for larger veins.[160,162] These are generally outpatient procedures. Common complaints include burning, stinging, itching, and muscle spasm with injection. Extravasation of the agent can cause fat or skin necrosis, ulcerations, and/or hyperpigmentation of the surrounding skin. Posttreatment veins are often a brown color as opposed to the blue-red pretreatment color. Microthrombectomy appears to reduce postsclerotherapy pigmentation especially in veins 1 mm or less in diameter.[164] Other potential complications of sclerotherapy include allergic reactions and toxicity if too many veins are treated at one sitting.[163] Therefore, a limited amount of sclerosing agent is typically injected during a single setting. Major venous insufficiency, if present, must be eliminated to prevent recurrence following branch varicosity sclerotherapy even with the use of high dose and foam sclerotherapy.[160,163,165]

Vein Stripping/Ablation

Duplex imaging of patients prior to invasive saphenous treatment has proven that not all saphenous veins are incompetent when varicosities exist. In such cases, saphenous preservation still leads to good results.[166] However, in the face of saphenous insufficiency, stripping can be employed. Deep venous obstruction was once thought an absolute contraindication to removal of the saphenous system but may actually be indicated in patients with mixed obstruction/reflux disease and in cases of combined deep and superficial insufficiency.[167,168] Vein stripping includes ligation and disconnection of the GSV at the saphenofemoral junction followed by complete removal of the vein to the knee. If the below knee greater saphenous vein is incompetent based on preoperative diagnostic studies, it is also excised. Preoperatively, with the patient standing to fully dilate the veins, the varicosities are marked with a permanent marker for later operative visualization. The method of vein removal may involve the introduction of long metal or plastic stripping wires with removable heads of varying size (i.e., Codman), the PIN stripper, or various others devices aimed at pulling the vein from the leg.[169,170] Both GSV and SSV can be treated by these methods taking into account required patient positioning and anatomic variability, especially of the SSV.[169] Another method of removing the GSV from the venous circulation is to thermally heat the inside with radiofrequency-generated heat (closure technique).[171,172] Placed percutaneously or by venous cut down, the probe is sequentially heated to 85°C throughout the length of the GSV. Often, a thermal sink and anesthetic is administered within the saphenous compartment via tumescent anesthesia. Alternatively, laser energy of various wavelengths delivered via a bare-tipped fiber will cause a focal thermal injury to the vein wall.[173–175] Some have found utility of this newer method for the SSV.[174] When delivering endoluminal therapy aimed at obliterating the vein lumen, energy is delivered beginning about 1 cm below the superficial epigastric vein to preserve lower abdominal wall venous drainage and to prevent thrombosis of the deep system.

In addition to eliminating axial reflux, branch varicosities are removed. This can be accomplished by making small incisions over the preoperatively marked branch varicosities, grasping the vein with a small hemostat or other small device and removing it bluntly. There are a number of such devices available.[176] Sclerotherapy can be used in conjunction with axial reflux surgery as an alternative.[177] A subcutaneous light assisted powered phlebectomy (cutter with suction) has been suggested for removal of long lengths of branch varicosities via minimal incisions.[178]

Complications of GSV surgery are rare, but include wound infection, DVT, nerve damage, and hematoma formation to mention the more prominent.[179–181] Saphenous nerve injury can result in an area of numbness around the knee or foot but is often clinically irrelevant.[82,99] Among properly selected patients undergoing vein stripping, recurrent saphenous varicosities will be noted in less than 15% of cases.[170,179] The SSV can be stripped if needed with similar results. Complications from this procedure are typically rare, but include bleeding, hematoma formation, sural nerve damage, DVT, and wound infection.[182] A complication unique to the radiofrequency and laser procedures are thermal damage to adjacent structures, such as nerve or skin that appear to be mitigated by tumescent anesthesia.[171] Complications and short-term freedom from recurrence for both radiofrequency and laser saphenous vein ablation compares favorably with standard stripping and may provide some early patient comfort benefit.[172,175]

Perforator Vein Ligation

Ligation of perforating veins can be an effective treatment for patients with isolated perforator vein incompetence. This procedure can be performed in conjunction with saphenous vein removal. Perforating vein ligation can be performed via an open or minimally invasive endoscopic technique. A Linton type procedure utilizes an incision along the medial or posterior lower leg and creation of subfascial flaps.[183] The perforating veins are directly ligated. If a skin ulcer is present, this can be débrided. If a large amount of soft tissue and/or fascia is involved, a skin graft can be placed to aid healing once the diseased tissues are removed.[183] Alternatively, an endoscopic technique [subfascial endoscopic perforator surgery (SEPS)] can be employed.[184] Following slight knee flexion, two small (10 to 15 mm) incisions are made on the medial aspect of the lower leg near the knee proximal to areas of induration and inflammation. Subfascial dissection is performed using sharp and blunt balloon dissection. Some surgeons place a tourniquet on the upper leg to be inflated prior to subfascial insufflation of carbon dioxide (CO_2) which is used to improve visualization and to prevent CO_2 emboli. Others feel this step is not necessary because the venous system is better visualized with blood within the perforator veins and because the risk of embolism is CO_2 minimal. Under direct video-enhanced vision, the perforating veins are ligated with clips and divided. Some physicians have utilized mediastinoscopes through which a long clip applier can be advanced, obviating the need for a second incision. Most surgeons preoperatively mark the perforating veins using duplex scanning to ensure that all offending veins are identified at the time of surgery. A current evaluation of patients undergoing SEPS demonstrates the patients to have decreased symptoms and a near 90% ulcer healing rate at 2 years.[185] Wound complications are less common after SEPS (0% to 10%) compared to the open method (12% to 53%) with comparable outcomes.[186] Whether SEPS is required in addition to saphenous surgery for advanced CVD when both systems demonstrate insufficiency remains debatable.[186]

Iliac Stenting and Venous Bypass

Endovascular stenting of iliac vein stenosis/obstruction has improved the symptoms of venous occlusive disease including decreased edema and pain.[88,105,120,187,188] The primary and assisted primary stent patency rates at 3 years are 75% and 92%, respectively.[189] Intervention was performed in the presence of significant clinical symptoms (>class 2 but always associated with pain if class 2) and greater than 50% morphologic stenosis found on transfemoral venography or intravascular ultrasonography.[105,189] Potential complications include DVT, access site complications, retroperitoneal hematoma, and other catheter- and balloon-related problems. Essentially no mortality is associated with the procedure.[144] If technically feasible, endovascular surgery is replacing more invasive approaches.

The open surgical procedures use native saphenous vein or polytetrafluoroethylene (PTFE) graft material as the conduit to bypass from a nondiseased distal vein to a disease-free proximal vein. Vena cava reconstructions often use PTFE grafts to allow a proper size match.[190] Preoperative venous pressure studies are often obtained to document venous hypertension.[191] Iliac vein decompression has been used in the instance of extrinsic compression by an overlying right iliac artery (e.g., May-Thurner syndrome). If the iliac vein is severely stenosed or occluded, cross-femoral venous bypass can be performed, but the procedure of choice is direct repair of the involved segment of iliac vein or balloon angioplasty with stenting.[135,192] If iliac vein compression is due to neoplastic growth, patient survival should be considered prior to aggressive intervention. The cross-femoral venous bypass (Palma procedure) is performed by passing a vein graft or graft material via a suprapubic subcutaneous tunnel to the contralateral femoral vein. The saphenous vein or prosthetic graft is then connected to the unaffected femoral vein by an end-to-side technique. The key to success of this surgery may be graft diameter. If the native vein is less than 4.5 mm in diameter, better success may be achieved with an 10-mm diameter PTFE graft, although others would question whether PTFE is superior to vein in this location.[190,191] An arteriovenous fistula can be created to increase flow through the graft in the immediate postoperative period. This fistula can then be ligated in 1 to 3 months. In one series, venous reconstruction for ileofemoral and IVC obstruction having a reported 62% 3-year patency with the saphenous vein Palma procedure have the overall best patency (83% 4-year).[190] Mortality was negligible and wound complications were rare.

Indications for a saphenopopliteal bypass are symptomatic patients with isolated femoral or popliteal vein occlusion, a patent common femoral and iliocaval system, a nonvaricosed saphenous vein, and femoral phlebitis inactive for at least 1 year. In addition, conservative therapy must have failed, and venous hypertension must be documented. These distal to proximal venous bypasses use autogenous vein as the conduit of choice and bypasses extend from distal to proximal nondiseased segments.[191] This operation is rarely performed.

Although not yet proved as a method of treating occlusive venous disease due to prior thrombosis, some data suggest that endophlebectomy (operative removal of synechiae and septa) of iliac, femoral, popliteal, and even tibial veins is possible and can result in a 77% primary patency rate at 8 months.[193]

Venous Valve Repair or Replacement

During the conduct of these operations, several observations influence what the surgeon does for a given patient. If operative handling of the suspect valve results in vasoconstriction and secondary competence (often determined by a standard "strip test"), an external valvuloplasty or a prosthetic sleeve technique may be viable options.[194] For a valve station requiring *in situ* repair, careful adventitial dissection of the valve attachment lines facilitates proper venotomy when required and helps to verify the feasibility of valve repair. [195] A lack of valve attachment lines may signify the destruction of the valve as a postthrombotic sequela, prompting other than an *in situ* repair.[195]

An internal valvuloplasty or an open direct valve repair has been a mainstay for the repair of primary venous valvular reflux for decades. This technique involves venotomy and suturing of the elongated valve leaflets under direct visualization with 7-0 polypropylene suture to tighten the valve cusps. Kistner[196] reported success with a longitudinal venotomy extending through the valve commissure in 1968 (Fig. 105.2). Raju[197] championed a supracommissural approach involving a transverse venotomy at least 2.5 cm above the valve. Sottiurai[198] devised a hybrid approach (a "T"-shaped venotomy,) using a supravalvular transverse venotomy with distal extension into the valve sinus. Recently, a "trapdoor" approach involving two transverse incisions (supravalvular and infravalvular) connected by a single vertical incision through the commissure has been described (see Fig. 105.2).[199] Regardless of the approach, the suturing of the valve leaflets remains essentially the same and plication of approximately 20% of the valve leaflet length tends to restore valve competency in the majority of cases.[200]

The technique of external valvuloplasty offers the advantage of valve repair without venotomy.[201] It is performed by placing sutures transmurally through the valve attachment lines and when tied reduces the commissural angle resulting in a competent valve. Reported results suggest that it maybe less durable than the more precise open valvuloplasty, but patient selection plays a key role.[147] A modification (limited anterior

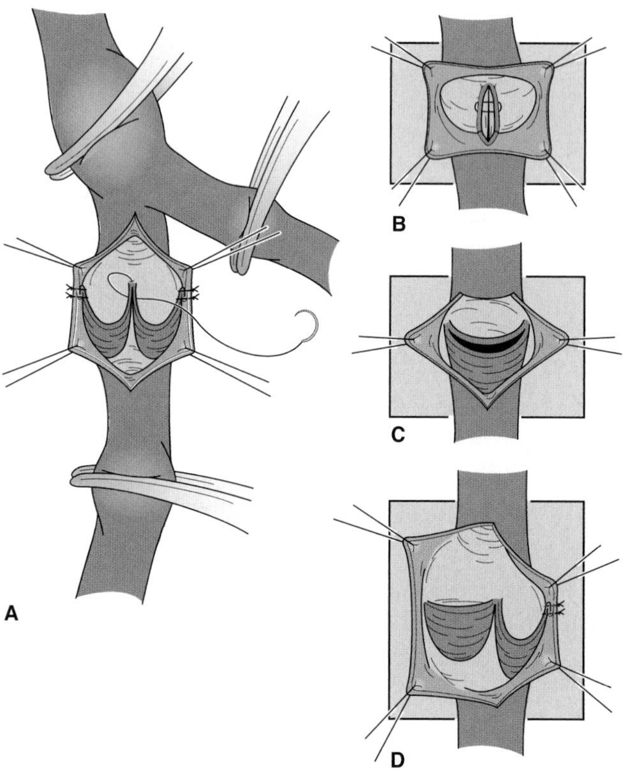

FIGURE 105.2 Open valvuloplasty to repair an insufficient valve can be accomplished by various venotomy incisions. (*A*) The method of Kistner. (*B*) The method of Raju. (*C*) The method of Sottiurai. (*D*) The method of Tripathi and his colleagues.

plication) involves only anterior vein dissection and then reefing of the cusps using a running mattress suture from a point 3 to 4 mm proximal to the angle of the valve cusp insertion lines up to the angle of valve cusp insertion.[202] About 3 mm of the vein wall is incorporated into the stitch to approximate the cusps. This technique was developed with the aim of decreasing vein dissection and potentially reducing the progressive dilatation of the postrepair vein that occurs in some cases of valvuloplasty. It has been described in conjunction with saphenous vein stripping and limited to the femoral vein valve. Results after 10-year follow-up demonstrated improved VRT and decreased AVPs in patients with moderate deep venous valvular incompetence.[202] Thus, it shows promise as a mode of therapy for highly selected patients. Another modification of this technique features the use of an angioscope.[203] A side branch of the GSV allows introduction of an angioscope, which is advanced into the femoral vein to a position above the incompetent valve and external sutures are then placed under direct vision. [203] Following a learning curve while using the angioscope, Raju et al.[204] demonstrated good clinical and competency data with the "transcommissural" technique without the use of the angioscope with 30 months of follow-up.

External banding has been employed when dissection vasospasm renders a valve spontaneously competent. The technique uses an external sleeve made of synthetic material wrapped circumferentially around the vein at the site of the valve and tightened to diminish the size of the vein lumen until the valve is competent. The sleeve is then anchored in place to the adventitia by sutures to avoid slippage. It has achieved good results when used in select patients.[147]

Venous valve transplantation is an option when the valve is absent or destroyed. This procedure was first reported clinically by Taheri in 1982.[205] A 2- to 3-cm segment of upper extremity vein containing a competent valve (or a reparable one) is first removed. The incompetent femoral vein valve is opened below the takeoff of the profunda femoris vein, and the axillary vein segment is sutured into place following the removal of an appropriate length of femoral vein. The popliteal location may be more appropriate if the femoral location does not control all axial reflux into the leg, for example, if the profunda femoral vein system is also incompetent. The proximal anastomosis may be accomplished first to confirm the competence of the newly transplanted valve and to allow distention and lengthening of the vein/valve to facilitate the distal anastomosis. For vein transplantation in trabeculated postthrombotic veins, investigators have described excision of intraluminal synechiae to create one acceptable lumen for transplantation.[206] Interrupted sutures are preferred to avoid suture line stenosis.[200] Valve competence is determined by the intraoperative strip test. An external sleeve can then be placed around the segment to prevent later dilatation of the segment. Because approximately 40% of axillary vein valves are incompetent at the time of explant, a bench repair may be required.[195,200] Should a bench repair be necessary, the transcommissural external valvuloplasty technique appears to have better results than the standard external valvuloplasty,[195] and some success has been achieved with internal valvuloplasty.[207]

Another option in management of the postthrombotic syndrome is valve transposition. If a venous valve is competent in one of the major thigh venous systems, then a transposition procedure can be performed placing the incompetent venous system below the competent valve. Most commonly, the femoral system is incompetent and the profunda femoris valve remains competent. Here, the incompetent femoral vein can be excised and reimplanted distal to the competent valve in the profunda femoris vein. Alternatively, the incompetent femoral system can be placed below a competent valve in the GSV or when the profunda femoris venous system is incompetent, it may be placed distal to a competent valve in either the femoral vein or the GSV. More recently, a technique has been described for transposition of the ipsilateral valve-competent GSV to the femoral vein and subsequent ligation of the femoral vein proximally yet distal to the takeoff of the profunda femoris vein to escape problems with diameter mismatch.[208] At 10 years, 55% of the patients were reported to be ulcer-free.

Aggressive venous valve surgery requires appropriate consideration of perioperative adjunctive care: prophylactic antibiotics, intraoperative heparin use especially if the vein is opened, the use of pneumatic compression devices postoperatively, and the use of low molecular weight heparin or intravenous heparin in the postoperative period. Some recommend closed suction drainage of wounds to avoid hematoma and seroma formation. Warfarin should have an initial target INR range of 2.0 to 2.5 for the first 6 weeks and some would advocate a subsequent decreased to 1.7 to 2.0 until 4 months when it is discontinued. Adjustments are made to accommodate those with an increased risk of thrombosis. One suggested long-term regimen is "minidose" warfarin, which utilizes daily doses of 1 to 2.5 mg to prevent thrombosis.[195,209] Although many surgeons encourage the use of compressive support, many patients do not comply, yet experience a good clinical response.[114,115]

Valve repair procedures are well tolerated by most patients and have a low morbidity, as well as essentially zero mortality in most series.[104] Hematoma and seroma formation is seen in up to 15% of cases, with some expected variation depending on the level of anticoagulation.[114,200,210,211] DVT occurs in less than 10% of cases in most series,[114,195,200,210,211] although one series had an incidence of clot noted in the extremity of repair (often not occlusive or extensive) of approximately 20% detected by ascending venogram 2 days postoperatively.[212] These events did not appear to have an impact on clinical results.[212] Wound infections have been seen in 2% to 4% of cases.[114,195,200]

In general, the results reported have been segregated by the method of deep venous reconstruction. Kistner et al. have followed patients requiring internal valvuloplasty for decades and have reported life-table clinical results (Fig. 105.3). Valve competency is 60% to 70% at 5 years in most series.[114,115,147,197,199,212–218] In general, a patent and competent valve translates into clinical improvement and a healed ulcer, whereas recurrent reflux is associated with clinical failure. A similar commentary can be made about all types of venous valvular reconstruction.

The technique of valve transposition has resulted in reported clinical improvement of 50% to 60% of patients after 3 to 5 years of follow-up.[104,114,208,217] The valve competency rate varies from 30% to 80% and is reflected in the clinical improvement noted.[104,114,208,217]

Valve transplantation is undertaken in the most complex and difficult conditions. Clinical improvement is seen in about 50% of patients even at 8 years of follow-up, and it remains a good option in cases where other techniques are not possible.[103,104,200] There does not appear to be a difference between reported competency rates or clinical results when considering the location of valve repair (femoral vs. popliteal), but, in general, the competency rates reported are inferior to internal valvuloplasty.[197,205,217,219–224]

In general, patients with postthrombotic reflux tend to have more problems maintaining healed ulcers than those with a primary etiology of reflux, as noted from the results of internal valvuloplasty (generally a primary etiology) versus those requiring transplantation or a transposition operative approach.[114] Although, Raju et al.[147] find little difference between the postthrombotic and primary patient results in their series, this may simply reflect a delay in the appearance

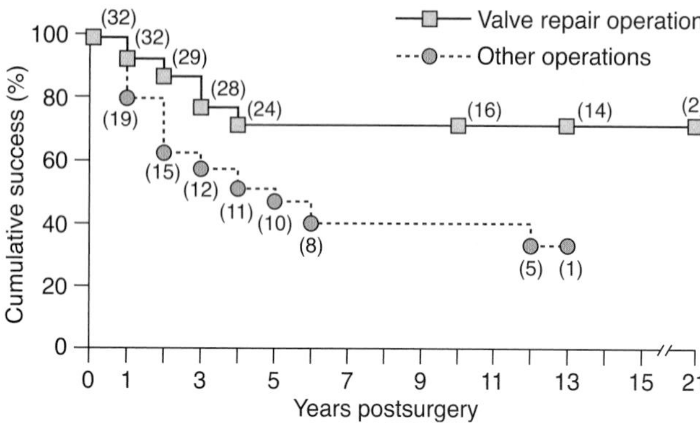

FIGURE 105.3 This life-table demonstrates the cumulative clinical success rate based on type of valve reconstruction procedure. The valve repair operation is valvuloplasty as preformed by Kistner and associates via the Kistner technique. "Other operations" refer to valve transpositions ($n = 14$), superficial femoral vein valve transplantations ($n = 2$), and combined valve repair and transposition procedures ($n = 3$). Numbers in parentheses indicate the number of valve repairs remaining in the study at that time point. Significant difference exists between valve repair versus other operations. (After Masuda EM, Kistner RL. Long-term results of venous valve reconstruction: a four to twenty-one year follow-up. *J Vasc Surg*. 1994;19:391.)

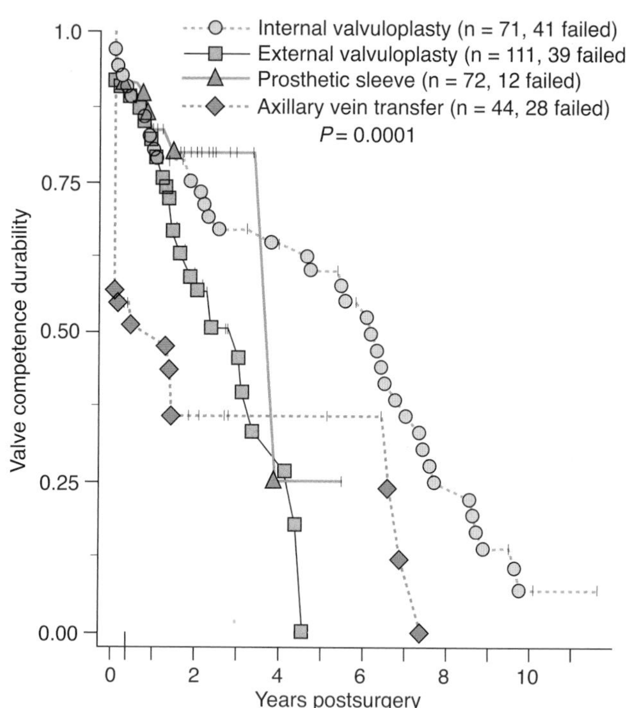

FIGURE 105.4 This life-table method of presentation demonstrates the actuarial durability of various valve reconstruction techniques assessed by serial duplex examination for competence. (After Raju S, Fredericks RK, Neglen PN, et al. Durability of venous valve reconstruction techniques for "primary" and postthrombotic reflux. *J Vasc Surg*. 1996;23:357.)

of ulceration following valve failure. These same investigators are one of a few with a high volume experience in a variety of venous valve repairs and do report a difference in valve competence based on method of repair (Fig. 105.4). It would appear that there is decreasing durability as one progresses from internal valvuloplasty, to external valvuloplasty, and finally, to a need for transplantation.

Valve Substitutes

For those unfortunate patients with chronic DVI and no autogenous valve available, only the hope of finding a valve substitute exists. Raju and associates have a small series of patients who received de novo valve reconstruction procedures with acceptable clinical results.[195] These procedures involve the use of donor vein tissue from which semilunar cusps are fashioned after trimming adventitia and part of the media. The valve "cusps" are sutured into the recipient vein with the nonendothelial surface directed toward the lumen to decrease the risk of thrombosis. Another attempt to use autogenous vein as a valve substitute has been reported by Plagnol et al.[225] This approach invaginates a stump of the long saphenous vein into the femoral vein to fashion a bicuspid valve. They report 19 of 20 reconstructions to be patent and competent at a mean of 10 months with one valve demonstrating reflux. The invagination of an adventitial surface into the venous lumen is of some concern but was not substantiated in this report.

Psathakis reported on a substitute "valve" operation using a Silastic tendon designed to produce an external compression of the popliteal valve (to prevent popliteal reflux) with relaxation of the calf muscles.[226] The technique has not gained wide acceptance. To date, only one other study reports comparable results after 2 years of follow-up.[227] Perrin[212] has attempted this procedure in nine patients, but poor clinical and hemodynamic results were obtained. He stopped using this procedure after 1 year.

Many experimental attempts using allografts and synthetics have been unsuccessful.[228] A clinical attempt to use cryopreserved venous valve-containing allografts for the treatment of CVI demonstrated poor patency rates and minimal clinical improvement in patients receiving the valve in mid-term follow-up.[229] A new cell-free cryopreserved allograft is available (Cryolife, Inc.) that appears to incite very little antigenic response as monitored by panel reactive antibody (PRA) levels.[230] This may prove to be a viable option as a venous valve substitute but may require endothelial seeding.[231] Cadaveric cryopreserved pulmonary monocusp patch has been described as well, with reasonable clinical results in a small group of patients studied over several years.[232]

Most recently, a bioprosthetic (small intestinal submucosa architecture), bicuspid square stent-based venous valve was developed and placed percutaneously in the external jugular vein of sheep.[233] The valve appears to be somewhat resistant to thrombosis and becomes repopulated with recipient endothelial cells following implantation.[233,234] This technique shows promise as a minimally invasive synthetic valve.

The Pelvic Congestion Syndrome

This distressing clinical condition can result from gonadal vein and/or hypogastric vein reflux. Pelvic pain is a constant complaint. Superficial varicosities are managed in ways similar to saphenous vein branch varicosities. Gonadal vein reflux may be best managed with gonadal vein excision due to its many areas of potential reflux, whereas hypogastric vein reflux may best be managed by percutaneous embolization.[235]

KEY POINTS

- **The diagnosis and treatment of acute and chronic venous disease has made significant advances in the last few years.**
- **New drug therapies exist or on the verge of impacting the treatment of acute DVT.**
- **Chronic venous disease has experienced a resurgence of interest in the United States with new endoluminal and surgical interventions being investigated and utilized clinically.**

- **Even characterization of the disease is being scrutinized to allow for a better understanding of how treatment truly impacts patient outcomes.**
- **The care of venous disease is an active and maturing discipline within the realm of the surgical disciplines.**

References

1. **Heit JA, Silverstein MD, Mohr DN, et al. The epidemiology of venous thromboembolism in the community. *Thromb Haemost.* 2001;86:452.**
2. Bauer KA, Rosendaal FR, Heit JA. Hypercoagulability: Too many tests, too much conflicting data. *Hematology* 2002;1:353.
3. **Henke PK, Schmaier A, Wakefield TW. Thrombosis due to hypercoagulable states. In: Rutherford R ed. *Rutherford's textbook of vascular surgery,* 6th ed. Philadelphia: Elsevier; 2005, pp. 560–578.**
4. Goldhaber SZ, Tapson VF, DVT Free Screening Committee. A prospective registry of 5,451 patients with ultrasound confirmed deep vein thrombosis. *Am J Cardiol.* 2004;93:259.
5. Andre P, Hartwell D, Hrachovinova I, et al. Pro-coagulant state resulting from high levels of soluble P-selectin in blood. *Proc Natl Acad Sci.* 2000;97:13835.
6. Myers DD, Hawley AE, Farris DM, et al. P-selectin and leukocyte microparticles are associated with venous thrombogenesis. *J Vasc Surg.* 2003;38:1075 [erratum *J Vasc Surg* 2004;39:188].
7. Hrachovinova I, Cambien B, Hafezi-Moghadam A, et al. Interaction of P-selectin and PSGL-1 generates microparticles that correct hemostasis in a mouse model of hemophilia A. *Nat Med.* 2003;9:1020.
8. Himber J, Wohlgensinger C, Roux S, et al. Inhibition of tissue factor limits the growth of venous thrombus in the rabbit. *J Thromb Haemost.* 2003;1:889.
9. Varma MR, Varga AJ, Knipp BS, et al. Neutropenia impairs venous thrombosis resolution in the rat. *J Vasc Surg.* 2003;38:1090.
10. Lin J, Proctor MC, Varma M, et al. Factors associated with recurrent venous thromboembolism in patients with malignant disease. *J Vasc Surg.* 2003;37:976.
11. Humphries J, McGuinness CL, Smith A, et al. Monocyte chemotactic protein-1 (MCP-1) accelerates the organization and resolution of venous thrombi. *J Vasc Surg.* 1999;30:894.
12. Northeast AD, Soo KS, Bobrow LG, et al. The tissue plasminogen activator and urokinase response in vivo during natural resolution of venous thrombus. *J Vasc Surg.* 1995;22:573.
13. Soo KS, Northeast AD, Happerfield LC, et al. Tissue plasminogen activator production by monocytes in venous thrombolysis. *J Pathol.* 1996;178:190.
14. Singh I, Burnand KG, Collins M, et al. Failure of thrombus to resolve in urokinase type plasminogen activator gene-knockout mice: rescue by normal bone marrow-derived cells. *Circulation* 2003;107:869.
15. Fowl RJ, Strothman GB, Bleabea J, et al. Inappropriate use of venous duplex scans: an analysis of indications and results. *J Vasc Surg.* 1996;23:881.
16. **Douglas MG, Sumner DS. Duplex scanning for deep vein thrombosis: has it replaced both phlebography and noninvasive testing? *Semin Vasc Surg.* 1996;9:3.**
17. Schellong SM, Schwarz T, Halbritter K, et al. Complete compression ultrasonography of the leg veins as a single test for the diagnosis of deep venous thrombosis. *Thromb Haemost.* 2003;89:228.
18. **Wells PS, Anderson DR, Rodger M, et al. Evaluation of D-Dimer in the diagnosis of suspected deep-vein thrombosis. *N Engl J Med.* 2003;349:1227.**
19. Kucher N, Goldhaber SZ. Cardiac biomarkers for risk stratification of patients with acute pulmonary embolism. *Circulation* 2003;108:2191.
20. **Hull RD, Raskob GE, Brant RF, et al. Relation between the time to achieve the lower limit of the APTT therapeutic range and recurrent venous thromboembolism during heparin treatment for deep vein thrombosis. *Arch Intern Med.* 1997;157:2562.**
21. Prandoni P, Lensing AW, Cogo A, et al. The long-term clinical course of acute deep venous thrombosis. *Ann Intern Med.* 1996;125:1.
22. van den Belt AGM, Prins MH, Lensing AWA, et al. Fixed dose subcutaneous low molecular weight heparins versus adjusted dose unfractionated heparin for venous thromboembolism. *Cochrane Peripheral Vascular Diseases Group Cochrane Database of Systematic Reviews* 1, 2003.
23. Ageno W, Turpie AG. Low-molecular-weight heparin in the treatment of pulmonary embolism. *Semin Vasc Surg.* 2000;13:189.
24. Hyers TM, Agnelli G, Hull RD, et al. Antithrombotic therapy for venous thromboembolic disease. *Chest* 2001;119[1 suppl]:176S.
25. **Ridker PM, Goldhaber SZ, Danielson E, et al. Long-term, low-intensity warfarin therapy for the prevention of recurrent venous thromboembolism. *N Engl J Med.* 2003;348:1425.**
26. Kearon C, Ginsberg JS, Kovacs MJ, et al. Comparison of low-intensity warfarin therapy with conventional-intensity warfarin therapy for long-term prevention of recurrent venous thromboembolism. *N Engl J Med.* 2003;349:631.
27. Hull RD, Marder VJ, Mah AF, et al. Quantitative assessment of thrombus burden predicts the outcome of treatment for venous thrombosis. A systematic review. *Am J Med* 2005;118:456.
28. Levine MN, Raskob G, Landefeld S, et al. Hemorrhagic complications of anticoagulant treatment. *Chest* 1998;114[5 suppl]:511S.
29. Almeida JI, Coats R, Liem TK, et al. Reduced morbidity and mortality rates of the heparin-induced thrombocytopenia syndrome. *J Vasc Surg.* 1998;27:309.
30. Greinacher A, Michels I, Mueller-Eckhardt C. Heparin-associated thrombocytopenia: the antibody is not heparin specific. *Thromb Haemost.* 1992;67:545.
31. Laster J, Silver D. Heparin-coated catheters and heparin-induced thrombocytopenia. *J Vasc Surg.* 1988;7:667.
32. Alving BM. How I treat heparin-induced thrombocytopenia and thrombosis. *Blood* 2003;101:31.
33. Greinacher A, Volpel H, Janssens U, et al. Recombinant hirudin (lepirudin) provides safe and effective anticoagulation in patients with heparin-induced thrombocytopenia: a prospective study. *Circulation* 1999;99:73.
34. Lopez-Beret P, Orgaz A, Fontcuberta J, et al. Low molecular weight heparin versus oral anticoagulants in the long-term treatment of deep venous thrombosis. *J Vasc Surg.* 2001;33:77.
35. Lee AY, Levine MN, Baker RI, et al. Low-molecular-weight heparin versus a coumarin for the prevention of recurrent venous thromboembolism in patients with cancer. *N Engl J Med.* 2003;349:146.
36. van Dongen CJ, Mac Gillavry MR, Prins MH. Once versus twice daily LMWH for the initial treatment of venous thromboembolism. *Cochrane Peripheral Vascular Disease Group Cochrane Database of Systematic Reviews* 1, 2003.
37. Schulman S, Wahlander K, Lundstrom T, et al. Secondary prevention of venous thromboembolism with the oral direct thrombin inhibitor ximelagatran. *N Engl J Med.* 2003;349:1713.
38. Matisse Investigators. The Matisse-DVT and PE trials. *J Thromb Haemost.* 2003;1:[suppl 1 July]:abstracts OC331, OC332.
39. Bueller HR, Davidson BL, Decousus H, et al. Subcutaneous fondaparinux versus intravenous unfractionated heparin in the initial treatment of pulmonary embolism. *N Engl J Med.* 2003;349:1695.
40. Eriksson BI, Bauer KA, Lassen MR, et al. Fondaparinux compared with enoxaparin for the prevention of venous thromboembolism after hip-fracture surgery. *N Engl J Med.* 2001;345:1298.
41. Bauer KA, Eriksson BI, Lassen MR, et al. Fondaparinux compared with enoxaparin for the prevention of venous thromboembolism after elective major knee surgery. *N Engl J Med.* 2001;345:1305.
42. Turpie AG, Bauer KA, Eriksson BI, et al. Fondaparinux vs enoxaparin for the prevention of venous thromboembolism in major orthopedic surgery. *Arch Intern Med.* 2002;162:1833.
43. Eriksson BI, Lassen MR, for the PENTasaccharide in hip-fracture surgery plus (PENTHIFRA Plus). Investigators. *Arch Intern Med.* 2003; 613:1337.
44. Arnesen H, Hoiseth A, Ly B, et al. Streptokinase or heparin in the treatment of deep vein thrombosis: follow-up results of a prospective study. *Acta Med Scand.* 1982;211:65.
45. Elliot MS, Immelman EJ, Jeffery P, et al. A comparative randomized trial of heparin versus streptokinase in the treatment of acute proximal venous thrombosis: an interim report of a prospective study. *Br J Surg.* 1979;66:838.
46. **Comerota AJ. Quality-of-life improvement using thrombolytic therapy for iliofemoral deep vein thrombosis. *Rev Cardiovasc Med.* 2002;3:S61.**
47. Meissner MH. Thrombolytic therapy for acute deep vein thrombosis and the venous registry. *Rev Cardiovasc Med.* 2002;3:S53.
48. Semba CP, Dake MD. Iliofemoral deep vein thrombosis: aggressive therapy with catheter-directed thrombolysis. *Radiology* 1994;191:487.
49. Mewissen MW. Catheter-directed thrombolysis for lower extremity deep vein thrombosis. *Tech Vasc Intervent Radiol.* 2001;4:111.
50. Bjarnason H, Kruse JR, Asinger DA, et al. Iliofemoral deep vein thrombosis: safety and efficacy outcome during 5 years of catheter-directed thrombolytic therapy. *J Vasc Interv Radiol.* 1997;8:405.
51. Goldhaber SZ. Thrombolytic therapy in venous thromboembolism. Clinical trials and current indications. *Clin Chest Med.* 1995;16:307.
52. Konstantinides S, Geibel A, Heusel G, et al. Heparin plus alteplase compared with heparin alone in patients with submissive pulmonary embolism. *N Engl J Med.* 2002;347:1143.
53. Comerota AJ, Aldridge SC, Cohen G, et al. A strategy of aggressive regional therapy for acute iliofemoral venous thrombosis with contemporary venous thrombectomy or catheter-directed thrombolysis. *J Vasc Surg.* 1994;20:244.
54. Sharafuddin MJ, Sun S, Hoballah JJ. Endovascular management of venous thrombotic diseases of the upper torso and extremities. *J Vasc Interv Radiol.* 2002;13:975.
55. Meier GH, Pollak JS, Rosenblatt M, et al. Initial experience with venous stents in exertional axillary-subclavian vein thrombosis. *J Vasc Surg.* 1996;24:974.
56. Plate G, Eklof B, Norgren L, et al. Venous thrombectomy for iliofemoral vein thrombosis—10-year results of a prospective randomized study. *Eur J Vasc Endo Surg.* 1997;14:367.
57. Juhan CM, Alimi YS, Barthelemy PJ, et al. Late results of iliofemoral venous thrombectomy. *J Vasc Surg.* 1997;25:417.
58. Rhodes JM, Cho JS, Gloviczki P, et al. Thrombolysis for experimental deep venous thrombosis maintains valvular competence and vasoreactivity. *J Vasc Surg.* 2000;31:1193.

59. Gandini R, Maspes F, Sodani G, et al. Percutaneous ilio-caval thrombectomy with the Amplatz device: preliminary results. *Eur Radiol.* 1999;9:951.
60. Kasirajan K, Gray B, Ouriel K. Percutaneous Angiojet thrombectomy in the management of extensive deep venous thrombosis. *J Vasc Interv Radiol.* 2001;12:179.
61. Brandjes DP, Buller HR, Heijober H, et al. Randomized trial of effort of compression stockings in patients with symptomatic proximal-vein thrombosis. *Lancet* 1997;349:759.
62. **Prandoni P, Frulla M, Mosena L, et al. Benefit of below knee elastic compression stockings for prevention of the post-thrombotic syndrome in patients with proximal-vein thrombosis. A prospective controlled randomized study. *Pathophysiol Haemost Thromb.* 2002;32[suppl 2]:72.**
63. Schellong SM, Schwarz T, Kropp J, et al. Bed rest in deep vein thrombosis and the incidence of scintigraphic pulmonary embolism. *Thromb Haemost.* 1999;82[suppl 1]:127.
64. Aschwanden M, Labs KH, Engel H, et al. Acute deep vein thrombosis: early mobilization does not increase the frequency of pulmonary embolism. *Thromb Haemost.* 2001;85:42.
65. Partsch H, Kaulich M, Mayer W. Immediate mobilization in acute vein thrombosis reduces postthrombotic syndrome. American Venous Forum, San Diego, February 2004.
66. Vitti MJ, Barnes RW. Nonoperative treatment of acute superficial thrombophlebitis and deep femoral venous thrombosis. In: Ernst CB, Stanley JC, eds. *Current therapy in vascular surgery.* St. Louis: Mosby; 1995, p. 888.
67. Belcaro G. Nicolaides AN, Errichi BM, et al. Superficial thrombophlebitis of the legs: a randomized, controlled, follow-up study. *Angiology* 1999;50:523.
68. Krause U, Kock HJ, Kroger K, et al. Prevention of deep venous thrombosis associated with superficial thrombophlebitis of the leg by early saphenous vein ligation. *Vasa* 1998;27:34.
69. Lutter KS, Kerr TM, Roedersheimer LR, et al. Superficial thrombophlebitis diagnosed by duplex scanning. *Surgery* 1991;110:42.
70. Hafner CD, Cranley JP, Krause RJ, et al. A method of managing superficial thrombophlebitis. *Surgery* 1964;55:201.
71. Ascer E. Lorensen E, Pollina RM, et al. Preliminary results of a nonoperative approach to saphenofemoral junction thrombophlebitis. *J Vasc Surg.* 1995;22:616.
72. Chengelis DL, Bendick PJ, Glover JL, et al. Progression of superficial venous thrombosis to deep vein thrombosis. *J Vasc Surg.* 1996;24:745.
73. Jorgensen JO, Hanel KC, Morgan AM, et al. The incidence of deep venous thrombosis in patients with superficial thrombophlebitis of the lower limbs. *J Vasc Surg.* 1993;18:70.
74. Blumbenberg RM, Barton E, Gelfand ML, et al. Occult deep venous thrombosis complicating superficial thrombophlebitis. *J Vasc Surg.* 1998;27:338.
75. Sover ER, Brarnmer HM, Rowedder AM. Thrombosis of the proximal greater saphenous vein: ultrasonographic diagnosis and clinical significance. *J Ultrasound Med.* 1997;16:113.
76. Gjores J. Surgical therapy of ascending thrombophlebitis in the saphenous system. Angiology 1962;13:241.
77. Husni EA, Williams WA. Superficial thrombophlebitis of lower limbs. *Surgery* 1982;91:70.
78. Williams RD, Zollinger RW. Surgical treatment of superficial thrombophlebitis. *Surg Gynecol Obstet.* 1964;118:775.
79. Lohr JM, McDevitt DT. Lutter KS, et al. Operative management of greater saphenous thrombophlebitis involving the saphenofemoral junction. *Am J Surg.* 1992;164:269.
80. Sullivan V, Denk PM, Sonnad SS, et al. Ligation versus anticoagulation: treatment of above-knee superficial thrombophlebitis not involving the deep venous system. *J Am Coll Surg.* 2001;193:556.
81. **Caggiati A, Bergan JJ, Gloviczki P, et al. Nomenclature of the veins of the lower limbs: An international interdisciplinary consensus statement. *J Vasc Surg.* 2002;36:416.**
82. Morrison C, Dalsing MC. Signs and symptoms of saphenous nerve injury after greater saphenous vein stripping: prevalence, severity, and relevance for modern practice. *J Vasc Surg.* 2003;38:886.
83. Corrales NE, Irvine A, McGuinness CL, et al. Incidence and pattern of long saphenous vein duplication and its possible implications for recurrence after varicose vein surgery. *Br J Surg.* 2002;89:323.
84. Caggiati A, Bergan JJ. The saphenous vein: derivation of its name and its relevant anatomy. *J Vasc Surg.* 2002;35:172.
85. Caggiati A. Fascial relationship of the short saphenous vein. *J Vasc Surg.* 2001;34:241.
86. Mozes G, Gloviczki P, Menawat SS, et al. Surgical anatomy for endoscopic subfascial division of perforating veins. *J Vasc Surg.* 1996;24:800.
87. Browse NL, Burnand KG, Thomas ML. *Disease of the veins: pathology, diagnosis, and treatment.* London: Edward Arnold; 1988:53–69.
88. Goidano JM, Trout HH. Anomalies of the inferior vena cava. *J Vasc Surg.* 1986;3:924.
89. Nehler MR, Moneta GL. The lower extremity venous disease Part 1 anatomy and physiology. *Perspect Vasc Surg.* 1991;4:104.
90. Moreno AH, Katz AL, Gold LD, Reddy RV. Mechanics of distension of dog veins and other thin walled tubular structures. *Circ Res.* 1970;27:1069.
91. Moneta GL, Bedford G, Beach K, et al. Duplex ultrasound assessment of venous diameters, peak velocities, and flow patterns. *J Vasc Surg.* 1988; 8:286.
92. **Lurie L, Kistner RL, Eklof B, et al. Mechanism of venous valve closure and role of the valve in circulation: a new concept. *J Vasc Surg.* 2003; 38:955.**
93. vanBemmelen PS, Bedford G, Beach K, et al. Quantitative segmental evaluation of venous valvular reflux with duplex ultrasound scanning. *J Vasc Surg.* 1989;10:425.
94. Mattos MA, Summer D. Direct noninvasive tests (duplex scan) for the evaluation of chronic venous obstruction and valvular incompetence. In: Gloviczki P, Yao JST, eds. *Handbook of venous disorders.* London: Arnold; 2001, pp. 120–131.
95. Van Bemmelen PS, Beach K, Bedford G, Strandness DE. The mechanism of venous valve closure. *Arch Surg.* 1990;125:617.
96. Raju S, Fredericks R, Lishman P, et al. Observation on the calf venous pump mechanism: determinants of postexercise pressure. *J Vasc Surg.* 1993;17:459.
97. Brand FN, Dannenberg AL, Abbott RD, Kannel WB. The epidemiology of varicose veins: the Framingham Study. *Am J Prev Med.* 1988;4:96.
98. Coon WW, Willis PW, Keller JB. Venous thromboembolism and other venous disease in the Tecumseh community health study. *Circulation* 1973;48:839.
99. Dale WA, Cranley JJ, DeWeese JA, et al. Symposium: management of varicose veins. *Contemp Surg.* 1975;6:86.
100. Baker SR, Stacey MC, Jopp-McKay AG, et al. Epidemiology of chronic venous ulcers. *Br J Surg.* 1988;78:864.
101. Heit JA, Rooke TW, Silverstein MD, et al. Trends in the incidence of venous stasis syndrome and venous ulcer: a 25-year population-based study. *J Vasc Surg.* 2001;33:1022.
102. **Nicolaides AN. Investigation of chronic venous insufficiency: a consensus statement. *Circulation* 2000;102:126.**
103. O'Donnell TF. Chronic venous insufficiency: an overview of epidemiology, classification, and anatomic considerations. *Semin Vasc Surg.* 1988;1:60.
104. Eklof BG, Kistner RL, Masuda E. Venous bypass and valve reconstruction: long-term efficacy. *Vasc Med.* 1998;3:157.
105. Neglen P, Thrasher TL, Raju S. Venous outflow obstruction: an underestimated contributor to chronic venous disease. *J Vasc Surg.* 2003;38:879.
106. Lalka, SG. Management of chronic obstructive venous disease of the lower extremity. In: Rutherford RB, ed. *Vascular surgery*, 4th ed. Philadelphia: WB Saunders; 1995:1862–1882.
107. Crockett FB, Thomas ML. The iliac compression syndrome. *Br J Surg.* 1965;52:816.
108. Browse NL, Burnand KG, Thomas ML. *Disease of the veins: pathology, diagnosis, and treatment.* London: Edward Arnold; 1988, pp. 271–287.
109. Martin-Pedrosa JM, Del Blanco I, Carrera S, et al. Intravascular lipoma of the external iliac vein and common femoral vein. *Eur J Vasc Endovasc Surg.* 2002;23:470.
110. Plate G, Brodin L, Eklof B, et al. Physiologic and therapeutic aspects in congenital vein valve aplasia of the lower limb. *Ann Surg.* 1983; 198:229.
111. Rose SS, Ahmed A. Some thoughts on the etiology of varicose veins. *J Cardiovasc Surg.* 1986;27:534.
112. Clarke H, Smith SR, Vasdekis SN, et al. Role of venous elasticity in the development of varicose veins. *Br J Surg.* 1989;76:577.
113. Kistner RL, Eklof B, Masuda EM. Deep venous valve reconstruction. *Cardiovasc Surg.* 1995;3:129.
114. Masuda EM, Kistner RL. Long-term results of venous valve reconstruction: a four to twenty-one year follow-up. *J Vasc Surg.* 1994;19:391.
115. **Raju S, Fredericks RK, Hudson CA, et al. Venous valve station changes in "primary" and postthrombotic reflux: an analysis of 149 cases. *Ann Vasc Surg.* 2000;14:193.**
116. Killewich LA, Bedford GR, Beach KW, Strandness DE Jr. Spontaneous lysis of deep venous thrombi: rate and outcome. *J Vasc Surg.* 1989;9:89.
117. Pappas PJ, Duran WN, Hobson RW. Pathology and cellular physiology of chronic venous insufficiency. In: Gloviczki P, Yao JST, eds. *Handbook of venous disorders.* New York: Arnold; 2001, pp. 58–67.
118. Stanley AC, Park H Y, Phillips TJ, et al. Reduced growth of dermal fibroblasts from chronic venous ulcerations can be stimulated with growth factors. *J Vasc Surg.* 1997;26:994.
119. Killewich LA, Martin R, Cramer M, et al. Pathophysiology of venous claudication. *J Vasc Surg.* 1984;1:507.
120. **Raju S, Owen S, Neglen P. The clinical impact of iliac venous stents in the management of chronic venous insufficiency. *J Vasc Surg.* 2002;35:8.**
121. Labropoulos N, Volteas M, Leon M, et al. The role of venous outflow obstruction in patients with chronic venous dysfunction. *Arch Surg.* 1997;132:46.
122. Prepared by the Executive Committee, chaired by Andrew N. Nicolaides, of the ad hoc committee, American Venous Forum, 6th Annual Meeting. February 22–25, 1994, Maui, Hawaii. Classification and grading of chronic venous disease in the lower limbs: a consensus statement. In: Gloviczki P, and Yao JST, eds. *Handbook of venous disorders.* New York: Arnold; 2001, pp. 521–525.
123. Porter JM, Moneta GL, an International Consensus Committee on Chronic Venous Disease. Reporting standards in venous disease: an update. *J Vasc Surg.* 1995;21:634.
124. Rutherford, RB, Padberg FT Jr, Comerota AJ, et al. Venous severity scoring: an adjunct to venous outcome assessment. *J Vasc Surg.* 2000; 31:1307.

125. Lamping DL, Schroter S, Kurz X, et al. Evaluation of outcomes in chronic venous disorders of the leg: Development of a scientifically rigorous, patient-reported measure of symptoms and quality of life. *J Vasc Surg.* 2003;37:410.
126. Wong JK, Duncan JL, Nichols DM. Whole-leg duplex mapping for varicose veins: observations on patterns of reflux in recurrent and primary legs, with clinical correlation. *Eur J Vasc Endovasc Surg.* 2003;25:267.
127. Mercer KG, Scott DJ, Berridge DC. Preoperative duplex imaging is required before all operations for primary varicose veins. *Br J Surg.* 1998;85:1495.
128. Labropoulos N, Mansour MA, Kang SS, et al. New insights into perforator vein incompetence. *Eur J Vasc Endovasc Surg.* 1999;18:228.
129. Labropoulos N, Tiongson J, Pryor L, et al. Definition of venous reflux in lower-extremity veins. *J Vasc Surg.* 2003;38:793.
130. Lynch TG, Dalsing MC, Ouriel K, et al. Developments in diagnosis and classification of venous disorders: non-invasive diagnosis. *Cardiovasc Surg.* 1999;7:160.
131. Labropoulos N, Giannoukas AD, Delis K, et al. The impact of isolated lesser saphenous vein system incompetence on clinical signs and symptoms of chronic venous disease. *J Vasc Surg.* 2000;32:954.
132. Danielsson G, Eklof B, Grandinetti A, et al. Deep axial reflux, an important contributor to skin changes or ulcer in chronic venous disease. *J Vasc Surg.* 2003;38:1336.
133. Mantoni M, Larsen L, Lund JO, et al. Evaluation of chronic venous disease in the lower limb: comparison of five diagnostic methods. *Br J Surg.* 2002;75:578.
134. Stanson AW, Breen JF. Computed tomography and magnetic resonance imaging in venous disorders. In: Gloviczki P, Yao JST, eds. *Handbook of venous disorders.* London: Arnold; 2001, pp. 153–176.
135. Wolpert LM, Rahmani O, Stein B, et al. Magnetic resonance venography in the diagnosis and management of May-Thurner syndrome. *Vasc Endovasc Surg.* 2002;36:51.
136. Butty S, Hagspiel KD, Leung DA, et al. Body MR venography. *Radiol Clin North Am.* 2002;40:899.
137. Kibbe MR, Ujiki M, Goodwin AL, et al. Iliac vein compression in an asymptomatic patient population. *J Vasc Surg.* 2004;39:937.
138. Coakley FV, Varghese SL, Hricak H. CT and MRI of pelvic varices in women. *J Comput Assisted Tomogr.* 1999;23:429.
139. Bays RA, Healy DA, Atnip RG, et al. Validation of air plethysmography, photoplethysmography, and duplex ultrasonography in the evaluation of severe venous stasis. *J Vasc Surg.* 1994;20:721.
140. Nicolaides AN, Christopoulos D. Quantification of venous reflux and outflow obstruction with air-plethysmography. In: Bernstein EF, ed. *Vascular diagnosis.* St. Louis: Mosby; 1993, pp. 915–921.
141. Criado E, Farber MA, Marston WA, et al. The role of air plethysmography in the diagnosis of chronic venous insufficiency. *J Vasc Surg.* 1998;27:660.
142. Araki CT, Back TL, Padberg FT, et al. The significance of calf muscle pump function in venous ulceration. *J Vasc Surg.* 1994;20:872.
143. Cordts PR, Hartono C, LaMorte WW, et al. Physiologic similarities between extremities with varicose veins and with chronic venous insufficiency utilizing air plethysmography. *Am J Surg.* 1992;164:260.
144. Neglen P, Raju S. Proximal lower extremity chronic venous outflow obstruction: recognition and treatment. *Semin Vasc Surg.* 2002;15:57.
145. Neglen P, Raju S. Intravascular ultrasound scan evaluation of the obstructed vein. *J Vasc Surg.* 2002;35:694.
146. Kistner RL, Feuier EB, Randhawn F, et al. A method of performing descending venography. *J Vasc Surg.* 1986;4:464.
147. Raju S, Fredericks RK, Neglen PN, et al. Durability of venous valve reconstruction techniques for "primary" and postthrombotic reflux. *J Vasc Surg.* 1996;23:357.
148. Cheatle TR, Perrin M. Venous valve repair: early results in fifty-two cases. *J Vasc Surg.* 1994;19:404.
149. Kistner RL, Sparkuhl MD. Surgery in acute and chronic venous disease. *Surgery* 1979;85:31.
150. **Nicolaides AN, Hussein MK, Szendro G, et al. The relation of venous ulceration with ambulatory venous pressure measurements. *J Vasc Surg.* 1993;17:414.**
151. Raju S. New approaches to the diagnosis and treatment of venous obstruction. *J Vasc Surg.* 1986;4:42.
152. Erickson CA, Lanza DJ, Karp DL, et al. Healing of venous ulcers in an ambulatory care program: the roles of chronic venous insufficiency and patient compliance. *J Vasc Surg.* 1995;22:629.
153. Nicoloff AD, Moneta GL, Porter JM. Compression treatment of chronic venous insufficiency. In Gloviczki P, Yao JST, eds. *Handbook of venous disorders*, 2nd ed. London: Arnold; 2001, pp. 303–308.
154. Padberg FT Jr, Johnson MV, Sisto SA. Structured exercise improves calf muscle pump function in chronic venous insufficiency: a randomized trial. *J Vasc Surg.* 2004;39:79.
155. Neumann H, van den Broek M. A comparative clinical trail of graduated compression stockings and O-(beta-hydroxyethyl)rutosides in the treatment of patients with chronic venous insufficiency. *Phlebology* 1995;24:78.
156. Jull A, Waters J, Arroll B. Pentoxifylline for treatment of venous leg ulcers: a systemic review. *Lancet* 2002;359:1550.
157. Guilhou JJ, Dereue O. Efficacy of Daflon 500mg in venous leg ulcer healing: a double blind randomised, controlled versus placebo trial in 107 patients. *Angiology* 1997;48:77.
158. Schmeller W, Gaber Y. Surgical removal of ulcer and lipodermatosclerosis followed by split-skin grafting (shave therapy) yields good long-term results in "non-healing: venous leg ulcers. *Acta Derm Venereol.* 2000; 80:267.
159. Falanga V, Sabolinski M. A bilayered living skin construct accelerates complete closure of hard to heal venous ulcers. *Wound Repair Regen.* 1999;7:201.
160. Belcaro G, Cesarone MR, Di Renzo A, et al. Foam-sclerotherapy, surgery, and combined treatment for varicose veins: a 10-year, prospective, randomized, controlled, trial (VEDICO trial). *Angiology* 2003;54:307.
161. Miyazaki K, Nishibe T, Sata F, et al. Stripping operation with sclerotherapy for primary varicose veins due to greater saphenous vein reflux: three-year results. *World J Surg.* 2003;27:551
162. Hamel-Desnos C, Desnos P, Wollman JC, et al. Evaluation of the efficacy of polidocanol in the form of foam compared with liquid form in sclerotherapy of the greater saphenous vein: initial results. *Dermatol Surg.* 2003;29:1170.
163. Villavicencio JL. Sclerotherapy guidelines. In Gloviczki P, Yao JST, eds. *Handbook of venous disorders*, 2nd ed. New York: Arnold; 2001, pp. 253–266.
164. Scultetus AH, Villaviciencio JL, Kao TC, et al. Microthrombectomy reduces postsclerotherapy pigmentation: multicenter randomized trial. *J Vasc Surg.* 2003;38:896.
165. Neglen P, Einarsson E, Eklof B. The functional long-term value of different types of treatment for saphenous vein incompetence. *J Cardiovasc Surg.* 1993;34:295.
166. Criado E, Salvador L, Luis I, et al. Conservative hemodynamic surgery for varicose veins. *Semin Vasc Surg.* 2002;15:27.
167. Raju S, Easterwood L, Fountain T, et al. Saphenectomy in the presence of chronic venous obstruction. *Surgery* 1998;123:637.
168. Padberg FT Jr, Pappas PJ, Araki CT, et al. Hemodynamic and clinical improvement after superficial vein ablation in primary combined venous insufficiency with ulceration. *J Vasc Surg.* 1997;26:169.
169. Dalsing MC. Lower extremity varicose vein disease. In Cameron JL, ed. *Current surgical therapy,* 7th ed. St. Louis: Mosby; 2001, pp. 992–998.
170. **Dwerryhouse S, Davies B, Harradine K, et al. Stripping the long saphenous vein reduces the rate of reoperation for recurrent varicose veins: five-year results of a randomized trial. *J Vasc Surg.* 1999;29:589.**
171. Chandler JG, Pichot O, Sessa C, et al. Treatment of primary venous insufficiency by endovenous saphenous vein obliteration. *Vasc Surg.* 2000; 34:201.
172. Lurie F, Creton D, Eklof B, et al. Prospective randomized study of endovenous radiofrequency obliteration (Closure procedure) versus ligation and stripping in a selected patient population (EVOLVeS Study). *J Vasc Surg.* 2003;38:207.
173. Navarro L, Min RJ, Bone' C. Endovenous laser: a new minimally invasive method of treatment for varicose veins—preliminary observations using an 810 nm diode laser. *Dermatol Surg.* 2001;27:117.
174. Proebstle TM, Gul D, Kargl A, et al. Endovenous laser treatment of the lesser saphenous vein with a 940-nm diode laser. *Dermatol Surg.* 2003;29:357.
175. Min RJ, Khilnani N, Zimmet SE. Endovenous laser treatment of saphenous vein reflux: long-term results. *J Vasc Intervent Radiol.* 2003;14:991.
176. Bergan JJ. Varicose veins: hooks, clamps, and suction. Application of new techniques to enhance varicose vein surgery. *Semin Vasc Surg.* 2002;15:21.
177. Iwamoto S, Masataka I, Kawasaki T, et al. Treatment of varicose veins: an assessment of intraoperative and postoperative compressive sclerotherapy. *Am Vasc Surg.* 2003;17:290.
178. Spitz GA, Braxton JM. Outpatient varicose vein surgery with transilluminated powered phlebectomy. Proceedings from the American Venous Forum 12th Annual Meeting. Phoenix, Arizona, February 2–6, 2000.
179. Larson RA, Toftgren EP, Myers TT, et al. Long-term results after vein surgery: study of 1000 cases after 10 years. *Mayo Clin Proc.* 1974;49:114.
180. Keith LM Jr, Smead WL. Saphenous vein stripping and its complications. *Surg Clin North Am.* 1983;63:1303.
181. Ramsheyi A, Soury P, Saliou C, et al. Inadvertent arterial injury during saphenous vein stripping: three cases and therapeutic strategies. *Arch Surg.* 1998;133:1120.
182. Seror P. Sural nerve neuropathy (external saphenous) linked to a disease of the small saphenous vein. *J Maladies Vasculaires* 2000;25:128.
183. DePalma RG. Management of incompetent perforators: conventional techniques. In: Gloviczki P, Yao JST, eds. *Handbook of venous disorders,* 2nd ed. London: Arnold; 2001, pp. 384–390.
184. Gloviczki P, Bergan JJ, Menawat SS, et al. Safety, feasibility, and early efficacy of subfascial endoscopic perforator surgery: a preliminary report from the North American registry. *J Vasc Surg.* 1997;25:94.
185. **Gloviczki P, Bergan JJ, Rhodes JM, et al. Mid-term results of endoscopic perforator vein interruption for chronic venous insufficiency: lessons learned from the North American subfascial endoscopic perforator surgery registry. The North American Study Group. *J Vasc Surg.* 1999;29:489.**
186. Kalra M, Gloviczki P. Subfascial endoscopic perforator vein surgery: who benefits? *Semin Vasc Surg.* 2002;15:39.
187. Raju S, Owen S, Neglen P. Reversal of abnormal lymphoscintigraphy after placement of venous stents for correction of associated venous obstruction. *J Vasc Surg.* 2001;34:779.
188. Raju S, McAllister S, Neglen P. Recanalization of totally occluded iliac and adjacent venous segments. *J Vasc Surg.* 2002;36:903.

189. Neglen P, Raju S. In-stent recurrent stenosis in stents placed in the lower extremity venous outflow tract. *J Vasc Surg.* 2004;39:181.
190. Corey JJ, Gloviczki P, Cherry KJ, et al. Surgical reconstruction of iliofemoral veins and the inferior vena cava for nonmalignant occlusive disease. *J Vasc Surg.* 2001;33:320.
191. Lalka SG. Autogenous venous bypass grafts for chronic iliac or infrainguinal venous occlusive disease. In: Gloviczki P, Yao JST, eds. *Handbook of venous disorders*, 2nd ed. London: Arnold; 2001, pp. 362–373.
192. Akers DL, Creado B, Hewitt RL. Iliac vein compression syndrome: case report and review of the literature. *J Vasc Surg.* 1996;24:477.
193. Puggioni A, Kistner RL, Eklof B, et al. Surgical disobliteration of postthrombotic deep veins—endophlebectomy—is feasible. *J Vasc Surg.* 2004; 39:1048.
194. Camilli S, Guarnera G. External banding valvuloplasty of the superficial femoral vein in the treatment of primary deep valvular incompetence. *Int Angiol.* 1994;13:218.
195. Raju S, Hardy JD. Technical options in venous valve reconstruction. *Am J Surg.* 1997;173:301.
196. Kistner RL. Surgical repair of a venous valve. *Straub Clin Proc.* 1968; 24:41.
197. Raju S. Venous insufficiency of the lower limb and stasis ulceration: changing concepts and management. *Ann Surg.* 1983;197:688.
198. Sottiurai VS. Technique in direct venous valvuloplasty. *J Vasc Surg.* 1988;8:646.
199. Tripathi R, Ktenidis KD. Trapdoor internal valvuloplasty: a new technique for primary deep vein valvular incompetence. *Eur J Vasc Endovasc Surg.* 2001;22:86.
200. Raju S, Fredericks R. Valve reconstruction procedures for nonobstructive venous insufficiency: rationale, techniques, and results in 107 procedures with two- to eight-year follow-up. *J Vasc Surg.* 1988;7:301.
201. Kistner RL. Surgical technique of external venous valve repair. *Straub Found Proc.* 1990;55:15.
202. Belcaro G, Nicolaides AN, Ricci A, et al. External femoral vein valvuloplasty with limited anterior plication (LAP): a 10-year randomized, follow-up study. *Angiology* 1999;50:531.
203. Gloviczki P, Merrell SW, Bower TC. Femoral vein valve repair under direct vision without venotomy: a modified technique with use of angioscopy. *J Vasc Surg.* 1991;14:645.
204. Raju S, Berry MA, Neglen P. Transcommissural valvuloplasty: technique and results. *J Vasc Surg.* 2000;32:969.
205. Taheri SA, Lazar L, Elias SM, et al. Vein valve transplant. *Surgery* 1982;91:28.
206. Raju S, Neglen P, Doolittle J, Meydrech EF. Axillary vein transfer in trabeculated postthrombotic veins. *J Vasc Surg.* 1999;29:1050.
207. Sottiurai VS. Supravalvular incision for valve repair in primary valvular insufficiency. In: Bergan JJ, Kistner RL, eds. *Atlas of venous surgery.* Philadelphia: WB Saunders, 1992, pp. 137–138.
208. Cardon JM, Cardon A, Joyeux A, et al. Use of ipsilateral greater saphenous vein as a valved transplant in management of post-thrombotic deep venous insufficiency: long-term results. *Ann Vasc Surg.* 1999;13:284.
209. Poller L, McKernan A, Thomson JM, et al. Fixed minidose warfarin: a new approach to prophylaxis against venous thrombosis after major surgery. *Br Med J.* 1987;295:1309.
210. Welch H, McLaughlin RL, O'Donnell TF. Femoral vein valvuloplasty: intraoperative angioscopic evaluation and hemodynamic improvement. *J Vasc Surg.* 1992;16:694.
211. Jamieson WG, Chinnick B. Clinical results of deep venous valvular repair for chronic venous insufficiency. *Can J Surg.* 1997;40:294.
212. Perrin M. Reconstructive surgery for deep venous reflux: a report on 144 cases. *Cardiovasc Surg.* 2000;8:246.
213. Kistner RL. Surgical repair of the incompetent femoral vein valve. *Arch Surg.* 1975;110:1336.
214. Ferris EB, Kistner RL. Femoral vein reconstruction in the management of chronic venous insufficiency: a 14-year experience. *Arch Surg.* 1982;117:1571.
215. Eriksson I, Almgren B. Influence of the profunda femoris vein on venous hemodynamics of the limb. Experience from thirty-one deep vein valve reconstructions. *J Vasc Surg.* 1986;4:390.
216. Lurie F, Makarova NP, Hmelniker SM. Results of deep-vein reconstruction. *Vasc Surg.* 1997;31:275.
217. Perrin MR. Results of deep-vein reconstruction. *Vasc Surg.* 1997;31:273.
218. Perrin M, Hiltbrand B, Bayon JM. Results of valvuloplasty in patients presenting deep venous insufficiency and recurring ulceration. *Ann Vasc Surg.* 1999;13:524.
219. Taheri SA, Elias SM, Yacobucci GN, et al. Indications and results of vein valve transplant. *J Cardiovasc Surg.* 1986;27:163.
220. O'Donnell TF, Mackey WC, Shepard AD, et al. Clinical, hemodynamic, and anatomic follow-up of direct venous reconstruction. *Arch Surg.* 1987;122:474.
221. Nash T. Long term results of vein valve transplants placed in the popliteal vein for intractable post-phlebitic venous ulcers and pre-ulcer skin changes. *J Cardiovasc Surg.* 1988;29:712.
222. Rai DB, Lerner R. Chronic venous insufficiency disease. Its etiology. A new technique for vein valve transplantation. *Int Surg.* 1991;76:174.
223. Bry JD, Muto PA, O'Donnell TF, et al. The clinical and hemodynamic results after axillary-to-popliteal vein valve transplantation. *J Vasc Surg.* 1995;21:110.
224. Sottiurai VS. Results of deep-vein reconstruction. *Vasc Surg.* 1997; 31:276.
225. Plagnol P, Ciostek P, Grimaud JP, et al. Autogenous valve reconstruction technique for post-thrombotic reflux. *Ann Vasc Surg.* 1999;13:339.
226. Psathakis ND, Psathakis DN. Surgical treatment of deep venous insufficiency of the lower limb. *Surg Gynecol Obstet.* 1988;166:131.
227. Sun JM, Zhang PH. The substitute valve operation on the popliteal vein in the treatment of deep venous incompetence of the lower extremity. *Vasc Surg.*
228. Dalsing MD, Ricotta JJ, Wakefield T, et al. Animal models for the study of lower Extremity chronic venous disease: lessons learned and future needs. *Ann Vasc Surg.* 1998;12:487.
229. Neglen P, Raju S. Venous reflux repair with cryopreserved vein valves. *J Vasc Surg.* 2003;37:552.
230. Madden R, Lipkowitz G, Benedetto B, et al. Decellularized cadaver vein allografts used for hemodialysis access do not cause allosensitization or preclude kidney transplantation. *Am J Kidney Dis.* 2002;40:1240.
231. Teebken OE, Puschmann C, Aper T, et al. Tissue-engineered bioprosthetic venous valve: a long-term study in sheep. *Eur J Vasc Endovasc Surg.* 2003;25:305.
232. Garcia-Rinaldi R, Soltero E, Gaviria J, et al. Implantation of cryopreserved allograft pulmonary monocusp patch: to treat nonthrombotic femoral vein incompetence. *Tex Heart Inst J.* 2002;29:92.
233. Pavcnik D, Uchida BT, Timmermans HA, et al. Percutaneous bioprosthetic venous valve: a long-term study in sheep. *J Vasc Surg.* 2002;35:598.
234. Brountzos E, Pavcnik D, Timmersmans HA, et al. Remodeling of suspended small intestinal submucosa venous valve: an experimental study in sheep to assess the host cells' origin. *J Vasc Intervent Radiol.* 2003; 14:349.
235. Scultetus AH, Villavicencio JL, Gillespie DL, et al. The pelvic venous syndrome: analysis of our experience with 57 patients. *J Vasc Surg.* 2002;36:881.

SECTION O
PEDIATRICS

CHAPTER 106 ■ SURGICAL PHYSIOLOGY OF INFANTS AND CHILDREN

DAVID K. MAGNUSON

This chapter introduces a variety of physiologic issues relevant to the care of infants and children with surgical disease. Reviewed are some of the basic physiologic concepts that govern clinical management, delineating some of the differences between pediatric and adult patients. These differences may be merely quantitative when comparing adults with adolescents and older children. The distinction between neonates and older patients, however, is frequently of a more dramatic and qualitative nature. These differences are the consequences of two unique conditions: the functional immaturity of organ systems during the transition from fetal to neonatal life and the demands placed on the physiologic machinery of the neonate by the overriding priority of growth. Whereas homeostasis is a valid concept on a small scale, in a larger sense the concept of a "steady state" is paradoxical in the newborn infant. Virtually every physiologic function in the infant is influenced in some way by the exponential growth that occurs during the first year of life. That growth, and the metabolic activity it demands, is perhaps the single most important property that differentiates the neonatal patient from the adult.

GROWTH AND METABOLISM

Growth, Development, and Prematurity

The 40-week gestational period is divided by convention into an 8-week embryonic period and a 32-week fetal period. During the embryonic period, developmental events occur that transform a fertilized egg into a "preorganism" that comprises all the specialized tissues and organ systems required for future independent life. The subsequent fetal period is characterized by accelerated growth and continuous organ maturation, both of which are required to translate embryonic potential into biologic reality. Many of the congenital defects encountered in the practice of pediatric surgery have their beginnings in some developmental miscue during the embryonic period that prevents normal growth and maturation during the fetal period. At birth, the consequences of these antecedent events often are manifested by serious physiologic derangements.

Fetal maldevelopment is complicated frequently by prematurity, that is, entry into the extrauterine world before fetal growth and maturation have been completed. Most fetal growth and organ maturation occur in the third trimester, and so premature birth interrupts development at a time when the rate of biological change is most rapid. In many cases, prematurity is the direct consequence of intrauterine developmental abnormalities, such as those that produce polyhydramnios (excess amniotic fluid that results in increased uterine size and early labor). In others, prematurity occurs in an otherwise normal fetus and is the result of maternal factors. In both cases, prematurity causes significant morbidity by forcing the neonate to contend with extrauterine challenges using physiologic systems that are not yet prepared to do so and also forces the neonate to complete simultaneously a schedule of preprogrammed fetal tasks.

Although the "normal" gestational period is generally agreed to be 40 weeks, infants are considered to be full-term at 37 weeks. Neonates born before 37 weeks are referred to as *premature* or *preterm*. A normal-term birthweight is defined as 2,500 g or more. Infants born at less than 2,500 g are considered to be low birthweight, regardless of gestational age. More precise classifications include moderately low birthweight (1,500–2,500 g), very low birthweight (1,000–1,500 g), and extremely low birthweight (<1,000 g).

Mortality rates are directly related to both gestational age and birthweight. As neonatal support technologies continue to improve, survival is being attained at birthweights recently considered to be incompatible with life. The current thresholds for survival appear to be approximately 22 weeks' gestation and 350 g birthweight. Above this threshold, survival rates increase rapidly, achieving 50% survival at approximately 24 to 25 weeks' gestation and 700 g.[1] Continued gains in survival have come at an increasingly high cost of long-term morbidity.

The most common types of serious long-term morbidity resulting from prematurity are neurodevelopmental conditions (e.g., cerebral palsy, mental retardation, seizure disorders) and chronic lung disease.

Although virtually all premature infants are born at low birthweights, a distinction is drawn between those whose weights are appropriate for their gestational age and those who are *small for gestational age* (SGA). SGA infants are defined as those in the 10th percentile or less with respect to age-adjusted birthweight. Normal intrauterine growth is a sensitive indicator of fetal well-being. Infants who qualify as SGA, whether term or preterm, are presumed to have experienced some intrauterine event that has compromised development. This phenomenon, referred to as *intrauterine growth retardation* (IUGR), can be caused by a plethora of factors that either reduce oxygen and nutrient delivery to the fetus or result in their decreased utilization. These abnormalities include maternal factors (tobacco, alcohol, and drug use; malnutrition; systemic disease), fetal factors (congenital defects, genetic or chromosomal anomalies), and placental factors (vascular anomalies, placental infarction, placental separation).

Both prematurity and IUGR may have detrimental consequences for the newborn. Both groups are challenged by insufficient energy reserves, poor thermal insulation, and increased heat and water loss. The premature infant must confront the extrauterine world with physiologically immature organ systems but may have a good eventual outcome if properly supported. Prenatal development may have been otherwise normal but prematurely terminated by maternal factors. On the other hand, the full-term SGA infant may have functionally mature organ systems and not require extensive physiologic support. When IUGR is the result of maternal or placental factors, premature birth separates the fetus from those factors and often results in compensatory growth and a good prognosis. When IUGR results from fetal or genetic factors, however, a poor prognosis may be anticipated. In general, an SGA infant has a better prognosis than a premature infant of the same birthweight because physiologic immaturity is less pronounced in the former.[2]

The rapid somatic growth and maturation occurring during the last trimester continues into the postnatal period and accounts for many of the unique metabolic events and nutritional requirements of the newborn surgical patient. This explosive growth phase is regulated largely by growth hormone *(somatotropin)* and its peptide intermediates, insulinlike growth factors 1 (IGF-1) and -2, but it also is influenced by insulin and thyroid hormone. Recently defined mediators of growth and metabolic activity such as leptin and ghrelin have also been implicated in fetal and neonatal growth. Ghrelin, a 28-amino acid peptide produced by the stomach and intestinal tract and linked to appetite has been shown to be active in fetuses and may play a role in prenatal programming of behavioral activities such as sucking and swallowing in preparation for postnatal feeding. Ghrelin levels peak in late infancy and decline to puberty, coinciding with the rapid growth rate that characterizes early childhood.[3] Leptin, a hormone produced by adipocytes, also appears to regulate metabolicic rate and substrate utilization in fetuses and neonates. Both ghrelin and leptin stimulate the secretion of growth hormone.

The normal term baby will nearly double its birthweight by 4 months of age and will triple it by 1 year. The near-exponential rate of growth declines gradually thereafter until late adolescence. This pattern of growth is so constant in normal infants that significant departures from it are commonly the earliest indication of previously unrecognized disease. Any metabolic stress contributed by an acute disease or injury event will therefore be superimposed on the existing stringent demands for energy substrates.

As the neonate transitions to later infancy, childhood, and adolescence, its metabolic processes and responses gradually approximate those of the adult. As this transition represents a continuum, no clear delineation between these stages can be made. It is reasonable, however, to consider the metabolic responses of the neonate to starvation and stress as being qualitatively different from those of the adult, whereas those of older infants and children should be considered as only quantitatively different.

Basic Patterns of Energy Metabolism

In general, two basic patterns of energy metabolism are recognized: anabolic and catabolic. Anabolic processes characterize growth and involve the consolidation of nutrient substrates into structural and storage molecules. Catabolic processes involve the breakdown and redistribution of preexisting reserves to meet the short-term needs of specific tissues for specific substrates. Although persistent catabolism is pathologic and ultimately fatal, short-term catabolism is a necessary adaptive response to both starvation and stress.

The endocrine and cytokine environments that promote these two states are likewise distinct. Anabolic metabolism is mediated principally by insulin, IGF-1, and growth hormone. These mediators promote conversion of circulating glucose into glycogen *(glycogenesis)*, storage of excess carbohydrate as fat *(lipogenesis)*, and synthesis of new structural proteins from amino acids. The presence of available substrate and the absence of physiologic stress elicit a neuroendocrine environment conducive to these processes.

Catabolic metabolism is mediated by "counterregulatory" cytokines and hormones that have effects that are diametrically opposed to the anabolic mediators. These agents include tumor necrosis factor, interleukins, glucagon, cortisol, and catecholamines. These mediators promote an increase in glucose availability through hepatic glycogenolysis and gluconeogenesis and by inhibition of the peripheral effects of insulin on target organs. The objective of short-term catabolism is to generate adequate substrate for critical glucose-obligate tissues such as the brain, red and white blood cells, and renal medulla.

Gluconeogenesis requires a supply of three-carbon fragments that reenter the glycolytic pathway under conditions that favor the reverse flow of intermediates and the synthesis of glucose. These three-carbon fragments are supplied by amino acids from protein breakdown (especially alanine and glutamine) and by glycerol from the hydrolysis of triglycerides. An additional source of gluconeogenic substrate is the Cori cycle, in which lactate from anaerobic metabolism in compromised tissues (e.g., surgical or traumatic wounds) is transported to the liver and converted directly back to glucose.

Catabolic metabolism can be separated into two distinct patterns: simple starvation and the stress response. In simple starvation, the brain (which accounts for the greatest demand for glucose) undergoes a gradual process called *ketoadaptation*, in which receptors and enzymes are expressed that allow for the utilization of ketone bodies as fuel (Fig. 106.1). Fatty acid metabolism then is altered to allow for the diversion of some fatty acids away from oxidative energy production and into the production of ketone bodies. The increased production of ketone bodies *(ketogenesis)*, and their utilization by brain and myocardium, gradually reduces the demand for glucose and the degradation of visceral protein to gluconeogenic precursors.

In stress metabolism, however, the transition to the chronic starvation response of ketoadaptation is inhibited, and an ongoing requirement for glucose drives the continued breakdown of proteins to amino acids. Most of the amino acids produced by proteolysis during stress catabolism are rechanneled into gluconeogenesis (Fig. 106.2). The remainder is used

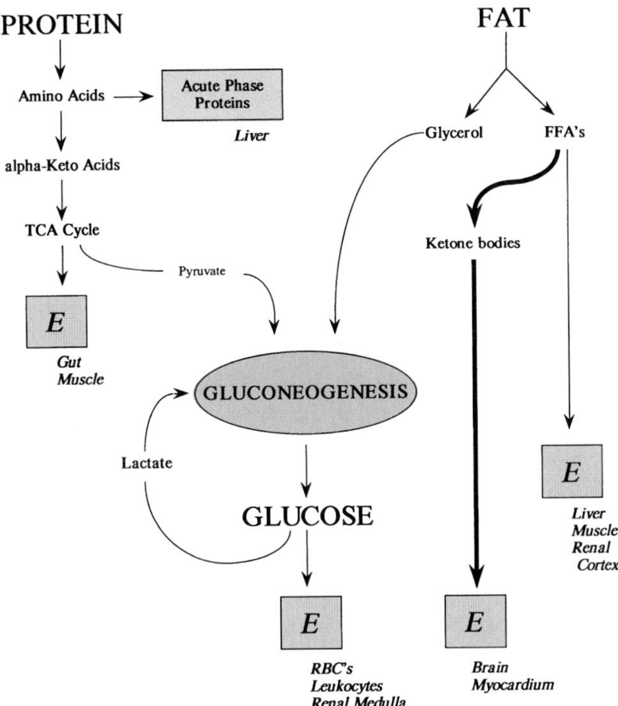

FIGURE 106.1 Energy production (E) during simple starvation. Ketoadaptation by brain and other glucose-obligate tissues allows free fatty acids (FFA) to be used for energy production and limits the requirement for protein catabolism to generate gluconeogenic precursors via the tricarboxylic acid (TCA) cycle. (From Magnuson DK, Maier RV. In: Eichelberger MR, ed. *Pediatric trauma: prevention, acute care, rehabilitation.* St. Louis: Mosby, 1993, with permission.)

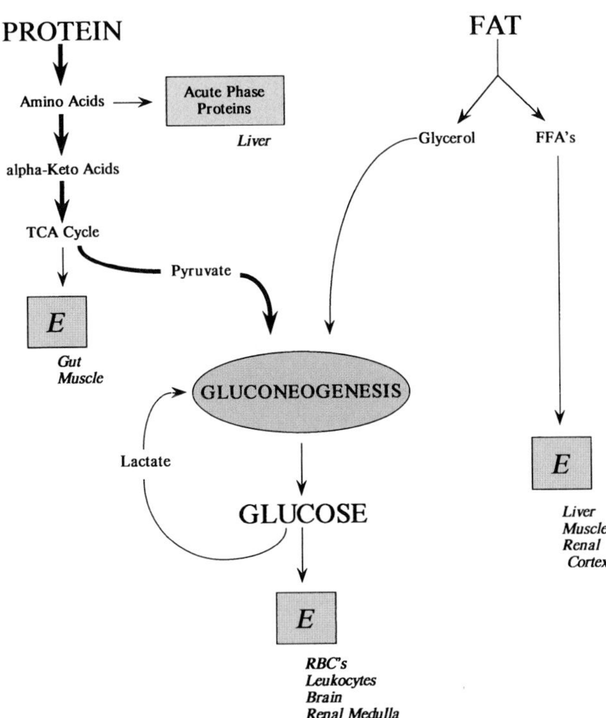

FIGURE 106.2 Energy production (E) during stress catabolism. Inhibition of ketoadaptation results in persistent protein catabolism to produce gluconeogenic precursors for glucose-obligate tissues. (From Magnuson DK, Maier RV. In: Eichelberger MR, ed. *Pediatric trauma: prevention, acute care, rehabilitation.* St. Louis: Mosby, 1993, with permission.)

in the synthesis of acute phase proteins, the synthesis of structural proteins for tissue repair, and for direct energy production by conversion to α-keto acids and entry into the tricarboxylic acid cycle. The mechanism of this inhibition is not well defined but most likely involves the persistence of stress-related neuroendocrine and cytokine mediators.

Metabolic Patterns in Neonates

The fetus utilizes glucose as its primary energy substrate. Transplacental movement of glucose by facilitated diffusion maintains fetal glucose levels at about 75% of maternal levels. At birth, the neonate experiences an abrupt withdrawal of placental support and plasma glucose levels fall. In response to hypoglycemia, secretion of catecholamines, cortisol, and glucagon mediates a shift to acute stress metabolism, relying initially on glycogenolysis because the capacity for gluconeogenesis is markedly decreased in newborns. Hepatic glycogen stores are limited in the neonate, and available glycogen reserves are depleted within 2 to 3 hours. Thereafter, gluconeogenesis is the sole supply of endogenous glucose until feeding provides new substrate. Protein and triglyceride breakdown provide direct energy substrates and gluconeogenic precursors, but fetal adipose and muscle mass are relatively modest, and this endogenous supply of fuel is also soon depleted. At this point, plasma glucose levels of 40 to 50 mg/dL are expected. As the infant begins to feed, absorption of exogenous substrates reverses the catabolic pattern, and an anabolic phase mediated by insulin begins. Plasma glucose levels usually rebound to 70 to 80 mg/dL by 3 days of age.

Neonatal demand for exogenous glucose is therefore immediate, and the provision of enteral or parenteral glucose soon after birth is critical. Not only does the neonate have a higher relative energy demand than older children and adults but a much greater proportion of the total caloric demand is generated by glucose-obligate tissues, and the availability of endogenous glucose from glycogen and gluconeogenesis is limited. Furthermore, fat stores and lipolytic pathways are both poorly developed at birth, requiring more metabolically versatile tissues to utilize glucose as well.

The metabolic priorities of the premature or SGA infant are identical to those of the full-term neonate, but striking differences in substrate stores and biochemical maturity make the preterm infant even more vulnerable to the risks of starvation and hypoglycemia. The time between birth and access to exogenous glucose tolerated by the preterm infant is inversely proportional to the degree of prematurity and may be measured in minutes instead of hours in extreme cases. In fact, one of the most striking differences between the normal-term infant and the preterm or SGA infant is the increased risk for hypoglycemic crisis in the latter: 50% in infants who are both premature and SGA.

Several factors contribute to this added vulnerability. Glycogen synthetase-b activity increases steadily in the last trimester. At 36 weeks' gestation, hepatic glycogen stores are only 30% of term levels; most glycogen deposition occurs after 36 weeks. Glycogen storage is therefore even more limited in preterm infants than in term infants, whose stores are depleted in a few hours. Additionally, skeletal muscle and fat constitute about 1% of body weight in a 1,000-g premature newborn, compared with about 15% in term infants, and so reserves of alternative energy substrates and gluconeogenic precursors are more limited as well. The ability to carry out β-oxidation of fatty acids and to produce ketone bodies also is depressed more severely in premature infants.[4] Ketogenesis is impaired even when given an exogenous source of lipid.

Thermoregulation

Temperature governs the kinetics of complex biochemical processes that have evolved to be maximally efficient within a narrow temperature range. Regulation of core body temperature has a high priority in the metabolic activities of the neonate and is a significant contributor to energy consumption. The fetal environment is one of thermal constancy: maternal and placental mechanisms maintain an optimal temperature for fetal development and obviate the need for fetal energy expenditure to regulate temperature. In fact, the net heat produced by fetal metabolic activity must be transferred away from the fetal environment to avoid a rise in temperature.

Thermal equilibrium is a balance between heat production and heat loss. Newborns, particularly premature newborns, are characterized both by diminished capacity for heat production and by increased vulnerability to heat loss compared with older children and adults. The surface area-to-volume ratio of the neonate is greater than that of older patients, and so the area across which heat can be lost is disproportionately large compared with the mass of metabolically active tissue generating energy. The body surface area-to-mass ratio averages approximately 250 cm^2/kg in the adult and may be as high as 1,400 cm^2/kg in the premature infant.[5] The paucity of insulating fat and the lower muscular activity level contribute to the problem.

Heat loss in the neonate occurs chiefly through four mechanisms. *Conduction* refers to the transfer of heat by direct contact with another static heat acceptor. The rate and direction of heat flow depend on the heat gradient and the heat capacities of the two objects. *Convection* refers to the transfer of heat from the skin surface to a fluid, such as air, which carries heat energy away from the body. *Radiation* is the loss of heat as electromagnetic energy in the infrared spectrum. *Evaporation* of water at the skin surface consumes heat energy by transforming water from liquid into gas.

The physical environment surrounding the sick neonate provides limitless opportunities for heat loss. Contact with cold surfaces, particularly wet sheets and blankets, is a principal cause of heat loss. The flow of cold air over exposed skin surfaces transfers heat by both convection and evaporation. Evaporation is exacerbated by radiant warmers and phototherapy lights. Premature infants with nonkeratinized epidermis are particularly susceptible to transepithelial water loss and may lose as much as 120 mL/kg of water each day. Evaporation consumes about 0.6 kcal/mL of water, which results in a metabolic cost of about 3 kcal/h. Means of reducing heat loss include the use of thermoneutral incubators and radiant warmers, removal of wet blankets and towels in contact with the skin, and covering the infant with impermeable barriers to evaporation.

Heat production is a consequence of the thermodynamic inefficiency of chemical reactions; wasted energy is dissipated as heat. Basal heat production normally results from both metabolic processes and muscular work. Two additional mechanisms have evolved to provide heat energy when basal heat production is insufficient to maintain thermal stability: shivering and nonshivering thermogenesis. The temperature threshold for initiating thermogenesis in adults is 26°C to 28°C, but it ranges from 32°C in term newborns to 35°C in preterm infants.

Shivering thermogenesis is the production of heat by rapid, cyclical skeletal muscle contractions. The heat produced as a by-product of this muscular "work" is transferred to blood circulating through the muscles and is redistributed throughout the body. Shivering thermogenesis is the major heat production mechanism in older infants, children, and adults.

Nonshivering thermogenesis is a process unique to the neonate and depends on the presence of brown adipose tissue (BAT). BAT is a unique tissue that is found transiently in the cervical, shoulder, axillary, and retroperitoneal regions of the neonate, and it is distinguished by its ability to generate metabolic heat by the inefficient metabolism of fatty acids. Sympathetic activation by cold stress causes norepinephrine to be released in BAT, bind to β-adrenergic receptors on adipocyte membranes, and initiate the hydrolysis of fatty acids. This process is facilitated by the presence of thyroid hormone. The fatty acids are shuttled into mitochondria where b-oxidation takes place. Normally, fatty acid oxidation is coupled to the phosphorylation of adenosine diphosphate (ADP) to adenosine triphosphate (ATP), preserving potential energy in the high-energy phosphate bond. In brown adipocytes, however, a unique peptide called *uncoupling protein 1 (UCP1)* "uncouples" the oxidative phosphorylation of ADP, allowing energy liberated by oxidation to be released as heat. The high density of mitochondria present in brown adipocytes attests to its role in heat production. Leptin also modulates UCP1, suggesting that BAT may play a role in overall energy balance regulation in infants.[6]

Nonshivering thermogenesis is the principal means of heat production in neonates, but it has severe limitations. It is a costly means of producing heat from a metabolic standpoint and rapidly depletes precious energy stores in term infants. Premature and SGA infants, with relatively reduced fat composition, are poorly equipped to use this strategy effectively. In term neonates, BAT constitutes about 10% of body fat and is gradually replaced by white adipose tissue in later infancy.

NUTRITIONAL SUPPORT

Energy Requirements

Neonates and children have significantly higher energy requirements than adults. These requirements diminish gradually throughout childhood, but they do not reach adult levels until physical maturity is attained. The two principal reasons for this discrepancy are a higher basal metabolic rate (BMR) and an additional energy requirement for growth. The total energy expenditure (TEE) comprises the BMR, the energy required to process substrates, energy for activity, energy for thermoregulation, and the energy cost of growth. The resting energy expenditure (REE), which may be substituted for BMR, is estimated to be 45 to 50 kcal/kg per day in term neonates and 50 to 60 kcal/kg daily in premature infants.[7,8] This compares with an REE of 20 to 25 kcal/kg daily in adolescents and adults.

Neonates and infants expend a much higher percentage of their total energy production on somatic growth than do older children. Growth consumes 35% to 40% of an infant's caloric intake during the first 6 months of life, a value that declines to about 5% at 2 years of age.[9] The energy cost of growth, which includes the energy used in new tissue synthesis plus the energy content of the synthesized tissue, approximates 40 to 50 kcal/kg daily in the neonate and progressively less in the older child. Add to these the energy requirements for nutrient processing, cold stress, and activity, and the baseline energy requirements for a term neonate are about 100 to 110 kcal/kg daily. The preterm neonate may require 120 kcal/kg/day or more to sustain growth. Caloric requirements for intravenous nutrition are perhaps 10% less because of the absence of obligate energy loss in fecal output.

The energy requirements of older infants and children gradually approach adult levels of 30 to 35 kcal/kg daily as BMR, cold stress, and rate of growth all decline with age (Table 106.1). This downward trend is moderated somewhat

TABLE 106.1

AGE-SPECIFIC ENERGY REQUIREMENTS

Age (y)	Energy requirement (kcal/kg/d)
0–1	120–90
1–7	90–75
7–12	75–60
12–18	60–30
>18	30

by an increase in energy expended in physical activity. Although many methods of estimating caloric requirements exist, the most straightforward estimation simply uses a weight-based calculation of caloric needs (Table 106.2).

It is important to recognize that these guidelines represent estimates for unstressed children. Energy requirements are altered in a variety of clinical settings commonly encountered in pediatric surgical patients. Both congenital heart disease and pulmonary disease can be associated with reduced pulmonary compliance and increased work of breathing, which can substantially increase energy expenditure. The healing of wounds related to major surgical procedures, trauma, and burns also increase caloric requirements. Sepsis, pancreatitis, and other conditions associated with generalized inflammatory activation may increase energy requirements dramatically.

It is equally important to appreciate that, in certain circumstances, caloric requirements in stressed children may be decreased because of changes in REE and the energy consumption related to growth. As opposed to older children and adults, infants actually may experience a decrease in REE during periods of postsurgical stress.[10,11] As previously discussed, the metabolic pattern that characterizes acute stress states is one of catabolism and growth postponement. This temporary growth inhibition is a consequence of, among other things, a cytokine and neuroendocrine environment that opposes the anabolic actions of insulin. Because 30% to 40% of a healthy neonate's caloric requirement represents energy required for growth, administration of the same caloric load to the stressed infant or child may result in significant overfeeding. The complications of overfeeding are not commonly recognized but include fluid overload, hepatic steatosis, and increased lipogenesis. Lipogenesis is associated with increased CO_2 production and is reflected in an increased respiratory quotient. Increased CO_2 production requires an increase in minute ventilation that may not be tolerated by critically ill neonates and children with respiratory disease and limited ventilatory reserve.

In the stressed infant or child, therefore, it may be prudent to reduce caloric administration transiently by as much as 25% to 30% during the acute stress phase, when growth is inhibited and the metabolic rate depressed. Determining when the metabolic environment has reverted back to one more permissive for growth and caloric utilization can be difficult. Direct calculation of the respiratory quotient by indirect calorimetry and measurement of nitrogen balance may be helpful in detecting a capacity to utilize more energy substrate. More frequently, however, a clinical judgment must be based on resolution of the hyperdynamic response to adrenergic stimulation or infection and the restoration of normal hemodynamics and fluid requirements.

TABLE 106.2

WEIGHT-SPECIFIC ENERGY REQUIREMENTS

Weight (kg)	Energy requirement (kcal/d)
0–10	100/kg
10–20	1,000 + 50/kg over 10
>20	1,500 + 20/kg over 20

Substrate Requirements

Carbohydrates

Carbohydrates constitute the major source of energy substrate for infants and older children, although they have a lower caloric density (3.4 kcal/g of intravenous hydrated dextrose, 4 kcal/g of enteral glucose) than either proteins (4 kcal/g) or fats (9 kcal/g). As discussed, glucose is the preferred fuel in a variety of tissues, including brain and blood cells. The obligate glucose consumption rate in neonates is about 4 to 6 mg/kg/min. This compares with a glucose utilization rate of about 1 mg/kg/min in adults. The discrepancy is explained in part by the fact that the neonatal brain accounts for 10% of body weight in the newborn and only 2% of body weight in adults. This contrast is even more striking in SGA infants whose brain growth is preserved in the face of generalized IUGR. In these infants, brain size and glucose consumption are even more disproportionately large. Most of the demand for glucose in newborns is for brain energy production, with relatively little remaining available for other tissues. Consequently, prolonged hypoglycemia may cause profound neurologic impairment.

The addition of small amounts of glucose to intravenous fluids prevents protein catabolism by providing a fuel source for glucose-obligate tissues and obviating gluconeogenesis. In adults, this protein-sparing glucose requirement is about 1 mg/kg/min and is conveniently provided by administering 5% dextrose in water (D_5W) intravenously at maintenance fluid rates. In neonates, who require 4 to 6 mg/kg/min of glucose to avoid protein catabolism, it is usually necessary to administer maintenance intravenous fluids as 10% dextrose in water ($D_{10}W$). The relatively higher fluid administration rate and dextrose concentration provide the increased glucose supply necessary to avert protein catabolism in the short term.

Normal plasma glucose values are variable and depend on gestational age, weight, and postnatal age. The definition of hypoglycemia is therefore somewhat fluid, but it is generally agreed that plasma glucose levels less than 35 mg/dL in term infants and less than 25 mg/dL in preterm infants constitute metabolic emergencies and require immediate intervention. Full-term infants of appropriate birthweight rarely develop hypoglycemia. Infants at risk for hypoglycemia include those who are premature, SGA infants, multiple gestations, infants of diabetic mothers, infants of toxemic mothers, and infants who are critically ill for some other reason. Neurologic injury resulting from an inadequate supply of substrate to brain cells depends on both the degree and duration of hypoglycemia. Signs of hypoglycemia are nonspecific and include respiratory irregularity, apnea, bradycardia, hypothermia, cyanosis, irritability, tremors, seizures, lethargy, hypotonia, and coma.

Mild, asymptomatic hypoglycemia usually can be managed simply by initiating early oral feedings with breast milk or $D_{10}W$. Severe or symptomatic hypoglycemia requires intravenous dextrose administration. Dextrose concentrations of 10% to 12.5% are the maximum that can be tolerated by peripheral veins; higher concentrations of dextrose require a central (e.g., umbilical) venous catheter. Treatment consists of administering glucose at a rate of 6 to 8 mg/kg/min

(3.6 to 4.8 mL/kg/h of $D_{10}W$). Profoundly hypoglycemic infants may require an initial dextrose "minibolus" of 200 mg/kg (2 mL/kg $D_{10}W$) over 1 to 2 minutes. The dextrose infusion rate then is increased by 2 mg/kg/min every 3 to 4 hours until stable plasma glucose levels of 40 to 50 mg/dL are achieved.

Most neonatal hypoglycemia is transient, allowing dextrose administration to be weaned down as feeding or intravenous nutritional support is begun. Persistent hypoglycemia, particularly in infants requiring more than 12 to 15 mg/kg/min of dextrose, may indicate a pathologic cause for hypoglycemia. Causes of pathologic hypoglycemia in neonates include hyperinsulinism (Beckwith-Wiedemann syndrome, nesidioblastosis or islet cell dysmaturation syndrome), congenital adrenal insufficiency, and other inborn errors of metabolism. In these circumstances, treatment options include corticosteroids, glucagon, epinephrine, somatostatin analogs, diazoxide, calcium channel blockade, intramuscular growth hormone, and near-total pancreatectomy.[12]

Fats

Lipids are the other main source of energy substrate. Nutrient lipids consist primarily of triglycerides—a glycerol backbone to which three fatty acids are esterified. During energy metabolism, the fatty acids are cleaved off the glycerol moiety and transported into mitochondria, where they undergo b-oxidation to produce energy stored in ATP. In addition to providing an energy source of high caloric density (9 kcal/g), lipids are essential for cell membrane structure, steroid hormones, the synthesis of inflammatory mediators such as prostaglandins and leukotrienes, and thermal insulation.

Most dietary triglycerides contain long-chain fatty acids 16 to 18 carbons long. Most fatty acids derived from animal sources have no double bonds within the carbon chain (saturated), whereas those derived from fish and vegetables have one or more double bonds (unsaturated). Because most fatty acids can be synthesized from carbohydrate precursors, there is no absolute dietary requirement for most fats as long as adequate calories are being provided from sugars. Two polyunsaturated fatty acids, linoleic and linolenic acid, are considered to be "essential" from a dietary standpoint because they cannot be synthesized *de novo*. Linoleic acid deficiency is marked by dryness and thickening of the skin, hair loss, and delayed wound healing. Linolenic acid deficiency has been associated with neurologic dysfunction, which suggests a role for linolenic acid in brain development.

Proteins

Although amino acids can be converted to their keto acid counterparts, enter the tricarboxylic acid cycle, and yield useable energy (4 kcal/g), they are ideally reserved for the synthesis of new structural and functional proteins. The need for protein precursors is particularly acute in the neonate who is undergoing accelerated somatic growth. As the infant ages and the rate of growth declines, the requirements for dietary protein diminish somewhat. Recommendations for protein requirements in infants and children are variable. Premature infants may require 3 to 4 g/kg each day, whereas term newborns require 2 to 3 g/kg each day, older infants 1.5 to 2 g/kg per day, and children and adolescents 1 to 1.5 g/kg daily. These recommendations are somewhat controversial given that healthy newborn infants on a breast milk diet maintain normal growth with an average protein intake of 1.5 to 2 g/kg daily.

Eight of the 20 amino acids are unable to be produced by enzymatic conversion of other existing amino acids and therefore must be obtained from dietary sources. These essential fatty acids are threonine, leucine, isoleucine, valine, lysine, methionine, phenylalanine, and tryptophan. Several other amino acids may be considered essential in the neonate because the specific enzyme systems for their conversion are consistently slow to mature in the postnatal period. These include histidine, tyrosine, cysteine, taurine, and possibly proline. Although clinical consequences of deficiencies in these amino acids have not been clearly defined, amino acid formulations designed for administration to adults may not contain them (especially cysteine and taurine), and specialized pediatric formulations supplemented with these amino acids are available.

Although not usually considered an essential amino acid, glutamine is of critical importance to many tissues and has been the subject of intense investigation.[13] Glutamine is produced from glutamate by the enzyme glutamine synthetase and has many physiologic functions. It participates in nitrogen transport in both the ammonia and urea cycles. It serves as a precursor for nucleic acid synthesis and an energy source in tissues with rapid cell proliferation. Intestinal epithelium is the primary consumer of glutamine, extracting a significant fraction from the circulation as well as the intestinal lumen. Within the continuously dividing enterocytes, glutamine is a necessary precursor to nucleic acid synthesis as well as the principal energy substrate. Maintenance of mucosal health and barrier function is directly dependent on the availability of glutamine for enterocyte metabolism.

Because glutamine synthetase is present in both infants and adults, and because glutamine is unstable in solution, this amino acid is not included in commercial amino acid formulations. During episodes of physiologic and metabolic stress, glutamine levels may fall despite the intravenous administration of other amino acids, suggesting a stress-induced alteration in glutamine synthesis. Intestinal mucosal atrophy and loss of barrier function may occur during prolonged periods of intestinal rest when only parenteral nutrition is administered. The addition of glutamine modified to increase stability in standard intravenous amino acid formulations, as well as enteral administration of glutamine-containing formulas in subnutritive quantities, are being investigated as strategies for improving mucosal function and promoting intestinal growth in infants and children with severe gut injury.

Types of Nutritional Support

Enteral Support

The provision of all fluids, electrolytes, and substrates through the gastrointestinal tract is the ultimate goal of nutritional therapy. Using the gastrointestinal tract, even if only for a fraction of the patient's needs, provides trophic substances and enteroendocrine stimulation for intestinal growth and development, maintains the integrity of intestinal barrier function, and mitigates against the cholestatic liver complications of prolonged gut rest. Enteral feeding is associated with significantly fewer complications than parenteral nutrition and can be administered at a much lower cost. Equally important, early institution of oral feeding is crucial for the maintenance of an intact suck and swallow reflex and the prevention of behavioral feeding aversion.

Breast milk is the optimal nutritional vehicle. Human milk is a complex mixture of macromolecules that evolves over time as the growing infant's needs change. The usable energy content of milk is divided almost equally between carbohydrates and lipids. The carbohydrate fraction is predominately lactose, but it includes more than 100 other oligosaccharides that have putative immunologic functions. A variety of lipids constitute the fat component, including both linoleic and linolenic acids. The protein content of human milk is relatively low compared with cow's milk and commercial formulas. As opposed to cow's milk, human milk has more whey than casein. The whey fraction includes many proteins, some with antibacterial functions, including the lactalbumins, albumin, lactoferrin, lysozyme, secretory immunoglobulin A (IgA), enzyme, growth factors, and hormones. In addition to these macromolecules, human milk contains a variety of cellular elements, including B- and T-lymphocytes, macrophages, and neutrophils.

When human breast milk is not available, a wide variety of commercial formulations are available from which to chose (Table 106.3). The nutritional compositions of these formulas are modeled on breast milk, but they differ with respect to the specific carbohydrate, protein, and fat content. Commercial formulas contain slightly more protein and less fat as a percentage of total calories than breast milk. Considerable variation in the specific nutritional components provides multiple options for optimizing nutrition in neonates with gastrointestinal derangements.

Most of the available formulas have a caloric density equal to that of human milk: 20 kcal/oz (0.67 kcal/mL). Formulas with higher caloric densities are available for infants with restrictions on fluid intake, or may be provided by fortifying standard formulas with polymeric glucose or other additives. Children between 6 months and 1 year of age may be transitioned to pediatric formulas with a higher caloric density of 30 kcal/oz.

The amount of formula required to supply adequate energy substrate to the growing infant can be estimated easily. Assuming an energy requirement of 110 kcal/kg daily, a feeding regimen of eight feedings per day, and a caloric density of 20 kcal/30 mL, the calculation of the required feeding volume can be reduced to a single "nutritional coefficient" of 22:

$$\text{Wt (kg)} \times 22 = \text{Volume of breast milk or formula required every 3 h}$$

This coefficient reduces to 7.3 for 24-hour continuous drip feedings.

A number of specialized formulas are available for infants with specific abnormalities of substrate absorption. The most important carbohydrate source for infants is lactose, the predominant disaccharide in human milk, which is hydrolyzed by intestinal lactase to glucose and galactose. Lactase and other disaccharidases are sensitive to changes in the villous environment and exhibit reduced activity in the setting of mucosal disease. Lactase is the most labile of brush-border enzymes, being among the first to exhibit decreased activity in disease and the last to increase during recovery. Inflammatory disorders that cause increased epithelial turnover result in a population of immature enterocytes with reduced lactase activity. Prolonged gut rest also results in reduced disaccharidase activity as a result of villous atrophy and mucosal loss.

Term infants with lactose intolerance may be given soy-based formulas that are lactose free. Premature infants have reduced intestinal brush-border enzyme activity as a result of epithelial immaturity, especially with respect to lactase, but they also have deficiencies in fat and protein absorption for the same reason. Premature-specific formulas provide carbohydrates largely as glucose polymers (corn syrup) with or without lactose. They also provide a fat mixture of long-chain and medium-chain triglycerides to improve fat absorption. In the extremely premature or stressed infant, formulations providing hydrolyzed proteins *(oligopeptides)* have advantages over those that contain complex, intact proteins. Formulas for premature infants also provide increased concentrations of various other components, such as calcium and phosphorous, to meet the needs of accelerated bone mineralization (a fetal task under normal circumstances).

Hypersensitivity to bovine protein antigens may cause inflammation of the gastrointestinal tract and malabsorption in some infants. Soy-based formulas are usually the initial option for infants with cow's milk protein allergy because the protein content derives exclusively from soy proteins. As many as 30% of these infants will develop hypersensitivity to soy proteins as well and may require the use of a formula containing only protein hydrosylates which are less allergenic than intact proteins.

Synthetic medium-chain triglycerides (MCTs) containing fatty acid moieties 8 to 10 carbons long are commercially available and have some advantages over long-chain triglycerides in certain clinical settings. MCTs are efficiently metabolized in the gut lumen to their constituent parts, are readily absorbed, and produce a nearly identical caloric yield. More importantly, they appear to have the capability of being transported directly into the enterocyte without prior degradation to glycerol and fatty acid. Hence, they offer the advantage of improved absorption in prematurity and other conditions that impair lipid digestion. These states include biliary obstruction (e.g., biliary atresia), bile salt insufficiency (e.g., ileal resection), pancreatic insufficiency (e.g., cystic fibrosis), and decreased absorptive surface area (e.g., short-gut syndrome). Because they bypass lymphatic absorption, they also may be useful in reducing lymphatic flow in treating chylous ascites and chylothorax. Because MCTs do not contain the essential fatty acids, periodic supplementation is necessary to avoid deficiency states.

Total Parenteral Nutrition

Few developments in clinical medicine have had a more profound impact on the survival of premature and critically ill neonates than the capability of administering hypertonic solutions of nutritional substrates by central venous catheter. The management of total parenteral nutrition (TPN) is complicated and covered more thoroughly elsewhere. Several issues related specifically to the management of TPN in infants and children are discussed here.

Indications for TPN depend on age, size, and clinical condition. In general, the younger the patient, the more intolerant of the effects of prolonged fasting. Although a healthy child or adolescent may tolerate a week or longer of inadequate nutrition, the infant and neonate are not so resilient. It is reasonable to consider initiating TPN in any neonate expected to fast for at least 2 to 3 days. Extremely premature neonates with multiple medical problems are commonly started on TPN within the first 2 days of life. Substrate concentrations are initially low and are gradually weaned up to calculated maintenance values over several days to avoid hyperglycemia and acidosis.

Estimations of caloric needs are made using the same assumptions discussed in the previous section. It is reasonable to divide total caloric requirements between carbohydrates and fats. The energy content of proteins should not be calculated to contribute to caloric requirements because the exogenous amino acids are expected to be used primarily for new protein synthesis. The appropriate distribution of calories between carbohydrates and fats may differ between individual patients, but in general fats should account for 40% to 50% of nonprotein calories, and carbohydrates usually account for 50% to 60%. Carbohydrates are administered as dextrose, and standard lipid emulsions containing essential fatty acids also are used. Although essential fatty acids can be supplied in adequate quantities with once-weekly lipid infusions, the high caloric density and low respiratory quotient characteristic of intravenous lipids make them attractive as a primary energy source for most neonates who may have difficulty handling large fluid and CO_2 loads.

TABLE 106.3

COMPOSITION OF SPECIALIZED INFANT FORMULAS (PER 100 mL)

Formula	Carbo	Grams	% kcal	Protein	gm	% kcal	Fat	Grams	% kcal	Osm	Uses
Human milk	Lactose	7.2	42	Casein 20% Whey 80%	1.1	6	Human	3.9	52	290	Infants
Cow's milk	Lactose	4.8	30	Casein 80%	3.4	21	Butterfat	3.4	49	260	Older Children
COW'S MILD BASED											
Enfamil 20 Similac 20 SMA	Lactose	7.3	43	Nonfat cow's milk	1.5	9	Coconut, soy oils	3.6	48	300	Healthy infants
SOY BASED											
Isomil	Corn syrup	6.9	41	Soy isolate	1.7	10	Coconut,	3.7	49	240	Lactose intolerance
Prosobee		6.7	40		2.0	12	soy	3.5	48	200	milk protein allergy
PREMATURE											
Enfamil premature	Corn syrup + lactose	7.4	44	Nonfat cow's milk	2.0	12	MCT 40% + coconut, soy	3.4	44	260	Premature infants
Similac special care	Cornstarch + lactose	7.2	42				MCT 50% + coconut, soy	3.7	47	250	
PROTEIN HYDROSYLATES											
Pregestamil	Corn syrup, cornstarch + dextrose	6.9	41	Hydrolyzed casein + cystein, tyrosine, tryptophan	1.9	11	MCT 60% + corn, safflower	3.8	48	320	Malabsorption
Nutramigen	Corn syrup. Cornstarch	7.4	44	Hydrolyzed casein + amino acid mix	1.9	11	Corn oil	3.4	45	320	
Alimentum	Tapioca starch + sucrose	6.9	41	Hydrolyzed casein	1.9	11	MCT 50% + corn, safflower	3.8	48	370	
ELEMENTAL DIET											
Neocate	Corn syrup	7.9	47	L-amino acids	2.1	12	Safflower, vegetable oils	3.1	41	342	Malabsorption
HIGH MCT											
Portagen	Corn syrup + sucrose, lactose	7.7	46	Sodium caseinate	2.3	14	MCT 85% + corn oil	3.1	40	220	Lymphatic leak

MCT, medium chain triglycerides.

Protein requirements in parenteral nutrition are age dependent because of the changing requirements for somatic growth. As discussed previously, premature infants typically require 3 to 4 g/kg daily, whereas term newborns require 2 to 3 g/kg daily, and older infants 1.5 to 2 g/kg daily. To promote efficient utilization of amino acids for protein synthetic purposes, the nonprotein calorie-to-nitrogen ratio should be 150:1 to 200:1. Special formulations, including amino acids thought to be essential specifically in neonates, are widely available. Pediatric requirements for electrolytes, fat- and water-soluble vitamins, and trace elements must be provided as well.

The administration of both enteral and parenteral nutrition involves many assumptions and estimations. One of the most important aspects of nutritional management, then, is monitoring the response to therapy. In the older child and adolescent, maintenance of weight is an important goal. In the rapidly growing neonate, measurable nonedema weight gain is the objective. A daily weight gain of about 0.5% to 1% is a reasonable goal (15 to 30 g daily in the average term neonate). Measurements of serum albumin, prealbumin, and transferrin are helpful in assessing protein synthetic status in the neonate, just as they are in the adult. Routine surveillance of serum electrolytes, plasma and urine glucose, and liver function studies are mandatory to recognize metabolic complications of TPN administration.

FLUID, ELECTROLYTE, AND RENAL PHYSIOLOGY

Fluid Compartments

Like the adult, but to a greater degree, the infant and child are composed primarily of water. This simple fact influences many clinical phenomena, ranging from fluid balance to the volume of distribution for electrolytes and drugs. The percentage of body weight that is water, as well as its distribution within physiologic compartments, is in a state of rapid flux during the fetal and neonatal period. Body fluid distribution approaches a steady state by approximately 1 year of age and remains reasonably constant thereafter.

The greatest changes in total body water (TBW) occur during fetal development. At 12 weeks' gestation, water constitutes 95% of fetal mass. This percentage declines to about 80% by 32 weeks' gestation and to 75% at term. Prematurity results in the birth of a fetus at a stage of rapid change in water content, a fact that needs to be appreciated when caring for the preterm surgical patient. A further decline in TBW occurs in a roughly linear fashion over the first year of life and reaches a plateau of about 65% by 1 year of age (Fig. 106.3).

Within the body, water is distributed between two main compartments: intracellular and extracellular. Although the extracellular compartment predominates early in fetal life, continued cellular proliferation and growth cause the intracellular and extracellular compartments to approach equivalence (about 40% each) at term. Postnatal diuresis of extracellular fluid causes the extracellular compartment to be reduced further within the first few weeks. Continued growth and fat deposition cause extracellular fluid to decline to about 25% at 1 year of age, whereas at the same time the intracellular compartment rises to a plateau of 40% to 45%.

The extracellular compartment is divided further into the interstitial and intravascular compartments. Generally, intravascular water accounts for only 25% of extracellular water, but this value is highly variable and depends on changeable factors, such as hematocrit and oncotic pressure. Blood volume itself is relatively high in the fetus because it includes blood circulating in the umbilical-placental vessels. At term, the normal fetal blood volume after cord occlusion is about 90 mL/kg (higher in premature infants). Blood volume declines gradually to 80 mL/kg in toddlers, 75 mL/kg in school-aged children, and 65 mL/kg in adolescents.

Fetal stress is often accompanied by the generalized accumulation of extracellular fluid, a condition referred to as *hydrops fetalis*. Fluid accumulates both as soft tissue edema and as effusions in the peritoneal, pleural, and pericardial spaces. This condition is readily diagnosed by prenatal ultrasound, which can detect cavitary fluid accumulations and quantify soft tissue edema by measuring the increased thickness of cervical soft tissues between the spine and the skin *(nuchal thickening)*.

The mechanism of fluid accumulation is ill defined but most likely involves hydrostatic forces related to *in utero* congestive heart failure and venous hypertension. A principal cause of hydrops fetalis is autoimmune hemolytic anemia secondary to maternofetal Rh antigen incompatibility *(erythroblastosis fetalis)*. The high fetal oxygen demand continues in the face of ongoing red cell destruction, resulting in a compensatory increase in cardiac output and the eventual development of high-output cardiac failure. Other causes of hydrops

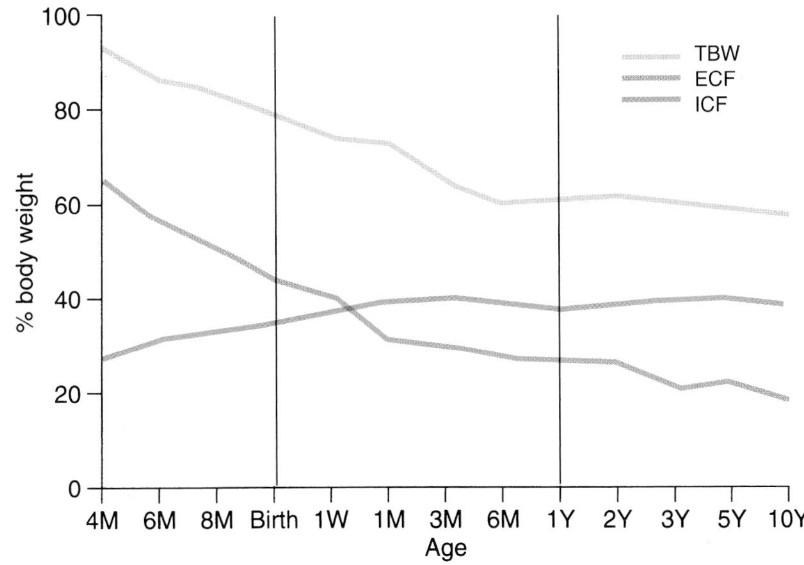

FIGURE 106.3 Changes in total body water distribution during prenatal and postnatal growth and development. (After Friis-Hansen B. Changes in body water compartments during growth. *Acta Pediatr.* 1957;46[suppl 110]:1, with permission.)

PEDIATRICS

fetalis also involve congestive heart failure: fetal arrhythmias, structural heart defects, mediastinal shift resulting from diaphragmatic hernia or developmental lung anomalies, and arterial "steal" syndromes caused by fetal tumors such as giant sacrococcygeal teratomas and hemangiomas. These later causes of fetal extracellular fluid accumulation are referred to as *nonimmune hydrops* and carry a poor prognosis. About 80% of fetuses identified with this condition die *in utero*, and only half of those that are liveborn survive beyond the neonatal period.

Renal Physiology

Maintenance of water and electrolyte balance within the body's fluid compartments is the responsibility of the kidney. Renal function in infants and children relies on the same physiologic principles as adults, but it differs in the relative capacities to excrete and conserve water and solutes. These differences mainly affect infants and small children; by the age of 2 years, a child's renal function approaches that of the adult.

Renal function depends on two interrelated processes: the glomerular ultrafiltration of plasma and the tubular modification of the ultrafiltrate by selective reabsorption of water and solutes. Glomerular filtration is a passive event in which water and low–molecular-weight solutes percolate through the glomerular capillary membrane into the glomerular lumen. About 20% of renal plasma flow is filtered through the glomeruli in this fashion. The glomerular filtration rate (GFR) is dependent on renal blood flow, which is autoregulated by a tubuloglomerular feedback mechanism between specialized renal tubular cells *(macula densa)* and proximal arterioles. Modification of the ultrafiltrate occurs in the tubular system and collecting ducts through active transport of some solutes and passive diffusion of water and other solutes. A detailed description of these physiologic events is beyond the scope of this chapter, but certain generalizations can be made regarding age-related differences in renal function.

Urine output in the immediate postnatal period is characterized by three distinct phases: prediuretic, diuretic, and postdiuretic. The *prediuretic phase* occupies the first 24 hours and is marked by a fixed, low urine output of 1 mL/kg/h or less. Urine output during the second and third day of life increases dramatically, to 5 to 10 mL/kg/h, and is largely insensitive to exogenous fluid administration. Much of the rapid reduction in TBW seen in the postnatal period occurs during this diuretic phase. The unloading of excess water has an extremely high priority and is observed even in premature infants.[14] Beginning on the fourth day of life, urine output begins to display an appropriate responsiveness to fluid balance.

Renal blood flow (RBF) and GFR are both markedly reduced in the neonate because of elevated renovascular resistance. In the newborn, RBF represents only 6% of cardiac output, compared with 25% in the older child and adult. As resistance falls, RBF increases by fourfold in the first 3 months and doubles again to adult levels (indexed to body surface area) by 1 or 2 years of age. Changes in GFR correspond roughly to those in RBF. Because of this pre-exisiting diminished RBF and GFR, and the delicate balance between vasconstrictive and vasodilatory forces, neonates are highly susceptible to the development of renal insufficiency under certain circumstances. Both acute tubular necrosis (ATN) and vasomotor nephropathy (VMNP) can occur secondary to reductions in renal perfusion because of hypovolemia, hypotension, sepsis, neonatal asphyxia, and administration of indomethicin and angiotensin-converting enzyme inhibitors. Treatment mainstays include dopamine administration for infants with congestive heart failure and furosemide in infants with indomethicin- induced ATN.

Tubular function also varies according to age. The ability to concentrate urine is dependent on mechanisms that cause reabsorption of free water in renal collecting ducts to regulate serum osmolarity. Free water absorption is governed by the actions of antidiuretic hormone (ADH), which is secreted by the posterior pituitary in response to increased serum osmolarity and decreased blood pressure, and which acts on tubular epithelium in the collecting ducts to increase permeability to water. Water diffuses out of the ductal lumen and into the interstitium and capillary network, as directed by the concentration gradient.

Although the capacity to produce ADH is fully developed both in preterm and term infants, the sensitivity of tubular epithelium to ADH appears to be diminished in all neonates. The mechanism for reduced sensitivity appears to be related to the diminished production and increased degradation of prostaglandin E_2. On stimulation by ADH, renal collecting duct cells increase the expression of aquaporin-2 transmembrane water channels, increasing the translocation of water from the collecting duct lumen to the interstium. The expression aquaporin-2 in neonates is diminished as well.[15] These differences account for the fact that infants have a reduced capability to excrete concentrated urine relative to adults. The neonatal kidney can concentrate urine to a maximum of 500 to 600 mOsm/L. By 1 year of age, maximum concentrating capacity reaches about 1,000 mOsm/L, and by 2 years of age, the concentrating capacity attains adult levels of 1,200 to 1,400 mOsm/L. In contrast, the ability of the neonate to excrete free water and to produce dilute urine appears to exceed that of the adult. Maximal urine dilution capacity in the preterm and term neonate is about 30 to 50 mOsm/L, compared with 70 to 100 mOsm/L in the adult.

The other primary tubular function is the regulation of sodium balance, which in turn determines TBW and affects intravascular volume. Sodium regulation is governed largely by two counterregulatory hormones: aldosterone and atrial natriuretic peptide (ANP). Aldosterone is secreted by the adrenal cortex in response to activation of the renin angiotensin system, and it acts on renal tubular epithelium to increase active sodium resorption and passive water resorption. Active sodium resorption is tightly coupled to potassium excretion. ANP is secreted in response to atrial distension and increased levels of ADH, catecholamines, and corticosteroids, and it promotes increased sodium excretion and water diuresis through enhanced GFR and reduced sodium resorption.

Both these systems appear to be active in the neonate. The term infant is able to conserve sodium effectively, like the adult, but it appears to be less effective in excreting an excess sodium load. In contrast, the preterm infant is a "salt waster," and demonstrates a marked inability to conserve sodium in the face of sodium restriction. Additionally, because sodium excretion occurs at an increased but relatively fixed rate in preterm infants, these patients are unable to excrete a sodium load by increasing sodium clearance beyond the preprogrammed rate. This relative inability to regulate sodium excretion makes the neonate particularly susceptible to changes in intravascular and extravascular volume resulting from inappropriate fluid management.

Sodium handling can be expressed in terms of the fractional excretion of sodium (FE_{Na}) or the percentage of sodium filtered that is actually excreted in the urine. Calculation of FE_{Na} requires measurement of plasma (P) and urine (U) concentrations of both sodium (Na) and creatinine (Cr) (sodium excretion is indexed to creatinine excretion because creatinine is not reabsorbed):

$$FE_{Na}\% = (U_{Na})(P_{Cr})/(U_{Cr})(P_{Na}) \times 100$$

Under normal circumstances, the FE_{Na} for both term infants and adults is 1% or less. Premature infants normally have elevated FE_{Na} values of 3% to 9%. Calculation of the FE_{Na} can be helpful in assessing the cause of oliguria by determining whether renal tubular function indicates increased sodium resorption. Recent diuretic use invalidates the FE_{Na} as an indicator of tubular function. Oliguria associated with an appropriately low FE_{Na} implies renal hypoperfusion. Oliguria associated with an abnormally high FE_{Na} (>1 in term infants, >3 in preterms) indicates inappropriate sodium excretion and suggests a renal parenchymal cause for the oliguria (e.g., ischemic acute tubular necrosis).

Fluid and Electrolyte Management

Neonates and young children are exquisitely sensitive to small changes in body chemistry and do not have mature homeostatic mechanisms to compensate for rapid changes in fluid and electrolyte flux and to maintain internal balance. Additionally, the requirements for chemical homeostasis in the neonate are superimposed on a background of ongoing change. Iatrogenic alterations of body chemistry in the child are therefore quickly and easily produced by inattention to the details of fluid and electrolyte administration, causing impairments of cardiovascular, pulmonary, neurologic, and gastrointestinal function.

The systematic approach to fluid and electrolyte management requires an estimate of maintenance requirements, which then are adjusted to take into account both preexisting imbalances and abnormal ongoing losses. Once therapy is initiated, frequent reassessment and readjustment are necessary to ensure that the patient is responding as initially predicted. This involves documenting reversal of the symptoms and signs of dehydration, correction of any electrolyte or acid-base abnormalities, and normalization of urine output.

When normal renal function is present, the most reliable and easily measured indicator of adequate hydration is urine output. In the adult, the production of urinary output at a rate of 0.5 mL/kg/h (30 to 40 mL/h) is adequate to excrete a normal renal solute load, given the concentrating capacity of the adult kidney. Because the immature kidney has diminished concentrating capacity compared with that of the adult, and because the pediatric solute load requiring excretion is relatively higher owing to the increased requirements for energy metabolism and growth, normal urinary outputs in children are higher. A desirable urine output in preterm infants is 3 to 4 mL/kg/h, dropping to 2 mL/kg/h in neonates and infants, and 1 mL/kg/h in toddlers and school-age children.

Maintenance Requirements

Maintenance fluid and electrolyte requirements are those required to replenish normal, anticipated losses. Obligate fluid losses can be estimated by considering water lost in the excretion of solutes in the urine, excretion of stool, transepithelial water and sweat lost by evaporation, water lost through respiration, water utilized in anabolic metabolism for growth, and water gained through oxidation of nutrient substrates. Obviously, the actual "maintenance" fluid requirements in individual patients will vary widely according to the variables listed, but certain generalizations can be helpful in estimating requirements and initiating therapy.

Maintenance fluid requirements are related primarily to patient size and can be estimated by the Holliday-Segar method (Table 106.4). Many neonates, however, will require much higher maintenance fluid volumes (100 to 150 mL/kg daily) as a result of increased obligatory losses from a variety of causes. Increased transepithelial losses occur with fever, the use of radiant warmers, exposure to phototherapy for hyperbilirubinemia, and in premature infants with thin, nonkeratinized skin.

TABLE 106.4

HOLLIDAY-SEGAR METHOD FOR ESTIMATING FLUID REQUIREMENTS

Weight (kg)	Fluid requirement (mL/d)
0–10	100/kg
10–20	1,000 + 50/kg over 10
>20	1,500 + 20/kg over 20

Neonates with tachypnea or those undergoing mechanical ventilation may have increased lung water loss despite inspired gas humidification. It is common practice to reduce the fluid volumes for the first 2 to 3 days of life to about 70% of maintenance to accommodate the obligatory diuresis of extracellular fluid.

Maintenance requirements of sodium are about 2 to 3 mEq/kg daily in term infants and children. This value may be somewhat higher in premature infants who cannot conserve sodium as effectively. Potassium requirements are also approximately 2 mEq/kg daily. Requirements for exogenous calcium are uncommon in older infants and children with adequate skeletal stores, but calcium supplementation may be necessary in the premature infant with little skeletal ossification, particularly in those with cardiac disease, and in all children receiving prolonged TPN. As discussed in the preceding section, glucose is administered along with maintenance fluids to provide sufficient caloric support to meet the needs of glucose-obligate tissues and to prevent protein catabolism for gluconeogenesis.

Taking these requirements into consideration, maintenance fluids composed of one-fourth normal saline in 10% dextrose (D_{10}1/4NaCl) should be appropriate for most healthy neonates. Half-normal saline in 10% dextrose may be required in the premature infant. After the infant transitions into the postnatal diuretic phase on the second or third day of life, 10 to 20 meq/L of KCl may be added to replenish obligate potassium losses and avoid hypokalemia. Depending on prior nutritional status and ongoing illness, it may be appropriate to reduce glucose intake to 5% dextrose after 1 to 2 weeks.

Preexisting Imbalances

Frequently, maintenance fluid administration must be superimposed on a significant preexisting deficit or excess. A complete history and physical examination are invaluable in detecting evidence of fluid imbalance and understanding its cause. Protracted vomiting or diarrhea, copious enterostomal output, chronic diuretic therapy, mechanical ventilation, phototherapy, and the like are all clues to extraordinary fluid losses. Physical examination is paramount in assessing current fluid status in all children. Because of the absence of comorbidity in most cases, physical signs of volume status are frequently more reliable in children than in adults.

Signs of both intravascular and extravascular fluid imbalance should be sought. Signs of extravascular fluid deficit, which are apparent with mild to moderate dehydration (<10%), include poor skin turgor, recessed eyes, sunken or soft fontanelle, dry mucous membranes, absence of tears, and orthostatic hypotension and tachycardia. Signs of intravascular fluid deficit, which usually indicate more severe dehydration (>10%), include resting tachycardia and hypotension, oliguria, delayed capillary refill, reduced extremity temperature, thready or absent peripheral pulses, and altered mental status.

Signs of intravascular volume depletion usually indicate a need for intravenous resuscitation, which is usually initiated before proceeding with maintenance therapy. Isotonic crystalloid resuscitation with serial boluses of lactated Ringer's solution (10 to 20 mL/kg) is usually appropriate and followed by careful assessment of the response to therapy. For dehydration associated with hyponatremia and hypochloremia, normal saline boluses may be preferable. In most conditions, however, repeated boluses of saline may be associated with iatrogenic hypernatremia and a normal anion gap metabolic acidosis resulting from hyperchloremia with a compensatory decrease in serum bicarbonate anion.

Preexisting fluid excesses are encountered less frequently in children, but it is important to recognize them to avoid exacerbating the underlying condition by instituting ill-advised maintenance therapy. Fluid excesses occur most frequently as a result of iatrogenic mismanagement, but they also may be seen in acute renal failure and congestive heart failure. Signs may include peripheral and pulmonary edema, hypertension, and increased heart size on chest radiography. Obviously, maintenance therapy may need to be postponed until euvolemia is achieved through diuresis.

Ongoing Losses: Body Secretion Compositions

Before a final strategy can be established, it is important to anticipate and account for the presence of extraordinary ongoing fluid losses. These losses usually result from increased gastrointestinal losses caused by nasogastric suction, enterostomal output, diarrhea, pancreatic or biliary drainage, or drainage of chylous ascites or chylothorax. Another common, although "occult" cause of ongoing fluid loss is the unavoidable sequestration of extracellular fluid in regions of surgical, inflammatory, or traumatic injury, often referred to as *third spacing*.

Because gastrointestinal secretions from various levels of the gastrointestinal tract have differing electrolyte profiles, they are most safely replaced on an equal volume (mL per mL) basis with fluid of similar composition. This can be accomplished by periodically measuring the electrolyte composition of the lost fluid or by estimating the composition according to known values (Table 106.5). In practice, upper gastrointestinal secretions in the setting of paralytic ileus or mechanical obstruction frequently approach isotonicity and may be safely replaced with lactated Ringer's solution as long as careful monitoring of serum electrolytes is maintained. Pancreatic, biliary, and some ileostomy-related fluids are safely replaced with 0.45% NaCl supplemented with sodium bicarbonate at a concentration of 25 to 50 mEq/L. Chylous drainage may require the addition of albumin to avoid a progressive decrease in serum oncotic pressure over time. Third-space losses are best replaced with lactated Ringer's solution administered by intermittent bolus (10 to 20 mL/kg), because the exact rate of fluid loss is not measurable and adequacy of resuscitation can be judged best by physiologic response.

Specific Examples

Abnormalities of Sodium Concentration

Changes in serum sodium concentration reflect changes in free water balance. Mild hyponatremia (serum sodium of 125 to 135 mEq/L) is a common electrolyte abnormality in children and is seen frequently in postoperative patients with excessive ADH secretion in response to perceived intravascular volume depletion. It is also seen in patients with chronic conditions associated with fluid retention, such as cirrhosis, nephrotic syndrome, and congestive heart failure. Severe, acute hyponatremia (serum sodium <120 mEq/L) usually is associated with volume contraction from hypertonic fluid loss, as can occur with vomiting, diarrhea, or excessive stomal output.

Acute hyponatremia can cause severe neurologic symptoms, including headache, nausea, vomiting, lethargy, seizure activity, and coma. These symptoms are referred to as *water intoxication* and result from diffusion of water into relatively hypertonic brain cells, causing cerebral edema and intracranial hypertension. Treatment of severe or symptomatic hyponatremia involves administration of hypertonic saline (3% NaCl) over 30 to 60 minutes to correct serum sodium to about 125 mEq/L, followed by a more gradual elevation of serum sodium levels to normal over the ensuing 24 to 48 hours. The sodium deficit can be calculated by using a volume of distribution for sodium of 0.6:

$$\text{Sodium deficit} = [\text{Na}^+_{\text{target}} - \text{Na}^+_{\text{measured}}] \times \text{weight (kg)} \times 0.6$$

Hyponatremia of a more chronic, gradual nature should be corrected more slowly, particularly if asymptomatic. When hyponatremia develops gradually, compensatory loss of osmotic agents from brain cells prevents water intoxication. Rapid normalization of serum sodium levels may therefore cause a rapid fluid shift out of compensated brain cells, occasionally causing permanent neurologic injury. This is referred to as *central pontine myelinosis (demyelination)* and can manifest as quadriparesis or pseudobulbar palsy. Mild, chronic hyponatremia in conditions associated with fluid retention usually can be corrected with free water restriction alone.

Hypernatremia is an uncommon electrolyte abnormality in children. Neurologic symptoms are related to brain-cell dehydration and shrinkage, causing disruption of bridging veins

TABLE 106.5

COMPOSITION OF BODY FLUIDS

Source	Na* (mEq/L)	K* (mEq/L)	Cl⁻ (mEq/L)	HCO⁻ (mEq/L)	Protein (g/dL)	Suggested replacement
Gastric	20–80	5–20	100–150	—	—	0.45% NaCl + 10 mEq/L Cl
Pancreatic	120–140	5–15	40–80	115	—	LR or 0.45% NaCl + 50 mEq/L $NaHCO_3$
Bile	120–140	5–15	80–120	100–115	—	LR or 0.45% NaCl + 50 mEq/L $NaHCO_3$
Ileostomy	45–135	3–15	20–115	30–50	—	LR or 0.45% NaCl + 25 mEq/L $NaHCO_3$
Diarrhea	10–90	10–80	10–110	30–50	—	LR or 0.45% NaCl + 25 mEq/L $NaHCO_3$
Pleural or peritoneal	140	5	100	25	6–8	LR 5% albumin or plasmanate

LR lactated Ringer's solution.

and intracranial hemorrhage. Recommendations for correction include calculation of the free water deficit and slow correction with D_5W over 24 to 48 hours. As a result of the production of cytoplasmic osmotic substances *(ideogenic osmoles)* by brain cells to offset increased extracellular sodium concentration, chronic hypernatremia is usually well tolerated and should be corrected gradually to avoid precipitating acute cerebral edema.

Abnormalities of Acid-Base Status

Metabolic acidosis can be categorized as having an increased anion gap or normal anion gap. The causes of an increased anion gap metabolic acidosis in children are the same as in adults: lactic acidosis or ketoacidosis accounts for most cases. Their implications and management in children do not differ from that in the adult. Normal anion gap metabolic acidosis, however, is much more common in infants than in older children and adults. The immature kidney is less efficient both at bicarbonate reclamation in the proximal tubule and at hydrogen ion excretion in the distal nephron. These functional deficits are considered a transient form of renal tubular acidosis type II (proximal), which is one of a heterogeneous group of disorders characterized by abnormal hydrogen ion and bicarbonate handling in the nephron. The vast majority of neonates outgrow this condition in the first year of life.

One of the most commonly encountered acid–base abnormalities in infants is metabolic alkalosis associated with hypochloremia, hypokalemia, and volume contraction. This pattern is typical of that seen in infants with protracted vomiting resulting from hypertrophic pyloric stenosis. Persistent vomiting of acidic gastric secretions causes the progressive depletion of both hydrogen and chloride ions. The loss of hydrogen ions results in alkalosis. Hypochloremia is associated with an increase in serum bicarbonate ion to maintain electroneutrality and with a decrease in renal hydrogen ion excretion. Renal tubular sodium resorption increases to reverse extracellular volume contraction. Sodium resorption is coupled with excretion of potassium. This potassium loss is facilitated by systemic alkalosis, which drives hydrogen ions out of renal tubular cells in exchange for potassium, raising renal tubular availability of potassium. As potassium becomes progressively depleted, a shift to hydrogen excretion occurs, resulting in the creation of urine with an inappropriately low pH: paradoxical aciduria. Treatment is directed at restoring extracellular fluid volume, chloride and potassium ions, and correcting the underlying pathology.

RESPIRATORY PHYSIOLOGY AND SUPPORT

Pulmonary Development

Abnormal or incomplete pulmonary development accounts for much of the clinical pathophysiology observed in infants with respiratory distress syndrome, bronchopulmonary dysplasia, and pulmonary hypoplasia related to congenital diaphragmatic hernia or cystic adenomatoid malformation. All these conditions manifest physiologic disturbances related to immature or altered development of the tracheobronchial tree, pulmonary vasculature, or alveolar parenchyma. A general knowledge of normal lung development is therefore necessary to understand these pathologic entities and their management.

Normal lung development can be described as occurring in roughly five phases. The *embryonic phase* begins in the third week of gestation, when a ventral diverticulum appears in the proximal foregut. This lung bud grows caudally, undergoing a series of bir… the lobar a… comprise e… epitheliun… bud bran… ate into… This pha…

The… and is… the pri… airwa… appea… phou… bror… diff… sue… co… tic… complete.

The *canalicular p*… characterized by development o… of the lung parenchyma. Primitive epithelia… into more complex groupings, interstitial tissue dimin… and capillary ingrowth occurs. Alveolar epithelial cells differentiate into type I and II pneumocytes. Type I pneumocytes make up the alveolar wall and have a flattened morphology with scant cytoplasm, which is appropriate for the diffusion interface between the alveolar lumen and the capillary blood. Type II pneumocytes contain cytoplasmic lamellar bodies that identify these cells as future surfactant producers. A considerable body of evidence suggests that type I pneumocytes differentiate from existing type II pneumocytes. The earliest time at which functional gas exchange is possible is at the end of the canalicular phase.

The *terminal saccular phase* follows the canalicular phase at 24 weeks and lasts until the end of gestation. Two principal events occur during this time: (a) further morphologic change in the gas-exchange units with thinning of the interstitium and increased exposure of capillaries to the epithelial interface and (b) production of surfactant in preparation for extrauterine life. At this stage, each capillary is exposed to only one respiratory surface.

At birth, each lung contains approximately 20 million immature gas-exchange units, referred to as *terminal sacs.* In the postnatal *alveolar phase,* these structures proliferate and mature, reaching 300 million mature alveoli by the time the child is 8 years old. The terminal sacs multiply in number and mature morphologically. During this final phase, the respiratory membrane thins out further and presents more surface area to the capillary network. In the mature alveolus, each capillary is exposed simultaneously to at least two alveolar surfaces. After the end of this phase, when the child is 8 years of age, further lung growth occurs only by increasing individual alveolar size.

Apoptosis, the process of programmed cell death without inflammation, plays an important role in both prenatal and postnatal lung development. As the airway epithelium proliferates into the mesenchym, apoptosis is involved in the formation of branch points. As the airways develop further, mesenchymal apoptosis is necessary for the thinning out of the interstitial connective tissue and the creation of the blood–alveolar interface. Apoptosis is also involved in the consolidation of the micorvascular network into a single capillary layer between alveoli. Apoptosis in the developing lung appears to be up-regulated by transforming growth factor β and insulinlike growth factor, and down-regulated by nitric oxide.[16]

Lung growth during prenatal development appears to be linked to the secretion of fetal lung liquid. Fetal breathing movements provide for amniotic fluid flow into and out of the pears to be outward, how- ecreted into the airway and atory cycle. The effect of lung be one of growth stimulation, ositive distending pressure in the e mechanism by which physical dis- liferation or apoptosis is referred to as . This process appears to depend on cell anges in cell-cell and cell-matrix adhesion, uced into cytoskeletal changes and activation kinases.

lmonary Physiology in the Neonate

Lung Volumes

otal lung capacity comprises four distinct lung volumes: *tidal* volume, *inspiratory* and *expiratory reserve* volumes, and *residual* volume (Fig. 106.4). Residual volume is the volume of gas left in the lung after complete, forced expiration. The sum of the three lung volumes above residual volume (expiratory reserve, tidal, and inspiratory reserve) is the *vital capacity*, or the maximal volume of gas that can be voluntarily inspired or expired. Two functional parameters with great relevance to the physiologic management of lung pathophysiology are the functional residual capacity (FRC), which is the total volume of gas remaining in the lung after passive expiration during tidal breathing when alveolar pressure has equilibrated to atmospheric pressure, and the closing capacity (CC), which is the volume below which small conducting airways and alveoli begin to collapse.

Alterations in FRC occur in many pathologic states and significantly impact the efficiency of gas exchange. Normally, FRC exceeds CC, and alveoli in most regions of the lung remain open for gas exchange during tidal breathing. In disease states in which FRC is reduced, usually because of diminished compliance, FRC may drop below CC, causing regional atalectasis and impaired gas exchange. Common conditions associated with reduced FRC include respiratory distress syndrome (RDS), adult respiratory distress syndrome (ARDS), cardiogenic pulmonary edema, pneumonia, and postoperative hypoventilation caused by pain and splinting. Management focuses on recruiting collapsed alveoli by restoring and maintaining a higher FRC. This usually entails applying positive intraalveolar distending pressure in the form of positive end-expiratory pressure (PEEP) or continuous positive airway pressure (CPAP).

Mechanical Properties and Their Effects on Ventilation

The bulk flow of gas can be described by the simple equation:

$$\Delta P = VR$$

where ΔP is the pressure gradient, V is volume flow per unit time, and R is resistance. The mechanical properties that govern clinically important aspects of lung ventilation include compliance, elastic recoil, and airway resistance. Compliance describes the distensibility of lung tissue and reflects the energy required to effect a volume change. *Compliance* is defined as the change in lung volume per unit change in pressure: $\Delta V/\Delta P$, with higher values signifying greater distensibility. Dynamic compliance (C_{dyn}) uses peak inspiratory pressure (PIP) in the calculation, whereas static compliance (C_{st}) uses plateau inspiratory pressure; hence, C_{dyn} is always lower than C_{st}. From a clinical standpoint, compliance is a critical determinant of lung volume, which in turn determines the efficiency of ventilation/perfusion matching and gas exchange. Conditions that reduce compliance make it more difficult to maintain volumes above closing capacity and therefore promote atalectasis. Low compliance states are caused by increased structural wall tension (edema or fibrosis), increased alveolar surface tension (surfactant deficiency), or decreased alveolar radius (reduced FRC).

Compliance is the inverse of *elastic recoil,* defined as the tendency for stretched tissue to return to its prestretched state. Whereas elastic recoil depends in part on intrinsic properties of lung and chest wall tissue structure, the elastic recoil of lung parenchyma is closely related to alveolar wall tension. Wall tension tends to cause collapse of the alveolus unless opposed by some internal "splinting" pressure within the alveolus. The interaction between wall tension, alveolar radius, and pressure is defined by the Laplace relationship:

$$P = 2T/R$$

where P equals the splinting pressure, T the wall tension, and R the alveolar radius. This relationship states that the internal distending pressure required to counteract alveolar collapse is directly proportional to wall tension and inversely proportional to alveolar radius. At low alveolar radii (volumes), higher splinting pressures are required to counteract wall tension and oppose alveolar collapse. This explains both the tendency for low lung volumes to promote regional atalectasis and the high energy investment required to reopen collapsed

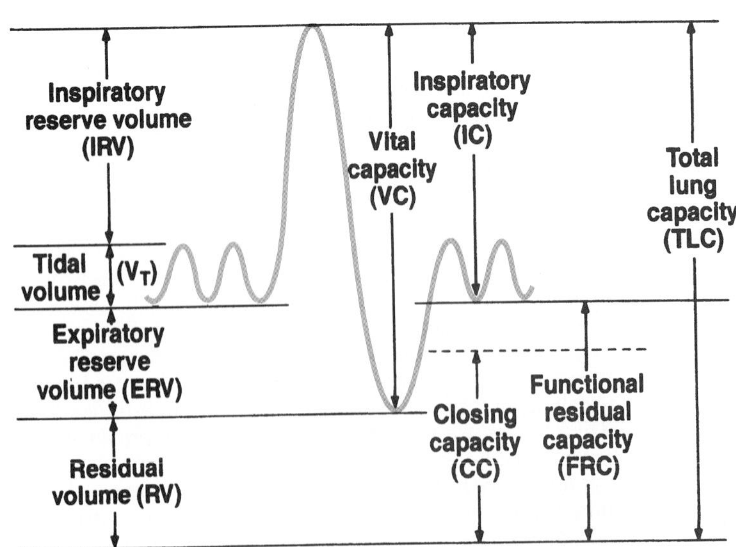

FIGURE 106.4 Lung volumes and capacities. (From Wilson JM, DiFiore JW. In: O'Neill JA, Rowe MI, Grosfeld JL, et al., eds. *Pediatric surgery*, 5th ed. St. Louis: Mosby, 1998, with permission.)

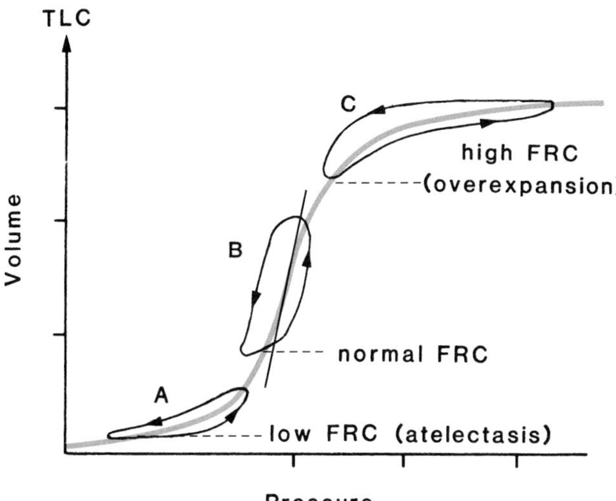

FIGURE 106.5 Static compliance curve. Nonlinear relationship between inflation pressure and volume change illustrated at low, normal, and high functional residual capacities (FRC). Volume represented as fraction of total lung capacity (TLC). (From Harris TR, Wood BR. In: Goldsmith JP, Karotkin EH, eds. *Assisted ventilation of the neonate*, 3rd ed. Philadelphia: WB Saunders, 1996, with permission.)

alveoli. The most important component of total wall tension in the neonate is surface tension, which is the tension created by the physiochemical properties of the gas–liquid interface. In the mature lung, surface tension is dramatically reduced by surfactant, a phospholipid that coats the alveolar surface and stabilizes it against collapse. Therefore, alveolar collapse is facilitated both by small lung volumes and by surfactant insufficiency.

The relationship between pressure and lung volume, referred to as the *static compliance curve*, is not linear (Fig. 106.5). At low lung volumes, atalectatic alveoli initially require a large energy input to reopen. As more alveoli are recruited, further increases in pressure bring about much larger increases in lung volume. At high lung volumes, alveoli are overdistended and less compliant. Pulmonary management aims at maintaining FRC in the steep portion of the static compliance curve, where lung compliance is optimal.

Extrinsic compliance refers to the component of lung compliance related to extrapulmonary structures, primarily chest wall, diaphragm, and abdomen. Under normal circumstances, chest wall compliance in the infant is high and contributes little to total compliance, which then is determined mostly by intrinsic lung compliance. In some instances, such as increased chest wall edema caused by sepsis, persistent fetal circulation, or superior vena caval thrombosis, reduced extrinsic compliance can have a significant impact on total compliance and ventilation. Chest wall compliance also can decrease with the use of intravenous fentanyl, which affects muscle tone. Extrinsic compliance also decreases when intraabdominal pressures are increased (e.g., ileus, closure of abdominal wall defects) and after diaphragmatic plication or diaphragmatic hernia repair.[17]

Ventilation is inversely related to resistance, which has both viscous and airway components. *Viscous resistance* is the friction generated by contiguous tissues moving against each other. It accounts for up to 40% of total resistance in neonates and is increased with conditions of high tissue density caused by edema (e.g., RDS, bronchopulmonary dysplasia, and anatomic left-to-right shunts). Airway resistance, on the other hand, reflects friction caused by gas molecules interacting with each other and with the airway walls.

Airway resistance is related to length, radius, turbulence, and density. According to Poiseuille's Law, resistance is directly related to the length of the conducting tube and inversely related to the fourth power of radius:

$$\Delta P = V8\text{h}L/\text{p}r^4$$

where h is viscosity, L is tube length, and r is radius. Radius is a powerful determinant of resistance in simple tubes, but in the branching bronchial tree, the impact of progressively smaller radii is offset by the large total cross-sectional area of the distal airways. This is particularly true for older children and adults, in whom occult small-airway disease may exist without affecting total resistance. The small airways in infants contribute a much larger percentage of total airway resistance, however; so conditions affecting these airways, such as bronchospasm and bronchiolitis, have a more significant effect on airflow. Although tube length has few important clinical ramifications, it is interesting to note that infants with pulmonary hypoplasia resulting from congenital diaphragmatic hernia have truncated development of the bronchial tree and lower airway resistance than normal infants.[18]

Turbulence refers to the random swirling of gas molecules during bulk flow, in contrast to laminar flow, which is characterized by organized streaming of gas molecules along the same axis. Turbulence is induced as flow rates increase, and it makes ventilation less efficient because it consumes energy. Gas density is directly and linearly related to resistance. Although this has little clinical relevance in most settings, the use of low-density gas mixtures improves ventilation with anatomic abnormalities that produce high resistance, such as tracheal stenosis and bronchopulmonary dysplasia. Heliox, a mixture of 80% helium and 20% oxygen, has a density one third that of room air and therefore generates one third the resistance.[19]

The calculated product of resistance and compliance is a useful parameter that integrates two of the primary determinants of airflow and is referred to as the *time constant* (TC):

$$TC = RC_{dyn}$$

where R is resistance, and C_{dyn} is dynamic compliance. The *time constant* reflects the time required for pressure equilibration to occur as air flows down a pressure gradient. During one time constant, 63% of an inspiratory or expiratory tidal volume can occur, whereas about four time constants are required for completion of flow. Conditions that increase either resistance or compliance will increase the time constant. During mechanical ventilation, consideration of this effect is required to allow adequate expiratory time before initiation of the next ventilatory cycle. Inadequate expiratory time results in "breath stacking" and overdistention of alveoli. Additionally, most focal lung diseases result in considerable inhomogeneity in regional time constants. Inspiratory times need to be adjusted to allow for the longest time constants to ensure even distribution of ventilation. Conditions associated with low compliance result in short time constants. Therefore, an increase in minute ventilation is accomplished more efficiently by increasing ventilatory rate, which is permitted by the short time constant, than by increasing tidal volume, which requires high pressures in low-compliance lungs.

Pulmonary Blood Flow

Although the pathophysiology of pulmonary hypertension is covered more thoroughly in the subsequent section, the basic principles governing the regulation of pulmonary vascular resistance and flow are introduced here because they determine the matching of ventilation and perfusion, and hence the efficiency of gas exchange. Blood flow in the lung is influenced by a variety of mechanical and vasoreactive phenomena, which combine to determine local vascular resistances and, therefore, the regional distribution of blood flow.

As discussed, resistance is inversely related to the fourth power of vessel radius, making vessel caliber the most important determinant of resistance and flow. Pulmonary vascular caliber is determined both by mechanical factors acting on vessel walls and by muscular contraction within vessel walls. The mechanical factors that influence vessel caliber include radial traction on larger vessels produced by parenchymal expansion and compressive pressure imparted on microvessels within the alveolar walls by air pressure within the alveolus.

These mechanical forces come into play primarily at the extremes of lung volume. At low lung volumes, the lack of radial traction reduces caliber and increases resistance within the larger parenchymal vessels. At high volumes, excessive intraalveolar pressures are imparted to the alveolar arterioles, capillaries, and venules as they transit through the alveolar unit. If this lateral pressure exceeds downstream pulmonary venous pressure (or pulmonary capillary wedge pressure), it becomes a determinant of the pressure gradient driving flow across the alveolar capillary. Normally, the pressure gradient is determined by the difference between mean pulmonary arterial pressure (P_{PA}) and pulmonary venous pressure (P_{PV}) ($\Delta P = P_{PA} - P_{PV}$). When alveolar pressure exceeds P_{PV}, it acts as the downstream pressure ($\Delta P = P_{PA} - P_{Alv}$). The anatomic arrangement of vessels "suspended" within the alveolar unit and influenced by external alveolar pressures is referred to as a *Starling resistor*. The phenomenon of the Starling resistor allows the lung to be viewed as a continuum of zones in which capillary blood flow depends on the relationship between hydrostatic venous pressure and intraalveolar pressure.

In addition to mechanical forces, the distribution of blood flow within the pulmonary circulation is affected by a variety of vasoconstrictive stimuli. Extensive autoregulation of pulmonary blood flow ensures that perfusion is directed toward capillaries adjoining well-ventilated alveoli and away from collapsed or fluid-filled alveoli. This autoregulation is accomplished by increasing pulmonary vascular tone in vessels leading to poorly ventilated alveoli with low partial pressures of oxygen, a process referred to as *hypoxic pulmonary vasoconstriction* (HPV).

Factors that influence HPV include (a) the partial pressure of oxygen within the alveolus (P_AO_2), (b) the partial pressure of oxygen within arteriolar blood (P_aO_2), (c) the partial pressure of carbon dioxide in arteriolar blood (P_aCO_2), and (d) the pH of arteriolar blood. Pulmonary vascular tone is inversely related to the partial pressure of oxygen in both the alveolus and the capillary blood, but P_AO_2 appears to be a more important factor. In fact, alveolar hypoxia is the single most powerful stimulus to pulmonary vasoconstriction. The pH of capillary blood also affects blood flow; local acidosis is an important stimulus to pulmonary vasoconstriction. Increased P_aCO_2 increases vascular tone both by lowering pH and also by acidosis-independent mechanisms.

Physiologic mediators of vascular smooth-muscle contraction common to these stimuli have not yet been fully identified. The caliber of pulmonary vessels at any given time is dependent on the balance of mediators causing vascular smooth-muscle contraction and relaxation. Mediators of vasodilatation include bradykinin, prostaglandins E_1 and A_1 (PGE_1, PGA_1), prostacyclin (PGI_2), and nitric oxide. Mediators of vasoconstriction include the leukotrienes, endothelin-1 (ET-1), prostaglandin D_2 (PGD_2), and histamine. Histamine, ET-1, and PGD_2 appear to have biphasic effects mediated by different receptor populations, causing vasodilatation in the fetal and early neonatal periods and vasoconstriction after the first few days of life.[20–22] Most of these mediators originate from local sources, such as pulmonary endothelial cells and mast cells).

Gas-exchange Determinants

The ultimate goal of respiratory function is gas exchange, which is the transfer of oxygen from inspired air to capillary blood and the reciprocal transfer of carbon dioxide from blood to alveolar gas. The principal determinants of gas exchange are total alveolar ventilation, ventilation/perfusion matching, diffusion, and extrapulmonary shunt. The mechanical properties discussed previously affect gas exchange primarily by determining the amount and distribution of ventilation. Regulation of pulmonary blood flow determines ventilation/perfusion matching and the efficiency of gas exchange. Extrapulmonary shunt occurs primarily through cardiac septal defects and the ductus arteriosus and is discussed in the section on cardiac physiology. Diffusion abnormalities are uncommon causes of gas exchange problems in children. Total ventilation and ventilation/perfusion matching are the most important causes of impaired gas exchange and merit further discussion.

Ventilation

Tidal volume is divided into two separate volumes: *alveolar ventilation*, which participates in gas exchange, and *physiologic dead space*, which does not. Physiologic dead space is further divided into *anatomic dead space*, which describes the volume of the prealveolar conducting airways, and *alveolar dead space*, which includes the ventilated but nonperfused alveoli. Normally, alveolar dead space is negligible, and total physiologic dead space approximates one third of tidal volume. In some diseases, such as ARDS, alveolar dead space may be increased. During mechanical ventilation, anatomic dead space is increased by the addition of ventilator tubing. Effective alveolar ventilation is best monitored by measuring PCO_2, which is relatively insensitive to abnormalities of ventilation/perfusion matching. Alveolar hypoventilation results in both inadequate oxygenation and inadequate carbon dioxide removal.

Ventilation/Perfusion Matching

The appropriate matching of ventilation and perfusion is the single most important determinant of gas exchange in the normal lung. Most disease states that cause abnormal gas exchange do so by promoting an imbalance between ventilation and perfusion. Perfusion is matched to regional ventilation by the mechanisms governing pulmonary blood flow discussed above. When the normal mechanisms of pulmonary vascular autoregulation are impaired, ventilation/perfusion ratio ($\dot{V}/\dot{Q}$) mismatch ensues.

Normal alveoli with matched ventilation and perfusion are considered to have a $\dot{V}/\dot{Q}$ ratio of 1. Those with relatively less ventilation have a $\dot{V}/\dot{Q}$ less than 1, and those with relatively less perfusion have a $\dot{V}/\dot{Q}$ greater than 1. Those with ventilation but no perfusion define alveolar dead space, whereas those with perfusion but no ventilation contribute to *intrapulmonary shunt*, which is microcirculatory bypass of alveolar exchange. Between these two extremes lies a spectrum of $\dot{V}/\dot{Q}$ relationships that may contribute to abnormal gas exchange. $\dot{V}/\dot{Q}$ mismatch generally results in hypoxemia with normocarbia. Because carbon dioxide diffuses through the capillary–alveolar interface much more readily than does oxygen, $\dot{V}/\dot{Q}$ mismatch has relatively little effect on PCO_2 levels.

Mismatching of ventilation and perfusion is responsible for the hypoxemia encountered in most clinical settings. These include the disease states in which lung compliance is reduced, FRC drops below closing volume, and regional alveolar collapse occurs: pneumonitis, aspiration, RDS, ARDS, cardiogenic pulmonary edema, postoperative splinting, and others. Simply increasing forced inspiratory oxygen (F_IO_2) does little to rectify the situation because the venous admixture of blood passing through low $\dot{V}/\dot{Q}$ units remains low in oxygen saturation, and blood passing through normal $\dot{V}/\dot{Q}$ units cannot further increase oxygen content to compensate. Therapeutic efforts must be directed at reopening closed alveoli and restoring homogenous alveolar ventilation.

Although diuresis, antibiotic therapy, and chest physiotherapy may have important roles in restoring FRC and matched ventilation and perfusion, perhaps the most effective therapeutic intervention is the use of continuous positive intraalveolar distending pressure: CPAP or PEEP, which recruit and maintain previously closed or underventilated alveoli and improve $\dot{V}/\dot{Q}$ matching and oxygenation. They also shift ventilation up on the static compliance curve, producing a higher tidal volume with less pressure trauma.

The use of positive-pressure mechanical ventilation and PEEP must be managed judiciously because they can have both beneficial and deleterious effects on $\dot{V}/\dot{Q}$ matching. It is important to remember that positive airway pressure is transmitted to the alveolar capillaries that carry blood flow through the alveolar network. The alveolar pressure surrounding these capillaries acts as a Starling resistor and can impede capillary blood flow if it exceeds downstream venous pressure. The use of high peak ventilatory pressures without the use of PEEP, or the excessive use of PEEP itself, can cause overdistention of alveoli, reduced compliance, increased alveolar capillary resistance, and diminished alveolar capillary perfusion. The result is redirection of blood flow to underventilated alveoli, which actually worsens $\dot{V}/\dot{Q}$ mismatch. Similarly, the use of PEEP in focal lung disease may be counterproductive because its effects are preferentially directed to the normal, more compliant alveoli. This causes overdistention of normal $\dot{V}/\dot{Q}$ units and redistribution of blood flow to diseased alveoli, cancelling the benefits of hypoxic pulmonary vasoconstriction.

Surfactant and Respiratory Distress Syndromes

Respiratory distress syndrome, or hyaline membrane disease (HMD), is the most common causes of respiratory distress in neonates and one of the primary causes of neonatal mortality in developed countries. RDS occurs as a direct result of pulmonary immaturity and surfactant deficiency. Because surfactant is not produced and secreted by type II alveolar epithelial cells until the third trimester, prematurity causes newborns to rely on lungs of variable maturity to support extrauterine respiration. Preterm infants born during the terminal saccular phase of lung development face the challenge of supporting gas exchange with lungs characterized by relatively thicker epithelial barriers, suboptimal capillary architecture, and a tendency toward alveolar collapse. This last feature is the most important cause of respiratory failure in premature infants and is directly related to the lack of surfactant, which lowers surface tension at the alveolar liquid–gas interface.

Surfactant is a complex substance composed of phospholipids (80%), proteins (10%), and cholesterol (10%). The phospholipid profile changes during lung maturation, but phosphotidylcholine predominates and is the principal substance responsible for the surface-tension lowering properties of surfactant. Phosphotidylinositol is present in immature surfactant, but it is largely replaced by phosphotidylglycerol in mature lungs, a useful fact when assessing fetal lung maturity. Surfactant also contains at least four specific proteins: surfactant protein-A (SP-A), SP-B, SP-C, and SP-D. The functions of these proteins have not been defined completely, but together they help promote the spreading, organization, and adherence of the phospholipid layer. They also have important roles in surfactant recycling and host immune defense.

The physiologic role of surfactant is to stabilize alveolar units against collapse and thereby to facilitate homogeneous lung ventilation and $\dot{V}/\dot{Q}$ matching. *LaPlace's law* states that the pressure required to overcome the retracting force of surface tension in a sphere is inversely related to radius. In clinical terms, this means that smaller alveoli actually require greater distending pressure to maintain stability. This is analogous to the phenomenon one experiences when trying to inflate a balloon: the initial pressure required to begin inflation is high and becomes progressively less as the balloon radius increases. Because the lung is a collection of alveoli of varying sizes, and all alveoli are exposed to the same atmospheric pressure through a shared network of airways, the natural tendency is for the smaller alveoli to collapse and transfer their volume of air to larger neighboring alveoli, which become overdistended. In both cases, the effect on compliance is deleterious: FRC declines, the work of breathing increases, $\dot{V}/\dot{Q}$ matching is compromised, and respiratory failure ensues. Surfactant not only reduces absolute surface tension, but it does so in a graded fashion. In small radius alveoli, the phospholipid layer is condensed and its effect on surface tension is great. As the alveolus expands, the phospholipid molecules spread out and impart a gradually decreasing effect on surface tension. This differential efficiency of surfactant function allows alveoli of different sizes to coexist in a stable fashion.

Surfactant composition is an important determinant and predictor of fetal lung maturity. By the 20th week of gestation, collections of surfactant appear in type II cells within cytoplasmic granules called *lamellar bodies*. Thereafter, surfactant begins to appear in the developing terminal sacs. Infants born at 25 weeks occasionally survive without respiratory support; at 30 weeks, the risk of respiratory distress approaches 50%, and by 35 weeks' gestation nearly all fetuses are capable of unassisted extrauterine respiration. There is considerable variability with respect to the timing of lung maturity, however, and clinical indices that assess lung maturity are useful in planning early delivery. The most common index of lung maturity is the amniotic fluid ratio of lecithin (phosphotidylcholine) to sphingomyelin, that is, the L/S ratio. Because amniotic phosphotidylcholine is derived solely from surfactant and sphingomyelin derives from all cell membranes, this provides a convenient self-indexed measurement of surfactant production that is independent of changes in amniotic fluid volume. An L/S ratio of 2.0 is achieved in the normal fetus by 35 weeks' gestation and is associated with an extremely low risk of RDS. Values of 1.5 to 2.0 are considered "immature" but of low risk. Values below 1.5 are associated with increased risk, and those below 1.0 are considered high risk. A more detailed test, the Lung Profile, utilizes the L/S ratio as well as percentages of phosphotidylglycerol and phosphotidylinositol to predict more accurately the risk of RDS.

The fact that some infants born before 35 weeks' gestation do not manifest RDS led to the idea of stress-induced lung maturation. Fetal stress that promotes preterm labor also appears to promote accelerated lung maturation. This observation prompted the use of exogenous maternal corticosteroid administration to promote early lung maturation in fetuses expected to deliver early because of preterm labor or induced delivery. Exogenous corticosteroids appear to accelerate the maturation of surfactant phospholipids as well as increasing the synthesis of surfactant proteins.[23]

Postnatal administration of exogenous surfactant has become a mainstay of treatment not only for prematurity-associated RDS but also for a wide variety of neonatal lung diseases associated with reduced compliance. Surfactant replacement therapy has been proved to decrease the incidence and severity of RDS, especially when used in conjunction with antenatal maternal corticosteroids, and it appears to be efficacious in both prophylactic and rescue strategies. The two most commonly used preparations are a synthetic phospholipid–alcohol mixture (Exosurf) and a bovine surfactant extract supplemented with phospholipids and surfactant proteins (Surventa). Modified recombinant preparations are expected to become available in the near future. These preparations are aerosolized into the airway through an endotracheal tube with positive pressure ventilation. Although initially designed for treatment of RDS, they appear to reduce ventilatory requirements and complications in a variety of diseases characterized by reduced compliance, including congenital diaphragmatic hernia, meconium aspiration, persistent pulmonary hypertension of the newborn (PPHN), and ARDS in older patients.[24]

Pulmonary Hypoplasia

Pulmonary hypoplasia refers to a condition in which pulmonary parenchymal tissue is abnormally reduced relative to body size. It is defined pathologically by reduced lung dry weight or DNA content relative to body mass and reduced alveolar number per unit volume. Although pulmonary hypoplasia may occur rarely as a primary disease, it is usually a stereotypical consequence of mechanical compression during lung development. Clinically, secondary pulmonary hypoplasia is associated most commonly with congenital diaphragmatic hernia, giant omphaloceles, and oligohydramnios caused by fetal renal dysfunction or urinary obstruction. Whether the true cause of pulmonary hypoplasia is mechanical compression, some alteration in fetal lung fluid dynamics, or a combination of both has not yet been elucidated.

Whatever the cause, pulmonary hypoplasia results from arrested development of the tracheobronchial tree and pulmonary vasculature. Depending on the severity of compression, the sequential binary branching of the developing airway may be arrested well before the usual 22 or 23 divisions, resulting in fewer respiratory units and a reduced pulmonary capillary network. The pulmonary arterial tree is not just quantitatively diminished, but it is histologically and functionally abnormal as well. The pulmonary arterioles in affected lungs are characterized by thickening of the muscular media, abnormal extension of the muscular media into terminal arterioles, and hyperreactivity of the vascular smooth muscle cells to vasoconstrictive stimuli. Endothelin is a potent vasoconstrictor that also acts as a smooth muscle mitogen, and may have a role in the development of fetal pulmonary vascular hyperplasia.[25] The pathophysiologic effects of pulmonary hypoplasia, therefore, include both inadequate gas exchange and persistent pulmonary hypertension.

In most cases of pulmonary hypoplasia, the life-threatening consequences of hypoplasia are related to persistent pulmonary hypertension, not to inadequate gas exchange. Most patients with congenital diaphragmatic hernia, for instance, have one or more blood gas measurements that document the potential for adequate gas exchange. Subsequent physiologic deterioration (and death) result from progressive, refractory pulmonary hypertension, extrapulmonary right-to-left shunting, and global hypoxemia. These subjects are covered more thoroughly in the discussion of persistent fetal circulation.

Ventilatory Support

Ventilatory management of pediatric patients has become increasingly complex as technologic innovation has expanded the number of available options. These advances have been motivated by a need to improve gas distribution in diseased lungs, to avoid complications associated with barotrauma, and to provide better synchronized and tolerated ventilation. Although conventional positive-pressure ventilation remains the mainstay of management for most infants and children requiring ventilatory support, a number of nonconventional technologies have gained increasing acceptance in certain situations where conventional techniques have proved inadequate.

Conventional Mechanical Ventilation

Conventional positive pressure ventilators deliver a bulk flow of oxygen-enriched gas to the lungs through an endotracheal tube. In general, they are classified according to the method used to initiate and terminate a single ventilatory cycle. Volume-cycled ventilators deliver a predetermined tidal volume of gas. Respiratory rate (cycles/min), flow rate (L/min), inspiratory-to-expiratory ratio, and inspired oxygen concentration are manipulated to achieve certain respiratory goals, but the actual termination of the positive-pressure breath occurs when the preset tidal volume has been delivered. Volume-cycled ventilation has the advantage of providing precise control of minute ventilation regardless of lung compliance, and it is used routinely in adults and older children.

Infants and small children historically have not been managed with volume-cycled ventilators. Although control of minute ventilation is equally important in this group, the risks of barotrauma are high, particularly in neonates with pulmonary immaturity. A reduction in compliance will result in a reciprocal increase in pressure during volume-cycled ventilation, leading to overdistention of ventilated alveoli, $\dot{V}/\dot{Q}$ mismatching, alveolar rupture and pneumothorax, and the chronic lung changes observed with barotrauma. For this reason, precise control of inspiratory pressure is preferable to volume control.

The vast majority of neonatal pediatric ventilators used today are technically not pressure-cycled, but instead are time-cycled and pressure-limited. Instead of ventilatory flow ceasing when a preset pressure is reached, flow continues at a plateau pressure until the inspiratory time is reached. This improves tidal volume consistency and distribution. Constant monitoring of respiratory function (e.g., continuous transcutaneous oximetry) is imperative to prevent hypoventilation in the event of a sudden decrease in compliance and tidal volume.

The usual options for ventilatory modes in pediatric ventilator management are essentially identical to those used in adults: control, assist control, intermittent mandatory ventilation (IMV), synchronized IMV, and pressure support. The function and utility of these modes in children are similar to their use in adults. Pressure support, in which each spontaneous breath is assisted by supplemental positive pressure, is becoming the preferred mode in many settings where the patient is conscious and breathing spontaneously. It is particularly effective in the weaning of mechanical ventilation and restoring respiratory muscle strength.

For most modes, parameters are selected that determine gas exchange: F_iO_2, respiratory rate, PIP, and PEEP. Inspiratory flow rates may need to be adjusted to provide an appropriate inspiratory/expiratory ratio within the constraints of the preset respiratory rate. PEEP is adjusted to optimize compliance and FRC; PIP is adjusted to provide an adequate tidal volume. Flow rates are adjusted with an appreciation of the different time constants observed in various clinical settings. The F_iO_2 is minimized to avoid pulmonary oxygen toxicity and retinopathy. The mean airway pressure (MAP), which is measured and represents the area under the time-pressure curve, is probably the single best parameter to follow for monitoring changes in the level of ventilatory support required as well as the risk of barotrauma.

With advances in ventilator technology, volume-controlled ventilation has become safer for use in neonatal and pediatric patients and may have some distinct advantages over pressure-limited ventilation in certain circumstances. Small tidal volumes and high respiratory rates can produce equivalent minute ventilation with less alveolar trauma, particularly if levels of PEEP are used that maximize pulmonary compliance. Some newer ventilators allow pressure-regulated volume control (PRVC) ventilation in which tidal and minute volumes are preset, and which the ventilator delivers in a pressure-limited fashion. The ventilator calculates compliance changes continuously and adjusts flow rates to minimize inspiratory pressure with each breath. The resulting ventilation mode is a hybrid of volume- and pressure-regulated techniques and may be helpful in infants with bronchopulmonary dysplasia and rapidly changing compliance who are at risk for alveolar injury.[26]

Unconventional Mechanical Ventilation

Conventional breathing and mechanical ventilation both involve the bulk transport of air through conducting airways to gas exchange chambers *(alveoli)*, where diffusion occurs across the alveolar–capillary membrane. The altered gas then is expired by bulk transport, and a new cycle begins. This type of bulk flow is implied when describing the ventilatory properties of the lung in terms of "bellows" function. In many disease states associated with reduced lung compliance, the high positive pressures necessary to produce this bulk flow of gas during mechanical ventilation result in considerable iatrogenic lung injury. This injury is manifested both by parenchymal changes and edema, which further reduce compliance and diffusion, as well as mechanical disruption of small bronchi and alveoli, resulting in mediastinal emphysema, pneumothorax, and bronchopleural fistulae. Excessively high inspiratory pressures also impair venous return to the right atrium, thereby reducing preload, lung perfusion, gas exchange, and global cardiac output.

Whether ventilation-induced acute lung injury is caused primarily by the pressure itself or by overdistention of the more compliant alveoli is a subject of considerable ongoing debate. Current evidence seems to favor the structural overdistention of alveoli as the principal cause of iatrogenic lung injury, leading some to prefer the term *volutrauma* to the more accepted term *barotrauma*.[27–29] The consequences of alveolar overdistension include impaired endothelial and epithelial barrier function, increased permeability, and interstitial edema. In reality, both mechanisms probably contribute to lung injury, as do excessive oxygen concentrations and preexisting inflammatory conditions. Whatever the underlying cause, peak inspiratory pressure seems to be the parameter that correlates best with induced lung injury.

Several novel ventilatory techniques have emerged recently that attempt to mitigate barotrauma and hemodynamic compromise by providing effective ventilation without excessive PIP. These techniques employ extremely high ventilatory rates and tidal volumes less than or equal to anatomic dead space. Although numerous variations exist, the most popular modes are high-frequency jet ventilation (HFJV) and high-frequency oscillatory ventilation (HFOV). In HFJV, a small cannula is advanced through the endotracheal tube and used to deliver rapid, low-volume bursts of inspired gas. Ventilation does not require bulk flow, but it relies on several poorly defined physical processes, the most important of which is probably coaxial flow. In coaxial flow, the jet stream induces continuous rotational flow of inspired gas down the center of the airway and reverse rotational flow of expired gas along the perimeter of the airway (Fig. 106.6). In HFOV, ventilation is driven by the oscillations of a diaphragm within a closed noncompliant system. The cyclical compression and expansion of gas within the system generate high-velocity, streaming flow patterns that are similar to the coaxial flow seen in HFJV. The major difference between the two is that the expiratory phase is active in HFOV, as opposed to the passive expiration seen in both HFJV and conventional ventilation. This difference may make HFOV more effective in reducing air leaks from bronchopleural fistulae and less likely to cause air trapping and overdistention in lungs with longer and more heterogeneous time constants.

In both modalities, ventilator management is often unpredictable and counterintuitive. For instance, in HFOV the F_iO_2, MAP, frequency (cycles per second, or Hz), and *amplitude* (volume displacement caused by oscillation of the diaphragm) are preset. The amplitude is not truly reflective of the tiny tidal volume produced at the end of the endotracheal tube and is therefore useful as a relative, "unitless" measurement only. In practice, the adequacy of the amplitude can be

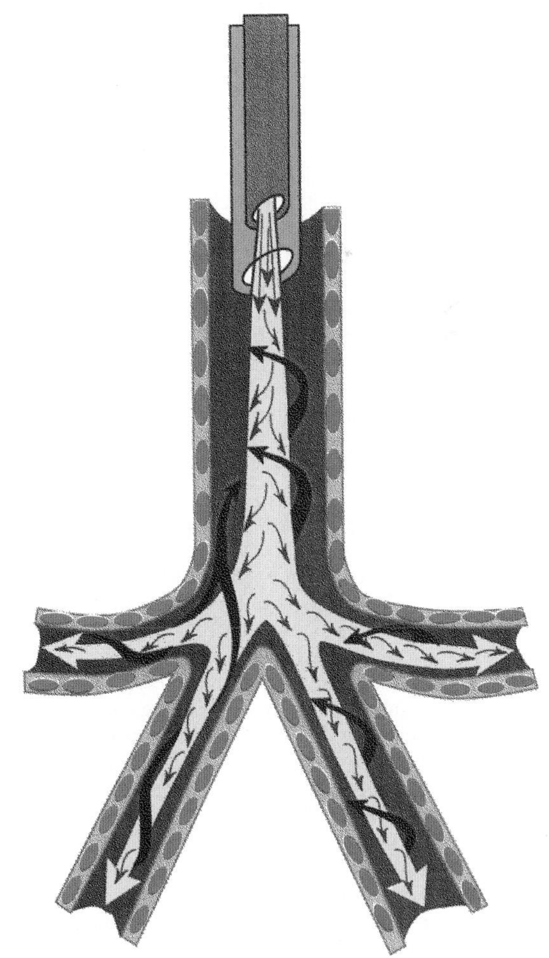

FIGURE 106.6 Proposed coaxial flow pattern during high-frequency jet and oscillatory ventilation. Gas inflow is confined to the center of the airway lumen, and outflow is confined to the periphery. (From Harris TR, Wood BR. In: Goldsmith JP, Karotkin EH, eds. *Assisted ventilation of the neonate*, 3rd ed. Philadelphia: WB Saunders, 1996, with permission.)

judged subjectively by observing chest wall vibration. Increasing P_aO_2 usually requires increasing the F_iO_2 or the MAP, which recruits alveoli and increases FRC similar to the use of PEEP. In some conditions, the MAP required actually may be higher than that required in conventional ventilation, but the PIP is far less. Reducing P_aCO_2 actually may require reducing the oscillatory rate to allow more time for gas displacement and more effective gas streaming.

In general, high-frequency ventilatory techniques are effective at promoting improved CO_2 elimination at lower pressures than conventional ventilation. Improved oxygenation is less reliable. HFJV and HFOV are both helpful in providing respiratory support in infants with preexisting barotrauma and air leaks. The ability of HFOV to support enhanced CO_2 removal and generate a respiratory alkalosis at lower pressures has made it useful in managing infants with persistent pulmonary hypertension, particularly those with congenital diaphragmatic hernia.

Liquid ventilation is a novel, experimental approach to respiratory support that currently is undergoing clinical trials in a variety of settings. In this approach, a liquid perfluorocarbon solution is instilled into the lungs instead of a gas mixture. Because many forms of respiratory failure are associated with surfactant insufficiency and reduced compliance, the substitution of liquid for gas in the alveolus eliminates the liquid–gas interface, reduces surface tension, and improves compliance. The improvement of mechanical properties in the perfluorocarbon-filled lung allows ventilation to occur at lower pressures and less barotrauma. The solubility of oxygen and carbon dioxide in perfluorocarbon solutions is extremely high, allowing respiratory gases to diffuse easily across the alveolar–capillary membrane.

Although total liquid ventilation requires a closed circuit and is clinically impractical, a partial liquid ventilation technique has been developed that is logistically feasible and promises to provide ventilatory benefits to some patients with reduced lung compliance.[30] In partial liquid ventilation, perfluorocarbon is instilled at a volume equal to FRC, and conventional ventilation then is superimposed on the liquid-phase FRC. In essence, this is analogous to providing "liquid PEEP," and improves pulmonary mechanics with little increase in alveolar distending pressure. The optimal role for partial or total liquid ventilation remains a subject for further investigation.

Extracorporeal Support

In certain situations, conventional and nonconventional ventilatory techniques are inadequate to provide gas exchange in the face of overwhelming pulmonary dysfunction. Under these circumstances, the use of extracorporeal membrane oxygenation (ECMO) may succeed in sustaining oxygen delivery and carbon dioxide removal until the underlying cause of respiratory failure is reversed and physiologic improvement occurs. It is important to recognize that, like conventional ventilation, ECMO is a supportive rather than therapeutic technique and has a limited window of utility imposed by the adverse effects of the technology itself.

Several variations of ECMO technology exist, but all share the same underlying principles: the partial diversion of blood from the patient to an external membrane oxygenator, *ex vivo* exchange of oxygen and carbon dioxide, and return of blood to the circulatory system. The circuit is driven by a roller pump that is similar to that used for routine cardiopulmonary bypass. Systemic anticoagulation is necessary to prevent thrombosis from occurring in the extracorporeal circuit.

Two basic methods of providing ECMO support are currently available: venoarterial (VA) and venovenous (VV). In VA ECMO, the right common carotid artery and jugular vein are cannulated. Venous inflow to the system results from passive drainage of the right atrium; arterial flow back to the patient occurs in the aortic arch (Fig. 106.7). As return flow is into the aorta, partial cardiac bypass occurs, which may provide significant benefit when respiratory failure is accompanied by compromised cardiac performance. The pump flow rate is advanced to 100 to 120 mL/kg/min, which approximates 60% to 80% of cardiac output. Although VA ECMO provides significant cardiac support, the return of oxygenated blood to the descending aorta and the flow of desaturated blood throught the left ventricle into the aortic root may result in a lower oxygen delivery to the coronary arteries.

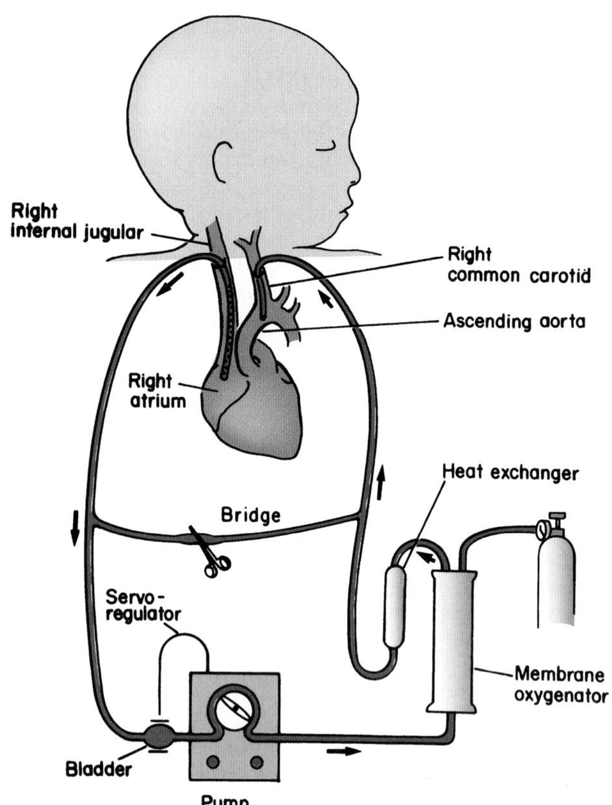

FIGURE 106.7 Components of a standard venoarterial extracorporeal membrane oxygenation (ECMO) circuit. (From O'Rourke PP. In: Holbrook PR, ed. *Textbook of pediatric critical care.* Philadelphia: WB Saunders, 1993, with permission.)

In VV ECMO, the circuit is interposed into the venous side of the circulation, with blood returning to the right atrium. This mode of extracorporeal support is less efficient than VA ECMO, resulting in a lower maximal SaO_2 dbecause of the phenomenon of recirculation. Because both cannulae are positioned on the venous side, some of the oxygenated perfusate will be siphoned back into the venous return instead of flowing forward to perfuse end organs. The degree of recirculation is monitored by comparing oygen saturations of the venous drainage and the arterial blood: the venous drainage saturation should be less than the arterial saturation. Although it provides no direct support of cardiac output, this method obviates the ligation and sacrifice of a carotid artery, avoids some of the risk of arterial embolization, and provides well-oxygenated blood for pulmonary and coronary circulation. Even in patients with decreased cardiac contractility, the improvement in oxygen delivery to the myocardium afforded by VV ECMO results in significant enhancement of cardiac output and may obviate VA ECMO. For most infants and children with adequate cardiac function, VV ECMO may become the modality of choice for extracorporeal support.[31]

Indications for ECMO vary among institutions. Because of the high cost and potential for complications, ECMO is justifiable only when all other available therapies for respiratory failure have proved inadequate and when quantifiable parameters predict a mortality rate of 80% or greater with conventional management. Several methods of providing a quantitative estimate of respiratory failure have been used to predict mortality with conventional ventilation and guide the use of ECMO. Perhaps the most widely used index is the oxygenation index (OI), which compares ventilatory support parameters (MAP and F_iO_2) with gas exchange results (postductal P_aO_2):

$$OI = (MAP)(F_iO_2)/P_aO_2 \times 100$$

An OI greater than 40 predicts a mortality rate 80% and is a commonly cited threshold indicator for the use of ECMO. Another useful, although more burdensome, parameter for quantifying respiratory failure and predicting mortality is the alveolar–arterial oxygen gradient (P_AO_2–P_aO_2), which when greater than 600 predicts a mortality rate of 80%. Other inclusion criteria for ECMO include the absence of a major intrinsic cardiac defect, chromosomal abnormality, or significant intraventricular hemorrhage, a gestational age greater than 33 weeks, weight greater than 2 kg, and an underlying respiratory pathology that is judged to be reversible.

Results for extracorporeal support are age and diagnosis dependent. Infants with respiratory failure (meconium aspiration syndrome, RDS, sepsis) appear to benefit most from extracorporeal support. This is most likely because neonatal respiratory failure often is associated with reversible pulmonary hypertension, and ECMO allows for the normalization of PO_2, PCO_2, pH, and pulmonary vascular resistance without the aggressive ventilatory support that frequently causes iatrogenic lung injury and chronic lung disease. Neonates with reversible, idiopathic PPHN benefit from ECMO for the same reasons. Neonates with respiratory failure and pulmonary hypertension attributable to congenital diaphragmatic hernia and pulmonary hypoplasia appear to benefit from ECMO, but the improvement in survival over conventional management is not as significant. This may reflect the irreversible problems related to inadequacy of alveolar number and microvascular development associated with pulmonary hypoplasia. The results of ECMO in children and adolescents with respiratory failure resulting from ARDS, trauma, bronchopleural fistula, viral pneumonia, or aspiration are less convincing, and the role of ECMO in these diseases is not yet well defined.[32]

CARDIOVASCULAR PHYSIOLOGY AND SUPPORT

Fetal Circulation

Fetal circulation has evolved to utilize an external organ of gas exchange, the placenta, while maintaining the anatomic relationships that will later be necessary in extrauterine life when responsibility for gas exchange transitions abruptly to the lungs. The fetal circulatory system is characterized by asymmetric ventricles that function in parallel, an arrangement made possible by two anatomic shunts—the foramen ovale and the ductus arteriosus. These shunts make possible the nonrandom distribution of blood of varying oxygen contents

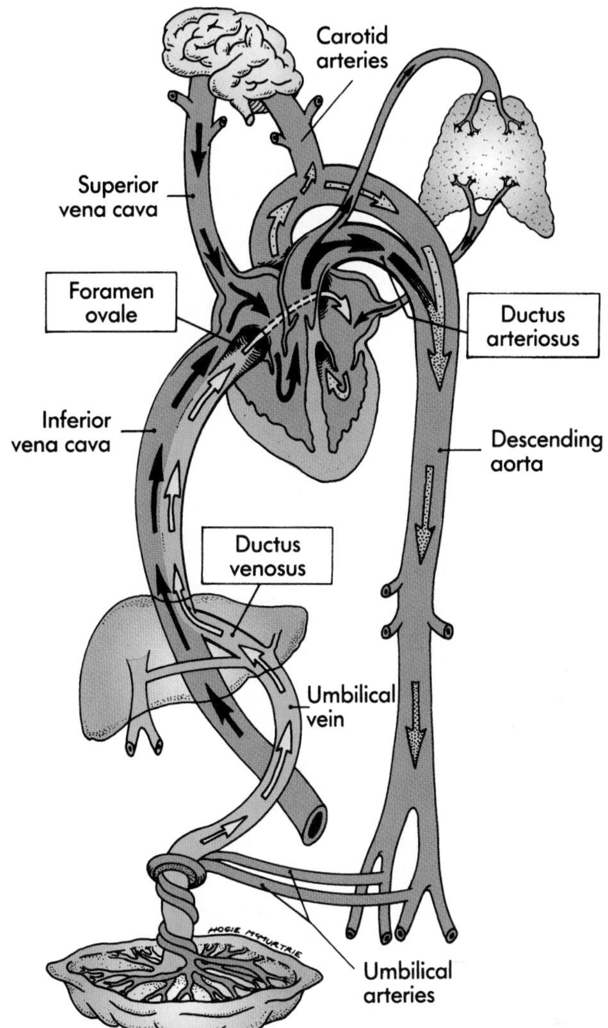

FIGURE 106.8 Fetal circulation. (From Bloom RS. In: Faranoff AA, Martin RJ, eds. *Neonatal–Perinatal Medicine: Diseases of the fetus and infant*, 6th ed. St. Louis: Mosby, 1997, with permission.)

and the delivery of adequate amounts of oxygen and substrate to developing organs (Fig. 106.8).

Well-oxygenated blood returning from the placenta and umbilical cord passes through the hepatic ductus venosus, into the inferior vena cava (IVC) and immediately into the right atrium. Ductus venosus blood mixes little with the less-oxygenated blood in the infrahepatic IVC and flows relatively undisturbed (in a laminar fashion referred to as *streaming*) along the medial wall of the IVC, through the right atrium, across the foramen ovale, and into the left atrium. This oxygen-rich blood then is pumped by the left ventricle into the aortic arch, where it is distributed to the developing heart, brain, and upper body (Fig. 106.9). The less-oxygenated blood in the IVC and superior vena cava (SVC) flows preferentially through the right atrium to the right ventricle and is pumped into the pulmonary artery, where most of it is shunted through the ductus arteriosus into the descending aorta. A small amount of pulmonary artery flow provides substrate to the lungs. Descending aortic flow is distributed to the developing organs of the lower body, with most of the flow being diverted back to the placenta through the two umbilical arteries. Flow through the placental circulation approximates 40% of cardiac output.

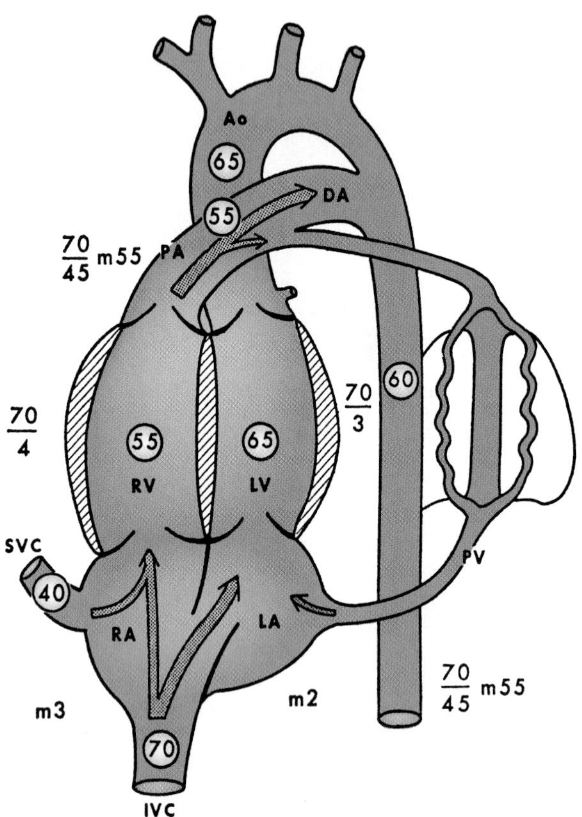

FIGURE 106.9 Oxyhemoglobin saturations in the fetal circulation. Preferential flow of saturated blood from the inferior vena cava (IVC) into the left atrium (LA) and desaturated blood from the superior vena cava (SVC) into the right atrium (RA) results in the distribution of blood with higher oxygen content to the aortic arch (Ao) and developing brain. (From Rudolph AM. Changes in the circulation after birth. In: Rudolph AM, ed. *Congenital diseases of the heart.* Chicago: Year Book Medical, 1974, with permission.)

The fetal pattern of blood flow is made possible by high pulmonary vascular resistance, which directs the flow of oxygen-poor blood from the pulmonary artery into the descending aorta. Only 5% to 10% of pulmonary artery flow actually traverses the pulmonary capillary bed. This minimizes the return of less-oxygenated blood through the pulmonary veins and prevents mixing with the oxygen-rich blood in the left ventricle destined for the heart and brain. The relatively low afterload presented to the right ventricle by the low-resistance shunt across the ductus arteriosus accounts for the fact that fetal right ventricular output exceeds left ventricular output, in some estimates by 40% to 100%.[33,34] Mechanisms of increased pulmonary resistance in the fetus include mechanical compression of pulmonary vessels in the fluid-filled lung and vasoconstriction secondary to hypoxemia, leukotrienes, and the peptide mediator endothelin-1.[35]

Transitional Circulation

At birth, profound changes in circulatory patterns, hemodynamics, and gas exchange occur as a result of the abrupt withdrawal of placental support. Transitional physiology is characterized by the cessation of placental blood flow and gas exchange and the simultaneous increase in blood flow and gas exchange in the lungs. As amniotic fluid is expelled from the lungs by compression during birth and the lungs expand with the infant's first breath, alveolar expansion causes an immediate reduction in pulmonary vascular resistance secondary to increased traction on larger parenchymal vessels and decreased intraalveolar pressure transmitted to alveolar microvessels. These purely mechanical changes account for a fourfold reduction in pulmonary vascular resistance (PVR), contributing significantly to the 15-fold overall reduction in PVR that occurs at birth. Pulmonary artery pressures fall more slowly over the first weeks of life and may approximate systemic pressures for the first several days of life.

Increased local oxygen concentrations reduce hypoxic pulmonary vasoconstriction through mechanisms mediated by endothelial-derived intermediates, such as nitric oxide (NO) and prostacyclin.[36,37] The enzymes responsible for the production of NO and prostacyclin in the pulmonary circulation, NO synthase and cyclooxygenase, undergo developmental maturation late in gestation, and their activity increases rapidly in response to birth-related stimuli, ventilation, and oxygenation. NO and prostacyclin act on pulmonary vascular smooth muscle cells to increase intracellular concentrations of cyclic guanosine monophosphate (GMP) and cyclic adenosine monophosphate (cAMP), respectively, which results in relaxation and vasodilation. ATP, released directly from oxygenated red blood cells in the pulmonary circulation is also a potent mediator of vasodilation. These vasodilatory mediators are counterregulated by vasoconstrictor substances such as endothelin, thromboxane, and cytochrome P450 pathway products.

The sudden decrease in pulmonary vascular resistance causes a dramatic increase in pulmonary blood flow and left atrial return. Left ventricular preload increases, resulting in increased left ventricular stroke volume and output. Right atrial return is reduced as placental flow ceases. Elevated left atrial pressure and reduced right atrial pressure cause closure of the flaplike foramen ovale, eliminating one of the fetal extrapulmonary shunts.

The other shunt, the ductus arteriosus, begins to close by vasoconstriction immediately. This process is mediated by both a withdrawal of placental-derived prostaglandins and an increase in oxygen tension, a potent vasoconstrictive stimulus for ductal tissue. Physiologic duct closure usually occurs by 24 hours but may take up to 3 days. Anatomic duct obliteration resulting from thrombosis and fibrosis may take several weeks or months. When spontaneous closure of the ductus arteriosus does not occur, as often happens in the premature infant whose immature ductal tissue is unresponsive to vasoconstrictive mediators, significant physiologic problems may occur. If pulmonary artery pressures remain abnormally high, an anatomic right-to-left shunt may occur that diverts desaturated blood around the pulmonary system, drastically lowering systemic oxygen delivery. If pulmonary artery pressure falls normally, a left-to-right shunt will occur, increasing pulmonary blood flow above cardiac output. Pulmonary overcirculation causes pulmonary edema and congestive heart failure in the short term and irreversible pulmonary hypertension in the long term, if uncorrected. Indomethicin administration, which inhibits prostaglandin synthetase, is effective in promoting ductal closure in most premature infants if given within the first 2 weeks of life. Failure of medical therapy indicates the need for surgical duct ligation.

Another event in the transition to extrauterine circulation involves vasoconstrictive or mechanical occlusion of the cord vessels. The abolishment of this "shunt" increases left ventricular afterload and systemic blood pressure and, along with increased left ventricular preload, accounts for an immediate increase in blood flow to target organs. Ductus venosus closure occurs by stasis and thrombosis as return flow through the umbilical vein ceases.

Postnatal Circulation and Cardiac Performance

Following the transition from fetal to neonatal life, the circulatory system is characterized by two separate cardiovascular circuits operating in a "series" configuration. By definition, right and left heart cardiac outputs are identical and can be considered symmetrical despite discrepancies in system pressures and contractile properties. The series configuration has great significance in that it imposes a degree of interdependence on the two circuits that does not exist *in utero.* Pathologic changes in one circuit necessarily impact the other circuit by virtue of alterations in the other circuit's preload or afterload. Failure of complete separation of the two circuits results in the deleterious shunting of blood from the pulmonary to systemic circuit or vice versa.

Cardiac output is determined by the same parameters in the neonate as is in the adult: heart rate and stroke volume. Stroke volume, in turn, is dependent on three factors: preload, contractility, and afterload. Although a detailed discussion of these four determinants of cardiac performance is beyond the scope of this chapter, it is instructive to consider some of the differences between pediatric and adult cardiac function relative to these four variables. These differences account for the fact that, in general, neonatal and pediatric patients have less cardiovascular reserve than do adolescents and young adults.

Heart rate, an important determinant of cardiac output in infants, becomes less important in childhood and adolescence. In fact, neonates are commonly referred to as *rate dependent.* The normal range for heart rate in neonates is higher than that in adults and decreases gradually throughout childhood to adult levels (Table 106.6). In adults, changes in heart rate result in little change in cardiac output because of compensatory changes in other parameters. When heart rate decreases, ventricular filling and stroke volume increase, and cardiac output is minimally altered. Reciprocal changes occur when heart rate increases. In neonates and, to a lesser extent, in children, these compensatory changes are less effective and changes in heart rate produce corresponding changes in cardiac output. The explanation for this observation lies in the fact that increased ventricular filling times and pressures fail to generate increased end-diastolic and stroke volumes because of decreased myocardial compliance and a blunted Frank-Starling mechanism, as discussed later.

The sympathetic innervation of the heart is relatively underdeveloped in the neonate, resulting in an autonomic imbalance with respect to cardiac function. Neonates respond to physiologic challenges in a predominantly vagal, or parasympathetic, fashion. Sinus bradycardia is therefore a common stereotypical response in the critically ill neonate to many stimuli, including hypoxemia, acidosis, hypoglycemia, intracranial hypertension, abdominal distention, and pulmonary aspiration. Because bradycardia is also more likely to result in an uncompensated decrease in cardiac output, prompt recognition and treatment of bradycardia are more urgent in these patients.

Preload refers to the myocardial fiber stretch at end diastole. *Fiber stretch* is related to end-diastolic volume, which in turn is related to end-diastolic pressure. The Frank-Starling mechanism describes this relationship: An increase in end-diastolic volume and fiber length produces an increase in stroke volume (Fig. 106.10). This phenomenon most likely is explained by changes in contractile fiber geometry that result from increased stretch. The Frank-Starling mechanism is not synonymous with an increase in contractility, which would produce an increased stroke volume at the same preload. This mechanism is less effective in neonates than in adults in producing an increase in myocardial performance. The immature heart is less compliant than the adult heart; so increases in end-diastolic pressure therefore do not produce similar increases in end-diastolic volume and fiber length. Furthermore, neonatal and infant hearts operate at a higher baseline end-diastolic volume (nearer the maximal fiber length) under normal circumstances, leaving less reserve for further effective increases in preload. These observations explain why the neonatal cardiovascular response to preload enhancement is less pronounced than in adults and why the neonate is generally more susceptible to congestive failure when challenged with a volume load.

Contractility refers to the magnitude and velocity of tension development by the cardiac myocytes in response to contractile stimuli. The contractile, or inotropic, state of the heart is influenced by many factors, including the availability of oxygen, calcium, and catecholamines. An increase in contractility does not result in a shift upward along the Frank-Starling curve, but rather it results in a shift of the entire curve to reflect a greater stroke volume generated at every preload. The neonatal heart is immature in several respects compared with the adult heart. Most importantly, the neonatal heart has a lower concentration of contractile fibers, generating less tension during contraction.[38] This is reflected in the lower mean arterial pressures observed throughout childhood. About 60% of the adult cardiac myocyte mass comprises contractile myofibrils, compared with 30% in fetal myocytes. Additional causes of reduced contractility include an underdeveloped sarcoplasmic reticulum and t-tubule system for releasing calcium, a lower concentration of myocyte cell surface β-adrenergic receptors, and

TABLE 106.6

NORMAL RANGE OF VITAL SIGNS

Age	Heart rate (beats/min)	Systolic blood pressure (mm Hg)	Diastolic blood pressure (mm Hg)	Respiratory rate (breaths/min)
Premature infant				
1 kg	120–140	36–58	18–38	40
3 kg	120–140	50–72	26–46	40
Term infant	120	65–80	30–50	40
0–12 mo[a]	100–120	105	65	40
1–6 y	100	105–110	70	30
6–12 y	80	110–125	70–80	20

[a]90th percentile.
Adapted from Horan MU. Report of the Second Task Force on Blood Pressure Control in Children—1987. *Pediatrics* 1987;79:1.

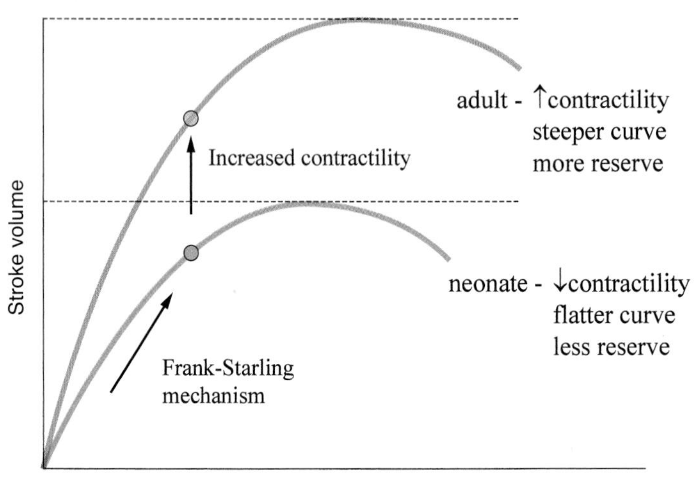

FIGURE 106.10 Conceptual differences in cardiac performance between neonates and adults. The neonatal heart displays reduced contractility, a reduced response to augmented preload, and a less reserve compared with the adult heart.

decreased sympathetic innervation.[39] The structural and functional immaturity of the infant heart account for the relatively greater sensitivity to negative inotropic stimuli, the greater requirement for calcium to maintain the inotropic state, and the requirement for higher concentrations of inotropic agents to achieve measurable hemodynamic effects. In contrast, the neonatal heart is more resistant to the negative inotropic effects of hypoxemia and acidosis than the adult heart, possibly conferring some advantage with respect to the success of cardiopulmonary resuscitation.[40]

Afterload refers to the resistance (or impedance) to ventricular output and is directly related to mean arterial pressure. During the transitional phase of circulation, afterload drops abruptly in the right ventricle as pulmonary vascular resistance drops. Left ventricular afterload increases immediately as the placental shunt is abolished but then falls as its output distributes to both the upper and lower body and a larger vascular bed. After the transitional phase, left ventricular afterload slowly increases throughout infancy and childhood, stimulating asymmetrical growth of the left ventricle compared with that of the right. This growth is caused primarily by hyperplasia until 2 to 3 months of age, when hypertrophy becomes more important. Before adaptive left ventricular growth occurs, the neonatal heart is exquisitely sensitive and decompensates rapidly when exposed to increases in afterload, such as those that occur in aortic stenosis and aortic coarctation.

Oxygen Content and Delivery

Oxygen delivery is the product of cardiac output and oxygen content. Arterial oxygen content (C_aO_2) is determined by the same set of variables in children as in adults:

$$C_aO_2 = (\text{Hb})(1.34 \text{ mL } O_2/\text{g Hb})(\% \text{ Hb saturation}) + \text{Dissolved } O_2$$

where Hb = hemoglobin.

Under most circumstances, dissolved oxygen is negligible. The main difference in the oxygen-carrying capacity of blood between neonates and older patients is the presence of fetal hemoglobin (HbF). The fetal red blood cell contains primarily HbF, a hemoglobin isomer with a higher affinity for oxygen than hemoglobin A (HbA), which predominates in adults. This gives HbF a lower P_{50} (the partial pressure of oxygen at which hemoglobin saturation is 50%), which is reflected in a leftward shift of the oxyhemoglobin dissociation curve relative to HbA (Fig. 106.11). This difference in affinities promotes the transfer

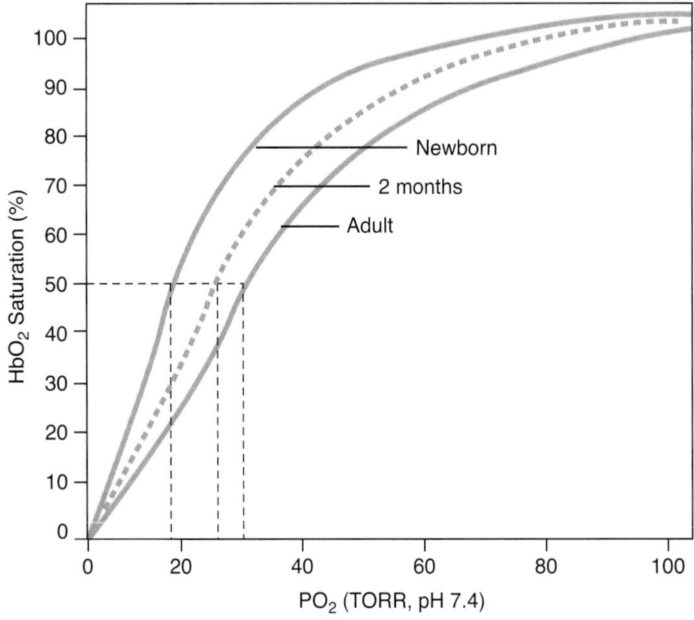

FIGURE 106.11 Representative oxyhemoglobin (HbO_2) saturation curves for newborn, infant, and adult. (From Hodson WA, Truog WE. In: Avery GB, Fletcher MA, MacDonald MG, eds. *Neonatology: pathophysiology and management of the newborn*, 5th ed. Philadelphia: Lippincott Williams & Wilkins, 1999, with permission.)

of oxygen from maternal to fetal hemoglobin in the placenta. Following birth, neonatal red blood cells gradually accumulate HbA at the expense of HgF, which disappears by 4 months of age.

The presence of HbF in the neonate has several clinical consequences. Adequate hemoglobin saturation may occur at lower P_aO_2 levels, but the benefits of this in the *ex utero* environment are deceiving. Greater oxygen affinity makes the unloading of oxygen in peripheral tissues more difficult. Increasing oxygen extraction during periods when oxygen demand temporarily exceeds supply is therefore less efficient. Increased difficulty in extracting oxygen from hemoglobin in peripheral tissues makes the neonate less tolerant than the older child of decreased oxygen delivery resulting from reduced hemoglobin concentration, hemoglobin saturation, or cardiac output. Constant attention to adequate oxygen content and cardiac output is therefore of paramount importance in the stressed neonate.

Pulmonary Hypertension and Persistent Fetal Circulation

In the older infant and child, PVR is normally low, which allows right ventricular output to equal that of the left ventricle at considerably lower pressure and contractile work. The instability of PVR in the neonate during the transitional period, along with the presence of anatomic connections between the pulmonary and systemic circuits, accounts for severe derangements in respiratory and hemodynamic performance in a wide variety of clinical disorders. These include acquired conditions (e.g., sepsis and meconium aspiration syndrome), congenital conditions (e.g., pulmonary hypoplasia), idiopathic abnormalities in pulmonary vascular function (e.g., PPHN), and chronic microangiopathy, alveolar-capillary dysplasia, and fibrosis ("fixed" pulmonary hypertension secondary to uncorrected anatomic left-to-right shunting and pulmonary overcirculation).

The common denominator in these conditions is an abnormally high PVR, which may be caused by inappropriate vasoconstriction, reduced total capillary cross-sectional area, or fibrotic arterioles of fixed caliber. Not uncommonly, increased PVR results from a combination of these factors. For example, pulmonary hypoplasia not only causes decreased cross-sectional area but also results in hyperreactive arterioles prone to vasospasm. In "fixed" pulmonary hypertension, both fibrosis and decreased vessel numbers have been demonstrated. In perinatal aspiration of meconium or blood, ventilation is delayed and pulmonary hypertension ensues. Fetal exposure to maternally ingested nonsteroidal anti-inflammatory drugs causes spasm of the ductus arteriosus, increased fetal pulmonary flows and pressures, diminished NO synthase activity, and harmful pulmonary vascular remodeling.

Whatever the cause, increased PVR has several deleterious consequences. Increased right ventricular afterload results in decreased output, diminished pulmonary perfusion, and reduced left ventricular preload. Hypoxemia, hypercarbia, and globally decreased cardiac output result, which in turn cause metabolic acidosis. Increased PVR also promotes anatomic right-to-left shunting at the levels of the patent ductus arteriosus (PDA) and foramen ovale, a phenomenon referred to as *persistent fetal circulation* (PFC). This profoundly exacerbates the hypoxemia, hypercarbia, and acidosis already present. Because hypoxemia, hypercarbia, and acidosis are all potent mediators of pulmonary vasoconstriction, PVR is further increased. For this reason, pulmonary hypertension and PFC in the neonate frequently deteriorate into a vicious cycle that culminates in circulatory and metabolic collapse.

Therapy for pulmonary hypertension and PFC is directed at treating the underlying cause, removing the physiologic stimuli for pulmonary vasoconstriction, and introducing pharmacologic mediators of pulmonary vasodilatation. Analgesia, sedation, and neuromuscular blockade are commonly used to decrease endogenous stimulation of pulmonary vasoconstriction by catecholamines. The mainstays of management include aggressive ventilatory support to maximize P_aO_2 and minimize P_aCO_2, and systemic alkalinization (pH 7.50 to 7.60) with sodium bicarbonate or tris-hydroxymethylaminomethane (THAM) if an adequate respiratory alkalosis cannot be induced. Because severe respiratory failure frequently precedes and causes pulmonary hypertension and PFC, attempts to achieve these objectives through conventional ventilatory support alone are often unsuccessful. Oscillatory ventilation has been of occasional benefit in neonates with PFC by achieving increased oxygenation and respiratory alkalosis in circumstances when conventional ventilatory support has failed. Pharmacologic agents with the ability to promote direct pulmonary vasodilatation would obviously be desirable.

Selective pulmonary vasodilatation is presently unrealistic from a clinical standpoint. No pharmacologic substance has yet been identified that has vasodilatory effects specifically limited to the pulmonary circulation. Intravenous administration of nitroprusside, nitroglycerine, and PGE_1 all produce systemic vasodilatation as well, negating the reduction of resistance and pressure in the pulmonary circuit, and resulting in unaltered right-to-left shunt. Tolazoline hydrochloride was commonly used in the past as a pulmonary vasodilator in neonates with pulmonary hypertension. Its vasodilatory effects can be ascribed both to a-adrenergic blockade as well as stimulation of pulmonary vascular histamine receptors.[41] Unfortunately, responses to tolazoline are unpredictable and nonselective, and no consistent clinical benefit has been convincingly demonstrated.

Perhaps the most promising pharmacologic approach to pulmonary vasodilatation is the administration of inhaled nitric oxide (INO). NO is a ubiquitous, potent vasodilator that serves as the final common pathway for vascular smooth-muscle relaxation induced by a wide variety of other agents with known vasodilatory properties.[42,43] Endogenous NO is generated from L-arginine by the action of NO synthase in endothelial cells (eNOS) and diffuses to adjacent smooth-muscle cells, where it promotes muscular relaxation via a cyclic guanosine monophosphate (GMP)-dependent mechanism.[44] Although smooth muscle relaxation induced by NO is not specific for the pulmonary circulation, vasodilatation is limited to the pulmonary circulation because INO is immediately scavenged and inactivated in the pulmonary bloodstream by binding to hemoglobin and forming methemoglobin. Thus, INO is able to bind to pulmonary vascular smooth-muscle cell receptors and induce relaxation before it diffuses into the capillary lumen and becomes inactivated. The fact the INO diffuses directly to the smooth muscle cells makes this therapy ideal in the presence of endothelial cell injury, which is commonly seen in PPHN.

INO is administered by mixing minute quantities of NO (5 to 20 ppm) into the gas mixture during mechanical ventilation. Although toxicity from methemoglobin has been suggested as a potential adverse effect, clinically significant methemoglobinemia has not been observed when NO is delivered at such low concentrations. A more significant difficulty with inhaled NO therapy is the development of tachyphylaxis, which frequently occurs after as little as 2 to 3 days of treatment.[45] Despite this potential obstacle, this novel strategy of selective delivery of a potent, nonspecific vasodilator to the pulmonary circulation represents a major new development in the treatment of pulmonary hypertension in infants.

Better understanding of mechanisms of pulmonary vasoreactivity have suggested alternate approaches to INO therapy for PPHN.[46] Direct infusion of L-arginine provides both increased substrate for endogenous NO generation as well as stimulation of increased eNOS activity. Phosphodiesterase inhibitors such as sildenafil delay the degradation of both cyclic AMP and cyclic GMP, resulting in higher intracellular concentations of these vasodilatory compounds. Sildenafil use may be limited by systemic hypotension, and studies are currently ongoing to establish the safety and efficacy of this drug in PPHN. Adenosine and ATP may also produce selective pulmonary vasodilation when infused intravenously, though their use in neonates with PPHN has not been studied.

Failure to promote pulmonary vasodilatation through physiologic or pharmacologic manipulation may indicate a need to use extracorporeal techniques to reverse hypoxemia, hypercarbia, hypoperfusion, and acidosis. As discussed, ECMO has become a widely accepted therapy for refractory pulmonary hypertension associated with a variety of causes. It is important to recognize that extracorporeal support for pulmonary hypertension (or respiratory failure) is indicated only when the underlying cause is thought to be reversible.

GASTROINTESTINAL AND HEPATIC PHYSIOLOGY

Most mechanisms of physiologic control in the gastrointestinal tract are present at birth, although continued postnatal maturation results in ongoing adjustments over time. Prematurity, however, is associated with a delay in gastrointestinal function, just as it is in the cardiovascular and pulmonary systems. For example, immaturity of gastrointestinal motility and digestive enzyme activity in the preterm infant frequently results in early feeding intolerance. The functional immaturity of small intestinal "brush-border" enzymes in premature infants has already been mentioned with respect to the particular nutritional requirements of preterm infants. Normal intestinal motility, as measured by the appearance of migrating motor complexes, has been documented to appear by 36 to 38 weeks of gestation. Whereas 95% of term infants will pass a meconium stool within 24 hours of birth (and virtually 100% by 48 hours), it is not unusual for premature infants to have a significant delay in the passage of meconium that is dependent on the degree of prematurity.

The extraordinarily complex physiology of the gastrointestinal tract, including the control of motility, digestion, absorption, neurologic function, and enteroendocrine feedback, is beyond the scope of this chapter. Several specific topics in gastrointestinal physiology are relevant, however, because they relate to functional problems commonly encountered in pediatric patients. These topics include the physiology of gastrointestinal growth and adaptation, the pathophysiology of inadequate gastrointestinal length (short gut syndrome), and neonatal jaundice.

Physiology of Intestinal Growth and Adaptation

To meet the needs of the growing child for energy and structural substrates, the absorptive surface area of the intestinal tract must increase along with somatic growth. The small intestine increases from a length of about 200 to 300 cm and a diameter of about 1.5 cm at birth to a length of 600 to 800 cm and a diameter of 4 cm at maturity. Further growth and maturation of the villous architecture and the development of plicae circulares increase the total absorptive surface area from approximately 900 cm^2 to 7,500 cm^2 over the same period.[47]

After growing to full length in childhood, the small intestine enters a state of dormancy and remains quiescent unless some major change occurs. Following massive intestinal resection, various adaptive responses occur in the small intestine; these responses are designed to enhance the absorptive function of the remaining bowel. These adaptive changes include an increase in diameter, an increase in the number and size of the plicae circulares, and epithelial hyperplasia manifested as increased villous height and crypt depth. These changes augment absorptive surface area significantly, but they do not constitute a physiologically equivalent substitute for intestine of normal length and caliber. The markedly dilated, adapted intestine displays abnormal motility as a result of muscular hypertrophy and an inability to sustain normal peristalsis by coaptation. These dyskinetic contractions do not provide consistent, unidirectional flow and, therefore, allow stasis and bacterial colonization of the proximal intestine.

Although the factors governing stimulation of intestinal growth and adaptation are poorly understood, it is becoming increasingly clear that trophic stimulation from both enteroendocrine mediators and intraluminal substances is necessary. The gastrointestinal mucosa is richly populated with a variety of peptide-secreting enteroendocrine cells that produce local signaling and mediator molecules in response to specific stimuli (Fig. 106.12). Some of these enteroendocrine peptides are expressed only during fetal development. Virtually every known postnatal enteroendocrine cell is present and functionally mature at term.[48] The levels of many of these peptides rise sharply in the first days of life in fed infants, but not in fasting infants.[49] The observation that intestinal growth and maturation are inhibited by withholding enteral feeds suggests that enteroendocrine stimulation is one of the processes responsible for normal postnatal intestinal growth. Glucagon, glucagon-like peptides 1 and 2, and gastrin are present in the fetal and

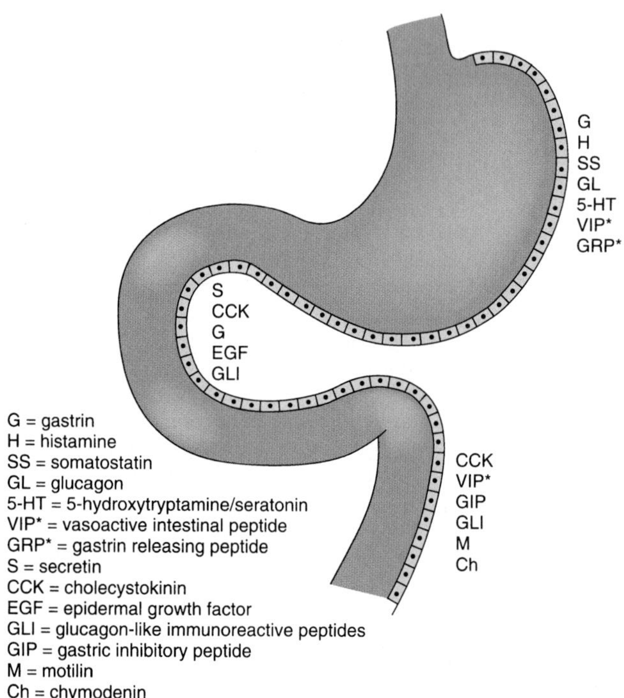

FIGURE 106.12 Distribution of selected enteroendocrine and neuroendocrine (*asterisks*) cells and their products in the proximal gastrointestinal tract. (From Magnuson DK, Schwartz MZ. In: Oldham KT, Colombani PM, Foglia RP, eds. *Surgery of infants and children*. Philadelphia: Lippincott–Raven, 1997, with permission.)

neonatal gut, and appear to be leading candidates for the principal enteroendocrine mediators of epithelial proliferation and overall gut growth, both by direct stimulation and through generation of other mediators such as insulin.[50–52]

Direct stimulation of mucosal growth by luminal nutrients plays a major role in intestinal adaptation. The fact that villous height and absorptive capacity are greatest in the proximal jejunum and gradually decrease through the remaining jejunum and ileum suggests that progressive depletion of luminal nutrients results in relatively diminished growth of the distal intestine. Reciprocal transposition of ileal and jejunal segments results in hypertrophy of the proximally transposed ileal segment and atrophy of the distally transposed jejunal segment. The "underdevelopment" of the distal small bowel may be viewed, to a certain extent, as built-in reserve potential.

In various experimental models, adaptive growth will not occur after resection unless some level of luminal nutrition is provided. Studies in animal models have shown that complex nutrients that require enzymatic degradation (e.g., long-chain fatty acids, disaccharides, and complex proteins) are more potent stimulators of growth than are more elemental nutrients.[53–55] This effect may result from the trophic properties of pancreaticobiliary secretions, which are stimulated by complex nutritional substrates. The amino acid glutamine is the preferred energy substrate for enterocytes and a necessary constituent of growth-promoting enteral nutrition formulas. It is not clear whether glutamine acts in a permissive fashion only by providing energy substrate for growth or whether it also has trophic properties separate from its energy content. Intravenous glutamine administration can preserve intestinal mucosal health in the absence of enteral glutamine, but whether it can promote long-term gut adaptation and growth also is not known. Epidermal growth factor (EGF), present in duodenal and biliary secretions, and growth hormone are both potent growth stimuli. The administration of enteral glutamine and EGF (or growth hormone or both) may have a therapeutic benefit in stimulating intestinal growth after bowel resection.

Clinical Aspects of Short-gut Syndrome

Although intestinal growth is commonly taken for granted in health, its importance is brought into sharp focus by conditions in which inadequate intestinal length causes malabsorption and malnutrition: *the short-gut syndrome*. This syndrome usually occurs after massive intestinal resection for a variety of diseases. The most common causes in the neonatal period are necrotizing enterocolitis and midgut volvulus, although gastroschisis also may be associated with decreased intestinal length in the absence of resection.[56,57] In older children, volvulus and inflammatory bowel disease predominate.[58] The extent of resection likely to result in short-gut syndrome is difficult to quantify and is influenced by patient age, site of intestinal loss, and status of the ileocecal valve (ICV). It is commonly held that a term newborn who retains at least 25 cm of small intestine with an intact ICV, or 40 cm without an ICV, has a reasonable potential for resuming full enteral feedings at some point. In older patients, loss of 75% to 80% of intestinal length may be tolerated as long as the ICV is preserved.

The loss of intestinal surface area diminishes absorptive capacity, brush-border digestive enzyme activity, and enteroendocrine mediator production. These deficiencies all lead to malnutrition and weight loss. Unabsorbed sugars pass through to the colon and produce an osmotic diarrhea. Presentation of undigested carbohydrates to the colon also provides fuel for bacterial proliferation. The bacteria metabolize the undigested sugars to lactate and short-chain fatty acids, which stimulate colonic secretion of water and electrolytes. Thus, a secretory diarrhea exacerbates the osmotic one. After ileal resections, bile salt recirculation is impaired and bile salts reach the colon, providing more bacterial fuel and further stimulating the secretory diarrhea. Bile salt wasting eventually depletes the hepatic bile salt pool, resulting in fat malabsorption and steatorrhea and producing lithogenic bile and gallstones. Extensive ileal resections also result in impaired absorption of vitamin B_{12} and the fat-soluble vitamins A, D, E, and K.

Bacterial overgrowth in the residual small intestine occurs in most patients with short-gut syndrome. It is related primarily to the loss of the ICV and reflux of colonic bacteria into the small intestine. Overgrowth also is promoted by stasis and hypomotility, which occur in adapted, dilated, dyskinetic intestine. Bacterial overgrowth in the proximal intestine leads to further increases in carbohydrate, protein, and fluid and electrolyte loss caused by diarrhea.

Gastric hypersecretion of fluid and acid is well documented in short-gut syndrome. Acid hypersecretion has been linked to hypergastrinemia, possibly because of the loss of somatostatin and gastrin-inhibiting peptide production. Gastric hypersecretion results in peptic complications, reduced enzymatic digestion caused by low intraluminal pH, and further exacerbation of diarrhea.

Management of short-gut syndrome is complex and may include any combination of the following: parenteral nutrition, limited enteral feeding with easily absorbed substrates (glucose polymers, medium-chain triglycerides, protein hydrosylates), judicious enteral exposure to trophic substrates (complex carbohydrates, intact protein, long-chain triglycerides, and glutamine), antibiotic suppression of bacterial overgrowth, supplementation of vitamins and minerals, and control of diarrhea with antimotility agents. Surgical treatment of short-gut syndrome by intestinal lengthening procedures and transplantation has been disappointing.

Neonatal Jaundice

Hepatic function in the older child is essentially the same as in the adult. In the neonatal period, however, liver function may be altered in a number of ways by hepatocyte immaturity. Although fetal hepatocytes begin to manifest synthetic capabilities early in gestation, the quantitative capacity to produce, modify, and detoxify various substances develops gradually and is often incompletely developed at birth, particularly in premature infants. This functional immaturity affects a range of processes, including glycogen metabolism and the biotransformation of many drugs, but most notably it affects the excretion of bilirubin.

Bilirubin Metabolism

Bilirubin is produced by the degradation of heme-containing compounds, primarily hemoglobin from senescent red blood cells, but also myoglobin, cytochromes, catalases, and other molecules. Because infants have a relatively greater red cell mass than adults, as well as a shorter red cell life span and higher turnover, bilirubin production is proportionately greatest in the first weeks of life. The conversion of heme to bilirubin occurs in reticuloendothelial cells in the liver, spleen, and elsewhere. In the first step, the ring structure of heme is opened by the oxidative removal of a carbon atom through heme oxygenase, which also releases a reduced iron atom. The resulting product, biliverdin, is a linear molecule that is further reduced by biliverdin reductase to bilirubin. Bilirubin is held in a tightly folded configuration by extensive hydrogen bonding, resulting in a highly hydrophobic and insoluble molecule. As such, transport of bilirubin from sites of production to the liver for excretion requires binding to albumin as a carrier molecule.

Bilirubin is extracted from hepatic sinusoidal blood and transported by a specific membrane carrier protein into the hepatocyte, where it is attached to the cytoplasmic carrier protein ligandin (glutathione S-transferase). Within the cytoplasm, bilirubin is conjugated with glucuronic acid by bilirubin glucuronosyltransferase (BGT) to form bilirubin monoglucuronides (BMG) and diglucuronides (BDGs). Both BMGs and BDGs then are transported into the bile canaliculi and excreted via the bile ducts into the duodenum. Normally, a small amount of conjugated bilirubin is found in the blood because of back-diffusion across the sinusoidal membrane. In pathologic states where the excretion of BMGs and BDGs cannot keep pace with production, serum levels of conjugated bilirubin rise. Hepatocyte excretion of BMGs and BDGs is the rate-limiting step in bilirubin clearance after 1 week of age, before which time conjugation of bilirubin is rate limiting because of diminished activity of BGT.

Within the intestinal lumen, bilirubin conjugates can have several fates. Most are metabolized by resident bacteria into a variety of compounds, including the urobilinogens and the urobilinoids, which are excreted in the feces. The conversion of conjugated bilirubin into urobilinoids prevents the reabsorption, or enterohepatic recirculation, of bilirubin. Other bacteria, as well as mucosal cells, contain b-glucuronidase capable of deconjugating BMG and BDG. Deconjugated bilirubin is hydrophobic and easily reabsorbed across the epithelial barrier and back into the circulation. Neonates are particularly susceptible to bilirubin reabsorption that results from increased levels of endogenous b-glucuronidase and decreased bacterial flora. The relative paucity of resident bacteria results in less successful conversion of bilirubin conjugates to urobilinoids, whereas the increased activity of b-glucuronidase deconjugates the bilirubin. Meconium contains a high concentration of conjugated bilirubin, which readily undergoes deconjugation if impaired motility delays its excretion.

Neonatal Hyperbilirubinemia

Transient, unconjugated hyperbilirubinemia is a ubiquitous finding in neonates and represents a normal stage in early postnatal life. For this reason, it is often referred to as *physiologic jaundice*. The exact cause of physiologic jaundice is unclear, but it appears to involve a combination of increased enterohepatic circulation of bilirubin and decreased BGT activity.[59] Both the duration and magnitude of the hyperbilirubinemia are variable but, in general, plasma levels of unconjugated bilirubin peak at about 5 to 6 mg/dL at 3 days of life and resolve by 7 to 10 days in healthy term infants.

In addition to physiologic jaundice, numerous conditions are associated with more severe unconjugated hyperbilirubinemia in the early postnatal period. These include breast-milk jaundice, hemolytic diseases (ABO or Rh incompatibility, hemoglobinopathies), reabsorption of extravascular blood, neonatal hepatitis, inborn errors of metabolism, and sepsis. Unconjugated hyperbilirubinemia can cause both a reversible encephalopathy and an irreversible neurologic injury termed *kernicterus*. The predilection of unconjugated bilirubin for neural tissue is related to its nonpolar structure, which makes it highly hydrophobic and lipophilic. Deposition of bilirubin in the basal ganglia and cranial nerve nuclei is the most common pathologic feature, although clinical manifestations include a wide variety of cognitive, developmental, motor, and sensory dysfunction. The risks of neurologic injury are related to peak sustained bilirubin levels; kernicterus is likely when sustained plasma levels exceed 30 mg/dL and is virtually unknown when levels do not exceed 20 mg/dL. Between 20 and 30 mg/dL, the incidence of reversible encephalopathy is greatest, but increasing risk of kernicterus is a concern.

Indications for intervention include early onset or prolonged duration of jaundice and exaggerated absolute levels of unconjugated bilirubin. The precise level at which therapeutic intervention is considered depends on postnatal and gestational age, weight, and presence of comorbidity, and is the subject of considerable debate. First-line therapies include stimulation of intestinal motility by oral feeding and rectal stimulation to promote the passage of meconium and reduce enterohepatic circulation. When levels become high or sustained enough to elicit genuine concern, the treatment of choice is phototherapy. Light in the blue spectrum with wavelengths of 420 to 480 nm is absorbed by unconjugated bilirubin. The absorbed energy alters the double bond structure of bilirubin in a process termed *photoisomerization*. The new isomers are less capable of forming internal hydrogen bonds and, therefore, become unfolded and more polar. This configurational change makes them more soluble, promotes their mobilization from central nervous system tissues, and allows their excretion in the bile without further conjugation. When extremely high levels of bilirubin are encountered and phototherapy is deemed insufficiently rapid, exchange transfusion provides the most reliable method of rapidly reducing serum bilirubin levels into a nontoxic range.

In contrast to unconjugated hyperbilirubinemia, elevation of serum conjugated bilirubin is always pathologic and mandates expeditious evaluation. The presence of isolated conjugated hyperbilirubinemia in the first weeks of life usually suggests the presence of a condition associated with reduced bile excretion. These include extrahepatic biliary atresia, Alagille's syndrome (arteriohepatic dysplasia or intrahepatic biliary hypoplasia), nonsyndromic intrahepatic bile duct paucity, Byler's syndrome (progressive familial intrahepatic cholestasis), choledochal cyst, and TPN-related cholestasis. Not all episodes of conjugated hyperbilirubinemia result from biliary obstruction, however. Because hepatocyte excretion of BMGs and BDGs is rate limiting after the first week of life, increased bilirubin loads generated by hemolysis or reabsorption may result in the production of bilirubin conjugates at a rate exceeding the hepatocyte's ability to excrete them into the canaliculi. Intracellular buildup results in back-diffusion of conjugated bilirubin into the sinusoidal and systemic circulation.

KEY POINTS

- **During the 8-week embryonic period, developmental events transform a fertilized egg into a "preorganism" that comprises all the specialized tissues and organ systems required for future independent life; the subsequent 32-week fetal period involves accelerated growth and continuous organ maturation.**
- **The fetus utilizes glucose as its primary energy substrate.**
- **Maternal and placental mechanisms maintain an optimal temperature for fetal development; the net heat produced by fetal metabolic activity must be transferred away from the fetal environment to avoid a rise in temperature.**
- **Neonates and children have significantly higher energy requirements than adults.**
- **Breast milk is a complex mixture of macromolecules that changes as the growing infant's needs change; the usable energy content of milk is divided almost equally between carbohydrates and lipids.**
- **At 12 weeks' gestation, water constitutes 95% of fetal mass; this declines to about 80% by 32 weeks' gestation and to 75% at term.**
- **The determinants of gas exchange are total alveolar ventilation, ventilation/perfusion matching, diffusion, and extrapulmonary shunt; the mechanical properties of the lung affect gas exchange primarily by determining the amount and distribution of ventilation. Regulation of pulmonary blood flow determines ventilation/perfusion matching and the efficiency of gas exchange.**

- **Respiratory distress syndrome, or hyaline membrane disease, is the most common causes of respiratory distress in neonates and one of the primary causes of neonatal mortality in developed countries.**
- **The variations of ECMO share underlying principles: the partial diversion of blood from the patient to an external membrane oxygenator, *ex vivo* exchange of oxygen and carbon dioxide, and return of blood to the circulatory system.**
- **At birth, circulatory patterns, hemodynamics, and gas exchange transition are characterized by the cessation of placental blood flow and gas exchange and the simultaneous increase in blood flow and gas exchange in the lungs.**
- **Most mechanisms of physiologic control in the gastrointestinal tract are present at birth, although continued postnatal maturation results in ongoing adjustments over time.**

References

1. **Bottoms SF, Paul RH, Mercer BM, et al. Obstetric determinants of neonatal survival: antenatal predictors of neonatal survival and morbidity in extremely low birth weight infants. *Am J Obstet Gynecol.* 1999;180(Pt 1):665–669.**
2. Horbar JD, Onstad L, Wright E. Predicting mortality risk for infants weighing 501 to 1,500 grams at birth. *Crit Care Med.* 1993;21:12–18.
3. Soriano-Guillen L, Barrios V, Chowen JA, et al. Ghrelin levels from fetal life through early adulthood: relations with endocrine and metabolic and anthropometric measures. *J Pediatr.* 2004; 144:30–35.
4. Hawdon JM, Ward Platt MP. Metabolic adaptation in small for gestational age infants. *Arch Dis Child.* 1993;68:262–268.
5. Lee H, Jain L. Physiology of infants with very low birth weight. *Semin Pediatr Surg.* 1990;9:50–55.
6. Sell H, Deshaies Y, Richard D. The brown adipocyte: update on its metabolic role. *Int J Biochem Cell Biol.* 2004;36:2098–2104.
7. Whyte RK, Campbell D, Stanhope R, et al. Energy balance in low birth weight infants fed formula of high or low medium chain triglyceride content. *J Pediatr.* 1986;108:964–971.
8. Sauer PJ, Dane HF, Visser HK. Longitudinal studies on metabolic rate, heat loss, and energy cost of growth in low birth weight infants. *Pediatr Res.* 1984;18:254–259.
9. Holliday MA. Body composition and energy needs during growth. In: Faulkner F, Tanner JM, eds. *Human growth: a comprehensivetreatise*, 2nd ed. New York: Plenum Press, 1986, pp. 101–117.
10. Groner JI, Brown MF, Stallings VA, et al. Resting energy expenditure in children following major operative procedures. *J Pediatr Surg.* 1989;24:825–827.
11. Mitchell IM, Davies PS, Day JM, et al. Energy expenditure in children with congenital heart disease, before and after cardiac surgery. *J Thorac Cardiovasc Surg.* 1994;107:374–380.
12. **Dekelbab BH, Sperling MA. Hyperinsulinemic hypoglycemia of infancy: the challenge continues. *Diabetes Metab Res Rev.* 2004;20:189–195.**
13. Souba WW, Herskowitz K, Austgen TR, et al. Glutamine nutrition: theoretical considerations and therapeutic impact. *JPEN J Parenter Enteral Nutr.* 1990;14(5 suppl):237S–243S.
14. Lorenz JM, Kleinman LI, Ahmed G, et al. Phases of fluid and electrolyte homeostasis in the extremely low birth weight infant. *Pediatrics* 1995;96(3 Pt 1): 484–489.
15. Bonilla-Felix M. Development of water transport. *Am J Physiol Renal Physiol.* 2004;287:F1093–101.
16. Del Riccio V, Van Tuyl M, Post M. Apoptosis in lung development and neonatal lung injury. *Pediatr Res.* 2004;55:183–189.
17. Nakayama DK, Motoyama EK, Tagge EM. Effect of preoperative stabilization on respiratory system compliance and outcome in newborn infants with congenital diaphragmatic hernia. *J Pediatr.* 1991;118:793–799.
18. Helms P, Stocks J. Lung function in infants with congenital pulmonary hypoplasia. *J Pediatr.* 1982;101:918–922.
19. Wolfson MR, Bhutani VK, Shaffer TH, et al. Mechanics and energetics of breathing helium in infants with bronchopulmonary dysplasia. *J Pediatr.* 1984;104:752–757.
20. Cassin S, Tod M, Philips J, et al. Effects of prostaglandin D2 in the perinatal circulation. *Am J Physiol.* 1981;240:H755–H760.
21. Chatfield BA, McMurtry IF, Hall SL, et al. Hemodynamic effects of endothelin-1 on the ovine fetal pulmonary circulation. *Am J Physiol.* 1991;261: R182–R187.
22. Ivy DD, Kinsella JP, Abman SH. Physiologic characterization of endothelin A and B receptor activity in the ovine fetal pulmonary circulation. *J Clin Invest.* 1994;93:2141–2148.
23. **Bunt JE, Carnielli VP, Darcos Wattimena JL, et al. The effect in premature infants of prenatal corticosteroids on endogenous surfactant synthesis as measured with stable isotopes. *Am J Respir Crit Care Med.* 2000;162:844–849.**
24. Gregory TJ, Steinberg KP, Spragg R, et al. Bovine surfactant therapy for patients with acute respiratory distress syndrome. *Am J Respir Crit Care Med.* 1997;155:1309–1315.
25. Galie N, Manes A, Branzi A. The endothelin system in pulmonary arterial hypertension. *Cardiovasc Res.* 2004;61:227–237.
26. Marraro GA. Innovative practices of ventilatory support with pediatric patients. *Pediatr Crit Care Med.* 2003;4:1–26.
27. Dreyfuss D, Soler P, Basset G, et al. High inflation pulmonary edema. *Am Rev Respir Dis.* 1988;137:1159–1164.
28. Hernandez LA, Peevy KJ, Moise AA, et al. Chest wall restriction limits high airway pressure-induced lung injury in young rabbits. *J Appl Physiol.* 1989;66:2364–2368.
29. Dreyfuss D, Saumon G. Role of tidal volume, FRC, and end-inspiratory volume in the development of pulmonary edema following mechanical ventilation. *Am Rev Respir Dis.* 1993;148:1194–1203.
30. Leach CL, Fuhrman BP, Morin FC III, et al. Perfluorocarbon-associated gas exchange (partial liquid ventilation) in respiratory distress syndrome: a prospective, randomized, controlled study. *Crit Care Med.* 1993;21: 1270–1278.
31. **Hansell DR. Extracorporeal membrane oxygenation for perinatal and pediatric patients. *Resp Care* 2003;48:352–362.**
32. Moler FW, Custer JR, Bartlett RH, et al. Extracorporeal life support for severe pediatric respiratory failure: an updated experience 1991–1993. *J Pediatr.* 1994;124:875–880.
33. St. John Sutton MG, Raichlen JS, Reichek N, et al. Quantitative assessment of right and left ventricular growth in the human fetal heart: a pathoanatomic study. *Circulation* 1984;70:935–941.
34. Rudolph AM, Heymann MA. Circulatory changes during growth in the fetal lamb. *Circ Res.* 1970;26:289–299.
35. Fineman JR, Soifer SJ, Heymann MA. Regulation of pulmonary vascular tone in the perinatal period. *Annu Rev Physiol.* 1995;57:115–134.
36. Shaul PW, Farrar MA, Magness RR. Oxygen modulation of pulmonary arterial prostacyclin synthesis is developmentally regulated. *Am J Physiol.* 1993;265(2 pt 2):H621–H628.
37. Shaul PW, Farrar MA, Zellers TM. Oxygen modulates endothelium-derived relaxing factor production in fetal pulmonary arteries. *Am J Physiol.* 1992;262(2 pt 2):H355–H364.
38. Anderson P. Physiology of the fetal, neonatal, and adult heart. In: Polin RA, Fox WW, eds. *Fetal and neonatal physiology*. Philadelphia: WB Saunders, 1992, pp. 722–758.
39. Artman M, Graham TP Jr, Boucek RJ Jr. Effects of postnatal maturation on myocardial contractile responses to calcium antagonists and changes in contraction frequency. *J Cardiovasc Physiol.* 1985;7:850–855.
40. Talner NS, Lister G, Fahey JT. Effects of asphyxia on the myocardium of the fetus and newborn. In: Polin RA, Fox WW, eds. *Fetal and Neonatal Physiology*. Philadelphia: WB Saunders, 1992, pp. 759–769.
41. Goetzman BG, Milstein JM. Pulmonary vasodilator action of tolazoline. *Pediatr Res.* 1979;13:942–944.
42. Palmer RMJ, Ferrige AG, Moncada S. Nitric oxide release accounts for the biological activity of endothelium-derived relaxing factor. *Nature* 1987;327: 524–526.
43. Ignarro LJ, Byrns RE, Buga GM, et al. Endothelium-dependent relaxing factor from pulmonary artery and vein possesses pharmacologic and chemical properties identical to those of nitric oxide radical. *Circ Res.* 1987;61:866–879.
44. Moncada S, Palmer RMJ, Higgs EA. Nitric oxide: physiology, pathophysiology, and pharmacology. *Pharmocol Rev.* 1991;43:109–142.
45. Kinsella JP, Nelsh SR, Ivy DD, et al. Clinical responses to prolonged treatment of persistent pulmonary hypertension of the newborn with low doses of inhaled nitric oxide. *J Pediatr.* 1993;123:103–108.
46. **Konduri GG. New approaches for persistent pulmonary hypertension of newborn. *Clin Perinatol.* 2004;31:591–611.**
47. Klish WJ, Putnam TC. The short gut. *Am J Dis Child.* 1981;135:1056–1061.
48. Bryant MG, Buchan AM, Gregor M, et al. Development of intestinal regulatory peptides in the human fetus. *Gastroenterology* 1982;83(1 pt 1):47–54.
49. Lucas A, Bloom SR, Aynsley-Green A. Metabolic and endocrine consequences of depriving preterm infants of enteral nutrition. *Acta Paediatr Scand.* 1983;72:245–249.
50. Bloom SR. Gut hormones in adaptation. *Gut* 1987;28[suppl 1]:31–35.
51. Fuller PJ, Beveridge DJ, Taylor RG. Ileal proglucagon gene expression in the rat: characterization in intestinal adaptation using in situ hybridization. *Gastroenterology* 1993;104:459–466.
52. Drucker DJ, Ehrlich P, Asa SL, et al. Induction of intestinal epithelial proliferation by glucagon-like peptide 2. *Proc Natl Acad Sci. USA* 1996;93:7911–7916.
53. Lentze MJ. Intestinal adaptation in short-bowel syndrome. *Eur J Pediatr.* 1989;148:294–299.
54. Weser E, Babbitt J, Hoban M. Intestinal adaptation: different growth responses to disaccharides compared with monosaccharides in rat small bowel. *Gastroenterology* 1986;91:1521–1527.
55. Vanderhoof JA, Grandjean CJ, Burkley KT, et al. Effect of casein versus casein hydrosylate on mucosal adaptation following massive small bowel resection in infant rats. *J Pediatr Gastroenterol Nutr.* 1984;3:262–267.
56. Grosfeld JL, Rescorla FJ, West JW. Short bowel syndrome in infancy and childhood. *Am J Surg.* 1986;151:41–46.
57. Grosfeld JL, Rescorla FJ, West JW, et al. Gastrointestinal injuries in childhood: analysis of 53 patients. *J Pediatr Surg.* 1989;24:580–583.
58. Ricour C, Duhamel JF, Arnaud-Battendier F, et al. Enteral and parenteral nutrition in the short-bowel syndrome in children. *World J Surg.* 1985;9: 310–315.
59. Kawade N, Onishi S. The prenatal and postnatal development of UDP-glucuronyltransferase activity towards bilirubin and the effect of premature birth on this activity in the human liver. *Biochem J.* 1981;196:257–260.

CHAPTER 107 ■ FETAL INTERVENTION

DARRELL L. CASS

Fetal surgery has emerged as an independent subspecialty of pediatric surgery. It is a field that has arisen from clinical necessity. Pediatric surgeons and perinatologists became frustrated with the management of a number of congenital structural anomalies in which the baby died or suffered severe life-long disability despite all efforts at treatment. With the advent of prenatal ultrasound in the 1970s, these conditions were diagnosed before birth. Fetuses were followed, and the prenatal natural history was elucidated. It became clear that a component of organ failure was acquired because of ongoing alterations in fetal development caused by the anomaly. Thus, it made sense that fetal interventions may be of benefit—to correct the pathophysiology to restore normal fetal development, survival, and good quality of life.

The first successful fetal intervention was reported by Sir A. W. Liley who successfully transfused a hydropic fetus for Rh disease.[1] Although a few attempts were made at exchange transfusion by an open technique in the 1960s, modern fetal surgery was envisioned and developed by Dr. Michael Harrison at the University of California, San Francisco (UCSF) in the late 1970s.[2] It was at UCSF that the concept of a fetal treatment program was developed, permitting a true multidisciplinary perspective on fetal disease. The first open fetal operation was performed in 1982, at which bilateral ureterostomies were performed in a 21-week gestation fetus with obstructive uropathy.[3] In the intervening years, tremendous progress has been made in the development of fetal surgery techniques, including advances in maternal–fetal anesthesia, tocolysis (prevention of preterm labor), and the development of less-invasive surgical techniques. During this same period there have been significant advances in neonatal surgical critical care that has improved the outcome of fetuses with congenital anomalies. Thus, fetal surgery indications must be continually reassessed. What may be an appropriate indication for fetal surgery in one decade, may not be in the next. At the present time there are only four fetal conditions that show clear benefit from fetal intervention: congenital cystic adenomatoid malformation (CCAM), fetal sacrococcygeal teratoma (SCT), a fetus with airway obstruction from a giant neck mass or laryngeal atresia, and twin-to-twin transfusion syndrome (TTTS). Fetal interventions, both open and videoscopic, have been used to treat a number of other fetal disorders, such as congenital diaphragmatic hernia, myelomeningocele, urologic obstruction, and most recently congenital heart malformations, but significant questions remain regarding the natural history of these disorders, whether we can accurately select those fetuses who may benefit from intervention, and whether fetal intervention can improve on the natural history of the disease.

FETAL IMAGING AND PRENATAL DIAGNOSIS

To consider any fetal therapy it is critical that: (a) one can accurately diagnose the condition and any associated anomalies that may have an impact on outcome; (b) one can reliably predict which individual fetuses will die or suffer serious long-term morbidity without fetal intervention; and (c) the procedure improves the outcome of the fetus with little to no maternal risk.

Most of the congenital defects that pediatric surgeons treat can now be detected before birth with the use of high-resolution ultrasound, color Doppler, and fetal magnetic resonance imaging (MRI). Frequently diagnosed anomalies include diaphragmatic hernia (Fig. 107.1), congenital lung lesions (Fig. 107.2), obstructive uropathy, neural-tube defects, neck masses (Fig. 107.3), congenital heart defects, and sacrococcygeal teratoma, as well as other surgical disorders, such as abdominal-wall defects (gastroschisis and omphalocele), intestinal atresias, and cystic and solid abdominal masses. Prenatal detection and serial ultrasonographic evaluation of these disorders has enhanced our understanding of their natural history, and has significantly improved perinatal management. Pediatric surgeons familiar with the management of congenital malformations before and after birth, along with obstetricians, neonatologists, geneticists, and other specialists, participate in family counseling and together contribute to optimal maternal—fetal management. Such multidisciplinary teams may recommend that the timing, mode (cesarean versus vaginal delivery), or location of delivery be altered. Furthermore, in rare circumstances prenatal diagnosis permits *in utero* treatment of the developing fetus to prevent, reverse, or minimize fetal organ injury or death.

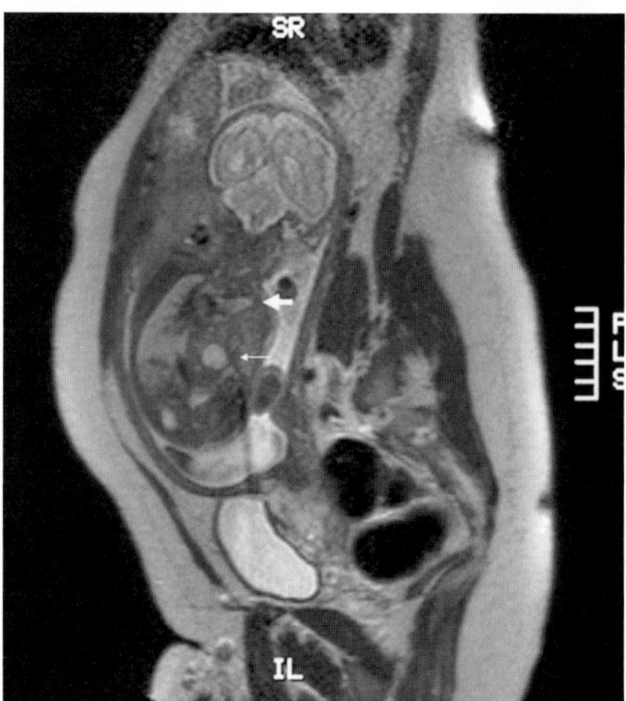

FIGURE 107.1 Coronal section of fetal magnetic resonance image (MRI) of a 30-week fetus with left congential high airway obstruction syndrome (CDH). The stomach (*small arrow*) and intestines are herniated into the left chest. The left lung is severely hypoplastic (*large arrow*).

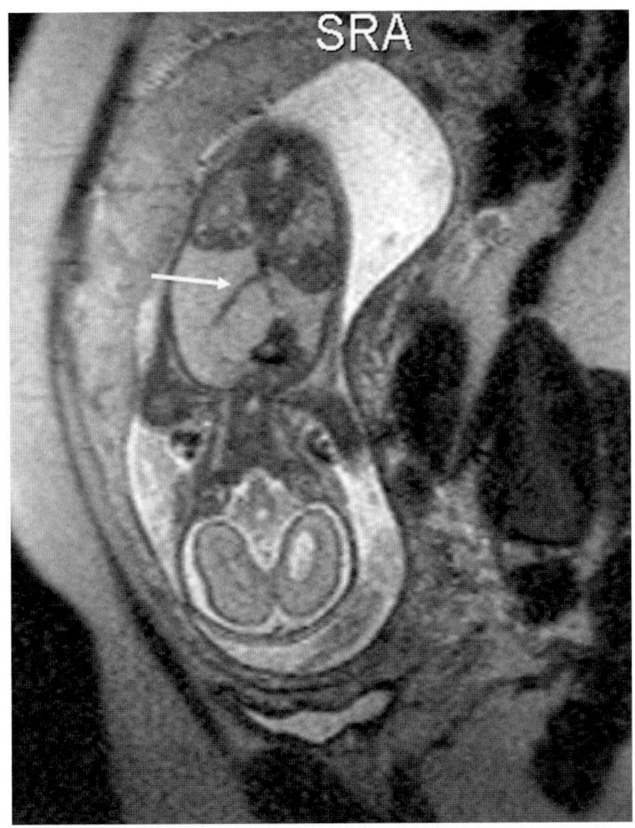

FIGURE 107.2 Coronal section of a fetal magnetic resonance image (MRI) of a 24-week fetus with a large left lung mass (bronchopulmonary sequestration). The left diaphragm is flattened and there is moderate dextroposition of the heart. A large vessel is seen coming from the low thoracic aorta (*arrow*). The congenital cystic adenomatoid malformation volume ratio (CVR) was 1.96; however, hydrops did not develop and the baby "grew around" the mass.

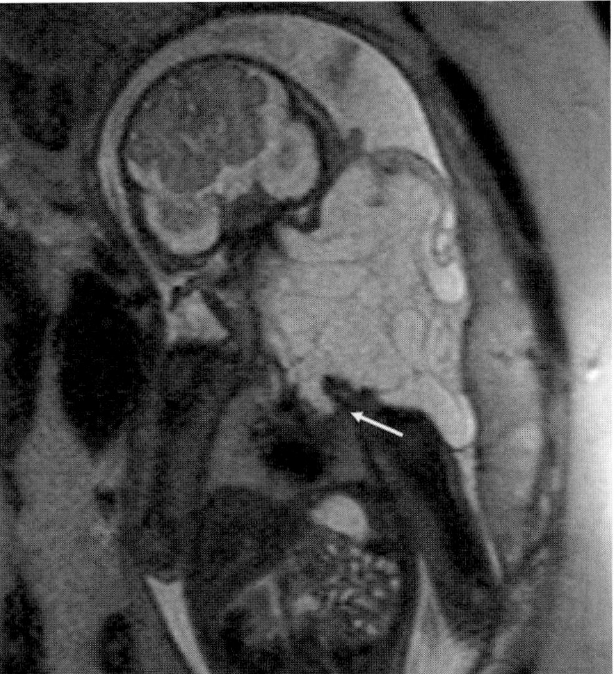

FIGURE 107.3 Coronal section of a fetal magnetic resonance image (MRI) of a 31-week fetus with a large left neck lymphatic malformation. The mass extends to the apex of the left chest (*arrow*). There is moderate left to right tracheal deviation. This fetus was delivered with an *ex utero* intrapartum treatment (EXIT) procedure.

In one study, prenatal consultation led to a change in pregnancy management in 67% of 221 pregnancies, of which 11 patients (5% of total) benefited from fetal intervention.[4]

Although most congenital anomalies are best managed with the use of appropriate medical and surgical therapy after delivery at term, rare life-threatening fetal anomalies may benefit from surgery before birth. The innovation of fetal surgery required the development of new surgical, anesthetic, and tocolytic techniques, as well as the resolution of such ethical issues as the safety of the mother and her future reproductive potential.[5–7]

MATERNAL—FETAL RISKS

Fetal surgery is unlike all other surgical specialties in that it involves two patients, and to accomplish it surgeons must pass through a healthy patient to fix a disease in the other patient. This paradigm presents challenging moral and ethical conflicts that must be considered and balanced in each circumstance. Chervenak and McCullough[8] and others have helped to provide an ethical framework within which fetal surgery should exist. The keys to this framework are that (a) the fetal operation has significant chance of being life-saving or of preventing serious or irreversible disease in the fetus; (b) the procedure involves low mortality and morbidity risk to the fetus; and (c) the operation has very low mortality and morbidity risk to the pregnant woman, including risks to future pregnancies. In light of these considerations, a number of contraindications to fetal intervention exist, including chromosomal abnormalities, the presence of other major anomalies, and significant maternal comorbidities.

There are significant maternal and fetal risks associated with fetal surgery that must be weighed for each patient. For the fetus, there is risk of preterm delivery, fetal death or survival with poor outcome. Most indications for fetal surgery, however, are ones in which the fetus would die without it, and therefore the risk-to-benefit ratio is very favorable. For those interventions aimed at improving the outcome of fetuses with nonlethal conditions the risk-benefit ratio is much more difficult to assess. Thus, the efficacy of fetal surgery for spina bifida is being evaluated with a prospective, randomized trial. For the mother, the risks and benefits are more challenging to assess, though the risks appear to be low. Benefits to the mother include the psychological reward from doing everything possible to improve the condition of the unborn baby. Also, there is physiologic benefit in preventing the possibility of "mirror syndrome," a preeclampsia-like condition in which the mother's condition "mirrors" that of a sick or dying fetus.[9] In the presence of this syndrome, fetal surgery is contraindicated and urgent fetal delivery is important to ensure maternal health. For the mother, fetal surgery adds the discomfort of one or two operations that would not have been required otherwise. For mothers who have hysterotomy other than low transverse, and for all mothers having fetal surgery, there are theoretical risks to subsequent pregnancies and future fertility. When maternal fertility following fetal surgery was studied, however, it was found that 32 of 35 mothers were able to achieve successful subsequent pregnancies and 31 live births resulted.[7] Postoperatively, nonhydrostatic pulmonary edema may occur in the mother. This problem was more prevalent in the early experience of open fetal repair approaches, but it persists. In a recent trial reported by Harrison et al.,[10] 3 of 11 mothers developed pulmonary edema and required oxygen after fetal surgery. In each of these patients the symptoms were mild and resolved within 48 hours. The cause of this phenomenon remains unclear, but is likely related to uterine manipulation and the release of prostaglandins or thromboplastins that alter maternal lung vascular permeability.[11] As with all obstetric surgery, blood loss may be significant and mothers undergoing fetal surgery occasionally require blood transfusion.[12] Chorioamniotic membrane separation and preterm labor remain the Achilles' heel of fetal interventions.[13,14] Surgical approaches that involve a smaller hysterotomy and more minimally invasive techniques appear to lower these risks.[15] Thus far, no maternal deaths have occurred at the major fetal surgery centers in the United States and Europe.

SURGICAL TECHNIQUES: OPEN AND VIDEOSCOPIC APPROACHES

Numerous technical aspects of fetal surgical procedures have evolved over 20 years of experimental and clinical work, and have been reviewed in detail elsewhere.[16–19] The comprehensive care of the fetal surgery patient is labor intensive and requires multidisciplinary cooperation between all team members. In the operating room, the leader of the fetal surgery team is a pediatric surgeon with specific training in fetal surgical techniques. Responsibility for the patient's anesthesia is usually shared between an obstetric and pediatric anesthesiologist with special interest in fetal anesthesia. A high-resolution ultrasound machine with color and enhanced Doppler is essential and used throughout the procedure to assess fetal and placental position, to monitor fetal heart rate, cardiac function and volume status, and to assess amniotic fluid replacement. A surgical nursing team trained in the specific aspects of fetal surgical procedures and instrumentation is mandatory.

Though some fetal interventions have been accomplished with local anesthesia, most are performed with general and epidural anesthesia. Epidural delivery of a fentanyl/ bupivacaine mixture provides optimal postoperative analgesia, and minimizes uterine irritability. Intraoperatively, inhaled isoflurane titrated to an end-tidal concentration of 2% or higher is used to achieve uterine relaxation, which is critical to successful outcomes. Because of the risk of postoperative pulmonary edema, the mothers are fluid restricted during these procedures and receive as little as 500 mL crystalloid. The patient is positioned supine with a roll under the right side to avoid compression of the inferior vena cava by the gravid uterus. The uterus is exposed through a low transverse abdominal incision. If the placenta is positioned posteriorly, subcutaneous flaps and a midline incision from the umbilicus to the pubis permit adequate uterine exposure. In cases of an anterior placenta, the fascia and rectus muscles are divided transversely so that the uterus can be tilted forward for a posterior hysterotomy. A large abdominal ring retractor is useful for abdominal wall retraction. After uterine relaxation is confirmed by palpation, the orientation of the fetus and placenta is confirmed by ultrasound. Two opposing traction sutures are placed with ultrasound guidance to provide hemostasis and to secure the fetal membranes to the uterine wall. The myometrium is then incised, and a modified uterine stapler is used to open the uterine wall in both directions. A rubber catheter connected to a rapid infuser is inserted into the amniotic space to replace egress of amniotic fluid with warmed Ringer's lactate. Infusion of warmed fluids is critical to maintain fetal temperature and amniotic volume and to minimize the risk of uterine contractions and umbilical cord compression.

One of the unique requirements of fetal surgery is that the surgeon must operate on the fetus, and then return the fetus to the amniotic environment in such a way as to minimize disturbance to the continuing pregnancy. The uterine closure must have adequate strength to prevent rupture, must have membrane reapproximation to prevent amniotic fluid leakage, and must limit risks for preterm labor or future infertility. Currently, the uterus is closed in two layers using an outer layer of full-thickness 0 polydioxanone (PDS) retention sutures, and an inner running layer of 2-0 PDS to close the myometrium and membranes. Before the closure is complete, the rapid infuser is used to restore amniotic volume and give antibiotics. An omental pedicle is secured over the hysterotomy to seal any small leaks from the full-thickness sutures.

Preterm labor is the single biggest concern during the operation and in the postoperative period. The mother receives a 50-mg indomethacin suppository 4 hours before surgery, and remains on indomethacin for 48 hours postoperatively. Daily echocardiography is essential; if there is evidence of patent duct arteriosus (PDA) restriction, then the indomethacin is stopped. During the operation terbutaline or nitroglycerin infusion can be used to help control uterine irritability and enhance relaxation. During closure of the hysterotomy, the mother is given a 6-g bolus dose of magnesium sulfate followed by a continuous infusion of 2 to 4 g per hour. Postoperatively the mother is observed in an intensive care unit (ICU) setting for close monitoring for pulmonary edema, fluid management, and uterine irritability. The magnesium sulfate is continued for 48 to 72 hours with close monitoring of magnesium levels and signs of toxicity. On the second to third postoperative day, usually the magnesium and indomethacin can be weaned, and the patient is converted to subcutaneous terbutaline or oral nifedipine. The patient is maintained on bedrest until the time of delivery. Postoperatively, daily ultrasound examinations help to assess the ductus arteriosus, amniotic fluid index (estimate of fetal urine output or of amniotic fluid leak), and fetal movement (marker of fetal well-being).

Videoscopic fetal surgery has been used most recently to permit a number of fetal surgical interventions, such as fetoscopic tracheal occlusion, laser ablation of communicating vessels in twin-to-twin transfusion syndrome, and fetoscopic ablation of posterior urethral valves for fetuses with obstructive uropathy. Initially, these procedures were done by exposing the uterus through a maternal laparotomy. More recently, surgeons have placed trocars into the uterus through the intact maternal abdominal wall. As with all videoscopic procedures the number and size of trocars have been reduced as surgeon experience and instrumentation increases. Visualization with amniotic fluid endoscopy requires continuous irrigation using a high-flow urology-type irrigation system. This permits maintenance of constant uterine fluid volume, avoids risk of air embolus with gas distention of the uterus, ensures a continuously washed operative field, improves visibility by exchanging the cloudy amniotic fluid with lactated Ringer's solution, and keeps the fetus warm.

RATIONALE AND OUTCOME OF FETAL SURGERY FOR SPECIFIC CONGENITAL ANOMALIES

Lung Malformations

Congenital cystic adenomatoid malformation (CCAM) and bronchopulmonary sequestration are the most common congenital lung malformations, and the most common fetal thoracic lesions that may benefit from fetal intervention.[20] The incidence of these lesions has been estimated at 1 in 25,000 to 35,000 pregnancies[21]; however, current referral patterns to our center suggest they may occur more frequently. Grossly, a CCAM is a discrete, space-occupying intrapulmonary mass that contains variable-sized cysts. These lesions do not function in normal gas exchange; however, airspaces within these masses communicate with the tracheobronchial tree. Histologically, CCAM is distinguished from other lesions and normal lung by (a) polypoid projections of the mucosa, (b) an increase in smooth muscle and elastic tissue within cyst walls, (c) an absence of cartilage (except that found in "entrapped" normal bronchi), (d) the presence of mucus-secreting cells, and (e) the absence of inflammation. In contrast, bronchopulmonary sequestrations (BPS) (intralobar or extralobar) are masses of nonfunctioning lung tissue that are supplied by an anomalous systemic artery and do not have connection to the native tracheobronchial tree. The pathogenesis of both lesions is unknown, but they are thought to arise during the fifth to sixth week in embryonic development, and may result from abnormalities in growth signals between the branching airway epithelium and pulmonary mesenchyme.[22,23] Congenital lung lesions are commonly diagnosed by prenatal ultrasound as an echogenic solid, or cystic and solid thoracic mass. Not infrequently these lesions may be seen to have a systemic blood supply on Doppler ultrasound. Although CCAM and BPS have been distinguished prenatally in the past by the presence or absence of a systemic vessel, it is now recognized that these lung lesions represent a continuum of pulmonary maldevelopment and there are lesions that have clinicopathologic features of both.[24,25] Fetal MRI may enhance diagnostic accuracy in examining these lesions and distinguishing them from other thoracic abnormalities, such as congenital lobar emphysema, bronchial atresia, bronchogenic cyst, and congenital diaphragmatic hernia.[26,27]

The natural history and clinical spectrum of these anomalies are variable, but they appear to depend mostly on the size of the mass and the secondary physiologic derangement. Most smaller lesions remain asymptomatic throughout fetal and postnatal life. In contrast, larger lesions produce significant mass effect, which can lead to pulmonary hypoplasia, impaired fetal swallowing and polyhydramnios, and impaired fetal circulation and heart failure. Congestive heart failure in the fetus, known as nonimmune fetal hydrops, is defined by the presence of skin or scalp edema, or by fluid accumulation in one or more serous cavities (ascites, or pericardial or pleural effusions). The risk of hydrops appears to depend on the size and rate of growth of the mass, and results from kinking of the superior vena cava and impaired cardiac venous return.[28] It has been demonstrated that hydrops is a harbinger of fetal demise, and is associated with near 100% mortality.[29] Rarely, hydrops is associated with hydrothorax and extralobar sequestration. As a prognostic factor, the CCAM volume ratio (CVR) has been developed to correlate the relative size of these lesions with fetal and postnatal outcome.[30] In one series in which 58 fetuses with a lung mass were followed prospectively, 75% of fetuses (12 of 16) with CVR greater than 1.6 developed hydrops, whereas only 17% (7 of 42) with CVR 1.6 or less had this complication.

For a fetus with a lung mass, the only indication for fetal intervention is the presence of hydrops. Most commonly, hydrops occurs in the period of rapid growth of these lesions between 19 and 26 weeks gestation.[20,29,30] Fetuses with a lung mass should be followed closely. It is recommended that those with a CVR less than 1.6 receive weekly ultrasound up to about 28 weeks' gestation, whereas those with CVR greater than 1.6 should be examined as frequently as two to three times per week. If signs of hydrops appear, the treatment options include percutaneous placement of a thoracoamniotic shunt for lesions with a dominant cyst, and open fetal thoracotomy and mass resection for more solid lesions. Use of the laser or radiofrequency ablation to debulk a large CCAM cannot be recommended now because of technical limitations and inability to control energy distribution and postprocedure swelling.[31,32]

Fetal surgery for fetal lung masses requires open hysterotomy (Fig. 107.4). Intraoperative echocardiography is important to assess fetal intravascular volume and right ventricle filling. These fetuses have tamponade physiology, and generally benefit from a fluid bolus before thoracotomy. A relatively large thoracotomy is required to permit adequate exposure, and the mass is delivered slowly to prevent rapid decreased cardiac venous return. At resection, the presence of a systemic vessel must be considered.

The first successful open fetal surgery for CCAM was reported in 1990 by Harrison et al. at UCSF.[33] Since then, there have been reports of 22 open fetal resections of lung masses, with 50% survival.[20] Delays in referral and intervention, the presence of maternal "mirror" syndrome, preterm labor, chorioamnionitis, and technical difficulties associated with the procedure have limited outcomes in half of the cases. Recently, results from a small series of patients suggest maternal administration of betamethasone should be considered for all fetuses with a large lung mass, and for those with hydrops who are not candidates for fetal intervention.[34]

Sacrococcygeal Teratoma

Sacrococcygeal teratoma (SCT) is the most common neonatal tumor, with an incidence of 1 in 35,000 live births.[35,36] Thought to arise from totipotent somatic cells originating in the caudal cell mass, this tumor contains multiple neoplastic tissues that lack organ specificity, are foreign to the sacrococcygeal region, and are derived from all three germ layers. The postnatal mortality of SCT is low, despite that about 10% of neonatal lesions are malignant. The prenatal mortality from SCT is more than 50%, however. The causes of death in fetal SCT are multifactorial, but primarily involve dystocia with tumor rupture and bleeding at the time of delivery, or high-output cardiac failure and hydrops from high blood flow within the mass.[37] The evolution of heart failure, placentomegaly and hydrops in a fetus with SCT is a harbinger of fetal demise, and is the sole indication for fetal surgical intervention. Furthermore, SCT may lead to maternal mirror syndrome (Ballantine syndrome).[38] In this condition, the mother experiences progressive preeclampsia-like symptoms, including vomiting, hypertension, peripheral edema, proteinuria, and pulmonary edema caused by the release of placental vasoactive factors or endothelial cell toxins from the edematous placenta. This syndrome is reversed only by delivering the child and the placenta, but not by removing the SCT prenatally.

The diagnosis of SCT can be made by fetal ultrasound as early as 14 weeks' gestation.[39] The sonographic appearance may be cystic, solid, or mixed, and may demonstrate irregular echogenic patterns secondary to areas of tumor necrosis, cystic degeneration, internal hemorrhage, or calcification. Ultrasound is important to assess abdominal or pelvic extension, evidence of bowel or urinary tract obstruction, assessment of the integrity of the fetal spine, and documentation of lower extremity function. Fetal MRI may be useful to help distinguish these lesions from myelomeningocele, meconium pseudocyst, and obstructive uropathy. Fetal echocardiography and Doppler ultrasound measurements are important in the diagnostic assessment and follow-up of fetuses with these conditions. The presence of hydrops, increased aortic velocity, increased combined cardiac output, increased cardiac-to-thoracic ratio, a dilated inferior vena cava, or reversed end-diastolic umbilical blood flow appear to be sensitive early predictors of impending hydrops and fetal demise.[40,41] For fetuses greater than 28 weeks' gestation, these findings are indication of emergency cesarean delivery and postnatal resection. For fetuses less than 28 weeks, open fetal surgery and resection is the treatment of choice. Minimally invasive approaches to interrupt the tumor's blood supply with radiofrequency ablation have had limited success,[42] but may be alternatives for a fetus that is a poor candidate for open fetal resection.

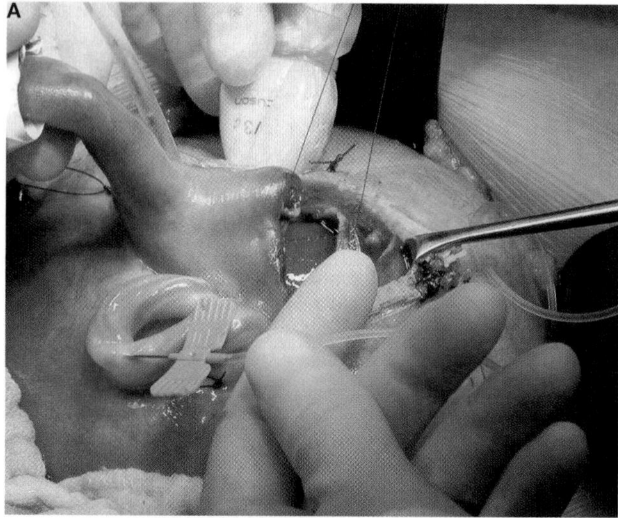

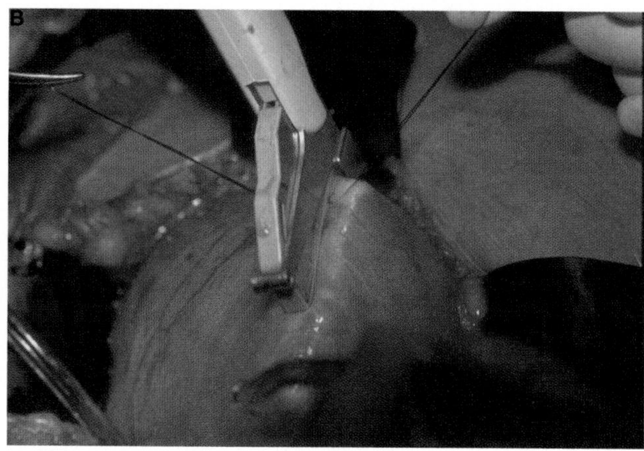

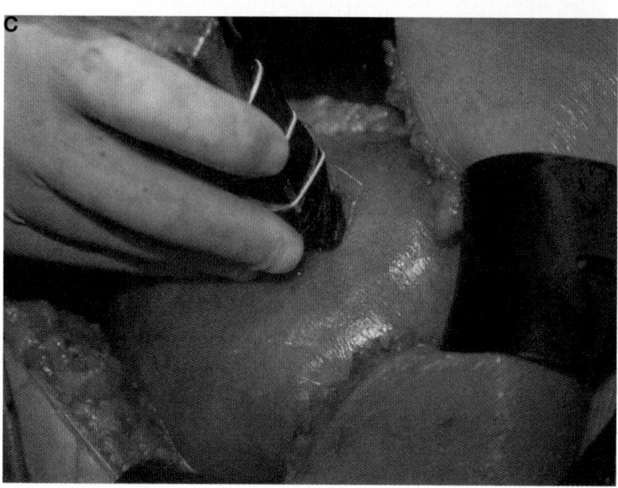

FIGURE 107.4 Fetal surgery of a hydropic 24-week fetus with a large left lung mass. (*A*) Intraoperative ultrasound to locate the placenta and fetus. (*B*) Uterine stay sutures are elevated to facilitate the use of the uterine stapler. (*C*) The mass has been removed and the remaining normal left lung is evident. A bolus of crystalloid is given into the umbilical vein, and the chest is being closed.

Adzick et al.[43] reported the first successful outcome for fetal surgery resection of a fetus with a large SCT and hydrops in 1997. More recently, investigators from that center have reported 75% survival (3 of 4) for fetal resection of SCT. A similar high-output heart failure physiology can occur with teratomas in other locations. A fetus with a cervical teratoma and hydrops had successful fetal resection of the lesion at 24 weeks' gestation.[44]

Congenital Diaphragmatic Hernia

At present, the role of fetal intervention in the management of fetuses with congenital diaphragmatic hernia (CDH) is not clear. A hole in the posterolateral diaphragm, left-sided in 80% to 85% of cases, permits abdominal viscera to herniate into the chest during fetal development. Severe pulmonary hypoplasia leads to mortality rates of more than 40% for fetuses with this condition. In current practice, more than half of the infants with CDH are diagnosed before birth. At times it can be difficult to distinguish CDH from a cystic lung mass or other cystic lesions. In these patients, fetal MRI has been useful to enhance diagnostic accuracy and to further exclude associated anomalies.[45,46]

Outcome for patients with CDH varies widely, depending on when the disease is diagnosed.[47] Fetuses with CDH have lower survival rates than those for live born infants, or for infants presenting to a neonatal surgical center. This paradigm has been termed the "hidden mortality" by Harrison et al.,[48] and has been confirmed by multiple investigators.[49–51] In 2000, Dillon et al.[52] reviewed the outcomes from a large series of fetuses with CDH registered in the Northern Region Congenital Abnormality Survey in the United Kingdom. Between 1985 and 1997, 201 fetuses were evaluated for diaphragmatic problems, of which 187 had congenital diaphragmatic hernia (14 had diaphragm eventration). From this cohort 38 pregnancies were terminated, 26 of which had "multiple abnormalities"; and 14 pregnancies (7%) were complicated by spontaneous miscarriage or stillbirth. The overall 1-year survival was 37%, but for live born fetuses the survival was 50%. Furthermore, for those live born babies with isolated CDH, the overall survival was 59%.

Ultrasound (and more recently MRI) can be used to predict fetal CDH severity. Herniation of the liver into the fetal chest and marked lung hypoplasia as estimated by a lung-to-head ratio (LHR) less than 1.0 are strong predictors of perinatal death.[53,54] Fetuses without liver herniation through the diaphragm have a reported survival rate between 75% and 93%, whereas those with "liver-up" have a survival rate as low as 43%.[55] In a recent report that included evaluation of 174 patients with CDH, LHR less than 0.9 was associated with only 13% survival, whereas survival was 68% for LHR 0.9 to 1.2, and 88% for LHR greater than1.2.[56]

For select infants with severe CDH, fetal surgery has been performed in an attempt to reverse the high mortality rate.

Initially, complete *in utero* repair of the diaphragmatic defect was attempted.[57] This approach, however, led to fetal bradycardia and immediate death after attempts to reduce the liver from the fetal chest resulted in kinking of the ductus venosus.[58] Subsequently, *in utero* tracheal occlusion has been used to treat fetuses with severe CDH. It has been shown that temporary tracheal occlusion, performed either as an open procedure or fetoscopically, can prevent the normal outflow of lung fluid and enhance growth of the fetal lungs.[59] In a review of 15 patients treated by open fetal tracheal occlusion at Children's Hospital of Philadelphia (CHOP), survival was 100% for patients with right-sided defects (2 of 2) and 23% for patients with left-sided defects (3 of 13), compared with 0 survival for a matched group of 7 infants with left-sided lesions managed by conventional treatment alone. Endoscopic approaches to fetal tracheal occlusion, termed "fetoscopic" or "FETENDO," showed more promising outcomes.[60] Recently, however, Harrison et al.[10] from UCSF reported results from a National Institutes of Health (NIH)-sponsored, prospective randomized trial that compared fetoscopic tracheal occlusion with standard postnatal care for fetuses with left-sided CDH, "liver-up" and LHR less than 1.4. Twenty-four fetuses were randomized, but at this point the trial was stopped because of an unexpected high survival in the standard treatment group, and the expectation that fetal therapy in this design would show no benefit. In this study of fetuses with liver-up CDH, the overall 90-day survival rate was 75%, a number much higher than those reported previously. Whereas 8 of 11 (73%) fetuses survived following fetoscopic tracheal occlusion, 10 of 13 (77%) survived with postnatal treatment alone, thus showing no benefit to fetal therapy in this study. As expected, a striking difference in the gestational ages was noted between the two groups. Whereas, the standard treatment group delivered at a mean gestation of 37 weeks, the tracheal occlusion group delivered at a mean of 30.8 (range of 28 to 34) weeks' gestational age. Although fetoscopic tracheal occlusion likely had an effect on lung growth, this response may have been limited by preterm labor, early delivery, and associated lung immaturity. As has been demonstrated in the treatment of other conditions, chorioamniotic membrane separation and preterm labor limit outcomes from fetal surgery.[13,14] The lack of benefit from fetal therapy may also result from the excellent outcomes that were achieved in the control group. These results certainly suggest that a standardized protocol involving prenatal steroids, and expert pre- and postnatal care may improve outcome for fetuses with severe CDH.

Most recently Deprest et al. from Europe[15] have reported initial results from the fetoscopic tracheal occlusion (FETO) task group, an ongoing prospective, multicenter study of patients with severe CDH treated by fetoscopic approaches. This study involves patients with isolated CDH, liver up, and a LHR of less than 1.0. Using either general or more recently local anesthesia, a single 10F cannula is placed through the intact maternal abdominal wall and uterus. A specially designed fetoscope is placed; the fetus is endotracheally intubated; and, a detachable balloon is deployed in the midtrachea of these patients. Initially, fetuses were delivered by an *ex utero* intrapartum therapy (EXIT) procedure; however, more recently investigators have performed a second fetoscopic procedure later in gestation to remove the balloon and permit vaginal delivery. Results from the first 21 patients treated between April 2002 and October 2003 showed 47% overall survival in the treatment group, with a mean gestation of 34 weeks. In comparison, a matched cohort of fetuses with severe CDH had only 8% survival (1 of 12). The results from this trial are limited because of lack of a randomized design and lack of standardized, centralized postnatal care in the control group of fetuses.

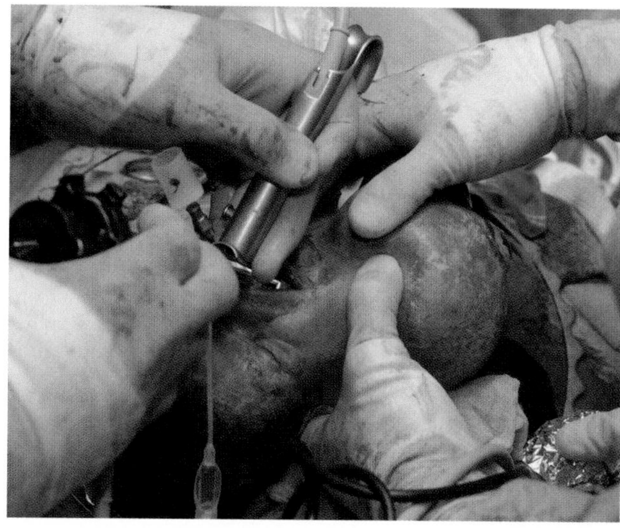

FIGURE 107.5 A 38-week fetus with large left neck teratoma (yolk sac tumor) at *ex utero* intrapartum treatment (EXIT) procedure. The trachea was severely deviated to the left and was intubated with a 2.5 reinforced endotracheal tube slid over a 1.8-mm bronchoscope.

It is likely that fetal intervention may play a role in the management of a small cohort of fetuses with the most severe form of CDH. Current work is directed at accurate identification of this cohort, and optimizing minimally invasive treatment approaches.

Giant Neck Masses and Laryngeal Atresia

As an outgrowth of the fetal-intervention efforts, *ex utero* intrapartum therapy (EXIT procedure) was devised to treat fetal airway obstruction caused by large neck masses or intrinsic airway problems.[61] This approach involves a planned hysterotomy and delivery with preservation of the maternal—fetal placental circulation for oxygenation of the fetus. While on "placental bypass," up to 65 minutes is available for direct laryngoscopy, bronchoscopy, endotracheal intubation, tumor resection, or tracheostomy to secure the airway (Fig. 107.5). The umbilical cord is then divided, and the fetus delivered. Indications for an EXIT procedure include the presence of a large cervical mass with evidence of airway deviation or compression. Polyhydramnios, caused by esophagus compression, is one marker for fetal tracheal compression. Recently, the tracheoesophageal displacement index (TEDI) has been described to assess the degree of tracheal deviation on fetal MRI.[62] Multiple centers have used the EXIT procedure to stabilize the airway in fetuses with large cervical tumors (e.g., teratomas or lymphatic malformations) with excellent fetal outcomes and very little additional maternal risk.[63–65]

An EXIT procedure is the treatment of choice for fetuses with congenital high airway obstruction syndrome (CHAOS). This syndrome is usually caused by laryngeal or tracheal atresia, tracheal stenosis, or a mucosal web. A fetus with this condition develops overdistended, echogenic lungs, which may compress the mediastinum, flatten or evert the diaphragms and cause hydrops because of compromise of central venous return. Fetuses with CHAOS should be delivered with an EXIT procedure to permit tracheostomy and airway control while maintaining the placental maternal—fetal circulation. For fetuses with CHAOS who develop hydrops, early delivery or prenatal tracheostomy are treatment options, depending on gestational age.[66–68]

Myelomeningocele

Myelomeningocele (MMC) was the first nonlethal anomaly to be treated by fetal surgery.[69–71] MMC, or spina bifida, is a midline defect of the spine and spinal cord that leads to exposure of the contents of the neural canal. It is relatively common, and occurs in 1 of every 2,000 live births. The natural history of fetuses with this condition is variable, but generally mortality is low. Instead, affected newborns suffer life-long disabilities, which include a combination of paraplegia, abnormalities in bowel or bladder control, sexual dysfunction, skeletal deformations, hydrocephalus, and mental impairment. More than 80% of fetuses with MMC can be identified before birth by maternal serum α-fetoprotein screening. Fetal ultrasound may detect the characteristic spine abnormalities as early as 16 weeks' gestation.

The rationale for fetal intervention for MMC is based on compelling evidence that associated neurologic deficits do not simply result from incomplete neurulation but rather from chronic mechanical and chemical trauma caused by exposure of the neural tissue to the amniotic environment. Support for this conclusion includes the observation that fetal leg movements decrease with advancing gestational age. Furthermore, in animal models of MMC *in utero* repair leads to improved neurologic function and reversal of hindbrain herniation.[72]

Human fetal interventions for MMC were initially designed to reduce intrauterine exposure of neural elements. Both fetoscopic and open techniques were attempted; however, open methods are considered the current standard. The first successful outcome of fetal surgery repair of MMC was reported by Adzick in 1998.[69] Since that time multiple centers have reported positive outcomes that suggest that surgical repair of MMC before 25 weeks' gestation can preserve neurologic function, reverse the hindbrain herniation, decrease the incidence of clubfoot, and obviate the need for postnatal placement of a ventriculoperitoneal shunt compared with historical controls.[70,71,73] No consistent improvement was seen in neurologic or bladder function, however, and these interventions did come at the cost of fetal prematurity (preterm labor) and increased maternal risk. Furthermore, lack of accurate prenatal indicators of neurologic function and absence of matched controls and long-term follow-up hamper evaluation of this approach. To better assess the merit of fetal surgery for this condition, an NIH-sponsored multicenter prospective, randomized trial is currently under way.

Urinary Obstruction

Obstructive uropathy, one of the most common fetal structural anomalies, occurs in about 1 of 1,000 live births. Of all fetuses with urinary tract dilatation, as many as 90% do not require fetal intervention, such as those with low-pressure dilation, continued good urine output, adequate amniotic fluid volume, unilateral urinary obstruction, or advanced irreversible renal dysplasia.[74,75] Fetuses with urethral obstruction, severe bilateral hydronephrosis, and preserved renal function may be candidates for fetal intervention. Urethral obstruction, usually caused by posterior urethral valves in a male fetus, leads to decreased fetal urine output, oligohydramnios, and eventually pulmonary hypoplasia, which is often the most important factor affecting postnatal outcome. Fetuses with oligohydramnios present in the early second trimester have mortality rates in excess of 90%.[76,77]

Prenatal ultrasound is very accurate in the detection of fetal hydronephrosis and in determining the level of urinary obstruction. Because most of the amniotic fluid in middle and late pregnancy is the product of fetal urination, the presence of a normal amniotic fluid index implies the excretion of urine from at least one kidney. Decreasing amniotic fluid volume on serial ultrasound usually indicates deteriorating renal function. Furthermore, renal function can be assessed by the sonographic appearance of the renal parenchyma and by the laboratory analysis of fetal urine via percutaneous bladder aspiration. The presence of cortical cysts or increased echogenicity is highly predictive of renal dysplasia, but the absence of these findings does not exclude it.[78] Normal fetal urine chemistry includes a urinary sodium less than 100 mEq/dL, chloride less than 90 mEq/dL, osmolarity less than 200 mOsm/L, and β2-microglobulin less than 4 mg/dL. Values greater than these suggest that the fetal kidney is unable to reabsorb these molecules and predicts poor postnatal renal function.

The greatest challenge is selecting fetuses that have severe urinary obstruction, yet reversible or salvageable renal function. Presently, selection criteria for fetal intervention are a male fetus less than 30 weeks' gestation with evolving oligohydramnios, normal renal function, and no associated anomalies. Fetuses older than this are best treated by postnatal approaches. If there is evidence of lung maturation, then early delivery is recommended. The goal of fetal therapy is to adequately drain the urinary obstruction and to restore normal amniotic fluid volume. Methods of urinary tract decompression include percutaneous vesicoamniotic shunt placement, fetoscopic or open vesicostomy, and fetoscopic fulguration of posterior urethral valves.[79,80] Open fetal surgery, including vesicostomy or ureterostomy, has resulted in 50% survival, with two of eight children in one series having normal renal function.[81] Today, the most widely used and accepted means of treating bladder outlet obstruction is percutaneous insertion of a double-J vesicoamniotic shunt. Placement of a vesicoamniotic shunt is associated with 50% survival, but shunt complication rates as high as 45% may result. Direct fetoscopic ablation of posterior urethral valves holds promise for the future, though currently limited data are available to assess selection criteria and outcomes for fetuses treated by this approach.

Twin-to-Twin Transfusion Syndrome

Twin-to-twin transfusion syndrome (TTTS), present in 5% to 35% of monochorionic twin pregnancies, occurs when there is unequal sharing of the monochorionic placenta. Generally, this finding can be made on prenatal ultrasound, and often the communicating placental vessels can be characterized by Doppler. Arteriovenous anastomoses lead to a net shunting of blood from the donor to recipient. The donor twin often suffers intrauterine growth retardation, cardiac failure, and oligohydramnios, whereas the recipient twin may suffer polyhydramnios, cardiomyopathy and fetal hydrops. The smaller twin's placental cord insertion is often marginal or velamentous, whereas the larger twin's cord inserts into the placenta centrally.[82] Quintero et al.[83] have described a staging system for this condition. In stage 1, polyhydramnios and oligohydramnios occur, but the donor bladder is still visible. In stage 2, the bladder is no longer visible, and in stage 3 abnormal Doppler signals are detected in the respective umbilical arteries or veins. Stage 4 is characterized by findings of hydrops, and stage 5 is fetal death. Overall, TTTS before 26 weeks' gestation is associated with a high rate of fetal loss, perinatal death, and a high incidence of brain damage in survivors.[84,85] In severe forms of TTTS, perinatal mortality rates of up to 90% have been reported.[86]

Treatment options include amniocenteses of the recipient sac, amniotic membrane septostomy, and fetoscopic ablation of communicating vessels.[87–89] Recently, endoscopic laser coagulation has become the treatment of choice for severe

TTTS diagnosed before 26 weeks' gestation.[85] In a multicenter European trial, twins with severe TTTS of all Quintero stages were randomized to undergo fetoscopic laser ablation or standard amnioreduction therapy. The trial was stopped after 142 women were randomized, because of the clear benefit of the laser approach. Endoscopic laser ablation led to improved outcomes in all variables examined, including increased fetal survival and decreased incidence of neurologic complications.

Congenital Heart Defects

Fetal intervention may play a role in the management of some fetuses with rare congenital heart defects, including those with severe aortic or pulmonary stenosis, and hypoplastic left heart syndrome with intact or highly restrictive atrial septum.[90–92] There is evidence that fetuses with aortic or mitral valve stenosis may progress to hypoplastic left heart syndrome, presumably as a result of decreased ventricular filling. Furthermore, critical pulmonary stenosis or atresia with intact ventricular septum may progress to the so-called "hypoplastic right heart syndrome." Staged palliative surgery is the only therapeutic option for newborns with these conditions, and mortality remains significant. The goals of fetal intervention for these anomalies are to relieve the obstruction, restore normal cardiac physiology, and reverse the progression toward ventricular hypoplasia. Although this hypothesis is physiologically sound, to date there is little data to support this assertion. In an initial report from investigators at Children's Hospital, Boston, in which 20 fetuses underwent balloon dilation of a stenotic aortic valve at 21 to 29 weeks' gestation, 5 fetuses died following the procedure.[90] Of 14 who were thought to have a technically successful procedure, three have evidence of a two-ventricle heart postnatally, thus supporting the experimental rationale. It is likely that a prospective, randomized trial will be needed to prove the efficacy of fetal intervention for this disorder.

Fetal Intervention for Other Anomalies

Fetal intervention is indicated for a number of other fetal conditions, including amniotic band syndrome and twin reversed arterial perfusion (TRAP) sequence. Fetoscopic lysis of constricting amniotic bands may lead to limb salvage and improved outcome.[93–95] Similarly, in the TRAP sequence, fetoscopic ligation or ablation of the acardiac twin's umbilical cord is the treatment of choice.[96]

FUTURE OF FETAL INTERVENTION

There will always be a role for fetal intervention in the treatment of certain specific congenital structural abnormalities. The exact nature of this role, however, is under constant reevaluation and change. The primary goal of fetal therapy is to improve the outcome of the affected fetus while minimizing maternal risks. If fetal outcomes can be improved by alternative means, such as lung liquid ventilation or other postnatal therapies that pose no risks to the mother, then indications for fetal therapy will decrease. On the other hand, as the risks and complications of fetal surgery continue to decrease, such as those related to preterm labor and chorioamniotic membrane separation, then the role for fetal interventions may increase. Increased miniaturization of videoscopic equipment and optics, advances in robotics, newer approaches to closure of the uterus and fetal membranes, and advances in our understanding and treatment of preterm labor will enhance our ability to change the outlook for an increased number of fetuses with congenital malformations.

KEY POINTS

- **Four fetal conditions clearly benefit from fetal intervention: congenital cystic adenomatoid malformation (CCAM), fetal sacrococcygeal teratoma (SCT), a fetus with airway obstruction from a giant neck mass or laryngeal atresia, and twin-to-twin transfusion syndrome (TTTS).**
- **Any fetal therapy requires (a) accurate diagnosis of the condition and any associated anomalies that may have an impact on outcome; (b) reliable prediction of which individual fetuses will die or suffer serious long-term morbidity without fetal intervention; and (c) that the procedure improves the outcome of the fetus with little to no maternal risk.**
- **Preterm labor is the single biggest concern during the operation and in the postoperative period.**
- **For a fetus with a lung mass the only indication for fetal intervention is the presence of hydrops.**
- **For a fetus with sacrococcygeal teratoma, increased aortic velocity, increased combined cardiac output, increased cardiac-to-thoracic ratio, a dilated inferior vena cava, or reversed end-diastolic umbilical blood flow are sensitive early predictors of impending hydrops and fetal demise; before 28 weeks gestation, open fetal surgery and resection is the treatment of choice.**
- **Fetal intervention may play a role in the management of a small cohort of fetuses with the most severe form of congenital diaphragmatic hernia.**
- **An EXIT procedure is the treatment of choice for fetuses with congenital high airway obstruction syndrome.**

References

1. Liley AW. Intrauterine transfusion of foetus in haemolytic disease. *BMJ* 1963;5365:1107–1109.
2. Bruner JP. In their footsteps: a brief history of maternal-fetal surgery. *Clin Perinatol.* 2003;30:439–447.
3. Harrison MR, Golbus MS, Filly RA, et al. Fetal surgery for congenital hydronephrosis. *N Engl J Med.* 1982;306:591–593.
4. Crombleholme TM, D'Alton M, Cendron M, et al. Prenatal diagnosis and the pediatric surgeon: the impact of prenatal consultation on perinatal management. *J Pediatr Surg.* 1996;31:156–162; discussion 162–163.
5. **Myers LB, Cohen D, Galinkin J, et al. Anaesthesia for fetal surgery. *Paediatr Anaesth.* 2002;12:569–578.**
6. Howell LJ, Adzick NS. Establishing a fetal therapy center: lessons learned. *Semin Pediatr Surg.* 2003;12:209–217.
7. Farrell JA, Albanese CT, Jennings RW, et al. Maternal fertility is not affected by fetal surgery. *Fetal Diagn Ther.* 1999;14:190–192.
8. Chervenak FA, McCullough LB. A comprehensive ethical framework for fetal research and its application to fetal surgery for spina bifida. *Am J Obstet Gynecol.* 2002;187:10–14.
9. Longaker MT, Golbus MS, Filly RA, et al. Maternal outcome after open fetal surgery. A review of the first 17 human cases. *JAMA* 1991;265:737–741.
10. **Harrison MR, Keller RL, Hawgood SB, et al. A randomized trial of fetal endoscopic tracheal occlusion for severe fetal congenital diaphragmatic hernia. *N Engl J Med.* 2003;349:1916–1924.**
11. DiFederico EM, Burlingame JM, Kilpatrick SJ, et al. Pulmonary edema in obstetric patients is rapidly resolved except in the presence of infection or of nitroglycerin tocolysis after open fetal surgery. *Am J Obstet Gynecol.* 1998;179:925–933.
12. Harrison MR. Fetal surgery. *Am J Obstet Gynecol.* 1996;174:1255–1264.
13. Sydorak RM, Hirose S, Sandberg PL, et al. Chorioamniotic membrane separation following fetal surgery. *J Perinatol.* 2002;22:407–410.
14. Wilson RD, Johnson MP, Crombleholme TM, et al. Chorioamniotic membrane separation following open fetal surgery: pregnancy outcome. *Fetal Diagn Ther.* 2003;18:314–320.
15. Deprest J, Gratacos E, Nicolaides KH. Fetoscopic tracheal occlusion (FETO) for severe congenital diaphragmatic hernia: evolution of a technique and preliminary results. *Ultrasound Obstet Gynecol.* 2004;24:121–126.
16. Bianchi DW, Crombleholme TM, D'Alton ME. *Fetology: diagnosis and management of the fetal patient.* New York: McGraw-Hill, 2000, p. 1081.

17. Adzick NS, Harrison MR, Glick PL, et al. Fetal surgery in the primate. III. Maternal outcome after fetal surgery. *J Pediatr Surg.* 1986;21:477–480.
18. Harrison MR, Adzick NS. Fetal surgical techniques. *Semin Pediatr Surg.* 1993;2:136–142.
19. Harrison MR, Evans MI, Adzick NS, et al. *The Unborn Patient: The art and science of fetal therapy.* Philadelphia: WB Saunders, 2001.
20. **Adzick NS. Management of fetal lung lesions. *Clin Perinatol.* 2003;30: 481–492.**
21. Laberge JM, Flageole H, Pugash D, et al. Outcome of the prenatally diagnosed congenital cystic adenomatoid lung malformation: a Canadian experience. *Fetal Diagn Ther.* 2001;16:178–186.
22. Cass DL, Quinn TM, Yang EY, et al. Increased cell proliferation and decreased apoptosis characterize congenital cystic adenomatoid malformation of the lung. *J Pediatr Surg.* 1998;33:1043–1046; discussion 1047.
23. Liechty KW, Crombleholme TM, Quinn TM, et al. Elevated platelet-derived growth factor-B in congenital cystic adenomatoid malformations requiring fetal resection. *J Pediatr Surg.* 1999;34:805–809; discussion 809–810.
24. Cass DL, Crombleholme TM, Howell LJ, et al. Cystic lung lesions with systemic arterial blood supply: a hybrid of congenital cystic adenomatoid malformation and bronchopulmonary sequestration. *J Pediatr Surg.* 1997;32:986–990.
25. Langston C. New concepts in the pathology of congenital lung malformations. *Semin Pediatr Surg.* 2003;12:17–37.
26. Olutoye OO, Coleman BG, Hubbard AM, et al. Prenatal diagnosis and management of congenital lobar emphysema. *J Pediatr Surg.* 2000;35:792–795.
27. Hubbard AM, Adzick NS, Crombleholme TM, et al. Congenital chest lesions: diagnosis and characterization with prenatal MR imaging. *Radiology* 1999;212:43–48.
28. Rice HE, Estes JM, Hedrick MH, et al. Congenital cystic adenomatoid malformation: a sheep model of fetal hydrops. *J Pediatr Surg.* 1994;29:692–696.
29. Adzick NS, Harrison MR, Crombleholme TM, et al. Fetal lung lesions: management and outcome. *Am J Obstet Gynecol.* 1998;179:884–889.
30. **Crombleholme TM, Coleman B, Hedrick H, et al. Cystic adenomatoid malformation volume ratio predicts outcome in prenatally diagnosed cystic adenomatoid malformation of the lung. *J Pediatr Surg.* 2002;37:331–338.**
31. Milner R, Kitano Y, Olutoye O, et al. Radiofrequency thermal ablation: a potential treatment for hydropic fetuses with a large chest mass. *J Pediatr Surg.* 2000;35:386–389.
32. Bruner JP, Jarnagin BK, Reinisch L. Percutaneous laser ablation of fetal congenital cystic adenomatoid malformation: too little, too late? *Fetal Diagn Ther.* 2000;15:359–363.
33. Harrison MR, Adzick NS, Jennings RW, et al. Antenatal intervention for congenital cystic adenomatoid malformation. *Lancet* 1990;336:965–967.
34. Tsao K, Hawgood S, Vu L, et al. Resolution of hydrops fetalis in congenital cystic adenomatoid malformation after prenatal steroid therapy. *J Pediatr Surg.* 2003;38:508–510.
35. Grosfeld JL, Ballantine TV, Lowe D, et al. Benign and malignant teratomas in children: analysis of 85 patients. *Surgery* 1976;80:297–305.
36. Berry CL, Keeling J, Hilton C. Teratomata in infancy and childhood: a review of 91 cases. *J Pathol.* 1969;98:241–252.
37. Langer JC, Harrison MR, Schmidt KG, et al. Fetal hydrops and death from sacrococcygeal teratoma: rationale for fetal surgery. *Am J Obstet Gynecol.* 1989;160:1145–1150.
38. Kuhlmann RS, Warsof SL, Levy DL, et al. Fetal sacrococcygeal teratoma. *Fetal Ther.* 1987;2:95–100.
39. Holzgreve W, Mahony BS, Glick PL, et al. Sonographic demonstration of fetal sacrococcygeal teratoma. *Prenat Diagn.* 1985;5:245–257.
40. Olutoye OO, Johnson MP, Coleman BG, et al. Abnormal umbilical cord Doppler sonograms may predict impending demise in fetuses with sacrococcygeal teratoma. A report of two cases. *Fetal Diagn Ther.* 2004;19: 35–39.
41. **Hedrick HL, Flake AW, Crombleholme TM, et al. Sacrococcygeal teratoma: prenatal assessment, fetal intervention, and outcome. *J Pediatr Surg.* 2004;39:430–438; discussion 430–438.**
42. Paek BW, Jennings RW, Harrison MR, et al. Radiofrequency ablation of human fetal sacrococcygeal teratoma. *Am J Obstet Gynecol.* 2001;184:503–507.
43. Adzick NS, Crombleholme TM, Morgan MA, et al. A rapidly growing fetal teratoma. *Lancet* 1997;349:538.
44. Hirose S, Sydorak RM, Tsao K, et al. Spectrum of intrapartum management strategies for giant fetal cervical teratoma. *J Pediatr Surg.* 2003;38:446–450; discussion 446–450.
45. Walsh DS, Hubbard AM, Olutoye OO, et al. Assessment of fetal lung volumes and liver herniation with magnetic resonance imaging in congenital diaphragmatic hernia. *Am J Obstet Gynecol.* 2000;183:1067–1069.
46. Hubbard AM, Crombleholme TM, Adzick NS, et al. Prenatal MRI evaluation of congenital diaphragmatic hernia. *Am J Perinatol.* 1999;16: 407–413.
47. Doyle NM, Lally KP. The CDH Study Group and advances in the clinical care of the patient with congenital diaphragmatic hernia. *Semin Perinatol.* 2004;28:174–184.
48. Harrison MR, Bjordal RI, Langmark F, et al. Congenital diaphragmatic hernia: the hidden mortality. *J Pediatr Surg.* 1978;13:227–230.
49. Betremieux P, Lionnais S, Beuchee A, et al. Perinatal management and outcome of prenatally diagnosed congenital diaphragmatic hernia: a 1995–2000 series in Rennes University Hospital. *Prenat Diagn.* 2002;22:988–994.
50. Stege G, Fenton A, Jaffray B. Nihilism in the 1990s: the true mortality of congenital diaphragmatic hernia. *Pediatrics* 2003;112:532–535.
51. Skari H, Bjornland K, Haugen G, et al. Congenital diaphragmatic hernia: a meta-analysis of mortality factors. *J Pediatr Surg.* 2000;35:1187–1197.
52. Dillon E, Renwick M, Wright C. Congenital diaphragmatic herniation: antenatal detection and outcome. *Br J Radiol.* 2000;73:360–365.
53. Metkus AP, Filly RA, Stringer MD, et al. Sonographic predictors of survival in fetal diaphragmatic hernia. *J Pediatr Surg.* 1996;31:148–51; discussion 151–152.
54. Lipshutz GS, Albanese CT, Feldstein VA, et al. Prospective analysis of lung-to-head ratio predicts survival for patients with prenatally diagnosed congenital diaphragmatic hernia. *J Pediatr Surg.* 1997;32:1634–1636.
55. Albanese CT, Lopoo J, Goldstein RB, et al. Fetal liver position and perinatal outcome for congenital diaphragmatic hernia. *Prenat Diagn.* 1998;18: 1138–1142.
56. Cohen MS, Rychik J, Bush DM, et al. Influence of congenital heart disease on survival in children with congenital diaphragmatic hernia. *J Pediatr.* 2002;141:25–30.
57. Harrison MR, Adzick NS, Longaker MT, et al. Successful repair in utero of a fetal diaphragmatic hernia after removal of herniated viscera from the left thorax. *N Engl J Med.* 1990;322:1582–1584.
58. Harrison MR, Adzick NS, Flake AW, et al. Correction of congenital diaphragmatic hernia in utero: VI. Hard-earned lessons. *J Pediatr Surg.* 1993;28:1411–1417; discussion 1417–1418.
59. Hedrick MH, Estes JM, Sullivan KM, et al. Plug the lung until it grows (PLUG): a new method to treat congenital diaphragmatic hernia in utero. *J Pediatr Surg.* 1994;29:612–617.
60. Harrison MR, Sydorak RM, Farrell JA, et al. Fetoscopic temporary tracheal occlusion for congenital diaphragmatic hernia: prelude to a randomized, controlled trial. *J Pediatr Surg.* 2003;38:1012–1020.
61. **Mychaliska GB, Bealer JF, Graf JL, et al. Operating on placental support: the ex utero intrapartum treatment procedure. *J Pediatr Surg.* 1997;32:227–230; discussion 230–231.**
62. Cass DL, Cassady CI, O'Day MP, et al. Predictors of airway obstruction and outcome of fetuses with giant neck masses. Surgical Section, American Academy of Pediatrics, San Francisco, CA, October 8–10, 2004.
63. Hedrick HL. Ex utero intrapartum therapy. *Semin Pediatr Surg.* 2003; 12:190–195.
64. **Hirose S, Farmer DL, Lee H, et al. The ex utero intrapartum treatment procedure: looking back at the EXIT. *J Pediatr Surg.* 2004;39:375–380; discussion 375–380.**
65. Noah MM, Norton ME, Sandberg P, et al. Short-term maternal outcomes that are associated with the EXIT procedure, as compared with cesarean delivery. *Am J Obstet Gynecol.* 2002;186:773–7777.
66. Crombleholme TM, Sylvester K, Flake AW, et al. Salvage of a fetus with congenital high airway obstruction syndrome by ex utero intrapartum treatment (EXIT) procedure. *Fetal Diagn Ther.* 2000;15:280–282.
67. Paek BW, Callen PW, Kitterman J, et al. Successful fetal intervention for congenital high airway obstruction syndrome. *Fetal Diagn Ther.* 2002; 17:272–276.
68. DeCou JM, Jones DC, Jacobs HD, et al. Successful ex utero intrapartum treatment (EXIT) procedure for congenital high airway obstruction syndrome (CHAOS) owing to laryngeal atresia. *J Pediatr Surg.* 1998;33:1563–1565.
69. Adzick NS, Sutton LN, Crombleholme TM, et al. Successful fetal surgery for spina bifida. *Lancet* 1998;352:1675–1676.
70. Bruner JP, Tulipan N, Paschall RL, et al. Fetal surgery for myelomeningocele and the incidence of shunt-dependent hydrocephalus. *JAMA* 1999;282: 1819–1825.
71. Sutton LN, Adzick NS, Bilaniuk LT, et al. Improvement in hindbrain herniation demonstrated by serial fetal magnetic resonance imaging following fetal surgery for myelomeningocele. *JAMA* 1999;282:1826–1831.
72. Meuli M, Meuli-Simmen C, Hutchins GM, et al. In utero surgery rescues neurological function at birth in sheep with spina bifida. *Nat Med.* 1995;1:342–347.
73. Farmer DL, von Koch CS, Peacock WJ, et al. In utero repair of myelomeningocele: experimental pathophysiology, initial clinical experience, and outcomes. *Arch Surg.* 2003;138:872–878.
74. Glick PL, Harrison MR, Golbus MS, et al. Management of the fetus with congenital hydronephrosis. II: Prognostic criteria and selection for treatment. *J Pediatr Surg.* 1985;20:376–387.
75. Harrison MR, Golbus MS, Filly RA, et al. Management of the fetus with congenital hydronephrosis. *J Pediatr Surg.* 1982;17:728–742.
76. Crombleholme TM, Harrison MR, Golbus MS, et al. Fetal intervention in obstructive uropathy: prognostic indicators and efficacy of intervention. *Am J Obstet Gynecol.* 1990;162:1239–1244.
77. Mandelbrot L, Dumez Y, Muller F, et al. Prenatal prediction of renal function in fetal obstructive uropathies. *J Perinat Med.* 1991;19[suppl 1]: 283–287.
78. Mahony BS, Filly RA, Callen PW, et al. Fetal renal dysplasia: sonographic evaluation. *Radiology* 1984;152:143–146.
79. Quintero RA, Shukla AR, Homsy YL, et al. Successful in utero endoscopic ablation of posterior urethral valves: a new dimension in fetal urology. *Urology* 2000;55:774.
80. Quintero RA, Johnson MP, Romero R, et al. In-utero percutaneous cystoscopy in the management of fetal lower obstructive uropathy. *Lancet* 1995;346:537–540.

81. Cortes RA, Farmer DL. Recent advances in fetal surgery. *Semin Perinatol.* 2004;28:199–211.
82. Fries MH, Goldstein RB, Kilpatrick SJ, et al. The role of velamentous cord insertion in the etiology of twin-twin transfusion syndrome. *Obstet Gynecol.* 1993;81:569–574.
83. Quintero RA, Morales WJ, Allen MH, et al. Staging of twin-twin transfusion syndrome. *J Perinatol.* 1999;19:550–555.
84. Ville Y, Hyett J, Hecher K, et al. Preliminary experience with endoscopic laser surgery for severe twin-twin transfusion syndrome. *N Engl J Med.* 1995;332:224–227.
85. **Senat MV, Deprest J, Boulvain M, et al. Endoscopic laser surgery versus serial amnioreduction for severe twin-to-twin transfusion syndrome. *N Engl J Med.* 2004;351:136–144.**
86. De Lia JE. Surgery of the placenta and umbilical cord. *Clin Obstet Gynecol.* 1996;39:607–625.
87. Hecher K, Plath H, Bregenzer T, et al. Endoscopic laser surgery versus serial amniocenteses in the treatment of severe twin-twin transfusion syndrome. *Am J Obstet Gynecol.* 1999;180:717–724.
88. De Lia JE, Kuhlmann RS, Harstad TW, et al. Fetoscopic laser ablation of placental vessels in severe previable twin-twin transfusion syndrome. *Am J Obstet Gynecol.* 1995;172:1202–1208; discussion 1208–1211.
89. Feldstein VA, Machin GA, Albanese CT, et al. Twin-twin transfusion syndrome: the 'select' procedure. *Fetal Diagn Ther.* 2000;15:257–261.
90. **Tworetzky W, Wilkins-Haug L, Jennings RW, et al. Balloon dilation of severe aortic stenosis in the fetus: potential for prevention of hypoplastic left heart syndrome: candidate selection, technique, and results of successful intervention. *Circulation* 2004;110:2125–2131.**
91. Marshall AC, van der Velde ME, Tworetzky W, et al. Creation of an atrial septal defect in utero for fetuses with hypoplastic left heart syndrome and intact or highly restrictive atrial septum. *Circulation* 2004;110:253–258.
92. Tworetzky W, Marshall AC. Fetal interventions for cardiac defects. *Pediatr Clin North Am.* 2004;51:1503–1513, vii.
93. Crombleholme TM, Dirkes K, Whitney TM, et al. Amniotic band syndrome in fetal lambs. I: Fetoscopic release and morphometric outcome. *J Pediatr Surg.* 1995;30:974–978.
94. Quintero RA, Morales WJ, Phillips J, et al. In utero lysis of amniotic bands. *Ultrasound Obstet Gynecol.* 1997;10:316–320.
95. Keswani SG, Johnson MP, Adzick NS, et al. In utero limb salvage: fetoscopic release of amniotic bands for threatened limb amputation. *J Pediatr Surg.* 2003;38:848–851.
96. Farmer DL, Hirose S. Fetal intervention for complications of monochorionic twinning. *World J Surg.* 2003;27:103–107.

CHAPTER 108 ■ PEDIATRIC HEAD AND NECK SURGERY

JOHN AIKEN AND KEITH OLDHAM

Surgical lesions of the head and neck are common in children and include a broad spectrum of congenital and acquired disorders. Most lesions of the head and neck in children are benign and the etiology is congenital or inflammatory, but a few lesions are neoplastic. They can present clinically as asymptomatic masses or as life-threatening emergencies as a result of airway obstruction. This chapter focuses on the general principles and management of airway obstruction in infants and children and the most common head and neck lesions seen in pediatric surgical practice.

AIRWAY OBSTRUCTION

Many lesions, both congenital and acquired, can produce airway obstruction in infants and children. They may be intrinsic or extrinsic to the airway and vary from clinically insignificant to universally fatal.[1]

Airway obstruction is the most serious complication of neck masses in children. Often the first significant sign of respiratory distress in an infant is restlessness, followed by tachypnea, dyspnea, chest wall retractions and respiratory arrest if the obstruction is not relieved. It is crucial to establish an adequate airway and administer respiratory support while proceeding with the diagnostic evaluation. These interventions may include simple measures, such as repositioning the infant, clearing or suctioning the nose and mouth, and administering supplemental oxygen, or more extreme measures, such as endotracheal intubation or tracheostomy. Evaluation includes a careful history and physical examination, chest radiography, and arterial blood gas analysis. A nasogastric tube should be passed into the stomach, as gastric distension limits excursion of the diaphragm and can significantly contribute to respiratory compromise. Laryngoscopy and bronchoscopy are employed as needed.

Because infants are obligate nasal breathers, congenital lesions that obstruct the nasal passages or nasopharynx (choanal atresia, encephalocele, teratoma) typically cause early respiratory distress. These disorders are readily identified by physical examination, and emergent management is usually placement of an oropharyngeal airway. Airway obstruction at the level of the oral cavity in newborn infants is often a consequence of macroglossia or structural abnormalities such as micrognathia. Macroglossia may be a consequence of muscular hyperplasia and hypertrophy, as in Beckwith-Wiedemann syndrome and congenital hypothyroidism, or of diffuse involvement of the tongue with tumor (hemangiopericytoma, lymphangioma, neurofibromatosis).[2] Structural abnormalities, such as Pierre Robin syndrome (hypoplastic mandible with cleft palate), cause respiratory distress as the tongue falls posteriorly and obstructs the airway. Cysts or tumors of the pharynx or a mass arising at the base of the tongue, such as a lingual thyroid, may also obstruct the airway.[3] Clinically, upper airway obstruction, above the glottis or larynx, is characterized by dyspnea, tachypnea, and suprasternal, intercostal and costal margin retractions, but the child has no significant difficulty exhaling, and the voice and cry are normal. Emergency management consists of placing an oropharyngeal airway. Placing the infant in a prone position allows the tongue to fall forward and often provides significant relief. The infant may be fed through an orogastric feeding tube pending definitive correction of the obstruction. In extreme cases, a tracheostomy may be necessary.

Laryngeal obstruction can result from congenital or acquired vocal cord paralysis or tumors or cysts originating in the neck. Hemangiomas, lymphangiomas, cystic hygromas, and teratomas are the most common cervical tumors in infants and children. Laryngoscopy is usually required to differentiate these lesions. Emergency management of such malformations frequently requires placement of an endotracheal tube or tracheostomy. Endotracheal intubation can be difficult in the setting of a large neck mass, possibly causing displacement of the larynx, and bronchoscopy may be necessary with passage of the tube over a flexible bronchoscope. After the airway is stabilized, further diagnostic evaluation may include neck and chest radiography, computerized tomography (CT), magnetic resonance imaging, and laryngobronchoscopy. Tracheostomy may be necessary at the time of definitive surgical excision, and placement of a gastrostomy tube may also be indicated if feeding problems are anticipated. Hemangiomas are the most common tumors involving the larynx; they often respond to intralesional or systemic steroids, or may regress spontaneously.[4]

Acquired Obstruction

Foreign body aspiration and acute epiglottitis are common causes of acquired airway obstruction in children. Acute epiglottitis most commonly occurs in children 2 to 4 years of age, and *Haemophilus influenza* type B can be isolated in more than 90% of cases. Since the introduction of *Haemophilus influenza* type b vaccine in 1991, the incidence of this illness has been reduced in children.[5] Pneumococci and β-hemolytic streptococci are also causative organisms in epiglottitis. Acute epiglottitis typically presents as a rapidly progressive illness with symptoms of severe stridor, airway obstruction, drooling and difficulty swallowing, and with signs of systemic toxicity, including an elevated temperature and white blood cell count, tachypnea and tachycardia. Prolonged inspiratory stridor that worsens in the supine position is characteristic. In advanced cases, the child usually sits erect and leans forward, is anxious, drools, and becomes increasingly exhausted with air hunger. Attempts to examine or visualize the larynx may result in sudden airway occlusion with aspiration and respiratory arrest and therefore should be performed only in the operating room with personnel prepared to perform endotracheal intubation or tracheostomy. If the child's condition permits, lateral neck radiographs with soft-tissue techniques are obtained and should confirm the diagnosis by demonstrating edema of the epiglottis and ballooning of the hypopharynx.

The most important aspect of management is establishing a definitive diagnosis without delay. Once the diagnosis is established, maintaining an adequate airway is vital. Because of the high risk for progressive airway obstruction, standard therapy often involves short-term endotracheal intubation performed in the operating room under general anesthesia. The surgeon should be prepared to perform a tracheostomy in the event that the airway cannot be secured with an endotracheal tube or flexible bronchoscope. The inflammatory process typically resolves rapidly with administration of intravenous antibiotics, and intubation is seldom required beyond 3 days. Ampicillin is no longer recommended because of the high incidence of resistant *Haemophilus*. The drug of choice is usually a third-generation cephalosporin, such as cefoxitin or cefuroxime. The timing of extubation should be based on resolution of the clinical signs and symptoms and direct visualization of the supraglottic area by fiberoptic nasopharyngoscopy. In the past, tracheostomy was the standard therapy, but comparative reviews demonstrate that short-term endotracheal intubation is associated with less morbidity and fewer complications.[6]

BRANCHIAL CLEFT REMNANTS

Remnants of the embryonic branchial apparatus (cysts, sinuses, fistulas, and cartilaginous rests) are common in children. Although congenital by definition, they are often unrecognized or misdiagnosed until symptoms or complications initiate an evaluation. Sinuses, fistulas, and cartilaginous remnants are usually apparent at birth and noticed early in life. Cysts are more likely to present later in childhood as a neck mass when they fill with secretions. All of these lesions have a risk of infection and can present as an abscess or with drainage and surrounding erythema. Rarely, the remnants may harbor malignancy.[7]

Anatomy and Embryology

During the fourth to eighth week after fertilization, four pairs of well-developed ridges (branchial arches) and associated clefts (externally) and pouches (internally) are prominent in the lateral cervicofacial region of the human embryo. The mature structures of the head and neck are derivatives of these paired branchial arches, clefts and pouches in the embryo.[8] The contributions of the branchial arches and clefts to the structures of the neck and jaw are summarized in Fig. 108.1. Incomplete closure or resorption of these primitive branchial clefts and arches may result in development of cysts, sinuses, fistulae, and masses. The first branchial arch forms the mandible and a portion of the upper jaw, and part of the first branchial cleft remains open as the eustachian tube and external auditory canal. Abnormal development results in anomalies such as cleft lip and palate, abnormal shape and contour of the external ear, and malformation of the internal ossicles. The second branchial arch forms the hyoid bone and cleft of the tonsillar fossa. Remnants of the first branchial cleft are found along the base of an imaginary fold extending from the auditory canal behind and below the angle of the mandible to

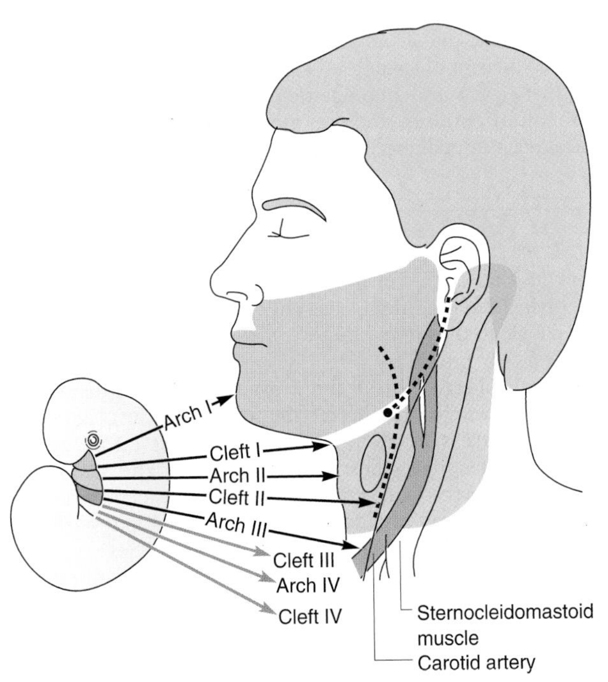

FIGURE 108.1 Derivation of various areas of the head and neck from the branchial arches and clefts of the embryo.

just below the midpoint of the mandible. Second branchial cleft remnants are found along any part of a line extending from the tonsillar fossa inferiorly to a point on the lower third of the anterior border of the sternocleidomastoid muscle. The third cleft migrates low in the neck to form the inferior parathyroid glands and the thymus. The fourth cleft also migrates but stops higher up in the neck and forms the superior parathyroid glands and C-cells of the thyroid gland.

Clinical Aspects

All abnormal branchial remnants are congenital abnormalities and therefore are present at birth. Branchial cleft sinuses present as cutaneous openings and are most often noted in infancy or at an early age, whereas cysts typically appear later in childhood when they accumulate secretions. Branchial cleft sinuses and fistulae frequently produce mucoid drainage from the skin opening, and the cutaneous openings are occasionally marked by skin tags or subcutaneous cartilaginous remnants. First branchial cleft remnants present as a sinus opening near the angle of the mandible in the region of the submandibular triangle or preauricular region. These sinus tracts extend from their submandibular opening superficial to the mandible up to the external auditory canal. The tract is intimately associated with the parotid gland and facial nerve.[9] First branchial anomalies are less common than those of the second cleft and are often misdiagnosed. A history of recurrent infection, often leading to incision and drainage, is generally present. A key to the diagnosis is a history of non-purulent drainage before infection. Second branchial anomalies are six times more common than first branchial anomalies and present as an opening along the anterior border of the sternocleidomastoid muscle in its lower third; they may be bilateral (10% of cases) (Figs. 108.2 and 108.3). The sinus tract of a second branchial anomaly passes over the bifurcation of the carotid artery between the external and internal carotid arteries and communicates with the tonsillar fossa. Cysts or infections arising from the third and fourth branchial arch and cleft are rare and much more challenging to diagnose and treat than first and second branchial remnants.[10–12] For both third and fourth remnants, the internal opening is located in the piriform sinus (Fig. 108.4). Radiographic imaging is typically not necessary for first and second branchial anomalies, but barium studies and CT may be useful in demonstrating a piriform sinus fistula. The third branchial cleft sinus presents as a mass lower in the neck than the second branchial sinus. Its course is superior and posterior to the carotid sheath, most commonly on the left side. Third and fourth branchial anomalies generally present before age 10 years, often as left thyroid lobe abscess. Contrast esophagram may demonstrate the fistula between the piriform sinus and neck.[13,14] Because of the risk of the development of infection in any of the branchial cleft anomalies, excision is recommended at diagnosis of a noninfected lesion. Surgery in infants may be delayed until age 3 to 6 months.

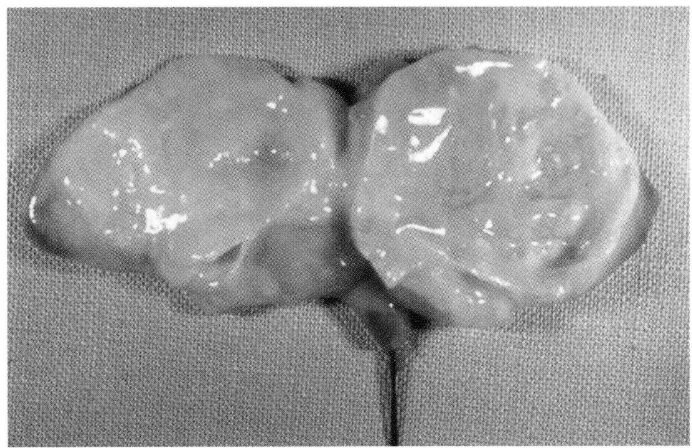

FIGURE 108.3 Branchial cyst. Most of these cysts arise from the second branchial cleft and occur laterally in the neck. The cysts have a thin wall, contain turbid fluid, and are lined by stratified squamous or respiratory-type epithelium. (From Rubin E, Farber JL. *Pathology*, 3rd ed. Philadelphia: Lippincott Williams & Wilkins, 1999, with permission).

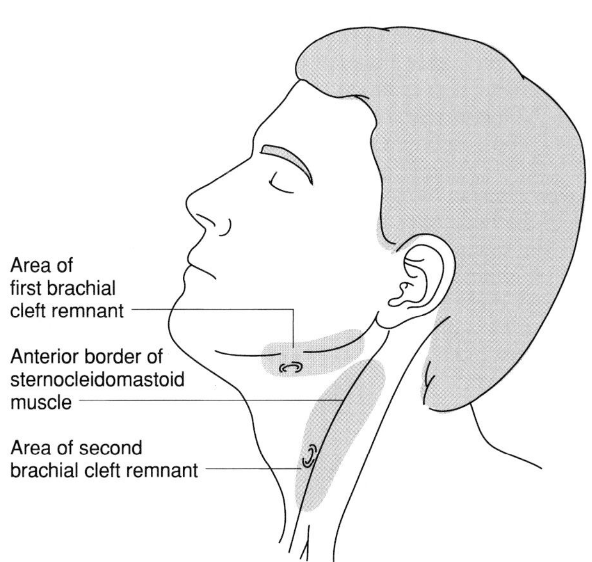

FIGURE 108.2 Areas of the neck in which cysts and sinuses originating from the first and second branchial clefts are usually found.

Treatment and Outcome

The goal of treatment of any branchial cleft remnant is complete surgical excision. The operation is usually performed once the diagnosis is secure, provided no active inflammation or infection is present. If infection is found, antibiotics are administered initially, and the operation is delayed several weeks to allow the inflammation to resolve. This approach provides the best opportunity for complete excision of the tract. Abscesses are managed initially with limited incision and drainage to control infection. Formal excision of branchial cleft lesions in the presence of active inflammation or infection is associated with a higher recurrence rate secondary to incomplete excision, [15] and an increased likelihood of injury to nerves (facial, hypoglossal) and other vital structures.

The operation is performed under general anesthesia. The patient is positioned with the head and neck slightly extended. An elliptical transverse incision along Langer's lines incorporates the sinus opening. The tract is identified and dissection continues cephalad immediately along the tract to avoid injury to contiguous structures. The dissection for a second branchial remnant penetrates the platysma muscle and cervical fascia, ascends along the carotid sheath to the level of the hyoid bone, turns medially between the branches of the carotid artery, courses behind the posterior belly of the digastric muscle and stylohyoid muscle and in front of the

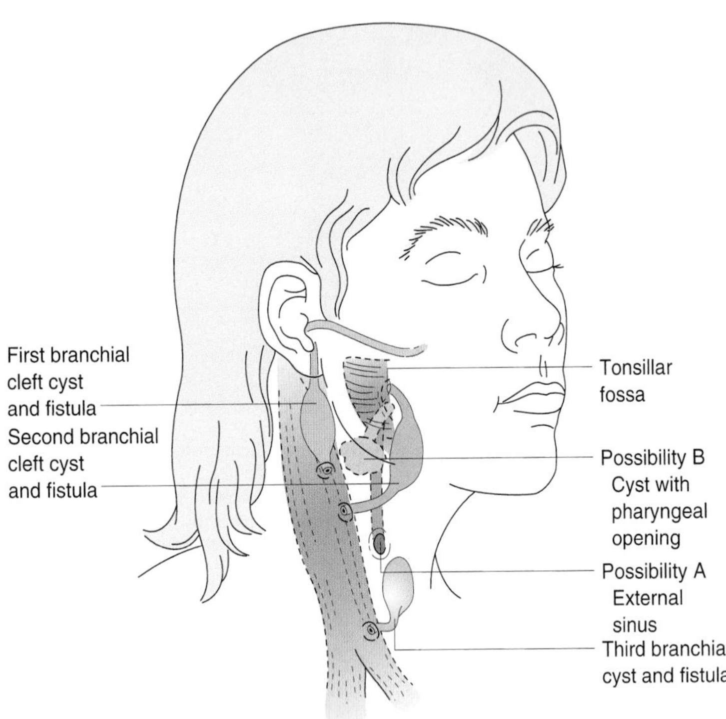

FIGURE 108.4 Types of first, second, and third branchial cleft remnants. Sinuses and fistulae are seen most often in infants and young children, whereas cysts usually appear at a later age.

hypoglossal nerve before ending in the pharynx, most often in the tonsillar fossa. A finger in the mouth pressing downward gently in the tonsillar fossa helps identify the endpoint of the dissection, where the tract is suture ligated with absorbable suture and divided (Fig. 108.5). Occasionally, in older patients with a long tract, a second, "stepladder" incision may be required to complete the dissection.

The tract for a first branchial cleft remnant typically courses from its sinus opening along the angle of the mandible cephalad in proximity to the parotid gland and facial nerve and ends at the external auditory canal (Fig. 108.6).[16] Draping should allow visualization of the lateral aspect of the eye and corner of the mouth. A nerve stimulator may be helpful in the effort to avoid injury to the facial nerve branches. The superficial lobe of the parotid gland may need to be reflected upward to expose the tract, or may require excision in cases of chronic infection.

For third and fourth branchial remnants, the dissection follows the tract to its termination in the piriform sinus. Endoscopy at the start of the operation may enable cannulation of the tract from above with a Fogarty catheter or small feeding tube, which greatly facilitates localization of the tract during excision.[14] The thyroid gland is exposed through a standard collar incision, and the appropriate lobe is mobilized. The recurrent and superior laryngeal nerves and parathyroid glands should be identified and protected. If no discrete cyst or tract is found, the fistula may be located at the laryngeal level near the cricothyroid membrane. The fibers of the inferior constrictor muscle are bluntly spread to expose the piriform recess. Extreme caution should be exercised in this region to preserve the external branch of the superior laryngeal nerve. The tract typically passes inferior and external to the recurrent laryngeal nerve along the trachea to the superior pole of the thyroid gland. It may end blindly near the gland or penetrate the capsule to terminate in the parenchyma of the left thyroid lobe. Thyroid lobectomy or resection of the superior pole is carried out as indicated by the extent of the cyst (Fig. 108.7).[17] Once surgical extirpation is complete, the wound is closed in layers with absorbable suture. Drainage is only used if infection is encountered during the dissection. Recurrence is rare and implies that the entire epithelium-lined tract was not excised.

When remnants of the branchial apparatus persist as cartilaginous rests, these masses are generally small and present subcutaneously along the anterior border of the sternocleidomastoid muscle. The lesion is typically visible and palpable on physical examination and may be bilateral (10% of cases). An accompanying sinus or cyst is uncommon and infection is rare. Excision is for cosmetic reasons.

Preauricular cysts and sinuses are also common in infants and children. They are believed to arise as a result of anomalies in the formation of the external ear and represent vestiges of the first two branchial arches. They differ from first branchial cleft cysts in that they are more common, often bilateral, often inherited, and only rarely are complicated by infection, involvement of the facial nerve, or entrance into the external auditory canal.[18] Operative excision is recommended only for symptomatic lesions. Draining sinuses and infected cysts require antibiotic treatment, incision and drainage for failure to resolve, and delayed excision to prevent recurrence. Complete surgical excision of the sinus tract and cyst to the level of the temporalis fascia is the treatment of choice in the uninfected draining sinus. The cyst or sinus may have multiple branches making complete resection difficult, and some clinicians have advocated an extended incision and removal of a small portion of adjacent cartilage to reduce the risk of missing one of these branching tracts.[19,20]

THYROGLOSSAL DUCT CYST

Anatomy and Embryology

Thyroglossal duct cysts are common midline neck lesions in children. Thyroglossal duct cysts or remnants arise when embryonic elements persist along the tract of descent of the thyroid gland.

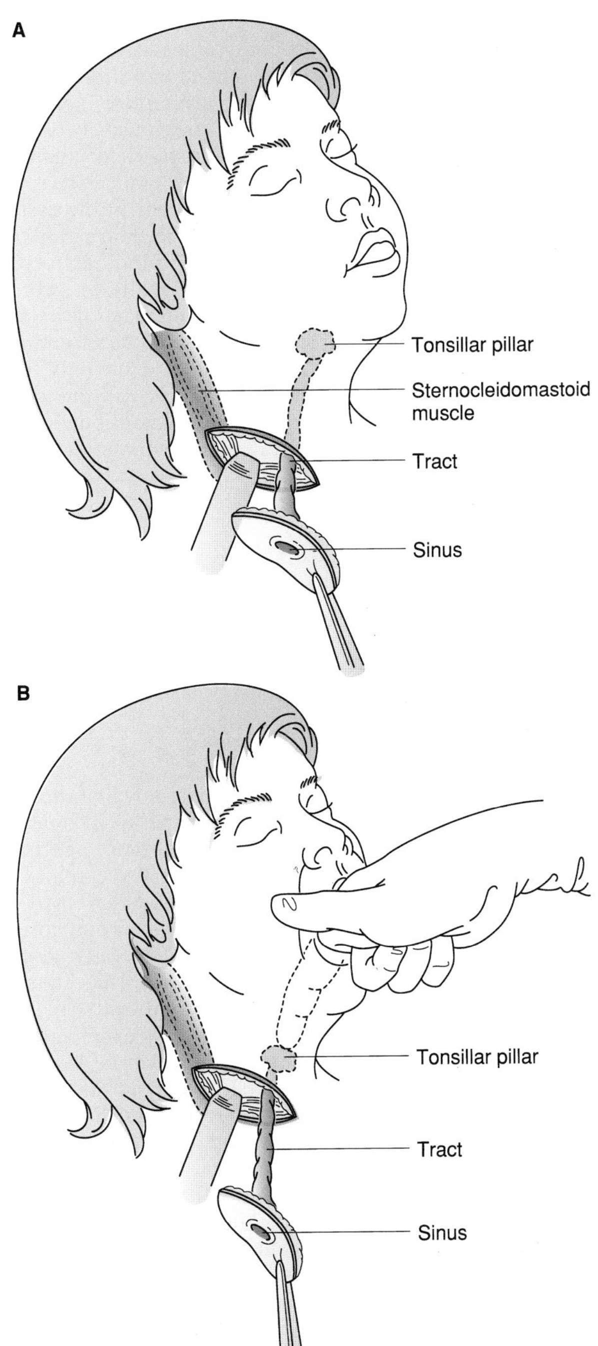

FIGURE 108.5 (*A*) Single incision in the lower part of the neck with the sinus tract developed to usual length. (*B*) The anesthesiologist's finger depresses the tonsillar fossa to facilitate complete dissection of the sinus tract through the single incision.

The thyroid gland starts as a diverticulum at the foramen cecum at the base of the tongue and descends in the sixth week of fetal life to its pretracheal position in the neck. In its descent, the tract most often passes through the central portion of the hyoid bone, but it may pass in front or behind the hyoid. Thyroglossal duct cysts may develop anywhere along the tract (Fig. 108.8). Ectopic thyroid tissue is identified within the thyroglossal duct remnant in about 25% to 35% of cases, and papillary adenocarcinoma has been described in up to 10% of patients undergoing thyroglossal duct excision in adulthood.[21–23]

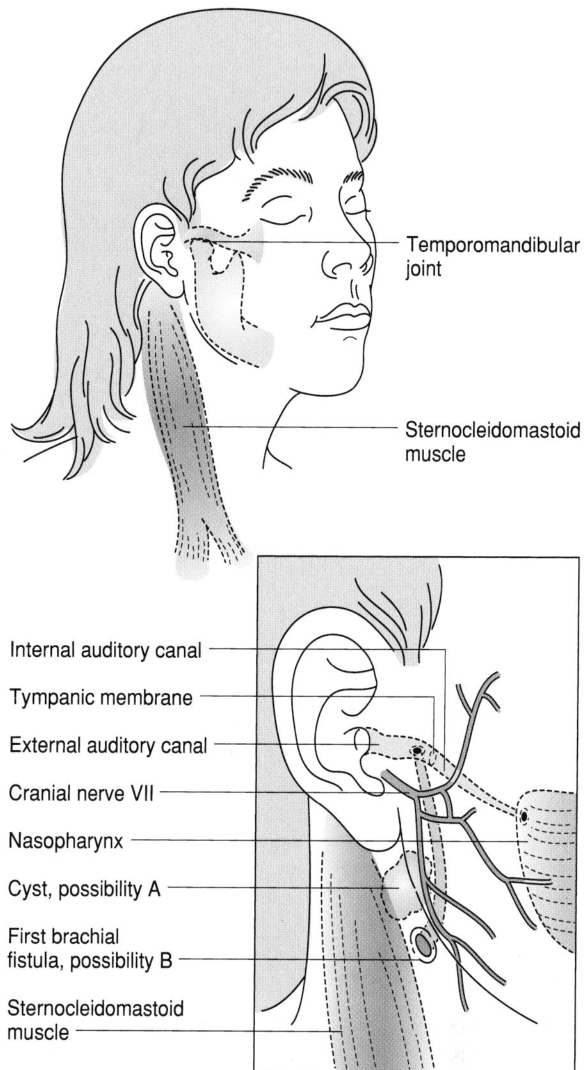

FIGURE 108.6 Relations of cyst or sinus of the first branchial cleft. Note especially the proximity to the facial nerve and external auditory canal.

Clinical Aspects

Thyroglossal duct cysts are present at birth but rarely present clinically in early infancy. The most common presentation is a midline cystic neck mass (Fig. 108.9) or draining sinus in early

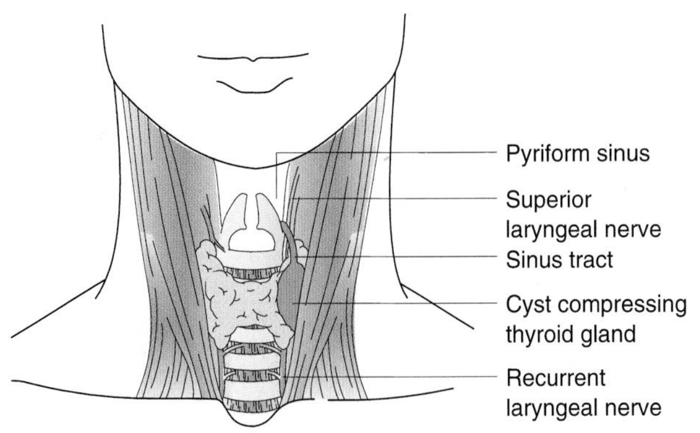

FIGURE 108.7 Relations of a third or fourth branchial cleft cyst or sinus to the thyroid gland and piriform sinus.

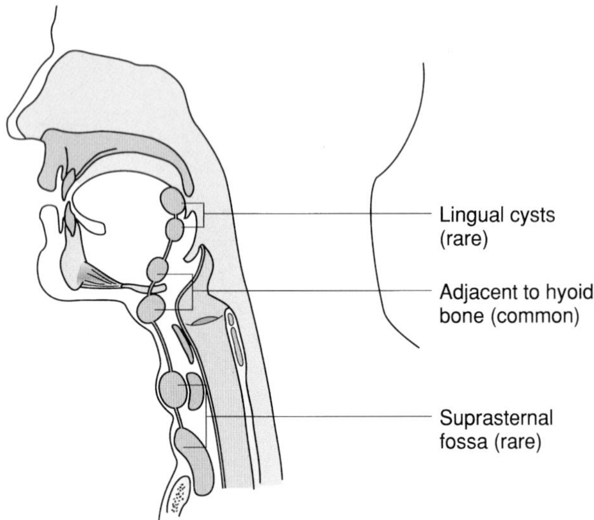

FIGURE 108.8 Locations of thyroglossal duct cysts.

childhood, most by age 5 years.[24, 25] Infection and abscess formation frequently arises because of communication with the mouth and contamination by oral flora. If it is not infected, the cyst is usually apparent by palpation. The cyst is at or near the midline, most commonly overlying the hyoid bone, but may be found at any level from the submental region to the upper trachea.[15] It is typically smooth, soft, and nontender in the absence of infection. Because the cyst and tract are attached to the foramen cecum of the tongue, the cyst often moves with protrusion of the tongue and swallowing. In contrast to branchial cleft remnants, a thyroglossal duct cyst does not have a sinus opening to the skin unless infection has resulted in spontaneous drainage or an incomplete excision or incision and drainage procedure has previously been performed. The cyst and duct are lined with stratified squamous or pseudostratified columnar epithelium with mucus-secreting glands. Ectopic thyroid tissue may be present in the cyst or tract, and in rare cases this may represent the child's only thyroid tissue. Preoperative thyroid scans with radioactive isotopes have been employed by some, but usually one can be reassured by simple palpation of the thyroid gland in its normal pretracheal location. Furthermore, even in the exceptional cases in which the thyroid tissue in the cyst is the only functional thyroid tissue, excision of the cyst is still mandated because of the risk for infection and the malignant potential of the dysgenetic thyroid tissue.[26] Review of the pathologic specimen after excision is important. If thyroid tissue is present in the specimen, thyroid function tests should then be performed and thyroid replacement therapy prescribed as indicated. As with branchial cleft remnants, definitive excision should not be performed in the presence of infection or inflammation because of the increased risk for incomplete excision and injury to contiguous structures. Preoperative preparation may require incision and drainage or a period of antibiotics.

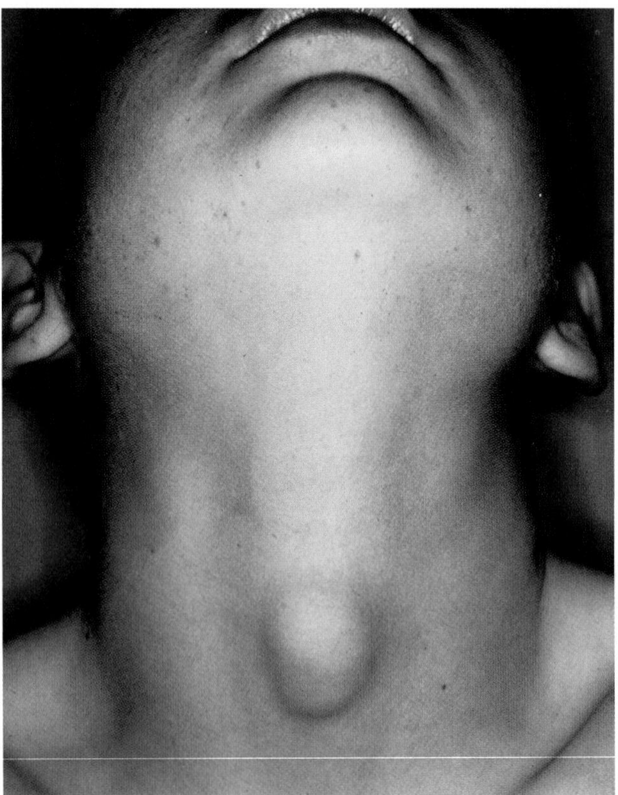

FIGURE 108.9 A thyroglossal duct cyst. (Courtesy of L. Thompson.)

Treatment

Successful management requires complete removal of the cyst, its entire tract and the central portion of the hyoid bone. In 1920, Sistrunk[27] not only described the importance of removing the central portion of the hyoid bone but also emphasized the possible existence of multiple tracts and therefore the importance of an *en bloc* dissection and removal of a core of tissue to the base of the tongue. Before these operative principles were elucidated, most series reported a recurrence rate of 20% or higher. The operation is performed under general endotracheal anesthesia. The patient's neck is extended, and often a roll is placed beneath the shoulders. A transverse skin incision is made directly over the cyst, usually in the infrahyoid region. If a sinus opening exists to the skin from prior infection or surgery, an elliptical incision to include the sinus is used. The cyst is easily identified beneath the platysma muscle. Dissection adjacent to the cyst wall mobilizes the cyst, and the tract is identified. Dissection is continued cephalad up to the hyoid bone. The muscular attachments to the superior and inferior portions of the body of the hyoid bone are divided, and the central portion of the hyoid bone is removed in continuity with the cyst and tract. Beyond the hyoid bone, a core of tissue 5 to 10 mm in diameter is excised through the muscles of the base of the tongue to the foramen cecum, where the tract is suture ligated with absorbable suture.[28,29] Identification of the end point of the dissection at the foramen cecum may be facilitated by having the anesthesiologist place downward pressure on the base of the tongue with a gloved finger. The ends of the hyoid bone are not reapproximated. The wound is copiously irrigated and closed in layers. A drain may be used, particularly if the patient has a history of infection, but most often it is not required. Complete excision of a thyroglossal duct cyst is generally curative. Contemporary recurrence rates generally are less than 10% and usually related to prior infection or incomplete surgical excision. Thyroid neoplasia (<1%) has been described in ectopic thyroid tissue, both associated and unassociated with thyroglossal duct cysts.[21–23]

Other midline neck masses that occur in children include dermoid and epidermoid inclusion cysts, pathologic lymph nodes, cervical thymic cysts and bronchogenic cysts. Dermoid and epidermoid cysts consist of ectodermal elements that were trapped beneath the skin or failed to separate from the neural tube.[30,31] Dermoids are distinguished histologically from epidermoids by the accessory glandular structures they possess, including sebaceous glands, hair follicles, connective tissues, and papillae. The most common location of dermoids in infants and children is the lateral orbital ridge. Midline dermoid cysts probably represent entrapment of epithelium of branchial arch origin at the time of embryologic midline fusion.[32,33] Differentiation from thyroglossal duct cysts can usually be accomplished on physical exam, with dermoid cysts typically more superficial and do not move with protrusion of the tongue. In atypical cases, ultrasound, CT, or magnetic resonance imaging helps to make the diagnosis and define the extent of the lesion. Complete surgical excision is recommended for these lesions. This is generally performed as an open operation, although increasing experience is accruing using endoscopic minimally invasive techniques.[34]

LYMPHADENOPATHY

Benign cervical lymphadenopathy is the most common neck mass in childhood.[35] The anterior cervical, occipital, retroauricular, and submandibular nodal groups are the ones most often enlarged. Bacterial and viral infections, particularly upper respiratory tract infections, otitis media and pharyngitis, are the most common cause, with bacterial infections most likely to progress to acute suppurative lymphadenitis. Other important inflammatory causes of cervical lymphadenopathy include cat-scratch disease, mononucleosis, atypical mycobacterial infection, and tuberculosis. Enlarged cervical or supraclavicular lymph nodes may also be the presenting manifestation of certain malignancies, particularly lymphoma.[36]

Acute suppurative cervical lymphadenitis most frequently occurs in young children between 6 months and 3 years of age. Typically, enlargement of the lymph node is preceded by an episode of pharyngitis or an upper respiratory tract infection. The most common organisms are penicillin-resistant *Staphylococcus aureus* and group A beta-hemolytic streptococci.[37] The enlarged node initially becomes erythematous and tender with surrounding cellulitis. Systemic signs of infection are usually present—fever, tachycardia, and an elevated white blood cell count with a leftward shift. Fluctuance develops as the abscess forms. Management includes systemic antibiotics to cover *Streptococcus* and *Staphylococcus* organisms. Fluctuant nodes require drainage. Occasionally, aspiration of the purulent and necrotic material with a large-bore needle provides fluid for culture, and in combination with antibiotics, may effect resolution without formal incision and drainage. More frequently, fluctuant nodes require incision and drainage, with the use of either conscious sedation and local anesthesia or general anesthesia in the operating room. The most important consideration when performing incision and drainage of a fluctuant neck mass is control of the airway. A skin line incision is made over the area of maximal fluctuance and the abscess cavity is drained, with care taken to break up any loculations. The incision should be designed with concern for complete drainage, avoidance of vital structures, particularly the branches of the facial nerve, and cosmesis. The wound is loosely packed open and covered with a dry gauze dressing. Drains may be used in cases of deep or complex neck abscesses, but are not generally necessary in uncomplicated cases. Recurrence is rare and should prompt evaluation for an underlying congenital anomaly. Viral infections are also associated with the development of acute cervical lymphadenitis, which is typically bilateral, rarely suppurative, and generally self-limited with spontaneous resolution.

Lymphadenitis is chronic or subacute when enlargement of lymph nodes persists long after any evidence of infection has disappeared or the patient has no history or evidence of a precipitating infectious illness. The child may have a history of frequent upper respiratory infections, otitis media, tonsillitis, sinusitis, or allergic rhinitis or eczema. Systemic signs of infection are not present. The nodes are usually solitary, nontender, mobile and soft. Enlarged nodes that are asymptomatic, less than 1 cm in diameter, and soft and that have been present for less than 8 weeks do not require treatment. Excisional biopsy should be performed for any node that is larger than 2 cm in diameter, persists beyond 8 weeks, or demonstrates worrisome characteristics, such as firmness, immobility or rapid growth. The child should be evaluated for tuberculosis, atypical mycobacterial infection, and cat-scratch disease. Most of the lymph nodes that come to biopsy are benign and the histologic examination reveals "reactive hyperplasia."

Mycobacterial lymphadenitis and cat-scratch disease also commonly cause lymphadenopathy in children.[38] Mycobacterial lymphadenitis is usually caused by atypical mycobacteria of the *Mycobacterium avium-intracellulare-scrofulaceum* (MAIS) complex.[39–41] The portal of entry is the oropharynx. Unlike *Mycobacterium tuberculosis*, person-to-person transmission of MAIS has not been demonstrated. Infection with *Mycobacterium tuberculosis* is uncommon in children in the United States, and when present, it is usually accompanied by positive findings on chest radiographs because the lung is the site of entry for this organism. Atypical mycobacterial lymphadenitis is typically asymptomatic with enlarged but nontender nodes and no associated fever or leukocytosis. If no treatment is given, drainage and sinus formation may occur spontaneously. The child with tuberculous scrofula is typically symptomatic with pulmonary tuberculosis. The results of chest radiography and skin testing with purified protein derivative-standard are usually positive. For *M. tuberculosis* infection, a trial of anti-tuberculosis chemotherapy is recommended. Current treatment regimens consist of multiple-agent chemotherapy with isoniazid and rifampin for 9 to 12 months and a third drug, (pyrazinamide, streptomycin, or ethambutol) for the first 2 months.[42] Atypical mycobacterial infections generally respond poorly to chemotherapy. When a lymph node biopsy is planned, if tuberculosis or atypical mycobacterial infection is suspected, complete excision is required. Incision and drainage or incomplete nodal excision in cases of atypical mycobacterial infection invariably leads to recurrence or cutaneous draining sinuses. Complete excision is generally curative, although there may be a role for adjunctive antimicrobial therapy with clarithromycin and rifabutin.[43]

Cat scratch disease is a common cause of lymphadenitis in children in western countries.[44] In most cases, the history reveals direct contact with a cat. The site of inoculation is most commonly an extremity, resulting in inguinal, epitrochlear, or axillary adenopathy; however, cervical nodes are involved in as many as 25% of cases.[45,46] The disease is believed to be caused by a gram-negative bacillus, *Bartonella henselae*, and typically begins as a superficial infection at the inoculation site on a limb. The diagnosis can be confirmed by skin test antigen. The clinical presentation usually is lymphadenopathy with only mild tenderness and without systemic symptoms. No treatment is necessary if the diagnosis is secure (positive skin test result) because the illness is generally self-limited and lymphadenopathy resolves in most cases in 6 to 8 weeks without specific treatment. Antibiotics are not generally effective despite in vitro sensitivities. If the diagnosis is in doubt, complete excision is recommended and curative.

Although most lymphadenopathy in children is benign, malignant conditions such as Hodgkin disease and non-Hodgkin lymphoma are also common in children and frequently present as primary neck lymphadenopathy. Any case of a neck mass that has concerning examination characteristics, or that persists despite appropriate antibiotic therapy, requires excisional biopsy for definitive diagnosis.

VASCULAR MALFORMATIONS AND CYSTIC HYGROMA

Hemangioma

Hemangiomas can occur anywhere in the body and involvement of the tongue, subglottic area and parotid glands is common. Except for intradermal capillary lesions, most hemangiomas are not obvious at birth but become clinically evident in the first few weeks of life. The lesions may be extensive. Typically, they have a blue coloration and a spongy or rubbery texture on palpation. The presenting symptom for subglottic hemangioma is often stridor that is not present at birth but presents at age 1 to 3 months. Parotid hemangioma typically develops in early infancy as an enlarging soft mass in the parotid gland. Cutaneous capillary hemangiomas may be present on the face, neck, or chest. Biopsy of these lesions was recommended in the past but is no longer routinely performed in most centers. Evaluation by ultrasonography with Doppler-flow studies is usually diagnostic.[47] CT with intravenous contrast and magnetic resonance angiographic imaging are very useful for the evaluating the extent of tissue involvement. Angiography is invasive and rarely necessary. The natural history of these lesions is one of significant growth in the first 6 to 12 months of life, followed by a period of minimal growth, after which involution and spontaneous resolution occurs by thrombosis and epithelialization.[48] If involution takes place, it is complete by age 5 years in 80% of patients. Lesions that because of their location or growth are obstructing the airway, involving the eye, or destroying tissue are generally treated with intralesional steroid injection or systemic steroids (Fig. 108.10). The response is typically excellent.

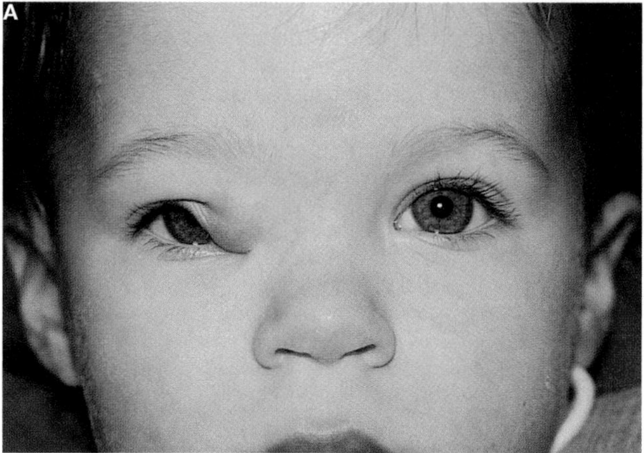

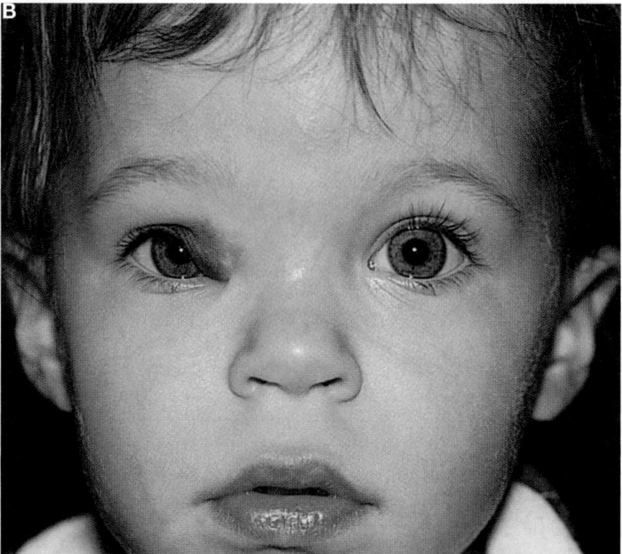

FIGURE 108.10 Capillary hemangioma. (*A*) The lesion of the upper lid is large enough to partially occlude the visual axis and induced a significant astigmatic error and strong visual preference for the left eye, requiring occlusion therapy. Because it is located in the deeper tissue layers, this hemangioma appears more bluish than more superficially located lesions. (*B*) Three days after intralesional steroid injection, the hemangioma has shrunk out of the visual axis. (From Tasman W, Jaeger E. The Wills Eye Hospital Atlas of Clinical Ophthalmology, 2e. Lippincott Williams & Wilkins, 2001, with permission.)

Lymphangioma and Cystic Hygroma

Anatomy and Embryology

At about the sixth week of gestation, a system of clefts develops in the cervical mesenchyme that subsequently form lymph channels. These channels give rise to jugular lymph sacs that become the cervical lymph nodes and lymphatics, ultimately draining into the internal jugular venous system (Fig. 108.11). Lymphangiomas are masses of disorganized, dilated lymph channels that arise when communications with the internal jugular system fail to develop in portions of the lymphatic channels. Lymphatic malformations can vary in size from a few centimeters in diameter to massive tumor-like lesions extending into the mediastinum. The larger lesions with macrocystic dilated lymphatic channels are often referred to as *cystic hygromas*. They are most commonly found in the lateral cervical and submandibular region. Other locations for lymphatic malformations are the extremities, the mediastinum, retroperitoneum and trunk. Most lymphatic malformations are evident early in life with 65% present at birth, 80% evident within the first year of life, and 90% diagnosed by the age of 2 years.[49] They typically present as an asymptomatic mass lesion and can be located anywhere in the body. Hemorrhage can occur within the lesion and is often the reason for the rapid enlargement sometimes noted clinically. The lesions have a significant tendency to become infected and also frequently present as an area of cellulitis or an abscess (Fig. 108.12). Symptoms such as pain or discomfort are rare unless the lesion has hemorrhaged or been infected. In the newborn, the lesions may cause significant airway compromise or esophageal and pharyngeal obstruction. Approximately 10% of cervical lymphatic malformations extend into the chest. Lymphatic malformations can be diagnosed by prenatal ultrasonography, but most are detected on routine examination after birth. The physical examination findings of a soft, cystic, multiloculated mass are often sufficient for a definitive diagnosis. Ultrasonography, particularly with Doppler-flow studies, is often very useful to confirm the diagnosis. CT with intravenous contrast or magnetic resonance angiography is used selectively to evaluate extension of the lesion from one body space to another and delineate associated vital structures when resection is being planned.

Treatment

Complete surgical excision is the optimal treatment for lymphatic malformations. Because these lesions are benign, radical extirpation resulting in loss of function or severe deformity is not indicated. Spontaneous regression is unusual but may occur after acute inflammation. Only two thirds of lymphatic malformations are amenable to complete excision. One third requires partial excision or, in the case of extensive or complex

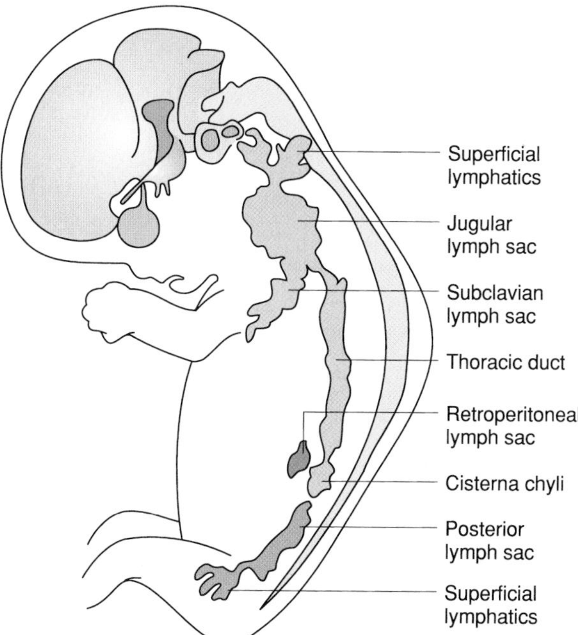

FIGURE 108.11 Lymphatic system in an 8-week-old human embryo. Development of the major and minor lymphatic sacs is well under way. The jugular lymphatic sac in the neck is prominent. Sequestration of tissue from any of the developing lymphatic structures leads to formation of a lymphangioma or cystic hygroma.

lesions, staged excision because of involvement of vital structures within the lesion. Needle aspiration of cysts is no longer recommended except to decompress a cyst emergently and relieve airway obstruction. Radiation treatment has not been of benefit in the treatment of lymphatic malformations and

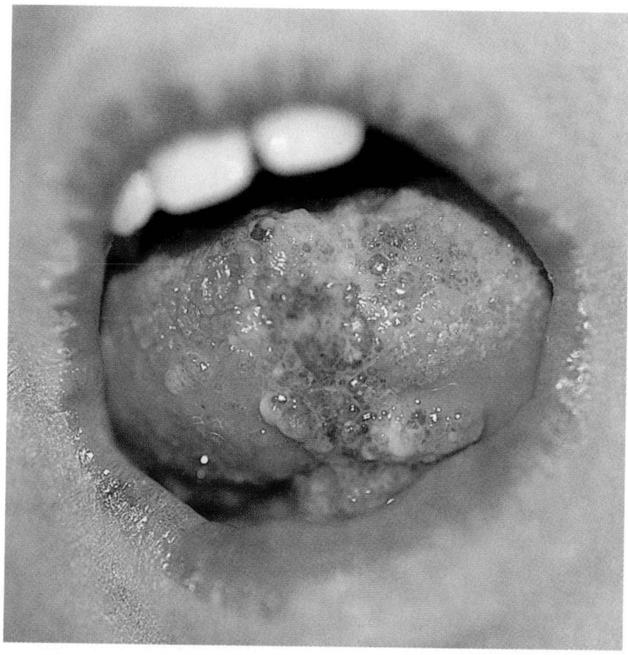

FIGURE 108.12 Infected cystic hygroma of the tongue. (From Fleisher GR, MD, Ludwig W, MD, Baskin MN, MD. Atlas of Pediatric Emergency Medicine. Philadelphia: Lippincott Williams & Wilkins, 2004, with permission.)

causes significant morbidity in the growing child. Injection of sclerosing agents, most commonly bleomycin, has been used but is associated with significant potential complications of infection, gastrointestinal problems, and pulmonary fibrosis.[50] More recently, large cystic lesions in locations difficult to manage surgically have been treated by injection of OK-432, a monoclonal antibody produced by incubation and interaction of *Streptococcus pyogenes* with penicillin.[51] At present this treatment remains experimental but has demonstrated success in some difficult cases.

KEY POINTS

- **Airway obstruction is the most serious complication of neck masses in children, and in infants presents with restlessness, followed by tachypnea, dyspnea, chest wall retractions, and respiratory arrest.**
- **Infants are obligate nasal breathers, thus congenital lesions that obstruct the nasal passages or nasopharynx (choanal atresia, encephalocele, teratoma) typically cause early respiratory distress.**
- **Acute epiglottitis presents as a rapidly progressive illness with severe stridor, airway obstruction, drooling and difficulty swallowing, and with signs of systemic toxicity, including an elevated temperature and white blood cell count, tachypnea, and tachycardia.**
- **Branchial cleft sinuses present as cutaneous openings and are most often noted in infancy or at an early age, whereas cysts typically appear later in childhood when they accumulate secretions; treatment is complete surgical removal.**
- **Thyroglossal duct cysts or remnants arise when embryonic elements persist along the tract of descent of the thyroid gland; treatment requires complete removal of the cyst, its entire tract and the central portion of the hyoid bone.**
- **Benign cervical lymphadenopathy is the most common neck mass in childhood**
- **Lymphangiomas are masses of disorganized, dilated lymph channels that arise when communications with the internal jugular system fail to develop in portions of the lymphatic channels; the larger lesions with macrocystic dilated lymphatic channels are often referred to as *cystic hygromas*.**

References

1. DeLorimer AA. Congenital malformations and neonatal problems of the respiratory tract. In: Welch KJ, Randolph JG, Ravitch MM, et al., eds. *Pediatric surgery,* 4th ed. Chicago: Year Book, 1986, p. 631.
2. Alpers CE, Rosenau W, Finkbeiner WE, et al. Congenital (infantile) hemangiopericytoma of the tongue and sublingual region. *Am J Clin Pathol.* 1984;81:377–382.
3. Weider DJ, Parker W. Lingual thyroid: review, case reports, and therapeutic guidelines. *Ann Otol Rhinol Laryngol.* 1977:86:841–848.
4. Fonkalsrud EW. Malformations of the lymphatic system and hemangiomas. In: Holder TM, Ashcraft KW, eds. *Pediatric surgery*. Philadelphia: WB Saunders, 1980, p. 1042.
5. Adams WG, Deaver KA, Cochi SL, et al. Decline of *Haemophilus influenzae* type B (HIB) disease in the HIB vaccine era. *JAMA.* 1993;269:221–226.
6. Kinnefors A, Olofsson J. Acute epiglottitis in children: experience with tracheostomy and intubation. *Clin Otolaryngol Allied Sci.* 1983:25–30.
7. Soper RT, Pringle KC. Cysts and sinuses of the neck. In: Welch KJ, Randolph JG, Ravitch MM, et al., eds. *Pediatric surgery,* 4th ed. Chicago: Year Book, 1986, p. 539.
8. Gray SW, Skandalakis JE. The pharynx and its derivatives. In: *Embryology for surgeons: the embryological basis for the treatment of congenital defects*. Philadelphia: WB Saunders, 1972.
9. Triglia JM, Nicollas R, Dueroz V, et al. First branchial cleft anomalies. A study of 39 cases and a review of the literature *Arch Otolaryngol Head Neck Surgery.* 1998;124:291–295.
10. Lin JN, Wang KL. Persistent third branchial apparatus. *J Pediatr Surg.* 1991;26:663–665.
11. Brown RL, Azizkhan RG. Pediatric head and neck lesions. *Pediatr Clin North Am.* 1998;45:889–905.

12. Rosenfeld RM, Biller HF. Fourth branchial pouch sinus: diagnosis and treatment. *Otolaryngol Head Neck Surg.* 1991;105:44–50.
13. Roback SA, Telander RL. Thyroglossal duct cysts and branchial cleft anomalies. *Semin Pediatr Surg.* 1994; 3:142–46.
14. Godin MS, Kearns DB, Pransky SM, et al. Fourth branchial pouch sinus: principles of diagnosis and management. *Laryngoscope* 1990;100: 174–178.
15. Rowe MI. Neck lesions. In: O'Neill JA, Grosfeld JL, Fonkalsrud EW, et al., *Essentials of pediatric surgery*. St. Louis, Mosby-Year Book, 1998.
16. **D'Souza AR, Uppal HS, De R, et al. Updating concepts of first branchial cleft defects: a literature review. *Int J Pediatr Radiol.* 200262:103–109.**
17. Miller D, Hill JL, Sun CC, et al. The diagnosis and management of pyriform sinus fistulae in infants and young children. *J Pediatr Surg.* 1983;18: 377–381.
18. Burge D, Middleton A. Persistent pharyngeal pouch derivatives in the neonate. *J Pediatr Surg.* 1983;18:230–4.
19. Singer R. A new technique for extirpation of preauricular cysts. *Am J Surg.* 1966;111:291–295.
20. **Currie AR, King WW, Vlantis AC, et al. Pitfalls in the management of preauricular sinuses. *Br J Surg.* 1996;83:1722–1724.**
21. LiVolsi VA, Perzin KH, Safetsky L. Carcinoma arising in ectopic thyroid tissue (including thyroglossal duct tissue). *Cancer* 1974;34:1303–1315
22. Page CP, Kemmerer WT, Hatt RC, et al. Thyroid carcinoma arising in thyroglossal ducts. *Ann Surg.* 1974;180:799–803.
23. Brown RI, Azizkhan RG. Pediatric Head and Neck lesions. *Pediatr Clin North Am.* 1998;45:889–905.
24. Guarisco JL. Congenital head and neck masses in infants and children: Part 1. *Ear Nose Throat J.* 1991;70:40–47.
25. Guarisco JL. Congenital head and neck masses in infants and children: Part I. *Ear Nose Throat J.* 70:75–82, 1991.
26. Radkowski D, Arnold J, Healy GB, et al. Thyroglossal duct remnants: Preoperative evaluation and management. *Arch Otolaryngol Head Neck Surg.* 1991;117:1378–1381.
27. Sistrunk WE. The surgical management of cysts of the thyroglossal tract. *Ann Surg.* 1920;71:121–122.
28. Hoffman MA, Schuster SR. Thyroglossal duct remnants in infants and children: Reevaluation of histopathology and methods for resection. *Ann Otol Rhinol Laryngol.* 1988;97:483–486.
29. Ein SH, Shandling B, Stephens CA, et al. Management of recurrent thyroglossal duct remnants. *J Pediatr Surg.* 1984;19:437–439.
30. Gold BC, Skeinkopf DE, Levy B. Dermoid, epidermoid, and teratomatous cysts of the tongue and floor of the mouth. *J Oral Surg.* 1974;32: 107–111.
31. Smirniotopoulos JG, Chiechi MV. Teratomas, dermoids, and epidermoids of the head and neck. *Radiographics* 1995;15:1437–1455.
32. McAvoy JM, Zuckerbraun L. Dermoid cysts of the head and neck in children. *Arch Otolaryngol.* 1976;102:529–531.
33. Waldhausen JA, Tapper D. Head and Neck Sinuses and Masses. *Ped Clin North Am.* 1998;45:889–905.
34. Huang MG, Cohen SR, Burstein FD, et al. Endoscopic pediatric plastic surgery. *Ann Plastic Surg.* 1997;38:1–8.
35. Telander RL, Filston HC. Review of head and neck lesions in infancy and childhood. *Surg Clin North Am.* 1992;72:1429–1447.
36. LaQuaglia MP. Non-Hodgkin lymphoma of the head and neck in childhood. *Semin Pediatr Surg.* 1994;3:207-215.
37. Bodenstein L, Altman RP. Cervical lymphadenitis in infants and children. *Semin Pediatr Surg.* 1994;3:134–141.
38. Zitelli BJ. Neck masses in children: adenopathy and malignant disease. *Pediatr Clin North Am.* 1981;28:813–821.
39. Altman RP, Margileth AW. Cervical lymphadenopathy from atypical mycobacteria: Diagnosis and surgical management. *J Pediatr Surg.* 1975; 10:419–422.
40. Taha AM, Davidson PT, Bailey WC. Surgical treatment of atypical mycobacterial lymphadenitis in children. *Pediatr Inf Dis J.* 1985;4:664–667.
41. Sigalet D, Lees G, Fanning A. Atypical tuberculosis in the pediatric patient: implications for the pediatric surgeon. *J Pediatr Surg.* 1992;27: 1381–1384.
42. Speck WT. Tuberculosis. In: Behrman RE, Kliegman R, Nelson W, eds. *Nelson textbook of pediatrics,* 14th ed. Philadelphia: WB Saunders, 1992.
43. **Starke JR. Management of nontuberculous mycobacterial cervical adenitis. *Pediatr Infect Dis J.* 2000;19:674–676.**
44. Jackson LA, Perkins BA, Wenger JD. Cat-scratch disease in the United States: an analysis of three national databases. *Am J Public Health.* 1993;83: 1707–11.
45. Carithers HA. Cat-scratch disease: an overview based on the study of 1,200 patients. *Am J Dis Child.* 1985;139:1124–1133.
46. Committee on Infectious diseases. Summaries of infectious diseases. In: Dickering CK, Baker CJ, Overturf GD, et al., eds. *Red book*, 26th ed. Elk Grove Village, IL: American Academy of Pediatrics, 2003, pp. 232–234.
47. Welch KJ. The salivary glands. In: Welch KJ, Randolph JG, Ravitch MM, eds. *Pediatric surgery,* 4th ed. Chicago: Year Book, 1986.
48. Mulliken JB, Young AE. *Vascular birthmarks: hemangiomas and malformations*. Philadelphia: WB Saunders, 1988.
49. Bill AH, Sumner DS. A unified concept of lymphangioma and cystic hygroma. *Surg Gynecol Obstet.* 1965;120:79–86.
50. Tanaka K, Inomata Y, Utsunomiya H, et al. Sclerosing therapy with bleomycin emulsion for lymphangioma in children. *Pediatr Surg Int.* 1990;5:270.
51. **Ogita S, Tsuto T, Deguchi E, et al. OK-432 therapy for unresectable lymphangiomas in children. *J Pediatr Surg.* 1991;26:263–270.**

CHAPTER 109 ■ PEDIATRIC CHEST

ROBERT E. CILLEY AND PETER W. DILLON

CHEST WALL DEFORMITIES

Deformities of the chest wall may be obvious at birth, but they often become more noticeable at the time of preadolescent and adolescent growth. The physical appearance may vary from barely detectable to grotesquely deforming. Although there may be some physiologic benefit from surgical correction of these deformities, restoration of a more normal appearance is equally important in the decision to operate. The impact of these deformities on normal psychosocial development and the less certain evidence of cardiorespiratory impairment constitute adequate justification for the correction of such deformities in the affected child.

Embryology, Development, and Etiology of Chest Wall Deformities

In the embryo, the ribs are derived from individual somites as mesoderm differentiates into cartilage and advances ventrally toward the developing sternum. The rib cartilage eventually approaches the sternum. The sternum itself is derived independently from two parallel bands of mesoderm that develop away from the midline. The two sternal bands fuse in a cranial to caudal direction and become progressively chondrified. Transverse divisions of the cartilaginous sternum differentiate into segments opposite each end of the rib pairs. At birth, small ossification centers are present in the sternum and the ribs have largely ossified. Final ossification is usually complete by midadolescence. The process is sufficiently predictable that sternal ossification is a reliable method of determining bone age. There is a sharp demarcation in each rib between the ossified portion and the cartilaginous portion, the latter becoming ossified only much later in life. The cause of chest wall deformities is poorly understood.[1] Explanations include abnormal intrauterine pressure applied to the chest, abnormalities of diaphragmatic development, connective tissue abnormalities, and genetic predisposition. Abnormal, excessive, or asymmetric growth of the costal cartilages associated with ribs three to ten is most implicated. Sternal clefts are understood as a failure of fusion of some portion of the sternal bands.

Pectus Excavatum

Pectus excavatum results from abnormal regulation of the growth of the costal cartilages. There is a corresponding posterior curve in the body of the sternum beginning at the manubrium and extending to the xiphoid. The deformity is rarely precisely symmetric, with one side (usually the right) slightly more curved in than the other. Asymmetry may be pronounced with the sternum rotated nearly to the sagittal plane. The deformity may be apparent at birth, but may become more apparent during growth and development, particularly during adolescence. Pectus excavatum occurs more frequently in boys than in girls. Another affected relative, most often a father or uncle, is found in one third of cases. Scoliosis is present at increased incidence in this population, but it rarely requires surgical correction. Patients often have an asthenic build and stoop-shouldered posture. Marfan syndrome predisposes to pectus excavatum. The diagnosis of Marfan syndrome may be made when patients are referred for evaluation of a chest wall deformity.

At the time of surgical consultation, concerns about the cardiopulmonary implications of the chest wall deformity are often paramount in the mind of the referring physician as well as the family. Many patients have complaints of chest pain or shortness of breath. Most patients are disturbed by the appearance of the deformity, and some may be profoundly depressed and dysfunctional. The physiologic consequences of the deformity are less certain. Invasive and echocardiographic assessment of cardiovascular performance has demonstrated improvement in cardiac function and resolution of mitral valve prolapse in some patients following surgical correction of pectus excavatum.[2–6] There is no consensus on the exact nature of the cardiopulmonary impairment caused by this common chest wall deformity.

Clinical assessment of the severity of the deformity has included chest radiographs, computerized tomography, caliper measurements, and contrast volume measurements of the cavity. The "pectus index" is defined as the ratio of the maximum internal transverse diameter of the thorax to the minimum sternovertebral distance.[7] If cardiac disease is suspected on the basis of the history and physical examination, an echocardiogram may be indicated. Pulmonary function testing is rarely helpful.

Surgical Correction of Pectus Excavatum

The timing of surgical correction for pectus excavatum has become more uniform since the mid-1990s. Infants and young children should not undergo surgical correction because of the risk of acquired thoracic dystrophy.[8,9] Most pediatric surgeons agree that the optimal timing is in late childhood and in adolescence.

Traditional Operations

Surgical correction[3,10] is performed through a transverse incision centered on the defect in the line of the inframammary crease (Fig. 109.1). The necessary incision is quite small and may be kept well within the nipple lines. An alternative that may be useful, especially in older girls, uses a small incision in each inframammary crease. Endoscopic techniques have been

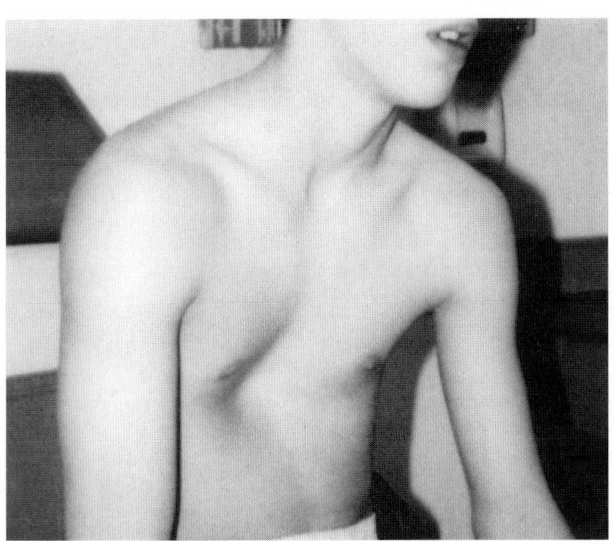

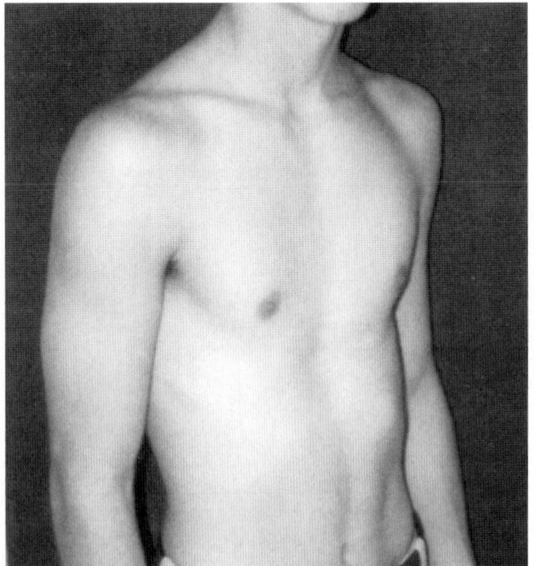

FIGURE 109.1 Pectus excavatum. (*A*) Appearance of an adolescent male with a typical depression deformity. Note "stoop-shouldered" posture. (*B*) Postoperative appearance at 6 months. Erect posture and subpectoral incision give a good cosmetic result.

reported.[11] The operation requires exposure of the costal cartilages by elevation of the pectoral muscles from the chest wall. The involved costal cartilages are excised subperiochondrially. The third through seventh cartilages are excised along with portions of the eight, ninth, or tenth cartilages if particularly prominent flaring of the costal margin is present. The xiphoid is detached from the sternum and the rectus muscles are detached inferiorly. The undersurface of the sternum is dissected free from the pericardium and pleura. An anterior osteotomy is created in the sternum just below the manubrium and the posterior cortex is fractured. Closure of the osteotomy elevates the lower sternum. Asymmetric deformities may require alternative placement of the osteotomy or more than one osteotomy to achieve a flat sternum. Some degree of overcorrection is usually performed to help maintain the correction across time. A strut is usually placed beneath or through the sternum to maintain the corrected sternal position. The choice of material and configuration for the strut is variable. Struts may be left in place permanently but are usually removed after an interval of 2 to 12 months. The pectoral and rectus muscles are reattached. Closed suction drains are used to drain the substernal, submuscular, or subcutaneous spaces. Patients are discharged when they are able to tolerate a diet and their pain is controlled by oral analgesics. Drains are removed on either an inpatient or an outpatient basis. In current practice, patients are often discharged on the second postoperative day. Multimodal pain management, including regional anesthesia, postoperative epidural analgesia, nonsteroidal antiinflammatory agents, and narcotics, is used. Complications are generally limited to wound infections and pneumothorax that rarely requires tube drainage. Recurrence rates in large series with long-term follow-up range from 5% to 15%.[3] Migration of implanted struts and bars has caused the most serious problems, including cardiac injury.

The Lorenze Bar/Nuss Procedure

This procedure has gained widespread popularity. A rigid U-shaped bar inserted transversely across the chest that pushes the deformity back into place (Fig. 109.2).[12] The procedure is best performed in late childhood and early adolescence, when the costal cartilages are more pliable. The addition of thoracoscopic guidance to the technique of bar insertion has added to the safety of the procedure. Long-term follow-up data are encouraging.[13] Complications have been reported as the procedure has become more widely practiced, including pneumothorax, cardiac injury, bar displacement, chronic pain, pericarditis, and extraosseous bone formation.[14,15] The bar is left in place for up to 2 years during a period of development when most children are active and may engage in contact sports. Activity restrictions that are necessary while the bar is in place are not well defined. This technique is an important addition to the surgical treatment of chest wall deformities. Modifications of the procedure include concurrent or metachronous insertion of second bars in severe deformities. The procedure may also be used for recurrence after traditional open procedures.

Other Techniques

Implantation of submuscular Silastic molds to alter the chest contour may result in a very acceptable appearance.[16,17]

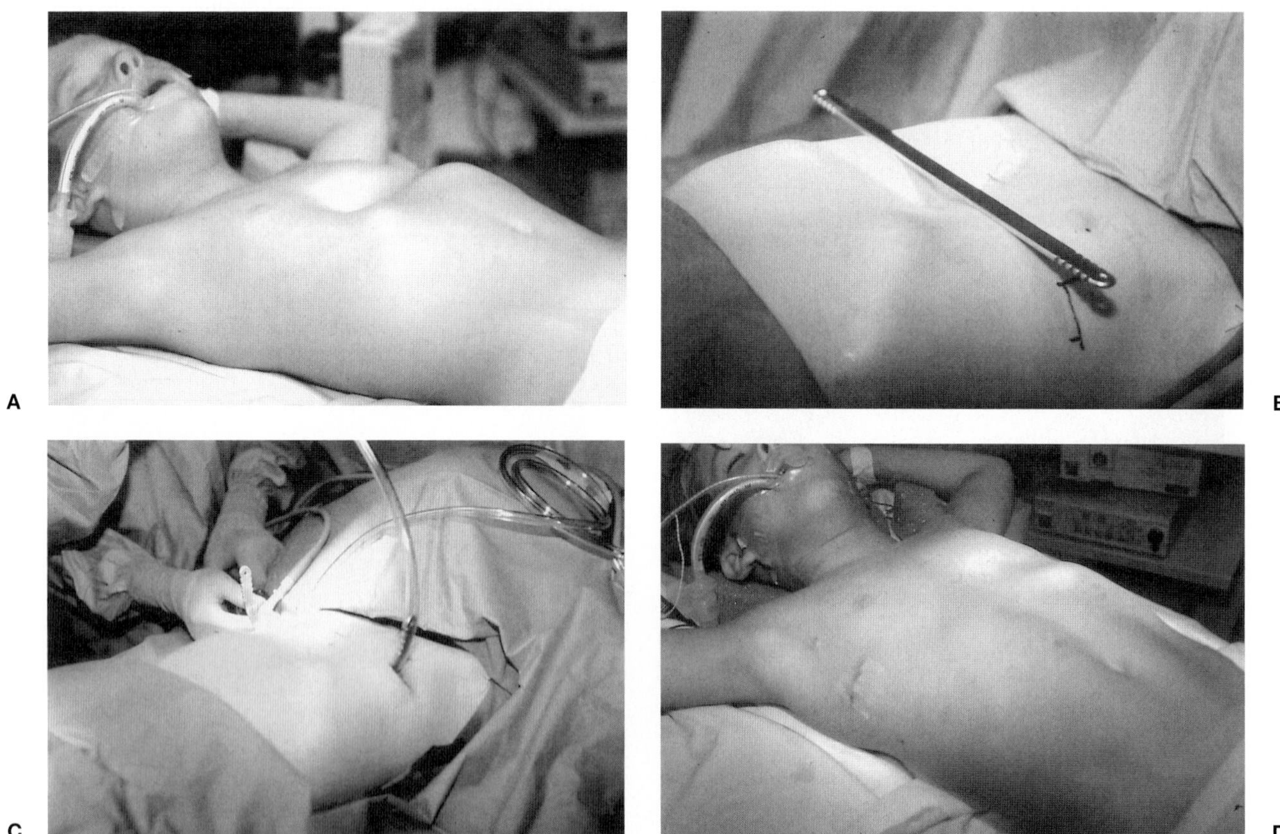

FIGURE 109.2 Thoracoscopically assisted Lorenz bar insertion (Nuss procedure). (*A*) Preoperative appearance with symmetrical depression deformity. (*B*) Lorenz bar. (*C*) Lorenz bar inserted with thoracoscopic guidance. (*D*) Immediate postoperative appearance. (Courtesy of William Hardin, M.D., University of Alabama.)

This technique does not address any of the potential physiologic problems associated with pectus excavatum and has not been used widely. Externally applied suction may also be used to treat depression deformities of the chest wall.[18]

Pectus Carinatum

The term *pectus carinatum* derives from *carina*, Latin for "keel" and also used to describe the protruding sternum of a bird; hence, "pigeon-breast." This deformity occurs less frequently than pectus excavatum and does not cause physiologic impairment. The concern for appearance may be even greater than with depression deformities of the chest wall. Protrusion deformities can be very difficult to hide even when the child is fully clothed. Rapid growth of the costal cartilages that occurs during puberty makes the deformity more pronounced at that time. The operative correction of a pectus carinatum deformity is similar to that described for pectus excavatum. The osteotomies and sternal fracture are performed in such a way as to depress the sternum. A strut is usually not required to maintain sternal position. Postoperative course and results are similar to those for pectus excavatum. In the immediate postoperative period, cardiac pulsation may be particularly visible. With healing, this finding disappears. External compression is also effective in treating protrusion deformities.[19] Success depends on prolonged application of the compression device.

Poland Syndrome

Poland described the features of this rare abnormality in 1841 in a cadaveric dissection. These features include absence of the sternal portions of the pectoralis major muscle; absence of the pectoralis minor muscle; absence of portions of the serratus anterior and external oblique muscles; forearm and hand deformities; ipsilateral hypoplasia of the nipple, breast, and chest wall subcutaneous tissues; absence or deformity of the second to fifth costal cartilages; and absence of axillary hair on the affected side. Surgical correction requires modification of the techniques used for other chest wall deformities.

Sternal Clefts

Congenital sternal clefts result from failure of midline fusion of the paired sternal bands. The cleft is usually in the superior portion of the sternum and may extend to, but not include, the xiphoid. These defects are rare and are usually repaired in the neonatal period to protect the underlying mediastinal structures. After subcutaneous mobilization, the fibrocartilaginous sternal bars are approximated in the midline. If the cleft is incomplete, it must be completed by dividing the intact portion so that closure does not lead to buckling of the inferior portion of the sternum. Cantrell pentology refers to a distal sternal cleft, omphalocele, diaphragmatic defect, pericardial defect, and intracardiac defect. *Thoracic ectopia cordis* (exstrophy of the heart) may occur as a part of this abnormality and until recently has been uniformly fatal.

Jeune Asphyxiating Thoracic Dystrophy

This rare developmental abnormality results in the failure of chest wall growth. Surgical correction involves the expansion of thoracic cavity by rib resection or the placement of expandable prosthetic ribs to promote chest enlargement.

The Slipping Rib Syndrome

This unusual abnormality has been ascribed to abnormal development of the costal cartilages along the costal margin such that the ninth or tenth rib is free floating. Particular movements that result in the involved rib crossing the costal margin may be painful. Marked disability has been described, which is relieved by excision of the involved rib and cartilage.

Flaring of the Costal Margin

Patients are sometimes referred for surgical opinions regarding unusual prominence of the costal margin. This finding is most pronounced when the patient is supine. This finding represents a variation of the normal development of the chest wall. Surgical correction should be avoided.

Costochondral Tumor

Prominence of a single costal cartilage may present as a concern of a tumor of cartilage or bone. This abnormality is usually found in preadolescents and adolescents. Patients may have undergone a diagnostic workup that included chest radiographs and computed tomography (CT) or magnetic resonance imaging (MRI) before surgical consultation. This abnormality most likely represents a minor variation of a chest wall deformity, such as a pectus carinatum. The area of enlargement is rarely tender, so that costochondritis is an unlikely explanation. Excision of the involved cartilage is rarely helpful. Plain radiographs are usually sufficient to exclude a tumor.

CONGENITAL CYSTIC DISEASE OF THE LUNG

The most common congenital cystic lesions of the lung result from abnormalities of lung embryogenesis.[20,21] These lesions include pulmonary sequestration (PS), congenital cystic adenomatoid malformation (CCAM), bronchogenic cyst (BC), and congenital lobar overinflation (CLO). The first three (PS, CCAM, and BC) are part of the spectrum of bronchopulmonary foregut malformations. The abnormality may be primarily characterized by aberrant blood supply (PS), hamartomatous lung parenchyma (CCAM), or an isolated epithelial cyst (BC). Mixed or intermediate forms that contain elements of more than one abnormality are common.[22] The coexistence of these malformations with congenital diaphragmatic hernia and congenital heart defects emphasizes that they may be part of a generalized problem with organogenesis. CLO is more likely a secondary response of the developing lung to abnormal compression or obstruction of a bronchus. The retention of fetal lung fluid during critical phases of lung development adversely affects the development of the lung.

Pulmonary Sequestration

Pulmonary sequestrations are divided into intralobar or extralobar lesions based on their relationship with the investing visceral pleura and adjacent normal lung tissue. Structurally, sequestrations represent abnormal lung tissue with anomalous systemic blood supply. They do not communicate normally with the trachea or a bronchus.

An intralobar sequestration lies within a lobe of the lung and is invested by its visceral pleura. They are most common in the posterior segment of the left lower lobe but can occur elsewhere. The anomalous arterial blood supply comes from either the thoracic or abdominal aorta and may traverse the diaphragm to supply the sequestration. Venous drainage from this aberrant tissue may be either pulmonary or systemic but is usually into the pulmonary vein. Aberrant air space connections with adjacent normal lung tissue may permit air trapping within the sequestration, causing it to be too aerated on radiographs. Though most often asymptomatic at birth, intralobar pulmonary sequestration may present during childhood as recurrent localized pneumonia because of these aberrant air space connections.

Extralobar sequestrations occur outside the pleura of the normal lung. They are most common in the lower left side of the chest but have been reported in various locations, including in the retroperitoneum below the diaphragm.[23] In this location they may be difficult to distinguish from an intraabdominal tumor, such as neuroblastoma. Rarely, extralobar sequestration is associated with congenital diaphragmatic hernias. In extralobar sequestration, both the arterial and venous blood supplies are usually systemic, and the arterial blood supply frequently arises from the aorta below the diaphragm. The lesion itself is usually a spongy consolidated mass with no aeration. Though infection is rarely present, these lesions can be associated with hemorrhage, arterial-venous shunting, or mediastinal compression. Occasionally the amount of blood shunted through the lesion is sufficient to result in symptomatic congestive heart failure. Pulmonary malignancies have occurred within these lesions. CCAM tissue may occur in sequestrations.

Radiographic evaluation of these lesions involves plane films of the chest and CT scans. Intralobar sequestrations are usually treated with thoracotomy and lobectomy (Fig. 109.3A, B). Extralobar sequestrations may be removed with minimally invasive surgical techniques (Fig. 109.3C). In dealing with both lesions, particular attention must be paid to the vascular supply.

Congenital Cystic Adenomatoid Malformations

Congenital cystic adenomatoid malformations (CCAMs) result from excessive proliferation of bronchial structures without the development of the corresponding alveoli. These malformations have a normal vascular supply and communicate with the normal tracheobronchial tree. On gross appearance they can be solid, cystic, or both. CCAMs have been classified into three types based on size, shape, spacing of the cysts, and histologic appearance.[24] Type I CCAMs are composed of cysts with large, irregular, and widely dispersed spaces larger than 2 cm in diameter or a single large cyst with small cysts surrounding it. Type II CCAMs consist of multiple cysts less than 1 cm in diameter that are closely packed together and resemble dilated bronchioles. Type III CCAMs are made up of small cysts less

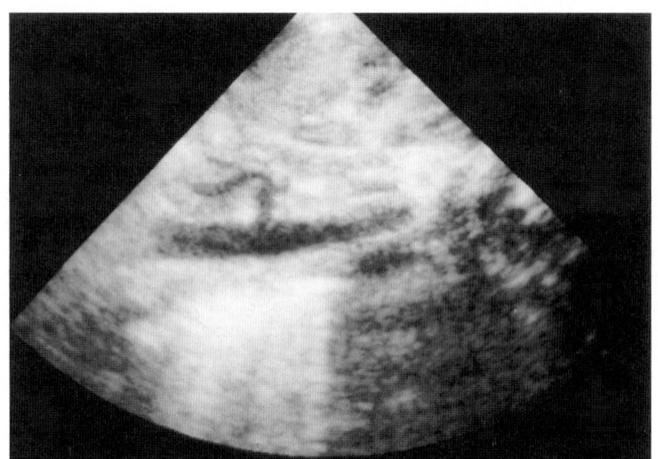

A

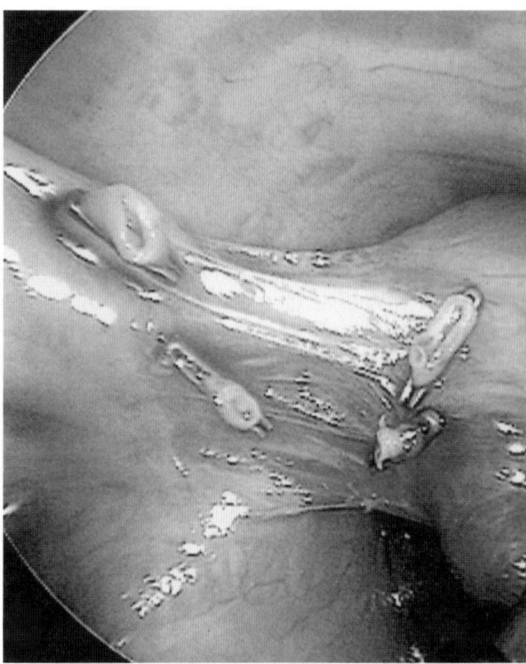

C

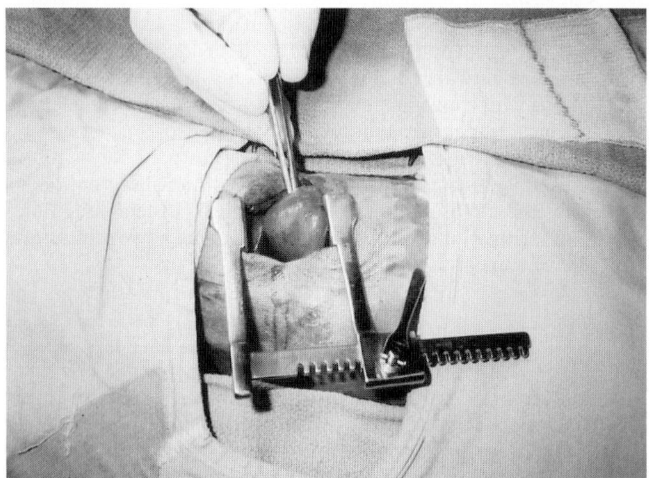

B

FIGURE 109.3 Pulmonary sequestration. (*A*) Sagittal ultrasound view of aortic branch supplying an extralobar pulmonary sequestration. (*B*) Left-sided extralobar pulmonary sequestration excised via a muscle-sparing thoracotomy. (*C*) Intraoperative view of extralobar sequestration removed thoracoscopically. Note main blood supply with clips.

than 0.5 cm in diameter, and the parenchymal tissue represents late gestational age fetal lung. Cartilage is usually lacking in all three types of CCAMs. Type I cysts account for almost 50% of cases, and Type II cysts make up an additional 40%. CCAMs usually affect only one lobe, but multilobar and bilateral involvement also occurs.

Cystic adenomatoid malformations may present as acute respiratory distress in the neonatal period. The usual radiologic appearance after birth is that of a solid mass because of retained fetal lung fluid (Fig. 109.4A). As ventilation occurs and fluid is reabsorbed, the mass appears larger and cystic and may begin to impinge on surrounding structures (Fig. 109.4B). A less common presentation is the appearance of recurrent pneumonia later in life. Prenatal diagnosis is common. The fetus may develop life-threatening hydrops. Open fetal surgical resection and thoracoamniotic shunting has resulted in survival of some of these severely affected fetuses.[25] As a result of serial prenatal ultrasounds, spontaneous *in utero* resolution has been observed to occur in as many as one third of these infants.[26] In these cases, a CT scan of the chest should be obtained after birth to document residual parenchymal abnormalities.

Infants with symptomatic lesions after birth require resection of the involved lobe. Asymptomatic lesions can be followed closely to allow for growth and development. Operation is recommended if symptoms occur. Although recommendations among pediatric surgeons differ, most recommend elective resection because of the concern about future symptoms and the possibility of malignancy (see later).[27,28] A CT scan at age 6 months confirms the diagnosis and assists in surgical planning in infants with asymptomatic lesions (Fig. 109.4C). Elective resection is then performed. When bilateral or multilobar involvement is found, CT scans may assist in planning lung-conserving resections and in follow-up of residual disease. Lung-preserving resections should be used for cystic adenomatoid malformations that involve multiple lung lobes.[29]

Bronchogenic Cysts

Bronchogenic cysts represent groups of epithelial cells from the developing trachea and lung that have become separated from the tracheobronchial tree. These cysts exist as discrete masses usually in the paratracheal region and do not incorporate pulmonary mesenchyme on which further lung development is dependent. If cells separate from the bronchopulmonary foregut structures early in development, these cysts tend to originate from the esophageal portion of the foregut. Separation that occurs later in development is from the ventral

A
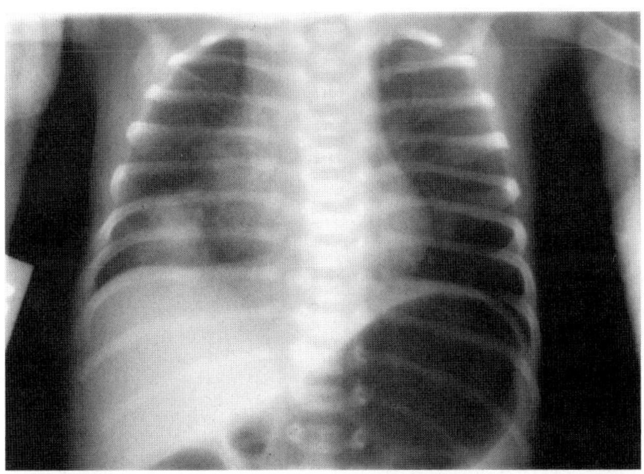

B
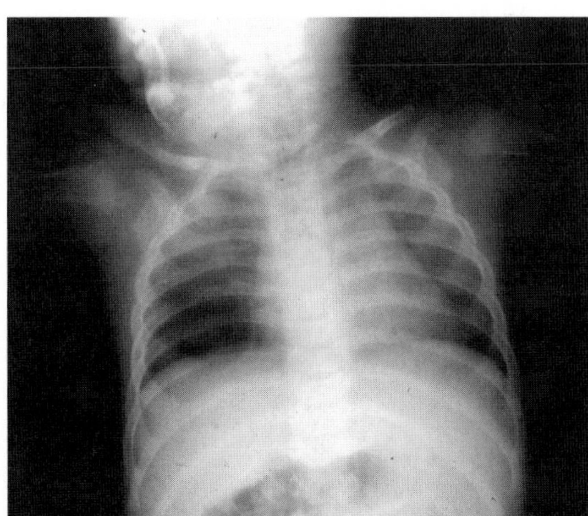

C
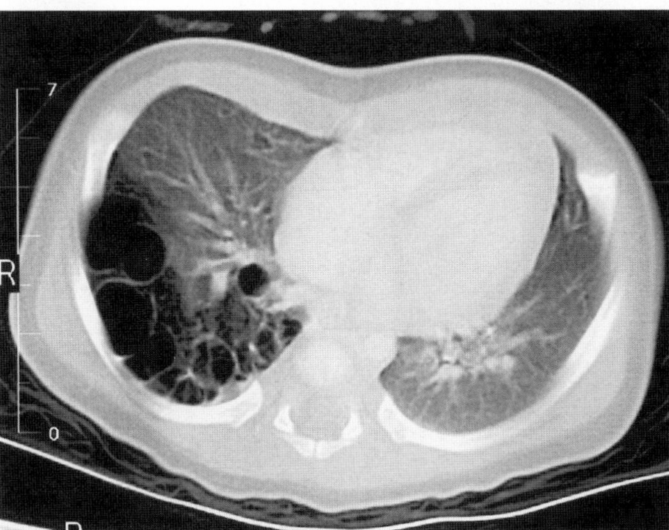

FIGURE 109.4 Congenital cystic adenomatoid malformation. (*A*) Newborn chest radiograph of a patient with prenatal diagnosis of congenital cystic adenomatoid malformation (CCAM.) Note that immediately after birth the mass is fluid filled and appears as a density in the right hemithorax. (*B*) Chest radiograph of the same child at 5 months of age prior to surgical excision. Note air-filled cystic appearance of CCAM. (*C*) Transverse thoracic computed tomographic view of CCAM.

or tracheal portion of the foregut, resulting in bronchogenic cysts. Bronchogenic cysts are usually extrapulmonary masses that do not communicate with the normal tracheobronchial tree. They do not have a unique blood supply. Resection of these lesions with either a thoracotomy or video-assisted thoracoscopy is recommended because of the risk of bleeding, infection, or enlargement with compression of adjacent mediastinal structures (Fig. 109.5).[30,31]

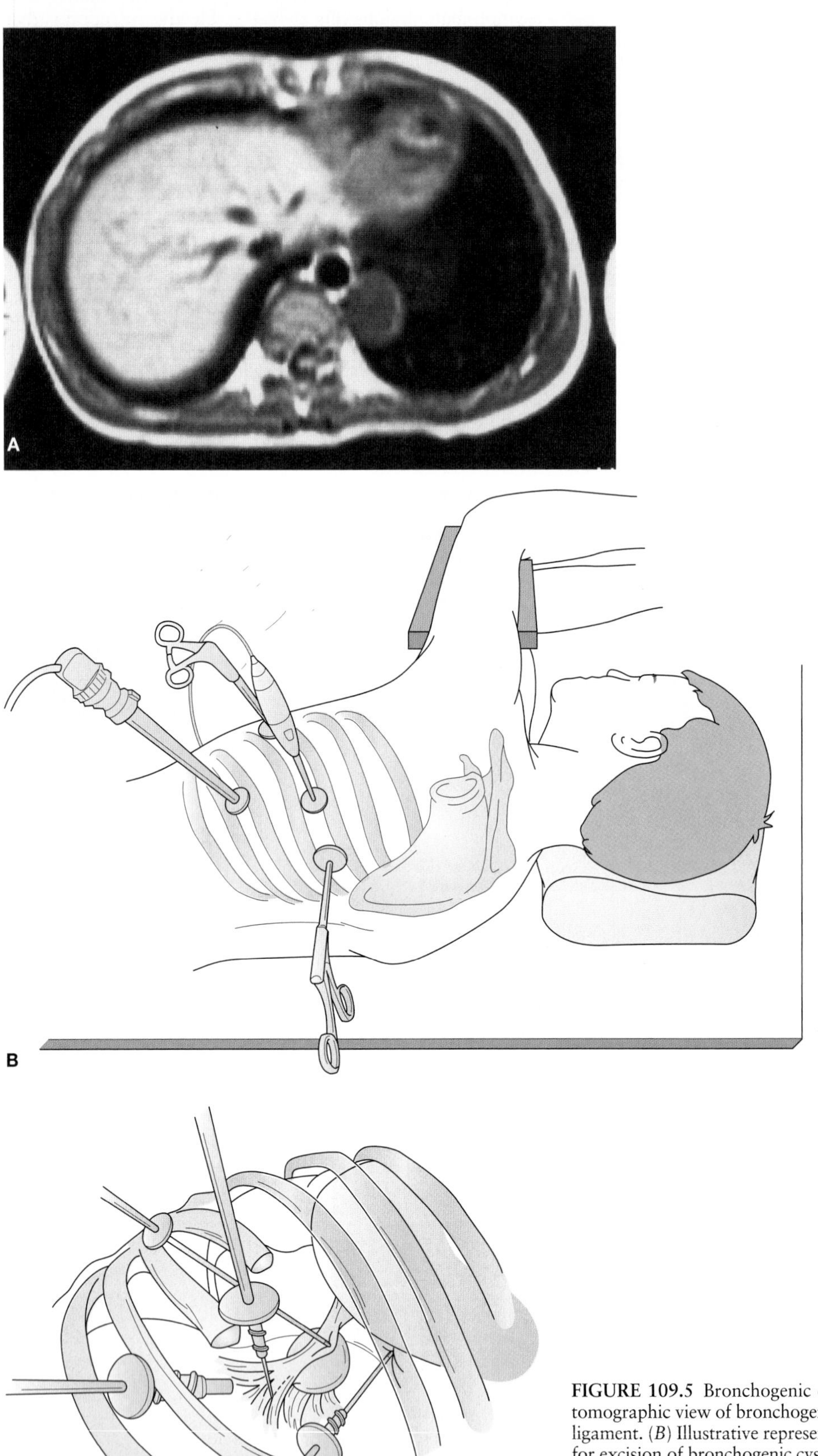

FIGURE 109.5 Bronchogenic cyst. (*A*) Transverse thoracic computed tomographic view of bronchogenic cyst located in the inferior pulmonary ligament. (*B*) Illustrative representation of thoracoscopic instrumentation for excision of bronchogenic cyst. (C) Operative detail. (After Dillon PW, Cilley RE, Krummel TM. Video assisted thoracoscopic excision of intrathoracic masses in children: report of two cases. *Surg Laparosc Endosc.* 1993;3:433436.)

Congenital Lobar Overinflation

Congenital lobar overinflation (previously referred to as congenital lobar emphysema) is caused by abnormal development or compression of a lobar bronchus resulting in retention of fluid during fetal lung development and subsequent air-trapping and overinflation after birth. The lung tissue is intrinsically normal but has been secondarily altered by the trapping of fluid and gas. The vascular supply is normal. The condition can result from a deficiency of bronchial cartilage that leads to focal airway collapse and bronchial obstruction. Congenital lobar overinflation can also result from extraluminal bronchial compression from a bronchogenic cyst, an enteric duplication cyst, lymphadenopathy, a mediastinal tumor, a vascular abnormality, or congenital heart disease.[32] In more than half the cases, no obstruction is identified. Usually the upper lobe of either lung field is involved, but multilobar involvement has been reported. Lobar overinflation presents as worsening respiratory distress caused by progressive emphysematous enlargement of the involved lobe with compression of normal adjacent tissue and mediastinal shift (Fig. 109.6A). Infants with symptomatic congenital lobar overinflation require complete resection of the affected lobe. In selected circumstances, bronchoplasty, bronchial suspension, or relief of an extrinsic bronchial obstruction may be useful. Great care must be taken at the time of anesthetic induction in these infants, because the institution of positive pressure ventilation may exacerbate the lobar overinflation. Immediate thoracotomy may be necessary to relieve the compression of the mediastinum and prevent cardiopulmonary collapse (Fig. 109.6B). Up to half of the cases identified will resolve during infancy with observation alone as the lung develops.[33–35] Surgery is reserved for symptomatic patients.

Diagnosis

With the routine use of prenatal ultrasound, many cystic lesions of the lung are now detected and followed prior to birth.[25,36] Many of these lesions are completely asymptomatic in the postnatal period. Standard chest radiographs remain the cornerstones of diagnosis and follow-up for these lesions. Rapid thoracic CT scanning provides definitive mapping of these lesions with IV contrast. When properly performed, such dynamic images show the aberrant systemic arterial supply when dealing with a pulmonary sequestration. Contrast esophagrams are indicated for children with dysphagia and serve to outline the possibility of an abnormal communication with the gastrointestinal tract. If aberrant vascular supply is suspected but not demonstrated on a CT scan, then MRI angiography of the chest can be obtained.

Treatment

Asymptomatic pulmonary cysts should be removed because of the possibility of infection. Additionally, it has been proposed that these cysts be removed because of the rare association of malignant pulmonary neoplasms in these congenital cysts. Any cyst that is enlarging on serial chest radiographs should be resected because of the respiratory compromise that may ensue and the possibility of infection either in the cyst or in the surrounding lung tissue. The only reason for following a lesion over the long term is when serial CT scans demonstrate progressive resolution, indicating the possibility of an acquired infectious cyst that has the potential for resolution.

Cysts of the Mediastinum

Benign cysts of the mediastinum are relatively common in pediatric patients. Although most of them are completely asymptomatic and are discovered incidentally, surgical resection is usually recommended because of the possibility of progressive enlargement with compression, hemorrhage, or infection. When symptoms do develop, they may include chest pain, cough, stridor, hemoptysis, or dysphasia. The common cystic lesions include thymic cysts, enterogenous cysts, dermoid cysts, pericardial cysts, and lymphatic malformations (cystic hygromas).

Thymic Cysts

Thymic cysts are usually asymptomatic and generally have both mediastinal and cervical components being located in the superior aspect of the mediastinum. These are benign lesions composed of ciliated epithelium with lymphocytes and cholesterol crystals imbedded in the cyst wall. Clinical problems are

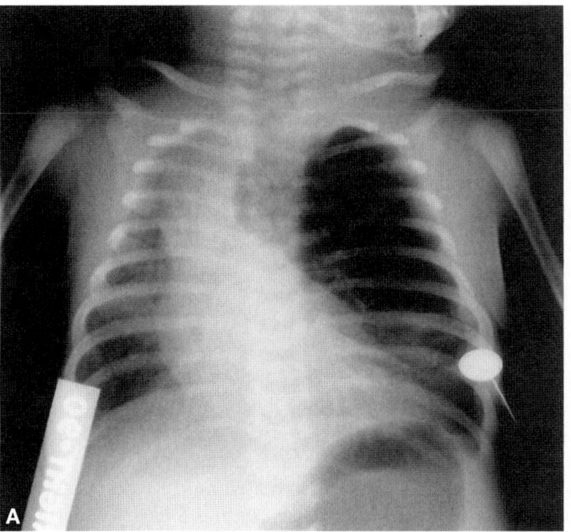

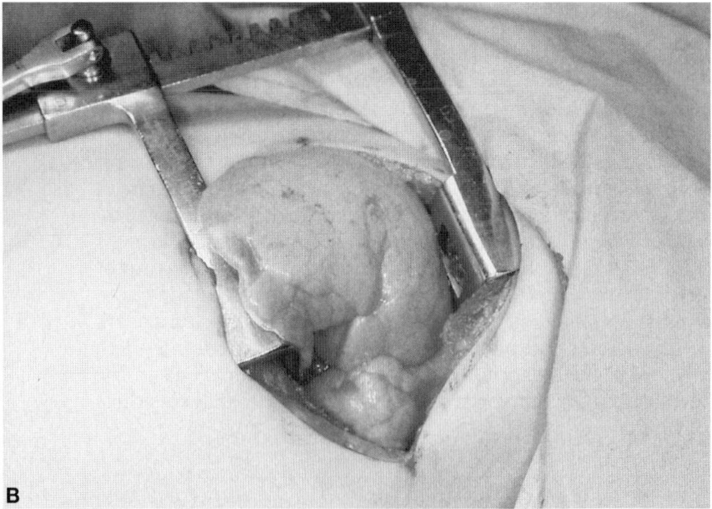

FIGURE 109.6 Congenital lobar overinflation. (*A*) Chest radiograph demonstrating overinflation of left upper lobe in an infant. Note mediastinal shift. (*B*) Operative photograph demonstrating overexpanded left upper lobe decompressing through the incision.

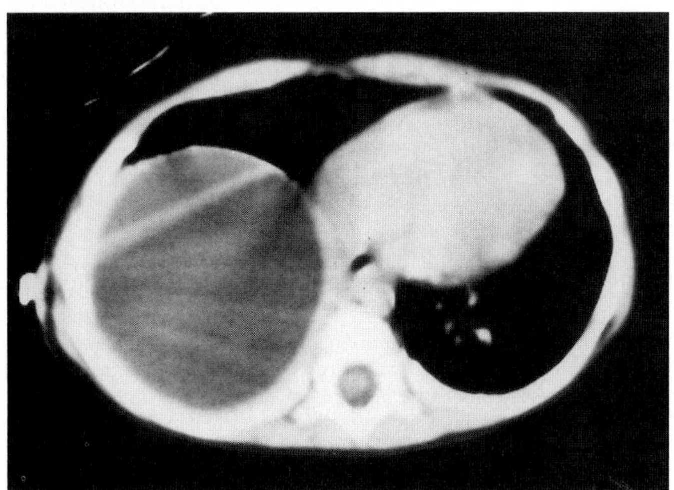
A

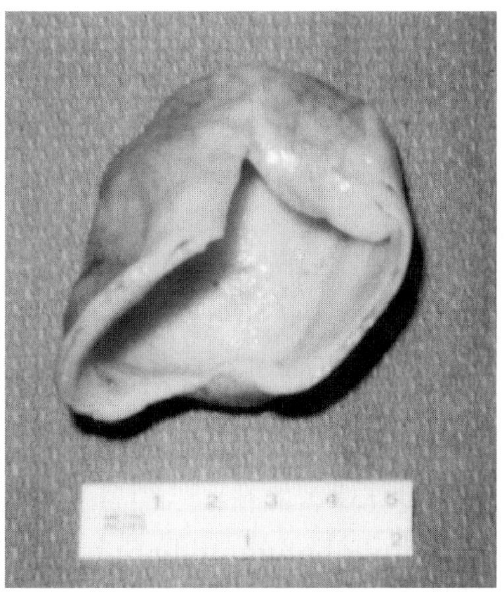
B

FIGURE 109.7 Enterogenous cyst. This represents another abnormality in the spectrum of bronchopulmonary foregut malformations. (*A*) Computed tomography scan demonstrating a large mass occupying the right hemithorax. (*B*) Surgical specimen.

usually the result of rapid expansion from either hemorrhage or infection.

Enteric Duplication Cysts/Enterogenous Cysts

Enteric duplication cysts usually occur in the posterior mediastinum and are composed of esophageal or gastric epithelium surrounded by smooth muscle (Fig. 109.7). They are part of the spectrum of bronchopulmonary foregut malformations that include bronchogenic cysts (see earlier), and esophageal duplications (addressed later). They may exist completely separately from the structure of origin, or they may communicate with the gastrointestinal tract above or below the diaphragm. In rare instances they may attach to or communicate with the spinal canal. A number of large thoracoabdominal enteric cysts have been reported. These cysts may penetrate the diaphragm and end blindly in the peritoneal cavity or communicate with the gastrointestinal tract. When gastric mucosa is present within the cyst, peptic ulceration with erosion and bleeding has been reported. Therefore, removal of these cysts is recommended to avoid these possible complications.

Lymphatic Malformations

Lymphatic malformations in the head, neck, and mediastinal region have been classically referred to as cystic hygromas. They are multilocular, thin-walled cysts derived from primitive, aberrant lymphatic sacs. Their mediastinal involvement can be extensive, because they insinuate around the great vessels and nervous structures of the superior mediastinum. As with other cystic structures, these lesions are usually asymptomatic. However, with enlargement, hemorrhage, or infection, symptoms may develop with life-threatening potential. Surgical resection of these lesions is usually recommended, without sacrificing important anatomic structures within the mediastinum. Recurrence develops in approximately one third of cases.

Pericardial Cysts

Pericardial cysts are almost always asymptomatic lesions discovered as incidental findings on chest radiographs. They appear in the cardiophrenic sulcus as small, discrete masses. They are thin-walled cysts containing clear fluid and lined by mesothelium. Resection can be performed with either an open thoracotomy or video-assisted thoracoscopy.

THORACIC TUMORS IN CHILDREN

Thoracic tumors in children are rare. Neoplasms originate from the chest wall, the mediastinum, and the lung. Lung metastases from extrathoracic cancers are more common than primary neoplasms. Surgical treatment may involve removal of the primary tumor, resection of adjacent structures, chest wall reconstruction, lung resection (including wedge resection, lobectomy, pneumonectomy), and tracheobronchial resection and reconstruction. The role of minimally invasive surgery and thoracoscopic surgery is increasing in both the diagnosis and treatment of thoracic tumors in children.[37]

Metastatic Lung Tumors

For surgical excision of metastatic lung tumors to be beneficial, the primary tumor must be eradicated and the patient should be free of other metastatic disease. Osteogenic sarcoma, other soft tissue sarcomas, and Wilms tumor are the tumors with lung metastases that are most often considered for surgical treatment.[38,39]

Osteogenic Sarcoma

Although the reported experience in the treatment of metastatic osteogenic sarcoma to the lung is based on retrospective review, there is good evidence that resection of lung metastases is beneficial. The success of surgical removal of metastatic lung disease depends on effective chemotherapy to eliminate other micrometastatic disease. The metastases are calcified and palpable, which facilitates their surgical removal. Fewer than four nodules, complete resection of all disease, and lack of penetration through the parietal pleura favor survival. Treatment failures and late recurrence are common, mandating careful follow-up. Available data support aggressive attempts at surgical resection, including the removal of many metastatic nodules and multiple resections.

Soft Tissue Sarcoma

Chemotherapy- and radiation-resistant tumors (e.g., liposarcoma, leiomyosarcoma, synovial sarcoma, fibrosarcoma, neurogenic sarcoma, epithelioid sarcoma, alveolar soft parts sarcoma) may benefit from resection when the primary tumor has been controlled.[39] Rhabdomyosarcoma and Ewing sarcoma are chemosensitive and radiation sensitive. Lung excision for metastatic disease is generally not helpful. Surgery may aid in diagnosis and may be beneficial in removing a large focus of residual disease.

Wilms Tumor

There is little advantage to excision of lung metastases in Wilms tumor. Chemotherapy is required for treatment, and surgical removal offers no added benefit. The role of whole-lung radiation (previously used for lung metastases) will be evaluated in the next phase of the National Wilms Tumor Study under the auspices of the Children's Oncology Group. Some special cases may benefit from surgery, including very young patients (in whom radiation therapy causes the most lung injury) with few or solitary lesions. Surgery may also be necessary for diagnostic purposes and to determine the effects of therapy.

Primary Lung Tumors

Reviews by Hartman and Shochat in 1983 and Hancock et al. in 1993 have catalogued fewer than 500 reported primary lung neoplasms in children (Table 109.1).[40,41]

TABLE 109.1 CLASSIFICATION

PRIMARY PULMONARY NEOPLASMS IN CHILDREN

Type of tumor	No. (%)
Benign	92
Inflammatory	48 (52.2)
Hamartoma	22 (23.9)
Neurogenic tumor	9 (9.8)
Leiomyoma	6 (6.5)
Mucous gland adenoma	3 (3.3)
Myoblastoma	3 (3.3)
Benign teratoma	1 (1.1)
Malignant	291
Bronchial adenoma	118 (40.5)
Bronchogenic	49 (16.8)
Pulmonary blastoma	45 (15.5)
Fibrosarcoma	28 (9.6)
Rhabdomyosarcoma	17 (5.8)
Leiomyosarcoma	11 (3.8)
Sarcoma	6 (2.1)
Hemangiopericytoma	4 (1.4)
Plasmacytoma	4 (1.4)
Lymphoma	3 (1.0)
Teratoma	3 (1.0)
Mesenchymoma	2 (0.7)
Myxosarcoma	1 (0.3)

(Modified from Hancock BJ, DiLorenzo M, Youssef S, et al. Childhood primary pulmonary neoplasms. *J Pediatr Surg.* 1993;28:1133–1136.)

Bronchial Adenomas

These are the most common primary lung tumors in children. Despite the name they carry, these tumors represent true malignancies. They are better described as low-grade adenocarcinomas of the lung. The incidence of metastasis is low. Histologically, there are three types: carcinoid (85%), mucoepidermoid (10%), and adenoid cystic carcinoma (5%). Bronchial adenomas most commonly arise in primary and secondary bronchi. Presenting symptoms include cough, hemoptysis, airway obstruction, pneumonia, atelectasis, and reactive airway disease. The chest radiographs may show air-trapping or pneumonia and atelectasis. The clinical presentation may be most suspicious for an airway foreign body. CT scan may demonstrate the lesion. Bronchoscopy is required for diagnosis. Biopsy must be done with great care and with some peril because life-threatening bleeding may result from biopsy attempts. Surgical resection with clean intraoperative margins is the treatment of choice. It may involve lobectomy, bilobectomy, pneumonectomy, or sleeve resection, as well as regional lymphadenectomy. Bronchial carcinoids are radiosensitive if residual disease remains.

Bronchogenic Carcinomas

These lesions are uncommon in children and are highly lethal, with a mortality rate of 90%. Unlike in adults, squamous cell carcinoma is rare; undifferentiated cancers and adenocarcinoma predominate. Disease is usually widespread at the time of diagnosis, compromising survival. Rarely, with early discovery and localized disease, cure is possible. Bronchoalveolar carcinoma is a rare lung tumor in children that caries a good prognosis with surgical resection.[42] This tumor is particularly associated with development in congenital cystic lung lesions.[43]

Pulmonary Blastoma

This is a malignant lung tumor that occurs most often in adults but occasionally in children. It comprises cells that histologically resemble fetal lung. They are usually peripherally located in the lung, and patients present with cough, chest pain, and hemoptysis. They are treated by lobectomy, with half of patients being long-term survivors.

Other malignant tumors

Sarcomas, including fibrosarcoma, rhabdomyosarcoma, and leiomyosarcoma, are the next most common primary malignant lung neoplasms found in children. They arise endobronchially as well as peripherally. It is also of note that 9% of all reported malignant lung neoplasms in children were associated with previously documented cystic lung disease.[41]

Inflammatory Pseudotumor

This is the most common benign lung tumor in children. Variable nomenclature relates to the description of the inflammatory cells involved. The terms *plasma cell granuloma, histiocytoma, xanthofibroma, fibroxanthoma,* and *inflammatory myofibroblastic tumor* have been used to describe these tumors. They may present as peripheral lesions or as obstructing endobronchial masses. Symptoms include cough, chest pain, hemoptysis, fever, and airway obstruction (Fig. 109.8). Although there may be some tendency for spontaneous resolution, aggressive local invasion and recurrence are often seen. It may be more accurate to describe these lesions as low-grade malignancies.[44] Complete surgical resection is usually preferred. Unresectable tumors may respond to nonsteroidal anti-inflammatory agents[45] even if extensive in nature should be undertaken because no adjuvant therapies have proved efficacy.

Hamartoma

Hamartomatous lung nodules are usually discovered in adults, but may be large enough or calcified to be discovered on chest

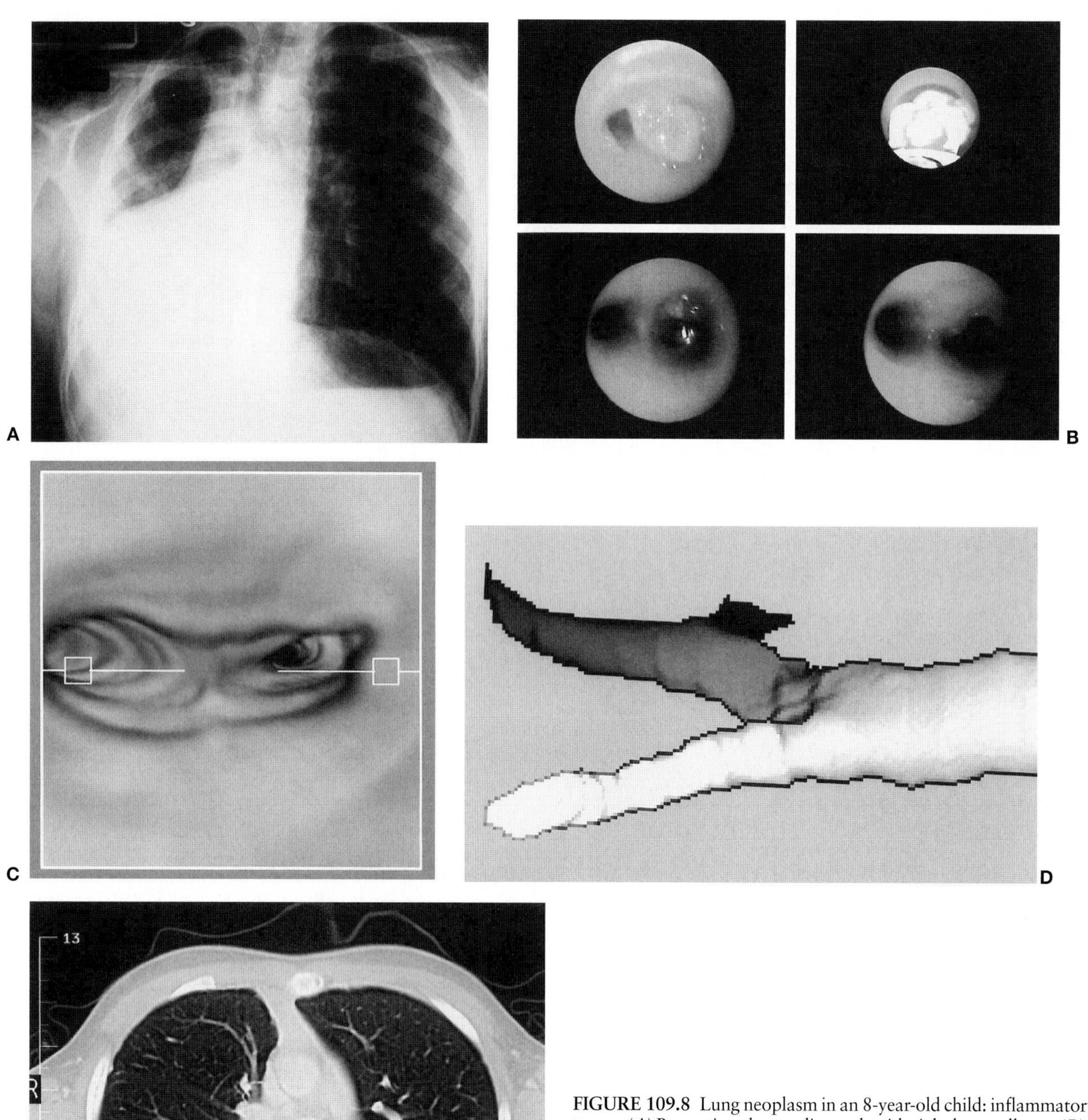

FIGURE 109.8 Lung neoplasm in an 8-year-old child: inflammatory pseudotumor. (*A*) Presenting chest radiograph with right lung collapse. (*B*) Biopsy of obstructing endobronchial mass demonstrates inflammatory pseudotumor (inflammatory myofibroblastic tumor). (*C*) Computed tomographic (CT) virtual bronchoscopy image after initial biopsy demonstrates deformation of the right main stem bronchus and carina resulting from tumor infiltration. (*D*) CT reconstruction of external appearance of airways demonstrating the deformation of the carina and right main stem bronchus. The child underwent excision of the right main stem bronchus and carina and tracheobronchial reconstruction. (*E*) Postoperative transverse thoracic CT image at the level of the reconstruction of the carina.

radiographs in children.[46] These tumors may be endobronchial and result in airway obstruction, or more commonly, peripheral and asymptomatic unless very large. Conservative pulmonary resection is the best treatment, but large lesions may require lobectomy or even pneumonectomy.

Mediastinal Tumors

Mediastinal tumors in children may be benign or malignant. Certain tumors have a predilection for arising from the anterior, middle, or posterior mediastinum.[47]

Neurogenic Tumors

These are the most common thoracic tumors in the pediatric population (Fig. 109.9). The tumors originate in the posterior mediastinum, often from elements of the sympathetic chain. They may grow very large before detection and may be found incidentally. Symptoms of Horner syndrome or tracheal displacement may be apparent. Intraspinal extension occasionally results in symptoms of spinal cord compression. They may be malignant (neuroblastoma, ganglioneuroblastoma) or benign (ganglioneuroma). Neuroblastoma originating in the mediastinum has a better prognosis than in other sites. The tumors

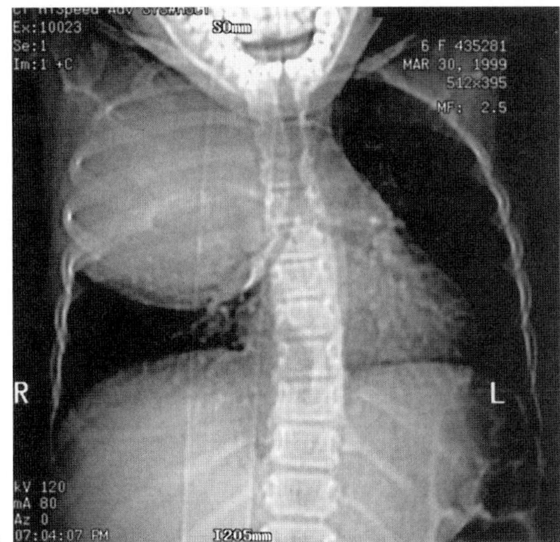

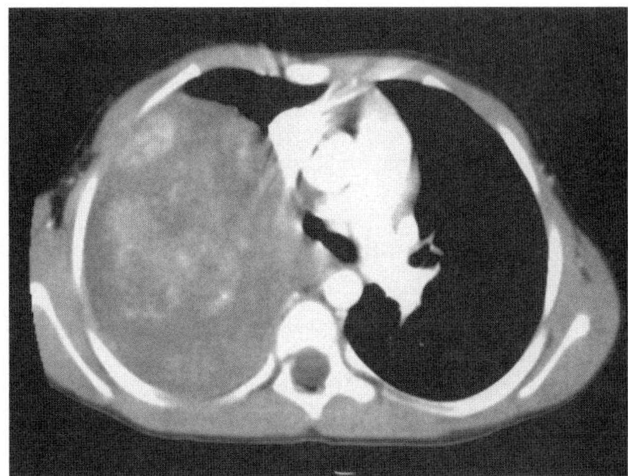

FIGURE 109.9 (*A*) Large neural tumor (ganglioneuroma arising from right sympathetic chain). (*B*) Calcification is apparent on computed tomography scan.

are lower stage and often have more favorable biologic activity. CT and MRI scanning provide anatomic definition of the mass and assess intraspinal extension. Widening of the intercostal spaces and enlargement of the spinal foramina at the level of origin of the tumor are often seen. All require removal for diagnosis. Large tumors are removed using a traditional muscle-sparing incision. Smaller tumors are removed thoracoscopically.

Neurofibromas

Neurofibromas arise from nerves in the posterior mediastinum, such as the intercostal nerves, the phrenic nerve, the vagus nerve, or the sympathetic chain. They may occur as isolated tumors or in association with neurofibromatosis. Scoliosis is particularly common in patients with thoracic neurofibromas. Isolated tumors are readily removed, but tumors associated with neurofibromatosis tend to extend along nerve sheaths so as to preclude complete removal. Recurrence is to be expected in neurofibromatosis, and malignant degeneration can occur in large tumors, mandating periodic monitoring.

Hodgkin and Non-Hodgkin Lymphomas

These may present as an anterior or middle mediastinal mass. Surgical removal is not required, but the pediatric surgeon often participates in the diagnostic workup.[48] Tissue sampling from cervical lymph nodes, mediastinoscopy, thoracoscopy, or open biopsy may be needed for diagnosis. Special anesthetic risks, including difficulty with ventilation and loss of airway, exist in the case of bulky central tumors that compress the large airways.

Teratomas

Teratomas arise in the anterior mediastinum and may contain elements of all three embryonic germ layers. The lesions are either solid or cystic. The most common form of a cystic teratoma, known as a dermoid cyst, consists of mature ectodermal elements. This lesion is characterized by a thick-walled fibrous sac with squamous epithelium in which various skin appendages, including hair and teeth, that can be found. Occasionally they are found within the pericardium. The tumors may be large (Fig. 109.10). Surgical removal of these

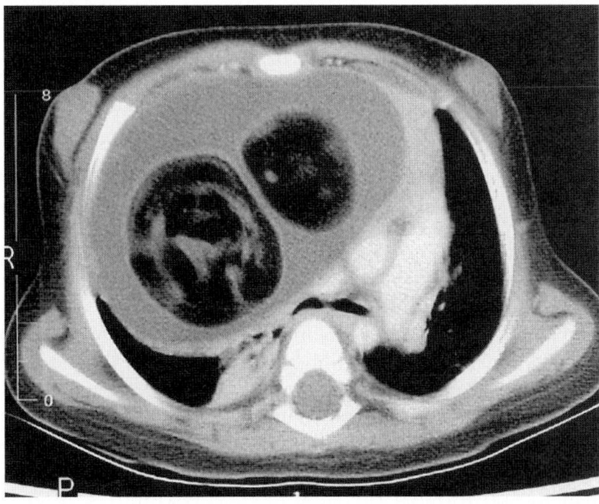

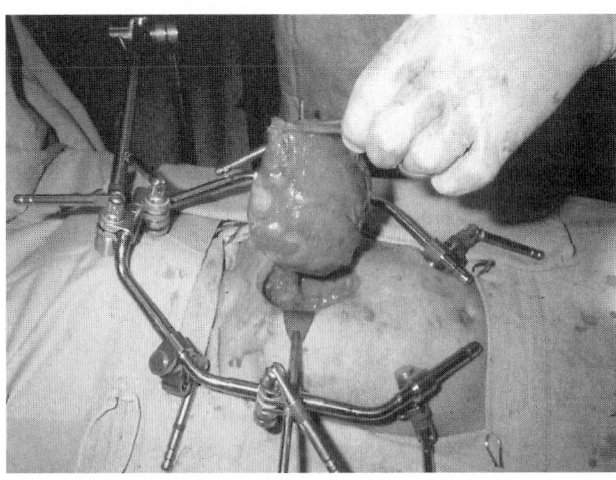

FIGURE 109.10 Mediastinal teratoma. (*A*) Transverse thoracic computed tomography scan of a large anterior mediastinal teratoma presenting with airway compression symptoms in a 9-month-old female. (*B*) Tumor removal via a median sternotomy.

cysts is indicated because of the risk of infection, erosion into the pleura or pericardium, and local compression. The rare occurrence of malignant components within the tumor mandates their removal.

Other neoplasms of the mediastinum are very rare in children but often require surgical biopsy or extirpation. These include neurilemmoma, pheochromocytoma, primitive neuroectodermal tumors, germ cell tumors, mesenchymal tumors including rhabdomyosarcoma, and thymic tumors.

Chest Wall Tumors

Ewing sarcoma, chondrosarcoma, and liposarcoma are malignant tumors that may originate from the chest wall. Local control of disease may require extensive chest wall excision and prosthetic reconstruction. Primitive neuroectodermal tumors are malignant small-cell tumors that carry a poor prognosis and may involve the chest wall and surrounding tissues and. Multimodal therapy with surgery, chemotherapy, and radiation may be of benefit.[49,50]

Respiratory Papillomatosis

Recurrent respiratory papillomatosis is a viral-induced disorder caused by the same human papilloma viruses that causes genital condylomata.[51] It is likely transmitted at birth, and there may be some protective prophylactic benefit from cesarean section in selected high-risk expectant mothers. Airway-obstructing papillomas develop in the first several years of life and are treated with laser ablation. Often many sessions are required to clear the airways. Children who develop symptoms before age 3 years are more likely to have severe disease.[52]

ESOPHAGEAL ATRESIA/TRACHEOESOPHAGEAL FISTUAL

Developmental disorders of the esophagus have been recognized and described in postmortem examination since the seventeenth century. Harald Hirschsprung, the Danish pediatrician remembered for the disease that carries his name, also described the most common form of esophageal atresia in 1861. Initial attempts at both corrective and palliative surgery in the early part of the twentieth century were unsuccessful. Surgeons understood the anatomy and physiology of the disorder and continued attempts at surgical correction, resulting in successful palliation and ultimately in successful primary repair of the defect. On March 15, 1941, Dr. Cameron Haight performed the first successful primary repair of esophageal atresia at the University of Michigan.[53] Refinements in surgical technique and postoperative care have resulted in a steady improvement in survival for such patients over the ensuing 5 decades.[54] In the modern era, survival is determined almost exclusively by the presence of associated anomalies, and not by the esophageal abnormality itself.

Embryology

Development of the human respiratory tract begins as primitive epithelial cells branch off the ventral foregut of the embryo into the surrounding mesenchyme at the beginning of the fourth week of gestation. Ongoing processes involve both elongation and separation of the foregut (esophagus) and the airway (trachea). By the end of the fourth week of gestation, the esophagus and trachea have completely separated to the level of the larynx. This developmental program is under the control of master regulatory genes that are turned on and off in an orderly fashion. Interruption of this developmental process during the fourth week of gestation probably results in the various forms of esophageal atresia with or without tracheoesophageal fistula. By the end of the sixth week of gestation, the circular muscular coat of the esophagus develops, followed by vagal innervation. The segmental blood supply from the aorta appears by the seventh week and the muscular coat has differentiated into two layers by the ninth week. The malformation can be recapitulated in an animal model by the administration of doxorubicin at specific times and doses to pregnant rats during organogenesis.[55,56]

Classification

Descriptive terminology is used to indicate the anatomic configuration of a patient with esophageal atresia (Fig. 109.11). Esophageal atresia with proximal pouch and distal tracheoesophageal fistula is by far the most common type encountered by the pediatric surgeon, accounting for 85% to 95% of all cases. Esophageal atresia without fistula (pure atresia) occurs in 5% to 7% of patients. Tracheoesophageal fistula without esophageal atresia (so-called H-type or N-type fistula) occurs in 2% to 6% of patients. The rarer forms of this anomaly include esophageal atresia with proximal tracheoesophageal fistula and esophageal atresia with both proximal and distal tracheoesophageal fistula. The frequency of these rare forms is less than 1% in most reports. Alphabetical and numeric classification schemes, devised by Haight, Gross, and Kluth, are of historical interest.[57–59] The most common variety (proximal pouch, distal fistula) is still commonly referred to as Gross type C.

Incidence and Epidemiology

The incidence of esophageal atresia varies among populations and races in the range of 1 in 2,500 to 1 in 20,000 births. The overall incidence is about 1 in 5,000. There is a slight male preponderance of 1.26:1. First pregnancy, advanced maternal age, hormonal exposure in pregnancy, an affected parent, and affected siblings are risk factors. Chromosomal abnormalities, twinning, and associated anomalies are more common than expected.

Clinical Findings, Diagnosis, and Pathophysiology

The diagnosis of esophageal atresia may be suspected by the finding of maternal polyhydramnios. Specific ultrasonic identification of the blind-ending upper pouch may be diagnostic, but many patients go undiagnosed until after birth. Most infants are asymptomatic in the first hours of life. Excessive drooling may be noted. Choking, coughing, and regurgitation may be present and worsened by attempts at feeding. Respiratory distress and cyanosis caused by aspiration may occur. Occasionally, in the breastfed infant, the diagnosis may be unrecognized for more than a day because the volume of feeding associated with colostrum ingestion prior to milk flow may be very low. The inability to pass a nasogastric or orogastric tube is confirmatory of the diagnosis. Radiographs confirm the position of the tube in the proximal blind-ending pouch. Injection of air during the radiograph outlines the pouch. The child with esophageal atresia and a tracheoesophageal fistula will have a full abdomen and gas visible

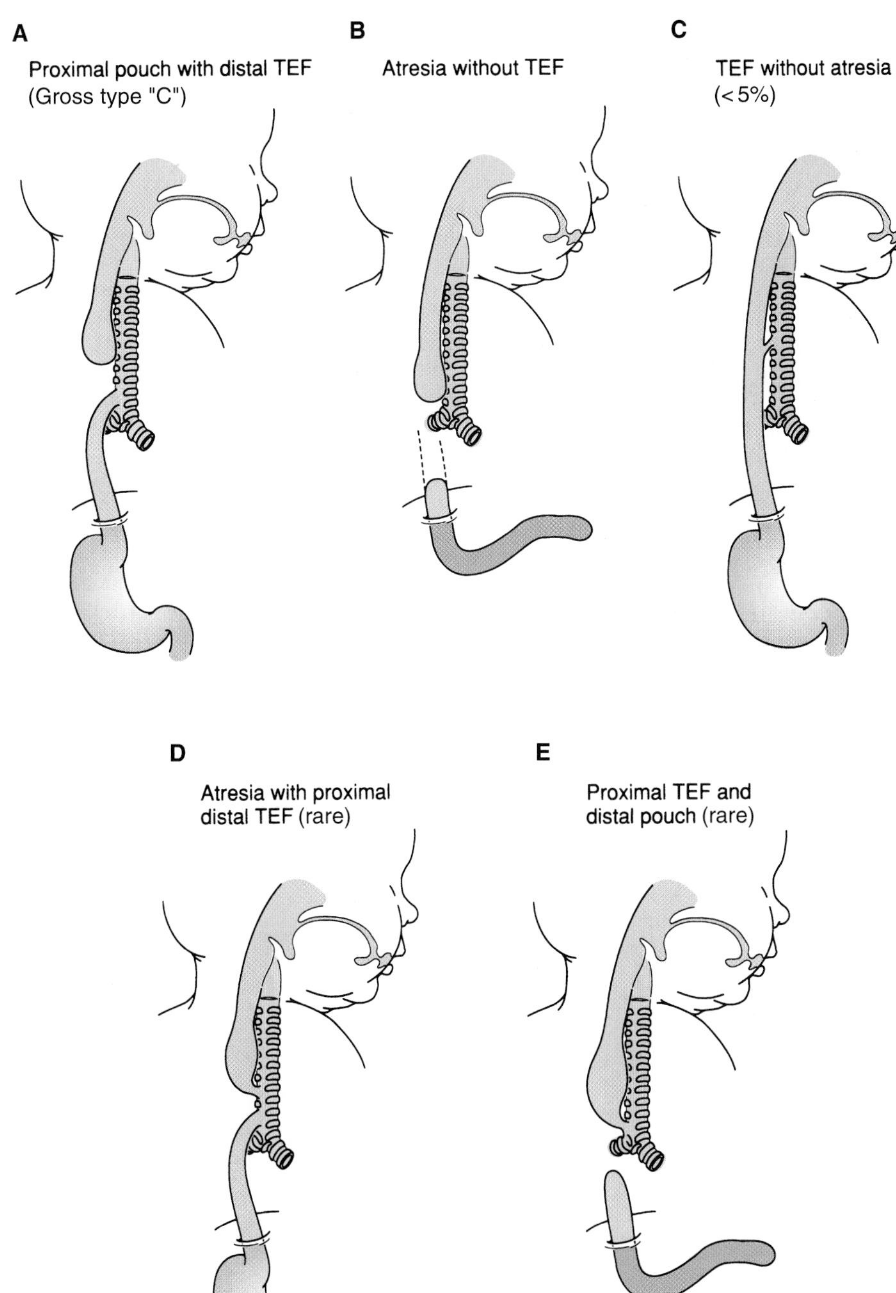

FIGURE 109.11 The anatomy of the variants of esophageal atresia (EA) and tracheoesophageal fistula (TEF). (*A*) Proximal pouch with distal TEF (most common type, occurring in 85% of patients; Gross type C). (*B*) Esophageal atresia without TEF (5%). (C) TEF without esophageal atresia (<5%). (*D*) Esophageal atresia with proximal and distal TEF (rare). (*E*) Proximal TEF and distal pouch (rare). (After Manning PB, Morgan RA, Coran AG, et al. Fifty years experience with esophageal atresia and tracheoesophageal fistula. *Ann Surg.* 1988; 204:446.)

throughout the bowel on the abdominal radiograph. A scaphoid abdomen and gasless radiograph indicate pure esophageal atresia with no fistula. Isolated tracheoesophageal fistula without esophageal atresia does not result in esophageal obstruction and therefore is diagnosed later in infancy or childhood as a result of respiratory symptoms such as aspiration pneumonia and choking with feeds. Exact delineation of the anatomy may require endoscopic evaluation at the time of surgical correction (Fig. 109.12). If a distal fistula is present, gastroesophageal reflux into the respiratory tract will result in chemical pneumonitis. This may be made worse by air distention of the stomach through the fistula. This is less of a problem if the respiratory tract is mature and the infant can breath normally. If significant respiratory failure is present, lung compliance is decreased, and positive pressure mechanical ventilation is required, ventilating gases may flow preferentially through the fistula into the gastrointestinal tract. Progressive abdominal distention may preclude adequate ventilation requiring emergency decompression of the stomach and control of the fistula.

Associated Anomalies

Associated anomalies are present in about half of newborns with esophageal atresia, indicating that other systems are affected by the early organogenic insult that disturbs the development of the trachea and esophagus. The most common associated anomalies are cardiovascular defects. Genitourinary, gastrointestinal, skeletal, neurologic, and craniofacial defects are found with increased frequency in patients with esophageal atresia as well.

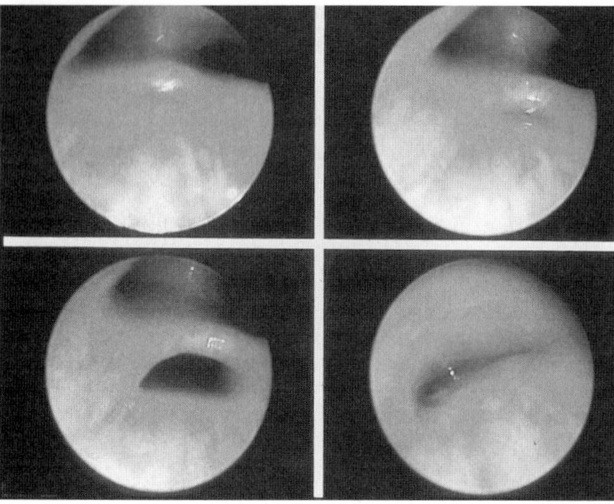

FIGURE 109.12 Bronchoscopic view of the trachea in a patient with common esophageal atresia and tracheoesophageal fistula. Note that during the inspiratory phase of positive pressure ventilation the fistula opens widely, demonstrating the face of TEF (*lower left*). The more proximal view in the trachea demonstrates tracheomalacia with coaptation of the anterior trachea and posterior membranous trachea (*lower right*).

The particular occurrence of vertebral anomalies, anorectal malformations, and cardiac, tracheoesophageal, renal, and (radial) limb defects is known as the VACTERL association. Two or more of these defects may be present.

Preoperative Treatment

Attempts at feeding are stopped. Intravenous fluids and antibiotics are started. Further aspiration is minimized by placement of a sump catheter in the upper esophageal pouch. The infant is positioned either upright "semiseated" or head up. Endotracheal intubation is avoided unless absolutely necessary because positive pressure ventilation may result in preferential flow of ventilatory gases through the fistula. Ventilation strategies that avoid filling the stomach with gas should be employed if respiratory failure is associated with decreased lung compliance. Early use of surfactant to improve lung compliance should be considered in premature infants with respiratory failure. High-frequency oscillatory ventilation may be useful. Bedside decompressive gastrostomy may be needed if gastric distention compromises ventilation or a prolonged interval is planned prior to surgery. Although rarely necessary, the surgeon must be prepared to control the fistula by emergency operative ligation or the bronchoscopic placement of an occluding balloon if ventilation cannot be maintained.

The goal of modern operative treatment is to correct the anomaly completely with a single operation, avoiding a gastrostomy if possible. Immediate surgery is rarely required, and a day or two may be used to complete the assessment of the infant, including the echocardiographic evaluation to determine the position of the aortic arch and the presence of structural heart disease. Respiratory hygiene, positioning, and antibiotics may improve the infant's overall condition, and the transition from fetal circulation is more complete.

High-risk infants who cannot safely undergo surgical correction of their esophageal abnormality may be treated with delayed repair. A decompressive gastrostomy, proximal pouch suctioning, and parenteral nutrition are used until the infant is ready for operation. Severe respiratory failure (usually from prematurity) and structural heart disease are the most common reasons to delay esophageal surgery. A staged repair that employs gastrostomy and surgical division of the tracheoesophageal fistula, followed by esophageal anastomosis as a second thoracic operation, is rarely used today.

In the case of pure esophageal atresia without fistula, a prolonged period of delay before repair may be used to improve the likelihood of completing a primary repair of the esophagus. A feeding gastrostomy is performed initially. This may be technically challenging because microgastria is present with pure atresia. Intragastric feeding and somatic growth result in shortening of the interval between the upper pouch and lower esophageal segment over the course of several weeks. The upper pouch may be stretched by daily or twice-daily passage of a blunt flexible bougie. Radiographic determination of the distance between the two esophageal ends guides the timing of operation (Fig. 109.13).

Waterson's classification stratified infants into good, moderate-risk, and high-risk groups based on birth weight, pneumonia, and associated anomalies.[60] Risk group was used to help determine the timing and staging of surgical correction and to compare the results at different centers. Low birth weight or prematurity has less of an impact on survival than in the past. Currently, the presence of major cardiac disease and chromosomal abnormalities is the most important predictor of survival.[61–64]

Surgical Technique

In most patients, it is unnecessary to perform a gastrostomy at the time of repair. With typical anatomy (left aortic arch),

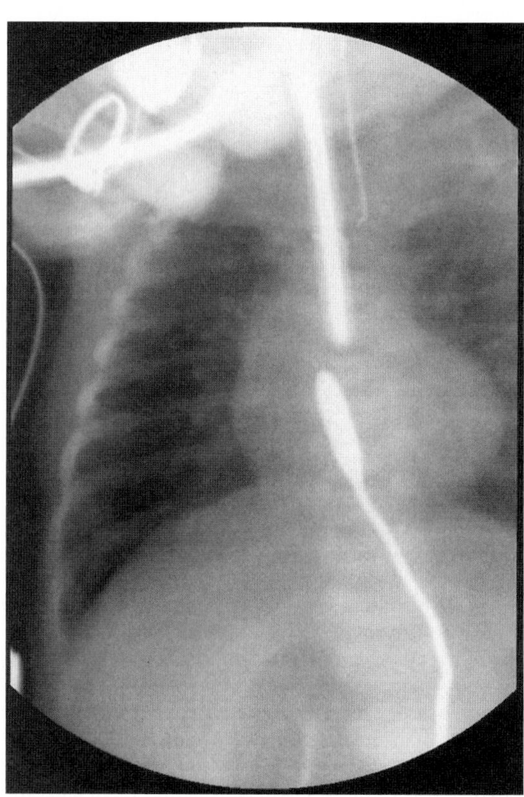

FIGURE 109.13 Patient with pure esophageal atresia treated initially with feeding gastrostomy and proximal pouch stretching. This gap-o-gram demonstrates close approximation of a dilator in the proximal pouch and a probe placed in the distal esophagus via the gastrostomy. The child subsequently underwent primary repair of the esophagus.

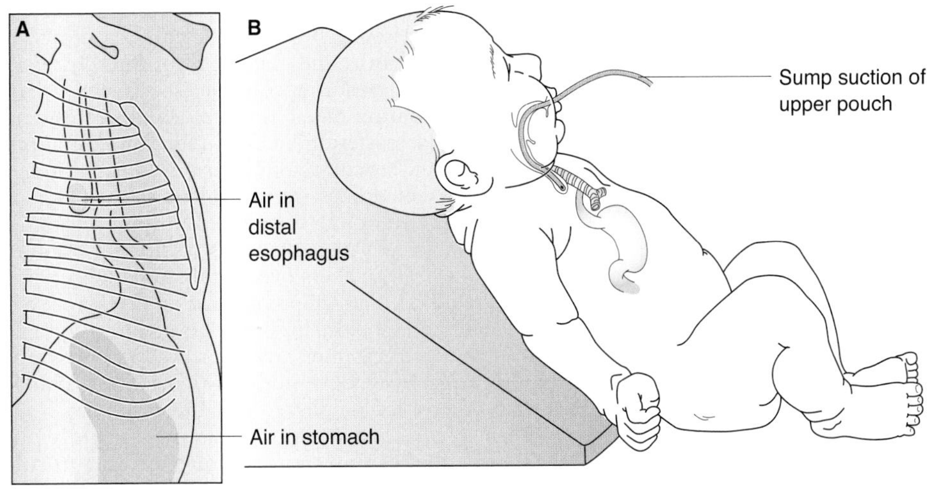

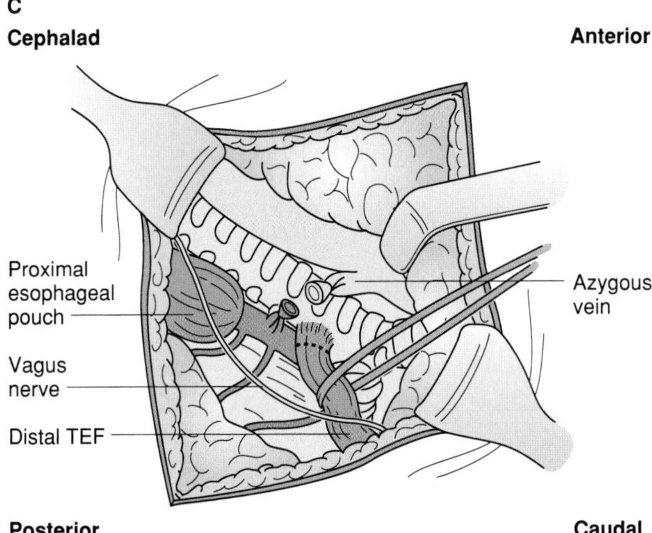

FIGURE 109.14 (*A*) Schematic illustration of esophageal atresia with distal tracheoesophageal fistula. (*B*) The initial management of this anomaly includes upright or prone posture, sump suction of the blind esophageal pouch. (*C*) The right extrapleural operative approach. After division and closure of the fistula, primary esophagoesophagostomy is performed. (After Coran AG. Congenital abnormalities of the esophagus. In: Zuidema GD, Orringer MD, eds. *Shackelford's surgery of the alimentary tract*, 2nd ed. Philadelphia, WB Saunders, 1990.)

the repair is performed via a right thoracotomy (Fig. 109.14). Although the approach may be either transpleural or extrapleural, most pediatric surgeons prefer the extrapleural approach. A standard posterolateral right thoracotomy may be used. There is no need to divide the latissimus or serratus muscles, and a muscle-sparing approach may have long-term benefits.[65] A more posterior approach through the auscultatory triangle affords excellent exposure with a very small skin incision. The extrapleural plane is established at the fourth intercostal space and developed sufficiently to allow control of the fistula and adequate mobilization of the proximal pouch. The distal tracheoesophageal fistula is divided and closed. The proximal pouch is identified and mobilized to whatever extent is needed to bring the ends together for anastomosis. If a proximal fistula is present it is closed.

Various lengthening techniques may be used when the gap is long between the esophageal ends. These techniques include circular myotomies, spiral myotomies, flap tubularization of the proximal pouch, and extensive mobilization of the proximal pouch through a supplementary cervical incision. Contrary to earlier teaching, the distal esophagus may be mobilized as well when there is a long distance between the upper pouch and lower esophagus or in the case of pure esophageal atresia. Distal mobilization may extend to the stomach. An anastomosis may heal, even under tension. One-layer, two-layer, and end-to-side repairs have been used. Most surgeons use a single-layer end-to-end anastomosis.

A staged repair has been described that has been successfully employed in pure and long-gap esophageal atresia.[66] Traction sutures are initially placed in the upper pouch and lower segment. Daily tensioning results in lengthening of the esophagus that allows anastomosis within 2 weeks (Fig. 109.15).

In the worst cases of long-gap atresia, pure atresia, or failed initial operative repairs, esophageal replacement may be performed at a later date using stomach, gastric tube, or colon.[67–69] Such conditions are temporized with a cervical esophagostomy ("spit fistula") and gastrostomy.

Tracheoesophageal fistula without esophageal atresia is referred to as H-type atresia. The orientation of the fistula is such that the opening into the trachea is always proximal to the esophageal entry site. Repair is performed through a cervical approach after bronchoscopically stenting the fistula with a small catheter. The catheter aids in the precise identification of the fistula during dissection in the neck. Care must taken to stay in the plane of the esophagus to avoid injury to the recurrent laryngeal nerves.

Minimally invasive techniques using modifications of thoracoscopy may be used to treat esophageal atresia.[70,71] It is uncertain whether such techniques will have an added advantage in the treatment of the disease. All attempts must be

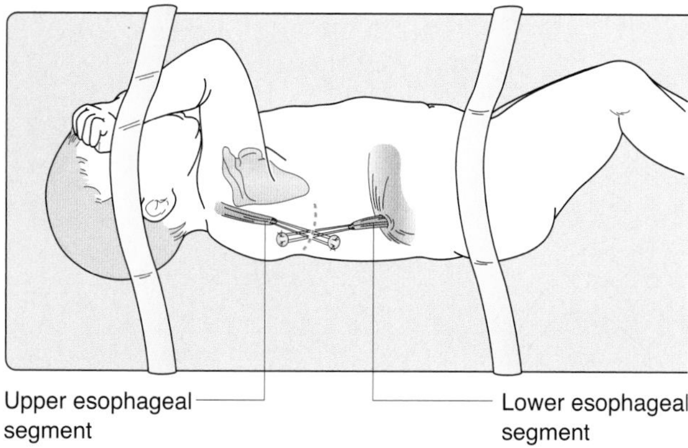

FIGURE 109.15 In patients with ultralong-gap esophageal atresia, traction sutures are placed on the upper pouch and lower segment. Tension is increased daily until the segments lengthen, allowing primary repair. (After Foker JE, Kendall TC, Catton K, et al. A flexible approach to achieve a true primary repair for all infants with esophageal atresia. *Semin Pediatr Surg.* 2005;14:815.)

closely monitored and results compared with current practices and not simply with historic controls.

Results, Complications, and Outcomes

Technical mishaps during the procedure occur when the anatomy is misidentified or dissection is carried out improperly. Unplanned pleural entry or injury to the vagus nerves, recurrent laryngeal nerves, posterior trachea, and adjacent vessels are all significant risks.

Anastomotic leak is said to occur in 10% to 20% of patients. The vast majority of such leaks heal spontaneously. The presence of a leak prolongs hospitalization and increases the likelihood of stricture formation at the anastomotic site. When a leak is detected, the retropleural chest tube is left in place, the infant is not fed by mouth, and antibiotics may be administered. Repeat contrast scans document healing before the initiation of feeds.

Esophageal stricture at the site of the repair is found in as many as 40% of patients after repair. Many strictures respond to a few sessions of dilation. Dilations are performed in the operating room with endoscopic and fluoroscopic assistance, as necessary, to ensure the safe traverse of the narrowing by guide wires and dilators. More recalcitrant strictures may require many dilation sessions, steroid injection, and medical or surgical control of gastroesophageal reflux for resolution. Occasionally reoperation, with resection of the stricture and reanastomosis of the esophagus, may be needed.

Recurrent tracheoesophageal fistula is reported to occur in up to 10% of patients. Recurrent fistulas may respond to endoscopic ablation or require operative division with interposition of pleura, muscle, or pericardium.

Gastroesophageal reflux is present in nearly all infants with esophageal atresia. It is symptomatic in many and may contribute to respiratory symptoms and stricture formation. Medical treatment consists of thickened feedings, upright positioning after feeds, frequent burping, small frequent feeds, and acid reduction and prokinetic agents. In many infants, medical treatments are inadequate to control symptoms and surgical control of reflux is required.

Esophageal dysmotility is present to some degree in all patients with esophageal atresia. Dysmotility contributes to gastroesophageal reflux and may be responsible for dysphagia and recurrent respiratory problems.

Tracheomalacia may result in symptoms after the correction of esophageal atresia. Bronchoscopically the trachea appears oval rather than round. The anterior and posterior walls coapt during the respiratory cycle (see Fig. 109.12). Fluoroscopic examination of the trachea demonstrates narrowing in the anterior-posterior dimensions during expiration. Tracheomalacia "fits" occur as the infant becomes agitated and develops worsening chest retractions with inspiration. The condition may deteriorate to complete inspiratory block and unconsciousness. When spontaneous respiration resumes in a quiet fashion, the "spell" is over. Intubation and resuscitation may be required. The symptoms are completely relieved by endotracheal intubation. Infants with less severe symptoms may improve over time as the trachea grows. Severe symptoms require either tracheostomy or tracheal suspension. Tracheal suspension is accomplished with an aortopexy.

Long-term results have improved in patients with esophageal atresia. Most children can look forward to survival with a normal existence.[72–76] Overall survival rates are reported in the 85% to 95% range. However, some subsets of infants do not fare as well. Mortality rate is high for infants with severe congenital heart defects and chromosomal abnormalities. Late deaths related to respiratory disease (tracheomalacia, reactive airway disease, gastroesophageal reflux, aspiration) can occur.[62] The very long-term outcomes for children with repaired esophageal atresia are not known. Disordered peristalsis and chronic esophagitis may have long-term implications such that periodic endoscopic surveillance of the esophagus should be performed in selected patients.[77]

OTHER CONGENITAL ABNORMALITIES OF THE TRACHEA AND ESOPHAGUS

Laryngotracheoesophageal cleft

Laryngotracheoesophageal cleft (LTEC) abnormalities represent the most severe anomalies of development of the trachea and esophagus. Type I abnormalities communicate at the level of the larynx and cricoid cartilage. Type II abnormalities extend beyond the cricoid cartilage into the cervical trachea. Type III LTEC involves the entire trachea from the larynx to the carina. The embryogenesis of LTEC is poorly understood but likely represents a disruption similar to, but more severe than, the more common EA/TEF abnormality. Associated abnormalities of the cardiovascular, genitourinary, and gastrointestinal tract are common. In patients with type I and II defects, esophageal atresia and a distal tracheoesophageal fistula are present about one third of the time.

Type I clefts may be approached endoscopically or translaryngeally. Type II clefts require cervical exposure, either laterally or by dividing the larynx and trachea in the midline. This anterior midline laryngofissure approach provides excellent exposure and avoids injury to the recurrent laryngeal nerves. Type III clefts extending to the carina, or beyond, require direct exposure through a right extrapleural thoracotomy, as well as cervical exposure. The trachea and esophagus are separated longitudinally in such a way as to leave a remnant of the esophagus with the trachea to be used in reconstructing the posterior membranous portion of the trachea. The esophagus is then tubularized. A multilayered repair of the larynx is completed through the cervical exposure. Breakdown of the repair and prolonged need for tracheostomy are common. Oromotor dysfunction and chronic aspiration are long-term problems. Most children will require a gastrostomy for feedings. Gastroesophageal reflux is common and may require surgical control.

Congenital esophageal stenosis

Acquired peptic strictures of the esophagus are relatively common and may occur early in life. True congenital stenosis is very uncommon. The stenotic areas may be (a) a membranous, web-like diaphragm, (b) fibromuscular thickening characterized by submucosal proliferation of smooth muscle cells and connective tissue, or (c) caused by sequestration of respiratory tract remnants in the form of respiratory epithelium and cartilage. The cartilage remnants may form a complete nondistensible ring in the esophagus. Dysphagia may be present from infancy or become apparent when solid foods are introduced. The diagnosis is confirmed by esophagoscopy. Stenoses are initially treated with dilations. Stenosis resulting from respiratory tract remnants is more likely to require segmental resection of the involved area.

Esophageal duplication

Esophageal duplications are found in the posterior mediastinum and are covered by a muscular wall that is in continuity with the muscular wall of the esophagus. The epithelial lining is usually intestinal, often gastric mucosa, and does not usually communicate with the esophagus. These cysts may also have a respiratory epithelium lining, underscoring the relatedness of the various bronchopulmonary foregut malformations. Neurenteric cysts communicate with the spinal canal. Masses are discovered incidentally or as a result of compression on adjacent organs. Acid-peptic ulceration from gastric mucosawithin the cyst may result in symptoms such as pain, bleeding, or erosion into adjacent structures (e.g., lung parenchyma, bronchus, esophagus). Excision is recommended. Thoracoscopic techniques allow excision with minimal morbidity (Fig. 109.16).

Vascular rings

Vascular rings result from faulty embryogenesis of the aortic arch and great vessels. In these abnormalities, the esophagus and trachea are surrounded by vascular structures and dense connective tissue that results in symptoms of airway or esophageal obstruction. Symptoms include wheezing, noisy breathing, coughing, stridor, pneumonia, and dysphagia (often when solid foods are started). A barium swallow may be suggestive or diagnostic. CT and MRI are used to define the anatomic abnormality. Echocardiography is used to rule out structural heart disease.

The most common abnormality encountered is a double aortic arch, resulting from the persistence of both the left and the right embryologic aortic arches. The ascending aorta bifurcates, surrounding the trachea and esophagus, then rejoins as the descending aorta. Other developmental abnormalities may result in complete or incomplete rings that compress the trachea or the esophagus or both. When the vascular ring is symptomatic, the patient should be treated surgically by appropriate division of the ring and the lysis of the fibrous bands that surround the trachea and esophagus.

Congenital tracheal stenosis

Failure of tracheal growth and development results in a wide variety of abnormalities. Short segments of the trachea may be narrowed or the entire trachea may be hypoplastic. Often complete tracheal cartilaginous rings are present. Short stenotic areas may respond to balloon dilation, which splits the complete tracheal rings. Segmental stenoses may be amenable to resection and anastomosis. Longer stenoses may be corrected with placement of a graft to widen the lumen of the trachea or by the slide tracheoplasty technique.[78,79]

FOREIGN BODIES OF THE TRACHEOBRONCHIAL TREE

Foreign body ingestion and aspiration occur commonly in the pediatric population.[80] Any foreign body that could obstruct the airway represents a potentially life-threatening problem. The National Safety Council estimates that 200 deaths (most in children under age 5 years) occur each year in persons under the age of 15 years as a result of suffocation by an ingested object.[81] The Hopkins rod lens optical system with fiberoptic illumination, developed in the 1970s, and the incorporation of the lens system into rigid pediatric bronchoscopes and specialized grasping devices has resulted in a safe and reliable method for airway foreign body extraction.

Pathophysiology

Complete obstruction of the airway and asphyxiation can occur at the level of the laryngeal inlet, the subglottis, or the trachea. Back blows (recommended in infants), abdominal

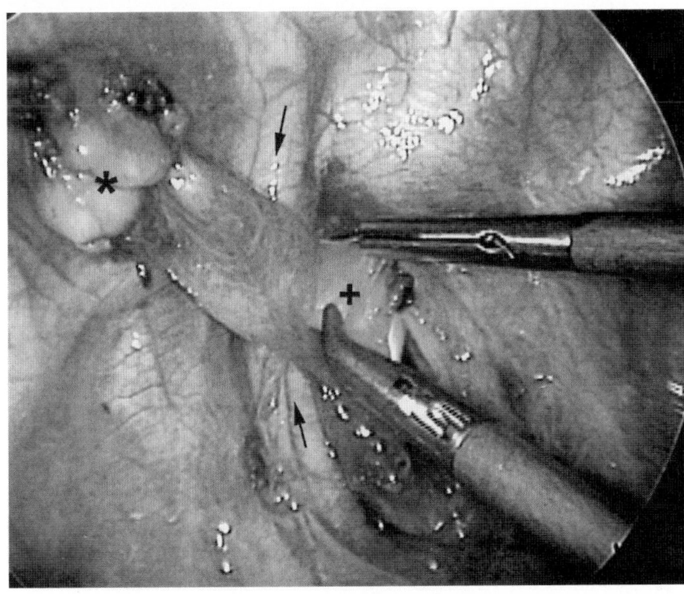

FIGURE 109.16 Thoracoscopic excision of an esophageal duplication cyst in a patient presenting with dysphagia. Video endoscopic view of the left superior hemithorax. (+) indicates site of original esophageal duplication cyst. Light from intraesophageal endoscope can be seen. Arrows demonstrate subclavian artery. The mass (*) is nearly excised.

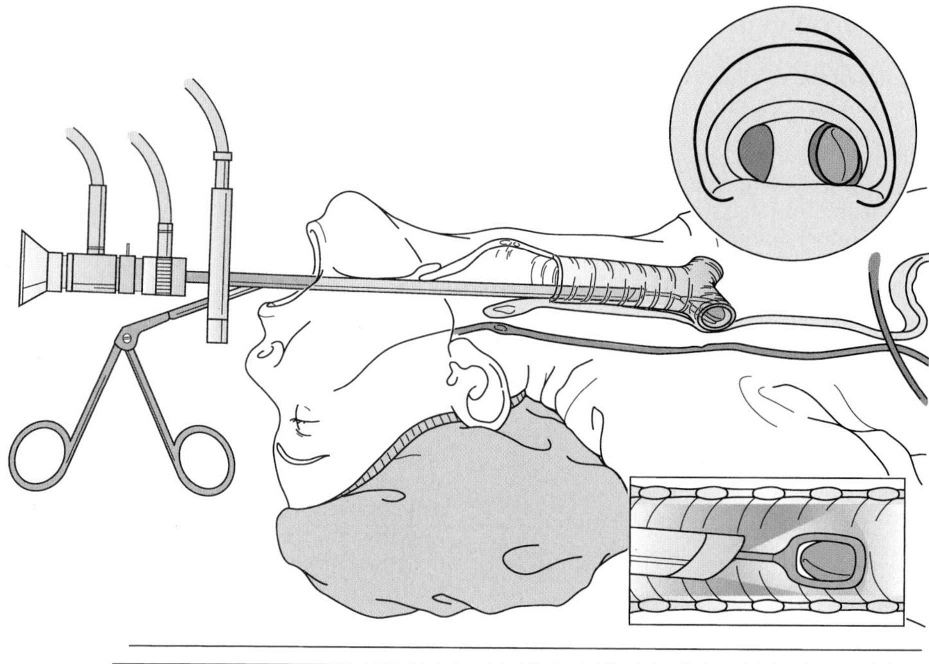

FIGURE 109.17 Schematic illustration of a peanut foreign body being extracted from the right main stem bronchus under direct vision.

thrust, or the Heimlich maneuver may dislodge the obstruction and save a life. An inhaled foreign body that lodges at the bronchial level can create a ball-valve phenomenon in the affected bronchus, allowing bidirectional but unequal flow of air. Air-trapping and hyperinflation in the affected lobe or lung lead to mediastinal shift to the opposite side. Complete blockage of the bronchus by the foreign body results in loss of volume in the affected lobe or lung. In this case, the resulting volume loss from atelectasis will shift the mediastinum to the ipsilateral side.

Clinical Presentation

Most affected children are less than 4 years of age, with a peak incidence between 1 and 2 years. Of foreign body aspirations, 20% occur after the age of 4 years. Foreign bodies are more likely to lodge in the right side of the tracheobronchial tree. Most will be found in the main stem bronchus.[80] Peanuts are commonly aspirated and particularly troublesome. They become soft, fracture readily, and may require piecemeal removal. Other types of food, such as carrots and popcorn, or inorganic material, such as pins, wood, paper, or metallic and plastic parts, may be aspirated.

The aspiration event may have been witnessed or suggested by a history of a coughing or choking spell. The most common symptoms include cough, wheezing, dyspnea, and fever, and the most common signs are unilateral decreased breath sounds, unilateral wheezing, and rhonchi. A foreign body may also masquerade as pneumonia. Inspiratory and expiratory chest radiographs (or bilateral decubitus views in the case of children too young to cooperate) may demonstrate hyperinflation on the affected side due to air-trapping. Although physical signs and symptoms and radiographic findings are often present, a suggestive history alone is an adequate indication to proceed with bronchoscopy.

Management

Bronchoscopic evaluation and foreign body removal are performed in the operating room under general anesthesia (Fig. 109.17). The rigid bronchoscope with optical forceps can be used to remove most aspirated foreign bodies safely. The flexible grasper and Fogarty balloon catheter can be useful, especially when the foreign body has migrated distally. Fluoroscopic assistance has been used for radiopaque objects that have migrated into the peripheral airways.

Occasionally, foreign body aspiration that presents as chronic lung infection requires surgical resection of the destroyed portion of the lung. Figure 109.18 shows the fluoroscopically assisted thoracoscopic removal of an aspirated pin that migrated to the peripheral lung surface.

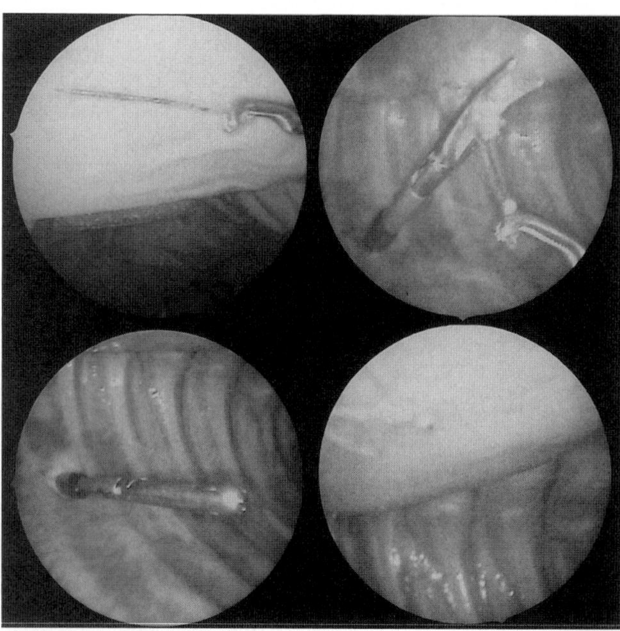

FIGURE 109.18 Four-panel operative photograph of removal of pin from lung periphery. Tip of pin seen on lung surface. Thoracoscopic instrumentation. Grasping pin. Pin removed.

CONGENITAL ABNORMALITIES OF THE DIAPHRAGM

Developmental defects of the diaphragm are of great interest to pediatric surgeons. Advances in the treatment of newborn respiratory failure, fetal surgery, and lung developmental biology have grown directly out of the clinical and laboratory investigation of congenital diaphragmatic hernia (CDH, Bochdalek hernia). These topics are fertile areas of clinical and basic science research.

McCauley described the clinical course and postmortem anatomy of an infant with CDH in 1754.[82] Although Bochdalek's understanding of the embryology was incorrect, this congenital defect continues to carry his name.[83] Successful repair of CDH remained rare prior to 1940.[84] In 1946 Gross reported the first infant less than 24 hours old surviving operative repair of the defect.[85] The standard of care remained immediate neonatal surgery until the 1980s. CDH was considered to be an anatomic derangement that was treated by an anatomic correction (i.e., the surgical solution was to "get the bowel out of the chest" and "prevent further lung compression from the intestines").

During the last 25 years greater emphasis has been placed on the physiologic behavior of the lungs in CDH. Lung function, as determined by the degree of pulmonary hypoplasia and pulmonary hypertension, is the most important determinant of survival in CDH. With endotracheal and orogastric intubation and positive pressure ventilation at low ventilator pressures, there is very little consequence to the presence of the abdominal viscera in the chest. Surgery may be delayed almost indefinitely, if necessary. Pulmonary hypertension is aggressively treated by whatever means necessary, including high-frequency oscillatory ventilation, nitric oxide, and extracorporeal membrane oxygenation (ECMO). Surgical repair is performed when labile pulmonary hypertension has resolved. Improved survival of infants with CDH has resulted from a better understanding of the physiology of postnatal pulmonary hypertension and changes in the timing of surgery. Better treatments for pulmonary hypertension and therapies aimed at augmenting the development of hypoplastic lungs will no doubt result in further improvements in the survival and long-term morbidity of infants with CDH.[86]

Embryology of the Lung and Diaphragm

Mammalian lung development occurs *in vivo* as a coordinated developmental process that includes (a) airway and acinar development, (b) cellular differentiation, (c) biochemical maturation, (d) interstitial development including vasculature and extracellular matrix, and (e) physical growth or enlargement. These parallel developmental processes occur in such a fashion that at any one time during development there are characteristic relationships among components that define the so-called stages of lung development.[87–89] Pulmonary development is marked by a series of programmed events regulated by master genes such as the homeobox genes, nuclear transcription factors, hormones, and growth factors. These processes involve genes regulating epithelial and endothelial interactions as well as temporal and spatial interactions of several hormones and growth factors.[90,91] Hormones such as the glucocorticoids, thyroid hormone, and retinoic acid have been shown to regulate several of the crucial cellular interactions required for proper pulmonary organogenesis and differentiation. In the human embryo, respiratory tract development begins in the fourth week of gestation as a ventral outpouching of the foregut, which soon has bifurcated and begun branching into the surrounding mesenchyme. The primitive, pluripotent epithelial cells differentiate into both bronchial and alveolar cell lines under the control of the surrounding mesenchyme. By a process of asymmetric branching, the divisions are complete by the 16th week of gestation. Lung at this phase has columnar epithelium with thick mesenchyme, giving rise to the descriptive term *pseudoglandular* phase of development because of its histologic appearance. The canalicular phase that follows and continues up to about the 24th gestational week is characterized by flattening of the epithelium of the distal airways, thinning of the mesenchyme, and the growth of the capillary network that surrounds the terminal airways. Gas exchange becomes functionally possible at the end of this phase. The terminal sac period that follows refers to the appearance of a thin respiratory epithelium in apposition to a capillary network capable of supporting gas exchange. True alveolar formation in humans begins shortly before or around the time of birth. Alveolar maturation and multiplication takes place after birth and may continue up to 8 years of age.

The precursors of the diaphragm begin to form during the fourth week of gestation with the appearance of the peritoneal folds from lateral mesenchymal tissue. At the same time, the septum transversum forms from the inferior portion of the pericardial cavity and serves to delineate the thoracic from the abdominal cavities. Eventually the septum transversum leads to the formation of the central tendinous area of the fully developed diaphragm. The pleuroperitoneal folds extend from the lateral body wall and grow medially and ventrally until they fuse with the septum transversum and dorsal mesentery of the esophagus during the sixth gestational week. Complete closure of the canal takes place during the eighth week of gestation, with the right side closing before the left.[92] Muscularization of the diaphragm appears to develop from the innermost layer of thoracic mesoderm, although other mechanisms have been proposed.[93] A contribution from cervically derived myoblasts is also present as evidenced by the innervation of the diaphragm by the phrenic nerve originating from the third, fourth, and fifth cervical nerve roots. Posterolaterally, at the junction of the lumbar and costal muscle groups, the fibrous lumbocostal trigone remains as a small remnant of the pleuroperitoneal membrane and relies for its strength on the fusion of the two muscle groups in the final stages of development. It is in this area that the defect of CDH occurs (Fig. 109.19).

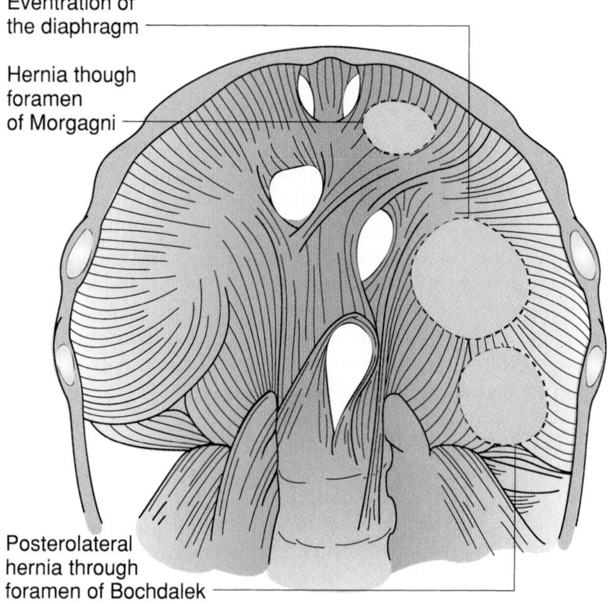

FIGURE 109.19 Anatomy of the diaphragm showing the location of congenital diaphragmatic defects.

Congenital Diaphragmatic Hernia Pathology and Pathophysiology

The reported incidence of CDH is estimated to be between 1 in 2,000 to 1 in 5,000 births, making it one of the most common congenital abnormalities.[94] Approximately one third of infants with CDH are stillborn, but these deaths are usually to the result of associated fatal anomalies such as neural tube defects (anencephaly, myelomeningocele, hydrocephalus, and encephaloceles) and cardiac defects. Defects are more common on the left side (80% left, 20% right). Bilateral CDH defects are rare. CDH is thought to represent a sporadic developmental anomaly, although a number of familial cases have been reported. The expected recurrence risk in a first-degree relative has been estimated to be 1 in 45.[94] One third of affected infants have associated major defects.[95] The combination of CDH and an abnormal karyotype is associated with a poor outcome.

The cause of CDH is unknown, but it is presumed that some combination of intrinsic predisposition (genetic factors) and environmental insult (teratogen or deficiency) results in abnormal diaphragm and lung development. Exposure to a number of pharmacologic agents has been implicated in its development, including certain drugs and insecticides such as phenmetrazine, thalidomide, quinine, and nitrofen.[94] Vitamin A deficiency in infants with CDH and the effects of vitamin A administration in nitrofen-induced pulmonary hypoplasia have strengthened the evolving hypothesis that alterations in retinoid-regulated target genes may be responsible for CDH development.[96] Diaphragmatic hernia and pulmonary hypoplasia can be created in animal models, both surgically and pharmacologically.[97–100]

During the early development of the diaphragm, the midgut is largely extracoelomic. If closure of the pleuroperitoneal canal has not occurred by the time the midgut returns to the abdomen during the ninth and tenth weeks of gestation, the abdominal viscera herniate through the lumbocostal trigone into the ipsilateral thoracic cavity. The resulting abnormal position of the bowel prevents its normal counterclockwise rotation and fixation. No hernia sac is present if the event occurs before complete closure of the pleuroperitoneal canal, but a nonmuscularized membrane forms a hernia sac in 10% to 15% of patients with CDH. In addition to small bowel, other intraabdominal organs, such as the spleen, stomach, colon, and liver, may also herniate through the diaphragmatic defect.

Left-sided CDH is a 2- to 4-cm posterolateral defect in the diaphragm through which the abdominal viscera have translocated into the ipsilateral thoracic cavity. Through a right-sided defect, the large right lobe of the liver can occupy most of the hemithorax. The hepatic veins may drain ectopically into the right atrium, and the liver and lung may be fused.[101]

The pathophysiology of CDH has been attributed to pulmonary parenchymal compression by the herniated organs and its effect on growth and maturation of the lung. An emerging school of thought attributes the pulmonary hypoplasia to an early developmental insult to the lung and diaphragm.[90,91,102] Unilateral diaphragmatic hernia is associated with both ipsilateral and contralateral abnormal pulmonary development, although hypoplasia is more severe on the ipsilateral side. The lung on the side of the hernia is much smaller than its normal counterpart (Fig. 109.20). The pulmonary vascular bed is abnormal in lungs from patients with CDH. There is a reduction in the total number of arterial branches in both the ipsilateral and contralateral pulmonary parenchyma. The small preacinar and intraacinar arterioles feature inappropriate and significant medial muscular hyperplasia (Fig. 109.21). The physiologic consequence of this abnormal arteriolar muscularization may be an increased susceptibility to development of pulmonary hypertension.

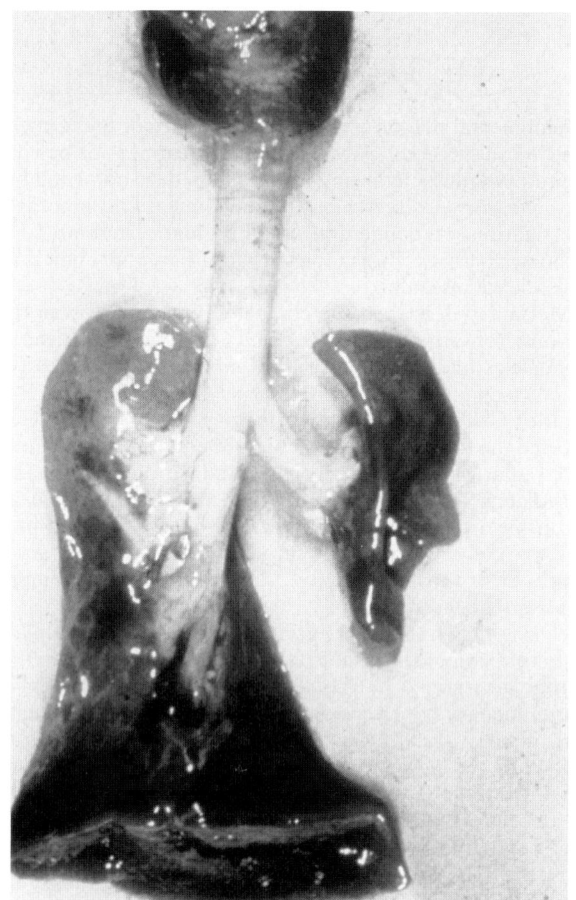

FIGURE 109.20 Autopsy specimen of an infant with severe pulmonary hypoplasia secondary to congenital diaphragmatic hernia. Pulmonary hypoplasia is bilateral, but the left lung is most severely affected.

Pulmonary blood flow accounts for only 7% of cardiac output during normal fetal development. Pulmonary vascular resistance is high. The fetus preferentially shunts oxygenated blood from the placenta through the foramen ovale and ductus arteriosus in a right-to-left direction into the systemic circulation. With the institution of breathing at birth, pulmonary vascular resistance falls, permitting an increase in pulmonary blood flow. Increased arterial oxygen tension then induces spontaneous closure of the ductus arteriosus. *Persistent fetal circulation* may develop if this process is interrupted. Elevated pulmonary vascular resistance results in right-to-left shunting of blood at either the atrial or ductal level with the delivery of unsaturated blood into the systemic circulation. As shunting increases, the oxygen saturation in the systemic circulation falls. The resulting hypoxia further increases pulmonary vascular resistance and compromises pulmonary blood flow while increasing the right-to-left shunt flow.

Factors that contribute to the persistence of high pulmonary vascular resistance in CDH lungs are thought to be the structural changes of decreased total arteriolar cross-sectional area in the involved lungs and the increased muscularization of the arterial structures that are present. Additional exacerbations of pulmonary vascular resistance may be induced by the known stimulators of pulmonary hypertension, which include hypoxia, acidosis, hypothermia, and stress. Alternations in the levels of prostaglandins, leukotrienes, catecholamines, and the renin angiotensin system had been implicated as mediators of this complex process.

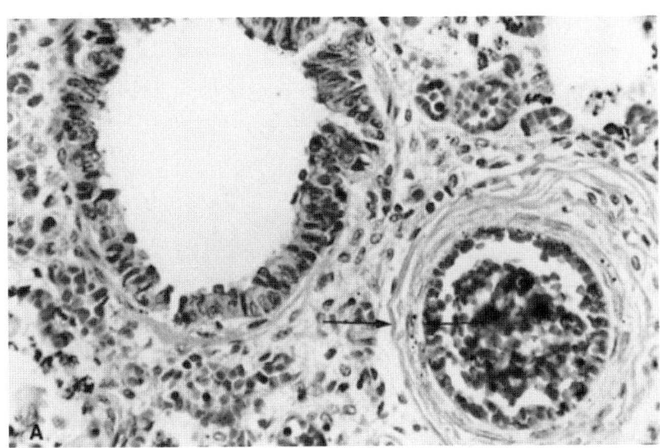
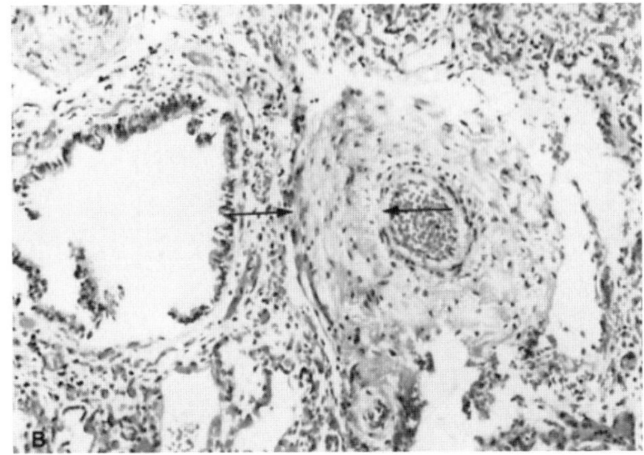

FIGURE 109.21 Histology of pulmonary arteries. Pulmonary artery branches of similar size and location are shown in a normal infant (*A*) and in an infant with Bochdalek diaphragmatic hernia (*B*). There is increased muscle mass associated with the arterial wall in *B* (*arrows*). This vascular smooth muscle is exquisitely sensitive to chemical, hormonal, and paracrine mediators in the neonatal period. Pulmonary arterial vasospasm is an important cause of persistent fetal circulation and respiratory failure. Treatment of pulmonary hypertension is the primary objective in the immediate care of the newborn with congenital diaphragmatic hernia.

Diagnosis

The diagnosis of CDH is often made on a prenatal ultrasound examination. Polyhydramnios is common. Prenatal MRI evaluation is being used with increasing frequency when obstetric sonography has detected a complex fetal anomaly and is ideally suited for fetuses with CDH.[103,104] After birth, the spectrum of respiratory symptoms in an infant with CDH is determined by the degree of pulmonary hypoplasia and reactive pulmonary hypertension. Severely affected infants develop respiratory distress at birth, and most demonstrate respiratory symptoms within the first 24 hours of life. On physical examination, these infants have a scaphoid abdomen. A plain chest radiograph that demonstrates loops of intestines in the chest confirms the diagnosis of a CDH (Fig. 109.22). The location of the stomach is confirmed by placement of a nasogastric tube. The chest radiograph shows angulation of the mediastinum and a shifting of the cardiac silhouette into the contralateral thorax. Chest radiographs are unreliable for estimating the degree of pulmonary hypoplasia. Once the diagnosis of a CDH is confirmed, additional radiographic and ultrasonographic examination should be carried out to search for associated anomalies. Echocardiography should also be obtained. Approximately 10% to 20% of infants are diagnosed after the first day of life. The diagnosis of a CDH can be confused with a number of other congenital thoracic conditions, including eventration of the diaphragm, anterior diaphragmatic hernia of Morgagni, congenital cystic disease of the pulmonary parenchyma, unilateral pulmonary effusion, and primary agenesis of the lung.[105]

Prognostic Factors

Attempts to define clinically relevant prognostic factors to predict the outcome of infants with CDH have largely been unsuccessful. A prenatal anatomic parameter that appears to have predictive correlation is the determination of the lung-to-head ratio (LHR). The ratio is determined from simultaneous sonographic measurements of the lung and head, and ratios less than 1.0 have been associated with poor outcomes.[106–109] Anatomic factors such as the position of the stomach either above or below the diaphragmatic rim and the size of the diaphragmatic defect itself are also unreliable in predicting outcome. Physiologic parameters have been difficult to define and are limited to variations of arterial blood gas analyses.

Treatment

The fetus and mother should be referred to an appropriate tertiary perinatal center where the full array of respiratory care strategies, including NO, oscillating ventilators, and ECMO, are immediately available. Anything less may potentially compromise the best possible outcome. A spontaneous vaginal delivery is preferred unless obstetric issues supervene. CDH is a *physiologic* emergency and not a *surgical* emergency. The respiratory distress associated with a CDH in newborn infants results from a combination of uncorrectable pulmonary hypoplasia and potentially reversible pulmonary hypertension. The balance between these two factors determines the response to therapy and ultimately the outcome.

Resuscitation should begin with endotracheal intubation and nasogastric tube insertion. Bag-mask ventilation is contraindicated to avoid distention of the stomach and intestines that may be in the thoracic cavity. Meticulous attention must be paid to maintaining proper temperature regulation, glucose homeostasis, and volume status in the neonate. Systemic hypotension and inadequate tissue perfusion may be reversed with intravenous fluid administration including crystalloid, blood products, and colloid. Inotropic drugs such as dopamine or dobutamine may be required. Most infants can be successfully managed with a simple pressure-cycled ventilator with the goal of ventilatory support being a preductal $p_aO_2 > 60$ (S_aO_2 90% to 100%) with a corresponding p_aCO_2 of less than 60.[110,111] The extremes of hyperventilation, particularly with high rates and high ventilatory pressures, should be avoided to prevent ventilator-induced lung injury. If conventional mechanical ventilatory techniques cannot reverse the hypoxemia or hypercarbia, high-frequency techniques using either the jet ventilator or the oscillating ventilator may be required.

A broad spectrum of drugs and antihypertensive agents has been used in attempts to modify the pulmonary vascular resistance in infants with CDH and respiratory failure. Agents

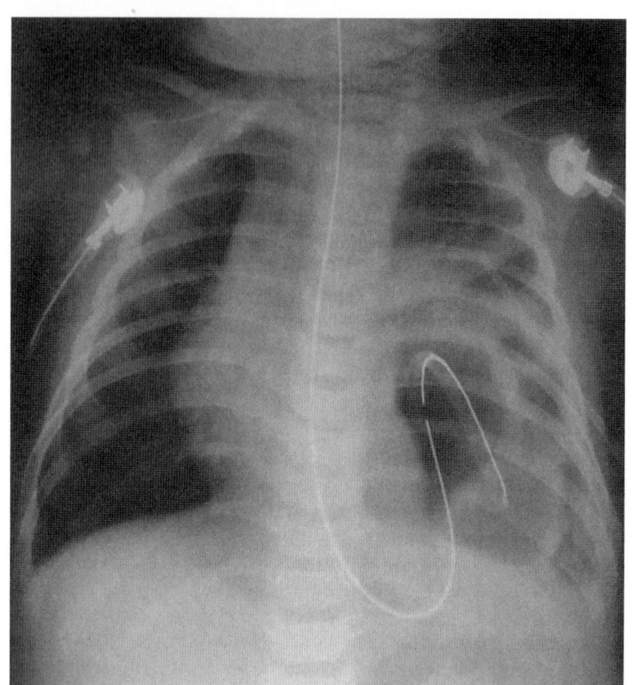

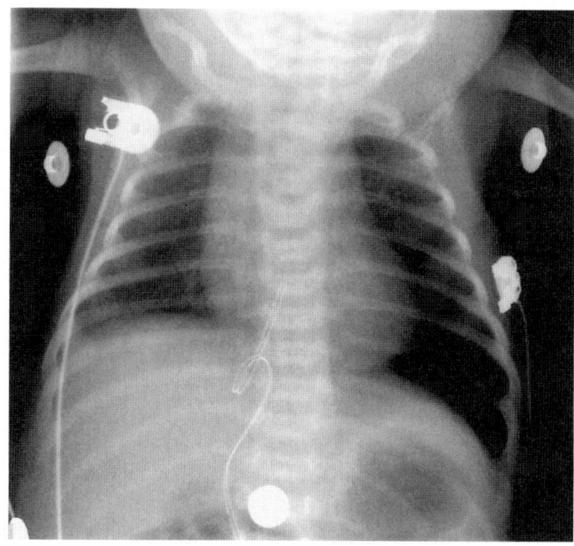

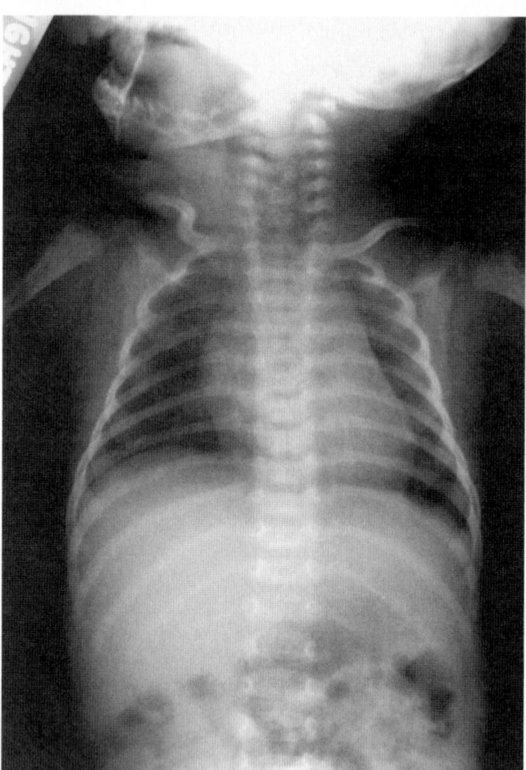

FIGURE 109.22 (*A*) Chest radiograph of a newborn with a left congenital diaphragmatic hernia. Mediastinal structures shifted to the right. Abdominal viscera occupy the left hemithorax. Nasogastric tube locates the stomach. The child underwent repair of the congenital diaphragmatic hernia after treatment and resolution of pulmonary hypertension. (*B*) Immediate postoperative photograph demonstrates return of mediastinal structures to a more normal position. The hypoplastic left lung is apparent. (*C*) Chest radiograph 1 month later is unremarkable.

such as tolazoline (α-receptor blocker) have had marginal benefit in affected infants. Other drugs, such as nitroprusside, isoproterenol, nitroglycerin, and captopril, have not been effective. The administration of various prostaglandin derivatives, including prostaglandin D_2 (PGD_2), prostaglandin 1 (PGE_1), and prostacyclin, and the cyclooxygenase inhibitor indomethacin has also been disappointingly unsuccessful. Clinical and experimental studies have demonstrated surfactant deficiencies in infants with CDH. A multicenter review of surfactant administration in CDH patients showed no overall benefit to its use and demonstrated a lower survival rate in preterm infants compared with full-term infants.[112] At this time, no clinical data support the administration of surfactant in the management of infants with CDH. NO is a potent mediator of vasodilatation and particularly suited for administration to the pulmonary vasculature using inhalation techniques. It has been shown to be effective in improving oxygen saturation levels in neonates with respiratory failure resulting from prematurity and persistent pulmonary hypertension of the newborn. Unfortunately, its effects in infants with CDH and respiratory failure have been mixed. No data show that NO administration improves survival or decreases the requirement for ECMO.[113] Patients who do not respond to conventional treatments, high-frequency oscillatory ventilation (HFOV), and NO are considered for ECMO treatment (see later).

Surgery

Multiple single-institutional studies have reported improved survival rates with delayed surgery as part of their treatment protocols, whereas others have found no changes in overall outcome. No study has shown a decrease in survival rates with this technique. Though delayed surgical repair is now widely practiced, no statistical evidence supports this approach over immediate repair at this time.[114]

To avoid the stresses of transport and sudden changes in ventilation parameters imposed by a trip to the operating room, a number of centers have adopted the policy of performing surgical repair of these infants in the neonatal intensive care unit (NICU).

The diaphragm defect is usually approached through a subcostal incision, although the repair can be performed through a thoracotomy incision (Fig. 109.23). Both thoracoscopic and laparoscopic techniques have been used to repair these defects. Ideally suited for older infants with delayed presentation, minimally invasive techniques may have a higher incidence of technical and physiologic consequences in the newborn.[115] Once the abdominal contents are reduced, the defect in the diaphragm in the posterolateral position can be examined. In some patients, a hernia sac formed by parietal pleura and peritoneum is present and must be excised. Usually, there is an anterior rim of diaphragm of varying size, while the posterior rim must be exposed in the retroperitoneal tissue. When diaphragmatic tissue is adequate, a primary repair with nonabsorbable

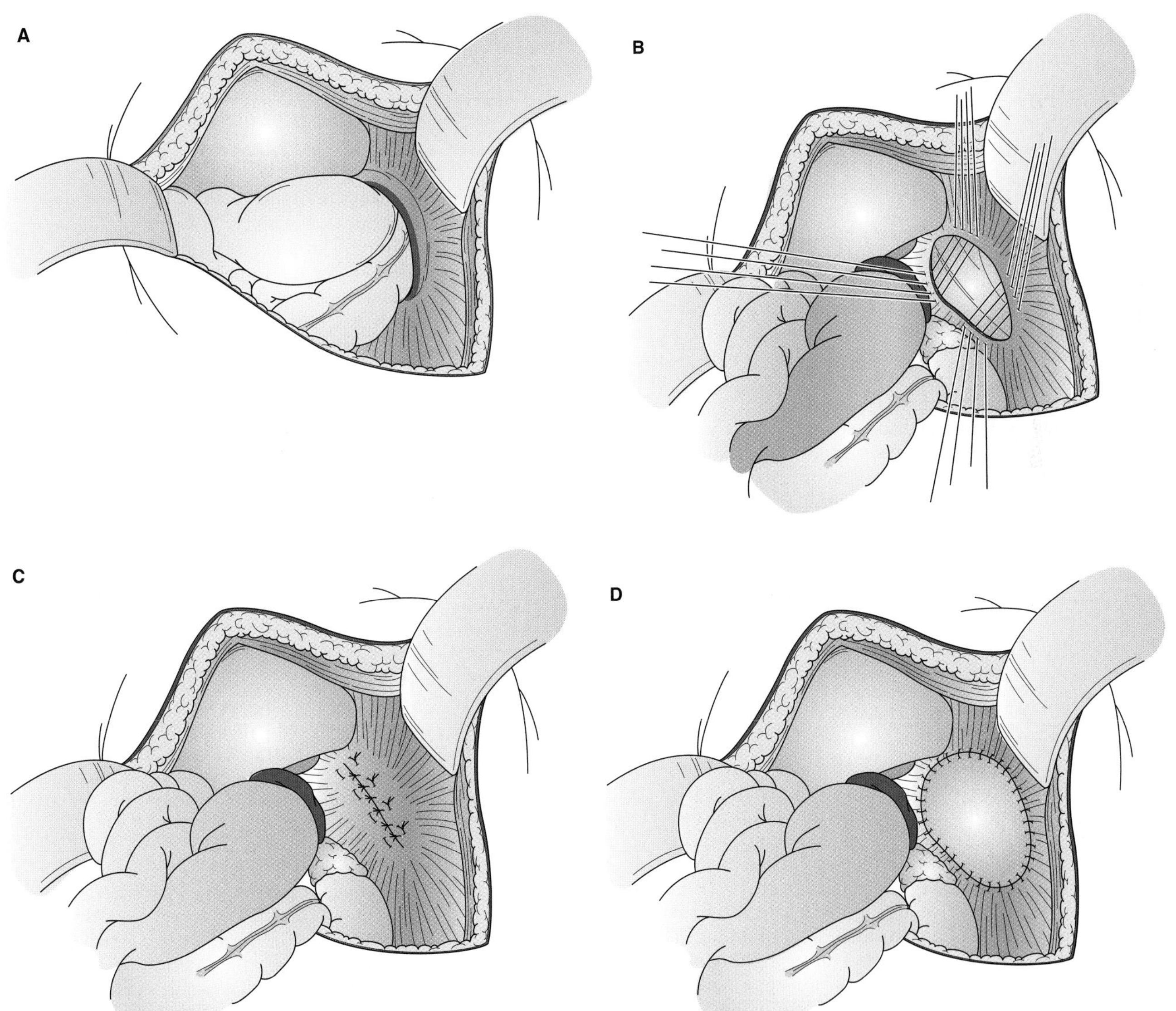

FIGURE 109.23 Repair of congenital diaphragmatic hernia. (*A*) Operative appearance of congenital diaphragmatic hernia. (*B*) Placement of sutures for repair of typical left posterolateral diaphragmatic defect. (*C*) Completed repair. (*D*) Prosthetic material may be used for large defects to avoid tension. (After Stollar CJH. Congenital diaphragmatic hernia. In: Spitz and Coran AG, eds. *Rob and Smith's Operative surgery: pediatric surgery*, 5th ed. London: Chapman and Hall, 1995.)

suture material can be performed. If the defect is too large to be closed in a primary fashion, a number of reconstructive techniques have been described using nearby prerenal fascia, rib structures, latissimus dorsi muscle, and abdominal wall muscle flaps. The use of prosthetic material to complete the diaphragmatic closure has gained widespread acceptance. A floppy, tension-free diaphragmatic repair can be accomplished that may lessen the degree of intraabdominal pressure when closing the abdominal wall. The major drawback to using a prosthetic patch closure is the risk of infection as well as the risk of dislodgment and subsequent reherniation. Tissue engineering may offer new materials for repair.[116]

With the loss of intraabdominal domain, abdominal wall closure may not be possible. In this situation, simple closure of the skin can be accomplished with repair of the ventral wall defect some months later. Drainage of the chest cavity on the repaired side with a tube thoracostomy is not usually necessary.

Postoperative management should continue the goals established before surgery. Meticulous attention to fluid status must be maintained, particularly in the immediate postoperative period. If respiratory decompensation develops, therapeutic interventions including nitric oxide, high-frequency ventilation, and ECMO may be employed. Weaning from ventilator support should be slow and deliberate as tolerated by the infant.

Extracorporeal Membrane Oxygenation

ECMO is a form of partial cardiopulmonary bypass with the goal of maintaining oxygen delivery to the body for an extended period of time when ventilator therapy has failed. It has become the cornerstone for managing infants with life-threatening respiratory failure with CDH.[117] ECMO allows respiratory support without the risks of barotrauma and oxygen toxicity associated with conventional ventilation. Initially, infants were placed on ECMO after developing respiratory failure following the immediate repair of the diaphragmatic defect. With the evolution of delayed surgical repair ECMO is now considered a part of the preoperative stabilization process. Failure to improve in the setting of severe pulmonary hypertension and progressive hypoxemia despite maximum medical intervention remains a valid qualifying criterion for ECMO support. As a result of the acceptance of delayed surgical repair as a treatment strategy, more than 90% of infants with CDH requiring ECMO support are placed on bypass before undergoing surgical repair.[118]

Outcome

Survival rates (discharge to home) for infants born with an isolated CDH have improved dramatically over the past decade when compared with the historical values of approximately 50%. Survival rates greater than 90% are being reached with current treatment modalities.[119] Resolution of pulmonary hypertension is predictive of survival.[120] Long-term studies have shown that many surviving infants have normal pulmonary function measurements including total lung capacity, vital capacity, and carbon monoxide diffusing capacity. In the last decade, as survival rates have improved, a new group of survivors is emerging with different patterns of long-term morbidities.[121] Chronic lung disease has been reported in survivors of CDH, particularly in those requiring ECMO.[122] Long-term problems that have been identified with increasing frequency include chronic lung disease, neurologic abnormalities with developmental delay, skeletal deformities, and nutritional and growth-related problems.

Evolving Therapies

Even with the increasing success of current treatment strategies, such as permissive hypercapnea, delayed surgery, antihypertensive pharmacology, and advanced ventilatory techniques, a cohort of infants refractory to these interventions continue to be candidates for novel treatments.

In Utero Repair of Diaphragmatic Hernia

The concept of fetal surgical intervention evolved from the experimental observation in lambs that reduction of compressive forces on the lung resulted in continued pulmonary growth and development.[123] Although technically and theoretically exciting, the clinical results have been disappointing.[124,125] A direct advancement of these initial attempts at *in utero* repair was the observation that fetal tracheal ligation accelerated fetal lung growth and reversed pulmonary hypoplasia.[126,127] Tracheal occlusion or PLUG (plug the lung until it grows) therapy resulted in improved oxygenation and ventilation after birth when compared with untreated control animals.[128] A randomized clinical trial that compared fetal endoscopic tracheal occlusion with current standard postnatal care for severe CDH showed no benefit in survival.[129] This intervention is being used in European centers.[130] Future research will determine whether fetal intervention has a role in the treatment of this process.

Liquid Ventilation

Liquid ventilation using perfluorocarbons has now advanced to the point of clinical applicability.[131] Partial liquid ventilation has been attempted in a small number of infants with CDH while they are on ECMO. Improvements in oxygenation levels and pulmonary function tests were noted. A prospective, controlled study is required to examine this form of ventilation before its clinical efficacy can be judged.

Pulmonary Transplantation

Successful neonatal lung transplantation for CDH has been achieved, but there is no long-term experience at this time to recommend this form of treatment. Neonatal single-lung or segmental pulmonary transplantation is feasible.

Pharmacology

New management strategies for treating persistent pulmonary hypertension now undergoing clinical evaluation include various calcium channel blockers, prostacyclin derivatives, endothelin receptor antagonists, and phosphodiesterase-5 inhibitors such as sildenafil.[132,133] The combined administration of thyrotropin-releasing hormone and glucocorticoid therapy has been demonstrated to have positive effects on lung growth.[134] In the future, the selective administrative of one or several pharmacologic agents or growth factors may be able to reverse the pulmonary hypoplasia and intractable pulmonary hypertension of CDH.

Foramen of Morgagni Hernia

The anterior diaphragmatic hernia of Morgagni is located anteromedially on either side of the junction of the septum transversum and the thoracic wall. Typically, a sac is present, and herniation of the colon, small bowel, or liver is usually discovered to the right or left of the midline. Morgagni hernias account for less than 2% of diaphragmatic defects and usually occur in older children or adults. The hernia is often discovered incidentally as a mass or air-fluid level on chest radiograph. Because of the risk of segmental intestinal volvulus or obstruction, surgical repair of the defect is recommended. Operative correction may be performed through an upper transverse abdominal incision or laparoscopically. The diaphragm is sutured to the undersurface of the posterior rectus sheath at the costal margin.

Eventration of the Diaphragm

Eventration of the diaphragm may be either congenital or acquired. The congenital form may be indistinguishable from a diaphragmatic hernia with a sac, and symptoms are similar. The acquired form results from paralysis of the phrenic nerve. The phrenic nerve is vulnerable to surgical trauma from a wide variety of cervical, thoracic, and diaphragmatic procedures. Phrenic nerve injuries and a variety of neuromuscular disorders, including primary myopathies and degenerative diseases, may produce diaphragmatic paralysis and require operative plication of the diaphragm in infants and young children. The most common cause of phrenic nerve injury in children is associated with thoracic and mediastinal surgery. Cervical stretching at birth may result in phrenic nerve injury. The diaphragmatic muscle is usually present in its normal distribution but is attenuated and nonfunctional.

An eventration may be completely asymptomatic and noted only on chest radiograph. Clinical findings may range from mild respiratory compromise with wheezing, frequent respiratory infections, and exercise intolerance to extreme respiratory distress. Diagnosis is usually made by fluoroscopic examination of the chest with examination of diaphragmatic motion. In such cases, the diaphragm moves paradoxically with respiration. A small or asymptomatic eventration may be left untreated and observed. An eventration that involves a large area of the diaphragm may adversely affect pulmonary function and lung growth and should be repaired. When an acquired nerve palsy is present, initial treatment may be expectant. However, if the respiratory status of the infant remains compromised after several weeks of observation, surgical intervention should be considered. Repair may be through either the abdomen or the chest, but in most cases a low thoracotomy is preferred.[135] The procedure may be performed with minimally invasive techniques. The diaphragm is plicated with nonabsorbable sutures placed in a radial pattern. The redundant diaphragmatic tissue is reefed up until it is taut. Proper suture placement is important to prevent additional injury to the phrenic nerve branches within the diaphragmatic tissue.

Diaphragm Pacing

Ventilator-dependent children with spinal cord injury or central hypoventilation syndromes may benefit from diaphragm pacing.[136] The application of repetitive stimulus patterns to the phrenic nerves causes rhythmic contractions of the diaphragm. Phrenic nerve electrodes are implanted at the cervical or intrathoracic level. Receivers are implanted in subcutaneous pockets, and an external microprocessor-controlled transmitter-antenna assembly activates the receiver. Patients with injured phrenic nerves (high spinal cord injury) may benefit from diaphragm pacing after intercostal to phrenic nerve transfer.[137]

PLEURAL DISEASES

Empyema

Empyema is an accumulation of purulent material within the pleural space. In children empyema occurs most often as a sequela of bacterial pneumonia. Empyema develops when a parapneumonic effusion becomes infected or necrotizing pneumonia erodes through the lung into the pleural space. Empyema may also develop after penetrating thoracic trauma, intrathoracic or cervical esophageal perforation, or surgery on the chest. Empyema is divided into three stages (i.e., *exudative:* thin free-flowing fluid with a low cell count; *fibrinopurulent:* thick purulent material resulting in multiple loculations and encasement of the lung parenchyma; *organizing:* fibroblasts have grown into the exudate and produced a fibrotic peel). *Haemophilus influenzae, Streptococcus pneumonia,* and *Staphylococcus aureus* are the most common pathogens in pediatric pneumonia, and anaerobes, gram-negative bacteria, and atypical organisms also occasionally are found. The signs and symptoms of an empyema in a child are usually those of worsening pneumonia with fever, tachypnea, shortness of breath, and sometimes cyanosis. Abdominal pain with distention and ileus may intensify the respiratory difficulty. Diagnosis is confirmed by the presence of pleural fluid on conventional chest radiographs (Fig. 109.24A). CT scan of the chest cavity is the best method for determining the extent of loculated effusion and underlying parenchymal involvement (Fig. 109.24B). Diagnostic paracentesis may be helpful.

When a small parapneumonic effusion develops, it may resolve with antibiotics alone. Larger effusions require adequate pleural space drainage with a tube thoracostomy in addition to antibiotic therapy. Instillation of intrapleural streptokinase or urokinase has been utilized for loculated effusions, but the failure rate is high.

In patients who do not respond to such therapy, surgical débridement of infected material surrounding the lung may be required. Video-assisted thoracoscopic decortication/pneumolysis and pleural débridement has proved to be very effective in the treatment of pediatric empyema (Fig. 109.24C,D). Early treatment with video-assisted thoracoscopic surgery (VATS) may shorten hospitalization and result in more rapid recovery.[138,139]

Pneumothorax

Spontaneous pneumothorax is seen in previously healthy older children and teenagers who are usually tall and thin. They often have apical blebs seen on chest radiographs. CT scanning is more sensitive to detect bleb disease. Pneumothorax may also complicate advanced pulmonary disease resulting from cystic fibrosis. Other causes include both blunt and penetrating thoracic trauma, severe asthmatic attack, and pulmonary infection. The classic presentation of a spontaneous pneumothorax is the sudden onset of chest pain and shortness of breath.

Diagnosis is best confirmed by chest radiograph. In patients with significant symptoms, tube thoracostomy should be performed immediately and the chest tube placed to water seal suction drainage.

Recurrent pneumothoraces can be treated nonoperatively with the intrapleural instillation of various sclerosing agents such as talc or tetracycline through the chest tube. Patients with recurrent pneumothorax and apical blebs are treated with apicectomy and pleurodesis/pleurectomy. This may be performed through a standard thoracotomy or with VATS.

Chylothorax

In the newborn, chylothorax may occur in association with manipulation during a difficult delivery, from a malformation of the thoracic duct, or spontaneously without an obvious cause. In older infants and children, cardiothoracic procedures can be complicated by postoperative chylothorax in 0.5% of cases. The thoracic duct has also been known to

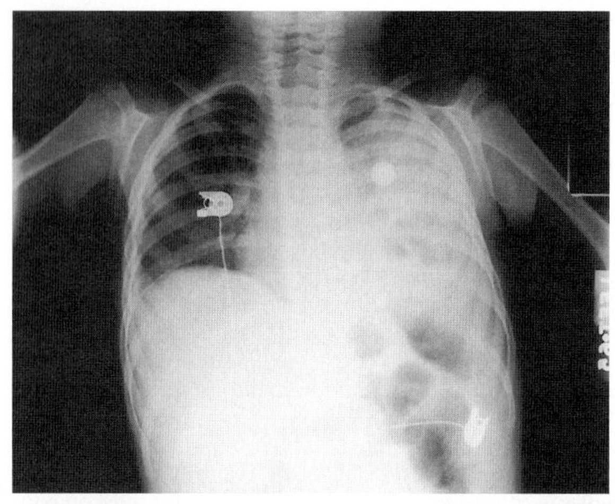
A

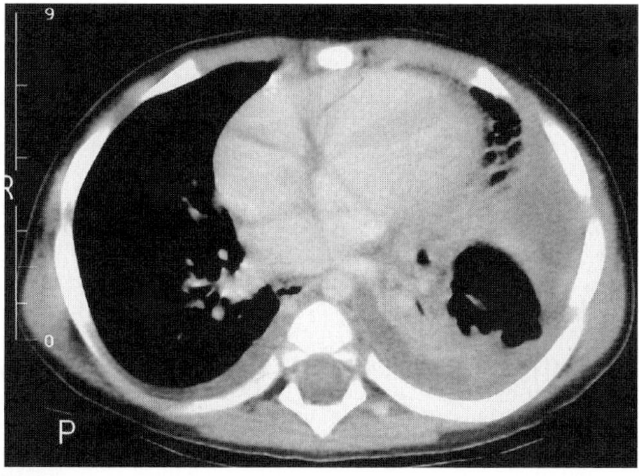

B

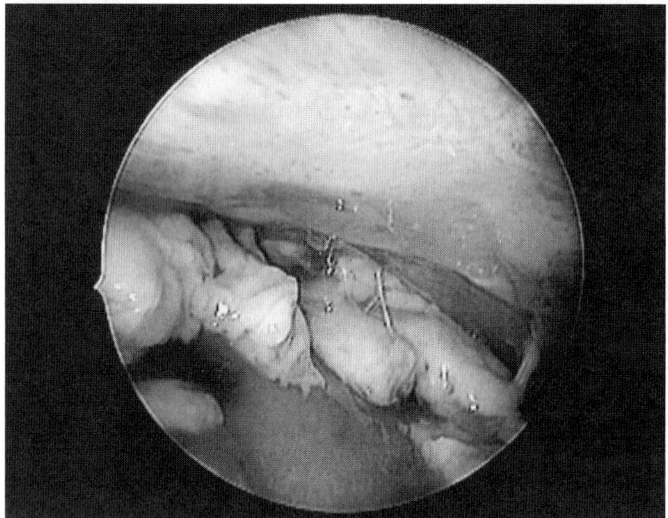
C

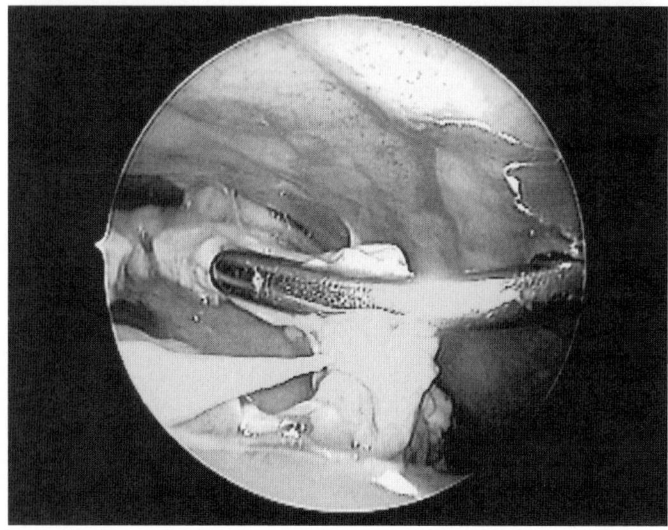
D

FIGURE 109.24 Video-assisted thoracoscopic treatment of complicated empyema in children. (*A*) Chest radiograph of a 2-year-old child presenting with pneumonia and pleural effusion. (*B*) Computed tomography image demonstrates complicated pneumonia with loculated empyema. (*C*) Video endoscopic view of organized empyema debris. (*D*) Decortication procedure includes removal of all loculated, organized debris from the hemithorax. All surfaces of the visceral and parietal pleura are accessible using video-endoscopic techniques. (*E*) Immediate postoperative chest radiograph shows the expected residual parenchymal lung disease. (*F*) Chest radiograph findings have resolved 1 month later.

rupture during violent bouts of coughing or with hyperextension of the spine. Obstruction or erosion of the duct may occur as a result of malignant disease, such as lymphoma, within the mediastinum. Other causes include inflammatory processes, subclavian vein thrombosis, and misplaced central venous devices.

A defect in the lower portion of the duct frequently results in an effusion into the right pleural space, whereas an effusion on the left results from a defect in the upper region of the duct. Clinically, the patient presents with a large pleural effusion resulting in pulmonary compression, mediastinal displacement, and the progressive development of respiratory distress. Radiographs generally show a massive effusion on the evolved side. The diagnosis should be suspected at the initial thoracentesis with the retrieval of milky, lipid-laden fluid.

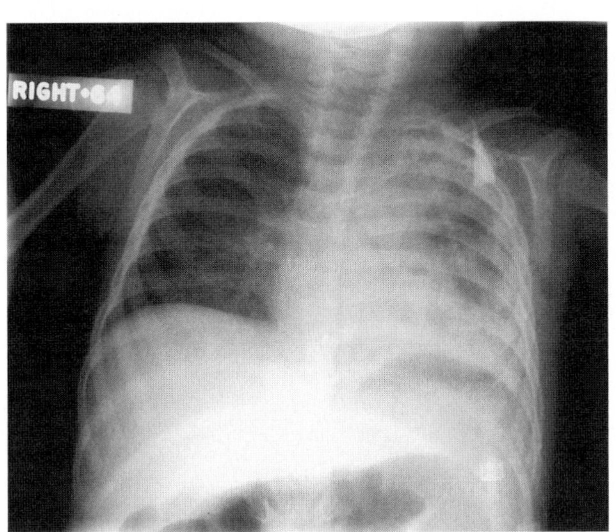

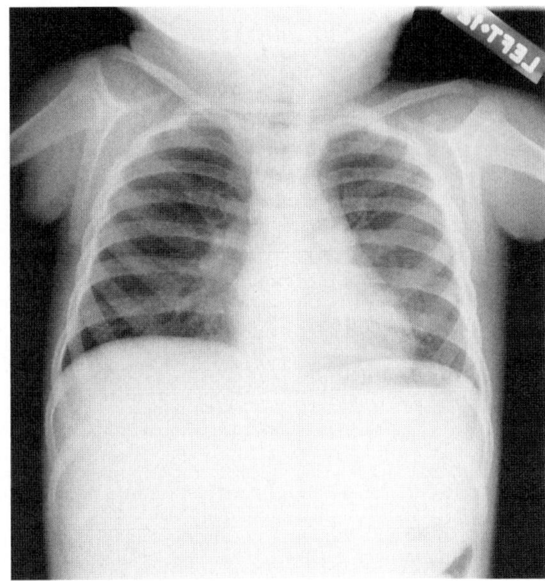

E F

FIGURE 109.24 (*Continued*)

Initial treatment consists of tube thoracostomy for evacuation of the chylous fluid and expansion of the collapsed lung. Minimizing the flow of lymph within the thoracic duct by placing the patient on complete bowel rest using parenteral nutrition has been shown to permit healing of the thoracic duct lymph fistula over time. With newborns, spontaneous chylothorax usually ceases spontaneously with adequate drainage. If no improvement is noted after conservative therapy, then surgical intervention can be considered. Through either an open thoracotomy or with VATS, the surgical therapy involves ligation of the thoracic duct just above the diaphragm within the right chest. This goal can be accomplished with surgical ligation, direct clipping, the use of fibrin glue, and pleurodesis. For intractable conditions, pleural peritoneal shunting can be considered. Somatostatin analogue has been useful in the treatment of chylothorax.[140]

KEY POINTS

- Pectus excavatum results from abnormal regulation of the growth of the costal cartilages with a corresponding posterior curve in the body of the sternum beginning at the manubrium and extending to the xiphoid; the deformity is rarely precisely symmetric, with one side (usually the right) slightly more curved in than the other.
- Pectus excavatum repair should occur in late childhood or adolescence and is now most frequently performed with a rigid transversely oriented bar (Lorenze bar) that pushes the deformity back into place.
- Pectus carinatum occurs less frequently than pectus excavatum and does not cause physiologic impairment; for operative repair, osteotomies and sternal fracture are performed in such a way as to depress the sternum.
- Pulmonary sequestrations are abnormal lung tissue with anomalous systemic blood supply that can be either intralobar or extralobar lesions based on their relationship with the investing visceral pleura and adjacent normal lung tissue. They do not communicate normally with the trachea or a bronchus.
- Congenital cystic adenomatoid malformations (CCAMs) have a normal vascular supply and communicate with the normal tracheobronchial tree. They result from excessive proliferation of bronchial structures without the development of the corresponding alveoli.
- Benign cysts of the mediastinum are relatively common and include thymic cysts, enterogenous cysts, dermoid cysts, pericardial cysts, and lymphatic malformations (cystic hygromas); resection is usually recommended because of the possibility of progressive enlargement with compression, hemorrhage, or infection.
- Primary lung tumors in children include bronchial adenoma, rarely bronchogenic carcinoma, pulmonary blastoma, inflammatory pseudotumor (composed of inflammatory cells), and hamartoma. Resection is generally appropriate initial therapy.
- Mediastinal tumors include neurogenic tumors (usually from the sympathetic chain), lymphoma (Hodgkin or non-Hodgkin), teratoma, neurilemmoma, sarcoma, and thymic tumors.
- Tracheoesophageal fistula can occur as esophageal atresia with proximal pouch and distal tracheoesophageal fistula (most common—at 85% to 95%); esophageal atresia without fistula (5% to 7%); tracheoesophageal fistula without esophageal atresia H-type—(2% to 6%), and rarer forms of this anomaly including esophageal atresia with proximal tracheoesophageal fistula and esophageal atresia with both proximal and distal tracheoesophageal fistula.
- Vascular rings result from faulty embryogenesis of the aortic arch and great vessels resulting in vascular structures and dense connective tissue that surround the esophagus and trachea and can result in symptoms of airway or esophageal obstruction.
- Approximately 200 children die from foreign body aspiration or ingestion each year. Bronchoscopic evaluation and foreign body removal are performed in the operating room under general anesthesia where the rigid bronchoscope with optical forceps can be used to remove most aspirated foreign bodies safely.
- Left-sided congenital diaphragmatic hernia is a 2- to 4-cm posterolateral defect in the diaphragm through which the abdominal viscera have translocated into the ipsilateral thoracic cavity. Through a right-sided defect, the large right lobe of the liver can occupy most of the hemithorax.
- Congenital diaphragmatic hernia (CDH) is a *physiologic* emergency, and not a *surgical* emergency. The newborn with CDH should be stabilized by nonsurgical means and delayed, well-planned surgical repair undertaken subsequently.

References

1. Sadler TW. Embryology of the sternum. *Chest Surg Clin North Am.* 2000;10:237–244.
2. Kowalewski J, Brocki M, Dryjanski T, et al. Pectus excavatum: increase of right ventricular systolic, diastolic, and stroke volumes after surgical repair. *J Thorac Cardiovasc Surg.* 1999;118:87–93.
3. Shamberger RC. Congenital chest wall deformities. In O'Neill JA Jr, Rowe MI, Grosfeld JL, et al., eds. *Pediatric surgery*, 5th ed. St. Louis: Mosby, 1998.
4. Sigalet DL, Montgomery M, Harder J. Cardiopulmonary effects of closed repair of pectus excavatum. *J Pediatr Surg.* 2003;38:380–385.
5. Shamberger RC. Cardiopulmonary effects of anterior chest wall deformities. *Chest Surg Clin North Am.* 2000;10:245–252.
6. Malek MH, Fonkalsrud EW, Cooper CB. Ventilatory and cardiovascular responses to exercise in patients with pectus excavatum. *Chest* 2003;124: 870–882.
7. Haller JA Jr, Scherer LR, Turner CS, et al. Evolving management of pectus excavatum based on a single institutional experience of 664 patients. *Ann Surg.* 1989;209:578–582.
8. Haller JA Jr, Colombani PM, Humphries CT, et al. Chest wall constriction after too extensive and too early operations for pectus excavatum. *Ann Thorac Surg.* 1996;61:1618–1625.
9. Weber TR, Kurkchubasche AG. Operative management of asphyxiating thoracic dystrophy after pectus repair. *J Pediatr Surg.* 1998;33:262–265.
10. Ravitch MM. The chest wall. In Welch KJ, Randolph JG, Ravitch MM, et al., eds. *Pediatric surgery*, 4th ed. Chicago: Year Book.
11. Komuro Y, Masuda T, Kobayashi S, et al. Endoscopic correction of pectus excavatum. *Ann Plastic Surg.* 1999;43:232–238.
12. **Nuss D, Kelly RE Jr, Croitoru DP, et al. A 10-year review of a minimally invasive technique for the correction of pectus excavatum. *J Pediatr Surg.* 1998;33:545–552.**
13. **Croitoru DP, Kelly RE Jr, Goretsky MJ, et al. Experience and modification update for the minimally invasive Nuss technique for pectus excavatum repair in 303 patients. *J Pediatr Surg.* 2002;37:437–445.**
14. Moss RL, Albanese CT, Reynolds M. Major complications after minimally invasive repair of pectus excavatum: case reports. *J Pediatr Surg.* 2001;36:155–158.
15. Ostlie DJ, Marosky JK, Spilde TL, et al. Evaluation of pectus bar position and osseous bone formation. *J Pediatr Surg.* 2003;38:953–956.
16. Horch RE, Springer O. Minimally-invasive endoscopic correction of funnel chest deformity via an umbilical incision. *Aesthetic Plast Surg.* 2002; 26:295–298.
17. Marks MW, Iacobucci J. Reconstruction of congenital chest wall deformities using solid silicone onlay prostheses. *Chest Surg Clin North Am.* 2000;10:341–355.
18. Schier F, Bahr M, Klobe E. The vacuum chest wall lifter: an innovative, nonsurgical addition to the management of pectus excavatum. *J Pediatr Surg.* 2005;40:496–500.
19. Egan JC, DuBois JJ, Morphy M, et al. Compressive orthotics in the treatment of asymmetric pectus carinatum: a preliminary report with an objective radiographic marker. *J Pediatr Surg.* 2000;35:1183–1186.
20. Luck SR, Reynolds M, Raffensperger JG. *Curr Probl Surg.* Chicago, Year Book Medical Publishers, 1986.
21. Coran AG, Drongowski R. Congenital cystic disease of the tracheobronchial tree in infants and children. *Arch Surg.* 1994;129:521–527.
22. Conran RM, Stocker JT. Extralobar sequestration with frequently associated congenital cystic adenomatoid malformation, type 2: report of 50 cases. *Pediatr Dev Pathol.* 1999;2:454–463.
23. Gross E, Chen MK, Lobe TE, et al. Infradiaphragmatic extralobar pulmonary sequestration masquerading as an intra-abdominal, suprarenal mass. *Pediatr Surg Int.* 1997;12:529–531.
24. Stocker JT, Madewell JE, Drake RM. Congenital cystic adenomatoid malformation of the lung: classification and morphologic spectrum. *Hum Pathol.* 1977;8:155–171.
25. Adzick NS, Flake AW, Crombleholme TM. Management of congenital lung lesions. *Semin Pediatr Surg.* 2003;12:10–16.
26. Adzick NS, Harrison MR, Crombleholme TM, et al. Fetal lung lesions: management and outcome. *Am J Obstet Gynecol.* 1998;179:884–889.
27. van Leeuwen K, Teitelbaum DH, Hirschl RB, et al. Prenatal diagnosis of congenital cystic adenomatoid malformation and its postnatal presentation, surgical indications, and natural history. *J Pediatr Surg.* 1999;34: 794–798.
28. Bagolan P, Nahom A, Giorlandino C, et al. Cystic adenomatoid malformation of the lung: clinical evolution and management. *Eur J Pediatr.* 1999;158:879–882.
29. Mentzer SJ, Filler RM, Phillips J. Limited pulmonary resections for congenital cystic adenomatoid malformation of the lung. *J Pediatr Surg.* 1992;27:1410–1413.
30. Merry C, Spurbeck W, Lobe TE. Resection of foregut-derived duplications by minimal-access surgery. *Pediatr Surg Int.* 1999;15(3-4):224–226.
31. Dillon PW, Cilley RE, Krummel TM. Video assisted thoracoscopic excision of intrathoracic masses in children: report of two cases. *Surg Laparosc Endosc.* 1993;3:433–436.
32. Scully RE, Mark EJ, McNeely WF, et al. Case records of the Massachusetts General Hospital—Case 30-1997. *N Engl J Med.* 1997;337:916–924.
33. Nuchtern JG, Harberg FJ. Congenital lung cysts. *Semin Pediatr Surg.* 1994;3:233–243.
34. Stigers KB, Woodring JH, Kanga JF. The clinical and imaging spectrum of findings in patients with congenital lobar emphysema. *Pediatr Pulmonol.* 1992;14:160–170.
35. Karnak I, Senocak ME, Ciftci AO, et al. Congenital lobar emphysema: diagnostic and therapeutic considerations. *J Pediatr Surg.* 1999;34:1347–1351.
36. **Davenport M, Warne SA, Cacciaguerra S, et al. Current outcome of antenally diagnosed cystic lung disease. *J Pediatr Surg.* 2004;39:549–556.**
37. Rothenberg SS. Thoracoscopy in infants and children. *Semin Pediatr Surg.* 1998;7:194–201.
38. Black CT. Current recommendations for the resection of pulmonary metastases of pediatric malignancies. *Pediatr Pulmonol.* 1997;16(suppl):181.
39. La Quaglia. The surgical management of metastases in pediatric cancer. *Semin Pediatr Surg.* 1993;2:75–82.
40. Hartman GE, Shochat SJ. Primary pulmonary neoplasms of childhood: a review. *Ann Thorac Surg.* 1983;36:108–119.
41. Hancock BJ, DiLorenzo M, Youssef S, et al. Childhood primary pulmonary neoplasms. *J Pediatr Surg.* 1993;28:1133–1136.
42. Ohye RG, Cohen DM, Caldwell S, et al. Pediatric bronchioloalveolar carcinoma: a favorable pediatric malignancy? *J Pediatr Surg.* 1998;33: 730–732.
43. Granata C, Gambini C, Balducci T, et al. Bronchioloalveolar carcinoma arising in congenital cystic adenomatoid malformation in a child: a case report and review on malignancies originating in congenital cystic adenomatoid malformation. *Pediatr Pulmonol.* 1998;25:62–66.
44. Mentzel T, Fletcher CDM. Recent advances in soft tissue tumor diagnosis. *Am J Clin Pathol.* 1998;110:660–670.
45. Su W, Ko A, O'Connell TX, et al. Treatment of pseudotumors with nonsteroidal antiinflammatory drugs. *J Pediatr Surg.* 2000;35:1635–1637.
46. Eggli KD, Newman B. Nodules, masses and pseudomasses in the pediatric lung. *Radiol Clin North Am.* 1993;31:651.
47. Grosfeld JL, Skinner MA, Rescorla FJ, et al. Mediastinal tumors in children: experience with 196 cases. *Ann Surg Oncol.* 1994;1:121–127.
48. Glick RD, LaQuaglia MP. Lymphomas of the anterior mediastinum. *Semin Pediatr Surg.* 1999;8:69–77.
49. Taneli C, Genc A, Erikci V, et al. Askin tumors in children: a report of four cases. *Eur J Pediatr Surg.* 1998;8:312–314.
50. Sawin RS, Conrad EU III, Park JR, et al. Preresection chemotherapy improves survival for children with Askin tumors. *Arch Surg.* 1996;131: 877–880.
51. Kashima HK, Mounts P, Shah K. Recurrent respiratory papillomatosis. *Obstet Gynecol Clin North Am.* 1996;131:877–880.
52. **Armstrong LR, Derkay CS, Reeves WC. Initial results from the national registry for juvenile-onset recurrent respiratory papillomatosis. RRP Task Force. *Arch Otolaryngol Head Neck Surg.* 1999;125:743–748.**
53. Haight C, Towsley HA. Congenital atresia of the esophagus with tracheoesophageal fistula: extrapleural ligation of fistula and end-to-end anastomosis of esophageal segments. *Surg Gynecol Obstet.* 1943;76:672–688.
54. Manning PB, Morgan RA, Coran AG, et al. Fifty years' experience with esophageal atresia and tracheoesophageal fistula. Beginning with Cameron Haight's first operation in 1935. *Ann Surg.* 1986;204:446–451.
55. Oi BQ, Beasley SW. Pathohistological study of adriamycin-induced tracheal agenesis in the fetal rat. *Pediatr Surg Int.* 1999;15:17–20.
56. Possogel AK, Diez-Pardo JA, Morales C, et al. Embryology of esophageal atresia in the adriamycin rat model. *J Pediatr Surg.* 1998;33:606–612.
57. Haight C. Congenital esophageal atresia and trachesophageal fistula. In: Mustard WT, et al., eds. *Pediatric surgery.* Chicago: Year Book Medical Publishers, 1969.
58. Gross RE. *The surgery of infancy and childhood.* Philadelphia: WB Saunders, 1953.
59. Kluth D. Atlas of esophageal atresia. *J Pediatr Surg.* 1976;11:901–919.
60. Waterson DJ, Bonham-Carter RE, Aberdeen E. Esophageal atresia: tracheo-oesophageal fistula. A study of survival in 218 infants. *Lancet* 1962;1:819–822.
61. Randolph JG, Newman KD, Anderson KD. Current results in repair of esophageal atresia with tracheoesophageal fistula using physiologic status as a guide to therapy. *Ann Surg.* 1989;209:526–530.
62. Choudhury SR, Ashcraft KW, Sharp RJ, et al. Survival of patients with esophageal atresia: influence of birth weight, cardiac anomaly, and late respiratory complications. *J Pediatr Surg.* 1999;34:70–74.
63. Dunn JC, Fonkalsrud EW, Atkinson JB. Simplifying the Waterston's stratification of infants with tracheoesophageal fistula. *Am Surg.* 1999; 65:908–910.
64. **Deurloo JA, de Vos R, Ekkelkamp S, et al. Prognostic factors for mortality of oesophageal atresia patients: Waterston revived. *Eur J Pediatr.* 2004;163:624–625.**
65. Cilley RE, Dillon PW. Pulmonary resection and thoracotomy. In Stringer MD et al., eds. *Pediatric surgery and urology: long term outcomes.* London: W B Saunders Company Limited, 1998.
66. **Foker JE, Kendall TC, Catton K, et al. A flexible approach to achieve a true primary repair for all infants with esophageal atresia. *Semin Pediatr Surg.* 2005;14:8–15.**

67. Spitz L, Kiely E, Pierro A. Gastric transposition in children—a 21 year experience. *J Pediatr Surg.* 2004;39:276–281.
68. Puri P, Khurana S. Delayed primary esophageal anastomosis for pure esophageal atresia. *Semin Pediatr Surg.* 1998;7:126–129.
69. Othersen HB Jr, Hebra A, Tagge EP. Esophageal replacement for atresia without fistula. *Semin Pediatr Surg.* 1998;7:134–136.
70. Lobe TE, Rothenberg S, Waldschmidt J, et al. Thoracoscopic repair of esophageal atresia in an infant: a surgical first. *Pediatric Endosurgery and Innovative Techniques* 1999;3:141–148.
71. Rothenberg SS. Thoracoscopic repair of tracheoesophageal fistula in newborns. *J Pediatr Surg.* 2002;37:869–872.
72. Spitz L. Esophageal atresia: past, present, and future. *J Pediatr Surg.* 1996;31:19–25.
73. Bouman NH, Koot HM, Hazebroek FW. Long-term physical, psychological, and social functioning of children with esophageal atresia. *J Pediatr Surg.* 1999;34:399–404.
74. Tonz M, Kohli S, Kaiser G. Oesophageal atresia: what has changed in the last 3 decades? *Pediatr Surg Int.* 2004;20:768–772.
75. Orford J, Cass DT, Glasson MJ. Advances in the treatment of oesophageal atresia over three decades: the 1970s and the 1990s. *Pediatr Surg Int.* 2004; 20:402–407.
76. **Little DC, Rescorla FJ, Grosfeld JL, et al. Long-term analysis of children with esophageal atresia and tracheoesophageal fistula. *J Pediatr Surg.* 2003;38:852–856.**
77. Beasley SW. Esophageal atresia: surgical aspects. In: Stringer MD et al, eds. *Pediatric surgery and urology: long term outcomes.* London: WB Saunders, 1998.
78. Rutter MJ, Cotton RT, Azizkhan RG, et al. Slide tracheoplasty for the management of complete tracheal rings. *J Pediatr Surg.* 2003;38: 928–934.
79. Backer CL, Mavroudis C, Holinger LD. Repair of congenital tracheal stenosis. *Semin Thorac Cardiovasc Surg. Pediatr Card Surg Annu.* 2002; 5:173–186.
80. **Manning PB, Wesley JR, Polley TZ, et al. Esophageal and tracheobronchial foreign bodies in infants and children. *Pediatr Surg Int.* 2:346, 1987.**
81. National Safety Council Accident Facts. http://www.nsc.org. February, 2000.
82. McCauley G. An account of viscera herniation. *Phil Trans R Coll Phys.* 1754;6:25.
83. Bochdalek VA. Einige Betrachtungen uber die Enstehung des angeborenen Zwerfekkbruches. *Als Bietrag Zur pathologischen Anatomie der Hernien vjscher Prakt Heilk* 1848;18:89.
84. Ladd WE, Gross RE. Congenital diaphragmatic hernia. *N Engl J Med.* 1940;223:917.
85. Gross RE. Congenital hernia of the diaphragm. *Am J Dis Child.* 1946;71:579.
86. Cilley RE. Invited commentary. Weber TR, Kountzman B, Dillon PA, et al. Improved survival in congenital diaphragmatic hernia with evolving therapeutic strategies. *Arch Surg.* 1998;133:503.
87. Cilley RE. Respiratory physiology and extracorporeal life support. In: Oldham KT, Foglia RP, Colombani PM, eds. *Surgery of infants and children: scientific principles and practice.* Philadelphia: Lippincott-Raven Publishers, 1997, pp. 183–222.,
88. DiFiore JW, Wilson JM. Lung development. *Semin Pediatr Surg.* 1994;3:221–232.
89. Davies GM, Reid L. Growth of the alveoli and pulmonary arteries in childhood. *Thorax* 1970;25:669–681.
90. Chinoy MR. Lung growth and development. *Front Biosci.* 2003;8:d392.
91. Chinoy MR. Pulmonary hypoplasia and congenital diaphragmatic hernia: advances in the pathogenetics and regulation of lung development. *J Surg Res.* 2002;106:209.
92. Moore KL. *The developing human,* 3rd ed. Philadelphia: WB Saunders, 1982.
93. Iritani I. Experimental study on embryogenesis of congenital diaphragmatic hernia. *Anat Embryol.* 1984;169:133–139.
94. Stolar CJH, Dillon PW. Congenital diaphragmatic hernia and eventration. In: O'Neill JA, Rowe MI, Grosfeld JL, et al. ed. *Pediatric surgery,* 5th ed. St. Louis: Mosby-Year Book, 1998.
95. **Dott MM, Wong LY, Rasmussen SA. Population-based study of congenital diaphragmatic hernia: risk factors and survival in Metropolitan Atlanta, 1968–1999. *Birth Defects Res A Clin Mol Teratol.* 2003; 67:261.**
96. Greer JJ, Babiuk RP, Thebaud B. Etiology of congenital diaphragmatic hernia: the retinoid hypothesis. *Pediatr Res.* 2003;53:726.
97. deLorimer AA, Tierney DF, Parker HR. Hypoplastic lungs in fetal lambs with surgically produced congenital diaphragmatic hernia. *Surgery* 1967;62:12–17.
98. Harrison MR, Jester JA, Ross NA. Correction of congenital diaphragmatic hernia *in utero.* I. The model: intrathoracic balloon produces fatal pulmonary hypoplasia. *Surgery* 1980;88:174–182.
99. Brandsma AE. *Lung development in congenital diaphragmatic hernia.* Rotterdam: Offsetdrukkerij Ridderprint B.V., 1995.
100. Cilley RE, Zgleszewski SE, Krummel TM, et al. Nitrofen dose-dependent gestational day-specific murine lung hypoplasia and left-sided diaphragmatic hernia. *Am J Physiol.: 272 (Lung Cell. Mol. Physiol.* 16): L362–L371, 1997.
101. Keller RL, Aaroz PA, Hawgood S, et al. MR imaging of hepatic pulmonary fusion in neonates. *AJR Am J Roentgenol.* 2003;180:438.
102. Tibboel D, Hazebroek F, Mooi W, eds. Pathogenetic and experimental aspects of congenital diaphragmatic hernia. Netherlands Symposium, Erasmus University Rotterdam May 3–5, 1999.
103. Hubbard AM, Crombleholme TM, Adzick NS, et al. Prenatal MRI evaluation of congenital diaphragmatic hernia. *Am J Perinatol.* 1999; 16:407.
104. Leung JW, Coakley FV, Hricak H, et al. Prenatal MR imaging of congenital diaphragmatic hernia. *AJR Am J Roentgenol.* 2000;174:1607.
105. Kasales CJ, Coulson CC, Meilstrup JW, et al. Diagnosis and differentiation of congenital diaphragmatic hernia from other noncardiac thoracic fetal masses. *Am J Perinatol.* 1998;15:623–628.
106. Keller RL, Glidden DV, Paek BW, et al. The lung-to-head ratio and fetoscopic temporary tracheal occlusion: prediction of survival in severe left congenital diaphragmatic hernia. *Ultrasound Obstet Gynecol.* 2003;21:244.
107. Laudy JA, Van Gucht M, Van Dooren MF, et al. Congenital diaphragmatic hernia: evaluation of the prognostic value of the lung-to-head ratio and other prenatal parameters. *Prenat Diagn.* 2003;23:634.
108. Lipshutz GS, Albanese CT, Feldstein VA, et al. Prospective analysis of lung-to-head ratio predicts survival for patients with prenatally diagnosed congenital diaphragmatic hernia. *J Pediatr Surg.* 1997;32:1634.
109. Harrison MR, Mychaliska GB, Albanese CT, et al. Correction of congenital diaphragmatic hernia in utero X: fetuses with poor prognosis (liver herniation and low lung-to-head ratio) can be saved by fetoscopic temporary tracheal occlusion. *J Pediatr Surg.* 1998;33:1017–1023.
110. Wung JT, Sahni R, Moffitt ST, et al. Congenital diaphragmatic hernia: survival treated with very delayed surgery, spontaneous respiration, and no chest tube. *J Pediatr Surg.* 1995;30:406–409.
111. Boloker J, Bateman DA, Wung JT, et al. Congenital diaphragmatic hernia in 120 infants treated consecutively with permissive hypercapnea/spontaneous respiration/elective repair. *J Pediatr Surg.* 2002;37:357.
112. Lally KP, Lally PA, Langham MR, et al. Congenital Diaphragmatic Hernia Study Group: Surfactant does not improve survival rate in preterm infants with congenital diaphragmatic hernia. *J Pediatr Surg.* 2004;39:829.
113. Finer NN, Barrington KJ. Nitric oxide for respiratory failure in infants born at or near term. *Cochrane Database Syst Rev.* 2001;CD 000399.
114. Moyer V, Moya F, Tibboel R, et al. Late versus early surgical correction for congenital diaphragmatic hernia in newborn infants. *Cochrane Database Syst Rev.* 2002;CD001695.
115. Arca MJ, Barnhart DC, Lelli JL Jr, et al. Early experience with minimally invasive repair of congenital diaphragmatic hernias: results and lessons learned. *J Pediatr Surg.* 2003;38:1563.
116. Fuchs JR, Kaviani A, Oh JT, et al. Diaphragmatic reconstruction with autologous tendon engineered from mesenchymal amniocytes. *J Pediatr Surg.* 2004;39:834–838.
117. Cilley RE, Bartlett RH. Extracorporeal life support for respiratory failure. In: Gravlee GP, ed. *Principles and practice of cardiopulmonary bypass.* Baltimore: Williams and Wilkins, 1993.
118. Lally KP, The CDH Study Group. The use of ECMO for stabilization of infants with congenital diaphragmatic hernia—a report of the CDH Study Group. Presented at the 20th Annual Meeting of the Surgical Section of the American Academy of Pediatrics, October 2002, Boston, MA.
119. Reickert CA, Hirschl RB, Atkinson JB, et al. Congenital diaphragmatic hernia survival and use of extracorporeal life support at selected level III nurseries with multimodality support. *Surgery* 1998;123:305–310.
120. **Dillon PW, Cilley RE, Mauger D, et al. The relationship of pulmonary artery pressure and survival in congenital diaphragmatic hernia. *J Pediatr Surg.* 2004;39:307.**
121. Iocono JA, Cilley RE, Mauger DT, et al. Postnatal pulmonary hypertension after repair of congenital diaphragmatic hernia: predicting risk and outcome. *J Pediatr Surg.* 1999;34:349–353.
122. Muratore CS, Kharasch V, Lund DP, et al. Pulmonary morbidity in 100 survivors of congenital diaphragmatic hernia monitored in a multidisciplinary clinic. *J Pediatr Surg.* 2001;36:133.
123. Kitano Y, Flake AW, Crombleholme TM, et al. Open fetal surgery for life-threatening fetal malformations. *Semin Perinatol.* 1999;23:448–461.
124. Harrison MR, Adzick NS, Flake AW, et al. Correction of congenital diaphragmatic hernia *in utero.* VI. Hard earned lessons. *J Pediatr Surg.* 1993;28:1411–1418.
125. Harrison MR, Adzick NS, Bullard KM, et al. Correction of congenital diaphragmatic hernia in utero VII: a prospective trial. *J Pediatr Surg.* 1997;32:1637–1642.
126. DiFiore JW, Fauza DO, Slavin R, et al. Experimental fetal tracheal ligation reverses the structural and physiological effects of pulmonary hypoplasia in congenital diaphragmatic hernia. *J Pediatr Surg.* 1994;29: 248–257.
127. DiFiore JW, Fauza DO, Slavin R, et al. Experimental fetal tracheal ligation and congenital diaphragmatic hernia: a pulmonary vascular morophometric analysis. *J Pediatr Surg.* 1995;30:917–924.
128. Hedrick MH, Estes JM, Sullivan KM, et al. Plug the lung until it grows (PLUG): a new method to treat congenital diaphragmatic hernia *in utero.* *J Pediatr Surg.* 1994;29:612–617.

129. **Harrison MR, Keller RL, Hawgood SB, et al. A randomized trial of fetal endoscopic tracheal occlusion for severe fetal congenital diaphragmatic hernia. *N Engl J Med.* 2003;349:1916.**
130. Deprest J, Gratacos E, Nicolaides KH, et al. FETO Task Group: Fetoscopic tracheal occlusion (FETO) for severe congenital diaphragmatic hernia: evolution of a technique and preliminary results. *Ultrasound Obstet Gynecol.* 2004;24:121.
131. Hirschl RB. Respiratory failure: current status of experimental therapies. *Semin Pediatr Surg.* 1999;8:155–170.
132. Farber HW, Loscalzo J. Pulmonary arterial hypertension. *N Engl J Med.* 2004;351:1655.
133. Rashid A, Ivy D. Severe paediatric pulmonary hypertension: new management strategies. *Arch Dis Child.* 2005;90:92.
134. Suen HC, Losty P, Donahoe PK, et al. Combined antenatal thyrotropin-releasing hormone and low-dose glucocorticoid therapy improves the pulmonary biochemical immaturity in congenital diaphragmatic hernia. *J Pediatr Surg.* 1994;29:359–363.
135. Cilley RE, Coran AG . Eventration of the diaphragm. In: Spitz L, Coran AG, eds. *Operative surgery*. London: Butterworth-Heinemann, 1995.
136. Dobelle WH, D'Angelo MS, Goetz BF, et al. 200 cases with a new breathing pacemaker dispel myths about diaphragm pacing. *ASAIO J* 1994; 40:M244–252.
137. Krieger LM, Krieger AJ. The intercostal to phrenic nerve transfer: an effective means of reanimating the diaphragm in patients with high cervical spine injury. *Plast Reconstr Surg.* 2000;105:1255–1261.
138. Kalfa N, Allal H, Montes-Tapia F, et al. Ideal timing of thoracoscopic decortication and drainage for empyema in children. *Surg Endosc.* 2004;18:472–477.
139. Gates RL, Caniano DA, Hayes JR, et al. Does VATS provide optimal treatment of empyema in children? A systematic review. *J Pediatr Surg.* 2004;39:381–386.
140. Rasiah SV, Oei J, Lui K. Octreotide in the treatment of congenital chylothorax. *J Paediatr Child Health* 2004;40:585–588.

CHAPTER 110 ■ PEDIATRIC ABDOMEN

THOMAS T. SATO AND KEITH T. OLDHAM

ABDOMINAL WALL DEFECTS

Gastroschisis

Gastroschisis occurs with an incidence rate of 1 in 3,000 to 8,000 live births, and for unknown reasons, the incidence rate is increasing. Infants with gastroschisis tend to be born prematurely, have lower birth weights, and have younger mothers.[1,2] Familial cases of gastroschisis have been reported and are distinctly rare.[3] Associated congenital anomalies are uncommon and occur in about 10% of cases, most commonly intestinal atresia or stenosis. These anomalies are thought to reflect mechanical or vascular compromise to the herniated bowel. Rarely, infants with gastroschisis have complete loss of small bowel secondary to *in utero volvulus*.

The pathophysiology of gastroschisis remains unknown. In normal fetal development, there are two paired umbilical veins; as the intestine returns to the abdominal cavity through the umbilicus, the right umbilical vein undergoes resorption, leaving the left umbilical vein intact. Weakness of the umbilical membrane at the site of umbilical vein resorption may evolve into a hernia, and, in the case of membrane rupture, evisceration of the intestine through the defect may occur. This explanation is consistent with the clinical observation that the abdominal wall defect in gastroschisis almost always is located to the right of the umbilicus. With the advent of routine antenatal ultrasonography, the sequential development of a typical gastroschisis has been documented as a consequence of a ruptured hernia of the umbilical cord in utero.[4] Therefore, this observation suggests that gastroschisis is an isolated mechanical defect of the developing umbilical cord rather than a global defect in embryogenesis.

The amount of bowel eviscerated in gastroschisis can be extensive because the bowel has not undergone complete mesenteric rotation and fixation. Typically, the bowel is thickened and the mesentery may be foreshortened secondary to the inflammatory response induced by direct exposure to amniotic fluid. Given the typical small size of the abdominal wall defect, herniation of the liver in gastroschisis is distinctly unusual (Fig. 110.1).

Omphalocele

Anatomy, Embryology, and Pathophysiology

The incidence rate of omphalocele is estimated to be 1 in 6,000 to 10,000 live births and has been stable over the past several decades. *Omphalocele* is an abdominal wall defect of varying size that is characterized by the presence of herniated visceral contents into a translucent sac. The sac is composed of amniotic membrane, mesenchymal tissue known as

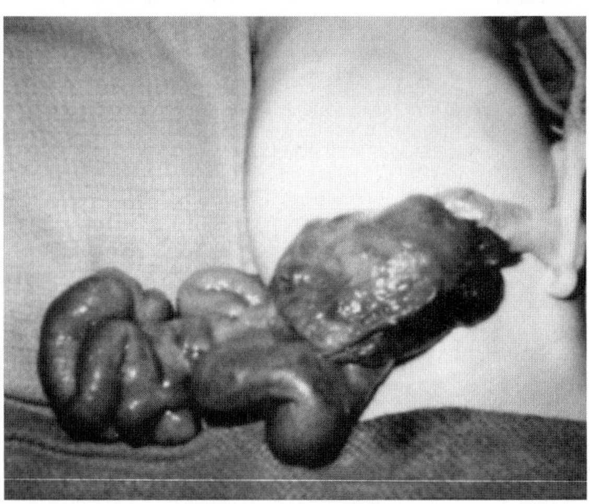

FIGURE 110.1 Gastroschisis. The defect is to the right of the normal umbilicus, and the bowel is thickened and inflamed.

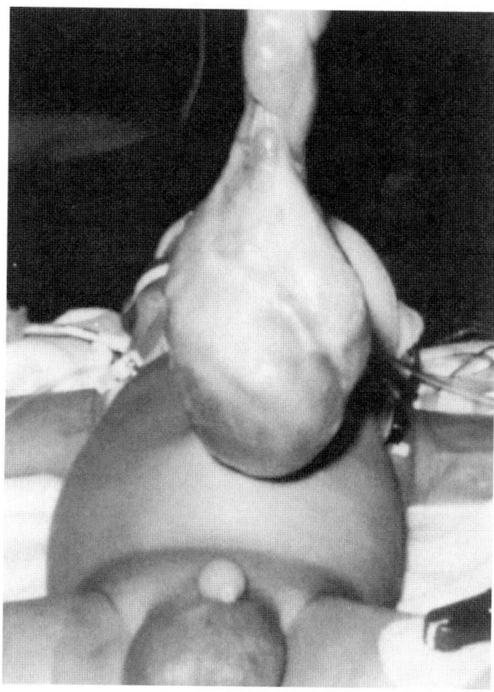

FIGURE 110.2 Omphalocele. The herniated intestines and liver are visible inside the sac. The umbilical cord attaches to the sac.

Wharton's jelly, and peritoneum. The umbilical cord typically attaches to the sac and may be eccentric in origin (Fig. 110.2). The sac may be inadvertently ruptured before or during delivery, but it is always present. Similar to gastroschisis, intestinal malrotation is present. Unlike gastroschisis, the bowel is typically normal in appearance because it has not been directly exposed to the amniotic fluid. Small omphaloceles are typically abdominal wall defects 2 to 5 cm in diameter and may have only a small amount of herniated bowel within the sac. Giant omphaloceles larger than 10 cm in diameter can lead to massive and extensive herniation of the stomach, bowel, liver, and spleen, with subsequent underdevelopment of the abdominal cavity (Fig. 110.3).

Omphalocele is a result of incomplete closure of the anterior abdominal wall at the umbilicus during embryogenesis. During week 4 of gestation, the midgut undergoes progressive elongation in the yolk sac outside the embryonic coelomic cavity. The midgut returns to the abdominal cavity during week 10 of gestation, where it undergoes normal rotation and fixation of its mesentery to the posterior abdominal wall. Normal closure of the anterior abdominal wall requires return of the midgut to the abdominal cavity, along with growth and fusion of the anterior body folds (cephalic, caudal, and two lateral) at the base of the umbilicus. Failure of growth, migration, or fusion of the lateral body folds leads to omphalocele. Failure of growth and fusion of the cephalic folds may lead to either a supraumbilical omphalocele associated with a midline sternal defect and a herniated heart, termed *ectopia cordis*, or a constellation of defects known as the *pentalogy of Cantrell.*[5] This sequence includes a sternal cleft, an absence of the septum transversum of the diaphragm, a pericardial defect, a cardiac defect, and an epigastric omphalocele (Fig. 110.4). Infants born with either ectopia cordis or pentalogy of Cantrell have significant morbidity, and often these conditions are lethal.

Associated anomalies are much more common in infants with omphalocele than with gastroschisis, reflecting the more global abnormality of embryogenesis in omphalocele compared with the simple mechanical defect in gastroschisis. About 50% to 60% of infants with omphalocele have at least one associated congenital anomaly.[6,7] These infants are at moderate to high risk for anomalies of the skeleton, gastrointestinal tract, nervous system, genitourinary system, and cardiopulmonary system. In addition, infants with omphalocele have a higher incidence of chromosomal abnormalities and other conditions, such as Beckwith-Wiedemann syndrome. A comparison of gastroschisis and omphalocele is summarized in Table 110.1.

Perioperative Management for Gastroschisis and Omphalocele

In the absence of fetal distress, whether elective cesarean section improves neonatal outcome in infants with gastroschisis or omphalocele remains controversial.[8,9] Some investigators advocate elective delivery of infants with gastroschisis following the establishment of lung maturity. A prospective study that alternated vaginal delivery with elective cesarean section for infants with gastroschisis demonstrated no significant differences in outcome.[10] To prevent birth-related hepatic injury, cesarean section is preferable for prenatally diagnosed infants with giant omphaloceles.

After delivery, infants with either gastroschisis or omphalocele have similar initial management priorities. Attention must be given to the establishment of an adequate airway with effective ventilation and oxygenation. The infant should be maintained under either an external warmer or a humidified incubator. A nasogastric or orogastric sump tube should be inserted early and placed on suction to prevent further intestinal

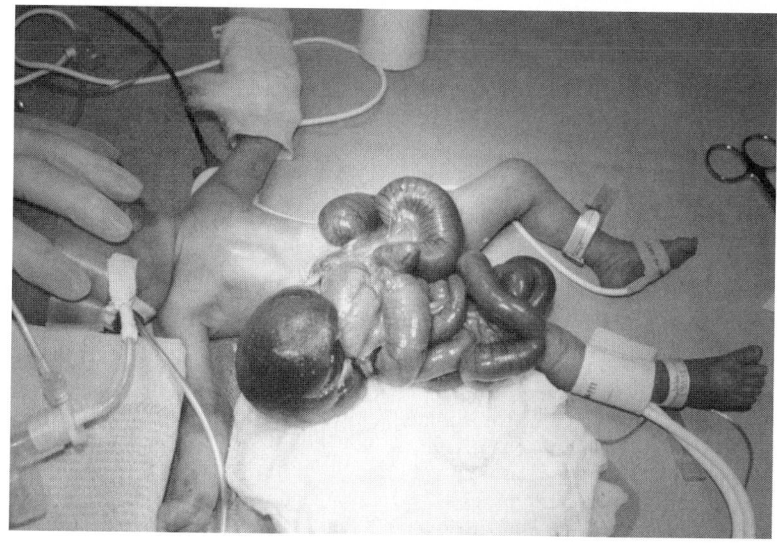

FIGURE 110.3 Ruptured omphalocele. Although the bowel is relatively normal in appearance, the abdominal cavity is extremely underdeveloped.

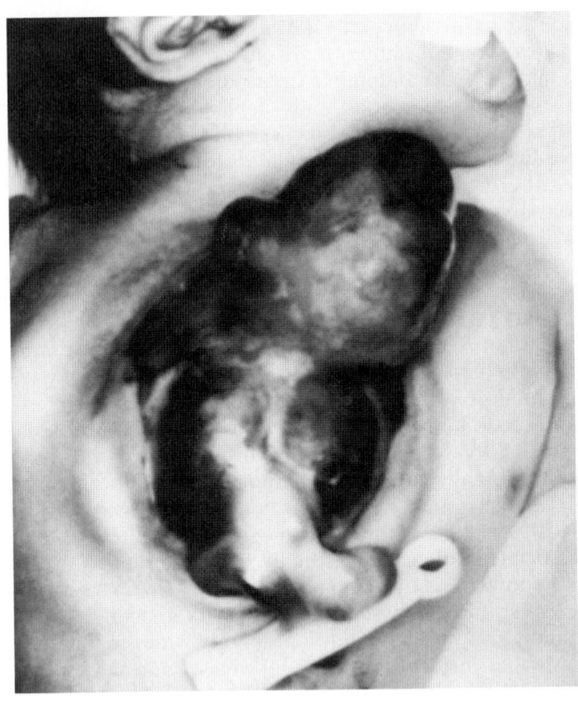

FIGURE 110.4 Pentalogy of Cantrell: sternal cleft, absence of the septum transversum of the diaphragm, pericardial defect, cardiac defect, and an epigastric omphalocele.

distention. The herniated viscera should be covered with warm, saline-soaked gauze and covered with plastic wrap to prevent further contamination; this maneuver also helps to prevent hypothermia and volume depletion. Alternatively, the infant's entire lower torso can be placed inside a plastic bowel bag. Regardless of the method, the initial therapeutic goal is to provide rapid, effective temporary coverage of the viscera. Adequate support of the herniated viscera must be provided to prevent intestinal ischemia. With large omphaloceles, the position of the infant's liver and viscera may impair venous return from the inferior vena cava when the infant is supine, and these infants may preferentially require a left-side-down position to maintain hemodynamic stability. An intravenous catheter should be placed early, and 10% intravenous dextrose, along with broad-spectrum antibiotics, should be administered. Infants with gastroschisis may have higher intravenous fluid requirements secondary to the inflammatory nature of the intestine. If the infant is not delivered at a center

TABLE 110.1 DIAGNOSIS

COMPARISON OF GASTROSCHISIS AND OMPHALOCELE

Characteristic	Gastroschisis	Omphalocele
Defect size (diameter)	2–3 cm	2–15 cm
Sac	Never	Always, may be ruptured
Gestational age	Prematurity	Term common common
Umbilical cord	Left of defect	Attached to sac
Herniated viscera	Small bowel, stomach, colon	Small bowel. stomach, colon, liver
Malrotation	Yes	Yes
Bowel character	Inflammatory, edematous	Normal
Enteral nutrition	Delayed	Normal
Associated anomalies	Uncommon (10% atresia)	Common (50%)

where definitive surgical care can be provided, urgent transport should be arranged.

Given the high incidence of associated anomalies, infants with an intact omphalocele should undergo diagnostic investigation preoperatively, guided by the clinical presentation and physical examination of the infant. These studies include a chest film, echocardiogram, and renal ultrasound, in addition to baseline blood work. Until the decision is made with respect to the timing and method of repair, the omphalocele should remain covered and protected with a dressing. If the omphalocele is ruptured or torn, immediate closure or coverage is necessary.

Once the infant has been stabilized and assessment for other anomalies is complete, the infant is taken to the operating room for correction of the abdominal wall defect. Reduction of the herniated viscera with primary fascial closure of the abdominal wall is an achievable goal in approximately 60% to 70% of infants with either gastroschisis or omphalocele. Gentle but definitive stretching of the abdominal wall is performed, and proximal decompression of the bowel is maintained with nasogastric or orogastric decompression. The defect may require enlargement to evaluate fully the intestinal tract. With omphalocele, the sac is usually resected. The limiting factor in primary closure of an abdominal wall defect is the increased intraabdominal pressure generated by the reduction of the herniated viscera. Increased intraabdominal pressure can lead to a clinical situation known as *abdominal compartment syndrome*. Features of neonatal abdominal compartment syndrome include impaired venous return caused by compression of the inferior vena cava, reduction of sphlanic blood flow leading to mesenteric ischemia, and respiratory compromise secondary to impaired diaphragmatic excursion. Intraoperative measurement of intragastric or intravesical pressure, end-tidal CO_2, or central venous pressure may be helpful in determining the safety of primary abdominal wall closure.[11] If the herniated viscera cannot be reduced primarily, a Silastic pouch or silo is constructed and daily partial reduction of the silo is performed. This technique allows more gradual reduction of the herniated viscera into the abdominal cavity, and complete reduction usually is obtained within 3 to 7 days. The infant then can return to the operating room for removal of the temporary silo with delayed primary closure of the abdominal

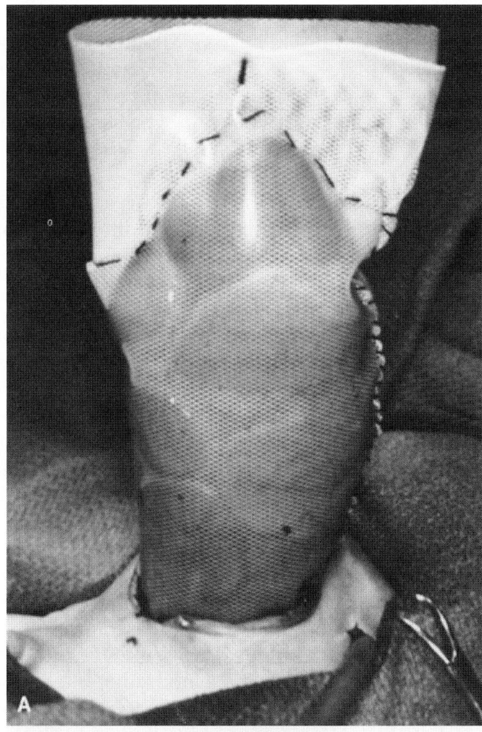

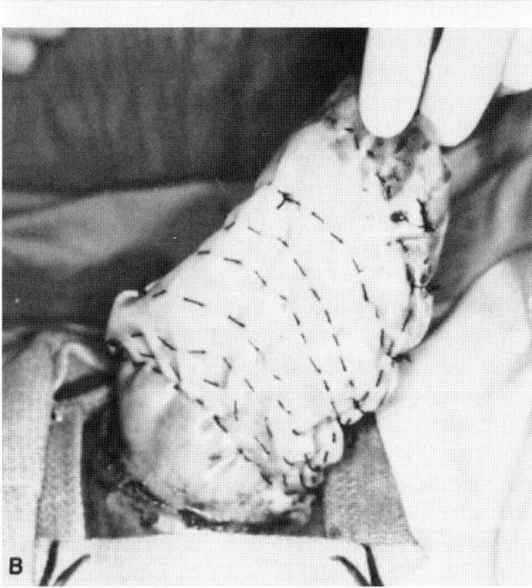

FIGURE 110.5 Silastic chimney or silo for temporary coverage of giant omphalocele.

wall defect (Fig. 110.5). Staged closure of gastroschisis using commercially available Silastic silos has been reported to decrease the risk of long-term bowel dysfunction and need for reoperation by avoiding abdominal compartment syndrome.[12] Alternatively, a large abdominal wall defect may be covered with abdominal skin flaps with delayed repair of the ventral hernia months to years later.

Infants with giant omphaloceles may also be managed nonoperatively. The sac can be physically supported and left intact, allowing epithelialization of the sac over several weeks to months. Antibiotic solutions or ointments are usually applied to control desiccation. Delayed repair of the ventral hernia is required. This delay is particularly useful in the infant with a giant omphalocele and a small, underdeveloped abdominal cavity that prohibits primary closure.

Infants with repaired omphalocele usually have relatively prompt return of bowel function after definitive repair. In comparison, nearly all infants with gastroschisis have a delay in intestinal function following closure. The use of total parenteral nutrition (TPN) is essential in the treatment of these infants because it allows nutritional support while the bowel inflammatory process resolves. It is not unusual for these infants to require up to 4 weeks after repair to have bowel function normalize, and time taken to achieve full enteral feeding is not affected by the use of erythromycin as a prokinetic agent.[13] Approximately 15% of infants with gastroschisis develop necrotizing enterocolitis (NEC), a diffuse, often life-threatening inflammatory complication of the neonatal intestinal tract.[14] In addition, infants with gastroschisis are at risk for nutrient malabsorbtion and intestinal dysmotility with inability to tolerate full enteral feeding. This latter situation can evolve into a long-term condition termed *pseudoobstruction* and may require long-term, sometimes lifelong, dependence on TPN for caloric intake.

Long-term outcome of infants operated on for gastroschisis or omphalocele is usually dependent on the morbidity and mortality of associated conditions rather than the abdominal wall defect itself. Surgical conditions such as undescended testicles, Meckel's diverticulum, and adhesive small bowel obstruction are encountered with moderate frequency. Most children with repaired abdominal wall defects enjoy satisfactory health and quality of life, although they have been reported to have a lower degree of physical fitness measured by exercise time and maximal oxygen consumption.[15]

Umbilical Hernia

Anatomy and Embryology

Congenital umbilical hernia is the most common abdominal wall defect in infants and children. The umbilical ring begins to contract circumferentially after birth and normally is reinforced by the paired lateral umbilical ligaments (the obliterated umbilical arteries), the singular round ligament (the obliterated umbilical vein), the urachus, and the transversalis fascia. Incomplete growth or impaired development of any one of these structures can lead to weakness at the umbilical ring and cause a congenital umbilical hernia.

Clinical Issues and Management

Congenital umbilical hernias generally do not pose significant problems during childhood. Rarely, an umbilical hernia presents with incarceration of intraabdominal contents within the sac.[16] Infants and children may also present with infection or drainage at the umbilicus from associated urachal or vitelline duct remnants. The incidence rate of congenital umbilical hernia has been reported to be 25% to 50% in black infants and 4% to 9% in white infants in the first few months of life.[17] There is an increased incidence of umbilical hernia in premature infants, and there is a tendency for familial inheritance.

Diagnosis of umbilical hernia is usually made after separation of the umbilical cord remnant from the umbilicus and is often initially noted by parents or pediatrician. The defect size may vary from a few millimeters to several centimeters and is typically reducible and asymptomatic. Most umbilical hernias spontaneously close within the first 2 to 3 years of life. Parents should be reassured that complications related to untreated umbilical hernia are rare. Given the high rate of spontaneous closure and the relatively asymptomatic nature of most umbilical hernias, operative repair is generally not performed during the first 2 years of life. Symptoms referable to the hernia, skin maceration, or an episode of incarceration should prompt earlier repair. Large defects with significant protrusion may necessitate surgery, and parents may desire repair if the child appears to be self-conscious about the hernia.

Nearly all umbilical hernia repairs can be performed as outpatient surgical procedures. An incision is made along the umbilicus, and the hernia sac is dissected free circumferentially. The sac is completely excised and primary fascial closure is performed. The umbilical skin is typically preserved and sutured to the fascial closure, and an acceptable cosmetic result is almost always achievable. Large umbilical hernias with redundant skin may require umbilicoplasty. The incidence of complications such as wound infection and recurrence is low.

Inguinal Hernia and Hydrocele

Anatomy, Embryology, and Pathophysiology

Inguinal hernias constitute one of the major surgical problems of infancy and childhood. Inguinal hernia repair is the most common elective general surgical procedure performed by pediatric surgeons. Three distinct anatomic types of inguinal hernias are observed in children: congenital or indirect (99% of infants and children), direct (0.5%), and femoral (<0.5%). An *indirect inguinal hernia* is an abnormal, patent continuation of the peritoneum through the internal inguinal ring. The hernia sac originates lateral to the deep inferior epigastric vessels and descends along the spermatic cord within the cremasteric fascia. The sac can reside completely within the inguinal canal or descend through the external inguinal ring into the scrotum. A *direct inguinal hernia* originates medial to the deep inferior epigastric vessels and is external to the cremasteric fascia. The hernia sac protrudes directly through the posterior wall of the inguinal canal and can descend through the external inguinal ring and into the scrotum. A *femoral hernia* originates medial to the femoral vein and descends inferior to the inguinal ligament along the femoral canal. A femoral hernia never enters the scrotum or labia.

The developing testicle is initially adjacent to the mesonephros and subsequently descends to the scrotum during the third trimester of gestation. The peritoneal extension that descends alongside the chorda gubernaculum of the testicle is called the processus vaginalis. A slightly higher incidence rate of right-sided indirect inguinal hernia is thought to reflect delay of right-sided testicular descent from the developing inferior vena cava and right external iliac vein. As the testicle descends into the scrotum, the processus vaginalis forms a serous covering around the testicle known as the tunica vaginalis. Normally, the patent processus vaginalis undergoes obliteration, closing the communication between the peritoneal cavity and the inguinal canal. A patent processus vaginalis can lead to a variety of anatomic conditions of the inguinal region (Fig. 110.6).

The incidence of patent processus vaginalis has been reported to be as high as 80% to 94% in newborn infants undergoing autopsy,[18] whereas in adulthood, the incidence is 20% to 30%. Infants with unilateral inguinal hernias have been found to have a patent contralateral processus vaginalis in 60% during the first few months of life. By the age of 2 years, 20% of these hernias were obliterated, and half of the remaining 40% became clinical hernias.[19] At least 30% of infants requiring placement of a ventriculoperitoneal shunt for hydrocephalus have been observed to have a patent processus vaginalis in the first few months of life, with a rapid decline in patency in older children.[20] These studies demonstrate that although a patent processus vaginalis is common in infancy, there is some degree of obliteration that occurs with increasing age, and a patent processus vaginalis by itself does not constitute a clinical inguinal hernia.

Clinical Issues

Inguinal hernias occur in 1% to 3% of all children and in 3% to 5% of premature infants. There is no known inheritance pattern, but there is an increased incidence of inguinal hernia in children with connective tissue disorders such as Ehlers-Danlos syndrome and Marfan syndrome. There is a 6:1 predominance of males to females. At least 30% of these children are younger than 6 months of age at the time of operative repair. Inguinal hernia more commonly presents as right-sided (56.2%) compared with left-sided (27.5%) or bilateral (16.2%).[21]

Most infants and children have a history of an intermittent inguinal mass or bulge that may descend into the scrotum or labia. The hernia may become more pronounced during times of increased intraabdominal pressure, such as crying or having a bowel movement. Most inguinal hernias in children reduce spontaneously or are reducible with gentle, manual pressure along the inguinal canal. Female infants may have an ovary and fallopian tube in the hernia sac, identified clinically as a firm, slightly mobile, nontender mass in the labia or inguinal canal. Most parents or pediatricians give a characteristic history that is sufficient to warrant inguinal exploration, even in children in whom the hernia cannot be clinically demonstrated at the time of examination. Depending on institution and surgeon preference, infants and children with a strong history consistent with inguinal hernia and an equivocal clinical examination can be offered either ultrasound[22] or diagnostic laparoscopy to effectively confirm the diagnosis before groin exploration.

Incarceration is a common consequence of untreated inguinal hernia and presents as a nonreducible mass in the inguinal canal, scrotum, or labia.[23] Clinical symptoms and signs are related to the duration of incarceration. If the incarceration has been present for several hours, the infant may be inconsolable and have feeding intolerance, pain, abdominal distention, vomiting, and lack of flatus or stool, signaling complete intestinal obstruction. The affected groin may become quite edematous, and a reactive scrotal hydrocele may evolve. Elevation of the infant's lower extremities with a pillow may help to encourage spontaneous reduction. Attempts at manually reducing an incarcerated inguinal hernia should be performed by an experienced surgeon. If necessary, sedation to calm the infant before attempting manual reduction may be used with caution. Ice packs should be avoided in infants and children. Following successful reduction of an incarcerated hernia, expedient elective repair of the hernia should be performed after the edema has subsided. If reduction of an incarcerated hernia requires several attempts and is difficult, overnight inpatient observation is warranted to rule out reduction of strangulated bowel; fortunately, this is an uncommon occurrence in the pediatric population. Inability to reduce an incarcerated hernia is a clear indication for urgent operative exploration and repair. Incarcerated inguinal hernia must be differentiated from an acute, noncommunicating hydrocele or inguinal lymphadenitis. With acute hydrocele, it is usually possible to transilluminate the hydrocele and palpate normal cord structures above the scrotal mass. Acute lymphadenitis typically is associated with fever, erythema, and tenderness, and there may be a history of lower-extremity infection on the ipsilateral side. If the inguinal mass is not reducible and an incarcerated hernia cannot be excluded, urgent groin exploration is required.

Operative Considerations and Outcome

The diagnosis of inguinal hernia in an infant or child is an indication for operative repair. The rationale for elective repair is to prevent the complications associated with incarceration. At least 71% of infants who require operative reduction of incarcerated inguinal hernia are younger than 11 months.[24] Therefore, an approach emphasizing timely elective repair of inguinal hernia is warranted, particularly during infancy. Delay of elective repair may be necessary in premature,

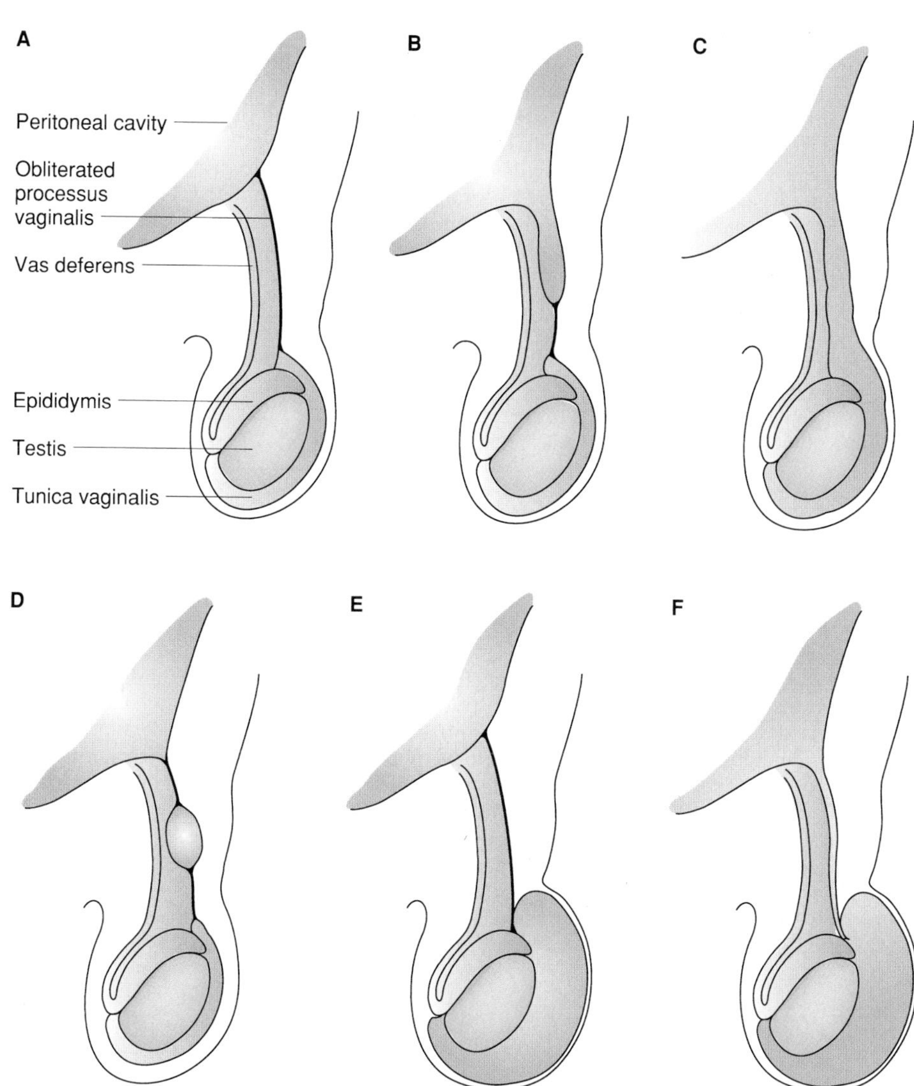

FIGURE 110.6 Diagrammatic representation of the anatomic variations that occur with different degrees of obliteration of the processus vaginalis. (*A*) Normal; obliterated processus vaginalis. (*B*) Proximal hernia sac; distal obliterated processus. (*C*) Hernia sac extending into scrotum; no obliteration. (*D*) Proximal and distal obliteration with hydrocele of the cord. (*E*) Hydrocele of the scrotum, obliterated processus. (*F*) Patent processus with communicating hydrocele.

extremely low birth weight (<1,500 g) infants and in children with other conditions such as congenital heart disease, pulmonary disease, infection, or metabolic disease. The risk of using general anesthesia in these children may be significant enough to defer inguinal hernia repair until the coexisting conditions are corrected.

Elective inguinal hernia repair in the pediatric age group is usually performed as an outpatient surgical procedure using general anesthesia, although spinal anesthesia is an effective alternative in selected high-risk infants.[25] A regional caudal block or local inguinal nerve block using local anesthetic is useful to diminish perioperative pain and increase patient comfort. These techniques, along with the use of rapid-acting general anesthetics, allow the vast majority of children to be discharged home within hours of operation. Overnight observation and monitoring are required for high-risk infants and children, including premature infants, infants less than 50 weeks postconceptual age, or children with significant cardiac, pulmonary, or other disorders that increase anesthetic risk.

Repair of pediatric inguinal hernia relies on high ligation of the hernia sac at the level of the internal inguinal ring. Sensory nerves deep to the external oblique aponeurosis should be identified and preserved. Careful visualization, identification, and dissection of the vas deferens and the testicular blood supply from the hernia sac must be performed; operative magnifying loupes are extremely helpful in this regard. The vas deferens must be carefully dissected free from the sac, and direct handling or pinching of the vas with forceps is avoided. The absence of a vas deferens or a blind-ending vas may be observed in children with cystic fibrosis (CF). In female infants, opening the hernia sac to visualize the ovary and fallopian tube may help to avoid inadvertent injury to these structures during high suture ligation of the sac. The distal component of the hernia sac is opened widely, and any fluid in the sac is evacuated. If the internal inguinal ring is attenuated or enlarged from a large hernia, it can be repaired with a few sutures. The testicle is returned to its scrotal position by gentle traction on the gubernaculum, and the spermatic cord is carefully aligned along the inguinal canal. The skin incisions are typically closed with absorbable, subcuticular sutures and covered with either collodion or a waterproof dressing for the first few postoperative days. Postoperative pain is handled with oral acetaminophen for 24 to 48 hours; older children may require acetaminophen with codeine.

Operative exploration of the asymptomatic contralateral groin remains controversial but is often performed in infants younger than 2 years because of the reported 60% to 70% incidence of a patent processus vaginalis on the opposite side.[26] In a survey of the surgical section of the American Academy of Pediatrics, 65% of the respondents perform contralateral exploration in male patients younger than 2 years, and 84% perform exploration for female infants up to age 4 years.[27] Direct visualization of the contralateral groin can be performed using a laparoscope inserted either through a small, separate abdominal incision or through a side-viewing laparoscope inserted through the hernia sac. Experience with diagnostic laparoscopy has demonstrated that approximately one third to one half of children have a patent processus vaginalis on the contralateral, asymptomatic groin, with higher rates in infants younger than 1 year.[28–30] This approach avoids unnecessary contralateral groin exploration in about half of all children who undergo surgery for unilateral inguinal hernia.

The major risk of inguinal hernia repair in infants and children is related to general anesthesia, and this risk is usually well tolerated. Complications in pediatric inguinal hernia repair include wound infection, injury to the vas deferens or testicular vessels, injury or displacement of the testicle, and recurrence. Fortunately, all these complications are infrequent. The overall complication rate is higher for children requiring emergent operation for incarcerated or strangulated hernia. Recurrent inguinal hernia following elective repair is unusual and may be an indication of an underlying connective tissue disorder such as Ehlers-Danlos syndrome.

Hydrocele

A *hydrocele* is a fluid collection that resides in the tunica vaginalis in the scrotum or the processus vaginalis in the inguinal canal. A hydrocele may be present at birth, or it may occur acutely as a result of an incarcerated hernia or torsion of the appendix testis. On examination, a hydrocele transilluminates with a bright hand-held light. A hydrocele is described as either *communicating* or *noncommunicating* depending on whether there is direct patency between the hydrocele and the peritoneal cavity. A history of intermittent fluctuation in the size of the scrotal fluid mass is generally diagnostic for communicating hydrocele. A communicating hydrocele is synonymous with a patent processus vaginalis, and therefore, a communicating hydrocele is treated operatively in the same fashion. In male patients, a hydrocele of the cord is a collection of fluid in the processus vaginalis separate from the tunica vaginalis. In female patients, fluid trapped in the processus vaginalis is considered a hydrocele of the canal of Nuck. In noncommunicating hydrocele, the isolated fluid collection is typically asymptomatic and tends to spontaneously resolve before age 12 months. Operative management of noncommunicating hydrocele is usually reserved for lesions that persist after this age, acute enlargement of the hydrocele, or if there is any question of undiagnosed communication. In children, an inguinal approach is used to treat hydrocele. Transcrotal needle aspiration of a hydrocele is not widely used or advocated as definitive treatment.

GASTROINTESTINAL DISORDERS

Neonatal Intestinal Obstruction

A variety of congenital anatomic defects, inherited metabolic diseases, and acquired physiologic disorders may present as intestinal obstruction in a newborn infant. Neonatal intestinal obstruction is characterized clinically by bilious emesis and is often associated with abdominal distention. Bilious emesis in a neonate must be considered to be the result of an acute mechanical intestinal obstruction until proven otherwise. Emergent surgical evaluation is warranted for any newborn with bilious emesis. Table 110.2 provides differential diagnoses for neonatal intestinal obstruction along with salient features of the history, physical examination, and diagnostic studies.

The clinical presentation of neonatal intestinal obstruction depends, in part, on the site of obstruction and the age of the infant. Clinical examination of the infant typically provides the

TABLE 110.2 DIAGNOSIS

NEONATAL INTESTINAL OBSTRUCTION

Diagnosis	History	Physical examination	Diagnostic studies
Intestinal atresia or stenosis	Bilious emesis Failure to pass meconium	Abdominal distention Acholic meconium	Plain abdominal film Contrast enema
Duodenal atresia or stenosis	Bilious emesis	Gastric distention Trisomy 21	Plain abdominal film Upper GI contrast study
Imperforate anus	Failure to pass meconium Bilious emesis (late)	Absent anus or visible fistula Abdominal distention VACTERL association	Plain chest, abdominal film Ultrasound kidneys, sacrum, rectum Echocardiogram
Necrotizing enterocolitis	High-risk, premature infant Bilious emesis	Abdominal distention Hematochezia, guaiac-positive stool	Plain abdominal film
Meconium ileus	Cystic fibrosis (10%) Bilious emesis	Acholic meconium Abdominal distention	Plain abdominal film Contrast enema
Malrotation	Bilious emesis Term, healthy infant	No abdominal distention	Plain abdominal film Upper GI contrast study
Hirschsprung disease	Delayed passage of meconium Bilious emesis	Abdominal distention Trisomy 21	Plain abdominal film Contrast enema
Uncommon causes of obstruction (intussusception, Meckel's diverticulum, duplication)		Abdominal mass, incarcerated hernia	Variable
Medical conditions associated with ileus	Bilious emesis	Sepsis, hypothyroidism, etc.	Plain abdominal film

GI , gastrointestinal; VACTERL, vertebral, anal, cardiac, tracheal, esophageal, renal, and limb anomalies.

surgeon with a preliminary diagnosis and helps to guide further diagnostic studies. Abdominal distention is a characteristic physical finding with distal bowel obstruction, whereas the abdomen may be flat in proximal obstruction. The presence of bile in the gastric contents or stool provides clinical evidence of the location of an obstruction relative to the ampulla of Vater. Bilious emesis in an infant or child should be considered an anatomic obstruction requiring surgical evaluation until proven otherwise. An infant with bilious emesis who has already passed meconium and has tolerated feeding is unlikely to have intestinal atresia and more likely to have malrotation with midgut volvulus. If volvulus is suspected, emergent evaluation must be done diagnose and potentially prevent catastrophic bowel injury or death.

In general, the diagnosis of neonatal intestinal obstruction relies on a clear history, thorough clinical examination, and adjunctive radiologic studies. Definitive diagnosis of neonatal intestinal obstruction may often be made by physical examination and readily available radiologic studies. Incarcerated inguinal hernia is an important cause of neonatal bowel obstruction, and examination leads to a straightforward diagnosis. Some congenital conditions have clearly recognizable features and may be associated with anatomic lesions causing intestinal obstruction. For example, infants with trisomy 21 have a higher probability of having duodenal atresia or Hirschsprung disease than the general population. The approach to imaging the neonate suspected of having an intestinal obstruction is to obtain a plain abdominal radiograph, followed by either a contrast enema or an upper gastrointestinal series. Plain films of the newborn abdomen can be extremely useful and diagnostic because swallowed air acts as a contrast agent. An illustrative example is duodenal atresia, which gives rise to a dilated, air-filled stomach and duodenum proximal to the obstruction; the remainder of the bowel remains gasless, giving rise to the double-bubble appearance on plain abdominal films. Other causes of proximal intestinal obstruction may lead to finding a microcolon on contrast enema, which is a small and unused but otherwise normal colon. If a retrograde contrast enema does not pass into the dilated segment of bowel, an upper gastrointestinal series may be useful to identify a more proximal obstruction. An upper gastrointestinal series is also the diagnostic procedure of choice in suspected malrotation with obstruction caused by volvulus.

Several medical conditions of the newborn appear clinically similar to mechanical intestinal obstruction (see Table 110.2). In particular, bilious emesis from an ileus secondary to neonatal sepsis is not uncommon. Congenital hypothyroidism is an infrequent and medically treatable condition that can produce delayed intestinal motility that mimics mechanical intestinal obstruction in a neonate.

Intestinal Atresia or Stenosis

Embryology and Anatomy

The embryonic intestine undergoes segmental development as early as week 3 of gestation. The septum transversum demarcates the developing foregut from the midgut. The hindgut develops in the primitive tail fold. Developmental issues relevant to the discussion that follows are limited to the midgut.[30] The midgut can be considered a tubular structure that progressively undergoes several predictable, developmental stages: (a) elongation; (b) herniation from and reduction into the coelomic cavity; (c) rotation; and (d) fixation of the mesentery to the posterior body wall.

Several different types of intestinal atresia are clinically observed (Fig. 110.7) and reflect common patterns of abnormal embryogenesis.[31] *Type I* atresia is an intraluminal web or diaphragm that can either be complete or fenestrated. The

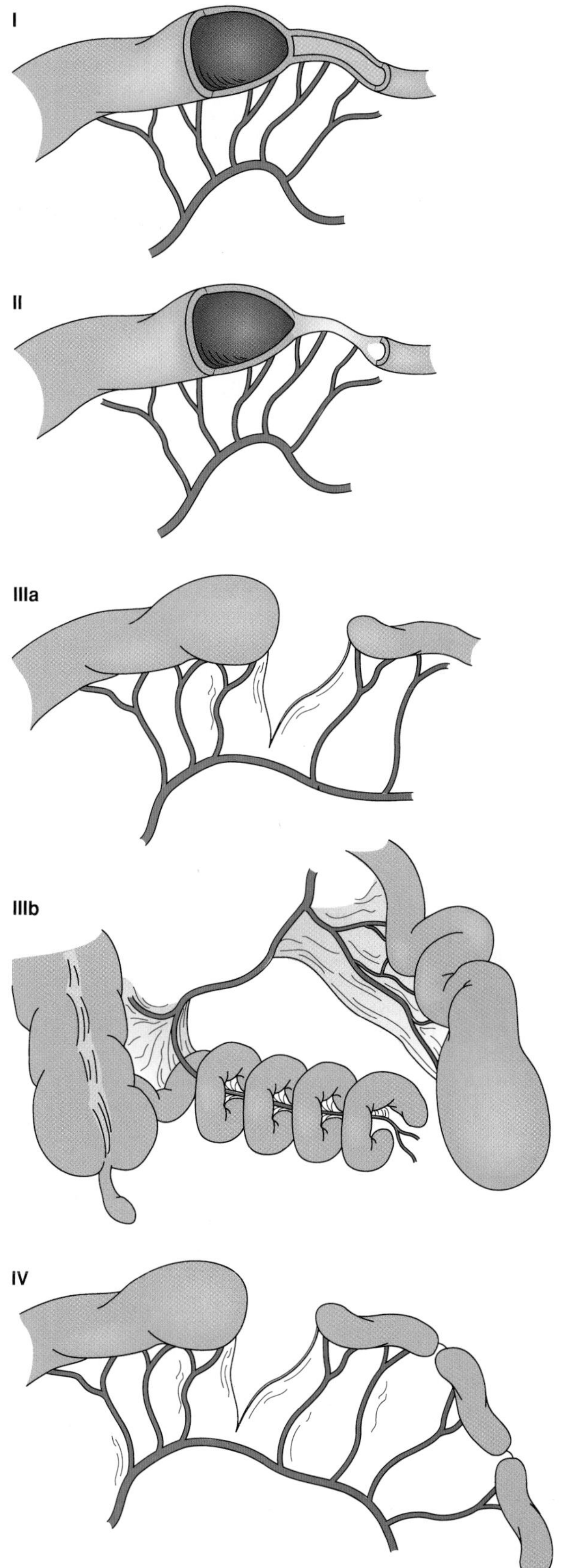

FIGURE 110.7 Classification of intestinal atresia. Type I, muscular continuity with a complete web. Type II, mesentery intact, fibrous cord. Type IIIa, muscular and mesenteric discontinuous. Type IIIb, apple-peel deformity. Type IV, multiple atresias. (After Grosfeld JL. Jejunoileal atresia and stenosis. In: O'Neill JA Jr, Rowe MI, Grosfeld JL, et al., eds. *Pediatric surgery,* 5th ed. St. Louis: Mosby, 1998, pp. 1145–1158 with permission.)

seromuscular layers of bowel remain intact. *Types II* and *IIIa* atresia are believed to be a result of in utero mesenteric vascular accidents. Experimental interruption of the fetal mesenteric blood supply in utero leads to this type of atresia.[32] *Type IIIb* atresia, also known as the *apple-peel* or *Christmas tree deformity,* has complete mesenteric discontinuity, with the distal bowel concentrically surrounding a singular mesenteric blood supply. *Type IV* atresia has multiple segmental areas of discontinuous bowel. Type IIIb and IV atresia are thought to be consequences of major and multiple vascular interruptions, respectively, of fetal mesenteric blood flow.

At least 90% of infants with congenital intestinal obstruction of the small bowel have complete atresia, whereas the remaining children have either stenoses or fenestrated intraluminal webs. The most common location is the distal ileum, and multiple areas of atresia are discovered in 3.6% to 20% of these infants.[33] Infants with fenestrated intraluminal webs may have a small, often eccentric opening that is only millimeters in diameter. These infants may not have obstructive symptoms until the introduction of solid food at 6 to 12 months of age. Occasionally, these children present much later in life with failure to thrive, abdominal pain, or feeding intolerance.

Congenital colonic atresia is a distinctly unusual condition. In a contemporary series of 277 infants treated with intestinal atresia, only 21 children had colonic atresia.[33] Similar to small bowel atresia, colonic atresia is believed to reflect fetal mesenteric vascular injury. Given the distal nature of colonic atresia, initial feeding may be well tolerated and definitive diagnosis may be delayed for several days. The diagnostic evaluation and surgical treatment of colonic atresia is essentially identical to the approach used for small bowel atresia. Colonic atresia may be associated with abdominal wall defects, skeletal or cardiac defects, or coexisting intestinal atresia.

Clinical Presentation

The actual incidence rate of congenital intestinal atresia is unknown. Reported estimates in the United States are 3.5 to 3.75 cases per 10,000 total births.[34] Infants with jejunal or ileal atresia generally have a low incidence rate of significant associated anomalies. Conversely, about 10% of infants with gastroschisis have intestinal atresia or stenosis secondary to mechanical interruption of the mesenteric vascular supply.

Detection of maternal polyhydramnios on routine prenatal ultrasound screening can be an indication of proximal bowel obstruction caused by the interruption of normal amniotic fluid absorption in the fetal gut.[35] Following delivery, the classic clinical presentation of intestinal atresia is bilious emesis, abdominal distention, and failure to pass meconium. The degree of abdominal distention depends on the site of obstruction, the infant's age, and the efficacy of proximal decompression. Abdominal distention may be absent with proximal intestinal atresia. Distal intestinal atresia may lead to abdominal distention with visible or palpable intestinal loops on examination. Rectal examination and evaluation of stool character remains important when intestinal obstruction is suspected.

Diagnosis

Following history and physical examination, plain radiographic abdominal films should be obtained. Plain films in jejunal or ileal atresia demonstrate marked gaseous distention of the proximal intestine with gasless distal small bowel and colon. Haustral markings are normally not apparent in the neonatal colon, and therefore discrimination between small bowel and colon in the newborn is difficult without intraluminal contrast. A contrast enema is generally obtained to confirm the diagnosis of jejunoileal atresia. A diminutive, unused but otherwise normal microcolon is typical of proximal intestinal obstruction. The inability to reflux contrast into the proximal, dilated small bowel segment is diagnostic for congenital intestinal obstruction. This radiographic finding, in conjunction with the clinical setting, warrants operative exploration. An upper gastrointestinal series is generally unnecessary and may increase the risk of further emesis and aspiration in the newborn with obstruction. Incomplete obstruction from a fenestrated intraluminal web may require more sophisticated imaging techniques, such as catheter-directed enteroclysis.

Treatment

Anatomic lesions causing neonatal intestinal obstruction require operative treatment. Whereas malrotation with midgut volvulus requires emergent diagnostic work-up and operative intervention to prevent bowel loss and death, obstruction resulting from intestinal atresia is generally not associated with life-threatening physiologic disturbances. Therefore, initial treatment is aimed at treating any other associated problems, confirming diagnosis, and preparing the infant for an operation under general anesthesia. During this period, the infant always should have an orogastric or nasogastric tube in place and on suction to provide proximal decompression of the obstructed bowel.

The operative strategy in treating intestinal atresia is to restore gastrointestinal tract continuity while preserving as much intestinal length as possible. The operation is straightforward and an end-to-end or end-to-oblique (end-to-back) anastomosis is typically performed (Fig. 110.8). Short segmental

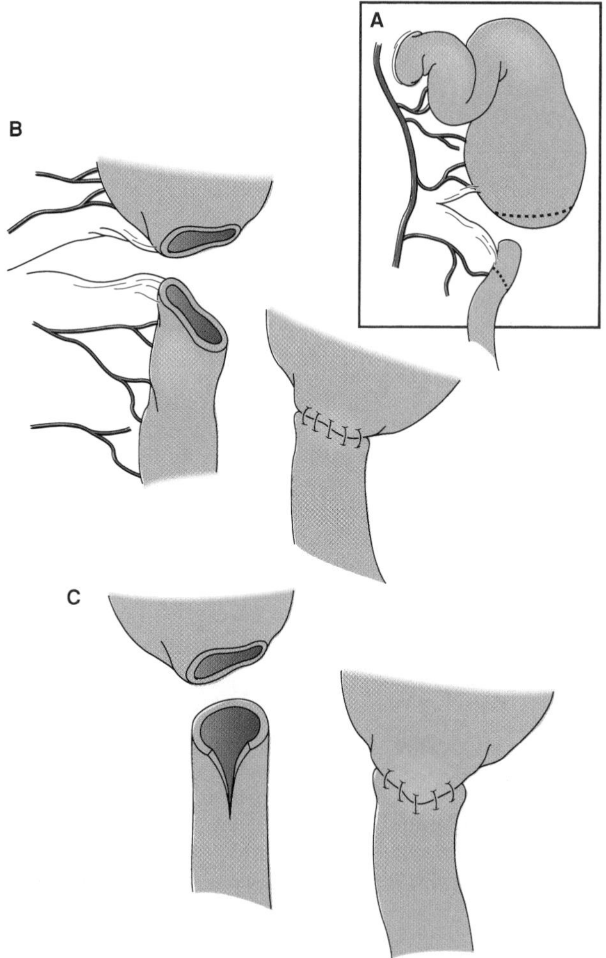

FIGURE 110.8 (*A,B*) The end-to-oblique anastomosis for small bowel atresia. (C) An extension of the distal enterostomy along the antimesenteric border may be used to create proximal and distal lumens of equal size for anastomosis.

bowel resection and excision of an intraluminal web or diaphragm are used when necessary. Visual inspection and instillation of intraluminal saline or air to exclude distal atresia or web prior to anastomosis is important to evaluate patency of the downstream bowel. The size discrepancy between the proximal and distal bowel is usually considerable, and delay of postoperative bowel motility is common. Some surgeons advocate the use of technical procedures to improve emptying of the proximal bowel by reducing overall bowel diameter. These procedures include resection, plication, and tapering enteroplasty. Complex atresia associated with apple-peel deformity or multiple segmental atresias may require multiple serial anastomoses to preserve as much bowel length as possible. The ileocecal valve is preserved whenever possible, allowing improved tolerance of enteral nutrition in infants with limited small bowel length. It is estimated that approximately 40 cm of small bowel without an ileocecal valve, compared with 15 to 20 cm with an ileocecal valve, is sufficient for long-term enteral feeding tolerance in the neonate.[36] The treatment of colonic atresia is essentially identical to small bowel atresia. Contemporary management of colonic atresia includes primary anastomosis when technically possible.

Results and Outcome

Currently, the overall survival rate for infants treated for intestinal atresia or stenosis (including duodenal atresia) exceeds 93% in most large series[33,37] Mortality in these infants is generally related to cardiac anomalies and other associated congenital defects. Infants with a limited amount of intestinal length for nutritional absorption (short bowel syndrome with less than 40 cm) usually require long-term TPN and are at moderate to high risk for sepsis and liver injury. Infants with normal gastrointestinal length may still have prolonged gut dysfunction and delayed return of gastrointestinal motility for several days to weeks. Whether this dysfunction is related to physiologic abnormalities in the proximally dilated segment of bowel[38] or the distal microbowel[39] is unknown. During this period, the development of cholestatic jaundice related to TPN may occur and usually is reversible with the establishment of enteral feeding.

Congenital Duodenal Obstruction

Causes of duodenal obstruction in the newborn include duodenal atresia or stenosis, duodenal intraluminal web, and annular pancreas. Because of the common embryologic basis, clinical presentation, and treatment, these entities are considered jointly.

Embryology and Anatomy

The duodenum is derived from both the caudal segment of the foregut and the cranial segment of the midgut. Duodenal development is intimately related to the developing pancreaticobiliary system. The process of epithelial proliferation and recanalization are similar in the duodenum and midgut. The fetal pancreas arises from paired dorsal and ventral foregut diverticula during week 6 of gestation. The dorsal anlage gives rise to the body and tail of the pancreas as well as the main pancreatic duct. The ventral anlage migrates 180 degrees to fuse with the dorsal gland, forming the uncinate process and the distal portion of the duct of Wirsung (Fig. 110.9). An annular pancreas is characterized by glandular persistence surrounding the duodenum at the site of the embryonic ventral anlage. It is invariably associated with intrinsic duodenal obstruction, and a patent accessory pancreatic duct is common (Fig. 110.10).[40]

It is believed that the vast majority of congenital duodenal obstructions result from abnormalities of pancreatic development, failure of duodenal recanalization, or vascular compromise to the duodenum. In contrast to jejunoileal atresia, congenital duodenal obstruction divided nearly evenly between

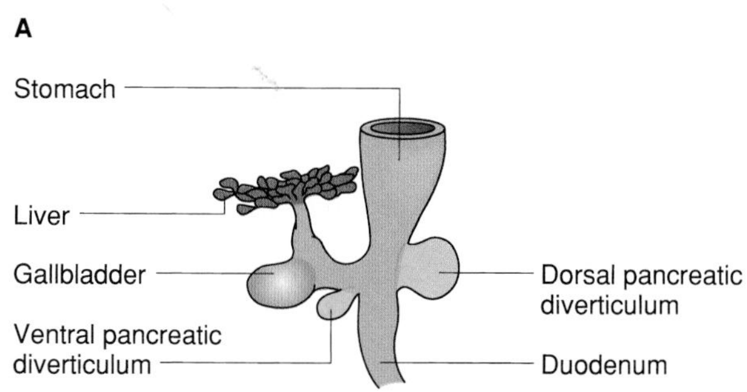

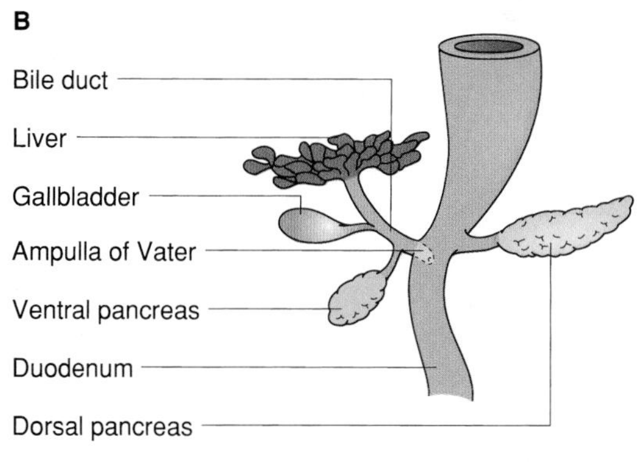

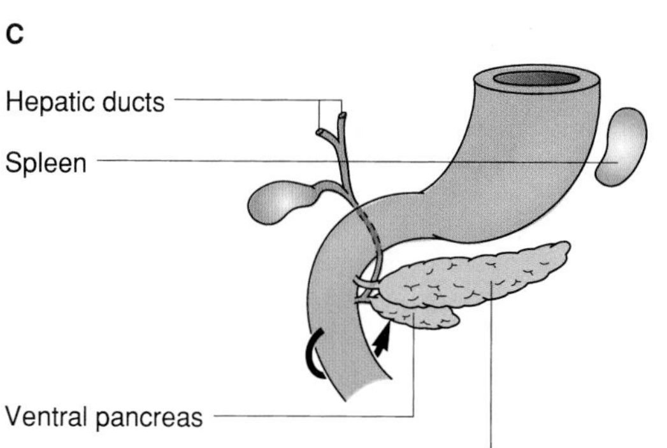

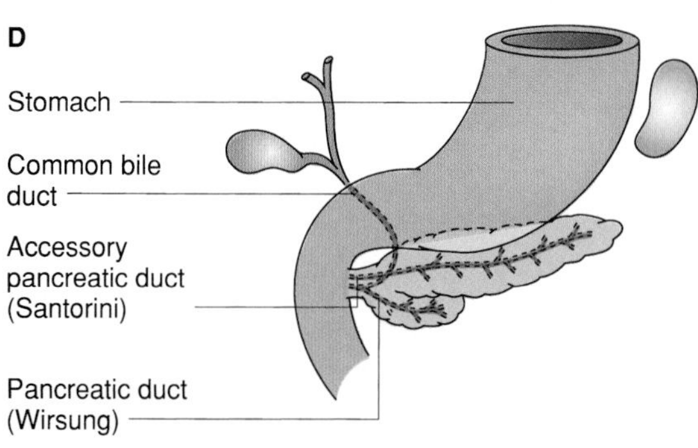

FIGURE 110.9 Normal embryologic development of the duodenum, pancreas, and bile ducts. (*A*) Fifth gestational week. (*B*) Sixth week. (*C*) Seventh week. (*D*) Eighth week.

PEDIATRICS

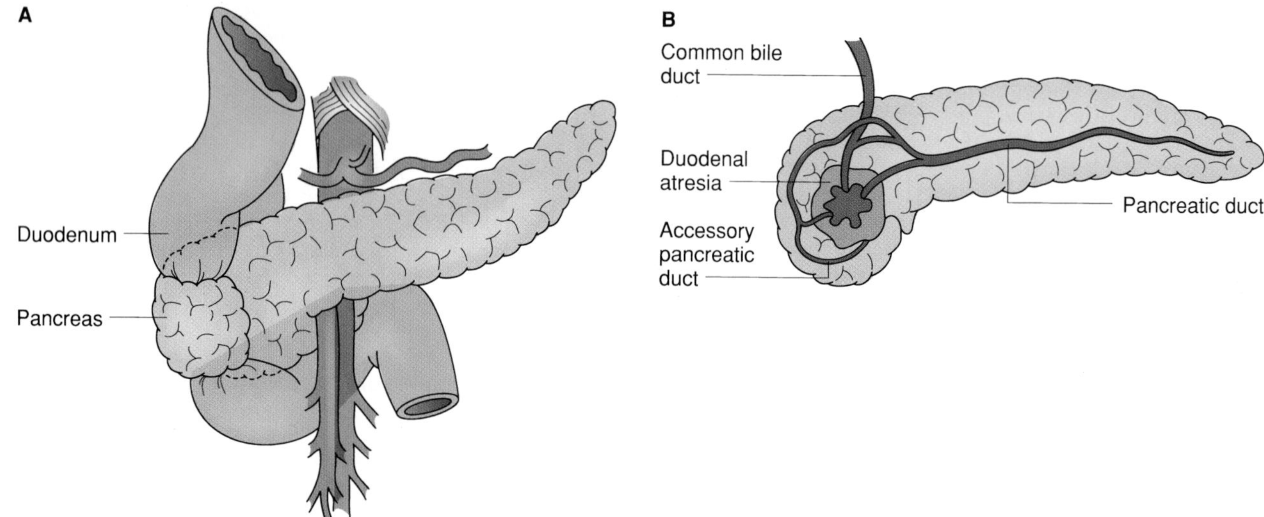

FIGURE 110.10 Annular pancreas. (*A*) The associated duodenal atresia is shown. (*B*) The relationships of the annular pancreas to the common bile duct and main and accessory pancreatic ducts are shown in cross-section.

intraluminal webs or stenoses and complete atresia. Duodenal atresia may occur with or without seromuscular continuity, and an intraluminal duodenal web may occur with or without fenestration. The most frequent location for duodenal atresia is in the descending duodenum distal to the ampulla of Vater. Most series report a 5% to 10% incidence of duodenal atresia proximal to the ampulla, giving rise to nonbilious gastric contents and emesis. Another important variant is a periampullary web that projects distally into the duodenal or jejunal lumen, forming a wind-sock deformity (Fig. 110.11). In this instance, the ampulla must be clearly identified before excision and repair because of the proximity of the ampulla to the web and even incorporation of the ampulla into the web.

Clinical Presentation

The incidence rate of congenital duodenal obstruction is estimated to be about 1 in 6,000 to 10,000 births.[41] About 30% of these infants have trisomy 21.[42] Infants born with duodenal atresia should be examined with a high degree of suspicion for trisomy 21 and undergo routine karyotype analysis. Other associated anomalies such as congenital heart disease, genitourinary tract malformations, and musculoskeletal disorders are common in these infants, and appropriate preoperative work-up is necessary.

Congenital duodenal obstruction most commonly presents in the first 24 to 48 hours of life with feeding intolerance and bilious emesis; duodenal obstruction proximal to the ampulla of Vater results in nonbilious emesis. On physical examination, infants with untreated duodenal obstruction may have a palpable epigastric mass, and gastric peristaltic waves may be visible. The collapsed and unused distal small intestine typically does not produce diffuse abdominal distention. Partial duodenal obstruction from a fenestrated web may not produce symptoms in the newborn period, and delayed diagnosis is common.

Diagnosis

Prenatal diagnosis of duodenal atresia is possible given contemporary fetal ultrasound techniques. Following birth, infants with suspected duodenal atresia should undergo plain abdominal radiographs. The classic radiographic finding of duodenal atresia is a double bubble from the air-filled stomach and duodenum (Fig. 110.12). In complete duodenal obstruction, no gas is seen distal to the duodenum; in this setting, the plain film is sufficiently diagnostic that no further imaging of the gastrointestinal tract is necessary. If there is incomplete obstruction, gas may be seen distally in the small or large intestine. Infants with suspected incomplete obstruction at the duodenal level may have either a fenestrated web or volvulus secondary to malrotation. Given the need for emergent operative intervention in malrotation with acute volvulus, an urgent upper gastrointestinal series with contrast should be strongly considered to exclude a neonatal surgical emergency. Importantly, all anatomic lesions causing neonatal duodenal obstruction require operative repair using a similar approach.

Treatment

Following expedient treatment of any associated life-threatening medical conditions and preoperative evaluation, infants with congenital duodenal obstruction are explored promptly. Because the differential diagnosis of duodenal obstruction includes duodenal atresia versus malrotation with obstructive Ladd's bands (as discussed later), prompt surgical exploration is advised. The operative goals are to restore gastrointestinal continuity without sacrificing intestinal length or absorptive surface area. Because most obstructive duodenal lesions are near the ampulla of Vater, great care must be exercised in their treatment to avoid inadvertent injury to the ampulla or pancreas.

Congenital duodenal atresia is treated by duodenoduodenostomy. Usually, duodenojejunostomy is avoided to prevent exclusion of the distal duodenum; currently, this procedure generally is reserved for obstructive lesions of the distal duodenum. Duodenal obstruction secondary to annular pancreas is also treated by duodenoduodenostomy. Direct division of annular pancreas is not performed because this does not address the underlying intraluminal duodenal obstruction, and there is significant risk of injury to the accessory pancreatic duct (see Fig. 110.10).

Duodenoduodenostomy is performed by making a transverse incision in the dilated, proximal duodenum and a longitudinal incision in the unused, downstream duodenum. The lumens are sutured together to form a diamond-shape anastomosis (Fig. 110.13).[43] Downstream duodenal patency should be demonstrated by passing a catheter or infusing saline or air distally to avoid overlooking a synchronous intestinal atresia.

Duodenal webs are excised through a longitudinal duodenotomy. The wind-sock duodenal web must be clearly identified

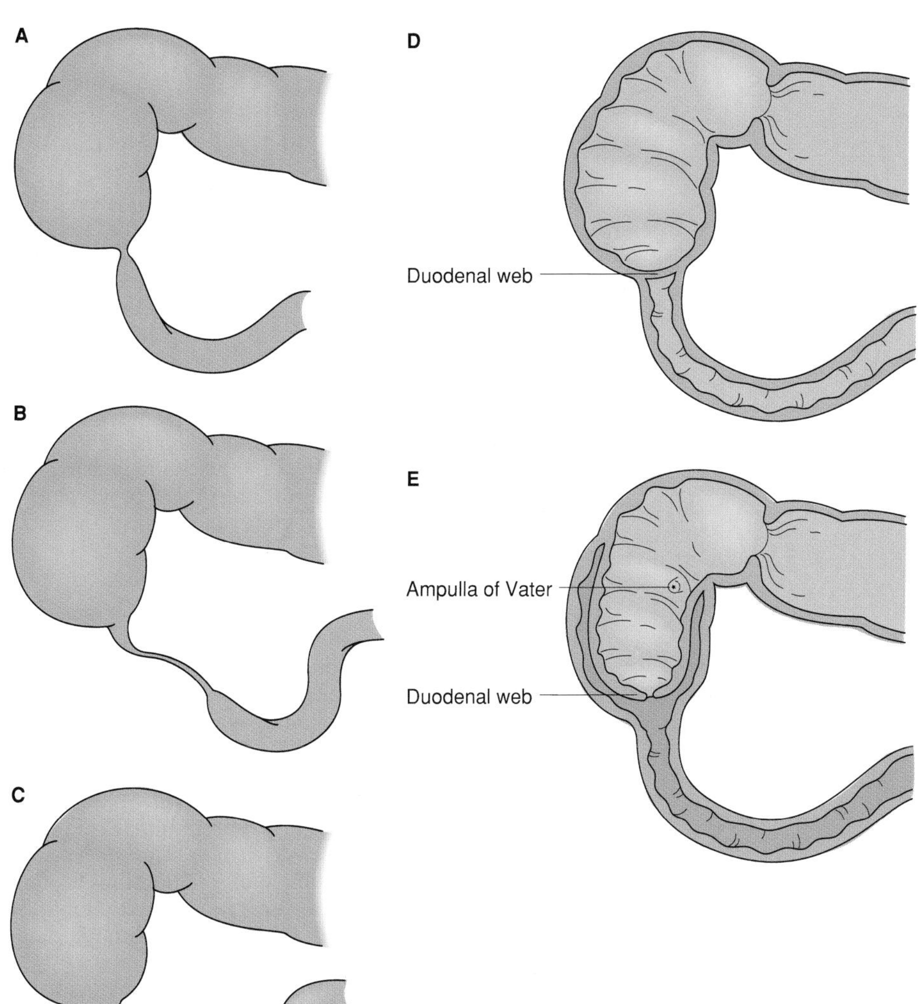

FIGURE 110.11 Anatomic forms of duodenal atresia (*A–C*) and webs (*D,E*). In particular, (*E*) demonstrates the unique windsock deformity. This lesion is important and potentially confusing because the point of obstruction is not at the apparent point of change in luminal diameter.

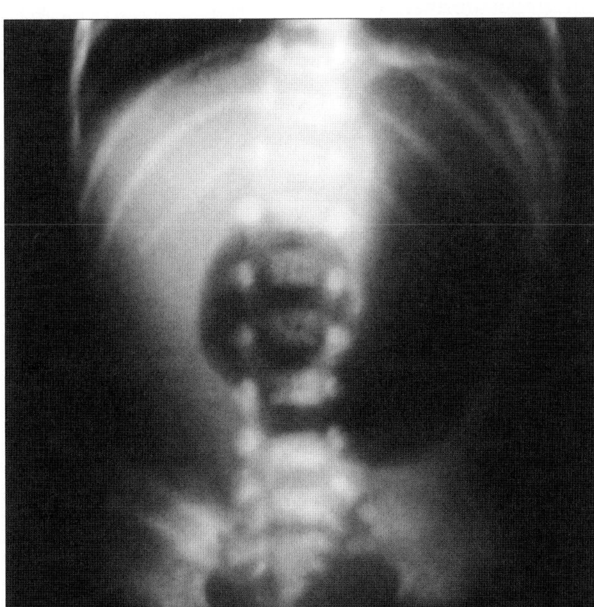

FIGURE 110.12 Classic radiographic appearance of duodenal atresia. There is a double bubble of gas in the stomach and proximal duodenum, with no gas in the distal intestinal tract.

because the visible transition from the distended, proximal duodenum to the small, downstream duodenum may be several centimeters distal to the base of the web. Traction applied at the apex of the web deforms the duodenum at its point of attachment and allows complete excision at the base. The ampulla of Vater must be unequivocally identified before duodenal web excision to avoid injury. Closure of the longitudinal duodenotomy is performed transversely to avoid narrowing of the duodenum.

There is usually great size discrepancy between the dilated, proximal pouch and the distal duodenal lumen, leading some surgeons to advocate procedures designed to reduce the diameter of the proximal duodenum in an effort to facilitate improved postoperative bowel motility. The efficacy of these procedures, which include tapering duodenoplasty and duodenal plication, have been described in anecdotal fashion without randomized comparison.

Results and Outcome

After successful operative repair of duodenal atresia or stenosis, delayed gastric emptying is common and typically manifests as enteral feeding intolerance. Patience and persistence are essential during the postoperative period. Surgical outcomes after repair of congenital duodenal obstruction are excellent,[42–44] with perioperative survival exceeding 95%.

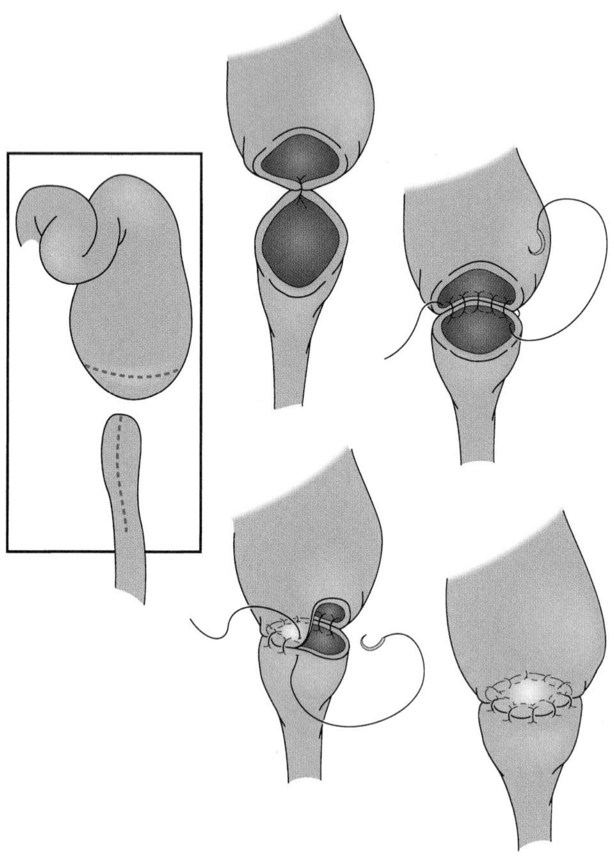

FIGURE 110.13 Diamond-shaped duodenoduodenostomy for repair of duodenal atresia.

Perioperative mortality generally is related to associated anomalies, and in particular, in infants with trisomy 21 with congenital heart defects. Other late problems may be encountered that reflect gastroduodenal motility issues such as poor gastric emptying, gastroesophageal reflux, and duodenal dilatation. These symptoms may appear several months to years following repair and therefore, long-term surgical follow-up remains important.

Anorectal Malformations (Imperforate Anus)

Embryology

By week 5 of gestation, the fetal cloaca is identifiable with the adjacent hindgut, allantois, and vestigial tailgut (Fig. 110.14). The mesoderm of the urorectal septum extends caudally to fuse with the cloacal closing plate.[30] Fusion of the lateral cloacal ridges completes division of the cloaca into the rectum and the urogenital sinus. The caudal aspect of the urorectal septum forms the perineal body. The anal membrane normally ruptures during week 8 of gestation, completing the patency of the distal rectum to the skin. Further development of the urogenital sinus leads to the formation of the urethra and bladder. In female infants, the uterus and portions of the vagina develop from the müllerian ducts. The diverse anatomic variation observed with anorectal malformations is thought to reflect anomalous or interrupted development of these structures during normal embryogenesis.

Anatomy and Classification

The normal anatomy of the anus and rectum is reviewed in previous chapters. Normally, the rectum descends to the perineum and ultimately, to the anal orifice through a striated muscle complex in the pelvis resembling a funnel. The striated muscle complex is under voluntary control and is responsible for providing fecal continence (Fig. 110.15). Contiguous portions of the *levator ani,* the *external sphincter,* and the *puborectalis* muscles compose the *striated muscle complex*. These anatomically indistinct components of the muscle complex act together to provide control of defecation. The concept of the striated muscle complex and anatomic relationships leading to normal fecal continence with respect to anorectal malformations has evolved from both clinical and anatomic data as described by Peña.[45]

Because of the variety of anorectal malformations observed, different classification systems have been proposed in an attempt to characterize the defects. A summary of the 1984 Wingspread Classification is provided in Table 110.3. This anatomically descriptive, well-accepted, classification scheme is useful in planning the operative management of anorectal malformations.

In male subjects, the two most common anorectal malformations observed are low imperforate anus with a perineal fistula

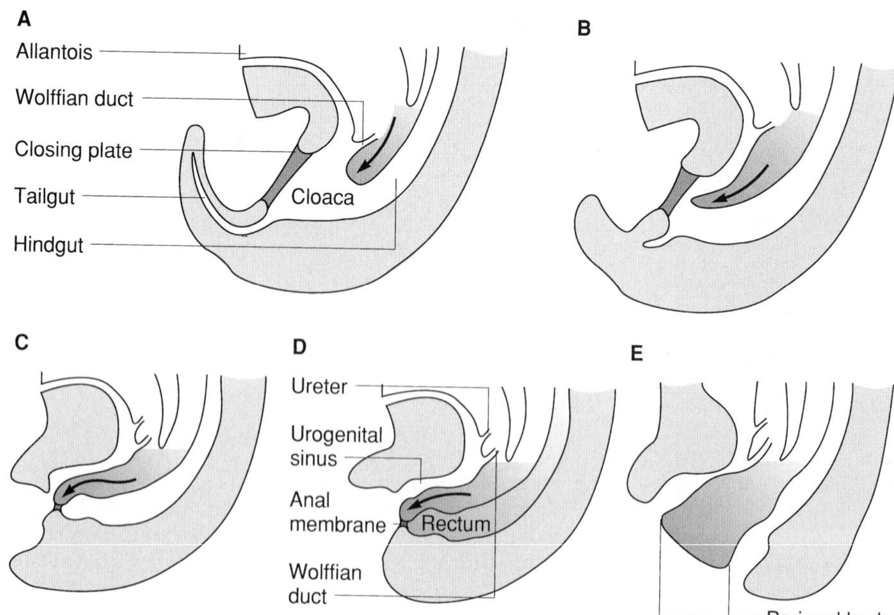

FIGURE 110.14 Normal embryologic division of the cloaca by the urorectal septum into the ventral urinary tract and the dorsal rectum. This process is normally completed by the ninth or tenth week of gestation.

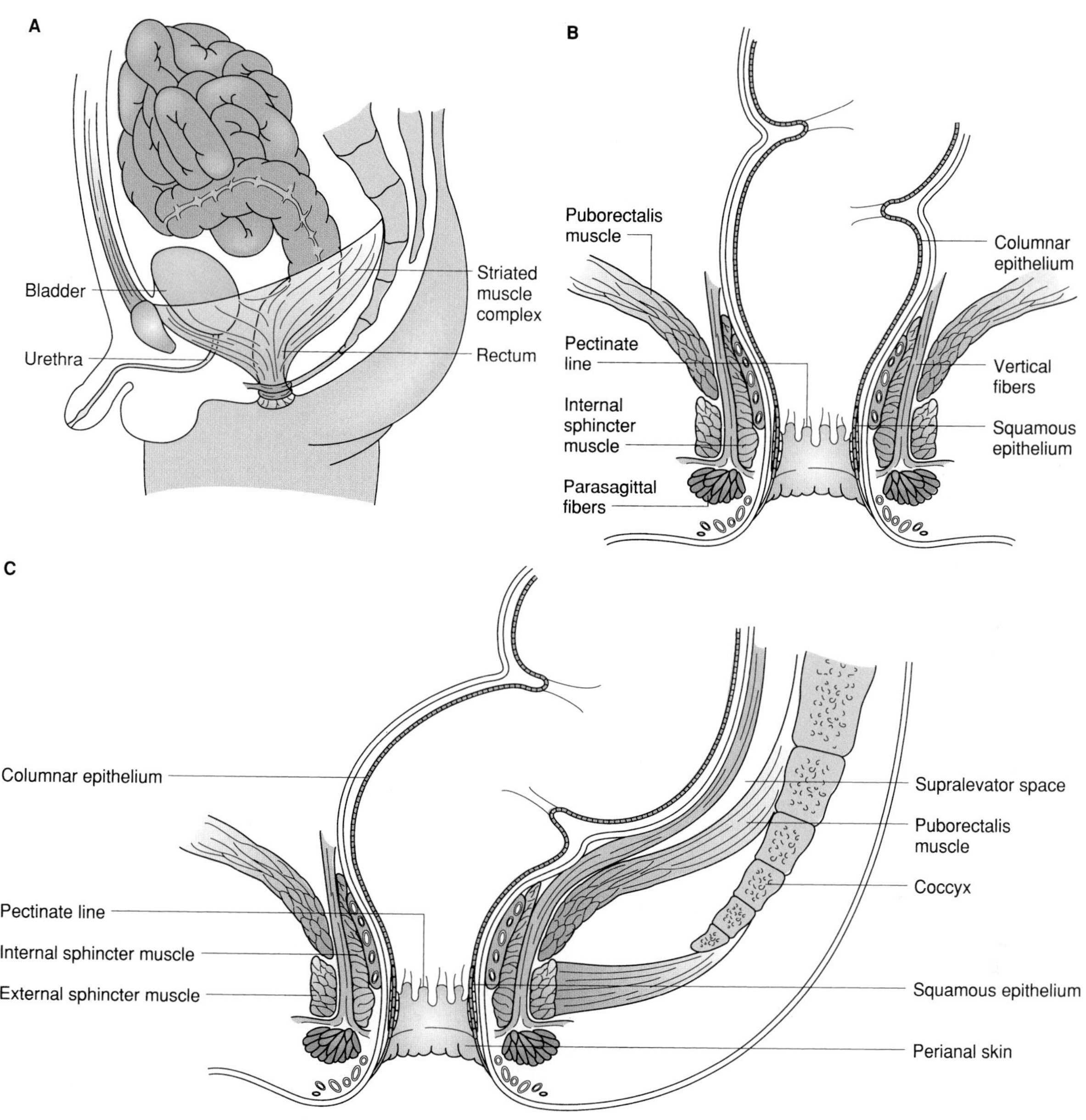

FIGURE 110.15 The normal relations of the pelvic striated muscle complex and the rectum. (*A*) Normal male anatomy. (*B*) Coronal view showing individual components of the striated muscle complex. (*C*) Sagittal view of normal anatomy.

(Fig. 110.16) and high anorectal agenesis with a rectoprostatic urethral fistula (Fig. 110.17). Male patients without a visible perineal fistula are assumed to have high imperforate anus with a rectourethral fistula until proven otherwise. In female subjects, the most common malformation encountered is low imperforate anus with a fistula from the rectum to either the perineal body or the vaginal vestibule (Fig. 110.18). As these malformations result from developmental arrest at various times during migration of the urogenital septum, considerable anatomic variability exists in both male and female subjects.

A common anatomic feature of imperforate anus is incomplete descent of the rectum to the perineum. Consequently, the rectum is not completely within the striated muscle complex. Therefore, the caudal portion of the striated muscle complex remains a solid mass of striated muscle, whereas the cephalad portion may be normally positioned circumferentially around the rectal pouch. In low imperforate anus, the rectum nearly reaches the perineum, and the configuration of the striated muscle complex surrounding the rectum more closely approximates normal. With high imperforate anus, less striated muscle surrounds the rectal pouch. All anorectal malformations are considered to have some component of striated muscle complex hypoplasia and dysfunction, although the physiologic effects are variable. Low anorectal lesions have a more favorable prognosis for fecal continence than intermediate or high lesions.

The classic delineation between low and high anorectal malformations is made anatomically at the pubococcygeal line. Low imperforate anus describes a rectal pouch descending within the striated muscle complex below the inferior border of the ossified ischium and the pubococcygeal line. The vast majority of low lesions have associated perineal or vestibular fistulas. High imperforate anus has a blind-ending rectal pouch above the pubococcygeal line and, therefore, above the striated muscle complex (or levator ani). Some

TABLE 110.3 CLASSIFICATION

ANATOMIC CLASSIFICATION OF ANORECTAL MALFORMATIONS

Female	Male
HIGH	HIGH
Anorectal agenesis with rectovaginal fistula without fistula	Anorectal agenesis with rectoprostaticurethral fistula* without fistula
Rectal atresia	Rectal atresia
INTERMEDIATE	
Rectovestibular fistula	Rectobulbar urethral fistula
Rectovaginal fistula	Anal agenesis without fistula
Anal agenesis without fistula	
LOW	
Anovestibular fistula[a]	Anocutaneous fistula[a]
Anocutaneous fistula[a,b]	Anal stenosis[a,c]
Anal stenosis[c]	Rare malformations
Cloacal malformations[d]	
Rare malformations	

[a]Relatively common lesion.
[b]Includes fistulas occurring at the posterior junction of the labia minora, often called *fourchette fistulas* or *vulvar fistulas.*
[c]Previously called *covered anus.*
[d]Previously called *rectocloacal fistulas.* Entry of the rectal fistula into the cloaca may be high or intermediate, depending on the length of the cloacal canal.

lesions have a variable degree of descent into the striated muscle complex and are described anatomically as intermediate malformations.

Associated Anomalies

Associated anomalies in infants with anorectal malformations are very common, and may be found in more than 70% of patients. The VACTERL (vertebral, anal, cardiac, tracheal, esophageal, renal and limb) association is important and requires consideration in any infant with imperforate anus. *Vertebral anomalies* are common and include sacral dysplasia and agenesis. Infants with sacral anomalies commonly have high imperforate anus and sacral autonomic dysfunction that can lead to poor long-term fecal continence and neurogenic bladder. A variety of spinal cord malformations also can be observed in these infants, including tethered spinal cord syndromes and some myelodysplastic syndromes. During the neonatal period, these spinal lesions may be detected by using ultrasound or magnetic resonance imaging (MRI), and surgical treatment may be necessary within the first 8 to 18 months of life. *Anorectal malformations* include lesions discussed in this section. *Tracheoesophageal* fistula with or without esophageal atresia is estimated to occur in about 10% of infants with anorectal malformations. *Renal anomalies* are the most common associated abnormalities with anorectal malformations and include both upper and lower tract conditions. Genitourinary screening in the form of a renal ultrasound and voiding cystourethrogram is routinely performed. *Cardiac* anomalies are common and screening echocardiography is clinically indicated. *Limb abnormalities,* in particular, involvement of the radius, complete the associated anomalies defined by the acronym.

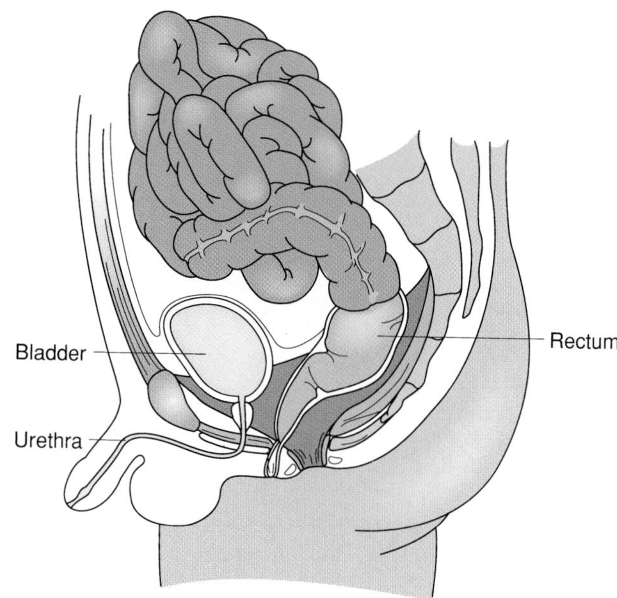

FIGURE 110.16 Male infant with low imperforate anus and perineal fistula. Note that the fistula is anterior to the striated muscle complex.

Clinical Presentation

The incidence rate of anorectal malformations is estimated at 1 in 2,524 to 5,000 live births,[46] with a slightly rate in male neonate. High lesions are also twice as common in male neonates as in female neonates. Careful examination of the neonatal perineum reveals the diagnosis. If unrecognized and left untreated, high imperforate anus eventually leads to signs and symptoms of complete bowel obstruction characterized by abdominal distention, feeding intolerance, and bilious emesis. Because of the nearly uniform rectourethral or rectovesicular fistula in high imperforate anus, some of these infants pass meconium or gas through the urethra during urination. In contrast, infants with low malformations typically pass meconium through a perineal or vestibular fistula within the first 24 hours of life. Occasionally, infants with low lesions associated with large fistulas are not diagnosed with imperforate anus until difficulty passing stool is noticed weeks to months after birth, particularly at the time of progressing to solid foods.

Delineation of high versus low anorectal malformation is generally made by physical examination. In male infants, more than 95% of low malformations are associated with either a thin anal membrane or a fistula to the perineum or scrotal raphe. The presence of a "bucket-handle" skin deformity at the presumptive anal dimple is also diagnostic of a low lesion. Infants with high malformations typically lack anal skin dimpling, have a flat gluteal contour, and may have little or absent contraction of the external sphincter with cutaneous stimulation. In female infants, 90% to 95% of low malformations have a perineal or vestibular fistula. In both male and female infants, a perineal fistula may not become apparent in the first 12 to 24 hours of life until meconium progresses distally through the rectum into the fistula.

Diagnosis

From a clinical standpoint, intermediate lesions are treated as high malformations; thus, the two groups are considered jointly. Because surgical treatment of a high or intermediate anorectal malformation is different from that for low lesion, a

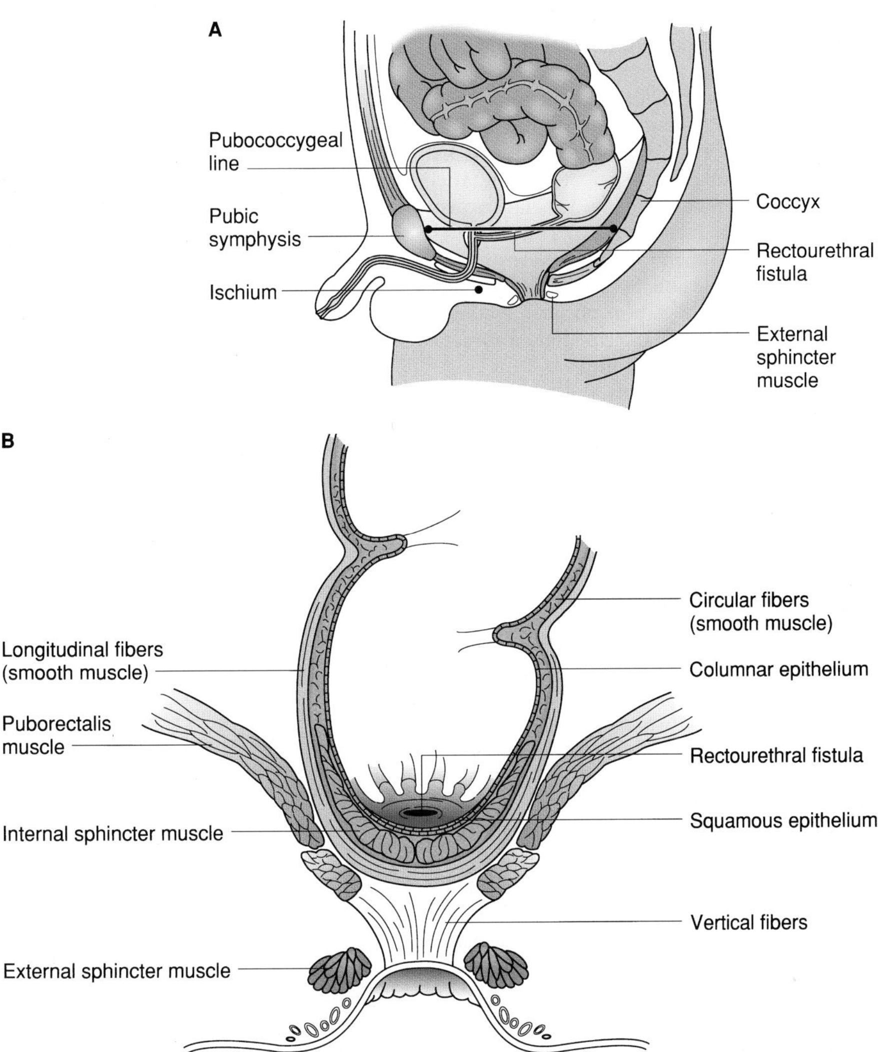

FIGURE 110.17 Male infant with high imperforate anus, showing the pubococcygeal line, ischium, and striated muscle complex. (*A*) The rectal pouch ends cephalad to the pubococcygeal line. This location of the rectourethral fistula is typical. (*B*) Coronal view showing incomplete development of the rectal pouch within the striated muscle complex. The rectourethral fistula is shown.

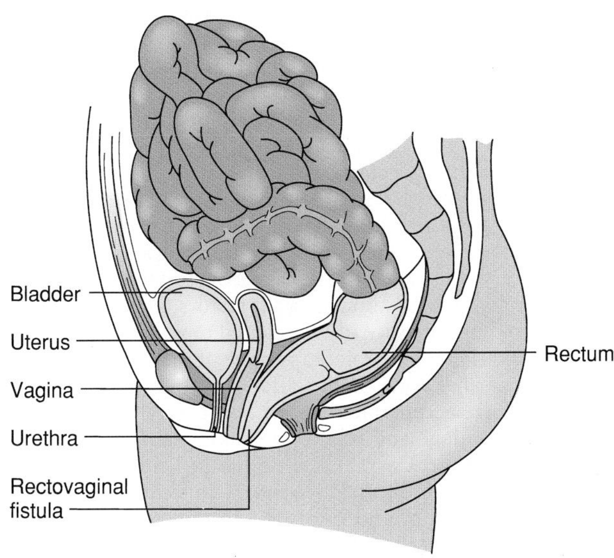

FIGURE 110.18 Female infant with low imperforate anus and vestibular fistula.

primary diagnostic goal is to determine whether an infant with imperforate anus has a high or low malformation. A secondary diagnostic goal is to determine the specific anorectal malformation as it relates to the rectourethral or rectourinary fistula. The infant with imperforate anus also must be assessed in comprehensive fashion for associated congenital anomalies.

Clinical examination of an infant with low imperforate anus almost always reveals an external fistula to the perineum or vestibule. The classic radiographic study of newborns with imperforate anus is the Wangensteen-Rice invertogram, with a lateral view of the pelvis obtained 12 to 24 hours after birth with the infant in a head-down position. Swallowed air serves as intraluminal contrast, and using a radiodense perineal skin marker, the relationship of the rectal pouch to the perineum, pubococcygeal line, and the ischium is assessed. The procedure is accurate if conducted by a technically skilled and experienced examiner; however, incomplete distention of the distal rectum with gas may decrease the accuracy of this technique. Other diagnostic modalities to define high versus low lesions include the prone cross-table lateral view as well as ultrasound.[47] Real-time ultrasound is currently well-accepted as an accurate method of determining the distal extent of the rectal pouch. Computed tomography (CT) imaging and MRI can be extremely useful in evaluating the pelvic striated muscle complex. MRI is also useful in evaluation of the distal spinal cord in these infants.

If there is a suspected perineal fistula or covered anus, diagnostic needle aspiration under anesthesia may be useful. Aspiration of meconium not only localizes the rectum or fistula, but it also can provide an estimation of the distance between the perineum and the rectum or the fistula. In general, low lesions are within 1 to 2 cm of the perineum; high lesions are greater than 2 cm from the perineum. Any infant not clearly found to have a low lesion by physical examination, radiographic studies, or examination under anesthesia should be considered to have a high or intermediate anorectal malformation and should be treated accordingly.

A voiding cystourethrogram is generally the procedure of choice for defining the rectourethral or rectovesical fistula. In some instances, cystoscopy is a useful adjunct before repair of high imperforate anus. For example, an infant with a large rectourethral fistula may require cystoscopic guidance of a urinary catheter to avoid inadvertent placement of the catheter through the fistula and into the rectum.

Treatment

Imperforate anus by itself is not a life-threatening condition, and, in many instances, observation for 12 to 24 hours may help to delineate the presence or absence of a fistula. The surgical management of anorectal malformations has been well described elsewhere[45] and a brief summary follows below.

Low Malformations. Definitive repair of most low anorectal malformations can be performed in the newborn period with perineal procedures that do not require a diverting colostomy. Simple dilatation of the fistula or unroofing of a covered anus may relieve the anatomic obstruction. For more complex anal stenoses or anterior perineal fistulas, a formal perineal anoplasty may be required. A common perineal procedure performed is cutback anoplasty, in which the anterior fistula or anal orifice is opened posteriorly by dividing the perineum to the external sphincter. More complex alternative approaches may be preferred in female infants with low vaginal or anterior perineal fistulas. These lesions generally require circumferential mobilization of the anterior fistula with transposition to the center of the external sphincter. Anterior reconstruction of the perineal body is then performed. The transposition anoplasty is designed to position the neoanus within the center of the external sphincter and separate the neoanus from the vaginal introitus.

Intermediate and High Malformations. Infants determined to have an intermediate, high, or indeterminate anorectal malformation generally require diverting colostomy as initial surgical management. Care must be taken to ensure that the proximal diverting colostomy provides adequate length and mobility of the distal colon in anticipation of eventual anorectoplasty. A divided colostomy is preferred over a loop colostomy by many surgeons to provide maximal fecal diversion from the downstream rectourinary fistula. Following diverting colostomy, a distal contrast study into the rectal pouch can also define the fistula and delineate the position of the rectum relative to the perineum.

Anorectoplasty is generally performed when the infant is approximately 8 to 12 months of age or weighs of about 8 kg. Many different approaches have been described, and considerable personal and institutional variation is common. No single approach has superior results, and all have technical merits and difficulties. The common surgical objectives in the treatment of anorectal malformations include: (a) relief of the rectal obstruction; (b) creation of a new anus; (c) position the rectum as normally as possible within the striated muscle complex; and (d) divide the rectourinary fistula. In addition, preservation of the surrounding structures (prostate, urethra, seminal vesicles, vaginal wall) is essential.

For repair of high and intermediate anorectal malformations, the most widely used procedure in the United States is the posterior sagittal anorectoplasty described in detail by Peña.[45] The infant is placed prone and a posterior sagittal incision following the gluteal crease is used. The external sphincter and the striated muscle complex are divided posteriorly along the midline to expose the rectal pouch. A muscle stimulator is used to define and map the striated muscle complex and to confirm symmetric dissection along the midline. Typically, the rectal pouch can be adequately dissected by this approach to allow enough length to reach the perineum. Infrequently, a combined abdominoperineal approach is required. The mobilized rectal pouch is opened and the rectourinary fistula identified and closed directly. The rectal pouch is placed centrally within the striated muscle complex, which is reconstructed circumferentially around the rectum. The neoanus is centered within the external sphincter and the mucosa is sutured to the perineum.

Other accepted and practiced surgical approaches to imperforate anus include a sacroperineal approach as proposed by Stephens,[48] and an approach that uses components of endorectal dissection as attributed to Rehbein.[49] Both these surgical procedures are characterized by blind pull-through of the distal rectum to the perineum without direct visualization of the striated muscle complex. Experience with laparoscopic dissection and division of the rectourinary fistula with perineal pull-through reconstruction has been reported.[50] It appears that personal preference, experience, and familiarity rather than differences in outcome dictate the selection of procedure. In general, diverting colostomy in all of these procedures is maintained until the anorectoplasty has completely healed, after which the colostomy is closed electively.

Results, Complications, and Outcome

Mortality following anorectoplasty is related to the presence of associated congenital anomalies other than imperforate anus. A careful review of 284 infants undergoing repair of anorectal malformations observed an 18.7% mortality,[51] suggesting that this group is at moderate to high risk for complications and death secondary to coexisting congenital anomalies.

Complications are similar to other gastrointestinal surgical procedures and include infection or leak. Leak or stricture formation is observed in 5% to 10% of infants undergoing tapering rectoplasty during posterior sagittal anorectoplasty. Anorectal strictures are treated by gradual postoperative anal dilatation for weeks to months. Recurrent rectourethral fistula or urethral stricture is uncommon.

Long-term functional outcome in infants with low malformations is generally excellent given the relatively normal descent of the distal rectum within the striated muscle complex. Infants with intermediate or high lesions have a less predictable prognosis and are much more likely to have difficulty with fecal continence. Currently, the outcomes appear to be independent of the type of surgical reconstruction performed and more related to anatomic patient factors, including degree of rectal descent, integrity of the striated muscle complex, and sacral innervation. Few or perhaps none of these children have completely normal bowel habits after operation. About half of the infants have acceptable to good results with few episodes of accidental soilage and relatively simple management using enemas and cathartics.[52,53] The remaining children require major adjustments in lifestyle secondary to fecal incontinence, chronic constipation, and odor. In some instances, socially acceptable continence can be assisted by the use of daily antegrade enemas via a cecostomy or appendicostomy. In other situations, a permanent diverting colostomy may be desirable.

Necrotizing Enterocolitis

Pathophysiology

NEC is a neonatal disease characterized by an initial intestinal mucosal injury that may ultimately progress to transmural bowel necrosis. NEC is the most frequently encountered neonatal surgical emergency and a major cause of morbidity and mortality in the premature infant. Despite its frequency and extensive study, the pathogenesis remains obscure, and surgical treatment is directed largely at controlling the complications of intestinal necrosis. The development of NEC occurs in association with a variety of associated conditions, including perinatal stress, sepsis, respiratory failure, hypoxemia, hypotension, and congenital cardiac defects. In general, NEC is observed in the premature infant with multiple risk factors and potential etiologic events and conditions. Current clinical and experimental data support the concept that the pathophysiology of NEC remains enigmatic and multifactorial.

The intestinal mucosal injury observed in NEC is likely to be the end result of an ischemic insult in a susceptible host. Normally, the neonatal pulmonary and systemic vascular smooth muscle undergoes rapid structural and physiologic changes shortly after birth. The premature infant appears to be particularly vulnerable to vasoconstriction. With regard to NEC, it is hypothesized that hypoperfusion and ischemia of the premature neonatal intestinal tract may be the result of uncontrolled splanchnic vasoconstriction. This situation may be worsened in critically ill premature infants with low cardiac output states and relatively high circulating red cell mass leading to hyperviscosity. Perinatal stress such as acidosis, hypoxemia, and hypothermia also are associated with acute pulmonary vascular hypertension and right-to-left shunting via a patent ductus arteriosus. This shunting can significantly decrease oxygen delivery to areas of already marginal tissue perfusion in the neonatal intestine.

A common characteristic of NEC is the host inflammatory response to the initiating mucosal injury. Experimental data are consistent with an important role for oxygen-derived free radicals and inflammatory mediators in the propagation of intestinal injury in NEC.[54–56] Although the local inflammatory response is necessary for repair of injured tissue, an uncontrolled or exaggerated systemic inflammatory response may be elicited in a vulnerable host, ultimately causing multiorgan dysfunction and failure.

More than 90% of cases of NEC occur after the initiation of enteral feeding, and several studies document that the osmolarity or rate of initial feeding may be important. Although controversy exists, most neonatal centers now avoid rapid advancement of hyperosmolar enteral feedings and attempt to prevent excessive fluid volume in premature infants.[57,58] Episodic clustering of cases of NEC has been reported, and infectious etiologic agents such as *Clostridium* species (including *C. difficile*), *Pseudomonas aeruginosa, Enterobacter cloacae, Staphyloccocus aureus,* and *Klebsiella* species have been implicated. These normal intestinal flora may be more opportunistic in the face of intestinal mucosal injury; whether they are directly responsible for the initiation of NEC remains unclear.

The most common site of involvement of NEC is the terminal ileum and right colon. NEC may be localized, segmental, or it may involve the entire gastrointestinal tract. Histopathologic examination of intestinal tissue from infants with NEC demonstrates submucosal edema, hemorrhage, and microvascular thrombosis leading to transmural necrosis. The histopathology of NEC resembles that of experimental intestinal ischemia, with areas of reversible mucosal injury adjacent to areas of transmural necrosis (Fig. 110.19). Dissection of intraluminal gas through the injured mucosa leads to gas within the bowel wall, known as *pneumatosis intestinalis*. The finding of pneumatosis intestinalis is a classic radiographic and pathologic feature of NEC. Initially, the gas may be localized in the submucosa or lymphatic vessels, but it may dissect into the muscularis, the portal venous tract, or into the subserosa. Intestinal perforation, inflammatory phlegmon, and diffuse peritonitis are common with advanced NEC.

Clinical Presentation

Over the past three decades, advancements in technology, prenatal care, and neonatology have improved overall outcome in premature infants that were previously unable to survive. In the United States alone, low birth weight infants (less than 2,500 g) account for approximately 281,015 births (7.41% of all live births), with 67% of these infants born prematurely.[59] At least half of all infants with NEC are extremely low birth weight infants weighing less than 1,500 g. In a study of 302 infants with NEC treated over two decades, the average birth weight fell from 1,645 to 1,505 g, and in similar fashion, the mean gestational age fell from 32.4 weeks to 30.4 weeks.[60] NEC is estimated to occur in 1 to 3 of 1,000 live births and in

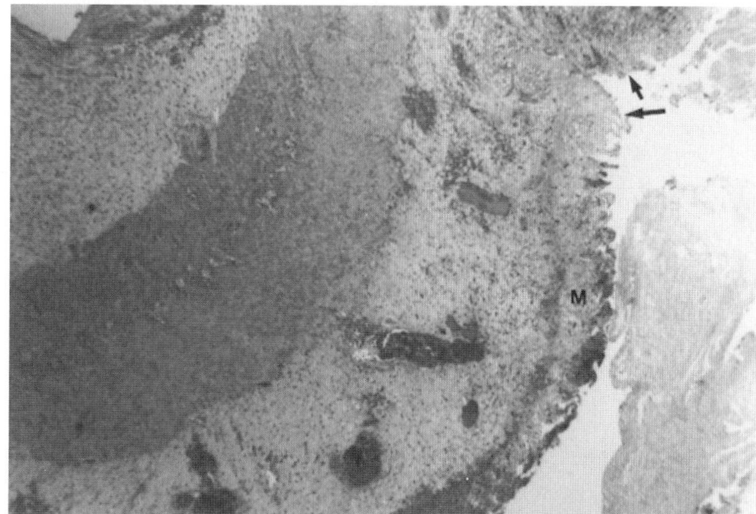

FIGURE 110.19 Photomicrograph of intestine in an infant with necrotizing enterocolitis. An area of epithelial slough is adjacent to injured but surviving mucosa (M). Despite the obvious injury, the muscular mucosa is not infarcted.

TABLE 110.4 STAGING

NECROTIZING ENTEROCOLITIS

STAGE I NEC (SUSPECTED)
Any one or more historical factors producing perinatal stress
Systemic manifestations
- Temperature instability
- Lethargy
- Apnea
- Bradycardia

Gastrointestinal manifestations
- Poor feeding
- Increasing pregavage residuals
- Emesis
- Mild abdominal distention
- Occult blood in stool

Abdominal radiographs showing distention with mild ileus

STAGE II NEC (DEFINITE)
Any one or more historical factors
Above signs and symptoms, plus:
- Persistent occult or gross gastrointestinal bleeding
- Marked abdominal distention

Abdominal radiographs showing significant intestinal distention with:
- Ileus
- Small bowel edema
- Pneumatosis intestinalis
- Portal venous gas

STAGE III NEC (ADVANCED)
Any one or more historical factors
Above signs and symptoms, plus: Deterioration of vital signs
- Evidence of septic shock
- Marked gastrointestinal hemorrhage
- Abdominal radiographs showing pneumoperitoneum in addition to findings listed for stage II

From Bell MJ, Kosloske AM, Benton C, et al. Neonatal necrotizing enterocolitis: prevention of perforation. *J Pediatr Surg*. 1973;8:601–605, with permission.

30 per 1,000 low birth weight births.[61] NEC may also occur in term infants, and in this group, it has a tendency to involve the colon and may present without classic signs.[62] The actual incidence of NEC remains difficult to determine because the diagnosis is subjective; classic signs on physical examination and diagnostic imaging are not always uniformly present. The classic clinical signs of NEC include abdominal distention, feeding intolerance, bilious emesis, and either occult or gross blood in the stool. Gastrointestinal mucosal bleeding is present in the vast majority of cases (80% to 90%) but is rarely significant from a hemodynamic standpoint. On physical examination, abdominal tenderness with distention is common, and individual loops of thickened or fixed bowel may be palpable. Edema, erythema, crepitus, or discoloration of the abdominal wall suggests intestinal necrosis, perforation, or intraabdominal abscess. Hematochezia or guaiac-positive stool is typical. Systemic signs of inflammation and sepsis such as temperature instability, apnea, bradycardia, hypoxemia, acidosis, and thrombocytopenia are also common. The primary diagnostic goal during initial clinical evaluation is to determine whether irreversible, transmural intestinal necrosis is present. There is no single physical finding or laboratory test that makes this distinction, but some clinically relevant observations useful in determining the need for operative intervention are discussed later.

Diagnosis

The diagnosis of NEC relies on clinical evaluation and judgment based on symptoms and signs in the appropriate setting. Table 110.4 summarizes diagnostic criteria and a staging system for NEC most commonly used in the United States.[63] Radiographic confirmation of NEC requires only plain abdominal films. During the acute inflammatory phase, contrast studies may be hazardous and are contraindicated. The classic radiographic finding of pneumatosis intestinalis (Fig. 110.20) confirms the diagnosis in the appropriate clinical setting but is variably present. Other radiographic findings consistent with NEC include thickened bowel loops, ascites, and portal venous gas. Serial abdominal films, including a left lateral decubitus or upright film, should be obtained every 6 to 8 hours during the early course of the disease. These sequential studies help to document the progression or resolution of the inflammatory process and, importantly, evaluate for the presence of intestinal perforation presenting as free intraperitoneal gas or pneumoperitoneum. The presence of pneumoperitoneum mandates operative intervention; however, up to half of infants with perforated NEC do not have discernible pneumoperitoneum on plain films.

Treatment

Nonoperative. The vast majority of infants with NEC can be managed medically. Initial management of NEC includes proximal decompression with a nasogastric or orogastric tube, bowel rest, and broad-spectrum intravenous antibiotics. Prompt correction of hypotension, hypoxemia, and inadequate ventilation must be undertaken. Intravenous fluid management, with particular attention to electrolytes and acid–base status, is essential. Central venous access is secured and TPN is initiated. Oxygen delivery and cardiac performance must be maintained, which in a premature neonate may require operative closure of a patent ductus arteriosus; this approach is preferable over the use of indomethacin in the setting of NEC.[64] Serial physical examinations and blood work are useful in monitoring disease progress.

Most infants with NEC improve with the relatively simple medical management outlined previously. Typically, reversal

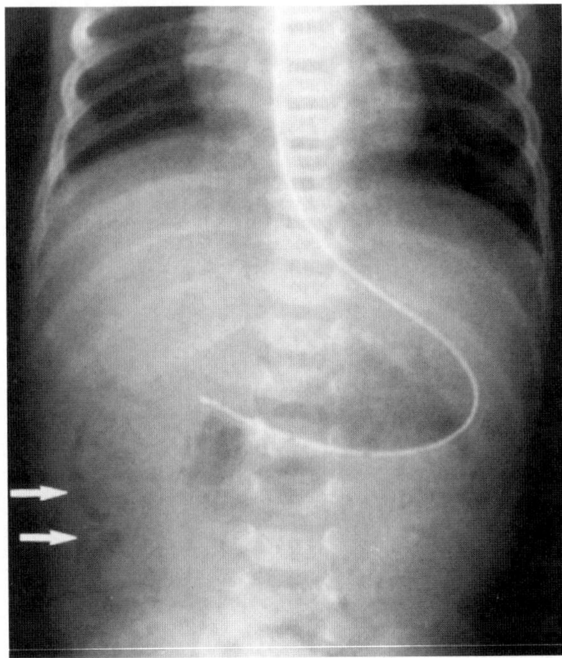

FIGURE 110.20 Plain abdominal film demonstrating *pneumatosis intestinalis* (*arrows*) in an infant with necrotizing enterocolitis.

of the systemic inflammatory response occurs rapidly, and the abdominal distention and ileus resolve over a period of days. Nasogastric tube decompression and intravenous antibiotics are usually continued for 7 to 14 days. Enteral feeding usually is resumed once antibiotics have been discontinued and there has been return of gastrointestinal function. The usual course of medically treated NEC is rapid clinical response and stabilization in the first 24 to 36 hours. Infants with significant intestinal necrosis typically have signs of either pneumoperitoneum or clinical deterioration during the initial 24 to 72 hours of treatment.

Indications to abandon medical management and escalate surgical therapy include evidence of intestinal perforation or clinical deterioration with persistent or progressive systemic illness despite maximal medical therapy. Evidence of persistent or progressive systemic sepsis includes temperature instability, refractory hypotension, acidosis, hypoglycemia, neutropenia, and thrombocytopenia. Local findings such as portal venous gas, abdominal wall cellulitis, or crepitus also may signal intestinal necrosis and the need for operative intervention. A palpable, fixed abdominal mass consistent with intestinal perforation with an inflammatory phlegmon or abscess also may be a relative indication for operation. Because there is not complete agreement on what constitutes clinical deterioration, some controversy exists regarding operative indications for NEC in the absence of pneumoperitoneum. Because the interpretation of clinical deterioration criteria remains subjective, the decision to operate remains a multifactorial clinical judgment. In equivocal situations, abdominal paracentesis of ascitic fluid may be helpful in diagnosing intestinal necrosis with perforation in the absence of pneumoperitoneum if the aspirate contains bacteria or stool.[65]

Operative. Operative indications in NEC include the presence of intestinal necrosis with or without frank intestinal perforation. Conventional operative intervention is aimed at treating the complications of NEC (i.e., intestinal necrosis) rather than preventing or stopping the factors that cause the disease. In general, resection of intestine involved with NEC does not prevent further extension of disease in other involved areas of the bowel. For isolated segmental disease, the traditional surgical treatment of NEC is resection of necrotic bowel with proximal enterostomy and distal mucous fistula placement. In infants with diffuse NEC, multiple resections with several enterostomies may be required. The primary operative goal is an expedient operation with preservation of as much intestinal length as possible, including the ileocecal valve. Because the risk of developing short-gut syndrome is substantial in infants with diffuse disease, preservation of marginal areas of involved intestine with a planned second-look operation to reevaluate intestinal viability may be useful. Accurate measurement of the remaining bowel length is important from a diagnostic and prognostic standpoint, with the length of bowel resected determined by the extent of transmural intestinal necrosis. Resection with primary anastomosis in selected infants with NEC has been reported,[66] with a recent study observing recurrent NEC in 22% and strictures in 17% of 18 treated infants following primary anastomosis.[67] Complete intestinal necrosis of the small intestine and colon is uncommon and is not compatible with long-term survival without the sequelae of short-gut syndrome and the potential need for intestinal transplantation (Fig. 110.21).

Infants with NEC are typically fragile and premature and complications in this population are not well tolerated. For the high-risk, low birth weight infant, some data suggest that initial management with primary peritoneal drainage rather than laparotomy and bowel resection may be useful as either a temporizing measure or, in some instances, a definitive procedure.[68]

Complications, Results, and Outcome

Most infants with NEC are treated successfully without operative intervention. Morbidity and mortality for this group are related primarily to problems associated with prematurity. Given the delay of bowel function and the need for TPN, cholestatic jaundice commonly occurs but is generally reversible. Infants placed on broad-spectrum antibiotics for an extended period are at risk for developing fungal sepsis. For infants with intestinal necrosis from NEC, infectious complications, including peritonitis, systemic sepsis, and intraabdominal abscess formation may occur. Progression of disease may also occur after surgical therapy, particularly if marginally viable bowel is preserved.

The overall surgical complication rate in infants with NEC is at least 20% to 40%. Virtually every infant with NEC has a significant complication, an associated medical problem, or both. Immediate technical complications in treating NEC include intestinal leak, fistula formation, stoma necrosis, bleeding, and liver injury during exploration. These complications

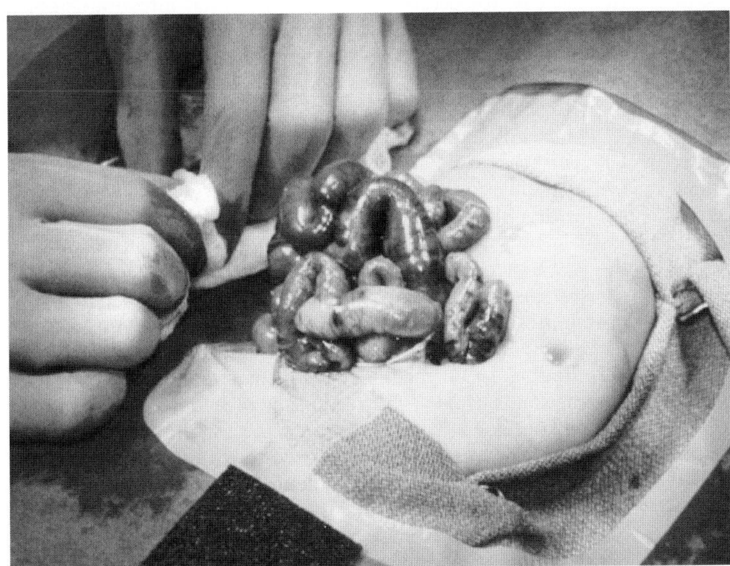

FIGURE 110.21 Fulminant necrotizing enterocolitis involving the entire gastrointestinal tract in a premature infant. Note the presence of pneumatosis intestinalis.

are obviously magnified in the extremely low birth weight infant with preexisting intestinal injury. Fluid and electrolyte losses from proximal diverting enterostomies can be significant and even life threatening in extremely low birth weight infants whose circulating blood volume is less than 50 to 100 mL. A review of 68 infants treated surgically for NEC observed a 26% mortality rate and a 68% complication rate related to the stoma or its closure in the perioperative survivors.[69] Complications included intestinal stricture, incisional or parastomal hernia, stoma prolapse, intussusception, wound dehiscence or infection, small bowel obstruction, and anastomotic failure. The complications associated with diverting enterostomy in this unique population provide a compelling rationale for early enterostomy closure once the inflammation from peritonitis has resolved. A prospective, randomized trial comparing resection and enterostomy with resection and primary anastomosis in the treatment of NEC has not been reported.

Intestinal stricture formation following NEC, whether managed operatively or nonoperatively, is not uncommon. This consequence usually results from a normal host inflammatory response to transmural intestinal injury. As host mechanisms begin to heal and repair the injured intestine, submucosal fibrosis may occur. The degree of fibrosis and subsequent stricture formation are clearly related to the severity and extent of disease. Less frequently, mesenteric vascular compromise secondary to an intraabdominal adhesion may lead to stricture formation. Although stricture can develop anywhere in the gastrointestinal tract involved with NEC, a higher rate of demonstrable stricture is observed in the left colon, occurring in as many as 36% of medically treated infants.[70] Routine contrast enema 4 to 6 weeks after clinical resolution of NEC treated operatively or nonoperatively has been advocated in some institutions. Symptomatic strictures generally require segmental resection with anastomosis, although fluoroscopically guided balloon catheter dilatation has been reported.

Overall survival rates for infants with NEC have improved significantly over the past three decades and is currently about 60% to 80% for both operative and nonoperative groups.[68] The observed improvement in survival is thought to reflect improved neonatal intensive care, the use of TPN, and early, aggressive treatment for suspected NEC. Most neonatal intensive care units initiate aggressive medical treatment in any infant with suspected NEC. Whether surgical interventions such as resection with primary anastomosis or limited primary peritoneal drainage can improve morbidity and mortality in these critically ill infants remains to be fully determined. Long-term outcome for NEC survivors generally reflects associated problems of prematurity. In particular, many of these infants have persisting neurodevelopmental, ophthalmologic, and pulmonary disease, but morbidity from the gastrointestinal system generally is limited to infants with short-gut syndrome following extensive bowel resection. These infants present complex ethical and management issues beyond the scope of this review. Most NEC survivors (75%) enjoy a good to excellent quality of life, suggesting that the treatment cost relative to the potential benefit for these infants is worthwhile.[71]

Meconium Ileus

Meconium ileus is a descriptive term for small bowel obstruction in a newborn infant with cystic fibrosis (CF). About 10% to 20% of infants with CF initially present with meconium ileus. A review of CF is useful to understand the pathophysiology and treatment of meconium ileus.

CF is the most common fatal hereditary disease in Europe and North America. It is an autosomal recessive disorder found with a heterozygous carrier incidence rate of 1 in 20 to 25 in white populations. The estimated incidence rate of homozygous gene expression and phenotypic manifestation of CF is about 1 in 2,000 to 2,500 in this population.[72] The CF gene has been cloned and the single most common mutation characterized.[73,74] The most common point mutation is a three-base-pair deletion found in 70% to 75% of the carrier population. This mutation leads to deletion of a phenylalanine residue in amino acid position 508 of the CF transmembrane conductance regulator (*CFTR*) gene. In addition, there are about 200 more infrequent mutations of the *CFTR* gene that lead to clinical CF. The molecular heterogeneity of *CFTR* gene mutations produces practical implications in the development and use of carrier screening tests in the general population. Currently, widespread use of molecular genetic screening tests in the general population to identify asymptomatic carriers and at-risk couples without a family history of CF is not recommended; there are significant technical, ethical, and social issues that must be prospectively addressed.[75] Screening of at-risk couples with a family history of CF is recommended, however, and in this setting, carrier discovery approaches 100% so that appropriate genetic counseling can be provided. Molecular genetic screening also should be offered to parents and infants with clinically suspected CF as well as asymptomatic infants born to at-risk couples. This approach allows rapid identification and confirmation of virtually all infants homozygous for CF.

Pathophysiology

The clinical manifestations of CF are caused by an epithelial electrolyte transport defect that results in impermeability to the chloride (Cl^-) ion.[76] The epithelial defect occurs in apocrine sweat glands and the tracheobronchial tree as well as the pancreas, gastrointestinal tract, and liver. In sweat glands, failure of normal Cl^- ion reabsorption following beta-adrenergic stimulation leads to an obligate sodium chloride loss despite a normal adenosine triphosphate (ATP)-dependent sodium-potassium pump. This mechanism is the basis for the traditional diagnostic *sweat chloride test*.

Reduction of Cl^- permeability in the tracheobronchial tree leads to diminished secretion volume as well as increased absorption of sodium chloride. As a result, airway secretions in CF patients are low in volume and particularly viscous. Because of the tenacious nature of the airway secretions, airway clearance is impaired, which leads to chronic, recurrent infection with bronchitis and pneumonia. As the disease advances, bronchiectasis and progressive pulmonary parenchymal destruction ensues. Recurrent pulmonary bacterial infection is common, and airway colonization by *P. aeruginosa* is predictable. Chronic pulmonary disease accounts for more than 90% of the deaths in advanced CF, with a mean life expectancy approaching 30 years.

Pancreatic exocrine function is also affected by impaired Cl^- permeability. Pancreatic duct obstruction resulting from inspissated viscous secretion is followed by glandular autolysis, acinar atrophy, and pancreatic fibrosis. Pancreatic exocrine insufficiency is a classic early clinical feature of CF and is thought to account for many of the gastrointestinal manifestations of the disease. In particular, the deficiency of pancreatic proteinases leads to meconium ileus in the newborn, characterized by abnormally thick and viscid, protein-laden meconium that causes mechanical gastrointestinal obstruction. The obstruction is usually observed in the terminal ileum just proximal to the ileocecal valve (Fig. 110.22). Infants with meconium ileus have small pellets, or concretions, of pale, nonbilious meconium in the terminal ileum with a distal microcolon. Proximal to the obstruction, the meconium is variably mixed with gas and often is thick and tarry in consistency. The bowel containing the thick meconium is often grossly distended and

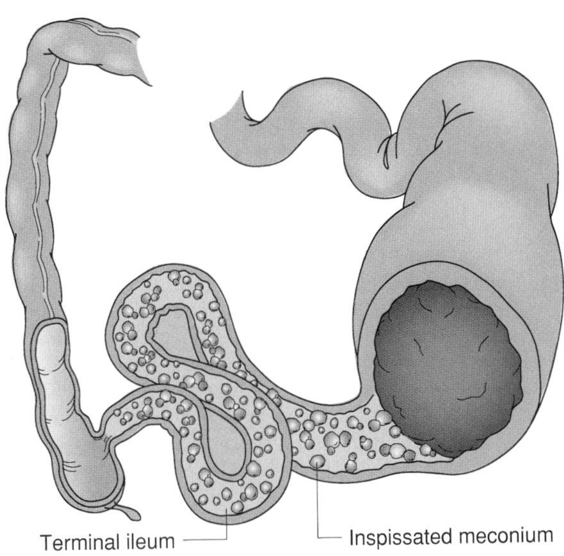

FIGURE 110.22 Meconium ileus causing obstruction of the terminal ileum from abnormally thick, inspissated meconium.

thickened. Microscopically, the muscularis is hypertrophied; distended mucous glands with prominent goblet cells may be present. The most proximal jejunum is typically normal.

In utero events such as proximal volvulus of the dilated segment of ileum, perforation from distention, or atresia occur in approximately one third to one half of fetuses with meconium ileus. These clinical entities are characterized together as *complicated meconium ileus*. A classic clinical presentation of complicated meconium ileus is in utero intestinal perforation with sterile meconium peritonitis and formation of a calcified pseudocyst (Fig. 110.23). Gastrointestinal conditions presenting later in life occur in 10% of children with CF and include acute appendicitis, recurrent rectal prolapse, and intussusception. These conditions reflect abnormal transit of thick, inspissated stool causing proximal distention or obstruction of the bowel lumen. Small-bowel obstruction in CF outside the neonatal period is termed *meconium ileus equivalent*. Treatment of meconium ileus equivalent is similar to initial nonoperative management of uncomplicated meconium ileus in the newborn and is discussed below. Prevention of meconium ileus equivalent relies on conscientious pancreatic enzyme replacement. Finally, children with CF are at risk to cholestasis secondary to obstruction of small intrahepatic bile ducts. Chronic hepatic inflammation can occur with subsequent fibrosis and cirrhosis, causing hepatic failure and portal hypertension in approximately 5% of CF patients.

Diagnostic Evaluation

In nearly all newborns with CF, the diagnosis is clinically apparent by the presence of meconium ileus, a family history of CF in a sibling, or a positive newborn screening test. Laboratory confirmation of *CFTR* gene dysfunction is performed in several ways. The historical standard for detection of CF has been analysis of the sodium chloride content of the sweat. The most commonly used and reliable technique uses pilocarpine iontophoresis, with positive sweat test results showing sodium and chloride concentrations exceeding 60 mEq/L.[77] This test is less useful during the first 4 to 6 weeks of age because normal neonates do not reliably conserve sodium chloride in sweat. Generally, abnormal *CFTR* gene is documented by two elevated sweat chloride tests obtained on separate days. With the emergence of genetic technology capable of providing accurate assessment of *CFTR* gene mutations, the sweat test is

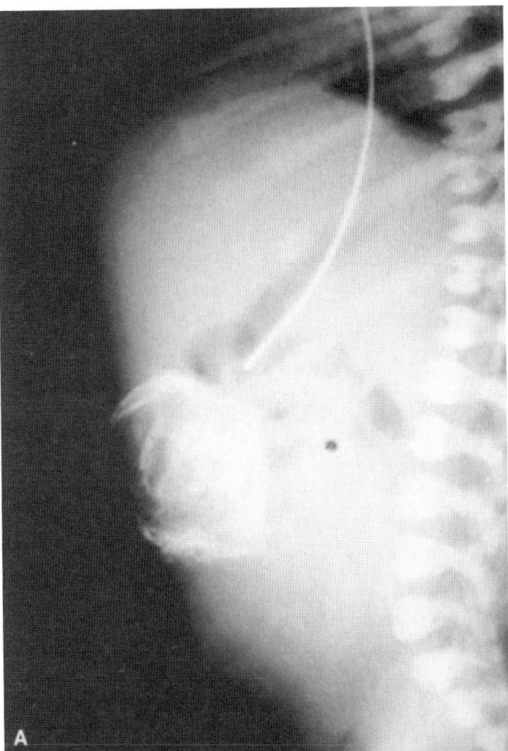

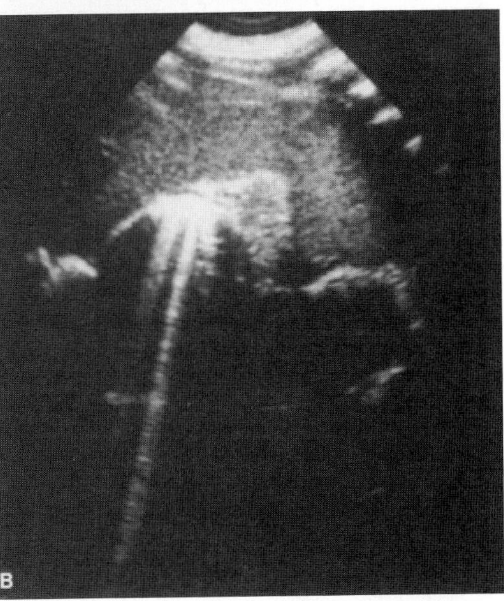

FIGURE 110.23 (*A*) Plain film radiograph of calcified pseudocyst in complicated meconium ileus. (*B*) *In utero* ultrasound demonstrating calcified pseudocyst.

now largely used to provide clinical confirmation of *CFTR* gene dysfunction along with molecular diagnosis of CF.

Clinical Presentation

With routine prenatal ultrasound practices along with selected fetal DNA screening, the prenatal diagnosis of CF or meconium ileus is feasible, potentially allowing for improved management of anticipated clinical problems following delivery.[78] Initial signs of meconium ileus include neonatal bowel obstruction with abdominal distention, bilious emesis, and failure to pass meconium. On examination, the neonate may have palpable loops of meconium-filled intestine with a texture on palpation described as "doughy." Similar to other causes of proximal neonatal intestinal obstruction, rectal examination and evaluation of the meconium typically reveals clear white mucus or thick gray meconium. In utero intestinal perforation with pseudocyst formation in complicated meconium ileus may cause a palpable abdominal mass that is not particularly tender. On plain films or ultrasound, calcifications is visible in the pseudocyst wall. In contrast, volvulus or intestinal perforation secondary to meconium ileus following birth generally results in diffuse peritonitis and sepsis. Intestinal atresia also may be seen as a consequence of complicated meconium ileus.

Diagnosis

Abdominal plain films may be diagnostic in meconium ileus, demonstrating multiple, distended loops of bowel (Fig. 110.24A). Fluid- or meconium-filled loops of bowel mixed with gas give a characteristic "soap-bubble" or "ground-glass" appearance. Classic air-fluid levels seen in other causes of intestinal obstruction are not expected because of the tenacious, sticky intraluminal meconium. The presence of intraperitoneal calcifications or a calcified cyst is consistent with prenatal intestinal perforation of sterile meconium.

A contrast enema is useful in the evaluation and treatment of simple meconium ileus. This study usually demonstrates an unused but functionally normal microcolon (Fig. 110.24B). Reflux of contrast into the terminal ileum may confirm the presence of inspissated meconium pellets. In conjunction with a family history and plain films, this finding is sufficient evidence to confirm the diagnosis of neonatal meconium ileus. Upper gastrointestinal contrast studies are generally unnecessary and may complicate further therapeutic efforts.

Treatment

Nonoperative. Nonoperative management of simple meconium ileus is achieved in about 60% to 70% of newborns. Once the diagnosis of meconium ileus is confirmed, the initial treatment of choice is to perform retrograde irrigation of the terminal ileum with one of several solutions designed to dissipate the obstructing meconium. In the United States, several different enema techniques and a variety of contrast media have been described, including normal saline, hyperosmolar contrast agents, and dilute N-acetylcysteine. Initially, it was believed that using hyperosmolar contrast material was necessary to create an osmolar gradient. The resultant influx of fluid into the intestinal lumen was thought to solubilize the inspissated meconium. Recent data suggest that successful meconium clearance is not necessarily related to the osmolality of the contrast agent; however, a significantly higher overall success rate is reported with the use of Gastrografin (sodium and meglumine amidotrizoate) and the use of other solubilizing agents such as Tween-80 and N-acetylcysteine.[79] As long as clinical progress is being made, sequential enemas may be required to disimpact the inspissated meconium from the terminal ileum. In similar fashion, children and older patients presenting with meconium ileus equivalent are treated with retrograde enemas until the obstruction resolves. The distinct advantage of this treatment approach is the avoidance of general anesthesia and exploratory laparotomy. Reported complications with this approach include rare intestinal perforation, intestinal mucosal injury, and persistent obstruction resulting from meconium concretions.

Operative. The major indications for operative intervention are either failure to clear the obstruction by retrograde enema or complicated meconium ileus with cyst formation, volvulus, atresia, or perforation. For simple meconium ileus with persistent obstruction despite contrast enemas, the operative goals are meconium disimpaction from the ileum and evacuation of the remaining stool from the small intestine. These steps can be accomplished by either milking the intraluminal meconium downstream into the colon or solubilizing the meconium by transmural needle instillation of irrigant. In general, however, enterotomy or enterostomy and direct irrigation of the bowel lumen are required to completely clear the inspissated, sticky meconium. Simple closure of the enterotomy is preferred, but segmental resection may be required if marginal or compromised intestine is found. End-to-end anastomosis is the appropriate reconstruction technique following segmental bowel resection. A temporary enterostomy may be required, and several historical techniques have been described. Another surgical option is the placement of a T-tube into the ileum for continued irrigation with dilute N-acetylcysteine. Following clearance of

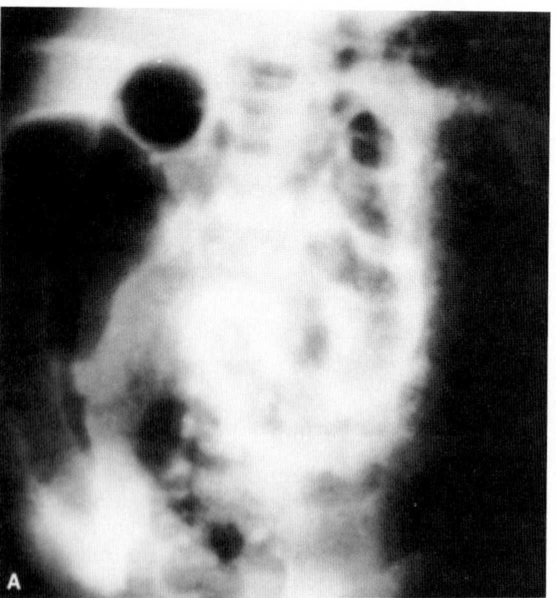

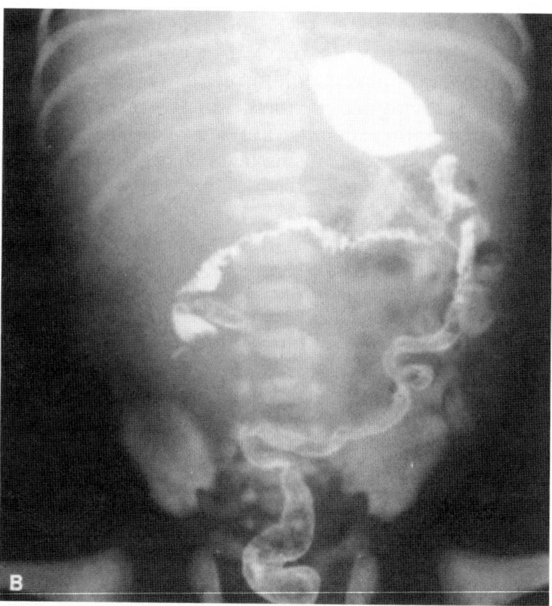

FIGURE 110.24 (*A*) Plain radiograph of neonate with meconium ileus. (*B*) Contrast enema in an infant with meconium ileus demonstrating an unused but intrinsically normal microcolon.

meconium from the intestine and the return of bowel function, the T-tube can be safely and simply removed.[80]

Complicated meconium ileus occurs in about one third of patients and includes segmental volvulus, intestinal atresia or stenosis, necrosis, perforation, and meconium cyst formation. The surgical management of these entities is individualized. Intestinal atresia is not uncommon in meconium ileus, and the entire length of the intestine must be inspected for patency. When possible, resection of nonviable, stenotic, or perforated intestine is performed with immediate reconstruction via primary anastomosis. Patency of the downstream bowel must be confirmed to prevent anastomotic leak resulting from distal obstruction. If the infant is critically ill or has diffuse peritonitis, a safe primary anastomosis may not be possible and a diverting enterostomy is required. Stoma closure may be performed promptly after the resolution of the underlying problems. Appendectomy usually is performed during laparotomy for meconium ileus because of the potential for appendicitis following luminal obstruction and possible confusion during future episodes of meconium ileus equivalent.

Postoperative Care and Results. If the meconium has been successfully cleared without opening the intestine, dilute N-acetylcysteine may be given through the nasogastric tube or by enema. Alternatively, if a T-tube has been placed, dilute N-acetylcysteine or other irrigant can be used directly into the ileum. These efforts are aimed at keeping the meconium soluble and preventing recurrent ileal obstruction. Following return of bowel function, enteral feeding using an elemental formula is started along with oral pancreatic enzyme replacement. Aggressive pulmonary therapy is routine and includes percussion and postural drainage, mucolytics, and antibiotics when indicated. Nutritional assessment and support are essential in the long-term management of these infants and children.

Successful nonoperative management of simple meconium ileus historically was associated with a more favorable outcome; however, the operative mortality rates of infants with meconium ileus have improved dramatically over the past several decades, and current short-term operative survival rates of 70% to 100% are reported.[81,82] Long-term survival following meconium ileus is generally determined by the course of the underlying pulmonary disease. Contemporary management of CF has produced a mean survival age that approaches 30 years in most centers. With the exception of the development of portal hypertension in about 5% of patients, the intestinal manifestations of the CF are treatable. Future medical and surgical efforts to improve the long-term outcome in these patients include direct replacement of the diseased pulmonary system by lung transplantation, manipulation of the epithelial chloride transport defect with pharmacologic agents, and gene therapy directed at *CFTR* gene transfer into respiratory epithelial cells.

Meconium Plug Syndrome

Meconium plug syndrome is characterized by functional obstruction of the colon or rectum by a meconium plug. It affects both normal and premature infants with immature gastrointestinal motility and must be differentiated from other causes of neonatal intestinal obstruction. Unlike meconium ileus, in meconium plug syndrome the colon is of normal caliber and the meconium is not inspissated. The infant's symptoms within the first few days of life are abdominal distention and bilious emesis. Spontaneous passage of meconium is often absent. On examination, the infant is normal with a patent anus and a distended abdomen. Digital rectal examination may deliver the meconium plug. Plain films of the abdomen demonstrate dilated loops of bowel consistent with distal bowel obstruction. The diagnosis is confirmed by contrast enema, which is also therapeutic in helping the meconium plug pass. The meconium plug is followed by bile-stained meconium of normal consistency. Importantly, although the vast majority of these infants are normal, a few have Hirschsprung disease or CF. Therefore, infants presenting with meconium plug syndrome should undergo routine rectal suction biopsy and have CF screening tests performed.

Malrotation

Embryology

Normal midgut fixation requires sequential growth, elongation, and rotation of the intestine beginning as early as week 5 of gestation and illustrated in Figure 110.25. Three distinct events occur during normal midgut fixation. The first stage involves herniation of the primary midgut loop into the base of the umbilical cord, where it remains until week 10 of gestation. The axis of the midgut loop is the superior mesenteric artery (SMA), with the omphalomesenteric duct at the apex of the midgut loop. The midgut loop rotates 180 degrees counterclockwise so that the proximal half passes posterior to the SMA. The proximal portion gives rise to the proximal duodenum, which lies to the right of midline. A portion of this segment becomes the third and fourth portions of the duodenum. The distal duodenum is normally fixed to the left of the aorta at the ligament of Treitz, having rotated 270 degrees counterclockwise from its original position. The jejunoileal segment undergoes dramatic elongation, forming about six primary intestinal loops. The distal midgut loop gives rise to the cecum and the right colon, which also undergoes growth and elongation with concomitant rotation 270 degrees counterclockwise. Therefore, the cecum is initially positioned to the left, then anterior, and finally to the right of the SMA before reaching its final location.[30]

Reduction of the extracoelomic gut is the second stage of midgut development and fixation, occurring between weeks 10 and 12 of gestation. By this time, the duodenojejunal junction has passed posterior to the SMA and the midgut has rotated 180 degrees counterclockwise; however, the small intestine initially remains to the right side of midline, and the cecum and ascending colon are anterior to the SMA after return of the gut into the abdomen. Many common abnormalities of intestinal fixation occur as a result of arrested development during this 2-week period.

The final stage of midgut development is fixation of the intestine to the posterior body wall, occurring after week 12 of gestation. Cecal descent occurs at this time. Normal points of fixation include the cecum in the right iliac fossa and the duodenojejunal junction at the ligament of Treitz just to the left of the aorta and anterior to the left renal vein (Fig. 110.26). Therefore, the normal intestinal mesentery is fixed with a broad base extending from the ligament of Treitz to the cecum. This broad-based mesenteric attachment prevents volvulus from occurring. In contrast, in disorders of intestinal rotation, the base of the mesentery is neither fixed nor broad, placing the entire midgut at risk for volvulus.

Anatomy

The normal sequence required for intestinal positioning and fixation can be interrupted at any developmental stage, producing a diverse spectrum of rotational abnormalities. Some neonatal surgical conditions are uniformly associated with abnormal intestinal rotation resulting from displacement of the midgut from the abdominal cavity during embryologic development. These anomalies include omphalocele, gastroschisis, and congenital diaphragmatic hernia. The term

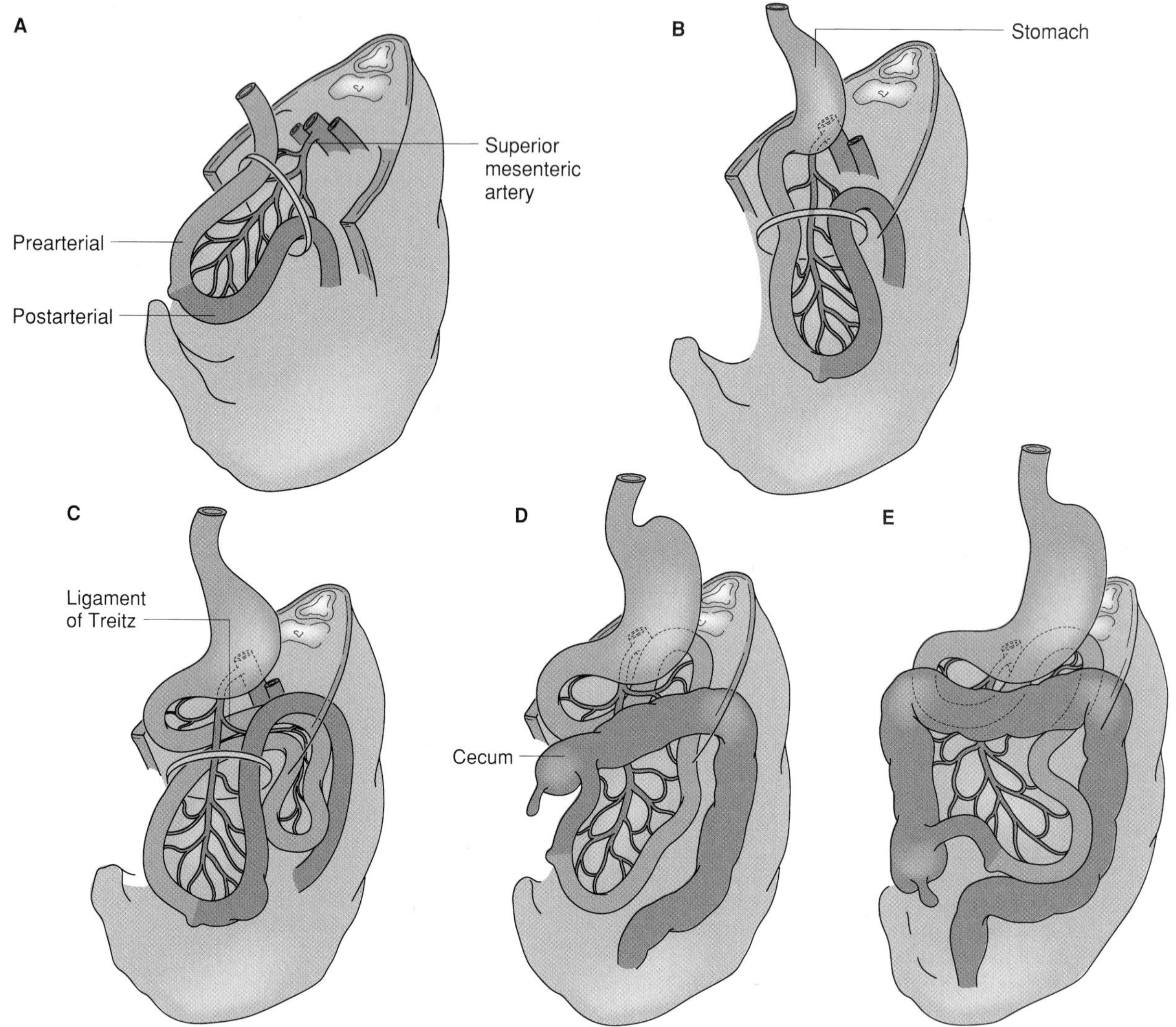

FIGURE 110.25 Normal midgut rotation is shown with appropriate positioning of the stomach, duodenum, small intestine, and cecum from the fifth gestational week (*A*) through completion by the 12th week (*E*).

malrotation has been applied generically to describe disorders of intestinal rotation and fixation, although specific definitions of the more commonly encountered lesions are provided in the following sections.

Nonrotation. This common anomaly is characterized by inadequate counterclockwise rotation of the midgut around the SMA. Instead of the normal 270-degree arc, rotation is either absent or arrested before exceeding 90 degrees (Fig. 110.27). The small intestine resides on the right side of midline, the colon resides on the left, and the cecum is anterior and near the midline. The duodenojejunal junction is to the right of midline and more caudal and anterior in position. Nonrotation carries a significant clinical risk of midgut volvulus because the mesenteric vascular pedicle is narrow. Duodenal obstruction also may occur as a result of peritoneal attachments known as *Ladd's bands*. These peritoneal bands fix the cecum to the posterior body wall by passing anterior and lateral to the distal duodenum.

Mixed or Incomplete Rotation. This rotational abnormality is characterized by arrest of the normal rotation at or near 180 degrees rather than the normal 270 degrees (Fig. 110.28). Instead of rotating posterior and to the left of the SMA, incomplete or arrested rotation of the prearterial segment leaves the duodenojejunal junction to the right of midline. The cecum also does not complete its counterclockwise passage anterior to the SMA; it usually resides in the upper abdomen just to the left of the SMA. Similar to nonrotation, fixation of the cecum to the posterior body wall by Ladd's bands places the duodenum at risk for compression or obstruction. Additionally, the SMA pedicle is narrow and places the midgut at risk for volvulus.

Mesocolic Hernias. Mesocolic hernias are rare but important anomalies characterized by failure of fixation of either the right or left mesocolon to the posterior body wall. Small bowel can become entrapped in the resulting potential cavities on either side of the abdomen. A right-sided mesocolic defect (paraduodenal hernia) is associated with nonrotation of the proximal midgut segment. Small bowel entrapment posterior to the right colon and cecum may occur. Similar entrapment of small bowel may occur from an incompletely fixed left mesocolon but is associated with normal colonic and cecal position. Entrapped small bowel in a left mesocolic hernia usually is contained within a hernia sac with the neck composed of the inferior mesenteric vein and peritoneal bands extending to the posterior body wall. Both left and right mesocolic hernias

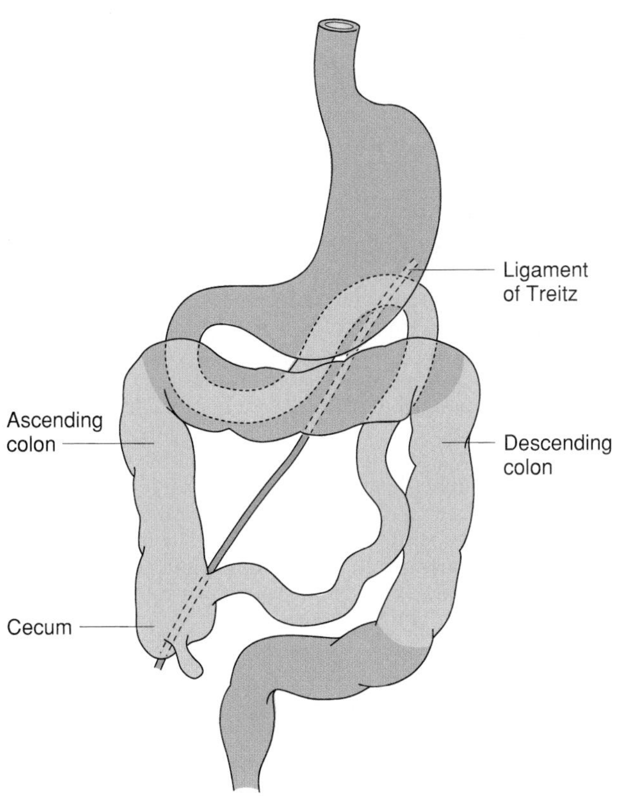

FIGURE 110.26 Normal oblique fixation of the midgut mesentery at the ligament of Treitz and in the right lower quadrant. The blue portions of the colon are extraperitoneal.

carry the potential risks of obstruction, incarceration, and strangulation of bowel.

Clinical Presentation

Abnormalities of intestinal rotation are estimated to be present in about 1% of the population. Most persons with intestinal

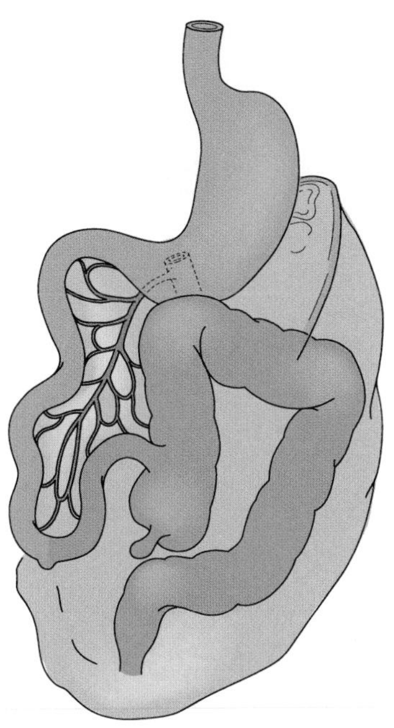

FIGURE 110.27 Nonrotation. The proximal segment of the small intestine resides on the right side of the abdomen, and the distal segment (*colon*) is on the left. Neither has rotated normally.

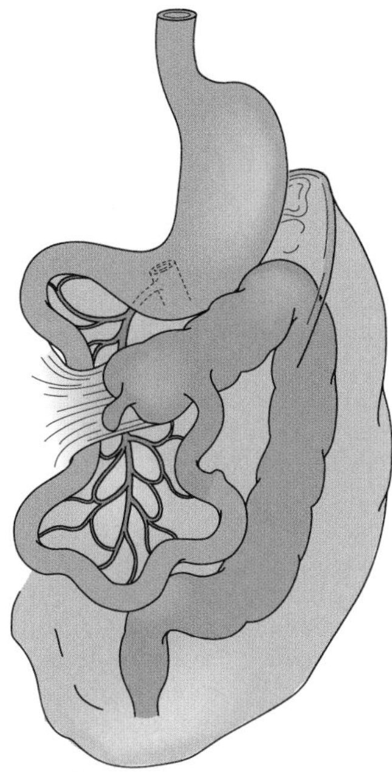

FIGURE 110.28 Incomplete rotation. The proximal segment has failed to rotate and is on the right. The distal segment has rotated to reside anterior to the duodenum so that cecal bands to the posterior abdominal wall may compress and obstruct the duodenum.

rotational anomalies are clinically asymptomatic; therefore, some children are found to have malrotation incidentally by upper gastrointestinal contrast studies conducted for other reasons. Symptomatic malrotation usually is encountered clinically in the setting of duodenal obstruction or midgut volvulus. As previously discussed, duodenal obstruction may occur as a result of Ladd's bands fixing the abnormally positioned cecum to the posterior body wall. These peritoneal bands cause duodenal obstruction by extrinsic compression. Children with symptomatic duodenal obstruction present with bilious emesis and distention of the stomach and proximal duodenum. Similar to proximal neonatal intestinal obstruction, newborn infants may present with bilious emesis without abdominal distention secondary to partial duodenal obstruction. A paucity of small bowel gas may be seen on plain abdominal films.

A potential consequence of intestinal malrotation is midgut volvulus. Midgut volvulus should be considered in any infant or child presenting with bilious emesis. The clinical outcome of midgut volvulus is time dependent, which is the fundamental reason that signs and symptoms of acute intestinal obstruction in an infant or child must be pursued aggressively until a clear diagnosis is made. The devastating, life-threatening consequence of midgut volvulus is vascular insufficiency, gut ischemia, and, if untreated, infarction of the entire bowel supplied by the SMA. The initial symptoms may be subtle and limited to feeding intolerance, abdominal pain, and irritability followed by bilious emesis. Guaiac-positive stool from mucosal injury is a common early finding. Late findings include progressive abdominal distention, hematemesis, and hypotension. Metabolic acidosis, coagulopathy, and shock may become prominent clinical features. If unrecognized or left untreated, transmural necrosis of the entire midgut will occur.

At least 50% to 75% of intestinal rotational abnormalities are discovered within the first month of life, and about 90% occur in children younger than 1 year.[83,84] Symptomatic infants and children require emergent surgical exploration and correction. Older children and adults initially may present with acute volvulus but also may have a history of vague symptoms of episodic intestinal obstruction and chronic abdominal pain. It is essential to recognize that, regardless of age or chronicity of symptoms, midgut volvulus from malrotation occurs in a completely unpredictable manner.[85] Therefore, it is recommended that patients with incidentally discovered, asymptomatic malrotation undergo operative management to reduce the risk of volvulus.

Diagnosis

As with other forms of neonatal intestinal obstruction, the diagnostic evaluation begins with a plain abdominal radiograph. Classic findings with malrotation include gastric and proximal duodenal distention with a paucity or absence of distal small bowel gas (Fig. 110.29A). The plain film alone may not differentiate malrotation from duodenal atresia or stenosis. In most cases of suspected duodenal obstruction with concern of malrotation, an upper gastrointestinal series is the second and conclusive imaging study (Fig. 110.29B). Malrotation with volvulus typically produces incomplete duodenal obstruction with a corkscrew or coiled appearance in the distal duodenum. Extrinsic compression of the duodenum by Ladd's bands may be visible on contrast study. Duodenal atresia and stenosis may occur anywhere within the duodenum but tends to be more proximal. Complete absence of small bowel gas is typical of duodenal atresia, whereas diminished but discernable distal gas is characteristic of duodenal stenosis or malrotation with volvulus.

Other radiographic findings in malrotation include incorrect position of the duodenojejunal junction, particularly to the right of midline. Failure to achieve normal cephalad and posterior fixation is typical in malrotation and may be best appreciated on lateral views. The small bowel resides in the right side of the abdomen, the colon and cecum on the left (Fig. 110.29C). In a symptomatic infant or child, radiographic evidence of malrotation alone is enough to warrant emergent exploration. Whether or not volvulus is present may be difficult to differentiate radiographically, therefore, efforts to do so may be hazardous in clinical practice. A contrast enema is helpful in the evaluation of neonatal intestinal obstruction, although it may not be the initial study of choice if malrotation is suspected. The classic finding on contrast enema for malrotation is cecal malposition, usually in the left abdomen or near the midline. Finally, the relative position of the SMA to the superior mesenteric vein may be assessed by ultrasound. Normally, the superior mesenteric vein is to the right of the SMA on transverse sonograms. Abnormal position of the superior mesenteric vein either ventral or to the left of the SMA is associated with malrotation.[86]

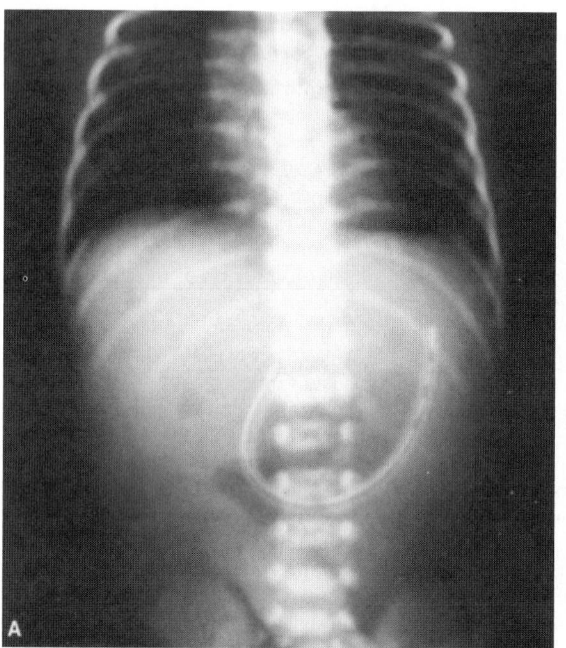

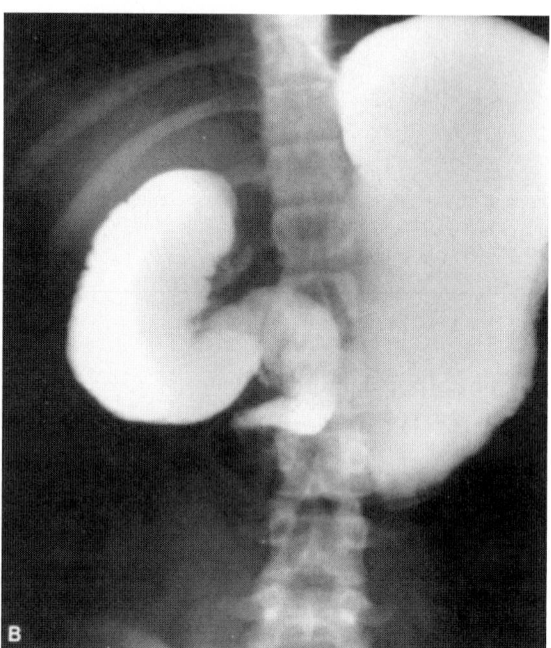

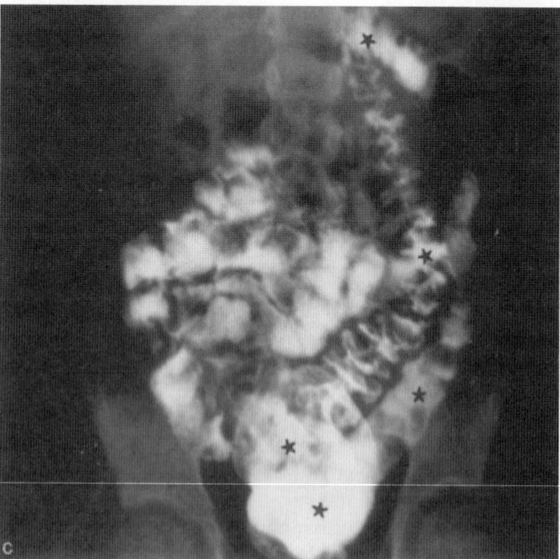

FIGURE 110.29 (*A*) Plain radiograph of an infant with malrotation. There is a paucity of small-bowel gas. (*B*) Upper gastrointestinal contrast study demonstrating malrotation with midgut volvulus and duodenal obstruction. The position of the duodenojejunal junction is abnormal. (C) Plain film showing a contrast-filled colon and cecum on the patient's left (*asterisks*). The entire small bowel is to the right of midline. These are typical radiographic findings of malrotation.

Treatment

The management of bowel obstruction from malrotation or an internal hernia in a neonate is operative. Initial assessment, resuscitation, and preoperative preparation in a symptomatic newborn should be conducted simultaneously so that confirmation of malrotation can be followed immediately by laparotomy. Urgent laparotomy is required because even a minimal delay may represent the difference between viable or infarcted intestine. Volvulus with complete infarction of the midgut, if not immediately lethal, is survivable only with enterectomy followed by permanent or long-term TPN support. In older, asymptomatic children with incidentally discovered malrotation, operative repair is somewhat controversial. Given the devastating consequences of midgut volvulus, however, elective surgical correction appears to be warranted.

Operative repair of malrotation is performed by Ladd's procedure.[87] The first objective is to relieve the midgut volvulus, if present. This is accomplished by delivery and detorsion of the affected midgut, usually in a counterclockwise direction. Recurrent volvulus is prevented by broadening the base of the mesenteric vascular pedicle by dividing the peritoneal bands that tether the cecum, small bowel mesentery, mesocolon, and duodenum around the base of the SMA (Fig. 110.30). Once completed, the mesentery and mesocolon open widely and the mesenteric pedicle is at low risk for recurrent volvulus.

The second objective of Ladd's procedure is to divide the abnormal peritoneal attachments between the cecum and the abdominal wall. A modified Kocher maneuver involving meticulous and complete mobilization of the entire duodenum with division of all anterior, lateral, and posterior attachments is performed. Duodenal and distal small bowel patency should be demonstrated using intraluminal air or saline because concurrent cases of atresia have been reported. An appendectomy is usually performed to eliminate potential confusion from acute appendicitis developing in an abnormally positioned appendix. Performance of laparoscopic Ladd's procedure has been demonstrated to be feasible and may help to reduce time

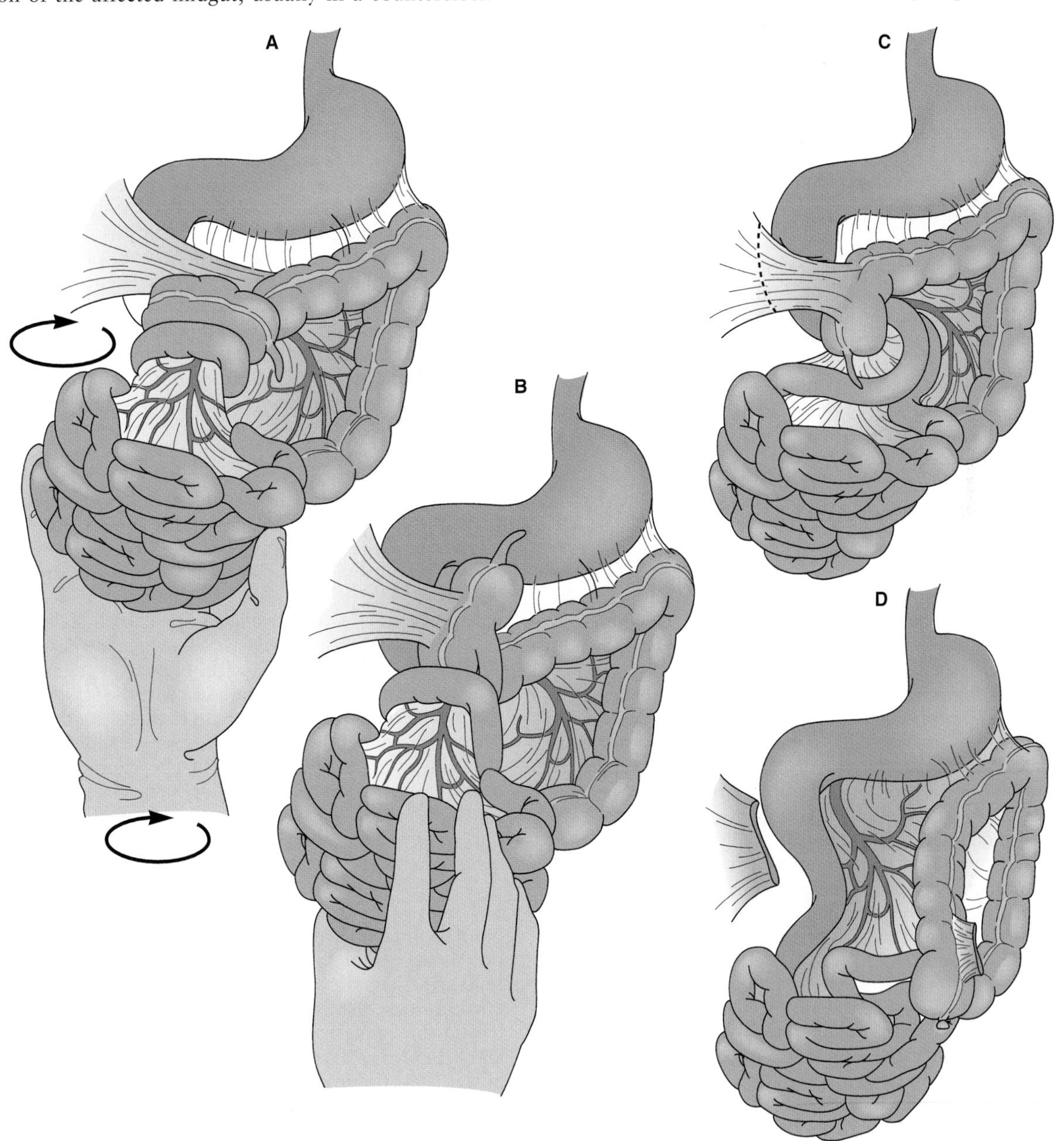

FIGURE 110.30 Correction of malrotation. (*A,B*) Detorsion of midgut. (*C,D*) Division of peritoneal attachments (Ladd's bands) of cecum to abdominal cavity.

to enteral feeding and hospital length of stay; however, the long-term efficacy of this approach has been debated.[88] Fixation of the mesentery by cecal or duodenal plication to the body wall has been abandoned for lack of data supporting efficacy. Postoperative small bowel obstruction secondary to adhesions is reported in about 10% of patients.

Volvulus with intestinal necrosis is treated by preserving as much bowel length as possible. If bowel viability is unclear during initial exploration, a second-look procedure may be helpful to delineate reversible from irreversible injury. The management of nonviable bowel from volvulus is not different from other situations in which intestinal necrosis is encountered, and clinical decisions regarding resection, exteriorization, and anastomosis are necessarily individualized. In situations where the entire small intestine is lost and long-term survival doubtful, difficult ethical decisions must be made with the family.

Surgical management of right mesocolic hernia is directed at dividing the lateral peritoneal attachments of the cecum and right colon to eliminate the hernia. In addition, given the associated nonrotation of the proximal bowel, the vascular pedicle should be broadened as much as possible. Left mesocolic hernia is treated by mobilization of the inferior mesenteric vein, reduction of the small bowel from the hernia sac, and closure of the neck of the hernia sac to eliminate the potential space.

Results and Complications

Results following surgical correction of intestinal rotational abnormalities should be excellent, and life expectancy should be normal in the absence of intestinal necrosis. Recurrent volvulus and recurrent duodenal obstruction are distinctly unusual if the initial procedure is technically complete. Adhesive small bowel obstruction following Ladd's procedure is reported in 1% to 10% of patients. Long-term outcome is obviously less favorable in patients with intestinal necrosis at the time of exploration.

Congenital Aganglionosis (Hirschsprung Disease)

Embryology

Congenital aganglionosis of the intestine (Hirschsprung disease) is characterized by the absence of intestinal ganglion cells. The exact pathogenesis of aganglionosis remains unknown. In normal development, neuroblasts derived from neural crest precursors become evident by week 5 of gestation. The neuroblasts begin maturation and caudal migration along with vagal nerve fibers. The initial caudal migration in an intermuscular plane is followed by intramural dispersal into both superficial and deep submucosal nerve plexuses. Ultimately, the neuroblasts give rise to the ganglion cells of the myenteric nervous system, with functional maturation continuing well into infancy. The orderly migration pathway of myenteric innervation has been documented in human embryos; normally, ganglion cells can be identified in the esophagus at week 6 of gestation, in the transverse colon at week 8 of gestation, and in the rectum by week 12 of gestation.[89]

Anatomy

Hirschsprung disease is characterized by a lack of ganglion cells in the distal intestine. The length of aganglionosis is variable but most commonly involves the distal rectosigmoid colon in 75% to 80% of affected infants. In about 5% of cases, the transition zone between the normal, proximal bowel and the distal, aganglionic segment occurs in the small intestine.[90] Discontinuous aganglionosis has been reported but is considered distinctly unusual. Therefore, in virtually all cases, the aganglionic intestinal segment is continuous with the distal rectum to the anal verge and also includes the internal sphincter. Because of this distribution, the pathogenesis of congenital aganglionosis is often attributed to failure of neuroblast migration. The characteristic lesion in the distal bowel is the absence of ganglion cells in the intermuscular and submucosal plexuses. Large, hypertrophied, nonmyelinated nerve fibers are present within the muscularis mucosa, lamina propria, submucosa, and Auerbach intermuscular plexus. These are both postganglionic fibers from normal, proximal ganglion cells and disordered preganglionic parasympathetic fibers without discernable synaptic connections. Both adrenergic and cholinergic fibers are prominent in the aganglionic segment, and acetylcholinesterase staining is useful diagnostically. The aganglionic segment also has a decrease or absence of nonadrenergic inhibitory fibers that are thought to be functionally important.[91] Abnormalities in the peptidergic nervous system, including vasoactive intestinal peptide, substance P, and neurotensin immunoreactive fibers, also are described in the aganglionic bowel segment.[92] Recent studies have demonstrated deficient neuronal nitric oxide synthase mRNA and subsequent decreased local nitric oxide synthase activity in the aganglionic bowel.[93] These experimental data are consistent with the concept that a defect in nitric oxide-mediated smooth-muscle relaxation may account for some of the characteristic clinical features of Hirschsprung disease.

The transition zone between the normal, proximal bowel and the aganglionic distal bowel is distinguished grossly by distention of the proximal bowel with histologic evidence of muscular hypertrophy. The transition zone often becomes evident to direct inspection or on contrast enema during the first few weeks of life as functional obstruction leads to progressive proximal dilatation and development of congenital megacolon. On gross inspection, the transition zone may appear as a short funnel or cone-shaped colonic segment. The discrepancy in bowel lumen diameter is somewhat age dependent and may be subtle in a newborn or in a child with total colonic aganglionosis. Therefore, it may be difficult for the surgeon or radiologist to define the exact transition zone site based on gross inspection or contrast enema. Gross examination alone is not sufficient for surgical decision making, and histologic confirmation of the level of ganglion cell transition is required. Given the continuous nature of aganglionosis, a rectal biopsy performed 1 to 1.5 cm above the dentate line demonstrating ganglion cells effectively excludes Hirschsprung disease.

Neuronal intestinal dysplasia is a clinically described entity similar to or associated with Hirschsprung disease.[94,95] Despite the presence of ganglion cells, dysplastic changes in the myenteric nervous system affect bowel motility in similar fashion to aganglionosis. Clinical presentation and treatment are similar to those of classic Hirschsprung disease. There is considerable controversy regarding neuronal intestinal dysplasia, but it is reasonable to suggest that this entity represents one variant in the spectrum of abnormalities of the intestinal myenteric nervous system.

Pathophysiology

Normal intestinal motility depends on coordinated propagation of segmental contraction waves immediately preceded by relaxation of the enteric smooth muscle. Patients with Hirschsprung disease lack a functional myenteric nervous system in the aganglionic segment; therefore, both propulsion and reflexive relaxation is disordered or absent in the distal bowel. This finding appears to result from neuronal dysfunction of cholinergic (propulsive) innervation as well as from diminished or absent adrenergic and nonadrenergic inhibitory signaling pathways. Loss of neuronal nitric oxide synthase activity appears to play an important role. The internal sphincter is aganglionic and lacks the normal reflexive relaxation following rectal distention. In fact, patients with Hirschsprung disease may exhibit a paradoxical increase in sphincter tone in response to rectal distention. The functional result is tonic contraction of the aganglionic segment of bowel with ineffective peristalsis. Clinically, this presents as incomplete, distal intestinal obstruction in the newborn or as chronic constipation in the older child or adult.

Hirschsprung disease has been associated with mutations in at least three specific genes: the *RET* protooncogene, the endothelin B receptor (*EDNRB*) gene,[96] and the endothelin 3 (*EDN3*) gene. Additionally, several other candidate genes are under investigation. In mice, natural and in vitro induced mutations affecting the *RET, EDNRB,* and *EDN3* genes generate intestinal aganglionosis identical to Hirschsprung disease.[97,98] Although widely accepted, it is still unknown whether the primary event in aganglionosis is failure of neuroblast migration to the distal bowel. Alternatively, ineffective microenvironmental support of neuroblasts that have already migrated may fail to promote normal neuroblast development and survival.[99]

Clinical Features

Incidence and Associations. The incidence rate of Hirschsprung disease is estimated at 1 per 5,000 live births with a marked male-to-female (4:1) preponderance. Most cases are sporadic, but long-segment and total colonic aganglionosis and female gender are strongly associated with familial inheritance. Genetic chromosomal analysis suggests that multiple loci may be involved, including chromosomes 13q22, 21q22, and 10q, among others.[100,101] Familial Hirschsprung disease has been clearly associated with *RET* protooncogene mutations. From a clinical standpoint, mutations of the *RET* protooncogene are associated with disorders of neural crest development, namely, multiple endocrine neoplasia (MEN) types IIA and IIB as well as familial medullary thyroid carcinoma. These are occasionally associated with Hirschsprung disease. Congenital cardiac defects are present in 2% to 5% of patients with Hirschsprung disease. Other rare congenital anomalies have been reported, but a consistent and important association is a 5% to 15% incidence of trisomy 21.[102] For unknown reasons, aganglionosis in a premature infant is uncommon. Infants presenting with meconium plug syndrome or neonatal appendicitis should undergo rectal suction biopsy because these are the initial clinical manifestations in a small number of infants with Hirschsprung disease.

Presentation. Most infants with Hirschsprung disease fail to pass meconium within the first 24 to 48 hours of life. Nonspecific signs of neonatal intestinal obstruction (feeding intolerance, abdominal distention, and bilious emesis) may develop. About half of patients with Hirschsprung disease are diagnosed as neonates, with the remainder discovered before the age of 2 years. Infrequently, older children or adults are diagnosed with aganglionosis during evaluation for chronic constipation. In this setting, symptoms may be minimal to disabling, and parents or patients often develop elaborate strategies to deal with the chronic constipation. Abdominal distention is characteristic, and sometimes failure to thrive and malnutrition may occur. Physical examination is nonspecific. Digital rectal examination may demonstrate spasm. In the presence of enterocolitis, forceful expulsion of foul-smelling, liquid stool may occur with digital rectal examination.

Enterocolitis occurs in about 10% to 30% of infants and children with Hirschsprung disease and may be the presenting clinical manifestation. Enterocolitis associated with Hirschsprung disease has an unknown pathophysiology, but obstructive stasis and bacterial overgrowth are thought to be important factors. *C. difficile* and rotavirus have been implicated as important pathogenic organisms; diagnostic and treatment plans should consider these possibilities. The early presenting symptoms and signs of enterocolitis include fever, abdominal distention, and diarrhea, which may be explosive, foul-smelling, and bloody. Systemic sepsis, transmural intestinal necrosis, and perforation are all possible later findings. The clinical progression can be rapid, with death occurring in as few as 12 to 24 hours if treatment is not initiated. Infants are particularly vulnerable to this complication, which continues to have a 25% to 30% mortality rate, accounting for virtually all mortality directly related to Hirschsprung disease in modern pediatric surgical practice. Infants with known Hirschsprung disease and suspected enterocolitis should be treated aggressively. Initial treatment includes resuscitation, broad-spectrum antibiotics, cessation of feeding, and rectal irrigation. If the enterocolitis does not respond promptly, emergent intestinal decompression with an enterostomy proximal to the transition zone is indicated.

Diagnosis

A high index of suspicion for Hirschsprung disease should be maintained for any newborn infant with abdominal distention that fails to pass meconium in 24 to 48 hours. The signs of neonatal intestinal obstruction should lead to a stereotypical work-up. In the presence of characteristic findings on history, examination, or radiographic studies, any infant suspected of having Hirschsprung disease should undergo rectal biopsy.

Plain Abdominal Radiographs. Plain film radiographs of the neonate with Hirschsprung disease are nonspecific and typically demonstrate distended, air-filled loops of bowel throughout the abdomen. It is often difficult to discriminate between small and large intestine on plain films at this age, but the pattern is consistent with distal intestinal obstruction. Older children or adults may have a stool-filled megacolon on plain radiographs, but this finding is also nonspecific. In the presence of enterocolitis, thickened, dilated intestinal loops and pneumatosis intestinalis may be present.

Contrast Enema. When distal neonatal intestinal obstruction is suspected on plain abdominal films, a contrast enema should be performed. With an experienced pediatric radiologist, findings consistent with Hirschsprung disease can be accurately detected in most instances. Neonatal contrast enema is performed without a rectal balloon to minimize the risks of perforation or obstructing rectal findings. The classic radiographic finding in Hirschsprung disease is a transition zone (Fig. 110.31A). As previously mentioned, a definitive transition zone may not be apparent in a neonate because proximal dilatation takes some time to develop. Additionally, infants with short-segment disease or total colonic aganglionosis may not have obvious transition zones on contrast enema. In these instances, a lateral view of the rectum may show abnormal spasm (Fig. 110.31B). Contrast remaining in the rectum more than 24 hours following a study is suggestive of Hirschsprung disease.

Rectal Biopsy. The diagnostic standard for aganglionosis is the rectal biopsy. Several commercially available instruments capable of performing rectal suction biopsies are in widespread use. The rectal suction biopsy can be performed at bedside or in clinic without anesthesia in all newborns and most children up to several years of age. The desire for neonatal diagnosis and the technical simplicity of the procedure allow liberal use of this technique in all suspected or at-risk infants. When applied liberally, the vast majority (85% to 90%) of infants undergoing this procedure have normal ganglion cells on biopsy, effectively excluding Hirschsprung disease. Using the

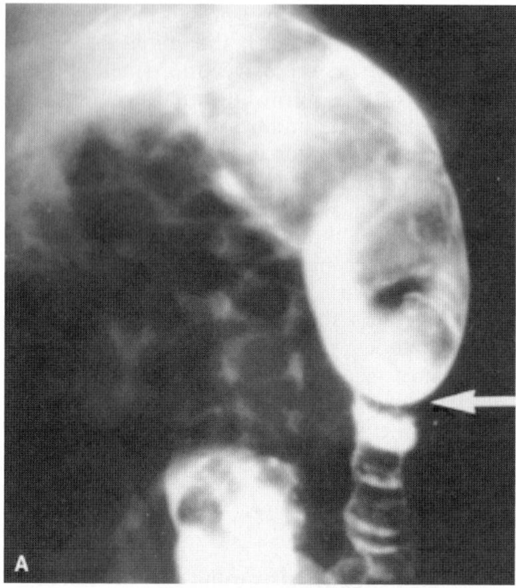

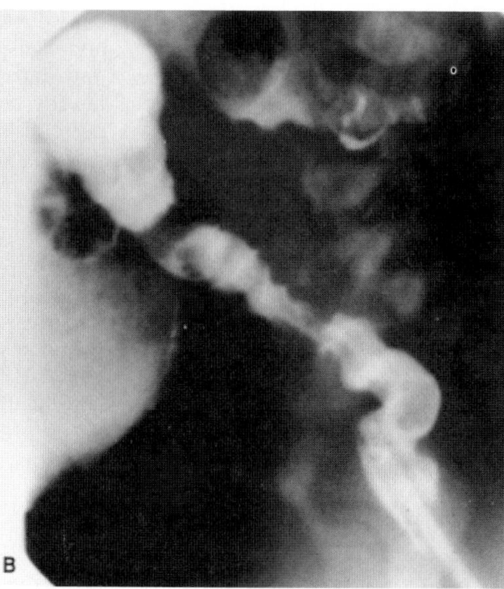

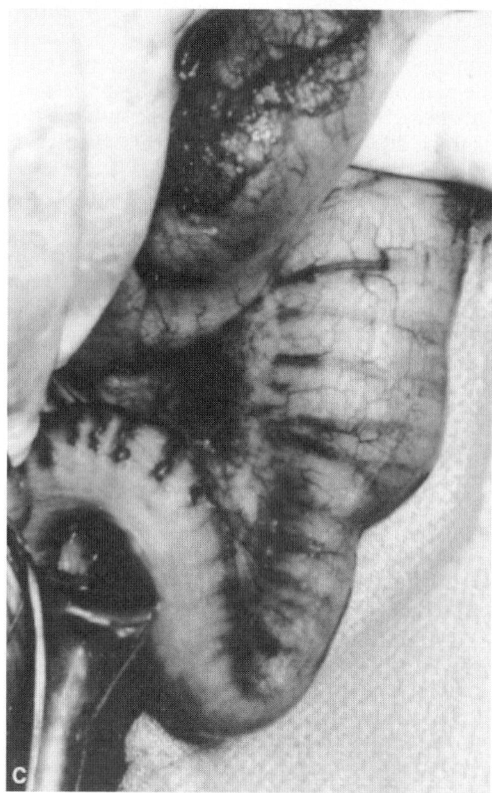

FIGURE 110.31 (*A*) Contrast enema demonstrating a classic rectosigmoid transition zone in Hirschsprung's disease. (*B*) Lateral view of rectum illustrates typical distal spasm of rectum. (*C*) Operative photograph of rectosigmoid transition zone.

rectal suction biopsy technique, a biopsy of the mucosa and submucosa is obtained. This is sufficient to establish the diagnosis because ganglion cells are absent from all intramural plexuses in Hirschsprung disease. The biopsy must be taken 1 to 1.5 cm proximal to the dentate line. Complications of infection, perforation, and bleeding with rectal suction biopsy are infrequent. Full-thickness rectal biopsy under general anesthesia is reserved for older children and in infants in whom suction biopsy has been inadequate. An experienced pediatric pathologist must read the biopsies for maximal diagnostic accuracy. Evaluation for ganglion cells and the axons of the myenteric neurons must be performed (Fig. 110.32), which may be accomplished using conventional hematoxylin-eosin staining or histochemical staining for acetylcholinesterase. Similar histochemical staining for nitric oxide synthase can be performed. These adjunctive techniques are used routinely in some centers and can help to provide additional evidence of Hirschsprung disease rather than simply demonstrating aganglionosis in the biopsy specimen. Communication between the pathologist and the surgeon is essential to correlate clinical data with histologic findings. Diagnostic accuracy for Hirschsprung disease is excellent with a correctly obtained rectal suction biopsy and an experienced pediatric pathologist.[103]

Anorectal Manometry. Characteristic manometric findings of Hirschsprung disease include an abnormal response of the internal sphincter to balloon-induced rectal distention. The absence of sphincter relaxation in response to rectal dilatation is consistent with Hirschsprung disease. Because of the relative ease and accuracy of rectal suction biopsy, anorectal manometry is not widely used in the United States for the primary diagnosis of Hirschsprung disease in infancy; however, this is

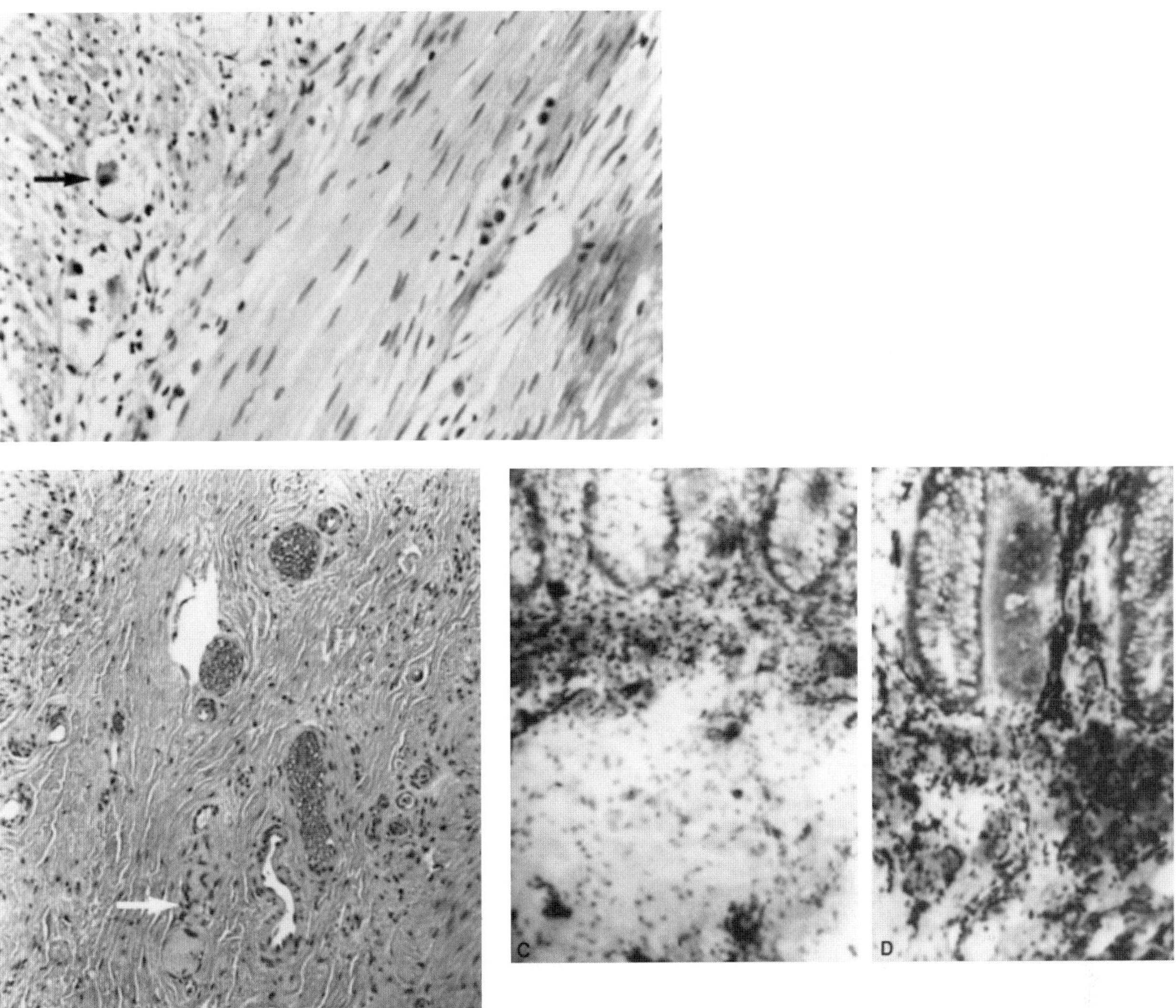

FIGURE 110.32 (*A*) Normal rectal biopsy with ganglion cells indicated by arrow (hematoxylin-eosin). (*B*) Rectal biopsy specimen with aganglionosis (hematoxylin-eosin). Note the characteristic thickened nerve fiber (*arrow*). (C) Normal rectal biopsy using acetylcholinesterase histochemical staining. (*D*) Similarly stained specimen from a patient with Hirschsprung disease. Many thickened submucosal nerve fibers stain densely black.

used in some centers around the world and, when applied carefully with an appropriate transduction probe, accurate manometric diagnosis is achievable in 85% to 90% of cases.

Treatment

Diverting colostomy should be considered for a newborn infant with Hirschsprung disease who has enterocolitis or multiple associated medical problems or anomalies. In the presence of enterocolitis, rectal irrigation and decompression can be an effective temporizing measure while resuscitation and broad-spectrum antibiotics are being instituted. Prompt proximal diversion in all likelihood will be required once the patient has stabilized. In the neonate, the traditional approach following diagnosis is to perform proximal diversion by means of a colostomy (or enterostomy) placed in normal, ganglionated intestine. The diverting colostomy must be proximal to the histologic transition zone, and a series of biopsies examined by frozen section may be necessary to find the correct level for diversion. For classic rectosigmoid disease, a leveling colostomy is placed just proximal to the transition zone. Alternatively, some surgeons prefer a right transverse colostomy following confirmation of ganglion cells at the site. This approach is generally done in two stages, with takedown of the stoma and definitive pull-through operation performed together weeks to months later, typically when the infant reaches 9 to 12 months of age. In older children, definitive pull-through is deferred until the colon has decompressed to relatively normal caliber.

Recently, a single-stage approach in selected infants, which eliminates the diverting colostomy, has been advocated.[104,105] Despite a number of different operative techniques in performing a single-stage pull-through, results and outcomes appear nearly equivalent. Definitive repair of Hirschsprung disease with a single operation is desirable from technical and economical standpoint and essentially eliminates the complications associated with neonatal stomas. As with most aspects

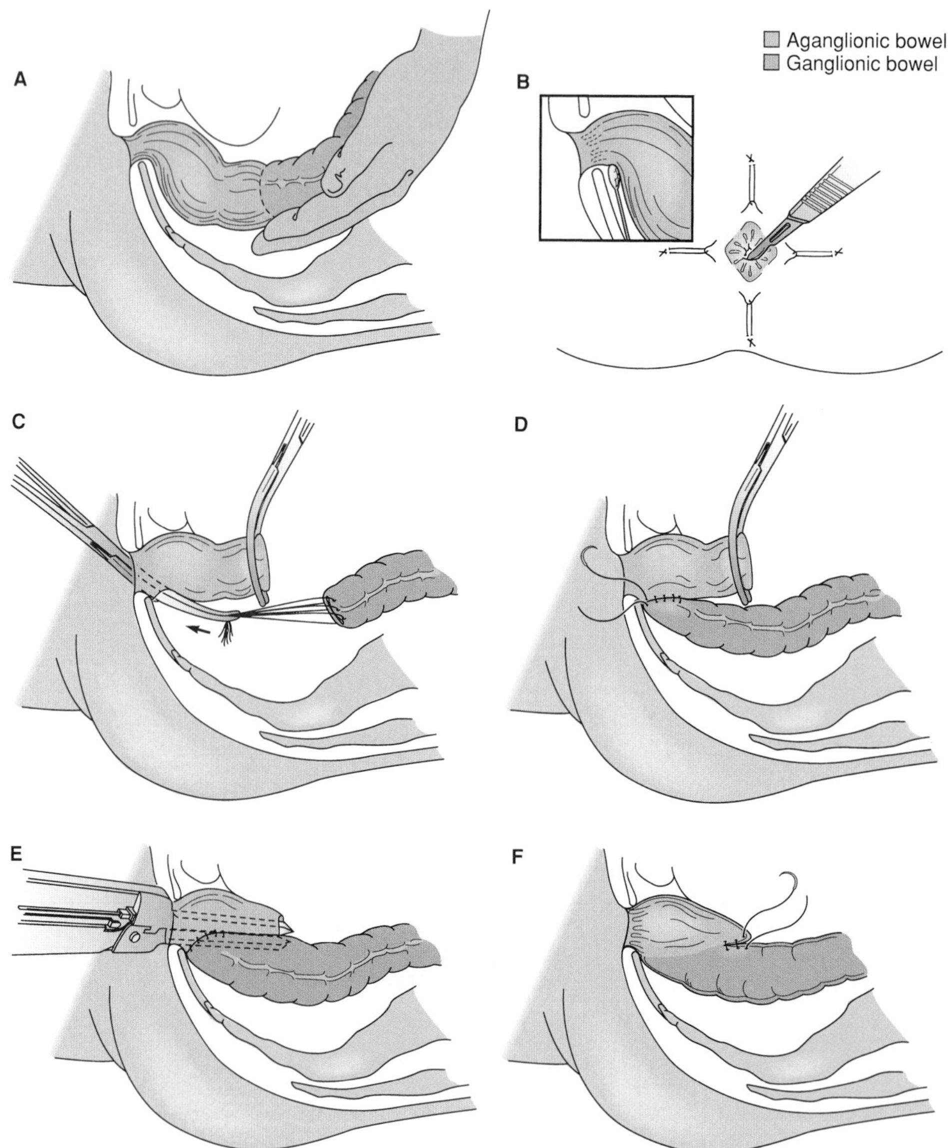

FIGURE 110.33 Duhamel procedure (Martin modification). (*A*) Blunt retrorectal dissection. (*B*) Incision in the posterior wall of the aganglionic rectum. (*C*) Retrorectal pull-through after resection of the proximal aganglionic segment. (*D*) End-to-side colorectal anastomosis preserving aganglionic rectum (as originally described). (*E*) Stapled conversion of anastomosis into an extended side-to-side colorectal anastomosis (Martin modification). (*F*) Completed procedure.

of pediatric surgery, an increasing experience with laparoscopically assisted, single-stage pull-through operations has been reported.[106] The contemporary, laparoscopic single-stage approach in the management of Hirschsprung disease has gained wide acceptance in the pediatric surgical community and is considered by many surgeons as the current standard of care for most infants and children.

Definitive Operations for Hirschsprung Disease

The major goal of operative therapy in the treatment of Hirschsprung disease is to provide resection or bypass of the distal aganglionic rectum with the performance of a low rectal anastomosis with normally innervated proximal intestine. Numerous definitive procedures were designed to treat Hirschsprung disease, and a brief description of the principal procedures in use follows. In general, the selection of a procedure depends on a surgeon's individual training and preference rather than compelling differences in outcome.[107,108]

Duhamel Procedure (Martin Modification). The key elements of the Duhamel procedure are illustrated in Fig. 110.33. After minimal pelvic dissection, resection of the aganglionic colon is performed. The aganglionic rectum is left in situ. Normal proximal colon is brought caudad to the retrorectal space, and a colorectal anastomosis is performed about 1 cm above the dentate line. The original operation left the defunctionalized rectal pouch as shown, which proved problematic. The procedure has been modified by Martin to include a longer side-to-side colorectal anastomosis, now considered standard. Advantages of this procedure include its relative technical ease and limited pelvic dissection. Adoption of the stapled anastomosis has simplified this procedure significantly.

Soave Procedure. The Soave procedure is illustrated in Fig. 110.34. Following resection of aganglionic colon, an endorectal dissection in the submucosal plane is performed from proximal rectum to anus. The endorectal dissection is started in the extraperitoneal rectum. This dissection is typically

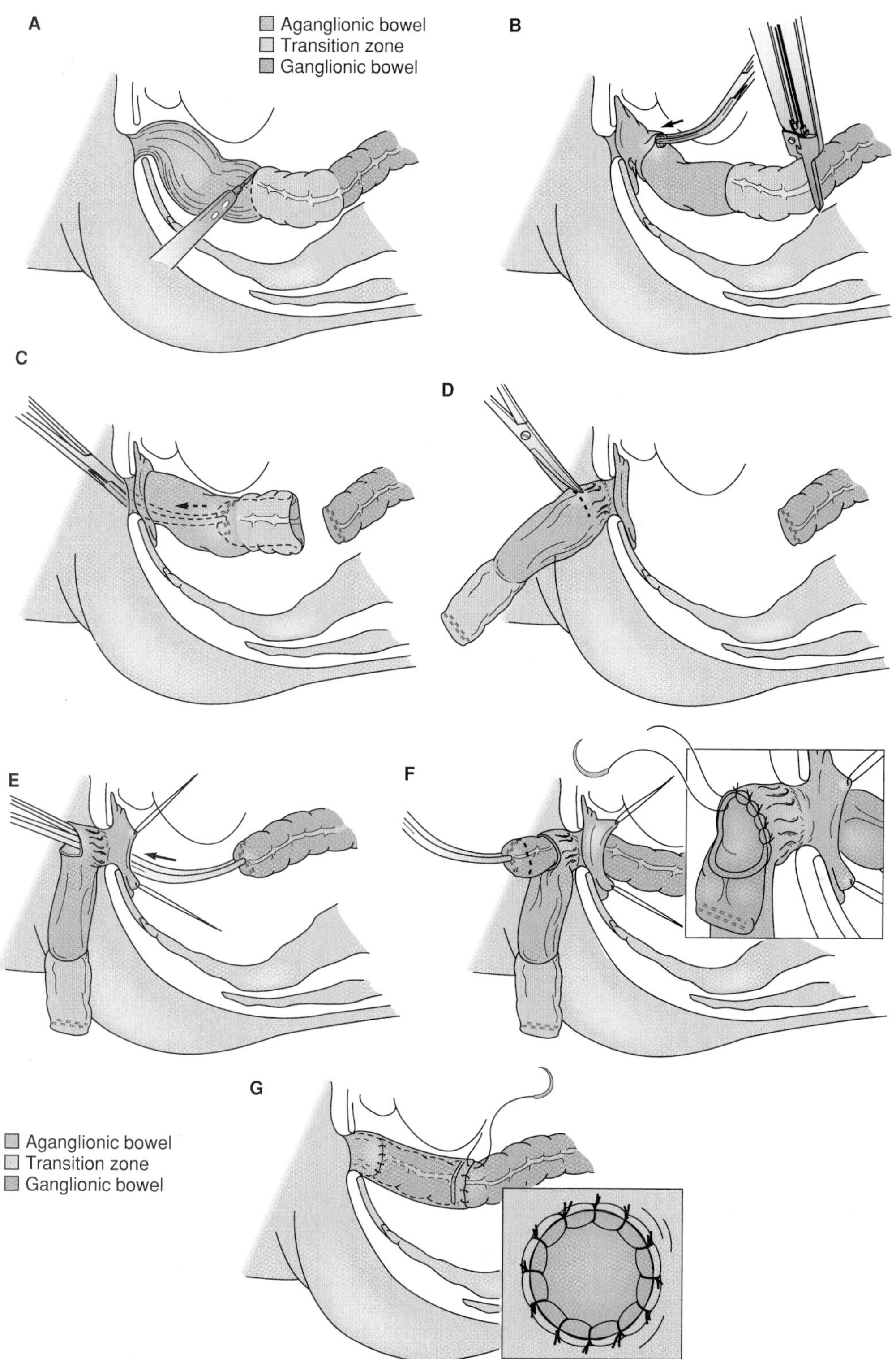

FIGURE 110.34 Soave endorectal procedure. (*A*) Endorectal dissection initiated. (*B*) Endorectal dissection complete. (*C*) Eversion of the aganglionic segment and rectal mucosal tube. (*D*) Incision of everted rectal tube. (*E*) Endorectal pull-through. (*F*) Colorectal anastomosis. (*G*) Completed procedure.

much easier than similar dissection for ulcerative colitis. The dissected rectal mucosal tube is everted through the anus and onto the perineum. The mucosal tube is excised, and normal proximal bowel is pulled through the rectal muscular cuff. The original operation did not suture the pull-through segment of proximal bowel to the rectum. A formal sutured colorectal anastomosis is now universally performed. Care must be taken to ensure that the pull-through segment is not obstructed by the muscular cuff. This procedure is essentially equivalent to the Duhamel procedure in terms of technical ease, operative time, and outcome.

Swenson Procedure. The Swenson procedure is the original definitive procedure for the treatment of Hirschsprung disease.

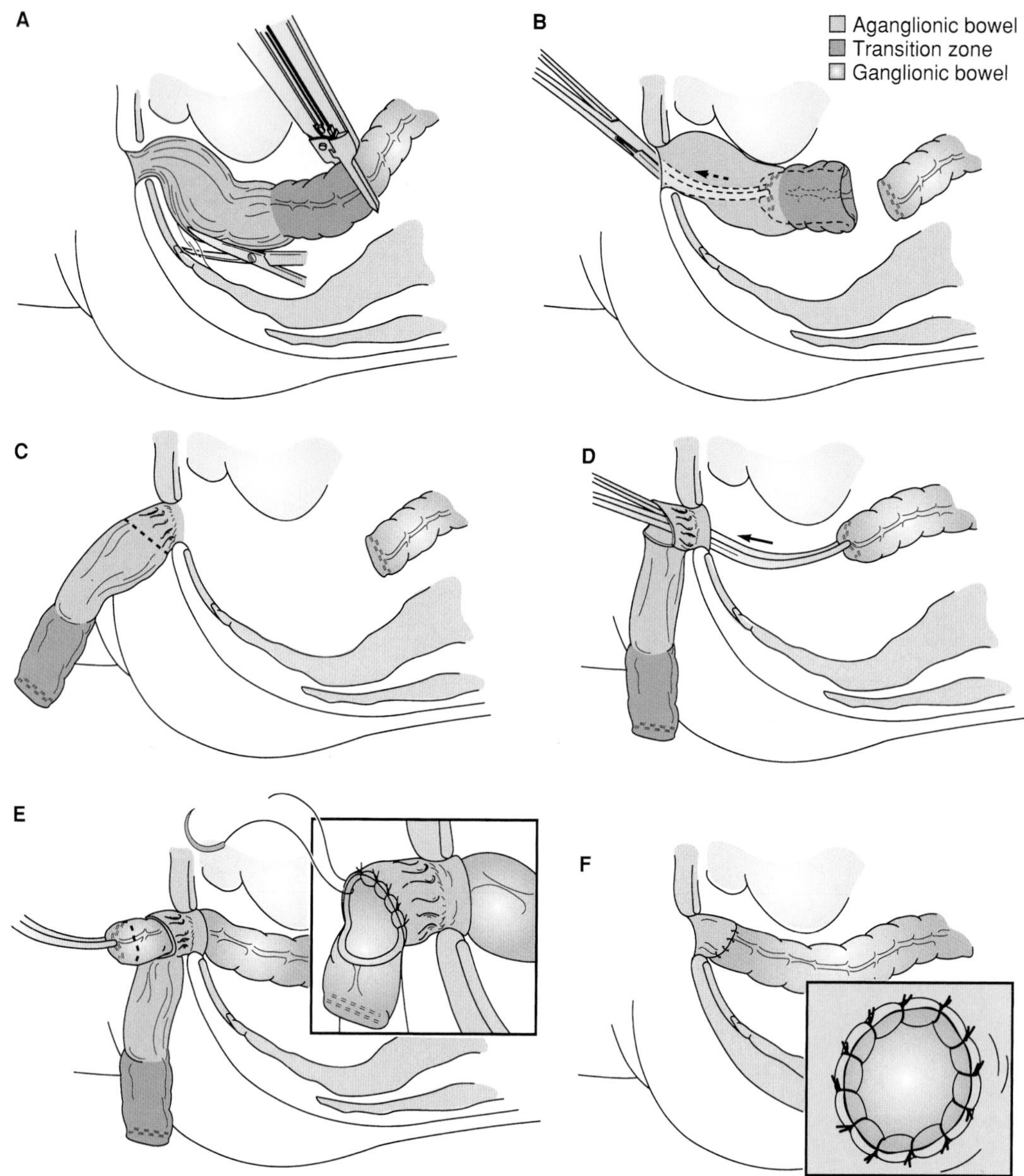

FIGURE 110.35 Swenson procedure. (*A*) Extramural rectal dissection. (*B* and *C*) Eversion of aganglionic segment and full-thickness rectum. (*D*) Pull-through of normal, ganglionic bowel. (*E*) Colorectal anastomosis. (*F*) Completed procedure.

It is somewhat more demanding from a technical standpoint, and, as such, it has been reported to have a slightly higher incidence of postoperative complications. However, long-term outcome in children who undergo a properly performed Swenson procedure is equivalent to other procedures. The basic strategy is outlined in Fig. 110.35. The aganglionic segment of colon is resected and a careful, nearly complete extramural dissection of the distal rectum is performed. Care must be taken to avoid inadvertent injury to the seminal vesicles, vas deferens, ureters, and pelvic splanchnic nerves. The dissected rectum is everted through the anus onto the perineum and excised. Normal proximal bowel is pulled through and a colorectal anastomosis is performed.

Laparoscopically Assisted Endorectal Pull-through. A multi-institutional clinical experience with a laparoscopically assisted endorectal pull-through technique for the treatment of Hirschsprung disease has been reported.[106] Potential advantages of this approach include excellent visibility of the distal rectum during dissection, early return of postoperative bowel function, and decreased length of hospital stay. The early results report outcomes similar to the other established procedures. The procedure is reviewed in Fig. 110.36.

Rectal Myectomy. Resection of a longitudinal strip of the posterior rectal muscular wall has been used for definitive management of ultrashort-segment Hirschsprung disease. This procedure can be performed via transanal approach combined with submucosal dissection or by a posterior sagittal approach. Although controversial, the use of rectal myectomy as a definitive operation for Hirschsprung disease may be considered most useful in the selected older child identified with ultrashort segment disease.[109]

Total Colonic Aganglionosis. Total colonic aganglionosis is complex and, fortunately, relatively rare. Several different operative procedures have been described and treatment must be individualized. The endorectal pull-through with ileoanal anastomosis has been used with good success when most or all of the small bowel is normal. For extensive small bowel aganglionosis,

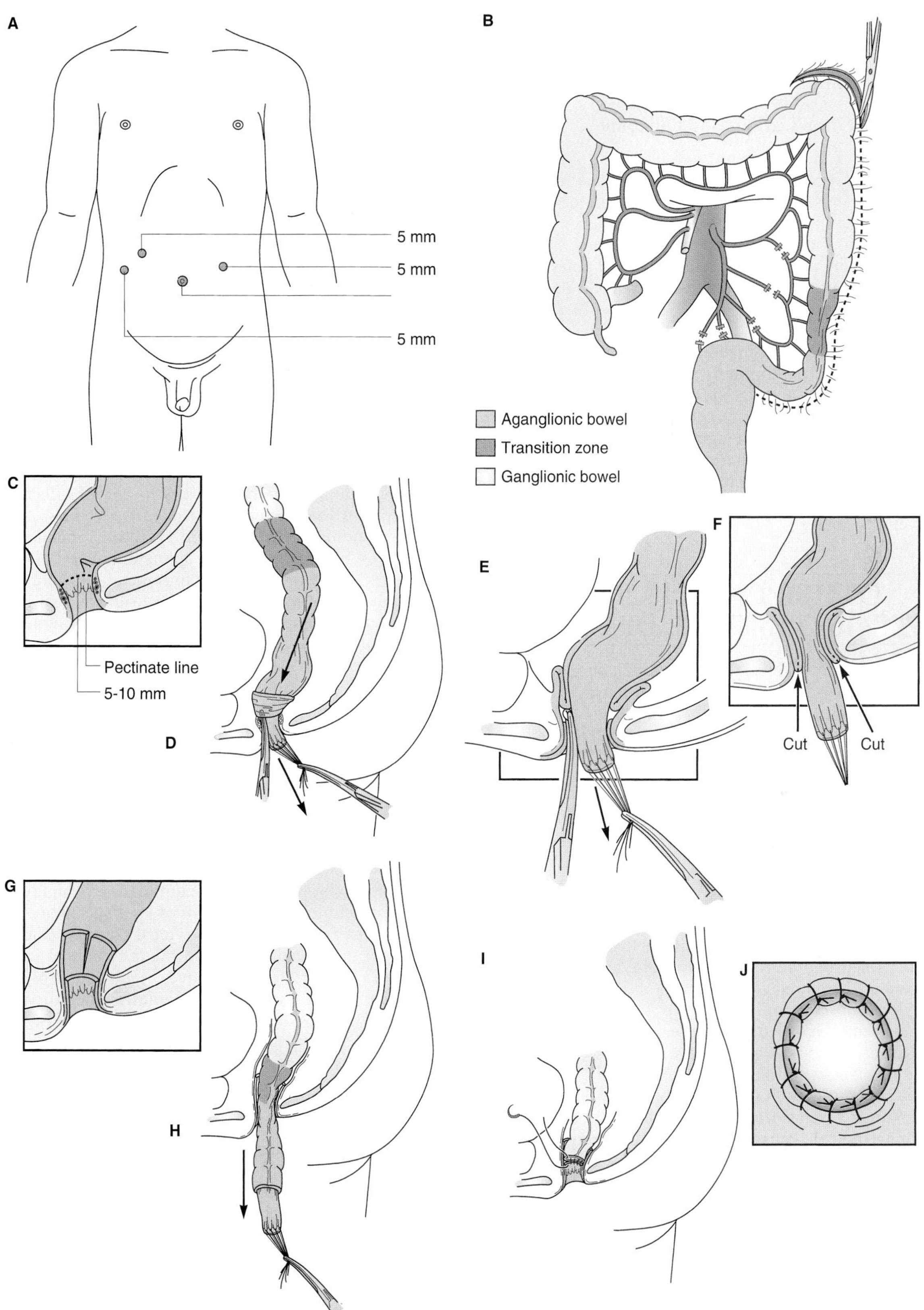

FIGURE 110.36 Laparoscopically assisted pull-through for Hirschsprung disease. (*A*) Sites for operative trocar placement. (*B*) Division of colon and rectal mesentery with mobilization of proximal colon. (*C*) Circumferential incision in rectal mucosa 5 to 10 mm cephalad to the pectinate line. (*D*) Mucosal traction sutures to facilitate further dissection from rectal muscular cuff. (*E*) Transanal submucosal dissection is continued cephalad to meet the caudal extent of the transperitoneal rectal dissection. (*F*) Circumferential incision of rectal muscular cuff. (*G*) Rectal muscular cuff is split posteriorly to accommodate the pull-through segment (the pull-through segment is not shown here to clarify this maneuver). (*H*) Rectum and sigmoid colon are pulled through the rectal muscular cuff to the anastomotic site. (*I*) Colon is transected at appropriate site with confirmation of ganglion cells by frozen section. (*J*) Transanal, end-to-end single layer colorectal anastomosis.

an extended side-to-side anastomosis of normally innervated proximal small bowel to the aganglionic colon has been successfully performed. For complete intestinal aganglionosis, extended intestinal myectomy has been described.

Complications and Outcome

Complications resulting from definitive procedures for Hirschsprung disease include anastomotic leak, stricture, pelvic or rectal muscular cuff abscess, intestinal obstruction, and wound infection. These occur with a frequency of 1% to 10% with most experienced pediatric surgeons. Mortality from Hirschsprung disease is distinctly unusual unless enterocolitis is the presenting feature or associated medical problems or anomalies are present.

A unique complication following definitive repair of Hirschsprung disease is postoperative enterocolitis. The clinical presentation and pathogenesis have been discussed, and it remains an important and significant cause of morbidity. The incidence of postoperative enterocolitis ranges from 10% to 30% in most large series. Although rare, Hirschsprung enterocolitis can occur even in the presence of a diverting colostomy. Long-term outcomes appear quite good for all the procedures used, with 80% to 90% of patients maintaining good to excellent bowel function.

OTHER CHILDHOOD GASTROINTESTINAL DISORDERS

This review is limited to relatively common surgical conditions that are either congenital in origin or unique in children. For other surgical conditions that can affect both children and adults, the reader is referred to other chapters in this text.

Infantile Hypertrophic Pyloric Stenosis

Anatomy and Pathophysiology

The pathogenesis of infantile hypertrophic pyloric stenosis is unknown, but current data suggest that local deficiency of neuronal nitric oxide synthase in the pylorus may be responsible for the clinical manifestations of the disease.[110,111] The deficiency of neuronal nitric oxide synthase leads to a lack of nitric oxide-mediated relaxation of smooth muscle and subsequent pyloric obstruction. Luminal narrowing occurs as a result of concentric hypertrophy of the pyloric smooth muscle. Clinically, this presents as progressive gastric outlet obstruction that becomes symptomatic by 2 to 4 weeks of age. The maximal narrowing and clinical symptoms of hypertrophic pyloric stenosis occurs between 4 and 8 weeks of age. The hypertrophic pyloric muscle ultimately undergoes gradual involution over a period of weeks to months. Anatomic evidence of the hypertrophied pylorus is absent if surgical exploration is performed for other reasons at a later date.

Clinical Presentation

The reported incidence rate of hypertrophic pyloric stenosis is approximately 0.1% to 0.4% among white infants and is slightly lower in the black population. There is a distinct familial predisposition with an approximate 7% incidence rate in children of parents with a history of pyloric stenosis. The incidence rate is about four times higher in males than females and is higher in first-born infants.[112] There is an apparent increased risk of hypertrophic pyloric stenosis in infants receiving oral erythromycin for pertussis prophylaxis.[113] Association of pyloric stenosis in infants treated for esophageal atresia and in infants with Smith-Lemli-Opitz syndrome has been reported.[114]

Infants with hypertrophic pyloric stenosis have a history of nonbilious, postprandial emesis that becomes progressively projectile. The infant otherwise appears well and will feed vigorously until late in the clinical course. The typical age at diagnosis is between ages 2 and 12 weeks . A history of identified feeding intolerance and formula change is common.

The definitive clinical finding on examination is a palpable, hypertrophied pylorus in the right upper quadrant to midepigastric region, often described as a firm, mobile "olive" on examination. This is a pathognomonic finding, and in the correct clinical setting no further diagnostic imaging studies are required. An experienced clinician should be able to palpate a hypertrophied pylorus in nearly all cases. A successful physical examination requires an empty stomach, a quiet infant, and patience; repeated examinations may be necessary. Inability to palpate the pyloric mass in a quiet or anesthetized infant should place the diagnosis of hypertrophic pyloric stenosis in question. Other physical findings include visible or palpable gastric peristaltic waves, which also can be seen with any cause of gastric or duodenal obstruction. Transient indirect hyperbilirubinemia occurs in 1% to 2% of affected infants and typically resolves with postoperative feeding.

Late findings with advanced symptoms include dehydration and a hypochloremic, hypokalemic metabolic alkalosis from gastric fluid losses. Profound metabolic alkalosis is less common in current practice but occasionally can be encountered in an extremely dehydrated infant with a long-standing history of emesis. The intravascular volume depletion and chloride-responsive alkalosis must be corrected prior to operative repair. The serum chloride should be restored to at least 90 to 95 mEq/L, and the measured CO_2 should be less than 30 mEq/L prior to induction of general anesthesia.

Diagnosis

Surgical repair of pyloric stenosis should be proposed for any infant with an appropriate history and characteristic findings on physical examination. If the diagnosis is equivocal or confirmation desirable, either an upper gastrointestinal contrast series or a pyloric ultrasound examination is highly accurate. Both examinations have sensitivity and specificity exceeding 95% in experienced hands. A typical contrast study demonstrating a narrowed, elongated pyloric channel is shown in Fig. 110.37. Contrast studies have the advantage of evaluating other causes of symptomatic emesis, including gastroesophageal reflux disease, malrotation, and antroduodenal webs. The disadvantage of this approach is the presence of contrast in a poorly emptying stomach before general anesthesia is administered. In general, lavage and removal of the gastric contrast can be safely performed prior to anesthesia to minimize the risk of aspiration. Ultrasound examination of the pylorus can effectively demonstrate both elongation and thickening consistent with hypertrophy and is a preferred diagnostic test in many institutions. In general, the diagnosis of hypertrophic pyloric stenosis is being made at an earlier stage of the disease compared with several decades ago.

Treatment

Hypertrophic pyloric stenosis is a progressive situation that subsequently resolves over several weeks to months. Nonoperative treatment during this period requires either long-term parenteral or enteral nutrition and is not practical from a risk or cost standpoint. The Ramstedt pyloromyotomy has achieved universal acceptance because it offers definitive, rapid cure in virtually all infants, and morbidity rates have been negligible (Fig. 110.38). The operation is performed once the infant is rehydrated and the serum electrolytes are corrected.

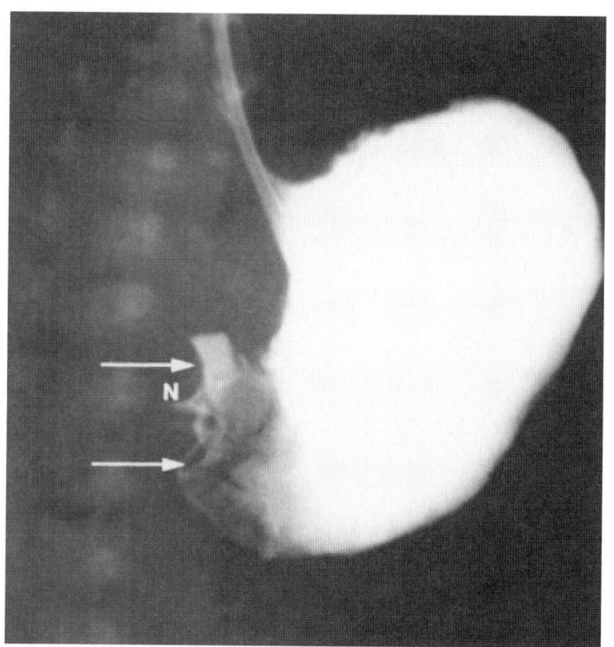

FIGURE 110.37 Infantile hypertrophic pyloric stenosis demonstrated by barium upper gastrointestinal series showing pyloric channel narrowing (N) and elongation with antral shouldering or cushioning (*arrows*).

Typically, the pylorus is delivered through a transverse right upper quadrant incision. A single longitudinal incision is made in the hypertrophied pyloric muscle. The hypertrophied circular pyloric muscle must be meticulously divided from the stomach to the junction of the proximal duodenum. An adequate pyloromyotomy is achieved when the submucosa bulges into the myotomy site and both edges of the divided pyloric muscle are freely mobile. Increasing experience with laparoscopic pyloromyotomy has been reported to be successful with similar operative times and outcome to the open repair.[115]

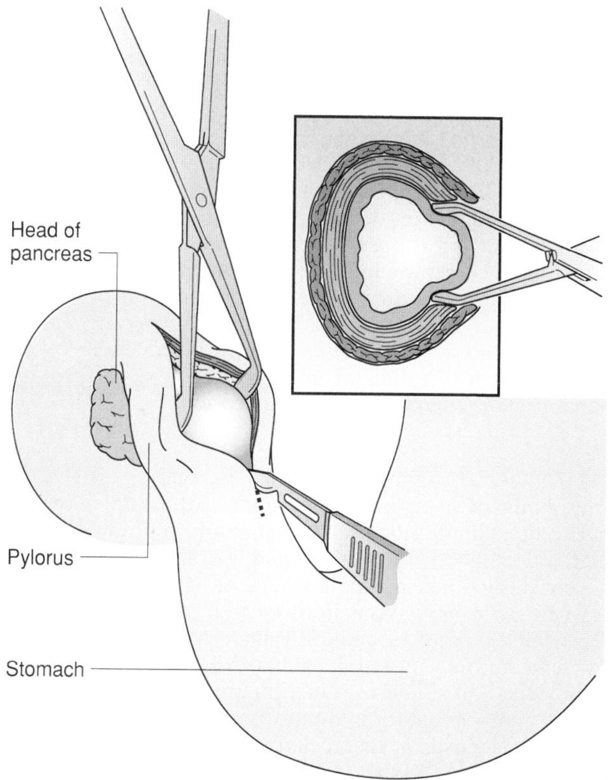

FIGURE 110.38 Ramstedt pyloromyotomy for infantile hypertrophic pyloric stenosis. The cross-sectional view shows herniation of the submucosa into the myotomy site, indicative of an adequate myotomy.

Nasogatric suction is not required. Postoperative feeding typically is started within 6 to 8 hours after recovery from anesthesia. Most infants are tolerant of enteral feeding and can be discharged home safely within 24 hours of operation. The surgical treatment of pyloric stenosis is straightforward, and the recovery is typically uncomplicated. A population-based study reviewing 1777 infants with pyloric stenosis demonstrated a shorter length of stay and a lower overall complication rate in infants operated on by specialty-trained pediatric surgeons compared to general surgeons.[116] Mortality following pyloromyotomy is distinctly unusual in the absence of concomitant medical problems. Complications are rare and usually represent either wound infection, technical failures related to an inadequate pyloromyotomy, or inadvertent entry into the duodenum or stomach. Rarely, infants with inadequate pyloromyotomy may require reexploration and a second myotomy on the posterior pyloric wall. Inadvertent duodenotomy or gastrotomy must be recognized and repaired.

Intussusception

Anatomy and Physiology

Intussusception is defined as the invagination or telescoping of a proximal segment of intestine into an adjacent distal segment and is the most common cause of intestinal obstruction in infants and children age 3 months to 3 years (Fig. 110.39). The invaginated proximal bowel is referred to as the *intussusceptum* and the recipient distal bowel is called the *intussuscipiens*. This process most commonly originates in the small intestine either at or near the ileocecal valve, with the terminal ileum passing into the cecum and colon (ileocolic intussusception). In the pediatric population, the vast majority (95%) of cases are considered idiopathic because of a lack of an identifiable anatomic lesion causing the intussusception. Older children are more likely to have a pathologic lead point causing the intussusception. In similar fashion, infants and children with repeated episodes of intussusception have a greater probability of a pathologic lead point. Table 110.5 describes several factors that have been associated with the development of intussusception.

Many cases of idiopathic intussusception in infants are probably caused by the normally prominent intramural lymph nodes (Peyer's patches) in the terminal ileum acting as functional lead points. The anatomic consequence of intussusception is obstruction of the distal bowel. As bowel edema and inflammation progress, mesenteric vascular insufficiency from compression and congestion may occur. Incarceration, strangulation, and intestinal perforation ultimately may result if this condition remains unrecognized or untreated.

Clinical Presentation

Intussusception is estimated to occur with an incidence rate of 1 to 4 cases per 1,000 children. There is a slight (3:2) male predominance; in a large retrospective series of children with intussusception, 79% were younger than 12 months, and seasonal variation in incidence was not observed.[117] There is an association between the development of intussusception and the administration of a previously available, tetravalent rhesus-based rotavirus vaccine (RotaShield, Wyeth Laboratories, Inc., Marietta, PA).[118]

Otherwise healthy infants who develop intussusception have a characteristic clinical history. The classic triad of abdominal pain, vomiting, and bloody stool is diagnostic but

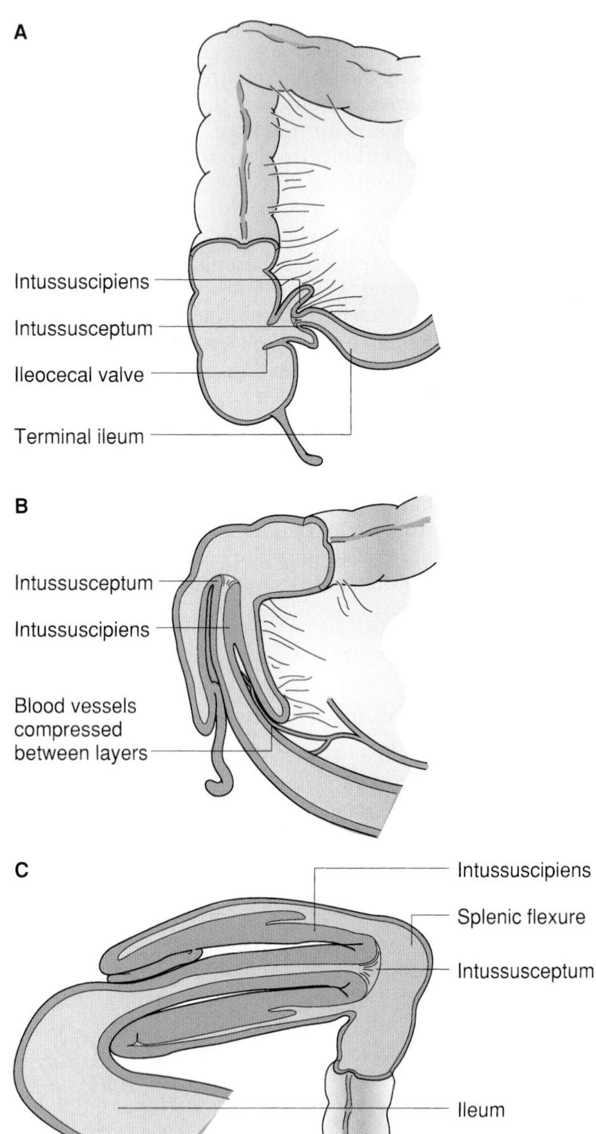

FIGURE 110.39 Ileocolic intussusception with the intussusceptum and intussuscipiens indicated.

variably present. The typical infant develops the acute onset of severe, colicky abdominal pain. Intermittent episodes of irritability and crying may be associated with drawing the legs up to the abdomen for several minutes. Between bouts of colic, the infant is often lethargic or sleepy. During periods of relative exhaustion, the abdominal examination may not be impressive; however, on careful physical examination, a palpable mass in the right abdomen may be appreciated in 80% to 90% of cases. On occasion, the intussusceptum is palpable on digital rectal examination and may present with prolapse through the anus. Emesis is common and is often the presenting complaint. As intestinal obstruction progresses, intractable vomiting with abdominal distention and intravascular volume depletion may occur. Guaiac-positive stool is present in 90% to 95% of infants as a result of the ischemic mucosal injury to the intussusceptum. The passage of bloody stool mixed with mucus, classically described as *currant-jelly stool*, may be observed.

Diagnosis

Plain radiographs of the abdomen are generally nonspecific and may show a paucity of gas in the right lower quadrant

TABLE 110.5

PREDISPOSING FACTORS LEADING TO INTUSSUSCEPTION

ANATOMIC LEAD POINTS
Meckel's diverticulum
Polyp
Lymphatic hypertrophy (Peyer's patch)
Appendix
Duplication or enteric cyst
Lymphoma
Other neoplasm
Heterotopic pancreatic tissue
ASSOCIATED INFECTIONS
Adenovirus
Rotavirus
Parasitic infestation
Other
BLEEDING DISORDERS[a]
Henoch-Schönlein purpura
Hemophilia
Leukemia
TRAUMAA
Blunt abdominal trauma
Major retroperitoneal dissections
OTHERS
Cystic fibrosis

[a]These factors are more likely to be associated with small bowel-to-small bowel intussusception than with ileocolic intussusception.

with a mass effect in the ascending colon. Late findings demonstrate mechanical small-bowel obstruction with proximal distention, air–fluid levels, and a decrease or absence of gas distally. Diagnostic enema techniques using either air or contrast approach 100% accuracy with typical ileocolic intussusception (Fig. 110.40). An approach using retrograde enemas allows therapeutic reduction of intussusception as well. Ultrasound examination typically reveals a mass resembling a bull's eye or target sign, corresponding to the intussusceptum within the intussuscipiens. The target sign of intussusception also may be demonstrated by CT scan imaging. Both these latter modalities do not allow for potential therapeutic reduction and may be more useful in diagnosing suspected cases of proximal jejunoileal or enteroenteral intussusception.

Treatment

Any infant with suspected intussusception in the absence of peritonitis should undergo diagnostic retrograde enema. A high index of clinical suspicion and liberal application of this approach should be maintained. The incidence of normal contrast enema examinations in this setting may exceed 75% in most pediatric centers, and this is justified by the considerable risk inherent in a missed diagnosis. An experienced pediatric radiologist and surgical evaluation are essential. Intravenous access and resuscitation should occur before attempts are made at diagnostic or therapeutic enemas.

Successful hydrostatic or pneumatic reduction of ileocolic intussusception is achieved in 60% to 80% of infants in most pediatric centers in the United States. Some centers prefer pneumatic enema using air as a contrast agent, and this technique

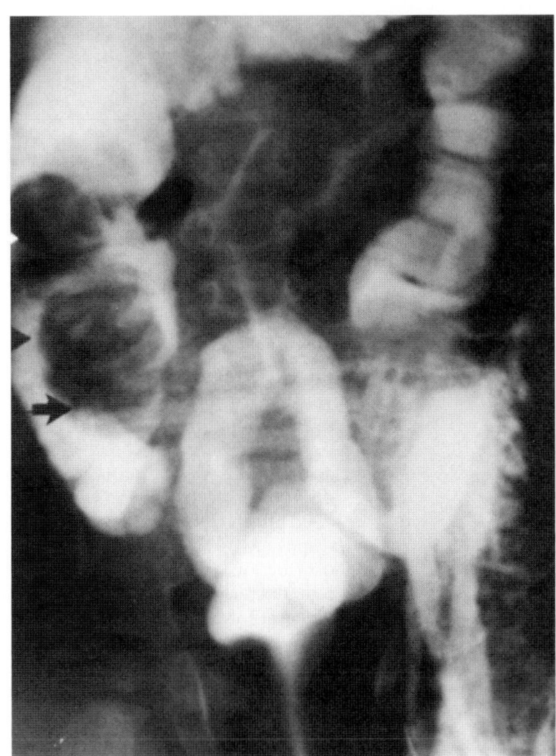

FIGURE 110.40 Contrast enema demonstrating classic ileocolic intussusception with the intussusceptum visible in the ascending colon (*arrows*).

appears comparable to the hydrostatic approach in both diagnosis and therapeutic reduction of intussusception. The ability to reduce intussusception using these techniques is time dependent and diminishes substantially after the duration of symptoms exceeds 24 hours. In this setting, a contrast enema is still diagnostic and potentially therapeutic if carefully performed.[119] With most experienced pediatric radiologists, the risk of perforation or reduction of a strangulated intussusceptum is quite low.

The technique of retrograde reduction of intussusception is straightforward. Contrast or air is introduced into the rectum by a balloon catheter, with the height of the hydrostatic column 1 m or less. Most centers use three attempts at reduction, with each attempt no longer than 3 minutes in duration. As long as progress is being made, however, attempts can be repeated until reduction is achieved. Successful reduction of ileocolic intussusception is demonstrated by observing retrograde flow of contrast or air into the terminal ileum. Inability to demonstrate retrograde flow into the ileum suggests incomplete reduction requiring surgical exploration.

Operative Management. Infants presenting with peritonitis and small-bowel obstruction with a clinical diagnosis of intussusception should undergo immediate resuscitation and exploration without attempts at retrograde enema. Surgical exploration also is required immediately after incomplete retrograde enema reduction of intussusception or in the relatively infrequent situation of bowel perforation during diagnostic or therapeutic enema. The operative strategy is dictated by the findings. Spontaneous reduction of the intussusception is reported to occur in up to 20% to 30% of infants following induction of general anesthesia. In this situation, exploration confirming the reduction and examining the bowel for a pathologic lead point is sufficient. With persistent intussusception and viable bowel, the bowel is manually reduced, generally pushing the intussusceptum out of the distal bowel. If manual reduction cannot be performed or the intussusceptum is strangulated, then segmental resection with primary anastomosis is performed. Attempts at reducing intussusception with clearly necrotic bowel should be avoided. Diverting enterostomy as a result of peritoneal contamination usually is not required. Appendectomy is routinely performed in all infants undergoing operative exploration for intussusception. As with many aspects of pediatric surgery, a laparoscopic approach to the diagnosis and management of intussusception has been reported successful in approximately two thirds of selected patients.[120]

Complications and Outcome

Retrograde enema techniques are successful at reducing idiopathic ileocolic intussusception in 60% to 80% of cases. Following successful enema reduction, the infant is given intravenous fluids and usually observed for 24 hours. Tolerance of oral feeding is predictably rapid. Recovery from operative reduction or bowel resection is generally no different than from other similar gastrointestinal procedures. Most infants enjoy a complete recovery with minimal or no morbidity. Recurrent intussusception after either nonoperative or operative reduction occurs in about 5% of infants and usually can be treated definitively with repeat enema. Mortality from intussusception is rare and is almost always the result of systemic sepsis and shock from unrecognized, strangulated intestine.

Meckel's Diverticulum and Related Disorders

Embryology and Anatomy

The most frequently encountered congenital anomaly of the gastrointestinal tract is Meckel's diverticulum, representing one of several malformations resulting from persistence of the yolk stalk (synonymous with *vitelline duct* and *omphalomesenteric duct*) and its components. The embryonic yolk stalk connects the yolk sac and the developing midgut (Fig. 110.41). Between weeks 5 and 7 of gestation, the yolk sac involutes and the stalk fuses with the umbilical cord. Developmental failure or arrest of yolk sac involution creates a spectrum of clinical malformations as outlined in Figure 110.42, with Meckel's diverticula constituting greater than 95% of these anomalies. Meckel's diverticulum is a true diverticulum of variable size derived from the intestinal remnant of the yolk stalk. Typically, it is found on the antimesenteric border of the terminal ileum

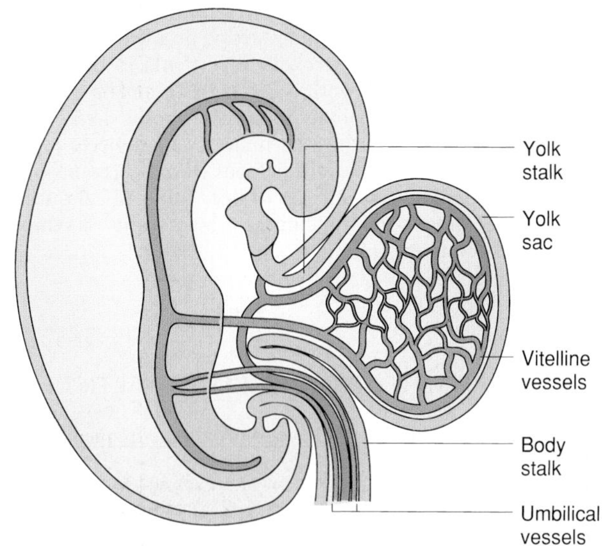

FIGURE 110.41 Normal embryonic relations of the yolk sac, yolk stalk, and developing gut.

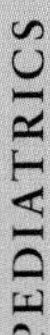

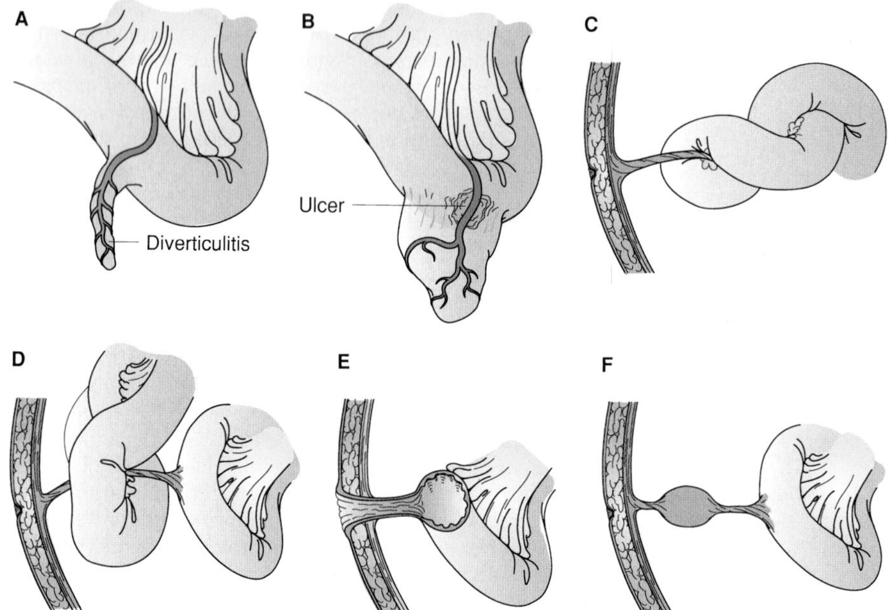

FIGURE 110.42 Common variants of yolk stalk malformations. (*A,B*) Meckel's diverticulum can manifest with inflammation (diverticulitis) or hemorrhage from acid-induced ulceration. (*C,D*) Meckel's diverticulum in association with abnormal band attached to the abdominal wall predisposing to volvulus and intestinal obstruction. (*E*) Patent omphalomesenteric duct. (*F*) Omphalomesenteric sinus and cyst formation.

approximately 40 to 50 cm from the ileocecal valve in adults. The blood supply is derived from persistent vitelline vessels supplied from the SMA. About 25% of the diverticula have a fibrous or vascular attachment to the anterior abdominal wall at the umbilicus (Fig. 110.42C). Heterotopic gastric mucosa or pancreatic tissue is found in about half of the diverticula examined at autopsy. In about 75% of patients with symptomatic diverticula, gastric mucosa is present. When symptoms occur, bleeding or perforation is generally the result of peptic ulceration of the adjacent ileal mucosa, not from the diverticulum itself.

Clinical Presentation

Symptomatic yolk stalk anomalies are usually diagnosed by history and clinical examination. Umbilical drainage from a persistent fistula or sinus tract may be noted in a newborn following separation of the umbilical cord. Intestinal prolapse or passage of stool from the umbilicus signifies a patent omphalomesenteric duct. Small bowel obstruction in an otherwise healthy infant without a history of laparotomy may be a result of volvulus around an omphalomesenteric band or intussusception from a Meckel's diverticulum acting as a lead point.

The incidence rate of Meckel's diverticula in the general population is about 2%, with a 2:1 male-to-female predominance. The risk of developing symptoms from the diverticulum decreases with age, and the vast majority of subjects remain asymptomatic. About half of the persons who do become symptomatic are younger than 2 years of age. Table 110.6 outlines several of the more common clinical presentations of symptomatic Meckel's diverticulum.

TABLE 110.6 DIAGNOSIS

SIGNS AND SYMPTOMS OF MECKEL'S DIVERTICULUM

Clinical presentation	Approximate frequency (%)
Hemorrhage	30–35
Small bowel obstruction	30–35
Diverticulitis	20–25
Umbilical fistula	10
Other	Uncommon

Hemorrhage. Gastrointestinal bleeding related to Meckel's diverticulum generally results from peptic ulceration of the adjacent ileal mucosa. Clinically, it manifests as painless, episodic hemorrhage that is typically bright red to maroon in color; melena is not characteristically seen. Bleeding from Meckel's diverticulum is generally not hemodynamically significant or exsanguinating, but it can be persistent enough to require transfusion. The diagnostic test of choice is the ^{99m}Tc-pertechnetate radioisotope scan (Meckel's scan) because of the high affinity of the isotope for gastric mucosa and the high probability of gastric mucosa within a symptomatic Meckel's diverticulum. Diagnostic accuracy is reported to be as high as 90% for Meckel's-related bleeding. Contrast studies and endoscopy have a limited role when the problem is hemorrhage from a Meckel's diverticulum.

Obstruction. Intestinal obstruction associated with omphalomesenteric duct anomalies usually results from either intussusception or volvulus around an abnormal attachment between the bowel and the abdominal wall. In about 5% to 10% of persons with symptomatic Meckel's diverticula, intussusception is the initial symptom. In patients with Meckel's diverticula whose initial symptom is small bowel obstruction, about half have intussusception, and the remainder have volvulus, internal hernias, or other mechanical causes. Intussusception secondary to a Meckel's diverticula has a decreased likelihood for successful enema reduction. Small bowel obstruction from volvulus around an omphalomesenteric band requires operative exploration and treatment.

Diverticulitis. bout one third of patients with symptomatic Meckel's diverticulum have acute diverticulitis. Similar to appendicitis, intraluminal obstruction at the base of a Meckel's diverticulum can lead to distal inflammation, gangrene, and subsequent perforation. Peptic ulceration also can lead to local inflammation and perforation with the development of peritonitis. The signs and symptoms of Meckel's diverticulitis are virtually indistinguishable from appendicitis, and exploration is both diagnostic and therapeutic.

Umbilical Anomalies. About 10% of patients with yolk stalk or persistent omphalomesenteric duct anomalies have umbilical problems. The usual clinical presentation is persistent drainage or intestinal mucosa found at the umbilicus. The diagnosis can be confirmed by contrast sonogram of the umbilical orifice or tract. Occasionally, ultrasound examination may be useful to demonstrate omphalomesenteric cysts. Ultimately, surgical exploration may be required for both diagnosis and treatment.

Meckel's Diverticulum as an Incidental Finding. The management of an incidentally discovered Meckel's diverticulum during abdominal exploration for other reasons is controversial. The risk of resecting an asymptomatic diverticulum must be weighed against the reasons for the operative exploration, patient age, and the potential for future symptoms from the diverticulum. Infants younger than 2 years are at greater probability of becoming symptomatic from Meckel's diverticula. Resection is clearly indicated with demonstration of heterotopic gastric mucosa in the diverticulum to prevent peptic ulceration. This finding may occasionally be determined by direct palpation because the gastric mucosa is thicker than ileal mucosa. Abnormal omphalomesenteric bands to the abdominal wall also should be excised. If clinical judgment suggests that the diverticulum is at risk for luminal obstruction, resection is warranted.

Treatment

Infants and children with symptomatic umbilical abnormalities from yolk stalk remnants are usually well, and umbilical exploration with possible laparotomy can be undertaken electively. The yolk stalk remnant is excised, and, if present, the communication with the ileum is closed primarily with minimal morbidity and mortality. Operative exploration is required for patients with symptomatic Meckel's diverticula. Typically, exploration can be accomplished through a variety of incisions. The treatment of choice is resection through either antimesenteric wedge excision or segmental bowel resection with primary closure or anastomosis. Laparoscopic diagnosis and management of Meckel's diverticulum has also been described.[121] In the absence of associated medical problems, excellent functional outcome is expected with minimal morbidity and essentially no mortality unless intestinal necrosis has occurred.

Foreign Bodies

Ingestion of foreign bodies by infants and children is common. Toddlers in the age range of 9 months to 2 years are at particular risk given the newly acquired mobility and the tendency for oral exploration. The type of foreign body and the location in the gastrointestinal tract on discovery dictates overall management.

Esophagus

Typical foreign bodies found in the esophagus include coins and small toys. In normal children, these objects become impacted at predictably narrow portions of the esophagus, including the cricopharyngeus, the esophagus at the level of the left mainstem bronchus, and the gastroesophageal junction. Previous areas of esophageal repair or injury predispose to points of obstruction. In particular, infants and children with repaired esophageal atresia, gastroesophageal reflux, or caustic esophageal injury are at risk for impaction at these sites.

Esophageal foreign bodies produce clinical symptoms of drooling, feeding intolerance (particularly to solids), dysphagia, and pain. Unrecognized foreign bodies with unusual configuration or sharp points and edges may cause esophageal perforation and mediastinitis. The diagnosis is straightforward on plain radiographs if the object is metallic or radiopaque. If a radiolucent object is suspected, an upper gastrointestinal contrast study is usually required to confirm the diagnosis. Lateral plain films of the neck or chest may be useful to differentiate between small foreign bodies in the esophagus or trachea.

Foreign bodies impacted in the esophagus cause partial esophageal obstruction and can cause complications including aspiration, erosion, perforation, and late stricture formation. Therefore, all esophageal foreign bodies should be removed. Extraction of foreign objects can be accomplished by using balloon catheter retrieval under fluoroscopic guidance or direct visualization using endoscopy. Performed within 24 hours of ingestion, balloon catheter retrieval of esophageal foreign bodies is relatively straightforward. This technique is limited to smooth radiopaque objects such as coins to minimize the risk of esophageal perforation. The most significant risk with balloon catheter retrieval is potential aspiration from an unprotected airway, and this must be anticipated as the foreign body traverses the pharynx. Alternatively, for esophageal coin impaction of less than 24 hours' duration in children without a history of esophageal surgery or injury, esophageal bougienage with clearance of the coin into the stomach has been successful.[122]

Retrieval of esophageal foreign bodies under direct endoscopic vision requires general anesthesia. Either flexible or rigid endoscopy systems are widely available and used with individual and institutional preferences. Esophageal perforation, the major risk, occurs in fewer than 5% of cases in most reported series. Longstanding esophageal foreign bodies may erode into the aorta and cause life-threatening hemorrhage from aortoesophageal fistula.[123]

Distal Gastrointestinal Tract

More than 95% of foreign bodies that pass beyond the gastroesophageal junction proceed uneventfully through the gastrointestinal tract. The transit time for an asymptomatic foreign body is highly variable and can take hours to weeks. Progress of an asymptomatic radiopaque foreign body can be followed by abdominal plain films, but this is rarely useful from a clinical standpoint unless it is a battery. The stool may also be screened to confirm passage of a known foreign body.

Operative exploration or endoscopic retrieval of distal gastrointestinal foreign bodies is generally reserved for clinical symptoms related to either obstruction or intestinal injury heralded by abdominal pain, vomiting, fever, or peritonitis. Additionally, persistence of an asymptomatic foreign body in the stomach for several weeks is a relative indication for upper endoscopic retrieval, particularly with foreign bodies with irregular shape, configuration, or sharpness. This is a clinical judgment that is best reserved for an experienced pediatric surgeon because remarkably complex and improbable objects may pass uneventfully through the gastrointestinal tract. For asymptomatic foreign bodies lodged distal to the stomach, a relative indication for operative removal is a fixed, persistent location in the intestine longer than 1 week in duration.

Ingested batteries, in particular alkaline disc batteries, are a potentially serious hazard to children and require a more aggressive approach. Disruption of the battery casing and spillage of the contents have been reported to cause intestinal injury and perforation, presumably because of leakage of potassium or sodium hydroxide. Esophageal impaction of a battery warrants prompt removal when recognized because the risk of acquired esophageal injury, perforation, and development of traumatic tracheoesophageal fistula is present.[124] In the distal bowel, cathartics, lavage, and enemas may be helpful to expedite passage of the battery. Operative removal may be necessary if the battery fails to progress distally over a few days or if symptoms related to the battery occur. Notably, the vast majority of batteries pass through the gastrointestinal tract uneventfully.

TABLE 110.7 ETIOLOGY

CAUSES OF UPPER GASTROINTESTINAL HEMORRHAGE[a]

Patient age group	Common causes	Less common causes
Neonatal (0 to 30 days)	Gastritis Esophagitis Ingested maternal blood Peptic ulcer	Iatrogenic trauma Primary coagulopathy Vascular malformation (hemangioma, telangiectasia, arteriovenous malformation) Nasal or pharyngeal bleeding Miscellaneous (leiomyoma, gastric polyp, duplication)
Infant (30 days to 1 year)	Gastritis Esophagitis Peptic ulcer	Same as neonate, with addition of: Drugs (steroids, nonsteroidal antiinflammatory drugs) Foreign body, caustic ingestion Esophageal varices
Child (1 to 12 years)	Esophageal varices Esophagitis Peptic ulcer	Same as infant, with addition of: Acquired thrombocytopenia (chemotherapy)
Older child (12 years to adult)	Esophageal varices Esophagitis Peptic ulcer	Same as for child

[a]Order in appearance approximates clinical frequency.
(Modified from Oldham, KT, Lobe TE. Gastrointestinal hemorrhage in children. A pragmatic update. *Pediatr Clin North Am.* 1985;32:1247–1263, with permission.)

Gastrointestinal Hemorrhage

The subject of gastrointestinal hemorrhage and general principles of management are discussed elsewhere this book. The following section reviews some of the important and age-dependent clinical causes and unique issues of gastrointestinal bleeding in pediatric population. These causes are age dependent and are summarized in Tables 110.7 and 110.8.

Diagnostic work-up of an infant or child with gastrointestinal hemorrhage requires coordinated participation between

TABLE 110.8 ETIOLOGY

CAUSES OF LOWER GASTROINTESTINAL HEMORRHAGE[a]

Patient age group	Common causes	Less common causes
Neonatal (0 to 30 days)	Benign anorectal lesions (fissure) Upper gastrointestinal hemorrhage Milk allergy Necrotizing enterocolitis Midgut volvulus	Iatrogenic trauma Primary coagulopathy Vascular malformations Enterocolitis (Hirschsprung disease, other) Miscellaneous (duplication, lymphoma, lymphangiectasia)
Infant (30 days to 1 year)	Incarcerated inguinal hernia Benign anorectal lesions Idiopathic intussusception Meckel's diverticulum Infectious diarrhea Upper gastrointestinal hemorrhage Milk allergy	Same as neonate, with addition of: Acquired thrombocytopenia Ingestion of colored foodstuff (pseudohematochezia)
Child (1 to 12 years)	Benign anorectal lesions Juvenile polyps Intussusception Meckel's diverticulum Infectious diarrhea Upper gastrointestinal hemorrhage	Same as infant, with addition of: Juvenile polyposis coli/Familial polyposis coli Hemolytic uremic syndrome Henöch-Schonlein purpura Systemic vasculitis (dermatomyositis, lupus) Acquired thrombocytopenia (as above plus idiopathic thrombocytopenic purpura)
Older child (12 years to adult)	Juvenile polyps Benign anorectal lesions Inflammatory bowel disease Upper gastrointestinal hemorrhage	Same as child, except: Henöch-Schonlein purpura and hemolytic uremic syndrome less likely Meckel's diverticulum

[a]Order in appearance approximates clinical frequency.
(Modified from Oldham, KT, Lobe TE. Gastrointestinal hemorrhage in children. A pragmatic update. *Pediatr Clin North Am.* 1985;32:1247–1263, with permission.)

pediatricians, surgeons, gastroenterologists, and radiologists. Several general principles governing the diagnostic approach to gastrointestinal bleeding in infants and children follow:

a. A clear diagnosis can be made in most situations; given the current technology available to assist with diagnosis, an aggressive approach is warranted. Diagnostic procedures such as flexible fiberoptic endoscopy, radioisotope imaging, and angiography are widely available, safe, and applicable to any age group, including the newborn. Despite these measures, in approximately 16% of cases, the cause of guaiac-positive stools in a neonate or infant remains unknown,[125] and the bleeding is self-limited.
b. The primary diagnostic investigation of choice for upper gastrointestinal bleeding is esophagogastroduodenoscopy. This procedure is optimally performed within the first 24 hours after cessation of active hemorrhage and may require general anesthesia. Imaging studies for active upper gastrointestinal hemorrhage are usually limited in their ability to aid with diagnosis.
c. Infants and children presenting with minor lower gastrointestinal bleeding are best evaluated by a careful perineal and digital rectal examination followed by anoscopy.
d. Massive lower gastrointestinal hemorrhage in an infant or child outside the newborn period is most likely the result of a bleeding Meckel's diverticulum.
e. If a definitive source for lower gastrointestinal hemorrhage is not found on colonoscopy, evaluation for an upper gastrointestinal source, including upper endoscopy and diagnostic laparoscopy, is warranted.
f. Pain is an uncommon symptom with pediatric gastrointestinal hemorrhage and implies a more complex problem such as volvulus, ischemic bowel, or inflammatory bowel disease. Painful gastrointestinal hemorrhage in pediatric patient requires urgent evaluation and prompt diagnostic work-up.
g. In contrast to that in adults, gastrointestinal bleeding in children is rarely a symptom or sign of gastrointestinal neoplasm.

Neonates (0–30 Days of Age)

The most common cause of gastrointestinal hemorrhage in a neonate is gastritis. Endoscopic evaluation of newborns with symptomatic upper gastrointestinal hemorrhage demonstrates gastritis or esophagitis in 50% to 75% of cases. About 10% to 15% have swallowed maternal blood during birth, and 10% of newborns are found to have an underlying coagulopathy. Anatomic lesions requiring operative control are distinctly unusual in this age group. Significant and sometimes massive upper gastrointestinal hemorrhage may occur in a neonate without a definable anatomic lesion despite endoscopic evaluation. This finding is usually the result of gastritis, and treatment is directed at blood and volume replacement, evaluation for and correction of any underlying coagulopathy, and supportive care.

Significant conditions responsible for lower gastrointestinal bleeding in the newborn include NEC, malrotation with volvulus, enterocolitis, or bowel obstruction secondary to an incarcerated inguinal hernia. These clinical entities present with characteristic histories, findings on clinical examination, and surgical treatment guidelines previously discussed. Anorectal fissure is also common in neonates, and bleeding is typically self-limited.

Infants (30 Days to 1 Year)

Infants with upper gastrointestinal bleeding deserve comprehensive evaluation, including endoscopy, to identify potential lesions requiring operative intervention. The most common causes of lower gastrointestinal hemorrhage in this age group include infectious diarrhea, intussusception, food allergy, and bleeding Meckel's diverticulum. Most of these lesions have distinct symptoms, signs, and diagnostic findings to facilitate diagnosis. Infectious diarrhea is usually accompanied by a history of fever, feeding intolerance, possibly emesis, and abdominal pain. Fecal leukocytes may be present on stool examination, and enteric pathogens or their toxins can be identified by stool culture.

Children (1 to 12 Years)

An important surgical cause of upper gastrointestinal bleeding in this age group includes esophageal variceal bleeding from portal hypertension. Children with biliary atresia or extrahepatic portal venous obstruction account for most cases of variceal bleeding in this age group. In the acute setting, endoscopic sclerotherapy is used as a temporizing measure for hemorrhage control; some investigators advocate maintenance sclerotherapy. Ultimately, for these children, orthotopic liver transplantation may offer definitive surgical treatment. The use of operative portosystemic shunts for acute variceal hemorrhage are not widely used in pediatric surgical practice in the United States.

Conditions causing lower gastrointestinal bleeding in this age group include juvenile polyps. These are benign, hamartomatous polyps and represent the single most common cause of lower gastrointestinal bleeding in children. About 20% to 30% of the polyps are palpable on digital rectal examination. A history of painless, bright red blood per rectum during a bowel movement is typical. The bleeding results from mucosal irritation, involution, and sloughing of a pedunculated polyp and is usually not associated with hemodynamically significant hemorrhage. Tissue may be passed or the pedunculated polyp may prolapse out the anus. A hypochromic, microcytic anemia may be present. Diagnostic work-up generally involves a contrast enema to identify the polyp and evaluate the colon for synchronous lesions. Colonoscopy may require general anesthesia in this age group, and endoscopic snare polypectomy is the treatment of choice for appropriate sized polyps. Infrequently, transanal excision or open resection of larger polyps is required. In the case of multiple juvenile polyps not amenable to endoscopic polypectomy, management may be expectant based on the benign natural history characterized by involution during adolescence. Histologic confirmation is necessary to differentiate these lesions from adenomatous polyps seen in familial polyposis syndromes or Gardner's syndrome.

Older Children and Adolescents (Older Than 12 Years)

Causes of both upper and lower gastrointestinal hemorrhage in this age group include most etiologic conditions found in adults. Importantly, inflammatory bowel disease is significant in this age group.

Intestinal Duplication

The embryologic origin of enteric duplication formation remains controversial, but duplication likely represents abnormal development of either a diverticulum or adjacent portion of the developing gut. In some cases, duplication cysts of the upper gastrointestinal tract may be associated with thoracic spinal cord or vertebral defects; this association appears to reflect abnormal sequestration and integration of developing primitive notochord elements in addition to duplication. The resulting lesions are described as either *cystic* or *tubular* based on their gross appearance (Fig. 110.43). All types of gastrointestinal-derived epithelia are found, but the clinically relevant

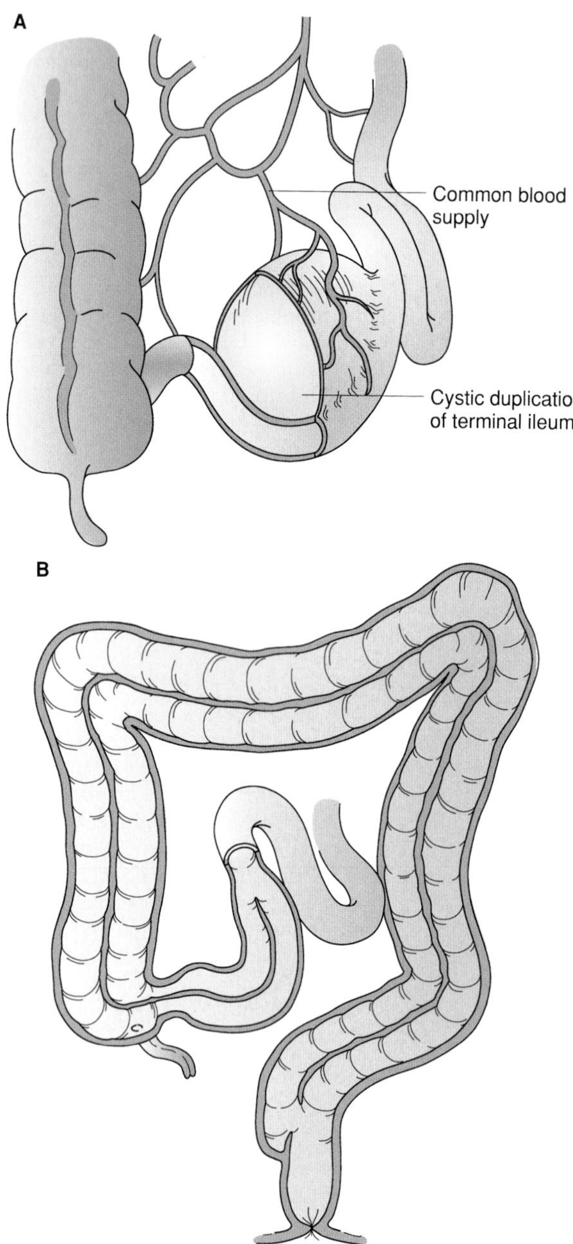

FIGURE 110.43 Enteric duplication. (*A*) Cystic duplication of the terminal ileum. (*B*) Tubular duplication of the terminal ileum and colon.

finding is ectopic gastric mucosa. Duplications are commonly found along the mesenteric border of the native bowel. The muscular wall is typically well developed and intimately attached to the functional bowel. Additionally, the blood supply is also shared with the functional intestine, an important surgical consideration.

Cystic Duplications

Cystic duplications may be found throughout the gastrointestinal tract. They are frequently located in the esophagus and the hindgut, particularly the rectum. Direct communication between a duplication cyst and the functional gut lumen is unusual. Typically, asymptomatic duplications are discovered as incidental mass lesions during diagnostic imaging studies, particularly when the location is the thoracic cavity or the rectum. Duplications also may present as symptomatic lesions from ectopic gastric mucosa leading to ulceration and bleeding. Other potential presenting symptoms of enteric duplication include obstruction, intussusception, perforation or traumatic rupture, torsion, infection, and occasional malignant degeneration. Useful examinations to define the extent of the lesion include ultrasound, CT scanning, MRI studies, and contrast studies. The identification of enteric duplication on routine prenatal ultrasound examination has been reported.

The treatment for all cystic duplications is operative. Even in asymptomatic infants and children, uncertainty regarding the nature of the mass and the potential for subsequent problems dictates surgical exploration. Esophageal and rectal duplication cysts are generally amenable to simple excision. In contrast, duplication cysts of the small intestine usually require segmental resection and primary anastomosis, given the intimate attachment and shared blood supply with the native bowel. For large cystic duplications involving longer segments of native bowel, individualized treatment strategies are required. One option is cyst marsupialization with resection of the duplication cyst wall with preservation of the common blood supply and wall between the cyst and native bowel. This technique is combined with submucosal dissection and stripping of the remaining epithelium from the cyst wall. Another approach is internal drainage of the cyst into the adjacent native intestine, for example, creation of a cyst-duodenostomy for duodenal duplication not amenable to local resection and anastomosis. This is usually unnecessary, however, and long-term drainage is a potential problem.

Tubular Duplications

Tubular duplications may be found anywhere along the length of the gastrointestinal tract. They are less frequent than cystic duplications and have a tendency to involve the ileum and the colon. It is believed that tubular duplication generally reflects abnormal, disordered recanalization of the gastrointestinal tract after epithelial proliferation and obliteration of the intestinal lumen during weeks 6 and 7 of gestation. Similar to cystic duplications, tubular lesions share a common wall and blood supply with the native bowel. Communication between the tubular duplication and native bowel lumen is common. Tubular duplications may be extensive and can involve the entire length of terminal ileum and colon. Malformations of the entire colon and rectum are associated with genitourinary anomalies, particularly duplications of the external genitalia or bladder. These latter anomalies embryologically appear to represent an interrupted twinning process.

Tubular duplications manifest clinically in similar fashion to cystic lesions. Symptomatic lesions most commonly present with gastrointestinal bleeding or obstruction. Treatment is operative, and an individualized strategy is required that is based on the location and nature of the duplication. Resection with primary anastomosis may require removal of an unacceptable length of normal bowel. Marsupialization with submucosal stripping of the duplication epithelium may be particularly helpful if ectopic gastric mucosa is suspected or found. Obstruction from a long, blind-ending parallel duplication that communicates with the functional gut lumen can be treated effectively with a reentry procedure such as a distal enteroenterostomy. This approach avoids a potentially complex resection of a significant length of bowel.

The outcomes of surgical management of enteric duplications are generally excellent in the absence of other associated anomalies or medical problems. Mortality attributable to the duplication itself is distinctly unusual. Postoperative morbidity is generally dependent on the nature and location of the duplication.

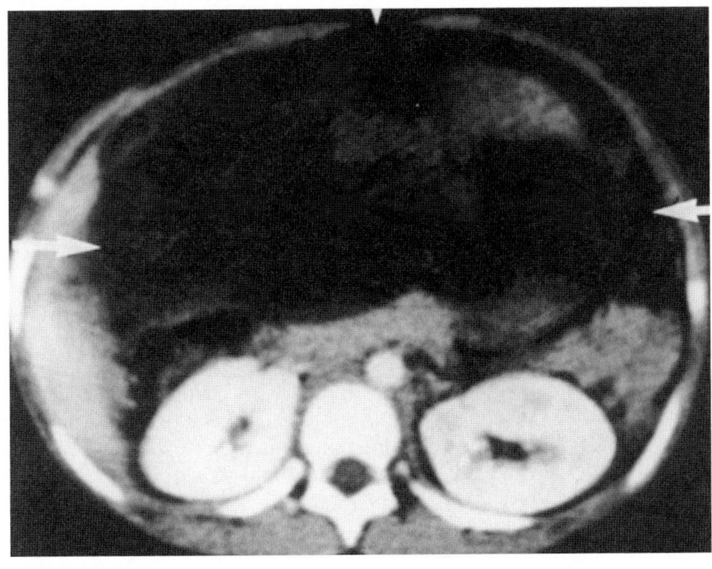

FIGURE 110.44 Computed tomography scan image from a child after abdominal trauma. Hemorrhage into large omental cyst is apparent (*arrows*).

Mesenteric and Omental Cysts

Mesenteric and omental cysts are rare lesions thought to result from the sequestration of lymphatic tissue during development. Mesenteric cysts are twice more common than omental cysts. Both are characterized by thin and often incomplete walls lined with endothelial cells without surrounding smooth muscle. They may be filled with either serous lymphatic fluid or chyle and may be unilocular or multilocular. These cysts may become extraordinarily large before producing symptoms.

Most infants and children with mesenteric or omental cysts are diagnosed prior to adolescence. Asymptomatic children are usually diagnosed incidentally during studies for other reasons. Symptomatic children present with abdominal pain, and, on examination, a soft, mobile abdominal mass is characteristic. Bleeding, rupture, obstruction, torsion, or cyst infection may be observed. Most of these lesions can be diagnosed by ultrasound or CT scan, although specific diagnosis may not be apparent. Ascites, duplication cysts, pancreatic pseudocysts, and large ovarian cysts may have a similar appearance on diagnostic imaging. Peripheral calcification and evidence of recent hemorrhage may be seen in mesenteric or omental cysts (Fig. 110.44).

The treatment for these lesions is simple excision, if possible. Total excision of mesenteric or omental cysts is generally preferable over partial excision with marsupialization. Limited resection with primary anastomosis may be required for a mesenteric cyst located adjacent to the intestinal wall, particularly if there is concern that the cyst actually may be an enteric duplication. Morbidity and mortality are generally limited to concurrent problems associated with the intestine. In particular, volvulus of a mesenteric cyst may cause vascular compromise and infarction of the adjacent intestine.

Primary Peritonitis

Bacterial peritonitis without a specific, identifiable cause is referred to as *primary peritonitis,* which now accounts for fewer than 1% of all cases of childhood peritonitis. Use of the term now includes children who develop peritonitis secondary to a clearly identifiable cause, such as an indwelling peritoneal dialysis catheter or a ventriculoperitoneal shunt. Spontaneous bacterial peritonitis in children with ascites or nephrosis is generally included in this group. It is thought that hematogenous seeding of the protein-rich ascitic fluid is responsible for the development of spontaneous bacterial peritonitis. The infecting bacterial organisms were classically gram-positive with a variety of staphylococcal, streptococcal, and other species accounting for most cases. In a contemporary series of infants and children with primary peritonitis, more than two thirds of the cases were caused by gram-negative organisms such as *Escherichia coli.*[126]

The other etiologic mechanism for the development of primary peritonitis is believed to involve retrograde inoculation of the peritoneal cavity via the genitourinary tract. This etiology is characteristic of prepubertal girls 5 to 10 years of age, accounting for as many as half of the cases of primary peritonitis. The initial signs and symptoms in these children are virtually identical to children with perforated appendicitis: fever, emesis, abdominal pain, and tenderness on examination. Leukocytosis is characteristic, and an ileus is observed on plain abdominal films. On exploration, these children have inflammatory peritonitis without an identifiable enteric cause. Gram-negative enteric organisms are commonly cultured from the peritoneal fluid.

Infants and children with primary peritonitis in association with an indwelling peritoneal dialysis catheter or ventriculoperitoneal shunt are occasionally treated successfully with intravenous broad-spectrum antibiotics. The catheter or shunt should be removed or exteriorized promptly if peritonitis does not resolve within 24 to 48 hours. In association with ascites or nephrosis, diagnostic paracentesis should be performed and the peritoneal fluid examined by Gram stain and culture. If there is any diagnostic uncertainty, laparoscopic or open operative exploration may be required to exclude a gastrointestinal source. If the appendix is normal, peritoneal cultures should be obtained and a thorough, complete abdominal exploration for other causes should be performed. Appendectomy is generally performed when the diagnosis of primary peritonitis is established by a right lower-quadrant incision. Other than perforated appendicitis, distinct causes of intestinal perforation or peritonitis in this age group include perforated Meckel's diverticulum, duodenal ulcer, and acute pancreatitis. About half of the peritoneal fluid cultures are positive for a single organism. Treatment with specific antibiotics is continued until the patient is afebrile with a normal white blood cell count and normal clinical examination. Following operative exploration in primary peritonitis, the morbidity is no different than that for appendectomy, and the recovery is generally uneventful.

TABLE 110.9 ETIOLOGY

COMMON CAUSES OF NEONATAL ASCITES

Maternal-fetal Rh incompatibility (rare)
Structural malformations
- Urinary obstruction
- Congenital heart disease
- Malrotation, duplications, cyst (associated with intestinal volvulus)
- Biliary perforation
- Ovarian ascites
- Pulmonary abnormalities

Chylous ascites
Hematologic disorders
- (α-Thalessemia

Infection
- Toxoplasmosis
- Cytomegalovirus

Others
- α_1-Antitrypsin deficiency
- Idiopathic

Ascites

The common causes of neonatal and childhood ascites are listed in Tables 110.9 and 110.10. The clinical presentation is that of abdominal distention with bulging flanks and demonstrable fluid on palpation and percussion. Ultrasound or CT scan imaging may be useful to confirm the clinical diagnosis. Paracentesis and routine examination of the fluid for Gram stain, cell count, cytology, protein, chemistries, and culture should be performed. Chylous ascites is characterized by a white milky appearance, high lymphocyte count, and high triglyceride content. Bile-stained fluid in the absence of demonstrable bowel perforation is characteristic of biliary ascites. High fluid amylase content is seen in pancreatic ascites, and a low protein count (<3 g/dL) is consistent with serous ascites. Elevated urea nitrogen or creatinine in the fluid may suggest urinary ascites, particularly in a male patient. Cytology should be performed to exclude peritoneal ascites secondary to malignancy, particularly in pubertal and adolescent females.

If the initial fluid does not provide a diagnosis in an otherwise normal-appearing child, a comprehensive diagnostic imaging evaluation is warranted. An echocardiogram should be performed and either ultrasound or CT scan imaging performed to evaluate the genitourinary system, the hepatobiliary system, and the pancreas. A voiding cystourethrogram may also be indicated.

Treatment of neonatal or childhood ascites depends on the establishment of a specific diagnosis. In the absence of anatomic lesion or injury, spontaneous resolution of chylous ascites occurs in 50% to 75% of cases with the cessation of enteral feeding and administration of parenteral nutrition. Persistence of chylous ascites for longer than 4 to 6 weeks is an indication for operative attempts to repair or ligate the cisterna chyli. Neonatal biliary ascites may result from spontaneous bile duct perforation, in which case, a diagnosis of CF must be considered. Transient bile duct obstruction typically leads to perforation at the junction of the cystic duct with the common duct. Simple external drainage is the treatment of choice, and complex hepatobiliary tract reconstruction in this setting is unnecessary and potentially hazardous. Urinary ascites in a male patient requires a work-up that includes a voiding cystourethrogram to exclude posterior urethral valves. Urinary ascites resolves with treatment of obstructive uropathy. Pancreatic ascites is typically self-limited, and treatment by drainage procedures is generally not required or limited for relief of persistent symptoms.

Massive neonatal ascites may cause hypoventilation secondary to impairment of diaphragmatic excursion, and therapeutic paracentesis may be required. Childhood ascites generally responds to adequate treatment of the underlying problem and occasionally requires medical therapy. The need for placement of a peritoneovenous shunt in children for intractable ascites is rare.

Rectal Prolapse

Spontaneous rectal prolapse is relatively common in toddlers and preschool-age groups. A peak incidence occurs at or near the time of toilet training. There is an association between straining during bowel movement and rectal prolapse; it may

TABLE 110.10 ETIOLOGY

COMMON CAUSES OF CHILDHOOD ASCITES

SEROUS ASCITES
Cirrhosis
Budd-Chiari syndrome
Nephrosis
Right-sided heart failure
Postoperative ascites (after renal transplantation, peritoneal dialysis, ventriculoperitoneal shunt)
α_1-Antitrypsin deficiency
Other rare metabolic disorders

CHYLOUS ASCITES
Malrotation with volvulus
Small bowel obstruction
Incarcerated hernia
Lymphangioma
Trauma (includes operative trauma)

BILIARY ASCITES
Neonatal bile duct perforation
Cystic fibrosis
Biliary atresia
Hepatitis
Cytomegalovirus infection

URINARY ASCITES (7:1 MALE PREDOMINANCE)
Urinary obstruction
Posterior urethral valves
Bladder perforation
Ureterocele
Neurogenic bladder

PANCREATIC ASCITES
Acute pancreatitis (drugs, trauma, gallstones, infection)
Pancreatic pseudocysts

OVARIAN ASCITES
Cysts (torsion, rupture)
Tumors

MALIGNANT ASCITES

Intraabdominal neoplasm

IDIOPATHIC

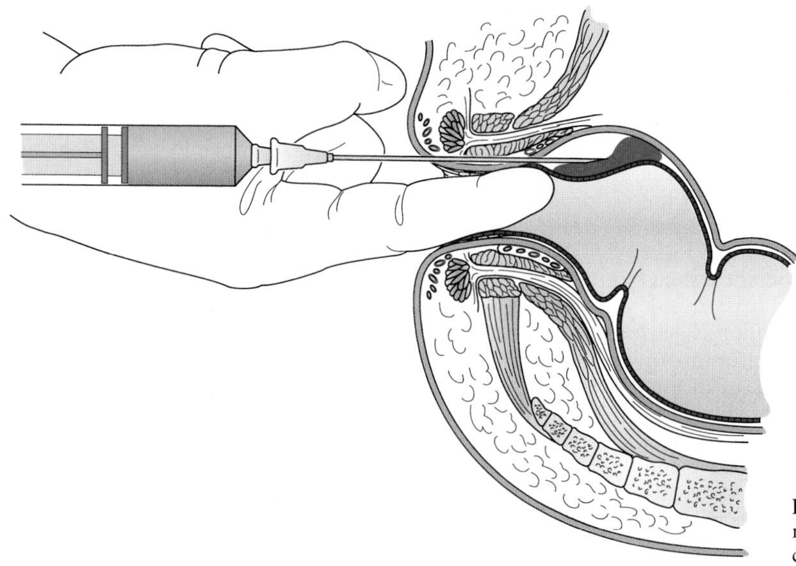

FIGURE 110.45 Four-quadrant injection of sclerosant into the rectal submucosa for the treatment of childhood rectal prolapse.

be more commonly observed in children with CF, myelodysplasias with sacral neuropathy, congenital anorectal malformations, Hirschsprung disease, and colorectal polyps. However, most children presenting with rectal prolapse are normal.

A history of protrusion of mucosa or full-thickness rectum with or without bleeding is usually described. Other lesions of childhood that have a similar appearance are either prolapse of an intussusceptum or passage of a polyp through the anus. The rectal examination is diagnostic. If the protruding intestine is an intussusceptum, a finger can be placed adjacent to it within the rectum; this action is not possible with rectal prolapse.

Nonoperative management using manual reduction is successful in most infants and children. Sedation may be required in some instances. Therapeutic interventions include stool softeners and parental instruction on manual reduction, and spontaneous resolution over a few weeks is typical. For persistent rectal prolapse in children, operative intervention is generally governed by doing the least invasive procedure possible. Unlike adults, complex operations involving bowel resection and pelvic suspension are generally unnecessary in children with rectal prolapse. The most useful and commonly used procedure is rectal submucosal injection using a sclerosant (Fig. 110.45). With the patient under general anesthesia, injection with 5% sodium morrhuate has been performed successfully on an outpatient basis. About 90% of children can be treated successfully with a single four-quadrant sclerosant technique, but on occasion further sclerosis is necessary. Submucosal dissection or cauterization is also successful but may have a higher incidence of postoperative bleeding or stricture formation and usually requires a short period of hospitalization. The major objective in treating childhood rectal prolapse is to create a local extraperitoneal inflammatory process in the perirectal space. Morbidity is low and the long-term outcome is excellent.

PEDIATRIC LIVER

Tumors of the Liver

Primary hepatic tumors are rare in children; however, at least 60% to 70% are malignant.[127,128] Table 110.11 reviews the incidence rates and types of hepatic tumors presenting during infancy and childhood. Pediatric hepatic tumors often manifest as asymptomatic abdominal masses discovered by parents or pediatrician. Symptoms related to the tumor, such as pain, hemorrhage, hypertension, and precocious puberty, are less frequent. Initial diagnostic imaging studies include plain abdominal radiographs and ultrasound to assist in early determination as to whether the mass is cystic or solid and whether calcifications are present. CT scan imaging and MRI remain definitive in the ability to discern anatomic characteristics of the mass and its relationship to adjacent structures. Most children require operative exploration for either definitive excision or for diagnostic incisional biopsy in lesions deemed unresectable.

Benign Tumors

Of all primary liver tumors of childhood, 30% are benign. The most common benign tumors are hemangiomas, hemangioendotheliomas, mesenchymal hamartomas, cysts, focal nodular hyperplasia, and hepatic adenoma. In most large series, hemangiomas constitute about 50% of the benign hepatic tumors observed.[129]

TABLE 110.11

INCIDENCE OF LIVER TUMORS IN CHILDHOOD

Tumor type	Incidence rate (%)
BENIGN	
Vascular tumors	13
Hemangioma	9
Hemangioendothelioma	4
Mesenchymal hamartoma	6
Focal nodular hyperplasia	2
Adenoma	2
Teratoma	2
OTHER	3
MALIGNANT	
Hepatoblastoma	43
Hepatocellular carcinoma	23
Malignant mesenchymal tumor	4
Sarcoma	2
Embryonal cell carcinoma	2
Angiosarcoma	1

Vascular Tumors. Hemangiomas are disordered and dilated vascular channels and are often described as *cavernous hemangiomas*. Cavernous hemangiomas represent the most common benign vascular hepatic tumor in the pediatric age group. Infantile hemangioendotheliomas are vascular tumors derived from endothelial cells that have formed vascular channels but maintain a diffuse, hypercellular pattern.[130] Infantile hemangioendotheliomas have a tendency to manifest in the first few months to years of life, whereas hemangiomas present in the adolescent and young adult population. Both these vascular lesions of the liver are typically asymptomatic lesions.

Most benign vascular lesions of the pediatric liver do not require operative management. Operative intervention is generally reserved for bleeding secondary to traumatic rupture or the evolution of high-output congestive heart failure or thrombocytopenia. Treatment strategies remain highly individualized given the relatively common, spontaneous involution of these lesions over time. In the face of congestive heart failure and thrombocytopenia secondary to sequestration, medical treatment with corticosteroid therapy may be useful. More invasive procedures such as irradiation, selective hepatic arterial ligation or angiographic embolization remain useful in selected patients with uncontrollable symptoms. Chemotherapeutic agents, including recombinant alpha-interferon, low-dose vincristine, and cyclophosphamide have been used for life-threatening vascular lesions. Hepatic resection is generally reserved for mass lesions of unknown diagnosis, ruptured vascular lesions with signs of active hemorrhage, or for symptomatic, locally resectable lesions. Infants with large hemangiomas should be screened for treatable hypothyroidism secondary to endogenous production of iodothyronine deiodinase[131]

Hemangioendotheliomas are most important in the infant age group and vary in size from 1 cm to several cm in diameter and may be multiple (Fig. 110.46). Presenting symptoms and signs in a neonate include an abdominal mass, hepatomegaly, and congestive heart failure. These infants may also experience spontaneous rupture and hemoperitoneum. Symptomatic infants present with tachycardia, tachypnea, and cyanosis or, in the instance of rupture, hypovolemic shock. On examination, the infant may have other cutaneous hemangiomas visible on the skin. About half of these infants develop thrombocytopenia secondary to platelet sequestration in the vascular malformation (*Kasabach-Merritt syndrome*). CT scan imaging or MRI is diagnostic. Treatment is directed at controlling symptoms using medical management principles as discussed previously; however, hemangioendotheliomas tend to be more problematic than hemangiomas because of the tendency to occur during infancy and the more extensive, symptomatic nature of the lesions.

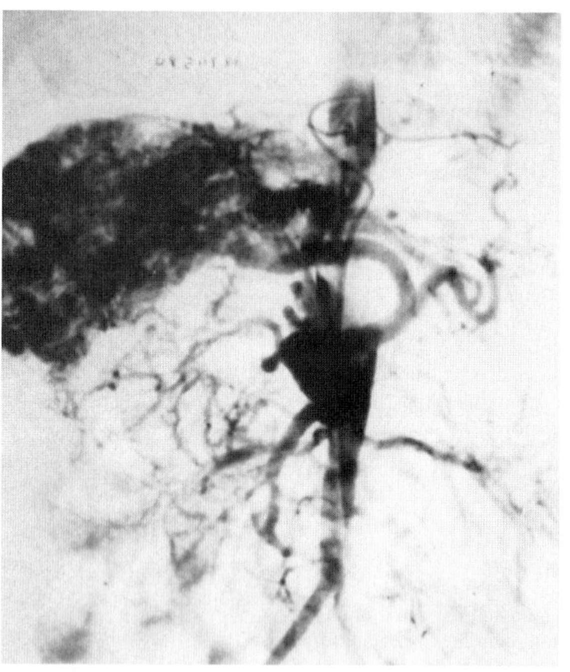

FIGURE 110.46 Selective visceral angiogram demonstrating large hepatic vascular malformation in a neonate with congestive heart failure. This finding is consistent with a bilobar hemangioendothelioma.

Mesenchymal Hamartomas. Approximately one third of benign hepatic tumors in children are mesenchymal hamartomas. A mesenchymal hamartoma is often quite large and typically presents within the first year of life as an asymptomatic, solitary abdominal mass. CT scan imaging or MRI studies are usually diagnostic and show a solid mass that may have cystic components within the liver parenchyma. Definitive diagnosis may require open tissue biopsy, and the therapy of choice is complete excision, although spontaneous involution has been described. Simple enucleation may be adequate because these tumors tend to be well circumscribed. On occasion, formal hepatic resection may be required.[132] Recurrence is low after adequate resection.

Focal Nodular Hyperplasia. This tumor occurs primarily in female children and in adults and may be associated with the use of oral contraceptives or focal hepatic injury. Focal nodular hyperplasia is usually a well defined, solitary mass that has characteristic findings on CT scan imaging. Open or percutaneous biopsy may be required to differentiate the lesion from hepatic adenoma. As the name implies, this lesion results from a focal inflammatory response of normal hepatic parenchyma surrounded by areas of micronodular fibrosis and cirrhosis. Operative management is generally unnecessary unless there is a question of diagnosis or active hemorrhage from the lesion.

Hepatic Adenoma. Adenomas are rare in infants and children and constitute less than 5% of all benign hepatic lesions in the pediatric age group. There is an association between the use of oral contraceptives, exogenous anabolic steroid use, and glycogen storage disease type I (von Gierke disease). These tend to be large, solitary lesions located in the right hepatic lobe. The typical presentation is an asymptomatic abdominal mass, although symptoms are seen more commonly than with focal nodular hyperplasia. About 20% to 25% of patients with hepatic adenoma present with hemoperitoneum from tumor rupture. On histologic examination, these lesions are composed of normal hepatocytes without evidence of dysplasia. Operative therapy is usually directed at either making a definitive diagnosis or treating hemorrhage. Enucleation or local resection is adequate, and recurrence rates are low.

Hepatic Cysts. Congenital cysts of the liver may be either solitary or multiple. These cysts are thought to result from failure of the intralobular or interlobular biliary ducts to fuse during development. They may be lined with cuboidal, columnar, or squamous epithelium.[133] The presence of multiple hepatic cysts is associated with polycystic kidney disease, and future development of hepatic and renal failure are potential problems with this disease. The vast majority of children with hepatic cysts are asymptomatic. Adjunctive diagnostic imaging, including ultrasound and CT scan imaging, may be useful.

Asymptomatic congenital hepatic cysts do not require surgical therapy. Operative therapy is reserved for symptomatic cysts, and resection or drainage by marsupialization or hepaticocystenterostomy may be required. If patency to the biliary tract is present on contrast injection study of the cyst, internal drainage will be necessary.

The differential diagnosis includes hydatid disease of the liver, which is suggested by calcification and loculation of the cyst wall. Hydatid disease can be diagnosed using specific serologic tests, which is an important surgical consideration prior to exploration. Patients with echinococcal cysts should be treated with mebendazole and undergo cyst injection with hypertonic saline or other scolicidal agents into the parent cyst before surgical excision. Careful control of the cyst contents is required during echinococcal cyst excision or marsupialization.

Teratomas. Teratomas of the liver are exceedingly rare and have potential for harboring immature elements capable of transforming into malignancy. Surgical resection on discovery is recommended.

Malignant Tumors

Two thirds of childhood hepatic tumors are malignant, with hepatoblastoma constituting half of the malignancies, followed by hepatocellular carcinoma, malignant mesenchymal tumors, and sarcoma.[127] Malignant hepatic tumors are fortunately rare, and effective treatment requires a multidisciplinary approach that is best achieved in an experienced pediatric center.

Hepatoblastoma. Most hepatoblastomas are discovered in children younger than 2 years of age. There is a 2:1 male-to-female predominance. Hepatoblastomas usually are found as either an asymptomatic abdominal mass on examination or because of gastrointestinal obstructive symptoms from extrinsic compression by the mass. There is an association of hepatoblastoma in patients with Beckwith-Wiedemann syndrome and hemihypertrophy. On examination, a firm, palpable upper abdominal mass is notable. Obstructive jaundice is unusual. More than 90% of children with hepatoblastoma have elevated levels of alpha-fetoprotein, which is useful serum tumor marker for postoperative surveillance. In few instances, children have initial symptoms and signs of excess androgen secretion, including virilization and precocious puberty. Diagnostic imaging with CT scan imaging or MRI is essential to evaluate the extent of the tumor and evaluate for metastatic disease (Fig. 110.47). Given the increased resolution of current imaging modalities, preoperative diagnostic angiography is no longer commonly used.

Most children presenting with hepatoblastoma initially have unresectable disease. In the absence of metastatic disease, however, an aggressive surgical approach is used. Cure and long-term survival with hepatoblastoma requires complete surgical excision of the primary lesion. Therefore, localized, resectable tumors usually are excised by formal hepatic lobectomy or extended trisegmentectomy. Children with hepatoblastomas considered initially unresectable or with metastatic disease should undergo percutaneous or incisional biopsy to confirm the histologic diagnosis, followed by multiagent chemotherapy to reduce the size of the primary tumor and control metastases. Delayed resection is appropriate if enough functional, normal hepatic parenchyma remain after resection. More than half of the patients who initially have unresectable hepatoblastoma can be rendered disease-free with the combination of chemotherapy and subsequent surgery.[134] Cure rates for hepatoblastoma range from 60% to 75% if histologically clear margins and no metastatic disease are present. All patients with hepatoblastoma, regardless of stage, receive chemotherapy after resection. Unfortunately, cure cannot be expected in children treated with chemotherapy and radiation therapy alone without complete surgical resection.

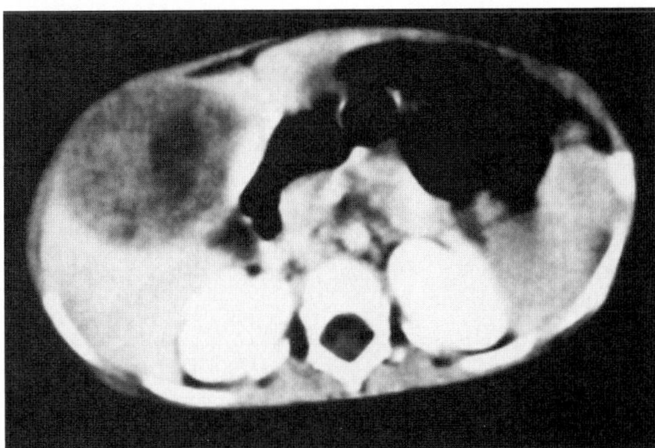

FIGURE 110.47 Computed tomography scan of the abdomen demonstrating an infant with hepatoblastoma of the right hepatic lobe.

Hepatocellular Carcinoma. Hepatocellular carcinoma is significantly more common in adults but is seen occasionally in older children and adolescents. There is a male predilection (2:1) and, except for the age at diagnosis, the clinical presentation is similar to that for hepatoblastoma. Children with hepatocellular carcinoma are more likely to have jaundice and abnormal liver enzymes. The high association of cirrhosis in adults (80%) is not seen in children with hepatocellular carcinoma; only 5% of children develop hepatocellular carcinoma in the background of cirrhosis. An increased risk of hepatocellular carcinoma is seen in children with Beckwith-Wiedemann syndrome, hemihypertrophy, von Gierke disease, hepatitis B, and Fanconi syndrome. Exposure to oral contraceptives, anabolic steroids, and some chemotherapeutic agents also has been associated with hepatocellular carcinoma. This malignancy carries a poor prognosis with an overall survival rate of 10% to 20% despite aggressive surgical resection and multiagent chemotherapy. A histologic variant, fibrolamellar hepatocellular carcinoma, carries a more favorable prognosis. As with hepatoblastoma, complete surgical resection with clear histologic margins is necessary for long-term survival and cure.

Malignant Mesenchymal Tumors. These rare hepatic malignancies occur in children 5 to 10 years of age; initial signs are fever, pain, and an abdominal mass, which is usually quite large on diagnosis and may have both solid and cystic components. Multidisciplinary treatment, including complete surgical resection, multiagent chemotherapy, and radiation therapy is required for cure. In general, the prognosis of primary malignant mesenchymal tumors of the liver remains poor.

Sarcomas. Children may rarely have a primary sarcoma of the liver. Embryonal rhabdomyosarcoma of the biliary tract is distinctly unusual. It may manifest with obstructive jaundice attributable to both extrinsic and intrinsic biliary tract obstruction. Undifferentiated, embryonal sarcoma of the liver is also seen. Angiosarcoma developing in the liver may be associated with exposure to toxins such as arsenic. Aggressive surgical resection may be required, but long-term survival is uncommon. Despite radical surgery, chemotherapy, and radiation therapy, the prognosis and long-term survival of children with these malignancies remains poor, and data regarding effective drug regimens are limited.[135]

Liver Resection

Operative principles and techniques for hepatic resection are discussed elsewhere in this book. Several unique issues in the safe performance of hepatic resection in children should be emphasized.[136] Contemporary management of hepatic resection for tumors in children requires adequate preoperative assessment and the liberal use of intraoperative monitoring techniques.

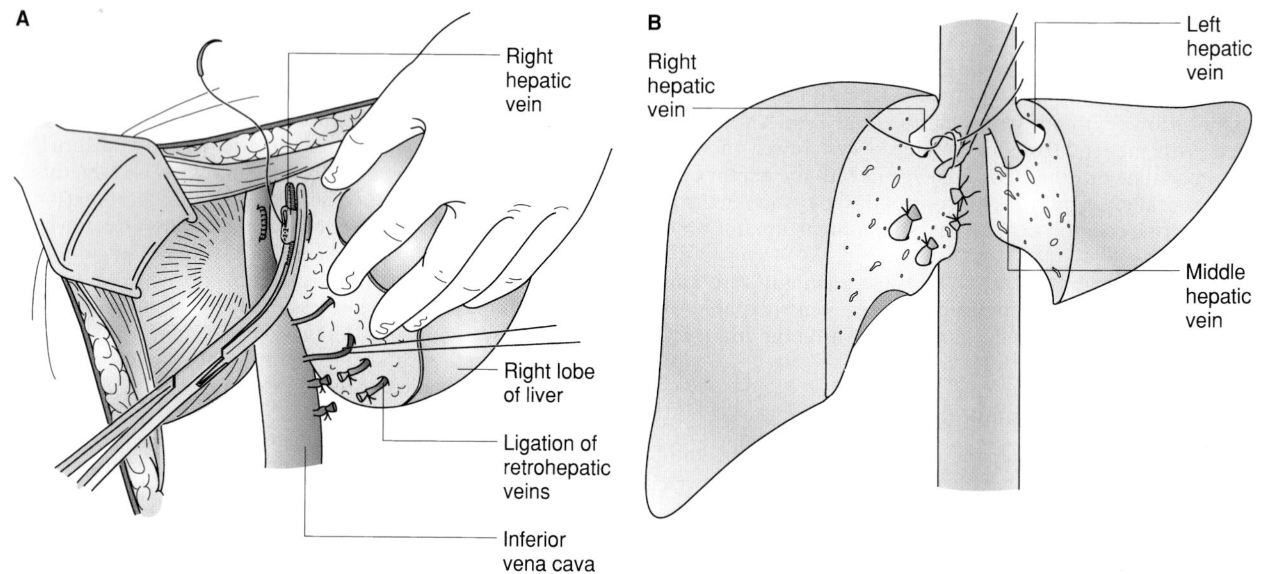

FIGURE 110.48 (*A*) The hepatic veins in infants and children may be extremely short, making extrahepatic control impossible or dangerous. (*B*) Intrahepatic control of the hepatic veins via an anterior approach may be safer in infants and children.

The circulating blood volume of an infant or child is small compared with that of an adult, and children are sensitive to compression of the inferior vena cava causing decreased right heart venous return. Blood must be available for transfusion. Resection can be performed through either a subcostal or a right thoracoabdominal incision; in general, the ability to perform the operation safely should not be limited by the size of the incision. In children, the right and left hepatic veins are difficult to control near the inferior vena cava because of their short lengths, and intraparenchymal control from an anterior approach may be safer (Fig. 110.48). Resection may be performed using total hepatic vascular isolation by controlling the hepatic and portal inflow, the suprahepatic inferior vena cava, and the suprarenal inferior vena cava caudal to the liver. This may help to reduce blood loss during parenchymal dissection, but adequate upper-extremity and central venous access must be maintained to provide adequate intravascular volume expansion, right heart filling and cardiac output. When extrahepatic biliary duct reconstruction is required, T-tube drainage is not routinely performed given the small diameter of the ducts in most children.

Hepatic Infections

Hepatic infections are generally rare in the pediatric population, and their management is similar to that used in adults. An important issue is the development of hepatic abscess in an immunocompromised child, and in particular, the association of chronic granulomatous disease with pyogenic hepatic abscess formation.

Pyogenic Abscess

The most common cause of pyogenic liver abscess before the advent of antibiotic therapy was perforated appendicitis. Now the most common causative factor in the development of pyogenic hepatic abscess in children is chronic granulomatous disease and other causes of immunosuppression.[137] Chronic granulomatous disease is an inherited disorder characterized by a defect in oxidative burst-mediated bacterial killing by neutrophils. These children develop abscesses in skin and soft-tissue structures as well as in the solid organs. About 40% of children with pyogenic liver abscesses have chronic granulomatous disease. Another third of these children are immunosuppressed either as a primary or acquired immunodeficiency. Liver abscesses are infrequently seen as a complication of umbilical vein catheterization, omphalitis, biliary tract disease, and hepatobiliary operations.

Patients with pyogenic liver abscesses present with fever, jaundice, and leukocytosis. Hepatosplenomegaly and a tender liver may be found on physical examination. Diagnostic imaging with ultrasound, CT scan imaging, or MRI is useful. Common responsible organisms include staphylococcal species, streptococcal species, and *E. coli*. Gram-negative organisms and anaerobic bacteria are becoming increasingly prevalent. Treatment involves the use of broad-spectrum antibiotics. Large abscess cavities may require image-guided percutaneous drainage to expedite resolution of sepsis. Currently, few hepatic abscesses require open operative drainage. The outcome is dependent upon the disease process giving rise to the hepatic abscess. Recovery from the abscess is predictably good following adequate antibiotic therapy and drainage when indicated.

Amebic Abscess

Amebic abscess of the liver is uncommon in the United States, but it is endemic to areas of Central and South America. It is caused by infection with the parasite *Entamoeba histolytica*. Children with amebic dysentery develop hepatic infection as the parasite travels through the portal circulation. Patients have a history of chronic illness, fever, and abdominal pain. Examination typically demonstrates a tender right upper quadrant. Infection can be confirmed by a serum antibody test, and amebic abscess can be demonstrated by ultrasound or CT scan. Spontaneous rupture of amebic abscess is reported in as many as 10% of patients in some series.[138] The treatment of choice is the antibiotic metronidazole. Surgical resection or drainage of amebic abscess of the liver is typically not required for resolution.

PEDIATRIC BILIARY TRACT

Common biliary tract problems including infectious, inflammatory, and gallstone-related problems are managed similarly in both children and adults, and the management principles are discussed elsewhere in this text. Two congenital problems of the biliary tract, namely, biliary atresia and congenital cystic disease of the biliary tract (choledochal cyst), are somewhat unique to infants and children in presentation and management and are reviewed in the following discussion.

Embryology

The fetal liver and biliary tract develop between weeks 4 and 10 of gestation, representing the fusion of an endodermal foregut diverticulum with a mesodermal component from the septum transversum.[30] The hepatocytes are derived from cords of endodermal cells in the hepatic diverticulum and ultimately give rise to the hepatic sinusoidal endothelium. The proximal hepatic diverticulum gives rise to the extrahepatic biliary tract, including the gallbladder, cystic duct, and common bile duct. As the intrahepatic and extrahepatic ductal systems develop, they unite to form a connected, arborizing system of cords composed of primitive ductular epithelial cells. These epithelial cells assume tubular configuration with ductal patency established between weeks 6 and 12 of gestation. Bile flow from the hepatocytes and into the biliary duct system is apparent by the beginning of the second fetal trimester.

This embryologic sequence appears to take place normally in infants who develop biliary atresia. In fact, the term *biliary atresia* does not reflect embryologic atresia resulting from failure of recanalization of the biliary tree. Rather, biliary atresia is believed to be caused by a sclerosing, inflammatory process that produces progressive obliteration of the normally developed extrahepatic biliary tract.

Biliary Atresia

Anatomy

The overall incidence rate of biliary atresia is about 1 in 8,000 to 12,000 live births and is the most common cause of chronic cholestasis in infants and children as well as the most frequent indication for pediatric liver transplantation.[139] Extrahepatic biliary atresia must be differentiated from biliary hypoplasia. Biliary hypoplasia describes a diminutive but patent biliary system and can result from many underlying situations such as neonatal hepatitis and alpha$_1$-antitrypsin deficiency. Biliary hypoplasia involves both intrahepatic and extrahepatic ductal systems. Because of this diffuse defect, procedures designed to improve extrahepatic biliary drainage alone, such as portoenterostomy, are not useful with biliary hypoplasia.

Microscopic Anatomy. Biliary atresia is characterized by replacement of the extrahepatic biliary tract with dense, fibrous inflammatory tissue. In most cases, complete obliteration of the extrahepatic biliary tract, including the gallbladder, occurs. There appears to be gradual progression of the inflammatory process with advancing age. The common hepatic duct and common bile duct are almost uniformly obliterated by the inflammatory process. Few or absent patent ductal remnants and an absence of portal inflammation may be associated with a less favorable prognosis.[140] Intraoperative evaluation for duct patency by frozen section analysis has historically been used help guide the extent of proximal resection at the porta hepatis (Fig. 110.49), however, this is no longer in widespread use. The presence of bile ducts at the porta hepatis with diameter greater than 150 (μm has been reported to be associated with postoperative bile flow in up to 90% to 95% of cases.[141] Histologic features of biliary atresia reflect hepatic parenchymal injury. Neocholangiogenesis, or biliary duct proliferation of disorganized and nonpatent ducts within the liver, is considered highly suggestive but not specific for biliary atresia (Fig. 110.50). Other findings include bile pigment deposition throughout the liver. Multinucleated giant cell formation and periductal inflammation are commonly seen but also may be present in neonatal hepatitis. These features within the liver appear to be age related but may be highly variable. Characteristic early findings in biliary atresia include evidence for acute inflammation with neutrophil predominance in the periportal regions. Older infants and children typically have chronic inflammatory changes with considerable fibrosis. Periportal bridging fibrosis is commonly seen in intermediate stages of the disease. Ultimately, progressive biliary atresia leads to intractable cirrhosis. Nearly all patients with biliary atresia have histologic evidence of liver injury. The severity and extent of liver damage may be the most important predictors of long-term outcome and survival in biliary atresia.

Pathophysiology

Despite numerous investigations, the exact pathogenic mechanism causing biliary atresia remains unknown. The current, widely accepted concept is that the normally developed biliary tract undergoes inflammatory sclerosis and subsequent obliteration. This process appears to occur over a course of months during the newborn period. Infants who develop biliary atresia are rarely jaundiced at birth, and biliary atresia is either rare or nonexistent in fetal autopsy studies. Clinical data are consistent with the fact that biliary atresia appears to be a progressive, dynamic inflammatory response that is acquired during the perinatal period and targets the extrahepatic biliary tract. Early establishment of biliary drainage via portoenterostomy within the first 2 to 4 months of age may be associated with reversal of liver injury and subsequent long-term survival. Conversely, infants operated on after 120 days of life typically have obliterated bile ducts. Neonatal biliary atresia shares some clinical and morphologic features of sclerosing cholangitis in adults. Data supporting an infectious etiologic agent, and in particular reoviruses, rotaviruses, and hepatitis C, have been reported and may play a role in some cases. Previous interest in reovirus 3 as an etiologic agent has waned because of the inability to find evidence for its presence by using reverse transcriptase-mediated polymerase chain reaction analysis.[142,143] Additionally, other noninfectious stimuli may trigger an inflammatory response directed at the neonatal extrahepatic bile duct.[144] The actual mechanism(s) may reflect a stereotypical inflammatory response that is initiated by a variety of different stimuli and directed preferentially against the neonatal bile duct. An inflammatory response directed against the biliary tract may explain the progression of intrahepatic biliary tract injury and liver disease observed in many patients with biliary atresia, despite apparently successful portoenterostomy.

Clinical Presentation and Diagnosis

The cardinal sign of biliary atresia is progressive neonatal jaundice with an onset during the first few weeks of life. Dark urine and acholic stools are expected findings. Infants are discovered as progressive hyperbilirubinemia produces clinical jaundice around 2 to 4 weeks of age. The physical examination is generally unremarkable except for jaundice and possibly mild hepatomegaly. Alagille syndrome, which presents with neonatal jaundice, can usually be distinguished from biliary atresia on physical examination. Children with Alagille syndrome have biliary hypoplasia and commonly abnormal facies, growth retardation, vertebral defects, and pulmonic stenosis.

A characteristic laboratory finding is conjugated hyperbilirubinemia consistent with obstructive jaundice. Generally, a direct fraction of bilirubin greater than 50%, or greater than 2 mg/dL, requires investigation. Mild elevation of hepatic transaminases are commonly seen. The alkaline phosphatase

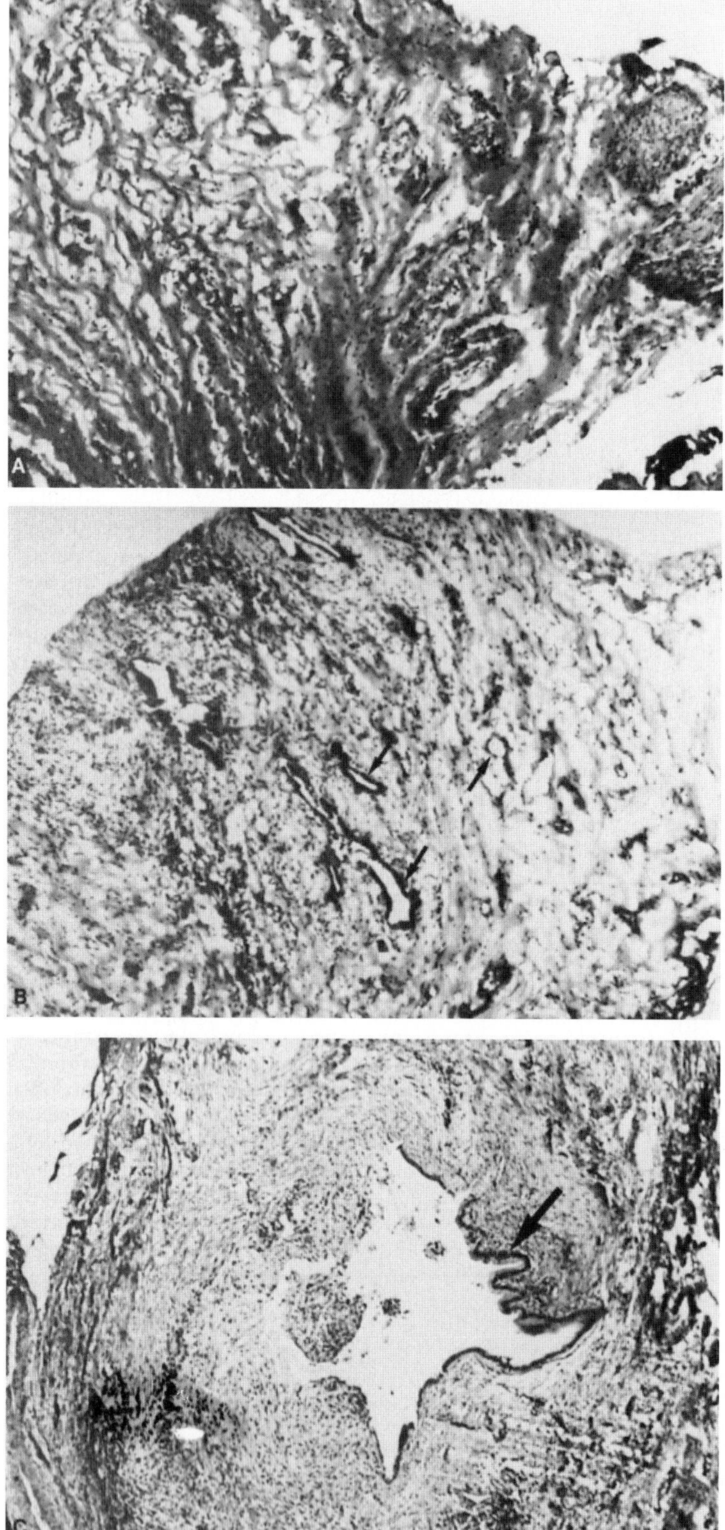

FIGURE 110.49 Frozen sections of the fibrous biliary tract remnant at the proximal point of transection. (*A*) Complete absence of patent bile ducts with fibrous obliteration of the extrahepatic biliary tract. (*B*) Several patent but small ducts (*arrows*). (*C*) Larger duct with periductal inflammatory response and fibrosis with loss of normal biliary epithelium (*arrow*). (Courtesy of K. Heidelberger, M.D., University of Michigan, Ann Arbor.)

is significantly elevated, often in the range of 500 to 1,000 IU/L. There are no specific biochemical markers for biliary atresia, as these serum profiles can be seen in other causes of neonatal cholestasis. Late findings in biliary atresia include failure to thrive, feeding intolerance, stigmata of portal hypertension, and fat-soluble vitamin deficiency.

Table 110.12 is a partial list of the causes of neonatal cholestatic syndromes. Neonatal physiologic jaundice is commonly encountered. This condition is self-limited once the glucuronyl transferase system matures, allowing the hepatocytes to conjugate bilirubin efficiently. Because of the numerous causes of neonatal jaundice and the relative infrequency of biliary atresia, a delay in diagnosis is not unusual. The jaundiced neonate is subject to a number of diagnostic tests with longitudinal follow-up, and frequently the delay in diagnosis of biliary atresia can be 1 to 2 weeks in duration. Given the age-sensitive nature

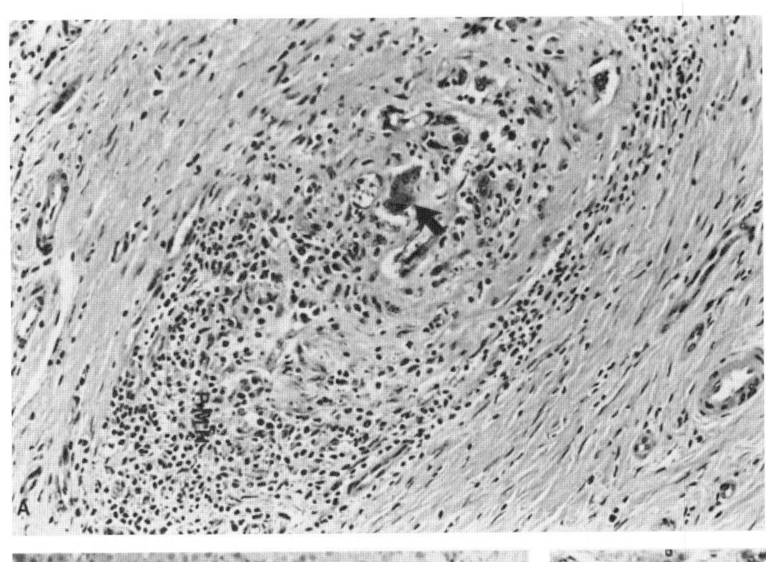

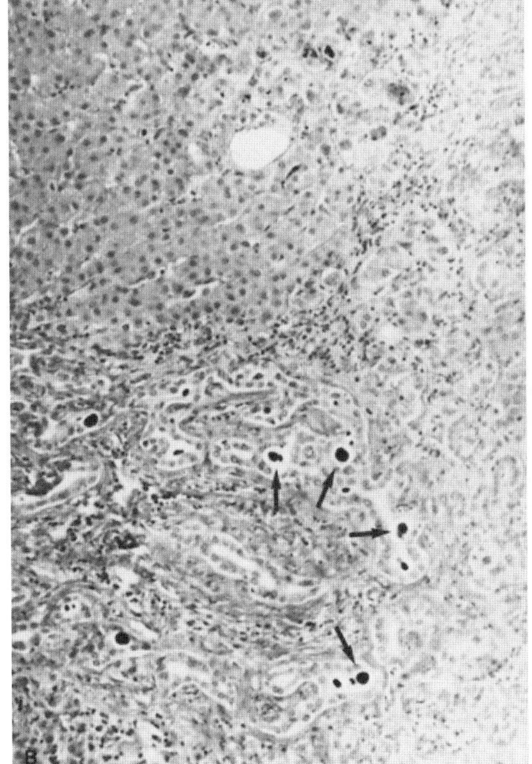

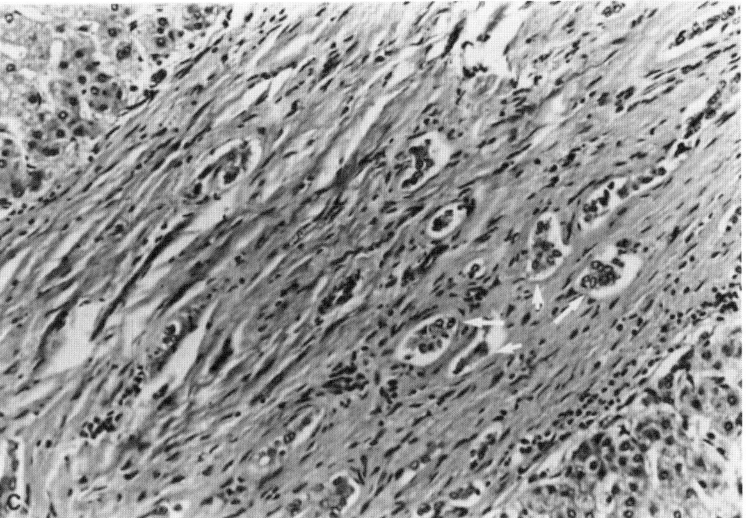

FIGURE 110.50 Liver morphology of patients with biliary atresia shows evidence of neocholangiogenesis, or bile duct proliferation, and bile plugs. The degree of inflammation and cirrhosis varies greatly. (*A*) Liver histology at an early stage characterized by acute periportal neutrophil infiltration and giant cell formation (*arrow*). (*B*) Classic bile plug formation (*arrow*). Liver histology from an older child with biliary atresia and cirrhosis. There is almost complete replacement of normal hepatocytes with fibrosis and prominent bile duct proliferation (*arrows*).

of biliary atresia and the improved outcome in younger infants, the diagnostic work-up should be expedient.

Radioisotope Scanning. Pertechnetate 99m–iminodiacetic acid (^{99m}Tc-IDA) analogues are widely used for hepatobiliary imaging and provide the basis for a sensitive and specific test for biliary atresia. The sensitivity of this diagnostic examination for biliary atresia can be 100% with a specificity of 94%.[139] To improve sensitivity, infants are administered a 2- to 7-day course of oral phenobarbital (5 mg/kg daily) to induce hepatic microsomal enzymes and increase hepatocyte processing of ^{99m}Tc-IDA. Both hepatic uptake of radionuclide and excretion into the gastrointestinal tract are evaluated over a timed interval. Infants with primary hepatocellular disorders characteristically have impaired hepatocyte uptake of radionuclide, whereas normal infants and infants with biliary atresia have prompt uptake. Normal infants excrete the isotope rapidly into the gut through the biliary tract. In biliary atresia, there is no excretion into the gut because of the obliteration of the extrahepatic bile ducts (Fig. 110.51). The hepatobiliary scan is a rapid test that can be performed simultaneously with other diagnostic examinations, for example, ultrasound. This test reliably identifies infants with choledochal cyst as well.

Other Diagnostic Tests. Several other diagnostic tests are of interest in the work-up of an infant with conjugated hyperbilirubinemia in whom obstructive jaundice is suspected. The important management principle is that prompt operative exploration, liver biopsy, and cholangiogram should be performed in any infant in whom biliary atresia is suspected. An aggressive approach is warranted in that unnecessary delay in definitive drainage may lead to a less favorable outcome.

Ultrasound. A standard examination of the jaundiced infant is a comprehensive abdominal ultrasound, with particular

TABLE 110.12 ETIOLOGY

CAUSES AND ASSOCIATIONS OF NEONATAL CHOLESTASIS

CONGENITAL INFECTIOUS CAUSES
Cytomegalovirus[a]
Rubella virus[a]
Herpes virus
Hepatitis virus B[a]
Echovirus 14, 19
Coxsackievirus B
Toxoplasmosis
Syphilis

GENETIC ASSOCIATIONS
Galactosemia
Tyrosinemia
Congenital fructose intolerance
alpha$_1$-Antitrypsin deficiency
Cystic fibrosis
Niemann-Pick disease
Trisomy 17, 18, 21
Turner syndrome
Menkes syndrome
Zellweger syndrome
Polysplenia syndrome[b]

MISCELLANEOUS ASSOCIATIONS
Hemolytic disease
Bacterial sepsis
Pyelonephritis
Total parenteral nutrition (prolonged)
Congestive heart failure
Hypoplastic left heart syndrome
Necrotizing enterocolitis, gastroschisis, omphalocele
Neonatal hypopituitarism
Inspissated bile syndrome (without hemolysis) neonatal shock, respiratory distress syndrome, acidosis

[a]Rarely associated with biliary atresia.
[b]Frequently associated with biliary atresia.

attention given to the liver and biliary tract. The most common ultrasonographic finding in biliary atresia is a diminutive or absent gallbladder without associated intrahepatic duct dilatation. Biliary tract obstruction from a choledochal cyst also can be reliably identified by ultrasound. Other rare causes of extrahepatic biliary duct obstruction are associated with proximal duct dilatation.

Liver Biopsy. Because the histologic findings in biliary atresia are not specific, about 20% to 25% of infants who undergo percutaneous liver biopsy remain undiagnosed. Liver biopsy is often performed in conjunction with the work-up of conjugated hyperbilirubinemia following hepatobiliary scanning and ultrasonography, but in the setting of biliary atresia, it has limited utility. The histologic examination of a percutaneous liver biopsy is probably most helpful in diagnosing nonoperative causes of neonatal jaundice, thus avoiding anesthesia and operative exploration.

Alpha1-Antitrypsin Deficiency. Alpha$_1$-antitrypsin deficiency is perhaps the single most important medical condition that may be difficult or impossible to differentiate from biliary atresia. All jaundiced infants should have plasma alpha$_1$-antitrypsin levels determined before operative exploration for suspected biliary atresia. Infants with alpha$_1$-antitrypsin deficiency do not benefit from operative exploration or portoenterostomy.

Treatment

It is well accepted that infants with biliary atresia require surgical therapy as the initial management intervention. Medical therapy is directed to the postoperative management of the chronic liver disease. The role of portoenterostomy versus orthotopic liver transplantation for biliary atresia are more complementary than competitive. In general, the use of sequential surgical treatment, using portoenterostomy in infancy and orthotopic liver transplantation for children with progressive hepatic failure, provides improvement in overall survival.[145,146] Limited organ availability and a higher rate of perioperative complications limit primary liver transplantation for biliary atresia in infants younger than 1 year. In the rare instance of unrecognized biliary atresia in an older child with established hepatic dysfunction, primary orthotopic liver transplantation may be a reasonable option.

Portoenterostomy. The recommended initial procedure for the treatment of biliary atresia is portoenterostomy. Before the development of portoenterostomy in Japan during the late 1950s, all infants with biliary atresia died of chronic liver disease and cirrhosis. Current management dictates that operative exploration and portoenterostomy be performed promptly in the management of biliary atresia. Early intervention by portoenterostomy to provide biliary drainage has been

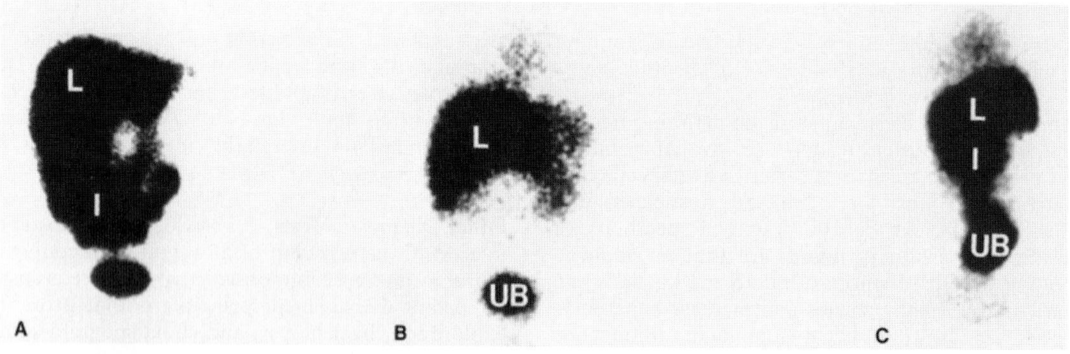

FIGURE 110.51 (*A*) Normal scan using p-isopropylacetanilidoiminodiacetic acid (PIPIDA) as the hepatobiliary scanning agent. At 45 minutes, isotope is clearly visible in the liver (L) and intestine (I). (*B*) Scan after phenobarbital administration in infant with biliary atresia. Even after 8 hours, isotope is apparent only in the liver and urinary bladder (UB). (C) Patient with cholestatic jaundice. At 65 minutes, isotope is visible in the liver (L) and intestine (I). Hepatocyte uptake is variable but usually decreased or normal, whereas excretion into the gut is predictably present with cholestatic jaundice or hepatocellular disease.

proposed to arrest or reverse the parenchymal liver injury, but the point at which the liver injury becomes irreversible remains unknown. From a clinical standpoint, most long-term success with portoenterostomy alone appears to be achieved in infants younger than 2 to 3 months, whereas infants older than 3 to 4 months appear to have a less favorable prognosis. Portoenterostomy for this "late" group has been reported successful in approximately one third of infants, however, and should be considered a potential alternative in the absence of available liver transplant donors.[147]

The initial approach to the infant with suspected biliary atresia is to perform an operative cholangiogram. If the diagnosis is confirmed, a portoenterostomy is constructed (Fig. 110.52). To maximize the potential for effective biliary drainage with portoenterostomy, several technical caveats are worthy of mention. An open liver biopsy is routinely performed to document the state of parenchymal injury. The cholangiogram is generally attempted through the gallbladder. In the 10% to 15% instance of a patent distal biliary tree, treatment still requires portoenterostomy. A nonpatent, fibrous cord rather than a normal common bile duct is found in the hepatoduodenal ligament. This cord is dissected free proximally to the level of the porta hepatis between the portal vein bifurcation. The fibrous remnant is sharply transected at this level to preserve any patent bile ducts. A short, 15- to 25-cm retrocolic, jejunal Roux-Y limb is constructed. There has been no clear advantage with longer or modified conduits with intussusception-type antireflux valves in the prevention of cholangitis.[148,149]

Some surgeons prefer to exteriorize the biliary conduit (Fig. 110.53). With an exteriorized biliary conduit, postoperative bile flow is directly visible. The diverting stoma must be closed, however, and there is potential to develop parastomal variceal hemorrhage from progressive portal hypertension. Additionally, fluid and electrolyte losses from the biliostomy can be significant, and there are no reported survival differences between patients with exteriorized and closed biliary conduits following portoenterostomy. Because many of these infants may ultimately require liver transplantation, there is a trend toward using a simple, closed biliary conduit with portoenterostomy.

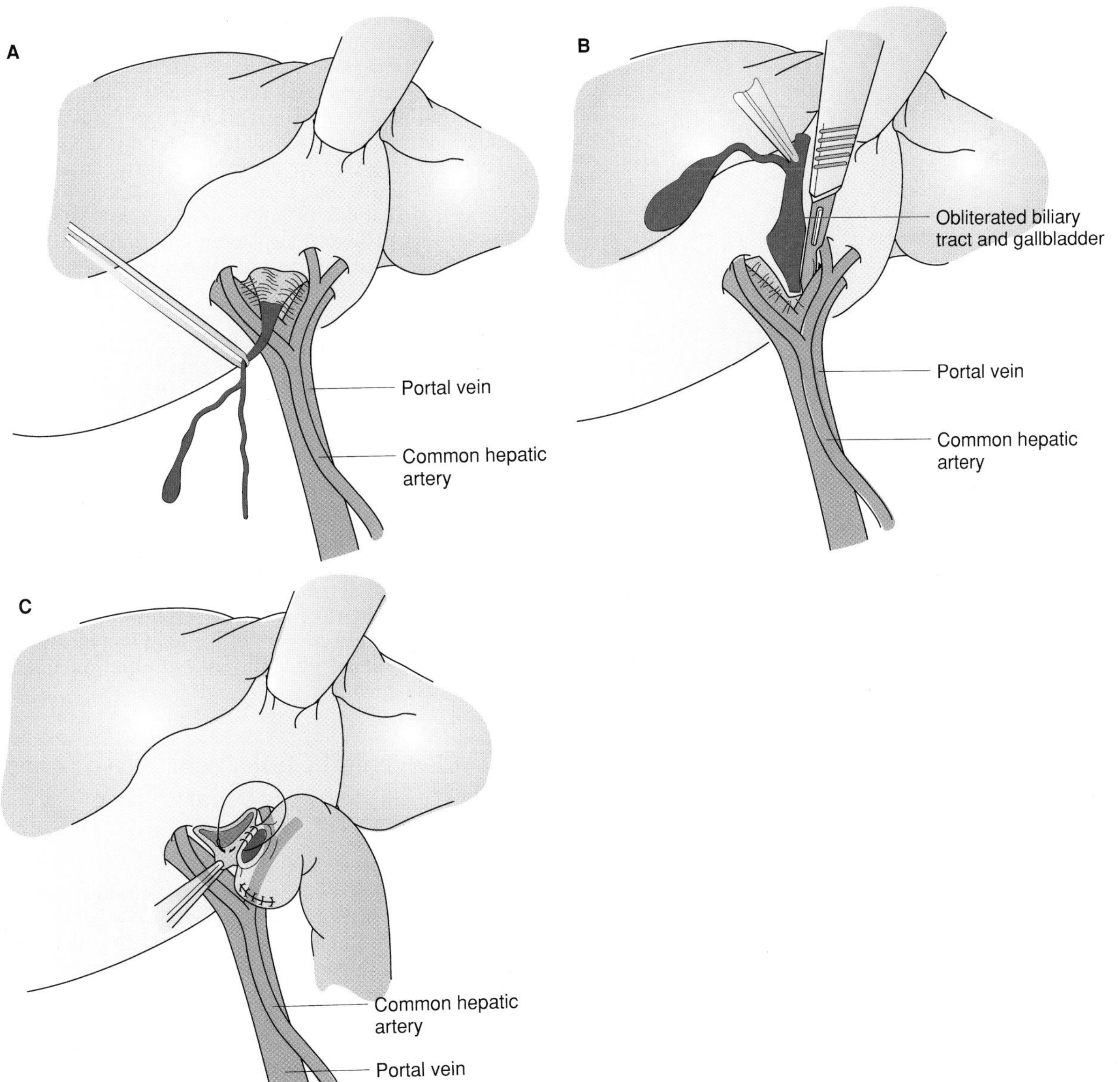

FIGURE 110.52 The essential features of the portoenterostomy for biliary atresia include appropriate mobilization (*A*) and transection (*B*) of the fibrous biliary tract remnant. (*C*) Creation of a Roux-Y jejunal conduit with biliary enteric anastomosis completes the procedure.

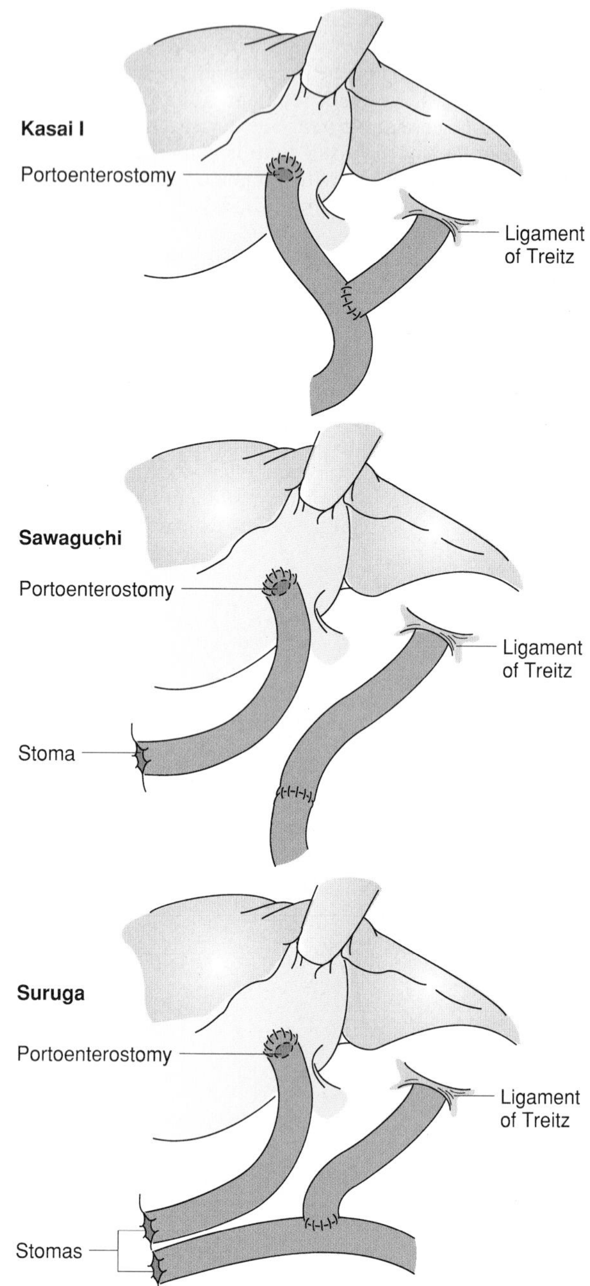

FIGURE 110.53 Several types of conduits have been used for biliary drainage following portoenterostomy. There are relatively few data to help in selecting from among them, and current trends emphasize simplicity. These are the three most commonly used conduits. The primary importance of this issue is that the reoperative surgeon must be familiar with the anatomic variations.

Therefore, the use of a stoma to divert the bile flow in the Roux limb has been largely abandoned.

Results and Complications. Following portoenterostomy, bile flow occurs in about 66% to 75% of all infants when operated on at less than 60 days of age; however, establishment of bile flow may take weeks to months. The probability of bile flow appears related to age at the time of operation. Bile flow appears less likely to occur in infants older than 120 days of age,[150] although some infants may still benefit from portoenterostomy as previously mentioned.

Cholangitis is a constant concern and an important postoperative problem after portoenterostomy. The clinical signs include fever, leukocytosis, and decreased bile flow in the absence of other systemic illness. All patients are at risk for the development of postoperative cholangitis, but reported postoperative rates of cholangitis are as low as 40% to 50%. Cholangitis following portoenterostomy is characterized by a systemic inflammatory response and may be associated with progressive liver injury. Treatment is generally intravenous fluid resuscitation and broad-spectrum antibiotics. Occasionally, steroids or other antiinflammatory agents may be helpful, whereas reoperation or endoscopic revision of the portoenterostomy usually is not.[151] In an effort to determine the optimal treatment of infants with biliary atresia, a group of investigators have recently formed the Biliary Atresia Research Consortium.[152] The primary objectives of the consortium are to establish a clinical database and establish a blood and tissue repository. Studies examining the role and efficacy of postoperative prophylactic antibiotics and steroids in preventing progressive liver disease in biliary atresia are being prospectively addressed by the consortium.

Nearly all patients with biliary atresia have residual liver injury. Hepatic synthetic failure, portal hypertension with esophageal variceal bleeding, hypersplenism, and fat-soluble vitamin deficiencies can be problematic. Most institutions report 5-year survival rates between 30% and 50% for portoenterostomy alone. About 25% to 35% of patients undergoing a portoenterostomy survive more than 10 years without liver transplantation. The remaining two thirds of children with biliary atresia ultimately require liver transplantation for survival. Although the failure rate for portoenterostomy is high, the possibility of long-term success is notable. Additionally, the limited availability of infant donor organs and the technical limitations of liver transplantation in infants younger than 1 year of age make portoenterostomy an accepted initial treatment of biliary atresia in most centers.

Hepatic Transplantation. Hepatic transplantation is discussed in detail elsewhere in this text. For biliary atresia, transplantation offers a means of long-term survival in children with failed portoenterostomies. The current 5-year survival of children with biliary atresia who undergo liver transplantation ranges from 75% to 82%.[146,153,154] Additionally, with the use of reduced-size cadaveric donor livers as well as living-related donor livers, the mortality rate for infants on transplant waiting lists may be decreasing. Indications for liver transplantation in biliary atresia include progressive hepatic failure despite portoenterostomy, growth retardation, and complications of portal hypertension. It is important to consider the consequences of life-long immunosuppression in these children, including the risks of infection and treatment-related malignancy.

Congenital Choledochal Cystic Disease of the Biliary Tract

Anatomy

The anatomic description and classification scheme for choledochal cystic disease initially proposed by Alonso-Lej et al. in 1959 and modified by Todani et al. are illustrated in Fig. 110.54.[155,156] The most frequently encountered are type I cysts, accounting for approximately 85% to 90% of the lesions in most series. Type I cysts typically are characterized by fusiform dilatation of the entire common bile duct with only mild dilatation of the common hepatic duct; the intrahepatic ducts are normal. Type II cysts represent true diverticula of the common bile duct. These lesions are rare and account for only 1% to 2% of all cases. Type III cysts are also uncommon and sometimes are referred to as *choledochoceles.* Type III cysts constitute fewer than 2% of the observed lesions

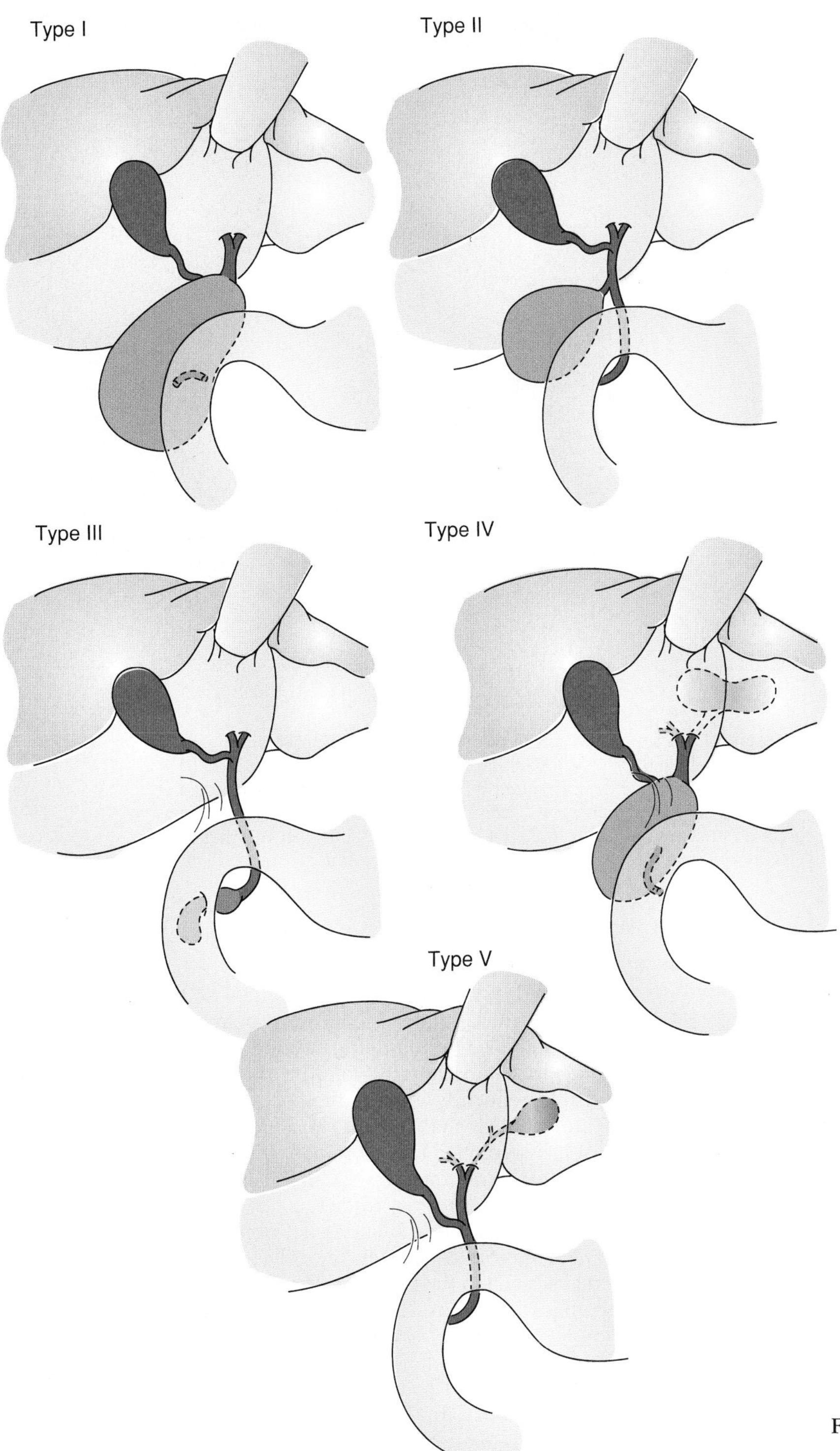

FIGURE 110.54 Classification of choledochal cyst.

and are defined as local dilatation of the distal, intramural portion of the common bile duct. Type IV cystic disease is characterized by the presence of multiple cysts typically involving both intrahepatic and extraheptic ducts. Type IV cysts are observed with an incidence of 15% in some series. Type V disease is rare and represents cystic malformation of the intrahepatic ducts. Variations are common, and biliary atresia is occasionally seen in association with choledochal cystic disease.

Type I cysts are generally quite large and often cause displacement of neighboring viscera. The fusiform dilatation usually begins at the origin of the common bile duct, generally sparing the common hepatic ducts. The distal common bile duct is diminutive and typically is distorted mechanically by the large cyst, leading to the common clinical presentation of obstructive jaundice. The junction of the distal common bile duct and the pancreatic duct is not within the normal intramural duodenum but rather is extrinsic and proximal to the duodenal wall and the sphincter of Oddi (Fig. 110.55). It remains unknown whether the configuration of a long, extramural common channel allows greater pancreatic secretion reflux into the common bile duct.

Microscopic examination of the choledochal cyst wall reveals that the normal biliary epithelium is either absent or replaced by abnormal and occasionally dysplastic columnar

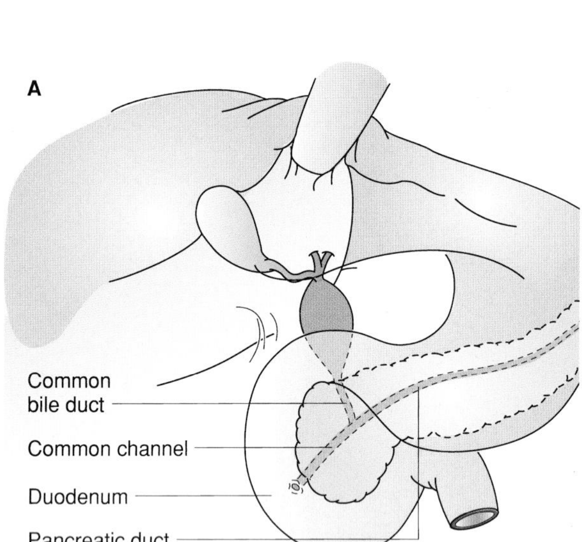

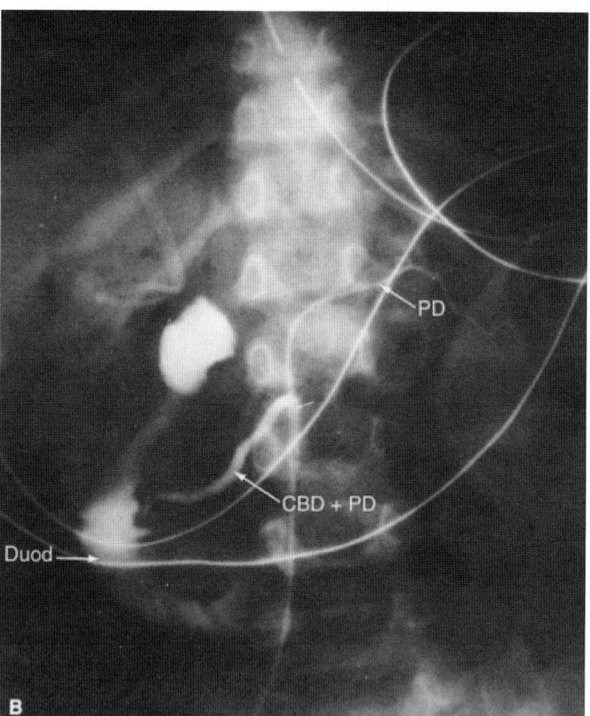

FIGURE 110.55 An anomalous, extramural junction between the distal common bile duct and the pancreatic duct is characteristic of type I choledochal cyst. (*A*) Schematic depiction of this anatomy. (*B*) Operative cholangiogram from a patient with a long extramural common channel. It has been suggested that the long common channel may allow reflux of pancreatic secretions into the common bile duct resulting in inflammation and proteinase-mediated injury to the common duct, possibly contributing to the development of the cyst itself. Duod, duodenum; CBD + PD, common bile duct and pancreatic duct; PD, pancreatic duct.

epithelium. The cyst wall has normal smooth muscle with variable degrees of inflammation and fibrosis. The exception to this common histologic characteristic is the type III cyst. The choledochocele is generally lined by normal duodenal mucosa. Choledochal cysts tend to have less inflammation in infancy and early childhood. In contrast, there is generally well-established inflammation involving the cyst and surrounding structures in the hepatoduodenal ligament in adolescents and adults. From a surgical standpoint, extensive inflammation in and around the choledochal cyst can produce significant technical and management issues as discussed later in this chapter.

Pathophysiology

The pathophysiologic mechanism for the development of cystic lesions of the biliary tract is unclear. Choledochal cysts have been identified accurately by prenatal ultrasound, and it appears likely that these lesions represent abnormalities in the developing biliary tract. Several hypotheses for the development of choledochal cyst have been proposed. Whether the cystic dilatations result from abnormal recanalization of the primitive bile duct cords or from inflammation caused by reflux of pancreatic secretions into the common bile duct remains unknown. The pathophysiology of choledochal cyst is that of obstructive jaundice. The obstruction may be primarily the result of mechanical outflow obstruction of a diminutive distal common bile duct with a large, dilated choledochal cyst. Alternatively, a large inflammatory cyst can cause obstruction of the biliary tract and of neighboring viscera by extrinsic compression. When discovered during infancy, obstructive jaundice is usually the initial clinical finding. The liver injury is typically reversible, and progression to biliary cirrhosis is rare. The exception to this situation is type V disease, which is associated with a high incidence of hepatic fibrosis.

Other initial clinical situations include cholelithiasis and acute bacterial cholangitis secondary to diminished bile drainage. Children with type III cysts may have acute pancreatitis. Infrequently, extrinsic compression of the portal vein by a large choledochal cyst may produce symptoms and signs of portal hypertension. Abdominal pain and tenderness following minor injury may lead to an incidental diagnosis of choledochal cyst on imaging studies.

Carcinoma of the biliary tract occurs in about 3% to 5% of patients with choledochal cyst. The number of reported cases remains small in the literature, but the incidence for biliary tract neoplasm is about 1,000 times that of the normal population.[157,158] Patients with choledochal cyst are at increased risk for the development of biliary tract carcinoma in adolescence or early adulthood. The dysplastic cyst epithelium may be susceptible to malignant change from chronic inflammation. Interestingly, there appears to be an increased risk of malignancy to develop anywhere in the biliary tract, gallbladder, or pancreas, and not just the choledochal cyst itself.[159] Therefore, current treatment emphasis is on complete cyst excision or the cyst epithelium while providing adequate biliary drainage to prevent stasis and chronic inflammation. Infants and children treated for choledochal cyst should have long-term follow-up for complications and potential malignancy.

Clinical Presentation and Diagnosis

Choledochal cysts are encountered infrequently, but they are important lesions when evaluated and treated in pediatric tertiary care centers. Presentation is now most common in infancy and early childhood. The characteristic presentation

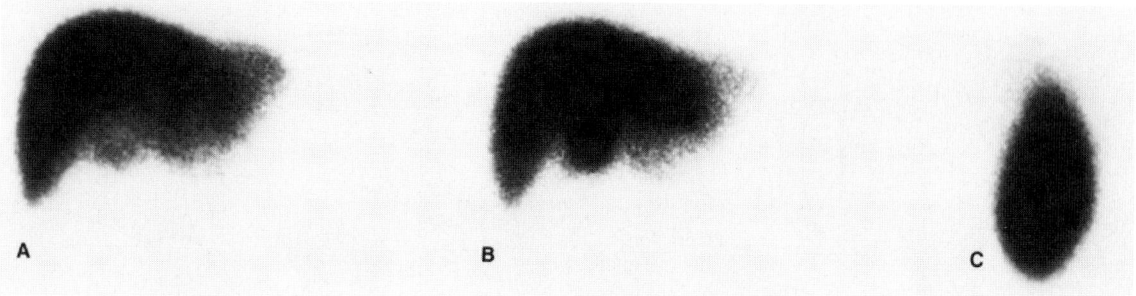

FIGURE 110.56 Typical ^{99M}Tc-N-substituted-2,6-dimethylphenyl carbamoylethyl iminodiacetic acid (HIDA) scan from a child with a type I choledochal cyst. Images were made in 5 minutes (*A*), 30 minutes (*B*), and 3 hours (*C*), after isotope injection. The isotope is retained within the choledochal cyst more than 24 hours, and the pattern of hepatocyte uptake is normal.

of choledochal cyst in the neonate is obstructive jaundice. In older children and adults, the classic clinical triad of episodic abdominal pain, a palpable right upper-quadrant mass, and jaundice occurs in fewer than 50% of patients. Adults occasionally present with hepatomegaly or evidence of portal hypertension. The diagnosis in infants and most children can be confirmed by ultrasound examination and ^{99m}Tc-IDA imaging studies (Figs. 110.56 and 110.57). In older children, endoscopic retrograde cholangiopancreatography (ERCP) is highly sensitive and specific in confirming diagnosis. These lesions also are diagnosed incidentally during radiologic imaging studies for other reasons. Partial duodenal obstruction may lead to an upper gastrointestinal series that may show extrinsic compression from a large type I cyst or an intraluminal filling defect from a type III cyst. CT imaging of the abdomen following blunt trauma may lead to the diagnosis of biliary tract dilatation. Liver biopsy is not specific in choledochal cyst and has little diagnostic role other than to document the extent of liver injury.

Treatment

Type I Cysts. Definitive management of choledochal cyst is operative, and the operation must be tailored to the specific anatomic defect. The initial operative strategy for a type I choledochal cyst is exploration and cholangiography, usually through the gallbladder, but occasionally contrast injection must be made directly into the common bile duct. Cholecystectomy is routinely performed. Historically, internal drainage procedures without cyst excision were widely used. These procedures have been associated with a higher rate of failure because of stricture, stone formation, pancreatitis, and cholangitis. Additionally, the potential development of biliary tract carcinoma in the retained cyst is a serious concern. Therefore, internal drainage procedures without cyst excision have been abandoned. The current consensus for the surgical management of type I choledochal cyst is performance of primary cyst excision with Roux-Y hepaticojejunostomy reconstruction (Fig. 110.58). Primary cyst excision is performed as total transmural excision that is accomplished routinely in infants and children.[160] For adults with severe inflammation and fibrosis, dissection may be present problems resulting from inflammation and adhesion of the cyst wall to the hepatoduodenal ligament. A safer approach in this situation may be intramural cyst dissection and removal of the cyst wall epithelium, leaving the posteromedial outer cyst wall adjacent to the portal vein and hepatic artery intact.

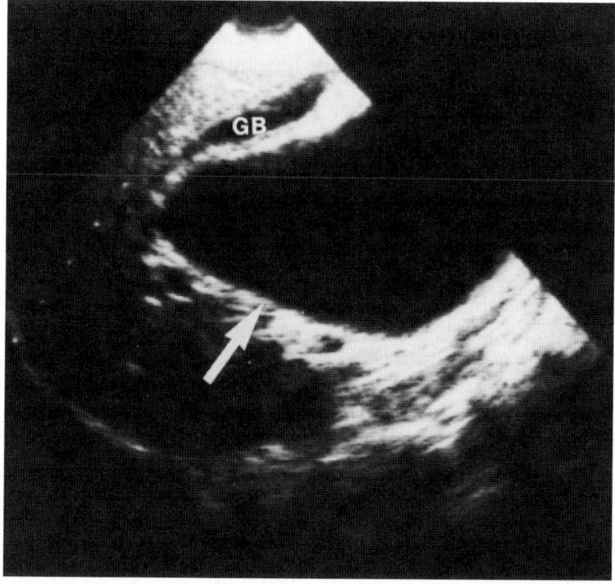

FIGURE 110.57 Ultrasound image of a type I choledochal cyst (*arrow;* longitudinal image). The gallbladder (GB) is also shown.

Other Types of Cysts. Type II cysts are excised completely and the choledochotomy closed primarily. Type III choledochoceles require a transduodenal approach with either marsupialization or excision of the cyst. Care must be taken to identify the ampulla, and a formal sphincteroplasty may be required to ensure adequate drainage from the biliary tract and the pancreas. Types IV and V intrahepatic cystic disease must be approached on an individualized basis. In general, unilobar or focal cystic disease can be either resected or drained with a Roux-Y jejunostomy reconstruction. Bilobar intraparenchymal disease, particularly in the setting of hepatic fibrosis, may be difficult, if not impossible, to obtain complete, adequate drainage.

Complications and Outcome. The major complications associated with operative repair of choledochal cyst include cholangitis, stricture formation, choledocholithiasis, and development of biliary tract malignancy. A summary of the incidence of complications, mortality, and reoperation for the different procedures in 955 cases reported in the literature demonstrated a clear advantage for primary cyst excision in terms of morbidity and need for reoperation, and no significant increase in mortality occurred using this approach.[161] Subsequent to this analysis in 1975, internal drainage procedures without cyst excision have been essentially replaced by primary cyst excision with hepaticojejunostomy reconstruction. Currently, several series have reported excellent results with little or no mortality using total transmural excision of choledochal cysts.[162] Primary transmural excision with biliary

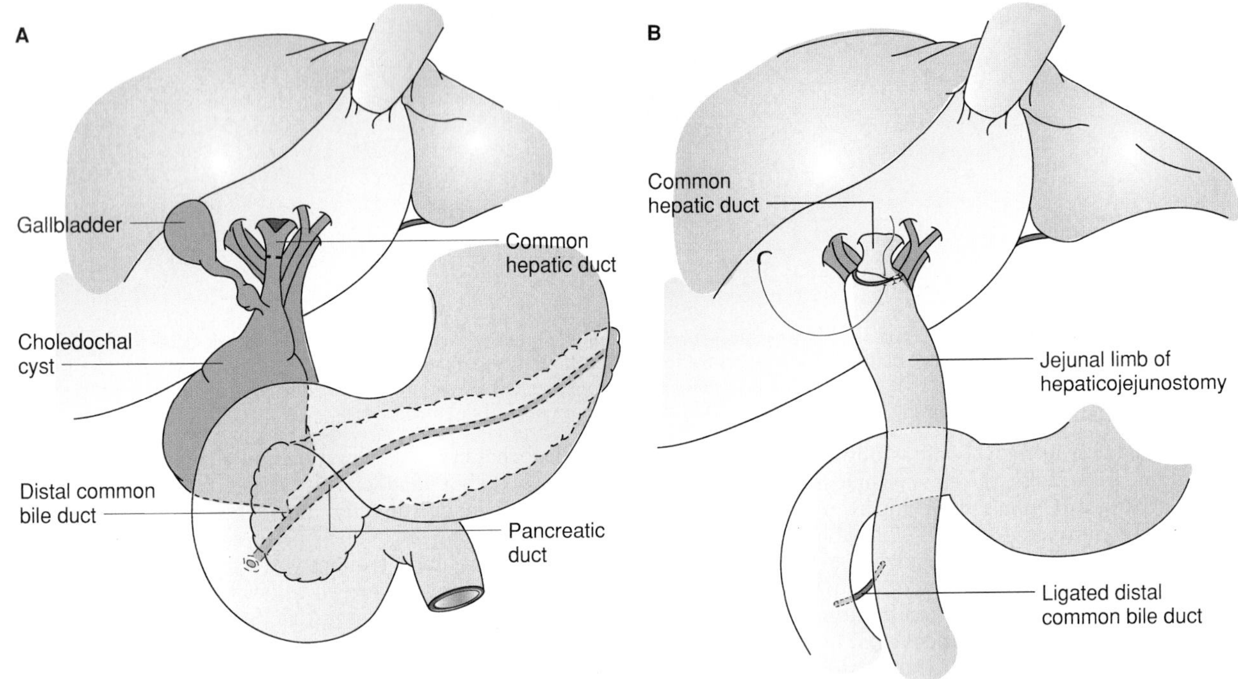

FIGURE 110.58 The preferred operative treatment of type I choledochal cyst consists of primary total transmural cyst excision with Roux-Y hepaticojejunostomy.

tract reconstruction continues to be a safe and desirable operative approach for cystic lesions of the biliary tract.

PEDIATRIC PANCREAS

Disorders of the pancreas are uncommon in infants and children. Pancreatic disorders in children include congenital anatomic disorders, inflammatory pancreatitis, rare neoplastic lesions, and pancreatic endocrinopathies.[163] Several significant issues are relative to the pancreatic problems in the pediatric age group, and a brief overview is presented in the following discussion.

Embryology

The embryologic development of the pancreas was reviewed in the preceding section with respect to duodenal atresia and annular pancreas. Briefly, the fetal pancreas arises from the paired dorsal and ventral foregut diverticular buds during the sixth week of gestation. The dorsal pancreatic anlage gives rise to the body and tail of the pancreas as well as the main pancreatic duct. The ventral pancreatic anlage migrates 180 degrees to fuse with the dorsal gland, forming the uncinate process and the distal portion of the duct of Wirsung (Fig. 110.59). The independent ductal systems of the developing pancreatic anlage fuse. The dorsal (Santorini) duct opens directly into the duodenum, and this anatomy is persistent in 10% to 15% of normal subjects. The ventral (Wirsung) duct opens into the duodenum by fusion with the common bile duct. Normally, the dorsal duct fuses with the ventral duct just to the right of the mesenteric vessels. Failure of the dorsal and ventral ducts to fuse normally leads to two separate pancreatic ducts, a condition known as *pancreatic divisum*. Occasionally, the ventral duct regresses and the entire pancreatic gland is drained by the accessory duct of Santorini.

Primitive duct cells of the pancreas give rise to both the acinar cells and the islet cells of the normal pancreas. Primary islet cells become apparent at week 8 of gestation within the interlobular tissue, with acini becoming visible shortly thereafter. The primary islet cells regress after the fifth month of gestation and are usually nonexistent by term. Secondary islet cells arise from centroacinar proliferation during the third month of gestation. These intralobular cells migrate out of the acini in which they were formed and develop into islets that remain connected to the duct by a thin cellular stalk (the tubule of Bensley).

Exocrine pancreatic anomalies generally arise from defective development during embryogenesis. As previously discussed, the most common of these conditions is annular pancreas. The circumferential distribution of pancreatic tissue around the duodenum is thought to result from interrupted migration of the ventral pancreatic anlage. Less common defects include pancreatic ductal abnormalities, pancreatic duplications, heterotopic pancreatic tissue, and congenital agenesis of portions of the pancreas.

Acute Pancreatitis

Acute pancreatitis is often overlooked as a cause of abdominal pain in children; however, it is the most common disorder of the pancreas in both infants and children. Adult pancreatitis is often caused by either alcohol ingestion or gallstones. In contrast, 50% to 80% of cases in children, particularly adolescents, are posttraumatic or idiopathic in origin. There are many other causal agents and events associated with the development of acute pancreatitis in children. An important clinical condition seen with moderate frequency is acute pancreatitis in the setting of immunosuppression, in particular, high-dose corticosteroids. Steroid-induced acute pancreatitis typically accounts for the third most common cause of pancreatitis in most children's hospitals. Other causes of acute pancreatitis include gallstones, CF, hyperlipidemia, juvenile diabetes mellitus, mumps, coxsackievirus infection, infectious mononucleosis, collagen vascular diseases, and anatomic lesions such as choledochal cyst. Medications significantly associated with acute pancreatitis include oral contraceptives, chlorothiazide, tetracyclines. azathioprine, and L-asparaginase. Valproic acid, an anticonvulsant useful in some children with seizure disorders, is associated with a particularly virulent form of acute necrotizing pancreatitis that may be life threatening.

Clinical manifestation of acute pancreatitis in a child typically reveals a history of midepigastric abdominal pain with anorexia and emesis. On examination, the child usually has a tender abdomen with distention. Fever and leukocytosis are common. Serum amylase and lipase levels usually are elevated, although significant pancreatitis can occur despite a normal amylase level. Conversely, the lipase may be mildly elevated in the absence of clinical symptoms or signs of acute pancreatitis. Ultrasonography and CT imaging of the abdomen are probably the most commonly used adjunctive diagnostic tests. CT imaging is particularly useful in demonstrating enlargement and edema of the gland as well as evaluating for peripancreatic fluid collections. While usually deferred during the acute phase of pancreatitis, ERCP may be useful to evaluate the hepatobiliary tract anatomy once the inflammatory process has resolved. Recently, MRI techniques have been able to provide cholangiopancreatograms (MRCPs) of high resolution. This alternative may be particularly useful in the infant or small child in whom ERCP (which usually requires general anesthesia) is more technically difficult.

Treatment principles for childhood acute pancreatitis are not different from strategies used in adults. The vast majority of children have simple edematous pancreatitis. Hemorrhagic and necrotizing pancreatitis are distinctly unusual in this age group but can be seen in immunosuppressed patients. Therefore, initial therapy is designed to be supportive and nonoperative in approach. Endotracheal intubation and mechanical ventilation may be required. Intravenous fluid resuscitation, pancreatic rest by nasogastric tube decompression, analgesia, and TPN are provided. No clinical efficacy data are available to support the widespread use of anticholinergics or somatostatin analogues for acute pancreatitis in children. Operative intervention is reserved for complications of pancreatitis, such as hemorrhage, infected pancreatic necrosis, or pancreatic pseudocyst.

Recurrent pancreatitis in a child usually is associated with an anatomic abnormality or specific physiologic problem. Following recovery from the acute inflammatory event, an aggressive diagnostic work-up, including consideration of ERCP or MRCP to define ductal anatomy, should be performed. In particular, the presence of pancreas divisum with stenosis of the accessory papilla should be considered. Children with pancreatitis in the setting of cholelithiasis should undergo laparoscopic cholecystectomy after resolution of the pancreatitis.

Pancreas Divisum

Pancreas divisum occurs with failure of normal fusion between the dorsal and ventral pancreatic ducts. About 10% to 15% of normal persons have two separate pancreatic ducts, and up to 10% of asymptomatic persons undergoing ERCP have two complete ductal systems. The anatomic variant of pancreas divisum is not necessarily pathologic, but if the orifice of the accessory papilla is stenotic or obstructed, pancreatitis can occur.[164] About 25% of these persons are thought to be at risk for developing pancreatitis. Because pancreas divisum is characterized by a dominant dorsal duct system dependent on secretion through the accessory papilla, stenosis of the accessory (lesser) papilla is probably necessary to produce pancreatic symptoms. Most of the experience with surgical treatment of pancreas divisum is reported in adults.[165] Successful surgical management of children presenting with recurrent pancreatitis secondary to accessory papilla stenosis with pancreas divisum also has been reported.[166]

To diagnose pancreas divisum, ERCP is required. Endoscopic visualization of the major and accessory papillae is essential. Radiographic findings with pancreas divisum demonstrate a short or absent duct of Wirsung that does not communicate with the duct of Santorini (see Fig. 110.59). A definitive diagnosis of pancreas divisum is made by demonstrating two separate, parallel ductal systems. Whether or not this anatomic abnormality is contributing to the physiologic problem causing pancreatitis for a specific patient has been

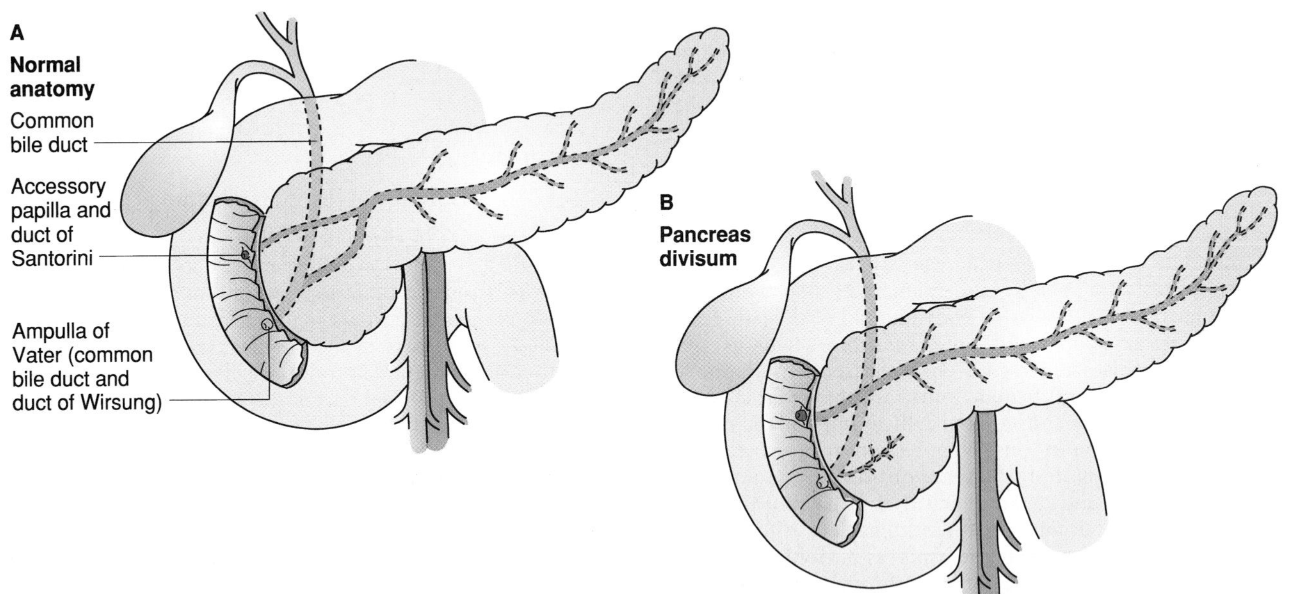

FIGURE 110.59 (*A*) Normal pancreatic ductal anatomy. (*B*) Pancreas divisum. There is no communication between the duct of Wirsung and the duct of Santorini. The duct of Wirsung is short or absent. Most of the pancreas is drained by the duct of Santorini through the accessory papilla. This anatomy is found in about 10% to 15% of normal individuals.

investigated using real-time ultrasonography and intravenous secretin stimulation. Functional stenosis of the accessory papilla with secretin-induced proximal ductal dilatation on ultrasound is thought to be indicative of clinically significant pancreas divisum in a patient with a history of pancreatitis.

Few pediatric patients with pancreatitis and pancreas divisum requiring operation have been reported. Most of these children were female patients who had a history of recurrent pancreatitis. The primary operative goal is to provide adequate drainage of the duct of Santorini by performing a sphincterotomy of the accessory duct.[167] An open dorsal duct sphincterotomy appears to be more durable than endoscopic sphincterotomy. Some surgeons advocate sphincterotomy of the main papilla as well, but dorsal duct sphincterotomy alone appears effective in preventing acute pancreatitis associated with pancreas divisum. The reported surgical outcome in the limited number of children treated for pancreatitis associated with pancreas divisum is favorable.

Pancreatic Cysts

Pancreatic pseudocysts are uncommon in the pediatric age group and are usually the result of blunt traumatic abdominal injury or acute pancreatitis. Children typically present with abdominal pain, nausea, emesis, and weight loss. There may be a palpable midepigastic mass on examination. Diagnosis usually is made with ultrasound or CT imaging of the abdomen. The serum amylase and lipase are usually elevated.

In children, many small asymptomatic pseudocysts regress spontaneously with resolution of the pancreatic inflammation. Larger or symptomatic pseudocysts may require drainage. Symptoms and potential complications of untreated pseudocysts include hemorrhage, infection, perforation, gastrointestinal or biliary tract obstruction, or, rarely, development of pancreaticoenteric fistula. The decision to use either external or internal drainage procedures for a pseudocyst depends on the status of the pancreatic duct. In many centers, definitive external drainage of a large or symptomatic pseudocyst is performed with acceptable morbidity and mortality rates by an ultrasound- or CT-guided percutaneous approach.[168] Pseudocyst recurrence or persistent external drainage without resolution suggests significant pancreatic duct injury or complete ductal transection. Determination of whether a major pancreatic ductal injury is associated with a pseudocyst may be made by either percutaneous contrast injection of the pseudocyst or ERCP.[169] Pseudocysts associated with pancreatic duct injury may not resolve with percutaneous external drainage; so internal drainage procedures such as cystgastrostomy or cystjejunostomy with or without distal pancreatectomy are required.[170]

Epithelial cysts of the pancreas are rare in children. Congenital cysts are lined by epithelium and acinar tissue and are seen most commonly in the body and tail of the pancreas. They may be associated with other syndromes such as von Hippel-Lindau disease, which is characterized by hereditary cerebellar cysts, retinal hemangioma, and pancreatic cysts. Congenital pancreatic cysts are typically asymptomatic unless they are large enough to cause compression or obstruction of the stomach or colon. In the absence of trauma, spontaneous rupture of a pancreatic epithelial cyst is rare. Treatment is cyst excision or internal drainage into the stomach or jejunum.

Other rare cystic lesions of the pancreas in children include retention cysts. These cysts result from chronic ductal obstruction. They are characteristically lined by epithelium unless inflammatory obliteration has occurred. Enteric duplication cysts of the stomach or duodenum can also be associated intimately with the pancreas and communicate with the pancreatic duct. Treatment of both retention cysts and enteric duplication cysts either within or associated with the pancreas includes excision, occasionally internal drainage, and, if necessary, distal pancreatectomy. Not all pancreatic cysts in children can be uniformly considered benign. Suspicious lesions should be investigated thoroughly and biopsy performed. Cystadenoma, cystadenocarcinoma, and rhabdomyosarcoma associated with a pancreatic cyst have been reported. These neoplasms are treated by anatomic pancreatic resection following histologic confirmation on biopsy.

Pancreatic Neoplasms

Childhood malignant neoplasms of the pancreas are uncommon. Typically, pancreatic malignancy in childhood is found on discovery of an asymptomatic abdominal mass. Infrequently, the lesion may be found incidentally or during a diagnostic imaging work-up for abdominal trauma. Jaundice may occur with a lesion in the pancreatic head causing common bile duct obstruction. The most frequently encountered lesions include islet cell carcinoma and adenocarcinoma. The treatment of choice for localized malignant neoplasms of the pancreas is surgical resection.[171] Pancreaticoduodenectomy in children can successfully control some malignancies of the pancreatic head. To promote adequate nutrient absorption and growth, children undergoing pancreaticoduodenectomy should be considered for oral pancreatic enzyme replacement and fat-soluble vitamin supplementation.[172]

Two pancreatic neoplasms seen in childhood and adolescence deserve further discussion. The *papillary cystic neoplasm* of the pancreas occurs predominantly in younger female children, is typically slow growing with low malignant potential, and is highly curable with surgical resection.[173] This tumor is thought to be a neoplasm of the ductuloacinar primordial cells of the pancreas. The other lesion is the *pancreatoblastoma,* also referred to as *juvenile adenocarcinoma of the pancreas.* Pancreatoblastoma is somewhat more common in boys than girls and typically has slow growth with low malignant potential as well. Histologic examination demonstrates undifferentiated ductular and acinar areas with nodules of squamous epithelium, suggesting that these tumors arise from primordial pancreatic cells. Both papillary cystic neoplasm and pancreatoblastoma have more favorable prognoses than adenocarcinoma following surgical resection.

Endocrine Lesions of the Pancreas

Zollinger-Ellison Syndrome

Childhood tumors of the endocrine pancreas are exceedingly rare. The diagnosis and management of these tumors do not differ greatly from the adult population. The most common of these lesions include gastrinoma and insulinoma. The functional endocrine tumors of the pancreas typically are characterized by secreted peptide products such as glucagon, vasoactive intestinal peptide, somatostatin, and pancreatic polypeptide.

Similar to adults, children with Zollinger-Ellison syndrome clinically present with symptoms related to gastric hypersecretion. Peptic ulcer disease with or without gastrointestinal hemorrhage, abdominal pain, and diarrhea is a common presenting symptoms. The diagnosis is confirmed by finding elevated serum gastrin levels. The basal acid output typically is elevated as well. A paradoxical increase in serum gastrin levels is found following intravenous administration of secretin (secretin stimulation test).

Contemporary management of Zollinger-Ellison syndrome in children relies on control of gastric acid hypersecretion with the oral administration of a proton-pump inhibitor. Diagnostic imaging studies, including helical CT scanning and MRI, are useful in localization of a primary gastrinoma and evaluating for metastatic disease before exploration. Definitive treatment relies on complete excision of the primary gastrinoma, which typically is found in the right of the superior mesenteric vessels in the head of the pancreas or the duodenum. The growth and progression of gastrinoma appear to be less aggressive in children than in adults; however, total gastrectomy occasionally is required in a child to control intractable symptoms related to persistent hypergastrinemia or metastatic disease.[174]

About 25% of gastrinomas occur in the setting of MEN syndrome, reviewed elsewhere in this book. At least 90% of patients with MEN type I have hyperparathyroidism secondary to hyperplasia. Additionally, 30% to 80% of patients have pancreatic islet cell tumors, and 15% to 50% have pituitary tumors. In contrast, sporadic tumors, pancreatic tumors associated with MEN I, are typically multicentric and are more frequently malignant.

Hypoglycemia

There are diverse metabolic causes for hypoglycemia in infancy and childhood. These include endocrinopathies such as panhypopituitarism, hypothyroidism, adrenal insufficiency, and congenital adrenal hyperplasia (adrenogenital syndrome). Several inborn errors of metabolism interrupt normal glucose regulatory mechanisms. Systemic disease states, perinatal stress, and sepsis can predispose an otherwise normal infant to low blood glucose levels. Infants who remain unresponsive to glucose infusion typically have inappropriately high circulating insulin levels for a given blood glucose level. Hyperinsulinemia should be suspected in any infant or child younger than 1 year of age who has significant, persistent hypoglycemia. There are heterogeneous causes for hyperinsulinemic hypoglycemia, but the most common historical cause in infancy is nesidioblastosis, which is characterized by uncontrolled development of the pancreatic endocrine tissue, in particular, beta cell mass, which functions abnormally beyond birth or during infancy.[175,176] Clinically, these cells secrete inappropriately high amounts of insulin, typically causing clinical hypoglycemia in infants (Fig. 110.60). Two distinct histologic lesions appear to be responsible for congenital hyperinsulinism. Mutations in the beta cell K_{ATP} channel genes may lead to either focal, adenomatous hyperinsulinism or diffuse hyperinsulinism; both genotypes lead to phenotypic hypoglycemia if left untreated.

Infants with congenital hyperinsulinism usually become symptomatic from hypoglycemia within the first few hours or days of life. These infants commonly present with neurologic symptoms such as lethargy or generalized seizures and have corresponding fasting blood glucose levels below 40 mg/dL. The diagnosis of hyperinsulinemia is supported by the clinical features of Whipple's triad, which includes (a) neurologic changes with fasting or activity, (b) fasting blood glucose levels below 40 to 50 mg/dL, and (c) neurologic symptoms reversed by the administration of glucose. The diagnosis is made by demonstrating inappropriately high levels of circulating insulin for a given level of blood glucose. An insulin (IU/mL) to glucose (mg/dL) ratio that is greater than 0.5 in a fasting patient is consistent with hyperinsulinemic hypoglycemia. In infants and children, an absolute insulin level greater than 5 IU/ml in the presence of a blood glucose less than 40 mg/dL is generally diagnostic. Ketone body production is impaired in infants with congenital hyperinsulinism.

The initial management of a hypoglycemic infant with congenital hyperinsulinism is to provide adequate glucose concentrations to prevent permanent neurologic injury. Dextrose-containing intravenous solutions are titrated to maintain blood glucose levels greater than 40 mg/dL and may require a central venous catheter. The short-term administration of somatostatin analogues to increase blood glucose levels in hyperinsulinemic states has been demonstrated to be useful.[177] Other pharmacologic agents used to reduce insulin levels and raise blood glucose concentration include diazoxide (15 mg/kg daily). The use of streptozocin to control hyperinsulinemia most often is reserved for adults with metastatic islet cell carcinoma and is not widely used in infants because of the potential side effects.

Following initial control of blood glucose and clinical confirmation of hyperinsulinemia, operative intervention should be considered a means of providing definitive control of hypoglycemia. Diagnostic imaging using CT scanning may be useful either to identify or to exclude a focal lesion. Localization of focal lesions via selective arterial calcium stimulation with venous sampling is extremely important in that this approach may lead to effective glucose control with selective partial pancreatectomy and allow for preservation of normal pancreatic tissue and function.[178,179]

Operatively, the abdomen is explored thoroughly, and the entire pancreas must be exposed. Preoperative localization data guided by intraoperative ultrasound and frozen section analysis may identify focal lesions amenable to partial resection. In the

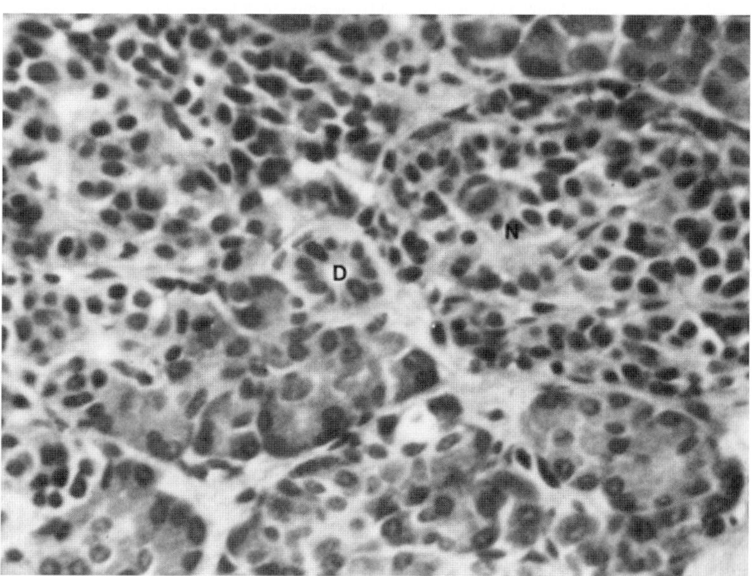

FIGURE 110.60 Nesidioblastosis demonstrating neoislet formation (N) from primitive pancreatic ductules.

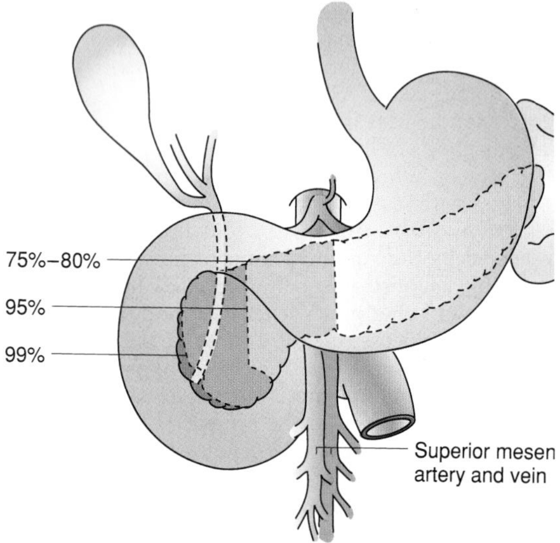

FIGURE 110.61 Illustration of the various degrees of pancreatic resection.

absence of a focal lesion, the infant is presumed to have diffuse islet cell hyperplasia. In this setting, the general operative strategy is total or near total pancreatectomy.[180–182] Lesser procedures such as subtotal (80%) pancreatectomy do not effectively treat diffuse congenital hyperinsulinism. Near-total pancreatectomy involves resection of the distal 95% of the gland with preservation of the spleen. The entire distal pancreas, including the uncinate process, is resected, leaving a small rim of pancreatic tissue adjacent to the duodenum (Fig. 110.61). Total pancreatectomy is usually reserved for persistent or recurrent hypoglycemia following lesser procedures. Near-total pancreatectomy controls hypoglycemia in about 90% of infants with diffuse congenital hyperinsulinism. The remaining infants with persistent hypoglycemia may require further pancreatic resection. With extensive pancreatic resection, the typical postoperative course is a transient period of hyperglycemia with subsequent stabilization of blood glucose levels. Pancreatic exocrine function also is decreased and oral replacement therapy is indicated. Despite clinical remission following resection, however, diabetes mellitus may occur as a long-term consequence in children treated either medically or surgically for diffuse congenital hyperinsulinism.[183] Therefore, these infants need long-term metabolic follow-up for both pancreatic endocrine and exocrine function.

KEY POINTS

- **Gastroschisis occurs with an incidence rate of 1 in 3,000 to 8,000 live births, and for unknown reasons the incidence rate is increasing; the sequential development of a typical gastroschisis is an *in utero* ruptured hernia of the umbilical cord.**
- **Omphalocele is an abdominal wall defect of varying size characterized by herniated visceral contents in a translucent sac; the incidence of omphalocele is 1 in 6,000 to 10,000 live births and has been stable over the past several decades.**
- **An indirect inguinal hernia is an abnormal, patent continuation of the peritoneum through the internal inguinal ring; repair of this hernia is the most common elective procedure in pediatric surgery.**
- **Bilious emesis in a neonate is the result of an acute mechanical intestinal obstruction until proved otherwise; emergent surgical evaluation is warranted for any newborn with bilious emesis. Diagnosis relies on a clear history, thorough clinical examination, and adjunctive radiologic studies.**
- **Necrotizing enterocolitis (NEC) is characterized by initial intestinal mucosal injury that may progress to transmural bowel necrosis and is the most frequently encountered neonatal surgical emergency. Development of NEC occurs in association with a variety of conditions, including perinatal stress, sepsis, respiratory failure, hypoxemia, hypotension, and congenital cardiac defects.**
- **Hirschsprung disease is characterized by a lack of ganglion cells involving the distal rectosigmoid colon in 75% to 80% of affected infants. Without a functional myenteric nervous system in the aganglionic segment, both propulsion and reflexive relaxation is disordered or absent in the distal bowel leading to incomplete, distal intestinal obstruction in the newborn or as chronic constipation in the older child or adult.**
- **Intussusception is the invagination or telescoping of a proximal segment of intestine into an adjacent distal segment and is the most common cause of intestinal obstruction in infants and children 3 months to 3 years of age**
- **The incidence of biliary atresia is 1 in 8,000 to 12,000 live births and is the most common cause of chronic cholestasis in infants and children as well as the most frequent indication for pediatric liver transplantation.**

References

1. Nichols CR, Dickinson JE, Pemberton PJ. Rising incidence of gastroschisis in teenage pregnancies. *J Matern Fetal Med.* 1997;6:225–229.
2. Blakelock RT, Upadhyay V, Pease PW, et al. Are babies with gastroschisis small for gestational age? *Pediatr Surg Int.* 1997;12:580–582.
3. Torfs CP, Curry CJ. Familial cases of gastroschisis in a population-based registry. *Am J Med Genet.* 1993;45:465–467.
4. Glick PL, Harrison MR, Adzick NS. The missing link in the pathogenesis of gastroschisis. *J Pediatr Surg.* 1985;20:406–407.
5. Cantrell JR, Haller JA Jr, Ravitch MM. A syndrome of congenital defects involving the abdominal wall, sternum, diaphragm, pericardium, and heart. *Surg Gynecol Obstet.* 1958;107:602–605.
6. Calzolari E, Bianchi F, Dolk H, et al. Omphalocele and gastroschisis in Europe: a survey of 3 million births 1980–1990. EUROCAT Working Group. *Am J Med Genet.* 1995;58:187–194.
7. Boyd PA, Bhattacharjee A, Gould S, et al. Outcome of prenatally diagnosed anterior abdominal wall defects. *Arch Dis Child Fetal Neonatal Ed.* 1998;78:F209–F213.
8. Lurie S, Sherman D, Bukovsky I. Omphalocele delivery enigma: the best mode of delivery still remains dubious. *Eur J Obstet Gynecol Reprod Biol.* 1999;82:19–22.
9. Sipes SL, Weiner CP, Sipes DR, et al. Gastroschisis and omphalocele: does either antenatal diagnosis or route of delivery make a difference in perinatal outcome? *Obstet Gynecol.* 1990;76:195–199.
10. Bethel CA, Seashore JH, Touloukian RJ. Cesarean section does not improve outcome in gastroschisis. *J Pediatr Surg.* 1989;24:1–4.
11. Puffinbarger NK, Taylor DV, Tuggle DW, et al. End-tidal carbon dioxide for monitoring primary closure of gastroschisis. *J Pediatr Surg.* 1996;31:280–282.
12. **Kidd JN Jr, Jackson RJ, Smith SD, et al. Evolution of staged versus primary closure of gastroschisis. *Ann Surg.* 2003;237:759–65.**
13. **Curry JJ, Lander AD, Stringer MD, et al. A multicenter, randomized, double-blind, placebo-controlled trial of the prokinetic agent erythromycin in the postoperative recovery of infants with gastroschisis. *J Pediatr Surg.* 2004;39:565–569.**
14. Jayanthi S, Seymour P, Puntis JW, et al. Necrotizing enterocolitis after gastroschisis repair: a preventable complication? *J Pediatr Surg.* 1998;33:705–707.
15. Zaccara A, Iacobelli BD, Calzolari A, et al. Cardiopulmonary performances in young children and adolescents born with large abdominal wall defects. *J Pediatr Surg.* 2003;38:478–481.
16. Papagrigoriadis S, Browse DJ, Howard ER. Incarceration of umbilical hernias in children: a rare but important complication. *Pediatr Surg Int.* 1998;14:231–232.
17. Evans A. The comparative incidence of umbilical hernias in colored and white infants. *J Natl Med Assoc.* 1941;33:158–162.
18. Snyder WH Jr, Greanly EM Jr. Inguinal hernia. In: Benson CD, Mustard WT, Ravitch MM, et al., eds. *Pediatric surgery.* Chicago: Year Book Medical, 1962.
19. Rowe MI, Copelson LW, Clatworthy HW. The patent processus vaginalis and the inguinal hernia. *J Pediatr Surg.* 1969;4:102–107.

20. Clarnette TD, Lam SK, Hutson JM. Ventriculo-peritoneal shunts in children reveal the natural history of closure of the processus vaginalis. *J Pediatr Surg.* 1998;33:413–416.
21. Wesley JR. Abdominal wall defects. In: Greenfield LJ, Mulholland MW, Oldham KT, et al., eds. *Surgery: scientific principles and practice,* 2nd ed. Philadelphia: Lippincott–Raven, 1997, pp. 2028–2034.
22. Chou TY, Chu CC, Diau GY, et al. Inguinal hernia in children: US versus exploratory surgery and intraoperative contralateral laparoscopy. *Radiology* 1996;201:385–388.
23. Palmer BV. Incarcerated inguinal hernia in children. *Ann R Coll Surg Engl.* 1978;60:121–124.
24. Rowe MI, Clatworthy HW. Incarcerated and strangulated hernias in children: a statistical study of high-risk factors. *Arch Surg.* 1970;101:136–139.
25. Somri M, Gaitini L, Vaida S, et al. Postoperative outcome in high-risk infants undergoing herniorrhaphy: comparison between spinal and general anesthesia. *Anaesthesia* 1998;53:762–766.
26. Hrabovszky Z, Pinter AB. Routine bilateral exploration for inguinal hernia in infancy and childhood. *Eur J Pediatr Surg.* 1995;5:152–155.
27. Wiener ES, Touloukian RJ, Rodgers BM, et al. Hernia survey of the Section on Surgery of the American Academy of Pediatrics. *J Pediatr Surg.* 1996;31:1166–1169.
28. Tackett LD, Breuer CK, Luks FI, et al. Incidence of contralateral inguinal hernia: a prospective analysis. *J Pediatr Surg.* 1999;34:684–687.
29. Wolf SA, Hopkins JW. Laparoscopic incidence of contralateral patent processus vaginalis in boys with clinical unilateral inguinal hernias. *J Pediatr Surg.* 1994;29:1118–1120.
30. Owings EF, Georgeson, KE. A new technique for laparoscopic exploration to find contralateral patent processus vaginalis. *Surg Endosc.* 2000;14:114–116.
30. Skandalakis JE, Gray SW. *Embryology for Surgeons: The embryological basis for the treatment of congenital anomalies,* 2nd ed. Baltimore: Williams & Wilkins, 1994, pp. 184–241.
31. Haller JA Jr, Tepas JJ, Pickard LR, et al. Intestinal atresia: current concepts of pathogenesis, pathophysiology, and operative management. *Am Surg.* 1983;49:385–391.
32. Koga Y, Hayashida Y, Ikeda K, et al. Intestinal atresia in fetal dogs produced by localized ligation of mesenteric vessels. *J Pediatr Surg.* 1975;10:949–953.
33. Dalla Vecchia LK, Grosfeld JL, West KW, et al. Intestinal atresia and stenosis: a 25-year experience with 277 cases. *Arch Surg.* 1998;133:490–496.
34. James LM, Erickson JD, McClean AB. *Prevalence of birth defects.* Atlanta: Centers for Disease Control, 1992.
35. Filkins K, Russo J, Flowers WKD. Third trimester ultrasound diagnosis of intestinal atresia following clinical evidence of polyhydramnios. *Prenat Diagn.* 1985;5:215–220.
36. Wilmore DW. Factors correlating with a successful outcome following extensive intestinal resection in newborn infants. *J Pediatr.* 1972;80:88–95.
37. Touloukian RJ. Intestinal atresia. *Clin Perinatol.* 1978;5:3–18.
38. Masumoto K, Suita S, Nada O, et al. Abnormalities of enteric neurons, intestinal pacemaker cells, and smooth muscle in human intestinal atresia. *J Pediatr Surg.* 1999;34:1463–1468.
39. Doolin EJ, Ormsbee HS, Hill JL. Motility abnormality in intestinal atresia. *J Pediatr Surg.* 1987;22:320–324.
40. Menardi G. Duodenal atresia, stenosis, and annular pancreas. In: Freeman NV, Burge DM, Griffiths M, et al., eds. *Surgery of the newborn.* Edinburgh: Churchill Livingstone, 1994, pp. 107–115.
41. Stauffer UG, Schwoebel M. Duodenal atresia and stenosis–annular pancreas. In: O'Neill JA Jr, Rowe MI, Grosfeld JL, et al., eds. *Pediatric surgery.* St. Louis: Mosby, 1998, pp. 1133–1143.
42. Stauffer UG, Irving I. Duodenal atresia and stenosis—long-term results. *Prog Pediatr Surg.* 1977;10:49–60.
43. Kimura K, Mukohara N, Nishijima E, et al. Diamond-shaped anastomosis for duodenal atresia: an experience with 44 patients over 15 years. *J Pediatr Surg.* 1990;25:977–979.
44. Weber TR, Lewis JE, Mooney D, et al. Duodenal atresia: a comparison of techniques of repair. *J Pediatr Surg.* 1986;21:1133–1136.
45. Peña A. *Atlas of surgical management of anorectal malformations.* New York: Springer-Verlag, 1990.
46. Spouge D, Baird PA. Imperforate anus in 700,000 consecutive liveborn infants. *Am J Med Genet.* 1986;2(suppl):151–161.
47. Schuster SR, Teele RL. An analysis of ultrasound scanning as a guide in determination of "high" or "low" imperforate anus. *J Pediatr Surg.* 1979;14:798–800.
48. Ong NT, Beasley SW. Long-term continence in patients with high and intermediate anorectal anomalies treated by sacroperineal (Stephens) rectoplasty. *J Pediatr Surg.* 1991;26:44–48.
49. Ito Y, Yokoyama J, Hayashi A, et al. Reappraisal of endorectal pull-through procedure. I. Anorectal malformations. *J Pediatr Surg.* 1981;16:476–483.
50. Georgeson KE, Inge TH, Albanese CT. Laparoscopically assisted anorectal pull-through for high imperforate anus—a new technique. *J Pediatr Surg.* 2000;35:927–930.
51. Kiesewetter WB, Hoon A. Imperforate anus: an analysis of mortalities during a 25-year period. *Prog Pediatr Surg.* 1979;13:211–220.
52. Kiesewetter WB, Chang JH. Imperforate anus: a five- to thirty-year follow-up perspective. *Prog Pediatr Surg.* 1977;10:111–120.
53. Bliss DP Jr, Tapper D, Anderson JM, et al. Does posterior sagittal anorectoplasty in patients with high imperforate anus provide superior fecal continence? *J Pediatr Surg.* 1996;31:26–30.
54. Parks DA, Bulkley GB, Granger DN. Role of oxygen-derived free radicals in digestive tract diseases. *Surgery* 1983;94:415–422.
55. Clark DA, Fornabaio DM, McNeill H, et al. Contribution of oxygen-derived free radicals to experimental necrotizing enterocolitis. *Am J Pathol.* 1988;130:537–542.
56. Muguruma K, Gray PW, Tjoelker LW, et al. The central role of PAF in necrotizing enterocolitis development. *Adv Exp Med Biol.* 1997;407:379–382.
57. Anderson DM, Kliegman RM. The relationship of neonatal alimentation practices to the occurrence of endemic necrotizing enterocolitis. *Am J Perinatol.* 1991;8:62–67.
58. Rayyis SF, Ambalavanan N, Wright L, et al. Randomized trial of "slow" versus "fast" feed advancements on the incidence of necrotizing enterocolitis in very low birth weight infants. *J Pediatr.* 1999;134:293–297.
59. Center for Disease Control and Prevention, National Center for Health Statistics. *National vital statistics report. 1999.* April 29, 1999. Report No. 47:(18).
60. Grosfeld JL, Cheu H, Schlatter M, et al. Changing trends in necrotizing enterocolitis: experience with 302 cases in two decades. *Ann Surg.* 1991;214:300–306.
61. Pokorny WJ, Garcia-Prats JA, Barry YN. Necrotizing enterocolitis: incidence, operative care, and outcome. *J Pediatr Surg.* 1986;21:1149–1154.
62. Andrews DA, Sawin RS, Ledbetter DJ, et al. Necrotizing enterocolitis in term neonates. *Am J Surg.* 1990;159:507–509.
63. Bell MJ, Kosloske AM, Benton C, et al. Neonatal necrotizing enterocolitis: prevention of perforation. *J Pediatr Surg.* 1973;8:601–605.
64. Grosfeld JL, Chaet M, Molinari F, et al. Increased risk of necrotizing enterocolitis in premature infants with patent ductus arteriosus treated with indomethacin. *Ann Surg.* 1996;224:350–355.
65. Ricketts RR. The role of paracentesis in the management of infants with necrotizing enterocolitis. *Am Surg.* 1986;52:61–65.
66. Cooper A, Ross AJ, O'Neill JA Jr, et al. Resection with primary anastomosis for necrotizing enterocolitis: a contrasting view. *J Pediatr Surg.* 1988;23:64–68.
67. Ade-Ajayi N, Kiely E, Drake D, et al. Resection and primary anastomosis in necrotizing enterocolitis. *J R Soc Med.* 1996;89:385–388.
68. Sato TT, Oldham KT. Abdominal drain placement versus laparotomy for necrotizing enterocolitis with perforation. *Clin Perinatol.* 2004;31:577–589.
69. O'Connor A, Sawin RS. High morbidity of enterostomy and its closure in premature infants with necrotizing enterocolitis. *Arch Surg.* 1998;133:875–880.
70. Schwartz MZ, Hayden CK, Richardson CJ, et al. A prospective evaluation of intestinal stenosis following necrotizing enterocolitis. *J Pediatr Surg.* 1982;17:764–770.
71. Patel JC, Tepas JJ III, Huffman SD, et al. Neonatal necrotizing enterocolitis: the long-term perspective. *Am Surg.* 1998;64:575–579.
72. Statement from the National Institutes of Health workshop on population screening for the cystic fibrosis gene. *N Engl J Med.* 1990;323:70–71.
73. Riordan JR, Rommens JM, Kerem B, et al. Identification of the cystic fibrosis gene: cloning and characterization of complementary DNA. *Science* 1989;245:1066–1073.
74. Kerem B, Rommens JM, Buchanan JA, et al. Identification of the cystic fibrosis gene: genetic analysis. *Science* 1989;245:1073–1080.
75. Rosenstein BJ, Cutting GR. The diagnosis of cystic fibrosis: a consensus statement. Cystic Fibrosis Foundation Consensus Panel. *J Pediatr.* 1998;132:589–595.
76. Quinton PM. Cystic fibrosis: a disease in electrolyte transport. *Faseb J.* 1990;4:2709–2717.
77. Quinton PM, Bijman J. Higher bioelectric potentials due to decreased chloride absorption in the sweat glands of patients with cystic fibrosis. *N Engl J Med.* 1983;308:1185–1189.
78. Irish MS, Ragi JM, Karamanoukian H, et al. Prenatal diagnosis of the fetus with cystic fibrosis and meconium ileus. *Pediatr Surg Int.* 1997;12:434–436.
79. Kao SC, Franken EA Jr. Nonoperative treatment of simple meconium ileus: a survey of the Society for Pediatric Radiology. *Pediatr Radiol.* 1995;25:97–100.
80. Mak GZ, Harberg FJ, Hiatt P, et al. T-tube ileostomy for meconium ileus: four decades of experience. *J Pediatr Surg.* 2000;35:349–352.
81. Del Pin CA, Czyrko C, Ziegler MM, et al. Management and survival of meconium ileus: a 30-year review. *Ann Surg.* 1992;215:179–185.
82. Docherty JG, Zaki A, Coutts JA, et al. Meconium ileus: a review 1972–1990. *Br J Surg.* 1992;79:571–573.
83. Andrassy RJ, Mahour GH. Malrotation of the midgut in infants and children: a 25-year review. *Arch Surg.* 1981;116:158–160.
84. Ford EG, Senac MO Jr, Srikanth MS, et al. Malrotation of the intestine in children. *Ann Surg.* 1992;215:172–178.
85. Powell DM, Othersen HB, Smith CD. Malrotation of the intestines in children: the effect of age on presentation and therapy. *J Pediatr Surg.* 1989;24:777–780.
86. Weinberger E, Winters WD, Liddell RM, et al. Sonographic diagnosis of intestinal malrotation in infants: importance of the relative positions of the superior mesenteric vein and artery. *AJR Am J Roentgenol.* 1992; 159:825–828.
87. Ladd WE, Gross RE. *Abdominal surgery of infancy and childhood.* Philadelphia: WB Saunders, 1941.
88. Bass KD, Rothenberg SS, Chang JH. Laparoscopic Ladd's procedure in infants with malrotation. *J Pediatr Surg.* 1998;33:279–281.

89. Fujimoto T, Hata J, Yokoyama S, et al. A study of the extracellular matrix protein as the migration pathway of neural crest cells in the gut: analysis in human embryos with special reference to the pathogenesis of Hirschsprung's disease. *J Pediatr Surg.* 1989;24:550–556.
90. Kleinhaus S, Boley SJ, Sheran M, et al. Hirschsprung's disease—a survey of the members of the Surgical Section of the American Academy of Pediatrics. *J Pediatr Surg.* 1979;14:588–597.
91. Lolova I, Davidoff M, Itzev D, et al. Histochemical, immunocytochemical, and ultrastructural data on the innervation of the smooth muscle of the large intestine in Hirschsprung's disease. *Acta Physiol Pharmacol Bulg.* 1986;12:55–62.
92. Tomita R, Munakata K, Kurosu Y. Peptidergic nerves in Hirschsprung's disease and its allied disorders. *Eur J Pediatr Surg.* 1994;4:346–351.
93. Kusafuka T, Puri P. Altered mRNA expression of the neuronal nitric oxide synthase gene in Hirschsprung's disease. *J Pediatr Surg.* 1997;32:1054–1058.
94. Puri P, Wester T. Intestinal neuronal dysplasia. *Semin Pediatr Surg.* 1998;7:181–186.
95. Meier-Ruge WA, Ammann K, Bruder E, et al. Updated results on intestinal neuronal dysplasia (IND B). *Eur J Pediatr Surg.* 2004;14:384–391.
96. Tanaka H, Moroi K, Iwai J, et al. Novel mutations of the endothelin B receptor gene in patients with Hirschsprung's disease and their characterization. *J Biol Chem.* 1998;273:11378–11383.
97. Kusafuka T, Puri P. Genetic aspects of Hirschsprung's disease. *Semin Pediatr Surg.* 1998;7:148–155.
98. Robertson K, Mason I, Hall S. Hirschsprung's disease: genetic mutations in mice and men. *Gut* 1997;41:436–441.
99. Puri P, Ohshiro K, Wester T. Hirschsprung's disease: a search for etiology. *Semin Pediatr Surg.* 1998;7:140–147.
100. Puffenberger EG, Kauffman ER, Bolk S, et al. Identity-by-descent and association mapping of a recessive gene for Hirschsprung disease on human chromosome 13q22. *Hum Mol Genet.* 1994;3:1217–1225.
101. Romeo G, Ronchetto P, Luo Y, et al. Point mutations affecting the tyrosine kinase domain of the RET protooncogene in Hirschsprung's disease. *Nature* 1994;367:377–378.
102. Quinn FM, Surana R, Puri P. The influence of trisomy 21 on outcome in children with Hirschsprung's disease. *J Pediatr Surg.* 1994;29:781–783.
103. Qualman SJ, Jaffe R, Bove KE, et al. Diagnosis of Hirschsprung disease using the rectal biopsy: multi-institutional survey. *Pediatr Dev Pathol.* 1999;2:588–596.
104. Ramesh JC, Ramanujam TM, Yik YI, et al. Management of Hirschsprung's disease with reference to one-stage pull-through without colostomy. *J Pediatr Surg.* 1999;34:1691–1694.
105. Albanese CT, Jennings RW, Smith B, et al. Perineal one-stage pull-through for Hirschsprung's disease. *J Pediatr Surg.* 1999;34:377–380.
106. Georgeson KE, Cohen RD, Hebra A, et al. Primary laparoscopic-assisted endorectal colon pull-through for Hirschsprung's disease: a new gold standard. *Ann Surg.* 1999;229:678–682.
107. Skinner MA. Hirschsprung's disease. *Curr Probl Surg.* 1996;33:389–460.
108. **Saleh W, Rasheed K, Al Mohaidly M, et al. Management of Hirschsprung's disease: a comparison of Soave's and Duhamel's pull-through methods. *Pediatr Surg Int.* 2004;20:590–593.**
109. Sawin R, Hatch E, Schaller R, et al. Limited surgery for lower-segment Hirschsprung's disease. *Arch Surg.* 1994;129:920–924.
110. Vanderwinden JM, Mailleux P, Schiffmann SN, et al. Nitric oxide synthase activity in infantile hypertrophic pyloric stenosis. *N Engl J Med.* 1992;327:511–515.
111. Saur D, Vanderwinden J, Seidler B, et al. Single-nucleotide promoter polymorphism alters transcription of neuronal nitric oxide synthase exon 1c in infantile hypertrophic pyloric stenosis. *Proc Natl Acad Sci.* 2004; 101:1662–1667.
112. Rasmussen L, Green A, Hansen LP. The epidemiology of infantile hypertrophic pyloric stenosis in a Danish population, 1950–84. *Int J Epidemiol.* 1989;18:413–417.
113. Honein MA, Paulozzi LJ, Himelright IM, et al. Infantile hypertrophic pyloric stenosis after pertussis prophylaxis with erythromycin: a case review and cohort study. *Lancet* 1999;354:2101–2105.
114. Schechter R, Torfs CP, Bateson TF. The epidemiology of infantile hypertrophic pyloric stenosis. *Paediatr Perinat Epidemiol.* 1997;11:407–427.
115. **Hall NJ, Van Der Zee J, Tan HL, et al. Meta-analysis of laparoscopic versus open pyloromyotomy. *Ann Surg.* 2004;240:774–778.**
116. Langer JC, To T. Does pediatric surgical specialty training affect outcome after Ramstedt pyloromyotomy? A population-based study. *Pediatrics* 2004;113:1342–1347.
117. Kim YS, Rhu JH. Intussusception in infancy and childhood: analysis of 385 cases. *Int Surg.* 1989;74:114–118.
118. From the Centers for Disease Control and Prevention. Withdrawal of rotavirus vaccine recommendation. *JAMA* 1999;282:2113–2114.
119. Okuyama H, Nakai H, Okada A. Is barium enema reduction safe and effective in patients with a long duration of intussusception? *Pediatr Surg Int.* 1999;15:105–107.
120. Poddoubnyi IV, Dronov AF, Blinnikov OI, et al. Laparoscopy in the treatment of intussusception in children. *J Pediatr Surg.* 1998;33:1194–1197.
121. Schier F, Hoffmann K, Waldschmidt J. Laparoscopic removal of Meckel's diverticula in children. *Eur J Pediatr Surg.* 1996;6:38–39.
122. Bonadio WA, Jona JZ, Glicklich M, et al. Esophageal bougienage technique for coin ingestion in children. *J Pediatr Surg.* 1988;23:917–918.
123. Stuth EA, Stucke AG, Cohen RD, et al. Successful resuscitation of a child after exsanguination due to aortoesophageal fistula from undiagnosed foreign body. *Anesthesiology* 2001;95:1025–1026.
124. Maves MD, Carithers JS, Birck HG. Esophageal burns secondary to disc battery ingestion. *Ann Otol Rhinol Laryngol.* 1984;93:364–369.
125. Thompson EC, Brown MF, Bowen EC, et al. Causes of gastrointestinal hemorrhage in neonates and children. *South Med J.* 1996;89:370–374.
126. McDougal WS, Izant RJ Jr, Zollinger RM Jr. Primary peritonitis in infancy and childhood. *Ann Surg.* 1975;181:310–313.
127. Newman KD. Malignant liver tumors of children. *Semin Pediatr Surg.* 1992;1:145–151.
128. Bowman LC, Riely CA. Management of pediatric liver tumors. *Surg Oncol Clin N Am.* 1996;5:451–459.
129. Luks FI, Yazbeck S, Brandt ML, et al. Benign liver tumors in children: a 25-year experience. *J Pediatr Surg.* 1991;26:1326–1330.
130. Coran AG. Pediatric liver. In: Greenfield LJ, Mulholland MW, Oldham KT, et al., eds. *Surgery: scientific principles and practice,* 2nd ed. Philadelphia: Lippincott–Raven, 1997, pp. 2078–2083.
131. Huang SA. Tu HM, Harney JW, et al. Severe hypothyroidism caused by type 3 iodothyronine deiodinase in infantile hemangioma. *N Engl J Med.* 2000;343:185–187.
132. Yandza T, Valayer J. Benign tumors of the liver in children: analysis of a series of 20 cases. *J Pediatr Surg.* 1986;21:419–423.
133. Ein SH, Stephens CA. Benign liver tumors and cysts in childhood. *J Pediatr Surg.* 1974;9:847–851.
134. Pazdur R, Bready B, Cangir A. Pediatric hepatic tumors: clinical trials conducted in the United States. *J Surg Oncol.* 1993;3(suppl):127–130.
135. Urban CE, Mache CJ, Schwinger W, et al. Undifferentiated (embryonal) sarcoma of the liver in childhood: successful combined-modality therapy in four patients. *Cancer* 1993;72:2511–2516.
136. Randolph JG, Altman RP, Arensman RM, et al. Liver resection in children with hepatic neoplasms. *Ann Surg.* 1978;187:599–605.
137. Larsen LR, Raffensperger J. Liver abscess. *J Pediatr Surg.* 1979; 14:329–331.
138. Jessee WF, Ryan JM, Fitzgerald JF, et al. Amebic liver abscess in childhood. *Clin Pediatr (Phila).* 1975;14:134–146.
139. Balistreri WF, Grand R, Hoofnagle JH, et al. Biliary atresia: current concepts and research directions. *Hepatology* 1996;23:1682–1692.
140. Tan CE, Davenport M, Driver M, et al. Does the morphology of the extrahepatic biliary remnants in biliary atresia influence survival? A review of 205 cases. *J Pediatr Surg.* 1994;29:1459–1464.
141. Chandra RS, Altman RP. Ductal remnants in extrahepatic biliary atresia: a histopathologic study with clinical correlation. *J Pediatr.* 1978;93:196–200.
142. Bates MD, Bucuvalas JC, Alonso MH, et al. Biliary atresia: pathogenesis and treatment. *Semin Liver Dis.* 1998;18:281–293.
143. Steele MI, Marshall CM, Lloyd RE, et al. Reovirus 3 not detected by reverse transcriptase-mediated polymerase chain reaction analysis of preserved tissue from infants with cholestatic liver disease. *Hepatology* 1995;21:697–702.
144. Schmeling DJ, Oldham KT, Guice KS, et al. Experimental obliterative cholangitis: a model for the study of biliary atresia. *Ann Surg.* 1991;213:350–355.
145. Ryckman FC, Alonso MH, Bucuvalas JC, et al. Biliary atresia—surgical management and treatment options as they relate to outcome. *Liver Transpl Surg.* 1998;4(5 suppl 1):S24–S33.
146. **Visser BC, Suh I, Hirose S, et al. The influence of portoenterostomy on transplantation for biliary atresia. *Liver Transpl.* 2004;10:1279–1286.**
147. **Davenport M, Puricelli V, Farrant P, et al. The outcome of the older (>100 days) infant with biliary atresia. *J Pediatr Surg.* 2004;4:575–581.**
148. Sartorelli KH, Holland RM, Allshouse MJ, et al. The intussusception antireflux valve is ineffective in preventing cholangitis in biliary atresia. *J Pediatr Surg.* 1996;31:403–406.
149. Ogasawara Y, Yamataka A, Tsukamoto K, et al. The intussusception antireflux valve is ineffective for preventing cholangitis in biliary atresia: a prospective study. *J Pediatr Surg.* 2003;38:1826–1829.
150. Kasai M, Suzuki H, Ohashi E, et al. Technique and results of operative management of biliary atresia. *World J Surg.* 1978;2:571–579.
151. Rothenberg SS, Schroter GP, Karrer FM, et al. Cholangitis after the Kasai operation for biliary atresia. *J Pediatr Surg.* 1989;24:729–732.
152. Dolgin, SE. Answered and unanswered controversies in the surgical management of extra hepatic biliary atresia. *Pediatr Transplant.* 2004;8:628–631.
153. Chardot C, Carton M, Spire-Bendelac N, et al. Prognosis of biliary atresia in the era of liver transplantation: French national study from 1986 to 1996. *Hepatology* 1999;30:606–611.
154. Goss JA, Shackleton CR, Swenson K, et al. Orthotopic liver transplantation for congenital biliary atresia: an 11-year, single-center experience. *Ann Surg.* 1996;224:276–284.
155. Alonso-Lej F, Revor WB, Pessagno DJ. Congenital choledochal cyst, with a report of 2, and an analysis of 94 cases. *Surg Gynecol Obstet.* 1959;108:1–30.
156. Todani T, Watanabe Y, Narusue M, et al. Congenital bile duct cysts: classification, operative procedures, and review of thirty-seven cases including cancer arising from choledochal cyst. *Am J Surg.* 1977;134:263–269.
157. Todani T, Tabuchi K, Watanabe Y, et al. Carcinoma arising in the wall of congenital bile duct cysts. *Cancer* 1979;44:1134–1141.
158. Komi N, Tamura T, Miyoshi Y, et al. Histochemical and immunohistochemical studies on development of biliary carcinoma in forty-seven patients with choledochal cyst—special reference to intestinal metaplasia in the biliary duct. *Jpn J Surg.* 1985;15:273–278.

159. Fieber SS, Nance FC. Choledochal cyst and neoplasm: a comprehensive review of 106 cases and presentation of two original cases. *Am Surg.* 1997;63:982–987.
160. Miyano T, Yamataka A, Kato Y, et al. Hepaticoenterostomy after excision of choledochal cyst in children: a 30-year experience with 180 cases. *J Pediatr Surg.* 1996;31:1417–1421.
161. Flanigan PD. Biliary cysts. *Ann Surg.* 1975;182:635–643.
162. Lipsett PA, Pitt HA, Colombani PM, et al. Choledochal cyst disease: a changing pattern of presentation. *Ann Surg.* 1994;220:644–652.
163. Werlin SL. Disorders of the pancreas in children. *Curr Opin Pediatr.* 1998;10:507–511.
164. Warshaw AL, Richter JM, Schapiro RH. The cause and treatment of pancreatitis associated with pancreas divisum. *Ann Surg.* 1983;198:443–452.
165. Warshaw AL, Simeone JF, Schapiro RH, et al. Evaluation and treatment of the dominant dorsal duct syndrome (pancreas divisum redefined). *Am J Surg.* 1990;159:59–64.
166. Adzick NS, Shamberger RC, Winter HS, et al. Surgical treatment of pancreas divisum causing pancreatitis in children. *J Pediatr Surg.* 1989;24:54–58.
167. Keith RG, Shapero TF, Saibil FG, et al. Dorsal duct sphincterotomy is effective long-term treatment of acute pancreatitis associated with pancreas divisum. *Surgery* 1989;106:660–666.
168. Kagan RJ, Reyes HM, Asokan S. Pseudocyst of the pancreas in childhood: current advances in diagnosis. *Arch Surg.* 1981;116:1200–1203.
169. Rescorla FJ, Plumley DA, Sherman S, et al. The efficacy of early ERCP in pediatric pancreatic trauma. *J Pediatr Surg.* 1995;30:336–340.
170. Cooney DR, Grosfeld JL. Operative management of pancreatic pseudocysts in infants and children: a review of 75 cases. *Ann Surg.* 1975;182:590–596.
171. Grosfeld JL, Vane DW, Rescorla FJ, et al. Pancreatic tumors in childhood: analysis of 13 cases. *J Pediatr Surg.* 1990;25:1057–1062.
172. Shamberger RC, Hendren WH, Leichtner AM. Long-term nutritional and metabolic consequences of pancreaticoduodenectomy in children. *Surgery* 1994;115:382–388.
173. Wang KS, Albanese C, Dada F, et al. Papillary cystic neoplasm of the pancreas: a report of three pediatric cases and literature review. *J Pediatr Surg.* 1998;33:842–845.
174. Wilson SD. Zollinger-Ellison syndrome in children: a 25-year follow-up. *Surgery* 1991;110:696–702.
175. Sempoux C, Poggi F, Brunelle F, et al. Nesidioblastosis and persistent neonatal hyperinsulinism. *Diabetes Metab.* 1995;21:402–407.
176. Aynsley-Green A, Polak JM, Bloom SR, et al. Nesidioblastosis of the pancreas: definition of the syndrome and the management of the severe neonatal hyperinsulinaemic hypoglycaemia. *Arch Dis Child.* 1981;56:496–508.
177. Hirsch HJ, Loo S, Evans N, et al. Hypoglycemia of infancy and nesidioblastosis: studies with somatostatin. *N Engl J Med.* 1977;296:1323–1326.
178. Fekete CN, de Lonlay P, Jaubert F, et al. The surgical management of congenital hyperinsulinemic hypoglycemia in infancy. *J Pediatr Surg.* 2004; 39:267–269.
179. Adzick NS, Thornton PS, Stanley CA, et al. A multidisciplinary approach to the focal form of congenital hyperinsulinism leads to successful treatment by partial pancreatectomy. *J Pediatr Surg.* 2004;39:270–275.
180. Warden MJ, German JC, Buckingham BA. The surgical management of hyperinsulinism in infancy due to nesidioblastosis. *J Pediatr Surg.* 1988;23:462–465.
181. Willberg B, Muller E. Surgery for nesidioblastosis—indications, treatment, and results. *Prog Pediatr Surg.* 1991;26:76–83.
182. Parashar K, Upadhyay V, Corkery JJ. Partial or near-total pancreatectomy for nesidioblastosis? *Eur J Pediatr Surg.* 1995;5:146–148.
183. Leibowitz G, Glaser B, Higazi AA, et al. Hyperinsulinemic hypoglycemia of infancy (nesidioblastosis) in clinical remission: high incidence of diabetes mellitus and persistent beta-cell dysfunction at long-term follow-up. *J Clin Endocrinol Metab.* 1995;80:386–392.
184. Grosfeld JL. Jejunoileal atresia and stenosis. In: O'Neill JA Jr, Rowe MI, Grosfeld JL, et al., eds. *Pediatric surgery,* 5th ed. St. Louis: Mosby, 1998, pp. 1145–1158.

CHAPTER 111 ■ PEDIATRIC GENITOURINARY SYSTEM

EUGENE MINEVICH AND CURTIS A. SHELDON

THE NEPHRIC SYSTEM

The nephric system develops progressively through three stages. The initial stage, *the pronephros*, disappears completely by the fourth week of embryonic life. *The mesonephros*, the second stage, degenerates as well, although part of it becomes associated with the reproductive system. The caudal portion of the mesonephric duct communicates with the cloaca and forms a ureteral bud between the fourth and sixth week of gestation. The cranial portion of the ureteral bud joins with the metanephric blastema, branching into the renal pelvis and the calyces and inducing nephron formation during the final stage of development, *metanephros*. The kidneys undergo ascent and rotation before assuming their final position.

ANOMALIES OF THE KIDNEYS

Supernumerary Kidney

The supernumerary kidney is a very rare anomaly of the urinary system and represents a distinct extra kidney (or kidneys). Embryologically, an additional ureteral bud develops a separate metanephric mass, resulting in the formation of an extra kidney, which is usually caudal to the dominant kidney. This anomaly is rarely discovered at birth. It is usually an incidental finding on abdominal imaging for unrelated reasons, although some adults occasionally present with abdominal pain, hypertension, or urinary tract infections (UTI).

Renal Agenesis

Absence of a ureteral bud or its failure to join the metanephric blastema results in renal agenesis. A bilateral anomaly occurs in approximately 1 per 4,000 births (*Potter's syndrome*). This is manifested by characteristic faces, pulmonary hypoplasia, and orthopedic abnormalities.[1] These infants are stillborn or rapidly die of respiratory failure.

The incidence of unilateral renal agenesis is about 1 in 1,200 births. The ipsilateral ureter is absent in more than 50% of cases, although an adrenal gland is usually present. The most common contralateral anomalies are vesicoureteral reflux (30%), renal malrotation, or renal ectopia (15%). Genital anomalies are more often observed in girls (25% to 50%) than in boys (10% to 15%); malformations of the rectum, anus, and lower spine frequently occur in both sexes. Other associated congenital anomalies may involve the cardiovascular, gastrointestinal or musculoskeletal systems. Unilateral renal agenesis is usually asymptomatic and found incidentally.

Renal Ectopy

Failure of the *metanephros* to ascend leads to an ectopic kidney, which occurs in about 1 in 1,100 people. An ectopic kidney may be on the ipsilateral side (*simple ectopy*) or on the contralateral side (*crossed ectopy*) with or without fusion. The adrenal gland develops separately from the kidney and is therefore found in its normal position, despite anomalies in renal position. Further classification of renal ectopia is based on the position of the kidney in the retroperitoneum: abdominal, lumbar, or pelvic kidney. Rarely, the kidney is located above the ipsilateral diaphragm (intrathoracic kidney) because of delayed closure of the diaphragm or accelerated kidney ascent.

Most ectopic kidneys are asymptomatic and detected incidentally. Almost half of ectopic kidneys have hydronephrosis secondary to malrotation, aberrant renal vessels compressing the renal pelvis, or ureteropelvic junction (UPJ) obstruction.[2] If surgical correction of the obstructed kidney is required, the anomalous renal vasculature may be important. Ectopic kidney function should be preserved because the contralateral kidney is abnormal in up to 50% of cases, with hydronephrosis or vesicoureteral reflux (VUR) most common. Genital anomalies have been reported in 15% to 45% of patients with renal ectopia.

Horseshoe Kidney

Horseshoe kidney is the most common renal fusion, occurring in 0.25% of population. Patients with Turner's syndrome and trisomy 18 have a significantly higher incidence. The anomaly consists of two renal masses connected by the isthmus at the midline, usually at the lower poles. The isthmus, which consists of renal parenchyma or fibrous tissue, lies just below the junction of the inferior mesenteric artery and aorta and anterior to the great vessels. The pelvises and ureters of horseshoe kidney are usually anteriorly placed, crossing the isthmus ventrally.

The horseshoe kidney does not usually produce symptoms unless it is associated with other anomalies. The most commonly associated abnormality is VUR and UPJ obstruction, which can lead to UTI or urolithiasis, with corresponding symptomatology. If surgical repair of UPJ obstruction is required, a standard dismembered pyeloplasty with or without division of the renal isthmus is recommended. The retroperitoneal flank approach is usually successful but the surgeon should be prepared for transperitoneal approach as well. The incidence of Wilms tumor seems to be increased in patients with horseshoe kidney.[3]

Cystic Disease of the Kidney

Renal cystic disease, congenital or acquired, is one of the most common causes of pediatric abdominal mass. Several classifications have been proposed, based on the clinical or radiological presentation, pathologic studies, and genetic associations.[4]

Autosomal recessive ("infantile") polycystic kidney disease results from dilated collecting ducts and has a spectrum of severity, with the severest forms appearing in infancy. This congenital disorder affects both kidneys and liver (ranging from biliary ectasia to congenital hepatic fibrosis). The affected infant usually presents with large flank masses. Renal ultrasound demonstrates enlarged, homogeneously hyperechogenic kidneys. Most children develop progressive renal or hepatic failure, or both. No cure has been found for this disease.

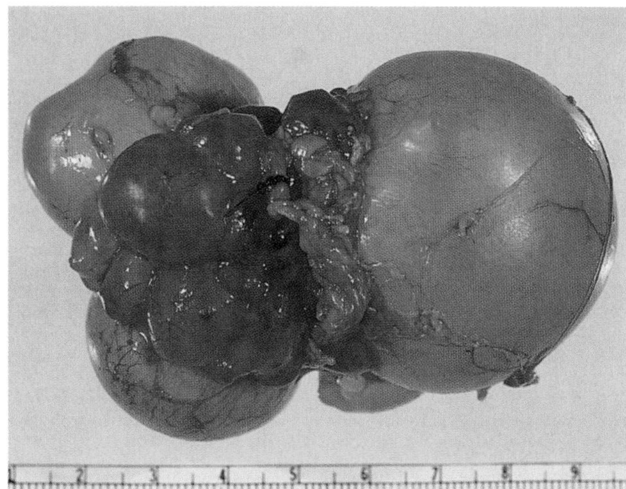

FIGURE 111.1 Multicystic dysplastic bladder. (From Rubin E, Farber JL. *Pathology*, 3rd ed. Philadelphia, Lippincott Williams & Wilkins, 1999, with permission.)

Multicystic dysplastic kidney (MCDK) is the most common type of renal cystic disease. This anomaly represents a severe form of renal dysplasia with complete replacement of renal parenchyma by different-sized cysts (Fig. 111.1). Renal ultrasound is usually definitive in making the correct diagnosis, although renal scintigraphy is necessary to demonstrate the absence of renal function in the involved kidney and occasionally differentiate MCDK from severe obstructed hydronephrosis. The high incidence of vesicoureteral reflux in the solitary functioning contralateral kidney (18% to 43%) makes a voiding cystourethrogram (VCUG) an essential part of the evaluation. Involution of MCDK may occur to the point that the involved kidney disappears from subsequent sonograms. Potential long-term sequelae of retained MCDK, including hypertension, infection and pain, are very rare. Sporadic reports of renal cell carcinoma and Wilms' tumor in MCDK raise concern of the persistent potential for malignant degeneration in the dysplastic kidney. The latest recommendation for management of the patient with MCDK is strict ultrasonic surveillance, especially in early childhood.[5] Nephrectomy is reserved for the patient with equivocal radiologic appearance, MCDK that fails to regress, or the patient who proves to be noncompliant with follow-up.[6]

Ureteropelvic Junction Obstruction

The UPJ is the most common site of obstruction in the urinary tract and the most common cause of neonatal hydronephrosis. The pathogenesis of this disorder is variable. Of the intrinsic factors, an adynamic segment is most often associated with classic UPJ obstruction. This obstruction is a congenital absence or abnormal arrangement of the muscular fiber at the transition zone of the upper ureter and renal pelvis leading to failure of peristaltic wave propagation. Extrinsic causes include fibrous bands, aberrant accessory vessels, and various organ-compressing factors. Most cases of UPJ obstruction are diagnosed *in utero* and such patients are initially asymptomatic. Some children present with abdominal or flank pain, hematuria, or UTI. Occasionally, previously asymptomatic UPJ

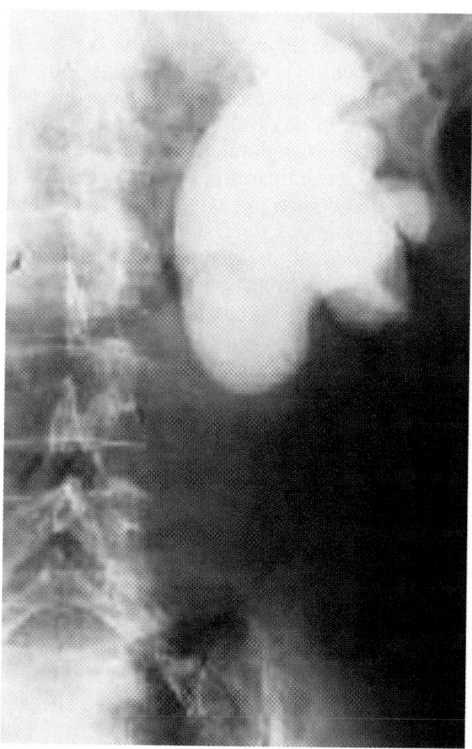

FIGURE 111.2 Intravenous pyelogram showing hydronephrosis secondary to ureteropelvic junction (UPJ) obstruction.

obstruction is discovered in the patient with renal injury following relatively minor abdominal trauma.

Renal ultrasound is the test of choice to determine the degree of renal pelvic dilatation, parenchymal thickness, and associated abnormalities of the bladder and the ureter. Diuretic renography and occasionally Whitaker antegrade pressure perfusion studies are necessary to confirm UPJ obstruction. The VCUG and occasional excretory urogram (intravenous pyelogram, or IVP) may define anatomic details (Fig. 111.2). Retrograde pyelography is used to rule out other causes of obstruction and is usually performed just before surgery.

A dismembered pyeloplasty, with removal of an adynamic segment, remains the surgical treatment of choice because it provides dependent drainage of the renal pelvis. With utilization of optical magnification and careful attention to surgical technique, a successful outcome is expected in over 95% of cases.[7]

ANOMALIES OF THE URETER

Ureteral Duplication

Ureteral duplication is the most common anomaly of the urinary tract. Early branching of the single ureteral bud results in *incomplete (partial) duplication* with a single ureteral orifice and bifid proximal ureters (1 in 125 individuals). An accessory ureteral bud creates *complete duplication* (1 in 500 individuals), with the upper ureter usually inserting into the bladder more medially and inferiorly than the lower ureter. The upper ureter is more likely to be associated with ectopic insertion, ureterocele, or obstruction, whereas the lower ureter is frequently associated with VUR. Most patients with ureteral duplication are asymptomatic, though they occasionally present with UTI.

Ureteral Ectopia and Ureterocele

The ectopic ureteral orifice lies in a position caudal to the normal insertion of the ureter on the bladder trigone. Ureteral ectopia is much more common in association with complete ureteral duplication. In the boy, ectopic ureteral orifices are most frequently found at the prostatic urethra and even along the course of the male genital ductal system. In the girl, ectopic ureters can be found draining into the bladder neck, urethra, vagina, or even the uterus. Boys with bilateral anomaly and girls with termination of an ectopic ureter below the external urinary sphincter usually present with urinary incontinence.

Ureteroceles are congenital cystic dilatations of the distal ureter. Those associated with a single ureter (simple ureterocele) are usually located in an orthotopic trigonal position. Ureteroceles found in association with duplicated ureters usually drain the upper pole kidney and are located in an ectopic position. Ectopic ureteroceles are commonly associated with obstruction and varying degrees of dysplasia of the affected renal segment. Decompression of the obstructed renal moiety from above (ureteropyelostomy) or from below (excision of ureterocele with ureteral reimplantation) is usually successful. Transurethral puncture of an ureterocele is usually reserved for infants, whereas a severely dysplastic moiety can be managed by partial nephrectomy. Large ureteroceles obstructing other renal moieties and the bladder neck will most likely require secondary procedures to restore normal urinary tract anatomy.[8]

Vesicoureteral Reflux

Vesicoureteral reflux refers to the retrograde passage of urine from the bladder into the ureter. The incidence of VUR in otherwise normal children is approximately 1%; a much higher incidence of up to 40% is reported in patients undergoing evaluation for UTI. A significant familial association has been encountered. A sufficient tunnel length of submucosal ureter is the most important component of the competent ureterovesical junction. This provides a predominantly passive valve mechanism compression of the ureter, preventing retrograde passage of urine. Marginal tunnel pressure can be made to reflux primarily or secondarily because of loss of compliance of the valve roof (during UTI), structural weakness of the detrusor floor (bladder diverticulum, ureterocele), or excessively high intravesical pressure caused by neurovesical dysfunction or bladder outlet obstruction. VUR is graded according to the International Classification System based on the proximal extent of retrograde urine flow, ureteral and pelvic dilatation, and the resultant anatomy of the calyceal fornices.

Reflux-induced renal injury is usually caused by the association of VUR with UTI and may range from clinically silent focal scar formation to generalized scarring and renal atrophy (reflux nephropathy) with hypertension and even end-stage renal failure. Children of either sex should be investigated at the time of the initial infection. The diagnosis of VUR is accomplished by cyclic VCUG, with either contrast medium or isotope (Fig. 111.3). Imaging of the upper tracts (kidneys and ureters) is extremely important and can be accomplished by ultrasonography, isotope renography or, rarely, intravenous urography. Ultrasonography is helpful in quantifying renal growth or atrophy, whereas isotope renography is particularly sensitive in detecting focal scarring. Patients with voiding dysfunction should be considered strongly for urodynamic studies.

Because the submucosal ureter tends to lengthen with age, the ratio of tunnel length to ureteral diameter increases, and

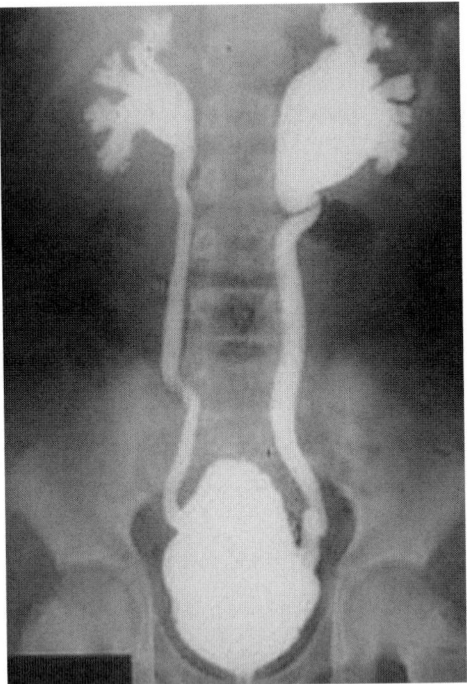

FIGURE 111.3 Voiding cystourethrogram of bilateral vesicoureteral reflux (VUR).

the propensity for reflux may disappear. In general, a lower reflux grade correlated with a better chance of spontaneous resolution. Nonoperative management of VUR (which is successful in most patients) requires prevention of UTI with suppression antibiotics, treatment of symptomatic voiding dysfunction, and long-term strict surveillance. Patients with breakthrough UTIs, significant renal injury, high-grade reflux, pubertal age, or who fail to respond to 4 to 5 years of suppression therapy may require surgical correction. The principle of open ureteral reimplantation is the creation of a capacious subepithelial tunnel with the ratio of its length to ureteral diameter equal to 5:1. In general, excellent results are attained with most open intravesical or extravesical procedures. The extravesical approach, which preserves the integrity of the bladder lumen as well as not requiring an ureteral anastomosis, eliminates postoperative hematuria, minimizes bladder spasms, decreases the risk of postoperative obstruction, and shortens hospital stay.[9] Since the initial report of successful endoscopic subureteral injection of polytetrafluoroethylene (Teflon) for correction of VUR, this minimally invasive technique has been widely used worldwide with different injectable materials. The most promising injectable substance to date is dextranomer/hyaluronic acid copolymer (Deflux).[10]

Megaureter

The term megaureter refers to an enlarged ureter, of which there are four categories: refluxing, obstructing, refluxing or obstructing, and nonrefluxing or nonobstructing with an additional subdivision of each group into primary or secondary. Most patients are asymptomatic with an incidental finding of hydroureteronephrosis on screening renal ultrasound. The most common clinical presentation is UTI. The VCUG is necessary to rule out VUR, although its presence does not exclude the possibility of a coexistent obstruction. Diuretic renography is helpful to establish the presence of ureteral obstruction, which is usually at the level of ureterovesical junction.

Megaureter secondary to severe VUR or obstruction is usually managed with ureteral reimplantation to prevent deterioration of renal function. Reduction of ureteral caliber by excision of the distal redundant ureter to achieve a satisfactory antireflux mechanism is usually necessary. Patients without reflux or obstruction may demonstrate radiographic improvement of the megaureter with preservation of renal function without surgical intervention. Therefore, initial nonoperative management with close follow-up of patients with nonobstructing or nonrefluxing megaureters is advisable.[11]

VESICOURETHRAL SYSTEM

The cloaca forms from the blind caudal end of the hindgut. The division of the cloaca by the urorectal septum into a ventral portion—the urogenital sinus (UGS)—and a dorsal portion (rectum) is completed by the seventh week of gestation. Simultaneously, the mesodermal growth of the lower abdominal wall separates the umbilical cord from the genital tubercle. The mesonephric duct and ureteral bud have independent opening sites. The mesonephric duct (which will become the ejaculatory duct) migrates downward and medially, whereas the opening of ureteral bud (which will become the ureteral orifice) migrates upward and laterally. The UGS can be divided into two segments at the point where the müllerian ducts join the dorsal wall of the UGS. The ventral portion forms the bladder, part of the prostatic urethra in male, and the entire female urethra. The caudal portion gives rise to a portion of the prostatic and the entire membranous urethra in males and forms the lower part of vagina and the vaginal vestibule in females.

ANOMALIES OF THE BLADDER

Urachal Abnormality

Embryologically, the urachus represents the apical attachment of the cloaca to the allantois. During fetal development it is obliterated and eventually represented by a fibrous retroperitoneal cord extending from the dome of the bladder to the umbilicus. Symptomatic urachal anomalies are rare and clinical syndromes most often arise from a patent urachus or an urachal cyst. The former condition is suggested by a persistently wet umbilicus and may be seen in patients with bladder outlet obstruction. Excision of the urachus with bladder closure is usually necessary.

The urachal cyst is an inclusion cyst lined with transitional epithelium. If infected, it can present with abdominal pain and tenderness as well as fever, nausea, and leucocytosis, closely mimicking the acute abdomen. Radiologic evaluation should include abdominal ultrasound, computed tomography (CT), or both. The infected urachal cyst is best managed by initial drainage of the abscess and delayed excision of the urachal remnant. Exploratory laparotomy is indicated if signs of peritonitis are present[12] (Algorithm 111.1).

Exstrophy–Epispadias Complex

The overgrowth and delayed rupture of the cloacal membrane prevents medial mesenchymal migration and proper lower abdominal wall development. Depending on the extent of the infraumbilical defect and the stage of development at which rupture occurs, bladder exstrophy, epispadias or cloacal exstrophy results.

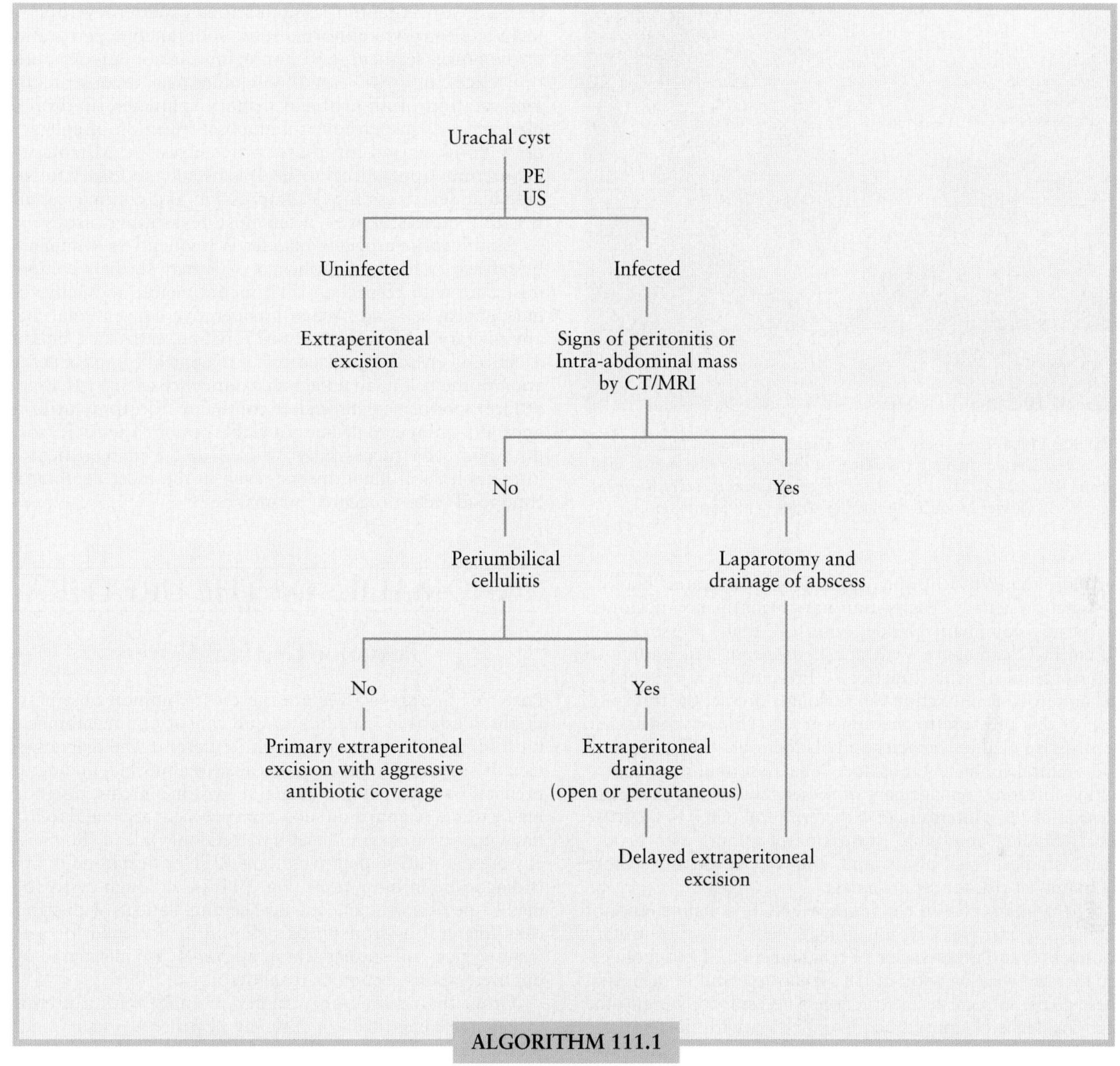

ALGORITHM 111.1 Surgical management of urachal cyst. PE, physical examination. US, ultrasound. (After Minevich E, Wacksman J, Lewis AG, et al. The infected urachal cyst: primary excision versus a staged approach. *J Urol.* 1997;157:1869, with permission.)

Epispadias in boys, as an isolated defect, consists of a dorsally placed urethral meatus and the degree of penile deformity is related to the extent of the meatal displacement. Most often, epispadias are associated with exstrophy of the bladder (Fig. 111.4). This defect usually involves pubic diastasis with separation of the rectus abdominis muscles, inguinal hernias, and anterior displacement of the anus. Male external genitalia have a characteristic epispadiac appearance, whereas females have a bifid clitoris with a stenotic and short vagina. Complete primary closure of the bladder plate with simultaneous repair of epispadias within the first 72 hours of life is the most appropriate treatment of this complicated anomaly.[13]

Cloacal exstrophy is the most severe defect that can occur in the formation of the ventral abdominal wall. Anatomically, there is exstrophy of the shortened hindgut or cecum, which displays its bulging mucosa between the two hemibladders. There is no anus or rectum, and omphalocele is present (Fig. 111.5). The initial surgical approach (in the neonatal period) includes closure of omphalocele, separation of the bladder from the bowel, and closure of the bladder. Considerable reconstructive surgery remains to be done later to restore acceptable anatomic appearance and functioning urinary and intestinal tracts.

Neurogenic Bladder

An abnormal spinal column development affecting spinal cord function (myelodysplasia) is the most common cause of neurogenic bladder (NGB) in children. Myelomeningocele accounts

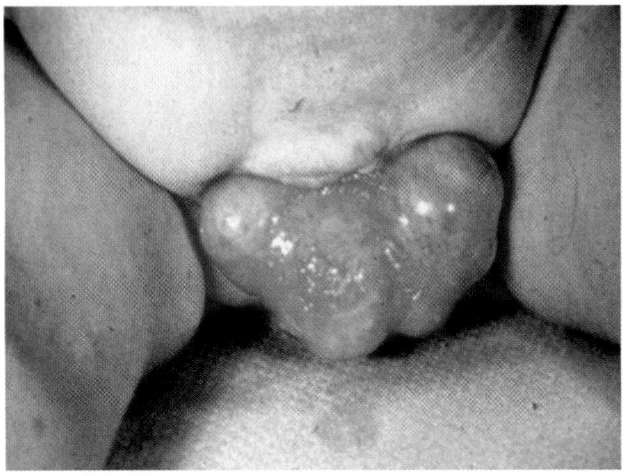

FIGURE 111.4 Exstrophy of the urinary bladder. The bladder mucosa is everted through the defect in the anterior abdominal wall. (From Weiss MA, Mills SE. *Atlas of genitourinary tract diseases.* New York: Gower Medical Publishing, 1988, with permission.)

for more than 90% of open spinal dysraphic states. Bladder dysfunction usually results in urinary incontinence, although the poorly compliant bladder with leak point pressure over 40 cm H_2O can cause VUR and hydronephrosis, leading to deterioration of renal function.[14] Presumably at this point, the ureterovesical junction can no longer protect the transmission of this pressure to the upper tracts. Urinary continence depends on bladder capacity and bladder outlet (bladder neck and urethral sphincter) resistance. The most important contribution affecting management of these children was the introduction of clean intermittent catheterization (CIC) to facilitate timely bladder emptying. Evaluation of infants with urodynamic studies, renal ultrasound, and VCUG identifies those ultimately at risk for renal damage.

The primary goal in children with NGB is maintenance of safe intravesical pressure, the ultimate achievement of urinary continence, and preservation of renal function. If anticholinergic therapy with or without CIC is unsuccessful in achieving these goals, surgical reconstruction is necessary. Owing to the high incidence of upper tract deterioration with time and the significant sequelae of altered body image following cutaneous urinary diversion, incontinent diversion is no longer considered an acceptable alternative to reconstruction in the pediatric population. The goals of reconstructive surgery are to achieve a large capacity, low-pressure reservoir, adequate bladder outlet resistance, and easy access for catheterization. A variety of donor tissues sources, including bowel segments, stomach or ureter, are available for bladder augmentation (Fig. 111.6). Potential complications of enterocystoplasty include electrolyte abnormalities, spontaneous perforation of the bowel segment, and tumor formation. Bladder outlet resistance can be increased by bladder neck reconstruction, implantation of an artificial urinary sphincter, urethral or bladder neck suspension, submucosal injection of collagen, or a combination of these procedures. A Mitrofanoff neourethra (appendiceal or ileal) is usually necessary to provide bladder access for decompression and continence, and is highly successful in even the most devastating cases.[15]

Significant neurogenic bladder is frequently accompanied by refractory fecal incontinence. This may severely compromise care with respect to UTI, incontinence, and achieving independent self-care. When preoperative conventional therapy (dietary modification, timed toileting, cathartics, bulking agents and enemas) is unsuccessful to control complete evacuation of the colon, an antegrade continence enema (ACE procedure), performed through a continent cecostomy utilizing appendix or tapered ileum, is a viable option. The ACE procedure has been successfully utilized in the management of intractable fecal incontinence, even in the most debilitating childhood recto-urogenital anomalies.[16]

ANOMALIES OF THE URETHRA

Posterior Urethral Valves

Posterior urethral valves are the most common obstructive urethral lesions in male infants and consist of a membrane or mucosal leaflet within the prostatic urethra. The diagnosis is usually suspected in neonates because of abnormal findings on prenatal hydronephrosis (bilateral hydronephrosis, distended bladder) and oligohydramnios. Some of them are found to have flank masses, ascites, and urinary retention. Older children usually present with voiding symptoms, UTI, or hematuria. VCUG is diagnostic in most cases (Fig. 111.7), although cystoscopy may be necessary in an equivocal setting. Patients with significant bilateral hydronephrosis should be screened for renal insufficiency, and nuclear scintigraphy may be indicated to rule out ureteral obstruction or renal dysplasia.

Other than temporary urinary drainage with a urethral catheter (feeding tube), in critically ill patients primary endoscopic valve ablation is the preferred approach and can be accomplished safely in most instances. Initial temporary cutaneous vesicostomy is useful in occasional circumstances. High upper urinary tract diversion may on rare occasion be necessary in infants who demonstrate a rising creatinine level despite a lower tract drainage. Long-term follow-up is necessary, with special attention directed to the possible development of a poorly compliant, high-pressure bladder.[17] Careful urodynamic

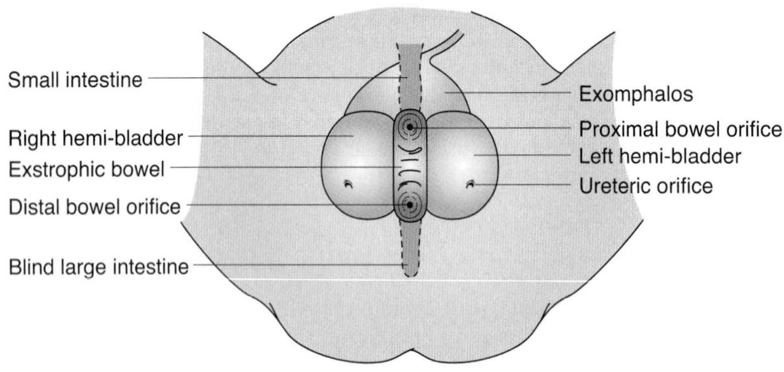

FIGURE 111.5 Diagram depicting cloacal exstrophy.

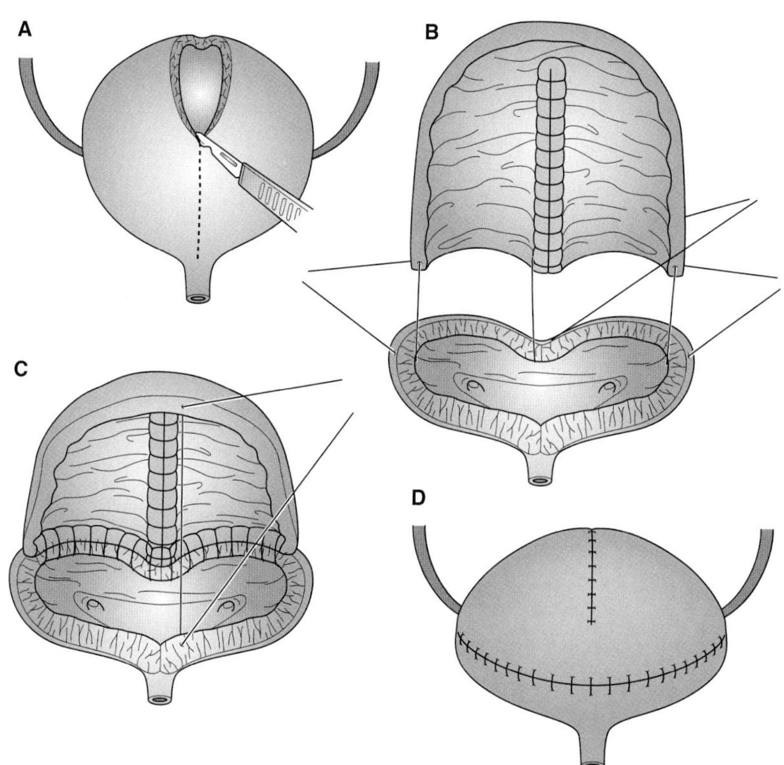

FIGURE 111.6 Bladder augmentation employing an intestinal segment. (*A*) The bladder is opened as a "clam shell." (*B*) The intestinal segment is detubularized by longitudinal incision along the antimesenteric border. A cup-patch is fashioned by suturing one edge of the resultant rectangle to itself. (*C*) The cup-patch is sutured to the remnant bladder plate. (*D*) Final appearance. (After Sheldon CA and Bukowski T. Bladder function. In: Rowe MI, O'Neal JA, Grosfeld JL, et al., eds. *Essentials of pediatric surgery*. St. Louis: Mosby-Year Book, 1995, with permission.)

evaluation and timely treatment of the "valve bladder" with anticholinergics, CIC, and very selective vesical reconstruction (including enterocystoplasty) as well as prevention of UTI ensure the best chance for successful prevention or management of chronic renal failure.

Hypospadias

Hypospadias is a common congenital defect resulting from incomplete tubularization of the urethral plate and closure of the genital folds. The cause of this anomaly is unknown, but is probably related to inadequate androgenization before the 20th week of gestation. The meatus can be located anywhere from the perineum to the glans penis, although in more than 85% of cases it is distal to the midshaft. Typically, the ventral prepuce is deficient and ventral penile chordee occurs more frequently with proximal hypospadias.

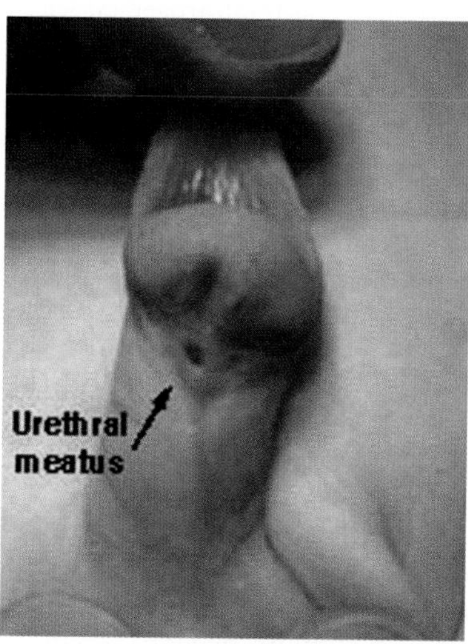

FIGURE 111.7 Voiding cystourethrogram showing dilated posterior urethra secondary to posterior urethral valves.

Principles of hypospadias repair include meticulous surgical technique with sufficient optical magnification to advance the urethral meatus to a normal glanular position and to correct penile chordee, if necessary. Numerous operations have been described for surgical correction of hypospadias and the surgeon treating this anomaly should be familiar with all possible approaches. An outpatient one-stage procedure can be safely performed after 6 months of age in most cases. Whereas local skin flaps are used in repairs of more distal hypospadias, vascularized preputial pedicle flaps or a tube-graft may be necessary in more proximal hypospadias. Patients with hypospadias should not be circumcised until an experienced pediatric urologist evaluates them. If sufficient penile skin is not available, bladder mucosal or buccal mucosal grafts can be utilized. Although rare, complications after hypospadias surgery include urethrocutaneous fistula, urethral strictures, and meatal stenosis.

GENITAL SYSTEM

The development of the genital tract follows a sequential pattern and is initially determined by chromosomal composition of the fertilizing sperm, resulting in 46 XY (male genotype) or 46 XX zygote (female genotype). The genetic material necessary for the development of the testis is found on the short arm of the Y chromosome and is known as the SRY gene. The presence of this gene determines an aggregation of primitive indifferent germ cells and Sertoli cells into the testicular cord. Thereafter, the endocrine effect on sexual development is most crucial in male phenotype development. Testosterone, produced by Leydig cells, result in *wolffian duct* (remnant of mesonephric duct) differentiation into the vas deferens, the seminal vesicles, and the epididymis. In addition, testosterone converted at the end-organ target sites to dihydrotestosterone (DHT) by 5a-reductase, regulates the virilization of the urogenital sinus and external genitalia around the ninth week of gestation. Only at this point, the previously indifferent genital tubercle starts to differentiate into a penis while the genital swelling fuses to form the scrotum. At the same time, müllerian-inhibiting substance (MIS) produced by testicular Sertoli cells results in an almost complete regression of the müllerian ducts.

In the absence of the SRY gene, the primitive gonads differentiate into an ovary. The female development of the müllerian (paramesonephric) duct system into fallopian tube, uterus, and cervix; the feminization of the external genitalia; and involution of the wolffian ducts are automatic processes in the absence of testosterone and MIS.

AMBIGUOUS GENITALIA

The term *ambiguous genitalia* refers to genitalia in the spectrum of sexual development that are not clearly male or female. This situation represents a true medical and social emergency. Rapid but careful determination of the genetic composition, gonadal sex, and genitourinary anatomy of the affected newborn is essential to enable gender assignment, acceptance of the child by the family, and ultimately surgical reconstruction.

The condition of patients with ambiguous genitalia can be divided into four categories: female and male pseudohermaphroditism, true hermaphroditism, and gonadal dysgenesis. Table 111.1 lists the elements of complete evaluation of the infant with ambiguous genitalia. Occasionally diagnostic laparoscopy and gonadal biopsy are necessary to guide the gender assignment. After the chromosomal and gonadal composition is established, sex assignment is determined, based mostly on the potential for sexual function. Surgical reconstruction is aimed at matching the external genitalia to the gender assigned to the child and is usually undertaken at 6 to 12 months of age.[18]

Female Pseudohermaphroditism

Female pseudohermaphroditism is the largest diagnostic category and, within this category, the leading cause is congenital adrenal hyperplasia (CAH). CAH results from a deficiency in the enzymes responsible for the synthesis of mineralocorticosteroids and glucocorticosteroids, resulting in overproduction of adrenal androgens. A deficiency of 21-hydroxylase represents 95% of patients with CAH. All of these patients are genetic females (46, XX karyotype, ovarian gonads) with masculinization of the external genitalia ranging from an enlarged clitoris to a normal appearing male phallus with complete labial fusion (Fig. 111.8). These patients are potentially fertile regardless of how severe the degree of virilization.

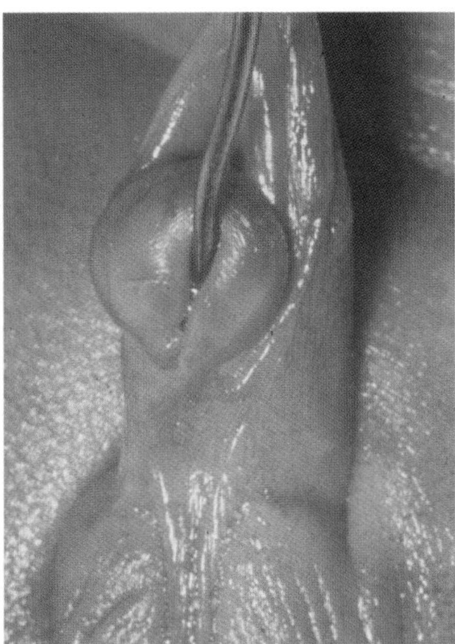

FIGURE 111.8 Severe masculinization of the external genitalia in a girl with congenital adrenal hyperplasia (CAH).

A high index of suspicion allows for early diagnosis of this condition and initiation of hormonal replacement (glucocorticosteroids and mineralocorticosteroids) to prevent adrenal insufficiency, salt-wasting syndrome, and continued virilization. Because internal müllerian structures are always present, these children are reared as females and feminizing genitoplasty is performed to correct the cosmetic and functional deformities of external genitalia. If the vagina enters the urogenital sinus distally, a cutback or flap vaginoplasty can be combined with clitoroplasty (reduction and relocation of the clitoris with preservation of glanular sensation) and labioplasty in a single procedure. If the vagina enters the urogenital sinus more proximally, a total urogenital sinus mobilization, pedicle skin flap, or a segmental bowel interposition vaginoplasty is deferred to a later date.

TABLE 111.1 DIAGNOSIS

EVALUATION OF AMBIGUOUS GENITALIA

- Thorough physical examination (special attention to palpable gonads, phallic structure, vaginal orifice, and anus)
- Complete family history (genital anomalies in other family members, unexplained neonatal death in previous children)
- Evaluation of the pregnancy (especially maternal exposure to androgenic agents)
- Blood karyotype
- Biochemical evaluation (serum electrolytes, adrenal steroids and precursors, serum gonadotropins, and testosterone)
- Radiologic evaluation (renal and pelvic ultrasound, genitogram)

Male Pseudohermaphroditism

Male pseudohermaphrodites are genetic males (46XY) with decreased virilization of the external genitalia. This anomaly can result from abnormal testosterone synthesis, 5a-reductase deficiency leading to decreased levels of DHT, and androgen insensitivity syndrome (defect of the androgen receptor). The phallic structure may be inadequate for the male gender role. In this setting, consideration should be given to female gender assignment.

Testicular feminization syndrome (complete androgen insensitivity) is the most common form of male pseudohermaphroditism, although affected individuals appear as normal phenotypic females with a short vagina. They are usually diagnosed at puberty with primary amenorrhea, although infrequently diagnosis is made during routine childhood herniorrhaphy, at which time testes are found. Bilateral gonadectomy is indicated because of increased risk of gonadoblastoma development in the intraabdominal testis. It can be delayed till puberty in selected cases. Short vagina can be managed with vaginal dilatation but vaginal reconstruction or vaginal replacement will be necessary in some patients.

True Hermaphroditism

In true hermaphroditism, patients have both ovarian and testicular tissue (ovary and testis, ovotestis, or a combination of these). True hermaphroditism is the rarest form of intersex abnormality. The internal genital structures conform with the ipsilateral gonad. The most common karyotype is 46XX, although mosaicism and a 46XY karyotype may be seen as well. The appearance of external genitalia varies widely. After gender is assigned, gonadal tissue of the opposite sex is removed and surgical reconstruction is undertaken.

Mixed Gonadal Dysgenesis

Mixed gonadal dysgenesis is the second most frequent cause of genital ambiguity. Most neonates with this condition exhibit a 45XO/46XY mosaic karyotype. They generally present with a dysgenetic testis on one side and a streak of gonads on the other. The appearance of external genitalia is variable; however, most are poorly virilized and consequently most infants will be raised as females. Appropriate genital reconstruction is required. Early gonadectomy is indicated because of the high risk of malignant degeneration (gonadoblastoma, seminoma, and dysgerminoma) of the dysgenetic gonad.

ANOMALIES OF MALE GENITALIA

Anomalies of the Foreskin

At birth, the prepuce is retractable in only 4% of boys. No special care of the uncircumcised penis is required. During the first years of life, spontaneous separation occurs physiologically in most boys secondary to intermittent erections and epithelialization of the inner prepuce. It is unnecessary to retract the prepuce on any routine basis to promote retractability or to hasten physiologic separation. This usually results in pain, bleeding, and, occasionally, paraphimosis.

Much confusion exists as to the indications for neonatal circumcision. The most important arguments are those of custom and tradition. In infants, circumcision may be performed using the Gomko clamp under local penile block. The most important principles of neonatal circumcision are complete lysis of penile adhesions, adequate but not excessive excision of outer and inner preputial layers, hemostasis, and protection of the glans penis.

Truly pathologic phimosis, paraphimosis, and recurrent balanitis are definitive indications for circumcision. It is estimated that as many as 18% of uncircumcised boys may develop one of the aforementioned indications by 8 years of age. Phimosis is a fibrotic contraction of the foreskin preventing its retraction over the glans. This pathologic condition should be differentiated from physiologic phimosis of infancy. Paraphimosis is the entrapment of a phimotic prepuce proximal to the coronal sulcus. The skin ring causes venous congestion initially but as the condition progresses, arterial occlusion and necrosis of the glans penis may occur. If persistent manual compression does not reduce paraphimosis, emergency circumcision or the creation of a dorsal slit is indicated. Circumcision in infancy undoubtedly prevents cancer of the penis. If the decision is made not to circumcise a male infant, there must be a life time commitment to genital hygiene to minimize the risks of developing penile cancer. Circumcision should be encouraged in boys with a history of UTI, VUR, or other urinary abnormalities to decrease the chance of ascending infection. Patients with hypospadias, penile chordee, penile torsion, epispadias, buried penis, or megalourethra are not candidates for routine circumcision. A sufficient amount of foreskin must be available to correct these conditions.

Cryptorchidism

Descend of the testis from its original position near the kidney into the cooler scrotum is necessary for its normal development and production of fertile sperm. Various mechanisms, including gubernacular traction and intraabdominal pressure, have been proposed to be responsible for testicular descent, but endocrine factors of the hypothalamic-pituitary-testicular axis also play a major role in this process. Between the 12th and 17th weeks of gestation, the testis undergoes transabdominal migration to a location near the internal inguinal ring. It is not until the seventh month of gestation that transinguinal migration of the testis to its final position takes place.

True undescended testes fail to reach the scrotum despite following a normal line of descent. Ectopic testes follow the usual course of descent until they emerge from the external inguinal ring, but are then misdirected to an ectopic position (superficial inguinal pouch, perineal, femoral, transverse scrotal). Although approximately 3.4% of full-term boys have undescended testes, 30% of premature infants have this anomaly. By 1 year of age, the incidence of cryptorchidism is about 1% and remains at this level thereafter. Actually, most cryptorchid testes descending during the first year of life do so within the first 3 months after birth. The diagnosis of cryptorchidism relies on gentle and patient genital examination. Relaxation of the patient and warming of the examiner's hand aid in successful examination. Reexamination of the child in the cross-legged position may also reveal the gonad. A functional classification that provides a practical approach to therapy is based on whether the testis is palpable or impalpable (20%). Whereas endocrine testing is reliable in predicting bilateral anorchidism, radiologic means, including abdominal sonography, CT, magnetic resonance imaging, or gonadal arteriography, are inaccurate in localization of nonpalpable testes. Diagnostic laparoscopy will provide diagnosis of vanishing testis by identification of blind-ending spermatic vessels or accurate localization of the intraabdominal testis in this situation.[19] Undescended testes must be distinguished from retractile testes that may reside above the scrotum but, with careful positioning, can be made to stay within the lower scrotum without continuous traction.

Although the correction of undescended testes eliminates any coexisting inguinal hernia (found in 95% of cases) and prevents possible testicular injury or torsion (the risk of which is increased in these patients), the central issues in managing these patients revolve around future fertility and the risk of developing a testicular neoplasm. There is an increased risk of testicular carcinoma in undescended testes and orchidopexy facilitates self-examination and early detection of the cancer. Because germ cell count of the infant undescended testis deteriorates after 1 year of life, correction of cryptorchidism is indicated between 6 and 12 months of age. For palpable undescended testes, routine inguinal orchidopexy is successful in most patients. For high intraabdominal testes, testicular microsurgical autotransplantation[20] provides the highest success rate among different surgical options.[21]

Torsion of the Testis and Appendages

Torsion of the testicle is classified as a surgical emergency because it causes strangulation of gonadal blood supply with subsequent testicular necrosis and atrophy. Testicular salvage is likely if the duration of torsion is less than 6 to 8 hours.[22] Torsion presenting in the neonatal period most commonly develops prenatally in the spermatic cord proximal to the attachments of the tunica vaginalis (extravaginal torsion). Although possible at any age, testicular torsion is most common in adolescents, being distal to the insertion of the tunica vaginalis (intravaginal torsion). A bell-clapper deformity predisposes to this condition.

Prenatal torsion presents with a firm, hard scrotal mass that does not transilluminate in an otherwise asymptomatic newborn male. Salvage of the testis is extremely rare,[23] but timely surgical exploration is indicated to anchor the contralateral testis, because bilateral (synchronous or asynchronous) neonatal testicular torsion has been described. In older boys, sudden onset of severe testicular pain followed by scrotal swelling is the classic presentation of testicular torsion. On physical examination, a swollen, tender testis with shortening of the cord is noticed. If testicular torsion is clinically suspected, an immediate surgical scrotal exploration is indicated. A negative exploration of the scrotum is more acceptable than the loss of a testis that might have been salvaged. In situations with a low suspicion of testicular torsion, scrotal color Doppler ultrasound or testicular nuclear scan can be helpful to differentiate torsion from acute epididymitis. At surgical exploration, the testis is untwisted and observed for viability. A frankly necrotic testis is removed, whereas viable gonads (return of color, return of Doppler flow, signs of arterial blood after incision of tunica albuginea) are fixed to the scrotal wall to prevent subsequent torsion. Exploration and anchoring of the contralateral testis, which can be done through the same incision, is mandatory to prevent its subsequent torsion. Manual detorsion of the torsed testis is usually difficult because of acute pain during manipulation but, if successful (and confirmed by color Doppler ultrasound in a patient with complete resolution of symptoms), definitive surgical fixation of the testes should be performed before the patient leaves the hospital as an urgent rather than emergency procedure.

The testicular appendix, a müllerian duct remnant, is the most common genital appendage susceptible to torsion. Although frequently presenting with symptoms similar to testicular torsion, this condition can usually be diagnosed by a finding of a tender focal induration or a blue dot near the upper pole of the testis. Appendix testis torsion is best managed by several days of bedrest and oral preventive antibiotics. If a reliable diagnosis cannot be made, scrotal color Doppler ultrasound or even surgical exploration is indicated to rule out testicular torsion.

Prepubertal Testicular Tumor

In boys presenting with a painless palpable scrotal mass, a testicular tumor should be included in the differential diagnosis. Prepubertal testis tumors account for approximately 2% of all testicular tumors, with a peak patient age of approximately 2 years. The most common lesion is a yolk sac tumor, which is a variant of embryonal cell carcinoma. When spread occurs, it is usually a hematogenous spread to the lungs and, less commonly, lymphatic spread to the retroperitoneal nodes. Scrotal ultrasound is usually definitive in visualizing an intratesticular mass, whereas abdominal and chest CT scans are necessary for metastatic evaluation. Tumor markers (α-fetoprotein and β-human chorionic gonadotropin [β-HCG]) are helpful for initial evaluation and also during follow-up. In young children, prognosis is excellent and the radical inguinal orchiectomy is the initial treatment. Retroperitoneal lymph node dissection and multidrug chemotherapy are necessary in cases of disseminating disease. In the absence of metastasis or elevated tumor marker levels, the applicability of these treatment modalities remains controversial.

Varicocele

Varicocele is a dilation of the veins of the spermatic cord and is reported to occur at a 15% incidence in adolescent boys, which correlates with that in general male population. In most adolescents the varicocele is grade I, whereas in 35% it is grade II or III. Varicocele is generally visible or palpable in the upright position. Most urologists agree that scrotal discomfort and ipsilateral testicular growth failure are reliable indications for varicocele surgery in this population. Additionally, some authors have advocated surgical repair in patients demonstrating a progressive increase in varicocele size, bilateral varicoceles, or a large varicocele associated with a change in testicular consistency. Incisional surgery with an inguinal, retroperitoneal, or modified approach is the basis of varicocelectomy in adolescents. The optical magnification allows reliable identification and preservation of the testicular artery and lymphatics during ligation of the venous channels. As a result, the postoperative development of hydrocele or recurrence of the varicocele may be prevented.[24]

VAGINAL ANOMALIES AND UROGENITAL SINUS MALFORMATIONS

The urogenital sinus is apparent by 6 weeks of gestation. After it receives the fused müllerian ducts, the distal potion of UGS forms the lower third of the vagina, whereas the fused müllerian ducts form the upper two thirds of vagina and uterus. Although most vaginal anomalies occur in conjunction with intersex disorders, isolated vaginal anomalies or those occurring in association with a urogenital sinus are also seen (Table 111.2). Vaginal agenesis may occur in isolation or as a component of the Mayer-Rokitansky syndrome, which refers to normal phenotypic females with vaginal and occasional uterine dysgenesis. Because the distal vagina is normally formed in most of these patients, the diagnosis is not usually made until puberty, at which time the patient presents with amenorrhea. Approximately one third of these patients have urologic anomalies, the most common being unilateral renal agenesis. Vaginoplasty is indicated in almost all patients and depends on the anatomy present. Several techniques using tubularized skin flaps, skin grafts, and bowel segments have been described for vaginal reconstruction.[25] Careful preoperative counseling and evaluation of patient's and parents' motivation are essential for a good result because

TABLE 111.2 CLASSIFICATION

CLASSIFICATION OF VAGINAL ANOMALIES

Vaginal agenesis
Urogenital sinus
Duplication anomalies
Canalization anomalies
Cloacal anomalies
Intersex or isolated

long-term vaginal dilatation is occasionally required until the patient is old enough to participate in sexual intercourse.

Urogenital sinus anomalies occur because of a failure of the urethra and the vagina to separate. These children have two perineal openings, including the anus, because the rectum is usually normal. Many of these girls have some degree of bladder dysfunction and CIC may be necessary. If CIC of the bladder is not possible, temporary vesicostomy may be indicated. To separate the urethral and vaginal orifices, urethral lengthening or vaginal pull-through procedures are required.[25–27]

OTHER GENITOURINARY DISORDERS

Eagle-Barrett Syndrome

The Eagle-Barrett syndrome, also referred to as prune-belly syndrome (PBS) is a set of genitourinary malformations with a deficiency or absence of the abdominal wall musculature accompanied by a broad spectrum of associated organ system anomalies. It was theorized that delayed canalization of the urethral membrane resulted in a temporary total urinary obstruction causing massive dilatation of the ureters, a large bladder frequently associated with a patent urachus, and a dilated proximal urethra with hypoplastic prostate. The wrinkled, prunelike skin of the abdominal wall in the newborn is a characteristic manifestation. Renal dysplasia is frequently seen and in severe cases it is associated with pulmonary hypoplasia, resulting in stillbirth or death in the neonatal period. Bilateral cryptorchidism with intraabdominal testes is a characteristic feature of PBS. Extraurinary problems are associated with this syndrome in 73% of patients and usually involve defects of the cardiovascular, musculoskeletal, respiratory, or central nervous systems.[28] Because the dilatation of the urinary tract is usually nonobstructive, a favorable outcome in these patients can be expected with a conservative approach of observation, prevention of UTI, and surgical drainage, with reconstruction only being performed when absolutely required.

Urologic Implications of Imperforate Anus

Anorectal malformations (ARM) encompass a broad spectrum of abnormalities of termination of the hindgut and urogenital sinus, ranging from the simple covered anus to complex cloacal malformations involving the gastrointestinal, urinary, and genital tracts. Morbidity and mortality in these cases are largely attributed to associated structural and functional genitourinary anomalies, ranging from vesicoureteral reflux (57%) to renal dysplasia and agenesis (65%). Therefore, neonatal screening with renal ultrasound and VCUG is essential in all patients with ARM.[29] The assessment of bladder function is also critical because of a reportedly high incidence of occult neurovesical dysfunction.[30] The combination of rectourinary fistula and neurovesical dysfunction or bladder outlet obstruction predisposes to critical neonatal illness.

Cases of cloaca should never be managed by initial anorectal reconstruction alone, which necessitates extensive and complicated subsequent surgery. A fully diverting colostomy with complete evacuation of the distal limb should initially be considered. The goals of management in the first few years of life are to protect the upper urinary tract, ensure low-pressure urinary drainage, normalize anorectal anatomy, and minimize any neurologic deficit that may arise from treatable spinal pathology. A comprehensive, integrated approach with posterior sagittal anorectalurethrovaginoplasty at approximately 6 to 12 months of age is the most appropriate definitive surgical procedure yielding excellent results in such cases. If bladder outlet obstruction or neurovesical dysfunction is detected or suspected, incidental appendectomy is contraindicated. The goals of management of the preschool and school-aged child with ARM are to ensure social urinary and fecal continence and to promote self-esteem and self-care.[25]

KEY POINTS

- **The initial nephric system development stage, *the pronephros*, disappears completely by the fourth week of embryonic life. *The mesonephros* degenerates, though part is associated with the reproductive system. The cranial portion of the ureteral bud joins with the metanephric blastema, branching into the renal pelvis and the calyces and inducing nephron formation during the final stage of development, *metanephros*.**
- **Horseshoe kidney is the most common renal fusion, occurring in 0.25% of population.**
- **The ureteropelvic junction (UPJ) is the most common site of obstruction in the urinary tract and the most common cause of neonatal hydronephrosis.**
- **Ureteral duplication is the most common anomaly of the urinary tract.**
- **The incidence of vesicoureteral reflux in otherwise normal children is approximately 1%; the incidence is up to 40% patients undergoing evaluation for UTI.**
- **Epispadias in boys consists of a dorsally placed urethral meatus and the degree of penile deformity is related to the extent of the meatal displacement.**
- **Posterior urethral valves are the most common obstructive urethral lesions in male infants and consist of a membrane or mucosal leaflet within the prostatic urethra.**
- **Descend of the testis from its original position near the kidney into the cooler scrotum is necessary for its normal development and production of fertile sperm. True undescended testes fail to reach the scrotum despite following a normal line of descent.**
- **Prepubertal testis tumors account for approximately 2% of all testicular tumors, with a peak patient age of approximately 2 years.**

References

1. Potter EL. Bilateral absence of ureters and kidneys: a report of 50 cases. *Obstet Gynecol.* 1965;25:3.
2. Gleason PE, Kelalis PP, Husman DA, et al. Hydronephrosis in renal ectopia: incidence, etiology and significance. *J Urol.* 1994;151:1660.
3. Mesrobian HJ, Kelalis PP, Hrabovsky E, et al. Wilms tumor in horseshoe kidneys: a report from the National Wilms Tumor Study. *J Urol.* 1985;133:1002.
4. Glassberg KI, Stephens, FD, Lebowitz, RL, et al. Renal dysgenesis and cystic disease of the kidney: a report of the Committee on Terminology, Nomenclature and Classification. *J Urol.* 1987;138:1085.
5. **Minevich E, Wacksman J, Phipps L, et al. Importance of accurate diagnosis and early close follow-up in patients with suspected MCDK. *J Urol.* 1997; 158:1301.**
6. Wacksman J, Sheldon CA. Multicystic kidney disease. In: Kelalis PP, King LR, Belman AB, eds. *Clinical pediatric urology*. Philadelphia: WB Saunders, 1992:780.
7. Minevich E, Wacksman J. Pyeloplasty. In: Graham, SD, ed. *Glenn's urologic surgery*. Philadelphia: Lippincott-Raven, 1998.
8. **DeFoor W, Minevich E, Tackett L, et al. Ectopic ureterocele: clinical application of classification based on renal unit jeopardy. *J Urol.* 2003;169: 1092–1094.**
9. Sheldon CA, Minevich E, Wacksman J. Urinary tract infection and vesicoureteral reflux. In: Ascraft K, Holder T, eds. *Pediatric surgery*. Philadelphia: WB Sanders, 1999.
10. Puri P, Chertin B, Velayudham M, et al. Treatment of vesicoureteral reflux by endoscopic injection of dextranomer/hyaluronic acid copolymer: preliminary results. *J Urol.* 2003;170(Pt 2):1541–1544.
11. Keating MA, Escola J, Snyder HM, et al. Changing concepts in management of primary obstructive megaureter. *J Urol.* 1989;142:636.
12. **Minevich E, Wacksman J, Lewis AG, et al. The infected urachal cyst: primary excision versus a staged approach. *J Urol.* 1997;157:1869.**

13. Grady RW, Mitchell ME. Complete primary closure of the bladder exstrophy. *Urol Clin North Am.* 1999;26:95.
14. McGuire EJ, Woodside JR, Borden TA, et al. Prognostic value of urodynamic testing in myelodysplastic patients. *J Urol.* 1981;126:205.
15. Minevich E, Sheldon CA. Urinary tract reconstruction for continence and renal preservation. In: Ziegler MM, Azizkhan RG, Weber TR, eds. *Operative pediatric surgery.* McGraw-Hill, 2003.
16. Sheldon CA, Minevich E, Wacksman J, et al. Role of the antegrade continence enema in the management of the most debilitating childhood recto-urogenital anomalies. *J Urol.* 1997;158:1277.
17. Peters CA, Bolkier M, Bauer SB, et al. The urodynamic consequences of posterior urethral valves. *J Urol.* 1990;144:122.
18. Sheldon CA. Intersex states. In: Oldham KT, Colombani PM, Foglia RT, eds. *Surgery of infants and children: scientific principles and practice.* Philadelphia: Lippincott-Raven, 1997.
19. Weiss RM, Seashore JH. Clinical implications of laparoscopy in the management of a nonpalpable undescended testis. *J Urol.* 1986;135:332.
20. Tackett LD, Wacksman J, Billmire D, et al. The high intra-abdominal testis: technique and long-term success of laparoscopic testicular autotransplantation. *J Endourol.* 2002;16:359–361.
21. **Docimo SG. Results of surgical therapy for cryptorchidism: literature review and analysis. *J Urol.* 1995;154:1148.**
22. Ransler CW, Allen TD. Torsion of the spermatic cord. *Urol Clin North Am.* 1982;9:245.
23. Brandt MT, Sheldon CA, Wacksman J, et al., Prenatal testicular torsion: principles of management. *J Urol.* 1992;147:670.
24. Minevich E, Wacksman J, Lewis AG, et al. Inguinal microsurgical varicocelectomy in the adolescent: technique and preliminary results. *J Urol.* 1998;159:1022.
25. Sheldon CA. Imperforate anus, urogenital sinus and cloaca. In: Kelalis PP, King LR, Belman AB, eds. *Clinical pediatric urology.* Philadelphia: WB Sanders, 2000.
26. Jenak R, Ludwikowski B, Gonzalez R. Total urogenital sinus mobilization: a modified perineal approach for feminizing genitoplasty and urogenital sinus repair. *J Urol.* 2001;165:2347–2349.
27. Sheldon CA, Gilbert A, Lewis AG. Vaginal reconstruction: critical technical principles. *J Urol.* 1994;152:190.
28. Geary DF, MacLusky IB, Chirchill BM, et al. A broader spectrum of abnormalities in the prune belly syndrome. *J Urol.* 1986;135:324.
29. **Sheldon CA, Gilbert A, Lewis AG, et al. Surgical implications of genitourinary tract anomalies in patients with imperforate anus. *J Urol.* 1994; 152: 196.**
30. Sheldon CA, Cormier M, Crone K, et al. Occult neurovesical dysfunction in children with imperforate anus and its variants. *J Pediatr Surg.* 1991;26:49.

CHAPTER 112 ■ CHILDHOOD TUMORS

MICHAEL P. LAQUAGLIA

The focus of this chapter is malignant solid tumors of infancy, childhood, and adolescence. Fortunately, these conditions are rare, especially compared with the incidence of major adult malignancies like breast and lung cancer. This rarity, however, poses special problems to the clinical and basic science cancer researcher. For the clinician studying the effectiveness of a particular drug or surgical technique, the number of patients available for randomized trials is drastically reduced. Similarly, the basic scientist wishing to analyze the effect of a particular genetic mutation on the development or virulence of a tumor is limited in the material available for study. The solution to this problem has been the establishment of cooperative groups for the clinical and basic scientific study of pediatric malignancies. Previously, these included the Children's Cancer Group (CCG; formerly Children's Cancer Study Group, or CCSG) and the Pediatric Oncology Group (POG) in the United States, and the Societé Internacionale Oncologique Pediatrique in Europe. These agencies were originally focused on the study of hematologic malignancies. Collaboration was later extended to the study of pediatric solid tumors, and cooperation between groups allowed prospective protocols to be done on some rare tumors. The Intergroup Rhabdomyosarcoma Study (IRS) was established as a collaborative effort between POG and CCG to address the special problems posed by childhood sarcomas, most importantly rhabdomyosarcoma. The National Wilms Tumor Study (NWTS) enrolls most Wilms tumors diagnosed in the United States. This organization has made significant progress in increasing the cure rate from Wilms tumors and in developing therapies with minimal early and late toxicity. This and other cooperative studies, combined with pioneering single-institutional efforts, have resulted in a 40% increase in the overall survival rate for pediatric cancer since the 1970s. Overall 5-year survival rates for all stages are approximately 85% for Wilms tumor, 70% for hepatoblastoma, and 60% (83% to 31% by stage, age, and site[1]) for rhabdomyosarcoma. In comparison, the survival rate was less than 20%, and closer to zero, respectively, for these malignancies before the advent of multidisciplinary therapy.

Despite this progress, less than 30% of children with high-risk neuroblastomas survive more than 5 years. Of children with lymphomas and germ cell tumors, 10% to 30% relapse or become resistant to treatment. Less than 10% of children with hepatocellular carcinomas survive more than 5 years after diagnosis, and almost no patients who have rhabdoid tumor, pediatric colon cancer, or renal cell carcinoma in childhood survive more than 5 years. Because of lack of progress in these rare pediatric malignancies, the four American cooperative groups—CCG, POG, IRS, and NWTS—merged in 2000 into a single national pediatric cooperative group, the Children's Oncology Group (COG). As in the past, the pediatric surgical oncologist will be instrumental to advances in the field.[2–4]

Future progress will depend on myriad biologic analyses done on each tumor system. The pediatric surgical oncologist is the first line of defense in tumor diagnosis and staging. It is crucial that biopsy specimens be adequate both in size and quality. Snap freezing of portions of a tumor biopsy should become more routine. Molecular biologic studies often require a biopsy that exceeds 1 cm^3, and this factor should be kept in mind when planning the operative approach.

INCIDENCE OF SOLID TUMORS IN CHILDHOOD

The percent distribution for all races and sexes of various pediatric solid tumors of interest to pediatric surgeons are compared in Figure 112.1.[5] Neuroblastoma is the most common

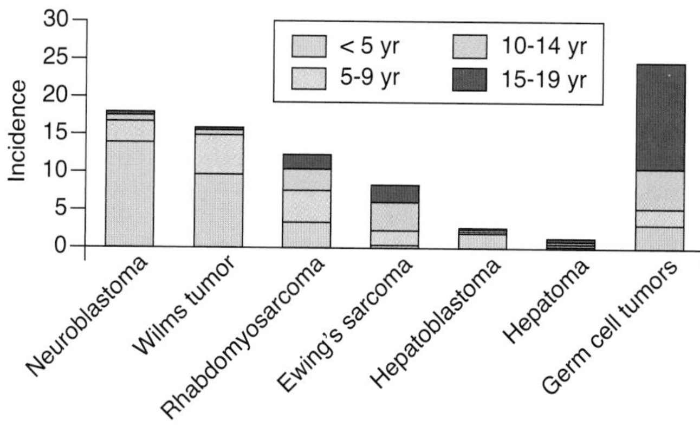

FIGURE 112.1 Percentage distribution of common pediatric solid tumors by age group.

extracranial solid tumor, followed in incidence by Wilms tumors. Rhabdomyosarcomas are about three quarters of the percentage of the previous two but have a biphasic age distribution with 40% of cases occurring in the 10- to 19-year-old age range. Hepatoblastomas are much less frequent and hepatocellular carcinomas are, fortunately, extremely rare. Many germ cell tumors occur in adolescents or young adults.

NEUROBLASTOMA

Epidemiology and Associated Conditions

Neuroblastoma is the most common extracranial solid tumor and the most common abdominal malignancy of childhood. High-risk neuroblastoma remains one of the central problems of pediatric oncology. The overall incidence rate of sympathetic nervous system cancers in children and adolescents younger than 20 years of age is 7.8%, and 97% of these are neuroblastomas.[6] This rate translates into approximately 650 new cases in the United States per year, and sympathetic nervous system tumors comprise 7.8% of all cancers among children younger than 15 years of age. The age-adjusted incidence rate for boys younger than 15 years of age was 9.4 per million, and that for girls was 9.1 per million. The ratio of white to black incidence rates was 1.7:1 for boys and 1.9:1 for girls among infants.[6] The overall male to female ratio is approximately 1.2:1, and the incidence is uniform throughout the world.[7] Neuroblastoma is much more likely to occur in infancy, with a combined male to female incidence of 64 per million compared with 29 per million during the second year of life. The overall incidence of neuroblastoma has remained stable over a 21-year period of observation. Rates, however, have increased somewhat among infants during recent years. This increase may be a result of the use of mass screening in certain areas. The median age at diagnosis is approximately 2 years, and 80% of children are younger than 4 years of age at diagnosis.[8]

Case reports associating neuroblastoma with fetal exposures, including the fetal alcohol syndrome, or hydantoin or phenobarbital exposure have not been supported by larger studies.[9,10] The occurrence of neuroblastoma has also been associated with neurofibromatosis type I (NF1), Beckwith-Wiedemann syndrome, Hirschsprung disease, musculoskeletal and cardiovascular malformations, Turner syndrome, and neurodevelopmental abnormalities.[11–13] However, none of these associations has been rigorously proved, and data remain conflicting. Possible but unproven environmental risk factors include parental exposure to solvents or electromagnetic fields, maternal hormone use during pregnancy, and parental cigarette smoking.[6]

Basic Science

Neuroblastoma was the first tumor in which molecular biologic advances in the field of oncogenes were translated into a clinically useful tool. The *MYCN* oncogene (formerly N-myc), whose function and mechanism of action remain the subject of investigation, was empirically shown to be a useful predictor of survival and risk. Patients with an increased number of copies of the *MYCN* gene have a much worse prognosis.[14] Most authorities consider a copy number of more than 10 to be significant. It has also been shown that when *MYCN* is amplified in the primary tumor, the same is true for metastatic deposits or recurrent tumors. More recent research has uncovered a more nuanced role for *MYCN* as a prognostic factor in neuroblastoma. In one report, *MYCN* amplification was not shown to be an independent predictor of outcome in infants with neuroblastoma, although it remained a strongly adverse prognostic indicator in children diagnosed after 12 months of age. This finding is supported by the results of an Italian study that showed that *MYCN* amplification was an adverse prognostic factor except in patients with stage 4S disease.[15]

Rapid assessment of the *MYCN* copy number can be performed using the process of *in situ* fluorescent hybridization, whereas the traditional method using Southern blotting takes longer. An example of a tumor analysis from a patient is presented in Figure 112.2. The mechanism of *MYCN* amplification in neuroblastoma remains unknown. *MYCN* is a DNA-binding protein and has been shown to increase the levels of endogenous MDM2 mRNA and protein with consequent p53 inhibition. Modulation of MDM2 levels by *MYCN* may partially explain its role in neuroblastoma resistance to therapy.[16, 17]

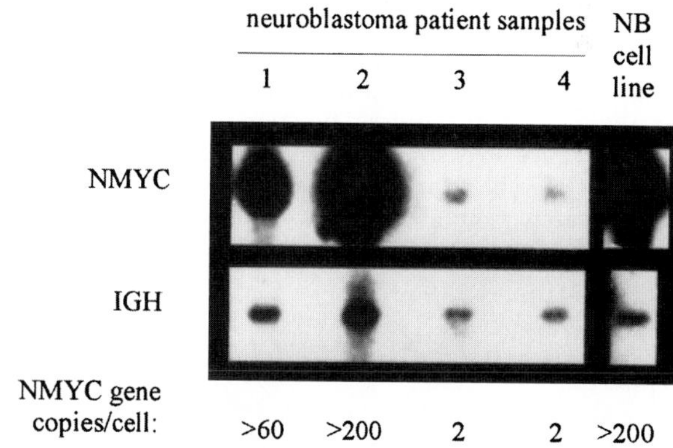

FIGURE 112.2 Example of *MYCN* amplification analysis by Southern blotting in neuroblastoma samples from four patients. The Southern blot hybridization signal obtained with the *MYCN* probe is normalized to that obtained on the same blot with a control probe for a gene not subject to amplification, such as the immunoglobulin heavy chain gene (IGH). The signals are then normalized to a negative control (placental DNA, not illustrated). A neuroblastoma cell line with *MYCN* amplification is used as a positive control. The IGH signals show that similar amounts of DNA are present in each lane, but the *MYCN* signals are grossly different from each other, indicating amplification in cases 1 and 2 and in the control cell line. Samples 1 and 2 show high-level *MYCN* amplification, exceeding 60 and 200 copies of *MYCN* per cell, respectively, which corresponds to greater than 30-fold and 100-fold amplification. Samples 3 and 4 contain two copies of *MYCN* per cell, as expected in diploid cells without amplification. (Courtesy of Marc Ladanyi, M.D., Department of Pathology, Memorial Sloan-Kettering Cancer Center.)

The most common cytogenetic abnormalities in neuroblastoma are 1p deletion, and a gain of genetic material on 17q [18] The presence of a 1p deletion correlates with a worse outcome in neuroblastoma and has been used as a prognostic factor.[19–21] It has been shown using cell fusion that replacement of this deleted segment is associated with a marked reduction in tumorigenicity.[22] More recently, interest has focused on another common cytogenetic abnormality observed in neuroblastoma: an unbalanced gain of genetic material on the long arm of chromosome 17. In one multivariate analysis, a gain at 17q was a significant predictor of outcome and was associated with a worse prognosis.[23] This factor had a greater impact on outcome than either stage or 1p status.

Another active area of neuroblastoma research is the relation of nerve growth factor receptors to differentiation and clinical risk. The low-affinity nerve growth factor receptor gene *LNGFR* and the *TRK* proto-oncogene, which is a component of the high-affinity nerve growth factor receptor, are expressed in human neuroblastoma tissue. A number of authors have shown that *LNGFR* and *TRK* (*TRK-A*) expression are inversely correlated with *MYCN* amplification and are associated with lower stage at diagnosis and improved prognosis.[24–26] The absence of *TRK-A* expression has been highly correlated with *MYCN* amplification in one study, in which 96% of *MYCN*-amplified tumors lacked *TRK-A* expression.[27] *TRK-C* expression is also a favorable prognostic factor in neuroblastoma, whereas *TRK-B* expression is associated with poor survival.[28] One recent study used microarray analysis to identify targets affected by Trk gene expression. In this report, TrkA expression was associated with up-regulation of proapoptotic factors and angiogenesis inhibitors. In contrast, TrkB expression correlated with the up-regulation of genes involved with invasion and therapy resistance.[29]

Pathology

Neuroblastoma cells are derived from the primitive neural crest, as are melanocytes, Schwann cells, neuroendocrine or amine precursor uptake and decarboxylation (APUD) cells, C cells of the thyroid gland, the autonomic nervous system, and adrenal medulla. Neuroblastoma cells are thought to arise from primitive sympathoblasts functioning as stem cells and sometimes called *I cells*.[30] Under certain circumstances, these pluripotential cells demonstrate an ability to differentiate along a separate neural crest lineage. For instance, pure ganglioneuroma is thought to arise from complete differentiation of primitive neuroblasts into ganglion cells. Schwann cell differentiation is also clearly and frequently observed in these tumors. It is also possible to identify melanocytic differentiation in certain rare but well-reported neuroblastomas. Finally, because the sympathetic nervous system extends along the entire neuraxis, neuroblastoma can arise from cervical, thoracic, abdominal (retroperitoneal), and pelvic primary sites.

Neuroblastoma falls into the category of a small, round, blue cell tumor of childhood characterized by sheets of cells staining with hematoxylin. Other tumors that fall into this category include primitive neuroectodermal tumors (PNET) and Ewing's sarcoma, non-Hodgkin lymphomas, and undifferentiated sarcomas (certain rhabdomyosarcomas). Light microscopic diagnosis depends on the identification of Homer-Wright pseudorosettes, ganglion cells, neuropil and neuritic processes, and schwannian stroma (Fig. 112.3). Homer-Wright pseudorosettes consist of rings of dark-staining neuroblasts surrounding an eosinophilic core of neuropil. The diagnosis can be aided by immunohistochemical staining that is positive for neurofilament proteins (S-100), synaptophysin, and neuron-specific enolase. PNETs may express neuron-specific enolase but not the other neural markers.[31]

At presentation, most neuroblastomas are highly cellular and have a uniform appearance. After chemotherapy, the tumor often appears to have rests of neuroblasts contained in a schwannian stroma. This histologic appearance is called *ganglioneuroblastoma,* and although it is appears more differentiated, there is no impact on clinical risk, which is determined by the findings at initial diagnosis. It is also possible for tumors to contain significant amounts of stroma at diagnosis, and this finding is associated with improved outcome. This observation is the basis of the Shimada grading system, which is summarized in Table 112.1.[32] To help predict risk, all neuroblastomas should undergo Shimada classification at diagnosis.

Neuroblastoma metastasizes to regional lymph nodes and distant sites, most frequently bone marrow and cortical bone. The liver and, rarely, lungs can also be sites of metastatic spread. Cortical bone involvement as manifested by a positive bone scan is a particularly poor prognostic indicator.[33]

Presentation, Workup, and Staging

Clinical presentation depends on site of origin, age at diagnosis, and the biologic aggressiveness of the tumor. The proportion of patients with cervical or pelvic tumors is increased in patients younger than 1 year of age compared with older children.

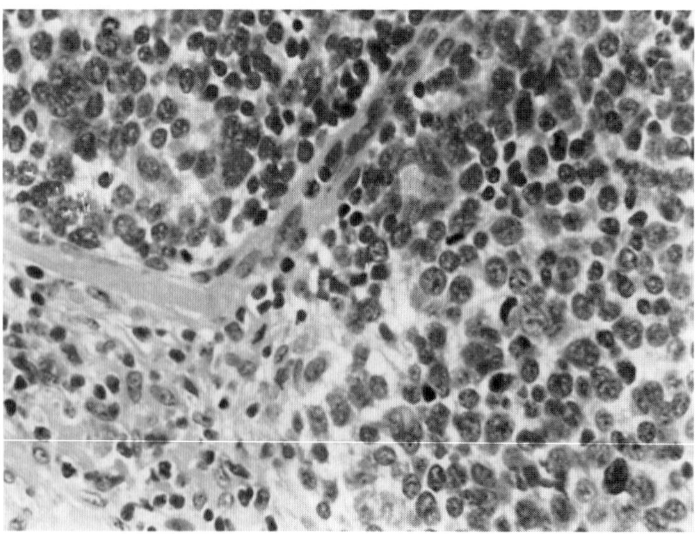

FIGURE 112.3 Typical neuroblastoma with monotonous cellular patterns. Note the mitotic figure (*center*) (X450).

TABLE 112.1 CLASSIFICATION

SHIMADA HISTOPATHOLOGIC CLASSIFICATION OF NEUROBLASTOMA

FAVORABLE
Stroma rich, all ages, no nodular pattern
Stroma poor, age 1.5–5 y, MKI < 100
C , 1.5 y, MKI , 200
UNFAVORABLE
Stroma rich, all ages, nodular pattern
Stroma poor, age >5 y
Stroma poor, age 1.5–5 y, undifferentiated
Stroma poor, age 1.5–5 y, differentiated, MKI >100
Stroma poor, age > 1y, MKI >200

MKI, mitosis–karyorrhexis index (number of mitoses and karyorrhexis per 5,000 cells).

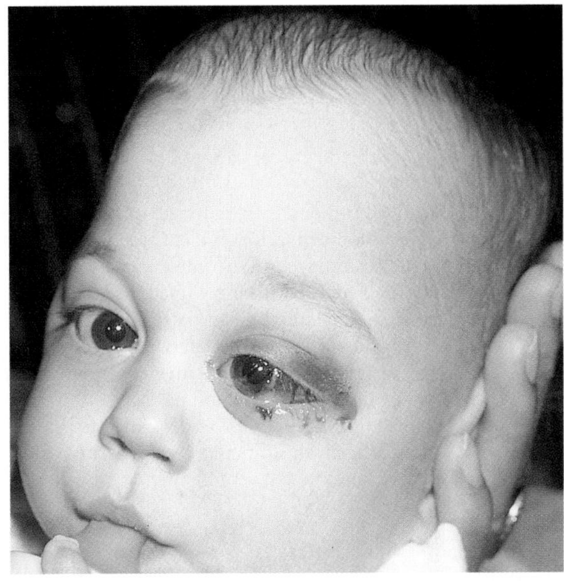

FIGURE 112.4 Periorbital neuroblastoma. (From Fleisher GR, Ludwig W, Baskin MN. *Atlas of pediatric emergency medicine*. Philadelphia: Lippincott Williams & Wilkins, 2004, with permission.)

Cervical tumors present as a lateral neck mass, and airway compromise is not usually observed. Because they arise from cervical sympathetic ganglia, cervical tumors may be associated with Horner's syndrome, which is often permanent after resection and should be discussed before surgery with the parents. Regional nodal involvement is common, but distant metastases are rare, and most tumors are of low risk.

Pelvic tumors usually are diagnosed after a parent or caretaker palpates a mass. Bladder and bowel symptoms such as recurrent urinary tract infections and chronic constipation can occur when pelvic tumors reach great size and compress these organs. Hydronephrosis secondary to ureteral compression is often observed with large tumors and usually resolves after resection. Epidural extension to the sacrum can also be noted, and neurologic evaluation documenting somatic motor and sphincter function is mandatory.

In all age groups, the most common presentation is an abdominal tumor that is often hard and fixed. The tumor arises from the midline sympathetic nerves or the adrenal. Often, regional nodal echelons are involved along the aorta. These involved nodes can be bulky and may extend distally to the aortic bifurcation and proximally into the mediastinum, overshadowing the primary tumor. Patients with metastatic or large, bulky tumors, especially if older than 1 year of age, may appear generally ill or anemic.

Several syndromes are particularly associated with neuroblastoma: periorbital ecchymoses (raccoon eyes), opsoclonus–myoclonus syndrome, and the secretory diarrhea syndrome. Periorbital ecchymoses are caused by orbital metastases with subsequent obstruction and rupture of veins in the periorbital skin (Fig. 112.4). The optic nerve and vision are not usually threatened, and the ecchymoses often take months to resolve even after the orbital tumors have regressed. Opsoclonus–myoclonus is a paraneoplastic syndrome thought to be autoimmune in nature; it is caused by development of antibodies against the tumor that cross-react with Purkinje cells in the cerebellum. Unfortunately, the symptoms may not regress after resection of the neuroblastoma, and the condition can result in devastating neurologic injury. Secretory diarrhea in this condition is caused by release of vasoactive intestinal peptide by the tumor. The watery diarrhea may require intravenous support but usually resolves with treatment. This condition is an indication of tumor differentiation and is associated with low-risk lesions.

The workup is directed toward delineation of tumor extent in the primary site and identification of metastatic deposits. The primary site is usually evaluated by computed tomography (CT) or magnetic resonance imaging (MRI); no reported analyses compare the two in neuroblastoma. If CT scans are used, they should be performed with both gastrointestinal and intravenous contrast. This is true even for cervical and thoracic primaries so that the position and course of the pharynx and esophagus are precisely determined. The volume scanned should include not only the primary tumor but also the regional lymphatics. The lower chest should be included in scans of cervical primaries, the upper abdomen and lower neck in thoracic tumors, and the entire abdomen, pelvis, and lower chest for abdominal primaries. Because of the high incidence of cortical bone involvement, especially in children older than 1 year of age, bone scans or radiographic series should also be performed routinely. The bone marrow is assessed by bone marrow aspiration at four iliac crest sites and bone biopsy at two sites. If CT or MRI scans include the liver, appropriate windows can be used to identify hepatic metastases. Ultrasound can also be used in this regard, and plain chest films are used to identify pulmonary metastases. If pulmonary metastases are present, Doppler ultrasonography can be used to identify intracaval tumor extension. It is also useful to perform a ^{131}I (or ^{123}I) metaiodobenzylguanidine scan to assess metastatic sites and as a baseline for evaluation of therapeutic response in the primary site. ^{123}I scans are more sensitive and preferable for imaging. About 10% of neuroblastomas do not take up metaiodobenzylguanidine (MIBG) and a useful surrogate is a positron emission tomography (PET) scan.[34] Finally, a 24-hour urine collection for measurement of metanephrine, dopamine, and vanillylmandelic acid may help diagnostically and as a tumor marker to assess therapeutic response.

The diagnosis of neuroblastoma requires histologic confirmation either by direct tumor biopsy or by demonstration of malignant cells in bone marrow samples. Because of the wide range of molecular biologic studies that have prognostic importance, many groups attempt to obtain enough tissue at diagnosis to allow full molecular biologic and cytogenetic analysis in addition to histologic diagnosis. When possible, several grams of tumor tissue should be obtained, and a portion should be snap frozen. Given the seriousness of this tumor, this is a reasonable objective. The application of biologic studies to determine risk

TABLE 112.2 STAGING

INTERNATIONAL STAGING CRITERIA FOR NEUROBLASTOMA

Stage	Criteria	3-Year Survival Rate (%)	
		Overall	Relapse free
1	Localized tumor confined to site of origin; complete gross resection with or without microscopic margin; all identifiable regional nodes negative, including contralateral	97	88
2A	Unilateral tumor with incomplete gross excision; nodes negative	87	72
2B	Unilateral tumor with incomplete or complete gross excision with positive ipsilateral but negative contralateral nodes	86	63
3	Infiltration across the midline with or without regional nodal involvement; unilateral tumor with positive contralateral nodes, midline tumor with bilateral	62	58
4	Distant metastases to lymph nodes, (4N), bone, bone marrow, liver, or other organs	<40	<40
4S	Localized primary tumor as described for stage 1 or 2 with distant metastases limited to liver, skin, and bone marrow (<10% involvement)	−75	−75

status and therapy makes adequate tumor biopsies mandatory. Biopsy can usually be achieved through a mini laparotomy or laparoscopic approach. Some groups have questioned the ethics of open biopsy when the diagnosis can be obtained by examination of the bone marrow and assessment of urinary catecholamines. Some groups have tried to avoid initial mini laparotomy and base the diagnosis on elevation of urinary catecholamines and bone marrow aspirates. In this situation biologic studies are dependent on the number of tumor cells in the aspirate with *MYCN* copy number assessed by fluorescent *in situ* hybridization.

The most widely used staging system for neuroblastoma is based on the international system, which is listed in Table 112.2.[35–37] This system evolved from previous systems developed by Evans et al. and the POG.[38] Tumor size and location with regard to the midline remain important determinants of stage, as does the presence and degree of metastatic disease. The present system is also highly dependent on surgical resection of the primary tumor in patients with nonmetastatic disease.

Risk Groups

As a result of insights gained through cooperative group studies, as well as the work done by several single institutions, it is possible to categorize patients with neuroblastoma into high-, intermediate-, and low-risk groups at diagnosis. This assessment is based on age, stage, Shimada classification, and the results of specialized studies, including flow cytometry, analysis for *MYCN* amplification, cytogenetics, and *TRK* gene expression. Ancillary criteria include serum ferritin, lactate dehydrogenase, and neuron-specific enolase determinations at diagnosis and before blood transfusion. Table 112.3 lists criteria for high-, intermediate-, and low-risk patients. Risk assignment is important because it strongly determines therapy. The COG is currently revising this risk assessment. In particular, stage 4 patients less than 18 months of age who are not *MYCN*-amplified will receive a reduction in treatment, as will other specific groups.

Treatment

Neuroblastoma treatment depends on degree of risk, as noted earlier. In general, low-risk tumors do not require chemotherapy or radiation. Resection of the primary lesion to obtain the diagnosis and biologic markers is followed by observation. Serial imaging studies of the primary and possible metastatic sites in low-risk patients are performed. Urinary catecholamines should fall to normal levels and remain there.

High-risk neuroblastoma remains one of the central problems in pediatric oncology, with overall survival rates below 30% despite multidisciplinary therapy and the use of multiagent chemotherapy and myeloablative regimens. Initial surgery should be confined to acquisition of diagnostic tissue, staging,

TABLE 112.3

RISK STATUS DETERMINANTS IN NEUROBLASTOMA

Parameters	Low risk	High risk
Age	<1 y (especially <6 mo)	>1 y at diagnosis
Stage	1, 2A, 2B, 4S	3, 4
Shimada classification	Favorable	Unfavorable
N-myc amplification	<3 Copies	>3 Copies
Expression of TRK	TRK Expressed	No TRK expression
Flow cytometry	Hyperdiploid, triploid	Diploid
Cytogenetics	No 1p abnormality	1p Deletion
Ferritin at diagnosis	<142 ng/mL	≥142 ng/mL
Lactate dehydroqenase	≤1,500 U/mL	>1,500U/mL
Neuron-specific enolase	≤100 ng/ml	>100 ng/mL

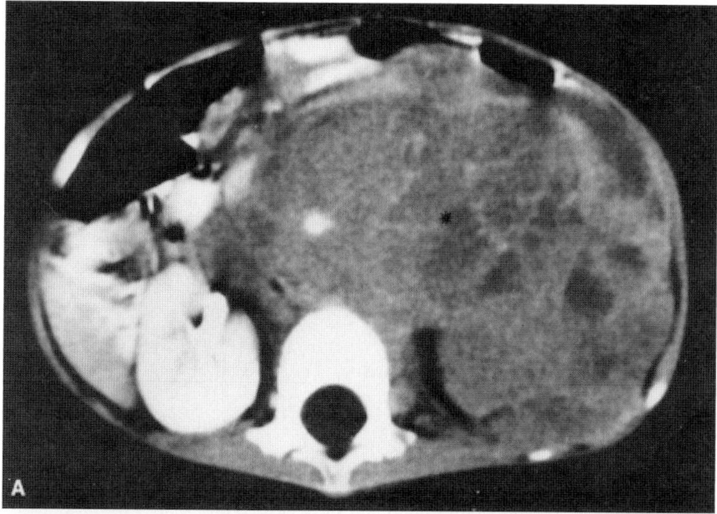

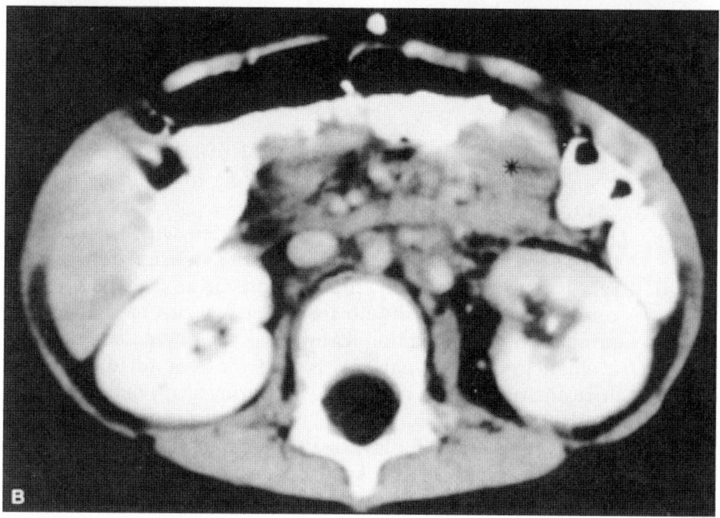

FIGURE 112.5 (*A*) Initial computed tomography (CT) scan of a child with stage 4 neuroblastoma. (*B*) CT scan of the same child after incisional biopsy and cytoreductive chemotherapy. Residual tumor is present despite dramatic reduction in overall tumor size.

and placement of a vascular access device. It has been noted that surgical complications are higher with initial attempts at complete resection without impact on survival.[39] After a course of chemotherapy, usually four or five cycles, second-look surgery is performed (Fig. 112.5). Although controversy surrounds the issue of resection in high-risk patients, most authorities agree that complete gross resection should be the goal of second-look procedures. Gross total resection of the primary tumor is associated with excellent local control.[40] The approach is dictated by the particular properties of the primary tumor. For upper abdominal lesions, especially those involving major midline branches of the abdominal aorta or the vena cava, thoracoabdominal exposure is helpful and well tolerated. The goal of resection is a complete vascular dissection and should encompass not only the primary but also all involved regional nodal echelons.

Chemotherapy for neuroblastoma has evolved toward higher dose intensities of multiple agents. *Dose intensity* is defined as the drug dose, usually normalized to surface area, divided by the time interval over which it is administered. In one meta-analysis, increased dose intensity correlated with improved overall and disease-free survival rates. In another report, primary tumor resectability correlated with increased chemotherapy intensity. There is no widely accepted regimen, and the major cooperative groups as well as larger single institutions have differing protocols. The COG is planning to base the induction phase of its new high-risk neuroblastoma protocol (called the *N7 protocol*) on a regimen developed at Memorial Sloan-Kettering Cancer Center. This protocol includes cyclophosphamide, 70 mg/kg per day for 2 days; doxorubicin, 75 mg/m^2 over 72 hours; and vincristine, 2 mg/m^2 over 72 hours, given as cycles 1, 2, 4, and 6. These cycles alternate with cisplatin, 50 mg/m^2 per day for 4 days, and etoposide, 200 mg/m^2 per day for 3 days, for cycles 3, 5, and 7. Second-look surgery is performed after cycle 4. This regimen has resulted in a 45% disease-free survival rate at 2 years from diagnosis in high-risk patients with stage 4 disease. After induction and local control with second-look resection, patients will receive a stem cell transplant, and randomization will be based on whether the stem cells are purged to remove possible contamination with circulating neuroblastoma cells or remain unpurged. The study is designed to determine whether purging is necessary. This approach is based on randomized data from the former CCG showing a significant survival improvement in patients with neuroblastoma who underwent autologous bone marrow transplantation as part of therapy.[41] This important study also indicated that treatment with 13-*cis*-retinoic acid after bone marrow transplantation was associated with an improved survival rate. The roles of dose-intensive chemotherapy, autologous stem cell or bone marrow transplantation, retinoids, and marrow support with colony-stimulating factors are now well established in the treatment of high-risk neuroblastoma. A randomized comparison of one versus two tandem stem cell transplants for patients with high-risk disease is in the planning stages.

TABLE 112.4

WILMS TUMOR–ASSOCIATED SYNDROMES AND CONDITIONS

Syndrome	Syndrome components	Wilms tumor risk
Beckwith-Wiedemann	Macroglossia, somatic gigantism, visceromegaly, hypoglycemia, abdominal wall defects	~5% (500-fold increase)
WAGR	Wilms tumor, aniridia, ambiguous genitalia, mental retardation, WTI deletion	40%–50% (40,000-fold to 50,000-fold increase)
Neurofibromatosis	Café au lait spots, plexiform neurofibromas, predisposition to multiple tumors	~0.26% (26-fold increase)
Denys-Drash	Pseudohermaphroditism, glomerulopathy, gonadal tumors or dysgenesis	~60%–70% (60,000-fold to 70,000-fold increase)
Perlman's familial nephroblastomatosis	Bilateral renal hamartomas, macrosomia, islet cell hypertrophy, unusual facies, mental retardation	~60%[a]
Genital anomalies	Cryptorchidism, hypospadias, gonadal dysgenesis, pseudohemaphroditism	Increased

[a]There is an increased risk of nephroblastoma in patients with the Denys-Drash and Perlman's syndromes, but these cases are very rare, with less than 10 cases of Perlman's syndrome reported. The incidence of Wilms tumor in the general population is 1 in 10,000; therefore, the incidence of Wilms tumor in Beckwith-Wiedemann syndrome is 5/100 / 1/10,000, which is a 500-fold increase.

Future Directions

Treatment with radiolabeled or cold monoclonal antibodies is also undergoing trial. These antibodies are usually of the immunoglobulin G (IgG) class and recognize the surface ganglioside GD2 that is usually highly expressed on the surface of human neuroblastoma cells. Current strategies include induction of antibody-dependent, cell-mediated cytotoxicity by cold antibody, usually of the IgG3 class, and direct cell killing by attachment of ^{131}I to the antibody that then specifically recognizes a tumor cell. More sophisticated approaches involve stimulation of a host antitumor response by vaccination with antiidiotypic monoclonal antibodies versus anti-GD2. Tumor vaccines and techniques of adoptive immunotherapy are being evaluated in clinical trials but so far are not curative. Biologic agents, such as N-(4-hydroxyphenyl)retinamide (4-HPR) or fenretinide, and various antiangiogenic agents have been proposed for use in minimal disease states and are undergoing clinical trials. In intermediate risk neuroblastoma there is a strong trend to eliminate or minimize chemotherapy.

WILMS TUMOR

Epidemiology and Associated Conditions

Malignancies of the kidney represent 6.3% of all cancer diagnoses among children younger than 15 years of age, with an incidence of 7.9 per million.[42] In the United States, approximately 550 children per year younger than 20 years of age are diagnosed with a renal cancer, and 500 of these are Wilms tumors. The overall incidence of Wilms tumor or nephroblastoma is 7 per 1 million children (1 per 10,000) younger than the age of 16 years.[43] The incidence is highest for African-Americans and lowest for patients of East Asian descent. Whites have an intermediate incidence. The sex ratio is approximately 1:1, and the peak incidence occurs between 2 and 3 years of age.[44] Most Wilms tumors occur in patients younger than 5 years of age. Median ages reported from the NWTS were 36 months for boys and 43 months for girls with unilateral disease, whereas boys and girls with bilateral disease presented at a median age of 23 and 30 months, respectively.[45] Rhabdoid tumors of the kidney, clear cell sarcomas, and renal cell carcinomas make up 1.0%, 1.6%, and 2.6%, respectively, of renal cancers occurring in children younger than 15 years of age [42]

Table 112.4 lists conditions associated with the development of Wilms tumor in addition to the associated increase in relative risk. In general, the presence of any of these conditions or syndromes should initiate a workup to rule out the presence of Wilms tumor. Known risk factors include race (the incidence in Asian patients is half that found in whites or African-Americans), aniridia, genitourinary anomalies, WAGR syndrome (Wilms tumor, aniridia, genitourinary anomalies, mental retardation), Beckwith-Wiedemann syndrome, Perlman's syndrome, Denys-Drash syndrome, and the Simpson-Golabi-Behmel syndrome.[42]

Basic Science

In Wilms tumor, cytogenetic abnormalities have been identified on chromosomes 11p13, 1p, and 16q.[46–48] A gene called *WT1* was cloned from the site on the 11th chromosome and has been shown to bind to DNA, suggesting that it functions to control gene expression. Furthermore, *WT1* has been shown to be linked to the gene locus associated with aniridia but was not linked to the occurrence of Wilms tumor in three separate, multiple-case kindreds.[49] This finding suggests that the Wilms tumor suppressor is probably not *WT1,* but may reside on a locus at 1p or especially 16q. NWTS-5 is directed to determining which genetic locus is associated with the development of Wilms tumor and is the most likely candidate for the Wilms tumor suppressor gene.

Pathology

The study of Wilms tumor has benefited greatly from a central pathology review performed at the NWTS Pathology Center. Much progress in defining Wilms tumor risk categories has ensued, underscoring the need for accurate and adequate histologic analysis of all Wilms tumor specimens.

It is hypothesized that Wilms tumor arises from primitive metanephric blastema, and individual tumors often contain primitive metanephric cells but also cartilage, skeletal muscle, and squamous epithelium. Most tumors arise unifocally within the kidney, but approximately 7% of unilateral Wilms tumors are multicentric.[44] The proportion of synchronous bilateral tumors among all patients with nephroblastoma ranges from 4.4% to 7%, whereas that of metachronous tumors is 1.0% to 1.9%.[50] Wilms tumors are equally distributed with regard to the left and right side and may occur with no apparent connection to the kidneys. Usually, extrarenal Wilms tumor occurs in the retroperitoneal area, but other reported sites include the pelvis, scrotum, and inguinal region.

Grossly, the tumors are globular or spherical and uniformly pale-gray or tan on sectioning. Calcification is not usually apparent, but "egg-shell" calcification can be observed in tumors that have undergone significant spontaneous hemorrhage. This finding differs from the stippled calcifications associated with neuroblastoma. Cysts may be present, and in infants, polypoid extension into the pelvicalyceal system may cause confusion with botryoid rhabdomyosarcoma. Also, a pseudocapsule of compressed renal parenchyma is often found. Most tumors, unless composed of a large proportion of stromal elements, are friable and easily ruptured. This is of great significance to the operating surgeon, who must determine whether preoperative rupture has occurred and must avoid intraoperative spillage. The consequence of either of these events is upstaging of the lesion and the need for whole-abdomen radiation therapy with its attendant morbidity.

Microscopically, these tumors demonstrate a triphasic pattern of blastemic, stromal, and epithelial cells. Biphasic tumors with blastemic and stromal cells are common, and some specimens consist of only a single type (see Fig. 112.5). A major parameter predictive of tumor aggressiveness and patient survival is the histologic finding of anaplasia. This finding is defined by the presence of hyperdiploid mitotic figures, threefold or greater nuclear enlargement, and hyperchromasia of enlarged nuclei. The effect of anaplasia on prognosis is so marked that tumors with these findings are designated "unfavorable histology" by the NWTS. Anaplastic tumors, which comprise approximately 5% of all Wilms tumors, are rare in the first 2 years of life, but their incidence increases to 13% of patients diagnosed at 5 years of age or older.

Presentation, Workup, and Staging

Most Wilms tumors are first diagnosed after appreciation of an asymptomatic abdominal mass, which can attain great size. This finding usually occurs during routine pediatric examination or while the children are handled by a relative. Parents are usually surprised and feel guilty that such a mass could have gone unnoticed, and they need reassurance. In a subset of patients, rapid abdominal enlargement develops, associated with pain, fever, and gross hematuria. This is attributed to intratumoral hemorrhage and may be associated with spontaneous rupture.

The NWTS recommends the following workup for patients with suspected nephroblastoma. An excretory urogram is obtained to identify the tumor site; pelvicaliceal distortion is demonstrated, thus localizing the process to the kidney; and the function of the contralateral kidney is assessed. It is acceptable to substitute CT scanning of the abdomen with intravenous and oral contrast for excretory urography (Fig. 112.6). Indeed, almost every center performs this study routinely. Abdominal, real-time Doppler ultrasonography is performed to identify intracaval tumor extension, liver metastases, or enlarged retroperitoneal lymph nodes. Finally, good posteroanterior and oblique plain films of the chest are obtained to identify pulmonary metastases. All data concerning stage IV patients in the NWTS studies are based on the diagnosis being made by plain chest radiographs. Several studies have been performed that support the validity of this approach. In particular,

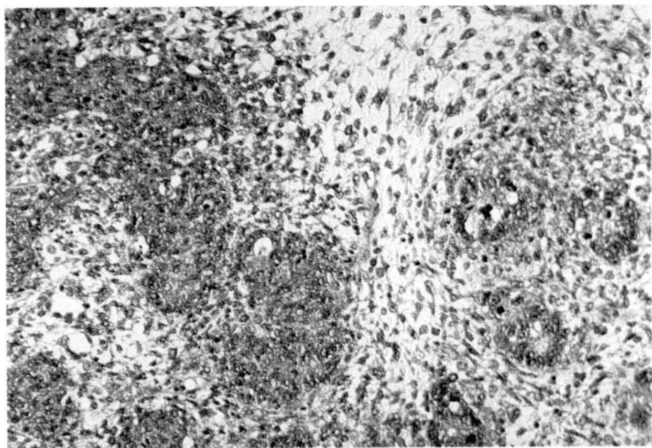

FIGURE 112.6 Wilms tumor (nephroblastoma). This photomicrograph of the tumor shows highly cellular areas composed of undifferentiated blastema, loose stroma containing undifferentiated mesenchymal cells, and immature tubules. (From Rubin E, Farber JL. *Pathology*, 3rd ed. Philadelphia: Lippincott Williams & Wilkins, 1999, with permission.)

patients with pulmonary metastases diagnosed by CT but not by plain chest films did as well as patients with nonmetastatic disease when staged and treated on the basis of their abdominal tumor alone. It is recommended that patients with pulmonary nodules identified by CT scan but not plain chest radiographs undergo biopsy to verify the diagnosis. This has obvious cost-of-care and quality-of-life implications. Some effort to resolve this controversy is needed, given the prevalence of CT scanning.

In the United States, this initial workup is followed by surgical resection of the tumor if possible (Fig. 112.7). This approach then allows surgical and histologic parameters to be included in staging. The surgeon must pay strict attention to the local tumor extent or tumor rupture and status of the regional periaortic, interaortocaval, paracaval, and perirenal lymph nodes. Previously, direct visualization and manual palpation of the contralateral kidney was considered mandatory in all cases, even when CT scans do not indicate involvement. *Surgeons should be aware that the Renal Tumor Committee of the COG no longer recommends this approach.* Preoperative assessment of the contralateral kidney is inaccurate in one

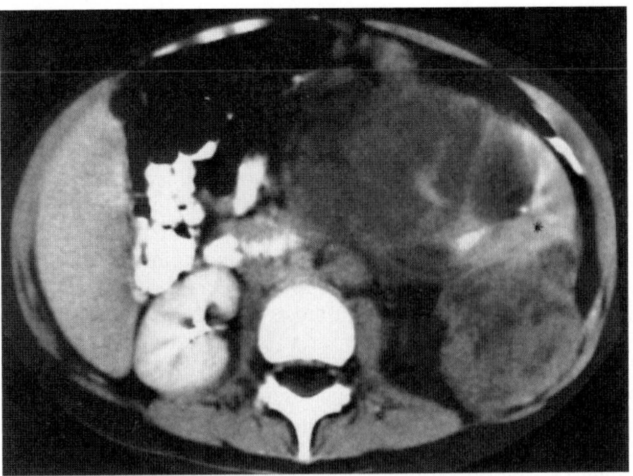

FIGURE 112.7 Initial computed tomography scan of a child with a left-sided Wilms tumor. The distortion of the calyceal system is characteristic of intrinsic renal tumor. A kidney (*asterisk*) is identifiable.

TABLE 112.5 STAGING

STAGING CRITERIA FOR WILMS TUMOR

Wilms tumor staging system*		4-Year survival rate (%)
Stage 1	Tumor limited to kidney and completely excised; surface intact with no evidence of rupture	97
Stage 2	Tumor extends beyond kidney but completely excised; infiltration through the renal capsule, or extension into vessels outside the kidney substance, or local open biopsy or spillage confined to the flank; no residual tumor	95
Stage 3	Residual nonhematogenous tumor	91
Stage 4	Hematogenous metastases to lung, liver, bone, brain, etc.	78
Stage 5	Bilateral renal involvement at diagnosis	Same as for highest-stage unilateral

*Survival based on outcome for patients with favorable histologic-types in the National Wilms Tumor Study–3

third of cases. Finally, the liver should be carefully palpated and the peritoneal and diaphragmatic surfaces inspected for metastases. Recently, in cases of bilateral Wilms tumor, and patients who have significant vascular invasion, initial treatment with chemotherapy has been recommended and is discussed later in this chapter.

Once the imaging and surgical and pathologic data are acquired, a tumor stage is assigned; the current NWTS staging schema is listed in Table 112.5. Stage is basically an assessment of risk group and has been validated by previous NWTS studies. Its importance lies in defining the least morbid treatment that results in long-term remission or cure.

Treatment

The standard of care in the United States is initial surgical resection. Exceptions to this rule include extensive intracaval tumors that require cardiopulmonary bypass for extraction, obviously unresectable tumors with documented invasion of contiguous structures, and possibly bilateral tumors, especially if it is unclear which side is most heavily involved. These special cases are discussed later in this chapter. For most patients, exploration and resection should be performed through a wide transverse incision that allows comfortable inspection and palpation of the contralateral kidney. As noted earlier, complete sampling of regional nodal echelons is mandatory, as is careful assessment of the tumor margins and possible areas of metastases. Most authors recommend early ligation of the renal vein, but most surgeons admit to not performing this maneuver because it is often difficult or unsafe owing to the size of the tumor. The available data indicate that later ligation of the renal vein after tumor mobilization does not adversely affect prognosis. After the kidney and accompanying Gerota fascia is mobilized, the renal artery is most easily identified by posterior dissection. Radical ureterectomy does not affect outcome, but the ureter should be divided well distal to the calyceal system to ensure any polypoid pelvicalyceal extensions are encompassed.

All patients with resectable Wilms tumor receive postoperative chemotherapy. There may be one exception to this rule, as reported by the Dana Farber Group. This group consists of patients with stage I favorable histology disease who are younger than 24 months of age at diagnosis and have tumors weighing less than 250 g at resection. Beckwith suggested a further refinement of histologic criteria to identify low-risk stage I patients: no vascular invasion beyond the renal hilar plane and absence of capsular invasion. Unfortunately, in a recent NWTS study, the local recurrence rate for stage I patients treated by surgery alone was higher than expected, and the current recommendation is to give two-drug chemotherapy to all patients with stage I disease.[51]

A major effort by the NWTS was the development of chemotherapy protocols for Wilms tumor that minimize toxicity while maintaining efficacy. Data accumulated from these studies have shown that in patients with stage I or II favorable histology disease, survival is improved when combination chemotherapy with vincristine and actinomycin D is used. The current 4-year relapse-free and overall survival for favorable histology stage I Wilms tumors is 94%, and 98%, respectively. Recommended treatment is initial nephrectomy and lymph node sampling followed by 18 weeks of vincristine and dactinomycin chemotherapy. The treatment regimen is the same for favorable histology patients with stage II disease and results in an 85% relapse-free, and 96% overall survival 4-year survival. Dactinomycin is given in pulse-intensive fashion. For stage I patients with focal or diffuse anaplasia a similar regimen is used and the 2-year relapse-free and overall survival is about 86%. Stage II patients with focal anaplasia receive vincristine, dactinomycin, and doxorubicin for 24 weeks as well as abdominal radiation. Stage II patients with diffuse anaplasia are treated with vincristine, cyclophosphamide, doxorubicin, etoposide, and mesna for 24 weeks and also receive abdominal radiation. Four-year survival is 70% in this group.[52,53] Favorable histology stage III tumors or those with focal anaplasia are treated with nephrectomy, lymph node sampling, 24 weeks of chemotherapy and abdominal radiation. The chemotherapy consists of vincristine, doxorubicin, and pulse-intensive dactinomycin.[52] This regimen results in a 90%, 4-year, relapse-free survival and 95% 4-year overall survival. For stage III patients with diffuse anaplasia nephrectomy, lymph node sampling, abdominal radiation, and 24 weeks of vincristine, doxorubicin, cyclophosphamide, and etoposide are given, resulting in a 56% 4-year survival.[54]

External beam radiation therapy is delivered to patients with stage III favorable histology disease. One study that analyzed the effect of the time between nephrectomy and flank radiation for favorable histology stage II to IV patients (included patients from NWTS III and IV) found no difference in the rate of abdominal or flank recurrence in patients treated within 9 days or less compared to those initiating radiation in more than 10 days.[55] The usual dose is 1,080 cGy given in daily fractions of 150 to 180 cGy. The entire kidney bed, as well as areas of gross residual disease, is targeted, and radiation is delivered to the entire vertebral column at the level of involvement to minimize the risk of scoliosis. Patients with stage IV disease should have their primary tumor staged as if metastases were not present. If the primary kidney tumor is stage I or II, no local radiation is delivered; the previously noted guidelines are followed for primary stage III tumors. Pulmonary metastases are treated with whole-thorax external beam radiation therapy to a total dose of 1,200 cGy given in 150-cGy fractions. The mediastinum is not shielded to prevent recurrence in central lymphatics or the lung margins. Nonresectable liver metastases are treated to a total dose of 1,980 cGy. Localized liver lesions may receive focal radiation, but diffuse hepatic metastases require treatment of the entire hepatic volume. Supplemental boosts to localized areas of

500 to 1,000 cGy may also be used. Bulky nodal, brain, and skeletal metastases receive 3,060 cGy and supplemental focal boosts as necessary.

Bilateral Wilms Tumor

The overall survival rate of patients who have bilateral Wilms tumor is 87%.[56] The survival rate for this disease is high because 90% of cases are of favorable histology, most kidneys are stage I when considered individually, and advances have made treatment more successful. Because of the danger of debilitating loss of renal function, it is acceptable to administer preoperative chemotherapy. It is no longer felt necessary to perform a renal biopsy in obvious cases of bilateral involvement based on imaging studies. After tumor shrinkage, a second-look procedure and nephron-sparing renal resection can be performed. Using this strategy, survival rates have been achieved that are equivalent to those obtained with the more traditional approach. The latter involves an initial nephrectomy of the most heavily involved kidney, followed by chemotherapy, and then reexploration.[57]

Renal Vein and Inferior Vena Cava Involvement

A study reported from NWTS-3 included 164 patients with gross involvement and 47 patients with microscopic involvement of the renal vein beyond the kidney (11.3%). Two-year survival rates were 90%, 79%, and 72%, respectively, for patients with stages I, II, and III disease. Important predictors of outcome were histologic pattern and stage. The authors suggested that complete *en bloc* resection of the primary tumor and the renal vein extension constituted the most effective initial management.[58] In a second report from the NWTS, 165 of 2731 Wilms tumor patients were found to have intravascular extension (6%).[59] Vascular extension involved the inferior vena cava in 134 cases and the atrium in 31. Of these, 69 patients received preoperative neoadjuvant chemotherapy for a median of 8 weeks; 55 were treated for caval extension and 14 for atrial extension. The intravascular extension was noted to regress in 39 of 49 patients with comparable preoperative and postoperative imaging studies. In particular, seven of 12 patients with atrial extension at diagnosis realized regression into the inferior vena cava obviating the need for cardiopulmonary bypass. The overall complication rate in patients undergoing neoadjuvant chemotherapy compared with those treated with immediate surgery was not statistically different and occurred in 36.7% of patients with atrial extension compared with 17.2% of those with tumors localized to the inferior vena cava. The authors suggest that neoadjuvant chemotherapy be used in most patients with vascular extension.

The 3-year relapse-free survival rates of patients with intravascular tumor extension (76.9%) do not statistically differ from those for Wilms tumor as a whole (80.3%).[59] It has been suggested that a complicated operation involving cardiopulmonary bypass can be safely avoided by administration of preoperative chemotherapy. A second-look procedure should then be performed and all residual tumors resected. Second-look surgery is usually less complicated, and resection can be accomplished using conventional means when this approach is taken. Tumor shrinkage usually is rapid when cytotoxic drugs are first administered, but stabilizes after four to five cycles of therapy. At this point, no further tumor reduction can be expected and resection should be planned with appropriate preoperative consultation from other services (e.g., cardiovascular) as indicated. Nevertheless, a preoperative workup that includes Doppler ultrasonography should always be performed before operation. Contrast vena cavography has become less crucial with advances in contrast-enhanced CT or MRI techniques, which now provide detailed information concerning the vascular anatomy. Nevertheless, an accurate picture of the anatomic extent of the tumor thrombus must be determined before surgery. If tumor thrombus continues to extend to the proximal vena cava or right atrium, resection should be coordinated and performed under cardiopulmonary bypass. If resection is not done, intraoperative tumor embolism, which is often fatal, may be the result.

Extrarenal Wilms Tumor

Wilms tumors can arise from areas other than the kidney, but this is extremely rare. The most common site is the retroperi-

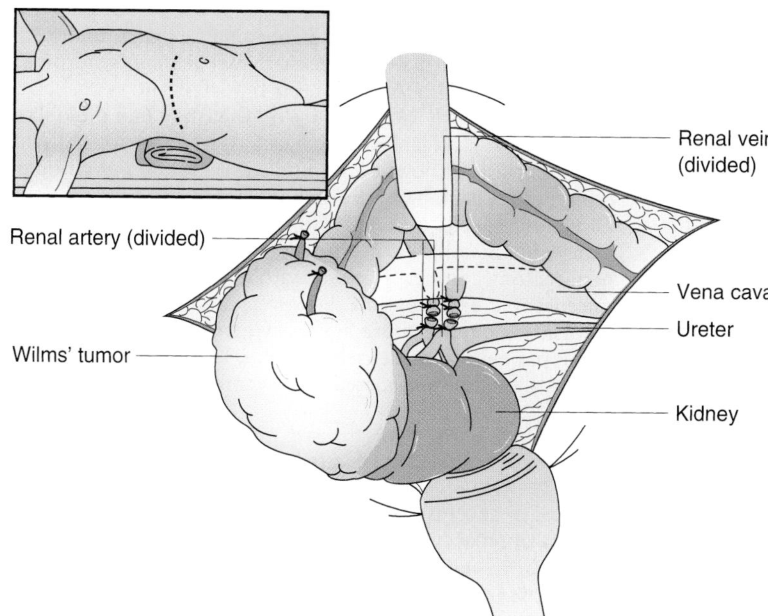

FIGURE 112.8 Operative approach to resection of a right renal Wilms tumor.

toneum, followed by the pelvis and inguinal canal. Two mechanisms for this phenomenon have been proposed. In the first theory, the tumor is thought to arise from the rests of metanephric tissue. The second theory suggests that Wilms tumor develops from germinal tissue present in a teratoma. It is possible that both mechanisms are operative. Stage for stage, extrarenal Wilms tumors have a prognosis similar to that of renal primary tumors, and therapy should be guided by principles developed by NWTS.[60–62]

Adult and Neonatal Wilms Tumor

Wilms tumors that occur at both ends of the age spectrum are rare.[63, 64] In a report by Hrabovsky et al.,[64] 27 of 3,340 (0.8%) patients with renal tumors were younger than 30 days of age at presentation. Of these 27 patients, 18 had mesoblastic nephroma, 1 had a malignant rhabdoid tumor, and 4 had nonneoplastic lesions. The remaining four patients had Wilms tumor, and all had favorable histology. Also, none of the patients with Wilms tumor had metastases at diagnosis, and all have survived. Adult Wilms tumors are associated with worse outcomes, even in patients with favorable histology. A 3-year overall survival rate has been reported by NWTS and supports the use of aggressive therapy in all adult patients with Wilms tumor.[65–67]

Future Directions

The NWTS-5 will not ask a clinical question but, rather, will focus on the predictive effect on outcome of cytogenetic abnormalities of chromosomes 1, 16, and 11. This is testimony to the progress achieved by previous NWTS studies. Other areas of investigation include the role of autologous bone marrow transplantation in patients with relapsed favorable and unfavorable histology disease, and attempts to improve outcome in the non-Wilms renal tumors that occur in childhood. In this regard, sarcoma-like protocols, using agents such as cisplatin, ifosfamide, and etoposide, are being evaluated.

NON-WILMS RENAL TUMORS OF CHILDHOOD AND ADOLESCENCE

Clear Cell Sarcoma

Clear cell sarcoma of the kidney is considered a distinct histopathologic and clinical entity from Wilms tumor.[68] It has an age distribution similar to that observed in Wilms tumor but a markedly worse prognosis. This tumor is characterized by a proclivity to metastasize to bones and has been called the *bone-metastasizing renal tumor of childhood* by British workers. Histopathologically, the tumor consists of cords and nests of pale-stained tumor cells separated by vascular structures. Confusion with classic Wilms tumor is possible, however, and central pathologic review is recommended. Clear cell sarcoma can metastasize not only to bone but also to brain. Bony metastases are usually polyostotic, but the skull is almost invariably involved. A CT scan of the abdomen or intravenous urogram, chest radiograph, MRI of the brain, and bone scan are recommended as part of the workup. The staging system is similar to that for Wilms tumor, but high rates of tumor relapse are associated with even stage I tumors, supporting the use of aggressive systemic chemotherapy in all stages. Relapse and death occur in 75% of patients treated with actinomycin-D and vincristine alone, with more than half dying within 1 year of diagnosis. The addition of doxorubicin to the treatment regimen for these children has resulted in significant survival improvement with a 6-year relapse-free survival of 64.6%.[69] Treatment recommendations include radical resection of the primary tumor when possible as well as involved regional lymph nodes, followed by a postoperative chemotherapy regimen that includes doxorubicin, actinomycin D, and vincristine. In one randomization, a 15-month course of chemotherapy compared with 6 months improved relapse-free survival but not overall survival.[70] Postoperative radiation therapy to the tumor bed is recommended regardless of stage. Usually, 1,080 cGy of postoperative flank irradiation is administered. Patients should be followed with serial chest radiographs or CT scans and 6-monthly brain MRI scans and bone scans for at least 3 years after treatment.

Rhabdoid Tumor

Rhabdoid tumors are rare malignancies that most commonly involve the kidney in childhood; they also can occur primarily in the mediastinum or brain.[71–73] Outcome is particularly poor, and there is no proved chemotherapy regimen. The tumor is characterized histopathologically by a rhabdomyosarcomatoid or myoblastic appearance, but the tumors do not express muscle markers and are not myoblastic in origin. Rhabdoid tumors of the kidney occur in infancy, with a median age at presentation of 13 months (range 2 months to 5 years). Some rhabdoid tumors may be associated with the coincident development of PNETs of the brain. Extrarenal rhabdoid tumors occur in older patients. The survival rate is almost zero, and even patients with stage I disease fare poorly. Therefore, aggressive therapy is warranted that includes surgical resection, local radiation therapy, and systemic chemotherapy. Because these tumors have been refractory to historical protocols, use of experimental dose-intensive chemotherapy regimens or new chemotherapeutic agents is warranted.

CONGENITAL MESOBLASTIC NEPHROMA

Congenital mesoblastic nephroma was first described by Bolande[74] in 1969 and differentiated from Wilms tumor. This tumor usually occurs in infants and typically follows a benign course; however, well-documented cases have resulted in metastases and death. Mesoblastic nephroma has been reported in adults and in patients with Beckwith-Wiedemann syndrome. A translocation, t(12;15), has been reported and is associated with an *ETV6–NTRK3* gene fusion that may link mesoblastic nephroma to congenital fibrosarcoma.[75] Histologically, the tumor consists of bundles of spindle cells, tubules of basophilic cells, and invasion into the renal parenchyma or perinephric soft tissue. The cells resemble fibroblasts or smooth muscle. Congenital mesoblastic nephroma is usually curable by radical nephrectomy alone. Tumors with high cellularity on light microscopic examination, however, and those with evident metastases require more aggressive treatment. In particular, older patients with densely cellular lesions or high mitotic indices should be considered for systemic chemotherapy.

Renal Cell Carcinoma

There are several reported series as well as scattered case reports of renal cell carcinoma occurring in childhood, adolescence, and young adults. In one study,[76] the median age was 15.5 years (range 3 to 21 years). Histologically, the tumor is an adenocarcinoma similar to that seen in older patients. Most reported cases are of the clear cell variant of renal adenocarcinoma. There is no predilection for the right or left side, and the tumors are equally distributed between upper and lower poles and mid-kidney. Sites of metastases include lung (64%), liver (57%), bone (42%), and pleura or brain (7%). Staging is based on the adult staging system and survival is stage dependent. Unfortunately, many of these patients present with stage IV disease. Outcome analysis has shown a correlation of survival with complete resection, although resectability was also associated with adverse prognostic factors like lymph node involvement or distant metastases. Recommended therapy is complete resection by radical nephrectomy, if feasible. The role of chemotherapy is undefined, but given the poor outcome associated with higher-stage disease, it is reasonable to administer postoperative chemotherapy as an experimental protocol. This should probably be performed as part of a national cooperative study.

RHABDOMYOSARCOMA

Epidemiology and Associated Conditions

In the United States, 850 to 900 children and adolescents younger than 20 years of age are diagnosed with soft tissue sarcoma each year, and approximately 350 of these are rhabdomyosarcomas.[77] Rhabdomyosarcoma is the most common soft tissue sarcoma in children younger than 14 years of age, comprising almost 50% of soft tissue sarcomas in this age group. There are two major histologic subtypes occurring in childhood, embryonal and alveolar. Embryonal rhabdomyosarcoma constitutes approximately 75% of cases.[77] The alveolar subtype is more common in older children and extremity lesions. The incidence of rhabdomyosarcoma in the United States is 4 cases per 1 million white children younger than 15 years and approximately half that rate for black children.[78] The male to female ratio is 1.4:1, and 80% of patients are white, 12% are black, and 8% fall into other categories.

Rhabdomyosarcoma has been observed in patients with neurofibromatosis and Beckwith-Wiedemann syndrome. The Li-Fraumeni cancer family syndrome involves the occurrence of sarcoma, in particular rhabdomyosarcoma, in addition to breast, bone, or brain cancer, lung and laryngeal cancer, and adrenocortical neoplasia. In this syndrome, children with rhabdomyosarcoma have first-degree relatives with the other malignancies. In an autopsy study from the IRS, 32% of patients with rhabdomyosarcoma had congenital anomalies that included (in order of frequency) genitourinary, central nervous system, and cardiovascular malformations.[79] Also, basal cell carcinoma has been observed in conjunction with rhabdomyosarcoma.

Basic Science

Myogenic cell differentiation can be arbitrarily divided into three broad stages: (a) commitment of a multipotent stem cell to a monopotent myoblast; (b) differentiation of a monopotent myoblast into a multinucleated myofiber expressing muscle-specific genes; and (c) maturation, during which the expression of specific cellular proteins progresses through embryonic, fetal, neonatal, and adult patterns. Genetic determinants of the first stage of myogenic cell differentiation were identified first. It was initially observed that fibroblasts briefly exposed to 5-azacytidine developed a myoblastic phenotype manifested by the presence of myotubes. Genomic DNA transfection experiments verified that myoblast but not fibroblast DNA could convert fibroblasts into stably determined myoblasts, and the frequency of conversion was consistent with a single genetic locus. This finding allowed the first identification of a myogenic determination gene, *MyoD1*.[80] *MyoD* is expressed exclusively in skeletal muscle as well as myoblasts derived from 5-azacytidine-treated fibroblasts. When this gene is transfected, under the control of a viral promoter, into a variety of cell types (i.e., fibroblast, melanoma cells, neuroblastoma, hepatic cells, and adipocytes), expression of the *MyoD* cDNA induces myogenesis with expression of muscle-specific structural genes.

Pathology

Rhabdomyosarcomas are malignant tumors that arise from the ubiquitously distributed primitive mesenchyme found in the fetus. These tumors display characteristics of striated muscle, including immunohistochemical expression of skeletal muscle myosin and actin, desmin, myoglobin, and Z-band protein. Electron microscopy may show actin–myosin bundles or Z-band material. Expression of the DNA-binding protein, MyoD1, has been shown to be a lineage marker for rhabdomyosarcoma.[81]

Based on classic pathology, rhabdomyosarcoma has been divided into four main histopathologic subtypes: embryonal, alveolar, botryoid, and pleomorphic. The most common type in children is embryonal (75%). Botryoid tumors are really of the embryonal subtype but growing into a hollow space (e.g., vagina, bladder) so that they assume a characteristic grapelike appearance. Alveolar tumors are so named because of a resemblance to the microscopic structure of the lung (Fig. 112.8). Rhabdomyosarcomas are identified as alveolar if any alveolar elements are found in the tumor. Pleomorphic tumors usually occur in older adults. For all histologic types, sites of occurrence include: (a) head and neck (orbit, infratemporal fossa); (b) genitourinary tract, including perineum and perianal area; (c) extremities; (d) trunk (chest wall, paraspinal area); (e) retroperitoneum; and (f) biliary tract.

The initial biopsy should be generous enough for cytogenetic and immunohistochemical studies. Light microscopy alone is no longer adequate to secure the diagnosis and establish histopathologic subtype. For instance, the alveolar subtype is currently characterized by a t(2;13) or t(1;13) translocation in which the *FKHR* gene on chromosome 13 is translocated onto either a *PAX3* (chromosome 2) or *PAX7* (chromosome 1) gene.[82] Thus, even if minimal alveolar elements are noted on light microscopy, a tumor with either of these translocations would be classified as alveolar. Embryonal rhabdomyosarcoma is associated with hyperdiploidy and loss of heterozygosity at chromosome 11p15 or other genes.[77, 83] An initial clinical application of these findings is the detection of minimal residual disease by polymerase chain reaction.[84]

Presentation and Workup

The incidence of rhabdomyosarcoma is biphasic, with one peak in infancy followed by a second peak in the adolescent years. Presentation is site dependent. Head and neck lesions can cause facial or cervical swelling and associated pain or skin discoloration. Sinusitis or middle ear infections can occur because the tumor blocks the normal drainage from these sites (i.e., sinusal ostia, eustachian tubes). Epistaxis, proptosis, or cranial nerve palsies may also be evident in head and neck lesions. Genitourinary tumors can present with gross or microscopic hematuria, a suprapubic mass, and urinary tract infection or obstruction. Vaginal and cervical primary tumors often prolapse through the vaginal orifice as a friable polypoid mass

TABLE 112.6 DIAGNASIS

DIAGNOSTIC EVALUATION FOR SUSPECTED RHABDOMYOSARCOMA[a]

Examination or test	Rationale
History and physical examination	Search for lymph nodes, size of primary mass, general condition, underlying conditions
Complete blood count	Bone marrow replacement associated with anemia or thrombocytopenis; bone marrow toxicity is the major side effect of chemotherapy
Electrolytes, renal and hepatic function tests, creatinine clearance	Renal toxicity associated with cisplatin and other alkylators; genitourinary tumors may obstruct ureters; hepatic toxicity with dactinomycin
Four-site bone marrow aspirations, two-site bone biopsies	Bone marrow metastases reported in up to 6% of patients at diagnosis (29% of stage 4 patients have marrow involvement); bone marrow assessment before chemotherapy
Bone scan	Possibility of bone and bone marrow metastases
CT scan of the primary site	Evaluation of tumor size, invasiveness, enlargement of regional nodes, and complicating ureteral, biliary, bowel, or airway patency
CT scan of possible metastatic sites	CT scanning of the lungs and liver should be done to rule out parenchymal metastases. CT scanning is superior to MRI in assessing the degree of bone destruction in paraspinal, extremity, and head and neck (base of skull) lesions.
MRI	MRI is done for the same rationale as CT scanning. It may give more detailed information regarding the extent of viable tumor (T2-weighted imaging) and the presence of hepatic metastases. It is also the most useful tool for evaluation of the epidural space in paraspinal or base of skull primaries.
Gallium scanning	Both the primary tumor and metastatic deposits may be identified by gallium scanning

[a]The same workup is applicable to other high-grade sarcomas.
CT, computed tomography; MRI, magnetic resonance imaging.

and may hemorrhage. Paratesticular lesions are most often observed in adolescence as a hard mass above and separable from the testis. Extremity tumors present as a painless or painful expanding mass, and there may be an associated limp or overlying skin change. Local bony invasion may result in pathologic fractures.

Rational management depends on a thorough pretreatment workup that completely defines local tumor extent as well as evaluating regional and distant sites of metastases. Table 112.6 lists the standard workup for pediatric patients with sarcoma. An extensive history, including a family history of breast cancer or other forms of sarcoma, and a thorough physical examination are elementary. Radiographic staging has been markedly facilitated by modern imaging methods. Even greater progress in this area is promised by current efforts in the field of positron emission tomographic scanning, which allows determination of the metabolic activity of a tumor mass. Figure 112.9 is a CT scan of a large pelvic rhabdomyosarcoma originating from the bladder.

Staging

An evolution in sarcoma staging has occurred since the late 1980s, with most groups adopting the tumor, node, metastasis (TNM) system defined by the International Union Against Cancer. This staging system, which is used with the older IRS grouping, is listed in Table 112.7. The TNM schema attempts to divide each stage into definable clinical components. It is applied before any therapeutic interventions (although a second staging based on histologic findings of the primary tumor and regional lymph nodes after resection can also be performed). The IRS grouping schema is retained as well, although it remains operator dependent.

Local tumor invasiveness is the result of cellular and molecular phenotypic properties, which are rapidly being defined by molecular analyses. The ability of cells to invade surrounding basement membranes depends on manufacture of a spectrum of lytic enzymes as well as cellular motility. Furthermore, regional or distant metastasis is not possible without initial cellular invasion. The gross invasiveness assessed for TNM staging is a rough measure of these cellular events. In this sense, the TNM system begins to relate macroscopic tumor behavior to the properties and interactions of individual tumor cells. Future directions include more precise definitions of the invasive process. Assays of collagenolytic activity and assessment of growth and invasion in nude mice are intermediate steps in this regard. Eventually, genetic determinants of invasion and metastases that are the final determinants of prognosis will be identified.

Using the TNM system, the reported overall percentage of patients with tumors greater than 5 cm ranges from 50% to 68%. The proportions of other staging variables include invasive tumors, 37% to 71%; regional nodal involvement, 7% to 28%; and distant metastases at diagnosis, 20% to 23%.

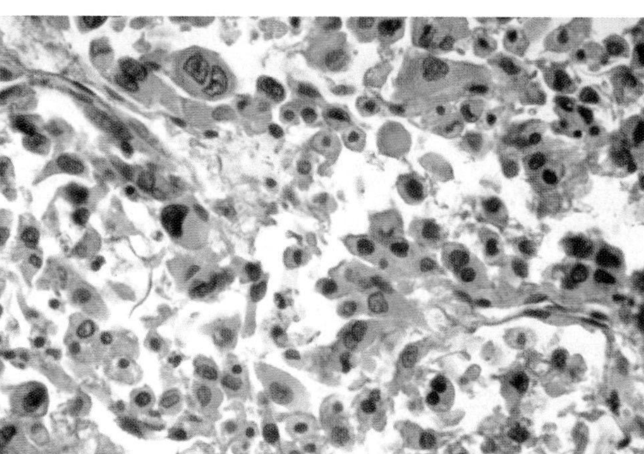

FIGURE 112.9 Photomicrograph illustrating the typical lung-like appearance of an alveolar rhabdomyosarcoma. (From Rubin E, Farber JL. *Pathology*, 3rd ed. Philadelphia: Lippincott Williams & Wilkins, 1999, with permission.)

TABLE 112.7 STAGING

TNM STAGING SYSTEM FOR RHABDOMYOSARCOMA

Clinical stage	Invasiveness	Size	Status of nodes	Distant metastases
I	T1	a or b	N0	M0
II	T2	a or b	N0	M0
III	T1 or T2	a or b	N1	M0
IV	T1 or T2	a or b	N0 or N1	M1

T1, noninvasive; T2, invasive; £5cm; Tb, >5cm; N0, regional nodes negative; N1, nodes positive; M0, no distant metastases at diagnosis; M1, metastases present.

A sarcoma is adequately staged when the following criteria are met: (a) the primary tumor pathologic type and histopathologic subtype have been determined by biopsy, and (b) all components in the TNM staging system are known with reasonable certainty. It is preferable to sample metastatic regional lymph nodes, but extensive nodal dissections are not indicated. In the special case of paratesticular rhabdomyosarcoma, a limited dissection of ipsilateral, periaortic nodes is used as a determinant of the need for nodal radiation. The use of prechemotherapy nodal sampling in paratesticular rhabdomyosarcoma is controversial because many European groups favor chemotherapy along with radical orchiectomy as sole primary treatment. Most North American groups favor lymph node biopsy with consequent periaortic nodal radiation if N1 status is proved. Laparoscopic biopsy may prove a useful alternative in this regard.

Small, accessible primary lesions should undergo excisional biopsy. If biopsy is performed, the surgeon should attempt to obtain a clear microscopic margin. Patients with larger infiltrating lesions or lesions for which removal would cause debilitation or deformity (i.e., amputation or cystectomy) should undergo limited incisional or endoscopic biopsy. It is acceptable to perform transperineal needle core biopsies for bladder neck or perineal primary tumors. Enough biopsy material for light and electron microscopic analysis, immunohistochemistry, and cytogenetics should be obtained. It is preferable to freeze extra tissue to facilitate further specialized studies. Even though such investigations do not have direct short-term benefit for the patient, they are crucial in expanding knowledge concerning rhabdomyosarcoma. Tissue should be frozen in liquid nitrogen as soon as possible after biopsy.

Risk Status

Presently the soft tissue sarcoma committee of the COG, the successor of the IRS, uses risk group assessment to determine therapy. Risk status is dependent on IRS group or stage but also age, anatomic location, and histopathology.[85–87] Favorable anatomic sites include the orbit, nonparameningeal head and neck, paratestis, vagina and nonbladder-prostate genitourinary sites, and the biliary tract.[88–90] High-risk sites include extremities, retroperitoneum, bladder-prostate, and parameningeal primaries.

Low-risk patients have embryonal rhabdomyosarcoma at favorable anatomic sites (stage 1, groups I, II, or II), or embryonal rhabdomyosarcoma occurring at unfavorable sites but completely resected, or resected with only a positive microscopic margin (groups I or II). Intermediate-risk patients have embryonal rhabdomyosarcoma occurring at unfavorable sites with residual gross disease (group III). The intermediate-risk group also includes patients with metastatic rhabdomyosarcoma who are younger than 10 years of age, and patients with localized disease who have alveolar histology or undifferentiated sarcoma. High-risk patients have metastatic rhabdomyosarcoma or undifferentiated sarcoma at presentation, excepting patients younger than 10 years of age.

Treatment

The modern treatment of rhabdomyosarcoma is multidisciplinary and includes multiagent chemotherapy, judicious resection, and radiation therapy. The intensity of therapy should be tailored to the risk of subsequent relapse, which is a function of TNM stage. In general, agents are combined to limit drug resistance while attaining a synergistic antitumor effect. A major surgical responsibility during chemotherapy is maintenance of adequate vascular access both for administration of medications as well as blood drawing. An external or implanted vascular access device usually can be inserted at the time of diagnostic biopsy.

Surgical resection of the primary tumor was the mainstay of treatment 30 years ago but resulted in overall survival rates of only approximately 20%. This rate improved to 50% with the addition of chemotherapy and resulted in uncertainty regarding the role of tumor resection in rhabdomyosarcoma. It is difficult to prove that surgical removal of the primary tumor affects survival. One reason is that a significant proportion of patients present with distant metastases, which so profoundly influences survival that the effect of other variables is obscured. Also, most tumors that can be readily removed without serious disfigurement or disability are resected. Thus, the effect of leaving a tumor in situ cannot readily be evaluated. With current survival rates, it would be unethical to randomize patients with nonmetastatic, resectable tumors to a non-surgical arm. Complete resection of primary tumors should be undertaken either before chemotherapy for small, noninvasive lesions or after documented response with more formidable primary tumors. An example of the operative approach for a lower extremity rhabdomyosarcoma involving anterior thigh muscles is depicted in Figure 112.10. In certain situations in which chemotherapy results in complete or very good tumor regression, external beam irradiation may be used as a primary means of local control. Even in these circumstances, it is important to obtain biopsy specimens to document complete tumor eradication. Debilitating or disfiguring surgery should be performed only if residual tumor is present after both chemotherapy and therapeutic irradiation. Amputation of extremity rhabdomyosarcomas does not enhance cure and should be performed only when lesions are bulky, invade bone or neurovascular structures, or are recurrent. Similarly, radical cystectomy is reserved for situations in which complete tumor eradication has not been accomplished by chemotherapy and external beam irradiation. The guiding principle of rhabdomyosarcoma surgery is complete tumor resection, but

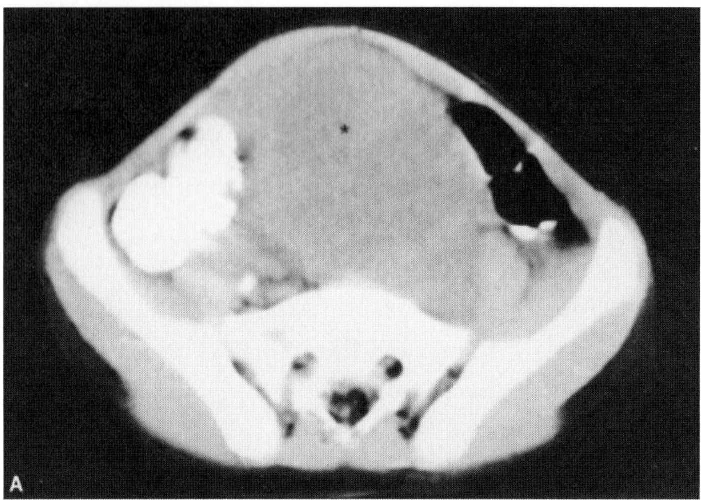

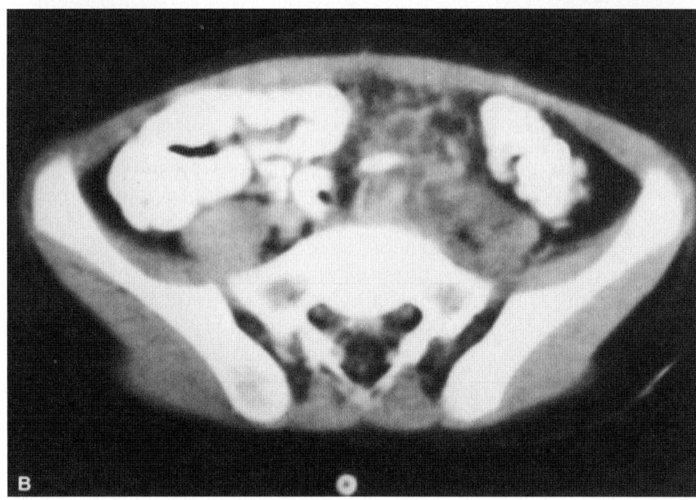

FIGURE 112.10 (*A*) Initial computed tomography (CT) scan of a child with a large pelvic rhabdomyosarcoma. (*B*) CT scan of the same child after biopsy and cytoreductive chemotherapy. No tumor was demonstrable by diagnostic imaging.

removal of large amounts of normal tissue (i.e., muscle group resection, amputation) alone does not affect outcome.

Most patients with low-risk rhabdomyosarcoma are treated with vincristine and dactinomycin. Intermediate-risk patients also receive cyclophosphamide in addition to these two drugs. High-risk patients have a very poor outlook and new therapies are in development. These include the use of irinotecan, melphalan, ifosfamide, and etoposide.

External beam radiation therapy of the primary site or involved regional nodal echelons has contributed to locoregional control. Orbital and genitourinary primaries receive radiation therapy as the primary means of local control with surgery reserved for very specific indications in patients with refractory or recurrent disease. Clinical data suggest that control of microscopic rhabdomyosarcoma can be accomplished with doses of 4,000 cGy, and gross deposits require in excess of 5400 cGy for sterilization.[91]

Outcome

The overall 5-year survival for children with rhabdomyosarcoma is approximately 64%. Table 112.8 lists the results of studies analyzing the effects of various prognostic factors on outcome in rhabdomyosarcoma.[92–97] As expected, the presence of distant parenchymal metastases at diagnosis has an overwhelming adverse effect on survival. Because of this, some groups have analyzed the effect of prognostic parameters in nonmetastatic subsets. Site and invasiveness of the primary tumor have also been independent predictors of outcome in some studies. Regarding site, most authors agree that orbital, paratesticular, and vaginal primary tumors are associated with improved outcome, whereas extremity, parameningeal, and truncal and retroperitoneal sites carry a worse prognosis. Survival is stage dependent. If all cases (both high and low risk) are included, the overall survival rate from rhabdomyosarcoma is approximately 50%.

Most studies conclude that overall and disease-free survival rates in rhabdomyosarcoma are equivalent; this means that salvage after initial relapse is low and may depend on initial stage and histopathologic subtype. Therefore, primary therapy is crucial for long-term survival.[98] This suggests that, after risk assessment by staging, therapy should be as intense as possible to eradicate the tumor.

Special Considerations for Specific Anatomic Sites

Head and Neck

Rhabdomyosarcoma can occur anywhere in the head and neck. Orbital sites in young children have a favorable outlook, but this is not true for older children. Parameningeal involvement has a very poor outcome. Tumor size (>5 cm), regional lymph node involvement, and age at diagnosis have been found to influence survival.[99] There is a high frequency of regional nodal involvement in head and neck rhabdomyosarcoma and

TABLE 112.8 RESULTS

COLLECTED INDICATORS OF OUTCOMES FOR RHABDOMYOSARCOMA

Institution	Ref.	Year	Patients	Predictors of outcome
Memorial Sloan-Kettering Cancer Center	(70)	1994	290	Age at diagnosis, invasion, metastases, histology, regional lymph nodes
Italian Cooperative Group	(71)	1991	145	Site, size, alveolar histology, clinical group
International Rhabdomyosarcoma Workshop	(72)	1991	951	Invasiveness, site, interaction between inva siveness and site
Cooperative Soft Tissue Sarcoma Study (CWS -81)	(73)	1991	131	Site, degree of tumor regression after 7 wks of four-drug chemotherapy
Societé Internacionale Oncologique Pediatrique (SIOP)	(74)	1988	253	Site, stage, sex
Second Intergroup Rhabdomyosarcoma	(75)	1993	1115	Site, stage, alveolar histology
IRS-3	(76)	1995	1062	Site, stage

regional node sampling may be important in determination of risk status.[100] Resection of localized and anatomically accessible tumors may allow a reduction in radiation dosage with equivalent cure.[101,102]

Bladder and Bladder–Prostate

Bladder-prostate rhabdomyosarcomas have a worsened prognosis compared with other genitourinary sites, including the dome of the bladder. The trend since the early 1990s has been to minimize treatment toxicity for genitourinary rhabdomyosarcoma.[103–107] Currently, all patients with these tumors receive neoadjuvant chemotherapy after cystoscopic or transperineal biopsies confirm the diagnosis. This therapy is followed by repeat evaluations, including cystoscopic or percutaneous biopsies as well as imaging studies. A complete response after chemotherapy may obviate the need for external beam radiation therapy in some cases, but most patients require local radiation. Surgery is reserved for recurrent or poorly responsive cases with residual gross tumor.[108] Partial cystectomy, when anatomically feasible, is effective and preserves bladder function.[106] Newer techniques of urinary reconstruction involving stomas that can be catheterized may add to the patient's quality of life.

Paratesticular Rhabdomyosarcoma

An important point of discussion concerning patients with paratesticular rhabdomyosarcoma is the necessity of retroperitoneal lymph node dissection. Initially, this had been a formal recommendation for patients treated in North America. More recently, the IRS embarked on a study that used radiographic imaging rather than retroperitoneal nodal dissection to determine lymph node involvement.[109,110] Patients with positive lymph nodes receive radiation therapy to the retroperitoneum. Unfortunately, results from these types of studies have shown an increased rate of recurrence in older patients who did not undergo surgical staging. The current recommendation is for ipsilateral, nerve-sparing lymph node dissection, especially in boys more than 10 years of age at diagnosis. This was the age group that was seriously understaged by imaging studies alone. Patients 10 years of age or younger are still staged with computed axial tomography.

Future Directions

The results of myeloablative regimens with bone marrow or peripheral stem cell rescue have not improved overall outcome in patients with recurrent or metastatic disease.[111–114] Biologic or immunologic therapy for rhabdomyosarcoma is not available. There is great interest in reducing the intensity of therapy for patients with low-risk tumors. In the worst-risk cases, the thrust of most clinical research has been the development of new chemotherapeutic regimens with activity against this tumor. There is also an interest in combining the use of chemotherapy and radiotherapy and in using preresection radiotherapy.

NONRHABDOMYOMATOUS SOFT TISSUE SARCOMAS

Fibrosarcoma

Epidemiology

Fibrosarcomas, although rare, are the most common nonrhabdomyomatous sarcomas of infancy, childhood, and adolescence. A biphasic age incidence similar to that observed with rhabdomyosarcoma is characteristic, with one peak before 5 years of age and a second peak in the 10- to 15-year age group. Fibrosarcomas are most frequently encountered on the extremities, with 70% of congenital fibrosarcomas occurring distally. Cases are equally distributed between the sexes. Most reports suggest that prognosis is better in younger children.[115]

Pathology

Fibrosarcomas are spindle cell tumors characterized by a herringbone or interweaving pattern of tumors cells with a large amount of stromal collagen putatively arising from a fibroblastic lineage. Fibrosarcomas can be difficult, if not impossible, to distinguish from desmoid tumors or aggressive fibromatoses. For practical purposes, desmoids, fibromatoses, and low-grade fibrosarcomas can be thought of as a spectrum of similar and related neoplasms. Important characteristics of malignancy include nuclear pleomorphism, mitotic index, and basophilia. The tumor must be distinguished from undifferentiated rhabdomyosarcomas, neurofibrosarcoma, nodular fasciitis, myositis ossificans, and inflammatory pseudotumor. Infantile fibrosarcomas sometimes demonstrate a t(12;15) (ETV6-NTRK3) translocation.[116]

Presentation and Diagnostic Evaluation

Congenital fibrosarcomas and those diagnosed in early childhood are usually located on the distal upper or lower extremity. The trunk is a secondary site. A hard, often infiltrating mass is appreciated, and there may be skin or deep fixation.

Fibrosarcomas in the head and neck associated with swallowing and airway problems are also occasionally observed and may require lifesaving tracheostomy. High-grade lesions may invade bony or neural structures and metastasize to lung or liver. Multifocal lesions with multiple primary tumors affecting an extremity are sometimes seen. Bone marrow metastases do not develop. Workup is similar to that for rhabdomyosarcoma except that bone marrow aspiration and biopsy are not required.

Staging

The TNM schema is used, although lymph node metastases from fibrosarcoma are uncommon except with high-grade lesions. An adequate incisional or excisional biopsy, depending on the extent and invasiveness of the primary lesion, should be performed.

Treatment

The primary treatment of fibrosarcoma is surgical resection with negative microscopic margins if this can be done without significant debilitation or deformity. Patients occasionally present with rapidly progressive or extensive lesions. Under these circumstances, an initial trial of systemic chemotherapy may result in gratifying tumor regression.[117–119] In very young children (usually younger than 5 years of age), these tumors can be indolent and may regress spontaneously. In cases in which complete resection requires mutilating surgery like amputation or laryngectomy, a plan of simple observation may be best. Often, the tumor mass is dormant for years, allowing growth of the affected part and the possibility of a less debilitating or deforming resection later. These tumors should also undergo pathologic review to make certain that what is called fibrosarcoma is not simply infantile fibromatosis. A margin of greater than 1 cm has been associated with a reduced rate of recurrence.[98] Heroic resections should be performed only if the tumor is progressive or otherwise causing severe symptoms.

High-grade lesions, especially in very young children, respond to a variety of agents. Chemotherapy may be tried for unresectable, symptomatic, and progressive lesions as noted above. Effective chemotherapeutic agents include doxorubicin, actinomycin D, vincristine, and cyclophosphamide, in various combinations. The combination of ifosfamide and etoposide has been shown effective in the treatment of metastatic fibrosarcoma. In summary, systemic chemotherapy may be useful for extensive or progressive lesions or in patients with congenital fibrosarcoma. A common initial regimen includes actinomycin D and vincristine, which are less toxic than alkylating agents.

In the only prospective, randomized trial, use of external beam radiation therapy was associated with a lower local recurrence rate for margin-positive low-grade sarcomas, including fibrosarcoma.[120] Interstitial brachytherapy has been shown to lower local recurrence rates with margin-positive or margin-negative high-grade lesions. Despite this, most patients should initially be treated by wide surgical excision.

Outcome

The survival rate for low-grade nonmetastatic fibrosarcomas occurring in infancy is greater than 90%. Patients with metastatic disease have a guarded prognosis and require multidisciplinary therapy.

Tendosynovial Sarcoma

Epidemiology

Tendosynovial sarcoma is the third most common malignant pediatric soft tissue tumor. In large combined adult and pediatric series, tendosynovial sarcomas constitute approximately 8% of all soft tissue sarcomas. In a report of nonrhabdomyomatous soft tissue sarcomas, this histologic type was identified in 29% of patients. The male to female distribution is 1:1.2 to 1.6. Most patients present in the early teenage years, but there is also a small incidence spike centered on 5 years of age, giving the familiar bimodal age distribution observed with other sarcomas.

Pathology

Tendosynovial sarcomas arise from the synovial tissue, which is ubiquitous in the body and helps compose tendons, joint membranes, and bursae. Synonyms include *synovioma* or *tendosynovioma, pseudoglandular synovial sarcoma, clear cell sarcoma,* and *chordoid sarcoma.* The lower extremity is the most common site of origin, with an equal distribution between the thigh, foot, and posterior knee. The shoulder and forearm are also relatively common areas of involvement. Tendosynovial sarcomas close to bone may incite a periosteal reaction. Other possible primary sites include the abdominal wall and trunk, and the head and neck, with the tongue and retropharyngeal or hypopharyngeal areas being the most common.

The most common metastatic sites are lung and pleura. Tendosynovial sarcomas are known to relapse in lung even decades after resection of the primary tumor. Metastases to regional lymph nodes and subcutaneous sites have been described but are rare. Terminally, metastases to multiple organs are possible.

Microscopically, tendosynovial sarcoma is divided into two subtypes, monophasic and diphasic. In the diphasic form, epithelioid cells and stromal spindle cells are observed. The epithelioid component is arranged in glandlike structures resembling true epithelial cells but devoid of basement membrane. The diphasic subtype has been associated with a better prognosis, but some studies have not verified this finding. The monophasic variant is the most common and consists of sheets and parallel cords of spindle-shaped cells with little cytoplasm and cigar-shaped nuclei. Prognosis has been reported to be worse with the monophasic histologic type. In synovial sarcoma, the t(X;18) translocation has been identified and is useful in diagnosis.[121,122]

Presentation and Diagnostic Evaluation

An enlarging extremity mass brings most patients to medical attention. Pain may be prominent if bony or neural invasion is present. Regional lymph node metastases occur in 3% and distant metastases (lung) in 6% of patients at diagnosis. A workup similar to that described for rhabdomyosarcoma is appropriate. Adequate radiographic imaging of the primary site is crucial because of the impact of complete resection on outcome.

Treatment

Chemotherapy has historically been ineffective, and the primary treatment of tendosynovial sarcoma is surgical. The goal is clear microscopic margins, and every effort should be made to accomplish this, including use of amputation. Limb-sparing procedures are acceptable if complete resection is accomplished but incomplete removal results in a high rate of local recurrence.

There has been a recent, renewed interest in the use of adjuvant or neoadjuvant chemotherapy in selected patients with synovial sarcoma. Rosen et al.[123] have reported on the use of high-dose ifosfamide in the treatment of metastases from tendosynovial sarcoma. All 13 patients treated in this study had objective responses. Chemotherapy is reserved for patients who present with metastatic disease or in whom complete resection with clear microscopic margins cannot be accomplished.

Outcome

Overall survival rates are in the range of 43% to 75%. Important prognostic indicators are large primary tumor size and high nuclear grade with extensive tumor necrosis (high grade), as well as the presence of metastases at diagnosis. Worse survival rates are correlated for patients with tumors greater than 10 cm in diameter at diagnosis, compared with tumors less than 5 cm, with 86% versus 22% 5-year survival rates, respectively. Studies have shown no effect of monophasic versus biphasic histologic type on outcome.[124]

Peripheral Primitive Neuroectodermal Tumor

Epidemiology, Pathology, and Clinical Presentation

Peripheral PNET (peripheral neuroepithelioma, Askin's tumor, peripheral neuroblastoma) is a small, round blue cell malignancy distinguished from Ewing sarcoma only by ultrastructural and immunocytochemical features. This tumor shares the t(11;22)(q24;q12) translocation with Ewing sarcoma and esthesioneuroblastoma. The incidence is low, with 54 patients treated during a 20-year period reported from a major cancer center. Approximately two thirds of patients are 19 years of age or younger at diagnosis, and 57% are male. The disease affects predominantly white people, and 82% of tumors are localized at diagnosis. Common sites of involvement include chest wall (33%), pelvis (22%), paraspinal areas (13%), retroperitoneum (11%), limbs (9%), and abdomen (7%). In one study, epidural extension from the primary tumor was noted in 24% of patients at diagnosis, and 18% had distant metastases.[125] None of the patients in this series who had chest wall primary tumors had distant metastases at diagnosis. All primary tumors were greater than 5 cm in diameter in at least one dimension. Urinary catecholamines are not elevated in peripheral PNET. There is no familial or sex predilection.

Light microscopic criteria include fairly uniform, poorly differentiated round cells arranged in cords, nests, or clusters; no spindle cells with fine reticular or collagenous processes; no ganglionic or schwannian differentiation; and positive immunostaining for neuron-specific enolase. Ultrastructurally, neurosecretory-like granules and tapering ("neuritic") cytoplasmic processes are evident.

Treatment

The outcome of PNET has been historically poor, whereas survival rates for Ewing sarcoma, which is a related neoplasm sharing the typical t(11;22) translocation, have approached 60% to 65% in patients presenting without distant metastases. There may be underlying differences in fundamental biology, but the data also suggest that the uniform, multidisciplinary approach used for Ewing sarcoma and including multiagent chemotherapy may have utility in the treatment of PNET. The diagnosis should be established by incisional biopsy and the patient quickly started on an intensive multiagent chemotherapy regimen. A dose–response effect of cyclophosphamide has been observed. Occasionally, the tumor can be completely resected before chemotherapy; resection should be performed, if feasible, without an extensive procedure or the requirement for complicated reconstruction techniques. In most cases, definitive resection should be deferred until after administration of several cycles of systemic treatment. In general, surgery is required because complete responses to chemotherapy do not occur. External beam radiation therapy using 4,500 to 6,000 cGy can shrink but not cure macroscopic tumors. Radiation may be effective in improving local control after resection, especially if margins are microscopically positive.

Outcome

In patients with localized PNET at diagnosis, complete resection of all gross disease within 3 months resulted in improved progression-free survival (p = .0003).[125] The effect of myeloablative therapy with autologous bone marrow rescue is being evaluated.

Desmoplastic Small Round Cell Tumor

The desmoplastic small round cell tumor is a distinctive malignant neoplasm with a predilection for boys and young men. Eighty percent of patients present before the age of 30 years, and approximately half are 5 to 20 years of age at diagnosis.[126,127] There is a striking male predominance (male to female ratio, 4.1:1), and most of the patients are white. A striking feature is the frequent occurrence of divergent, multilineage differentiation with expression of epithelial, neural, and myogenic immunophenotypes. The tumor is characterized by the t(11;22)(p13;q12) translocation.

Common presenting complaints include abdominal or back pain, abdominal distention or mass, acute abdomen, and bowel, biliary, or ureteral obstruction. Small nodules found in hernia sacs during repair have been the first indication the tumor. CT of the chest and abdomen using both gastrointestinal and vascular contrast is the most useful diagnostic procedure. Initial laparoscopic biopsy is adequate to establish the diagnosis and assess the extent of abdominal disease. Small serosal nodules not detected by imaging studies can be identified using laparoscopic magnification. A careful pelvic and serosal inspection should be carried out. Adequate tissue for immunohistochemistry, electron microscopy, and molecular biologic studies should be obtained.

Because desmoplastic small round cell tumor is a diffuse serosal malignancy, systemic chemotherapy using a dose-intensive sarcoma regimen is the initial treatment. Serial abdominal CT scans can be followed to judge response, remembering that small mucosal implants may escape detection with imaging studies. After four to seven cycles, exploratory laparotomy with resection of all gross disease is attempted. Consolidation chemotherapy and external beam radiation therapy to the primary site are then used. If diffuse peritoneal seeding is identified either at diagnostic or second-look laparotomy or laparoscopy, whole-abdomen irradiation is required. Myeloablative chemotherapy with autologous marrow reconstitution may also be necessary.

Of 19 reported patients with adequate follow-up, only two were disease free 2 and 3.5 years after diagnosis. The other 17 died from progressive disease within 6 months to 4 years after presentation. A recent report, however, suggests that outlook may be improved using a dose-intensive, multiagent chemotherapy regimen including cyclophosphamide, ifosfamide, etoposide, and doxorubicin.[128] This justifies aggressive treatment for these patients, including extensive surgical debulking.[129]

Neurofibrosarcoma

Neurofibrosarcomas (neurogenic sarcomas, malignant schwannomas, malignant nerve sheath tumor, malignant neurilemoma) constitute 5% to 10% of nonrhabdomyomatous soft tissue sarcomas in childhood. Approximately 20% of all patients (children and adults) with neurofibrosarcoma have von Recklinghausen disease (NF1), and a neurofibrosarcoma develops in 5% to 16% of patients with NF1. The incidence of NF1 in children with neurofibrosarcomas is as high as 66%.[130] Neurofibrosarcomas have been reported as secondary tumors after external beam radiation therapy. Malignant peripheral nerve sheath tumors can be differentiated from their benign variant by the occurrence of more complex chromosomal abnormalities.[131]

The most common sites in children are extremity (42%), retroperitoneum (25%), and trunk. Less than 10% of patients present with metastatic disease. Microscopically, the tumor resembles fibrosarcoma but is differentiated by the presence of schwannian elements. Whorl, storiform, and tactile body-like formations are observed, and the S-100 stain is positive in approximately 60% of cases. Ultrastructural findings are important distinguishing criteria, and in all suspected cases, a specimen should be sent for electron microscopy. Electron microscopic findings include the presence of schwannian differentiation with cytoplasmic concavities lacking neurites. Primary neurofibrosarcoma of skin and subcutaneous tissues has also been described.

Two thirds of patients have associated NF1, and aggressive diagnostic procedures, including biopsy, are warranted when enlarging extremity or truncal masses are observed. Pain may be prominent depending on location. Radicular or sciatic pain is reported with paraspinal or retroperitoneal tumors causing sciatic pressure. Spontaneous hemothorax has been reported with chest wall primary tumors. Pelvic tumors may present as a perineal or perianal mass. The primary treatment of neurofibrosarcoma is wide local excision. In one series of 20 patients (14 with NF1), local recurrence developed in 8 of 12 patients undergoing local tumor excision plus radiation or chemotherapy but in only 1 of 6 patients treated with radical excision as well as chemotherapy or irradiation.[130] Unfortunately, a significant proportion had distant metastases despite local control. Patients with intermediate or high-grade neurofibrosarcomas should undergo radical local excision followed by chemotherapy and irradiation.

Leiomyosarcoma

Leiomyosarcoma accounts for 7% of soft tissue sarcomas in adults but less than 2% of childhood sarcomas. The gastrointestinal (oropharynx to anus) or genitourinary tract, retroperitoneum, lungs, pulmonary artery, vascular wall (i.e., middle third of the inferior vena cava, saphenous or femoral vein), popliteal artery, sinonasal area, and peripheral soft tissues (i.e., extremities) are reported sites of involvement.[132] Most cases are gastrointestinal in origin. The lungs are the most common site for metastases. Regional lymph node involvement occurs in 14% of gastric (perigastric nodes) and 5% of small intestinal leiomyosarcomas at diagnosis. Dissemination to liver and brain has also been reported. Also, tumors arising from gastrointestinal structures can disseminate throughout the peritoneal cavity. Leiomyosarcoma has been reported in patients with von Recklinghausen disease and coincident with the occurrence of neurofibrosarcoma.

True leiomyosarcomas are derived from smooth muscle and are often pseudoencapsulated. Cytologically, they demonstrate uniform, elongated cells with cigar-shaped nuclei. An epithelioid variant with more aggressive behavior is reported to arise in up to 40% of cases. Bone marrow metastases are not reported.

The usual presentation is pain (up to 80%) or gastrointestinal bleeding (60%). There are also reports of presentation with intussusception and perforation of a Meckel's diverticulum. Congenital leiomyosarcoma associated with hydrops fetalis has also been reported. Double-contrast CT scans, gastrointestinal contrast studies, and endoscopy may aid in diagnosis.

The most effective treatment of leiomyosarcoma is complete surgical resection, which should be accomplished even when resection requires amputation or results in other disability because chemotherapy and radiation are ineffective. Reports have been made of long-term survival with resection in cases with hepatic and cerebral metastases. For gastrointestinal tumors, a 10-cm margin of bowel should be obtained in addition to a wide mesenteric resection. For gastric primary tumors, omentectomy is advised as well.

Overall, approximately half of gastrointestinal primary tumors can be resected for cure at diagnosis; in these patients, survival rates are 50% at 5 years and 35% at 10 years. In a series of gastrointestinal leiomyosarcomas reported by Ng et al.,[133] overall survival was stage dependent; survival rates were 75% for stage I disease, 52% for stage II, 28% for stage III, and 7% to 12% for stage IV. Important determinants of disease-free survival in multivariate analysis included tumor rupture (P = 0.002), contiguous organ invasion (P = 0.02), and high tumor grade (P = 0.02). Size (>5 cm) and location have been found to predict outcome in other analyses. Pediatric colorectal leiomyosarcomas, although extremely rare, are reported to have a relatively favorable prognosis.

Liposarcoma and Alveolar Soft Parts Sarcoma

Liposarcomas are one of the most common types of soft tissue sarcomas in adults but are extremely rare in childhood. The peak incidence is in the second decade of life, and there is equal distribution between the sexes. Most childhood tumors are of the myxoid histopathologic subtype and are low grade. The most common sites are, in order, the lower extremity, upper extremity, and retroperitoneum. A t(12;16) translocation has been described.[134] The usual presenting complaint is a mass, which is often painless. Metastases are uncommon, with the lung being the most common site. Lymph node metastases are possible but extremely rare. The treatment of choice is complete surgical excision with negative microscopic margins.

Alveolar soft parts sarcoma is a rare tumor; only 102 cases were reported during a 50-year period. A t(X;17) translocation has been noted to occur in these tumors.[135] The tumor is associated with skeletal muscle and fascial planes, and the thigh and buttocks are the most common sites of occurrence (39.5%), followed by abdominal and chest walls. The cell of origin is unknown and some have argued both for and against a skeletal muscle ontogeny. Approximately one third of patients have metastases at diagnosis, with the most common sites being lung, bone, and brain, in that order.

The primary treatment is surgical, and the roles of chemotherapy and radiation therapy remain undefined. Unfortunately, most patients experience relapse in distant sites and die from progressive disease, although this may take 20 years or longer.

HEPATIC TUMORS

Hepatoblastoma Versus Hepatocellular Carcinoma

From 1960 to the early 1970s, there were sporadic reports of survival from hepatoblastoma after successful surgical resection. The risks of major hepatic surgery were great, however, with operative and early postoperative mortality rates approaching 25%. Approximately two thirds of patients with hepatoblastoma had potentially resectable tumors, and complete surgical removal was associated with a 60% long-term survival rate. Systemic relapse was the most frequent cause of failure, and patients with locally unresectable disease or systemic spread at the outset were essentially incurable.

In 1975, the first consistent reports of success with doxorubicin appeared.[136] Before this, many agents had been tested with only sporadic responses. Since then, major advances have occurred in both adjuvant chemotherapy for patients with resectable disease and cytoreductive therapy for unresectable disease. In 1982, the CCSG and Southwest Oncology Group reported a significant reduction in relapse rates after complete resections of hepatoblastoma using combination chemotherapy with vincristine, cyclophosphamide, doxorubicin, and 5-fluorouracil.[137] The long-term relapse-free survival rate in patients with stage I disease was reported at 94%.

Shortly thereafter, reports appeared of dramatic tumor necrosis and cure in patients with unresectable tumors and metastatic disease using doxorubicin and cisplatin as single or combined agents, with delayed resection.[138] Prospective trials with combinations of doxorubicin and cisplatin have confirmed these results, and patients with initially unresectable hepatoblastoma can now achieve long-term survival rates in the range of 60% to 70%.[139] In another study the 5-year event-free survival was 66% and the overall survival 75% in patients treated with cisplatin and doxorubicin.[140]

Despite this period of progress in the treatment of hepatoblastoma, the treatment of children with hepatocellular carcinoma remains problematic and their outcome poor. A complete resection is initially possible in only 10% to 20% of patients, and the problems of local and systemic relapse remain. Despite response to chemotherapy in some instances, children with unresectable disease usually remain unresectable or relapse after resection. In one study, the response rate to chemotherapy was less than 50%, with many patients having disease progression despite systemic chemotherapy.[141] Event-free and overall survival were 17% and 28%, respectively. In another report, there was no difference between patients with fibrolamellar versus non-fibrolamellar hepatocellular carcinoma with respect to advanced disease at diagnosis, resectability, and 5-year event-free survival.[142] Early diagnosis by screening of patients with genetic defects and families with hepatitis B is unlikely to have a major impact in Western nations. In Taiwan a program of early vaccination significantly reduced the incidence of hepatocellular carcinoma.[143,144]

Epidemiology

In Europe and North America, primary liver tumors constitute approximately 1.1% of childhood malignant neoplasms (1.4 cases per 1 million children in the United States).[145] The ratio of hepatoblastoma to hepatocellular carcinoma is variously reported from 1.3:1 to 6.5:1, but in areas endemic for hepatitis B, the ratio may be reversed and as low as 0.2:1. No geographic clustering of cases of hepatoblastoma has been noted. A male predominance is usually reported for both tumors, the ratio ranging from 1.5:1 to 3.1:1 for hepatoblastoma and from 1.3:1 to 3.2:1 for hepatocellular carcinoma. Between 1973 and 1997, 67% of hepatic malignancies in patients under 20 years of age were hepatoblastomas and 33% hepatocellular carcinomas.[146] Among children less than five years of age hepatoblastoma comprised 91%. In children 15 to 19 years of age hepatocellular carcinoma comprised 87%.

Hepatoblastoma has been reported to occur sporadically in adults, but the tumor usually presents in the first 3 years of life. Congenital presentation and antenatal diagnosis have also been reported.[147] Hepatocellular carcinoma, in contrast, is rare in infancy. In one large series of children and adults with hepatic tumors, no cases of hepatocellular carcinoma occurred in patients age 4 years or younger in a cohort of 2,286 patients. Historical series without pathologic review may report a higher rate of infantile hepatoma because of misdiagnosis of some early hepatoblastomas.

CLINICAL PRESENTATION

Children with hepatoblastoma most commonly present with abdominal mass or diffuse abdominal swelling. Not infrequently, the child is in good health and the lesion may be discovered by an observant parent or a clinician on routine examination. Accompanying symptoms, such as pain, irritability, minor gastrointestinal disturbances, fevers, and pallor, occur in smaller numbers of patients. Significant weight loss is unusual, although patients may fail to thrive.

In contrast, although children and adolescents with hepatocellular carcinoma frequently present with palpable abdominal masses, these are rarely incidental. Pain is a frequent accompaniment and can occur in the absence of an obvious mass. Constitutional disturbances, such as anorexia, malaise, nausea and vomiting, and significant weight loss, occur with greater frequency. Jaundice is an uncommon feature of either disease.

In most series of hepatoblastoma and hepatocellular carcinoma, small numbers of patients present acutely with tumor rupture. Hepatoblastoma can present with sexual precocity caused by androgen synthesis, although this is rare.

LABORATORY STUDIES

Mild anemia is common in both conditions, and thrombocytosis is most often seen in patients with hepatoblastoma, but this finding has also been reported in occasional patients with hepatocellular carcinoma.[148] The cause for thrombocytosis in these conditions is unknown but may be related to release of tumor-derived cytokines.

Liver function test results are usually nonspecifically deranged in both conditions. A high serum cholesterol level is present in 50% to 60% of cases, and there is evidence to suggest that higher elevations may correlate with a poorer prognosis. The most useful tumor marker is the serum α-fetoprotein (AFP). Elevation, often extreme, occurs in approximately 84% to 91% of cases of hepatoblastoma. Fewer patients with hepatocellular carcinoma have elevated AFP levels, and the elevation tends to be less marked. Although nonspecific for epithelial liver tumors, the AFP marker is used extensively to monitor both disease reduction in patients undergoing nonoperative therapy and disease recurrence in treated patients. Some reports concluded that a rise in AFP above normal in a patient with quiescent disease is more sensitive than radiology or surgical exploration at detecting recurrence.

IMAGING STUDIES

Abdominal CT scanning is the investigation of choice both for diagnostic discrimination and to assess operability. The chest should be included to identify pulmonary metastases. The typical appearance of hepatoblastoma is that of a solitary mass with lower attenuation values than normal liver (Fig. 112.11). Dramatic contrast enhancement (as in benign vascular neoplasms), invasion of the portal vein, and lymph node involvement are unusual. Hepatocellular carcinomas have a similar appearance but are more likely to be multifocal, invade the portal vein, and metastasize to draining lymph nodes. Distinction between the two lesions cannot be definite because the pattern of disease may be atypical in either instance.

The diagnostic ability of MRI is similar to that of CT. The particular features of both hepatoblastoma and hepatocellular carcinoma on MRI are low signal intensity on T_1-weighted images and high intensity on T_2-weighted images. The two lesions cannot be distinguished by appearance alone.

Plain radiographs and liver–spleen scans usually indicate abnormalities but do not often contribute to diagnosis or assist

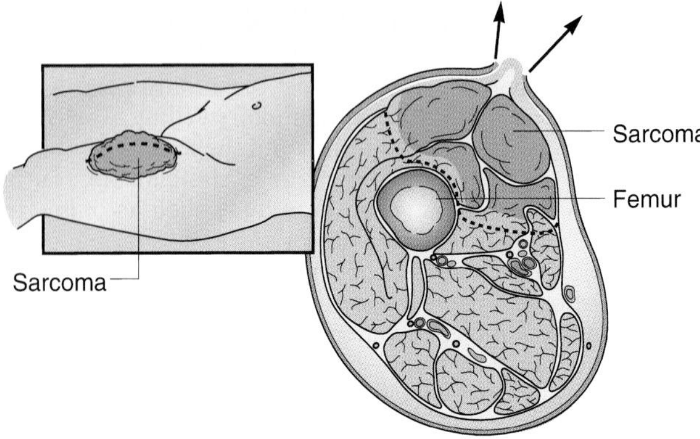

FIGURE 112.11 Technique for resection of a proximal lower-extremity rhabdomyosarcoma. Longitudinal incisions are always used. It is important to excise the tumor completely, with a surrounding 1- to 2-cm margin if feasible.

in planning therapy. Angiography is indicated if embolization or infusion chemotherapy is contemplated, but this test is invasive, technically difficult in childhood, and not universally available. Similar information is available from dynamic CT scan or MRI such that these methods are considered adequate in most instances.

An abdominal ultrasound, in view of the low cost and ready accessibility, is probably the most useful screening investigation for children with large livers. This technique allows distinction between space-occupying lesions and diffuse hepatomegaly. Anatomic detail of the tumor margin is not usually sufficiently well delineated to assess resectability. Doppler ultrasound is also useful to evaluate patency of the inferior vena cava and hepatic veins, but extreme compression of these vessels may prevent useful interpretation.

The ability of imaging studies to predict resectability is questionable. Resectable lesions must usually be confined to the right lobe, right lobe plus medial left lobe, or the left lobe; in addition, the hepatic veins, inferior vena cava, and portal vein must be free of disease. On occasion, the distinction between compression versus invasion of liver adjacent to the lesion cannot be made, nor can the patency of vessels be established with certainty. In rare instances, it may be obvious that metastases in the remaining liver, portal or periaortic nodes, or other intraabdominal organs preclude complete resection.

The available data do not establish any superiority of MRI or CT scan for evaluating the resectability of hepatic malignancies in children. In view of the possible advantage of primary resection, a more reliable option is to judge resectability at formal laparotomy.

STAGING

A staging system was derived by the CCG and the Southwest Oncology Group to compare prognosis and outcome in various intergroup study protocols. Modifications have occurred, and the system in most frequent use is shown in Table 112.9. Stage is best determined operatively in most instances. Alternatively, a TNM classification has been proposed by the International Union Against Cancer and the American Joint Committee on Cancer and another by the Japanese Society for Pediatric Surgery. More recently, the PRETEXT (PRETreatment EXTent of disease) system has been advocated by SIOPEL (International Society of Pediatric Oncology Liver Tumor Group). This is a pretreatment staging system that emphasizes the anatomic site of involvement as well as the number of involved Couinaud hepatic segments.[149]

PATHOLOGY

Hepatoblastoma usually presents as a single, pseudoencapsulated lesion, often reaching large proportions before becoming clinically apparent. The tumor grows in an expansive fashion such that the umbilical fissure usually is not breached. Thus, despite a 30% to 40% incidence of bilobar disease, successful extended resection may still be possible. Multicentricity or massive diffuse disease within the liver occurs in less than 20% of patients, and cirrhosis of the surrounding liver is unusual.

In contrast, hepatocellular carcinoma usually lacks a distinct capsule. The tumor spreads diffusely through the liver in up to 70% of patients, often with satellite nodules well separated from the main tumor mass. Bilobar involvement occurs in 50% to 70% of cases, and the umbilical fissure does not constitute a barrier to spread. As a result, hepatocellular carcinoma is usually unresectable. Finally, because of the association of hepatocellular carcinoma with hepatitis B infection, cirrhosis may be present in the surrounding nonneoplastic liver. This may preclude complete tumor resection if the volume of liver to be removed is likely to compromise liver function further.

The epithelial element of hepatoblastoma can display a range of differentiation from a frankly anaplastic form (indistinguishable on light microscopy from other small cell neoplasms of childhood) to embryonal differentiation (cellular arrangement resembles early ducts of embryonal liver) or fetal differentiation (cells resemble normal but small hepatocytes). In addition to the epithelial element, hepatoblastoma may contain varying amounts of immature stromal tissue, often containing osteoid.

TABLE 112.9

RELATION OF STAGING TO PROGNOSIS FOR HEPATOBLASTOMA

Clinical group	Criteria	Relative risk for death of disease
I	Complete resection of tumor as initial treatment, regardless of resectional technique	0.16
IIA	Complete resection after irradiation or chemotherapy	0.57[a]
IIB	Residual disease confined to one lobe	—
III	Disease involving both hepatic lobes	2.87
IIIB	Regional nodal involvement	—
IV	Distant metastases, regardless of the extent of the hepatic tumor	3.51

[a]Relative risk was assessed for stage II and III patients collectively. The relative risk is compared with other stages.

TABLE 112.10

COMPARISON OF RELATIVE RISK OF DEATH FOR HISTOLOGIC SUBTYPES OF HEPATOBLASTOMA

Histopathologic subtype	Relative risk for death of disease[a]
Fetal	1.07
Embrycnal	1.74
Mixed	0.53
Macrotrabecular pattern	1.20
Small cell undifferentiated	3.71

[a]Risk of death adjusted for age, sex, and stage compared with other histologic subtypes

A pure fetal pattern is said to be favorable and the presence of embryonal or undifferentiated histologic types unfavorable; for example, pure fetal histologic type has been associated with improved resectability and better long-term survival. One analysis showed that resected patients with pure fetal histologic type have a 2-year survival rate of 92%, which is significantly better than that for patients with embryonal or anaplastic tumor components (63% and zero 2-year survival rates, respectively).[150] In contrast, anaplastic histologic type is unfavorable and may not be chemoresponsive. A comparison of the relative mortality risks for subtypes of hepatocellular carcinoma is listed in Table 112.10.

The fibrolamellar subtype of hepatocellular carcinoma is characterized by broad fibrous septa that separate the cellular component into nodules and is most commonly seen in late childhood and adolescence. It is associated with a better prognosis and a higher resection rate. This difference, however, may not be independent of stage. Of patients with hepatoblastoma, 10% to 20% present with distant metastases. The locations of metastases at autopsy in 46 patients in one report were the lungs in 46%, portal and periaortic nodes in 11%, brain in 7%, and peritoneum and diaphragm in 4% each.[151] The incidence of metastases is reportedly higher in patients with embryonal and anaplastic histologic types (80% and 100%, respectively) compared with fetal differentiation (29%).

Hepatocellular carcinoma presents with metastatic disease in 30% to 50% of patients. The location of metastases at autopsy was reported by the Liver Cancer Study Group of Japan.[152] The lungs were involved in 48% of patients, lymph nodes in 37%, intraperitoneal organs in 16%, peritoneum in 15%, adrenal in 11%, bone in 10%, brain in 2%, and skin in 1%. Tumor emboli were detected in the portal vein in 59.7% and in the hepatic vein in 26.6% of patients. The higher incidence of lymphatic and intraabdominal spread in hepatocellular carcinoma is relevant to local resectability and recurrence. Nodal disease in the porta hepatis and periaortic region is not readily resectable, and recurrence is inevitable if such disease is present.

TREATMENT

Hepatoblastoma

Complete surgical resection remains the major objective of therapy for hepatoblastoma (Fig. 112.12). At presentation, approximately 60% of patients with hepatoblastoma have resectable tumors, and one review reported no survivors among children who underwent biopsy only or incomplete resection. More recently, sporadic patients who received nonoperative treatments have achieved complete response,[153,154]

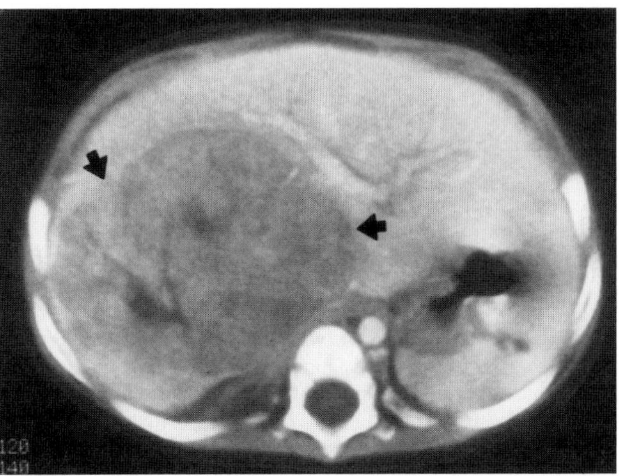

FIGURE 112.12 Computed tomography scan of a 2-year-old child with a large right lobar hepatoblastoma (*arrows*). Despite the large size, these lesions can often be completely resected before chemotherapy. Hepatocellular carcinoma, in contrast, often involves multiple hepatic segments, and there is a significant incidence of extrahepatic extension.

and chemotherapy and radiation therapy have been able to salvage some patients whose tumors were incompletely resected at the primary site.

A nonanatomic resection, wedging out the tumor with a satisfactory margin, may be feasible in the uncommon instance of a small peripheral or pedunculated lesion. More often, a major anatomic resection is required, depending on tumor location and extent. As much as 85% of hepatic substance may be removed, with subsequent full and rapid regeneration despite the administration of postoperative chemotherapy.[155] The principles of safe hepatic resection are now well developed, and a considerable reduction in operative mortality rates has been possible since the 1970s. In two historical series, the mortality rate was reported to be approximately 22%, but in more recent series, it was as low as 0% to 3%.[156,157] Invasive monitoring during anesthesia allows the precise control of central venous and arterial blood pressure to the advantage of minimizing blood loss. Clotting factors and platelets are more readily available. Postoperative measures, such as respiratory and hemodynamic support, antibiotics, and total parenteral nutrition, have all made significant contributions to overall patient care.

The surgical principles include wide exposure using a generous bilateral subcostal incision and dissection at the liver hilum with isolation of vascular and ductal structures of the segment or lobe to be resected. After hepatic arterial and portal venous inflow to the relevant area is ligated, a color demarcation acts a guide to the correct plane of division of liver substance and allows this to proceed with minimal blood loss. Technologic advances such as the Cavitron Ultrasonic Surgical Aspirator (CUSA; Cooper Lasersonics, Santa Clara, CA) and metallic clip applicators have made this step less hazardous in terms of hemorrhage, although finger-fracture technique with individual vessel and duct suture–ligation remains an acceptable alternative. Hemostasis of the transected surface can be completed with use of the argon beam coagulator or electrocautery and topical agents such as thrombin and Gelfoam (Pharmacia & Upjohn, Kalamazoo, MI). A trend to eliminate use of abdominal drains in uncomplicated cases has emerged.

Approximately 40% of patients with hepatoblastoma have inoperable tumors at presentation. Bilaterality, diffuse multicentricity, and metastatic lesions may all preclude resection. Various techniques have been used to increase the resectability rates, including preoperative chemotherapy, profound hypothermia with circulatory arrest, and total hepatic vascular occlusion. These maneuvers are a useful part of the surgical armamentarium in selected instances. For truly unresectable disease, aside from transplantation, chemotherapy is the major treatment option available. During the 1990s, it became evident that some of these tumors may be rendered resectable by preoperative therapy. A randomized trial performed through an intergroup collaboration of the CCG and POG showed that survival was equivalent when either doxorubicin plus cisplatin or a combination of vincristine, cisplatin, and 5-fluorouracil was administered. In contrast, toxic side effects were significantly increased in patients receiving the former regimen. It is recommended that all patients with hepatoblastoma undergo initial treatment with vincristine, cisplatin, and 5-fluorouracil.

The role of radiation therapy is not clearly defined. In treating patients with bulky disease, the tolerance of normal liver is not compatible with the doses that would be required for tumor ablation, although temporary stability may be achieved. Hepatic toxicity has been described at doses to the whole liver of greater than 25 Gy. Focal radiation up to 45 Gy can be administered with safety. There may be a place for radiation in a dose range of 25 to 45 Gy combined with chemotherapy in inoperable hepatoblastoma and in patients with postresectional residual disease. In one report, eight patients were treated after incomplete resections (four with gross and four with microscopic residual disease) with combined irradiation and chemotherapy; six of these patients were free of disease at 4 to 83 months' follow-up.[153]

Other treatments with encouraging results are in developmental phases. Intraarterial infusion chemotherapy and orthotopic liver transplantation may extend the definition of resectability as clear indications emerge. The intraarterial route allows the administration of agents directly to the tumor with the theoretic advantage of less systemic toxicity. Some agents with a high hepatic extraction (e.g., doxorubicin, cisplatin, and fluorodeoxyuridine) have been shown to be useful in hepatoblastoma. Several anecdotal reports exist of dramatic responses in unresectable disease, allowing subsequent resection. Yokomori et al.[158] reported on the treatment of a 4-month-old infant with fetal hepatoblastoma using intraarterial therapy consisting of 5-fluorouracil, vincristine, doxorubicin, and cisplatin for 18 months. Total tumor regression occurred, and the child remained well at 6 years' follow-up. The technique, although promising, is not without hazards, such as catheter infection, thrombosis, and displacement. Also, it is technically difficult in children. In a large review of recurrence and survival rates in 597 patients who received liver transplants, a recurrence rate of 40% was found in patients with hepatoblastoma, with 2- and 5-year survival rates of only 32% and 7%, respectively.[154] Until prospective studies of arterial infusion, including chemoembolization, or hepatic transplantation are available, these modalities should be considered investigational.

With improving management of the primary lesion, mortality is increasingly the result of metastatic relapse in the lungs. If metastases demonstrate progression or relapse on therapy, surgical resection is an option. Cure of pulmonary metastatic disease has not been demonstrated with radiation therapy. One series reported the operative treatment of five cases of pulmonary metastatic disease that developed after successful management of the primary tumor.[159] All lesions developed during or soon after chemotherapy. Four patients were free of disease at 8 to 83 months' follow-up, despite having multiple lesions and requiring more than one resection in two cases. No patients with hepatoblastoma with metastases to sites other than lung or regional nodes have been reported cured.

Hepatocellular Carcinoma

Analogous to hepatoblastoma, complete surgical resection is a prerequisite for cure in hepatocellular carcinoma of childhood. Patients with incompletely resected tumors do not survive. Although patients undergoing resection survive longer than those who do not undergo resection, the gain is small owing to the high local and systemic relapse rates. The Japanese Liver Cancer Study Group reported a 40% 1-year survival rate for resectable disease and 10% for unresectable lesions.

Stage for stage, the prognosis of hepatocellular carcinoma is said to be no worse than that for hepatoblastoma. Many more patients present with advanced hepatocellular carcinoma, however, because the prevalence of bilobar and multicentric tumors and extrahepatic extension renders them unresectable. Nodal and systemic metastatic disease is more common at the outset. The liver may be cirrhotic in some instances, precluding an extensive resection short of transplantation.

Most series report the percentage of children with resectable hepatocellular carcinoma to be approximately 10% to 20%. Patients with fibrolamellar histologic pattern may be an exception, with a resection rate of 48% to 60%. Relapse after resection is common. A POG and CCG intergroup study showed no impact of either cisplatin plus doxorubicin or cisplatin, vincristine, and 5-fluorouracil on outcome in patients with hepatocellular carcinoma. The overall survival rate in the pediatric age group for hepatocellular carcinoma is rarely reported to exceed 20% and more realistically approaches zero. A role for external beam radiation therapy has not been established. Only temporary stability of bulky disease has been demonstrated, and radiation has also failed to decrease the relapse rate in patients with minimal disease after surgical resection.

In view of poor results for conventional therapy, there may be a place for liver transplantation. In one report, treatment of nine patients who had hepatocellular carcinoma by transplantation resulted in four survivors with a median follow up of 2.3 years. Longer follow-up will be necessary to recognize the true recurrence rate and intercurrent mortality rate.

OUTCOME

After a successful complete surgical resection and without further treatment, long-term survival can be expected in approximately 60% to 80% of patients with hepatoblastoma. Local relapse is unusual, and the most frequent cause of failure in the remaining 20% to 40% is systemic relapse. The overall cure rate with surgery alone is approximately 35%, and all patients should receive preoperative or postoperative systemic chemotherapy.

KEY POINTS

- **In childhood, neuroblastoma is the most common extracranial solid tumor, followed in incidence by Wilms tumor; rhabdomyosarcoma is less common than neuroblastoma and Wilms tumor but has a biphasic age distribution, with 40% of cases occurring in the age range 10 to 19 years.**
- **Patients with neuroblastoma and an increased number of copies of the *MYCN* gene have a much worse prognosis.**
- **High-risk neuroblastoma remains one of the central problems in pediatric oncology, with overall survival rates below 30% despite multidisciplinary therapy and the use of multiagent chemotherapy and myeloablative regimens.**
- **The standard of care for Wilms tumor in the United States is initial surgical resection, with exceptions to this rule only for**

extensive intracaval tumors that require cardiopulmonary bypass for extraction, obviously unresectable tumors with documented invasion of contiguous structures, and possibly bilateral tumors, especially if it is unclear which side is most heavily involved; all patients with resectable Wilms tumor receive postoperative chemotherapy.

- **Clear cell sarcoma of the kidney is a distinct histopathologic and clinical entity from Wilms tumor with an age distribution similar to that observed in Wilms tumor but a markedly worse prognosis; it has been called the *bone-metastasizing renal tumor of childhood.***
- **The modern treatment of rhabdomyosarcoma is multidisciplinary and includes multiagent chemotherapy, judicious resection, and radiation therapy; the intensity of therapy should be tailored to the risk of subsequent relapse as a function of tumor, node, or metastasis stage.**

References

1. **Punyko JA, Mertens AC, Baker KS, et al. Long-term survival probabilities for childhood rhabdomyosarcoma. *Cancer* 2005;103:1475–1483.**
2. Miller RW, Dalager NA. U.S. childhood cancer deaths by cell type, 1960–68. *J Pediatr.* 1974;85:664–668.
3. Kramer S, Meadows AT, Jarrett P, et al. Incidence of childhood cancer; experience of a decade in a population-based registry. *J Natl Cancer Inst.* 1983;70:49–55.
4. Bleyer WA. The U.S. pediatric cancer clinical trials programmes: international implications and the way forward. *Eur J Cancer.* 1997;33:1439–1447.
5. **Ries LAG, Bunin GR. Introduction. In: Ries LAG, Gurney JG, Linet M, et al., eds. *Cancer incidence and survival among children and adolescents: United States SEER Program 1975–1995.* Bethesda, MD: National Cancer Institute SEER Program, 1999, pp. 1–15.**
6. Goodman MT GJ, Smith MA, Olshan AF. Sympathetic nervous system tumors. In: Ries LAG, Gurney JG, Linet M, et al, eds. *Cancer incidence and survival among children and adolescents: United States SEER Program 1975–1995.* Bethesda, MD: National Cancer Institute SEER Program. NIH Pub. No.99-4649; 1999, pp. 65–72.
7. Young JL Jr, Ries LG, Silverberg E, et al. Cancer incidence, survival and mortality for children younger than 15 years. *Cancer* 1986;58(suppl 2):598.
8. Brodeur GM, Castleberry RP. Neuroblastoma. In: Pizzo PA, Poplack DG, eds. *Principles and practice of pediatric oncology.* 2nd ed. Philadelphia: JB Lippincott, 1993, p. 739.
9. Allen RW Jr, Ogden B, Bentley FL, et al.. Fetal hydantoin syndrome neuroblastoma and hemorrhagic disease in a neonate. *JAMA.* 1980;244: 1464–1465.
10. Kinney H, Faix R, Brazy J. The fetal alcohol syndrome and neuroblastoma. *Pediatrics* 1980;66:130–132.
11. Blatt J, Olshan AF, Lee PA, et al. Neuroblastoma and related tumors in Turner's syndrome *J Pediatr.* 1997;131:666–670. [Erratum appears in *J Pediatr.* 1998;133:312.]
12. Pivnick EK, Furman WL, Velagaleti GV, et al. Simultaneous adrenocortical carcinoma and ganglioneuroblastoma in a child with Turner syndrome and germline p53 mutation. *J Med Genet.* 1998;35:328–332.
13. Geraci AP, de Csepel J, Shlasko E, et al. Ganglioneuroblastoma and ganglioneuroma in association with neurofibromatosis type I: report of three cases. *J Child Neurol.* 1998;13:356–358.
14. Brodeur GM, Schwab M, Varmus HE, et al. Amplification of N-*myc* in untreated human neuroblastomas correlates with advanced disease stage. *Science* 1984;224:1121–1124.
15. Tonini GP, Boni L, Pession A, et al. MYCN oncogene amplification in neuroblastoma is associated with worse prognosis, except in stage 4s: the Italian experience with 295 children. *J Clin Oncol.* 1997;15:85–93.
16. Slack A, Chen Z, Tonelli R, et al. The p53 regulatory gene MDM2 is a direct transcriptional target of MYCN in neuroblastoma. *Proc Natl Acad Sci USA.* 2005;102:731–736.
17. Tweddle DA, Pearson AD, Haber M, et al. The p53 pathway and its inactivation in neuroblastoma. *Cancer Lett.* 2003;197:93–98.
18. Caron H, van Sluis P, de Kraker J, et al. Allelic loss of chromosome 1p as a predictor of unfavorable outcome in patients with neuroblastoma. *N Engl J Med.* 1996;334:225–230.
19. Maris JM, Weiss MJ, Guo C, et al. Loss of heterozygosity at 1p36 independently predicts for disease progression but not decreased overall survival probability in neuroblastoma patients: a Children's Cancer Group study. *J Clin Oncol.* 2000;18:1888–1899.
20. Maris JM, White PS, Beltinger CP, et al. Significance of chromosome 1p loss of heterozygosity in neuroblastoma. *Cancer Res.* 1995;55:4664–4669.
21. **Rubie H, Delattre O, Hartmann O, et al. Loss of chromosome 1p may have a prognostic value in localised neuroblastoma: results of the French NBL 90 Study. Neuroblastoma Study Group of the Societe Francaise d'Oncologie Pediatrique (SFOP). *Eur J Cancer.* 1997;33:1917–1922.**
22. Bader SA, Fasching C,, Brodeur GM, et al. Dissociation of suppression of tumorigenicity and differentiation in vitro effected by transfer of single human chromosomes into human neuroblastoma cells. *Cell Growth Differ.* 1991;2:245–255.
23. Bown N, Lastowska M, Cotterill S, et al. 17q gain in neuroblastoma predicts adverse clinical outcome. U.K. Cancer Cytogenetics Group and the U.K. Children's Cancer Study Group. *Med Pediatr Oncol.* 2001;36: 14–19.
24. Kogner P, Barbany G, Dominici C, et al. Coexpression of the messenger for RNA for TRK protooncogene and low affinity nerve growth factor receptor in neuroblastoma with favorable prognosis. *Cancer Res.* 1993; 53:2044–2050.
25. Nakagawara A, Arima M, Azar CG, et al. Inverse relationship between TRK expression and N-myc amplification in human neuroblastomas. *Cancer Res.* 1992;52:1364–1368.
26. Nakagawara A, Arima-Nakagawara M,, Scavarda NJ, et al. Association between high levels of expression of the TRK gene and favorable outcome in human neuroblastoma. *N Engl J Med.* 1993;328:847–854.
27. Kramer K, Cheung NK, Gerald WL, et al. Correlation of MYCN amplification, Trk-A and CD44 expression with clinical stage in 250 patients with neuroblastoma. *Eur J Cancer* 1997;33:2098–2100.
28. Ryden M, Sehgal R, Dominici C, et al. Expression of mRNA for the neurotrophin receptor trkC in neuroblastomas with favourable tumour stage and good prognosis. *Br J Cancer* 1996;74:773–779.
29. **Schulte JH, Schramm A, Klein-Hitpass L, et al. Microarray analysis reveals differential gene expression patterns and regulation of single target genes contributing to the opposing phenotype of TrkA- and TrkB-expressing neuroblastomas. *Oncogene* 2005;24:165–177.**
30. Walton JD, Kattan DR, Thomas SK, et al. Characteristics of stem cells from human neuroblastoma cell lines and in tumors. *Neoplasia* 2004;6: 838–845.
31. Triche TJ, Askin FB, Kissane JM. Neuroblastoma, Ewing's sarcoma, and the differential diagnosis of small-, round-, blue-cell tumors. In: *Pathology of neoplasia in children and adolescents.* Philadelphia: WB Saunders, 1986, p. 145.
32. **Shimada H, Ambros IM, Dehner LP, et al. The International Neuroblastoma Pathology Classification (the Shimada system). *Cancer* 1999;86:364–372.**
33. Katzenstein HM, Cohn SL, Shore RM, et al. Scintigraphic response by 123I-metaiodobenzylguanidine scan correlates with event-free survival in high-risk neuroblastoma. *J Clin Oncol.* 2004;22:3909–3915.
34. Kushner BH, Yeung HW, Larson SM, et al. Extending positron emission tomography scan utility to high-risk neuroblastoma: fluorine-18 fluorodeoxyglucose positron emission tomography as sole imaging modality in follow-up of patients. *J Clin Oncol.* 2001;19:3397–3405.
35. Ikeda H, Iehara T, Tsuchida Y, et al. Experience with International Neuroblastoma Staging System and Pathology Classification. *Br J Cancer* 2002;86:1110–1116.
36. Brodeur GM, Pritchard J, Berthold F, et al. Revisions of the international criteria for neuroblastoma diagnosis, staging, and response to treatment. *J Clin Oncol.* 1993;11:1466–1477.
37. Brodeur GM, Seeger RC, Barrett A, et al. International criteria for diagnosis, staging, and response to treatment in patients with neuroblastoma [see comments]. *J Clin Oncol.* 1988;6:1874–1881.
38. Evans AE, Albo V, D'Angio GJ, et al. Factors influencing survival of children with nonmetastatic neuroblastoma. *Cancer* 1976;38:661–666.
39. Shamberger RC, Allarde-Segundo A, Kozakewich HP, et al. Surgical management of stage III and IV neuroblastoma: resection before or after chemotherapy? *J Pediatr Surg.* 1991;26:1113–1117; discussion 1117– 1118.
40. **La Quaglia MP, Kushner BH, Su W, et al. The impact of gross total resection on local control and survival in high-risk neuroblastoma. *J Pediatr Surg.* 2004;39:412–417; discussion 412-417.**
41. Matthay KK, Villablanca JG, Seeger RC, et al. Treatment of high-risk neuroblastoma with intensive chemotherapy, radiotherapy, autologous bone marrow transplantation, and 13-cis-retinoic acid. Children's Cancer Group. *N Engl J Med.* 1999;341:1165–1173.
42. Bernstein L, Linet M, Smith MA, et al. Renal tumors. In: Ries LAG, Smith MA, Gurney JG, et al, eds. *Cancer incidence and survival among children and adolescents: United States SEER Program 1975–1995.* Bethesda, MD: National Cancer Institute SEER Program. NIH Pub. No. 99-4649; 1999, pp. 79–90.
43. Crist WM, Kum LE. Common solid tumors of childhood. *N Engl J Med.* 1991;324:461–471.
44. Breslow N, Beckwith JB, Ciol M, et al. Age distribution of Wilms' tumor. *Cancer Res.* 1988;48:1653–1657.
45. Breslow NE, Beckwith JB.. Epidemiological features of Wilms' tumor: results of the national Wilms' tumor study. *J Natl Cancer Inst.* 1982;68: 429–436.
46. Maw MA Grundy PE, Millow LJ, et al. A third Wilms' tumor locus on chromosome 16q. *Cancer Res.* 1992;52:3094–3098.
47. Francke U, Holmes LB, Atkins L et al. Aniridia-Wilms' tumor association: evidence for specific deletion of 11p13. *Cytogenet Cell Genet.* 1979;24: 185–192.

48. Rose EA, Glaser T, Jones C, et al. Complete physical map of the WAGR region of 11p13 localizes a candidate Wilms' tumor gene. *Cell* 1990;60: 495–508.
49. Grundy P, Koufos A, , Morgan K, et al. Familial predisposition to Wilms' tumor does not map to short arm of chromosome 11. *Nature* 1988;336: 374–376.
50. Horwitz JR, Ritchey ML, Moksness J, et al. Renal salvage procedures in patients with synchronous bilateral Wilms' tumors: a report from the National Wilms' Tumor Study Group. *J Pediatr Surg.* 1996;31: 1020–1025.
51. **Green DM, Breslow NE, Beckwith JB, et al. Treatment with nephrectomy only for small, stage I/favorable histology Wilms' tumor: a report from the National Wilms' Tumor Study Group. *J Clin Oncol.* 2001;19: 3719–3724.**
52. Green DM, Breslow NE, Beckwith JB, et al. Comparison between single-dose and divided-dose administration of dactinomycin and doxorubicin for patients with Wilms' tumor: a report from the National Wilms' Tumor Study Group. *J Clin Oncol.* 1998;16:237–245.
53. Green DM, Breslow NE, Beckwith JB, et al. Effect of duration of treatment on treatment outcome and cost of treatment for Wilms' tumor: a report from the National Wilms' Tumor Study Group. *J Clin Oncol.* 1998;16:3744–3751.
54. Green DM, Beckwith JB, Breslow NE, et al. Treatment of children with stages II to IV anaplastic Wilms' tumor: a report from the National Wilms' Tumor Study Group. *J Clin Oncol.* 1994;12:2126–2131.
55. Kalapurakal JA, Li SM, Breslow NE, et al. Influence of radiation therapy delay on abdominal tumor recurrence in patients with favorable histology Wilms' tumor treated on NWTS-3 and NWTS-4: a report from the National Wilms' Tumor Study Group. *Int J Radiat Oncol Biol Phys.* 2003;57:495–499.
56. Malcolm AW, Jaffe N, Folkman MJ, et al.. Bilateral Wilms' tumor. *Int J Radiat Oncol Biol Phys.* 1980;6:167–174.
57. Montgomery BT, Kelalis PP, Blute ML, et al. Extended followup of bilateral Wilms tumor: results of the National Wilms Tumor Study. *J Urol.* 1991;146:514–518.
58. Ritchey ML, Othersen HB Jr, de Lorimier AA, et al. Renal vein involvement with nephroblastoma: a report of the National Wilms' Tumor Study-3. *Eur Urol.* 1990;17:139–144.
59. Shamberger RC, Ritchey ML, Haase GM, et al. Intravascular extension of Wilms tumor. *Ann Surg.* 2001;234:116–121.
60. Ward SP, Dehner LP. Sacrococcygeal teratoma with nephroblastoma (Wilms' tumor): a variant of extragonadal teratoma in childhood: A histologic and ultrastructural study. *Cancer* 1974;33:1355–1363.
61. Luchtrath H, de Leon F, Giesen H, et al. Inguinal nephroblastoma. *Virchows Arch A Pathol Anat Histopathol.* 1984;405:113–118.
62. Naito K, Yokoyama O, Yamaguchi K, et al. Extrarenal nephroblastoma: report of a case and review of the literature. *Hinyokika Kiyo.* 1985;31: 1773–1780.
63. Wexler HA, Poole CA, Fojaco RM. Metastatic neonatal Wilms' tumor, a case report with review of the literature. *Pediatr Radiol.* 1975;3: 179–181.
64. Hrabovsky EE, Othersen HB Jr, deLorimier A, et al. Wilms' tumor in the neonate: a report from the national Wilms' Tumor Study. *J Pediatr Surg.* 1986;21:385–387.
65. Babaian RJ, Skinner DG, Waisman J. Wilms' tumor in the adult patient: diagnosis, management, and a review of the world medical literature. *Cancer* 1980;45:1713–1719.
66. Byrd RL, Evans AE, D'Angio GJ. Adult Wilms' tumor: effects of combined therapy on survival. *J Urol.* 1982;127:648–651.
67. Hupperets PS, Havenith MG, Blijham GH. Recurrent adult nephroblastoma: long-term remission after surgery plus adjuvant high-dose chemotherapy, radiation therapy, and allogenic bone marrow transplantation. *Cancer* 1992;69:2990–2992.
68. **Argani P, Perlman EJ, Breslow NE, et al. Clear cell sarcoma of the kidney: a review of 351 cases from the National Wilms Tumor Study Group Pathology Center. *Am J Surg Pathol.* 2000;24:4–18.**
69. Green DM, Breslow NE, Beckwith JB, et al. Treatment of children with clear-cell sarcoma of the kidney: a report from the National Wilms' Tumor Study Group. *J Clin Oncol.* 1994;12:2132–2137.
70. **Seibel NL, Li S, Breslow NE, et al. Effect of duration of treatment on treatment outcome for patients with clear-cell sarcoma of the kidney: a report from the National Wilms' Tumor Study Group. *J Clin Oncol.* 2004;22:468–473.**
71. Eftekhari F, Erly WK, Jaffe N. Malignant rhabdoid tumor of the kidney: imaging features in two cases. *Pediatr Radiol.* 1990;21:39–42.
72. Weeks DA, Beckwith JB, Mierau GW, et al. Rhabdoid tumor of kidney. A report of 111 cases from the National Wilms' Tumor Study Pathology Center. *Am J Surg Pathol.* 1989;13:439–458.
73. Beckwith JB. Histopathology as a prognostic indicator in tumors of childhood. *Prog Clin Biol Res.* 1983;132E:159–164.
74. Bolande RP. Congenital mesoblastic nephroma of infancy. *Perspect Pediatr Pathol.* 1973;1:227–1250.
75. Knezevich SR, Garnett MJ, Pysher TJ, et al. ETV6-NTRK3 gene fusions and trisomy 11 establish a histogenetic link between mesoblastic nephroma and congenital fibrosarcoma. *Cancer Res.* 1998;58:5046– 5048.
76. Aronson DC, Medary I, Finlay JL, et al. Renal cell carcinoma in childhood and adolescence: a retrospective survey for prognostic factors in 22 cases. *J Pediatr Surg.* 1996;31:183–186.
77. Gurney JG, Roffers SD, Smith MA, et al. Soft tissue sarcomas. In: Ries LAG, Gurney JG, Linet M, et al, eds. *Cancer incidence and survival among children and adolescents: United States SEER Program 1975–1995.* Bethesda, MD: National Cancer Institute SEER Program. NIH Pub. No.99-4649; 1999, pp. 111–123.
78. Young JL Jr, Miller RW.. Incidence of malignant tumors in U.S. children. *J Pediatr.* 1975;86:254–258.
79. Ruymann FB, Maddux HR, Ragab A, et al. Congenital anomalies associated with rhabdomyosarcoma: an autopsy study of 115 cases. A report from the Intergroup Rhabdomyosarcoma Study Committee (representing the Children's Cancer Study Group, the Pediatric Oncology Group, the United Kingdom Children's Cancer Study Group, and the Pediatric Intergroup Statistical Center). *Med Pediatr Oncol.* 1988;16:33–39.
80. Davis RL, Weintraub H, Lassar AB. Expression of a single transfected cDNA converts fibroblasts to myoblasts. *Cell* 1987;51:987–1000.
81. Dias P, Parham DM, Shapiro DN, et al. Myogenic regulatory protein (MyoD1) expression in childhood solid tumors: diagnostic utility in rhabdomyosarcoma. *Am J Pathol.* 1990;137:1283–1291.
82. Barr FG, Fitzgerald JC, Ginsberg JP, et al. Predominant expression of alternative PAX3 and PAX7 forms in myogenic and neural tumor cell lines. *Cancer Res.* 1999;59:5443–5448.
83. Bridge JA, Liu J, Weibolt V, et al. Novel genomic imbalances in embryonal rhabdomyosarcoma revealed by comparative genomic hybridization and fluorescence in situ hybridization: an intergroup rhabdomyosarcoma study. *Genes Chromosomes Cancer* 2000;27:337–344.
84. Kelly KM, Womer RB, Barr FG. Minimal disease detection in patients with alveolar rhabdomyosarcoma using a reverse transcriptase-polymerase chain reaction method. *Cancer* 1996;78:1320–1327.
85. La Quaglia MP, Heller G, Ghavimi F, et al. The effect of age at diagnosis on outcome in rhabdomyosarcoma. *Cancer* 1994;73:109–117.
86. Joshi D, Anderson JR, Paidas C, et al. Age is an independent prognostic factor in rhabdomyosarcoma: a report from the Soft Tissue Sarcoma Committee of the Children's Oncology Group. *Pediatr Blood Cancer* 2004;42:64–73.
87. **Raney RB, Anderson JR, Barr FG, et al. Rhabdomyosarcoma and undifferentiated sarcoma in the first two decades of life: a selective review of Intergroup Rhabdomyosarcoma Study Group experience and rationale for Intergroup Rhabdomyosarcoma Study V. *J Pediatr Hematol Oncol.* 2001;23:215–220.**
88. Spunt SL, Lobe TE, Pappo AS, et al. Aggressive surgery is unwarranted for biliary tract rhabdomyosarcoma. *J Pediatr Surg.* 2000;35:309–316.
89. Crist W, Gehan EA, Ragab AH, et al. The Third Intergroup Rhabdomyosarcoma Study. *J Clin Oncol.* 1995;13:610.
90. Crist WM, Anderson JR, Meza JL, et al. Intergroup rhabdomyosarcoma study-IV: results for patients with nonmetastatic disease. *J Clin Oncol.* 2001; 19:3091–3102.
91. Mandell L, Ghavimi F, Peretz T, et al. Radiocurability of microscopic disease in childhood rhabdomyosarcoma with radiation doses less than 4000 cGy. *J Clin Oncol.* 1990;8:1536–1542.
92. Rodary C, Gehan EA, Flamant F, et al. Prognostic factors in 951 children with non-metastatic rhabdomyosarcoma: a report from the International Rhabdomyosarcoma Workshop. *Med Pediatr Oncol.* 1991;19:89–95.
93. Maurer HM, Gehan EA, Beltangady M, et al. The Intergroup Rhabdomyosarcoma Study-II. *Cancer* 1993;71:1904–1922.
94. Suder J, Stienen U, Kaatsch P, et al. Analysis of prognostic factors in rhabdomyosarcoma: preliminary univariate and multivariate results of the Soft Tissue Sarcoma Study (CWS-81). *Klin Padiatr.* 1986;198:218–223.
95. Neville HL, Andrassy RJ, Lobe TE, et al. Preoperative staging, prognostic factors, and outcome for extremity rhabdomyosarcoma: a preliminary report from the Intergroup Rhabdomyosarcoma Study IV (1991–1997). *J Pediatr Surg.* 2000;35:317–321.
96. LaQuaglia MP, Ghavimi F, Penenberg D, et al. Factors predictive of mortality in pediatric extremity rhabdomyosarcoma. *J Pediatr Surg.* 1990;25:238–243.
97. LaQuaglia MP. Extremity rhabdomyosarcoma: biological principles, staging, and treatment. *Semin Surg Oncol.* 1993;9:510–519.
98. Blakely ML, Spurbeck WW, Pappo AS, et al. The impact of margin of resection on outcome in pediatric nonrhabdomyosarcoma soft tissue sarcoma. *J Pediatr Surg.* 1999;34:672–675.
99. Simon JH, Paulino AC, Smith RB, et al. Prognostic factors in head and neck rhabdomyosarcoma. *Head Neck.* 2002;24:468–473.
100. Kraus DH, Saenz NC, Gollamudi S, et al. Pediatric rhabdomyosarcoma of the head and neck. *Am J Surg.* 1997;174:556–560.
101. Pappo AS, Meza JL, Donaldson SS, et al. Treatment of localized nonorbital, nonparameningeal head and neck rhabdomyosarcoma: lessons learned from intergroup rhabdomyosarcoma studies III and IV. *J Clin Oncol.* 2003;21:638–645.
102. Daya H, Chan HS, Sirkin W, et al. Pediatric rhabdomyosarcoma of the head and neck: is there a place for surgical management? *Arch Otolaryngol Head Neck Surg.* 2000;126:468–472.
103. LaQuaglia M. Genitourinary rhabdomyosarcoma in children. *Urol Clin North Am.* 1991;18:575–580.

104. Corpron CA, Andrassy RJ, Hays DM, et al. Conservative management of uterine pediatric rhabdomyosarcoma: a report from the Intergroup Rhabdomyosarcoma Study III and IV pilot. *J Pediatr Surg*. 1995;30:942–944.
105. Andrassy RJ, Hays DM, Raney RB, et al. Conservative surgical management of vaginal and vulvar pediatric rhabdomyosarcoma: a report from the Intergroup Rhabdomyosarcoma Study III. *J Pediatr Surg*. 1995;30:1034–1036.
106. Hays DM, Raney RB, Wharam MD, et al. Children with vesical rhabdomyosarcoma (RMS) treated by partial cystectomy with neoadjuvant or adjuvant chemotherapy, with or without radiotherapy. A report from the Intergroup Rhabdomyosarcoma Study (IRS) Committee *J Pediatr Hematol Oncol*. 1995;17:46–52. [Erratum appears in *J Pediatr Hematol Oncol*. 1995 Nov;17:356.]
107. Andrassy RJ, Wiener ES, Raney RB, et al. Progress in the surgical management of vaginal rhabdomyosarcoma: a 25-year review from the Intergroup Rhabdomyosarcoma Study Group. *J Pediatr Surg*. 1999;34:731–734.
108. Lobe TE, Wiener E, Andrassy RJ, et al. The argument for conservative, delayed surgery in the management of prostatic rhabdomyosarcoma. *J Pediatr Surg*. 1996;31:1084–1087.
109. Wiener ES, Lawrence W, Hays D, et al. Retroperitoneal node biopsy in paratesticular rhabdomyosarcoma. *J Pediatr Surg*. 1994;29171–29177.
110. Wiener ES, Anderson JR, Ojimba JI, et al. Controversies in the management of paratesticular rhabdomyosarcoma: is staging retroperitoneal lymph node dissection necessary for adolescents with resected paratesticular rhabdomyosarcoma? *Semin Pediatr Surg*. 2001;10:146–152.
111. **Carli M, Colombatti R, Oberlin O, et al. European intergroup studies (MMT4-89 and MMT4-91) on childhood metastatic rhabdomyosarcoma: final results and analysis of prognostic factors. *J Clin Oncol*. 2004;22:4787–4794.**
112. Koscielniak E, Klingebiel TH, Peters C, et al. Do patients with metastatic and recurrent rhabdomyosarcoma benefit from high-dose therapy with hematopoietic rescue? Report of the German/Austrian Pediatric Bone Marrow Transplantation Group. *Bone Marrow Transplant*. 1997;19:227–231.
113. Boulad F, Kernan NA, LaQuaglia MP, et al. High-dose induction chemoradiotherapy followed by autologous bone marrow transplantation as consolidation therapy in rhabdomyosarcoma, extraosseous Ewing's sarcoma, and undifferentiated sarcoma. *J Clin Oncol*. 1998;16:1697–706.
114. Carli M, Colombatti R, Oberlin O, et al. High-dose melphalan with autologous stem-cell rescue in metastatic rhabdomyosarcoma. *J Clin Oncol*. 1999;17:2796–2803.
115. Soule EH, Pritchard DJ. Fibrosarcoma of infants and children: a review of 110 cases. *Cancer* 1977;40:1711–1721.
116. Bourgeois JM, Knezevich SR, Mathers JA, et al. Molecular detection of the ETV6-NTRK3 gene fusion differentiates congenital fibrosarcoma from other childhood spindle cell tumors. *Am J Surg Pathol*. 2000;24:937–946.
117. Ferguson WS. Advances in the adjuvant treatment of infantile fibrosarcoma. *Expert Rev Anticancer Ther*. 2003;3:185–191.
118. Loh ML, Ahn P, Perez-Atayde AR, et al. Treatment of infantile fibrosarcoma with chemotherapy and surgery: results from the Dana-Farber Cancer Institute and Children's Hospital, Boston. *J Pediatr Hematol Oncol*. 2002;24:722–726.
119. Kurkchubasche AG, Halvorson EG, Forman EN, et al. The role of preoperative chemotherapy in the treatment of infantile fibrosarcoma. *J Pediatr Surg*. 2000;35:880–883.
120. Pisters PW, Harrison LB, Woodruff JM, et al. A prospective randomized trial of adjuvant brachytherapy in the management of low-grade soft tissue sarcomas of the extremity and superficial trunk. *J Clin Oncol*. 1994;12:1150–1155.
121. Birdsall S, Osin P, Lu YJ, et al. Synovial sarcoma specific translocation associated with both epithelial and spindle cell components. *Int J Cancer* 1999;82:605–608.
122. Inagaki H, Murase T, Otsuka T, et al. Detection of SYT-SSX fusion transcript in synovial sarcoma using archival cytologic specimens. *Am J Clin Pathol*. 1999;111:528–533.
123. Rosen G, Forscher C, Lowenbraun S, et al. Synovial sarcoma: uniform response of metastases to high dose ifosfamide. *Cancer* 1994;73:2506–2511.
124. Brodsky JT, Burt ME, Hajdu SI, et al. Tendosynovial sarcoma: clinicopathologic features, treatment and prognosis. *Cancer* 1992;70:484–489.
125. Kushner BH, Hajdu SI, Gulati SC, et al. Extracranial primitive neuroectodermal tumor. *Cancer* 1991;67:1825–1829.
126. Gerald WL, Ladanyi M, de Alava E, et al. Clinical, pathologic, and molecular spectrum of tumors associated with t(11;22)(p13;q12): desmoplastic small round-cell tumor and its variants. *J Clin Oncol*. 1998;16:3028–3036.
127. Gerald WL, Rosai J. Desmoplastic small round cell tumor with multiphenotypic differentiation. *Zentrabl Pathol*. 1993;139:141–151.
128. Kushner BH, LaQuaglia MP, Wollner N, et al. Desmoplastic small round-cell tumor: prolonged progression-free survival with aggressive multimodality therapy. *J Clin Oncol*. 1996;14:1526–1531.
129. Schwarz RE, Gerald WL, Kushner BH, et al. Desmoplastic small round cell tumors: prognostic indicators and results of surgical management. *Ann Surg Oncol*. 1998;5:416–422.
130. Riccardi VM, Powell PP. Neurofibrosarcoma as a complication of von Recklinghausen neurofibromatosis. *Neurofibromatosis* 1989;2:152–165.
131. Mertens F, Dal Cin P, De Wever I, et al. Cytogenetic characterization of peripheral nerve sheath tumours: a report of the CHAMP study group. *J Pathol*. 2000;190:31–38.
132. Swanson PE, Wick MR, Dehner LP. Leiomyosarcoma of the somatic soft tissues in childhood: an immunohistochemical analysis of six cases with ultrastructural correlation. *Hum Pathol*. 1991;22:569–577.
133. Ng EH, Pollock RE, Munsell MF, et al. Prognostic factors influencing survival in gastrointestinal leiomyosarcomas: implications for surgical management and staging. *Ann Surg*. 1992;215:68–77.
134. Rabbitts TH, Forster A, Larson R, et al. Fusion of the dominant negative transcription regulator CHOP with a novel gene FUS by translocation t(12;16) in malignant liposarcoma. *Nat Genet*. 1993;4:175–180.
135. Joyama S, Ueda T, Shimizu K, et al. Chromosome rearrangement at 17q25 and xp11.2 in alveolar soft-part sarcoma: a case report and review of the literature. *Cancer* 1999;86:1246–1250.
136. Olweny CL, Toya T, Kantongole-Mbidde E, et al. Treatment of hepatocellular carcinoma with Adriamycin. *Cancer* 1975;36:1250–1257.
137. Evans AE, Land VJ, Newton WA, et al. Combination chemotherapy (vincristine, adriamycin, cyclophosphamide and 5-flourouracil) in the treatment of children with malignant hepatoma. *Cancer* 1982;50:821–826.
138. Quinn JJ, Altman AJ, Robinson HT, et al. Adriamycin and cisplatinum for hepatoblastoma. *Cancer* 1985;56:1926–1929.
139. Ortega JA, Krailo MD, Haas JE, et al. Effective treatment of unresectable or metastatic hepatoblastoma with cisplatinum and continuous infusion doxorubicin chemotherapy: a report from the children's cancer study group. *J Clin Oncol*. 1991;9:2167-2176.
140. Pritchard J, Brown J, Shafford E, et al. Cisplatin, doxorubicin, and delayed surgery for childhood hepatoblastoma: a successful approach–results of the first prospective study of the International Society of Pediatric Oncology. *J Clin Oncol*. 2000;18:3819–3828.
141. Czauderna P, Mackinlay G, Perilongo G, et al. Hepatocellular carcinoma in children: results of the first prospective study of the International Society of Pediatric Oncology group. *J Clin Oncol*. 2002;20:2798–27804.
142. **Katzenstein HM, Krailo MD, Malogolowkin MH, et al. Fibrolamellar hepatocellular carcinoma in children and adolescents. *Cancer* 2003;97:2006–2012.**
143. Chang MH, Shau WY, Chen CJ, et al. Hepatitis B vaccination and hepatocellular carcinoma rates in boys and girls. *JAMA* 2000;284:3040–3042.
144. Huang K, Lin S. Nationwide vaccination: a success story in Taiwan. *Vaccine* 2000;18(suppl 1):S35–S38.
145. Ni Y, Hsu H, et al. Hepatocellular carcinoma in childhood: clinical manifestations and prognosis. *Cancer* 1991;68:1737–1741.
146. Darbari A, Sabin KM, Shapiro CN, et al. Epidemiology of primary hepatic malignancies in U.S. children. *Hepatology* 2003;38:560–566.
147. Weinberg AG. Primary hepatic tumors of childhood. *Hum Pathol*. 1983;14:512–537.
148. Nickerson HJ, Silberman TL, McDonald TP.. Hepatoblastoma, thrombocytosis, and increased thrombopoietin. *Cancer* 1980;45:315–317.
149. **Aronson DC, Schnater JM, Staalman CR, et al. Predictive value of the pretreatment extent of disease system in hepatoblastoma: results from the International Society of Pediatric Oncology Liver Tumor Study Group SIOPEL-1 study. *J Clin Oncol*. 2005;23:1245–1252.**
150. Haas JE, Muczynski KA, Krailo M, et al. Histopathology and prognosis in childhood hepatoblastoma and hepatocellular carcinoma. *Cancer* 1989;64:1082–1095.
151. Lack EE, Neave C, Vawter GF. Hepatocellular carcinoma: review of 32 cases in childhood and adolescence. *Cancer* 1983;52:1510–1515.
152. The Liver Cancer Study Group of Japan. Primary liver cancer in Japan. *Cancer* 1987;60:1400.
153. Habrand JL, Nehme D, Kalifa C, et al. Is there a place for radiation therapy in the management of hepatoblastomas and hepatocellular carcinoma in children? *Int J Radiat Oncol Biol Phys*. 1992;23:525–531.
154. Weinblatt ME, Siegel SE, Siegel MM, et al. Preoperative chemotherapy for unresectable primary hepatic malignancies in children. *Cancer* 1982;50:1061–1064.
155. Taylor PH, Filler RM, Nebesar RA, et al. Experience with hepatic resection in childhood. *Am J Surg*. 1969;117:435–441.
156. Lee CS, Sung JL, Hwang LY, et al. Surgical treatment of 109 patients with symptomatic and asymptomatic hepatocellular carcinoma. *Surgery* 1986;99:481–490.
157. Exelby PR, Filler RM, Grosfeld JL. Liver tumors in children in the particular reference to hepatoblastoma and hepatocellular carcinoma: American Academy of Pediatrics Surgical Section Survey-1974. *J Pediatr Surg*. 1975;10:329–337.
158. Yokomori K, Hori T, Asoh S, et al. Complete disappearance of unresectable hepatoblastoma by continuous infusion therapy through the hepatic artery. *J Pediatr Surg*. 1991;26:844–846.
159. Black CT, Luck SR, Musemeche CA, et al. Aggressive excision of pulmonary metastases is warranted in the management of childhood hepatic tumors. *J Pediatr Surg*. 1991;26:1082–1086.

SECTION P
MUSCULOSKELETAL SYSTEM

CHAPTER 113 ■ ORTHOPEDIC SURGERY

H. DAVID MOEHRING

Rapid developments in the field of molecular biology and tissue engineering promise great advances in the near future and will modify or radically change current orthopedic philosophies. Minimally invasive techniques and "biologic fixation" will continue to evolve for fracture treatment. Anatomically contoured plates have been developed for the treatment of periarticular fractures. Threaded screw holes in these plates provide a locked construct and more rigid fixation for comminuted fractures. Arthroscopic applications and innovations will expand outpatient treatment of joint disease. Endoscopic-assisted spine surgery, biodegradable implants, and artificial joint lubricants will experience increasing evolution. Gene therapy and the development of chondroprotective agents hold promise for the prevention and treatment of osteoporosis and arthritis.

Osteogenic proteins, also referred to as *bone morphogenetic proteins,* are low-molecular-weight polypeptides that have been isolated from the bones of a variety of mammalian species and also reproduced by recombinant techniques. They have been shown to be capable of osteoinduction and the healing of gap defects and frank nonunions of bone and promise accelerated healing of problem fractures and more effective bone graft substitutes.[1]

Angiogenic growth factors are considered promising candidates for the induction of neovascularization of the ischemic myocardium and in the promotion of wound and bone healing. Similarly, endothelial progenitor cells involved in physiologic and pathologic neovascularization can be isolated from bone marrow and peripheral blood. Pluripotent stem cells exist in the connective tissue of postnatal mammals, including humans, and have the capacity to self-renew and form multiple tissue types throughout their life span.

Growth factors can be introduced directly or gene therapy techniques can be used to introduce genetically modified cells that are capable of producing the programmed growth factors in vivo. As the field of tissue engineering develops, generating three-dimensional tissue structures will become a reality, and cells grown on a biocompatible scaffold will allow for development of tissues in vitro or in vivo. Such tissues can replace a functional tissue or stimulate repair. Articular cartilage repair using cartilage constructs grown in vitro with in vivo remodeling is a current example. Chondrocytes are isolated, grown in culture, and successfully implanted into small chondral defects in the knee. Future tissue engineering techniques can be expected to be directed at chondral resurfacing of large joints, creation of small joints, and, eventually, the modification or replacement of mechanical joint arthroplasty by biologic constructs. Anatomically correct bones have been produced experimentally, and it is likely that entire bones with articular cartilage can be made through advanced tissue engineering.[2]

Neural stem cells and new biomaterials hold promise for reconstruction and repair of spinal cord injury. Exciting advances in tissue engineering, stem cell biology, and gene therapy promise great benefits in the near future. The next decade will see increased focus on the biologic aspects of soft tissue and fracture healing as more is learned about the multiple factors involved in this process.[3]

HISTORICAL PERSPECTIVES

Fracture treatment began in ancient Egypt with splints made of sticks or pieces of wood wrapped with linen bandages to immobilize the fracture and reduce pain. Hippocrates advocated stiffening the bandages with lard mixed with wax, resin, or pitch. Little attention was paid to reduction, and fractures often healed in a malaligned position. Later, through trial and error, various types of splints were discovered that improved functional results after fracture healing.[4]

Casting techniques as we know them today were developed in 1851. The first external fixator was developed in the 1840s using percutaneous methods and a claw-and-screw construct to treat a nonunited patellar fracture. The technique of "pins in plaster," whereby pins inserted above fracture fragments were incorporated in a plaster cast to immobilize a reduced fracture, and the first attempt at open reduction and internal fixation of the tibia were both reported in approximately 1900. These techniques were defeated by the metallurgy of the time and the high complication rate of infection, nonunion, and even death.[4,5]

Reconstructive procedures for the treatment of posttraumatic, congenital, and arthritic disorders evolved, broadening the orthopedic armamentarium. Plating techniques for the treatment of fractures were introduced in the first half of the 20th century. However, the wide acceptance of the principles of open reduction and internal fixation awaited the introduction of sound surgical methodology and implant technology developed in the 1960s by the Swiss Arbeitsgemeinschaft fur Osteosynthesefragen (Association of the Study of Internal Fixation). These techniques are especially valuable in the treatment of the polytrauma patient with multiple fractures.[4]

The need for surgical specialization according to anatomic region and specific organ systems became apparent in the early part of the 20th century. Some of the most famous contributors to orthopedic knowledge were general surgeons. It was their interest in developing orthopedics as a specialty that led to the formation of the American Board of Orthopaedic Surgery in 1934. As in other surgical specialties, appropriate subspecialization has occurred, focusing the wide spectrum of musculoskeletal disease into distinct regional areas that are discussed in this chapter. The interested reader is referred to a selected bibliography for an in-depth focus on areas of particular interest.

ORTHOPEDIC ASPECTS OF POLYTRAUMA

Musculoskeletal trauma remains a continuing problem in modern society, and prompt diagnosis and emergent treatment of fractures and dislocations is crucial to optimal patient outcomes (Fig. 113.1). It is vitally important to recognize the potential for associated neurovascular injury, occult or frequently missed injuries, and other pitfalls in diagnosis. Although minor soft tissue injuries and many isolated fractures are adequately treated without surgery, advanced surgical techniques have resulted in improved treatment of major soft tissue and bone injuries. Early coverage of exposed bone, neurovascular, and tendinous structures with local muscle flap, skin grafts, or remote microvascular grafts and advanced techniques for the treatment of extremity and spine trauma have been developed in the 1990s. Aggressive surgical treatments of intraarticular fractures and modern implant technology have resulted in shortened healing times and improved results. A significant portion of the aggressive approach to orthopedic injuries can be attributed to safer anesthesia and improved patient monitoring and postoperative care.

Orthopedic injuries fall into two basic types: blunt and penetrating. The latter are readily diagnosed, usually more localized, and infrequently associated with fracture, except for gunshot wounds. Penetrating trauma is more likely to cause neurovascular injury, whereas blunt trauma results in greater energy absorption over a wider area, with fractures, dislocations, and associated systemic trauma.[4]

Diagnosis

Isolated displaced fractures or dislocations are readily diagnosed on physical examination. The classic findings are pain, deformity, crepitus, and inability to bear weight or use an extremity. Undisplaced or minimally displaced fractures are diagnosed by radiography. Polytrauma patients frequently present a greater diagnostic challenge because resuscitation, treatment of life-threatening injuries, and orthopedic assessment proceed simultaneously.

Initial Survey

The initial survey is discussed more fully elsewhere in this book (see Chapter 16). After the establishment of an airway, venous access, and volume replacement, a rapid orthopedic evaluation is made by palpation of the entire spine for stepoffs and assessment of the pelvis for instability and the extremities for deformity or open injury. A cervical collar should always be provided and spine precautions continued until injury has been ruled out clinically and radiographically.

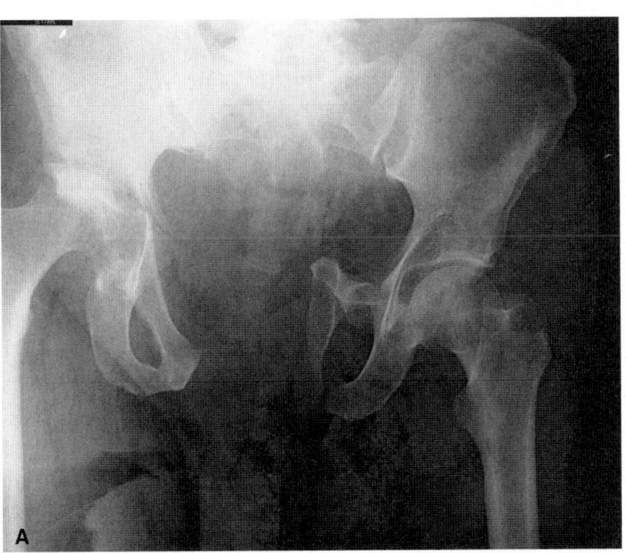

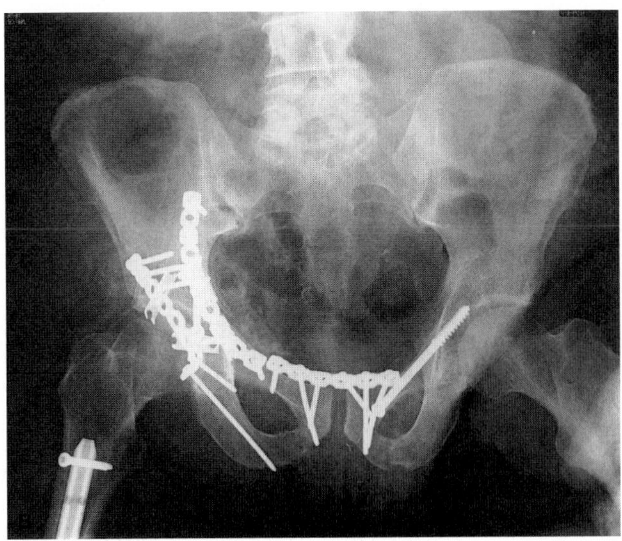

FIGURE 113.1 Polytrauma victim. *(A)* Grade III open pelvic disruption with associated urogenital injury. Orthopedic injuries include pubic diastasis, left sacroiliac dislocation, left superior and inferior pubic rami fractures, right acetabular fracture and hip dislocation, and right femoral fracture. *(B)* The same patient, 6 weeks after staged open reduction and internal fixation of right acetabular fracture and pubic diastasis with pelvic reconstruction plates, retrograde left superior ramus lag screw, and retrograde interlocked intramedullary rod for associated right femoral fracture.

TABLE 113.1 CLASSIFICATION

GUSTILLO AND ANDERSON CLASSIFICATION OF OPEN FRACTURES.*

Grade	Wound size	Soft tissue
I	<1 cm	No or minimal tissue damage
II	>1 cm	Moderate tissue damage
III	>10 cm	Major tissue damage
		Soft-tissue loss
		Bone loss
		Gross contamination
IIIa		Bone can be covered
IIIb		Bone cannot be covered
IIIc		Vascular injury requiring repair

*Interobserver variation occurs, but this is the most widely accepted and useful classification.

Extremity bleeding is controlled by direct pressure, avoiding tourniquets or direct ligation except in uncontrollable hemorrhage. Deformities should be corrected and fractures splinted before radiographic evaluation. Emergent radiographic evaluation includes a lateral view of the cervical spine to include the C-7 vertebra, and anteroposterior radiographs of the chest and pelvis.

Secondary Survey

After stabilization of the patient, more specific examination for spinal and orthopedic injuries can be undertaken. The patient should be log rolled gently to inspect the spine and sacral areas and to detect occult or open fractures of the pelvis or extremities.[4] Areas suspect for fracture undergo standard regional radiographs. Computed tomography (CT) scans are extremely valuable in evaluating head, spinal, abdominal, and pelvic trauma.[6] Occasionally, magnetic resonance imaging (MRI) is indicated to detect acute disc herniation as a cause of quadriplegia or other spinal cord injury in the absence of other obvious causes.

Open Fractures

Open fractures have significantly greater incidences of infection and nonunion, especially when they involve the tibia.[7–9] Clinically, the diagnosis is usually obvious; however, small punctures or wounds at a distance from the fracture can be overlooked. The most important determinants of outcome with open fractures are the size of the open wound, the degree of soft tissue damage, and the extent of contamination (Table 113.1).[7] Uncomplicated grade I open fractures have a prognosis similar to that of closed fractures, but require débridement, especially if they occur in an organically contaminated environment.

Treatment

In the emergency department, open fractures should be irrigated with sterile saline solution and a gauze dressing applied, followed by alignment and splinting of the fracture. Formal irrigation and débridement in the operating room should be rapidly accomplished. Open fractures that are irrigated and débrided more than 6 hours after injury have a higher incidence of infection. Coincident with emergent splinting and sterile dressing, tetanus toxoid and a broad-spectrum intravenous (IV) antibiotic should be administered. A first-generation cephalosporin is administered for low-grade (grades I and II) open injuries, an aminoglycoside is added for more extensive injury, and anaerobic coverage (triple antibiotics) for highly contaminated open fractures (Table 113.2).[8]

TABLE 113.2 MANAGEMENT

ANTIBIOTIC REGIMEN FOR OPEN FRACTURES*

Grade	Antibiotic regimen
I	Cefazolin 1 g q4th while in OR, q8h thereafter
II	Cefazolin as for grade I fractures
III	Cefazolin as for grade I fractures
	Penicillin-G 2 million U q4h
	Gentamicin 2.0 mg/kg load for young and healthy patients, 1.6 mg/kg load q8h maintenance

*Intravenous antibiotics should be begun as soon as possible after open fracture. Local antibiotic beads should also be considered in grade III open fractures.

The operating room débridement removes all devitalized soft tissue and small fragments of bone without vascular attachments and allows lavage of the open fracture with pulsed saline irrigation. The wound is left open or packed with antibiotic beads and loosely approximated with sutures. Alternatively, an oxygen-permeable membrane can be applied over the open wound, which is packed with antibiotic beads, until the patient is returned to the operating room in 48 to 72 hours for repeat irrigation and débridement. Local antibiotic beads elute high levels of antibiotics and are used in conjunction with IV antibiotics.[10] When the wound appears clean and there is no evidence of necrotic tissue, delayed primary closure or split-thickness skin grafting may be undertaken. Two or three débridements may be necessary. Extensive areas of exposed bone should be covered by local or regional muscle flaps or, if necessary, microvascular free flap. The goal is to have a closed wound within the first 5 to 7 days if at all possible.

Stabilization of Open Fractures

Controversy exists regarding the best form of stabilization after open fracture. In the lower extremity, most grade II and certain grade III open shaft fractures can be treated with intramedullary fixation, either initially or within the first week of injury.[11] Grade III fractures with a high degree of contamination are best treated by external fixation, but it is difficult to produce definitive fracture healing. External fixation can be converted to intramedullary fixation within the first week or two, and in the tibia, external fixation may also be followed by cast immobilization once soft tissue considerations permit.[9]

Plating of open tibial shaft fractures should rarely if ever be performed in the acute setting, although it is mandatory to fix open articular injuries internally. Bulky implants should be avoided because soft tissue necrosis resulting in exposed metal and bone may ensue. Hybrid external fixation is used for intraarticular fractures with associated traumatized soft tissue and high-grade open fractures, especially those involving the knee and ankle. This type of fixation uses tensioned Kirschner wire–ring constructs connected by external carbon rods to pins placed in the diaphysis of a long bone (Fig. 113.2). Using ligamentotaxis and indirect techniques or limited open reduction and cannulated subarticular screws, a reasonable reconstruction of the joint surface can usually be obtained.[12] The use of locked plating and minimally invasive techniques is an increasingly popular alternative.

In contrast to the lower extremity, most open fractures of the humerus, radius, and ulna can be treated by open reduction and compression plating, either initially or at subsequent washout.

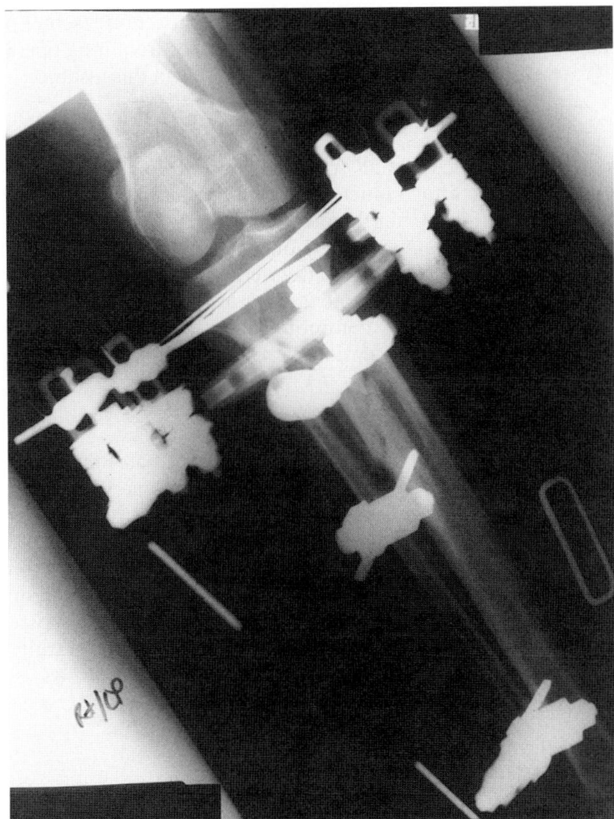

FIGURE 113.2 Hybrid fixation of a comminuted proximal tibial fracture associated with grade III open injury and fracture blisters. Open reduction and internal fixation is too risky in this situation.

Summary

Open fractures are an orthopedic emergency and must be treated promptly to prevent the serious complications of infection and nonunion. The principles of treatment involve thorough débridement, IV and local antibiotics, and fracture stabilization. Coverage of exposed bone by viable soft tissue must be achieved.

Chronic osteomyelitis and infected nonunions are notoriously difficult to treat, often requiring radical débridement of all dead bone and soft tissue and prolonged administration of IV and local antibiotics. Union is frequently difficult to obtain and may require massive bone grafts when the site is aseptic, or bone transport through distraction osteogenesis according to the method of Ilizarov. Amputation may be necessary for refractory infected tibial nonunions.

Arterial Injuries

Arterial injuries of the extremities are occasionally associated with an open fracture (Fig. 113.3). Knee dislocations and scapulothoracic disassociations are also frequently accompanied by arterial injury. The Vietnam experience has shown that internal fixation of fractures after arterial repair is not necessary in the acute setting. Nevertheless, in nonbattlefield situations, there is great benefit from stabilizing these injuries, especially when the diaphysis is fractured. Bone stabilization can precede or follow arterial repair, depending on the warm ischemia time.

Arterial repair should not be delayed significantly regardless of the type of fracture stabilization elected. External fixation can be rapidly applied to shaft fractures of the tibia, femur, or humerus. Skeletal traction, usually temporary, can be effectively used for femur fractures. Internal fixation with a compression plate can be used, but may not provide good stabilization in the presence of comminution.

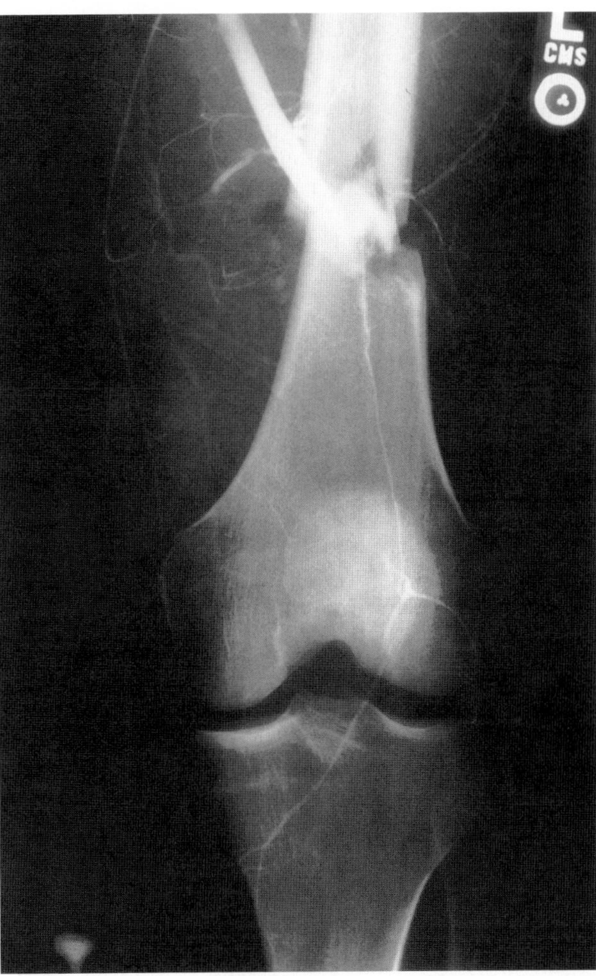

FIGURE 113.3 Distal femoral fracture associated with disruption of the femoral artery. Retrograde or antegrade intramedullary fracture stabilization can be accomplished rapidly and is the fixation of choice. Alternatively, through a separate lateral incision, a compression plate may be applied and functions as a tension band. A medial plate should not be used.

Retrograde femoral rods inserted through a small knee incision (Fig. 113.1) or small-diameter antegrade tibial rods can be rapidly applied and interfere less with vascular access than external fixation. In the upper extremity, compression plates are an effective means of stabilization. Minimally displaced or relatively stable articular and metaphyseal fractures can be treated electively after successful vascular repair.[4] Compartment syndrome may be associated with arterial injury or follow vascular repair, and prophylactic fasciotomy should be considered in patients with prolonged ischemic time, and compartment pressure monitoring used in high-risk injuries.

Dislocations

Shoulder: Anterior Dislocation

The shoulder is one of the most frequently dislocated joints, with anterior presentation accounting for more than 95% of dislocations. Frequently it is an isolated injury, often occurring in athletic events or falls. Occasionally, an axillary nerve palsy may be present. The prognosis for recovery is good for neuropraxic injuries. Reduction usually is not difficult and can be accomplished by one of numerous mechanisms. One of the most reliable methods is that of gentle external rotation of the shoulder beyond the midcoronal plane. In middle-aged or elderly people, rotator cuff injuries may be associated with dislocation, although recurrent dislocation is less likely than in young adults. In the latter group and adolescents, recurrent dislocation rates are very high, presumably because of the continued activities that place the shoulder at risk. In this group, surgical repair of recurrent dislocation is often necessary and highly successful.[13]

Shoulder: Posterior Dislocation

Posterior dislocation of the shoulder is uncommon and is one of the most frequently missed diagnoses in orthopedics. It is often associated with seizure disorder. Clinically, the shoulder is held in fixed internal rotation. Radiographically, the findings are subtle because the humeral head is directly posterior on the anteroposterior view and appears to be located. An axillary or transcapsular "Y" view is necessary to demonstrate the posterior dislocation. A high index of suspicion is necessary if permanent disability is to be prevented. A computed tomography (CT) scan is most helpful in evaluating complex shoulder injuries. After reduction, the patient's shoulder is immobilized in external rotation in the so-called gunslinger's position.[13] Late presentation often necessitates open reduction. A large impaction fracture of the humeral head may render the joint unstable requiring operative treatment. The prognosis is less favorable in this instance.

Elbow

Elbow dislocation is usually posterior or posterolateral in direction and stable after reduction. It is important to begin early, protected motion within the range of stability. Recurrent dislocation of the elbow is extremely uncommon, but some residual loss of terminal extension is frequently encountered despite immediate or early mobilization of the reduced joint. Fracture–dislocation is common and usually requires open reduction and internal fixation to restore anatomy and render the joint stable.[13]

Hip

Dislocations of the hip are also common and frequently accompany motor vehicle accidents and other high-energy injuries. Posterior hip dislocation is much more common than anterior dislocation. The patient presents clinically with an adducted, flexed, and internally rotated extremity (Fig. 113.4A). Reduction should be effected promptly by appropriate sedation and traction in line with the extremity. After reduction of a posterior hip dislocation, the hip should be checked for stability

A

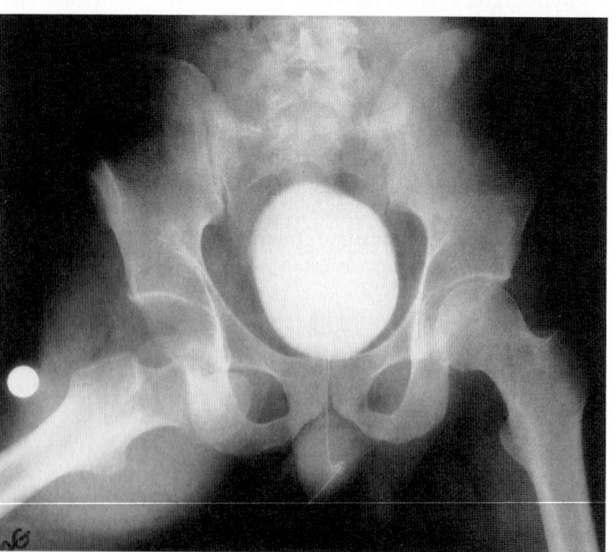

B

FIGURE 113.4 (*A*) Posterior dislocation of the hip. The thigh is flexed adducted and internally rotated. (*B*) Anterior dislocation of the hip. The thigh is abducted and externally rotated. There is an associated fracture of the femoral head. A cystogram is negative.

at 90 degrees of flexion in neutral rotation. The presence of a significant posterior wall acetabular fracture may render the hip irreducible or unstable, necessitating open reduction and internal fixation of the acetabulum and hip dislocation. A high incidence of avascular necrosis of the femoral head has been reported with dislocations that are reduced late.

Anterior dislocation of the hip, although less common, is more frequently associated with fracture of the femoral head or indentation deformation (Fig. 113.4B). Small osteochondral fragments associated with a symmetric hip joint may occasionally be observed. They usually require excision or, if large enough, open reduction and internal fixation through an anterior approach. Large femoral head fractures and those associated with acetabular or femoral neck fractures have a high incidence of avascular necrosis and hip arthritis.

The clinical presentation of anterior hip dislocation is characterized by abduction and external rotation. Radiographically, the femoral head is often located over the obturator foramen. Reduction can be attempted under appropriate sedation in the emergency department, but often requires anesthesia in the operating room. Almost all pure dislocations reduce quite easily under general anesthesia and muscle relaxation.[14]

Knee

Anterior or posterior dislocation of the knee is frequently associated with injury to the popliteal neurovascular bundle. Reduction is not difficult because all of the capsule and ligamentous structures are usually severely disrupted. Absent pulses may be restored after reduction, but an arteriogram is frequently indicated to rule out associated intimal injury that could progress to thrombosis. Arterial repair requires an interposed vein graft and may need to be protected with an external fixator spanning the knee.[4]

Associated peroneal nerve palsy is common and results in loss of dorsiflexion, which can be accommodated by an orthosis. However, if the posterior tibial nerve is avulsed, the prognosis is quite dismal, with eventual amputation being likely secondary to an anesthetic foot.

Ligamentous repair is usually undertaken immediately or in the first 10 days. Wherever possible, the menisci, at least one cruciate, and both collateral ligaments should be repaired. The prognosis is guarded for this severe injury, which usually does not permit the return to competitive athletics. A knee dislocation equivalent may present with less dramatic radiographic signs because of either spontaneous relocation or incomplete dislocation. This dislocation carries essentially the same clinical implications and caveats regarding neurovascular injury.

Ankle

Pure ankle dislocation is very uncommon; most ankle injuries are fracture–dislocations. Gross deformity is present with bone protruding or palpable through a gaping wound. Associated avulsion of neurovascular structures may be present. The vital posterior tibial neurovascular bundle is usually spared, however, because of the direction of dislocation. Most pure ankle dislocations are posteromedial in direction and widely open, and require irrigation and débridement, open reduction, and ligamentous repair. If the articular surface is intact and there is no fracture, the prognosis is surprisingly good if the ankle mortise is restored.[15]

Subtalar Joint

Dislocations are relatively uncommon and usually present with the foot displaced medially. Clinical presentation is dramatic, with the foot at right angles to the ankle and the skin severely tented over bony prominences opposite the direction of dislocation. Immediate reduction is indicated to prevent skin slough and restore circulation to the foot. The foot is usually stable after reduction and the functional results are good after a brief period of immobilization. Lateral subtalar dislocation is uncommon and more frequently associated with fracture. Open reduction may be necessary to extract entrapped neurovascular and tendinous structures as well as internally fix associated tarsal fractures.[16,17]

Fracture–Dislocations

Pure dislocations of the major joints are discussed in the preceding sections. Most displaced fractures are treated by orthopedists, in contrast to dislocations, which are not infrequently treated by emergency and family physicians, or occasionally by the patient or companions in an emergent situation. Fracture–dislocations result from higher-energy forces and frequently involve major joints. Fracture reduction by open technique is usually necessary to restore anatomy of the bone and obtain reduction of the joint.

FRACTURE ASSESSMENT AND TREATMENT

The goal of contemporary fracture treatment is to stabilize and restore bony anatomy, promote fracture healing, and ultimately restore function. Although closed treatment is indicated and effective for many isolated or nondisplaced fractures, patients may have to accept minor degrees of shortening or malalignment, which are of little functional consequence. There is no risk of infection or anesthetic complications with closed treatment, but this method cannot consistently produce the same number of good and excellent results as precise open reduction and internal fixation of selected fractures. Operative treatment is especially valuable for polytrauma victims and patients with multiple, bilateral, or articular fractures.[4,6,18,19] In these patients, relief of pain, correction of deformity, and ease of nursing care are distinct advantages. Open reduction and internal fixation also reduces the incidence and severity of pulmonary complications such as adult respiratory distress syndrome and pulmonary embolism. Prompt stabilization of fractures permits early joint motion, mobilization of the patient, and improved functional results. Ultimately, events occurring at the cellular level determine outcomes, and thus a fundamental understanding of the biology of fracture and soft tissue healing is necessary.

Biology of Fracture Healing and Soft Tissue Repair

After traumatic fracture, the acute hematoma becomes organized and invaded by cells recruited from the bone itself and, more important, from the periosteum. Pluripotent osteoprogenitor cells undergo differentiation into osteoblasts that begin to lay down the woven bone of the provisional callus. This phase is orchestrated and influenced by a host of recently identified growth factors. These osteogenic proteins are a family of bone matrix polypeptides (bone morphogenetic proteins) capable of inducing a sequence of cellular events leading to bone formation and repair. The process of osteoinduction continues through a combination of mechanisms, including enchondral ossification involving a cartilage intermediate stage, and direct bone apposition similar to intramembranous bone formation in the embryo. Woven bone is gradually converted to lamellar bone with secondary osteoclastic remodeling occurring under physiologic stresses, according to Wolff's law.[20]

Fracture healing is significantly influenced by fracture characteristics, including displacement, comminution, presence or absence of open injury, and methods of fracture stabilization. It is the external callus that contributes most to the restoration of strength and continuity after diaphyseal fractures. This type of healing response is predominant in fractures treated by intramedullary nailing, closed reduction and casting, or traction. The cells and blood vessels responsible for this phase appear to arise from the periosteum, and this type of fracture healing can be greatly diminished or totally abolished by fixation systems that impose total rigidity on the fracture. Late medullary callus is less tolerant of motion and forms more slowly. Primary cortical bone union occurs when a fracture has been anatomically reduced and rigidly plated. In this instance, no external callus appears. Healing is very slow and depends on osteonal penetration and the development of haversian systems.[21] After biologic stabilization of a fracture by the initial woven callus, continued mineralization and bone formation by osteocytes is accompanied by osteoclastic remodeling. Ultimate fracture healing produces bone that is mechanically and histologically identical to normal bone. Interruption of the healing process at any phase can result in delayed union or nonunion. Factors that contribute to nonunion are open soft tissue injury and devascularization, infection, smoking, and systemic disease.

The skeleton provides a framework over which the soft tissue is draped. Therefore, healing of damaged skin and neurovascular, ligamentous, and tendinous injuries is paramount for a satisfactory functional result. Soft tissue coverage of bone may be accomplished by delayed primary closure, split-thickness skin grafting, or local or remote microvascular flaps. Soft tissues are composed of collagen, elastin, and a hydrophilic ground substance. The latter contains mucopolysaccharides, proteoglycans, glycosaminoglycans, and water. The most important structural component of connective tissue is collagen, by virtue of its high mechanical integrity. The three-dimensional organization and relative amounts of these constituents determine the physical property of the tissue. Because the function of connective tissue is primarily mechanical, the cells provide a low level of homeostatic activity, except when faced with injury or damage.

The first stage in the repair of soft tissue involves formation of vascularized granulation tissue in which collagen fibers are randomly oriented. As healing progresses, and especially under the influence of early mobilization and a good vascular supply, orientation becomes functionally organized. Alignment of the collagen fibers along the lines of stress results in increased tensile strength and a more normal structure. Remodeling and adaptation of the soft tissue structures occurs under the normal physiologic loading conditions.

After nerve injury, wallerian degeneration occurs distal to the injury; repair involves regeneration of axons at the rate of approximately 1 mm per day. Ultimate reinnervation and restoration of muscle strength depend on the inherent regenerative potential, which varies from nerve to nerve, the type of injury, and the distance of the injury from the final innervation site[20]

PELVIC AND LOWER EXTREMITY FRACTURES

Pelvic Fractures

Pelvic fractures vary considerably in terms of severity, treatment, and prognosis. Only in recent decades has the concept of surgical stabilization been extended to pelvic fractures.[4,6,22,23] Minimally displaced fractures of the pubic rami and anterior portion of the pelvic ring are usually treated symptomatically, whereas major pelvic ring disruption has a significant mortality rate because of massive retroperitoneal hemorrhage and requires emergent stabilization as a lifesaving measure (Fig. 113.5). The incidence of pelvic fractures in fatal motor vehicle accidents is as high as 24% and approaches 50% for fatal pedestrian accidents.[4] Anatomically, the pelvis can be conceptualized as a ring. It consists of the two innominate bones and the sacrum joined together by strong ligaments. Considerable force is necessary to disrupt the posterior pelvic ring through fracture of the ilium or sacrum or pure ligamentous disruption, as described by Joseph François Malgaigne in his classic fracture text of 1847.

Diagnosis

Physical examination of the pelvis requires palpation and compression for the detection of instability and localization of pain. Repeated examinations should be avoided. In the presence of hypovolemic shock secondary to retroperitoneal hemorrhage a temporary pelvic binder should be applied to stabilize the pelvis. Emergent arterial embolization of the internal iliac vessels can be most valuable in the presence of massive retroperitoneal hemorrhage Urologic examination, inspection of soft tissues, and vaginal and rectal examination should be performed to rule out communication of the fracture with these areas. Open pelvic fractures are associated with a high mortality rate and may require diverting colostomy or a suprapubic cystostomy (Fig. 113.6). Bleeding at the urethral meatus in the male patient requires a urethrogram before passing a Foley catheter. A cystogram is often indicated by the presence of hematuria or wide pubic diastasis. Speculum examination of the vagina is required in the presence of bleeding, and sigmoidoscopy may be necessary to ascertain the presence of rectal tear.

Radiography

Standard anteroposterior radiography of the pelvis is part of the initial trauma evaluation. At secondary survey, a pelvic inlet and outlet view and, ultimately, a pelvic CT scan should be obtained. The latter can frequently be performed at the time of abdominal CT with fine 3-mm cuts through the acetabulum if indicated. CT scan is very valuable for assessing minor degrees of sacroiliac joint subluxation, sacral fractures, incarcerated acetabular fracture fragments, and other more subtle injuries to the pelvic ring.[4,6]

Classification

There are several different classifications of pelvic injury, according to the location of fractures and implied vectors of force. Pelvic fractures may be divided into three types (Fig. 113.7).[6] Minimally displaced fractures of the pelvis that are stable are classified as *type A fractures, type B fractures* are rotationally unstable, and *type C fractures* are vertically unstable (Figs. 113.1, 113.8). The latter two types are the clinically relevant disruptions and are often associated with visceral injury and polytrauma. Type C fractures or widely displaced type B fractures may be associated with life-threatening retroperitoneal hemorrhage.

Treatment

External Fixation. Pelvic external fixation can be rapidly applied when necessary to stabilize a disrupted pelvis associated with hemorrhagic shock. It is most effective in pubic diastasis and disruption of the anterior portion of the pelvic ring. It cannot be used in the presence of a major fracture of the iliac wing and may accentuate associated posterior pelvic disruption and bleeding. In addition to being a resuscitative tool, it may be used definitively in association with posterior fixation or in open fractures not amenable to internal stabilization (Fig. 113.8). Localized pin reaction or occasionally frank infection limits external fixation use to 10 to 12 weeks or

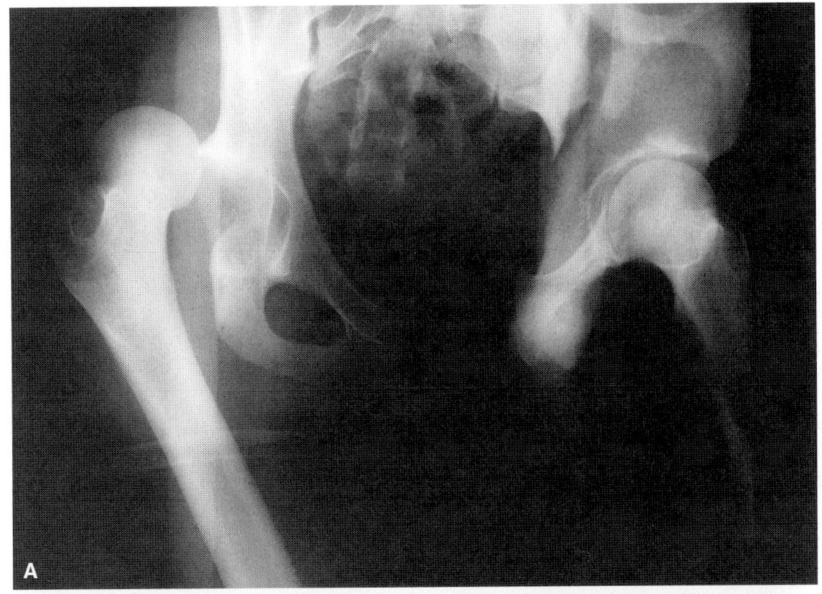

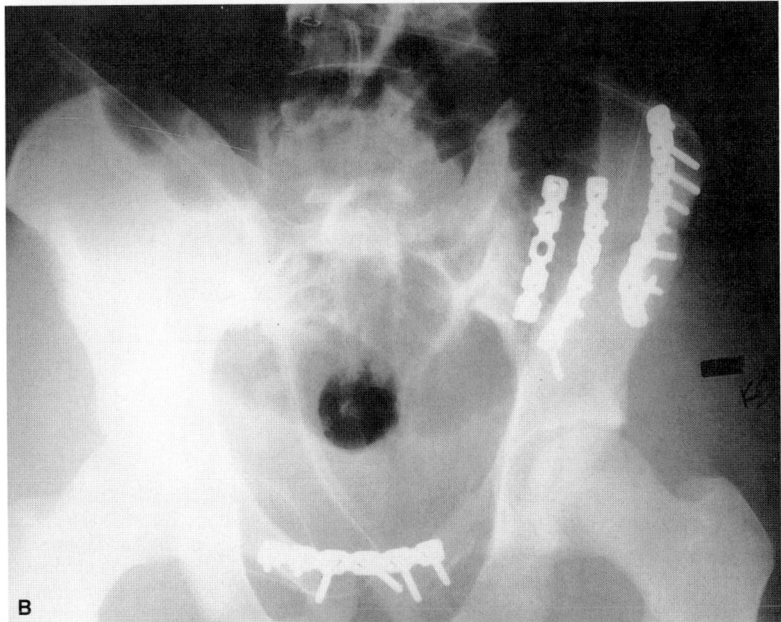

FIGURE 113.5 (*A*) Gross pelvic disruption associated with hemorrhagic shock in a young motor vehicle accident victim. There is posterior dislocation of the right hip, wide pubic diastasis, and comminuted fracture of left iliac wing. (*B*) Anteroposterior radiograph after open reduction and plating of pubic diastasis and associated iliac wing fracture and reduction of dislocated hip.

less.[6,23] Balanced skeletal traction of 20 to 25 pounds should be provided until definitive stabilization by external or internal fixation is accomplished.

Internal Fixation. Pure ligamentous disruption of the sacroiliac joint is best treated by open reduction and internal fixation accomplished through an anterior approach.[6] Pubic diastasis with or without bladder rupture is commonly treated by pubic plating. Displaced fractures of the posterior ileum and certain sacral fractures can be treated by open reduction from a posterior approach.

Ileosacral Screws. Ileosacral screws can be used in conjunction with open reduction and internal fixation or inserted independently by closed technique using cannulated screws and monitoring by fluoroscopic image intensification (Fig. 113.8). They are valuable adjuncts to anterior fixation such as pubic plating. The safe window for insertion of these screws is narrow, and occasional violation of the sacral foramina or neural canal may occur in even the most experienced hands. Fortunately, if malpositioned screws are detected and removed promptly, permanent sequelae rarely occur.[22]

Acetabulum Fractures

Fractures of the acetabulum can be isolated or associated with pelvic disruption and systemic polytrauma (Fig. 113.9). They are usually high-energy injuries secondary to motor vehicle accidents or falls from a height. Displaced fractures require surgical treatment to restore stability and congruency of the hip joint and allow mobilization of the patient. Classification systems have conceptually divided the acetabulum into anterior and posterior columns. The anterior column consists of the iliac wing, anterior wall and dome of the acetabulum, as well as the superior pubic ramus. The posterior column comprises the sciatic notch, posterior wall of the acetabulum, quadrilateral plate, and ischium. Fractures can involve the anterior, posterior, or both columns of the acetabulum. Radiographic evaluation includes anteroposterior and 45-degree oblique

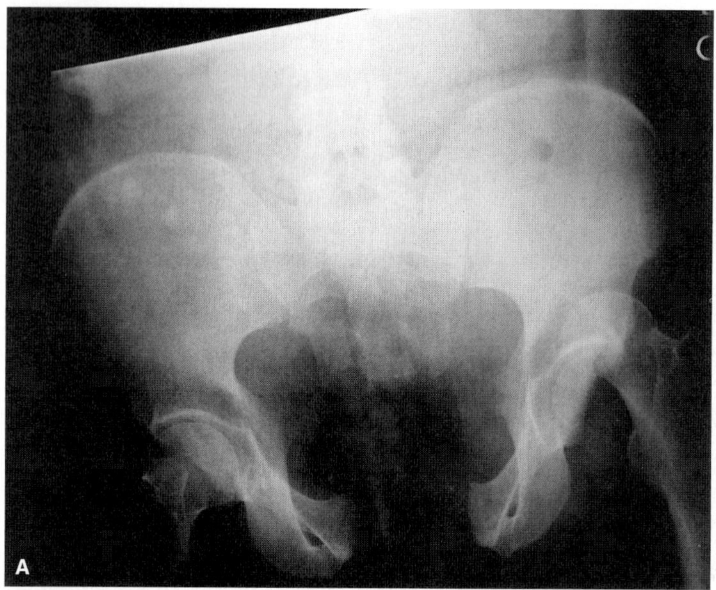

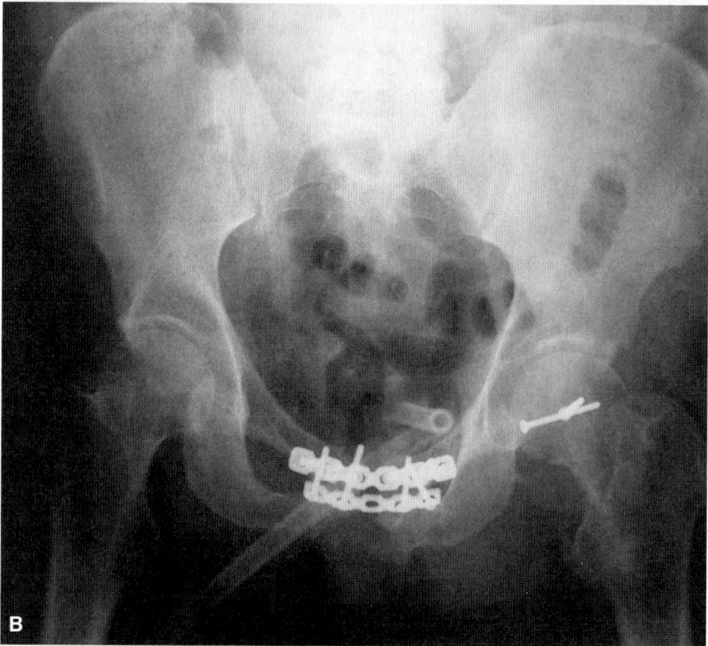

FIGURE 113.6 (*A*) Wide pubic diastasis, characteristic of "open book" horizontally unstable pelvis (type B), with associated femoral head fracture and hip dislocation. (*B*) Anteroposterior radiograph after open reduction and dual plating of pubic diastasis and open reduction and internal fixation of femoral head fracture. The patient had associated bladder rupture requiring repair and suprapubic cystostomy.

(Judet) views of the acetabulum. A CT scan is helpful in identifying joint fragments, marginal impaction, femoral head fractures, and sacroiliac joint involvement.[6,24]

Treatment

Surgical treatment is technically demanding and may require anterior, posterior, or combined approaches. Treatment is designed to allow mobilization of the patient and restoration of articular congruency. The ileoinguinal approach requires isolation of the spermatic cord, external iliac vessels, femoral nerve, and psoas muscle. This approach provides three windows for exposure, reduction, and fixation of the fracture. The posterior and straight lateral approaches release portions of the gluteus maximus and medius and short external rotators to expose the sciatic nerve and notch, posterior wall, column, and ischial tuberosity. Extensile approaches such as the extended ileofemoral, may be used but are associated with higher morbidity, wound problems, and residual muscle weakness.[25]

Special reduction techniques and pelvic instrumentation 0struction, and buttress plates provide internal fixation. Postoperative management includes deep vein thrombosis (DVT) precautions, early motion, and delayed weight bearing. Reported results vary considerably, and range from approximately 40% to 80% good and excellent. In many patients, however eventual posttraumatic arthritis occurs and may require hip replacement. Postoperative complications of infection or sciatic nerve injury seriously jeopardize functional outcome.

Operative treatment and anatomic reduction correlate with optimal patient outcomes but do not preclude subsequent chondrolysis, avascular necrosis, or posttraumatic arthritis (Fig. 113.10).[6,23–25]

LONG-BONE FRACTURES

Long-bone and open fractures were fatal injuries in ancient times, depriving a person of the ability to escape danger, defend himself or herself, or obtain nourishment. Subsequently, reduction and maintenance of length of femoral fractures was achieved by providing traction. Initially described in the 1300s, traction consisted of a weight attached to the leg by a cord that was

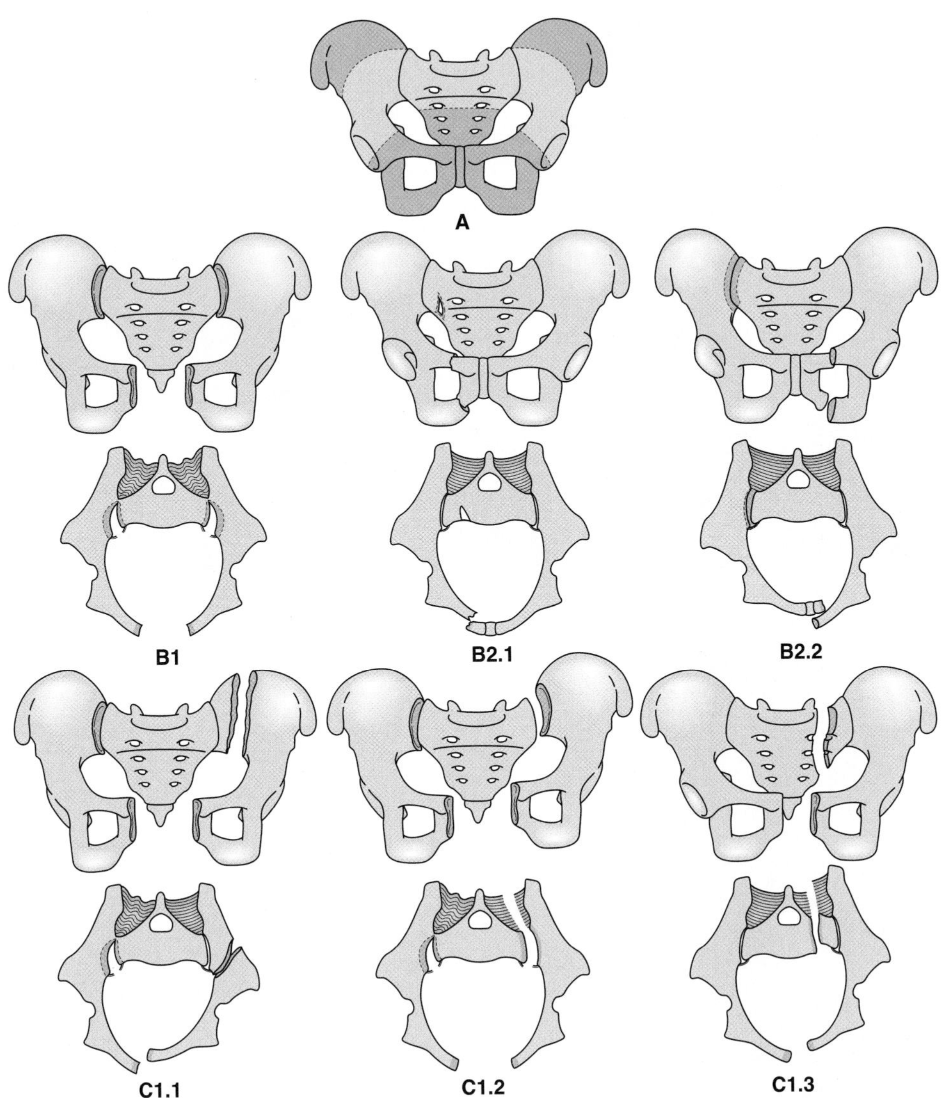

FIGURE 113.7 The AO classification of pelvic injuries. Type A fractures are undisplaced and do not result in instability. Type B fractures are horizontally unstable. Type B1 is commonly known as the *open book* fracture and is characterized by diastasis of the symphysis pubis and disruption of the anterior sacroiliac ligaments. Type C fractures are vertically unstable. They can involve pure ligamentous disruption through the pubis and sacroiliac joint, a fracture characteristically through the sacral foramina, or a posterior iliac fracture. All three mechanisms result in varying degrees of cephalad migration of the hemipelvis (Malgaigne).

strung over a pulley. Traction changed little over the next 500 years, but in the 1800s became somewhat more sophisticated through the use of various splints, frames, or slings. During the Civil War, skin traction (Buck's traction) for femoral fractures was popularized. Skin traction is still used today for temporary immobilization of adult hip fractures before surgery and as definitive treatment of pediatric lower extremity fractures or hip disorders. Skeletal traction allowed greater weight to be applied, with subsequent better control of the fracture. Steinmann began to use this method in 1907, and skeletal traction is used today for the temporary or definitive treatment of pelvic, acetabular, or femoral fractures.[4,5]

Intramedullary fixation was attempted very early, as evidenced by the skeletal remains of ancient peoples. The Aztecs and Incas treated long bone nonunions with resinous intramedullary pegs in the 16th century. Short ivory pegs were used in femoral fractures in the late 1800s and long metal nails during World War I. Open war injuries treated in this fashion before the era of antibiotics predictably resulted in infection and gas gangrene, leading to abandonment of this technique.[4,5]

Kúntscher introduced modern intramedullary nailing in Germany during the early days of World War II. His technique used large, stainless steel cloverleaf intramedullary nails.[26] The advantages of this method were compromised by problematic intramedullary infection. Development of the image intensifier not only decreased radiation exposure but permitted closed reduction and intramedullary fixation of fractures, greatly reducing the rate of infection and nonunion.

Long-bone fractures involve the diaphyseal regions of the femur, tibia, humerus, radius, and ulna and can be treated successfully by closed methods when minimally displaced or isolated; however, long-bone fractures in polytrauma victims, especially with femur and tibia fractures, are best stabilized surgically. Closed reduction and insertion of an intramedullary rod using a guide pin and fluoroscopic control greatly minimizes surgical trauma and reduces the incidence of infection and nonunion by keeping the fracture site closed. Modest reaming of the medullary canal is usually performed, but is limited or omitted in high-grade open fractures, polytrauma, and in patients with significant pulmonary contusions, in whom embolic marrow contents can worsen respiratory problems.

Femoral Fractures

Closed interlocked intramedullary fixation is the treatment of choice for fractures from just below the subtrochanteric to the high supracondylar region. The rods may be inserted antegrade (Fig. 113.10) or retrograde through the intercondylar notch of the femur and knee joint (see Fig. 113.1).[27,28] The latter method is useful for polytrauma victims for whom rapidity of treatment is essential. A fracture table is not necessary

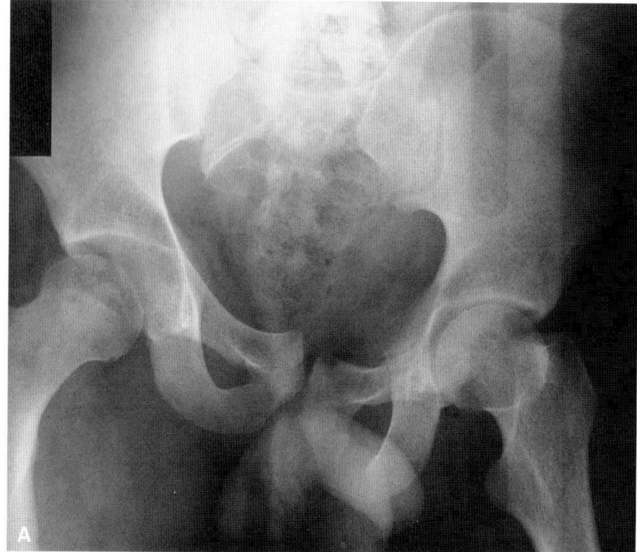

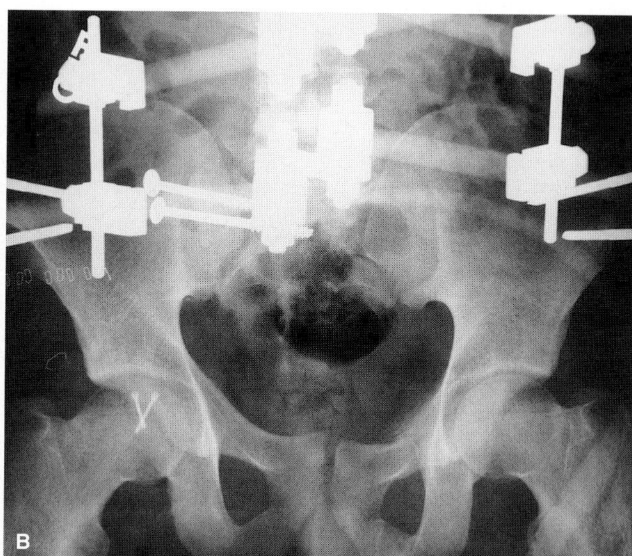

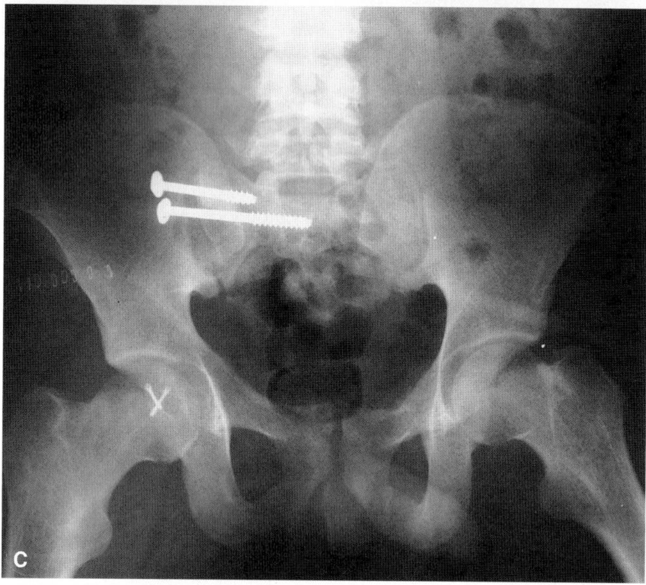

FIGURE 113.8 (*A*) Anteroposterior radiograph of pelvis showing open dislocation of the sacroiliac joint and symphysis pubis with vertical migration (type C). (*B*) Anteroposterior radiograph of open pelvic injury showing pelvic external fixation and iliosacral screw stabilization of the sacroiliac joint, as well as open reduction and internal fixation of associated femoral head fracture. (*C*) Iliosacral screws allowed early removal of the external fixation applied for open pelvic injury emergently. Note residual impaction of sacral fracture.

(see Fig. 113.1). This technique is also indicated for bilateral fractures, morbid obesity, and certain ipsilateral fractures of the tibia. Interlocking screws prevent loss of fracture reduction. Comminuted fractures require accurate assessment of length to avoid leg length discrepancy. Approximately 5% of femur fractures have an associated fracture at the femoral neck that may be overlooked without a high index of suspicion. The current treatment of choice for this combination is retrograde nailing of the shaft and cannulated screw fixation of the femoral neck.

Femur fractures were formerly treated by traction for 6 to 8 weeks followed by a unilateral walking spica cast; however, the advantages of rapid mobilization, decreased hospitalization costs, and better fracture reduction provided by intramedullary stabilization make it the treatment of choice.

Tibial Fractures

The vulnerable subcutaneous border predisposes tibial fractures to open injury and higher complication rates (Algorithm 113.1). Isolated, minimally displaced fractures of the tibial diaphysis can be treated with a long leg cast followed by a patellar tendon-bearing cast to allow knee motion at approximately 4 to 6 weeks. Minor malalignment is common after fracture healing (typically 4 to 6 months), but usually of little functional significance.[29,30] Closed intramedullary interlocked fixation is the treatment of choice for most other tibial fractures, those associated with ipsilateral femur fractures or polytrauma, and all segmental fractures (Fig. 113.11).[11,16] Compartment syndrome occurs most commonly in the calf, and therefore fractures of the tibia require careful and repeated examination.

Compartment Syndrome

Compartment syndrome is caused by the rapid accumulation of blood or interstitial fluid in a swollen, tense compartment, usually in the leg. Common causes are fractures, local trauma, crush injury, and positional hypoxia or ischemia and reperfusion swelling after vascular injury and reconstruction. Prolonged surgical procedures and tourniquet times are notorious iatrogenic causes. Elevated pressure occurs in the involved compartments, impeding cellular perfusion at the microvascular level. If the pressure is unrelieved, tissue necrosis may occur with ischemic contracted muscles as the final result.[31] These sequelae can usually be prevented in patients with tense compartments by prompt fascial decompression.[4]

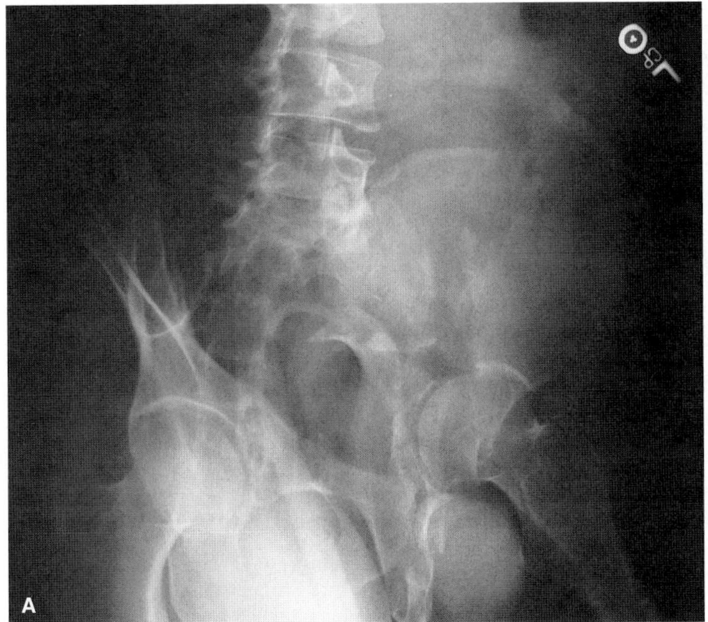

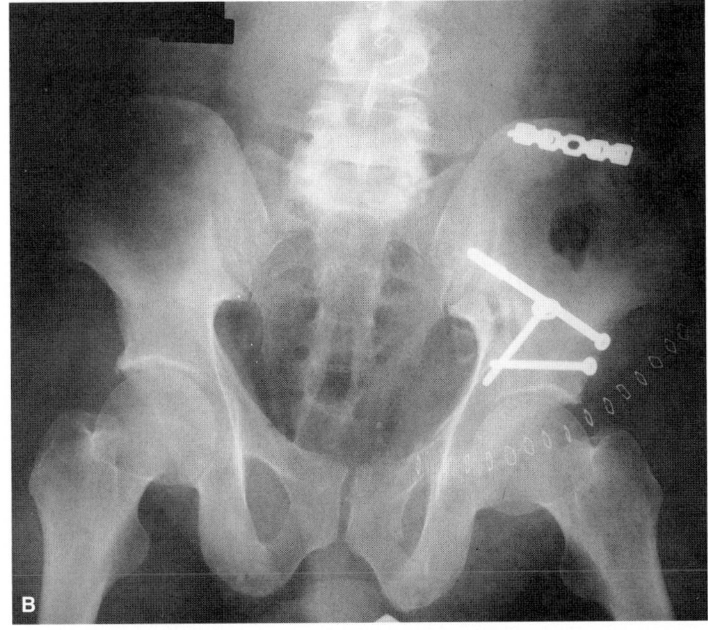

FIGURE 113.9 (*A*) Polytrauma victim with markedly displaced left acetabular fracture, associated with severe retroperitoneal hemorrhage. Hemorrhage was from bone and avulsed superior gluteal vessels. (*B*) Anteroposterior radiograph of pelvis after anatomic open reduction and internal fixation. Patient died 10 days after surgery from adult respiratory distress syndrome.

Diagnosis

In a cooperative and awake patient, the diagnosis can often be made on a clinical basis. Classically, there is pain out of proportion to the injury that increases with gentle passive stretch of the involved joint, paresthesias, and a very tense, tender fascial compartment. The classic signs however are not always present or complete and are highly subjective in nature. Most compartment syndromes occur in the leg, although the thigh, forearm, hand, or foot can also be involved. Pulses are present unless there is a concomitant arterial injury. After arterial repair, compartment syndrome is not infrequent and prophylactic fasciotomy is often indicated. Differentiating compartment syndrome from neurovascular injury can occasionally be problematic because they may coexist (Table 113.3). Compartment pressure measurements can be easily obtained to objectively document the clinical diagnosis and are especially helpful in equivocal cases.

Compartment pressures can be measured with a hand-held unit or by a pressure transducer connected by sterile tubing to a side-ported needle inserted into the suspected compartments. Pressure measurements are most valuable in unconscious or uncooperative patients in whom clinical evaluation is unreliable. Pressures in the 35- to 40-mm Hg range are suspect for compartment syndrome, and those significantly higher than this range are diagnostic. The closer the compartment pressure is to the patient's diastolic pressure, the greater the sensitivity to compartment syndrome. When this pressure differential is less than 30 mm Hg (Delta p), compartment syndrome is likely.[32]

Treatment

The treatment of compartment syndrome is immediate fasciotomy. Even though compartment pressures may be abnormally high in only one compartment, it is best to decompress all four compartments. In the leg, this can be accomplished by a lateral parafibular incision or the two-incision technique. If the latter method is selected, the incisions should be at least 20 cm

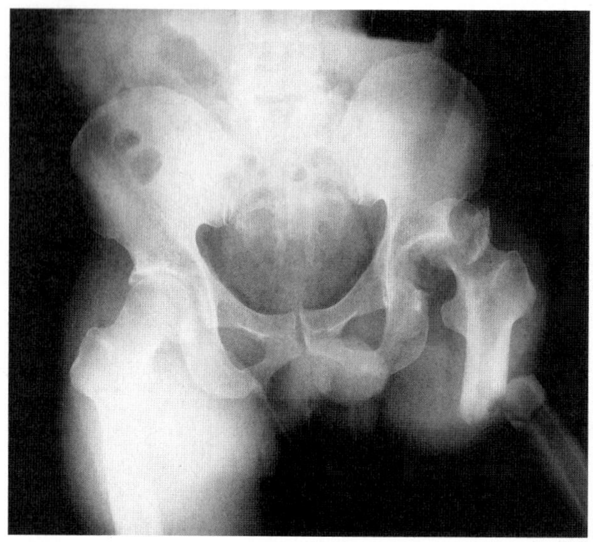

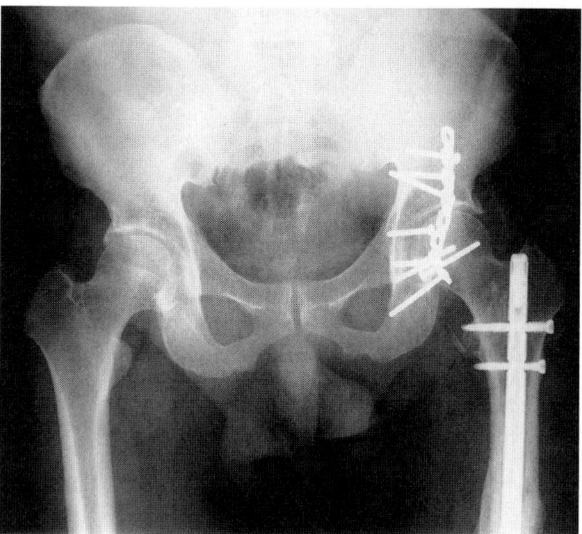

FIGURE 113.10 (*A*) Unusually severe injury secondary to a motor vehicle accident, with femoral head fracture, posterior wall acetabular fracture, hip dislocation, and subtrochanteric fracture of the femur. (*B*) Three-year follow-up after open reduction and internal fixation of femoral head and acetabular fractures and interlocked intramedullary fixation of the subtrochanteric femur fracture. All fractures have healed. The joint space is preserved and the patient has a surprisingly good result, with no avascular necrosis and full range of motion.

long and centered over the anterolateral and posteromedial aspects of the calf.[33] The fasciotomy incisions can usually be closed by delayed primary closure at 5 to 6 days, but occasionally necessitate split-thickness skin grafting. In the upper extremity, the carpal tunnel should always be decompressed at the time of forearm fasciotomy, but usually this portion can be closed after release of the transverse carpal ligament.[4]

Humeral Fractures

Most humeral shaft fractures are treated by closed methods with a coaptation splint, sling, or fracture brace, but fractures in obese patients or distal-third, distracted, or angulated fractures require surgical treatment.[34]

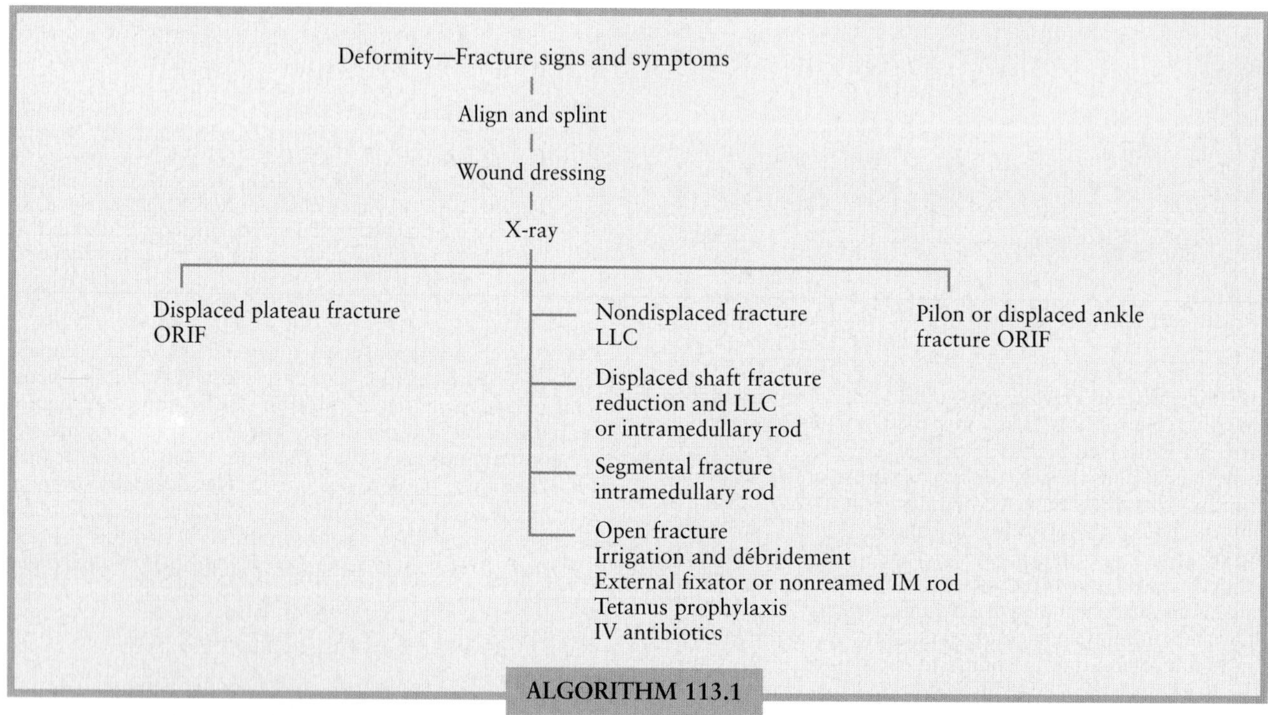

ALGORITHM 113.1 Management of tibial fractures. ORIF, open reduction and internal fixation; LLC, long leg cast.

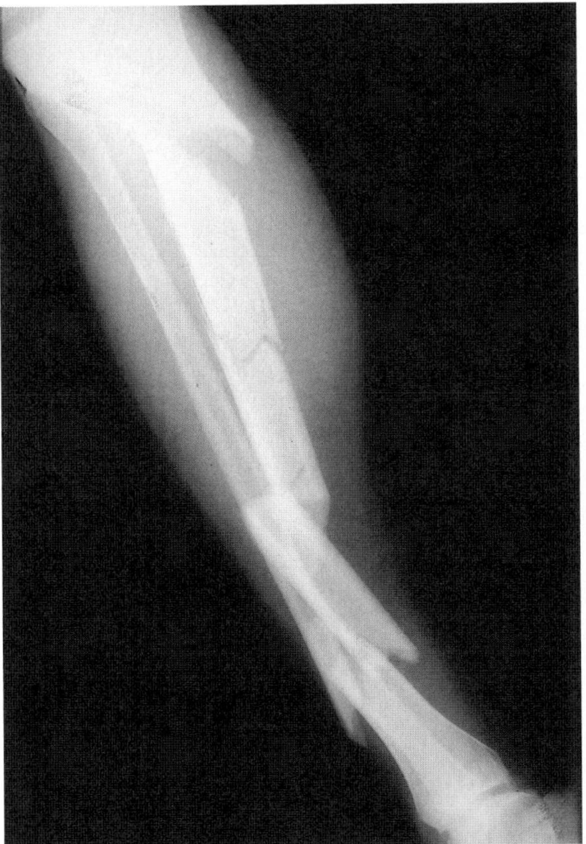

A

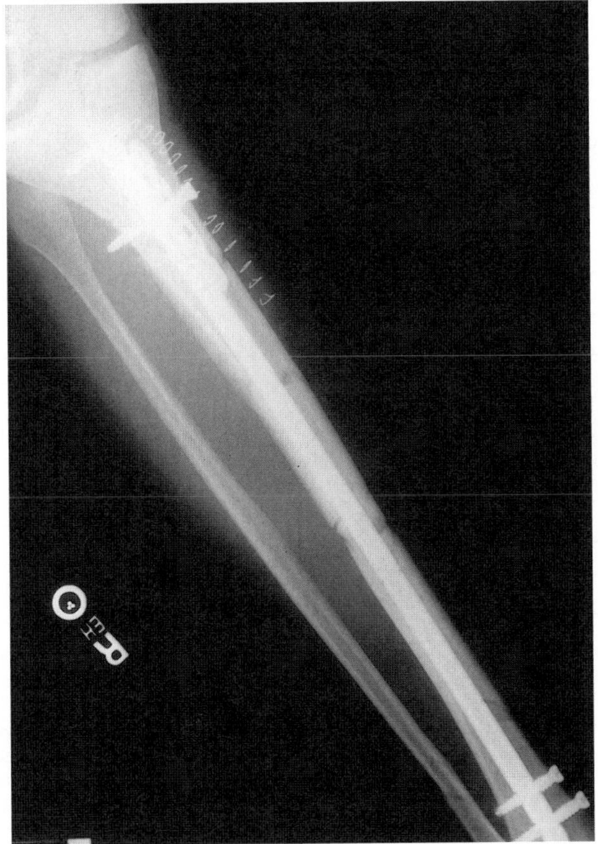

B

FIGURE 113.11 (*A*) Comminuted displaced segmental fracture of the tibia. (*B*) Anteroposterior radiograph after open reduction and plating of the proximal segment and intramedullary fixation of the multisegmented tibial fracture.

TABLE 113.3 DIAGNOSIS

COMPARTMENT SYNDRME FINDINGS

Finding	Compartment syndrome*	Arterial injury	Nerve injury
Pressure increase	+	−	−
Pain with motion	+	+	−
Paresthesia	+	+	+
Pulses intact	+	−	+

*Compartment syndrome occurs most often in the leg. A high index of suspicion and repeated examination, including compartment pressure measurements where indicated, are necessary. Fascial compartments released early have the most favorable prognosis, whereas those released after more than 6 hours usually have varying degrees of muscle necrosis. Occassionally, below-knee leg amputation is necessary.

Operative stabilization with an intramedullary rod or plate is indicated for associated ipsilateral fractures, open fractures with or without radial nerve palsy, bilateral fractures, and polytrauma victims (Fig. 113.12B). Somewhat greater degrees of angulation and shortening can be accepted in the humerus than in the lower extremity. Radial nerve palsy is present in 10% to 15% of fractures, especially spiral fractures of the distal third, where the nerve winds around the bone and can become stretched or entrapped. Laceration of the nerve is distinctly uncommon and recovery is the rule. Surgical exploration is indicated with persistent displacement, interposed soft tissue, and open injuries. A secondary radial nerve palsy that occurs as a result of manipulation or that arises during treatment may cautiously be observed provided that fracture alignment is maintained. Nonunion is more common with smokers, morbid obesity, and distracted fractures. It is treated by compression plating and iliac bone graft.

Radial and Ulnar Fractures

"Both-bone" forearm fractures in adults are optimally treated by open reduction and compression plating of both fractures (Fig. 113.13A and C) to ensure union and restoration of function of the hand and upper extremity. Isolated, minimally displaced fractures of the distal third of the ulna are exceptions and can be treated satisfactorily by closed reduction and casting.

Monteggia fractures are fractures of the ulna in association with a dislocation of the radial head. The radial head may be dislocated anteriorly (most common), posteriorly, or laterally, or dislocated and fractured, which are termed, respectively, *type 1, type 2, type 3, and type 4.*[18,19,35]

Galeazzi fractures are fractures of the distal radial shaft associated with a dislocation of the distal radioulnar joint. Reduction of dislocation is achieved by anatomic surgical reduction and internal fixation of the fracture and maintained by splinting or fixing the joint in the position of maximal stability. The distal radioulnar joint is reduced in full wrist supination.

Open both-bone fractures are stabilized by rigid plating as for closed fractures except for extremely contaminated fractures, which require external fixation. The latter is converted to internal plating when the soft tissue is receptive.[4,18,35]

METAPHYSEAL AND ARTICULAR FRACTURES

Displaced articular fractures are severe injuries that require open reduction and internal fixation to restore joint congruency and stability. Most metaphyseal or periarticular fractures, because of their proximity to the joint, also require internal

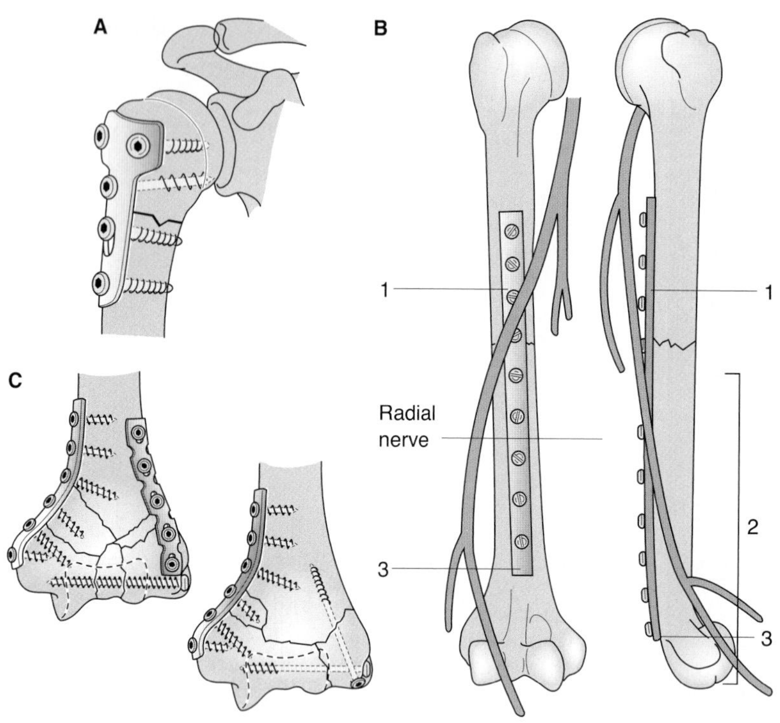

FIGURE 113.12 Operative treatment of humeral fractures. (*A*) Most fractures of the proximal humerus are treated nonoperatively with a hanging cast, or "sling and swathe." When displaced or associated with other fractures, they are best stabilized surgically. This approach allows for early range of motion of the joints involved. (*B*) Isolated shaft fractures are usually treated nonoperatively. With multiple, widely displaced, or open fractures, surgical treatment is indicated. An intramedullary rod may be used, but a plate is preferred in the humerus. The radial nerve should be identified and protected as it winds around the spiral groove of the humerus. (*C*) Supracondylar fractures of the humerus are frequently intraarticular. In adults, they require open reduction and internal fixation through a posterior triceps-splitting approach.

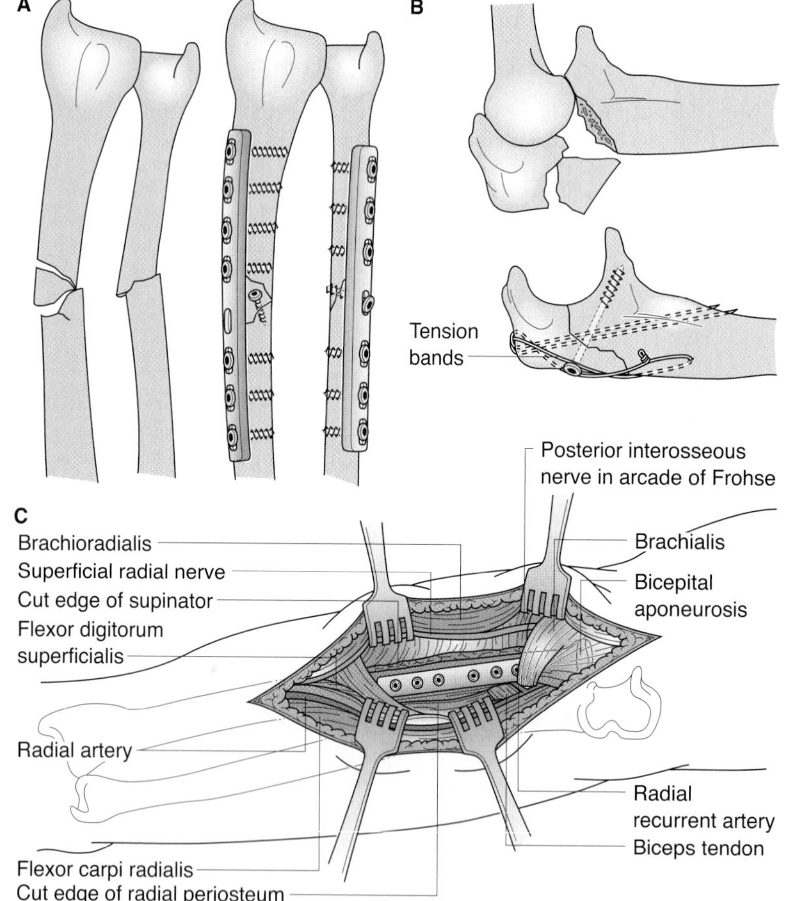

FIGURE 113.13 (*A*) Both-bone fractures of the radius and ulna in adults are best treated by anatomic open reduction and internal fixation. (*B*) Displaced fractures of the olecranon require open reduction and internal fixation. Tension-band technique and interfragmentary fixation are illustrated. (*C*) Open reduction and internal fixation of a proximal radius fracture. This fracture may be associated with a dislocation of the radial head (Monteggia fracture). An anterior approach is illustrated, although a posterior approach is more commonly used. The posterior interosseous branch of the radial nerve is at risk because it lies in the supinator muscle. It must be carefully identified and protected.

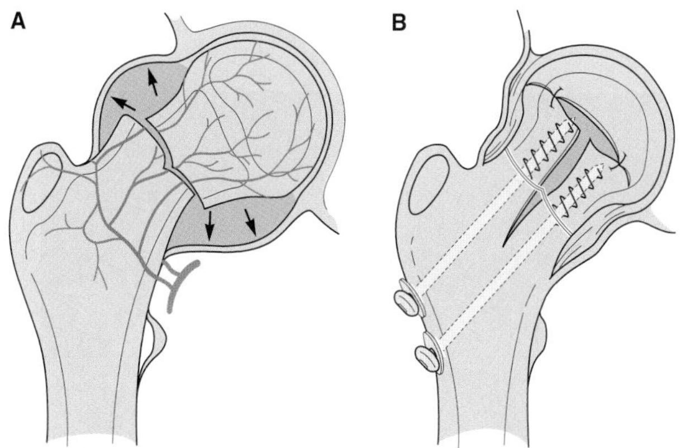

FIGURE 113.14 (*A*) Anteroposterior radiograph of the hip showing displaced femoral neck fracture in a child. (*B*) Urgent open reduction and accurate internal fixation is necessary to unkink the retinacular vessels and prevent their occlusion from vascular tamponade caused by the fracture hematoma. The screws should be accurately inserted and avoid crossing the growth plate. Even with these techniques, a significant incidence of avascular necrosis of the femoral head and growth disturbance may occur. In adults, closed reduction is usually effective and the screws are advanced to the subchondral bone of the femoral head.

fixation when displaced. The more common fractures are described in the following sections.

Femoral Neck Fractures

Intracapsular fractures of the femoral neck usually occur in elderly osteoporotic patients, but occasionally occur in young patients as a result of high-energy trauma. Whenever the fracture can be reduced, especially in younger patients, it should be treated by reduction and multiple pin fixation, usually using cannulated screws and image intensification (Fig. 113.14). When the fracture is completely displaced and is immediately subcapital in an elderly patient, it is best treated by hemiarthroplasty and prosthetic replacement of the femoral head. This approach to treatment allows immediate weight bearing and eliminates concerns over nonunion and avascular necrosis, which are notoriously common.[36]

Intertrochanteric Fractures

Intertrochanteric femoral fractures are also common in elderly patients and are best treated by compression screws and side plates, yielding high rates of healing and satisfactory results (Fig. 113.15).[37] The complications of avascular necrosis and nonunion are rarely seen in this extracapsular fracture, in contradistinction to intracapsular femoral neck fractures. In the elderly, both types of hip fractures are associated with a 10% to 25% mortality rate in the first year, and up to 25% of patients may require long-term nursing care.

The complications of hip fractures are usually related to preexisting medical problems. In elderly patients, it is imperative surgically to stabilize hip fractures as rapidly as possible to decrease pain, allow mobilization, and prevent exacerbation of medical problems.

Subtrochanteric Fractures

These fractures are higher-energy fractures associated with more bleeding, difficulty with surgical stabilization, and postoperative morbidity. Because of high stress acting on implants, they are often best treated with an intramedullary device that also captures the femoral head and neck.[38] These special intramedullary devices are known as *reconstruction rods* (Fig. 113.16). Alternatively, blade plates or standard compression screws with longer side plates can be used, but have a higher risk of cyclic fatigue failure.[18]

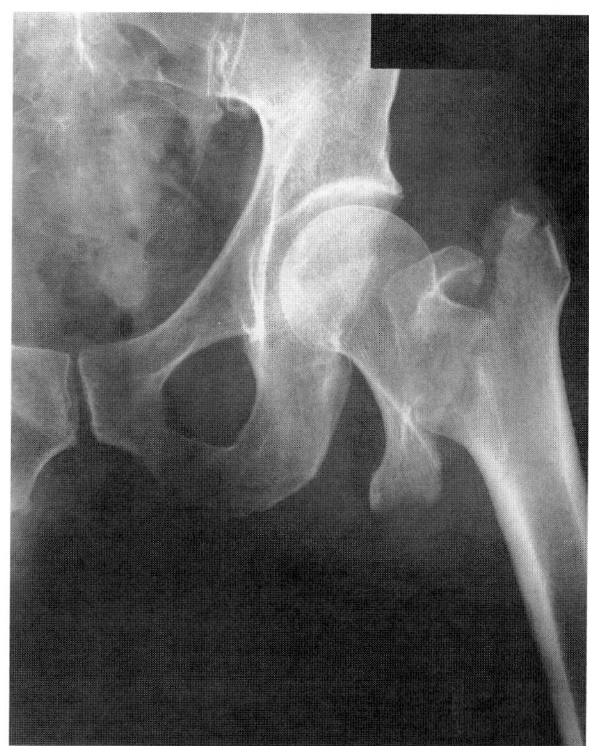

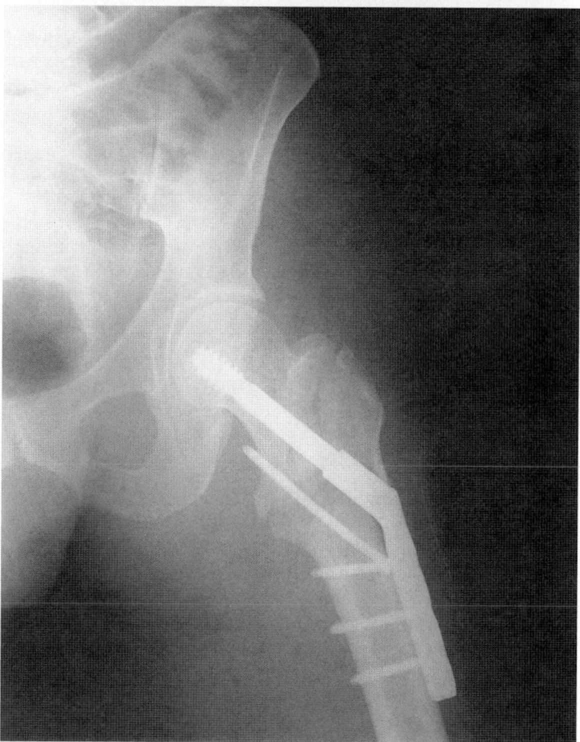

FIGURE 113.15 (*A*) Anteroposterior radiograph of irreducible intertrochanteric fracture of the femur, necessitating formal open reduction. (*B*) Anteroposterior radiograph of intertrochanteric fracture of the femur after open reduction and internal fixation with a compression lag screw and a side plate.

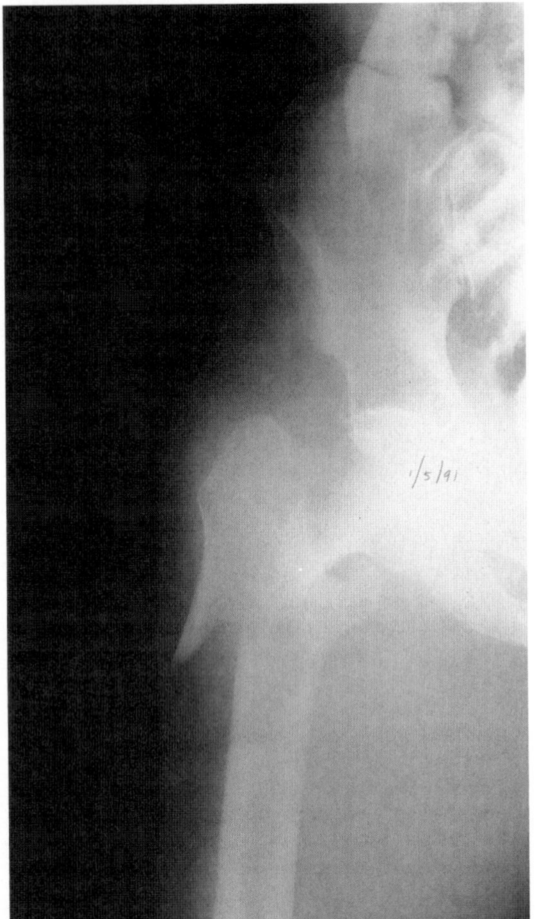

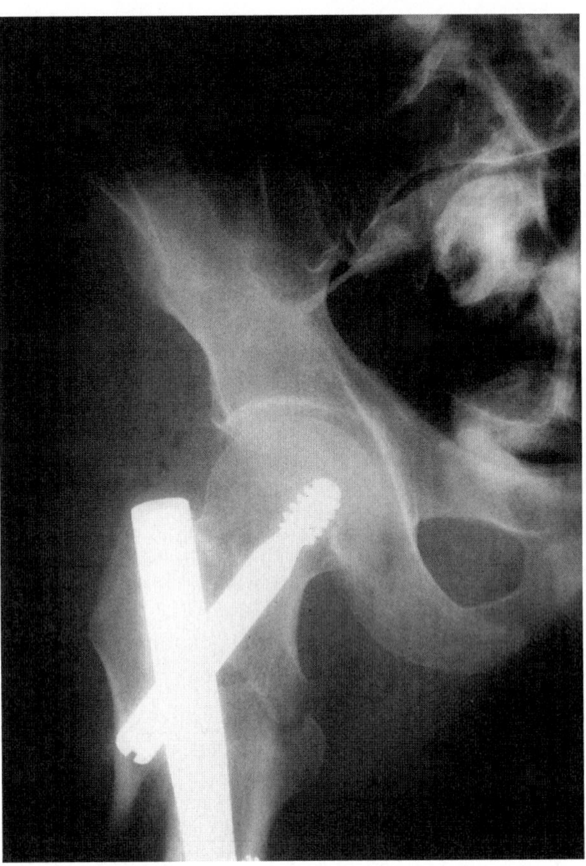

FIGURE 113.16 (*A*) Reverse-obliquity intertrochanteric femoral fracture. (*B*) Anteroposterior radiograph after Gramma reconstruction nailing. Failure of fixation is significantly less likely than with compression screw and side plate. This implant is also used for subtrochanteric fractures and for femoral shaft and ipsilateral femoral neck fractures.

Supracondylar Fractures of the Femur

Supracondylar fractures are challenging intraarticular fractures that are often significantly displaced. They require accurate open reduction and internal fixation, usually with a compression screw and side plate. Locking plates and jigs allow less invasive treatment utilizing limited joint exposure and percutaneous plate fixation to the shaft. More proximal supracondylar fractures can be treated with interlocked intramedullary rods, often inserted retrograde to ensure centering of the rod in the knee and correct alignment with the femoral shaft. Comminuted fractures oriented in the coronal plane require interfragmentary fixation and buttress plating (Fig. 113.17). Occasionally with extremely comminuted fractures in elderly, osteoporotic patients, distal femoral resection and modular total knee replacement may be indicated[12,18] (Fig. 113.18). Postoperative continuous passive motion, early joint mobilization, and delayed weight bearing are used.

Fractures of the Tibial Plateau

These challenging intraarticular fractures require open reduction, elevation of depressed fragments, bone grafting, and appropriate plating (Fig. 113.19). The lateral plateau is more frequently involved and somewhat more forgiving if healing occurs without valgus malalignment. Bicondylar fractures may require dual plating. Complications include skin slough over the subcutaneous medial plateau and avascular necrosis—the so-called "dead bone sandwich." Contemporary treatment with locked, less-invasive plating techniques has decreased this complication. The meniscus should be saved and repaired if injured. Intraarticular fractures with extension into the tibial shaft or traumatized skin are particularly problematic and may require hybrid fixation. After surgery, all intraarticular fractures require judicious mobilization or continuous passive motion to prevent adhesions. Weight bearing is restricted until fracture healing at 10 to 12 weeks.[12,18]

Patellar Fractures

Displaced fractures of the patella disrupt the extensor mechanism of the knee and patellofemoral articulation. They require open reduction and fixation with tension-band wiring, intrafragmentary lag screws, or both. Excision of the distal pole or patellectomy is occasionally necessary for comminuted fractures. Postoperative protected motion is desirable for most fractures.[12,19]

Pilon Fractures

Pilon fractures are severe injuries that involve the intraarticular surface (plafond) of the distal tibia and ankle and are often

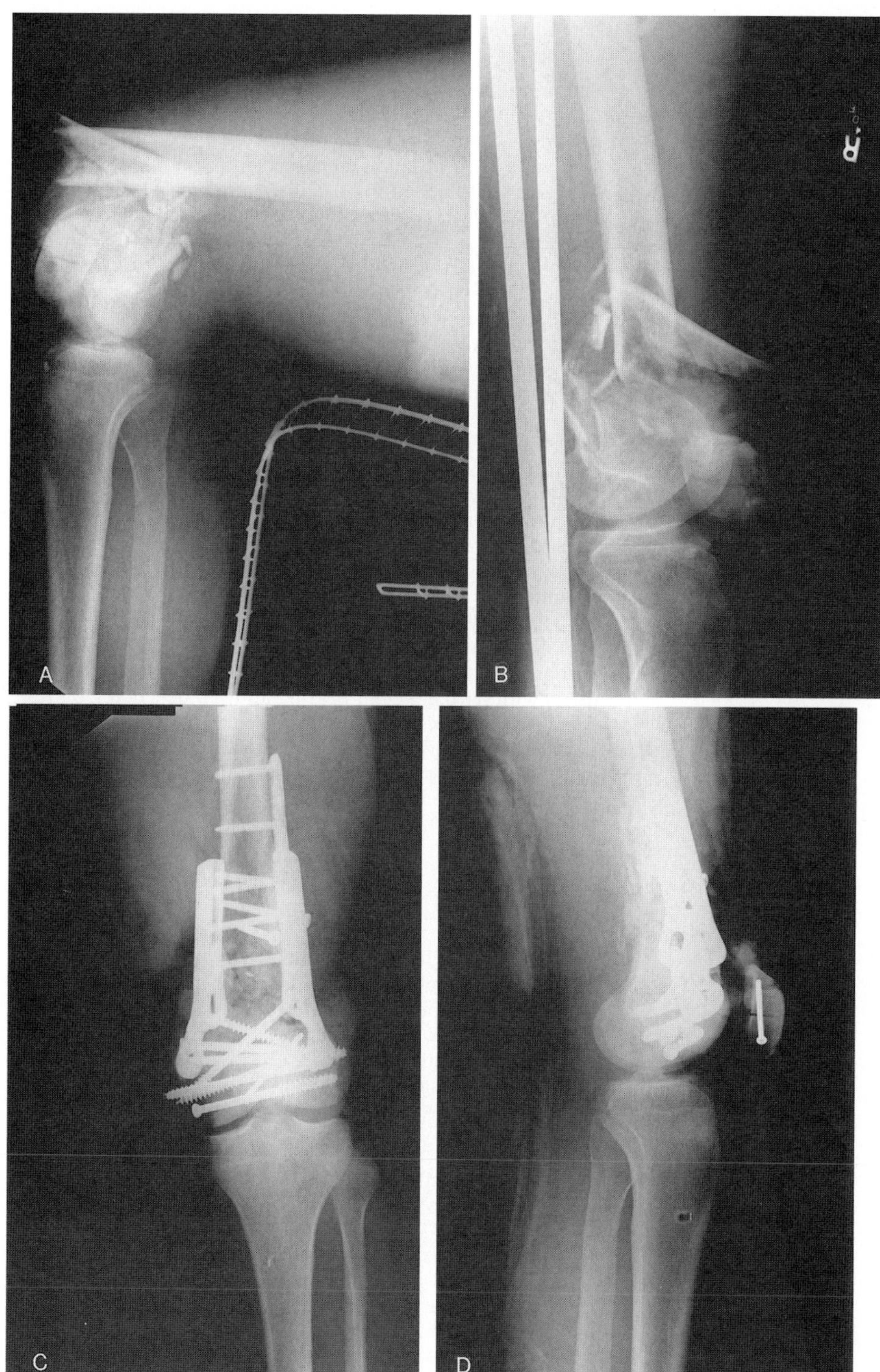

FIGURE 113.17 (*A*) Markedly comminuted, displaced open supra-condylar fracture of the right femur. Note inappropriate splinting. (*B*) Lateral radiograph of same fracture. (*C*) Postoperative radiograph of supracondylar fracture of the femur after dual-buttress plating and iliac crest bone grafting. (*D*) Lateral view of the same patient showing good restoration of the knee joint cartilage space and also satisfactory reduction of an associated patellar fracture.

accompanied by marked swelling and fracture blisters that may preclude early operative treatment. In this instance, temporary external fixation across the ankle joint is indicated. The fibula often may be safely surgically stabilized, restoring correct length and secondary ankle alignment. When the swelling has subsided and the soft tissue is receptive, open treatment is necessary for displaced articular fractures (Fig. 113.20). An anterior approach is used and the articular surface elevated, reconstructed, and frequently bone grafted. Low-profile plates, atraumatic surgical technique, and low tourniquet time are necessary to avoid the disastrous results of skin slough, infection, and exposed hardware. Even with microvascular free flap a suboptimal result is likely in this event, and amputation may eventually be necessary. In expert hands, the results are satisfactory in approximately 75% of cases. Nevertheless, a significant number of pilon fractures go on to posttraumatic arthritis and require eventual ankle arthrodesis despite restoration of anatomy.[4,16,18]

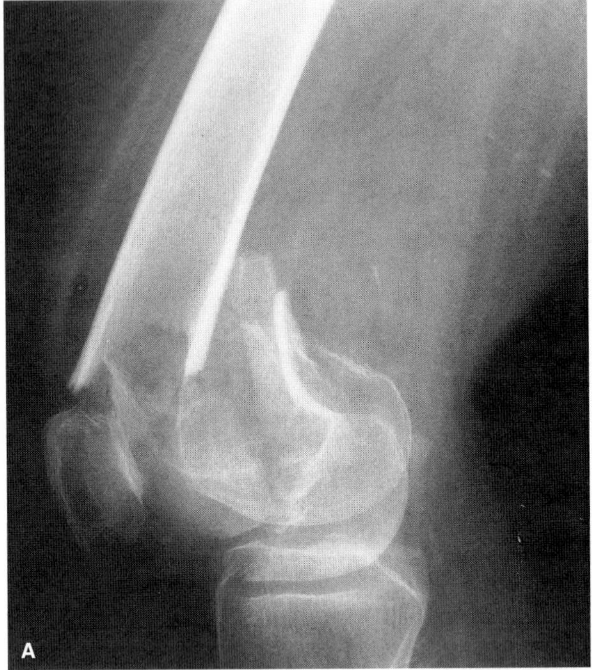

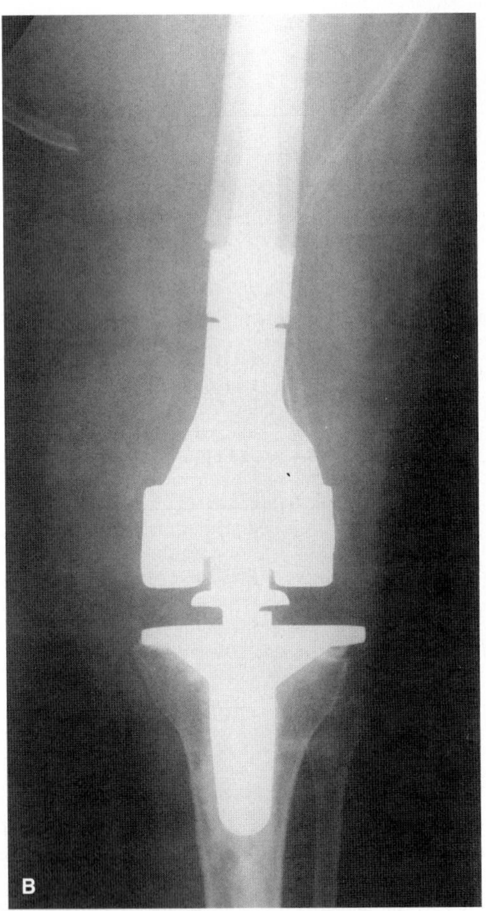

FIGURE 113.18 (*A*) Comminuted, displaced supracondylar femoral fracture in an elderly patient with poor bone quality. (*B*) Anteroposterior radiograph of knee after distal femoral replacement and modular total knee arthroplasty. This implant is more commonly used for tumors of the distal femur or complex revision total knee arthroplasty.

Ankle Fractures

Ankle fractures are common injuries and, when displaced, require anatomic restoration of the ankle mortise for a good functional result. In contrast to the axial articular impaction seen with pilon fractures, torsional forces result in malleolar fractures that largely spare the tibial articular surface (plafond). These fractures may involve the distal fibula, the medial malleolus, or both (bimalleolar). If the posterior tibial malleolus is involved, these injuries are known as *trimalleolar fractures*. Closed treatment is effective for certain isolated lateral malleolar or undisplaced fractures.

Frequently, operative reduction is the only way to guarantee restoration of anatomy. Typically, a low-profile plate is used for the fibula and two 3.5-mm lag screws for the medial malleolus for the common inversion injury.

A more severe injury occurs when the foot is in pronation as the talus rotates laterally, producing in addition an injury to the tibiofibular syndesmosis. Characteristically, a high fibular fracture occurs several centimeters above the ankle, but may occur as far proximal as the knee—the Maisonneuve fracture. Therefore, "isolated" fractures of the proximal fibula require examination of the ankle. In addition to fracture fixation, a fibulotibial syndesmosis screw is required to approximate the torn syndesmosis and restore the ankle mortise (Fig. 113.21). A short leg cast is worn for 6 to 8 weeks for most ankle fractures, with partial weight bearing allowed depending on fracture characteristics and stability. Typically, ankle fractures do not involve the weight-bearing articular surface of the tibial plafond to any extent, heal rapidly, and are unassociated with arthritic sequelae if anatomic reduction of the ankle has been maintained.[4,16,18]

Foot Fractures

Fractures of the foot are frequently treated closed, with the exception of displaced fractures of the calcaneus and talus. Dislocation of the tarsometatarsal joints or Lisfranc injury requires reduction and pinning or screw fixation. Most metatarsal fractures can be treated closed; however, displaced multiple metatarsal fractures can be treated by open reduction and Kirschner wire intramedullary fixation.[17]

UPPER EXTREMITY FRACTURES

Fractures of the clavicle are usually treated with a sling or figure-of-eight bandage and rarely require operative treatment. An exception is associated fracture of the scapula, which renders the shoulder unstable. In this instance, plating of the clavicle alone can help restore some stability. Widely displaced fractures, which tent the skin, may also require open reduction and internal fixation.[4,19]

Scapulothoracic Dissociation

This uncommon injury is devastating, resulting in an internal degloving injury usually associated with fractures of the clavicle or scapula. The shoulder is literally ripped from the thorax, avulsing the subclavian or axillary vessels and portions of the brachial plexus. The injury may be open or closed, and partial or incomplete. In complete lesions, the patient presents with a pulseless flail arm. Hypovolemic shock is frequently present, as well as associated injuries, and a 20% mortality rate has been reported. Resuscitation is followed by arterial

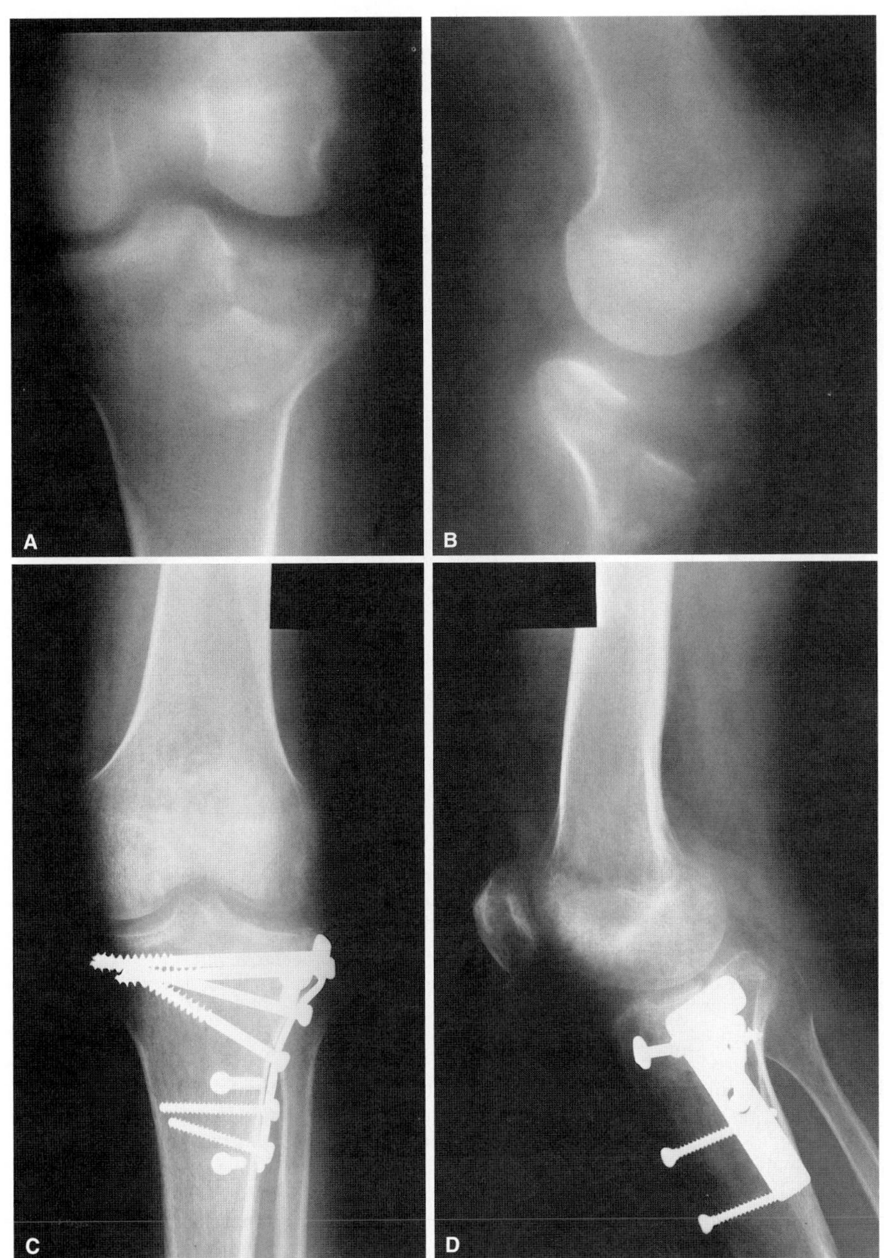

FIGURE 113.19 (*A*) Anteroposterior tomogram of markedly depressed lateral tibial plateau fracture, extending into the intercondylar notch and including the tibial tubercle. (*B*) Lateral tomogram of same fracture showing marked displacement and depression of the articular surface. (*C*) Anteroposterior radiograph after open reduction, elevation of depressed fragments, bone grafting and internal fixation. (*D*) Postoperative lateral radiograph of same fracture.

repair and exploration of the brachial plexus. The latter is frequently unrepairable. The protocol for brachial plexus injuries is followed and the clavicle can be plated to provide some stabilization to the thorax. The prognosis is poor with amputation likely for complete lesions.[39]

Scapular Fractures

Most scapular fractures do not violate the articular surface of the shoulder joint. They are often associated with other fractures and polytrauma and are treated symptomatically with a sling or shoulder immobilizer and graduated mobilization. Displaced intraarticular fractures of the glenoid, although uncommon, require operative fixation. A posterior approach between the infraspinatus and teres minor along the axillary border of the scapula is usually selected. The axillary and suprascapular nerves need to be identified and protected. The posterior approach provides good visualization of the fracture and has low postoperative morbidity. The results are surprisingly good when anatomic restoration of the glenoid has been accomplished.[40]

Fractures of the proximal humerus are usually treated closed unless significantly displaced and associated with multiple fractures, polytrauma, or ipsilateral injury. Displaced fractures of the tuberosities, as well as three-part and certain four-part fractures in active patients, may require open reduction (Fig. 113.12A). Four-part fractures in older patients are frequently treated by hemiarthroplasty and prosthetic replacement because they are associated with a significant incidence of avascular necrosis.[18,41]

Supracondylar fractures of the humerus frequently involve the articular surface and require open reduction and internal fixation through a posterior triceps splitting approach and plating of both the medial and lateral columns of the distal humerus.[42] The ulnar nerve should be protected but does not usually require anterior transposition. Early postoperative motion is important for all intraarticular fractures.[42,18]

Fractures of the olecranon that are displaced require open reduction and internal fixation. Small fractures can be ignored

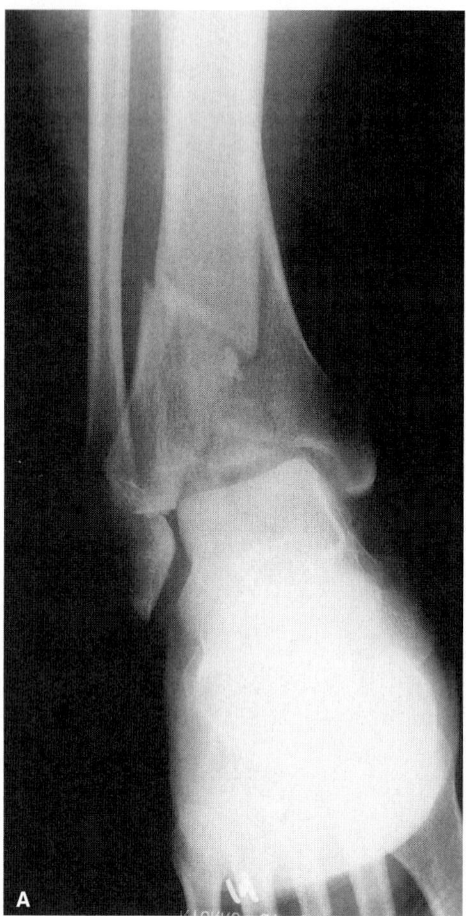

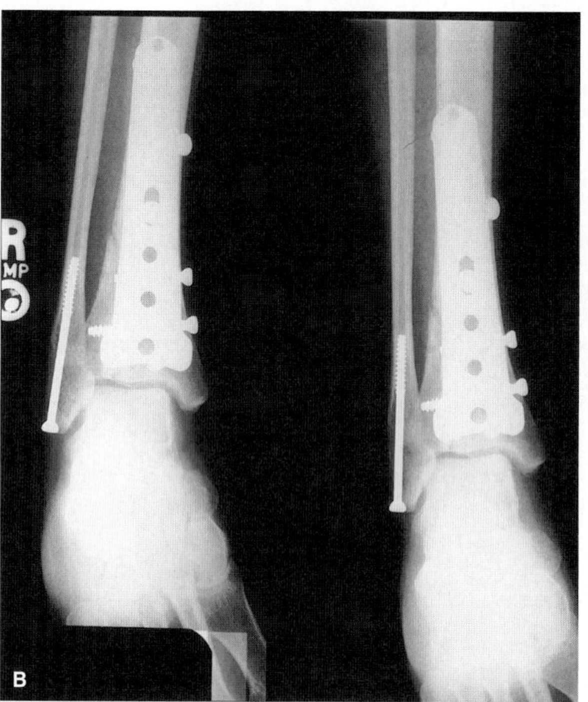

FIGURE 113.20 (*A*) Pilon impaction fracture of the distal tibial articular surface. (*B*) Postoperative film of pilon fracture after closed intramedullary fixation of the fibula and open reduction and internal fixation of the distal tibia, restoring the ankle joint.

or excised if comminuted.[4,18,19] Tension-band fixation, interfragmentary screws, or reconstruction plates may be used depending on fracture characteristics (Fig. 113.13B).

Radial head fractures are treated nonoperatively unless comminuted and displaced. Excision is performed for comminuted fractures, and occasionally radial head replacement is necessary for associated elbow instability because of coexisting coronoid fracture of the ulna. Where amenable, open reduction and internal fixation using small or miniature fragment fixation plates is indicated.[18,19,43]

Fractures of the distal radius (Colles' fracture) are common. They occur most often in elderly patients, especially osteoporotic postmenopausal women. When displaced, they present with the classic "dinner fork" deformity.[44] Fracture of the ulnar styloid is often present. They usually can be treated by closed reduction and casting. In the 1990s, external fixation and percutaneous pinning have been added to the orthopedist's armamentarium and are indicated for unstable fragments or inadequate closed reduction (Fig. 113.22A). Open reduction and buttress plating are increasingly indicated for certain displaced intraarticular fractures (e.g., Barton fractures) and higher energy injuries in younger patients.[44,45]

Scaphoid Fractures

The scaphoid is the most frequently fractured carpal bone and is injured as a result of a fall on an outstretched, dorsiflexed hand. This fracture is a known diagnostic pitfall that often is misdiagnosed as a sprain. Repeat examination and radiography may be necessary to rule out this fracture. In patients with tenderness over the tubercle or anatomic snuff box, thumb spica cast immobilization is indicated followed by repeat examination and radiography at 10 to 14 days to confirm or rule out fracture. Healing may take place slowly and prolonged immobilization may be necessary. Scaphoid fractures that are unstable or displaced are usually treated surgically (Fig. 113.22C). Distal pole and waist fractures are approached palmarly and proximal pole fractures dorsally. Nonunion and avascular necrosis are known complications of scaphoid fractures, especially when diagnosis and treatment have been delayed. Disability is best avoided by a high index of suspicion and awareness of this common fracture.[4,18,19,46]

SPINE

Orthopedic spine surgery encompasses the diagnosis and treatment of discogenic disease, stabilization of degenerative spine disease, correction of deformity, and treatment of fractures and associated spinal cord injury.

Spinal Cord Injury and Spinal Fractures

The immediate stabilization and protection of a potentially injured spine by paramedical and transport personnel has reduced the incidence of neurologic injury. Quadriplegia and paraplegia are among the most dreaded of all injuries, and

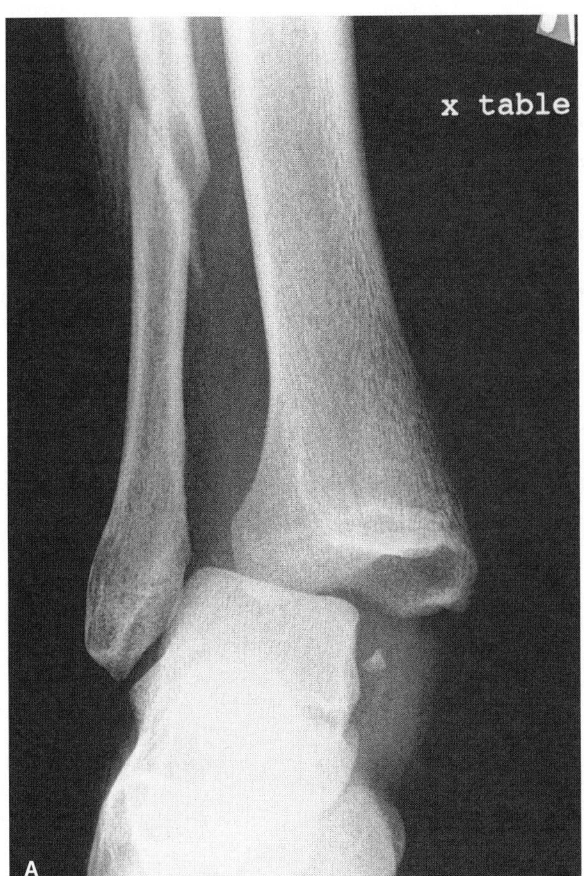

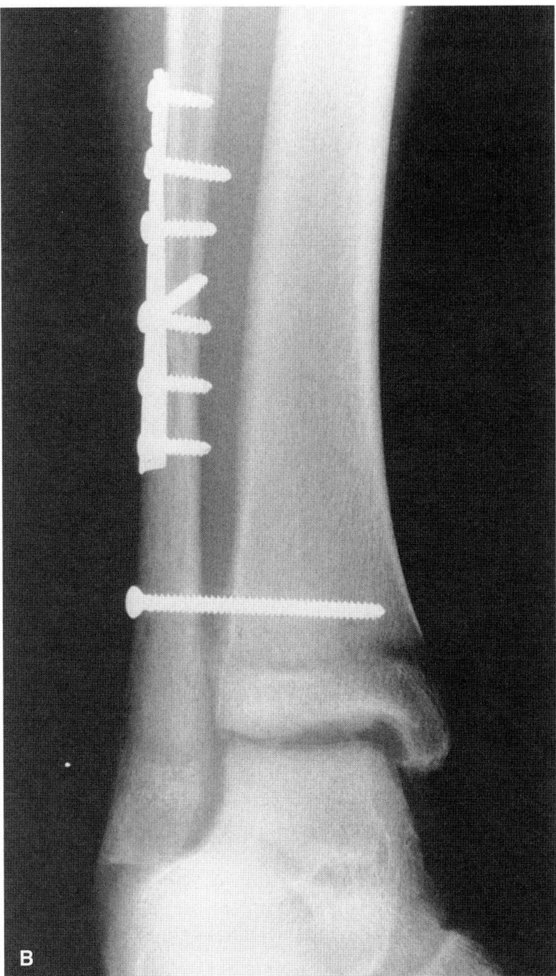

FIGURE 113.21 (*A*) Fracture—dislocation of the ankle secondary to a pronation–lateral rotation injury. The syndesmosis is completely disrupted from the fibular fracture to the ankle. The deltoid ligament is completely torn, along with an avulsion fracture of the medial malleolus. (*B*) The fibula has been stabilized by open reduction and internal fixation. The ligamentous syndesmosis has been stabilized by a screw passing from the fibula to the tibia—the "syndesmosis screw."

simple principles must be followed to avoid precipitating catastrophic spinal cord trauma. Spinal precautions dictate that a backboard and cervical collar be applied to all trauma victims with potential spinal injury and maintained until the spine is cleared clinically and radiographically. A cervical spine lateral radiograph should be obtained of the C-7 to T-1 disc spaces. In uncooperative or comatose patients, a cervical collar should be continued until a satisfactory clinical evaluation of the spine can be performed. Standard radiographs are usually diagnostic, although CT scans are extremely valuable and almost always indicated in polytrauma victims with any question of spine injury. MRI studies may also be indicated to evaluate the disc, nerve roots, and paraspinous soft tissues. In the cervical spine, dynamic flexion and extension views are also helpful to rule out occult instability. The fracture is then characterized and classified and a treatment plan established.[47,48]

Stable Injuries

Stable injuries consist of sprains, minor tears of the posterior ligamentous structures and related soft tissues that induce muscle spasm and pain. The patient is neurologically intact and has no radicular symptoms. Radiographic analysis is negative or reveals isolated spinous process, undisplaced laminar, or minor compression fractures. Dynamic flexion and extension views are obtained to ensure stability in equivocal cases.

Unstable Injuries

By definition, a spinal fracture with associated neurologic deficit is unstable. Radiographically, a fracture or fracture–dislocation may reveal obvious instability, but it is important to look for subtle signs of instability such as widened interpedicular distance or deviation of the spinous processes. In the cervical spine, extensive retropharyngeal hemorrhage seen on the lateral radiograph as well as apparent "minor" subluxations at contiguous levels may be present. Small anterior avulsion or so-called teardrop fractures may be stable or associated with a highly unstable hyperextension injury of the cervical spine. CT scan and MRI are extremely helpful in identifying potentially unstable fractures. Limited cone-beam spiral CT has resulted in a dramatic decrease in scan times with obvious beneficial implications for trauma victims.

Anatomy and Classification

Conceptually, the spine can be thought of as a three-column structure. The anterior column consists of the anterior longitudinal ligament and anterior two thirds of the vertebral body,

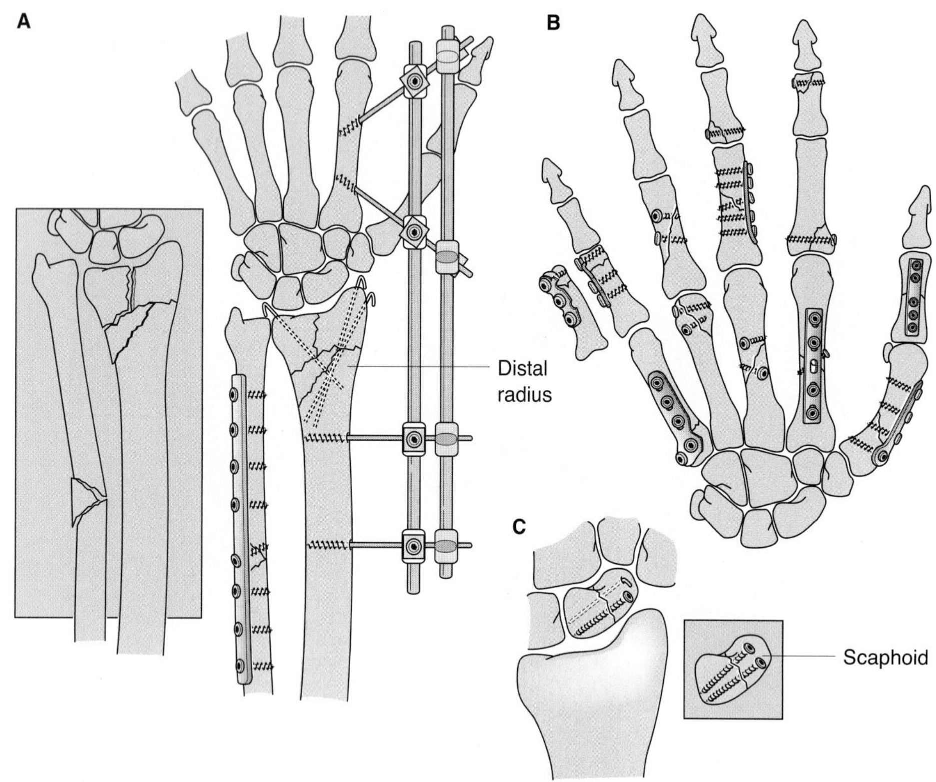

FIGURE 113.22 (*A*) Most fractures of the distal radius are treated by closed reduction and casting for 5 or 6 weeks. With significant displacement, inadequate closed reduction, or intraarticular fragments, percutaneous pinning, limited open reduction or external fixation across the wrist joints is indicated. The distal ulna was internally plated, but when isolated and minimally displaced, can be treated satisfactorily by closed reduction and casting. (*B*) Most isolated, minimally displaced fractures of the phalanges or metacarpals can be treated nonoperatively by appropriate reduction and splinting. When significantly displaced, intraarticular, or involving multiple digits, these fractures are best stabilized surgically. Mini-fragment plates and screws are illustrated; however, Kirschner wire fixation can be used very effectively. (*C*) Undisplaced scaphoid fractures are treated by thumb spica cast immobilization for 8 weeks or longer. When displaced, open reduction and internal fixation is indicated. With nonunion, bone grafting is also performed.

and the anterior portion of the intervertebral disc. The middle column includes the posterior portion of the body and disc, the posterior longitudinal ligament, and the lateral ligament and masses. The posterior column includes the facet and facet capsules, the lamina and spinous processes, the ligamentum flavum, and the interspinous and supraspinous ligaments.[49]

Compression fractures typically injure the anterior column, occur secondary to flexion and compression forces, and are common in osteoporotic vertebrae. Unless severely wedged, these injuries are considered stable. When the middle column is involved, as in burst fractures, instability is usually present. Burst fractures usually display some degree of retropulsion of the posterior body into the spinal canal as viewed on the lateral radiograph and transpedicular widening on the anteroposterior view. All three columns may be fractured and have highly unstable lesions.

General Principles of Treatment

Stable injuries are treated symptomatically. A soft cervical collar may be worn for comfort. For minor injuries in the thoracolumbar region, a thoracolumbosacral orthosis also may be indicated. Occasionally, the subsequent development of increased kyphosis or deformity requires surgical treatment.

Operative Treatment

The absolute indication for operative intervention in spinal injuries is a progressive neurologic deficit in the presence of identified fracture or proven spinal cord compression. The relative indications include irreducible fractures and dislocations, open spinal injuries, and polytrauma. Uncooperative or restless patients may be at risk for neurologic complications, and stabilization is justified in these instances. in general, stabilization is performed for all unstable patterns or deformities that are likely to become clinically symptomatic because of deformity, even in the absence of neurologic injury. The most effective method of achieving neurologic decompression is anatomic reduction and alignment of the spinal fracture. Laminectomy is not indicated as an isolated procedure and may further destabilize the spine. A relative exception to this rule is acute disc herniation with neurologic deficit.[47,48]

Injuries above the level of C-4 may result in death caused by respiratory paralysis in the acute setting. The examining physician must distinguish between a complete and incomplete injury, as well as between root and spinal cord trauma. Obviously, any neurologic progression is an emergency and needs to be acted on immediately. Dual-crush, multilevel fractures, or associated systemic trauma may make diagnosis difficulty.

The presence of spinal shock may mask some incomplete cord injuries. After spinal shock has resolved in 24 to 72 hours, accurate diagnosis is possible. If there has been no neurologic recovery at this time, quadriplegia is permanent although some important root recovery may occur. Extensive hemorrhage or complete cord transection can be identified on MRI, as well as severe edema and of specific nerve root lesions. The goal of treatment in any spinal cord injury is protecting uninjured cord or root function by decompression of the spinal cord using closed or open spinal column realignment and stabilization. Protection of residual function also requires restoration of hemodynamics, treatment of other associated injuries, and maintenance of adequate perfusion pressures. High-dose steroids are indicated in acute spinal cord injury, especially in incomplete lesions. After recovery from spinal shock, high-dose steroids are of no use in patients who are permanently quadriplegic.[47]

Cervical Spine Fixation Modalities

Posterior wiring techniques using the spinous processes or the facet joints provide good stability; however, lateral mass plating is also very effective. Anterior corpectomy, bone grafting, and plate stabilization are necessary for certain teardrop or other comminuted body fractures in the cervical spine. In this instance, the plate functions as a tension band in extension and as a buttress plate in flexion of the neck. It is used most often after severe wedge compression or burst fracture. A cannulated screw can be inserted for odontoid fractures using an image intensifier and minimally invasive anterior technique.

Upper Cervical Spine Fractures

Fracture of C-1 (Jefferson fracture). Fractures of the ring of the atlas (C-1) can be diagnosed on the open-mouth anteroposterior radiograph, which shows lateral displacement of the lateral masses. CT reveals undisplaced fractures or subtle atlantoaxial abnormality. Treatment with a halo brace usually suffices. Uncommonly, a myelopathy develops on a chronic basis and a C-1 laminectomy followed by fusion from occiput to C-2 may be necessary.[47]

Odontoid (Dens) fracture. Odontoid (C-2) fractures are among the most frequently missed spinal fractures. An adequate open-mouth view can be difficult to obtain, and an axial CT section may miss the axially oriented fracture line that lies in the same plane. For this reason, reformatted images in the coronal and sagittal planes are mandatory. Undisplaced fractures at the base of the odontoid (type 3) can be treated in a halo vest. Fractures through the waist (type 2) and above frequently do not heal and require posterior sublaminar wiring (Fig. 113.23A). Alternatively, in younger patients with a reducible fracture, odontoid screw fixation can be effective. This preserves rotation at C-1 to C-2 (Fig. 100.24B).

Hangman fracture (fracture of the neural arch of C-2). Traumatic atlantoaxial spondylolisthesis is a well-known and common injury in the upper cervical spine. Patients who survive this injury are neurologically intact. The injury results in decompression or widening of the neural canal so that even in unstable injuries, spinal cord injury is not common. For minor degrees of displacement, a rigid cervical orthosis may be all that is necessary. Usually a period of halo traction followed by halo vest immobilization for 10 to 12 weeks is necessary. Occasionally, reduction cannot be obtained by traction or the C-2/C-3 facet joint is dislocated, requiring open reduction and facet wiring.

C-1 to C-2 Subluxation. Instability at C-1/C-2 may occur rarely in the absence of a fracture owing to traumatic rupture

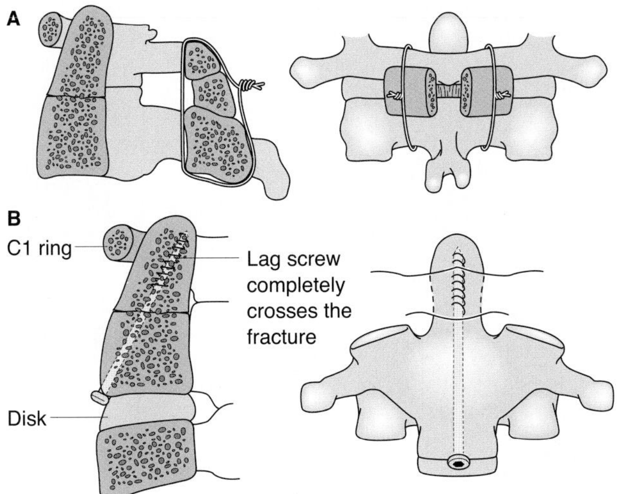

FIGURE 113.23 Stabilization of fractures of the odontoid. (*A*) Posterior sublaminar wiring of C-1 to C-2 with incorporated bone graft is the most common method for treating displaced or nonunited fractures of the odontoid. (*B*) This method preserves rotation at the C-1 to C-2 level. An anterior cervical exposure and fluoroscopic control is used to insert an odontoid screw.

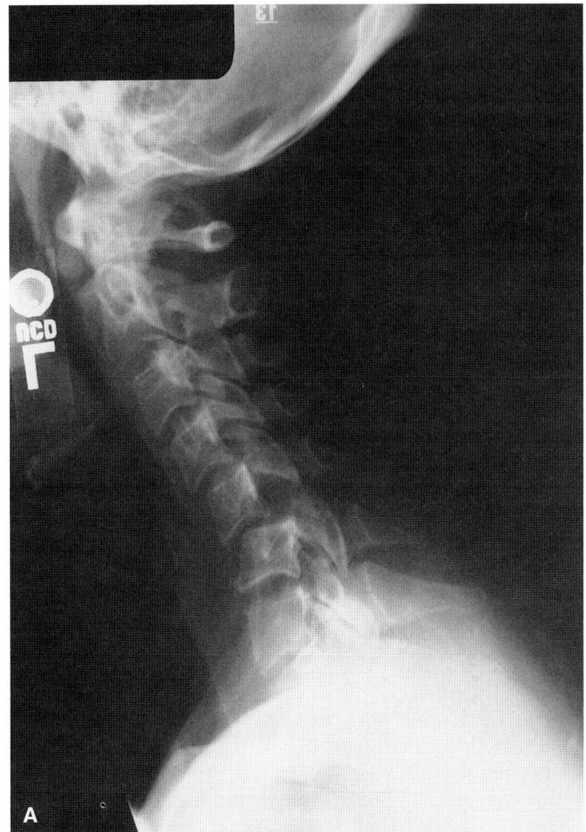

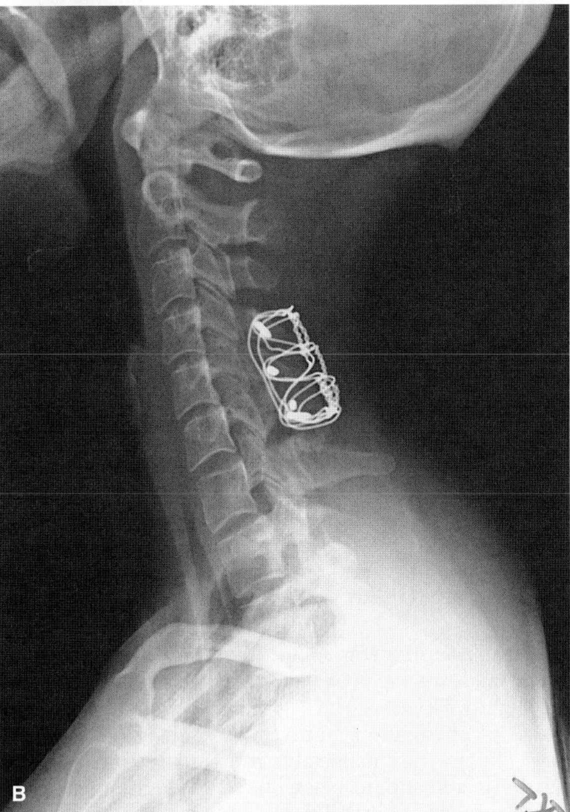

FIGURE 113.24 (*A*) Lateral cervical spine radiograph demonstrating unilateral facet dislocation. (*B*) Lateral radiograph after open reduction and sublaminar wiring with posterior bone grafting. After reduction, these injuries are often stable, and immobilization in a halo vest may suffice.

of the transverse and apical ligaments. The rheumatoid spine is prone to such injuries. These ligaments stabilize and control the relationships between the ring of C-1 and the odontoid (dens). In the upper cervical spine, the normal atlantodens interval as seen on the lateral radiograph is up to 3 to 4 mm, and greater than 6 to 7 mm is clearly abnormal. In the latter case, chronic and progressive instability is common because these ligamentous injuries frequently do not heal well. Treatment is usually a halo brace, but subsequent instability frequently requires C-1 to C-2 fusion and sublaminar wires or transarticular screws across the lateral masses. If instability is allowed to progress, spinal cord compression can lead to myelopathy, global weakness, respiratory depression, and ultimately death. These patients—justifiably so—have a sense of "impending doom."

Lower Cervical Spine Fractures

Unilateral Facet Dislocation. Radiographic diagnosis is made by the presence of a mild anterior subluxation on the lateral radiograph (approximately 25%) and a subtle shift of the spinous process at the level of injury seen on the anteroposterior radiograph. Oblique views may show a "perched facet." Closed reduction is the treatment of choice, but may require gradually increasing traction forces of up to 60 to 90 pounds. Before undertaking this degree of traction, an MRI scan should be obtained to rule out the uncommon but potentially disastrous extruded herniation that might cause cord compression with reduction of the deformity. If the dislocation does not reduce in traction, open reduction followed by interspinous wiring and bone grafting is required (Fig. 113.24).

Bilateral Facet Dislocation. The radiographic diagnosis is more obvious, with usually greater than 50% displacement of one vertebra on the other. In addition, local kyphosis is present. This injury cannot occur unless the posterior annulus and longitudinal ligament are disrupted, rendering the spine very unstable. The dislocation is easily reduced but very unstable, requiring posterior cervical stabilization.

In patients with incomplete injury or certainly with progressive neurologic signs, urgent operative reduction should be undertaken. This is warranted even in the quadriplegic patient because the salvage of a cervical root has a major impact on upper extremity function.

Burst Fracture. These injuries are unstable to varying degrees and they are usually treated with surgery or a halo brace. In a neurologically intact patient or one who has an incomplete lesion, an anterior approach is often necessary, with corpectomy decompression, strut grafting, and anterior plating. Highly unstable lesions involving the posterior column and elements may also require supplementation with posterior fusion or a halo vest. Failure to recognize a three-column injury can lead to major complications secondary to residual or recurrent instability.

Teardrop Fracture. Some minor compression fractures can cause a small fragment of the anterior vertebral body to displace slightly. However, the true teardrop fracture represents a somewhat uncommon but very unstable hyperextension injury. This fracture is unstable rotationally and sagittally in an orthosis and should be stabilized through anterior interbody fusion and plating (Fig. 113.25).

Fracture—Dislocation. This injury is essentially a progression in severity of a burst fracture, is usually highly unstable, and has a significant incidence of spinal cord injury. All three mechanical columns are disrupted through soft tissue res-traints, fracture, or dislocation. Treatment is by anterior vertebrectomy,

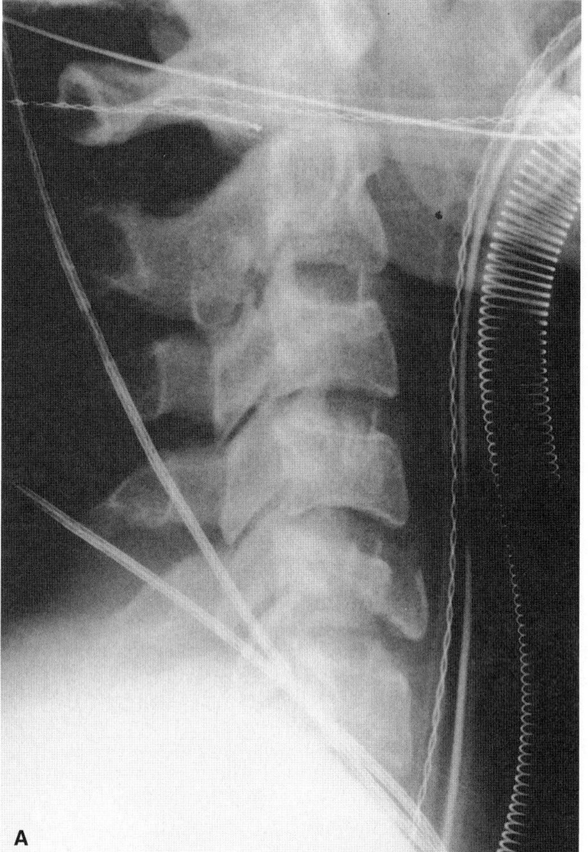

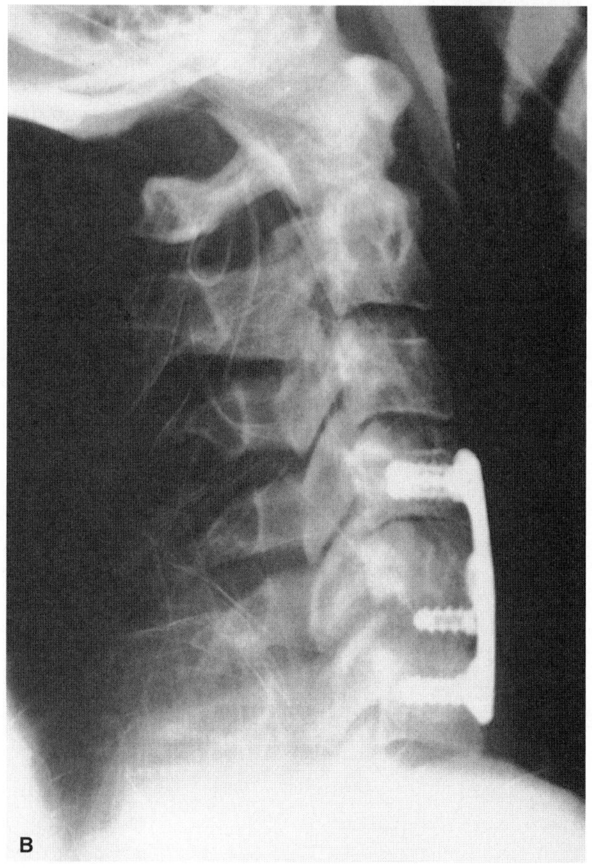

FIGURE 113.25 (*A*) Teardrop fracture of the anterior body of C-5. (*B*) Postoperative lateral radiograph after open reduction and anterior cervical fusion from C-4 to C-6 stabilized by a low-profile titanium plate.

bone grafting, and plating, augmented by halo immobilization or, in more severe multilevel injuries, combined anterior and posterior fusion providing immediate 360-degree circumferential stability and spinal cord decompression.[47]

Fracture of the Posterior Elements and Lateral Masses. Isolated fractures of the spinous process, lamina, and facets are frequently stable. Treatment is either a cervical orthosis or halo vest. Facet injuries vary in degree of instability. Some displaced facet fractures can impinge on the neural foramen, producing nerve root symptoms and associated neurologic deficits. In this instance, the most appropriate treatment is reduction of the fracture followed by posterior fusion. Lateral mass fractures are usually stable and respond to immobilization and bracing.

Thoracic Spine

The thoracic spinal canal is less capacious than the cervical spine above or lumbar spine below, and therefore any significant displacement is likely to result in paraplegia. The conceptual anatomy is the same as described for the cervical spine in terms of classification and radiographic definitions of instability. In the thoracic spine, the rib cage and sternum, if intact, tend somewhat to splint or stabilize thoracic spine fractures. Pure compression fractures in the thoracic spine are common and may involve contiguous vertebrae. Unless associated with signs of instability or severe kyphosis, they are usually treated nonoperatively with appropriate bracing. With involvement of only the anterior column, neurologic loss is uncommon. With highly unstable lesions, transthoracic anterior decompression, grafting, and plating may be indicated, and this usually prevents later deformity and pain. Unstable fracture dislocations may require posterior instrumentation and stabilization.[47]

Thoracolumbar Spine

Because of changes in the anatomic configuration of the facet joints and the increased mobility at the thoracolumbar junction, fractures and fracture–dislocations are more common in this region. T-12 and L-1 and contiguous vertebrae are frequently involved. The spinal cord terminates at the lower border of L-1, and therefore injuries at this level and above involve the conus or cord and injuries below involve the cauda equina nerve roots.[48]

Diagnosis is by physical examination, with palpation for defect or malalignment of the spinal column, localized pain, or neurologic deficit. A rectal examination is mandatory, noting the sphincter tone and presence of bulbocavernous reflex. Recovery of this reflex usually occurs within 24 to 48 hours and signals the end of spinal shock. Residual neurologic deficit beyond this point is usually permanent when the cord is involved; however, some root recovery may occur with cauda equina lesions. A CT scan provides an accurate assessment of canal compromise and occult fractures involving the posterior elements. Where neurologic deficit exists with no apparent fracture, such as when a vascular cause is suspected, an MRI is indicated to assess the cord, disc, and related soft tissues.

Compression Fractures. Involvement of the anterior column alone without severe kyphosis can be treated symptomatically with a brace. If there is greater than 50% anterior wedging or contiguous vertebrae are involved, a hyperextension body cast may be indicated or, occasionally, posterior segmental spinal stabilization may be required using pedicle screws, sublaminar hooks, and rod constructs.

Burst Fractures. Axial compression injuries and burst fractures are common in the thoracolumbar junction and characteristically display local kyphosis with retropulsion of bone into the spinal canal. Fortunately, the canal is more capacious at this level, and a surprisingly large degree of retropulsed bone is compatible with intact neurologic function.

Burst fractures always involve the anterior and middle columns and are unstable to varying degrees. These fractures are some of the most common spinal injuries that require operative stabilization. Usually this is performed semielectively while continuing spinal precautions until after the patient has been stabilized and life-threatening injuries attended to. Important exceptions to this are incomplete lesions or any progressive neurologic deficit. These patients require urgent decompression and stabilization. With significant retropulsion and disruption of the anterior and middle columns, an anterior approach with corpectomy, interbody fusion, and plating is indicated (Fig. 113.26). The cord is best decompressed anteriorly in these instances because laminectomy only adds further to instability. Posterior stabilization is usually performed simultaneously or sequentially in this instance. In paraplegic patients, surgical stabilization is indicated if there is significant kyphosis to prevent progressive late deformity and chronic pain.[48]

Fracture—Dislocation. As in the cervical spine, these injuries are highly unstable and frequently cause neurologic compromise or frank paraplegia. All three spinal columns are involved as well as soft tissue restraints to varying degrees. Patients who are fortunate enough to have intact neural function or incomplete lesions need to be handled extremely carefully with this highly unstable injury. Anterior decompression, corpectomy, and fusion, in addition to simultaneous or subsequent posterior segmental instrumentation, are necessary to ensure circumferential decompression and stabilization.

Flexion—Distraction Injuries. Flexion—distraction injuries are a distinct variant that classically occur in seat belt injuries when the person is subjected to sudden deceleration and the body flexes forward over the restraining belt. Failure of the posterior and middle columns occurs in tension. The anterior column may fail in tension or flexion depending on the location of the fulcrum and center of rotation. If the failure is anterior to the spine, all three columns may fail in tension and the spine is literally pulled apart, producing a highly unstable injury associated with paraplegia. The Chance fracture is a unique flexion–distraction injury, sometimes referred to as the *all-bone fracture,* in which there is a horizontal splitting of the neural arch, pedicles, and vertebral bodies. This fracture is usually unassociated with any neural compromise and can be treated with hyperextension body cast or orthosis, unless significantly displaced.[48]

Fixation Modalities. Anterior decompression in the thoracolumbar spine is accompanied by structural bone grafting to prevent collapse and recurrence of deformity. Tricortical iliac crest, ribs, allograft bone rings, or, alternatively, cancellous bone in titanium mesh cages may be used. Anterior plates or local neutralization constructs are often used where additional support is needed.

Powerful posterior fixation systems are available. Segmental instrumentation, using pedicle screws in the lumbar and lower thoracic spine and sublaminar hooks in the thoracic spine connected to contoured rods, is commonly used. When possible, short segment instrumentation should be used to save motion segments. Compressive or, more commonly, neutralization–distraction modes may be used.

Discogenic Disease

Disc herniation or degeneration is common in both the cervical and lumbar areas. Many herniations produce only minor symptoms or are asymptomatic. Most disc herniations respond to "tincture of time" and conservative treatment. Those that produce significant symptoms or progressive deficit frequently

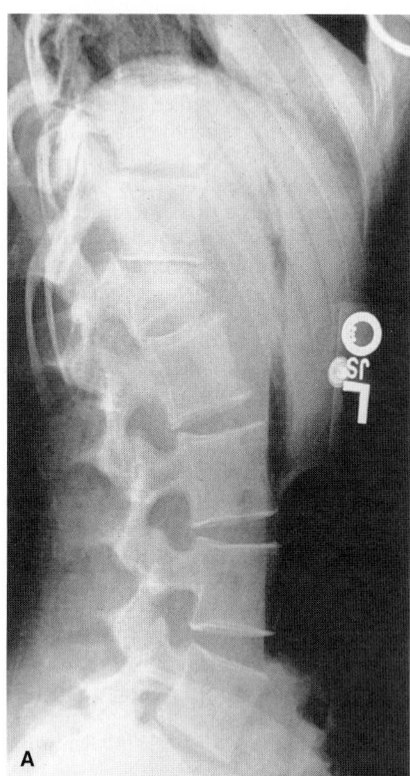

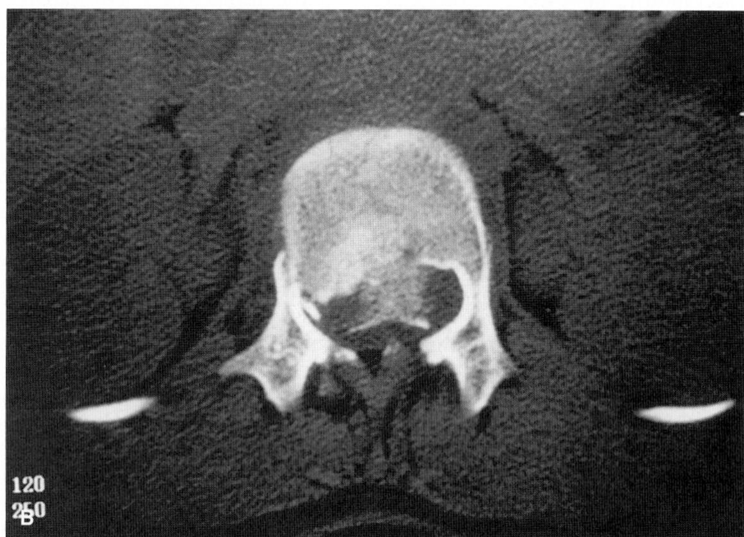

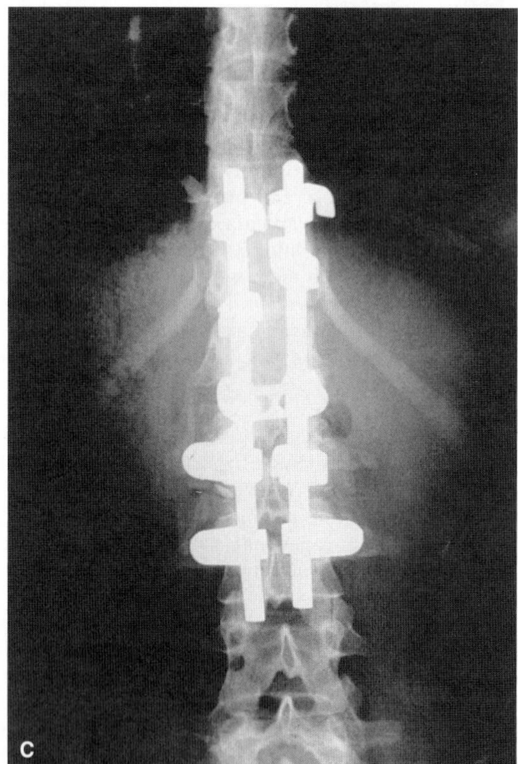

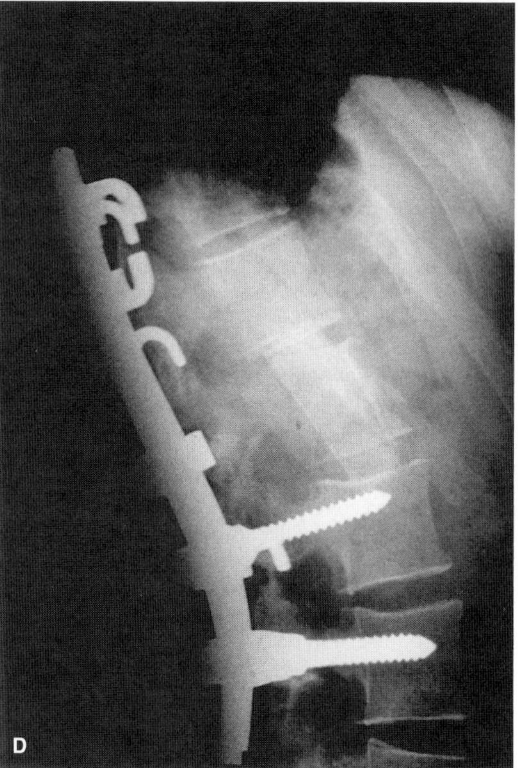

FIGURE 113.26 (*A*) Burst fracture of L-1, secondary to motor vehicle accident. Patient had incomplete neurologic injury. (*B*) Computed tomography scan showing marked retropulsion of bone into the spinal canal. (*C*) Anteroposterior radiograph of thoracolumbar junction after reduction and stabilization using contoured rods, proximal hooks, and inferiorly placed pedicle screws. (*D*) Postoperative lateral radiograph. Note improved restoration of spinal canal and sagittal contours after open reduction, corpectomy, and anterior bone grafting of L-1 burst fracture.

require operative treatment. In both the cervical and lumbosacral spine, nerve roots are invariably involved, producing characteristic symptoms and signs. Rarely, massive herniations in the cervical spine may produce myelopathy or quadriparesis. In this instance, long tract signs such as hyperreflexia and clonus are present. Similarly, a large disc extrusion in the lumbosacral region can produce cauda equina syndrome with loss of bladder and bowel function. In these situations, prompt diagnosis and treatment are mandatory to prevent sequelae. Otherwise, surgical treatment is elective and usually instituted only after appropriate and prolonged nonoperative treatment has failed.[19]

Cervical Spine

Cervical disc herniations usually involve the C-5 to C-6 or C-6 to C-7 discs, but can occur at other levels as well. Neck pain and paraspinous muscle spasm is usually present. Cervical radiculopathy commonly produces shoulder or scapular pain with varying degrees of radiation into the upper extremity. Disc herniation at C-5 to C-6 produces a C-6 radiculopathy, which may be characterized by a weakness of wrist extension or sensory deficits along the C-6 dermatome. The brachioradialis reflex may be asymmetric compared with the opposite side. A C-7 radiculopathy is produced by herniation of the disc at the C-6 to C-7 level and is characterized by triceps weakness and, to a lesser degree, weakness of wrist flexion and digital extension. The classic hypesthesia involves the third digit. Most of the surgery for discs, both in the cervical and lumbar regions, is done for relief of pain, and with the exceptions noted previously, the neurologic deficits are usually not profound.

Treatment. Surgical treatment of cervical disc disease is anterior discectomy and fusion. The spine is readily and safely approached anteriorly from C-2 to T-1 with minimal postoperative morbidity.[18,50,51] Alternatively, for posterolateral herniations associated with spur formation or foraminal stenosis, a keyhole laminotomy can be performed to decompress the nerve root completely. When anterior interbody fusion is performed, the graft may be inlayed and locked in place or secured with a low-profile plate. In general, surgical treatment of cervical disc disease is more predictable and results in greater patient satisfaction than lumbar discectomy.

Degenerative disc disease may be present at contiguous levels. MRI evaluation is extremely helpful in determining the levels to be fused. Two-level disc involvement is treated by standard anterior fusion. Rheumatoid spines with steplike subluxation frequently require longer fusions. Three-level disease or greater is often associated with spinal stenosis or a myelopathy and is best treated by posterior expansion laminoplasty.

Thoracic Spine

Thoracic disc herniation is uncommon but should be included in a differential diagnosis of atypical chest and back pain. Operative treatment is uncommon and usually involves anterior transthoracic discectomy because posterior laminectomy has been associated with paraplegia. Disc herniation is not common in this area and, when neurologic involvement is absent, difficult to diagnose because of its rarity.

Lumbar Spine

Low back pain, with or without sciatica, is one of the most common maladies affecting humankind. It is sometimes difficult to determine whether low back pain is caused by muscle spasms, degenerative disc disease and arthritic changes, or disc herniation. With disc herniations producing nerve root compression, radicular leg pain becomes predominant. Patients who have mild neurologic deficits, such as foot drop or reflex change, may be initially treated nonoperatively. An obvious exception is progressive neurologic deficit or cauda equina syndrome, which requires urgent laminectomy and decompression.

Most disc herniations occur at the L-4 to L-5 and L-5 to S-1 levels. A disc herniation at the latter level may produce an S-1 radiculopathy with loss of the Achilles reflex, decreased plantar flexion strength, and varying degrees of dysesthesia or numbness in S-1 distribution. Disc herniation at the L-4 to L-5 level may produce a foot drop or weakness of dorsiflexion of the great toe. The patellar reflex so frequently tested may not be diminished or asymmetric when either of these two common disc levels is involved. Considerable overlap in neurologic findings can exist. The major indication for surgery is severe radicular pain, especially when associated with a neurologic deficit. MRI is highly sensitive and can help corroborate the diagnosis. It is somewhat nonspecific, however, with frequent disc bulges found incidentally or at asymptomatic levels. MRI has no known biologic hazard and has essentially replaced myelography for the diagnosis of discogenic disease.

Treatment. When indicated by progression of symptoms or neurologic findings, laminectomy and discectomy are the surgical treatments of choice in the lumbar spine. This treatment can be performed by a standard posterior approach or through microdiscectomy using a microscope and small, atraumatic incision. Paraspinal decompression using image intensification and fiberoptic visualization is a third, less common option. It is difficult to remove large amounts of disc by this method. Injection of chymopapain, which enzymatically dissolves the disc, is no longer used extensively because of the few case reports of neurologic deficit or paraplegia. A few patients also had severe anaphylactic reactions. Nevertheless, this modality was successful in a significant number of patients and it is still used in some countries.[52]

Spondylolisthesis. The most common form of spondylolisthesis is characterized by a defect in the pars interarticularis that allows variable anterior slipping of L-5 on S-1. Spondylolysis is a defect alone without forward subluxation. The etiology is unknown, but trauma and familial predisposition may be factorial. Elongation and fatigue fracture of the pars interarticularis occurs. Subluxation or "listhesis" may range from mild to severe. Radiographs reveal a break in the pars the neck of the "Scotty dog" seen on oblique views of the lumbosacral spine. Lateral views reveal the degree of forward slip and inclination or slip angle. CT or MRI scans are also obtained.

Symptoms are variable and may begin in childhood or adolescence. Rapid slip progression may occur during growth spurts and cease or slow significantly at skeletal maturity. Low back pain and muscle spasm are common. Children may exhibit hamstring tightness or fatigue. High-grade slips may carry neurologic symptoms, severe pain, and deformity. Complete displacement of L-5 on S-1 can occur and, rarely, with high slip angles L-5 may descend into the pelvis (spondyloptosis), producing cauda equina syndrome. The rib cage abuts or slips over the iliac crests.

Treatment is symptomatic in most cases. It is estimated that less than 10% of patients require surgery. Chronic or progressive pain is the usual surgical indication. In situ posterolateral fusion is used for intermediate slips (Fig. 113.27). Patients with moderate to severe slips frequently need discectomy, decompression of nerve roots, and resection of a loose neural arch. Because progression of slip and pseudoarthrosis is common in these cases, anterior fusion may also be indicated. In severe slips, it is difficult to reduce the slip or improve alignment and attempts to do so may result in neural compromise. In spondyloptosis, resection of the body of L-5 and fusion of L-4 to the sacrum may be the best choice because it does not lengthen the spine and is less likely to stretch the nerve roots or cauda equina.

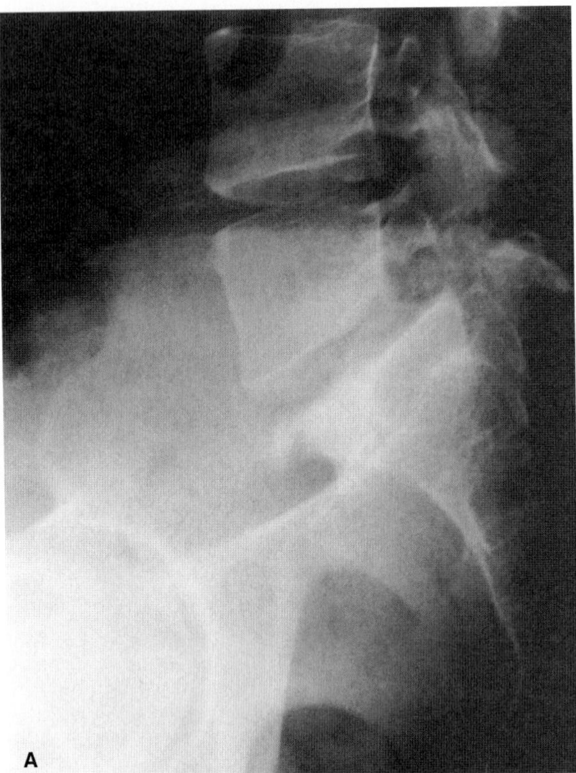

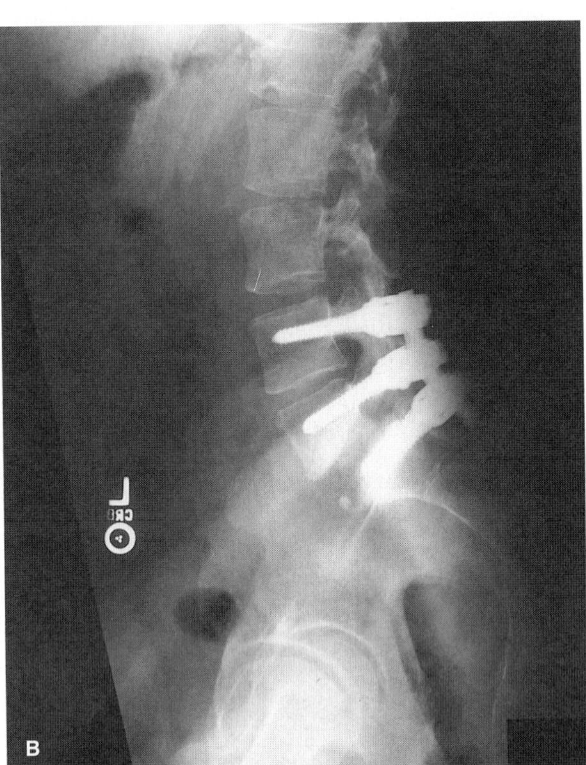

FIGURE 113.27 (*A*) Symptomatic grade II spondylolisthesis of L-5 to S-1. (*B*) Postoperative lateral radiograph of the lumbosacral spine after posterior lumbar interbody fusion and posterior instrumentation with pedicle screw construct at L-4 to the sacrum.

A pararectal, retroperitoneal, or transperitoneal surgical approach is usually necessary to gain exposure. Injury to the superior hypogastric plexus may result in retrograde ejaculation in male patients, and an attempt to preserve this structure should always be made.

Degenerative spondylolisthesis occurs in adults at L-4 to L-5 and is associated with modest subluxation, a narrowed disc space, facet arthrosis, and arthritic changes. It is a frequent source of chronic low back syndrome.

Ankylosing Spondylitis. Ankylosing spondylitis is a seronegative spondyloarthropathy characterized by a chronic inflammatory process affecting the axial skeleton. It is also known as *Marie-Strümpell disease* and is grouped with other spondyloarthropathies associated with psoriasis, colitis, and Reiter syndrome. The articulations of the spine, and frequently the hip and shoulder, are principally involved. Most patients are human leukocyte antigen B27 positive. Treatment with antiinflammatory medication suffices for most patients. However, progressive flexion deformity of the spine may produce severe kyphosis and "chin on chest" deformity, requiring corrective osteotomy. Hip replacement may be required. A proclivity for spinal fracture and neurologic sequelae is present, and orthotic protection or surgical stabilization often is required.

Anterior Spinal Approaches

Thoracic Spine: T-4 to T-11

A transthoracic approach is used to gain access to the anterior thoracic spine from T-4 to T-11. Exposure of the thoracic spine above this level is difficult and may require resection or osteotomy of the medial head of the clavicle. Common indications include scoliosis, kyphosis, tumors, and infection. In idiopathic scoliosis, the convexity is almost always to the right. Thoracotomy on the side of the convexity, usually with rib resection, provides adequate exposure and the resected rib may be used for bone graft. The thoracotomy is centered two ribs higher than the apex of the lesion. In scoliosis, the large thoracic vessels are found on the concave side of the curve. Thus, with a left-sided thoracotomy for left-convex scoliosis, the aorta usually is found on the right side of the spinal column.

Blood flow to the spinal cord is supplied by the anterior and posterior spinal arteries; branches from the posterior intercostal arteries reach the spinal cord through the interspinal foramina and anastomose with the anterior spinal artery. A critical watershed lies between T-4 and T-9. Dissection in this region must be meticulous and, where possible, the segmental feeders spared. Ligation of the segmental arteries should be performed on the vertebral bodies as far anteriorly as possible and subsequent posterior dissection limited so that arterial arcades joining the segmental arteries in the region of the vertebral canal are preserved.

Thoracolumbar Junction

A transpleural—retroperitoneal thoracoabdominal approach with transection of the diaphragm can be used to expose the anterior spine from T-9 to L-5. Approaches to the thoracolumbar junction are principally indicated for vertebral fractures and also for scoliosis, kyphosis, tumors, or infection. This approach is used when it is necessary to expose several contiguous vertebrae in the region of the thoracolumbar junction (Fig. 113.28).

Lumbar and Lumbosacral Spine

The lumbar spine and lumbosacral junction from L-2 to L-5 is approached retroperitoneally, preferentially from the left. Access to L-2 may require resection of the 12th rib. Principal indications are kyphosis, tumors, or spondylitis.

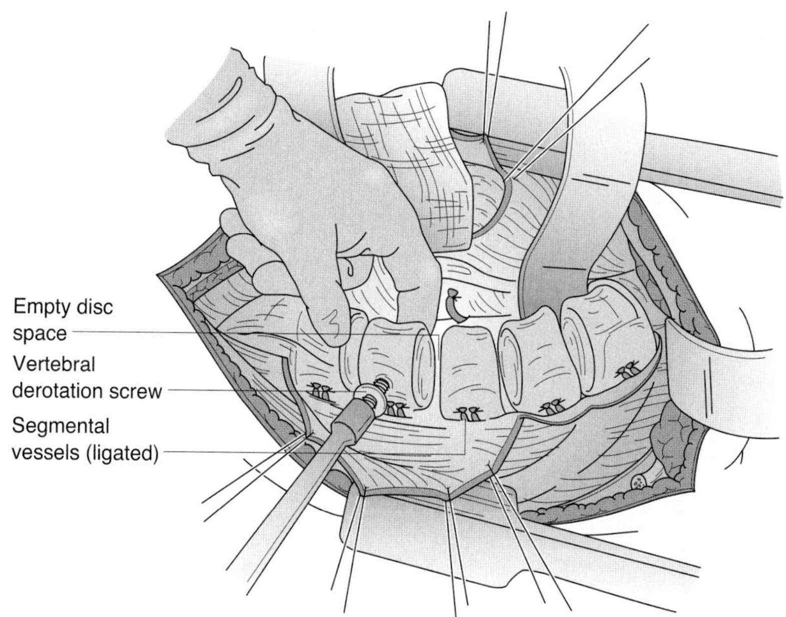

FIGURE 113.28 Thoracoabdominal retroperitoneal approach to the thoracolumbar spine for correction of a lumbar curve. The segmental vessels have been ligated and the disc space cleared, and a vertebral derotation screw is being inserted. Sequential screws are inserted and connected to a solid rod, allowing derotation and correction of the deformity. Structural bone graft is placed in the disc spaces to enhance fusion and prevent postoperative kyphotic deformity. This surgical approach is also used for thoracolumbar spine fractures, infection, and tumors.

Lumbosacral Junction and Sacrum

A pararectal retroperitoneal approach to the lumbar spine and sacrum from L-3 to S-2 can be accomplished with the patient in the supine position. At the inferior margin of L-4, the ureter crosses the common iliac artery, accompanied by the testicular vessels. The superior hypogastric plexus courses above the aortic bifurcation and is responsible for the innervation of the genitourinary system. Injury to this plexus may lead to retrograde ejaculation in the male patient.

A transperitoneal approach to the lumbosacral junction is principally indicated for high-grade spondylolisthesis or tumor. This approach can expose the lumbosacral disc space fairly rapidly, but injury to the superior hypogastric plexus is more frequent.

Chronic Low Back Syndrome

There are many causes of low back pain. Beginning in middle age, spondylolisthesis, facet arthrosis, degenerative arthritis, and disc disease are common. Lumbar or lumbosacral fusion is recommended for severely symptomatic patients and those with instability who have not responded to nonoperative treatment. Pedicle screws connected to rods ensure stability and increase the rate of fusion. Posterior lumbar interbody fusion can be very successful in stabilizing unstable arthritic lumbar spines[53] (Fig. 113.27).

Acquired lumbar spinal stenosis may present in middle or old age and is characterized by neurogenic claudication and occasionally bladder and bowel disturbance. In contrast to vascular claudication, peripheral pulses are usually present and back and leg pain is relieved by recumbency. The cause is narrowing and hypertrophy of the posterior elements of the spine, including the pedicles, facet joints, and laminae. Treatment is by wide laminectomy.

Spinal Infection

Disc space infection is usually accompanied radiographically by destruction of both end plates or the presence of a paraspinal or psoas abscess. Extensive destruction of vertebral bodies may occur with tuberculosis, which is more common in developing nations. Disc space infections or vertebral osteomyelitis also occur in IV drug abusers, diabetic patients, or immunocompromised individuals. Infection can mimic neoplasms, old trauma, or congenital abnormality.[54] MRI and CT scan are extremely helpful in evaluating and differentiating spinal abnormalities. Chronic low back pain can be caused by infection, often with unusual organisms such as *Coccidioides, Brucella,* or *Cryptococcus*. Diagnostic work-up frequently includes bone scan, gallium scan, erythrocyte sedimentation rate, C-reactive protein, serologic titers where indicated, and skin tests. Blood cultures may be positive in bacterial infections and DNA amplification techniques helpful. Specific enzyme-linked immunosorbent assay may be necessary with unusual infections such as brucellosis.

The specific diagnosis is made by aspiration or biopsy and culture and sensitivity of the disc space or vertebral bodies. Fungal organisms may be identified microscopically. Treatment is appropriate decompression or specific antimicrobial therapy, or both. Disc space infection frequently responds to antimicrobial treatment alone. Extensive bone destruction, instability, or neurologic loss requires judicious spinal stabilization.

ARTHRITIS AND JOINT REPLACEMENT

Coincident with the natural aging process is an increased instance of degenerative arthritis. Presumably this disease is caused by repetitive microdamage occurring over a lifetime. Age, sex, body weight, and familial predisposition are other factors that influence the development of degenerative changes. The onset of symptoms is typically in the sixth or seventh decade, but can be much earlier. The gradual onset of joint pain, usually increasing in severity and associated with varying amounts of deformity and loss of motion, is typical. Radiographs reveal loss of joint space and cartilage, subchondral sclerosis, and cyst formation. Early treatment with analgesics, antiinflammatory agents, or joint injections is helpful in alleviating the severity of symptoms. A cane or a walker may mechanically unload the involved joint. Unfortunately, in a significant number of patients symptoms progress to the

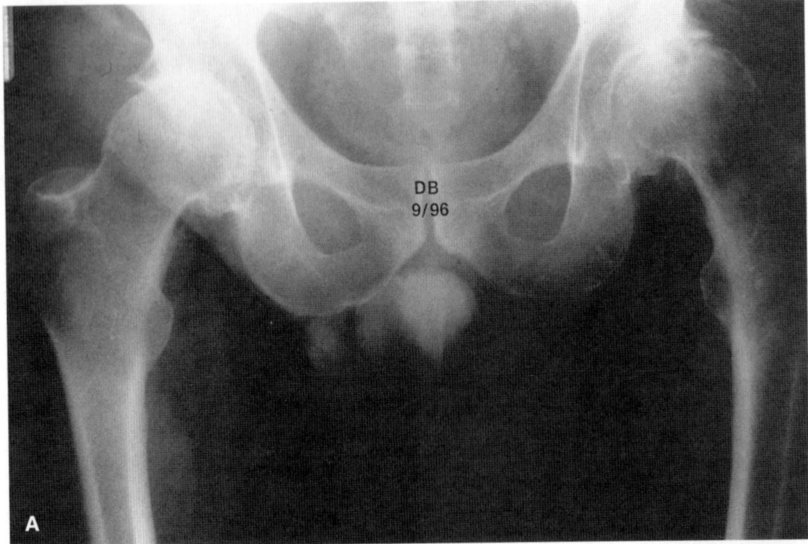

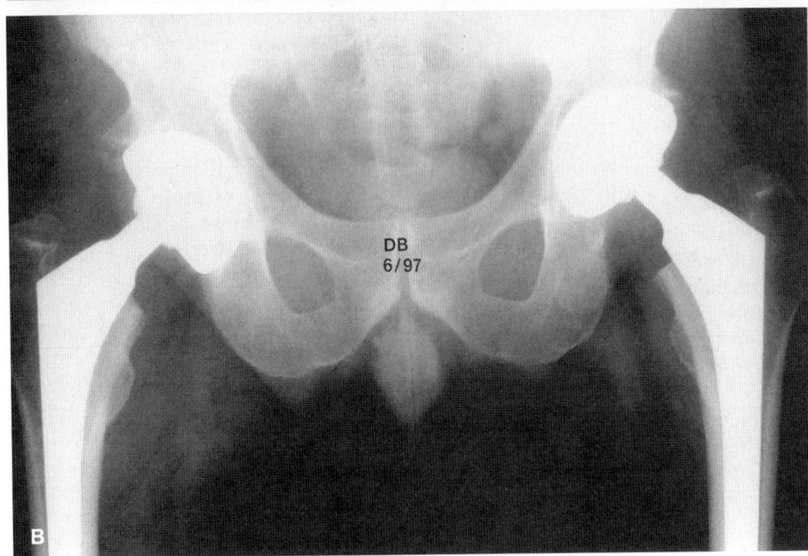

FIGURE 113.29 (*A*) Anteroposterior radiograph of the pelvis showing bilateral advanced degenerative arthritis of the hip. (*B*) Postoperative radiograph after bilateral total hip arthroplasty, which successfully relieved the patient's pain and restored function.

point at which joint replacement is necessary. In the United States alone, an estimated 300,000 total joint arthroplasties are performed annually. In the hip and knee, this procedure is highly successful in restoring pain-free ambulation and improved motion. Joint replacement is capable of providing dramatic improvement in the quality of life and restoration of function[55] (Fig. 113.29).

Under favorable circumstances, the longevity of total hip and knee arthroplasty can be 15 to 20 years. Frequently, however, radiographic evidence of bone resorption at the implant interfaces appears and may or may not be symptomatic. With progressive bone resorption, mechanical loosening occurs and the patient again becomes symptomatic.

Periprosthetic fractures may occur, requiring long-stem revision, strut allografts, and cerclage cable plates or megaprostheses in the femur. When the knee is involved, supracondylar femur fracture is invariably present.

Revision surgery, which requires removal and reimplantation of articulating components, is complex and associated with somewhat less satisfactory outcomes. In younger and more active patients, the wear rate is increased and failure may occur earlier. It is therefore more important in these patients to maximize and exhaust all nonoperative modalities before embarking on joint replacement.

Total Hip Arthroplasty

Joint replacement is most commonly performed for degenerative and posttraumatic arthritis, rheumatoid disease, avascular necrosis of the femoral head, and residua of congenital or acquired pediatric hip disorders. The modern era of joint replacement began in the early 1960s with Sir John Charnley, who defined and implemented the scientific principles on which the procedure is based. He emphasized a low-friction bearing surface, use of biocompatible material, and the intimate interfacing of the implants with bone through the use of polymethylmethacrylate cement. High-density polyethylene remains the material of choice for the metal-backed acetabular component. Polished metal alloys of chrome cobalt or titanium are used for the femoral component. Significant advances have improved the longevity of artificial joints.[20] For younger patients, metal or ceramic components offer reduced wear characteristics and longer survival of implants.

One of the main causes of aseptic loosening appears to be a macrophage foreign body reaction and osteoclastic resorption of bone, and noncemented implants are recommended in younger patients. The femoral component is manufactured to produce a porous surface that allows for biologic ingrowth and fixation of the implant. Technically, it is important to obtain precise filling of the femoral canal to prolong longevity. Primary total hip arthroplasty for degenerative arthritis is straightforward and can be performed through one of several different surgical approaches. Immediate weight bearing as tolerated is allowed after surgery.[20]

The incidence of postoperative complications is low, but of serious consequence. Infection occurring early in the postoperative period is treated by evacuation of hematoma, IV antibiotics, and institution of a suction irrigation system. Late-occurring infection usually requires removal of all components and meticulous débridement of cement particles from the femoral canal and acetabulum. Antibiotic beads or a cement spacer are then implanted for several months, and if repeat aspiration of the joint is negative for organisms, reimplantation may be considered. Postoperative dislocation is usually preventable by appropriate precautions. Recurrent dislocation frequently indicates component malposition and may require revision.

Deep venous thrombosis is common and frequently asymptomatic. Pulmonary embolism can be prevented in most cases by the use of sequential compression devices on the lower extremities and carefully monitored anticoagulation. In high-risk patients or when anticoagulation is contraindicated, a vena caval filter should be considered.

Revision total hip arthroplasty is much more complex, usually because of loosening of components, bone loss, and occasionally the presence of previous infection. Revision frequently requires long-stem or custom implants. Preoperative planning may include three-dimensional modeling of the pelvis and acetabulum. Bulk allografts may be used but have been associated with catastrophic late failure. With severe loss of bone, bone grafting of defects and special acetabular cages or modified components are frequently necessary. Revision hip surgery is complex, complication rates are higher, and functional results less satisfying than in primary total hip arthroplasty.[53]

Total Knee Arthroplasty

Artificial replacement of the knee joint is based on principles similar to those developed for the hip. Precisely sized components and custom jigs align the surfaces and allow for exact surgical resection of femoral, tibial, and patellar bone to accept the components. The femoral component is metal and articulates with the polyethylene metal-backed tibial component. The components are cemented in place and appropriate ligament balancing is necessary to achieve stability. Progressive weight bearing as tolerated is usually permitted. Cementless designs are available for younger patients but are otherwise less commonly used. Posterior stabilized systems are increasingly used in primary replacement or when some ligamentous deficiency exists. Constrained total knee arthroplasty is occasionally necessary for complex revisions or major ligamentous deficiency (Fig. 113.18). Although in ideal cases the longevity of total knee arthroplasty approaches that of the total hip procedure, impact or sports activity is always discouraged and associated with a high rate of loosening in younger patients.[20,53,56]

Other Joints

Historically, total ankle replacement has not been as successful in relieving pain and restoring function as ankle arthrodesis, but there is a resurgence of interest in this procedure because of improved design and implant techniques.

Prosthetic replacements of the shoulder and elbow are less commonly indicated procedures except in patients with rheumatoid or other inflammatory arthritis. These patients frequently have multiple joint involvement, so it is important to restore as much mobility as possible.

Wrist arthrodesis is more predictable and generally preferable to total wrist joint arthroplasty. Proximal row carpectomy may be indicated in certain low-demand patients.

In patients with severe rheumatoid hand deformities, metacarpophalangeal arthroplasty is an excellent technique to restore alignment and improve function.[56]

Arthritis in the Younger Patient

Most arthritic conditions in younger patients are posttraumatic and often occur as a result of fractures involving joints of the lower extremity (Fig. 113.30). Avascular necrosis of the hip due to steroid use, alcoholism, or idiopathic factors is also common. Joint replacement is not a good option in young and middle-aged patients, and modification of activities and nonoperative treatment is always indicated as a first option but frequently fails to address symptoms adequately.

Osteotomy to realign limbs and redistribute forces across arthritic joints is modestly successful in relieving symptoms for a period of several years delaying joint replacement. Osteotomies are most frequently indicated about the knee and usually performed for a varus or bow-legged deformity associated with unicompartmental arthritis. Periacetabular pelvic osteotomies are very useful in patients with hip subluxation and acetabular dysplasia.

Arthroscopic débridement, especially of the knee, is also beneficial. Where indicated, it can be accompanied with abrasion chondroplasty and microfracture, or newer cartilage grafting techniques. More severe and localized arthritic changes confined to one compartment of the knee can be treated with unicompartmental knee replacement.

Posttraumatic arthritis of the hip can be treated with arthrodesis, which in the past has been recommended for people who intend to engage in heavy physical activity or hard labor. Short-term results are satisfactory, but many problems eventually arise, including chronic low back pain and degenerative changes in the ipsilateral knee or contralateral extremity. When given a choice, most young patients prefer total hip arthroplasty even through it is not a permanent solution. Other alternatives include resection arthroplasty of the head and neck (Girdlestone procedure), which results in a foreshortened but reasonably functional limb and adequate relief of pain, and, most important, delays the need for total joint replacement.

Arthrodesis of the knee is even less satisfactory but may be necessary in the presence of severe deformity, instability, and pain, or for failed total knee replacement or infection.

Posttraumatic arthritis of the ankle is best prevented by anatomic open reduction and internal fixation of fractures. Nevertheless, with severe involvement of the tibial plafond or fractures of the body of the talus, advanced arthritic changes may necessitate ankle arthrodesis, which is well accepted and predictable in relieving pain and providing satisfactory function. Similarly, subtalar arthrodesis, usually performed for malunited calcaneal fractures, is also associated with a high percentage of good results.[55]

CORRECTION OF DEFORMITY AND NONUNION

Malunited fractures are treated by corrective osteotomy and internal fixation or occasionally external fixation techniques. They are more common and problematic in the lower extremity, especially in the tibia. Malunited fractures of the femur are less common when an intramedullary rod is used and, when

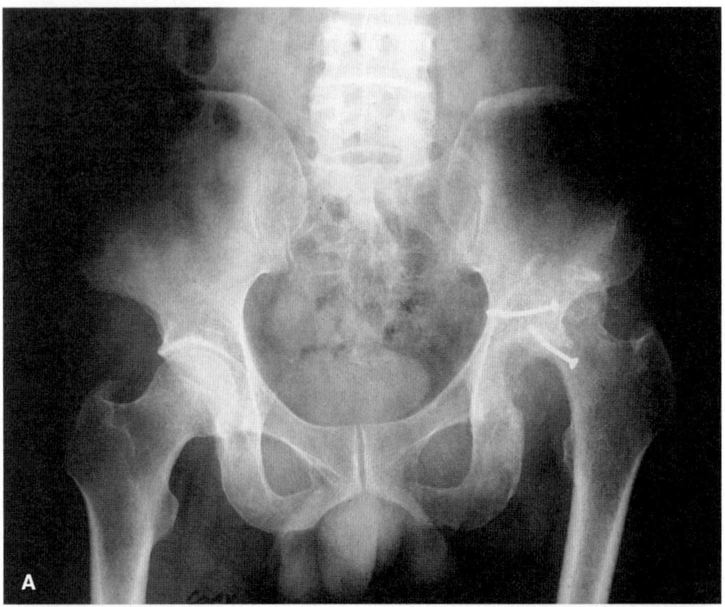

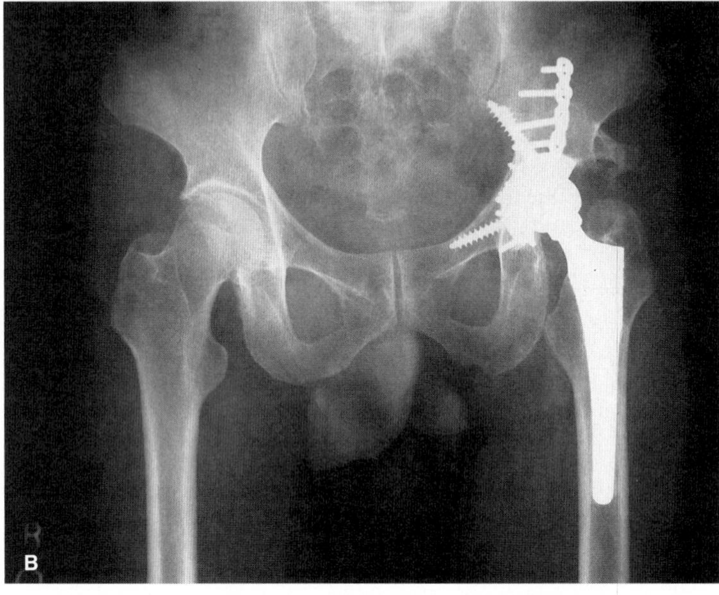

FIGURE 113.30 (*A*) Avascular necrosis and loss of fixation after inadequate treatment of posterior wall acetabular fracture. (*B*) Anteroposterior radiograph after bone grafting of posterior wall defect and total hip arthroplasty.

they occur, are less likely to be angulatory and more likely to be related to excessive shortening or rotational abnormality.

Leg length discrepancy in the femur is best treated by contralateral closed femoral shortening of the normal femur, unless the discrepancy is large (Fig. 113.31). In this situation, lengthening of the shortened femur may be considered, although it is less predictable. Torsional malrotation and angular deforming of the femur are corrected by derotation osteotomy and maintenance of correction by an interlocked intramedullary device. Alternatively, single or dual compression plates can be used with autogenous iliac crest bone grafting.

Fortunately, posttraumatic shortening usually does not exceed 2 to 3 cm, which can be accommodated by a shoe lift. Tibial lengthening is less problematic than in the femur. Congenital shortening or dwarfism can require bilateral lengthening. As much as 25 cm of length has been obtained in the latter group of young patients by distraction osteogenesis and Ilizarov methods.

Malunited fractures of the tibia in well-vascularized, healthy legs are treated by corrective osteotomy and compression plating or, less commonly, by intramedullary fixation. Unfortunately, a significant number of tibial malunions are associated with open fractures, soft tissue damage, and infection. These more complex injuries are best treated by atraumatic osteotomy through a small incision (corticotomy) and application of external devices consisting of the classic wire-and-ring Ilizarov fixator, hybrid fixators combining both a ring and rod construct, or monolateral external fixators. Using the Ilizarov apparatus, excessive shortening and deformity can be corrected simultaneously using appropriate placement of hinges and distraction osteogenesis techniques (Fig. 113.32). Gradual lengthening proceeds, usually over four equally spaced 0.25-mm increments per day. As the bone separates at the corticotomy site, immature bone is evident by radiography and progresses to eventual maturation. When the desired length has been achieved, the frame is continued for an additional time, usually equal to the period of lengthening. Protection is then provided within a cast or a removable orthosis as further maturation of new-formed bone takes place.[57] Monolateral external fixators in the tibia are easier to manage but are somewhat less versatile than the classic Ilizarov ring frame. The goal of all corrective osteotomies, regardless of

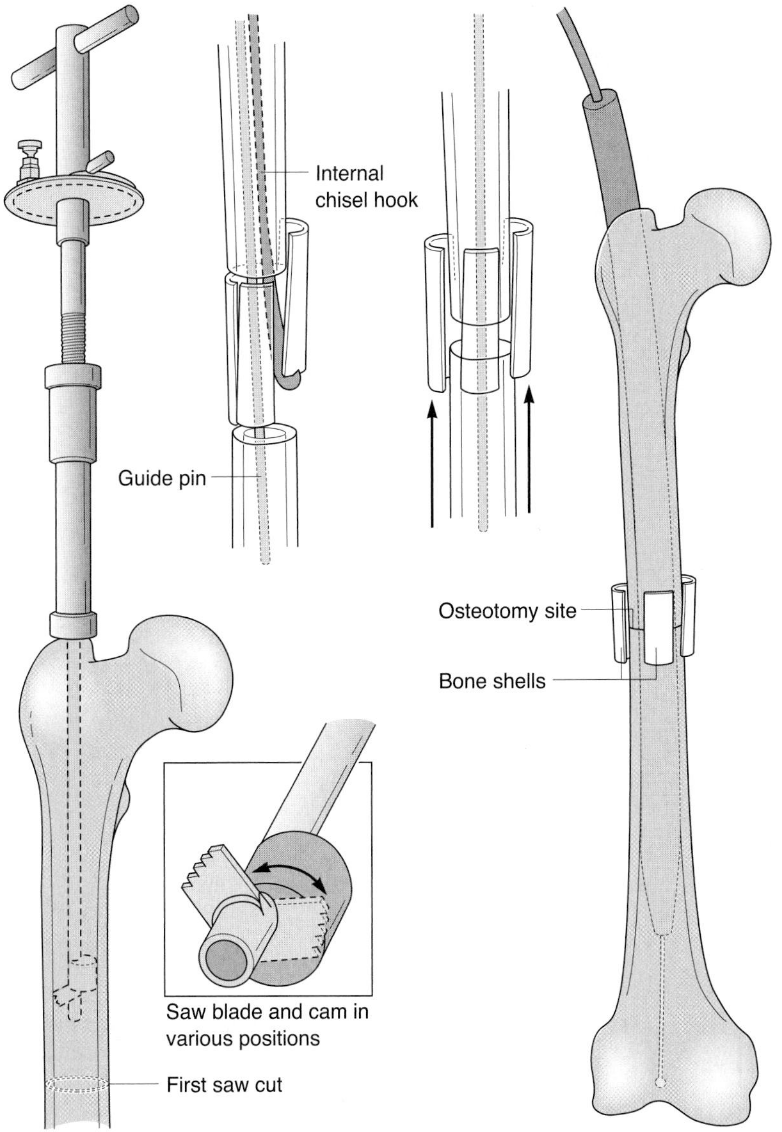

FIGURE 113.31 Closed femoral shortening. Treatment of leg length inequality of 6 to 8 cm or less is most predictably accomplished by contralateral closed femoral shortening. The osteotomy is performed in closed technique with a special intramedullary saw. After the osteotomized segment is split and pushed out of the way, the osteotomy is compressed and fixed with an interlocked intramedullary rod.

technique, is realignment of the limb, correction of length, and restoration of a normal mechanical joint axis.

Nonunion

Failure of fracture to heal within the expected time frame is termed *nonunion*. Nonunion and malunion frequently coexist. Nonunion is characterized by gross motion across the fracture site and a paucity of callus formation at 4 to 6 months or greater. Nonunion may occur after any fracture, but it is most common in the tibia, the femoral neck, and the humerus. Nonunion may be accompanied by avascular necrosis, especially when it occurs in the talus, femoral neck, or humeral head and scaphoid. In diaphyseal fractures, the most common cause of nonunion is open injury with associated soft tissue damage or infection. In closed fractures, a history of smoking, severe diabetes, or immunocompromise may be contributory. Nonunion may also occur in otherwise healthy people without any known risk factors.[11,16,19]

Delayed union may be treated with dynamization of intramedullary rods by removing the distal or proximal interlocking screws, allowing bone-to-bone load transfer. This method is most applicable in the tibia. External electrical stimulation using pulsed electromagnetic fields has been shown to be useful in so-called vascular nonunions unassociated with bone loss or fracture gap.

The most common nonunion treatment method is autologous iliac crest bone graft. In the humerus and upper extremity, it is usually accompanied by compression plating.

Posterolateral bone grafting is the treatment for most tibial nonunions, with the graft placed across the posterior fibula, interosseous membrane, and tibial nonunion site.[55] With large defects and deficient donor bone, demineralized bone allograft or artificial bone substitutes, and growth factors such as bone morphogenetic proteins 1 or 7 can be used to augment autogenous bone. For segmental defects accompanied by low-grade infection or deficient soft tissue, bone transport can be utilized *vis-à-vis* Ilizarov technique and distraction osteogenesis. This method is also useful in chronic osteomyelitis after resection of significant amounts of necrotic bone (Fig. 113.33).[30,57]

A time-honored method of treatment of tibial nonunion is fibular osteotomy and compression weight bearing in a cast. The patient usually must accept minor degrees of angulation and shortening for the goal of fracture union. Although controversial, ultrasound has been used to stimulate fracture healing in vascularized low-grade nonunion.

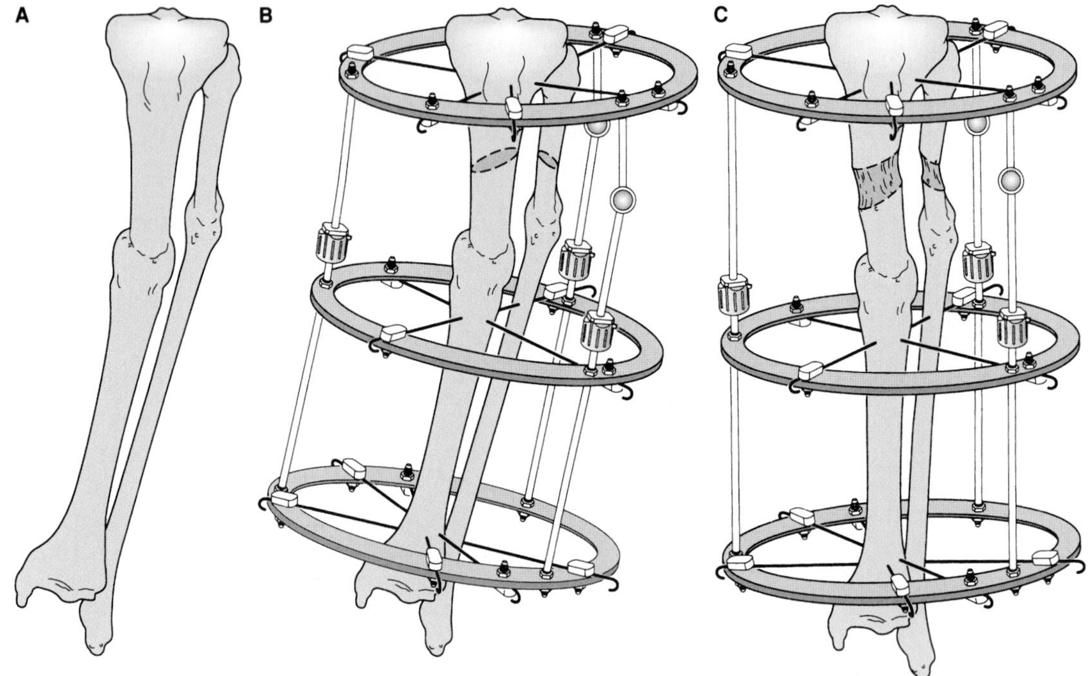

FIGURE 113.32 Malunion. (*A*) Schematic depiction of malunited fractures of the tibia and fibula with unacceptable shortening and varus deformity. (*B*) The use of the Ilizarov technique, proximal corticotomies, and appropriate positioning of external fixator rings with transfixation pins followed by gradual distraction (1 mm/d) and simultaneous correction of malunion. (*C*) The angulation and shortening were both corrected, and healing of the histogenesis site has occurred.

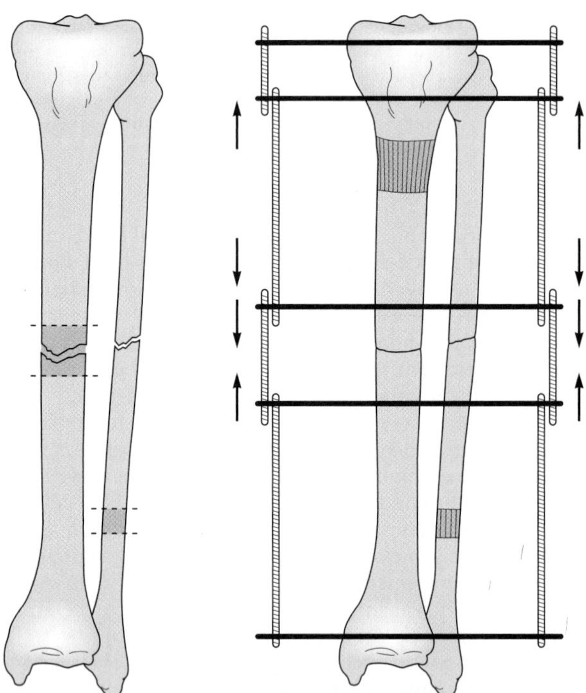

FIGURE 113.33 Ilizarov method of distraction osteogenesis used for treatment of infected pseudoarthrosis of the tibia. Infected bone has been resected, and transport of bone segment to close the resultant defect is illustrated. Distraction occurs at the proximal corticotomy at a rate of 1 mm/d, and this area gradually fills in with new bone. This method can be used to treat segmental bone loss from other causes.

SPORTS MEDICINE

Treatment of recreational or athletic injuries in otherwise healthy people constitutes a significant portion of orthopedic surgery. Most minor injuries, sprains, contusions, and incomplete ligament tears are treated nonoperatively. Ice, elevation, and rest are the usual modalities for acute injury. Physical therapy may be indicated to restore motion and strength, especially in the injured athlete. Unstable major ligamentous injuries are treated surgically, especially in the professional athlete with ligamentous injury of the knee.

Arthroscopy

Arthroscopy has added an effective low-morbidity procedure that addresses a variety of traumatic degenerative joint problems. Arthroscopy began as a diagnostic adjunct to clinical evaluation of patients with knee problems. Through small stab incisions, using fiberoptic scopes, the entire joint can be visualized better than with standard surgical approaches. The logical development of various small instruments and motorized shavers ushered in operative arthroscopy. The procedure was expanded to include other joints, including the shoulder, wrist, elbow, ankle, and hip.

Meniscal tears of the knee can be repaired in young patients or débrided to a stable edge in older patients with degenerative tears. Total meniscectomy, commonly performed in the past, is hardly ever indicated as an isolated procedure because the meniscus is an important stabilizer, shock absorber, and modulator of knee kinematics. Removal of loose bodies, drilling of chondral defects, resection of symptomatic synovial plicae, and abrasion chondroplasty are common knee arthroscopic procedures. Assessment of articular fracture reductions is possible when closed or limited open techniques are used. In the shoulder, débridement, rotator cuff repair, subacromial decompression, labral repair, capsular shifts, and recurrent dislocation are often arthroscopically assisted. After arthroscopic procedures, rapid rehabilitation is possible because of the small size of incisions, irrigation of inflammatory products, and instillation of long-acting local anesthetics.[58]

Knee Injury

Meniscal tears are common injuries and may present acutely in conjunction with ligamentous injury or as chronic tears characterized by intermittent locking, catching, and localized joint pain. Examination may reveal joint line tenderness and reproduction of the patient's symptoms by compression–rotation of the flexed knee (McMurray sign). Incomplete knee extension may be present the "locked knee." Medial meniscal tears are more common than lateral tears. MRI accurately identifies and characterizes the meniscal injury.

Ligamentous Knee Injuries

Incomplete ligamentous injuries are characterized by a stable knee examination and respond to nonoperative modalities and rehabilitation. One of the most significant and common athletic and recreational knee injuries is rupture of the anterior cruciate ligament (ACL). Classically, a loud "pop" and subsequent hemarthrosis accompany the injury. Examination immediately after injury reveals a positive anterior drawer sign and Lachman test indicative of excessive anterior excursion of the tibia on the femur. There may be associated injuries to the lateral or medial menisci. In the subacute phase, disruption of the ACL may be somewhat more difficult to diagnose because of guarding by the patient in the presence of a hemarthrosis. A tense hemarthrosis is best aspirated to relieve pain, followed by a temporary immobilization of the joint, elevation, and application of ice. Gradual rehabilitation of the knee is attempted and with incomplete tears is usually effective.[59] Complete tears are usually reconstructed at 4 to 6 weeks to allow for resolution of the acute injury and institution of early rehabilitation.

Chronic insufficiency of the ACL is characterized by a giving-way of the knee, especially when the patient attempts to turn suddenly or cut. Clinically, this phenomenon can be demonstrated by the lateral pivot shift test in which the examiner reproduces the anterolateral subluxation of the tibia on the femur. Diagnosis can be confirmed by MRI, which also evaluates for associated injuries to the menisci or other structures. Surgical treatment consists of arthroscopically assisted autogenous tendon graft using either quadruple hamstring, patellar tendon, or allograft substitution (Fig. 113.34). Results are good to excellent in most instances and are better for acute repairs than for chronic cases. Neglected ACL insufficiency can lead to meniscal tears, joint space narrowing, and early degenerative arthritis.[60,61]

Rupture of the posterior cruciate ligament can usually be treated by rehabilitation and nonoperative methods, except in the high-demand patient. The most common mechanisms are a direct "dashboard" blow or impact from a fall on a flexed knee. Surgical repair is most often performed in athletes or when other associated ligamentous injury produces instability, as in knee dislocation. Results after posterior cruciate repair are not as predictable as ACL repair.[62]

Isolated ligamentous tears of the medial collateral ligament can also be treated nonoperatively; however, if they involve the posterior oblique corner of the knee and are associated with cruciate injury, they should be repaired. Likewise, acute ligamentous injuries to the posterolateral corner and arcuate complex of the knee should be repaired primarily because late repair is difficult and associated with suboptimal results.

Complete knee dislocation is frequently associated with popliteal neurovascular injury and has already been discussed. Ligamentous repair should usually be undertaken acutely or after arterial repair. Ideally, all torn structures should be repaired, including the menisci wherever possible. External fixation across the knee joint may be necessary to protect the ligamentous and arterial repair.[59]

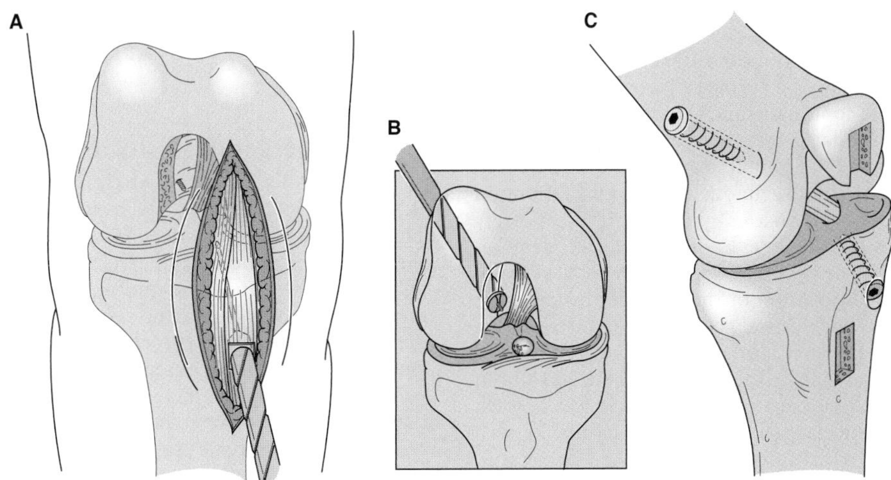

FIGURE 113.34 Arthroscopic-assisted anterior cruciate ligament (ACL) reconstruction. (*A*) Reaming of tibial tunnel over precisely placed guide pin, monitored arthroscopically. (*B*) Intraarticular view of femoral tunnel reaming. Posterior placement of tunnel must be immediately adjacent to posterior cortex. (C) Appropriately tensioned ACL: graft secured with interference screws. Precise positioning achieves appropriate isometry throughout full range of knee motion. Bone–patellar tendon–bone graft is illustrated, although quadrupled hamstrings or allograft may be used. (*A* and *B* From Hardin GT, Bach BR Jr, Bush-Joseph C, et al. Endoscopic single incision ACL reconstruction using patellar tendon autograft: surgical technique. *Am J Knee Surg.* 1991;5:144–155, with permission. C from Nogalski MN, Bach BR Jr. Acute anterior cruciate ligament injuries. In: Fu F, Harner C, Vince K, eds. *The knee.* Baltimore: Williams & Wilkins, 1994, pp. 717–718, with permission.)

Ruptures of the patellar tendon occur most commonly in younger people and are repaired primarily. Rupture of the quadriceps mechanism, on the other hand, more frequently occurs in middle-aged or older men, usually through a degeneratively weakened area of the tendon. Surgical repair is indicated and usually produces satisfactory results.

Ankle

Most injuries to the lateral ligamentous complex produce typical ankle sprain that is best treated by ice, elevation, and compression bandaging. Temporary splinting with an air cast may be appropriate, followed by early institution of protected weight bearing and range of motion. This method allows the most rapid restoration of tensile strength and integrity to the ligamentous complex. Occasionally, more severe injuries may require a brief period of cast immobilization. Rarely, complete tears of the lateral ligamentous complex result in pure ankle dislocation requiring operative repair.[15] Recurrent ankle sprain occasionally results in elongation of the lateral ligamentous complex. Subluxation can be demonstrated on stress radiographs of the ankle. Operative reconstruction predictably yields good results.

Osteochondritis dissecans can involve the talus. Small lesions respond to arthroscopic débridement or drilling. Large lesions are more problematic and have an unfavorable prognosis regardless of treatment

Shoulder

Tendinitis and inflammatory bursitis frequently exist with impingement syndrome of the shoulder. Most tendinitis occurs in middle-aged or elderly men and responds to conservative treatment. Injection of the shoulder with local anesthetic and cortisone is effective in relieving symptoms for a significant period.

Rotator cuff tears are diagnosed by shoulder pain and difficulties with initiating abduction, weakness on isolation testing of the supraspinatus muscle, and a positive MRI. Although acute traumatic tears can occur in athletes and younger patients, most are degenerative, chronic tears occurring in older men. They may require rotator cuff repair and subacromial decompression, usually performed through a small open incision or with arthroscopic assistance.[58] Small or incomplete tears respond to occasional cortisone injection, physical therapy, and tincture of time. Complete tears should be repaired promptly with suture anchor techniques before cuff retraction or progression occurs. Occasionally the cuff is severely retracted and repair is not possible. In these instances, débridement of the inflamed tissue produces satisfactory relief of pain.

Recurrent anterior dislocation of the shoulder usually presents in young people and responds well to operative treatment. Classically, the Bankart labral lesion is repaired along with capsular plication. Many different techniques have been advocated, and overall success rates approach 95%. With multiple dislocations, the classic Hill-Sachs defect may be seen in the humeral head. Arthroscopic repair can be successful, but open surgery has more predictable success.[19]

Elbow

Chronic inflammation or tears of the medial collateral ligament of the elbow may occur in throwing athletes. This injury is usually considered a repetitive valgus overload syndrome and can produce instability, chronic pain, and ulnar neuropathy. Surgical repair may be indicated, as well as decompression or transposition of the ulnar nerve.

Biceps Tendon Rupture

Degenerative tears of the long head of the biceps usually occur proximally in middle-aged men. They do not result in significant disability and are treated symptomatically. In weight lifters or athletes, surgical repair may be indicated because the quality of the tendon is better and the disability relatively greater. Distal ruptures occur in younger people and if diagnosed acutely are surgically repaired. Supination strength and endurance are significantly reduced in unrepaired distal biceps rupture.

Achilles Tendon Rupture

This injury occurs in athletes, active people, and deconditioned middle-aged patients. In the latter group, tears are degenerative and occur with lower-energy forces. Nonoperative treatment with a gravity equinus cast for 8 weeks followed by gradually decreasing heel lifts produces satisfactory results in lower-demand patients and nonathletes. Surgical treatment is recommended for athletes and active people. Results are usually satisfactory with both treatment methods, but greater tensile strength is claimed for surgically repaired ruptures. Even when successful, this is a career-threatening injury in the professional athlete.[19,55]

HAND SURGERY

Knowledge of the kinematics and pathophysiology of the hand and wrist historically lagged behind that of other areas of the body. The advent of radiography allowed precise diagnosis and understanding of fractures and injury patterns involving the wrist and hand. Sterling Bunnell's comprehensive book, *Surgery of Hand,* was published in 1944 and was predicated on advances in the treatment of military casualties with severe hand injuries.[4,60] Subsequently, the development of hand surgery as a specialty and measured advances in the treatment of pathologic processes involving the hand and upper extremity occurred. Microvascular techniques, arthroplasty or replacement of arthritic joints, tendon transfers, nerve grafting, and appropriate arthrodesis have produced significant benefit for patients.[4,60]

Fractures and Dislocations of the Hand: General Principles

The diagnosis of injury depends on a thorough knowledge of the functional anatomy and careful physical examination of the hand and wrist. The hand and wrist should be carefully examined and gently palpated for acute injury. Obvious swelling or deformity may direct the clinician to an injured digit, but should not preclude examination of the remaining hand. Neurovascular status, including two-point discrimination and range of motion, both active and passive, should be tested and recorded. Deformity or open injury is obvious, but subtle injury is notorious for the potential to produce permanent disability. Sprains of the fingers are common but may represent avulsion fractures with the subsequent development of joint instability, restricted motion, or tendon imbalance. Tenderness in the anatomic snuffbox or over the scaphoid tubercle should be treated as a fracture until radiographically ruled out. Open injury associated with fracture should be documented, aseptically irrigated, bandaged, and splinted before obtaining radiographs. The minimal radiographic requirement is two views at 90 degrees opposed. Additional radiographs may be indicated to rule out acute carpal or ligamentous injury.[60,61]

Open fractures require formal irrigation of the bone or joint in the operating room. Tetanus prophylaxis and IV antibiotics are administered and should include anaerobic coverage if the open fracture occurred as a result of a human bite or is contaminated by organic material (Fig. 113.22B). Fingers should be immobilized in the position of function and the "intrinsic plus" position used to splint the hand so that the collateral ligaments are appropriately elongated, thereby decreasing the likelihood of ligament contracture and subsequent joint stiffness. This position is approximately 80 to 90 degrees of metacarpal phalangeal joint flexion and 10 to 20 degrees at the interphalangeal joints.

Fracture of the Digits

Crush injuries of the fingers or thumb are common and usually involve the nail, nail bed, and tuft of the distal phalanx. They are usually treated nonoperatively. If the nail is avulsed, the nail bed should be carefully repaired. A tense subungual hematoma should be decompressed with an 18-gauge needle or heated paperclip. Avulsion of the tip of the finger is best treated open unless significant volar soft tissue is lost, in which case local advancement of soft tissue may be indicated. Judicious resection of exposed bone may be necessary to avoid a painful digital tip.[63,64]

Distal Phalanx

Dorsal phalangeal avulsion fracture of the distal phalanx is a common injury that is usually secondary to a hyperflexion or extension injury. A mallet finger deformity may be present with or without fracture because of disruption of the terminal extensor mechanism. Treatment is extension splinting of the distal joint for 6 weeks. Open reduction is indicated when the articular fragment is large or the joint is subluxed.

When bone is avulsed from the flexor aspect of the distal joint, the patient cannot flex the terminal phalanx and has a palpable mass at the base of the finger or in the palm. Radiographs may show the bone fragment. Operative treatment is required to reattach the flexor tendon to the base of the proximal phalanx with fine wire or nonabsorbable suture.

Middle Phalanx and Proximal Interphalangeal Joint

Stable fractures that do not involve the joint can be initially immobilized in a splint in position of function and "buddy taped" to the adjacent finger. Protected motion is begun at 3 weeks. Avulsion fractures of the base of the middle phalanx usually include the volar plate and result in dorsal dislocation, frequently misdiagnosed as a "sprained finger." If the joint is unstable after reduction, it may need to be pinned. Dislocation of the proximal interphalangeal joint with or without fracture usually disrupts the central slip and dorsal capsule in addition to the palmar plate. If active extension of the joint is absent after reduction, the central slip should be repaired, followed by immobilization of the joint for 5 to 6 weeks in extension. If the fracture–dislocation is irreducible, open reduction should be performed. Late presentation reveals a chronic boutonniere deformity that is difficult to treat.[65]

Proximal Phalanx and Metacarpals

If minimally displaced and nonarticular, these fractures can usually be treated by appropriate splinting and early range of motion. Grossly displaced fractures that are unstable and fractures with significant articular involvement should be treated by open reduction and internal fixation. Other surgical indications include multiple fractures, mangled hands, and open fractures. Metacarpophalangeal joint dislocation usually follows a hyperextension force. Dorsal dislocation is most frequent and occasionally may be irreducible by closed methods. Open reduction, when necessary, if performed through a palmar approach, freeing the entrapped volar plate.[65] Fractures of the fifth metacarpal neck are common and are known as *boxer's fractures*. Because of increased excursion of the fourth and fifth rays, fractures involving the metacarpal necks of these bones can usually be treated by closed reduction and ulnar gutter splinting with the metacarpophalangeal joint flexed 50 to 70 degrees for approximately 4 weeks, followed by a removable splint and protected motion. Displaced fractures of the index and long finger metacarpals, however, often require open reduction.

Thumb metacarpal fractures are usually caused by a fall on the hand and frequently result in an intraarticular fracture of the proximal end. The fracture can almost always be treated by closed reduction and percutaneous pinning for 4 to 6 weeks. If the fragment is large and widely displaced, open reduction and internal fixation are indicated. A comminuted fracture at the base of the metacarpal may be treated by thumb spica splint if minimally displaced or by percutaneous pinning. Occasionally, open reduction is necessary.

Injuries to the metacarpophalangeal joint of the thumb are common, including avulsion fractures in association with ulnar collateral ligament tear, or "gamekeeper's thumb." These are usually initially treated by splinting but may require ligament repair. Metacarpophalangeal joint dislocation of the thumb may cause serious articular or vascular injury. The metacarpal protrudes through a tear in the capsule and occasionally the volar plate may be interposed in the joint, making it irreducible and requiring open reduction.

Summary of Treatment Principles

Stable fractures are, by definition, minimally displaced or reducible. A brief period of splinting followed by buddy taping allows early, protected motion. Potentially unstable injuries require radiographic and clinical follow-up during the first 7 to 10 days to detect loss of reduction. Percutaneous pinning may be indicated in this instance. Large articular fragments and unstable oblique or open fractures require open reduction and surgical stabilization[63–66] (Fig. 113.22B).

Carpal Fractures and Wrist Dislocations

Displaced intercarpal fracture–dislocations require accurate reduction and surgical stabilization. Isolated fractures of carpal bones other than the scaphoid are less common. When undisplaced, these fractures are treated by cast immobilization. Dorsal chip fractures of the triquetrum are relatively benign injuries unless associated intercarpal instability. Capitate fractures require open reduction when displaced and are often associated with other wrist lesions. Fractures of the lunate are less common than dislocation, but traumatic compressive injury may precede avascular necrosis. Fractures of the hamate may involve the body or hamulus. The latter often requires carpal tunnel views, tomography, or CT for diagnosis. Because of proximity to the motor branch of the ulnar nerve, neuropathy may be present. Pisiform fractures are uncommon and usually do not result in significant disability. Excision is infrequently performed.[64,65]

Perilunate Dislocation

Perilunate dislocation encompasses a spectrum of pathologic processes. Pure dorsal dislocation of the capitate, an associated fracture, or an oblique fracture of the radial styloid may occur individually or in combination. Radiography of the wrist may show carpal overlap, a "signet ring" sign over the scaphoid, or a wide gap between the scaphoid and lunate.

Initial treatment requires prompt reduction. Median nerve neuropathy is not uncommon because of the displaced lunate or stretching of the median nerve. If post reduction radiographs show satisfactory reduction without residual displacement of the carpus, immobilization in plaster cast is appropriate. Residual abnormalities present on postreduction radiographs dictate open reduction and internal stabilization. Late sequelae of intercarpal injury and instability include chronic pain and weakness. Scapholunate ligament reconstruction, selected intercarpal arthrodesis, or complete radiocarpal arthrodesis (wrist fusion) may be indicated to relieve pain and provide stable function.[46,65]

Tendon Injury and Repair

Tendon injury in the hand and digits may frequently be suspected or diagnosed by the abnormal position of a digit in complete disruptions. Partial lacerations, however, may have normal appearance and range of motion. Inability to move the involved digit or joint is indicative of tendon disruption, usually caused by laceration, but associated digital nerve or vascular injury may coexist. The diagnosis is secured by testing for active motion, sensation, two-point discrimination, and capillary refill.[64,67]

Extensor Tendon Injuries

The diagnosis of most extensor lesions is straightforward and surgical repair usually is not as technically demanding as that for flexor tendons. However, the extensor tendons are thin and intimately proximate to the interphalangeal joints and bones. The swan neck and boutonniere deformities are classic examples of residua from extensor tendon injury. The latter deformity results from disruption of the central slip of the tendon from its insertion at the base of the middle phalanx. Laceration of extensor tendons in the forearm may be accompanied by injury to sensory branches of the radial or ulnar nerves. After repair of extensor tendons in the digits or dorsum of the hand, extension splinting of the wrist at 45 degrees and the digit(s) at 10 degrees of flexion for 4 to 5 weeks is necessary. When motion is begun, the digits are protected by a removable splint.[66,67]

Flexor Tendon Injuries

Anatomy. The flexor system consists of two tendons for each finger and one for the thumb. The flexor digitorum superficialis divides into two tendon slips in the palm and inserts on the middle phalanx of each digit. The flexor digitorum profundus and flexor pollicis longus tendons insert on the base of the distal phalangeals of the figures and thumb, respectively. It is useful to divide the hand into zones in differentiating one tendon laceration from another, and also for determining how to treat lacerations in the current different zones (Fig. 113.35A).

Flexor Tendon Repair. Tendon repair should be performed under optimal conditions, providing satisfactory anesthesia, appropriate lighting, and hemostasis. Appropriate extension of the traumatic wound is necessary to visualize the injury adequately. In the finger, this usually indicates a zigzag extension. Lacerations in zone I involve the flexor digitorum profundus; in zone II, "no man's land," lacerations frequently involve both flexor tendons within the fibroosseous tunnel, and this is the most critical and most challenging zone to treat surgically.[68,69] Zone V, which extends from the proximal transverse carpal ligament at the wrist to the musculotendinous junction of the flexor tendons in the distal third of the forearm, contains the median nerve and the ulnar neurovascular bundle as well as the wrist flexors and all of the deep and superficial digital flexors. All lacerated structures should be repaired. Repair of both tendons in zone II should be performed in clean wounds (Fig. 113.35B). Delayed repair is necessary for poor-quality skin or contamination. Crush injuries may require tendon grafting when the soft tissue is receptive. Laceration of the profundus tendon in zone I is repaired by advancing the tendon slightly and securing it to its insertion on the base of the distal phalanx. Associated injuries to the median or ulnar nerves require repair with fine nylon sutures using an operating microscope.[67–70]

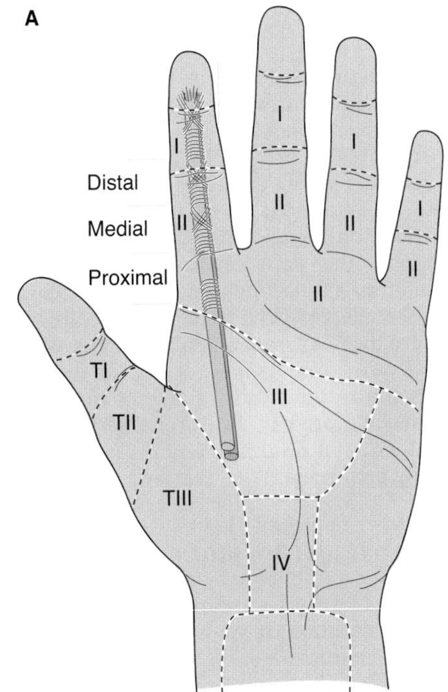

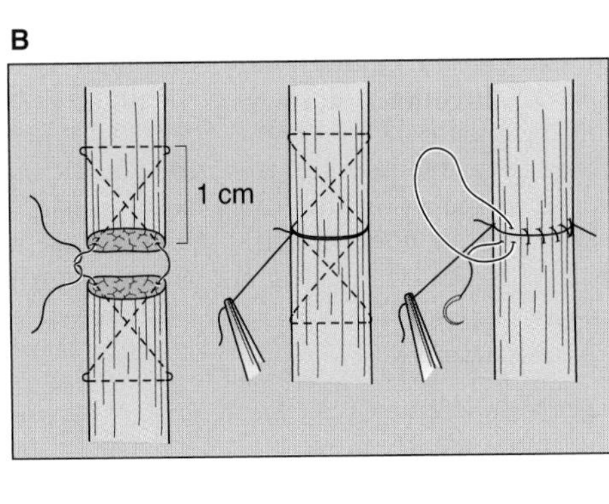

FIGURE 113.35 (*A*) Zone 1, distal to the sublimis; zone 2, "no-man's land"; zone 3, region of the lumbrical origin; zone 4, carpal tunnel; zone 5, proximal to carpal tunnel. (*B*) Many methods of flexor tendon suture repair exist, but most involve a core suture followed by a running peripheral suture through the epitenon.

Postoperative Care. After surgery, the wrist is splinted in flexion for approximately 4 weeks. Supervised rehabilitation should begin immediately after surgery. Gentle passive motion can be started early. Careful supervision is necessary during the postoperative period because rupture of repaired tendons is likely to produce a suboptimal result even if recognized and repaired.

Tendon Grafting. Tendon grafting is indicated for late injuries, extensive loss of motion due to adherent tendons, or failed primary repair. Grafting requires reasonable motion and an intact pulley system. The palmaris longus, toe extensors, or ring finger sublimis may be used as the donor tendon graft depending on availability and the size of the flexor tendon needed. After surgery, the wrist and fingers are splinted in flexion for 4 to 5 weeks, followed by protective splinting for an additional several weeks. Gentle passive motion is allowed during the first period and graduated active-assisted and active motion during the second period.[70]

When the finger is stiff, the gliding surface fibrotic, and the pulley system severely damaged, a Silastic rod (Hunter) is inserted after resection of the fibrosed tendon and scar.[71] The Silastic rod is secured distally but left free in the proximal palm or wrist to permit passive motion. The pulleys over the distal end of the proximal phalanx (A2) and mid-middle phalanx (A4) are reconstructed. A pseudosheath forms over the rod as passive motion is produced and swelling subsides, which may require 3 to 6 months before grafting. A tendon graft using the second or third long toe extensor is harvested, attached to the detached distal Silastic rod, and pulled proximally under the new sheath. The latter can be modified to form or augment pulleys and to permit free gliding of the graft. Tension is carefully adjusted and postoperative care proceeds.[70,71]

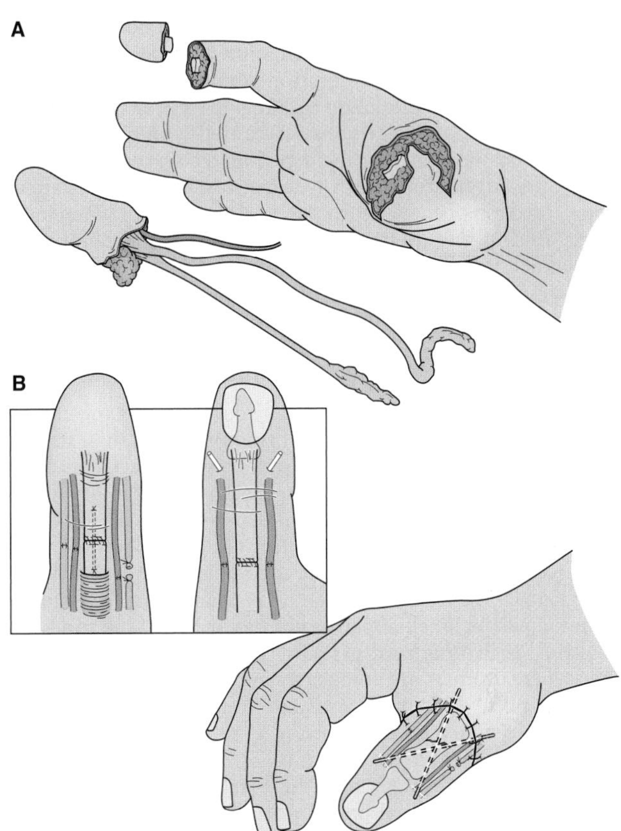

FIGURE 113.36 Digital replantation. Whenever possible, the thumb should always be replanted because its loss results in major hand dysfunction.

Replantation of Amputated Limbs and Digits

Replantation is the reattachment of a part that has been completely severed (Fig. 113.36). The indications for replantation proceed according to the following priorities: (a) thumb; (b) multiple digits; (c) partial hand amputation through the palm; (d) amputation in a child; (e) wrist or forearm; (f) above-elbow amputation unassociated with crush or avulsion; and (g) isolated digit distal to the superficiales insertion. General replantation of thumbs, multiple digits, or the complete hand produces the best results.[72,73] Crushed, avulsed, or severely mangled parts or those associated with extensive contamination or greater than 6 hours of ischemia are not replantable.

Surgical Technique

The sequence of replantation is (a) locate vessels and nerves, (b) débride the amputated part of the stump, (c) securely fix the bone with an intramedullary pin, (d) repair extensor tendons, (e) repair flexor tendons, (f) repair arteries, (g) repair nerves, (h) repair veins, and (i) obtain loose skin coverage. Arterial repair takes precedence if warm ischemia time is prolonged.[72,73]

Postoperative Management

Appropriate splinting is provided, and adjusted-dose heparin and IV antibiotics are administered for 5 to 7 days. Most major replantation centers report an approximately 80% viability rate. Functional results vary according to the replanted structure. Replanted thumbs produce the best functional results, followed by replants of digits distal to the superficial tendon insertion. Replantation of amputated digits at the base of the finger usually produces poor functional results.

Nerve Injury

Physical examination may reveal complete or, more frequently, incomplete motor and sensory loss below the level of the injury. With lacerations or injuries of tendons or adjacent structures, therefore, injury to peripheral nerves should be suspected. This is especially so for penetrating injuries about the wrist and antecubital fossa. Bleeding from these areas should be controlled by direct pressure because attempts to clamp or ligate actively bleeding vessels under suboptimal visualization may damage nearby nerves.

Primary repair of lacerated nerves is accomplished under a bloodless field using an operating microscope. Intrafascicular or epineural repairs with fine nonabsorbable sutures may be indicated depending on the size of the nerve and its location. Postoperative splinting is used for 3 to 4 weeks depending on the location and type of repair, as well as associated tendon injuries.[73,74]

Nonpenetrating Nerve Injuries

Nerve injuries associated with fractures or fracture—dislocations are frequently injuries in continuity, producing a neurapraxia. Exploration of these nerves is not indicated unless it is incidental to the open treatment of fracture. A relatively high incidence of radial nerve palsy is present with fractures of the humeral shaft. Recovery usually occurs within 10 to 12 weeks, but can take as long as 6 months. Ulnar and median nerve injuries are usually secondary to fractures about the elbow, forearm, or wrist. Treatment is by appropriate fracture reduction and observation. Nerve regeneration occurs at approximately 1 mm/day and is evidence by an advancing Tinel sign signifying an intact and recovering nerve. Electromyographic and nerve conduction velocities are helpful in determining the type of injury and potential for recovery. Exploration is indicated if there is no evidence of returning function by 3 to 4 months. An additional 6 to 8 weeks of observation is warranted with closed radial nerve palsies because the incidence of recovery approaches 90%. Surgical treatment involves neurolysis, release of adhesions, resection of small neuromas, and nerve repair when indicated. End-to-end anastomosis is preferred, although with segmental crush or defect, nerve grafting may be indicated. The most commonly used graft is the sural nerve, whose absence causes only hypesthesia along the lateral border of the foot.

Brachial Plexus Injuries

Brachial plexus injuries are potentially devastating. Low-energy injuries or sports accidents have a better prognosis than stab or gunshot wounds. Motorcycle and motor vehicle accidents are a frequent cause of severe injury. The mechanism of injury in the latter is usually severe and forceful depression of the shoulder with simultaneous forceful movement of the head in the opposite direction, producing traction. A complete palsy involves all five roots (C-5, C-6, C-7, C-8, T-1). There are two types of more common partial brachial plexus injuries. In type 1, all roots are involved but in differing degrees. In type 2, some roots are damaged whereas others are completely intact. Injury may occur to roots, trunks, divisions, cords, or branches (Fig. 113.37). Frequently a mixed picture evolves.[75]

Upper brachial plexus lesions (C-5, C-6) result in paralysis of the shoulder muscles and the biceps brachia. With the extended upper brachial plexus or middle trunk lesion, there is paralysis of muscles innervated by the radial nerve. Lower brachial plexus lesions (C-8, T-1) result in paralysis of ulnar-innervated and most median-innervated muscles.[74–76]

Treatment. Except for open injuries, exploration, neurolysis, or nerve grafting is performed on a delayed basis to allow for any spontaneous recovery to occur. Exposure of the structures involved is technically demanding and requires meticulous dissection and the use of nerve stimulators and appropriate magnification. The sural, intercostal, medial cutaneous antebrachial, and occasionally a superficial branch of the radial nerve may be used as nerve grafts.

Prognosis. Prognosis depends on the severity of the nerve injury and location of the lesion. Avulsion of cervical roots from the spinal cord has a dismal prognosis and no spontaneous recovery occurs. Incomplete lesions or complete lesions in continuity have varying degrees of return. Minor stretch injuries may have complete recovery. Appropriately timed tendon transfers and arthrodesis may be helpful. Because of the long distance from the plexus to the ulnar-innervated muscles, only partial recovery can be expected, and intrinsic hand function required for fine movements is never restored. One of the main goals of surgery is return of elbow flexion so that the arm can function as a "helper." Neurogenic pain develops in a significant number of patients, and a completely anesthetic and functionless limb requires above-elbow amputation.[74–76]

Tendon Transfers

Tendon transfers are performed to restore power or balance to a partially paralyzed hand. This operation requires transfer of an expendable musculotendinous unit resulting in a redistribution of remaining functional parts into the best possible working combination. In general, when one of the three major nerves of the arm (median, ulnar, or radial) is lost, excellent functional restoration can be achieved, but with the loss of two of the three, a substantial functional impairment is inevitable.[67,74]

Preoperative Planning

Precise assessment of the patient's need and functioning parts is required. Muscle transfers must be expendable, of normal strength, and free of spasticity. They also should have adequate amplitude of excursion and suitable anatomic location for rerouting in a straight line of pull between the origin and new attachment. In-phase transfers are preferable but often not available. Retraining of transferred tendons requires considerable patient motivation and effort.

There are many types of tendon transfers described for different paralytic conditions.[67,74] Radial nerve palsy is a common indication and has predictably good results. The goal is to restore wrist and digital extension. A variety of motors are available if the ulnar and median nerves are normal. Closed radial nerve palsy, frequently secondary to fracture, has an

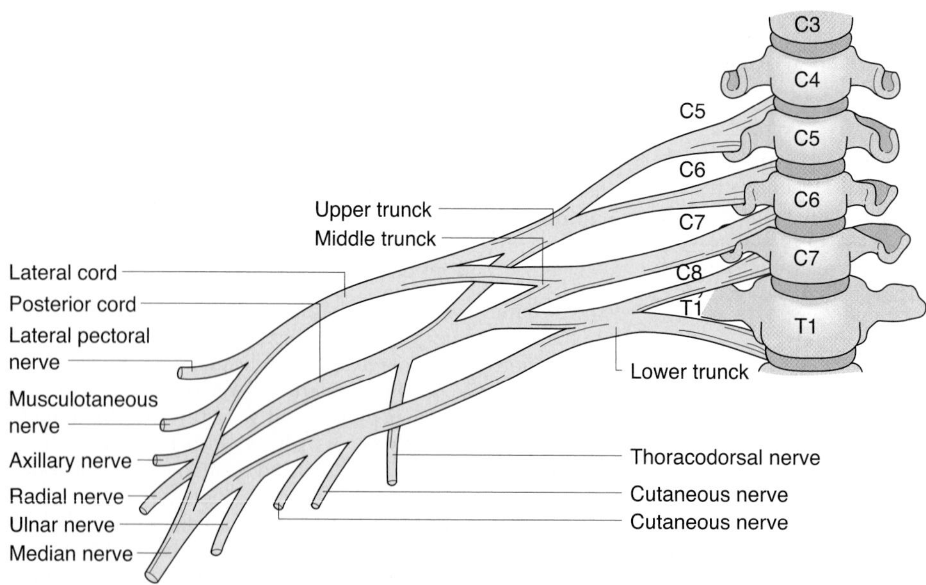

FIGURE 113.37 Anatomy of the brachial plexus.

TABLE 113.4 DIAGNOSIS

FINDINGS OF UPPER EXTREMITY PERIPHERAL NERVE INJURY

Nerve	Sensory	Motor
Brachial plexus	Spotty, mixed or complete loss	Mixed weakness, arm, forearm, and hand
Median	Palmar hand, thumb, index, long. and radial fingers; dorsal thumb, index, long, and radial fingertips only	Below elbow: loss of opposition of thumb with fingers, thenar muscle palsy Above elbow: inability to flex distal thumb and index fingers, inability to pronate forearm, flex wrist
Radial	Dorsal hand to mid-fingers, thumb, index, long, and radial half of ring finger	Below elbow: wrist drop, inability to extend fingers at MP joint High arm: inability to extend elbow
Ulnar	Ulnar wrist, hand, and fingers, ulnar ring, and all of fifth finger	Inability to spread fingers or flex MP joints without phalangeal flexion Clawing of fourth and fifth fingers

MP, metacarpophalangeal.

excellent prognosis for spontaneous recovery, and therefore tendon transfers should be delayed 6 to 8 weeks past the usual arbitrary 4- to 6-month time frame.

Ulnar nerve palsy resulting in intrinsic muscle paralysis in the hand has many described tendon transfers, depending on the location of the lesion and the etiology. The goal is to correct claw deformity, loss of grip strength, and asynchronous motion, as well as loss of abduction–adduction control of the digits.

Complete median nerve palsy due to proximal laceration or brachial plexopathy is fortunately not common. It results in profound motor loss involving all of the superficial flexors; the radial half of the deep flexors, including the flexor pollicis, pronator teres and quadratus, and flexor carpi radialis; the entire thenar group; and radial two lumbricals and the palmaris longus (Table 113.4).

Thenar weakness secondary to carpal tunnel compression at the wrist is relatively common. Long-standing or profound weakness results in loss of opposition of the thumb and can be treated by opponensplasty, which substitutes for the paralyzed abductor pollicis brevis.[67]

In biceps paralysis, weakness or loss of elbow flexion results from injury to the musculocutaneous nerve, or is secondary to spinal cord or brachial plexus injury. Loss of elbow flexion results in serious loss of hand and forearm function and is frequently an indication of one of many described tendon transfers.

Injuries resulting in combined nerve palsy are more complex because there is typically greater loss of sensation, proprioception, and residua of soft tissue or vascular injury. There are fewer motor units available for transfer, and retraining is more problematic. Transfers for combined palsies, however, can provide important restoration of function in these severely injured extremities.[67,74,76]

Arthroplasty and Arthrodesis: Upper Extremity

The upper extremity does not have the imposition of weight bearing, and therefore degenerative arthritis and subsequent joint replacements are less common.[55]

Shoulder

Tendinitis and other soft tissue inflammation is a much more common cause of morbidity, chronic pain, and loss of function than degenerative arthritis. Total shoulder arthroplasty is a satisfactory solution for arthritic pain, although normal function is rarely achieved. Frequently there are associated injuries or degeneration of the rotator cuff, which compromise motion and strength to some degree.

Hemiarthroplasty may also be indicated if the glenoid is less involved. The most common indication for its use is a four-part fracture of the humeral head in which avascular necrosis is inevitable. Reattachment of the greater and lesser tuberosities with the rotator cuff, as well as appropriate height of the prosthesis are necessary to restore balance and function to the shoulder.

Arthrodesis may be indicated for younger patients with paralysis of the shoulder muscles or global instability associated with arthritic changes. The desired position of arthrodesis is the so-called "sloppy salute position," approximately 25 degrees of flexion, abduction, and 35 to 40 degrees of internal rotation.[62]

Elbow

Elbow arthroplasty is performed primarily in patients with rheumatoid or other inflammatory arthritis and multiple joint involvement.[53] It is best used in low-demand patients because the prosthetic components are less capable of resisting cyclic fatigue and failure. Arthrodesis of the elbow is not frequently performed or necessary. Most patients tolerate a moderate degree of arthritic symptoms or instability for retention of some motion. The position of fusion is usually a right angle, although occasionally an extended position may be indicated. An example of the latter would be a person who must fire a weapon or otherwise function with the elbow in an extended position.

Wrist

Except in rheumatoid arthritis, wrist joint arthroplasty is rarely performed. Arthrodesis of the wrist is a sound and satisfactory treatment for symptomatic arthritis or instability. Desired position of fusion is approximately 15 to 20 degrees of dorsiflexion, which is the best compromise between the power and precision grip positions. Proximal-row carpectomy preserves motion and is an alternative procedure for low-demand patients.[46]

Hand

Interposition arthroplasty has been used for the trapezium, scaphoid, and capitate but is not frequently indicated or as useful as soft tissue procedures. Selected intercarpal arthrodesis may be useful in certain cases. One of the most useful types of arthroplasty in the rheumatoid hand is done for severe metacarpophalangeal deformity, ulnar drift, and joint destruction. The metacarpophalangeal joints are replaced with Silastic or titanium implants and a pseudocapsule develops about the resected joints. The appearance and function are greatly improved. It is essential to centralize the extensor mechanism and treat any tendon ruptures by tenodesis or grafting.[64]

Infection

Digits

Purulent flexor tenosynovitis requires prompt diagnosis and treatment if loss of motion and function is to be avoided. Classic signs of infection of the flexor sheet are exquisite tenderness, a semiflexed position of the finger, exquisite pain on extension, and associated symmetric fusiform swelling of the entire finger. This infection can develop from puncture wounds or abrasions. Treatment is by two incisions, one in the palm proximal to the first annular (A1) pulley, and a second, mid-lateral incision on the ulnar side of the distal interphalangeal joint crease. Through these wounds, the flexor tendon sheet can be carefully exposed and drained. A small pediatric feeding tube or rubber catheter can be used to irrigate the sheath after surgery.[77] Appropriate IV antibiotics to include anaerobic coverage where indicated are administered for 2 to 5 days. Oral antibiotics for an additional 5 to 7 days may also be indicated.

Hand

Infection of the radial and ulnar bursa or midpalm space is characterized by pain, erythema, induration, and tenderness in the particular anatomic location. Subtendinous infection in the distal forearm may occur between the flexor tendons and the pronator quadratus and may coexist with digital purulent tenosynovitis. Surgical irrigation and débridement is indicated for abscess formation and for equivocal cases that do not respond to elevation and intravenous antibiotics.

Septic Joints

Small septic joints in the fingers, as well as the wrist, can occasionally be treated by aspiration and irrigation. Elevation of the hand and intravenous antibiotics may result in resolution of early infection or cellulitis. When significant swelling and signs of infection are present, it is usually necessary to proceed promptly with open irrigation and débridement.

Human Bites

Human bite injuries usually involve tooth puncture wounds over the dorsum of the hand, frequently in the region of the fourth and fifth metacarpal heads. Treatment is usually delayed until the patient realizes that he may not actually have won the fight. Human mouth organisms inoculated in tissue are quite virulent. Frequently they are anaerobic or mixed. Aggressive débridement is required, as is the administration of broad-spectrum antibiotics with both gram-positive and gram-negative activity. Anaerobic coverage should be provided by penicillin, clindamycin, or metronidazole. Similar treatment is indicated for animal bites, although they are less problematic.[54,77]

Necrotizing Fasciitis

Necrotizing fasciitis, a devastating infection, is a limb- and potentially life-threatening problem. It frequently begins as an innocuous puncture wound, abrasion, or laceration in a digit. It is also commonly seen in intravenous drug abusers. Presentation is usually late after a period of erythema has progressed to induration, swelling, pain, or drainage.

A high index of suspicion is necessary to differentiate this from less virulent forms of soft tissue infection or more common cellulitis. A diffuse swelling and erythema over the digits, hand, forearm, or upper arm characterize necrotizing fasciitis. It is usually rapidly progressive. The patient may initially be only moderately symptomatic, but becomes toxic and septicemic within hours.

Treatment. Once the diagnosis of necrotizing fasciitis has been made, immediate surgical débridement is indicated. The incision should be extended proximally in the extremity until normal-appearing tissue is encountered. The boundaries between normal and abnormal are frequently blurred, but infection can be assumed to be present as far proximally as the swelling and erythema exist. Frequently only watery pus and necrotic fascia and subcutaneous tissue are found. Infections that spread onto the chest wall are often fatal. Repeat débridement may be necessary. Hyperbaric oxygen may be helpful if used early as an adjunct to radical débridement. Anaerobic streptococci, other anaerobes, or mixed organisms are usually responsible. Antibiotics should include gram-positive, gram-negative, and anaerobic coverage in full therapeutic dosages. Despite aggressive therapy, amputation is often necessary. Necrotizing fasciitis is more frequently seen than clostridial myonecrosis, but both infections are limb and life threatening.[54,77]

Miscellaneous Soft Tissue Disorders of the Hand

Carpal Tunnel Syndrome

Carpal tunnel syndrome is a common compressive neuropathy of the median nerve at the wrist. It occurs most frequently in middle-aged women engaged in repetitive activities of the upper extremity. Dysesthetic pain, numbness, and tingling involving the volar aspects of the thumb, index, long, and radial half of the ring finger are present to variable degrees. Nocturnal symptoms are particularly bothersome. Physical findings include hypesthesia and decreased two-point discrimination over the median nerve distribution. Provocative testing with the wrists firmly pressed in full flexion (Phalen test) reproduces the patient's syndromes. Tapping over the carpal tunnel produces paresthesias in the involved digit (Tinel sign). Weakness of opposition of the thumb and thenar atrophy may be present in long-standing cases.

Nonoperative treatment includes soft night splints, antiinflammatory medication, and occasional steroid injection of the carpal tunnel. Avoidance of repetitive motion of the hand and wrist is very important and may result in resolution of symptoms. Electromyographic and nerve conduction studies can document median neuropathy. These studies are frequently ordered, but not necessary in clear-cut cases.

Surgical decompression by section of the transverse carpal ligament yields predictably good results and should be offered early on to patients unresponsive to conservative measures. It is performed under outpatient local or regional anesthesia through a small incision paralleling the thenar crease. Some surgeons prefer endoscopic release, but the open technique has low morbidity and has withstood the test of time.

Tendinitis

Tenosynovitis is a common and bothersome entity that is frequently associated with repetitive activities. It is more common in women and frequently seen in secretaries and keypunch and computer operators. Tendinitis may precede or accompany carpal tunnel syndrome. Symptoms may be prolonged and are treated with antiinflammatory drugs, modification of activities, splinting, and occasional steroid injections. Tendinitis is associated with significant lost work time and Workers' Compensation claims.

Trigger Digit

Repetitive trauma may produce inflammation of a flexor tendon, resulting in localized swelling or a nodule that prevents movement of the flexor tendon beneath the A1 pulley in the hand. The patient has difficulty straightening out the finger, which then characteristically snaps painfully or triggers when it is forcibly straightened or flexed. Restriction of repetitive activities and use of antiinflammatory drugs or local injection of cortisone may result in a cure. If not, surgical treatment is simple and rewarding by incising the A1 pulley to allow the tendon to move smoothly. This procedure can be performed under local anesthesia. When the thumb is involved, care must be taken to identify the digital nerves because they are close to the flexor tendon. The triggering occurs at the interphalangeal joint; however, the nodule is palpable over the metacarpophalangeal joint.

DeQuervain Disease

Tendinitis involving the abductor pollicis longus and the extensor pollicis brevis in the first dorsal compartment was first described by DeQuervain in 1895.[4] There is tenderness along the sheath over the first dorsal compartment and radial aspect of the wrist. Hyperflexion of the first ray with ulnar deviation of the wrist reproduces pain during physical examination. Conservative treatment is usually effective in relieving symptoms. Otherwise, surgical excision of the thickened tendon sheath of the first dorsal compartment is curative.

Ganglion

Ganglion formation is common, particularly over the dorsum of the wrist, and is likely traumatic in origin. The cyst contains a typical gelatinous fluid and the stalk usually extends down to the related joint. Most ganglions are small and minimally symptomatic and can be ignored. They may spontaneously change in size. Diagnosis can be confirmed by aspiration of the typical jelly-like material. Simultaneous injection of a small amount of corticosteroid and appropriate splinting may be curative. Recurrence is common and surgical excision is reserved for symptomatic lesions. Dissections should carefully include the stalk to prevent recurrence.

Lateral Epicondylitis

Often referred to as *tennis elbow,* lateral epicondylitis is a very common inflammation caused by repetitive activity and less frequently to tennis. Wrist extension against resistance causes pain at the lateral epicondyle. Throwing and wringing motions may be painful, as well as backhand racquet movements. Treatment is by rest, application of ice, and use of nonsteroidal antiinflammatory drugs. A proximal forearm tennis strap may be helpful. The condition is usually benign and responds to restriction or modification of activities. Surgery is indicated in recalcitrant cases and consists of excision of granulation tissue involving the extensor carpi radialis brevis or any localized calcification that may be present. Postoperative splinting is instituted for 2 to 3 weeks.

Dupuytren's Contracture

Dupuytren's contracture is a rather common condition without any obvious etiology, and characterized by hypertrophy and contracture of the palmar and digital fascia. Typically, the small and ring fingers are involved, but extension can involve other digits as well. Deep cords of fascia can develop that produce progressive flexion of the metacarpophalangeal joint by the deep attachments to the volar plate. So-called spiral cords can wind around the neurovascular bundles, rendering them vulnerable at surgical dissection.

Most Dupuytren's contractures are minimally progressive or nonprogressive with minimal functional impairment. When the contracture is progressive, flexion begins to develop, and it is best to treat the patient early before extensive flexion contracture evolves.[60]

Surgical Treatment. Simple fasciotomy may be effective for patients with thin palmar fascial cords and primarily involvement of the metacarpophalangeal joint. Simple fasciotomy is also useful in elderly or chronically ill patients who might do less well with a more extensive procedure.[78] The usual treatment is fasciectomy, which involves careful preoperative planning of Z-plasty and skin flaps, careful dissection of thin skin, avoidance of digital nerve injury, and complete resection of diseased palmar fascia. Transection of contracting skin and fascial cords, followed by full-thickness skin grafting, may be attempted in an effort to interrupt the contiguity of the cord.[79] Complications of surgery include digital nerve damage, skin necrosis, and recurrence. Digital joint capsulectomy may be necessary for severe or recurrent contracture.[60]

FOOT

The three main functional requirements for the foot are that it fits in a shoe, strikes the floor flat, and is pain free. The symptomatic foot can be a source of great disability. Causes for this include fractures, acquired and degenerative deformities, and arthritic conditions. Peripheral neuropathies associated with diabetes or malnutrition are also problematic.[19]

Fracture of the Talus

Closed reduction and casting or percutaneous screw fixation can treat fractures of the neck of the talus when they are undisplaced. Open injuries and associated fractures in the foot and ankle may be present. Displaced fractures of the body of the talus have a very poor prognosis with a high incidence of avascular necrosis or nonunion. It is mandatory to obtain as accurate a reduction of the articular surface as possible (Fig. 113.38A).These injuries frequently require an osteotomy of the medial malleolus of the tibia to gain exposure and, despite anatomic reduction, chondral damage and interference with blood supply frequently lead to avascular necrosis or arthritis even if the fracture unites. Weight bearing should be restricted for a minimum of 8 weeks or longer after surgery.[16,17]

Calcaneal Fractures

Fractures of the calcaneus are common and potentially disabling injuries resulting usually from a fall from a height. A lumbar compression fracture is a frequent associated injury, although usually not requiring operative treatment.

Open reduction and internal fixation to restore the anatomy and articular facets of the subtalar joint is usually used to treat the joint depression fractures involving the calcaneus (Fig. 113.38B). Occasionally, extremely comminuted fractures warrant consideration for primary subtalar arthrodesis because normal motion and pain relief are not likely to be accomplished by open reduction and internal fixation (Fig. 113.16).

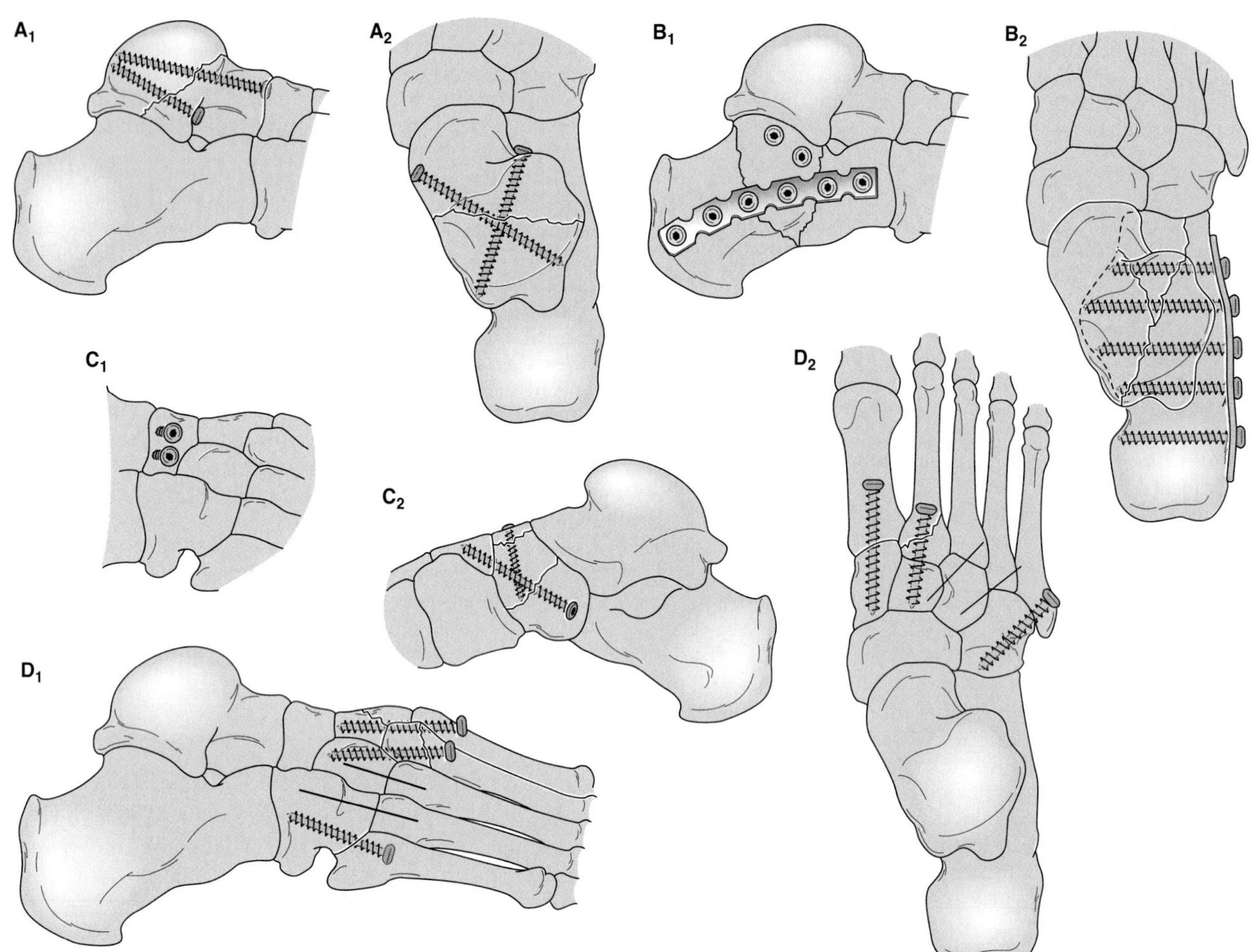

FIGURE 113.38 (*A*) Displaced joint fractures of the calcaneus can be treated by open reduction and internal fixation provided that the soft tissue is in good condition. After surgery, early subtalar motion is encouraged and weight bearing is delayed for 10 to 12 weeks. (*A2*) Axial view of internally fixed calcaneal fracture. (*B1*) Lateral view of the ankle after open reduction and internal fixation of a fracture of the talar neck with interfragmentary screw. (*B2*) Anteroposterior radiograph of same fracture. (*C1*) Anteroposterior view of surgical stabilization of a fractured navicular. (*C2*) Lateral view of the foot after open reduction and screw stabilization of same fracture. Occasionally, bone graft is necessary for comminuted fractures to buttress the articular surfaces. (*D*) Lisfranc fracture–dislocation of tarsometatarsal joints. The second metatarsal base–cuneiform articulation is a good key to reduction. Frequently, all five articulations are involved. Significant swelling and soft tissue injury occurs with this injury. Treatment is by open reduction and internal fixation, or occasionally closed reduction and percutaneous fixation as indicated. (*D2*) Anteroposterior view of Lisfranc fracture–dislocation after surgical stabilization.

Severe swelling and blister formation may preclude immediate operation. It is best to elevate the foot and wait until the soft tissue has healed, frequently 7 to 10 days and occasionally longer, before operation. Surgical treatment allows the restoration of normal architecture, avoiding the broad, flattened heel that accompanies nonoperative treatment. The flattened heel frequently is difficult to fit in a shoe and is associated with entrapment or irritation of the peroneal tendons. Despite operative treatment, subtalar motion is frequently diminished. After surgery, weight bearing is restricted for 10 to 12 weeks until fracture healing has occurred. Results are usually satisfactory with accurate reduction; however, an unpredictable number of patients require eventual subtalar arthrodesis because of pain.

Nonoperative treatment consists of molding the fracture and a period of immobilization in a cast, followed by rehabilitation. Symptomatic patients can be treated with subtalar fusion, although this procedure is somewhat more problematic because of the broadened configuration, loss of height, and proximity of the calcaneus to the talus.[16,17,19]

Midfoot Fractures

Fractures of the navicular, cuboid, and cuneiforms are less common. The midfoot is relatively rigid, with the linked articulations firmly bound by ligamentous structures, and therefore significant force is necessary to produce injury. Other associated foot injuries may be present. Fractures of the navicular and cuboid are often associated with lesions involving the talus, calcaneus, or subtalar joint.[16] Injuries involving the cuneiforms invariably involve their articulation with the metatarsal bases. Displaced fractures and dislocations need to be reduced and appropriately immobilized, which often requires open reduction and internal fixation[16] (Fig. 113.38C).

Lisfranc's Fracture—Dislocation

Fracture—dislocation of the tarsometatarsal joints may be associated with severe swelling and potential neurovascular compromise of the distal foot. Usually all five joints are dislocated, and associated fracture of the base of the metatarsal or cuneiforms may be present. A key to diagnosis is loss of the recessed keystone appearance of the second metatarsal—cuneiform articulation. Treatment is by closed or, more frequently, open reduction and transarticular pin or screw fixation. The latter is more secure (Fig. 113.38D). There is little motion at the tarsometatarsal joints, so the security of fixation warrants a transarticular screw placement if necessary to maintain reduction.[17]

Metatarsal and Toe Fractures

Most metatarsal fractures are treated closed. Multiple metatarsal fractures that are displaced or displaced fractures of the metacarpal neck may require open reduction and internal fixation. Dislocations of the toes are easily overlooked and can be a source of late disability or medical—legal problems. These should be reduced promptly and are usually stable. Buddy taping to a fellow toe is usually all that is necessary. Intraarticular fractures of the metatarsal heads or adjacent phalanges should be treated by open reduction if they involve significant portions of the joint. This is especially true for the great toe.

Hallux Valgus

Bunion formation and hallux valgus are common in modern society. Most patients who desire surgical correction are women who have subjected their feet to high-heeled or tight shoes. Hallux valgus observed in cultures where shoes are not worn is largely asymptomatic. When indicated, a number of different surgical procedures may be used. The simplest procedures are exostectomy or cheilectomy. Soft tissue realignment procedures or osteotomies involving the base or distal aspects of the first metatarsal may be required for severe degrees of hallux valgus. Partial proximal phalangectomy and temporary Kirschner wire pinning frequently can correct claw and hammertoe deformities. Syndactyly occasionally may be indicated.

Posterior Tibial Tendon Rupture

Posterior tibial tendon rupture is a potentially disabling condition that develops from overload of the posterior tibial tendon and longitudinal arch. Characteristically it begins as tendinitis and progresses to partial or complete rupture. If the latter occurs, a severe acquired flat foot or pes plano valgus deformity occurs as the heel slides out from underneath the talus and most of the weight is born on the medial column of the foot. Early treatment is by appropriate splinting, arch support, and medications during the inflammatory stage. Once a tendon is ruptured, treatment is surgical by débridement, repair, or frequently tendon transfer of the flexor hallucis longus or flexor digitorum longus tendons.

This is a frequently overlooked condition that can be diagnosed by typical symptoms of discomfort along the posterior tibial tendon and inability to do a heel lift without producing valgus displacement of the hindfoot. Variable weakness of the posterior tibial muscle results in difficulties with plantar flexion and inversion. Occasionally, triple or subtalar arthrodesis is necessary to realign the foot and relieve the symptoms.

PEDIATRIC ORTHOPEDICS

The term *orthopaedy* is derived from two Greek words, *orthos,* meaning "straight, upright, or free from deformity," and *paidos,* "a child." It was originally used by Nicholas André in 1741. Musculoskeletal disorders present at birth, arising during growth and development, or secondary to trauma are unique and distinct. Because they are often asymptomatic, diagnosis depends on a fundamental knowledge of their existence, a high index of suspicion, and careful examination.[80]

Developmental Dysplasia of the Hip

Formally known as *congenital dislocation of the hip,* the diagnosis of developmental dysplasia of the hip can readily be made at birth. It has also been detected *in utero* by ultrasound methods. Girls are usually affected, and the left hip is most commonly involved. It frequently occurs in otherwise healthy infants, but can be associated with other congenital abnormalities. Diagnosis is made by noting asymmetric abduction of the flexed hips, foreshortening of the flexed thigh (Galeazzi sign), or asymmetric skin folds. A click or sensation of reduction and dislocation (Ortolani and Barlow signs) may be present. Regular radiographs are not helpful at this stage because of immature development of the acetabulum and the absence of the proximal femoral ossific nuclei.

Problems can arise in diagnosis of bilateral dislocation because of lack of asymmetry. Nevertheless, abduction is limited, a click may be present on examination, and ultrasound reveals bilateral dislocated hips. The latter is the preferred diagnostic adjunct for diagnosis at birth. Treatment is by closed reduction and the application of triple diapers or a simple Pavlik harness, which holds the hips flexed at greater than 90 degrees in midabduction, the so-called "human position." Previously, hips were immobilized in spica casts in full abduction, resulting in a significant incidence of avascular necrosis occasionally involving the uninvolved hip. Appropriate splinting allows for normal development of the hip, which can be monitored clinically and after a few months radiographically. Well recognized radiographic criteria such as the center-edge angle, acetabular index, and Shenton's line are measured and evaluated.[80]

If the diagnosis of developmentally dislocated hip is not made until a child is walking, treatment is much more problematic, frequently requiring open reduction accompanied by varus osteotomy and femoral shortening. Subsequent innominate osteotomy may be necessary if the acetabulum is vertical or shallow and fails adequately to contain the femoral hip.

Adult residua of degenerative dysplasia of the hip include a waddling gait as a result of dislocation of the hip and weak abductors, and ultimately the development of symptomatic arthritic symptoms. Joint replacement in adults with long-standing developmental dysplasia of the hip is difficult because a false acetabulum is frequently present. The hip is high riding, the extremity short, and the femoral canal small. Special acetabular and femoral components are usually needed. Frequently, adult patients with developmental dysplasia of the hip do not become significantly symptomatic until the third or fourth decade.[55,81]

Legg-Calvé-Perthes Disease

Legg-Calvé-Perthes disease is an idiopathic hip disorder occurring in children, usually between 4 and 8 or 9 years of age. It may be detected incidentally in younger children or be characterized by mild discomfort and an intermittent limp. The source of discomfort may be referred to the knee. Physical findings are usually normal unless the process is advanced and a mild limp and limitation of motion, especially abduction, may be present. Radiographs characteristically show variable degrees of avascular changes in the femoral head. The entire head may appear to be involved, only to become revascularized at the completion of the healing phase. Treatment is controversial but has involved efforts to limit weight bearing, use of an abduction brace, or surgical osteotomy of the proximal femur or acetabulum to provide containment of the head with "at-risk" signs radiographically. The younger the child at presentation, the better the prognosis. The older child presenting at 7 or 8 years of age is more likely to have some permanent residua, which can lead to degenerative arthritis in early or middle adult life.[80,81]

Slipped Capital Femoral Epiphysis

The typical presentation of slipped capital femoral epiphysis is in an obese young adolescent lacking secondary sex characteristics and complaining of mild knee pain and a limp. A sudden increase in the pain may occur with acute slip. Bilateral involvement is common, although symptoms may be unilateral. The etiology is unknown, but endocrine and mechanical factors have been suspected.

Treatment for acute slipped capital femoral epiphysis is gentle reduction and percutaneous pinning, and for chronic slips, in situ pinning. Attempts to reduce acute or chronic slips may result in increased damage to the growth plate or kinking of the retinacular vessels, leading to avascular necrosis. A single cannulated screw is placed across the physis. Because the epiphysis is located posteriorly and the metaphysis has actually "slipped" anterolaterally, the starting point is often more proximal and located anteriorly on the femoral neck. Titanium screws should not be used because of their biologic affinity for bone and the great difficulty in removing them should this be necessary. After successful pinning, the physis closes over 3 to 6 months and further slipping is prevented. Because the children are approaching skeletal maturity and the process is often bilateral, leg length discrepancy is not a significant factor.[80]

Club Foot

The diagnosis of talipes equinovarus, or club foot, is readily apparent at birth. This deformity is more rigid and pronounced than the more common metatarsus adductus, which is supple and easily correctable by the examiner. The deformity occurs frequently in otherwise normal infants, but can accompany other developmental abnormalities. Physical examination should include careful spinal evaluation for a hair patch, dimple, or evidence of myelomeningocele, and other spinal or neurologic disorders. Treatment consists of taping the corrected foot and subsequent corrective cast application initially. A percutaneous heel cord lengthening is often indicated after the talonavicular subluxation has been corrected and residual equinus remains to be addressed. For rigid club feet or for those that do not respond to manipulation, taping, or cast treatment, early operative correction is warranted. This correction can be safely performed as early as 6 weeks of age through a (Cincinnati) posterior incision, which allows exposure and release of tethered ligaments, tendons, and joint capsules of the ankle and subtalar joint. Early correction allows the foot to be in a normal position at the time the child begins to ambulate. It also avoids some of the iatrogenic consequences of prolonged casting, false correction, and development of rocker-bottom foot deformity. It is especially valuable in arthrogryposis and other rigid types of flat feet.

Scoliosis

Idiopathic scoliosis is now detected earlier by nearly universal screening methods. Subtle cases of scoliosis or balanced curves may be difficult to detect. Physical findings include shoulder asymmetry or rib hump in pronounced cases with obvious deviation of the spine. Less obvious curves may be missed unless a high index of suspicion is maintained. A screening anteroposterior spinal radiograph centered at T-12, and in cases of obvious kyphosis, a lateral radiograph, should be obtained on initial suspicion of scoliosis. Subsequently, supine side-bending films may be indicated to evaluate the rigidity of the curve and its correctability. Curves of less than 15 degrees require only observation. Curves beyond 20 degrees should be considered for bracing. Some patients have progressive curves, however, ultimately requiring surgical correction. Most patients are girls and have thoracic curves that are convex to the right. The younger the patient at presentation, the more likely is the curve to progress. Although some progression of curves continues slowly in adulthood, rapid progression ceases at skeletal maturity. Indications for surgery are usually relative, but include curves of greater than 35 to 40 degrees, rapidly progressive curves, and symptomatic scoliosis in some adult patients (Fig. 113.39). Curves that are convex to the left should give raise the suspicion of congenital vertebral abnormalities, intraspinal disease, or neuromuscular disease.

Congenital scoliosis may require anterior exposure and resection of a hemivertebra or other associated spinal abnormalities, followed by anterior fusion and usually simultaneous or staged posterior instrumentation. Neurogenic curves frequently require stabilization, especially when they are unbalanced and severe. Large curves can eventually cause respiratory compromise, especially if they exceed 50 to 60 degrees. Curves beyond this level may require anterior release before posterior instrumentation and correction. Long fusions extending to the sacrum with anterior instrumentation may also be necessary for certain curve patterns[56] (Fig. 113.37).

The treatment of scoliosis, kyphosis, and related spinal deformity has undergone extensive evolution. Fortunately, most curves are small or moderate and nonprogressive, requiring only observation or occasionally bracing. If surgery is indicated, powerful systems have been developed to ensure maximum stability while fusion occurs. These include various anterior instrumentation methods, posterior sublaminar wiring and Luque rod techniques, or pedicle screws and segmental instrumentation methodologies (Fig. 113.39).

Neuromuscular Disease

Myelomeningocele

Patients with spina bifida and an open neural arch frequently are first seen after neurosurgical closure of the dural sac. Depending on the level of the myelomeningocele and the extent of neurologic involvement, various neurologic deficits in the lower extremities exist. Patients with high-level myelomeningoceles with absent motor and sensory function from the hips on down are not candidates for ambulation. Patients with preservation of the quadriceps will usually be at least household and sometimes community ambulators. Low-level or sacral myelomeningocele may produce only minor deformity or neurologic deficits in the foot or toes. A high arch or cavus foot and claw toe deformity should alert the examiner to the possibility of spinal or other neurologic problem. Treatment is designed to optimize ambulatory function by appropriate physical therapy, bracing, or, where indicated, surgical procedures. These procedures may include operations

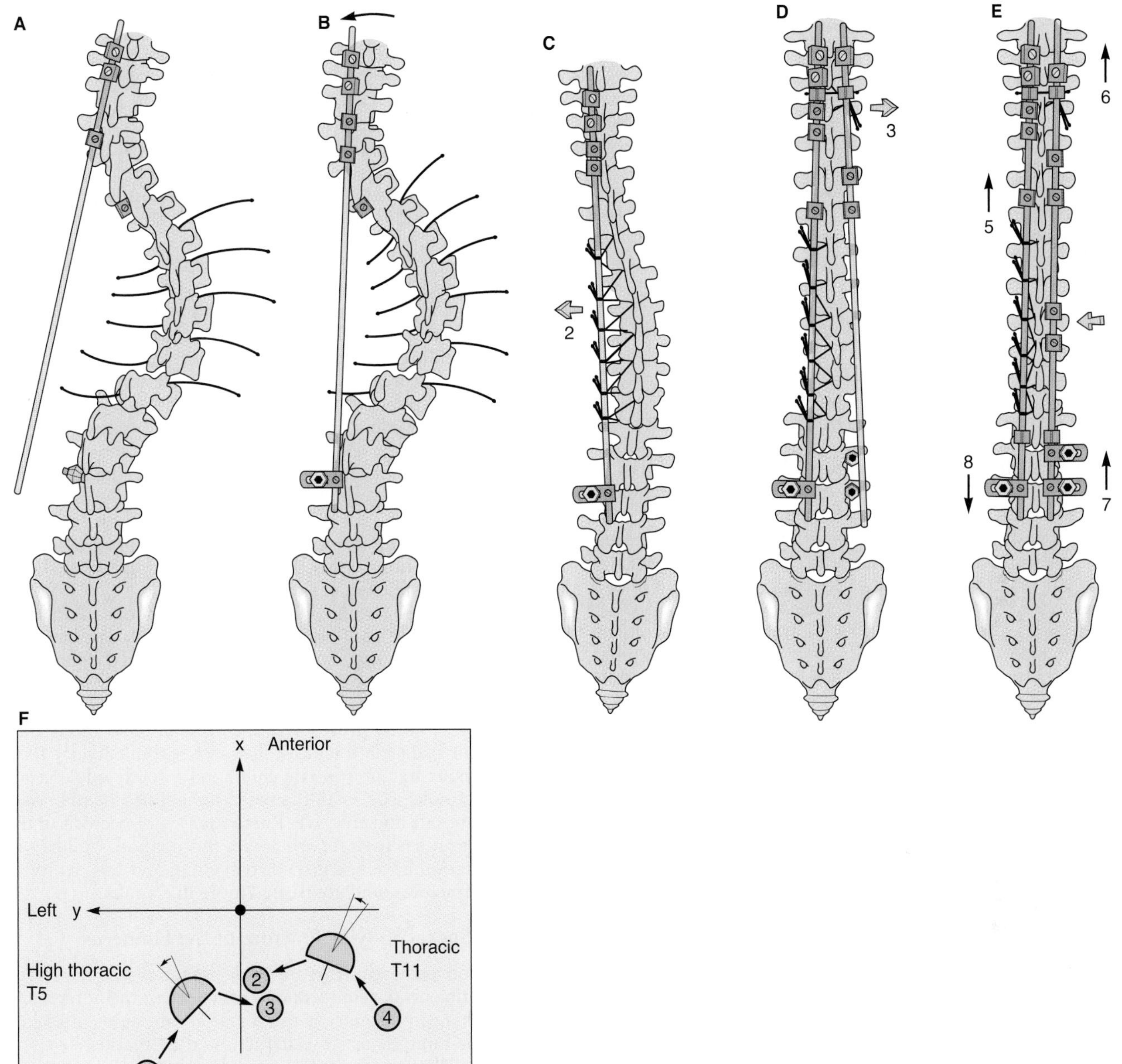

FIGURE 113.39 Idiopathic scoliosis, double thoracic curve. (*A*) After placement of the left anchors and initial placement of longitudinal member (note that the low hook of the claw is placed sublaminar). (*B*) After securing of convex longitudinal member to the lower anchor, resulting in T-2 coronal plane angular position correction. (*C*) Low thoracic curve requiring medial and, if necessary, posterior translation. (*D*) Initial placement of right-side rod, during which the T-2 coronal plane force couple is completed. (*E*) After construct completion. (*F*) Drawing of transverse plane apex force couples. In reality, application of a transverse plane high thoracic curve apex force couple is difficult because of the constraints placed by the rib cage.

to treat dislocated hips, unless they are bilateral, release contractures, and correct deformities in the foot. Tendon lengthening and occasionally tendon transfers may be helpful in select cases. Stretching and splinting exercises by the parents, physical therapists, and occupational therapists are an important part of the treatment regimen.[80]

Cerebral Palsy

Affected children usually have undergone anoxia at birth. Difficult labor and delivery, prematurity, and low birth weight are frequently found in the history of children with cerebral palsy. Acquired cases may be secondary to head injury, near drowning, or congenital and familial syndromes. The disease is characterized by developmental delay, psychomotor retardation, and, usually, spasticity. Intellectual capacity may range from normal or superior to profoundly deficient. Many of the latter children are totally dependent for all activities of daily living and have no ambulatory potential.

Treatment is designed to optimize function and neuromuscular control. Much of the treatment and care of these children involves physical therapists, occupational therapists, and special education teachers through a coordinated program. Parents become heavily involved in the adaptive and developmental needs of these children. Orthotists are important to fashion and fabricate appropriate splints and to modify wheelchairs.

Orthopedic treatment consists of orchestrating many of the child's musculoskeletal needs and, where indicated, appropriate surgery to release contracted joints, occasional tendon transfers, and the prevention and treatment of hip subluxation or dislocation. Spinal curves should be appropriately followed and treated with bracing or spinal fusion when indicated. Stretching exercises and night splints such as ankle—foot orthoses or knee immobilizers are helpful in preventing contractures or maintaining postoperative correction.

Pediatric Fractures

Fractures in children are unique in several ways. The blood supply to the developing skeleton and the thick periosteum covering long bones results in rapid and predictable fracture healing. Nonunion is extremely rare. Most pediatric fractures can be treated by closed reduction and casting techniques. In the case of femur fractures, skin traction in younger children for a few days can be followed by the application of a spica cast. Some shortening and deformity can be accepted because slight overgrowth and subsequent remodeling result in an excellent functional and cosmetic result. The time in plaster varies for the involved fracture, but usually is 5 to 6 weeks.[81,82]

In contradistinction, injuries or fractures involving the growth plate (physis) can produce permanent disability, deformity, and joint destruction unless treated appropriately. Salter and Harris have developed a classification of injuries to the growth plate (Fig. 113.40). Types I and II injuries do not cross the growth plate and heal well after closed reduction, with no residua in most cases. Type III fractures involve the physis (growth plate) and epiphysis and require accurate reduction if displaced by more than 2 mm (Fig. 113.41). Type IV injuries cross the metaphysis, growth plate, and epiphysis.

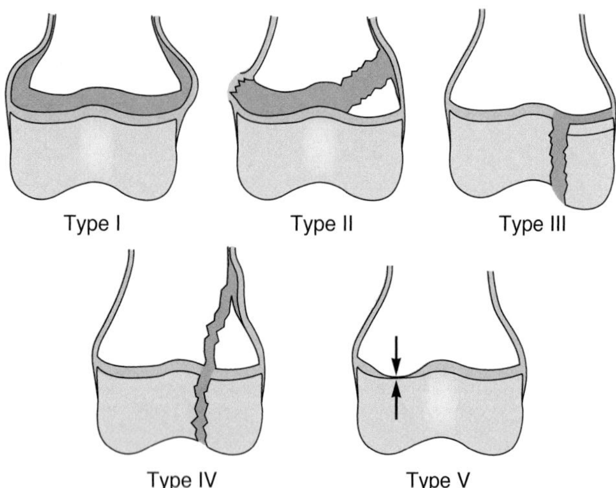

FIGURE 113.40 Salter-Harris classification of epiphyseal injuries. Type I injury is an epiphyseolysis of the involved growth plate without associated fracture. Type II has an additional metaphyseal fracture fragment. Type I and II injuries have a good prognosis and are usually treated with closed reduction and casting. Type III injury results in a fracture through the growth plate and epiphysis. Type IV fracture crosses the epiphysis, growth plate (physis), and metaphysis. Type III and IV injuries require careful open reduction and internal fixation if displaced. Type V injury involves a crush of the growth plate without a fracture and is usually detected late by asymmetric or premature closure of the growth plate.

They demand careful and accurate open reduction and internal fixation, and are associated with potential for growth arrest and subsequent deformity. Type V injuries involve a crush of the growth plate that usually is not visible on plain radiographs, but is determined subsequently by growth arrest and shortening, or deformity of the site of injury.[16,81,82]

Computed tomographic evaluation of fractures involving the growth plate can be helpful. Juvenile Tillaux and triplane fractures occur in adolescence because of a closing distal tibial growth plate and require open reduction if closed reduction is not successful.

After open reduction and internal fixation, stabilization of type III and IV fractures is by Kirschner wire or screw fixation, avoiding the growth plate. The prognosis is usually good when atraumatic anatomic reduction has been achieved. Nevertheless, in young children, types III and IV injuries must be watched closely. Treatment of subsequent growth arrest may require completion of epiphyseodesis to prevent asymmetric deformity. Contralateral stapling or epiphyseodesis may be appropriately timed to prevent leg length discrepancy. In very short patients, or those with significant discrepancies, lengthening using distraction osteogenesis and Ilizarov techniques may be attempted (Figs. 113.31, 113.32). These operations require accurate assessment of the rate of growth inhibition, progression of deformity, amount of growth remaining, and anticipated discrepancy at completion of skeletal growth.

In infants and young children, fractures about joints may be difficult to evaluate because the epiphysis is cartilaginous and anlage of the ossific nuclei has not appeared. Obtaining radiographs of the opposite site for comparison is helpful in these situations.

Except as noted previously, open reduction is rarely performed for pediatric fractures; however, intramedullary fixation of femur fractures in late childhood or early adolescence is usually indicated. Small-diameter, nonreamed flexible rods (Ender) are safe and effective. Rarely, avascular necrosis of the femoral head has been reported with this method. Children in this age group have less growth remaining and less ability to remodel fractures, and are treated more like adults.[82]

Supracondylar Fracture of the Humerus

A common pediatric fracture with potential for disastrous complications is the supracondylar fracture of the humerus.[83] The mechanism of injury is usually a fall on the outstretched hand. The injury is usually characterized by marked swelling about the elbow with associated deformity and occasionally neurologic deficits. Treatment of choice is closed reduction and cross-pinning with fine Kirschner wires followed by splinting for 3 weeks, at which time the fracture is usually healed (Fig. 113.42). Open reduction infrequently is necessary. Volkmann ischemic contracture is not encountered with this form of treatment; rather, this complication is related to closed reduction and splinting in acute flexion that kinks off neurovascular structures and leads to compartment syndrome, fibrosis, and a permanent withered hand.

Fractures of the Lateral and Medial Epicondyles of the Humerus

Fractures of the lateral epicondyle of the humerus in children have potential for misdiagnosis, with radiographic displacement appearing slight because the epicondyle is largely cartilaginous. These injuries are usually type IV epiphyseal injuries and require accurate open reduction and internal fixation. Even with this treatment, cubitus valgus deformity develops in a certain percentage of patients owing to growth plate closure on the lateral side. This closure can lead to tardy ulnar nerve palsy later in life because of deformity and chronic stretching of the nerve.[81,82] Fractures of the medial epicondyle may also

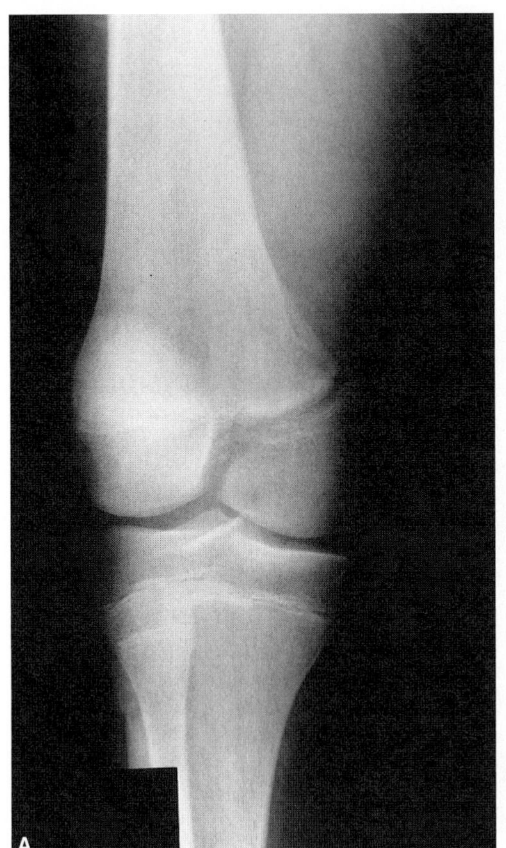

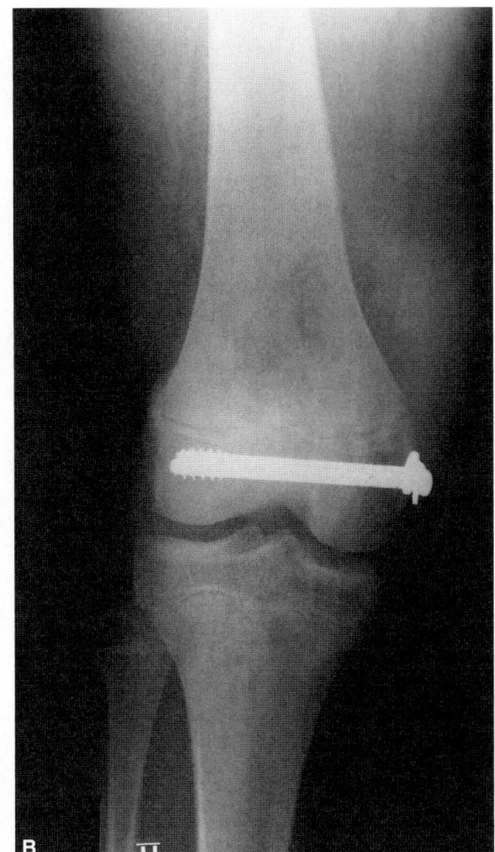

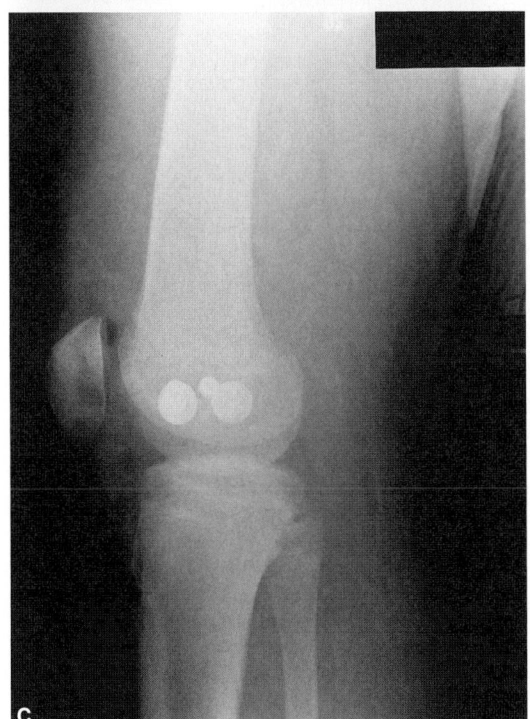

FIGURE 113.41 (*A*) Salter-Harris type III epiphyseal fracture of the medial femoral condyle in 14-year-old boy. (*B*) Anteroposterior radiograph after anatomic open reduction and internal fixation with cannulated lag screws. (*C*) Postoperative lateral radiograph of type III medial femoral condylar epiphyseal fracture. Note that lag screws avoid the growth plate on both views. Premature closure of the medial portion of distal femoral growth could produce a varus deformity of the knee. Complete symmetric closure of the growth plate would result in slight shortening. Both deformities are likely to be less problematic because the patient is approaching skeletal maturity. Primary indication for surgery was restoration of articular congruity as in adults.

require open reduction if significantly displaced. They are occasionally entrapped in the joint when associated with elbow dislocation and may render the joint irreducible by closed methods. Other pediatric elbow fractures that may require surgical treatment include open fractures, fractures of the ulna associated with radial head dislocation (Monteggia fractures), and unstable fracture–dislocations.

Femoral Neck Fractures

Femoral neck fractures in children are fortunately very uncommon, because they have a significant risk of avascular necrosis and growth disturbance. This risk may occur with closed or open treatment. Closed reduction and percutaneous pinning for minimally displaced fractures or careful open

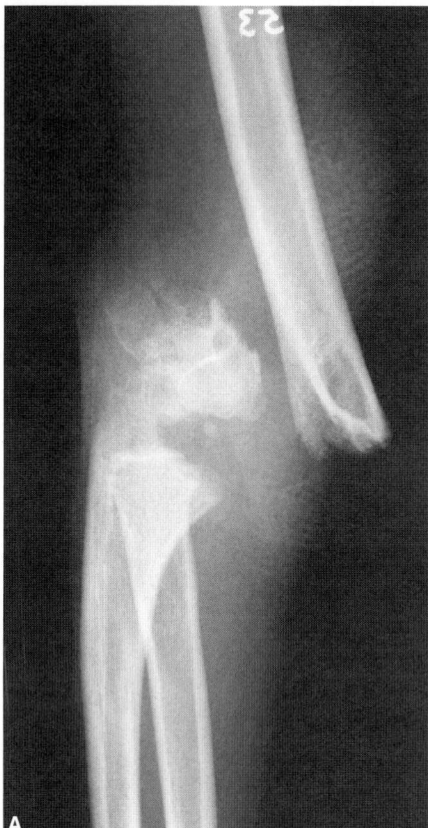

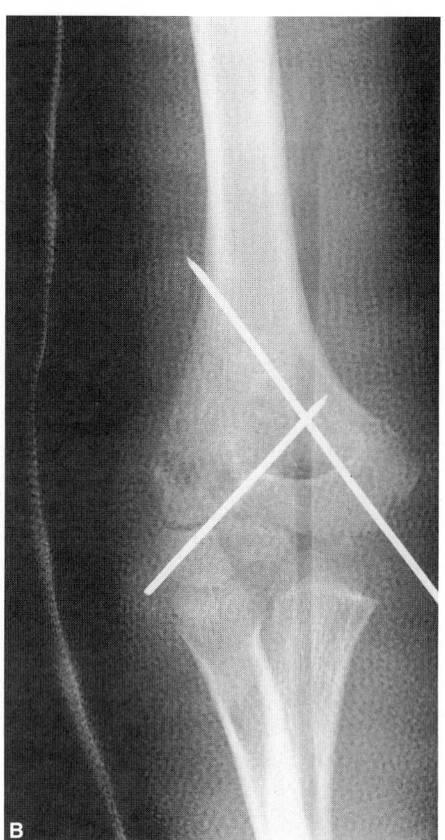

FIGURE 113.42 (*A*) A 10-year-old patient with a severely displaced supracondylar fracture of the humerus associated with brachial artery avulsion but a viable, well perfused hand, good collateral flow, and intact neurologic function. (*B*) Anteroposterior radiograph. Fracture healed rapidly with an excellent functional result.

reduction for displaced fractures is indicated (Fig. 113.14). Femoral neck fracture is a serious injury with potential for permanent disability, especially in young children with much growth remaining.[81,82]

Closed Reduction and Casting

Children requiring reduction of fractures should usually be seen for a cast check the next day. Admission for observation may be indicated for severely displaced fractures or whenever significant swelling is anticipated. Casts applied to the extremities should be split anteriorly and spread slightly to accommodate any swelling. Should this occur after discharge, the parents can be instructed in the method of spreading the split cast to relieve pressure. Children younger than 5 years of age may have difficulty using crutches after lower extremity fracture and may be treated for a brief period in a wheelchair until the fracture has healed. Older children usually are able to manage crutches or pediatric walkers. With appropriate diagnosis and treatment, as well as attention to the caveats and pitfalls noted previously, most children with fractures have excellent results.

Pediatric Bone and Joint Infection

In contrast to adults, septic arthritis or acute hematogenous osteomyelitis frequently occurs in otherwise healthy children. There may be an antecedent sore throat or upper respiratory illness, or a history of minor trauma. The latter can be a diagnostic pitfall because radiographic evaluation of a swollen extremity reveals no fracture and no evidence of bone infection for at least the first 10 to 14 days. Clearly, diagnosis must be made well before this period if permanent sequelae are to be avoided.

Septic Arthritis

It is urgent that the diagnosis of septic arthritis be made promptly in infants, especially when it involves the hip joint. In neonates, the classic signs of infection such as elevated temperature and white blood cell count may be absent. Pseudoparalysis or apparent inability to move a limb, associated with crying or irritability with passive motion, is frequently present. Ultrasound may be helpful in revealing fluid in the joint or capsular edema. The diagnosis is secured by aspiration of infected fluid or frank pus, yielding organisms on Gram strain and subsequent culture and sensitivity. *Staphylococcus aureus* is the most frequent organism encountered, although in neonates gram-negative organisms and in young children *Haemophilus* species may be encountered. Once the diagnosis has been made, immediate surgical drainage is indicted, followed by administration of appropriate antibiotics dictated by culture and sensitivity. Late diagnosis frequently results in hip dislocation, chondrolysis, and ultimate joint destruction.

Involvement of other joints is somewhat more forgiving, but still demands surgical irrigation and débridement if the joint is distended. The knee joint may be aspirated for small effusions, and local installation of antibiotics in addition to IV administration may suffice. In older children and adolescents, arthroscopic irrigation as with adults is indicated.[84,85]

Hematogenous Osteomyelitis

The diagnosis of hematogenous osteomyelitis is secured as for septic arthritis. In addition, there may be obvious tenderness, swelling, and erythema over a long bone. When these findings are present over a subcutaneous border such as the tibia, osteomyelitis is present until ruled out by aspiration. The latter is the diagnostic procedure of choice and should be performed promptly. In children and adolescents, systemic signs of infection such as elevated temperature, white blood cell count, and, in particular, erythrocyte sedimentation rate are present. The differential diagnosis may include insect stings, rheumatoid arthritis, and especially minor trauma. Osteomyelitis may accompany septic arthritis; therefore, at the time of surgical decompression of infected joints, the metaphysis should also be drilled to rule out or drain an associated focus of osteomyelitis. This is especially true in the hip and shoulder joint, where the physis is intraarticular.[81,85]

Multifocal osteomyelitis may present with several sites of involvement and be confused with inflammatory arthritis. These children are frequently desperately ill and rapidly become septic. Early surgical drainage and appropriate antibiotic treatment yields excellent results. Delayed diagnosis may lead to systemic complications such as bacterial endocarditis or local destruction of the physis with resultant growth arrest. The sequelae of this are severe, especially in the younger child with considerable growth remaining.

Most musculoskeletal infections are bacterial, although viral and fungal infections can occur. Likewise, tuberculosis should be suspected in children who are born in or who have lived in areas of the developing world where tuberculosis is endemic.[86] Tuberculous arthritis of the hip has been mistakenly diagnosed as Legg-Calvé-Perthes disease with disastrous results. The spine may also be involved. Tuberculous arthritis has a longer prodrome and symptoms present gradually so that radiographic changes are usually apparent at the time of presentation but can easily be misinterpreted. Treatment is surgical decompression and antituberculous or other antimicrobial agents as indicated.

ORTHOPEDIC ONCOLOGY

Cancer is a leading cause of death in the United States and throughout the world. As a result, metastatic disease of bone is much more commonly encountered than primary malignant tumors of bone. The latter are dreaded tumors that appear primarily in children and young adults, whereas metastatic disease is more common in middle-aged and elderly people.

In general, treatment for primary bone tumors involves limb salvage procedures or amputation. The former is elected if the tumor is confined or involves a specific compartment of an extremity. Primary malignant bone tumors frequently present in healthy, active adolescents and young adults and thus have significant associated psychosocial implications. Therefore, whenever feasible, limb salvage is the procedure of choice because 5-year survival rates for appropriately selected cases are similar to those with amputation. CT and especially MRI scans are an essential part of preoperative planning. Adjunctive chemotherapy or radiation is administered as dictated by the oncologist.[87,88]

METASTATIC DISEASE OF BONE

Metastatic disease of bone is the most common cause of neoplastic bone lesions. Many different types of cancer can metastasize, but the most common sources are breast, prostate, and renal cell cancer. Increased survival is a result of early detection and the institution of chemotherapy. This, however, results in a clinically increased incidence of bony metastasis and related pathologic long bone fractures. Metastatic carcinoma is the most common malignancy of bone, affecting more than 40 times as many patients as are affected by all other types of bone cancer combined. The goals of treatment are the alleviation of pain, preservation of function, and prevention of pathologic fracture.

Specific Treatment

Impending fractures of long bones are best treated by closed intramedullary fixation. It is extremely important to detect impending fractures before they occur because open treatment is associated with greater morbidity due to infection, bleeding, and dissemination of tumor cells. Polymethylmethacrylate cement may be necessary to stabilize areas of bone loss. Because survival is usually limited, fracture healing is less important than stability.[88] Metastases involving joints frequently require resection and customized total joint arthroplasty. Often, polymethylmethacrylate cement is necessary to fill defects and anchor prosthetic components. Preoperative workup includes CT, MRI, and, where indicated, arteriography.

Metastatic Disease of the Spine

Impending paraplegia may require anterior decompression, resection of tumor, and insertion of titanium cages, local distraction constructs, or other means supplemented by polymethylmethacrylate cement to create an immediately stable situation. Posterior stabilization may also be necessary. Bony fusion is not expected or required in this case because treatment is entirely palliative.[88]

Soft Tissue Sarcomas of Extremities

Soft tissue sarcomas are derived from mesodermal tissues, and pseudoencapsulation by surrounding fibrous connective tissue is consistent finding. Metastatic spread to the lungs by the hematogenous route is present in approximately 10% of cases at diagnosis. In general, sarcomas tend to remain well confined to an anatomic compartment until late in the course of the disease or on destruction by surgical procedure. Preoperative workup includes CT or MRI scans to determine the fine extent of the tumor. Depending on the location and histologic grade, wide or radical excision is indicated, followed by limb salvage procedures or amputation where necessary[88]

BENIGN BONE TUMORS

Benign bone tumors are more common and may range from small, incidental lesions in asymptomatic patients to large lesions capable of producing pathologic fracture. Except in the latter instance, most benign bone tumors are minimally symptomatic. They are often diagnosed by their characteristic radiographic appearance. Frequently, this is an isolated lesion of bone, usually with elliptical and well circumscribed sclerotic borders. The cortex of a long bone may be expanded but usually is not violated, and there is no invasion of soft tissue. Unusual appearing or atypical lesions may warrant biopsy for definitive diagnosis (Table 113.5). Differential diagnosis includes infection, which can mimic many bone tumors, as well as congenital, developmental, or acquired bone lesions.[89]

TABLE 113.5

COMMON SKELETAL NEOPLASMS

Type	Bone	Cartilage	Fibrous	Marrow
Benign	Osteoid osteoma Osteoblastoma	Osteochondroma Enchondroma Chondroblastoma	Nonossifying fibroma Giant cell tumor Desmoplastic fibroma	Eosinophilic granuloma
Malignant	Osteosarcoma Periosteal osteosarcoma	Primary chondrosarcoma Secondary chondrosarcoma	Fibrosarcoma Fibrous histiocytoma	Ewing's sarcoma Lymphoma Myeloma

Osteochondroma

Osteochondroma is a cartilage-capped bony projection involving primarily the metaphyseal regions of long bones. It is the most common of all benign tumors (45%). Most tumors are located about the knee, shoulder, or ankle and are minimally symptomatic. The stalk projects away from the adjacent joint. Malignant transformation is extremely uncommon for isolated lesions (Fig. 113.43A). Multiple lesions are seen in the hereditary form known as *multiple hereditary osteochondromatosis*

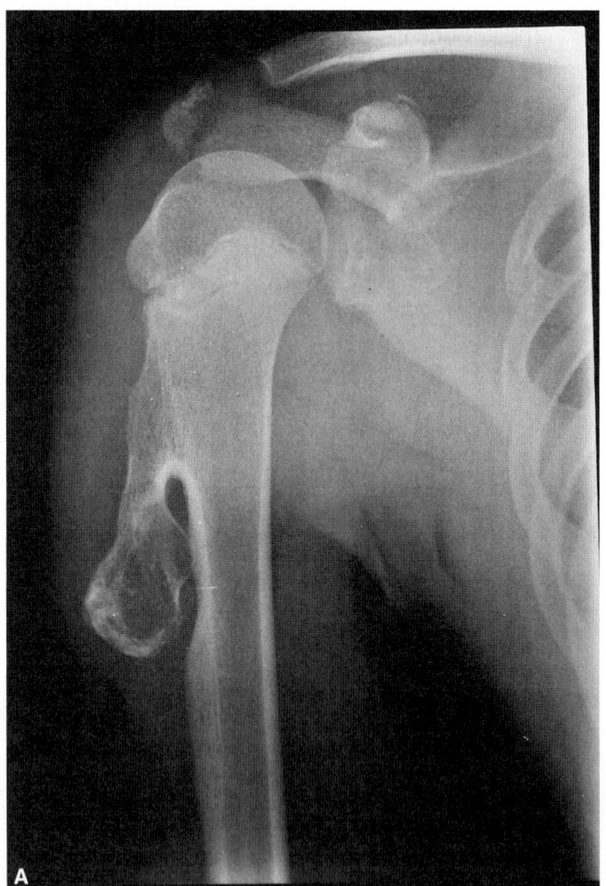

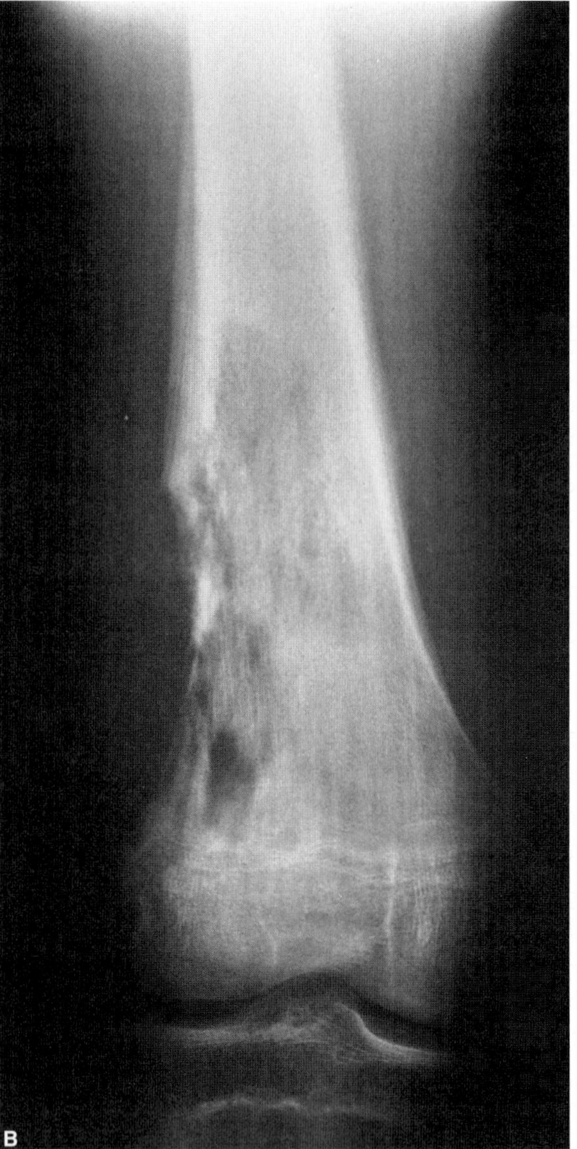

FIGURE 113.43 (*A*) Osteochondroma: typical appearance of a benign lesion. Osteochondroma is the most common benign bone tumor, representing 45% of all benign tumors. (*B*) Characteristic appearance of a malignant tumor in an adolescent patient. Note destruction of bone, cortical erosion, invasion of soft tissue, and subperiosteal new bone formation. Treatment in this case was amputation.

or *multiple exostosis*. Defective longitudinal growth and deformation of affected bones is present, producing variable symptoms. Malignant transformation is more common (5% to 15%) than in solitary lesions. Surgical resection is indicated only occasionally for large lesions or to rule out rare malignant transformation.

Enchondroma

Enchondroma is the second most common benign bone tumor and accounts for 10% of all benign lesions. Round or ovoid tumors exhibiting fine cartilage stippling or "popcorn" appearance are seen on plain radiographs. The short tubular bones of the hands and feet are the most common locations. Most tumors are asymptomatic and are found incidentally. Larger tumors in atypical locations may be difficult to differentiate from low-grade chondrosarcoma.

Ollier's disease is a nonhereditary disseminated form also known as *multiple enchondromatosis*. Large numbers of cartilaginous tumors are present and have a significant risk (30% to 50%) of malignant degeneration to chondrosarcoma. Maffucci syndrome is characterized by associated multiple soft tissue angiomas in the skin and subcutaneous tissues.

Osteoid Osteoma

Osteoid osteoma is a relatively common, curious lesion of bone characterized by nocturnal pain relieved by aspirin. The classic presentation is present in most cases, strongly suggesting the diagnosis by history. Histologically, a small (<1 cm) osteoid nidus usually surrounded by a zone of reactive bone formation is present. The ends of long bones are frequently but not exclusively affected. Bone scans are strongly positive. CT is often the diagnostic study of choice and helps with preoperative planning. Surgical resection is dramatically curative but must include complete excision of the nidus.

Osteoblastoma

Osteoblastoma accounts for 3% of all benign bone tumors, and most present in the second and third decades. Because of similar histologic characteristics, it has been referred to as *giant osteoid osteoma*. The lesion has a distinct predilection for the axial skeleton and vertebral column; approximately 30% to 40% involve the posterior elements. Conventional tomography and CT scan are helpful in localization and surgical planning. Resectable tumors are treated by excision and curettage as for osteoid osteoma. Reported recurrence rates are less than 20%. Radiation has been used for large symptomatic lesions that are unresectable.

Unicameral Bone Cyst

Of unicameral bone cysts, 80% to 90% of these circumscribed lytic lesions are found in the metaphysis of the proximal humerus or femur. Most benign bone cysts occur in children. Current treatment involves interlesional steroid injections with an approximately 50% to 80% healing rate, which is comparable with that of surgical curettage and bone graft. The latter procedure, obviously, has greater morbidity but is indicated for large lesions, especially near the hip joint, with impending or frank pathologic fracture.

Aneurysmal Bone Cyst

Aneurysmal bone cyst has a slight female predilection and occurs most frequently in adolescents. The cyst is blood filled and presents as a painful swelling, usually over a long bone. Treatment is by curettage and bone graft, although steroid injection can be tried. Radiation therapy or adjunctive cryotherapy is used for recurrent cysts, especially those that have some degree of soft tissue extension. Occasionally, preoperative arterial embolization may be helpful.

Nonossifying Fibroma

Most lesions in nonossifying fibroma are asymptomatic and are discovered incidentally. They are frequently found in the metaphyseal regions of long bones in adolescents or young adults. Radiographically, the appearance is characteristic, revealing a small, eccentrically located lytic region with a scalloped, thin, sclerotic border. Rarely, curettage and bone grafting may be necessary for symptomatic legions.

Fibrous Dysplasia

Fibrous dysplasia is a disease of childhood that may be monostotic or polyostotic. It is a benign developmental condition usually discovered as an incidental radiographic finding on examination. Some patients, however, may have pain and progressive deformity, especially with lesions about the proximal femur, where the characteristic "shepherd's crook" is present. Treatment is indicated for pathologic or impending pathologic fracture and consists of curettage, bone grafting, and frequently surgical stabilization. Albright syndrome is a triad of polyostotic fibrous dysplasia, endocrinopathy, and café au lait skin lesions.

Eosinophilic Granuloma

Radiographically, this condition appears as a solitary or occasionally multifocal lytic lesion of bone and is characteristically found in long bones, skull, and ribs. The margins of the lesions are usually well defined, although some periosteal reaction may be present, making differentiation from malignant tumors difficult. Small or asymptomatic lesions require observation only, and larger lesions are treated by curettage, cryosurgery, or low-dose radiation therapy. Histologically, the lesion contains multinucleated giant cells, eosinophils, and mononuclear Langerhans cells. Multifocal lesions may be associated with other manifestations similar to the spectrum of diseases termed *histiocytosis X,* with diabetes insipidus, adenopathy, and hepatosplenomegaly.

Chondroblastoma

Chondroblastoma is an uncommon cartilaginous tumor of adolescents and young adults. Symptoms are variable, but because of the typical location, joint complaints predominate. This lesion, along with giant cell tumor, occurs specifically in the epiphysis as a lytic round hole in bone. Fine cartilaginous stippling may be present. Treatment is thorough curettage and bone grafting, which is usually curative. The tumor is usually considered to be benign, although very rare metastases have been reported.

Giant Cell Tumor

This tumor is usually eccentric and located in the metaphysis or epiphysis of long bones, with 50% of lesions occurring about the knee. Proximal humerus and distal radius are also common locations, and the sacrum may be involved. Typically, the lesions present with a painful, slowly enlarging mass. The tumor frequently extends to the subchondral bone of the adjacent joint, rendering treatment with preservation of function difficult. Curettage and bone grafting may be appropriate for small lesions. More aggressive lesions, which demonstrate expansion and thinning of the cortices, may require filling of the cavity with polymethylmethacrylate, either definitively or as a temporary measure, followed by bone grafting in 4 to 6 months. Lesions with extension into adjacent soft tissue require *en bloc* resection.[88] The recurrence rate is significant for larger, more aggressive lesions. Occasionally, *en bloc* resection with modified arthrodesis, allograft, or prosthetic reconstruction is indicated. In the knee, this operation may require distal femoral resection and total knee replacement (Fig. 113.18).

Malignant Bone Tumors

Malignant Myeloma

Myeloma is the most common primary tumor of bone, accounting for 40% to 50% of all malignant bone tumors. It is largely a disease of middle age and beyond, with most patients between the ages of 50 and 70 years. Isolated lesions may occur, but eventual dissemination or progression to widespread skeletal involvement is more common. Multiple lytic lesions may involve the axial skeleton, skull, or vertebral column.

Diagnosis may first be made by the occurrence of pathologic fracture from a trivial injury. Pain is prominent and often severe, and is usually associated with systemic symptoms of malaise and fatigue. Most patients are anemic because of replacement of hematopoietic marrow. Classically, a monoclonal gammopathy demonstrated on serum protein electrophoresis is present. So-called light-chain disease may occur and be detected by urine electrophoresis. Very rarely, a hypogammaglobulinemia may be present with the so-called "nonsecretory" form of the disease.

Treatment is chemotherapy, with most protocols using melphalan and other antineoplastic agents. Steroids are used occasionally to relieve symptoms. Solitary lesions may be treated by radiation, and surgical intervention is indicted for impending or acute pathologic fractures. Long bones should be rodded before fracture whenever possible. Vertebral involvement with neurologic symptoms dictates decompression and stabilization, usually through an anterior approach. The overall prognosis is poor, with a mean survival of 32 months. Death is usually caused by to intercurrent infection, pancytopenia, and renal failure.[88]

Osteogenic Sarcoma

Osteogenic sarcoma is the second most common primary malignant bone tumor, accounting for approximately 20% of all malignant tumors. Adolescents or young adults are most frequently affected. The long bones are more frequently involved, with approximately half the cases occurring about the knee. Patients present clinically with a brief history of pain and swelling, or occasionally with a pathologic fracture. Depending on the type of tumor cells elaborated, osteoblastic, chondroblastic, or fibroblastic subtypes may be present.

Radiographically, the lesion appears as mixed lytic and blastic lesion with aggressive, indistinct margins, cortical destruction, and subperiosteal new bone formation (Fig. 113.43B), giving rise to its typical "sunburst" appearance. An uncommon variant is the parosteal sarcoma that rises on the surface of the bone. This tumor has a better prognosis than conventional osteosarcomas, and has a well differentiated histologic appearance.

Careful preoperative staging and a multidisciplinary approach are essential to developing a treatment plan. A staging classification for malignant tumors is shown in Table 113.6. For high-grade osteosarcoma, amputation is the treatment of choice and has a 5-year survival rate of approximately 20%. Neoadjuvant chemotherapy is used and is especially important in limb salvage, where its preoperative administration reduces the tumor mass.

The goal of limb salvage surgery is to provide local control of the tumor comparable with amputation while maintaining reasonable functional status of the extremity. Reconstruction techniques after resection depend on the location of the tumor. They include allograft replacement, custom prosthesis, or arthrodesis. Current 5-year survival rates with a multidisciplinary approach range from 40% to 60%. Overall survival with limb salvage surgery is comparable with that of amputation in appropriately selected cases. Death results from metastatic disease, frequently involving the lungs. Selective pulmonary metastases may be treated by surgical resection.[90]

TABLE 113.6 STAGING

STAGING FOR MALIGNANT TUMORS (ENNEKING)

Stage	Grade	Site	Metastasis
IA	Low	Intracompartmental	None
IB	Low	Extracompartmental	None
IIA	High	Intracompartmental	None
IIB	High	Extracompartmental	None
III	Any	Any	Present

Chondrosarcoma

Chondrosarcoma accounts for approximately 10% of malignant tumors and tends to occur in older people. Approximately 75% of the lesions are located in the pelvis or proximal portions of the humerus or femur. Frequently, they are slow growing, and variable symptoms may be present for months or years before treatment. Local recurrence is common, but metastases occur infrequently. Chondrosarcomas have a characteristic radiographic appearance, presenting predominantly lytic lesions containing stippled calcification and usually cortical destruction.

High-grade lesions may require amputation; however, wide excision with or without prosthetic replacement may be indicated, especially when the proximal femur or humerus is involved. Internal hemipelvectomy and fusion may be indicated for pelvic lesions.[90] The survival rate for low-grade lesions after 5 years approaches 50%. Highly malignant chondrosarcoma has a poor prognosis despite treatment, with a 5-year survival rate of less than 10%.[89]

Malignant Fibrous Histiocytoma and Fibrosarcoma

These tumors account for less than 5% of primary osseous malignancies and affect both sexes equally. They occur over a wide age distribution, and have a skeletal distribution similar to that of osteosarcoma. Clinical symptoms may be present for significant periods, including variable degrees of pain, swelling, and functional loss. Radiographically, the lesion appears as an osteolytic area of bone destruction with frequent soft tissue extension, and cortical erosion. As with other malignant tumors, CT and MRI are essential to determine the extent of the tumor. Histologically, the tumors are characterized by spindle-shaped cells of fibrous origin arranged in a herringbone pattern. Considerable variation in the degree of anaplasia exists.

Surgical treatment depends on the location and size of the tumor. Low-grade lesions are treated by minimal to limb-sparing surgery, whereas high-grade lesions require radical excision, or amputation. The overall 5-year survival rate is approximately 30% and is correlated to histologic grade of the tumor, with the well differentiated lesions having a distinctly better prognosis.

Ewing's Sarcoma

Ewing's sarcoma accounts for approximately 5% of primary bone tumors, and more than 90% of the patients are younger than 30 years of age. Histologically, this is a highly anaplastic, small round cell tumor, possibly of neuroectodermal origin.

Any bone may be involved, but typically the metaphysis is involved with extension onto the shaft of the long bone.

Radiographically, a moth-eaten appearance results from combined lytic and blastic foci. Periosteal new bone formation may form multiple layers, giving rise to the classic "onion skin" appearance. In the past, recommended treatment consisted of radiation and chemotherapy. Surgical resection is indicated, especially for involvement of expendable bones. One of the most lethal sarcomas, Ewing's tumor historically had a 5-year survival rate of less than 20%. However, with contemporary protocols using surgery, radiation, and chemotherapy, 5-year survival rates have improved to approximately 40%.[91]

Malignant Lymphoma

Malignant lymphoma is an uncommon neoplasm of the reticuloendothelial system. It accounts for less than 5% of primary bone malignancies. Although any age group can be affected, it is more common in the fifth, sixth, and seventh decades. Histologically, the tumor consists of small cells containing a fine reticulum network. Multinucleated Reed-Sternberg cells may be present, especially with Hodgkin disease. Radiographically, a lytic lesion with distinct margins and cortical destruction may be present, or occasionally a sclerotic appearance may be seen. Differentiation from metastatic carcinoma, osteomyelitis, or Ewing's sarcoma may be difficult. Radiation therapy is the mainstay of treatment. Like other round cell tumors, bone lymphoma is radiosensitive. Surgical treatment is reserved for impending or frank pathologic fractures. The overall 5-year survival rate is approximately 50%, significantly better than with Ewing's sarcoma, despite histologic similarity.

Chordoma

Chordoma originates from primitive notochord remnants, accounts for approximately 1% to 4% of primary bone tumors, and often presents late. These tumors arise in the midline of the axial skeleton. Approximately half are located in the sacral coccygeal region of the pelvis and are notoriously difficult to visualize radiographically. Approximately 35% are at the base of the skull, and the remainder arise in the vertebrae. Peak incidence is in the fifth to sixth decades, with men affected twice as often as women. Evidence of osseous destruction may be seen on plain film; CT and MRI scans enhance visualization.[89] Treatment is surgical resection and radiation therapy, with survival closely related to the location of the tumor and the ability to achieve a wide surgical margin. When that is possible, a 10-year survival rate of approximately 85% is reported. The survival rate with sacral chordoma is approximately 40% at 10 years.

Adamantinoma

Adamantinoma is a rare tumor has a distinct tendency to occur in the tibial diaphysis, accounting for more than 90% of lesions. Adamantinoma occurs most often in the second to fifth decades and presents with pain and a palpable bony mass. On radiography, the lesion is usually seen in the mid-diaphysis of the tibia with a blistered, expanded, thin cortex. Treatment is by wide *en bloc* resection, if possible, and otherwise by amputation.[89] Pathologically, epithelial cells oriented in palisaded fashion are seen, with center islands of spindle cells.

BONE AND JOINT INFECTIONS IN ADULTS

Infections involving bone and joints have historically been among the most feared and difficult of clinical problems. Because of the rigid structure, vulnerable vascularity, and unique anatomy of bone, infection is often hard to treat and in some cases cannot be completely eradicated—hence the emphasis on strict aseptic surgical technique, avoidance of hematomas, and use of prophylactic antibiotics. The prevention of bone and joint infection is a far easier task than the treatment of established osteomyelitis and related complications.

Exogenous Osteomyelitis

Open fractures, especially when they involve the lower extremity, are the most common cause of infection and chronic osteomyelitis.[7,8] Treatment of early postoperative orthopedic infection is prompt return to surgery, evacuation of hematomas, and irrigation and débridement of the wound, followed by appropriate antimicrobial therapy.

In the absence of drainage, subacute or chronic infection can be more difficult to diagnose. It is frequently associated with pain, delayed or absent fracture healing, loss of fixation, and abnormal laboratory values. Definitive diagnosis is established by aspiration or culture and sensitivity studies of surgical specimens.

Treatment requires irrigation and débridement and, at times, resection of significant portions of necrotic bone. The resultant segmental defects are dealt with as discussed earlier. Long-standing cases of chronic osteomyelitis may be associated with soft tissue ulcerations, induration, and foul-smelling sinus drainage. Radiographs may show extensive destruction of bone or sclerotic appearance of dead bone. Sequestrum consisting of variably sized necrotic bone fragments may be present. With long-standing infection, nonunion, and painful, nonfunctional joints, amputation may be indicated.[54,55]

Septic Arthritis and Hematogenous Osteomyelitis

In contrast to children, most adults who acquire bone and joint infection by hematogenous spread are likely to be malnourished, systemically ill, immunocompromised, or diabetic. The source of infecting bacteria may be lung, oral cavity, urinary tract, or frequently an unidentified endogenous source. Intravenous drug abuse is a frequent source of cellulitis and often contiguous septic arthritis secondary to inoculation from unsterile needles. Many of these people are also malnourished, and positive for hepatitis and human immunodeficiency virus antigens. Infection can also occur at sites remote from the primary injection, especially the intervertebral disc spaces.

Diagnosis

Symptoms may be acute or chronic, resulting in delayed diagnosis. A history of recent bacterial infection, endemic exposure, or immunocompromise may be obtained. Disc space infection is associated with acute or chronic back pain, frequently located in the lumbar or thoracic spine. Physical findings are variable and can be compatible with acute trauma, remote injury, or degenerative processes. Systemic signs of infection may be absent, but the erythrocyte sedimentation rate is universally elevated. Radiographic changes are highly variable, ranging from normal to extensive joint or bone destruction. MRI is helpful in detecting soft tissue edema, inflammation, or abscess formation. Blood cultures may be positive, especially with acute presentations. Definitive diagnosis is made by culture and sensitivity after aspiration or open biopsy of the involved bone or joint.

Treatment requires a minimum of 6 weeks of culture-specific antimicrobial therapy. Surgery consists of arthroscopic or open irrigation and débridement of septic joints, evacuation of abscesses, or resection of necrotic bone. Most bacterial infections that are diagnosed and treated promptly have a satisfactory prognosis; however, chronic infections have a poor prognosis because of extensive destruction of bone or joints.[54] The adequacy of treatment is determined by a clinical response and a falling erythrocyte sedimentation rate.

Tuberculous Infection

Skeletal involvement in patients with tuberculosis is not uncommon, especially in underdeveloped parts of the world, and is usually, but not exclusively, associated with pulmonary tuberculosis. Involvement of the spine (Pott disease) can produce vertebral destruction and paraplegia. The hip, knee, or other extremity locations may also be involved. Symptoms are often indolent and may have been present for months or years. History of endemic exposure is usually present.[54]

Radiographically, tuberculosis produces rarefaction of bone, joint destruction, and bony erosion of the involved areas. Workup includes sputum cultures, skin tests where appropriate, and open biopsy for histologic and culture and sensitivity studies. Surgical débridement must be complete but judicious because a surprising amount of healing and restoration of bony architecture can occur after prolonged antituberculous therapy.[92]

Fungal Osteomyelitis

Fungal osteomyelitis is not common, but is characterized by delay in diagnosis and confusion with other causes of bone pain or radiographic changes, such as degenerative arthritis, remote trauma, or neoplasms. A high index of suspicion and the inclusion of infection in the differential diagnosis of obscure musculoskeletal complaints is most important.

Coccidioidomycosis

This fungal disease is endemic in the San Joaquin Valley of California, and is caused by the inhalation of spores of *Coccidioides immitis,* with resultant respiratory tract infection. The disease is more likely to be found in farmers, migrant workers, the elderly, or those with immunocompromise secondary to diabetes, corticosteroid administration, or AIDS. Skin tests or serologic tests are usually positive. Fungal organisms may be seen on microscopic analysis of infected granulomas and the fungus may be grown in culture. Treatment is surgical débridement and appropriate antifungal drugs, including ketoconazole, itraconazole, or amphotericin B.[57]

Blastomycosis

Blastomycosis frequently begins as a respiratory infection and spreads hematogenously to the bones and synovial tissue. Clinically, the appearance is similar to other granulomatous diseases and the diagnosis is made as described previously. Treatment is surgical débridement and antifungal therapy.

Sporotrichosis

Sporotrichosis produces an indolent inflammatory process frequently involving the wrist, digits, or elbows. It may be confused with arthritis or bacterial infection. Inoculation is frequently from contaminated soil, benign-appearing puncture wounds, or thorn penetration. The organisms may be difficult to culture, but are grown on Sabouraud agar and have a characteristic cigar-shape histologic appearance. Treatment consists of surgical débridement and antifungal therapy.

Cryptococcosis

Cryptococcosis may occur in immunocompromised patients and usually begins as a pulmonary infection that spreads to the central nervous system and then, through the bloodstream, to various sites in the axial skeleton, vertebrae, and pelvis. Diagnosis is made serologically and by the characteristic histologic appearance and growth on Sabouraud's culture medium.

Histoplasmosis

Histoplasmosis is quite common and frequently asymptomatic. Rarely, it may be a source of bone and joint infection, primarily in immunocompromised or immunosuppressed patients. Diagnosis is by direct microscopic examination and identification of characteristic organisms or by culturing the organism on Sabouraud's agar. Skin and serologic tests may also be helpful in establishing the diagnosis.

Brucellosis

Brucellosis is uncommon in the United States, although it remains endemic in many parts of the world. Signs and symptoms of the disease are highly variable, with musculoskeletal complaints occurring frequently. The combination of an uncommon infection presenting with protean manifestations often results in missed or delayed diagnosis in the Western world. *Brucella* organisms are gram-negative coccobacilli, and infection is the result of direct contact with sick animals in approximately 80% of cases, or by ingestion of contaminated by-products. In the United States, the disease is primarily occupational, occurring in people involved in dairy farming, veterinary medicine, or meat processing. Musculoskeletal complaints are frequent, but radiographic changes are notoriously slow to appear, and may be confused with previous trauma or degenerative arthritis. The most common site of skeletal involvement is the spine, especially the lumbar region. The sacroiliac joints may also be involved, as well as the long bones. It is difficult to grow the organism on culture medium, and special laboratory techniques are necessary for its isolation. Diagnosis is frequently made immunoserologically. Treatment is usually nonoperative. In some cases, bone or joint destruction dictates débridement of necrotic material. The organism responds to rifampin or tetracycline administration, which is highly effective in most cases.[93]

KEY POINTS

- **Open fractures are an orthopedic emergency and must be treated promptly to prevent the serious complications of infection and nonunion. The principles of treatment involve thorough débridement, intravenous and local antibiotics, and fracture stabilization. Coverage of exposed bone by viable soft tissue must be achieved.**
- **Fracture–dislocations result from higher-energy forces and frequently involve major joints. Fracture reduction by open technique is usually necessary to restore anatomy of the bone and obtain reduction of the joint. The goal of contemporary fracture treatment is to stabilize and restore bony anatomy, promote fracture healing, and ultimately restore function.**
- **Fracture healing is significantly influenced by fracture characteristics, including displacement, comminution, presence or absence of open injury, and methods of fracture stabilization.**
- **Coincident with the natural aging process is an increased instance of degenerative arthritis. Presumably this disease is caused by repetitive microdamage occurring over a lifetime. Age, sex, body weight, and familial predisposition are other factors that influence the development of degenerative changes.**

- **Stable fractures are, by definition, minimally displaced or reducible. A brief period of splinting followed by buddy tapping allows early protected motion. Potentially unstable injuries require radiographic and clinical follow-up during the first 7 to 10 days to detect loss of reduction. Percutaneous pinning may be indicated in this instance. Large articular fragments and unstable oblique or open fractures require open reduction and surgical stabilization.**
- **Injuries or fractures involving the growth plate can produce permanent disability, deformity, and joint destruction unless treated appropriately.**
- **Metastatic disease of bone is much more commonly encountered than primary malignant tumors of bone.**

References

1. Cook SD. Preclinical and clinical evaluations of osteogenic protein-1, BMP-7 in bony sites. *Orthopaedics* 1999;7:669–671.
2. Reddi AH, Shushan MA, Cunningham NS. Induction and maintenance of new bone formation by growth and differentiation factors. *Ann Chir Gynaecol.* 1988;77:189–192.
3. **Spector M. Tissue engineering: the next revolution in orthopaedic surgery? *Harvard Orthop J.* 1999;1:103–105.**
4. Kennedy JP, Blaisdell WF, eds. *Extremity trauma.* New York: Thieme, 1992.
5. Garrison FH. *History of medicine.* Philadelphia: WB Saunders, 1929.
6. Tile M. *Fractures of the pelvis and acetabulum,* 2nd ed. Baltimore: Williams & Wilkins, 1995.
7. Gustilo RB, Simpson L, Nixon RA, et al. Analysis of 511 open fractures. *Clin Orthop.* 1969;66:148–154.
8. Patzakis MJ, Wilkins J, Moore TM. Use of antibiotics in open tibial fractures. *Clin Orthop.* 1983;178:31–35.
9. Behrens F, Comfort TH, Searls K, et al. Treatment of severe open tibial fractures: prospective evaluation. *Orthop Trans.* 1983;7:528.
10. Moehring HD, Gravel CA, Chapman MW, et al. Comparison of antibiotic beads and intravenous antibiotics in open fractures. *Clin Orthop.* 2000;372:254–261.
11. Russell TS. Fractures of the tibial shaft. In: Moehring HD, Greenspan A, eds. *Fractures: current diagnosis and treatment.* Philadelphia: Current Medicine, 2000, pp. 165–171.
12. Moehring HD. Regional fractures of the knee. In: Larson RL, Grana WA, eds. *The knee: form, function, pathology, and treatment.* Philadelphia: WB Saunders, 1993, pp. 147–201.
13. Moehring HD. Acute dislocations of the shoulder girdle and elbow. In: Chapman MW, Madison M, eds. *Operative orthopaedics,* 2nd ed. Philadelphia: Lippincott–Raven, 1993.
14. **Moehring HD. Hip dislocations femoral head fractures. In: Chapman MW, Madison M, eds. *Operative orthopaedics,* 2nd ed. Philadelphia: Lippincott–Raven, 1993.**
15. Moehring HD, Tan RT, Marder RA, et al. Ankle dislocation. *J Orthop Trauma.* 1994;8:167–172.
16. **Moehring HD. Fractures of the tibia, fibula, ankle, and foot. In: Callahm BC, ed. *Current practices of emergency medicine.* Philadelphia: Decker, 1991.**
17. Hansen S, Levine D. Foot fractures. In: Moehring HD, Greenspan A, eds. *Fractures: current diagnosis and treatment.* Philadelphia: Current Medicine, 2000, pp. 198–201.
18. Müller ME, Allgöwer M, Schneider R, et al. *Manual of internal fixation: techniques,* 3rd ed. Berlin: Springer-Verlag, 1991.
19. Browner BD, Jupiter JB, Levine AM, et al. *Skeletal trauma,* vol 1. Philadelphia: WB Saunders; 1992.
20. Matthews LS, Goldstein SA. In: Greenfield LJ, et al., eds. *Orthopaedic surgery: principles and practice.* Philadelphia: Lippincott–Raven, 1997.
21. McKibbin B. The biology of fracture healing in long bones. *J Bone Joint Surg Br.* 1978;60:150–162.
22. **Egol KA, Kellam JF. Diagnosis and management of pelvic ring fractures. In: Moehring HD, Greenspan A, eds. *Fractures: current diagnosis and treatment.* Philadelphia: Current Medicine; 2000:71–78.**
23. Mears DC, Rubash H. *Pelvic and acetabular fractures.* Thorofare, NJ: Slack, 1986.
24. Letournel E. *Fractures of the acetabulum.* New York: Springer, 1981.
25. Moehring HD. Fractures of the acetabulum. In: Moehring HD, Greenspan A, eds. *Fractures: current diagnosis and treatment.* Philadelphia: Current Medicine, 2000, pp. 79–88.
26. Kuntscher G, ed. *Practice of intramedullary nailing.* Springfield, IL: Charles C Thomas, 1962.
27. Brumback RJ, Stibling Ellision P, Poka A, et al. Intramedullary nailing of open fractures of the femoral shaft. *J Bone Joint Surg Am.* 1989;71:1324–1331.
28. Moed BR, Watson JT. Retrograde nailing of the femoral shaft. *J Am Acad Orthop Surg.* 1999;7:209–215.
29. Dehne E, Metz CW, Deffer PA. Nonoperative treatment of the fractured tibia by immediate weight bearing. *J Trauma* 1961;1:514–535.
30. Moehring HD, Voightlander JR. Compartment pressure monitoring during intramedullary reaming of tibial fractures. *Orthopaedics* 1995;18:7:631–636.
31. Whitesides TE, Haney TC, Morimoto K, et al. Tissue pressure measurements as a determinant for the need of fasciotomy. *Clin Orthop.* 1975;113:43.
32. Mubarak SJ, Hargens AR. *Compartment syndromes and Volkmann's contracture.* Philadelphia: WB Saunders; 1981.
33. Mubarak SJ, Owen CA. Double-incision fasciotomy of the leg for decompression in compartment syndromes. *J Bone Joint Surg Am.* 1977;59: 184–187.
34. Sarmiento A, Watson JT. Functional bracing of diaphyseal humeral fractures and operative management of humeral shaft fractures. In: Moehring HD, Greenspan A, eds. *Fractures: current diagnosis and treatment.* Philadelphia: Current Medicine, 2000, pp. 225–239.
35. Weiss LE, Osterman L. Fractures of the radius and ulna. In: Moehring HD, Greenspan A, eds. *Fractures: current diagnosis and treatment.* Philadelphia: Current Medicine, 2000, pp. 257–266.
36. Teague DC, Swiontkowski MF. Femoral neck fractures. In: Moehring HD, Greenspan A, eds. *Fractures: current diagnosis and treatment.* Philadelphia: Current Medicine, 2000, pp. 91–95.
37. Kyle RF, Ellis TJ. Intertrochanteric hip fractures. In: Moehring HD, Greenspan A, eds. *Fractures: Current Diagnosis and Treatment.* Philadelphia: Current Medicine, 2000, pp. 95–105.
38. Lindsey R. Subtrochanteric fractures of the femur. In: Moehring HD, Greenspan A, eds. *Fractures: current diagnosis and treatment.* Philadelphia: Current Medicine, 2000, pp. 107–115.
39. Ebraheim NA, Pearlstein SR, Savolaine ER, et al. Scapulothoracic dissociation (closed avulsion of the scapula, subclavian artery, and brachial plexus): a newly recognized variant, a new classification and a review of the literature and treatment options. *J Orthop Trauma* 1987;1:18–23.
40. Goss TP. Fractures of the scapula. In: Moehring HD, Greenspan A, eds. *Fractures: current diagnosis and treatment.* Philadelphia: Current Medicine, 2000, pp. 209–215.
41. Torchia MD. Fractures of the humeral head and neck. In: Moehring HD, Greenspan A, eds. *Fractures: current diagnosis and treatment.* Philadelphia: Current Medicine, 2000, pp. 217–219.
42. Vrahas MS, Leddy MJ III. Supracondylar fractures of the humerus. In: Moehring HD, Greenspan A, eds. *Fractures: current diagnosis and treatment.* Philadelphia: Current Medicine, 2000, pp. 243–246.
43. Mason MB. Some observations on fractures of the head of the radius with a review of one hundred cases. *Br J Surg.* 1954;42:123.
44. Colles A. On the fracture of the carpal extremity of the radius. *Edinb Med Surg J.* 1814;10:181.
45. Whipple T, Padgett LR. Fractures of the distal radius. In: Moehring HD, Greenspan A, eds. *Fractures: current diagnosis and treatment.* Philadelphia: Current Medicine, 2000, pp. 269–272.
46. Slater RR. Fracture dislocations of the wrist. In: Moehring HD, Greenspan A, eds. *Fractures: current diagnosis and treatment.* Philadelphia: Current Medicine, 2000, pp. 281–286.
47. **Mclain RF. Cervical spine fractures. In: Moehring HD, Greenspan A, eds. *Fractures: current diagnosis and treatment.* Philadelphia: Current Medicine, 2000, pp. 49–56.**
48. Gupta MC, Benson DR. Thoracolumbar fractures and fracture-dislocations. In: Moehring HD, Greenspan A, eds. *Fractures: current diagnosis and treatment.* Philadelphia: Current Medicine, 2000, pp. 59–68.
49. Denis F. The three column spine and its significance in classification of acute thoracolumbar spinal injuries. *Spine* 1983;8:817–831.
50. Bailey RW, Badgley CE. Stabilization of the cervical spine by anterior fusion. *J Bone Joint Surg Am.* 1960;42:565.
51. Robinson RA, Walker AE, Ferlic DC, et al. The results of an anterior interbody fusion of the cervical spine. *J Bone Joint Surg Am.* 1962;44:1569.
52. McCullouch JA, McNab I, eds. *Sciatica and chymopapain.* Baltimore: Williams & Wilkins, 1983.
53. Greenwald AS, ed. *Concepts in joint replacement.* Thorofare, NJ: Orthopaedics, 1999.
54. Esterhai JL Jr, Gristina AG, Poss R, eds. *Musculoskeletal infection.* Park Ridge, IL: American Academy of Orthopaedic Surgeons, 1992.
55. Rockwood CA, Green DP, Bucholz RW, eds. *Fractures in adults,* 3rd ed. Philadelphia: JB Lippincott, 1991.
56. Morrey BF, ed. *Joint replacement arthroplasty.* New York: Churchill-Livingstone, 1991.
57. Catagni MA, Malzev V, Kirienko A. Advances in Ilizarov apparatus assembly, treatment of fractures, pseudoarthroses: lengthening and deformity correction. Milan: Medicalplastic srl, 1994.
58. Parisien JS, ed. *Current techniques in arthroscopy,* 2nd ed. Philadelphia: Current Medicine, 1996.
59. Larson RL. Acute ligamentous injury, chronic anterior instability. In: Larsen RL, Grana WA, eds. *The knee.* Philadelphia: WB Saunders, 1993, pp. 493–620.
60. Boyes JH. *Bunnell's surgery of the hand,* 4th ed. Philadelphia: JB Lippincott, 1964.
61. Bunnell S. Splinting the hand. *Instr Course Lect.* 1952;9:233.
62. Grana WA. Chronic posterior and posterolateral laxity. In: Larsen RL, Grana WA, eds. *The knee.* Philadelphia: WB Saunders, 1993, pp. 621–679.
63. Lewis DS, Jebson PJL. Current management of selected problem fractures of the phalanges and metacarpals. In: Moehring HD, Greenspan A, eds.

Fractures: current diagnosis and treatment. Philadelphia: Current Medicine, 2000, pp. 293–299.

64. Green DP. General principles in operative hand surgery. In: *Operative hand surgery.* New York: Churchill Livingstone, 1982, pp. 1–21.
65. Green DP, Rowland SA. In: Rockwood CA, Green DP, eds. *Fractures and dislocations of the hand.* Philadelphia: JB Lippincott, 1991.
66. American Academy of Orthopaedic Surgeons, ed. Symposium on tendon surgery in the hand. Philadelphia: American Academy of Orthopaedic Surgeons, 1974.
67. Green DP, Anderson JR. Closed reduction and percutaneous pin fixation of fractured phalanges. *J Bone Joint Surg Am.* 1973;55:1651–1654.
68. Verdan CE. Primary repair of flexor tendons. *J Bone Joint Surg Am.* 1960; 42:647–657.
69. Kleinert HE, Kutz JE, Ashbell TS, et al. Primary repair of lacerated flexor tendons in "no man's land." *J Bone Joint Surg Am.* 1967;49:577.
70. Nunley JA, Goldner LJ. Tendon injury and repair. In: Sabiston DC, Lyerly HK, eds. *Textbook of surgery,* 15th ed. Philadelphia: WB Saunders, 1997, pp. 1470–1479.
71. Hunter JM, Salisbury RE. Flexor-tendon reconstruction in severely damaged hands. A two-stage procedure using a silicone-Dacron reinforced gliding prosthesis prior to tendon grafting. *J Bone Joint Surg Am.* 1971;53:829.
72. Urbaniak JR. Replantation of amputated limbs and digits. In: Sabiston DC, Lyerly HK, eds. *Textbook of surgery,* 15th ed. Philadelphia: WB Saunders; 1997, pp. 1487–1491.
73. Urbaniak JR. Digital replantation: a 12-year experience. In: Urbaniak JR, ed. *Microsurgery for major limb reconstruction.* St. Louis: Mosby, 1987, p. 12.
74. Dolenc VV. Contemporary treatment of peripheral nerve and brachial plexus lesions. *Neurosurg Rev.* 1986;9:149.
75. Millesi H. Brachial plexus injuries. In: Chapman MW, Madison M, eds. *Operative orthopaedics,* 2nd ed. Philadelphia: JB Lippincott, 1993.
76. Sedel L. The results of surgical repair of brachial plexus lesions. *J Bone Joint Surg (Am).* 1982;64:54.
77. Szabo RM, Spiegel JD. Infections of the hand. In: Chapman MW, Madison M, eds. *Operative orthopaedics,* 2nd ed. Philadelphia: JB Lippincott, 1993.
78. Lubahn JD, Lister GD, Wolfe T. Fasciectomy and Dupuytren's disease: a comparison between the open-palm technique and wound closure. *J Hand Surg.* 1984;9:53.
79. Open fasciotomy and full thickness skin graft in the Gonzalez correction of digital flexion deformity. In: Hueston JT, Tubiana R, eds. *Dupuytren's disease.* New York: Churchill Livingstone, 1985.
80. Tachdjian MO, ed. *Pediatric orthopaedics,* vol 1. Philadelphia: WB Saunders, 1972.
81. Rang M. *Children's fractures,* 2nd ed. Philadelphia: JB Lippincott, 1983, p. 24.
82. Weber BG, Brunner C, Freuler F. *Treatment of fractures in children and adolescents.* New York: Springer, 1980.
83. Worlock PH, Colton CL. Severely displaced supracondylar fractures of the humerus in children. *J Pediatr Orthop.* 1987;7:49–53.
84. Morrey BF, Peterson HA. Hematogenous pyogenic osteomyelitis in children. *Orthop Clin North Am.* 1975;6:935.
85. Griffin PP. *Septic arthritis in children.* Orthopedic surgery update series. Princeton, NJ: CPEC, 1982.
86. Marmor L, Chan KB, Ho KC, et al. Surgical treatment of tuberculosis of the hip in children. *Clin Orthop.* 1969;67:135.
87. Simon MA. Current concepts review: limb salvage for osteosarcoma. *J Bone Joint Surg Am* 1988;70:307.
88. Enneking WF. *Musculoskeletal tumor surgery.* New York: Churchill Livingstone, 1983.
89. Greenspan A, Remagen W. *Differential diagnosis of tumors and tumor-like lesions of bone and joints.* Philadelphia: Lippincott–Raven, 1998.
90. Dahlin DC, Coventry MB. Osteogenic sarcoma: a study of 600 cases. *J Bone Joint Surg Am.* 1967;49:1001–1010.
91. Bacci G, Toni A, Avella M, et al. Long-term results in 144 localized Ewing's sarcoma patients treated with combined therapy. *Cancer* 1989;63: 1477.
92. Centers for Disease Control. Leads from the MMWR: tuberculosis United States, 1985. *JAMA* 1986;256:3335.
93. Moehring HD. *Brucella sacroiliitis. Orthopaedics* 1985;8:499–502.

CHAPTER 114 ■ NEUROSURGERY

JEAN-CHRISTOPHE LEVEQUE AND JULIAN T. HOFF

A detailed history and physical examination are the foundations of neurosurgical diagnosis. Headache, altered consciousness, memory impairment, speech difficulty, visual disturbance, weakness, paresthesia, and incoordination are symptoms suggestive of central nervous system (CNS) disease. The examination should include an assessment of mental status, thorough cranial nerve testing, optic funduscopy, and motor, sensory, cerebellar, and reflex testing. The history may reveal the etiology (e.g., traumatic, neoplastic, vascular, infectious, degenerative, or metabolic), whereas neurologic examination permits anatomic localization of the lesion. For patients with nervous system disorders, an accurate history need be taken only once, but the examination must be repeated and recorded often to gauge the course of the illness and to judge the urgency of other diagnostic steps necessary before treatment can be given.

DIAGNOSTIC STUDIES

Once a differential diagnosis is formulated with the information gathered from the history and examination, it is necessary to confirm the principal diagnosis by use of diagnostic aids. Studies helpful in the practice of neurosurgery include plain film radiography, myelography, angiography, computed tomography (CT), magnetic resonance imaging (MRI), ultrasonography, electromyography (EMG) and nerve conduction velocity testing, evoked potentials (visual, auditory, and somatosensory), positron emission tomography, and electroencephalography.

Plain films, especially of the spine, are useful in trauma and degenerative disorders. Myelography, both with and without CT, is useful for the evaluation of radiculopathies and, when MRI is not available, myelopathies due to trauma, tumor, and degenerative spine disease. CT and MRI provide detailed imaging of both cranial and spinal contents. They are useful in combination for visualization of bone and soft tissues, respectively. Both magnetic resonance and CT angiography are noninvasive alternatives to conventional angiography. Angiography provides detailed information about aneurysms, vascular malformations, and atherosclerotic disease. It is an essential tool in the evaluation of cerebral hemorrhage and embolic and thrombotic stroke and in preoperative planning for tumor surgery. Ultrasound is an important adjunct in the operating room, providing visualization of tumors, cysts, vascular malformations, and congenital anomalies lying beneath the exposed surface. It is also extensively used in brain and spinal cord imaging in the newborn.

EMG and nerve conduction velocity testing are helpful in evaluating peripheral nerve and nerve root lesions. They are also used to monitor brachial plexus and peripheral nerve recovery after traumatic injury. Visual and auditory evoked potentials can be used in comatose patients to monitor the severity of head injury. Auditory potentials are useful in surgical excision of tumors of the eighth cranial nerve. Somatosensory evoked potentials continually monitor spinal cord (dorsal column) function during surgical manipulation of spinal fractures and tumors. Functional MRI allows for some localization of functional brain areas by measuring blood flow through a region during specific motor, sensory, or verbal tasks. Positron emission tomography scans play an important role in epilepsy surgery, in preembolization assessment of skull-based tumors involving the cavernous sinus and surgically untreatable vascular anomalies, and in brain tumor follow-up. Electroencephalography helps delineate structural and metabolic disorders and can be used during cerebrovascular surgery as a guard against irreversible ischemia. Transcranial Doppler sonography allows noninvasive evaluation of blood flow velocity in intracranial arteries, which is useful in monitoring patients with cerebral ischemia caused by vascular spasm.

TRAUMA

Trauma is the single most common cause of death in children, adolescents, and young adults. Most accidents involving motor vehicles and falls include injury to the brain and spinal cord and their surrounding structures.[1]

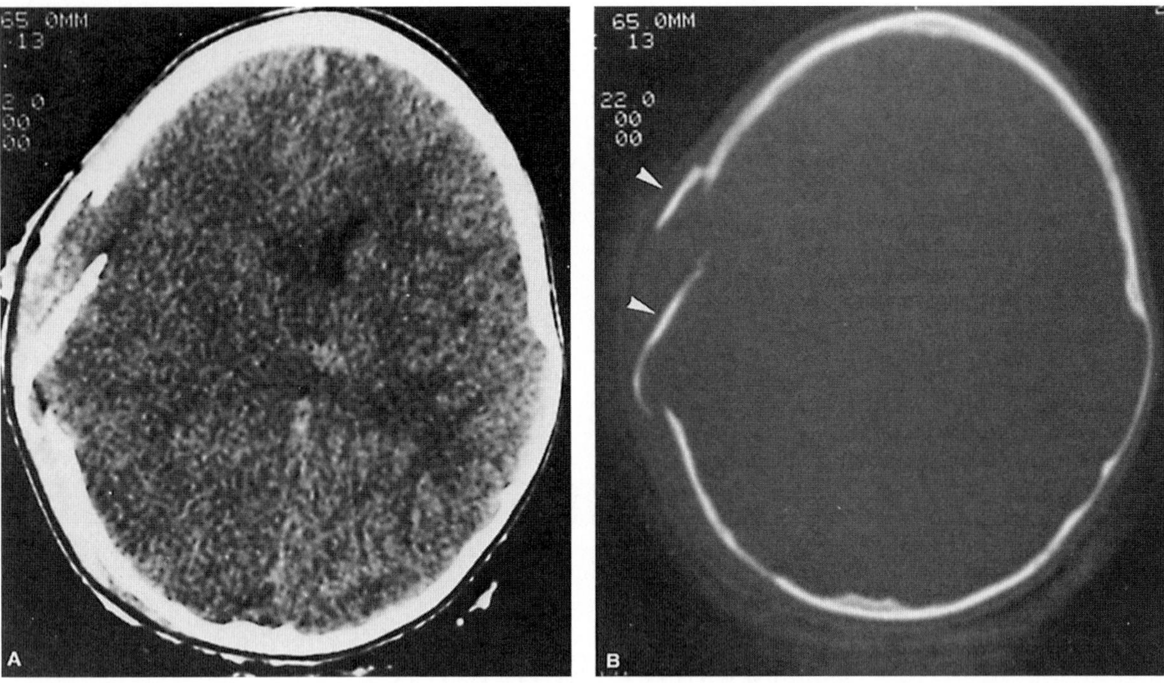

FIGURE 114.1 A compound, comminuted, depressed skull fracture imaged by noncontrast computed tomography with the use of soft tissue (*A*) and bone windows (*B*). Multiple fracture fragments are visible (*arrowheads*).

Scalp Injury

Scalp injury can cause serious hemorrhage and subsequent shock if not promptly treated. Bleeding can usually be controlled with a simple pressure dressing, by firm finger pressure, or by hemostats applied to the galea (the aponeurosis of the scalp). Scalp wounds should be closed as soon as possible. Lacerations that overlie a depressed fracture or a penetrating wound of the skull require debridement in the operating room.

Simple scalp lacerations should be débrided of foreign matter, copiously irrigated, and closed primarily, taking care to approximate both the galea and skin. Scalp avulsions typically include all layers of the scalp, with sparing of the underlying periosteum. If the avulsion is small, closure can often be accomplished primarily. Replantation with the use of microsurgical technique is the preferred method of repair for large scalp avulsions.

If the injured scalp is not viable but the periosteum is intact, split-thickness skin grafts can be used to close the defect. When the periosteum is absent or desiccated, closure is more difficult because it is through the periosteal layer that the outer skull table receives its blood supply. In this instance, closure can be accomplished with vascular flaps of greater omentum or muscle.

Skull Fracture

Skull fractures are classified according to whether the skin overlying the fracture is intact (closed) or disrupted (open or compound); whether there is a single fracture line (linear), several fractures radiating from a central point (stellate), or fragmentation of bone (comminuted); and whether the edges of the fracture line have been driven below the level of the surrounding bone (depressed) or not (nondepressed).

Simple skull fractures (linear, stellate, or comminuted nondepressed) require no specific treatment. They are potentially serious, however, and can be fatal if they cross major vascular channels in the skull, such as the groove of the middle meningeal artery or the dural venous sinuses. If these structures are torn, epidural or subdural hematomas can form. A simple skull fracture that extends into the accessory nasal sinuses or the mastoid air cells is considered open because it communicates with an external body surface.

Depressed skull fractures often require surgery to elevate the depressed bone fragments (Fig. 114.1). If there are no adverse neurologic signs and the fracture is closed, repair can be done electively. During surgery, the dura should be inspected and repaired as described later.

Open skull fractures also require surgical intervention. Linear or stellate, nondepressed open fractures can be treated by simple closure of the scalp after thorough cleansing. Open fractures with severe comminution of underlying bone should be treated in the operating room. The dura should be inspected to ensure that a laceration has not been overlooked. Dural tears should be closed either primarily or with a fascial patch graft to reduce the risk of infection. Preoperative preparations should be made for craniotomy, in case broader exposure of underlying injured dura and brain is necessary.

Basal skull fractures involve the floor of the calvarium. Bruising can occur about the eye (raccoon sign) or behind the ear (Battle's sign), suggesting a fracture involving the anterior or middle fossa, respectively. Isolated cranial nerve deficits are associated with this fracture type. The facial nerve is frequently affected, with injury due to laceration (acute deficit) or swelling (delayed deficit). Almost all facial nerve deficits resolve spontaneously, especially with incomplete or delayed lesions. No specific therapy is warranted. On the other hand, complete lesions should be explored, although the timing of exploration remains a matter of debate. Patients with a fracture through the temporal bone should have a fine-cut temporal bone CT study and may require a consultation from the otolaryngology service if deficits are noted.

Any associated cerebrospinal fluid (CSF) rhinorrhea or otorrhea should be treated expectantly. Traumatic CSF leaks typically stop within the first 7 to 10 days. Should a leak persist, lumbar CSF drainage with bed rest can be implemented to seal the leak by lowering CSF volume and intracranial pressure (ICP). If this therapy fails, surgical exploration and oversewing of the defect with a fascial patch graft are indicated. Less than 5% of patients actually require surgical repair. Prophylactic antibiotics are no longer used because prospective studies have failed to demonstrate any significant benefit from their use.

Brain Injury

Injury to the brain is caused by the rapid deceleration, acceleration, and rotation associated with a blow to the head. The initial impact can produce neuronal and axonal disruption, which constitutes the primary injury. Any subsequent complication, such as an intracranial hematoma, cerebral edema, hypoxia, hypotension, hydrocephalus, or endocrine disturbance, characterizes secondary injury and always compounds the initial insult.[2]

Mild head injury is usually not associated with significant primary brain injury, and neurologic deficits are limited to temporary loss of consciousness (concussion). Moderate to severe head injury, on the other hand, is typically associated with deficits that may or may not be reversible. Moreover, this degree of injury is usually accompanied by secondary injury.

Distortional forces causing the primary injury can produce diffuse axonal injury or tear intraparenchymal capillaries, superficial subdural bridging veins, or epidural vessels, thus producing uncontained blood. Vasogenic cerebral edema occurs in response to vasodilation and disruption of the blood—brain barrier. Ischemia from hypotension or hypoxia can produce cell death and consequent cytotoxic edema. Disruption of CSF absorption pathways by uncontained subarachnoid blood can lead to hydrocephalus. Cerebral salt wasting, in which brain injury causes intravascular volume loss and hyponatremia, or diabetes insipidus can aggravate cerebral edema by fluid and electrolyte imbalance. Severe head injury can also lead to vasomotor dysregulation and an abnormal increase in cerebral blood flow, or hyperemia. These changes, either in part or in combination, result in an elevation of ICP.

Elevated ICP contributes to secondary brain injury by reducing cerebral perfusion pressure, which is the difference between the mean arterial blood pressure and the cerebral venous pressure. For all clinically relevant purposes, the cerebral venous pressure is identical to ICP. Thus, when ICP increases and mean arterial blood pressure remains stable, cerebral perfusion pressure decreases. When the cerebral perfusion pressure falls below 70 mm Hg, cerebral blood flow is compromised, producing cerebral ischemia and compounding the primary brain injury with secondary insult.

In studies of head injury mortality, intracranial hypertension appears to be one of the most important factors affecting outcome. For this reason, aggressive management to circumvent cerebral blood flow reduction and secondary injury is imperative. Early resuscitative therapy should be initiated in the accident field with airway control and hyperventilation. In the absence of hypotension, osmotherapy can also be used.

Rapid clinical assessment is essential. Although extensive neurologic testing is limited in uncooperative or unresponsive patients, certain features of the examination are crucial. The Glasgow Coma Scale score, established in 1974, uses a numeric score to evaluate eye opening and verbal and motor behavior, both spontaneously and in response to stimulation (Table 114.1). This scale is useful for determining the patient's neurologic status and provides information regarding the ultimate outcome of the head-injured patient.

The initial neurologic examination determines whether diagnostic testing is indicated. Patients without headache, lethargy, or a focal neurologic deficit are not likely to experience a secondary complication from their injury, and imaging studies usually are not indicated. Conversely, symptomatic patients with or without a focal deficit should undergo a CT scan of the head. Should CT fail to disclose a lesion despite high clinical suspicion, further imaging with MRI and/or angiography may be necessary.

TABLE 114.1

GLASGOW COMA SCALE

Parameter	Score
EYE OPENING	
Spontaneously	4
To voice stimulus	3
To pain	2
No eye opening	1
MOTOR RESPONSE	
Follows commands	6
Localizes a pain stimulus	5
Withdraws from pain	4
Flexor posturing to pain	3
Extensor posturing to pain	2
No response to pain	1
VERBAL RESPONSE	
Oriented	5
Confused	4
Inappropriate words	3
Incomprehensible sounds	2
No sounds	1

[a]The Glasgow Coma Scale assigns a numeric value to the responses in each of three categories, with the score equal to the sum of the three responses.

After emergent surgical removal of any traumatic cerebral mass lesion, the goals of medical management are normalization of cerebral perfusion pressure and prevention of secondary injury to the already damaged brain.[3] ICP monitoring may be indicated, especially in patients with marked depression or deterioration in neurologic function. In general, patients with a severe head injury (Glasgow Coma Scale †8) and evidence of a brain injury on CT (e.g., a mass lesion, contusions, subarachnoid hemorrhage) have greater than a 50% chance of having elevated ICP and should receive an ICP monitor or a ventriculostomy to allow drainage of CSF. Factors with a significant negative effect on outcome in severe head injury are hypotension (systolic blood pressure <90 mm Hg) or hypoxia (PaO_2 <60 mm Hg). A patient with a severe head injury, a negative head CT, and a single observation of either hypotension or hypoxia has the same risk of elevated ICP (>50%) as a similar patient with a positive head CT and should also receive ventriculostomy or ICP monitoring. Comatose patients who require emergent surgery (e.g., abdominal, thoracic, orthopedic) should also be monitored because frequent neurologic examination is not possible during general anesthesia. Elevation of the head of bed with the cervical spine in a neutral position facilitates venous drainage. Sedation reduces posturing and reflexive combative activity, both of which worsen ICP. Moderate hyperventilation with $PaCO_2$ levels between 30 and 35 mm Hg lowers cerebral blood volume and ICP without provoking cerebral ischemia. Prophylactic use of anticonvulsants prevents cerebral injury from seizures. Prevention of hypotension reduces the extent of ischemic injury, whereas aggressive treatment of hypertensive episodes reduces cerebral blood volume and further disruption of the blood—brain barrier. Avoidance of hyperthermia minimizes the brain's metabolic demands.

An additional measure for control of ICP is mannitol, an osmotic diuretic that reduces cerebral blood volume and cerebral edema. Deep sedation with narcotics and the use of paralyzing agents such as pancuronium or atracurium can be helpful. Barbiturate coma can be effective for patients with refractory ICP elevation despite these measures. Corticosteroids have no proven benefit in the management of severe head injury.

The outcome in head injury depends on many factors. Age is the single most important predictive factor in head injury; elderly patients fare significantly worse than younger patients. Penetrating injuries, particularly gunshot wounds, have a poorer outcome compared with blunt trauma. The presence of an intracranial hemorrhage also indicates a less favorable outcome. Subdural hematoma has a poorer prognosis than epidural hematoma. Other important factors include delay in treatment, multiple trauma, and systemic insults such as acidosis, hypoxia, and hypotension. Predictors of poor prognosis also include evidence of brainstem dysfunction on initial examination and refractory intracranial hypertension.

Epidural Hematoma

Hemorrhage between the inner table of the skull and the dura mater most commonly arises from a tear of the middle meningeal artery or one of its branches (Fig. 114.2). Arterial bleeding strips the dura from the undersurface of the bone and produces still more bleeding because the small bridging veins from the dura to the skull are torn. The hematoma rapidly increases in size and compresses the cerebral cortex. An epidural hematoma can also arise from torn venous channels in the bone at a point of fracture or from lacerated major dural venous sinuses. Because venous pressure is low, epidural venous hematomas usually form only when a depressed skull fracture has stripped the dura from the bone and left a space in which the hematoma can develop.

Epidural hematoma classically follows a blow to the head that causes a brief period of unconsciousness. After the patient regains consciousness, there may be a lucid interval during which there are no abnormal neurologic symptoms or signs. As the hematoma enlarges, hemispheric compression occurs. With time, the medial portion of the temporal lobe is forced over the edge of the tentorium, causing compression of the oculomotor nerve and subsequent dilatation of the ipsilateral pupil. Similarly, compression of the ipsilateral cerebral peduncle causes contralateral hemiparesis, which can progress to decerebrate posturing. Coma, fixed and dilated pupils, and decerebration is the classic triad suggestive of transtentorial herniation.

Epidural hematomas are curable lesions, but the mortality rate remains high because the severity of injury often is not recognized early. A patient may be seen during the lucid interval and discharged. Later, the patient can become unconscious because of progressive brain compression by the expanding hematoma.

Because of the danger of misdiagnosis, any patient with a history of a blow to the head leading to a period of unconsciousness should have a CT scan. If a symptomatic expanding epidural hematoma is found, emergent craniotomy is indicated. If the hematoma is small and the patient has a normal neurologic examination, the patient can be followed in an intensive care unit, with the understanding that any change in neurologic status may necessitate surgical clot evacuation. If the CT is negative and the patient's examination is nonfocal, the patient can be discharged, although a reliable person should be instructed to awaken the patient frequently during the next 24 hours to be certain that he or she remains arousable. Any deterioration should prompt quick return for repeat evaluation.

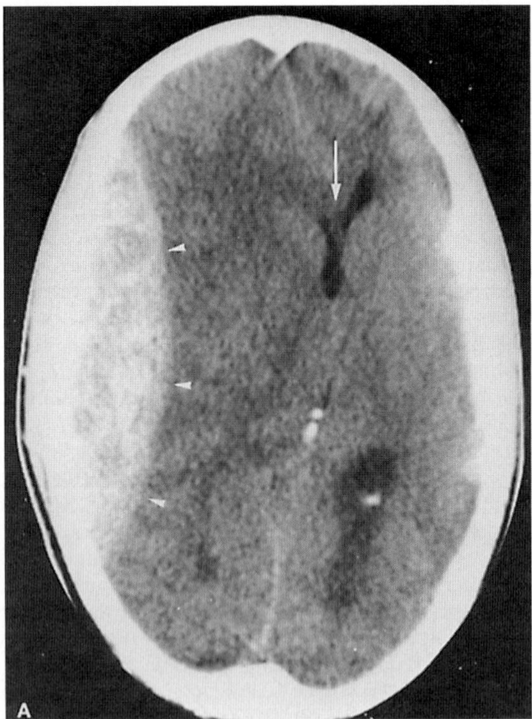

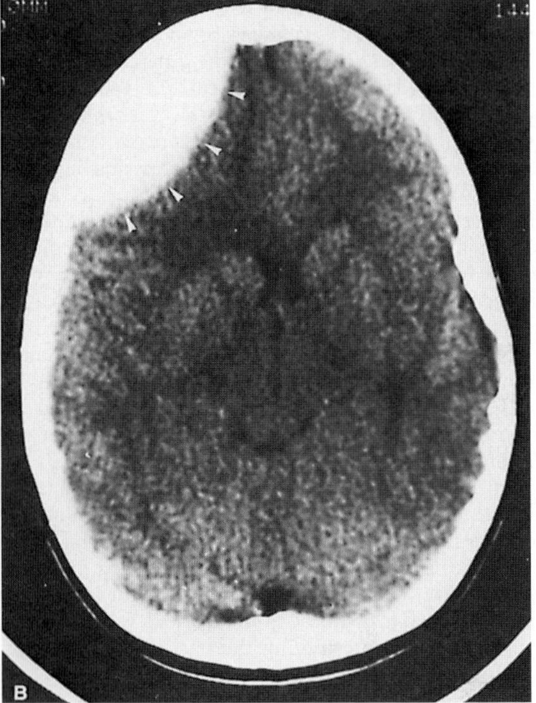

FIGURE 114.2 Two examples of acute epidural hematoma imaged by noncontrast computed tomography. The increased attenuation of the lenticular mass (arrowheads) indicates that it is an acute lesion in the epidural space. There is a marked midline shift in *A* (*arrow*) compared with *B*. The patient in *A* was comatose and had little brainstem function on examination. The patient in *B* was awake and conversant.

Subdural Hematoma

When veins bridging from the cortex to the dura or venous sinuses are torn or when an intracerebral hematoma extends into the subdural space, subdural hematomas can develop. They can be large, even though the bleeding is of venous (low-pressure) origin.

Acute subdural hematomas are associated with severe head injury and arise from a combination of torn bridging veins, disruption of cortical arteries, and laceration of the cortex. The hematoma is best imaged with CT (Fig. 114.3). Evacuation of the clot can result in significant improvement, but often a major neurologic deficit remains because of the accompanying widespread neuronal and axonal injury. Subacute subdural hematomas become apparent several days after injury and are associated with progressive lethargy, confusion, hemiparesis, or other hemispheric deficits. Removal of the hematoma usually produces striking improvement. Chronic subdural hematomas arise from tears in bridging veins, often after a minor head injury. Initially, the hematoma is small. Later, it becomes encased in a fibrous membrane, liquefies, then gradually enlarges. These lesions are more common in infants and the elderly. Typical presentation includes progressive mental status changes, with or without focal signs such as hemiparesis or aphasia. Papilledema may be present. The diagnosis is confirmed by CT scanning. Treatment consists of bur-hole drainage, and craniotomy may be necessary if the fluid reaccumulates.

Subdural hygromas are collections of clear or xanthochromic fluid in the subdural space. They develop when CSF escapes into the potential subdural space through a tear in the arachnoid, becomes trapped, and cannot be absorbed. The resulting fluid mass can cause the same signs and symptoms as chronic subdural hematomas. Like their hematoma counterparts, hygromas are treated by bur-hole drainage.

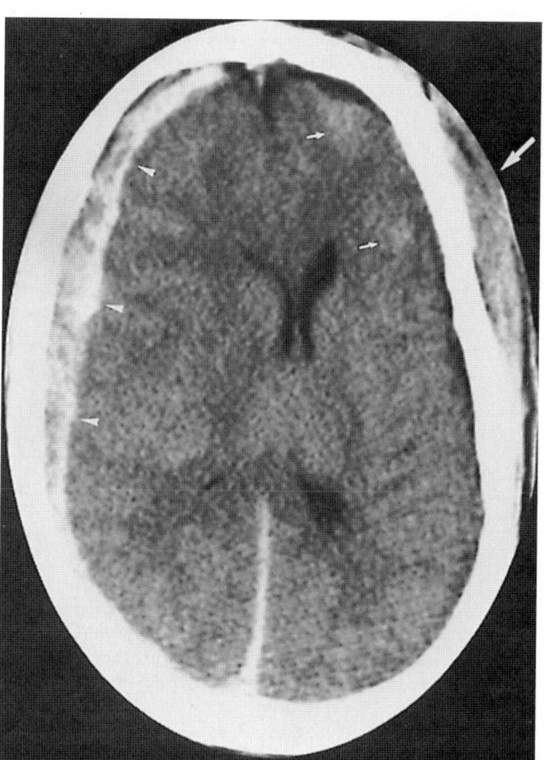

FIGURE 114.3 Acute subdural hematoma imaged by noncontrast computed tomography. The high-attenuation, crescent-shaped lesion (*arrowheads*) indicates acute hemorrhage in the subdural space. Scalp swelling is visible on the contralateral side (*large arrow*), suggesting that the hematoma is due to a contrecoup injury. There are small hemorrhagic contusions in the contralateral frontal lobe as well (small arrows). These often accompany subdural hematomas in head trauma and signify severe injury. Midline shift is apparent.

Spinal Cord Injury

Traumatic injury of the spinal cord can result from vertebral fracture, subluxation, hyperextension, herniation of intervertebral disc material into the canal, and penetrating injuries. Neurologic involvement ranges from mild and transient to severe and permanent. Spinal fracture and cord injury should be suspected in head-injured patients with or without coma and in those with multiple injuries. It is best to assume that the spine is unstable and to immobilize the patient on a backboard with a hard cervical collar until proper examination and diagnostic testing rule out injury.

Clinical findings can include spinal tenderness, extremity weakness, numbness or paresthesia, respiratory compromise, and hypotension. Spinal root involvement produces a radiculopathy characterized by motor and sensory impairment in the corresponding myotome and dermatome. Spinal cord involvement produces a myelopathy of variable manifestations.

Complete lesions, signifying total loss of function below the level of injury, are often referred to as *transections* of the cord. Acute transections are characterized by areflexia, flaccidity, anesthesia, and autonomic paralysis below the level of the lesion. Arterial hypotension is invariably present when the transection is above T-5 because of the loss of sympathetic vascular tone.

Incomplete lesions can result in the Brown-Séquard syndrome, which is manifested by ipsilateral loss of motor function and position–vibratory sensation with contralateral loss of pain and temperature sensation below the level of injury. Anatomically, this presentation is explained by hemisection of the cord (Fig. 114.4A). The central cord syndrome is characterized by bilateral loss of motor function and pain and temperature sensation in the upper extremities, with relative preservation of these functions in the lower extremities. Typically, the distal upper extremities are more severely affected because the most medial portions of the corticospinal and spinothalamic tracts subserve these areas (Fig. 114.4B). This deficit can be seen after a hyperextension injury of the cervical spine, with or without fracture. The anterior spinal artery syndrome involves the bilateral loss of motor function and pain and temperature sensation below the level of the lesion, with sparing of position–vibratory and light touch sensation. This incomplete lesion develops when the anterior spinal artery is occluded. This renders the cord ischemic within the anterior spinal artery distribution, affecting the anterior and lateral columns bilaterally (Fig. 114.4C). One common cause is an acutely ruptured cervical disc (Fig. 114.5).

Trauma to the lumbar spine can produce signs and symptoms of cauda equina compression. Presentation consists of multiple lumbosacral radiculopathies of variable severity. Lower extremity motor, sensory, and reflex functions can be affected, producing variable degrees of weakness, sensory loss (all modalities in the specific distribution of the roots involved), and diminution or absence of reflexes. Bladder distention from detrusor muscle paralysis, flaccidity of the anal sphincter, and loss of perineal sensation are common in severe injuries.

In addition to the neurologic deficit, acute spinal cord injury is accompanied by many systemic responses. If the spinal cord is damaged above C-3, respiratory efforts cease, accounting for this injury's high mortality rate at the scene of the accident. Although spontaneous ventilatory efforts can be initiated with injuries involving C-4 to C-6, tidal volumes are often insufficient, accounting for progressive hypoxia and

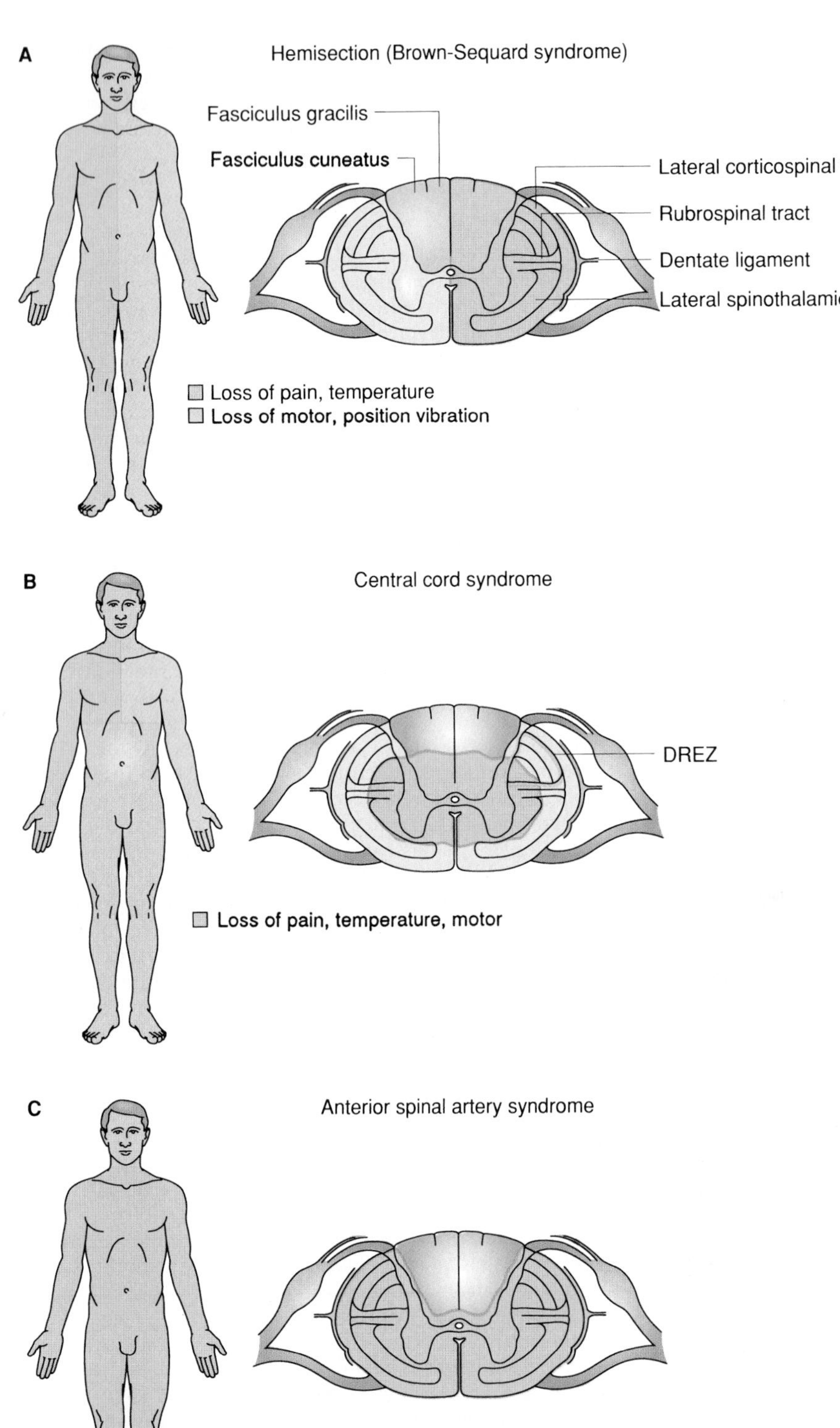

FIGURE 114.4 Schematic cross-sections of the spinal cord, showing hemisection (*A*), central cord syndrome lesion (*B*), and anterior spinal artery syndrome lesion (*C*). The figure diagrams demonstrate the neurologic deficits. DREZ, dorsal route entry zone.

carbon dioxide retention. Airway obstruction, atelectasis, and pneumonia are common complications. Assisted ventilation may be indicated, especially early after injury.

Blood pressure is usually low if the cord injury is above the T-5 level, as such a lesion effectively denervates the sympathetic nervous system, leading to increased venous capacitance and decreased venous return. The resulting hypotension is controlled by the administration of intravenous (IV) fluids. Colloid is preferred to reduce the threat of vascular overload and iatrogenic pulmonary edema. Postural changes that will drop the blood pressure precipitously should be avoided.

Tachycardia is a common compensatory response to hypotension, but bradycardia is the rule when the cervical cord is damaged and the sympathetic input to the heart is lost. This bradycardia does not require treatment unless the patient is symptomatic or at risk for myocardial infarction or stroke

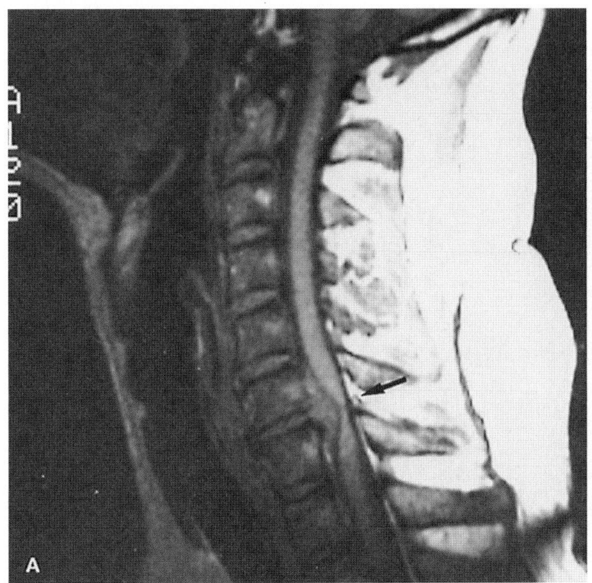

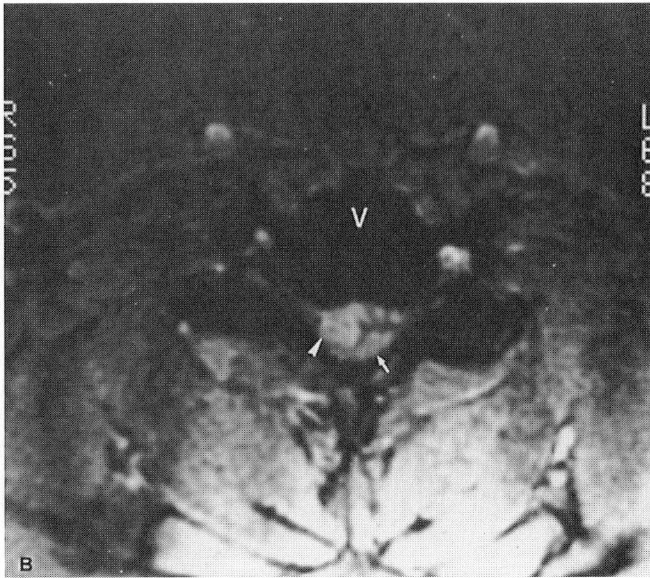

FIGURE 114.5 This patient experienced severe neck pain and quadriparesis when he stood from a squatting position. (*A*) Sagittal cervical spine magnetic resonance imaging (MRI) scan reveals an acute herniated disc with marked cord compression (*arrow*). (*B*) Axial MRI scan shows the compressed cord (*arrow*) at the level of the herniation (arrowhead). V, vertebral body.

because of age or other debilitating illness. If necessary, treatment with atropine and fluids is effective.

Once the patient is hemodynamically stable, spine radiographs are essential, but only while the patient remains immobilized on a backboard with a hard cervical collar firmly secured. Standard views are obtained, ensuring good visualization of the cervicothoracic junction (Fig. 114.6A). Comatose and severely injured patients with multiple trauma should have good plain film imaging of the complete spine. Fractured areas are further studied with CT, using both axial and sagittal views (Figs. 114.6B and C). Recent protocols in many hospitals include CT scanning of the C-spine in patients with altered consciousness even if no abnormality is detected on plain films, as CT scanning has been shown to be virtually 100% sensitive in detecting bony spine injury. If no abnormality is found despite a neurologic deficit that localizes to the spinal cord, MRI or myelography followed by CT must be used to look for traumatic intervertebral disc rupture, spinal epidural hematoma, ligamentous spine injuries, or spinal cord contusions (see Fig. 114.5).

The goals of treatment are to correct spinal alignment, to protect undamaged neural tissue, to restore function to reversibly damaged neural tissue, and ultimately to achieve permanent spinal stability.[4] Reduction and immobilization of any fracture or dislocation must receive top priority to meet these objectives. Solu-Medrol has been shown to improve outcome in spinal cord injury, although its use is still somewhat controversial, and use greater than 24 hours has been shown to increase risk of pneumonia without a significant increase in neurologic benefit.

Cervical spine malalignment can almost always be reduced by skeletal traction applied with skull tongs or halo apparatus. The patient is placed in cervical traction with frequent lateral-view radiographs to ensure good reduction and to prevent overdistraction, which can lead to further cord injury. Once the spinal injury is reduced, traction should be maintained. Cervical traction should never be performed in a patient who is comatose or unable to comply with a neurologic examination. Sometimes a cervical fracture cannot be reduced by traction alone without jeopardizing spinal cord function. Open reduction, usually through a posterior approach, combined with a fusion procedure may be necessary in those instances. This especially pertains to unilaterally or bilaterally locked facets.

Indications for early operation on patients with spinal cord injury include the inability to reduce the fracture or dislocation satisfactorily by closed methods, neurologic deterioration in a patient with an initially incomplete cord lesion, severe compression of the spinal cord by an intraspinal mass, and a penetrating injury with or without a CSF leak. Open wounds, such as stab and gunshot wounds, should be débrided and closed whether the cord injury is complete or incomplete. Early operation to stabilize the spine is warranted because this translates into early mobilization and rehabilitation. If closed reduction is successful and the fracture is stable, external immobilization is necessary for a minimum of 3 months to ensure proper healing. For the cervical spine, this involves a halo vest. Exceptions include anterior and posterior metal plating procedures, for which a hard cervical collar may suffice. The thoracic and upper lumbar spines usually require a plastic body jacket or plaster cast for a minimum of 3 months. The lower lumbar spine may require a thoracolumbar orthosis with leg extension if there is a concern for postfixation instability. Plain films are used to monitor spinal alignment and extent of fusion after immobilization during the recovery period.

If any cord function is preserved immediately after injury, additional function usually returns if the cord and spine are protected from secondary injury. Sometimes the patient with an incomplete cord injury can walk again if early care is protective and rehabilitation is aggressive and well planned. Patients with complete injuries rarely recover function below the level of the lesion. Rehabilitation for them is directed toward self-care and vocational readjustment. Most people with these handicaps can eventually achieve independence. Life expectancy is shortened slightly in paraplegic and significantly in quadriplegic patients.

Peripheral Nerve Injury

Peripheral nerve injuries can be categorized functionally. Neurapraxia is a temporary loss of function without axonal or structural injury. The foot that "goes to sleep" after crossing

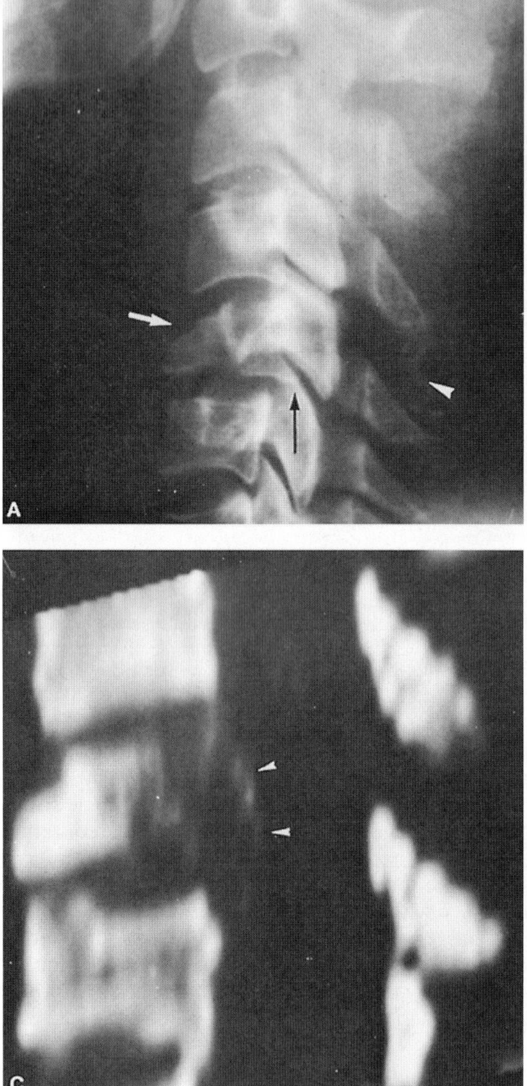

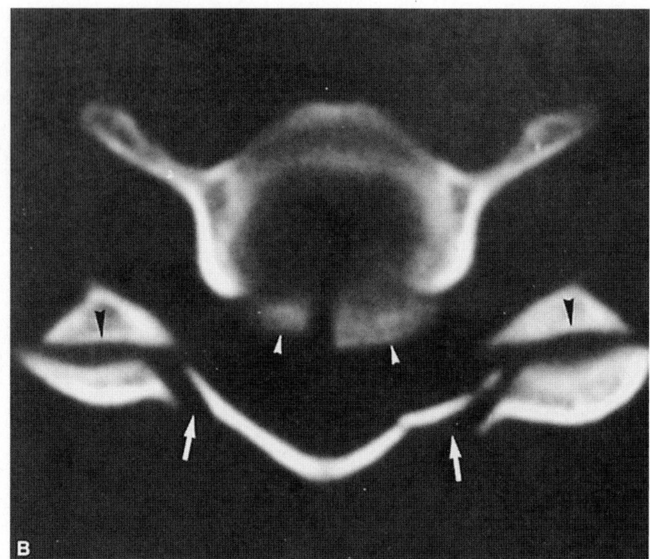

FIGURE 114.6 (*A*) Lateral cervical spine radiograph showing a C-5 fracture in a patient who was an unrestrained passenger in a motor vehicle accident. C-5 vertebral body compression (*white arrow*), retropulsion of a fracture fragment into the spinal canal (*black arrow*), and posterior interspinous widening (arrowhead) are visible. These findings are consistent with a hyperflexion injury. (*B*) Axial computed tomography (CT) scan through the C-5 level reveals fractures of the vertebral body (*white arrowheads* indicate the retropulsed fragments) and the laminae (*arrows*) as well as disruption of both facet joints (*black arrowheads*). (*C*) Sagittal CT scan offers another view of the compromised spinal canal by the retropulsed fragments (*arrowheads*).

the legs is an example of neuropraxia. Axonotmesis is a disruption of the axon with preservation of the axon sheath. Wallerian degeneration of the distal axon fragment occurs. Stretch or prolonged compression causes this functional and structural loss. Regeneration of the proximal axon occurs, but functional recovery depends on associated injuries, the amount of healthy proximal axon remaining after injury, and the age of the patient. Neurotmesis is disruption of both the axon and axon sheath with corresponding loss of function and is caused by transection of a nerve. Regeneration occurs, but function rarely returns to normal.

Clinically, sensory and motor changes correspond to the peripheral nerve involved. A detailed history and a precise neurologic examination can localize the site of injury with accuracy. Sensory findings are usually accurate early and remain so until regeneration is nearly complete. Compensatory motor function is rarely seen acutely. A crude but clinically helpful sign of sensory regeneration is Tinel's sign, in which percussion of the skin overlying the length of the injured nerve elicits paresthesias at the site where regeneration is occurring. Radiographs of the injury site help find fractures or foreign bodies. EMG is not useful within the first 3 weeks of injury but is highly effective for monitoring the status of the degeneration and regeneration process that occurs later.

Treatment of a lacerated nerve consists of primary repair when the wound is clean and uncomplicated, as in stab wounds, lacerations from glass, and surgical incisions. Secondary or delayed repair is indicated when the wound is dirty or complicated and is best accomplished a few weeks after injury, when tissue viability is obvious, the likelihood of infection is reduced, and dissection planes are distinct.

Nerve injuries in continuity (i.e., resulting from contusion or compression without laceration) are often explored if they do not improve within 6 weeks of injury, whether loss of function is complete or incomplete. Intraneural and extraneural scar tissue at the site of the lesion can prevent axonal regrowth by its constricting effect. Neurolysis releases the regenerating nerve fibers from the impinging scar and can improve functional recovery.

Prompt institution of physical therapy is also indicated for improvement of muscle function and maintenance of joint motion. It is the best means of minimizing the complications of denervation. The denervated portion of the limb is subject to muscle atrophy and fibrosis, joint stiffness, motor end plate atrophy, and trophic skin changes. The longer the denervation persists, the less likely it is that good function will result. Regeneration in a peripheral nerve occurs at 1 mm per day (roughly 1 inch each month), so improvement may not be obvious for many months. Unfortunately, incomplete neurologic recovery is often the rule.

NEOPLASMS

Nervous system tumors represent almost 10% of all neoplasms. Nearly 70% of adult tumors are found above the tentorium (supratentorial), whereas 70% of childhood tumors are found below (infratentorial). CNS tumors are the most common solid tumors in children. Of pediatric cancers, they are second only to leukemia in prevalence.[5]

The incidence of nervous system neoplasia decreases in late adolescence and begins to peak again by middle age. By then, only 25% of intracranial tumors are benign. This percentage rises to 50% in the older patient because of the increasing incidence of meningiomas and schwannomas. Overall, there is a slightly greater prevalence of tumors in men (55%), but schwannomas and meningiomas are more common in women. Of all CNS neoplasms, spinal tumors constitute approximately 15%.

INTRACRANIAL TUMORS

The Monroe-Kelly doctrine states that the intracranial size is of a fixed volume and is filled by three components: CSF, blood, and cranial tissue. Any increase in the size of one of these components will lead to an increase in ICP. Intracranial tumors therefore exert both local and generalized effects by their presence in a closed bony structure, either arising from within or on the surface of a noncompliant brain. A tumor's local influence consists of either irritative or destructive effects. Focal seizures occur because of irritation of adjacent cortex, whereas a focal neurologic deficit develops because of compressive forces on nearby functional brain. More generalized effects consist of raised ICP because of the presence of the abnormal mass. This may be in the form of obstructive hydrocephalus, tumor hemorrhage, or cerebral edema, or it may simply be the result of the added volume imparted by the tumor in the closed bony compartment of the skull.

These tumor effects can present as headache, occasional nausea and vomiting, decreased level of consciousness, and slowed cognitive function. A full discussion of neurologic tumors is beyond the scope of this chapter, but the more common types are discussed later.[6]

Astrocytoma

Tumors arising from the glial cells of the brain make up more than 60% of all intracranial tumors. Low-grade astrocytomas (grades I and II) constitute 10% to 20% of all brain tumors in adults and 8% to 25% in children. In adults they typically arise during the fourth decade and present with a 1- to 2-year history of signs and symptoms that include headaches, seizures, vomiting, mental status changes, papilledema, and focal neurologic deficits relevant to the hemisphere involved. On CT, they appear as low-attenuation lesions with minimal to mild contrast enhancement. These tumors are infiltrative and rarely can be totally excised. Surgery is usually performed for diagnosis and debulking and is usually followed by radiation therapy (RT). The 5-year survival rate with surgery and subsequent radiation is greater than 65%. Some low-grade astrocytomas can become anaplastic and, as such, become high-grade gliomas (see later).

Low-grade astrocytomas of the cerebellum typically occur in the pediatric population as a subtype of astrocytoma known as the *pilocytic astrocytoma*. They are often cystic and carry a favorable prognosis. These tumors are often totally resectable. RT is reserved for incomplete resections when follow-up has demonstrated continued tumor growth. The 10-year survival rate is more than 80%.

Brainstem gliomas are also posterior fossa tumors that occur most often in childhood. Most are benign astrocytomas. Patients may present with cranial nerve palsies, hemiparesis, and headache, often attributable to hydrocephalus. These tumors cannot be removed surgically because of significant risk of neurologic injury to the brainstem. They are treated with RT once a diagnosis is established through either open or stereotactic biopsy. Unfortunately, prognosis is a function of their location, and 5-year survival rates are 17% to 50%.

High-grade astrocytomas (grades III and IV) are the most common primary intracranial tumor, constituting 35% to 45% of all adult brain tumors and 50% of all gliomas. Age at discovery ranges from 45 to 65 years. Because of their infiltrative nature, many of these high-grade neoplasms involve both cerebral hemispheres by invading across the corpus callosum and are called *butterfly gliomas*. Patients present with a short history of headache, focal neurologic deficit, mental status changes, or seizures. The tumors are readily seen on CT scan as low-attenuation lesions with marked peritumoral edema and mass effect (Fig. 114.7), and classically enhance with IV contrast. Despite aggressive surgery, radiation, and chemotherapy, which can extend survival and improve quality of life, these tumors are nearly uniformly fatal. The average survival with surgery plus adjuvant therapy is approximately 12 months.

Chemotherapy is often used when tumor recurs, when the brain can no longer be irradiated, or when the tumor is not radiosensitive. It can be delivered intravenously, intraarterially, and intrathecally. Most drugs are directed at the tumor cells, whereas others indirectly attack the cells by sensitizing them to subsequent radiation. Although still in the early stages of development, immunotoxins toward tumor cells use antibodies to tumor antigens, thus using the host immune system as a means of destroying the cancerous tissue.

Meningioma

Most meningiomas are benign tumors that arise from the arachnoid layer of the meninges. The incidence of meningiomas increases through life, reaching its peak at age 85 years. The male-to-female ratio for symptomatic meningiomas is 1 to 2.3. Together, symptomatic meningiomas constitute approximately 20% of all intracranial tumors.

Parasagittal (falcine) and convexity (hemispheric surface) meningiomas tend to present with seizures, focal neurologic deficits, and signs of intracranial hypertension. Sphenoid ridge tumors can present with proptosis, decreased visual acuity, cranial nerve (III, IV, V, VI) palsies, seizures, or the more generalized effects of increased ICP. Posterior fossa tumors present with cerebellar signs, hydrocephalus, lower cranial nerve palsies, or long tract signs. Tuberculum sellae tumors are often

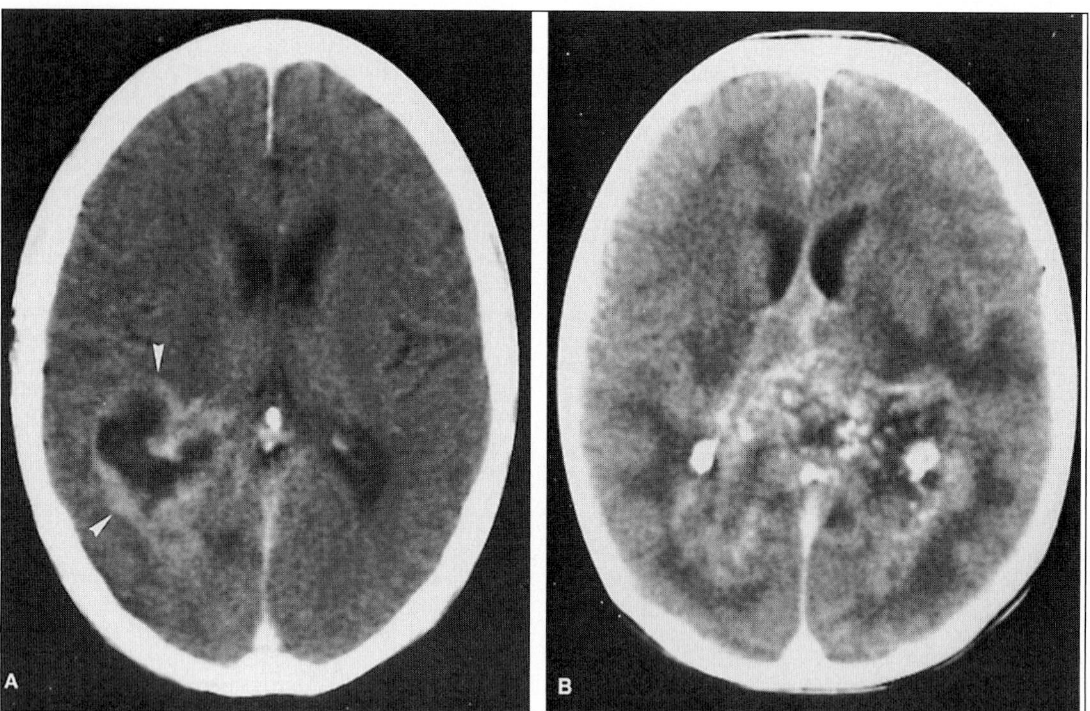

FIGURE 114.7 Glioblastoma multiforme (astrocytoma grade IV) discovered on contrast-enhanced computed tomography. (*A*) Typical appearance is that of a low-attenuation lesion with peripheral enhancement (*arrowheads*). (*B*) A more complex lesion demonstrating invasion across the corpus callosum.

accompanied by decreasing vision. Olfactory groove meningiomas can present with the classic Foster-Kennedy syndrome of ipsilateral optic nerve atrophy and central scotoma with contralateral papilledema and bilateral loss of smell. Foramen magnum tumors can be difficult to recognize and are often misdiagnosed—as multiple sclerosis, syringomyelia, or cervical spondylosis. Patients complain of neck pain, clumsiness, sensory disturbances in the upper extremities, and gait difficulties.

Either CT or MRI is the principal means of diagnosis (Fig. 114.8). Homogeneous pathologic contrast enhancement is characteristic of these neoplasms. Calcification and hyperostosis are apparent on CT, and MRI often demonstrates a characteristic "dural tail," or region of thickened, enhancing dura representing invasion of the tumor in the surrounding dura. Meningiomas are highly vascularized, and angiography classically shows a blush in the late arterial phase.

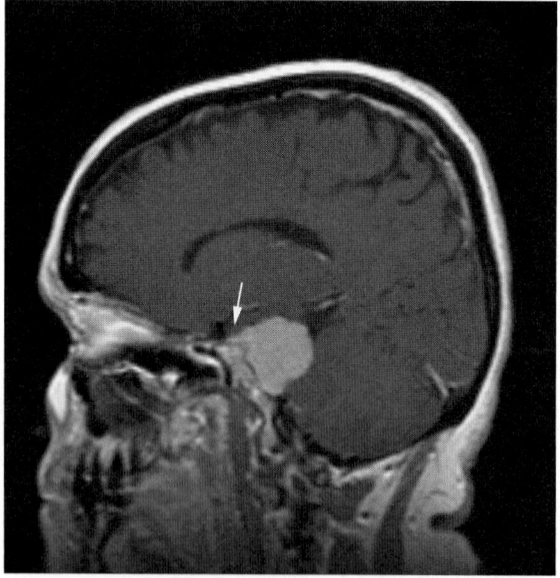

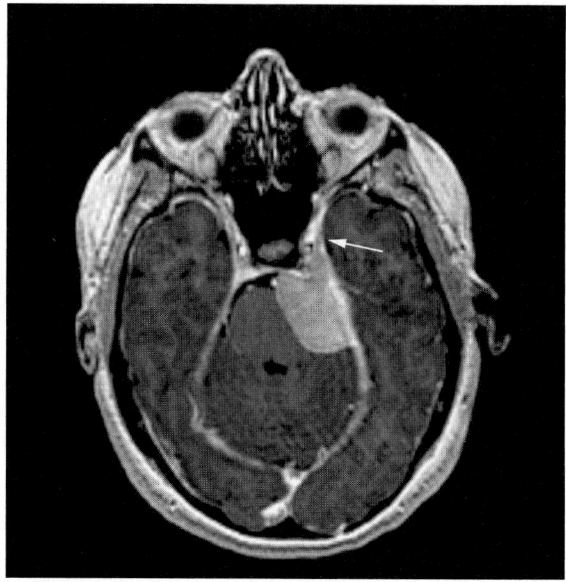

FIGURE 114.8 Large petroclival meningioma in a patient who presented with headaches exacerbated by Valsalva maneuver, imaged by magnetic resonance imaging. In the sagittal image (*A*), minimal compression of the cerebellum is seen, whereas the axial image (*B*) demonstrates moderate compression of the brainstem from this extraaxial lesion. The dural tail is observed in both images (*arrow*) and can be seen extending into the left cavernous sinus on the axial image.

The treatment for meningiomas is surgical. The techniques and goals are individualized for each tumor location, taking into account the patient's age and symptoms. In general, the goal is total excision, including the dura at the site of the tumor's attachment. If the meningeal origin cannot be excised, it is usually cauterized generously. Some meningiomas, such as those along the sphenoid ridge, may be en-plaque tumors (i.e., flat and tending to spread along the inner table of the skull). This feature often precludes total resection.

The recurrence rate of meningiomas after surgery depends primarily on the degree of excision and the presence of malignant histologic features. If the tumor is totally removed, including its dural attachment, the recurrence rate for nonmalignant meningiomas is less than 10%. With subtotal resection, the recurrence rate is approximately 60%. Malignant meningiomas have a 73% recurrence rate with gross total resection. RT is usually reserved for malignant meningiomas, although it can be used for incompletely removed benign meningiomas. After subtotal resection, RT decreases the recurrence rate from 60% with surgery alone to 32%.

Medulloblastoma

Medulloblastomas are part of the primitive neuroectodermal classification of brain tumors. They are thought to arise from primitive cells of the cerebellum. Two thirds of medulloblastomas occur in children, with a peak incidence in the first decade of life. In children, these tumors are more likely to occur in the midline, usually within the fourth ventricle, whereas adult tumors are frequently positioned more laterally. They commonly metastasize throughout the subarachnoid space by way of the CSF and are rarely found outside the CNS.

Children with medulloblastomas commonly present with elevated ICP secondary to hydrocephalus. Cerebellar signs may be prominent, with truncal ataxia and nystagmus. The diagnosis usually is made by seeing an enhancing mass on CT, although MRI provides the best images of this common posterior fossa tumor. Cytologic examination of the CSF is often positive for neoplastic cells.

Treatment involves aggressive surgical removal of the tumor, followed by radiation of the brain. If CSF cytology is positive or if staging spinal myelography or MRI is positive, the spinal axis is included in the radiated field. The 5-year survival rate varies from 30% to 70% and depends on the extent of tumor resection and the efficacy of RT.

Schwannoma

Schwannomas are benign tumors and arise from the Schwann cells that surround axons as they leave the CNS by way of cranial nerves. Schwannomas constitute 8% of all intracranial tumors and are more common in women. They occur usually in the middle decades of life. If associated with von Recklinghausen's disease, they can be multiple and are often associated with other intracranial tumors such as meningiomas, astrocytomas, and ependymomas.

Schwannomas usually occur on sensory cranial nerves. The vestibular portion of the acoustic nerve is by far the most common site (Fig. 114.9). Depending on their size, these acoustic neuromas usually produce hearing loss. As they enlarge, they can create facial numbness by compression of the trigeminal nerve and loss of coordination by compression of the adjacent cerebellar hemisphere. Only very late in their course do they cause facial weakness. Symptoms of increased ICP from obstructive hydrocephalus can also present late.

Much less commonly, schwannomas arise from the trigeminal nerve itself, presenting as a mass in the middle fossa that is associated with facial numbness. Some patients complain of lancinating, burning, and episodic pain similar to trigeminal neuralgia. Only rarely do other cranial nerves serve as the primary site of origin for schwannomas.

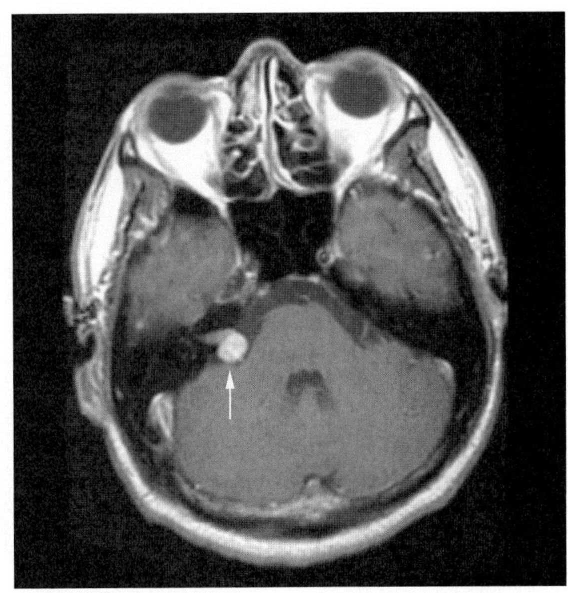

FIGURE 114.9 Small intracanalicular acoustic neuroma observed on axial magnetic resonance imaging (*arrow*). The patient is a 42-year-old man who had reported progressive hearing loss in the right ear. Given his profound preoperative hearing loss, he had this lesion resected through a translabyrinthine approach without preservation of hearing function.

The treatment of schwannomas is surgical, and total resection is curative. Microsurgical techniques have reduced the risks of surgery and have allowed preservation of cranial nerve function. The decision regarding approach is made on the basis of size and existing hearing function. Hearing preservation is usually attempted in patients with good preoperative hearing and tumors less than 1.5 cm in size; preservation of hearing is unlikely in tumors greater than 1.5 cm.

Pituitary Adenoma

Tumors arising from the pituitary gland are usually benign histologically and constitute 10% of intracranial tumors. The presentation, diagnosis, and treatment of these tumors are addressed fully elsewhere in this text (see Chapter 80).

Ependymoma

Ependymomas originate in the glial cells that line the ventricular system. The mean age at diagnosis is 5 years. They arise below the tentorium (usually in the fourth ventricle) in two thirds of cases and are far more common in children. When they occur above the tentorium, 50% are intraventricular. The presenting symptoms are related to the tumor location. Typically, children harboring fourth ventricular tumors present with headache and vomiting related to the associated obstructive hydrocephalus. They also tend to have ataxia secondary to cerebellar compression. Patients with supratentorial tumors present with signs of raised ICP as well, but this is usually because of brain edema. Focal neurologic deficits are common. These tumors are usually well circumscribed on CT scans as enhancing masses. MRI is the study of choice when the tumor involves the posterior fossa because MRI far surpasses the imaging capabilities of CT in this region.

Treatment involves aggressive surgical excision. Unfortunately, fourth ventricular tumors can rarely be totally removed

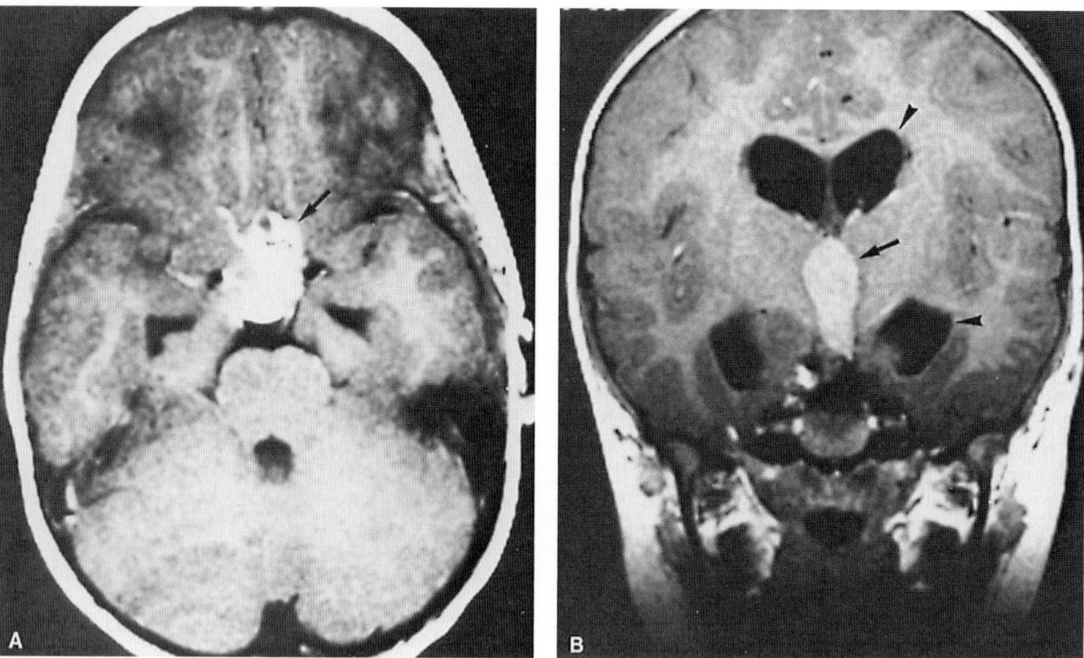

FIGURE 114.10 This 5-year-old child presented with decline in visual acuity and papilledema. (*A*) Axial magnetic resonance imaging scan with gadolinium reveals an enhancing mass (*arrow*) in the region of the sella turcica. (*B*) A coronal view shows a large cyst (*arrow*) extending up into the third ventricle. There is hydrocephalus (*arrowheads*). At surgery, a craniopharyngioma was removed.

because of invasion of the fourth ventricular floor. They are radiosensitive, so this modality clearly prolongs survival. The average 5-year survival rate with surgery and irradiation for both children and adults is in the range of 50%, with children faring less well overall. Chemotherapy is reserved for the higher-grade neoplasms. All ependymomas have a propensity to recur despite aggressive management.

Metastatic Tumor

The percentage of intracranial tumors representing metastases approaches 25%. Malignant cells invade the CNS hematogenously and tend to lodge at the gray and white matter junction. Metastatic tumors occur singly or multiply and can involve virtually any portion of the brain or spinal cord. The most common primary sites are the lung, breast, kidney, testis, colon, and skin. The presenting symptoms are determined by the site or sites of the metastases and commonly include headache, mental status changes, seizures, and hemiparesis. Metastatic lesions are best imaged with MRI. If a metastasis is suspected, an extensive workup to find the primary source is recommended. If the primary site is not identified, an excisional biopsy is indicated.

In general, a symptomatic, solitary lesion that is surgically accessible should be removed. Surgery should not be undertaken for multiple lesions or in patients who are severely afflicted by their primary disease. Treatment should also include preoperative dexamethasone to reduce adjacent brain edema. Whole-brain irradiation is almost always indicated. Prognosis depends on tumor type, with median survival ranging from 1 to 2 years. Chemotherapy is useful in some metastatic tumors such as breast, lung, testicular, and ovarian cancer and choriocarcinoma. Stereotactic radiosurgery plays an increasing role in the treatment of metastatic tumors.

Tumor metastasis to the leptomeninges (meningeal carcinomatosis) is also common, particularly in the childhood leukemias and in adults with lymphoma, breast and lung cancer, and melanoma. Patients can present with cranial nerve palsies, radiculopathies, or obstructive hydrocephalus. They often have signs and symptoms suggestive of meningitis. Analysis of the CSF is usually critical, often revealing an increased opening pressure, elevated white blood cell count and protein levels, and a decreased glucose. There may or may not be identifiable malignant cells, but cytologic examination should always be performed. Treatment of meningeal carcinomatosis usually involves RT and intraventricular chemotherapy. The outlook for patients with leptomeningeal tumor spread is in general poor, but a few long-term survivors emerge.

Other Intracranial Tumor Types

Other common intracranial tumors include craniopharyngiomas (Fig. 114.10), which often mimic pituitary mass lesions in their presentation, and pineal region tumors, which are typically diagnosed when they cause obstructive symptoms such as hydrocephalus or Parinaud's syndrome, a midbrain disorder characterized by upward gaze paresis, loss of convergence, and small unreactive pupils. Teratoma, dermoid, and epidermoid tumors arise from retained embryonic tissues and are usually treated surgically. Hemangioblastomas are benign vascular lesions most commonly associated with von-Hippel Lindau disease, an autosomal dominant disorder consisting of CNS hemangioblastomas, retinal angiomatosis, renal and pancreatic cysts, and renal cell carcinoma.

SPINAL TUMORS

Spinal tumors constitute approximately 20% of all CNS tumors. They are classified as intradural or extradural. Of the intradural type, approximately 70% are outside the spinal cord (extramedullary). Intradural tumors are almost always primary CNS tumors, whereas most extradural tumors are either metastatic or primary bone tumors of the spine. Most intradural spinal neoplasms are benign and can often be totally excised surgically. Tumors occurring within the cord (intradural-intramedullary) tend to produce weakness, increased tone, usually in the form of spasticity, and sensory loss. Extramedullary lesions present with radicular pain from nerve root (lower motor neuron) compression as well as long tract (upper motor neuron) signs from cord compression. Patients with spinal tumors involving the conus region may have early loss of bladder and bowel function; those with tumors in the cauda equina present primarily with leg pain and only later experience sphincter disturbances.

The definitive study for spinal tumors is MRI, although abnormal plain films and myelograms can be diagnostic. Plain films may show widening of the interpeduncular distance, bony erosion, enlargement of the neural foramina, or a paraspinous mass. Myelography helps determine the tumor's relation to the spinal cord and dura, whereas postmyelography CT can further define that relation.

Neurilemoma and Neurofibroma

Typically benign, neurilemomas and neurofibromas are the most common spinal cord tumors, making up almost 30% of the total. They are usually extramedullary intradural tumors. Of these, 13% have extradural extension through an adjacent foramen, producing the classic dumbbell shape of the neurofibroma. The extradural component tends to enlarge the involved foramen. Treatment is surgical removal. Adjacent or involved spinal nerve roots (usually the dorsal ones) may need to be sacrificed to obtain total excision. Multiple neurofibromas are associated with von Recklinghausen's disease. In those instances, only the symptomatic tumors are removed.

Meningioma

Meningiomas constitute 26% of spinal tumors, are benign, and are usually extramedullary intradural tumors. Two thirds arise in the thoracic spine, affecting women in their fourth through sixth decades in 80% of cases. Surgical excision is the treatment of choice.

Ependymoma

Arising from the ependymal cells of the CNS, ependymomas are intramedullary tumors and constitute 13% of all spinal tumors. They occur more frequently in men. Nearly 60% are found in the conus region. Ependymomas should be surgically excised, and their distinct borders often allow complete resection. RT is usually used when total removal is not possible.

Astrocytoma

These glial tumors are derived from astrocytes and are often intramedullary. Their incidence is approximately equal to that of spinal ependymomas. Total excision is rarely possible because of their infiltrative nature. Low-grade astrocytomas, if recurrent, are usually reoperated. RT is reserved for malignant astrocytomas but is usually only palliative. Although the growth rate of spinal cord astrocytomas is slow, prognosis is poor.

Hemangioblastoma

Hemangioblastomas are rare tumors and are intramedullary 60% of the time. Up to 25% of patients have von Hippel-Lindau syndrome. They are benign and well encapsulated and should be surgically excised.

Dermoid

Dermoids are congenital lesions usually found in the lumbosacral area. They often have an associated sinus tract to the skin surface and can present with infection. The treatment is surgical resection, including the sinus tract. The resection of the portion entering the spinal cord is usually incomplete. The long-term prognosis is good.

Metastatic Tumor

Up to 25% of all spinal neoplasms are metastatic in origin, and most appear in an extradural location. Common primary sites include the breast, lung, prostate, and kidney. Treatment is surgical decompression with biopsy if the primary site is not known or if the neurologic decline is rapid. Otherwise, local RT is the treatment of choice. Other extradural malignant tumors include lymphoma, myeloma, plasmacytoma, chordoma, and osteogenic sarcoma. When significant bone destruction or surgical decompression renders the spine unstable, surgical stabilization through an anterior or posterior route is necessary.

PERIPHERAL NERVE TUMORS

The peripheral nervous system includes the peripheral and cranial nerves, spinal roots, and autonomic nervous system. Tumors can arise from any of these elements. The more common tumors are discussed in the following sections. More unusual tumors include gangliogliomas, neuroblastomas, paragangliomas, chemodectomas, and pheochromocytomas.

Schwannoma

Schwannomas arise from the peripheral nerve Schwann cells, which provide the myelin sheaths for axons. Schwannomas tend to displace the nerve of origin and thus usually present as a painless mass. With continued growth, they can create pain in the distribution of the nerve. As they enlarge, nerve function deteriorates. They tend to arise from sensory nerves but can also be found on motor nerves. The treatment is surgical excision. The nerve of origin can usually be preserved. At times, total excision may mean division of the parent nerve. If the nerve serves a significant function, it is preferable to leave a portion of the tumor to spare the nerve. Malignant transformation is rare.

Neurofibroma

Neurofibromas differ from schwannomas in that they actually engulf the nerve of origin within the tumor because they arise from the nerve itself. They are often cutaneous, making it difficult to identify one specific nerve of origin. When associated with von Recklinghausen's disease, they are usually multiple. When found alone, treatment is resection. When multiple tumors are present, only the symptomatic ones need to be resected. Removal requires sacrifice of the nerve, should that nerve be expendable. If the function of the nerve of origin is critical, a portion of tumor should be left attached to the nerve. Unlike patients with schwannomas, patients with neurofibromas should be followed closely because these tumors have a higher incidence of malignant transformation.

Malignant Nerve Sheath Tumor

These tumors typically occur beyond the third decade. The treatment of choice is radical wide resection. If there is evidence of muscle or soft tissue invasion, amputation of the involved extremity is recommended. These tumors are usually resistant to RT.

CEREBROVASCULAR DISEASE

Cerebrovascular disease is the third most common cause of death in the United States and is an equally significant cause of chronic disability.[7,8] Death and disability are the result of either ischemia causing focal or diffuse infarction or hemorrhage causing compressive mass lesions. Cerebrovascular problems producing infarction can become hemorrhagic, and hemorrhagic lesions can lead to infarction.

Ischemic Vascular Disease (Stroke)

Ischemia and subsequent infarction of the brain can occur in the distribution of any of the cerebral vessels. Because the carotid circulation provides the greatest blood supply to the brain, ischemia and infarction are most common within its distribution. Ischemia can be the result of diminished flow secondary to stenosis or occlusion of major arteries or can result from transient or permanent occlusion of smaller arterioles from intravascular emboli.

The most common cause of stenosis or occlusion of large vessels is atherosclerosis. This often occurs extracranially at the origin of the internal carotid artery in the neck but can occur in the carotid siphon (that portion of the artery within the cavernous sinus), the distal internal carotid, or even the proximal middle cerebral artery.

The primary role of the neurosurgeon in the management of stroke is to identify stroke-prone patients and reduce their risk of cerebral ischemia. High-risk patients are usually identified by a history of transient ischemic attacks (TIAs), presenting as either transient cerebral ischemia or amaurosis fugax. Transient cerebral ischemia in the carotid circulation usually consists of temporary hemianesthesia, hemiparesis, or aphasia. Amaurosis fugax is transient loss of vision in one eye, usually in the form of an ascending or descending shade effect. Ischemia in the vertebrobasilar system can consist of transient diplopia, dizziness, dysarthria, dysphagia, weakness, numbness, loss of vision, or even loss of memory.

Most ischemic episodes last seconds to minutes; rarely do they last longer than 30 minutes. As long as the neurologic deficit resolves within 24 hours, the episode is a TIA. An ischemic deficit that lasts 24 hours to 1 week is termed a *reversible ischemic neurologic deficit (RIND)*. Ischemic deficits lasting longer than this are considered completed strokes. Patients with TIAs and even those with slow-onset strokes are potential candidates for preventive surgical intervention. Surgical procedures to prevent stroke are directed at either removing a source of emboli or providing increased blood flow to the brain. The primary neurosurgical procedure for treatment of this condition is carotid endarterectomy. Potential candidates usually undergo a CT or MRI scan of the brain to evaluate any degree of cerebral infarction and to rule out other diagnoses such as tumor, subdural hematoma, or subarachnoid hemorrhage. Patients then undergo careful angiography including the aortic arch and carotid, vertebral, and cerebral arteries (Fig. 114.11). Noninvasive studies of the carotid circulation remain less accurate, although they are useful as screening procedures.

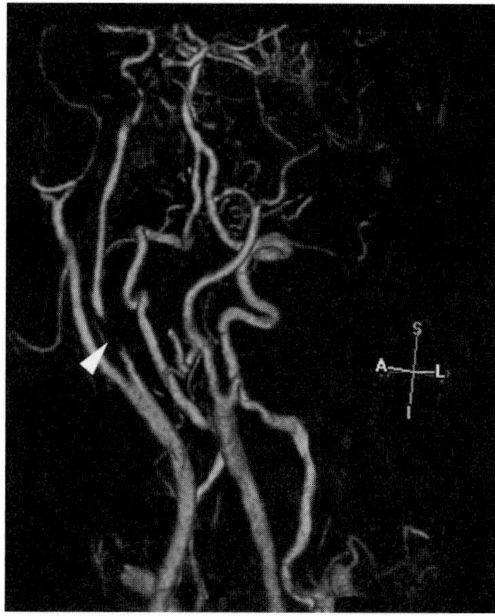

FIGURE 114.11 Three-dimensional reconstruction of carotid computed tomography angiogram demonstrating a region of stenosis in the right internal carotid (*arrowhead*). This patient presented with a history of episodic left-sided weakness and subsequently underwent carotid endarterectomy of the right internal carotid artery.

Carotid endarterectomy is indicated when ipsilateral symptoms of cerebral ischemia exist and angiography demonstrates either significant stenosis (>70%) or ulceration in the accessible portions of the common and proximal internal carotid arteries. The procedure consists of opening the affected portion of the carotid artery and removing the atherosclerotic plaque. Blood flow during the procedure may or may not be continued to the distal internal carotid artery by an internal shunt system. The mortality rate from carotid endarterectomy is approximately 1%, and the neurologic morbidity rate is 1% to 5% in experienced hands.

Advances in interventional radiology capabilities have led to the use of carotid stents for treatment of symptomatic carotid stenosis. Although the use of these stents is relatively new, initial phase 1 trials have reported no difference in mortality and stroke rate at 30 days. These stents are currently used more often in high-risk patients who might not be medically stable for surgery or those who have contralateral carotid occlusion. It is likely that the use of these stents in lower risk patients will increase in upcoming years.

Some patients have cerebral ischemia ipsilateral to an occluded internal carotid artery or stenosis of the internal carotid or middle cerebral artery that is not surgically accessible. For patients with inadequate collateral cerebral circulation, a microvascular bypass procedure is sometimes indicated. The most common of these is the superficial temporal artery to middle cerebral artery anastomosis.

Intracranial Aneurysms

Intracranial aneurysms are diseased dilatations of the cerebral arteries consisting of ballooned-out intima, media, and adventitia with a variable degree of intraluminal or mural thrombus. Most are congenital, evolving and developing during life. They can become atherosclerotic. Aneurysms typically are found at the bifurcation of the major vessels of the circle of Willis (Fig. 114.12). Up to 20% of patients with aneurysms have multiple aneurysms, and 1% demonstrate an associated arteriovenous malformation (AVM). If aneurysms are found

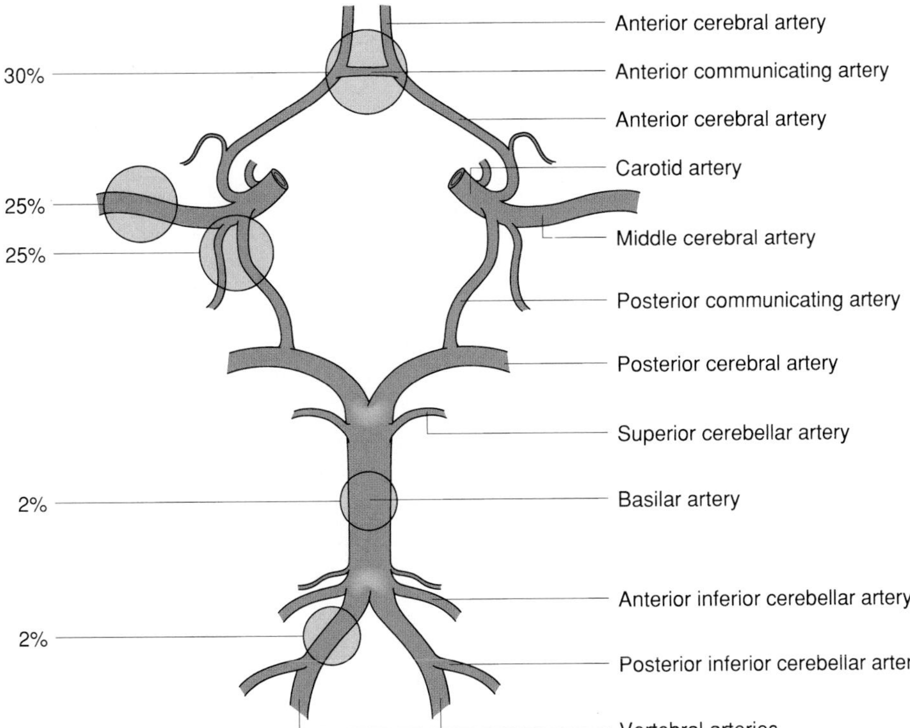

FIGURE 114.12 Locations of aneurysms of the circle of Willis and their relative occurrence.

more peripherally in the cerebrovasculature, a secondary cause such as trauma or infection must be considered.

More than 85% of cerebral aneurysms occur in the carotid or anterior circulation. Approximately 30% arise from the intracranial portion of the internal carotid artery, usually at or near the origin of the posterior communicating artery (Fig. 114.13). Another 30% occur in the region of the anterior communicating artery. Aneurysms of the vertebrobasilar or posterior circulation are most frequently found at the tip of the basilar artery but can occur more proximally along its trunk.

Patients with intracranial aneurysms most commonly present with signs and symptoms of subarachnoid hemorrhage. In fact, 80% of nontraumatic subarachnoid hemorrhages are caused by aneurysm rupture. The victim typically reports a sudden, severe headache commonly followed by neck stiffness and photophobia due to associated meningeal irritation caused by the subarachnoid blood. Transient loss of consciousness can occur. Some patients acquire a focal neurologic deficit or become comatose because of the acute rise in ICP. The severity of the subarachnoid hemorrhage can be graded

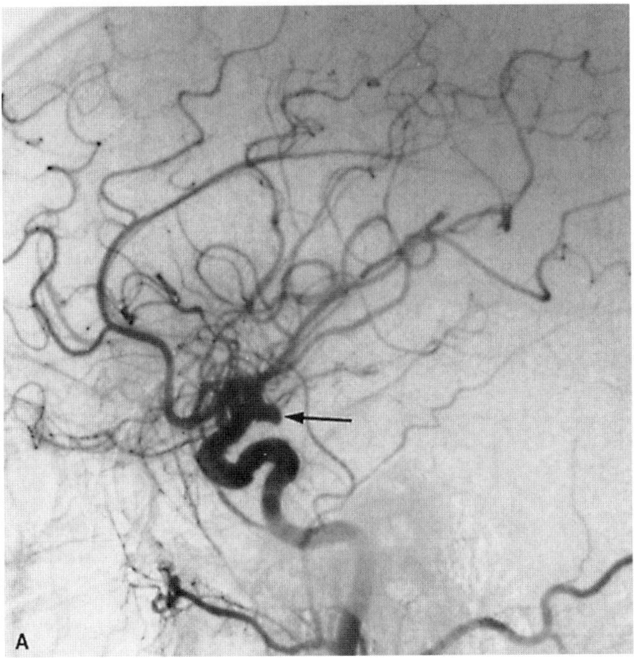

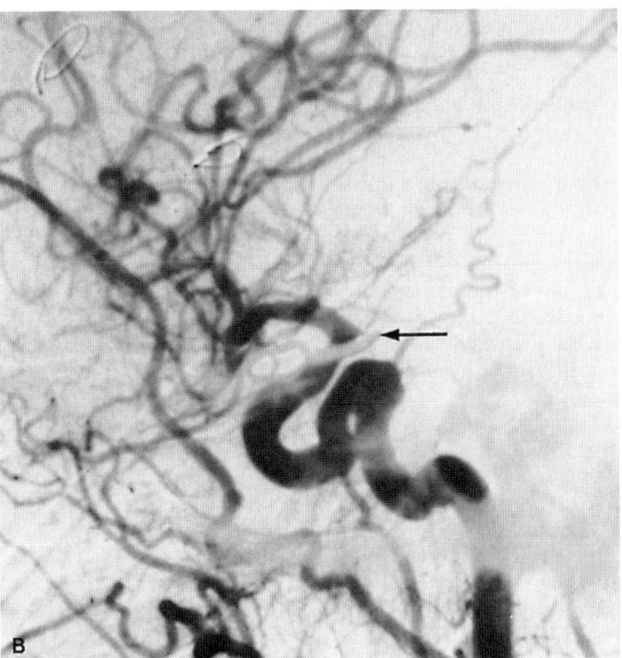

FIGURE 114.13 (*A*) Cerebral angiogram of the internal carotid artery shows an aneurysm near the posterior communicating artery (*arrow*). (*B*) Follow-up angiogram after craniotomy demonstrates obliteration of the aneurysm by a metal clip (*arrow*).

TABLE 114.2 CLASSIFICATION

HUNT-HESS CRITERIA FOR GRADING OF PATIENTS WITH SUBARACHNOID HEMORRHAGE

Grade	Description
I	No symptoms or minimal headache and slight nuchal rigidity
II	Moderate to severe headache and nuchal rigidity; no neurologic deficit other than a cranial nerve palsy
III	Lethargy, confusion, and mild focal neurologic deficit
IV	Stupor, moderate to severe hemiparesis, possible early decerebrate posturing, and vegetative disturbances
V	Deep coma, decerebrate posturing, and moribund appearance

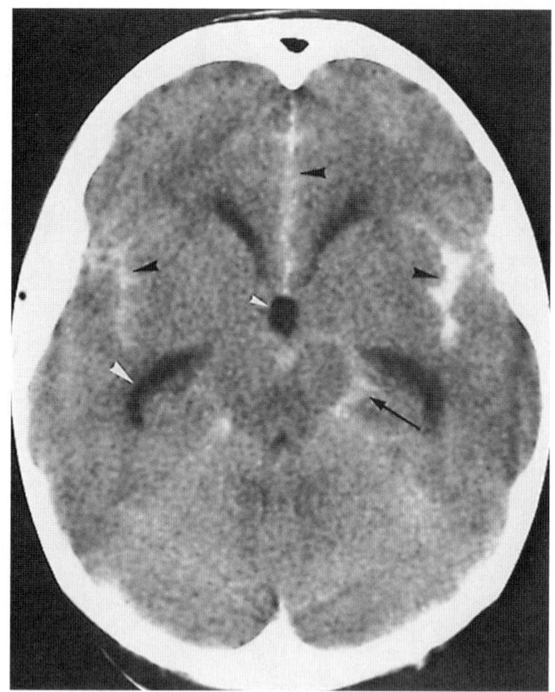

FIGURE 114.14 This patient presented with severe headache, nausea, and lethargy of acute onset. A noncontrast computed tomography scan reveals diffuse subarachnoid hemorrhage with blood in the interhemispheric and bilateral sylvian fissures (*black arrowheads*) and in the subarachnoid spaces around the brainstem (*arrow*). Early hydrocephalus is evidenced by the rounding of the third ventricle (*small white arrowhead*) and visualization of the temporal horns (*large white arrowhead*).

on the Hunt and Hess criteria (Table 114.2). In general, the lower the grade, the better the outcome.

Not all patients with aneurysms present with symptoms related to rupture. Through mass effect, an internal carotid artery aneurysm can compress the third cranial nerve, producing a palsy characterized by diplopia, ptosis, and dilated pupil. An internal carotid artery aneurysm in the cavernous sinus can compress the sixth cranial nerve and create diplopia. A giant aneurysm (>25 mm in diameter) of the basilar tip can block the cerebral aqueduct and create hydrocephalus. Rarely, an aneurysm can be large enough to be mistaken for a tumor due to its mass effect.

The diagnosis of subarachnoid hemorrhage is usually made clinically and confirmed either by noting blood in the subarachnoid spaces on CT or by finding bloody CSF with xanthochromia on a lumbar puncture (Fig. 114.14). The CT scan should be obtained first because it usually spares the patient a lumbar puncture and also eliminates the potential risk of brainstem compression from herniation if an unsuspected mass lesion is present. Complete cerebral angiography is then used to identify and delineate the aneurysm and, at the same time, rule out multiple aneurysms or an associated AVM. Typically conventional angiography is used, but in unstable patients, CT angiography can be used to identify an aneurysmal rupture rapidly (Fig. 114.15).

Once the diagnosis of aneurysmal rupture is confirmed, the patient is placed on a medical regimen to reduce the risk of rebleeding. This includes strict bed rest with the head elevated. Stimulation is kept to a minimum. Blood pressure is tightly controlled below 150 mm Hg systolic. Careful observation is necessary to watch for signs of raised ICP, which may be attributable to delayed hydrocephalus. Anticonvulsants are started for seizure prophylaxis. The ultimate treatment of aneurysms is obliteration, usually by placement of a metallic clip on the aneurysm's neck by way of a craniotomy (see Fig. 114.13B). The timing of surgery depends on the clinical grade of the patient. Patients with a good grade (I and II) should undergo operation within 72 hours of rupture. Those with a poor grade (III and IV) should continue intensive medical management until they improve to a lower grade. Aneurysms that are surgically inaccessible, or ruptured aneurysms with high-grade subarachnoid hemorrhage, can be effectively treated by embolization with detachable metal coils using interventional neuroradiologic techniques. The International Subarachnoid Aneurysm Trial attempted to determine whether endovascular treatment compared with neurosurgical treatment reduced the proportion of patients dependent or dead posttreatment. The results showed a 6.9% absolute risk reduction at 1 year in the disability outcome of patients who were treated with coiling. The long-term risk of rebleeding and the need for repeat procedures was higher within the coiling group, however. These results are still controversial, and most experts recommend that the treatment of ruptured intracranial aneurysms

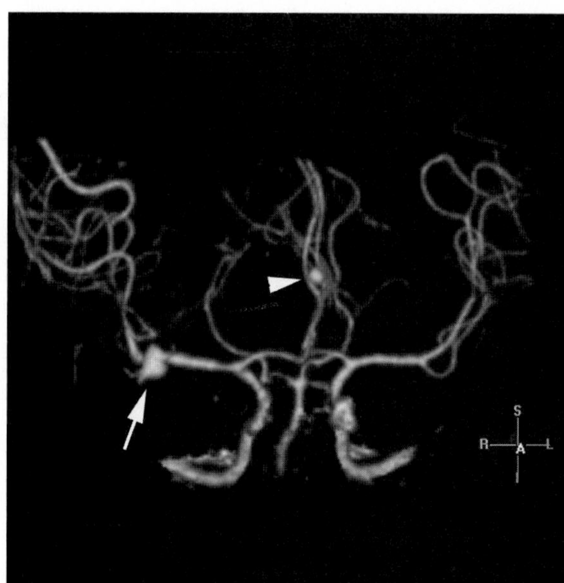

FIGURE 114.15 Three-dimensional reconstruction of computed tomography angiogram in a patient with a right middle cerebral artery trifurcation aneurysm (*arrow*) and a smaller anterior communicating artery aneurysm (*arrowhead*). Although not as detailed as conventional angiograms, these reconstructions allow the treating surgeon to preoperatively analyze the aneurysm from multiple angles and can aid in planning the operative approach.

should be addressed by a multidisciplinary team composed of neurosurgeons and interventional neuroradiologists.

Complications of aneurysmal rupture include a 30% rebleeding rate within the first 8 weeks if the lesion remains unrepaired, hydrocephalus from obstruction of the arachnoid villi by subarachnoid clot, vasospasm, intracerebral hematomas, raised ICP, and seizures. The most significant and least understood of these is cerebral vasospasm. This phenomenon occurs most frequently within 4 to 7 days of the hemorrhage and results in narrowing of adjacent cerebral arteries. Vasospasm may be seen on angiography without any untoward clinical effects, or it may produce profound and life-threatening cerebral ischemia in the distribution of the involved vessels. Symptomatic vasospasm can be treated with measures to increase cerebral blood flow. This can be accomplished by increasing systemic blood pressure with inotropic support and intravascular volume expansion. Vasospasm that persists despite medical intervention can be treated with cerebral angioplasty.

Patients with unruptured aneurysms should undergo elective treatment of these aneurysms, as these patients do better than those with ruptured aneurysms because the brain has not been injured by the subarachnoid hemorrhage. Smaller unruptured aneurysms can be followed with serial imaging. In general, unruptured aneurysms larger than 10 mm should be treated definitively, whereas those less than 5 mm may be monitored. In addition, aneurysms of the internal carotid artery carry less risk than those of the vertebrobasilar system, with the exception of complex anterior communicating artery aneurysms. In general, if the aneurysm can be treated and vasospasm avoided or effectively overcome, most patients do well.

Arteriovenous Malformations

AVMs occur within the CNS as congenital abnormalities in which blood is directly shunted from arteries to veins. AVMs can be small with only a single feeding artery, or they can encompass several lobes of the brain, incorporating arterial feeders from multiple sources. They can occur in almost any portion of the brain, including the cerebellum and brainstem. Rarely, AVMs occur in the spinal cord, or they can exclusively involve the dura.

Diagnosis of AVMs usually occurs before 30 years of age. The most common presentation is hemorrhage (50% of cases and 10% of all intracerebral hemorrhages, second only to aneurysms). Bleeding usually occurs in the brain substance but can occur in the ventricular system or subarachnoid space. The patient experiences a sudden headache, often associated with loss of consciousness and a neurologic deficit. The next most common presenting symptom is a seizure. In a few cases, seizures are frequent and refractory to medical therapy. AVMs can present with the insidious onset of a focal neurologic deficit as a result of mass effect, increased venous pressure, or vascular steal phenomenon. Occasionally, young patients with severe, unrelenting headaches are found to be harboring an AVM.

The risk of hemorrhage for unruptured AVMs is 2% to 4% per year, with an associated mortality rate of 1% per year. Once an AVM has bled, the risk of rebleeding is increased to 5% per year. With each hemorrhage, the risk of death is approximately 10%; morbidity is at least 15%. Smaller AVMs are more likely to bleed than larger ones. Most AVMs remain stable in size, but some enlarge with time. Up to 10% have an associated aneurysm on a feeding artery. In these cases, hemorrhage is usually due to rupture of the aneurysm.

An AVM can be identified on contrast-enhanced CT scanning as a hyperdense mass, part of which has a serpentine configuration related to the presence of large draining veins. Their configuration and extent is more easily delineated with MRI (Fig. 114.16A). After hemorrhage, an unenhanced CT scan usually demonstrates intracerebral or subarachnoid blood. AVMs may be too small to be seen on CT, so careful angiography may be necessary to identify the source of hemorrhage.

In all cases of suspected or proven AVM, complete cerebral angiography must be undertaken to define carefully the extent of the malformation (see Fig. 114.16B and C). All feeding arteries, including any from the external carotid system, as well as the draining veins, must be evaluated. A treatment decision can be reached only with angiography. Should angiography fail to delineate a lesion despite suspicion, MRI can identify the angiographically occult abnormality.

The treatment of AVMs depends on the size, location, and venous drainage of the lesion, combined with the presenting symptoms, age, and condition of the patient[9] (Table 114.3). Because of the risk of rebleeding, an AVM that has bled should be surgically excised if possible. In the patient who presents with seizures, the treatment decision is more difficult. In general, if the patient is young and the malformation is readily accessible, surgical resection is recommended, especially when the seizures are medically refractory. Surgery involves the microsurgical dissection and resection of the entire malformation, rather than simple ligation of feeding arteries. The results of surgery are related to the size and location of the malformation.

Alternate or adjunctive methods of treatment include intraarterial embolization and RT. With the use of interventional neuroradiologic techniques, particulate matter or glues can be introduced into AVMs by way of feeding vessels in an attempt to occlude the arteriovenous shunt. It is rarely possible to completely obliterate these lesions with this method. This technique can reduce flow through the AVM before direct surgical intervention. Ionizing radiation, on the other hand, can completely obliterate selected small to medium AVMs. Focused gamma or proton beam irradiation has demonstrated the best results, but an occasional success with conventional irradiation has been reported. Ionizing radiation causes endothelial proliferation and can take 6 months to 2 years to obliterate the lesion. The patient is still at risk for hemorrhage during the time period until complete obliteration. Focused irradiation is usually recommended for deep, surgically inaccessible AVMs.

Brain Hemorrhage

Spontaneous hemorrhage is most commonly associated with systemic hypertension and occurs in predictable locations, including the putamen, thalamus, cerebellum, and pons. Hemorrhage can also occur in the various lobes of the brain. Nonhypertensive causes of brain hemorrhage were discussed earlier, such as rupture of AVMs and aneurysms, and hemorrhage into areas of ischemia. Additional causes include induced or endogenous coagulopathies, primary or metastatic brain tumors, and rare conditions such as amyloid angiopathy.

Although brain hemorrhage is often devastating, it can be surprisingly well tolerated. The hematoma tends to dissect along axonal planes, separating rather than destroying vital structures. If the resultant mass is tolerated by the patient, the blood is slowly resorbed by macrophages along the periphery, leaving only a hemosiderin-stained slit in the brain. Patients can worsen clinically after the initial hemorrhage because of associated edema formation.

Hemorrhage into the putamen accounts for most hypertensive bleeds. Presentation is characterized by lack of headache and the gradual development of hemiparesis progressing to hemiplegia. This can be associated with a hemisensory loss, aphasia, hemianopia, or ipsilateral deviation of the eyes, depending on the size of the hematoma and its direction of dissection. The patient can, of course, progress into a coma if the lesion is large. Similarly, thalamic hemorrhage presents initially with a hemisensory loss and a hemiparesis. Localizing

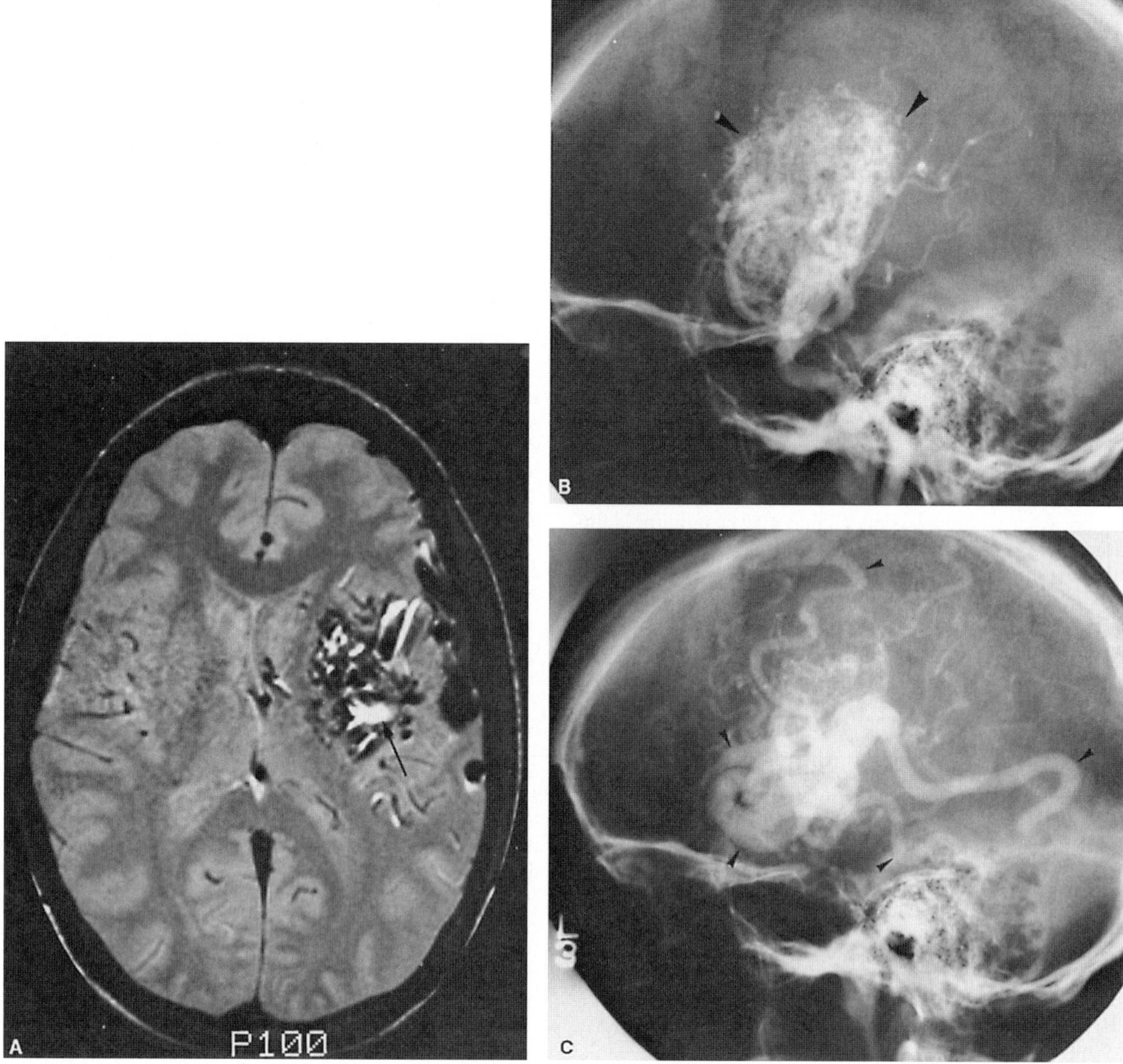

FIGURE 114.16 This young woman presented with a history of right arm clumsiness and seizures. (*A*) Magnetic resonance imaging scan without gadolinium shows a complex collection of tortuous blood vessels in the basal ganglia and temporal lobe consistent with an arteriovenous malformation (AVM). The bright signals in the lesion suggest previous hemorrhage (*arrow*). (*B*) Cerebral angiography (lateral view) on the same patient demonstrates a large AVM in the middle cerebral artery distribution (*arrowheads*). (*C*) Later phase of the angiogram reveals multiple draining veins (*arrowheads*).

features include downward eye deviation with limitation of vertical gaze and small, sluggish pupils due to involvement of the nearby mesencephalon. Headache is uncommon.

Cerebellar hemorrhage is sudden in onset and presents with headache. Vomiting, ataxia, and dizziness are accompanying features. This hemorrhage is extremely dangerous in that it can cause coma and ultimately death because of brainstem compression and acute hydrocephalus. Brainstem hemorrhage (usually pontine) is the most devastating and often presents with quadriparesis, decerebrate posturing, pinpoint pupils, and coma. Most patients do not survive if the hematoma is larger than 1 cm. Those who do survive have a high degree of morbidity. The symptoms depend on the area of brain involved.

CT scanning has become an invaluable tool in diagnosing and defining brain hemorrhage (Fig. 114.17). CT not only delineates the hemorrhage but also assesses the ventricular size and the presence of edema and often suggests the cause of the hemorrhage (e.g., AVM, tumor, aneurysm). The hematoma appears hyperdense in the acute phase. As the blood breaks down, the clot progresses to a hypodense lesion. After days or weeks, the hematoma may demonstrate an enhancing ring. If a vascular lesion is suspected, careful angiography is indicated. In all cases, appropriate coagulation studies should be obtained.

The treatment of brain hemorrhage can be medical or surgical depending on the size of the lesion, its location, and the condition of the patient. In general, if a hematoma is more than 3 cm in diameter, surgical resection is strongly considered. Surgical resection is recommended if the patient is deteriorating

TABLE 114.3 CLASSIFICATION

SPETZLER ARTERIOVENOUS MALFORMATION GRADING SCALE

Grading criteria	Points
SIZE	
Small (<3 cm)	1
Medium(3—6 cm)	2
Large(<6 cm)	3
ELOQUENCE OF ADJACENT CORTEX	
Noneloquent	0
Eloquent	1
VENOUS DRAINAGE	
Superficial (all drainage is through cortical venous system)	0
Deep (any or all drainage is through deep veins)	1

The total grade is the sum of the above and ranges from minimum of 1 to maximum of 5.
Inoperable lesions are graded a 6.
Grade I or II patients should undergo surgery, whereas grade IV or V should be treated surgically only in the event of repetitive or severe hemorrhage or progressive neurologic dysfunction.

neurologically, no matter what the size of the hematoma. Because a high percentage of these hemorrhages occur in older patients with a history of hypertension and vascular disease, however, the overall condition of the patient must be taken into account when recommending surgical treatment. Cerebellar hematomas are particularly important to remove because a small change in surrounding reactive edema can result in life-threatening brainstem compression, hydrocephalus, or both.

Because hematomas are mass lesions, medical management is directed at keeping the ICP under control. If the hemorrhage renders the patient unconscious, hyperventilation and hyperosmolar agents may be required to meet this goal. ICP monitoring can be a helpful adjunct to direct treatment. Steroids are useful in controlling brain edema if the patient bled into a tumor. Blood pressure needs close observation and tight control. Coagulopathies should be corrected. Despite medical and surgical therapy, mortality and morbidity remain high for all types of brain hemorrhage.

DEGENERATIVE SPINE DISEASE

Anatomy

The spinal column is composed of 33 vertebrae divided into the cervical (7), thoracic (12), lumbar (5), sacral (5 fused), and coccygeal (4 fused) regions. Each vertebra consists of a body, which bears weight, and the posterior elements (pedicles, laminae, spinous and transverse processes), which impart flexibility and stability to the vertebral column. Most spine movement occurs in the cervical and lumbar regions. Flexion and extension are greatest in the lower cervical and lumbar segments, whereas maximal rotation occurs predominantly in the upper cervical and lumbar segments.

The intervertebral disc lies between two adjacent vertebral bodies and provides support and cushioning. Its location is described by the two surrounding bodies; the C-4/C-5 disc lies between the C-4 and C-5 vertebral bodies, for example. The disc itself consists of two parts. The circumferential annulus making up the outer portion is composed of dense fibrous tissue of great strength. The central nucleus consists of fibrocartilage with little tensile strength but substantial elasticity. The nucleus is approximately 80% water at birth but gradually dehydrates with age, a process that leads to loss of elasticity. The fibrocartilage can then fragment acutely or degenerate gradually. It heals poorly because of limited blood supply. The annulus heals well and is buttressed by heavy anterior and posterior longitudinal ligaments for added strength. Intervertebral disc disease can occur at any level from C-1 to S-1. The lower segments of the cervical and lumbar areas are affected most often.

The spinal cord extends from the cervicomedullary junction at the base of the skull to the conus or spinal cord tip at the L-1 to L-2 vertebral level. The blood supply is provided by the radicular arteries, which arise from the vertebral arteries and thyrocervical trunks in the neck, from the intercostal arteries in the thorax, and from the lumbar arteries in the low back. An arterial confluens, the artery of Adamkiewicz, is typically found in the T-10 to L-2 region, usually on the left side. It supplies the lower thoracic cord and conus medullaris.

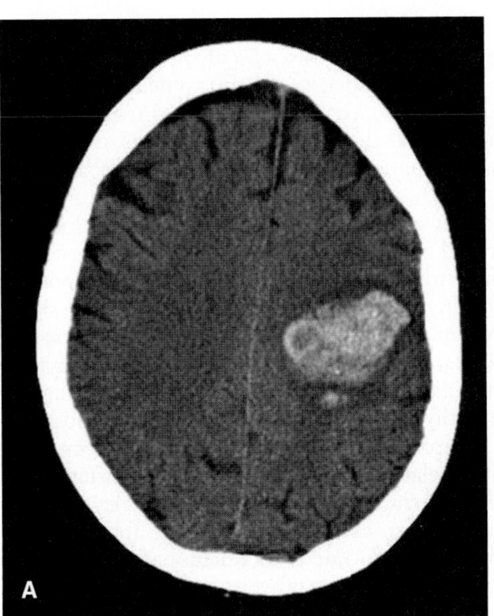

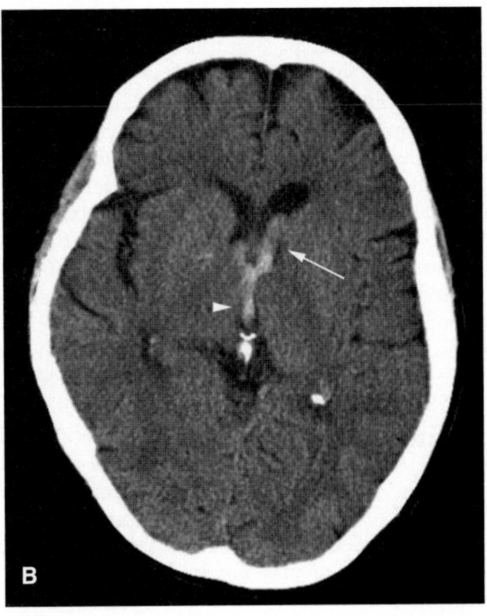

FIGURE 114.17 (*A*) Noncontrast computed tomography scan showing a spontaneous frontal lobe hemorrhage in a patient who complained of acute onset headache. Examination revealed weakness in the right arm. (*B*) Note the extension of blood into the lateral ventricles (arrow) and third ventricle (*arrowhead*).

Three fiber tracts of the spinal cord are important clinically. The laterally positioned corticospinal tracts carry motor fibers from the cortical upper motor neurons to the spinal lower motor neurons located in the ventral horns of the spinal cord. These tracts cross the midline at the pyramidal decussation in the lower medulla. The spinothalamic tract, also positioned laterally, transmits pain and temperature sensation from the contralateral side of the body. Within two or three segments of each dorsal root entry zone, the axons cross through the anterior commissure of the cord and ascend to the ipsilateral thalamus through this tract. The dorsal columns carry sensory fibers conveying position, vibratory, and light touch sensation from the dorsal roots to the opposite cerebral cortex through a decussation in the brainstem.

Dorsal and ventral nerve roots emerge from the spinal cord separately, pass to their respective intervertebral foramina, and exit from the spinal canal. The roots join to form a spinal nerve within the neural foramen. In the cervical spine, the roots exit above the corresponding vertebrae. For instance, the C-5 root exits above the C-5 pedicle. Because there are eight cervical roots, C-7 exits above the C-7 pedicle, and C-8 exits above the T-1 pedicle. Consequently, all roots below C-8 exit below the pedicle of the corresponding vertebrae. Below the conus, the lumbar and sacral roots form the cauda equina, which surrounds the filum terminale, the pial-arachnoid structure that anchors the distal cord to the caudal end of the spinal canal.

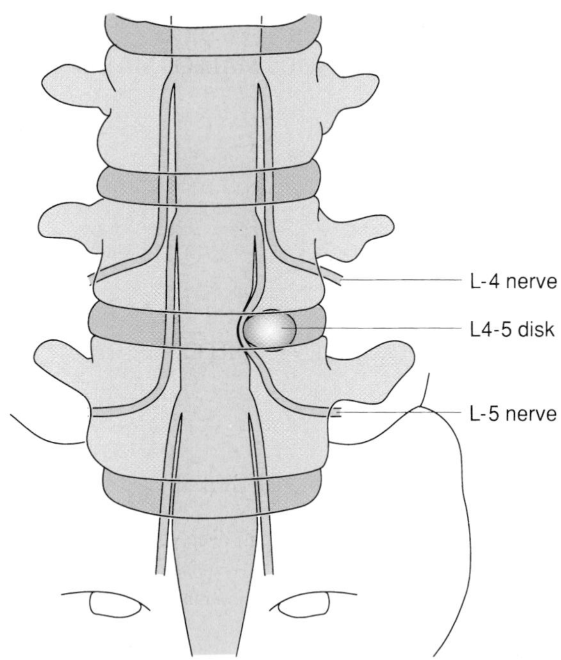

FIGURE 114.18 Relation between lumbar disc and nerve root exiting foramen.

Pathology

If the nucleus of an intervertebral disc extrudes (herniates) through the annulus, adjacent neural structures may be compressed. The pattern of compression defines the symptoms that are experienced by the patient. In the cervical and thoracic spine, compression of the spinal cord can result in paraparesis or quadriparesis, depending on the spinal segment involved. At all levels, compression of a spinal root can cause weakness and sensory loss in structures innervated by that root. The severity of the clinical syndrome depends on the site and severity of compression by the displaced disc fragment. Because a lumbar root (e.g., L-4) enters the neural foramen to exit the spinal canal above the level of the adjacent disc (e.g., L-4/L-5), a more central disc herniation will affect the nerve root one level lower (e.g., L-5), whereas a far lateral disc herniation at this same level can affect the upper root (e.g., L-4) after its exit from the foramen (Fig. 114.18). Often the nucleus does not extrude but simply fragments in response to the forces exerted on the spinal column. This is intensified by the concomitant dehydration of the disc with loss of elasticity as it ages. The disc space gradually narrows, the joint becomes loose, and the cartilaginous end plates of the adjacent vertebral bodies abut and wear more quickly. Bony spurs (osteophytes) develop at the joint in reaction to the increased mobility and decreased elasticity.

Formation of osteophytes around the joints of vertebrae is termed *spondylosis,* a common disorder that is considered by some investigators to represent the normal process of aging. If an osteophyte forms in a neural foramen, the nerve root passing through can be chronically irritated and compressed. If the osteophyte develops in the cervical or lumbar canal, the cord or cauda equina can be compromised.

Cervical Spine

Clinical Presentation

The onset of symptoms and signs of an extruded disc fragment can be acute or chronic. Acute symptoms may or may not be related to trauma. In the cervical spine, neck and radicular discomfort occur simultaneously. Spinal cord symptoms are rare. There is usually limitation of neck motion, with loss of the normal cervical lordosis. With foraminal osteophytes, episodes of cervical discomfort recur over many months or years before radicular symptoms appear. Interscapular aching, suboccipital headaches, and even chest pain are common complaints. Nerve root compression produces a radiculopathy often characterized by pain and hypesthesia in the distribution of the involved root. Associated deep tendon reflex loss with or without weakness may be seen on examination. Cervical cord compression causes myelopathy characterized by progressive spastic paraparesis, mild to moderate sensory changes in the lower extremities and trunk with cervical dermatomal sensory loss, weak upper extremity musculature, hyperreflexia, and plantar extensor responses.

Diagnosis

Cervical disc disease must be differentiated from other ailments, including inflammatory diseases of the soft tissues and joints of the arm and shoulder, nerve entrapment syndromes, and neoplasms. The pain must be distinguished from the pain that accompanies cardiac disease. Spinal infections, congenital lesions, and posttraumatic disorders are other important considerations.

Plain radiographs typically demonstrate loss of the lordotic curve of the cervical spine with narrowing of one or more disc spaces. Osteophyte formation may be seen. In cervical spondylosis, there is usually radiologic evidence of osteophytes and disc space narrowing at multiple levels. In most cases, the anteroposterior diameter of the cervical spinal canal is narrowed. MRI is the diagnostic procedure of choice in evaluating cervical radiculopathy or myelopathy (Fig. 114.19). In addition to defining the compressive lesion, MRI often shows intrinsic cord abnormalities related to the compression, consistent with edema or myelomalacia, a finding of clinical relevance. In patients who are unable to have an MRI, myelography with CT is useful in the diagnostic workup of a radiculopathy. The use of intrathecal contrast enhances the power of CT to delineate the lesion. EMG can confirm the diagnosis and localize the lesion

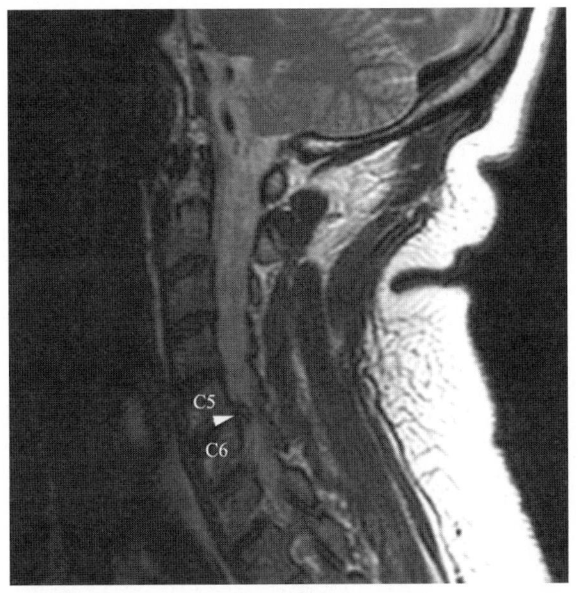

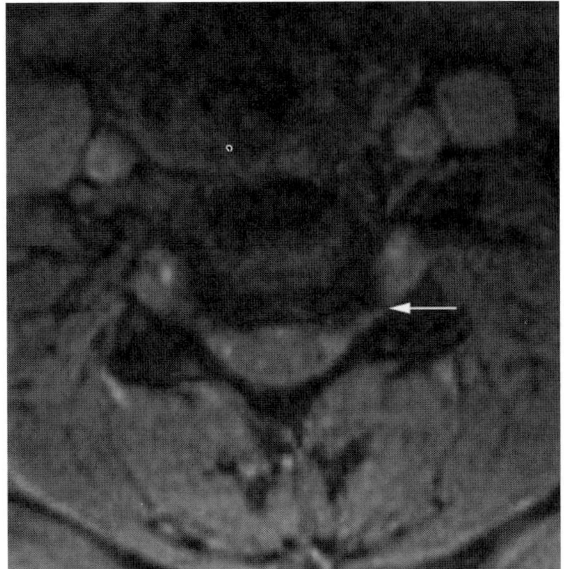

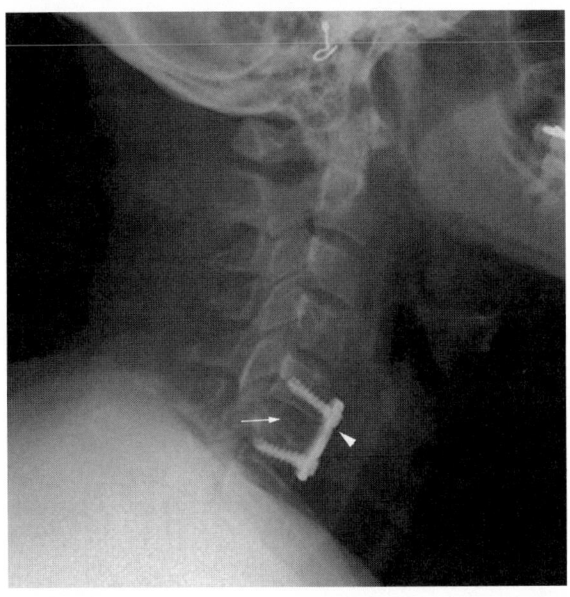

FIGURE 114.19 MRI images of a patient with posterior cervical pain with radiation of pain down the left arm into the thumb and index finger. Sagittal images (*A*) demonstrate a C5/6 disc herniation (*arrowhead*), which is seen to be eccentric towards the left and compressing the neural foramen (*small arrow*) on axial images (*B*). The patient underwent anterior cervical diskectomy and fusion (*C*); note the anterior plate (*arrowhead*) and interbody fusion (*arrow*). The C5 and C6 bodies will fuse over the next few months.

more specifically, particularly when myelographic defects are multiple. EMG is not often useful early in the course of disease, however (<3 weeks).

Treatment

Painful cervical disc disease can be treated medically as long as there is no evidence of a progressive neurologic deficit (motor loss and bowel and bladder dysfunction being most important). Adequate medical therapy includes immobilization of the neck with a soft or hard cervical collar, analgesics, muscle relaxants, and local heat. Most patients with cervical disc disease improve after an adequate trial (10 to 14 days) of medical therapy. Some have recurrence of radicular symptoms on return to full activity. In many cases, these patients can be managed for years with intervals of cervical traction and a cervical collar, but some require surgical therapy. There are essentially two approaches to the surgical treatment of cervical disc disease. Anteriorly, nerve roots, spinal cord, or both can be decompressed through discectomy with or without bone graft fusion (see Fig. 114.19). The other approach is posteriorly through a laminectomy, foraminotomy, or both. The choice of operative direction should be based on a particular patient's anatomic lesion. Regardless of approach, improvement follows operative treatment of symptomatic cervical disc disease in approximately 80% of patients who fail to respond to medical treatment. Surgical treatment of cervical spondylotic myelopathy results in improvement in approximately 60% of cases, although the primary goal of decompression for myelopathy is arrest of the progressive myelopathic deficit.

Thoracic Spine

In the thoracic spine, forceful trauma can cause the nucleus of a disc to extrude into the spinal canal. Because the canal is small relative to the spinal cord in it, cord compression readily occurs. Paraplegia is often abrupt and can be permanent. More often, osteophyte formation secondary to thoracic disc degeneration accounts for spinal canal narrowing. Development of thoracic myelopathy is more gradual. Primary treatment for both acute and chronic thoracic disc disease is surgical. The offending disc fragment or spur is best removed by an anterior or lateral approach.

Lumbar Spine

Herniated lumbar intervertebral discs often produce some degree of nerve root compression. The severity of the syndrome depends on the degree of root compression. Occasionally, the entire cauda equina is involved, resulting in loss of motor and sensory function, including bowel and bladder sphincter control. Sometimes disc rupture can occur in the midline, compressing centrally positioned sacral roots preferentially, without involvement of laterally placed lumbar roots.

Fragmentation of a lumbar disc can occur without extrusion of the nucleus, as described earlier for cervical disc disease. Because of loss of elasticity in the disc, mobility of the intervertebral joint is increased. The annulus may simply bulge without tearing. With time, osteophytes can form around the degenerated disc and encroach on the spinal canal and neural foramina. This degenerative hypertrophy involves the ligamentous structures as well. Stenosis of the lumbar spinal canal is the end result, a spondylotic condition common in the elderly.

Clinical Presentation

In the lumbar spine, more than 90% of clinical problems arise from the L-4/L-5 and L-5/S-1 intervertebral discs. Pain is usually chronic, but its onset can be acute when associated with frank herniation. There may be back pain, leg pain, or both. This radiating lower extremity pain can be exacerbated by coughing, sneezing, or straining. Bending and sitting accentuate the discomfort, whereas lying down characteristically relieves it. The pain is typically described as aching but frequently has a sharp or shooting element and is limited to one lower extremity. With lumbar stenosis, patients are unable to extend their spine without developing pain, numbness, or weakness, usually in both lower extremities. With upright posture, either standing or walking, the cauda equina becomes ischemic, producing neurogenic claudication. Relief is obtained by sitting or flexing forward. This condition must be distinguished from vascular claudication, which is caused by insufficient blood supply to the lower extremities. One simple discerning characteristic is that neurogenic claudication can be brought on by standing or walking, whereas vascular claudication is elicited by walking but not standing.

Palpation usually reveals tenderness over the sciatic notch, popliteal fossa, or both. Paravertebral muscles can be in spasm. With true nerve root compression, straight leg raising produces leg pain that is accentuated by dorsiflexion of the foot. Ipsilateral leg pain produced by contralateral straight leg raising is highly suggestive of lumbar disc herniation. Other signs include the lower motor neuron findings associated with the specific root or roots involved. Sensory loss, weakness, and loss of tendon jerks can occur in many combinations and to variable degrees.

Diagnosis

Back pain with radiation to the leg has many causes besides lumbar disc disease. The differential diagnosis includes bony abnormalities such as subluxation, degenerative facet fracture, and osteophyte formation; primary and metastatic tumors of the cauda equina, spine, and pelvis; inflammatory disorders, including abscess, arachnoiditis, ankylosing spondylitis, and rheumatoid arthritis; degenerative lesions of the spinal cord; peripheral neuropathies; peripheral vascular occlusive disease, including abdominal aortic aneurysm; and gynecologic problems such as endometriosis.

Plain films of the lumbosacral spine can identify congenital or acquired bony changes. Disc space narrowing is an unreliable sign of symptomatic disease because narrowing of the disc space can occur without clinical symptoms. Flexion and extension lateral views reveal any concomitant instability. MRI without contrast has replaced myelography and CT at most centers in the workup of lumbar radiculopathy (Fig. 114.20).

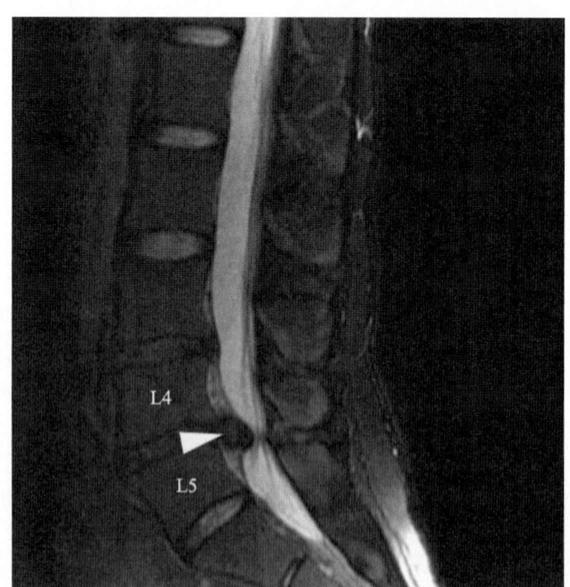

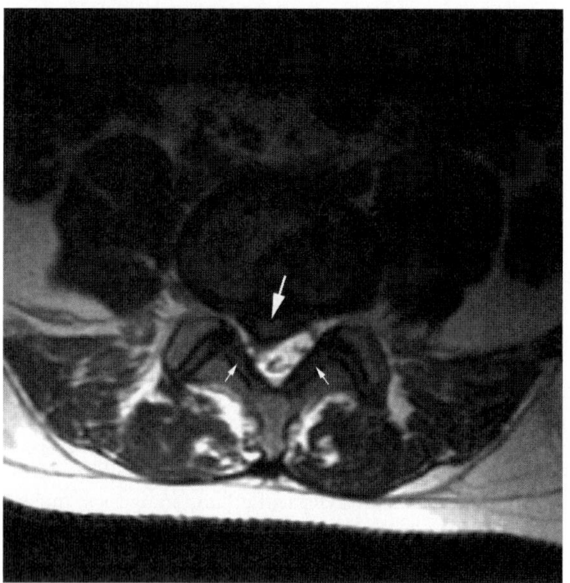

FIGURE 114.20 Sagittal (*A*) and axial (*B*) Magnetic resonance imaging of a patient presenting with acute low back and right lower extremity pain. The sagittal image demonstrates an L-4/L-5 disc herniation (*arrowhead*), whereas the axial slice through the L-4/L-5 level demonstrates a right paramedian herniation (*arrow*) into the spinal canal with compression of the descending L5 nerve root in the thecal sac. The short arrows identify the ligamenta flava.

With IV contrast, it can be extremely helpful in differentiating scar tissue from recurrent herniated discs in previously operated cases. EMG can confirm the diagnosis, especially when physical examination is unable to localize the involved level.

Treatment

Initially, medical treatment is indicated in all patients who do not have neurologic deterioration. Bed rest, local heat, analgesics, and skeletal muscle relaxants are usually effective within a few days. Physical therapy and limited exercise often help when the acute episode passes. A back brace partially immobilizes the patient and can prevent recurrent muscle spasm. With aggressive conservative management, most patients improve sufficiently to return to full activity. Recurrent symptoms can be treated in a similar fashion, often successfully. Surgical treatment is reserved for the patient with an acute or progressive neurologic deficit, chronic disabling pain, or both. The acute onset of weakness or sphincter disturbance constitutes an emergency, demanding prompt diagnosis and early operation.

Surgery usually entails a unilateral partial laminectomy with removal of the offending disc fragment. With lumbar stenosis, multilevel laminectomy is curative. If the imaging studies demonstrate an extruded disc fragment that accounts for the clinical signs and symptoms, 85% to 90% of patients recover with surgical treatment. If the syndrome is atypical, the myelogram equivocal, or the patient poorly motivated, operation is less effective. The next few years will see the introduction of the artifical disc, which is designed to replace a degenerated spinal disc that is generating chronic back pain. Clinical trials of these devices are currently underway in the United States, although they have been used in Europe during the past few years with impressive results.

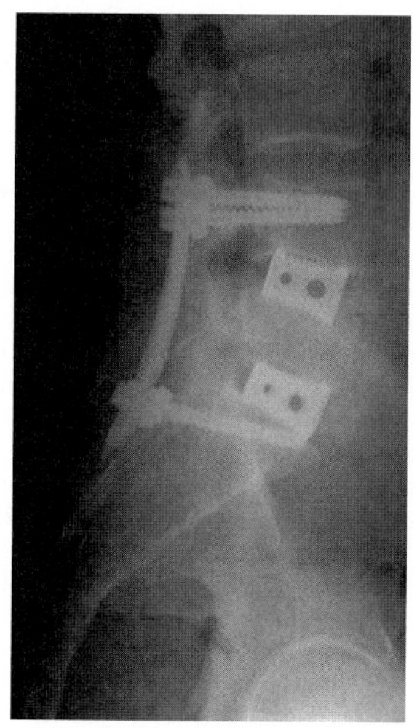

FIGURE 114.21 Postoperative plain film of patient who underwent posterior spinal fusion for the treatment of low back pain with radiation into the right leg. Note the pedicle screw fixation, which provides posterior support, and the interbody grafts, which provide anterior stability and assist in maintaining lumbar lordosis.

Instability, Scoliosis, and Pain

In some patients, back pain is a result of spinal instability. This commonly takes the form of a spondylolisthesis, a condition in which one vertebral body shifts relative to the vertebral body beneath it. This slippage is usually a result of a congenital or acquired fracture in the pars interarticularis, a bony bridge between the lamina and facet. Back pain is usually the presenting symptoms, but if the slippage is severe enough to cause a compromise of the neural foramen, the exiting nerve root at this level can be compressed, leading to a radiculopathic syndrome similar to that seen in disc herniation. Initial treatment for this condition is medical, as in lumbar disc herniation. For patients with refractory or progressive symptoms, a lumbar fusion may be warranted. The goal of surgery is to create a situation that will, over time, lead to new bone growth between the affected vertebral bodies and thereby fuse them into one solid bone. Surgical treatment can consist of anterior or posterior fusion, with or without instrumentation (Figs. 114.21 and 114.22).

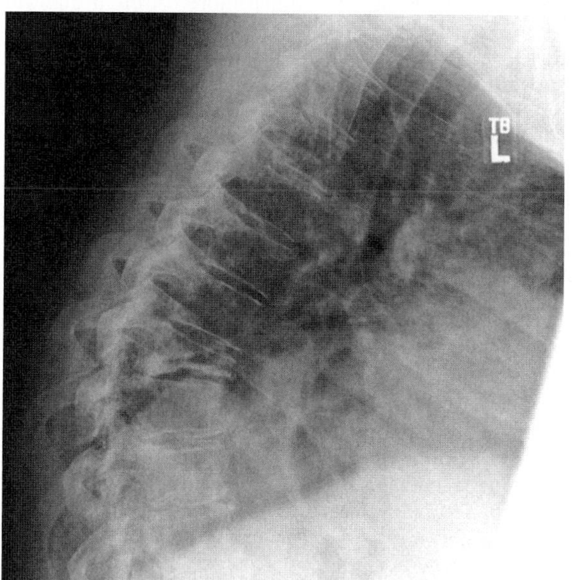

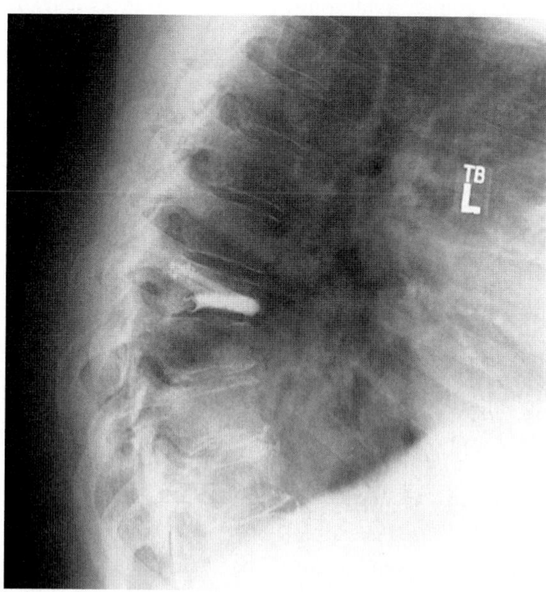

FIGURE 114.22 Plain films of a patient who presented with onset of back pain after jumping from a 10-foot ledge. Initial films show a wedge compression fracture (*A*), which was treated with percutaneous kyphoplasty (*B*). The patient had immediate relief of his pain postoperatively.

In all cases, bone material or a suitable substitute is laid down over unstable areas to promote long-term growth. Instrumentation is used to provide a temporary scaffolding for support until more solid bone growth takes place. Classically, lumbar fusion has been accomplished from a posterior approach, but the development of small lumbar interbody cages and supports has led to a boom in combined or anterior-only approaches.

The use of lumbar fusion for the treatment of back pain only is somewhat controversial. A large part of the difficulty in evaluating these patients is determining the actual pain generator. It is thought that motion of the vertebral bodies relative to one another may lead to pain, even when such movement cannot be identified on plain films or with other diagnostic tests. Unfortunately, some patients who have had multiple spine operations for the treatment of disc herniations or stenosis develop a condition known as failed back syndrome. These patients often have a fusion performed at some point in their clinical course, but relief of pain varies widely. The use of anterior procedures may provide some benefit over posterior approaches in such patients.

Scoliosis is a curvature of the spine in the sagittal and/or coronal planes. Childhood forms are most commonly idiopathic, whereas adult patients often have a history of trauma or other destabilizing condition such as a neuromuscular disorders. Patients are often targeted initially with conservative management and bracing. In patients who begin to develop progressive pain or neurologic dysfunction, however, surgical treatment may be warranted. In some patients, the curvature in the thoracic region progresses to such a degree that lung capacity is compromised. Such patients can also be aided by surgical correction of their scoliosis. Surgical fixation is typically accomplished by a posterior approach with rod and screw placement. The extent of fusion is dependent on the degree of curvature and the length over which this curvature occurs. If the curvature is especially acute, some correction may be accomplished by combining an anterior approach to bolster the vertebral bodies and a pedicle subtraction osteotomy to reduce the curvature posteriorly. These patients typically require workup with full-spine bending plain films and CT scan.

With advancing age, vertebral body bone density often declines. When placed under a loading stress, the vertebral body may compress acutely, leading to a compression fracture. Although this fracture may compress adjacent neural elements and cause neurologic symptoms, in many instances it leads only to back pain in the region of the affected vertebrae. In the past, these patients were managed conservatively, with open surgical fusion reserved only for progressive symptoms or significant pain. The development of kyphoplasty and vertebroplasty has allowed for a relatively noninvasive surgical treatment of these fractures. In these procedures, a percutaneous cannula is advanced into the vertebral body under fluoroscopic guidance. Vertebroplasty involves the injection of a bone cement material into the vertebral body through this cannula, whereas in kyphoplasty a balloon is first placed into the vertebral body through the cannula and inflated. The expanding balloon displaces bone in the vertebral body and is often able to restore some vertebral body height. The balloon is then removed and the cavity is filled with bone cement as in vertebroplasty. These procedures may be performed under local anesthesia, and patients often have immediate relief of pain.

INFECTIONS

The CNS can be infected by viruses, bacteria, fungi, and parasites. Development of infection depends on the host's resistance (i.e., immune defenses) and on the infecting agent's virulence. Bone, brain, spinal cord, meninges, and CSF can be involved separately or in combination. The routes of infection include hematogenous dissemination, local extension from a neighboring source, and direct contamination through an open wound. The infection can be diffuse, as in meningitis, or focal, as in brain abscess.

The clinical spectrum of signs and symptoms of CNS infection varies from nonspecific (fever, confusion, and lethargy) to highly specific focal neurologic deficits. Consequently, CNS infections present difficult diagnostic and therapeutic problems. Early diagnosis and treatment are crucial to a successful outcome.

Bacterial Infections

Subgaleal Abscess

Localized infection between the galea of the scalp and the pericranium constitutes subgaleal abscess. Usually, the process is initiated by contamination of an open scalp wound by staphylococci, streptococci, or anaerobic cocci. Localized scalp tenderness, warmth, and swelling are signs of abscess formation. Osteomyelitis of the skull can occur secondarily. Subgaleal infections rarely extend intracranially, unless the skull has been penetrated. Treatment includes open drainage, débridement, and systemic antibiotics.

Osteomyelitis

Osteomyelitis can develop from extension of a localized infection, such as sinusitis or mastoiditis, from direct contamination at operation or after trauma, or, rarely, by hematogenous spread from a distant source such as the respiratory or urinary tract. An established skull or spine infection can extend to the epidural space and produce a localized abscess. The usual osteomyelitis pathogens are staphylococci and anaerobic streptococci. Occasionally, gram-negative organisms and fungi are responsible. Treatment consists of drainage, débridement of infected bone, and appropriate antibiotics for a prolonged period, usually 6 weeks. Patients should be followed even after the infection has cleared to monitor for the development of any spinal instability secondary to bone destruction.

Epidural Abscess

Spinal epidural abscess is much more common than intracranial epidural abscess. It is characterized by fever, local spinal tenderness, and rapid progression of neurologic deficits, often constituting a medical and surgical emergency. Radicular pain and impairment of cord function, with early motor and sensory deficits including sphincter disturbances, occur within a few days. Most epidural abscesses are caused by local extension of osteomyelitis or by hematogenous spread from a distant suppurative focus. The diagnosis is suggested by the clinical presentation. Lumbar puncture is discouraged, as it can cause spread of the infection into the intradural space and lead to meningitis. Instead, the diagnosis is typically made on the basis of clinical symptoms and confirmed with imaging. Contrast-enhanced MRI defines the extent of the epidural mass. If the dura is intact, infection rarely extends across it.

The most common causative organisms are *Staphylococcus aureus* and *Streptococcus* species. Treatment should be immediate, beginning with broad antibiotic coverage until the offending agent is identified. Specific antibiotic therapy must be continued for a prolonged period, often up to 6 weeks. Surgical drainage is necessary when neurologic deficits progress despite aggressive medical therapy. Decadron in the perioperative period is beneficial in reducing localized edema, although prolonged use can reduce the host immune response to the infection. Recovery of neurologic function is directly related to the duration and severity of impairment before treatment.

Subdural Empyema

Subdural empyema is a purulent infection of the subdural space. It accounts for approximately 25% of all intracranial infections and is usually a complication of sinusitis, meningitis, or open contamination of the subdural space at operation or after trauma.

With sinusitis, infection can spread intracranially by transcranial emissary vein thrombophlebitis. Staphylococci, streptococci, and anaerobic cocci are commonly responsible. Once the subdural space is violated, infection can spread over the convexity of the brain. The accumulation of purulent material may be sufficient to produce an intracranial mass, provoking adjacent brain swelling. The clinical result is rapid neurologic deterioration, often with lateralizing signs, coma, and death. Treatment includes craniotomy with débridement, drainage, and IV antibiotics. The source of the infection must be treated aggressively. A sinus or mastoid drainage procedure is often required if this is the source. The mortality rate from acute fulminant subdural empyema from a paranasal source remains approximately 25%.

The diagnosis of intracranial subdural empyema is made readily by CT scan but can be difficult to distinguish from subacute or chronic subdural hematoma. The mass itself may be isodense, necessitating the administration of IV contrast. Including the sinuses on the CT scan can demonstrate the source of infection. Lumbar puncture is contraindicated, as its results are often nonspecific and it carries a high risk of herniation or neurologic deterioration in patients with subdural empyema. A head CT is therefore the first test of choice in a patient suspected of harboring an intracranial mass.

Spinal subdural empyema is rare. It usually develops from local extension transdurally or through the arachnoid in the presence of meningitis. Spinal cord compression and transverse myelitis can develop. Treatment is emergent, consisting of surgical drainage and prolonged antibiotic administration.

Meningitis

Bacterial meningitis is an acute, purulent infection of the leptomeninges. It is manifested by fever, lethargy, headache, nausea, vomiting, and nuchal rigidity. Coma can develop in up to 10% of patients with missed diagnoses, heralding a poor prognosis. Untreated bacterial meningitis is almost always fatal.

A CSF Gram stain demonstrates the offending organism in 75% of cases. Cultures provide a diagnosis 90% of the time. CSF pleocytosis with a preponderance of polymorphonuclear cells is typical of untreated bacterial meningitis. CSF glucose is almost always reduced, whereas the protein content is typically increased.

Meningitis that develops after a penetrating wound or a neurosurgical procedure is usually caused by staphylococcal, streptococcal, or gram-negative organisms. Meningitis occurring after closed head trauma with either a skull fracture or CSF rhinorrhea is most often caused by *Streptococcus pneumoniae*. Ventricular shunt and reservoir infections leading to meningitis are more likely due to *Staphylococcus epidermidis* or *S. aureus*.

The treatment for acute bacterial meningitis depends on the causative organism, its antibiotic sensitivity, and the primary source of infection from which the meninges were contaminated. The presumed diagnosis is made clinically, a sample of CSF is obtained by lumbar puncture, and broad-spectrum IV antibiotics are immediately started. The extent of antibiotic penetration into the CNS varies, depending on the degree of meningeal inflammation. Intrathecal administration of those antibiotics that do not readily cross the blood–CSF barrier may be necessary, especially when an artificial substance such as a ventricular shunt is present. Shunt removal is often necessary despite IV and intrathecal antibiotic administration.

Complications of bacterial meningitis include communicating hydrocephalus, brain abscess, subdural empyema, and subdural effusions, particularly after *Haemophilus influenzae* meningitis in infants. The risk of complications is significantly reduced by prompt, early treatment.

Brain Abscess

Brain abscess is a purulent lesion of brain tissue, beginning as a focal infection, usually in the white matter, surrounded by a typical inflammatory response. The blood–brain barrier becomes disrupted. Necrosis and liquefaction follow the acute inflammatory stage. Eventually, either the process is encapsulated by fibrous granulation tissue or the infection spreads through the parenchyma to the subarachnoid spaces and the ventricular system.

Brain abscess is usually secondary to focal infection elsewhere. Abscesses that develop by direct intracranial extension are usually solitary and are typically found in the frontal and temporal lobes. Multiple brain abscesses that develop in the septic patient are often related to bacterial endocarditis, pneumonia, and diverticulitis. Abscess formation is frequent among patients with compromised immunity from an underlying illness or pharmacologic immunosuppression.

Signs and symptoms of brain abscess are related to its mass effect. Headache, focal neurologic deficits, and impaired mentation are often observed. There may be little or no evidence of systemic infection and the patient may be afebrile. Conversely, the patient can be gravely ill from bacteremia with fever, hypotension, and a markedly elevated white blood cell count. Seizures can occur. Progressive mass effect leads to brain shifts, followed by coma.

Contrast CT and MRI are highly accurate in detecting brain abscesses. As with abscesses elsewhere in the CNS, lumbar puncture is typically discouraged. Instead, every attempt should be made to biopsy the abscess directly, as the causative organism can be identified and cultured from the abscess itself in 60% to 80% of cases, provided cultures are processed carefully for both aerobic and anaerobic organisms. Blood cultures are also helpful, particularly if the abscess is secondary to systemic infection.

In cases of early abscess formation or high surgical risk, medical therapy alone with the appropriate parenteral antibiotic may be sufficient. The most effective therapy is drainage of the purulent material with simultaneous administration of appropriate IV antibiotics. Although needle aspiration can be successful, craniotomy with evacuation and removal of the abscess wall may be necessary. Surgical drainage reduces the mass effect, thereby reducing the most critical and dangerous aspect of the infection, and also allows for accurate bacteriologic analysis.

Results of treatment for brain abscess depend on the patient's neurologic status on presentation, the efficacy of the antibiotic used, the extent to which the intracranial mass is controlled by surgery, and the effective treatment of the primary source of the abscess. Despite aggressive surgical and medical management, mortality rates associated with brain abscess approach 40%, especially in the malnourished, chronically debilitated, or immunosuppressed patient.

Postoperative Infection

Any or all of the pyogenic infections described earlier can develop after operation. Once identified, characterized, and treated with appropriate antibiotics, the infection almost always subsides. Commonly isolated organisms include *S. aureus* and *S. epidermidis*. If a foreign body such as prosthetic material or a ventricular shunt is involved, eradicating the infection becomes more difficult, often requiring a combination of IV and intrathecal antibiotics with removal of the artificial material. Infrequently, infections can be satisfactorily treated in the presence of retained foreign bodies, such as spinal hardware, provided the infection is indolent.

Fungal Infections

As a rule, fungi are opportunistic organisms. They can become pathogenic because of depression of the host immune system, prolonged systemic antibiotic therapy, or severe systemic illness. When the CNS becomes infected, it is usually associated with pulmonary fungal infection and depressed host resistance. The CNS involvement can be a diffuse meningitis or a focal abscess. At times, multiple abscesses are present. Treatment requires long-term, systemic antifungal chemotherapy. Surgical intervention is reserved for drainage of abscesses and resection of symptomatic mass lesions.

Parasitic Infestations

Although uncommon in North America and western Europe, parasitic diseases of the CNS are a major cause of neurologic disability and death worldwide. Control of these diseases remains a public health problem. A major emphasis is placed on their prevention, because once the CNS is infested, therapeutic options are limited. Treatment, both medical and surgical, is usually ineffective or palliative at best. The two most common parasitic infections encountered in the United States are cysticercosis, caused by *Taenia solium,* and echinococcosis, caused by infection with *Echinococcus granulosus.* Cysticercosis (the pork tapeworm) infests the human CNS by transmission of its larvae through the blood after ingestion. Its presence can take one or all of four forms: meningeal, parenchymal, ventricular, or spinal. Echinococcosis (the dog tapeworm) causes infection after larval ingestion. Humans serve as intermediate hosts for the organism. The liver and lungs are preferentially involved through hematogenous dissemination with subsequent formation of hydatid cysts. When the CNS is involved, cysts are usually solitary, large, and confined to white matter. In both of these infections, diagnosis rests on serologic and radiologic testing. Newer anthelmintic agents can be effective in the treatment of cysticercosis, but long-term prognosis is poor. Treatment of echinococcus consists of isolating the patient from the source and surgical removal of symptomatic cysts. Hydatid disease of the CNS is disabling but rarely fatal if the cysts are removed when they become symptomatic.

CONGENITAL AND DEVELOPMENTAL ABNORMALITIES

Approximately 2% of newborns possess some type of congenital abnormality.[10] Sixty percent of these involve the CNS, and over half of those are related to defective development or closure of the dorsal midline structures. Many have associated hydrocephalus. The commonly encountered neurologic malformations include congenital lesions such as Arnold-Chiari malformation, Dandy-Walker malformation, spinal dysraphism, meningocele, myelomeningocele, lipomyelomeningocele, diastematomyelia, dermal sinus, and myeloschisis

Spinal Dysraphism

Between days 18 and 28 of embryonic development, the neural groove closes posteriorly in the midline to form the neural tube. This tube becomes encircled by bone derived from adjacent somites and is covered superficially by skin derived from ectoderm. Abnormal closure of the neural groove, failure of fusion of the adjacent bone, or maldevelopment of the overlying ectoderm can lead to many spinal dysraphic states. Thus, dysraphism implies an abnormal fusion of normally united parts.

Failure of the bony structures to close with normal closure of the neural groove is called *spina bifida occulta.* These patients have normal spinal cords and normal cord function. The abnormality usually goes unnoticed unless seen on plain radiographs. Should the meninges fail to close, a meningocele develops, producing an obvious cutaneous abnormality. The underlying neural structures develop normally, so there is no compromise of neurologic function.

Failure of the underlying neural tissue to fuse has been called *spina bifida cystica* or, more recently, *spina bifida aperta.* Myelomeningocele, the more common form, involves incomplete closure of the neural groove, usually in the lumbar region, with the abnormal, unfused neural tissue on the dorsal surface exposed through an associated defect in the spinal column. This can be partially or totally covered with epithelium. The accompanying neurologic deficit usually consists of complete absence of motor and sensory function below the level of spinal cord involvement.

The most severe form of spinal dysraphism is myeloschisis, which is much less common than myelomeningocele. The spinal cord is unfused and presents directly on the surface of the back without overlying meninges or epithelium. It usually occurs at the thoracolumbar region and is virtually always associated with paraplegia and absence of bladder function.

Both myelomeningocele and myeloschisis are associated with hydrocephalus. The hydrocephalus is caused by a developmental abnormality of the hindbrain called *Arnold-Chiari malformation,* which is associated with the more severe forms of spinal dysraphism (Fig. 114.23). This malformation consists

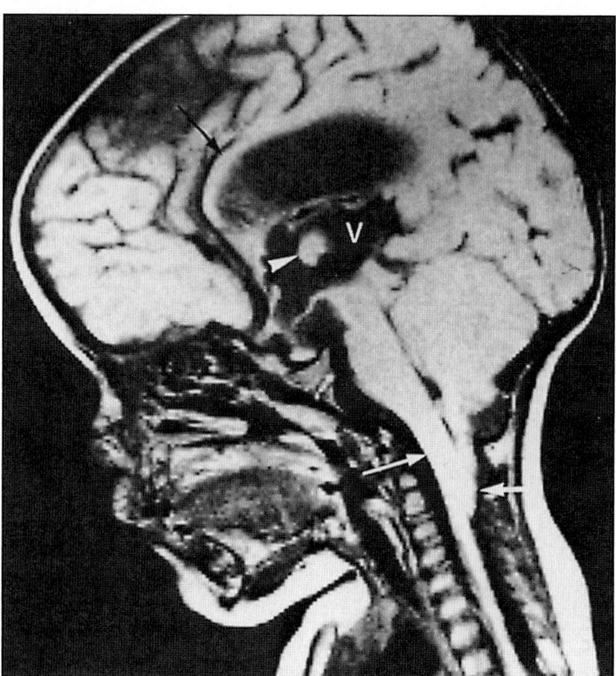

FIGURE 114.23 Sagittal magnetic resonance imaging scan of the brain and upper cervical spine demonstrates some of the features of the Arnold-Chiari type II malformation. Note the herniation of the cerebellum through the foramen magnum to the level of C-4 (*short arrow*), the downward displacement of the medulla and fourth ventricle (*long arrow*), the absence of the corpus callosum, the hydrocephalus with enlargement of the third ventricle (V), and the enlarged massa intermedia (arrowhead).

of caudal displacement of the cerebellar tonsils, vermis, inferior fourth ventricle, and medulla. There is a dorsal kink in the cervicomedullary junction and beaking of the quadrigeminal plate. Associated features include agenesis of the corpus callosum and obstructive hydrocephalus.

The treatment of spinal dysraphism is surgical. Meningoceles are excised and the skin is closed primarily after watertight closure of the posterior meningeal defect. Myelomeningoceles and myeloschises are closed as early as possible to reduce the risk of superficial infection and subsequent meningitis. Surgical repair is usually undertaken within 36 hours. The goal is to preserve as much neural tissue as possible, to untether the spinal cord from surrounding soft tissue, and to fashion a dural closure to prevent CSF leakage. Accompanying hydrocephalus is treated with shunting (see later discussion).

Survival of infants with these dysraphic states continues to improve. Despite a devastating neurologic deficit, they usually do well. Newborns with lower-level lesions do better overall than do those with higher-level lesions. The more severe the dysraphic state, the higher the morbidity and mortality rates. Timely revision of failed shunts placed for hydrocephalus preserves the potential for intellectual development.

In 1999, Vanderbilt University published its 10-year experience with intrauterine repair of myelomeningoceles. The early closure of myelomeningoceles may help reduce the development of hydrocephalus and hindbrain herniation. This closure typically takes place between 24 and 30 weeks of gestation. Although such procedures are technically difficult and do carry risk to the fetus, early results suggest that intrauterine repair may provide a clinical benefit to the affected fetus beyond that which can be achieved by standard postnatal repair.

Cranial Dysraphism

Cranial dysraphic states are one tenth as common as their spinal counterparts. Encephaloceles, although rare, are most commonly seen. They consist of a midline skull defect through which a small portion of brain protrudes. Most encephaloceles are covered with skin. Associated hydrocephalus occurs in up to 65% of patients with occipital encephaloceles but is uncommon in patients with anterior encephaloceles. Once thought to arise from defects in the closure of the primitive neural tube, they probably develop because of an overlying mesodermal abnormality with subsequent perturbation of underlying cerebral tissue. In North America and Europe, 85% of encephaloceles occur in the posterior cranial vault; the remainder are found in the anterior cranial vault. In Southeast Asia, this distribution is reversed for unknown reasons.

The surgical repair involves early resection of malformed and devitalized brain with dural closure. The mortality rate of patients with encephaloceles varies greatly. Prognostic factors include the size and location of the anomaly, the extent of brain protrusion, and the presence of associated hydrocephalus, seizure disorder, or cerebral dysgenesis. The smaller and more anterior defects usually have a better outcome. Whereas 83% of patients with occipital encephaloceles have significant mental and physical impairment, most patients with anterior encephaloceles have normal or near-normal intelligence.

Hydrocephalus

The term *hydrocephalus* implies an increase in the amount of CSF in the ventricular system. This is almost always due to a decrease in the absorption of fluid, although there are rare cases of choroid plexus papillomas causing hydrocephalus by an increase in CSF production. Hydrocephalus is traditionally referred to as *communicating* or *noncommunicating*. In the former, the ventricular system continues to communicate with the subarachnoid spaces outside the brain through the fourth ventricular foramina of Luschka and Magendie. In the noncommunicating type, often termed *obstructive*, it does not. *Hydrocephalus ex vacuo* is a term used to describe an increase in the size of the ventricles and CSF spaces secondary to a reduction in the amount of brain tissue, as that often seen in elderly patients. The common causes of hydrocephalus vary with age and include congenital causes (Arnold-Chiari, Dandy-Walker malformation, aqueductal stenosis, developmental cyst, encephalocele, neoplasm) or acquired ones (infectious meningitis or ventriculitis, intraventricular or subarachnoid hemorrhage, neoplasm).

Infantile Hydrocephalus

Hydrocephalus occurs most frequently between birth and 2 years of age and is most commonly due to congenital abnormalities of the brain. These abnormalities typically produce noncommunicating hydrocephalus. Stenosis of the cerebral aqueduct is one such common congenital anomaly. Another is the Arnold-Chiari malformation described previously, consisting of caudal displacement of the cerebellar tonsils into the upper cervical spine and at times an associated spinal syrinx. The Dandy-Walker malformation produces a markedly enlarged fourth ventricle as a result of congenital obstruction of CSF outflow from the fourth ventricle, with resultant hydrocephalus. Other, less common congenital lesions include arachnoid cysts, vascular anomalies, and congenital tumors.

Acquired hydrocephalus in the infant is often the result of meningitis or intracranial hemorrhage, both potentially causing obstruction of either the CSF absorptive mechanism or the intraventricular pathways (Fig. 114.24). Aqueductal stenosis can develop well after birth because of infection or hemorrhage and thus is termed *acquired*. Tumors can also obstruct the outflow of CSF, resulting in noncommunicating hydrocephalus. This obstruction is typically present at the foramen of Monro but may also be related to a tumor within or adjacent to the fourth ventricle or cerebral aqueduct.

Infants with hydrocephalus usually but not invariably present with an enlarging head circumference. They often have a tense, bulging anterior fontanelle with distended scalp veins and split cranial sutures. They may appear to have so-called sun setting of the eyes with only the tops of the irises visible (Parinaud's syndrome). The head may transilluminate because of lack of cerebral substance. Neurologically, the hydrocephalus usually does not cause deficits initially because of the open cranial sutures that allow for cranial vault expansion (assuming absence of any underlying brain dysgenesis). In the more chronic forms, or in older infants with closed sutures, optic atrophy and sixth nerve palsies may be seen.

Childhood Hydrocephalus

Hydrocephalus in children older than 2 years can have a more acute presentation because of the decreased ability of the more mature brain and skull to accommodate the increase in CSF. Consequently, the raised ICP can acutely cause headache, nausea, vomiting, lethargy, coma, and even death. Slower onset can result in decreased mentation, behavioral changes, diminished performance in school, sixth nerve palsies, optic atrophy, paralysis of upward gaze, spastic leg weakness, and endocrine (hypothalamic) disorders. Causes of hydrocephalus in this age group include tumors, meningitis, intracranial hemorrhage (both spontaneous and traumatic), and aqueductal stenosis. Ventricular shunt malfunction can cause acute hydrocephalus in the shunt-dependent patient, regardless of the patient's age or the underlying cause.

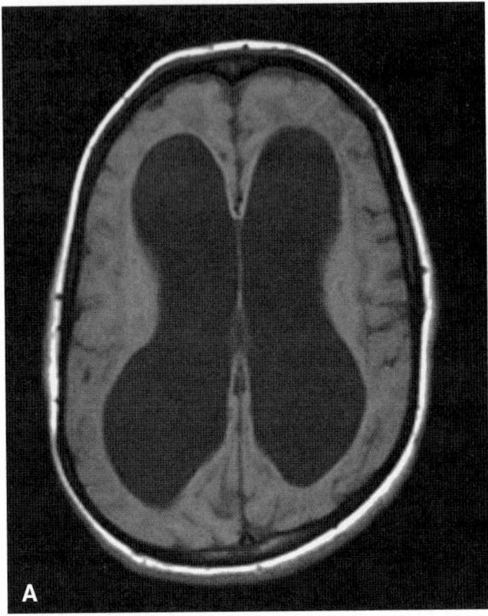

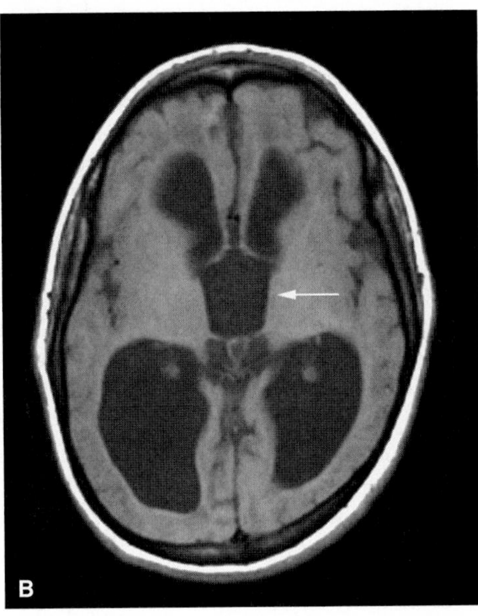

FIGURE 114.24 This 7-year-old patient had a history of neonatal intraventricular hemorrhage and later developed hydrocephalus. Note the grossly dilated lateral ventricles (*A*) and the dilated occipital horns (*B*). The third ventricle is rounded and bulbous (*arrow*), a classic finding in long-standing hydrocephalus.

Adult Hydrocephalus

Hydrocephalus in adults can also result from obstructive tumors, meningitis, and intracranial hemorrhage but can also be more insidious in onset. An entity called *normal-pressure hydrocephalus* occurs in the older population and involves a communicating hydrocephalus with a normal intraventricular pressure. The cause remains unknown but is thought to be due to subclinical hemorrhage or infection in the patient's remote past. The classic clinical triad described by Hakim in 1965 includes ataxia, urinary incontinence, and cognitive decline.

Regardless of cause, the treatment of hydrocephalus is essentially the same. Either the cause must be removed or a shunting procedure must be performed to divert accumulated CSF. Sometimes, both measures are necessary. The most commonly used procedure is a lateral ventricle to peritoneal shunt with a one-way pressure-regulating valve in the system. If the peritoneal cavity is not suitable for shunting, the distal catheter can be placed in the right atrium of the heart or, rarely, in the pleural cavity. In selected cases of communicating hydrocephalus, a lumbar subarachnoid to peritoneal shunt can be used. Common complications of indwelling shunts include shunt obstruction and infection. Any suspicion of infection or failure should be investigated promptly, because progressive neurologic deficits and even death can result secondary to increasing ICP.

Craniosynostosis

Craniosynostosis is the premature closure of one or more cranial sutures typically manifested within the first 6 months of life. Because the brain doubles in size during the first 6 months of life and grows another 50% by age 2 years, the cranial sutures must remain open to allow for skull expansion to accommodate this growth. Usually, when one suture fuses prematurely, the brain is not compressed to a deleterious degree, but the skull develops in a distinctly abnormal shape. If more sutures are fused, the brain can be damaged from restricted growth.

The sagittal suture is most commonly involved, with a male-to-female ratio of 4:1. The skull develops an elongated shape with a narrow biparietal diameter, often referred to as *scaphocephaly*. The supraorbital ridge may be square shaped as a result of overexpansion of the open metopic suture. Associated congenital anomalies are rare.

The next most common suture involved is the coronal, which can close prematurely on one or both sides. Unilateral involvement produces an asymmetrically shaped forehead with flattening on the affected side and compensatory enlargement on the opposite side. This is called *plagiocephaly* and is not usually associated with other abnormalities. Bilateral coronal synostosis produces a more severe foreshortening of the entire anterior fossa and is often manifested by shallow orbits with exophthalmos and hypertelorism. This entity is often associated with inherited congenital disorders such as Crouzon's disease and Apert's and Carpenter's syndromes.

Less common forms of craniosynostosis include premature closure of the lambdoid suture or the metopic suture. With unilateral synostosis of the lambdoid suture, the skull appears flattened in the affected occipital area, which can be confused with birth molding. With premature closure of the metopic suture, the forehead takes on a triangular shape (trigonocephaly). Neither of these forms is associated with other congenital anomalies.

The treatment of craniosynostosis is surgical and usually involves opening the affected suture along its entire length. This should be carried out as soon as possible after the diagnosis is made because early surgical intervention provides the best cosmetic result. In cases of multiple suture involvement, prompt treatment provides early skull expansion to accommodate brain growth. Long-term cosmetic results can be impressive, with many patients having a normal or near-normal appearance after correction.

STEREOTACTIC NEUROSURGERY

Stereotactic neurosurgery is a discipline devoted to spatial localization of intracranial structures.[11] Stereotactic neurosurgery is based on the principle that any point in the brain can be referenced to a specific coordinate system using precise measurements. Most stereotactic systems are based on the cartesian coordinate system, although a polar coordinate system is also common. In its original forms, a rigid frame is attached to the patient's head, and a coordinate system based on the frame is correlated with CT or MRI images of the patient's brain.

Stereotactic brain lesion biopsy is a common application. Stereotactic guidance is used to place a bur hole in an optimal location to permit passage of a needle into the lesion for a tissue sample. Stereotactic craniotomy permits optimal design of a craniotomy flap and access to underlying tumors or other lesions. Stereotactic guidance is also used for a variety of functional neurosurgery procedures.

Frameless stereotactic navigation is a recently developed technique that obviates the need for a frame. Preacquired CT or MRI brain images are reconstructed into a three-dimensional image in a computer in the operating room. A variety of recognizable landmarks on the patient's head, such as the ears, nose, and other facial features, are used as reproducible marker locations called fiducials. These fiducials are registered with the computer, allowing the system to triangulate between the patient, a reference area containing a set of signal emitters, and a hand-held instrument that also contains a set of signal emitters. This system allows planning of the operation based on the three-dimensional image of the patient and can provide assistance with navigation as the operation proceeds. Recent incarnations of these devices have allowed for intraoperative updating of the three-dimensional model through the use of intraoperative MRI or ultrasound.

Stereotactic radiosurgery is a technique for producing sharply delimited lesions in the brain by focusing multiple external sources of radiation on a single target. It is based on the principle that a large number of low-radiation beams traveling through normal brain tissue from a variety of angles can deliver a high dose of radiation to the region where the beams converge, putting the surrounding normal brain at minimal risk of radiation injury. It is noninvasive and a useful adjunct for management of a variety of tumors and vascular malformations when standard craniotomy and resection of the lesion is hazardous or impossible. Limitations of radiosurgery include the treatable lesion size and the time required for ablation of the lesion.

FUNCTIONAL NEUROSURGERY

Functional neurosurgery involves operations to alter the function of the CNS. The most common uses are for the treatment of pain syndromes, epilepsy, and movement disorders.

Neurosurgical Management of Pain

Most neurosurgical patients have pain either as their primary complaint or as a secondary manifestation of their disease process.[2] These painful conditions can be categorized as acute processes, such as arm pain from a herniated cervical disc, or chronic processes, such as extremity pain from an invasive neoplasm. For most acute pain states, the cause can be identified and treated, but for chronic pain there often is no ready solution. The more common neurosurgical procedures available to manage chronic pain are described here.

At one time, the perception of pain was thought to involve a simple system of pathways extending from the peripheral receptors to the brain. It has subsequently been shown that this system is a complex network of pathways, with a considerable amount of modification at multiple synaptic levels. Impulses from pain receptors reach the spinal cord by way of the dorsal root ganglion and can receive significant modification in the various laminae of the dorsal horn. This information is then relayed to the thalamus but again can undergo considerable modification in the area of the brainstem reticular formation. This sensory input is subsequently relayed to the cortex for conscious interpretation.

Traditionally, neurosurgical procedures for chronic pain have been ablative or destructive, but many neuromodulating or neurostimulating procedures have been developed. These procedures are usually reserved for those chronic pain conditions that medical therapy has failed to alleviate.

Cranial Nerves

Trigeminal neuralgia (tic douloureux) is one of the most common neuropathic conditions. It presents as an intermittent, shocklike pain in one or more divisions of one trigeminal nerve. It typically involves the second (maxillary) or third (mandibular) divisions of the nerve, or both, and rarely is bilateral. The pain usually lasts for seconds, is severe, and can be incapacitating. It is often triggered by touching the face, talking, or chewing. The pain can be present for weeks or months and then spontaneously disappear, only to return with increased severity. Most patients can be initially controlled with phenytoin or carbamazepine, but eventually many require surgical intervention. A small percentage of patients can have a posterior fossa tumor causing the pain, so evaluation should include a CT or MRI scan before therapy.

In the past, surgical treatment involved ablation of the involved branches of the trigeminal nerve. Pain control through these neurectomies was usually short-lived. Experience found that preganglionic lesions must be made for more permanent relief. Retrogasserian rhizotomy is typically performed percutaneously by placing a radiofrequency electrode through the foramen ovale. Percutaneous rhizolysis is safe, effective, and widely used. If performed properly, it has the advantage of destroying pain fibers only, leaving a variable amount of touch sensation intact.

A popular nonablative approach involves microvascular decompression of the trigeminal nerve in the posterior fossa. The theory behind this approach is that trigeminal neuralgia is caused by external pressure on the nerve by vascular structures (an artery or vein) near its entry into the brainstem. This procedure has a higher success rate and a longer duration of symptomatic relief than the percutaneous method but carries more risk. An advantage is that the nerve's function remains intact.

Glossopharyngeal neuralgia is similar to trigeminal neuralgia but much less common. Symptoms consist of lancinating paroxysmal pain, most commonly in the throat and at the base of the tongue, triggered by swallowing, chewing, or talking. Medical therapy is the same as that for trigeminal neuralgia. Should this fail, surgical intervention is warranted.

Spinal Cord

As with other surgical procedures for chronic pain, those involving the spinal cord have traditionally been ablative. Cordotomy, designed to obliterate the spinothalamic tract, can be performed openly or percutaneously. The percutaneous method creates a functional cordotomy at the C-1 to C-2 level with a radiofrequency lesion generator. Anterolateral cordotomy can provide excellent temporary relief of pain for patients with terminal malignancies, but it is rarely effective for chronic benign conditions such as low back, postherpetic, or phantom limb pain.

For selected cases of severe pain of peripheral nerve origin, ablative lesions can be made at the dorsal root entry zones of the spinal cord. These lesions are made with a radiofrequency lesion generator or laser through an open exposure of the cord by use of a laminectomy. Several levels are usually included. An effective result is obtained in 80% to 90% of patients.

Intrathecal morphine can also be given temporarily or permanently by infusion of minute but effective doses. This method of pain control is particularly effective in debilitated patients with terminal illnesses. The procedure involves the subcutaneous implantation of a constant infusion pump that can be recharged periodically. Morphine is delivered by this device into the CSF in small amounts sufficient to control severe pain.

In chronic nonmalignant pain conditions, such as failed back syndrome, reflex sympathetic dystrophy, and phantom limb pain, spinal cord stimulation can be effective. This nonablative neuromodulation technique involves direct stimulation of the dorsal surface of the spinal cord. Electrodes are placed percutaneously to lie within the dura, over the dorsal surface of the spinal cord. An impulse generator is placed subcutaneously in the flank or abdominal region. The precise mechanism of action for spinal cord stimulation is not understood but is thought to involve activation of inhibitory pathways in the spinal cord that suppress conduction of pain impulses.

Peripheral Nerve

Many chronic painful states can arise from peripheral nerve or major plexus injuries. Pain from a partial or complete nerve injury usually involves the sensory distribution of the nerve but can include the whole extremity. Chronic pain developing after an amputation can be present in the remaining portion of the limb at the site of the amputation (stump pain) or in the nonexistent amputated portion (phantom pain). The cause of the pain can be related to the sensory component of the nerve or to its associated sympathetic nerve supply.

With partial or complete peripheral nerve transection, a painful neuroma can form. A neuroma is a mass of misdirected axons that can develop from an injured nerve's attempt to regenerate. These axons can become sensitive to external stimuli or they can generate spontaneous pain. The usual treatment is excision of the neuroma, with prevention of recurrent formation by burying the nerve end in bone or muscle or by wrapping it in tantalum or Silastic. Neuromodulation techniques can also be applied in cases of painful neuromas. These include transcutaneous stimulation and implanted devices that directly stimulate the proximal nerve.

Chronic pain resulting from peripheral nerve injury can be significantly altered by interruption of the sympathetic nerve supply to the affected extremity. The classic example of this dysautonomic state is major causalgia. This term implies a partial injury to a major nerve in an extremity. Minor causalgia is reserved for an injury to a more distal minor sensory nerve, which can also become a source of significant pain. It is also well recognized that a dysautonomic state can be created by major or minor trauma to an extremity that does not involve a peripheral nerve. These have been labeled *major* and *minor traumatic dystrophies*. The entire collection of causalgias and traumatic dystrophies makes up a syndrome termed *reflex sympathetic dystrophy*.

The treatment of these dysautonomic states is complex. They can be helped by disruption of the sympathetic nerve supply to the extremity accomplished temporarily with a chemical sympathectomy by use of a local anesthetic or permanently by a surgical sympathectomy. Sympathetic denervation can be rewarding in major causalgia but less so in minor causalgia and the traumatic dystrophies.

Less severe and more easily treated pain can arise from chronic compression of selected peripheral nerves. The most common are compression of the median nerve at the wrist (carpal tunnel syndrome) and compression of the ulnar nerve at the elbow. Chronic compression can result in pain, paresthesias, numbness, and eventually weakness and atrophy of muscles in the distribution of the affected nerve. These compression syndromes are diagnosed clinically and confirmed by finding denervation and slowed nerve conduction on EMG and nerve conduction velocity testing. Treatment is surgical decompression of the involved nerve, with prompt and long-lasting relief in most cases.

Epilepsy

Approximately 2 million people in the United States have epilepsy. Seizures can usually be categorized as generalized, characterized by loss of consciousness with tonic-clonic movements, or partial, manifested by involuntary movements but no loss of consciousness. Most seizure disorders are idiopathic; known causes of epilepsy include congenital anomalies, traumatic brain injury, vascular lesions, infection, and tumors. Mesial temporal sclerosis, involving atrophy and cell loss in the hippocampus, is a common cause of epilepsy in adults. In the developing world, cysticercosis is a leading cause of epilepsy.

Medical management of epilepsy is successful for approximately 70% of patients. Patients with symptomatic epilepsy despite anticonvulsant medication are potential candidates for surgery. The goal of most surgery for seizure disorders is to resect the area of brain responsible for generating or propagating epileptic activity. Therefore, the preoperative workup of a patient with medically refractory epilepsy must identify the seizure focus, as well as regions of the brain that subserve language, vision, and sensory or motor functions (eloquent cortex).

A number of brain imaging and testing modalities have been introduced that assist with patient selection and operative planning in epilepsy surgery. Electroencephalography, both interictal and long-term (inpatient) monitoring, can help localize the seizure focus. CT and MRI can identify brain lesions that may be epileptogenic. Cerebral angiography in which sodium amobarbital is injected selectively into either the left or right hemisphere, followed by language testing (Wada test), can identify the side of language dominance. Positron emission tomography scanning can be useful for localizing the seizure focus, and functional MRI can help identify eloquent cortex. Invasive monitoring techniques include stereotactically placed hippocampal depth electrodes and subdural electrodes placed through a bur hole.

Epilepsy surgery is often done with the patient awake under local anesthesia. This condition permits further localization of the seizure focus and eloquent cortex. Stimulation mapping, in which a stimulating electrode is applied to the surface of the brain, is particularly useful for identifying language areas. The most common surgical procedure for epilepsy is resection of the anterior part of the temporal lobe. Vagal nerve stimulation, involving placement of an electrode in contact with the left vagus nerve and powered by an implanted subcutaneous pulse generator, can be effective for patients with refractory partial seizures. The mechanism for suppression of seizures is unknown.

Approximately two thirds of patients with temporal lobe epilepsy are seizure free after temporal lobectomy, and one fourth are improved in terms of seizure frequency or intensity. Vagal nerve stimulation is most effective at reducing seizure frequency; 50% of patients report at least a 50% reduction in seizures. The results of other epilepsy operations vary widely with type of seizure disorder, location of seizure focus, and etiology.

Movement Disorders

The basal ganglia are a complex group of subcortical nuclei that are concerned with control of motor function: organization and execution as well as learning and cognition related to movement. Movement disorders are disorders of motor control that manifest primarily as tremor, athetosis (slow, writhing movements of the extremities), chorea (abrupt movements of the limbs and facial muscles), ballism (violent, flailing movements), and dystonia (persistent, distorted posture). Most movement disorders are referable to a lesion in the basal ganglia. The prototypical movement disorder is Parkinson's disease. In Parkinson's disease, selective degeneration of dopaminergic neurons in the substantia nigra leads to an imbalance of inhibitory and excitatory circuits in the basal ganglia and the characteristic symptom complex of tremor, rigidity, and slowness of movement. Other disorders of the basal ganglia include Huntington's disease, which is typified by chorea, decreased muscle tone, and dementia; hemiballismus, in which damage to the subthalamic nucleus causes severe involuntary movement; and tardive dyskinesia, in which an acquired hyper-sensitivity to dopamine in the basal ganglia leads to abnormal involuntary movements. A common movement disorder that is not identified with a known basal ganglia abnormality is essential tremor, an idiopathic kinetic tremor syndrome.

Stereotactic pallidotomy, consisting of making a radiofrequency lesion in the globus pallidus, can be effective in treating rigidity, dystonia, choreoathetosis, and hemiballismus. Thalamotomy, with lesioning of the ventral intermediate nucleus of the thalamus (Vim), is useful for the treatment of tremor. Patients for whom tremor is the primary feature of their movement disorder, such as some patients with Parkinson's disease, essential tremor, and intention tremor associated with multiple sclerosis, are potential candidates for thalamotomy. More recently, deep brain stimulation for movement disorders has been used. Thalamic stimulation for tremor is the most common. An electrode implanted in the Vim and powered by a subcutaneous pulse generator can deliver stimulation in a variety of amplitudes, pulse widths, and frequencies. These stimulation parameters can be fine-tuned to optimize treatment of the patient's symptoms.

KEY POINTS

- **Injury to the brain is caused by the rapid deceleration, acceleration, and rotation associated with a blow to the head. Mild head injury is usually not associated with significant primary brain injury, and neurologic deficits are limited to temporary loss of consciousness (concussion). Moderate to severe head injury, on the other hand, is typically associated with deficits that may or may not be reversible.**
- **Intracranial size is of a fixed volume and is filled by three components: cerebrospinal fluid, blood, and cranial tissue. Any increase in the size or volume of one of these components will lead to an increase in intracranial pressure.**
- **Intracranial aneurysms are diseased dilatations of the cerebral arteries consisting of ballooned-out intima, media, and adventitia with a variable degree of intraluminal or mural thrombus. Most are congenital, evolving and developing during life.**
- **The most common cause of stenosis or occlusion of large vessels is atherosclerosis.**
- **Initially, medical treatment is indicated in patients with ruptured intervertebral discs who do not have neurologic deterioration. Surgical treatment is reserved for the patient with an acute or progressive neurologic deficit, chronic disabling pain, or both.**
- **Approximately 2% of newborns possess some type of congenital abnormality. Of these, 60% involve the CNS, and more than half of those are related to defective development or closure of the dorsal midline structures. Many have associated hydrocephalus.**

References

1. Apuzzo MLJ. *Brain injury: complications, avoidance, and management.* New York: Churchill Livingstone, 1993, p. 2365.
2. Narayan RK, Wilberger JE Jr, Povlishock JT, eds. *Neurotrauma.* New York: McGraw-Hill, 1995.
3. **The Brain Trauma Foundation. *Guidelines for the management of severe head injury.* Park Ridge, IL: American Association of Neurological Surgeons, 1995.**
4. Menezes AH, Sonntag VKH, Benzel EC, et al., eds. *Principles of spinal surgery.* New York: McGraw-Hill, 1996.
5. Russell DS, Rubinstein LJ. *Pathology of tumors of the nervous system,* 5th ed. Baltimore: Williams & Wilkins, 1989.
6. Greenberg HS, Chandler WF, Sandler HM, eds. *Brain tumors.* New York: Oxford University Press, 1999.
7. **Crockard A, Hayward R, Hoff JT, eds. *Neurosurgery: the scientific basis of clinical practice,* 3rd ed. Boston: Blackwell Scientific, 1999.**
8. Batjer HH, Caplan LR, Friberg L, et al., eds. *Cerebrovascular disease.* Philadelphia: Lippincott—Raven, 1997.
9. Hamilton, MG, Spetzler RF. The prospective application of a grading system for arteriovenous malformations. *Neurosurgery* 1994;34:2.
10. Albright AL, Pollack IF, Adelson PD, eds. *Principles and practice of pediatric neurosurgery.* New York: Thieme, 1999.
11. Gildenberg PL, Tasker RR, eds. *Textbook of stereotactic and functional neurosurgery.* New York: McGraw-Hill, 1998.

SECTION R
GENITOURINARY SYSTEM

CHAPTER 115 ■ MALE GENITOURINARY ANATOMY AND PHYSIOLOGY

DAVID Y. CHAN, ARTHUR L. BURNETT, RONALD RODRIGUEZ, AND THOMAS W. JARRETT

This chapter is an introduction to clinical disorders of the male genitourinary system. As a framework for understanding their causes and characteristics, the principles of normal genitourinary anatomy and physiology are initially discussed. Next, common disease states are presented with particular emphasis placed on diagnosis and treatment.

LOWER URINARY TRACT

The lower urinary tract refers to the urinary bladder and outlet region of the anterior pelvis, which carry out the orderly functions of urine collection and elimination. Discrete anatomic structures include the distal ureter, bladder, ureterovesical junction, trigone, prostate, external urinary sphincter, and anterior urethra. The lower urinary tract also functionally relates to pelvic floor supporting structures.

The bladder is superbly designed for storage and expulsive functions. With an adult capacity of approximately 500 mL, this spheroid organ is designed as follows: an interior lining of transitional epithelium as much as six cells thick resting on a basement membrane; a surrounding layer of fibroelastic connective tissue termed *lamina propria* and *muscularis mucosae* that mainly permits the passive filling of the bladder; and an exterior bladder wall consisting of an inner longitudinal, middle circular, and outer longitudinal detrusor muscle arrangement that ideally suits the emptying properties of the organ. At the bladder neck, the radially oriented inner longitudinal fibers form the inner longitudinal layer of the smooth muscle of the urethra. The middle layer forms a circular preprostatic sphincter, so called because it is more robust in the man than the woman, and is thought to provide urinary continence at the level of the bladder neck. The outer longitudinal fibers form a thick backboard posteriorly at the bladder base with the lateral fibers encircling the bladder neck and contributing to the continence mechanism. This backboard supports the trigone, a triangular, essentially nondeformable portion of the bladder bounded by the two ureteral orifices and the internal urethral meatus.

The ovoid (~3 cm on the long axis) prostate is situated at the bladder base and encircles the urethra; the base abuts the bladder neck proximally and the apex is continuous with the striated urethral sphincter distally. Situated distally to the prostate and ending at the perineal membrane is the membranous urethra, spanning approximately 2.5 cm in length. This location represents the primary region of urinary continence, structurally associated with a surrounding tubular sleeve of musculature identified as the striated external urinary sphincter. Further distally, the anterior urethra, consisting of a proximal bulbar portion and a distal pendulous portion, provides a conduit for the passage of urine from the body. The anterior urethra is formed by smooth muscle and a urothelial lining that changes from transitional epithelium to nonkeratinized stratified squamous epithelium along its course toward the external urethral meatus.

The normal physiologic function of the lower urinary tract is to contain urine in the bladder after its drainage from the upper urinary tracts and, on command and on proper social occasions, to empty urine completely from the bladder with only a low resistance to its passage. Both autonomic and somatic nervous system mechanisms, involving central and peripheral pathways, control these functions.[1] Although these mechanisms are extensive and still incompletely known, the basic central regulation of micturition occurs at the cerebral cortex, with inhibitory control of reflexive voiding involving the pontine micturition center.[2] At the peripheral level, bladder emptying is mediated by excitatory cholinergic innervation of the bladder, with effects exerted principally by acetylcholine released from local nerve terminals that act on postjunctional muscarinic receptors. Adrenergic innervation characterizes the predominant nervous system control of the bladder neck and urethra. α-Adrenergic receptors are activated by the local neuronal release of norepinephrine and mediate contraction of smooth muscle in the urethra, thereby contributing to closure during bladder filling. This classic definition of lower urinary tract neurotransmission is undergoing modification, however, with the more recent findings that nonadrenergic, noncholinergic factors (e.g., nitric oxide) and sensory neurotransmitters contribute significantly to control of lower urinary tract function.

OBSTRUCTIVE UROPATHY

A wide variety of conditions associated with symptoms of urinary obstruction or bladder irritability result from structural, biochemical, and functional changes of the lower urinary tract. Benign prostatic hyperplasia (BPH) is understood to be the most common cause of anatomic bladder outlet obstruction in men older than 50 years of age. Autopsy studies have shown that 50% to 60% of men older than 50 years have significant benign enlargement of the prostate, with a prevalence proportionate to increasing age.[3] In clinical practice, however, symptoms experienced by older men are not always caused by an obstructive prostate but may reflect other age-related phenomena of the structural components of the lower urinary tract. Assorted other conditions may also be associated with symptoms of bladder outlet obstruction in the man, including urethral stricture disease, prostate cancer, neurogenic bladder, bladder calculus, prostatitis, bladder neck contracture, and bladder cancer. Functional obstruction is a consequence of such nonanatomic disorders as chronic bladder overdistention, debilitating disease, psychogenic retention, or side effects of medication.

Diagnosis

History and physical examination, combined with appropriate laboratory testing, represent the cornerstone of diagnosis. Bladder outlet obstruction is characterized by symptoms of urinary hesitancy, diminished force and caliber of the urinary stream, intermittency, sensation of incomplete emptying, and postmicturition dribbling. The symptoms of urinary frequency, urgency, and nocturia are experienced as the bladder attempts to compensate for the obstruction, resulting in a diminished functional bladder capacity, bladder muscle hypertrophy, and bladder instability. Bladder decompensation develops over time, producing such complications as residual urine, infection, hematuria, hydronephrosis, and renal failure.

Certain typical features revealed during history taking may suggest the cause of urinary obstruction. Patients with urethral stricture usually have a history of prior urethral trauma, instrumentation, or infection. Those with advanced prostate cancer may present with obstructive urinary symptoms, along with back or bone pain, anorexia, or weight loss. Patients with a neurogenic bladder often exhibit other symptoms of neurologic disease, including concomitant bowel or sexual dysfunction, or present with known neurologic diseases or injuries that regularly cause bladder dysfunction, such as diabetes mellitus, stroke, multiple sclerosis, and spinal cord injury. Medications should be reviewed in all patients to discern whether any may be associated with voiding dysfunction (Table 115.1). Agents that depress bladder muscle contractility (e.g., anticholinergic agents, antispasmodic drugs, and antidepressant drugs) or increase bladder outlet resistance (e.g., sympathomimetics) are known to disturb normal micturition.

During physical examination of the patient with symptoms of bladder outlet obstruction, the clinician should be alert for abdominal, genital, rectal, and neurologic abnormalities suggestive of the extent and possible cause of the problem. Preliminary laboratory testing may include urinalysis, urine culture (if pyuria is present), and measurement of serum creatinine. A prostate-specific antigen (PSA) test has been recommended to screen for an elevated level that might warrant prostate biopsy to exclude a prostate cancer diagnosis.[4] The urinary flow rate, represented by the amount of urine voided during a timed period, is a simple, valuable tool; normal men have 5-second volumes exceeding 75 mL, whereas men with urinary obstruction have flows less than 50 mL in 5 seconds. More extensive tests may be done as part of a urologic investigation if significant complications such as hematuria, urinary tract infection, or renal failure) are confirmed or if an invasive therapy is considered. Available diagnostic tests include intravenous urography (IVU) or renal ultrasonography to evaluate the upper urinary tracts, bladder catheterization for postmicturition volume, cystourethroscopy to visualize directly the lower urinary tract, and cystometrography to assess the function of the bladder and urinary outlet during filling and emptying phases of the micturition cycle. Symptomatic urinary obstruction alone does not require specialized testing, particularly if a nonsurgical, reversible intervention with surveillance is planned.

TABLE 115.1 ETIOLOGY

PHARMACOLOGIC AGENTS WITH KNOWN INFLUENCE ON BLADDER FUNCTION

Drugs that increase bladder tone and contractility
- Bethanecol (Urecholine)

Drugs that decrease bladder contractility
- Anticholinergic drugs (e.g., propantheline, belladonna, oxybutynin, tolterodine)
- Calcium antagonists (e.g., verapamil, nifedipine, diltiazem)
- Prostaglandin inhibitors (e.g., ibuprofen)
- Tricyclic antidepressants (e.g., imipramine, nortriptyline)
- Beta adrenergic agonists (e.g., terbutaline)

Drugs that increase bladder outlet resistance
- β-Sympathomimetic drugs (e.g., ephedrine, phenylpropanolamine, Ornade)
- β-Adrenergic antagonists (e.g., propranolol)
- Estrogens

Drugs that decrease outlet resistance
- α-Adrenergic antagonists (e.g., terazosin, doxazosin, tamsulosin)
- Antispasticity drugs (e.g., diazepam, baclofen)

Treatment

The management of BPH has rapidly expanded in recent years to include a variety of medical and surgical options. Both surgical prostatectomy (i.e., transurethral resection of the prostate) or open surgical enucleation of adenomatous tissue through suprapubic, retropubic, or perineal incisions have been long available and remain the standard interventions in the setting of significant anatomic urinary obstruction with risks of bladder decompensation. The preferred approach follows an assessment of the condition of the patient and the size and configuration of the prostate gland. Novel, alternative surgical therapies include transurethral microwave thermotherapy, transurethral needle ablation, transurethral electrovaporization of the prostate, interstitial laser coagulation, holmium laser enucleation of the prostate, transurethral incision of the prostate, intraprostatic stent insertion, and photoselective vaporization of the prostate. U.S. Food and Drug Administration approval has been given to medications that appear increasingly attractive to use, particularly when lower urinary tract symptoms provide the primary indication for intervention. These include α_1-adrenergic blockers (e.g., doxazosin, terazosin, tamsulosin) and 5-α-reductase inhibitors (e.g., finasteride), which may be offered alternatively, depending on patient desires and clinical circumstances. Interest in alternative medical therapies has led to increasing public use of phytotherapeutic agents such as saw palmetto to treat lower urinary tract symptoms.

Urethral stricture disease may be treated with urethral dilatation, transurethral incision, urethral stent insertion, or open urethral reconstructive surgery. The selected approach usually depends on the severity and location of the stricture and the patient's overall health and expected longevity. Other anatomic abnormalities such as bladder calculus or bladder neck contracture are commonly managed with transurethral surgical techniques. The neurogenic bladder is primarily managed by intermittent catheterization, although sphincterotomy, vesicostomy, suprapubic or urethral catheterization, or urinary diversion (i.e., surgical reconstruction using bowel segments to drain the urinary system) has been applied in certain situations.

PROSTATITIS

Prostatitis is commonly identified as an inflammatory condition of the prostate, although its reference may be more broadly associated with a symptom complex characterized by pain in the pelvic or perineal region combined with variable voiding. It is the most common urologic diagnosis in men younger than 50 years of age,[5] with prevalence estimates that range from 5% to 8.8%.[6] Categories of prostatitis derive from the National Institutes of Health classification system[7]: acute bacterial prostatitis, a relatively rare diagnosis involving an acute infection of the prostate gland; chronic bacterial prostatitis, a frequent, chronic condition that results from recurrent infection of the prostate; and chronic abacterial prostatitis, otherwise termed *chronic pelvic pain syndrome* or *prostatodynia,* which describes chronic symptoms in the absence of demonstrable prostatic infection. Evidence suggests that some men with symptoms of chronic prostatitis may actually have interstitial cystitis (i.e., bladder condition characterized by severe pain and urinary frequency and considered to have a female predominance).[8]

Diagnosis

Clinical diagnosis largely hinges on recognition of symptoms. Pain sensations may be associated with the perineal region, although localizations also include the suprapubic, scrotal, penile, or lower back regions. Voiding symptoms of variable degree include urinary urgency, nocturia, weak urinary stream, frequency, dysuria, hesitancy, dribbling after micturition, and interrupted urinary flow. Acute prostatitis can usually be confirmed by a positive voided urine culture showing typically gram-negative organisms. Among the chronic forms of prostatitis, distinction is made by demonstration of a positive bacterial culture of expressed prostatic secretions in the bacterial form. The cause of abacterial prostatitis is unclear, but autoimmunity may be involved.[9]

Treatment

Treatment is aimed at relieving symptoms and eliminating documented infection. Systemically administered antimicrobial drugs are routinely offered, directed toward either a known positive culture or otherwise suspected prostatic pathogen. The most appropriate antibiotics are the fluoroquinolones, trimethoprim (or trimethoprim—sulfamethoxazole), carbenicillin, and doxycycline. For chronic bacterial prostatitis, treatment may extend for 8 to 12 weeks. A 50% cure rate is generally expected with this form of treatment, whereas patients with relapsing or refractory prostatitis should be considered for ancillary investigations such as urinary cytology, cystoscopy, transrectal ultrasound, and urodynamics to exclude masquerading urologic conditions ranging from a bladder malignancy to interstitial cystitis. If findings are negative, low-dose antibiotic prophylaxis may be offered for frequently recurrent episodes. Antimicrobial therapy is often empirically given for 8 to 12 weeks in cases of chronic abacterial prostatitis. These patients may respond in the presence of a non-culturable infectious process. In others, therapy may then extend to α_1-adrenergic blocker medications or amitriptyline, which have been shown to relieve sympathetically maintained genitourinary pain syndromes, or antiinflammatories or analgesics or pentosan polysulfate sodium.[10] Some experts have also recommended muscle relaxants such as diazepam, prostatic massage, sitz baths, and biofeedback (training the patient to contract and relax the pelvic floor muscles to interrupt the myofascial pain attacks), although the roles of these therapies remain unproved. Transurethral surgeries such as prostate resection or microwave thermotherapy and even radical prostatectomy have been applied, although these are considered options of last resort.

URINARY INCONTINENCE

Urinary incontinence, more accurately understood as a symptom rather than an actual diagnosis, refers to the involuntary loss of urine through the external urethral meatus. The term generally excludes rare congenital anomalies and fistulae, in which involuntary urine loss may also occur. The condition most commonly affects women, with a prevalence as high as 10% to 20% of women between 15 and 64 years of age.[11] American men also experience urinary incontinence, in the range of 1.5% to 5% for the similar age range. In elderly people (i.e., >60 years of age), the incontinence prevalence rates approximately double.[12] Stress urinary incontinence is commonly associated with anatomic deformities or disorders of either urethral sphincteric support or closure. In women, underlying factors include postpartum structural effects, postmenopausal tissue atrophy, and prior surgical trauma. In men, local trauma, as seen after prostatectomy, can compromise urethral sphincteric closure, and is classified as type III stress urinary incontinence or intrinsic sphincteric deficiency. Clinical history, cystoscopic evaluation, and urodynamic measurement of sphincteric integrity usually suffice to make the diagnosis. Treatment options in men typically include pelvic floor strengthening exercises, administration of sympathomimetic agents, transurethral collagen injections, and artificial urinary sphincter implantation.

Another form of urinary incontinence, known as urge urinary incontinence, usually pertains to involuntary urine loss associated with an overactive bladder disorder. Unstable bladder contractions and poor bladder storage function are characteristic features of the disorder. Known causes include various neurologic disorders, urinary tract infection, urethral obstruction, bladder calculus, and bladder or prostate carcinoma, although in many instances an underlying cause cannot be found. Classic irritative voiding symptoms such as urinary frequency and urgency may accompany urge urinary incontinence. The diagnosis is determined by clinical history and physical examination, which may identify a particular causative, treatable condition. Pharmacologic therapy with either anticholinergic or antispasmodic medications represents the usual initial course of management, often in combination with micturition behavioral modification.

MALE GENITALIA AND REPRODUCTIVE SYSTEM

The penis consists of the paired, dorsally located corpora cavernosa and the midline ventral corpus spongiosum that surrounds the urethra and distally forms the glans penis. The corpora cavernosa, the primary erectile bodies of the penis, are invested by a collagenous sheath called the tunica albuginea and contain a spongelike meshwork of trabecular smooth muscle and fibroelastic tissue lined by vascular endothelium. The cavernous arteries provide the main vascular supply to the penis, coursing from the internal pudendal arteries and feeding into branches in the corpora cavernosa called *helicine arteries*. Subtunical venules provide vascular drainage from the corpora cavernosa, forming the emissary veins as they pierce the tunica albuginea and eventually drain into the main venous tributaries of the penis, the dorsal and crural veins.

The fundamental physiology of the penis relates to blood flow in the organ as determined by the degree of vascular and corporal smooth muscle tone. Penile flaccidity is considered to be a tonic, low blood-flow state resulting from corporal smooth muscle contraction governed locally primarily by the sympathetic division of the autonomic nervous system through its classic neurotransmitter norepinephrine. Other vasocontractile factors, however, have been identified as contributing to this physiology, such as endothelin, a substance released from the vascular endothelium. Penile erection, conversely, involves corporal smooth muscle relaxation, whereupon blood engorgement occurs; this process is under the control of nitric oxide as well as other vasodilatory mediators locally released from nerve endings originating from the parasympathetic division of the autonomic nervous system. The central nervous system (CNS) also influences this function, processing "psychogenic" stimuli and other regulatory information.

The remainder of the external male reproductive system consists of the contents of the scrotum, a multilayered structure separated by a septum into two compartments. These bilateral compartments each provide a receptacle for the testis, the spermatic cord, and the related excurrent duct system, consisting of the epididymis, vas deferens, and ejaculatory ducts. The internal male reproductive system comprises the accessory glands, including the prostate and seminal vesicles. The testes and excurrent duct system structures provide for the creation, maturation, and collection of sperm before seminal emission and ejaculation.

ERECTILE DYSFUNCTION

Erectile dysfunction, commonly referred to as *impotence,* is defined as the consistent inability to attain and maintain penile erection sufficient to permit satisfactory sexual intercourse. This condition may affect as many as 18 million American men, most often men older than 65 years of age, although approximately 30% of all men between the ages of 40 and 70 years are affected.[13] Various diseases, injuries, and drugs have been associated with erectile dysfunction (Table 115.2). These circumstances may produce alterations in the endocrine, neurologic, vascular, and end-organ requirements for normal penile erection. It has also been suggested that there is a gradual loss of erectile tissue integrity with aging that is unrelated to other medical problems. The rapidly evolving understanding that actual organic factors underlie as much as 80% of presentations of erectile difficulty has reinforced the clinical relevance of this condition.

Diagnosis

It is recommended that the diagnostic evaluation for erectile dysfunction be performed such that it facilitates treatment objectives without being unnecessarily costly or invasive. Goals of the basic evaluation are to determine the nature of the problem and, once it is confirmed, to identify and immediately address causative factors. A proper sexual function history (involving patient and partner) should begin the evaluation (Table 115.3). It may yield findings that suggest an organic basis for the erectile dysfunction, such as reports of erectile difficulty after physical trauma to the pelvic region, gradual deterioration of erectile function, a consistent inability to maintain an erection once it is attained, and the absence of erections on awakening from sleep.

Additional components of the basic evaluation include general medical and psychosocial history, drug history, physical examination, and basic laboratory testing. Clinical history may reveal certain past medical conditions or use of drugs that are known to be associated with erectile dysfunction. Physical

TABLE 115.2 ETIOLOGY

COMMON ORGANIC CAUSES OF ERECTILE DYSFUNCTION

Category	Examples
Systemic disorders	Atherosclerosis, hypertension, peripheral vascular disease, diabetes mellitus, renal failure
Neurogenic disorders	Diabetes, cardiovascular accidents, Parkenson's disease, multiple sclerosis
Endocrine disorders	Hypogonadism, hyperprolactinemia, hyperthyroidism, hypothyroidism
Penile disorders	Peyronie's disease, priapism
Injuries	Perineal, pelvic, or nervous system trauma; radiation or surgery to the pelvis or retroperitoneum
Medications	Antihypertensives, antidepressants, antiandrogens, nonsteroidal antinflammatory drugs
Substances of abuse	Alcohol, tobacco, recreational drug

TABLE 115.3 DIAGNOSIS

ERECTILE PROBLEMS: COMPREHENSIVE SEXUAL FUNCTION HISTORY

Element	Specific questions
Onset, duration, evolution of erectile dysfunction	Gradual or sudden?
Type of dysfunction	Failure to attain or maintain erections?
Current quality of erections	Sufficient for sexual intercourse: Under certain circumstances? With certain positions?
Stimulus for achievable erections	Sexual encounters? Self-stimulation? On awakening?
Sexual issues distinct from erectile dysfunction	Libido Ejaculation Orgasm
Other issues	Availability, interest, health of partner Changes in medical status or other events relating to onset of dysfunction All prior attempts to manage the problem by the patient or another caregiver

examination attending to development of primary and secondary sex characteristics, genital anatomy, and neurologic and vascular functioning may suggest alterations consistent with the diagnosis. A basic laboratory investigation involving routine urinalysis, blood count, and serum chemistries may lead to the detection of commonly associated metabolic disorders such as diabetes mellitus and renal insufficiency.

The value of routine endocrinologic testing remains controversial because endocrinopathy may occur in only 2% of patients presenting with erectile dysfunction, and reportedly pertains more to decreased sexual libido than to erectile dysfunction.[14] Because sexual function may improve in some men receiving hormonal replacement therapy, a reasonable recommendation is to screen for hypogonadism by obtaining a morning serum total testosterone level. An abnormal testosterone level or other clinical indications of an endocrine disorder may prompt further endocrinologic testing. In the event that prostatic disease might be stimulated by exogenously administered testosterone, treatment may reasonably be withheld and thus diagnostic evaluation deemed unnecessary. Accordingly, both a PSA level and digital rectal examination (DRE) should be completed to assess for abnormalities.

Beyond the basic clinical evaluation, further specialized hormonal, neurologic, and vascular testing may be conducted in selected patients, usually by a urologist who specializes in erectile dysfunction. Such extensive testing in clinical practice usually follows the need to establish the exact cause and extent of the problem, often because of a patient's request or before initiating surgical interventions. Sleep-related penile tumescence and rigidity monitoring, performed either in a sleep laboratory or at home with a portable testing device, is often used as a minimally invasive technique that can graphically record the frequency, duration, and quality of erection. In-office assessments of erectile response to intracavernosal vasoactive drug injection can be done either by clinical rating or by diagnostic measurement of blood flow response (e.g., with penile duplex ultrasonography). Radiographic contrast injection into the penis or the surrounding pelvic vasculature can be used to locate an obstructive lesion or leak.

Treatment

Treatment of erectile dysfunction usually is based on the findings of the clinical evaluation and treatment preferences of the individual patient. Initial efforts are directed at addressing any medical conditions associated with erectile dysfunction, including treating medical diseases and exploring a change in or discontinuation of drugs with adverse effects on erectile function. Several physical interventions are available, and a perspective of them should be presented to the patient in a balanced and complete way. Discussion should include the efficacy and complication profiles, patient and partner satisfaction rates, and expected patient and partner involvement with regard to each treatment option. Given the relative minimal invasiveness of many of the available options, one or more may be explored regardless of the physical cause for the erectile dysfunction. An option may otherwise be considered in light of the type and severity of the underlying physical cause, presumably with greater treatment success. Even if a physical intervention is planned, referral for sex therapy or counseling may be useful whether the dysfunction is mainly psychogenic or organic. The contribution of emotional factors to any presentation should not be underestimated.

In addition to sexual counseling, physical interventions for erectile dysfunction include pharmacologic therapies, mechanical devices, vascular reconstruction, and penile prosthesis implantation surgery. Nonhormonal pharmacologic therapies include oral, intracavernosal, and intraurethral treatments. Traditional oral therapies such as yohimbine (Yocon; Palisades Pharmaceuticals, Tenafly, NJ) and trazodone HCl (Desyrel; Bristol-Meyers Squibb, Princeton, NJ) have been found to have limited efficacy profiles and have given way to newly emerging, highly effective oral therapies such as sildenafil (Viagra; Pfizer, New York, NY), vardenafil (Levitra, Bayer, Leverkusen, Germany), and tadalafil (Cialis, Lilly ICOS, Indianapolis, IN). These phosphodiesterase (PDE) 5 inhibitors appear to produce erections useful for intercourse in more than 50% of patients.[15] Prescribers, however, must be aware of the significant drug interactions between PDE 5 inhbitors and nitrates and α-blockers. Intracavernosal or penile injection therapy remains the gold standard of pharmacologic treatment options. The therapy requires the insertion of a small needle into the side of the penis for injecting vasoactive medications that stimulate the erectile tissue to relax and expand with blood. Various vasoactive drugs have been applied, including prostaglandin E_1 (alprostadil [Caverject; Pharmacia & Upjohn, Kalamazoo, MI]), papaverine, and phentolamine. These agents can be used as monotherapy or in combination, with the expectation of producing a satisfactory, functional erection in approximately 90% of patients.[16] Intraurethral therapy, made available since 1996, requires the insertion of an applicator into the distal urethra to deliver a suppository of vasoactive medication. Currently, only prostaglandin E_1 [alprostadil (MUSE) (VIVUS, Inc., Mountain View, CA)] is commercially available, with efficacy in producing erections in approximately 40% of patients with erectile dysfunction.[17]

Externally applied erection devices offer a nonpharmacologic and noninvasive alternative therapy for erectile dysfunction. A plastic cylinder is placed over the penis to create a closed chamber, and is connected by tubing to a vacuum that withdraws air from around the penis to facilitate penile engorgement with blood. A constrictive ring is then positioned at the base of the penis to contain the blood. An erectionlike state is obtained in 98% of users, according to manufacturers. Surgical implantation of a semirigid malleable or hydraulic inflatable device into the penis has long been an available treatment, with success achieved in approximately 95% of cases.[18] Although such surgery is ostensibly more invasive than other alternatives, it may be indicated after diagnostically confirmed severe hemodynamic dysfunction of the penis and on lack of success with alternative therapies. Penile vascular reconstruction represents another surgical intervention. Surgical procedures include both arterial revascularization and venous ligation, offered chiefly to patients who are documented to have a focal vascular lesion, usually as a result of pelvic trauma. Success is noted in 40% to 60% of cases.[19]

PEYRONIE'S DISEASE

Peyronie's disease is a benign, inflammatory fibrosis of the tunica albuginea of the corpora cavernosa that produces a deformity of the erect penis and occasionally erectile dysfunction. The disorder is common, with a prevalence that approaches 1% of adult men, although it is seen primarily in men between 45 and 60 years of age.[20] Hypothesized causes for the disorder include chronic irritation, inherited trait, autoimmune defect, delamination injury, and superoxide injury.

Diagnosis

The diagnosis is usually based on the patient presentation of penile pain that usually resolves over time, penile angulation with an often palpable plaque involving the penile shaft, and occasionally impaired erectile function. Recollections of penile trauma and descriptions of fibrotic conditions elsewhere in the body can sometimes be elicited with a clinical history, although frequently no discernible associations can be found. Further diagnostic assessment can be done to evaluate the severity of the deformity, which may limit the physical act of sexual intercourse and the extent of erectile dysfunction. Commonly used modalities include photographic documentation of a naturally occurring erection and penile duplex ultrasonography after vasoactive drug pharmacostimulation.

Treatment

Treatment is conservative in most presentations, particularly during the first 12 months after disease onset, to ascertain its resolution with either spontaneous improvement or stabilization of plaque formation. For the patient's condition to resolve with only minimal to moderate curvature, no penile pain, and continued normal sexual activity, no invasive diagnostic procedure or treatment is indicated. Medical therapies such as vitamin E and colchicine may be tried early with the intent to decrease the inflammatory process and fibrosis. After 12 months, patients with significant impairment may be offered more invasive interventions. Techniques for reducing fibrosis include intralesional injection therapy and radiation therapy. Treatments for impaired sexual function include intracavernosal self-injection therapy and surgery involving either penile straightening or penile prosthesis insertion.

DISORDERS OF THE SCROTUM AND ITS CONTENTS

Pathologic conditions arising in the scrotum are frequently challenging to diagnose and treat. A hydrocele is the most common benign scrotal mass lesion. The pathologic process consists of the accumulation of serous fluid secreted by the tunica vaginalis layer of the scrotum, occurring secondary to tumor, trauma, or inflammation, or idiopathically. Epididymitis is a common intrascrotal lesion that is associated with a mass effect and pain. This disorder usually begins with a bacterial or chemical insult to the vas deferens, epididymis, and testis that leads to an inflammatory response. Varicocele, or a dilated vein of the pampiniform plexus, is the most common mass arising from the spermatic cord. Other major intrascrotal conditions include neoplasia, cystic lesions, testicular torsion, ruptured testicle, and scrotal abscess.

Discriminating between different scrotal disorders and initiating treatment promptly in emergent situations are the charges of the clinician whose patient presents with scrotal symptomatology. A focused clinical history should provide immediate information about the occurrence of scrotal or perineal trauma, symptoms of a lower urinary tract infection, and the presence of pain. Urinalysis is routinely performed, and the presence of bacteria and pyuria suggests an inflammatory cause. The physical examination constitutes the most important part of the diagnostic evaluation. The normal hemiscrotum and inguinal region should be examined first to provide a reference with which to compare abnormal findings.

The important differentiation of scrotal masses as solid or cystic may require scrotal transillumination or color Doppler ultrasonography. A solid mass suggests neoplasia and usually warrants radical orchiectomy. A cystic mass is atypical for a malignancy, and treatment may range from observation with reassurance to surgical excision if the mass is large and symptomatic. Epididymitis and related inflammatory conditions of the scrotum usually are treated medically with antibiotics, antiinflammatory medications, analgesics, and supportive measures, including heating pads and scrotal elevation. The diagnosis of a scrotal abscess mandates surgical drainage, but it also dictates prompt evaluation of the lower urinary tract for a cause that may require immediate attention as well (e.g., urethral stricture disease, trauma with infectious urine extravasation). Clinical suspicion of testicular torsion or rupture should lead to surgical exploration and orchiopexy (testicular fixation), testicular salvage procedures, or orchiectomy, depending on testicular viability.

MALE INFERTILITY

Infertility, defined as the inability to conceive a pregnancy within 1 year of unprotected sexual intercourse, affects approximately 15% of couples in the United States.[21] Male factors are thought to contribute to approximately half of the instances. Although the condition is poorly understood, new information continues to emerge to provide insight into its complexity. Along with this improved understanding, new diagnostic and therapeutic techniques have been developed to assist in the management of the problem.

Diagnosis

An informative and cost-effective initial evaluation should begin with a complete history taking, physical examination, and appropriate laboratory tests. Information should be obtained about duration of infertility, current sexual practices, erectile and ejaculatory functions, and fertility history. Medical history should be obtained to identify congenital anomalies, endocrine disorders, systemic illness, prior surgeries (e.g., herniorrhaphy and bladder or scrotal surgeries), and infections or trauma of the genital and urinary tracts. It is important to identify exposures to gonadotoxins, including recreational drugs, anabolic steroids, chemotherapeutic agents, chemical pesticides, and even environmental toxins that affect spermatogenesis. The physical examination is focused on the genitalia. Scrotal contents should be carefully assessed to evaluate whether the testes are abnormal (measuring <4 cm in length and having a consistency other than moderately firm), whether the vas deferens on either side is absent, and whether a varicocele is present. Rectal examination should be performed to determine whether the seminal vesicles are abnormally palpable or a midline prostatic cyst is detectable that would suggest ejaculatory duct obstruction. General physical characteristics relative to virilization should be assessed for abnormal sexual maturation, which may be the manifestation of an endocrinopathy.

The semen analysis represents the cornerstone of the male infertility evaluation. Normal standards are available that refer to the amount, morphology, and function of sperm and conditions of the ejaculate (Table 115.4). Three separate specimens collected at least 2 but not more than 5 days after the last ejaculation are required before instituting therapy. Serum levels of follicle-stimulating hormone (FSH), luteinizing hormone (LH), and testosterone should be obtained in patients with abnormal semen analysis parameters or evidence of an endocrinopathy to assess the hypothalamic–pituitary–gonadal axis. Tests to evaluate spermatogenesis and the presence of excurrent duct system obstruction include testicular biopsy, vasography, and transrectal ultrasonography. A variety of tests can be applied to assess sperm function, including sperm penetration assays, postcoital testing, and antisperm antibody testing.

Treatment

Therapy in the field of male infertility is evolving toward identifying a treatable cause and rationally initiating therapy that has a high likelihood of success. Oligospermia (low sperm

TABLE 115.4

NORMAL SEMEN PARAMETERS

Volume	2–5 mL
Sperm concentration	$>20 \times 10^6$/mL
Total sperm	$>60 \times 10^6$
Motility	>60%
Forward progression	>75%
Normal morphology	>60%
Fructose	Present
Agglutination	Absent
White blood cells	<5 WBCs/HPF

count) usually receives empiric treatment with clomiphene citrate to raise gonadotropin levels and, in theory, stimulate the testes to function better. Varicocelectomy through laparoscopic ligation or open microsurgical techniques has in some instances improved sperm counts and function, supported by the hypothesis that varicoceles cause disordered scrotal temperature regulation and retrograde flow of adrenal hormones and renal toxins. Other surgical applications include microsurgical reconstruction to treat vas deferens and epididymal obstructions, transurethral resection to treat the obstructed ejaculatory duct orifice, and microsurgical sperm aspiration of the epididymides for use with assisted reproduction techniques for the diagnosis of absent or atretic excurrent duct structures. Hormone replacement may be appropriately offered when specific endocrine disorders have been defined. Complete testicular failure, as determined by testicular biopsy showing no sperm production or a markedly elevated FSH level, has been considered untreatable in the past. However, recently developed assisted reproduction techniques have been applied to treat this disorder as well as others in which goal-directed therapies cannot be offered.

UROLITHIASIS

Urolithiasis (also termed *urinary stones* or *calculi*) has always afflicted humankind and has been documented in Egyptian mummies from 4800 BC. Hippocrates was quoted as saying, "I will not cut even for the stone, but leave such procedures to the practitioners of the craft." It is a significant health problem, because the overall cost of the disease is approximately $2 billion per year in the United States.[22]

Urolithiasis affects a significant portion of the population. Today, most urinary stones in industrialized countries are renal (nephrolithiasis), with bladder stones being relatively uncommon. An understanding of the disorder's epidemiology is important for identification of patient risk factors and prevention. Each year, 0.1% to 0.4% of the population is believed to have kidney stones, with a peak incidence between the ages of 45 and 64 years in the United States and Europe[23] (even though most people report the onset of disease in their teenage years). In addition, men have a threefold higher incidence of the disease than women,[24] and patients with a family history of stone disease have a 25-fold higher incidence of new stone formation.

There are geographic variations in the risk for development of a stone, with a higher risk in mountainous, desert, and tropical areas. In the United States, the southeastern region has a higher incidence compared with the rest of the nation. It is unclear whether this difference is caused by the hot weather, hydrational status, or other factors (e.g., increased vitamin D production from sunlight exposure).[25] International variability is also evident, with the whole-population lifetime risk for development of kidney stone disease at 2% to 5% in Asia, 8% to 15% in Europe and North America, and 20% in Saudi Arabia.[23] In addition to geographic variations, there is seasonal variation because the incidence increases in the summer months in both the northern and southern hemispheres.

The incidence of stone recurrence is significant, with 50% of all patients with nephrolithiasis experiencing a recurrence within 5 to 10 years[24] and 75% recurring during the first 20 years.[26] These factors commit the patient and physician to a lifetime of follow-up and awareness of the possibility of recurrent episodes.

TABLE 115.5

TYPES OF KIDNEY STONES

Stone composition	Frequency (x)	Degree of radiopacity
Calcium stones (total)	82	Opaque
Calcium oxalate ± calcium phosphate	75	Very opaque
Pure calcium phosphate	7	
Magnesium ammonium phosphate	12	Opaque
Uric acid	7	Lucent
Cystine	2	Slightly opaque

Stone Compositions

Most stones found in patients in industrialized countries contain calcium and usually consist of calcium oxalate (Table 115.5). The remaining 20% of stones are composed of uric acid, struvite or carbonate apatite, cystine, and other rare precipitates.[27] Cystine stones form only in patients with a rare congenital defect called *cystinuria.* In addition, medicines such as indinavir sulfate, used in the treatment of HIV infection, have been reported to crystallize in the urinary tract,[28] leading to symptoms similar to those with conventional urolithiasis.

Pathophysiology

Stone formation is the end result of a complex interaction of many different factors that results in the crystallization of stone-forming salts. There are several different theories regarding which factors lead to the formation and progression of renal calculi. Nucleation is a process whereby stone formation is initiated by the presence of a crystal or foreign body, which promotes the growth of salt crystals only in supersaturated urine. Often, the nidus is composed of a substance other than the stone crystal itself (heterogeneous nucleation). Examples of heterogeneous nucleation are crystallization on injured surfaces of renal tubular cells or a different solute (i.e., uric acid, matrix). Nucleation requires the presence of transiently or intermittently supersaturated urine. Other factors such as low concentrations of crystallization inhibitors (e.g., citrate, nephrocalcin, pyrophosphate, acidic glycopeptides, uropontin, magnesium) as well as altered pH may have a significant effect on solubility and crystallization.

Most crystals pass through the urinary system unless they are adherent to the renal collecting system or are retained by urinary stasis. In some instances, kidney stones can be attached to Randall's plaques or sites of previous renal injury, preventing distal passage. Furthermore, anatomic factors such as distal obstruction (i.e., ureteral stricture) or location in the lower pole may lead to stasis and subsequent stone formation or propagation.

Diagnosis

It is generally accepted that stones initially form in the proximal urinary tract. As stones grow on the surfaces of the renal papillae or calyces, they usually do not produce symptoms and may be discovered only incidentally. Most symptoms occur as the stone traverses the renal pelvis and ureter, which leads to intermittent obstruction. The most common presentations of nephrolithiasis are pain and hematuria. Lateralizing pain from urolithiasis or renal colic is usually intermittent and can be located anywhere from the flank to the loin as the stone moves distally in the urinary tract. The presence of pain signifies obstruction and distention of the ureter or renal pelvis. However, the severity of pain is not usually related to the amount of distention but rather to the rapidity with which it develops. Sudden distention causes severe pain, whereas gradual distention may have no symptoms whatsoever. Associated nonrenal symptoms are the result of the autonomic innervation of the kidneys and may include nausea, vomiting, and ileus.

A thorough physical examination is required to rule out other causes of abdominal pain. Patients are usually in obvious distress and frequently have some costovertebral angle tenderness. Fever is usually absent unless there is concomitant infection. The urinalysis usually reveals hematuria but may be negative in approximately 5% of cases.[29] The urinary pH is frequently helpful in assessing risk factors for stone disease because uric acid stones tend to form in acidic urine (pH <6.0) and struvite in alkaline urine (pH >7.0). The diagnosis of nephrolithiasis is confirmed by characteristic radiographic findings or stone passage.

Radiographic Examination

There is no perfect radiographic examination for the evaluation of kidney stones and the chosen study depends on availability, patient factors (i.e., age, pregnancy, allergies, renal function), and situation (elective or emergency). The most commonly used studies are listed in Table 115.6, with their characteristic advantages and disadvantages.

Intravenous Urography

Intravenous urography has been the mainstay of imaging for stone disease because the study has a high sensitivity and specificity for the diagnosis of stones. A well-prepared (with a mechanical bowel preparation) study provides information not only about the presence of stones but also about renal function, upper tract anatomy, and the presence or absence of obstruction. Important anatomic information, such as ureteral duplication or calyceal diverticulum, may be seen only on an IVU study. The major limitations of the study are an unprepared study (without a prior mechanical bowel preparation) in the emergency department because of poor visualization of retroperitoneal strictures. Other limitations include failure to visualize radiolucent stones, risks of contrast reaction and nephrotoxicity, and the prolonged examination time, especially with an obstructing stone. For these reasons, spiral computed tomography (CT) has supplanted the IVU in the emergency setting.[30] IVU still provides the most information when done electively for preoperative planning.[31]

Ultrafast Spiral Computed Tomography

Spiral CT has gained popularity in the evaluation of acute flank pain in the emergency department setting, for obvious reasons. The study is quick, does not require intravenous contrast or bowel preparation, and is the most sensitive test for detection of ureteral stones. Additional advantages are the ability to determine stone compositions (except for indinavir sulfate) and the ability to detect an extrarenal pathologic process that may be the primary cause of lateralizing pain (e.g., aortic aneurysm).[32] There are, however, several significant limitations, including the lack of functional information. Also, spiral CT does not accurately delineate the anatomy of the ureter and renal collecting system. Detection of anomalies such as calyceal diverticulum or ureteral duplication is critical for proper preoperative planning. In addition, follow-up of stone disease is usually done using plain films. In many instances, comparison of plain films with spiral CT is difficult in assessing for stone movement or passage.

TABLE 115.6 DIAGNOSIS

IMAGING STUDIES FOR THE EVALUATION OF NEPHROLITHIASIS

Imaging study	Advantages	Disadvantages
Plain abdominal film	■ Readily accessible ■ Good sensitivity for detection of renal stones ■ Best study for routine follow-up of opaque stones	■ Radiation exposure ■ Low sensitivity for ureteral stones ■ Radiolucent stones (uric acid) ■ Cannot evaluate function or obstruction
Sonography	■ Radiation free ■ Usually accessible ■ High sensitivity in kidney and distal ureter (UVJ) ■ Detects hydronephrosis ■ Detects all stone types	■ Poor sensitivity mid and proximal ureter ■ Operator dependent
Intravenous urogram	■ Assesses entire urinary tract for presence of stones, renal function and ureteral obstruction ■ Anatomic information of upper urinary tract ■ Best study for preoperative planning	■ Risk of contrast reaction and ■ Radiolucent stones ■ Optimally requires prep ■ Contrast nephrotoxicity
Spiral computed tomography	■ Fast ■ No bowel preparation required ■ Accurately detects all stone types ■ Evaluates adjacent pathology ■ No contrast required ■ Best study to evaluate flank pain in emergency department setting	■ Radiation exposure ■ Lack of function ■ Does not assess upper urinary tract anatomy (i.e., duplicated system)

Ultrasonography

The use of ultrasound for evaluation of the upper urinary tract has steadily increased because of improved technology and user comfort. The study is noninvasive and available in both the hospital and outpatient setting. Ultrasound has become the procedure of choice in the pediatric population and with pregnant women. The study presents no radiation risk, detects stones in the kidney and ureterovesical junction with reasonable accuracy, and gives some anatomic information such as about the presence of hydronephrosis.[33] The shortcomings of the study are its poor sensitivity for stone detection in the middle and upper ureter, lack of functional information, and limited visualization of renal anatomy.

Plain Imaging

The kidneys–ureters–bladder plain radiograph is readily available and most useful in the follow-up of patients with stones, especially when it can be compared with a previously obtained IVU. The examination is reasonably accurate in the detection of radiopaque renal stones. The limitations of the study are its poor sensitivity in detection of ureteral stones, which may be superimposed on the bony pelvis, its inability to display renal anatomy and function, and its inability to visualize all stone compositions.

Management

After the diagnosis is confirmed, the situation is assessed for size, location, degree of obstruction, and complicating factors. Most stones (<6 mm) pass spontaneously and the patient can be followed conservatively. In the emergency setting, intravenous hydration and analgesics are usually sufficient to treat the acute attack. The patient can be discharged with outpatient urology follow-up when pain and associated symptoms have been controlled. Immediate intervention usually involves stone removal or bypassing the ureteral obstruction with stenting or placement of a percutaneous nephrostomy tube. Indications for intervention are listed in Table 115.7 and are usually related to associated pyelonephritis, unremitting pain, and deterioration of renal function or presence of high-grade obstruction. Other relative indications for intervention are large stones (>1 cm) that are unlikely to pass spontaneously or occupations that require stone-free status (e.g., airline pilots).

Patients not requiring acute intervention are sent home and told to strain their urine. Even stones with significant ureteral obstruction can be safely observed for up to a month. In the absence of infection, most studies have shown no evidence of renal damage even with complete obstruction at 1 month. Elective intervention can be planned for failure of stone passage.

TABLE 115.7 INDICATIONS/CONTRAINDICATIONS

INDICATIONS FOR IMMEDIATE INTERVENTION IN PATIENTS WITH UROLITHIASIS

Absolute
Obstructive pyelonephritis (true emergency)
Unremitting pain
Deterioration of renal function
Anuria due to ureteral obstruction
Bilateral stones
Solitary kidney
Relative
Large ureteral stones (>7 mm) that are unlikely to pass spontaneously
Occupational requirements (i.e., airline pilot)
Transplant kidney

Treatment Options

The safest management for patients with ureteral stones is spontaneous passage, providing there are no complicating factors. The chance of spontaneous stone passage is related to stone size and anatomic features of the upper urinary tract. The American Urological Association Clinical Guidelines Panel on ureteral stones determined that over 95% of stones less than 5 mm in diameter pass spontaneously.[34] Another factor determining stone passage is impedance at the three narrowest portions of the ureter: the ureteropelvic junction, ureterovesical junction, and the crossing of the iliac vessels. In some cases, anatomic abnormalities (e.g., ureteral stricture) prevent passage.

For stones that are unlikely to pass or that have failed conservative management, acceptable options are described in the following sections.

Extracorporeal Shock Wave Lithotripsy

The first shock wave lithotripsy (SWL) was reported in 1984 by Chaussy et al.[35] and revolutionized the treatment of nephrolithiasis. The field of stone management was changed from largely surgical procedures to image-guided therapy. SWL is a truly noninvasive, image-guided therapy whereby shock waves are generated and focused on the target stone, usually requiring only intravenous sedation. The effect of these shock waves is to pulverize the stone into smaller fragments that can easily pass through the urinary tract. The major risks of the procedure are ecchymosis, perinephric hematoma, renal colic and ureteral obstruction from fragments, and sepsis.

Ureterorenoscopy

Advances in technology have led to the design of endoscopes that can be safely passed to all parts of the urinary tract in a retrograde fashion. Larger stones can be fragmented using intracorporeal lithotripsy, and smaller stones can be grasped and removed under direct vision. Available lithotripsy devices include holmium and pulsed-dye lasers and electrohydraulic, electromechanical, and ultrasonic devices. The major risks of the procedure are anesthesia, ureteral injury, sepsis, stricture formation, bleeding, and sepsis.

Percutaneous Nephrolithotomy

Percutaneous techniques for stone removal were developed in the 1980s and quickly supplanted open surgical techniques for treatment of stones. Their use greatly decreased after the development of SWL, which provided a less invasive alternative. The procedure involves establishment of a nephrostomy tract directly into the renal collecting system from the flank, through which large-diameter instruments are passed, resulting in the ability to remove large amounts of stone from the kidney and upper ureter efficiently. The procedure is more invasive than ureteroscopy or SWL and thus has higher complication and morbidity rates.

Open Surgery or Laparoscopy

Open surgery and laparoscopy are rarely required but may be necessary for the removal of larger staghorn calculi, for stones refractory to conventional, minimally invasive options, or for patients with anatomic limitations that prevent a minimally invasive procedure. Stone removal may also be done concomitantly with repair of an anatomic defect (e.g., a ureteropelvic junction obstruction).[36,37]

Location-specific Treatment Options

Renal Calculi

In general, SWL therapy is the procedure of choice for renal stones less than 2 cm in size. Treatment-related failure and complication rates increase significantly for larger and staghorn calculi.[38] Additional factors that significantly influence the success of SWL therapy are stone location, stone composition, and anatomic factors. With regard to stone location, stones in the upper and middle calyces pass more readily than stones in the lower calyx, especially if there is an unfavorable acute angle in relation to the renal pelvis. Stones composed of calcium oxalate monohydrate and cystine tend to fragment into fewer pieces (if at all) and are less likely to be successfully treated. Last, any anatomic factor that inhibits distal stone passage such as distal obstruction (i.e., stricture, ureteropelvic junction obstruction), stone location in a calyceal diverticulum, or hydronephrosis provides a relative contraindication.

Patients who have failed SWL therapy or possess factors making success of SWL unlikely (e.g., staghorn calculus, lower pole location, cystine composition) should be considered for percutaneous stone removal. Percutaneous nephrolithotomy has the ability to both fragment and remove stones without depending on spontaneous passage of fragments. Ureteroscopy has gained more popularity for treatment of stones in the kidney and distal ureter. Optimal candidates are patients who have failed SWL therapy and are not good candidates for percutaneous nephrolithotomy.

Proximal and Mid-ureteral Calculi

Shock wave lithotripsy and ureteroscopy are both acceptable options for treatment of stones in the proximal and middle ureter. Because of limitations in stone localization, SWL has lower success rates for calculi appearing in this location than it does for renal calculi. Ureteroscopy in this portion of the ureter usually requires flexible techniques. A ureteroscopic approach can be technically difficult but highly successful in competent hands.[39] In some instances, antegrade ureteroscopy through an established nephrostomy tract is an acceptable alternative. The choice is largely dependent on physician experience or preference and on patient preference. Blind basketing is not acceptable, and open surgery should be reserved as a salvage procedure.

Distal Ureteral Calculus

There has been an ongoing debate over whether ureteroscopy or SWL is the optimal treatment for distal stones. SWL has less morbidity than ureteroscopy but has somewhat lower success rates because of difficulty with stone localization. Ureteroscopy is technically straightforward using rigid or semirigid endoscopes, and has success rates of more than 95% in most series, with minimal complications.[34] The choice depends largely on patient and urologist preference.

Evaluation of the Stone-forming Patient

The most important initial step in evaluating the stone-forming patient is to gather the stone for analysis. Although most stones contain calcium, approximately 20% are composed of other minerals and require different long-term management plans. Other important factors in evaluation of the stone-forming patient are a careful history with emphasis on family members with urolithiasis, factors contributing to dehydration, diet, bowel disease (e.g., sprue, ulcerative colitis), previous bowel surgery, and fluid intake. A complete physical examination and baseline laboratory evaluation consisting of urinalysis, urine culture, serum electrolytes, blood urea nitrogen, creatinine, uric acid, and calcium should be done. If the stone was not collected, a screening test for cystinuria should be done. The goal of the initial evaluation is to identify uncommon but treatable causes of nephrolithiasis.

The presence of normocalcemia and normouricemia, plus the absence of urinary tract infection, bowel disease, or marked hyperoxaluria, can usually differentiate uncomplicated calcium stone disease from other types. For the first-time uncomplicated calcium stone former, no further evaluation is warranted. The patient is counseled on a low-oxalate diet, told to drink enough fluid to produce more than 2,000 mL of urine per day, and followed up on a regular basis for evaluation of stone recurrence.

Metabolically active stone disease is characterized by formation of new stones, enlargement of an old stone, or passage of gravel. For patients with noncalcium or metabolically active stone disease, a complete evaluation is indicated. Complete metabolic evaluation is directed at identifying specific factors that influence the crystallization of stone-forming salts. These protocols include analysis of 24-hour urine collection, complete serum panels, and further evaluation for risk factors. Pak characterized urinary risk factors (Table 115.8) and specific treatments directed at correcting the underlying abnormalities (Table 115.9).[40]

ENDOUROLOGY

Endourology is a term coined in 1978 at the Annual Meeting of the American Urological Association that refers to the endoscopic evaluation of and intervention in the urinary tract. Although urologists have always been endoscopists, procedures were usually limited to endoscopic evaluation of the lower urinary tract. At that meeting, a poster highlighted advanced techniques performed in all parts of the urinary tract, mostly in patients not viewed as candidates for open surgical approaches. The discipline of endourology is a natural progression of minimally invasive surgery that is the result of the creative efforts of urologists, radiologists, and engineers. Current endoscopic techniques can safely access the upper urinary tract by retrograde ureteropyeloscopy and antegrade percutaneous approaches, and the retroperitoneum by laparoscopic and retroperitoneoscopic approaches. These advances were significant enough to require special expertise and, thus, launch the subspecialty of endourology.

Ureterorenoscopy

Ureterorenoscopy is the endoscopic evaluation of the upper urinary tract through a retrograde (transurethral) approach. The technique involves accessing the ureter through the urethra and bladder. Hugh Hampton Young[41] performed the first ureteroscopy in 1912 when he passed a cystoscope into the distal ureter of a child with massive hydronephrosis from vesicoureteral reflux, owing to posterior urethral valves. Subsequent advances in techniques and ureteroscope technology have allowed us to reach all portions of the urinary tract with minimal morbidity.

Flexible and rigid ureteroscopes are available in sizes less than 8 French. This caliber of instrument allows for passage into the ureter with minimal or no dilation. Semirigid ureteroscopes are available is sizes as small as 4.9F, with working ports of sufficient size to admit a variety of lithotripsy devices and working instruments. These ureteroscopes can be reliably passed into the distal ureter and, in some patients, can be further advanced into the middle and upper ureter. Advancement of the ureteroscope may not be possible in all patients (especially

TABLE 115.8 DIAGNOSIS

PATHOPHYSIOLOGY AND DIAGNOSIS OF STONE DISEASE

Condition	Primary defect	Stone composition	Minimum diagnostic criteria
Resorptive hypercalciuria	Hyperparathyroidism	Ca oxalate, Ca phosphate	Hypercalcemia and elevated PTH
Absorptive hypercalciuria			
Type I	High intestinal Ca absorption	Ca oxalate, Ca phosphate	Hypercalciuria on random and restricted diet, normal serum Ca and PTH
Type II	High intestinal Ca absorption	Ca oxalate, Ca phosphate	Hypercalciuria on random diet, normacalciuria on restricted diet, normal serum Ca and PTH
Renal hypercalciuria	Renal Ca leak	Ca oxalate, Ca phosphate	Normal serum Ca, high serum PTH, hypercalciuria
Hypocitraturic Ca nephrolithiasis	Acidosis or excess of dietary acid	Ca oxalate	Hypocitraturia
Distal renal tubular acidosis	Renal acid retention	Ca phosphate	Hypocitraturia
Hyperuricosuric Ca nephrolithiasis	Diet rich in animal protein	Ca oxalate	Urinary pH >5.5, hyperuricosuria
Gouty diathesis	Excessive urinary acidification	Uric acid, Ca oxalate, Ca phosphate	Urinary pH ,<5.5 without diet rich in animal protein or diarrhea
Enteric hyperoxaluria	Ileal disease or resection	Ca oxalate, uric acid	Hyperoxaluria, hypocitraturia, pH <5.5
Cystinuria	Impaired cystine transport	Cystine	Urinary cystine >250 mg/g, creatinine
Infection stones	Excessive urease activity	Struvite, carbonate apatite	Urinary pH>7.5, positive culture for urea-splitting organisms

PTH, parathyroid hormone.
(Adapted from Pak CY. Kidney stones. *Lancet* 1998;351:1797–1801.)

TABLE 115.9 TREATMENT

MEDICAL MANAGEMENT OF NEPHROLITHIASIS

Condition	Specific treatments	Simplified treatments
Resorptive hypercalciuria	Surgical parathyroidectomy	
Absorptive hypercalciuria		Thiazide + potassium citrate
Type I	Thiazide + potassium citrate (sodium cellulose phosphate)	
Type II	Low calcium diet	Potassium citrate
Renal hypercalciuria	Thiazide + potassium citrate	Potassium citrate
Gouty diathesis	Potassium citrate	Potassium citrate
Dietary hyperoxaluria		Restrict dietary oxalate Avoid severe calcium restriction
Hypocitraturic Ca nephrolithiasis and distal renal tubular acidosis	Potassium citrate	Potassium citrate
Hyperuricosuric Ca nephrolithiasis	Allopurinol, potassium citrate	Potassium citrate
Enteric hyperoxaluria	Potassium citrate, calcium citrate, magnesium citrate	Potassium citrate, Ca citrate, Mg citrate
Cystinuria potassium citrate		
Mild (250–500 mg/d)	Chelating agents, potassium citrate	Chelating agents
>500 mg/d	Tiopronin (thiola) Antibiotic, acetohydroxamic acid	High fluid intake Potassium citrate Antibiotic, acetohydroxamic acid
Infection stones	Complete removal of all stones	

(Adapted from Pak CY. Kidney stones. *Lancet* 1998;351:1797–1801.)

TABLE 115.10

APPLICATIONS OF URETEROSCOPY

Ureteroscopic diagnosis and biopsy of ureteral and renal lesions
Removal of ureteral and renal calculi
Primary therapy
Failed or contraindications to shock wave lithotripsy
Treatment of upper urinary tract transitional cell carcinoma
Incisional procedure
Ureteral stricture
Ureteropelvic junction obstruction
Renal calyceal diverticulum or infundibular stenosis

male patients) because of the course of the more proximal ureter. Flexible ureteroscopes bypass some of the limitations of rigid ones by conforming to the course of the ureter, allowing for reliable passage to the upper ureter and kidney. Flexible ureteroscopes are available in sizes as small as 7F and have a working channel to allow for passage of a variety of instruments and lithotripsy devices without the need for significant dilation of the ureter.

The applications for ureterorenoscopy are listed in Table 115.10. By far the most common application is in the treatment of ureteral and renal calculi. SWL is the least invasive of the options for treating stones but may be unsuccessful because of stone size, composition, or location, or anatomic limitations. In such cases, ureteroscopy is an attractive option. Other applications, in order of decreasing frequency, include diagnosis and biopsy, incisional procedures such as endopyelotomy, and treatment of transitional cell carcinoma of the upper urinary tract.

PERCUTANEOUS RENAL SURGERY

The first percutaneous nephrostomy tube was placed by Goodwin[42] in 1955. The concept that the kidney could be accessed in an antegrade fashion without the morbidity of an open incision revolutionized the treatment of upper urinary tract disease. The application expanded beyond simple drainage to removal of renal and upper ureteral stones. Shortly after the development of techniques for percutaneous stone removal, SWL revolutionized the field, decreasing the applications and impact of the technique. Percutaneous renal surgery, however, still plays a large role in urologic surgery.

The applications of percutaneous renal surgery are listed in Table 115.11. By far the most common application is removal of renal stones. It is unquestionably the treatment of choice for large or staghorn calculi. Other applications include management of congenital abnormalities such as calyceal diverticulum, incisional procedures such as endopyelotomy, treatment of renal cysts, and surgical management of transitional cell carcinoma of the upper urinary tracts.

TABLE 115.11

APPLICATIONS OF PERCUTANEOUS RENAL SURGERY

Removal of renal and upper ureteral stones
Stone burden >2 cm
Staghorn calculi
Lower pole stones >1 cm
Failed shock wave lithotripsy
Anatomic abnormalities—calyceal diverticulum, hydronephrosis
Treatment of transitional cell carcinoma
Incisional procedures
Ureteropelvic junction obstruction
Infundibular stenosis
Ablative procedures
Calyceal diverticulum
Renal cysts

LAPAROSCOPIC SURGERY OF THE RETROPERITONEUM

Kelling[43] reported the first laparoscopy in 1901 when he used air insufflation in a canine model and viewed the peritoneal cavity through a cystoscope. It was not until 1976, when Cortesi et al.[44] evaluated cryptorchid testes and Wickham[45] performed ureterolithotomy, that laparoscopy was used for urologic purposes. Laparoscopic techniques remained underused until 1989, when Reddick and Olsen[46] reported on laparoscopic cholecystectomy, marking the transition from a predominantly diagnostic to a therapeutic modality. In response to this landmark achievement in general surgery, many potential urologic applications were quickly identified and performed with varying degrees of difficulty. Currently accepted applications of laparoscopy are listed in Table 115.12.

A retroperitoneal or transperitoneal approach can be used for most procedures, depending on the disease process, patient considerations (e.g., body habitus, previous surgeries, presence of infection), and surgeon familiarity. The basic advantage of the retroperitoneal approach is avoidance of the peritoneal cavity, but at the expense of a limited working space. The transperitoneal approach provides a larger working space but requires mobilization of the colon and carries the risk of various bowel-related complications (e.g., visceral hernia, adhesions, perforation). The retroperitoneal approach is generally favored for removal of smaller, nonmalignant kidneys. To date, no overall advantage has been clearly identified between the two approaches,[47] and choice largely depends on surgeon preference and the clinical situation. More recently, the use of an intraabdominal sleeve to allow the surgeon to use his or her hand for manually assisted laparoscopy has shown promise in decreasing complications and improving surgical results.[48]

Laparoscopic techniques show benefits beyond improved cosmesis and decreased postoperative morbidity. Studies have shown results comparable with those of open surgery for radical

TABLE 115.12

APPLICATION OF LAPAROSCOPY

Diagnostic
Nonpalpable testes
Lymph node sampling
Pelvic for prostate, bladder, penile malignancies
Retroperitoneal for testicular cancer
Nephrectomy for renal donation
Simple for benign disease
Radical for renal cell carcinoma
Nephroueterectomy
Transitional cell carcinoma of upper urinary tract
Nonfunctioning kidney with reflux
Radical prostatectomy
Adrenalectomy
Pyeloplasty
Pyelolithotomy
Ureterolithotomy
Calyceal diverticulum
Nephropexy

nephrectomy,[49] pyeloplasty,[50] adrenalectomy,[51] and simple nephrectomy for benign disease.[52] Results from laparoscopic radical prostatectomy are comparable with the open radical retropubic technique technqiue.[53] The steep learning cure and high positive margin rates in the early series, however, remain the primary concern. As the techniques and technology improve, acceptance and applications will increase.

UROTHELIAL CARCINOMA

Tumors derived from the urothelial lining of the urinary system, commonly referred to as *transitional cell epithelium,* account for almost 63,000 newly diagnosed cancers in 2005 in the United States. Bladder cancer is the fourth most common cause of cancer death in men.[54] The most common type of urothelial cancer is transitional cell carcinoma (90%), although other histologic types can occur, including squamous cell carcinoma (5%), adenocarcinoma (2%), lymphoma (<1%), and sarcoma (<1%). Development of squamous cell carcinoma appears to be related to chronic irritation secondary to stone or a foreign body, or in the case of certain developing countries, from urinary schistosomiasis.[55] Adenocarcinoma of the urinary bladder may originate from the bladder or urachal remnant as a primary lesion, or from a gastrointestinal metastasis. Transitional cell carcinomas can be broadly categorized as superficial or invasive. The precise cause of these tumors is unknown, although genetic alterations are common.[56] Superficial transitional cell carcinoma is most commonly associated with trisomy or deletion of chromosome 9(9p21), whereas invasive transitional cell carcinoma is most commonly associated with 17p chromosomal aberrations (especially *p53* mutations). Although multiple factors have been identified with the development of these urothelial tumors[57] (Table 115.13), the single most important of these is a prior exposure to tobacco smoke. Thus, the demographics of the development of bladder cancer mirrors cigarette use in the United States. Men have urothelial tumors three times as often as women, and whites acquire these tumors approximately twice as often as African Americans. The peak incidence of these tumors is typically in the sixth or seventh decade of life, but can vary over a considerable range.

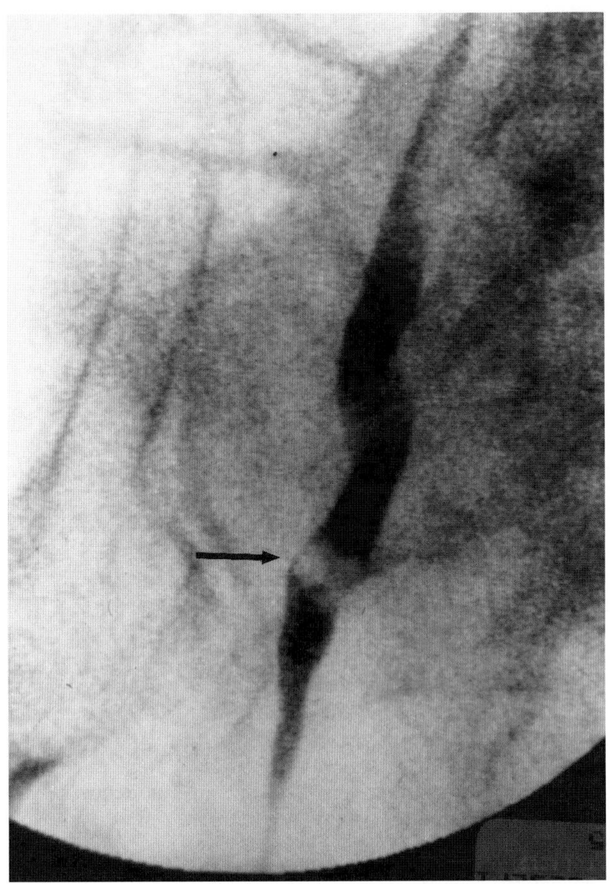

FIGURE 115.1 Retrograde pyelogram demonstrating a distal transitional cell carcinoma (stage T1) (*arrow*) in a 65-year-old white woman. The patient presented with painless hematuria and a positive urinary cytologic analysis. Her risk factors for this disease included a long-standing history of tobacco use and prior pelvic radiation as part of treatment for a low-grade cervical neoplasm 20 years earlier.

Diagnosis

Cancers of the urothelial lining may occur anywhere from the kidney to the bladder. Fig. 115.1 shows an example of a distal ureteral transitional cell carcinoma presenting with painless hematuria, which is the most common method of presentation for patients with any urothelial malignancy. Significant voiding symptoms do not usually occur unless there is profuse disease, as might be seen with carcinoma *in situ* or invasive disease. In the case of advanced disease, the patient may experience significant frequency, urgency, stranguria, and marked gross hematuria. Widespread urinalysis screening for hematuria enables most of these tumors to be found at an early stage. Patients who present with persistent microhematuria require evaluation with urinalysis, urinary culture, urinary cytology, and radiographic imaging of the upper urinary tract, either by IVU or contrast-enhanced CT. Although radiographic imaging also may demonstrate the presence of bladder tumors (Fig. 115.2), cystoscopy is always indicated to confirm this diagnosis. If the patient presents with active gross hematuria, cystoscopy may be undertaken immediately to identify the source. Otherwise, the radiographic evaluation is performed in conjunction with the cystoscopy. Newer methods of urine screening with fluorescence *in situ* hybridization (FISH)[58] and dipstick tests such as NMP22[59] are changing the evaluation of bladder cancer. Their precise roles, however, have yet to be determined. They are likely to prove most useful in monitoring patients with previously treated urothelial tumors.

Once the diagnosis of a urothelial malignancy is made, further staging is necessary. Clinicopathologic staging is outlined in Table 115.14. Because patients with urothelial tumors have already undergone radiographic imaging of the urinary system as part of their hematuria evaluation, subsequent imaging, if

TABLE 115.13

FACTORS ASSOCIATED WITH THE DEVELOPMENT OF UROTHELIAL TUMORS

Aniline dyes
2-Naphthlylamine
Nitrosamines
Cyclophosphamide
Acrolein
Phenacetin
Schistosomiasis (e.g., *Schistosoma haematobium*)
Chronic irritation (stones or hardware such as a catheter)
Radiation exposure
Tobacco exposure

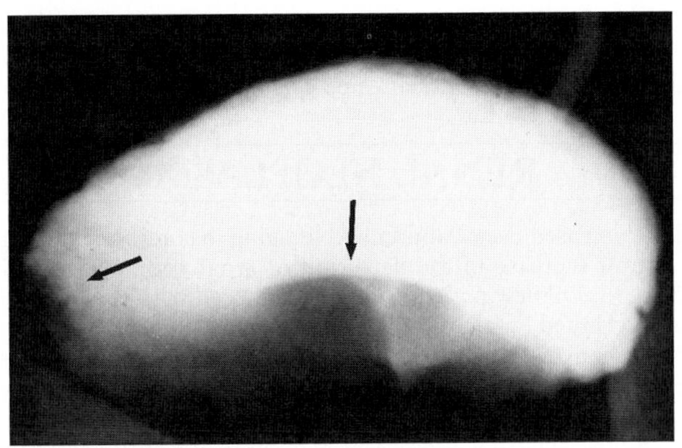

FIGURE 115.2 Intravenous pyelogram demonstrating a small lateral bladder filling defect (*arrow*). The midline defect (*arrow*) is most consistent with an enlarged prostate in this elderly African American man. Cystoscopy confirmed the filling defect was in fact a bladder tumor. Subsequent resection revealed that this was a low-grade urothelial cancer (stage Ta). This patient's risk factor for the disease was a history of tobacco use.

necessary, is focused on completing the staging evaluation. The first step in this process is obtaining a tissue diagnosis with adequate deep muscle tissue to distinguish muscle-invasive disease from superficial disease. If there is a high suspicion of invasive disease based on the initial cystoscopy, then a preoperative staging CT of the abdomen and pelvis is worthwhile because a postoperative study may be unable to distinguish tissue reaction and local artifact related to endoscopic resection of the primary tumor with deep biopsies. Superficial disease (Ta) is usually low grade and associated with only a 10% rate of progression to invasive carcinoma. Unfortunately, this low-grade disease is prone to recurrence (up to 60%) and requires close surveillance with urinary cytology and cystoscopy every 3 months and periodic radiographic imaging (IVU or CT) at least annually. T1 disease and carcinoma *in situ* are more likely to progress to a frankly invasive malignancy (roughly one third of the time) and similarly require close surveillance. Of the T1 lesions, high-grade disease (grade 3) carries the worst prognosis, with progression rates in excess of 50%, such that many urologists advocate treating patients with extensive high-grade disease (T1G3) as if they had muscle-invasive disease.[60] Patients who are thought to be candidates for surgical therapy require completion of their staging with chest radiography and laboratory studies, including complete blood count (CBC), coagulation profile, serum metabolic panel, and serum chemistries.

TABLE 115.14 STAGING

CLINICOPATHOLOGIC STAGING OF UROTHELIAL TUMORS[a]

Clinicopathologic staging	Urothelial tumors
Ta	Superficial papillary
Tis	Carcinoma *in situ*
T1	Invasive, limited to lamina propria
T2	Invasive, limited to superficial muscle (muscularis propria)
T3	Deeply invasive urothellal carcinoma
T3a	Invasion limited to deep muscle
T3b	Invasion limited to perivesical fat
T4	Advanced urothelial carcinoma
T4a	Involvement limited to prostate/uterus/vagina
T4b	Involvement limited to pelvic or abdominal wall
Nx	Nodal status cannot be assessed
N0	None
N1	Single lymph node <2 cm
N2	Lymph node involvement 2–5 cm
N3	Lymph node involvement <5 cm
Mx	Cannot be assessed
M0	No metastasis
M1	Distant metastasis

[a]Based on the American Joint Committee on Cancer. *American Joint Committee on Cancer (AICC) manual for staging of cancer,* 5th ed. 1997.

Treatment

Treatment options for superficial urothelial carcinoma include endoscopic local resection with or without intravesical chemotherapy. In rare cases, superficial carcinoma can be best treated with a partial cystectomy, but extreme care must be taken to prevent conversion of a Ta or T1 lesion to T4 from tumor spillage. Unlike many other tumors, even low-grade transitional cell carcinoma can readily implant and grow locally.

The use of adjuvant intravesical chemotherapy is largely restricted to recurrent superficial transitional cell carcinoma and carcinoma *in situ*.[60] Various agents have been tested, including mitomycin C, thiotepa, doxorubicin, and bacillus Calmette-Guérin (BCG) without or with inteferon. BCG therapy appears to be the most effective method of treatment in the adjuvant setting; however, emerging data suggest that immediate postoperative adjuvant with intravesical epirubicin results in similar complete response rates.[61] Although many institutions have slightly different protocols for BCG administration, BCG is usually administered as an intravesical instillation, once a week for a total of 6 weeks. Maintence BCG regimens have also been recommended. Patient tolerance, however, limits its wide spread acceptance. Use of intravesical BCG with interferon has also been proposed to salvage BCG failures.[62]

Muscle-invasive transitional cell carcinoma is most appropriately treated with radical cystoprostatectomy in men or anterior exenteration in women, provided the patient is a reasonable surgical candidate. Patients who are not candidates for radical surgery can be offered bladder salvage therapy consisting of endoscopic resection, local radiation therapy, and systemic chemotherapy; however, the long-term outcomes from such an approach are still under investigation.[63] Radical surgery involves the removal of local regional lymph nodes, the bladder, prostate, and seminal vesicles and a portion of the vas deferens. In women, the bladder and anterior vagina are resected *en bloc.* The urinary stream therefore must be diverted either into a continent neobladder or through an intestinal conduit to a cutaneous stomal apparatus. The choice of reconstruction depends on patient preference, extent of disease, and the surgeon's technical expertise.

Continent cutaneous neobladders (e.g., Koch pouch) can obviate the need for a stomal appliance and preserve the patient's perception of body image, but do not fully recapitulate the original anatomy and voiding process. They are also prone to recurrent infections, metabolic abnormalities, and urinary stone formation.[64] Orthotopic neobladder more closely approximates the original voiding process, but requires a negative urethral margin with focal disease, and a motivated patient who is willing to perform intermittent self-catheterization if necessary to ensure complete emptying and irrigation of mucus from the neobladder.

Because these reconstructions are less common, they are probably best performed in tertiary care centers specializing in that type of surgery.[65] Typically, such reconstructions are performed with ileum or terminal ileum/proximal colon. The use of the colon segment allows implantation of the ureters in a tunneled (nonrefluxing) fashion, although this is not always necessary. Removing the ileocolic valve from the fecal stream may also place the patient at increased risk for diarrhea and poorly formed stools. Moreover, removing the terminal ileum is associated with vitamin B_{12} deficiency. Ileal neobladders circumvent some of these problems, but their construction requires longer intestinal segments (60 cm). The basic tenets of neobladder reconstruction are to provide a moderate-capacity reservoir with low filling pressure and a continence mechanism. The intestinal segment used determines the capacity. The low filling pressure is achieved by detubularizing the bowel segment, and continence is achieved either by using the intact external urethral sphincter (orthotopic neobladder) or by creating a continent cutaneous stoma that is catheterized periodically to empty the pouch. Although neobladder diversions are gaining in popularity, they do have higher complication rates than simple conduit diversions and these patients require closer follow-up, not just for cancer recurrence, but for metabolic monitoring, infection risk assessment, and adequate emptying and protection of the upper urinary tracts.

Simple conduit urinary diversion can be performed with virtually any segment of bowel. The most common method uses distal ileum, as described initially by Bricker.[66,67] These ileal loop conduits are technically easy to create, result in minimal metabolic abnormalities, and provide a durable and reliable method of urinary diversion. As long as the stoma is positioned such that it does not interfere with the patient's beltline, placement of a stomal appliance is usually well tolerated. Alternative conduits derived from jejunum or colon have higher rates of metabolic abnormalities and are usually reserved for situations that preclude the use of ileum (e.g., short gut, or pelvic radiation exposure to ileum).

Metastatic bladder cancer is largely an incurable disease. Multiple approaches have been studied, but durable responses are uncommon. Chemotherapy is the mainstay of treatment, usually with cisplatin-based regimens. M-VAC [methotrexate, vinblastine, doxorubicin (Adriamycin), cisplatin], the best-studied regimen to date, has a complete remission rate of less than 40%. Newer regimens that include paclitaxel and gemcitabine may have higher response rates, but the cancer commonly recurs and progresses.[68] Surgical intervention in these patients is usually directed at palliation only.

RENAL NEOPLASMS

The increased use of abdominal imaging has resulted in a significant increase in the detection of renal neoplasms. More than 36,000 new patients will be diagnosed with renal tumors in the United States and more than 13,000 Americans will die from renal cell carcinoma (RCC) in 2005.[54] When the disease becomes advanced, the prognosis is poor despite aggressive treatment regimens.[69,70] Although renal neoplasms can occur at almost age, they are most common in the fifth to seventh decades of life. Fig. 115.3 shows a case of a large left-sided RCC presenting as flank fullness in a 17-year-old man. It occurs in men twice as often as women, and although genetic syndromes associated with RCC are well described, most of these cases are sporadic.

The most common type of renal cancer is a clear cell renal cell carcinoma, commonly referred to as RCC (>75%); it is thought to be derived from the proximal convoluted tubule. These cancers tend to have a significant degree of tumor vascularity (i.e., tend to enhance with intravenous contrast) and were once referred to as *hypernephromas,* in the incorrect belief that they were derived from the adrenal gland. Fuhrman's grading system (1 is well-differentiated, 4 is highly undifferentiated) is commonly used when evaluating these cancers because the more anaplastic cancers tend to carry a poorer prognosis. Other, less common tumors of the kidney include the papillary RCC (10%), chromophobe cell carcinoma (3% to 5%), oncocytoma (5%), angiomyolipoma (<2%), and sarcomatoid carcinoma (<1%).

Compared with transitional cell carcinoma, relatively little is known about environmental risk factors in the promotion of RCC.[57] Proposed risk factors include acquired renal cystic disease (typically in patients with end-stage renal disease on hemodialysis), exposure to lead or cadmium, asbestosis, high-fat diet, obesity, hypertension, and tobacco exposure.[71] Genetic risk factors include von Hippel-Lindau (VHL) disease, tuberous sclerosis, polycystic kidney disease (especially the autosomal recessive form), and hereditary papillary RCC. VHL disease is an autosomal dominant genetic defect that

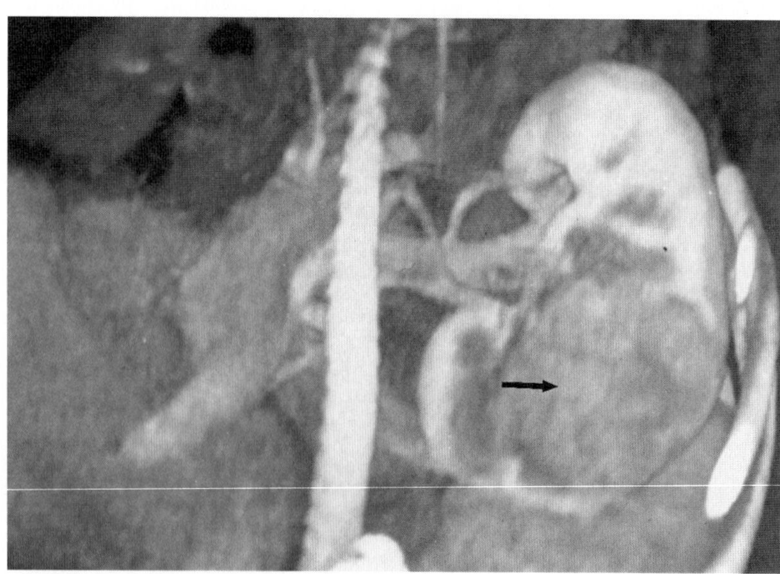

FIGURE 115.3 Computed tomography scan with three-dimensional reconstruction demonstrating a large (>7 cm) lower pole renal cell carcinoma in a 17-year-old patient presenting with flank pain and microscopic hematuria.

manifests as CNS hemangioblastomas, retinal angiomatosis, cysts of certain organs (kidney, epididymis, and pancreas), and RCC.[72] It is caused by a mutation in the *VHL* tumor suppressor gene. RCC develops in fully 50% of these patients, and is now the most common cause of death in this population. Most of the sporadic RCC studied to date either have mutations in the *VHL* gene or inactivation of *VHL* gene expression.[73] Tuberous sclerosis is also an autosomal dominant genetic syndrome that often manifests with seizures (from benign CNS tumors, referred to as *tubers*), adenoma sebaceum, mental retardation (variable), renal cysts, and increased risk of either renal angiomyolipoma or RCC.[74] It is caused by a mutation in one of two tumor suppressor genes (*TSC1* and *TSC2*) that are thought to be evolutionarily related through gene duplication.

The risk of RCC originally was thought to be increased in patients with autosomal dominant polycystic kidney disease (ADPKD). Now that the genes responsible for both VHL and ADPKD have been identified, however, it seems more likely that the cases of RCC originally attributed to ADPKD were in fact subtle forms of VHL. The autosomal recessive form of polycystic kidney disease, however, does still seem to carry approximately a 30-fold elevated risk for development of RCC over the general population. Hereditary papillary RCC is a recently described syndrome, and the details of this entity are still being evaluated. Early work in this area suggests that papillary RCCs are associated with a high incidence of activation of the *c-Met* protooncogene.[75] A recently described renal medullary carcinoma appears to be a highly anaplastic cancer found in young African Americans with hemoglobin gene sickle cell trait or hemoglobin sickle cell disease.[76]

Diagnosis

The decreasing costs of radiographic imaging have resulted in a marked increase in the number of incidentally discovered renal masses (approximately 40% to 50%), with a resultant migration to lower-stage disease at discovery. As a result, the classic triad of flank pain, flank fullness or mass, and hematuria now occurs in less than 10% of patients diagnosed with RCC.[77] Constitutional symptoms are still common and weight loss may occur in as many as a third of the patients. Others symptoms include fever of unknown origin, renally mediated hypertension, new-onset varicocele (especially left side), malaise, and anemia. Paraneoplastic syndromes are common with RCC, as outlined in Table 115.15. These paraneoplastic syndromes typically resolve spontaneously after resection of the primary mass. Because most patients present with incidentally discovered renal tumors, the subsequent evaluation is typically directed at accurate staging and preoperative planning. The criteria for staging are outlined in Table 115.16. CT appears to be the best overall modality for assessing clinical stage and has supplanted the more traditional IVU as a means of diagnosis and staging. CT allows determination of tumor size, location, extension, and adrenal involvement, and provides preliminary information regarding nodal involvement. RCC has a predilection for invading into the renal vein and inferior vena cava (IVC), although this is not usually a direct invasion into the vessels themselves, but rather a tumor thrombus. Renal vein and IVC tumor thrombus involvement does not necessarily portend a poorer prognosis and should not be a deterrent to definitive surgical management.[78]

Renal cystic masses detected by CT are confirmed by ultrasound for evaluation of any solid components. The risk of cancer progression in complex renal cysts has been extensively studied by Bosniak, who developed a classification system (Table 115.17) to help distinguish the risk of underlying malignancy.[79] Bosniak class I and II cysts are typically followed conservatively, whereas class III and IV cysts are explored and resected surgically if the patients are otherwise surgical candidates.

Completion of the staging evaluation typically involves a chest radiograph, CBC, coagulation profile, screening chemistries, and metabolic panel (including renal function and liver function tests, alkaline phosphatase, and serum calcium). In patients with large tumors (T2), a CT scan of the chest is often done because this is more sensitive for detecting occult pulmonary metastasis. Magnetic resonance imaging angiography or venocavography may be used if there is any concern over the possibility of an IVC tumor thrombus (approximately 5%) or in patients with azotemia, which precludes them from a contrast-enhanced CT scan. In addition, the azotemic patient may also be a candidate for nuclear renography to assess differential renal function.

TABLE 115.15

PARANEOPLASTIC SYNDROMES ASSOCIATED WITH RENAL CELL CARCINOMA

Hypercalcimia
Erythrocytosis
Anemia
Amyloidosis
Elevated sedimentation rate
Elevated liver function test results (Stauffer's syndrome)
Elevated serum alkaline phosphatase
Elevated serum ferritin

TABLE 115.16 STAGING

CLINICOPATHOLOGIC STAGING OF RENAL TUMORS[a]

Clinicopathologic staging	Renal tumor
Tx	Primary tumor cannot assessed
T0	No evidence of primary tumor
T1	Tumor 7.0 cm, limited to kidney
T2	Tumor >7.0 cm, limited to kidney
T3	Locally extensive disease
T3a	Tumor invades adrenal gland or perinephric tissues, but limited to Gerota's fascia
T3b	Tumor grossly extends into renal vein or vena cava below the diaphragm
T3c	Tumor extends into vena cava above the level of the diaphragm
T4	Tumor invades beyond Gerota's fascia
Nx	Regional nodes cannot be assessed
N0	No regional node involvement
N1	Metastasis into a single regional lymph node
N2	Metastasis into more than a single regional lymph node
Mx	Distant metastasis cannot be assessed
M0	No distant metastasis
M1	Distant metastasis

[a]Based on the American Joint Committee on Cancer. *American Joint Committee on Cancer (AICC) manual for staging of cancer*, 5th ed. 1997.

TABLE 115.17 CLASSIFICATION

BOSNIAK RENAL CYSTIC MASS CLASSIFICATION[a]

Classification	Type of cystic mass	Management
I	Simple cyst	No follow-up necessary
II	Minimal complex (usually benign) Curvilinear Calcification Thin septa Hyperdense cyst	Observe
III	Equivocal cyst Irregular calcification Thick septa Heterogeneity of cyst fluid	Consider surgery
IV	Frankly malignant Nodular/solid components Lesion enhances with contrast	Surgical excision

[a]These criteria require a contrast-enhanced spiral computed tomography scan.

Treatment

In 1963, Robson showed a significant increase in 5-year survival rates after radical nephrectomy for RCC.[80] Despite rapid changes in the practice of radiation and medical oncology, stage for stage there has not been a significant improvement in survival since that time. Thus, whenever feasible, surgery remains the treatment of choice for renal malignancies. Traditionally, the radical nephrectomy procedure is performed through a flank incision, and involves removal of the kidney, adrenal gland, and proximal ureter, *en bloc* and with Gerota's fascia. The adrenal gland, however, is infrequently involved and does not necessarily need to be removed in small, lower pole masses, unless it is enlarged. Although advocated by some, the role of extended lymphadenectomy is limited and it usually is not performed.[81] Patients with a solitary kidney or with underlying renal insufficiency can still be candidates for curative resection by a partial nephrectomy. Provided the primary tumor is less than 4 cm, the local recurrence rate is very low (<5%).[82] Indeed, the results of partial nephrectomies have been so encouraging that many now advocate partial nephrectomy for all patients with small peripheral renal masses, even with a normal contralateral kidney. Another recent development has been the use of laparoscopy to perform a radical or even a partial nephrectomy.[49] Early data regarding outcomes with this approach show a significant decrease in morbidity without compromising disease-free survival. When performing a laparoscopic nephrectomy, care must be taken to prevent tumor spillage during morcellation of the kidney. Alternatively, a small midline incision, just large enough to permit retrieval of the specimen, can be performed at the end of the procedure.

Small RCCs (<3 cm) are known to have a low propensity to metastasize, and thus experimental nephron-sparing techniques have been developed to try to treat these tumors in a minimally invasive manner. Aside from the more traditional methods of partial nephrectomy, minimally invasive methods using high-frequency ultrasound, radiofrequency thermal ablation, and cryosurgery have all been attempted. Currently, laparoscopically directed cryosurgery and percutaneous applied radiofreqency or cryoablation have been gaining popularity for the small, peripheral renal mass, although the long-term efficacy of such an approach remains to be determined.[83]

Advanced RCC is a devastating disease. Because of the ready access of these tumors to the venous vasculature, hematogenous metastasis can occur to a wide number of sites, including adrenal gland, lung, liver, brain, bone, and the contralateral kidney. When widespread disease occurs, treatment can be difficult. Factors that improve prognosis include a long interval between the time of original treatment and detectable metastasis, good performance status (rare), and metastasis limited to one portion of the lung. Patients with a solitary metastasis may still be candidates for surgical resection. Patients with a synchronous solitary metastasis carry a poorer prognosis than those with a delayed solitary metastasis. Nonetheless, surgical resections in this scenario have been associated with a 5-year survival rate of approximately 30%, although most of these patients are not cancer free.

Because spontaneous regression of advanced RCC occurs in approximately 1% to 2% of patients, there has been a great deal of enthusiasm for the development of immunologically based therapy for advanced disease.[84] Multiple strategies have been used, including the use of autologous harvested tumor-infiltrating lymphocytes, interferon administration, interleukin-2 administration, and *ex vivo* gene therapy. Combination protocols involving both immunotherapy and surgery have also been developed as a method of consolidation in those patients who are responders.[85] Even in the best of circumstances, the response rate for immunotherapy of RCC has been poor, with complete remission rates of approximately 6% and total response rates (partial response plus complete response) of approximately 30%. Chemotherapy has also been largely ineffective for RCC because multiple drug resistance appears to be a common finding in these cancers. Despite these poor early outcomes, immunotherapy and gene therapy remain active and exciting areas of research for the eventual treatment of advanced RCC.

PROSTATE CANCER

Prostate cancer is the most common cancer in men and the second most common cause of cancer-related deaths in American men. Approximately 30,000 prostate cancer-related deaths occurred in the United States in 2005.[54] Unlike many other malignancies, prostate cancer typically does not become symptomatic until the advanced stages. Increased interest in screening and the availability of the serum marker, PSA, have resulted in an improvement in the diagnosis of early-stage disease.[87] In widespread use as a diagnostic marker since 1987,[88] PSA is one of at least two serine proteases present in the blood and semen. It is thought that this protease lyses the seminal coagulum at the appropriate time to allow subsequent fertilization.

Prostate-specific antigen circulates in sera predominantly bound to carrier proteins such as $_1$-antichymotrypsin. Both the total and the free forms of PSA can be measured in most clinical laboratories with commercially available kits. The total PSA is commonly used as a screening test, with a typical cutoff of 4 ng/mL considered as the upper limit of normal. The unbound form is referred to as free PSA. Although formal cutoffs for percentage free PSA have not yet been determined, in general, patients with prostate cancer have a lower percentage of free PSA than patients without prostate cancer. Using a cutoff of less than 25% free PSA, coupled with a total PSA of 4 to 10 ng/mL, allows detection of approximately 95% of prostate cancers and reduces the proportion of unnecessary biopsies by 20%.[89] Lower cutoffs result in higher specificity of detection but poorer sensitivity.

Diagnosis

Staging

Prostate cancer staging has undergone numerous revisions. The earliest commonly used staging system was devised by Whitmore and Jewett and is still in use by many institutions. In 1992, the American Joint Committee on Cancer (AJCC) developed the more commonly used tumor, necrosis, metastasis (TNM) classification system, which has now become the standard for staging prostate cancer. The AJCC revised the classification system in 1997, eliminating the distinction between a unilateral nodule that occupies less than half of that side from a substantially larger unilateral nodule. Thus, in the newer classification, a unilateral nodule is classified as stage T2a, whereas bilateral bilateral disease is classified as stage T2b, and the size of the nodule in relation to the gland is ignored. The newer TNM classification is still not in widespread use, and some reports suggest that the older TNM classification retains better prognostic value.[90] A comparison of the various staging criteria is show in Table 115.18.

Screening

The diagnosis of prostate cancer is determined histopathologically after prostatic biopsy, typically performed under transrectal ultrasound guidance. Most men undergo prostatic biopsy because of an abnormality on rectal examination, or PSA elevation. However, the routine use of DRE and PSA testing in asymptomatic men as a means of reducing prostate cancer mortality by early detection and treatment is controversial.[91] The American Cancer Society and the American Urological Association recommend the routine use of DRE and PSA in asymptomatic men older than 50 years of age. Men with an increased risk of prostate cancer (e.g., African Americans or those with a family history of prostate cancer) should start screening at an earlier age.[92] The Canadian Task Force on the Periodic Health Examination does not support the routine use of PSA for prostate cancer screening.[93] Arguments for prostate cancer screening are based on the belief that early detection will decrease disease mortality rates, particularly because effective treatments are available for early-stage disease. Arguments against prostate cancer screening are based on the belief that early detection could result in excessive treatment of many cancers with low risks of progression rather than improvement of health in large populations.

Although no randomized trials have been performed to demonstrate the value of prostate cancer screening, population trends after the onset of widespread PSA testing suggest that screening may reduce mortality rates. Since 1987, large populations of otherwise asymptomatic men have undergone PSA screening, in combination with DRE, followed by prostatic

TABLE 115.18 STAGING

CLINICOPATHOLOGIC STAGING OF PROSTATE TUMORS: WHITMORE-JEWETT (W-J)AND TNM CLASSIFICATION FOR THE STAGING OF PROSTATE CANCER AS DEFINED BY THE AMERICAN JOINT COMMITTEE ON CANCER (1992 AND 1997)

W-J	1992	1997	Prostate tumor
—	TX	TX	Primary tumor cannot be assessed
—	T0	T0	No evidence of primary tumor
A	T1	T1	Clinically inapparent tumor no palpable or visible by imaging
A1	T1a	T1a	Tumor incidental histologic finding in ≤5% of tissue resected[a]
A2	T1b	T1b	Tumor incidental histologic finding in >5% of tissue resected[a]
—	T1c	T1c	Tumor identified by needle biopsy[b]
B	T2	T2	Organ-confined, palpable prostate cancer
BIN	T2a	T2a	Unilateral nodule, less than half the lobe
B1	T2b	T2a	Unilateral nodule, more than half the lobe
B2	T2c	T2b	Bilateral palpable disease
C	T3	T3	Tumor extends through the prostatic capsule
C1	T3a	T3a	Unilateral extracapsular extension
C1	T3b	T3a	Bilateral extracapsular extension
C1	T3c	T3b	Tumor extends into seminal vesicle(s)
C2	T4	T4	Tumor is fixed or invades adjacent structures other than seminal vesicles: bladder neck, external sphincter, rectum, levator, pelvic wall
—	NX	NX	Regional lymph nodes cannot be assessed
—	N0	N0	No regional lymph node metastases
D1	N1	N1	Metastasis in regional lymph node(s)
—	MX	MX	Distant metastases cannot be assessed
—	M0	M0	No distant metastases
D2	M1	M1	Distant metastases
D2	M1a	M1a	Nonregional lymph nodes
D2	M1b	M1b	Bone
D2	M1c	M1c	Other distant sites
D3	—	—	Hormone-refactory disease

[a]Incidental prostate cancer detected during resection of the prostate for presumed benign disease (e.g., transurethral resection of the prostate).
[b]Nonpalpable prostate cancer that was evaluated by prostate needle biopsy because of prostate-specific antigen elevation or ultrasonographic abnormality.

biopsy when indicated. Three observations since the onset of PSA screening suggest that early disease detection results in a decreased mortality rate. First, introduction of a successful screening test should result in an increased incidence, as the prevalent cases are detected, followed by a decreased incidence to near prescreening levels. Second, a successful screening test should result in stage migration to early-stage disease, with a decreased rate of detection of advanced disease. Third, the mortality rate should decline. Early analyses of the prostate cancer population statistics have indeed revealed a sharp increase in prostate cancer diagnoses, which peaked approximately 1992.[86,87] Subsequently, there has been a steady decline in the rate of prostate cancer diagnosis, so that the current rate of detection is approaching the pre-PSA screening era.[92] Multiple studies have now also documented a migration of stage to earlier forms of the disease, so that stage T1c cancers, detected by PSA screening alone (negative DRE), account for a substantial proportion of locally treated cancers.[94] Also noted is an age migration, so that prostate cancers are being diagnosed in men at an earlier age. Cancer-specific survival for stage T1c disease is better than for stage T2 disease (palpable, but organ confined). Whether this stage migration and subsequent treatment translates into a population-based improvement in cancer-specific survival remains to be determined. Before 1991, however, mortality rates for prostate cancer were steadily rising, and since that time the rates have leveled off and currently appear to be decreasing at the rate of approximately 1% per year.[86] Although many would argue that the jury is still out regarding the efficacy of prostate cancer screening, the early population trends suggest PSA testing in combination with DRE may successfully reduce prostate cancer mortality rates.

Treatment

Localized Disease

Because advanced prostate cancer remains essentially incurable, the diagnosis and treatment of localized prostate cancer (clinical stages T1 and T2) represents a unique opportunity for cure. Just because a cancer can be cured, however, does not mean cure is necessary. What needs to be distinguished is which cancers are clinically significant and are likely to progress and which ones are at low risk of progression and can be followed conservatively. Small-volume, latent prostate cancer in older men may not affect overall health because of the long natural history of the disease and the limited life expectancy of older men. Risk assessment is currently practiced by stratifying the most important clinical parameters relating to risk of disease progression. These parameters include grade of the cancer as defined by Gleason, stage, PSA, and DRE. The Gleason grade can range from 1 (well differentiated) to 5 (poorly differentiated), and a score is given as the sum of the two highest grades determined for the specimen. Thus, the Gleason score can range from 2 to 10. Because time at risk in part determines the chance of disease progression, men older than 65 years of age thought to have small-volume disease represent the target group for watchful waiting. Our current practice is to offer watchful waiting to patients with stage T1c disease, who are 65 years or older, whose PSA density is 0.15 ng/mL/g (PSA divided by ultrasound-estimated prostate size) or less, and whose biopsy results are scored as Gleason 6 or less with no more than two cores involved with cancer and less than 50% involvement of any one core.[95] In those situations where watchful waiting is deemed reasonable, yearly surveillance biopsies and twice-yearly DRE and PSA are still performed, and the patient's eligibility for watchful waiting reassessed.

Patients with local but clinically significant disease (i.e., higher-grade or larger-volume disease), on the other hand, require intervention as long as they otherwise have life expectancies of more than 10 years. Age and comorbid disease should be considered together when assessing the need for treatment. The two conventional modes of therapy are radiation and surgery.

Of the radiation-based options, the most commonly used method consists of external beam radiation, typically with a conformal apparatus.[96] Brachytherapy using radioactive implants has been gaining widespread popularity; however, the data regarding outcomes in terms of biochemical progression suggest that brachytherapy fails to control localized prostate cancer, particularly in the palpable disease stage (T2), compared with conventional therapies.[97] However, although many studies purport to compare radiation outcomes with surgical outcomes directly, the data are collected by different methods. After treatment, PSA is the most sensitive indicator of freedom from disease. An undetectable PSA after surgery indicates eradication of cancer. A stable PSA (not rising) of less than 0.5 ng/mL after radiation therapy is thought to be consistent with a disease-free state. The American Society for Therapeutic Radiology and Oncology (ASTRO) definition of treatment failure after external beam radiation is three consecutive PSA rises after the nadir PSA is reached. The median time to a nadir PSA is between 2 and 3 years. Because PSAs are often measured every 6 months, it may take up to 4.5 years before a treatment failure is recognized. This ASTRO definition results in backdating and early censoring of events and artificially improves the biochemical survival rates and is highly biased for favorable outcomes for radiation therapy.[98]

Surgical therapy of local prostate cancer is most commonly performed as an anatomically radical retropubic prostatectomy. This procedure, pioneered by Walsh, has resulted in significantly reduced morbidity in terms of recovery of urinary continence and maintenance of erectile function. Outcomes data from both institutional series (single surgeon)[99] and hospital cancer registries[100] suggest that a radical retropubic prostatectomy can be performed safely, with low morbidity for most men. Outcomes data from the Medicare population[101] suggest that morbidity is higher in older men (Table 115.19).

Perineal prostatectomy offers no apparent advantage with regard to cancer control, continence, or erectile function. Moreover, initial claims of improved pain control and lower

TABLE 115.19 — RESULTS

SURGICAL MORBIDITY OF RADICAL RETROPUBIC PROSTATECTOMY FOR THE JOHNS HOPKINS HOSPITAL (JHH), AMERICAN COLLEGE OF SURGEONS (ACC), AND MEDICARE PATIENT POPULATIONS

Variable	JHH (1982–1988)	ACS (1993)	Medicare (1988–1990)
Age (y)	Mean—59	40% <65	50% >70
Mortality	<1%	<1%	—
Potency (maintenance of preoperative erectile function)	68%	30%	12%
Continence (not requiring any urinary pads)	92%	80%	70%

blood loss no longer appear to be as significant compared with the current method of radical retropubic prostatectomy. Finally, some recent evidence suggests that patients who undergo radical perineal prostatectomy have a significantly elevated risk of fecal incontinence.[102] Our current practice is to offer a radical retropubic prostatectomy to those patients who have the highest likelihood of organ-confined disease with minimized morbidity (i.e., those patients who are most likely to benefit from surgery). The probability of organ-confined disease can be most easily determined by referring to nomograms combining PSA, histologic grade of the cancer, and DRE findings.[103] These tables, when combined with the clinical picture, are extremely useful for patient counseling.

Neoadjuvant therapy with hormonal ablation has been gaining widespread use in both radiation therapy and surgical therapy. Success with conventional external beam conformal radiation may be augmented by pretreatment with hormone-based therapy.[104] In certain cases where surgical therapy has revealed locally advanced disease (T3), as might be manifested by a positive surgical margin but negative lymph node dissection, adjuvant therapy with external beam radiation may also play a role in preventing or delaying biochemical progression and consequently cancer progression. Prospective studies of this type of treatment practice are needed to determine fully the role of adjuvant radiation therapy in margin-positive disease.

The role of neoadjuvant hormonal therapy with surgical treatment remains controversial. Initial results from such trials have revealed a significant decrease in the number of positive surgical margins. The significance of this finding, however, is not clear. No current evidence suggests that such an approach causes any decrease in biochemical progression or survival.

Advanced Disease

Hormonal therapy is the mainstay of palliative treatment for advanced prostate cancer. The discovery that male sex hormones are required to maintain the size and function of the prostate led to the development of treatments designed to interfere with this effect. It is well known that androgen deprivation results in a significant involution of the prostate gland with a particularly marked glandular progression to apoptosis (programmed cell death). Not all of the cells are affected by this process because reconstitution of the hormonal supply results in substantial regrowth. Similarly, prostate cancer regresses secondarily to an apoptotic pathway. Invariably, however, the cancer selects out an androgen-independent or insensitive population, which clonally expands and progresses until death. Thus, hormonal therapy is useful, but not curative. The process of selection and expansion, however, can take as long as 2 or more years and may provide a significant window of cancer regression for the patient. Indeed, for some elderly patients, this type of delay in progression may be sufficient to render their disease clinically insignificant compared with their comorbid diseases.

Current options for hormonal therapy include orchiectomy, LH-releasing hormone (LHRH) agonists, and antiandrogen therapy. Orchiectomy is the most cost-effective method of hormonal ablation, but is often unacceptable to the patient. Alternatives include LHRH agonists, which act by disrupting the normal cyclic pattern of secretion of LHRH, thus leading to insignificant levels of LH in the serum. Because LH is required for testosterone synthesis by the Leydig cells, the result is a castrate level of testosterone synthesis. The current LHRH agonists (e.g., goserelin) can now be administered subcutaneously at 3-month intervals.

Although castration, either by medical or surgical means, leads to a low level of androgen synthesis, it does not completely abolish it. Adrenal synthesis of androgens occurs to a limited degree. As a result, there has been some concern that castration alone is inadequate in obtaining maximal benefit from hormonal ablation. Total androgen ablation is achieved, therefore, by adding an antiandrogen in addition to medical or surgical castration. Antiandrogens act at the peripheral target tissues and block the action of androgens at the level of the androgen receptor. Subsequent analyses, however, of this combined modality have failed to demonstrate any significant benefit.[105]

When LHRH agonists are administered, there is an initial increase in testosterone production followed by a rapid nadir as a result of an initial LH surge. To prevent this temporary surge in testosterone from allowing prostate cancer growth, an antiandrogen typically is added for the first few weeks of therapy. Newer-generation antiandrogens (e.g., bicalutamide, nilutamide) can now be administered by once-daily dosing with little or no significant differences in side effects compared with the older agents, such as flutamide. Thus, although advanced prostate cancer is incurable, many of its symptoms can be palliated with hormonal therapy.

Prostate cancer, unlike most other malignancies, progresses while maintaining a relatively low proliferation rate. It is estimated that only 2% to 3% of prostate cancer cells in a given patient are actively dividing at any given moment. Because most chemotherapeutic agents are directed at rapidly proliferating cells, prostate cancer is relatively resistant to these agents when used as monotherapy. Multiple agents, including suramin, liarozole, paclitaxel, estramustine, and doxorubicin, have shown mild activity over short periods, but a significant survival benefit has not been demonstrated. Combination chemotherapy may have a slightly better activity against prostate cancer. The results, however, are still rather poor and the survival benefit, if any, is limited. Moreover, these agents have yet to demonstrate significant improvements in quality of life. After hormonal therapy has failed, conventional treatment is directed at ameliorating symptoms when possible.

TESTIS CANCER

Although testis cancer is the most common cancer in men between the ages of 15 and 34 years, it is nonetheless a rare tumor, accounting for only approximately 1% of all cancers in American men. The testes start as a pair of undifferentiated intraabdominal organs that become primitive testes around the seventh week of gestation. With time, the testes migrate to a more caudal position and eventually descend out of the abdomen into the scrotum near the time of the completion of gestation. The factors important for testicular descent are complex but include, at a very minimum, hormonal stimulation, neuronal support, and mechanical support. Because the testes are originally retroperitoneal organs, they derive their blood, lymphatic, and nerve supply from the retroperitoneum. The gonadal artery is a direct branch of the aorta, and the lymphatic drainage pattern is directly into the retroperitoneal nodes surrounding the IVC and aorta. Thus, the primary lymphatic drainage of the right testis is to the interaortocaval, precaval, and preaortic lymph nodes. The lymphatic drainage of the left testis is into the paraaortic, preaortic, and interaortocaval nodes.

The factors most commonly associated with an increased risk for development of testis cancer are listed in Table 115.20. Foremost among these risk factors is a history of cryptorchidism. Approximately 15% of men with testis cancer have had a prior history of cryptorchidism, although only 75% of those tumors occurred in the testis that failed to descend. The fact that the cancer formed in the normally descended

TABLE 115.20

RISK FACTORS FOR THE DEVELOPMENT OF TESTICULAR CANCER

Age	
Pediatric	Nonseminomatous tumor (e.g., yolk sac tumors)
Young adults	Seminoma > nonseminomatous tumors
Geriatric	Spermatocytic seminoma, lymphoma
Race (whites at highest risk)	
Cryptorchidism	
Family history	
HIV infection/AIDS (lymphoma)	
Presence of carcinoma *in situ* (e.g., testicular biopsy for infertility)	
Prior history of testicular cancer in contralateral testis	
Occupational risks (nonseminomatous tumors only)	
Miners, oil and gas workers, leather workers, food and beverage processing workers, janitors, and utility workers	

testis with a 25% incidence suggests that cryptorchidism is not the direct cause of testis cancer, but merely a manifestation of some other cause. Many cases of cryptorchidism resolve spontaneously, usually within the first year of life. Subsequent to that, many advocate surgical correction (i.e., orchiopexy) to allow better self-examination and surveillance for a subsequent testis cancer.

Because the testes contain both germ cells and supportive cells (i.e., Sertoli and Leydig cells), tumors derived from the testes can occur from either source. Sex cord stromal tumors (i.e., Sertoli or Leydig cell tumor) are far less common than germ cell tumors and often present with signs of hormonal secretion[106] (e.g., gynecomastia). Germ cell tumors can be broadly categorized as seminoma and nonseminoma. Seminomas are the most common type of testicular tumors, although mixed tumors are common.[107]

Nonseminomatous tumors may secrete certain marker proteins that allow both preoperative and postoperative assessment. Endodermal sinus cancer (i.e., yolk sac tumor) is known to secrete α-fetoprotein (AFP), and choriocarcinoma is known to secrete β-human chorionic gonadotropin (β-HCG). Pure seminoma does not secrete AFP, but may secrete β-HCG in up to 10% of cases. Thus, if these tumor markers are elevated before surgery, they are useful markers to follow after surgery for recurrence or progression. Typically, at least five times the biologic half-life ($t_{1/2}$) should elapse before a postoperative tumor marker is measured, to allow adequate clearance from the body. Because the $t_{1/2}$ for AFP is approximately 5 days, five half-lives corresponds to roughly 1 month. The $t_{1/2}$ of β-HCG is approximately 1 day, so follow-up measurements can be started as early as 1 week after surgery. β-HCG shares a common a subunit with LH and FSH (as well as thyroid-stimulating hormone); thus, elevations in any of these gonadotropins may result in spuriously elevated β-HCG measurements if the assay method used cannot distinguish them adequately. Most currently used commercial laboratories can easily distinguish these different peptide hormones. Historically, however, it is recommended that the other gonadotropins be assessed when a postoperative (β-HCG is slightly elevated.

Diagnosis

Most cases of testis cancer are brought to clinical attention from self-examination. The most common finding is an abnormally enlarged testis or firm nodule. Often, scrotal trauma precedes the diagnosis because it prompts either the patient or his physician to examine the testes. Occasionally, the patient may present with orchialgia, but this is more the exception than the rule. The first step to diagnosis is scrotal ultrasonography, which is very helpful in documenting a testicular mass, particularly when a thorough examination is difficult. Scrotal enlargement may also result from benign processes such as a hydrocele, which can also be easily distinguished by ultrasonography. If there is a suspicion of a testicular mass, then surgical exploration with orchiectomy is indicated. Preoperative evaluation should include CBC, serum tumor markers including lactate dehydrogenase, AFP, and β-HCG, coagulation profile, and chest radiography. Once a pathologic diagnosis is made, then the staging is completed and subsequent treatment recommendations are made.

Treatment

Initial treatment and definitive diagnosis occur contemporaneously by orchiectomy through an inguinal surgical incision. Transscrotal orchiectomy carries the theoretic risk of altering the lymphatic drainage, and is discouraged. Once a definitive diagnosis is made, staging can be completed. Radiographic staging requires a CT scan of the chest, abdomen, and pelvis with oral and intravenous contrast. The criteria for staging are outlined graphically in Fig 115.4.

Seminomas are known to be highly radiosensitive. Thus, patients with stage I or II seminomas are treated with adjuvant radiation therapy to the paraaortic and paracaval areas below the diaphragm, as well as the ipsilateral inguinal and pelvic regions. Higher-stage seminomas require adjuvant chemotherapy with a cisplatin-based regimen.

Nonseminomatous tumors are less radiosensitive and, thus, require either surgical resection or chemotherapy, or both. Stage I tumors (limited to the testes) may be treated by either watchful waiting with close surveillance, limited chemotherapy with close surveillance, or a retroperitoneal lymph node dissection (RPLND). The choice is driven mainly by patient preference, institutional preference, and physician experience. Currently, there is no clear consensus on how to proceed in these patients with limited disease. The advent of laparoscopic retroperitoneal lymphadenectomy has allowed a minimally invasive technique for achieving the same goal (i.e., diagnostic assessment, potential therapeutic resection) with minimal morbidity. When an RPLND is performed (open or laparoscopic), a template dissection is recommended to allow partial preservation of the sympathetic chain and thus allow antegrade postoperative ejaculation. Regardless of which approach is taken, these patients require close follow-up and observation with serum tumor markers and chest radiographs on at least an every-other-month basis for 2 years and periodic CT scans performed with alternate visits.

Small stage II nonseminomatous tumors (<5 cm) are treated initially with RPLND, followed by adjuvant cisplatin-based chemotherapy if cancer is discovered in the final pathologic specimen. Bulky stage II and III nonseminomatous tumors are often treated initially with chemotherapy and then, if a residual retroperitoneal mass is seen on subsequent imaging with normalization of the tumor markers, a postchemotherapy RPLND is performed. If residual cancer is found on the subsequent RPLND, additional chemotherapy is indicated. Because of advances in chemotherapy, metastatic testis cancer is still a treatable disease.[108] Survival rates of greater than 70% are reported for patients with advanced disease and greater than 90% for lower-stage disease. Long-term surveillance is indicated in these patients because remote recurrences as long as 20 years after initial treatment have been described.

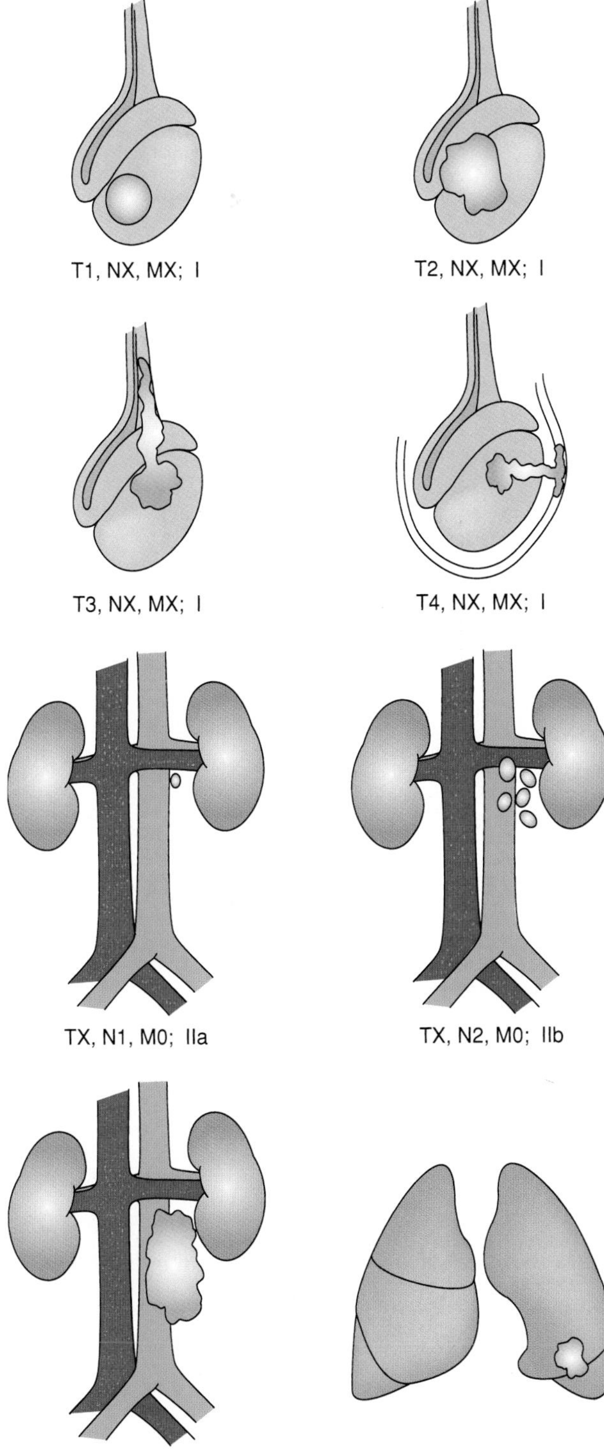

FIGURE 115.4 Staging of testis cancer. Both the tumor necrosis metastasis (TNM; American Joint Committee on Cancer, 1997) and a commonly used descriptive system are shown.

KEY POINTS

- Urinary incontinence most commonly affects women, with a prevalence as high as 10% to 20% of women between 15 and 64 years of age.
- Erectile dysfunction, commonly referred to as *impotence,* is defined as the consistent inability to attain and maintain penile erection sufficient to permit satisfactory sexual intercourse.
- Infertility, defined as the inability to conceive a pregnancy within 1 year of unprotected sexual intercourse, affects approximately 15% of couples in the United States. Male factors are thought to contribute to approximately half of the instances.
- Most kidney stones contain calcium and usually consist of calcium oxalate.
- The most common presentations of nephrolithiasis are pain and hematuria.
- The most common type of urothelial cancer is transitional cell carcinoma, and the most frequent type of renal cancer is a clear cell renal cell carcinoma.
- Prostate cancer is the most common cancer in men and the second most common cause of cancer-related deaths in American men.

References

1. Burnett AL, Wesselmann U. Neurobiology of the pelvis and perineum: principles for a practical approach. *J Pelvic Surg*, 1999;4:224.
2. Chai TC, Steers WD. Neurophysiology of micturition and continence. *Urol Clin North Am.* 1996;23:221.
3. Roehrborn CG, McConnell JD. Etiology, pathophysiology, epidemiology, and natural history of benign prostatic hyperplasia. In: Walsh PC, Retik AB, Vaughan D, et al., eds. *Campbell's urology*, 8th ed. Philadelphia: WB Saunders, 2002, pp. 1297–1336.
4. AUA Guideline on the Management of Benign Prostatic Hyperplasia: Diagnosis and Treatment Recommendations. http://www.auanet.org/timss-net/products/guidelines/main_reports/bph_management/chapt_1_appendix.pdf. 2005. Accessed
5. Collins MM, Stafford RS, O'Leary P, et al. How common is prostatitis? A national survey of physician visits. *J Urol.* 1997;157:243A.
6. Roberts RO, Lieber MM, Bostwick DG, et al. A community-based study on the prevalence of prostatitis. *J Urol.* 1997;157:242A.
7. Hua VN, Schaeffer AJ. Acute and chronic prostatitis. *Med Clin North Am.* 2004;88:483.
8. Miller JL, Rothman I, Bavendam TG, et al. Prostatodynia and interstitial cystitis: one and the same? *Urology* 1995;45:587.
9. Alexander RB, Mann DL, Borkowski AA, etal. Granulomatous prostatitis linked to HLA-DRB1*1501. *J Urol.* 2004;171(6 Pt 1):2326.
10. Nickel JC, Forrest JB, Tomera K etal. Pentosan polysulfate sodium therapy for men with chronic pelvic pain syndrome: a multicenter, randomized placebom controlled study. *J Urol.* 2005;173:1252.
11. Thomas TM, Plymat KR, Blann J, et al. Prevalence of urinary incontinence. *BMJ* 1980;281:1243.
12. Diokno AC, Brock BM, Brown MB, et al. Prevalence of urinary incontinence and other urological symptoms in the noninstitutionalized elderly. *J Urol.* 1986;136:1022.
13. NIH Consensus Conference. Impotence. NIH Consensus Development Panel on Impotence [Review]. *JAMA* 1993;270:83.
14. Johnson AR, Jarow JP. Is routine endocrine testing of impotent men necessary? *J Urol.* 1992;147:1542.
15. Nehra A, Steers WD, Althof SE, etal. Third International Conference on the Management of Erectile Dysfunction: Linking Pathophysiology and Therapeutic Response. *J Urol.* 2003;170(Pt 2):S3.
16. Fallon B. Intracavernous injection therapy for male erectile dysfunction. *Urol Clin North Am.* 1995;22:833.
17. **Padma-Nathan H, Hellstrom WJ, Kaiser FE, et al. Treatment of men with erectile dysfunction with transurethral alprostadil: Medicated Urethral System for Erection (MUSE) Study Group. *N Engl J Med.* 1997; 336:1.**
18. Montague DK, Angermeier KW. Current status of penile prosthesis implantation. *Curr Urol Rep.* 2000;1:291.
19. Goldstein I, Hatzichristou DG, Pescatori ES. Pelvic, perineal, and penile trauma-associated arteriogenic impotence: pathophysiologic mechanisms and the role of microvascular arterial bypass surgery. In: Bennett AH, ed. *Impotence: diagnosis and management of erectile dysfunction.* Philadelphia: WB Saunders, 1994, p. 213.
20. Dean RC, Lue TF. Peyronie's disease: advancements in recent surgical techniques. *Curr Opin Urol.* 2004;14:339.
21. Greenhall E, Vessey M. The prevalence of subfertility: a review of the current confusion and a report of two new studies. *Fertil Steril.* 1990;54:978.
22. Clark JY, Thompson IM, Optenberg SA. Economic impact of urolithiasis in the United States. *J Urol.* 1995;154:2020.
23. Robertson WG. Urinary tract calculi. In: Nordin BEC, Need AG, Morris HA, eds. *Metabolic bone and stone disease.* New York: Churchill Livingstone, 1993.

24. Rotolo JE, O'Brien WM, Pahira JJ. Urinary tract calculi. *Consultant* 1989;29:129.
25. Preminger GM. Cost and time effective outpatient metabolic stone evaluation. *Probl Urol.* 1987;36:181.
26. Sutherland JW, Parks JH, Coe FL. Recurrence after a single renal stone in a community practice. *Miner Electrolyte Metab.* 1985;11:267.
27. Daudon M, Dosimoni R, Hennequin C, et al. Sex and age related composition of 10,617 calculi analyzed by infrared spectroscopy. *Urol Res.* 1995;23:319.
28. Gentle DL, Stoller ML, Jarrett TW, et al. Protease inhibitor-induced urolithiasis. *Urology* 1997;50:508.
29. Press SM, Smith AD. Incidence of negative hematuria in patients with acute urinary lithiasis presenting to the emergency room with flank pain. *Urology* 1995;45:753.
30. Gottlieb RH, La TC, Erturk EN. CT in detecting urinary tract calculi: influence on patient imaging and clinical outcomes. *Radiology* 2002;225:441.
31. Liberman SN, Halpern EJ, Sullivan K, et al. Spiral computed tomography for staghorn calculi. *Urology* 1997;50:519.
32. **Pfister SA, Deckart A, Laschke S, et al. Unenhanced helical computed tomography vs intravenous urography in patients with acute flank pain: accuracy and economic impact in a randomized prospective trial. *Eur Radiol.* 2003 Nov;13(11):2513.**
33. Hill MC, Rich JI, Mardiat JG, et al. Sonography vs. excretory urography in acute flank pain. *AJR Am J Roentgenol.* 1985;144:1235.
34. **Segura JW, Preminger GM, Assimos DG, et al. Ureteral Stones Clinical Guidelines Panel summary report on the management of ureteral calculi. The American Urological Association. *J Urol.* 1997;158: 1915.**
35. Chaussy C, Schmeidt E, Jocham D, et al. First clinical experience with extracorporeally induced destruction of kidney stones by shock waves. *J Urol.* 1982;127:417.
36. Micali S, Moore RG, Averch TD, et al. The role of laparoscopy in the treatment of renal and ureteral calculi. *J Urol.* 1997;157:463.
37. Zafar FS, Lingeman JE. Value of laparoscopy in the management of calculi complicating renal malformations. *J Endourol.* 1996;10:379.
38. Segura JW, Preminger GM, Assimos DG, et al. Nephrolithiasis Clinical Guidelines Panel summary report on the management of staghorn calculi. The American Urological Association Nephrolithiasis Clinical Guidelines Panel. *J Urol.* 1994;151:1648.
39. Grasso M, Loisides P, Beaghler M, et al. The case for primary endoscopic management of upper urinary tract calculi: I. A critical review of 121 extracorporeal shock-wave lithotripsy failures. *Urology* 1995; 45:363.
40. Pak CY. Kidney stones. *Lancet* 1998;351:1797.
41. Young HH, McKay RW. Congenital valvular obstruction of prostatic urethra. *Surg Gynecol Obstet.* 1929;43:435.
42. Goodwin WE, Casey WC, Woolf W. Percutaneous trocar (needle) nephrostomy in hydronephrosis. *JAMA* 1955;157:891.
43. Kelling G. Zur Colioskopie. *Arch Klin Chir.* 1923;126:226.
44. Cortesi N, Ferrari P, Zambardae A, et al. Diagnosis of bilateral abdomen cryptorchidism by laparoscopy. *Endoscopy* 1976;8:33.
45. Wickham JEA. The surgical treatment of renal lithiasis. In: Wickham JEA, ed. *Urinary calculus disease.* New York: Churchill Livingstone, 1979, p. 145.
46. Reddick EJ, Olsen DO. Laparoscopic laser cholecystectomy: a comparison with mini-lap cholecystectomy. *Surg Endosc.* 1989;3:131.
47. McDougall EM, Clayman RV. Laparoscopic nephrectomy for benign disease: comparison of the transperitoneal and retroperitoneal approaches. *J Endourol.* 1996;10:45.
48. Wolf JS, Moon TD, Nakada SY. Hand assisted laparoscopic nephrectomy: a comparison to standard laparoscopic nephrectomy. *J Urol.* 1998; 160:22.
49. Ono Y, Hattori R, Gotoh M, Yoshino Y, et al. Laparoscopic radical nephrectomy for renal cell carcinoma: the standard of care already? *Curr Opin Urol.* 2005;15:75.
50. Jarrett TW, Chan DY, Charambura TC, et al. Laparoscopic pyeloplasty: the first 100 cases. *J Urol.* 2002;167:1253–1256.
51. Winfield HN, Hamilton BD, Bravo EL, et al. Laparoscopic adrenalectomy: the preferred choice? A comparison to open adrenalectomy. *J Urol.* 1998;160:325.
52. Rassweiler J, Fornara P, Weber M, et al. Laparoscopic nephrectomy: the experience of the Laparoscopy Working Group of the German Urologic Association. *J Urol.* 1998;160:18.
53. Trabulsi EJ, Guillonneau B. Laparoscopic radical prostatectomy. *J Urol.* 2005;173(4):1072.
54. **Jemal A, Murray T, Ward E, et al. Cancer statistics, 2005. *CA Cancer J Clin.* 2005;55:10.**
55. Badawi AF. Molecular and genetic events in schistosomiasis-associated human bladder cancer: role of oncogenes and tumor suppressor genes. *Cancer Lett.* 1996;105:123.
56. Strohmeyer T. Urothelial cancers: cytogenetic and molecular biology principles [in German]. *Urologe A.* 1994;33:122.
57. Morrison AS. Epidemiology and environmental factors in urologic cancer. *Cancer* 1987;60:632.
58. Lubbe L, Nowack R, May M, et al. FISH—a new noninvasive method for the diagnosis of urinary bladder carcinomas. *Clin Lab.* 2004; 50:395.
59. Grossman HB, Messing E, Soloway M, et al. Detection of bladder cancer using a point-of-care proteomic assay. *JAMA* 2005;293:810.
60. Sarosdy MF. Principles of intravesical chemotherapy and immunotherapy. *Urol Clin North Am.* 1992;19:509.
61. de Reijke TM, Kurth KH, Sylvester RJ, et al. Bacillus Calmette-Guerin versus epirubicin for primary, secondary or concurrent carcinoma in situ of the bladder: results of a European Organization for the Research and Treatment of Cancer—Genito-Urinary Group Phase III Trial (30906). *J Urol.* 2005;173:405.
62. O'Donnell MA, Lilli K, Leopold C, et al.. Interim results from a national multicenter phase II trial of combination bacillus Calmette-Guerin plus interferon alfa-2b for superficial bladder cancer. *J Urol.* 2004; 172:888.
63. Herr HW, Bajorin DF, Scher HI. Neoadjuvant chemotherapy and bladder-sparing surgery for invasive bladder cancer: ten-year outcome. *J Clin Oncol.* 1998;16:1298.
64. Mills RD, Studer UE. Metabolic consequences of continent urinary diversion. *J Urol.* 1999;161:1057.
65. Eisenberger CF, Schoenberg M, Fitter D, et al. Orthotopic ileocolic neobladder reconstruction following radical cystectomy: history, technique, and results of the Johns Hopkins experience, 1986–1998. *Urol Clin North Am.* 1999;26:149, ix.
66. Bricker EM. Pelvic exenteration. *Adv Surg.* 1970;4:13.
67. Levallois M, Granier B. Bricker's operation: simplified technic [in French]. *J Urol Nephrol (Paris)* 1968;74:287.
68. Mead GM, Roberts JT. The role of the nonsurgical oncologist in the management of advanced transitional cell cancer. Part I: Locally advanced disease. *BJU Int.* 2004;94:977.
69. Gelb AB. Renal cell carcinoma: current prognostic factors. Union Internationale Contre le Cancer (UICC) and the American Joint Committee on Cancer (AJCC). *Cancer* 1997;80:981.
70. Motzer RJ, Bacik J, Schwartz LH, Reuter V, et al. Prognostic factors for survival in previously treated patients with metastatic renal cell carcinoma. *J Clin Oncol.* 2004;22:454.
71. Godley PA, Stinchcombe TE. Renal cell carcinoma. *Curr Opin Oncol.* 1999;11:213.
72. Wagner JR, Linehan WM. Molecular genetics of renal cell carcinoma. *Semin Urol Oncol.* 1996;14:244.
73. Gnarra JR, Glenn GM, Latif F, et al. Molecular genetic studies of sporadic and familial renal cell carcinoma. *Urol Clin North Am.* 1993;20:207.
74. Sampson JR. The kidney in tuberous sclerosis: manifestations and molecular genetic mechanisms. *Nephrol Dial Transplant.* 1996;11(suppl 6):34.
75. Fleming S. Genetics of kidney tumours. *Forum (Genova)* 1998;8:176.
76. Avery RA, Harris JE, Davis CJ Jr, et al. Renal medullary carcinoma: clinical and therapeutic aspects of a newly described tumor. *Cancer* 1996;78:128.
77. Rodriguez R, Fishman EK, Marshall FF. Differential diagnosis and evaluation of the incidentally discovered renal mass. *Semin Urol Oncol.* 1995;13:246.
78. Mattos RM, Libertino JA. Survival of patients with renal cell carcinoma invading the inferior vena cava. *Semin Urol Oncol.* 1996;14:223.
79. Bosniak MA. The current radiological approach to renal cysts. *Radiology* 1986;158:1.
80. Robson CJ. Radical nephrectomy for renal cell carcinoma. *J Urol.* 1963;89:37.
81. Bono AV, Lovisolo JA. Renal cell carcinoma—diagnosis and treatment: state of the art. *Eur Urol.*997;31[suppl 1]:47.
82. Novick AC. Nephron-sparing surgery for renal cell carcinoma. *Br J Urol* 1998;82:321.
83. Ankem MK, Nakada SY.. Needle-ablative nephron-sparing surgery. *BJU Int.* 2005;95[suppl 2]:46.
84. Figlin RA. Renal cell carcinoma: management of advanced disease. *J Urol.* 1999;161:381; discussion, 386.
85. Linehan WM, Walther MM, Alexander RB, et al. Adoptive immunotherapy of renal cell carcinoma: studies from the Surgery Branch, National Cancer Institute. *Semin Urol.* 1993;11:41.
86. Mettlin CJ, Murphy GP, Rosenthal DS, et al. The National Cancer Data Base report on prostate carcinoma after the peak in incidence rates in the U.S. The American College of Surgeons Commission on Cancer and the American Cancer Society. *Cancer* 1998;83:1679.
87. **Cooperberg MR, Park S, Carroll PR. Prostate cancer 2004: insights from national disease registries. *Oncology (Huntingt).* 2004;18:1239; discussion 1248.**
88. Partin AW, Carter HB, Chan DW, et al. Prostate specific antigen in the staging of localized prostate cancer: influence of tumor differentiation, tumor volume, and benign hyperplasia. *J Urol.* 1990;143:747.
89. Partin AW, Catalona WJ, Southwick PC, et al. Analysis of percent free prostate-specific antigen (PSA) for prostate cancer detection: influence of total PSA, prostate volume, and age. *Urology* 1996;48:55.
90. Han M, Walsh PC, Partin AW, et al. Ability of the 1992 and 1997 American Joint Committee on Cancer staging systems for prostate cancer to predict progression-free survival after radical prostatectomy for stage T2 disease. *J Urol.* 2000;164:89.

91. Collins MM, Barry MJ. Controversies in prostate cancer screening: analogies to the early lung cancer screening debate [see comments]. *JAMA* 1996;276:1976.
92. Farkas A, Schneider D, Perrotti M, et al. National trends in the epidemiology of prostate cancer, 1973 to 1994: evidence for the effectiveness of prostate-specific antigen screening. *Urology* 1998;52:444; discussion, 448.
93. Feightner JW. The early detection and treatment of prostate cancer: the perspective of the Canadian Task Force on the Periodic Health Examination [see comments] [Review]. *J Urol.* 1994;152:1682.
94. Stephenson RA, Stanford JL. Population-based prostate cancer trends in the United States: patterns of change in the era of prostate-specific antigen. *World J Urol.* 1997;15:331.
95. Allaf ME, Carter HB.. Update on watchful waiting for prostate cancer. *Curr Opin Urol.* 2004;14:171.
96. Nilsson S, Norlen BJ, Widmark A.. A systematic overview of radiation therapy effects in prostate cancer. *Acta Oncol.* 2004;43:316.
97. D'Amico AV, Whittington R, Malkowicz SB, et al. Biochemical outcome after radical prostatectomy, external beam radiation therapy, or interstitial radiation therapy for clinically localized prostate cancer [see comments]. *JAMA* 1998;280:969.
98. Gretzer MB, Trock BJ, Han M, et al. A critical analysis of the interpretation of biochemical failure in surgically treated patients using the American Society for Therapeutic Radiation and Oncollogy criteria. *J Urol.* 2002;168(4 Pt 1):1419.
99. Walsh PC, Partin AW, Epstein JI. Cancer control and quality of life following anatomical radical retropubic prostatectomy: results at 10 years [see comments]. *J Urol.* 1994;152:1831.
100. Mettlin CJ, Murphy GP, Sylvester J, et al. Results of hospital cancer registry surveys by the American College of Surgeons: outcomes of prostate cancer treatment by radical prostatectomy. *Cancer* 1997;80: 1875.
101. Fowler FJ Jr, Barry MJ, Lu-Yao G, et al. Patient-reported complications and follow-up treatment after radical prostatectomy. The National Medicare Experience: 1988–1990 (updated June 1993). *Urology* 1993; 42:622.
102. Bishoff JT, Motley G, Optenberg SA, et al. Incidence of fecal and urinary incontinence following radical perineal and retropubic prostatectomy in a national population. *J Urol.* 1998;160:454.
103. Partin AW, Mangold LA, Lamm DM, et al. Contemporary update of prostate cancer staging nomograms (Partin Tables) for the new millennium. *Urology* 2001;58:843.
104. D'Amico AV, Manola J, Loffredo M. 6-month androgen suppression plus radiation therapy vs radiation therapy alone for patients with clinically localized prostate cancer: a randomized controlled trial. *JAMA* 2004;292(7):821.
105. Eisenberger MA, Blumenstein BA, Crawford ED, et al. Bilateral orchiectomy with or without flutamide for metastatic prostate cancer. *N Engl J Med.* 1998;339:1036.
106. Cortez JC, Kaplan GW. Gonadal stromal tumors, gonadoblastomas, epidermoid cysts, and secondary tumors of the testis in children. *Urol Clin North Am.* 1993;20:15.
107. Levin HS. Prognostic features of primary and metastatic testis germ-cell tumors. *Urol Clin North Am.* 1993;20:39.
108. **Einhorn EH. Testicular cancer: an oncological success story. *Clin Cancer Res.* 1997;3:2630.**

CHAPTER 116 ■ FEMALE GENITOURINARY ANATOMY AND PHYSIOLOGY

ROBERT L. GIUNTOLI II, GEOFFREY CUNDIFF, AND ROBERT E. BRISTOW

It is appropriate that surgeons at The Johns Hopkins Hospital author a surgical treatise addressing the female pelvis. American gynecologic pelvic surgery had its inception and subsequent codification at this institution under Howard Kelly, Richard Telinde, Cullen Richards, Howard Jones, Jr., and numerous others. Many of the landmark advances in gynecologic surgical management originated at the facility, which was the legacy of a Quaker bachelor grocer.

Our presentation of gynecologic disease processes focuses on diseases that are commonly, if not predominantly, treated surgically. For each of the entities discussed, we cursorily summarize the pertinent nonsurgical options and highlight those realities that led to surgical therapy being the preferred treatment modality. This chapter is structured in a specific format in which each anatomic site is individually addressed. Pathologic processes are catalogued under congenital, infectious, traumatic, and neoplastic diseases. The latter topic encompasses both malignant and nonmalignant processes.

SURGICAL ANATOMY

This section does not provide a meticulous review of the pelvic anatomy because there are numerous, excellent atlases that can refresh the memory of the pelvic surgeon. We do, however, focus on those details of pelvic anatomy that are necessary for the surgeon to know to perform the full array of complex procedures.

Pelvic Compartments and Spaces

The female pelvis is usually envisioned as having three compartments and eight potential spaces. The compartments are self-evident, but often forgotten by the neophyte pelvic surgeon when defining sources of disease, rational surgical techniques, and sources of comorbidity.

Compartments

Traditionally, the female pelvis is divided into three functional compartments: the anterior compartment (distal ureters, bladder, and urethra), the middle compartment (ovaries, fallopian tubes, uterine corpus and cervix, vagina, and perineum), and the posterior compartment (distal sigmoid colon, rectum, and anus; Fig. 116.1). Although the pelvic organs can be divided into these compartments, a rigid separation is fallacious because all three compartments are integrally intertwined in function, vascular and lymphatic supply and drainage, enervation, and support.

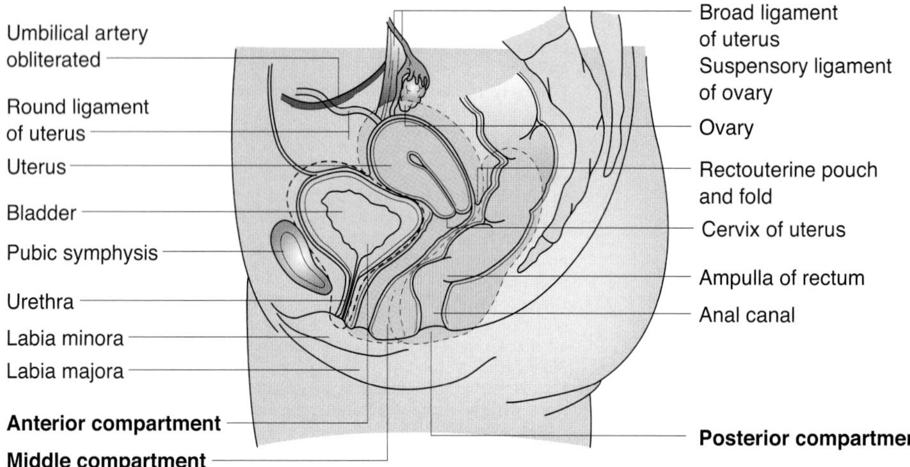

FIGURE 116.1 The three pelvic compartments: lateral view.

Spaces

Knowledge of the eight major pelvic spaces (Fig. 116.2) is of great value not only in performing pelvic surgery but also in effectively managing intraoperative misadventures. In a ventral-dorsal sequence, the spaces are the retropubic space (space of Retzius), the vesicovaginal space, the rectovaginal septum, and the retrorectal (presacral) space. Lateral to these midline spaces are the paravesical and pararectal spaces. It is evident that these spaces are potential, being coapted in the natural state; devoid of major vascular or visceral structures, although these structures encompass the spaces; and valuable for defining pelvic anatomy in those settings where anatomic anomalies exist.

In addition to the eight pelvic spaces, we have found two other compartments to be of great value while performing ureteral dissection or lysis. These are the space of Morrow and the tunnel of Wertheim (Fig. 116.3). Using these spaces as routes of dissection facilitates complete ureteral lysis throughout the pelvis without necessitating entrance into the ureteral sheath with associated devascularization.

Blood Supply

The rich, highly collateral blood supply in the pelvis is the proverbial double-edged sword: it facilitates healing and return of function to remaining pelvic organs after extensive dissection, but can do so at a high intraoperative cost in blood loss. Our experience has confirmed what the great Italian anatomists noted 5 centuries ago: the pelvic blood supply is remarkably consistent and predictable, with minimal interpatient variation. Numerous anatomic texts offer excellent reviews of the pelvic blood supply.

Ureteral Course

Gynecologic pelvic surgery is the most common source of an iatrogenic ureteral injury. This phenomenon is the end result of the numerous inflammatory and neoplastic diseases that occur in the pelvis and cause the ureter to adhere to surrounding structures from which it is developmentally free, or deviate

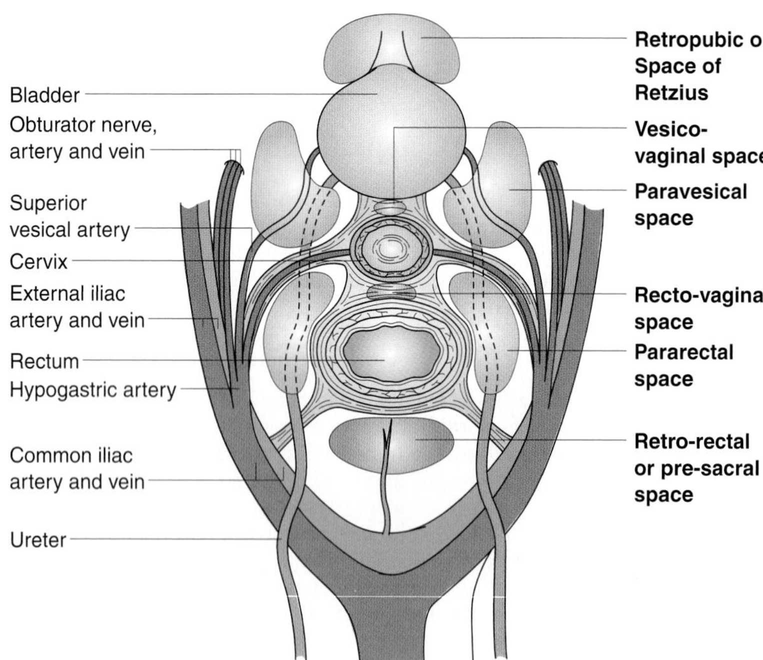

FIGURE 116.2 The eight pelvic spaces: transverse view.

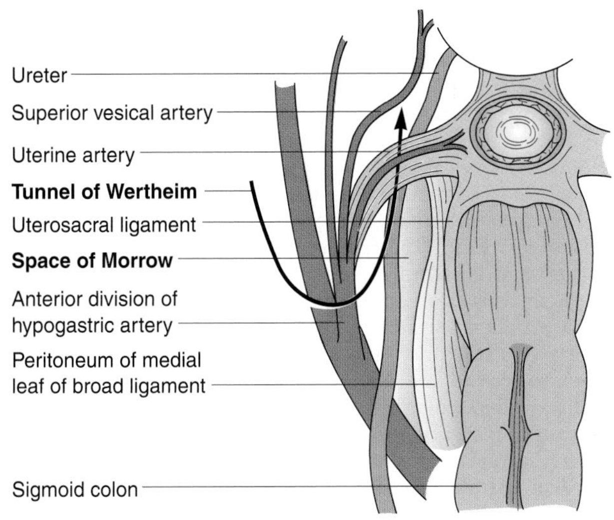

FIGURE 116.3 The space of Morrow and the tunnel of Wertheim.

from its anticipated course. At the time of gynecologic surgery, ureteral injury occurs most commonly at three locations: first as the ureter enters the pelvis under the infundibulopelvic ligament and on top of the bifurcation of the common iliac artery, second as the ureter runs under the uterine artery as that vessel supplies the uterus, and third as the ureter enters the bladder wall.

PHYSIOLOGY

Reproductive physiology is a complex discipline about which entire textbooks have been written. However, an essential understanding of the anatomic changes that occur in parallel with the reproductive physiologic changes associated with menarche, menopause, and the gravid state, as well as with the "normal" and "dysfunctional" estrus cycle, must be possessed by the pelvic surgeon. Before menarche, the ovary is a small, almond-shaped structure. As the ovary becomes more biologically active (Fig. 116.4), it doubles or triples in size. Subsequently, with the onset of the climacteric, the ovary returns to its premenarche size, although it is more fibrotic and has surface irregularities. The latter findings may appear aberrant to the naive pelvic surgeon and should be appreciated as normal end results of years of ovulation. The changes that occur during the menstrual cycle mimic, to a significant degree, those that occur during a woman's reproductive life. The dominant follicle measures approximately 2.5 cm immediately before ovulation at day 14 of the idealized 28-day cycle. Superimposing this normal follicle onto a 2 × 2 × 3 cm ovary makes it easy to appreciate why there are numerous adnexal "masses" identified when pelvic examinations are performed in the mid-cycle. Postovulation, with the development of the corpus luteum, there may be a persistent adnexal mass. Failure to appreciate the normality of these physiologic changes leads to unnecessary imaging and surgical intervention.

Just as there are changes in the size of the ovary that reflect its role as a source of sex steroids and oocytes, a parallel change occurs in the other reproductive structures that reflects hormonal effect on the gravid uterus. In general, the female reproductive tract organs demonstrate shrinkage, fibrosis, and epithelial thinning when estrogenic stimulation is removed, with the opposite effects occurring after stimulation. The greater the estrogen stimulation, the more physiologic engorgement occurs. This axiom is taken to its extreme during pregnancy, when the circulating levels of endogenous estrogen are the highest that occur in a nonpathologic state. Last, the growing gravid uterus can represent a "pelvic mass." As the embryo and subsequent fetus grows and pregnancy-associated physiologic changes occur, the uterus rises out of the pelvis, displacing those other pelvic organs that are freely mobile and compressing those that are not. Important general rules of reference are that a uterus with a 12-week gestation reaches the pelvic brim, a 20-week gestation the umbilicus, and a 40-week full-term gestation the xiphoid process.

VULVA

Congenital

Labial Fusion

Labial fusion in association with a nonperforate hymen is the end results of abnormalities of müllerian duct fusion and junction between the perineal plate and the developing vagina. To understand fully this continuum of congenital abnormalities, it is essential to remember that the normal female genital tract is the end result of midline fusion of the müllerian ducts and their attachment to and subsequent fenestration of the perineal plate. In the most extreme degrees of midline nonfusion, a complete duplication of the vagina, cervix, and uterine corpus occurs. Depending on the extremity of nonfusion, there

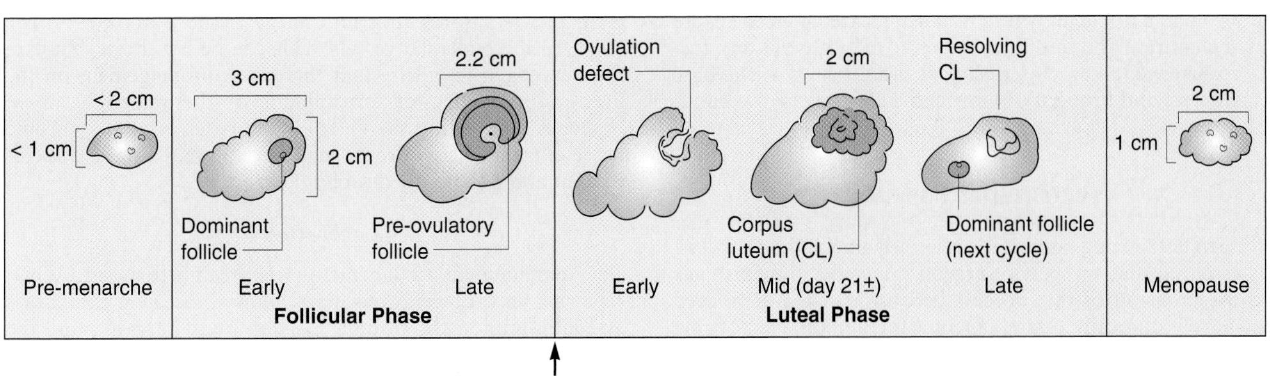

FIGURE 116.4 Physiologic structural changes in the ovary during reproductive life.

may be as much as a 60% chance of an associated congenital abnormality in the kidneys, ureters, or bladder.

Labial fusion may be a congenital or acquired abnormality, with the latter the result of some degree of inflammation caused by trauma, radiation, or menopause. In almost all cases, a combination of local estrogenic creams (1 g applied locally on a daily basis for 6 weeks, followed by the same dosage administered two to three times a week) improves epithelial integrity and strength and decreases inflammation. Thereafter, surgical separation with either reapproximation of the vulvar epithelium to the vagina or, in the most severe cases, placement of a split-thickness skin graft, is necessary to minimize risk of recurrence.

Inguinal Hernias and Patent Canals of Nuck

Inguinal hernias, the end result of trauma on a congenitally deficient support system, are not reviewed here. A condition that can lead to a diagnostic dilemma (the patent canal of Nuck), however, must be remembered. The round ligaments decussate in the labia majora, running through the canal of Nuck. If this canal maintains patency, collections of peritoneal fluid, direct hernias, or even inclusionlike cysts can develop. The latter can present as masses on the labia majora that have a tendency to enlarge with time and may worsen during the luteal phase. The diagnosis is verified if there is enlargement of the mass and increased associated symptoms with the patient in the upright position. Resection of any masses and ligation of the canal of Nuck, through a transvulvar approach, are the preferred surgical modalities.

Infectious

The vulva may present with all of the infectious processes that are found on the other cutaneous surfaces. Uniquely, vulvar infections can develop in the major (Bartholin's) and minor vestibular glands. These are usually a result of sexually transmitted organisms (predominantly gonorrhea). An end result of these infections is occlusion of the draining ducts. This obstruction can lead to a distention of the proximal gland duct. This loculation of effluxing fluid may be sterile or have a superimposed infection (Bartholin's duct abscess). Initial therapy is always antimicrobial [1] and antiinflammatory (e.g., medicinal and topical using sitz baths). Commonly, there is a degree of scarring and fibrosis that makes the condition recalcitrant to conservative therapy, and surgical intervention then becomes warranted. Surgical management options include drainage or marsupialization versus excision. Marsupialization is effective in 65% to 85% of cases. Complete resection of the affected gland and duct is performed in those instances where marsupialization has been repeatedly tried and failed. When resection is undertaken, it is preferable that the surgery be completed in a not acutely inflamed state, care taken to ensure that the entire gland and duct are removed to avoid any further recurrence, and a closed suction drain be left at the base of the defect and brought out through a separate stab wound.

Necrotizing Fasciitis

Although necrotizing fasciitis is a relatively uncommon process, it is essential that the pelvic surgeon remember the existence and presentation of this process because if it is not treated aggressively surgically, a fatal outcome is common. Necrotizing fasciitis, which most commonly occurs in women with the comorbidities of diabetes mellitus or atherosclerosis (70%), is also more common in people taking long-term nonsteroidal antiinflammatory drugs or glucocorticoids, or with underlying immune disease. Usually this infectious process is caused by *Streptococcus pyogenes* (group A *Streptococcus*) with or without *Staphylococcus aureus*, or it can be of polymicrobial cause as a result of anaerobic and facultative aerobic bacteria. Most frequently, necrotizing fasciitis starts as a relatively insignificant infection in a hair follicle, pilonidal cyst, vestibular gland or duct, or surgical site (episiotomy or vulvar resection). The clinical findings that require the surgeon to proceed to adequate surgical resection are those of necrosis (which may in the early stages simply be represented by a purple-blue discoloration) and anesthesia at the site. Once the disease is diagnosed, therapy is a combination of systemic support (fluids, blood products), systemic antibiotics, and radical excision. Radicality of the dissection must be emphasized because hesitation to extend the dissection until reaching a margin of healthy, well-vascularized, and vigorously bleeding tissue with oxygenated (i.e., bright red) blood at best leads to the need for repeated surgical excision. Histologic confirmation of the disease demonstrates vascular occlusion and thrombosis, intense leukocyte infiltration, and necrosis.

Traumatic

Trauma has a "field effect" and depending on the source of the insult, may include the vulva, perineum, vagina, anus, rectum, distal sigmoid colon, urethra, bladder, distal ureters, and even the cervix, if the injury was sexual assault with a rigid instrument. Fistulae are discussed in the section on vaginal diseases and abnormalities, whereas abnormalities of support are presented under cervical diseases.

Hematomas

Hematomas are most commonly the result of blunt trauma to the pudendal vessels or their terminal branches secondary to a straddle injury (e.g., bicycle seat, gym bar, horse back riding). In women who are on anticoagulant medications, however, what would be considered an insignificant degree of trauma can be sufficient to induce a significant hematoma. The overriding dictum when managing hematomas is to support the patient and avoid attempts at evacuation and vessel ligation unless the patient is hemodynamically unstable or symptomatically uncontrolled. Local care with hot sitz baths and concomitant narcotic analgesics is frequently all that is needed. Prophylactic antibiotics, particularly for women at increased risk for development of necrotizing fasciitis, are of theoretic, if not proved, benefit. In cases of inability to void, anterior or periurethral hematomas may necessitate urethral catheterization (which should be left *in situ* for 72 hours). In some cases, surgical intervention is necessary. Any attempt at drainage is best undertaken in the operating theater. It is common for no specific bleeding site to be identified and, therefore, the surgeon places sutures that take large tissue purchases in the locale of the pudendal vessels. This can be beneficial, but care must be taken to ensure that there is no impingement on the urethra or ureters or entrapment of the pudendal nerve branches innervating the vulva. If the latter occurs, a chronic nerve entrapment syndrome may develop that can be difficult to treat and potentially disabling.

Lacerations

The management of lacerations is straightforward. When repairing vulvar lacerations, particularly those near the clitoris and labia minor, the trauma surgeon must keep in mind the critical role that body image plays in sexual function. The patient should be taken to the operating room, adequately anesthetized, and have the microarchitecture reestablished with the same degree of care that would be taken when repairing a

TABLE 116.1 TREATMENT

UNIQUE FEATURES OF THE MANAGEMENT OF PERIPARTUM LACERATIONS

- Lacerations are usually multifocal. Therefore, a thorough inspection of the entire lower pelvis is essential to guarantee that no unappreciated injuries that may be the source of delayed morbidity are present.
- The site of the laceration is contaminated with bacteria. Copious lavage and appropriate antibiotic prophylaxis are valuable in minimizing subsequent wound breakdown and infection.
- Repair must focus on a complete, layered reapproximation of all the disrupted tissue planes and structures to minimize the chance of a subsequent functional or supporting abnormality. It is essential to assess and repair any injury to the rectal mucosa, anal sphincter, transverse perineal muscles, the levator ani, and the overlying epithelium and subepithelial connecting tissue.

TABLE 116.2

ESTIMATED NEW CANCER CASES, UNITED STATES, 2000

Uterine corpus	36,100
Ovary	23,100
Uterine cervix	12,800
Vulva	3,400
Vagina and others	2,100

(From Greenlee RT, Murray T, Bolden S, et al. Cancer statistics, 2000. *CA Cancer J Clin.* 2000;50:7–33, with permission).

facial laceration in a young woman. Butterfly bandages and similar nonsuture techniques are rarely useful in vulvar lacerations because of their three-dimensional nature and the constant moistness and motion that is present.

Peripartum. Perineal lacerations and episiotomies are classified based on their extent and depth. First-degree lacerations or episiotomies affect only the vulvar and vaginal cutaneous dermis. Second-degree lacerations or episiotomies extend into the subdermal tissue. Third-degree lacerations or episiotomies extend into (partial) or through (complete) the rectal sphincter, and fourth-degree lacerations (episioproctotomies) extend into the anorectal lumen. A few features unique to the management of peripartum lacerations to the vulva, perineum, anus, rectum, and vagina are listed in Table 116.1.

Neoplastic

Vulvar Intraepithelial Neoplasia

Vulvar intraepithelial neoplasia (VIN), as with all of the preinvasive squamous lesions of the lower genital tract, is graded based on the degree of abnormal (dysplastic) cells involving the epithelium: VIN I, 33%; VIN II, 33% to 66%; and VIN III, greater than 66%.[2] There is a natural continuum of degrees of dysplasia. Only approximately 30% of the lesser-grade lesions develop into full-thickness dysplasia, however, and of those that do, probably only 5% ever become invasive lesions. In younger women, VIN is usually associated with human papillomavirus (HPV) infection most commonly type 18. Whereas in older women, especially those with comorbidities (e.g., diabetes mellitus, chronic steroid use), VIN usually results from chronic inflammation.[3,4]

Typically, VIN is associated with nonspecific presenting symptoms, predominantly pruritus but also bleeding, a palpable lesion, and discharge. Similarly, the appearance of VIN is highly variable, with raised lesions of variable coloration (pink, white, gray, red, melanotic) predominating. The diagnosis of VIN is made by biopsy of an evident lesion in a patient at risk. VIN has a tendency to be multicentric as well as part of a multifocal disease entity affecting the vagina and cervix as well. Therefore, evaluation must include, as a minimum, cytologic screening of the cervix and, preferably, microscopic (colposcopic) surveillance. Numerous therapeutic regimens have been used to treat VIN. We prefer excisional biopsy for small lesions that are not located where there could be a potential negative functional or cosmetic outcome. Larger lesions or those not treated with wide excision are best treated with a combination of numerous colposcopically directed biopsies and laser vaporization to a depth of the third dermal layer. Depending on the extent of the lesion and the degree of keratinization, initial therapy may be as much as 90% effective at eliminating all disease, although persistence and recurrence rates in the range of 30% to 40% are probably more accurate. There is a subset of patients for whom a skinning vulvectomy with split-thickness skin graft is the preferred therapy.

Vulvar Cancer

Vulvar cancer is a relatively uncommon gynecologic cancer [5] (Table 116.2), predominantly affecting women in their seventh and eighth decades of life. Risk factors and presenting symptoms for vulvar cancer are the same as those for VIN. Reflecting insufficient vigilance for possibility of vulvar cancer, the average woman at time of diagnosis of her vulvar cancer has been evaluated by three antecedent physicians for the same symptom complex without a diagnostic biopsy being performed.

As with all gynecologic malignancies, therapy of vulvar cancer is predicated on the stage, with the classification set forth by the Federation Internationale de Gynecologie et d'Obstetrique (FIGO) being most widely used (Table 116.3). The current standard includes adequate local radical resection of the primary lesion and removal of at-risk lymph nodes.[6] The principle of radical local excision is to remove the primary lesion and a 2-cm margin in all three planes. Lesions for which this cannot be accomplished without loss of function (near the clitoris, urethral sphincter, or anal sphincter) are best treated with local radiation after directed node sampling. For lesions that have more than a 1-mm depth of invasion (a finding that may not be determined until after the radical local excision is performed), a directed node sampling is indicated. This includes unilateral superficial (above the fossa ovalis) groin node dissections with the femoral artery serving as the lateral margin if the lesion is well lateralized (≥2 cm), or bilateral if not. Deep groin and pelvic dissections should be performed only in a setting of grossly positive superficial groin nodes. Grossly positive nodes are best resected because they have been demonstrated to be radioresistant. There are limited but encouraging data regarding sentinel node sampling in women with vulvar cancer.[7] This technique has yet to be proved beneficial in a large, heterogeneous patient population. Once the vulvar lesion is resected, it is essential to ensure that the surgical defect is repaired or covered, using tension-free, well-vascularized tissue. Because of the significant consequences of a poorly healing vulvar wound, we have a very low

TABLE 116.3 STAGING

STAGING OF GYNECOLOGIC CANCER AS RECOMMENDED BY THE INTERNATIONAL FEDERATION OF GYNECOLOGY AND OBSTETRICS

Stage	Description
VULVAR CANCER	
0	
Tis	Carcinoma *in situ*; intraepithelial carcinoma
I	
T1, N0, M0	Tumor confined to vulva or perineum, 2 cm or less in greatest dimension. No nodal metastasis
II	
T2 N0, M0	Tumor confined to vulva or perineum, more than 2 cm in greatest dimension. No nodal metastasis
III	
T3, N0, M0	Tumor of any size with:
T3, N1, M0	(1) Adjacent spread to lower urethra, vagina, anus, or
T1, N1, M0	(2) Unilateral regional lymph node metastasis
T2, N1, M0	
IVA	
T1, N2, M0	Tumor invades any of the following:
T2, N2, M0	Upper urethra, bladder mucosa, rectal mucosa, pelvic bone, or bilateral regional node metastasis
T3, N2, M0	
T4, any N, M0	
IVB	
Any T, any N, M1	Any distant metastasis including pelvic lymph nodes
Note	
N (regional lymph nodes)	
N0	No lymph node metastasis
N1	Unilateral regional lymph node metastasis
N2	Bilateral regional lymph node metastasis
M (distant metastasis)	
M0	No clinical metastasis
M1	Distant metastasis (including pelvic lymph node metastasis)
VAGINAL CANCER	
0	Carcinoma *in situ*; intraepithelial
carcinoma	
I	Carcinoma limited to vaginal mucosa
II	Carcinoma involving subvaginal tissue but not onto pelvic wall
III	Carcinoma onto pelvic wall or pubic symphysis
IV	Carcinoma beyond true pelvis; involvement of bladder or rectal mucosa
CERVICAL CANCER	
0	Carcinoma *in situ*; intraepithelial carcinoma
I	Carcinoma confined to cervic
IA	Preclinical carcinoma; diagnosed microscopically
IA1	Minimal microscopic evidence of stromal invasion
IA2	Microscopic invasion from base of epithelium of 5 mm or less and lateral spread of 7 mm or less
IB	Lesions of greater dimensions than stage IA2
II	Carcinoma beyond cervix but not to pelvic wall. Cancer involves vagina but not lower third
IIA	Obvious parametrial involvement
IIB	Obvious parametrial involvement
III	Carcinoma to pelvic wall. No cancer-free space between tumor and pelvic wall. Tumor involves lower third of vagina. Hydronephrosis or nonfunctioning kidney not due to another cause
IIIA	No extension to pelvic wall
IIIB	Extension to pelvic wall or hyronephrosis of nonfunctioning kidney
IV	Carcinoma beyond true pelvis or involving mucosa of bladder or rectum
IVA	Spread to adjacent organs
IVB	Spread to distant organs
UTERINE CORPUS CANCER	
IA	Tumor limited to endometrium
G123	
IB	Invasion to less than half the myometrium
G123	
IC	Invasion to more than half the myometrium
G123	
IIA	Endocervical glandular involvement only
G123	
IIB	Cervical stromal invasion
G123	
IIIA	Tumor invades serosa or adnexa, or presence of positive peritoneal cytology
G123	
IIIB	Vaginal metastases
G123	
IIIC	Metastases to pelvic or paraaortic lymph nodes
G123	
IVA	Tumor invasion of bladder or bowel mucosa
G123	
IVB	Distant metastases including intraabdominal or inguinal lymph nodes
Note:	
G1	5% or less of a nonsquamous or nonmorular solid growth pattern
G2	6%–50% of a nonsquamous or nonmorular solid growth pattern
G3	More than 50% of a nonsquamous or nonmorular solid growth pattern
OVARIAN CANCER	
I	Growth limited to ovaries
IA	One ovary; no tumor on external surfaces; capsule intact; no ascites present containing malignant cells
IB	Both ovaries; no tumor on external sufaces; capsules intact; no ascites present containing malignant cells

TABLE 116.3 (CONTINUED) STAGING

STAGING OF GYNECOLOGIC CANCER AS RECOMMENDED BY THE INTERNATIONAL FEDERATION OF GYNECOLOGY AND OBSTETRICS

Stage	Description	Stage	Description
IC	IA or IB but with tumor on surface of one or both ovaries; or with capsule ruptured; or with ascites containing malignant cells or with positive peritoneal washings	IIIA	Tumor limited to true pelvis with negative nodes but with histologically confirmed seeding of peritoneal surfaces
II	Growth involving one or both ovaries with pelvic extension	IIIB	Tumor limited to one or both ovaries with histologically confirmed implants of peritoneal surfaces, none greater than 2 cm in diameter; nodes negative
IIA	Extension or metastases to uterus or fallopian tubes	IIIC	Abdominal implants greater than 2 cm in diameter or positive retroperitoneal or inguinal nodes
IIB	Extension to other pelvic tissues		
IIC	IIA or IIB but with tumor on surface of one or both ovaries; or with capules ruptured; or with ascites containing malignant cells or with positive peritoneal washings	IV	Growth involving one or both ovaries with distant metastasis; pleural effusion with positive with positive cytology; parenchymal liver metastasis
III	Tumor involving one or both ovaries with peritoneal implants outside pelvis or positive retroperitoneal or inguinal nodes; superficial liver metastases; tumor limited to pelvis but with histologically verified malignant extension to small bowel or omentum		
		INVASIVE GESTATIONAL TROPHOBLASTIC NEOPLASIS	
		I	Tumor confined to uterine corpus
		II	Tumor to adnexa but limited to genital structures
		III	Tumor to lungs with or without genital involvement
		IV	Metastasis to other sites

threshold for undertaking plastic reconstruction of the vulvar defect. Our preference is to perform vascular pedicle grafts such as vertical rectus abdominis muscle (VRAM) or island flaps using surrounding tissue. If radiation therapy is chosen as part of the therapeutic armamentarium for squamous cell carcinoma, concomitant chemosensitization using a platinum-containing regimen should be considered given the survival advantage demonstrated in prospective, randomized, clinical trials administered by the Gynecologic Oncology Group (GOG).[8–10] Long-term outcomes of vulvar and other gynecologic cancer therapies are demonstrated in Table 116.4.

VAGINA

Congenital

Septa

Septa may either be transverse or longitudinal to the vaginal axis. Transverse septa occur at the site of the junction of the upper vagina and the perineal plate. Longitudinal septa are the result of a müllerian fusion defect.

Transverse septa are usually first appreciated during menarche, when the adolescent acquires secondary sex characteristics but remains amenorrheic secondary to outflow obstruction. In women who become sexually active in the perimenarcheal period, the presenting symptom may be coital dysfunction. Obstruction of menstrual flow results in clinical finding including a bulging tissue plate at the hymen, a lower abdominal mass palpable on rectal examination, and lower abdominal pain secondary to retrograde menstruation. Therapy is surgical, with the placement of a cruciate incision in the septum, resection of the central cross-hatch, and approximation of the vaginal edges in a cephalad-caudad manner. If there is an area of nonjunction of the descending vagina and the perineal plate is greater than a few millimeters, some degree of undermining of the cephalad vaginal tube or placement of a split-thickness skin graft over the nonepithelialized supporting tissue is necessary. Postreconstruction, the use of an indwelling vaginal stent is mandatory to minimize constriction and fibrosis until healing has progressed to the point that coitus can be resumed.

Longitudinal vaginal septa are frequently completely asymptomatic, although they may be associated with coital dysfunction or a variety of other presentations based on other concomitant structural defects. Removal is straightforward, with a resection of the septum leaving an approximately 1-cm margin around the perimeter that can be approximated in a side-to-side fashion to facilitate healing. Dilator or stent use is rarely necessary in these women.

Agenesis (Rokitansky-Küster-Hauser Syndrome)

Vaginal agenesis is surgically a more elaborate and difficult entity than simple septa. Vaginal agenesis as an independent finding (i.e., with a normal cervix and upper genital tract) is very rare. This condition is more commonly a part of a complicated müllerian abnormality. Typically, there is a total loss of the upper two thirds of the vagina, cervix, uterus, and proximal fallopian tubes, the so-called Rokitansky-Küster-Hauser syndrome. This process is usually identified when a woman experiences thelarche and pubarche without menarche. In contradistinction to a transverse vaginal septum or imperforate

TABLE 116.4 RESULTS

OUTCOMES OF GYNECOLOGIC CANCER THERAPY: OVERALL SURVIVAL AT 5 YEARS

Stage	5-year survival rate (%)
CERVIX	
Ia1	95.1
Ia2	94.9
Ib	80.1
IIa	66.3
IIb	63.5
IIIa	33.3
IIIb	38.7
IVa	17.1
IVb	9.4
CORPUS UTERI	
Ia	90.9
Ib	88.2
Ic	81.0
IIa	76.9
IIb	67.1
IIIa	60.3
IIIb	41.2
IIIc	31.7
IVa	20.1
IVb	5.3
FALLOPIAN TUBE	
I	83.6
II	51.6
III	35.9
IV	15
OVARY	
Ia	86.9
Ib	71.3
Ic	79.2
IIa	66.6
IIb	55.1
IIc	57.0
IIIa	41.1
IIIb	24.9
IIIc	23.4
IV	11.1
VAGINA	
0	83.5
I	62.7
II	45.0
III	21.8
IV	18.8
VULVA[a]	
I	71.4
II	61.3
III	43.8
IV	8.3

[a]Epidermoid invasive cancer only.
(From Federation Internationale de Gynecologie et d'Obstetrique. Annual report on the results of treatment in gynaecological cancers. *J. Epidemiol Biostat.* 1998;3:1–168, with permission.)

hymen, no cyclic pain, hematocolpos, hematometra, or endometriosis is present. Clinical finding include a normal distal one third of the vagina, an absent upper tract except for the distal two thirds of the fallopian tubes and ovaries, and, in as many as 60% of patients, some degree of upper urinary tract abnormality (e.g., duplication, pelvic kidney, congenital absence). These women have normal gonadal function.

Correction of the agenesis can be accomplished by one of two major methods: sequential upward dilation and extension of the extant vagina using the so-called Mackenrodt technique or dissection of the fibrotic tissue at the apex of the distal vagina and placement of some form of graft, such as a split-thickness skin graft with or without an omental J-flap to facilitate neovascularization, a pedicle flap, or, our least favorite, a segment of large intestine that is attached to the remnant of the vagina. Our preferred method (split-thickness skin graft with omental J-flap) has the advantages of being able to make a capacious vagina without removing a segment of the anterior abdominal wall, has an acceptable amount of discharge, and has a very high success rate when used in this and similar settings.[11] After the neovagina is developed, the patient must make a serious commitment to comply with the recommendations of repeated and serial vaginal dilations and use of a prosthesis until frequent vaginal intercourse is allowed.

Traumatic

A discussion of traumatic injury to the vagina has been incorporated in our summary on traumatic vulvar injuries. Additionally, findings related to traumatic processes (e.g., birth, age, physical activity) that lead to abnormalities of vaginal support are discussed in the section on cervical trauma.

Although fistulae have become progressively less common in the industrialized world secondary to changes in obstetric practice, genital fistulae remain a common source of morbidity for women. Historically, the most common source of a vaginal fistula was as a residuum of birth trauma. In the modern era, however, the most common antecedent event is surgical trauma. The decision about how best to manage a fistula involving the pelvic organs is based on the cause of the fistula, prior attempts, underlying vascular integrity (including cigarette smoking), and patient preferences. In general, in the setting where the patient has not previously received radiation therapy, has not had a prior attempt at repair, and does not have an underlying vascular abnormality, a primary layered repair with meticulous attention paid to establishing tension-free closure is the preferred method. In all other settings, it is meritorious to bring in a new source of blood supply through either a VRAM flap, pedicle graft (e.g., a Martius flap), or an omental J-flap. An exhaustive discussion of the operative techniques and options is beyond the scope of this chapter.

Infectious

Infectious processes affecting the vagina are extremely rarely managed surgically except for in the setting of necrotizing fasciitis, as described previously.

Neoplastic

Vaginal neoplasms and malignancies are some of the least common of all such lesions occurring in the genital tract.

Benign Neoplasms

Nonmalignant or nonprecancerous tumors that occur in the vagina and surrounding tissues can arise from any of the cell types found in these environs. The three most commonly identified space-occupying lesions are posttraumatic inclusion cysts, paramesonephric duct remnants, and leiomyomata uteri. The former two entities are usually small, cystic, and relatively mobile, with paramesonephric cysts being less fixed than posttraumatic inclusion cysts. Paramesonephric cysts are almost universally noted along the lateral aspects of the vagina, following the course of their embryonic progenitors. Inclusion cysts, of course, can be located anywhere that prior trauma has occurred, usually near the perineum or sulci. Myomata are similar to inclusion cysts with regard to their nonspecific location. Myomata, however, are firm and usually mobile. Therapy for all of these lesions includes excision, with care taken to ensure that there is neither entry into nor injury to the bladder or distal ureters. We almost universally perform cystoscopy at time of resection, after closure of the subepithelial dead space and before approximation of the vaginal epithelium.

Vaginal Intraepithelial Neoplasia

From a pathophysiologic and treatment perspective, vaginal intraepithelial neoplasia (VAIN) has more in common with cervical intraepithelial neoplasia (CIN; discussed later) than it does with VIN. Therefore, the bulk of the essential information regarding VAIN is presented in the section on CIN. A few unique points, however, must be highlighted. Of women who have VAIN, 60% have previously been diagnosed with CIN. It has become evident that HPV is the causative agent in the vast majority of instances. Therapy of VAIN, because of the significant potential for inducing undesirable scarring, contraction, and subsequent dysfunction of the vagina, must be undertaken cautiously. Small lesions are best simply surgically excised, whereas larger lesions are treated with multiple colposcopic biopsies to ensure the absence of invasive disease, followed by laser vaporization. Locally caustic agents (5-fluorouracil) or immune modulators (imiquimod) have been used, although the latter only outside of U.S. Food and Drug Administration-approved labeling. In general, despite the effectiveness of these therapies, we are hesitant to use them because of the significant inflammatory response that can occur. In the worst case, epithelial sloughing and chemical vaginitis leads to coaptation of the vagina, secondary amenorrhea, and coital dysfunction. Similarly, a chronic inflammatory process associated with copious discharge and dyspareunia has been reported.

Vaginal Cancer

Vaginal cancer, as with the precancerous changes described previously, has much in common with cervical cancer. As a general staging rule, if a malignancy involves the vagina and the cervix, it is classified and staged as a cervical cancer. The same is true if the lesion involves the vagina and the vulva (i.e., it is classified and staged as a vulvar cancer; see FIGO staging in Table 116.3).

Two special histologic types of vaginal cancer deserve special comment (Table 116.5). Vaginal clear cell carcinoma has been noted to occur in a disproportionate number of women who were exposed *in utero* to diethylstilbestrol (DES). This exposure leads to a delay in squamous metaplasia in the upper vagina with the presence of endocervical-like glands (vaginal adenosis). The adenosis appears to be a site from which a series of oncogenic events can give rise to clear cell carcinomas. During the period when women were exposed *in utero* to DES (1943 to 1971) and developed to maturity, approximately two thirds of all clear cell cancers of the vagina were allegedly associated with this exposure. In contradistinction, only approximately one third of the clear cell carcinomas of the cervix during that same period were presumed to be DES related. The rates of DES-related clear cell carcinoma have, obviously, significantly decreased because most of the affected women have reached their late 30s and beyond.

TABLE 116.5 CLASSIFICATION

HISTOLOGIC CELL TYPES OF VAGINAL CANCER

Epidermoid squamous
Adenocarcinomas
Diethylstilbestrol-related clear cell
Melanoma
Metastatic disease
- Local
- Cervical
- Vulvar
- Anorectal
- Distal
- Endometrial
- Gestational trophoblastic disease
- Breast
- Others

Besides being a source of primary malignancy, the vagina is a common site of metastasis, particularly when the primary lesion arises in an adjoining organ (see earlier). Most notable is the proclivity of both endometrial cancer and gestational trophoblastic disease to have associated vaginal metastases. This is an important clinical phenomenon that may lead to the diagnosis of an otherwise occult primary after biopsy of a symptomatic (usually bleeding) vaginal lesion.

The guiding principle of therapy for vaginal cancers is that lesions involving the upper one third of the vagina are best treated as a similar-sized cervical lesion would be treated, whereas lesions of the distal two thirds are treated like vulvar cancer. This difference is based on both anatomic realities and lymphatic drainage.

CERVIX

Congenital

As has been repeatedly emphasized, congenital abnormalities of the female reproductive tract are best understood as a continuum of one disease entity. Cervical agenesis as an isolated abnormality is unheard of. Duplication of the cervix is discussed in the section on congenital abnormalities of the uterine corpus.

Traumatic

As with congenital abnormalities, the cervix is rarely the sole organ affected by genital trauma. Blunt object assault is much more likely to lead to trauma to the posterior vaginal fornix and retrocervical cul-de-sac (i.e., a posterior colpotomy). Although the cervix is generally resilient, it may be lacerated if an assault occurs with a sharp foreign object.

The two most common sources of cervical trauma are attempted or completed vaginal delivery and postexcision for cervical dysplasia. Peripartum cervical lacerations may occur independent of, or simultaneously with a vulvar, perineal, or vaginal birth injury. In contradistinction to the distal vagina, which may go from a relatively nonexpanded state to the passage of a term infant in a short time, the cervix usually dilates slowly over many hours and is therefore less susceptible to lacerations. Cervical tears are more likely to result from a "precipitous" labor with rapid cervical dilatation, from a dysfunctional labor leading to fetal instrumentation with either forceps or vacuum extraction, or from direct iatrogenic injury at time of cesarean section. In a setting where there has been an operative delivery, a precipitous birth, or the occurrence of a vulvar/ perineal/vaginal laceration, it is essential that the clinician thoroughly inspect the cervix. Lacerations of the cervix are common and do not require repair unless they are bleeding or extend to the cervicovaginal reflection. Repair can be effected by a simple, single-layer, running-locked number 0 or 1 delayed absorbable suture. When the laceration extends to the cervical vaginal reflection, further evaluation must be undertaken to ensure that there has been no injury to surrounding structures, particularly the bladder, distal ureters, and uterine artery complex. The former can lead to fistula formation and chronic urinary tract dysfunction, and the latter can lead to significant occult blood loss into the potential space of the broad ligament (see Fig. 116.2). Injury to the urinary tract should be assessed by immediate cystoscopy with administration of intravenous indigo carmine (10 mL) followed by 5 mg of furosemide to speed nephric clearance of the dark blue dye. Further surgical management depends on site and degree of injury, and is usually directed by a gynecologic oncologist, urogynecologist, or urologist who specializes in the care of the female patient.

Postcone Biopsy

By definition, a cervical excision procedure, whether in the form of a cold-knife cone, laser cone, or loop electrical excision procedure (LEEP), is a form of traumatic injury to the cervix. All of these procedures have an associated rate of delayed, postprocedural bleeding (from as high as 8% to 10% for a cold-knife cone to as low as 1% to 2% for a LEEP). Bleeding has a tendency to occur anywhere from 72 hours to 7 to 10 days after the performance of the procedure. Because of the high number of these procedures performed each year, postexcision bleeding is commonly encountered, although the optimal method of management has yet to be described. When bleeding occurs, usually an indolent soft tissue infection has developed (directly affecting the cervical stroma) in the presence of a foreign body (suture). Our preferred therapeutic protocol is to (a) institute intravenous broad-spectrum antibiotics that give adequate coverage for both vaginal flora and anaerobes; (b) take the patient to a procedure room where adequate analgesia may be induced; and (c) remove all extant sutures and replace with directed sutures, using them sparingly simply to obtain hemostasis. We prefer to use a long-acting, monofilament, absorbable suture in gauge 0. Further use of electrical cautery or of fulgurating agents (silver nitrate or Monsol's solution) is of limited value and may actually be counterproductive by inducing further foreign body and inflammatory reaction, leading to another bleeding episode.

Deficiencies of Support

It is not the intent of this chapter to give an exhaustive description of the diagnosis and operative management of abnormalities of pelvic support. As with many topics covered in this general chapter, numerous excellent, in-depth textbooks are available to the reader desiring further education, and only a brief summary is presented here.

As was emphasized in the opening sections of this chapter that discussed the intertwined nature of the anatomy and physiology of the female reproductive tract, a deficiency in support of one pelvic structure (with associated functional failure) is rarely an isolated event. To understand these processes fully, the clinician must reflect on the three pelvic compartments. A well-standardized and validated terminology of female pelvic organ prolapse and pelvic floor dysfunction has been developed and should be used when quantifying these abnormalities.[12]

Anterior compartment support failure leads to urethrocele, hypermobile urethrovesical junction, and cystocele. Often, these anatomic findings are associated with symptoms of a mass effect at the vaginal introitus, a sensation of pelvic heaviness, coital laxity, and urinary incontinence in stressful activity. Paradoxically, the more severe degrees of loss of mobility may actually be accompanied by obstruction as a result of severe urethral kinking; if residual urine volumes increase and remain high, overflow incontinence may result.

Midcompartment support abnormalities lead to descent of the cervix and uterine corpus (or vaginal vault, if the cervix and corpus are absent) and associated enterocele. Associated symptoms are similar to those of anterior support failure, with a preponderance of symptoms caused by the mass effect of the prolapsing uterus.

Posterior compartment support abnormalities can lead to the findings of a descending perineal body, rectocele, or enterocele. Symptomatology is as described previously, with the added symptom complex of either fecal incontinence (if the rectal sphincter is either anatomically disrupted or physiologically nonfunctional) or constipation and difficulty with evacuation, which is treated with "splinting" (digital dorsal displacement of the rectocele) to allow for adequate transmission of Valsalva pressure vectors and evacuation of the lower gastrointestinal tract. The diagnosis of these processes is usually straightforward and is made during physical examination of the patient who has not undergone prior attempts at surgical repair or has a concomitant neurologic (either distal or proximal) dysfunction.

Women who present with symptoms of urinary incontinence are more likely than not to have a mixed pattern of dysfunction, that is, one that involves both failure of the continence mechanism secondary to anatomic or intrinsic sphincter insufficiency and a degree of loss of detrusor muscle control. Because of this reality, a thorough urodynamic evaluation by cystometrography is mandatory except in those settings in which (a) a thorough and meticulous history has identified symptoms of urinary loss that occur only immediately after a stress activity, (b) the patient has no history of prior attempts at surgical urinary incontinence correction, and (3) urethrovesical junction hypermobility is demonstrated.[13] Thorough pretreatment assessment is even more strongly encouraged for those women who present with fecal incontinence because it is highly probably that these patients have a mixed anatomic and neurologic cause for their symptoms. Rectal sphincter dynamic ultrasonography, defecography, pelvic floor electromyography, and even dynamic pelvic floor magnetic resonance imaging may be required to make an accurate diagnosis that leads to appropriate patient counseling and treatment.

Numerous surgical and nonsurgical therapeutic options are available to the physician caring for the patient with a pelvic floor defect and functional abnormality. Estrogen can both increase the collagen content of the supporting ligaments and help to reestablish the normal, premenopausal hermetic seal of the urethra and tone of the perineal and vaginal tissues. Neuromuscular stimulation and exercise, in the form of Kegel's exercises, vaginal weights, or direct electrical stimulator application, are beneficial and minimally invasive. Apparatuses that support the pelvic structures or fill the coital hiatus (pessaries) may be useful, particularly in the patient who is not a surgical candidate but has failed other noninvasive therapies. Unfortunately, there is a very high rate of patient-initiated discontinuation of pessary use secondary to pain, pressure, or simple inconvenience of repeated removal, cleaning, and replacement.

The past 125 years has seen an almost innumerable array of surgical procedures proposed and used in the management of pelvic support deficiencies. Since the early 1980s, however, the randomized clinical trial has been applied to procedure selection. Although the extant evidence, as for most surgical procedures, is suboptimal, recommendations can be made based on current knowledge[14] (Table 116.6).

Infectious

Surgical therapy for an isolated acute cervical infection has never been reported because these entities are treated pharmacologically.[1] The cervix may be, although it does not need to be, removed as part of the definitive surgical management of tuboovarian abscess (TOA), which is presented in the section on ovarian diseases.

TABLE 116.6 TREATMENT

RECOMMENDATIONS FOR THE MANAGEMENT OF PELVIC SUPPORT DEFICIENCIES

1. All compartments must be evaluated and treated.
2. ISD should be treated with a sling procedure, preferably using fascia lata, Allo-derm, or nonreactive synthetic materials (i.e., polypropylene mesh [tension-free vaginal tape] or PTFE [Gore-Tex]).
   - For patients with recurrent disease, periurethral collagen injections can be used.
3. Genuine SUI secondary to an anatomic defect (the hypermobile urethra) is best repaired using a modified RPUP (Burch procedure).
   - A concomitant anterior colporrhaphy should be performed if there is residual cystocele after the RPUP.
   - As sling procedures appear to be successful in the treatment of both the hypermobile urethra and ISD, they have become increasingly popular in the treatment of uncomplicated SUI.
4. Potential vaginal vault prolapse should be addressed prophylactically by use of the Mayo modification of the McCall culdoplasty.
5. Documented vaginal vault prolapse should be treated with either a Mayo-modified McCall culdoplasty or a sacral colpopexy using a noninflammatory, closed-pore prosthesis (fascia lata, PTFE).
6. Enteroceles should invariably be repaired as part of the management of vault suspension.
   - Occurring as isolated postsurgical findings, these are best treated with a culdoplasty.
7. Rectoceles are best treated with posterior colporrhaphy with specific attention paid to reconstruction of the perineal body, the major source of posterior support.
8. Rectal sphincter failure is managed by a multimodality approach, including repair of anatomic defects, neosphincter reconstruction using levator ani muscles, and physiotherapy.

ISD, intrinsic sphincter deficiency; SUI, stress urinary incontinence; PTFE, polytetrafluoroethylene; RPUB, retropubic urethropexy.

Nabothian cysts, the end result of chronic cervicitis, are sometimes inadvertently treated because of naiveté on behalf of the treating surgeon. These cysts, which are caused by inflammatory or benign metaplastic occlusion of the cervical gland ducts and subsequent dilatation (at times massive) secondary to buildup of cervical mucus, may appear neoplastic to the inexperienced physician. Clinically, nabothian cysts may enlarge to 1 cm or more in diameter, are rarely symptomatic, and are best left untreated.

Neoplastic

The relative importance of cervical cancer is demonstrated in Table 116.2. Although cervical cancer is relatively uncommon as a source of morbidity and mortality in the United States, it ranks as the number two cause of cancer-related death in women in the developing world, and in selected countries, it is number one.

Fifty years ago, a highly effective screening tool, the Papanicolaou (Pap) smear, entered into broad use in the United States. It was the institution of common, although not universal, screening of at-risk women that has led to a 75% fall in the incidence of cervical cancer over the last 70 years.

Although cervical cancer has become a less important public health entity, cervical dysplasia remains a significant burden to the U.S. healthcare system. Every year, approximately 3.5 million minimally abnormal [atypical squamous cells of undetermined significance (ASCUS) and low-grade squamous epithelial lesion (LGSIL)] Pap smears are collected in the United States. Approximately 15% to 20% of these women have an associated, unappreciated, precancerous lesion (CIN II or III), with a significant, if not the largest, percentage of precancerous lesions eventually identified in that group of women who present with minimally abnormal Pap smears. These lesions are called *precancerous* because they have approximately a 30% chance of progressing to invasive disease if left untreated, in contradistinction to the histologic changes that are reflected in the minimal abnormalities that have, at most, a 1% to 2% chance of developing into a malignant disease.

Evaluation of the abnormal Pap smear is based on recommendations by the American Society for Colposcopy and Cervical Pathology hosted consensus conference (Algorithm 116.1).[15] The pathways are confined to the management of squamous cell abnormalities. The most remarkable change in the triage and assessment algorithm has been the integration of HPV typing. As HPV is a responsible coagent in nearly 100% of women with cervical precancerous lesions or cancer, the capacity to identify accurately the oncogenic strains of HPV has led to the incorporation of hybrid capture testing into the aforementioned algorithm.

Treatment of Cervical Dysplasia

Only precancerous lesions require therapy; patients with lesser lesions are more likely to experience a deleterious side effect from therapy than progress to cancer. The goal of therapy is twofold: to ensure that there is no underlying, occult cancer (a finding in 3% to 10% of patients with CIN II to III)[2]; and to eliminate the lesion in its entirety such that the chance of recurrence is minimized. Our preferred modality for treatment is the loop electrosurgical excisional procedure (LEEP), during which a 0.0001-inch tungsten wire loop carrying low-energy electrical current is used to excise the abnormal tissue. Because there is a small, but real risk that the surgical margins will be uninterpretable secondary to thermal artifact, in those settings in which subtleties of pathologic interpretation will make a significant difference in subsequent therapy (e.g., glandular dysplasias, microinvasive disease), we recommend that a

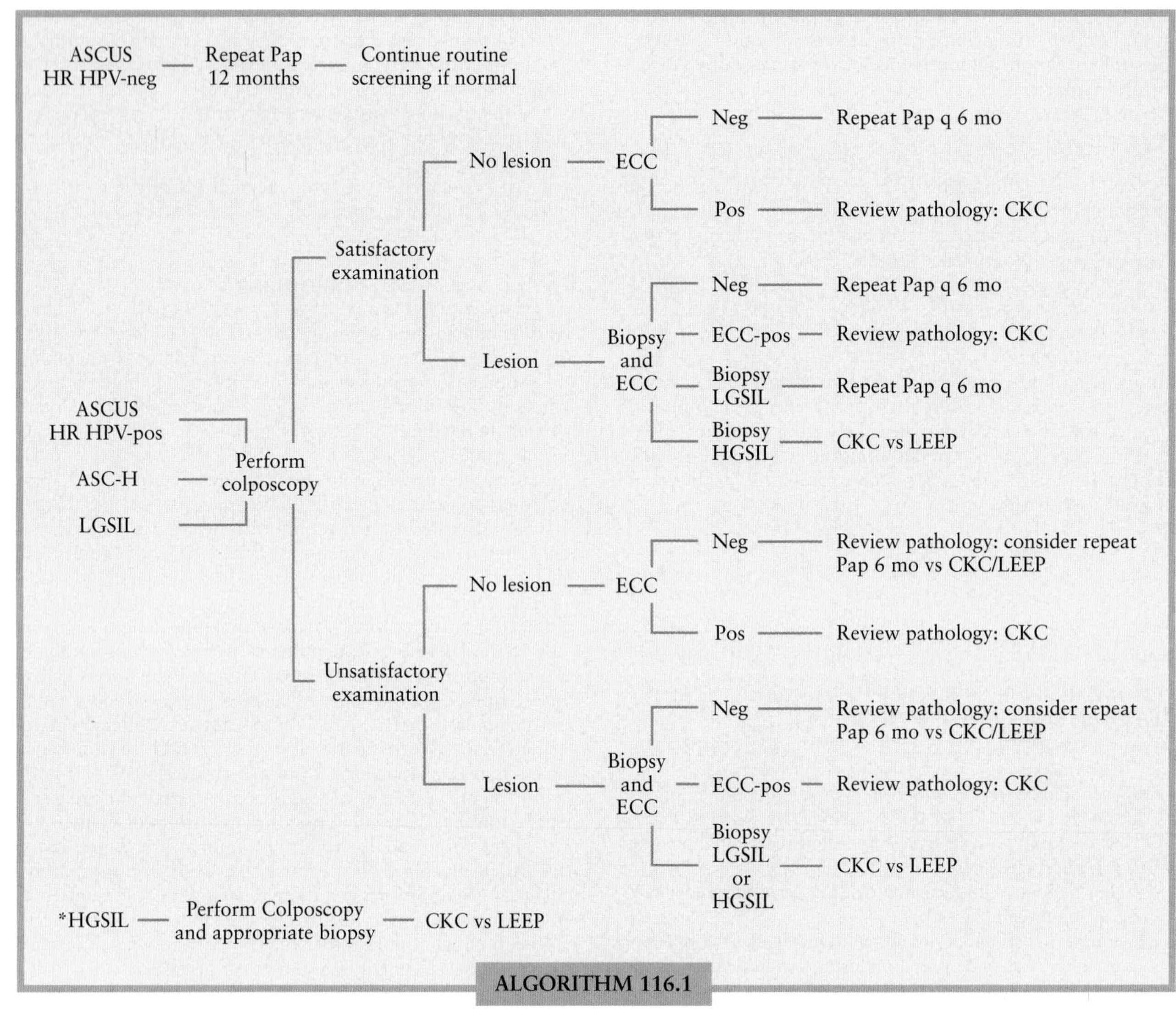

ALGORITHM 116.1 ASCUS/LGSIL Pap smear management. LGSIL, low-grade squamous intraepithelial lesion; HGSIL, high-grade squamous intraepithelial lesion; ASCUS, atypical squamous cells of undetermined significance, ASC-H, atypical squamous cells, cannot exclude HGSIL; HR HPV, high-risk human papillomavirus; ECC, endocervical curettage; CKC, cold-knife cone; LEEP, loop electrosurgical excisional procedure. *Ultimately, HGSIL Pap smears typically require LEEP or CKC. (From Wright TC, Cox JT, Massad LS, et al. Consensus guidelines for the management of women with cervical cytological abnormalities. *JAMA* 2002;287:2120–2129, with permission.)

cold-knife cone (CKC) biopsy be performed in a surgical center under systemic analgesia.

Cervical Cancer

Cervical cancer, as emphasized previously, has become a less significant source of morbidity for North American and European women. This disease occurs uncommonly in people who have been compliant with recommended exfoliative cytologic screening (Pap smear). Depending on the community surveyed, between 40% and 60% of all women in whom cervical cancer develops have either never had a Pap smear or have been suboptimally screened.

Most cervical cancers are of the squamous cell type and have been demonstrated to be caused in part by an infection with high-risk HPV types, as noted previously. Adenocarcinomas have become more common and comprise 15% to 25% of all cervical cancers. The cervix can also be a site of metastatic disease, with endometrial cancer being the most common primary site.

Cervical cancer, when not first appreciated by Pap smear, is symptomatic in approximately 75% of cases, with abnormal bleeding, vaginal discharge, and pain predominating. By FIGO criteria, cervical cancer is clinically staged (see Table 116.3). The most critical element in the staging process is a thorough and accurate pelvic examination searching for findings consistent with extracervical spread. To be optimal, this examination often must be performed under analgesia. A chest radiograph and, in women with suspected disease extension, an intravenous pyelogram, cystoscopy, and, rarely, proctosigmoidoscopy, may be included. More advanced radiographic studies can be performed (computed tomography and magnetic resonance imaging), although the information they provide, except for the finding of hydronephrosis, cannot be used to "upstage" patients. Algorithm 116.2 gives the Kelly Gynecologic Oncology Service guidelines for management of cervical cancer.

Radical Hysterectomy

Cervical cancer's natural proclivity is for local advancement and spread and systematic, stepwise involvement of sequential draining lymph nodes. These phenomena were appreciated over 150 years ago and led to the development of a new surgical procedure: the radical hysterectomy. This procedure was first developed and performed in the United States by J. Goodrich Clark, a resident surgeon under the tutelage of Dr. Howard A. Kelly at The Johns Hopkins Hospital in 1895. The driving principle was to develop a surgical procedure that could safely remove the primary lesion *en bloc* with a margin of surrounding tissue that was grossly devoid of tumor and included the first-level lymphatic drainage while leaving the adjoining vital organs (urinary bladder, ureter, and rectum) intact and functional. Meigs added to this procedure a systematic resection of the secondary and tertiary lymphatic drainage, with both a therapeutic and diagnostic intent. Over the decades, this procedure has been refined and classified[16] (Fig. 116.5), and specific indications for use of each of the types of radical hysterectomy described (see Algorithm 116.2). Although various approaches (transvaginal, transabdominal, laparoscopically assisted, and complete laparoscopic) to the performance of radical hysterectomy

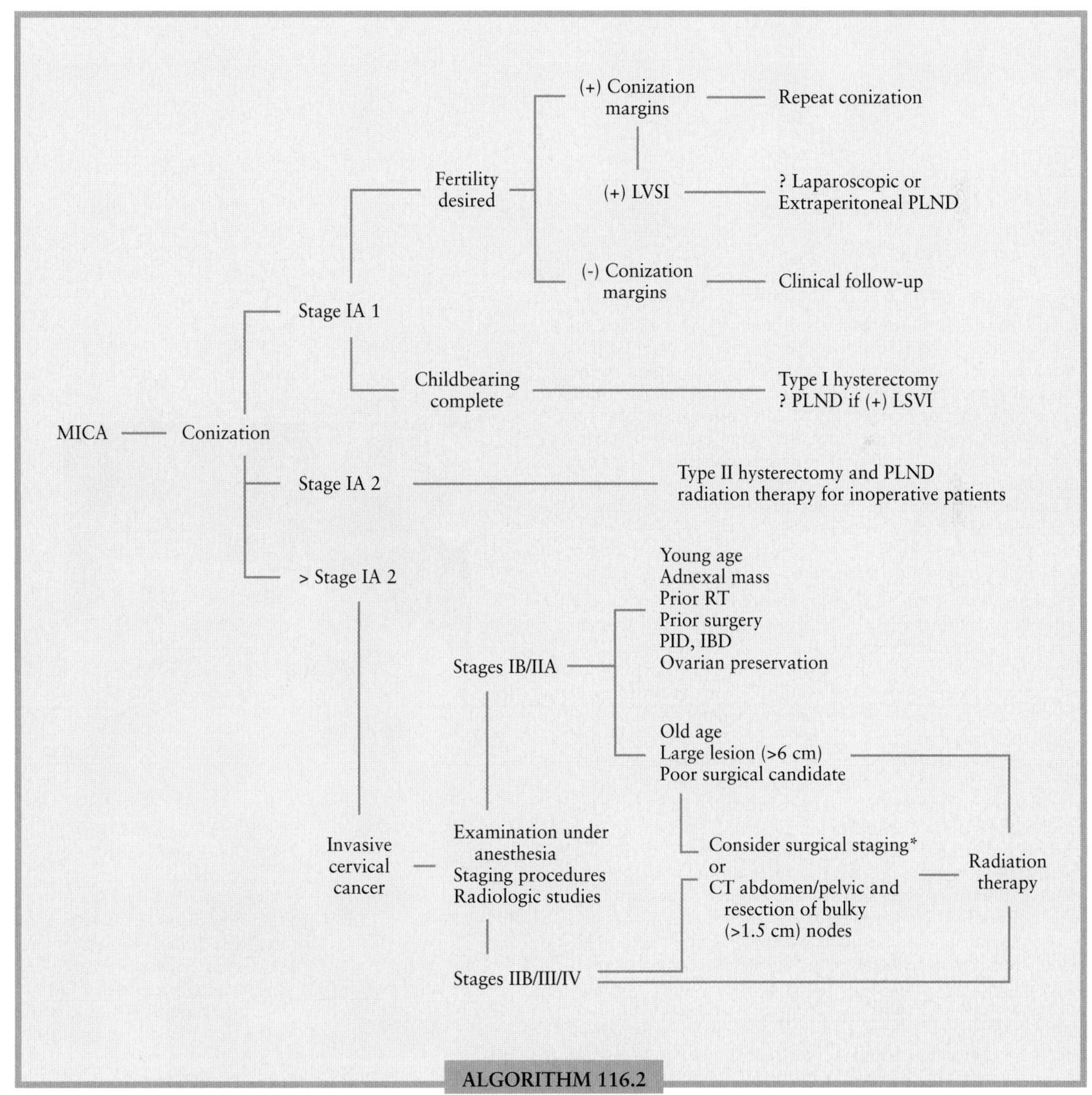

ALGORITHM 116.2 Cervical cancer management.

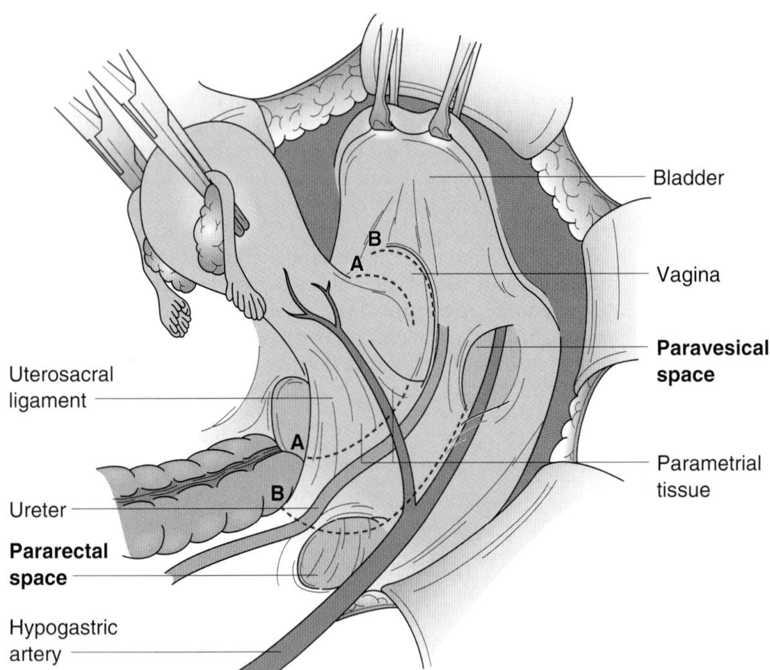

FIGURE 116.5 Illustration of differences between a class II and III radical hysterectomy.

have been and still are used, because of the general familiarity with the surgical procedure, the thoroughness of the resection possible, and the comorbidity profile, the transabdominal approach is the most commonly used. A new variation of the procedure is the performance of a radical vaginal trachelectomy with a concomitant laparoscopic lymph node dissection for women with early localized disease (stage Ia2 to Ib1) who desire preservation of fertility. A growing database supports not only that this procedure can be performed safely and with acceptable disease control rates but also that most women who wish to preserve fertility are able to do so.[17]

Pelvic Exenteration Even with advances in radiation therapy techniques and the administration of radiosensitizing doses of cytotoxic chemotherapy, a significant proportion of women with locally advanced cervical cancer have a recurrence. For these women, who had only local persistent or recurrent disease, no curative option existed until the work of Bruecher et al. in the 1940s. They described the performance of an ultraradical extirpation of the pelvic organs (bladder, urethra, distal ureters, uterus, fallopian tubes, ovaries, vagina, parametria and paracolpos, distal sigmoid and rectum, and, when performed in an infralevatory fashion, segments of the levator ani muscles, perineum, and anal sphincter) and development of a urinary conduit and colostomy. This procedure, called *pelvic exenteration*, has led to salvage rates as high as 60% in selected subgroups of patients, with average long-term cure rates in the 35% to 40% range. These cures were not obtained without significant losses in both physiologic and psychological domains. Over the intervening 50 years, the focus has been on refining the procedure in an attempt to reestablish urinary and fecal continence and coital function and to maintain a healthy body image. The current standard[18] calls for establishment of a continent urinary diversion, anastomosis of the resected margins of the large intestine, and construction of a dynamic vagina using cutaneous island flaps, with a VRAM or transverse rectus abdominis muscle flap being our preference. This leads to a cosmetic outcome that offers a significant advantage (Fig. 116.6).

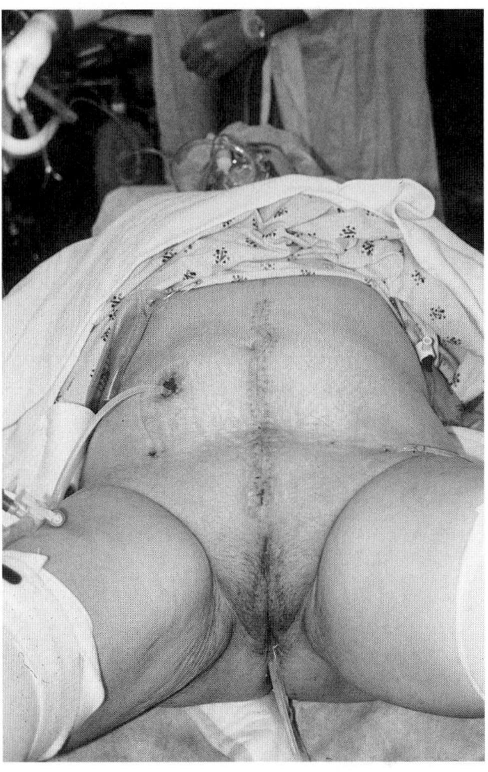

FIGURE 116.6 Patient after total pelvic exenteration with rectosigmoid anastomosis, neovagina formation, and development of continent urinary diversion (Miami pouch). Note single, small stoma in the right lower quadrant, which is used only for intermittent catheterization.

UTERUS

Congenital

Congenital abnormalities of the female reproductive organs, as noted in the discussion of vaginal abnormalities, lie along a continuum related to the degree of nonfusion of the paired müllerian-derived structures or failure of one half of the müllerian system to develop. A formal classification system was developed by the American Fertility Society (now called the American Society for Reproductive Medicine) and is commonly used.[19] The most severe cases are those of didelphic or unobstructed double uterus, whereas the least severe are subseptate uteri. The didelphic uterus does not require surgical unification, although patients with a septate uterus, because of significant difficulties with reproductive failure, are candidates for such a procedure. Rudimentary and noncommunicating uterine horns are best treated with resection.

There are numerous metroplasty techniques and methods for transcervical hysteroscopic resection, a complete discussion of which is beyond the scope of this chapter. A critical point, however, is that women who have undergone metroplasty and become pregnant must, because of the inordinate risk of uterine rupture, undergo cesarean delivery before labor.

Traumatic

The most common traumatic injury to the uterine corpus is perforation. This can occur during office endometrial biopsy, intrauterine device (IUD) placement, dilation and curettage, operative pregnancy termination, or diagnostic or operative hysteroscopy. Perforation is uncommon in the premenopausal, nonpregnant patient except when operative resection of uterine disease (e.g., septum, myoma) is being undertaken. However, in the edematous (pregnant or infected) uterus or, paradoxically, the fibrotic, nonelastic, postmenopausal uterus, perforation may occur in up to 10% of instrumentations. Fortunately, morbidity associated with perforation is uncommon except in selected circumstances. If perforation is suspected, consideration must be given not only to sequelae that result from direct injury to the uterine wall, but also to those of injury to the surrounding structures. When perforation has occurred with a blunt object (sound, probe, plastic cannula) and without negative pressure being applied (i.e., suction), significant bleeding from the uterine defect and injury to surrounding structures are rare. If a sharp instrument (curette) or negative pressure has been used, however, some reparative action probably will be needed. In the former setting, observation for signs and symptoms of bleeding in the immediate postoperative period is advised. In the latter settings, we recommend that a diagnostic laparoscopy be performed at a minimum, with a low threshold for exploratory celiotomy.

Asherman's Syndrome

Asherman's syndrome, or intrauterine synechia, is usually a result of endometrial trauma (curettage) in the setting of endometritis. The presentation is one of secondary amenorrhea or infertility. Diagnosis is made by hysterosalpingogram or hysteroscopy, and therapy consists of resection of the intrauterine adhesions, placement of a device to keep the uterine walls separate (either an IUD or pediatric Foley catheter with concomitant antibiotic prophylaxis), and estrogenic stimulation to reestablish the endometrium. The rate of successful correction is approximately 80% using this multimodality approach.

Hematomucometria and Pyomucometria

Hematomucometria and pyomucometria are phenomena that result from the near-total or total occlusion of the cervix and production of cervical mucus or endometrial blood, which can become superinfected. These processes are almost universally the end result of surgical trauma (cone biopsy, LEEP, cryotherapy, birth trauma), radiation or chronic atrophic changes, or an obstructive cervical malignancy. Surgically, simple dilation of the cervix, cervical conical excision, and, rarely, hysterectomy are the mainstays of therapy.

Infectious

Rarely are infectious processes of the uterine corpus surgically managed. The exceptions are infected degenerating fibroids, which are probably the result of inoculation of the hypo-oxygenated necrotic fibroid by instrumentation, and TOAs in which the uterus may be involved with microabscesses. Historically, before the modern era of antibiotics and the abandonment of the use of braided IUD strings, emergent hysterectomy for the management of myometrial infection was a standard and often lifesaving practice.

Neoplastic

Leiomyomata Uteri

Leiomyomata, or fibroids, are benign, nonmalignant, and nonprecancerous overgrowths of the smooth muscle of the uterine wall, the cause of which is unknown. Women with fibroids may have one or more of a constellation of symptoms. The most common symptoms are abnormalities of bleeding, pain (specifically dysmenorrhea and dyspareunia), and the effects of the large uterus pressing on surrounding structures (e.g., urinary frequency and incontinence, rectal frequency, low back pain). It has been well demonstrated that fibroids are estrogen responsive, and this has been taken into consideration in the creation of treatment algorithms. Antiestrogenic therapy is variably effective depending on the degree of blockage or suppression of estrogen and the size of the fibroids. In general, using the most effective agents [gonadotropin-releasing hormone (GnRH) antagonists], up to 70% of myomata that are less than 7 to 9 cm in maximal diameter undergo a 70% shrinkage in volume (not diameter).[20] This therapy results in almost universal hypoestrogenic symptomatology. The long-term morbidity and potential mortality associated with postmenopausal estrogen levels in young women (e.g., osteoporosis, heart disease), limits the use of GnRH antagonists. Therefore, these agents are most frequently used for a short time to stop bleeding so that a patient can be autotransfused before surgical management.

Surgical management of fibroids can be divided into definitive (i.e., hysterectomy) or nondefinitive (either myomectomy or hysteroscopic resection of submucosal myomata). The advantage of myomectomy is that fertility is spared, although approximately 15% of women require further surgical management of the myoma. Myomectomy may be performed by open or laparoscopic techniques, although there are significant concerns about the reestablishment of uterine wall integrity and the safety of subsequent pregnancy in the latter setting. Blood loss at time of myomectomy, which can be massive, can be limited with the use of tourniquets, vascular "bulldog" clamps, vasoconstrictive agents, and hemostatic dissecting instruments (electrocautery, laser, or, our preference, the argon beam coagulator). At time of myomectomy, meticulous closure is needed to enhance myometrial healing to minimize the

TABLE 116.7 CLASSIFICATION

CLINICAL CLASSIFICATION OF UTERINE SARCOMAS

Endometrial stromal sarcomas (ESS)
Leiomyosarcomas (LMS)
Carcinosarcomas or malignant mixed mesodermal tumors (MMMT)
  Malignant glandular and stromal elements
Adenosarcomas
  Benign glandular elements and malignant stromal elements

potential for intrapartum uterine rupture. Hysteroscopic resection offers the advantage of a minimally invasive procedure, although one with the potentially lethal associated morbidity of intravascular fluid overload, pulmonary edema, and congestive heart failure. Pregnancy is not recommended after hysteroscopic resection and may be impossible because of endometrial adhesions. Uterine artery embolization has been used with increasing frequency in the treatment of uterine fibroids.[21,22] The safety of this investigational procedure in women interested in future fertility is unproved.

Sarcomas

Uterine sarcomas are uncommon but aggressive and frequently fatal diseases that have a complex and at times confusing histologic classification (Table 116.7). The basis of treatment of uterine sarcomas is hysterectomy with bilateral salpingo-oophorectomy. There may be merit in the performance of a thorough surgical staging such as is recommended for endometrial adenocarcinomas (see later), although no high-level evidence supports this belief, mostly because the use of adjuvants is of unproved benefit. Previously identified myomata that are noted to grow rapidly probably do not represent malignant degeneration, and such growth is not typically in itself a justification for surgical intervention. A perimenopausal or postmenopausal woman, however, who does not have a known history of fibroids and acquires a single, rapidly growing uterine mass, is of sufficient concern to justify resection and pathologic assessment.

Endometrial Hyperplasia

In most settings, endometrial hyperplasia is the result of an endocrinopathy and not a demonstrable genetic oncogenic abnormality. The constant and inadequately opposed or unopposed estrogen stimulation of the endometrium leads to development of these lesions. It is critical to appreciate this when discussing therapeutic options. Endometrial hyperplasias have the same risk factors as endometrial cancers (Table 116.8). As with endometrial cancer, the most common presenting symptom is abnormal vaginal bleeding, in most cases occurring in the menopause. Endometrial cancer can also present with a putrid vaginal discharge or pain; these latter symptoms are more common in the setting of advanced disease.

Therapy for endometrial hyperplasia is based on the risk of a malignancy developing if left untreated and the probability that the patient will experience a significant complication from the definitive, surgical therapy. Women with endometrial hyperplasia devoid of nuclear atypia or those desiring future fertility can be treated with continuous progestins; our preference is megestrol (40 mg/d) for 90 days. Thereafter, the patient undergoes a repeat endometrial sampling in the office. If the hyperplasia has resolved, the patient can be treated with cyclic progestins (for 14 days of the month) or birth control pills. If the hyperplasia persists, a longer period of megestrol therapy (up to 9 months) may be needed. If the hyperplasia is not reversed by that time, it is unlikely that further progestin therapy will be effective, and the patient should proceed to definitive therapy (hysterectomy).

TABLE 116.8

RISK FACTORS FOR THE DEVELOPMENT OF ENDOMETRIAL HYPERPLASIAS AND CANCERS

Characteristic	Relative risk
Nulliparity	2–3
Late menopause	2.4
Obesity	
21–50 lbs	3
>50 lbs	10
Diabetes mellitus	2.8
Unopposed estrogen therapy	4–8
Tamoxifen	2–3
Atypical endometrial hyperplasia	8–29

(Adapted from Lurain J. Endometrial cancer. In Berek JS, Adashi EY, Hillard PA, eds. *Novak's gynecology,* 12th ed. Baltimore: Williams & Wilkins, 1996, p. 1058.)

Endometrial Cancer

Endometrial cancer is the most common gynecologic malignancy in North America (see Table 116.2). Because early symptoms often lead to early assessment and diagnosis, however, most lesions are identified before extracorporeal spread has occurred and are successfully treated. This is in contradistinction to ovarian cancers.

Numerous unresolved controversies surround the management of endometrial cancers. The treatment approach set forth in Algorithm 116.3, however, reflects both the modern understanding of this disease and the recommended FIGO guidelines for staging and the National Comprehensive Cancer Network guidelines for therapy. We recommend surgical staging for all women who have more than a 5% statistical chance of having extrauterine disease, a position that is both evidence based and widely held among academic gynecologic oncology surgeons.

ADNEXA

Although the adnexa include both the ovary and the fallopian tube, it is the former structure that is the primary source of pathologic processes, excluding salpingitis or tuboovarian abscess.

Congenital

Paramesonephric Duct Cysts

When the paramesonephric or wolffian duct system fails to develop and undergoes resorption, remnants may remain that, over time, can expand with clear serous fluid and become evident. Only very rarely are these small cysts appreciated clinically. They usually are either an incidental finding at the time of surgery or are detected with imaging. These cysts can distend or may undergo torsion incorporating the adnexa, however. Treatment is surgical resection, with the degree dependent on the age of the patient and her wishes regarding further fertility. Very rarely (<1%) are these cysts associated with malignant

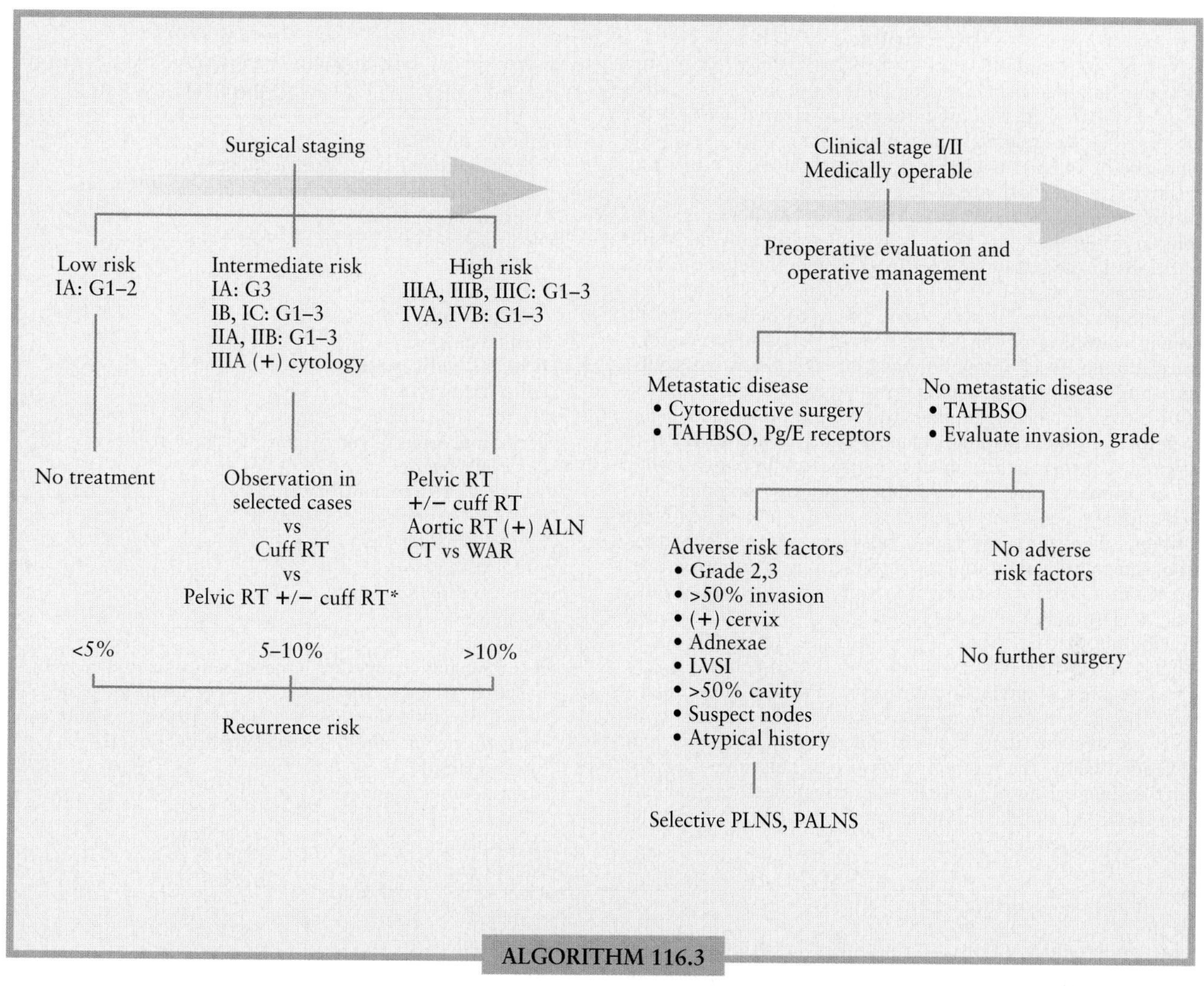

ALGORITHM 116.3 Endometrial cancer management. *Radiation therapy should be considered for intermediate-risk endometrial cancer, especially with increasing grade, increasing depth of invasion, or tumor size larger than 2 cm. Megace may be considered for patients with positive cytology.

degeneration and are best treated exactly like an ovarian malignancy.

Traumatic

Torsion

Adnexal torsion is a relatively rare but, from the perspective of maintenance of optimal fertility, potentially disastrous side effect. Those processes that predispose to adnexal torsion include an elongated infundibulopelvic or uteroovarian ligament, an adnexal mass (although large masses are actually less likely to undergo torsion), and the absence of the attachment to the uterus. Adnexal torsion commonly presents as an intermittent and often progressively worsening unilateral pain. Historically, therapy has been to remove that segment of the adnexa that has undergone torsion because of a fear that "untwisting" the adnexa would lead to the occurrence or propagation of clot up the ovarian veins with the potential formation of a pulmonary embolus. This philosophy is no longer universally held, and except in the most extreme cases of necrosis or in the paramenopausal age or later, the torsion is reversed, the adnexa is fixed, usually to the psoas muscle tendon, and return of oxygenated blood flow is awaited.

Uterine Perforation

The other common traumatic insult to the adnexa is injury during uterine perforation associated with pregnancy termination. Because of the retrouterine location of the adnexa and the cul-de-sac, it is not uncommon for the adnexal structures to be involved when a perforation-associated extracorporeal injury occurs. The adnexa may be drawn into the uterine cavity if a suction dilation and curettage was being undertaken. More potentially dangerous is the laceration of the ovarian vessels in their retroperitoneal location. This can lead to massive, ascending, retroperitoneal, and dangerously unappreciated blood loss. A posttermination patient who has symptoms and findings of hypovolemia that are not explicable by intraprocedure blood loss must be assumed to have a major adnexal or retroperitoneal vessel injury until proved otherwise. Our preference remains surgical evaluation via laparotomy through a midline incision or laparoscopy with a vascular surgery consultant on standby.

Infectious

Although salpingo-oophoritis remains a not uncommon disease in North America, the surgically treated associated process, TOA, is relatively uncommon. This decrease in the incidence of TOA is caused by numerous factors: improved sensitivity to the existence of salpingo-oophoritis by primary care physicians and, therefore, earlier treatment; newer generations of antibiotics that are effective at clearing mixed floral infections in the setting of decreased tissue oxygenation; and the decreasing use of IUD for contraception. TOA present like salpingo-oophoritis, but are more likely to be identified in women who have had prior episodes of pelvic inflammatory disease, received suboptimal therapy, or have persistent symptoms and signs despite adequate therapy. The suspicion of TOA is confirmed radiographically, with our preferences being a vaginal probe ultrasound. Once TOAs are identified, it is essential that their natural history be tracked. In patients who fail to experience disease improvement (either symptomatically or because of persistent hyperpyrexia) in the face of adequate antibiotic therapy, consideration must be given to either surgical or interventional radiology-based therapy. In young women for whom gonadal preservation is a priority, we prefer to use either ultrasound or computed tomography–directed drainage, a technique that has become popular since the mid-1980s.[23] When conservative management is unsuccessful, we prefer definitive surgical intervention, which usually includes a bilateral salpingo-oophorectomy at a minimum. In patients who have an abscess that has distended the cul-de-sac and descended below the internal cervical os, transvaginal colpotomy drainage is an option. Only an experienced vaginal surgeon should undertake this technique because of the potential for significant rectosigmoid injury.

Pelvic Tuberculosis

Pelvic tuberculosis (TB) is a rare entity in all but the new immigrant to North America. Because of the endemicity of gastrointestinal TB in parts of Mexico and Central America as well as the Indian subcontinent, however, this process must always be included in the differential diagnosis of a pelvic mass in women from those geographic locales. Pelvic TB is not treated surgically because of the significant potential sequelae and inability to totally remove the innumerable tubers.

Neoplastic

Adnexal Mass

The evaluation and management of the female adnexal mass is a treatise in itself. Certain caveats, however, allow a relatively easy understanding of the classification and management of this extremely heterogeneous entity (Tables 116.9 and 116.10).

Ovarian Nonmalignant Neoplasms

Regardless of the patient's age (see Table 116.9), ovarian lesions must be followed intensively to ensure either regression or lack of progression. Laparoscopy has become the preferred surgical modality for investigation of a persistent adnexal mass. Diagnostic and therapeutic laparoscopy can be performed in most instances in the outpatient setting with very low rates of associated morbidity. It is important that adequate surgical instrumentation be available to perform the most common adnexal laparoscopic procedures. Our preference is to use a direct trocar insertion technique. When there is significant likelihood of the presence of subumbilical

TABLE 116.9 DIAGNOSIS

DIFFERENTIAL DIAGNOSIS OF THE ADNEXAL MASS STRATIFIED BY PATIENT'S REPRODUCTIVE AGE

Newborn and infants
Congenital anomalies (e.g., pelvic kidney)
Physiologic residuum of maternal hormones
- Ovarian theca—luteum cysts

Neoplasms
- Germ cell
  - Benign (dermoids)
  - Malignant (predominant)

Premenarchal
Functional ovarian cysts
- Follicular
- Hemorrhagic corpus luteum
- Persistent corpus luteum
- Polycystic ovaries

Neoplastic (predominant)
- Germ cell neoplasms
- Epithelial neoplasms

Reproductive age
Functional (predominant)
- As above

Neoplastic
- As above and below (the closer the patient is to the age of menarche, the more likely that the neoplasm is of germ cell origin; the closer the patient is to menopause, the more likely the neoplasm is of ovarian epithelial origin).

Postmenopausal
Neoplastic (predominant)
- Benign "simple" cysts
- Epithelial neoplasm (benign and malignant)
- Metastatic
- Primary colorectal cancer

Inflammatory
- Diverticular disease

TABLE 116.10 DIAGNOSIS

CAVEATS ABOUT EVALUATING AND MANAGING ADNEXAL MASSES

- Remember all the structures that are found in the female pelvis. The appendix and sigmoid colon are both pelvic structures and potential sources for adnexal masses. The same is true of an aberrantly located kidney.
- The closer the patient is to a reproductive milestone, the more likely that the mass represents a physiologic or functional change in the gonad.
- Congenital abnormalities, such as pelvic or horseshoe kidneys, are commonly not appreciated until menarche. Failure to rule out the presence of these structures can lead to life-threatening surgical error.
- Except in the immediate newborn period, when the female infant can manifest residuum of maternal hormone effects, adnexal masses presenting at the extremes of life are malignancies until proved otherwise.
- During the reproductive years, adnexal masses are nonmalignant until proved otherwise.
- A gonad, once removed, cannot be replaced; it is therefore better to reexplore a patient than castrate her under questionable circumstances.

adhesions, we use an alternative site for access, such as the left infracostal margin lateral to the superior epigastric artery. To minimize the potential for postoperative wound complications, we use 5-mm ports for all sites except one, where a 10- to 12-mm trocar is placed. This larger trocar can be used for placement of linear stapling devices and removal of the mass. At the completion of intraperitoneal surgery, care is taken to ensure complete closure of all 8-mm or larger port sites, closing both the peritoneum and the fascia *en bloc* to minimize the occurrence of Richter's hernia.

A common clinical dilemma faced by the general surgeon is how to manage the finding of an incidental adnexal mass at the time of exploratory celiotomy for a presumed nongynecologic disease process. Remembering the caveats set forth previously and the age-dependent differential diagnosis, the decision about how to proceed should be based on the answers to the following questions.

1. *What does the lesion look like?* Small masses (<8 cm in maximal diameter, in addition to the size of the gonad) that are freely mobile and have a smooth surface are unlikely to represent any neoplasm, much less a malignant one. These masses are best left alone in the premenopausal patient unless the surgeon is skilled at ovarian cystectomy and reconstruction. The exception to this recommendation is the patient who has a benign-appearing cyst that has led to adnexal torsion. There is no hard – and fast rule as to whether the torsion should be reversed, viability ensured, and the ovary fixed into the ovarian fossa, or whether adnexectomy should be performed. Clinical judgment as well as the degree of torsion and necrosis is important. The threshold for consultation with an experienced gynecologic surgeon must be very low. In contradistinction, masses that have surface papillae or excrescences are highly suspect for malignancy, although this presentation does occur in ovarian cystadenofibromas. Excisional biopsy of the surface irregularity followed by frozen-section analysis is valuable in deciding how to proceed (see section on ovarian cancer, later).
2. *What is the patient's age?* In those patients who have definitively completed their childbearing, the removal of a single adnexa has little and probably no meaningful effect on age of menopause. Removal of one of the adnexa, however, decreases fertility rates by 15% and must be avoided if there is any question regarding the patient's desires. Women older than 45 years of age are best served by a bilateral adnexectomy, even if the mass is apparently benign and unilateral. The long-term effects of the induction of surgical menopause, even in the average-risk patient, are offset by the benefits of ovarian cancer prevention.
3. *Why is the surgery being performed?* When operating on a young patient with presumed appendicitis, and a normal appendix but an abnormal ovary are found, the ovarian lesion, even though it is probably physiologic, is best removed by cystectomy because it is probably not optimal medical care to explore a patient, find a potential source for her symptoms, and elect to do nothing. In contradistinction, when a postmenopausal woman is undergoing exploration for surgical management of colon cancer and a small (1- to 4-cm), simple cystic mass is identified in a single ovary (a mass that has less than a 0.5% chance of representing a malignancy), both adnexa should be removed as prophylaxis against ovarian cancer or pathologic processes and gonadal metastasis from the gastrointestinal primary. These two scenarios, which represent extremes of the clinical continuum, serve to illustrate the need for a global clinical perspective. As noted previously, if ever doubt exists about how to proceed, gynecologic surgical consultation must be obtained.

TABLE 116.11 CLASSIFICATION

PATHOLOGIC TYPES OF OVARIAN CANCER

EPITHELIAL
Serous (mimics fallopian tube)
Mucinous (mimics endocervix)
Endometrioid (mimics endometrium)
Brenner's tumor (mimics urothelium)
GERM CELL
Primary gonadal choriocarcinoma
Immature teratoma
Dysgerminoma
Yolk sac tumor
SPECIALIZED GONADAL STROMAL LESIONS
Female directed
Granulosa-thecal cell tumors
Male directed
Sertoli-Leydig cell tumors
NONSPECIALIZED STROMAL TUMORS
Fibromas
Sarcomas
Mixed mesodermal tumors (carcinosarcoma)
METASTATIC LESIONS
Krukenberg's tumor (gastrointestinal)
Breast
Endometrium

Ovarian Cancer

Ovarian cancer, most commonly arising from the surface epithelium (Table 116.11), is the number one cause of death from a gynecologic malignancy in North America.[5] In the united States, this disease affects 1 of 70 American women who live into their ninth decade. Despite the lack of accurate screening methods, specific factors are known to uniquely increase the probability of epithelial ovarian cancer development (Table 116.12).

TABLE 116.12

RISK FACTORS FOR AND PREVENTION OF OVARIAN CANCER

INCREASES RISK
Early menarche
Late menopause
Long-term (>12 cycles) and high-dose ovulation induction
Lack of oral contraceptive use
Low parity
Advanced age (>30 y) at time of first term delivery
Lack of or late (>30 y of age) breast feeding
Personal or family history of breast, colon, or endometrial cancer
Perineal talc use
DECREASES RISK
Opposite of above, plusTubal ligation

TABLE 116.13 DIAGNOSIS

PRESENTING SYMPTOMS OF OVARIAN CANCER

Abdominal bloating and distention
Abdominal or pelvic pain
Pelvic pressure
Change in stool habits
Change in urinary habits
Abnormal vaginal bleeding

Of those women affected by ovarian cancer, most have the disease diagnosed when it has extended beyond the female reproductive tract and eventually succumb to their disease. The delay in diagnosis is secondary to several factors. First, the ovaries lie in a cavernous potential space (the female pelvis) where large structures can be hidden. Second, the ovaries are usually freely mobile, and symptoms of malignancy usually occur late. Last, as outlined in Table 116.13, the symptoms associated with ovarian cancer are nonspecific and commonly associated with other, significantly less morbid diseases (e.g., diverticulitis, degenerative joint disease). The lack of specific symptoms typically results in delay in referral to a gynecologic oncologist.

The classic findings of ovarian cancer are a fixed, tender, cystic, and solid pelvic mass in the woman at risk. Many women, however, lack these findings and present only with ascites or abdominal distention. Radiographic and invasive studies (i.e., colonoscopy) are more beneficial in eliminating the disease from the differential diagnosis than they are at definitively making the diagnosis of ovarian cancer. Diagnosis is made during surgical exploration, preferably in a setting where a skilled pelvic surgeon is available to perform an optimal procedure. The two critical guidelines for the surgical management of ovarian cancer are remove as much of the disease, if not all of the disease, as is possible; and if the disease appears to be limited to the pelvis, perform complete surgical staging (Table 116.14).

TABLE 116.14 DIAGNOSIS

STAGING PROCEDURES IN OVARIAN CANCER

Pelvic fluid collection (washings)
Bilateral paracolic gutter fluid collection (washings)
Upper abdomen (diaphragm surface) fluid collection (washings)
Bilateral ovarian fossa peritoneum biopsy
Cul-de-sac peritoneum biopsy
Bladder peritoneum biopsy
Bilateral paracolic gutter peritoneum biopsy
Appendectomy
Bilateral pelvic lymph node sampling (from the mid common iliac artery to the circumflex iliac artery in the cephalad—caudad dimension and from the genitofemoral nerve to the obturator nerve in the lateromedial dimension)
Bilateral paraaortic lymph node sampling (from the mid common iliacartery to the renal vein in the caudocephalad dimension, lateral to aorta and medial to the ureter)
Infracolic omentectomy
Diaphragm surface scrape (taken as a Papanicolaou smear)

It is imperative that the clinician remember that the only surgical variable that can have a direct effect on patient curability is the degree of debulking that was accomplished.[24] Although in cases with massive extrapelvic metastasis (>10 cm) controversy remains regarding the benefits of aggressive debulking, adequate data support its merit in all settings. The smaller the amount of tumor that is visibly left at the completion of the initial surgery, the more likely it is that cure will be obtained, once the surgeon has been able to debulk such that the maximal tumor nodule size is less than 2 cm. When residual disease is greater than 2 cm, the amount of disease remaining does not appear to make a difference because eventual failure is inevitable. Debulking frequently includes multiple bowel resections and the performance of retrograde radical hysterectomy, in which the entire pelvic tumor mass, including bladder, sidewall, cul-de-sac, peritoneum, and rectosigmoid, as needed, are removed in an extraperitoneal, ventral-to-dorsal technique. Splenectomy, total omentectomy, hepatic resection, diaphragm peritoneal stripping, and the like may all be necessary to obtain optimal debulking. The patient who has undergone extensive debulking for metastatic ovarian cancer is often critically ill after the procedure, with numerous abnormalities of fluid volume, blood components, and electrolytes. Just as there must be a commitment to adequate aggressive surgery, an intensive care unit and skilled intensivist must be available to help maintain the patient in the postoperative period.

Secondary Cytoreductive Surgery Recently published reviews have led to the development of guidelines for the use of secondary cytoreductive surgery.[25] This procedure, which has the potential for lengthening patients' lives in a meaningful way with acceptable operative morbidity, requires the utmost in surgical skill and judgment[26] (Table 116.15). If attempted in inappropriately selected patients or performed by less skilled surgeons, the procedure is more likely than not to lead to both a shortening of the patient's life and deterioration in the quality of that remaining life.

Second-look Procedures After completion of aggressive first-line therapy for epithelial ovarian cancer, accurate knowledge of the patient's disease status is beneficial. Symptom complexes, physical examinations, radiographic imaging, and biochemical markers are less than 60% accurate for determining actual disease status. Therefore, many experts believe that surgery is justified to obtain such data. The controversy surrounds not whether surgery is more accurate at making the diagnosis, but whether changes in treatment based on surgical findings make a difference in the patient's eventual outcome. We prefer to perform second-look procedures laparoscopically. The patient must be fully prepared to have the procedure converted to an open approach, either because of an operative complication or inability to perform the complete procedure using laparoscopic technique. At the time of a second-look

TABLE 116.15 TREATMENT

GUIDELINES FOR SECONDARY CYTOREDUCTIVE SURGERY

1. No prior "adequate" attempts at optimal cytoreductive surgery, *or*
2. Isolated lesion
3. Acceptable performance status
4. If disease is recurrent, a 6-month disease-free interval
5. Presence of further medical or radiotherapeutic options
6. Adequate informed consent

procedure, consideration should be given to the placement of an intraperitoneal access catheter so that further therapy, if deemed necessary or appropriated, can be administered directly into the peritoneal space.

Chemotherapy In all but the rarest cases, multiagent chemotherapy is not curative for ovarian cancer when administered without surgical debulking. Yet aggressive, adequate chemotherapy is an essential part of the algorithm for the successful management of ovarian cancer. Standards for ovarian cancer chemotherapy are fluid. As of the writing of this chapter, taxane or a platinum-containing regimen for six to nine cycles is the community standard.

KEY POINTS

- **A Bartholin's duct abscess is usually the result of infection with a sexually transmitted organism (predominantly gonorrhea) with the initial treatment consisting of antibiotics and antiinflammatory measures.**
- **The standard treatment of vulvar carcinoma includes local radical resection of the primary lesion (2-cm margin) and removal of at-risk lymph nodes with a unilateral superficial groin dissection**
- **Deficiencies of pelvic support may involve the anterior compartment (urethrocele, hypermobile urethrovesical junction, cystocele), mid-compartment (descent of the cervix or uterine corpus) or posterior compartment (enterocele or rectocele) and may frequently have a mixed pattern of dysfunction.**
- **Human papillomavirus (HPV) infection is a responsible co-agent in nearly 100% of cervical precancerous lesions or cancer.**
- **Women with precancerous lesions of the uterine cervix (CIN II or III) have a 3% to 10% chance of harboring occult cancer and a 30% chance of progressing to invasive disease if untreated.**
- **Uterine perforation can result in direct injury both to the uterine wall and to surrounding structures (bowel, vessels, adnexa).**
- **Uterine leiomyomata are nonmalignant, nonprecancerous overgrowths of uterine smooth muscle that can be treated by hormonal therapy, either definitive (hysterectomy) or nondefinitive (myomectomy) surgical treatment, or more recently uterine artery embolization.**
- **The treatment of adnexal torsion in the premenopausal woman, in all but extreme cases of necrosis, is to reverse the torsion and fix the adnexa usually to the psoas muscle tendon.**
- **Adnexal masses presenting in the extremes or life should be considered malignant until proved otherwise, whereas during the reproductive years they should be considered benign.**
- **Critical guidelines of surgical management of ovarian cancer include (a) remove as much of, if not all of, the disease as possible; and (b) if the disease appears limited to the pelvis, perform complete surgical staging.**

References

1. Sexually transmitted diseases treatment guidelines 2002. Centers for Disease Control and Prevention. *MMWR Recomm Rep.* 2002;51:1–78.
2. Kiryu H, Ackerman AB. A critique of current classifications of vulvar diseases. *Am J Dermatopathol.* 1990;12:377–392.
3. Basta A, Adamek K, Pitynski K. Intraepithelial neoplasia and early stage vulvar cancer. Epidemiological, clinical and virological observations. *Eur J Gynaecol Oncol.* 1999;20:111–114.
4. Junge J, Poulsen H, Horn T, et al. Human papillomavirus (HPV) in vulvar dysplasia and carcinoma in situ. *APMIS* 1995;103:501–510.
5. Greenlee RT, Murray T, Bolden S, Wingo PA. Cancer statistics, 2000. *CA Cancer J Clin.* 2000;50:7–33.
6. **Morgan MA, Mikuta JJ. Surgical management of vulvar cancer. *Semin Surg Oncol.* 1999;17:168–172.**
7. **Levenback C. Intraoperative lymphatic mapping and sentinel node identification: gynecologic applications. *Recent Results Cancer Res.* 2000;157:150–158.**
8. Keys HM, Bundy BN, Stehman FB, et al. Cisplatin, radiation, and adjuvant hysterectomy compared with radiation and adjuvant hysterectomy for bulky stage IB cervical carcinoma. *N Engl J Med.* 1999;340:154–161.
9. Rose PG, Bundy BN, Watkins EB, et al. Concurrent cisplatin-based radiotherapy and chemotherapy for locally advanced cervical cancer. *N Engl J Med.* 1999;340:1144–1153.
10. Whitney CW, Sause W, Bundy BN, et al. Randomized comparison of fluorouracil plus cisplatin versus hydroxyurea as an adjunct to radiation therapy in stage IIB-IVA carcinoma of the cervix with negative para-aortic lymph nodes: a Gynecologic Oncology Group and Southwest Oncology Group study. *J Clin Oncol.* 1999;17:1339–1348.
11. Wheeless CR Jr. Neovagina constructed from an omental J flap and a split thickness skin graft. *Gynecol Oncol.* 1989;35:224–226.
12. Bump RC, Mattiasson A, Bo K, et al. The standardization of terminology of female pelvic organ prolapse and pelvic floor dysfunction. *Am J Obstet Gynecol.* 1996;175:10–17.
13. Videla FL, Wall LL. Stress incontinence diagnosed without multichannel urodynamic studies. *Obstet Gynecol.* 1998;91:965–968.
14. **Keane DP, Eckford SD, Abrams P. Surgical treatment and complications of urinary incontinence. *Curr Opin Obstet Gynecol.* 1992;4:559–564.**
15. Wright TC Jr, Cox JT, Massad LS, et al. 2001 Consensus Guidelines for the management of women with cervical cytological abnormalities. *JAMA* 2002;287:2120–2129.
16. **Piver MS, Rutledge F, Smith JP. Five classes of extended hysterectomy for women with cervical cancer. *Obstet Gynecol.* 1974;44:265–272.**
17. Dargent D, Martin X, Sacchetoni A, et al. Laparoscopic vaginal radical trachelectomy: a treatment to preserve the fertility of cervical carcinoma patients. *Cancer* 2000;88:1877–1882.
18. Estape R, Angioli R. Surgical management of advanced and recurrent cervical cancer. *Semin Surg Oncol.* 1999;16:236–241.
19. The American Fertility Society classifications of adnexal adhesions, distal tubal occlusion, tubal occlusion secondary to tubal ligation, tubal pregnancies, mullerian anomalies and intrauterine adhesions. *Fertil Steril.* 1988;49:944–955.
20. Barbieri RL. Ambulatory management of uterine leiomyomata. *Clin Obstet Gynecol.* 1999;42:196–205.
21. Spies JB, Ascher SA, Roth AR, et al. Uterine artery embolization for leiomyomata. *Obstet Gynecol.* 2001;98:29–34.
22. Goodwin SC, McLucas B, Lee M, et al. Uterine artery embolization for the treatment of uterine leiomyomata midterm results. *J Vasc Interv Radiol.* 1999;10:1159–1165.
23. Worthen NJ, Gunning JE. Percutaneous drainage of pelvic abscesses: management of the tubo-ovarian abscess. *J Ultrasound Med.* 1986;5:551–556.
24. **Dauplat J, Le Bouedec G, Pomel C, et al. Cytoreductive surgery for advanced stages of ovarian cancer. *Semin Surg Oncol.* 2000;19:42–48.**
25. Roberts WS. Cytoreductive surgery in ovarian cancer: why, when, and how? *Cancer Control.* 1996;3:130–136.
26. Eisenkop SM, Friedman RL, Spirtos NM. The role of secondary cytoreductive surgery in the treatment of patients with recurrent epithelial ovarian carcinoma. *Cancer* 2000;88:144–153.
27. Federation Internationale de Gynecologie et d'Obstetrique. Annual report on the results of treatment in gynaecological cancers. *J Epidemiol Biostat.* 1998;3:1–168.
28. Lurain J. Endometrial cancer. In: JS Berek EA, PA Hillard, eds. *Novak's gynecology.* Baltimore: Williams & Wilkins, 1996.

CHAPTER 117 ■ THE PREGNANT PATIENT

N. SCOTT ADZICK AND ALEXANDER S. KRUPNICK

Four million pregnancies occur annually in the United States. Despite the continuous presence of this patient population, little emphasis has been placed on educating the general surgeon in the diagnosis and treatment of surgical problems in the pregnant patient. Although obstetricians routinely deal with pregnancy-related maternal disease and gynecologic surgery, few training programs expose the gynecologist to the wide array of surgical problems of the alimentary tract or the signs and symptoms of nongynecologic disease. The general surgeon is often called on in this situation, and it is imperative that he or she understands the normal physiologic changes occurring during pregnancy as well as the presentation of surgical disease. Often the surgeon is the first person to evaluate a pregnant patient with abdominal pain, or learns of the pregnancy during the initial workup. Because the incidence of surgical disease does not disappear in pregnancy but simply changes its frequency and nature of presentation, the surgeon must be aware of these variations as well as conversant with the safety and utility of diagnostic tests and imaging modalities. Pathways and algorithms for diagnosis and treatment of diseases in the nonpregnant woman must be altered to ensure the safety and well-being of the fetus as well as that of the mother. The purpose of this chapter is to review the current data on the presentation, frequency, and treatment of some common surgical diseases during pregnancy, as well as their adverse effects on the pregnancy. Pregnancy is the only time when surgical decisions directly affect the lives of two people, and although mistakes can be twice as costly, rewards can double.

FETAL DEVELOPMENT

Human development begins immediately on fertilization of the oocyte by the sperm, but because it is impossible to determine the exact time of fertilization, the age of development is calculated from the first day of the last menstrual period. The *embryonic period* refers to these earliest stages of development and extends to the end of the eighth week, by which time organogenesis has occurred. Although the rudimentary precursors of all major organ systems are present at this point, only the circulatory system and the heart are functional. The fetal period lasts from the ninth week to birth. During this period, growth and development of tissues formed during embryogenesis occur in preparation for birth.[1] The effect of teratogenic drugs or radiation can vary drastically, depending on the period of exposure.

Survival outside the womb depends on the adaptation of fetal organ systems for independent function at the time of birth. Because oxygen exchange and respiration are critical to immediate survival, the functional status of the respiratory system is crucial in determining fetal viability. Surfactant, a complex mixture of phospholipids consisting mostly of phosphatidylcholine, is necessary for reduction of surface tension at the alveolar–air interface and proper oxygen exchange. Surfactant production begins by the 20th week of gestation but is present in only small amounts before 24 weeks.[1] Although the survival rate of infants born at 24 weeks of development is dismal, the mortality rate before that time is nearly 100% (Fig. 117.1). The delivery of a fetus before this period of potential viability, whether spontaneous or induced, is termed an *abortion,* whereas delivery after this period is defined as a *premature birth.*

One of the most significant advances in the reduction of morbidity of prematurity has been the use of corticosteroids to accelerate organ maturation. Binding of corticosteroids in the fetal lung not only increases secretion of phosphatidylcholine but also induces morphologic development of pulmonary epithelial cells and increases neonatal lung compliance. Corticosteroids stimulate development of other organ systems as well, decreasing the incidence of necrotizing enterocolitis in the premature intestine and intraventricular hemorrhage of the premature brain. The maximum developmental effects can be seen as early as 24 hours after maternal administration of dexamethasone or betamethasone, and administration at the first sign of premature onset of labor can improve survival.[2]

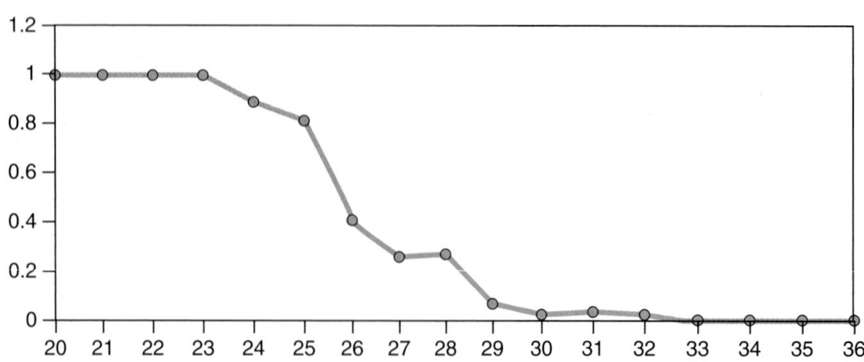

FIGURE 117.1 Multicenter analysis of preterm mortality based on gestational age. (After Copper RL, Goldenberg RL, Creasy RK, et al. A multicenter study of preterm birth weight and gestational age-specific neonatal mortality. *Am J Obstet Gynecol.* 1993;168:78–84, with permission.)

UTERINE ANATOMY AND PHYSIOLOGY OF LABOR

The uterus is a muscular organ responsible for reception, implantation, development, and expulsion of the fetus. In the nonpregnant woman, the uterus is an exclusively pelvic organ weighing approximately 70 g with a cavity volume of 10 mL. During pregnancy, the uterus gradually becomes an intraabdominal organ weighing close to 1,100 g and expanding to a total volume of 5 L.

By the 12th week of gestation, the uterus becomes too large to reside exclusively in the pelvis and extends into the abdominal cavity. By the 20th week, the uterine fundus reaches the umbilicus, and by the third trimester it reaches almost to the liver[3] (Fig. 117.2). As the uterus continues to rise, it exerts pressure on the anterior abdominal wall, displaces the intestines superiorly and laterally, and changes the relationship between the abdominal visceral organs. In the upright position, the uterus is supported by the anterior abdominal wall and usually undergoes a dextrorotation because of the presence of the rectosigmoid on the left. In the supine position, most of the uterine weight falls on the spinal column, but compression of the surrounding great vessels, especially the flaccid inferior vena cava, also occurs.

Uterine activity and contractions are coupled to the electrical changes in the myometrium, which is physiologically arranged to maximize the efficiency of uterine contraction and expulsion of the fetus at term. The resting membrane potential of the uterine myocyte ranges from –40 to –60 mV. It becomes more negative (–60 mV) early in gestation and increases to –40 mV near term. Early in pregnancy, the myometrium exhibits irregular electrical activity termed *slow waves*. These rhythmic alterations in the membrane potential occasionally reach the threshold potential and lead to an action potential at the top of the slow wave. Entry of Ca^{2+} through voltage-sensitive Ca^{2+} channels allows for actin—myosin interaction and electromechanical coupling, leading to uterine contraction. By the second trimester, these irregular contractions can be palpated through the abdominal wall and are known as *Braxton Hicks contractions*.[4] Irregular contractions during pregnancy lead to relatively small increases in uterine pressure, but at term are replaced by coordinated, purposeful contractions generating pressures up to 80 mm Hg. Gap junctions allow for electrical and metabolic communication between uterine myocytes, and the onset of labor is preceded by an increase in the number of gap junctions.

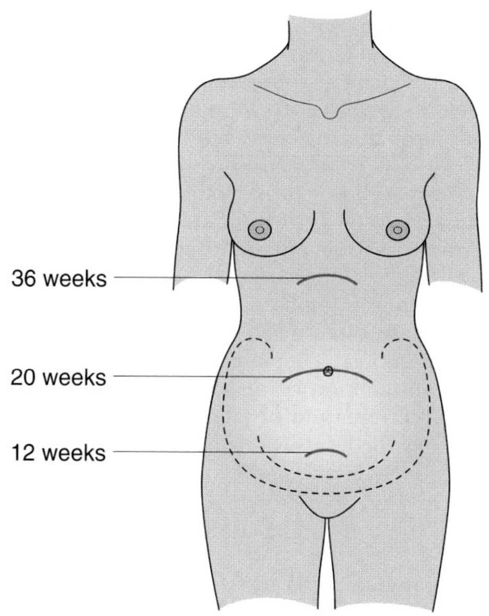

FIGURE 117.2 Enlarging uterus during gestation. At 12 weeks, the uterus rises out of the pelvis into the abdomen. At 20 weeks, the fundus is at the height of the umbilicus, and at 36 weeks the uterus reaches to the upper abdomen.

TABLE 117.1

MEDIATORS OF UTERINE ACTIVITY

Stimulates uterine activity	Down-regulates uterine activity
Estrogen Oxytocin PGE_2, $PGF_{2\alpha}$ IL-1, IL-6	Progesterone

IL, interleukin; PG, prostaglandin.

The mechanisms behind human parturition are being unraveled. Numerous hormones, peptides, and local mediators act on the myometrium both to stimulate and down-regulate its activity (Table 117.1). Parturition begins when forces favoring uterine activity override those of quiescence and tip the balance toward contraction and birth. Progesterone maintains uterine relaxation during most of pregnancy by blocking Ca^{2+} flux through cell membranes and opposing the action of estrogen. Close to term, the concentration of estrogen increases relative to that of progesterone, leading to uterine activation. Synthesis and surface expression of contraction-associated proteins, including gap junctions, ion channels, and oxytocin receptors, is initiated and the uterus is transformed from its pliable, relaxed state to one of responsiveness and excitability. A shift in arachidonic acid metabolism from lipoxygenase products to those of cyclooxygenase, especially prostaglandin (PG) E_2 and PGF_{2a}, favors activation of the uterine musculature as well as the onset of uterine contractions. Prostaglandins raise local Ca^{2+} concentrations by increasing Ca^{2+} flux across cell membrane and stimulating Ca^{2+} release from intracellular stores. Inflammatory cytokines, especially interleukin (IL)-1 and IL-6, are produced locally by placental tissues and act in concert with other stimulatory factors to propagate uterine activity.[5,6]

Oxytocin is a nonapeptide synthesized in the hypothalamus and secreted from the posterior pituitary. Its name means "quick birth," and it was the first uterotonin to be implicated in parturition. Oxytocin stimulates Ca^{2+} flux across myometrial plasma membranes and has distinct receptors located in the myometrium and other reproductive tissues. Uterine responsiveness to oxytocin is directly related to receptor concentration, which can increase 300-fold during pregnancy. The surface expression of oxytocin receptors is increased by maternal estrogen and opposed by progesterone. Although it was originally isolated from the posterior pituitary, the placental content of oxytocin is approximately five times that of the pituitary, and the placenta is most likely the main source of oxytocin during pregnancy and parturition.[5]

The timing of birth is regulated by an internal placental clock based on corticotropin-releasing hormone (CRH). CRH is a 41-amino-acid peptide normally found in the hypothalamus. Its action on the pituitary causes secretion of adrenocorticotropic hormone, which in turn increases secretion of cortisol from adrenal tissue. In the nonpregnant woman, cortisol forms part of a negative feedback system acting on the hypothalamus and pituitary to dampen CRH secretion and down-regulate cortisol levels. In the pregnant woman, CRH seems to

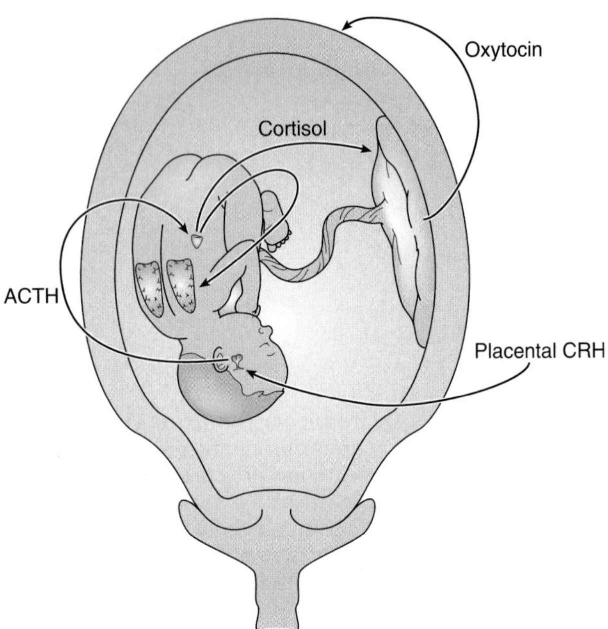

FIGURE 117.3 Positive feedback loops initiated by corticotropin-releasing hormone potentiate parturition.

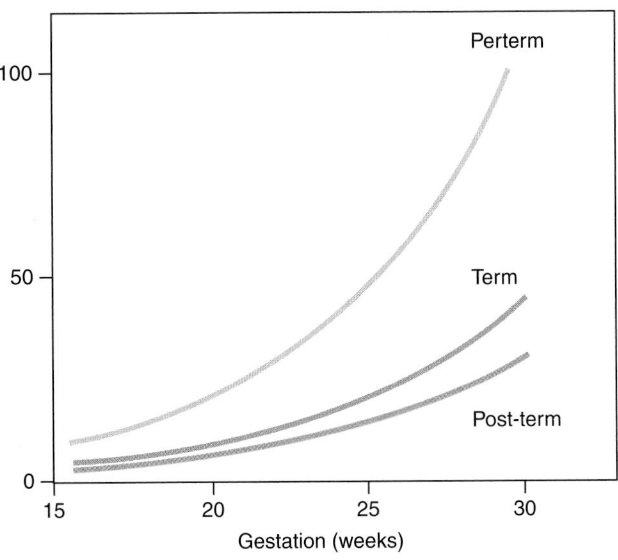

FIGURE 117.4 Corticotropin-releasing hormone concentration (pmol/L) varies during gestation based on timing of delivery. (From McLean M, Bisits A, Davies J, et al. A placental clock controlling the length of human pregnancy. *Nat Med.* 1995;1:460–463, with permission.)

have a different function. During pregnancy, the concentration of CRH gradually rises. Although it is produced by both the fetal and the maternal hypothalamus, most of the CRH orchestrating delivery originates from the placenta itself. Placental CRH is in a perfect position to coordinate timing of fetal lung maturity and uterine preparation for delivery. Once concentration reaches a critical level, CRH acts on the fetal hypothalamic–pituitary–adrenal (HPA) axis to increase fetal cortisol production. Increased levels of cortisol stimulate fetal lung maturation and surfactant production in preparation for oxygen exchange. Fetal cortisol also acts on placental tissue, increasing the expression of enzymes responsible for production of estrogen, shifting the balance of steroidogenesis away from progesterone production.[6] Rather than acting in a negative feedback fashion, as would be expected in the hypothalamus, cortisol actually up-regulates placental CRH production as part of a positive feedback loop. CRH and cortisol also increase prostaglandin and oxytocin production by the placenta, and these substances in turn act locally to up-regulate CRH secretion further, forming another positive feedback loop (Fig. 117.3). CRH itself contributes to uterine contractions and can potentiate contractions by other substances such as oxytocin. The culmination of these actions leads to expected uterine activation and parturition.

Secretion of CRH is regulated by an internal clock, with production increasing steadily throughout pregnancy. Maternal levels of CRH detected as early as 16 to 20 weeks of pregnancy can be used to predict when the woman will give birth (Fig. 117.4). Mothers with the highest levels tend to deliver prematurely, whereas those with the lowest levels are more likely to deliver past term.[7] Although proper coordination between the placenta and fetal HPA axis can lead to the timely birth of a fetus able to survive outside the womb, maternal illness or intraabdominal inflammation can disturb the system.

PREMATURE ONSET OF LABOR

Premature labor consists of premature uterine contractions producing cervical change. A premature birth is defined as one occurring before 37 weeks from the first day of the last menstrual period.[8] Although only 10% of all births fit this criterion, prematurity is responsible for 83% of all neonatal mortality and most of the morbidity and cost of neonatal care.[9] Survival has increased with improvement in neonatal intensive care units, but the premature infant still experiences a wide variety of ailments with long-term sequelae in many organ systems. The cause of preterm labor is often multifactorial, but the onset of labor from fetal and uterine stress during surgical manipulation or intraabdominal inflammatory processes is of most concern to the surgeon.

Early activation of the fetal HPA axis can take place in response to fetal stress. An adverse uterine environment caused by hypoxemia or maternal shock leads to increased expression of CRH in the fetal hypothalamus. Levels of cortisol rise and its activity on the local environment leads to uterine activation along with fetal lung maturation. Increased prostaglandin production in the presence of an infective process can also activate preterm labor. Bacterial infection of the amniotic tissues or peritoneum leads to a local increase in eicosanoids and the onset of labor.[10] Endotoxin acts on inflammatory cells to increase production of IL-1 and IL-6, which also amplify local prostaglandin production. All these factors can act in concert to initiate and propagate preterm labor. Uterine activation and increased expression of gap junctions as well as oxytocin receptors can be induced by uterine stretch.[6,11] Uterine trauma caused by surgical manipulation could affect these same mechanisms, leading to premature uterine contractions. The interrelations at various levels between the inflammatory response, uterine and maternal trauma, and the initiation of labor can represent the body's attempt to expel the fetus from a hostile uterine environment.

Tocolysis

Tocolytic therapy attempts to reverse or alleviate the premature onset and progression of labor while the underlying inflammatory cause is corrected. By understanding the basic physiology of both premature and term labor, pharmacologic manipulation of the system can be attempted to prevent the progression of premature uterine contractions to premature labor and premature delivery. Even if delivery cannot be avoided, simply extending gestation by 1 or 2 days can allow exogenous steroids to promote fetal lung development and surfactant secretion, decreasing the risk of respiratory distress syndrome and multiorgan failure in the preterm neonate. Prostaglandin synthesis inhibitors, magnesium sulfate, β-adrenergic agonists, and calcium channel blockers are the four most common pharmacologic agents used as tocolytics.

Because of the importance of prostaglandins in the initiation of uterine contraction, prostaglandin synthetase inhibitors, especially nonsteroidal antiinflammatory drugs, are used to stop premature labor. Indomethacin is the nonsteroidal drug used most frequently for tocolysis because of its quick onset of action and ease of dosing. Studies report a 95% tocolytic success rate at 48 hours and a potential delay in delivery of 1 week in 80% of patients.[12] Magnesium sulfate, long used in the treatment of preeclampsia, has now gained acceptance as a tocolytic agent. It is often the first-line agent used once the onset of premature contractions is documented. Most data support the theory that magnesium exerts its effects by calcium antagonism. High intracellular magnesium concentrations inhibit Ca^{2+} entry into myometrial cells, interfering with actin–myosin coupling. High magnesium concentrations also increase the sensitivity of K^+ channels, favoring hyperpolarization and uterine relaxation. Maternal serum levels necessary to inhibit myometrial contractility range between 4 and 9 mg/dL, two to six times normal levels, and are difficult to achieve with oral administration alone. Success with magnesium tocolysis for 24 hours is possible in 96% of patients, 48 hours in 70% of patients, and up to 1 week in 49% of patients.[13] β_2-Adrenergic agonists used in the treatment of preterm labor include ritodrine and terbutaline. Stimulation of uterine β_2 receptors leads to activation of adenylate cyclase and an increase in intracellular cyclic adenosine monophosphate (cAMP) concentration. Activation of cAMP-dependent protein kinase A inhibits myosin light-chain phosphorylation and actin–myosin coupling. Protein kinase A activity is also associated with increased Ca^{2+} efflux, decreased Ca^{2+} influx, and increased K^+ conductance. All these actions lead to myometrial relaxation.[4] Calcium channel blockers inhibit entry of calcium through voltage-dependent Ca^{2+} channels. The use of oral nifedipine can abolish uterine activity and prevent delivery with minimal toxicity and side effects.[14]

Although the success of tocolysis in preventing or delaying premature birth varies based on cause, no foolproof combination of drugs has been globally successful in all cases of premature labor. Maternal and fetal side effects can be serious and close observation is necessary with all forms of tocolysis. Premature constriction of the fetal ductus arteriosus with the use of indomethacin has been reported and can result in fatal neonatal pulmonary hypertension.[15] Maternal cardiovascular side effects, including pulmonary edema, can occur in 5% of β_2 agonist users and 10% of those treated with magnesium. Although this complication is rare, it can result in maternal death. Serum concentrations of magnesium needed for tocolysis (4 to 9 mg/dL) are not far from levels causing ablation of deep tendon reflexes (9 to 13 mg/dL) or respiratory depression (14 mg/dL). The decision to use tocolytics must be made only after the diagnosis of premature onset of labor is confirmed and the benefits of prolonging gestation outweigh the risks of tocolysis. Initiation of tocolytic therapy for potential but unconfirmed preterm labor is discouraged.[8]

FETAL MONITORING

Perioperative fetal monitoring as well as the monitoring of premature uterine contractions is based on technology developed for fetal monitoring during birth. As early as 1862, it was suspected that fetal distress during birth and prolonged, difficult labor led to infantile spastic palsies. Experimental data in primate fetuses have shown that prolonged hypoxemia and acidemia produces anatomic lesions in the brain similar to those seen in human cerebral palsy.[16] Sublethal asphyxia of the fetus can also lead to multisystem dysfunction, including conduction defects of the heart, ischemic mucosal injury to the gastrointestinal tract, necrotizing enterocolitis, and impaired surfactant production and respiratory distress of the newborn. Interventions to reduce the incidence of fetal hypoxemia and acidemia reduce the incidence of these and other disorders.[17]

Evaluation of fetal oxygenation and acid–base status is possible by direct sampling of arterial pH from the umbilical artery or capillary blood sampling of the fetal scalp. Both techniques demand access to the fetus through a dilated, open cervix with crowning of the scalp, through a hysterotomy during fetal surgery, or through the maternal abdomen during percutaneous umbilical blood sampling. Because such exposure is not available during most surgical procedures, monitoring of fetal oxygenation is based on other indirect methods. In the late 1950s and early 1960s, the relationship between fetal heart rate patterns and fetal stability was demonstrated.[18] Established heart rate patterns and variable cardiac responses to fetal and maternal stimuli reflect an intact, well oxygenated central nervous system (CNS). Deviation from these patterns can indicate fetal distress or impending compromise.

Electronic fetal heart rate monitoring has gained wide acceptance and as of the early 1990s was used in 79% of all pregnancies.[17] Direct fetal monitoring is used intrapartum and relies on analysis of fetal cardiac patterns from electrocardiogram leads placed directly on the exposed part of the fetus. A transcervical intrauterine pressure catheter is concurrently placed to monitor the strength of uterine contractions. Indirect monitoring methods are used when access to the uterine cavity and fetus is not available, and fetal heart rate analysis is performed with Doppler ultrasound applied to the maternal abdomen or transvaginally while a surface tocodynamometer detects uterine contractions (Fig. 117.5). Both tracings are printed on a continuous strip of paper, with the fetal heart rate plotted at the top of the graph and uterine activity at the bottom.

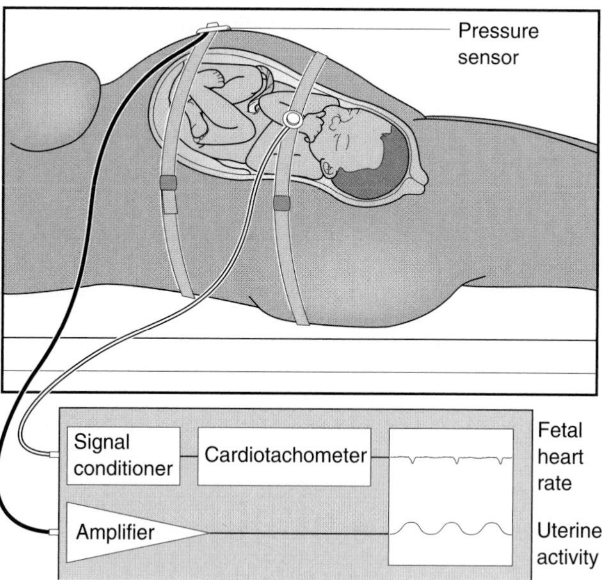

FIGURE 117.5 Intraoperative and postoperative fetal monitoring using noninvasive surface Doppler and pressure sensor to monitor uterine contractions.

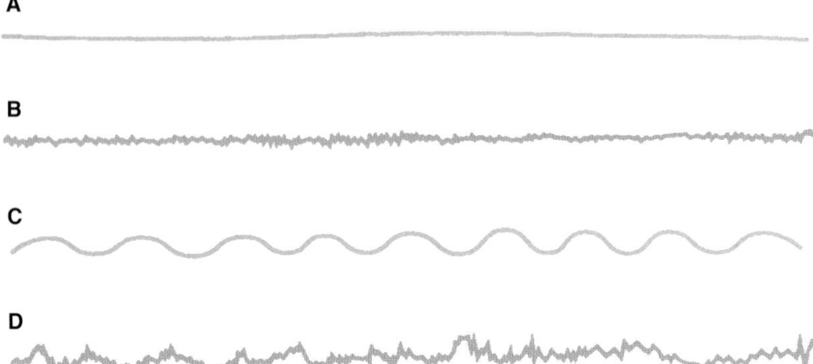

FIGURE 117.6 Fetal heart variability. (*A*) Short-term and long-term variability both absent: abnormal. (*B*) Short-term variability present, long-term variability absent: abnormal. (*C*) Long-term variability present, short-term variability absent: abnormal. (*D*) Both short- and long-term variability present: normal.

Fetal Heart Rate

Normal fetal heart rate during pregnancy ranges between 120 and 160 beats/min. A prolonged baseline above 160 beats per minute is considered a tachycardia, whereas that below 120 beats per minute is a bradycardia. These terms refer to long-term patterns, and minute-to-minute variability in the heart rate away from baseline is known as *acceleration* and *deceleration*. Changes in blood pressure and oxygenation are detected by the chemoreceptors and baroreceptors of the aortic arch and carotid bodies, resulting in a change in the heart rate to maintain a steady state. Normal, healthy fetal heart rate tracings express continuous adjustment in the vagal tone through variability in the heart rate. Short-term, or beat-to-beat, variability is superimposed on broader, long-term variability of the baseline by 3 to 5 beats per minute. The fetal heart rate response governed by a nonacidotic, well-functioning vagal conduction system manifests both long-term and short-term variability with fluctuations of peaks and troughs ranging from 6 to 25 beats per minute (Fig. 117.6). Decreased heart rate variability, either long or short term, can signal diminished CNS activity. Although this can be a physiologic response of the fetal sleep–wake cycle or maternal medication and sedatives, persistently decreased reactivity can signal CNS acidosis. This is particularly true if combined with other findings suggestive of hypoxia. Fetal heart rate accelerations are normal findings in the second half of pregnancy and occur as a result of increased sympathetic stimulation and decreased parasympathetic stimulation with fetal movements. Vibroacoustic stimulation of the fetus for 5 seconds at 2,000 Hz through the mother's abdomen can provoke fetal movement with resultant heart rate acceleration.[19] Failure of this response suggests fetal hypoxia. A sinusoidal heart rate pattern is an uncommon baseline abnormality also suggestive of fetal distress. It has the characteristics of a smooth sine wave with little beat-to-beat variability, long-term variability with a frequency of 2 to 5 cycles per minute, and amplitude of 5 to 15 beats per minute. This pattern has been associated with anencephaly, fetal anemia, and hypoxia (Fig. 117.7).

Fetal heart rate decelerations are usually encountered during uterine contractions of the intrapartum period. Evaluation of decelerations during birth and as part of postoperative fetal monitoring can give clues to the status of the placental blood supply. Early decelerations are uniform, shallow drops in the fetal heart rate that mirror uterine contractions and reflect increased vagal tone from a transient increase in intracranial pressure. This pattern is considered a benign physiologic manifestation of a functioning autonomic nervous system, and has no adverse outcome. Variable decelerations result from umbilical cord compression by uterine contractions. Isolated variable decelerations have little clinical significance, but if persistent with inadequate recovery between contractions, fetal hypoxemia and acidosis can occur. Variable decelerations can also indicate pathologic cord compression from either a prolapsed or nuchal cord. Late decelerations signify a significant deficit in fetal oxygen supply; causes can range from maternal hypotension caused by inferior vena cava compression to hypoxia or anemia. Persistent late decelerations warrant quick investigation to correct the cause or emergently deliver the child by cesarean section.[17]

Fetal heart rate patterns offer noninvasive clues to uterine oxygenation and fetal blood supply. Utility of both fetal heart rate and uterine contraction monitoring lies in the ability to intervene based on the acquired information. Progression of premature labor despite maximum tocolysis may necessitate adding a second tocolytic agent or starting corticosteroids to assist fetal lung maturation before the premature birth. Intraoperative fetal distress as indicated by an ominous heart rate tracing must be treated by correcting maternal hypotension or increasing oxygen delivery with increased fraction of inspired oxygen (Fio_2), blood transfusion, or more aggressive fluid resuscitation. The inability to improve the intrauterine milieu can necessitate an emergent cesarean section to prevent fetal demise. Continuous fetal monitoring is unnecessary if the ability to intervene is limited. Because the chances of survival before 24 weeks of gestation are close to zero, emergent delivery at this stage is not warranted. The inability to improve uterine perfusion because of maternal extremis could make fetal monitoring futile, simply adding an extra variable to the care of an already complicated patient. By understanding the principles and indications for intraoperative and postoperative fetal monitoring, the surgeon can provide an improved level of care for both mother and unborn child.

IMAGING MODALITIES IN THE PREGNANT PATIENT

Advances in radiology have revolutionized surgical practice. By visualizing the lesion before exploration, surgical intervention can focus on the area of disease or avoid it altogether. The choice of imaging modalities in the pregnant patient is difficult because of the real and perceived danger to the developing fetus. Risks of ionizing radiation can force the physician to avoid the definitive diagnostic study of choice and inadvertently put both the mother and fetus in greater danger from misdiagnosis. Although experimental data regarding the effects of ionizing radiation on the developing human fetus are impossible to obtain, animal exposure and follow-up of those inadvertently exposed to radiation have provided some information. Retrospective studies of atomic bomb survivors in Hiroshima and Nagasaki have also allowed for evaluation of the effects of massive radiation exposure *in utero*.

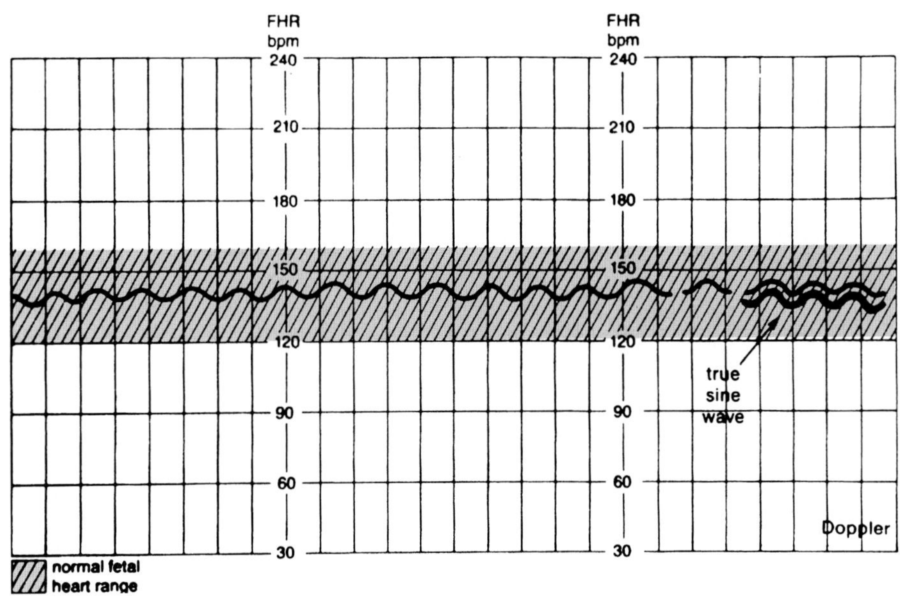

FIGURE 117.7 A sinusoidal pattern is one of several heart rate patterns indicating potential fetal hypoxia.

Ionizing Radiation

Fetal effects of ionizing radiation depend on the dose absorbed by the fetal tissue and the stage of fetal development during exposure. Exposure is defined as the amount of ionic charge created by the radiation on passing through a defined mass of air. The roentgen is a common unit of exposure, producing 0.26 millicoulomb per kilogram of air or 2 billion ion pairs per cubic centimeter of exposed air.[20] Although exposure is useful for measuring radiation output, the absorbed dose is the radiation imparted to tissue that creates a biologic effect. One gray (Gy) is strictly defined as the deposition of 1.0 joule of energy per kilogram of tissue, and 1 rad, another measure of absorbed dose, is 1% of 1 Gy. As a gross estimate, exposure to 1 roentgen gives an absorbed dose of 1 rad or 10 mGy.

It is a misconception to assume that the radiation absorbed by the mother is the same as that absorbed by the fetus. Dosing of radiation to the uterus and conceptus can vary severalfold based on abdominal wall depth, the anteverted or retroverted position of the uterus, or whether the exposure is in the anteroposterior or posteroanterior direction. Radiographic evaluation of the abdomen and pelvis is most likely to expose the fetus to direct ionizing radiation, whereas examination of the extremities and chest leads to exposure from scatter radiation only[20] (Table 117.2).

TABLE 117.2

RADIATION DOSING TO THE CONCEPTUS AND UTERUS FROM SELECTED RADIOGRAPHIC EXAMINATIONS

Examination	Dose (mrad)
Routine chest radiograph	8–50
Routine mammography	<50
Computed tomography, chest (uterus shielded and not exposed)	25–1,000
Computed tomography, upper abdomen (uterus shielded and not exposed)	670–3,000
Computed tomography, abdomen	2,000–3,000
Abdomen (flat plate)	250–300
Endoscopic retrograde cholangiopancreatography with no permanent films and shielding of abdomen	4

Radiation-induced ionization of vital cellular structures can result in cellular death or lasting genetic mutations in the DNA. Cellular destruction either leads to the death of the embryo if a significant amount of tissue is affected or has no effect if the damaged cells are replaced by healthy ones. Growth impairment of organs occurs if the population of cells cannot be replaced or damage occurs to a small population of progenitor cells at a vital stage of development. All these effects are produced at threshold doses, and exposure to radiation levels below the threshold does not have biologic consequences compared with control populations.[21] The outcome of radiation exposure depends on the absorbed dose and the stage of development during exposure, with potential death early in gestation, teratogenesis during organogenesis, and growth retardation or leukemic potential at later gestational stages.

Lethal Effects

The multicellular embryo, before the blastocyst stage, is most sensitive to the lethal effects of radiation but resistant to teratogenesis and growth retardation if it survives. The cause of this phenomenon is uncertain but could relate to the totipotent nature of the embryo at this stage and its ability indiscriminately to replace a specific volume of tissue below the lethal threshold. Because 50% to 75% of all human pregnancies abort, mostly without any recognition that fertilization has even occurred,[22] determining the lethal dose of radiation at this stage is difficult. Exposure of rat embryos to ionizing radiation at various stages of gestation reveals a maximum 10% mortality rate at 30 rads and 65% mortality rate at 150 rads. The lethal effects of 30 rads are seen only before implantation, returning to baseline levels after 1 week (Fig. 117.8). Both of these doses are orders of magnitude higher than those used for most diagnostic studies.

Teratogenic Effects

Teratogenic effects of radiation can be seen during early organogenesis in animal studies. Exposure of rats to 100 rads at various points of development reveals a very narrow window for teratogenesis (Fig. 117.9). This window corresponds to weeks 2 to 4 in human development, consistent with early organ formation. Despite these experimental data, it is difficult to link any specific human malformation with radiation exposure other than those of the CNS. Microcephaly, pigmentary changes in the retina, hydrocephalus, and optic nerve atrophy have been reported at a significantly higher rate after exposure

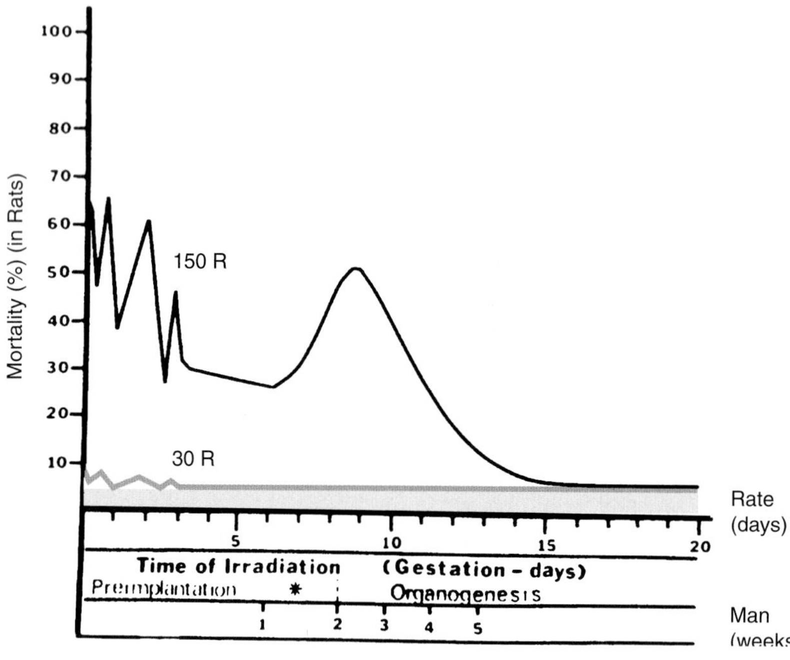

FIGURE 117.8 Mortality in rats exposed to 150 and 30 rads during various points in gestation. The embryo is most sensitive early in gestation. Human embryonic timetable is provided for comparison purposes only. (From Brent RL. The effects of embryonic and fetal exposure to x-ray, microwaves, and ultrasound. *Clin Obstet Gynecol.* 1983;26:488, with permission.)

to radiation in pregnancy.[23] All patients were exposed to a minimum estimated dose of 100 rads, and no visceral, limb, or other malformations were found unless the child also exhibited CNS abnormalities. One explanation for this discrepancy is that the developmental period of the CNS is much longer, continuing throughout gestation and into the neonatal period, whereas other organs have a very narrow period during which morphologic alterations can be produced. Exposure to high doses of radiation during this narrow window is rare, and even if an isolated congenital abnormality were to occur, it would be difficult to separate this event from the background malformation rate. The extended period for CNS sensitivity to teratogenesis increases the prevalence of CNS malformation. CNS malformation also occurs at threshold doses, however, and low levels of exposure to 10 to 20 rads of radiation do not increase the incidence of microcephaly in experimental animals over baseline.[21]

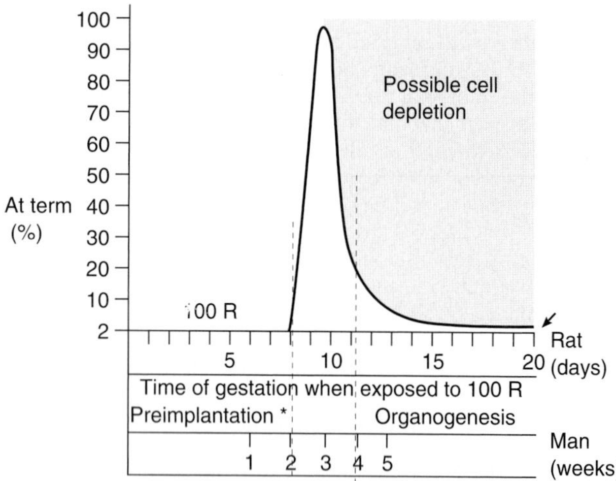

FIGURE 117.9 Relative incidence of gross congenital malformation in the rat when exposed to 100 rads during gestation. A very large increase in congenital malformations occurs during the early organogenetic period, corresponding to the third and fourth weeks of human gestation. Although gross malformations return to the background rate outside of this time frame, an irreversible loss of cells can occur. (From Brent RL. The effects of embryonic and fetal exposure to x-ray, microwaves, and ultrasound. *Clin Obstet Gynecol.* 1983;26:488, with permission.)

Growth Retardation

Growth retardation results from radiation-induced cellular depletion. Although catch-up growth can occur if exposure happens early in gestation, permanent cell depletion and growth retardation occur with exposure during later fetal stages.[24] Wood et al.[25,26] studied growth retardation of children exposed *in utero* to the Japanese atomic blasts. Those within 1,500 m from the center of the explosion were exposed to over 25 rads and, when followed through age 17 years, were 2 to 3 cm shorter and 3 kg lighter, and had a head circumference 1 cm smaller than normal. Those beyond 1,500 m from the blast received less than 25 rads and had a normal head circumference, height, and weight.[20,25,26] Further animal and human data support the contention that exposures of less than 5 rads should not cause either anatomic malformation or growth retardation.[21]

Oncogenic Potential

The correlation between childhood cancer and *in utero* exposure to radiation has been demonstrated. Steward in 1970 demonstrated an increased incidence of cancer with exposures of approximately 2 rads.[20] Although conclusions regarding the cause-and-effect relationship of this correlation cannot be definitively established, further studies using twins[27] and extensive data analysis[28] have strengthened the argument that *in utero* radiation can increase the rate of childhood cancer even at doses of 1 rad. The current increase in childhood cancer is estimated at 1 to 2 cases per 3,000 children exposed to 1 rad *in utero*.[20] Although these risks are very small, the patient must be counseled regarding this potential danger. By reviewing the current data, it is obvious that exposure to diagnostic levels of radiation carries little chance for spontaneous abortion, teratogenesis, or growth retardation. The increased risk of future cancer, however, does exist and must be weighed against the utility of the information provided by the study.

Ultrasound

Ultrasonography uses high-frequency, nonionizing, acoustic radiation to create images. A surface transducer sets up vibratory motions that are transmitted through matter as acoustic waves. The boundaries between different densities of tissue reflect some of these sound waves back to be detected by a transducer. Ultrasonic images therefore detect acoustic boundaries between different biologic materials in the body. Audible sound ranges from 20 to 20,000 vibrations per second, whereas ultrasonography uses frequencies of 1 to 10 million vibrations per second. Since its initial use in the 1950s, diagnostic ultrasonography has not produced fetal damage or harmful effects;[20,29] however, theoretic dangers do exist. Rapid compression and decompression of tissue by sound waves could cause tissue damage. Conversion of mechanical energy to thermal energy, especially at the bone–soft tissue interface, could lead to local hyperthermia, whereas the phenomenon known as *cavitation* could cause microscopic bubbles already present in tissues to grow in size because of absorption of surrounding diffused gases. Despite all these theoretic concerns, no consistent evidence exists that properly used diagnostic ultrasound is detrimental to the conceptus.[31,37]

Magnetic Resonance Imaging

Like ultrasonography, magnetic resonance imaging (MRI) uses no ionizing radiation, instead relying on the magnetic properties of tissues to create images. Four magnetic fields interact during an MRI examination to create the image. The intrinsic magnetic field of an atomic nucleus, usually that of a hydrogen proton, is combined with a strong, uniformly applied external magnetic field and a weaker magnetic field gradient. In addition, a magnetic field is intermittently generated by pulsed radiofrequency waves.[20] When this external radiofrequency is applied to nuclei in an existing magnetic field, the nuclei absorb some of the energy and change their orientation. When the radiofrequency ceases, the nuclei return to their previous orientation and emit the radiofrequency they absorbed. These signals are detected, stored, and processed by a computer to create an image.

Based on current data, it is unlikely that magnetic fields of the intensity used for diagnostic MRI pose any danger to the developing fetus, but biologic mechanisms do exist that could, at least theoretically, lead to damage. Charged particles and molecules moving in a strong magnetic field create an electrostatic potential difference, and normal red blood cells can alter their shape and create a charge when moving within an electric field.[31] Changing magnetic fields can induce visual light flashes because of magnetic effects on the photoreceptors in the eye,[31,32] and heat can be generated during the application of radiofrequencies. All these effects, however, occur with applications well above those used for diagnostic purposes. Based on these and other data, the International Radiation Protection Association has concluded that, despite the lack of evidence that mammalian embryos are sensitive to the magnetic fields encountered during MRI examination, elective examination of pregnant women by MRI should be postponed until after the first trimester and completion of organogenesis. Ultrasonography should be the diagnostic modality of choice during pregnancy, with MRI limited to cases in which unique diagnostic information is required.[33] MRI, however, is not absolutely contraindicated even in the first trimester when ultrasound will not suffice.

PHYSIOLOGIC CHANGES OF PREGNANCY THAT MIMIC DISEASE

Pregnancy physiology reflects the changes necessary for fetal gestation. It is characterized by the enlarging, gravid uterus and a changing hormonal milieu. These conditions predispose to certain diseases and change maternal physiology to mask the diagnosis of others.

The cardiovascular system is affected by pregnancy. The cardiac output increases by 30% to 50%, as does the total blood volume. The corresponding red blood cell volume increases only by 20% to 30%, leading to a decrease in the hematocrit. Although the maternal oxygen-carrying capacity is increased and the rheologic properties of blood are optimized for maximum nutrient delivery to the fetus, a physiologic anemia develops that can be confused with a pathologic state.[34] Diagnosis of anemia caused by chronic blood loss, as occurs with cancers of the gastrointestinal tract, may be delayed as the gradually decreasing hematocrit is attributed to pregnancy. Other laboratory evaluations also can mask various disease states (Table 117.3). Serum alkaline phosphatase levels gradually increase because of production of an alkaline phosphatase isozyme by the placenta. This does not reflect biliary or bone disease. Albumin levels, commonly used to measure hepatic synthetic function, decrease, and a relative leukocytosis mimics a systemic infection.

TABLE 117.3

CHANGE IN LABORATORY VALUES DURING PREGNANCY

Parameter	Change	Normal nonpregnant value	Late pregnancy value
Albumin (g/dL)	↓	3.2–3.8	2.4–3.1
Alkaline phosphatase (IU/L)	↑	30–115	100–210
Total biliburin (mg/dL)	↔	0.26–1.00	Unchanged
Aspartate aminotransferase (IU/L)	↔	0–31	Unchanged
Hemoglobin (g/dL)	↓	12.0–16.0	10.5–14
Leukocyte count ($\times 10^3$/mm^3)	↑	4.5–11.0	6.0–16.0

(From Martin C, Varner MW. Physiologic changes in pregnancy surgical implications. *Clin Obstet Gynecol.* 1994;37:241–255.)

The gastrointestinal tract undergoes a state of relaxation and decreased smooth muscle activity during pregnancy. The lower esophageal sphincter tone gradually decreases, as does gastric emptying. Prolonged small bowel transit time and decreased colonic emptying work to maximize nutrient and water absorption but also contribute to the constipation reported by 38% of pregnant women.[35] Although multifactorial, the actions of progesterone have been linked to inhibition of gut smooth muscle activity both *in vitro* and *in vivo*. Because this dose-dependent inhibition can be blocked by increasing the extracellular concentration of Ca^{2+}, at least *in vitro*, it is proposed than progesterone works by limiting the effective Ca^{2+} available for actin–myosin coupling.[36,37] This same mechanism contributes to uterine relaxation early in pregnancy, decreased intestinal motility, and the concurrent decrease in gallbladder tone and rate of emptying. The gallbladder empties more slowly during pregnancy and undergoes a gradual increase in residual volume, both during fasting and after meals. With these changes, combined with supersaturation of bile by cholesterol, pregnancy becomes a lithogenic state.[38] These effects of pregnancy are transient and gallbladder motility and volumes return to normal as early as 2 weeks after pregnancy, but the gallstones, if formed, may persist.

Nausea and vomiting of pregnancy is a common occurrence affecting between 50% and 90% of all women.[39,40] Its correlation with pregnancy was documented as early as 2000 B.C.E., and although a clear cause has not been established, it rarely extends beyond the first trimester. Other causes must be investigated if the nausea and vomiting occur later in pregnancy. Abdominal pain, although often related to a surgical pathologic process, can have many causes. Round ligament pain is described as an aching, dragging pain more often felt on the right side. It is a common occurrence until 31 weeks of gestation. Pain in the hypochondrium can result from uterine pressure on the lower ribs, and lower abdominal pain may be psychogenic, related to anxiety about the pregnancy or insecurity over the social situation.[41] The surgeon must determine the cause of abdominal pain in the pregnant patient and decide the course of diagnosis and intervention.

APPENDICITIS IN THE PREGNANT PATIENT

Appendicitis affects 250,000 patients every year in the United States. Because it is a disease of the young, its peak incidence corresponds to the childbearing years. Appendicitis is the most common nonobstetric indication for surgery during pregnancy, with an average incidence of 1 in 1,500 deliveries. Although some smaller studies have suggested this condition is more common later in gestation,[42–44] larger series show an equal distribution throughout pregnancy.[45] The incidence is similar to that in nonpregnant women, but the anatomic and physiologic changes of the gravid state make the diagnosis difficult.

Classic appendicitis in the nonpregnant patient presents with a constellation of signs and symptoms suggesting the disorder. Luminal obstruction of the appendiceal orifice, whether by fecalith or lymphoid hyperplasia, leads to an increase in intraluminal pressure by blocking the normal egress of mucus. Progressive obstruction of venous outflow followed by capillary and arterial thrombosis leads to mucosal ulceration, transmural wall necrosis, and, if unabated, perforation. Because early appendiceal distention is relayed by stretch receptors to the 10th thoracic ganglion, referred pain is perceived in the distribution corresponding to the epigastric region. Once the ongoing inflammation extends to involve the parietal peritoneum, the pain localizes to the right lower quadrant. Anorexia, nausea, and vomiting, initiated by visceral mechanisms similar to those responsible for the referred pain, follow the onset of pain. Findings on physical examination arise from this pathophysiologic process. Voluntary guarding of the right lower quadrant reflects the patient's anticipation of pain with palpation in the area. Rigidity or involuntary guarding indicates reflex spasm of the abdominal musculature caused by the nearby inflammatory process, whereas psoas and obturator signs indicate respective irritation of these muscles. Tenderness on rectal examination can be elicited with a low-lying appendix, whereas fever and leukocytosis indicate systemic inflammation. Although none of these signs or symptoms is 100% diagnostic, the presence of right lower quadrant pain, rigidity, and migration of pain was found to have the highest likelihood ratio for the presence of appendicitis in a large multifactorial analysis.[46] All of the aforementioned signs and symptoms are altered by pregnancy (Table 117.4).

TABLE 117.4

VARIATION IN SIGNS AND SYMPTOMS OF APPENDICITIS DURING PREGNANCY

Signs and symptoms	First trimester (%)	Second trimester (%)	Third trimester (%)
Right lower quadrant pain	100	50	14
Right upper quadrant pain	0	17	57
Guarding (muscle spasm)	80	50	43
Nausea and vomiting	53	60	23
Tenderness on rectal examination	60	17	0
Perforation rate	20	49	70

In a classic 1932 study, Baer et al.[47] evaluated the migration of the appendix through the duration of pregnancy with barium enemas. Beginning in the third month of pregnancy, the appendix and cecum are gradually displaced by the uterus and start a craniad migration out of the pelvis into the upper abdomen. By the third trimester, the appendiceal tip can abut the gallbladder (Fig. 117.10). The vague, referred epigastric pain caused by early appendiceal obstruction is not changed by this anatomic consideration, but the location of the somatic pain is. In a large study of pregnant women with proved appendicitis, abdominal pain was present in all patients. Location of pain in the right lower quadrant, however, was common only early in gestation, and a portion of patients reported pain in the right upper quadrant. This change in symptomatology is easily understood if the anatomic changes of the appendix are taken into consideration.[45] Both guarding and rigidity are valuable findings on physical examination but are common only in the first trimester. Elevation of the abdominal wall from the more laterally placed, upward-directed appendix and the laxity of the abdominal wall musculature caused by this distention decrease the reliability of these findings. Only 42.9% of patients in the third trimester are reported to have abdominal spasm and guarding, compared with 80% during the first trimester.[55] Psoas and obturator signs are similarly obscured as the appendix is moved from its normal location.

Anorexia, nausea, and vomiting occur in 58% to 77% of pregnant patients with appendicitis.[45,48] Although nausea and vomiting in the first trimester is common, its occurrence during the later stages of pregnancy should raise suspicion. Anorexia, nausea, and vomiting during the second and third

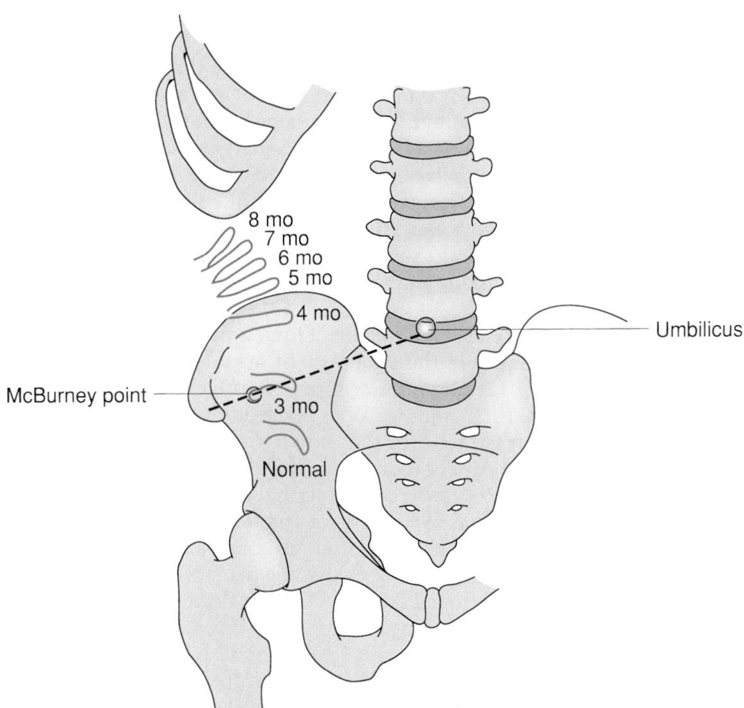

FIGURE 117.10 Changing location of the appendix throughout gestation. (From Baer JL, Reis RA, Arens RA. Appendicitis in pregnancy. *JAMA* 1932;98:1963, with permission.)

trimester, especially if associated with abdominal pain, require a thorough investigation.

The results of laboratory examinations commonly used to assist in the diagnosis of appendicitis are also obscured by pregnancy. The physiologic leukocytosis of pregnancy, ranging from 5,000 to 12,000 white blood cells (WBCs)/mL, overlaps that of appendicitis. In one collected series, the WBC counts of pregnant patients with proved appendicitis was not significantly elevated over these values, and only 25% of patients had a WBC count over 15,000. Most patients (50%) had WBC counts ranging between 10,000 and 15,000, and 25% had less than 10,000 WBCs/mL.[45] Urinalysis is a useful adjunct in the workup of appendicitis, but again presents a dilemma in pregnancy. Urinary tract infection is common in pregnancy as the enlarging uterus compresses the right ureter. Dilatation and stagnant flow in the right collecting system can contribute to bacterial overgrowth and infection, and an inflamed and enlarging appendix can contribute to the urinary tract infection by further compressing this system. Pyuria without bacteria can also indicate involvement of the right ureter in the appendiceal inflammatory process. Pus or bacteria in the urine does not rule out appendiceal inflammation because the two conditions often coexist. Attributing abdominal pain to pyelonephritis and choosing a course of antibiotics rather than further investigation only leads to a delay in diagnosis and missed appendicitis.[44]

All these complicating factors and the physician's fear of surgically induced premature labor contribute to delayed appendectomy in pregnancy. One series documents a correlation between a delay in the diagnosis and gestational age. In the first trimester, all of the diagnoses were made promptly and timely surgical intervention undertaken. A delay in diagnosis occurred in 18% of patients presenting in the second trimester, but in the third trimester delay was the rule. Numerous patients were discharged from the emergency room with various misdiagnoses ranging from false labor, nausea and vomiting of pregnancy, to gastroenteritis. All presented with vague signs and symptoms obscuring the true diagnosis.[49] Other series document the same delay in operation with a high rate of perforation, as high as 49% in the second trimester and 70% in the third.[45,48] Patients with perforated appendicitis usually experienced symptoms more than 24 hours before operation.[43]

Perforated appendicitis presents a greater infectious risk in the pregnant patient than in the population as a whole. The large uterus interferes with proper omental migration throughout the abdominal cavity and prevents the walling off of the inflammatory process. Braxton Hicks contractions disrupt adhesion formation, and the general increase in vascularity of the abdomen with greater lymphatic drainage allows rapid dissemination of infection. The high circulatory levels of adrenocorticoids in pregnancy have also been hypothesized to diminish the tissue inflammatory response and hinder containment of infection.[50,51] Perforated appendicitis in pregnancy rapidly leads to diffuse peritonitis, premature labor, and fetal loss. The rate of preterm labor and fetal loss with perforated appendicitis ranges from 26% to 66%, compared with 0% to 5% for uncomplicated appendicitis.[45,48,52]

Although history and clinical examination for suspected appendicitis during pregnancy are not ideal, they are still the best tools for detecting the disease. A patient with appendicitis during the first trimester might present with right lower quadrant pain, guarding, and nausea and vomiting, whereas a women in the third trimester would most likely have pain in another location and a more confusing clinical picture. The adage "If you cannot rule it out, take it out" applies in pregnancy as well as the nongravid state.[45] In applying this principle, the average negative laparotomy rate is 19% to 35% in the pregnant patient, a rate similar to that in the population as a whole.[53] Negative laparotomy rates as high as 75% in the third trimester, however, have been reported.[54] Although complication rates are low for negative explorations, fetal loss does occur. Imaging studies offer the potential of increasing the accuracy of the diagnosis of appendicitis.

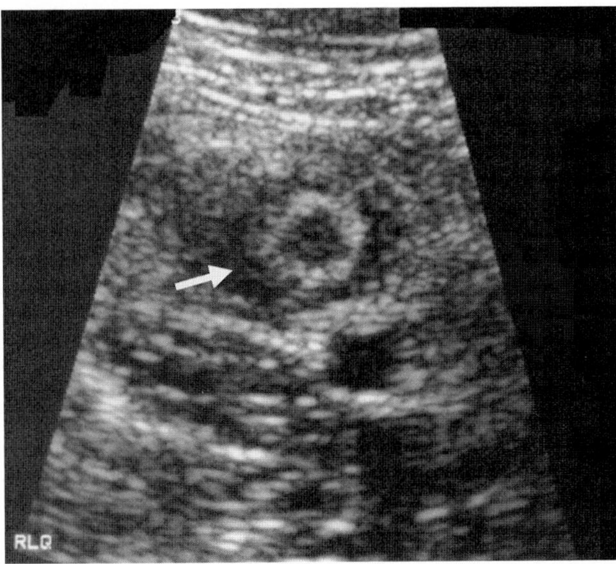

FIGURE 117.11 Ultrasonographic appearance of appendicitis. The appendix appears as a thick, noncompressible tubular structure with central hypoechogenicity. The walls are 5 mm thick, over the 3-mm limit for a normal appendix. (Courtesy of Dr. Beverly Coleman, Department of Radiology, Hospital of the University of Pennsylvania, Philadelphia, PA.)

Imaging Modalities

Ultrasonography is safe for the developing fetus and the study of choice in the pregnant patient. Findings suggesting appendicitis include visualization of a tubular structure with a diameter greater than 6.0 mm, a wall thickness above 3.0 mm,[54] and lack of peristalsis (Fig. 117.11). Because a normal appendix is difficult to visualize, simply seeing the appendix combined with tenderness on palpation with the ultrasound probe is suggestive of appendicitis. Ultrasonography, however, has been criticized for being operator dependent and situation specific. Sensitivity varies widely, from 68% to 89%,[55,56] and examination can be prohibitive because of abdominal guarding, pain during examination, and a thick abdominal wall. Distortion of anatomic landmarks and the displacement of the appendix by the gravid uterus complicate the diagnosis. Other structures such as an inflamed salpinx can also mimic appendicitis on ultrasound,[57] and a dilated uterine vein during pregnancy has been mistaken for an acutely inflamed appendix.[56] Despite these limitations, ultrasound is readily available in the emergency department or office and often can add diagnostic information to a confusing clinical picture. If the patient's history and physical examination do not warrant an immediate operation, abdominal ultrasonography should be the first study obtained.

Computed tomography (CT) has emerged as a highly reliable modality in the diagnosis of appendicitis. Appendiceal CT, using rectally administered contrast, can be performed within 10 to 20 minutes, does not require a waiting period for oral contrast to progress down through the cecum, and exposes the patient to only one third the radiation of a regular CT scan.[58] Results at one center have indicated that CT interpretation can be 98% sensitive and 98% specific for the diagnosis of appendicitis. Routine use of this modality has been shown to reduce costs, expedite the diagnosis, and reduce perforation rates from 22% to 14% while decreasing the incidence of negative laparotomy from 20% to 7%.[59,60] Although radiation risks to the developing fetus do exist, it is unlikely that fetal loss or malformations will occur with the dosing needed for an abdominal CT. Because even low levels of radiation *in utero* can increase the incidence of childhood cancer, widespread use of this modality in the pregnant patient with abdominal pain may be detrimental. Reserving the CT scan for those cases where the clinical history, physical examination, and ultrasonography are indeterminate should decrease the rate of perforation and negative exploration, just as it has in the nonpregnant population (Fig. 117.12).

Magnetic resonance imaging uses no ionizing radiation and, like CT, has the potential to image the whole abdomen. It is generally considered safe in pregnancy, and initial experimentation has shown that the higher water content of an inflamed appendix can be detected by MRI.[61] Reported sensitivity for appendicitis approaches 100%, at least in children.[62] Routine use of MRI may be hindered by availability and limited experience for detecting appendicitis using this modality. Future studies of MRI in appendicitis are warranted.

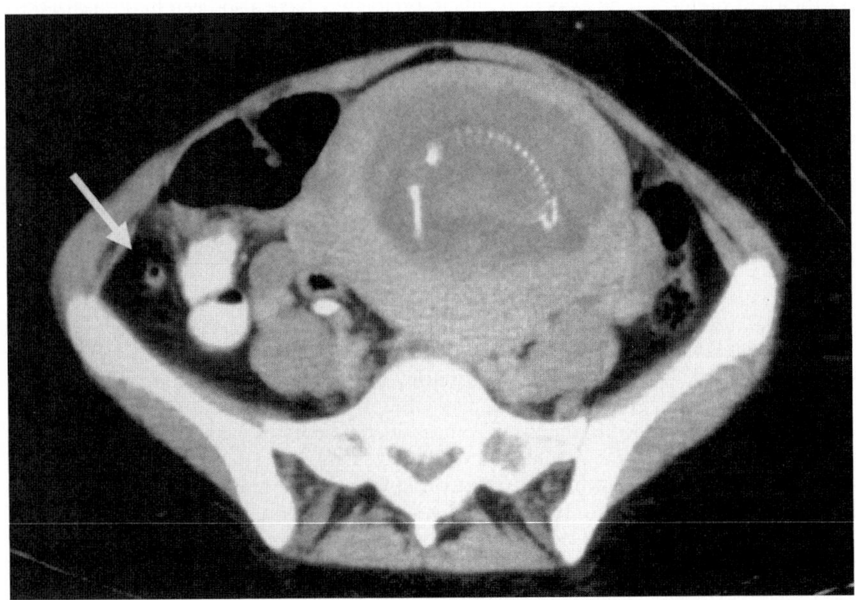

FIGURE 117.12 Computed tomography (CT) scan of a woman in the 18th week of gestation presenting with a 12-hour history of right-sided abdominal pain. Abdominal examination on presentation revealed significant tenderness and, after a nondiagnostic ultrasound, a laparotomy is considered for presumed appendicitis. A CT scan is obtained instead, revealing a normal, air-filled appendix with no sign of periappendiceal inflammation *(arrow)*. The laparotomy was postponed, and 12 hours later the patient aborted a septic fetus. An unnecessary laparotomy for an atypical presentation of chorioamnionitis was avoided by the judicious use of the CT scan. (Courtesy of Dr. David Weiss, Chestnut Hill Hospital, University of Pennsylvania Health System, Chestnut Hill, PA.)

Laparoscopy

Pregnancy is no longer a contraindication to laparoscopy. Although earlier studies reported a high rate of fetal and maternal complications, it is likely the underlying pathologic process rather than laparoscopy contributed to maternal morbidity and fetal demise.[63] Fetal acidosis with experimental maternal CO_2 pneumoperitoneum has been reported but can be minimized in the clinical setting with arterial blood gas monitoring and careful attention to maternal ventilation and acid-base balance.[64] Concerns regarding the effect of increased intraabdominal pressure are questionable considering the high uterine pressures during delivery. Experimental pneumoperitoneum in itself does not alter hemodynamics in the fetus until pressures of 20 mm Hg are reached.[64] Reduced insufflation pressures of 8 to 12 mm Hg should not contribute to fetal morbidity and mortality. Patients undergoing nongynecologic laparoscopic surgery begin a regular diet sooner, have lower narcotic requirements, and are discharged from the hospital earlier than patients undergoing open surgery.[65]

Laparoscopy to evaluate the appendix is a feasible diagnostic modality during pregnancy but may be difficult during later gestation. Anatomic changes alter placement of trocars above the gravid uterus[66] and require the use of the open Hasson technique of trocar placement under direct visualization rather than blind insufflation with a Veress needle. Maneuvers to enhance operative safety of laparoscopy in pregnancy have been outlined by the Society of American Gastrointestinal Endoscopic Surgeons[67] (Table 117.5)

Appendectomy

Once the diagnosis of appendicitis is made, treatment is strictly surgical. The type of incision can vary based on surgeon preference but becomes an issue during later pregnancy. Because of the migration of the appendix, an incision over McBurney's point in the late second and third trimester is inadequate. A low midline incision is favored by some to allow treatment of other conditions that mimic appendicitis, but may require excessive retraction of the uterus.[49] A right-sided transverse incision over the point of maximal tenderness is usually the safest approach because the appendix customarily lies beneath that point.[43,45,48] A similar incision at the level of the umbilicus allows good exposure of most of the right upper and lower abdomen. By tilting the patient 30 degrees to the left, the uterus is shifted away from the operative field and off the inferior vena cava. A right paramedian incision usually necessitates medial retraction of the uterus for exposure and increases the risk of precipitating premature labor. The laparoscopic approach, although useful for both diagnosis and treatment, might be difficult in later gestation. Although the potential benefits over the open appendectomy include less uterine manipulation and decreased incidence of preterm labor, its utility depends heavily on surgeon experience and comfort with the procedure.[65,66]

If exploration reveals a normal appendix, an appendectomy still should be performed. Although some authors question this approach because of the suggested high rate of preterm labor with a normal appendectomy,[68] most believe this to be untrue. Taking out the normal appendix adds little to morbidity while eliminating potential confusion if symptoms should recur.[45] Perforated appendicitis or pus in the abdominal cavity demands thorough peritoneal toilet along with the appendectomy. Drainage of the perforated appendectomy bed was avoided in the past because of fears that foreign material increased the risk of premature labor,[47] but these fears have not been substantiated and drainage of the appendiceal stump has been performed without complications.

TABLE 117.5 TREATMENT

GUIDELINES FOR LAPAROSCOPIC SURGERY DURING PREGNANCY

1. Defer operative intervention until the second trimester, when the fetal risk is lowest, whenever possible.
2. Pneumatic compression devices must be used because of the enhancement of lower venous stasis with pneumoperitoneum and pregnancy-induced hypercoagulable state.
3. Fetal and uterine status, as well as maternal end-tidal CO_2 and arterial blood gases, should be monitored.
4. Use fluoroscopy selectively and protect the uterus with lead shield if intraoperative cholangiography is possible.
5. Given enlarged gravid uterus, abdominal access should be obtained using open technique.
6. Dependent positioning should be used to shift the uterus off the inferior vena cava.
7. Pneumoperitoneum pressures should be minimized (to 8–12 mm Hg) and not allowed to exceed 15 mm Hg.
8. Obstetric consultation should be obtained before operation.

(From SAGES Committee on Standards Practice. Guidelines for laparoscopic surgery during pregnancy. *Surg Endosc.* 1998;12:189–190.)

BILIARY TRACT DISEASE IN PREGNANCY

Acute cholecystitis is the second most common general surgery diagnosis during pregnancy. Progesterone-induced relaxation of the gallbladder combined with estrogen-induced supersaturation of bile predispose to gallstone formation.[38,69] The risk for development of gallstones is related to the number of pregnancies, doubling after two pregnancies and nearly quadrupling after four.[69–71] Although gallstones are found in approximately 4% of all pregnant patients undergoing routine ultrasonography early during pregnancy, the rate can be as high as 12.2% immediately after delivery in high-risk populations.[70] Despite this high prevalence of gallstones, the incidence of acute cholecystitis during pregnancy is relatively low, 1 to 8 in 10,000 pregnancies (0.01% to 0.08%).[72,73] Inhibition of gallbladder contraction by progesterone is most likely the reason for this discrepancy. Although gallstones and sludge can form, weaker contractions prevent cystic duct obstruction until delivery. Postpartum, the progesterone concentrations decrease and the increased force of gallbladder contraction potentiates gallstone-induced cystic duct obstruction. An increased prevalence of cholecystitis in the year after childbirth has been noted.[74–76]

Symptoms of cholecystitis or biliary colic caused by cystic duct obstruction are similar in the pregnant and nonpregnant patient. Crampy right upper quadrant or epigastric pain after a meal can last several minutes to hours. The pain may radiate to the back and accompany nausea and vomiting. Tenderness on palpation of the right upper quadrant is usually present with acute cholecystitis, but laboratory evaluation may be obscured by the normal leukocytosis and elevated alkaline phosphatase during pregnancy. Increased bilirubin or visible jaundice, however, is unlikely without common bile duct obstruction.[73]

The differential diagnosis for cholecystitis during pregnancy includes hepatitis, acute fatty liver of pregnancy, and appendicitis. The diagnosis can be strengthened by the history and physical examination, and confirmed by abdominal ultrasound. Ultrasonography is more than 97% accurate in detecting cholecystitis, with typical findings of echogenic shadowing, gallbladder wall thickening, and pericholecystic fluid.[77] Pain on palpation with the ultrasound transducer, or sonographic Murphy's sign, is confirmatory of inflammation.

Historically, medical management was the definitive treatment of cholecystitis during pregnancy. The pregnant patient was given nothing orally, maintained on intravenous hydration, and treated with antibiotic for signs of infection. A low-fat diet was started once symptoms abated, antibiotics discontinued, and the patient discharged to home. Most women had initial relief of symptoms with this management and surgery was reserved for those with persistent symptoms, severe toxicity, and sepsis, peritonitis, or obstructive jaundice.[78] Fear of surgical complications prompted some to place pregnant patients with disabling biliary symptoms on total parenteral nutrition until delivery.[65,79] Analysis of patient outcomes throughout the course of pregnancy, however, has put strict medical management into question. Between 57% and 70% of patients treated for gallstone disease during pregnancy have recurrence at some time during gestation.[80,81] This risk is close to 92% for those who present in the first trimester, 64% for those presenting during the second trimester, and 44% for those who present during the third. Of these patients, 90% require hospitalization for management of the relapse,[80] and a significant portion of those presenting in the first trimester experience pregnancy loss as a complication of the disease.[79,82] Complications of gallstones such as choledocholithiasis and pancreatitis can also arise with future attacks and have been associated with a maternal mortality rate of 15% and a 60% chance of fetal demise.[78,83–85]

Laparoscopic cholecystectomy is a safe and reliable modality to treat gallstone disease during pregnancy. Numerous reports and case-control studies comparing laparoscopic with open cholecystectomy have supported the laparoscopic approach. Overall, patients have a shorter postoperative stay, resume oral intake earlier, have fewer postoperative hernias, and experience less pain with lower narcotic requirements by avoiding a large open incision.[63,65,86] Because fetal loss is most likely related to the underlying maternal illness and extent of uterine manipulation during surgery,[81,87] laparoscopic cholecystectomy offers a solution to both problems. Removing the diseased gallbladder eliminates the potential for recurrence, and the minimal uterine retraction needed with laparoscopic access to the right upper quadrant should decrease the risk for preterm labor. Although no randomized studies exist, preliminary data seem to support these assumptions. The incidence of premature uterine contractions with laparoscopic cholecystectomy has been reported at 0% to 21%, but contractions are usually well controlled by tocolytics. Most series report rates of premature birth or spontaneous abortion ranging from 0% to 7% with the laparoscopic approach.[66,80,81,87] After an open cholecystectomy, the reported rate of premature labor ranges from 0% to 40%, based on trimester,[88] and a spontaneous abortion or premature birth rate of up to 22% has been reported.[7] Based on the available data, laparoscopic cholecystectomy is safe during pregnancy and is preferable to open cholecystectomy.[88] An isolated report of three laparoscopic cholecystectomies ending in abortion, however, has been published, emphasizing that this procedure is not without risk and careful attention must be paid to the timing, indications, and maternal physiology before any procedure.[96]

Because most biliary symptoms can be controlled, at least initially, with conservative management, the management of symptomatic gallstones varies based on the stage of gestation. The second trimester is the optimal time to perform an elective cholecystectomy. Organogenesis is complete and the gravid uterus is not yet large enough to impinge on the operating field.[85] Clinical studies of open cholecystectomy confirm that this is the safest time to perform the operation. Spontaneous abortion rates after an open cholecystectomy are 12% during the first trimester, whereas the incidence of premature labor can be as high as 40% during the third trimester. The second trimester offers the ideal compromise, with the low spontaneous abortion rate of 5.6%.[88] Laparoscopic cholecystectomy offers the potential to decrease fetal loss even further over these values. Suggested management for symptomatic cholelithiasis during the first trimester consists of conservative measures until elective cholecystectomy can be performed safely during the second trimester of gestation. Second trimester disease can be dealt with surgically, whereas those presenting later in gestation can probably be managed symptomatically until the postpartum period. If symptoms are unremitting and cannot be handled with diet alone, surgical intervention might be necessary regardless of the period of gestation.[76,81]

Fetal heart rate monitoring is an essential part of laparoscopic procedures. Because pneumoperitoneum can have detrimental physiologic effects on both the mother and fetus, any evidence of fetal distress should result in immediate desufflation.[67] Fetal heart rate aberrations can also be treated by increasing uterine perfusion with maternal intravascular volume and changing the mother's position on the operating room table to decrease uterine compression of the inferior vena cava. Because the transabdominal signal is lost with pneumoperitoneum, transvaginal monitoring should be used during surgery,[65] whereas an external tocodynamometer should be placed on the abdomen immediately after the completion of the operation to monitor for uterine contractions. Tocolytic agents need not be used prophylactically, but can be administered if the patient demonstrates uterine irritability or contractions. The rate of successful tocolysis after laparoscopic procedures with minimal uterine manipulation is close to 100%.[63,65,76,83,87,90]

Choledocholithiasis

Indications for evaluation of the common bile duct are no different in the pregnant patient from in the population as a whole, namely, a bilirubin above 1.5 mg/dL, a dilated common bile duct, or gallstone pancreatitis.[66] Endoscopic retrograde cholangiopancreatography (ERCP) can be performed safely in pregnancy. With proper lead shielding, judicious use of fluoroscopy time, and avoidance of permanent roentgenographic films, ERCP has been performed with no direct exposure of the fetus to radiation. Calculated scatter radiation on the order of 4 mrads during the whole examination presents the only risk from ionizing radiation.[84] Evaluation of the biliary tree, stone retrieval, and sphincterotomy can be performed under these conditions without maternal or fetal complications.[91] Other methods avoid radiation altogether and include imaging of choledocholithiasis with endoscopic ultrasonography,[92] endoscopic papillotomy under ultrasonographic control,[93] and magnetic resonance cholangiography for choledocholithiasis.[94] Success with all these modalities has been reported but can be limited by operator experience and availability.

INTESTINAL OBSTRUCTION DURING PREGNANCY

The incidence of intestinal obstruction during pregnancy rose throughout the 20th century. In the presurgical era, cases were cited as infrequently as 1 in every 68,000 deliveries. Since the 1940s, however, the incidence has increased to 1 in 2,500 to 3,500 deliveries.[95] This change reflects the increased number of laparotomies in young women and the prevalence of postoperative adhesions during pregnancy. Adhesions remain the most common cause of intestinal obstruction in the gravid

TABLE 117.6 ETIOLOGY

CAUSES OF INTESTINAL OBSTRUCTION COMPLICATING PREGNANCY AND THE PUERPERIUM IN 66 PATIENTS

Adhesions	39 (59%)
Volvulus	15 (23%)
Sigmoid	7
Cecal	3
Midgut	3
Volvulus around vitellointestinal band	2
Intussusception	3 (5%)
Hernia	2 (3%)
Carcinoma	1 (1%)
Appendicitis	1 (1%)
Idiopathic (ileus)	5 (8%)

(From Perdue PW, Johnson HW, Stafford PW, et al. Intestinal obstruction complicating pregnancy. *Am J Surg.* 1992;164:385.)

patient, but intestinal volvulus is a much more common complication than in the population as a whole. Intussusception, hernia, and carcinoma are responsible for a minority of cases of bowel obstruction (Table 117.6).

Obstruction during pregnancy classically presents during three peak periods because of the change in the interrelationship between the abdominal viscera caused by the gravid uterus. The first peak occurs during the fourth to fifth months of gestation as the uterus becomes an intraabdominal organ, stretching any previously formed adhesions. The second peak occurs during the eighth to ninth months, when the fetal head descends into the pelvis, decreasing the uterine size. The third peak occurs after delivery as the sudden decrease in uterine size drastically changes the association of adhesions to surrounding bowel. The incidence of adhesion-related obstruction is highest during the first pregnancy after an operation, when the association between the viscera and adhesions is initially tested.[95,96]

In the general population, incarceration of bowel in groin hernias is the second most common cause of small bowel obstruction, but in the pregnant patient volvulus becomes the number two cause. As the enlarging uterus displaces the bowel out of the pelvis and away from the inguinal region, symptomatic groin hernias diminish in frequency.[97] Volvulus increases in prevalence during pregnancy because of changes in colon and small bowel anatomy and causes one fourth of all bowel obstructions. Sigmoid volvulus normally occurs owing to a long and redundant sigmoid colon. In the United States, this is usually seen in debilitated, institutionalized, or chronically constipated people. In countries such as those of Africa, a high incidence of sigmoid volvulus has been attributed to the high-fiber vegetable diet characteristic of that population. Anatomic changes of pregnancy further exacerbate this condition by causing the redundant sigmoid colon to rise out of the pelvis and twist around its point of fixation.[98] It is the most common site of volvulus during pregnancy.[99]

Cecal volvulus occurs because of failure of lateral peritoneal fixation during development. As the uterus enlarges during pregnancy, it raises the redundant or abnormally mobile cecum out of the pelvis. If a transition point or distal obstruction should occur from uterine pressure or an adhesive band, the colonic distention raises the colon even higher, producing torsion around this fixed point.[100] Volvulus of the small bowel also results from a congenital abnormality of rotation and fixation. Because clinical presentation usually occurs in infancy or childhood, the true incidence of malrotation in adulthood is unknown. The enlarging uterus potentially predisposes to the presentation of this anomaly during pregnancy by pushing the nonfixed, mobile portions of the small bowel into the upper abdomen, initiating the volvulus.[101]

Presentation and Diagnosis

Symptoms of intestinal obstruction are similar to those in the nonpregnant patient and commonly include abdominal pain and vomiting. High small bowel obstruction results in short periods between vomiting episodes with poorly localized, crampy upper abdominal pain. Colonic obstruction can present with less frequent feculent vomiting and lower abdominal pain. Findings on physical examination such as abdominal distention are often difficult to evaluate because of the gravid uterus. Obstipation, although characteristic of low obstruction such as that of sigmoid volvulus, may not occur with high obstruction. Laboratory studies, although useful to rule out other conditions, are not reliable enough to be considered diagnostic of obstruction. Significant leukocytosis can occur with necrosis and bowel strangulation, but mild elevations are confusing because of the physiologic leukocytosis of pregnancy. Tachycardia and hypotension are also late signs suggesting bowel compromise and shock.

The murky clinical picture combined with the tendency to treat the progressive vomiting as a normal part of pregnancy and crampy abdominal pain as early contractions lead to a delay in presentation and diagnosis. The median time from the onset of symptoms to admission in one series was 48 hours, and the median time from admission to a necessary laparotomy was also 48 hours. This delay in diagnosis and treatment contributed to excessive maternal and fetal mortality.[97] Abdominal pain and vomiting in a pregnant patient with an abdominal scar should raise the serious suspicion of small bowel obstruction.

If intestinal obstruction is suspected, upright and flat films of the abdomen are the diagnostic studies of choice. Although some authors believe that radiographs are nonspecific early in obstruction, serial films obtained every 4 to 6 hours usually show progressive changes confirming the diagnosis.[95] Small bowel obstruction gives the appearance of a progressive stepladder formation with dilatation and multiple air–fluid levels. Large bowel obstruction can produce a similar picture or reveal a grossly dilated bowel loop suggestive of volvulus. Contrast studies are also useful, and a "bird's bill" shape of contrast with gradual narrowing after a barium enema can be diagnostic of colonic volvulus, whereas dilute Gastrografin or barium by mouth can usually differentiate partial from complete obstruction. Fetal radiation risks from the plain radiographs are negligible and greatly outweighed by those from the possibility of misdiagnosis.

Treatment

The initial treatment for bowel obstruction in the pregnant patient is no different from that of a nonpregnant patient. Nasogastric tube decompression and fluid resuscitation are the cornerstones of therapy. By the time an obstruction is visible on plain film, the fluid deficit from vomiting and intraluminal losses is estimated at 1,000 to 1,500 mL. In advanced cases of dehydration presenting with tachycardia and hypotension, fluid losses may be as high as 4 to 6 L.[95] Prompt fluid resuscitation is essential in the pregnant patient because compromise of uterine blood flow leads to fetal distress and demise.

Surgical intervention plays a more prominent and earlier role in the management of the pregnant patient with bowel obstruction. Although adhesion-related small bowel obstruction in the nonpregnant patient usually resolves with nasogastric decompression and fluid administration, numerous series have documented failure of conservative management of small bowel obstruction in the pregnant woman. Of patients, 89% to 100% eventually require an operation, and 13% to 23% require resection of gangrenous bowel at the time of laparotomy.[97,102] Based on these outcomes, some have stated that once the diagnosis of small bowel obstruction is made in a pregnant patient, the only role of nasogastric decompression and fluid resuscitation is to prepare the patient for an operation.[102] Cecal volvulus is also treated surgically, and although sigmoid volvulus in the nonpregnant patient can be managed with sigmoidoscopic decompression and placement of a rectal tube, the large gravid uterus may act as a mechanical impediment to detorsion. A laparotomy is usually necessary for treatment.[97,98]

A generous midline incision allows for maximum exposure of the abdomen with minimal manipulation of the uterus. During lysis of small bowel adhesions, bowel viability must be carefully assessed. Definitive management of cecal volvulus requires resection of necrotic cecum or detorsion and cecopexy. Sigmoid volvulus should also be treated by resection, if necrotic, but simple detorsion and placement of a rectal tube can be performed if the sigmoid is viable. Although resection of the redundant sigmoid is the definitive treatment for this disease, it can be delayed until the postpartum period. Aggressive surgical treatment has been credited with reducing the maternal and fetal mortality rates from 20% and 50%, respectively, in the 1930s to 6% and 26% today.[97] Increased awareness of this disease and expeditious management can reduce those rates even further.

COLORECTAL CANCER DURING PREGNANCY

Colon cancer is a rare disease during pregnancy but one with lethal consequences. The incidence of colon cancer was estimated as 1 in 50,000 pregnancies based on a 1955 report.[103] More recent reviews estimate the incidence as 1 in 13,000 deliveries,[104] with the increasing prevalence caused by increasing maternal age with the delay in pregnancy until later in life.[105] Presenting symptoms are similar to those in nonpregnant patients and include rectal bleeding, constipation, abdominal pain and distention, as well as nausea and vomiting.[106] All of these symptoms are common during pregnancy. Even the findings of occult blood in the stool and hematochezia are often attributed to pregnancy-related hemorrhoids and ignored.

The anatomic distribution and stage of colorectal cancer in the pregnant patient differ from those in the population as a whole. A nationwide survey of the members of the American Society of Colon and Rectal Surgeons who had cared for pregnant patients with colorectal cancer revealed a predominance of rectal cancer in this patient population. Of tumors, 64% were distributed below the peritoneal reflection and 36% were in the more proximal colon. A review of more than 200 pregnancy-associated colorectal cancers reported in the literature disclosed a similar distribution, with 86% of tumors located in the rectum and only 14% above the peritoneal reflection.[107] This is in contrast to the general population, where most tumors (69%) are located in the colon and only 31% in the rectum. This trend could reflect a presentation bias because of frequent rectal examinations during prenatal care, or the change in pelvic anatomy and symptoms of rectal compression by the gravid uterus.

Pregnant patients present with more advanced cancers than the population as a whole. In the previously mentioned study, no pregnant patient was Dukes stage A at presentation, whereas 41% were Dukes stage B, 44% stage C, and 15% stage D.[107] Although increased hormonal stimulation during pregnancy could cause rapid tumor growth and progression of disease,[107–109] not all colon cancers have estrogen or progesterone receptors and respond to this stimulation.[110] The advanced stage of disease on presentation most likely results from a delay in the diagnosis and the low clinical suspicion of malignancy in this patient population. This trend is similar to that in the young population as a whole, and although only 4% to 8% of all colon cancer occurs in those younger than 40 years of age, these patients also have a delayed presentation with more advanced disease.[111] The average interval between the onset of symptoms and diagnosis of colon cancer in those younger than 40 years is 6.4 months, and 32% of patients wait longer than 1 year before seeking medical attention for symptoms.[112] The stage of disease on presentation in this patient population is similar to that in the pregnant patient (Table 117.7), and colonic malignancy during gestation most likely represents pregnancy superimposed on colon cancer rather than a pregnancy-related disease.

TABLE 117.7 STAGING

STAGE AT PRESENTATION OF COLORECTAL CANCER DURING PREGNANCY AND THOSE YOUNGER THAN 40 YEARS OF AGE

Dukes Stage	Pregnant patients (%)	Patients <40 y (%)
A	0	2
B	41	30
C	44	45
D	15	23

(Data from Bernstein MA, Madoff RD, Caushaj PF, Colon and rectal cancer in pregnancy. *Dis Colon Rectum* 1993;36:172–178; and Smith C, Butler JA. Colorectal cancer in patients younger than 40 years of age. *Dis Colon Rectum* 1989;32:843–846.)

Diagnosis

Diagnosis of colorectal cancer during pregnancy demands a very high level of suspicion. Patients with rectal bleeding, occult blood-positive stools, and anemia below physiologic levels of pregnancy should be evaluated for a colonic malignancy. Sigmoidoscopy is not contraindicated during pregnancy and does not appear to induce labor or congenital malformations. Because most cancers are located below the peritoneal reflection, they can be easily accessed and sampled for biopsy through a limited sigmoidoscopic examination. Because of the 5% risk of a second, synchronous primary, a more extensive colonoscopic evaluation might be necessary, especially if findings were to change the treatment or extent of surgical resection. Colonoscopy during pregnancy is still considered experimental and may be technically difficult because of colonic compression by the gravid uterus. Maneuvers to increase safety include use of only gentle pressure when manipulating the colonoscope, maternal administration of supplemental oxygen, and fetal heart rate monitoring during the procedure.[113]

Transrectal ultrasonographic staging of rectal cancer is particularly helpful during pregnancy because of its ability to evaluate cancerous invasion of the uterus or encroachment on the cervix that could prevent vaginal delivery.[113] Serum carcinoembryonic antigen levels are not normally elevated during pregnancy and, although of limited use as a screening tool, levels can be obtained before resection for early detection of recurrence.[114] Evaluation of metastatic disease to the liver can be performed with transabdominal ultrasonography at no risk to the fetus, and a CT scan can be obtained in more difficult cases.

Treatment

Treatment of colorectal cancer during pregnancy presents as an ethical dilemma for both the patient and the physician. Aside from the difficulty in dealing with a potentially lethal disease in a young person, there is an inherent conflict between the treatment of the mother and fetus. Treatment of other surgical conditions encountered during pregnancy, such as appendicitis or cholecystitis, equally benefits both the mother and the unborn child. Treatment of colon cancer puts the two at odds. Although early tumor resection can improve the prognosis for the mother, this treatment might be detrimental to the fetus. Adjuvant chemotherapy or radiation therapy can improve survival of the mother but is generally contraindicated during pregnancy, especially early in gestation. Careful attention must be paid to the wishes of the family while explaining the risks and benefits for both the mother and child.

If the cancer is discovered in the first half of gestation, a definitive resection should be performed. Waiting months until adequate fetal maturation for delivery can allow cancer dissemination and disease progression.[106,113] In most cases, a colon resection can be handled without disturbing the pregnancy and resection of even low-lying tumors can be performed before 20 weeks of gestation.[110,114] Total abdominal hysterectomy is recommended only if tumor invasion into the uterus has occurred, a technically complete operation cannot be performed without it, or the mother's life expectancy is shorter than the time needed to reach fetal viability. If the tumor is unresectable, a colostomy is performed for palliation until fetal viability is documented.

Treatment of tumors discovered after the 20th week can be postponed until term or fetal viability. Vaginal delivery is not contraindicated unless the tumor is obstructing the birth canal or presents a risk of episiotomy entering the tumor bed. Tumor resection is undertaken several days after the birth to allow uterine involution and resolution of pelvic vascular congestion. If a cesarean section is performed for obstetric reasons or because of tumor impingement on the birth canal, resection can be performed immediately, but the operation may be technically easier if done as a separate procedure and postponed for several days. This is especially important with low rectal lesions, where decreased pelvic vasculature can facilitate a low anterior or abdominoperineal resection.[106]

Management of the ovaries is a controversial issue. The incidence of colon carcinoma metastasizing to the ovaries is estimated between 3% and 8%[115] in the general population, but can be as high as 25% during pregnancy and in young patients.[112,116] Bilateral salpingo-oophorectomy at the time of tumor resection has been advocated by some,[115] but during pregnancy carries a high chance of spontaneous abortion, especially during the first half of gestation. Although resection should be performed if the ovaries are grossly involved with tumor or a hysterectomy is undertaken, bilateral ovarian wedge biopsies with frozen-section evaluation can be safely carried out without disturbing the pregnancy. Salpingo-oophorectomy is then performed only if the ovaries are involved with tumor.[106]

Adjuvant chemotherapy conveys a survival advantage to patients with Dukes stage C colon cancer. The classic adjuvant chemotherapy includes 5-fluorouracil, an antimetabolite that inhibits DNA synthesis. The safety of this drug during pregnancy is questionable, and evidence of fetal toxicity exists in animal models. Limited data on the human fetal safety of this drug are available, and it is considered a category D drug during pregnancy by the U.S. Food and Drug Administration: generally unsafe during pregnancy, but the risk may be justifiable in certain circumstances. Chemotherapy during the first trimester is usually contraindicated and should be limited to those patients with Dukes stage C lesions who are willing to accept the risks of fetal teratogenesis or demise. Chemotherapy during the second and third trimesters is less teratogenic because of the completion of organogenesis, but still carries some risk for the fetus.[113,117]

Adjuvant radiation therapy reduces the local recurrence of rectal cancer. Because the most effective dose to eradicate microscopic disease is on the order of 50 Gy and the fetus cannot be effectively shielded from pelvic exposure, radiation therapy cannot be safely performed during pregnancy. Therapeutic pelvic radiation also results in permanent and irreversible female sterility, so the mother considering this form of therapy must be fully aware of the risks to the current and future pregnancies.[113,118]

KEY POINTS

- **Surfactant production begins by the 20th week of gestation, but is present in only small amounts before 24 weeks. Although the survival rate of infants born at 24 weeks of development is dismal, the mortality rate before that time is nearly 100%.**
- **By the 12th week of gestation, the uterus becomes too large to reside exclusively in the pelvis and extends into the abdominal cavity. By the 20th week, the uterine fundus reaches the umbilicus, and by the third trimester it reaches almost to the liver.**
- **Parturition begins when forces favoring uterine activity override those of quiescence. Close to term, the concentration of estrogen increases relative to that of progesterone, leading to uterine activation. Oxytocin from the posterior pituitary and placenta is the main stimulator of strong uterine contractions and parturition.**
- **Prostaglandin synthesis inhibitors, magnesium sulfate, β-adrenergic agonists, and calcium channel blockers are the four most common pharmacologic agents used as tocolytics.**
- **Fetal effects of ionizing radiation depend on the dose absorbed by the fetal tissue and the stage of fetal development during exposure.**
- **Perforated appendicitis in pregnancy rapidly leads to diffuse peritonitis, premature labor, and fetal loss. The rate of preterm labor and fetal loss with perforated appendicitis ranges from 26% to 66%, compared with 0% to 5% for uncomplicated appendicitis.**
- **Laparoscopic cholecystectomy is a safe and reliable modality to treat gallstone disease during pregnancy. Symptomatic cholelithiasis treatment during the first trimester includes conservative measures until elective cholecystectomy can be performed safely during the second trimester of gestation. Second trimester disease can be dealt with surgically, whereas that presenting later in gestation can probably be managed symptomatically until the postpartum period.**
- **Adhesions are the most common cause of intestinal obstruction in the gravid patient, but intestinal volvulus is a much more common complication than in the population as a whole. Intussusception, hernia, and carcinoma are responsible for a minority of cases of bowel obstruction**

References

1. Moore KL, Persaud TVN. *The developing human,* 6th ed. Philadelphia: WB Saunders, 1998.
2. Gardner MO, Goldstein RL. The clinical use of antenatal corticosteroids. *Clin Obstet Gynecol.* 1995;38:746–754.
3. Resnik R. Anatomic alterations in the reproductive tract. In: Creasy RK, Resnik R, eds. *Maternal–fetal medicine,* 4th ed. Philadelphia: WB Saunders, 1998, pp. 90–94.
4. Monga M, Sanborn BM. Uterine biology and the control of myometrial contractions. In: Creasy RK, Resnik R, eds. *Maternal–fetal medicine,* 4th ed. Philadelphia: WB Saunders, 1998, pp. 95–101.

5. Petraglia F, Florio P, Nappi C, et al. Peptide signaling in human placenta and membranes: autocrine, paracrine, and endocrine mechanisms. *Endocr Rev.* 1996;17:156–186.
6. Challis JRG. Characteristics of parturition. In: Creasy RK, Resnik R, eds. *Maternal–fetal medicine,* 4th ed. Philadelphia: WB Saunders, 1998, pp. 484–497.
7. McLean M, Bisits, Davies J, et al. A placental clock controlling the length of human pregnancy. *Nat Med.* 1995;1:460–463.
8. Kort B, Katz VL, Watson WJ. The effects of nonobstetric operation during pregnancy. *Surg Gynecol Obstet.* 1993;177:371–376.
9. Copper RL, Goldenberg RL, Creasy RK, et al. A multicenter study of preterm birth weight and gestational age-specific neonatal mortality. *Am J Obstet Gynecol.* 1993;168:78–84.
10. Romero R, Avila C, Brekus CA, et al. The role of systemic and intrauterine infection in preterm parturition. *Ann NY Acad Sci.* 1991;622:355–375.
11. Ou CW, Orsino A, Lye S. Expression of connexin-43 and connexin-26 in the rat myometrium during pregnancy and labor is differentially regulated by mechanical and hormonal signals. *Endocrinology* 1997;138: 5398–5407.
12. Gordon MC, Samuels P. Indomethacin. *Clin Obstet Gynecol.* 1995;38:697–705.
13. Gordon MC, Iams JD. Magnesium sulfate. *Clin Obstet Gynecol.* 1995;38:706–712.
14. Ray D, Dyson D. Calcium channel blockers. *Clin Obstet Gynecol.* 1995;38:713–721.
15. **Hill WC. Risks and complications of tocolysis. *Clin Obstet Gynecol.* 1995;38:725–745.**
16. Meyers RE. Two patterns of perinatal brain damage and their conditions of occurrence. *Am J Obstet Gynecol.* 1972;122:246–276.
17. Miller DA, Paul R. Antepartum–intrapartum monitoring. In: Scott JR, DiSaia PJ, Hammond CB, et al., eds. *Danforth's obstetrics and gynecology,* 8th ed. Philadelphia: Lippincott Williams & Wilkins, 1999, pp. 243–255.
18. Hon EH. The fetal heart rate patterns preceding death in utero. *Am J Obstet Gynecol.* 1959;78:47.
19. Smith CV. Vibroacoustic stimulation. *Clin Obstet Gynecol,* 1995;38: 68–77.
20. Wagner LK, Lester RG, Saldana LR. *Exposure of the pregnant patient to diagnostic radiation.* Madison, WI: Medical Physics Publishing, 1997.
21. Brent RL. The effects of embryonic and fetal exposure to x-ray, microwaves, and ultrasound: counseling the pregnant and non-pregnant patient about these risks. *Semin Oncol.* 1989;16:347–368.
22. **Boklage CE. Survival probability of human conceptions from fertilization to term. *Int J Fertil.* 1990;35:75–94.**
23. Brent RL. Radiation teratogenesis. *Teratology* 1980;21:281–298.
24. Brent RL. The effects of embryonic and fetal exposure to x-ray, microwaves, and ultrasound. *Clin Perinatol.* 1986;13:615–649.
25. Wood JW, Johnson KG, Omori Y, et al. Mental retardation in children exposed in utero to the atomic bombs in Hiroshima and Nagasaki. *Am J Public Health* 1967;57:1381–1390.
26. Wood JW, Keehan RJ, Kawamoto S, et al. The growth and development of children exposed in utero to the atomic bombs in Hiroshima and Nagasaki. *Am J Public Health* 1967;57:1374–1380.
27. Harvey EB, Boice JD, Honeyman M, et al. Prenatal x-ray exposure and childhood cancer in twins. *N Engl J Med.* 1985;312:541–545.
28. **Doll R, Wakeford. Risk of childhood cancer from fetal irradiation. *Br J Radiol.* 1997;70:130–139.**
29. Reece AE, Goldstein I, Hobbins JC. *Fundamentals of obstetric and gynecologic ultrasound.* Norwalk, CT: Appleton & Lange, 1994.
30. Brent RL, Jensh RP, Beckman DA. Medical sonography: reproductive effects and risks. *Teratology* 1991;44:123–146.
31. Kanal E, Shellock FG, Talagala L. Safety considerations in MR imaging. *Radiology* 1990;176:593–606.
32. Schenck JF, Dumoulin CL, Redington RW. Human exposure to 4.0-tesla magnetic fields in a whole-body scanner. *Med Phys.* 1992;19:1089–1098.
33. IRPA/INIRC. Protection of the patient undergoing a magnetic resonance examination. *Health Phys.* 1991;61:923–928.[AQ0]
34. Martin C, Varner MW. Physiologic changes in pregnancy: surgical implications. *Clinical Obstet Gynecol.* 1994;37:241–255.
35. Bonapace ES, Fisher RS. Constipation and diarrhea in pregnancy. *Gastroenterol Clin North Am.* 1998;27:197–211.
36. Gill RC, Bowes KL, YJ Kingma. Effects of progesterone on canine colonic smooth muscle. *Gastroenterology* 1985;88:1941–1947.
37. Katz PO, Castell DO. Gastroesophageal reflux during pregnancy. *Gastroenterol Clin North Am.* 1998;27:153–167.
38. Everson GT, McKinley C, Lawson M, et al. Gallbladder function in the human female: effect of the ovulatory cycle, pregnancy, and contraceptive steroids. *Gastroenterology* 1982;82:711–719.
39. Broussard CN, Richter JE. Nausea and vomiting of pregnancy. *Gastroenterol Clin North Am.* 1998;27:123–151.
40. Abel TL, Riely CA. Hyperemesis gravidum. *Gastroenterol Clin North Am.* 1992;21:835–849.
41. Baker PN, Madeley RJ, Symonds EM. Abdominal pain of unknown aetiology in pregnancy. *Br J Obstet Gynaecol.* 1989;96:688–691.
42. Al-Mulhim AA. Acute appendicitis in pregnancy. *Int Surg.* 1996;81:295–297.
43. **Tamir IL, Bongard FS, Klein SR. Acute appendicitis in the pregnant patient. *Am J Surg.* 1990;160:571–576.**
44. Masters K, Levine BA, Gaskill HV, et al. Diagnosing appendicitis during pregnancy. *Am J Surg.* 1984;148:768–771.
45. Babaknia A, Parsa H, Woodruff JD. Appendicitis during pregnancy. *Obstet Gynecol.* 1977;50:40–44.
46. Wagner JM, McKinney WP, Carpenter JL. Does this patient have appendicitis? *JAMA* 1996;276:1589–1594.
47. Baer JL, Reis RA, Arens RA. Appendicitis in pregnancy. *JAMA* 1932;98:1359–1364.
48. Weingold AB. Appendicitis in pregnancy. *Clin Obstet Gynecol.* 1983;26:801–809.
49. Cunningham FG, McCubbin JH. Appendicitis complicating pregnancy. *Obstet Gynecol.* 1975;45:415–420.
50. Black WP. Acute appendicitis in pregnancy. *BMJ* 1960;1:1938–1941.
51. Parker RB. Acute appendicitis in late pregnancy. *Lancet* 1954;1:1252–1257.
52. Horowitz MD, Gomez GA, Santiesteban R, et al. Acute appendicitis during pregnancy. *Arch Surg.* 1985;120:1362–1367.
53. Varner MW. Surgical diseases in pregnancy. *Clin Obstet Gynecol.* 1994;37:239–315.
54. Worrell JA, Drolshagen LF, Kelly TC, et al. Graded compression ultrasound in the diagnosis of appendicitis: a comparison of diagnostic criteria. *J Ultrasound Med.* 1990;9:145–150.
55. Schwerk WB, Wichtrup B, Rothmund M, et al. Ultrasonography in the diagnosis of acute appendicitis: a prospective study. *Gastroenterology* 1989;97:630–639.
56. Abu-Yousef MM, Phillips ME, Franken EA, et al. Sonography of acute appendicitis: a critical review. *Crit Rev Diagn Imaging* 1989;29: 381–408.
57. Paulman AA, Huebner DM, Forrest TS. Sonography in the diagnosis of acute appendicitis. *Am Fam Physician* 1991;44:465–468.
58. Rao PM, Rhea JT, Novelline RA, et al. Helical CT combined with contrast material administered only through the colon for imaging of suspected appendicitis. *AJR Am J Roentgenol.* 1997;169:1275–1280.
59. Rao PM, Rhea JT, Rattner DW, et al. Introduction of appendiceal CT impact on negative appendectomy and appendiceal perforation rates. *Ann Surg.* 1999;229:344–349.
60. Rao PM, Rhea JT, Novelline RA, et al. Effects of computed tomography of the appendix on treatment of patients and use of hospital resources. *N Engl J Med.* 1998;338:141–146.
61. Jacobs DO, Settle RG, Clarke JR, et al. Identification of human appendicitis by in vitro nuclear magnetic resonance. *J Surg Res.* 1990;48:107–110.
62. Hormann M, Paya K, Eibenberger K, et al. MR imaging in children with nonperforated acute appendicitis: value of unenhanced MR imaging in sonographically selected cases. *AJR Am J Roentgenol.* 1998;171: 467–470.
63. **Conron RW, Abbruzzi K, Cochrane SO, et al. Laparoscopic procedures in pregnancy. *Am Surg.* 1998;65:259–263.**
64. Hunter JG, Swanstrom L, Thornburg K. Carbon dioxide pneumoperitoneum induces fetal acidosis in a pregnant ewe model. *Surg Endosc.* 1995;9:272–279.
65. Curet MJ, Allen D, Josloff RK, et al. Laparoscopy during pregnancy. *Arch Surg.* 1996;131:546–551.
66. Gurbuz AT, Peetz ME. The acute abdomen in the pregnant patient. *Surg Endosc.* 1997;11:98–102.
67. SAGES. Guidelines for laparoscopic surgery during pregnancy. *Surg Endosc.* 1998;12:189–190.
68. Saunders P, Milton PJD. Laparotomy during pregnancy: an assessment of diagnostic accuracy and fetal wastage. *BMJ* 1973;3:165–167.
69. Everson GT. Gastrointestinal motility in pregnancy. *Gastroenterol Clin North Am.* 1992;21:751–776.
70. Valdivieso V, Covarrubias C, Siegel F, et al. Pregnancy and cholelithiasis: pathogenesis and natural course of gallstones diagnosed in early puerperium. *Hepatology* 1993;17:1–4.
71. Barbara L, Sama C, Morselli Labate AM, et al. A population study on the prevalence of gallstone disease: the Sirmione Study. *Hepatology* 1987;7:913–917.
72. Basso L, McCollum PT, Darling MN, et al. A study of cholelithiasis during pregnancy and its relationship with age, parity, menarche, breast-feeding, dysmenorrhea, oral contraception, and a maternal history of cholelithiasis. *Surgery* 1992;175:41–46.
73. Mayer IE, Hussain H. Abdominal pain during pregnancy. *Gastroenterol Clin North Am.* 1998;27:1–36.
74. Gerwig WH, Thistlethwaite JR. Cholecystitis and cholelithiasis in young women following pregnancy. *Surgery* 1950;28:983–996.
75. Scott LD. Gallstone disease and pancreatitis in pregnancy. *Gastroenterol Clin North Am.* 1992;21:803–815.
76. Steinbrook RA, Brooks DC, Datta S. Laparoscopic cholecystectomy during pregnancy review of anesthetic management: surgical considerations. *Surg Endosc.* 1996;10:511–515.
77. Epstein FB. Acute abdominal pain in pregnancy. *Emerg Med Clin North Am.* 1994;12:151–165.
78. Simon JA. Biliary tract disease and related surgical disorders during pregnancy. *Clin Obstet Gynecol.* 1983;26:810–821.

79. Dixon NP, Faddis DM, Silberman H. Aggressive management of cholecystitis during pregnancy. *Am J Surg.* 1987;154:292–294.
80. **Glasgow RE, Visser BC, Harris HW, et al. Changing management of gallstone disease during pregnancy. *Surg Endosc.* 1998;12:241–246.**
81. Graham G, Baxi L, Tharakan T. Laparoscopic cholecystectomy during pregnancy: a case series and review of the literature. *Obstet Gynecol Surv.* 1998;53:566–574.
82. Hiatt JR, Hiatt JCG, Williams RA, et al. Biliary disease in pregnancy: strategy for surgical management. *Am J Surg.* 1986;151:263–265.
83. Eichenberg BJ, Vanderlinden J, Miguel C, et al. Laparoscopic cholecystectomy in the third trimester of pregnancy. *Am Surg.* 1996;62:874–877.
84. Baillie J, Cairns SR, Cotton PB. Endoscopic management of choledocholithiasis during pregnancy. *Surgery* 1990;171:1–4.
85. Printen KJ, Ott RA. Cholecystectomy during pregnancy. *Am Surg.* 1978;44:432–434.
86. Pucci RO, Seed RW. Case report of laparoscopic cholecystectomy in the third trimester of pregnancy. *Am J Obstet Gynecol.* 1991;165:401–402.
87. Elerding SC. Laparoscopic cholecystectomy in pregnancy. *Am J Surg.* 1993;165:625–627.
88. McKellar DP, Anderson CT, Boynton CJ, et al. Cholecystectomy during pregnancy without fetal loss. *Surg Gynecol Obstet.* 1992;174:465–468.
89. Amos JD, Schorr SJ, Norman PF, et al. Laparoscopic surgery during pregnancy. *Am J Surg.* 1996;171:435–437.
90. Lanzafame RJ. Laparoscopic cholecystectomy during pregnancy. *Surgery* 1995;118:627–633.
91. Axelrad AM, Fleischer DE, Strack LL, et al. Performance of ERCP for symptomatic choledocholithiasis during pregnancy: techniques to increase safety and improve patient management. *Am J Gastroenterol.* 1994;89: 109–112.
92. Amouyal P, Amouyal G, Levy P, et al. Diagnosis of choledocholithiasis by endoscopic ultrasonography. *Gastroenterology* 1994;106:1062–1067.
93. Parada AA, Goncalves MOL, Tafner E, et al. Endoscopic papillotomy under ultra-sonographic control. *Int Surg.* 1991;76:75–76.
94. Yu-leung C, Chan ACW, Lam WWM, et al. Choledocholithiasis: comparison of MR cholangiography and endoscopic retrograde cholangiography. *Radiology* 1996;200:85–89.
95. Davis MR, Bohon CJ. Intestinal obstruction in pregnancy. *Clin Obstet Gynecol.* 1983;26:832–842.
96. Hill LM, Symmonds RE. Small bowel obstruction in pregnancy: a report and review of four cases. *Obstet Gynecol.* 1976;49:170–173.
97. **Perdue PW, Johnson HW, Stafford PW. Intestinal obstruction complicating pregnancy. *Am J Surg.* 1992;164:384–388.**
98. Lord SA, Boswell WC, Hungerpiller JC. Sigmoid volvulus in pregnancy. *Am Surg.* 1996;62:380–382.
99. Kantor HM. Midgut volvulus in pregnancy: a case report. *J Reprod Med.* 1990;35:577–580.
100. Pratt AT, Donaldson RC, Evertson LR, et al. Cecal volvulus in pregnancy. *Obstet Gynecol.* 1981;57:37S–40S.
101. Rothstein RD, Rombeau JL. Intestinal malrotation during pregnancy. *Obstet Gynecol.* 1993;81:817–819.
102. Meyerson S, Holtz T, Ehrinpreis M, et al. Small bowel obstruction in pregnancy. *Am J Gastroenterol.* 1995;90:299–302.
103. McLean DW, Arminski TC, Bradley GT. Management of primary carcinoma of the rectum diagnosed during pregnancy. *Am J Surg.* 1955;90:816–825.
104. Woods JB, Martin JN Jr, Ingram FH, et al. Pregnancy complicated by carcinoma of the colon above the rectum. *Am J Perinatol.* 1992;9:102–110.
105. Antonelli NM, Dotters DJ, Katz VL, et al. Cancer in pregnancy: a review of the literature, part 1. *Obstet Gynecol Surv.* 1996;51:125–142.
106. Nesbitt JC, Moise KJ, Sawyers JL. Colorectal carcinoma in pregnancy. *Arch Surg.* 1985;120:636–640.
107. Bernstein MA, Madoff RD, Caushaj PF. Colon and rectal cancer in pregnancy. *Dis Colon Rectum* 1993;36:172–178.
108. Francavilla A, Leo D, Polimeno L, et al. Nuclear and cytosolic estrogen receptors in human colon carcinoma and in surrounding noncancerous colonic tissue. *Gastroenterology* 1987;93:1301–1306.
109. Stedman KE, Moore GE, Morgan RT. Estrogen receptor proteins in diverse human tumors. *Arch Surg.* 1980;115:244–248.
110. Wobbes T, Beex LVAM, Koenders AMJ. Estrogen and progestin receptors in colonic cancer? *Dis Colon Rectum* 1984;27:591–592.
111. Smith C, Butler JA. Colorectal cancer in patients younger than 40 years of age. *Dis Colon Rectum* 1989;32:843–846.
112. Pitluk H, Poticha SM. Carcinoma of the colon and rectum in patients less than 40 years of age. *Surg Gynecol Obstet.* 1983;157:335–337.
113. Cappell MS. Colon cancer during pregnancy: the gastroenterologist's perspective. *Gastroenterol Clin North Am.* 1998;7:225–256.
114. McCall JL, Black RB, Rich CA, et al. The value of serum carcinoembryonic antigen in predicting recurrent disease following curative resection of colorectal cancer. *Dis Colon Rectum* 1994;37:875–881.
115. Mason MH III, Kovalcik PJ. Ovarian metastases from colon carcinoma. *J Surg Oncol.* 1981;17:33–38.
116. **Walsh C, Fazio VW. Cancer of the colon, rectum, and anus during pregnancy: the surgeon's perspective. *Gastroenterol Clin North Am.* 1998;27: 257–267.**
117. Zemlickis D, Lishner M, Degendorfer P, et al. Fetal outcome after in utero exposure to cancer chemotherapy. *Arch Intern Med.* 1992;152: 573–576.
118. Mayr NA, Wen B-C, Saw CB. Radiation therapy during pregnancy. *Obstet Gynecol Clin North Am.* 1998;25:301–321.

SECTION S
SKIN AND SOFT TISSUE

CHAPTER 118 ■ CUTANEOUS NEOPLASMS

ALFRED E. CHANG, TIMOTHY M. JOHNSON, AND AMY KIM GIRA

Cutaneous neoplasms are the most commonly diagnosed malignant tumors in the United States, with an incidence of approximately 1.4 million new cases annually.[1,2] One in five Americans born in 2004 will be diagnosed with skin cancer in their lifetime. More than half of all cancers diagnosed in the United States are skin cancers. The most common skin cancer types are basal and squamous cell carcinoma (BCC and SCC). Cutaneous melanoma accounts for 4% of skin cancer diagnoses but accounts for 75% of skin cancer deaths, with 7,910 deaths due to melanoma in 2004, or about one every hour. Approximately 95,880 new cases of melanoma will be diagnosed in the United States in 2004: 40,780 *in situ* and 55,100 invasive (29,900 men and 25,200 women). This represents a 4% increase in new cases of melanoma from 2003. The incidence of melanoma has more than tripled among Caucasians between 1980 and 2003. Invasive melanoma is the fifth most common cancer in men, seventh most common cancer in women, and the most common form of cancer of any type in women between 25 and 29 years of age.[1,3] The early diagnosis and surgical treatment of these skin cancers can be curative.

MELANOMA

Etiology and Risk Factors

Numerous environmental and genetic risk factors have been implicated in the development of cutaneous melanoma.[2] Risk factors include ultraviolet light (UVL) exposure, fair complexion/inability to tan, blue or green eyes, blonde or red hair, freckling, history of actinic keratosis or nonmelanoma skin cancer, history of blistering or peeling sunburns, immunosuppression, personal or family history of melanoma, CDKN2A/p16/MC1R mutation, xeroderma pigmentosa, atypical (dysplastic) nevus, more than 100 normal nevi, and giant congenital melanocytic nevus. Patients with a significant history of sun exposure are at particularly high risk, especially if they experienced peeling or blistering sunburns, even during childhood. Melanoma occurs infrequently in skin of color, suggesting that skin pigment plays a protective role. Melanoma incidence is subject to large geographic and ethnic variations, mainly because of an inverse correlation with latitude and with degree of skin pigmentation. Populations residing closer to the equator have a higher incidence of melanoma. Certainly UVL exposure from sun or artificial light sources is considered the best-known risk factor. However, UVL exposure does not cause all or even most melanomas.

Adults with more than 100 clinically normal-appearing nevi, children with more than 50 clinically normal-appearing nevi, and any patient with atypical or dysplastic nevi are at risk. A prior history of melanoma places a patient at increased risk, with 5% to 10% of individuals developing a second primary melanoma. This risk of developing a second primary is lifelong and can occur anywhere on the skin. Therefore, long-term surveillance with a thorough total body examination is recommended.

A genetic component has been implicated in the pathogenesis of melanoma. Of patients with melanoma, 10% to 15% report a positive family history. The most common chromosomal mutation associated with melanoma involves CDKN2A, also known as p16. However, the mutation accounts for only a small percentage of melanoma cases observed, estimated at 0.2%. A MC1R gene mutation is clearly a risk factor for cutaneous melanoma. The combination of MC1R mutation and red hair is associated with a very high risk of melanoma development. In addition, MC1R R151C has been shown to modify the effect of another cutaneous melanoma susceptibility gene, CDKN2A. The genetic etiology of melanoma represents an area of future discovery.

The hereditary nature of cutaneous melanoma was also noted in the 1970s.[4] Members afflicted with the "B-K mole syndrome," named after two families, acquired large, irregular, and dysplastic nevi, often in sun-protected regions of the body such as the scalp and trunk. During this time period, Lynch et al.[5] independently reported a familial association of melanoma among individuals with atypical nevi, which he termed "Familial Atypical Multiple Mole-Melanoma Syndrome," or FAMMM syndrome, with an autosomal dominant inheritance pattern. The 10-year melanoma risk in the setting of atypical mole syndrome is reported to be 10.7% compared with 0.62% in control patients. Greene et al.[6] approximated a 56% cumulative risk from age 20 to 59 years, with 100% of atypical mole syndrome patients developing melanoma by age 76. An atypical nevus is not a premelanoma but represents a genetic marker for increased risk of development of melanoma, which may occur anywhere on the skin surface including sun-protected sites. In fact more than 50% to 75% of melanomas develop on clinically normal skin de novo, not in preexisting melanocytic lesions.

Xeroderma pigmentosa (XP) is a rare autosomal recessive disorder associated with a reduced or absent ability to repair DNA damaged by ultraviolet light. Consequently, this disorder results in the development of multiple primary cutaneous malignancies, including melanoma as well as BCC and SCC. Individuals are usually diagnosed with their first cancer before the age of 10 years. Unfortunately, the development of skin cancers is relentless.

Congenital melanocytic nevi (CMN*)* are present at birth or appear within the first 6 months of infancy.[7] An estimated 1% to 6% of children are born with CMN. The nevi are classified by size. Small CMN measure less than 1.5 cm in diameter and account for the majority of lesions. Medium CMN measure between 1.5 and 19.9 cm in diameter. Large CMN, also termed giant congenital nevi, measure 20 cm or greater. This large size can lead to significant cosmetic and psychosocial implications. The risk of melanoma development in small and medium-size CMN is similar to any other area of skin. Melanoma development in small and medium CMN usually occurs after childhood and arises from the dermoepidermal junction, making early detection feasible. Routine prophylactic removal of small and medium CMN is rarely indicated in the absence of signs or symptoms for malignant progression. Conversely, giant congenital nevi carry an increased risk for melanoma, with an estimated rate of 5% to 20%. Of giant congenital nevi that progress to melanoma, 70% are diagnosed prior to age 10 years. Melanoma can originate deep in the epidermis in giant congenital nevi. Consequently, diagnosis within the setting of giant congenital nevi is challenging and may develop deep in the skin with a more advanced primary lesion.

Patients with a giant congenital nevus, especially on the posterior axis, or in conjunction with many satellite lesions are also at risk for neurocutaneous melanocytosis (NCM).[8,9] NCM is characterized by the presence of benign or malignant leptomeningeal tumors. Most patients present in the first 2 years of life with neurologic manifestations of increased intracranial pressure, mass lesions, or malignant transformation to melanoma. Magnetic resonance imaging (MRI) findings of NCM may be present, even in asymptomatic children. NCM is associated with an increased risk of development of central nervous system melanoma. Symptomatic NCM is associated with a poor prognosis, even in the absence of malignancy. Chemotherapy is not effective, but shunt placement to reduce intracranial pressure may be palliative.

Clinical Diagnosis and Classification

Melanoma may have a characteristic appearance (Fig. 118.1). Early detection is key. The ABCD rule, which outlines the warning signs of melanoma, was developed decades ago.[10] A stands for *a*symmetry—one half of the lesion does not match the other half when drawing an imaginary line through the center of the lesion. B is *b*order irregularity—the edges of the lesion are ragged, notched, or fuzzy. C is *c*olor—the pigmentation is not uniform throughout the lesion. Varying shades of tan, dark brown to black, or shades of red, white, and/or blue may be present with a mottled appearance. And D is *d*iameter—the width is greater than 6 mm (about the size of a pencil eraser). The seven-point checklist used in Europe incorporates several of the ABCD features with the addition of change. Another useful diagnostic aid is the "ugly duckling" sign. A pigmented lesion that is different from the others should be carefully approached with a high index of suspicion.

The goal of any diagnostic aid is early detection, the ability to differentiate between benign and malignant, with 100% sensitivity combined with high specificity. The ABCD rule, seven-point checklist, and ugly duckling sign all provide relatively highly sensitivity but none fulfills all of these criteria, especially with respect to specificity to distinguish melanoma from benign lesions.

The ABCD criteria may fail to detect an important subset of nodular melanoma, which often does not exhibit the ABCDs and is often less than 6 mm in early development. The ABCD rule is also relatively static without the important critical characteristic of change. Studies have documented early signs of a change in size, shape, or color and the early symptom of persistent itching. One of the best tools for diagnosis of early lesions that may fail to exhibit many of the standard melanoma features is the importance of *change*. Thus, we and others have used the D in the ABCD rule to signify "*d*ifference." A difference or change in lesions, especially with respect to size, shape, color, or persistent itching, warrants evaluation. Furthermore, the nevi on the body should globally share a common look or family resemblance. If one of the nevi seems different from the rest, it should be evaluated with a high index of suspicion. Additionally, if all of the nevi are atypical or irregular, but are morphologically similar to one another and are not changing, there may be no reason for individual lesion concern (atypical or dysplastic nevi). However, the presence of atypical nevi represents a risk factor for melanoma development anywhere on the skin surface with development in clinically normal skin, normal nevi, and dysplastic nevi with relatively equal frequency. Thus, excision of all atypical nevi does little for prevention. Education of the patient for early signs and symptoms, particularly change or difference, is key in this clinical scenario.

It must be emphasized that critical diagnostic decisions concerning skin lesions should still always be based on clinical assessments and the history, with attention to melanoma risk factors. The optimum diagnostic aid that combines 100% sensitivity and specificity currently does not exist. Use of all available means including the ABCD and seven-point checklists, ugly duckling sign, difference, photography, dermoscopy, and evolving digital and computer-assisted imaging technologies enhances the ability to diagnose melanoma at the earliest stage.[10] The result of using these multiple diagnostic aids is earlier detection of melanoma with higher overall survival rates.

Based on histological patterns and clinical characteristics, melanomas can be classified into four major subtype categories: lentigo maligna melanoma (LMM), superficial spreading melanoma (SSM), nodular melanoma (NM), and oral-acral lentiginous melanoma (ALM).[11] In general, these subtypes derive their prognostic biological behavior and risk of metastasis based on a secondary correlation with Breslow depth and are thus not independent prognostic factors. Invasive LMM constitutes 10% to 15% of cutaneous melanomas and typically occur on the chronically sun-exposed areas of the head and neck, most often in older inividuals. Clinically, the LMM pattern is associated with a significantly higher rate of often extensive and asymetrical subclinical growth several centimeters beyond the clinical lesion. Failure to completely excise the entire lesion with meticulous margin control results in higher recurrence rates with lethal potential. Additionally, amelanotic and desmoplastic melanoma with neurotropism is more frequent in the lentigo maligna lesion subtype. Lentigo maligna (LM) is not a benign disease as once thought. LM represents *in situ* melanoma and, with time, progresses to invasive LMM. LMM often begins as a flat brown lesion on

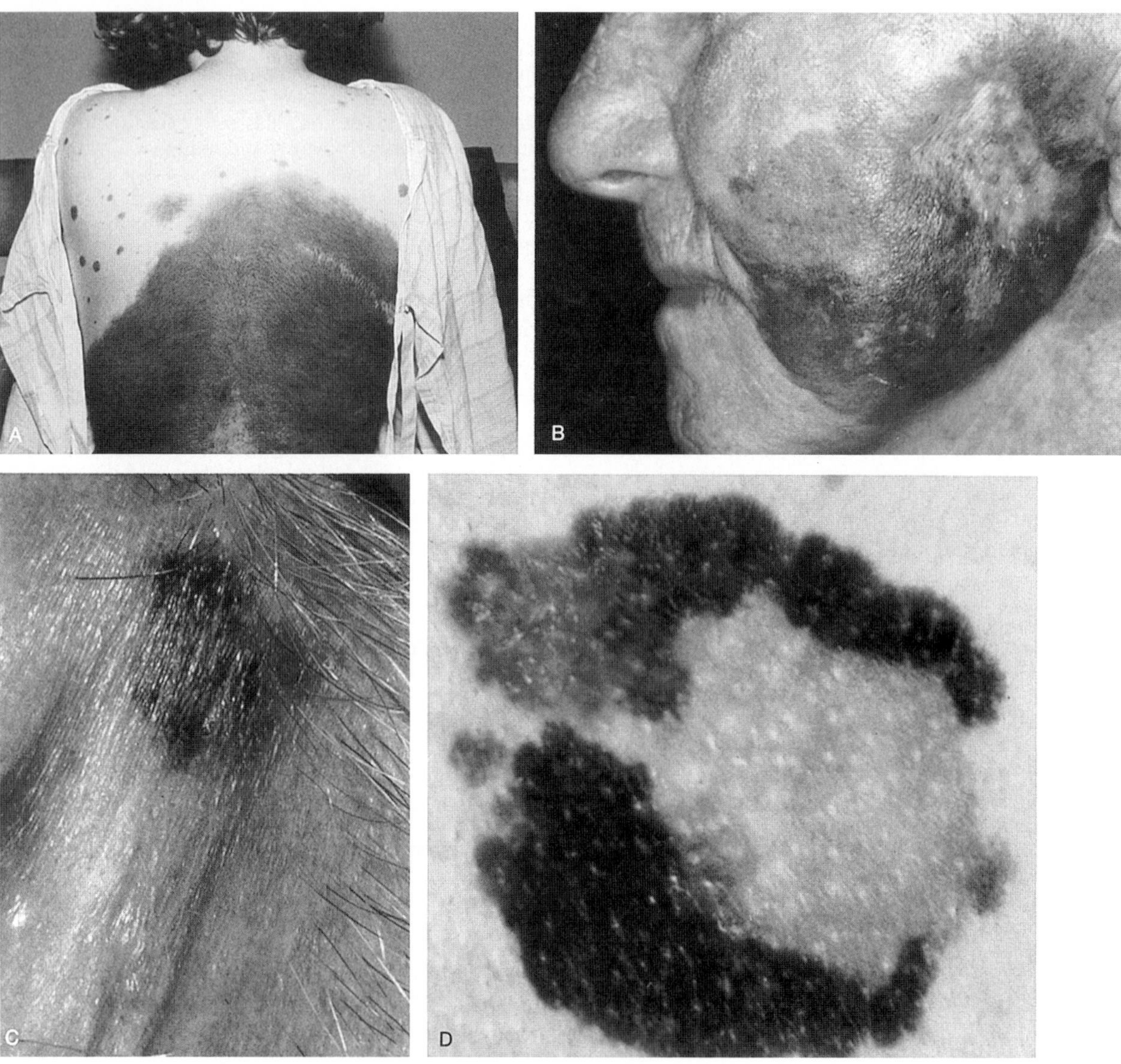

FIGURE 118.1 Examples of skin lesions. (*A*) Giant congenital nevus. (*B*) Lentigo maligna (Hutchinson freckle). (*C*) Melanoma arising in a lentigo maligna (lentigo maligna melanoma). (*D*) Superficial spreading melanoma. (*E*) Nodular melanoma. (*F*) Acral lentiginous melanoma (ulcerated nodular plantar melanoma with satellite lesions). (*G*) Subungual melanoma. (*H*) Pigmented basal cell carcinoma.

chronically sun-exposed areas with progression to black and other classic melanoma features over time.

SSM accounts for approximately 70% of cutaneous melanomas. This pattern is the most common in melanomas arising in a preexisting nevus. SSM is typically characterized by variation in color, irregular borders, and irregular surface and often exhibits the classic melanoma clinical features.

NM occurs in approximately 15% to 30% of patients with cutaneous melanoma and is often the most aggressive of the four types of melanoma because of later detection and rapid growth. In general, NM may be more uniform in coloration than the other types, have regular borders with size less than 6 mm in early lesions, and lack the classic melanoma features initially. Lesion change and difference is important for early detection.

ALM is a distinct clinicopathologic variant of melanoma that most commonly occurs on the hands, feet, fingers, and toes as well as in subungual locations (see Fig 118.1). ALM represents only 2% to 8% of melanoma in Caucasians but 35% to 60% in people of color. Later detection frequently occurs because of location that is not easily or routinely examined and a low index of suspicion. When corrected for Breslow depth, the overall prognosis for ALM is similar to the other subtype categories. In subungual locations, this phase can appear as an irregular, tan-brown streak in the nail that originates from the base of the nail bed. More than three fourths of subungual melanomas involve the great toe or thumb, and they can be confused with subungual hematoma.

Other rare melanoma subtypes deserve brief mention. Mucosal, anal, and vulvovaginal melanomas are associated with a poorer prognosis, possibly related to advanced disease at presentation with late detection and high vascularity at the lesion site. Desmoplastic melanoma is associated with a higher rate of neurotropism and local recurrence.[12] Small cell or nevoid melanoma often lacks any of the classic features, is difficult to accurately diagnose without expert dermatopathology interpretation, and thus may be initially more frequently misdiagnosed. And amelanotic melanoma, occuring in 3% to 4% of cases, is often associated with late detection due to lack of pigment and failure to diagnose early.

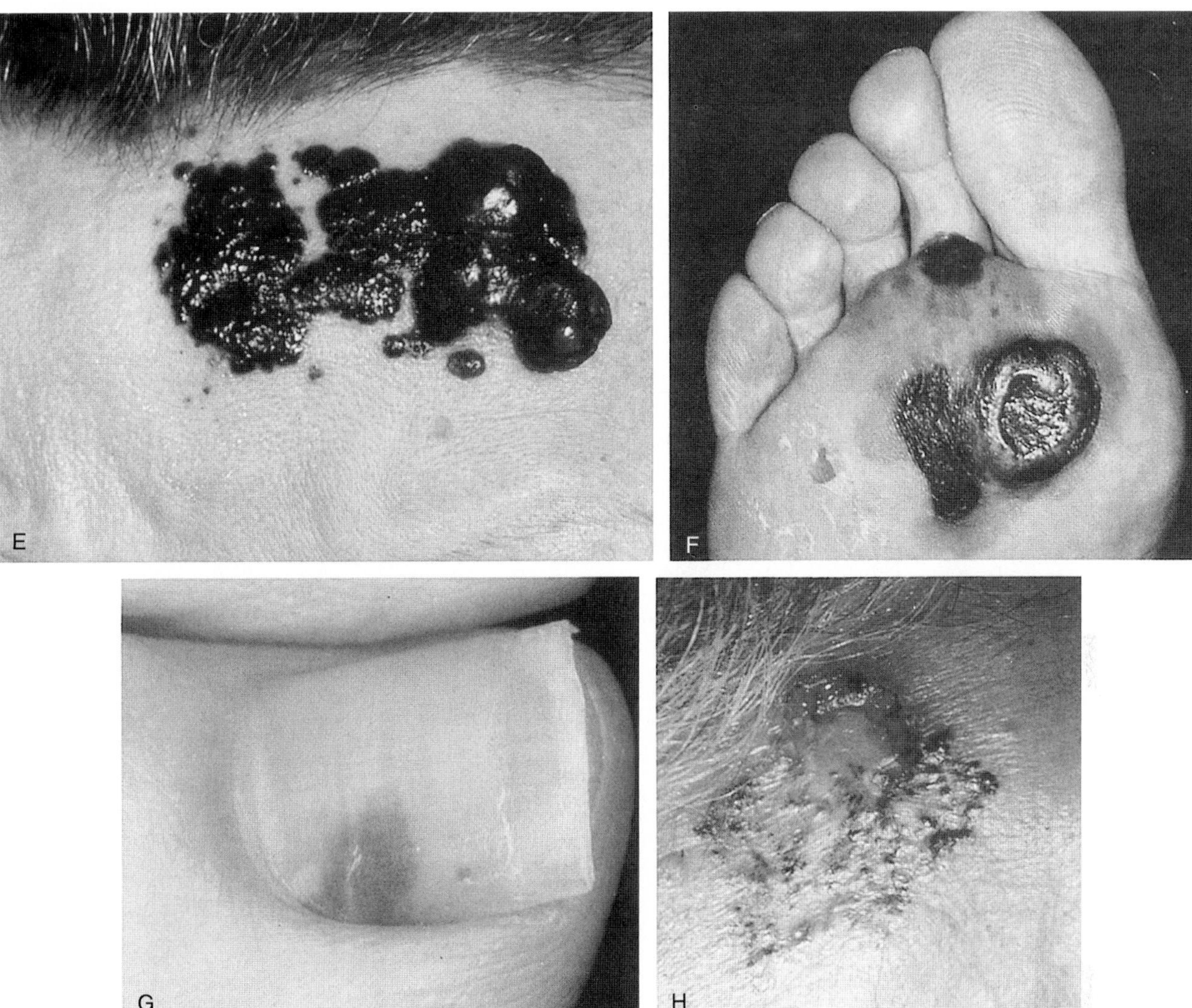

FIGURE 118.1 (*Continued*)

Staging and Prognostic Factors

A great deal of information is available regarding various factors that correlate with the clinical outcome of patients with melanoma. Some of these prognostic factors, such as microstaging and nodal status, are of sufficient independent significance to be incorporated into staging systems with known survival rates. Other prognostic factors, such as tumor ulceration and microscopic versus macroscopic nodal disease, have also been found to be significant variables that influence survival and have been incorporated into the staging system.

Microstaging

One of the most important prognostic features of cutaneous melanoma is the stage of development of the primary tumor. The microstaging method that is used routinely was originally described by Breslow.[13] This method classifies the primary tumor according to its thickness in millimeters, as measured with an ocular micrometer, from the top of the granular layer to the base of the tumor. Many investigators have documented an inverse correlation between tumor thickness and survival. The largest series of 17,600 patients reported by Balch et al.[14] is summarized in Table 118.1. The ulceration status and mitotic rate are also independent factors that are used to determine microstaging of the primary lesion.[14,15] Prior to the use of the Breslow microstaging method, melanomas were staged according to the level of invasion into the histologic layer of skin. This was known as Clark's level of invasion and comprised five levels (I = *in situ* lesions, V = subcutaneous involvement). Several studies have confirmed that Breslow thickness conveys more accurate prognostic information than does the determination of Clark level.[14,16]

The presence of regional lymph node metastases is associated with a worsening prognosis. The tumor burden (microscopic versus macroscopic disease) of involved lymph nodes has an inverse correlation with long-term survival.[14,16] The 5-year survival rate for patients with involved lymph nodes ranges from 70% to 25%, based primarily on tumor burden and ulceration status of the primary lesion (Table 118.2). The use of sentinel lymph node biopsy (SLNB) has identified a subgroup of patients with micrometastatic nodal disease who have a favorable prognosis compared with patients with macroscopic nodal involvement. This information has been incorporated in the staging system as well.

TABLE 118.1 RESULTS

SURVIVAL RATES FOR MELANOMA TNM AND STAGING CATEGORIES

Stage	TNM	Thickness (mm)	Ulceration	No. + Nodes	Nodal size	Distantmets	No. of pts.	Survival 1-Year	2-Year	5-Year	10-Year
IA	T1a	†1	No	0	—	—	4,510	99.7	99.0	95.3	87.9
IB	T1b	†1	Yes or level IV,V	0	—	—	1,380	99.8	98.7	90.9	83.1
	T2a	1.01–2.0	No	0	—	—	3,285	99.5	97.3	89.0	79.2
IIA	T2b	1.01–2.0	Yes	0	—	—	958	98.2	92.9	77.4	64.4
	T3a	2.01–4.0	No	0	—	—	1,717	98.7	94.3	78.7	63.8
IIB	T3b	2.01–4.0	Yes	0	—	—	1,523	95.1	84.8	63.0	50.8
	T4a	>4.0	No	0	—	—	563	94.8	88.6	67.4	53.9
IIC	T4b	>4.0	Yes	0	—	—	978	89.9	70.7	45.1	32.3
IIIA	N1a	Any	No	1	Micro	—	252	95.9	88.0	69.5	63.0
	N2a	Any	No	2–3	Micro	—	130	93.0	82.7	63.3	59.6
IIIB	N1a	Any	Yes	1	Micro	—	217	93.3	75.0	52.8	37.8
	N2a	Any	Yes	2–3	Micro	—	111	92.0	81.0	49.6	35.9
	N1b	Any	No	1	Macro	—	122	88.5	78.5	59.0	47.7
	N2b	Any	No	2–3	Macro	—	93	76.8	65.6	46.3	39.2
IIIC	N1b	Any	Yes	1	Macro	—	98	77.9	54.2	29.0	24.4
	N2b	Any	Yes	2–3	Macro	—	109	74.3	44.1	24.0	15.0
	N3	Any	Any	4	Micro/Macro	—	396	71.0	49.8	26.7	18.4
IV	M1a	Any	Any	Any	Any	Skin, SQ	179	59.3	36.7	18.8	15.7
	M1b	Any	Any	Any	Any	Lung	186	57.0	23.1	6.7	2.5
	M1c	Any	Any	Any	Any	Other	793	40.6	23.6	9.5	6.0
Total							17,600				

From Balch M, Buzaid AC, Soong SJ, et al. Final version of the American Joint Committee on Cancer Staging System for Cutaneous Melanoma. *J Clin Oncol* 2001;19:3635–3648. Reprinted with permission from the American Society of Clinical Oncology.

TABLE 118.2 RESULTS

FIVE-YEAR SURVIVAL RATES FOR PATIENTS WITH STAGE III MELANOMA STRATIFIED BY NUMBER OF NODES WITH METASTASIS, ULCERATION, AND TUMOR BURDEN

No. positive nodes	Nodal burden	Ulceration	% 5-year survival ± standard error	No. patients in study group
1	Microscopic	Absent	69 ± 3.7	252
1	Microscopic	Present	52 ± 4.1	217
2–3	Microscopic	Absent	63 ± 5.6	130
2–3	Microscopic	Present	50 ± 5.7	111
>3	Microscopic	Absent	27 ± 9.3	57
>3	Microscopic	Present	37 ± 8.8	46
1	Macroscopic	Absent	59 ± 4.7	122
1	Macroscopic	Present	29 ± 5.0	98
2–3	Macroscopic	Absent	46 ± 5.5	93
2–3	Macroscopic	Present	25 ± 4.4	109
>3	Macroscopic	Absent	27 ± 4.6	109
>3	Macroscopic	Present	13 ± 3.5	104

Modified from Balch M, Soong SJ, Gershenwald JE, et al. Prognostic factors analysis of 17,600 melanoma patients: validation of the American Joint Committee on Cancer Melanoma Staging System. *J Clin Oncol* 2001;19:3622–34.

Clinical and Pathologic Staging

The American Joint Committee on Cancer (AJCC) developed a five-stage system that divides melanomas according to tumor thickness (T), nodal status (N), and metastatic disease (M).[14,16] The current system was updated in 2002 and is summarized in Table 118.3. There are five stages based on prognosis: stage 0 (*in situ* melanoma), stage I (local disease), stage II (local disease), stage III (regional nodal, in-transit, or satellite metastases), and stage IV (distant metastases; Table 118.4). In general, increasing stage is associated with decreasing survival (see Table 118.1).

Other Prognostic Factors

The major prognostic factors that predict survival in melanoma patients have been accounted for in the AJCC staging system: namely, tumor microstaging, ulceration, nodal status, and distant metastases.[14,16] The presence of ulceration in a melanoma appears to be associated with a poorer prognosis. Men have a higher proportion of ulcerated lesions than women (27% vs. 19%, respectively). Although ulceration appears to correlate with thickness of the melanoma, the presence of ulceration has been shown to be an independent prognostic factor and has been included in the staging system.[14,16] Additionally, a higher mitotic rate of 1.0 mm^2 or greater has been shown to be an independent prognostic factor in one large study.[15]

Treatment of Primary Melanoma

Biopsy

For localized melanoma, the tumor thickness (Breslow depth of invasion) is the single variable that most accurately determines therapy and prognosis. The ulceration status and mitotic rate

TABLE 118.3 STAGING

AMERICAN JOINT COMMISSION ON CANCER MELANOMA STAGING SYSTEM, TNM DEFINITIONS

PRIMARY TUMOR

TX: Cannot be assessed (shave biopsy, regressed lesion)
T0: Unknown primary
Tis: *In situ* melanoma
T1: †1.0 mm Breslow thickness
- a. without ulceration
- b. with ulceration or Clark level IV or V

T2: 1.01 to 2.0 mm
- a. without ulceration
- b. with ulceration

T3: 2.01 to 4.0 mm
- a. without ulceration
- b. with ulceration

T4: >4.0 mm
- a. without ulceration
- b. with ulceration

REGIONAL LYMPH NODE INVOLVEMENT

NX: Cannot be assessed (previously removed)
N0: No regional node metastasis
N1: Metastasis in one regional node
- a. micrometastasis (diagnosed by SLNB or elective lymph node dissection)
- b. macrometastasis (clinically palpable or found on imaging studies, confirmed histologically, or gross extracapsular extension)

N2: Metastasis in two to three regional nodes
- a. micrometastasis
- b. macrometastasis
- c. in-transit or satellite metastasis without nodal metastasis

N3: Metastasis ‡4 regional nodes, matted nodes, or in-transit or satellite metastasis with positive metastatic nodes

DISTANT METASTASIS

MX: Cannot be assessed
M0: No distant metastasis
M1a: Distant skin, subcutaneous, or lymph node metastasis with normal LDH
M1b: Lung metastasis with normal LDH
M1c: All other distant metastasis or any distant site with elevated LDH

SLNB, sentinal lymph node biopsy; LDH, lactate dehydrogenase

TABLE 118.4 STAGING

STAGE GROUPINGS FOR CUTANEOUS MELANOMA

	Clinical staging[a]			Pathological staging[b]		
	T	N	M	T	N	M
0	Tis	N0	M0	Tis	N0	M0
IA	T1a	N0	M0	T1a	N0	M0
IB	T1b	N0	M0	T1b	N0	M0
	T2a	N0	M0	T2a	N0	M0
IIA	T2b	N0	M0	T2b	N0	M0
	T3a	N0	M0	T3a	M0	M0
IIB	T3b	N0	M0	T3b	N0	M0
	T4a	N0	M0	T4a	N0	M0
IIC	T4b	N0	M0	T4b	N0	M0
		N1				
III[c]	Any T	N2	M0			
		N3				
IIIA				T1-4a	N1a	M0
				T1-4a	N2a	M0
				T1-4b	N1a	M0
				T1-4b	N2a	M0
IIIB				T1-4a	N1b	M0
				T1-4a	N2b	M0
				T1-a/b	N2c	M0
				T1-4b	N1b	M0
IIIC				T1-4b	N2b	M0
				Any T	N3	M0
IV	Any T	Any N	Any M1	Any T	Any N	Any M1

[a]Clinical staging includes microstaging of the primary melanoma and clinical/radiologic evaluation for metastasis. By convention, it should be used after complete excision of the primary melanoma with clinical assessment for regional and distant metastases.
[b]Pathologic staging includes microstaging of the primary melanoma and pathologic information about the regional lymph nodes after partial or complete lymphadenectomy. Pathologic stage 0 or stage IA patients are the exception; they do not require pathologic evaluation of their lymph nodes.
[c]There are no stage III subgroups for clinical staging.
(From Balch M, Buzaid AC, Soong SJ, et al. Final version of the American Joint Committee on Cancer Staging System for Cutaneous Melanoma. *J Clin Oncol.* 2001;19:3635–3648. Reprinted with permission from the American Society of Clinical Oncology.)

also represent independent prognostic variables. A full-thickness biopsy with 1- to 2-mm margins only, to the adipose tissue, is preferred for any lesion highly suspect for melanoma.[17] If the melanoma is transected with a partial-thickness shave biopsy, the ability to obtain an accurate measurement of tumor thickness is lost. Therefore, a superficial shave biopsy is never recommended for a suspect pigmented lesion.

Excisional biopsy with 1- to 2-mm margins is the preferred method for suspect lesions to provide the pathologist a total specimen for histologic interpretation and accurate microstaging. Performing a wide excision as the first step, especially on the trunk or head and neck, is not recommended because of doing so may result in the inability to accurately perform SLNB. Formalin-fixed, paraffin-embedded, permanent sections should be used for biopsy diagnosis of primary cutaneous melanoma to determine accurately tumor thickness and other histopathologic prognostic variables. Frozen sections have no role in the diagnosis or microstaging of primary melanoma. If the lesion is a melanoma, the excisional biopsy represents the first stage of a two-stage procedure. The second stage is reexcision with margins generally ranging from 0.5 to 2 cm, with or without SLNB, depending primarily on the tumor thickness. The desired orientation of the biopsy on the extremity is parallel to the lymphatics.

For suspicious lesions that are too large for complete excision and those that are located where the amount of skin is critical in terms of functional or cosmetic results, an incisional biopsy may be performed with an eliptical incision, deep saucerization shave to adipose or deep dermis in thick skin areas, or a punch. Incisional biopsies for melanoma do not increase the risk of metastasis or affect patient survival. They should generally be performed on the most raised or most pigmented area of the lesion to maximize the obtainable diagnostic and prognostic information. The most raised area usually corresponds to the maximal thickness of the lesion, but not always. Several incisional biopsies can be obtained from different areas for large lesions with multiple morphologic features. In the scenario of incisional biopsy with significant remaining lesion, complete excision for accurate microstaging

TABLE 118.5 TREATMENT

FOLLOW-UP GUIDELINES: INTERVAL FREQUENCY AND TESTS

	NCCN	UMMC
In situ	Periodic skin exam for life	q6 mo for 1 yr, then annually
Local disease <1 mm or >1 mm with a negative SLNB and without ulceration	q3–12 mos	q6 mo for 3 yr, then annually
Local disease—1 mm. No SLNB or negative SLNB with ulceration	q3–12 mos for 3 yr, then 4–12 mos for 2 yr, then annually	q6 mo for 3 yr, then annually. Tests based on H&P
Regional disease	q3–12 mos for 3 yr, then 4–12 mos for 2 yr, then annually. CXR, LDH, CBC q3–12 mos (optional). Other imaging studies (optional)	q6 mo for 3 yr, then annually. Tests based on H&P
Distant disease	Medical oncology trials	Medical oncology trials

Shorter intervals with dysplastic nevus syndrome or patient difficulty with self-examination
Coordinate dermatologist and primary care provider/internist/or medical oncology team.
NCCN, National Comprehensive Cancer Network; UMMC, University of Michigan Multidisciplinary Melanoma Clinic; SLNB, sentinal lymph node biopsy; H&P, histology and pathology.

should be considered prior to definitive treatment, unless the lesion is already 1 mm or greater in Breslow depth.

Metastatic Workup

In an attempt to standardize staging workup for melanoma, the National Comprehensive Cancer Network (NCCN) has published guidelines.[18,19] There are three basic reasons to perform a metastatic workup following the diagnosis of primary cutaneous melanoma: (a) for staging and prognosis, (b) to detect an early metastasis with potential survival benefit, and (c) to avoid morbidity of an extensive surgical procedure by detection of a distant metastasis.[19] The best test for the staging workup still starts with a history (focused review of systems concentrating on constitutional, respiratory, neurologic, hepatic, musculoskeletal, gastrointestinal, skin, and lymphatic systems) and physical examination (total body skin examination, palpation of lymph nodes). Routine imaging and blood studies in asymptomatic patients are low in both sensitivity and specificity.[19–22] False-positive staging tests are common and lead to more tests and patient distress. SLNB represents the best baseline staging test, with both relatively high sensitivity and specificity in patients at significant risk for metastasis. The ability to detect stage IV disease with routine studies is small if the SLNB is negative. Ultrasound is perhaps the most sensitive noninvasive test to detect small nodal metastases. However, the sensitivity and specificity of ultrasound and PET scanning are inferior to tissue diagnosis with SLNB.

With respect to potential outcome benefit, unfortunately no satisfactory treatment exists and asymptomatic detection of stage IV melanoma has not resulted in impact on overall survival. Regional disease survival is based on the number of metastatic nodes, the tumor burden (microscopic vs. macroscopic), and the ulceration status of the primary melanoma. The potential clinical and survival benefit for early therapeutic lymph node dissection in patients with nodal disease is based on a large body of evidence.

In sum, the extent of the staging workup should be defined by the extent of local and regional disease and geared toward meaningful, early detection of additional primary melanomas and early lymph node metastasis. A high index of suspicion with symptom-directed workup is recommended to detect stage IV disease in asymptomatic patients with localized disease. Significant emotional distress has been demonstrated in up to 30% of patients with melanoma, independent of disease stage.[23] Thus, access to psychooncology intervention is also an important aspect of the overall management of the patient with melanoma.

Based on the best current evidence, with an unremarkable history and physical examination, the NCCN has recommended (a) no routine tests for local disease smaller than 1 mm, (b) no routine but still optional chest radiography and lactate dehydrogenase (LDH) plus SLNB (if indicated to follow) for local disease of 1 mm or greater, and (c) chest radiography, LDH, pelvic CT if groin nodes involved (vs. CT chest/abdomen/pelvis), and head MRI for regional disease. Workup for stage IV disseminated melanoma is often dictated by clinical trial protocols. Follow-up test guidelines are similar to these workup principles (Table 118.5).

Surgical Excision of Primary Melanoma

The primary purpose of a melanoma excision is to prevent local recurrence due to persistent disease.[24] For melanoma *in situ*, excision margins of 0.5 to 1 cm are indicated. For invasive melanoma, wide excision of the primary tumor, with margins generally ranging from 1 to 2 cm, is indicated for local control. The optimal margin width remains somewhat controversial. The historical approach of excising all primary melanomas with a 3- to 5-cm margin is extinct. At least five randomized controlled trials failed to demonstrate a difference in overall survival or local recurrence with narrow (1 to 2 cm) versus wide (3 to 5 cm) margins (Table 118.6).[24] Of note, one trial demonstrated an increased risk of locoregional recurrence with 1 versus 3 cm margins for melanoma more than 2 mm thick.[25] Hopefully, results from future randomized prospective trials will demonstrate how narrow a margin is truly safe and efficacious. Until more definitive data become available, current consensus guidelines recommend margins of 1 cm for melanoma of 1 mm or less thick, 1 to 2 cm for 1 to 2 mm thick, and at least 2 cm for greater than 2 mm thick (Table 118.7).

For the clinically ill-defined LMM, histological confirmation of negative margins is important and it should be empha-

TABLE 118.6 RESULTS

RANDOMIZED CONTROLLED TRIALS: NARROW VERSUS WIDE EXCISION MARGINS

Trial[a]	No. of subjects	Narrow resection margin (cm)	Wide resection margin (cm)	Tumor thickness (mm)	Tumor site	Median length follow-up (yr)
French 2003	326	2	5	<2.1	T, E, H&N (16)	10
Intergroup 1996	470	2	4	1–4	T, E	7.6
Swedish 2000	989	2	5	0.8–2	T, E	11
WHO 1991	612	1	3	<2	T, E	7.5
UK 2004	900	1	3	‡2	T, E	5

[a]No difference in any outcomes in first four trials. UK 2004 showed increased locoregional recurrence but no difference in local or in-transit recurrence.

sized that these margin recommendations may not apply to *in situ* LM and invasive LMM on the head and neck.[26,27] LM and LMM are often associated with extensive subclinical involvement to as much as several centimeters beyond the clinical component. Careful and complete margin control, including excision of the lesional trailing edge of atypical melanocytic hyperplasia, often beyond the standard margins. may be necessary for complete surgical resection of LM/LMM on the head and neck.

Treatment of Regional Metastatic Melanoma

Lymphadenectomy Results and Indications

Surgical excision of metastases to regional lymph nodes is potentially curative therapy. The 5-year survival rate for patients who undergo lymphadenectomy for clinically positive involved nodes (AJCC stage III) ranges from 25% to 70%. In addition, for those patients not cured by lymphadenectomy, resection can avoid potential pain associated with tumor enlargement, skin breakdown, and tumor necrosis (Fig. 118.2). Only 10% of patients who first present with the diagnosis of melanoma have clinical evidence of nodal metastases; approximately 85% have localized disease; the remaining 5% have distant metastases. In less than 3% of patients, a diagnosis of melanoma is made in the absence of a definable primary lesion.[28] When patients present with isolated nodal disease from an unknown primary site, the results of lymphadenectomy are similar to those for patients with known primary tumors. For patients with melanoma 1.0 mm thick or greater who present with clinically negative nodes, SLNB should be considered to determine whether therapeutic lymphadenectomy is indicated.[19]

TABLE 118.7 TREATMENT

RECOMMENDED SURGICAL MARGINS FOR MELANOMA EXCISION

Melanoma thickness (mm)	Clinical excision margin (cm)
In situ	0.5 to 1.0
†1.0	1.0
1.1 to 2.0	1.0 to 2.0
‡2.0	2.0

Margins may need to be modified based on anatomic considerations but still require histologic confirmation of tumor-free margins. For clinically ill-defined LM/LMM, wider margins may be required for histologic confirmation of tumor-free margins.

Sentinel Lymph Node Biopsy

Morton et al.[29] were the first to develop the concept of "sentinel lymph nodes" in the nodal basins draining cutaneous melanomas. They hypothesized that melanoma involvement of a nodal basin develops in an orderly fashion with metastasis to the sentinel lymph node as the first step in that process. With the intradermal injection of a blue dye, these investigators were able to identify sentinel lymph nodes 90% of the time. If the sentinel node was negative for melanoma, the remaining lymph nodes were also free of involvement in at least 96% of cases. These results have been confirmed by multiple other groups.[30,31]

Two techniques are available for identifying the sentinel lymph nodes, and they are often combined. These techniques use two different lymphatic tracers: a blue dye, 1% isosulfan blue (Lymphazurin); and a radiolabeled colloid solution. The blue dye is injected intradermally a few minutes before the procedure. The injection site is around the primary tumor site or excision site, taking care to avoid injecting directly into any residual tumor. Blue-stained lymphatics and lymph nodes can be directly

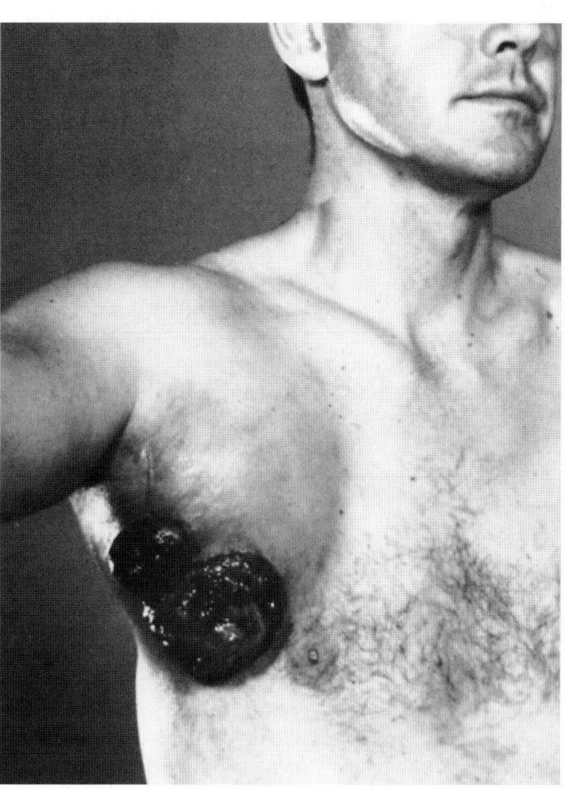

FIGURE 118.2 Patient with large melanoma axillary involvement with skin ulceration.

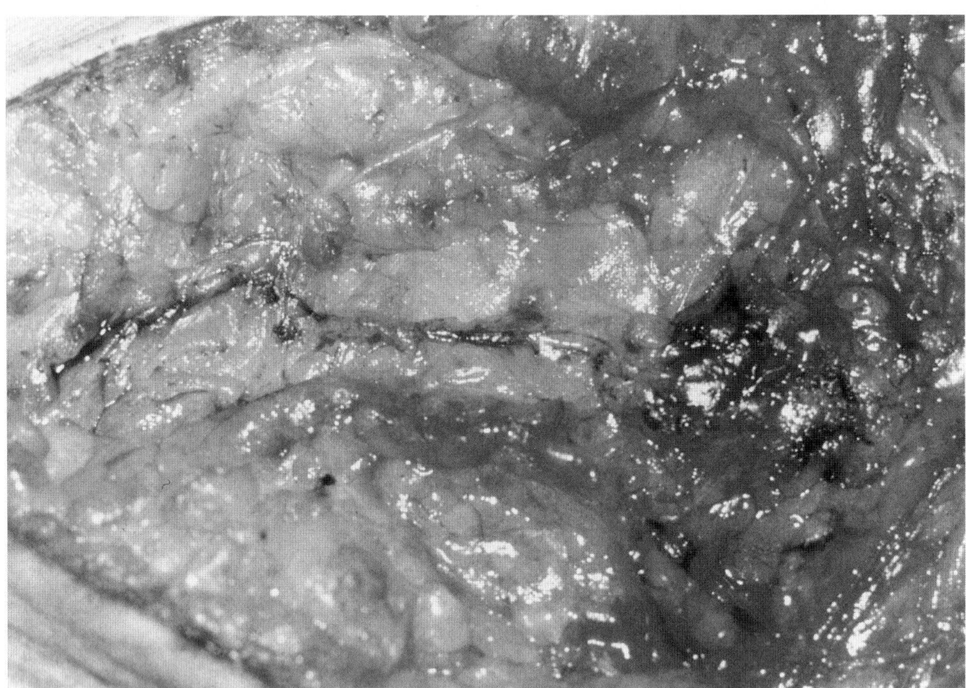

FIGURE 118.3 Blue dye tracking up a lymphatic vessel to a blue-stained lymph node.

visualized (Fig. 118.3). The other technique involves intradermal injection of a radiolabeled colloid solution, which is performed between 1 and 4 hours before surgery, also at the site of the primary tumor. Using a hand-held gamma detector probe, the surgeon is able to identify the sentinel lymph node location through the skin, thereby limiting the incision necessary to find the node. Furthermore, this technique allows lymphoscintigraphy imaging, which can identify sentinel nodes outside the traditional nodal basin. The combined use of the blue dye plus the radiolabeled colloid enables the detection of the sentinel node in more than 90% of cases.[30] The technique of SLNB is most often performed in conjunction with the wide excision of the primary tumor. It can routinely be performed as an outpatient procedure.

Once the sentinel lymph node is removed, it is processed by the pathologist by step-sectioning the entire node into multiple sections for routine hematoxylin and eosin staining. This is done to examine for micrometastases that could be missed by the standard approach to examining nodes, which involves bivalving the lymph node and performing an examination of only one section. If serial sectioning and staining are negative for metastasis, then immunohistochemical staining for melanoma markers such as S-100, Melan-A, and HMB-45 is performed.[32] These stains can identify microscopic clusters of tumor cells that are hard or impossible to identify by hematoxylin and eosin staining. The thoroughness of assessing the sentinel lymph nodes for metastatic disease has resulted in much more accurate staging of patients. Micrometastases to lymph nodes has been incorporated in the current staging system as described above. Clinical trials assessing the utility of reverse transcriptase-polymerase chain reaction to identify messenger RNA of melanoma-associated proteins in sentinel lymph nodes as a prognostic tool are currently being conducted.[33,34]

If the sentinel lymph node is positive for melanoma, regional therapeutic lymphadenectomy (Fig. 118.4) is indicated based on potential survival and clinical benefit. To date, no factors have been identified to determine who will have additional non–sentinel node metastasis. The patient is then eligible for consideration of adjuvant therapy, as discussed later. As noted above, patients with primary melanomas equal to or greater than 1 mm thickness and clinically negative nodes should be considered for SLNB. For some subgroups of patients with

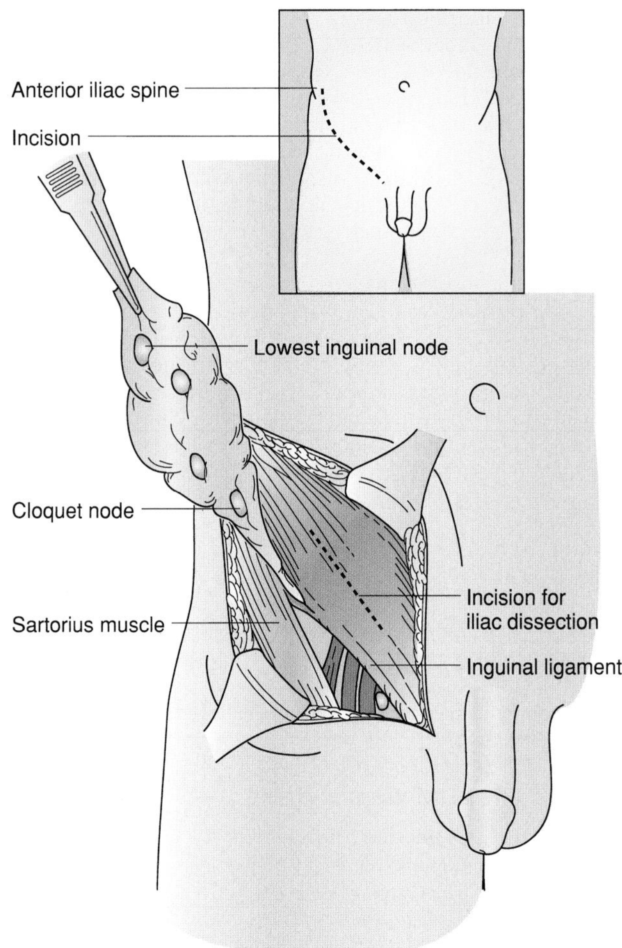

FIGURE 118.4 Technique of groin dissection.

melanoma Breslow depth of 0.75 to 1.0 mm, SLNB maybe considered. These subgroups include younger patients, evidence of ulceration, extensive dermal regression to 1.0 mm, or 1.0 mitosis/mm^2 or greater in the primary tumor.[35] Reasons not to perform SLNB include significant medical comorbidities, patient desire if the wide excision can be done with local anesthesia versus general or intravenous anesthesia required for SLNB, or the patient does not desire SLNB after an informed discussion.

Adjuvant Therapy

Although the prognosis for patients with early-stage cutaneous melanoma is quite good, less than 50% of patients with thick primaries (i.e., >4 mm) or regional node involvement are cured by surgery alone. The development of effective adjuvant therapy capable of increasing postsurgical survival in high-risk groups of patients has been a long-standing goal of clinicians.[36,37] Chemotherapy with dacarbazine (DTIC) has been evaluated as a postoperative adjuvant in a randomized study to be without effectiveness. Numerous randomized trials evaluating bacillus Calmette-Guerin (BCG) immunotherapy in the adjuvant setting have also been negative.

Interferon-α2b (IFN-α) has a variety of modulatory effects on the immune system that could enhance antitumor reactivity. IFN-α has been reported to have antitumor activity in patients with metastatic disease. In 1996, Kirkwood et al.[38] reported the effectiveness of IFN-α to improve disease-free and overall survival rates of patients with stage IIb (>4 mm) or III disease after surgery. In this multiinstitutional prospective randomized trial, 287 high-risk patients with deep primary (>4 mm) tumors or positive nodes were randomly assigned after surgery to either postoperative adjuvant treatment with IFN-α-2b or to observation. IFN-α-2b therapy significantly increased median overall survival, by 1 year, and produced a 24% improvement in the 5-year overall survival rate (46% for IFN-α-2b patients vs. 37% for observation patients). Based on these results, the U.S. Food and Drug Administration (FDA) approved the use of adjuvant IFN-α-2b after surgical resection of stage IIb or III melanoma. Follow-up studies have raised concerns about the relative efficacy of IFNα in this setting; however, in healthy melanoma patients at high risk of relapse this is the only known adjuvant therapy that should be considered.[36]

For localized melanomas measuring 1.5 to 4 mm in thickness, a vaccine trial has demonstrated interesting results in the adjuvant setting. In this trial, conducted by the Southwest Oncology Group, patients with intermediate-thickness melanomas were randomized to receive an allogeneic tumor vaccine (Melacine) versus observation after primary tumor resection.[39,40] A total of 689 patients were enrolled. Analysis of the randomized groups revealed no difference in survival. However, patients who were HLA-A2 or HLA-C3 positive who received the vaccine had significantly improved disease-free and overall survival compared with the randomized control group as well as patients who were HLA-A2 or HLA-C3 positive who did not receive the vaccine. These observations have opened the door to examine this vaccine in follow-up trials and also indicated that immunotherapy with tumor vaccines may have a clinical role in the future.

Treatment of Disseminated Melanoma

Evaluation for Metastatic Disease and Clinical Course

The follow-up evaluation for patients with AJCC stage I, II, or III melanoma who are rendered tumor free by surgery should include regular histories and physical examinations. The use of extensive and frequent radiographic studies and blood work in asymptomatic, clinically disease-free patients is rarely productive.[18–22] In 2004, the National Comprehensive Cancer Network issued guidelines for follow-up of patients with various stages of disease. For AJCC stage IA (≤1 mm), patients should undergo a history and physical examination with emphasis on skin and nodal examinations every 3 to 12 months as clinically indicated. For AJCC stage IB to III, patients should undergo a history and physical examination every 3 to 6 months for 3 years, then every 4 to 12 months for 2 years, then annually as clinically indicated (see Table 118.5). The use of chest radiographs and blood work, and other imaging scans are indicated when clinically indicated, is based on the history and physical examination.

Melanoma can disseminate to any organ. The most common sites of recurrence are skin, subcutaneous tissues, and distant lymph nodes, followed by visceral sites. Common visceral sites of metastasis, in order of decreasing occurrence, are lung, liver, brain, bone, and gastrointestinal tract. Most patients who die with disseminated disease have multiple organ involvement. Frequently, the cause of death is respiratory failure or brain complications. Patients with disseminated disease have a poor prognosis, with a mean survival of approximately 6 months. Cure with any treatment is rare. Selection of treatment or a decision against treatment should be based on several factors, including the patient's medical condition, the potential for palliation, and the impact of treatment on quality of life.

Surgery

Surgical excision of recurrent melanoma can be effective for palliation in patients with isolated recurrences in the skin, central nervous system, lung, or gastrointestinal tract.[20,41–47] Surgical excision of solitary brain metastases has been shown to provide improved palliation and quality of life compared with brain irradiation. Resection of isolated pulmonary metastases or of subcutaneous recurrences is usually not considered curative but can result in significantly prolonged disease-free survival. Gastrointestinal lesions causing obstruction or bleeding should be considered for resection or bypass to relieve these symptoms.

Radiation Therapy

Melanoma can respond to radiation therapy.[43,45–48] Radiation therapy is commonly used for palliation of bone pain secondary to metastatic disease or brain metastasis. The average survival after brain irradiation for melanoma is approximately 4 months.

Chemotherapy

Melanoma is responsive to few chemotherapeutic drugs.[49–53] The best single agents for treatment of melanoma are DTIC, the nitrosoureas, vinca alkaloids, and cisplatin, which have objective response rates in the range of 10% to 20%. Conventionally, objective responses have included complete disappearance of all known tumor sites (complete response) and reduction of more than half in all assessable tumor (partial response). Complete responses are rare and nearly always of brief duration (<6months). Responses are more frequently observed in patients with tumor in skin, subcutaneous tissue, lymph nodes, or lung. Combination chemotherapy with the potential of drug synergy has been used with limited success in the treatment of metastatic melanoma. No evidence indicates that combination chemotherapy offers better results than single-agent DTIC at this time.

Several centers have reported experience with isolated hyperthermic limb perfusion of chemotherapeutic agents to treat multiple subcutaneous (in-transit) or skin (satellitosis) metastases of the extremities. This technique requires the isolation and cannulation of the afferent and efferent vessels of the involved extremity to an extracorporeal pump. High doses of chemotherapeutic agents can be infused into the limb without systemic toxicity. Sometimes dramatic tumor responses can be obtained. A European study of hyperthermic limb perfusion

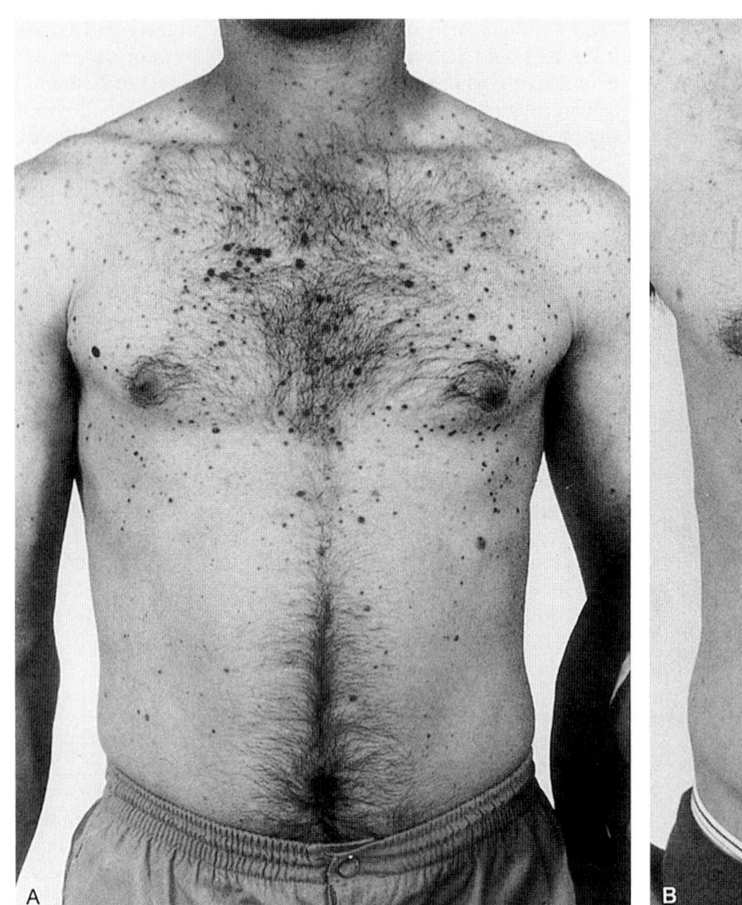

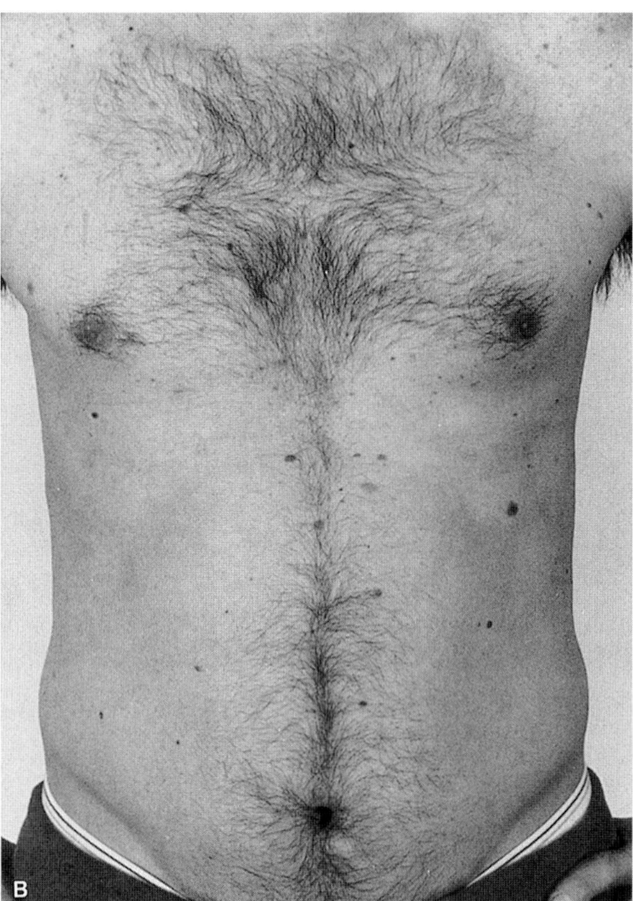

FIGURE 118.5 (*A*) Patient with disseminated melanoma metastatic to multiple cutaneous sites. (*B*) After several courses of therapy with lymphokine-activated killer cells and interleukin-2, the patient had a complete response. (Courtesy of Steven A. Rosenberg, M.D., Surgery Branch, National Cancer Institute, Bethesda, MD.)

with a combination of melphalan, TNF, and interferon-α reported partial and complete responses among patients with melanoma lesions.[54–56] TNF cannot be administered systemically because of its severe toxicity; the use of isolated perfusion to an extremity avoids this limitation. This approach appears to be effective in the small subgroup of patients with disease confined to an extremity, but confirmatory studies are needed.

Immunotherapy

The rapid evolution of recombinant DNA technology has resulted in the availability of cytokines, such as the interferons and interleukins, that can be administered to modulate a patient's immune response.[36–40] These biologic agents have been used in immunotherapeutic trials for metastatic melanoma and demonstrate that an antitumor immune response can be generated in selected patients.

IFN-α was one of the first cytokines used in tumor therapy. IFN-α was originally produced by virus-stimulated leukocytes and is now available in recombinant form. The interferons are known to induce macrophage cytotoxicity, enhance natural killer cell activity, upregulate major histocompatibility complex (MHC) antigens on tumors, and upregulate tumor-associated antigens. The objective response rates of melanoma to IFN-α administration range from 10% to 20%. As reviewed earlier, IFN-α has been approved by the FDA for adjuvant treatment of patients with stage III disease.[36–38]

The most significant advance in melanoma immunotherapy has been associated with the use of interleukin-2 (IL-2). IL-2 is a cytokine secreted by antigen-activated helper T cells and was initially discovered because it was a T-cell growth factor. Subsequently, it was found to have many other immunologic effects, and it appears to have an important role in the enhancement of immune responses. Mulé et al.[57] discovered that the *in vivo* administration of IL-2 in preclinical animal models resulted in dramatic tumor regression. In clinical studies, the administration of IL-2 resulted in a 15% to 20% response rate in patients with advanced melanoma. [58] Approximately 5% of patients have a complete response which has been durable for prolonged periods (Fig. 118.5). This latter result prompted the FDA to approve IL-2 for the treatment of metastatic melanoma.

IL-2 has been used in combination with other forms of immunotherapy. One example of this is the use of antitumor reactive T cells as reagents to treat tumor that is called *adoptive immunotherapy*. One source of these T cells is from the tumor itself, known as tumor-infiltrating lymphocytes. In clinical studies Rosenberg et al.[59–61] have reported that patients with advanced melanoma treated with the combination of tumor-infiltrating lymphocytes, IL-2, and chemotherapy can result in response rates between 35% and 50%.

Vaccines derived from melanoma tumor cells or extracts of tumor cells have been an emerging field in the treatment of melanoma.[40] The discovery of unique melanoma tumor–associated antigens has opened the door for the development of highly specific reagents for tumor vaccines. Rosenberg et al. [62] reported that the administration of a modified peptide antigen, gp100, given with incomplete Freund's adjuvant along with the concomitant administration of IL-2, resulted in a 42% response rate in patients with stage IV melanoma. Because this response rate was higher than that reported for IL-2 alone, it suggests that the vaccination with a tumor-associated peptide may have induced immunity to tumor cells and that the IL-2 was "helping" the response. Currently, there are many trials evaluating the use of vaccines in the therapy of melanoma.

Another development in the field of vaccines is the use of dendritic cells (DCs). DCs are potent antigen-presenting cells of the immune system that are capable of sensitizing naive T cells to respond against tumor antigen. DCs can be "pulsed" with tumor antigen in the form of peptides, whole tumor cells, lysates of tumor cells, or genes encoding antigen. Animal studies have shown that antigen-pulsed DC can cause the regression of established tumors by intradermal or intravenous administration. The administration of IL-2 with DC therapy has improved the antitumor response rate in animal studies.[63] In humans, antigen-pulsed DCs have resulted in complete responses in patients with stage IV melanoma.[64] Numerous studies are being conducted to evaluate DC vaccine therapy with or without the concomitant use of IL-2.

Biochemotherapy

Combinations of IL-2 and/or IFN-α with chemotherapy, known as biochemotherapy, have shown significant improved response rates compared with chemotherapy alone or cytokines alone. As might be expected, these regimens are more toxic than the component therapies by themselves. One of the biochemotherapy regimens that has demonstrated a significant response rate (i.e., 64%, including 21% complete and 43% partial) with moderate toxicity is a combination of cisplatin, vinblastine, dacarbazine, IL-2, and IFN-α .[49–53] A follow-up randomized trial comparing this biochemotherapy regimen to chemotherapy alone indicated that the addition of the cytokines significantly enhanced the antitumor activity of the chemotherapy.[53] Biochemotherapy should be considered in patients with advanced melanoma who are thought to be able to tolerate the toxicities of the therapy.

Gene Therapy

The technical feasibility of transfer of genetic material into somatic cells has established a new approach to the treatment of malignancies. Many of the gene therapy strategies for cancer have focused on modulating the host immune response by altering tumor cells to be more "immunogenic." A variety of preclinical studies have demonstrated that genetic engineering of tumor cells to secrete or express immunoregulatory peptides (i.e., cytokines, costimulatory molecules, or adhesion molecules) increases the host immune response to these tumors.[65] Several clinical studies are evaluating the efficacy of genetic modification of melanoma tumor cells to secrete cytokines that can be administered to patients as tumor vaccines.[64–71]

NONMELANOMA SKIN TUMORS

BCC and SCC account for 96% of new nonmelanoma skin cancers (NMSC). These tumors are derived from epithelial origin.[1–3] The ratio of BCC to SCC is approximately 4:1. The annual incidence of BCC and SCC in the United States alone exceeds 1 million cases. The public health burden on the U.S. population from NMSC, for which the incidence is rapidly rising, is highly significant. Patients with NMSC have an excellent prognosis with 90% to 99% curable with appropriate treatment and less than 1% resulting in death. SCCs account for 75% of NMSC deaths, which are estimated at 2,000 to 2,500 per year.

Etiology

Both BCC and SCC are most commonly induced by significant exposure to ultraviolet light from the sun or tanning booths.[2] These cancers are the predominant neoplasms on the head, neck, trunk, lower legs, and extensor arms and hands where sun exposure is common. Skin cancer is a significant occupational hazard for people who work outdoors. The phenotype at increased risk is one with fair skin who sunburns and freckles easily, blue eyes, and red or blonde hair. Melanin pigment in the skin appears to be the protective factor.

T number of genetic syndromes are associated with an increased risk of developing NMSC, including Gorlin syndrome, xeroderma pigmentosa, and albinism. Gorlin syndrome is an autosomal dominant disorder associated with multiple BCCs, palmoplantar pits, jaw cysts, frontal bossing, and hypertelorism. Albinism is a disorder characterized by a partial or complete deficiency in melanin production and, thus, loss of protective pigment. Another factor associated with NMSC, primarily SCC, is chronic exposure to chemicals such as aresenic and hydrocarbons (found in coal tars, soot, and asphalt). Cigarette smoking has been associated with SCC of the lip and mouth. Human papillomavirus has been associated with cutaneous SCC in the genital and acral/periungual areas. Radiation has been associated with both SCC and BCC.

Basal Cell Carcinoma

BCC is the most common form of skin cancer. These epithelial-derived tumors can be divided into various subtypes according to clinical appearance, histologic pattern, and biologic behavior. Although BCCs rarely metastasize, they are characterized by slow but relentless and destructive local invasion that results in high morbidity without treatment. The subclinical local invasion may be deep, extensive, and asymmetric, with fingerlike extensions several centimeters beyond the clinical borders.

The most common subtype of BCC is the well-circumscribed nodular variety. These tumors often present as pearly papules or nodules with telangiectases. They may be pruritic and bleed occasionally. With time, the center ulcerates to create peripheral "rolled" borders; such ulcerating BCCs are called rodent ulcers (Fig. 118.6). Occasionally, the lesions are deeply pigmented and nodular and can be confused with melanoma. This variant has been called a pigmented BCC (see Fig. 118.1H). The histologic features of these tumors demonstrate isolated areas of basaloid tumor islands arising from the

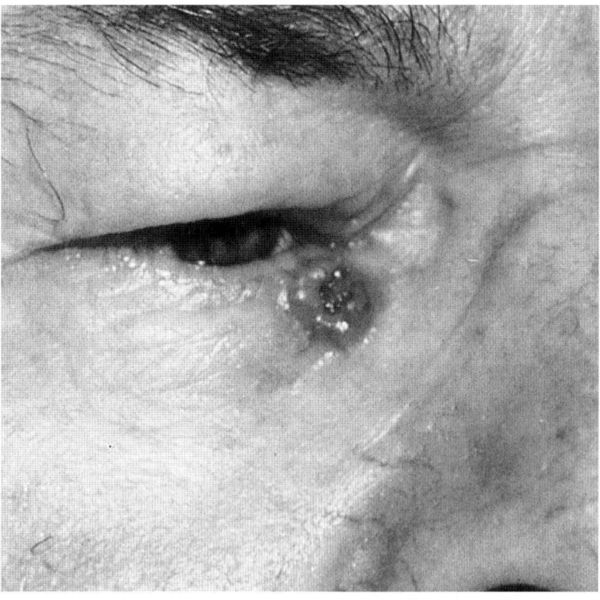

FIGURE 118.6 Basal cell carcinoma near the eye.

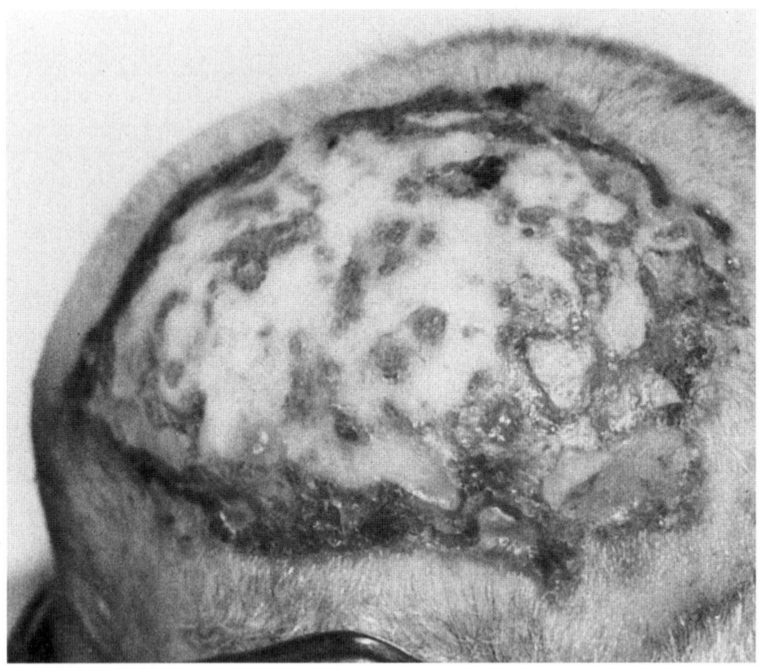

FIGURE 118.7 Morpheaform basal cell carcinoma of the scalp.

epidermis with peripheral palisading of nuclei and stromal retraction. In some cases, the BCC has histologic features of squamous metaplasia with keratinization. These tumors have basosquamous differentiation and can become more aggressive and develop regional lymphatic spread.

The most locally agressive type of BCC is characterized by a diagnostic histopathologic aggressive growth pattern, known as morpheaform, sclerosing, or fibrosing BCC (Fig. 118.7). Clinically, these tumors may be more subclinical, are flat, and appear to be scarlike. They have a significant incidence of recurrence because of the isolated, fingerlike fronds of basal cell tumor cells that may deeply invade the surrounding structures well beyond the clinical margins of the lesion. These small, fingerlike islands are often missed with standard histologic margin control.

Clinically, superficial BCCs are scaly pink to red lesions. Frequently, they are confused with psoriasis or other eczematous, scaly dermatoses. Although these tumors are usually relatively superficial, extensive superficial subclinical involvement is common. Numerous risk factors are associated with possible extensive subclinical invasion and increased rates of local recurrence for BCC after standard treatment, including surgical excision (Table 118.8).

Squamous Cell Carcinoma

SCC is the second most common form of skin cancer and is derived from the epithelial keratinocyte. SCC can deeply invade surrounding structures and metastasizes most commonly to regional lymph nodes. In immunosuppressed transplant individuals, SCC is the most common skin cancer, occurring 65 to 250 times more frequently than in the general population. SCC in these individuals tends to have more aggressive behavior.

Several precursor lesions to invasive SCC exist, most commonly actinic keratoses and Bowen's disease (*in situ* SCC). Erythroplasia of Queyrat, another precursor lesion, represents SCC *in situ* on the glans penis. Histologically, SCC shows malignant degeneration of epithelial cells with differentiation toward keratin formation. SCC often appears clinically as a nonhealing sore with ulceration and inflammatory pink borders or an erythematous papulonodule with overlying keratotic crust or ulceration (Figs. 118.8 and 118.9). These tumors most often arise in chronically actinically damaged skin or within an actinic keratosis, but they may also develop in burn scars or chronic inflammatory wounds. These lesions may infiltrate widely. Metastasis to regional lymph nodes accounts for approximately 80% to 90% of metastatic cases. Distant sites, such as lung, liver, brain, bone, and skin, account for the other 10% to 20%. Metastatic SCC portends a poor prognosis with a 10-year survival rate for regional lymph node disease of less than 20% and for distant disease of 10%.[72]

Accurate assessment of the higher-risk cutaneous SCCs is handicapped because of the lack of large prospective studies using multivariate analysis. Nine variables, however, have been identified as prognostic risk factors by retrospective analysis. Factors that may determine a higher risk for local recurrence, extensive subclinical invasion, and metastasis are noted in Table 118.9.

TABLE 118.8

BASAL CELL CARCINOMA: HIGHER RISK FACTORS FOR SUBCLINICAL INVASION AND RECURRENCE[79]

- Recurrent tumor
- Anatomic location
  - High risk: central face, eyelid, eyebrow, periorbital, nose, lip, chin, mandible, temple, ear, in front or behind the ear, genitalia, hand and foot
  - Medium risk: cheeks, forehead, scalp, and neck
  - Low risk: trunk, extremity (excluding hand/foot)
- Size
  - Lesions ≥6 mm on high-risk area
  - Lesions ≥10 mm on medium-risk area
  - Lesions ≥20 mm on low-risk area
- Histologic subtype pattern
  - Aggressive growth (morpheaform, fibrosing, sclerosing, infiltrating)
  - Micronodular
- Ill-defined clinical borders
- Perineural invasion
- Development in sites of prior radiation
- Immunosuppression

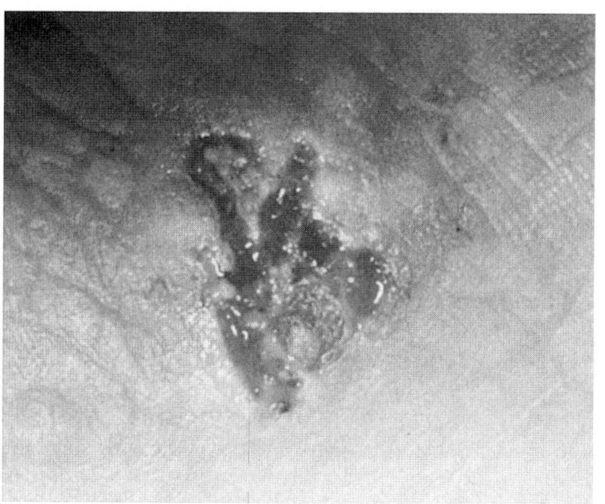

FIGURE 118.8 Squamous cell carcinoma of the hand secondary to exposure to arsenic in welding flux.

Other Tumors of Interest

Hundreds of cutaneous tumors exist, and their description is beyond the scope of this chapter. Tumors that may be encountered by the surgeon for further management include Merkel cell carcinoma, sweat gland carcinoma, and dermatofibrosarcoma protuberans.[73–78]

Merkel cell carcinoma is a malignant neuroendocrine tumor with features of epithelial differentiation. Merkel cell carcinoma is biologically aggressive, with a high incidence of local recurrence (36% to 50%), regional nodal metastasis (46% to 66%), and systemic metastasis (28%) based on reports primarily from tertiary care centers.[74] The 5-year survival rates are as follows: 88% for stage I (no nodal disease), 48% for stage II (regional nodal disease), and 0% for stage III (distant metastatic disease). Merkel cell carcinoma typically appears as a red to purple papulonodule or indurated plaque (Fig. 118.10). Approximately 50% of tumors arise on the head and neck, 40% on the extremities, and 10% on the trunk. Merkel cell carcinoma is a small cell tumor with characteristic positive immunocytochemical staining for CK-20, neuron-specific enolase, cytokeratin, and neurofilament protein. A chest radiograph is usually indicated to rule out cutaneous metastatic oat cell carcinoma, which may be similar in clinical and histologic appearance. Treatment consists of wide local excision with 1- to 2-cm margins. SLNB with immunostaining using CK-20 is recommended by the NCCN to stage the nodal basin and guide the consideration for nodal radiation.[75] Adjuvant radiation to the primary site and the primary draining nodal groups if SLNB is not performed should also be considered. Primary treatment

TABLE 118.9

SQUAMOUS CELL CARCINOMA: HIGHER RISK FACTORS FOR SUBCLINICAL INVASION AND RECURRENCE[79]

- Recurrent tumor
- Anatomic location
  - High risk: central face, eyelid, eyebrow, periorbital, nose, lip, chin, mandible, temple, ear, in front or behind the ear, genitalia, hand and foot
  - Medium risk: cheeks, forehead, scalp, and neck
  - Low risk: trunk, extremity (excluding hand/foot)
- Size
  - Lesions ≥6 mm on high-risk area
  - Lesions ≥10 mm on medium-risk area
  - Lesions ≥20 mm on low-risk area
- Histology
  - Poorly differentiated
- Depth of invasion
  - Clark's level IV (lesion that involves the reticular dermis), V (lesion that invades into subcutaneous fat), or ≥4 mm
- Perineural invasion
- Rapid growth
- Etiology
  - Scar, chronic ulcer or inflammatory process, sinus tract, sites of prior radiation therapy
- Immunosupression

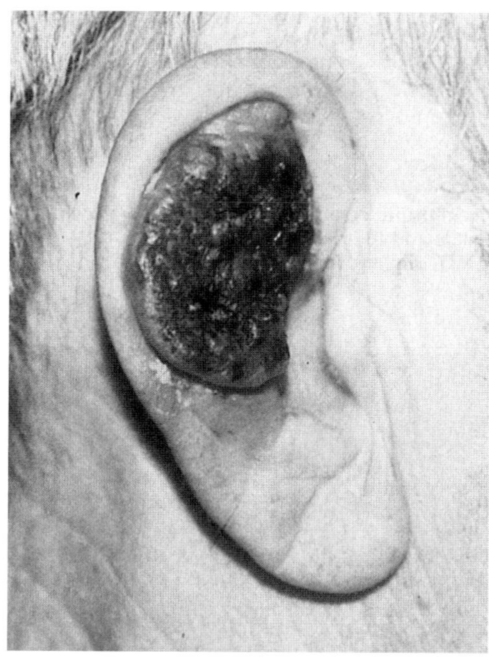

FIGURE 118.9 Ulcerative squamous cell carcinoma.

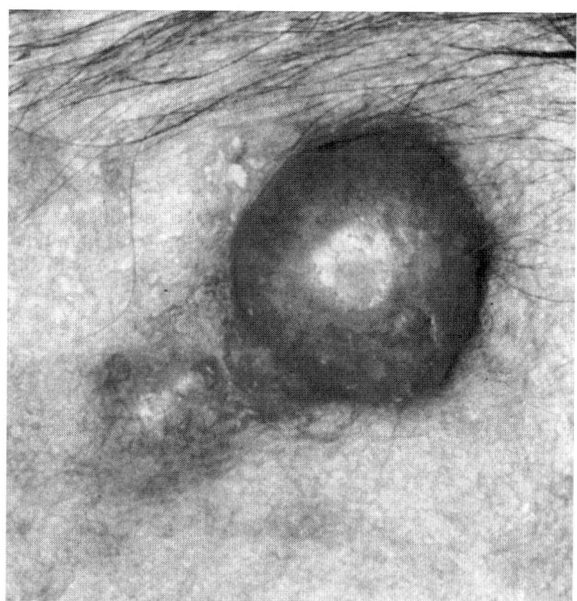

FIGURE 118.10 Merkel cell carcinoma.

with radiation therapy may also be considered. The role of adjuvant chemotherapy is unknown but may be considered for patients with lymph node metastasis.[73,75]

Sweat gland carcinomas represent a broad scope of neoplasms with variable risk for local and/or regional/distant metastasis, most commonly of eccrine or apocrine origin.[76] These are rare tumors (0.005% of skin malignancies) that have multiple histologic subtypes, giving rise to a diverse and confusing nomenclature. The aggressive types of sweat gland carcinomas have a propensity for both local recurrence and regional or systemic metastasis. Clinically, these tumors appear as indurated plaques, papules, or nodules commonly in the head and neck or extremity regions and are red, blue, pink, or skin colored. Histologic subtypes that are associated with a risk of regional lymph node or systemic metastatsis include aggressive digital papillary adenocarcinoma, hidradenocarcinoma, and eccrine carcinoma. Recommended treatments have included wide excision of the primary tumor with consideration of SLNB for high-risk lesions commonly based on size, mitotic rate, growth rate, or immunosuppression.[76] Postoperative radiation may also be considered as adjuvant therapy.

Dermatofibrosarcoma protuberans (DFSP) is a rare soft tissue sarcoma (1% of all soft tissue sarcomas) with a propensity for local recurrence rather than systemic metastasis. It is a spindle cell tumor that characteristicallly demostrates immunoreactivity to CD34.[77,78] Adults in their third to fifth decades are most commonly affected, but DFSP may occur in children to the elderly. These tumors appear as firm flesh-colored to dull red plaques that may be mistaken for keloids or hypertrophic scars. Although DFSPs may appear discrete, they characteristically demonstrate extensive subclinical involvement, which makes this sarcoma difficult to manage. Histologically, these sarcomas are identified by their fingerlike projections of spindle cells which likely account for tumor recurrence. Standard histologic processing makes it difficult to track these fingerlike projections. Treatment commonly consists of wide local excision with more comprehensive margin assessment or Mohs surgery, depending on patient and tumor factors. A multidisciplinary approach utilizing the expertise from several fields (Mohs surgery, surgical subspecialties, pathology) may be needed to achieve the goals of tumor excision and reconstructive repair. Radiation may also be beneficial in surgically unresectable cases.[77,78]

Surgical Treatment of Nonmelanoma Skin Cancers

A skin biopsy for diagnosis is important before treatment of any skin cancer. Fortunately, most nonmelanoma skin cancers are small, low-risk lesions that respond with 90% to 95% cure rates to standard treatment techniques, including curettage and electrodesiccation, cryosurgery, radiation therapy, and surgical resection.[79] Many skin cancers can be removed with elliptical excisions. Margins for low-risk SCC range from 0.5 to 1 cm. Margins for low-risk BCC range from 0.3 to 0.5 cm. Mohs surgery should be considered for BCCs and SCCs that exhibit the higher-risk factors in Tables 118.8 and 118.9. If Mohs surgery is not available, excision with careful frozen-section control (with permanent section confirmation) is indicated. The fundamental oncologic principle of tumor clearance first, reconstruction second should be followed.

Mohs Surgery

Mohs surgery was developed by Frederick E. Mohs, a general surgeon from the University of Wisconsin, in the 1940s. Initially, a chemical fixative paste was applied to the skin to fix the tissue *in situ*; hence, the now outdated term *Mohs chemosurgery*. The fresh tissue technique, which omitted the chemical paste, was developed and refined in the 1970s. Mohs micrographic surgery is most useful for the treatment of higher risk NMSC (see Tables 118.8 and 118.9). Mohs surgery is usually performed under local anesthesia in an outpatient Mohs surgical unit.[80–82] After removal of all gross tumor, the surgeon excises a thin layer of tissue with 2- to 3-mm margins. The tissue is mapped, color-coded for orientation, and sent to the technician for frozen-section processing. The specimen is flexible and flattened, with the beveled peripheral skin edge placed in the same horizontal plane with the deep margin. In this plane, both the deep and peripheral margins are examined in one horizontal cut by frozen-section analysis with total (theoretically 100%) margin control. Good-quality frozen sections may be achieved only by a skilled and experienced Mohs histotechnician. The Mohs surgeon functions as both surgeon and pathologist. After histologic interpretation of the frozen-section specimens, the precise anatomic location of any residual tumor can be identified and reexcised until all margins are tumor free (Fig. 118.11). The Mohs surgeon's ability microscopically to track subclinical tumor extensions results in the highest cure rate with maximal preservation of normal tissue. Soft tissue reconstruction can then be performed on the same day, after completion of Mohs surgical excision of the tumor (Fig. 118.12). A multidisciplinary approach involving Mohs, plastic, head and neck, and oculoplastic surgeons and radiation oncologists may be needed for extensive tumors. Mastering the Mohs technique is based on a steep learning curve. The American College of Mohs Micrographic Surgery and Cutaneous Oncology requires 1 to 2 years of fellowship training with a minimum of 500 to 600 cases before certification.

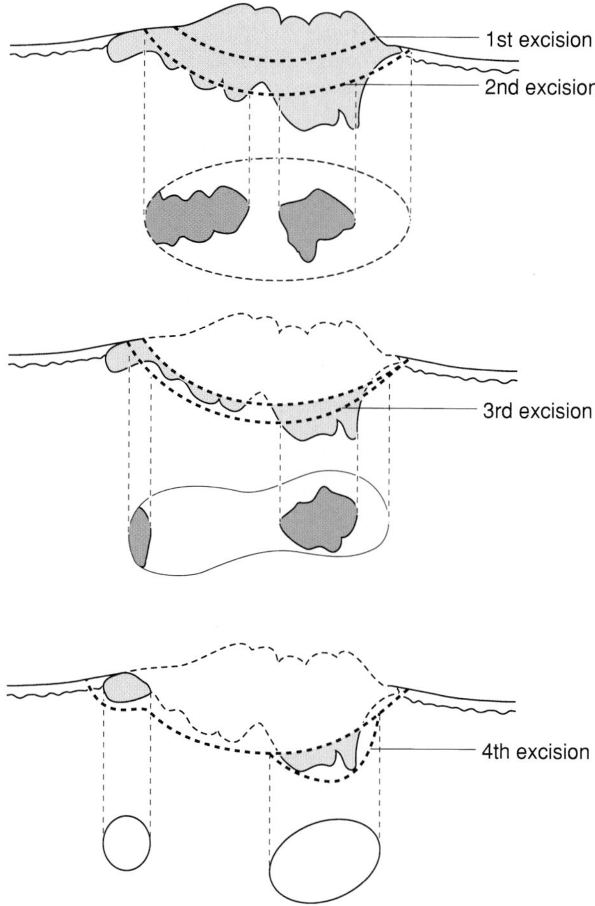

FIGURE 118. 11 Mohs micrographic surgical technique.

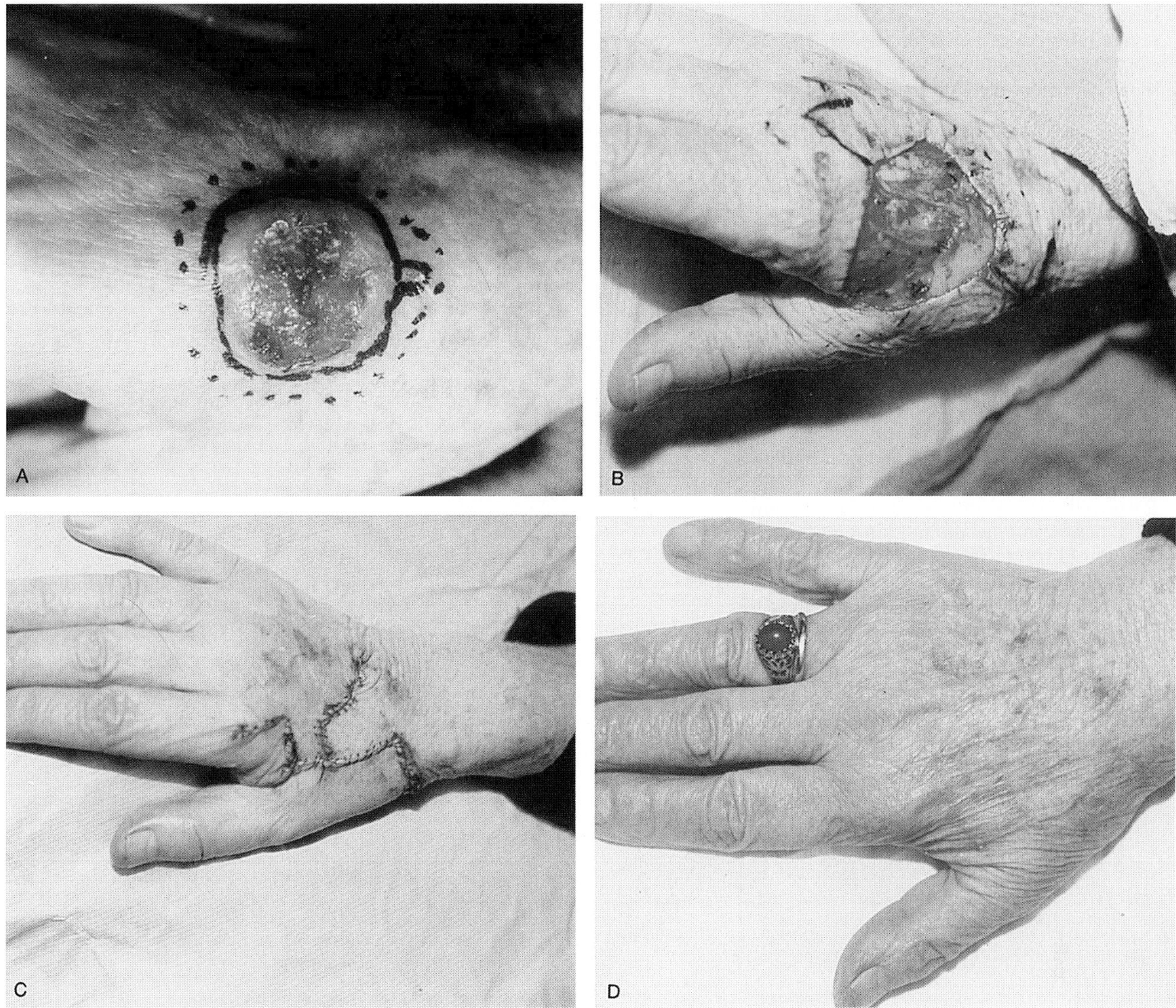

FIGURE 118.12 (*A*) Patient with a 3 × 3 cm basal cell carcinoma on the right dorsal hand with mixed nodular and aggressive growth histologic pattern. (*B*) Final Mohs surgery defect measuring 4 × 4.8 cm to the underlying tendon with preservation of tendon and nerve structures. Complete excision of the tumor required two Mohs stages (10 frozen sections). (I) The defect was reconstructed immediately after achievement of clear margins under local anesthesia in the Mohs surgery unit using birhombic flap soft tissue reconstruction. (I) Result 3 months after surgery.

Based on a review of all studies from all disciplines since 1950, the 5-year cure rate for treatment of previously untreated primary BCC by Mohs surgery is 99%, versus 90% to 93% for all non-Mohs modalities, including standard surgical excision.[83] For previously treated recurrent BCC, the 5-year cure rates are 94% for Mohs versus 60% to 84% for non-Mohs modalities.[84] In general, Mohs surgery should be considered for NMSCs that are associated with a higher risk of recurrence after standard treatment and for tumors for which conservation of normal tissue is important. Risk factors for recurrence after standard treatment have been previously mentioned. Tumors for which maximal conservation of tissue may be important include tumors in the high-risk locations and tumors in young patients.

Adjuvant and Primary Radiation Therapy

Radiation therapy may be useful for primary treatment of low-risk nonmelanoma skin cancers.[79] In experienced hands, primary radiation therapy may also be useful for higher risk tumors with high cure rates. For cutaneous SCC with many high-risk factors and for those with extensive neurotropism, adjuvant prophylactic radiation therapy to the primary site and the primary draining lymph nodes may decrease the risks of local recurrence and regional nodal metastasis. Prophylactic adjuvant radiation therapy should also be considered for highly aggressive, deeply invasive BCCs that exhibit extensive neurotropism.

KEY POINTS

- **Cutaneous neoplasms are the most commonly diagnosed malignant tumors in the United States, with an incidence of approximately 1.4 million new cases annually.**
- **Risk factors for development of cutaneous melanoma include ultraviolet light (UVL) exposure, fair complexion/inability to tan, blue or green eyes, blonde or red hair, freckling, history of actinic keratosis or nonmelanoma skin cancer, history of**

blistering or peeling sunburns, immunosuppression, personal or family history of melanoma, CDKN2A/p16/MC1R mutation, xeroderma pigmentosa, atypical (dysplastic) nevus, more than 100 normal nevi, and giant congenital melanocytic nevus.

- **The ABCD rule is used to assess skin lesions for melanoma risk: A is for *a*symmetry; B is *b*order irregularity; C is *c*olor, and D is *d*ifference greater than 6 mm.**
- **Melanoma prognosis is inverse correlated to tumor thickness; ulceration and increased mitotic rate are independent survival risk factors; nodal tumor burden (uninvoled versus microscopic versus macroscopic disease) has an inverse correlation with survival.**
- **For melanoma *in situ,* excision margins of 0.5 to 1 cm are indicated; for invasive melanoma, wide excision of the primary tumor with margins generally ranging from 1 to 2 cm is indicated for local control.**
- **Clinically involved lymph nodes should be resected; patients with primary melanomas of 1 mm thickness or greater and clinically negative nodes should be considered for sentinel lymph node biopsy.**
- **Basal cell and squamous cell skin carcinoma account for 96% of new nonmelanoma skin cancers.**
- **Dermatofibrosarcoma protuberans is a rare soft tissue sarcoma (1% of all soft tissue sarcomas) with a propensity for local recurrence rather than systemic metastasis.**

References

1. American Cancer Society. Cancer facts and figures 2004. Available from: URL: http://www.cancer.org. Accessed January 2005.
2.Diepgen TL, Mahler V. The epidemiology of skin cancer. *Br J Dermatol.* 2002;146:1–6.
3. Jemal A, Murray T, Samuels A, et al. Cancer statistics, 2003. *CA Cancer J Clin.* 2003;53:5–26.
4. Lynch HT, Shaw TG, Lynch JF. Inherited predisposition to cancer: a historical overview. *Am J Med Genet C Semin Med Genet.* 2004;129:5–22.
5. Lynch HT, Frichot BC, Lynch JF. Familial atypical multiple mole-melanoma syndrome. *J Med Genet.* 1978; 15:352–356.
6. Greene MH, Clark WH, Tucker MA, et al. High risk of malignant melanoma in melanoma-prone families with dysplastic nevi. *Ann Intern Med.* 1985;102:458.
7. Marghoob AA, Borrego JP, Halpern AC. Congenital melanocytic nevi: treatment modalities and management options. *Semin Cutan Med Surg.* 2003;22:21–32.
8. Di Rocco F, Sabatino G, Koutzoglou M, et al. Neurocutaneous melanosis. *Childs Nerv Syst.* 2004;20:23–28.
9. Bittencourt FV, Marghoob AA, Kopf AW, et al. Large congenital melanocytic nevi and the risk for development of malignant melanoma and neurocutaneous melanocytosis. *Pediatrics* 2000;106:736–741.
10. **Abbasi NR, Shaw HM, Rigel DS, et al. Early diagnosis of cutaneous melanoma: revisiting the ABCD criteria. *JAMA* 2004;292:2771-2776.**
11. Buettner PG, Leiter U, Eigentler TK, et al. Development of prognostic factors and survival in cutaneous melanoma over 25 years: an analysis of the Central Malignant Melanoma Registry of the German Dermatological Society. *Cancer* 2005;103:616–624.
12. Su LD, Fullen DR, Lowe L, et al. Desmoplastic and neurotropic melanoma. *Cancer* 2004;100:598–604.
13. Breslow A. Thickness, cross-sectional area, and depth of invasion in prognosis of cutaneous melanoma. *Ann Surg.* 1970;172:902–908.
14. Balch CM, Buzaid AC, Soong S, et al. Final version of the American Joint Committee on Cancer staging system for cutaneous melanoma. *J Clin Oncol.* 2001;19:3635–3648.
15. Azzola MF, Shaw HM, Thompson JF, et al. Tumor mitotic rate is a more powerful prognostic indicator than ulceration in patients with primary cutaneous melanoma: an analysis of 3661 patients from a single center. *Cancer* 2003; 97:1488–498.
16. **Balch CM, Soong S, Gershenwald JE, et al. Prognostic factors analysis of 17,600 melanoma patients: validation of the American Joint Committee on Cancer melanoma staging system. *J Clin Oncol.* 2001;19:3622–3634.**
17. Arca MJ, Biermann JS, Johnson TM, et al. Biopsy techniques for skin, soft-tissue, and bone neoplasms. *Surg Oncol Clin N Am.* 1995;4:157–174.
18. **National Comprehensive Cancer Network. Available from URL: http://www.nccn.org/professionals/physician_gls/PDF/melanoma.pdf. Accessed January 2005.**
19. Johnson TM, Bradford CR, Gruber SB, et al. Staging workup, sentinel node biopsy, and follow-up tests for melanoma: update of current concepts. *Arch Dermatol.* 2004;140:107–113.
20. Wang TS, Johnson TM, Cascade PN, et al. Evaluation of staging chest radiographs and serum lactate dehydrogenase for localized melanoma. *J Am Acad Dermatol.* 2004;51:399–405.
21. Tsao H, Feldman M, Fullerton JE, et al. Early detection of asymptomatic pulmonary melanoma metastases by routine chest radiographs is not associated with improved survival. *Arch Dermatol.* 2004;140:67–70.
22. Miranda EP, Gertner M, Wall J, et al. Routine imaging of asymptomatic melanoma patients with metastasis to sentinel lymph nodes rarely identifies systemic disease. *Arch Surg.* 2004;139:831–836.
23. Trask PC, Paterson AG, Hayasaka S, et al. Psychosocial characteristics of individuals with non-stage IV melanoma. *J Clin Oncol.* 2001;19:2844–2850.
24. Johnson TM, Sondak VK. Melanoma margins: the importance and need for more evidence-based trials. *Arch Dermatol.* 2004;140:1148–1150.
25. **Thomas JM, Newton-Bishop J, A'Hern R, et al. United Kingdom Melanoma Study Group; British Association of Plastic Surgeons; Scottish Cancer Therapy Network. Excision margins in high-risk malignant melanoma. *N Engl J Med.* 2004;350:757–766.**
26. Anderson KW, Baker SR, Lowe L, et al. Treatment of head and neck melanoma, lentigo maligna subtype: a practical surgical technique. *Arch Facial Plast Surg.* 2001;3:202–206.
27. Agarwal-Antal N, Bowen GM, Gerwels JW. Histologic evaluation of lentigo maligna with permanent sections: implications regarding current guidelines. *J Am Acad Dermatol.* 2002;47:743–748.
28. Chang AE, Karnell LH, Menck HR. The National Cancer Data Base report on cutaneous and noncutaneous melanoma: a summary of 84,836 cases from the past decade. The American College of Surgeons Commission on Cancer and the American Cancer Society. *Cancer* 1998;83:1664–1678.
29. Morton DL, Wen D-R, Wong JH, et al. Technical details of intraoperative lymphatic mapping for early stage melanoma. *Arch Surg.* 1992;127:392.
30. Gershenwald JE, Thompson W, Mansfield PF, et al. Multi-institutional melanoma lymphatic mapping experience: the prognostic value of sentinel lymph node status in 612 stage I or II melanoma patients. *J Clin Oncol.* 1999;17:976–983.
31. McMasters KM, Reintgen DS, Ross MI, et al. Sentinel lymph node biopsy for melanoma: controversy despite widespread agreement. *J Clin Oncol.* 2001;19:2851–2855.
32. Karimipour DJ, Lowe L, Su L, et al. Standard immunostains for melanoma in sentinel lymph node specimens: which ones are most useful? *J Am Acad Dermatol.* 2004;50:759–764.
33. Takeuchi H, Morton DL, Kuo C, et al. Prognostic significance of molecular upstaging of paraffin-embedded sentinel lymph nodes in melanoma patients. *J Clin Oncol.* 2004;22:2671–2680.
34. Kammula US, Ghossein R, Bhattacharya S, et al. Serial follow-up and the prognostic significance of reverse transcriptase-polymerase chain reaction–staged sentinel lymph nodes from melanoma patients. *J Clin Oncol.* 2004;22:3989–3996.
35. Sondak VK, Taylor JM, Sabel MS, et al. Mitotic rate and younger age are predictors of sentinel lymph node positivity: lessons learned from the generation of a probabilistic model. *Ann Surg Oncol.* 2004;11:247–258.
36. Sabel MS, Sondak VK. Pros and cons of adjuvant interferon in the treatment of melanoma. *Oncologist* 2003;8:451458.
37. Pawlik TM, Sondak VK. Malignant melanoma: current state of primary and adjuvant treatment. *Crit Rev Oncol Hematol.* 2003;45:245–264.
38. **Kirkwood JM, Strawderman MH, Ernstoff MS, et al. Interferon alpha-2b adjuvant therapy of high-risk resected cutaneous melanoma: the Eastern Cooperative Oncology Group trial EST 1684. *J Clin Oncol.* 1996;14:7–17.**
39. **Sondak VK, Liu PY, Tuthill RJ, et al. Adjuvant immunotherapy of resected, intermediate-thickness, node-negative melanoma with an allogeneic tumor vaccine: overall results of a randomized trial of the Southwest Oncology Group. *J Clin Oncol.* 2002;20:2058–2066.**
40. Sosman JA, Sondak VK. Melacine: an allogeneic melanoma tumor cell lysate vaccine. *Expert Rev Vaccines* 2003;2:353–368.
41. Rose DM, Essner R, Hughes TM, et al. Surgical resection for metastatic melanoma to the liver: the John Wayne Cancer Institute and Sydney Melanoma Unit experience. *Arch Surg.* 2001;136:950–955.
42. Leo F, Cagini L, Rocmans P, et al. Lung metastases from melanoma: when is surgical treatment warranted? *Br J Cancer* 2000;83:569–572.
43. Stone A, Cooper J, Koenig KL, et al. A comparison of survival rates for treatment of melanoma metastatic to the brain. *Cancer Invest.* 2004;22:492–497.
44. Panagiotou I, Brountzos EN, Bafaloukos D, et al. Malignant melanoma metastatic to the gastrointestinal tract. *Melanoma Res.* 2002;12:169–173.
45. Ang KK, Peters LJ, Weber RS, et al. Postoperative radiotherapy for cutaneous melanoma of the head and neck region. *Int J Radiat Oncol Biol Phys.* 1994;30:795–798.
46. Calabro A, Singletary SE, Balch CM. Patterns of relapse in 1001 consecutive patients with melanoma nodal metastases. *Arch Surg.* 1989;124:1051–1055.
47. Lee RJ, Gibbs JF, Proulx GM, et al. Nodal basin recurrence following lymph node dissection for melanoma: implications for adjuvant radiotherapy. *Int J Radiat Oncol Biol Phys.* 2000;46:467–474.
48. National Comprehensive Cancer Network. Available from URL: http://www.nccn.org/professionals/physician_gls/PDF/cns.pdf. Accessed January 2005.
49. Buzaid AC. Management of metastatic cutaneous melanoma. *Oncology (Huntingt).* 2004;18:1443–1450.
50. Legha SS, Ring S, Eton O, et al. Development of a biochemotherapy regimen with concurrent administration of cisplatin, vinblastine, dacarbazine,

interferon alfa, and interleukin-2 for patients with metastatic melanoma. *J Clin Oncol.* 1998;16:1752–1759.

51. Ridolfi R, Chiarion-Sileni V, Guida M, et al. Italian Melanoma Intergroup. Cisplatin, dacarbazine with or without subcutaneous interleukin-2, and interferon alpha-2b in advanced melanoma outpatients: results from an Italian multicenter phase III randomized clinical trial. *J Clin Oncol.* 2002;20:1600–1607.
52. Buzaid AC. Biochemotherapy for advanced melanoma. *Crit Rev Oncol Hematol.* 2002;44:103–108.
53. Eton O, Legha SS, Bedikian AY, et al. Sequential biochemotherapy versus chemotherapy for metastatic melanoma: results from a phase III randomized trial. *J Clin Oncol.* 2002;20:2045–2052.
54. Lienard D, Ewalenko P, Delmotte J-J, et al. High-dose recombinant tumor necrosis factor alpha in combination with interferon gamma and melphalan in isolation perfusion of the limbs for melanoma and sarcoma. *J Clin Oncol.* 1992;10:52
55. Grover A, Alexander HR Jr. The past decade of experience with isolated hepatic perfusion. *Oncologist* 2004;9:653–664.
56. **Fraker DL. Management of in-transit melanoma of the extremity with isolated limb perfusion. *Curr Treat Options Oncol.* 2004;5:173–184.**
57. Mulé JJ, Shu S, Schwartz SL, et al. Adoptive immunotherapy of established pulmonary metastases with LAK cells and recombinant interleukin-2. *Science* 1984;225:1487.
58. Rosenberg SA, Lotze MT, Muul LM, et al. A progress report on the treatment of 157 patients with advanced cancer using lymphokine-activated killer cells and interleukin-2 or high-dose interleukin-2 alone. *N Engl J Med.* 1987;316: 889.
59. Rosenberg SA, Spiess P, Lafreniere R. A new approach to the adoptive immunotherapy of cancer with tumor-infiltrating lymphocytes. *Science* 1986;233:1318.
60. Rosenberg SA, Yannelli JR, Yang JC, et al. Treatment of patients with metastatic melanoma with autologous tumor-infiltrating lymphocytes and interleukin 2. *J Natl Cancer Inst.* 1994;86:1159–1166.
61. **Rosenberg SA, Dudley ME. Cancer regression in patients with metastatic melanoma after the transfer of autologous antitumor lymphocytes. *Proc Natl Acad Sci USA.* 2004;101(suppl 2):14639–14645.**
62. Rosenberg SA, Yang JC, Schwartzentruber DJ, et al. Immunologic and therapeutic evaluation of a synthetic peptide vaccine for the treatment of patients with metastatic melanoma. *Nat Med.* 1998;4:269.
63. Shimizu K, Fields, RC, Giedlin M, et al. Systemic administration of interleukin 2 enhances the therapeutic efficacy of dendritic cell-based tumor vaccines. *Proc Natl Acad Sci USA* 1999;96:2268.
64. Nestle FO, Alijagic S, Gilliet M, et al. Vaccination of melanoma patients with peptide- or tumor lysate-pulsed dendritic cells. *Nat Med.* 1998;4:328.
65. Miller AR, McBride WH, Hunt K, et al. Cytokine-mediated gene therapy for cancer. *Ann Surg Oncol.* 1994;1:436.
66. Moiseyenko VM, Danilov AO, Baldueva IA, et al. Phase I/II trial of gene therapy with autologous tumor cells modified with tag7/PGRP-S gene in patients with disseminated solid tumors: miscellaneous tumors. *Ann Oncol.* 2005;16:162–168.
67. Ito F, Li Q, Shreiner AB, et al. Anti-CD137 monoclonal antibody administration augments the antitumor efficacy of dendritic cell-based vaccines. *Cancer Res.* 2004;64:8411–8419.
68. Ito F, Carr A, Svensson H, et al. Antitumor reactivity of anti-CD3/anti-CD28 bead-activated lymphoid cells: implications for cell therapy in a murine model. *J Immunother.* 2003;26:222–233.
69. Salas AP, Chang AE. Genetic approaches to adoptive cellular immunotherapy. *Surg Oncol Clin N Am.* 1998;7:487–503.
70. Shu S, Plautz GE, Krauss JC, et al. Tumor immunology. *JAMA* 1997;278: 1972–1981.
71. Nabel GJ, Gordon D, Bishop DK, et al. Immune response in human melanoma after transfer of an allogeneic class I major histocompatibility complex gene with DNA-liposome complexes. *Proc Natl Acad Sci USA* 1996;93:15388.
72. Johnson TM, Rowe DE, Nelson BR, et al. Squamous cell carcinoma of the skin (excluding lip and oral mucosa). *J Am Acad Dermatol.* 1992;26:467.
73. Su LD, Lowe L, Bradford CR, et al. Immunostaining for cytokeratin 20 improves detection of micrometastatic Merkel cell carcinoma in sentinel lymph nodes. *J Am Acad Dermatol.* 2002;46:661–666.
74. Ratner D, Nelson BR, Brown MD, et al. Merkel cell carcinoma. *J Am Acad Dermatol.* 1993;29:143–156.
75. National Comprehensive Cancer Network. Available from URL: http://www.nccn.org/professionals/physician_gls/PDF/mcc.pdf. Accessed January 2005.
76. Bogner PN, Fullen DR, Lowe L, et al. Lymphatic mapping and sentinel lymph node biopsy in the detection of early metastasis from sweat gland carcinoma. *Cancer* 2003;97:2285–2289.
77. **DuBay D, Cimmino V, Lowe L, et al. Low recurrence rate after surgery for dermatofibrosarcoma protuberans: a multidisciplinary approach from a single institution. *Cancer* 2004;100:1008–1016.**
78. National Comprehensive Cancer Network. Available from URL: http://www.nccn.org/professionals/physician_gls/PDF/dfsp.pdf. Accessed January 2005.
79. National Comprehensive Cancer Network. Available from URL: http://www.nccn.org/professionals/physician_gls/PDF/nmsc.pdf. Accessed January 2005.
80. Cook J, Zitelli JA. Mohs micrographic surgery: a cost analysis. *J Am Acad Dermatol.* 1998;39:698–703.
81. Vuyk HD, Lohuis PJ. Mohs micrographic surgery for facial skin cancer. *Clin Otolaryngol.* 2001;26:265–273.
82. Swanson NA. Mohs surgery: technique, indications, applications, and the future. *Arch Dermatol.* 1983;119:761.
83. Rowe DE, Carroll RJ, Day CL Jr. Long-term recurrence rates in previously untreated (primary) basal cell carcinoma: implications for patient follow-up. *J Dermatol Surg Oncol.* 1989;15:315–328.
84. Rowe DE, Carroll RJ, Day CL Jr. Mohs surgery is the treatment of choice for recurrent (previously treated) basal cell carcinoma. *J Dermatol Surg Oncol.* 1989;15:424.

CHAPTER 119 ■ SARCOMAS OF BONE AND SOFT TISSUE

MICHAEL S. SABEL

Sarcomas are a heterogeneous group of cancers that arise from mesoderm-derived elements, including bone, cartilage, connective tissue, fat, and muscle. Although the soft tissues and bony structures constitute almost two thirds of the mass of the human body, sarcomas are relatively uncommon. In 2004, an estimated 11,120 new soft tissue and bone sarcomas occurred, accounting for less than 1% of human cancers.[1] The relative rarity of sarcomas makes it difficult for any but a few specialized centers to gain wide experience with treating them. Still, sarcomas are sufficiently prevalent that a practicing surgeon will likely encounter them and must therefore be prepared to recognize them.

The behavior of carcinomas varies dramatically depending on their site of origin in the body. In contrast, sarcomas typically behave in a similar fashion wherever they arise. For example, very few histologic subtypes metastasize to the regional lymph nodes; the exceptions are synovial sarcoma, epithelioid sarcoma, clear-cell sarcoma, and rhabdomyosarcoma. Their behavior is determined by the depth (deep versus superficial), grade, and size of the tumor, with much less emphasis placed on histology.

Most soft tissue sarcomas arise in the limbs (legs more often than arms), followed by the retroperitoneum, trunk, and the head and neck (Table 119.1). The site of origin of a

TABLE 119.1

SITE OF ORIGIN OF SOFT TISSUE SARCOMAS IN ADULTS

Anatomic site	Percentage
Lower extremity	46.4
Trunk	17.9
Upper extremity	13.1
Retroperitoneum	12.5
Head and neck	8.9
Mediastinum	1.3

From Lawrence W Jr, Donegan WL, Natarajan A, et al. Adult soft tissue sarcomas: a pattern of care survey of the American College of Surgeons. *Ann Surg*. 1987;205:349–359, with permission.

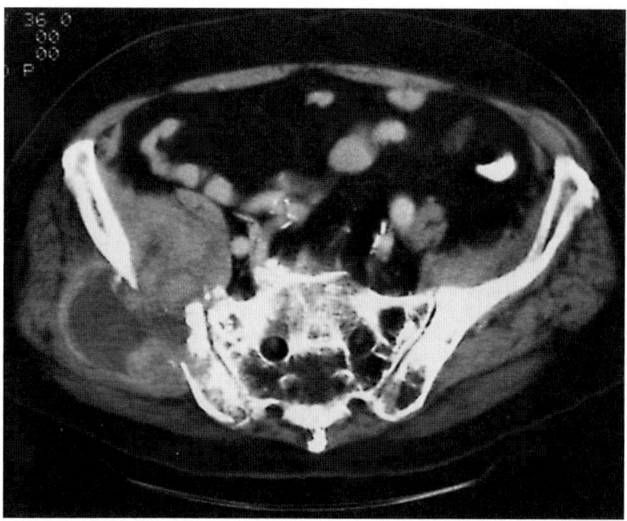

FIGURE 119.1 Osteosarcoma of the iliac bone that occurred 7 years after radiation therapy for cancer of the prostate and 30 years after radiation therapy for testicular cancer. The lesion was unresectable and associated with severe pain and lower extremity edema. The patient received significant palliation from two courses of intraarterial doxorubicin, after which the blood supply to the tumor was occluded by transcatheter embolization.

sarcoma does affect treatment, however, and hence outcome. For extremity sarcomas, emphasis is placed on wide resections while preserving a functional limb, although sometimes amputation is required. Sarcomas located in the retroperitoneum, however, are almost invariably situated near major organs and blood vessels, which precludes an extensive resection with a wide margin of normal tissue around the tumor. Thus, local recurrence is frequent. Depending on their size and location, sarcomas on the head and neck or the trunk are also difficult to excise with wide margins. Thus, although the basic biologic and clinical behavior of all sarcomas is similar, each type requires a somewhat different management approach.

Surgical resection remains the mainstay of treatment for patients with sarcoma, but surgery alone is rarely the treatment of choice. A multimodality approach that combines surgery, radiation, and, in some cases, chemotherapy is the rule. Because treatment is substantially better when provided in specialty centers,[2] a multidisciplinary team in a tertiary-care center should manage most sarcomas of bone or soft tissues.

EPIDEMIOLOGY

There is no classic profile of the sarcoma patient, and most sarcomas occur in patients who have no identifiable predisposing factors. Although they increase in frequency with age, sarcomas occur in all age groups and are among the most common cancers in children, adolescents, and young adults. The genders are generally equally affected, and there does not seem to be a strong tendency for sarcomas to occur in any particular ethnic or racial groups. Soft tissue sarcomas do not seem to result from malignant degeneration of benign soft tissue tumors.

Several agents are known to cause sarcoma, although they account for less than 10% of all cases.[3] Although it is a common belief that a history of trauma predisposes to sarcoma development, this theory does not seem to be true. Although many patients recall a trauma to the area, it is more likely the patient first notices a soft tissue or bony lesion after an unrelated minor trauma and associates the two events. Nonetheless, all patients presenting with soft tissue or bony tumors should be questioned about prior trauma because of the need to differentiate malignancy from a variety of benign posttraumatic lesions, such as myositis ossificans.

Radiation exposure is clearly linked to the development of sarcomas. Among factory workers who were exposed to ^{226}radium while coating watch dials with luminous paint, osteosarcomas developed in several. Radium is incorporated into bone in a manner analogous to calcium, and these workers were ingesting it when they used their tongues to wet the tips of their brushes. Once this practice was stopped, the epidemic ceased. The radioactive substance thorium dioxide (Thorotrast) was widely used as a contrast agent for radiologic procedures in the 1940s and 1950s. This agent predominantly accumulates in the liver where, with its half-life of more than 400 years and extremely low rate of excretion, it can deliver as much as 15,000 cGy (1 cGy = 1 rad) to the hepatic parenchyma. Hepatic angiosarcomas occur with an extremely high frequency in patients who have received thorium dioxide, after a latency period of 18 to 36 years.

With the increasing use of external beam radiation in cancer treatment, the connection between radiation and sarcoma became more apparent. The incidence of sarcoma is increased eightfold in patients treated with radiation for a variety of malignancies, depending on the dose of radiation.[4,5] Sarcomas occurring in irradiated tissues are most commonly osteosarcomas or malignant fibrous histiocytomas, and they usually arise after a latency period of 7 to 20 years (Fig. 119.1).

Certain chemicals that are not radioactive have also been implicated as causing sarcomas. They include arsenic and vinyl chloride, both of which are associated with hepatic angiosarcomas in exposed people. Some herbicides (phenoxyacetic acid compounds) have been linked to soft tissue sarcoma development. The highly toxic chemical dioxin is used in manufacturing these herbicides, and soft tissue sarcoma cases have been reported among workers who were exposed to dioxin and other chemicals in an industrial accident.[6] Dioxin (as well as some phenoxyherbicides) is present in small quantities in the defoliant Agent Orange, widely used during the Vietnam War. The Department of Veterans Affairs ruled that Vietnam veterans in whom soft tissue sarcomas develop are entitled to compensation for their treatment, although the epidemiologic data linking Agent Orange exposure with sarcoma development remain inconclusive.[7]

Long-standing lymphedema of an extremity predisposes to the development of lymphangiosarcomas. Originally described in patients with arm edema after radical mastectomy and postoperative radiation (Fig. 119.2), the subsequent lymphangiosarcoma is known as *Stewart-Treves syndrome*. Lymphangiosarcomas have been seen in patients with severe edema from other causes as well, including in the lower extremities.

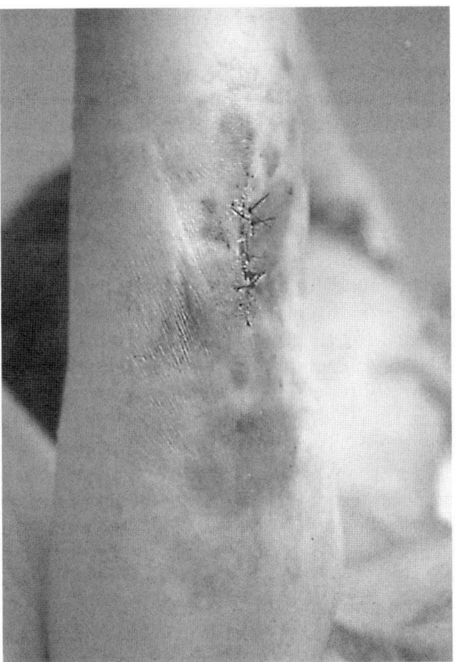

FIGURE 119.2 Lymphangiosarcoma of the right upper extremity occurring 21 years after a radical mastectomy and postoperative chest wall irradiation for breast cancer. At presentation, pulmonary metastases were already evident. The diffuse discoloration is more suggestive of ecchymosis than tumor. Although most instances of postmastectomy lymphangiosarcoma are associated with severe lymphedema, the extremity was relatively normal in this case.

Neurofibromatosis type 1 (von Recklinghausen's disease) represents a condition with a genetic predisposition to sarcoma development (Fig. 119.3). A sarcoma develops during their lifetime in an estimated 5% of patients with neurofibromatosis. These tumors are virtually all *neurofibrosarcomas* (sometimes called *malignant schwannomas* or *malignant peripheral nerve tumors*) and usually arise within preexisting neurofibromas. All patients presenting with a neurofibrosarcoma should be closely examined, and a thorough family history should be obtained for evidence of neurofibromatosis. Conversely, any rapidly enlarging or newly symptomatic lesion in a patient with neurofibromatosis should be suspected of malignancy.

MOLECULAR BIOLOGY

Numerous genetic alterations are associated with both bone and soft tissue sarcomas. One well-documented mechanism of sarcoma development is the inactivation of tumor suppressor genes. Initially, it was thought that the high incidence of osteosarcomas noted in the orbit after radiation therapy for primary retinoblastoma was secondary to the radiation. However, it was subsequently demonstrated that the incidence of all types of sarcomas is markedly increased in patients with retinoblastoma, particularly in those with the familial rather than the sporadic form. The precise genetic defect responsible is now understood: mutation in one copy of the retinoblastoma (*Rb*) gene.

The finding of a link between familial retinoblastoma and sarcoma led researchers to search for specific genetic changes responsible for the observed susceptibility to sarcoma development. Retinoblastoma, the most common childhood malignant tumor of the eye, has been associated with a genetic defect in the retinoblastoma gene (RB1) on the long arm of chromosome 13. RB1 is a recessive oncogene, or "tumor suppressor gene," which means that both alleles must be inactivated before malignant transformation can occur. The normal product of this gene is involved in regulating cell division. Losing both normal copies of the gene predisposes to tumor formation by removing this growth control. Patients with familial retinoblastoma inherit one inactivated RB1 gene. For retinoblastoma to develop in these individuals, they must undergo only one additional genetic mutation inactivating the normal gene, compared with two mutations (involving both normal RB1 genes) necessary for someone without the inherited defect. By virtue of the increased susceptibility, people inheriting one defective RB1 gene have multiple, bilateral retinoblastomas at an early age (often in the first year of life).

The RB1 gene appears to affect more than retinoblastoma development. The susceptibility to sarcoma formation in patients with familial retinoblastoma relates to the genetic defect in RB1 as well.[8] RB1 may also play a role in the pathogenesis of certain types of nonfamilial soft tissue sarcomas. In a study of soft tissue sarcomas in nonretinoblastoma patients, 3 of 69 cases had homozygous deletions of the RB1 gene.[9] Another five cases had evidence of heterozygous deletion. This finding illustrates an important principle of the genetics of cancer formation: it is frequently the case that the same gene involved in a familial cancer syndrome (in which one inherited copy of the gene is defective and the other is presumably lost later) is also important in the spontaneous development of the

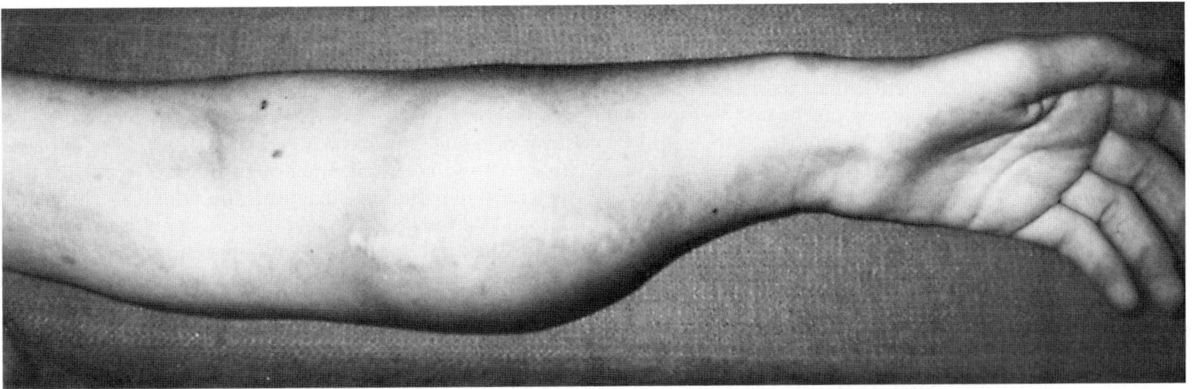

FIGURE 119.3 Large neurofibrosarcoma arising from the median nerve in a 17-year-old patient with neurofibromatosis. The incision is from a biopsy of the lesion 18 months before the diagnosis of malignancy. Since the earlier biopsy (which revealed only benign neurofibroma), the mass progressively enlarged and became painful, and the patient lost sensory and motor function in the median nerve distribution. Wasting of the thenar eminence is evident.

relevant tumor type (in which both normal copies of the gene must be lost to mutations or genetic deletions).

Another inherited defect of a tumor suppressor gene is associated with soft tissue sarcomas and breast cancer, as well as several other types of cancer. This condition, termed the *Li-Fraumeni syndrome*, is caused by an inherited mutation in the p53 gene (also referred to as *TP53*), a key growth-regulatory gene. Inactivation of the second, normal copy of the gene leaves the cell without the ability to regulate gene transcription, particularly after DNA damage.[10] This exposes affected family members susceptible to early-onset breast cancer, sarcomas (often in childhood), and a variety of other malignancies (notably brain tumors, adrenal cortical cancers, and leukemias).[11] Like the genetic defect in familial retinoblastoma, the p53 gene is also important in sporadic sarcoma development, observed in 30% to 60% of soft tissue sarcomas.[12, 13] One study found p53 abnormalities in approximately 60% of osteosarcomas and malignant fibrous histiocytomas, as well as approximately 33% of other sarcomas.[14] Interestingly, some sarcomas that do not show evidence of any p53 gene abnormalities have been found to possess amplifications of a gene called *MDM2*, which codes for a protein that inactivates the function of normal p53 protein.[15]

Several oncogenes that can induce malignant transformation and drive proliferation have also been associated with sarcoma development, including amplifications of N-myc, c-erbB2 and member of the *ras* family.[16]

Cytogenetic aberrations have been recognized in a number of soft tissue sarcomas, and some of these may be specific for certain sarcomas. Several histologic subtypes sarcomas have each been found to have characteristic chromosomal translocations that potentially could assist in the differentiation of these tumors from other sarcomas.[8] Examples include EWS-FLI-1 fusion in Ewing's sarcoma, EWS-ATF1 fusion in clear-cell sarcoma, PAX3-FHKR fusion in alveolar rhabdomyosarcoma, and SSX-SYT fusion in synovial sarcoma. Flow cytometric analysis of DNA from osteosarcomas has been shown to have prognostic importance, and similar analysis of soft tissue sarcomas suggests a correlation between histologic grade and ploidy status, with most high-grade lesions being aneuploid rather than diploid. Large, prospective trials of flow cytometry and cytogenetic analysis are needed to ascertain the importance of these studies in diagnosing and treating sarcomas.

One other important genetic change in some sarcomas is the presence of the multidrug-resistance (MDR1) gene, which is found in greater numbers of untreated sarcomas than most other tumor types.[17] The presence of this gene has been correlated *in vitro* with resistance to a number of cytotoxic drugs, many of which are routinely used in sarcoma chemotherapy. Experimental studies have shown the importance of MDR1 gene activation in the resistance of sarcoma cells to doxorubicin, probably the most commonly used drug for sarcoma treatment.[18] Although other genetic abnormalities are likely to prove important in sarcoma development and treatment, these carefully studied genes vividly demonstrate the rapidly evolving link between the research laboratory and the clinic as well as the extent to which the practicing physician must be aware of developments in molecular biology.

SOFT TISSUE SARCOMAS

Clinical Presentation

The most common presentation of a soft tissue sarcoma is an asymptomatic mass. Sarcomas tend to grow in a centrifugal fashion, pushing surrounding structures away rather than directly invading them. Rarely does this compression produce pain, swelling, or obstructive symptoms until the tumors are large. Tumors of the distal extremities tend to be detected at a small size, whereas tumors of the proximal extremities or retroperitoneum can grow to be quite large without causing symptoms. Retroperitoneal sarcomas most often present as a palpable abdominal mass in association with nonspecific abdominal symptoms including fullness, early satiety, or vague abdominal pain.

Even when a soft tissue mass is detected, the overwhelming propensity of these masses to be benign leads to prolonged delays before definitive treatment, secondary to both patient and physician delays. In a survey of more than 5,800 patients with sarcoma, roughly half waited 4 or more months before seeking medical treatment, and 20% waited at least 6 months after seeing a physician before a correct diagnosis was made.[19] Many patients with sarcoma undergo prolonged treatment for chronic hematomas or pulled muscles. In nonathletic adults, persistent soft tissue masses rarely develop from either of these causes in the absence of a history of unusually strenuous activity. Only in a setting of clear-cut local trauma should these diagnoses be entertained. If a soft tissue mass arises in a patient with no history of trauma or persists more than 6 weeks after local trauma, biopsy should be performed.

While evaluating any soft tissue mass, the physician must always remain cognizant of the possibility of malignancy. The differential diagnosis of a soft tissue mass includes not only benign lesions (lipomas, lymphangiomas, leiomyomas, epidermoid cysts, neuromas) but also other malignant lesions (primary or metastatic carcinoma, melanoma, lymphoma). Biopsy should be done for virtually all soft tissue masses larger than 5 cm as well as for any new, enlarging, or symptomatic lesions. Small, subcutaneous lesions that have not changed for many years may be safely observed. The decision of when, and how, to biopsy a soft tissue mass can have significant implications on the subsequent outcome of therapy.

Biopsy

Properly performed, a timely surgical biopsy is the critical first step in a multimodality treatment approach. Improperly done, it can markedly complicate the care of the patient with sarcoma and occasionally even eliminate treatment options. *Fine needle aspiration biopsy* is an excellent tool for the evaluation of enlarged lymph nodes, thyroid nodules, or breast masses. It is the procedure of choice when looking to confirm a local recurrence or metastatic foci in a patient with a known malignancy. The use of fine-needle aspiration biopsy in the primary diagnosis of soft tissue masses, however, is severely limited. The amount of material obtained by fine-needle aspiration biopsy is small, and the diagnostic accuracy is dependent on the experience and skill of a cytopathologist. It is rarely possible to establish grade, which is often essential for treatment planning.

Core-needle biopsy is the initial procedure of choice in diagnosing soft tissue masses. A core-needle biopsy retrieves a thin sliver of tissue (approximately 1×10 mm). Besides being safe, accurate and economical, enough tissue is typically obtained for accurate pathologic diagnosis, immunohistochemical staining, and where necessary, cytogenetic analysis or flow cytometry. Image-guided core-needle biopsy, using computed tomography (CT) or ultrasound, allows for the biopsy of deep masses that are only vaguely palpable and can help avoid biopsying necrotic areas of the tumor that are of no diagnostic value. Fears that core-needle biopsies would result in a significant number of hematomas, resulting in dissemination of tumor cells, appear to be groundless. Complications occur in less than 1% of patients who undergo core-needle biopsy.[20] Series comparing core-needle and open biopsies of soft tissue tumors have documented that both the histologic type and grade of a sarcoma could be correctly determined by core-needle biopsy in more than 90% of cases.[21] Ideally, the core biopsy should be performed at the center where the patient is being treated to avoid inappropriate placement of the biopsy site as well as the pitfalls of not handling the specimen correctly. A large sample from a viable area of sarcoma is required for definitive diagnosis and accurate grading. Even with adequate sampling, a core-needle biopsy may lead to nonspecific diagnoses such as "spindle-cell neoplasm, not otherwise specified."

Open surgical biopsy, or *incisional biopsy*, is utilized when core-needle biopsy specimens yield nondiagnostic findings. Several important technical factors must be considered when performing an incisional biopsy, and so it is preferable that the same surgeon who will perform the definitive surgery also perform the biopsy. For extremity lesions, the incision should be oriented along the long axis of the extremity. For truncal or retroperitoneal lesions, the biopsy incision should be situated so that it can be readily excised along with the tumor if a diagnosis of sarcoma is made. Any biopsy site should be placed directly over the tumor, at the point where the lesion is closest to the surface, and there should be no raising of flaps or disturbance of tissue planes superficial to the tumor (Fig. 119.4). A poorly oriented incision can result in an excessively large surgical defect from a wide excision. This can increase the size of the postoperative radiation field necessary to encompass all at-risk tissue, or necessitate the use of flaps or grafts to close the surgical defect. Most sarcomas possess a pseudocapsule, and attempts to enucleate the sarcoma within pseudocapsule to make a diagnosis should be strongly discouraged. Incisional biopsy leaving the bulk of the lesion undisturbed is preferable, with careful attention to hemostasis to avoid a hematoma that could disseminate tumor cells through normal tissue planes. At least a 1- to 2-cm^3 piece of fresh tissue should be obtained, which can be partitioned by the pathologist for special studies. Frozen-section pathologic analysis is often helpful, not to provide a definitive diagnosis, but to assure that enough diagnostic tissue has been obtained. Drains are not used routinely; in the uncommon case when a drain is required, it should exit either through or near the biopsy incision. If malignancy is diagnosed, the drain tract must be excised in continuity with the tumor mass.

In cases where the mass is easily accessible, such as small (<3 to 5 cm), superficial lesions on the trunk or extremity, excisional biopsy is appropriate, especially when the likelihood of malignancy is low. It is important to consider ahead of time whether complete excision would not jeopardize subsequent treatment in the event a sarcoma is discovered, and similar surgical principles as with incisional biopsies should be strictly followed.

Pathologic Classification

Sarcomas are classified by the type of tissue formed by the tumor (histogenic classification) rather than by the type of tissue in which the tumor arises. Thus, a malignant tumor arising in a skeletal muscle but composed of malignant smooth muscle cells is termed a *leiomyosarcoma*, and not a rhabdomyosarcoma. Bone tumors are not termed *osteosarcomas* unless the malignant cells clearly produce osteoid. Some bone tumors produce cartilage (chondrosarcomas); a few are fibrosarcomas or other histologic types. Occasionally, soft tissue neoplasms produce bone or cartilage; these lesions are termed *extraosseous osteosarcomas* or *chondrosarcomas*, as appropriate. The various types of benign and malignant soft tissue tumors are noted in Table 119.2, and the relative frequency of the different sarcomas is listed in Table 119.3.

The development of specialized markers for identifying individual types of sarcoma has led to greater precision in their classification. Available immunohistochemical stains include S-100, a marker for neural crest origin (positive in

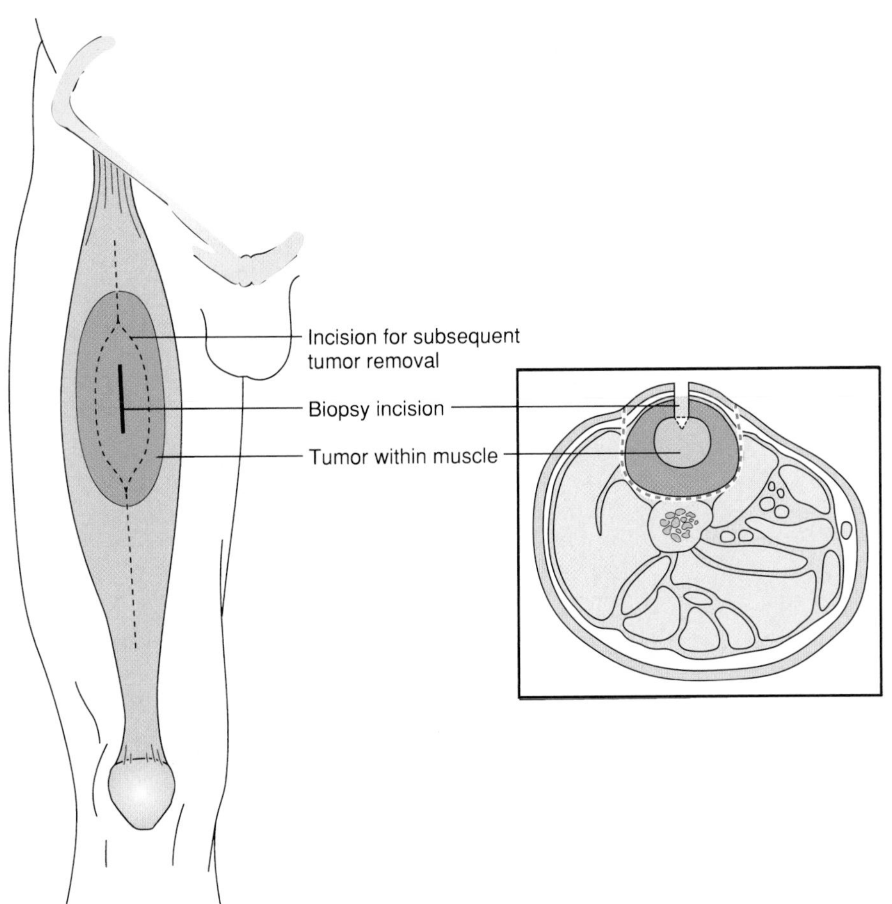

FIGURE 119.4 Technique for biopsy of an extremity soft tissue mass suspected of being a sarcoma. The incision should be oriented along the long axis of the extremity, at the point where the lesion is closest to the surface, and situated so that it can be readily excised along with the tumor if a diagnosis of sarcoma is made. There should be no raising of flaps or disturbance of tissue planes superficial to the tumor. The mass should not be enucleated within the pseudocapsule; rather, incisional biopsy leaving the bulk of the lesion undisturbed should be carried out. Before wound closure, hemostasis should be achieved to avoid a hematoma, which could disseminate tumor cells through normal tissue planes. Drains are not used routinely.

TABLE 119.2 CLASSIFICATION

HISTOGENIC CLASSIFICATION SCHEME FOR BENIGN AND MALIGNANT SOFT TISSUE TUMORS

Tissue formed	Benign soft tissue tumor	Malignant soft tissue tumor (histogenesis)
Fat	Lipoma	Liposarcoma
Fibrous tissue	Fibroma	Fibrosarcoma
Skeletal muscle	Rhabdomyoma	Rhabdomyosarcoma
Smooth muscle	Leiomyoma	Leiomyosarcoma
Bone	Osteoma	Osteosarcoma
Cartilage	Chondroma	Chondrosarcoma
Synovium	Synovioma	Synovial sarcoma
Blood vessel	Hemangioma hemangiopericytoma	Angiosarcoma; malignant
Lymphatics	Lymphangioma	Lymphangiosarcoma
Nerve	Neurofibroma	Neurofibrosarcoma
Mesothelium	Benign mesothelioma	Malignant mesothelioma
Tissue histiocyte	Benign fibrous histiocytoma	Malignant fibrous histiocytoma
Pluripotent	None recognized	Malignant mesenchymoma
Uncertain	None recognized sarcoma; epithelioid sarcoma	Ewing's sarcoma; alveolar soft parts

neurofibrosarcomas); factor VIII, which identifies cells of endothelial origin (positive in angiosarcomas); and myoglobin, which is found only in rhabdomyosarcomas. Although these stains are often helpful, they are not positive in every tumor of the appropriate type. Electron microscopy may reveal ultrastructural elements that are pathognomonic for a specific cell

TABLE 119.3

RELATIVE FREQUENCY OF HISTOLOGIC TYPES OF SOFT TISSUE SARCOMAS IN ADULTS (ALL SITES)

Histologic type	Percentage
Malignant fibrous histiocytoma	25.9
Liposarcoma	17.7
Leiomyosarcoma	14.8
Fibrosarcoma	6.6
Neurofibrosarcoma	4.0
Synovial sarcoma	3.6
Rhabdomyosarcoma	3.6
Angiosarcoma	2.9
Extraskeletal chondrosarcoma	1.2
Malignant mesenchymoma	1.0
Extraskeletal osteosarcoma	0.6
Unclassified	5.4
Other	12.7

Modified from Lawrence W Jr, Donegan WL, Natarajan A, et al. Adult soft tissue sarcomas; a pattern of care survey of the American College of Surgeons. *Ann Surg.* 1987;205:349, with permission.

type, but in most cases sarcomas are classified by their light microscopic appearance. In a small percentage of tumors (approximately 10% in most series), the tumor cells are so poorly differentiated that no specific histogenesis can be determined, even using the supportive diagnostic tools mentioned.

Although the exact histologic type is an important datum in the evaluation of the patient with sarcoma, it is not as influential in terms of prognosis and therapy as histologic grade. Histologic grade is assessed based on the degree of cellular atypia, the frequency of mitotic figures, and the presence or absence of spontaneous tumor necrosis (Fig. 119.5). Low-grade

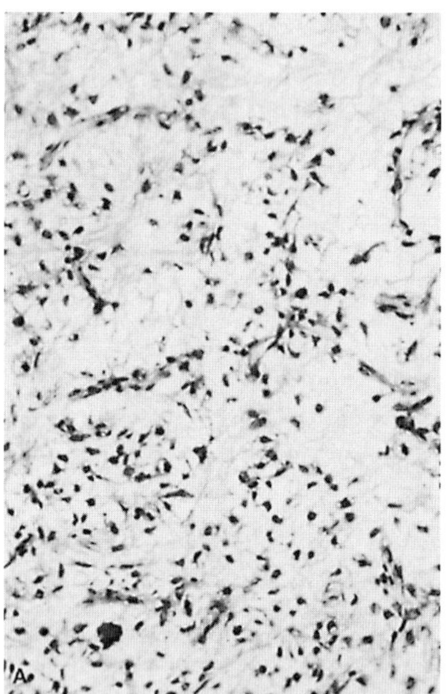

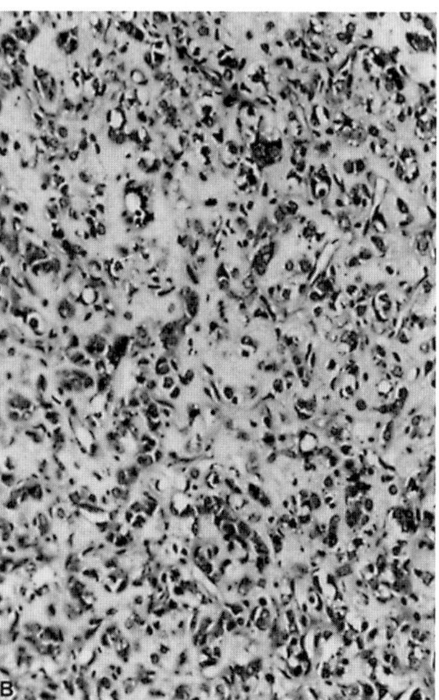

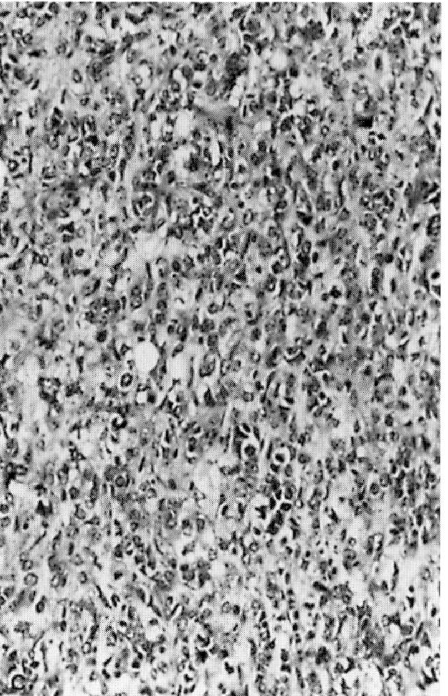

FIGURE 119.5 Photomicrographs of three fibrosarcomas illustrating the differing appearance of different grades of the same tumor type. (*A*) The low-grade fibrosarcoma shows relatively little cellular atypia, few mitoses, and no tumor necrosis, whereas (*B*) the intermediate-grade tumor has more atypia, numerous mitoses, and scant tumor necrosis. (*C*) The high-grade tumor shows a significant degree of necrosis in addition to atypia and frequent mitotic figures. (Courtesy of Sharon Weiss, M.D., Emory University, Atlanta, GA.)

tumors have relatively little cellular atypia, few mitoses, and no tumor necrosis. Intermediate-grade tumors have more atypia and numerous mitoses, but little or no tumor necrosis. High-grade tumors show a significant degree of necrosis in addition to atypia and frequent mitotic figures. A consistently applied grading system discriminates between tumors with good prognosis (low grade) and those with poorer prognosis (intermediate and high grade). Most studies also show an important distinction between intermediate-grade and high-grade lesions. The metastatic potential for low-grade lesions is approximately 5% to 10%, rising to 25% to 30% for intermediate-grade lesions and 50% to 60% for high-grade tumors.[22] The pathologist should assign a histologic grade to every sarcoma biopsy specimen. For lesions in which disparate areas exist, the highest grade encountered is generally used to categorize the tumor. Because sarcomas may be misdiagnosed or misclassified by a general pathologist in up to 25% to 40% of cases, it is prudent to defer treatment planning until experts in sarcoma pathology can review the cases.[23,24]

Imaging

Accurate radiologic imaging is critical in the management of sarcoma to provide information about the precise extent and diagnosis of the primary tumor, and in some cases provide reference for monitoring tumor changes after neoadjuvant treatment and detecting recurrences after resection. CT scanning and magnetic resonance imaging (MRI) are the most important studies for assessing the extent and resectability of soft tissue sarcomas, regardless of the site of origin.[25] Plain radiographs and radionuclide bone scans occasionally provide useful information regarding invasion of bone by tumor (Fig. 119.6), but these studies usually do not play a major role in evaluating a primary soft tissue sarcoma. Both CT and MRI can provide definition of the primary tumor in relation to bone, muscle, neurovascular structures, and adjacent organs, which is critical information when planning treatment. In most cases either study is sufficient, so the choice between them is based on availability, cost, and the experience of the radiologist. Each study has advantages and disadvantages, however, and these factors should be considered on a case-by-case basis.

CT scans are widely available, and both the primary site and the lungs (the major site of sarcoma metastasis) can be imaged at the same sitting. CT of the chest should be included for patients with high-grade lesions or tumors larger than 5 cm. CT of the abdomen and pelvis should be considered in any patient with a myxoid liposarcoma of an extremity because this subtype often metastasizes to the abdomen.[26] Tumor involvement of bone is often more clearly visible on CT scan, although bone marrow invasion may be better defined by MRI. CT is the preferred imaging technique for evaluating retroperitoneal sarcomas. Disadvantages of CT scanning include the ionizing radiation and the need for intravenous iodinated contrast administration.

MRI is the preferred imaging modality for extremity sarcomas.[27,28] It routinely involves axial T2-weighted and precontrast and postcontrast T1-weighted images. Contrast enhancement is crucial for detecting and characterizing lesions. MRI may help distinguish between benign and malignant lesions, such as lipomas versus liposarcomas.[29,30] Coronal, sagittal, and even oblique planes may be imaged with MRI. This modality can accurately delineate between muscle groups and distinguish among tumor and neurovascular structures better than CT.[25] Magnetic resonance angiography (MRA) can be performed if more accurate delineation of vascular structures is needed (Fig. 119.7). Because of the strong magnetic fields

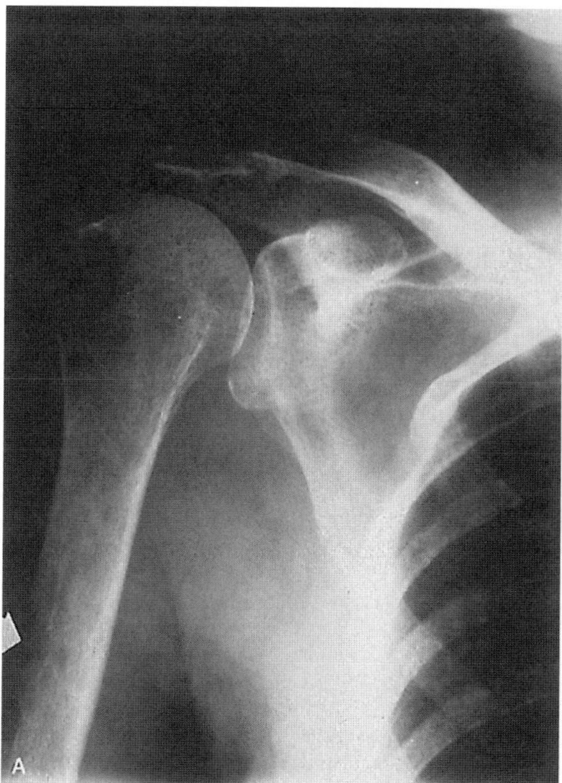

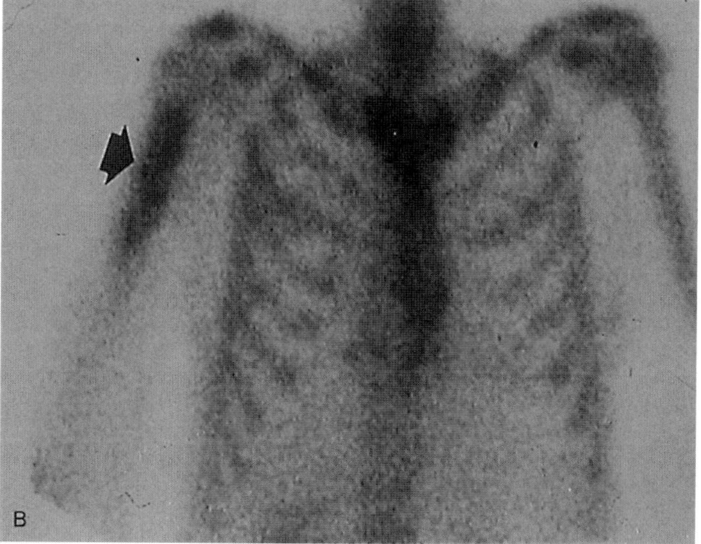

FIGURE 119.6 (*A*) Plain radiograph of the proximal humerus and shoulder joint, showing bony destruction (*arrow*) secondary to a large, high-grade soft tissue sarcoma adjacent to the humerus. (*B*) Radionuclide bone scan in the same patient reveals a much greater degree of involvement (*arrow*).

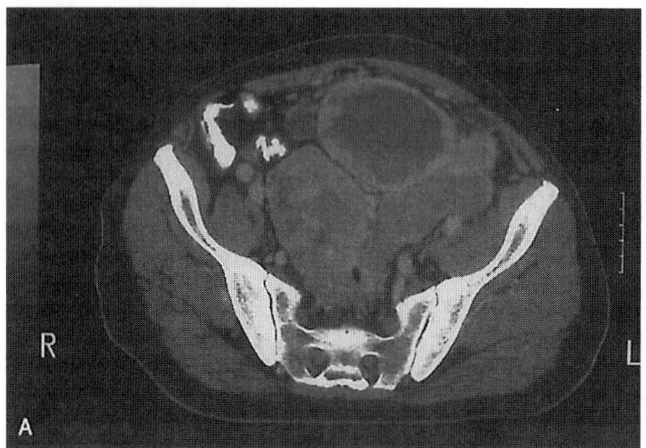

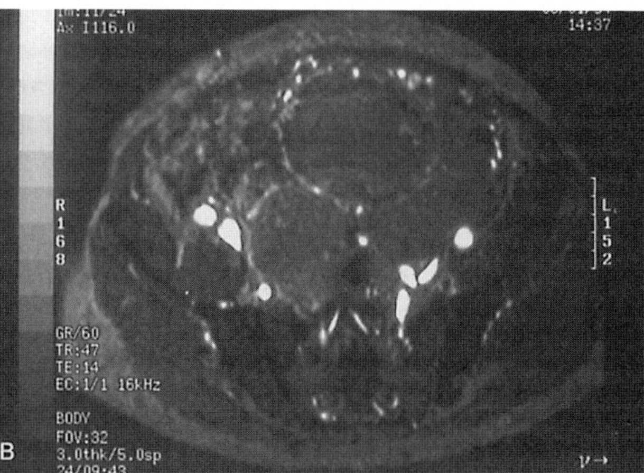

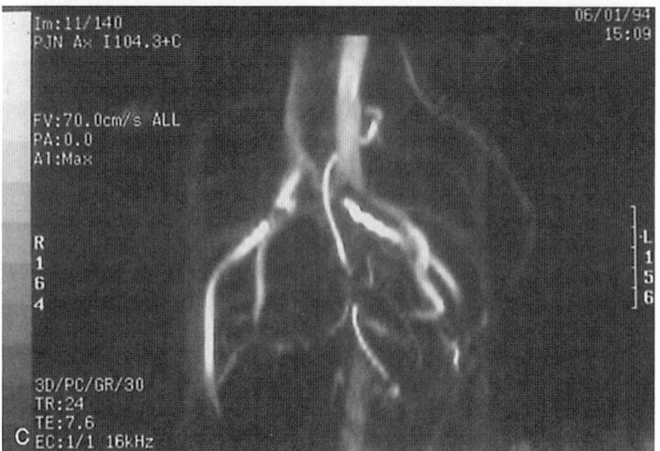

FIGURE 119.7 (*A*) Computed tomography scan of a large, high-grade pelvic sarcoma. There are multiple lobulations of tumor, with areas of spontaneous necrosis and a fluid–fluid level. The iliac vessels cannot be clearly distinguished as separate from the tumor mass. (*B*) Magnetic resonance angiogram (MRA)of the same region revealing the iliac arteries and veins as prominent white spots against the dark background of tumor. (*C*) Planar reconstruction demonstrating the distal aorta and vena cava and the iliac arteries and veins. The MRA suggested that the vessels were free of involvement, as indeed was the case at the time of resection.

required for imaging, patients with implanted metallic objects, such as pacemakers, artificial joints, and some vena cava filters, may not be able to undergo MRI.

Positron emission tomography (PET) scanning using fluoro-13-deoxyglucose also offers the potential for noninvasive analysis of tumor metabolism and has been shown to correlate with both tumor grade and response to treatment.[31] However, it does not allow for discrimination between low-grade tumors and benign lesions, nor does it hold any significant advantage in detecting recurrences.[32,33] Therefore its use should be limited to research purposes, assessing the biologic behavior of sarcomas in the context of neoadjuvant therapy.

Staging and Metastatic Workup

Because of the prognostic importance of histologic grade, the staging of the primary tumor is based on both clinical and histologic information. The usual TNM classification is modified according to a GTNM system (Table 119.4). This staging system is clinically useful because it assigns patients into groups with clearly differing prognoses (Fig. 119.8).

Four tumor grades are designated: well differentiated (G1), moderately differentiated (G2), poorly differentiated (G3), and undifferentiated (G4). For the purposes of staging, well-differentiated and moderately differentiated tumors (grades 1 and 2) are considered together as "low grade," whereas poorly differentiated and undifferentiated tumors (grades 3 and 4) are considered together as "high grade." One limitation of this system is that it does not recognize a difference between well-differentiated and moderately differentiated tumors, although significant data suggest that grade 2 tumors fare worse than grade 1 lesions.[34] Other grading systems have been proposed.[35,36]

The T stage is assigned based on size (<5 cm = T1, >5 cm = T2) and depth relative to the fascia (entirely above the fascia = a, invasion of or entirely below the fascia = b). The addition in 1998 of anatomic location to size added significant prognostic information to the staging system. One series of 215 patients with superficial extremity sarcomas documented a 10-year survival rate of 85% despite that 53% of tumors were high grade and 25% of tumors were 5 cm or larger.[37] Thus, a 5.5-cm sarcoma that is entirely located in the subcutaneous tissue above the muscular fascia would be categorized as T2a, whereas the same tumor involving the fascia would be T2b. All intraabdominal sarcomas are by definition "b" lesions. It is important to remember that although the GTNM size cut-off is 5 cm, tumors larger than 10 cm have an

TABLE 119.4 CLASSIFICATION AND STAGING

AMERICAN JOINT COMMISSION ON CANCER GTNM CLASSIFICATION AND STAGE GROUPING OF SOFT TISSUE SARCOMAS

Stage	Description
TUMOR GRADE	
GX	Grade cannot be assessed
G1	Well differentiated
G2	Moderately differentiated
G3	Poorly differentiated
G4	Undifferentiated
PRIMARY TUMOR	
TX	Primary tumor cannot be assessed
T0	No evidence of a primary tumor
T1	Tumor <5 cm in greatest diameter
T1a	Superficial tumor
T1b	Deep tumor
T2	Tumor <5 cm in greatest diameter
T2a	Superficial tumor
T2b	Deep tumor
LYMPH NODE INVOLVEMENT	
NX	Regional lymph nodes cannot be assessed
N0	No known metastases to lymph nodes
N1	Verified metastases to lymph nodes
DISTANT METASTASIS	
MX	Presence of distant metastasis cannot be assessed
M0	No known distant metastasis
M1	Known distant metastasis
STAGE GROUPING	
Stage I	G1-2, T1a, N0, M0
	G1-2, T1b, N0, M0
	G1-2, T2a, N0, M0
	G1-2, T2b, N0, M0
Stage II	G3-4, T1a, N0, M0
	G3-4, T1b, N0, M0
	G3-4, T2a, N0, M0
Stage III	G3-4, T2b, N0, M0
Stage IV	Any G, Any T, N1, M0
	Any G, Any T, N0, M1

Modified from the American Joint Committee on Cancer. *American Joint Committee on Cancer (AJCC) cancer staging manual*, 6th ed. 2002, with permission.

even worse prognosis.[38,39] When 316 patients with soft tissue sarcoma were grouped into four subgroups (<5 cm, 5 to 10 cm, 10 to 15 cm, and >15 cm) each subgroup had a distinct prognosis (84%, 70%, 50%, and 33%, respectively).[39]

Nodal metastasis of soft tissue sarcomas is rare (less than 5% of cases), with the exception of a few histologic subtypes for which the incidence of nodal involvement may be between 10% and 20%. These subtypes include rhabdomyosarcoma, epithelioid sarcoma, synovial sarcoma, and clear cell sarcoma. When node involvement occurs, it conveys essentially the same prognosis as distant metastatic disease and therefore is classified as stage IV. Nearly all patients who ever manifest nodal involvement have high-grade primary sarcomas (Fig. 119.9).

Distant metastatic disease is present in as many as 25% of patients with soft tissue sarcoma at the time of presentation. By far the most common site of metastasis is the lungs. In patients with sarcoma who have metastases, the lungs are involved more than 75% of the time. Approximately half of all patients with sarcoma who die of metastatic disease have lung metastases as their only site of distant spread. For this reason, all patients with newly diagnosed soft tissue sarcomas should have a chest radiograph and chest CT scan. Liver involvement is rare except in intraabdominal and retroperitoneal sarcomas, where it represents the second most common site of distant spread. In these cases, a CT scan that includes the liver should be done. Occasional patients have bone or central nervous system metastases; these sites of disease are uncommon in patients who do not already have lung metastases. Radionuclide bone scans, CT scanning, or MRI of the head, are not indicated in the absence of symptoms that suggest metastatic involvement.

In addition to size, depth, and grade, several other factors determine the prognosis of soft tissue sarcomas. Kattan et al.[40] created and validated a prognostic nomogram that predicts disease-specific death for patients with soft tissue sarcoma. (Fig. 119.10) This nomogram may be useful in counseling patients, deciding on the benefit of adjuvant therapy, and devising individual follow-up evaluations based on the patient's relative risk of recurrence.

SOFT TISSUE SARCOMAS OF EXTREMITIES

Principles of Surgical Resection

Historically, the wide local excision of an extremity soft tissue sarcoma resulted in local recurrence rates of 30% to 50%.[41,42] Amputation reduced local recurrence rates to less than 10% and became the standard of care. Radical amputation is amputation at least one joint space above the most proximal extent of tumor (Fig. 119.11). For a distal thigh tumor, a radical

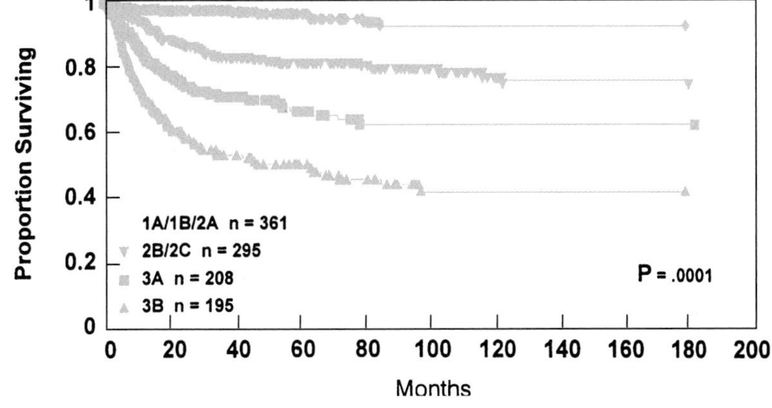

FIGURE 119.8 Survival rates of patients with soft tissue sarcoma categorized by tumor depth, grade, and size according to the American Joint Committee on Cancer staging system, with 3A designating stage III tumors of 5 to 10 cm and 3B designating tumors greater than 10 cm in size. (From Brennan MF. Staging of soft tissue sarcomas. *Ann Surg Oncol.* 1999;6:8–9, with permission.)

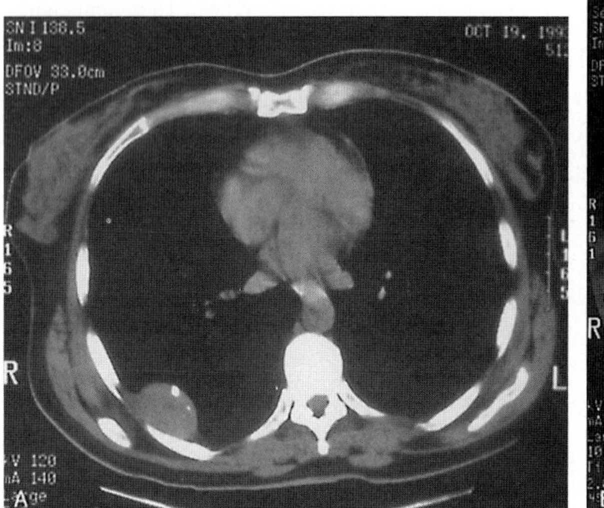

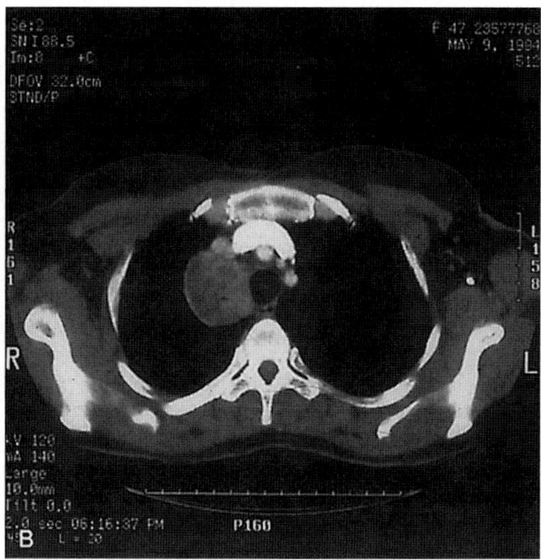

FIGURE 119.9 (*A*) High-grade malignant fibrous histiocytoma of the pleura. This tumor was treated with chest wall resection and postoperative radiation. (*B*) A follow-up computed tomography scan 7 months later revealed mediastinal adenopathy, which was subsequently confirmed to represent nodal metastasis from sarcoma.

amputation would be a hip disarticulation; for a high thigh lesion, a hemipelvectomy. At one time, more than 50% of all soft tissue sarcomas of the extremity were treated with radical amputations. Even with such extensive and mutilating procedures, however, local recurrence rates of up to 20% were seen.

In the 1970s, the concept of limb salvage through combining less radical surgery with radiation therapy emerged. In 1982, Rosenberg et al.[43] published the results of a randomized trial of limb-sparing resection plus adjuvant radiation therapy versus amputation. Both groups received adjuvant chemotherapy. No differences were found in the disease-free survival rates (71% versus 78%) or the overall survival rates (83% versus 88%) at 5 years between the limb-sparing group and the amputation group. This trial demonstrated that amputation was not mandatory, a finding confirmed by several additional studies.[44–46] In 1985 the National Institutes of

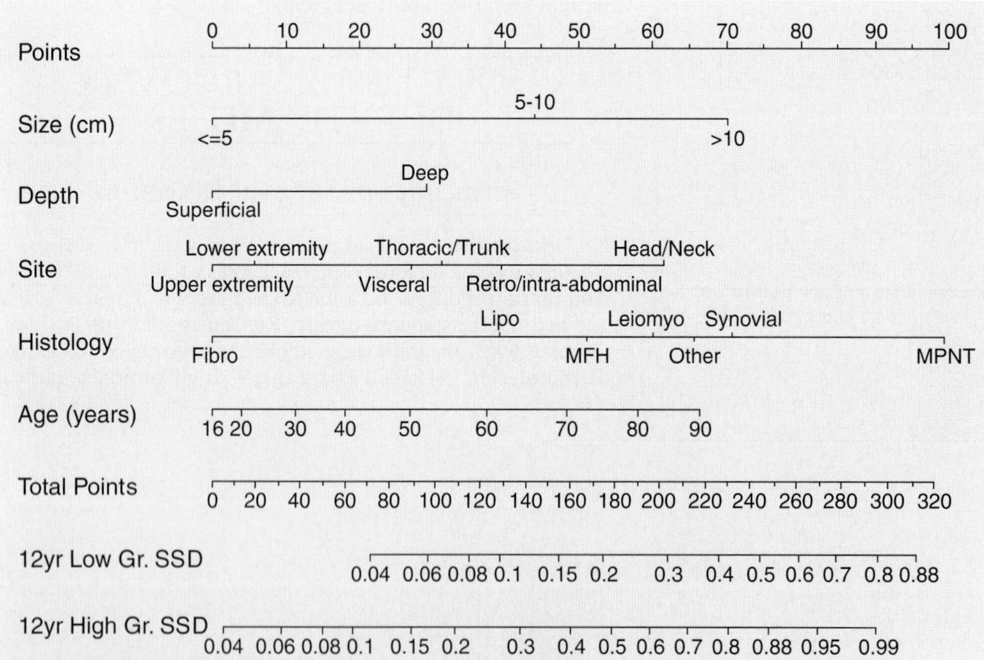

Instructions for Physician: Locate the patient's tumor size on the Size axis. Draw a line straight upwards to the Points axis t o determine how many points towards sarcoma-specific death the patient receives for his tumor size. Repeat this process for the other axes, each time drawing straight upward to the Points axis. Sum the points achieved for each predictor and locate this sum on the Total Points axis. Draw a line straight down to either the Low Grade or High Grade axis to find the patient 's probability of dying from sarcoma within 12 years assuming he or she does not die of another cause first.

Instruction to Patient: If we had 100 patients exactly like you, we would expect between <predi cted percentage from nomogram – 8%> and <predicted percentage + 8%> to die of sarcoma within 12 years if they did not die of another cause first, and death from sarcoma after 12 years is still possible."

FIGURE 119.10 Postoperative nomogram for 12-year sarcoma-specific death. Fibro 5 fibrosarcoma; Lipo 5 liposarcoma; Leiomyo 5 leiomyosarcoma; MFH 5 malignant fibrous histiocytoma; MPNT 5 malignant peripheral nerve tumor; Gr 5 Grade; SSD 5 sarcoma-specific death. (From Kattan MW, Leung DH, Brennan MF. Postoperative nomogram for 12 year sarcoma specific death. *J Clin Oncol.* 2002;20:791–796. Reprinted with permission from the American Society of Clinical Oncology.)

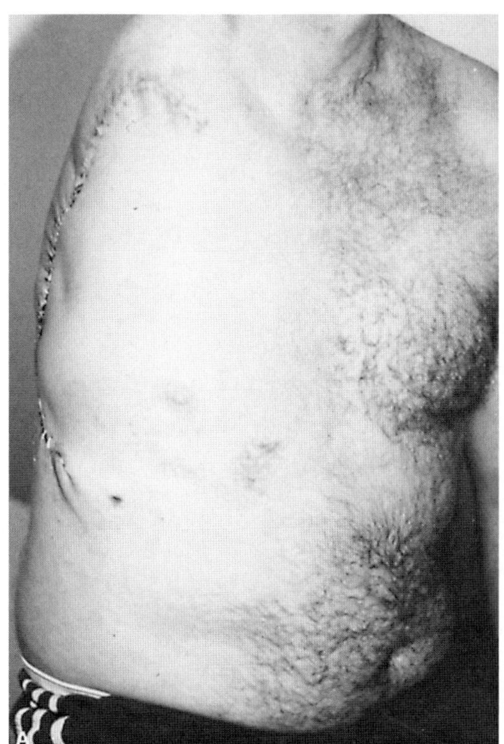

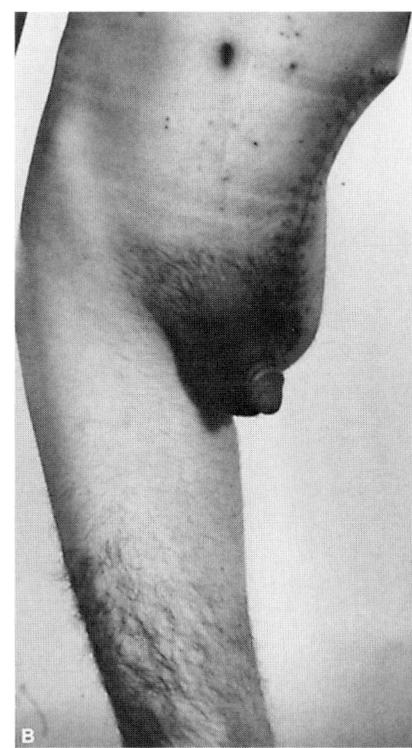

FIGURE 119.11 Radical amputations for extremity sarcomas include one joint above the most proximal extent of tumor. (*A*) In the upper extremity, the standard radical amputation for an upper arm tumor is a forequarter (interscapulothoracic) amputation. (*B*) In the lower extremity, the standard amputation for most tumors of the proximal thigh or buttock is a hemipelvectomy. Less extensive amputations are possible for more distal tumors.

Health released a consensus statement recommending limb-sparing surgery for most patients with high-grade extremity sarcomas.[47] Radical amputation now is reserved for patients who are not suitable candidates for limb-sparing approaches, usually because of bony invasion or large tumor size (Fig. 119.12), or for recurrence after previous limb-sparing surgery.

Today, the surgical approach of choice for most limb-sparing protocols is the wide radical excision (Fig. 119.13). Wide local excision involves gross total removal of the tumor with a wide margin of normal tissue. This approach is in contrast to compartment excision, which was based on the belief that sarcomas spread diffusely throughout one muscular compartment but are prevented by fascial boundaries from lateral spread provided the rationale for this procedure. Unfortunately, most sarcomas are not confined in a single muscular compartment, and those that are do not usually involve the muscles for more than 2 to 3 cm beyond the grossly visible boundaries. Long, origin-to-insertion skin incisions often cross one or even two joints, making postoperative radiation and rehabilitation more difficult, and compartment excisions are of historical interest only with the exception of rare cases when the tumor is large but remains confined to one compartment.

Rather, a margin of at least 2 to 3 cm of normal tissue is obtained proximally and distally. On the lateral and deep margins, at least one grossly uninvolved fascial plane is resected en bloc with the tumor whenever possible. For large or deep-seated tumors, resection of uninvolved periosteum or adventitia may represent the deep margin. If necessary, major vascular structures can be resected and reconstructed with autologous or other graft material (Fig. 119.14A). Having positive margins after resection nearly doubles the risk of local recurrence and increases the risk of distant recurrence and disease-related deaths.[48] If negative margins are not obtained on the first attempt at resection, a re-excision should be performed because this procedure improves both local recurrence and distant disease-free survival.[48,49]

Several important surgical principles bear mentioning. Soft tissue sarcomas are generally surrounded by a zone of compressed reactive tissue that forms a pseudocapsule. Surgeons inexperienced in sarcoma often mistakenly use this zone to guide the resection, in effect enucleating the tumor. This approach commonly results in microscopically positive margins and a significantly increased risk of local recurrence, ranging between 33% and 66%.[41,50,51] The tumor and its pseudocapsule should not be entered during the definitive excision. Patients seen after excisional biopsy should undergo wide reexcision, even if they have no clinical or radiographic evidence of residual tumor. Metallic clips placed in the tumor bed during surgery can help define the limits of resection and aid in radiation therapy planning.

On occasion, major nerves, such as the sciatic nerve, are sacrificed to preserve a functional, albeit neurologically compromised, extremity. When low-grade lesions are resected, because of their less aggressive nature, major vessels or nerves are not removed along with the tumor (Fig. 119.14B). Sometimes, negative margins around high-grade tumors cannot be achieved

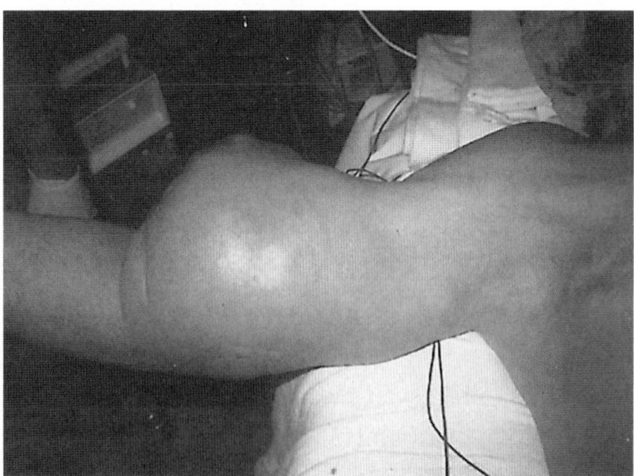

FIGURE 119.12 Enormous high-grade malignant fibrous histiocytoma circumferentially involving the upper arm just above the elbow. This tumor was treated with a radical amputation (shoulder disarticulation). Aggressive local or systemic treatment to shrink the tumor and avoid amputation was not used because of the patient's advanced age.

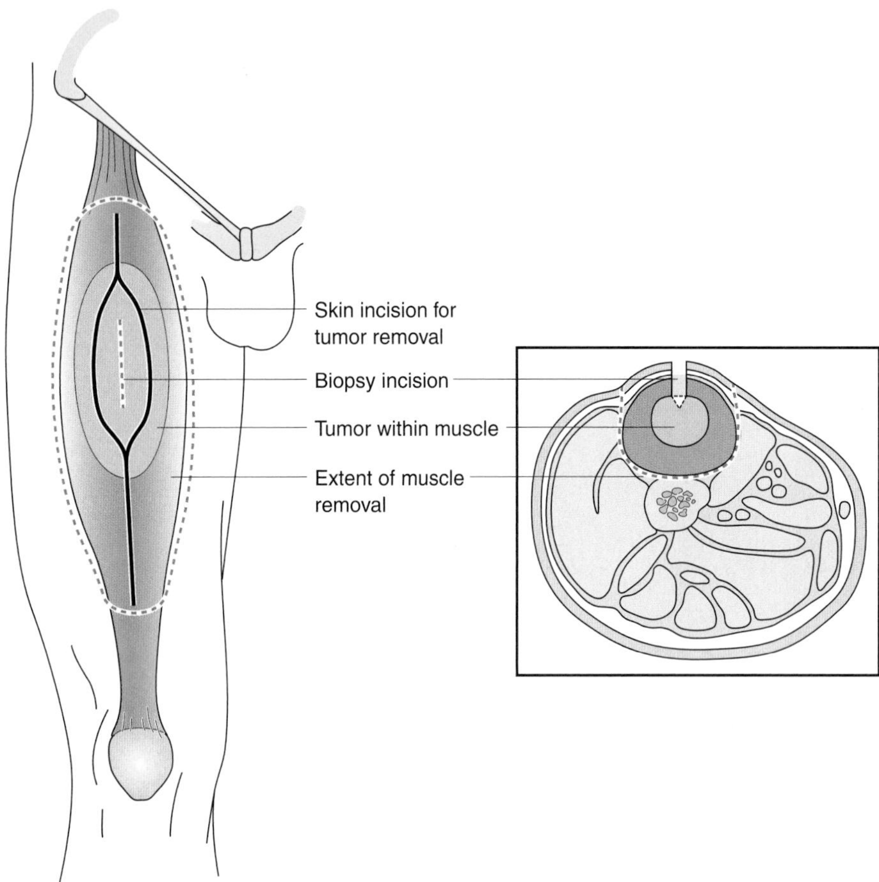

FIGURE 119.13 Wide excision involves removal of the tumor with a margin of normal tissue: 3 to 5 cm is obtained proximally and distally, and on the lateral and deep margins at least one grossly uninvolved fascial plane is resected *en bloc* with the tumor. No attempt is made to resect an entire muscle compartment. If necessary, major vascular structures or nerves may be resected.

because of the tumor's proximity to vital structures, and resection of these structures would result in substantial functional compromise. In these cases, it should be taken into consideration that neither a positive surgical margin nor a local recurrence has been shown to adversely affect overall survival, and the risks and benefits of more radical resection must be carefully balanced.[52,53]

A significant number of patients require an extensive removal of tissue, so simple wound closure is not possible. This is particularly true in patients who have had preoperative

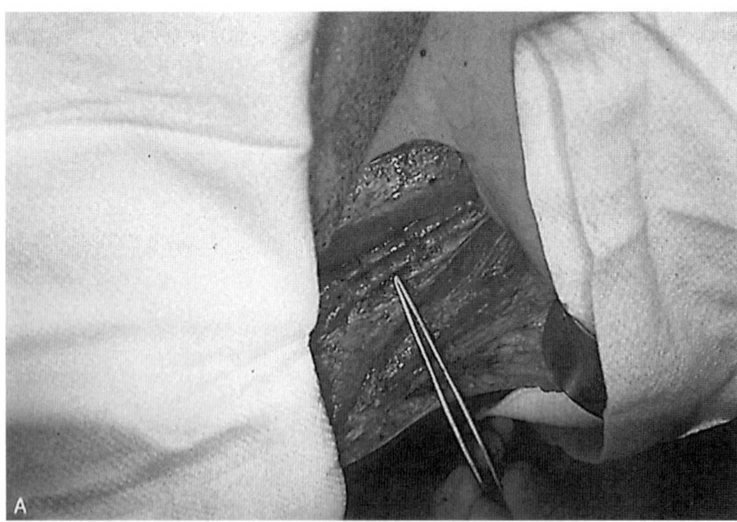

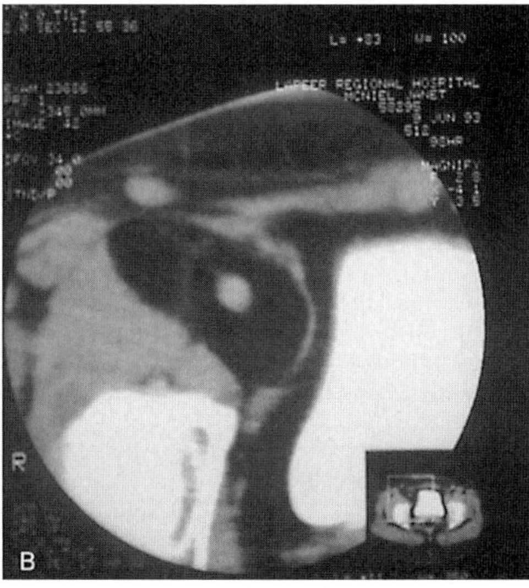

FIGURE 119.14 (*A*) Complete removal of a large, intermediate-grade synovial sarcoma of the right groin required resection of a small portion of the superficial femoral artery. This structure was reconstructed with an interposition graft of ipsilateral saphenous vein (at tip of forceps). The patient received postoperative irradiation and remains free of disease with excellent distal pulses 6 years later. (*B*) Contrast-enhanced computed tomography scan demonstrates a well-differentiated liposarcoma surrounding the right femoral artery (*central white dot*) in the groin. This tumor was resected without removal of the artery or vein by bisecting the tumor and peeling it free from the vascular structures.

radiation. In these cases, resection should be planned in conjunction with a plastic surgeon to provide reconstruction. Several advances in plastic surgery techniques now allow the plastic surgeon to transfer large amounts of tissue to provide closure.[54]

When discussing most cancers, the surgical therapy includes attention to the regional lymph nodes. Overall, sarcoma has an extremely low (2% to 3%) incidence of nodal metastases, and so there is no role for routine regional lymph node dissection. However, there are several subtypes that have an increased incidence of lymph node metastases. They include angiosarcoma, synovial, embryonal rhabdomyosarcoma, and epithelioid histiotypes. If lymphadenopathy is discovered on physical examination, a therapeutic lymphadenectomy should be performed, and although this is considered stage IV disease, in the absence of extranodal disease it may result in a 34% survival rate.[55] In patients with these subtypes who are clinically node negative, there may be a role for sentinel lymph node biopsy, although the benefits remain unproven.[56]

Postoperative Surveillance

The majority of soft tissue sarcoma recurrences occur in the first 2 years after therapy. Many patients with locally recurrent or even metastatic sarcomas can be cured by aggressive surgery, often combined with radiation and chemotherapy. For this reason, all patients with sarcoma should be observed carefully for recurrence. For high-grade lesions, follow-up should be directed toward detecting both local recurrence and metastases. Low-grade lesions rarely metastasize in the absence of local recurrence, and follow-up should focus on the original tumor site. Low-grade sarcoma can recur up to 20 years after original resection, however, so follow-up must be maintained over the long term.

The most useful component of follow-up is the history and physical examination, which should be performed every 3 months for the first 2 to 3 years. Chest radiography to look for pulmonary metastases should be obtained every 6 months for the first 2 to 3 years and yearly after that. CT scan of the chest should be reserved for evaluation of abnormal findings on the chest radiography.

Evaluation of the primary site for local recurrence is more controversial. Because aggressive resection can salvage many patients with a local recurrence, many clinicians have advocated an aggressive follow-up schedule. Part of this approach is dependent on the ease of physical examination. For regions that are more difficult to evaluate on physical examination, imaging with ultrasound, CT scan, or MRI is useful for evaluating for recurrence. MRI is particularly useful for both detecting recurrence or evaluating equivocal changes found on exam, with strict guidelines for distinguishing between recurrences and postoperative changes.[57] The choice of imaging study depends on availability, cost, and anatomic site being examined. A typical follow-up schedule consists of a study at 3 months for a baseline, followed by another every 6 months for the first 2 years, and then either every 6 months or annually for years 2 through 5. Other authors have advocated a more cost-efficient and conservative follow-up schedule.[58] It may be possible to tailor a follow-up schedule to each patient based on their relative risk of recurrence and death.[40] After 5 years, history, physical examination, and chest radiograph should be obtained yearly.

Multimodality Management

For patients with small, low-grade tumors, wide local excision alone is associated with a low rate of local recurrence, assuming adequate negative margins have been obtained. If a wide margin has been obtained around a small, low-grade sarcoma, observation may be appropriate. Most other patients undergoing surgical excision, however, receive additional therapy, primarily the use of radiation, to improve the chances for local control. Radiation also has some effectiveness as primary therapy for extremity sarcomas in patients who refuse or cannot tolerate surgery, although the results do not match the local control rates achieved with surgery alone.[59]

In general, in cases in which a low-grade sarcoma was excised with narrow margins or the margins were compromised to preserve major neurovascular structures, postoperative radiation is indicated. Intermediate- and high-grade extremity sarcomas almost always receive multimodality therapy, although this practice is being called into questioned. If the preoperative evaluation reveals a sarcoma smaller than 10 cm that can be resected with a satisfactory surgical margin, it is appropriate to proceed with wide excision plus postoperative radiation. Otherwise, for those tumors larger than 10 cm or for smaller tumors that cannot be adequately resected, patients should undergo preoperative treatment of the tumor consisting of radiation alone or with chemotherapy. Amputation should be reserved for tumors that extensively surround or involve bone, that recur after a limb-sparing approach and cannot be re-resected locally, or that fail to respond to preoperative therapy.

Postoperative Radiation

The optimal method of delivery and the timing and margin of postoperative radiation therapy are not completely defined. Postoperative radiation therapy planning is based on the anatomic location, tumor grade, and status of the surgical margins. Typically, doses of 6,000 to 7,000 cGy are required to ensure local control. The entire surgical scar and drain sites are included in the field, along with a typical radiation margin of 5 to 7 cm (although some centers advocate wider margins). It is important that the entire circumference of the extremity must not be irradiated because massive lymphedema results. A strip of skin and subcutaneous tissue surrounding the tumor usually is excluded from the treatment field to prevent this complication.

An alternate approach to postoperative radiation is brachytherapy. This therapy involves the placement of multiple catheters in the tumor resection bed to administer iridium[192] (Fig. 119.15). Unlike the 6 to 7 weeks needed for external beam radiation, brachytherapy is completed in 4 to 6 days. Brachytherapy also produces less radiation scatter in critical areas, improving functional outcome. Among the disadvantages are that brachytherapy is technically complex and requires an experienced radiation oncologist in the operating room, and an extended inpatient hospital stay and bed rest

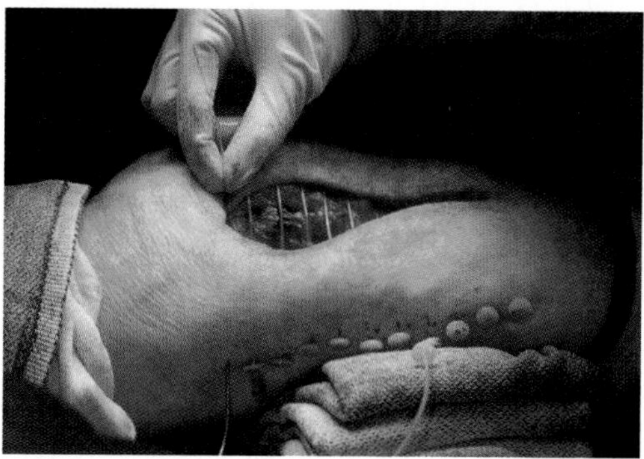

FIGURE 119.15 Brachytherapy catheters placed after resection of a soft tissue sarcoma.

are required. Despite these requirements, brachytherapy is not more expensive than external beam radiation and may be less costly.[60] From a therapeutic standpoint, brachytherapy and external beam radiation appear to be equivalent when properly administered.

Typically, postoperative radiation has been recommended for all patients with intermediate or high-grade tumors of any size. However, small tumors (<5 cm) have lower recurrence rates and radiation therapy may not be necessary.[22,39,61–63] With better preoperative imaging and improved surgical and pathologic techniques, local recurrence rates may be improved over past series. More importantly, two series demonstrated that postoperative radiation did not improve the 5-year local recurrence or survival rates in patients with small soft tissue sarcomas.[64,65] For patients with small soft tissue sarcomas, the benefits of adjuvant radiation must be balanced against the potential complications. The long-term complications of radiation are related to fibrosis, necrosis, edema, fractures, and contractures, all of which can impair function. Complications vary with the dose and field treated and tumor location, mandating an individual approach to each patient.

Preoperative Radiation

Experience with postoperative radiation therapy for large extremity sarcomas (10 cm or more) was more disappointing, with a high incidence of local failure. Subsequently, extensive investigations suggested that preoperative radiation offered significant advantages in this group of patients. Local control rates were considerably higher when large tumors were treated before surgery; in some cases, tumors initially considered unresectable without amputation shrank sufficiently to permit limb-sparing resection. Although these investigations were not randomized, the prospect of preoperative treatment for large extremity sarcomas broadened the spectrum of patients for whom limb-sparing surgery could be considered.

There are several potential advantages to delivering radiation therapy preoperatively in addition to facilitating surgical resection. There is no delay in delivering radiation, as may occur in the case of wound complications after surgery. Planning radiation while the tumor is in place is simpler and allows for smaller radiation fields and lower doses, including fewer joints in the field than with postoperative radiation. Although this approach has been suggested to result in improved functional outcome,[66] a randomized trial demonstrated that the timing of radiation had minimal impact on patient function and quality of life beyond the initial 6 weeks after surgery.[67] Radiation may be more effective when delivered to an undisturbed tumor bed because of improved tissue oxygenation.[68–70] However, delivering radiation preoperatively may affect the ability to accurately stage the sarcoma as well as assess the surgical margins. The radiation oncologist must completely rely on the imaging characteristics of the tumor to define the target volume, which may underestimate the true extent of the tumor. There can also be an increased rate of wound complications. In a randomized comparison of preoperative and postoperative radiation therapy, 190 patients were randomized to 50 Gy preoperatively or 66 Gy postoperatively.[71] Wound complications occurred in 35% of the preoperative group compared with 17% in the postoperative group ($P = .01$), the majority being in the lower extremity. Local control and progression-free survival were similar in both groups. The judgment about which approach is the most appropriate for resectable tumors is still a matter of debate,[72] but preoperative radiation therapy should be the choice for more adverse presentations in need of more extensive surgery.

Chemotherapy

Adjuvant Chemotherapy

The main cause of death in patients with soft tissue sarcoma is distant metastatic disease, particularly for those with high-grade tumors or extremity lesions.[73] As local control rates have improved, emphasis has been placed on eradicating metastatic disease with postoperative adjuvant systemic chemotherapy. The histologic subtypes of sarcoma run the gamut from being very responsive to cytotoxic chemotherapy to those that are completely resistant. Three agents are consistently associated with response rates of greater than 20%: doxorubicin, ifosfamide, and dacarbazine.

The use of adjuvant chemotherapy remains controversial because the risk of adverse toxic effects may not be outweighed by the minimal response. Much of the interest in adjuvant chemotherapy for extremity soft tissue sarcoma began with a randomized trial reported by Rosenberg et al.[74] that demonstrated an improvement in disease-free and overall survival with adjuvant doxorubicin, cyclophosphamide, and high-dose methotrexate. After a longer follow-up period (median follow-up 7.1 years), however, both disease-free and overall survival were not statistically significant.[75] Multiple randomized trials of postoperative chemotherapy have failed to demonstrate an improvement in disease-free or overall survival in soft tissue sarcoma.[76,77] The benefit that is seen might be only within the first year of therapy, without sustained benefit.[78] The Sarcoma Meta-analysis Collaboration evaluated the effect of adjuvant doxorubicin-based chemotherapy in 1,568 patients from 14 trials.[79] Although the time to local and distant recurrence, and recurrence-free survival rates, was significantly better in the treatment group, the overall survival advantage was only 4% and not statistically significant ($P = .12$). However, in patients with extremity sarcomas, there was a 7% overall survival benefit, which was significant ($P = 0.029$).

This meta-analysis compared doxorubicin containing regimens to controls. It is possible that the combination of the two most active agents, doxorubicin and ifosfamide, may provide increased clinical benefit. A randomized trial of both of these agents as postoperative adjuvant therapy for very-high-risk patients demonstrated a benefit in both disease-free and overall survival.[80] Additional trials are ongoing, but it is reasonable to conclude that postoperative adjuvant chemotherapy is an option that should be discussed with patients with high-risk soft tissue sarcoma.

Neoadjuvant Chemotherapy

As with radiation, there may be potential advantages to delivering systemic chemotherapy prior to surgical resection. It may help shrink tumors and allow less morbid surgical resection than otherwise would have been necessary. Another theoretical advantage is that it allows the treatment of occult micrometastatic disease as soon as possible after diagnosis, which may prevent the development of chemoresistance or prevent the postoperative growth of micrometastases. This theory has not yet been borne out in clinical trials, however. In one study of 65 patients with stage II or III soft tissue sarcoma, preoperative chemotherapy allowed a reduction of the scope of operation in only 12% of patients and did not allow for limb salvage in any of the patients who required amputation.[81] In a series of 76 patients treated at the M. D. Anderson Cancer Center, the event-free outcomes were comparable to those observed with postoperative chemotherapy.[82] Likewise, a prospective study from Memorial Sloan-Kettering Cancer Center failed to demonstrate any advantage to two cycles of doxorubicin over postoperative doxorubicin or local therapy alone.[83]

A significant potential advantage of systemic chemotherapy would be the ability to assess the tumor response *in situ*. By seeing whether the tumor responds to the chemotherapy, both radiologically and pathologically, it may be possible to spare patients prolonged therapy if they are not responding, and continue therapy postoperatively in patients who do respond, possibly improving outcome. However, this approach is still theoretical and has yet to be definitively established. The correlation of treatment-induced necrosis with clinical outcomes has not been well defined in soft tissue sarcoma. Complete pathologic necrosis occurs in only 5% to 15% of patients with doxorubicin-based induction chemotherapy.[84–86] Although patients who have a clinical or pathologic response may have improved local control and decreased distant disease-free survival, it is unclear whether this translates to an overall survival advantage.[87,88] In the M. D. Anderson series, comparison of responding patients to nonresponding patients did not reveal any significant differences in event-free outcome.[82] Continuing studies of aggressive neoadjuvant therapy are ongoing.[89] Using aggressive combinations of doxorubicin- and ifosfamide-based regimens, response rates may be higher.[90] Preliminary data suggest these regimens can be successfully delivered, they are still considered experimental, and neoadjuvant chemotherapy should be performed only in the context of a clinical trial.

An alternative approach for patients who have unresectable extremity sarcomas is the use of preoperative regional chemotherapy. Hyperthermic isolated limb perfusion (HILP) allows for the administration of high doses of chemotherapeutic agents to a limb. The limb circulation is isolated from the patient's systemic circulation by cannulating the artery and vein and connecting to a heart-lung machine. Extracorporeal circulation allows the delivery of drug concentrations 10 to 20 times higher than with systemic delivery. A large European study showed that for unresectable soft tissue sarcomas of the extremities, a limb-salvage rate of 71% could be obtained using HILP with melphalan and tumor necrosis factor-α.[91,92] Further research into the potential for isolated limb perfusion in the preoperative therapy for soft tissue sarcomas continues.

Neoadjuvant Chemoradiation

In an effort to improve on the results of chemotherapy alone, the use of preoperative chemoradiation has been examined. Patients with intermediate- and high-grade extremity sarcomas have been treated with preoperative radiation therapy combined with regional chemotherapy. Three days of intraarterial chemotherapy with doxorubicin, followed by large-fraction radiation (3,500 cGy in 10 days) and wide local excision, was successful in achieving local control and in preserving a functional extremity. Significant degrees of necrosis were commonly seen in the resected tumor specimen. Although the more direct route to the tumor made this the initially favored approach, it is more complex and expensive and has more complications than the intravenous route.[87] Local complications were frequent and proved to be the most common reason for subsequent amputation of the treated limb, which was necessary in approximately 5% of cases.[87] When a subsequent prospective randomized trial demonstrated no difference between preoperative intraarterial doxorubicin and intravenous doxorubicin, both followed by 28 Gy of radiation and then surgery, intraarterial chemotherapy fell out of favor.

Neoadjuvant chemoradiation continues to be an active area of research for soft tissue sarcoma. Several regimens investigated include radiation with doxorubicin alone,[93,94] in combination with ifosfamide, mesna and dacarbazine,[95] and actinomycin D.[45] These trials appear encouraging, but until the results from prospective, randomized trials of chemoradiation demonstrate a survival advantage, neoadjuvant chemoradiation, either concurrent or sequential, should be performed only with clinical protocols at specialty centers.

RETROPERITONEAL SARCOMAS

Diagnosis and Prognosis

Retroperitoneal sarcomas account for approximately 15% of all sarcomas; liposarcoma and leiomyosarcoma are the two most common subtypes. Other, less common subtypes include fibrosarcoma, malignant fibrous histiocytoma, and unclassified sarcoma. Retroperitoneal sarcomas are generally large at presentation; more than half are larger than 20 cm at the time of diagnosis. Retroperitoneal tumors rarely cause significant symptoms until they achieve large size, and even then, symptoms usually are vague and nonspecific. Abdominal pain, weight loss, early satiety, and nausea and vomiting are the most common complaints. An abdominal mass can be felt in approximately 45% to 70% of patients at the time of presentation. Many patients have an increased abdominal girth. Neurologic symptoms related to direct neural involvement and compression can occur in up to one third of patients and can include paresthesia, dysesthesia, weakness, and swelling or varicosities in the lower extremities.

The differential diagnosis of a retroperitoneal mass includes benign masses such as lymphangioma, lipoma, or leiomyoma and other malignancies such as lymphoma, germ-cell tumors, and renal or adrenal tumors. In addition to a thorough history and physical examination, looking for the signs and symptoms of lymphoma (B symptoms, adenopathy), laboratory assessment should include lactate dehydrogenase (elevated in lymphoma) and β-human chorionic gonadotropin and α-fetoprotein levels (suggestive of a germ-cell tumor). Radiologic assessment should include a high-quality helical CT of the chest, abdomen, and pelvis, with enteric and intravenous contrast to define the extent of the tumor and look for lung or liver metastases. In addition, this approach documents the presence and extent of necrosis and document bilateral renal function in case a unilateral nephrectomy is required. CT-guided core-needle biopsy is the most appropriate first step in making the diagnosis. Open incisional biopsy should be reserved for cases in which the needle biopsy is inconclusive. The area of the biopsy should be isolated to prevent tumor spillage into the peritoneal cavity. If lymphoma or a germ-cell tumor can be ruled out and the diagnosis of retroperitoneal sarcoma is clear from the imaging studies, tissue sampling is not required prior to surgical resection other than when neoadjuvant therapy is contemplated.

MRI of the abdomen can provide improved tumor delineation as well as reconstruction in sagittal, coronal, and transaxial planes and delineate vascular involvement. If this information is not adequately provided by the CT scan and the resectability remains in question, then an MRI can be helpful in the preoperative workup. MRI should also be used in patients with contraindications to iodinated contrast material or pregnant patients.

Unfortunately, the overall prognosis for patients with retroperitoneal sarcomas remains poor. The significant advances in multimodality therapy of extremity sarcomas have not been matched by similar progress in the management of retroperitoneal tumors. The wide margins of resection routinely obtained for extremity sarcomas are difficult to achieve in the retroperitoneum, and the delivery of radiation is more limited. Most patients with retroperitoneal sarcomas die of their disease, frequently with locally recurrent tumor as the major or sole site of failure. Unlike the situation with extremity sarcomas, even patients with low-grade retroperitoneal sarcomas

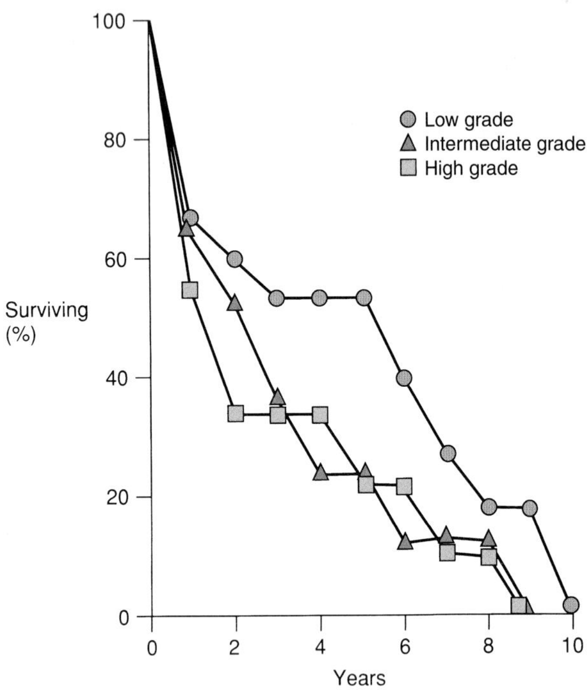

FIGURE 119.16 Survival rates of patients with retroperitoneal sarcoma classified by histologic grade. All patients had tumors larger than 5 cm in this series. (Storm FK, Eilber FR, Mirra J, et al. Retroperitoneal sarcomas: a reappraisal of treatment. *J Surg Oncol.* 1980;17:1, with permission.)

usually die of progressive tumor (Fig. 119.16). Approximately 75% of patients with retroperitoneal sarcomas ultimately die of locally recurrent disease with distant metastases.[96]

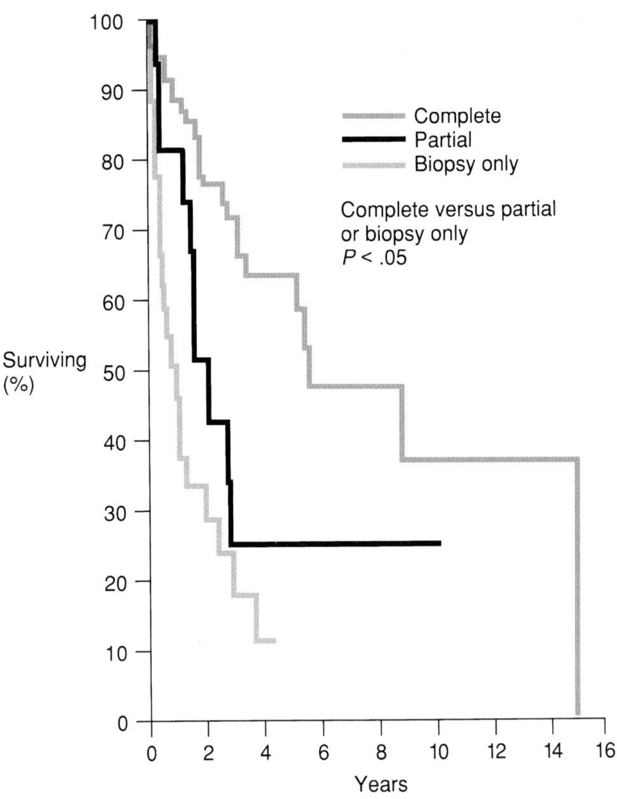

FIGURE 119.17 Survival rates of patients with retroperitoneal sarcoma classified by type of operation. Patients undergoing partial excision of their tumors had no improvement in survival compared with those deemed unresectable. (Jacques DP, Coit DG, Hajdu SI, et al. Management of primary and recurrent soft tissue sarcoma of the retroperitoneum. *Ann Surg.* 1990;212:51, with permission.)

Surgery

Complete excision of all gross tumor is essential for long-term disease-free survival. The goal of any potentially curative operation is *en bloc* resection of the tumor with a rim of normal tissue. In one series, median survival was 103 months for patients who underwent complete resection, compared with only 18 months for those who underwent incomplete resection.[97] Unfortunately, because these tumors often involve vital structures, it is rarely possible to obtain clearly negative margins. Even with an aggressive approach to *en bloc* resection, complete surgical excision is possible in only approximately 50% of cases.[98] Partial excisions or debulking procedures do not improve survival compared with biopsy alone (Fig. 119.17).

A transperitoneal approach is much more likely to allow complete resection than a flank approach. A midline abdominal incision is adequate for most tumors. A chevron-shaped incision can be used for upper abdominal tumors. In cases of extensive upper quadrant tumors, a thoracoabdominal incision is occasionally necessary. The abdominal cavity should be explored for sarcomatosis or liver metastases. Tumor respectability is then assessed, looking for extensive mesenteric or nerve root involvement, which may preclude resection. Debulking for palliation, where gross tumor is intentionally left in the patient, has a survival rate comparable to biopsy alone and should play minimal role in management.[97,99] Palliative resection may be useful in carefully selected patients, primarily to relieve urinary or gastrointestinal obstruction.

To remove all gross tumor, concomitant resection of adjacent organs is required more than 75% of the time, most commonly of the kidney and colon (Table 119.5). Although it is not common for retroperitoneal sarcomas to directly invade surrounding organs, the intense desmoplastic reaction makes this difficult to determine intraoperatively. The surgeon should opt to resect neighboring structures, rather than risk positive margins.[100]

The transperitoneal approach permits resection of adjacent organs and allows for early control of the vascular supply to the tumor. In the upper retroperitoneum, the blood supply to the tumor is frequently derived from multiple small branches, including lumbar arteries. In the pelvic retroperitoneum, one or

TABLE 119.5 TREATMENT

ORGANS RESECTED IN CONTINUITY WITH A PRIMARY RETROPERITONEAL SARCOMA

Organ	Cases in which organ is resected (%)
Kidney	46
Colon	24
Pancreas	15
Spleen	10
Major vessels (vena cava, iliac artery, or vein)	10

From Jacques DP, Coit DG, Hajdu SI, et al. Management of primary and recurrent soft tissue sarcoma of the retroperitoneum. *Ann Surg.* 1990;212:51, with permission.

both internal iliac arteries usually supply most of the tumor. Occasionally, the blood supply to a highly vascular pelvic retroperitoneal sarcoma may be occluded before surgery by angiographic embolization to minimize intraoperative blood loss. If the tumor involves the infrarenal inferior vena cava, this structure can be resected and ligated with minimal morbidity. If the tumor involves the suprarenal inferior vena cava, resection with primary repair or interposition grafting is performed.[101]

After surgery, postoperative surveillance should consist of history and physical examination every 3 months and chest radiograph every 6 months for the first 2 to 3 years. Abdominal imaging guidelines are less clear. CT scanning is useful for detecting both local recurrence and distant metastases in the liver and elsewhere in the abdomen and pelvis. For this reason, some surgeons have advocated that CT scans should be obtained every 3 to 6 months for the first 2 years and every 6 months until 5 years. However, there is no evidence that earlier detection improves survival,[97] so other surgeons believe that a less aggressive imaging schedule for asymptomatic patients is more appropriate, particularly after a second recurrence of retroperitoneal sarcoma.[53]

Radiation Therapy

Although radiation has had dramatic results in the management of extremity sarcomas, this success has not been equaled in the retroperitoneum, stressing the importance of complete surgical resection. Much of this difference is related to the difficulty of delivering the same doses to the abdomen because of normal tissue tolerance. Extremity tumors can frequently be treated with 6,000 cGy or more in conventional dose fractions. In contrast, the small bowel can tolerate only 4,500 to 5,000 cGy and the liver and kidney even less.

Because of the difficulty in achieving wide resection margins, however, radiation is frequently used as a postoperative adjuvant. The results have been mixed, with some retrospective studies demonstrating a benefit[102,103] and other studies failing to show much benefit.[104] The potential benefits in each individual case must be balanced against the potential toxicity of therapy.

As with extremity sarcoma, there is potential benefit to delivering preoperative radiation therapy. In addition to the advantages described for extremity sarcomas, preoperative radiation in the retroperitoneum capitalizes on the tumor bulk displacing the dose-limiting small bowel out of the high-dose region. This approach allows for higher doses to be delivered.[105] No data supports the concept that preoperative radiation for retroperitoneal sarcomas is superior to postoperative therapy. Another approach to limiting normal tissue toxicity is the use of intraoperative radiation therapy (IORT). This approach offers the advantage of allowing the bowel and other sensitive structures to be moved out of the field while a single high dose of radiation is administered directly to the tumor bed. Although some nonrandomized studies have suggested a benefit,[106] intraoperative radiation therapy is costly, logistically difficult, and associated with complications of its own, such as neurotoxicity. A randomized trial of IORT plus low-dose postoperative external beam radiation versus high-dose postoperative external beam radiation demonstrated an improvement in local recurrence but no effect on overall survival.[107]

Chemotherapy

Aggressive systemic chemotherapy is poorly tolerated in patients who have just undergone a major intraabdominal procedure with resection of multiple organs. Several trials of postoperative adjuvant chemotherapy do not show any benefit for patients with retroperitoneal sarcoma, and in one series, treated patients fared worse than those not receiving chemotherapy.[62] The meta-analysis of chemotherapy that demonstrated a survival benefit for the patients with extremity sarcoma failed to demonstrate the same benefit in retroperitoneal tumors.[79] In one trial of an aggressive multimodality approach, there was an improvement in locoregional control but no overall survival advantage and significant toxicity from the chemotherapy and radiation therapy.[108] Another study attempted to deliver the chemotherapy intraarterially, although this is often limited by the lack of a single feeder vessel in most retroperitoneal tumors. Nonetheless, a nonrandomized study suggested that preoperative doxorubicin (given intravenously in those patients without a single feeding artery) and external beam radiation followed by aggressive surgical resection led to longer survival times and lower local recurrence rates than those found in a historical cohort treated with surgery with or without postoperative radiation.[108] Additional studies of neoadjuvant chemotherapy and radiation therapy are ongoing.[109]

DESMOID TUMORS

Desmoid tumors are unusual soft tissue lesions with unique characteristics but definite similarities to low-grade soft tissue sarcomas. Although clinical reports of low-grade soft tissue sarcomas often include desmoid tumors,[110] in fact desmoid tumors virtually never metastasize even after multiple local recurrences.[111] Often they are referred to as *aggressive fibromatosis*, reflecting their potential for progressive growth and high recurrence rates. Desmoid tumors present in a fashion identical to soft tissue sarcomas, as an enlarging, often painless soft tissue mass. Clinically and radiographically, except for the special settings described later, there is nothing to distinguish a desmoid tumor from a soft tissue sarcoma. As with low-grade sarcomas, wide excision is the mainstay of treatment, but local recurrence after surgical treatment is very common. Deaths caused by desmoid tumors are infrequent because the tumors do not metastasize, but death can occur because of local recurrence in a critical area such as the neck.

Desmoids are classified by their location as abdominal, extraabdominal, intraabdominal, and mesenteric. Little is known about the etiology of desmoid tumors. There are two specific clinical settings in which desmoids arise, which have provided insights into both the cause of and the therapy for these lesions. The first is during or just after pregnancy. Desmoid tumors are more common in women than men and frequently present within 1 to 2 years of delivery, occasionally arising in the vicinity of a cesarean section scar. These facts, combined with isolated reports of spontaneous regression of desmoid tumors at menopause and the demonstration of estrogen receptors on some tumors, suggest a hormonal component to their development. Based on this knowledge, hormonal therapy with a variety of agents, most notably tamoxifen, has been used with occasional success. Complete disappearance, marked shrinkage, or stabilization of tumor growth combined with marked symptomatic improvement has been described after treatment with tamoxifen alone or in combination with other agents.[111,112]

Desmoid tumors occur with greatly increased frequency in patients with familial adenomatous polyposis. The link of familial polyposis with desmoid and other soft tissue tumors was originally given the eponym *Gardner syndrome*. It is now known, however, that all patients with familial polyposis are at risk for development of desmoid tumors and that the genetic defect in patients with polyposis, with or without desmoid tumors, is identical. Hence, the term *Gardner syndrome* has fallen into disuse. The desmoid tumors in patients with polyposis tend to occur in the abdomen, often in the colonic mesentery after total proctocolectomy has been performed to prevent the development of adenocarcinoma of the colon. Patients with familial polyposis are born with one defective copy of the apc gene, a tumor suppressor gene. As with the RB1 and p53 genes, the second, the normal copy must be lost for a tumor (either an adenomatous polyp or a desmoid) to develop. It is likely that, in a predisposed person, surgical trauma and the resultant stimulation of fibroblast growth increases the chance that a desmoid tumor will develop, which may explain the predilection for both mesenteric tumors in patients with polyposis and abdominal wall tumors in some women after cesarean section.

Another nonsurgical therapy for desmoid tumors, nonsteroidal anti-inflammatory drugs, was suggested by studies in patients with familial polyposis. Of the available drugs, the little-used arthritis medication sulindac (Clinoril; Merck & Co., West Point, PA) appears to be the most active. This drug has a relatively unique enterohepatic circulation, and at least some patients with familial polyposis have experienced significant reduction in the number of colonic polyps after treatment with oral sulindac. In the course of such treatment, anecdotal regressions of coexisting desmoid tumors have been seen. Alone or in combination with tamoxifen, objective regression of as many as 50% of polyposis-associated desmoid tumors has been reported.[112] Sporadic desmoids, not associated with familial polyposis, also occasionally respond to this combination. Other therapeutic modalities have been used to treat desmoid tumors. Radiation therapy has been used both as primary treatment and as postoperative adjuvant therapy.[110,111] Cytotoxic chemotherapy regimens have been used, with some successes reported with relatively nontoxic regimens.[112]

The surgical approach to resectable sporadic desmoid tumors has been similar to that used for low-grade soft tissue sarcomas: resect with a histologically negative margin if possible, but do not sacrifice major neurovascular structures or adjacent organs unless absolutely necessary. If pathologic analysis of the resected specimen reveals close approximation of tumor to the surgical margin, either reexcision or postoperative radiation is used. Unresectable or recurrent desmoid tumors, as well as those associated with familial polyposis, are treated first with the combination of tamoxifen and sulindac. Resection or radiation is used for failures of this therapy or to eliminate residual disease after partial responses. Chemotherapy is usually reserved as a last resort in patients who have failed all other therapies and who have severe symptoms or who are in danger of dying because of compression of vital structures by tumor.

OSTEOSARCOMAS

More than 70% of bone malignancies are metastatic from another site or are of hematologic origin (lymphoma or myeloma). A variety of primary bone tumors are known, both benign and malignant (Table 119.6). Primary sarcomas of bone, however, are relatively rare types of cancer. Osteosarcoma, the most common primary malignant tumor of bone, is extremely rare, with only approximately 1,000 cases per year in the United States.[113] The management of osteosarcoma poses certain unique challenges, but in many ways, osteosarcoma behavior is similar to that of soft tissue sarcoma. Lessons learned from the treatment of bone sarcomas provide important leads for improving soft tissue sarcoma therapy. For this reason, the general surgeon should be acquainted with the diagnosis and treatment of bone sarcomas.

Osteosarcomas occur most commonly around the knee, either in the distal femur or proximal tibia, but they can be encountered in any bone (Table 119.7). Osteosarcomas originate in the metaphyseal ends of the involved bone. Most osteosarcomas occur in childhood and adolescence; approximately 80% of patients are younger than 20 years, but a second peak begins after age 60 years. This latter peak corresponds to osteosarcomas arising in bones affected with Paget's disease, the most common condition predisposing to osteosarcoma development. Osteosarcomas arise in as many as 10% of patients with long-standing Paget disease. Other etiologic factors for bone sarcomas, such as exposure to radiation, have been discussed previously.

Like soft tissue sarcomas, osteosarcomas are graded using a three-part system. Most osteosarcomas are high grade, but low-grade variants exist. These less aggressive tumors are usually parosteal or periosteal in location, in contrast to the intramedullary origin of classic osteosarcoma. As with soft tissue sarcomas, a GTNM staging system is used. The stage groupings, however, are somewhat different from those for soft tissue tumors (Table 119.8). Involvement of regional lymph nodes is rare at the time of presentation (<3%). Pulmonary metastases are the most common type of distant spread and may be discovered in as many as 25% of patients at the time of presentation. Bone metastases are not uncommon in osteosarcoma, although they are less frequent than lung metastases.

TABLE 119.6 CLASSIFICATION

BENIGN AND MALIGNANT BONE TUMORS

Category	Benign	Malignant
Bone producing	Osteoid osteoma	Osteogenic sarcoma
	Osteoblastoma	Parosteal osteogenic sarcoma
Cartilage producing	Osteochondroma	Periosteal osteogenic sarcoma
	Endochondroma	Chondrosarcoma
	Chondroblastoma	Mesenchymal chondrosarcoma
Fibrous lesions	Benign fibrous histiocytoma	Malignant fibrous histiocytoma
	Giant cell tumor	Adamantinoma
	Fibrous dysplasia	Fibrosarcoma
Vascular	Aneurysmal bone cyst	Angiosarcoma
Other	Glomus tumor	Hemangiopericytoma
		Ewing's sarcoma

TABLE 119.7

SITE OF ORIGIN OF OSTEOSARCOMAS

Anatomic site	Percentage
Lower extremity	77.6
Upper extremity	12.9
Pelvis	6.0
Shoulder	2.6
Vertebrae	0.8

Modified from Eilber F, et al. Management of stage IIB osteogenic sarcoma: experience at the University of California, Los Angeles. *Cancer Treat Symp.* 1985;3:11B, with permission.

TABLE 119.8 CLASSIFICATION AND STAGING

AMERICAN JOINT COMMISSION ON CANCER GTNM CLASSIFICATION AND STAGE GROUPING OF PRIMARY BONE MALIGNANCIES

Stage	Description
TUMOR GRADE	
GX	Grade cannot be assessed
G1	Well differentiated
G2	Moderately well differentiated
G3	Poorly differentiated
G4	Undifferentiated
PRIMARY TUMOR	
TX	Primary tumor cannot be assessed
T0	No evidence of primary tumor
T1	Tumor ≤8 cm in greatest dimension
T2	Tumor >8 cm in greatest dimension
T3	Discontinuous tumors in the primary bone site
LYMPH NODE INVOLVEMENT	
NX	Regional lymph nodes cannot be assessed
N0	No regional lymph node metastasis
N1	Regional lymph node metastasis
DISTANT METASTASIS	
MX	Presence of distant metastasis cannot be assessed
M0	No distant metastasis
M1	Distant metastasis
STAGE GROUPING	
Stage IA	G1-2, T1, N0, M0
Stage IB	G1-2, T2, N0, M0
Stage IIA	G3-4, T1, N0, M0
Stage IIB	G3-4, T2, N0, M0
Stage III	Any G, T3, N0, M0
Stage IVA	Any G, any T, N0, M1a
Stage IVB	Any G, any T, N1, any M
	Any G, any T, any N, M1b

Modified from the American Joint Committee on Cancer. *American Joint Committee on Cancer (AJCC) cancer staging manual*, 6th ed. 2002, with permission.

Clinical Evaluation

A painful mass is the most common presenting complaint with an extremity osteosarcoma. The tumor may also present as a painless mass, particularly when it originates in the axial skeleton. Limitation of motion is often present when the tumor arises near or involves a joint. A history of trauma is not uncommon, but traumatic injury has never been linked with sarcoma development. It is more likely that the trauma alerted the patient to the sarcoma. Patients occasionally present with pathologic fracture of the involved bone.

Plain radiographs of the affected bone are the first step in evaluating a suspected osteosarcoma. High-grade osteosarcomas lead to rapid destruction of bone with new bone formation and periosteal reaction. These changes manifest radiographically by an extensive, poorly defined destructive bony lesion, often with an extraosseous component (Fig. 119.18). Codman's triangles, indicative of periosteal reaction, are characteristic but not pathognomonic of osteosarcoma. If the radiographic picture suggests an osteosarcoma, further radiologic evaluation should be done before proceeding with biopsy to allow the full anatomic extent of tumor to be defined without postsurgical artifact. More important, the radiologic evaluation allows the biopsy incision to be planned with an understanding of subsequent limb-sparing surgical options.

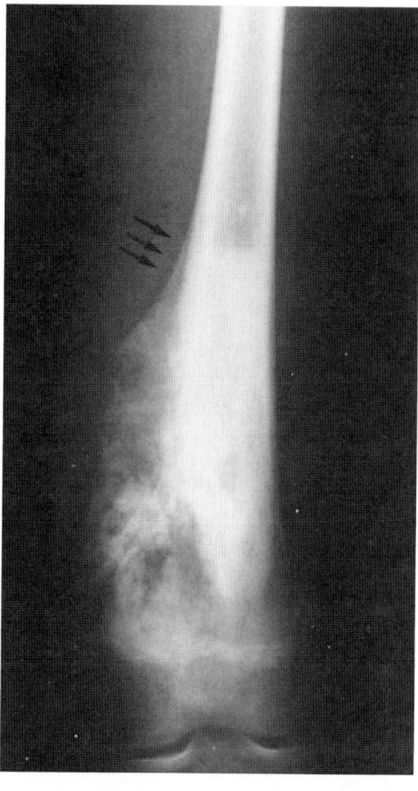

FIGURE 119.18 Plain radiograph of the femur showing a high-grade osteosarcoma. The tumor is an ill-defined destructive lesion with an extensive soft tissue component. Codman's triangles are present (*arrows*).

Radionuclide bone scanning using ^{99}technetium pyrophosphate can identify distant metastases to other bones as well as define skip areas of involvement in the bone of origin. Gallium-67 and 201-thallium scans may be useful for assessing the response of a primary osteosarcoma to preoperative chemotherapy. More recently, PET scanning and MRI spectroscopy have been used in this role.[31,114]

CT scanning is the most important modality in evaluating a bone sarcoma. It is excellent for assessing the degree of bony destruction, the extent of soft tissue involvement, and the relation of the tumor to adjacent neurovascular structures. The entire affected bone, including the complete joint above and below the tumor, should be visualized on the scan. A chest CT scan can provide evidence of pulmonary metastases too small to be seen on chest radiograph.

MRI is an important adjunct to CT scans in some patients, particularly those who are being considered for limb-sparing surgery. The excellent definition of marrow involvement by tumor allows for accurate planning of the proximal extent of the tumor resection. Angiography, although accurate in defining the relation of tumor to vessels, is rarely necessary unless intraarterial chemotherapy is used.

Biopsy

After the radiologic evaluation establishes the extent of the bony lesion, an incisional biopsy should be performed.[115] The biopsy incision should be carefully planned to avoid jeopardizing subsequent efforts at limb sparing. A vertical incision, oriented along the long axis of the extremity, is always used for arm or leg tumors. For tumors situated close to the knee, the incision is placed medially or laterally because a posterior incision can compromise the functional result of subsequent surgery. When the primary tumor is located in the pelvis or shoulder girdle, the biopsy should be performed in a location that allows its ready inclusion in the subsequent definitive operation incision.

Subject to the aforementioned constraints, the biopsy incision is usually placed over the most superficial portion of the tumor, and dissection is kept to a minimum. Any tissue planes entered during the biopsy are considered contaminated by tumor and must be excised in the subsequent definitive resection. If an adequate amount of tissue can be obtained by sampling the extraosseous component, this is preferable to biopsy of the bone itself. If the cortex of bone is entered, a plug of methylmethacrylate can be used to seal the bone and prevent hemorrhage or tumor spillage. Hemostasis should be achieved before closure; a drain should almost never be necessary. After the biopsy, weight bearing on the affected limb should be restricted to minimize the chance of pathologic fracture.

Preoperative Chemotherapy

In contrast to soft tissue sarcomas, preoperative (neoadjuvant) chemotherapy is sufficiently well established to be considered standard treatment for patients with osteosarcoma.[116] Historically, patients with clinically localized osteosarcoma treated by surgery alone had a 5-year survival rate of approximately 20%. Adjuvant systemic chemotherapy after surgery improved that figure to 55% to 70% in randomized trials (Fig. 119.19). Contemporary protocols that incorporate preoperative chemotherapy into the regimen have been associated with 5-year survival rates in excess of 80%, and most of these long-term survivors have been cured of their cancer.[117]

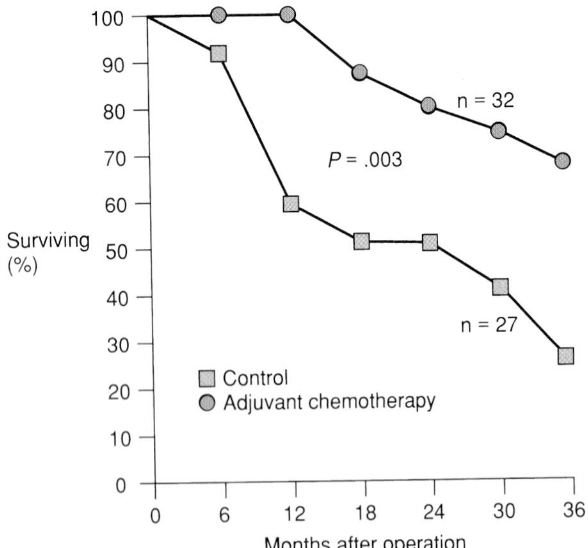

FIGURE 119.19 Survival rates of patients with surgically resected osteosarcoma treated with or without postoperative adjuvant chemotherapy in a randomized, controlled clinical trial. (Eilber F, Giuliano A, Eckardt J, et al. Adjuvant chemotherapy for osteosarcoma: a randomized prospective trial. *J Clin Oncol.* 1987;5:21–26.)

Several significant advantages of preoperative chemotherapy for osteosarcomas have emerged. The preoperative therapy makes limb-sparing surgery more successful by decreasing the extent of soft tissue involvement and allowing time for the creation of a custom-made bone replacement. Furthermore, the tumor's response to the preoperative chemotherapy may identify patients who require more intensive postoperative chemotherapy.

Preoperative response to chemotherapy is monitored in several ways. A serum alkaline phosphatase level should be obtained before initiating therapy, because many patients with osteosarcomas have an elevated level, which should decline if therapy is effective. Serial scans, such as 201-thallium scans, can be used to document decreasing tumor uptake. Failure of serum markers or scans to improve during preoperative therapy may be an indication to switch to more intensive therapy even before surgery. At the time of tumor resection, assessing the viability of the excised tumor provides the best measure of tumor response. A good response is defined as either complete absence of viable tumor cells or presence of only microscopic foci of viable cells, without any confluent areas of viable tumor. Attempts at scoring the percentage of necrosis have been less consistent, but at least 95% necrosis is necessary before a response can be considered good. Indeed, the histologic definition of a good response outlined previously correlates more nearly with 98% to 99% necrosis. Patients who achieve a good response require only a short course of postoperative chemotherapy; those who do not are treated with a longer postoperative regimen that includes doxorubicin and cisplatin.

Surgery

Extremity osteosarcomas may be treated surgically either by radical amputation (amputation at least one joint above the most proximal extent of tumor) or by *en bloc* resection with limb sparing. Limb-sparing approaches can be considered for most patients with extremity sarcomas and no evidence of neurovascular involvement. Patients presenting initially with pathologic fractures are at higher risk for local recurrence and are less suitable candidates for limb sparing. Virtually all limb-sparing protocols for osteosarcoma incorporate some form of preoperative chemotherapy.

Essential to any limb-sparing operation is complete removal of the affected bone and soft tissues. The old biopsy site is taken in continuity with the tumor, and the adjacent joint is also resected. A proximal bone margin of 6 to 7 cm usually is taken beyond the highest area of abnormality on preoperative, pretherapy scans. Even if pretreatment induces some degree of tumor shrinkage, the operation should remove all areas where disease was noted at initial presentation. The marrow at the level of bony transection is curetted and sent for frozen-section analysis to verify the adequacy of the proximal bone margin. For extensive lesions of the femur, resections of the entire femur with limb sparing can be performed.

A variety of reconstructive techniques are available after resection of an extremity osteosarcoma. Autografts (such as vascularized or nonvascularized fibular grafts), cadaver allografts, and simple arthrodeses have all been used (Fig. 119.20). Custom-made titanium endoprostheses are often used (Fig. 119.21), but their use is limited by the size of bone that can accommodate them (the distal tibia is often too small to accept the prosthesis and still have adequate strength to bear weight after proximal tibial resection), the fact that many patients with osteosarcoma are children who continue to grow on the unoperated side, and the long-term stresses that an

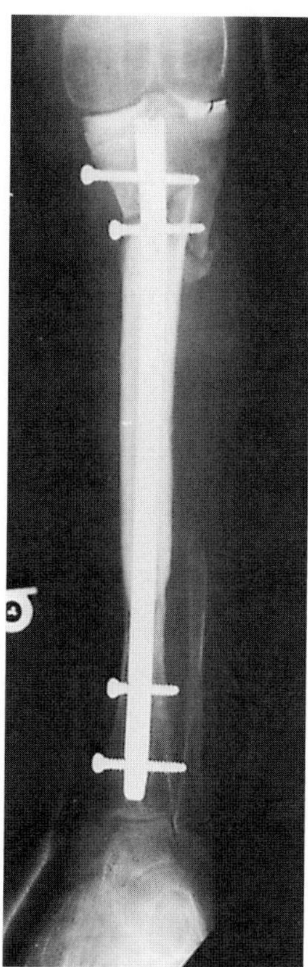

FIGURE 119.20 Allograft reconstruction after resection of an osteosarcoma of the proximal tibia.

active young adult puts on a prosthetic bone and joint. Technologic advances are addressing some of these issues. A new modular distal femoral prosthesis has been developed that can be periodically expanded, progressively lengthening the limb as the other leg grows. Newer materials and cementless prostheses that promote bony ingrowth rather than rely on fixative cements may provide better long-term functional results.

Some pelvic osteosarcomas can also be resected with limb sparing. Small or low-grade tumors of the bony pelvis can be removed by internal hemipelvectomy.[118] Virtually the entire hemipelvis and hip joint can be resected, leaving the neurovascular supply to the leg intact (Fig. 119.22A). Although the leg on the affected side is significantly shortened, weight bearing is eventually possible secondary to fibrous adhesion of the femur to the resection site (Fig. 119.22B). Alternatively, allograft reconstruction of the hemipelvis can be performed to shorten the length of time until full weight bearing is possible.

Postoperative Chemotherapy

Adjuvant postoperative chemotherapy has been proved to increase survival of patients with osteosarcoma after amputation or limb-sparing surgery.[119] As previously discussed, most limb-sparing regimens now incorporate preoperative chemotherapy as well. Preoperative chemotherapy does not replace postoperative treatment but may influence the duration and type of postoperative chemotherapy given. The so-called T12 regimen (Fig. 119.23) is an example: patients with total or near-total tumor necrosis receive a short course of the same chemotherapy after surgery (total duration of preoperative and postoperative treatment is 15 weeks). Those with lesser degrees of necrosis are switched to a more intensive regimen of doxorubicin and cisplatin lasting 27 weeks. Overall

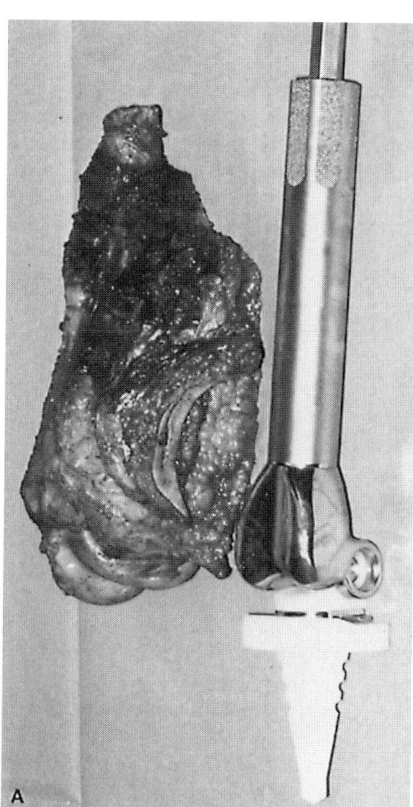

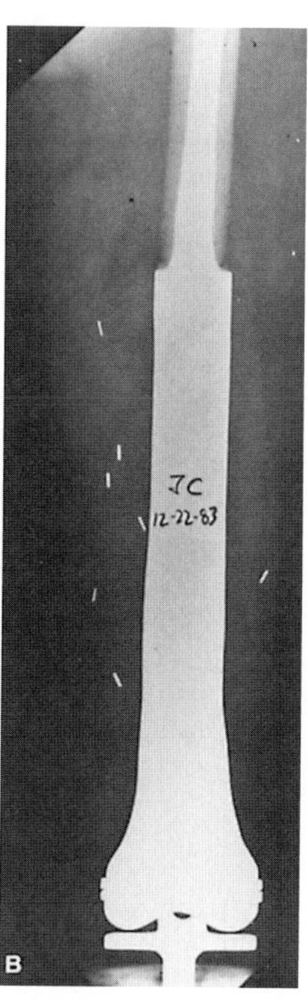

FIGURE 119.21 *(A)* Custom-made titanium prosthesis for replacement of the distal femur and knee joint. *(B)* Postoperative radiograph showing the prosthesis in place.

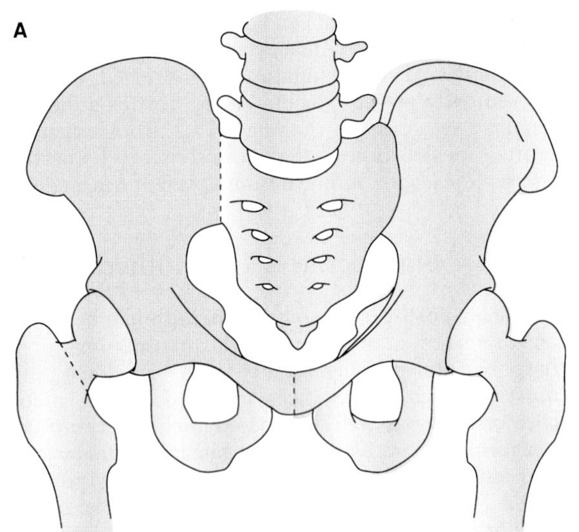

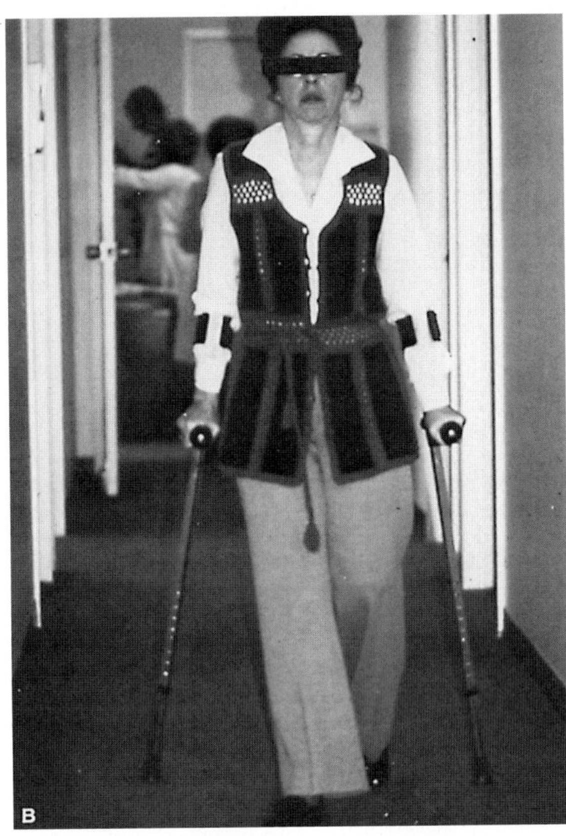

FIGURE 119.22 (*A*) Depiction of the bony structures removed in the conduct of an internal hemipelvectomy. (*B*) Postoperative photograph showing the ability of the patient to bear weight on the noticeably shorter operated side.

results of this regimen have been as good as those in which all patients receive more toxic chemotherapy. It remains to be determined, however, whether the more aggressive chemotherapy is in fact improving the outcome for patients with poor initial tumor necrosis.[48] Although the optimal regimen for adjuvant chemotherapy of osteosarcoma has yet to be defined, combined preoperative and postoperative chemotherapy regimens, in which the postoperative therapy is tailored to the initial histologic response, are state of the art, particularly for patients undergoing limb-sparing surgery.

GASTROINTESTINAL STROMAL TUMORS

A more unusual subtype of sarcoma is gastrointestinal stromal tumor (GIST). Originally, most gastrointestinal mesenchymal tumors were thought to be of smooth muscle origin. However, many of these tumors were relatively resistant to doxorubicin-based treatment regimens and lacked immunohistochemical or electron microscopic characteristics of smooth muscle.[120,121] The

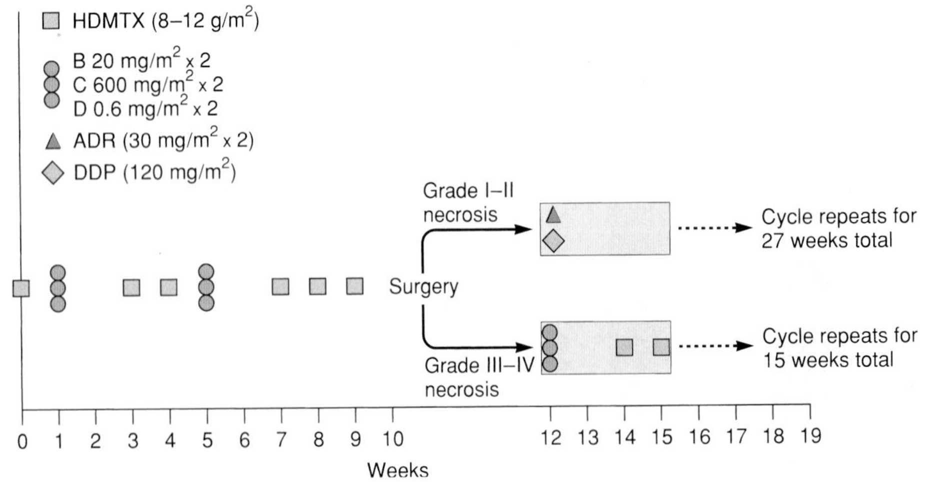

FIGURE 119.23 The T12 protocol used by Rosen for resectable osteosarcoma of the extremity. HDMTX, high-dose methotrexate; B, bleomycin; C, cyclophosphamide; D, dacarbazine; ADR, doxorubicin (Adriamycin); DDP, cisplatin (cis-diammine-dichloroplatinum). (Rosen G. Preoperative [neoadjuvant] chemotherapy for osteogenic sarcoma: a 10-year experience. *Orthopaedics* 1985; 8:659–664, with permission.)

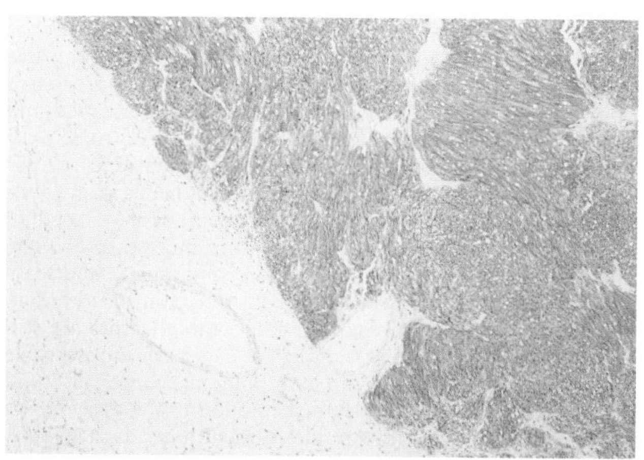

FIGURE 119.24 Strong and diffuse kit immunoreactivity in a gastrointestinal stromal tumor. (From Kelsen DP, Daly JM, Kern SE, et al. *Gastrointestinal oncology: principles and practice*. Philadelphia: Lippincott Williams & Wilkins, 2002, with permission.)

term *gastrointestinal stromal tumors* was adopted for a specific category of mesenchymal neoplasms of the gastrointestinal tract. It soon became apparent that these tumors had more in common with the interstitial cell of Cajal, a pacemaker cell within the gastrointestinal tract.[122] Both the interstitial cells of Cajal and GIST cells express the hematopoietic progenitor cell marker CD34 and the growth factor receptor c-Kit (CD117) (Fig. 119.24).[122–124] It is still unclear whether all GISTs arise from these cells, however, because some come from the mesentery or omentum where there are no interstitial cells of Cajal. This finding suggests an origin in multipotential mesenchymal stem cells.[125]

GISTs demonstrate no gender difference and occur predominately in middle-aged and older patients, with a median age of 60 years.[126] They are rare before age 40 years. Nearly 70% occur in the stomach, 20% to 30% occur in the small bowel, and 10% elsewhere.[127,128] Clinical presentation is dependent on the location but is generally nonspecific. Signs and symptoms include nausea, vomiting, abdominal pain, abdominal mass, anemia, or melena.

The diagnosis of GIST is often strongly suggested by CT scan findings. In these cases, a preoperative percutaneous biopsy is not necessary and may risk peritoneal seeding or tumor rupture. Otherwise, core-needle biopsy should be used when a lymphoma or germ-cell tumor cannot be ruled out or when preoperative therapy is contemplated. About half of GISTs have evidence of metastases at diagnosis, most commonly to the liver or peritoneum.[126] If there is no evidence of metastases and the tumor appears resectable, GISTs should be approached with the intent of performing complete *en bloc* removal with negative margins. The 5-year survival rate is 75% for patients with early-stage tumors that have been completely excised.[126] Lymph node dissection is not warranted because GISTs very rarely metastasize to regional nodes. Incomplete resection should be used only for the palliation of bleeding or obstruction.

GISTs are remarkably resistant to both radiation and chemotherapy. However, the treatment of GISTs has been dramatically altered with the development of imatinib (formerly referred to as *STI571* and now manufactured as Gleevac [Novartis Pharma AG, Basel, Switzerland]), a selective c-Kit inhibitor. The expression of c-Kit is an important, defining feature of GISTs. c-Kit is a transmembrane glycoprotein receptor with an internal tyrosine kinase component that, when activated, triggers a cascade of intracellular signals regulating cell growth and survival.[129–131] This process may be responsible for the pathogenesis of GISTs. This gain of function c-Kit mutation occurs in up to 90% of GISTs, and the constitutive tyrosine kinase activity has been shown to promote tumor growth *in vitro*.[123,132,133] GISTs with mutant c-Kit are more likely to be high-grade tumors, with more frequent recurrences and a lower survival.[134]

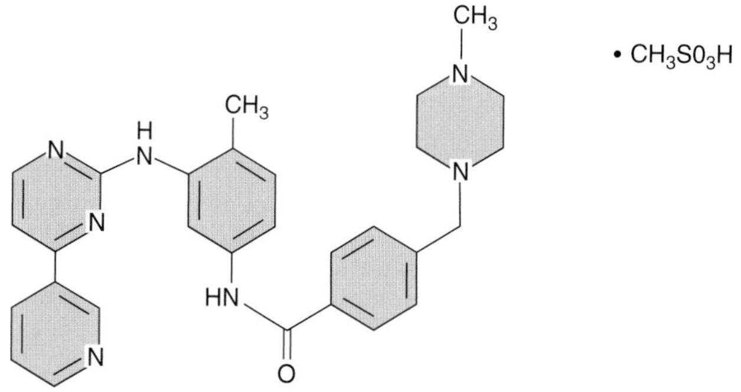

FIGURE 119.25 Molecular structure of imatinib mesylate (STI-571, Gleevac). 4-[(4-methyl-1-piperazinyl)methol]-N-[4-methyl-3-[[4-(3-pyridinyl)-2-pyrimidinyl]amino-]-phenyl]benzamide methanesulfonate. (Courtesy of Novartis Pharma AG, Basel, Switzerland.)

Imatinib is a powerful competitive inhibitor of tyrosine kinase. It is a multiringed molecule (Fig. 119.25) that binds to the adenosine triphosphate binding site of the target kinase and inhibits downstream signaling, switching the balance toward reduced cellular proliferation and increased apoptosis. Approved in 2002 by the U.S. Food and Drug Administration, imatinib is the first effective systemic therapy for patients with metastatic or locally advanced GISTs. It can produce impressive clinical responses in a large percentage of patients, with more than 50% responding to treatment and only 10% to 15% experiencing progressive disease.[135,136] Imatinib may be useful in the management of metastatic disease, as well as the neoadjuvant treatment of tumors determined to be unresectable at presentation. Gleevac is still relatively new, and the long-term effect of therapy, the optimum timing of delivery, and the optimum duration of treatment are unknown. Clinical trials of neoadjuvant and adjuvant use are ongoing.

RECURRENT AND METASTATIC SARCOMAS

Local Recurrence

Despite aggressive multimodality therapy, local recurrence remains a major mode of failure in patients with sarcoma. Most soft tissue sarcomas that recur do so within 2 to 3 years of treatment. The risk of local recurrence after surgical treatment of soft tissue sarcomas varies based on a number of factors. The most significant of these is the site of origin of the tumor, with lesions of the head and neck, trunk, and retroperitoneum all associated with a higher risk of local recurrence than lesions of the extremities. Local and regional failure is the site of first recurrence after definitive resection in 50% of head, neck, and truncal sarcomas and in 75% of retroperitoneal tumors but in only 15% of extremity lesions.[137] Other factors influencing recurrence rates include the size and histologic grade of the primary tumor, deep versus superficial location, and local failure of prior surgery.

If a recurrence is suspected, a biopsy is necessary to confirm this as well as determine any change in tumor grade from the original. In cases of a long interval between the primary tumor and the recurrence, it is possible that this may represent a second primary tumor. Previous specimens should be retrieved for comparison. The same approach to both local and distant staging examinations should be performed as with a primary sarcoma. It is not unusual to detect concurrent metastatic disease when a local relapse is discovered. In this case, the management of the local recurrence is directed by the patient's symptoms and aggressive surgery is rarely indicated.

In the absence of distant disease, an aggressive surgical approach is warranted with the goal being the same as with a primary sarcoma: control of the tumor and preservation of as much function as possible. Limb-sparing approaches can control and even cure local recurrence in the absence of distant metastases. For patients who were initially treated with surgery alone and who failed locally, multimodality treatment with repeat resection, radiation, and sometimes chemotherapy is associated with survival rates close to those of previously untreated patients [138–141] (Fig. 119.26). Patients with recurrence after surgery and radiation are more likely to require radical amputation to control recurrence in an extremity but are still candidates for salvage surgery. Locally recurrent retroperitoneal sarcomas, particularly low-grade tumors, can sometimes be resected on multiple occasions with long-term survival, but few of these patients are cured.[142] In a large series of retroperitoneal tumors, an adequate resection was obtainable more than half of the time after the first recurrence, but only 20% after a second recurrence and 10% after the third.[97]

Distant Metastases

The lungs are the most frequent site of distant spread for sarcomas and are often the only site of metastasis.[73] Unresectable metastatic soft tissue sarcomas are fatal, and chemotherapy is given primarily for palliation, to prolong life, and to improve quality of life. Therefore an aggressive surgical approach to both solitary and multiple lung metastases is warranted and can be associated with cure in approximately 25% to 35% of patients.[143] Even patients with bilateral metastases are candidates for surgery, which can be performed either as staged thoracotomies or, preferably, as one procedure using a median sternotomy. Patients with three or fewer metastases, a long doubling time of the metastatic tumors, and unilateral disease have the best prognosis after surgical resection,[144] although patients lacking one or all of these favorable factors are still candidates for curative resection. Patients with unresectable pulmonary metastases or with extrapulmonary metastases are usually treated with cytotoxic chemotherapy. Active agents include doxorubicin, ifosfamide, gemcitabine, dacarbazine, high-dose methotrexate, and cisplatin.[145,146] Radiation therapy may be useful as palliation for the occasional patient with bony or cerebral metastases. Notwithstanding that occasional patients with metastatic sarcoma are cured by surgery with or without chemotherapy, the best hope for increasing survival in patients with sarcoma remains the prompt initiation of aggressive, multimodality therapy before clinically detectable metastatic disease develops. For the foreseeable future, surgeons will therefore retain their prominent role in treating these complex and challenging patients.

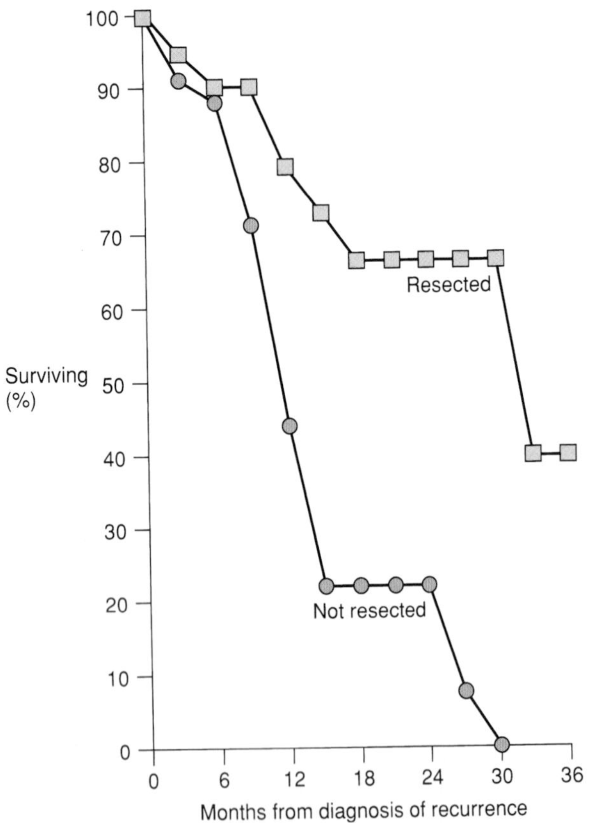

FIGURE 119.26 Survival of patients after resection of isolated local recurrence of an extremity soft tissue sarcoma. (From Huth J, Eilber FR. Patterns of metastatic spread following resection of extremity soft tissue sarcomas and strategies for treatment. *Semin Surg Oncol.* 1988;4:20, with permission.)

KEY POINTS

- **Sarcomas are a heterogeneous group of cancers that arise from mesoderm-derived elements, including bone, cartilage, connective tissue, fat, and muscle.**
- **Radiation exposure, some chemicals, chronic lymphedema, and some heritable genetic defects are clearly linked to the development of sarcomas.**
- **Core-needle biopsy is the initial procedure of choice in diagnosing soft tissue masses. Open surgical biopsy, or incisional biopsy, is used when core-needle biopsy specimens yield nondiagnostic findings.**
- **Sarcomas are classified by the type of tissue formed by the tumor (histogenic classification) rather than by the type of tissue in which the tumor arises.**
- **Computed tomography scanning and magnetic resonance imaging are the most important studies for assessing the extent and resectability of soft tissue sarcomas, regardless of the site of origin.**
- **Wide local excision, with gross total removal of the tumor including a wide margin of normal tissue, is the standard operative management of extremity soft tissue sarcoma. For most patients, postoperative radiation treatment is also added.**
- **Neoadjuvant chemotherapy or radiation therapy is useful for some patients.**
- **Removal of all gross tumor is the basis for operative treatment of retroperitoneal sarcomas; concomitant resection of adjacent organs is required more than 75% of the time, most commonly of the kidney and colon.**
- **The management of gastrointestinal stromal tumors has been revolutionized by the availability of imatinib, a selective tyrosine kinase inhibitor, as an effective systemic agent.**

References

1. Jemal A, Tiwari RC, Murray T, et al. Cancer statistics, 2004. *CA Cancer J Clin.* 2004;54:8–29.
2. Clasby R, Tilling K, Smith MA, et al. Variable management of soft tissue sarcoma: regional audit with implications for specialist care. *Br J Surg.* 1997;84:1692–1696.

3. McClay EF. Epidemiology of bone and soft tissue sarcomas. *Semin Oncol.* 1989;16:264–272.
4. Brady MS, Gaynor JJ, Brennan MF. Radiation-associated sarcoma of bone and soft tissue. *Arch Surg.* 1992; 127:1379–1385.
5. Zahm SH, Fraumeni J, F.H. The epidemiology of soft tissue sarcoma. *Semin Oncol.* 1997;24:504–514.
6. Collins JJ, Strauss ME, Levinskas GJ, et al. The mortality experience of workers exposed to 2,3,7,8-tetrachlorodibenzo-p-dioxin in a trichlorophenol process accident. *Epidemiology* 1993;4:7–13.
7. Wolfe WH, Michalek JE, Miner JC, et al. Health status of Air Force veterans occupationally exposed to herbicides in Vietnam: I. physical health. *JAMA* 1990;264:1824–1831.
8. Bennicelli JL, Barr FG. Genetics and the biologic basis of sarcomas. *Curr Opin Oncol.* 1999;11:267–274.
9. Stratton MR, Williams S, Fisher C, et al. Structural alterations of the RB1 gene in human soft tissue tumours. *Br J Cancer* 1989;60:202–205.
10. Greenblatt MS, Bennett WP, Hollstein M, et al. Mutations in the p53 tumor suppressor gene clues to cancer etiology and molecular pathogenesis. *Cancer Res.* 1994;54:4855–4878.
11. Malkin D, Li FP, Strong LC, et al. Germ line p53 mutations in a familial syndrome of breast cancer, sarcomas, and other neoplasms. *Science* 1990;250:1233–1238.
12. Latres E, Drobnjak M, Pollack D, et al. Chromosome 17 abnormalities and TP53 mutations in adult soft tissue sarcomas. *Am J Pathol.* 1994;145:345–355.
13. Heiken TJ, Das Gupta TK. Mutant p53 expression: a marker of diminished survival in well-differentiated soft tissue sarcoma. *Clin Cancer Res.* 1996;2:1391–1395.
14. Andreassen A, Oyjord T, Hovig E, et al. p53 abnormalities in different subtypes of human sarcomas. *Cancer Res.* 1993;53:468–471.
15. Oliner JD, Kinzler KW, Meltzer PS, et al. Amplification of a gene encoding a p53-associated protein in human sarcomas. *Nature* 1992;358:80–83.
16. Levine EA. Prognostic factors in soft tissue sarcoma. *Semin Surg Oncol.* 1999;17:23–32.
17. Gerlach JH, Bell DR, Karakousis C, et al. P-glycoprotein in human sarcoma: evidence for multidrug resistance. *J Clin Oncol.* 1987; 5:1452–1460.
18. Jimenez RE, Zalupski MM, Frank JJ, et al. Multidrug resistance phenotype in high grade soft tissue sarcoma: correlation of P-glycoprotein immunohistochemistry with pathologic response to chemotherapy. *Cancer* 1999; 86:976–981.
19. Lawrence W Jr., Donegan WL, Natarajan N, et al. Adult soft tissue sarcomas: a pattern of care survey of the American College of Surgeons. *Ann Surg.* 1987; 205:349–359.
20. Dupay DE, Rosenberg AE, Punyaratabandhu T, et al. Accuracy of CT-guided needle biopsy of musculoskeletal neoplasms. *AJR* 1998; 171:759–762.
21. Heslin MJ, Lewis JJ, Woodruff JM, et al. Core needle biopsy for diagnosis of extremity soft tissue sarcoma. *Ann Surg Oncol.* 1997;4:25–31.
22. Coindre JM, Terrier P, Bui NB, et al. Prognostic factors in adult patients with locally controlled soft tissue sarcoma. A study of 546 patients from the French Federation of Cancer Centers Sarcoma Group. *J Clin Oncol.* 1996;14:869–877.
23. Presant CA, Russell WO, Alexander RW, et al. Soft tissue and bone sarcoma histopathology peer review: the frequency of disagreement in diagnosis and the need for second pathology opinions. The Southeastern Cancer Study Group experience. *J Clin Oncol.* 1986;4:1658–1661.
24. Alvegard TA, Berg NO. Histopathology peer review of high-grade soft tissue sarcoma: the Scandinavian Sarcoma Group experience. *J Clin Oncol.* 1989;7:1845–51.
25. Arca MJ, Sondak VK, Chang AE, et al. Diagnostic procedures and pretreatment evaluation of soft tissue sarcomas. *Semin Surg Oncol.* 1994;10:323–331.
26. Pearlstone DB, Pisters PW, Bold RJ, et al. Patterns of recurrence in extremity liposarcoma: implications for staging and follow-up. *Cancer* 1999;85:85–92.
27. Hanna SL, Fletcher BD. MR imaging of malignant soft tissue tumors. *Magn Reson Imaging Clin North Am.* 1995;3:629–650.
28. Demas BE, Heelan RT, Lane J, et al. Soft tissue sarcomas of the extremities: comparison of MR and CT in determining the extent of disease. *AJR* 1988;150:615–620.
29. Jelinek JS, Kransdorf MJ, Shmookler BM, et al. Liposarcoma of the extremities: MR and CT findings in the histologic subtypes. *Radiology* 1993;186:455–459.
30. Fenstermacher MJ. Imaging evaluation of patients with soft tissue sarcoma. *Surg Oncol Clin North Am.* 2003;12:305–332.
31. Jones DN, McCowage GB, Sostman HD, et al. Monitoring of response to neoadjuvant therapy of soft tissue and musculoskeletal sarcomas using F18-FDG PET. *J Nucl Med.* 1996;37:1438–1444.
32. Israel-Mardirosian N, Adler LP. Positron emission tomography of soft tissue sarcomas. *Curr Opin Oncol.* 2003;15:327–330.
33. Ioannidis JPA, Lau J. 18F-FDG PET for the diagnosis and grading of soft tissue sarcoma: A meta-analysis. *J Nucl Med.* 2002;44:717–724.
34. Myhre Jensen O, Kaae S, Madsen EH, et al. Histopathologic grading in soft tissue tumors: relation to survival in 261 surgically treated patients. *Acta Path Microbiol Immunol Scand.* 1983;91A:145–150.
35. Guillou L, Coindre JM, Bonichon F, et al. Comparative study of the National Cancer Institute and French Federation of Cancer Centers Sarcoma Group grading system in a population of 410 adult patients with soft tissue sarcoma. *J Clin Oncol.* 1997;15:350–362.
36. Costa J, Wesley RA, Glatstein E, et al. The grading of soft tissue sarcomas. Results of a clinicohistopathologic correlation in a series of 163 cases. *Cancer* 1984;53:530–541.
37. Brooks AD, Heslin MJ, Leung DH, et al. Superficial extremity soft tissue sarcoma: an analysis of prognostic factors. *Ann Surg Oncol.* 1998;5:41–47.
38. Brennan MF. Staging of soft tissue sarcomas. *Ann Surg Oncol.* 1999;6:8–9.
39. Ramanathan RC, A'Hern R, Fisher C, et al. Modified staging system for extremity soft tissue sarcomas. *Ann Surg Oncol.* 1999;6:57–69.
40. Kattan MW, Leung DH, Brennan MF. Postoperative nomogram for 12 year sarcoma specific death. *J Clin Oncol.* 2002;20:791–796.
41. Cantin J, McNeer GP, Chu FC, et al. The problem of local recurrence after treatment of soft tissue sarcoma. *Ann Surg.* 1968;168:47–53.
42. Rosenberg SA, Glatstein EJ. Perspectives on the role of surgery and radiation therapy in the treatment of soft tissue sarcomas of the extremities. *Semin Oncol.* 1981;8:190–200.
43. Rosenberg SA, Tepper J, Glatstein E, et al. The treatment of soft tissue sarcomas of the extremities: prospective randomized evaluations of (1) limb-sparing surgery plus radiation therapy compared with amputation and (2) the role of adjuvant chemotherapy. *Ann Surg.* 1982;196:305–315.
44. Potter DA, Kinsella T, Glatstein E, et al. High-grade soft tissue sarcomas of the extremities. *Cancer* 1986;58:190–205.
45. Abbatucci JS, Boulier N, de Ranieri J, et al. Radiotherapy as an integrated part of the treatment of soft tissue sarcomas. *Radiother Oncol.* 1984;2:115–121.
46. Leibel SA, Tranbaugh RF, Wara WM, et al. Soft tissue sarcomas of the extremities: survival and patterns of failure with conservative surgery and postoperative irradiation compared to surgery alone. *Cancer* 1982;50:1076–1083.
47. National Institutes of Health. NIH consensus development panel on limb-sparing treatment of adult soft tissue sarcoma and osteosarcomas. *Cancer Treat Symp.*; 3:1.
48. Stojadinovic A, Leung DHY, Hoos A, et al. Analysis of the prognostic significance of microscopic margins in 2,084 localized primary adult soft tissue sarcomas. *Ann Surg.* 2002;235:424–434.
49. Lewis JJ, Leung DH, Espat J, et al. The effect of re-resection in extremity soft tissue sarcoma. *Ann Surg.* 2000;231:655–663.
50. Bowden L, Booher RJ. The principles and techniques of resection of soft parts for sarcoma. *Surgery* 1958;44:963–977.
51. Gerner RE, Moore GE, Pickren JW. Soft tissue sarcomas. *Ann Surg.* 1975; 181:803–808.
52. Tanabe KK, Pollock RE, Ellis LM, et al. Influence of surgical margins on outcome in patients with preoperatively irradiated extremity soft tissue sarcomas. *Cancer* 1994;73:1652–1659.
53. Cormier JN, E. PR. Soft tissue sarcomas. *CA Cancer J Clin.* 2004; 54:94–109.
54. Langstein HN, Robb GL. Reconstructive approaches in soft tissue sarcoma. *Semin Surg Oncol.* 1999;17:52–65.
55. Fong Y, Coit DG, Woodruff JM, et al. Lymph node metastasis from soft tissue sarcoma in adults. Analysis of data from a prospective database of 1772 sarcoma patients. *Ann Surg.* 1993;217:272–277.
56. Blazer DG, Sabel MS, Sondak VK. Is there a role for sentinel lymph node biopsy in the management of sarcoma? *Surg Oncol.* 2003; 12:201–206.
57. Vanel D, Shapeero LG, De Baere T, et al. MR imaging in the follow-up of malignant and aggressive soft tissue tumors: results of 511 examinations. *Radiology* 1994;190:263–268.
58. Whooley BP, Mooney MM, Gibbs JF, et al. Effective follow-up strategies in soft tissue sarcoma. *Semin Surg Oncol.* 1999;17:83–87.
59. Suit HD, Mankin HJ, Wood WC, et al. Treatment of the patient with stage M0 soft tissue sarcoma. *J Clin Oncol.* 1988;6:854–862.
60. Janjan NA, Yasko AW, Reece GP, et al. Comparison of charges related to radiotherapy for soft tissue sarcomas treated by preoperative external beam irradiation versus interstitial implantation. *Ann Surg Oncol.* 1994;1:415–422.
61. Pisters PW, Leung DH, Woodruff JM, et al. Analysis of prognostic factors in 1,041 patients with localized soft tissue sarcomas of the extremities. *J Clin Oncol.* 1996;14:1679–1689.
62. Singer S, Corson JM, Gonin R, et al. Prognostic factors predictive of survival and local recurrence for extremity soft tissue sarcoma. *Ann Surg.* 1994;219:165–173.
63. Collin C, Godbold J, Hadju S, et al. Local extremity soft tissue sarcoma: an analysis of factors affecting survival. *J Clin Oncol.* 1987;5:601–612.
64. Geer RJ, Woodruff JM, Casper ES, et al. Management of small soft tissue sarcoma of the extremity in adults. *Arch Surg.* 1992;127:1285–1289.
65. Karakousis CP, Emrich LJ, Rao U, et al. Limb salvage in soft tissue sarcomas with selective combination of modalities. *Eur J Surg Oncol.* 1991;17:71–80.
66. Nielson OS, Cummings B, O'Sullivan B, et al. Preoperative and postoperative irradiation of soft tissue sarcomas: effect of radiation field size. *Int J Radiat Oncol Biol Phys.* 1991;21:1595–1599.
67. Davis AM, O'Sullivan B, Bell RS, et al. Function and health status outcomes in a randomized trial comparing preoperative and postoperative radiotherapy in extremity soft tissue sarcoma. *J Clin Oncol.* 2002;20:4472–4477.

68. Wilson AN, Davis A, Bell RS, et al. Local control of soft tissue sarcoma of the extremity: the experience of a multidisciplinary sarcoma group with definitive surgery and radiotherapy. *Eur J Cancer* 1994;30A:746–751.
69. Suit HD, Mankin HJ, Wood WC, et al. Preoperative, intraoperative and postoperative radiation in the treatment of primary soft tissue sarcoma. *Cancer* 1985;55:2659–2667.
70. Sadoski C, Suit HD, Rosenberg A, et al. Preoperative radiation, surgical margins and local control of extremity sarcoma of soft tissues. *J Surg Oncol.* 1993;52:223–230.
71. O'Sullivan B, Davis AM, Turcotte R, et al. Preoperative versus postoperative radiotherapy in soft tissue sarcoma of the limbs: a randomised trial. *Lancet* 2002;359:2235–2241.
72. Robinson MH, Deus RB, Shasha D, et al. Is preoperative radiotherapy superior to postoperative radiotherapy in the treatment of soft tissue sarcoma? *Eur J Cancer* 1998;27:1091–1099.
73. Huth JF, Eilber FR. Patterns of metastatic spread following resection of extremity soft tissue sarcomas and strategies for treatment. *Semin Surg Oncol.* 1988;4:20–26.
74. Rosenberg SA, Tepper J, Glatstein E, et al. Prospective randomized evaluation of adjuvant chemotherapy in adults with soft tissue sarcomas of the extremities. *Cancer* 1983;52:424–434.
75. Chang AE, Kinsella T, Glatstein E, et al. Adjuvant chemotherapy for patients with high-grade soft tissue sarcomas of the extremity. *J Clin Oncol.* 1988;6:1491–1500.
76. Antman K, Crowley J, Balcerzak SP, et al. An intergroup phase III randomized study of doxorubicin and dacarbazine with or without ifosfamide and mesna in advanced soft tissue and bone sarcomas. *J Clin Oncol.* 1993;11:1276–1285.
77. Bramwell V, Rouesse J, Steward W, et al. Adjuvant CYVADIC chemotherapy for adult soft tissue sarcoma-reduced local recurrence but no improvement in overall survival: a study of the European Organization for Research and Treatment of Cancer Soft Tissue and Bone Sarcoma group. *J Clin Oncol.* 1994;12:1137–1149.
78. Cormier JN, Huang X, Thall PF, et al. Cohort analysis of patients with localized, high-risk extremity soft tissue sarcoma treated at two cancer centers: Chemotherapy-associated outcomes. *J Clin Oncol.* 2004;22:4567–4574.
79. Tierney JF, Stewart LA, Parmat MKB, et al. Adjuvant chemotherapy for localised resectable soft tissue sarcomas of adults: meta-analysis of individual data. Sarcoma Meta-analysis Collaboration. *Lancet* 1997;350:1647–1654.
80. Frustaci S, Gherlinzoni F, De Paoli A, et al. Adjuvant chemotherapy for adult soft tissue sarcomas of the extremities and girdles: results of the Italian randomized cooperative trial. *J Clin Oncol.* 2001;19:1238–1247.
81. Meric F, Hess KR, Varma DG, et al. Radiographic response to neoadjuvant chemotherapy is a predictor of local control and survival in soft tissue sarcomas. *Cancer* 2002;95:1120–1126.
82. Pisters PW, Patel S, Varma DG, et al. Preoperative chemotherapy for stage IIIB extremity soft tissue sarcomas. Long term results from a single institution. *J Clin Oncol.* 1997;15:3481–3487.
83. Casper ES, Gaynor JJ, Harrison LB, et al. Preoperative and postoperative adjuvant combination chemotherapy for stage IIIB extremity soft tissue sarcoma: long term results from a single institution. *Cancer* 1994; 73:1644–1651.
84. Ottaino A, De Chiara A, Fazioli F, et al. Neoadjuvant chemotherapy for intermediate/high-grade soft tissue sarcomas: five-year results with epirubicin and ifosfamide. *Anticancer Res.* 2002;22:3555–3559.
85. Henshaw RM, Priebat DA, Perry DJ, et al. Survival after induction chemotherapy and surgical resection for high-grade soft tissue sarcoma. Is radiation necessary? *Ann Surg Oncol.* 2001;8:484–495.
86. Rahoty P, Konya A. Results of preoperative neoadjuvant chemotherapy and surgery in the management of patients with soft tissue sarcoma. *Eur J Surg Oncol.* 1993;19:641–645.
87. Eilber FC, Eckardt J, Rosen G, et al. Preoperative therapy for soft tissue sarcomas. *Hematol Oncol Clin North Am.* 1995;9:817–823.
88. Eilber FC, Rosen G, Eckardt J, et al. Treatment-induced pathologic necrosis: a predictor of local recurrence and survival in patients receiving neoadjuvant therapy for high-grade extremity soft tissue sarcomas. *J Clin Oncol.* 2001;19:3203–3209.
89. Kraybill W, Spiro I, Harris J, et al. Radiation Therapy Oncology Group (RTOG) 95-14: a phase II study of neoadjuvant chemotherapy and radiation therapy in high-risk, high-grade soft tissue sarcomas of the extremities and body wall: a preliminary report (abstract). *Proc Am Soc Clin Oncol.* 2001;29:38a.
90. Patel SR, Vadhan-Raj S, Papadopoulus NJ, et al. High-dose ifosfamide in bone and soft tissue sarcomas: results of phase II and pilot studies dose response and schedule dependence. *J Clin Oncol.* 1997;15:2378–2384.
91. Eggermont AM, Schraffordt-Koops H, Lienard D, et al. Isolated limb perfusion with high-dose tumor necrosis factor-alpha in combination with interferon gamma and melphalan for nonresectable extremity soft tissue sarcomas: a multicenter trial. *J Clin Oncol.* 1996;14:2653–2665.
92. Hoekstra HJ, van Ginkel RJ. Hyperthermic isolated limb perfusion in the management of extremity sarcoma. *Curr Opin Oncol.* 2003;15:300–303.
93. Wanebo HJ, Temple WJ, Popp MB, et al. Preoperative regional therapy for extremity sarcoma. A tricenter update. *Cancer* 1995;75:2299–2306.
94. Temple WJ, Temple CLF, Aurthur K, et al. Prospective cohort study of neoadjuvant treatment in conservative surgery of soft tissue sarcomas. *Ann Surg.* 1997;4:586–590.
95. DeLaney TF, Spiro IJ, Suit HD, et al. Neoadjuvant chemotherapy and radiotherapy for large extremity soft tissue sarcomas. *Int J Radiat Oncol Biol Phys.* 2003;56:1117–1127.
96. Goffman T, Tochner Z, Glatstein E. Primary treatment of large and massive adult sarcomas with iododeoxyuridine and aggressive hyperfractionated irradiation. *Cancer* 1991;67:572–576.
97. Lewis JJ, Leung DH, Woodruff JM, Brennan MF. Retroperitoneal soft tissue sarcoma: analysis of 500 patients treated and followed at a single institution. *Ann Surg.* 1998;228:355–365.
98. Storm FK, Mahvi DM. Diagnosis and management of retroperitoneal soft tissue sarcoma. *Ann Surg.* 1991;214:2–10.
99. Jaques DP, Coit DG, Hadju SI, et al. Management of primary and recurrent soft tissue sarcoma of the retroperitoneum. *Ann Surg.* 1990;212:51–59.
100. Russo P, Kim Y, Ravindram S, et al. Nephrectomy during operative management of retroperitoneal sarcoma. *Ann Surg Oncol.* 1997;4:421-424.
101. Mingoli A, Sapienza P, Cavallaro A, et al. The effect of extent of caval resection in the treatment of inferior vena cava leiomyosarcoma. *Anticancer Res.* 1997; 17:3877–3881.
102. Bose B. Primary malignant retroperitoneal tumors: analysis of 30 cases. *Can Surg.* 1979;22:215–221.
103. Harrison LB, Guitierrez E, Fisher JJ. Retroperitoneal sarcoma: the Yale experience and a review of the literature. *J Surg Oncol.* 1986;32:159–165.
104. Karakousis CP, Velez AF, Gerstenbluth R, et al. Resectablility and survival in retroperitoneal sarcomas. *Ann Surg Oncol.* 1996;3:150–158.
105. Wylie JP, O'Sullivan B, Catton CN, et al. Contemporary radiotherapy for soft tissue sarcoma. *Semin Surg Oncol.* 1999;17:33–46.
106. Willet CG, Suit HD, Tepper JE, et al. Intraoperative electron beam radiation therapy for retroperitoneal soft tissue sarcoma. *Cancer* 1991; 8:278–284.
107. Sindelar WF, Kinsella T, Chen PW, et al. Intraoperative radiotherapy in retroperitoneal sarcomas: final results of a prospective, randomized clinical trial. *Arch Surg.* 1993;128:402–410.
108. Glenn J, Sindelar WF, Kinsella T, et al. Results of multimodality therapy of resectable soft tissue sarcomas of the retroperitoneum. *Surgery* 1985; 97:316–325.
109. Rajput A, Kraybill WG. Clinical trials and soft tissue sarcomas. *Surg Oncol Clin North Am.* 2003;12:485–497.
110. Yang JC, Chang AE, Baker AR, et al. Randomized prospective study of the benefit of adjuvant radiation therapy in the treatment of soft tissue sarcomas of the extremity. *J Clin Oncol.* 1998;16:197–203.
111. Hayry P, Scheinin TM. The desmoid (Reitamo) syndrome: etiology, manifestations, pathogenesis, and treatment. *Curr Probl Surg.* 1988;25:225–320.
112. Church JM. Desmoid tumors in familial adenomatous polyposis. *Surg Oncol Clin North Am.* 1994;3:435.
113. Arndt CAS, Crist WM. Common musculoskeletal tumors of childhood and adolescence. *N Engl J Med.* 1999;341:342–352.
114. Brenner W, Bohuslavizki KH, Eary JF. PET imaging of osteosarcoma. *J Nucl Med.* 2003;44:930–942.
115. Arca MJ, Biermann JS, Johnson TM, et al. Biopsy techniques for skin, soft tissue and bone neoplasms. *Surg Oncol Clin North Am.* 1995; 4:157–174.
116. Bielack SS, Machatschek J-N, Flege S, et al. Delaying surgery with chemotherapy for osteosarcoma of the extremities. *Expert Opin Pharmachother.* 2004;5:1243–1256.
117. Baker L, Crowley J, Ryan J, et al. Long-term follow-up in the cure of osteogenic sarcoma. *Proc Am Soc Clin Oncol.* 1989; 8:320.
118. Apffelstaedt JP, Zhang PJ, Driscoll DL, et al. Various types of hemipelvectomy for soft tissue sarcomas: complications, survival, and prognostic factors. *Surg Oncol.* 1995;4:217–222.
119. Eilber FR, Guiliano AE, Eckhardt JJ, et al. Adjuvant chemotherapy for osteosarcoma: a randomized prospective trial. *J Clin Oncol.* 1987; 5:21.
120. Edmonson J, Marks R, Buckner J, et al. Contrast of response to D-MAP + Sargramostim between patients with advanced malignant gastrointestinal stromal tumors and patients with other advanced leiomyosarcomas. *Proc Am Soc Clin Oncol.* 1999;18:541A.
121. Mazur MT, Clark HB. Gastric stromal tumors. Reappraisal of histogenesis. *Am J Surg Pathol.* 1983; 7:507–519.
122. Kindblom LG, Remotti HE, Aldenborg F, et al. Gastrointestinal pacemaker cell tumor (GIPACT): gastrointestinal stromal tumor show phenotypic characteristics of the interstitial cells of Cajal. *Am J Pathol.* 1998;152:1259–1269.
123. Hirota S, Isozaki K, Moriyama Y, et al. Gain of function mutations of c-Kit in human gastrointestinal stromal tumors. *Science* 1998;279:577–580.
124. Sarlomo-Rikala M, Kovatich AJ, Barusevicius A, et al. CD117: a sensitive marker for gastrointestinal stromal tumors that is more specific for CD34. *Mod Pathol.* 1998;11:728–734.
125. Connoly EM, Gaffney E, Reynolds JV. Gastrointestinal stromal tumors. *Br J Cancer* 2003;90:1178–1186.
126. DeMatteo RP, Lewis JJ, Leung DH, et al. Two hundred gastrointestinal stromal tumors: recurrence patterns and prognostic factors for survival. *Ann Surg.* 2000;231:51–58.
127. Graadt van Roggen JF, van Velthuysen MLF, Hogendoorn PCW. The histopathological differential diagnosis of gastrointestinal stromal tumors. *J Clin Pathol.* 2001;54:96–102.
128. Miettinen M, Sarlomo-Rikala M, Lasota J. Gastrointestinal stromal tumors: recent advances in understanding of their biology. *Hum Pathol.* 1999;30:1213–1220.

129. Zsebo KM, Williams DA, Geissler EN, et al. Stem cell factor is encoded at the SI locus of the mouse and is the ligand for the c-Kit tyrosine kinase receptor. *Cell* 1990;63:213–224.
130. Yarden Y, Kuang WJ, Yang-Feng T, et al. Human proto-oncogene c-Kit: a new cell surface receptor tyrosine kinase for an unidentified ligand. *EMBO J.* 1987;6:3341–3351.
131. Williams DE, Eisenman J, Baird A, et al. Identification of a ligand for the c-Kit protooncogene. *Cell* 1990;63:167–174.
132. Lux ML, Rubin BP, Biase TL, et al. KIT extracellular and kinase domain mutations in gastrointestinal stromal tumors. *Am J Pathol.* 2000; 156:791–795.
133. Joensuu H, Dimitreijevic S. Tyrosine kinase inhibitor imatinib (STI571) as an anticancer agent for solid tumours. *Ann Med.* 2001;33:451–455.
134. Connolly EM, Gaffney E, Reynolds JV. Gastrointestinal stromal tumors. *Br J Cancer* 2003;90:1178–1186.
135. van Oosterom AT, Judson I, Verweij J, et al. Safety and efficacy of imatinib (STI571) in metastatic gastrointestinal stromal tumours: a phase I study. *Lancet* 2001;358:1421–1423.
136. von Mehren M, Blanke C, Joensuu H, et al. High incidence of durable responses induced by imatinib mesylate (Gleevac) in patients with unresectable and metastatic gastrointestinal stromal tumors. *Proc Am Soc Clin Oncol.* 2002; abstract 1608.
137. Potter DA, Glenn J, Kinsella T, et al. Patterns of recurrence in patients with high-grade soft tissue sarcomas. *J Clin Oncol.* 1985;3:353–356.
138. Nori D, Schupak K, Shiu MH, et al. Role of brachytherapy in recurrent extremity sarcoma in patients treated with prior surgery and irradiation. *Int J Radiat Oncol Biol Phys.* 1991;20:1229–1233.
139. Midis GP, Pollock RE, Chen NP, et al. Locally recurrent soft tissue sarcoma of the extremities. *Surgery* 1998;123:666–671.
140. Karakousis CP, Proimakis C, Rao U, et al. Local recurrence and survival in soft tissue sarcomas. *Ann Surg Oncol.* 1996;3:255–260.
141. Guiliano AE, Eilber FR, Morton DL. The management of locally recurrent soft tissue sarcoma. *Ann Surg.* 1982;196:87.
142. Karakousis C, Gerstenbluth R, Kontzoglou K, et al. Retroperitoneal sarcomas and their management. *Arch Surg.* 1995;130:1104–1109.
143. Putnam JB, Roth JA. Resection of sarcomatous pulmonary metastases. *Surg Oncol Clin North Am.* 1993;2:673.
144. Casson AG, Putnam JB, Natarajan G, et al. Five-year survival after pulmonary metastatectomy for adult soft tissue sarcoma. *Cancer* 1992; 69:662–668.
145. Antmann KH, Elias AD. Chemotherapy of advanced soft tissue sarcomas. *Semin Surg Oncol.* 1988; 4:53–58.
146. von Mehren M. New therapeutic strategies for soft tissue sarcomas. *Curr Treat Options Oncol.* 2003; 4:441–451.

CHAPTER 120 ■ PLASTIC AND RECONSTRUCTIVE SURGERY

DAVID L. BROWN, STEVEN R. BUCHMAN, PAUL S. CEDERNA, KEVIN C. CHUNG, WILLIAM M. KUZON, AND EDWIN G. WILKINS

Plastic and reconstructive surgery can be defined as a discipline that addresses problem wounds using a diverse array of nonsurgical and, especially, surgical therapies. In this definition, the term *problem wounds* is taken in the broadest sense; plastic surgeons treat traumatic, congenital, developmental, and even psychological wounds. Perhaps it is this latter aspect of plastic surgery that most fully sets it apart from other surgical specialties:

> We restore and make whole those parts which nature or ill fortune have taken away, not so much to delight the eye but to buoy up the spirit of the afflicted.
>
> —Gaspare Tagliacozzi, 1597

In more concrete terms, plastic surgery is an approach to surgical problems. Plastic surgeons operate "from the top of the head to the tip of the toes," and they envision themselves as surgical innovators. Plastic surgeons have been instrumental in the development of microvascular surgery, craniofacial surgery, head and neck reconstruction, nerve grafting, and even renal transplantation.[1] Although the field of plastic surgery can be arbitrarily divided into "cosmetic" surgery (surgery to improve the appearance of a normal phenotype) and "reconstructive" surgery (repair of damaged anatomy or an abnormal phenotype), in many circumstances, both functional reconstruction and aesthetic improvement are paramount. Plastic surgery is truly "general surgery," with a broad and growing list of subspecialties (Table 120.1).

TABLE 120.1

THE SPECTRUM OF PLASTIC SURGERY

Aesthetic surgery
Burns: acute and reconstructive surgery
Craniofacial surgery
Cutaneous and soft tissue oncology
Hand and upper extremity surgery
Head and neck oncology
Microvascular surgery
Maxillofacial and orthognathic surgery
Peripheral nerve surgery
Reconstructive surgery
Face (ear, lip, nose, eyelid)
Breast
Trunk
Lower extremity

PRINCIPLES OF MANAGEMENT FOR PROBLEM WOUNDS

Regardless of the etiology or location of a wound, the principles of management are universal and can be embodied by a straightforward algorithm:

1. Evaluate and, if possible, eliminate the factors contributing to the presence of the wound.
2. Control or optimize the wound prior to closure.
3. Close the wound using the simplest method, unless specific factors mitigate a more complex approach.

Although it is the nature of surgeons to focus on the technical details of operative procedures, the first two steps in this algorithm are most critical for the successful reconstruction of problem wounds. This algorithmic approach allows plastic surgeons to treat diabetic foot ulcers, infected sternotomy wounds, major defects after composite resection of the head and neck, pressure ulcers, lower extremity wounds after open tibial fractures, venous stasis ulcers, and other difficult defects with a high degree of success. *This rational approach is the core of plastic surgery.* In plastic surgery there is no one-to-one correlation between a surgical problem and a specific operation. There is no "right" way to reconstruct a given defect, and a spectrum of options must be considered for every reconstructive problem. Selecting the best option for a given patient is the challenge.

TABLE 120.2

LOCAL AND SYSTEMIC FACTORS THAT AFFECT WOUND MANAGEMENT

LOCAL FACTORS
Infection
Local malignancy
Foreign bodies
Local toxins
Radiation
Ischemia
Venous insufficiency
Lymphatic insufficiency
Repetitive trauma
Reduced sensation
SYSTEMIC FACTORS
Immune deficiencies
Distant malignancy
Diabetes mellitus
Cigarette smoking
Chemotherapeutic agents
Hereditary healing disorders
Nutritional deficiency
Old age
Uremia
Glucocorticoid therapy, immunosuppressive agents

Evaluation of Problem Wounds

The evaluation of patients with difficult wounds is best approached by considering local and systemic (or intrinsic and extrinsic) contributing factors for each phase of the workup. In the history, local factors of importance include the mechanism that resulted in the wound, symptoms such as pain or loss of function, the time course and progression of the wound, any previous nonsurgical or surgical treatments for the wound, and any history of previous injury, irradiation, malignancy, or other local factors that contributed to the presence of the wound. The history should also uncover systemic factors that impair wound healing, including immunosuppression (e.g., chemotherapy, immune deficiencies), medical conditions known to impair healing (e.g., diabetes, renal failure), medications (e.g., steroids, cyclosporin A), cigarette smoking, and general debility (e.g., nutritional deficiencies, old age).

The physical examination of patients with problem wounds should be focused on local and systemic signs that affect wound healing. For the wound itself, the location, size, depth, exposure of deep or vital structures, presence of necrotic material, presence of foreign bodies, or signs of any neoplastic processes should be carefully noted. Because all open wounds are contaminated, the designation of a wound as "infected" should be contingent on the physical examination findings of local inflammation: erythema, pain, swelling, fluctuance, purulence, and loss of function. Physical examination should be the primary criterion for the diagnosis of local wound infection; surface swabs indicating the presence of pathogenic bacteria do not correlate with clinically significant infection.[2] In addition to the wound itself, surrounding tissue should be examined for signs of injury (e.g., actinic changes), previous irradiation, arterial or venous insufficiency, lymphedema, loss of sensation, and dermal thinning (e.g., aging, steroid therapy). For all wounds on an arm or leg, a careful neurovascular examination for the entire limb is mandatory. In addition to the local examination, a focused systematic physical examination is mandatory in patients with problem wounds. Systemic signs of infection (e.g., fever, hypotension) are of particular importance. Obesity is a major risk factor that impairs wound healing. The general physical examination should focus on the systemic factors that affect wound healing as noted previously. Table 120.2 lists some of the local and systemic factors that impair wound healing; history and physical examination are the principal modalities for diagnosing these problems.

Laboratory examinations can be invaluable in the management of problem wounds. However, laboratory tests are often misused in wound patients, and a rational, evidence-based approach is necessary to efficiently utilize this expensive resource. Again, the local-systemic paradigm is useful in determining which laboratory examinations are warranted.

For local evaluation, as already mentioned, wound swabs can be valuable for surveillance of the flora contaminating a wound but should not be used as a trigger to initiate therapy for wound infection. Wound biopsy and quantitative bacteriology have proved valuable in the management of burns and chronic wounds.[3,4] Bacterial loads in excess of 10^5/g tissue indicate contamination at a level that precludes skin graft take and jeopardizes wound closure of any kind. The use of quantitative cultures, however, is not justified for most acute or uncomplicated chronic wounds. In general, quantitative cultures are reserved for "high stakes" wounds, where a failure of closure on the initial attempt may leave an unreconstructable situation with grave consequences, such as amputation or death. Wound biopsies can be invaluable for diagnosing invasive burn wound infection and are preferred over quantitative culture for this purpose.[5] The presence of bacteria in the deep dermis on biopsy is highly correlated with the risk of systemic sepsis in burn patients. Bone biopsy demonstrating bacteria within the bone is the preferred test for making the diagnosis of osteomyelitis. Standard radiographs are most useful for diagnosing and delineating acute fractures and are much less useful in the setting of chronic, open wounds. Ultrasound, computed tomography (CT) scan, or magnetic resonance imaging (MRI) may be useful for delineating fluid collections, necrotic tissue, or inflammation in selected circumstances. In contrast, radionuclide bone scans have little role to play in patients with open wounds or fractures. In the face of an open wound or recent fracture, a "hot" bone scan (even a triple-phase bone scan) is not specific for osteomyelitis and has little value. Therefore, obtaining bone scans in patients with suspected sternal osteomyelitis after recent midline sternotomy, in pressure sore patients with exposed bone, or in other patients with open wounds overlying exposed bone is unwarranted. Under these circumstances, bone biopsy is preferred for making a diagnosis of osteomyelitis and for determining the responsible pathogen; MRI is preferred for delineating the extent of bony involvement. Magnetic resonance angiography (MRA)or standard angiography may be indicated if vascular insufficiency is suspected or if a free-tissue transfer is planned.

The use of systemic laboratory investigations should be limited to specific indications; "routine" blood work is not required for patients with acute or chronic wounds. White blood cell differential counts and blood cultures can confirm the diagnosis of systemic infection. Serum albumin and transferrin determinations may be valuable in determining nutritional status. A greatly elevated erythrocyte sedimentation rate can help confirm the diagnosis of osteomyelitis. Other laboratory tests to confirm the diagnosis and severity of associated medical conditions may be justified for specific indications.

Treatment of the Problem Wound

Once a wound has been fully evaluated, the treatments should be designed to achieve specific goals. In order of greatest priority, these goals are: (a) prevention of complications resulting from the wound, (b) preserving or restoring critical functions, (c) achieving wound closure, and (d) restoration of aesthetics. Again, each of these goals may require specific local or systemic interventions.

Preventive Treatment

The preventive measures that should be taken for patients with open wounds depend on the setting. For an acute laceration, tetanus prophylaxis should be considered. For patients with pressure sores, a strict adherence to pressure-relief protocols and an assessment of nutritional status take priority. In wounds caused by human or animal bites, prophylactic antibiotics are warranted. In addition, any associated medical conditions that are contributing to the wound must be aggressively optimized. It is the responsibility of the surgeon to ensure that a patient with a wound does not develop a complication from that wound and that the patient does not develop more wounds from the same mechanism. This is of particular importance in bedridden, obtunded, or paralyzed patients, in whom it should be possible to completely prevent pressure sores with proper nursing care.

Preservation of Function

Preserving joint motion must always be considered for patients with open wounds of the extremities. Aggressive physiotherapy to maintain or improve joint motion can be instituted in the presence of an open wound. Splinting should be used aggressively to minimize joint contractures and any plans for wound closure should include measures to maintain joint function. In the case of facial defects, especially if facial paralysis is present, oral competence and the maintenance of eye protection should weigh heavily into any reconstructive plan. Function takes precedence over form in the reconstructive algorithm.

Nonsurgical Therapy

After careful consideration of preventive measures and the preservation of critical function, a strategy for wound closure can be formulated. The basic tenet is: "débride dirty wounds, close clean wounds." Therefore, the first step in wound closure is achieving control of the wound by eliminating necrotic debris and controlling any infection present. Nonsurgical therapies are used in conjunction with surgical therapy to achieve a clean wound. The mainstay of local, nonsurgical therapy is the use of wound dressings. It is beyond the scope of this chapter to review the wide range of options available to dress wounds. Recent articles contain a contemporary review of this topic.[6–8] However, the basic principle is to employ débriding dressings for dirty wounds and occlusive dressings for clean wounds. The most commonly employed débriding dressing is the "wet-to-dry" dressing. Gauze made damp with normal saline, weak acetic acid, weak bleach, or various other solutions is applied to the wound. Over a period of hours, evaporation dries the dressing, which becomes slightly adherent to the wound surface. When the dressing is removed, necrotic debris is pulled off with the dressing, but healthy tissue is left behind. Wet-to-dry dressings work through *mechanical débridement*, and the most important component of their use is how often they are changed. Wet-to-dry dressings must be changed a minimum of three times per day; they should not be "soaked" off to reduce patient discomfort because this technique completely defeats their purpose. Enzymatic dressings have also been used to débride wounds, but their use is limited by patient tolerance to the pain they cause. Débriding dressings are indicated for infected wounds and wounds containing necrotic debris.

If a wound is "clean," meaning that it does not contain necrotic debris and has an acceptable bacterial load, a dressing to encourage wound healing can be used. In the case of many simple wounds, a nonadherent sterile dressing is all that is required. In the case of more complex wounds, occlusive dressings that maintain a moist environment to maximize wound healing are preferred. Options include hydrocolloid dressings, alginate dressings, and various hydrogels. Again, occlusive dressings must not be used on infected or dirty wounds. For many wounds, judicious application of hydrocolloid dressings may allow closure by secondary intention in a reasonable period of time.

Under some circumstances, it is appropriate to use antibiotic dressings. Burn wounds are most commonly dressed with silver sulfadiazine or mafenide Sulfamylon (Bertek Pharmaceuticals, Inc., Research Triangle Park, NC) dressings. Heavily contaminated wounds from other mechanisms may also benefit from antibiotic dressings. In general, however, antibiotic dressings are not required for clean wounds, even if they are chronic.

Last, it should be noted that we are entering a new era of nonsurgical wound management. A rapid advance in our understanding of wound healing has led to the development of growth factor therapy, cellular therapy, and new physical modalities for the treatment of chronic wounds. For pressure sores and diabetic ulcers in particular, recombinant platelet-derived growth factor appears to be a useful adjunct to the dressing regime.[9,10] Tissue-engineered dressings and skin substitutes are also poised to revolutionize wound care.[11] Negative pressure wound therapy and hyperbaric oxygen treatment have become widespread and have been demonstrated to be efficacious and cost effective when applied appropriately for complex wounds.[12] Nevertheless, the basic algorithm for evaluation and nonsurgical management of wounds will not change.

Surgical Therapy

Wound Preparation. For problem wounds, surgical therapy is primarily aimed at wound preparation and wound reconstruction. For dirty wounds with necrotic debris, a judicious but thorough surgical débridement can convert a contaminated, chronic wound into a fresh surgical wound ready for immediate closure. Although débriding dressings can prepare wounds for

TABLE 120.3

THE RECONSTRUCTIVE LADDER

1. Primary wound closure
2. Healing by secondary intention
3. Skin grafting
4. Local flaps
5. Regional flaps
6. Distant flaps

closure under some circumstances, an operative débridement is preferred to a long course of débriding dressings for most problem wounds. Consequently, most problem wounds require an operative débridement prior to definitive reconstruction. In the case of chronic osteomyelitis, a formal resection of the sequestrum is required before formal wound closure. Prolonged treatment with intravenous or oral antibiotics cannot clear bacteria from a focus of dead bone; chronic osteomyelitis is a surgical disease cured with a saw, rongeur, bur, or bone curette. Therefore, the common practice of placing patients with chronic osteomyelitis on 6 weeks of antibiotic therapy is irrational unless performed in conjunction with a formal sequestrectomy.

Reconstructive Principles. As stated earlier, there is no "right" way to close any given wound. Plastic surgeons use a straightforward set of principles in delineating the optimum way to close a given wound for a given patient. The predominant principle is that the simplest method to close a wound is usually the best choice. This principle is embodied in the "reconstructive ladder," which is a hierarchy of reconstructive options progressing from simple to complex (Table 120.3). Therefore, when engaging options for wound closure, plastic surgeons "climb" the reconstructive ladder, usually stopping on the lowest rung that will achieve a closed wound. However, other principles of reconstruction sometimes override a slavish adherence to the reconstructive ladder. The choice of a technique for wound closure should take into consideration the need for subsequent procedures and other factors that might mitigate skipping over simpler options for wound closure. An example would be an avulsion injury to the palm of the hand. Although it might be possible to close this wound with a skin graft, the need to restore flexor tendon function is preeminent in the hand, so that the use of a distant flap to provide a suitable bed for tendon grafting may be the preferred choice. In addition to the reconstructive ladder, other examples of guiding reconstructive principles are: function takes precedence over form, single-stage reconstructions are preferred over multistage approaches, and autologous tissue is preferred over alloplastic reconstructions. Other factors to be considered are the durability of the reconstruction over many years, the psychological impact on the patient, and data indicating that some options are sometimes preferred for specific reasons. For example, muscle flaps are known to be superior to skin flaps in their ability to resist or eradicate infection.[13] Therefore, a muscle flap may be chosen over a simpler option if the eradication of osteomyelitis or mediastinitis is the goal. As mentioned earlier, weighing this complex array of factors to arrive at the optimal reconstruction for a given patient is the true challenge in reconstructive surgery.

Reconstructive Techniques. Regardless of the reconstructive method chosen, plastic surgeons strive for technical virtuosity in the operating room. To maximize healing and minimize scar formation, atraumatic technique includes delicate tissue handling, the use of skin hooks and sharp rakes, bipolar electrocautery, sharp dissection, and loupe magnification. When reconstructing difficult wounds, the margin for error is very small, and small errors in technical execution can result in failure. The general surgical methods used by reconstructive surgeons are briefly considered in this chapter.

Primary closure. If a laceration or other wound can be closed primarily, consideration is given to a meticulous, layered closure. Emphasis is placed on eversion of skin edges without strangling tissue. Nonabsorbable skin stitches that provoke minimal inflammatory response are preferred, but they must be removed promptly to minimize cross-hatching. Therefore, for most wounds, deep dermal, absorbable stitches are placed to allow early removal of skin stitches while still providing prolonged support to the repair; this may minimize the chances of a dehiscence or scar spread. It is preferable to place a closed suction drain to eliminate dead space rather than suturing fat or other easily devascularized tissue. If a technically perfect, tension-free repair cannot be achieved with primary closure, it is preferable to use a more complex surgical option.

Skin grafting. Skin grafting was one of the foundations on which the specialty of plastic surgery was established. Skin grafts are classified by as either split thickness, in which epidermis and a portion of the dermis are harvested, or full thickness, in which the entire dermis is harvested. Both full-thickness and split-thickness skin grafts can be used to resurface open wounds in cases in which primary closure is not possible. Skin graft take is contingent on the successful revascularization of the graft within a narrow time window (48 to 72 hours). Initially, grafts are nourished by a process of plasmatic imbibition, wherein serum from the wound bed diffuses into the adjacent graft. Revascularization occurs by the process of inosculation. Vessels from the wound bed grow into the graft, forming functional circulatory connections with the vasculature of the graft. For plasmatic imbibition and inosculation to be successful, two criteria must be met. First, the wound bed must be appropriately vascularized. Therefore, skin grafts cannot be placed on poorly vascularized wound surfaces, including bone denuded of periosteum, tendon denuded of peritenon, or cartilage. Second, a bolster dressing or splint must be used to ensure absolute immobilization of the graft on the bed to prevent shearing of the nascent vascular connections during inosculation. If either of these criteria cannot be met, a more complex reconstructive option must be considered.

Random skin flaps. The use of tissue (usually skin) immediately adjacent to the defect as the tissue for reconstruction is referred to as a local flap reconstruction. Skin rearrangement can range in complexity from simple undermining to complex, geometric skin flaps. Which method is appropriate is dependent on multiple factors, including the etiology of the defect, the desired direction of the scar, the fragility or mobility of underlying structures, and the need to avoid distortion to adjacent free margins such as the lip or eyelid. Significant experience is required for the optimal utilization of skin rearrangement. When plastic surgeons think of "classical" skin flaps, they are referring to random skin flaps, without an axial blood supply. These skin flaps rely on a dermal plexus of vessels for their survival, and the perfusion of the distal end of the flap is inadequate to allow tissue survival if the flap design is inappropriate. It was previously thought that survival of the distal part of random skin flaps could be ensured by adhering to length-to-width ratios established for various areas of the body. It is now recognized that these ratios have no basis in circulatory physiology, and the surviving length of a random skin flap does not depend on flap width.[14] In practice, most of the commonly employed skin flaps have been developed empirically. There are three basic types of random skin flaps: rotation, advancement, and transposition, depending on how adjacent skin is shifted into the defect. Each type of flap has specific design criteria. Many eponyms are used to describe variations on these basic three flap designs; examples are the Romberg transposition flap, the Mustarde rotation flap, and the Rintala advancement flap. Excellent reviews of the use of skin flaps in reconstructive surgery are available.[15,16]

As mentioned, the concern with flap viability limits the utility of random skin flaps. Several strategies have been developed to circumvent this problem. The first of these is the concept of surgical delay. Delay is defined as the partial interruption of blood flow to a defined piece of tissue. At present, surgical delay is the only method available to augment the surviving length of random skin flaps (Fig. 120.1). Another strategy is the use of tissue expanders. Tissue expanders are implantable balloons that are inserted in a deflated state and are inflated with sterile saline via percutaneous injection into a self-sealing valve. Except for the scalp, where expanders are placed in the subgaleal plane, tissues expanders are usually placed subcutaneously. The insertion of the tissue expander into the effects a surgical delay, and the slow expansion has been demonstrated to result in the formation of new skin. However, the most important strategy to circumvent the use of random skin flaps has been to develop axial pattern flaps that do not rely on a random blood supply.

Flaps with axial blood supply. Regional flaps are defined as the transfer of tissue that is not immediately adjacent to the defect without the disruption of blood supply to the transferred tissue. For this approach to be practical, an axial blood supply to the transferred tissue must be present.

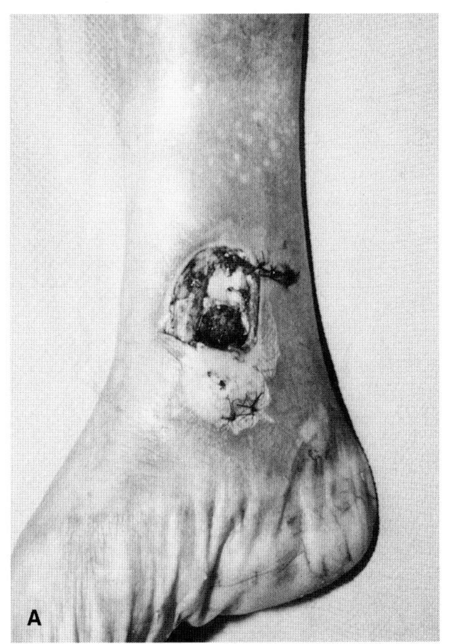

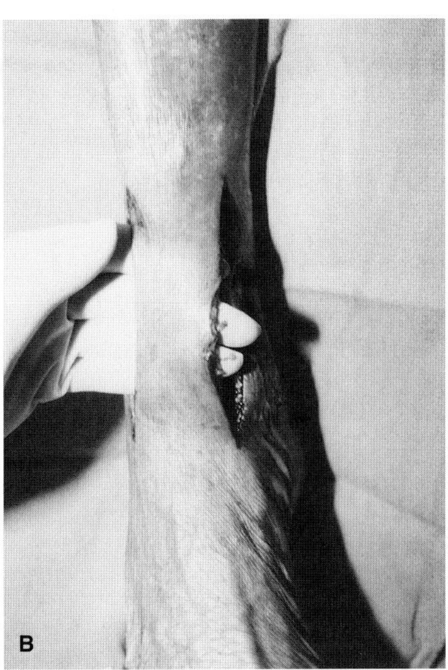

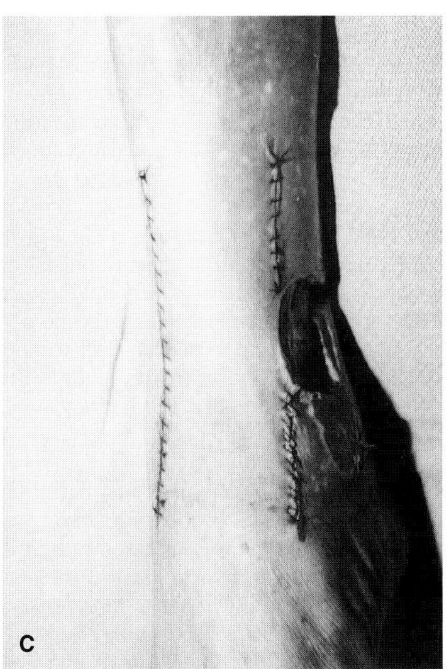

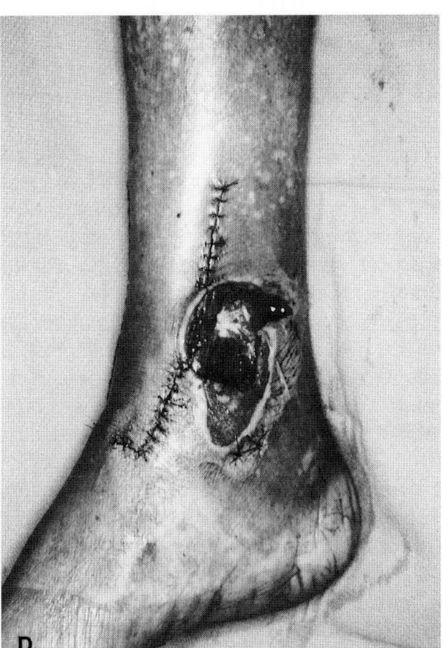

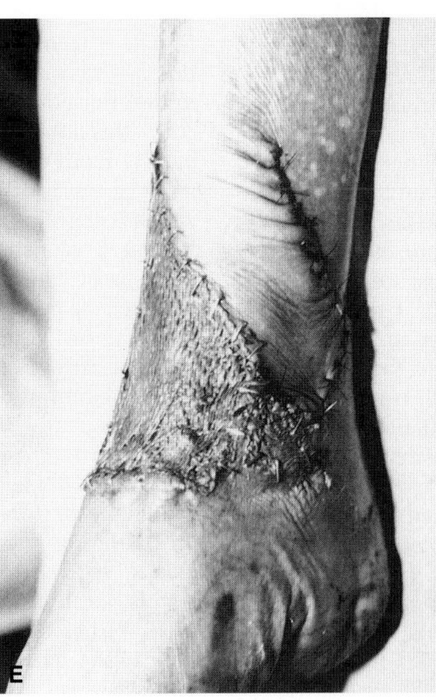

FIGURE 120.1 Example of surgical delay. Because of associated medical problems, the patient was not a candidate for microvascular tissue transfer. (*A*) Lower-third tibial defect secondary to an open ankle fracture. Note exposed bone, which precludes use of a skin graft. (*B*) In the first stage, a bipedicle flap was created anterior to the defect. The deep perforators to the skin of the flap were divided by full undermining. The flap is perfused only from the proximal and distal ends. (*C*) The incisions were repaired, and the wound was dressed. (*D*) After 5 days, the bipedicle flap was again elevated and part of the distal pedicle was divided (*arrow*). The incisions were again closed, and the wound was dressed. This procedure was repeated 10 days after the initial operation to leave only a small skin bridge at the distal end of the flap. (*E*) Fourteen days after the initial procedure, the remaining distal skin bridge was divided and the flap transferred. The donor site was skin-grafted. This photograph depicts full survival of the flap and complete take of the skin graft.

Axial skin flaps. The pioneering work of Bakamjian[17] and McGregor and Jackson[18] identified longitudinal blood vessels of large caliber traversing a defined region of skin. Their descriptions of the deltopectoral and groin flaps, respectively, opened a new era of reconstructive surgery. Surgeons were no longer constrained to the use of random skin flaps; any piece of tissue in the body with an axial blood supply could be transposed on a vascular pedicle with a high degree of assurance that the tissue would survive. Taylor and Palmer's[19] description of the angiosome concept solidified our ability to design flaps based on a sound knowledge of vascular anatomy. An angiosome is defined as a region of tissue supplied by an identifiable, and usually named, artery and its venae comitantes. Because of the ability of choke vessels crossing angiosome boundaries to enlarge, flaps can be designed to encompass an adjacent angiosome. However, flaps crossing two angiosome boundaries are destined to undergo partial necrosis. In practice, there are relatively few axial skin flaps, most being better classified as fasciocutaneous flaps.

Fasciocutaneous flaps. Cormack and Lamberty[20] further expanded our understanding of the blood supply to the skin with their description of fasciocutaneous flaps. They pointed out that the dermal plexus derives its inflow from vertically oriented vessels arising at the level of the deep fascia. The vessels at the deep facial level have horizontal orientation relative to the skin's surface and form a subfacial plexus. This subfacial plexus can form the basis for the design of fasciocutaneous flaps based on several defined anatomical patterns.[20] Several fasciocutaneous flaps have enjoyed widespread use. The radial forearm flap has become a workhorse for hand reconstruction and as a free flap for head and neck reconstruction. The osteoseptocutaneous fibula free flap has been widely used for intraoral reconstruction during reconstruction of oromandibular defects.

Muscle and myocutaneous flaps. Based on the knowledge that tissue with an axial blood supply can be reliably transferred, muscle and myocutaneous flaps came into widespread use in the 1980s, thanks in large part to the classification system by Mathes and Nahai.[21] Whole muscles can be transferred as a pedicled or free flap if a dominant vascular pedicle is present. Segmental muscle transfers are sometimes possible on minor vascular pedicles. Muscle flaps have enjoyed wide use for a diverse array of indications. As mentioned earlier, muscle flaps have an enhanced ability to eradicate infection and are preferred for contaminated or osteomyelitic wounds. For a given defect, muscle flaps are chosen by their size and arc of rotation.

The rediscovery of the musculocutaneous perforator as a predominant vascular supply to the skin in many areas of the body has led to the wide use of musculocutaneous flaps. These flaps derive their inflow from a major muscular artery. Perforators emanating vertically from the muscle surface supply the skin overlying the muscle. Table 120.4 lists "workhorse" muscle and myocutaneous flaps. Of particular note is the transverse rectus abdominis myocutaneous (TRAM) flap, based on periumbilical myocutaneous perforators from the rectus abdominis muscle has risen to preeminence for breast reconstruction.[22] Recently, "perforator" flaps have enjoyed a resurgence of use.[23] These flaps are derived from fasciocutaneous or myocutaneous flaps but are designed and dissected to minimize the loss of muscle in the donor site, thereby minimizing donor site morbidity.

Microvascular tissue transfer. Historically, pedicled flaps were used to reconstruct distant defects. The distant transfer was accomplished in one of two ways. Flaps could be moved to the defect in a series of pedicled transfers (waltzing or tumbling flaps). Alternatively, flaps could be attached directly to the defect with a temporary pedicle to the donor site being maintained temporarily. At a second stage the flap was detached from the donor site, after it had developed sufficient blood supply from the recipient bed (e.g., cross leg flaps, pedicled groin flaps). Although the distant transfer of pedicled flaps still has definitive indications (e.g., the median forehead flap for nasal reconstruction), reconstruction using distant tissue is now most commonly performed via microvascular tissue transfer, or "free" flaps. First described clinically by Daniel and Taylor,[24] free flaps have revolutionized reconstructive surgery. Any tissue with an axial blood supply with pedicle vessels 1 mm in diameter or larger can be reliably transferred microsurgically. Circulation in the transferred tissue is established via microvascular anastomoses between the axial flap vessels and vessels in the recipient site. Microvascular anastomoses are performed with 9-0 or 10-0 suture with the aid of an operating microscope; success rates for free flap transfers exceed 90%.[25] The greatest advantage of free flap reconstruction is that the surgeon is not restricted to the use of available, local tissues. By using composite tissue flaps, massive, complex tissue defects can be reconstructed replacing "like with like" [26] (Fig. 120.2). Bowel, skin, bone, muscle, fascia, and composite tissue can be transferred microsurgically. Free flaps

TABLE 120.4

WORKHORSE MUSCLE AND MYOCUTANEOUS FLAPS

Flap	Myocutaneous	Common uses
Temporalis	No	Orbital and intraoral reconstruction, facial reanimation (pedicled flap)
Pectoralis major	Yes	Intraoral and neck reconstruction; reconstruction of sternal defects (muscle only)
Latissimus dorsi	Yes	Breast reconstruction, neck reconstruction, free flap for very large defects
Rectus abdominis	Yes, including TRAM	Breast reconstruction, sternal reconstruction, reconstruction of groin defects, free flap for medium sized defects
Gluteus maximus	Yes	Ischial pressure sores, sacral pressure sores
Biceps femoris	Yes	Ischial pressure sores
Tensor fascia lata	Yes	Trochanteric pressure sores, abdominal wall reconstruction
Gracilis	Yes	Perineal reconstruction, vaginal reconstruction, facial reanimation (muscle free flap), free flap for small defects
Rectus femoris	Yes	Infected hip wounds, abdominal wall reconstruction
Medial gastrocnemius	Rarely	Knee defects, proximal third tibial defects
Soleus	No	Middle third tibial defects

TRAM, transverse rectus abdominis myocutaneous.

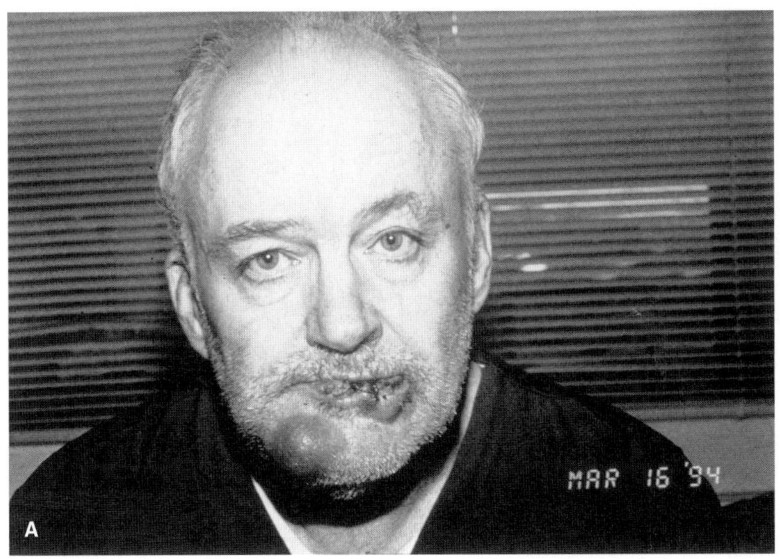

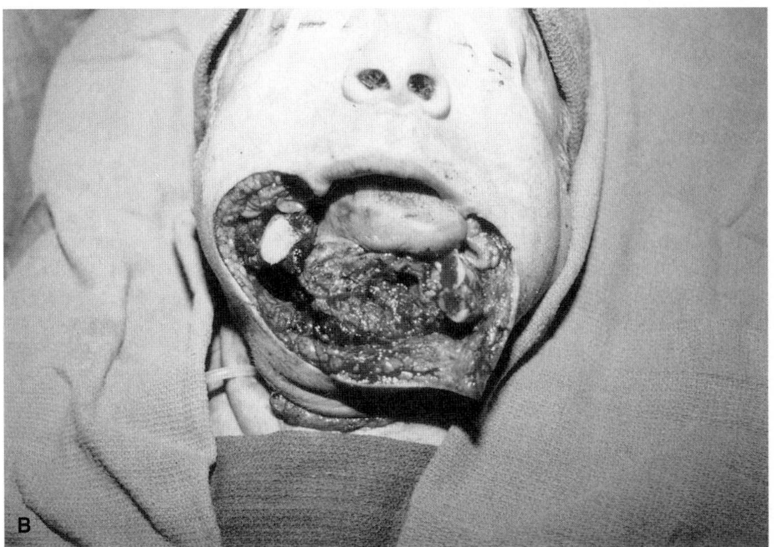

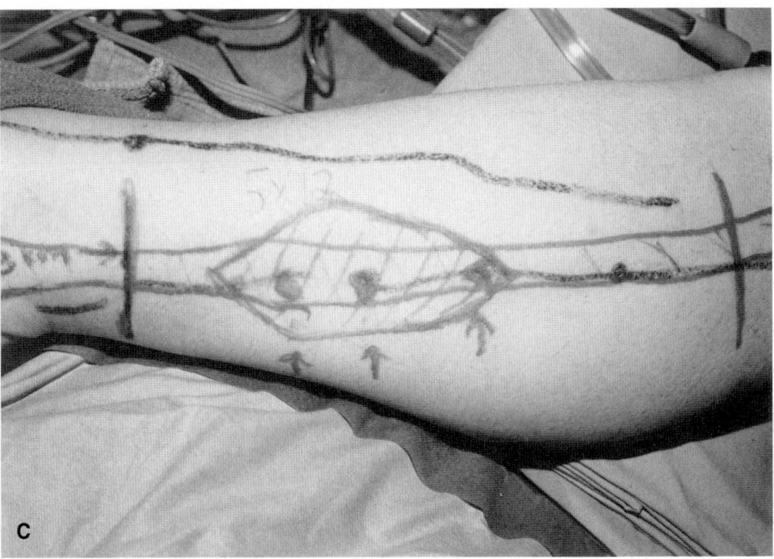

FIGURE 120.2 Double free-flap reconstruction of a massive, complex defect. (*A*) Squamous cell carcinoma of lip, chin, mandible, and floor of mouth after resection. Massive tissue defect encompasses skin of the chin, entire lower lip, mandible from midbody to midbody, and floor of the mouth. (*B*) Fibula free flap. Skin paddle is centered on fasciocutaneous perforators. (*C*) Fibula free flap elevated but still *in situ*. Osteotomies have been performed to conform to the mandibular contour. The skin paddle will form the floor of the mouth.

(*Continued*)

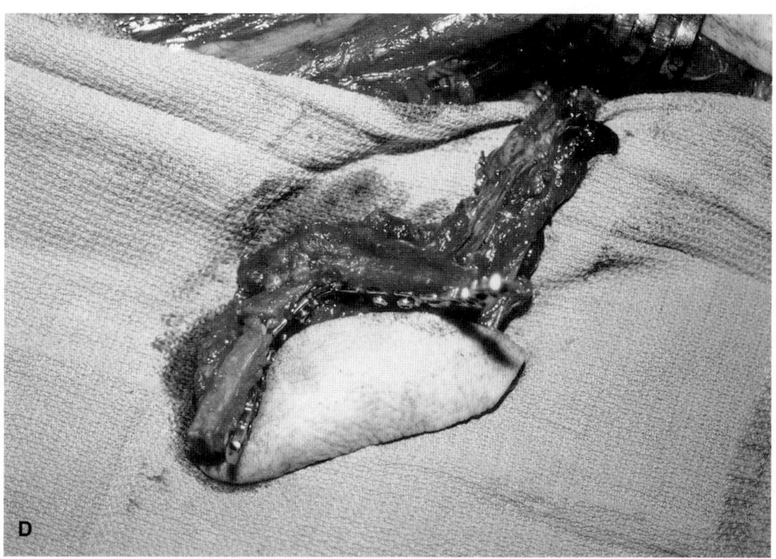

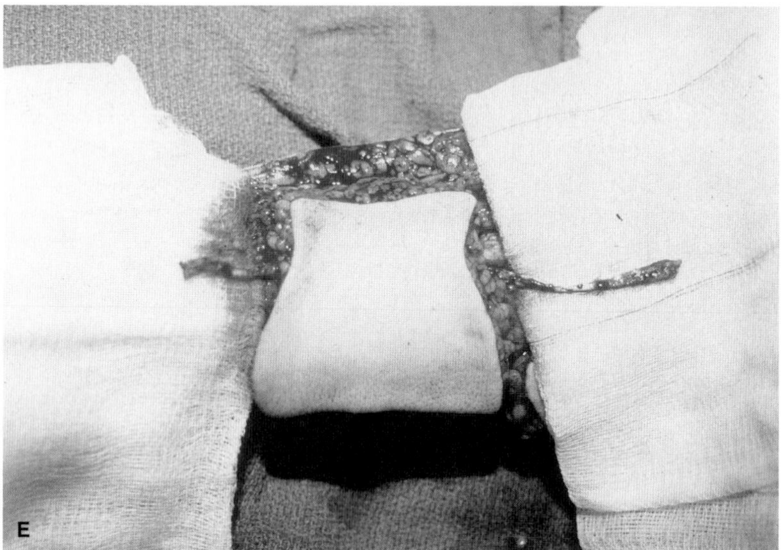

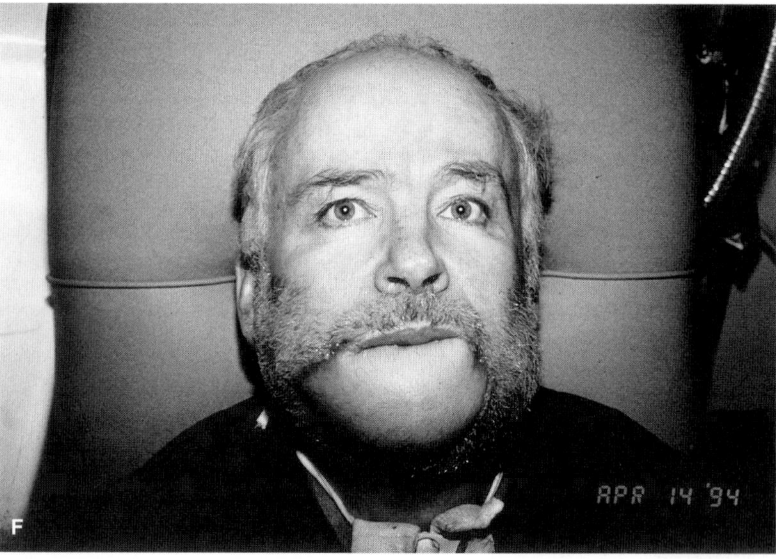

FIGURE 120.2 (*Continued*) (*D*) Radial forearm free-flap plan. Skin paddle will be harvested along with the palmaris longus tendon. The tendon will be attached to the modiolus on either side of the lower-lip defect, and the skin paddle will reconstruct the skin of the chin and lip. For the lip, the skin paddle will be draped over the tendon like a bed sheet on a clothesline. (*E*) Radial forearm flap elevated but *in situ*. (*F*) Postoperative result, mouth closed.

(*Continued*)

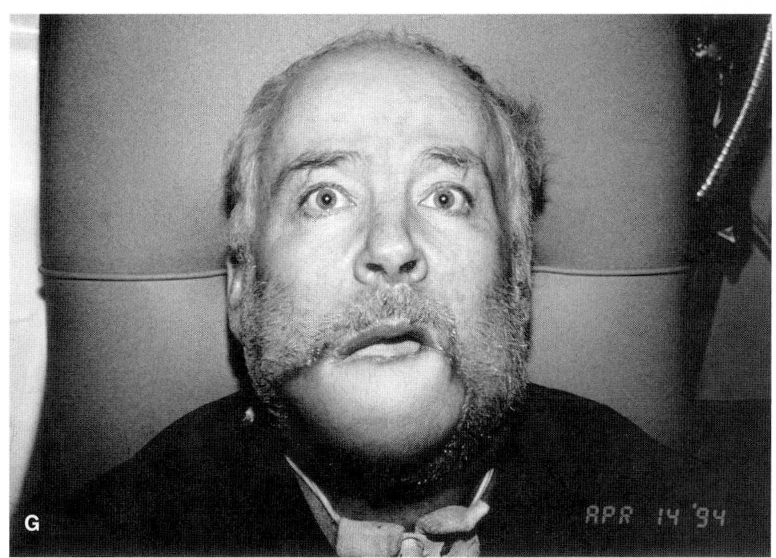

FIGURE 120.2 (*Continued*) (*G*) Postoperative result, mouth open. (From Kuzon WM Jr, Jejurikar S, Wilkins EG, et al. Double free-flap reconstruction of massive defects involving the lip, chin, and mandible. *Microsurgery* 1998;18:372–378.)

are the primary modality for reconstruction of major head and neck defects after composite resection of squamous cell carcinoma and for the reconstruction of traumatic defects in the distal foreleg.

RECONSTRUCTIVE AND AESTHETIC SURGERY OF THE BREAST

Plastic surgery of the female breast includes both reconstructive and aesthetic procedures. Breast reconstruction following mastectomy and reduction mammaplasty for macromastia (oversized breasts) are the most common examples of reconstructive breast surgery. By contrast, breast augmentation (enlargement) and mastopexy (breast lift) generally are performed for aesthetic reasons. Although some surgical approaches may be applicable to both categories of breast procedures, the relative benefits, risks, and costs of reconstructive versus aesthetic breast surgery may be quite different, particularly as viewed by patients, providers, and payers.

Before advising women on reconstructive or aesthetic breast procedures, the surgeon should carefully assess the patient's current preferences, concerns, history, and physical findings. Initially, any history of breast disease (as well as familial history of breast pathologies) should be evaluated. On physical examination, careful linear measurements and preoperative photographs should be taken to document existing contour deformities, asymmetries or other findings. A standard breast examination should be carried out to detect previously undiagnosed masses, nipple discharge, or lymphadenopathy. Finally, it is also advisable that women age 40 years or older undergo mammography unless this study has been performed in the previous 12 months.

Preoperative consultation should include a thorough discussion covering the relative benefits and risks of the various surgical options. The surgeon is well advised to provide comprehensive information in an understandable format. To enhance patient satisfaction with the eventual surgical result, providers should elicit patients' preferences and expectations for surgical outcomes and tailor treatment options accordingly. Because of the prevalence of breast cancer in North American women, the impact of reconstructive or aesthetic procedures on breast cancer monitoring also should be discussed.

Reconstructive Breast Surgery

Postmastectomy Reconstruction

A variety of operative procedures have been described for breast reconstruction following mastectomy. These approaches can be categorized as implant-based, autogenous (natural) tissue, and "hybrid" procedures. For purposes of this discussion, the term *hybrid* is applied to procedures combining elements of both implant and autogenous tissue techniques. This overview describes the advantages and disadvantages of the most common techniques. Ultimately, procedure selection is based on a range of patient variables, including size and shape of the desired reconstructed breast; availability of local, regional, and distant donor tissues; coexisting medical problems; and, perhaps most important, patient preferences.

Implant-Based Techniques. As most commonly practiced, the implant approach usually requires two operative procedures to reconstruct the female breast. In the first stage, a temporary tissue expander is placed in a soft tissue pocket, usually located deep to the pectoralis major muscle. The tissue expander is a deflated Silastic (silicone) envelope with an integrated or remote injection port through which saline solution can be percutaneously injected. Following expander placement and meticulous closure of the overlying muscle and skin, saline is periodically injected beginning at 10 to 21 days (Fig. 120.3A). As the device enlarges, growth is induced in the overlying skin, recreating soft tissue coverage for the new breast.[27]

Following completion of expansion, most surgeons delay the second stage of reconstruction for 1 to 4 months to allow for maximal skin growth. At the conclusion of this hiatus, the second procedure is performed, consisting of removal of the expander and placement of the reconstructive implant (Fig. 120.3B). Currently available breast implants include a range of options, including variations in shape (round versus "anatomic" or teardrop configurations), fill material (silicone gel versus saline), and surface configuration (smooth versus textured envelopes). The relative advantages and disadvantages of these options are discussed in the Breast Augmentation section later in this chapter. As the most common option for postmastectomy reconstruction in the United States, the expander-implant approach offers several advantages. The length of the surgical procedures associated with this approach usually are

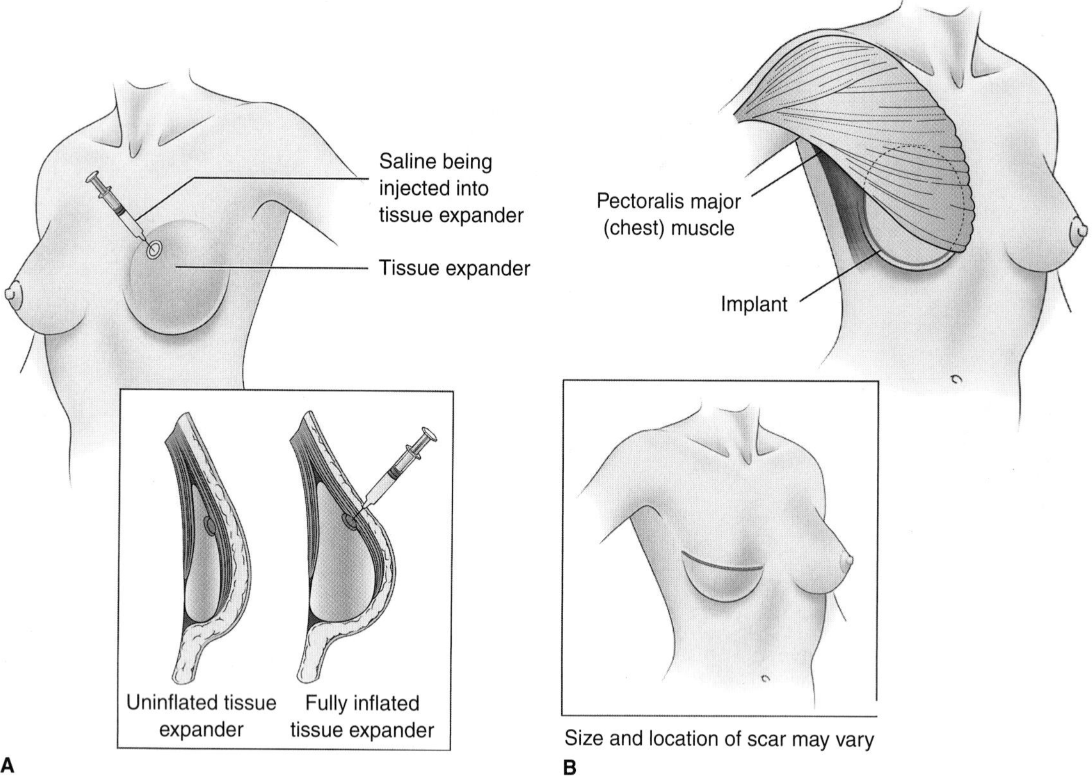

FIGURE 120.3 Expander—implant reconstruction.

relatively brief (often 1 hour or less) and are technically straightforward. Particularly when employed in concert with procedures on the contralateral breast (i.e., breast reduction, mastopexy, or augmentation), resulting symmetry and aesthetic outcomes are relatively good.

Patients considering implant reconstruction should also be mindful of the disadvantages of these procedures. The expander-implant approach usually requires two surgical procedures, multiple visits for expansion, and approximately 4 to 6 months to complete. For patients eager to return to a normal lifestyle following breast cancer treatment, this delay can be particularly frustrating. In addition, tissue expanders and reconstructive implants have been associated with a number of complications. Early in the postoperative period, these devices may be troubled by delays in wound healing, at times resulting in implant exposure and requiring explantation. Implant infections also may necessitate removal of the prosthetic device. Late complications include expander or implant leakage. Also, the development of excessive scar tissue surrounding the implant (termed a *capsular contracture*) can produce a hard, painful, or deformed breast requiring surgical revision.

Autogenous Tissue Reconstruction. A variety of autogenous (natural) tissue options have been described for postmastectomy breast reconstruction. Currently, the most commonly performed of these procedures is the TRAM flap. Originally popularized by Hartrampf et al.,[22] the TRAM flap is most commonly performed as a pedicle muscle flap, that is, the transferred rectus muscle is left partially attached to the costal margin, preserving the superior epigastric artery and vein as the flap's blood supply (Figs. 120.4A and B). In pedicle TRAM reconstruction, the rectus muscle serves as the vascular carrier for a large ellipse of lower abdominal skin and fat. These tissues are tunneled subcutaneously into the mastectomy defect, where they are sculpted into the desired breast size and shape. Meanwhile, the abdominal donor site is closed by reapproximating the anterior rectus sheath and by advancing the remaining superior skin edge of the donor site as a modified abdominoplasty (Fig. 120.4C).

Pedicle TRAM reconstruction offers several benefits. Because the TRAM flap usually provides a generous amount of lower abdominal adipose tissue for breast bulk, implants are rarely needed with this approach. The TRAM flap can be inset and sculpted in a virtually infinite number of ways, giving the reconstructive surgeon considerable latitude in the creation of breast shapes and sizes. Furthermore, in contrast to implant approaches, TRAM reconstruction is a one-stage technique, requiring only a single surgery to recreate the breast mound. An additional advantage of TRAM flaps is their tendency to gain or lose volume in association with weight changes and body mass, thereby maintaining better symmetry than implant reconstructions over time. Among reconstructive surgeons, there appears to be a growing consensus that TRAM flaps produce superior aesthetic results compared with other techniques.

Despite these advantages, TRAM flaps also are associated with several disadvantages. Compared with implant approaches, TRAM reconstruction requires longer operations, hospitalizations, and recovery times. Furthermore, TRAM procedures can produce a range of complications, including partial and total flap loss as a result of vascular compromise of the transferred tissue. Also, occurrences of postoperative abdominal hernias or (more commonly) abdominal wall laxity remain persistent issues for some patients choosing TRAM reconstruction.[28]

Although the pedicle TRAM flap is the most frequently employed option for autogenous tissue breast reconstruction,

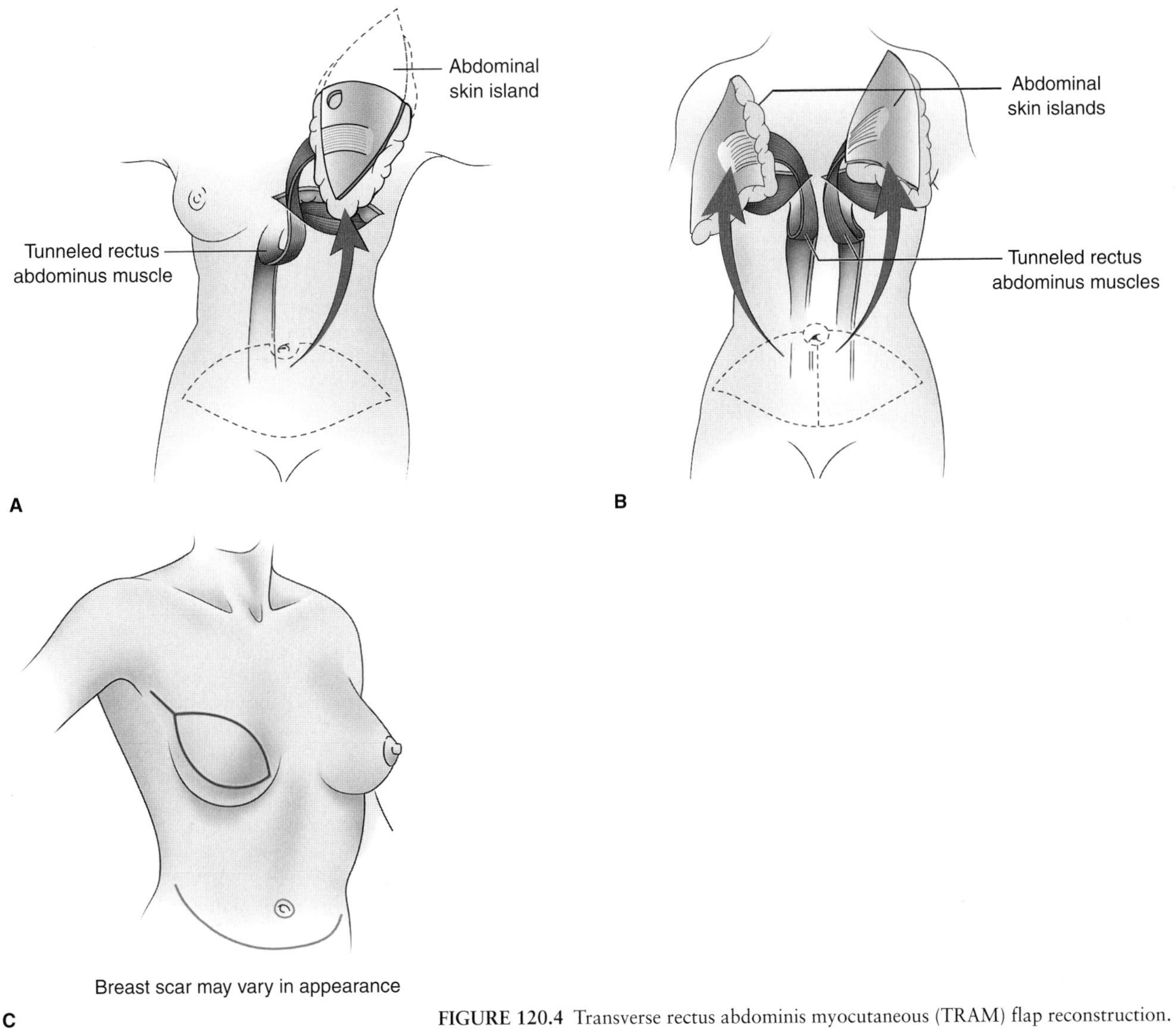

Abdominal skin island

Tunneled rectus abdominus muscle

A

Abdominal skin islands

Tunneled rectus abdominus muscles

B

Breast scar may vary in appearance

C

FIGURE 120.4 Transverse rectus abdominis myocutaneous (TRAM) flap reconstruction.

free tissue transfer has received growing attention as a potentially useful technique for recreating the breast mound. In particular, the free TRAM flap has been promoted by Kroll and Baldwin,[29] Grotting,[30] and others[31] as producing superior results compared with the pedicle version of the flap. With the free TRAM flap, a lower abdominal segment of skin and fat is harvested based on the deep inferior epigastric artery and vein. A small island of rectus abdominis muscle also is included with the flap, mainly to facilitate inclusion of small perforating vessels that travel from the deep inferior epigastric artery and vein into the overlying skin and fat (Fig. 120.5). Using microsurgical techniques, the flap's vascular pedicle is then anastomosed to recipient vessels (usually the thoracodorsal, subscapular, or internal mammary vessels) adjacent to the mastectomy site. In the views of Grotting[30] and other investigators,[29] free TRAM flaps offer the potential advantages of greater flap reliability, superior aesthetics, and preservation of abdominal wall integrity.

Allen and Treece and Allen and Tucker[32] have taken the free TRAM flap a step further with their development of the deep inferior epigastric perforator flap: by meticulously dissecting vascular perforators from the deep inferior epigastric pedicle into the overlying abdominal fat, these investigators have been able to avoid removal of any rectus abdominis muscle with free TRAM harvest, thereby minimizing disruption of

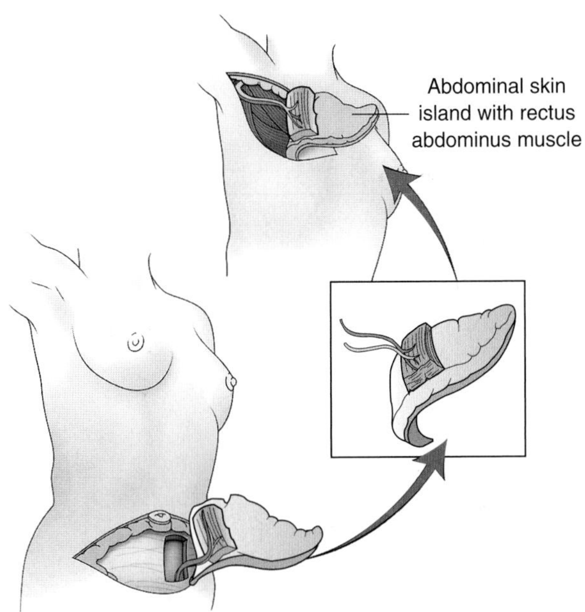

FIGURE 120.5 Free transverse rectus abdominis myocutaneous (TRAM) flap reconstruction.

abdominal wall structures.[31] The free perforator flap concept also has been applied to other donor sites for breast reconstruction, most notably the superior gluteal artery perforator flap.[32 33] Although they appear to avoid the functional deficits associated with muscle flap harvest, perforator flaps (like all free tissue transfers) entail long, technically difficult operations requiring special facilities, equipment, and expertise. Also, because the blood supply for the entire flap depends on two or three microsurgical anastomoses (each usually involving vessels no more than 2 to 3 mm in diameter), there is the potential for complete flap loss in the event of anastomotic thrombosis.

Hybrid" Breast Reconstruction Techniques. As an additional alternative for breast reconstruction, flaps can be used in concert with saline or silicone gel implants. Most commonly, the ipsilateral latissimus dorsi and a segment of overlying skin are harvested as a musculocutaneous pedicle flap and are tunneled anteriorly into the mastectomy defect (Figs. 6A to -C). Although the latissimus dorsi and its associated skin island constitute an extremely reliable flap when used for wound coverage, this approach usually provides insufficient bulk for breast volume. Tissue expanders or implants are often used to address this volume deficiency. The combination of a latissimus dorsi flap and tissue expansion may be particularly appropriate for cases in which the remaining mastectomy skin is of insufficient quality or quantity to tolerate tissue expansion. Following transfer and expansion of a latissimus dorsi musculocutaneous flap, an appropriately sized breast implant usually can be safely placed in a secondary operation.

Nipple-Areolar Reconstruction. Reconstruction of the nipple-areolar complex (NAC) can be accomplished at the conclusion of breast mound reconstruction or at a later date. Following recreation of the mound, many surgeons prefer to allow several months for tissue healing and settling before proceeding with nipple-areolar reconstruction. To recreate the papule, common options usually rely on local skin flaps or a segment of redundant contralateral papule. For the areola, a full-thickness skin graft or tattooing of the surrounding skin can be used.

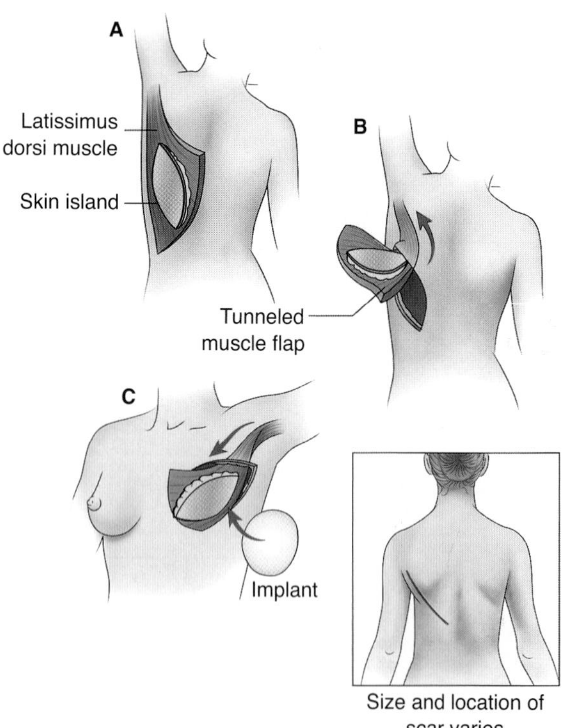

FIGURE 120.6 Latissimus dorsi flap reconstruction.

Breast Reduction (Reduction Mammaplasty)

Because reduction mammaplasty is intended to alleviate functional problems and symptoms of macromastia, this procedure is considered a reconstructive rather than an aesthetic operation. In general, appropriate candidates for reduction mammaplasty are women with macromastia and associated back, neck, or shoulder pain; limitations in daily work or recreational activities; or difficulties obtaining proper fit in bras or other clothing. Although reduction mammaplasty usually is a covered benefit by most health-care payers, patients' symptomatic and functional concerns must be carefully assessed and documented before proceeding with surgery. As noted earlier in this section, patients' preferences and expectations regarding postoperative breast size, shape, and functional results also should be carefully evaluated.

Although a variety of approaches have been described for breast reduction, common surgical options share a number of characteristics. Most techniques of breast reduction resect both breast parenchyma and redundant skin. Also, reduction procedures generally reposition the NAC to a more superior point on the breast mound. To maintain nipple viability and sensation, the NAC usually is mobilized as part of a pedicle of breast parenchyma or dermis. Following dissection of the nipple pedicle and reduction of the surrounding breast skin and parenchyma, the pedicle is transferred superiorly with its vascular and neural supplies intact, while the remaining breast is reapproximated around the nipple pedicle.

In categorizing reduction mammaplasty techniques, surgical options often are described in terms of the nipple pedicle design. For example, the most common approaches rely on an inferiorly or centrally based dermal-parenchymal pedicle to maintain vascular and nerve supplies to the NAC (Figs. 120.7A to C and 120.8A to C).[34–36] In designing skin incisions, traditional methods of reduction often have incorporated a modification of a pattern originally described by Wise.[37] While allowing considerable flexibility in resection of redundant breast skin, the modified Wise pattern produces an inverted T—shaped scar, the inferior portion of which runs along the inframammary fold (IMF). In an effort to eliminate the IMF scar, Lejour[38] and others[39] have described a vertical scar reduction mammaplasty.

Prospective outcome analysis of women undergoing reduction mammaplasty indicate that this surgical intervention produces considerable improvements in somatic pain and in functional status.[40,41] However, patients and providers also should be aware of the potential risks associated with reduction. Complications reported with these procedures include instances of nipple or skin loss, changes in levels of nipple sensation, hypertrophic scarring or keloid formation, contour deformities, and breast asymmetry.

Aesthetic Breast Surgery

Breast Augmentation (Augmentation Mammaplasty)

Augmentation or breast enlargement is one of the most commonly performed aesthetic procedures. Evaluation of patients seeking breast augmentation should follow the guidelines described earlier. Particular attention should be focused on thoroughly assessing several factors, including patient preferences for postoperative breast size and shape, history of breast disease, and physical findings. The preoperative examination

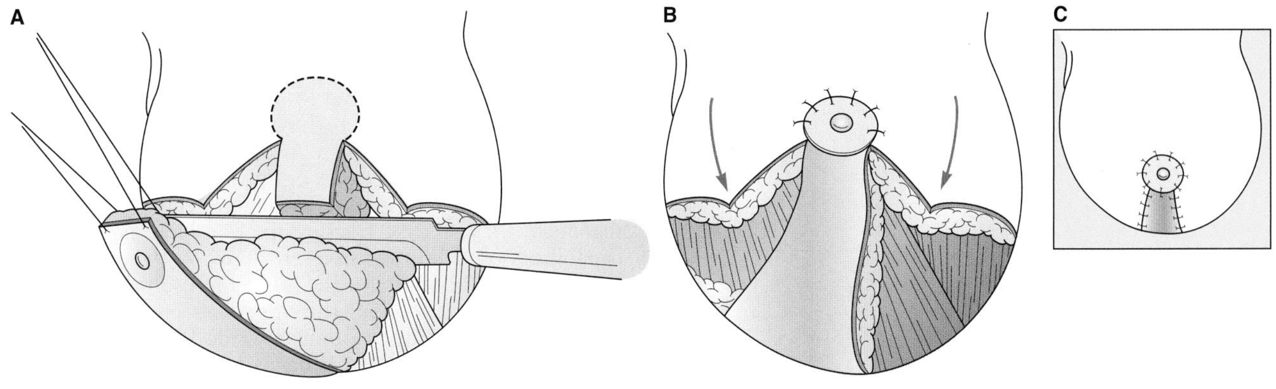

FIGURE 120.7 Inferior pedicle technique reduction mammaplasty.

should evaluate and document any possible breast masses as well as existing breast size, asymmetries, and contour deficits.

In planning augmentation mammaplasty, a variety of approaches and options are available. Decisions regarding these choices are often best reached in consultation with the patient. Implants can be placed through a variety of incisions including periareolar, inframammary fold, and transaxillary approaches. With the advent of endoscopic techniques in recent years, transaxillary augmentation now can be carried out with direct visualization of the implant pocket. This latter approach commonly produces excellent aesthetic results with minimal visible skin scarring.

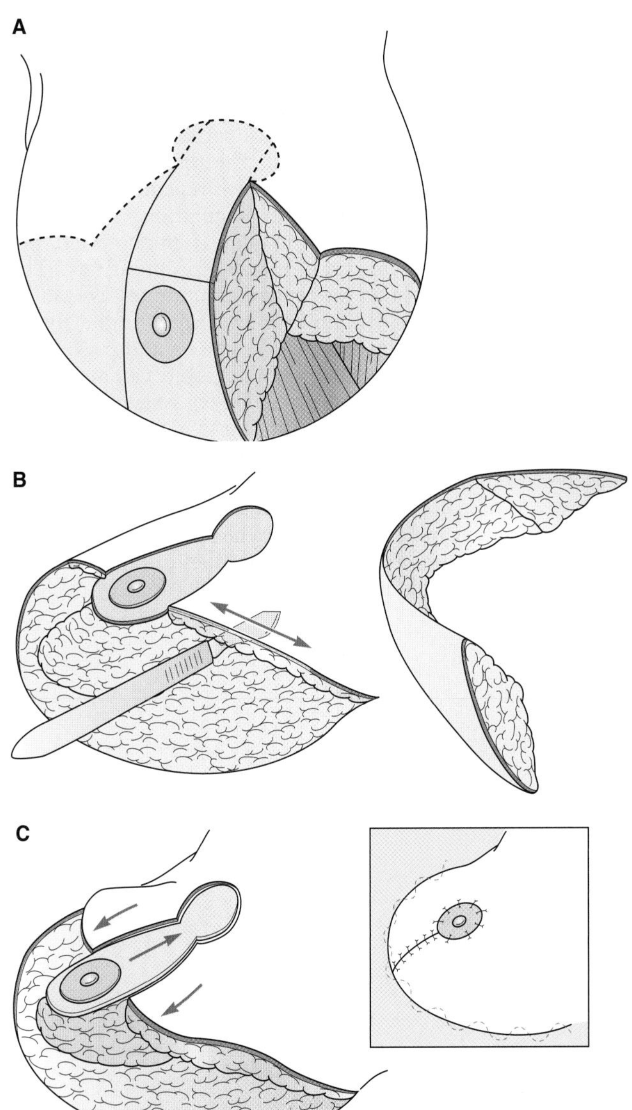

FIGURE 120.8 Central pedicle technique for reduction mammaplasty.

Location of the implant pocket is another critical decision in augmentation mammaplasty. Implants can be placed anterior to the pectoralis major muscle ("subglandular" location) or posterior to the muscle ("subpectoral" location). Subglandular placement usually results in less postoperative pain, but a submuscular implant location may produce lower rates of capsular contracture[42] and may pose fewer difficulties in obtaining subsequent mammograms.[43]

Several choices also exist in selection of implant types. Since the mid-1990s, many surgeons have relied the use of implants with textured surfaces to reduce capsular contracture rates. Although textured surfaces appear to lessen scar tissue contracture,[44] some patients and surgeons assert that, compared with the smooth-walled envelope, the thicker, less pliable textured envelope gives the augmented breast a less natural appearance and feel. With the recent reintroduction of silicone gel–filled implants under research protocols in selected centers, patients and providers also have a choice of implant fill materials. Although gel implants may produce aesthetically superior results compared with saline implants in some patients, diagnosis and surgical treatment of implant rupture may be more challenging with gel devices.

Whatever options are chosen for breast augmentation, surgeons should clearly communicate with patients about the potential risks of these procedures. The most commonly reported complications include implant rupture, capsular contracture, implant infection, contour deformities, and breast asymmetries.[45] Despite the potential for local complications, there currently is no substantial evidence that silicone gel filler material or implant envelopes are associated with increased risk for systemic disease. At this writing, concerns voiced in the early 1990s about adverse "health effects" of silicone breast implants appear to be unfounded.[46]

Mastopexy

Mastopexy (or "breast lift") describes a category of surgical procedures designed to address redundancy or laxity of the breast's skin envelope, a condition termed *ptosis of the breast*. Breast ptosis can be classified as mild, moderate, or severe, depending on the location of the NAC relative to the inframammary fold (Fig. 120.9). Ptosis occurs when an imbalance exists between the volume of breast parenchyma and the

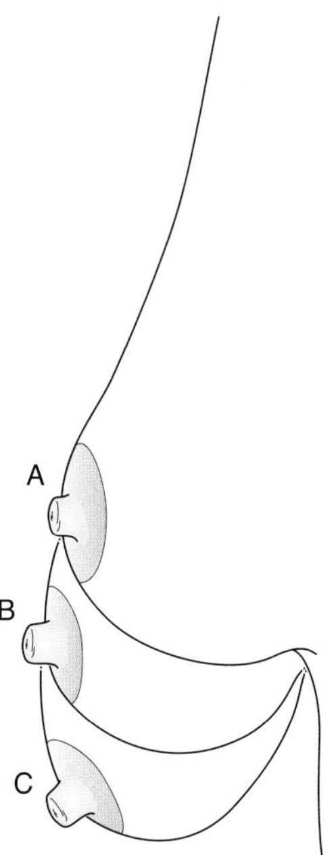

FIGURE 120.9 (*A*) Mild ptosis. (*B*) Moderate ptosis. (C) Severe ptosis.

quantity of overlying skin. Mastopexy procedures usually reduce ptosis by removing redundant breast skin and by relocating the NAC to a more superior position. These goals can be achieved through a variety of skin incisions and excisions, many of which closely resemble techniques described earlier for reduction mammaplasty. Fundamentally, mastopexy differs from breast reduction in that mastopexy removes redundant skin while leaving most or all of the breast parenchyma. Approaches to mastopexy range from minimal periareolar techniques to more extensive skin resections using more extensive vertical incisions (Fig. 120.10A and B). As always, patients considering this procedure must weigh the potential benefits of mastopexy (most notably, diminished ptosis) with the disadvantages (scars and risks of complications) associated with the operation. Although relatively rare, the potential complications of mastopexy closely parallel those described for reduction mammaplasty.

RECONSTRUCTIVE SURGERY OF THE HAND

Advances in plastic surgery have improved our ability to reconstruct hands that have been mutilated by trauma, destroyed by arthritic diseases, or impaired by congenital conditions. Innovations in microvascular techniques, wound management, and rigid fracture fixation have expanded the capabilities of plastic surgeons by allowing them to borrow tissues from other parts of the body and use them to reconstruct complex defects in the upper extremity in a single procedure. These innovations provide limitless technical possibilities for the restoration of hand function and the eventual return of patients as productive members of society. The following sections highlight the technical aspects of hand reconstruction and discuss indications for and applications of these techniques.

Trauma

Replantation

Since the first successful finger replantation by Komatsu and Tamai[47] in 1968, replantation surgery has flourished throughout the world. Thirty years of experience with replantation surgery has improved our understanding of this procedure and has resulted in the development of indication guidelines to ensure that replanted upper extremity parts not only survive, but have acceptable function as well. The absolute indications for replantation (i.e., situations in which replantation should always be attempted) are (a) thumb amputation, (b) multiple finger amputations, (c) pediatric population amputations, and (d) mid-hand, wrist, or distal forearm amputations. The absolute contraindications for replantation are (a) associated life-threatening injuries, (b) multiple-level injury in the amputated part, causing injuries along the vessels and preventing blood flow into the replanted part, and (c) severe contamination of the part, which carries a high probability of systemic infection if replanted. There are other situations in which the benefit of replantation is debatable because outcome data are not available. For example, single finger amputation at zone II (a tight fibroosseous tunnel extending from the insertion of the superficialis tendon at the middle phalange to the first annular pulley) is generally not recommended. Tendon adhesion after zone II replantation may result in a stiff finger, which can interfere with

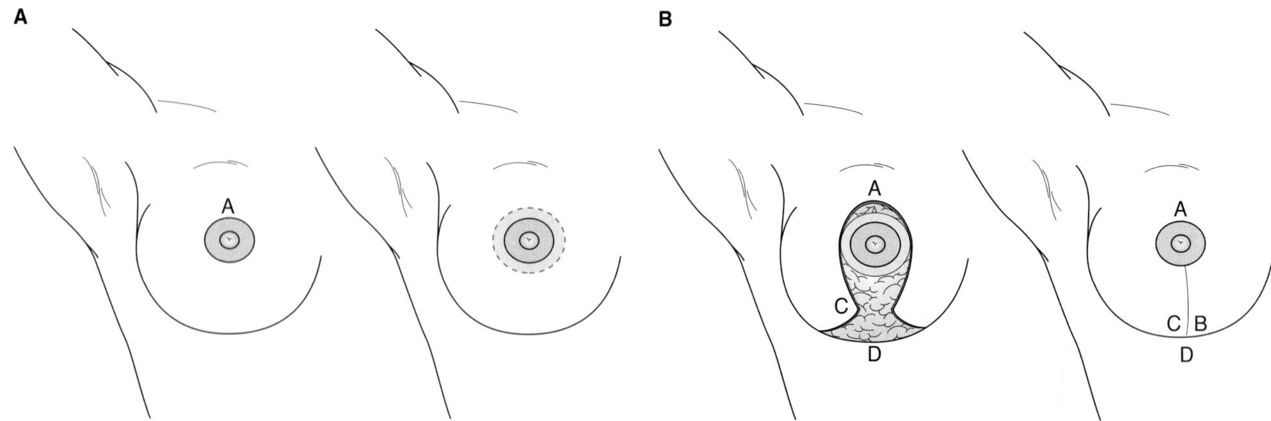

FIGURE 120.10 Mastopexy procedures. (Redrawn from Bostwick J. *Plastic and reconstructive breast surgery*. St. Louis: Quality Medical Publishing, 1990, with permission.)

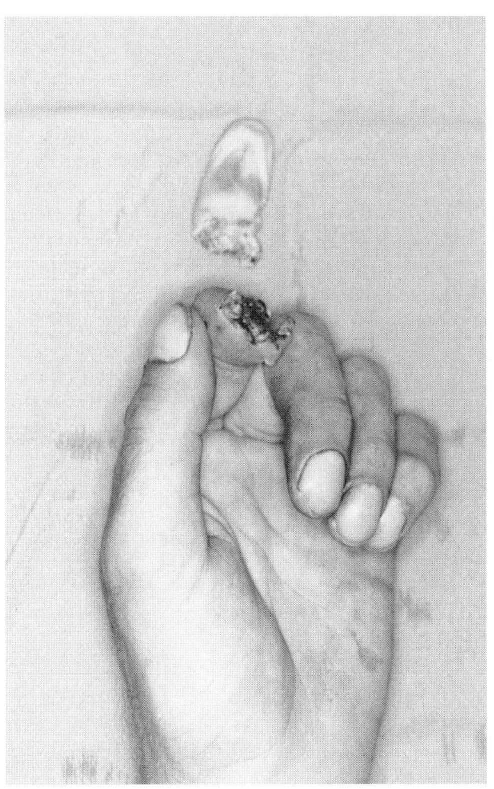

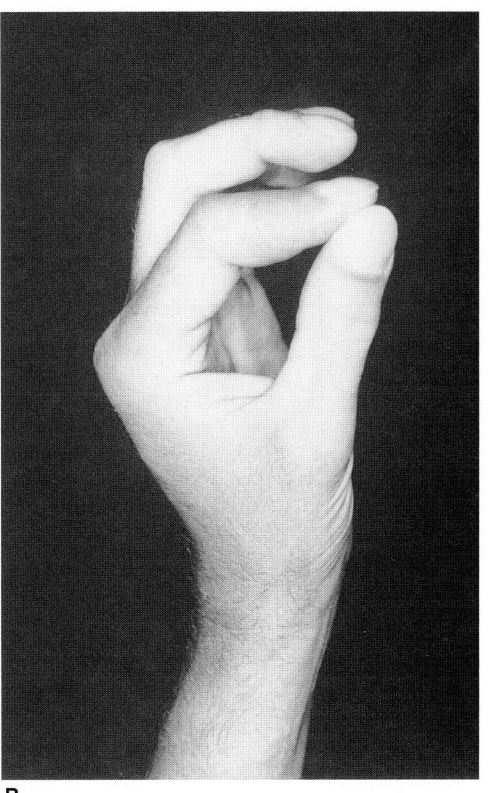

A B

FIGURE 120.11 (*A*) Amputation of the index finger at zone 1 in a mechanic. The patient requested replantation because his work requires fine manipulative tasks. (*B*) Successful replantation with good aesthetic outcome and function.

the overall performance of the hand. On the other hand, single-finger amputation at zone I (distal to the superficialis insertion) is often recommended (Fig. 120.11). A stiff distal interphalangeal joint generally does not cause much impairment, and nerve regeneration to the replanted part is quite rapid because of the short distance to the terminal sensory organs. Furthermore, the aesthetic appearance of zone I replantation is far superior to that of an amputation stump. In the future, the use of patient-related outcome instruments and an increased body of replantation experience among centers will help to define the utility of various digit replantation procedures.

Toe Transfer

When finger replantation is not possible or not successful, patients are left with significant functional loss. Disability is most severe when the thumb has been amputated at or proximal to the metacarpophalangeal joint or when all of the fingers have been amputated in machine injuries. In these cases, toe transfer to the hand is an effective procedure in restoring grasp and pinch function. Although a prosthesis is available to mimic the thumb, lack of sensation is a major drawback and often leads to disuse of the prosthesis. For a patient who has had a thumb amputation at or proximal to the metacarpophalangeal joint, big toe or second toe transfer to the thumb can create a sensate digit that will oppose to the other fingers. Big toe transfer is advantageous because it provides a broad contact surface and closely resembles the shape of the thumb, particularly when the big toe is trimmed and sculptured to match the size of the thumb. However, the disadvantage of the big toe transfer is the conspicuous donor site appearance in the foot and potential gait problems with foot push off if the head of the first metatarsal is taken along with the big toe. For these reasons, the second toe has become the preferred method of transfer in some centers (Fig. 120.12). The disadvantage of the second toe transfer procedure is the slender appearance of the digit as compared to the original thumb, but the donor site appearance is quite acceptable. A recent outcome study, using objective physical measurements and validated outcome questionnaires, demonstrated that toe-to-thumb transfer is an effective procedure in restoring hand function.[48] In addition, patients did not complain of gait difficulty after either big toe or second toe transfer.

One of the most complex problems in hand surgery is the reconstruction of a hand without digits. To create a new hand capable of tripod pinch, plastic surgeons can transfer multiple toes from both feet to the hand (Fig. 120.13). This type of reconstruction can restore function to an otherwise useless hand and has allowed two farmers who were treated at one center to return to heavy farm labor.

Complex Hand Injuries

Although crush injuries to the hand are common, injuries associated with sufficient force to disrupt the structural integrity of the wrist and to sever the blood supply to the hand are uncommon events (Fig. 120.14). Because multiple structures are traumatized in injuries of this kind, a systematic treatment approach is important in salvaging the hand and in restoring its function. Crucial steps in the management of this injury are: (a) ruling out other injuries, (b) aggressive débridement, (c) skeletal fixation, (d) decompression of fascial compartments in the hand, (e) revascularization, (f) tendon repair, (g) nerve repair, and (h) early soft tissue coverage (within 1 week of injury).

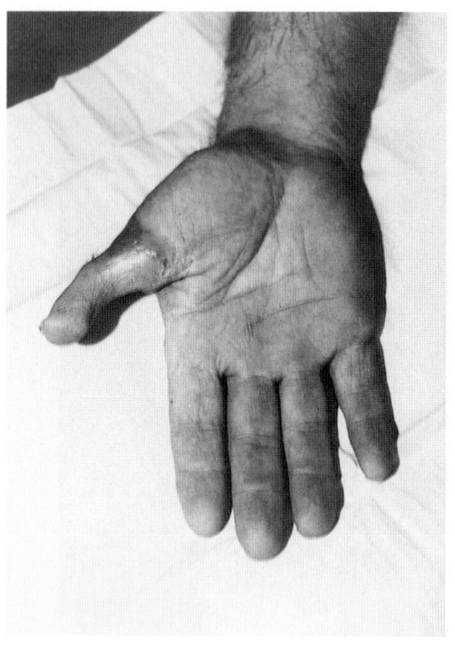

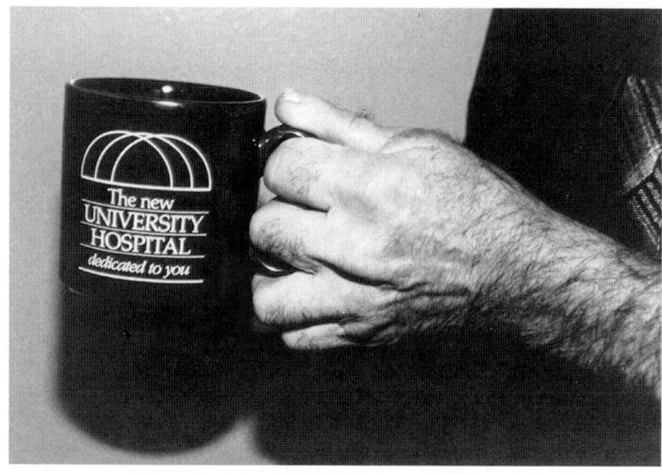

A B

FIGURE 120.12 (*A*) Second-toe transfer for thumb reconstruction in a carpenter. He sustained a thumb amputation at the metacarpophalangeal joint while using a saw at work. (*B*) Good function with restoration of fine pinch. The patient returned to work as a carpenter 3 months after the toe reconstruction.

Ruling Out Other Injuries

In devastating trauma, attention is often focused on the obvious injury, and injuries to other organ systems may be ignored. In a review of 1,100 patients referred for emergent microsurgery over a 7-year period, investigators found nine cases (0.8%) of unrecognized life-threatening injuries that required abandonment of the microsurgical procedures.[49] Therefore, systematic trauma evaluation and ruling out other associated injuries should precede treatment of the hand injury.

Débridement

Severe crush and blast injuries are associated with large zones of injury, and the wounds may be contaminated with foreign materials such as grease or paint, as in printing-press injuries. In these cases, aggressive débridement is important in preventing infection. Except for critical structures that include nerves and tendons, all devitalized soft tissues and bone fragments must be excised. The concept of radical débridement has been

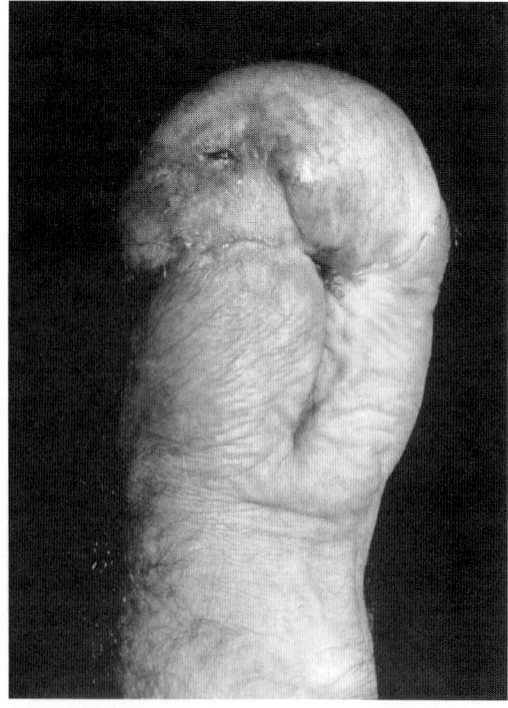

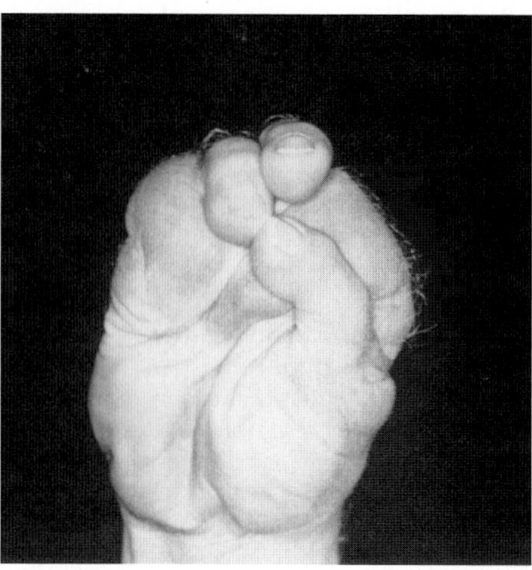

FIGURE 120.13 (*A*) A farmer who lost all his fingers when he was injured by a corn picker. A groin skin flap was used to cover the exposed metacarpal heads. (*B*) A second toe was removed from one foot to reconstruct the thumb, and the second and third toes were removed together from the other foot to reconstruct the fingers. Note the good opposition of the thumb and acceptable flexion of the digits. The patient returned to work on his dairy farm after the hand reconstruction.

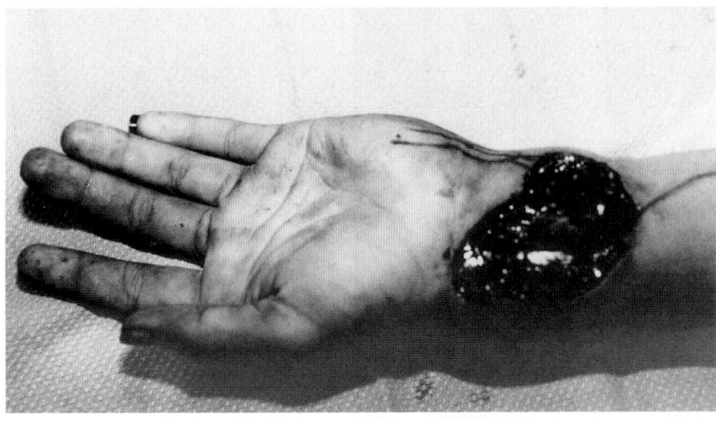

A

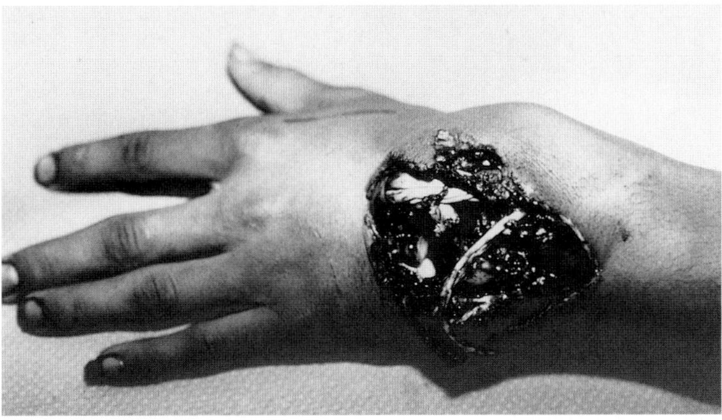

B

FIGURE 120.14 (*A*) Accidental shotgun blast injury in a 16-year-old boy. Both the radial and ulnar arteries were ruptured, and the hand was ischemic. The wrist was destroyed, and multiple tendons and nerves were severed. (*B*) Volar wrist wound. Markings show incision lines for ulnar artery exposure.

shown to decrease wound infection and improve success of microvascular reconstruction.[50]

Skeletal Fixation

After débridement, the next priority is to stabilize the wrist and to rigidly fix hand fractures. A stable wrist provides a platform for repairing other injured structures. If the crush injury is associated with comminuted fractures of multiple carpal bones and rupture of the intercarpal ligaments, wrist fusion may be the best option because it is often impossible to reconstitute the normal anatomy of the distal and proximal carpal rows in face of severe comminution of the carpal bones. To avoid possible bone graft contamination with primary wrist fusion, external fixators are placed for provisional fixation during the initial débridement. Definitive wrist fusion with bone grafting is performed after adequate débridements and during the flap coverage procedure. Two 2.7-mm fixator pins are placed through an incision along the radial index metacarpal, and two proximal 3.5-mm pins are placed into the radius using an incision along the radial border of the distal radius, between the brachioradialis and the extensor carpi radialis longus. The superficial radial nerve, which lies under the brachioradialis, is dissected free and retracted away from the pins. External fixator rods are then secured to the pins with nuts and screws. If the wound is clean during the second-look procedure at 24 or 48 hours, total wrist fusion is then undertaken (Fig. 120.15). Otherwise, the external fixator is left in place until the wound is suitable for fusion using internal plating and cancellous bone grafts. This stable skeletal fixation allows early hand therapy, usually instituted on postinjury day 7 when tissue edema is subsiding.

Revascularization

In a crush injury of the wrist, the zone of injury can be extensive. Use of vein grafts is essential in performing the arterial anastomosis away from the zone of injury. The ulnar artery is chosen for repair because it is the dominant artery in most patients and because it can be exposed readily in the hypothenar area. If the ulnar artery is contused in the palm, distal anastomosis can be performed to the superficial palmar arch. Because soft tissue bridges are often present, venous outflow is not a problem and venous anastomosis is not necessary.

Decompression of Fascial Compartments

Increased edema associated with crush injuries often raises the compartmental pressures in the intrinsic muscle compartments and in the carpal tunnel. Prior reviews have shown a high incidence of ischemia and resultant fibrosis of the intrinsic muscles following crushing trauma to the hand.[51] Consequently, surgeons perform prophylactic carpal tunnel releases and intrinsic muscle decompressions in severe crush injuries of this kind.

Soft Tissue Coverage

After aggressive débridement, a soft tissue defect is often present around the wrist. A split-thickness autograft is placed over the vein graft to prevent desiccation. Other open wounds can be covered temporarily with homografts. If wrist fusion is undertaken during the second-look procedure, primary wound closure can be achieved. For residual wound defects, split-thickness autografts are used to cover the exposed muscle bellies. However, if tendons or nerves are exposed, coverage with either fasciocutaneous or muscle free flaps will allow

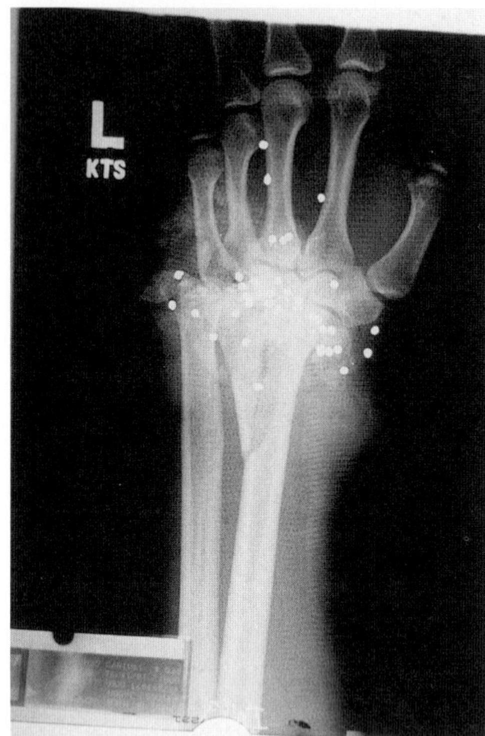

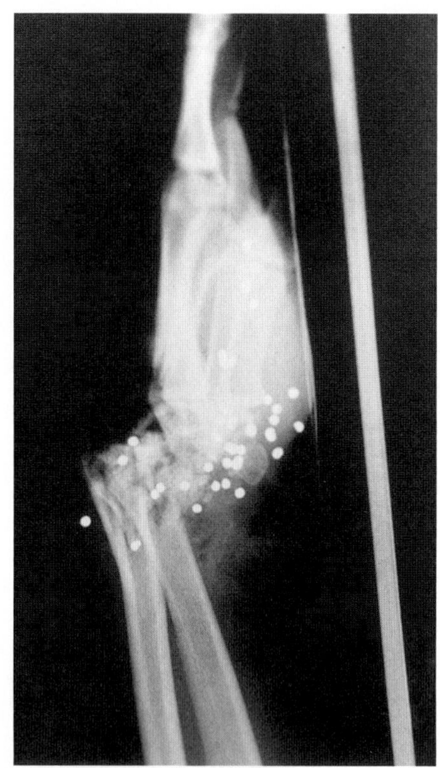

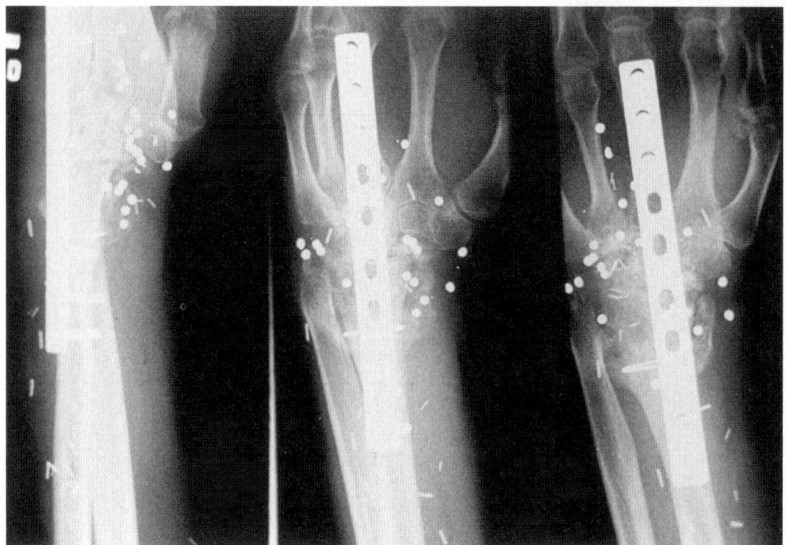

FIGURE 120.15 (*A* and *B*) Note destruction of the wrist joint, in addition to comminuted fractures of the distal ulna and radius. (C) Total wrist fusion was performed 48 hours after the initial injury.

earlier tendon mobilization and prevent tendon adhesions. Definitive early wound coverage is important in protecting vital structures and avoiding wound colonization with bacteria (Fig. 120.16).

Nerve Repair

When nerves are crushed, the delineation between viable and nonviable nerve fascicles is difficult to assess in the acute setting. Therefore, the traditional approach is to delay the nerve grafting procedures until 2 or 3 months after injury. To prevent retraction of the nerve ends, we suture the nerve ends to the surrounding soft tissues. However, secondary nerve grafting is often difficult because of the amount of scar in the wound. One way to primarily graft the nerve injury at the expense of more aggressive resection of the traumatized nerve ends.

In conclusion, rigid skeletal fixation, revascularization using vein grafts, and immediate wound coverage are crucial factors in successful limb salvage.

Congenital Anomalies

Syndactyly

Syndactyly is a condition in which the fingers are fused. It can be classified as complete or incomplete. Complete syndactyly is the union of the digits extending to the distal phalanx. Incomplete syndactyly is the union of the digits proximal to the distal phalanx but distal to the normal webbing at the midproximal phalanx. Syndactyly is further categorized as simple or complex. In simple syndactyly, there is no bony union between the digits, whereas complex syndactyly includes bony union.

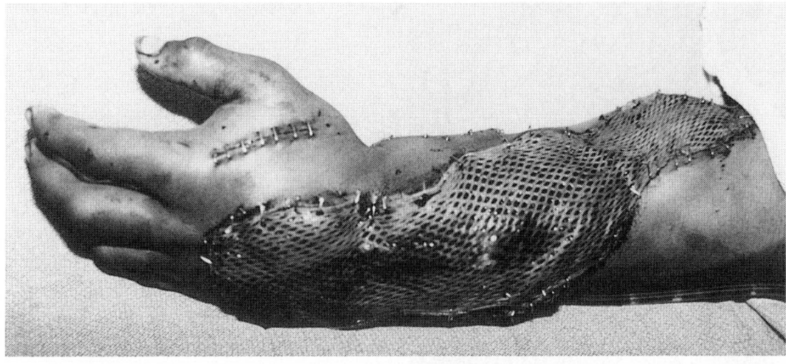

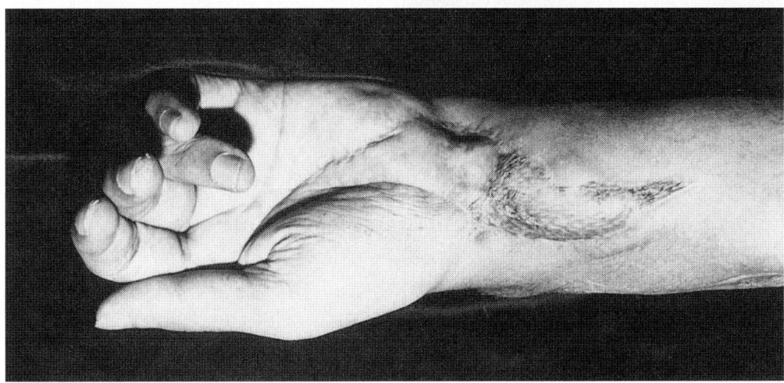

FIGURE 120.16 (*A*) A free rectus muscle was used for immediate coverage of the reconstructed wrist and tendons. (*B*) The hand was salvaged, and the patient has acceptable hand function after secondary nerve and tendon reconstruction.

Typically, syndactyly can be separated when the child is 1year of age. Surgery should be performed earlier if syndactyly affects the thumb–index finger or ring–little finger web space and causes deviation of the shorter digits during growth. Separating the fingers requires meticulous design of the skin flaps, and the dorsal skin flap is most crucial to creating a web space that is not prone to contracture (Fig. 120.17). Distally, triangular skin flaps are designed to drape the sides of the fingers. A full-thickness skin graft from the groin is often required to cover open areas in the fingers.

Thumb Duplication

Although thumb duplication does not often cause a functional problem for the child, the presence of this prominent hand malformation can have a significant impact on the child's psychosocial development. Surgery can be undertaken when the child is about 2 years old to prevent progressive deviation of the thumb during growth. Thumb duplication can be classified into seven groups, depending on the level of the duplication. Type I consists of a bifid distal phalanx, whereas type II is a complete duplication of the distal phalanx. Types III and IV involve the proximal phalanx, and Types V and VI involve the metacarpal. Type VII is triphalangeal thumb or a thumb with three phalanges. Usually the radial, less developed thumb is removed. Retention of the ulnar thumb has the added advantage of preserving the important stabilizing ulnar collateral ligament. The surgery requires a delicate reconstruction of the bone, ligament, and tendon structures to sculpture the remaining thumb as normally as possible (Fig. 120.18). After the immediate postsurgical period, these patients are followed once a year to evaluate potential growth abnormality.

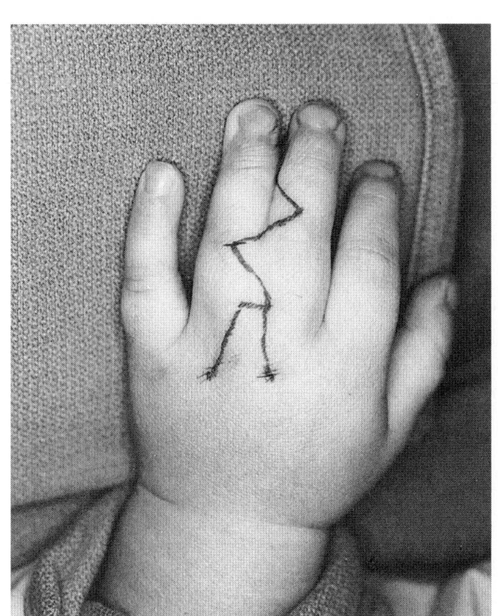

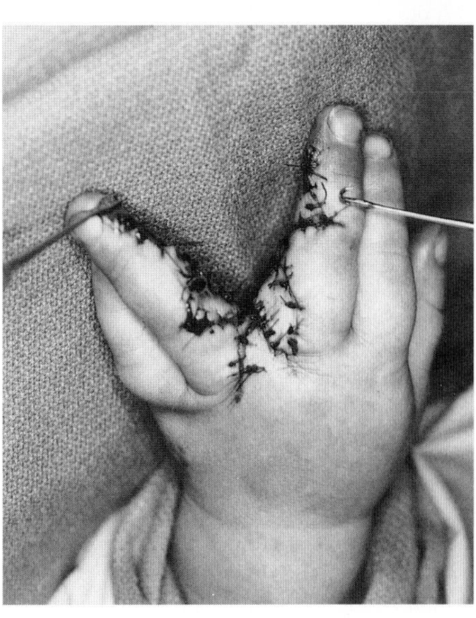

FIGURE 120.17 (*A*) A simple, complete syndactyly in a 1-year-old child. Note the design of the dorsal skin flap to reconstruct the web space and the interdigitating distal skin flaps. (*B*) Immediate postoperative photograph of the syndactyly release.

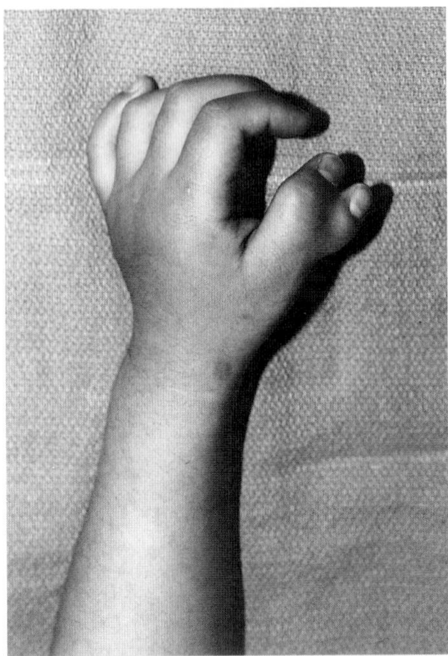

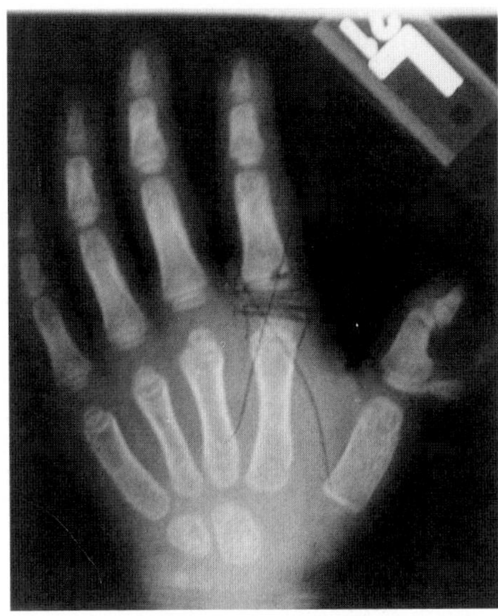

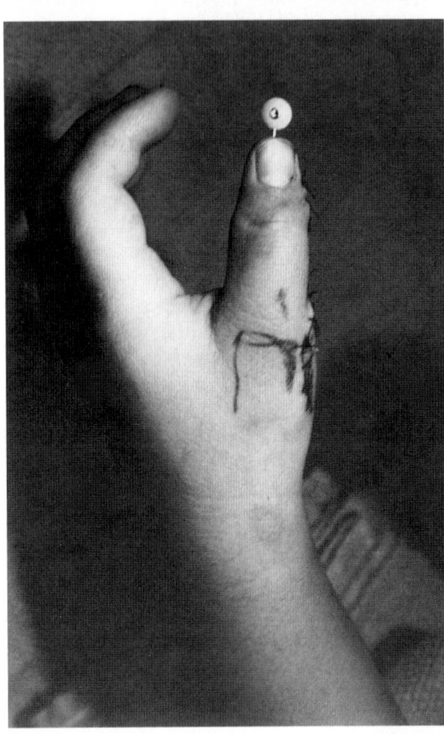

FIGURE 120.18 (*A*) Wassel type 3 duplication in a 2-year-old child. (*B*) The radial digit was hypoplastic and was removed. (C) Intraoperative picture shows the aesthetically pleasing reconstructed thumb.

Hypoplasia and Aplasia of the Thumb

The thumb contributes about 50% of hand function and is important in pinch and grip. Reconstruction of the underdeveloped thumb is critical in improving hand function for the child. Hypoplasia of the thumb can be classified into five grades, and treatment options are often based on this classification. Grade I consists of minor hypoplasia; all components of the thumb are present, but the thumb is smaller than normal. Grade II consists of adduction contracture of the first web space and laxity of the ulnar collateral ligament at the metacarpophalangeal joint; the thenar musculature is hypoplastic but the skeletal framework of the thumb is normal. Grade III includes severe hypoplasia of the thumb with absent intrinsic muscles and underdeveloped extrinsic tendons; the skeletal framework is hypoplastic and the carpometacarpal joint is vestigial. Grade IV is characterized by a floating, nonfunctional thumb (pouce flottant), with soft tissue attachment of the thumb at the metacarpophalangeal joint of the index finger. Grade V is defined by total absence of the thumb. Grade I hypoplasia does not require treatment and grades III, IV, and V require index pollicization (reconstructing a thumb using the index finger) for optimal function (Fig. 120.19). In grade II, the thumb can be reconstructed by using a combination of tendon, joint, and soft tissue procedures.

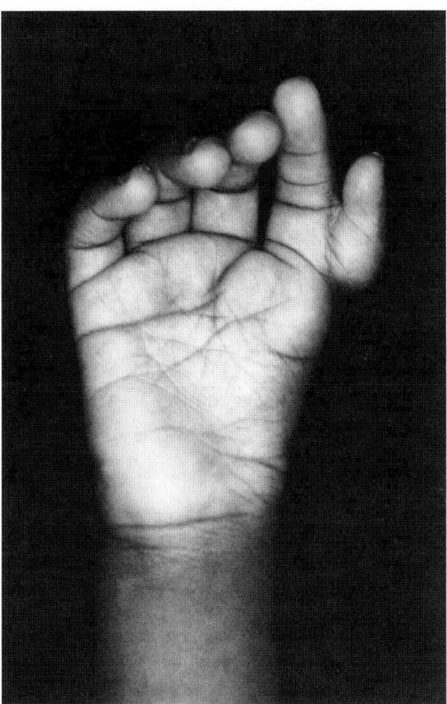

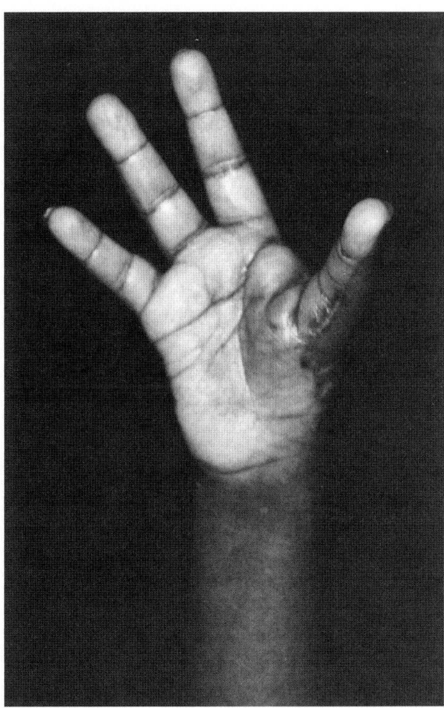

FIGURE 120.19 (*A*) Absence of a thumb in a 2-year-old child. Note the floating thumb attached to the index finger. (*B*) Three months after index pollicization, the child is able to use the new thumb for grasp and fine pinch.

Rheumatoid Arthritis

Rheumatoid arthritis (RA) is a crippling disease that severely affects the quality of life for millions of Americans. RA is postulated to be an autoimmune disease mediated by inflammatory cells that attack the synovial tissues in the body. Persistent synovitis in the joints causes erosion of the articular surfaces and disrupts their soft tissue supports.

Because the hand is often damaged by RA, effective surgical treatment of hand deformities can improve patient function and restore independence. The goals of surgery for the rheumatoid hand include: (a) pain control, (b) improvement or restoration of function, (c) prevention of disease progression, and (d) aesthetic improvement. To accomplish these goals, the surgeon must have good rapport with both the rheumatologist and the patient as priorities of treatment are determined. By listening to patients with RA describe their impairments and their goals, the surgeon can gain insight into the surgical plan that will offer the patient the most benefit.

Surgical treatment can be classified as preventive, corrective, or salvage.[52] Preventive procedures include tenosynovectomy to avoid tendon rupture and synovectomy to ameliorate ongoing joint destruction from erosive synovitis in the joints. Corrective procedures include tendon transfers for tendon ruptures and nerve decompression for carpal tunnel syndrome. Salvage procedures consist of joint arthroplasty and joint fusion.

A common hand deformity in RA consists of subluxation and ulnar deviation of the fingers at the level of the metacarpophalangeal joints (MPJs) (Fig. 120.20). Synovitis at the

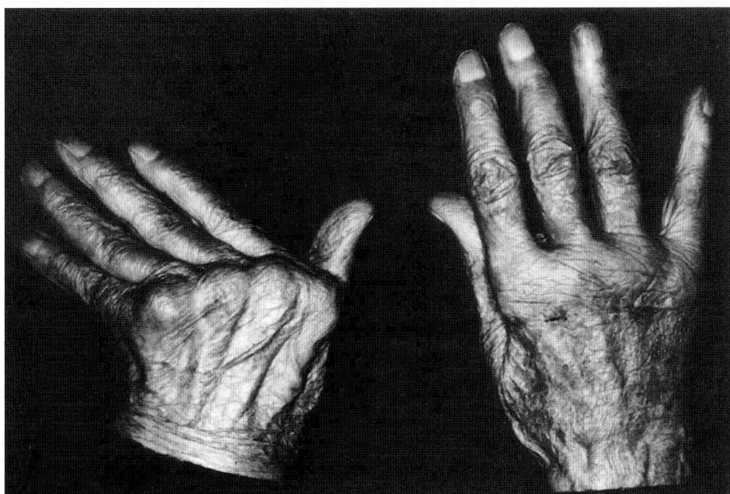

FIGURE 120.20 Severe destruction of the metacarpophalangeal joints with ulnar deviation of the fingers of the left hand. Note restoration of normal finger alignment of the right hand after Swanson metacarpophalangeal joint arthroplasty.

MPJs distends the joints and attenuates the supporting ligaments. Wrist destruction in RA contributes to the radial deviation of the metacarpals, which accentuates the ulnar deviation of the fingers. With progressive MPJ disease, patients have great difficulty opening their hands because of subluxation of the MPJs and difficulty with fine pinch because of the ulnar deviation of the fingers. In addition to pain at the MPJs secondary to their worn articular surfaces, RA patients often complain of the aesthetic appearance of their hands.

The Swanson metacarpophalangeal joint arthroplasty (SMPA) is an effective procedure that will meet all four goals of RA surgery. By replacing the arthritic joints with prosthetic spacers and realigning the soft tissue envelope around the MPJs, surgeons are able to markedly improve function and enhance the aesthetic appearance of RA hands. A recent systematic overview of the world's literature on this procedure showed that SMPA is an effective procedure in improving the health-related quality of life for RA patients.[53]

AESTHETIC SURGERY

Plastic surgery is a discipline that adapts broad surgical principles to a multitude of unique clinical problems by altering form and function. Plastic surgery not only restores physical function, it also enhances a patient's body image and self-esteem. In no other area of surgery is this truer than in aesthetic surgery. A blepharoplasty not only may improve the appearance of baggy, tired eyes, but also may treat visual field defects caused by eyelid ptosis. A rhinoplasty can improve the outward appearance of a nose as well as the nasal airflow.

Aesthetic surgery requires meticulous attention to detail, careful patient selection, rigorous procedural planning, and precise execution of technically challenging procedures. If patients are carefully selected and their goals are realistic, then the chances for a successful outcome are good. However, if a patient is poorly selected, then a technically successful operation may be a dismal failure in the eyes of the patient. The aesthetic surgeon not only must diagnose the clinical deformity, but also must carefully evaluate the patient's expectations and motivations for surgery. Through the application of sound surgical principles and technical expertise, the aesthetic surgeon can experience life-long career and personal satisfaction.

Cosmetic Procedures for the Head and Neck

Brow Lift

Brow ptosis is a natural consequence of the biologic process of aging. If left uncorrected, patients can appear angry or older than their chronologic age. If severe, brow ptosis may cause visual field obstruction; correction of this deformity can produce dramatic functional and aesthetic improvements. Patients frequently present with a chief complaint of looking tired or angry and request a blepharoplasty. In many cases, however, these patients require a brow lift to treat brow ptosis rather than a blepharoplasty.

Correction of brow ptosis can be achieved with either an open or endoscopic approach. The traditional open approach requires a long transcoronal incision with resection of excess scalp or forehead. Unfortunately, this approach results in a long scar and anesthesia of the scalp and forehead. In addition, an open brow lift in male patients with a receding hairline requires resection of hair-bearing scalp, which is an undesirable outcome. To reduce these complications, the endoscopic brow lift was developed and has become the primary approach for repair of brow ptosis.[54] The endoscopic brow lift requires only 3 to 5 1-cm incisions behind the hairline to gain access to the forehead and glabellar rhytids, producing less of an aesthetic deformity. There is also evidence to suggest that the endoscopic approach produces a more lasting result than the traditional approach.[55] As a result, there is a significant reduction in the amount of scarring that is needed for performance of a brow lift and reduced problems related to forehead and scalp anesthesia.

Endoscopic and open brow lifts may be performed under local or general anesthesia. Patients are marked preoperatively in the upright position. The desired brow position is at the level of the orbital rim in male patients and 1 cm above the orbital rim in female patients. During an open brow lift, a coronal incision is made and the entire forehead is mobilized in a subgaleal or subperiosteal plane down to the orbital rim. The supraorbital and supratrochlear nerves are dissected free of surrounding tissues and preserved. The corrugator and procerus muscles are resected if prominent glabellar rhytids are present. The forehead is then redraped posteriorly, the redundant scalp is resected, and the wound is closed. In an endoscopic brow lift, incisions are made within the hair-bearing scalp at the midpupillary line and over the temporal fossa. The entire forehead flap is elevated under endoscopic guidance, the procerus and corrugator muscles are resected as necessary, and the forehead is retracted posteriorly. The forehead and brow are then secured in their new position with nonabsorbable sutures attached to absorbable screws or plates or passed through cortical tunnels.[54–55]

Postoperatively, patients are instructed to avoid vigorous physical exercise for at least 6 weeks. Bruising and swelling are anticipated for the first 2 to 3 weeks following the procedure. The final result is not expected for at least 6 to 8 weeks following the procedure.

Rhytidectomy

The deleterious effects of aging, gravity, sun exposure, and smoking are particularly evident on the face. Ultraviolet radiation and tobacco use produce fine facial wrinkling and skin laxity as a result of poor elasticity. Aging and gravity result in gradual relaxation of the facial retaining ligaments producing midfacial ptosis, deepened nasolabial folds, "jowling" along the mandibular border, and redundancy of cervical skin.[56] Old family photographs are constant reminders of a more youthful appearance with high cheekbones and smooth skin. However, as the aging process marches on, patients may lose self-confidence and self-esteem in social, political, and business situations, encouraging them to seek facial rejuvenation surgery. If the patients are selected appropriately and the surgery is carefully planned and executed, the results will be gratifying for both patient and surgeon.[57]

During the preoperative evaluation, the patient's expectations and motivations are carefully evaluated and addressed. Surgeons need to be cautious of patients whose concerns about their appearance are out of proportion to their physical deformity. Under these circumstances, a perfectly designed and performed operation may still have a dismal outcome in the eyes of the patient.

Patients who smoke are at a significantly increased risk for developing postoperative complications, including skin flap necrosis, infection, or wound dehiscence, and are consequently instructed to quit. Older patients with coexisting medical illnesses are referred to a general practitioner for optimization of their medical condition preoperatively. If the patient is deemed a moderate or high risk for general anesthesia because of medical comorbidities, then the operation may be postponed until those medical conditions are optimized or cancelled if the risk of anesthesia is too high.

Younger patients (40 to 50 years old) with good skin quality, mild midfacial ptosis, and early "jowling" may benefit from a minimally invasive facelift. This operation is typically combined with an endoscopic brow lift to provide upper and lower facial rejuvenation with minimal scarring. The operation is performed under local or general anesthesia. Bilateral temporal and superior buccal sulcus incisions are made. The temporal fossa dissection is carried down to the level of the superficial layer of the deep temporal fascia. Under endoscopic guidance, the superficial layer of the deep temporal fascia is then incised to expose the temporal fat pad. The dissection then proceeds caudally until the zygomatic arch is identified. A subperiosteal plane of dissection provides access to the midface while preserving the integrity of the frontal branch of the facial nerve. The subperiosteal plane of dissection is continued into the midface with care taken to avoid the infraorbital nerves. The masseter is mobilized from its lateral attachments. The superior buccal sulcus incisions are made, and a midface subperiosteal dissection is performed under both direct visualization and endoscopic guidance. Once the dissection is completed, the entire midface is suspended in the desired position with 2-0 polydioxanone (PDS) sutures spanning from the superficial layer of the deep temporal fascia to the midface periosteum. Symmetry of the suspension is then confirmed and the wounds are closed in layers. This technique will nicely correct midface ptosis, mild jowling, and early nasolabial fold prominence, but if significant skin laxity exists, then a traditional rhytidectomy is required.[54,58]

In patients who require resection of excess skin, a traditional rhytidectomy can be performed under local or general anesthesia. The skin incision is made over the temporal fossa 4 to 5 cm cephalad to the root of the helix and extended caudally toward the apex of the ear. The incision is then extended anterior to the ear, behind the tragus, around the base of the earlobe into the retroauricular sulcus, across the mastoid, and caudally along the anterior hairline of the neck. The skin flap is then elevated just superficial to the superficial musculoaponeurotic system (SMAS) and platysma. This plane of dissection maintains a thin layer of subcutaneous fat on the skin flap to preserve viability, while avoiding injury to the facial nerve, parotid gland, and jugular vein. The flaps are elevated medially to the nasolabial fold in the face and to the midline in the neck. Occasionally a platysmal diastasis may exist which creates an obtuse cervicomental angle and prominent neck. Under these circumstances, a platysmal plication may be performed through a 2- to 3-cm submental incision to correct the diastasis and improve the appearance of the neck. Once the skin flaps are completely elevated, many plastic surgeons then mobilize the lateral SMAS and platysma to improve control of facial and cervical tightening, while reducing the tension on the skin closure. The SMAS and platysma are placed under tension and secured to create the desired facial appearance. The skin flaps are then redraped posteriorly, the patient is examined for symmetry, and a skin resection is performed. Hemostasis is obtained through judicious use of bipolar electrocautery. The wounds are closed in layers and a pressure dressing is applied. Drains are typically used in the face and neck.[59–63]

Postoperatively, the patient is evaluated in the recovery room for any evidence of a hematoma or facial nerve injury. It is crucial to identify a hematoma early to avoid overlying skin necrosis. Facial nerve injuries occur in only 2% to 3% of cases. On the first postoperative day, the pressure dressings and drains are removed and the patient is examined for evidence of a late hematoma, unrecognized facial nerve injury, or compromised skin flap. Patients should expect to have significant swelling and bruising for at least 2 weeks following the procedure. The final postoperative result is not realized until approximately 6 months following the procedure (Fig. 120.21).

Blepharoplasty

Eyelid surgery may be performed to correct functional or aesthetic deformities. Excessive skin and fat of the eyelids can give the patient an angry, aged, or tired look and may cause visual field obstruction. Older patients typically present with redundant skin and fine wrinkling, whereas younger patients commonly complain of persistent bags under their eyes or fine wrinkling ("crow's feet") at the lateral canthus. Treatment of each clinical entity requires a unique approach based on the diagnosis and presentation.[64] All patients being evaluated for blepharoplasty require a complete ophthalmologic examination preoperatively to evaluate visual acuity, upper eyelid ptosis, exophthalmos, lower eyelid laxity, and symptoms of "dry" eye. Meticulous attention to details is critical for the successful outcome of blepharoplasty surgery.[55] If there is lower lid laxity preoperatively, and a standard blepharoplasty is performed, the patient may develop a lower lid ectropion postoperatively. Symptoms of dry eye can also be significantly worsened by a blepharoplasty.

Once the diagnosis has been made and an operative plan has been formulated, the operation can be performed under local or general anesthesia. Older patients frequently require skin excisions and removal or repositioning of orbital fat. The blepharoplasty incisions are designed preoperatively with the patient in the upright position. Local anesthesia with epinephrine is then infiltrated for pain control and hemostasis. The upper eyelid blepharoplasty then begins with an elliptical excision of upper eyelid skin and orbicularis oculi muscle. Small openings are made in the orbital septum to gain access to the two compartments of periorbital fat. A conservative fat resection is performed to avoid a postoperative hollowed-out appearance. The skin is then redraped and the wounds are closed in a single layer with running subcuticular 6-0 Prolene sutures. If an upper lid blepharoplasty is being performed in conjunction with a brow lift, the brow lift should be performed first, so that the amount of excess upper eyelid skin can be determined after the brow has been elevated.

The traditional lower eyelid blepharoplasty begins with a subciliary incision. The dissection is then carried deep to the orbicularis oculi muscle until the orbital septum is identified. The orbital septum is then divided to gain access to the three compartments of periorbital fat in the lower lid. Fat may be resected in cases of prominent herniation, but overresection must be avoided. A trend in blepharoplasty surgery has emphasized periorbital fat repositioning rather than resection. Simply repositioning the herniated periorbital fat over the inferior orbital rim, rather than resecting fat, can dramatically improve the appearance of the lower eyelids.[65] Once the periorbital fat has been resected or repositioned, the skin/muscle flap is redraped superiorly and the redundant tissue is excised. The lower eyelid wounds are closed with interrupted sutures of 6-0 silk. Ancillary procedures may also be necessary to improve the position of the lower eyelid, including a medial canthoplasty, a lateral canthoplasty, or horizontal lid shortening. If a lower lid blepharoplasty is being performed in conjunction with a rhytidectomy, the rhytidectomy should be performed first, so that the amount of excess lower eyelid skin can be determined after the facial soft tissues have been elevated.

In younger patients, the tired appearance of the lower eyelids is commonly a result of excessive or herniated periorbital fat. A lower lid blepharoplasty through a transconjunctival approach allows removal or repositioning of the periorbital fat without an external scar. The conjunctiva is divided transversely 1 mm above the sulcus to gain access to the orbital septum. The septum is divided and the periorbital fat is removed or repositioned from all three compartments. The wound is then allowed to heal by secondary intention, allowing rejuvenation of the lower lids without an external incision.

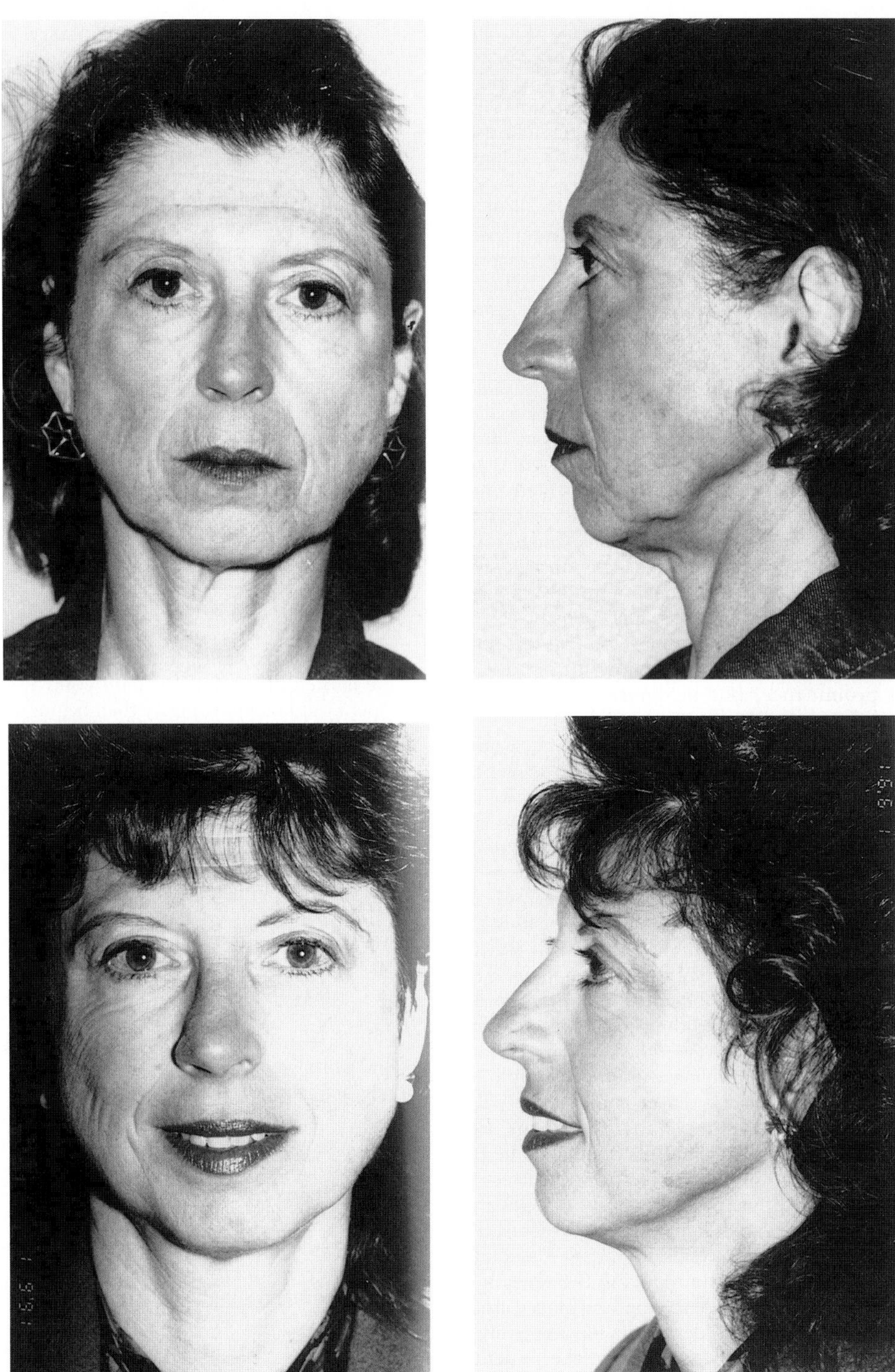

FIGURE 120.21 Rhytidectomy with superficial musculoaponeurotic system resection, platysmal plication, and endoscopic brow lift. (*A* and *B*) Preoperative appearance. (*C* and *D*) Postoperative appearance. Note the improved brow position above the orbital rim, malar prominence, flattened nasolabial folds, reduced "jowling" along the mandibular border, and improved cervicomental angle.

Postoperatively, patients are evaluated in the recovery room for corneal abrasions, changes in visual acuity, or hematomas, which may require emergent intervention. No vigorous physical exercise is permitted during the early postoperative period. Artificial tears are used to maintain appropriate lubrication. Sutures are removed 5 days postoperatively. Patients are informed that they will be bruised and swollen for approximately 2 weeks and that it will be approximately 6 to 8 weeks before the final result will be seen.

Rhinoplasty

Rhinoplasty is an exacting operation to alter the external appearance and internal anatomy of the nose. The nose may be aesthetically unappealing or functionally impaired as a result of trauma, surgery, or a congenital deformity. Clearly, many familial and ethnic traits result in a multitude of nasal appearances. As a result, it is crucial that the patient and surgeon discuss the goals of the procedure and the likelihood of achieving those goals. The patient must have realistic expectations and be prepared for the operation both physically and mentally.

To successfully achieve the goals of rhinoplasty, a complete nasal history is obtained with particular attention paid to nasal airway obstruction, allergies, trauma, and previous surgery. A photographic analysis is performed to evaluate facial and nasal dimensions. The photographs are examined with the patient, the operative plan is discussed, and the potential structural and functional outcomes are reviewed.[66]

Rhinoplasty may be performed under local or general anesthesia. The patient is prepared for surgery by intranasal injections of vasoconstrictors containing lidocaine and epinephrine. Topical vasoconstrictors (i.e., cocaine) are applied to the nasal lining and septum. The operation can be performed in an "open" or "closed" fashion. The open technique requires a transcolumellar incision extended intranasally to allow exposure of the cartilage and bones of the nose. Direct visualization of the structure of the nose allows greater precision in cartilaginous sculpting and nasal bone repositioning. The paired lower lateral cartilages create the shape and provide the support for the nasal tip. Any deformity involving the nasal tip requires manipulations of this cartilage, including resections for a bulbous or overprojecting tip, suturing to reposition an asymmetric nasal tip, or cartilage grafting to increase tip projection. The paired upper lateral cartilages and nasal bones define the shape of the nasal dorsum and control nasal airflow. A prominent dorsal hump may require resection of both upper lateral cartilage and nasal bone. Osteotomies of the nasal bones may be required to narrow nasal width by disconnecting the base of the nasal bones from the maxilla (Fig. 120.22). In contrast, "saddle nose" deformities may require cartilage or bone grafting to provide dorsal augmentation. Cartilage grafts may also be used to improve nasal airflow. By placing a "spreader graft" between the nasal septum and the upper lateral cartilage, the internal nasal valve area becomes less restrictive to nasal airflow.[67] The "closed" technique allows access to the nasal cartilage and bones through intranasal incisions. Many experienced rhinoplastic surgeons prefer this less invasive approach. However, many of the complicated cartilage grafting and suturing techniques can be difficult to perform with this limited exposure.

Postoperatively, the patient is instructed to keep the head elevated and apply ice packs. An external splint is used to maintain the position of the nasal bones and cartilage for 10 to 14 days. Patients should expect nasal swelling, pain, and bruising for 2 to 3 weeks; if osteotomies are performed, the patient may also experience periorbital ecchymosis. A full year is required for complete resolution of nasal tip swelling, particularly following an open tip rhinoplasty. Approximately 5% to 10% of patients require a revision rhinoplasty, which should not be performed for at least 1 year following the original procedure.

Genioplasty

Genioplasties are common plastic surgical procedures to manipulate the position of the chin and thereby improve facial appearance. Based on the design of the mandibular symphysis osteotomy, the vertical height and anterior projection of the chin can be adjusted.[68] Patients with a "weak" chin may undergo an advancement genioplasty to enhance chin projection and improve the cervicomental angle. Chin augmentation may also be accomplished with an alloplastic implant (i.e., Silastic), eliminating the need for an osteotomy. Patients with a very prominent chin can undergo a reduction genioplasty where the vertical height and anterior projection can be reduced. The dental occlusion is not affected by these procedures, but the lip position and neck appearance may be altered.[69]

A complete physical examination, photographic analysis, and radiographic evaluation are performed to evaluate facial harmony and determine the extent of the advancement or reduction. Dental occlusion is carefully examined to ensure that orthognathic surgery is not required to correct chin position.

Operations are typically performed under general anesthesia. Local anesthesia containing epinephrine is injected intraorally for hemostasis and postoperative pain control. Access to the mandibular symphysis is achieved through an inferior buccal sulcus incision. The osteotomy is measured and marked based on the preoperative photographs and lateral radiographs; the mental foramen is avoided. The bony segment is mobilized and secured in its new position with plates and screws. Postoperatively, swelling and pain persist for approximately 4 to 6 weeks. During this time, the patient should perform meticulous oral hygiene and avoid foods that may traumatize the inferior buccal sulcus incision.

Cosmetic Procedures of the Trunk and Extremities (Body Sculpting)

Abdominoplasty

Abdominoplasties encompass a wide array of surgical procedures used to correct abdominal deformities resulting from excess abdominal skin, fatty tissue, and abdominal wall laxity. Abnormalities in any of these tissue planes may produce an aesthetically unappealing abdomen. Surgical procedures are designed to correct the underlying pathology and include dermatolipectomy, liposuction, and abdominal wall plication. These procedures are often combined and tailored to fit the surgical needs and desires of the patient. It is critical to define the physical anomaly responsible for the abdominal deformity so that the appropriate operative procedure or combination of procedures can be performed.[70,71]

A standard abdominoplasty combines a dermatolipectomy, liposuction, and abdominal wall plication to correct deformity in each of the three previously mentioned abdominal wall layers. The operation is performed under general anesthesia through a bikini-line incision extending from the cephalad margin of the pubic escutcheon to the iliac crests bilaterally. The skin incisions are made and the abdominal flap is elevated off the underlying abdominal wall fascia. A circumferential incision is made around the umbilicus to allow complete elevation of the abdominal flap up to the costal margin. The patient is then placed in a flexed position, the abdominal flap is redraped caudally, and the elliptical-shaped redundant skin is resected. If any abdominal wall laxity is identified along with the skin redundancy, then a vertical, midline abdominal wall plication is also performed. Occasionally, suction-assisted lipectomy (SAL) is performed at the time of abdominoplasty to help recontour the abdomen and flanks. However, aggressive SAL of the abdominal flap may critically compromise flap vascularity and contribute to flap necrosis. Closed-suction drains are placed prior to wound closure (Fig. 120.23).

A "mini-abdominoplasty" is used to treat mild abdominal skin redundancy and abdominal wall laxity. The same approach is used as previously described for a standard abdominoplasty except the skin incision is limited to the central portion of the abdomen. A limited skin resection can be performed through this approach along with an abdominal wall plication. SAL can be used in combination with this procedure if necessary.

Endoscopic abdominoplasty can be used to treat abdominal wall laxity (i.e., postpartum rectus diastasis) and localized collections of fatty tissue. Patients who are candidates for this

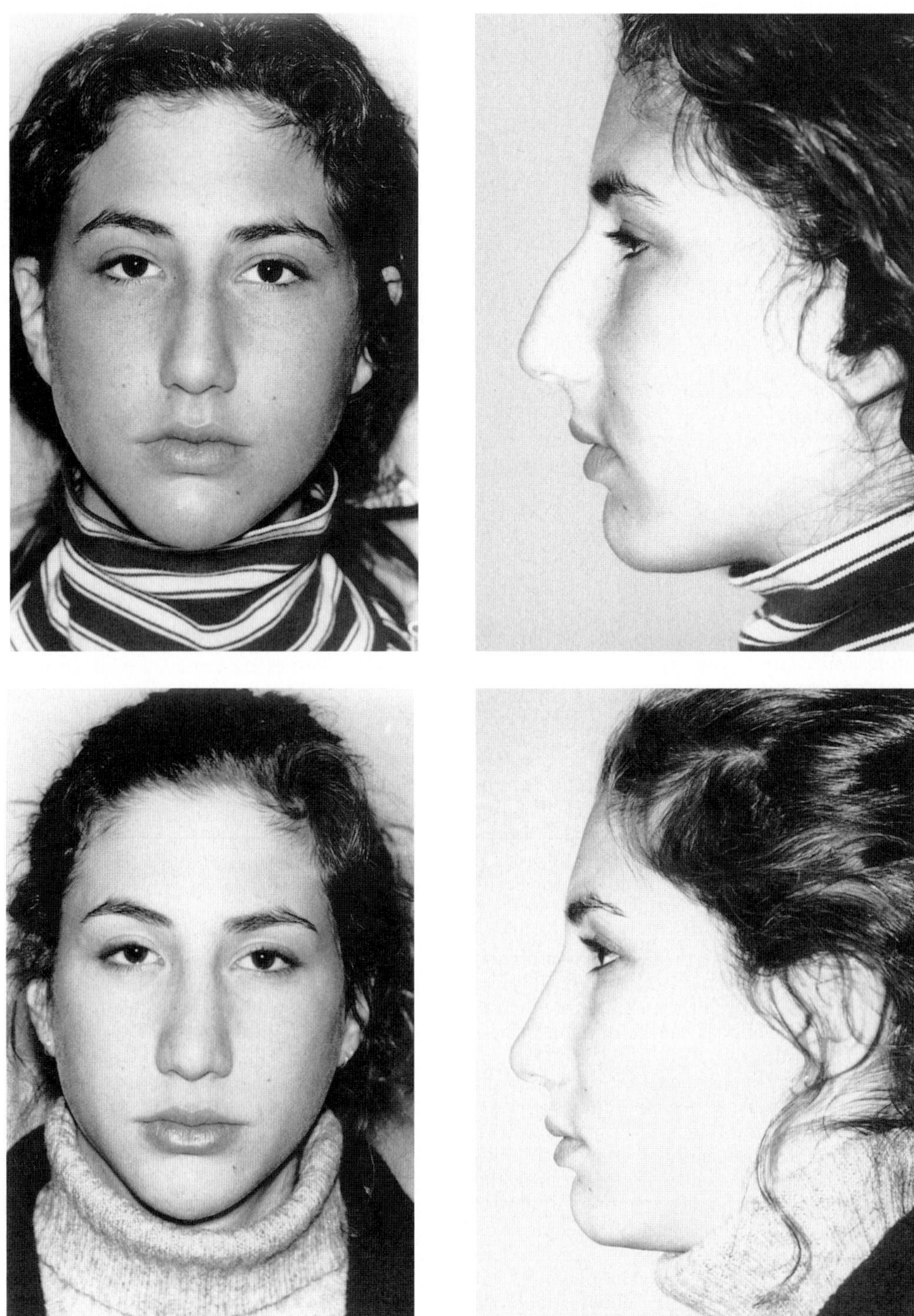

FIGURE 120.22 Open rhinoplasty with partial lower lateral cartilage resection, dorsal cartilage and bone resection, and nasal osteotomies. (*A* and *B*) Preoperative appearance. (*C* and *D*) Postoperative appearance. Note the dorsal hump reduction and slight supratip break.

operation must have good skin quality and only mild to moderate lipodystrophy. The endoscopic abdominoplasty is performed through two incisions, a 3-cm transverse incision within the pubic hair and a circumferential incision around the umbilicus. These incisions function as the two access ports through which the endoscopic instruments are passed. The entire abdominal wall is then elevated from the abdominal wall fascia under endoscopic visualization with electrocautery. The midline of the abdominal wall is plicated from pubis to xiphoid. The abdominal wall is then recontoured with SAL, which is performed through the two access ports.[54]

Liposuction

Liposuction is a surgical procedure designed to resect collections of fat from isolated anatomic regions. It is not a form of weight loss and is not indicated in obese patients. Liposuction is ideally suited to patients who are within 20% to 30% of

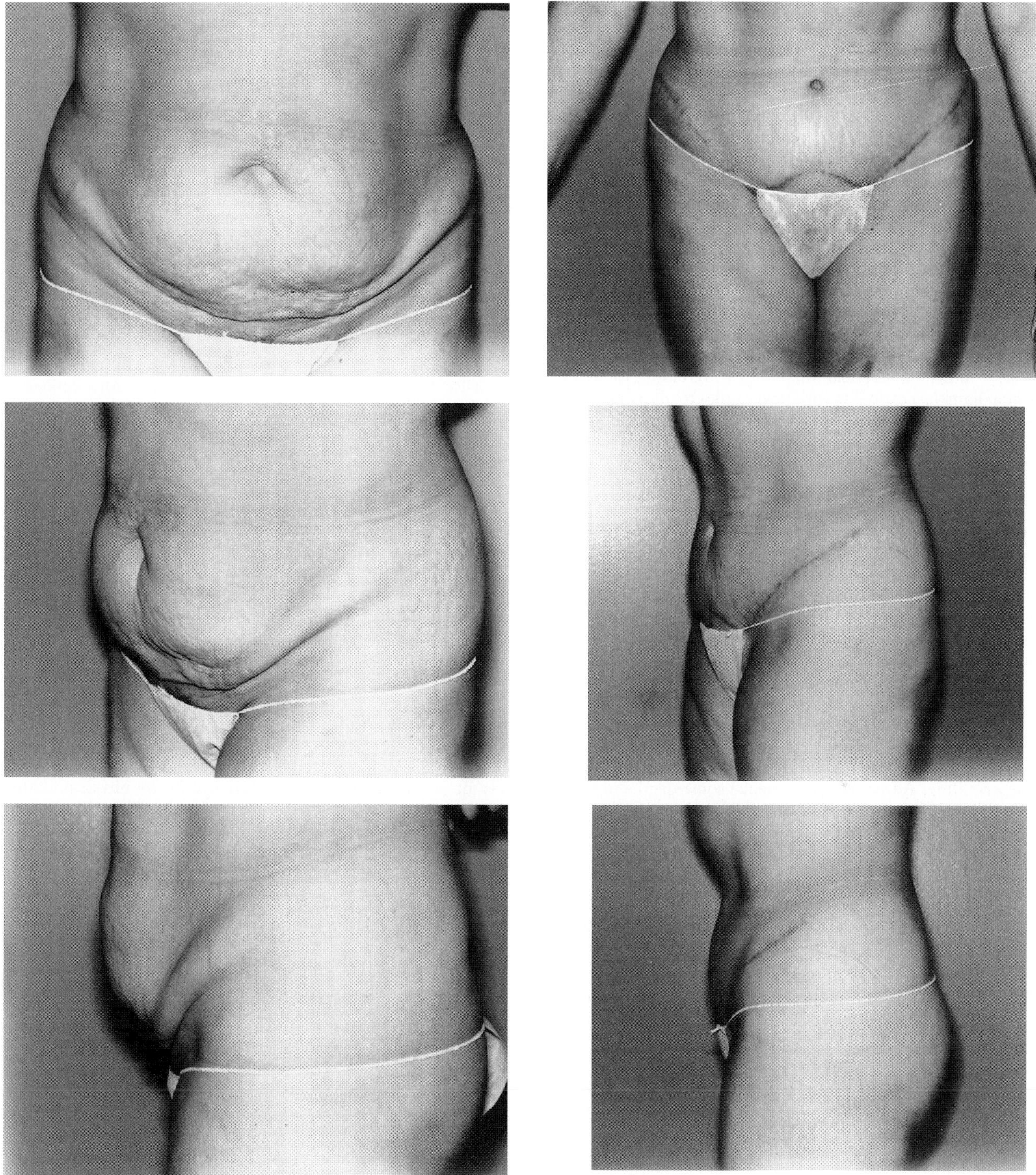

FIGURE 120.23 Abdominoplasty with dermatolipectomy, lateral liposuction, and abdominal wall plication. (*A–C*) Preoperative appearance. (*D–F*) Postoperative appearance. Note the reduced abdominal bulging and "hourglass" shape after lateral suction-assisted lipectomy and abdominal wall plication.

their ideal body weight and have localized collections of fat that are refractory to dietary modifications and exercise. A complete evaluation of skin elasticity is very important in patients considering liposuction because once fat is surgically removed, the skin must be able to contract down to the contour of the remaining subcutaneous tissue. If the skin quality is poor, then wrinkling, dimpling, or skin ptosis may severely compromise the aesthetic result.[70–72]

Two forms of liposuction are currently used: suction-assisted lipectomy (SAL) and ultrasonic assisted liposuction (UAL). SAL is used in all areas of the body but may not be as effective as UAL in more fibrous anatomic regions such as the flank, upper abdomen, or male breast. Treatment of lipodystrophy in these regions is more effective with UAL alone or UAL in combination with SAL.[73,74]

As with all aesthetic procedures, careful patient selection is of paramount importance. All patients must undergo a complete evaluation preoperatively to ensure that their goals can be achieved by performance of liposuction. Preoperative photographic documentation is performed on all patients. Markings are then made with the patient in the upright position. Access ports (6 to 8 mm), through which the SAL or UAL is performed, are marked in concealable areas. Intravenous sedation or general anesthesia is used. Tumescent fluid (1,000 mL of LR, 50 mL of 1% lidocaine, and 1 mg of epinephrine) is then infiltrated for pain control and hemostasis.

SAL is performed with metal cannulas connected to an aspirating device that generates a negative pressure of 1 atmosphere. Various cannula configurations are used to perform the resection. Fatty tissue is aspirated into the holes of the cannula and then resected by movement of the cannula tip. The operation is performed through multiple access ports, starting with large (6- to 8-mm diameter) cannulas and progressing to smaller (4-mm diameter) cannulas with fewer holes to allow more precise body contouring. Overlapping patterns of resection are used to avoid contour irregularities.

UAL is a surgical technique that allows body contouring through the liquefaction and aspiration of fatty tissue. When employed alone or in combination with traditional SAL, UAL is effective for treating lipodystrophy in fibrous anatomic regions such as the flank, upper abdomen, and male breast. The UAL probe tip produces sound waves at an ultrasonic frequency of 20 to 30 kHz. The effect of these sound waves is to cavitate and liquefy to low-density lipocytes. Low-power suction is then employed to remove the resultant fluid. If UAL is used inappropriately, patients may experience severe complications, including full-thickness skin loss from thermal injury.[75]

All patients are placed in a compressive garment 24 hours per day for 6 weeks postoperatively. Early postoperative compression reduces the chances of hematoma formation. Prolonged compression reduces swelling and the potential for skin wrinkling. All patients experience some degree of ecchymosis, swelling, and decreased sensibility. The end result will not be realized for approximately 2 to 3 months following the procedure.

PEDIATRIC PLASTIC SURGERY

The specialized area of pediatric plastic surgery focuses on the reconstruction of abnormalities in children with congenital malformations and acquired deformities. Utilizing a sound knowledge of embryology as well as the changes inherent during growth and development, pediatric plastic surgeons employ a combination of innovation and technical expertise to restore both form and function to their patients. Although the manifestations of congenital malformations may be diverse, the approach to reconstruction is always based on solid fundamental surgical principles. Similarly, the management of traumatic or other acquired maladies in the pediatric population is founded on essential surgical tenets influenced by the special considerations of maturation and growth. This section concentrates on the most salient aspects of pediatric plastic surgery to give the clinician an accurate grasp of the subspecialty.

Cleft Lip and Palate

Perhaps the area of expertise that best exemplifies the specialty of pediatric plastic surgery is the management of children with cleft lip and palate deformity. The cleft lip and palate pose a variety of structural and functional deficits that must be addressed with respect to growth and development as well as psychosocial concerns of the individual patient and family. The care of these children requires exacting surgical technique in combination with the efforts of a team of allied health professionals to effect a comprehensive level of rehabilitation.

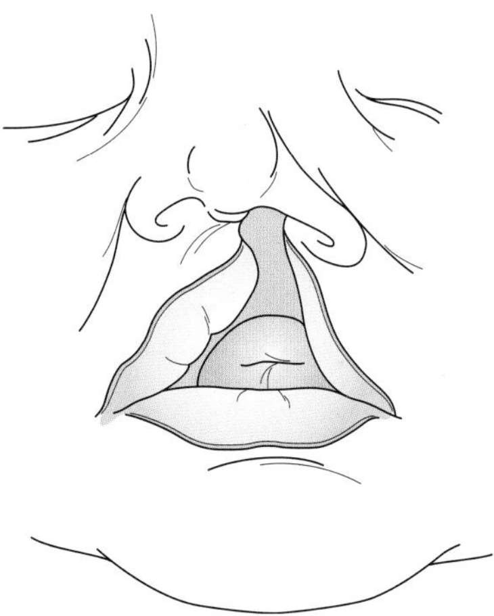

FIGURE 120.24 Left unilateral complete cleft lip. (After Jurkiewicz MJ, Krizek TJ, Mathes SJ, eds. *Plastic surgery: principles and practice*, vol. 1. St. Louis: Mosby, 1990, p. 64, with permission.)

The overall incidence of cleft lip and palate deformity is approximately 1 in 750 children. This incidence is significantly higher in the Asian population, 1 in 300, and significantly lower in the black population, 1 in 2,000.[76–78] The distribution of cleft types is approximately 46% combined cleft lip and palate, 21% isolated cleft lip, and 33% isolated cleft palate.[79] Almost 30% of children with cleft lip and palate deformity have associated birth defects that vary in scope and extent and therefore require vigilance in the physical examination.[80] The chance of having a second child with cleft lip and palate to unaffected parents is approximately 4% as is the chance of one affected parent producing an offspring with a cleft.[80–81] Genetic counseling is usually helpful in both educating the parents and screening for other associated congenital anomalies.

A cleft lip deformity can be bilateral or unilateral and is considered *complete* if it extends into the nose and *incomplete* if it does not (Fig. 120.24). The cleft lip can extend into the gum partially or completely through the alveolus, creating a bony defect. The cleft lip deformity affects the nose as well as the lip, and therefore both of these structures must be addressed in the reconstruction of the deformity. Although the timing of cleft lip repair is controversial, the repair of the cleft lip is most often addressed in about the third month of life, after the child shows sufficient weight gain. This timing permits a potentially safer anesthetic administration.

There are multitudes of cleft lip repairs, but the goals of the repairs remain the same: an anatomic reconstruction with minimal scarring and normal function. In general, the skin around the cleft is cut into flaps that are brought together in a way that will give adequate length to the lip and restore the continuity of the orbicularis musculature (Fig. 120.25). Symmetry is the mainstay of reconstructive procedures to the cleft lip, allowing the normal side of a unilateral cleft to serve as a template for restoration and insuring equal balance and proportion in a bilateral cleft repair.

The cleft palate can affect the soft palate alone or include the hard palate. A unilateral cleft of the hard palate exposes only one side of the vomer, whereas a bilateral cleft of the hard palate exposes both sides of the vomer (Fig. 120.26). The cleft of the hard palate can be continuous with an alveolar defect

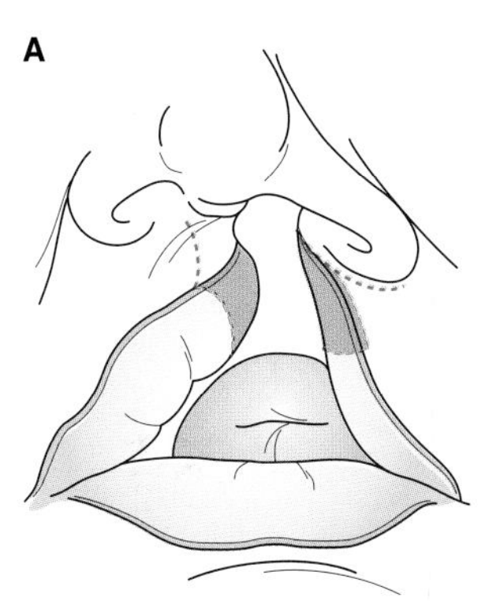

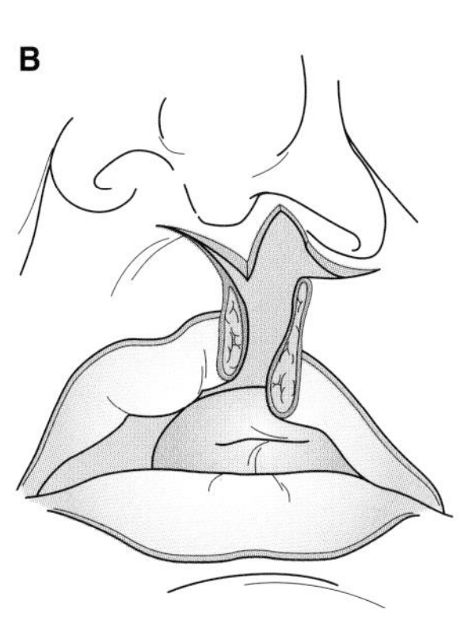

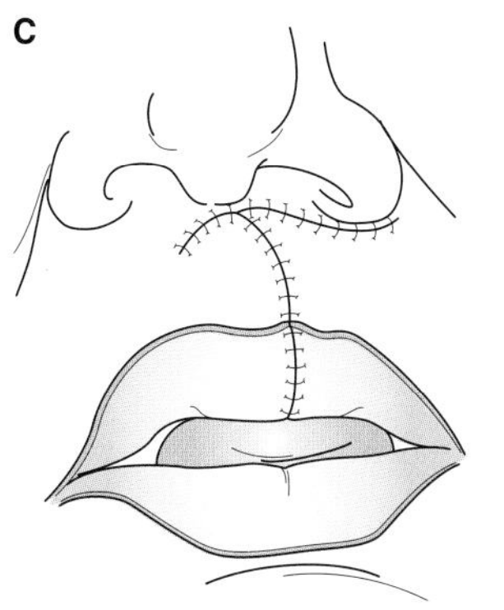

FIGURE 120.25 Millard rotation—advancement lip repair. (After Jurkiewicz MJ, Krizek TJ, Mathes SJ, et al. *Plastic surgery: principles and practice,* vol. 1. St. Louis: Mosby, 1990, p. 71, with permission.)

from a cleft lip, resulting in an opening that runs from the most anterior portion of the lip through to the back of the uvula. In some cases, a cleft palate may have no mucosal separation at all and display only a separation or clefting of the underlying musculature. This special situation is referred to as a submucous cleft palate and may also have functional consequences for the patient. Functionally, the hard palate acts as a structural barrier between the oropharynx and the nose. The soft palate moves superiorly and articulates with the posterior and lateral pharyngeal walls to effect a seal between the oropharynx and the nasopharynx during speech and swallowing. The coordinated activity of the soft palate prevents regurgitation of solids and liquids into the nose while eating and prevents hypernasal speech while producing strictly oral sounds. As with cleft lip, there are a multitude of cleft palate repairs but the goals of the repairs remain the same: an anatomic reconstruction with minimal scarring and normal function. Reconstructive procedures are based on reconstituting the oral and nasal lining of the palate and reapproximating and realigning the palatal musculature. A purely soft palatal cleft may require only the separation of the layers of the palate, reapproximation of the muscles, and simple closure. The wider clefts and many of the hard palatal clefts, however, require relaxing incisions and release of the mucosa from the underlying bone. The lateral mucosa from both sides is transposed over the midline cleft and sewn closed (Fig. 120.27). Flaps derived from the vomer may be required to achieve closure

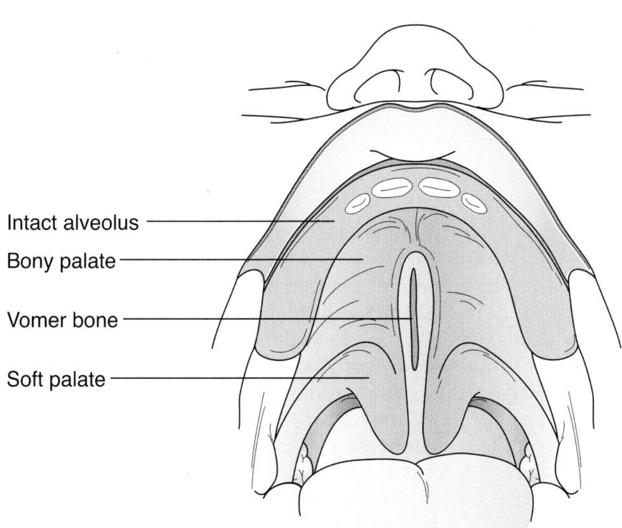

FIGURE 120.26 Cleft palate. (After Jurkiewicz MJ, Krizek TJ, Mathes SJ, et al. *Plastic surgery: principles and practice,* vol. 1. St. Louis: Mosby, 1990, p. 84, with permission.)

without tension, a chief precept for any repair of the palate. The dissection of mucosal tissue off the bone is thought to contribute to the severe growth restriction of the midface and bony palate exhibited by many of the children with this deformity.[82] A delay in the procedure is thought to enhance the growth of the midface and palate, whereas early intervention is thought to improve speech. For this reason, the timing of the repair of the cleft palate is controversial; however, the cleft palate repair is most often addressed by the age of 1 year.

Speech therapy is almost always required for children with a cleft palate and is instituted as soon as the child develops the necessary language skills. "Early on" programs have arisen for preschoolers, and speech programs are often available through local school systems. Unfortunately, the palate repair alone is successful in normalizing speech in only about 80% of patients.[83] The remainder of patients will require a supplemental operation to decrease residual hypernasality and improve speech. The operations directed at salvaging speech are performed early enough to have the most beneficial effect on speech development, while giving adequate time to ensure that the patient has been given ample opportunity for speech therapy to maximize the potential of the palate repair. The decision to operate is based on a perceptual analysis of speech and is aided by visualization of palatal function with nasoendoscopy and objective measures of function using nosometry techniques. Techniques vary, but the operative procedures are based on placement of either dynamic or static tissue near the velopharyngeal port to better regulate and impede the abnormal flow of air into the nasopharynx.

Orthodontics is a key portion of the comprehensive restoration of the cleft patient and requires close interaction between the pediatric plastic surgeon and the orthodontist. One of the early interactions involves the repair of any residual clefting of the alveolus. Bone grafting is required for reconstruction of the alveolar cleft to restore the continuity of the upper maxillary dental arch, allow the normal emergence of the canine tooth, close the persistent oral nasal fistula, and provide structural support for the recessed nasal alar base. The orthodontist will monitor tooth eruption and may institute early-phase therapy to align the teeth in preparation for bone grafting. The timing of alveolar bone grafting is also controversial but is mandatory for normal tooth emergence. Bone grafting is often performed at about 7 to 8 years of age and entails the surgical isolation and excision of the oral nasal fistula, the reconstruction of the adjacent nasal floor and palatal roof, the placement of bone graft in the alveolar defect, and coverage anteriorly with gingival flaps. The bone grafts are most often cancellous in composition and can be taken from the iliac crest or the cranial diploe.

Many patients respond favorably to the skilled implementation of a long-term orthodontic plan, but some patients display bony hypoplasia as mentioned earlier and require orthognathic surgery of the maxilla, and possibly the mandible, to

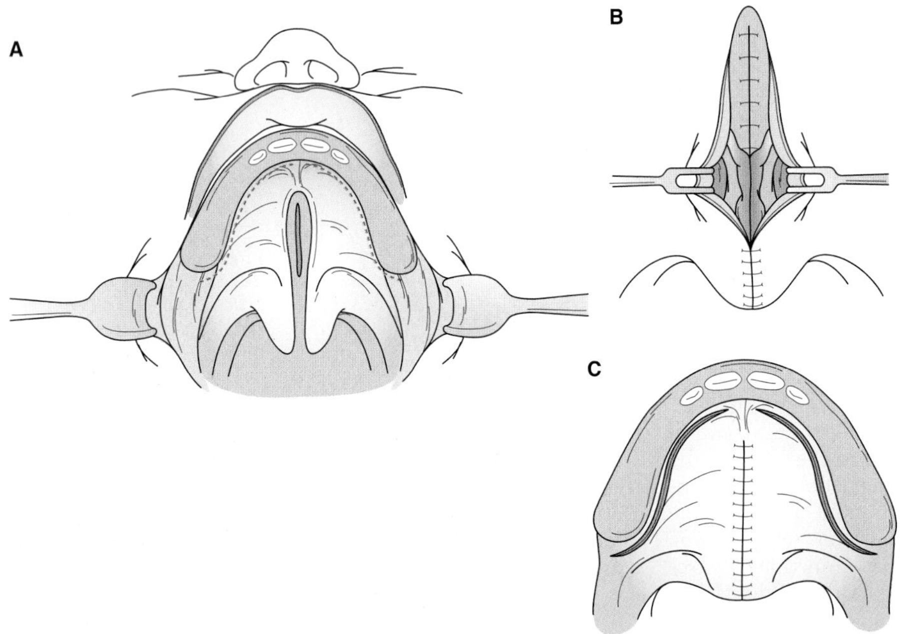

FIGURE 120.27 (*A*) Von Langenbeck palatoplasty. (*B*) Nasal mucosa and levator muscles approximated. (C) Layered closure of oral mucosa and lateral relaxing incisions. (After Jurkiewicz MJ, Krizek TJ, Mathes SJ, et al. *Plastic surgery: principles and practice*, vol. 1. St. Louis: Mosby, 1990, p. 91, with permission.)

assist in establishing normal occlusion. Operations to restore a normal occlusion should await the cessation of growth so that the surgical registration of occlusion will be permanent and not require additional procedures. The most common operation to address midfacial hypoplasia and restore occlusion in the cleft patient is the Le Fort I osteotomy. The orthodontist helps the pediatric plastic surgeon to determine the best postoperative occlusion for the patient based on the orthodontic plan, and an oral surgical splint is fashioned to allow easy registration intraoperatively. The patient undergoes a horizontal osteotomy above the level of the tooth roots and across the nasomaxillary and zygomaticomaxillary buttresses below the level of the zygomatic body (Fig. 120.28). The bones of the midface are separated from the cranial base by performing a pterygomaxillary disjunction, and the floating maxilla is then repositioned into the planned occlusion by registering the teeth in the splint. The bones of the maxilla are then fixed using plates and screws. In severe malocclusion cases, the mandible may also need to be cut and reregistered into a position that results in an anatomic orthognathic bite.

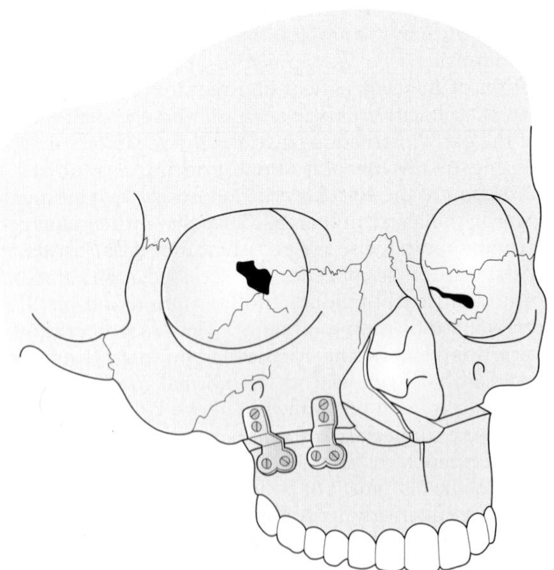

FIGURE 120.28 Le Fort I osteotomy in an advanced position. One side has been plated into position. (Jurkiewicz MJ, Krizek TJ, Mathes SJ, et al. *Plastic surgery: principles and practice,* vol. 1. St. Louis: Mosby, 1990, with permission.)

The last operation to be performed on the patient with a cleft lip and nasal deformity is often the formal rhinoplasty. There is almost always a septal deviation that must be addressed in these patients and is an important part of the procedure. Each rhinoplasty is necessarily individualized, but the procedure usually entails repositioning and trimming of the nasal tip cartilages, added support to the nasal tip and slumping lower lateral cartilages to achieve projection, straightening of the septum, and finally infracturing of the widened nasal bones.

Although, the care of the cleft patient requires interaction with the pediatric plastic surgeon and the cleft team throughout the patient's childhood, it should remain a small and unobtrusive part of life. The number of operations is kept to the minimum needed to attain an adequate reconstruction as deemed necessary by both the patient and the doctor. Revisional surgery is usually an important part of cleft care but should be done, as often as possible, *for* the child and not to the child, with an attempt to empower the patient as often as possible.

Craniosynostosis

Craniosynostosis is defined as the premature fusion of one or more of the cranial sutures. The child afflicted with craniosynostosis displays abnormalities in the size and shape of the cranial vault. Virchow's law proposes that the growth of the skull will be restricted in the direction perpendicular to a synostosed suture while compensatory growth occurs in a parallel direction.[84] The ensuing skull shape of the patient provides the nomenclature of the deformity and is primarily empiric in nature (Fig. 120.29). Synostosis of the metopic suture most often results in a triangular forehead and is referred to as *trigonocephaly*. Unilateral coronal suture involvement often results in a recessed or slanted supraorbital bar and forehead and is referred to as *plagiocephaly,* whereas bilateral coronal synostosis often results to a shortened and flattened forehead

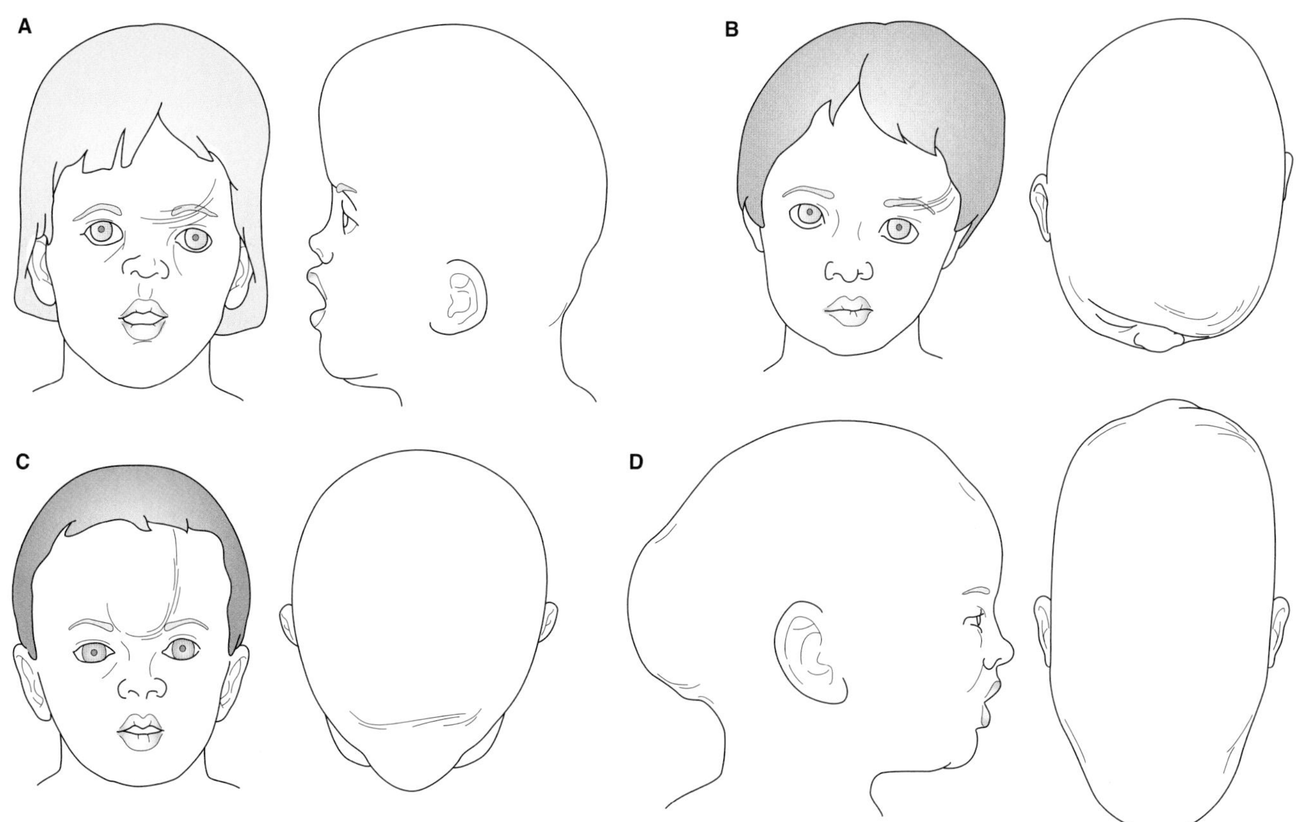

FIGURE 120.29 (*A*) Turribrachycephaly (short, flat head). (*B*) Plagiocephaly (slanted head). (*C*) Trigonocephaly (triangular head). (*D*) Scaphocephaly (keel-shaped head). (After Jurkiewicz MJ, Krizek TJ, Mathes SJ, et al. *Plastic surgery: principles and practice,* vol. 1. St. Louis: Mosby, 1990, p. 119, with permission.)

referred to as *brachycephaly*. The sagittal suture is the most commonly fused suture and results in a boat- or keel-shaped head referred to as *scaphocephaly*.

The abnormal shape of the affected skulls can often be severe and progressively worsen with time as the expanding brain reinforces and emphasizes the deformity. In addition, a small percentage of patients with a single-suture synostosis, and a much larger percentage of children with multiple-suture synostosis, are at risk for the development of increased intracranial pressure.[85–86] The care of these patients, therefore, requires close interaction between a pediatric neurosurgeon and a pediatric craniofacial plastic surgeon. A thorough clinical evaluation is mandatory, and an ophthalmologic evaluation to check for papilledema can be beneficial. A CT scan is also useful in these patients to assess the ventricular system as well as the neuroanatomy for possible associated developmental anomalies of the brain.

Once the functional aspects of craniosynostosis are evaluated and addressed, the operative strategy is then aimed at restoring normal morphology. The operation is tailored to the individual diagnosis and malformation, but the underlying surgical principles remain the same. A sinusoidal coronal incision is used to afford access to the cranium and to hide the scar. The pediatric neurosurgeon performs a craniotomy to provide access to the cranial vault. In the case of plagiocephaly and trigonocephaly, the craniofacial pediatric plastic surgeon removes the frontal bar by performing a bilateral osteotomy at the lateral orbital rim, and along the orbital roof meeting in the midline with a cut across the region just above the glabella. The frontal bar is removed, bent and reshaped, and replaced in an advanced position with interposition bone grafts placed to support the reconstruction. The bones of the forehead are similarly cut, bent and reshaped, and placed into a normal anatomic position. The bones are fixed with small metal or resorbable plates and screws (Fig. 120.30). A gap is left in the area of the coronal suture to allow growth and expansion of the brain. During infancy the open dura is osteogenic and fills in slowly with newly formed bone. In the case of a sagittal synostosis, the frontal bar often need not be removed; the operation entails the creation of barrel stave osteotomies in the parietal skull and outfracturing of the bone. The forehead is then backfractured and gently posteriorly compressed, the occipital bone is then fractured and gently anteriorly compressed, and the bones are then fixed into position with the aid of bone grafts. During gentle compression the brain takes on a rounder shape filling out behind the parietal bone outfracture. This arrangement encourages subsequent growth to fill out the parietal region and secure a more anatomic shape.

In the case of syndromic craniosynostosis patients, such as those with Apert, Crouzon, or Pfeiffer syndrome, similar reconstructions may be required for the cranial vault. Additional operations are often needed to address deformities of the orbits and midface. In contrast to the midfacial hypoplasia exhibited by the cleft patient, the patient with syndromic craniosynostosis has a much more severe deformity and therefore requires larger operations. Le Fort III and Monoblock operations that move the entire upper and midfacial region forward can be used to vastly improve the appearance of the patient while establishing a more normal functional

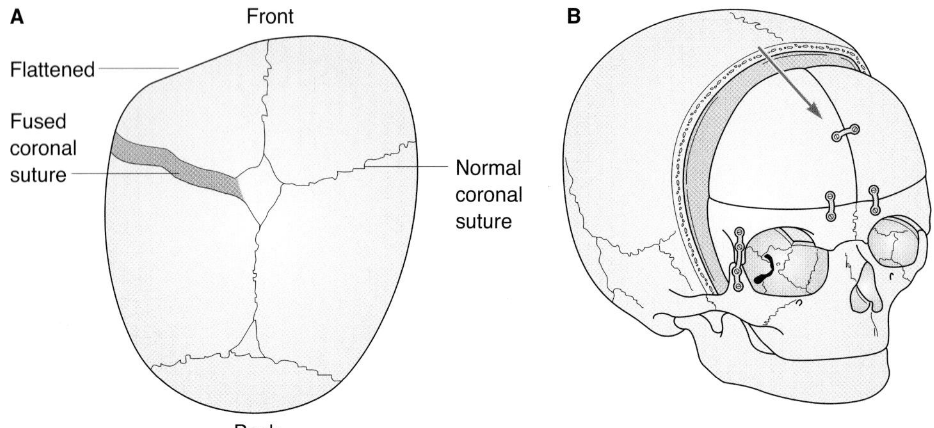

FIGURE 120.30 (*A*) Plagiocephalic head viewed from above. (*B*) The surgeon removes the bone of the forehead and advances the forehead to allow the brain to grow and the skull to resume a normal shape. (After Sidhu SR, Zang L, Schultz KL, et al. *Craniosynostosis and craniofacial surgery: a parent's guide*. Ann Arbor: University of Michigan, 1996, p. 9, with permission.)

anatomy (Fig. 120.31). These operations address the bulging eyes, malar hypoplasia, and recessed and diminutive nasopharyngeal airway of these patients, restoring normal eye position and opening up the breathing passages to relieve symptoms of sleep apnea.

Hemangiomas and Vascular Malformation

The pediatric plastic surgeon is often the primary care giver for children afflicted with hemangiomas and vascular malformations. These lesions may present at birth or in the neonatal period and require careful diagnosis and management. Hemangiomas are benign tumors that most often arise just after birth and undergo a spontaneous rapid growth phase followed by slow involutional stage.[87,88] In general, management of hemangiomas is nonoperative; however, ulceration or interference with function may require intervention. The use of systemic or local steroids may induce an involutional regression, but operative intercession may be necessary. Surgical strategies should strive to conserve tissue and function, avoiding the creation of significant deformities that would necessitate delayed reconstruction.

Vascular malformations are usually made up of veins, lymphatic vessels, or capillaries or a combination of each. The malformations are usually present at birth and grow in proportion to the patient. There is usually neither a growth phase, as in a hemangioma, nor an involutional stage. Small capillary hemangiomas such as port–wine stains are well treated with pulse dye laser therapy, and larger, more involved lesions may be better treated with a combination of surgical intervention and laser treatment. Lymphangiomas are difficult to treat because they are diffuse and often adjacent to vital structures. Staged partial excisions can be performed if there are functional indications for intervention.

Nevi

Congenital nevi are perhaps the most common benign tumor seen by the pediatric plastic surgeon. The small- to moderate-size nevi are usually of little consequence but need to be monitored closely for any significant changes in size, shape, color, bleeding, or ulceration. The potential for degenerative malignancy into a melanoma for small- to moderate-size congenital nevi is controversial. The figures reported in several studies range so widely as to make a reasonable estimation difficult.[89] Serial examination and even photographs can be helpful to document changes over time, and the gold standard for any doubtful skin lesion is still excisional biopsy.

Giant hairy congenital nevi are larger and rarer, but they can be quite devastating to a child and the family. These lesions can affect the entire body or vast areas, including vital structures such as the eyelids, anus, and external sexual organs. A

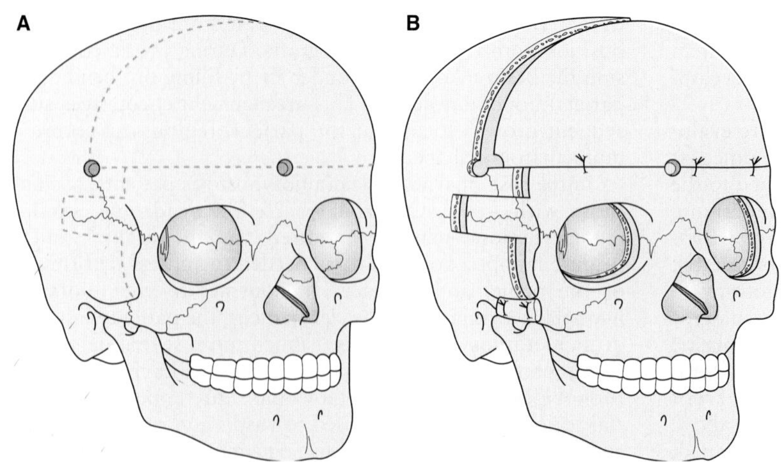

FIGURE 120.31 Monoblock frontofacial advancement. (After Jurkiewicz MJ, Krizek TJ, Mathes SJ, et al. *Plastic surgery: principles and practice*, vol 1. St. Louis: Mosby, 1990, p. 119, with permission.)

reasoned and conservative approach to such difficult cases is mandatory. It is often helpful to enlist the assistance of a dermatologist and the patient's pediatrician to assist in monitoring these lesions. Again, photographic documentation is helpful in serially assessing these lesions. Areas that show significant change warrant incisional biopsy and pathologic evaluation. The aesthetic consequences of these lesions often can be severe, and the parents often want them to be excised. The surgical approaches to benign giant hairy congenital nevi are varied and range from excision and grafting to serial excision and the use of tissue expansion.

The use of extensive skin grafting as a reconstructive option for the reconstruction of giant hairy congenital nevi is usually reserved for malignant or dysplastic lesions. Skin grafts are not a particularly durable long-term cover, and they are often aesthetically displeasing and require subsequent resection and reconstruction. Serial excision can be useful in limited giant hairy congenital nevi, especially in locations near tissues that stretch well. The tissues adjacent to the lesion are undermined and advanced over the nevus to determine the amount that can be resected, and then a portion of the nevus is excised and the tissues are then reapproximated and allowed to heal. After 4 to 6 months the same procedure is performed until the nevus is fully excised. Tissue expansion requires the placement of a tissue expander adjacent to the lesion with slow instillation of saline into the expander over time, allowing stretching and recruitment of new tissue near the nevus to assist in excision and closure. If the expansion is not adequate in size, it can be removed after full expansion and replaced with a larger expander to fully expand the tissue. The quality and thickness of the skin, the possibility of exposure and infection, and the cooperation of the young patient at times limit the usefulness of this technique.

Prominent Ears

Prominent ears are a deformity that is mainly in the domain of the pediatric plastic surgeon. Children with prominent ears are prone to ridicule by classmates in school, teasing by siblings, and thoughtless comments by insensitive adults. The deformity does not usually present with an enlarged ear but rather with a lack of an antihelical fold, either with or without conchal hypertrophy. The remedy is aimed specifically at the deformity. An incision is made on the posterior portion of the ear exposing the cartilage, and sutures are placed in a mattress fashion to reconstruct an antihelical fold. The stiff conchal cartilage can be shaved, and the conch is then secured to the mastoid fascia using permanent suture. A strict postoperative head-banding protocol is used to avoid trauma to the ear and allow undisturbed healing. Successful otoplasty is one of the most rewarding procedures performed by a pediatric plastic surgeon because the child usually wants the surgery and is rewarded with immense satisfaction.

Myelomeningocele

The interaction between the pediatric neurosurgeon and the pediatric plastic surgeon often extends beyond the realm of craniofacial surgery. A prime example of the symbiotic interaction between the two specialties is in the repair and reconstruction of the myelomeningocele. The neurosurgeon is often presented with an exposed dural sac and a wide-open skin defect. The neurosurgeon may be faced with a tenuous dural closure and often resorts to the use of a homograft to achieve an adequate repair. The pediatric plastic surgeon can assist by closing the defect over the dural repair with stable, reliable coverage using well-vascularized tissue, protecting the neurosurgeon's repair. The soft tissue coverage may require local paraspinous muscle flaps or various fasciocutaneous flaps, but the goal of a durable reconstruction with a normal contour is paramount so as to avoid persistent long-term complications both at the level of the skin and at the level of the dural repair (Fig. 120.32).

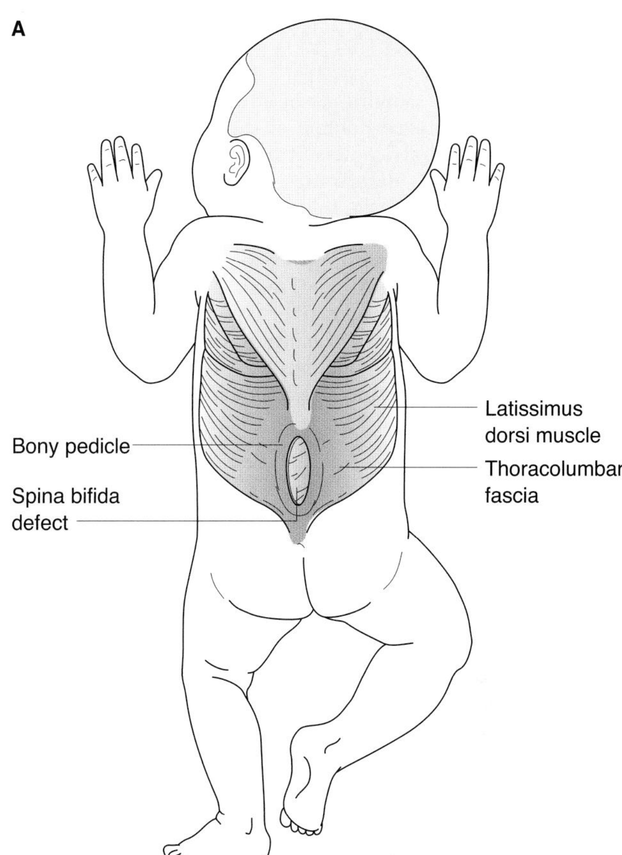

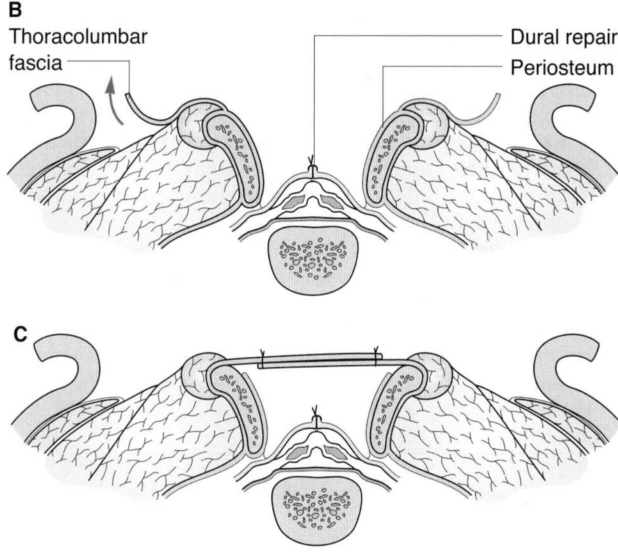

FIGURE 120.32 (*A*) Myelomeningocele defect. (*B*) Cross section of local flap coverage of myelomeningocele defect. (*C*) Durable closure over defect of muscle, fascia, and skin. This can be mobilized to complete repair. (After Fiala TGS, Buchman SR, Muraszko KM. Use of lumbar periosteal turnover flaps in myelomeningocele. *Neurosurgery* 1996;39 with permission.)

SUMMARY

Although there are a multitude of additional procedures and topics in the specialized domain of the pediatric plastic surgeon, such as pediatric facial trauma, facial reanimation surgery, and various deformities resulting from congenital hypoplasia and hyperplasia, this chapter has focused on some of the major and more common areas of patient management. In fact, the pediatric plastic surgeon is often a chief collaborator with many of the pediatric surgical services when presented with a case of challenging wound care or a reconstructive dilemma. Continuing innovation and technical advances combined with an appreciation for sound fundamental surgical principles allow the specialty to continue meeting that challenge.

KEY POINTS

- **Because all open wounds are contaminated, the designation of a wound as "infected" should be contingent on the physical examination findings of local inflammation: erythema, pain, swelling, fluctuance, purulence, and loss of function.**
- **Once a wound has been fully evaluated, the treatments should be designed to achieve specific goals. In order of greatest priority, these are: (a) prevention of complications resulting from the wound, (b) preserving or restoring critical functions, (c) achieving wound closure, and (d) restoration of aesthetics.**
- **Skin grafts are classified by as either split thickness, where epidermis and a portion of the dermis are harvested, or full thickness, where the entire dermis is harvested.**
- **The musculocutaneous perforator is the predominant vascular supply to the skin in many areas of the body; this organization has led to the wide use of musculocutaneous flaps. These flaps derive their inflow from a major muscular artery. Perforators emanating vertically from the muscle surface supply the skin overlying the muscle.**
- **A variety of operative procedures have been described for breast reconstruction following mastectomy. These approaches can be categorized as implant-based, autogenous (natural) tissue, and hybrid procedures.**
- **A variety of autogenous tissue options have been described for postmastectomy breast reconstruction. Currently, the most commonly performed of these procedures is the transverse rectus abdominis musculocutaneous (TRAM) flap, commonly performed as a pedicle muscle flap. The transferred rectus muscle is left partially attached to the costal margin, preserving the superior epigastric artery and vein as the flap's blood supply.**
- **A cleft lip deformity can be bilateral or unilateral and is considered complete if it extends into the nose and incomplete if it does not.**
- **Craniosynostosis is defined as the premature fusion of one or more of the cranial sutures. The child with craniosynostosis displays abnormalities in the size and shape of the cranial vault. Virchow's law proposes that the growth of the skull will be restricted in the direction perpendicular to a synostosed suture while compensatory growth occurs in a parallel direction.**

References

1. Murray JE. Reminiscences for the "50-year retrospective" of transplantation. *Transplant Proc.* 1999;34:3101–3102.
2. Brown DL, Smith DJ. Bacterial colonization/infection and the surgical management of pressure ulcers. *Ostomy Wound Manage.* 1999;45:109S–118S.
3. Robson M, Heggers J. Delayed wound closure based on bacterial counts. *J Surg Oncol.* 1970;2:379–384.
4. Pruitt BA Jr, McManus AT, Kim SH, et al. Burn wound infections: current status. *World J Surg.* 1998;22:135–145.
5. McManus AT, Kim SH, McManus WF, et al. Comparison of quantitative microbiology and histopathology in divided burn-wound biopsy specimens. *Arch Surg.* 1987;122:74–76.
6. Ladin DA. Understanding dressings. *Clin Plast Surg.* 1998;25:433–441.
7. Cho CY, Lo JS. Dressing the part. *Dermatol Clin.* 1998;16:25–47.
8. Lionelli GT, Lawrence WT. Wound dressings. *Surg Clin North Am.* 2003;83:617–638.
9. Rees RS, Robson MC, Smiell JM, et al. Becaplermin gel in the treatment of pressure ulcers: a phase II randomized, double-blind, placebo-controlled study. *Wound Repair Regen.* 1999;7:141–147.
10. Piascik P. Use of Regranex gel for diabetic foot ulcers. *J Am Pharm Assoc (Wash).* 1998;38:628–630.
11. Sefton MV, Woodhouse KA. Tissue engineering. *J Cutan Med Surg.* 1998;3 (suppl 1): 18–23.
12. **Hess CL, Howard MA, Attinger CE. A review of mechanical adjuncts in wound healing: hydrotherapy, ultrasound, negative pressure therapy, hyperbaric oxygen, and electrostimulation. *Ann Plast Surg.* 2003;51:210–218.**
13. Chang N, Mathes SJ. Comparison of the effect of bacterial inoculation in musculocutaneous and random-pattern flaps. *Plast Reconstr Surg.* 1982;70:1–10.
14. Milton SH. The effects of "delay" on the survival of experimental pedicled skin flaps. *Br J Plast Surg.* 1969;22:244–252.
15. Grabb WC, Myers MB, eds. *Skin flaps.* Philadelphia: Williams and Wilkins, 1975.
16. Jackson IT. *Flaps in head and neck reconstruction.* St. Louis: Harcourt Health Sciences Group, 1985.
17. Bakamjian VY. Total reconstruction of pharynx with medially based deltopectoral skin flap. *N Y State J Med.* 1968;68:2771–2778.
18. McGregor IA, Jackson IT. The groin flap. *Br J Plast Surg.* 1972;25:3–16.
19. Taylor GI, Palmer JH, The vascular territories (angiosomes) of the body: experimental study and clinical applications. *Br J Plast Surg.* 1987;40:113–141.
20. **Cormack GC, Lamberty BG. A classification of fascio-cutaneous flaps according to their patterns of vascularisation. *Br J Plast Surg.* 1984;37:80–87.**
21. Mathes SJ, Nahai F. Classification of the vascular anatomy of muscles: experimental and clinical correlation. *Plast Reconstr Surg.* 1981;67:177–187.
22. **Hartrampf CR, Scheflan M, Black PW. Breast reconstruction with a transverse abdominal island flap. *Plast Reconstr Surg.* 1982;69:216–225.**
23. Geddes CR, Morris SF, Neligan PC. Perforator flaps: evolution, classification, and applications. *Ann Plast Surg.* 2003;50:90–99.
24. Daniel RK, Taylor GI. Distant transfer of an island flap by microvascular anastomoses. A clinical technique. *Plast Reconstr Surg.* 1973;52:111–117.
25. Khouri RK, Cooley BC, Kunselman AR, et al. A prospective study of microvascular free-flap surgery and outcome. *Plast Reconstr Surg.* 1998;102: 711–721.
26. Kuzon WM Jr, Jejurikar S, Wilkins EG, et al. Double free-flap reconstruction of massive defects involving the lip, chin, and mandible. *Microsurgery* 1998;18:372–378.
27. Argenta LC. Reconstruction of the breast by tissue expansion. *Clin Plast Surg.* 1984;11:257–264.
28. Wilkins EG. Donor Site Morbidity in TRAM Breast Reconstruction. Presented at the Annual Meeting of the American Society of Plastic Surgeons; October, 1999; New Orleans.
29. Kroll SS, Baldwin B. A comparison of outcomes using three different methods of breast reconstruction. *Plast Reconstr Surg.* 1992;90:455–462.
30. Grotting JC, Urist MM, Maddox WA, et al. Conventional TRAM flap versus free microsurgical TRAM flap for immediate breast reconstruction. *Plast Reconstr Surg.* 1989;83:828–844.
31. Allen RJ, Treece P. Deep inferior epigastric perforator flap for breast reconstruction. *Ann Plast Surg.* 1994;32:32–38.
32. Allen RJ, Tucker C. Superior gluteal artery perforator free flap for breast reconstruction. *Plast Reconstr Surg.* 1995;95:1207–1212.
33. Blondeel PN. The sensate free superior gluteal perforator (S-GAP) flap: a valuable alternative in autologous breast reconstruction. *Br J Plast Surg.* 1999; 52:185–193.
34. Mandrekas AD, Zambacos GJ, Anastasopoulos A, et al. Reduction mammaplasty with the inferior pedicle technique: early and late complications in 371 patients. *Br J Plast Surg.* 1996;49:442–446.
35. Wallace WH, Thompson WOB, Smith RA, et al. Reduction mammaplasty with the inferior pedicle technique. *Ann Plast Surg.* 1998;40:235–240.
36. Hester TR Jr, Bostwick J, Miller L, et al. Breast reduction utilizing the maximally vascularized central breast pedicle. *Plast Reconstr Surg.* 1985; 76:890–900.
37. Wise RJ. Preliminary report on a method of planning the mammaplasty. *Plast Reconstr Surg.* 1956;17:367–375.
38. Lejour M. Vertical mammaplasty and liposuction of the breast. *Plast Reconstr Surg.* 1994;94:100–114.
39. Hammond DC. Short scar periareolar inferior pedicle (SPAIR) mammaplasty. *Plast Reconstr Surg.* 1999;103:890–901.
40. Mizgala CL, MacKenzie KM. Breast reduction outcome study. *Ann Plast Surg.* 2000;44:125–134.
41. Behmand RA, Tang DH, Smith DJ Jr. Outcomes in breast reduction surgery. *Ann Plast Surg.* 2000;45:575–580.
42. Gruber RP, Kahn RA, Lash H, et al. Breast reconstruction following mastectomy: A comparison of submuscular and subcutaneous techniques. *Plast Reconstr Surg.* 1981;67:312–317.

43. Handel N, Silverstein MJ, Gamagami P, et al. Factors affecting mammographic visualization of the breast after augmentation mammaplasty. JAMA 1992;268:1913–1917.
44. Maxwell GP, Falcone PA. Eighty-four consecutive breast reconstructions using a textured silicone tissue expander. *Plast Reconstr Surg*. 1992;89:1022–1036.
45. Gutowski KA, Mesna GT, Cunningham BL. Saline-filled breast implants: A plastic surgery educational foundation multicenter outcome study. *Plast Reconstr Surg*. 1997;100:1019–1027.
46. **Janowsky EC, Kupper LL, Hulka BS. Meta-analysis of the relation between silicone breast implants and the risk of connective-tissue diseases. *N Engl J Med*. 2000;342:781–790.**
47. Komatsu A, Tamai S. Successful replantation of a completely cut-off thumb. Case report. *Plast Reconstr Surg*. 1968;42:374–377.
48. Chung KC, Wei FC: An outcome study of thumb reconstruction using microvascular toe transfer. *J Hand Surg [Am]*. 2000;25:651–658.
49. Partington MT, Lineaweaver WC, O'Hara M, et al. Unrecognized injuries in patients referred for emergency microsurgery. *J Trauma* 1993;34: 238–241.
50. Godina M. Early microsurgical reconstruction of complex trauma of the extremities. *Plast Reconstr Surg*. 1986;78:285–292.
51. Weinzweig N, Sharzer LA, Starker I. Replantation and revascularization at the transmetacarpal level: long-term functional results. *J Hand Surg [Am]*. 1996;21:877–883.
52. Feldon P. Rheumatoid arthritis. In: Manske P, ed. *Hand surgery update*, vol. 1. Englewood, CO: American Society for Surgery of the Hand, 1994, pp. 1–10.
53. Chung KC, Kowalski CP, Kim HM, et al. Patient outcomes following Swanson Silastic metacarpophalangeal arthroplasty in the rheumatoid hand: systematic overview. *J Rheumatol*. 2000;27:1395–1402.
54. Bostwick J, Eaves F, Nahai F, eds. *Endoscopic plastic surgery*. St. Louis: Quality Medical Publishers, 1995.
55. Romo T 3rd, Sclafani AP, Yung RT. Endoscopic foreheadplasty: temporary vs. permanent fixation. *Aesthetic Plast Surg*. 1999;23:388–394.
56. Furnas D. Facial aesthetic surgery: art, anatomy, anthropometrics, and imaging. *Clin Plast Surg*. 1987;14:579–788.
57. Antell D, Taczanowski E. How environment and lifestyle choices influence the aging process. *Ann Plast Surg*. 1999;43:585–588.
58. Ramirez O, Pozner J. Subperiosteal endoscopic techniques in secondary rhytidectomy. *Aesthetic Surg*. 1997;17:22.
59. Barton FE Jr. Rhytidectomy and the nasolabial fold. *Plast Reconstr Surg* 1992;90:601–607.
60. Pitanguy I. Facial cosmetic surgery: a 30 year perspective. *Plast Reconstr Surg*. 2000;105:1517–1527.
61. Owsley J. Face lifting: problems, solutions, and an outcome study. *Plast Reconstr Surg*. 2000;105:302–315.
62. Rees T. In search of the perfect facelift: a personal odyssey. *Aesthetic Surg*. 1997;17:29.
63. Menick F, ed. Aesthetic surgery of the face. *Clin Plast Surg*. 1997;24:2
64. Smith B, ed. *Ophthalmic plastic and reconstructive surgery*. St. Louis: Mosby-Yearbook, 1987.
65. Goldberg R. Transconjunctival orbital fat repositioning: transposition of orbital fat pedicles into a subperiosteal pocket. *Plast Reconstr Surg*. 2000;105:743–51.
66. Constantian MB. Four common anatomic variations that predispose to unfavorable rhinoplasty results: a study based on 150 consecutive secondary rhinoplasties. Plast Reconstr Surg. 2000;105:316–333.
67. Godley FA, Nemeroff RF, Josephson JS. Current trends in rhinoplasty and the nasal airway. *Med Clin North Am*. 1993;77:643–656.
68. Zide BM, Pfeifer TM, Longaker MT. Chin surgery: I. Augmentation–the allures and the alerts. *Plast Reconstr Surg*. 1999;104:1843–1862.
69. Guyuron B, Kadi JS. Problems following genioplasty: diagnosis and treatment. *Clin Plast Surg*. 1997;24:507–514.
70. **Pitanguy I. Evaluation of body contouring surgery today: a 30-year perspective. *Plast Reconstr Surg*. 2000;105:1499–1516.**
71. Wang T, Vasconez LO Body contour surgery. In Jurkiewicz, MJ, Krizek TJ, Mathes SJ, et al., eds. *Plastic surgery: principles in practice*. St. Louis: Mosby-Year Book, 1990.
72. Rohrich R, Mathes S. Suction lipectomy. In: Jurkiewicz, MJ, Krizek TJ, Mathes SJ, et al., eds. *Plastic surgery: principles in practice*. St. Louis: Mosby-Year Book, 1990.
73. Zocchi M. Ultrasonic liposculpturing. *Aesthetic Plast Surg*. 1992;16:287–298.
74. Zocchi ML. Ultrasonic assisted lipoplasty. Technical refinements and clinical evaluations. *Clin Plast Surg*. 1996;23:575–598.
75. Troilius C. Ultrasound-assisted lipoplasty: is it really safe? *Aesthetic Plast Surg*. 1999;23:307–311.
76. Fogh-Andersen P. *Inheritance of harelip and cleft palate*. Copenhagen: Arnold Busck, 1942.
77. Millicovsky G, Johnston MC. Maternal hypoxia greatly reduces the incidence of phenytoin-induced cleft lip and palate in A/J mice, *Science* 1981;212:671.
78. Neel JV. A study of major congenital defects in Japanese. *Am J Hum Genet*. 1958;10:398–445.
79. Sando WC, Jurkiewicz MJ. Cleft lip. In: Jurkiewicz, MJ, Krizek TJ, Mathes SJ, et al., eds. *Plastic surgery: principles in practice*. St. Louis: Mosby-Year Book, 1990.
80. Byrd HS. Cleft lip I. *Selected Readings in Plastic Surgery* 1985;3:1.
81. Cohen MM Jr: Syndromes with cleft lip and cleft palate. *Cleft Palate J*. 1978;15:306.
82. Shinbashi T, O'Hata N, Hayashi Y, et al. Changes in bone remodeling after palatal surgery. *Ann Plast Surg*. 1985;14:267.
83. Morris HL. Velopharyngeal competence and primary cleft palate surgery 1960–1971: a critical review. *Cleft Palate J*. 1973;10:621.
84. Virchow R. Uber den cretinismus nametlich in franken, und uber pathologische schadelforamen. *Ver Phys Med Cesselsch (Wurzburg)* 1891;2:230.
85. Marchac D. Radical forehead remodeling for craniostenosis. *Plast Reconstr Surg*. 1978;61:823–835.
86. Renier D, Sainte-Rose C, Marchac D, et al. Intracranial pressure in craniostenosis. *J Neurosurg*. 1982;57:370.
87. Buchman SR, Smith DJ. Congenital vascular lesions in infancy and childhood in
88. Ernst CB Stanley JC, eds. *Current therapy and vascular surgery*. St. Louis: C.V. Mosby and Company, 1995.
89. Kaplan EN: The risk of malignancy in large congenital nevi. *Plast Reconstr Surg*. 1974;53:42153.

INDEX

Note: Page numbers followed by f indicate figures; those followed by t indicate tables.

Gum chewing, for ileus, 783, 784t